W9-AKT-037

The premier source of definitive medical information

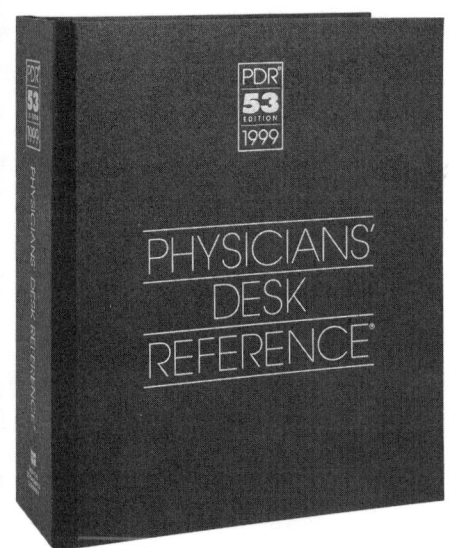

Medical Economics has long been the most respected, most trusted publisher of essential medical information in the country. Thousands of professionals regularly rely on these vital publications in their day-to-day work.

For over 50 years, *Physicians' Desk Reference*® has been universally recognized as the "last word" on prescription medicines and their effects. Medical Economics has proudly continued this tradition of providing resources for the entire healthcare industry in all its publications.

Every edition is guaranteed to be:

COMPREHENSIVE—Complete coverage of all the essential details assures you of getting all the facts.

AUTHORITATIVE—FDA-approved information gives you the confidence of always getting the official data you need.

UP-TO-DATE—We pride ourselves on our widespread network which allows us to constantly gather, organize and publish critical medical information in easy-to-use formats. Our full-time staff verifies all data before it is published.

EASY-TO-USE—Organized and indexed for quick, easy access, all publications are ready for fast reference.

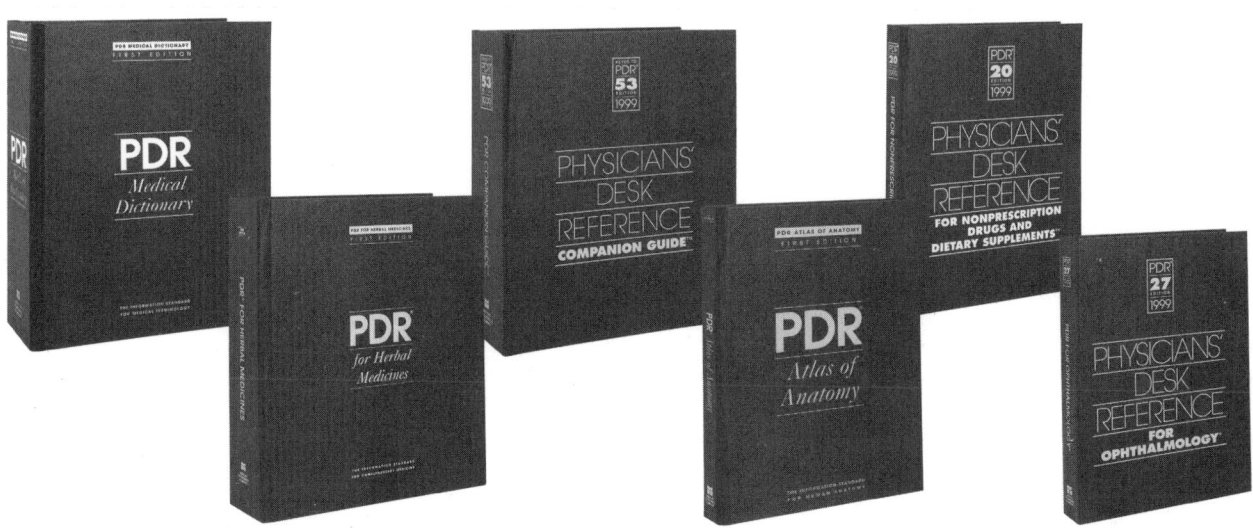

Keep Your Entire Drug Reference Library Completely Up-To-Date With These Key Volumes

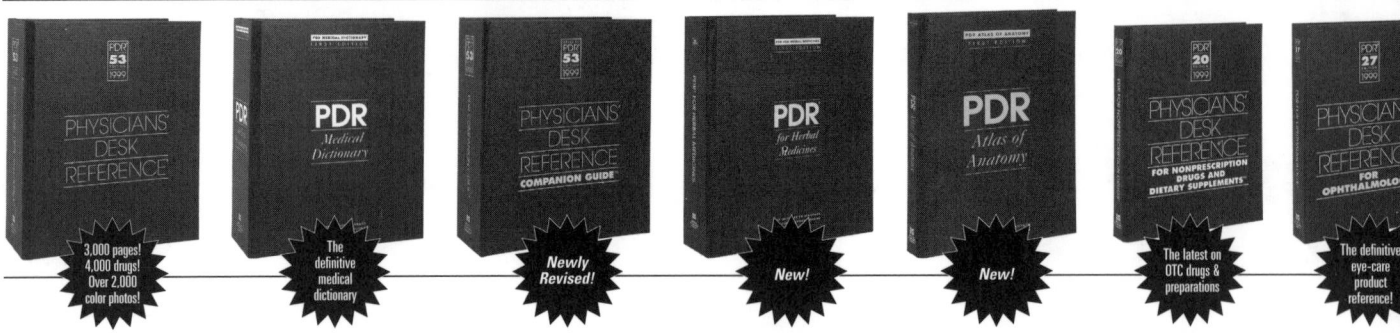

1999 Physicians' Desk Reference®

Physicians have turned to PDR for the latest word on prescription drugs for over 50 years! Today, PDR is still considered the standard prescription drug reference and can be found in virtually every physician's office, hospital, and pharmacy in the United States. The 53rd edition is more than 3,000 pages—our largest edition ever! And, a new manufacturing process has increased the margin width, thereby dramatically improving readability. PDR provides the most complete data on over 4,000 drugs by product and generic name (both in the same convenient index), manufacturer, and category. Also, product overviews that summarize listings with more than 2,000 full-size, full-color photos cross-referenced to complete drug information.

PDR® Medical Dictionary

More than 100,000 entries! 1,900+ pages include a complete medical etymology section to help the reader understand medical/scientific word formation. Includes a comprehensive cross-reference table of generic and brand-name pharmaceuticals and manufacturers, plus a 31-page appendix containing useful charts on scales, temperatures, temperature equivalents, metric and SI units, laboratory and reference values, blood groups and much more.

PDR® Companion Guide™

Formerly PDR Guide to Drug Interactions, Side Effects, Indications, Contraindications'

Now revised and renamed, this unique, all-in-one clinical reference assures safe, appropriate drug selection with nine critical checkpoints: **Interactions Index, Side Effects Index, Food Interactions Cross-Reference, Indications Index, Contraindications Index, Off-label Treatment Guide, Cost of Therapy Guide, International Drug Guide,** and a **Generic Availability Table** showing forms and strengths of brand-name drugs dispensed generically. This time-saving complement to your 1999 PDR, PDR for Nonprescription Drugs and PDR for Ophthalmology, will soon prove to be indispensable.

1999 PDR for Herbal Medicines

The most comprehensive prescribing reference of its kind, the PDR for Herbal Medicines is based upon the work conducted by renowned botanist Jöerg Grüenwald, Ph.D, and the German Federal Authority's Commission E, the governmental body widely recognized as having conducted the mo authoritative evaluation of herbs in the world. Entries include: the pharmacological effects of ea plant; applicable precautions, warnings, interactions and contraindications ; administration and dosage; adverse reactions and overdose data; plus much more.

1999 PDR Atlas of Anatomy

The PDR Atlas of Anatomy provides an innovative and unique visual representation of the human bod includes hundreds of full-color illustrations and photographs that present anatomical structures and interrelationships clearly and precisely, numerically labeled for easy use in practical examination revie

1999 PDR for Nonprescription Drugs and Dietary Supplements®

The acknowledged authority offers full FDA-approved descriptions of the most commonly used medicines, four separate indices and in-depth data on ingredients, indications, and drug interac Includes a valuable **Companion Drug Index** that lists common diseases and frequently encountered effects, along with the prescription drugs associated with them, plus OTC products recommende symptomatic relief. Newly expanded to include a section on supplements, vitamins, and herbal reme

1999 PDR for Ophthalmology®

The definitive reference filled with accurate, up-to-date information specifically for the eye professional. It provides detailed reference data on drugs and equipment used in the fiel ophthalmology and optometry. Its comprehensive coverage includes lens types and their us specialized instrumentation... color product photographs... a detailed encyclopedia of pharmaceutic ophthalmology... five full indices... an extensive bibliography... and much more.

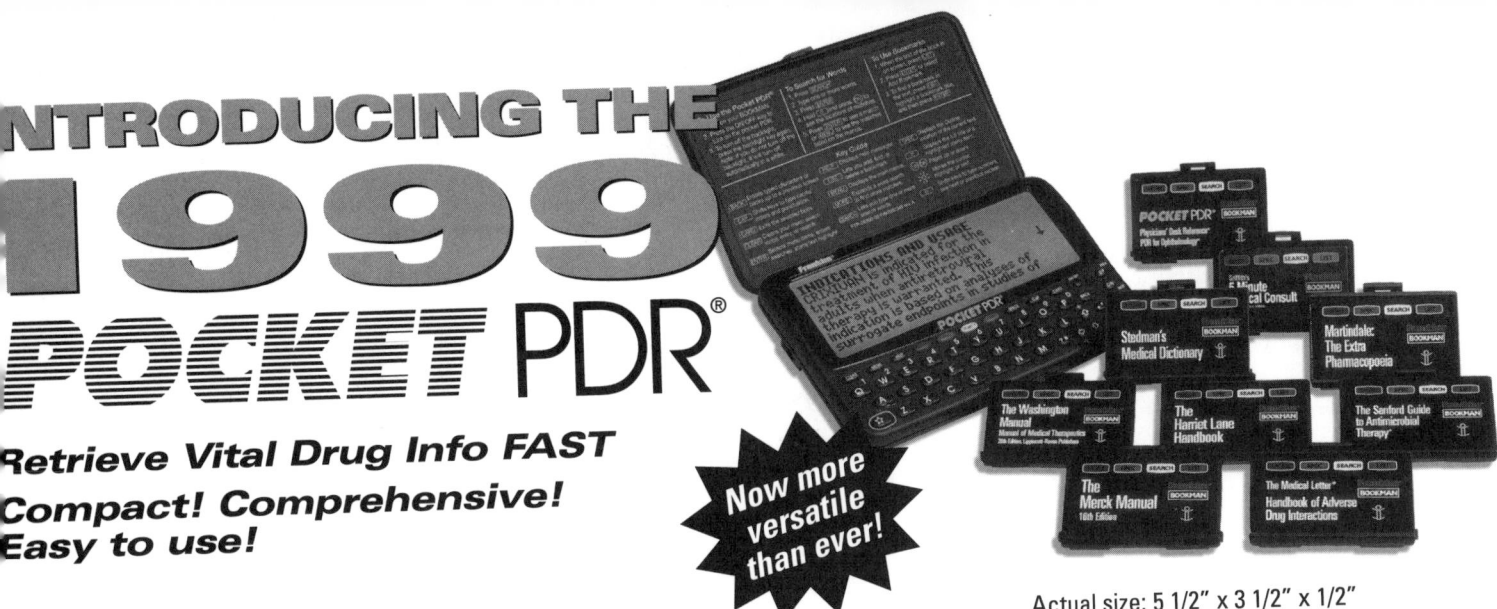

PDR® Electronic Library™ on CD-ROM

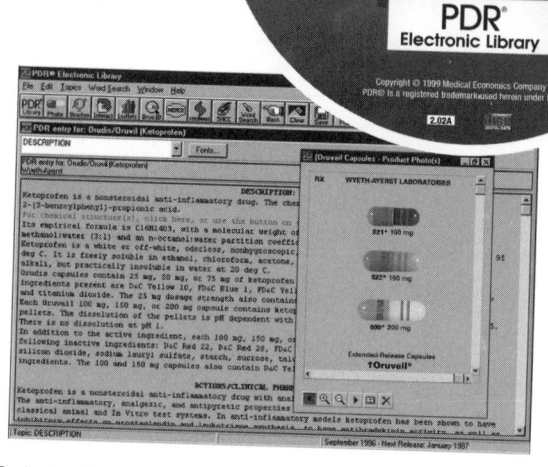

Speed diagnosis and prescribing with fast, flexible access to the medical references you need in one fully integrated system.

PDR Electronic Library on CD-ROM is a Windows-based system that instantly gives you all the information you need from the most current editions of Physicians' Desk Reference®. This powerful system lets you look products up 7 different ways—by brand name, generic name, manufacturer, therapeutic class, indication, side effects or drug interaction. The system also includes a powerful multi-drug interaction screening module. (Institutional version only)

Choose from these optional best selling titles available on the PDR Electronic Library CD-ROM:

The Merck Manual. The most widely-used medical text in the world integrated with PDR and Stedman's Medical Dictionary.

Stedman's Medical Dictionary. The most comprehensive medical dictionary available fully integrated with PDR and the Merck Manual.

Stedman's PLUS Spell Checker. 300,000+ medical and pharmaceutical terms added to your word processor's spell checker. (Not available for free trial.)

Reviewing the full prescribing information for any product alongside available product images and chemical structures is a snap with the new Windows version of PDR Electronic Library.

Equipment Required: IBM PC compatible computer, MS Windows 3.1 or higher, 8MB RAM, 10MB available on hard drive, VGA color monitor, Double-speed CD-ROM drive. Provided under terms of one-year single-user license agreement. Institutional version includes multi-drug interactive screening module and two updates.

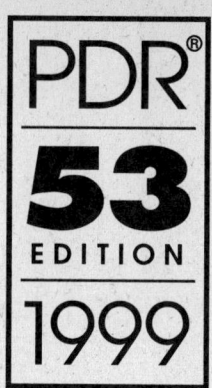

PDR® 53 EDITION 1999

PHYSICIANS' DESK REFERENCE®

Medical Consultant
Ronald Arky, MD, Charles S. Davidson Professor of Medicine and Master, Francis Weld Peabody Society, Harvard Medical School

Vice President of Directory Services: Stephen B. Greenberg

Director of Product Management: David P. Reiss
Senior Product Manager: Mark A. Friedman
Associate Product Manager: Bill Shaughnessy
Director of Sales: Dikran N. Barsamian
National Sales Manager: Anthony Sorce
National Account Manager: Don Bruccoleri
Account Managers:
Marion Gray, RPh
Lawrence C. Keary
Jeffrey F. Pfohl
Christopher N. Schmidt
Stephen M. Silverberg
Suzanne E. Yarrow, RN
National Sales Manager, Trade Group: Bill Gaffney
Director of Direct Marketing: Michael Bennett
Direct Marketing Manager: Lorraine M. Loening
Promotion Manager: Donna R. Lynn
Director, Professional Support Services: Mukesh Mehta, RPh

Senior Drug Information Specialist: Thomas Fleming, RPh
Drug Information Specialist: Maria Deutsch, MS, RPh, CDE
Editor, Special Projects: David W. Sifton
Vice President of Production: David A. Pitler
Director of Print Purchasing: Marjorie A. Duffy
Director of Operations: Carrie Williams
Manager of Production: Kimberly H. Vivas
Senior Production Coordinators: Amy B. Brooks, Dawn McCall
Production Coordinator: Mary Ellen R. Breun
PDR Data Manager: Jeffrey D. Schaefer
Senior Format Editor: Gregory J. Westley
Index Editors: Johanna M. Mazur, Robert N. Woerner
Art Associate: Joan K. Akerlind
Senior Digital Imaging Coordinator: Shawn W. Cahill
Digital Imaging Coordinator: Frank J. McElroy, III
Electronic Publishing Designer: Robert K. Grossman
Fulfillment Managers: Stephanie DeNardi, Kenneth Siebert

Officers of Medical Economics Company: *President and Chief Executive Officer:* Curtis B. Allen; *Vice President, New Media:* L. Suzanne BeDell; *Vice President, Corporate Human Resources:* Pamela M. Bilash; *Vice President and Chief Information Officer:* Steven M. Bressler; *Senior Vice President, Finance, and Chief Financial Officer:* Thomas W. Ehardt; *Vice President, Directory Services:* Stephen B. Greenberg; *Vice President, New Business Planning:* Linda G. Hope; *Executive Vice President, Healthcare Publishing and Communications:* Thomas J. Kelly; *Executive Vice President, Magazine Publishing:* Lee A. Maniscalco; *Vice President, Group Publisher:* Terrence W. Meacock; *Vice President, Production:* David A. Pitler; *Vice President, Group Publisher:* Thomas C. Pizor; *Vice President, Magazine Business Management:* Eric Schlett; *Senior Vice President, Operations:* John R. Ware

 Printed on recycled paper

ISBN: 1-56363-288-8

FOREWORD TO THE FIFTY-THIRD EDITION

In this, the final year of the 20th century, *PDR* is proud to present its largest edition ever, reflecting over 50 years of unprecedented progress in the field of pharmaceutical science. At the same time, we are pleased to announce the introduction of a unique and much-needed adjunct: the new *PDR® for Herbal Medicines™*.

Herbal remedies are no longer a minor fad to simply be ignored. Consumers are self-medicating with obscure botanical preparations to such an extent that the use of herbs in the United States is doubling every four years. Included among these largely unregulated products are some genuinely beneficial agents. But also lurking among them are a variety of untested nostrums with little if any genuine value.

Which herbals should be taken seriously and which dismissed? Until now, there had been no single, authoritative source to turn to for answers. But with the advent of *PDR for Herbal Medicines*, the void has been filled. Covering a total of over 600 botanicals, this important new medical reference includes detailed information on each plant's physical characteristics, chemical composition, and physiological effects, along with a summary of its accepted indications, contraindications, drug interactions, side effects, and dosage. When appropriate, symptoms and treatment of overdose are discussed as well.

Although botanical products are not officially regulated or monitored in the United States, *PDR for Herbal Medicines* provides you the closest analog to FDA-approved labeling—the findings of the German Regulatory Authority's herbal watchdog agency, Commission E—augmented with exhaustive literature reviews from the PhytoPharm U.S. Institute for Phytopharmaceuticals. These reports represent the most accurate, impartial, and reliable assessment of a botanical agent's safety and effectiveness currently available in medicine.

Now, when patients pepper you with questions about the latest "herb du jour," *PDR for Herbal Medicines* can provide you with a rational basis for response. It tells which botanicals to encourage—and which to avoid. It clearly distinguishes between valid indications and specious claims, warns of conflicting conditions and drugs, and provides you with an exhaustive bibliography of the relevant clinical literature on each medicinal plant. It is a truly indispensable reference in an era when more

and more patients are experimenting with "natural" remedies.

If you haven't already encountered a copy, you should also take a look at the new *PDR Companion Guide™*, an 1,800-page reference that augments *PDR* with a total of nine unique decision-making tools:

- **Interactions Index** identifies all pharmaceuticals and foods capable of interacting with a chosen medication.
- **Food Interactions Cross-Reference** lists the drugs that may interact with a given dietary item.
- **Side Effects Index** pinpoints the pharmaceuticals associated with each of 3,600 distinct adverse reactions.
- **Indications Index** presents the full range of therapeutic options for any given diagnosis.
- **Off-Label Treatment Guide** lists medications routinely used—but never officially approved—for treatment of nearly 1,000 specific disorders.
- **Contraindications Index** list all drugs to avoid in the presence of any given medical condition.
- **International Drug Index** names the U.S. equivalents of some 15,000 foreign medications.
- **Generic Availability Guide** shows which forms and strengths of a brand-name drug are also available generically.
- **Cost of Therapy Guide** provides a quick overview of the relative expense of the leading therapeutic options for a variety of common indications.

The *PDR Companion Guide* includes all drugs described in *PDR, PDR For Nonprescription Drugs®*, and *PDR For Ophthalmology®*. We're certain that you'll find it makes safe, appropriate drug selection faster and easier than ever before.

With the advent of the PDR Companion Guide and PDR for Herbal Medicines, the complete roster of PDR's medical references now includes:

- *Physicians' Desk Reference®*
- *PDR For Nonprescription Drugs®*
- *PDR For Ophthalmology®*
- *PDR Companion Guide™*
- *PDR® for Herbal Medicines™*
- *PDR® Medical Dictionary™*
- *PDR® Nurse's Handbook™*
- *PDR® Nurse's Dictionary™*
- *PDR® Atlas of Anatomy™*
- *PDR Supplements*

PDR and its major companion volumes are also found in the *PDR® Electronic Library™* on CD-ROM, now used in over 40,000 practices. This Windows-compatible disc provides users with a complete database of *PDR* prescribing information, electronically searchable for instant retrieval. A standard subscription includes *PDR's* sophisticated prescription-screening program and an extensive file of chemical structures, illustrations, and full-color product photographs. Optional enhancements include the complete contents of *The Merck Manual and Stedman's Medical Dictionary*, as well as a comprehensive database of billing codes. The disc is available for use on individual PCs and PC networks. Remember, too, that the contents of *PDR* and its main companion volumes can always be found on the Internet at **www.medecinteractive.com**.

For personal use—on rounds or on the go—there's also *Pocket PDR®*, a unique handheld electronic database of prescribing information that literally fits in your pocket. For facilities with large, mainframe-based information systems, *PDR* information is also available as a preformatted text file on magnetic tape. And for anyone who wants to run a fast double-check on a proposed prescription, there's the *PDR® Drug Interactions, Side Effects, Indications, Contraindications System™* — sophisticated software capable of automatically screening a 20-drug regimen for conflicts, then proposing alternatives for any problematic medication. For more information on these or any other members of the growing family of PDR products, please call, toll-free, 1-800-232-7379 or fax 201-573-4956.

Physicians' Desk Reference is published by Medical Economics Company in cooperation with participating manufacturers. Each full-length entry provides you with an exact copy of the product's FDA-approved labeling. Under the federal Food, Drug and Cosmetics (FD&C) Act, a drug approved for marketing may be labeled, promoted, and advertised by the manufacturer for only those uses for which the drug's safety and effectiveness have been established. The Code of Federal Regulations 201.100(d)(1) pertaining to labeling for prescription products requires that for *PDR* content "indications, effects, dosages, routes, methods, and frequency and duration of administration and any relevant warnings, hazards, contraindications, side effects, and precautions" must be *"same in language*

and emphasis" as the approved labeling for the products. The Food and Drug Administration (FDA) regards the words *same in language and emphasis* as requiring VERBATIM use of the approved labeling providing such information. Furthermore, information that is emphasized in the approved labeling by the use of type set in a box, or in capitals, boldface, or italics, must be given the same emphasis in *PDR*.

The FDA has also recognized that the FD&C Act does not, however, limit the manner in which a physician may use an approved drug. Once a product has been approved for marketing, a physician may choose to prescribe it for uses or in treatment regimens or patient populations that are not included in approved labeling. The FDA also observes that accepted medical practice includes drug use that is not reflected in approved drug labeling. For products that do not have official package circulars, the publisher has emphasized the necessity of describing such products comprehensively, so that physicians can have access to all information essential for intelligent and informed decision-making. Particularly in the case of over-the-counter dietary supplements, it should be remembered that this information has not been evaluated by the Food and Drug Administration, and that such products are not intended to diagnose, treat, cure, or prevent any disease.

The function of the publisher is the compilation, organization, and distribution of this information. Each product description has been prepared by the manufacturer, and edited and approved by the manufacturer's medical department, medical director, and/or medical consultant. In organizing and presenting the material in *Physicians' Desk Reference*, the publisher does not warrant or guarantee any of the products described, or perform any independent analysis in connection with any of the product information contained herein. *Physicians' Desk Reference* does not assume, and expressly disclaims, any obligation to obtain and include any information other than that provided to it by the manufacturer. It should be understood that by making this material available, the publisher is not advocating the use of any product described herein, nor is the publisher responsible for misuse of a product due to typographical error. Additional information on any product may be obtained from the manufacturer.

CONTENTS

SECTION 1

MANUFACTURERS' INDEX

Listed in this index are all manufacturers participating in PHYSICIANS' DESK REFERENCE. It is through their courtesy that PDR is brought to the medical profession.

Each company's entry includes the address, phone, and fax number of its headquarters and regional offices, as well as contacts for inquiries, orders, and medical emergency information. Products with entries in the Product Information or Diagnostic Product Information sections are listed with their page numbers. Other products available from the manufacturer are listed following the described products.

If an entry in the index lists multiple page numbers, the first ones shown refer to photographs of the product, the last one to its prescribing information.

- ■ **Bold page numbers** indicate full prescribing information.

- ■ *Italic page numbers* signify partial information.

- ■ The ◆ symbol marks drugs shown in the Product Identification Guide.

- ■ The ▣ symbol means product information is located in *PDR For Nonprescription Drugs and Dietary Supplements*.

- ■ The ⊙ symbol means product information is located in *PDR For Ophthalmology*.

◆ Shown in Product Identification Guide   *Italic Page Number* **Indicates Brief Listing**   ⊙ **Described in PDR For Ophthalmology**

Pentothal (Thiopental Sodium for Injection)
Pentothal Kit
Pentothal RTM Syringe
Physiosol Irrigation (Aqualite)
Plegisol
Potassium Acetate 40 mEq Vial, Pintop & Fliptop
Potassium Chloride Injection Ampoules & Vials, Pintop & Universal Additive Syringe
Potassium Phosphate 15 mM Vial & Fliptop
Potassium Phosphate 45 mM Vial
Procainamide Hydrochloride Injection, USP
Procaine Hydrochloride Injection 1% & 2% Vial
Quelicin (Succinylcholine Chloride Injection) Ampul & Vial, Pintop
Ringer's Injection, USP
Ringer's Irrigation, USP (Aqualite)
Sodium Acetate 40 mEq, 100 mEq and 200 mEq Vials
4.2% Sodium Bicarbonate Injection, 10 mEq in 10 mL Abboject (Neonatal)
5% Sodium Bicarbonate Injection, USP
7.5% Sodium Bicarbonate Injection, 44.6 mEq in 50 mL ampul or Abboject
8.4% Sodium Bicarbonate Injection, 10 mEq in 10 mL Abboject (Pediatric)
8.4% Sodium Bicarbonate Injection, 50 mEq in 50 mL Abboject or Fliptop Vial
5% Sodium Chloride
0.45% Sodium Chloride Injection, USP
0.9% Sodium Chloride Injection
0.9% Sodium Chloride Injection, USP (ADD-Vantage)
0.9% Sodium Chloride Injection, USP (Partial Fill)
0.45% Sodium Chloride Irrigation, USP (Aqualite)
0.9% Sodium Chloride Irrigation, USP (Flex and Aqualite)
Sodium Lactate Injection, USP, 1/6 Molar
Sodium Phosphate 45 mMoL
Sorbitol-Mannitol Irrigation (Flex & Aqualite)
Surbex 750 with Zinc Filmtab
Surbex with C Filmtab
Surbex-T Filmtab
Tham Solution
Theophylline in 5% Dextrose Injection (0.4, 0.8, 1.6, 2, 3.2, 4 mg/mL)
TPN Electrolytes
Tridione Dulcet Tablets
Tronothane Hydrochloride Cream
Tubocurarine Chloride Injection, USP
Ultane (Sevoflurane)
Ureaphil
Urologic G Irrigation (Aqualite)
Water for Injection Bacteriostatic 30 mL Fliptop
Water for Injection, Sterile, USP, Amps, Vial
Water for Irrigation, Sterile, USP (Flex and Aqualite)
Water for Respiratory Therapy, Sterile (Flex)
Zinc 10 mL (1 mg/1 mL)

ADAMS LABORATORIES, INC.
(See MEDEVA
PHARMACEUTICALS, INC.)

**ADVANCED NUTRITIONAL   483
TECHNOLOGY, INC.**
6988 Sierra Ct.
Dublin, CA 94568

Direct Inquiries to:
(925) 828-2128
FAX: (925) 828-6848

Products Described:
Nutr-E-Sol Liquid................483
SuperEPA Softgels...............483

**AGOURON   303, 484
PHARMACEUTICALS, INC.**
10350 North Torrey Pines Road
La Jolla, CA 92037-1020

Direct Inquiries to:
Customer Communications
(888) VIRACEPT
FAX: (619) 678-8266

For Medical Emergencies Contact:
Medical Affairs
(888) VIRACEPT
FAX: (619) 678-8245

Products Described:
◆Viracept Oral Powder............303, 484
◆Viracept Tablets.................303, 484

ALCON LABORATORIES, INC.   487
Alcon Laboratories, Inc.
And its affiliates
Corporate Headquarters
6201 South Freeway
Fort Worth, TX 76134

Direct Inquiries to:
Ophthalmic/VisionCare: (800) 451-3937
(Pharmaceuticals/Lens Care)
Surgical: (800) 862-5266
(Instrumentation/Surgical Meds)

For Medical Information Contact:
(817) 293-0450

Products Described:
Betoptic Ophthalmic Solution........487
Betoptic S Ophthalmic Suspension....489
Bion Tears.........................490
Ciloxan Ophthalmic Ointment........490
Ciloxan Ophthalmic Solution........490
Naphcon-A Ophthalmic Solution......491
Patanol Ophthalmic Solution........491
Tears Naturale Free Lubricant Eye Drops............................492
Tears Naturale II Lubricant Eye Drops............................492
TobraDex Ophthalmic Ointment.......492
TobraDex Ophthalmic Suspension.....492

Other Products Available:
A-OK Ophthalmic Knives
A.C.S. Closure System Needles and Sutures
Alcon Surgical System (Irrigation/ Aspiration Kits; Phacoemulsification Kits)
Alomide Ophthalmic Solution
Azopt Ophthalmic Solution
BSS and BSS Plus Irrigation Solution Administration Set
BSS Irrigation Solution (15 mL, 30 mL, 250 mL, 500 mL)
Cetamide Ointment
Cetapred Ointment
Cyclogyl Ophthalmic Solution
Cystitomes & Cannulas
Duovisc Viscoelastic System
Duratears Naturale Lubricant Eye Ointment
Emadine Ophthalmic Solution
Enucleane Cleaning/Lubricating Solution for Artificial Eyes
Epinal Ophthalmic Solution
Eye Pak Surgical Drape
Eye Stream Eye Irrigating Solution
Fluorescite Injection
Gonioscopic Prism Solution
I-Knife Ophthalmic Knife
I-Spear Surgical Eye Sponge
Intraocular Lenses
Iopidine Ophthalmic Solution
Ismotic Isosorbide Solution
Maxidex Ointment
Maxitrol Ointment
Microsponge Surgical Eye Sponge
Miostat Intraocular Miotic Solution
Natacyn Ophthalmic Suspension
Optemp Sterile Disposable Cautery
Osmoglyn Oral Osmotic Agent
Pilopine HS Gel
Post-Operative Kits
Procedure Packs
Profenal Ophthalmic Solution
ProSheild Corneal Collagen Shield
Provisc Viscoelastic Material
PTG, Alcon Applanation Pneumatonograph
SofGuard Flexible Eye Shield
Steri-Units Single Dose Surgical Drops
Vexol Ophthalmic Suspension
Viscoat Viscoelastic Solution

ALCON (PUERTO RICO) INC.
P.O. Box 3000
Humacao, Puerto Rico 00661

Direct Inquiries to:
Medical Department
P.O. Box 6380
Fort Worth, TX 76115
(817) 293-0450

Products Available:
Adsorbocarpine
Adsorbonac
Adsorbotear
Alcaine
Econopred
Econopred Plus
Glaucon
Isopto Atropine
Isopto Carbachol
Isopto Carpine
Isopto Cetamide
Isopto Cetapred
Isopto Homatropine
Isopto Hyoscine
Maxidex Suspension
Maxitrol Suspension
Mydfrin 2.5%

Mydrapred
Mydriacyl
Naphcon Forte
Zincfrin

ALLERGAN, INC.   303, 493
2525 Dupont Drive
P.O. Box 19534
Irvine, CA 92623-9534

Direct Inquiries to:
(714) 246-4500

Products Described:
Acular Ophthalmic Solution...........493
Acular PF Ophthalmic Solution........494
Alphagan Ophthalmic Solution........494
Azelex Cream........................495
Blephamide Ophthalmic Ointment.....496
Blephamide Ophthalmic Suspension...497
Botox Purified Neurotoxin Complex...498
Elimite Cream.......................499
Erygel Topical Gel..................499
Erymax Topical Solution.............500
Exsel Lotion/Shampoo................500
Fluonid Topical Solution............500
Fluoroplex Topical Cream............500
Fluoroplex Topical Solution.........500
Gris-PEG Tablets....................500
Maxiflor Cream......................501
Maxiflor Ointment...................501
Naftin Cream........................501
Naftin Gel..........................502
◆Ocuflox Ophthalmic Solution....303, 502
Opticrom Ophthalmic Solution........503
Penecort Cream......................504
Penecort Topical Solution...........504
Polytrim Ophthalmic Solution........504
Tazorac Gel.........................505

Other Products Available:
Albalon Ophthalmic Solution
Betagan Ophthalmic Solution with C Cap Compliance Cap Q.D. and B.I.D.
Bleph-10 Ophthalmic Ointment
Bleph-10 Ophthalmic Solution
Celluvisc Lubricant Eye Drops
Chloroptic Ophthalmic Ointment
Chloroptic Ophthalmic Solution
Epifrin Sterile Ophthalmic Solution
FML Forte Ophthalmic Suspension
FML Ophthalmic Suspension
FML S.O.P. Ophthalmic Ointment
FML-S Ophthalmic Suspension
Genoptic Ophthalmic Ointment
Genoptic Ophthalmic Solution
HMS Ophthalmic Suspension
Ocufen Ophthalmic Solution
Ophthetic Ophthalmic Solution
Poly-Pred Ophthalmic Suspension
Pred Forte Ophthalmic Suspension
Pred-G Ophthalmic Ointment
Pred-G Ophthalmic Suspension
Pred Mild Ophthalmic Suspension
Propine Ophthalmic Solution with C Cap Compliance Cap B.I.D.
Refresh Plus Lubricant Eye Drops
Refresh P.M. Lubricant Eye Ointment
Refresh Tears Lubricant Eye Drops

ALLERGAN SKIN CARE
(See ALLERGAN, INC.)

**ALPHA THERAPEUTIC   507
CORPORATION**
5555 Valley Boulevard
Los Angeles, CA 90032

Direct Inquiries to:
(213) 225-2221
(800) 421-0008
FAX: (213) 227-7027

For Medical Information Contact:
In Emergencies:
Medical Director
(213) 227-7419
After Hours Emergency Orders:
(800) 421-0008

Products Described:
Albutein 5% Solution................507
Albutein 25% Solution...............507
Alphanate Solvent Detergent/Heat Treated...........................507
AlphaNine-SD Solvent Detergent Treated/Virus Filtered..............507
Profilnine SD Solvent Detergent Treated............................507
Venoglobulin-S 5% Solution Solvent Detergent Treated..................507
Venoglobulin-S 10% Solution Solvent Detergent Treated...........507

ALPHARMA   507
U.S. Pharmaceuticals Division
7205 Windsor Blvd.
Baltimore, MD 21244

Direct Inquiries to:
Customer Service
(800) 638-9096

Products Described:
Lindane Lotion USP 1%..............507
Lindane Shampoo USP 1%...........508

ALRA LABORATORIES, INC.   510
3850 Clearview Court
Gurnee, IL 60031

Direct Inquiries to:
Professional Services
(847) 244-9440
(800) 248-ALRA
FAX: (847) 244-9464

Products Described:
Cholac Lactulose Solution............510
Constilac Lactulose Solution.........510
Eryzole Oral Suspension, USP.........510
Gelpirin Tablets.....................510
Gelpirin-M Tablets...................510
Gen-XENE Tablets.....................510
Ibu-Tab OTC Tablets, USP.............510
Ibu-Tab Rx Tablets, USP..............510
Infant Formula Multi-Vit/Fluoride Drops 0.25 mg.....................510
Infant Formula Multi-Vit/Fluoride Drops 0.50 mg.....................510
Infant Formula Tri-Vit/Fluoride Drops 0.25 mg.....................510
Infant Formula Tri-Vit/Fluoride Drops 0.50 mg.....................510
K + 8 Tablets........................510
K + 10 Tablets.......................510
K + Care ET..........................510
Silver Strength Female Geriatric Multi-Vit/Multi-Min Liquid.........510
Silver Strength Male Geriatric Multi-Vit/Multi-Min Liquid.........510

Other Products Available:
AZM-TAB, Acetazolamide Tablets
Chlordiazepoxide Capsules
Ferrous Sulfate Drops
Hydrochlorothiazide Tablets
IMP-TAB, Imipramine Tablets
Methalgen Cream
Multi Vitamin Drops
Multi Vitamin Drops With Fluoride
Multi Vitamin Drops With Iron
SS-TAB, Sulfisoxazole Tablets
TOL-TAB, Tolbutamide Tablets
Vitamin Drops With Fluoride

ALZA PHARMACEUTICALS   303, 510
A Division of Alza Corporation
950 Page Mill Road
P.O. Box 10950
Palo Alto, California 94303-0802

Direct Inquiries to:
Customer Service
(800) 227-9953
FAX: (415) 962-4212

For Medical Information or Emergencies Contact:
Medical Communications
(800) 634-8977
FAX: (415) 962-2488
For Ethyol:
Medical Communications
(800) 506-4959
FAX: (415) 962-2488

Products Described:
Bicitra.............................511
Ditropan Tablets and Syrup.........511
◆Elmiron Capsules...............303, 512
◆Ethyol for Injection...........303, 513
◆Mycelex Troche.................303, 515
Polycitra Syrup and Polycitra-LC Syrup............................515
Polycitra-K Crystals................516
Polycitra-K Oral Solution...........516
◆Testoderm Transdermal Systems......................304, 517

Other Products Available:
Progestasert Intrauterine Progesterone Contraceptive System

**AMERICAN LECITHIN   520
COMPANY**
115 Hurley Rd.
Unit 2 B
Oxford, CT 06478

Direct Inquiries to:
Randall E. Zigmont
(203) 262-7100
FAX: (203) 262-7101

For Medical Information Contact:
Randall E. Zigmont
(203) 262-7100
FAX: (203) 262-7101

Products Described:
PhosChol Concentrate..................520
PhosChol 900 Softgels...............520

Other Products Available:
PhosChol Gold

AMERICAN RED CROSS 520
National Headquarters
Biomedical Services
1616 Ft. Myer Dr., 17th Floor
Arlington, VA 22209-3100

Direct Inquiries to:
Professional Services Department:
(800) 293-5023
FAX: (703) 312-8742
Customer Service Department:
(800) 446-8883
FAX: (703) 312-8746

Products Described:
Albumarc 5% Solution...............520
Albumarc 25% Solution..............520
Monarc-M, Antihemophilic Factor
  (Human), Method M, Monoclonal
  Purified..........................520
Panglobulin Intravenous..............521
Polygam S/D..........................521

AMGEN INC. 304, 521
1840 Dehavilland Drive
Thousand Oaks, CA 91320-1789

Direct Inquiries to:
Customer Services Department
(800) 282-6436
FAX: (800) 292-6436

For Medical Information Contact:
Generally:
  Professional Services Department
  (800) 772-6436
  FAX: (805) 376-8556
In Emergencies:
  (800) 772-6436
After Hours and Weekends:
  (800) 772-6436

Sales and Ordering:
Customer Services Department
(800) 282-6436
FAX: (800) 292-6436

Products Described:
◆Epogen for Injection............. 304, 521
◆Infergen....................... 304, 528
◆Neupogen for Injection........... 304, 532

APOTHECON
(See BRISTOL-MYERS SQUIBB
COMPANY)

ARCO PHARMACEUTICALS, 545
INC.
105 Orville Drive
Bohemia, NY 11716

Direct Inquiries to:
Professional Service Department
(516) 567-9500

Products Described:
Arco-Lase Tablets....................545
Arco-Lase Plus Tablets...............545
Mega-B Tablets......................545
Megadose Tablets....................545

Other Products Available:
Arco-Cee Tablets
Arcoret Tablets
Arcoret w/Iron Tablets
Arcotinic Liquid
Arcotinic Tablets
C-B Time Capsules
C-B Time Liquid
C-B Time 500 Tablets
Co-Gel Tablets
Mega-B with C
Spantuss Liquid
Spantuss Tablets

ARMOUR PHARMACEUTICAL
COMPANY
(See CENTEON L.L.C.)

ASTRA MERCK INC.
(See ASTRA PHARMACEUTICALS,
L.P.)

ASTRA 304, 546
PHARMACEUTICALS, L.P.
725 Chesterbrook Boulevard
Wayne, PA 19087-5677

**For Medical Information,
Adverse Drug Experiences,
and Customer Service
Contact:**
(800) 236-9933

Products Described:
Albuterol Sulfate, USP Solution for
  Inhalation, Arm-a-Med..............546
Aquasol A Capsules, USP.............547
Aquasol A Parenteral.................548
Astramorph/PF Injection, USP
  (Preservative-Free)................548
◆Atacand Tablets................. 304, 550
Atropine Sulfate Injection, USP.......552
Bretylium Tosylate Injection..........552
Calcitonin-Salmon Injection,
  Synthetic........................552
Calcium Chloride 10% Injection,
  USP..............................552
Cocaine Hydrochloride Topical
  Solution.........................552
Dextrose 50% Injection, USP........553
Dobutamine Injection, USP..........553
Dopamine Hydrochloride Injection,
  USP..............................553
Doxorubicin Hydrochloride for
  Injection, USP....................553
Doxorubicin Hydrochloride
  Injection, USP....................553
Duranest Injection, USP..............555
Dyclone 0.5% and 1% Topical
  Solutions, USP....................558
◆EMLA Cream.................... 304, 559
◆EMLA Anesthetic Disc.......... 304, 559
Epinephrine Injection, USP...........562
Etoposide Injection..................562
Fentanyl Citrate and Droperidol
  Injection.........................563
Foscavir Injection...................564
Furosemide Injection, USP...........567
Hydromorphone HCl Injection.......567
Leucovorin Calcium Tablets..........568
◆Lexxel Tablets.................. 304, 568
Magnesium Sulfate Injection, USP....572
Mannitol Injection, USP, 25%........572
Meperidine Hydrochloride Injection,
  USP..............................572
Morphine Sulfate (Immediate
  Release) Concentrated Oral
  Solution.........................572
Morphine Sulfate Immediate
  Release Oral Solution..............573
Morphine Sulfate Injection, USP for
  Intravenous Infusion..............574
Morphine Sulfate Injection, USP for
  Intravenous Injection.............573
Morphine Sulfate Injection, USP for
  Intravenous Use After Dilution.....574
M.V.I.-12 Multi-Vitamin Infusion....575
M.V.I. Pediatric for Infusion.........575
Nalbuphine Hydrochloride Injection...575
◆Naropin Injection............... 304, 575
Nesacaine Injection..................579
Nesacaine-MPF Injection.............579
Pancuronium Bromide Injection.......581
◆Plendil Extended-Release
  Tablets.........................304, 581
Polocaine Injection, USP.............584
Polocaine-MPF Injection, USP.........584
◆Prilosec Delayed-Release
  Capsules........................304, 584
◆Pulmicort Turbuhaler
  Inhalation Powder..............304, 587
◆Rhinocort Nasal Inhaler......... 304, 591
◆Sensorcaine Injection 304, 593
◆Sensorcaine with Epinephrine
  Injection.......................304, 593
Sensorcaine-MPF Injection...........593
Sensorcaine-MPF Spinal Injection.....596
Sensorcaine-MPF with Epinephrine
  Injection.........................593
Sodium Bicarbonate Injection, USP....597
Streptase for Infusion................597
Tobramycin Sulfate Injection, USP....599
◆Tonocard Tablets............... 304, 599
◆Toprol-XL Tablets 304, 602
◆Xylocaine Injection............. 305, 603
Xylocaine Injection for Ventricular
  Arrhythmias......................606
◆Xylocaine 2% Jelly............. 305, 607
Xylocaine-MPF 1.5% Solution with
  Dextrose 7.5%....................606
Xylocaine-MPF 4% Sterile Solution...606
Xylocaine-MPF 5% with Glucose
  7.5%.............................607
Xylocaine 2.5% Ointment............607
Xylocaine 5% Ointment..............607
Xylocaine 10% Oral Spray...........607
Xylocaine 4% Topical Solution.......606
Xylocaine 2% Viscous Solution.......607
◆Xylocaine with Epinephrine
  Injection.......................305, 603

Other Products Available:
Aquasol E

ASTRA USA, INC.
(See ASTRA PHARMACEUTICALS,
L.P.)

ATHENA NEUROSCIENCES, 305, 607
INC.
800 Gateway Boulevard
South San Francisco, CA 94080

**For Medical Information or
To Report Adverse Events Contact:**
(888) NEURO-05
(888) 63876-05

Products Described:
◆Atamet Tablets.................. 305, 607
◆Atapryl Tablets................. *305, 609*
◆Diastat Rectal Delivery
  System..........................305, 609
Mysoline Suspension................614
◆Mysoline Tablets............... 305, 614
◆Permax Tablets................. 305, 614
◆Zanaflex Tablets............... 305, 617

AXCAN PHARMA U.S. INC. 305, 619
3940 Quebec Avenue North
Minneapolis, MN 55427

Direct Inquiries to:
Medical Department
(612) 417-0684 or
(800) 742-6706
FAX: (612) 417-9039

For Medical Emergencies Contact:
Medical Department
(612) 417-0684 or
(800) 742-6706
FAX: (612) 417-9039

Products Described:
◆Urso Tablets 250 mg........... 305, 619
Viokase Powder.....................620
◆Viokase Tablets................ 305, 620

AYERST LABORATORIES INC.
A Wyeth-Ayerst Company
(See listing under WYETH-AYERST
LABORATORIES for prescription products
and WHITEHALL-ROBINS
LABORATORIES INC. in PDR for
Nonprescription Drugs for nonprescription
products)

BARRE-NATIONAL INC.
(See ALPHARMA)

BAXTER HEALTHCARE 621
CORPORATION
Hyland Division
550 North Brand Boulevard
Glendale, CA 91203

Direct Inquiries to:
Product Management
(800) 423-2090

For Medical Emergencies Contact:
Edward Gomperts, M.D.
Medical Director,
Baxter Healthcare Corporation:
(818) 956-3200

Manufacturing and Distribution:
Coagulation Products Distributed By:
  Baxter Healthcare Corporation,
  Hyland Division
  Glendale, CA 91203
  (800) 423-2090

Plasma Expanders & Gamma Globulin
  Products Distributed By:
  Baxter Healthcare Corporation,
  Hyland Division
  Glendale, CA 91203
  (800) 423-2090

Products Described:
Buminate 5% Solution, USP.........621
Buminate 25% Solution, USP........621
Gammagard S/D.....................621
Hemofil M.........................623
Proplex T..........................623
Recombinate.......................623

BAXTER PHARMACEUTICAL 624
PRODUCTS INC.
110 Allen Road, P.O. Box 804
Liberty Corner, NJ 07938-0804

Direct Inquiries to:
Professional Services Department
(800) ANA-DRUG
(800) 262-3784

For Medical Emergencies Contact:
Raul Trillo, MD
Director, Medical Services
(800) ANA-DRUG
(800) 262-3784

Sales and Ordering:
To place an order between 7:00 AM and
  6:00 PM (Central):
(800) 345-2700

Products Described:
Atracurium Besylate Injection.........624
Atropine Sulfate Injection, USP.......624
Brevibloc Injection...................**624**
Bumetanide Injection, USP...........626
Diltiazem Hydrochloride Injection....627
Dobutamine Hydrochloride Injection..627
Duramorph Injection, USP...........627
Enlon Injection, USP.................627
Enlon-Plus Injection, USP............627
Ethrane Liquid for Inhalation, USP....627
Fentanyl Citrate Injection, USP.......627
Forane Liquid for Inhalation, USP.....628
Furosemide Injection, USP............628
Lidocaine HCl Injection, USP.........628
Meperidine Hydrochloride Injection
  Dosette, USP.....................628
Meperidine Hydrochloride Injection
  in Tubex, USP....................628
Metoclopramide Injection, USP......629
Morphine Sulfate Injection, USP......629
Naloxone HCl Injection, USP.........629
Neostigmine Methylsulfate
  Injection, USP....................629
Pancuronium Bromide Injection......629
Phenylephrine Hydrochloride
  Injection, USP....................629
Revex Injection.....................630
Sodium Nitroprusside Injection......630
Sufentanil Citrate Injection, USP......630
Suprane Liquid for Inhalation, USP... **630**
Thiopental Sodium for Injection,
  USP..............................634

BAYER CORPORATION 305, 674
PHARMACEUTICAL
DIVISION
ALLERGY PRODUCTS
400 Morgan Lane
West Haven, CT 06516

For Medical Information Contact:
Director, Medical Services
(800) 468-0894
(203) 812-2000

Products Described:
◆Ana-Kit Anaphylaxis
  Emergency Treatment Kit...... 305, 674

BAYER CORPORATION 305, 676
PHARMACEUTICAL
DIVISION
BIOLOGICAL PRODUCTS
400 Morgan Lane
West Haven, CT 06516

For Medical Information Contact:
Director, Clinical Services
(800) 468-0894
(203) 812-2000

Adverse Drug Experiences:
(888) 765-3203

Products Described:
BayHep B...........................**676**
BayRab.............................**678**
BayRho-D Full Dose................**681**
BayRho-D Mini-Dose...............**680**
BayTet.............................**682**
◆Gamimune N, 5% Solvent/
  Detergent Treated............. 305, 684
◆Gamimune N, 10% Solvent/
  Detergent Treated............. 305, 687
Koāte-HP..........................**690**
Kogenate..........................**691**
Konȳne 80.........................**693**
Prolastin...........................**695**
Thrombate III......................**696**

Other Products Available:
Plasbumin-5 Albumin (Human) 5%
Plasbumin-20 Albumin (Human) 20%
Plasbumin-25 Albumin (Human) 25%
Plasmanate Plasma Protein Fraction
  (Human) 5%

BAYER CORPORATION 305, 634
PHARMACEUTICAL
DIVISION
400 Morgan Lane
West Haven, CT 06516

For Medical Information Contact:
Director, Clinical Services
(800) 288-8371
(203) 812-2000

Adverse Drug Experiences:
(888) 765-3203

Products Described:
◆Adalat Capsules.................305, 634
◆Adalat CC Tablets.............305, 636
◆Baycol Tablets...................305, 638
◆Biltricide Tablets...............305, 641
◆Cipro HC Otic Suspension......305, 646
◆Cipro I.V.........................305, 647
◆Cipro I.V. Pharmacy Bulk
   Package.......................305, 651
◆Cipro Oral Suspension..........305, 641
◆Cipro Tablets....................305, 641
DTIC-Dome.........................656
Mezlin for Intravenous or
   Intramuscular Use..............657
Mezlin Pharmacy Bulk Package.......660
Mithracin for Intravenous Use.......663
◆Mycelex-G 500 mg Vaginal
   Tablets........................305, 664
◆Nimotop Capsules...............305, 665
Otic Domeboro Solution.............667
◆Precose Tablets..................305, 667
Trasylol Injection..................669
Tridesilon Cream 0.05%............673
Tridesilon Ointment 0.05%..........673

Other Products Available:
Cort-Dome High Potency Suppositories
Dome-Paste Bandage (Unna's Boot)
Mycelex Twin Pack
Stilphostrol Ampules

BEACH PHARMACEUTICALS 306, 698
Division of Beach Products, Inc.
5220 S. Manhattan Avenue
Tampa, FL 33611

Direct Inquiries to:
Richard Stephen Jenkins
(813) 839-6565
FAX: (813) 837-2511

Manufacturing and Distribution:
201 Delaware Street
Greenville, SC 29605
(800) 845-8210

Products Described:
◆Beelith Tablets...................306, 698
Citrolith Tablets....................698
◆K-Phos M.F. Tablets.............306, 698
◆K-Phos Neutral Tablets..........306, 698
◆K-Phos No. 2 Tablets............306, 698
◆K-Phos Original (Sodium
   Free) Tablets...................306, 699
◆Uroqid-Acid No. 2 Tablets.......306, 699

BEDFORD LABORATORIES 700
A Division of Ben Venue Laboratories, Inc.
300 Northfield Road
Bedford, OH 44146

Direct Inquiries to:
Customer Service
(800) 562-4797
FAX: (440) 232-6264

For Medical Emergencies Contact:
Professional Services
(800) 521-5169

Products Described:
Cerubidine for Injection..............700

Other Products Available:
Acetylcysteine Solution, USP
Acyclovir Sodium for Injection
Alprostadil Injection, USP
Amikacin Sulfate Injection, USP
Atracurium Besylate Injection
Azathioprine Sodium for Injection, USP
Bumetanide Injection, USP
Colchicine Injection, USP
Sterile Cytarabine, USP
Daunorubicin Hydrochloride Injection
Diltiazem Hydrochloride Injection
Dipyridamole Injection
Dobutamine Injection, USP
Doxorubicin Hydrochloride for Injection,
   USP
Doxorubicin Hydrochloride Injection, USP
Ephedrine Sulfate Injection, USP
Ergotrate Maleate
Etomidate Injection
Etoposide Injection
Fluphenazine Decanoate Injection, USP
Folic Acid Injection, USP
Haloperidol Decanoate Injection
Ketamine Hydrochloride Injection, USP
Leucovorin Calcium for Injection
Levothyroxine Sodium for Injection
Methotrexate Injection, USP
Mitomycin for Injection, USP
Papaverine Hydrochloride Injection, USP
Phentolamine Mesylate for Injection, USP
Sterile Polymyxin B Sulfate
Sterile Vinblastine Sulfate, USP

BEIERSDORF INC. 701
P. O. Box 5529
Norwalk, CT 06856-5529

Direct Inquiries to:
Medical Division
(203) 563-5800

Products Described:
Aquaphor Healing Ointment..........702
Aquaphor Original Ointment.........701
Eucerin Creme.....................702
Eucerin Lotion.....................702
Eucerin Facial Moisturizing Lotion
   SPF 25.........................702
Eucerin Light Moisture-Restorative
   Lotion.........................702
Eucerin Plus Creme................702
Eucerin Plus For The Face SPF 15....702
Eucerin Plus Lotion................702

Other Products Available:
Aquaphor Gauze
Coverlet
Coverlet Eye Occlusor
Coverlet O.R.
Cover-Roll
Cover-Strip
Cutinova Line - Advanced Wound Care
Elastomull
Elastoplast
Gelocast
Lightplast Pro
Mediplast

BERLEX LABORATORIES 306, 703
300 Fairfield Road
Wayne, NJ 07470

Direct Inquiries to:
(973) 694-4100

**For Medical Information and to Report
Drug Adverse Events Contact:**
Department of Epidemiology and Medical
Affairs
300 Fairfield Road
Wayne, NJ 07470
(888) BERLEX-4

Betaseron for SC Injection Only:
(Medical Information Only)
15049 San Pablo Avenue
P.O. Box 4099
Richmond, CA 94804-0099
(888) BERLEX-4

Fludara For Injection Only:
(Medical Information Only)
15049 San Pablo Avenue
P.O. Box 4099
Richmond, CA 94804-0099
(888) BERLEX-4

Products Described:
◆Betapace Tablets................306, 703
◆Betaseron for SC Injection.......306, 720
◆Climara Transdermal System.....306, 706
◆Fludara for Injection............306, 724
Levlen 21 Tablets..................713
◆Levlen 28 Tablets................306, 713
◆Quinaglute Dura-Tabs Tablets....306, 710
Tri-Levlen 21 Tablets...............713
◆Tri-Levlen 28 Tablets............306, 713

BERNA PRODUCTS, CORP. 306, 726
4216 Ponce de Leon Boulevard
Coral Gables, FL 33146

Direct Inquiries to:
Tina Pujals
(305) 443-2900, Ext. 232
(800) 533-5899

For Medical Information Contact:
Generally:
Andres Murai, Jr.
(305) 443-2900
(800) 533-5899
In Emergencies:
Andres Murai, Jr.
(305) 443-2900
(800) 533-5899

Products Described:
TE Anatoxal Berna..................726
◆Vivotif Berna....................306, 726

BERTEK PHARMACEUTICALS INC. 306, 728
10410 Corporate Drive
Sugar Land, TX 77478-2825

For Medical Information Contact:
Clinical Affairs Department
3711 Collins Ferry Road
Morgantown, WV 26504
(888) 823-7835
FAX: (304) 285-6453

Products Described:
◆Clorpres Tablets.................306, 728
Granulex Aerosol...................730
Kristalose for Oral Solution.........730
◆Maxzide Tablets.................306, 731

◆Maxzide-25 mg Tablets..........306, 731
Sulfamylon Cream..................733
Sulfamylon Topical Solution.........733

Other Products Available:
Biobrane Temporary Wound Dressing
Flexderm Hydrogel Wound Dressing
Flexzan Topical Wound Dressing
Hydrocol Hydrocolloid Wound Dressing
Sorbsan Topical Wound Dressing

BEUTLICH LP PHARMACEUTICALS 734
1541 Shields Drive
Waukegan, IL 60085-8304

Direct Inquiries to:
(847) 473-1100
(800) 238-8542 (in U.S. and Canada)
FAX: (847) 473-1122
E-mail: fjb1541@worldnet.att.com
World Wide Web: http://www.beutlich.com

Products Described:
Ceo-Two Evacuant Suppository.......734
Hurricaine Topical Anesthetic
   Aerosol Spray, 2 oz Wild Cherry....734
Hurricaine Topical Anesthetic Gel, 1
   oz Wild Cherry, Pina Colada,
   Watermelon, 1/8 oz Wild Cherry,
   Watermelon......................734
Hurricaine Topical Anesthetic
   Liquid, 1 oz Wild Cherry and
   Pina Colada .25 ml Dry Handle
   Swab Wild Cherry, 1/8 oz Wild
   Cherry..........................734
Hurricaine Topical Anesthetic Spray
   Extension Tubes (200)..............734
Hurricaine Topical Anesthetic Spray
   Kit.............................734
Peridin-C Tablets...................734

BIOGEN, INC. 306, 734
14 Cambridge Center
Cambridge, MA 02142

Direct Inquiries to:
Customer Service
(800) 456-2255
FAX: (617) 679-3100

For Medical Emergencies Contact:
Customer Service
(800) 456-2255
FAX: (617) 679-3100

Products Described:
◆Avonex..........................306, 734

BIOGLAN PHARMA, INC. 738
4902 Eisenhower Boulevard
Suite 150
Tampa, FL 33634

Direct Inquiries to:
(813) 243-8833
FAX: (813) 243-8832

Products Described:
Micanol 1% Cream..................738

BIO-TECHNOLOGY GENERAL CORP. 865
BTG Pharmaceuticals
70 Wood Avenue South
Iselin, N.J. 08830

Direct Inquiries to:
(732) 632-8800

**For Medical Information or Emergencies
Contact:**
(800) 741-2698

For Customer Service and Ordering:
(800) 741-2698
FAX: (800) 741-2696

Products Described:
Delatestryl Injection..................865
Oxandrin Tablets....................866

BLAINE COMPANY, INC. 739
1515 Production Drive
Burlington, KY 41005

**For Inquiries or Medical Information
Contact:**
(606) 283-9437
(800) 633-9353
FAX: (606) 283-9460

Products Described:
Mag-Ox 400 Tablets................739
Uro-Mag Capsules..................739

BLANSETT PHARMACAL CO., INC. 739
P.O. Box 638
North Little Rock, AR 72115

Direct Inquiries to:
Customer Service
(501) 758-8635
FAX: (501) 758-5369

Products Described:
Anolor 300 Capsules.................739
Cortane-B Otic Vials.................739
Nalex-A Tablets.....................739
Nalex Capsules.....................739
Nalex JR Capsules..................739
Nalex DH Liquid....................739

Other Products Available:
Cortane-B Otic Aqueous
Cortane-B Otic Lotion
Cortane-B Otic Plain
Nalex A Liquid
Nalex Expectorant
Prolex DH Liquid
Prolex DM Liquid

BLOCK DRUG COMPANY, INC. 739
257 Cornelison Avenue
Jersey City, NJ 07302

Direct Inquiries to:
Consumer Affairs
(201) 434-3000, Ext. 1308
FAX: (201) 434-5739

For Medical Information Contact:
Consumer Affairs
(800) 365-6500, Ext. 1308
FAX: (201) 434-5739

Products Described:
Aphthasol Oral Paste................739

BOCK PHARMACAL COMPANY
(See SANOFI
PHARMACEUTICALS, INC.)

BOEHRINGER INGELHEIM PHARMACEUTICALS, INC. 306, 740
A subsidiary of Boehringer Ingelheim
   Corporation
900 Ridgebury Road
P.O. Box 368
Ridgefield, CT 06877-0368
(203) 798-9988

For Medical Information Contact:
(800) 542-6257

Products Described:
◆Alupent Inhalation Aerosol.......306, 740
◆Alupent Inhalation Solution......306, 740
Alupent Syrup......................740
Alupent Tablets....................740
◆Atrovent Inhalation Aerosol......306, 742
◆Atrovent Inhalation Solution......306, 743
◆Atrovent Nasal Spray 0.03%......306, 744
◆Atrovent Nasal Spray 0.06%......306, 746
◆Catapres Tablets.................306, 747
◆Catapres-TTS....................306, 750
◆Combipres Tablets...............306, 750
◆Combivent Inhalation Aerosol....306, 752
◆Flomax Capsules................307, 755
◆Mexitil Capsules.................307, 758
◆Persantine Tablets...............307, 760
◆Prelu-2 Timed Release
   Capsules.......................307, 761
◆Respbid Tablets.................307, 762
Serentil Ampuls....................764
Serentil Concentrate................764
◆Serentil Tablets.................307, 764

BOEHRINGER MANNHEIM THERAPEUTICS
(See ROCHE LABORATORIES,
INC.)

BRAINTREE LABORATORIES, INC. 307, 766
P.O. Box 850929
Braintree, MA 02185-0929

Direct Inquiries to:
Harry P. Keegan, President
(781) 843-2202

For Medical Emergencies Contact:
Jack DiPalma, M.D.
(800) 874-6756

Products Described:
◆GoLYTELY for Oral Solution....307, 766
◆NuLYTELY for Oral Solution....307, 766
◆Cherry Flavor NuLYTELY for
   Oral Solution...................307, 766
◆PhosLo Tablets..................307, 767

◆ **Shown in Product Identification Guide**   *Italic Page Number* **Indicates Brief Listing**   ⚏ **Described in PDR For Nonprescription Drugs**

BRECKENRIDGE PHARMACEUTICAL, INC   767

P.O. Box 206
Boca Raton, FL 33429

Direct Inquiries to:
Customer Service Department
(561) 367-8512

Products Described:
Double Cap Cream 767
Prodium Tablets 768

BRISTOL LABORATORIES
(See BRISTOL-MYERS SQUIBB COMPANY)

BRISTOL-MYERS PRODUCTS
(See BRISTOL-MYERS SQUIBB COMPANY)

BRISTOL-MYERS SQUIBB   307, 817
COMPANY

P.O. Box 4500
Princeton, NJ 08543-4500
(609) 897-2000

For Medical Information Contact:
Generally:
Bristol-Myers Squibb Drug Information
Department
P.O. Box 4500
Princeton, NJ 08543-4500
(800) 321-1335
Adverse Drug Experiences
and Product Defects Reporting call
between 8:30 AM-6:00 PM EST:
(609) 818-3737

Sales and Ordering:
Orders may be placed by:

1. Calling your purchase orders toll-free
between 8:30 AM-6:00 PM EST:
(800) 631-5244

2. Mailing your purchase orders to:
Bristol-Myers Squibb U.S.
Pharmaceuticals
Attn: Customer Service
P.O. Box 5250
Princeton, NJ 08543-5250

3. Faxing your purchase orders to:
(800) 523-2965

4. Transmitting computer-to-computer on the
NWDA and UCS formats through Ordernet
Services use: DEA # PE0048579

Products Described:
◆Avapro Tablets.................... 307, 817
Azactam for Injection 820
◆BuSpar Tablets.................... 307, 823
Cefzil for Oral Suspension 825
◆Cefzil Tablets.................... 307, 825
◆Duricef Capsules.................. 307, 828
Duricef Oral Suspensions 828
◆Duricef Tablets.................. 307, 828
Estrace Vaginal Cream 830
◆Estrace Tablets.................. 307, 830
◆Glucophage Tablets.............. 307, 833
◆Maxipime for Injection.......... 307, 837
◆Monopril Tablets................ 307, 842
◆Ovcon 35 Tablets................ 307, 845
Ovcon 50 Tablets 845
◆Plavix Tablets.................. 307, 851
◆Pravachol Tablets.............. 307, 853
◆Questran Light for Oral
Suspension 307, 857
◆Questran Powder for Oral
Suspension 307, 857
◆Serzone Tablets................. 308, 859
◆Stadol NS Nasal Spray.......... 308, 863

APOTHECON   538
A Bristol-Myers Squibb Company
General Offices
P.O. Box 4500
Princeton, NJ 08543-4500

For Medical Information Contact:
Generally:
Bristol-Myers Squibb Drug Information
Department
P.O. Box 4500
Princeton, NJ 08543-4500
(800) 321-1335
Adverse Drug Experiences
and Product Defects Reporting call
between 8:30 AM-4:30 PM EST:
(609) 818-3737

Sales and Ordering:
Orders for Apothecon Products may be
placed by:

1. Calling toll-free between
8:30 AM - 6:00 PM EST:
(800) 631-5244

2. Mailing your purchase orders to:
Apothecon
Attn: Customer Service Department
P.O. Box 5250
Princeton, NJ 08543-5250

3. Faxing your purchase orders to:
Customer Service Department
(800) 523-2965

For listing of standard, purified, and human
insulins, see NOVO NORDISK
PHARMACEUTICALS INC.

Products Described:
Desyrel Tablets 539
Desyrel Dividose Tablets............. 539
Florinef Acetate Tablets............. 541
Nydrazid Injection 542
Stadol (See Bristol-Myers Squibb
Company)

Other Products Available:
Acyclovir Capsules & Tablets
Acyclovir Sodium for Injection
Albuterol Inhalation Aerosol
Amikin Injectable
Amoxicillin Capsules and Oral Suspension
(see Trimox)
Amoxicillin Tablets, USP (Chewable)
Ampicillin Capsules and Oral Suspension
(see Principen)
Ampicillin Sodium Injection USP and in
ADD-Vantage Vials
Buspirone Tablets, USP
Captopril Tablets, USP
Captopril/Hydrochlorothiazide Tablets,
USP
Cefaclor Capsules, USP
Cefaclor for Oral Suspension, USP
Cefadroxil Capsules, USP
Cefadyl for Injection
Cefazolin Sodium Injection USP
Cephalexin Capsules and for Oral
Suspension USP
Cholestyramine for Oral Suspension, USP
Cimetidine Tablets, USP
Cloxacillin Sodium Capsules, USP
Dicloxacillin Sodium Capsules and Oral
Suspension USP (See Dynapen)
Diltiazem Hydrochloride Tablets, USP
Doxycycline Hyclate Capsules & Tablets,
USP
Dynapen Oral Suspension
Enflurane, USP
Estradiol Tablets, USP
Fungizone Cream, Lotion and Ointment
Fungizone for Tissue Culture
Fungizone Intravenous
Isoflurane, USP
Kantrex Capsules
Kantrex Pediatric Injection
Kenalog Cream, Lotion, and Ointment
Kenalog in Orabase
Kenalog Spray Aerosol
Kenalog-10 and Kenalog-40 Suspension
Klotrix Tablets
K-Lyte Effervescent Tablets
K-Lyte DS Effervescent Tablets
K-Lyte/Cl Tablets
K-Lyte/Cl 50 Effervescent Tablets
Methylphenidate Hydrochloride
Extended-Release Tablets, USP
Methylphenidate Hydrochloride Tablets,
USP
Metoprolol Tartrate Tablets, USP
Mucomyst-10 and Mucomyst-20
Mycolog-II Cream and Ointment
Mycostatin Oral Suspension
Mycostatin Oral Tablets
Mycostatin Oral Tablets (Nystatin Tablets
USP)
Nadolol Tablets, USP
Nafcillin Sodium for Injection USP and in
ADD-Vantage Vials
Naldecon Syrup, Tablets, Pediatric Drops
and Pediatric Syrup
Naturetin-5 Tablets and Naturetin-10
Tablets
Niacin Tablets USP
Nitrazine Paper
Ophthaine Solution
Oxacillin Capsules USP and for Oral
Solution
Oxacillin for Injection USP and in
ADD-Vantage Vials
Penicillin G Potassium for Injection USP
Penicillin G Sodium for Injection USP
Pindolol Tablets, USP
Piroxicam Capsules, USP
Potassium Cl Extended Release Tablets
Principen Capsules, for Oral Suspension,
and Pediatric Drops
Prolixin Decanoate
Prolixin Elixir
Prolixin Enanthate
Prolixin Injection
Prolixin Oral Concentrate
Prolixin Tablets
Pronestyl Capsules, Tablets and Injection

Pronestyl-SR Tablets
Rauzide Tablets
Selegiline Hydrochloride Tablets, USP
SMZ-TMP Oral Solution and Tablets
Spec-T Sore Throat Anesthetic Lozenges
Spec-T Sore Throat/Cough Suppressant
Lozenges
Spec-T Sore Throat/Decongestant
Lozenges
Sumycin Tablets, Capsules and Syrup
Theragran Hematinic
Tobramycin Sulfate Injection USP
Trazodone Hydrochloride Tablets, USP
Trimox Capsules and for Oral Suspension
Tubocurarine Chloride Injection USP
Veetids Tablets and for Oral Suspension
Velosef Capsules and for Oral Suspension
Vesprin Injection

APOTHECON/INVAMED

Products Not Described:
Amantadine Hydrochloride Capsules, USP
Atenolol Tablets
Benztropine Mesylate Tablets, USP
Clomipramine Hydrochloride Capsules
Clonazepam Tablets, USP
Cyclobenzaprine Hydrochloride Tablets,
USP
Etodolac Capsules & Tablets
Gemfibrozil Tablets, USP
Glipizide Tablets, USP
Hydroxychloroquine Sulfate Tablets, USP
Indapamide Tablets, USP
Methazolamide Tablets, USP
Methylprednisolone Hydrochloride
Capsules, USP
Metoclopramide Tablets, USP
Naproxen Sodium Tablets, USP
Nortriptyline Hydrochloride Capsules, USP
Orphenadrine Citrate/Aspirin/Caffeine
Prochlorperazine Maleate Tablets, USP
Trifluoperazine Hydrochloride Tablets,
USP

BRISTOL-MYERS   307, 815
PRODUCTS
A Bristol-Myers Squibb Company
345 Park Avenue
New York, NY 10154

Direct Inquiries to:
Products Division
Consumer Affairs Department
1350 Liberty Avenue
Hillside, NJ 07207
(800) 468-7746

Products Described:
◆Aspirin Free Excedrin Caplets.... 307, 815
◆Aspirin Free Excedrin Geltabs.... 307, 815
◆Excedrin Extra-Strength
Caplets 307, 815
◆Excedrin Extra-Strength
Geltabs 307, 815
◆Excedrin Extra-Strength
Tablets......................... 307, 815
◆Excedrin Migraine Caplets 307, 816
◆Excedrin Migraine Tablets 307, 816
Excedrin P.M. Caplets 816
Excedrin P.M. Geltabs 816
Excedrin P.M. Tablets............. 816
◆Vagistat-1 Vaginal Ointment.... 307, 817

Other Products Available:
Alpha Keri Moisture Rich Cleansing Bar
Alpha Keri Moisture Rich Shower and
Bath Oil
Bufferin
Arthritis Strength Bufferin
Extra Strength Bufferin
Bufferin Low Dose (81 mg) Adult
Regimen
Comtrex Acute Head Cold & Sinus Relief
Comtrex Allergy-Sinus Treatment,
Maximum Strength
Comtrex Deep Chest Cold & Congestion
Relief Non-Drowsy
Comtrex Maximum Strength
Multi-Symptom Cold & Flu Relief
Comtrex Maximum Strength
Multi-Symptom Day/Night
Comtrex Maximum Strength
Multi-Symptom Non-Drowsy
Fostex 10% Benzoyl Peroxide Bar
Fostex 10% Benzoyl Peroxide (Vanish)
Gel
Fostex 10% Benzoyl Peroxide Wash
Fostex Medicated Cleansing Bar
Fostex Medicated Cleansing Cream
4-Way Fast Acting Nasal Spray - Regular
& Mentholated Formulas
4-Way Long Lasting Nasal Spray
4-Way Nasal Moisturizing Saline Mist
Keri Anti-bacterial Hand Lotion
Keri Cream
Keri Cort-10 Cream
Keri Lotion - Original Formula, Sensitive
Skin Fragrance - Free, and Silky Smooth
Minit-Rub Analgesic Ointment
No Doz Maximum Strength
Nuprin
Nuprin Backache
Pazo Hemorrhoid Ointment

Tempra 1 Aspirin Free Infant Drops,
Tempra 2 Aspirin Free Toddler Syrup
Tempra Quicklets Aspirin Free Junior and
Children's Strengths
Theragran, High Potency Multivitamins
Theragran, High Potency Multivitamin
Liquid with Minerals
Theragran Stress Formula High Potency
Multivitamins with Minerals and
Vitamin C & E
Theragran-M, High Potency Multivitamins
Therapeutic Mineral Ice
Therapeutic Mineral Ice Exercise Formula

BRISTOL-MYERS SQUIBB   308, 768
ONCOLOGY/
IMMUNOLOGY DIVISION
A Bristol-Myers Squibb Company
P.O. Box 4500
Princeton, NJ 08543-4500
(609) 897-2000

For Medical Information Contact:
Generally:
Bristol-Myers Squibb Drug Information
Department
P.O. Box 4500
Princeton, NJ 08543-4500
(800) 426-7644
Adverse Drug Experiences
and Product Defects Reporting call
during business hours only:
(609) 818-3737

Sales and Ordering:
Orders may be placed by:

1. Calling the following toll-free number
between 8:30 AM--6:00 PM EST:
Continental U.S.: (800) 631-5244
Alaska--Hawaii: (800) 631-5244

2. Mail orders and all inquiries should be
sent to:
Bristol-Myers Squibb Oncology Division
Attn: Customer Service
P.O. Box 5250
Princeton, NJ 08543-5250

3. Faxing your purchase orders to:
(800) 523-2965

4. Transmitting computer-to-computer on the
NWDA and UCS formats through Ordernet
Services use:
DEA # PE0048579

Products Described:
BiCNU............................ 768
◆Blenoxane 308, 769
CeeNU Capsules.................. 771
◆Cytoxan for Injection 308, 772
◆Cytoxan Tablets................. 308, 772
◆Droxia Capsules................ 308, 774
◆Etopophos for Injection 308, 776
Fungizone Oral Suspension 779
Hydrea Capsules.................. 779
◆Ifex for Injection.............. 308, 781
Lysodren Tablets................. 782
◆Megace Oral Suspension 308, 783
◆Megace Tablets................. 308, 785
◆Mesnex Injection............... 308, 786
◆Mutamycin for Injection 308, 787
Mycostatin Pastilles 788
◆Paraplatin for Injection......... 308, 789
Platinol for Injection 792
◆Platinol-AQ Injection 308, 794
Rubex for Injection 796
◆Taxol Injection................ 308, 798
Teslac Tablets................... 803
◆VePesid Capsules............... 308, 804
◆VePesid for Injection 308, 804
Videx Powder for Oral Solution 806
Videx Pediatric Powder for Oral
Solution 806
◆Videx Chewable Tablets........ 303, 806
Vumon for Injection............. 810
◆Zerit Capsules................. 308, 812
◆Zerit for Oral Solution......... 308, 812

WESTWOOD-SQUIBB   3242
PHARMACEUTICALS INC.
A Bristol-Myers Squibb Company
100 Forest Avenue
Buffalo, NY 14213
(716) 887-3400

For Medical Information Contact:
Generally:
Consumer Affairs Department
1-(800) 333-0950
Adverse Drug Experiences
and Product Defects Reporting
call during business hours only:
1-(800) 333-0950

Products Described:
Capitrol Shampoo 3242
Desquam-E 2.5 Emollient Gel........ 3242
Desquam-E 5 Emollient Gel......... 3242
Desquam-E 10 Emollient Gel........ 3242

◆ **Shown in Product Identification Guide**   *Italic Page Number* **Indicates Brief Listing**   ☉ **Described in PDR For Ophthalmology**

**BRISTOL-MYERS SQUIBB
ONCOLOGY/IMMUNOLOGY
DIVISION**
(See BRISTOL-MYERS SQUIBB
COMPANY)

**J. R. CARLSON LABORATORIES,   867
INC.**
15 College Drive
Arlington Heights, IL 60004-1985

Direct Inquiries to:
Customer Service
(847) 255-1600
FAX: (847) 255-1605

For Medical Emergencies Contact:
Customer Service
(847) 255-1600
FAX: (847) 255-1605

**CARNRICK   308, 867
LABORATORIES, INC.**
65 Horse Hill Road
Cedar Knolls, NJ 07927

Direct Inquiries to:
(973) 267-2670
FAX: (973) 267-2289

For Medical Information Contact:
Technical Service Dept.
(973) 267-2670
FAX: (973) 267-2289

CELGENE CORPORATION   309, 3457
7 Powder Horn Drive
Warren, NJ 07059

Direct Inquiries to:
(888) 423-5436

CENTEON L.L.C.   878
1020 First Avenue
King of Prussia, PA 19406-1310

Direct Inquiries to:
(610) 878-4000

For Medical Information Contact:
(800) 504-5434

Sales and Ordering:
Customer Support Center
(800) 683-1288
FAX: (610) 878-4888

CENTOCOR, INC.   309, 890
200 Great Valley Parkway
Malvern, PA 19355

Direct General Inquiries to:
(610) 651-6000
(888) 874-3083
FAX: (610) 651-6100

For Medical Emergencies Contact:
(800) 457-6399

**For Medical Information/Adverse
  Experience Reporting Contact:**
Medical Information and Product
  Surveillance
(800) 457-6399
FAX: 610-651-6197

Branch Office:
Centocor B.V.
Einsteinweg 101
2333 CB Leiden, The Netherlands

**CENTRAL PHARMACEUTICALS,
INC.**
(See SCHWARZ PHARMA, INC.)

**CETYLITE INDUSTRIES,   309, 894
INC.**
9051 River Road
Pennsauken, NJ 08110-3293
Mailing Address:
P.O. Box 90006
Pennsauken, NJ 08110-0700

Direct Inquiries to:
Mr. Stanley L. Wachman, President
(609) 665-6111
(800) 257-7740
FAX: (609) 665-5408

CHIRON CORPORATION   309, 894
4560 Horton Street
Emeryville, CA 94608-2997

For Medical Information Contact:
Generally:
Professional Services (6:00 AM to 5:00
  PM PST):
(800) CHIRON-8 selection #2
(800) 244-7668 selection #2
FAX: (510) 923-3435
E-mail: drug_info@cc.chiron.com
In Emergencies:
(6:00 AM to 5:00 PM PST):
(800) CHIRON-8 selection #3
(800) 244-7668 selection #3
After Hours & Weekend Emergencies:
(415) 885-8777

Sales and Ordering:
(800) CHIRON-8 selection #1
(800) 244-7668 selection #1
FAX: (510) 923-3434

**CIBAGENEVA
PHARMACEUTICALS**
(See NOVARTIS
PHARMACEUTICALS
CORPORATION for branded
products)
(See GENEVA
PHARMACEUTICALS, INC. for
branded generic products)

**COLGATE ORAL   902
PHARMACEUTICALS, INC.**
A subsidiary of Colgate-Palmolive
Company
One Colgate Way
Canton, MA 02021 USA

Direct Inquiries to:
Professional Services Department
(800) 226-5428

For Medical Emergencies Contact:
Pittsburgh Poison Control
(412) 692-5596

CONNETICS CORPORATION   309, 903
3400 West Bayshore Road
Palo Alto, CA 94303

Direct Inquiries to:
(650) 843-2800

COR THERAPEUTICS, INC.   309, 904
256 East Grand Avenue
South San Francisco, CA 94080

Direct Inquiries to:
(888) 267-4-MED

**CYPROS PHARMACEUTICAL   908
CORPORATION**
2714 Loker Avenue West
Carlsbad, CA 92008

Direct Inquiries to:
(800) 411-3065
(760) 929-9500
FAX: (760) 929-8038

**DAIICHI   309, 909
PHARMACEUTICAL
CORPORATION**
11 Phillips Parkway
Montvale, NJ 07645

Direct Inquiries to:
Medical Services Department
(877) 324-4244 (877-DAIICHI)
FAX: (888) 727-5666

**For Medical Emergencies and Product
  Information Contact:**
Medical Services Department
(888) 727-2500
FAX: (888) 272-7979

DERMIK LABORATORIES, INC.   910
500 Arcola Road
P.O. Box 1200
Collegeville, PA 19426-0107
(610) 454-8000

Direct Inquiries to:
QUALITY ASSURANCE QUESTIONS:
John Chiles, Manager, Quality Control
(610) 454-3130
REGULATORY AFFAIRS QUESTIONS:
Ron Panner, Director, Regulatory Affairs
(610) 454-3026

For Medical Information Contact:
PRODUCT INFORMATION/
  ADVERSE DRUG
  EXPERIENCES/EMERGENCIES:
Medical Information and Education
(800) 340-7502
(610) 454-8110

DEY   309, 916
2751 Napa Valley Corporate Drive
Napa, CA 94558
(800) 869-9005

Direct Inquiries to:
Russ Johnston
(800) 755-5560
FAX: (707) 224-8918

For Medical Emergencies Contact:
Cal McGoogan
(707) 224-3200
FAX: (707) 224-3235

**DISTA PRODUCTS   309, 917
COMPANY, DIVISION OF
ELI LILLY AND COMPANY**

For Medical Information Contact:
Lilly Research Laboratories
Lilly Corporate Center
Indianapolis, IN 46285
(800) 545-5979

Direct Inquiries to:
Lilly Corporate Center
Indianpolis, IN 46285
(317) 276-2000

AREA SALES OFFICES:
Atlanta, GA 30328
North Park Town Center
Building 500, Suite 710
1100 Abernathy Road, NE
(770) 551-5376
Bala Cynwyd, PA 19004
401 City Avenue
Suite 400
(610) 617-1157
Birmingham, AL 35243
3800 Colonade Parkway
Suite 250
(205) 969-4556
Anaheim, CA 92806
2400 East Katella Avenue
Suite 530
(714) 940-0800
Chicago, IL 60631
Suite 810, O'Hare Plaza
8725 West Higgins Road
(773) 693-1953
Dallas, TX 75248
15301 Dallas Parkway
Suite 960, Box 66
(972) 960-7637
Indianapolis, IN 46268
Suite 203, 10 Fortune Park
3905 Vincennes Road
(317) 276-5967
Stamford, CT 06902
300 First Stamford Place
(203) 316-2708

Products Described:

**DOW HICKAM
PHARMACEUTICALS**
(See BERTEK PHARMACEUTICALS
INC.)

DUPONT   **309, 929**
**PHARMACEUTICALS
COMPANY**
Chestnut Run Plaza
Hickory Run
P.O. Box 80723
Wilmington, DE 19880-0723
(302) 992-5000

Direct All Product-Related Inquiries to:
Medical Affairs Department

**For Product Information/Adverse Drug
Experience Reporting Contact:**
Product Information
(302) 992-4240

Products Described:

DURA PHARMACEUTICALS   **943**
7475 Lusk Boulevard
San Diego, CA 92121

**Direct Inquiries and
For Medical Information Contact:**
Medical Affairs Department
(888) 859-8583
FAX: (619) 657-0977

**For Sales Representatives Requests
Contact:**
(800) 859-8586

Products Described:

ECR PHARMACEUTICALS   **960**
Distributor of ECR Pharmaceuticals &
Wm. P. Poythress Products
3981 Deep Rock Road
P.O. Box 71600
Richmond, VA 23255

Direct Inquiries to:
Professional Services Department
(804) 527-1950
FAX: (804) 527-1959

For Medical Emergencies Contact:
Professional Services Department
(804) 527-1950
FAX: (804) 527-1959

Products Described:

EISAI INC.   **309, 960**
500 Frank W. Burr Boulevard
Teaneck, NJ 07666

Direct Inquiries to:
Eisai Medical Services
(888) 274-2378 (888-ARICEPT)
FAX: (201) 287-9744

For Medical Emergencies Contact:
(24 hours/day, 7 days/week):
(888) 274-2378 (888-ARICEPT)

Products Described:

ELKINS-SINN, INC.   **963**
2 Esterbrook Lane
Cherry Hill, NJ 08003-4099

Direct General Inquiries to:
(610) 688-4400

**For Emergency Medical Information
Contact:**
Day: (800) 934-5556 (8:30 AM to 4:30
PM, Eastern Standard Time, Weekdays
only)
Night: (610) 688-4400 (Emergencies only;
non-emergencies should wait until the
next day)

**For Medical/Pharmacy Inquiries on
Marketed Products Contact:**
(800) 934-5556 (8:30 AM to 4:30 PM,
Eastern Standard Time, Weekdays only)

Products Described:

Other Products Available:
Dipyramidole Injection
Dobutamine Hydrochloride Injection

ENDO PHARMACEUTICALS   **309, 971**
INC.
223 Wilmington West Chester Pike
Chadds Ford, PA 19317
(800) 462-3636
FAX: (302) 992-3006

Direct Inquiries to:
Customer Service
(800) 462-3636
FAX: (302) 992-3006

**For Medical Information/Adverse Drug
Experience Reporting Contact:**
Product Information:
(800) 462-3636

ENDO LABORATORIES

Products Described:

ENDO PHARMACEUTICALS INC.   **971**
223 Wilmington West Chester Pike
Chadds Ford, PA 19317
(800) 462-3636
FAX: (302) 992-3006

Direct Inquiries to:
Customer Service
(800) 462-3636
FAX: (302) 992-3006

**For Medical Information/Adverse Drug
Experience Reporting Contact:**
Product Information:
(800) 462-3636

ENDO GENERIC PRODUCTS

Products Described:

ENZON, INC.   **990**
20 Kingsbridge Road
Piscataway, NJ 08854

Direct Inquiries to:
Toni L. Klich
(732) 980-4619
FAX: (732) 980-5911

For Medical Emergencies Contact:
Anna T. Viau, Ph.D.
(732) 980-4677
FAX: (732) 980-9642

Products Described:

ESI LEDERLE INC.   **310, 992**
P.O. Box 41502
Philadelphia, PA 19101

Direct General Inquiries to:
(610) 688-4400

**For Emergency Medical Information
Contact:**
Medical Affairs
Day: (800) 934-5556 (8:30 AM to 4:30
PM, Eastern Standard Time, Weekdays
only)
Night: (610) 688-4400 (Emergencies only;
non-emergencies should wait until the
next day)

**For Medical/Pharmacy Inquiries on
Marketed Products Contact:**
(800) 934-5556 (8:30 AM to 4:30 PM,
Eastern Standard Time, Weekdays only)

Products Described:

Other Products Available:
Acebutolol Hydrochloride Capsules
Acyclovir Capsules
Acyclovir Injection
Acyclovir Tablets
Atracurium Besylate Injection
Cephalexin Oral Suspension
Etodolac Capsules
Etodolac Tablets
Griseofulvin
Griseofulvin Ultra
Guanfacine Hydrochloride Tablets
Hydrocodone Bitartrate and
Acetaminophen Tablets
Ketoprofen SR Capsules
Levothyroxine Sodium Tablets
Lorazepam Tablets
Methotrexate Sodium Tablets
Metoclopramide Tablets
Minocycline HCl Capsules
Oxazepam Capsules
Pentoxifylline ER Tablets
Prenatal Plus Tablets
Promethazine HCl and Codeine Phosphate
Syrup

Promethazine HCl and Dextromethorphan
Hydrobromide Syrup
Promethazine HCl and Phenylephrine HCl
Syrup
Promethazine HCl, Phenylephrine HCl and
Codeine Phosphate Syrup
Propanolol HCl Long-Acting Capsules
Quinidine Sulfate E-R
Selegiline HCl Tablets
Sulfamethoxazole and Trimethoprim
Tablets

ESI PHARMA, INC.
(See ESI LEDERLE INC.)

EVERETT LABORATORIES, INC.   994
29 Spring Street
West Orange, NJ 07052

Direct Inquiries to:
Professional Service Department
(973) 324-0200
FAX: (973) 324-0795

Products Described:
Cortic Ear Drops........................994
Strovite Forte Caplets..................994
Strovite Forte Syrup....................995
Tussafed-HC............................995
Vitafol Caplets........................995
Vitafol Syrup..........................995
Vitafol-PN Caplets.....................995

Other Products Available:
Florvite Drops .25 + .5 mg
Florvite + Iron Drops .25 + .5 mg
Florvite Tablets 0.5 + 1 mg
Florvite + Iron Tablets .5 + 1 mg
Repan-CF Tablets
Repan Tablets & Capsules
Strovite Plus Caplets
Strovite Tablets
Tussafed Drops
Tussafed Syrup

FAULDING LABORATORIES   310, 995
5511 Capital Center Drive
Suite P116
Raleigh, NC 27606

Direct Inquiries to:
Customer Service
(800) 432-8534
FAX: (908) 820-0142

Products Described:
◆Kadian Capsules.................310, 995

**FERNDALE LABORATORIES,   999
INC.**
780 West Eight Mile Road
Ferndale, MI 48220

Direct Inquiries to:
Mr. Thayer McMillan
(248) 548-0900
FAX: (248) 548-8427

For Medical Emergencies Contact:
Mr. Pravin M. Patel
(248) 548-0900
FAX: (248) 548-0708

Products Described:
Analpram HC Lotion 2.5%............999
Analpram-HC Rectal Cream 1% and
2.5%..................................999
Decubitene Oxygenated Oil...........999
Dermamist Spray......................1000
ELA-Max 5 Cream....................1001
ELA-Max Cream......................1000
Kronofed-A Kronocaps...............1002
Kronofed-A-Jr. Kronocaps...........1002
Locoid Cream........................1002
Locoid Lipocream Cream.............1003
Locoid Ointment......................1002
Locoid Topical Solution..............1002
Pramosone Cream....................1003
Pramosone Lotion....................1003
Pramosone Ointment.................1003
Prax Lotion..........................1004
Pro-Q Skin Protectant...............1004
SBR-Lipocream......................1004

Other Products Available:
Betuline Liniment
Capsaicin Cream 0.025%
Capsaicin-HP Cream 0.075%
Detachol Adhesive Remover
Liqui-Doss
Mastisol Liquid Adhesive
Tin-Ben Dispenser
Tin-Co-Ben Dispenser
Topiclude Occlusive Dressing

**FERRING PHARMACEUTICALS   1004
INC.**
120 White Plains Road
Suite 400
Tarrytown, NY 10591

Direct Inquiries to:
Ferring Pharmaceuticals Inc.
Customer Service Department
120 White Plains Road
Suite 400
Tarrytown, NY 10591
(888) FERRING (337-7464)

For Medical Emergencies Contact:
Ferring Pharmaceuticals Inc.
Professional Services Department
120 White Plains Road
Suite 400
Tarrytown, NY 10591
(888) 793-6367

Products Described:
Acthrel for Injection..........1004, 3468
Desmopressin Acetate Injection......1006
Desmopressin Acetate Rhinal Tube..1007
Repronex for Intramuscular
Injection..............................1009
Secretin-Ferring.....................3469
Thyrel TRH..........................3470

**THE FIELDING   1011
PHARMACEUTICAL
COMPANY, INC.**
P.O. Box 2186
112 Weldon Parkway
Maryland Heights, MO 63043

Direct Inquiries to:
Professional Services Department
(314) 567-5462

For Medical Emergencies Contact:
(314) 567-5462

Products Described:
Gerimed Tablets.....................1011
Irospan Capsules....................1011
Irospan Tablets......................1011
Lurline PMS Tablets.................1011
Nestabs CBF Tablets................1011

Other Products Available:
Duracid
Metric 21 Tablets
Nestabs Tablets
Nestrex Tablets

**FISONS CORPORATION
PRESCRIPTION PRODUCTS**
(See MEDEVA
PHARMACEUTICALS, INC.)

C. B. FLEET CO., INC.   1011
4615 Murray Place
Lynchburg, VA 24506-1349

Direct Inquiries to:
David Vaughan
Director of Quality Assurance
(804) 528-4000
FAX: (804) 847-4219

Products Described:
Fleet Bisacodyl Laxatives...........1011
Fleet Enema.........................1012
Fleet Enema for Children............1012
Fleet Mineral Oil Enema.............1012
Fleet Phospho-Soda.................1013
Fleet Prep Kits......................1013

FLEMING & COMPANY   1013
1600 Fenpark Dr.
Fenton, MO 63026

Direct Inquiries to:
H.C. Mansmann, Jr. M.D.
(314) 343-8200

Products Described:
Aerolate Liquid......................1013
Aerolate Jr. T.D. Capsules..........1013
Aerolate Sr. T.D. Capsules..........1013
Aerolate III T.D. Capsules..........1013
Chlor-3 Condiment..................1014
Congess Jr. T.D. Capsules..........1014
Congess Sr. T.D. Capsules..........1014
Extendryl Chewable Tablets.........1014
Extendryl Sr. & Jr. T.D. Capsules...1014
Extendryl Syrup.....................1014
Impregon Concentrate..............1014
Magonate Tablets and Liquid.......1014
Marblen Suspension Peach/Apricot....■□
Marblen Tablets........................■□
Nephrocaps..........................1014
Nephrox Suspension...................■□

Nicotinex Elixir.........................■□
Ocean Nasal Mist......................■□
Pima Syrup.........................1014
Purge Concentrate.....................■□
Rum-K Syrup.......................1014

Other Products Available:
Alumadrine Tablets

**FOREST   310, 1015
PHARMACEUTICALS,
INC.**
Subsidiary of FOREST LABORATORIES,
INC.
13622 Lakefront Drive
St. Louis, MO 63045

Direct Inquiries to:
Professional Affairs Department
13622 Lakefront Drive
St. Louis, MO 63045
(314) 344-8870

Products Described:
◆Aerobid Inhaler System.........310, 1015
◆Aerobid-M Inhaler System.......310, 1015
◆AeroChamber and
AeroChamber with Mask.....310, 1016
Antilirium Injectable.................1018
◆Armour Thyroid Tablets.......310, 1018
◆Cervidil Vaginal Insert.........310, 1019
Dalalone D.P. Injectable.............1020
Endal-HD...........................1020
◆Esgic Capsules..............310, 1020
Esgic Tablets.......................1020
◆Esgic-plus Capsules...............310
◆Esgic-plus Tablets.............310, 1021
Flumadine Syrup...................1022
◆Flumadine Tablets............310, 1022
◆Infasurf Intratracheal
Suspension...................310, 1023
◆Levothroid Tablets............310, 1025
◆Lorcet 10/650 Tablets.........310, 1027
Lorcet-HD Capsules................1026
◆Lorcet Plus Tablets............310, 1027
◆Monurol Sachet...............310, 1027
Sus-Phrine Injection................1029
◆Tessalon Perles...............310, 1029
◆Thyrolar Tablets...............310, 1030
◆Tiazac Capsules..............310, 1030

Other Products Available:
Adbcon Injectable
Almora Tablets
Ambenyl Cough Syrup
Ambenyl D Syrup
Andro L.A. "200" Injectable
Banalg Hospital Strength Arthritic Pain
Reliever
Banalg Liniment
Bancap HC Capsules
Banflex Injectable
Brompheniramine Maleate Injection
Bucet Capsules
Cebocap Capsules
Celexa Tablets
Cyomin Injectable
Dalalone Injectable
Dalalone L.A. Injectable
depAndrogyn Injectable
depGynogen Injectable
depMedalone "40" Injectable
depMedalone "80" Injectable
Disotate Injectable
Elixophyllin Elixir
Elixophyllin-GG Oral Solution
Elixophyllin-KI Elixir
Endafed Capsules
Endal Expectorant
Endal Tablets
Endal-HD Plus
Enzone Cream
Eudal SR Tablets
Feostat Drops
Feostat Suspension
Feostat Tablets
Gynogen LA "20" Injectable
Kay Ciel Oral Solution
Kay Ciel Powder Packets
Lidocaine 1% & 2% Injectable
Nitrogard Tablets
Pedameth Capsules
Pedameth Liquid
Theochron Tablets
Triad Capsules
Triamcinolone Diacetate Injectable
Triamonide "40" Injectable
UAD Otic Suspension
Zone A Forte Lotion
Zone A Lotion 1%

**FUJISAWA HEALTHCARE,   310, 1033
INC.**
Parkway North Center
3 Parkway North
Deerfield, IL 60015-2548

For Medical Information Contact:
Generally:
Medical and Scientific Information
(800) 727-7003

In Emergencies:
Medical and Scientific Information
(800) 727-7003

Products Described:
Adenocard Injection.................1033
Adenoscan.........................1034
AmBisome for Injection.............1035
Aristocort A 0.025% Cream.........1039
Aristocort A 0.1% Cream...........1040
Aristocort A 0.5% Cream...........1040
Aristocort A 0.1% Ointment........1040
Aristocort Suspension (Forte
Parenteral)........................1039
Aristocort Suspension
(Intralesional).....................1039
Aristospan Suspension
(Intra-articular)...................1040
Aristospan Suspension
(Intralesional).....................1040
Cefizox for Intramuscular or
Intravenous Use..................1041
Cefizox for Intramuscular or
Intravenous Use Pharmacy Bulk
Package..........................1043
Cefizox for Intravenous Infusion.....1043
Cefizox for Intravenous Use in
Galaxy Plastic Container..........1043
Cyclocort Topical Cream 0.1%.....1044
Cyclocort Topical Lotion 0.1%.....1044
Cyclocort Topical Ointment 0.1%....1044
◆Prograf........................310, 1044

**GALDERMA LABORATORIES,   1048
INC.**
P.O. Box 331329
Fort Worth, TX 76163

Direct Inquiries to:
(888) 898-DERM (3376)
8 a.m. to 5 p.m. Central (Monday through
Friday)

Products Described:
Benzac 5 & 10 Gel..................1048
Benzac AC 2 ½, 5 & 10 Gel.........1048
Benzac AC Wash 2 ½, 5 & 10......1048
Benzac W 2 ½, 5 & 10 Water
Base Gel..........................1048
Benzac W Wash 5 & 10.............1048
Cetaphil Gentle Cleansing Bar......1049
Cetaphil Antibacterial Gentle
Cleansing Bar.....................1049
Cetaphil Gentle Skin Cleanser......1049
Cetaphil Oily Skin Cleanser.........1049
Cetaphil Moisturizing Cream........1049
Cetaphil Moisturizing Lotion........1050
DesOwen Cream....................1050
DesOwen Lotion.....................1050
DesOwen Ointment..................1050
Differin Gel..........................1050
Differin Solution.....................1051
MetroCream........................1052
MetroGel...........................1052

**GATE PHARMACEUTICALS   310, 1053
A Division of TEVA
PHARMACEUTICALS USA**
650 Cathill Road
Sellersville, PA 18960

Direct Inquiries to:
(800) 292-4283
FAX: (215) 653-0839

Products Described:
Adipex-P Capsules..................1053
◆Adipex-P Tablets..............310, 1053
◆Orap Tablets..................311, 1054

GEBAUER COMPANY   1056
9410 St. Catherine Avenue
Cleveland, OH 44104

Direct Inquiries to:
(800) 321-9348
(216) 271-5252
www.gebauerco.com

For Medical Emergencies Contact:
(800) 321-9348
(216) 271-5252

After Hours and Weekend Emergencies:
Chemtrec
(800) 424-9300

Products Described:
Ethyl Chloride, U.S.P...............1056

Other Products Available:
Dr's. Cream
Fluori-Methane
Salivart

GENENTECH, INC.   311, 1057
1 DNA Way
South San Francisco, CA 94080-4990
(650) 225-1000

For Medical Information Contact:
Medical Information or Drug Experience Departments (24 hours):
(800) 821-8590
(650) 225-1000
Or write:
Medical Information or Drug Experience Departments:
Genetech, Inc.
1 DNA Way
South San Francisco, CA 94080-4990

Products Described:
◆Activase I.V. **311, 1057**
◆Nutropin AQ Injection **311, 1064**
◆Nutropin for Injection **311, 1061**
◆Protropin for Injection **311, 1067**
◆Pulmozyme Inhalation Solution **311, 1068**
◆Rituxan I.V. **311, 1070**

GENETICS INSTITUTE **311, 1073**
87 Cambridge Park Drive
Cambridge, MA 02140

Direct Inquiries to:
(888) NEUMEGA
(888) 638-6342

Products Described:
◆Neumega for Injection **311, 1073**

GENEVA PHARMACEUTICALS, INC. **1076**
2655 West Midway Boulevard
P.O. Box 446
Broomfield, CO 80038-0446

Direct Inquiries to:
Customer Support Department
(800) 525-8747
(303) 466-2400
FAX: (303) 469-6467

Products Described:
Albuterol Tablets *1076*
Alprazolam Tablets *1076*
Amitriptyline HCl Tablets *1076*
Amoxapine Tablets *1076*
Atenolol Tablets *1076*
Bromocriptine Mesylate Tablets *1076*
Captopril Tablets *1076*
Carisoprodol Tablets *1076*
Chlorpromazine HCl Tablets *1076*
Cimetidine Tablets *1076*
Clemastine Fumarate Syrup *1076*
Clemastine Fumarate Tablets *1076*
Clomipramine HCl Capsules *1076*
Cyclobenzaprine HCl Tablets *1076*
Desipramine HCl Tablets *1076*
Diclofenac Sodium Delayed-Release Tablets *1076*
Disobrom Tablets *1076*
Doxepin HCl Capsules *1076*
Ercaf Tablets *1076*
Etodolac Tablets *1076*
Fiorpap Tablets *1076*
Fiortal Capsules *1076*
Fiortal w/Codeine Capsules *1076*
Fluphenazine HCl Tablets *1076*
Flurbiprofen Tablets *1076*
Furosemide Tablets *1076*
Glipizide Tablets *1076*
Haloperidol Tablets *1076*
Hydroxychloroquine Sulfate Tablets *1076*
Imipramine HCl Tablets *1076*
Indomethacin Capsules *1076*
Isosorbide Dinitrate Tablets *1076*
Isoxsuprine HCl Tablets *1076*
Ketoprofen Capsules *1076*
Lonox Tablets *1076*
Loperamide HCl Capsules *1076*
Lorazepam Tablets *1076*
Meclizine HCl Tablets *1076*
Methazolamide Tablets *1076*
Methocarbamol Tablets *1076*
Metoprolol Tartrate Tablets *1076*
Mexiletine HCl Capsules *1076*
Naproxen Tablets *1076*
Naproxen Sodium Tablets *1076*
Nortriptyline HCl Capsules *1076*
Oxazepam Capsules *1076*
Perphenazine Tablets *1076*
Perphenazine/Amitriptyline HCl Tablets *1076*
Pindolol Tablets *1076*
Promethazine HCl Tablets *1076*
Propoxyphene HCl/Acetaminophen Tablets *1076*
Propoxyphene Napsylate/ Acetaminophen Tablets *1076*
Pseudoephedrine HCl Tablets *1076*
Quinidine Gluconate Extended-Release Tablets *1076*
Ranitidine HCl Capsules *1076*
Ranitidine HCl Tablets *1076*
Rimactane Capsules *1076*
Spironolactone Tablets *1076*
Sulindac Tablets *1076*
Temazepam Capsules *1076*
Thioridazine HCl Tablets *1076*
Thiothixene Capsules *1076*
Trazodone HCl Tablets *1076*
Triamterene/HCTZ 50mg/25mg Capsules *1076*
Triamterene/HCTZ (Dyazide) 37.5mg/25mg Capsules *1076*
Triamterene/HCTZ (mini-Maxzide) 37.5mg/25mg Tablets *1076*
Triamterene/HCTZ (Maxzide) 75mg/50mg Tablets *1076*
Trifluoperazine HCl Tablets *1076*
Verapamil HCl Tablets *1076*

GENZYME CORPORATION **1077**
One Kendall Square
Cambridge, MA 02139

Direct Inquiries to:
Clinical Services
(800) 745-4447
FAX: (617) 252-7700

For Medical Emergencies Contact:
(800) 745-4447

Products Described:
Ceredase Injection **1077**
Cerezyme for Injection **1078**

GILEAD SCIENCES **1079**
333 Lakeside Drive
Foster City, CA 94404

Direct Inquiries to:
Customer Service
(800) GILEAD5

For Medical Information or to Report an Adverse Event Contact:
Medical Information/Safety Surveillance
(800) GILEAD5
FAX: (650) 577-5477

Products Described:
Vistide Injection **1079**

GLAXO WELLCOME INC. **311, 1082**
Five Moore Drive
Research Triangle Park
North Carolina 27709
(919) 483-2100

For Medical Information for Healthcare Professionals Contact:
(888) Talk-2 GW or direct (919) 315-3272
Medical Information Department:
(800) 334-0089

In Emergencies:
Medical Information Department:
(800) 334-0089

For Consumer Inquiries Contact:
(888) Talk-2 GW

Products Described:
◆Aclovate Cream **311, 1082**
◆Aclovate Ointment **311, 1082**
◆Alkeran for Injection **311, 1083**
◆Alkeran Tablets **311, 1085**
◆Amerge Tablets **311, 1086**
◆Anectine Injection **311, 1090**
◆Beclovent Inhalation Aerosol and Refill **311, 1092**
◆Beconase Inhalation Aerosol **311, 1093**
◆Beconase AQ Nasal Spray **311, 1095**
◆Ceftin for Oral Suspension **311, 1096**
◆Ceftin Tablets **312, 1096**
◆Ceptaz **311, 1100**
◆Combivir Tablets **312, 1104**
◆Cutivate Cream **312, 1107**
◆Cutivate Ointment **312, 1108**
◆Daraprim Tablets **312, 1109**
◆Digibind **312, 1110**
◆Emgel 2% Topical Gel **312, 1112**
◆Epivir Oral Solution **312, 1112**
◆Epivir Tablets **312, 1112**
◆Exosurf Neonatal for Intratracheal Suspension **312, 1115**
◆Flolan for Injection **312, 1118**
◆Flonase Nasal Spray **312, 1122**
◆Flovent 44 mcg Inhalation Aerosol **312, 1124**
◆Flovent 110 mcg Inhalation Aerosol **312, 1124**
◆Flovent 220 mcg Inhalation Aerosol **312, 1124**
◆Flovent Rotadisk 50 mcg **312, 1126**
◆Flovent Rotadisk 100 mcg **312, 1126**
◆Flovent Rotadisk 250 mcg **312, 1126**
◆Fortaz **312, 1130**
◆Imitrex Injection **313, 1133**
◆Imitrex Nasal Spray **313, 1137**
◆Imitrex Tablets **313, 1141**
◆Imuran Injection **312, 1145**
◆Imuran Tablets **312, 1145**
◆Lamictal Tablets **313, 1148**
◆Lanoxicaps **313, 1153**
◆Lanoxin Elixir Pediatric **313, 1156**
◆Lanoxin Injection **313, 1160**
◆Lanoxin Injection Pediatric **313, 1164**
◆Lanoxin Tablets **313, 1167**
◆Leucovorin Calcium for Injection, Wellcovorin Brand **313, 1172**
◆Leukeran Tablets **313, 1171**
◆Mepron Suspension **313, 1174**
◆Mivacron Injection **313, 1177**
◆Mivacron Premixed Infusion **313, 1177**
◆Myleran Tablets **313, 1181**
◆Navelbine Injection **313, 1184**
◆Nimbex Injection **313, 1187**
◆Nuromax Injection **313, 1192**
◆Oxistat Cream **313, 1194**
◆Oxistat Lotion **313, 1194**
◆Purinethol Tablets **313, 1196**
◆Raxar Tablets **313, 1198**
◆Retrovir Capsules **313, 1202**
◆Retrovir IV Infusion **313, 1207**
◆Retrovir Syrup **313, 1202**
◆Retrovir Tablets **313, 1202**
◆Serevent Diskus **314, 1215**
◆Serevent Inhalation Aerosol **314, 1211**
◆Temovate Cream **314, 1220**
◆Temovate E Emollient **314, 1222**
◆Temovate Gel **314, 1221**
◆Temovate Ointment **314, 1220**
◆Temovate Scalp Application **314, 1222**
◆Thioguanine Tablets, Tabloid Brand **314, 1218**
◆Tracrium Injection **314, 1223**
◆Trandate Injection **314, 1226**
◆Trandate Tablets **314, 1229**
◆Tritec Tablets **314, 1231**
◆Ultiva for Injection **314, 1233**
◆Valtrex Caplets **314, 1239**
◆Vasoxyl Injection **314, 1241**
◆Ventolin Inhalation Aerosol and Refill **314, 1242**
◆Ventolin Inhalation Solution **314, 1244**
◆Ventolin Nebules Inhalation Solution **314, 1246**
◆Ventolin Rotacaps for Inhalation **314, 1247**
◆Ventolin Syrup **314, 1249**
◆Ventolin Tablets **314, 1250**
◆Wellbutrin Tablets **314, 1252**
◆Wellbutrin SR Sustained-Release Tablets **314, 1255**
◆Zantac 150 EFFERdose Granules **314, 1260**
◆Zantac 150 EFFERdose Tablets **314, 1260**
◆Zantac 150 GELdose Capsules **314, 1260**
◆Zantac 300 GELdose Capsules **315, 1260**
◆Zantac 150 Tablets **314, 1260**
◆Zantac 300 Tablets **315, 1260**
◆Zantac Injection **315, 1258**
◆Zantac Injection Premixed **315, 1258**
◆Zantac Syrup **315, 1260**
◆Zinacef **315, 1262**
◆Zofran Injection **315, 1265**
◆Zofran Injection Premixed **315, 1265**
◆Zofran Oral Solution **315, 1270**
◆Zofran Tablets **315, 1270**
◆Zovirax Capsules **315, 1272**
◆Zovirax Ointment 5% **315, 1274**
◆Zovirax Sterile Powder **315, 1275**
◆Zovirax Suspension **315, 1272**
◆Zovirax Tablets **315, 1272**
◆Zyban Sustained-Release Tablets **315, 1277**
◆Zyloprim Tablets **315, 1282**

GLENWOOD **315, 1284**
82 North Summit Street
Tenafly, NJ 07670

Direct Inquiries to:
Professional Services Department
(800) 542-0772
(201) 569-0050
FAX: (201) 567-4443

For Medical Emergencies Contact:
Professional Services Department
(800) 542-0772
(201) 569-0050
FAX: (201) 567-4443

Products Described:
Bichloracetic Acid Kahlenberg **1284**
◆Potaba Capsules **315, 1284**
◆Potaba Envules **315, 1284**
◆Potaba Tablets **315, 1284**
Scleromate Injection **1285**
Yocon Tablets **1285**
Yodoxin Tablets **1286**

Other Products Available:
Bar-Test
Boropak
Calphosan Injection
Carbiset
Isocom
PALS Internal Deodorant
X-Wax
ZBT Baby Powder

A.C. GRACE CO. **1286**
1100 Quitman Road
P.O. Box 570
Big Sandy, TX 75755

Direct Inquiries to:
Roy Erickson
(903) 636-4368
FAX: (903) 636-4051

For Medical Emergencies Contact:
Roy Erickson
(903) 636-4368
FAX: (903) 636-4051

Products Described:
Unique E Vitamin E Capsules **1286**

GRAY PHARMACEUTICAL CO. **1286**
Affiliate, The Purdue Frederick Company
100 Connecticut Avenue
Norwalk, CT 06850-3590

For Medical Information Contact:
Medical Department
(203) 853-0123

Products Described:
X-Prep Bowel Evacuant Liquid **1286**

Other Products Available:
X-Prep Kit 1
X-Prep Kit 2

GUARDIAN LABORATORIES **1286**
A Division of United-Guardian, Inc.
230 Marcus Boulevard
Hauppauge, NY 11788

Direct Inquiries to:
P.O. Box 18050
Hauppauge, NY 11788
(516) 273-0900
(800) 645-5566

For Medical Information Contact:
Director of Medical Research
(516) 273-0900
(800) 645-5566

Products Described:
Clorpactin WCS-90 .... **1286**
Renacidin Irrigation *1286*

HAUCK PHARMACEUTICALS
(See ROBERTS PHARMACEUTICAL CORPORATION)

HEALTHPOINT **315, 1287**
2600 Airport Freeway
Fort Worth, TX 76111

Direct Inquiries to:
(800) 441-8227

Products Described:
◆Accuzyme Debriding Ointment **315, 1287**

HEEL INC. **1287**
11600 Cochiti SE
Albuquerque, NM 87123

Direct Inquiries to:
Medical Department
(800) 621-7644, prompt 5
(505) 293-3843
FAX: (505) 275-1672
www.heelbhi.com

Products Described:
Traumeel Injection Solution **1287**
Traumeel Ointment *1287*
Traumeel Oral Drops *1287*
Traumeel Oral Liquid in Vials *1287*
Traumeel Tablets *1287*
Vertigoheel Liquid in Oral Vials **1288**
Vertigoheel Oral Drops **1288**
Vertigoheel Tablets **1288**

Other Products Available:
Engystol Tablets
Euphorbium Nasal Spray
Galium-Heel Liquid
Gripp-Heel Tablets
Lymphomyosot Liquid
Lymphomyosot Tablets
Zeel Ointment
Zeel Tablets

HIGH CHEMICAL CO. **1289**
3901-A Nebraska Street
Levittown, PA 19056

◆ **Shown in Product Identification Guide** *Italic Page Number* **Indicates Brief Listing** ⊙ **Described in PDR For Ophthalmology**

Direct Inquiries to:
Nalin Parikh
(800) 447-8792
FAX: (215) 788-3148

Products Described:
Sarapin.............................1289

HILL DERMACEUTICALS, INC. 1289
2650 So. Mellonville Avenue
Sanford, Florida 32773

Direct Inquiries to:
Rosario G. Ramirez
(407) 323-1887
FAX: (407) 649-9213

Products Described:
Derma-Smoothe/FS Topical Oil......*1289*
FS Shampoo.........................*1289*

**HOECHST MARION 315, 1289
ROUSSEL**
10236 Marion Park Drive
Mail: P.O. Box 9627
Kansas City, MO 64134-0627

Direct Inquiries to:
Customer Information Center, K1-MO928
P.O. Box 9627
Kansas City, MO 64134-0627
(800) 552-3656

For Medical Information Contact:
Generally:
Medical Informatics
P.O. Box 9627
Kansas City, MO 64134-0627
(800) 633-1610
After Hours and Weekend Emergencies:
(816) 966-5000

Products Described:
◆Allegra Capsules......... 315, 1289
◆Allegra-D Extended-Release
Tablets........................ 315, 1291
◆Altace Capsules............. 316, 1293
◆Amaryl Tablets............... 315, 1296
◆Anzemet Injection............ 316, 1299
◆Anzemet Tablets............. 316, 1302
◆A/T/S 2% Acne Topical Gel.... 315, 1305
◆A/T/S 2% Acne Topical
Solution................... 315, 1304
AVC Cream......................1305
AVC Suppositories..............1305
◆Bricanyl Subcutaneous
Injection.................. 316, 1306
◆Bricanyl Tablets.............. 316, 1307
Carafate Suspension............1308
◆Carafate Tablets............. 316, 1307
◆Cardizem CD Capsules......... 316, 1309
◆Cardizem Injectable......... 316, 1311
Cardizem Lyo-Ject Syringe.......1311
Cardizem Monovial..............1311
◆Cardizem SR Capsules........ 316, 1314
◆Cardizem Tablets............ 316, 1316
◆Claforan Sterile and Injection.. 316, 1318
◆Clomid Tablets.............. 316, 1321
◆DiaBeta Tablets............. 316, 1323
◆Lasix Tablets............... 316, 1325
◆Loprox Cream 1%............. 316, 1326
◆Loprox Lotion 1%............ 316, 1327
◆Nilandron Tablets........... 316, 1327
Nitro-Bid IV...................1329
Nitro-Bid Ointment.............1331
◆Norpramin Tablets........... 316, 1332
Priftin Tablets................1334
Refludan for Injection..........1338
◆Rifadin Capsules............ 316, 1341
Rifadin IV.....................1341
◆Rifamate Capsules........... 316, 1344
◆Rifater.................... 316, 1346
◆Teczem Tablets.............. 316, 1349
◆Topicort Emollient Cream
0.25%..................... 316, 1354
◆Topicort Gel 0.05%.......... 316, 1355
◆Topicort LP Emollient Cream
0.05%..................... 316, 1354
◆Topicort Ointment 0.25%...... 316, 1356
◆Trental Tablets............. 316, 1357

Other Products Available:
Bentyl Capsules, Tablets, Injectable, Syrup
Cantil Tablets
Cephulac Solution
Chronulac Solution
Hiprex
Novafed A Capsules
Pavabid Plateau Caps
Silvadene Cream 1%
Tenuate Tablets/Dospan
Tiamate Tablets

**HORIZON PHARMACEUTICAL 1358
CORPORATION**
1125 Northmeadow Parkway
Suite 130
Roswell, GA 30076

Direct Inquiries to:
Greg Hauck
(770) 442-9707
FAX: (770) 442-9594

For Medical Emergencies Contact:
(800) 849-9707
FAX: (770) 442-9594

Products Described:
Defen-L.A. Tablets................. *1358*
Mescolor Tablets................,.... *1358*
Protuss Liquid..................... *1358*
Protuss-D Liquid.................. *1358*
Protuss-DM Tablets............... *1358*
Tanafed Suspension............... *1358*
Zoto-HC Ear Drops............... *1358*

HYLAND DIVISION
(See BAXTER HEALTHCARE
CORPORATION)

**ICN PHARMACEUTICALS, 316, 1358
INC.**
ICN Plaza
3300 Hyland Avenue
Costa Mesa, CA 92626

For Medical Emergencies Contact:
Boanerges Rubalcava, Ph.D., M.D.
(800) 548-5100, Ext. 3531
FAX: (714) 641-7287

Products Described:
◆Ancobon Capsules............. 316, 1362
Android Capsules, 10 mg........... 1362
Benoquin Cream 20%.............. 1364
Efudex Cream.................... 1364
Efudex Topical Solutions........... 1364
◆8-MOP Capsules............... 317, 1358
Eldopaque Forte 4% Cream......... 1365
Eldoquin Forte 4% Cream......... 1365
Fototar Cream................... 1366
Levo-Dromoran Injectable......... 1366
◆Levo-Dromoran Tablets........ 316, 1366
◆Librium Capsules............. 316, 1368
Librium for Injection............. 1369
◆Limbitrol Tablets............ 316, 1370
◆Limbitrol DS Tablets......... 317, 1370
Mestinon Injectable.............. 1372
Mestinon Syrup.................. 1372
◆Mestinon Tablets............ 317, 1372
◆Mestinon Timespan Tablets.... 317, 1372
Oxsoralen Lotion 1%............. 1373
◆Oxsoralen-Ultra Capsules..... 317, 1374
Prostigmin Injectable............ 1377
◆Prostigmin Tablets.......... 317, 1378
Solaquin Forte 4% Cream......... 1365
Solaquin Forte 4% Gel........... 1365
Tensilon Injectable.............. 1379
◆Testred Capsules, 10 mg...... 317, 1380
◆Trisoralen Tablets.......... 317, 1381
Virazole....................... 1382

Other Products Available:
Eldopaque 2% Cream
Eldoquin 2% Cream
GlyDerm AHA's
Insta-Glucose
RVPaque Cream
Solaquin 2% Cream
Vitadye Lotion

**IDEC PHARMACEUTICALS 317, 1384
CORPORATION**
11011 Torreyana Road
San Diego, CA 92121

Direct Inquiries to:
(619) 550-8500

Products Described:
◆Rituxan for Infusion........... 317, 1384

IMMUNEX CORPORATION 1386
51 University Street
Seattle, WA 98101

Direct Inquiries to:
Customer Service
(800) 466-8639
FAX: (800) 441-6303

For Medical Information Contact:
Generally:
Professional Services
(800) 466-8639
FAX: (800) 221-6820
FAX: (206) 223-5525
In Emergencies:
Professional Services
(800) 466-8639
FAX: (800) 221-6820
FAX: (206) 223-5525

Products Described:
Amicar Syrup, Tablets, and
Injection.................... **1386, 1388**
Leucovorin Calcium for Injection.... **1389**
Leucovorin Calcium Tablets......... **1391**
Leukine........................ **1392**
Methotrexate Sodium Tablets,
Injection, for Injection and LPF
Injection................... **1397**
Novantrone for Injection......... **1401**
Thioplex for Injection........... **1404**

IMMUNO 1406
1200 Parkdale Road
Rochester, MI 48307

Direct Inquiries to:
(800) 423-2090

Products Described:
Albumin (Human) 5%.............. **1406**
Albumin (Human) 25%............. **1407**
Bebulin VH Immuno.............. **1408**
Feiba VH Immuno............... **1410**
Iveegam....................... **1411**

**INTERFERON SCIENCES, 317, 1413
INC.**
783 Jersey Avenue
New Brunswick, NJ 08901-3660

Direct Inquiries to:
J.R. Knill, M.D.
(732) 249-3250, Ext. 565
FAX: (732) 249-0623

For Medical Emergencies Contact:
J.R. Knill, M.D.
(732) 249-3250, Ext. 565
(800) 591-4483 (after business hours)

Products Described:
◆Alferon N Injection........... **317, 1413**

**JACOBUS PHARMACEUTICAL 1415
CO., INC.**
37 Cleveland Lane
P.O. Box 5290
Princeton, NJ 08540

Direct Inquiries to:
Professional Services
(609) 921-7447
FAX: (609) 799-1176

For Medical Emergencies Contact:
Medical Department
(609) 921-7447
FAX: (609) 799-1176

Products Described:
Dapsone Tablets USP................ **1415**
Paser Granules..................... **1417**

**JANSSEN 317, 1418
PHARMACEUTICA INC.**
1125 Trenton-Harbourton Road
P.O. Box 200
Titusville, NJ 08560-0200

For Medical Information Contact:
Monday through Friday 8am-8pm EST:
(800) JANSSEN
FAX: (609) 730-2461
After Hours & Weekends:
(800) JANSSEN
Holidays:
Emergencies: (800) JANSSEN

Products Described:
◆Duragesic Transdermal
System..................... 317, 1418
◆Ergamisol Tablets............ 317, 1422
◆Hismanal Tablets............ 317, 1423
◆Imodium Capsules............ 317, 1426
◆Nizoral 2% Cream............ 317, 1427
◆Nizoral 2% Shampoo.......... 317, 1427
◆Nizoral Tablets............. 317, 1428
◆Propulsid Suspension........ 317, 1430
◆Propulsid Tablets........... 317, 1430
◆Risperdal Oral Solution...... 317, 1432
◆Risperdal Tablets........... 317, 1432
◆Sporanox Capsules........... 317, 1436
◆Sporanox Oral Solution....... 317, 1439
◆Vermox Chewable Tablets..... 317, 1442

**JOHNSON & JOHNSON • 317, 1443
MERCK CONSUMER
PHARMACEUTICALS CO.**
7050 Camp Hill Road
Ft. Washington, PA 19034

Direct Inquiries to:
Consumer Affairs Department
Fort Washington, PA 19034
(215) 233-7000

For Medical Emergencies Contact:
(215) 233-7000

Products Described:
Mylanta AR Acid Reducer.......... **1443**
◆Children's Mylanta Upset
Stomach Relief Liquid........ 318, 1443
◆Children's Mylanta Upset
Stomach Relief Tablets....... 318, 1443
◆Mylanta Double Strength Tablets...... *317*
Fast-Acting Mylanta Antacid
Tablets..................... **1444**
Maximum Strength Fast-Acting
Mylanta Antacid Tablets...... **1444**
◆Fast-Acting Mylanta Liquid
Antacid................... 317, 1443
◆Maximum Strength
Fast-Acting Mylanta Liquid... 317, 1443
◆Mylanta Gas Relief Gelcaps.... 318, 1445
◆Mylanta Gas Relief Tablets..... 317, 1445
◆Maximum Strength Mylanta
Gas Relief Tablets.......... 317, 1445
◆Mylanta Gelcaps Antacid............ *318*
◆Mylanta Tablets................... *317*
◆Mylicon Infants' Drops....... 318, 1443
◆Pepcid AC Acid Controller..... 318, 1445

**JONES MEDICAL 318, 1445
INDUSTRIES, INC.**
1945 Craig Road
P.O. Box 46903
St. Louis, MO 63146

Direct Inquiries to:
Customer Service
(314) 576-6100
FAX: (314) 469-5749

Products Described:
Brevital Sodium for Injection, USP .. 1445
Cytomel Tablets................... *1445*
◆Levoxyl Tablets................ 318, 1445
Tapazole Tablets.................. *1447*
Thrombin-JMI.................... *1448*
Triostat Injection *1448*

**KEY PHARMACEUTICALS, 318, 1448
INC.**
Galloping Hill Road
Kenilworth, NJ 07033
(908) 298-4000

For Medical Information Contact:
Generally:
Drug Information Services
(800) 526-4099
(9:00 AM to 5:00 PM EST)
After Hours and Weekends:
(908) 298-4000

Products Described:
◆Imdur Tablets................ 318, 1448
Integrilin Injection.............. 1450
◆K-Dur Microburst Release
System E.R. Tablets......... 318, 1454
◆Nitro-Dur Transdermal
Infusion System........... 318, 1456
◆Theo-Dur Extended-Release
Tablets................... 318, 1457
◆Trinalin Repetabs Tablets...... 318, 1464
◆Uni-Dur Extended-Release
Tablets................... 318, 1465

KNOLL LABORATORIES 318, 1471
A Division of
Knoll Pharmaceutical Company
3000 Continental Drive North
Mount Olive, NJ 07828

Direct Inquiries to:
Knoll Pharmaceutical Company:
(973) 426-2600
Customer Operations Department:
(800) 526-0710

For Medical Information Contact:
(800) 526-0221

Products Described:
Akineton Injection.................. 1471
◆Akineton Tablets.............. 318, 1471
◆Collagenase Santyl Ointment... 318, 1472
Dilaudid Ampules................. 1473
Dilaudid Cough Syrup............. 1474
◆Dilaudid-HP Injection........ 318, 1475
◆Dilaudid-HP Lyophilized
Powder 250mg.............. 318, 1475
Dilaudid Injection................ 1473
Dilaudid Multiple Dose Vials
(Sterile Solution)............... 1473
Dilaudid Oral Liquid.............. 1477
Dilaudid Powder.................. 1473
Dilaudid Rectal Suppositories........ 1473
◆Dilaudid Tablets 2 mg and
4 mg..................... 318, 1473

KNOLL PHARMACEUTICAL COMPANY   319, 1491

3000 Continental Drive North
Mount Olive, NJ 07828

Direct Inquiries to:
Knoll Pharmaceutical Company:
(973) 426-2600
Customer Operations Department:
(800) 526-0710

For Medical Information Contact:
(800) 526-0221

KOS PHARMACEUTICALS, INC.   319, 1505

1001 Brickell Bay Drive
25th Floor
Miami, FL 33131

For Medical Information Contact:
Drug Information Services
(888) 4-LIPIDS
(888) 4-547437

KRAMER LABORATORIES INC.   1509

8778 S.W. 8th Street
Miami, FL 33174

Direct Inquiries to:
8778 S.W. 8th Street
Miami, FL 33174
(800) 824-4894

For Medical Emergencies Contact:
Professional Director
(800) 824-4894

LASER, INC.   1509

2200 W. 97th Place, P.O. Box 905
Crown Point, IN 46307

Direct Inquiries to:
Joseph N. Allegretti, R.Ph.
(219) 663-1165

LEDERLE LABORATORIES   319, 3471

Division of American Cyanamid Company
Pearl River, NY 10965

LEDERLE PARENTERALS, INC.
Carolina, Puerto Rico 00987

LEDERLE PIPERACILLIN, INC.
Carolina, Puerto Rico 00987

(For oncology products, please see
IMMUNEX CORPORATION)

For Medical Information Contact:
MARKETED ONCOLOGY PRODUCTS:
Immunex Corporation
Professional Services Department
51 University Street
Seattle, WA 98101
(800) IMMUNEX

OTHER MARKETED DRUG AND
BIOLOGICAL PRODUCTS:
Lederle Laboratories / Wyeth-Ayerst
Laboratories
Medical Affairs Department
P.O. Box 8299
Philadelphia, PA 19101
Day: (800) 934-5556 (8:30 AM to 4:30
   PM, Eastern Standard Time, Weekdays
   only)
Night: (610) 688-4400 (Emergencies only;
   non-emergencies should wait until the
   next day)
Distribution: See Wyeth-Ayerst
   Laboratories' listing

LEDERLE STANDARD PRODUCTS   320, 1562

P.O Box 41502
Philadelphia, PA 19101

Direct General Inquiries to:
(610) 688-4400

For Medical Information Contact:
Medical Affairs
Day: (800) 934-5556 (8:30 AM to 4:30
   PM, Eastern Standard Time, Weekdays
   only)
Night: (610) 688-4400 (Emergencies only;
   non-emergencies should wait until the
   next day)

ELI LILLY AND COMPANY   320, 1562

For Medical Information Contact:
Lilly Research Laboratories
Lilly Corporate Center
Indianapolis, IN 46285
(800) 545-5979

Direct Inquiries to:
Lilly Corporate Center
Indianapolis, IN 46285
(317) 276-2000

AREA SALES OFFICES:
Atlanta, GA 30328
   North Park Town Center
   Building 500, Suite 710
   1100 Abernathy Road, NE
   (770) 551-5376
Bala Cynwyd, PA 19004
   401 City Avenue
   Suite 400
   (610) 617-1157
Birmingham, AL 35243
   3800 Colonade Parkway
   Suite 250
   (205) 969-4556
Anaheim CA 92806
   2400 East Katella Avenue
   Suite 530
   (714) 940-0800
Chicago, IL 60631
   Suite 810, O'Hare Plaza
   8725 West Higgins Road
   (773) 693-1953
Dallas, TX 75248
   15301 Dallas Parkway
   Suite 960, Box 66
   (972) 960-7637
Indianapolis, IN 46268
   Suite 203, 10 Fortune Park
   3905 Vincennes Road
   (317) 276-5967
Stamford, CT 06902
   300 First Stamford Place
   (203) 316-2708

Other Products Available:
Atropine Sulfate Vials
Aventyl HCl Liquid
Aventyl Pulvules
Calcium Carbonate, USP
Dobutrex Sodium, USP
Dobutrex Vials
Morphine Sulfate Vials & Soluble Tablets
Opium Tincture, USP
Phenobarbital, USP
Quinidine Gluconate Vials
Sodium Bicarbonate Tablets
Sodium Chloride, USP
Tubocurarine Chloride Vials

THE LIPOSOME COMPANY, INC.   321, 1646

One Research Way
Princeton, NJ 08540-6619

Direct Inquiries to:
Professional Services
(800) 335-5476
FAX: (800) 236-4507

For Medical Emergencies Contact:
Professional Services
(800) 335-5476
(609) 452-7060
FAX: (609) 452-8512

LOTUS BIOCHEMICAL CORPORATION   1648

P.O. Box 3586
Radford, VA 24143
(800) 455-5525

Direct Inquiries to:
Iain Speirs
(800) 455-5525
FAX: (800) 962-2200

For Medical Emergencies Contact:
Lawrence P. Olon
(423) 989-9190
FAX: (423) 989-3532

LUNSCO, INC.   1649

Route 2, Box 62
Pulaski, VA 24301

Direct Inquiries to:
(540) 980-4358

For Medical Emergencies Contact:
(540) 980-4358

3M PHARMACEUTICALS   321, 1653

3M Center 275-3W-01
P.O. Box 33275
St. Paul, MN 55133-3275
WEBSITE: www.3M.com/pharma

For Medical Information Contact:
Generally:
   Medical Services Department
   3M Pharmaceuticals
   3M Center, Bldg. 275-2E-13
   P.O. Box 33275
   St. Paul, MN 55133-3275
   (800) 328-0255
In Emergencies:
   (651) 736-4930 (all hours)

Commercial Customers:
Orders, Returns, Accounting
(800) 447-4537

Trade and Government:
(800) 328-6523

MERICON INDUSTRIES, INC.　1926

8819 N. Pioneer Road
Peoria, IL 61615

Direct Inquiries to:
William R. Connelly
(309) 693-2150
E-mail: MONOCAL@aol.com
FAX: (309) 693-2158

Sales & Ordering:
(800) 242-6464

Products Described:

Other Products Available:
Chromium Picolinate 1.6 mg
Ginkgo Biloba Extract 60 mg
Hydrocortisone Lotion 1%
St. John's Wort 150 mg
Zinc Gluconate Lozenges
Zinc Oxide Ointment
Zinc Sulfate Tabs & Caps

MERZ PHARMACEUTICALS　1926

Division of Merz, Inc.
4215 Tudor Lane (27410)
P.O. Box 18806
Greensboro, NC 27419

Direct Inquiries to:
Director of Regulatory Affairs
(910) 856-2003
FAX: (910) 856-0107

For Medical Emergencies Contact:
Director of Regulatory Affairs
(910) 856-2003
FAX: (910) 856-0107

Manufacturing Facility:
4 Dundas Circle
Greensboro, NC 27407
(910) 292-5347
FAX: (910) 855-8011

Products Described:

Other Products Available:
Anamine Syrup
Anamine T. D. Capsules
Anatuss Syrup
Anatuss Tablets
Cyanoject-10
Cyanoject-30
Decaject-5
Depoject-40
Depoject-80
Flexoject
Kenaject-40
Phenoject-50
Tristoject

MGI PHARMA, INC.　321, 1650

Suite 300 E, Opus Center
9900 Bren Road East
Minnetonka, MN 55343-9667

For Medical Information Contact:
Generally:
Medical Affairs
(800) 562-5580
FAX: (612) 935-0468
In Emergencies:
Medical Affairs
(800) 562-5580
FAX: (612) 935-0468

Products Described:

MILEX PRODUCTS, INC.　1928

4311 N. Normandy
Chicago, IL 60634-1403

Direct Inquiries to:
(800) 621-1278
FAX: (800) 972-0696

Manufacturing and Distribution:
SHIPPING OFFICES:
Milex Carolinas
　4409 Lebanon Road
　Post Office Box 23060
　Charlotte, NC 28227
　(704) 545-4567
Milex Puerto Rico
　Post Office Box 360554
　San Juan, PR 00936-0554
　(787) 767-7358
Milex Southern
　1001 Palo Pinto Street

Weatherford, TX 76086
(817) 599-7604
Milex Western
Post Office Box 46305
639 N. Fairfax
Los Angeles, CA 90046
(213) 651-4301
Milex Hawaii
Box 6337
Honolulu, HI 96818
(808) 422-9581

Products Described:

**MISSION PHARMACAL　1928
COMPANY**

10999 IH 10 West, Suite 1000
San Antonio, TX 78230-1355

Direct Inquiries to:
P.O. Box 786099
San Antonio, TX 78278-6099
Toll Free: (800) 292-7364
(210) 696-8400
FAX: (210) 696-6010

For Medical Emergencies Contact:
George Alexandrides
(830) 249-9822
FAX: (830) 816-2545

Products Described:

Other Products Available:
Compete
Supac

**MONARCH　324, 1931
PHARMACEUTICALS**

355 Beecham Street
Bristol, TN 37620

Direct Inquiries to:
(800) 776-3637
FAX: (423) 989-6279

For Medical Emergencies Contact:
R. Henry Richards, M.D.
(800) 546-4906
FAX: (423) 989-6137

Products Described:

Other Products Available:
Adrenalin Chloride Solution
Chloromycetin Otic
Cortisporin Otic Solution Sterile
Cortisporin Otic Suspension Sterile
Histoplasmin, Diluted
Humatin
Ketalar
Mantadil Cream
Neosporin G.U. Irrigant Sterile
Neosporin Ophthalmic Ointment Sterile
Neosporin Ophthalmic Solution Sterile
Nucofed Capsules and Syrup CIII
Nucofed Expectorant Syrup CIII
Nucofed Pediatric Expectorant Syrup CV
Pitocin

Pitressin
Polysporin Ophthalmic Ointment Sterile
Proctocort Cream & Suppositories
Proloprim Tablets
Quibron Capsules
Quibron-T/SR Accudose Tablets
Tussend Tablets or Syrup CIII
Tussend Expectorant Syrup CIII

**MURO PHARMACEUTICAL,　1951
INC.**

an ASTA Medica company
890 East Street
Tewksbury, MA 01876-1496

Direct Inquiries to:
Professional Service Department
(800) 225-0974
(978) 851-5981

Products Described:

**MYLAN PHARMACEUTICALS　1955
INC.**

781 Chestnut Ridge Road
P.O. Box 4310
Morgantown, WV 26504-4310
(304) 599-2595

Direct Inquiries to:
(304) 599-2595

For Medical Information Contact:
Pharmacy Affairs Department
(800) 82-MYLAN

Sales and Ordering:
Sales Department
(800) RX-MYLAN

Products Described:

NABI   **1961**
5800 Park of Commerce Blvd., NW
Boca Raton, FL 33487

For Medical Information Contact:
Generally:
Immunotherapy Customer Service
(800) 458-HBIG (4244)
(305) 625-5303
(800) 4-WINRHO
(800) 327-7106 - AUTOPLEX
(800) 685-5579 - Medical
FAX: (305) 625-0925
In Emergencies:
Immunotherapy Customer Service
(800) 458-HBIG (4244)
(800) 4-WINRHO (494-6746)
(800) 327-7106 - AUTOPLEX
FAX: (305) 625-0925

Products Described:

NEUREX CORPORATION   **324, 1966**
3760 Haven Avenue
Menlo Park, CA 94025

Direct Inquiries to:
(888) 853-NXCO (6926)

Products Described:

NEUTROGENA   **324, 1969**
DERMATOLOGICS
5760 West 96th Street
Los Angeles, CA 90045

Direct Inquiries to:
Diane Foster
(310) 642-1150
FAX: (310) 337-2156

For Medical Emergencies Contact:
Kamran Mather, Ph.D.
(310) 642-1150
FAX: (310) 216-5399

Products Described:

Other Products Available:
Acne Mask
Neutrogena Antiseptic
Neutrogena Cleansing Bar for Acne-prone
   Skin
Neutrogena Cleansing Bar for Dry Skin
Neutrogena Cleansing Bar for Dry Skin
   fragrance-free
Neutrogena Cleansing Bar for Oily Skin
Neutrogena Cleansing Bar Original
   Formula
Neutrogena Cleansing Bar Original
   Formula fragrance-free
Neutrogena Cleansing Wash
Neutrogena Extra Gentle Cleanser
Neutrogena Extra Gentle Cleansing Bar
Neutrogena Healthy Skin Anti-Wrinkle
   Cream with Stabilized Retinol
Neutrogena Healthy Skin Face Lotion with
   SPF 15
Neutrogena Lip Moisturizer
Liquid Neutrogena
Liquid Neutrogena, fragrance free
Neutrogena Moisture
Neutrogena Moisture SPF 15 Untinted
Neutrogena Moisture SPF 15 with Sheer
   Tint
Neutrogena Non-Drying Cleanser
Neutrogena Norwegian Formula Emulsion
Neutrogena Norwegian Formula Hand
   Cream
Neutrogena Rainbath
Neutrogena Sensitive Skin Sunblock SPF
   17
Neutrogena Shampoo
Neutrogena Sunblock SPF 15
Neutrogena Sunblock SPF 30
Neutrogena T/Derm Tar Emollient
Neutrogena Vehicle/N
Neutrogena Vehicle/N Mild
Oil-Free Acne Wash
On-the-Spot Acne Treatment
Sunblock Stick SPF25
Sunless Tanning Lotion -- Body
Sunless Tanning Lotion -- Face
T/Gel Therapeutic Conditioner
T/Gel Therapeutic Shampoo (2% Neutar)
Maximum Strength T/Sal Therapeutic
   Shampoo (3% salicylic acid)

NEXSTAR PHARMACEUTICALS, 1970
INC.
650 Cliffside Drive
San Dimas, CA 91773

Direct Inquiries to:
Customer Service
(800) 403-3945

For Medical Information Contact:
(800) 403-3945

Products Described:

NICHE PHARMACEUTICALS, 1972
INC.
P.O. Box 449
200 N. Oak Street
Roanoke, Texas 76262

Direct Inquiries to:
Steve F. Brandon
(817) 491-2770
FAX: (817) 491-3533

For Emergency Medical Information
Contact:
Gerald L. Beckloff, M.D.
(817) 491-2770
FAX: (817) 491-3533

Products Described:

NORTH AMERICAN
BIOLOGICALS, INC.
(See NABI)

NORTH AMERICAN VACCINE, 1972
INC.
10150 Old Columbia Road
Columbia, MD 21046

Direct Inquiries to:
Stephen N. Keith, MD, MSPH, Vice
   President--Marketing and Sales
(410) 309-7200
FAX: (410) 381-3341

For Medical Emergencies Contact:
Helen Cicirello, MD
(888) 628-2829
(410) 309-7208
FAX: (410) 381-3372

Products Described:

NORTHAMPTON MEDICAL, INC.
(See UCB PHARMA, INC.)

NOVARTIS CONSUMER   **324, 1978**
HEALTH, INC.
560 Morris Avenue
Summit, NJ 07901-1312

Direct Product Inquiries to:
Consumer & Professional Affairs
(800) 452-0051
FAX: (800) 635-2801
or write to the above address

Products Described:

Other Products Available:
Arthritis Pain Ascriptin
Enteric Ascriptin
Maximum Strength Ascriptin
Regular Strength Ascriptin
Prescription Strength Cruex Cream
Cruex Spray Powder
Prescription Strength Cruex Spray Powder
Cruex Squeeze Powder
Desenex Foot and Sneaker Shake Powder
Desenex Foot and Sneaker Spray Powder
Desenex Ointment
Desenex Shake Powder
Desenex Spray Powder
Prescription Strength Desenex Spray
   Powder
Doan's Extra Strength Analgesic
Extra Strength Doan's P.M.
Doan's Regular Strength Analgesic
Maalox Anti-Gas Tablets, Regular Strength
   and Extra Strength
Nupercainal Hemorrhoidal and Anesthetic
   Ointment
Nupercainal Suppositories
Otrivin Nasal Drops
Otrivin Pediatric Nasal Drops
Otrivin Nasal Spray
Sunkist Children's Chewable
   Multivitamins - Complete
Sunkist Children's Chewable
   Multivitamins - Plus Extra C
Sunkist Vitamin C - Chewable
Sunkist Vitamin C Rolls

NOVARTIS   **324, 1987**
PHARMACEUTICALS
CORPORATION
Novartis Pharmaceuticals Corporation
59 Route 10
East Hanover, NJ 07936
(for branded products)
   For Information Contact:
   Customer Response Department
   (888) NOW-NOVARTIS (888-669-6682)
   Global Internet Address:
   http://www.novartis.com

Geneva Pharmaceuticals, Inc.
A Novartis Company
2655 West Midway Boulevard
P.O. Box 446
Broomfield, CO 80038-0446
(for branded generic product listing refer to
Geneva Pharmaceuticals, Inc.)
   For Information Contact:
   Customer Support Department
   (800) 525-8747
   (303) 466-2400
   FAX: (303) 469-6467

Products Described:

Tegretol Suspension **2088**
◆Tegretol Tablets................. **325, 2088**
◆Tegretol-XR Tablets............ **326, 2088**
◆Tofranil-PM Capsules........... **326, 2091**
◆Transderm-Nitro Transdermal
Therapeutic System........... **326, 2093**
◆Vivelle Transdermal System..... **326, 2095**
◆Voltaren Tablets **326, 2001**
◆Voltaren-XR Tablets **326, 2001**

Other Products Available:
Anturane Capsules
Anturane Tablets
Apresazide Capsules
Apresoline Hydrochloride Tablets
Bellergal-S Tablets
Brethaire Inhaler
Cafergot Suppositories
Esidrix Tablets
Hydergine Liquid
Hydergine LC Liquid Capsules
Hydergine Oral Tablets
Ismelin Tablets
Klorvess 10% Liquid
Klorvess Effervescent Granules
Lamprene Capsules
Lioresal Tablets
Ludiomil Tablets
Mellaril Concentrate
Mellaril Tablets
Mellaril-S Oral Suspension
Mesantoin Tablets
Methergine Injection
Methergine Tablets
Metopirone Capsules
Neo-Calglucon Syrup
PBZ Tablets
PBZ-SR Tablets
Priscoline Hydrochloride Ampuls
Rimactane Capsules
Sanorex Tablets
Sansert Tablets
Ser-Ap-Es Tablets
Slow-K Extended-Release Tablets
Syntocinon Injection
Tavist Syrup
Tavist Tablets
Tofranil Tablets
Visken Tablets

NOVO NORDISK PHARMACEUTICALS, INC. **326, 2098**
Suite 200
100 Overlook Center
Princeton, NJ 08540-7810

Direct Inquiries to:
Novo Nordisk Pharmaceuticals, Inc.
(800) 727-6500

In Emergencies After Hours & Weekends:
(609) 987-5800

Products Described:
Human Insulin Delivery Systems
(Durable, Disposable)............. *2101*
◆Norditropin for Injection......... **326, 2099**
◆NovoFine 30 Disposable
Needle........................ *326, 2103*
Novolin 70/30 Human Insulin 10
ml Vials......................... **2098**
◆Novolin 70/30 PenFill 1.5 ml
Cartridges.................... **326, 2101**
◆Novolin 70/30 Prefilled
Disposable Insulin Delivery
System........................ **326, 2103**
Novolin 70/30 PenFill 3 ml
Cartridges......................... *2101*
Novolin L Human Insulin 10 ml
Vials............................. **2106**
Novolin N Human Insulin 10 ml
Vials............................. **2100**
◆Novolin N PenFill 1.5 ml
Cartridges.................... **326, 2101**
Novolin N PenFill 3 ml Cartridges... *2101*
◆Novolin N Prefilled Syringe
Disposable Insulin
Delivery System.............. **326, 2103**
Novolin R Human Insulin 10 ml
Vials............................. **2101**
Novolin R PenFill 3 ml Cartridges... *2101*
◆Novolin R PenFill 1.5 ml
Cartridges.................... **326, 2101**
◆Novolin R Prefilled Syringe
Disposable Insulin Delivery
System........................ **326, 2103**
NovoPen 1.5 Insulin Delivery
Device........................... *2101*
◆NovoPen 3 Insulin Delivery
Device........................ *326, 2101*
Prandin Tablets (0.5, 1, and 2 mg)... **2107**
Purified Pork Lente Insulin.......... **2106**
Purified Pork NPH Isophane
Insulin........................... **2106**
Purified Pork Regular Insulin........ **2106**
Velosulin BR Human Insulin 10 ml
Vials............................. **2105**

NOVOPHARM, USA INC. **2110**
165 East Commerce Drive
Schaumburg, IL 60173-5326

Direct Inquiries to:
Robert J. Gunter, President & C.O.O.
(800) 635-5067
FAX: (847) 882-4232

Products Described:
Acyclovir Capsules and Tablets,
Caps 200 mg, Tabs 400 mg, 800
mg............................... *2110*
Albuterol Sulfate Inhalation
Aerosol, 90 mcg.................. *2110*
Albuterol Tablets, 2mg, 4mg......... *2110*
Amantadine HCl Syrup, 50 mg...... *2110*
Amoxicillin Capsules USP and
Oral Suspension, Caps 250 mg,
500 mg, O.S. 125 mg/5 mL, 250
mg/5 mL.......................... *2110*
Amoxicillin Tablets (Chewable),
125 mg, 250 mg................... *2110*
Atenolol Tablets, 50 mg, 100 mg..... *2110*
Captopril Tablets, 12.5 mg, 25 mg,
50 mg, 100 mg.................... *2110*
Cefaclor Capsules, 250 mg, 500
mg............................... *2110*
Cephalexin Capsules USP and Oral
Suspension, Caps 250 mg, 500
mg, O.S. 125 mg/mL, 250
mg/mL............................ *2110*
Cimetidine Oral Solution, 300 mg/
5 mL............................. *2110*
Cimetidine Tablets, 200 mg.......... *2110*
Cimetidine Tablets, 300 mg.......... *2110*
Cimetidine Tablets, 400 mg.......... *2110*
Cimetidine Tablets, 800 mg.......... *2110*
Clofibrate Capsules USP, 500 mg...... *2110*
Diclofenac Na Tablets, 75 mg........ *2110*
Flurbiprofen Tablets, 50 mg, 100
mg............................... *2110*
Glyburide Tablets USP, 1.25 mg,
2.5 mg, 5 mg..................... *2110*
Indomethacin Capsules, 25 mg, 50
mg............................... *2110*
Loperamide Hydrochloride
Capsules USP, 2 mg............... *2110*
Metoprolol Tartrate Tablets, 50 mg,
100 mg........................... *2110*
Mexiletine Capsules, 150 mg, 200
mg, 250 mg....................... *2110*
Naproxen Sodium Tablets, 275 mg,
550 mg........................... *2110*
Naproxen Tablets, 250 mg........... *2110*
Naproxen Tablets, 375 mg........... *2110*
Naproxen Tablets, 500 mg........... *2110*
Nifedipine Capsules, 10 mg.......... *2110*
Pindolol Tablets, 5 mg.............. *2110*
Pindolol Tablets, 10 mg............. *2110*
Ranitidine HCl Tablets, 150 mg,
300 mg........................... *2110*
Selegiline HCl Tablets, 5 mg........ *2110*
Timolol Maleate Tablets, 5 mg, 10
mg, 20 mg........................ *2110*
Tolmetin Sodium Capsules USP,
400 mg........................... *2110*

NUTRAMAX LABORATORIES, INC. **326, 2111**
5024 Campbell Boulevard
Baltimore, MD 21236

Direct Inquiries to:
(800) 925-5187
FAX: (410) 931-4009

Products Described:
◆Cosamin DS Capsules.......... **326, 2111**

OCLASSEN PHARMACEUTICALS, INC. **326, 2111**
A Division of Watson Laboratories, Inc.
311 Bonnie Circle
P.O. Box 1900
Corona, CA 91718-1900

Direct Inquiries to:
Customer Service Department
(800) 272-5525
FAX: (909) 270-1096

For Medical Emergencies Contact:
Customer Service Department
(800) 272-5525
FAX: (909) 270-1096

Products Described:
◆Condylox Gel................. **326, 2111**
◆Condylox Topical Solution...... **326, 2112**
◆Cordran Lotion................ **326, 2113**
◆Cordran Tape.................. **326, 2114**
◆Cormax Ointment............... **326, 2115**
◆Cormax Scalp Application...... **326, 2116**
◆Monodox Capsules.............. **326, 2117**

Other Products Available:
Cinobac Capsules, 250mg, 500mg
Cordran Ointment 0.025%, 30g, 60g
Cordran Ointment 0.05%, 15g, 30g, 60g
Cordran SP Cream 0.025%, 30g, 60g
Cordran SP Cream 0.05%, 15g, 30g, 60g

OHMEDA PHARMACEUTICAL PRODUCTS DIVISION INC.
(See BAXTER PHARMACEUTICAL PRODUCTS INC.)

ORGANON INC. **326, 2119**
375 Mt. Pleasant Ave.
West Orange, NJ 07052

Direct Inquiries to:
(973) 325-4500

For Medical Inquiries Contact:
(800) 631-1253
FAX: (973) 325-4699

Products Described:
Arduan for Injection................ *2119*
BCG Vaccine, USP (Tice) (see
Tice BCG Vaccine, USP)........... *2119*
◆Calderol Capsules.............. *326, 2119*
Cortrosyn for Injection.............. **2119**
◆Cotazym Capsules.............. **326, 2120**
◆Cotazym-S Capsules............ *326, 2121*
Deca-Durabolin Injection............ *2121*
◆Desogen Tablets............... **326, 2121**
◆Follistim for Injection......... **327, 2128**
◆Humegon for Injection.......... **327, 2132**
◆Mircette Tablets............... **327, 2134**
Norcuron for Injection.............. **2142**
◆Orgaran Injection.............. **327, 2144**
Pavulon Injection................... *2146*
Pregnyl for Injection................ **2146**
Regonol Injection................... *2147*
◆Remeron Tablets............... **327, 2147**
Reversol Injection.................. *2149*
Succinylcholine Chloride Injection... *2150*
◆Tice BCG Vaccine, USP......... **327, 2150**
◆Wigraine Tablets.............. **327, 2152**
◆Zemuron Injection............. **327, 2153**
◆Zymase Capsules............... **327, 2157**

ORTHO BIOTECH INC. **327, 2157**
P.O. Box 300
Raritan, NJ 08869-0602

Direct Inquiries to:
(800) 325-7504
Prompt #1, Customer Service
Prompt #2, Medical Information
FAX: (908) 526-9230
FAX: (908) 526-6457

Products Described:
◆Leustatin Injection............. **327, 2157**
Orthoclone OKT3 Sterile Solution... **2160**
◆Procrit for Injection........... **327, 2164**

ORTHO-CLINICAL DIAGNOSTICS, INC. **2171**
A Johnson & Johnson Company
1001 U.S. Hwy 202
Raritan, NJ 08869-0606

Direct Inquiries to:
Customer Service
(800) 322-6374

Products Described:
MICRhoGAM.......................... **2171**
RhoGAM............................. **2171**

ORTHO DERMATOLOGICAL **327, 2172**
199 Grandview Road
Skillman, NJ 08558

For Medical Information Contact:
Dermatological Medical Information
(800) 426-7762

Products Described:
◆Dermatop Emollient Cream..... **327, 2172**
◆Erycette Topical Solution....... **327, 2174**
◆Grifulvin V Tablets
Microsize and Oral
Suspension Microsize......... **327, 2174**
◆Monistat-Derm Cream.......... **327, 2175**
◆Renova Cream.................. **327, 2175**
◆Retin-A Cream/Gel/Liquid...... **327, 2177**
◆Retin-A Micro Microsphere,
0.1%.......................... **327, 2178**
◆Spectazole Cream.............. **327, 2179**

ORTHO DIAGNOSTIC SYSTEMS, INC.
(See ORTHO-CLINICAL DIAGNOSTICS, INC.)

ORTHO-McNEIL PHARMACEUTICAL **327, 2179**
A Division of Ortho Pharmaceutical
Corporation
1000 Route 202, P.O. Box 300
Raritan, NJ 08869-0602

For Medical Information Contact:
Generally:
(800) 682-6532
In Emergencies:
(908) 218-7325

Products Described:
Aci-Jel Therapeutic Vaginal Jelly..... **2179**
◆All-Flex Arcing Spring Diaphragm
(See Ortho Diaphragm Kits)......... *327*
◆Floxin I.V..................... **328, 2180**
◆Floxin Tablets.................. **327, 2184**
◆Floxin UroPak..................... *328*
◆Haldol Decanoate 50
Injection...................... **328, 2190**
◆Haldol Decanoate 100
Injection...................... **328, 2190**
◆Haldol Injection............... **328, 2188**
◆Levaquin Injection............. **328, 2192**
◆Levaquin Tablets............... **328, 2197**
◆Micronor Tablets............... **328, 2201**
Modicon 21 Tablets.................. **2221**
◆Modicon 28 Tablets............ **328, 2221**
◆Ortho-Cept 21 Tablets.......... **328, 2204**
Ortho-Cept 28 Tablets............... **2204**
Ortho Coil Spring Diaphragm (See
Ortho Diaphragm Kits)
◆Ortho-Cyclen 21 Tablets........ **328, 2229**
Ortho-Cyclen 28 Tablets............. **2229**
Ortho Diaphragm Kits -- All-Flex
Arcing Spring; Ortho Coil
Spring............................ **2211**
Ortho Dienestrol Cream.............. **2212**
◆Ortho-Novum 1/35 □ 21
Tablets....................... **328, 2221**
Ortho-Novum 1/35 □ 28 Tablets....... **2221**
Ortho-Novum 1/50 □ 21 Tablets....... **2215**
◆Ortho-Novum 1/50 □ 28
Tablets....................... **328, 2215**
Ortho-Novum 7/7/7 □ 21 Tablets..... **2221**
◆Ortho-Novum 7/7/7 □ 28
Tablets....................... **328, 2221**
Ortho-Novum 10/11 □ 21 Tablets.... **2221**
◆Ortho-Novum 10/11 □ 28
Tablets....................... **328, 2221**
◆Ortho Tri-Cyclen 21 Tablets..... **328, 2229**
Ortho Tri-Cyclen 28 Tablets......... **2229**
◆Pancrease Capsules............. **328, 2237**
◆Pancrease MT Capsules......... **328, 2238**
◆Parafon Forte DSC Caplets...... **328, 2239**
◆ParaGard T 380A Intrauterine
Copper Contraceptive......... **328, 2239**
◆Regranex Gel.................. **328, 2243**
Sultrin Triple Sulfa Cream.......... **2245**
◆Terazol 3 Vaginal Cream........ **328, 2245**
◆Terazol 3 Vaginal
Suppositories................. **328, 2246**
◆Terazol 7 Vaginal Cream........ **328, 2246**
◆Tolectin 200 Tablets........... **328, 2247**
◆Tolectin 600 Tablets........... **329, 2247**
◆Tolectin DS Capsules........... **329, 2247**
◆Topamax Tablets............... **329, 2249**
◆Tylenol with Codeine Elixir..... **329, 2252**
◆Tylenol with Codeine Tablets.... **329, 2252**
◆Tylox Capsules................. **329, 2253**
◆Ultram Tablets................. **329, 2254**
◆Vascor Tablets................. **329, 2257**

ORTHO PHARMACEUTICAL CORPORATION
(See ORTHO-McNEIL PHARMACEUTICAL)

PADDOCK LABORATORIES INC. **2260**
3940 Quebec Avenue North
Minneapolis, MN 55427

Direct Inquiries to:
David Chinnock, R.Ph.
(612) 546-4676
FAX: (612) 546-4842

For Medical Emergencies Contact:
Carol Anding, Regulatory Affairs
(800) 328-5113
FAX: (612) 546-4842

Products Described:
Actidose-Aqua Suspension............ *2260*
Actidose with Sorbitol Suspension... *2260*
Diabe-Tuss DM Syrup................. **2260**
Glutose 15, Glutose 45 (Oral
Glucose Gel)..................... *2260*
Kionex Powder....................... **2260**
Nystatin Paddock USP for
Extemporaneous Preparation of
Oral Suspension.................. *2261*
Nystop Topical Powder USP.......... **2261**
Podocon-25 Liquid................... **2261**

Other Products Available:
Acetaminophen Suppositories 120 mg, 650
mg
Acetaminophen Tablets 325 mg
Albuterol Sulfate USP Powder
Aluminum Paste
Aquabase
Aspirin Suppositories 300 mg, 600 mg
Aspirin Tablets, Enteric-Coated 325 mg,
650 mg
Bacitracin USP Micronized Powder

Belladonna and Opium Suppositories 16.2 mg/30 mg and 16.2 mg/60 mg CII
Benzoin Compound Tincture USP
Bisacodyl Suppositories 10 mg
Bisacodyl Tablets 5 mg
Castor Oil USP
Clinda-Derm Solution
Clindamycin Phosphate USP Powder
Colistin Sulfate USP Powder
Dermabase
Dexamethasone Acetate USP Micronized Powder
Dexamethasone Sodium Phosphate USP Powder
Docusate Sodium Capsules 100 mg, 250 mg
Emulsoil (Self-Emulsifying Castor Oil)
Erythra-Derm Solution
Erythromycin USP Powder
Fattibase
Ferrous Gluconate Tablets 324 mg
Ferrous Sulfate Tablets 324 mg
Gentamicin Sulfate USP Powder
Green Soap Tincture USP
Hydrocortisone USP Micronized Powder
Hydrocortisone Acetate USP Micronized Powder
Hydrocortisone Acetate Suppositories 25 mg
Hydrocream Base
Hydromorphone HCl USP non-sterile Powder CII
Hydromorphone HCl Suppositories 3 mg CII
Ipecac Syrup USP
Isoniazid Tablets 300 mg
Liqua-Gel
Liquaderm-A
Mesalamine (5-Aminosalicylic Acid)
Milk of Magnesia USP
Morphine Sulfate USP Powder CII
Morphine Sulfate Suppositories 5 mg, 10 mg, 20 mg, 30 mg CII
Neomycin Sulfate USP Micronized Powder
Ora-Plus
Ora-Sweet
Ora-Sweet SF
Polybase
Polymyxin B Sulfate USP Powder
Progesterone Injection USP
Progesterone USP Micronized Powder
Progesterone USP Wettable Microcrystalline Powder
Retinoic Acid USP Powder (Trans)
Sorbitol Solution USP 70%
Suspendol-S
Testosterone USP Micronized non-sterile Powder CIII
Testosterone Propionate USP Micronized non-sterile Powder CIII
Triamcinolone Acetonide USP Micronized Powder
Trimethobenzamide HCl Suppositories 100 mg, 200 mg
Zincate Capsules 220 mg

PAR PHARMACEUTICAL, INC. 2261

One Ram Ridge Road
Spring Valley, NY 10977

Direct Inquiries to:
Customer Service
(800) 828-9393
(914) 425-7100

Products Described:
Allopurinol Tablets ... *2261*
Alprazolam Tablets ... *2261*
Amiloride HCl Tablets ... *2261*
Amoxicillin Capsules ... *2261*
Amoxicillin Oral Suspension ... *2261*
Ampicillin Capsules ... *2261*
Ampicillin Oral Suspension ... *2261*
Atenolol Tablets ... *2261*
Benztropine Mesylate Tablets ... *2261*
Carisoprodol and Aspirin Tablets ... *2261*
Clonazepam Tablets ... *2261*
Dexamethasone Tablets ... *2261*
Doxepin HCl Capsules ... *2261*
Fluphenazine HCl Tablets ... *2261*
Flurazepam HCl Capsules ... *2261*
Haloperidol Tablets ... *2261*
Hydralazine HCl Tablets ... *2261*
Hydra-Zide Capsules ... *2261*
IBU Tablets ... *2261*
Ibuprofen Suspension ... *2261*
Ibuprofen Tablets ... *2261*
Imipramine HCl Tablets ... *2261*
Isosorbide Dinitrate Tablets ... *2261*
Meclizine HCl Tablets ... *2261*
Megestrol Acetate Tablets ... *2261*
Melatonin Caplets ... *2261*
Melatonin Tablets ... *2261*
Melatonin CR Capsules ... *2261*
Methocarbamol and Aspirin Tablets ... *2261*
Methylprednisolone Tablets ... *2261*
Minoxidil Tablets ... *2261*
Nicardipine Capsules ... *2261*
Nicotine Patch ... *2261*
Penicillin V Potassium Suspension ... *2261*
Penicillin V Potassium Tablets ... *2261*
Pindolol Tablets ... *2261*
Piroxicam Capsules ... *2261*
Prochlorperazine Tablets ... *2261*
SSD Cream ... *2261*
SSD AF Cream ... *2261*
Temazepam Capsules ... *2261*
TransZone Controlled Release Capsules ... *2261*
Triazolam Tablets ... *2261*
Zorprin Tablets ... *2261*

PARKEDALE PHARMACEUTICALS 329, 2262

870 Parkdale Road
Rochester, MI 48307

Direct Inquiries to:
(888) 401-2879
FAX: (423) 989-6279

For Medical Emergencies Contact:
Henry Richards, M.D.
(800) 546-4906
FAX: (423) 989-6137

Products Described:
◆Aplisol Injection ... **329, 2262**
◆Fluogen Injection ... **329, 2263**

PARKE-DAVIS 329, 2265

Division of Warner-Lambert Company
201 Tabor Rd.
Morris Plains, NJ 07950

For Medical Information Contact:
During working hours:
Customer Service
Product/Medical Information
(800) 223-0432
FAX: (973) 540-2248
After Hours and Weekend Emergencies:
(973) 540-6089

Products Described:
◆Accupril Tablets ... **329, 2266**
Benadryl Parenteral ... **2269**
◆Celontin Kapseals ... **329, 2269**
Cerebyx Injection ... **2270**
◆Cognex Capsules ... **329, 2274**
◆Dilantin Infatabs ... **329, 2280**
◆Dilantin Kapseals ... **329, 2278**
Dilantin-125 Suspension ... **2281**
Estrostep 21 Tablets ... **2283**
◆Estrostep Fe Tablets ... **329, 2283**
FemPatch ... **2291**
◆Lipitor Tablets ... **329, 2293**
◆Lopid Tablets ... **329, 2296**
◆Nardil Tablets ... **329, 2299**
◆Neurontin Capsules ... **329, 2301**
◆Nitrostat Tablets ... **329, 2304**
◆Omnicef Capsules ... **329, 2305**
Omnicef for Oral Suspension ... **2305**
Parcode Product List ... *2265*
◆Ponstel Kapseals ... **329, 2309**
◆Rezulin Tablets ... **329, 2310**
◆Zarontin Capsules ... **329, 2314**
Zarontin Syrup ... **2314**

Other Products Available:
Diphenhydramine Hydrochloride (see Benadryl)
Loestrin (21) 1/20
Loestrin (21) 1.5/30
Loestrin (Fe) 1/20
Loestrin (Fe) 1.5/30

PARNELL PHARMACEUTICALS, INC. 2315

P.O. Box 5130
Larkspur, CA 94977

Direct Inquiries to:
Customer Services
(800) 45-PHARM
(415) 256-1800
FAX: (415) 256-8099

For Medical Emergencies Contact:
Francis W. Parnell, M.D.
(415) 256-1800
FAX: (415) 256-8099

Products Described:
EarSol-HC Solution ... *2315*
Feminease Cream ... *2315*
MouthKote Oral Moisturizer ... *2315*
Oragesic Oral Analgesic Irrigating Solution ... *2315*
Pretz Irrigation Solution ... *2315*
Pretz Refill Solution ... *2315*
Pretz Spray ... *2315*
Pretz-D Spray ... *2315*
Tac-3 Suspension ... *2315*

PASTEUR MÉRIEUX CONNAUGHT 329, 3473

Swiftwater, PA 18370

For Medical Information Contact:
Generally:
Medical Affairs
(800) VACCINE
(800) 822-2463
Adverse Drug Experiences:
Medical Director
(717) 839-7187
(800) 835-3592

Sales and Ordering:
Pasteur Mérieux Connaught
Customer Service
(800) VACCINE
(800) 822-2463
(717) 839-7187

Products Described:
◆ActHIB ... **329, 2316**
◆Diphtheria and Tetanus Toxoids and Pertussis Vaccine Adsorbed USP (For Pediatric Use) ... **330, 2320**
◆Fluzone ... **330, 2324**
◆Imogam Rabies - HT ... **330, 2327**
◆Imovax Rabies I.D. Vaccine ... **330, 2331**
◆Imovax Rabies Vaccine ... **330, 2329**
◆Ipol ... **330, 2333**
◆JE-Vax ... **330, 2336**
◆Menomune-A/C/Y/W-135 ... **330, 2339**
◆Mono-Vacc Test (O.T.) ... *330, 3473*
◆MSTA Mumps Skin Test Antigen ... **330, 3473**
ProHIBiT ... *2345*
Tetanus and Diphtheria Toxoids Adsorbed For Adult Use ... *2340*
◆TheraCys ... **330, 2345**
◆TriHIBit (see ActHIB and Tripedia) ... *330*
◆Tripedia ... **330, 2340**
◆Tubersol ... **330, 3474**
◆Typhim Vi ... **330, 2348**
◆YF-Vax ... *330, 2350*

Other Products Available:
Diphtheria & Tetanus Toxoids Adsorbed USP (For Pediatric Use) (DT)
Tetanus Toxoid Adsorbed For Adult Use USP
Tetanus Toxoid USP

PATHOGENESIS CORPORATION 330, 2350

201 Elliott Avenue West
Seattle, WA 98119

Direct Inquiries to:
(888) 508-TOBI (8624)

Products Described:
◆TOBI Solution for Inhalation ... **330, 2350**

PEDINOL PHARMACAL INC. 2353

30 Banfi Plaza North
Farmingdale, NY 11735

Direct Inquiries to:
Director of Professional Services
(516) 293-9500

Products Described:
Breezee Mist Foot Powder ... *2353*
Castellani Paint Modified ... *2353*
CitraDerm Facial Complex Cream ... *2353*
Formalyde-10 Spray ... *2353*
Fungoid Creme ... *2353*
Fungoid Solution ... *2353*
Fungoid Tincture ... *2353*
Hydrisalic Gel ... *2353*
Hydrisinol Creme ... *2353*
Hydrisinol Lotion ... *2353*
Lactinol Lotion ... *2354*
Lactinol-E Creme ... *2354*
LazerCreme ... *2354*
Lazerformalyde Solution ... *2354*
Lazersporin-C Solution ... *2354*
Nail Scrub with Brush ... *2354*
Ony-Clear Solution ... *2354*
Ostiderm ... *2354*
Ostiderm Roll-On ... *2354*
Pedi-Boro Soak Paks ... *2354*
Pedi-Dri Topical Powder ... *2354*
Pedi-Pro Topical Powder ... *2354*
Sal-Acid Plasters ... *2354*
Sal-Plant Gel ... *2354*
Salactic Film ... *2354*
TI-Screen Sunscreens, Sunblocks, Sunless Tanning Creme, and Lip Protectant ... *2354*
Ureacin-10 Lotion & Ureacin-20 Creme ... *2354*

Other Products Available:
Alginate Styptic Gauze
Fungoid Tincture Topical Antifungal Treatment Kit
PNS Unna Boot
Wonder Ice

PENEDERM INCORPORATED 2354

320 Lakeside Drive, Suite A
Foster City, CA 94404-1146

Direct Inquiries to:
(800) 395-DERM
(650) 358-0100
E-mail: productinfo@penederm.com

Products Described:
Acticin Cream ... **2354**
Avita Cream ... **2355**
Avita Gel ... **2357**
Mentax Cream ... **2358**

PERSŌN & COVEY, INC 2360

616 Allen Avenue
P.O. Box 25018
Glendale, CA 91221-5018

Direct Inquiries to:
Frank Brisben, C.O.O.
(818) 240-1030
(800) 423-2341

Products Described:
Aquanil HC Lotion ... **2360**
DHS Tar Gel Shampoo ... **2360**
DHS Tar Shampoo ... **2360**
DHS Zinc Dandruff Shampoo ... **2360**
DML Facial Moisturizer with Sunscreen ... **2360**
DML-Forte Cream ... *2360*
DML-Lotion ... *2360*
Drysol Solution ... **2360**
Solbar PF Cream SPF 50 (PABA Free) ... **2361**
Solbar PF Liquid SPF 30 ... **2361**
Xerac AC Solution ... **2361**

PFIZER INC 330, 2362

235 East 42nd Street
New York, NY 10017-5755

For Medical Information Contact:
24 hours a day, seven days a week:
(800) 438-1985

Distribution:
Memphis, TN 38134
1855 Shelby Oaks Drive North
(901) 387-5200
Customer Service:
(800) 533-4535

EXPORT INQUIRIES:
Pfizer International Inc.
(212) 573-2323

Products Described:
Antivert, Antivert/25, & Antivert/50 Tablets ... **2363**
◆Aricept Tablets ... **330, 2364**
Atarax Tablets & Syrup ... **2367**
◆Cardura Tablets ... **330, 2368**
Cefobid Intravenous/Intramuscular ... **2372**
Cefobid Pharmacy Bulk Package - Not for Direct Infusion ... **2374**
Diabinese Tablets ... **2377**
◆Diflucan Tablets, Injection, and Oral Suspension ... **330, 2379**
◆Feldene Capsules ... **330, 2383**
Geocillin Tablets ... **2384**
◆Glucotrol Tablets ... **330, 2385**
◆Glucotrol XL Extended Release Tablets ... **330, 2387**
◆Lipitor Tablets ... **331, 2389**
Marax Tablets & DF Syrup ... **2393**
Minipress Capsules ... **2393**
Minizide Capsules ... **2394**
◆Navane Capsules ... **331, 2396**
Navane Concentrate ... **2396**
Navane Intramuscular ... **2397**
◆Norvasc Tablets ... **331, 2399**
Pfizerpen for Injection ... **2400**
◆Procardia Capsules ... **331, 2402**
◆Procardia XL Extended Release Tablets ... **331, 2404**
Renese Tablets ... **2406**
◆Sinequan Capsules ... **331, 2407**
Sinequan Oral Concentrate ... **2407**
Spectrobid Tablets ... **2409**
Streptomycin Sulfate Injection ... **2410**
Tao Capsules ... **2411**
Terra-Cortril Ophthalmic Suspension ... **2412**
Terramycin Intramuscular Solution ... **2412**
Terramycin with Polymyxin B Sulfate Ophthalmic Ointment ... **2414**
◆Trovan I.V. ... **331, 2414**
◆Trovan Tablets ... **331, 2414**
◆Unasyn for Injection ... **331, 2421**
Urobiotic-250 Capsules ... **2424**
◆Viagra Tablets ... **331, 2424**
Vibramycin Calcium Oral Suspension Syrup ... **2427**
Vibramycin Hyclate Capsules ... **2427**
Vibramycin Hyclate Intravenous ... **2429**
Vibramycin Monohydrate for Oral Suspension ... **2427**
Vibra-Tabs Film Coated Tablets ... **2427**
Vistaril Capsules ... **2430**
Vistaril Intramuscular Solution ... **2431**
Vistaril Oral Suspension ... **2430**
Zithromax Capsules, 250 mg ... **2431**
◆Zithromax for IV Infusion ... **331, 2440**

◆ **Shown in Product Identification Guide**　　　　*Italic Page Number* **Indicates Brief Listing**　　　　⊙ **Described in PDR For Ophthalmology**

**ROXANE LABORATORIES, 335, 2743
INC.**

1809 Wilson Road
Columbus, OH 43228-8601

Direct Inquiries to:
Professional Services Department
P.O. 16532
Columbus, OH 43216-6532
(800) 848-0120
(614) 276-4000

RUSS PHARMACEUTICALS, INC.
(See UCB PHARMA, INC.)

RYSTAN COMPANY, INC. 335, 2770
47 Center Avenue
P.O. Box 214
Little Falls, NJ 07424-0214

Direct Inquiries to:
Professional Services Department
(973) 256-3737

Other Products Available:
Chloresium Tablets
Chloresium Toothpaste
Prophyllin CCC Wet Dressing Powder

**SANDOZ PHARMACEUTICALS
CORPORATION**
(See NOVARTIS
PHARMACEUTICALS
CORPORATION)

**SANOFI 335, 2773
PHARMACEUTICALS,
INC.**
90 Park Avenue
New York, NY 10016

Direct Inquiries to:
(212) 551-4000

For Medical Information Contact:
Product Information Services
(800) 446-6267

Sales and Ordering:
East Coast: (800) 223-1062
West Coast: (800) 223-5511

SAVAGE LABORATORIES 336, 2810
A division of Altana Inc.
60 Baylis Road
Melville, NY 11747

Direct Inquiries to:
Customer Service
(800) 231-0206
FAX: (516) 454-0732

For Medical Information Contact:
Dr. Arnold Yeadon
(516) 454-9071
FAX: (516) 454-6389

SCANDIPHARM, INC. 336, 2815
22 Inverness Center Parkway
Birmingham, AL 35242

Direct Inquiries to:
Customer Services
(800) 950-8085
FAX: (205) 991-8426

For Medical Information Contact:
John R. Booth, R.Ph.
(205) 991-8085
FAX: (205) 991-9547

Other Products Available:
ADEKs Multivitamin Supplement
ADEKs Pediatric Drops
Flutter
ScandiCal
ScandiShake
ScandiShake--Lactose Free
ScandiShake--Sweetened with Aspartame

**SCHEIN 336, 2817
PHARMACEUTICAL, INC.**
100 Campus Drive
Florham Park, NJ 07932

Direct Inquiries to:
Customer Service Department
(800) 356-5790
FAX: (800) 760-9224

For Medical Information Contact:
(800) 548-6236 (24 Hours)

Other Products Available:
Acyclovir Tablets and Capsules
Atenolol Tablets
Atenolol and Chlorthalidone Tablets
Cefaclor Capsules, USP
Cefazolin Sodium (Sterile), USP
Cefuroxime Sodium (Sterile), USP
Cimetidine Tablets, USP
Clindamycin HCl Capsules, USP
Cyclobenzaprine HCl Tablets, USP
Dipivefrin HCl Ophthalmic Solution, USP
Doxepin HCl Capsules, USP
Levobunolol HCl Ophthalmic Solution,
  USP
Minocycline HCl Capsules, USP
Nadolol Tablets, USP

Neomycin and Polymyxin B Sulfates and Hydrocortisone Ophthalmic Suspension, USP
Neomycin and Polymyxin B Sulfates and Hydrocortisone Otic Suspension, USP
Nifedipine Capsules, USP
Nortriptyline HCl Capsules, USP
Penicillin Injection, USP
Piroxicam Capsules, USP
Primidone Tablets, USP
Tobramycin Ophthalmic Solution, USP
Trihexyphenidyl HCl Tablets, USP
Vecuronium Bromide for Injection
Verapamil Tablets, USP

SCHERING CORPORATION 336, 2819

A wholly-owned subsidiary of Schering-Plough Corporation
Galloping Hill Road
Kenilworth, NJ 07033
(908) 298-4000

Direct Inquiries to:
(908) 298-4000

Customer Service:
(800) 222-7579
FAX: (908) 820-6400

For Medical Information Contact:
Schering Laboratories
Drug/Information Services
2000 Galloping Hill Road
Kenilworth, NJ 07033
(800) 526-4099
FAX: (908) 298-2188

Manufacturing and Distribution:
Southeast Branch
5884 Peachtree Road, N.E.
Chamblee, GA 30341
(404) 457-6315
Midwest Branch
7500 N. Natchez Ave.
Niles, IL 60648
(708) 647-9363
Southwest Branch
1921 Gateway Drive
Irving, TX 75062
(214) 714-2200
West Coast Branch
14775 Wicks Blvd.
San Leandro, CA 94577
(510) 357-3125

Products Described:
◆Cedax Capsules................ 336, 2819
◆Cedax Oral Suspension......... 336, 2819
Celestone Soluspan Suspension...... 2823
◆Claritin Reditabs................ 336, 2825
◆Claritin Syrup................ 336, 2825
◆Claritin Tablets................ 336, 2825
◆Claritin-D 12 Hour Extended Release Tablets............ 336, 2827
◆Claritin-D 24 Hour Extended Release Tablets............ 336, 2829
◆Diprolene AF Cream 0.05%..... 336, 2831
◆Diprolene Gel 0.05%........... 336, 2832
Diprolene Lotion 0.05%.............. 2833
◆Diprolene Ointment 0.05%........ 336, 2833
Elocon Cream 0.1%................ 2834
Elocon Lotion 0.1%................ 2835
Elocon Ointment 0.1%.............. 2836
◆Etrafon 2-10 Tablets (2-10)..... 336, 2837
◆Etrafon Forte Tablets (4-25)..... 336, 2837
◆Etrafon Tablets (2-25)........... 336, 2837
◆Eulexin Capsules................ 336, 2840
◆Fareston Tablets................ 336, 2842
◆Fulvicin P/G Tablets............ 336, 2843
◆Fulvicin P/G 165 & 330 Tablets.................... 336, 2844
Garamycin Cream 0.1%............. 2845
Garamycin Injectable.............. 2845
Garamycin Ointment 0.1%........... 2845
Hyperstat I.V. Injection............ 2848
InspirEase Drug Delivery System.... *2849*
Intron A for Injection.............. 2850
Lotrimin Cream 1%................ 2859
Lotrimin Lotion 1%................ 2859
Lotrimin Solution 1%.............. 2859
Lotrisone Cream.................. 2859
Nasonex Nasal Spray.............. 2861
Netromycin Injection 100 mg/ml..... 2863
◆Normodyne Injection............ 336, 2866
◆Normodyne Tablets.............. 336, 2868
Proventil Inhalation Aerosol.......... 2871
◆Proventil HFA Inhalation Aerosol................... 318, 2877
Proventil Inhalation Solution 0.083%........................... 2873
◆Proventil Repetabs Tablets....... 336, 2875
Proventil Solution for Inhalation 0.5%............................. 2872
Proventil Syrup................... 2874
◆Proventil Tablets............... 336, 2875
Rebetron Combination Therapy...... 2880
Solganal Suspension.............. 2884
Trilafon Concentrate.............. 2886
Trilafon Injection................. 2886
◆Trilafon Tablets................ 336, 2886
◆Vancenase AQ Nasal Spray 0.042%.................... 336, 2889
◆Vancenase AQ Double Strength Nasal Spray 0.084%................... 336, 2890
◆Vancenase PocketHaler Nasal Inhaler...................... 336, 2888
◆Vanceril Inhaler................ 336, 2892
Vanceril Double Strength Inhalation Aerosol................ 2894

Other Products Available:
Celestone Phosphate Injection
Celestone Syrup
Celestone Tablets
Chlor-Trimeton Injection
Diprosone Cream 0.05%
Diprosone Lotion 0.05%
Diprosone Ointment 0.05%
Diprosone Topical Aerosol 0.1%
Estinyl Tablets
Fulvicin-U/F Tablets
Meticorten Tablets
Metimyd Ophthalmic Ointment--Sterile
Metimyd Ophthalmic Suspension--Sterile
Miradon Tablets
Naqua Tablets
Optimine Tablets
Oreton Methyl Buccal Tablets
Oreton Methyl Tablets
Otobiotic Otic Solution
Paxipam Tablets
Permitil Oral Concentrate
Permitil Tablets
Polaramine Expectorant
Polaramine Syrup
Polaramine Tablets
Polarmine Repetabs Tablets
Sebizon Lotion
Sodium Sulamyd Ophthalmic Ointment 10%-Sterile
Sodium Sulamyd Ophthalmic Solution 10%-Sterile
Sodium Sulamyd Ophthalmic Solution 30% Sterile
Valisone Cream, 0.1%
Valisone Lotion 0.1%
Valisone Ointment 0.1%
Valisone Reduced Strength Cream .01%

SCHWARZ PHARMA, INC. 336, 2896

5600 W. County Line Road
P.O. Box 2038
Milwaukee, WI 53201

For Medical Information Contact:
Drug Safety and Information
(414) 238-9994
(800) 558-5114

Products Described:
Calciferol Drops................... *2896*
Calciferol in Oil Injection........... *2896*
Calciferol Tablets.................. *2896*
Codiclear DH Syrup................ 2896
Codimal DH Syrup................. 2897
Codimal DM Syrup................. *2897*
Codimal PH Syrup................. *2897*
◆Colyte and Colyte-Flavored for Oral Solution........... 336, 337, 2897
◆Cortifoam...................... 337, 2898
◆Deponit Transdermal Delivery System.............. 337, 2899
Dilatrate-SR Capsules.............. 2900
◆Edex for Injection.............. 337, 2901
◆Epifoam...................... 337, 2906
Ku-Zyme Capsules................ 2907
Ku-Zyme HP Capsules............. 2908
Kutrase Capsules................. 2907
Levatol Tablets.................. 2908
◆Levbid Extended-Release Tablets.................... 337, 2910
Levsin Drops..................... 2910
Levsin Elixir..................... 2910
Levsin Injection.................. 2910
Levsin Tablets.................... 2910
◆Levsin/SL Tablets............... 337, 2910
Levsinex Timecaps................ 2910
◆Monoket Tablets................ 337, 2911
◆Nascobal Gel................... 337, 2913
◆Niferex-150 Capsules............ 337, 2916
◆Niferex-150 Forte Capsules....... 337, 2916
Niferex Elixir.................... 2915
Niferex Tablets................... 2915
◆Niferex-PN Tablets.............. 337, 2916
◆Niferex-PN Forte Tablets........ 337, 2917
◆ProctoCream-HC 2.5%........... 337, 2917
◆ProctoFoam-HC................. 337, 2918
◆Uniretic Tablets................ 337, 2919
◆Univasc Tablets................ 337, 2922
◆Urso Tablets................... 337, 2925

Other Products Available:
Co-Gesic Tablets
GG-Cen Capsules
Guaimax-D Extended-Release Tablets
Kudrox Suspension
Kutapressin Injection
Lactrase Capsules
Milkinol
Mono-Gesic Tablets
ProctoFoam-NS (Non-Steroid)

SCS PHARMACEUTICALS 2771

Box 5110
Chicago, IL 60680-5110

Direct Inquiries to:
(800) 323-1603

For Medical Information Contact:
Generally:
G.D. Searle & Co.
Healthcare Information Services
5200 Old Orchard Road
Skokie, IL 60077
In Emergencies:
Outside IL:
(800) 323-4204 (business hours)
(847) 982-7000 (at other times)
Within IL:
(847) 982-7000

Sales and Ordering:
(800) 323-1603

Products Described:
Flagyl I.V.......................... 2771
Flagyl I.V. RTU.................... 2771

Other Products Available:
Levora (levonorgestrel and ethinyl estradiol tablets USP)
Piroxicam Capsules USP

G.D. SEARLE & CO. 337, 2926

Box 5110
Chicago, IL 60680-5110

Direct Inquiries to:
(800) 323-1603

For Medical Information Contact:
Generally:
G.D. Searle & Co.
Healthcare Information Services
5200 Old Orchard Road
Skokie, IL 60077
In Emergencies:
Outside IL:
(800) 323-4204 (business hours)
(847) 982-7000 (at other times)
Within IL:
(847) 982-7000

Sales and Ordering:
(800) 323-1603

Products Described:
◆Aldactazide Tablets............ 337, 2926
◆Aldactone Tablets.............. 337, 2928
◆Ambien Tablets................ 337, 2929
◆Arthrotec Tablets.............. 337, 2933
◆Brevicon 21-Day Tablets........ 337, 2937
◆Brevicon 28-Day Tablets........ 337, 2937
◆Calan Tablets.................. 337, 2943
◆Calan SR Caplets............... 337, 2946
◆Covera-HS Tablets.............. 337, 2948
◆Cytotec Tablets................ 337, 2951
◆Daypro Caplets................ 337, 2953
◆Demulen 1/35-21 Tablets....... 338, 2955
◆Demulen 1/35-28 Tablets....... 338, 2955
◆Demulen 1/50-21 Tablets....... 338, 2955
◆Demulen 1/50-28 Tablets....... 338, 2955
◆Flagyl 375 Capsules............ 338, 2961
◆Flagyl ER Tablets.............. 338, 2963
◆Kerlone Tablets................ 338, 2965
Lomotil Liquid..................... 2968
◆Lomotil Tablets................ 338, 2968
◆Norinyl 1 + 35 21-Day Tablets................... 338, 2937
◆Norinyl 1 + 35 28-Day Tablets................... 338, 2937
◆Norinyl 1 + 50 21-Day Tablets................... 338, 2937
◆Norinyl 1 + 50 28-Day Tablets................... 338, 2937
◆Norpace Capsules............... 338, 2969
◆Norpace CR Capsules........... 338, 2969
Synarel Nasal Solution for Central Precocious Puberty................ 2972
Synarel Nasal Solution for Endometriosis..................... 2973
◆Tri-Norinyl 21 Tablets.......... 338, 2975
◆Tri-Norinyl 28 Tablets.......... 338, 2975

Other Products Available:
Flagyl Tablets

SEQUUS PHARMACEUTICALS, INC. 338, 2981

960 Hamilton Court
Menlo Park, CA 94025

Direct Inquiries to:
Department of Professional Services
(800) 323-9049

For Medical Emergencies Contact:
(800) 323-9049

Products Described:
◆Amphotec for Injection......... 338, 2981
◆Doxil Injection................ 338, 2984

SERONO LABORATORIES, INC. 2988

100 Longwater Circle
Norwell, MA 02061
www.seronousa.com

Direct Inquiries to:
Customer Service, Sales and Ordering
(888) 398-4567
(781) 982-9000

For Medical Information or to Report Adverse Drug Experiences Contact:
Drug Information and Surveillance Group
(888) 275-7376
(781) 982-9000 ext. 5562

Products Described:
Fertinex for Injection............... 2988
Geref for Injection................. 2989
Geref Diagnostic for Injection........ 2991
Gonal-F for Injection............... 2991
Pergonal for Injection............... 2995
Profasi for Injection............... 2997
Saizen for Injection............... 2998
Serophene Tablets.................. 2999
Serostim for Injection.............. 3001

SHIRE RICHWOOD INC. 338, 3003

7900 Tanners Gate Drive, Suite 200
Florence, KY 41042

Direct Inquiries to:
(606) 282-2100
FAX: (606) 282-2118

Products Described:
◆Adderall Tablets............... 338, 3003
◆Carbatrol Capsules............. 338, 3004
◆DextroStat Tablets............. 338, 3007

SIGMA-TAU PHARMACEUTICALS, INC. 3008

800 South Frederick Avenue, Suite 300
Gaithersburg, MD 20877

Direct Inquiries to:
TEL: (301) 948-1041
(800) 447-0169
E-mail: info@sigmatau.com
FAX: (301) 948-3194

Products Described:
Carnitor Injection.................. 3008
Carnitor Tablets and Solution........ 3009

SMITHKLINE BEECHAM CONSUMER HEALTHCARE, L.P. 3010

Unit of SmithKline Beecham Inc.
P.O. Box 1467
Pittsburgh, PA 15230

Direct Inquiries to:
Professional Services Department
(800) BEECHAM
PA Residents: (800) 242-1718

Products Described:
Cepastat Lozenges..................... ■□
Contac Continuous Action Decongestant/Antihistamine Capsules.......................... ■□
Contac Maximum Strength Continuous Action Decongestant/ Antihistamine Caplets............... ■□
Contac Severe Cold and Flu Formula Caplets............................ ■□
Contac Severe Cold & Flu Nighttime... ■□
Debrox Drops......................... ■□
Denavir Cream..................... 3010
Ecotrin Enteric Coated Aspirin Low Strength Tablets............. 3011
Ecotrin Enteric Coated Aspirin Maximum Strength Tablets.......... 3011
Ecotrin Enteric Coated Aspirin Regular Strength Tablets........... 3011
Feosol Caplets..................... 3013
Feosol Elixir....................... 3013
Feosol Tablets..................... 3013
Gaviscon Regular Strength Antacid Tablets............................ ■□
Gaviscon Extra Strength Antacid Tablets............................ ■□
Gaviscon Regular Strength Liquid Antacid............................ ■□
Gaviscon Extra Strength Liquid Antacid............................ ■□
Gly-Oxide Liquid..................... ■□
Massengill Douches, Towelettes and Cleansing Wash.................. ■□
Nicoderm CQ Patch................. 3014
Nicorette Gum..................... 3016
Os-Cal 250 + D, 500, 500 + D, and 500 Chewable Tablets............ ■□
Os-Cal Fortified Tablets.............. ■□
Singlet Tablets...................... ■□
Tagamet HB 200 Acid Reducer........ ■□
Tums Anti-gas/Antacid............... ■□

Tums, Tums EX, and Tums ULTRA Antacid/Calcium Supplement Tablets ... ⊡

SMITHKLINE BEECHAM PHARMACEUTICALS **338, 3018**
One Franklin Plaza
P.O. Box 7929
Philadelphia, PA 19101

For Medical Information Contact:
Medical Department
(800) 366-8900, Ext. 5231

Products Described:
◆Albenza Tablets ... **338, 3018**
◆Amoxil Capsules, Tablets and Chewable Tablets ... **338, 3019**
Amoxil Pediatric Drops, Powder for Oral Suspension ... **3019**
◆Ancef Injection ... **338, 3023**
◆Androderm Transdermal System ... **338, 3025**
◆Augmentin Powder for Oral Suspension and Chewable Tablets ... **338, 3028**
◆Augmentin Tablets ... **338, 339, 3031**
Bactroban Cream ... **3034**
Bactroban Nasal ... **3035**
Bactroban Ointment ... **3034**
◆Compazine Injection ... **339, 3036**
◆Compazine Multi-dose Vials ... **339, 3036**
◆Compazine Spansule Capsules ... **339, 3036**
◆Compazine Suppositories ... **339, 3036**
◆Compazine Syrup ... **339, 3036**
◆Compazine Tablets ... **339, 3036**
◆Coreg Tablets ... **339, 3039**
◆Dexedrine Spansule Capsules ... **339, 3043**
◆Dexedrine Tablets ... **339, 3043**
◆Dibenzyline Capsules ... **339, 3044**
◆Dyazide Capsules ... **339, 3045**
◆Dyrenium Capsules ... **339, 3047**
◆Engerix-B ... **339, 3048**
◆Eskalith Capsules ... **339, 3051**
◆Eskalith CR Controlled Release Tablets ... **339, 3051**
◆Famvir Tablets ... **339, 3052**
◆Fastin Capsules ... **339, 3055**
◆Havrix ... **339, 3056**
◆Hycamtin for Injection ... **339, 3058**
◆Infanrix ... **339, 3061**
◆Kytril Injection ... **339, 3066**
◆Kytril Tablets ... **339, 3068**
◆Monocid Injection ... **339, 3070**
◆OmniHIB ... **339, 3072**
◆Ornade Spansule Capsules ... **339, 3075**
◆Parnate Tablets ... **339, 3076**
Paxil Oral Suspension ... **3078**
◆Paxil Tablets ... **339, 3078**
◆Rabies Vaccine Adsorbed ... **340, 3083**
◆Relafen Tablets ... **340, 3085**
◆Requip Tablets ... **340, 3087**
◆Stelazine Concentrate ... **340, 3092**
◆Stelazine Multi-dose Vials ... **340, 3092**
◆Stelazine Tablets ... **340, 3092**
Tagamet Injection ... **3094**
Tagamet Liquid ... **3094**
◆Tagamet Tablets ... **340, 3094**
Tazicef for Injection ... **3098**
◆Thorazine Ampuls ... **340, 3101**
Thorazine Concentrate ... **3101**
◆Thorazine Multi-dose Vials ... **340, 3101**
◆Thorazine Spansule Capsules ... **340, 3101**
◆Thorazine Suppositories ... **340, 3101**
◆Thorazine Syrup ... **340, 3101**
◆Thorazine Tablets ... **340, 3101**
Ticar for Injection ... **3104**
◆Timentin for Injection ... **340, 3106**
◆Urispas Tablets ... **340, 3109**

Other Products Available:
Beepen-VK Powder for Oral Solution and Tablets

SMITHKLINE CONSUMER PRODUCTS
(See SMITHKLINE BEECHAM CONSUMER HEALTHCARE, L.P.)

SOLVAY PHARMACEUTICALS, INC. **340, 3110**
901 Sawyer Road
Marietta, GA 30062
(770) 578-9000

For Medical Information Contact:
Generally:
Medical Services Department
(770) 578-9000
FAX: (770) 578-5586
In Emergencies:
(770) 429-7110

Sales and Ordering:
Orders may be placed by calling this toll free number:
(800) 241-1643
FAX: (770) 578-5901
Ordernet access is available.
Mail orders should be sent to:
Solvay Pharmaceuticals
Order Entry Department
901 Sawyer Road
Marietta, GA 30062

Products Described:
Cortenema ... **3110**
◆Creon 5 Capsules ... **340, 3110**
◆Creon 10 Capsules ... **340, 3110**
◆Creon 20 Capsules ... **340, 3110**
Duphalac Solution ... **3111**
◆Estratab Tablets (0.3, 0.625, 2.5 mg) ... **340, 3112**
◆Estratest Tablets ... **340, 3116**
◆Estratest H.S. Tablets ... **340, 3116**
◆Lithobid Slow-Release Tablets ... **340, 3119**
◆Lithonate Capsules ... *340*
◆Lithotabs Tablets ... *340*
◆Luvox Tablets (25, 50, 100 mg) ... **340, 3121**
◆Prometrium Capsules (100 mg) ... **340, 3124**
◆Rowasa Rectal Suspension Enema 4.0 grams/unit (60 mL) ... **340, 3126**
◆Rowasa Suppositories, 500 mg ... **340, 3126**
◆Advanced Formula Zenate Tablets ... **340, 3128**

Other Products Available:
Dermacort Cream
Dermacort Lotion 1%
Dexone (0.5, 0.75, 1.5, 4 mg)
Orasone (1, 5, 10, 20, 50 mg)

SOMERSET PHARMACEUTICALS, INC. **340, 3128**
5215 W. Laurel Street, Suite 200
Tampa, FL 33607

For Medical Information Contact:
Generally:
Professional Services Department
(813) 288-0040
FAX: (813) 282-0287
In Emergencies:
(800) 892-8889
FAX: (813) 282-0287

Products Described:
◆Eldepryl Capsules ... **340, 3128**

SPEYWOOD PHARMACEUTICALS, INC. **3131**
27 Maple Street
Milford, MA 01757-3650

Direct Inquiries to:
Customer Service:
(800) 456-7322
Educational Information:
(508) 478-8900

For Medical Emergencies Contact:
(800) 456-7322

Sales and Ordering:
(800) 456-7322
Reimbursement Services:
(800) 334-1142

Products Described:
Hyate:C ... *3131*

STAR PHARMACEUTICALS, INC. **3131**
1990 N.W. 44th Street
Pompano Beach, FL 33064-8712

Direct Inquiries to:
Scott L. Davidson, President
(954) 971-9704

Sales and Ordering:
(800) 845-7827
FAX: (954) 971-7718
http://www.starpharmaceuticals.com

Products Described:
Aphrodyne Caplets ... *3131*
Prosed/DS Tablets ... *3131*
Uro-KP-Neutral Tablets ... *3131*
Urolene Blue Tablets ... *3131*
Virilon Capsules ... *3131*
Virilon IM Injection ... *3131*

STIEFEL LABORATORIES, INC. **3131**
255 Alhambra Circle
Coral Gables, FL 33134

BRANCH OFFICES:
Georgia
500 Satellite Blvd.
Suwanee, GA 30024
(770) 945-0101
Nevada
P.O. Box 2387
Sparks, NV 89432
New York
Route 145
Oak Hill, NY 12460
(518) 239-6901

Direct Inquiries to:
Professional Services Department
(305) 443-3800

Products Described:
Brevoxyl-4 Cleansing Lotion ... **3132**
Brevoxyl-8 Cleansing Lotion ... **3132**
Brevoxyl-4 Gel ... **3131**
Brevoxyl-8 Gel ... **3131**
Clindets Pledgets ... **3132**
LactiCare-HC Lotion, 1% ... *3133*
LactiCare-HC Lotion, 2 ½% ... *3133*
PanOxyl 5 Acne Gel ... *3133*
PanOxyl 10 Acne Gel ... *3133*
PanOxyl AQ 2 ½ Acne Gel ... *3133*
PanOxyl AQ 5 Acne Gel ... *3133*
PanOxyl AQ 10 Acne Gel ... *3133*
Sulfoxyl Lotion Regular ... *3133*
Sulfoxyl Lotion Strong ... *3133*

Other Products Available:
Benoxyl-10 Lotion
Brasivol Base
Brasivol Medium
Brasivol Rough
Epilyt Lotion
LactiCare Lotion
Oilatum Soap (Unscented)
PanOxyl Bar 10
Polytar Shampoo
Polytar Soap
Salicylic Acid & Sulfur Soap
Salicylic Acid Cleansing Bar
Sarna Lotion
SAStid Soap
SFC Lotion
Sulfur Soap
Zeasorb Powder
Zeasorb-AF Powder
ZNP Bar

STUART PHARMACEUTICALS
(See ZENECA PHARMACEUTICALS)

SUPERGEN, INC. **3133**
Two Annabel Lane, Suite 220
San Ramon, CA 94583

Direct Inquiries to:
Customer Service
(800) 905-5474
FAX: (800) 903-5474

For Medical Information Contact:
Generally:
Professional Services Department
(888) 43-SUPER
(888) 437-8737
FAX: (925) 327-7347
In Emergencies:
(415) 487-8441

Sales and Ordering:
Customer Service
(800) 905-5474
FAX: (800) 903-5474

Products Described:
Mitomycin for Injection, USP ... *3133*
Nipent for Injection ... **3133**

TAP PHARMACEUTICALS INC. **340, 3136**
2355 Waukegan Road
Deerfield, IL 60015

Direct Inquiries to:
Customer Service
(800) 621-1020

For Medical Information Contact:
Generally:
Medical Department
(800) 622-2011 (LUPRON)
(800) 478-9526 (PREVACID)
In Emergencies:
Medical Department
(800) 622-2011 (LUPRON)
(800) 478-9526 (PREVACID)

Products Described:
◆Lupron Depot 3.75 mg ... **341, 3139**
◆Lupron Depot 7.5 mg ... **340, 3141**
◆Lupron Depot--3 Month 11.25 mg ... **340, 3143**
◆Lupron Depot--3 Month 22.5 mg ... **340, 3145**
◆Lupron Depot--4 Month 30 mg ... **340, 3147**
Lupron Depot-PED 7.5 mg, 11.25 mg and 15 mg ... **3148**
Lupron Injection ... **3136**
Lupron Injection Pediatric ... **3137**
◆Prevacid Delayed-Release Capsules ... **341, 3150**
◆PREVPAC ... **341, 3155**

TAYLOR PHARMACEUTICALS **3159**
An Akorn Company
Corporate/Customer Service:
942 Calle Negocio
Suite 150
San Clemente, CA 92673
Sales:
150 S. Wyckles Road
Decatur, IL 62525

Direct Inquiries to:
Corporate/Customer Service:
(800) 223-9851

Sales:
(217) 428-1100

Products Described:
Alfenta Injection ... *3159*
Sufenta Injection ... *3159*

UAD LABORATORIES
(See FOREST PHARMACEUTICALS, INC.)

UCB PHARMA, INC. **341, 3159**
1950 Lake Park Drive
Smyrna, GA 30080

Direct Inquiries to:
(800) 477-7877

For Medical Information Contact:
Suzan E. Leake
Manager, Medical Affairs
(770) 437-5558
In Emergencies:
Medical Affairs
(800) 477-7877

Products Described:
◆Duratuss DM Elixir ... **341, 3160**
◆Duratuss G Tablets ... **341, 3160**
◆Duratuss HD Elixir ... **341, 3161**
◆Duratuss Tablets ... **341, 3159**
Fe-50 Caplets ... *3162*
◆Lortab 2.5/500 Tablets ... **341, 3162**
◆Lortab 5/500 Tablets ... **341, 3162**
◆Lortab 7.5/500 Tablets ... **341, 3162**
◆Lortab 10/500 Tablets ... **341, 3162**
◆Lortab ASA Tablets ... *341, 3163*
◆Lortab Elixir ... **341, 3162**
Precare Prenatal Multi-Vitamin/Mineral ... **3163**
◆Theo-24 Extended Release Capsules ... **341, 3164**
◆Trinsicon Capsules ... **341, 3170**
◆Vicon Forte Capsules ... **341, 3170**

Other Products Available:
Corticaine Cream
Vicon-C Capsules
Vi-Zac Capsules

UNIMED PHARMACEUTICALS, INC. **341, 3175**
2150 E. Lake Cook Road
Buffalo Grove, IL 60089-1862

Direct Inquiries to:
(847) 541-2525
FAX: (847) 541-2569

Products Described:
◆Anadrol-50 Tablets ... **341, 3175**
◆Marinol Capsules ... *341, 3177*
◆Maxaquin Tablets ... **341, 3177**

THE UPJOHN COMPANY
(See PHARMACIA & UPJOHN COMPANY)

UPSHER-SMITH LABORATORIES, INC. **341, 3181**
14905 23rd Avenue North
Minneapolis, MN 55447

For Medical Information Contact:
Write: Professional Services Department
or call: (800) 654-2299
(during business hours-8 a.m. to 5 p.m. CST)

Products Described:
Amlactin 12% Lotion and Cream ... *3181*
Klor-Con/EF Tablets ... *3181*
◆Klor-Con 8/Klor-Con 10 Tablets ... *341, 3181*
Klor-Con Powder ... *3181*
Klor-Con/25 Powder ... *3181*
Niacor Tablets ... *3181*

U.S. BIOSCIENCE, INC.   341, 3171
One Tower Bridge
100 Front Street
West Conshohocken, PA 19428

Direct Inquiries to:
U.S. Bioscience
(610) 832-0570

For Medical Information or Emergencies Contact:
(800) 872-4672

U.S. ETHICALS INC.
(See RHÔNE-POULENC RORER PHARMACEUTICALS INC.)

**U.S. PHARMACEUTICAL   3175
CORPORATION**
2401-C Mellon Court
Decatur, GA 30035
(800) 330-3040
FAX: (404) 987-4806

MAILING ADDRESS:
2401-C Mellon Court
Decatur, GA 30035

Direct Inquiries to:
Peter J. Krebs, Ph.D.
CEO, Management Unit
(800) 330-3040, or
Raymond F. Meyer, R.Ph.
Marketing Director (South East)
(800) 330-3040, or
Clayton W. Bishop
Director of Sales Development (South West)
(512) 847-3357

USANA, INCORPORATED   341, 3185
3838 West Parkway Boulevard
Salt Lake City, UT 84120-6336

Direct Inquiries to:
Technical Services Department
(801) 954-7860
FAX: (801) 954-7658

VITALINE CORPORATION   3186
385 Williamson Way
Ashland, OR 97520

Direct Inquiries to:
Jed D. Meese, Technical Director
(800) 648-4755
(541) 482-9231
FAX: (541) 482-9112
E-Mail: jmeese@vitaline.com

VIVUS, INC.   341, 3186
605 East Fairchild Drive
Mountain View, CA 94043

Direct Inquiries to:
(888) 345-6873

For Medical Information or Emergencies Contact:
Medical Services Department @ VIVUS:
(650) 934-5200
FAX: (650) 934-5209

**WAKEFIELD   3190
PHARMACEUTICALS, INC.**
310 Maxwell Road, Suite 100
Alpharetta, GA 30004

Direct Inquiries to:
(770) 664-1661
FAX: (770) 664-1126

WALLACE LABORATORIES   341, 3191
P.O. Box 1001
Cranbury, NJ 08512

For Medical Information Contact:
Generally:
Professional Services
(800) 526-3840
After Hours and Weekend Emergencies:
(609) 655-6474

Sales and Ordering:
Wallace Laboratories
Div. of Carter-Wallace, Inc.
P.O. Box 1001
Cranbury, NJ 08512

**WARNER CHILCOTT   3214
LABORATORIES**
Rockaway 80 Corporate Center
100 Enterprise Drive
Suite 280
Rockaway, NJ 07866
(800) 521-8813

Direct Inquiries to:
(800) 521-8813

For Product or Medical Information Contact:
(800) 521-8813
(973) 442-3236

For After Hours and Weekend Emergencies Contact:
(303) 739-1110

**WARNER CHILCOTT   342, 3208
LABORATORIES**
Professional Products Division
Rockaway 80 Corporate Center
100 Enterprise Drive
Suite 280
Rockaway, NJ 07866

Direct Inquiries to:
(800) 521-8813

For Product or Medical Information Contact:
(800) 521-8813
(973) 442-3236

For After Hours and Weekend Emergencies Contact:
(303) 739-1110

**WARNER-LAMBERT   3214
CONSUMER HEALTHCARE**
201 Tabor Road
Morris Plains, NJ 07950

Direct Inquiries and For Medical Information Contact:
Consumer Affairs
1-(800) 223-0182

WATSON LABORATORIES,   342, 3216
INC.

311 Bonnie Circle
Corona, CA 91720

Direct Inquiries to:
Customer Service Department
(800) 272-5525
FAX: (909) 735-2871

For Medical Emergencies Contact:
(800) 272-5525
FAX: (909) 735-2871

WE PHARMACEUTICALS, INC.   3241

P.O. Box 1142
Ramona, CA 92065

Direct Inquiries to:
(760) 788-9155

For Medical Emergencies Contact:
(760) 788-9155

WESTLAKE LABORATORIES,   3242
INC.

24700 Center Ridge Road
Cleveland, OH 44145
Internet: www.westlake-labs.com

Direct Inquiries to:
Customer Service
(888) WSTLAKE (978-5253)
FAX: (216) 835-2177

For Medical Information Contact:
Customer Service
(888) WSTLAKE (978-5253)
FAX: (216) 835-2177

Other Products Available:
Bona-Bacillus Capsules
Coenzyme Q-10 Chewable Tablets
GFS-2000 Capsules
Glutanac Capsules
Nutrision Capsules
Nutrisure OTC Tablets
Pantethine Capsules
Phosphatidyl-Serine Capsules
Total-E Softgels
Ultra G.I. Capsules
Ultra-Carotenoids Capsules

Ultra-Lipoic Forte Capsules
Uro-Pro Capsules

WESTWOOD-SQUIBB
PHARMACEUTICALS INC.
(See BRISTOL-MYERS SQUIBB
COMPANY)

WHITBY PHARMACEUTICALS,
INC.
(See UCB PHARMA, INC.)

WOMEN FIRST   343, 3253
HEALTHCARE, INC.

12220 El Camino Real
Suite 400
San Diego, CA 92130

Direct Inquiries to:
(888) 950-2246
FAX: (888) 950-2248

WYETH-AYERST   343, 3475
LABORATORIES

Division of American Home Products
  Corporation
P.O. Box 8299
Philadelphia, PA 19101

Direct Inquiries to:
(610) 688-4400

For Medical Information Contact:
  Medical Affairs
  Day: (800) 934-5556 (8:30 AM to 4:30
    PM, Eastern Standard Time, Weekdays
    only)
In Emergencies:
  Day: (800) 934-5556 (8:30 AM to 4:30
    PM, Eastern Standard Time, Weekdays
    only)
  Night: (610) 688-4400 (Emergencies
    only; non-emergencies should wait
    until the next day)

Manufacturing and Distribution:
(Do not use freight addresses for mailing
  of orders.)

Atlanta, GA--
  P.O. Box 1773
  Paoli, PA 19301-1773
  (800) 666-7248
  Freight address:
  1000 Union Court
  Kennesaw, GA 30144
  Mail DEA order forms to:
  P.O. Box 4365
  Atlanta, GA 30302-4365
Chicago, IL--
  P.O. Box 1773
  Paoli, PA 19301-1773
  (800) 666-7248
  Freight address:
  284 Lies Road
  Carol Stream, IL 60188
  Mail DEA order forms to:
  P.O. Box 140
  Wheaton, IL 60189-0140
Dallas, TX--
  P.O. Box 1773
  Paoli, PA 19301-1773
  (800) 666-7248
  Freight address:
  11240 Petal Street
  Dallas, TX 75238
  Mail DEA order forms to:
  P.O. Box 650231
  Dallas, TX 75265-0231
Philadelphia, PA--
  P.O. Box 1773
  Paoli, PA 19301-1773
  (800) 666-7248
  Freight address:
  31 Morehall Road
  Frazer, PA 19355
  Mail DEA order forms to:
  P.O. Box 61
  Paoli, PA 19301
Sparks, NV--
  P.O. Box 1773
  Paoli, PA 19301-1773
  (800) 666-7248
  Freight address:
  1802 Brierley Way
  Sparks, NV 89434
  Mail DEA order forms to:
  1802 Brierley Way
  Sparks, NV 89434
San Juan, Puerto Rico--
  GPO Box 362917
  San Juan, PR 00936
  (800) 462-4748

Freight address:
Wyeth-Ayerst Laboratories P.R. Inc.
Amelia Industrial Center
Street D
Lots 32-35
Guaynabo, Puerto Rico 00968
Mail DEA order forms to:
GPO Box 362917
San Juan, PR 00936-2917

◆ **Shown in Product Identification Guide**   *Italic Page Number* **Indicates Brief Listing**   ◎ **Described in PDR For Ophthalmology**

ZENECA   **345, 3402**
PHARMACEUTICALS
A Business Unit of Zeneca Inc.
Wilmington, DE 19850-5437 USA
General Number: (302) 886-3000

For Medical Information Contact:
  Generally:
  (302) 886-8000
  After Hours and Weekend Emergencies:
  (302) 886-3000
  Adverse Drug Experiences:
  (302) 886-8100

Sales Contact and Ordering:
(800) 842-9920

HOW TO USE THE BRAND AND GENERIC NAME INDEX

This index lists every product alphabetically by both brand and generic name. Generic names are underlined; brand names are not.

Under each generic name, you will find a list of the brands that contain it. This enables you to find a particular product by either of its names. For example, "Ativan Injection" is listed once alphabetically and again under its generic name, lorazepam.

Each time a brand name appears, it is followed by the manufacturer's name and the page to consult for further information. Under a generic heading, all fully described brands are listed first, followed by those with only partial information. In each case, the brands are listed alphabetically.

Brand name

ATIVAN INJECTION
(Wyeth-Ayerst) **3267**

◆ **ATIVAN TABLETS**
(Wyeth-Ayerst) **343, 3271**

ATIVAN IN TUBEX
(Wyeth-Ayerst) *3396*

Generic name

LORAZEPAM   Manufacturer
Ativan Injection
(Wyeth-Ayerst) **3267**

Bold page number
Indicates complete
prescribing information

Ativan Tablets
(Wyeth-Ayerst) **343, 3271**

Ativan in Tubex
(Wyeth-Ayerst) *3396*

Brands of lorazepam

Lorazepam Intensol *(Roxane)* ...*2743*
Lorazepam Tablets *(Geneva)*.....*1076*
Lorazepam Tablets *(Mylan)* *1955*
Lorazepam Tablets, USP
(Watson)..................................*3216*

Italic page number
Indicates partial
prescribing
information

Indicates photo in Product Identification Guide

◆ **LORCET 10/650 TABLETS**
(Forest)...............................*310, 1027*

◆ **LORCET-HD CAPSULES**
(Forest)..*1026*

◆ **LORCET PLUS TABLETS**
(Forest)...............................*310, 1027*

BRAND AND GENERIC NAME INDEX

This index includes all entries in the Product Information and Diagnostic Product Information sections. Products are listed alphabetically by brand and generic name.

■ An <u>underline</u> denotes a generic name.

■ **Bold page numbers** indicate full prescribing information.

■ *Italic page numbers* signify partial information.

■ The ◆ symbol marks drugs shown in the Product Identification Guide.

■ The ▣ symbol means product information is located in *PDR For Nonprescription Drugs and Dietary Supplements*.

■ The ⊙ symbol means product information is located in *PDR For Ophthalmology*.

If an entry in the index lists multiple page numbers, the first ones shown refer to photographs of the product, the last one to its prescribing information. For more on this index, see "How to Use the Brand and Generic Name Index" on the preceding page.

Otic Domeboro Solution (Bayer) ... 667
VōSoL Otic Solution (Wallace) ... 3207
VōSoL HC Otic Solution (Wallace) ... 3207
ACETOHYDROXAMIC ACID
Lithostat Tablets (Mission) ... 1930
ACETYLCYSTEINE
Acetylcysteine Solution (Roxane) ... 2743
Acetylcysteine Solution USP, Mucosil (Dey) ... 916
ACETYLSALICYLIC ACID (see under: ASPIRIN)
ACHROMYCIN V CAPSULES (Lederle Labs) ... 1514
ACI-JEL THERAPEUTIC VAGINAL JELLY (Ortho-McNeil Pharmaceutical) ... 2179
ACITRETIN
Soriatane Capsules (Roche Laboratories) ... 335, 2704
◆ ACLOVATE CREAM (Glaxo Wellcome) ... 311, 1082
◆ ACLOVATE OINTMENT (Glaxo Wellcome) ... 311, 1082
ACRIVASTINE
Semprex-D Capsules (Medeva) ... 1705
ACTH (see under: COSYNTROPIN)
HP ACTHAR GEL (Rhône-Poulenc Rorer) ... 2580
◆ ACTHIB (Pasteur Mérieux Connaught) ... 329, 2316
ACTHREL FOR INJECTION (Ferring) ... 1004, 3468
ACTICIN CREAM (Penederm) ... 2354
ACTIDOSE-AQUA SUSPENSION (Paddock) ... 2260
ACTIDOSE WITH SORBITOL SUSPENSION (Paddock) ... 2260
ACTIFED COLD & ALLERGY TABLETS (Warner-Lambert Consumer) ... 3214
ACTIFED COLD & SINUS CAPLETS AND TABLETS (Warner-Lambert Consumer) ... 3214
◆ ACTIGALL CAPSULES (Novartis) ... 324, 1987
◆ ACTIS VENOUS FLOW CONTROLLER (Vivus) ... 341, 3186
◆ ACTIVASE I.V. (Genentech) ... 311, 1057
◆ ACTONEL TABLETS (Procter & Gamble Pharmaceuticals) ... 332, 2531
ACULAR OPHTHALMIC SOLUTION (Allergan) ... 493
ACULAR PF OPHTHALMIC SOLUTION (Allergan) ... 494
ACYCLOVIR
Zovirax Capsules (Glaxo Wellcome) ... 315, 1272
Zovirax Ointment 5% (Glaxo Wellcome) ... 315, 1274
Zovirax Suspension (Glaxo Wellcome) ... 315, 1272
Zovirax Tablets (Glaxo Wellcome) ... 315, 1272
Acyclovir Capsules (Roxane) ... 2743
Acyclovir Capsules and Tablets (Mylan) ... 1955
Acyclovir Capsules and Tablets, Caps 200 mg, Tabs 400 mg, 800 mg (Novopharm) ... 2110
ACYCLOVIR SODIUM
Zovirax Sterile Powder (Glaxo Wellcome) ... 315, 1275
ADAGEN INJECTION (Enzon) ... 990
◆ ADALAT CAPSULES (Bayer) ... 305, 634
◆ ADALAT CC TABLETS (Bayer) ... 305, 636
ADAPALENE
Differin Gel (Galderma) ... 1050
Differin Solution (Galderma) ... 1051
◆ ADDERALL TABLETS (Shire Richwood) ... 338, 3003
ADENOCARD INJECTION (Fujisawa) ... 1033
ADENOSCAN (Fujisawa) ... 1034
ADENOSINE
Adenocard Injection (Fujisawa) ... 1033
Adenoscan (Fujisawa) ... 1034
ADIPEX-P CAPSULES (Gate) ... 1053
◆ ADIPEX-P TABLETS (Gate) ... 310, 1053
ADRENOCORTICOTROPIC HORMONE
HP Acthar Gel (Rhône-Poulenc Rorer) ... 2580
ADRIAMYCIN PFS/RDF FOR INJECTION (Pharmacia & Upjohn) ... 2451
ADULT STRENGTH PRODUCTS (see base product name)
◆ AEROBID INHALER SYSTEM (Forest) ... 310, 1015
◆ AEROBID-M INHALER SYSTEM (Forest) ... 310, 1015
◆ AEROCHAMBER AND AEROCHAMBER WITH MASK (Forest) ... 310, 1016
AEROLATE LIQUID (Fleming) ... 1013
AEROLATE JR. T.D. CAPSULES (Fleming) ... 1013
AEROLATE SR. T.D. CAPSULES (Fleming) ... 1013
AEROLATE III T.D. CAPSULES (Fleming) ... 1013
AGGRASTAT INJECTION (Merck) ... 1721
AGGRASTAT INJECTION PREMIXED (Merck) ... 1721
◆ AGRYLIN CAPSULES (Roberts) ... 334, 2620
AH-CHEW CHEWABLE TABLETS (We) ... 3241
AH-CHEW D CHEWABLE TABLETS (We) ... 3241
AIRET INHALATION SOLUTION (Medeva) ... 1692
AKINETON INJECTION (Knoll Labs) ... 1471
◆ AKINETON TABLETS (Knoll Labs) ... 318, 1471
ALATROFLOXACIN MESYLATE
Trovan I.V. (Pfizer) ... 331, 2414
ALBENDAZOLE
Albenza Tablets (SmithKline Beecham) ... 338, 3018
◆ ALBENZA TABLETS (SmithKline Beecham) ... 338, 3018
ALBUMARC 5% SOLUTION (American Red Cross) ... 520
ALBUMARC 25% SOLUTION (American Red Cross) ... 520
ALBUMIN (HUMAN)
Albumin (Human) 5% (Immuno) ... 1406
Albumin (Human) 25% (Immuno) ... 1407
Albuminar-5, U.S.P. (Centeon) ... 878
Albuminar-25, U.S.P. (Centeon) ... 878
Albumarc 5% Solution (American Red Cross) ... 520
Albumarc 25% Solution (American Red Cross) ... 520
Albutein 5% Solution (Alpha Therapeutic) ... 507
Albutein 25% Solution (Alpha Therapeutic) ... 507
Buminate 5% Solution, USP (Baxter Healthcare) ... 621
Buminate 25% Solution, USP (Baxter Healthcare) ... 621
ALBUMINAR-5, U.S.P. (Centeon) ... 878
ALBUMINAR-25, U.S.P. (Centeon) ... 878
ALBUTEIN 5% SOLUTION (Alpha Therapeutic) ... 507
ALBUTEIN 25% SOLUTION (Alpha Therapeutic) ... 507
ALBUTEROL
Proventil Inhalation Aerosol (Schering) ... 2871
Ventolin Inhalation Aerosol and Refill (Glaxo Wellcome) ... 314, 1242
Albuterol Inhalation Aerosol (Warner Chilcott) ... 3214
Albuterol Inhalation Aerosol (Dey) ... 309, 916
Albuterol Tablets (Mylan) ... 1955
ALBUTEROL SULFATE
Airet Inhalation Solution (Medeva) ... 1692
Albuterol Sulfate, USP Solution for Inhalation, Arm-a-Med (Astra) ... 546
Combivent Inhalation Aerosol (Boehringer Ingelheim) ... 306, 752
Proventil HFA Inhalation Aerosol (Schering) ... 318, 2877
Proventil Inhalation Solution 0.083% (Schering) ... 2873
Proventil Repetabs Tablets (Schering) ... 336, 2875
Proventil Solution for Inhalation 0.5% (Schering) ... 2872
Proventil Syrup (Schering) ... 2874
Proventil Tablets (Schering) ... 336, 2875
Ventolin Inhalation Solution (Glaxo Wellcome) ... 314, 1244
Ventolin Nebules Inhalation Solution (Glaxo Wellcome) ... 314, 1246
Ventolin Rotacaps for Inhalation (Glaxo Wellcome) ... 314, 1247
Ventolin Syrup (Glaxo Wellcome) ... 314, 1249
Ventolin Tablets (Glaxo Wellcome) ... 314, 1250
Volmax Extended-Release Tablets (Muro) ... 1953
Albuterol Sulfate Inhalation Aerosol, 90 mcg (Novopharm) ... 2110
Albuterol Sulfate Inhalation Solutions (Dey) ... 309, 916
Albuterol Sulfate Syrup (Watson) ... 3216
Albuterol Sulfate Tablets (Lederle Standard) ... 1562
Albuterol Tablets (Geneva) ... 1076
Albuterol Tablets, 2mg, 4mg (Novopharm) ... 2110
ALCLOMETASONE DIPROPIONATE
Aclovate Cream (Glaxo Wellcome) ... 311, 1082
Aclovate Ointment (Glaxo Wellcome) ... 311, 1082
◆ ALDACTAZIDE TABLETS (Searle) ... 337, 2926
◆ ALDACTONE TABLETS (Searle) ... 337, 2928
◆ ALDARA CREAM, 5% (3M) ... 321, 1653
ALDESLEUKIN
Proleukin for Injection (Chiron Corporation) ... 894
◆ ALDOCLOR TABLETS (Merck) ... 322, 1725
ALDOMET ORAL SUSPENSION (Merck) ... 1727
◆ ALDOMET TABLETS (Merck) ... 322, 1727
ALDOMET ESTER HCL INJECTION (Merck) ... 1729
◆ ALDORIL TABLETS (Merck) ... 322, 1731
ALENDRONATE SODIUM
Fosamax Tablets (Merck) ... 323, 1795
◆ ALESSE-21 TABLETS (Wyeth-Ayerst) ... 343, 3257
◆ ALESSE-28 TABLETS (Wyeth-Ayerst) ... 343, 3263
ALFENTA INJECTION (Taylor) ... 3159
ALFENTANIL HYDROCHLORIDE
Alfenta Injection (Taylor) ... 3159
◆ ALFERON N INJECTION (Interferon) ... 317, 1413
ALGLUCERASE
Ceredase Injection (Genzyme) ... 1077
◆ ALKERAN FOR INJECTION (Glaxo Wellcome) ... 311, 1083
◆ ALKERAN TABLETS (Glaxo Wellcome) ... 311, 1085
◆ ALL-FLEX ARCING SPRING DIAPHRAGM (SEE ORTHO DIAPHRAGM KITS) (Ortho-McNeil Pharmaceutical) ... 327
◆ ALLEGRA CAPSULES (Hoechst Marion Roussel) ... 315, 1289
◆ ALLEGRA-D EXTENDED-RELEASE TABLETS (Hoechst Marion Roussel) ... 315, 1291
ALLOPURINOL
Zyloprim Tablets (Glaxo Wellcome) ... 315, 1282
Allopurinol Tablets (Par) ... 2261
Allopurinol Tablets (Mylan) ... 1955
◆ ALORA TRANSDERMAL SYSTEM (Procter & Gamble Pharmaceuticals) ... 332, 2533
ALPHA TOCOPHERAL ACETATE (see under: VITAMIN E)
ALPHA$_1$-PROTEINASE INHIBITOR (HUMAN)
Prolastin (Bayer Biological) ... 695
ALPHAGAN OPHTHALMIC SOLUTION (Allergan) ... 494
ALPHANATE SOLVENT DETERGENT/HEAT TREATED (Alpha Therapeutic) ... 507
ALPHANINE-SD SOLVENT DETERGENT TREATED/VIRUS FILTERED (Alpha Therapeutic) ... 507
ALPRAZOLAM
Xanax Tablets (Pharmacia & Upjohn) ... 332, 2516
Alprazolam Tablets (Lederle Standard) ... 320, 1562
Alprazolam Tablets (Geneva) ... 1076
Alprazolam Tablets (Par) ... 2261
Alprazolam Tablets (Mylan) ... 1955
Alprazolam Tablets, USP (Watson) ... 3216
ALPROSTADIL
Edex for Injection (Schwarz) ... 337, 2901
MUSE Urethral Suppository (Vivus) ... 341, 3187
Caverject Sterile Powder (Pharmacia & Upjohn) ... 331, 2458
◆ ALTACE CAPSULES (Hoechst Marion Roussel) ... 316, 1293
ALTEPLASE, RECOMBINANT
Activase I.V. (Genentech) ... 311, 1057
ALTRETAMINE
Hexalen Capsules (U.S. Bioscience) ... 341, 3171
ALU-CAP CAPSULES (3M) ... 1655
ALU-TAB TABLETS (3M) ... 1655
ALUMINA AND MAGNESIA ORAL SUSPENSION (Roxane) ... 2743
ALUMINA, MAGNESIA, AND SIMETHICONE ORAL SUSPENSION I (Roxane) ... 2743
ALUMINUM ACETATE
Otic Domeboro Solution (Bayer) ... 667
ALUMINUM CHLORIDE
Drysol Solution (Persōn & Covey) ... 2360
Xerac AC Solution (Persōn & Covey) ... 2361
ALUMINUM HYDROXIDE
Amphojel Suspension (Wyeth-Ayerst) ... 3263
Amphojel Suspension without Flavor (Wyeth-Ayerst) ... 3263
Amphojel Tablets (Wyeth-Ayerst) ... 3263
Maalox Antacid Liquid (Novartis Consumer) ... 1982
Maalox Antacid/Anti-Gas Tablets (Novartis Consumer) ... 1983
Extra Strength Maalox Antacid/Anti-Gas Liquid (Novartis Consumer) ... 1983
Extra Strength Maalox Antacid/Anti-Gas Tablets (Novartis Consumer) ... 1983
Fast-Acting Mylanta Liquid Antacid (J&J • Merck) ... 317, 1443
Maximum Strength Fast-Acting Mylanta Liquid (J&J • Merck) ... 317, 1443
Alu-Cap Capsules (3M) ... 1655
Alu-Tab Tablets (3M) ... 1655
Alumina and Magnesia Oral Suspension (Roxane) ... 2743
Alumina, Magnesia, and Simethicone Oral Suspension I (Roxane) ... 2743
Aluminum Hydroxide Gel (Roxane) ... 2743
Aluminum Hydroxide Gel USP (Pharmaceutical Associates) ... 2450
Aluminum Hydroxide Gel Concentrate (Pharmaceutical Associates) ... 2450
Aluminum Hydroxide, Concentrate (Roxane) ... 2743
◆ ALUPENT INHALATION AEROSOL (Boehringer Ingelheim) ... 306, 740
◆ ALUPENT INHALATION SOLUTION (Boehringer Ingelheim) ... 306, 740
ALUPENT SYRUP (Boehringer Ingelheim) ... 740
ALUPENT TABLETS (Boehringer Ingelheim) ... 740
AMANTADINE HYDROCHLORIDE
Symmetrel Syrup (Endo Labs) ... 986
Symmetrel Tablets (Endo Labs) ... 310, 986
Amantadine HCl Syrup, 50 mg (Novopharm) ... 2110
Amantadine Hydrochloride Syrup USP (Pharmaceutical Associates) ... 2450
Amantadine Hydrochloride Syrup, USP (Endo Generics) ... 971
◆ AMARYL TABLETS (Hoechst Marion Roussel) ... 315, 1296
◆ AMBIEN TABLETS (Searle) ... 337, 2929

F

SECTION 3

PRODUCT CATEGORY INDEX

This index lists products by prescribing category, allowing you to quickly and easily identify all agents with a given therapeutic use or mechanism of action. Categories are based on the latest medical terminology and are comprehensively cross-referenced. Included are all fully described products in both the Product Information and Diagnostic Product Information sections of PDR.

If an entry in the index lists multiple page numbers, the first ones shown refer to photographs of the product, the last one to its prescribing information. The Quick-Reference Guide below gives you an overview of the categories.

PRODUCT CATEGORY QUICK-REFERENCE GUIDE

A

ACROMEGALY AGENTS
AIDS ADJUNCT AGENTS
ALCOHOL ABUSE PREPARATIONS
  ALCOHOL DEPENDENCE
  ALCOHOL WITHDRAWAL
ALTERNATIVE MEDICINE
ALZHEIMER'S DISEASE MANAGEMENT
AMYOTROPHIC LATERAL SCLEROSIS
  THERAPEUTIC AGENTS
ANALGESICS
  ACETAMINOPHEN & COMBINATIONS
  CENTRALLY ACTING ANALGESICS
  MISCELLANEOUS ANALGESIC AGENTS
  NARCOTICS
    NARCOTIC AGONIST-ANTAGONIST &
      COMBINATIONS
    NARCOTICS & COMBINATIONS
  NON-NARCOTIC & ANXIOLYTIC
    COMBINATIONS
  NONSTEROIDAL ANTI-INFLAMMATORY
    AGENTS (NSAIDS)
  SALICYLATES
    ASPIRIN & COMBINATIONS
    OTHER SALICYLATES &
      COMBINATIONS
ANESTHETICS
  GENERAL ANESTHETICS
  LOCAL ANESTHETICS
ANTICONVULSANTS
  BARBITURATES
  BENZODIAZEPINES
  GABA ANALOGUES
  HYDANTOINS
  MISCELLANEOUS ANTICONVULSANTS
  PHENYLTRIAZINES
  SUCCINIMIDES
ANTIDIABETIC AGENTS
  BIGUANIDES
  GLUCOSIDASE INHIBITORS
  INSULINS
    INTERMEDIATE ACTING INSULINS
    INTERMEDIATE AND RAPID ACTING
      INSULIN COMBINATIONS
    LONG ACTING INSULINS
    RAPID ACTING INSULINS
  MEGLITINIDES
  SULFONYLUREAS
  THIAZOLIDINEDIONES
ANTIDOTES
  ANTICHOLINERGIC ANTAGONISTS
  ANTICHOLINESTERASE ANTAGONISTS
  BENZODIAZEPINE ANTAGONISTS
  CHELATING AGENTS
    COPPER
    IRON
    LEAD
  DIGOXIN ANTAGONISTS
  FOLIC ACID DERIVATIVES
  HEPARIN ANTAGONISTS
  NARCOTIC ANTAGONISTS
  NONDEPOLARIZING MUSCLE
    RELAXANT ANTAGONISTS
ANTIFIBROSIS THERAPY, SYSTEMIC
ANTIHISTAMINES & COMBINATIONS
ANTI-INFECTIVE AGENTS, SYSTEMIC
  AIDS ADJUNCT ANTI-INFECTIVES
  AIDS CHEMOTHERAPEUTIC AGENTS
    NON-NUCLEOSIDE REVERSE
      TRANSCRIPTASE INHIBITORS

    NUCLEOSIDE REVERSE
      TRANSCRIPTASE INHIBITORS
    PROTEASE INHIBITORS
  AMEBICIDES
  ANTHELMINTICS
  ANTIBIOTICS
    AMINOGLYCOSIDES
    ββ-LACTAM ANTIBIOTICS,
      MISCELLANEOUS
    CEPHALOSPORINS
    MACROLIDES & COMBINATIONS
    MISCELLANEOUS ANTIBIOTICS
    PENICILLINS
    TETRACYCLINES
  ANTIFUNGALS
  ANTIMALARIAL AGENTS
  ANTITUBERCULOSIS AGENTS
  ANTIVIRALS
  LEPROSTATICS
  MISCELLANEOUS ANTI-INFECTIVES
  QUINOLONES
  SULFONAMIDES & COMBINATIONS
  URINARY ANTI-INFECTIVES &
    COMBINATIONS
ANTI-INFECTIVES, NON-SYSTEMIC
  SCABICIDES & PEDICULICIDES
ANTINEOPLASTICS
  ADJUNCT ANTINEOPLASTIC THERAPY
  ALKYLATING AGENTS
    MISCELLANEOUS ALKYLATING
      AGENTS
    NITROGEN MUSTARDS
    NITROSOUREAS
  ANTIBIOTICS
  ANTIMETABOLITES
  HORMONAL AGONISTS/ANTAGONISTS
    ANDROGENS
    ANTIANDROGENS
    ANTIESTROGENS
    ESTROGEN & NITROGEN MUSTARD
      COMBINATIONS
    ESTROGENS
    GONADOTROPIN RELEASING
      HORMONE (GNRH) ANALOGUES
    PROGESTINS
  IMMUNOMODULATORS
  MISCELLANEOUS ANTINEOPLASTICS
  PHOTOSENSITIZING AGENTS
ANTIPARKINSONIAN AGENTS
  ANTICHOLINERGIC AGENTS
  CATECHOL-O-METHYLTRANSFERASE
    INHIBITORS
  DOPAMINERGIC AGENTS
ANTIRHEUMATIC AGENTS
  GOLD COMPOUNDS
  MISCELLANEOUS ANTIRHEUMATIC
    AGENTS
APPETITE STIMULANTS
APPETITE SUPPRESSANTS

B

BIOLOGICAL RESPONSE MODIFIERS
BIOLOGICALS
  ALPHA₁-PROTEINASE INHIBITOR
  ANTITOXINS & ANTIVENINS
  IMMUNE SERUMS
  MISCELLANEOUS BIOLOGICALS
  SKIN TEST ANTIGENS
  TOXOIDS
  VACCINES
BLOOD MODIFIERS
  ANTICOAGULANTS

  ANTIPLATELET AGENTS
  COLONY STIMULATING FACTORS
    GRANULOCYTE (G-CSF)
    GRANULOCYTE MACROPHAGE
      (GM-CSF)
  HEMATINICS
    ANABOLIC STEROIDS
    CYANOCOBALAMIN (VITAMIN B₁₂) &
      COMBINATIONS
    ERYTHROPOIETIN
    FOLIC ACID DERIVATIVES &
      COMBINATIONS
    IRON & COMBINATIONS
    LIVER & COMBINATIONS
    MISCELLANEOUS BLOOD MODIFIERS
  HEMORRHEOLOGIC AGENTS
  HEMOSTATICS
    SYSTEMIC HEMOSTATICS
  HEPARIN ANTAGONISTS
  LEUKAPHERESIS ADJUNCT
  PLASMA EXTENDERS & EXPANDERS
  PLASMA FRACTIONS, HUMAN
    ALBUMIN
    ANTI-INHIBITOR COAGULANT
      COMPLEX
    ANTIHEMOPHILIC FACTOR
    ANTITHROMBIN III
    FACTOR IX COMPLEX
  THROMBIN INHIBITOR
  THROMBOLYTIC AGENTS
  VITAMIN K
BONE METABOLISM REGULATORS

C

CARDIOPROTECTIVE AGENTS
CARDIOVASCULAR AGENTS
  ADRENERGIC BLOCKERS, PERIPHERAL
    & COMBINATIONS
  ADRENERGIC STIMULANTS, CENTRAL &
    COMBINATIONS
  ALPHA/BETA ADRENERGIC BLOCKERS
  ANGIOTENSIN CONVERTING ENZYME
    (ACE) INHIBITORS
  ANGIOTENSIN CONVERTING ENZYME
    (ACE) INHIBITORS WITH CALCIUM
    CHANNEL BLOCKERS
  ANGIOTENSIN CONVERTING ENZYME
    (ACE) INHIBITORS WITH DIURETICS
  ANGIOTENSIN II RECEPTOR
    ANTAGONISTS
  ANGIOTENSIN II RECEPTOR
    ANTAGONISTS WITH DIURETICS
  ANTIARRHYTHMICS
    GROUP I
    GROUP II
    GROUP III
    GROUP IV
    MISCELLANEOUS ANTIARRHYTHMICS
  ANTILIPEMIC AGENTS
    BILE ACID SEQUESTRANTS
    FIBRIC ACID DERIVATIVES
    HMG-CoA REDUCTASE INHIBITORS
    NICOTINIC ACID
  BETA ADRENERGIC BLOCKING AGENTS
  BETA ADRENERGIC BLOCKING AGENTS
    WITH DIURETICS
  CALCIUM CHANNEL BLOCKERS
  DIURETICS
    CARBONIC ANHYDRASE INHIBITORS
    COMBINATION DIURETICS
    LOOP DIURETICS
    POTASSIUM-SPARING DIURETICS
    THIAZIDES & RELATED DIURETICS

  HYPERTENSIVE EMERGENCY AGENTS
  INOTROPIC AGENTS
  MISCELLANEOUS CARDIOVASCULAR
    AGENTS
  RAUWOLFIA DERIVATIVES &
    COMBINATIONS
  VASODILATORS
    CORONARY VASODILATORS
    PERIPHERAL VASODILATORS &
      COMBINATIONS
    VASOPRESSORS
CENTRAL NERVOUS SYSTEM
  STIMULANTS
  AMPHETAMINES
  MISCELLANEOUS CENTRAL NERVOUS
    SYSTEM STIMULANTS
CHOLINESTERASE INHIBITORS
CONTRACEPTIVES
  DEVICES
  IMPLANTS
  INJECTABLE CONTRACEPTIVES
  ORAL CONTRACEPTIVES
CYSTIC FIBROSIS MANAGEMENT

D

DEODORANTS
  INTERNAL DEODORANTS
DIAGNOSTICS
  ADRENOCORTICAL FUNCTION
  CUSHING'S SYNDROME
  GONADOTROPIC FUNCTION TEST
  HYPOTHALAMIC DYSFUNCTION TEST
  HYSTEROSALPINGOGRAPHY
  LYMPHOGRAPHY
  MYOCARDIAL PERFUSION
    SCINTIGRAPHY ADJUNCT
  PANCREATIC FUNCTION TEST
  PHEOCHROMOCYTOMA TEST
  RENAL FUNCTION TEST
  THYROID FUNCTION TEST
  TUBERCULIN TEST
    TUBERCULIN, OLD
    TUBERCULIN, P.P.D.
  ZOLLINGER-ELLISON SYNDROME
DOPAMINE RECEPTOR AGONISTS

E

EMERGENCY KITS
ENDOMETRIOSIS MANAGEMENT
ENZYMES
ERECTILE DYSFUNCTION THERAPY

F

FERTILITY AGENTS

G

GALACTORRHEA INHIBITORS
GASTROINTESTINAL AGENTS
  ANTACID & ANTIFLATULENT
    COMBINATIONS
  ANTACIDS
    ALUMINUM ANTACIDS &
      COMBINATIONS
    CALCIUM ANTACIDS &
      COMBINATIONS
    COMBINATION ANTACIDS
    MAGNESIUM ANTACIDS &
      COMBINATIONS

ANTIDIARRHEALS
ANTIEMETICS
ANTIFLATULENTS
ANTI-INFLAMMATORY AGENTS
ANTISPASMODICS &
ANTICHOLINERGICS
BOWEL EVACUANTS
CYTOPROTECTIVE AGENTS
DIGESTIVE ENZYMES
DUODENAL ULCER ADHERENT
COMPLEX
GALLSTONE DISSOLUTION AGENTS
GASTROINTESTINAL STIMULANTS
HISTAMINE (H₂) RECEPTOR
ANTAGONISTS
LAXATIVES
BULK-PRODUCING LAXATIVES
EMOLLIENT LAXATIVES
ENEMAS
FECAL SOFTENERS & COMBINATIONS
LAXATIVE COMBINATIONS
MISCELLANEOUS LAXATIVES
SALINE LAXATIVES
STIMULANT LAXATIVES &
COMBINATIONS
MISCELLANEOUS GASTROINTESTINAL
AGENTS
PROSTAGLANDINS
PROTON PUMP INHIBITORS

GAUCHER'S DISEASE MANAGEMENT

GOUT PREPARATIONS
MISCELLANEOUS GOUT PREPARATIONS
NONSTEROIDAL ANTI-INFLAMMATORY
AGENTS (NSAIDS)
URICOSURIC AGENTS & COMBINATIONS

H

HORMONES
ADRENAL CORTICAL STEROID
INHIBITORS
ANABOLIC STEROIDS
ANDROGEN & ESTROGEN
COMBINATIONS
ANDROGENS
CALCITONIN
ESTROGENS & COMBINATIONS
GLUCOCORTICOIDS
GLUCOSE ELEVATING AGENTS
GONADOTROPIN INHIBITORS
GONADOTROPIN RELEASING
HORMONES (GNRH)
GONADOTROPIN RELEASING
HORMONE (GNRH) ANALOGUES
GONADOTROPINS
CHORIONIC GONADOTROPIN
FOLLITROPINS
MENOTROPINS
GROWTH HORMONE
MINERALOCORTICOIDS
MISCELLANEOUS HORMONES
PROGESTIN & ESTROGEN
COMBINATIONS
PROGESTINS & COMBINATIONS
SOMATOSTATIN ANALOGUES
THYROID PREPARATIONS
ANTITHYROID AGENTS
SYNTHETIC T4
VASOPRESSIN & DERIVATIVES

HYPERCALCEMIA MANAGEMENT

HYPOCALCEMIA MANAGEMENT

HYPOGLYCEMIC AGENTS

I

IMMUNOMODULATORS

IMMUNOSUPPRESSIVES

L

**LEVOCARNITINE DEFICIENCY
MANAGEMENT**

M

MAST CELL STABILIZERS

MIGRAINE PREPARATIONS
BETA ADRENERGIC BLOCKING AGENTS
ERGOT DERIVATIVES & COMBINATIONS
ISOMETHEPTENE & COMBINATIONS

MISCELLANEOUS MIGRAINE
PREPARATIONS
SEROTONIN (5-HT) RECEPTOR
AGONISTS

MOTION SICKNESS PRODUCTS

MULTIPLE SCLEROSIS MANAGEMENT

MUSCLE RELAXANTS
NEUROMUSCULAR BLOCKING AGENTS
SKELETAL MUSCLE RELAXANTS &
COMBINATIONS
SMOOTH MUSCLE RELAXANTS

N

NARCOTIC DETOXIFICATION

NASAL PREPARATIONS
ANALGESICS
ANTIBIOTICS & COMBINATIONS
ANTICHOLINERGICS
ANTIHISTAMINES
ANTI-INFLAMMATORY AGENTS
STEROIDAL ANTI-INFLAMMATORY
AGENTS
HORMONES
SMOKING CESSATION AIDS

NUCLEOSIDE ANALOGUES

NUTRITIONALS
AMINO ACIDS & COMBINATIONS
MINERALS & ELECTROLYTES
CALCIUM & COMBINATIONS
FLUORIDE & COMBINATIONS
MAGNESIUM & COMBINATIONS
MULTIMINERALS & COMBINATIONS
ORAL ELECTROLYTE MIXTURES
PHOSPHORUS & COMBINATIONS
POTASSIUM & COMBINATIONS
MISCELLANEOUS NUTRITIONAL
SUPPLEMENTS
NUTRITIONAL THERAPY, ENTERAL
COMPLETE THERAPEUTIC
FIBER SUPPLEMENTS
VITAMINS & COMBINATIONS
GERIATRIC FORMULATIONS
MISCELLANEOUS VITAMIN
PREPARATIONS
MULTIVITAMINS & COMBINATIONS
MULTIVITAMINS WITH MINERALS
PRENATAL FORMULATIONS
RENAL FORMULATIONS
THERAPEUTIC FORMULATIONS
VITAMIN A & COMBINATIONS
B VITAMINS & COMBINATIONS
VITAMIN C & COMBINATIONS
VITAMIN D ANALOGUES &
COMBINATIONS
VITAMIN E & COMBINATIONS

O

OPHTHALMIC PREPARATIONS
ACETYLCHOLINE BLOCKING AGENTS
ANTIHISTAMINES & COMBINATIONS
ANTI-INFECTIVES
ANTIBIOTICS & COMBINATIONS
ANTIVIRALS
QUINOLONES
SULFONAMIDES & COMBINATIONS
ANTI-INFLAMMATORY AGENTS
NON-STEROIDAL
ANTI-INFLAMMATORY AGENTS
(NSAIDS)
STEROIDAL ANTI-INFLAMMATORY
AGENTS & COMBINATIONS
ARTIFICIAL TEARS/LUBRICANTS &
COMBINATIONS
BETA ADRENERGIC BLOCKING AGENT &
CARBONIC ANHYDRASE INHIBITOR
COMBINATIONS
BETA ADRENERGIC BLOCKING AGENTS
CARBONIC ANHYDRASE INHIBITORS
MAST CELL STABILIZERS
MIOTICS
CHOLINESTERASE INHIBITORS
MYDRIATICS & CYCLOPLEGICS
SYMPATHOMIMETICS & COMBINATIONS

OSTEOPOROSIS PREPARATIONS
BIPHOSPHONATES
HORMONAL AGENTS
CALCITONIN

ESTROGENS & COMBINATIONS
MISCELLANEOUS AGENTS

OTIC PREPARATIONS
ANALGESICS & ANESTHETICS
ANTIBIOTIC & STEROID COMBINATIONS
CERUMENOLYTICS
MISCELLANEOUS OTIC PREPARATIONS
STEROIDS & COMBINATIONS

OXYTOCICS
MISCELLANEOUS OXYTOCIC AGENTS

P

PARASYMPATHOLYTICS

PARASYMPATHOMIMETICS

PATENT DUCTUS ARTERIOSUS AGENTS

PHOSPHATE BINDERS

PORPHYRIA AGENTS

PROSTAGLANDINS

PSYCHOTHERAPEUTIC AGENTS
ANTIANXIETY AGENTS
BENZODIAZEPINES & COMBINATIONS
MISCELLANEOUS ANTIANXIETY
AGENTS
ANTIDEPRESSANTS
MISCELLANEOUS ANTIDEPRESSANTS
MONOAMINE OXIDASE INHIBITORS
(MAOI)
SELECTIVE SEROTONIN REUPTAKE
INHIBITORS (SSRI)
TRICYCLIC ANTIDEPRESSANTS &
COMBINATIONS
ANTIMANIC AGENTS
ANTIPANIC AGENTS
ANTIPSYCHOTIC AGENTS
MISCELLANEOUS ANTIPSYCHOTIC
AGENTS
PHENOTHIAZINES & COMBINATIONS
OBSESSIVE-COMPULSIVE DISORDER
MANAGEMENT
SELECTIVE SEROTONIN REUPTAKE
INHIBITORS (SSRI)
TRICYCLIC ANTIDEPRESSANTS

R

RADIOPAQUE AGENTS

RESINS, ION EXCHANGE

RESPIRATORY AGENTS
ANTI-INFECTIVE AGENTS
CYSTIC FIBROSIS MANAGEMENT
ANTI-INFLAMMATORY AGENTS
MISCELLANEOUS
ANTI-INFLAMMATORY AGENTS
STEROIDAL ANTI-INFLAMMATORY
AGENTS
ANTITUSSIVES
NARCOTIC ANTITUSSIVES &
COMBINATIONS
NON-NARCOTIC ANTITUSSIVES &
COMBINATIONS
BRONCHODILATORS
ANTICHOLINERGICS
ANTICHOLINERGICS WITH
SYMPATHOMIMETICS
SYMPATHOMIMETICS &
COMBINATIONS
XANTHINE DERIVATIVES &
COMBINATIONS
DECONGESTANTS & COMBINATIONS
DECONGESTANTS, EXPECTORANTS &
COMBINATIONS
ENZYMES
EXPECTORANTS & COMBINATIONS
LEUKOTRIENE ANTAGONISTS
LUNG SURFACTANTS
MISCELLANEOUS COLD & COUGH
PRODUCTS WITH ANALGESICS
MISCELLANEOUS RESPIRATORY
AGENTS
RESPIRATORY STIMULANTS

S

SALT SUBSTITUTES

SCLEROSING AGENTS

SEDATIVES & HYPNOTICS
BARBITURATES

BENZODIAZEPINES
MISCELLANEOUS SEDATIVES &
HYPNOTICS

SICKLE CELL ANEMIA MANAGEMENT

SKIN & MUCOUS MEMBRANE AGENTS
ACNE PREPARATIONS
ANALGESICS & COMBINATIONS
ANESTHETICS & COMBINATIONS
ANORECTAL PREPARATIONS
ANTIHISTAMINES & COMBINATIONS
ANTI-INFECTIVES
ANTIBIOTICS & COMBINATIONS
ANTIFUNGALS & COMBINATIONS
ANTIVIRALS
MISCELLANEOUS ANTI-INFECTIVES &
COMBINATIONS
SCABICIDES & PEDICULICIDES
ANTINEOPLASTICS
ANTIPERSPIRANTS
ANTIPRURITICS
ANTIPSORIATIC AGENTS
ANTISEBORRHEIC AGENTS
BURN PREPARATIONS
CAUTERIZING AGENTS
CLEANSING AGENTS
DEODORANTS
DEPIGMENTING AGENTS
DIAPER RASH PRODUCTS
EMOLLIENTS & MOISTURIZERS
ENZYMES & COMBINATIONS
HAIR GROWTH STIMULANTS
KERATOLYTICS
MISCELLANEOUS SKIN & MUCOUS
MEMBRANE AGENTS
MOUTH & THROAT PRODUCTS
CANKER SORE PREPARATIONS
COLD SORE PREPARATIONS
DENTAL PREPARATIONS
SALIVA PRODUCTS
PHOTOSENSITIZING AGENTS
POISON IVY, OAK OR SUMAC PRODUCTS
SHAMPOOS
SHAVE CREAMS
SKIN CONSTRUCT, HUMAN
STEROIDS & COMBINATIONS
SUNBURN PREPARATIONS
SUNSCREENS
TAR-CONTAINING PREPARATIONS
WART PREPARATIONS
WET DRESSINGS
WOUND CARE PRODUCTS

SMOKING CESSATION AIDS

SYMPATHOLYTICS

T

TOURETTE'S SYNDROME AGENTS

TREMOR PREPARATIONS

U

URINARY TRACT AGENTS
ACIDIFIERS
ALKALINIZERS
ANALGESICS & COMBINATIONS
ANTISPASMODICS
BENIGN PROSTATIC HYPERPLASIA
(BPH) THERAPY
CALCIUM OXALATE STONE
PREVENTION
CYTOPROTECTIVE AGENTS
ENURESIS MANAGEMENT
MISCELLANEOUS URINARY TRACT
AGENTS

V

VAGINAL PREPARATIONS
ANTI-INFECTIVES
ANTIFUNGALS & COMBINATIONS
MISCELLANEOUS ANTI-INFECTIVES &
COMBINATIONS
ESTROGENS
MISCELLANEOUS VAGINAL
PREPARATIONS
PROSTAGLANDINS

VASODILATORS
CEREBRAL VASODILATORS

VERTIGO AGENTS

W

WILSON'S DISEASE MANAGEMENT

PRODUCT CATEGORY INDEX

U

URICOSURIC AGENTS
(see under:
GOUT PREPARATIONS
URICOSURIC AGENTS & COMBINATIONS)

URINARY TRACT AGENTS
(see also under:
ANTI-INFECTIVE AGENTS, SYSTEMIC
URINARY ANTI-INFECTIVES &
COMBINATIONS)

ACIDIFIERS
K-Phos Neutral Tablets (Beach) 306, 698
K-Phos Original (Sodium Free)
Tablets (Beach) 306, 699

ALKALINIZERS
Bicitra (Alza) 511
Polycitra Syrup and Polycitra-LC Syrup
(Alza) 515
Polycitra-K Crystals (Alza) 516
Polycitra-K Oral Solution (Alza) 516
Urocit-K Tablets (Mission) 1929

ANALGESICS & COMBINATIONS
Elmiron Capsules (Alza) 303, 512
Prodium Tablets (Breckenridge) 768
Urised Tablets (PolyMedica) 2527
Urobiotic-250 Capsules (Pfizer) 2424

ANTISPASMODICS
Cystospaz Tablets (PolyMedica) 2526
Cystospaz-M Capsules (PolyMedica) 2526
Ditropan Tablets and Syrup (Alza) 511
Levbid Extended-Release Tablets
(Schwarz) 337, 2910
Levsin Drops (Schwarz) 2910
Levsin Elixir (Schwarz) 2910
Levsin Injection (Schwarz) 2910
Levsin Tablets (Schwarz) 2910
Levsin/SL Tablets (Schwarz) 337, 2910
Urised Tablets (PolyMedica) 2527
Urispas Tablets (SmithKline
Beecham) 340, 3109

BENIGN PROSTATIC HYPERPLASIA (BPH) THERAPY
Cardura Tablets (Pfizer) 330, 2368
Flomax Capsules (Boehringer
Ingelheim) 307, 755
Hytrin Capsules (Abbott) 303, 451
Proscar Tablets (Merck) 323, 1880

CALCIUM OXALATE STONE PREVENTION
Polycitra Syrup and Polycitra-LC Syrup
(Alza) 515
Polycitra-K Crystals (Alza) 516
Polycitra-K Oral Solution (Alza) 516
Urocit-K Tablets (Mission) 1929
Zyloprim Tablets (Glaxo Wellcome) . . . 315, 1282

CYTOPROTECTIVE AGENTS
Ethyol for Injection (Alza) 303, 513
Mesnex Injection (Bristol-Myers
Squibb Oncology/Immunology) 308, 786

ENURESIS MANAGEMENT
DDAVP Nasal Spray (Rhône-Poulenc
Rorer) 333, 2584
DDAVP Tablets (Rhône-Poulenc
Rorer) 333, 2586

IMPOTENCE AGENTS
(see under: ERECTILE DYSFUNCTION THERAPY)

MISCELLANEOUS URINARY TRACT AGENTS
Clorpactin WCS-90 (Guardian) 1286
Depen Titratable Tablets (Wallace) 3192
Detrol Tablets (Pharmacia &
Upjohn) 332, 2477
Urecholine Injection (Merck) 1905
Urecholine Tablets (Merck) 323, 1905

URICOSURIC AGENTS
(see under: GOUT PREPARATIONS:
URICOSURIC AGENTS
& COMBINATIONS)

UTERINE CONTRACTANTS
(see under:
OXYTOCICS)

V

VACCINES
(see under:
BIOLOGICALS
VACCINES)

VAGINAL PREPARATIONS
(see also under:
CONTRACEPTIVES
DEVICES)

ANTI-INFECTIVES
ANTIFUNGALS & COMBINATIONS
Mycelex-G 500 mg Vaginal Tablets
(Bayer) 305, 664
Terazol 3 Vaginal Cream
(Ortho-McNeil Pharmaceutical) . . 328, 2245
Terazol 3 Vaginal Suppositories
(Ortho-McNeil Pharmaceutical) . . 328, 2246
Terazol 7 Vaginal Cream
(Ortho-McNeil Pharmaceutical) . . 328, 2246
Vagistat-1 Vaginal Ointment
(Bristol-Myers Products) 307, 817

MISCELLANEOUS ANTI-INFECTIVES & COMBINATIONS
AVC Cream (Hoechst Marion Roussel) . . . 1305
AVC Suppositories (Hoechst Marion
Roussel) 1305
Betadine Medicated Douche (Purdue
Frederick) 2552
Cleocin Vaginal Cream (Pharmacia &
Upjohn) 2462
MetroGel-Vaginal Gel (3M) 321, 1661
Sultrin Triple Sulfa Cream
(Ortho-McNeil Pharmaceutical) 2245

ESTROGENS
Estrace Vaginal Cream (Bristol-Myers
Squibb) 830
Estrace Tablets (Bristol-Myers Squibb) . . 307, 830
Estring Vaginal Ring (Pharmacia &
Upjohn) 2483
Ortho Dienestrol Cream (Ortho-McNeil
Pharmaceutical) 2212
Premarin Vaginal Cream
(Wyeth-Ayerst) 344, 3371

MISCELLANEOUS VAGINAL PREPARATIONS
Aci-Jel Therapeutic Vaginal Jelly
(Ortho-McNeil Pharmaceutical) 2179
Amino-Cerv Creme (Milex) 1928

PROSTAGLANDINS
Cervidil Vaginal Insert (Forest) 310, 1019
Prepidil Gel (Pharmacia & Upjohn) 2503
Prostin E2 Suppository (Pharmacia &
Upjohn) 2504

VASODILATORS
(see also under:
CARDIOVASCULAR AGENTS
VASODILATORS)

CEREBRAL VASODILATORS
Nimotop Capsules (Bayer) 305, 665

VERTIGO AGENTS
Antivert, Antivert/25, & Antivert/50
Tablets (Pfizer) 2363
Traumeel Injection Solution (Heel) 1287

VITAMIN D ANALOGUES
(see under:
NUTRITIONALS
VITAMINS & COMBINATIONS
VITAMIN D ANALOGUES &
COMBINATIONS)

VITAMINS
(see under:
NUTRITIONALS
VITAMINS & COMBINATIONS)

W

WART PREPARATIONS
(see under:
SKIN & MUCOUS MEMBRANE AGENTS
WART PREPARATIONS)

WEIGHT CONTROL PREPARATIONS
(see under:
APPETITE SUPPRESSANTS
NUTRITIONALS
NUTRITIONAL THERAPY, ENTERAL)

WET DRESSINGS
(see under:
SKIN & MUCOUS MEMBRANE AGENTS
WET DRESSINGS)

WILSON'S DISEASE MANAGEMENT
Cuprimine Capsules (Merck) 323, 1766
Depen Titratable Tablets (Wallace) 3192
Syprine Capsules (Merck) 323, 1891

WOUND CARE
(see under:
SKIN & MUCOUS MEMBRANE AGENTS
WOUND CARE PRODUCTS)

X

X-RAY CONTRAST MEDIA
(see under:
RADIOPAQUE AGENTS)

DRUG INFORMATION CENTERS

ALABAMA

BIRMINGHAM
Drug Information Service University of
Alabama Hospital
619 S. 20th Street
1720 Jefferson Tower
Birmingham, AL 35233-6860
Mon.-Fri. 8 AM-5 PM
Tel: 205-934-2162
Fax: 205-934-3501

Global Drug Information Center
Samford University
McWhorter School of Pharmacy
800 Lakeshore Drive
Birmingham, AL 35229-7027
Mon.-Fri. 8 AM-5 PM
Tel: 205-870-2659
Fax: 205-414-4012

HUNTSVILLE
Huntsville Hospital Drug Information
Center
101 Sivley Road
Huntsville, AL 35801
Mon.-Fri. 8 AM-5 PM
Tel: 256-517-8288
Fax: 256-517-6558

ARIZONA

TUCSON
Arizona Poison and Drug Information
Center
Arizona Health Sciences Center
University Medical Center
1501 N. Campbell Ave.
Room 1156
Tucson, AZ 85724
7 days/week, 24 hours
Tel: 520-626-6016
     800-362-0101 (AZ)
Fax: 520-626-2720

CALIFORNIA

LOS ANGELES
Los Angeles Regional Drug and Poison
Information Center
LAC & USC Medical Center
1200 N. State Street
Room 1107 A & B
Los Angeles, CA 90033
7 days/week, 24 hours
Tel: 213-226-2622
     800-777-6476 (CA)
Fax: 213-226-4194
Poison Control Hotline:
     213-222-3212

SAN DIEGO
Drug Information
Analysis Service
Veterans Administration Medical
Center
3350 La Jolla Village Drive
San Diego, CA 92161
Mon.-Fri. 8 AM-4:30 PM
Tel: 619-552-8585
Fax: 619-552-7582

Drug Information Center
U.S. Naval Hospital
34800 Bob Wilson Drive
San Diego, CA 92134-5000
Mon.-Fri. 8 AM-4 PM
Tel: 619-532-8414

Drug Information Service
University of California
San Diego Medical Center
135 Dickinson Street
San Diego, CA 92103-8925
Mon.-Fri. 9 AM-5 PM
Tel: 900-288-8273
     619-543-6222
Fax: 619-692-1867

STANFORD
Drug Information Center
University of California
Stanford Health
Stanford Campus
300 Pasteur Drive
Room 80301
Stanford, CA 94305
Mon.-Fri. 9 AM-4 PM
Tel: 650-723-6422
Fax: 650-725-5028

COLORADO

DENVER
Rocky Mountain Drug Consultation
Center
8802 E. 9th Avenue
Denver, CO 80220
Mon.-Fri. 8 AM-4:30 PM
Tel: 303-893-3784
     900-370-3784
     (Outside Denver
     County, $1.99
     per minute)

Drug Information Center
University of Colorado
Health Science Center
4200 E. 9th Avenue, Box C239
Denver, CO 80262
Mon.-Fri. 8:30 AM-4:30 PM
Tel: 303-315-8489
Fax: 303-270-3353

CONNECTICUT

FARMINGTON
Drug Information Service
University of Connecticut Health
Center
263 Farmington Ave.
Farmington, CT 06030
Mon.-Fri. 8 AM-4:30 PM
Tel: 860-679-3783

HARTFORD
Drug Information Center Hartford
Hospital
P.O. Box 5037
80 Seymour Street
Hartford, CT 06102
Mon.-Fri. 8:30 AM-5 PM
Tel: 860-545-2221
     860-545-2961 (main
     pharmacy) after hours
Fax: 860-545-2415

NEW HAVEN
Drug Information Center
Yale-New Haven Hospital
20 York Street
New Haven, CT 06504
Mon.-Fri. 8:15 AM-4:45 PM
Tel: 203-688-2248
Fax: 203-737-4229

DISTRICT OF COLUMBIA

Drug Information Center
Washington Hospital Center
110 Irving St., NW, Room B147
Washington, DC 20010
Mon.- Fri. 7:30 AM-4 PM
Tel: 202-877-6646
Fax: 202-877-8925

Drug Information Service
Howard University Hospital
2041 Georgia Ave. NW
Washington, DC 20060
Mon.-Fri. 9 AM-5 PM
Tel: 202-865-1325
Fax: 202-745-3731

FLORIDA

GAINESVILLE
Drug Information &
Pharmacy Resource Center
Shands Hospital at
University of Florida
P.O. Box 100316
Gainesville, FL 32610-0316
Mon.-Fri. 9 AM- 5 PM
Tel: 352-395-0408
(for healthcare professionals only)
Fax: 352-338-9860

JACKSONVILLE
Drug Information Service
University Medical Center
655 W. 8th Street
Jacksonville, FL 32209
Mon.-Fri. 8 AM-5 PM
Tel: 904-549-4095
Fax: 904-549-4272

MIAMI
Drug Information Center (119)
Miami VA Medical Center
1201 NW 16th Street
Miami, FL 33125
Mon.-Fri. 7:30 AM-4:30 PM
Tel: 305-324-3237
Fax: 305-324-3394

GEORGIA

ATLANTA
Emory University Hospital
Dept. of Pharmaceutical Services-Drug
Information
1364 Clifton Rd. NE
Atlanta, GA 30322
Mon.-Fri. 8:30 AM-5 PM
Tel: 404-712-4640
Fax: 404-712-7577

Drug Information Service Northside
Hospital
1000 Johnson Ferry Road NE
Atlanta, GA 30342
Mon.-Fri. 9 AM-4 PM
Tel: 404-851-8676
Fax: 404-851-8682

AUGUSTA
Drug Information Center University of
Georgia
Medical College of GA
Room BIW201
1120 15th Street
Augusta, GA 30912-5600
Mon.-Fri. 8:30 AM-5 PM
Tel: 706-721-2887
Fax: 706-721-3827

IDAHO

POCATELLO
Idaho Drug Information Service
MFU 3 Box 8092
Pocatello, ID 83209
Mon.-Fri. 8 AM-5 PM
Tel: 208-236-4689
Fax: 208-236-4687

ILLINOIS

CHICAGO
Drug Information Center
Northwestern Memorial Hospital
250 E. Superior Street
Wesley 153
Chicago, IL 60611
Mon.-Fri. 8 AM-5 PM
Tel: 312-908-7573
Fax: 312-908-7956

Saint Joseph Hospital
2900 N. Lake Shore Drive
Chicago, IL 60657
8 AM-5 PM
Tel: 312-665-3140
Fax: 312-665-3462

Drug Information Services
University of Chicago
5841 S. Maryland Ave.
MC 0010
Chicago, IL 60637
Mon.-Fri. 8 AM-5 PM
Tel: 773-702-1388
Fax: 773-702-6631

Drug Information Center
University of Illinois at Chicago
Room C300, MC 883
1740 W. Taylor St.
Chicago, IL 60612
Mon.-Fri. 8 AM-4 PM
Tel: 312-996-0209
Fax: 312-413-4146

HARVEY
Drug Information Center
Ingalls Memorial Hospital
1 Ingalls Drive
Harvey, IL 60426
Mon.-Fri. 8 AM-4:30 PM
Tel: 708-333-2300
Fax: 708-210-3108

HINES
Drug Information Service
Hines Veterans Administration
Hospital
Inpatient Pharmacy (119B)
P.O. Box 5000
Hines, IL 60141-5000
Mon.-Fri. 8 AM-4:30 PM
Tel: 708-343-7200

PARK RIDGE
Drug Information Center
Lutheran General Hospital
1775 Dempster St.
Park Ridge, IL 60068
Mon.-Fri. 7:30 AM-4 PM
Tel: 847-696-8128

INDIANA

INDIANAPOLIS
Drug Information Center
St. Vincent Hospital
and Health Services
2001 W. 86th St.
P.O. Box 40970
Indianapolis, IN 46260
Mon.-Fri. 8 AM-4 PM
Tel: 317-338-3200
Fax: 317-338-3041

Indiana University Medical
Center/Pharmacy
Dept. OH1451
550 N. University Blvd.
Indianapolis, IN 46202
Mon.-Fri. 8 AM-4:30 PM
Tel: 317-274-0353
Fax: 317-274-2327

IOWA

DES MOINES
Regional Drug
Information Center
Mercy Hospital Medical Center
400 University Ave.
Des Moines, IA 50314
Mon.-Fri. 8 AM-6 PM
Tel: 515-247-3286 (answered
     7 days/week, 24 hours)
Fax: 515-247-3966

IOWA CITY
Drug Information Center
University of Iowa Hospitals and
Clinics
200 Hawkins Dr.
Iowa City, IA 52242
Mon.-Fri. 8 AM-5 PM
Tel: 319-356-2600
Fax: 319-356-4545

SIOUX CITY
Iowa Poison Center
2720 Stone Park Blvd.
Sioux City, IA 51104
Tel: 712-277-2222
       800-352-2222 (IA)
Fax: 712-279-7852

KANSAS
KANSAS CITY
Drug Information Center
University of Kansas
Medical Center
3901 Rainbow Blvd.
Kansas City, KS 66160
Mon.-Fri. 8 AM-6 PM
Tel: 913-588-2328
Fax: 913-588-2350

KENTUCKY
LEXINGTON
Drug Information Center
Chandler Medical Center College of
Pharmacy
University of Kentucky
800 Rose St., C-117
Lexington, KY 40536-0084
Mon.-Fri. 8 AM-5 PM
Tel: 606-323-5320
Fax: 606-323-2049

LOUISIANA
MONROE
Drug Information Center
St. Francis Medical Center
309 Jackson St.
Monroe, LA 71210-1901
Tel: 318-327-4250
Fax: 318-327-4125

NEW ORLEANS
Xavier University Drug Information
Center
Tulane University Hospital
and Clinic
Box HC12
1415 Tulane Ave.
New Orleans, LA 70112
Mon.-Fri. 9 AM-5 PM
Tel: 504-588-5670
Fax: 504-588-5862

MARYLAND
ANDREWS AFB
Drug Information Services
89th Med Gp/SGQP
1050 W. Perimeter Rd.
Suite F1-121
Andrews AFB, MD 20331
Mon.-Fri. 7:30 AM-6 PM
Tel: 301-981-4209
Fax: 301-981-4544

ANNAPOLIS
Drug Information Services
The Anne Arundel Medical Center
Franklin & Cathedral Streets
Annapolis, MD 21401
7 days/week, 24 hours
Tel: 410-267-1130
       410-267-1000
Fax: 410-267-1628

BALTIMORE
Drug Information Services
Franklin Square Hospital Center
9000 Franklin Square Dr.
Baltimore, MD 21237
7 days/week, 24 hours
Tel: 410-682-7744
Fax: 410-682-8181

Drug Information Service
Johns Hopkins Hospital
600 N. Wolfe St., Halsted 503
Baltimore, MD 21287-6180
Mon.-Fri. 8:30 AM-5 PM
Tel: 410-955-6348
Fax: 410-955-8283

Drug Information Center
University of Maryland at Baltimore
School of Pharmacy
506 W. Fayette, 3rd Floor
Baltimore, MD 21201
Mon.-Fri. 8:30 AM-5 PM
Tel: 410-706-7568
Fax: 410-706-0897

BETHESDA
Drug Information Service National
Institutes of Health
Building 10, Room 1S-259
10 Center Drive (MSC1196)
Bethesda, MD 20892-1196
Mon.-Fri. 8:30 AM-5 PM
Tel: 301-496-2407
Fax: 301-496-0210

EASTON
Drug Information Center Memorial
Hospital
219 S. Washington St.
Easton, MD 21601
7 days/week, 7 AM - Midnight
Tel: 410-822-1000
Fax: 410-820-9489

MASSACHUSETTS
BOSTON
Drug Information Services
Brigham and Women's Hospital
75 Frances St.
Boston, MA 02115
Mon.-Fri. 7 AM-3:30 PM
Tel: 617-732-7166
Fax: 617-732-7497

Drug Information Service
New England Medical
Center Pharmacy
750 Washington St., Box 420
Boston, MA 02111
Mon.-Fri. 9 AM-5 PM
Tel: 617-636-8985
Fax: 617-636-5638

WORCESTER
Drug Information Center U.M.M.C.
Hospital
55 Lake Ave. North
Worcester, MA 01655
Mon.-Fri. 8:30 AM-5 PM
Tel: 508-856-3456
       508-856-2775
Fax: 508-856-1850

MICHIGAN
ANN ARBOR
Drug Information Service
University of Michigan
Medical Center
1500 East Medical Center Dr.
UHB2 D301 Box 0008
Ann Arbor, MI 48109
Mon.-Fri. 8 AM-5 PM
Tel: 734-936-8200
       734-936-8251
Fax: 734-923-7027

DETROIT
Drug Information Services Harper
Hospital
3990 John R. St.
Detroit, MI 48201
Mon.-Fri. 8 AM-5 PM
Tel: 313-745-2006
       313-745-8216
       (after hours)
Fax: 313-745-1628

LANSING
Drug Information Center Sparrow
Hospital
1215 E. Michigan Ave.
Lansing, MI 48912
Mon.-Fri. 8 AM-4:30 PM
Tel: 517-483-2444
Fax: 517-483-2088

PONTIAC
Drug Information Center
St. Joseph Mercy Hospital
900 Woodward
Pontiac, MI 48341
Mon.-Fri. 8 AM-4:30 PM
Tel: 248-858-3055
Fax: 248-858-3010

ROYAL OAK
Drug Information Services
William Beaumont Hospital
3601 West 13 Mile Road
Royal Oak, MI 48073-6769
Mon.-Fri. 8 AM-4:30 PM
Tel: 248-551-4077
Fax: 248-551-4046

SOUTHFIELD
Drug Information Service
Providence Hospital
16001 West 9 Mile Rd.
P.O. Box 2043
Southfield, MI 48075
Mon.-Fri. 8 AM-4 PM
Tel: 248-424-3125
Fax: 248-424-5364

MINNESOTA
ROCHESTER
Drug Information Service
Mayo Clinic
1216 2nd St., SW
Rochester, MN 55902
Mon.-Fri. 8 AM-5 PM
Tel: 507-255-5062
       507-255-5732
       (after hours)
Fax: 507-255-7556

MISSISSIPPI
JACKSON
Drug Information Center
University of Mississippi Medical
Center
2500 N. State St.
Jackson, MS 39216
Mon.-Fri. 8 AM-5 PM
Tel: 601-984-2060
       (on call 24 hours)
Fax: 601-984-2063

MISSOURI
SPRINGFIELD
Drug Information & Clinical Research
Services
1235 E. Cherokee
Springfield, MO 65804
Mon.-Fri. 7:30 AM-4:30 PM
Tel: 417-885-3488
Fax: 417-888-7788

ST. JOSEPH
Drug Information Service
Heartland Hospital West
801 Faraon St.
St. Joseph, MO 64501
Mon.-Sat. 8 AM-8 PM
Tel: 816-271-7582
Fax: 816-271-7590

NEBRASKA
OMAHA
Drug Information Service
School of Pharmacy
Creighton University
2500 California Plaza
Omaha, NE 68178
Mon.-Fri. 8:30 AM-4:30 PM
Tel: 402-280-5101
Fax: 402-280-5149

Drug Information Center
Pharmacy Department, NHS
981090 Nebraska Medical
Center
Omaha, NE 68198-1090
Mon.-Fri. 8 AM-4:30 PM
Tel: 402-559-7205
       402-559-6747
Fax: 402-559-5463

NEW MEXICO
ALBUQUERQUE
New Mexico Poison & Drug
Information Center
University of New Mexico
Albuquerque, NM 87131-1076
7 days/week, 24 hours
Tel: 505-272-2222
       800-432-6866 (NM)
Fax: 505-272-5892

NEW YORK
BROOKLYN
International Drug
Information Center
Long Island University
Arnold & Marie Schwartz College of
Pharmacy
1 University Plaza
RM-Z509
Brooklyn, NY 11201
Mon.-Fri. 9 AM-5 PM
Tel: 718-488-1064
Fax: 718-780-4056

COOPERSTOWN
Drug Information Center
The Mary Imogene Bassett Hospital
1 Atwell Rd.
Cooperstown, NY 13326
Mon.-Fri. 8:30 AM-5 PM
Tel: 607-547-3686
Fax: 607-547-3629

NEW YORK CITY
Drug Information Center
Bellevue Hospital Center
462 1st Ave.
New York, NY 10016
Mon.-Fri. 9 AM-5 PM
Tel: 212-562-6504
Fax: 212-562-6503

Drug Information Center
Memorial Sloan-Kettering Cancer
Center
1275 York Ave.
RM S-702
New York, NY 10021
Mon.-Fri. 9 AM-5 PM
Tel: 212-639-7552
Fax: 212-639-2171

Drug Information Center
Mount Sinai Medical Center
1 Gustave Levy Place
New York, NY 10029
Mon.-Fri. 9 AM-5 PM
Tel: 212-241-6619
Fax: 212-348-7927

Drug Information Service
The New York Hospital
Cornell Medical Center
525 E. 68th St.
New York, NY 10021
Mon.-Fri. 9 AM-5 PM
Tel: 212-746-0741
Fax: 212-746-8506

ROCHESTER
Drug Information Service
Dept. of Pharmacy - Poison Division
University of Rochester
601 Elmwood Ave.
Rochester, NY 14642
24 HRS. 7 Days Week
Tel: 716-275-3718
       716-275-2681
       (after hours)
Fax: 716-473-9842

STONY BROOK
Suffolk Drug Information Center
University Hospital
S.U.N.Y. - Stony Brook
Room 3-559, Z7310
Stony Brook, NY 11794-7310
Mon.-Fri. 8 AM-3:00 PM
   No Holidays
Tel: 516-444-2672
       516-444-2680
       (after hours)
Fax: 516-444-7935

NORTH CAROLINA
BUIES CREEK
Drug Information Center
School of Pharmacy
Campbell University
P.O. Box 1090
Buies Creek, NC 27506
Mon.-Fri. 8:30 AM - 4:30 PM
Tel: 910-893-1478
       800-327-5467 (NC)
Fax: 910-893-1476

CHAPEL HILL
Drug Information Center
University of North Carolina Hospitals
101 Manning Drive
Chapel Hill, NC 27514
Mon.-Fri. 8 AM-4:30 PM
Tel: 919-966-2373
Fax: 919-966-1791

GREENSBORO
Triad Poison Center
Moses H. Cone Memorial Hospital
1200 N. Elm St.
Greensboro, NC 27401
7 days/week, 24 hours
Tel: 336-574-8105
Fax: 336-574-7198

GREENVILLE
Eastern Carolina Drug
Information Center
Pitt County Memorial Hospital
Dept. of Pharmacy Service
2100 Stantonsburg Rd.
Greenville, NC 27835
Mon.-Fri. 8 AM- 5 PM
Tel: 919-816-4257
Fax: 919-816-7425

WINSTON-SALEM
Drug Information
Service Center
Wake-Forest University
Baptist Medical Center
Medical Center Blvd.
Winston-Salem, NC 27157
Mon.-Fri. 8 AM-5 PM
Tel: 336-716-2037
Fax: 336-716-2186

OHIO
ADA
Drug Information Center
Raabe College of Pharmacy
Ohio Northern University
Ada, OH 45810
Mon.-Fri. 9 AM - 5 PM
Tel: 419-772-2307
Fax: 419-772-2289

CLEVELAND
Drug Information Center
Cleveland Clinic Foundation
9500 Euclid Avenue
Cleveland, OH 44195
Mon.-Fri. 8 AM - 5 PM
Tel: 216-444-6456
Fax: 216-445-6221

COLUMBUS
Central Ohio Poison Center
700 Children's Drive
Columbus, OH 43205
24 HRS. 7 Days/Week
Tel: 614-228-1323
800-682-7625 (OH)
Fax: 614-221-2672

Drug Information Center
Ohio State University Hospital
Dept. of Pharmacy
Doan Hall 368
410 W. 10th Avenue
Columbus, OH 43210-1228
Mon.-Fri. 8 AM - 4 PM
Tel: 614-293-8679
Fax: 614-293-3264

Drug Information Center
Riverside Methodist Hospital
3535 Olantangy River Road
Columbus, OH 43214
8 AM - 5 PM
Tel: 614-566-5425
Fax: 614-566-5447

OKLAHOMA
OKLAHOMA CITY
Drug Information Center
Integris Health
3300 Northwest Expressway
Oklahoma City, OK 73112
Mon.-Fri. 8 AM-4:30 PM
Tel: 405-949-3660
Fax: 405-951-8274

Drug Information Center
Presbyterian Hospital
700 NE 13th St.
Oklahoma City, OK 73104
Mon.-Fri. 7:30 AM-3:30 PM
Tel: 405-271-6226
Fax: 405-271-6281

TULSA
Drug Information Service
St. Francis Hospital
6161 S. Yale Ave.
Tulsa, OK 74136
Mon.-Fri. 9 AM-5:30 PM
Tel: 918-494-6339
Fax: 918-494-1893

PENNSYLVANIA
PHILADELPHIA
Drug Information Center
Temple University Hospital
Dept. of Pharmacy
Broad and Ontario St.
Philadelphia, PA 19140
Mon.-Fri. 8 AM-4:30 PM
Tel: 215-707-4644
Fax: 215-707-3463

Drug Information Center
Thomas Jefferson University Hospital
111 S. 11th
Philadelphia, PA 19107-5098
Mon.-Fri. 8 AM-5 PM
Tel: 215-955-8877
Fax: 215-923-3316

PITTSBURGH
The Pharmaceutical Information
Center
Mylan School of Pharmacy
Duquene University
431 Mellon Hall
Pittsburgh, PA 15282
Mon.-Fri. 8 AM-4 PM
Tel: 412-396-4600
Fax: 412-396-4488

Drug Information and
Pharmacoepidemiology Center
University of Pittsburgh Medical
Center
137 Victoria Hall
Pittsburgh, PA 15261
Mon.-Fri. 8:30 AM-4:30 PM
Tel: 412-624-3784
Fax: 412-624-6350

UPLAND
Drug Information Center
Crozer-Chester Medical Center
Dept. of Pharmacy
1 Medical Center Blvd.
Upland, PA 19013
Mon.-Fri. 8 AM-4:30 PM
Tel: 610-447-2851
610-447-2862 (after hours)
Fax: 215-447-2820

WILLIAMSPORT
Drug Information Center
Susquehanna Health System
Rural Avenue Campus
Williamsport, PA 17701
Mon.-Fri. 8 AM-4 PM
Tel: 717-321-3289
Fax: 717-321-3230

PUERTO RICO
SAN JUAN
Centro Information Medicamentos
Escuela de Farmacia RCM
P.O. Box 365067
San Juan, PR 00936-5067
Mon.-Fri. 8 AM-4:30 PM
Tel: 787-763-0196
Fax: 787-763-0196

RHODE ISLAND
PROVIDENCE
Drug Information Service
Dept. of Pharmacy
Rhode Island Hospital
593 Eddy Street
Providence, RI 02903
7 days/week, 24 hours
Tel: 401-444-5547
Fax: 401-444-8062

SOUTH CAROLINA
CHARLESTON
Drug Information Service
Medical University of
South Carolina
171 Ashley Ave.
Room 604-SFX
Charleston, SC 29425-0810
Mon.-Fri. 8 AM-5:30 PM
Tel: 803-792-3896
800-922-5250
Fax: 803-792-5532

SPARTANBURG
Drug Information Center
Spartanburg Regional
Medical Center
101 E. Wood St.
Spartanburg, SC 29303
Mon.-Fri. 8 AM-5 PM
Tel: 864-560-6910
Fax: 864-560-6017

SOUTH DAKOTA
SIOUX FALLS
Drug Information Center McKennan
Hospital
PLEASE NOTE:
THIS DRUG INFORMATION
CENTER HAS CLOSED

TENNESSEE
KNOXVILLE
Drug Information Center
University of Tennessee Medical
Center
1924 Alcoa Highway
Knoxville, TN 37920-6999
Mon.-Fri. 8 AM-4:30 PM
Tel: 423-544-9125

MEMPHIS
South East Regional Drug Information
Center
VA Medical Center
1030 Jefferson Ave.
Memphis, TN 38104
Mon.-Fri. 7:30 AM-4 PM
Tel: 901-523-8990

Drug Information Center
University of Tennessee
847 Monroe Avenue
Suite 238, Memphis, TN 38163
Mon.-Fri. 8:30 AM - 4:30 PM
Tel: 901-448-5555
Fax: 901-448-5419

TEXAS
GALVESTON
Drug Information Center
University of Texas
Medical Branch
301 University Blvd. - G01
Galveston, TX 77555-0701
Mon.-Fri. 8 AM-5 PM
Tel: 409-772-2734
Fax: 409-747-5222

HOUSTON
Drug Information Center
Ben Taub General Hospital
Texas Southern University/HCHD
1504 Taub Loop
Houston, TX 77030
Mon.-Fri. 8 AM-5 PM
Tel: 713-793-2917
Fax: 713-793-2937

Drug Information Center Methodist
Hospital
6565 Fannin (MSDB109)
Houston, TX 77030
Mon.-Fri. 8 AM-5 PM
Tel: 713-790-4190
Fax: 713-793-1224

LACKLAND A.F.B.
Drug Information Center
Dept. of Pharmacy
Wilford Hall Medical Center
2200 Berquist Dr., Suite 1
Lackland A.F.B., TX 78236
Mon.-Fri. 7:30 AM-5 PM
Tel: 210-292-7100

LUBBOCK
Methodist Hospital
Drug Information and Consultation
Service
3615 19th St.
Lubbock, TX 79410
Mon.-Fri. 8 AM-5 PM
Tel: 806-793-4012
(Attn: Pharmacy)
Fax: 806-784-5323

TEMPLE
Drug Information Center
Scott and White Memorial Hospital
2401 S. 31st St.
Temple, TX 76508
Mon.-Fri. 8 AM-6 PM
Tel: 254-724-4636
Fax: 254-724-1731

UTAH
SALT LAKE CITY
Drug Information Center
University of Utah Hospital
Dept. of Pharmacy Services
Room A-050
50 N. Medical Dr.
Salt Lake City, UT 84132
Mon.-Fri. 8:30 AM-4:30 PM
Tel: 801-581-2073
Fax: 801-585-6688

WEST VIRGINIA
MORGANTOWN
West Virginia Drug
Information Center
WV University-Robert C. Byrd
Health Sciences Center
1124 HSN, P.O. Box 9550
Morgantown, WV 26506
Tel: 304-293-6640
800-352-2501 (WV)
Fax: 304-293-7672

WISCONSIN
MADISON
University of Wisconsin Hospital &
Clinics
600 Highland Ave.
Madison, WI 53792
Voice mail/24 hrs. a day,
responses in 3 days
Tel: 608-262-1315
Fax: 608-263-9424

WYOMING
LARAMIE
Drug Information Center
University of Wyoming
P.O. Box 3375
Laramie, WY 82071
Mon.-Fri. 8 AM-5 PM
Tel: 307-766-6128
Fax: 307-766-2953

SECTION 4

PRODUCT IDENTIFICATION GUIDE

To aid in quick identification, this section provides full-color, actual-size photographs of tablets and capsules. A variety of other dosage forms and packages are shown at less than actual size. In all, the guide contains more than 2,400 photos.

Products in this section are arranged alphabetically by manufacturer. In some instances, not all dosage forms and sizes are pictured. If others are available, a † symbol precedes the product's name. Letters or numbers representing the manufacturer's identification code are followed by an asterisk.

For more information on any of the products in this section, please turn to the Product Information Section, or check directly with the manufacturer. The page number of each product's text entry appears with its photographs.

While every effort has been made to guarantee faithful reproduction of the photos in this section, changes in size, color, and design are always a possibility. Be sure to confirm a product's identity with the manufacturer or your pharmacist.

INDEX BY MANUFACTURER

This section is made possible through the courtesy of the manufacturers whose products appear on the following pages.

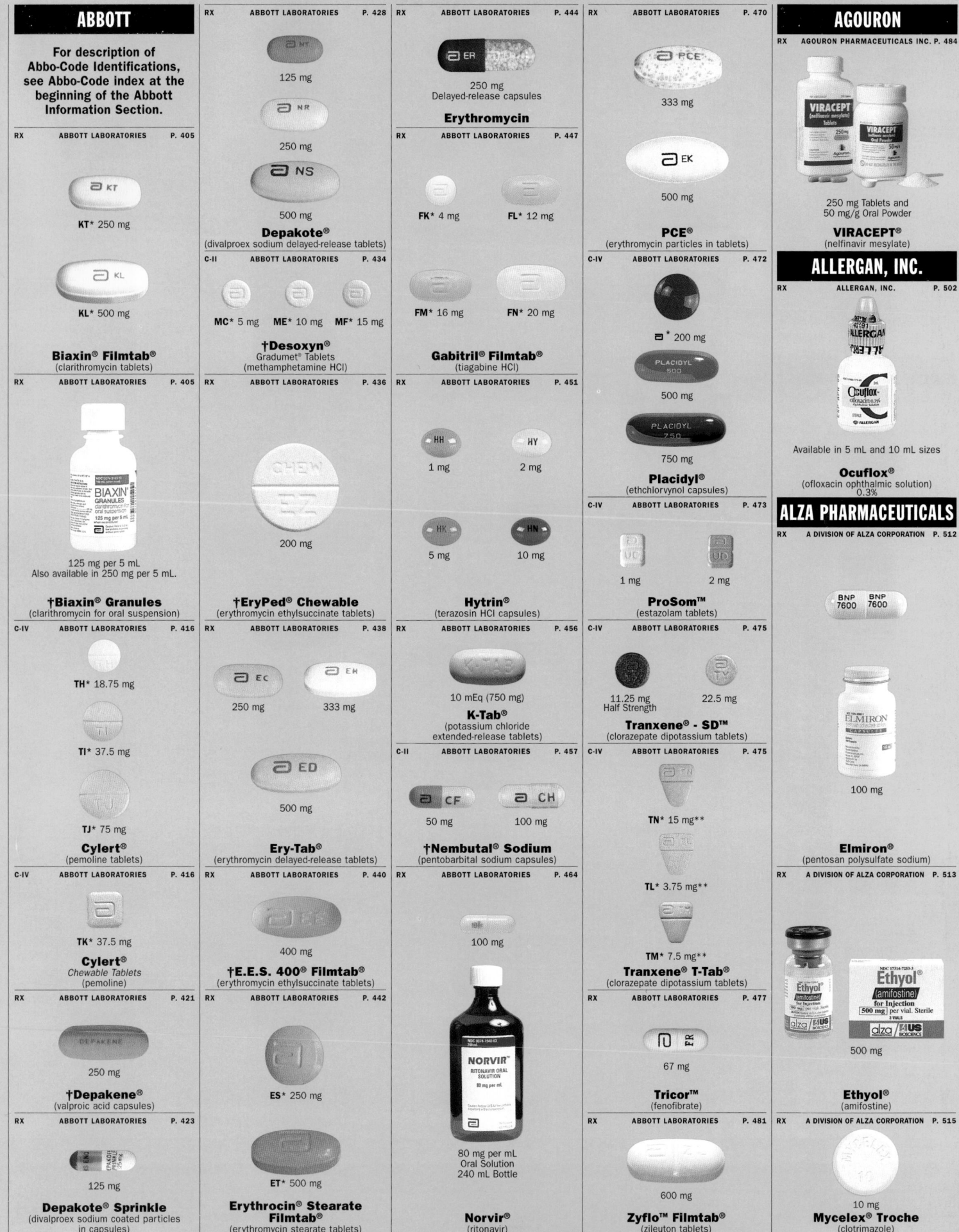

ABBOTT

For description of Abbo-Code Identifications, see Abbo-Code index at the beginning of the Abbott Information Section.

RX ABBOTT LABORATORIES P. 405

KT* 250 mg

KL* 500 mg

Biaxin® Filmtab®
(clarithromycin tablets)

RX ABBOTT LABORATORIES P. 405

125 mg per 5 mL
Also available in 250 mg per 5 mL.

†Biaxin® Granules
(clarithromycin for oral suspension)

C-IV ABBOTT LABORATORIES P. 416

TH* 18.75 mg

TI* 37.5 mg

TJ* 75 mg

Cylert®
(pemoline tablets)

C-IV ABBOTT LABORATORIES P. 416

TK* 37.5 mg

Cylert®
Chewable Tablets
(pemoline)

RX ABBOTT LABORATORIES P. 421

250 mg

†Depakene®
(valproic acid capsules)

RX ABBOTT LABORATORIES P. 423

125 mg

Depakote® Sprinkle
(divalproex sodium coated particles in capsules)

RX ABBOTT LABORATORIES P. 428

125 mg

250 mg

500 mg

Depakote®
(divalproex sodium delayed-release tablets)

C-II ABBOTT LABORATORIES P. 434

MC* 5 mg   ME* 10 mg   MF* 15 mg

†Desoxyn®
Gradumet® Tablets
(methamphetamine HCl)

RX ABBOTT LABORATORIES P. 436

CHEW EZ

200 mg

†EryPed® Chewable
(erythromycin ethylsuccinate tablets)

RX ABBOTT LABORATORIES P. 438

EC   250 mg   EK   333 mg

ED   500 mg

Ery-Tab®
(erythromycin delayed-release tablets)

RX ABBOTT LABORATORIES P. 440

400 mg

†E.E.S. 400® Filmtab®
(erythromycin ethylsuccinate tablets)

RX ABBOTT LABORATORIES P. 442

ES* 250 mg

ET* 500 mg

Erythrocin® Stearate Filmtab®
(erythromycin stearate tablets)

RX ABBOTT LABORATORIES P. 444

ER

250 mg
Delayed-release capsules

Erythromycin

RX ABBOTT LABORATORIES P. 447

FK* 4 mg   FL* 12 mg

FM* 16 mg   FN* 20 mg

Gabitril® Filmtab®
(tiagabine HCl)

RX ABBOTT LABORATORIES P. 451

HH 1 mg   HY 2 mg

HK 5 mg   HN 10 mg

Hytrin®
(terazosin HCl capsules)

RX ABBOTT LABORATORIES P. 456

K-TAB

10 mEq (750 mg)

K-Tab®
(potassium chloride extended-release tablets)

C-II ABBOTT LABORATORIES P. 457

CF 50 mg   CH 100 mg

†Nembutal® Sodium
(pentobarbital sodium capsules)

RX ABBOTT LABORATORIES P. 464

100 mg

Norvir®

NORVIR™
RITONAVIR ORAL SOLUTION
80 mg per mL

80 mg per mL
Oral Solution
240 mL Bottle

Norvir®
(ritonavir)

RX ABBOTT LABORATORIES P. 470

PCE

333 mg

EK

500 mg

PCE®
(erythromycin particles in tablets)

C-IV ABBOTT LABORATORIES P. 472

a * 200 mg

PLACIDYL 500

500 mg

PLACIDYL 750

750 mg

Placidyl®
(ethchlorvynol capsules)

C-IV ABBOTT LABORATORIES P. 473

UC 1 mg   UD 2 mg

ProSom™
(estazolam tablets)

C-IV ABBOTT LABORATORIES P. 475

11.25 mg
Half Strength   22.5 mg TY

Tranxene® - SD™
(clorazepate dipotassium tablets)

C-IV ABBOTT LABORATORIES P. 475

TN* 15 mg**

TL* 3.75 mg**

TM* 7.5 mg**

Tranxene® T-Tab®
(clorazepate dipotassium tablets)

RX ABBOTT LABORATORIES P. 477

FR

67 mg

Tricor™
(fenofibrate)

RX ABBOTT LABORATORIES P. 481

600 mg

Zyflo™ Filmtab®
(zileuton tablets)

AGOURON

RX AGOURON PHARMACEUTICALS INC. P. 484

VIRACEPT
(nelfinavir mesylate)
Tablets
250 mg

VIRACEPT
Oral Powder
50 mg/g

250 mg Tablets and
50 mg/g Oral Powder

VIRACEPT®
(nelfinavir mesylate)

ALLERGAN, INC.

RX ALLERGAN, INC. P. 502

ALLERGAN
Ocuflox
ofloxacin 0.3%

Available in 5 mL and 10 mL sizes

Ocuflox®
(ofloxacin ophthalmic solution)
0.3%

ALZA PHARMACEUTICALS

RX A DIVISION OF ALZA CORPORATION P. 512

BNP 7600   BNP 7600

ELMIRON

100 mg

Elmiron®
(pentosan polysulfate sodium)

RX A DIVISION OF ALZA CORPORATION P. 513

Ethyol
amifostine
for Injection
500 mg

Ethyol
amifostine
for Injection
500 mg per vial. Sterile

alza US BIOSCIENCE

500 mg

Ethyol®
(amifostine)

RX A DIVISION OF ALZA CORPORATION P. 515

10 mg

Mycelex® Troche
(clotrimazole)

*Abbott Abbo-Code identification letters. Filmtab® – Film sealed tablets, Abbott. **Grooved tablets.

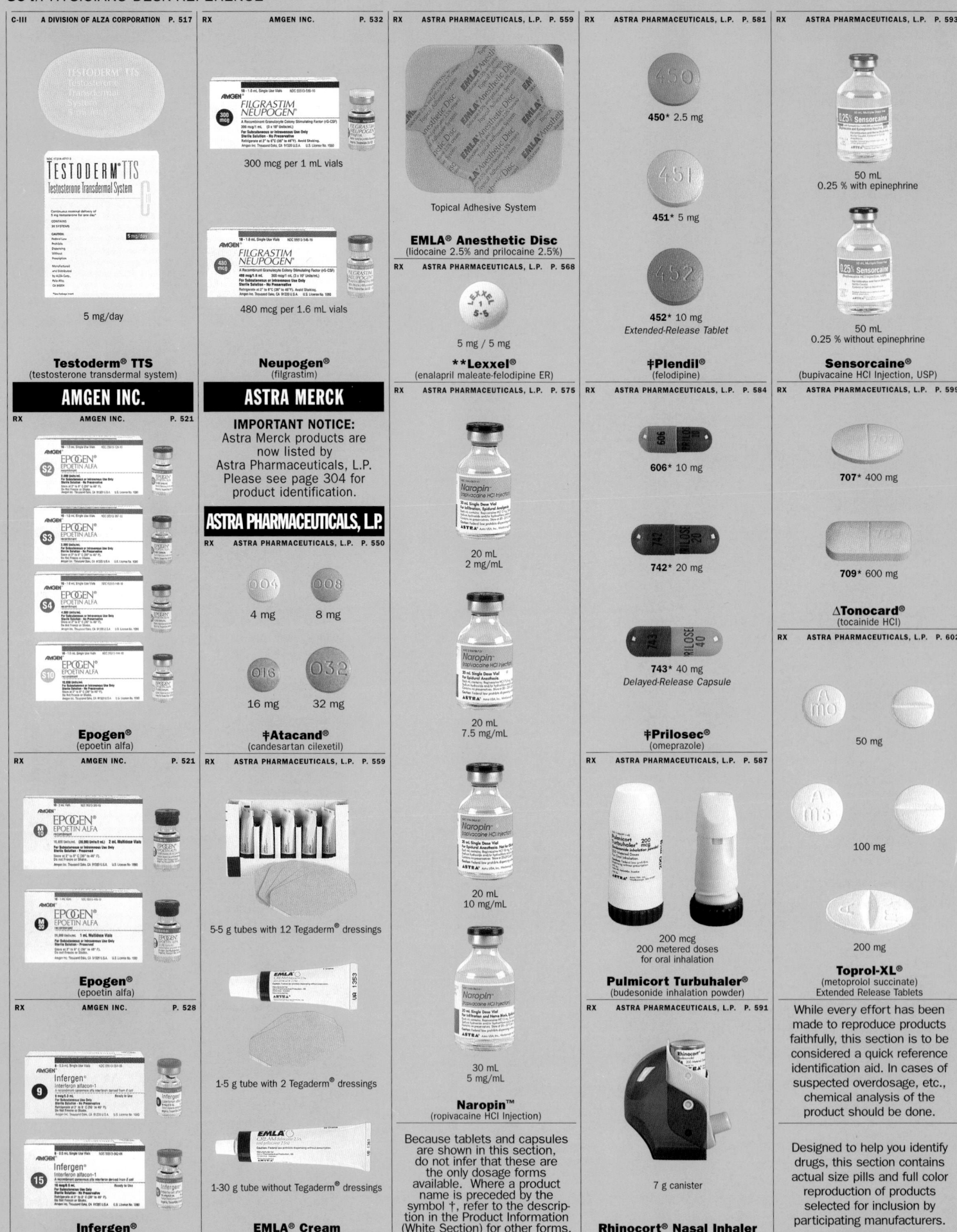

C-III   A DIVISION OF ALZA CORPORATION   P. 517

5 mg/day

Testoderm® TTS
(testosterone transdermal system)

AMGEN INC.

RX   AMGEN INC.   P. 521

Epogen®
(epoetin alfa)

RX   AMGEN INC.   P. 521

Epogen®
(epoetin alfa)

RX   AMGEN INC.   P. 528

Infergen®
(interferon alfacon-1)

RX   AMGEN INC.   P. 532

300 mcg per 1 mL vials

480 mcg per 1.6 mL vials

Neupogen®
(filgrastim)

ASTRA MERCK

IMPORTANT NOTICE:
Astra Merck products are
now listed by
Astra Pharmaceuticals, L.P.
Please see page 304 for
product identification.

ASTRA PHARMACEUTICALS, L.P.

RX   ASTRA PHARMACEUTICALS, L.P.   P. 550

004   4 mg   008   8 mg

016   16 mg   032   32 mg

†Atacand®
(candesartan cilexetil)

RX   ASTRA PHARMACEUTICALS, L.P.   P. 559

5-5 g tubes with 12 Tegaderm® dressings

1-5 g tube with 2 Tegaderm® dressings

1-30 g tube without Tegaderm® dressings

EMLA® Cream
(lidocaine 2.5% and prilocaine 2.5%)

RX   ASTRA PHARMACEUTICALS, L.P.   P. 559

Topical Adhesive System

EMLA® Anesthetic Disc
(lidocaine 2.5% and prilocaine 2.5%)

RX   ASTRA PHARMACEUTICALS, L.P.   P. 568

LEXXEL 1 5-5

5 mg / 5 mg

**Lexxel®
(enalapril maleate-felodipine ER)

RX   ASTRA PHARMACEUTICALS, L.P.   P. 575

20 mL
2 mg/mL

20 mL
7.5 mg/mL

20 mL
10 mg/mL

30 mL
5 mg/mL

Naropin™
(ropivacaine HCl Injection)

Because tablets and capsules
are shown in this section,
do not infer that these are
the only dosage forms
available. Where a product
name is preceded by the
symbol †, refer to the description in the Product Information
(White Section) for other forms.

RX   ASTRA PHARMACEUTICALS, L.P.   P. 581

450   450* 2.5 mg

451   451* 5 mg

452   452* 10 mg
Extended-Release Tablet

‡Plendil®
(felodipine)

RX   ASTRA PHARMACEUTICALS, L.P.   P. 584

606   606* 10 mg

742   742* 20 mg

743   743* 40 mg
Delayed-Release Capsule

‡Prilosec®
(omeprazole)

RX   ASTRA PHARMACEUTICALS, L.P.   P. 587

200 mcg
200 metered doses
for oral inhalation

Pulmicort Turbuhaler®
(budesonide inhalation powder)

RX   ASTRA PHARMACEUTICALS, L.P.   P. 591

7 g canister

Rhinocort® Nasal Inhaler
(budesonide)

RX   ASTRA PHARMACEUTICALS, L.P.   P. 593

50 mL
0.25 % with epinephrine

50 mL
0.25 % without epinephrine

Sensorcaine®
(bupivacaine HCl Injection, USP)

RX   ASTRA PHARMACEUTICALS, L.P.   P. 599

707   707* 400 mg

709   709* 600 mg

∆Tonocard®
(tocainide HCl)

RX   ASTRA PHARMACEUTICALS, L.P.   P. 602

50 mg

100 mg

200 mg

Toprol-XL®
(metoprolol succinate)
Extended Release Tablets

While every effort has been
made to reproduce products
faithfully, this section is to be
considered a quick reference
identification aid. In cases of
suspected overdosage, etc.,
chemical analysis of the
product should be done.

Designed to help you identify
drugs, this section contains
actual size pills and full color
reproduction of products
selected for inclusion by
participating manufacturers.

†Registered trademark of Astra AB and ∆Registered trademark of Astra Pharmaceutical Products, Inc.   **Registered Trademark of Astra Merck Inc.

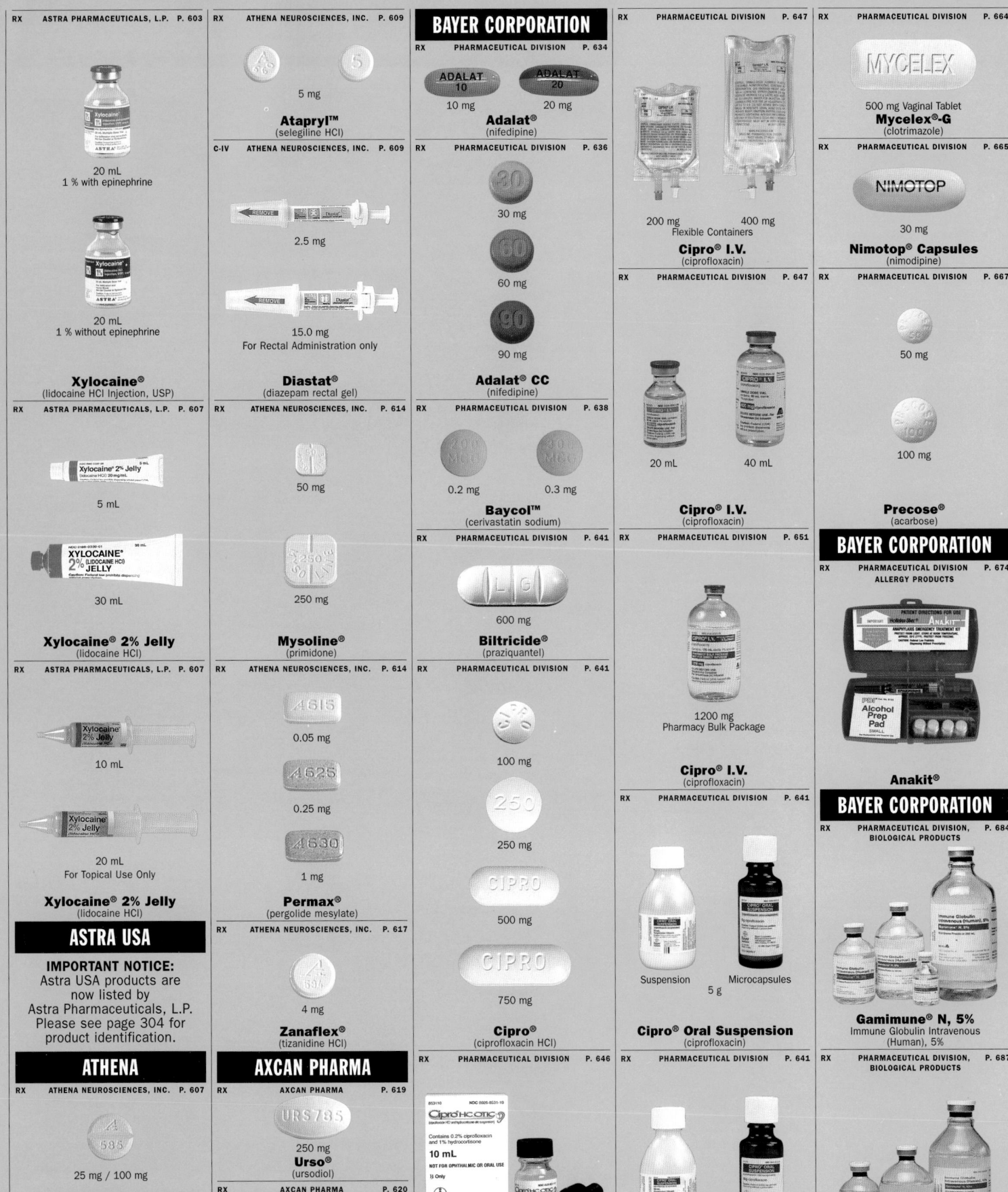

RX   ASTRA PHARMACEUTICALS, L.P.   P. 603

20 mL
1 % with epinephrine

20 mL
1 % without epinephrine

Xylocaine®
(lidocaine HCl Injection, USP)

RX   ASTRA PHARMACEUTICALS, L.P.   P. 607

5 mL

30 mL

Xylocaine® 2% Jelly
(lidocaine HCl)

RX   ASTRA PHARMACEUTICALS, L.P.   P. 607

10 mL

20 mL
For Topical Use Only

Xylocaine® 2% Jelly
(lidocaine HCl)

ASTRA USA

IMPORTANT NOTICE:
Astra USA products are
now listed by
Astra Pharmaceuticals, L.P.
Please see page 304 for
product identification.

ATHENA

RX   ATHENA NEUROSCIENCES, INC.   P. 607

25 mg / 100 mg

25 mg / 250 mg

Atamet®
(carbidopa, levodopa)

RX   ATHENA NEUROSCIENCES, INC.   P. 609

5 mg

Atapryl™
(selegiline HCl)

C-IV   ATHENA NEUROSCIENCES, INC.   P. 609

2.5 mg

15.0 mg
For Rectal Administration only

Diastat®
(diazepam rectal gel)

RX   ATHENA NEUROSCIENCES, INC.   P. 614

50 mg

250 mg

Mysoline®
(primidone)

RX   ATHENA NEUROSCIENCES, INC.   P. 614

4615
0.05 mg

4625
0.25 mg

4630
1 mg

Permax®
(pergolide mesylate)

RX   ATHENA NEUROSCIENCES, INC.   P. 617

4 mg

Zanaflex®
(tizanidine HCl)

AXCAN PHARMA

RX   AXCAN PHARMA   P. 619

URS785
250 mg

Urso®
(ursodiol)

RX   AXCAN PHARMA   P. 620

Viokase®
(pancrelipase, USP)

BAYER CORPORATION

RX   PHARMACEUTICAL DIVISION   P. 634

ADALAT 10
10 mg

ADALAT 20
20 mg

Adalat®
(nifedipine)

RX   PHARMACEUTICAL DIVISION   P. 636

30 mg

60 mg

90 mg

Adalat® CC
(nifedipine)

RX   PHARMACEUTICAL DIVISION   P. 638

0.2 mg

0.3 mg

Baycol™
(cerivastatin sodium)

RX   PHARMACEUTICAL DIVISION   P. 641

600 mg

Biltricide®
(praziquantel)

RX   PHARMACEUTICAL DIVISION   P. 641

100 mg

250 mg

500 mg

750 mg

Cipro®
(ciprofloxacin HCl)

RX   PHARMACEUTICAL DIVISION   P. 646

Contains 0.2% ciprofloxacin
and 1% hydrocortisone
10 mL
NOT FOR OPHTHALMIC OR ORAL USE

10 mL

Cipro® HC Otic
(ciprofloxacin HCl,
hydrocortisone otic suspension)

RX   PHARMACEUTICAL DIVISION   P. 647

200 mg   400 mg
Flexible Containers

Cipro® I.V.
(ciprofloxacin)

RX   PHARMACEUTICAL DIVISION   P. 647

20 mL   40 mL

Cipro® I.V.
(ciprofloxacin)

RX   PHARMACEUTICAL DIVISION   P. 651

1200 mg
Pharmacy Bulk Package

Cipro® I.V.
(ciprofloxacin)

RX   PHARMACEUTICAL DIVISION   P. 641

Suspension   Microcapsules
5 g

Cipro® Oral Suspension
(ciprofloxacin)

RX   PHARMACEUTICAL DIVISION   P. 641

Suspension   Microcapsules
10 g

Cipro® Oral Suspension
(ciprofloxacin)

RX   PHARMACEUTICAL DIVISION   P. 664

MYCELEX
500 mg Vaginal Tablet

Mycelex®-G
(clotrimazole)

RX   PHARMACEUTICAL DIVISION   P. 665

NIMOTOP
30 mg

Nimotop® Capsules
(nimodipine)

RX   PHARMACEUTICAL DIVISION   P. 667

50 mg

100 mg

Precose®
(acarbose)

BAYER CORPORATION

RX   PHARMACEUTICAL DIVISION   P. 674
ALLERGY PRODUCTS

Anakit®

BAYER CORPORATION

RX   PHARMACEUTICAL DIVISION,   P. 684
BIOLOGICAL PRODUCTS

Gamimune® N, 5%
Immune Globulin Intravenous
(Human), 5%

RX   PHARMACEUTICAL DIVISION,   P. 687
BIOLOGICAL PRODUCTS

Gamimune® N, 10%
Immune Globulin Intravenous
(Human), 10%

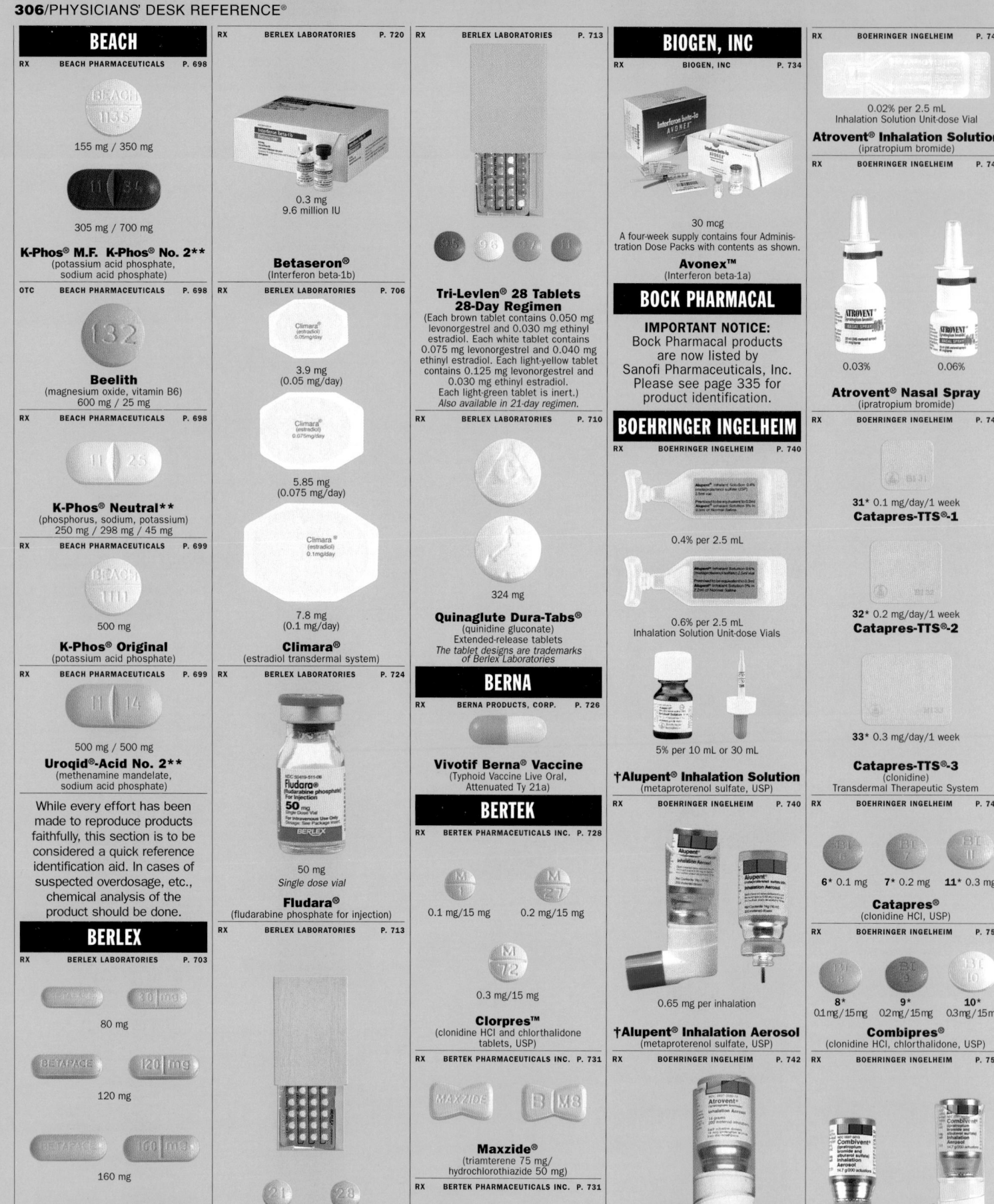

BEACH

RX — BEACH PHARMACEUTICALS — P. 698

155 mg / 350 mg

305 mg / 700 mg

K-Phos® M.F. K-Phos® No. 2
(potassium acid phosphate,
sodium acid phosphate)

OTC — BEACH PHARMACEUTICALS — P. 698

Beelith
(magnesium oxide, vitamin B6)
600 mg / 25 mg

RX — BEACH PHARMACEUTICALS — P. 698

K-Phos® Neutral
(phosphorus, sodium, potassium)
250 mg / 298 mg / 45 mg

RX — BEACH PHARMACEUTICALS — P. 699

500 mg

K-Phos® Original
(potassium acid phosphate)

RX — BEACH PHARMACEUTICALS — P. 699

500 mg / 500 mg

Uroqid®-Acid No. 2
(methenamine mandelate,
sodium acid phosphate)

While every effort has been
made to reproduce products
faithfully, this section is to be
considered a quick reference
identification aid. In cases of
suspected overdosage, etc.,
chemical analysis of the
product should be done.

BERLEX

RX — BERLEX LABORATORIES — P. 703

80 mg

120 mg

160 mg

240 mg

Betapace®
(sotalol HCl)

RX — BERLEX LABORATORIES — P. 720

0.3 mg
9.6 million IU

Betaseron®
(Interferon beta-1b)

RX — BERLEX LABORATORIES — P. 706

Climara®
(estradiol)
0.05mg/day

3.9 mg
(0.05 /day)

Climara®
(estradiol)
0.075mg/day

5.85 mg
(0.075 mg/day)

Climara®
(estradiol)
0.1mg/day

7.8 mg
(0.1 mg/day)

Climara®
(estradiol transdermal system)

RX — BERLEX LABORATORIES — P. 724

NDC 50419-511-06
Fludara®
(fludarabine phosphate)
For Injection
50 mg
Single Dose Vial
For Intravenous Use Only
Dosage: See Package Insert
BERLEX

50 mg
Single dose vial
Fludara®
(fludarabine phosphate for injection)

RX — BERLEX LABORATORIES — P. 713

21   28

**Levlen® 28 Tablets
28-Day Regimen**
(Each light-orange tablet contains 0.15
mg levonorgestrel and 0.03 mg ethinyl
estradiol. Each pink tablet is inert.)
Also available in 21-day regimen.

RX — BERLEX LABORATORIES — P. 713

**Tri-Levlen® 28 Tablets
28-Day Regimen**
(Each brown tablet contains 0.050 mg
levonorgestrel and 0.030 mg ethinyl
estradiol. Each white tablet contains
0.075 mg levonorgestrel and 0.040 mg
ethinyl estradiol. Each light-yellow tablet
contains 0.125 mg levonorgestrel and
0.030 mg ethinyl estradiol.
Each light-green tablet is inert.)
Also available in 21-day regimen.

RX — BERLEX LABORATORIES — P. 710

324 mg

Quinaglute Dura-Tabs®
(quinidine gluconate)
Extended-release tablets
*The tablet designs are trademarks
of Berlex Laboratories*

BERNA

RX — BERNA PRODUCTS, CORP. — P. 726

Vivotif Berna® Vaccine
(Typhoid Vaccine Live Oral,
Attenuated Ty 21a)

BERTEK

RX — BERTEK PHARMACEUTICALS INC. — P. 728

M
1
0.1 mg/15 mg

M
27
0.2 mg/15 mg

M
72
0.3 mg/15 mg

Clorpres™
(clonidine HCl and chlorthalidone
tablets, USP)

RX — BERTEK PHARMACEUTICALS INC. — P. 731

MAXZIDE   B M8

Maxzide®
(triamterene 75 mg/
hydrochlorothiazide 50 mg)

RX — BERTEK PHARMACEUTICALS INC. — P. 731

MAXZIDE   B M9

Maxzide®-25MG
(triamterene 37.5 mg/
hydrochlorothiazide 25 mg)

BIOGEN, INC

RX — BIOGEN, INC — P. 734

30 mcg
A four-week supply contains four Adminis-
tration Dose Packs with contents as shown.
Avonex™
(Interferon beta-1a)

BOCK PHARMACAL

IMPORTANT NOTICE:
Bock Pharmacal products
are now listed by
Sanofi Pharmaceuticals, Inc.
Please see page 335 for
product identification.

BOEHRINGER INGELHEIM

RX — BOEHRINGER INGELHEIM — P. 740

0.4% per 2.5 mL

0.6% per 2.5 mL
Inhalation Solution Unit-dose Vials

5% per 10 mL or 30 mL

†Alupent® Inhalation Solution
(metaproterenol sulfate, USP)

RX — BOEHRINGER INGELHEIM — P. 740

0.65 mg per inhalation

†Alupent® Inhalation Aerosol
(metaproterenol sulfate, USP)

RX — BOEHRINGER INGELHEIM — P. 742

14 gram vial
Atrovent® Inhalation Aerosol
18 mcg per inhalation (ipratropium bromide)

RX — BOEHRINGER INGELHEIM — P. 743

0.02% per 2.5 mL
Inhalation Solution Unit-dose Vial
Atrovent® Inhalation Solution
(ipratropium bromide)

RX — BOEHRINGER INGELHEIM — P. 744

0.03%   0.06%

Atrovent® Nasal Spray
(ipratropium bromide)

RX — BOEHRINGER INGELHEIM — P. 748

31* 0.1 mg/day/1 week
Catapres-TTS®-1

32* 0.2 mg/day/1 week
Catapres-TTS®-2

33* 0.3 mg/day/1 week
Catapres-TTS®-3
(clonidine)
Transdermal Therapeutic System

RX — BOEHRINGER INGELHEIM — P. 747

6* 0.1 mg   7* 0.2 mg   11* 0.3 mg

Catapres®
(clonidine HCl, USP)

RX — BOEHRINGER INGELHEIM — P. 750

8*
0.1mg/15mg

9*
0.2mg/15mg

10*
0.3mg/15mg

Combipres®
(clonidine HCl, chlorthalidone, USP)

RX — BOEHRINGER INGELHEIM — P. 752

Combivent® Inhalation Aerosol
(ipratropium bromide and albuterol sulfate)

**The name BEACH appears on the reverse side of these tablets.

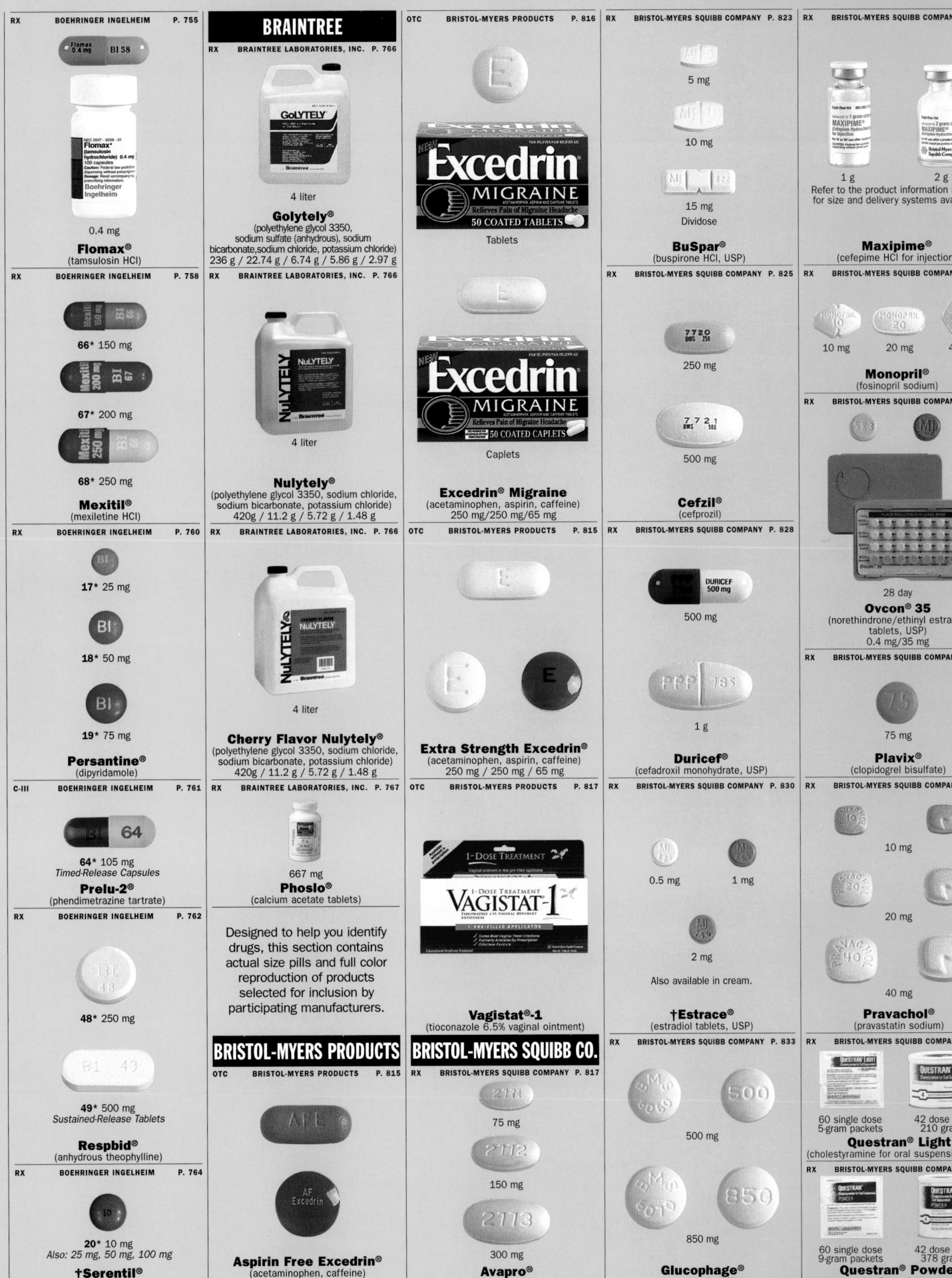

RX BOEHRINGER INGELHEIM P. 755

0.4 mg
Flomax®
(tamsulosin HCl)

RX BOEHRINGER INGELHEIM P. 758

66* 150 mg

67* 200 mg

68* 250 mg
Mexitil®
(mexiletine HCl)

RX BOEHRINGER INGELHEIM P. 760

17* 25 mg

18* 50 mg

19* 75 mg
Persantine®
(dipyridamole)

C-III BOEHRINGER INGELHEIM P. 761

64* 105 mg
Timed-Release Capsules
Prelu-2®
(phendimetrazine tartrate)

RX BOEHRINGER INGELHEIM P. 762

48* 250 mg

49* 500 mg
Sustained-Release Tablets
Respbid®
(anhydrous theophylline)

RX BOEHRINGER INGELHEIM P. 764

20* 10 mg
Also: 25 mg, 50 mg, 100 mg
†Serentil®
(mesoridazine besylate)

BRAINTREE

RX BRAINTREE LABORATORIES, INC. P. 766

4 liter
Golytely®
(polyethylene glycol 3350,
sodium sulfate (anhydrous), sodium
bicarbonate,sodium chloride, potassium chloride)
236 g / 22.74 g / 6.74 g / 5.86 g / 2.97 g

RX BRAINTREE LABORATORIES, INC. P. 766

4 liter
Nulytely®
(polyethylene glycol 3350, sodium chloride,
sodium bicarbonate, potassium chloride)
420g / 11.2 g / 5.72 g / 1.48 g

RX BRAINTREE LABORATORIES, INC. P. 766

4 liter
Cherry Flavor Nulytely®
(polyethylene glycol 3350, sodium chloride,
sodium bicarbonate, potassium chloride)
420g / 11.2 g / 5.72 g / 1.48 g

RX BRAINTREE LABORATORIES, INC. P. 767

667 mg
Phoslo®
(calcium acetate tablets)

Designed to help you identify
drugs, this section contains
actual size pills and full color
reproduction of products
selected for inclusion by
participating manufacturers.

BRISTOL-MYERS PRODUCTS

OTC BRISTOL-MYERS PRODUCTS P. 815

Aspirin Free Excedrin®
(acetaminophen, caffeine)
500 mg / 65 mg

OTC BRISTOL-MYERS PRODUCTS P. 816

Excedrin®
MIGRAINE
Relieves Pain of Migraine Headache
50 COATED TABLETS
Tablets

Excedrin®
MIGRAINE
Relieves Pain of Migraine Headache
50 COATED CAPLETS
Caplets

Excedrin® Migraine
(acetaminophen, aspirin, caffeine)
250 mg/250 mg/65 mg

OTC BRISTOL-MYERS PRODUCTS P. 815

Extra Strength Excedrin®
(acetaminophen, aspirin, caffeine)
250 mg / 250 mg / 65 mg

OTC BRISTOL-MYERS PRODUCTS P. 817

VAGISTAT-1
Vagistat®-1
(tioconazole 6.5% vaginal ointment)

BRISTOL-MYERS SQUIBB CO.

RX BRISTOL-MYERS SQUIBB COMPANY P. 817

75 mg

150 mg

300 mg
Avapro®
(irbesartan)

RX BRISTOL-MYERS SQUIBB COMPANY P. 823

5 mg

10 mg

15 mg
Dividose
BuSpar®
(buspirone HCl, USP)

RX BRISTOL-MYERS SQUIBB COMPANY P. 825

250 mg

500 mg
Cefzil®
(cefprozil)

RX BRISTOL-MYERS SQUIBB COMPANY P. 828

500 mg
Duricef®
(cefadroxil monohydrate, USP)

RX BRISTOL-MYERS SQUIBB COMPANY P. 830

0.5 mg   1 mg

2 mg
Also available in cream.
†Estrace®
(estradiol tablets, USP)

RX BRISTOL-MYERS SQUIBB COMPANY P. 833

500 mg

850 mg
Glucophage®
(metformin HCl)

RX BRISTOL-MYERS SQUIBB COMPANY P. 837

1 g   2 g
Refer to the product information section
for size and delivery systems available.
Maxipime®
(cefepime HCl for injection)

RX BRISTOL-MYERS SQUIBB COMPANY P. 842

10 mg   20 mg   40 mg
Monopril®
(fosinopril sodium)

RX BRISTOL-MYERS SQUIBB COMPANY P. 845

28 day
Ovcon® 35
(norethindrone/ethinyl estradiol
tablets, USP)
0.4 mg/35 mg

RX BRISTOL-MYERS SQUIBB COMPANY P. 851

75 mg
Plavix®
(clopidogrel bisulfate)

RX BRISTOL-MYERS SQUIBB COMPANY P. 853

10 mg

20 mg

40 mg
Pravachol®
(pravastatin sodium)

RX BRISTOL-MYERS SQUIBB COMPANY P. 857

60 single dose   42 dose cans
5-gram packets   210 grams
Questran® Light
(cholestyramine for oral suspension, USP)

RX BRISTOL-MYERS SQUIBB COMPANY P. 857

60 single dose   42 dose cans
9-gram packets   378 grams
Questran® Powder
(cholestyramine for oral suspension, USP)

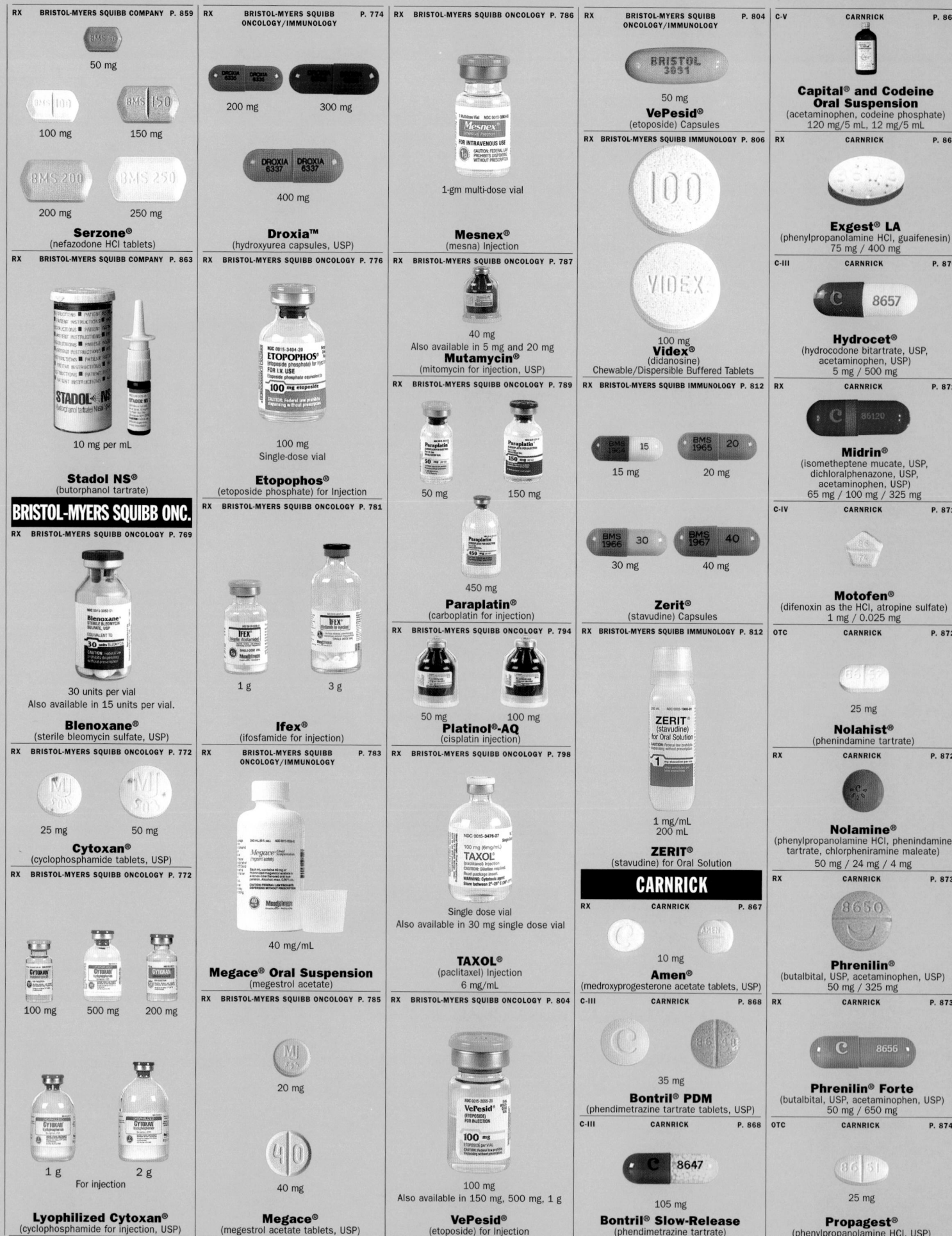

RX BRISTOL-MYERS SQUIBB COMPANY P. 859

50 mg

100 mg   150 mg

200 mg   250 mg

Serzone®
(nefazodone HCl tablets)

RX BRISTOL-MYERS SQUIBB COMPANY P. 863

10 mg per mL

Stadol NS®
(butorphanol tartrate)

BRISTOL-MYERS SQUIBB ONC.

RX BRISTOL-MYERS SQUIBB ONCOLOGY P. 769

30 units per vial
Also available in 15 units per vial.

Blenoxane®
(sterile bleomycin sulfate, USP)

RX BRISTOL-MYERS SQUIBB ONCOLOGY P. 772

25 mg   50 mg

Cytoxan®
(cyclophosphamide tablets, USP)

RX BRISTOL-MYERS SQUIBB ONCOLOGY P. 772

100 mg   500 mg   200 mg

1 g   2 g
For injection

Lyophilized Cytoxan®
(cyclophosphamide for injection, USP)

RX BRISTOL-MYERS SQUIBB ONCOLOGY/IMMUNOLOGY P. 774

200 mg   300 mg

DROXIA 6337   DROXIA 6337

400 mg

Droxia™
(hydroxyurea capsules, USP)

RX BRISTOL-MYERS SQUIBB ONCOLOGY P. 776

100 mg
Single-dose vial

Etopophos®
(etoposide phosphate) for Injection

RX BRISTOL-MYERS SQUIBB ONCOLOGY P. 781

1 g   3 g

Ifex®
(ifosfamide for injection)

RX BRISTOL-MYERS SQUIBB ONCOLOGY/IMMUNOLOGY P. 783

40 mg/mL

Megace® Oral Suspension
(megestrol acetate)

RX BRISTOL-MYERS SQUIBB ONCOLOGY P. 785

20 mg

40 mg

Megace®
(megestrol acetate tablets, USP)

RX BRISTOL-MYERS SQUIBB ONCOLOGY P. 786

1-gm multi-dose vial

Mesnex®
(mesna) Injection

RX BRISTOL-MYERS SQUIBB ONCOLOGY P. 787

40 mg
Also available in 5 mg and 20 mg

Mutamycin®
(mitomycin for injection, USP)

RX BRISTOL-MYERS SQUIBB ONCOLOGY P. 789

50 mg   150 mg

450 mg

Paraplatin®
(carboplatin for injection)

RX BRISTOL-MYERS SQUIBB ONCOLOGY P. 794

50 mg   100 mg

Platinol®-AQ
(cisplatin injection)

RX BRISTOL-MYERS SQUIBB ONCOLOGY P. 798

Single dose vial
Also available in 30 mg single dose vial

TAXOL®
(paclitaxel) Injection
6 mg/mL

RX BRISTOL-MYERS SQUIBB ONCOLOGY P. 804

100 mg
Also available in 150 mg, 500 mg, 1 g

VePesid®
(etoposide) for Injection

BRISTOL-MYERS SQUIBB ONCOLOGY/IMMUNOLOGY P. 804

50 mg

VePesid®
(etoposide) Capsules

RX BRISTOL-MYERS SQUIBB IMMUNOLOGY P. 806

100 mg

Videx®
(didanosine)
Chewable/Dispersible Buffered Tablets

RX BRISTOL-MYERS SQUIBB ONCOLOGY P. 812

15 mg   20 mg

30 mg   40 mg

Zerit®
(stavudine) Capsules

RX BRISTOL-MYERS SQUIBB IMMUNOLOGY P. 812

1 mg/mL
200 mL

ZERIT®
(stavudine) for Oral Solution

CARNRICK

RX CARNRICK P. 867

10 mg

Amen®
(medroxyprogesterone acetate tablets, USP)

C-III CARNRICK P. 868

35 mg

Bontril® PDM
(phendimetrazine tartrate tablets, USP)

C-III CARNRICK P. 868

105 mg

Bontril® Slow-Release
(phendimetrazine tartrate)

C-V CARNRICK P. 869

**Capital® and Codeine
Oral Suspension**
(acetaminophen, codeine phosphate)
120 mg/5 mL, 12 mg/5 mL

RX CARNRICK P. 869

Exgest® LA
(phenylpropanolamine HCl, guaifenesin)
75 mg / 400 mg

C-III CARNRICK P. 870

8657

Hydrocet®
(hydrocodone bitartrate, USP,
acetaminophen, USP)
5 mg / 500 mg

RX CARNRICK P. 871

86120

Midrin®
(isometheptene mucate, USP,
dichloralphenazone, USP,
acetaminophen, USP)
65 mg / 100 mg / 325 mg

C-IV CARNRICK P. 871

Motofen®
(difenoxin as the HCl, atropine sulfate)
1 mg / 0.025 mg

OTC CARNRICK P. 872

25 mg

Nolahist®
(phenindamine tartrate)

RX CARNRICK P. 872

Nolamine®
(phenylpropanolamine HCl, phenindamine
tartrate, chlorpheniramine maleate)
50 mg / 24 mg / 4 mg

RX CARNRICK P. 873

8650

Phrenilin®
(butalbital, USP, acetaminophen, USP)
50 mg / 325 mg

RX CARNRICK P. 873

8656

Phrenilin® Forte
(butalbital, USP, acetaminophen, USP)
50 mg / 650 mg

OTC CARNRICK P. 874

25 mg

Propagest®
(phenylpropanolamine HCl, USP)

8647

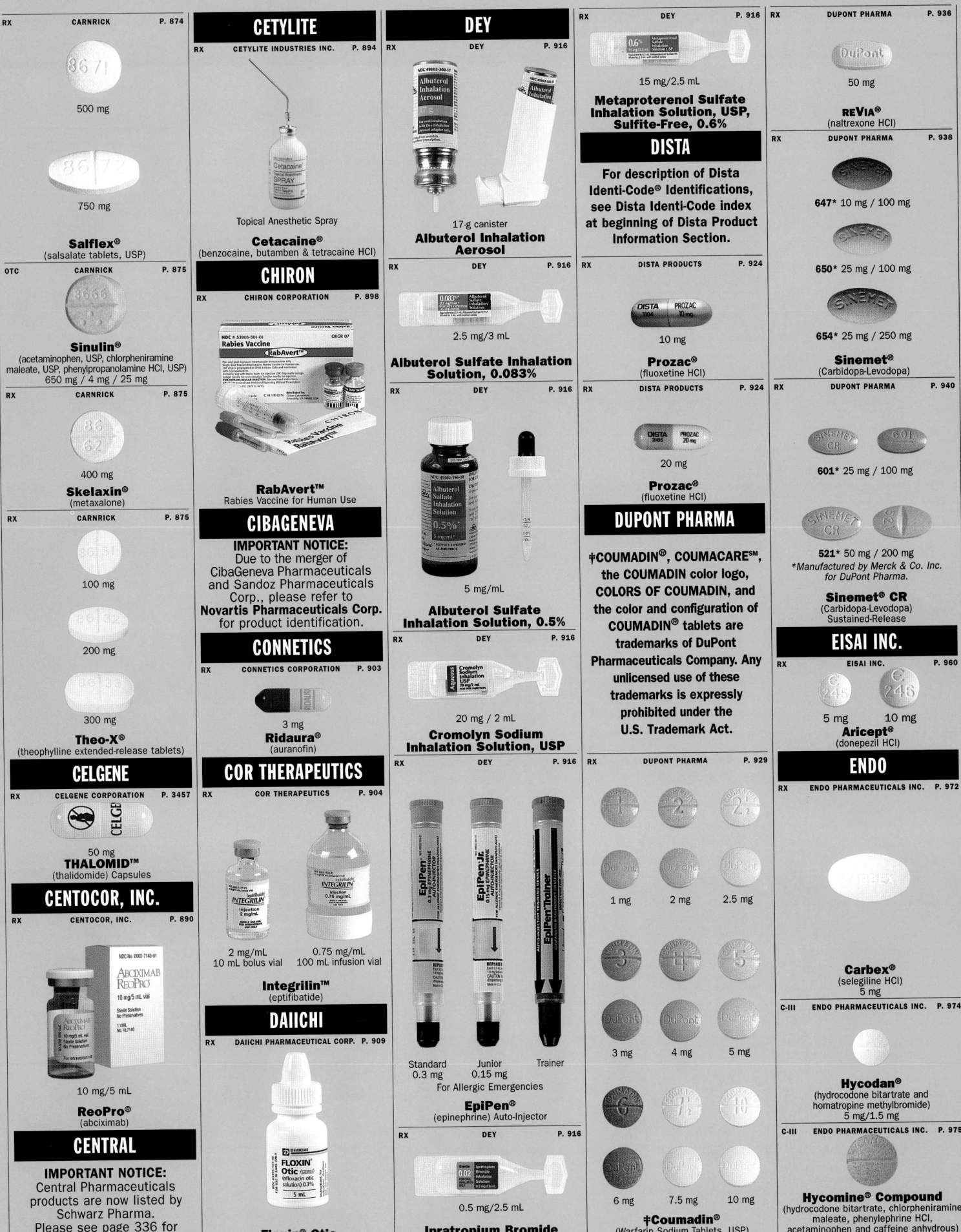

RX   CARNRICK   P. 874

500 mg

750 mg

Salflex®
(salsalate tablets, USP)

OTC   CARNRICK   P. 875

Sinulin®
(acetaminophen, USP, chlorpheniramine
maleate, USP, phenylpropanolamine HCl, USP)
650 mg / 4 mg / 25 mg

RX   CARNRICK   P. 875

400 mg

Skelaxin®
(metaxalone)

RX   CARNRICK   P. 875

100 mg

200 mg

300 mg

Theo-X®
(theophylline extended-release tablets)

CELGENE

RX   CELGENE CORPORATION   P. 3457

50 mg

THALOMID™
(thalidomide) Capsules

CENTOCOR, INC.

RX   CENTOCOR, INC.   P. 890

10 mg/5 mL

ReoPro®
(abciximab)

CENTRAL

IMPORTANT NOTICE:
Central Pharmaceuticals
products are now listed by
Schwarz Pharma.
Please see page 336 for
product identification.

CETYLITE

RX   CETYLITE INDUSTRIES INC.   P. 894

Topical Anesthetic Spray
Cetacaine®
(benzocaine, butamben & tetracaine HCl)

CHIRON

RX   CHIRON CORPORATION   P. 898

RabAvert™
Rabies Vaccine for Human Use

CIBAGENEVA

IMPORTANT NOTICE:
Due to the merger of
CibaGeneva Pharmaceuticals
and Sandoz Pharmaceuticals
Corp., please refer to
Novartis Pharmaceuticals Corp.
for product identification.

CONNETICS

RX   CONNETICS CORPORATION   P. 903

3 mg
Ridaura®
(auranofin)

COR THERAPEUTICS

RX   COR THERAPEUTICS   P. 904

2 mg/mL   0.75 mg/mL
10 mL bolus vial   100 mL infusion vial

Integrilin™
(eptifibatide)

DAIICHI

RX   DAIICHI PHARMACEUTICAL CORP.   P. 909

Floxin® Otic
(ofloxacin otic solution)

DEY

RX   DEY   P. 916

17-g canister
**Albuterol Inhalation
Aerosol**

RX   DEY   P. 916

2.5 mg/3 mL
**Albuterol Sulfate Inhalation
Solution, 0.083%**

RX   DEY   P. 916

5 mg/mL
**Albuterol Sulfate
Inhalation Solution, 0.5%**

RX   DEY   P. 916

20 mg / 2 mL
**Cromolyn Sodium
Inhalation Solution, USP**

RX   DEY   P. 916

Standard   Junior   Trainer
0.3 mg   0.15 mg
For Allergic Emergencies
EpiPen®
(epinephrine) Auto-Injector

RX   DEY   P. 916

0.5 mg/2.5 mL
**Ipratropium Bromide
Inhalation Solution, 0.02%**

RX   DEY   P. 916

15 mg/2.5 mL
**Metaproterenol Sulfate
Inhalation Solution, USP,
Sulfite-Free, 0.6%**

DISTA

For description of Dista
Identi-Code® Identifications,
see Dista Identi-Code index
at beginning of Dista Product
Information Section.

RX   DISTA PRODUCTS   P. 924

10 mg
Prozac®
(fluoxetine HCl)

RX   DISTA PRODUCTS   P. 924

20 mg
Prozac®
(fluoxetine HCl)

DUPONT PHARMA

‡COUMADIN®, COUMACARE℠,
the COUMADIN color logo,
COLORS OF COUMADIN, and
the color and configuration of
COUMADIN® tablets are
trademarks of DuPont
Pharmaceuticals Company. Any
unlicensed use of these
trademarks is expressly
prohibited under the
U.S. Trademark Act.

RX   DUPONT PHARMA   P. 929

1 mg   2 mg   2.5 mg

3 mg   4 mg   5 mg

6 mg   7.5 mg   10 mg

‡Coumadin®
(Warfarin Sodium Tablets, USP)
Crystalline

RX   DUPONT PHARMA   P. 936

50 mg
ReVia®
(naltrexone HCl)

RX   DUPONT PHARMA   P. 938

647* 10 mg / 100 mg

650* 25 mg / 100 mg

654* 25 mg / 250 mg

Sinemet®
(Carbidopa-Levodopa)

RX   DUPONT PHARMA   P. 940

601* 25 mg / 100 mg

521* 50 mg / 200 mg
*Manufactured by Merck & Co. Inc.
for DuPont Pharma.

Sinemet® CR
(Carbidopa-Levodopa)
Sustained-Release

EISAI INC.

RX   EISAI INC.   P. 960

5 mg   10 mg
Aricept®
(donepezil HCl)

ENDO

RX   ENDO PHARMACEUTICALS INC.   P. 972

Carbex®
(selegiline HCl)
5 mg

C-III   ENDO PHARMACEUTICALS INC.   P. 974

Hycodan®
(hydrocodone bitartrate and
homatropine methylbromide)
5 mg/1.5 mg

C-III   ENDO PHARMACEUTICALS INC.   P. 975

Hycomine® Compound
(hydrocodone bitartrate, chlorpheniramine
maleate, phenylephrine HCl,
acetaminophen and caffeine anhydrous)
5 mg/2 mg/10 mg/250 mg/30 mg

RX   ENDO PHARMACEUTICALS INC.   P. 978

5 mg

10 mg

25 mg

50 mg

100 mg

Moban®
(molindone HCl)

C-II   ENDO PHARMACEUTICALS INC.   P. 984

Percocet®
(oxycodone, acetaminophen, USP)
5 mg / 325 mg

C-II   ENDO PHARMACEUTICALS INC.   P. 985

Percodan®
(oxycodone, oxycodone
terephthalate, aspirin, USP)
4.5 mg/0.38 mg/325 mg

C-II   ENDO PHARMACEUTICALS INC.   P. 985

Percodan®-Demi
(oxycodone, oxycodone
terephthalate, aspirin)
2.25 mg/0.19 mg/325 mg

C-II   ENDO PHARMACEUTICALS INC.   P. 986

Percolone®
(oxycodone HCl, USP)
5 mg

RX   ENDO PHARMACEUTICALS INC.   P. 986

Symmetrel®
(amantadine HCl, USP)
100 mg

ESI LEDERLE

RX   ESI LEDERLE   P. 992

894* 5 mg
Aygestin®
(norethindrone acetate tablets, USP)

RX   ESI LEDERLE   P. 993

2.5 mg

5 mg

10 mg

Cycrin®
(medroxyprogesterone acetate tablets, USP)

FAULDING LABORATORIES

C-II   **FAULDING LABORATORIES**   P. 995

20 mg

50 mg

100 mg

Kadian®
(morphine sulfate sustained release)

FOREST

RX   FOREST PHARMACEUTICALS INC. P. 1015

250 mcg/per puff
7g 100 metered inhalations

Aerobid® Inhaler System
(flunisolide)

RX   FOREST PHARMACEUTICALS INC. P. 1015

250 mcg/per puff
7g 100 metered inhalations

AeroBid®-M Inhaler System
(flunisolide)

RX   FOREST PHARMACEUTICALS INC. P. 1016

AeroChamber®

AeroChamber®
with Mask

AeroChamber®
with Mask–Large

AeroChamber®
with Mask–Small

AeroChamber®

RX   FOREST PHARMACEUTICALS INC. P. 1018

1/4 gr.

1/2 gr.

1 gr.

1 1/2 gr.

2 gr.

3 gr.

4 gr.

5 gr.

Armour® Thyroid
(thyroid USP)

RX   FOREST PHARMACEUTICALS INC. P. 1019

Cervidil® Vaginal Insert
(dinoprostone 10 mg)

RX   FOREST PHARMACEUTICALS INC. P. 1020

G 535-12

Esgic®
(butalbital*, acetaminophen,
caffeine USP)
50 mg / 325 mg / 40 mg
*[Warning: May be habit forming]

RX   FOREST PHARMACEUTICALS INC. P. 1021

FOREST 0372   Esgic pl

Esgicplus™
(butalbital*, acetaminophen,
caffeine USP)
50 mg / 500 mg / 40 mg
*[Warning: May be habit forming]

RX   FOREST PHARMACEUTICALS INC. P. 1021

678

FOREST

Esgicplus™
(butalbital*, acetaminophen,
caffeine USP)
50 mg / 500 mg / 40 mg
*[Warning: May be habit forming]

RX   FOREST PHARMACEUTICALS INC. P. 1022

100 mg

Flumadine®
(rimantadine HCl)

RX   FOREST PHARMACEUTICALS INC. P. 1023

NDC 0456-4600-06
6 mL
INFASURF®
(calfactant)
Intratracheal Suspension
Sterile,
Non-Pyrogenic Suspension
for Intratracheal Use Only
Not for Injection

6 mL

Infasurf®
(calfactant)

RX   FOREST PHARMACEUTICALS INC. P. 1025

25 mcg

50 mcg

75 mcg

88 mcg

100 mcg

112 mcg

125 mcg

137 mcg

150 mcg

175 mcg

200 mcg

300 mcg

Levothroid®
(levothyroxine sodium tablet, USP)

C-III   FOREST PHARMACEUTICALS INC. P. 1027

UAD

63 50

Lorcet® 10/650
(hydrocodone* bitartrate,
acetaminophen USP)
10 mg/650 mg *[Warning: May be habit forming]

C-III   FOREST PHARMACEUTICALS INC. P. 1027

U U

Lorcet® Plus
(hydrocodone* bitartrate,
acetaminophen USP)
7.5 mg/650 mg *[Warning: May be habit forming]

RX   FOREST PHARMACEUTICALS INC. P. 1027

NDC 0456-4300-08
MONUROL™
(fosfomycin tromethamine)
(equivalent to 3 grams of fosfomycin)
Dissolve contents in 3 to 4 ounces
of water. Drink immediately.
CAUTION: Federal law prohibits
dispensing without prescription

Monurol®
(fosfomycin tromethamine)

RX   FOREST PHARMACEUTICALS INC. P. 1029

100 mg

Tessalon®
(benzonatate USP)

RX   FOREST PHARMACEUTICALS INC. P. 1030

1/4

1/2

1

2

3

Thyrolar®
(liotrix)

RX   FOREST PHARMACEUTICALS INC. P. 1030

Tiazac 120

120 mg

Tiazac 180

180 mg

Tiazac 240

240 mg

Tiazac 300

300 mg

Tiazac 360

360 mg

Tiazac™
(diltiazem HCl)
Extended-Release Capsules

FUJISAWA HEALTHCARE, INC.

RX   FUJISAWA HEALTHCARE, INC.   P. 1044

1 mg

5 mg

5 mg/mL
1 mL ampule

Prograf®
(tacrolimus)

GATE PHARMACEUTICALS

C-IV   GATE PHARMACEUTICALS   P. 1053

37.5 mg

†Adipex-P®
(phentermine HCl)

RX	GATE PHARMACEUTICALS	P. 1054

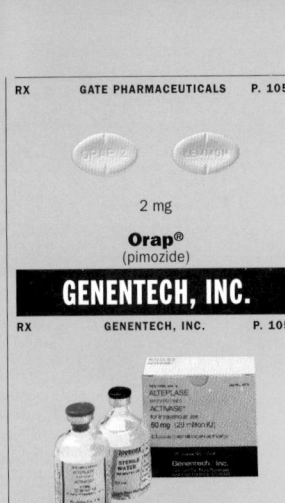

2 mg

Orap®
(pimozide)

GENENTECH, INC.

RX	GENENTECH, INC.	P. 1057

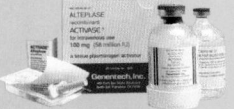

50 mg
29 million IU
Packaged with diluent

100 mg
58 million IU
Packaged with diluent and double-sided
sterile, siliconized transfer device

Activase®
(Alteplase, recombinant)

RX	GENENTECH, INC.	P. 1061

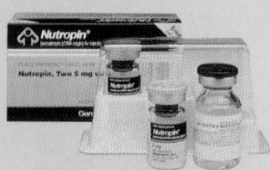

5 mg
approx. 15 IU
Packaged with 10 mL multi-dose vial of
bacteriostatic water
(benzyl alcohol preserved)

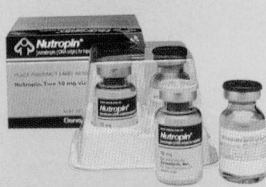

10 mg
approx. 30 IU
Packaged with 10 mL multi-dose vial of
bacteriostatic water
(benzyl alcohol preserved)

Nutropin®
(somatropin [rDNA origin] for injection)

RX	GENENTECH, INC.	P. 1064

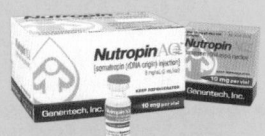

10 mg (5mg/mL)
approx. 30 IU
Each carton contains six (2 mL) vials

Nutropin AQ®
(somatropin [rDNA origin] injection)

RX	GENENTECH, INC.	P. 1067

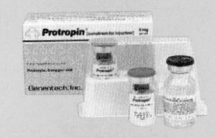

5 mg
approx. 15 IU
Packaged with 10 mL multi-dose vial of
bacteriostatic water
(benzyl alcohol preserved)

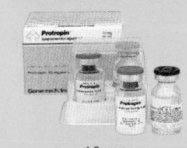

10 mg
approx. 30 IU
Packaged with 10 mL multi-dose vial of
bacteriostatic water
(benzyl alcohol preserved)

Protropin®
(somatrem for injection)

RX	GENENTECH, INC.	P. 1068

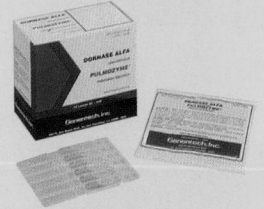

2.5 mL
(1.0 mg/mL dornase alfa)
Each carton contains 30 single-use
ampules

Pulmozyme®
(dornase alfa) recombinant,
Inhalation Solution

RX	GENENTECH, INC.	P. 1070

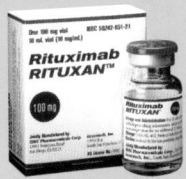

100 mg (10mg/mL)

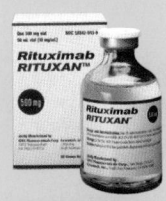

500 mg (10mg/mL)

Rituxan™
(Rituximab)
*Jointly marketed by IDEC Pharmaceuticals
Corp. and Genentech, Inc.*

Designed to help you identify
drugs, this section contains
actual size pills and full color
reproduction of products
selected for inclusion by
participating manufacturers.

Because tablets and capsules
are shown in this section,
do not infer that these are
the only dosage forms
available. Where a product
name is preceded by the
symbol †, refer to the description in the Product Information
(White Section) for other forms.

GENETICS INSTITUTE

RX	GENETICS INSTITUTE, INC.	P. 1073

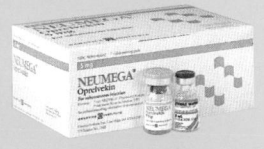

5 mg per vial
1 vial dispensing pack

5 mg per vial
7 vial dispensing pack

Neumega®
(Oprelvekin)

GLAXO WELLCOME

RX	GLAXO WELLCOME INC	P. 1082

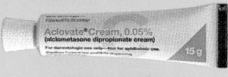

0.05% per 15 g

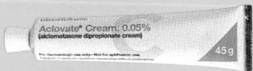

0.05% per 45 g
Also available in 60 g

Aclovate® Cream
(alclometasone dipropionate cream)

RX	GLAXO WELLCOME INC	P. 1082

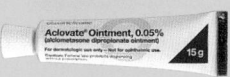

0.05% per 15 g

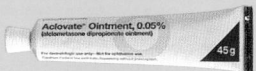

0.05% per 45 g
Also available in 60 g

Aclovate® Ointment
(alclometasone dipropionate ointment)

RX	GLAXO WELLCOME INC	P. 1083

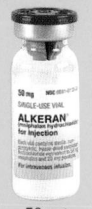

50 mg

Alkeran® for Injection
(melphalan HCl)

RX	GLAXO WELLCOME INC	P. 1085

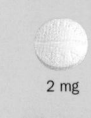

2 mg

Alkeran®
(melphalan)

RX	GLAXO WELLCOME INC	P. 1086

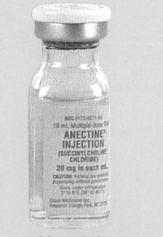

1 mg

2.5 mg

Amerge™
(naratriptan HCl)

RX	GLAXO WELLCOME INC	P. 1090

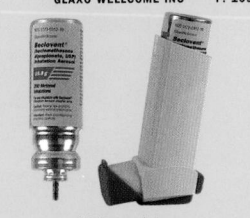

20 mg/mL
10-mL multiple-dose vial

**Anectine®
Injection, USP**
(succinylcholine chloride)

RX	GLAXO WELLCOME INC	P. 1092

16.8-g canister
200 metered inhalations
Also available in a 6.7-g canister
*The appearance of this inhaler is a
trademark of Glaxo Wellcome.*

**Beclovent®
Inhalation Aerosol**
(beclomethasone dipropionate, USP)

RX	GLAXO WELLCOME INC	P. 1092

16.8-g canister
200 metered inhalations

**Beclovent®
Inhalation Aerosol Refill**
(beclomethasone dipropionate, USP)

RX	GLAXO WELLCOME INC	P. 1093

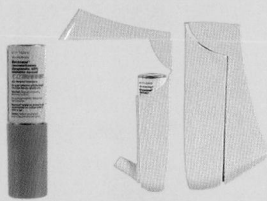

16.8-g canister
200 metered inhalations
Also available in a 6.7-g canister

**Beconase®
Inhalation Aerosol**
(beclomethasone dipropionate, USP)

RX	GLAXO WELLCOME INC	P. 1095

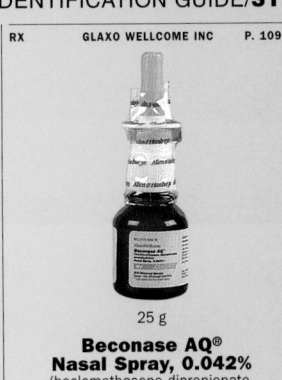

25 g

**Beconase AQ®
Nasal Spray, 0.042%**
(beclomethasone dipropionate,
monohydrate)

RX	GLAXO WELLCOME INC	P. 1100

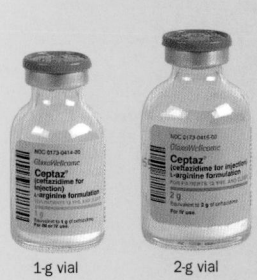

1-g vial   2-g vial

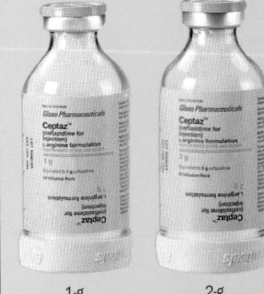

1-g   2-g
IV infusion pack IV infusion pack

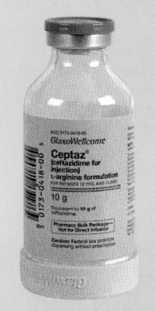

10-g
pharmacy bulk package

Ceptaz®
(ceftazidime for injection)
L-arginine formulation

RX	GLAXO WELLCOME INC	P. 1096

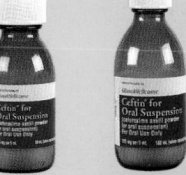

125 mg/5 mL   125 mg/5 mL
50 mL   100 mL

*Also available in 50- and 100-mL
bottles of 250 mg/5 mL.*

Ceftin® for Oral Suspension
(cefuroxime axetil powder for
oral suspension)

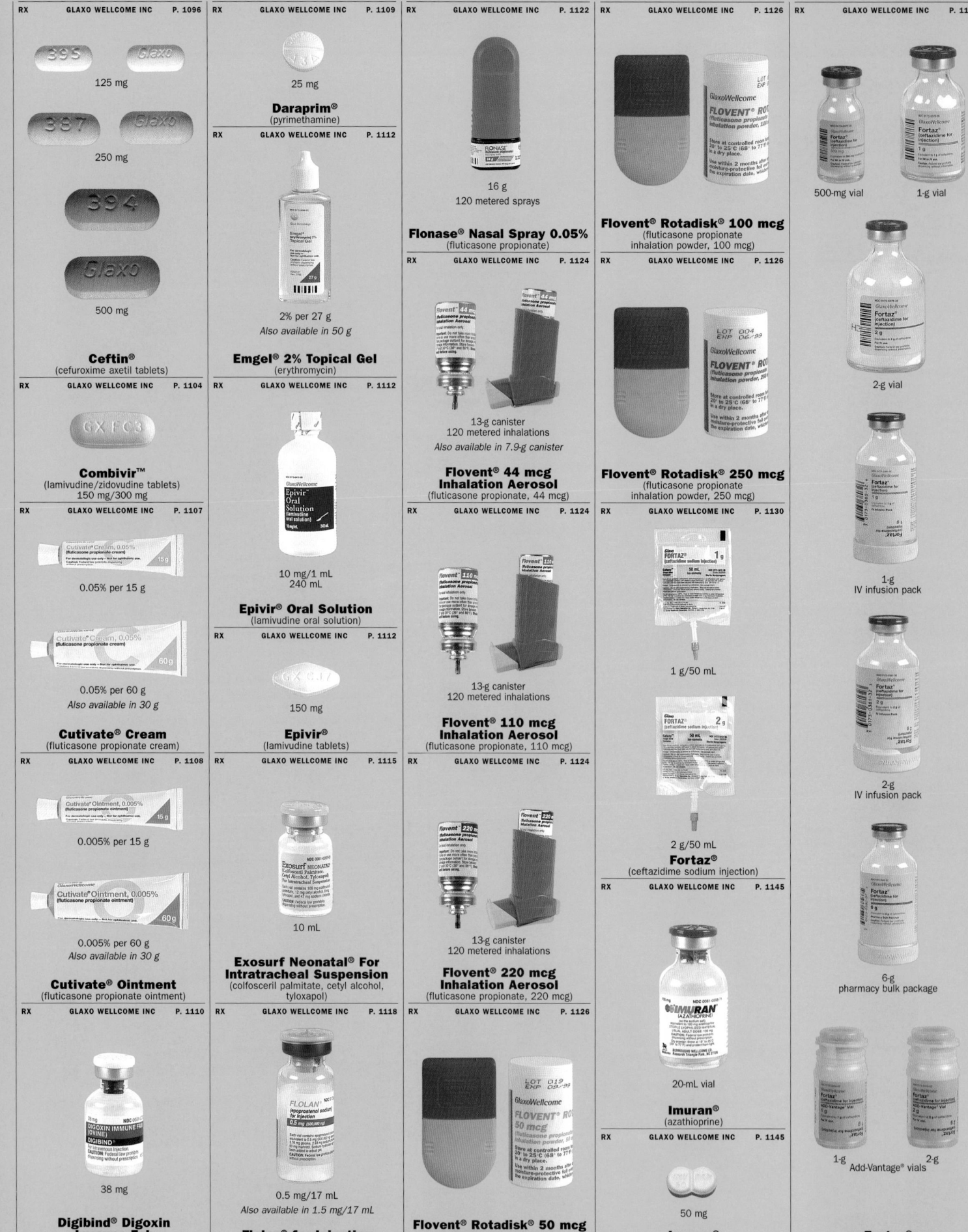

RX   GLAXO WELLCOME INC   P. 1096

125 mg

250 mg

500 mg

Ceftin®
(cefuroxime axetil tablets)

RX   GLAXO WELLCOME INC   P. 1104

GX FC3

Combivir™
(lamivudine/zidovudine tablets)
150 mg/300 mg

RX   GLAXO WELLCOME INC   P. 1107

0.05% per 15 g

0.05% per 60 g
Also available in 30 g

Cutivate® Cream
(fluticasone propionate cream)

RX   GLAXO WELLCOME INC   P. 1108

0.005% per 15 g

0.005% per 60 g
Also available in 30 g

Cutivate® Ointment
(fluticasone propionate ointment)

RX   GLAXO WELLCOME INC   P. 1110

38 mg

**Digibind® Digoxin
Immune Fab**
(Ovine)

RX   GLAXO WELLCOME INC   P. 1109

25 mg

Daraprim®
(pyrimethamine)

RX   GLAXO WELLCOME INC   P. 1112

2% per 27 g
Also available in 50 g

Emgel® 2% Topical Gel
(erythromycin)

RX   GLAXO WELLCOME INC   P. 1112

10 mg/1 mL
240 mL

Epivir® Oral Solution
(lamivudine oral solution)

RX   GLAXO WELLCOME INC   P. 1112

150 mg

Epivir®
(lamivudine tablets)

RX   GLAXO WELLCOME INC   P. 1115

10 mL

**Exosurf Neonatal® For
Intratracheal Suspension**
(colfosceril palmitate, cetyl alcohol,
tyloxapol)

RX   GLAXO WELLCOME INC   P. 1118

0.5 mg/17 mL
Also available in 1.5 mg/17 mL

Flolan® for Injection
(epoprostenol sodium)

RX   GLAXO WELLCOME INC   P. 1122

16 g
120 metered sprays

Flonase® Nasal Spray 0.05%
(fluticasone propionate)

RX   GLAXO WELLCOME INC   P. 1124

13-g canister
120 metered inhalations
Also available in 7.9-g canister

**Flovent® 44 mcg
Inhalation Aerosol**
(fluticasone propionate, 44 mcg)

RX   GLAXO WELLCOME INC   P. 1124

13-g canister
120 metered inhalations

**Flovent® 110 mcg
Inhalation Aerosol**
(fluticasone propionate, 110 mcg)

RX   GLAXO WELLCOME INC   P. 1124

13-g canister
120 metered inhalations

**Flovent® 220 mcg
Inhalation Aerosol**
(fluticasone propionate, 220 mcg)

RX   GLAXO WELLCOME INC   P. 1126

Flovent® Rotadisk® 50 mcg
(fluticasone propionate
inhalation powder, 50 mcg)

RX   GLAXO WELLCOME INC   P. 1126

Flovent® Rotadisk® 100 mcg
(fluticasone propionate
inhalation powder, 100 mcg)

RX   GLAXO WELLCOME INC   P. 1126

Flovent® Rotadisk® 250 mcg
(fluticasone propionate
inhalation powder, 250 mcg)

RX   GLAXO WELLCOME INC   P. 1130

1 g/50 mL

2 g/50 mL

Fortaz®
(ceftazidime sodium injection)

RX   GLAXO WELLCOME INC   P. 1145

20-mL vial

Imuran®
(azathioprine)

RX   GLAXO WELLCOME INC   P. 1145

50 mg

Imuran®
(azathioprine)

RX   GLAXO WELLCOME INC   P. 1130

500-mg vial   1-g vial

2-g vial

1-g
IV infusion pack

2-g
IV infusion pack

6-g
pharmacy bulk package

1-g   2-g
Add-Vantage® vials

Fortaz®
(ceftazidime for injection)

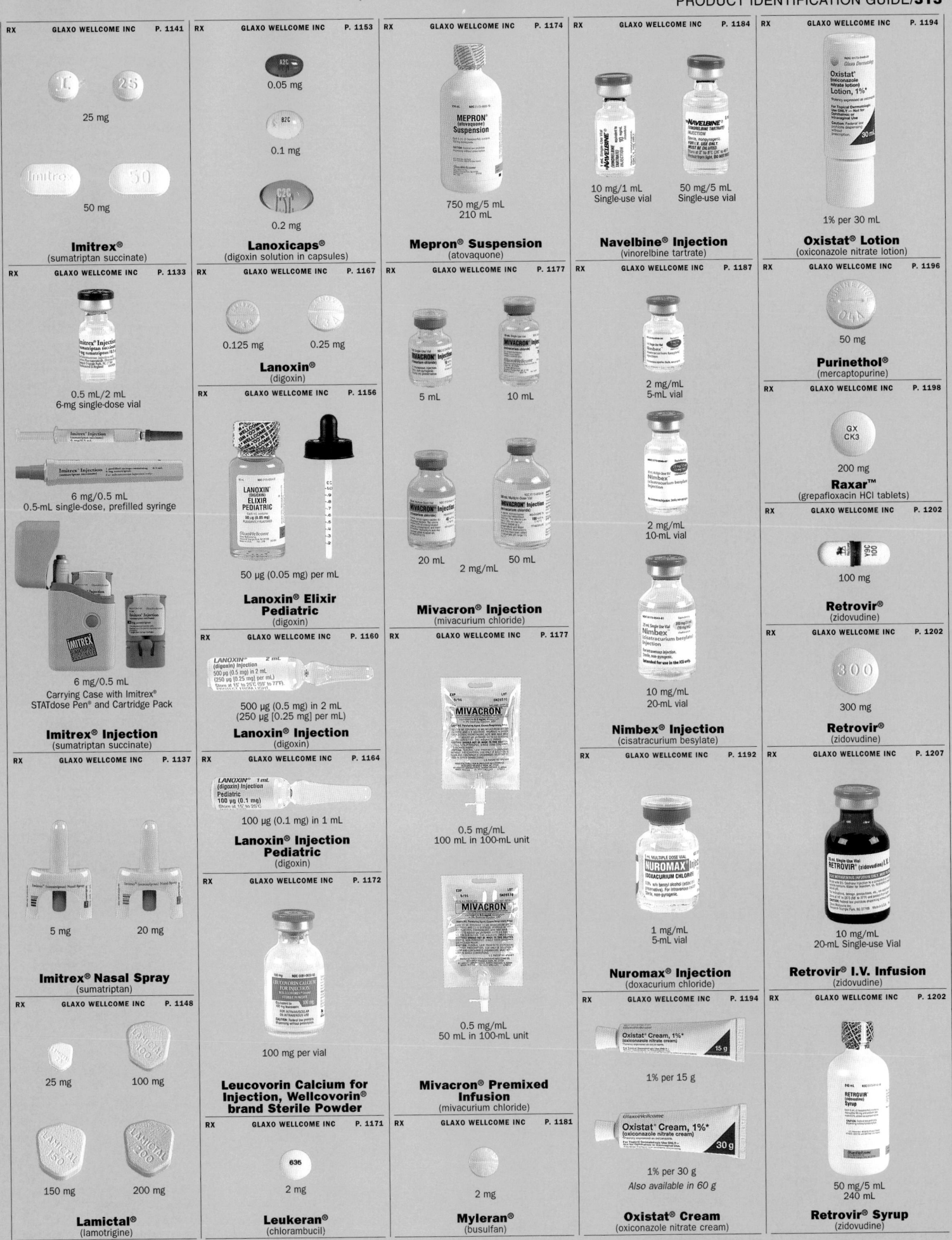

RX   GLAXO WELLCOME INC   P. 1141

25 mg

50 mg

Imitrex®
(sumatriptan succinate)

RX   GLAXO WELLCOME INC   P. 1133

0.5 mL/2 mL
6-mg single-dose vial

6 mg/0.5 mL
0.5-mL single-dose, prefilled syringe

6 mg/0.5 mL
Carrying Case with Imitrex®
STATdose Pen® and Cartridge Pack

Imitrex® Injection
(sumatriptan succinate)

RX   GLAXO WELLCOME INC   P. 1137

5 mg   20 mg

Imitrex® Nasal Spray
(sumatriptan)

RX   GLAXO WELLCOME INC   P. 1148

25 mg   100 mg

150 mg   200 mg

Lamictal®
(lamotrigine)

RX   GLAXO WELLCOME INC   P. 1153

0.05 mg

0.1 mg

0.2 mg

Lanoxicaps®
(digoxin solution in capsules)

RX   GLAXO WELLCOME INC   P. 1167

0.125 mg   0.25 mg

Lanoxin®
(digoxin)

RX   GLAXO WELLCOME INC   P. 1156

50 µg (0.05 mg) per mL

**Lanoxin® Elixir
Pediatric**
(digoxin)

RX   GLAXO WELLCOME INC   P. 1160

500 µg (0.5 mg) in 2 mL
(250 µg [0.25 mg] per mL)

Lanoxin® Injection
(digoxin)

RX   GLAXO WELLCOME INC   P. 1164

100 µg (0.1 mg) in 1 mL

**Lanoxin® Injection
Pediatric**
(digoxin)

RX   GLAXO WELLCOME INC   P. 1172

100 mg per vial

**Leucovorin Calcium for
Injection, Wellcovorin®
brand Sterile Powder**

RX   GLAXO WELLCOME INC   P. 1171

2 mg

Leukeran®
(chlorambucil)

RX   GLAXO WELLCOME INC   P. 1174

MEPRON®
(atovaquone)
Suspension

750 mg/5 mL
210 mL

Mepron® Suspension
(atovaquone)

RX   GLAXO WELLCOME INC   P. 1177

5 mL   10 mL

20 mL   50 mL
2 mg/mL

Mivacron® Injection
(mivacurium chloride)

RX   GLAXO WELLCOME INC   P. 1177

MIVACRON®

0.5 mg/mL
100 mL in 100-mL unit

MIVACRON®

0.5 mg/mL
50 mL in 100-mL unit

**Mivacron® Premixed
Infusion**
(mivacurium chloride)

RX   GLAXO WELLCOME INC   P. 1181

2 mg

Myleran®
(busulfan)

RX   GLAXO WELLCOME INC   P. 1184

10 mg/1 mL   50 mg/5 mL
Single-use vial   Single-use vial

Navelbine® Injection
(vinorelbine tartrate)

RX   GLAXO WELLCOME INC   P. 1187

2 mg/mL
5-mL vial

2 mg/mL
10-mL vial

Nimbex

10 mg/mL
20-mL vial

Nimbex® Injection
(cisatracurium besylate)

RX   GLAXO WELLCOME INC   P. 1192

NUROMAX®
DOXACURIUM CHLORIDE

1 mg/mL
5-mL vial

Nuromax® Injection
(doxacurium chloride)

RX   GLAXO WELLCOME INC   P. 1194

Oxistat® Cream, 1%*
(oxiconazole nitrate cream)
15 g

1% per 15 g

Oxistat® Cream, 1%*
(oxiconazole nitrate cream)
30 g

1% per 30 g
Also available in 60 g

Oxistat® Cream
(oxiconazole nitrate cream)

RX   GLAXO WELLCOME INC   P. 1194

Oxistat®
(oxiconazole
nitrate)
Lotion, 1%*

1% per 30 mL

Oxistat® Lotion
(oxiconazole nitrate lotion)

RX   GLAXO WELLCOME INC   P. 1196

50 mg

Purinethol®
(mercaptopurine)

RX   GLAXO WELLCOME INC   P. 1198

GX
CK3

200 mg

Raxar™
(grepafloxacin HCl tablets)

RX   GLAXO WELLCOME INC   P. 1202

100 mg

Retrovir®
(zidovudine)

RX   GLAXO WELLCOME INC   P. 1202

300 mg

Retrovir®
(zidovudine)

RX   GLAXO WELLCOME INC   P. 1207

RETROVIR® (zidovudine) I.V.

10 mg/mL
20-mL Single-use Vial

Retrovir® I.V. Infusion
(zidovudine)

RX   GLAXO WELLCOME INC   P. 1202

RETROVIR®
(zidovudine)
Syrup

50 mg/5 mL
240 mL

Retrovir® Syrup
(zidovudine)

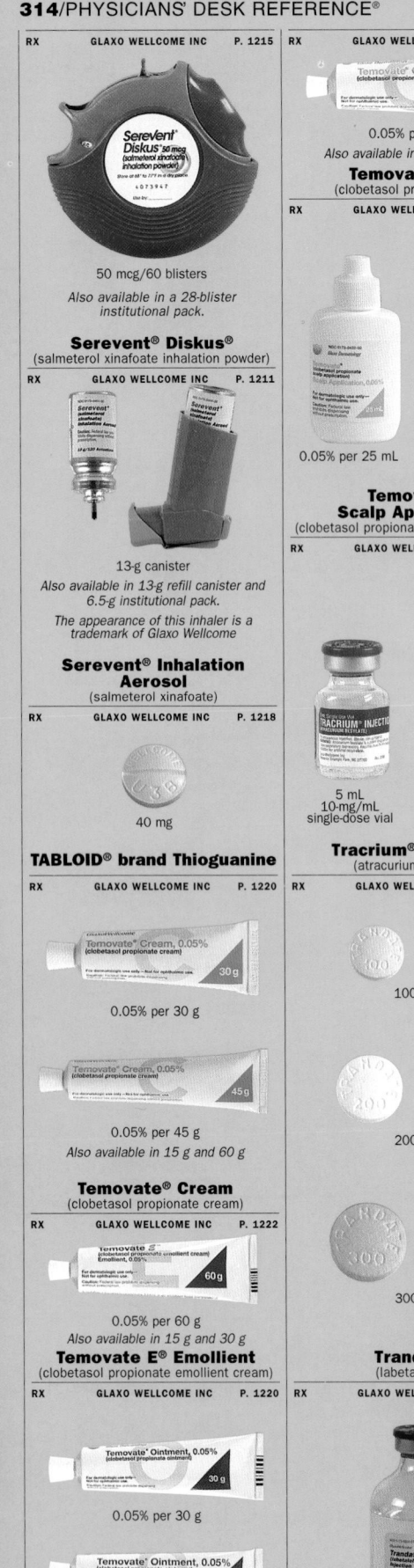

RX   GLAXO WELLCOME INC   P. 1215

50 mcg/60 blisters

Also available in a 28-blister institutional pack.

Serevent® Diskus®
(salmeterol xinafoate inhalation powder)

RX   GLAXO WELLCOME INC   P. 1211

13-g canister

Also available in 13-g refill canister and 6.5-g institutional pack.

The appearance of this inhaler is a trademark of Glaxo Wellcome

Serevent® Inhalation Aerosol
(salmeterol xinafoate)

RX   GLAXO WELLCOME INC   P. 1218

40 mg

TABLOID® brand Thioguanine

RX   GLAXO WELLCOME INC   P. 1220

30 g

0.05% per 30 g

45 g

0.05% per 45 g
Also available in 15 g and 60 g

Temovate® Cream
(clobetasol propionate cream)

RX   GLAXO WELLCOME INC   P. 1222

60 g

0.05% per 60 g
Also available in 15 g and 30 g

Temovate E® Emollient
(clobetasol propionate emollient cream)

RX   GLAXO WELLCOME INC   P. 1220

30 g

0.05% per 30 g

45 g

0.05% per 45 g
Also available in 15 g and 60 g

Temovate® Ointment
(clobetasol propionate ointment)

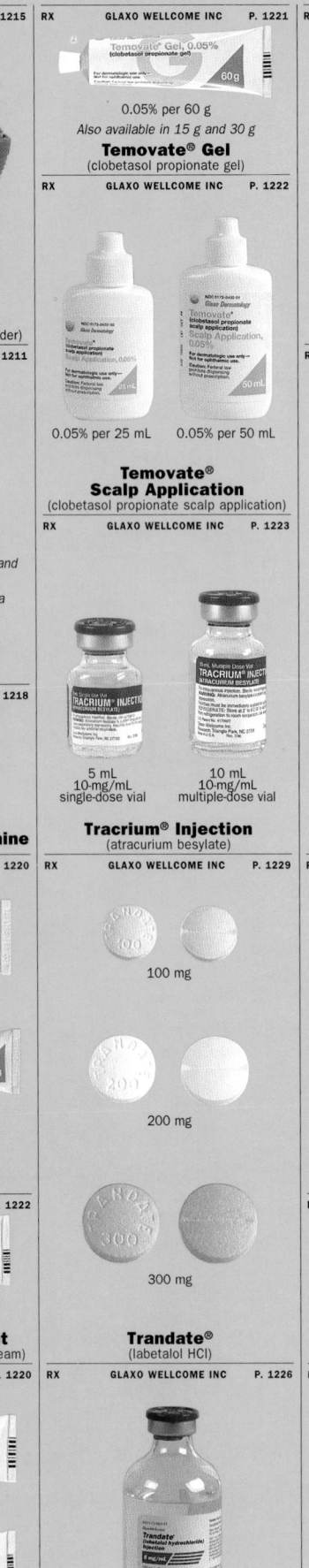

RX   GLAXO WELLCOME INC   P. 1221

60 g

0.05% per 60 g
Also available in 15 g and 30 g

Temovate® Gel
(clobetasol propionate gel)

RX   GLAXO WELLCOME INC   P. 1222

0.05% per 25 mL   0.05% per 50 mL

**Temovate®
Scalp Application**
(clobetasol propionate scalp application)

RX   GLAXO WELLCOME INC   P. 1223

5 mL
10-mg/mL
single-dose vial   10 mL
10-mg/mL
multiple-dose vial

Tracrium® Injection
(atracurium besylate)

RX   GLAXO WELLCOME INC   P. 1229

100 mg

200 mg

300 mg

Trandate®
(labetalol HCl)

RX   GLAXO WELLCOME INC   P. 1226

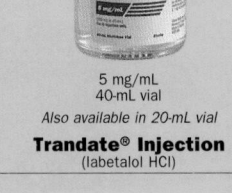

5 mg/mL
40-mL vial

Also available in 20-mL vial

Trandate® Injection
(labetalol HCl)

RX   GLAXO WELLCOME INC   P. 1231

400 mg

Tritec®
(ranitidine bismuth citrate)

RX   GLAXO WELLCOME INC   P. 1233

1 mg
3-mL vial

2 mg
5-mL vial   5 mg
10-mL vial

Ultiva™ for Injection
(remifentanil HCl)

RX   GLAXO WELLCOME INC   P. 1239

500 mg

1 g

Valtrex®
(valacyclovir HCl)

RX   GLAXO WELLCOME INC   P. 1241

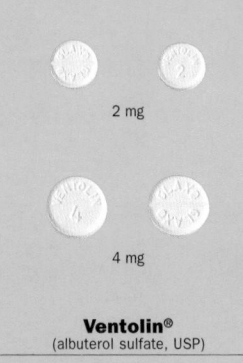

20 mg in 1 mL

Vasoxyl® Injection
(methoxamine HCl)

RX   GLAXO WELLCOME INC   P. 1250

2 mg

4 mg

Ventolin®
(albuterol sulfate, USP)

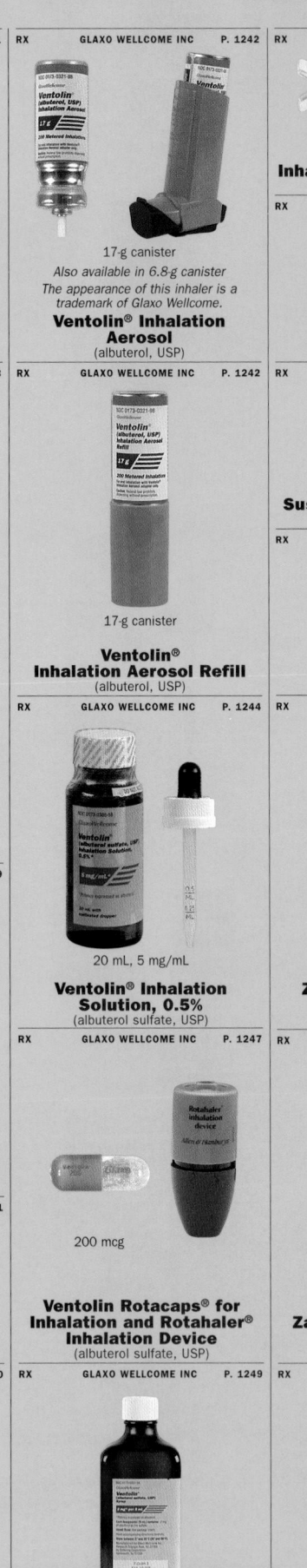

RX   GLAXO WELLCOME INC   P. 1242

17-g canister

*Also available in 6.8-g canister
The appearance of this inhaler is a
trademark of Glaxo Wellcome.*

**Ventolin® Inhalation
Aerosol**
(albuterol, USP)

RX   GLAXO WELLCOME INC   P. 1242

17-g canister

**Ventolin®
Inhalation Aerosol Refill**
(albuterol, USP)

RX   GLAXO WELLCOME INC   P. 1244

20 mL, 5 mg/mL

**Ventolin® Inhalation
Solution, 0.5%**
(albuterol sulfate, USP)

RX   GLAXO WELLCOME INC   P. 1247

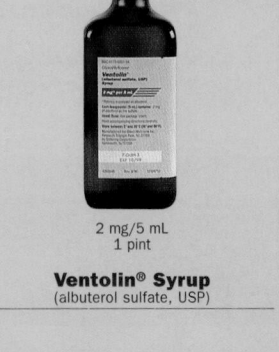

200 mcg

**Ventolin Rotacaps® for
Inhalation and Rotahaler®
Inhalation Device**
(albuterol sulfate, USP)

RX   GLAXO WELLCOME INC   P. 1249

2 mg/5 mL
1 pint

Ventolin® Syrup
(albuterol sulfate, USP)

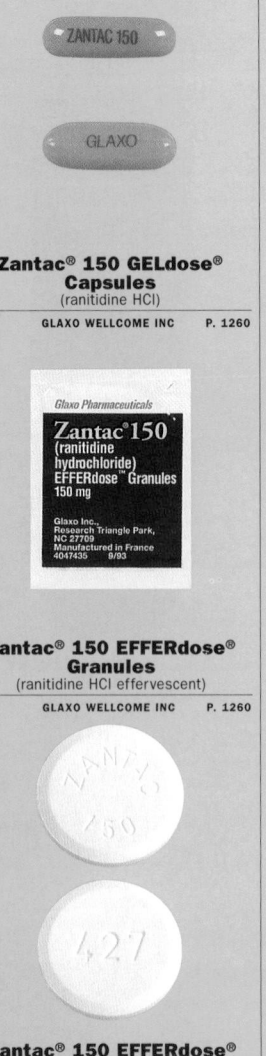

RX   GLAXO WELLCOME INC   P. 1246

2.5 mg/3 mL per 3-mL nebules

**Ventolin Nebules®
Inhalation Solution, 0.083%**
(albuterol sulfate, USP)

RX   GLAXO WELLCOME INC   P. 1252

75 mg   100 mg

Wellbutrin®
(bupropion HCl)

RX   GLAXO WELLCOME INC   P. 1255

100 mg   150 mg

**Wellbutrin SR®
Sustained-Release Tablets**
(bupropion HCl)

RX   GLAXO WELLCOME INC   P. 1260

150 mg

*The shape of this tablet is a
trademark of Glaxo Wellcome.*

Zantac® 150
(ranitidine HCl)

RX   GLAXO WELLCOME INC   P. 1260

ZANTAC 150

GLAXO

**Zantac® 150 GELdose®
Capsules**
(ranitidine HCl)

RX   GLAXO WELLCOME INC   P. 1260

Glaxo Pharmaceuticals

Zantac® 150
(ranitidine
hydrochloride)
EFFERdose™ Granules
150 mg

Glaxo Inc.,
Research Triangle Park,
NC 27709
Manufactured in France
4047435   9/93

**Zantac® 150 EFFERdose®
Granules**
(ranitidine HCl effervescent)

RX   GLAXO WELLCOME INC   P. 1260

427

Zantac® 150 EFFERdose®
(ranitidine HCl effervescent)

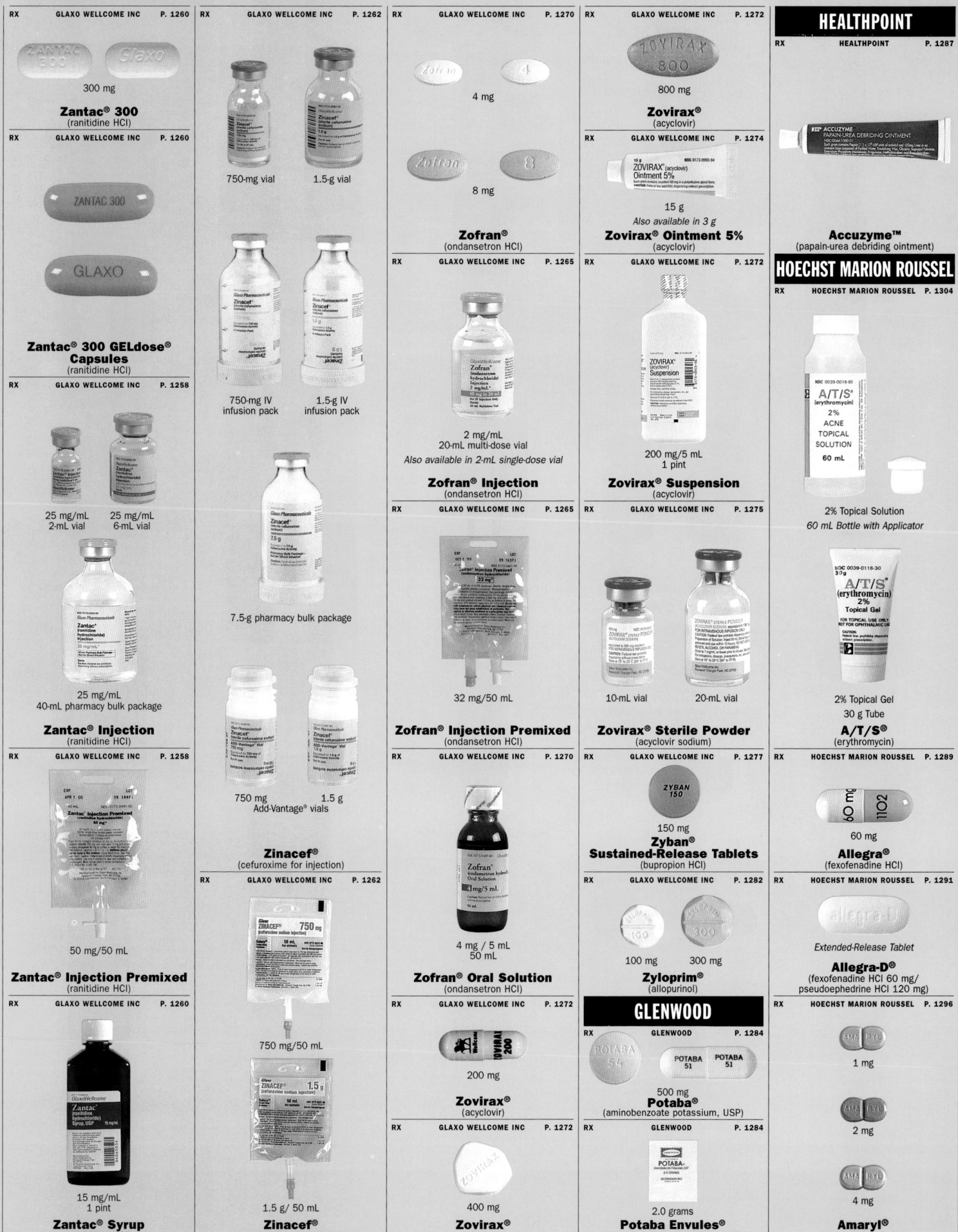

RX · GLAXO WELLCOME INC · P. 1260

300 mg
Zantac® 300
(ranitidine HCl)

RX · GLAXO WELLCOME INC · P. 1260

Zantac® 300 GELdose® Capsules
(ranitidine HCl)

RX · GLAXO WELLCOME INC · P. 1258

25 mg/mL 2-mL vial   25 mg/mL 6-mL vial

25 mg/mL 40-mL pharmacy bulk package
Zantac® Injection
(ranitidine HCl)

RX · GLAXO WELLCOME INC · P. 1258

50 mg/50 mL
Zantac® Injection Premixed
(ranitidine HCl)

RX · GLAXO WELLCOME INC · P. 1260

15 mg/mL 1 pint
Zantac® Syrup
(ranitidine HCl)

RX · GLAXO WELLCOME INC · P. 1262

750-mg vial   1.5-g vial

750-mg IV infusion pack   1.5-g IV infusion pack

7.5-g pharmacy bulk package

750 mg   1.5 g
Add-Vantage® vials
Zinacef®
(cefuroxime for injection)

RX · GLAXO WELLCOME INC · P. 1262

750 mg/50 mL

1.5 g/50 mL
Zinacef®
(cefuroxime injection)

RX · GLAXO WELLCOME INC · P. 1270

4 mg

8 mg
Zofran®
(ondansetron HCl)

RX · GLAXO WELLCOME INC · P. 1265

2 mg/mL
20-mL multi-dose vial
Also available in 2-mL single-dose vial
Zofran® Injection
(ondansetron HCl)

RX · GLAXO WELLCOME INC · P. 1265

32 mg/50 mL
Zofran® Injection Premixed
(ondansetron HCl)

RX · GLAXO WELLCOME INC · P. 1270

4 mg / 5 mL
50 mL
Zofran® Oral Solution
(ondansetron HCl)

RX · GLAXO WELLCOME INC · P. 1272

200 mg
Zovirax®
(acyclovir)

RX · GLAXO WELLCOME INC · P. 1272

400 mg
Zovirax®
(acyclovir)

RX · GLAXO WELLCOME INC · P. 1272

800 mg
Zovirax®
(acyclovir)

RX · GLAXO WELLCOME INC · P. 1274

15 g
Also available in 3 g
Zovirax® Ointment 5%
(acyclovir)

RX · GLAXO WELLCOME INC · P. 1272

200 mg/5 mL
1 pint
Zovirax® Suspension
(acyclovir)

RX · GLAXO WELLCOME INC · P. 1275

10-mL vial   20-mL vial
Zovirax® Sterile Powder
(acyclovir sodium)

RX · GLAXO WELLCOME INC · P. 1277

150 mg
**Zyban®
Sustained-Release Tablets**
(bupropion HCl)

RX · GLAXO WELLCOME INC · P. 1282

100 mg   300 mg
Zyloprim®
(allopurinol)

GLENWOOD

RX · GLENWOOD · P. 1284

500 mg
Potaba®
(aminobenzoate potassium, USP)

RX · GLENWOOD · P. 1284

2.0 grams
Potaba Envules®
(aminobenzoate potassium, USP)

HEALTHPOINT

RX · HEALTHPOINT · P. 1287

Accuzyme™
(papain-urea debriding ointment)

HOECHST MARION ROUSSEL

RX · HOECHST MARION ROUSSEL · P. 1304

2% Topical Solution
60 mL Bottle with Applicator

2% Topical Gel
30 g Tube
A/T/S®
(erythromycin)

RX · HOECHST MARION ROUSSEL · P. 1289

60 mg
Allegra®
(fexofenadine HCl)

RX · HOECHST MARION ROUSSEL · P. 1291

Extended-Release Tablet
Allegra-D®
(fexofenadine HCl 60 mg/
pseudoephedrine HCl 120 mg)

RX · HOECHST MARION ROUSSEL · P. 1296

1 mg

2 mg

4 mg
Amaryl®
(glimepiride tablets)

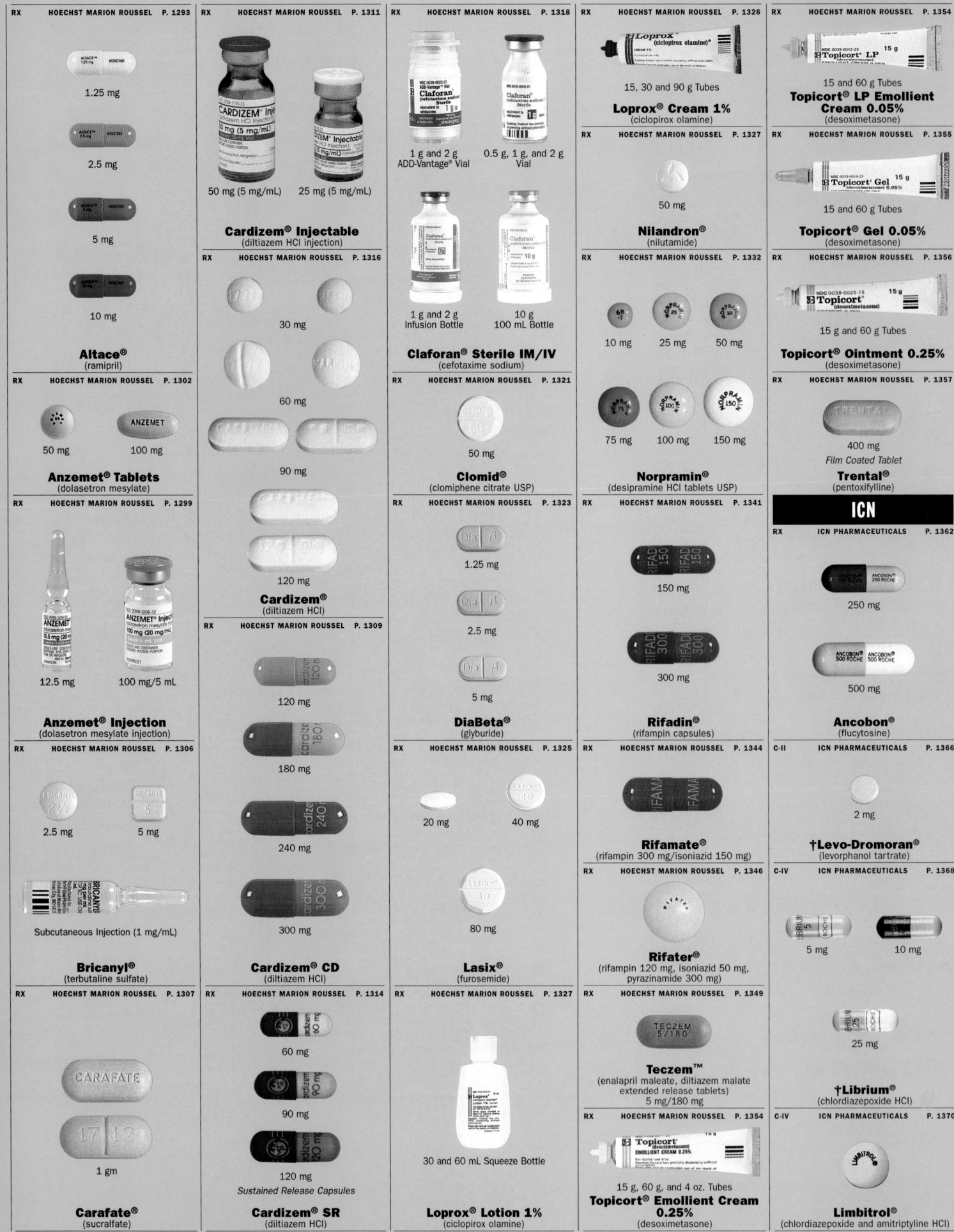

RX   HOECHST MARION ROUSSEL   P. 1293

1.25 mg

2.5 mg

5 mg

10 mg

Altace®
(ramipril)

RX   HOECHST MARION ROUSSEL   P. 1302

50 mg   100 mg

Anzemet® Tablets
(dolasetron mesylate)

RX   HOECHST MARION ROUSSEL   P. 1299

12.5 mg   100 mg/5 mL

Anzemet® Injection
(dolasetron mesylate injection)

RX   HOECHST MARION ROUSSEL   P. 1306

2.5 mg   5 mg

Subcutaneous Injection (1 mg/mL)

Bricanyl®
(terbutaline sulfate)

RX   HOECHST MARION ROUSSEL   P. 1307

CARAFATE

17 | 12

1 gm

Carafate®
(sucralfate)

RX   HOECHST MARION ROUSSEL   P. 1311

50 mg (5 mg/mL)   25 mg (5 mg/mL)

Cardizem® Injectable
(diltiazem HCl injection)

RX   HOECHST MARION ROUSSEL   P. 1316

30 mg

60 mg

90 mg

120 mg

Cardizem®
(diltiazem HCl)

RX   HOECHST MARION ROUSSEL   P. 1309

120 mg

180 mg

240 mg

300 mg

Cardizem® CD
(diltiazem HCl)

RX   HOECHST MARION ROUSSEL   P. 1314

60 mg

90 mg

120 mg

Cardizem® SR
(diltiazem HCl)

Sustained Release Capsules

RX   HOECHST MARION ROUSSEL   P. 1318

1 g and 2 g
ADD-Vantage® Vial

0.5 g, 1 g, and 2 g
Vial

1 g and 2 g
Infusion Bottle

10 g
100 mL Bottle

Claforan® Sterile IM/IV
(cefotaxime sodium)

RX   HOECHST MARION ROUSSEL   P. 1321

50 mg

Clomid®
(clomiphene citrate USP)

RX   HOECHST MARION ROUSSEL   P. 1323

1.25 mg

2.5 mg

5 mg

DiaBeta®
(glyburide)

RX   HOECHST MARION ROUSSEL   P. 1325

20 mg   40 mg

80 mg

Lasix®
(furosemide)

RX   HOECHST MARION ROUSSEL   P. 1327

30 and 60 mL Squeeze Bottle

Loprox® Lotion 1%
(ciclopirox olamine)

RX   HOECHST MARION ROUSSEL   P. 1326

15, 30 and 90 g Tubes

Loprox® Cream 1%
(ciclopirox olamine)

RX   HOECHST MARION ROUSSEL   P. 1327

50 mg

Nilandron®
(nilutamide)

RX   HOECHST MARION ROUSSEL   P. 1332

10 mg   25 mg   50 mg

75 mg   100 mg   150 mg

Norpramin®
(desipramine HCl tablets USP)

RX   HOECHST MARION ROUSSEL   P. 1341

150 mg

300 mg

Rifadin®
(rifampin capsules)

RX   HOECHST MARION ROUSSEL   P. 1344

Rifamate®
(rifampin 300 mg/isoniazid 150 mg)

RX   HOECHST MARION ROUSSEL   P. 1346

Rifater®
(rifampin 120 mg, isoniazid 50 mg,
pyrazinamide 300 mg)

RX   HOECHST MARION ROUSSEL   P. 1349

TECZEM
5/180

Teczem™
(enalapril maleate, diltiazem malate
extended release tablets)
5 mg/180 mg

RX   HOECHST MARION ROUSSEL   P. 1354

15 g, 60 g, and 4 oz. Tubes

**Topicort® Emollient Cream
0.25%**
(desoximetasone)

RX   HOECHST MARION ROUSSEL   P. 1354

15 and 60 g Tubes

**Topicort® LP Emollient
Cream 0.05%**
(desoximetasone)

RX   HOECHST MARION ROUSSEL   P. 1355

15 and 60 g Tubes

Topicort® Gel 0.05%
(desoximetasone)

RX   HOECHST MARION ROUSSEL   P. 1356

15 g and 60 g Tubes

Topicort® Ointment 0.25%
(desoximetasone)

RX   HOECHST MARION ROUSSEL   P. 1357

400 mg
Film Coated Tablet

Trental®
(pentoxifylline)

ICN

RX   ICN PHARMACEUTICALS   P. 1362

250 mg

500 mg

Ancobon®
(flucytosine)

C-II   ICN PHARMACEUTICALS   P. 1366

2 mg

†Levo-Dromoran®
(levorphanol tartrate)

C-IV   ICN PHARMACEUTICALS   P. 1368

5 mg   10 mg

25 mg

†Librium®
(chlordiazepoxide HCl)

C-IV   ICN PHARMACEUTICALS   P. 1370

Limbitrol®
(chlordiazepoxide and amitriptyline HCl)

ICN PHARMACEUTICALS

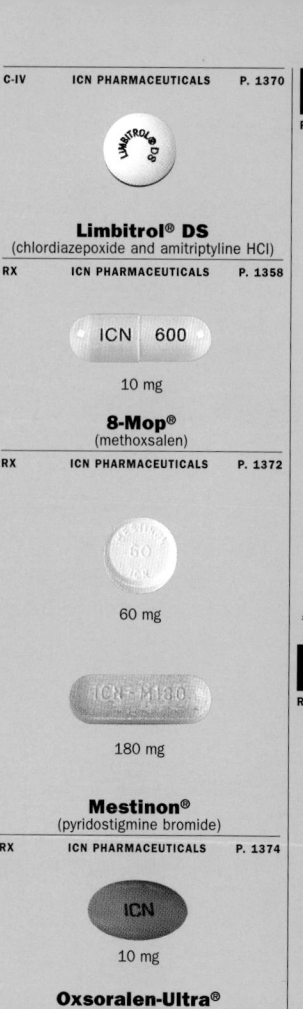

C-IV   ICN PHARMACEUTICALS   P. 1370

Limbitrol® DS
(chlordiazepoxide and amitriptyline HCl)

RX   ICN PHARMACEUTICALS   P. 1358

ICN 600

10 mg

8-Mop®
(methoxsalen)

RX   ICN PHARMACEUTICALS   P. 1372

60 mg

180 mg

Mestinon®
(pyridostigmine bromide)

RX   ICN PHARMACEUTICALS   P. 1374

ICN

10 mg

Oxsoralen-Ultra®
(methoxsalen)

RX   ICN PHARMACEUTICALS   P. 1378

15 mg

Prostigmin®
(neostigmine bromide)

C-III   ICN PHARMACEUTICALS   P. 1380

10 mg

Testred®
(methyltestosterone)

RX   ICN PHARMACEUTICALS   P. 1381

ICN

5 mg

Trisoralen®
(trioxsalen)

While every effort has been made to reproduce products faithfully, this section is to be considered a quick reference identification aid. In cases of suspected overdosage, etc., chemical analysis of the product should be done.

Designed to help you identify drugs, this section contains actual size pills and full color reproduction of products selected for inclusion by participating manufacturers.

IDEC

RX   IDEC PHARMACEUTICALS   P. 1384

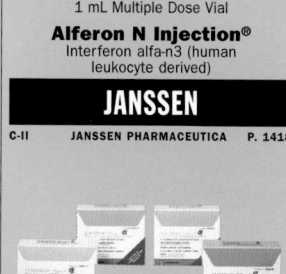

100 mg (10mg/mL)

500 mg (10mg/mL)

Rituxan™
(Rituximab)
Jointly marketed by IDEC Pharmaceuticals Corp. and Genentech, Inc.

INTERFERON SCIENCES

RX   INTERFERON SCIENCES, INC.   P. 1413

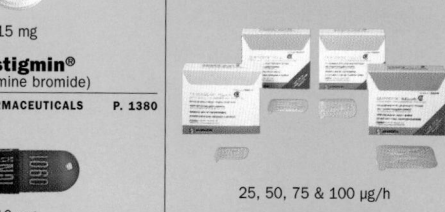

1 mL Multiple Dose Vial

Alferon N Injection®
Interferon alfa-n3 (human leukocyte derived)

JANSSEN

C-II   JANSSEN PHARMACEUTICA   P. 1418

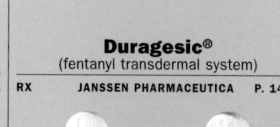

25, 50, 75 & 100 µg/h

Duragesic®
(fentanyl transdermal system)

RX   JANSSEN PHARMACEUTICA   P. 1422

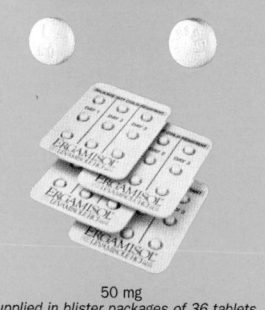

50 mg
Supplied in blister packages of 36 tablets

Ergamisol®
(levamisole HCl)

RX   JANSSEN PHARMACEUTICA   P. 1423

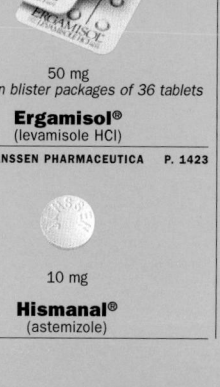

10 mg

Hismanal®
(astemizole)

JANSSEN (continued)

RX   JANSSEN PHARMACEUTICA   P. 1426

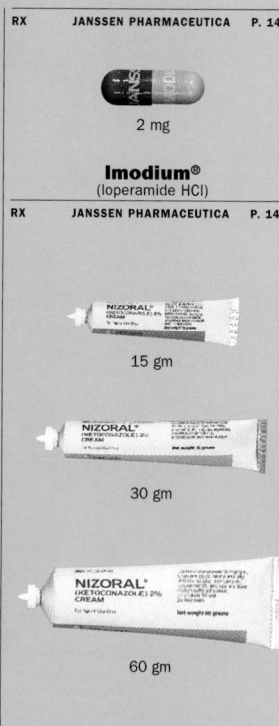

2 mg

Imodium®
(loperamide HCl)

RX   JANSSEN PHARMACEUTICA   P. 1427

15 gm

30 gm

60 gm

Nizoral® 2% Cream
(ketoconazole)

RX   JANSSEN PHARMACEUTICA   P. 1428

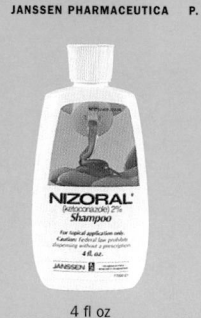

200 mg

Nizoral®
(ketoconazole)

RX   JANSSEN PHARMACEUTICA   P. 1427

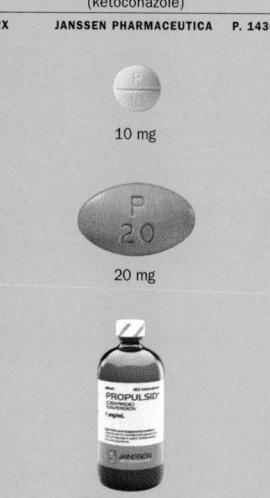

4 fl oz

Nizoral® 2% Shampoo
(ketoconazole)

RX   JANSSEN PHARMACEUTICA   P. 1430

10 mg

P 20

20 mg

Propulsid®
(cisapride)

450 mL 1 mg/mL

JANSSEN (continued)

RX   JANSSEN PHARMACEUTICA   P. 1432

R 1   R 2
1 mg   2 mg

R 3   R 4
3 mg   4 mg

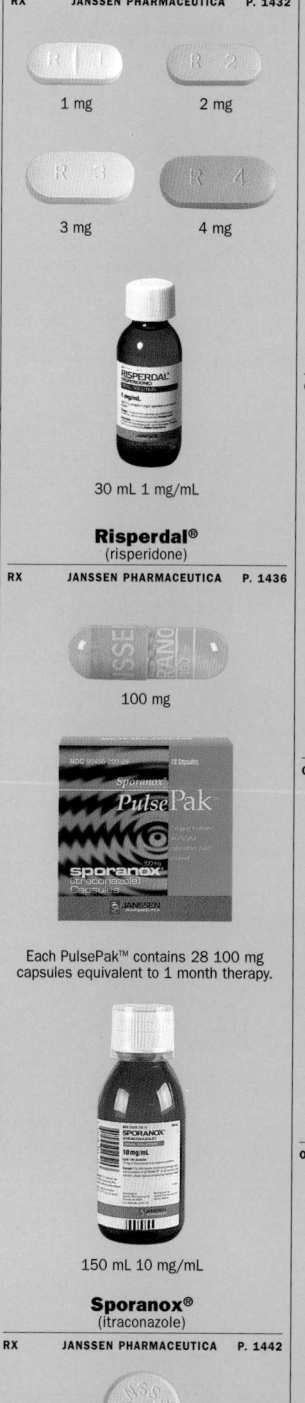

30 mL 1 mg/mL

Risperdal®
(risperidone)

RX   JANSSEN PHARMACEUTICA   P. 1436

100 mg

Sporanox PulsePak

Each PulsePak™ contains 28 100 mg capsules equivalent to 1 month therapy.

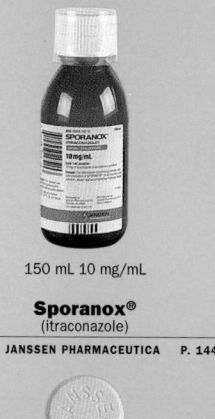

150 mL 10 mg/mL

Sporanox®
(itraconazole)

RX   JANSSEN PHARMACEUTICA   P. 1442

100 mg

Vermox®
(mebendazole)

J&J-MERCK CONSUMER

OTC   J&J-MERCK CONSUMER   P. 1443

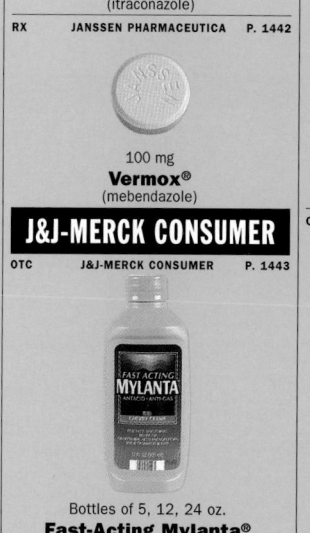

Bottles of 5, 12, 24 oz.

Fast-Acting Mylanta®
(aluminum hydroxide, magnesium hydroxide, simethicone)
200 mg / 200 mg / 20 mg

J&J-MERCK CONSUMER (continued)

OTC   J&J-MERCK CONSUMER   P. 1443

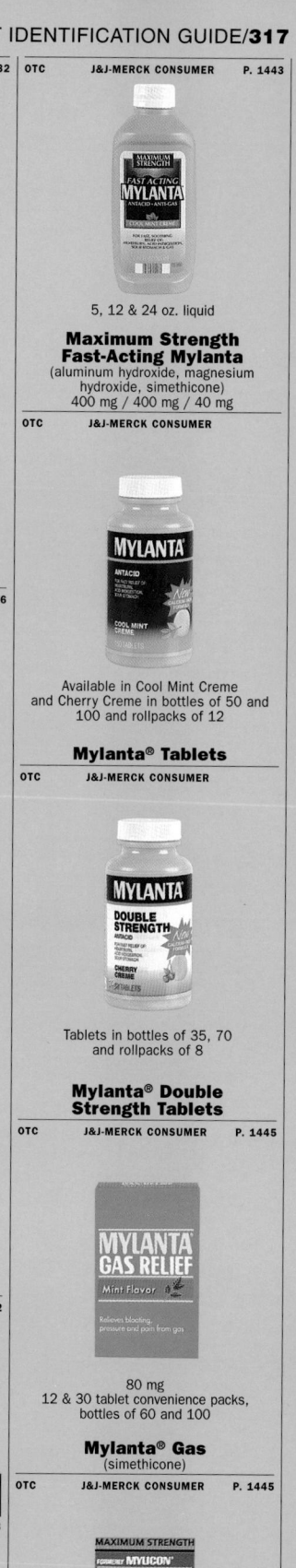

5, 12 & 24 oz. liquid

Maximum Strength Fast-Acting Mylanta
(aluminum hydroxide, magnesium hydroxide, simethicone)
400 mg / 400 mg / 40 mg

OTC   J&J-MERCK CONSUMER

Available in Cool Mint Creme and Cherry Creme in bottles of 50 and 100 and rollpacks of 12

Mylanta® Tablets

OTC   J&J-MERCK CONSUMER

Tablets in bottles of 35, 70 and rollpacks of 8

Mylanta® Double Strength Tablets

OTC   J&J-MERCK CONSUMER   P. 1445

80 mg
12 & 30 tablet convenience packs, bottles of 60 and 100

Mylanta® Gas
(simethicone)

OTC   J&J-MERCK CONSUMER   P. 1445

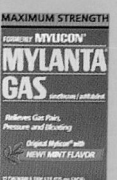

125 mg
12 & 24 tablet convenience packs

Maximum Strength Mylanta® Gas
(simethicone)

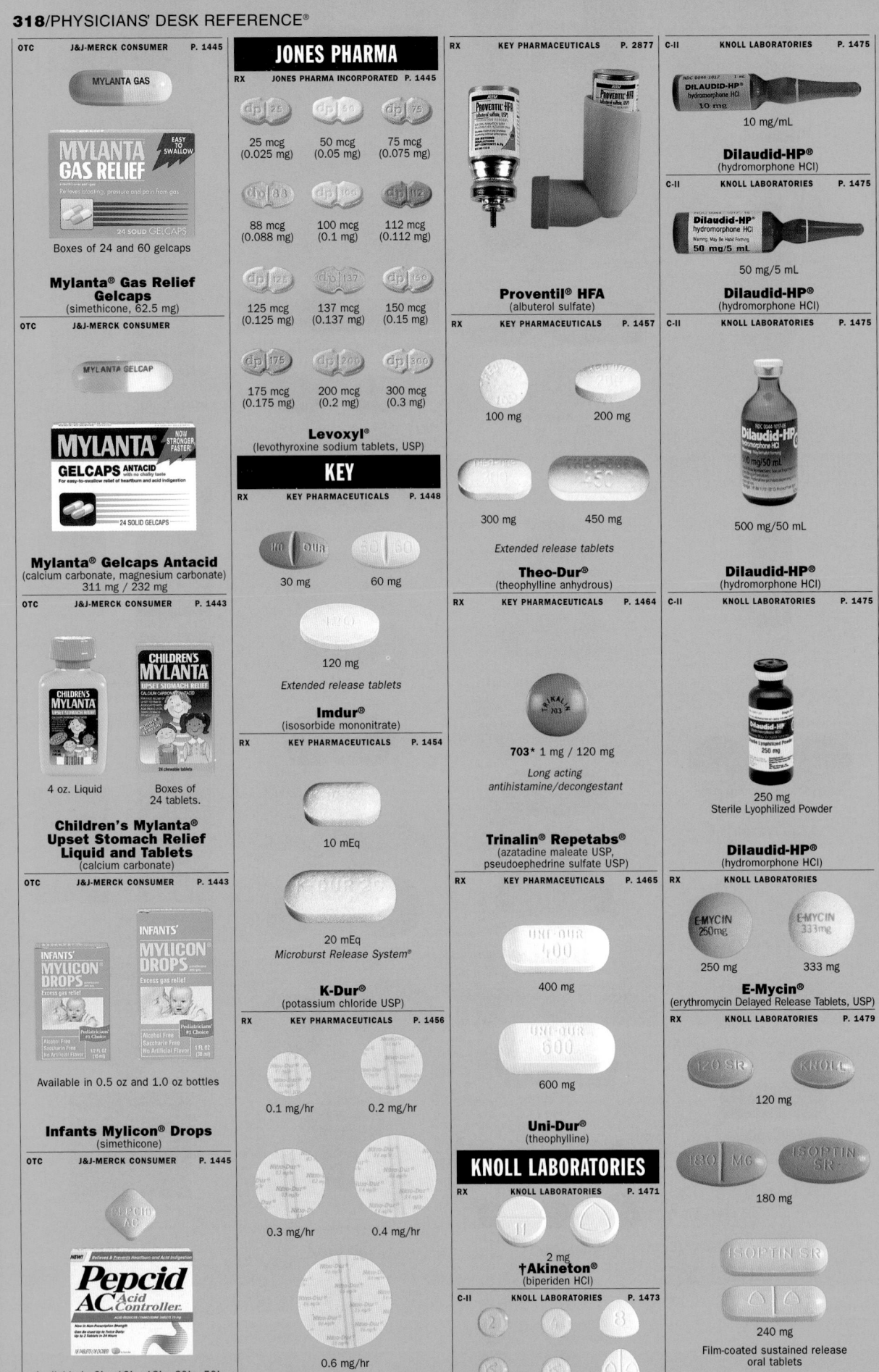

OTC J&J-MERCK CONSUMER P. 1445

MYLANTA GAS

MYLANTA GAS RELIEF
EASY TO SWALLOW

Boxes of 24 and 60 gelcaps

**Mylanta® Gas Relief
Gelcaps**
(simethicone, 62.5 mg)

OTC J&J-MERCK CONSUMER

MYLANTA GELCAP

MYLANTA
GELCAPS ANTACID

Mylanta® Gelcaps Antacid
(calcium carbonate, magnesium carbonate)
311 mg / 232 mg

OTC J&J-MERCK CONSUMER P. 1443

CHILDREN'S MYLANTA

4 oz. Liquid   Boxes of
24 tablets.

**Children's Mylanta®
Upset Stomach Relief
Liquid and Tablets**
(calcium carbonate)

OTC J&J-MERCK CONSUMER P. 1443

INFANTS' MYLICON DROPS

Available in 0.5 oz and 1.0 oz bottles

Infants Mylicon® Drops
(simethicone)

OTC J&J-MERCK CONSUMER P. 1445

**Pepcid
AC** Acid
Controller

Available in 6's, 12's, 18's, 30's, 50's
70's and 80's

Pepcid AC®
(famotidine)

JONES PHARMA

RX JONES PHARMA INCORPORATED P. 1445

25 mcg   50 mcg   75 mcg
(0.025 mg) (0.05 mg) (0.075 mg)

88 mcg   100 mcg   112 mcg
(0.088 mg) (0.1 mg) (0.112 mg)

125 mcg   137 mcg   150 mcg
(0.125 mg) (0.137 mg) (0.15 mg)

175 mcg   200 mcg   300 mcg
(0.175 mg) (0.2 mg) (0.3 mg)

Levoxyl®
(levothyroxine sodium tablets, USP)

KEY

RX KEY PHARMACEUTICALS P. 1448

30 mg   60 mg

120 mg

Extended release tablets

Imdur®
(isosorbide mononitrate)

RX KEY PHARMACEUTICALS P. 1454

10 mEq

20 mEq
Microburst Release System®

K-Dur®
(potassium chloride USP)

RX KEY PHARMACEUTICALS P. 1456

0.1 mg/hr   0.2 mg/hr

0.3 mg/hr   0.4 mg/hr

0.6 mg/hr

Transdermal Infusion System

Nitro Dur®
(nitroglycerin)

RX KEY PHARMACEUTICALS P. 2877

Proventil® HFA
(albuterol sulfate)

RX KEY PHARMACEUTICALS P. 1457

100 mg   200 mg

300 mg   450 mg

Extended release tablets

Theo-Dur®
(theophylline anhydrous)

RX KEY PHARMACEUTICALS P. 1464

703* 1 mg / 120 mg

*Long acting
antihistamine/decongestant*

Trinalin® Repetabs®
(azatadine maleate USP,
pseudoephedrine sulfate USP)

RX KEY PHARMACEUTICALS P. 1465

400 mg

600 mg

Uni-Dur®
(theophylline)

KNOLL LABORATORIES

RX KNOLL LABORATORIES P. 1471

2 mg
†Akineton®
(biperiden HCl)

C-II KNOLL LABORATORIES P. 1473

2 mg   4 mg   8 mg

†Dilaudid®
(hydromorphone HCl)

C-II KNOLL LABORATORIES P. 1475

10 mg/mL
Dilaudid-HP®
(hydromorphone HCl)

C-II KNOLL LABORATORIES P. 1475

50 mg/5 mL
Dilaudid-HP®
(hydromorphone HCl)

C-II KNOLL LABORATORIES P. 1475

500 mg/50 mL

Dilaudid-HP®
(hydromorphone HCl)

C-II KNOLL LABORATORIES P. 1475

250 mg
Sterile Lyophilized Powder

Dilaudid-HP®
(hydromorphone HCl)

RX KNOLL LABORATORIES

E-MYCIN
250 mg   333 mg

E-Mycin®
(erythromycin Delayed Release Tablets, USP)

RX KNOLL LABORATORIES P. 1479

120 mg

180 mg

240 mg

Film-coated sustained release
oral tablets

Isoptin® SR
(verapamil HCl)

RX KNOLL LABORATORIES P. 1481

150 mg

225 mg

300 mg

Rythmol®
(propafenone HCl)

RX KNOLL LABORATORIES P. 1472

15 Gm and 30 Gm Tubes

**Collagenase Santyl®
Ointment**
(collagenase)

C-III KNOLL LABORATORIES P. 1486

VICODIN

Vicodin®
(hydrocodone bitartrate, acetaminophen)
5 mg/500 mg

C-III KNOLL LABORATORIES P. 1487

VICODIN ES

Vicodin ES®
(hydrocodone bitartrate, acetaminophen)
7.5 mg / 750 mg

C-III KNOLL LABORATORIES P. 1484

VICODIN HP

Vicodin HP™
(hydrocodone bitartrate, acetaminophen)
10 mg/660 mg

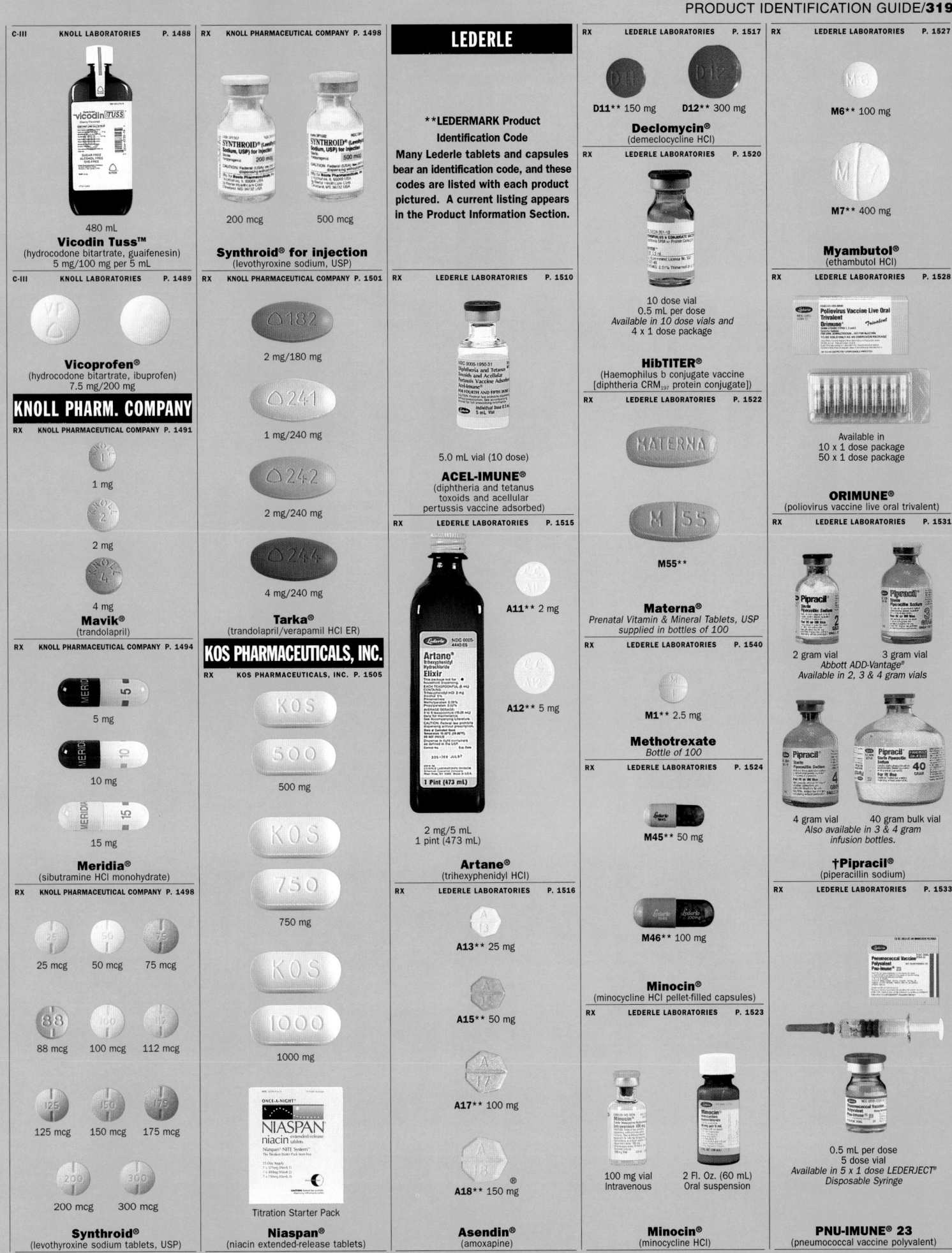

C-III   KNOLL LABORATORIES   P. 1488

480 mL

Vicodin Tuss™
(hydrocodone bitartrate, guaifenesin)
5 mg/100 mg per 5 mL

C-III   KNOLL LABORATORIES   P. 1489

Vicoprofen®
(hydrocodone bitartrate, ibuprofen)
7.5 mg/200 mg

KNOLL PHARM. COMPANY

RX   KNOLL PHARMACEUTICAL COMPANY   P. 1491

1 mg

2 mg

4 mg

Mavik®
(trandolapril)

RX   KNOLL PHARMACEUTICAL COMPANY   P. 1494

5 mg

10 mg

15 mg

Meridia®
(sibutramine HCl monohydrate)

RX   KNOLL PHARMACEUTICAL COMPANY   P. 1498

25 mcg   50 mcg   75 mcg

88 mcg   100 mcg   112 mcg

125 mcg   150 mcg   175 mcg

200 mcg   300 mcg

Synthroid®
(levothyroxine sodium tablets, USP)

RX   KNOLL PHARMACEUTICAL COMPANY   P. 1498

200 mcg   500 mcg

Synthroid® for injection
(levothyroxine sodium, USP)

RX   KNOLL PHARMACEUTICAL COMPANY   P. 1501

182
2 mg/180 mg

241
1 mg/240 mg

242
2 mg/240 mg

244
4 mg/240 mg

Tarka®
(trandolapril/verapamil HCl ER)

KOS PHARMACEUTICALS, INC.

RX   KOS PHARMACEUTICALS, INC.   P. 1505

KOS

500
500 mg

KOS
750
750 mg

KOS
1000
1000 mg

ONCE-A-NIGHT
NIASPAN
niacin
extended-release tablets

Titration Starter Pack

Niaspan®
(niacin extended-release tablets)

LEDERLE

****LEDERMARK Product
Identification Code**
Many Lederle tablets and capsules
bear an identification code, and these
codes are listed with each product
pictured. A current listing appears
in the Product Information Section.

RX   LEDERLE LABORATORIES   P. 1510

5.0 mL vial (10 dose)

ACEL-IMUNE®
(diphtheria and tetanus
toxoids and acellular
pertussis vaccine adsorbed)

RX   LEDERLE LABORATORIES   P. 1515

A11** 2 mg

A12** 5 mg

Artane®
Trihexyphenidyl
Hydrochloride
Elixir
1 Pint (473 mL)

2 mg/5 mL
1 pint (473 mL)

Artane®
(trihexyphenidyl HCl)

RX   LEDERLE LABORATORIES   P. 1516

A13** 25 mg

A15** 50 mg

A17** 100 mg

A18** 150 mg

Asendin®
(amoxapine)

RX   LEDERLE LABORATORIES   P. 1517

D11** 150 mg   D12** 300 mg

Declomycin®
(demeclocycline HCl)

RX   LEDERLE LABORATORIES   P. 1520

10 dose vial
0.5 mL per dose
*Available in 10 dose vials and
4 x 1 dose package*

HibTITER®
(Haemophilus b conjugate vaccine
[diphtheria CRM_{197} protein conjugate])

RX   LEDERLE LABORATORIES   P. 1522

MATERNA

M 55

M55**

Materna®
*Prenatal Vitamin & Mineral Tablets, USP
supplied in bottles of 100*

RX   LEDERLE LABORATORIES   P. 1540

M1** 2.5 mg

Methotrexate
Bottle of 100

RX   LEDERLE LABORATORIES   P. 1524

M45** 50 mg

M46** 100 mg

Minocin®
(minocycline HCl pellet-filled capsules)

RX   LEDERLE LABORATORIES   P. 1523

100 mg vial
Intravenous

2 Fl. Oz. (60 mL)
Oral suspension

Minocin®
(minocycline HCl)

RX   LEDERLE LABORATORIES   P. 1527

M6** 100 mg

M7** 400 mg

Myambutol®
(ethambutol HCl)

RX   LEDERLE LABORATORIES   P. 1528

Poliovirus Vaccine Live Oral
Trivalent
Orimune

Available in
10 x 1 dose package
50 x 1 dose package

ORIMUNE®
(poliovirus vaccine live oral trivalent)

RX   LEDERLE LABORATORIES   P. 1531

2 gram vial   3 gram vial
*Abbott ADD-Vantage®
Available in 2, 3 & 4 gram vials*

4 gram vial   40 gram bulk vial
*Also available in 3 & 4 gram
infusion bottles.*

†Pipracil®
(piperacillin sodium)

RX   LEDERLE LABORATORIES   P. 1533

0.5 mL per dose
5 dose vial
*Available in 5 x 1 dose LEDERJECT®
Disposable Syringe*

PNU-IMUNE® 23
(pneumococcal vaccine polyvalent)

****LEDERMARK Product Identification Code / ®: Unique tablet shapes are trademarks of American Cyanamid Company.

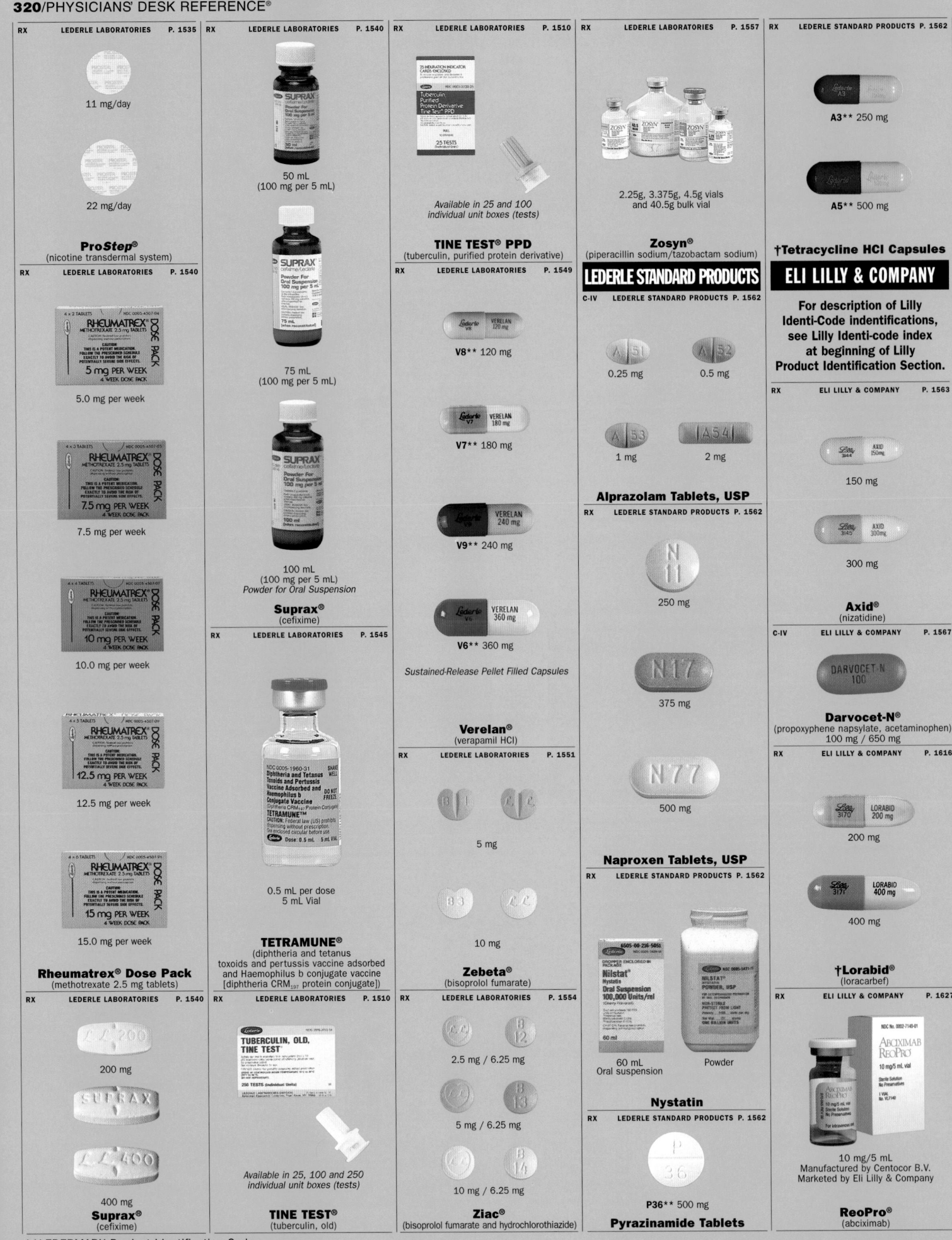

| RX | LEDERLE LABORATORIES | P. 1535 |

11 mg/day

22 mg/day

ProStep®
(nicotine transdermal system)

| RX | LEDERLE LABORATORIES | P. 1540 |

RHEUMATREX® DOSE PACK
METHOTREXATE 2.5 mg TABLETS
5 mg PER WEEK
4 WEEK DOSE PACK

5.0 mg per week

RHEUMATREX® DOSE PACK
METHOTREXATE 2.5 mg TABLETS
7.5 mg PER WEEK
4 WEEK DOSE PACK

7.5 mg per week

RHEUMATREX® DOSE PACK
METHOTREXATE 2.5 mg TABLETS
10 mg PER WEEK
4 WEEK DOSE PACK

10.0 mg per week

RHEUMATREX® DOSE PACK
METHOTREXATE 2.5 mg TABLETS
12.5 mg PER WEEK
4 WEEK DOSE PACK

12.5 mg per week

RHEUMATREX® DOSE PACK
METHOTREXATE 2.5 mg TABLETS
15 mg PER WEEK
4 WEEK DOSE PACK

15.0 mg per week

Rheumatrex® Dose Pack
(methotrexate 2.5 mg tablets)

| RX | LEDERLE LABORATORIES | P. 1540 |

LL 200

200 mg

SUPRAX

LL 400

400 mg

Suprax®
(cefixime)

| RX | LEDERLE LABORATORIES | P. 1540 |

50 mL
(100 mg per 5 mL)

75 mL
(100 mg per 5 mL)

100 mL
(100 mg per 5 mL)
Powder for Oral Suspension

Suprax®
(cefixime)

| RX | LEDERLE LABORATORIES | P. 1545 |

NDC 0005-1960-31
Diphtheria and Tetanus
Toxoids and Pertussis
Vaccine Adsorbed and
Haemophilus b
Conjugate Vaccine
TETRAMUNE™

0.5 mL per dose
5 mL Vial

TETRAMUNE®
(diphtheria and tetanus
toxoids and pertussis vaccine adsorbed
and Haemophilus b conjugate vaccine
[diphtheria CRM₁₉₇ protein conjugate])

| RX | LEDERLE LABORATORIES | P. 1510 |

**TUBERCULIN, OLD,
TINE TEST**

250 TESTS (Individual Units)

*Available in 25, 100 and 250
individual unit boxes (tests)*

TINE TEST®
(tuberculin, old)

| RX | LEDERLE LABORATORIES | P. 1510 |

25 INDURATION INDICATOR
CARDS ENCLOSED

Tuberculin,
Purified
Protein Derivative
Tine Test® PPD

25 TESTS
(Individual Units)

*Available in 25 and 100
individual unit boxes (tests)*

TINE TEST® PPD
(tuberculin, purified protein derivative)

| RX | LEDERLE LABORATORIES | P. 1549 |

Lederle V8 VERELAN
120 mg

V8✱✱ 120 mg

Lederle V7 VERELAN
180 mg

V7✱✱ 180 mg

Lederle V9 VERELAN
240 mg

V9✱✱ 240 mg

Lederle V6 VERELAN
360 mg

V6✱✱ 360 mg

Sustained-Release Pellet Filled Capsules

Verelan®
(verapamil HCl)

| RX | LEDERLE LABORATORIES | P. 1551 |

5 mg

10 mg

Zebeta®
(bisoprolol fumarate)

| RX | LEDERLE LABORATORIES | P. 1554 |

2.5 mg / 6.25 mg

5 mg / 6.25 mg

10 mg / 6.25 mg

Ziac®
(bisoprolol fumarate and hydrochlorothiazide)

| RX | LEDERLE LABORATORIES | P. 1557 |

2.25g, 3.375g, 4.5g vials
and 40.5g bulk vial

Zosyn®
(piperacillin sodium/tazobactam sodium)

LEDERLE STANDARD PRODUCTS

| C-IV | LEDERLE STANDARD PRODUCTS | P. 1562 |

A 51

0.25 mg

A 52

0.5 mg

A 53

1 mg

A54

2 mg

Alprazolam Tablets, USP

| RX | LEDERLE STANDARD PRODUCTS | P. 1562 |

N 11

250 mg

N 17

375 mg

N 77

500 mg

Naproxen Tablets, USP

| RX | LEDERLE STANDARD PRODUCTS | P. 1562 |

6505-00-236-5051
NDC 0005-3406-01
Nilstat®
Nystatin
Oral Suspesion
100,000 Units/ml

60 mL
Oral suspension

NDC 0005-3471-11
NILSTAT®
NYSTATIN
POWDER, USP

Powder

Nystatin

| RX | LEDERLE STANDARD PRODUCTS | P. 1562 |

P 36

P36✱✱ 500 mg

Pyrazinamide Tablets

| RX | LEDERLE STANDARD PRODUCTS | P. 1562 |

Lederle A3

A3✱✱ 250 mg

Lederle A5

A5✱✱ 500 mg

†Tetracycline HCl Capsules

ELI LILLY & COMPANY

For description of Lilly
Identi-Code indentifications,
see Lilly Identi-code index
at beginning of Lilly
Product Identification Section.

| RX | ELI LILLY & COMPANY | P. 1563 |

Lilly 3144 AXID
150mg

150 mg

Lilly 3145 AXID
300mg

300 mg

Axid®
(nizatidine)

| C-IV | ELI LILLY & COMPANY | P. 1567 |

DARVOCET-N
100

Darvocet-N®
(propoxyphene napsylate, acetaminophen)
100 mg / 650 mg

| RX | ELI LILLY & COMPANY | P. 1616 |

Lilly 3170 LORABID
200mg

200 mg

Lilly 3171 LORABID
400mg

400 mg

†Lorabid®
(loracarbef)

| RX | ELI LILLY & COMPANY | P. 1627 |

NDC No. 0002-7140-01
**ABCIXIMAB
ReoPro**
10 mg/5 mL vial

10 mg/5 mL
Manufactured by Centocor B.V.
Marketed by Eli Lilly & Company

ReoPro®
(abciximab)

✱✱LEDERMARK Product Identification Code

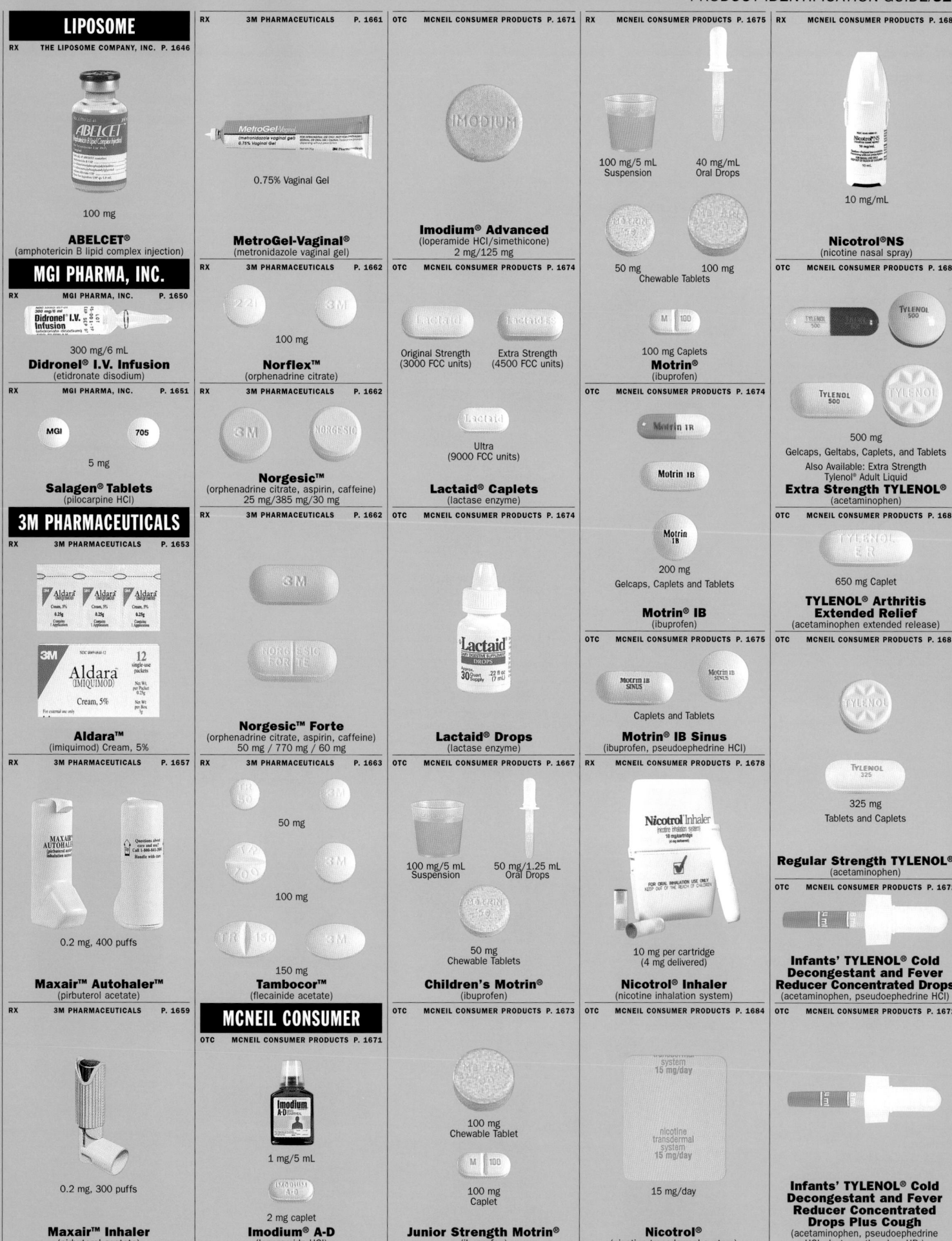

LIPOSOME

RX   THE LIPOSOME COMPANY, INC.   P. 1646

100 mg

ABELCET®
(amphotericin B lipid complex injection)

MGI PHARMA, INC.

RX   MGI PHARMA, INC.   P. 1650

300 mg/6 mL
Didronel® I.V. Infusion
(etidronate disodium)

RX   MGI PHARMA, INC.   P. 1651

5 mg

Salagen® Tablets
(pilocarpine HCl)

3M PHARMACEUTICALS

RX   3M PHARMACEUTICALS   P. 1653

Aldara™
(imiquimod) Cream, 5%

RX   3M PHARMACEUTICALS   P. 1657

0.2 mg, 400 puffs
Maxair™ Autohaler™
(pirbuterol acetate)

RX   3M PHARMACEUTICALS   P. 1659

0.2 mg, 300 puffs
Maxair™ Inhaler
(pirbuterol acetate)

RX   3M PHARMACEUTICALS   P. 1661

0.75% Vaginal Gel

MetroGel-Vaginal®
(metronidazole vaginal gel)

RX   3M PHARMACEUTICALS   P. 1662

100 mg

Norflex™
(orphenadrine citrate)

RX   3M PHARMACEUTICALS   P. 1662

Norgesic™
(orphenadrine citrate, aspirin, caffeine)
25 mg/385 mg/30 mg

RX   3M PHARMACEUTICALS   P. 1662

Norgesic™ Forte
(orphenadrine citrate, aspirin, caffeine)
50 mg / 770 mg / 60 mg

RX   3M PHARMACEUTICALS   P. 1663

50 mg

100 mg

150 mg

Tambocor™
(flecainide acetate)

MCNEIL CONSUMER

OTC   MCNEIL CONSUMER PRODUCTS   P. 1671

1 mg/5 mL

2 mg caplet
Imodium® A-D
(loperamide HCl)

OTC   MCNEIL CONSUMER PRODUCTS   P. 1671

Imodium® Advanced
(loperamide HCl/simethicone)
2 mg/125 mg

OTC   MCNEIL CONSUMER PRODUCTS   P. 1674

Original Strength   Extra Strength
(3000 FCC units)   (4500 FCC units)

Ultra
(9000 FCC units)

Lactaid® Caplets
(lactase enzyme)

OTC   MCNEIL CONSUMER PRODUCTS   P. 1674

Lactaid® Drops
(lactase enzyme)

OTC   MCNEIL CONSUMER PRODUCTS   P. 1667

100 mg/5 mL   50 mg/1.25 mL
Suspension   Oral Drops

50 mg
Chewable Tablets

Children's Motrin®
(ibuprofen)

OTC   MCNEIL CONSUMER PRODUCTS   P. 1673

100 mg
Chewable Tablet

100 mg
Caplet

Junior Strength Motrin®
(ibuprofen)

RX   MCNEIL CONSUMER PRODUCTS   P. 1675

100 mg/5 mL   40 mg/mL
Suspension   Oral Drops

50 mg   100 mg
Chewable Tablets

100 mg Caplets
Motrin®
(ibuprofen)

OTC   MCNEIL CONSUMER PRODUCTS   P. 1674

200 mg
Gelcaps, Caplets and Tablets

Motrin® IB
(ibuprofen)

OTC   MCNEIL CONSUMER PRODUCTS   P. 1675

Caplets and Tablets

Motrin® IB Sinus
(ibuprofen, pseudoephedrine HCl)

RX   MCNEIL CONSUMER PRODUCTS   P. 1678

10 mg per cartridge
(4 mg delivered)
Nicotrol® Inhaler
(nicotine inhalation system)

OTC   MCNEIL CONSUMER PRODUCTS   P. 1684

15 mg/day
Nicotrol®
(nicotine transdermal system)

RX   MCNEIL CONSUMER PRODUCTS   P. 1681

10 mg/mL

Nicotrol®NS
(nicotine nasal spray)

OTC   MCNEIL CONSUMER PRODUCTS   P. 1685

500 mg
Gelcaps, Geltabs, Caplets, and Tablets
Also Available: Extra Strength
Tylenol® Adult Liquid
Extra Strength TYLENOL®
(acetaminophen)

OTC   MCNEIL CONSUMER PRODUCTS   P. 1685

650 mg Caplet

**TYLENOL® Arthritis
Extended Relief**
(acetaminophen extended release)

OTC   MCNEIL CONSUMER PRODUCTS   P. 1685

325 mg
Tablets and Caplets

Regular Strength TYLENOL®
(acetaminophen)

OTC   MCNEIL CONSUMER PRODUCTS   P. 1672

**Infants' TYLENOL® Cold
Decongestant and Fever
Reducer Concentrated Drops**
(acetaminophen, pseudoephedrine HCl)

OTC   MCNEIL CONSUMER PRODUCTS   P. 1672

**Infants' TYLENOL® Cold
Decongestant and Fever
Reducer Concentrated
Drops Plus Cough**
(acetaminophen, pseudoephedrine
HCl, dextromethorphan HBr)

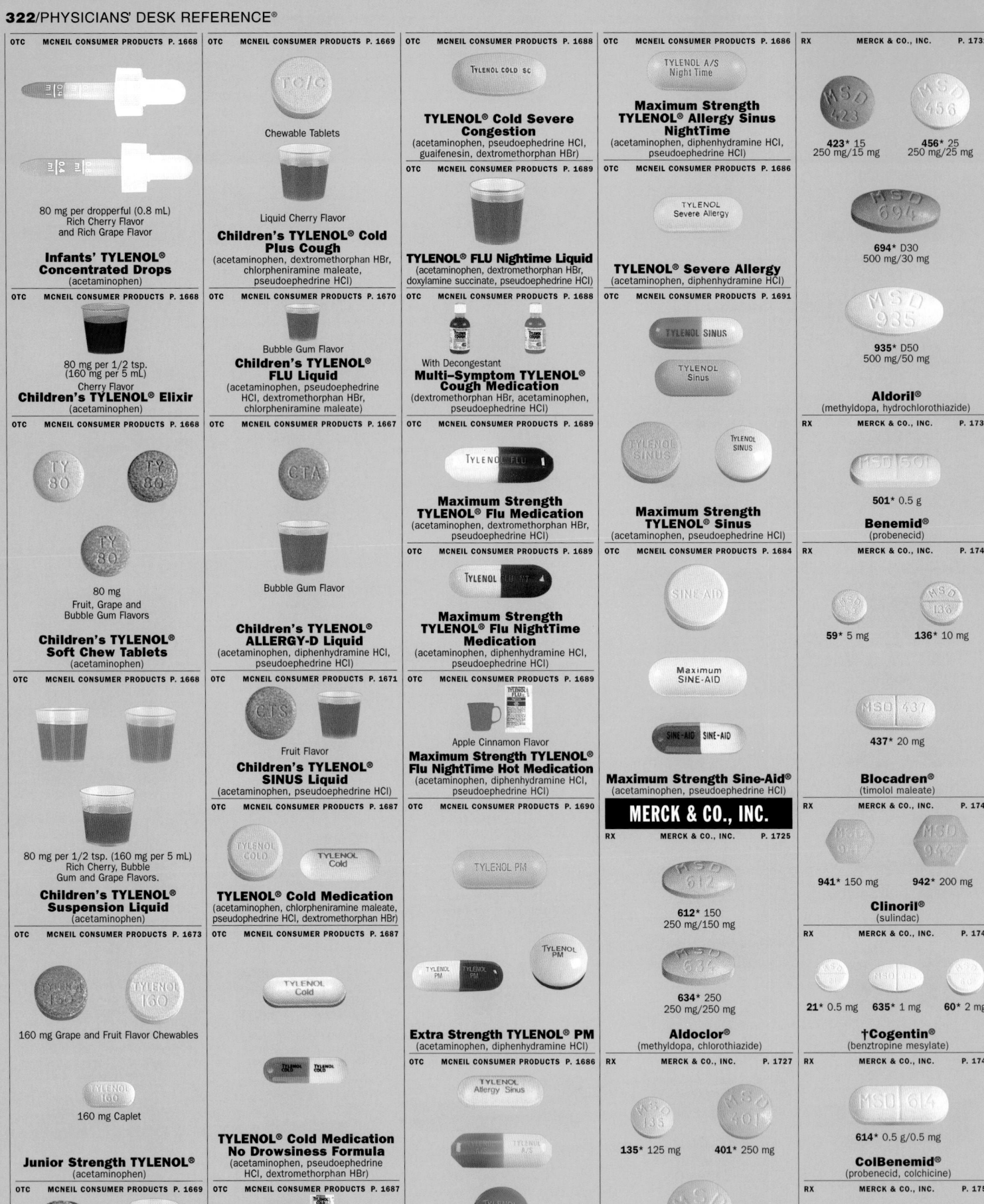

OTC   MCNEIL CONSUMER PRODUCTS P. 1668

80 mg per dropperful (0.8 mL)
Rich Cherry Flavor
and Rich Grape Flavor
**Infants' TYLENOL®
Concentrated Drops**
(acetaminophen)

OTC   MCNEIL CONSUMER PRODUCTS P. 1668

80 mg per 1/2 tsp.
(160 mg per 5 mL)
Cherry Flavor
Children's TYLENOL® Elixir
(acetaminophen)

OTC   MCNEIL CONSUMER PRODUCTS P. 1668

80 mg
Fruit, Grape and
Bubble Gum Flavors
**Children's TYLENOL®
Soft Chew Tablets**
(acetaminophen)

OTC   MCNEIL CONSUMER PRODUCTS P. 1668

80 mg per 1/2 tsp. (160 mg per 5 mL)
Rich Cherry, Bubble
Gum and Grape Flavors.
**Children's TYLENOL®
Suspension Liquid**
(acetaminophen)

OTC   MCNEIL CONSUMER PRODUCTS P. 1673

160 mg Grape and Fruit Flavor Chewables

160 mg Caplet

Junior Strength TYLENOL®
(acetaminophen)

OTC   MCNEIL CONSUMER PRODUCTS P. 1669

Chewable Tablets   Liquid Grape Flavor
Children's TYLENOL® Cold
(acetaminophen, chlorpheniramine
maleate, pseudoephedrine HCl)

OTC   MCNEIL CONSUMER PRODUCTS P. 1669

Chewable Tablets

Liquid Cherry Flavor
**Children's TYLENOL® Cold
Plus Cough**
(acetaminophen, dextromethorphan HBr,
chlorpheniramine maleate,
pseudoephedrine HCl)

OTC   MCNEIL CONSUMER PRODUCTS P. 1670

Bubble Gum Flavor
**Children's TYLENOL®
FLU Liquid**
(acetaminophen, pseudoephedrine
HCl, dextromethorphan HBr,
chlorpheniramine maleate)

OTC   MCNEIL CONSUMER PRODUCTS P. 1667

Bubble Gum Flavor
**Children's TYLENOL®
ALLERGY-D Liquid**
(acetaminophen, diphenhydramine HCl,
pseudoephedrine HCl)

OTC   MCNEIL CONSUMER PRODUCTS P. 1671

Fruit Flavor
**Children's TYLENOL®
SINUS Liquid**
(acetaminophen, pseudoephedrine HCl)

OTC   MCNEIL CONSUMER PRODUCTS P. 1687

TYLENOL® Cold Medication
(acetaminophen, chlorpheniramine maleate,
pseudophedrine HCl, dextromethorphan HBr)

OTC   MCNEIL CONSUMER PRODUCTS P. 1687

**TYLENOL® Cold Medication
No Drowsiness Formula**
(acetaminophen, pseudoephedrine
HCl, dextromethorphan HBr)

OTC   MCNEIL CONSUMER PRODUCTS P. 1687

Honey Lemon Flavor
**TYLENOL® Cold
Hot Medication**
(acetaminophen, chlorpheniramine
maleate, pseudoephedrine HCl,
dextromethorphan HBr)

OTC   MCNEIL CONSUMER PRODUCTS P. 1688

**TYLENOL® Cold Severe
Congestion**
(acetaminophen, pseudoephedrine HCl,
guaifenesin, dextromethorphan HBr)

OTC   MCNEIL CONSUMER PRODUCTS P. 1689

TYLENOL® FLU Nightime Liquid
(acetaminophen, dextromethorphan HBr,
doxylamine succinate, pseudoephedrine HCl)

OTC   MCNEIL CONSUMER PRODUCTS P. 1688

With Decongestant
**Multi–Symptom TYLENOL®
Cough Medication**
(dextromethorphan HBr, acetaminophen,
pseudoephedrine HCl)

OTC   MCNEIL CONSUMER PRODUCTS P. 1689

**Maximum Strength
TYLENOL® Flu Medication**
(acetaminophen, dextromethorphan HBr,
pseudoephedrine HCl)

OTC   MCNEIL CONSUMER PRODUCTS P. 1689

**Maximum Strength
TYLENOL® Flu NightTime
Medication**
(acetaminophen, diphenhydramine HCl,
pseudoephedrine HCl)

OTC   MCNEIL CONSUMER PRODUCTS P. 1689

Apple Cinnamon Flavor
**Maximum Strength TYLENOL®
Flu NightTime Hot Medication**
(acetaminophen, diphenhydramine HCl,
pseudoephedrine HCl)

OTC   MCNEIL CONSUMER PRODUCTS P. 1690

Extra Strength TYLENOL® PM
(acetaminophen, diphenhydramine HCl)

OTC   MCNEIL CONSUMER PRODUCTS P. 1686

**Maximum Strength
TYLENOL® Allergy Sinus**
(acetaminophen, chlorpheniramine
maleate, pseudoephedrine HCl)

OTC   MCNEIL CONSUMER PRODUCTS P. 1686

**Maximum Strength
TYLENOL® Allergy Sinus
NightTime**
(acetaminophen, diphenhydramine HCl,
pseudoephedrine HCl)

OTC   MCNEIL CONSUMER PRODUCTS P. 1686

TYLENOL® Severe Allergy
(acetaminophen, diphenhydramine HCl)

OTC   MCNEIL CONSUMER PRODUCTS P. 1691

**Maximum Strength
TYLENOL® Sinus**
(acetaminophen, pseudoephedrine HCl)

OTC   MCNEIL CONSUMER PRODUCTS P. 1684

Maximum Strength Sine-Aid®
(acetaminophen, pseudoephedrine HCl)

MERCK & CO., INC.

RX   MERCK & CO., INC.   P. 1725

612* 150
250 mg/150 mg

634* 250
250 mg/250 mg

Aldoclor®
(methyldopa, chlorothiazide)

RX   MERCK & CO., INC.   P. 1727

135* 125 mg   **401*** 250 mg

516* 500 mg

†Aldomet®
(methyldopa)

RX   MERCK & CO., INC.   P. 1731

423* 15   **456*** 25
250 mg/15 mg   250 mg/25 mg

694* D30
500 mg/30 mg

935* D50
500 mg/50 mg

Aldoril®
(methyldopa, hydrochlorothiazide)

RX   MERCK & CO., INC.   P. 1738

501* 0.5 g

Benemid®
(probenecid)

RX   MERCK & CO., INC.   P. 1741

59* 5 mg   **136*** 10 mg

437* 20 mg

Blocadren®
(timolol maleate)

RX   MERCK & CO., INC.   P. 1745

941* 150 mg   **942*** 200 mg

Clinoril®
(sulindac)

RX   MERCK & CO., INC.   P. 1747

21* 0.5 mg   **635*** 1 mg   **60*** 2 mg

†Cogentin®
(benztropine mesylate)

RX   MERCK & CO., INC.   P. 1749

614* 0.5 g/0.5 mg

ColBenemid®
(probenecid, colchicine)

RX   MERCK & CO., INC.   P. 1754

219* 25 mg

†Cortone®
(cortisone acetate)

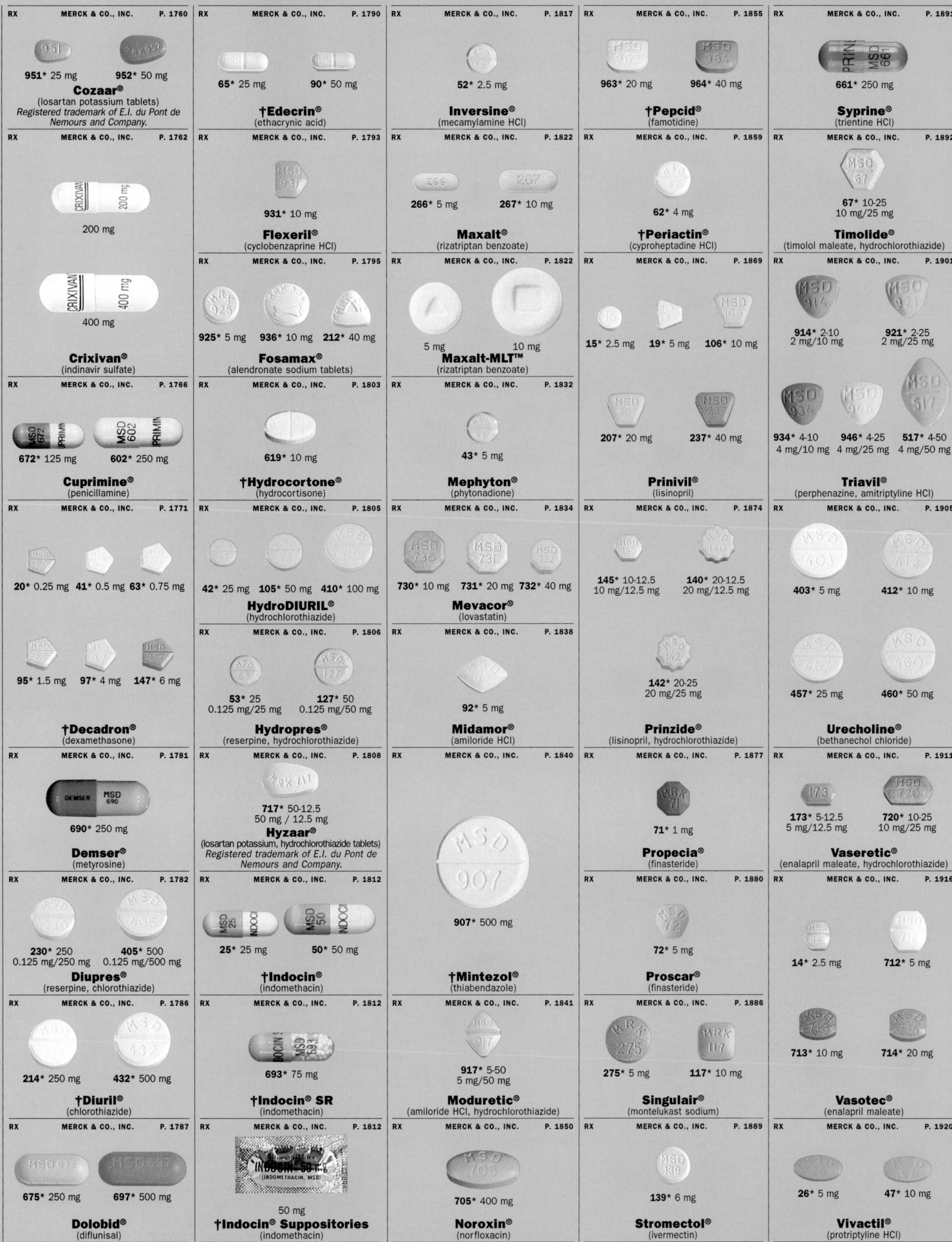

RX MERCK & CO., INC. P. 1760

951* 25 mg   **952*** 50 mg

Cozaar®
(losartan potassium tablets)
Registered trademark of E.I. du Pont de Nemours and Company.

RX MERCK & CO., INC. P. 1762

200 mg

400 mg

Crixivan®
(indinavir sulfate)

RX MERCK & CO., INC. P. 1766

672* 125 mg   **602*** 250 mg

Cuprimine®
(penicillamine)

RX MERCK & CO., INC. P. 1771

20* 0.25 mg **41*** 0.5 mg **63*** 0.75 mg

95* 1.5 mg   **97*** 4 mg   **147*** 6 mg

†Decadron®
(dexamethasone)

RX MERCK & CO., INC. P. 1781

690* 250 mg

Demser®
(metyrosine)

RX MERCK & CO., INC. P. 1782

230* 250   **405*** 500
0.125 mg/250 mg   0.125 mg/500 mg

Diupres®
(reserpine, chlorothiazide)

RX MERCK & CO., INC. P. 1786

214* 250 mg   **432*** 500 mg

†Diuril®
(chlorothiazide)

RX MERCK & CO., INC. P. 1787

675* 250 mg   **697*** 500 mg

Dolobid®
(diflunisal)

RX MERCK & CO., INC. P. 1790

65* 25 mg   **90*** 50 mg

†Edecrin®
(ethacrynic acid)

RX MERCK & CO., INC. P. 1793

931* 10 mg

Flexeril®
(cyclobenzaprine HCl)

RX MERCK & CO., INC. P. 1795

925* 5 mg   **936*** 10 mg   **212*** 40 mg

Fosamax®
(alendronate sodium tablets)

RX MERCK & CO., INC. P. 1803

619* 10 mg

†Hydrocortone®
(hydrocortisone)

RX MERCK & CO., INC. P. 1805

42* 25 mg   **105*** 50 mg   **410*** 100 mg

HydroDIURIL®
(hydrochlorothiazide)

RX MERCK & CO., INC. P. 1806

53* 25   **127*** 50
0.125 mg/25 mg   0.125 mg/50 mg

Hydropres®
(reserpine, hydrochlorothiazide)

RX MERCK & CO., INC. P. 1808

717* 50-12.5
50 mg / 12.5 mg

Hyzaar®
(losartan potassium, hydrochlorothiazide tablets)
Registered trademark of E.I. du Pont de Nemours and Company.

RX MERCK & CO., INC. P. 1812

25* 25 mg   **50*** 50 mg

†Indocin®
(indomethacin)

RX MERCK & CO., INC. P. 1812

693* 75 mg

†Indocin® SR
(indomethacin)

RX MERCK & CO., INC. P. 1812

50 mg

†Indocin® Suppositories
(indomethacin)

RX MERCK & CO., INC. P. 1817

52* 2.5 mg

Inversine®
(mecamylamine HCl)

RX MERCK & CO., INC. P. 1822

266* 5 mg   **267*** 10 mg

Maxalt®
(rizatriptan benzoate)

RX MERCK & CO., INC. P. 1822

5 mg   10 mg

Maxalt-MLT™
(rizatriptan benzoate)

RX MERCK & CO., INC. P. 1832

43* 5 mg

Mephyton®
(phytonadione)

RX MERCK & CO., INC. P. 1834

730* 10 mg   **731*** 20 mg   **732*** 40 mg

Mevacor®
(lovastatin)

RX MERCK & CO., INC. P. 1838

92* 5 mg

Midamor®
(amiloride HCl)

RX MERCK & CO., INC. P. 1840

907* 500 mg

†Mintezol®
(thiabendazole)

RX MERCK & CO., INC. P. 1841

917* 5-50
5 mg/50 mg

Moduretic®
(amiloride HCl, hydrochlorothiazide)

RX MERCK & CO., INC. P. 1850

705* 400 mg

Noroxin®
(norfloxacin)

RX MERCK & CO., INC. P. 1855

963* 20 mg   **964*** 40 mg

†Pepcid®
(famotidine)

RX MERCK & CO., INC. P. 1859

62* 4 mg

†Periactin®
(cyproheptadine HCl)

RX MERCK & CO., INC. P. 1869

15* 2.5 mg   **19*** 5 mg   **106*** 10 mg

207* 20 mg   **237*** 40 mg

Prinivil®
(lisinopril)

RX MERCK & CO., INC. P. 1874

145* 10-12.5   **140*** 20-12.5
10 mg/12.5 mg   20 mg/12.5 mg

142* 20-25
20 mg/25 mg

Prinzide®
(lisinopril, hydrochlorothiazide)

RX MERCK & CO., INC. P. 1877

71* 1 mg

Propecia®
(finasteride)

RX MERCK & CO., INC. P. 1880

72* 5 mg

Proscar®
(finasteride)

RX MERCK & CO., INC. P. 1886

275* 5 mg   **117*** 10 mg

Singulair®
(montelukast sodium)

RX MERCK & CO., INC. P. 1889

139* 6 mg

Stromectol®
(ivermectin)

RX MERCK & CO., INC. P. 1891

661* 250 mg

Syprine®
(trientine HCl)

RX MERCK & CO., INC. P. 1892

67* 10-25
10 mg/25 mg

Timolide®
(timolol maleate, hydrochlorothiazide)

RX MERCK & CO., INC. P. 1901

914* 2-10   **921*** 2-25
2 mg/10 mg   2 mg/25 mg

934* 4-10   **946*** 4-25   **517*** 4-50
4 mg/10 mg   4 mg/25 mg   4 mg/50 mg

Triavil®
(perphenazine, amitriptyline HCl)

RX MERCK & CO., INC. P. 1905

403* 5 mg   **412*** 10 mg

457* 25 mg   **460*** 50 mg

Urecholine®
(bethanechol chloride)

RX MERCK & CO., INC. P. 1911

173* 5-12.5   **720*** 10-25
5 mg/12.5 mg   10 mg/25 mg

Vaseretic®
(enalapril maleate, hydrochlorothiazide)

RX MERCK & CO., INC. P. 1916

14* 2.5 mg   **712*** 5 mg

Vasotec®
(enalapril maleate)

RX MERCK & CO., INC. P. 1920

26* 5 mg   **47*** 10 mg

Vivactil®
(protriptyline HCl)

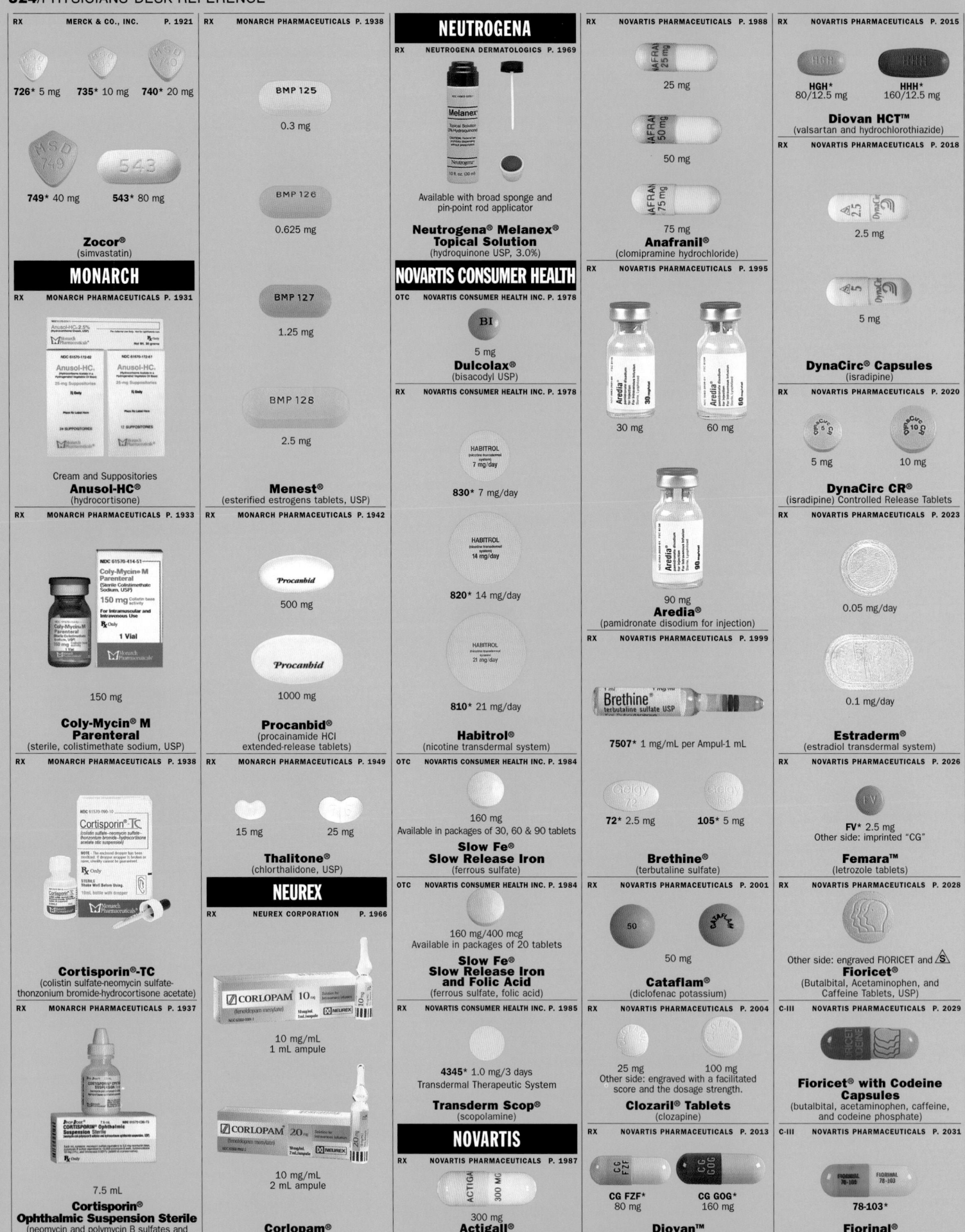

RX   MERCK & CO., INC.   P. 1921

726* 5 mg   **735*** 10 mg   **740*** 20 mg

749* 40 mg   **543*** 80 mg

Zocor®
(simvastatin)

MONARCH

RX   MONARCH PHARMACEUTICALS P. 1931

Cream and Suppositories
Anusol-HC®
(hydrocortisone)

RX   MONARCH PHARMACEUTICALS P. 1933

150 mg
**Coly-Mycin® M
Parenteral**
(sterile, colistimethate sodium, USP)

RX   MONARCH PHARMACEUTICALS P. 1938

7.5 mL
**Cortisporin®
Ophthalmic Suspension Sterile**
(neomycin and polymycin B sulfates and
hydrocortisone ophthalmic suspension, USP)

RX   MONARCH PHARMACEUTICALS P. 1938

BMP 125
0.3 mg

BMP 126
0.625 mg

BMP 127
1.25 mg

BMP 128
2.5 mg

Menest®
(esterified estrogens tablets, USP)

RX   MONARCH PHARMACEUTICALS P. 1942

Procanbid
500 mg

Procanbid
1000 mg

Procanbid®
(procainamide HCl
extended-release tablets)

RX   MONARCH PHARMACEUTICALS P. 1949

15 mg   25 mg
Thalitone®
(chlorthalidone, USP)

NEUREX

RX   NEUREX CORPORATION   P. 1966

10 mg/mL
1 mL ampule

10 mg/mL
2 mL ampule

Corlopam®
(fenoldapam mesylate)

NEUTROGENA

RX   NEUTROGENA DERMATOLOGICS P. 1969

Available with broad sponge and
pin-point rod applicator
**Neutrogena® Melanex®
Topical Solution**
(hydroquinone USP, 3.0%)

NOVARTIS CONSUMER HEALTH

OTC   NOVARTIS CONSUMER HEALTH INC. P. 1978

BI
5 mg
Dulcolax®
(bisacodyl USP)

RX   NOVARTIS CONSUMER HEALTH INC. P. 1978

HABITROL
(nicotine transdermal
system)
7 mg/day
830* 7 mg/day

HABITROL
(nicotine transdermal
system)
14 mg/day
820* 14 mg/day

HABITROL
(nicotine transdermal
system)
21 mg/day
810* 21 mg/day

Habitrol®
(nicotine transdermal system)

OTC   NOVARTIS CONSUMER HEALTH INC. P. 1984

160 mg
Available in packages of 30, 60 & 90 tablets
**Slow Fe®
Slow Release Iron**
(ferrous sulfate)

OTC   NOVARTIS CONSUMER HEALTH INC. P. 1984

160 mg/400 mcg
Available in packages of 20 tablets
**Slow Fe®
Slow Release Iron
and Folic Acid**
(ferrous sulfate, folic acid)

RX   NOVARTIS CONSUMER HEALTH INC. P. 1985

4345* 1.0 mg/3 days
Transdermal Therapeutic System
Transderm Scop®
(scopolamine)

NOVARTIS

RX   NOVARTIS PHARMACEUTICALS P. 1987

ACTIGA 300 MG
300 mg
Actigall®
(ursodiol USP)

RX   NOVARTIS PHARMACEUTICALS P. 1988

25 mg

50 mg

75 mg

Anafranil®
(clomipramine hydrochloride)

RX   NOVARTIS PHARMACEUTICALS P. 1995

30 mg   60 mg

90 mg
Aredia®
(pamidronate disodium for injection)

RX   NOVARTIS PHARMACEUTICALS P. 1999

Brethine
terbutaline sulfate USP
7507* 1 mg/mL per Ampul-1 mL

72* 2.5 mg   **105*** 5 mg
Brethine®
(terbutaline sulfate)

RX   NOVARTIS PHARMACEUTICALS P. 2001

50 mg
Cataflam®
(diclofenac potassium)

RX   NOVARTIS PHARMACEUTICALS P. 2004

25 mg   100 mg
Other side: engraved with a facilitated
score and the dosage strength.
Clozaril® Tablets
(clozapine)

RX   NOVARTIS PHARMACEUTICALS P. 2013

CG FZF*   CG GOG*
80 mg   160 mg
Diovan™
(valsartan)

RX   NOVARTIS PHARMACEUTICALS P. 2015

HGH*   HHH*
80/12.5 mg   160/12.5 mg
Diovan HCT™
(valsartan and hydrochlorothiazide)

RX   NOVARTIS PHARMACEUTICALS P. 2018

2.5 mg

5 mg

DynaCirc® Capsules
(isradipine)

RX   NOVARTIS PHARMACEUTICALS P. 2020

5 mg   10 mg
DynaCirc CR®
(isradipine) Controlled Release Tablets

RX   NOVARTIS PHARMACEUTICALS P. 2023

0.05 mg/day

0.1 mg/day

Estraderm®
(estradiol transdermal system)

RX   NOVARTIS PHARMACEUTICALS P. 2026

FV* 2.5 mg
Other side: imprinted "CG"
Femara™
(letrozole tablets)

RX   NOVARTIS PHARMACEUTICALS P. 2028

Other side: engraved FIORICET and ⚠
Fioricet®
(Butalbital, Acetaminophen, and
Caffeine Tablets, USP)

C-III   NOVARTIS PHARMACEUTICALS P. 2029

**Fioricet® with Codeine
Capsules**
(butalbital, acetaminophen, caffeine,
and codeine phosphate)

C-III   NOVARTIS PHARMACEUTICALS P. 2031

78-103*
Fiorinal®
(butalbital, aspirin, caffeine) Capsules, USP

RX   MONARCH PHARMACEUTICALS P. 1937

Cortisporin®-TC
(colistin sulfate-neomycin sulfate-
thonzonium bromide-hydrocortisone acetate)

C-III NOVARTIS PHARMACEUTICALS P. 2032

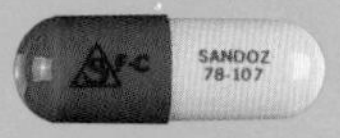

78-107*

Fiorinal® with Codeine Capsules, USP
(butalbital, aspirin, caffeine, and codeine phosphate)

RX NOVARTIS PHARMACEUTICALS P. 2038

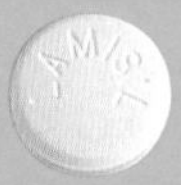

250 mg
Other side: imprinted "250"

Lamisil®
(terbinafine HCl tablets) Tablets

RX NOVARTIS PHARMACEUTICALS P. 2035

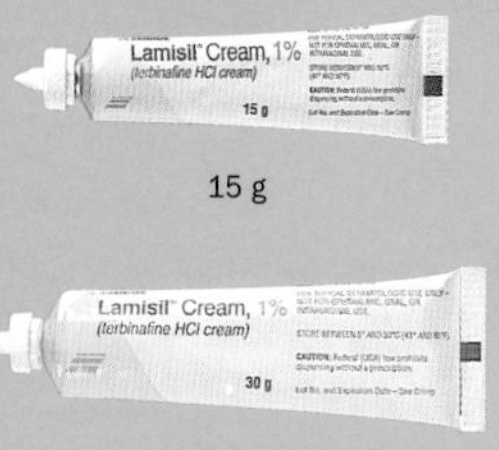

15 g

30 g

Lamisil® Cream, 1%
(terbinafine HCl cream)

RX NOVARTIS PHARMACEUTICALS P. 2036

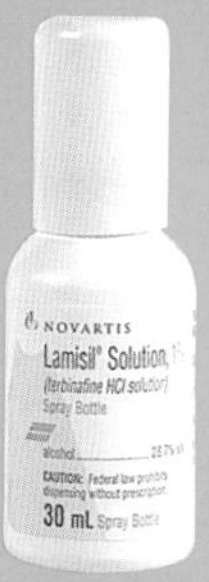

30 mL

Lamisil® Solution, 1%
(terbinafine HCl solution)

RX NOVARTIS PHARMACEUTICALS P. 2039

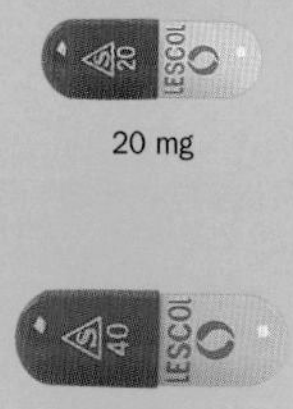

20 mg

40 mg

Lescol®
(fluvastatin sodium) Capsules

RX NOVARTIS PHARMACEUTICALS P. 2042

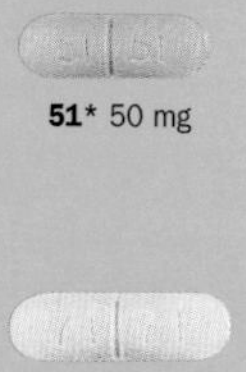

51* 50 mg

71* 100 mg

†Lopressor®
(metoprolol tartrate tablets, USP)

RX NOVARTIS PHARMACEUTICALS P. 2045

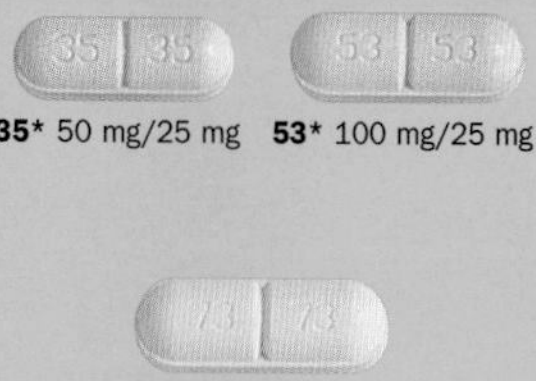

35* 50 mg/25 mg   **53*** 100 mg/25 mg

73* 100 mg/50 mg

Lopressor HCT®
(metoprolol tartrate USP and hydrochlorothiazide USP)

RX NOVARTIS PHARMACEUTICALS P. 2047

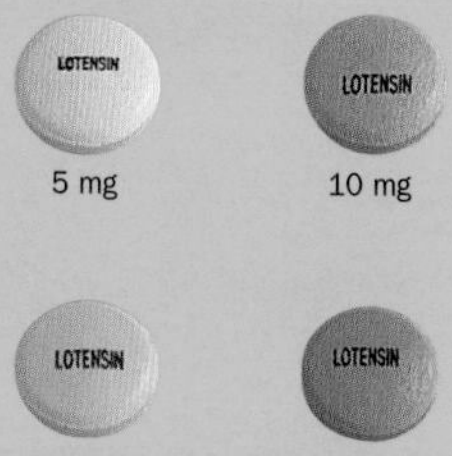

5 mg   10 mg

20 mg   40 mg

Lotensin®
(benazepril HCl)

RX NOVARTIS PHARMACEUTICALS P. 2049

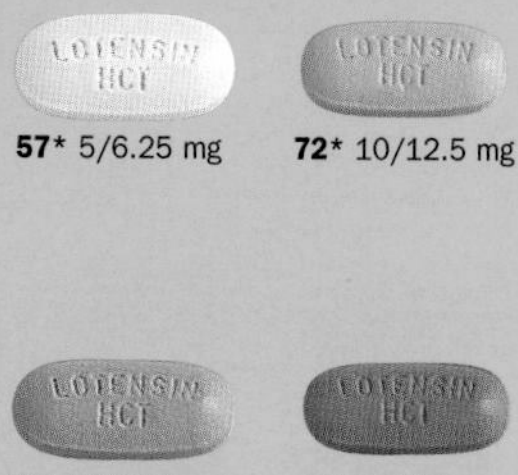

57* 5/6.25 mg   **72*** 10/12.5 mg

74* 20/12.5 mg   **75*** 20/25 mg

Lotensin HCT®
(benazepril HCl and hydrochlorothiazide USP)

RX NOVARTIS PHARMACEUTICALS P. 2053

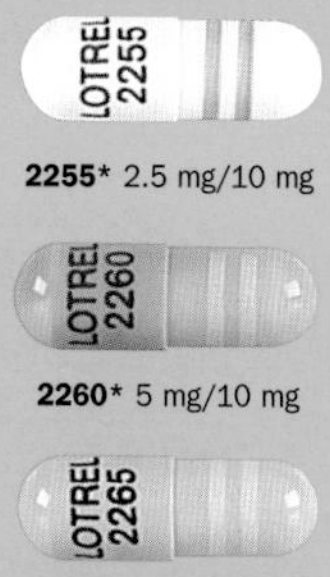

2255* 2.5 mg/10 mg

2260* 5 mg/10 mg

2265* 5 mg/20 mg

Lotrel®
(amlodipine and benazepril HCl)

RX NOVARTIS PHARMACEUTICALS P. 2057

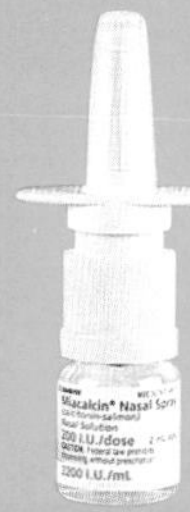

2200 I.U./mL

†Miacalcin® Nasal Spray
(calcitonin-salmon)
Nasal Solution

RX NOVARTIS PHARMACEUTICALS P. 2063

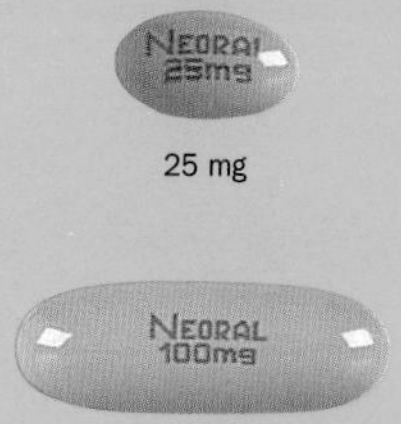

25 mg

100 mg

Neoral® Soft Gelatin Capsules
(cyclosporine capsules for microemulsion)

RX NOVARTIS PHARMACEUTICALS P. 2063

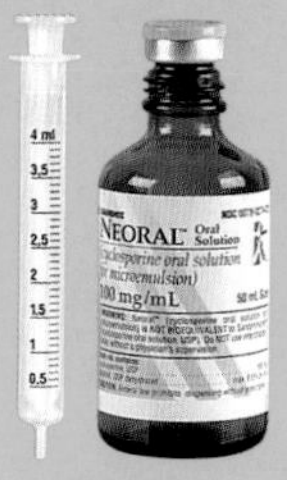

100 mg/mL

Neoral® Oral Solution
(cyclosporine oral solution for microemulsion)

RX NOVARTIS PHARMACEUTICALS P. 2070

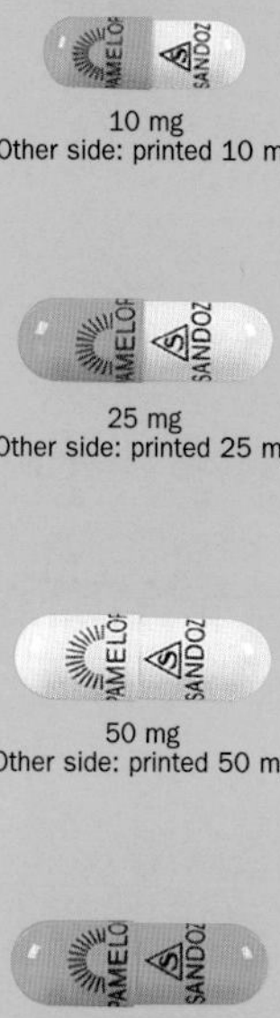

10 mg
Other side: printed 10 mg

25 mg
Other side: printed 25 mg

50 mg
Other side: printed 50 mg

75 mg
Other side: printed 75 mg

†Pamelor®
(nortriptyline HCl) Capsules, USP

RX NOVARTIS PHARMACEUTICALS P. 2072

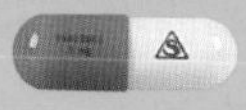

5 mg

Parlodel® Capsules
(bromocriptine mesylate) Capsules, USP

RX NOVARTIS PHARMACEUTICALS P. 2072

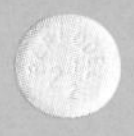

2 1/2 mg
Other side: scored

Parlodel® SnapTabs®
(bromocriptine mesylate) Tablets, USP

C-IV NOVARTIS PHARMACEUTICALS P. 2075

7.5 mg

15 mg

30 mg

Restoril®
(temazepam) Capsules, USP

C-II NOVARTIS PHARMACEUTICALS P. 2078

7* 5 mg

3* 10 mg

34* 20 mg

Ritalin® hydrochloride
(methylphenidate HCl tablets, USP)

C-II NOVARTIS PHARMACEUTICALS P. 2078

16* 20 mg
Sustained-release

Ritalin-SR®
(methylphenidate HCl, USP)

RX NOVARTIS PHARMACEUTICALS P. 2079

I.V. 5 mL (250 mg)   Oral Solution & Pipette
50 mL 100 mg/mL

Sandimmune®
(cyclosporine)

RX NOVARTIS PHARMACEUTICALS P. 2079

78-240* 25 mg

78-242* 50 mg

78-241* 100 mg

Sandimmune®
Soft Gelatin Capsules
(cyclosporine capsules, USP)

RX NOVARTIS PHARMACEUTICALS P. 2082

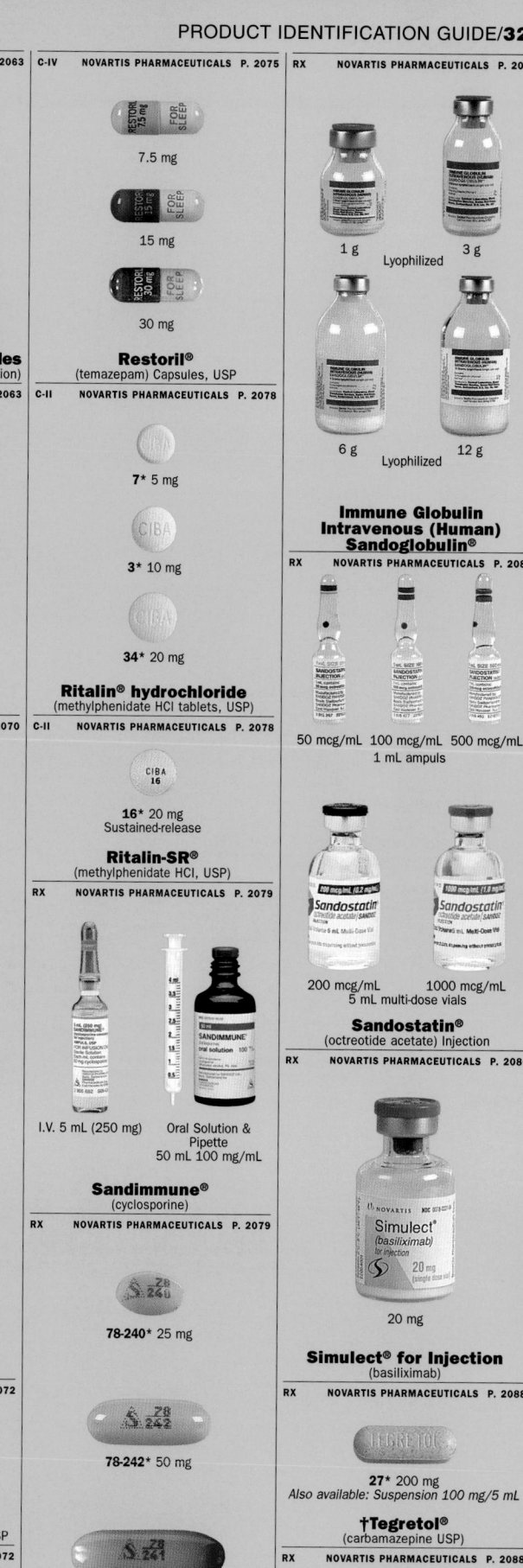

1 g   3 g
Lyophilized

6 g   12 g
Lyophilized

Immune Globulin Intravenous (Human) Sandoglobulin®

RX NOVARTIS PHARMACEUTICALS P. 2085

50 mcg/mL   100 mcg/mL   500 mcg/mL
1 mL ampuls

200 mcg/mL   1000 mcg/mL
5 mL multi-dose vials

Sandostatin®
(octreotide acetate) Injection

RX NOVARTIS PHARMACEUTICALS P. 2086

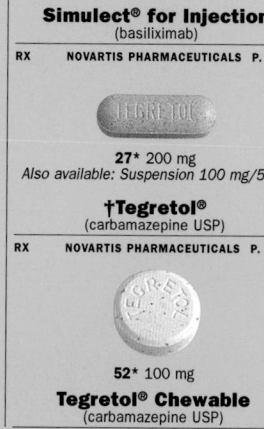

20 mg

Simulect® for Injection
(basiliximab)

RX NOVARTIS PHARMACEUTICALS P. 2088

27* 200 mg
Also available: Suspension 100 mg/5 mL

†Tegretol®
(carbamazepine USP)

RX NOVARTIS PHARMACEUTICALS P. 2088

52* 100 mg

Tegretol® Chewable
(carbamazepine USP)

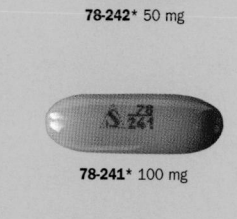

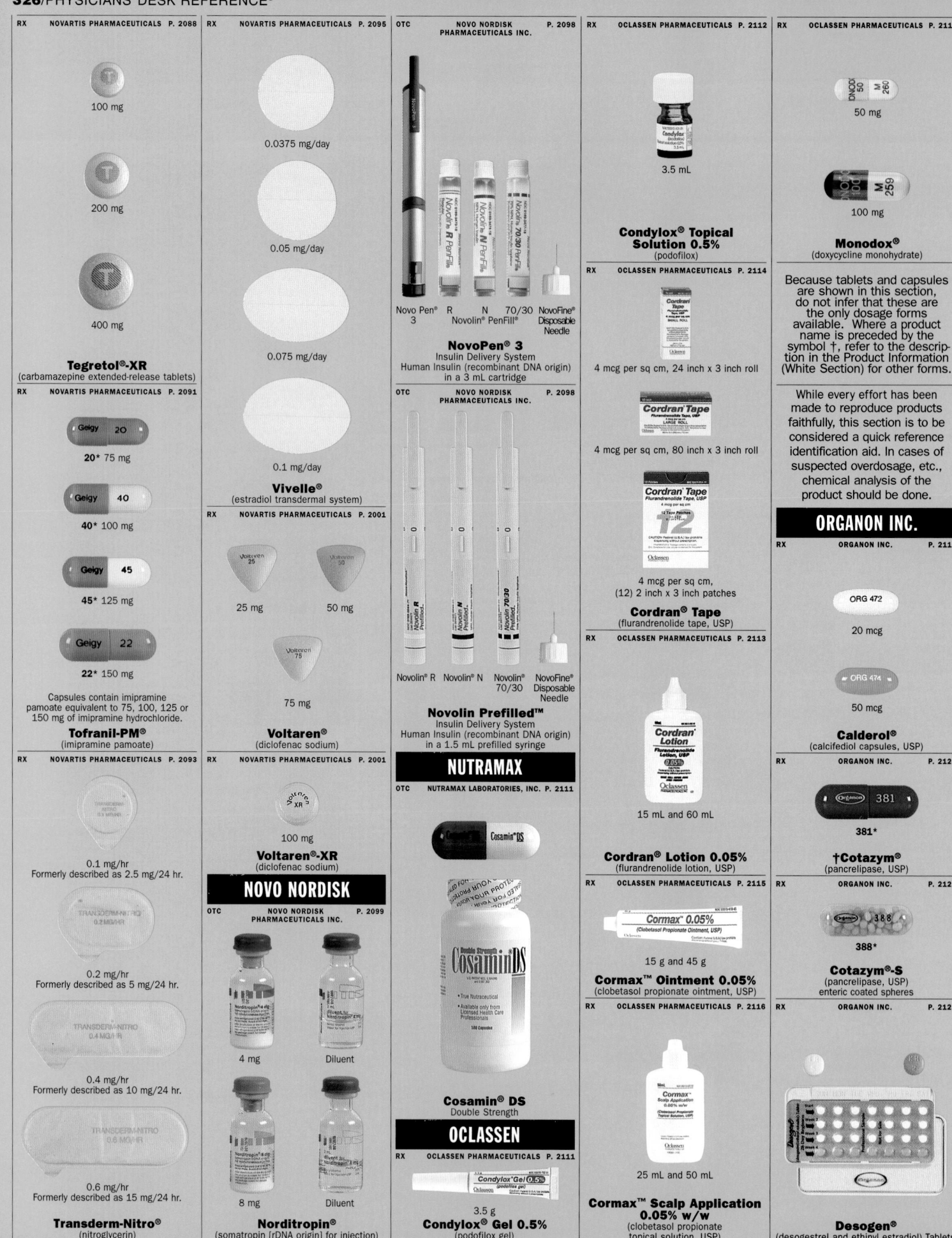

RX   NOVARTIS PHARMACEUTICALS   P. 2088

100 mg

200 mg

400 mg

Tegretol®-XR
(carbamazepine extended-release tablets)

RX   NOVARTIS PHARMACEUTICALS   P. 2091

20* 75 mg

40* 100 mg

45* 125 mg

22* 150 mg

Capsules contain imipramine
pamoate equivalent to 75, 100, 125 or
150 mg of imipramine hydrochloride.

Tofranil-PM®
(imipramine pamoate)

RX   NOVARTIS PHARMACEUTICALS   P. 2093

0.1 mg/hr
Formerly described as 2.5 mg/24 hr.

0.2 mg/hr
Formerly described as 5 mg/24 hr.

0.4 mg/hr
Formerly described as 10 mg/24 hr.

0.6 mg/hr
Formerly described as 15 mg/24 hr.

Transderm-Nitro®
(nitroglycerin)

RX   NOVARTIS PHARMACEUTICALS   P. 2095

0.0375 mg/day

0.05 mg/day

0.075 mg/day

0.1 mg/day

Vivelle®
(estradiol transdermal system)

RX   NOVARTIS PHARMACEUTICALS   P. 2001

25 mg   50 mg

75 mg

Voltaren®
(diclofenac sodium)

RX   NOVARTIS PHARMACEUTICALS   P. 2001

100 mg

Voltaren®-XR
(diclofenac sodium)

NOVO NORDISK

OTC   NOVO NORDISK   P. 2099
PHARMACEUTICALS INC.

4 mg   Diluent

8 mg   Diluent

Norditropin®
(somatropin [rDNA origin] for injection)

OTC   NOVO NORDISK   P. 2098
PHARMACEUTICALS INC.

Novo Pen®   R   N   70/30   NovoFine®
3   Novolin® PenFill®   Disposable
Needle

NovoPen® 3
Insulin Delivery System
Human Insulin (recombinant DNA origin)
in a 3 mL cartridge

OTC   NOVO NORDISK   P. 2098
PHARMACEUTICALS INC.

Novolin® R   Novolin® N   Novolin®   NovoFine®
70/30   Disposable
Needle

Novolin Prefilled™
Insulin Delivery System
Human Insulin (recombinant DNA origin)
in a 1.5 mL prefilled syringe

NUTRAMAX

OTC   NUTRAMAX LABORATORIES, INC. P. 2111

Cosamin® DS
Double Strength

OCLASSEN

RX   OCLASSEN PHARMACEUTICALS   P. 2111

3.5 g
Condylox® Gel 0.5%
(podofilox gel)

RX   OCLASSEN PHARMACEUTICALS P. 2112

3.5 mL

**Condylox® Topical
Solution 0.5%**
(podofilox)

RX   OCLASSEN PHARMACEUTICALS   P. 2114

4 mcg per sq cm, 24 inch x 3 inch roll

4 mcg per sq cm, 80 inch x 3 inch roll

4 mcg per sq cm,
(12) 2 inch x 3 inch patches

Cordran® Tape
(flurandrenolide tape, USP)

RX   OCLASSEN PHARMACEUTICALS   P. 2113

15 mL and 60 mL

Cordran® Lotion 0.05%
(flurandrenolide lotion, USP)

RX   OCLASSEN PHARMACEUTICALS   P. 2115

15 g and 45 g

Cormax™ Ointment 0.05%
(clobetasol propionate ointment, USP)

RX   OCLASSEN PHARMACEUTICALS   P. 2116

25 mL and 50 mL

**Cormax™ Scalp Application
0.05% w/w**
(clobetasol propionate
topical solution, USP)

RX   OCLASSEN PHARMACEUTICALS P. 2117

50 mg

100 mg

Monodox®
(doxycycline monohydrate)

Because tablets and capsules
are shown in this section,
do not infer that these are
the only dosage forms
available. Where a product
name is preceded by the
symbol †, refer to the description in the Product Information
(White Section) for other forms.

While every effort has been
made to reproduce products
faithfully, this section is to be
considered a quick reference
identification aid. In cases of
suspected overdosage, etc.,
chemical analysis of the
product should be done.

ORGANON INC.

RX   ORGANON INC.   P. 2119

20 mcg

50 mcg

Calderol®
(calcifediol capsules, USP)

RX   ORGANON INC.   P. 2120

381*

†Cotazym®
(pancrelipase, USP)

RX   ORGANON INC.   P. 2121

388*

Cotazym®-S
(pancrelipase, USP)
enteric coated spheres

RX   ORGANON INC.   P. 2121

Desogen®
(desogestrel and ethinyl estradiol) Tablets

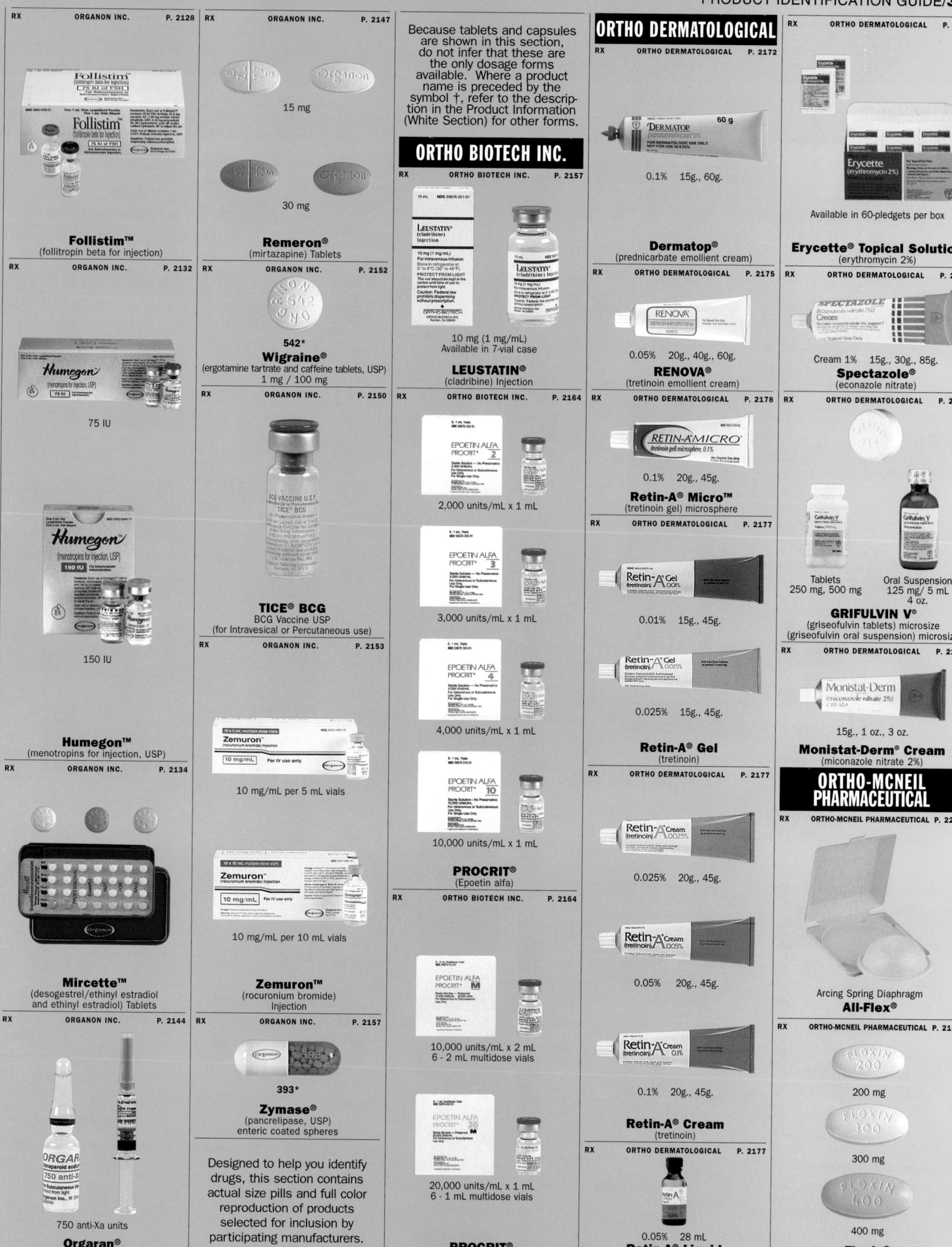

RX   ORGANON INC.   P. 2128

Follistim™
(follitropin beta for injection)

RX   ORGANON INC.   P. 2132

75 IU
Humegon™
(menotropins for injection, USP)

150 IU

RX   ORGANON INC.   P. 2134

Mircette™
(desogestrel/ethinyl estradiol
and ethinyl estradiol) Tablets

RX   ORGANON INC.   P. 2144

750 anti-Xa units
Orgaran®
(danaparoid sodium) Injection

RX   ORGANON INC.   P. 2147

15 mg

30 mg

Remeron®
(mirtazapine) Tablets

RX   ORGANON INC.   P. 2152

542*
Wigraine®
(ergotamine tartrate and caffeine tablets, USP)
1 mg / 100 mg

RX   ORGANON INC.   P. 2150

TICE® BCG
BCG Vaccine USP
(for Intravesical or Percutaneous use)

RX   ORGANON INC.   P. 2153

10 mg/mL per 5 mL vials

10 mg/mL per 10 mL vials

Zemuron™
(rocuronium bromide)
Injection

RX   ORGANON INC.   P. 2157

393*
Zymase®
(pancrelipase, USP)
enteric coated spheres

Designed to help you identify
drugs, this section contains
actual size pills and full color
reproduction of products
selected for inclusion by
participating manufacturers.

Because tablets and capsules
are shown in this section,
do not infer that these are
the only dosage forms
available. Where a product
name is preceded by the
symbol †, refer to the description in the Product Information
(White Section) for other forms.

ORTHO BIOTECH INC.

RX   ORTHO BIOTECH INC.   P. 2157

10 mg (1 mg/mL)
Available in 7-vial case
LEUSTATIN®
(cladribine) Injection

RX   ORTHO BIOTECH INC.   P. 2164

2,000 units/mL x 1 mL

3,000 units/mL x 1 mL

4,000 units/mL x 1 mL

10,000 units/mL x 1 mL

PROCRIT®
(Epoetin alfa)

RX   ORTHO BIOTECH INC.   P. 2164

10,000 units/mL x 2 mL
6 - 2 mL multidose vials

20,000 units/mL x 1 mL
6 - 1 mL multidose vials

PROCRIT®
(Epoetin alfa)

ORTHO DERMATOLOGICAL

RX   ORTHO DERMATOLOGICAL   P. 2172

60 g

0.1%   15g., 60g.
Dermatop®
(prednicarbate emollient cream)

RX   ORTHO DERMATOLOGICAL   P. 2175

0.05%   20g., 40g., 60g.
RENOVA®
(tretinoin emollient cream)

RX   ORTHO DERMATOLOGICAL   P. 2178

0.1%   20g., 45g.
Retin-A® Micro™
(tretinoin gel) microsphere

RX   ORTHO DERMATOLOGICAL   P. 2177

0.01%   15g., 45g.

0.025%   15g., 45g.

Retin-A® Gel
(tretinoin)

RX   ORTHO DERMATOLOGICAL   P. 2177

0.025%   20g., 45g.

0.05%   20g., 45g.

0.1%   20g., 45g.

Retin-A® Cream
(tretinoin)

RX   ORTHO DERMATOLOGICAL   P. 2177

0.05%   28 mL
Retin-A® Liquid
(tretinoin)

RX   ORTHO DERMATOLOGICAL   P. 2174

Available in 60-pledgets per box
Erycette® Topical Solution
(erythromycin 2%)

RX   ORTHO DERMATOLOGICAL   P. 2179

Cream 1%   15g., 30g., 85g.
Spectazole®
(econazole nitrate)

RX   ORTHO DERMATOLOGICAL   P. 2174

Tablets
250 mg, 500 mg

Oral Suspension
125 mg/ 5 mL
4 oz.

GRIFULVIN V®
(griseofulvin tablets) microsize
(griseofulvin oral suspension) microsize

RX   ORTHO DERMATOLOGICAL   P. 2175

15g., 1 oz., 3 oz.
Monistat-Derm® Cream
(miconazole nitrate 2%)

ORTHO-MCNEIL PHARMACEUTICAL

RX   ORTHO-MCNEIL PHARMACEUTICAL   P. 2211

Arcing Spring Diaphragm
All-Flex®

RX   ORTHO-MCNEIL PHARMACEUTICAL   P. 2184

200 mg

300 mg

400 mg

Floxin®
(ofloxacin tablets)

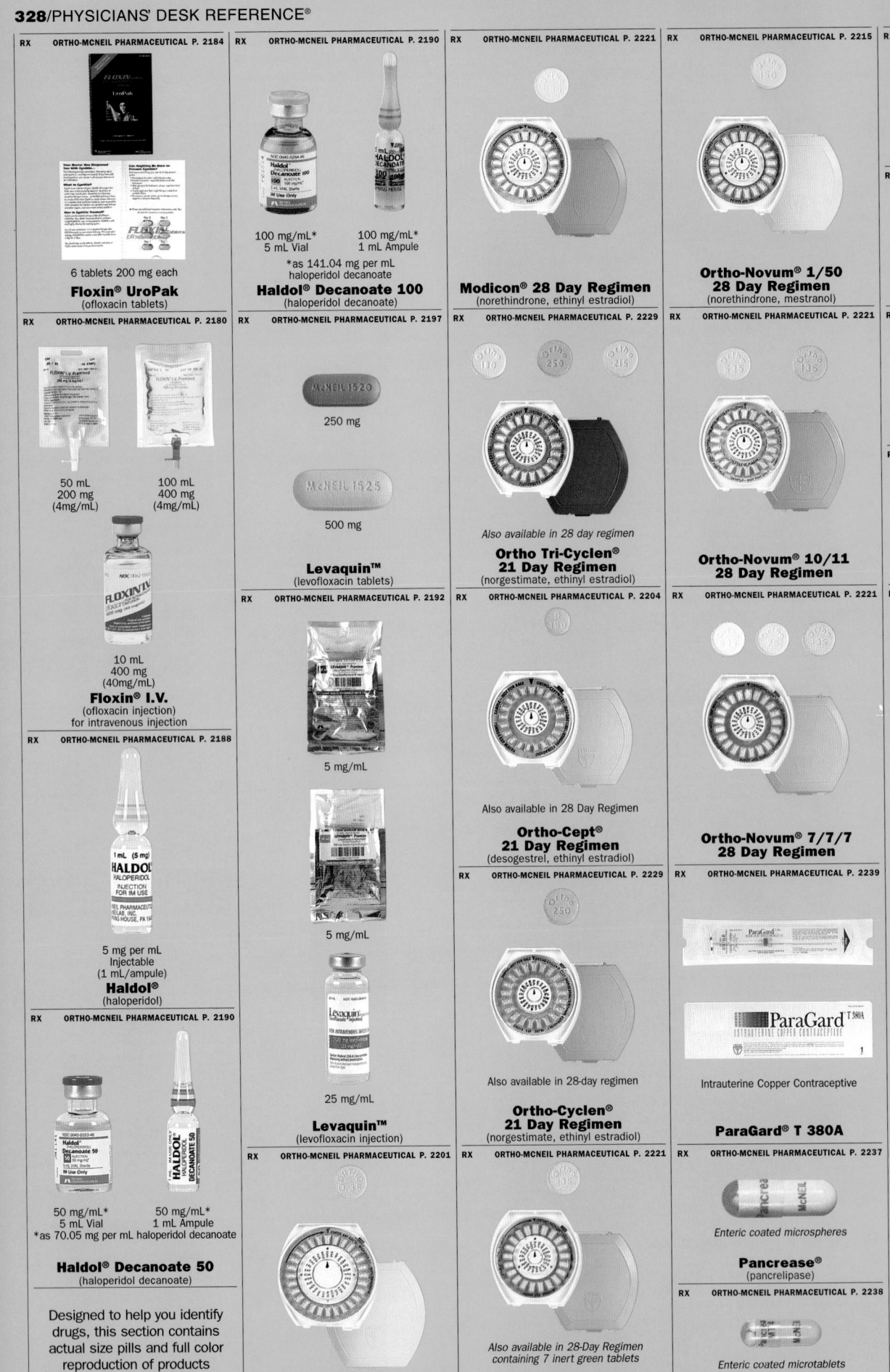

RX   ORTHO-MCNEIL PHARMACEUTICAL P. 2184

6 tablets 200 mg each

Floxin® UroPak
(ofloxacin tablets)

RX   ORTHO-MCNEIL PHARMACEUTICAL P. 2180

50 mL
200 mg
(4mg/mL)

100 mL
400 mg
(4mg/mL)

10 mL
400 mg
(40mg/mL)

Floxin® I.V.
(ofloxacin injection)
for intravenous injection

RX   ORTHO-MCNEIL PHARMACEUTICAL P. 2188

1 mL (5 mg)
HALDOL
HALOPERIDOL
INJECTION
FOR IM USE

5 mg per mL
Injectable
(1 mL/ampule)

Haldol®
(haloperidol)

RX   ORTHO-MCNEIL PHARMACEUTICAL P. 2190

50 mg/mL*
5 mL Vial

50 mg/mL*
1 mL Ampule
*as 70.05 mg per mL haloperidol decanoate

Haldol® Decanoate 50
(haloperidol decanoate)

Designed to help you identify
drugs, this section contains
actual size pills and full color
reproduction of products
selected for inclusion by
participating manufacturers.

RX   ORTHO-MCNEIL PHARMACEUTICAL P. 2190

100 mg/mL*
5 mL Vial

100 mg/mL*
1 mL Ampule

*as 141.04 mg per mL
haloperidol decanoate

Haldol® Decanoate 100
(haloperidol decanoate)

RX   ORTHO-MCNEIL PHARMACEUTICAL P. 2197

McNEIL 1520
250 mg

McNEIL 1525
500 mg

Levaquin™
(levofloxacin tablets)

RX   ORTHO-MCNEIL PHARMACEUTICAL P. 2192

5 mg/mL

5 mg/mL

25 mg/mL

Levaquin™
(levofloxacin injection)

RX   ORTHO-MCNEIL PHARMACEUTICAL P. 2201

0.35 mg
Micronor® 28 Day Regimen
(norethindrone)

RX   ORTHO-MCNEIL PHARMACEUTICAL P. 2221

Modicon® 28 Day Regimen
(norethindrone, ethinyl estradiol)

RX   ORTHO-MCNEIL PHARMACEUTICAL P. 2229

ortho 130   ortho 250   ortho 215

Also available in 28 day regimen

**Ortho Tri-Cyclen®
21 Day Regimen**
(norgestimate, ethinyl estradiol)

RX   ORTHO-MCNEIL PHARMACEUTICAL P. 2204

Also available in 28 Day Regimen

**Ortho-Cept®
21 Day Regimen**
(desogestrel, ethinyl estradiol)

RX   ORTHO-MCNEIL PHARMACEUTICAL P. 2229

ortho 250

Also available in 28-day regimen

**Ortho-Cyclen®
21 Day Regimen**
(norgestimate, ethinyl estradiol)

RX   ORTHO-MCNEIL PHARMACEUTICAL P. 2221

*Also available in 28-Day Regimen
containing 7 inert green tablets*

**Ortho-Novum® 1/35
21 Day Regimen**
(norethindrone, ethinyl estradiol)

RX   ORTHO-MCNEIL PHARMACEUTICAL P. 2215

**Ortho-Novum® 1/50
28 Day Regimen**
(norethindrone, mestranol)

RX   ORTHO-MCNEIL PHARMACEUTICAL P. 2221

ortho 835   ortho 135

**Ortho-Novum® 10/11
28 Day Regimen**

RX   ORTHO-MCNEIL PHARMACEUTICAL P. 2221

**Ortho-Novum® 7/7/7
28 Day Regimen**

RX   ORTHO-MCNEIL PHARMACEUTICAL P. 2239

ParaGard T 380A

ParaGard T 380A

Intrauterine Copper Contraceptive

ParaGard® T 380A

RX   ORTHO-MCNEIL PHARMACEUTICAL P. 2237

Enteric coated microspheres

Pancrease®
(pancrelipase)

RX   ORTHO-MCNEIL PHARMACEUTICAL P. 2238

Enteric coated microtablets

Pancrease® MT 4
(pancrelipase)

RX   ORTHO-MCNEIL PHARMACEUTICAL P. 2238

Enteric coated microtablets

Pancrease® MT 10
(pancrelipase)

RX   ORTHO-MCNEIL PHARMACEUTICAL P. 2238

Enteric coated microtablets

Pancrease® MT 16
(pancrelipase)

RX   ORTHO-MCNEIL PHARMACEUTICAL P. 2238

Enteric coated microtablets

Pancrease® MT 20
(pancrelipase)

RX   ORTHO-MCNEIL PHARMACEUTICAL P. 2239

PARAFON
FORTE DSC

500 mg

Parafon Forte® DSC
(chlorzoxazone)

RX   ORTHO-MCNEIL PHARMACEUTICAL P. 2243

REGRANEX GEL
(becaplermin)

REGRANEX GEL
(becaplermin)

15 g

Regranex® Gel 0.01%
(becaplermin)

RX   ORTHO-MCNEIL PHARMACEUTICAL P. 2245

0.8%, 20g

Terazol® 3
(terconazole)

RX   ORTHO-MCNEIL PHARMACEUTICAL P. 2246

Terazol 3   Terazol 3   Terazol
Terazol 3   Terazol 3

80 mg

Terazol® 3
(terconazole)

RX   ORTHO-MCNEIL PHARMACEUTICAL P. 2246

Net Weight 0.317 oz. (9g)

Terazol® 7
(terconazole)

RX   ORTHO-MCNEIL PHARMACEUTICAL P. 2247

200 mg

Tolectin® 200
(tolmetin sodium)

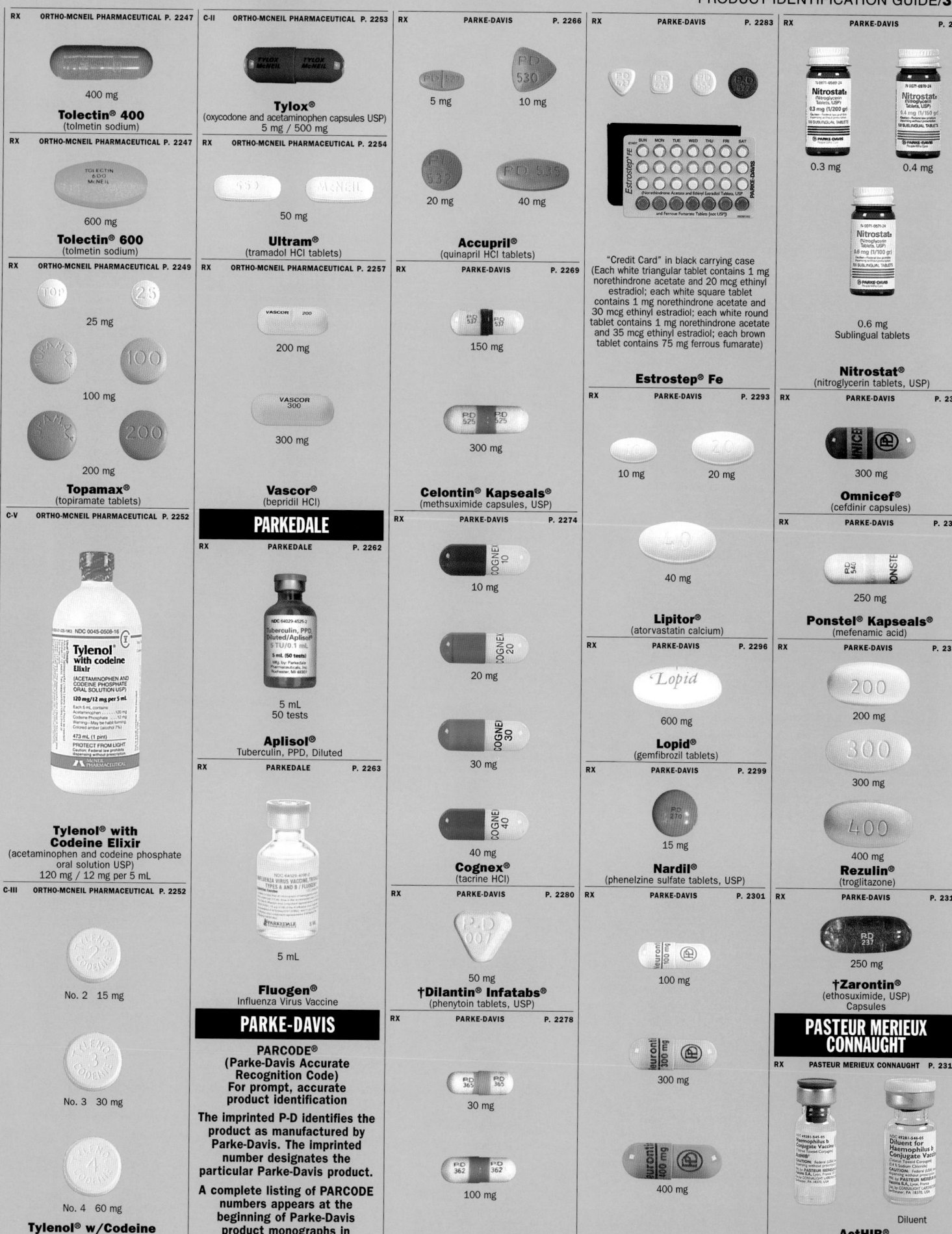

RX — ORTHO-MCNEIL PHARMACEUTICAL P. 2247

400 mg

Tolectin® 400
(tolmetin sodium)

RX — ORTHO-MCNEIL PHARMACEUTICAL P. 2247

600 mg

Tolectin® 600
(tolmetin sodium)

RX — ORTHO-MCNEIL PHARMACEUTICAL P. 2249

25 mg

100 mg

200 mg

Topamax®
(topiramate tablets)

C-V — ORTHO-MCNEIL PHARMACEUTICAL P. 2252

Tylenol® with codeine Elixir
(ACETAMINOPHEN AND CODEINE PHOSPHATE ORAL SOLUTION USP)
120 mg/12 mg per 5 mL

Tylenol® with Codeine Elixir
(acetaminophen and codeine phosphate oral solution USP)
120 mg / 12 mg per 5 mL

C-III — ORTHO-MCNEIL PHARMACEUTICAL P. 2252

No. 2   15 mg

No. 3   30 mg

No. 4   60 mg

Tylenol® w/Codeine
(acetaminophen and codeine phosphate tablets)

C-II — ORTHO-MCNEIL PHARMACEUTICAL P. 2253

Tylox®
(oxycodone and acetaminophen capsules USP)
5 mg / 500 mg

RX — ORTHO-MCNEIL PHARMACEUTICAL P. 2254

50 mg

Ultram®
(tramadol HCl tablets)

RX — ORTHO-MCNEIL PHARMACEUTICAL P. 2257

200 mg

300 mg

Vascor®
(bepridil HCl)

PARKEDALE

RX — PARKEDALE P. 2262

5 mL
50 tests

Aplisol®
Tuberculin, PPD, Diluted

RX — PARKEDALE P. 2263

5 mL

Fluogen®
Influenza Virus Vaccine

PARKE-DAVIS

PARCODE®
(Parke-Davis Accurate Recognition Code)
For prompt, accurate product identification

The imprinted P-D identifies the product as manufactured by Parke-Davis. The imprinted number designates the particular Parke-Davis product.

A complete listing of PARCODE numbers appears at the beginning of Parke-Davis product monographs in the white section.

RX — PARKE-DAVIS P. 2266

5 mg

10 mg

20 mg

40 mg

Accupril®
(quinapril HCl tablets)

RX — PARKE-DAVIS P. 2269

150 mg

300 mg

Celontin® Kapseals®
(methsuximide capsules, USP)

RX — PARKE-DAVIS P. 2274

10 mg

20 mg

30 mg

40 mg

Cognex®
(tacrine HCl)

RX — PARKE-DAVIS P. 2280

50 mg

†Dilantin® Infatabs®
(phenytoin tablets, USP)

RX — PARKE-DAVIS P. 2278

30 mg

100 mg

†Dilantin® Kapseals®
(extended phenytoin sodium capsules, USP)

RX — PARKE-DAVIS P. 2283

Estrostep® Fe

"Credit Card" in black carrying case (Each white triangular tablet contains 1 mg norethindrone acetate and 20 mcg ethinyl estradiol; each white square tablet contains 1 mg norethindrone acetate and 30 mcg ethinyl estradiol; each white round tablet contains 1 mg norethindrone acetate and 35 mcg ethinyl estradiol; each brown tablet contains 75 mg ferrous fumarate)

RX — PARKE-DAVIS P. 2293

10 mg

20 mg

40 mg

Lipitor®
(atorvastatin calcium)

RX — PARKE-DAVIS P. 2296

600 mg

Lopid®
(gemfibrozil tablets)

RX — PARKE-DAVIS P. 2299

15 mg

Nardil®
(phenelzine sulfate tablets, USP)

RX — PARKE-DAVIS P. 2301

100 mg

300 mg

400 mg

Neurontin®
(gabapentin capsules)

RX — PARKE-DAVIS P. 2304

0.3 mg

0.4 mg

0.6 mg
Sublingual tablets

Nitrostat®
(nitroglycerin tablets, USP)

RX — PARKE-DAVIS P. 2305

300 mg

Omnicef®
(cefdinir capsules)

RX — PARKE-DAVIS P. 2309

250 mg

Ponstel® Kapseals®
(mefenamic acid)

RX — PARKE-DAVIS P. 2310

200 mg

300 mg

400 mg

Rezulin®
(troglitazone)

RX — PARKE-DAVIS P. 2314

250 mg

†Zarontin®
(ethosuximide, USP)
Capsules

PASTEUR MERIEUX CONNAUGHT

RX — PASTEUR MERIEUX CONNAUGHT P. 2316

Diluent

ActHIB®
Haemophilus b Conjugate Vaccine
(Tetanus Toxoid Conjugate)

RX   PASTEUR MERIEUX CONNAUGHT   P. 2320

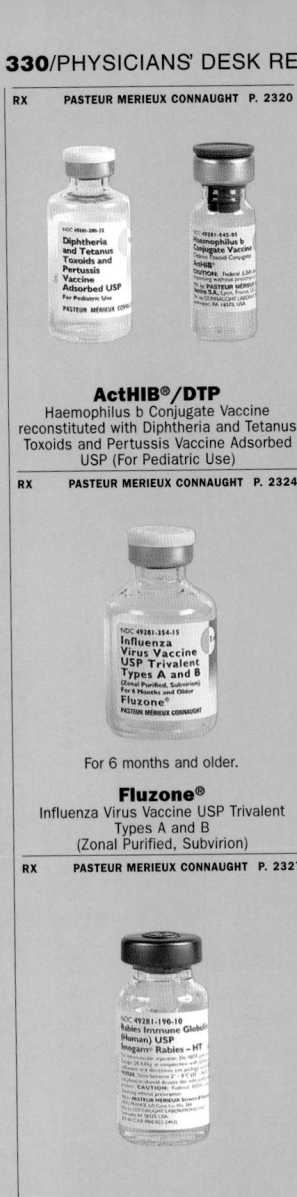

ActHIB®/DTP
Haemophilus b Conjugate Vaccine
reconstituted with Diphtheria and Tetanus
Toxoids and Pertussis Vaccine Adsorbed
USP (For Pediatric Use)

RX   PASTEUR MERIEUX CONNAUGHT   P. 2324

For 6 months and older.

Fluzone®
Influenza Virus Vaccine USP Trivalent
Types A and B
(Zonal Purified, Subvirion)

RX   PASTEUR MERIEUX CONNAUGHT   P. 2327

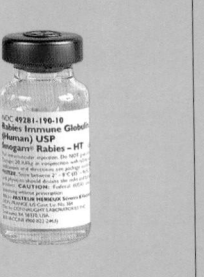

Imogam® Rabies - HT
Rabies Immune Globulin (Human) USP

RX   PASTEUR MERIEUX CONNAUGHT   P. 2329

Diluent
Pre- and post-exposure intramuscular
immunization only

Imovax® Rabies
Rabies Vaccine

RX   PASTEUR MERIEUX CONNAUGHT   P. 2331

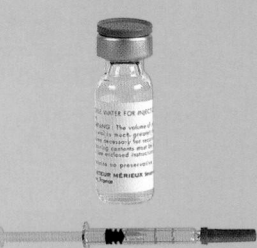

For pre-exposure intradermal
immunization only

Imovax® Rabies I.D.
Rabies Vaccine

RX   PASTEUR MERIEUX CONNAUGHT   P. 2333

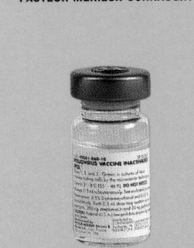

IPOL®
Poliovirus Vaccine Inactivated

RX   PASTEUR MERIEUX CONNAUGHT   P. 2336

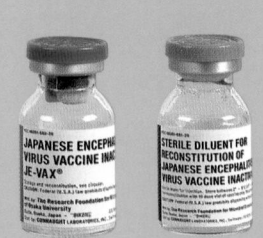

Diluent

JE-VAX®
Japanese Encephalitis Virus Vaccine
Inactivated

RX   PASTEUR MERIEUX CONNAUGHT   P. 2339

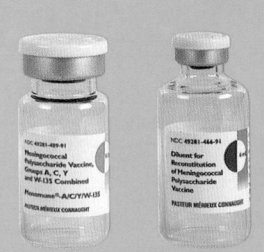

Diluent

Menomune® A/C/Y/W-135
Meningococcal Polysaccharide Vaccine,
Groups A,C,Y and W-135 Combined

RX   PASTEUR MERIEUX CONNAUGHT   P. 3473

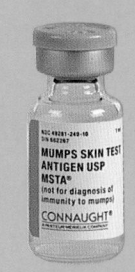

MSTA®
Mumps Skin Test Antigen USP

RX   PASTEUR MERIEUX CONNAUGHT   P. 3473

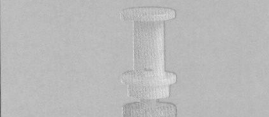

Mono-Vacc® Test (O.T.)
Tuberculin, Old

While every effort has been
made to reproduce products
faithfully, this section is to be
considered a quick reference
identification aid. In cases of
suspected overdosage, etc.,
chemical analysis of the
product should be done.

RX   PASTEUR MERIEUX CONNAUGHT   P. 2345

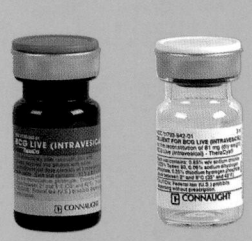

Diluent

TheraCys®
BCG Live (intravesical)

RX   PASTEUR MERIEUX CONNAUGHT   P. 2340

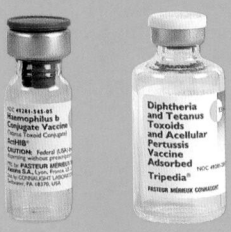

TriHIBit™
ActHIB, Haemophilus b Conjugate Vaccine
(Tetanus Toxoid Conjugate) reconstituted
with Tripedia, Diphtheria and Tetanus
Toxoids and Acellular Pertussis
Vaccine Adsorbed

RX   PASTEUR MERIEUX CONNAUGHT   P. 2340

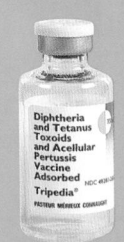

Tripedia®
Diphtheria and Tetanus Toxoids and
Acellular Pertussis Vaccine Adsorbed

RX   PASTEUR MERIEUX CONNAUGHT   P. 3474

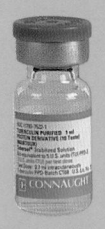

Tubersol®
Tuberculin Purified Protein Derivative
(Mantoux)

RX   PASTEUR MERIEUX CONNAUGHT   P. 2348

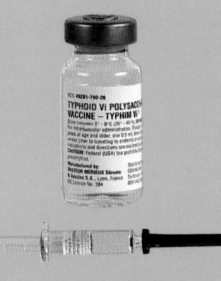

Typhim Vi®
Typhoid Vi Polysaccharide Vaccine

RX   PASTEUR MERIEUX CONNAUGHT   P. 2350

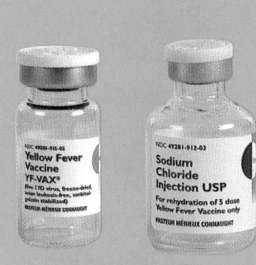

Diluent

YF-VAX®
Yellow Fever Vaccine

PATHOGENESIS

RX   PATHOGENESIS CORPORATION   P. 2350

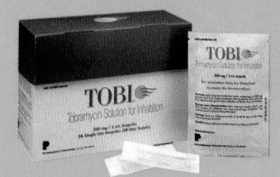

300 mg/5 mL Ampules

TOBI®
(tobramycin solution for inhalation)

PFIZER

RX   ROERIG DIVISION   P. 2364

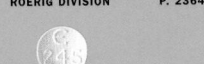

E245* 5 mg

E246* 10 mg

Aricept®*
(donepezil HCI)
*Registered trademark of Eisai Co., Ltd
Tokyo, Japan

RX   ROERIG DIVISION   P. 2368

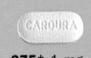

275* 1 mg   276* 2 mg

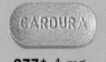

277* 4 mg   278* 8 mg

Cardura®
(doxazosin mesylate)

RX   ROERIG DIVISION   P. 2379

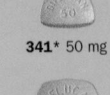

341* 50 mg

342* 100 mg

343* 200 mg

Diflucan®
(fluconazole)

RX   ROERIG DIVISION   P. 2379

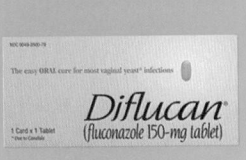

350* 150 mg

Diflucan®
(fluconazole)

RX   ROERIG DIVISION   P. 2379

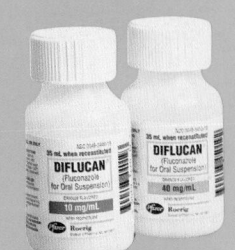

Available in 10 mg/mL
and 40 mg/mL

Diflucan®
(fluconazole for oral suspension)

RX   PRATT PHARMACEUTICALS   P. 2383

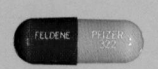

322* 10 mg

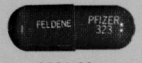

323* 20 mg

Feldene®
(piroxicam)

RX   PRATT PHARMACEUTICALS   P. 2385

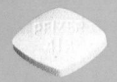

411* 5 mg   412* 10 mg

Glucotrol®
(glipizide)

RX   PRATT PHARMACEUTICALS   P. 2387

155* 5 mg

156* 10 mg

Glucotrol XL®
(glipizide)
Extended Release Tablets

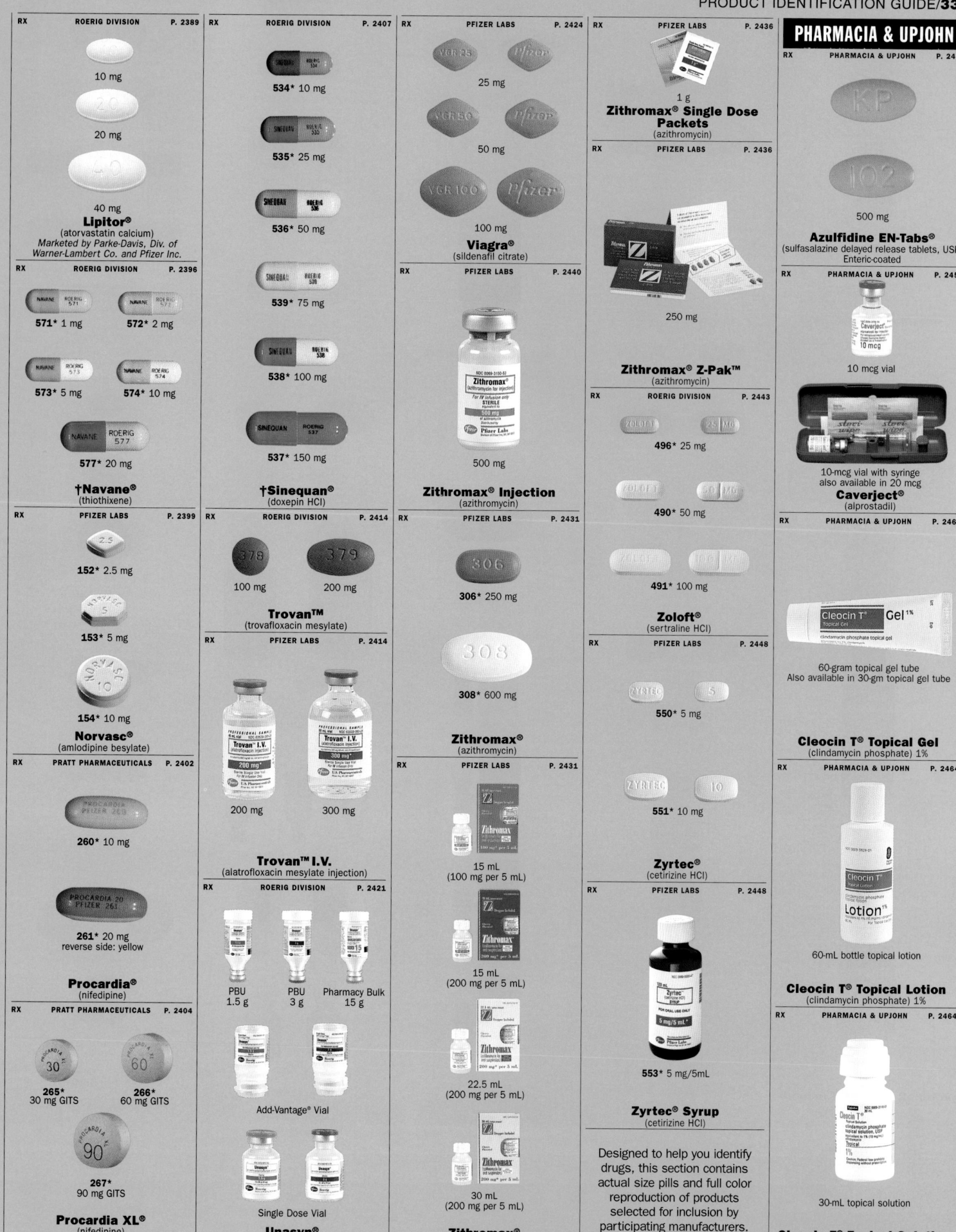

RX   ROERIG DIVISION   P. 2389

10 mg

20 mg

40 mg

Lipitor®
(atorvastatin calcium)
Marketed by Parke-Davis, Div. of
Warner-Lambert Co. and Pfizer Inc.

RX   ROERIG DIVISION   P. 2396

571* 1 mg   **572*** 2 mg

573* 5 mg   **574*** 10 mg

577* 20 mg

†Navane®
(thiothixene)

RX   PFIZER LABS   P. 2399

152* 2.5 mg

153* 5 mg

154* 10 mg

Norvasc®
(amlodipine besylate)

RX   PRATT PHARMACEUTICALS   P. 2402

260* 10 mg

261* 20 mg
reverse side: yellow

Procardia®
(nifedipine)

RX   PRATT PHARMACEUTICALS   P. 2404

265*
30 mg GITS   **266***
60 mg GITS

267*
90 mg GITS

Procardia XL®
(nifedipine)
Extended Release Tablets

RX   ROERIG DIVISION   P. 2407

534* 10 mg

535* 25 mg

536* 50 mg

539* 75 mg

538* 100 mg

537* 150 mg

†Sinequan®
(doxepin HCl)

RX   ROERIG DIVISION   P. 2414

100 mg   200 mg

Trovan™
(trovafloxacin mesylate)

RX   PFIZER LABS   P. 2414

200 mg   300 mg

Trovan™ I.V.
(alatrofloxacin mesylate injection)

RX   ROERIG DIVISION   P. 2421

PBU
1.5 g   PBU
3 g   Pharmacy Bulk
15 g

Add-Vantage® Vial

Single Dose Vial

Unasyn®
(ampicillin sodium/sulbactam sodium)

RX   PFIZER LABS   P. 2424

25 mg

50 mg

100 mg

Viagra®
(sildenafil citrate)

RX   PFIZER LABS   P. 2440

500 mg

Zithromax® Injection
(azithromycin)

RX   PFIZER LABS   P. 2431

306* 250 mg

308* 600 mg

Zithromax®
(azithromycin)

RX   PFIZER LABS   P. 2431

15 mL
(100 mg per 5 mL)

15 mL
(200 mg per 5 mL)

22.5 mL
(200 mg per 5 mL)

30 mL
(200 mg per 5 mL)

Zithromax®
(azithromycin for oral suspension)

RX   PFIZER LABS   P. 2436

1 g
Zithromax® Single Dose
Packets
(azithromycin)

RX   PFIZER LABS   P. 2436

250 mg

Zithromax® Z-Pak™
(azithromycin)

RX   ROERIG DIVISION   P. 2443

496* 25 mg

490* 50 mg

491* 100 mg

Zoloft®
(sertraline HCl)

RX   PFIZER LABS   P. 2448

550* 5 mg

551* 10 mg

Zyrtec®
(cetirizine HCl)

RX   PFIZER LABS   P. 2448

553* 5 mg/5mL

Zyrtec® Syrup
(cetirizine HCl)

Designed to help you identify
drugs, this section contains
actual size pills and full color
reproduction of products
selected for inclusion by
participating manufacturers.

PHARMACIA & UPJOHN

RX   PHARMACIA & UPJOHN   P. 2454

500 mg

Azulfidine EN-Tabs®
(sulfasalazine delayed release tablets, USP)
Enteric-coated

RX   PHARMACIA & UPJOHN   P. 2458

10 mcg vial

10-mcg vial with syringe
also available in 20 mcg
Caverject®
(alprostadil)

RX   PHARMACIA & UPJOHN   P. 2464

60-gram topical gel tube
Also available in 30-gm topical gel tube

Cleocin T® Topical Gel
(clindamycin phosphate) 1%

RX   PHARMACIA & UPJOHN   P. 2464

60-mL bottle topical lotion

Cleocin T® Topical Lotion
(clindamycin phosphate) 1%

RX   PHARMACIA & UPJOHN   P. 2464

30-mL topical solution

Cleocin T® Topical Solution
(clindamycin phosphate) 1%

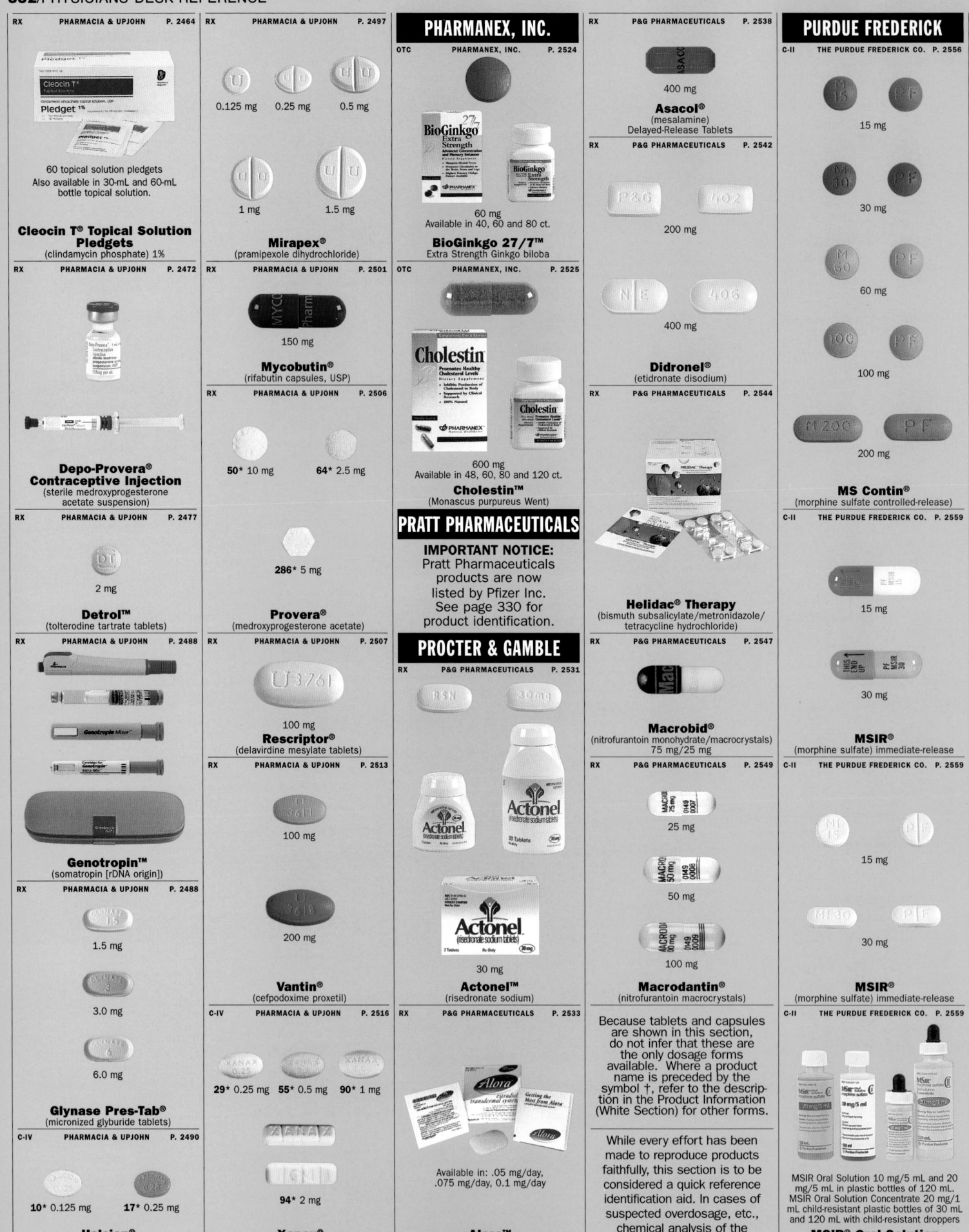

RX   PHARMACIA & UPJOHN   P. 2464

Cleocin T® Topical Solution Pledgets
(clindamycin phosphate) 1%

60 topical solution pledgets
Also available in 30-mL and 60-mL
bottle topical solution.

RX   PHARMACIA & UPJOHN   P. 2472

**Depo-Provera®
Contraceptive Injection**
(sterile medroxyprogesterone
acetate suspension)

RX   PHARMACIA & UPJOHN   P. 2477

2 mg

Detrol™
(tolterodine tartrate tablets)

RX   PHARMACIA & UPJOHN   P. 2488

Genotropin™
(somatropin [rDNA origin])

RX   PHARMACIA & UPJOHN   P. 2488

1.5 mg

3.0 mg

6.0 mg

Glynase Pres-Tab®
(micronized glyburide tablets)

C-IV   PHARMACIA & UPJOHN   P. 2490

10* 0.125 mg   **17*** 0.25 mg

Halcion®
(triazolam, USP)

RX   PHARMACIA & UPJOHN   P. 2497

0.125 mg   0.25 mg   0.5 mg

1 mg   1.5 mg

Mirapex®
(pramipexole dihydrochloride)

RX   PHARMACIA & UPJOHN   P. 2501

150 mg

Mycobutin®
(rifabutin capsules, USP)

RX   PHARMACIA & UPJOHN   P. 2506

50* 10 mg   **64*** 2.5 mg

286* 5 mg

Provera®
(medroxyprogesterone acetate)

RX   PHARMACIA & UPJOHN   P. 2507

100 mg

Rescriptor®
(delavirdine mesylate tablets)

RX   PHARMACIA & UPJOHN   P. 2513

100 mg

200 mg

Vantin®
(cefpodoxime proxetil)

C-IV   PHARMACIA & UPJOHN   P. 2516

29* 0.25 mg   **55*** 0.5 mg   **90*** 1 mg

94* 2 mg

Xanax®
(alprazolam)

PHARMANEX, INC.

OTC   PHARMANEX, INC.   P. 2524

60 mg
Available in 40, 60 and 80 ct.

BioGinkgo 27/7™
Extra Strength Ginkgo biloba

OTC   PHARMANEX, INC.   P. 2525

600 mg
Available in 48, 60, 80 and 120 ct.

Cholestin™
(Monascus purpureus Went)

PRATT PHARMACEUTICALS

IMPORTANT NOTICE:
Pratt Pharmaceuticals
products are now
listed by Pfizer Inc.
See page 330 for
product identification.

PROCTER & GAMBLE

RX   P&G PHARMACEUTICALS   P. 2531

30 mg

Actonel™
(risedronate sodium)

RX   P&G PHARMACEUTICALS   P. 2533

Available in: .05 mg/day,
.075 mg/day, 0.1 mg/day

Alora™
(estradiol transdermal system)

RX   P&G PHARMACEUTICALS   P. 2538

400 mg

Asacol®
(mesalamine)
Delayed-Release Tablets

RX   P&G PHARMACEUTICALS   P. 2542

200 mg

400 mg

Didronel®
(etidronate disodium)

RX   P&G PHARMACEUTICALS   P. 2544

Helidac® Therapy
(bismuth subsalicylate/metronidazole/
tetracycline hydrochloride)

RX   P&G PHARMACEUTICALS   P. 2547

Macrobid®
(nitrofurantoin monohydrate/macrocrystals)
75 mg/25 mg

RX   P&G PHARMACEUTICALS   P. 2549

25 mg

50 mg

100 mg

Macrodantin®
(nitrofurantoin macrocrystals)

Because tablets and capsules
are shown in this section,
do not infer that these are
the only dosage forms
available. Where a product
name is preceded by the
symbol †, refer to the description in the Product Information
(White Section) for other forms.

While every effort has been
made to reproduce products
faithfully, this section is to be
considered a quick reference
identification aid. In cases of
suspected overdosage, etc.,
chemical analysis of the
product should be done.

PURDUE FREDERICK

C-II   THE PURDUE FREDERICK CO.   P. 2556

15 mg

30 mg

60 mg

100 mg

200 mg

MS Contin®
(morphine sulfate controlled-release)

C-II   THE PURDUE FREDERICK CO.   P. 2559

15 mg

30 mg

MSIR®
(morphine sulfate) immediate-release

C-II   THE PURDUE FREDERICK CO.   P. 2559

15 mg

30 mg

MSIR®
(morphine sulfate) immediate-release

C-II   THE PURDUE FREDERICK CO.   P. 2559

MSIR Oral Solution 10 mg/5 mL and 20
mg/5 mL in plastic bottles of 120 mL.
MSIR Oral Solution Concentrate 20 mg/1
mL child-resistant plastic bottles of 30 mL
and 120 mL with child-resistant droppers

MSIR® Oral Solution
(morphine sulfate) immediate-release

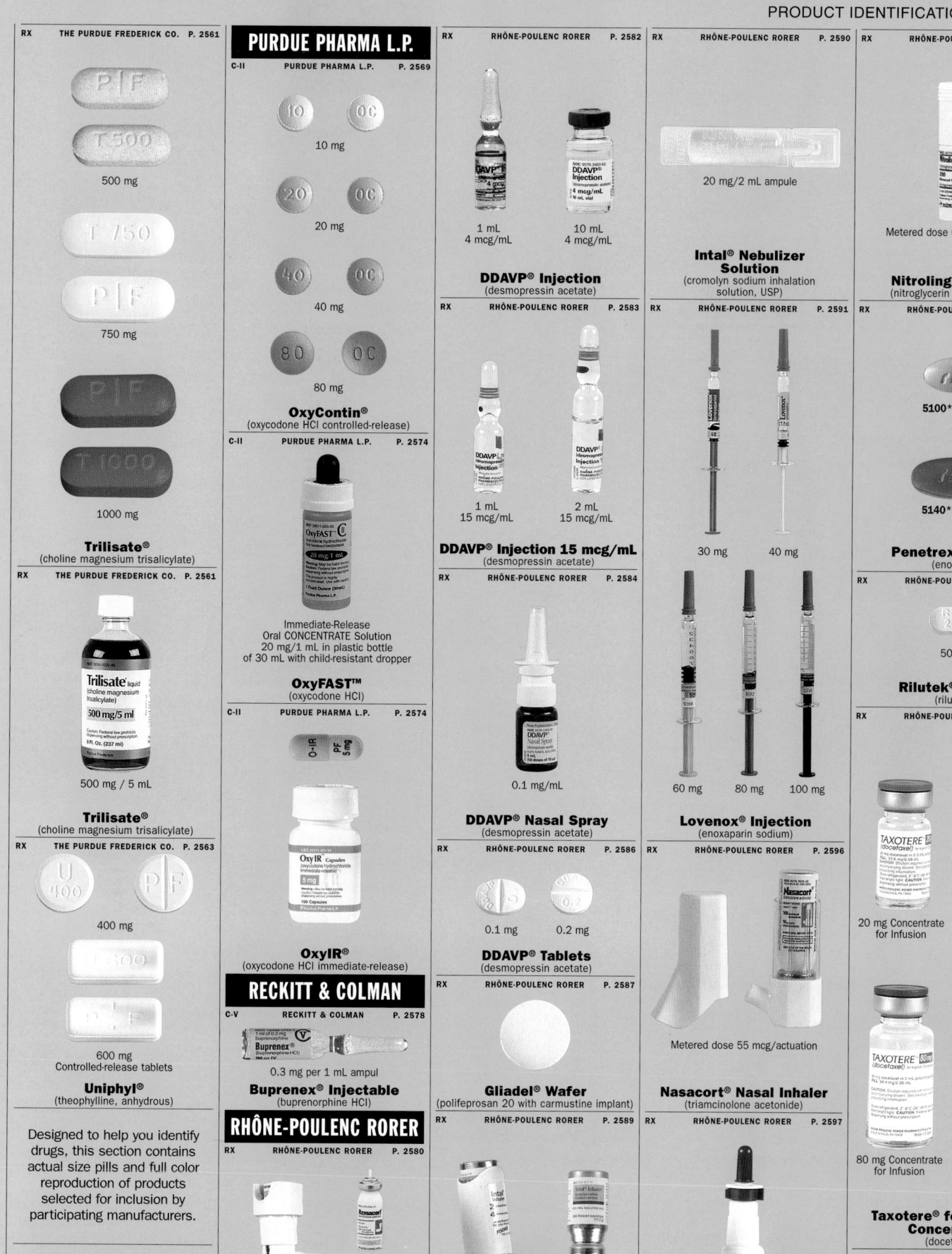

RX   THE PURDUE FREDERICK CO.   P. 2561

500 mg

750 mg

1000 mg

Trilisate®
(choline magnesium trisalicylate)

RX   THE PURDUE FREDERICK CO.   P. 2561

Trilisate® liquid
(choline magnesium trisalicylate)
500 mg/5 ml

500 mg / 5 mL

Trilisate®
(choline magnesium trisalicylate)

RX   THE PURDUE FREDERICK CO.   P. 2563

400 mg

600 mg
Controlled-release tablets

Uniphyl®
(theophylline, anhydrous)

Designed to help you identify drugs, this section contains actual size pills and full color reproduction of products selected for inclusion by participating manufacturers.

Because tablets and capsules are shown in this section, do not infer that these are the only dosage forms available. Where a product name is preceded by the symbol †, refer to the description in the Product Information (White Section) for other forms.

PURDUE PHARMA L.P.

C-II   PURDUE PHARMA L.P.   P. 2569

10 mg

20 mg

40 mg

80 mg

OxyContin®
(oxycodone HCl controlled-release)

C-II   PURDUE PHARMA L.P.   P. 2574

Immediate-Release
Oral CONCENTRATE Solution
20 mg/1 mL in plastic bottle
of 30 mL with child-resistant dropper

OxyFAST™
(oxycodone HCl)

C-II   PURDUE PHARMA L.P.   P. 2574

OxyIR®
(oxycodone HCl immediate-release)

RECKITT & COLMAN

C-V   RECKITT & COLMAN   P. 2578

0.3 mg per 1 mL ampul

Buprenex® Injectable
(buprenorphine HCl)

RHÔNE-POULENC RORER

RX   RHÔNE-POULENC RORER   P. 2580

60 mg/20 gram inhaler

**Azmacort®
Inhalation Aerosol**
(triamcinolone acetonide)

RX   RHÔNE-POULENC RORER   P. 2582

1 mL
4 mcg/mL

10 mL
4 mcg/mL

DDAVP® Injection
(desmopressin acetate)

RX   RHÔNE-POULENC RORER   P. 2583

1 mL
15 mcg/mL

2 mL
15 mcg/mL

DDAVP® Injection 15 mcg/mL
(desmopressin acetate)

RX   RHÔNE-POULENC RORER   P. 2584

0.1 mg/mL

DDAVP® Nasal Spray
(desmopressin acetate)

RX   RHÔNE-POULENC RORER   P. 2586

0.1 mg   0.2 mg

DDAVP® Tablets
(desmopressin acetate)

RX   RHÔNE-POULENC RORER   P. 2587

Gliadel® Wafer
(polifeprosan 20 with carmustine implant)

RX   RHÔNE-POULENC RORER   P. 2589

Metered dose 800 mcg/inhalation

Intal® Inhaler
(cromolyn sodium inhalation aerosol)

RX   RHÔNE-POULENC RORER   P. 2590

20 mg/2 mL ampule

**Intal® Nebulizer
Solution**
(cromolyn sodium inhalation
solution, USP)

RX   RHÔNE-POULENC RORER   P. 2591

30 mg   40 mg

60 mg   80 mg   100 mg

Lovenox® Injection
(enoxaparin sodium)

RX   RHÔNE-POULENC RORER   P. 2596

Metered dose 55 mcg/actuation

Nasacort® Nasal Inhaler
(triamcinolone acetonide)

RX   RHÔNE-POULENC RORER   P. 2597

Metered dose 55 mcg/actuation

Nasacort® AQ Nasal Spray
(triamcinolone acetonide)

RX   RHÔNE-POULENC RORER   P. 2599

Metered dose 0.4 mg/actuation

Nitrolingual® Spray
(nitroglycerin lingual aerosol)

RX   RHÔNE-POULENC RORER   P. 2602

5100* 200 mg

5140* 400 mg

Penetrex™ Tablets
(enoxacin)

RX   RHÔNE-POULENC RORER   P. 2604

50 mg

Rilutek® Tablets
(riluzole)

RX   RHÔNE-POULENC RORER   P. 2609

20 mg Concentrate
for Infusion   Diluent

80 mg Concentrate
for Infusion   Diluent

**Taxotere® for Injection
Concentrate**
(docetaxel)

While every effort has been made to reproduce products faithfully, this section is to be considered a quick reference identification aid. In cases of suspected overdosage, etc., chemical analysis of the product should be done.

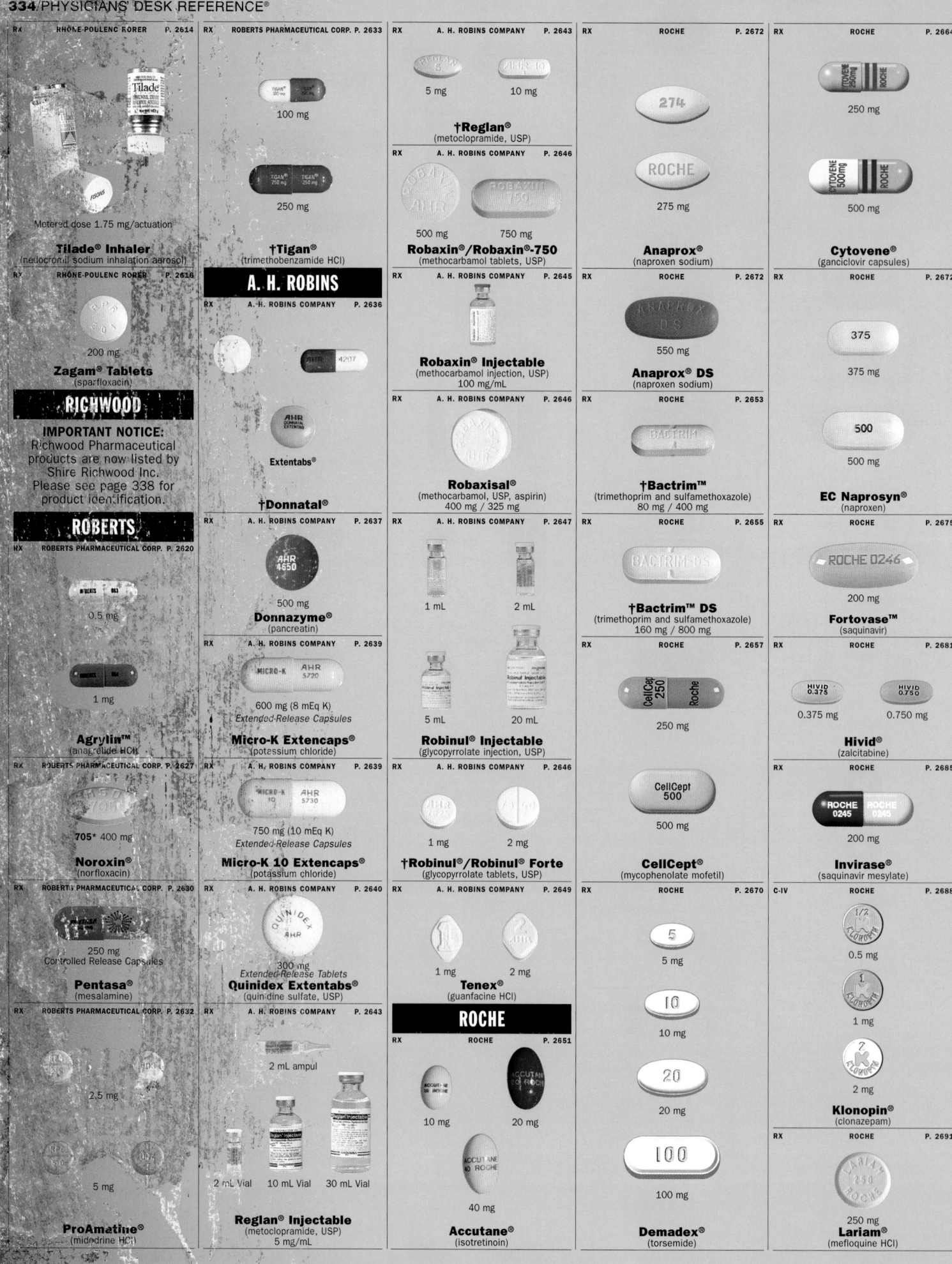

RX   RHÔNE-POULENC RORER   P. 2614

Metered dose 1.75 mg/actuation

Tilade® Inhaler
(nedocromil sodium inhalation aerosol)

RX   RHÔNE-POULENC RORER   P. 2618

200 mg

Zagam® Tablets
(sparfloxacin)

RICHWOOD

IMPORTANT NOTICE:
Richwood Pharmaceutical
products are now listed by
Shire Richwood Inc.
Please see page 338 for
product identification.

ROBERTS

RX   ROBERTS PHARMACEUTICAL CORP. P. 2620

0.5 mg

1 mg

Agrylin™
(anagrelide HCl)

RX   ROBERTS PHARMACEUTICAL CORP. P. 2627

705* 400 mg

Noroxin®
(norfloxacin)

RX   ROBERTS PHARMACEUTICAL CORP. P. 2630

250 mg
Controlled Release Capsules

Pentasa®
(mesalamine)

RX   ROBERTS PHARMACEUTICAL CORP. P. 2632

2.5 mg

5 mg

ProAmatine®
(midodrine HCl)

RX   ROBERTS PHARMACEUTICAL CORP. P. 2633

100 mg

250 mg

†Tigan®
(trimethobenzamide HCl)

A. H. ROBINS

RX   A. H. ROBINS COMPANY   P. 2636

4207

AHR
DONNATAL
EXTENTABS

Extentabs®

†Donnatal®

RX   A. H. ROBINS COMPANY   P. 2637

AHR
4650

500 mg

Donnazyme®
(pancreatin)

RX   A. H. ROBINS COMPANY   P. 2639

MICRO-K   AHR
5720

600 mg (8 mEq K)
Extended-Release Capsules

Micro-K Extencaps®
(potassium chloride)

RX   A. H. ROBINS COMPANY   P. 2639

MICRO-K   AHR
10   5730

750 mg (10 mEq K)
Extended-Release Capsules

Micro-K 10 Extencaps®
(potassium chloride)

RX   A. H. ROBINS COMPANY   P. 2640

QUINIDEX
AHR

300 mg
Extended-Release Tablets

Quinidex Extentabs®
(quinidine sulfate, USP)

RX   A. H. ROBINS COMPANY   P. 2643

2 mL ampul

2 mL Vial   10 mL Vial   30 mL Vial

Reglan® Injectable
(metoclopramide, USP)
5 mg/mL

RX   A. H. ROBINS COMPANY   P. 2643

5 mg   10 mg

†Reglan®
(metoclopramide, USP)

RX   A. H. ROBINS COMPANY   P. 2646

ROBAXIN
AHR

ROBAXIN
750

500 mg   750 mg

Robaxin®/Robaxin®-750
(methocarbamol tablets, USP)

RX   A. H. ROBINS COMPANY   P. 2645

Robaxin® Injectable
(methocarbamol injection, USP)
100 mg/mL

RX   A. H. ROBINS COMPANY   P. 2646

ROBAXISAL
AHR

Robaxisal®
(methocarbamol, USP, aspirin)
400 mg / 325 mg

RX   A. H. ROBINS COMPANY   P. 2647

1 mL   2 mL

5 mL   20 mL

Robinul® Injectable
(glycopyrrolate injection, USP)

RX   A. H. ROBINS COMPANY   P. 2646

AHR
7025

AHR
7150

1 mg   2 mg

†Robinul®/Robinul® Forte
(glycopyrrolate tablets, USP)

RX   A. H. ROBINS COMPANY   P. 2649

1   2

1 mg   2 mg

Tenex®
(guanfacine HCl)

ROCHE

RX   ROCHE   P. 2651

ACCUTANE
10 ROCHE

ACCUTANE
20 ROCHE

10 mg   20 mg

ACCUTANE
40 ROCHE

40 mg

Accutane®
(isotretinoin)

RX   ROCHE   P. 2672

274

ROCHE

275 mg

Anaprox®
(naproxen sodium)

RX   ROCHE   P. 2672

ANAPROX
DS

550 mg

Anaprox® DS
(naproxen sodium)

RX   ROCHE   P. 2653

BACTRIM

†Bactrim™
(trimethoprim and sulfamethoxazole)
80 mg / 400 mg

RX   ROCHE   P. 2655

BACTRIM-DS

†Bactrim™ DS
(trimethoprim and sulfamethoxazole)
160 mg / 800 mg

RX   ROCHE   P. 2657

CellCap
250   Roche

250 mg

CellCept
500

500 mg

CellCept®
(mycophenolate mofetil)

RX   ROCHE   P. 2670

5

5 mg

10

10 mg

20

20 mg

100

100 mg

Demadex®
(torsemide)

RX   ROCHE   P. 2664

CYTOVENE
250mg   ROCHE

250 mg

CYTOVENE
500mg   ROCHE

500 mg

Cytovene®
(ganciclovir capsules)

RX   ROCHE   P. 2672

375

375 mg

500

500 mg

EC Naprosyn®
(naproxen)

RX   ROCHE   P. 2675

ROCHE 0246

200 mg

Fortovase™
(saquinavir)

RX   ROCHE   P. 2681

HIVID
0.375

HIVID
0.750

0.375 mg   0.750 mg

Hivid®
(zalcitabine)

RX   ROCHE   P. 2685

ROCHE
0245   ROCHE
0245

200 mg

Invirase®
(saquinavir mesylate)

C-IV   ROCHE   P. 2688

1/2
KLONOPIN

0.5 mg

1
KLONOPIN

1 mg

2
KLONOPIN

2 mg

Klonopin®
(clonazepam)

RX   ROCHE   P. 2691

LARIAM
250
ROCHE

250 mg

Lariam®
(mefloquine HCl)

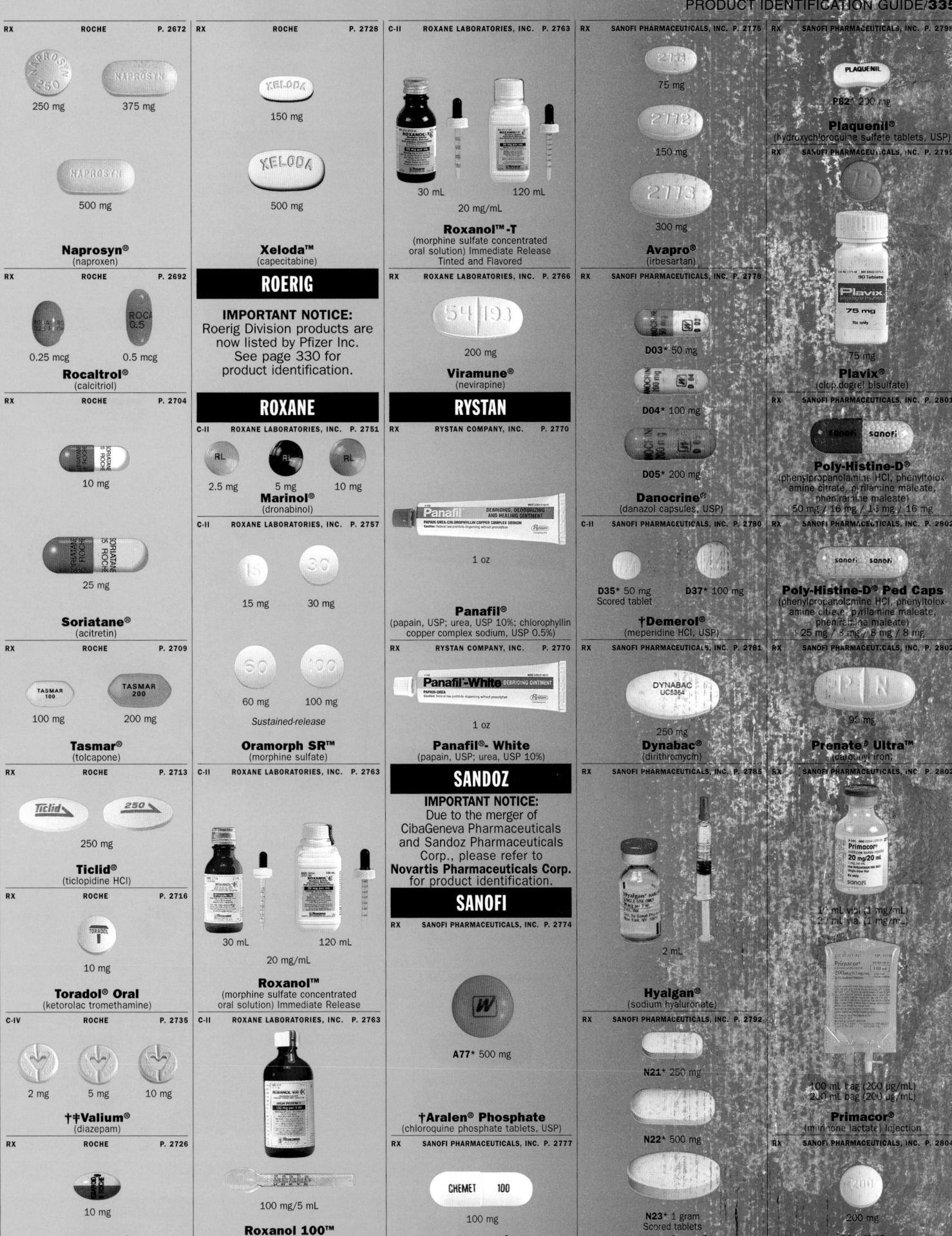

| RX | ROCHE | P. 2672 |

250 mg   **375 mg**

500 mg

Naprosyn®
(naproxen)

| RX | ROCHE | P. 2692 |

0.25 mcg   0.5 mcg

Rocaltrol®
(calcitriol)

| RX | ROCHE | P. 2704 |

10 mg

25 mg

Soriatane®
(acitretin)

| RX | ROCHE | P. 2709 |

TASMAR 100   TASMAR 200

100 mg   200 mg

Tasmar®
(tolcapone)

| RX | ROCHE | P. 2713 |

Ticlid   250

250 mg

Ticlid®
(ticlopidine HCl)

| RX | ROCHE | P. 2716 |

TORADOL

10 mg

Toradol® Oral
(ketorolac tromethamine)

| C-IV | ROCHE | P. 2735 |

2 mg   5 mg   10 mg

†‡Valium®
(diazepam)

| RX | ROCHE | P. 2726 |

10 mg

Vesanoid®
(tretinoin)

| RX | ROCHE | P. 2728 |

XELODA
150 mg

XELODA
500 mg

Xeloda™
(capecitabine)

ROERIG

IMPORTANT NOTICE:
Roerig Division products are
now listed by Pfizer Inc.
See page 330 for
product identification.

ROXANE

| C-II | ROXANE LABORATORIES, INC. | P. 2751 |

RL   RL   RL

2.5 mg   5 mg   10 mg

Marinol®
(dronabinol)

| C-II | ROXANE LABORATORIES, INC. | P. 2757 |

15   30

15 mg   30 mg

60   100

60 mg   100 mg

Sustained-release

Oramorph SR™
(morphine sulfate)

| C-II | ROXANE LABORATORIES, INC. | P. 2763 |

30 mL   120 mL

20 mg/mL

Roxanol™
(morphine sulfate concentrated
oral solution) Immediate Release

| C-II | ROXANE LABORATORIES, INC. | P. 2763 |

100 mg/5 mL

Roxanol 100™
(morphine sulfate concentrated
oral solution) Immediate Release

| C-II | ROXANE LABORATORIES, INC. | P. 2763 |

30 mL   120 mL

20 mg/mL

Roxanol™-T
(morphine sulfate concentrated
oral solution) Immediate Release
Tinted and Flavored

| RX | ROXANE LABORATORIES, INC. | P. 2766 |

54 193

200 mg

Viramune®
(nevirapine)

RYSTAN

| RX | RYSTAN COMPANY, INC. | P. 2770 |

Panafil DEBRIDING, DEODORIZING
AND HEALING OINTMENT
PAPAIN-UREA-CHLOROPHYLLIN COPPER COMPLEX SODIUM

1 oz

Panafil®
(papain, USP; urea, USP 10%; chlorophyllin
copper complex sodium, USP 0.5%)

| RX | RYSTAN COMPANY, INC. | P. 2770 |

Panafil®-White DEBRIDING OINTMENT
PAPAIN-UREA

1 oz

Panafil®- White
(papain, USP; urea, USP 10%)

SANDOZ

IMPORTANT NOTICE:
Due to the merger of
CibaGeneva Pharmaceuticals
and Sandoz Pharmaceuticals
Corp., please refer to
Novartis Pharmaceuticals Corp.
for product identification.

SANOFI

| RX | SANOFI PHARMACEUTICALS, INC. | P. 2774 |

W

A77* 500 mg

†Aralen® Phosphate
(chloroquine phosphate tablets, USP)

| RX | SANOFI PHARMACEUTICALS, INC. | P. 2777 |

CHEMET 100

100 mg

Chemet®
(succimer)

| RX | SANOFI PHARMACEUTICALS, INC. | P. 2775 |

2HH
75 mg

2772
150 mg

2773
300 mg

Avapro®
(irbesartan)

| RX | SANOFI PHARMACEUTICALS, INC. | P. 2778 |

D03* 50 mg

D04* 100 mg

D05* 200 mg

Danocrine®
(danazol capsules, USP)

| C-II | SANOFI PHARMACEUTICALS, INC. | P. 2780 |

D35* 50 mg
Scored tablet   **D37*** 100 mg

†Demerol®
(meperidine HCl, USP)

| RX | SANOFI PHARMACEUTICALS, INC. | P. 2781 |

DYNABAC
UC5364

250 mg

Dynabac®
(dirithromycin)

| RX | SANOFI PHARMACEUTICALS, INC. | P. 2785 |

Hyalgan sodium
SINGLE USE ONLY

2 mL

Hyalgan®
(sodium hyaluronate)

| RX | SANOFI PHARMACEUTICALS, INC. | P. 2792 |

N21* 250 mg

N22* 500 mg

N23* 1 gram
Scored tablets

†NegGram®
(nalidixic acid, USP)

| RX | SANOFI PHARMACEUTICALS, INC. | P. 2798 |

PLAQUENIL

P62* 200 mg

Plaquenil®
(hydroxychloroquine sulfate tablets, USP)

| RX | SANOFI PHARMACEUTICALS, INC. | P. 2799 |

75

Plavix
75 mg
Rx only

75 mg

Plavix®
(clopidogrel bisulfate)

| RX | SANOFI PHARMACEUTICALS, INC. | P. 2801 |

sanofi   sanofi

Poly-Histine-D®
(phenylpropanolamine HCl, phenyltoloxamine citrate, pyrilamine maleate,
pheniramine maleate)
50 mg / 16 mg / 16 mg / 16 mg

| RX | SANOFI PHARMACEUTICALS, INC. | P. 2802 |

sanofi   sanofi

Poly-Histine-D® Ped Caps
(phenylpropanolamine HCl, phenyltoloxamine citrate, pyrilamine maleate,
pheniramine maleate)
25 mg / 8 mg / 8 mg / 8 mg

| RX | SANOFI PHARMACEUTICALS, INC. | P. 2802 |

P N

90 mg

Prenate® Ultra™
(carbonyl iron)

| RX | SANOFI PHARMACEUTICALS, INC. | P. 2802 |

Primacor
20 mg/20 mL

1 mL vial (1 mg/mL)
2 mL vial (1 mg/mL)

Primacor
200 mg/100 mL

100 mL bag (200 µg/mL)
200 mL bag (200 µg/mL)

Primacor®
(milrinone lactate) Injection

| RX | SANOFI PHARMACEUTICALS, INC. | P. 2804 |

200

200 mg

Skelid®
(tiludronate disodium)

‡Roche Products Inc., Humacao, PR 00791

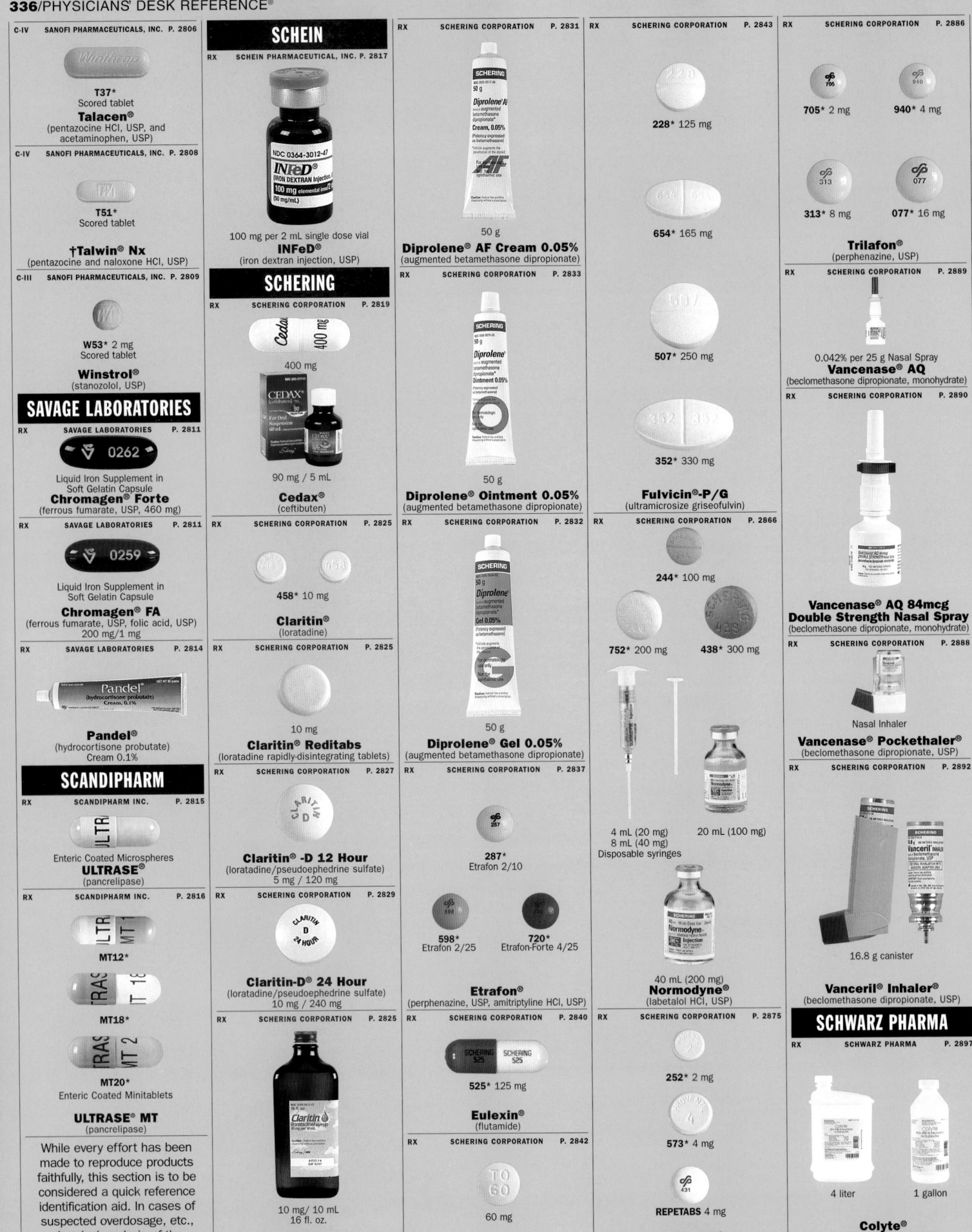

C-IV SANOFI PHARMACEUTICALS, INC. P. 2806

T37*
Scored tablet
Talacen®
(pentazocine HCl, USP, and
acetaminophen, USP)

C-IV SANOFI PHARMACEUTICALS, INC. P. 2808

T51*
Scored tablet
†Talwin® Nx
(pentazocine and naloxone HCl, USP)

C-III SANOFI PHARMACEUTICALS, INC. P. 2809

W53* 2 mg
Scored tablet
Winstrol®
(stanozolol, USP)

SAVAGE LABORATORIES

RX SAVAGE LABORATORIES P. 2811

0262
Liquid Iron Supplement in
Soft Gelatin Capsule
Chromagen® Forte
(ferrous fumarate, USP, 460 mg)

RX SAVAGE LABORATORIES P. 2811

0259
Liquid Iron Supplement in
Soft Gelatin Capsule
Chromagen® FA
(ferrous fumarate, USP, folic acid, USP)
200 mg/1 mg

RX SAVAGE LABORATORIES P. 2814

Pandel®
(hydrocortisone probutate)
Cream 0.1%

SCANDIPHARM

RX SCANDIPHARM INC. P. 2815

Enteric Coated Microspheres
ULTRASE®
(pancrelipase)

RX SCANDIPHARM INC. P. 2816

MT12*

MT18*

MT20*
Enteric Coated Minitablets
ULTRASE® MT
(pancrelipase)

While every effort has been
made to reproduce products
faithfully, this section is to be
considered a quick reference
identification aid. In cases of
suspected overdosage, etc.,
chemical analysis of the
product should be done.

SCHEIN

RX SCHEIN PHARMACEUTICAL, INC. P. 2817

NDC 0364-3012-47
INFeD®
(IRON DEXTRAN Injection, U.)
100 mg elemental iron/2
(50 mg/mL)
100 mg per 2 mL single dose vial
INFeD®
(iron dextran injection, USP)

SCHERING

RX SCHERING CORPORATION P. 2819

400 mg
Cedax®
(ceftibuten)
90 mg / 5 mL

RX SCHERING CORPORATION P. 2825

458* 10 mg
Claritin®
(loratadine)

RX SCHERING CORPORATION P. 2825

10 mg
Claritin® Reditabs
(loratadine rapidly-disintegrating tablets)

RX SCHERING CORPORATION P. 2827

Claritin® -D 12 Hour
(loratadine/pseudoephedrine sulfate)
5 mg / 120 mg

RX SCHERING CORPORATION P. 2829

Claritin-D® 24 Hour
(loratadine/pseudoephedrine sulfate)
10 mg / 240 mg

RX SCHERING CORPORATION P. 2825

10 mg/ 10 mL
16 fl. oz.
Claritin® Syrup
(loratadine)

RX SCHERING CORPORATION P. 2831

50 g
Diprolene® AF Cream 0.05%
(augmented betamethasone dipropionate)

RX SCHERING CORPORATION P. 2833

50 g
Diprolene® Ointment 0.05%
(augmented betamethasone dipropionate)

RX SCHERING CORPORATION P. 2832

50 g
Diprolene® Gel 0.05%
(augmented betamethasone dipropionate)

RX SCHERING CORPORATION P. 2837

287*
Etrafon 2/10

598*
Etrafon 2/25

720*
Etrafon-Forte 4/25

Etrafon®
(perphenazine, USP, amitriptyline HCl, USP)

RX SCHERING CORPORATION P. 2840

525* 125 mg
Eulexin®
(flutamide)

RX SCHERING CORPORATION P. 2842

60 mg
Fareston®
(toremifene citrate)

RX SCHERING CORPORATION P. 2843

228* 125 mg

654* 165 mg

507* 250 mg

352* 330 mg

Fulvicin®-P/G
(ultramicrosize griseofulvin)

RX SCHERING CORPORATION P. 2866

244* 100 mg

752* 200 mg

438* 300 mg

4 mL (20 mg)
8 mL (40 mg)
Disposable syringes

20 mL (100 mg)

40 mL (200 mg)
Normodyne®
(labetalol HCl, USP)

RX SCHERING CORPORATION P. 2875

252* 2 mg

573* 4 mg

REPETABS 4 mg
Proventil®
(albuterol sulfate, USP)

RX SCHERING CORPORATION P. 2886

705* 2 mg

940* 4 mg

313* 8 mg

077* 16 mg

Trilafon®
(perphenazine, USP)

RX SCHERING CORPORATION P. 2889

0.042% per 25 g Nasal Spray
Vancenase® AQ
(beclomethasone dipropionate, monohydrate)

RX SCHERING CORPORATION P. 2890

**Vancenase® AQ 84mcg
Double Strength Nasal Spray**
(beclomethasone dipropionate, monohydrate)

RX SCHERING CORPORATION P. 2888

Nasal Inhaler
Vancenase® Pockethaler®
(beclomethasone dipropionate, USP)

RX SCHERING CORPORATION P. 2892

16.8 g canister
Vanceril® Inhaler®
(beclomethasone dipropionate, USP)

SCHWARZ PHARMA

RX SCHWARZ PHARMA P. 2897

4 liter

1 gallon

Colyte®
(PEG-3350 & Electrolytes)
For Oral Solution

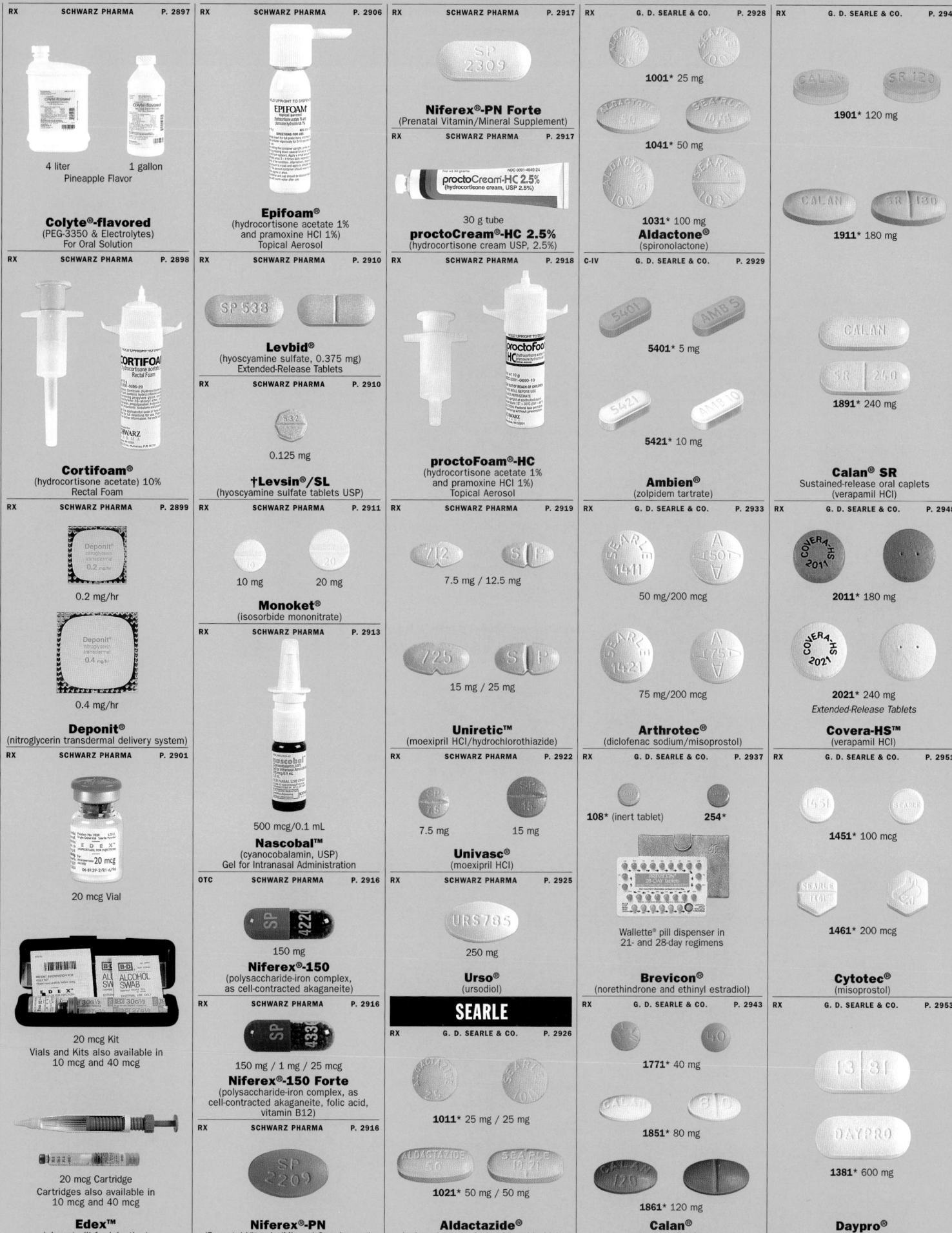

RX · SCHWARZ PHARMA · P. 2897

4 liter · 1 gallon
Pineapple Flavor

Colyte®-flavored
(PEG-3350 & Electrolytes)
For Oral Solution

RX · SCHWARZ PHARMA · P. 2898

Cortifoam®
(hydrocortisone acetate) 10%
Rectal Foam

RX · SCHWARZ PHARMA · P. 2899

0.2 mg/hr

0.4 mg/hr

Deponit®
(nitroglycerin transdermal delivery system)

RX · SCHWARZ PHARMA · P. 2901

20 mcg Vial

20 mcg Kit
Vials and Kits also available in
10 mcg and 40 mcg

20 mcg Cartridge
Cartridges also available in
10 mcg and 40 mcg

Edex™
(alprostadil for injection)

RX · SCHWARZ PHARMA · P. 2906

Epifoam®
(hydrocortisone acetate 1%
and pramoxine HCl 1%)
Topical Aerosol

RX · SCHWARZ PHARMA · P. 2910

SP 538

Levbid®
(hyoscyamine sulfate, 0.375 mg)
Extended-Release Tablets

RX · SCHWARZ PHARMA · P. 2910

0.125 mg

†Levsin®/SL
(hyoscyamine sulfate tablets USP)

RX · SCHWARZ PHARMA · P. 2911

10 mg · 20 mg

Monoket®
(isosorbide mononitrate)

RX · SCHWARZ PHARMA · P. 2913

500 mcg/0.1 mL

Nascobal™
(cyanocobalamin, USP)
Gel for Intranasal Administration

OTC · SCHWARZ PHARMA · P. 2916

SP 4220

150 mg

Niferex®-150
(polysaccharide-iron complex,
as cell-contracted akaganeite)

RX · SCHWARZ PHARMA · P. 2916

SP 4330

150 mg / 1 mg / 25 mcg

Niferex®-150 Forte
(polysaccharide-iron complex, as
cell-contracted akaganeite, folic acid,
vitamin B12)

RX · SCHWARZ PHARMA · P. 2916

SP 2209

Niferex®-PN
(Prenatal Vitamin/Mineral Supplement)

RX · SCHWARZ PHARMA · P. 2917

SP 2309

Niferex®-PN Forte
(Prenatal Vitamin/Mineral Supplement)

RX · SCHWARZ PHARMA · P. 2917

30 g tube

proctoCream®-HC 2.5%
(hydrocortisone cream USP, 2.5%)

RX · SCHWARZ PHARMA · P. 2918

proctoFoam®-HC
(hydrocortisone acetate 1%
and pramoxine HCl 1%)
Topical Aerosol

RX · SCHWARZ PHARMA · P. 2919

712 · SP

7.5 mg / 12.5 mg

725 · SP

15 mg / 25 mg

Uniretic™
(moexipril HCl/hydrochlorothiazide)

RX · SCHWARZ PHARMA · P. 2922

SP 7.5 · SP 15

7.5 mg · 15 mg

Univasc®
(moexipril HCl)

RX · SCHWARZ PHARMA · P. 2925

URS785

250 mg

Urso®
(ursodiol)

SEARLE

RX · G. D. SEARLE & CO. · P. 2926

1011* 25 mg / 25 mg

1021* 50 mg / 50 mg

Aldactazide®
(spironolactone, hydrochlorothiazide)

RX · G. D. SEARLE & CO. · P. 2928

1001* 25 mg

1041* 50 mg

1031* 100 mg

Aldactone®
(spironolactone)

C-IV · G. D. SEARLE & CO. · P. 2929

5401* 5 mg

5421* 10 mg

Ambien®
(zolpidem tartrate)

RX · G. D. SEARLE & CO. · P. 2933

50 mg/200 mcg

75 mg/200 mcg

Arthrotec®
(diclofenac sodium/misoprostol)

RX · G. D. SEARLE & CO. · P. 2937

108* (inert tablet) · 254*

Wallette® pill dispenser in
21- and 28-day regimens

Brevicon®
(norethindrone and ethinyl estradiol)

RX · G. D. SEARLE & CO. · P. 2943

1771* 40 mg

1851* 80 mg

1861* 120 mg

Calan®
(verapamil HCl)

RX · G. D. SEARLE & CO. · P. 2946

1901* 120 mg

1911* 180 mg

1891* 240 mg

Calan® SR
Sustained-release oral caplets
(verapamil HCl)

RX · G. D. SEARLE & CO. · P. 2948

2011* 180 mg

2021* 240 mg
Extended-Release Tablets

Covera-HS™
(verapamil HCl)

RX · G. D. SEARLE & CO. · P. 2951

1451* 100 mcg

1461* 200 mcg

Cytotec®
(misoprostol)

RX · G. D. SEARLE & CO. · P. 2953

1381* 600 mg

Daypro®
(oxaprozin)

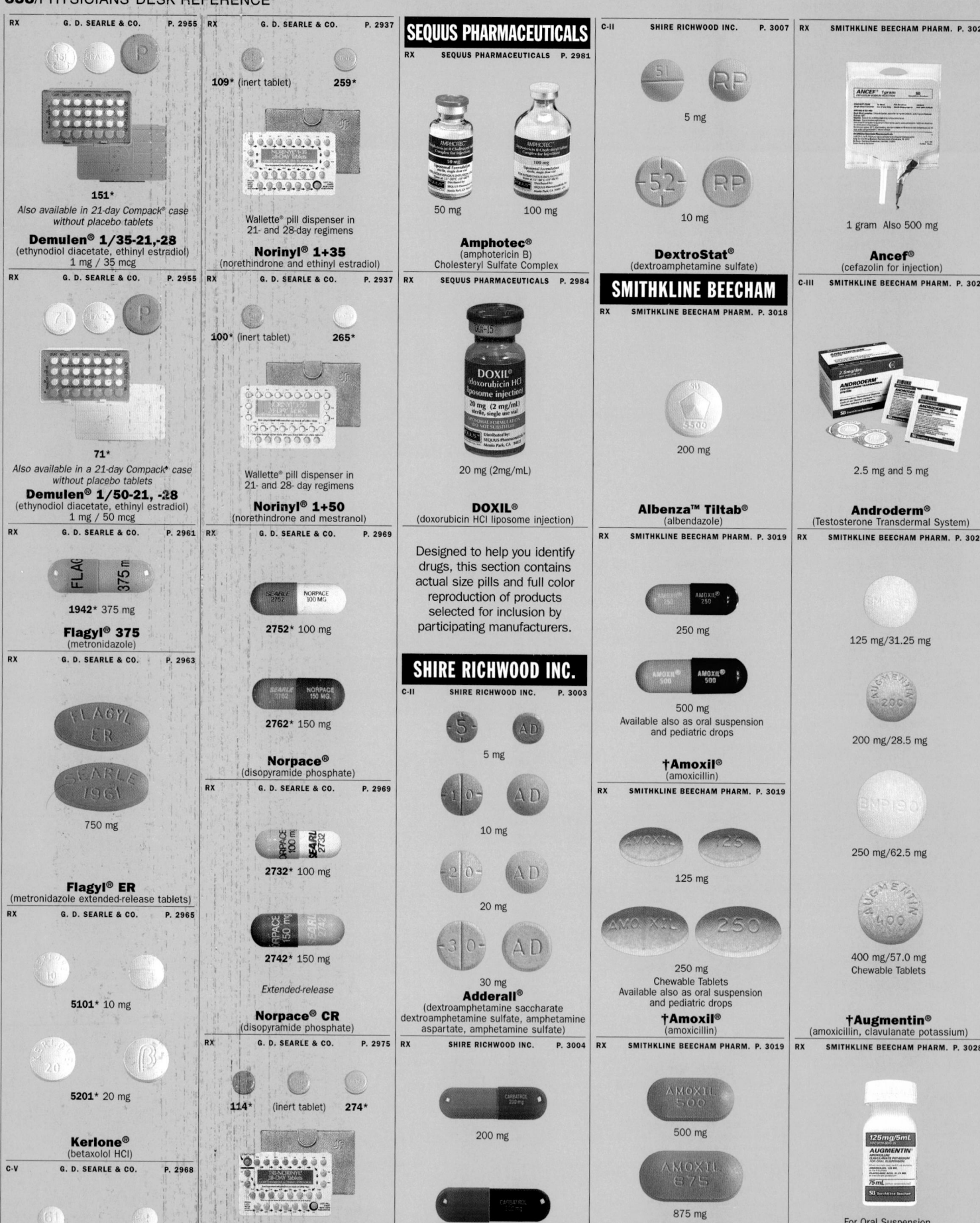

RX   G. D. SEARLE & CO.   P. 2955

151*

Also available in 21-day Compack® case without placebo tablets

Demulen® 1/35-21,-28
(ethynodiol diacetate, ethinyl estradiol)
1 mg / 35 mcg

RX   G. D. SEARLE & CO.   P. 2955

71*

Also available in a 21-day Compack® case without placebo tablets

Demulen® 1/50-21, -28
(ethynodiol diacetate, ethinyl estradiol)
1 mg / 50 mcg

RX   G. D. SEARLE & CO.   P. 2961

1942* 375 mg

Flagyl® 375
(metronidazole)

RX   G. D. SEARLE & CO.   P. 2963

750 mg

Flagyl® ER
(metronidazole extended-release tablets)

RX   G. D. SEARLE & CO.   P. 2965

5101* 10 mg

5201* 20 mg

Kerlone®
(betaxolol HCl)

C-V   G. D. SEARLE & CO.   P. 2968

61* 2.5 mg / 0.025 mg

†Lomotil®
(diphenoxylate HCl, atropine sulfate)

RX   G. D. SEARLE & CO.   P. 2937

109* (inert tablet)   **259***

Wallette® pill dispenser in 21- and 28-day regimens

Norinyl® 1+35
(norethindrone and ethinyl estradiol)

RX   G. D. SEARLE & CO.   P. 2937

100* (inert tablet)   **265***

Wallette® pill dispenser in 21- and 28- day regimens

Norinyl® 1+50
(norethindrone and mestranol)

RX   G. D. SEARLE & CO.   P. 2969

2752* 100 mg

2762* 150 mg

Norpace®
(disopyramide phosphate)

RX   G. D. SEARLE & CO.   P. 2969

2732* 100 mg

2742* 150 mg

Extended-release

Norpace® CR
(disopyramide phosphate)

RX   G. D. SEARLE & CO.   P. 2975

114* (inert tablet)   **274***

Wallette® pill dispenser in 21- and 28-day regimens

Tri-Norinyl®
(norethindrone and ethinyl estradiol)

50 mg   100 mg

Amphotec®
(amphotericin B)
Cholesteryl Sulfate Complex

RX   SEQUUS PHARMACEUTICALS   P. 2984

20 mg (2mg/mL)

DOXIL®
(doxorubicin HCl liposome injection)

Designed to help you identify drugs, this section contains actual size pills and full color reproduction of products selected for inclusion by participating manufacturers.

SHIRE RICHWOOD INC.

C-II   SHIRE RICHWOOD INC.   P. 3003

5 mg

10 mg

20 mg

30 mg

Adderall®
(dextroamphetamine saccharate
dextroamphetamine sulfate, amphetamine
aspartate, amphetamine sulfate)

RX   SHIRE RICHWOOD INC.   P. 3004

200 mg

300 mg

Carbatrol®
(carbamazepine extended-release capsules)

C-II   SHIRE RICHWOOD INC.   P. 3007

5 mg

10 mg

DextroStat®
(dextroamphetamine sulfate)

SMITHKLINE BEECHAM

RX   SMITHKLINE BEECHAM PHARM.   P. 3018

200 mg

Albenza™ Tiltab®
(albendazole)

RX   SMITHKLINE BEECHAM PHARM.   P. 3019

250 mg

500 mg

Available also as oral suspension
and pediatric drops

†Amoxil®
(amoxicillin)

RX   SMITHKLINE BEECHAM PHARM.   P. 3019

125 mg

250 mg
Chewable Tablets
Available also as oral suspension
and pediatric drops

†Amoxil®
(amoxicillin)

RX   SMITHKLINE BEECHAM PHARM.   P. 3019

500 mg

875 mg
Tablets
Available also as oral suspension
and pediatric drops

†Amoxil®
(amoxicillin)

RX   SMITHKLINE BEECHAM PHARM.   P. 3023

1 gram   Also 500 mg

Ancef®
(cefazolin for injection)

C-III   SMITHKLINE BEECHAM PHARM.   P. 3025

2.5 mg and 5 mg

Androderm®
(Testosterone Transdermal System)

RX   SMITHKLINE BEECHAM PHARM.   P. 3028

125 mg/31.25 mg

200 mg/28.5 mg

250 mg/62.5 mg

400 mg/57.0 mg
Chewable Tablets

†Augmentin®
(amoxicillin, clavulanate potassium)

RX   SMITHKLINE BEECHAM PHARM.   P. 3028

For Oral Suspension

†Augmentin®
(amoxicillin, clavulanate potassium)
125 mg/5 mL, 200 mg/5 mL,
250 mg/5 mL, and 400 mg/5 mL

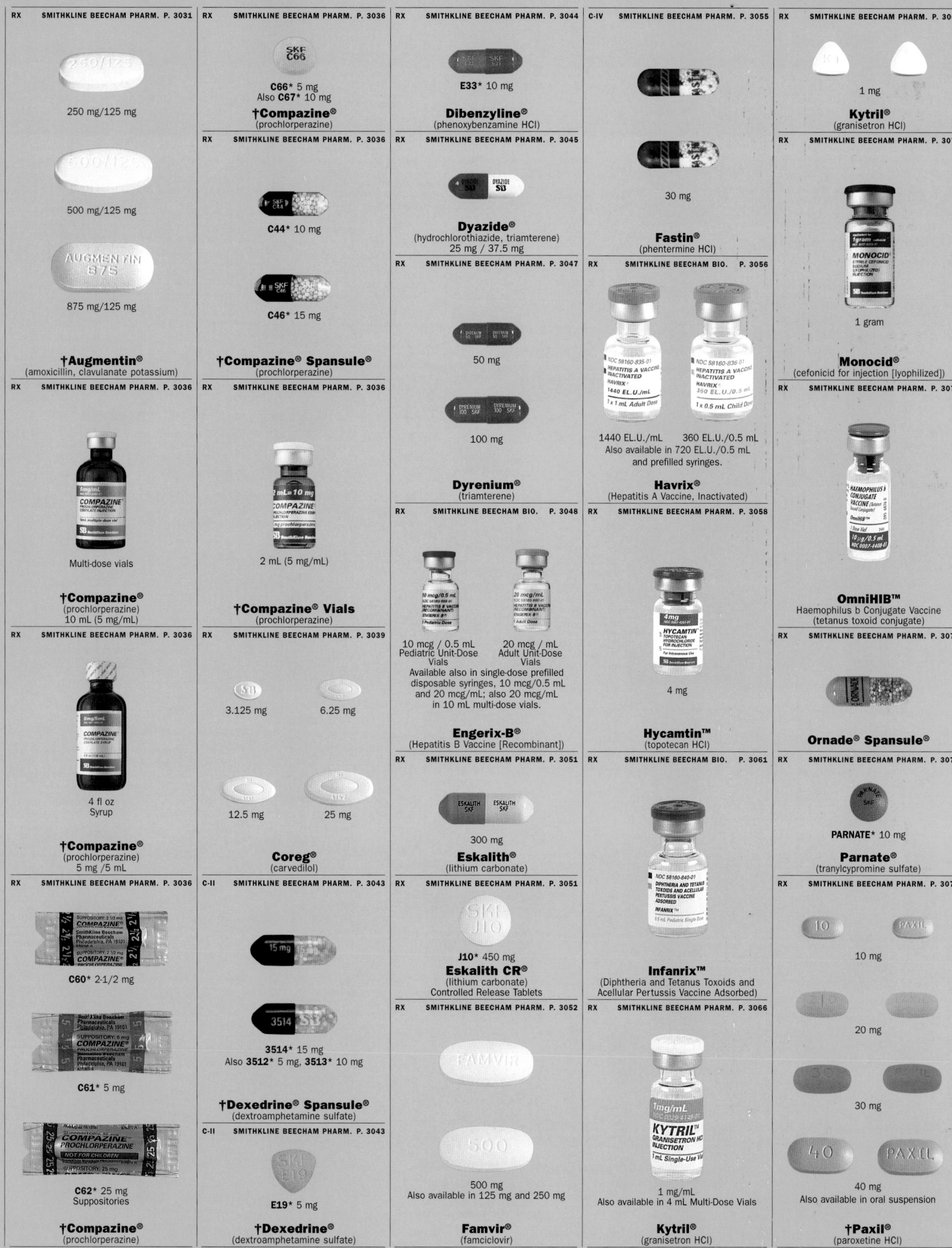

RX   SMITHKLINE BEECHAM PHARM. P. 3031

250 mg/125 mg

500 mg/125 mg

875 mg/125 mg

†Augmentin®
(amoxicillin, clavulanate potassium)

RX   SMITHKLINE BEECHAM PHARM. P. 3036

Multi-dose vials

†Compazine®
(prochlorperazine)
10 mL (5 mg/mL)

RX   SMITHKLINE BEECHAM PHARM. P. 3036

4 fl oz
Syrup

†Compazine®
(prochlorperazine)
5 mg /5 mL

RX   SMITHKLINE BEECHAM PHARM. P. 3036

C60* 2-1/2 mg

C61* 5 mg

C62* 25 mg
Suppositories

†Compazine®
(prochlorperazine)

RX   SMITHKLINE BEECHAM PHARM. P. 3036

C66* 5 mg
Also **C67*** 10 mg

†Compazine®
(prochlorperazine)

RX   SMITHKLINE BEECHAM PHARM. P. 3036

C44* 10 mg

C46* 15 mg

†Compazine® Spansule®
(prochlorperazine)

RX   SMITHKLINE BEECHAM PHARM. P. 3036

2 mL (5 mg/mL)

†Compazine® Vials
(prochlorperazine)

RX   SMITHKLINE BEECHAM PHARM. P. 3039

3.125 mg   6.25 mg

12.5 mg   25 mg

Coreg®
(carvedilol)

C-II   SMITHKLINE BEECHAM PHARM. P. 3043

15 mg

3514* 15 mg
Also **3512*** 5 mg, **3513*** 10 mg

†Dexedrine® Spansule®
(dextroamphetamine sulfate)

C-II   SMITHKLINE BEECHAM PHARM. P. 3043

E19* 5 mg

†Dexedrine®
(dextroamphetamine sulfate)

RX   SMITHKLINE BEECHAM PHARM. P. 3044

E33* 10 mg

Dibenzyline®
(phenoxybenzamine HCl)

RX   SMITHKLINE BEECHAM PHARM. P. 3045

Dyazide®
(hydrochlorothiazide, triamterene)
25 mg / 37.5 mg

RX   SMITHKLINE BEECHAM PHARM. P. 3047

50 mg

100 mg

Dyrenium®
(triamterene)

RX   SMITHKLINE BEECHAM BIO.   P. 3048

10 mcg / 0.5 mL   20 mcg / mL
Pediatric Unit-Dose   Adult Unit-Dose
Vials   Vials
Available also in single-dose prefilled
disposable syringes, 10 mcg/0.5 mL
and 20 mcg/mL; also 20 mcg/mL
in 10 mL multi-dose vials.

Engerix-B®
(Hepatitis B Vaccine [Recombinant])

RX   SMITHKLINE BEECHAM PHARM. P. 3051

300 mg

Eskalith®
(lithium carbonate)

RX   SMITHKLINE BEECHAM PHARM. P. 3051

J10* 450 mg

Eskalith CR®
(lithium carbonate)
Controlled Release Tablets

RX   SMITHKLINE BEECHAM PHARM. P. 3052

500 mg
Also available in 125 mg and 250 mg

Famvir®
(famciclovir)

C-IV   SMITHKLINE BEECHAM PHARM. P. 3055

30 mg

Fastin®
(phentermine HCl)

RX   SMITHKLINE BEECHAM BIO.   P. 3056

1440 EL.U./mL   360 EL.U./0.5 mL
Also available in 720 EL.U./0.5 mL
and prefilled syringes.

Havrix®
(Hepatitis A Vaccine, Inactivated)

RX   SMITHKLINE BEECHAM PHARM. P. 3058

4 mg

Hycamtin™
(topotecan HCl)

RX   SMITHKLINE BEECHAM BIO.   P. 3061

Infanrix™
(Diphtheria and Tetanus Toxoids and
Acellular Pertussis Vaccine Adsorbed)

RX   SMITHKLINE BEECHAM PHARM. P. 3066

1 mg/mL
Also available in 4 mL Multi-Dose Vials

Kytril™
(granisetron HCl)

RX   SMITHKLINE BEECHAM PHARM. P. 3068

1 mg

Kytril®
(granisetron HCl)

RX   SMITHKLINE BEECHAM PHARM. P. 3070

1 gram

Monocid®
(cefonicid for injection [lyophilized])

RX   SMITHKLINE BEECHAM PHARM. P. 3072

OmniHIB™
Haemophilus b Conjugate Vaccine
(tetanus toxoid conjugate)

RX   SMITHKLINE BEECHAM PHARM. P. 3075

Ornade® Spansule®

RX   SMITHKLINE BEECHAM PHARM. P. 3076

PARNATE* 10 mg

Parnate®
(tranylcypromine sulfate)

RX   SMITHKLINE BEECHAM PHARM. P. 3078

10   PAXIL

10 mg

20 mg

30 mg

40   PAXIL

40 mg
Also available in oral suspension

†Paxil®
(paroxetine HCl)

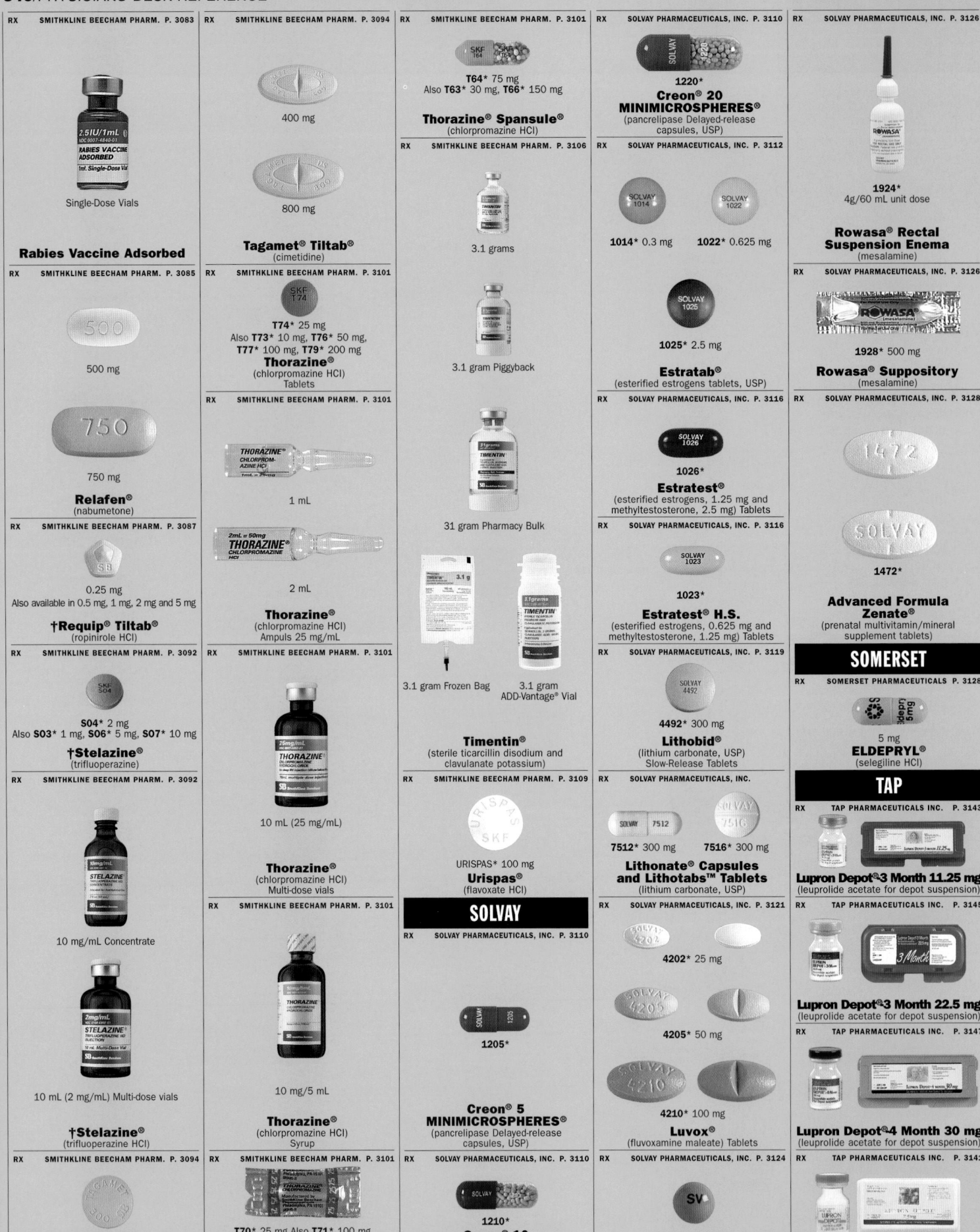

RX   SMITHKLINE BEECHAM PHARM. P. 3083

Single-Dose Vials

2.5IU/1mL
NDC 0007-4840-01
RABIES VACCINE ADSORBED
Iml Single-Dose Vial

Rabies Vaccine Adsorbed

RX   SMITHKLINE BEECHAM PHARM. P. 3085

500 mg

750 mg

Relafen®
(nabumetone)

RX   SMITHKLINE BEECHAM PHARM. P. 3087

0.25 mg
Also available in 0.5 mg, 1 mg, 2 mg and 5 mg

†Requip® Tiltab®
(ropinirole HCl)

RX   SMITHKLINE BEECHAM PHARM. P. 3092

S04* 2 mg
Also **S03*** 1 mg, **S06*** 5 mg, **S07*** 10 mg

†Stelazine®
(trifluoperazine)

RX   SMITHKLINE BEECHAM PHARM. P. 3092

10 mg/mL Concentrate

10 mL (2 mg/mL) Multi-dose vials

†Stelazine®
(trifluoperazine HCl)

RX   SMITHKLINE BEECHAM PHARM. P. 3094

300 mg

Tagamet®
(cimetidine)

RX   SMITHKLINE BEECHAM PHARM. P. 3094

400 mg

800 mg

Tagamet® Tiltab®
(cimetidine)

RX   SMITHKLINE BEECHAM PHARM. P. 3101

SKF
T 74

T74* 25 mg
Also **T73*** 10 mg, **T76*** 50 mg,
T77* 100 mg, **T79*** 200 mg

Thorazine®
(chlorpromazine HCl)
Tablets

RX   SMITHKLINE BEECHAM PHARM. P. 3101

THORAZINE®
CHLORPROM-
AZINE HCl

1 mL

2mL = 50mg
THORAZINE®
CHLORPROMAZINE
HCl

2 mL

Thorazine®
(chlorpromazine HCl)
Ampuls 25 mg/mL

RX   SMITHKLINE BEECHAM PHARM. P. 3101

25mg/mL
THORAZINE®
CHLORPROMAZINE
HYDROCHLORIDE

10 mL (25 mg/mL)

Thorazine®
(chlorpromazine HCl)
Multi-dose vials

RX   SMITHKLINE BEECHAM PHARM. P. 3101

THORAZINE®
CHLORPROMAZINE
HYDROCHLORIDE

10 mg/5 mL

Thorazine®
(chlorpromazine HCl)
Syrup

RX   SMITHKLINE BEECHAM PHARM. P. 3101

THORAZINE®
CHLORPROMAZINE

T70* 25 mg Also **T71*** 100 mg

Thorazine®
(chlorpromazine)
Suppositories

RX   SMITHKLINE BEECHAM PHARM. P. 3101

SKF
T64

T64* 75 mg
Also **T63*** 30 mg, **T66*** 150 mg

Thorazine® Spansule®
(chlorpromazine HCl)

RX   SMITHKLINE BEECHAM PHARM. P. 3106

TIMENTIN

3.1 grams

TIMENTIN

3.1 gram Piggyback

3.1 grams
TIMENTIN

31 gram Pharmacy Bulk

3.1 g

2.1 grams
TIMENTIN

3.1 gram Frozen Bag   3.1 gram
                       ADD-Vantage® Vial

Timentin®
(sterile ticarcillin disodium and
clavulanate potassium)

RX   SMITHKLINE BEECHAM PHARM. P. 3109

URISPAS
SKF

URISPAS* 100 mg

Urispas®
(flavoxate HCl)

SOLVAY

RX   SOLVAY PHARMACEUTICALS, INC. P. 3110

SOLVAY
1205

1205*

Creon® 5
MINIMICROSPHERES®
(pancrelipase Delayed-release
capsules, USP)

RX   SOLVAY PHARMACEUTICALS, INC. P. 3110

SOLVAY

1210*

Creon® 10
MINIMICROSPHERES®
(pancrelipase Delayed-release
capsules, USP)

RX   SOLVAY PHARMACEUTICALS, INC. P. 3110

SOLVAY
1220

1220*

Creon® 20
MINIMICROSPHERES®
(pancrelipase Delayed-release
capsules, USP)

RX   SOLVAY PHARMACEUTICALS, INC. P. 3112

SOLVAY 1014   SOLVAY 1022

1014* 0.3 mg   **1022*** 0.625 mg

SOLVAY 1025

1025* 2.5 mg

Estratab®
(esterified estrogens tablets, USP)

RX   SOLVAY PHARMACEUTICALS, INC. P. 3116

SOLVAY 1026

1026*

Estratest®
(esterified estrogens, 1.25 mg and
methyltestosterone, 2.5 mg) Tablets

RX   SOLVAY PHARMACEUTICALS, INC. P. 3116

SOLVAY 1023

1023*

Estratest® H.S.
(esterified estrogens, 0.625 mg and
methyltestosterone, 1.25 mg) Tablets

RX   SOLVAY PHARMACEUTICALS, INC. P. 3119

SOLVAY 4492

4492* 300 mg

Lithobid®
(lithium carbonate, USP)
Slow-Release Tablets

RX   SOLVAY PHARMACEUTICALS, INC.

SOLVAY 7512   SOLVAY 7516

7512* 300 mg   **7516*** 300 mg

Lithonate® Capsules
and Lithotabs™ Tablets
(lithium carbonate, USP)

RX   SOLVAY PHARMACEUTICALS, INC. P. 3121

SOLVAY 4202

4202* 25 mg

SOLVAY 4205

4205* 50 mg

SOLVAY 4210

4210* 100 mg

Luvox®
(fluvoxamine maleate) Tablets

RX   SOLVAY PHARMACEUTICALS, INC. P. 3124

SV

1708* 100 mg

Prometrium®
(progesterone, USP) Capsules

RX   SOLVAY PHARMACEUTICALS, INC. P. 3126

ROWASA

1924*
4g/60 mL unit dose

Rowasa® Rectal
Suspension Enema
(mesalamine)

RX   SOLVAY PHARMACEUTICALS, INC. P. 3126

ROWASA
(mesalamine)

1928* 500 mg

Rowasa® Suppository
(mesalamine)

RX   SOLVAY PHARMACEUTICALS, INC. P. 3128

1472

SOLVAY

1472*

Advanced Formula
Zenate®
(prenatal multivitamin/mineral
supplement tablets)

SOMERSET

RX   SOMERSET PHARMACEUTICALS P. 3128

Eldepryl
5mg

5 mg

ELDEPRYL®
(selegiline HCl)

TAP

RX   TAP PHARMACEUTICALS INC.   P. 3143

Lupron Depot®3 Month 11.25 mg
(leuprolide acetate for depot suspension)

RX   TAP PHARMACEUTICALS INC.   P. 3145

3 Month

Lupron Depot®3 Month 22.5 mg
(leuprolide acetate for depot suspension)

RX   TAP PHARMACEUTICALS INC.   P. 3147

Lupron Depot®4 Month 30 mg
(leuprolide acetate for depot suspension)

RX   TAP PHARMACEUTICALS INC.   P. 3141

Lupron Depot® 7.5 mg
(leuprolide acetate for depot suspension)

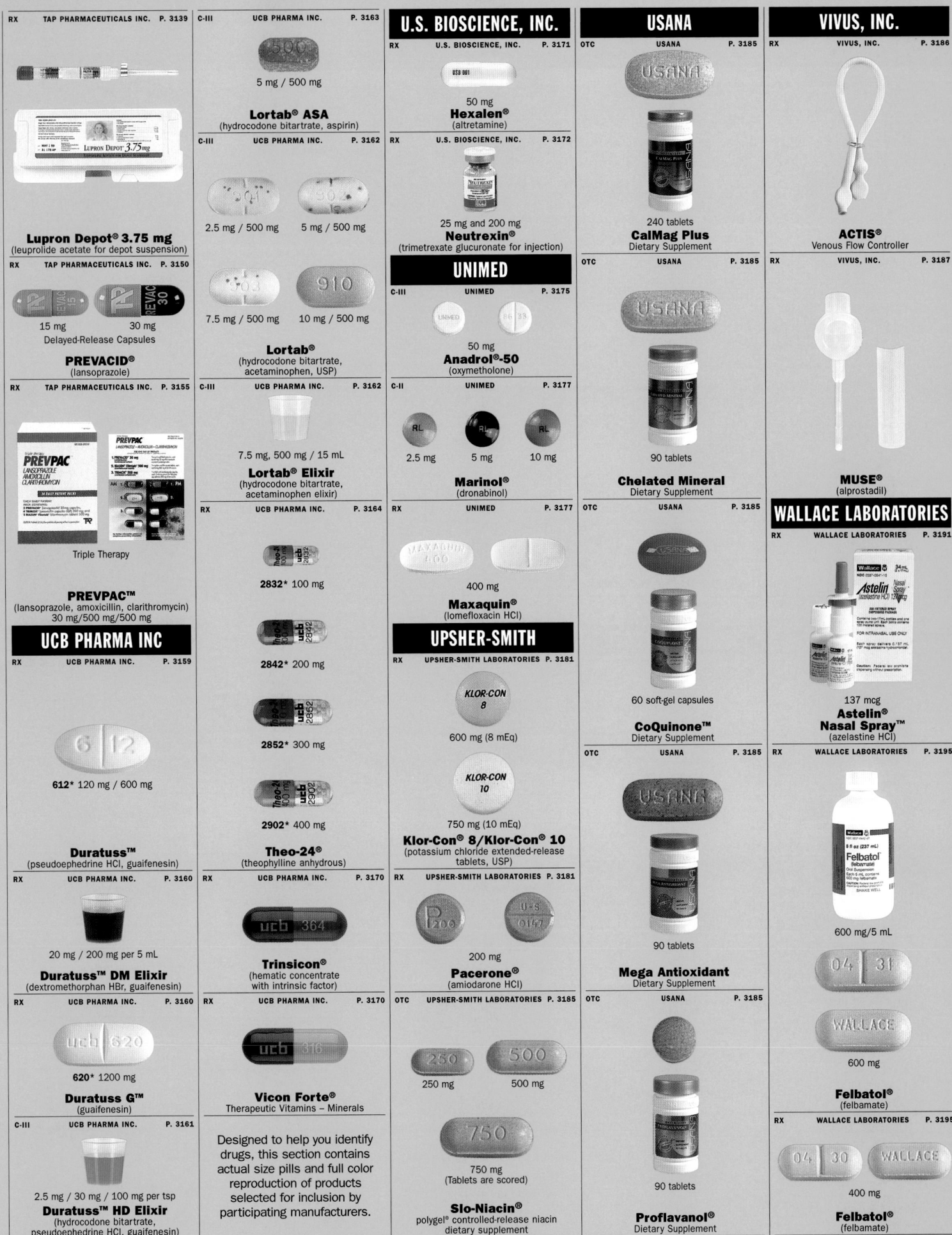

RX   TAP PHARMACEUTICALS INC.   P. 3139

Lupron Depot® 3.75 mg
(leuprolide acetate for depot suspension)

RX   TAP PHARMACEUTICALS INC.   P. 3150

15 mg   30 mg
Delayed-Release Capsules
PREVACID®
(lansoprazole)

RX   TAP PHARMACEUTICALS INC.   P. 3155

Triple Therapy
PREVPAC™
(lansoprazole, amoxicillin, clarithromycin)
30 mg/500 mg/500 mg

UCB PHARMA INC

RX   UCB PHARMA INC.   P. 3159

612* 120 mg / 600 mg
Duratuss™
(pseudoephedrine HCl, guaifenesin)

RX   UCB PHARMA INC.   P. 3160

20 mg / 200 mg per 5 mL
Duratuss™ DM Elixir
(dextromethorphan HBr, guaifenesin)

RX   UCB PHARMA INC.   P. 3160

620* 1200 mg
Duratuss G™
(guaifenesin)

C-III   UCB PHARMA INC.   P. 3161

2.5 mg / 30 mg / 100 mg per tsp
Duratuss™ HD Elixir
(hydrocodone bitartrate,
pseudoephedrine HCl, guaifenesin)

C-III   UCB PHARMA INC.   P. 3163

5 mg / 500 mg
Lortab® ASA
(hydrocodone bitartrate, aspirin)

C-III   UCB PHARMA INC.   P. 3162

2.5 mg / 500 mg   5 mg / 500 mg

7.5 mg / 500 mg   10 mg / 500 mg
Lortab®
(hydrocodone bitartrate,
acetaminophen, USP)

C-III   UCB PHARMA INC.   P. 3162

7.5 mg, 500 mg / 15 mL
Lortab® Elixir
(hydrocodone bitartrate,
acetaminophen elixir)

RX   UCB PHARMA INC.   P. 3164

2832* 100 mg

2842* 200 mg

2852* 300 mg

2902* 400 mg
Theo-24®
(theophylline anhydrous)

RX   UCB PHARMA INC.   P. 3170

Trinsicon®
(hematic concentrate
with intrinsic factor)

RX   UCB PHARMA INC.   P. 3170

Vicon Forte®
Therapeutic Vitamins – Minerals

Designed to help you identify
drugs, this section contains
actual size pills and full color
reproduction of products
selected for inclusion by
participating manufacturers.

U.S. BIOSCIENCE, INC.

RX   U.S. BIOSCIENCE, INC.   P. 3171

50 mg
Hexalen®
(altretamine)

RX   U.S. BIOSCIENCE, INC.   P. 3172

25 mg and 200 mg
Neutrexin®
(trimetrexate glucuronate for injection)

UNIMED

C-III   UNIMED   P. 3175

50 mg
Anadrol®-50
(oxymetholone)

C-II   UNIMED   P. 3177

2.5 mg   5 mg   10 mg
Marinol®
(dronabinol)

RX   UNIMED   P. 3177

400 mg
Maxaquin®
(lomefloxacin HCl)

UPSHER-SMITH

RX   UPSHER-SMITH LABORATORIES   P. 3181

600 mg (8 mEq)

750 mg (10 mEq)
Klor-Con® 8/Klor-Con® 10
(potassium chloride extended-release
tablets, USP)

RX   UPSHER-SMITH LABORATORIES   P. 3181

200 mg
Pacerone®
(amiodarone HCl)

OTC   UPSHER-SMITH LABORATORIES   P. 3185

250 mg   500 mg

750 mg
(Tablets are scored)
Slo-Niacin®
polygel® controlled-release niacin
dietary supplement

USANA

OTC   USANA   P. 3185

240 tablets
CalMag Plus
Dietary Supplement

OTC   USANA   P. 3185

90 tablets
Chelated Mineral
Dietary Supplement

OTC   USANA   P. 3185

60 soft-gel capsules
CoQuinone™
Dietary Supplement

OTC   USANA   P. 3185

90 tablets
Mega Antioxidant
Dietary Supplement

OTC   USANA   P. 3185

90 tablets
Proflavanol®
Dietary Supplement

VIVUS, INC.

RX   VIVUS, INC.   P. 3186

ACTIS®
Venous Flow Controller

RX   VIVUS, INC.   P. 3187

MUSE®
(alprostadil)

WALLACE LABORATORIES

RX   WALLACE LABORATORIES   P. 3191

137 mcg
**Astelin®
Nasal Spray™**
(azelastine HCl)

RX   WALLACE LABORATORIES   P. 3195

600 mg/5 mL

600 mg
Felbatol®
(felbamate)

RX   WALLACE LABORATORIES   P. 3195

400 mg
Felbatol®
(felbamate)

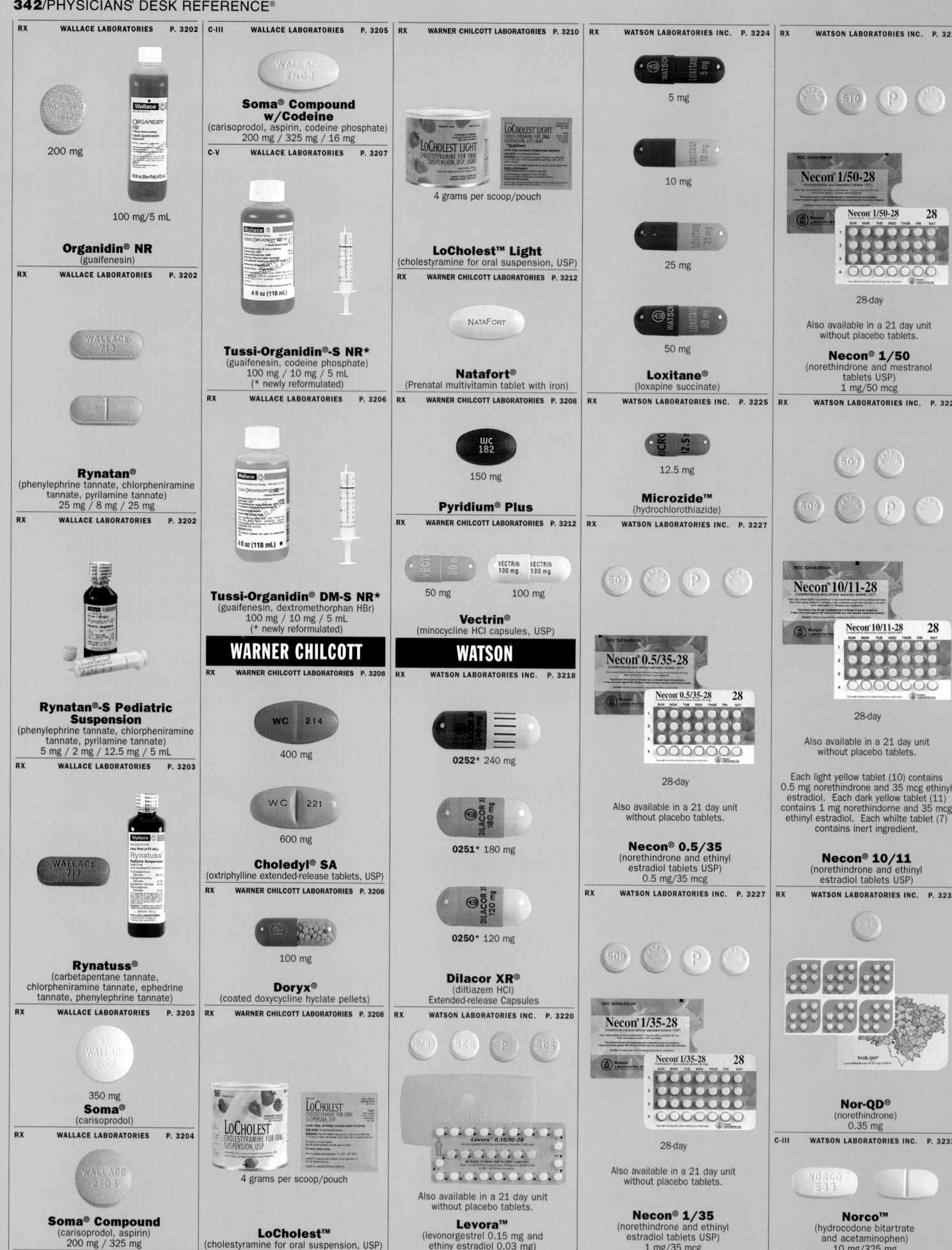

RX   WALLACE LABORATORIES   P. 3202

200 mg

100 mg/5 mL

Organidin® NR
(guaifenesin)

RX   WALLACE LABORATORIES   P. 3202

Rynatan®
(phenylephrine tannate, chlorpheniramine tannate, pyrilamine tannate)
25 mg / 8 mg / 25 mg

RX   WALLACE LABORATORIES   P. 3202

Rynatan®-S Pediatric Suspension
(phenylephrine tannate, chlorpheniramine tannate, pyrilamine tannate)
5 mg / 2 mg / 12.5 mg / 5 mL

RX   WALLACE LABORATORIES   P. 3203

Rynatuss®
(carbetapentane tannate, chlorpheniramine tannate, ephedrine tannate, phenylephrine tannate)

RX   WALLACE LABORATORIES   P. 3203

350 mg
Soma®
(carisoprodol)

RX   WALLACE LABORATORIES   P. 3204

Soma® Compound
(carisoprodol, aspirin)
200 mg / 325 mg

C-III   WALLACE LABORATORIES   P. 3205

Soma® Compound w/Codeine
(carisoprodol, aspirin, codeine phosphate)
200 mg / 325 mg / 16 mg

C-V   WALLACE LABORATORIES   P. 3207

4 fl oz (118 mL)

Tussi-Organidin®-S NR*
(guaifenesin, codeine phosphate)
100 mg / 10 mg / 5 mL
(* newly reformulated)

RX   WALLACE LABORATORIES   P. 3206

4 fl oz (118 mL)

Tussi-Organidin® DM-S NR*
(guaifenesin, dextromethorphan HBr)
100 mg / 10 mg / 5 mL
(* newly reformulated)

WARNER CHILCOTT

RX   WARNER CHILCOTT LABORATORIES   P. 3208

WC   214
400 mg

WC   221
600 mg

Choledyl® SA
(oxtriphylline extended-release tablets, USP)

RX   WARNER CHILCOTT LABORATORIES   P. 3208

100 mg
Doryx®
(coated doxycycline hyclate pellets)

RX   WARNER CHILCOTT LABORATORIES   P. 3208

4 grams per scoop/pouch

LoCholest™
(cholestyramine for oral suspension, USP)

RX   WARNER CHILCOTT LABORATORIES   P. 3210

4 grams per scoop/pouch

LoCholest™ Light
(cholestyramine for oral suspension, USP)

RX   WARNER CHILCOTT LABORATORIES   P. 3212

NATAFORT

Natafort®
(Prenatal multivitamin tablet with iron)

RX   WARNER CHILCOTT LABORATORIES   P. 3208

WC
182
150 mg

Pyridium® Plus

RX   WARNER CHILCOTT LABORATORIES   P. 3212

50 mg   100 mg

Vectrin®
(minocycline HCl capsules, USP)

WATSON

RX   WATSON LABORATORIES INC.   P. 3218

0252* 240 mg

0251* 180 mg

0250* 120 mg

Dilacor XR®
(diltiazem HCl)
Extended-release Capsules

RX   WATSON LABORATORIES INC.   P. 3220

Levora™
(levonorgestrel 0.15 mg and
ethiny estradiol 0.03 mg)

Also available in a 21 day unit
without placebo tablets.

RX   WATSON LABORATORIES INC.   P. 3224

5 mg

10 mg

25 mg

50 mg

Loxitane®
(loxapine succinate)

RX   WATSON LABORATORIES INC.   P. 3225

12.5 mg

Microzide™
(hydrochlorothiazide)

RX   WATSON LABORATORIES INC.   P. 3227

Necon® 0.5/35-28
28-day

Also available in a 21 day unit
without placebo tablets.

Necon® 0.5/35
(norethindrone and ethinyl
estradiol tablets USP)
0.5 mg/35 mcg

RX   WATSON LABORATORIES INC.   P. 3227

Necon® 1/35-28
28-day

Also available in a 21 day unit
without placebo tablets.

Necon® 1/35
(norethindrone and ethinyl
estradiol tablets USP)
1 mg/35 mcg

RX   WATSON LABORATORIES INC.   P. 3227

Necon® 1/50-28
28-day

Also available in a 21 day unit
without placebo tablets.

Necon® 1/50
(norethindrone and mestranol
tablets USP)
1 mg/50 mcg

RX   WATSON LABORATORIES INC.   P. 3227

Necon® 10/11-28
28-day

Also available in a 21 day unit
without placebo tablets.

Each light yellow tablet (10) contains
0.5 mg norethindrone and 35 mcg ethinyl
estradiol. Each dark yellow tablet (11)
contains 1 mg norethindrone and 35 mcg
ethinyl estradiol. Each white tablet (7)
contains inert ingredient.

Necon® 10/11
(norethindrone and ethinyl
estradiol tablets USP)

RX   WATSON LABORATORIES INC.   P. 3231

Nor-QD®
(norethindrone)
0.35 mg

C-III   WATSON LABORATORIES INC.   P. 3233

NORCO
533

Norco™
(hydrocodone bitartrate
and acetaminophen)
10 mg/325 mg

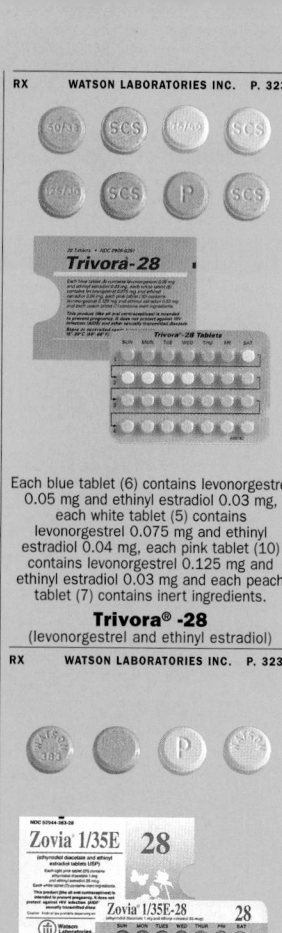

RX WATSON LABORATORIES INC. P. 3234

Trivora-28

Each blue tablet (6) contains levonorgestrel 0.05 mg and ethinyl estradiol 0.03 mg, each white tablet (5) contains levonorgestrel 0.075 mg and ethinyl estradiol 0.04 mg, each pink tablet (10) contains levonorgestrel 0.125 mg and ethinyl estradiol 0.03 mg and each peach tablet (7) contains inert ingredients.

Trivora® -28
(levonorgestrel and ethinyl estradiol)

RX WATSON LABORATORIES INC. P. 3237

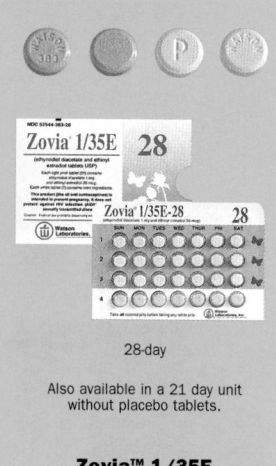

Zovia 1/35E 28

28-day

Also available in a 21 day unit without placebo tablets.

Zovia™ 1/35E
(ethynodiol diacetate and ethinyl estradiol tablets USP)
1 mg/35 mcg

RX WATSON LABORATORIES INC. P. 3237

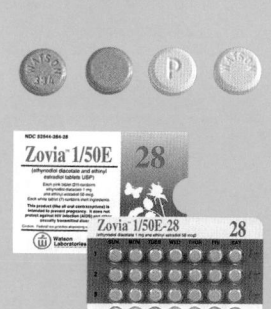

Zovia 1/50E 28

28-day

Also available in a 21 day unit without placebo tablets.

Zovia™ 1/50E
(ethynodiol diacetate and ethinyl estradiol tablets USP)

Because tablets and capsules are shown in this section, do not infer that these are the only dosage forms available. Where a product name is preceded by the symbol †, refer to the description in the Product Information (White Section) for other forms.

WOMEN FIRST HEALTHCARE, INC.

RX WOMEN FIRST HEALTHCARE, INC. P. 3253

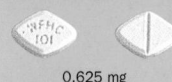

0.625 mg

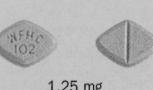

1.25 mg

Ortho-EST®
(estropipate)

WYETH-AYERST

RX WYETH-AYERST LABORATORIES P. 3257

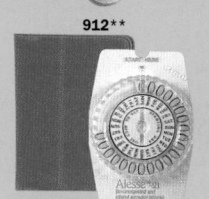

912**

Minipack™ Dispenser
Alesse™ -21
(levonorgestrel, ethinyl estradiol)
0.10 mg/0.02 mg

RX WYETH-AYERST LABORATORIES P. 3263

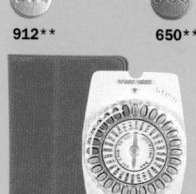

912** 650**

Minipack™ Dispenser
Alesse™ -28
(levonorgestrel, ethinyl estradiol)
0.10 mg/0.02 mg
and 7 green inert tablets

RX WYETH-AYERST LABORATORIES P. 3264

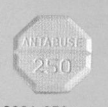

809* 250 mg   **810*** 500 mg

Antabuse®
(disulfiram)

C-IV WYETH-AYERST LABORATORIES P. 3271

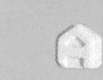

81* 0.5 mg   **64*** 1 mg   **65*** 2 mg

∆Ativan®
(lorazepam)

RX WYETH-AYERST LABORATORIES P. 3272

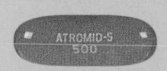

243* 500 mg

‡Atromid-S®
(clofibrate)

RX WYETH-AYERST LABORATORIES P. 3283

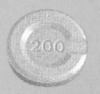 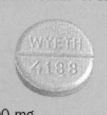

4188* 200 mg

Cordarone®
(amiodarone HCl)

RX WYETH-AYERST LABORATORIES P. 3289

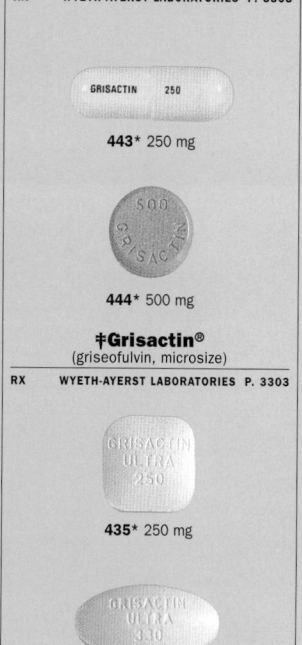

908*
For Vaginal Use Only
(Each single use, disposable vaginal applicator contains 2.6g of gel and delivers 1.125g of gel.)
Also available in Crinone™ 4%

Crinone™ 8%
(progesterone gel)

RX WYETH-AYERST LABORATORIES P. 3292

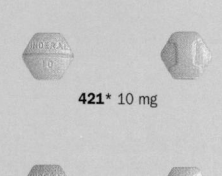

702* 50 mg

Diucardin®
(hydroflumethiazide)

RX WYETH-AYERST LABORATORIES P. 3293

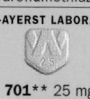

701* 25 mg

781* 37.5 mg

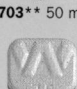

703* 50 mg

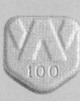

704* 75 mg

705* 100 mg

‡Effexor®
(venlafaxine HCl)

RX WYETH-AYERST LABORATORIES P. 3298

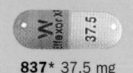

837* 37.5 mg

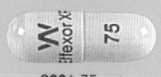

833* 75 mg

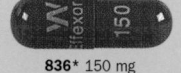

836* 150 mg
Extended-Release Capsules

‡Effexor® XR
(venlafaxine HCl)

RX WYETH-AYERST LABORATORIES P. 3303

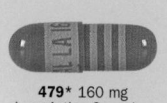

443* 250 mg

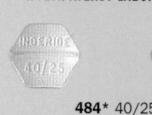

444* 500 mg

‡Grisactin®
(griseofulvin, microsize)

RX WYETH-AYERST LABORATORIES P. 3303

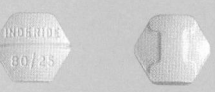

435* 250 mg

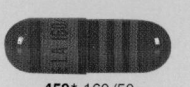

437* 330 mg

Grisactin® Ultra
(griseofulvin, ultramicrosize)

RX WYETH-AYERST LABORATORIES P. 3307

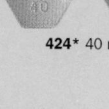

421* 10 mg

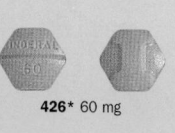

422* 20 mg

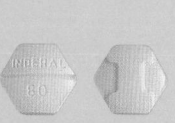

424* 40 mg

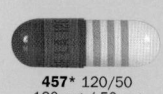

426* 60 mg

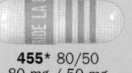

428* 80 mg

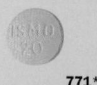

3265* 1 mg/mL
Injectable

∆Inderal®
(propranolol HCl)

While every effort has been made to reproduce products faithfully, this section is to be considered a quick reference identification aid. In cases of suspected overdosage, etc., chemical analysis of the product should be done.

RX WYETH-AYERST LABORATORIES P. 3309

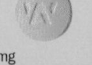

470* 60 mg

471* 80 mg

473* 120 mg

479* 160 mg
Long-Acting Capsules

∆Inderal® LA
(propranolol HCl)

RX WYETH-AYERST LABORATORIES P. 3311

484* 40/25
40 mg / 25 mg

488* 80/25
80 mg / 25 mg

∆Inderide®
(propranolol HCl, hydrochlorothiazide)

RX WYETH-AYERST LABORATORIES P. 3313

459* 160/50
160 mg / 50 mg

457* 120/50
120 mg / 50 mg

455* 80/50
80 mg / 50 mg
Long-Acting Capsules

∆Inderide® LA
(propranolol HCl, hydrochlorothiazide)

RX WYETH-AYERST LABORATORIES P. 3317

771* 20 mg

Ismo®
(isosorbide mononitrate)

---

† The appearance of these tablets and capsules is a trademark of Wyeth-Ayerst Laboratories.   ∆ The appearance of these tablets and capsules is a registered trademark of Wyeth-Ayerst Laboratories.

**Product identification number on reverse side

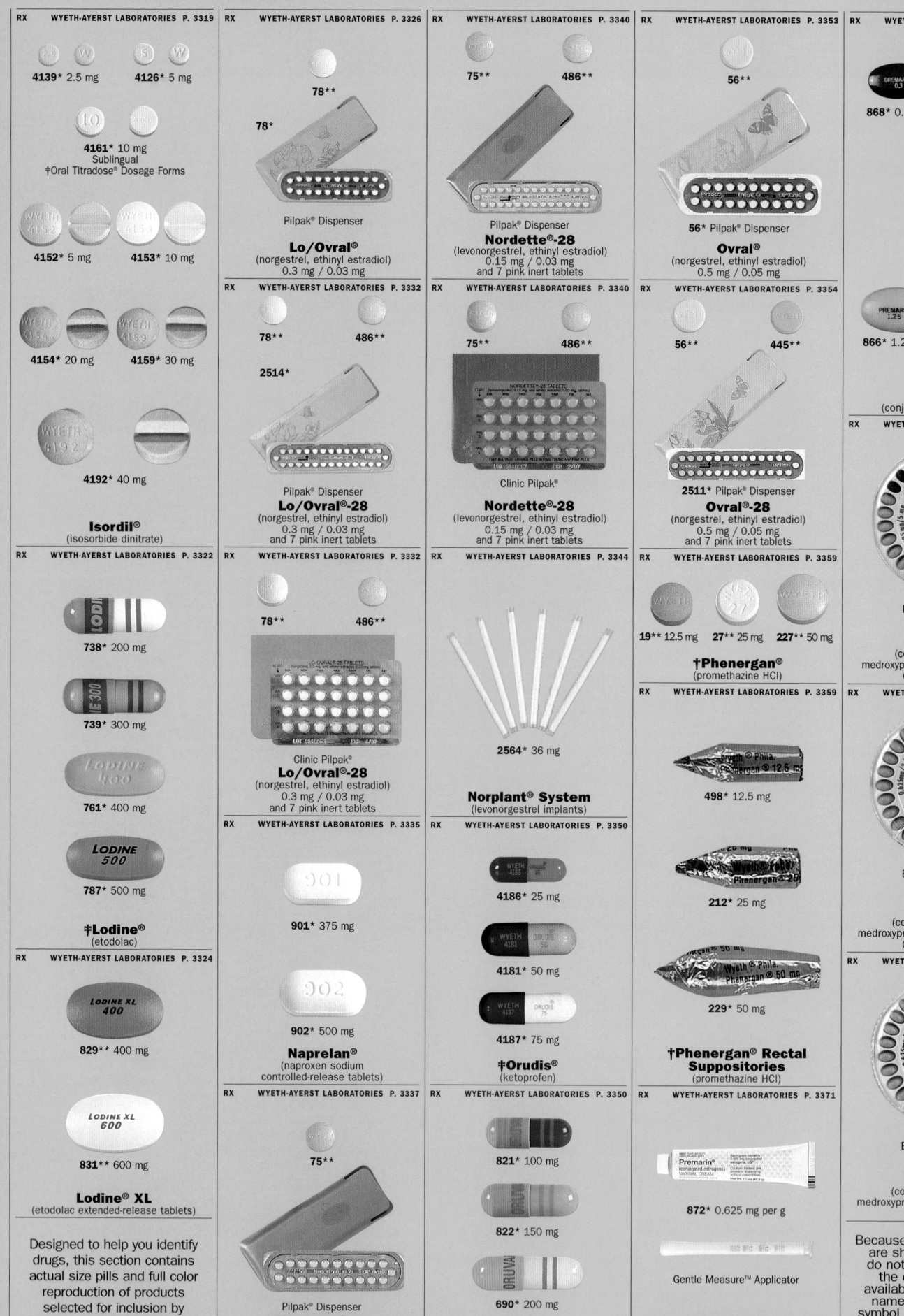

RX   WYETH-AYERST LABORATORIES   P. 3319

4139* 2.5 mg   **4126*** 5 mg

4161* 10 mg
Sublingual
†Oral Titradose® Dosage Forms

4152* 5 mg   **4153*** 10 mg

4154* 20 mg   **4159*** 30 mg

4192* 40 mg

Isordil®
(isosorbide dinitrate)

RX   WYETH-AYERST LABORATORIES   P. 3322

738* 200 mg

739* 300 mg

761* 400 mg

787* 500 mg

‡Lodine®
(etodolac)

RX   WYETH-AYERST LABORATORIES   P. 3324

829** 400 mg

831** 600 mg

Lodine® XL
(etodolac extended-release tablets)

Designed to help you identify
drugs, this section contains
actual size pills and full color
reproduction of products
selected for inclusion by
participating manufacturers.

RX   WYETH-AYERST LABORATORIES   P. 3326

78**

78*

Pilpak® Dispenser
Lo/Ovral®
(norgestrel, ethinyl estradiol)
0.3 mg / 0.03 mg

RX   WYETH-AYERST LABORATORIES   P. 3332

78**   **486****

2514*

Pilpak® Dispenser
Lo/Ovral®-28
(norgestrel, ethinyl estradiol)
0.3 mg / 0.03 mg
and 7 pink inert tablets

RX   WYETH-AYERST LABORATORIES   P. 3332

78**   **486****

Clinic Pilpak®
Lo/Ovral®-28
(norgestrel, ethinyl estradiol)
0.3 mg / 0.03 mg
and 7 pink inert tablets

RX   WYETH-AYERST LABORATORIES   P. 3335

901* 375 mg

902* 500 mg

Naprelan®
(naproxen sodium
controlled-release tablets)

RX   WYETH-AYERST LABORATORIES   P. 3337

75**

Pilpak® Dispenser
Nordette®-21
(levonorgestrel, ethinyl estradiol)
0.15 mg / 0.03 mg

RX   WYETH-AYERST LABORATORIES   P. 3340

75**   **486****

Pilpak® Dispenser
Nordette®-28
(levonorgestrel, ethinyl estradiol)
0.15 mg / 0.03 mg
and 7 pink inert tablets

RX   WYETH-AYERST LABORATORIES   P. 3340

75**   **486****

Clinic Pilpak®
Nordette®-28
(levonorgestrel, ethinyl estradiol)
0.15 mg / 0.03 mg
and 7 pink inert tablets

RX   WYETH-AYERST LABORATORIES   P. 3344

2564* 36 mg

Norplant® System
(levonorgestrel implants)

RX   WYETH-AYERST LABORATORIES   P. 3350

4186* 25 mg

4181* 50 mg

4187* 75 mg

‡Orudis®
(ketoprofen)

RX   WYETH-AYERST LABORATORIES   P. 3350

821* 100 mg

822* 150 mg

690* 200 mg

‡Oruvail®
(ketoprofen extended-release capsules)

RX   WYETH-AYERST LABORATORIES   P. 3353

56**

56* Pilpak® Dispenser**
Ovral®
(norgestrel, ethinyl estradiol)
0.5 mg / 0.05 mg

RX   WYETH-AYERST LABORATORIES   P. 3354

56**   **445****

2511* Pilpak® Dispenser**
Ovral®-28
(norgestrel, ethinyl estradiol)
0.5 mg / 0.05 mg
and 7 pink inert tablets

RX   WYETH-AYERST LABORATORIES   P. 3359

19** 12.5 mg   **27**** 25 mg   **227**** 50 mg

†Phenergan®
(promethazine HCl)

RX   WYETH-AYERST LABORATORIES   P. 3359

498* 12.5 mg

212* 25 mg

229* 50 mg

**†Phenergan® Rectal
Suppositories**
(promethazine HCl)

RX   WYETH-AYERST LABORATORIES   P. 3371

872* 0.625 mg per g

Gentle Measure™ Applicator

Premarin® Vaginal Cream
(conjugated estrogens)
Net Wt. 1 1/2 oz. (42.5 g)

RX   WYETH-AYERST LABORATORIES   P. 3369

868* 0.3 mg   **867*** 0.625 mg

864* 0.9 mg

866* 1.25 mg   **865*** 2.5 mg

‡Premarin®
(conjugated estrogens, USP)

RX   WYETH-AYERST LABORATORIES   P. 3374

EZ Dial™ Dispenser

Premphase®
(conjugated estrogens/
medroxyprogesterone acetate tablets)
0.625 mg / 2.5 mg

RX   WYETH-AYERST LABORATORIES   P. 3374

EZ Dial™ Dispenser

Prempro™
(conjugated estrogens/
medroxyprogesterone acetate tablets)
0.625 mg / 2.5 mg

RX   WYETH-AYERST LABORATORIES   P. 3374

EZ Dial™ Dispenser

Prempro™
(conjugated estrogens/
medroxyprogesterone acetate tablets)
0.625 mg / 5 mg

Because tablets and capsules
are shown in this section,
do not infer that these are
the only dosage forms
available. Where a product
name is preceded by the
symbol †, refer to the description in the Product Information
(White Section) for other forms.

† The appearance of these tablets and capsules is a trademark of Wyeth-Ayerst Laboratories.   Δ The appearance of these tablets and capsules is a registered trademark of Wyeth-Ayerst Laboratories.
**Product identification number on reverse side

RX   WYETH-AYERST LABORATORIES P. 3381

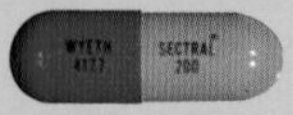

4177* 200 mg

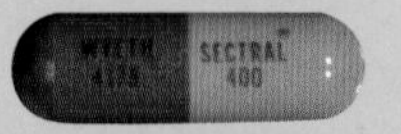

4179* 400 mg

‡†Sectral®
(acebutolol HCl)

C-IV   WYETH-AYERST LABORATORIES P. 3383

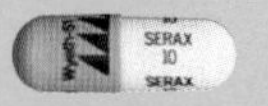

51* 10 mg

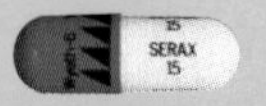

6* 15 mg

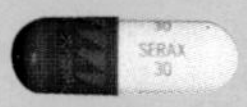

52* 30 mg

‡†Serax®
(oxazepam)

C-IV   WYETH-AYERST LABORATORIES P. 3383

317* 15 mg

‡†Serax®
(oxazepam)

RX   WYETH-AYERST LABORATORIES P. 3384

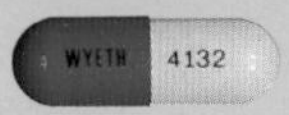

4132* 25 mg

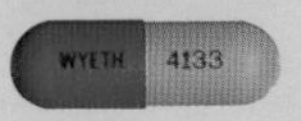

4133* 50 mg

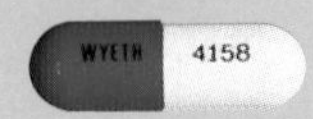

4158* 100 mg

†Surmontil®
(trimipramine maleate)

RX   WYETH-AYERST LABORATORIES P. 3389

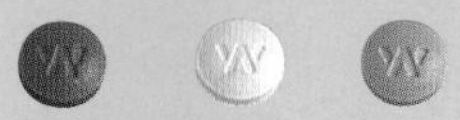

641**   **642****   **643****

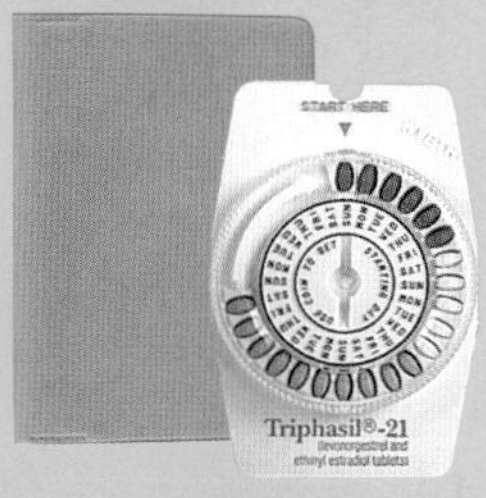

2535*

Triphasil®-21
(21 tablets containing the following: 6 brown tablets - 0.050 mg levonorgestrel + 0.030 mg ethinyl estradiol; 5 white tablets - 0.075 mg levonorgestrel + 0.040 mg ethinyl estradiol; 10 light-yellow tablets - 0.125 mg levonorgestrel + 0.030 mg ethinyl estradiol)

RX   WYETH-AYERST LABORATORIES P. 3394

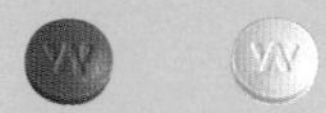

641**   **642****

643**   **650****

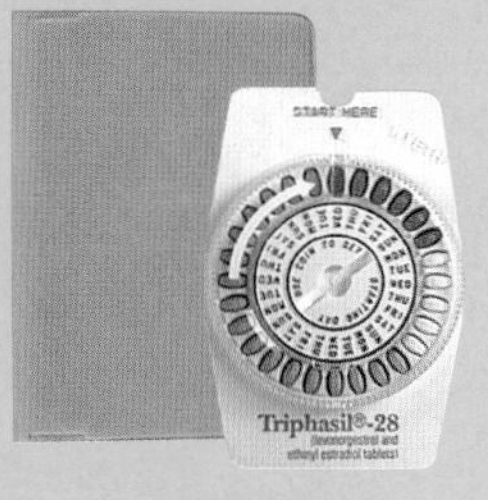

2536*

Triphasil®-28
(28 tablets containing the following: 6 brown tablets - 0.050 mg levonorgestrel + 0.030 mg ethinyl estradiol; 5 white tablets - 0.075 mg levonorgestrel + 0.040 mg ethinyl estradiol; 10 light-yellow tablets - 0.125 mg levonorgestrel + 0.030 mg ethinyl estradiol; 7 light-green inert tablets)

RX   WYETH-AYERST LABORATORIES P. 3394

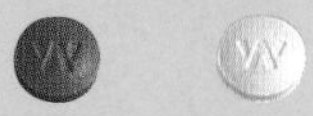

641**   **642****

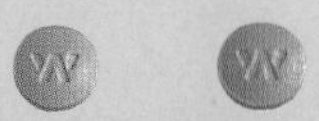

643**   **650****

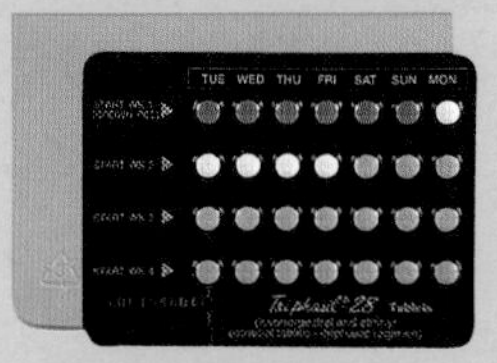

Clinic Pilpak®

Triphasil®-28
(28 tablets containing the following: 6 brown tablets - 0.050 mg levonorgestrel + 0.030 mg ethinyl estradiol; 5 white tablets - 0.075 mg levonorgestrel + 0.040 mg ethinyl estradiol; 10 light-yellow tablets - 0.125 mg levonorgestrel + 0.030 mg ethinyl estradiol; 7 light-green inert tablets)

C-IV   WYETH-AYERST LABORATORIES P. 3400

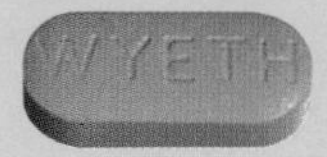

85**

Wygesic®
(propoxyphene HCl, USP, acetaminophen, USP)
65 mg /650 mg

RX   WYETH-AYERST LABORATORIES P. 3401

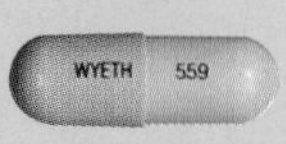

559* 250 mg

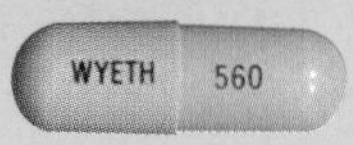

560* 500 mg

†Wymox®
(amoxicillin)

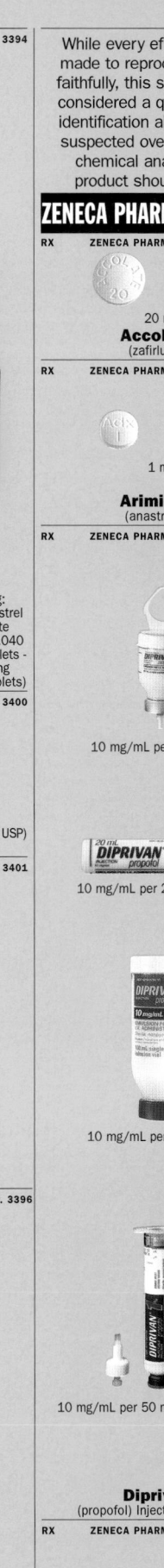

While every effort has been made to reproduce products faithfully, this section is to be considered a quick reference identification aid. In cases of suspected overdosage, etc., chemical analysis of the product should be done.

ZENECA PHARMACEUTICALS

RX   ZENECA PHARMACEUTICALS P. 3402

20 mg

Accolate®
(zafirlukast)

RX   ZENECA PHARMACEUTICALS P. 3404

1 mg

Arimidex®
(anastrozole)

RX   ZENECA PHARMACEUTICALS P. 3411

10 mg/mL per 50 mL vial

10 mg/mL per 20 mL ampules

10 mg/mL per 100 mL vial

10 mg/mL per 50 mL prefilled syringe

Diprivan®
(propofol) Injectable Emulsion

RX   ZENECA PHARMACEUTICALS P. 3406

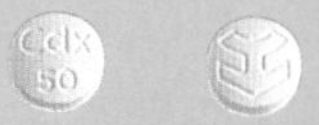

50 mg

Casodex®
(bicalutamide)

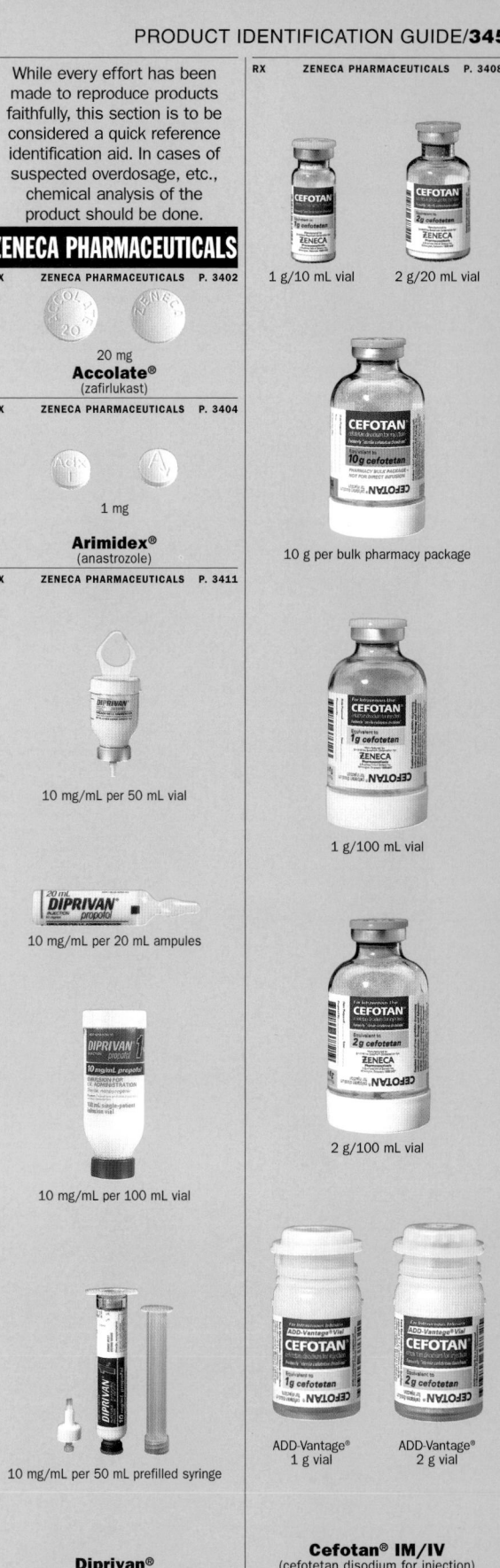

RX   ZENECA PHARMACEUTICALS P. 3408

1 g/10 mL vial   2 g/20 mL vial

10 g per bulk pharmacy package

1 g/100 mL vial

2 g/100 mL vial

ADD-Vantage®   ADD-Vantage®
1 g vial   2 g vial

Cefotan® IM/IV
(cefotetan disodium for injection)
formerly sterile cefotetan disodium

Designed to help you identify drugs, this section contains actual size pills and full color reproduction of products selected for inclusion by participating manufacturers.

RX   WYETH-AYERST LABORATORIES   P. 3396

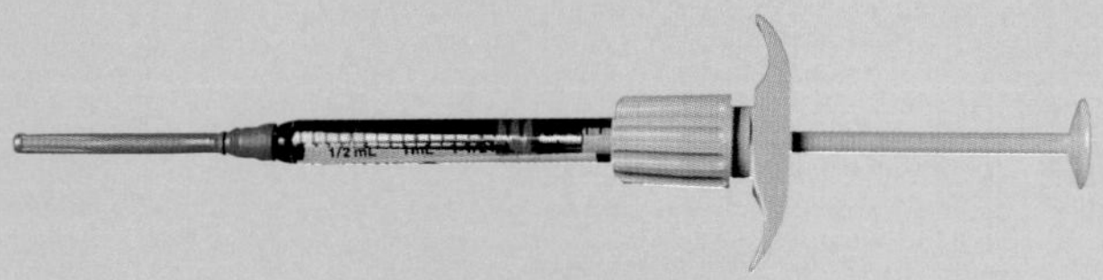

Tubex® Injector and Sterile Cartridge–Needle Unit
with hard cannula cover ready for injection.

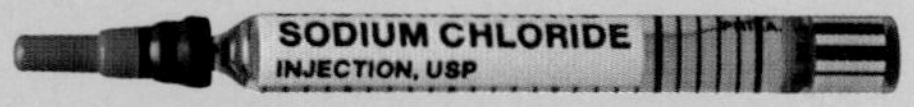

SODIUM CHLORIDE
INJECTION, USP

Tubex® Blunt Pointe™ Sterile Cartridge–Needle Unit
for use in selected "needle–less" IV port systems*

*(*Consult product prescribing information for compatibility
information in the Product Information section of this PDR.)*

Tubex® Closed Injection System
Examples of Tubex® Sterile Cartridge–Needle Units, Tubex® Blunt Pointe™ Sterile Cartridge–Unit, and Tubex® Injector, components of the Tubex Closed Injection System, the most comprehensive line of small–volume unit–dose prefilled syringe injectibles. For complete list of products available, consult Tubex listing in the Product Information Section.

† The appearance of these tablets and capsules is a trademark of Wyeth-Ayerst Laboratories.   Δ The appearance of these tablets and capsules is a registered trademark of Wyeth-Ayerst Laboratories.
**Product identification number on reverse side

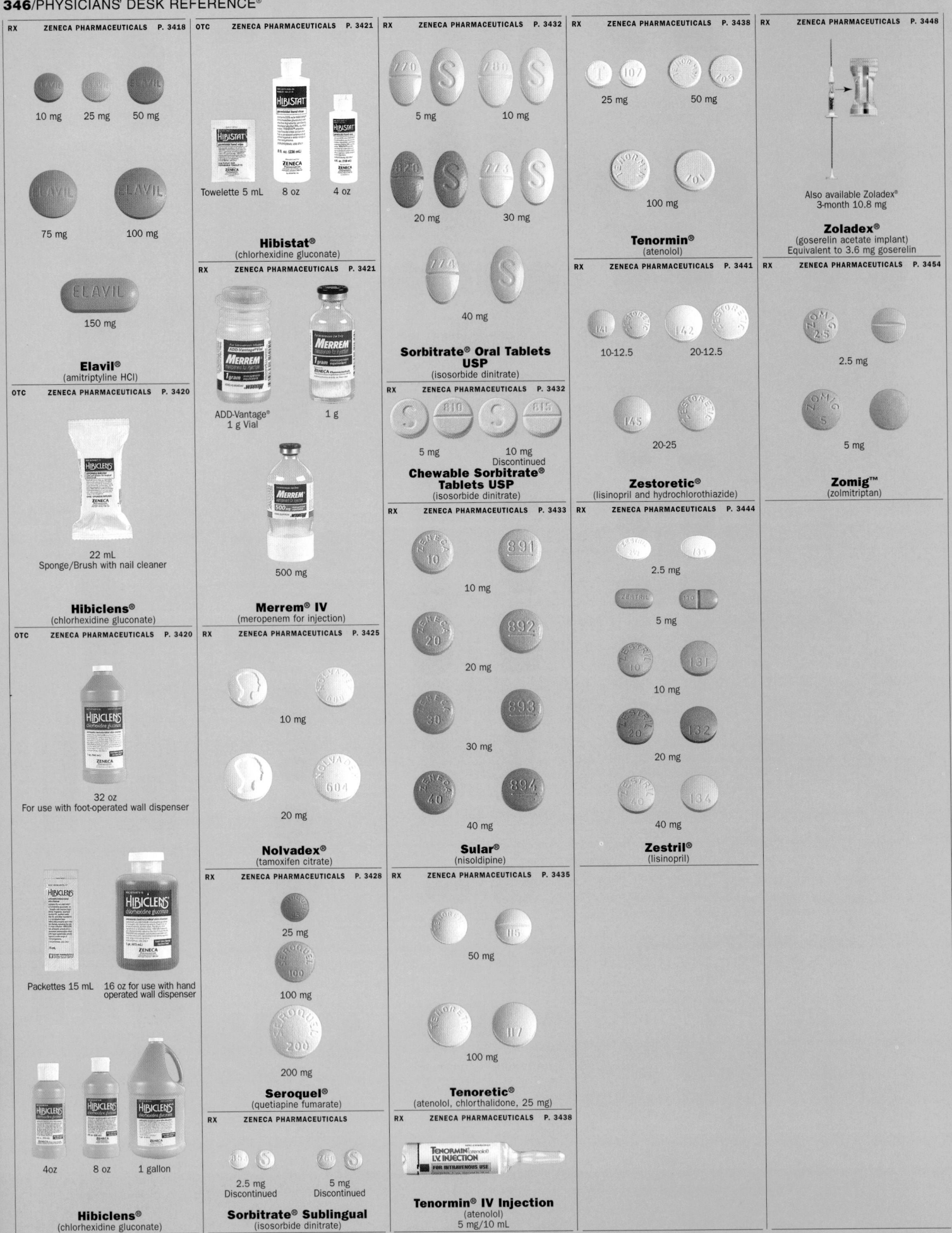

RX   ZENECA PHARMACEUTICALS   P. 3418

10 mg   25 mg   50 mg

75 mg   100 mg

150 mg

Elavil®
(amitriptyline HCl)

OTC   ZENECA PHARMACEUTICALS   P. 3420

22 mL
Sponge/Brush with nail cleaner

Hibiclens®
(chlorhexidine gluconate)

OTC   ZENECA PHARMACEUTICALS   P. 3420

32 oz
For use with foot-operated wall dispenser

Packettes 15 mL   16 oz for use with hand
operated wall dispenser

4oz   8 oz   1 gallon

Hibiclens®
(chlorhexidine gluconate)

OTC   ZENECA PHARMACEUTICALS   P. 3421

Towelette 5 mL   8 oz   4 oz

Hibistat®
(chlorhexidine gluconate)

RX   ZENECA PHARMACEUTICALS   P. 3421

ADD-Vantage®
1 g Vial   1 g

500 mg

Merrem® IV
(meropenem for injection)

RX   ZENECA PHARMACEUTICALS   P. 3425

10 mg

20 mg

Nolvadex®
(tamoxifen citrate)

RX   ZENECA PHARMACEUTICALS   P. 3428

25 mg

100 mg

200 mg

Seroquel®
(quetiapine fumarate)

RX   ZENECA PHARMACEUTICALS

2.5 mg
Discontinued   5 mg
Discontinued

Sorbitrate® Sublingual
(isosorbide dinitrate)

RX   ZENECA PHARMACEUTICALS   P. 3432

5 mg   10 mg

20 mg   30 mg

40 mg

Sorbitrate® Oral Tablets USP
(isosorbide dinitrate)

RX   ZENECA PHARMACEUTICALS   P. 3432

5 mg   10 mg
Discontinued

Chewable Sorbitrate® Tablets USP
(isosorbide dinitrate)

RX   ZENECA PHARMACEUTICALS   P. 3433

10 mg

20 mg

30 mg

40 mg

Sular®
(nisoldipine)

RX   ZENECA PHARMACEUTICALS   P. 3435

50 mg

100 mg

Tenoretic®
(atenolol, chlorthalidone, 25 mg)

RX   ZENECA PHARMACEUTICALS   P. 3438

Tenormin® IV Injection
(atenolol)
5 mg/10 mL

RX   ZENECA PHARMACEUTICALS   P. 3438

25 mg   50 mg

100 mg

Tenormin®
(atenolol)

RX   ZENECA PHARMACEUTICALS   P. 3441

10-12.5   20-12.5

20-25

Zestoretic®
(lisinopril and hydrochlorothiazide)

RX   ZENECA PHARMACEUTICALS   P. 3444

2.5 mg

5 mg

10 mg

20 mg

40 mg

Zestril®
(lisinopril)

RX   ZENECA PHARMACEUTICALS   P. 3448

Also available Zoladex®
3-month 10.8 mg

Zoladex®
(goserelin acetate implant)
Equivalent to 3.6 mg goserelin

RX   ZENECA PHARMACEUTICALS   P. 3454

2.5 mg

5 mg

Zomig™
(zolmitriptan)

Key to Controlled Substances Categories

Products listed with the symbols shown below are subject to the Controlled Substances Act of 1970. These drugs are categorized according to their potential for abuse. The greater the potential, the more severe the limitations on their prescription.

CATEGORY	INTERPRETATION
Ⓒ II	**HIGH POTENTIAL FOR ABUSE.** Use may lead to severe physical or psychological dependence. Prescriptions must be written in ink, or typewritten and signed by the practitioner. Verbal prescriptions must be confirmed in writing within 72 hours, and may be given only in a genuine emergency. No renewals are permitted.
Ⓒ III	**SOME POTENTIAL FOR ABUSE.** Use may lead to low-to-moderate physical dependence or high psychological dependence. Prescriptions may be oral or written. Up to 5 renewals are permitted within 6 months.
Ⓒ IV	**LOW POTENTIAL FOR ABUSE.** Use may lead to limited physical or psychological dependence. Prescriptions may be oral or written. Up to 5 renewals are permitted within 6 months.
Ⓒ V	**SUBJECT TO STATE AND LOCAL REGULATION.** Abuse potential is low; a prescription may not be required.

Key to FDA Use-in-Pregnancy Ratings

The U.S. Food and Drug Administration's use-in-pregnancy rating system weighs the degree to which available information has ruled out risk to the fetus against the drug's potential benefit to the patient. The ratings, and their interpretation, are as follows:

CATEGORY	INTERPRETATION
A	**CONTROLLED STUDIES SHOW NO RISK.** Adequate, well-controlled studies in pregnant women have failed to demonstrate a risk to the fetus in any trimester of pregnancy.
B	**NO EVIDENCE OF RISK IN HUMANS.** Adequate, well-controlled studies in pregnant women have not shown increased risk of fetal abnormalities despite adverse findings in animals, or, in the absence of adequate human studies, animal studies show no fetal risk. The chance of fetal harm is remote, but remains a possibility.
C	**RISK CANNOT BE RULED OUT.** Adequate, well-controlled human studies are lacking, and animal studies have shown a risk to the fetus or are lacking as well. There is a chance of fetal harm if the drug is administered during pregnancy; but the potential benefits may outweigh the potential risk.
D	**POSITIVE EVIDENCE OF RISK.** Studies in humans, or investigational or post-marketing data, have demonstrated fetal risk. Nevertheless, potential benefits from the use of the drug may outweigh the potential risk. For example, the drug may be acceptable if needed in a life-threatening situation or serious disease for which safer drugs cannot be used or are ineffective.
X	**CONTRAINDICATED IN PREGNANCY.** Studies in animals or humans, or investigational or post-marketing reports, have demonstrated positive evidence of fetal abnormalities or risk which clearly outweighs any possible benefit to the patient.

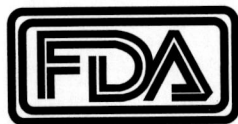

U.S. FOOD AND DRUG ADMINISTRATION

Medical Product Reporting Programs

MedWatch (24 hour service)...800-332-1088
   Reporting of problems with drugs, devices, biologics (except vaccines), medical foods, dietary supplements.

Vaccine Adverse Event Reporting System (24 hour service).................................800-822-7967
   Reporting of vaccine-related problems.

Mandatory Medical Device Reporting..301-594-3886
   Reporting required from User facilities regarding device-related deaths and serious injuries.

Veterinary Adverse Drug Reaction Program..888-FDA-VETS
   Reporting of adverse drug events in animals.

Medical Advertising Information..800-238-7332
   Inquiries from health professionals regarding product promotion.

USP Medication Errors...800-233-7767
   Reporting of medication errors or near-errors to help avoid future problems through improvement in product names and packaging.

Information for Health Professionals

Center for Drugs Information Branch...301-827-4573
   Information on human drugs including hormones.

Center for Biologics Executive Secretariat..301-827-2000
   Information on biological products including vaccines and blood.

Center for Devices and Radiological Health..301-443-4190
   Automated request for information on medical devices and radiation-emitting products.

Office of Orphan Products Development...301-827-3666
   Information on products for rare diseases.

Office of Health Affairs, Medicine Staff..301-827-6630
   Information for health professionals on FDA activities.

General Information

General Consumer Inquiries...800-532-4440
   Consumer information on regulated products/issues.   Local: 301-827-4420

Freedom of Information..301-827-6567
   Requests for publicly available FDA documents.

Office of Public Affairs..301-827-6250
   Interviews/press inquiries on FDA activities.

Seafood Hotline (24 hour service)..800-332-4010
   Prerecorded message/request information (English/Spanish).

SECTION 5

PRODUCT INFORMATION

This section is made possible through the courtesy of the manufacturers whose products appear in it. The information concerning each product has been prepared, edited, and approved by the medical department, medical director, and/or medical counsel of its manufacturer.

When a product appearing in *Physician's Desk Reference* has an official package circular, its description must be in full compliance with Food and Drug Administration (FDA) regulations pertaining to labeling for prescription drugs. These regulations require that in *PDR* "indications, effects, dosages, routes, methods, and frequency and duration of administration, and any relevant warnings, hazards, contraindications, side effects, and precautions" must be "*same in language and emphasis*" as those in the approved labeling for the product. The FDA regards the words "*same in language and emphasis*" as requiring VERBATIM use of the approved labeling providing such information. Furthermore, information in the approved labeling that is emphasized by the use of type set in a box or in capitals, boldface, or italics must be given the same emphasis in *PDR*.

For products that do not have official package circulars, the publisher has emphasized the necessity of describing such products comprehensively, so that physicians have access to all information essential for intelligent and informed decision making.

The product descriptions in *Physician's Desk Reference* include all information made available to *PDR* by the manufacturer. The publisher does not warrant or guarantee any product, and does not perform any independent analysis of the information provided. Inclusion of a product in *PDR* does not represent an endorsement, and the publisher does not necessarily advocate the use of any product listed.

This edition of *Physician's Desk Reference* contains the latest information available when the book went to press. As new drugs are released, and new research data and clinical findings become available throughout the year, the information in the *PDR* database is revised accordingly. These revisions are published twice annually in the *PDR* Supplements. To be certain that you have the most current data, always consult the supplements before prescribing or administering any product described in the following pages.

Abbott Laboratories Inc.
Pharmaceutical Products Division
NORTH CHICAGO, IL 60064, U.S.A.

Pharmaceutical Products Division—
Direct Inquiries to:
Customer Service:
(800) 255-5162
Technical Services:
(800) 441-4987
For Medical Information Contact:
Generally:
(800) 633-9110
Adverse Drug Experiences:
(800) 633-9110
Sales and Ordering:
(800) 255-5162

Hospital Products Division—
Direct Inquiries to:
Customer Service
(800) 222-6883
For Medical Information Contact:
(800) 615–0187
Sales and Ordering:
(800) 222-6883

ABBO–CODE™ INDEX

The Abbo-Code identification system provides positive identification of a drug and dosage strength. The following Abbott products are imprinted or debossed with an Abbo-Code designation:

PRODUCT	ABBO-CODE
Biaxin® Filmtab® Tablets (clarithromycin tablets)	
250 mg	KT
500 mg	KL
Cartrol® (carteolol hydrochloride) Filmtab® Tablets	
2.5 mg	IA
5 mg	IC
Cefol® Filmtab® Tablets B-complex vitamins with folic acid, vitamin E, and vitamin C	NJ
Colchicine Tablets, USP	
0.6 mg	AF
Cylert® Tablets Ⓘ (pemoline)	
18.75 mg	TH
37.5 mg	TI
75 mg	TJ
37.5 mg Chewable	TK
Depakene® Capsules (valproic acid capsules, USP)	
250 mg	DEPAKENE
Depakote® Sprinkle Capsules (divalproex sodium coated particles in capsules)	
125 mg	DEPAKOTE SPRINKLE
Depakote® Tablets (divalproex sodium delayed-release tablets)	
125 mg	NT
250 mg	NR
500 mg	NS
Desoxyn® Tablets Ⓘ (methamphetamine hydrochloride)	
5 mg Tablet	TE
5 mg Gradumet®	MC
10 mg Gradumet	ME
15 mg Gradumet	MF
Dicumarol Tablets	
25 mg	AN
E.E.S. 400® Filmtab® Tablets (erythromycin ethylsuccinate tablets, USP)	
400 mg erythromycin activity	EE
EryPed® Chewable Tablets (erythromycin ethylsuccinate tablets, USP)	
200 mg erythromycin activity	EZ
Enduron® Tablets (methyclothiazide tablets, USP)	
2.5 mg	ENDURON
5 mg	ENDURON
Enduronyl® Tablets	
5 mg methyclothiazide and 0.25 mg deserpidine	LS
Enduronyl® Forte Tablets	
5 mg methyclothiazide and 0.5 mg deserpidine	LT
Ery-Tab® Enteric-Coated Tablets (erythromycin delayed-release tablets, USP)	
250 mg	EC
333 mg	EH
500 mg	ED

PRODUCT	ABBO-CODE
Erythrocin® Stearate Filmtab® Tablets (erythromycin stearate tablets, USP)	
250 mg erythromycin activity	ES
500 mg erythromycin activity	ET
Erythromycin Base Filmtab® Tablets (erythromycin tablets, USP)	
250 mg	EB
500 mg	EA
Erythromycin Delayed-release Capsules, USP	
250 mg	ER
Fero-Folic-500® Filmtab® Tablets controlled-release iron, folic acid, and vitamin C	AJ
Gabitril™ Filmtab® Tablets (tiagabine HCl tablets)	
4 mg	FK
12 mg	FL
16 mg	FM
20 mg	FN
Hytrin® Capsules (terazosin hydrochloride capsules)	
1 mg	HH
2 mg	HY
5 mg	HK
10 mg	HN
Iberet-Folic-500® Filmtab® Tablets controlled-release iron, B-complex vitamins with folic acid, and vitamin C	AK
K ·Tab® Filmtab® Tablets (potassium chloride extended-release tablets, USP)	
10 mEq (750 mg)	K-TAB
Nembutal® Sodium Capsules Ⓘ (pentobarbital sodium capsules, USP)	
50 mg	CF
100 mg	CH
Norvir™ Capsules (ritonavir capsules)	
100 mg	PI
Oretic® Tablets (hydrochlorothiazide tablets, USP)	
25 mg	ORETIC
50 mg	ORETIC
PCE® Dispertab® Tablets (erythromycin particles in tablets)	
333 mg	PCE
500 mg	EK
Peganone® Tablets (ethotoin tablets, USP)	
250 mg	AD
500 mg	AE
Phenurone® Tablets (phenacemide tablets, USP)	
500 mg	I I
Placidyl® Capsules Ⓘ (ethchlorvynol capsules, USP)	
500 mg	PLACIDYL 500
750 mg	PLACIDYL 750
ProSom™ Tablets Ⓘ (estazolam tablets)	
1 mg	UC
2 mg	UD
Tranxene® T-Tab® Tablets Ⓘ (clorazepate dipotassium)	
3.75 mg Tablet	TL
7.5 mg Tablet	TM
15 mg Tablet	TN
Tranxene-SD™ Ⓘ (clorazepate dipotassium)	
Single Dose Tablets	
11.25 mg Half Strength	TX
22.5 mg	TY
Tricor™ (fenofibrate capsules), micronized	
67 mg	FR
Tridione® Dulcet® Tablets	
150 mg	LE
Zyflo™ Filmtab® Tablets (zileuton tablets)	
600 mg	ZL

ABBOKINASE®
UROKINASE FOR INJECTION ℞

ABBOKINASE (urokinase for injection) should be used in hospitals where the recommended diagnostic and monitoring techniques are available. Thrombolytic therapy should be considered in all situations where the benefits to be achieved outweigh the risk of potentially serious hemorrhage. When internal bleeding does occur, it may be more difficult to manage than that which occurs with conventional anticoagulant therapy.

Urokinase treatment should be instituted as soon as possible after onset of pulmonary embolism, preferably no later than seven days after onset. Any delay in instituting lytic therapy to evaluate the effect of heparin decreases the potential for optimal efficacy.[1]

When urokinase is used for treatment of coronary artery thrombosis associated with evolving transmural myocardial infarction, therapy should be instituted within six hours of symptom onset.

DESCRIPTION

Urokinase is an enzyme (protein) produced by the kidney, and found in the urine. There are two forms of urokinase differing in molecular weight but having similar clinical effects. ABBOKINASE (urokinase for injection) is a thrombolytic agent obtained from human kidney cells by tissue culture techniques and is primarily the low molecular weight form. It is supplied as a sterile lyophilized white powder containing mannitol (25 mg/vial), Albumin (Human) (250 mg/vial), and sodium chloride (50 mg/vial).

Thin translucent filaments may occasionally occur in reconstituted ABBOKINASE vials, but do not indicate any decrease in potency of this product. No clinical problems have been associated with these filaments. See "Dosage and Administration" section.

Following reconstitution with 5 mL of Sterile Water for Injection, USP, it is a clear, slightly straw-colored solution; each mL contains 50,000 IU of urokinase activity, 0.5% mannitol, 5% Albumin (Human), and 1% sodium chloride. The pH is adjusted with sodium hydroxide and/or hydrochloric acid prior to lyophilization.

ABBOKINASE is for intravenous and intracoronary infusion only.

CLINICAL PHARMACOLOGY

Urokinase acts on the endogenous fibrinolytic system. It converts plasminogen to the enzyme plasmin. Plasmin degrades fibrin clots as well as fibrinogen and other plasma proteins.

Intravenous infusion of urokinase in doses recommended for lysis of pulmonary embolism is followed by increased fibrinolytic activity. This effect disappears within a few hours after discontinuation, but a decrease in plasma levels of fibrinogen and plasminogen and an increase in the amount of circulating fibrin (ogen) degradation products may persist for 12–24 hours.[2,3] There is a lack of correlation between embolus resolution and changes in coagulation and fibrinolytic assay results.

Information is incomplete about the pharmacokinetic properties in man. Urokinase administered by intravenous infusion is cleared rapidly by the liver. The serum half-life in man is 20 minutes or less. Patients with impaired liver function (e.g., cirrhosis) would be expected to show a prolongation in half-life. Small fractions of an administered dose are excreted in bile and urine.

INDICATIONS AND USAGE
Pulmonary Embolism
ABBOKINASE (urokinase for injection) is indicated in adults:
— For the lysis of acute massive pulmonary emboli, defined as obstruction of blood flow to a lobe or multiple segments.
— For the lysis of pulmonary emboli accompanied by unstable hemodynamics, i.e., failure to maintain blood pressure without supportive measures.

The diagnosis should be confirmed by objective means, such as pulmonary angiography via an upper extremity vein, or non-invasive procedures such as lung scanning.

Angiographic and hemodynamic measurements demonstrate a more rapid improvement with lytic therapy than with heparin therapy.[4-8]

Coronary Artery Thrombosis
ABBOKINASE has been reported to lyse acute thrombi obstructing coronary arteries, associated with evolving transmural myocardial infarction.[9] The majority of patients who received ABBOKINASE by intracoronary infusion within six hours following onset of symptoms showed recanalization of the involved vessel.

IT HAS NOT BEEN ESTABLISHED THAT INTRACORONARY ADMINISTRATION OF ABBOKINASE DURING EVOLVING TRANSMURAL MYOCARDIAL INFARCTION RESULTS IN SALVAGE OF MYOCARDIAL TISSUE, NOR THAT IT REDUCES MORTALITY. THE PATIENTS WHO MIGHT BENEFIT FROM THIS THERAPY CANNOT BE DEFINED.

CONTRAINDICATIONS

Because thrombolytic therapy increases the risk of bleeding, urokinase is contraindicated in the following situations: (See WARNINGS.)
— Active internal bleeding
— History of cerebrovascular accident
— Recent (within two months) intracranial or intraspinal surgery
— Recent trauma including cardiopulmonary resuscitation
— Intracranial neoplasm, arteriovenous malformation, or aneurysm
— Known bleeding diathesis
— Severe uncontrolled arterial hypertension

WARNINGS

Bleeding

The aim of urokinase is the production of sufficient amounts of plasmin for lysis of intravascular deposits of fibrin; however, fibrin deposits which provide hemostasis, for example, at sites of needle puncture, will also lyse, and bleeding from such sites may occur.

Intramuscular injections and nonessential handling of the patient must be avoided during treatment with urokinase. Venipunctures should be performed carefully and as infrequently as possible.

Should an arterial puncture be necessary (except for intracoronary administration), upper extremity vessels are preferable. Pressure should be applied for at least 30 minutes, a pressure dressing applied, and the puncture site checked frequently for evidence of bleeding.

In the following conditions, the risks of therapy may be increased and should be weighed against the anticipated benefits:

— Recent (within 10 days) major surgery, obstetrical delivery, organ biopsy, previous puncture of non-compressible vessels
— Recent (within 10 days) serious gastrointestinal bleeding
— High likelihood of a left heart thrombus, e.g., mitral stenosis with atrial fibrillation
— Subacute bacterial endocarditis
— Hemostatic defects including those secondary to severe hepatic or renal disease
— Pregnancy
— Cerebrovascular disease
— Diabetic hemorrhagic retinopathy
— Any other condition in which bleeding might constitute a significant hazard or be particularly difficult to manage because of its location

Should serious spontaneous bleeding (not controllable by local pressure) occur, the infusion of urokinase should be terminated immediately, and treatment instituted as described under ADVERSE REACTIONS.

Use of Anticoagulants

Concurrent use of anticoagulants with intravenous administration of ABBOKINASE is not recommended. However, concurrent use of heparin may be required during intracoronary administration of ABBOKINASE. A clinical study[9] with concurrent use of heparin and ABBOKINASE during intracoronary administration has demonstrated no tendency toward increased bleeding that would not be attributable to the procedure or ABBOKINASE alone. Nevertheless, careful monitoring for excessive bleeding is advised.

Arrhythmias

Rapid lysis of coronary thrombi has been reported occasionally to cause atrial or ventricular dysrhythmias as a result of reperfusion requiring immediate treatment. Careful monitoring for arrhythmias should be maintained during and immediately following intracoronary administration of ABBOKINASE.

PRECAUTIONS

Laboratory Tests

Before commencing thrombolytic therapy, obtain a hematocrit, platelet count, and a thrombin time (TT), activated partial thromboplastin time (APTT), or prothrombin time (PT). If heparin has been given, it should be discontinued unless it is to be used in conjunction with ABBOKINASE for intracoronary administration. TT or APTT should be less than twice the normal control value before thrombolytic therapy is started.

During the infusion, coagulation tests and/or measures of fibrinolytic activity may be performed if desired. Results do not, however, reliably predict either efficacy or a risk of bleeding. The clinical response should be observed frequently, and vital signs, i.e., pulse, temperature, respiratory rate and blood pressure, should be checked at least every four hours. The blood pressure should not be taken in the lower extremities to avoid dislodgment of possible deep vein thrombi.

Following the intravenous infusion, *before (re)instituting heparin*, the TT or APTT should be less than twice the upper limits of normal. Following intracoronary infusion of ABBOKINASE, blood coagulation parameters should be determined and heparin therapy continued as appropriate.

Drug Interactions

The interaction of urokinase with other drugs has not been studied. Drugs that alter platelet function should not be used. Common examples are: aspirin, indomethacin and phenylbutazone.

Although a bolus dose of heparin is recommended prior to intracoronary use of urokinase, oral anticoagulants or heparin should not be given concurrently with large doses of urokinase such as those used for pulmonary embolism. Concomitant use of intravenous urokinase and oral anticoagulants or heparin may increase the risk of hemorrhage. (See "WARNINGS" section.)

Carcinogenicity

Adequate data are not available on the long-term potential for carcinogenicity in animals or humans.

TABLE I
Dose Preparation–Pulmonary Embolism

Weight (pounds)	Total Dose* Urokinase (IU)	Number Vials ABBOKINASE (urokinase for injection)	Volume of ABBOKINASE After Reconstitution (mL)**	+	Volume of Diluent (mL)	=	Final Volume (mL)
81–90	2,250,000	9	45		150		195
91–100	2,500,000	10	50		145		195
101–110	2,750,000	11	55		140		195
111–120	3,000,000	12	60		135		195
121–130	3,250,000	13	65		130		195
131–140	3,500,000	14	70		125		195
141–150	3,750,000	15	75		120		195
151–160	4,000,000	16	80		115		195
161–170	4,250,000	17	85		110		195
171–180	4,500,000	18	90		105		195
181–190	4,750,000	19	95		100		195
191–200	5,000,000	20	100		95		195
201–210	5,250,000	21	105		90		195
211–220	5,500,000	22	110		85		195
221–230	5,750,000	23	115		80		195
231–240	6,000,000	24	120		75		195
241–250	6,250,000	25	125		70		195

Infusion Rate:	Priming Dose 15 mL/10 min***	Dose for 12-Hour Period 15 mL/hr for 12 hrs

*Priming dose + dose administered during 12-hour period.
**After addition of 5 mL of Sterile Water for Injection, USP, per vial. (See Preparation.)
***Pump rate = 90 mL/hr

Pregnancy

Pregnancy category B. Reproduction studies have been performed in mice and rats at doses up to 1,000 times the human dose and have revealed no evidence of impaired fertility or harm to the fetus due to urokinase. There are, however, no adequate and well-controlled studies in pregnant women. Because animal reproduction studies are not always predictive of human response, this drug should be used during pregnancy only if clearly needed.

Nursing Mothers

It is not known whether this drug is excreted in human milk. Because many drugs are excreted in human milk, caution should be exercised when urokinase is administered to a nursing woman.

Pediatric Use

Safety and effectiveness in children have not been established.

ADVERSE REACTIONS

The following adverse reactions have been associated with intravenous therapy but may also occur with intracoronary artery infusion.

Bleeding

The type of bleeding associated with thrombolytic therapy can be placed into two broad categories:

— Superficial or surface bleeding, observed mainly at invaded or disturbed sites (e.g., venous cutdowns, arterial punctures, sites of recent surgical intervention, etc.).
— Internal bleeding, involving, e.g., the gastrointestinal tract, genitourinary tract, vagina, or intramuscular, retroperitoneal, or intracranial sites.

Several fatalities due to intracranial or retroperitoneal hemorrhage have occurred during thrombolytic therapy. Should serious bleeding occur, urokinase infusion should be discontinued and, if necessary, blood loss and reversal of the bleeding tendency can be effectively managed with whole blood (fresh blood preferable), packed red blood cells and cryoprecipitate or fresh frozen plasma. Dextran should not be used. Although the use of aminocaproic acid (ACA, AMICAR®) in humans as an antidote for urokinase has not been documented, it may be considered in an emergency situation.

Allergic Reactions

In vitro tests with urokinase, as well as intradermal tests in humans, gave no evidence of induced antibody formation. Relatively mild allergic type reactions, e.g., bronchospasm and skin rash, have been reported. When such reactions occur, they usually respond to conventional therapy. In addition, rare cases of anaphylaxis have been reported.

Miscellaneous

Fever and chills, including shaking chills (rigors), nausea and/or vomiting, transient hypotension or hypertension, dyspnea, tachycardia, cyanosis, back pain, hypoxemia, and acidosis have been reported together and separately. Rare cases of myocardial infarction have also been reported. A cause and effect relationship has not been established. Aspirin is not recommended for treatment of fever.

DOSAGE AND ADMINISTRATION

ABBOKINASE IS INTENDED FOR INTRAVENOUS AND INTRACORONARY INFUSION ONLY.

A. Pulmonary Embolism:

Preparation

Reconstitute ABBOKINASE (urokinase for injection) by aseptically adding 5 mL of Sterile Water for Injection, USP, to the vial. (It is important that ABBOKINASE be reconstituted *only* with Sterile Water for Injection, USP, *without* preservatives. Bacteriostatic Water for Injection should *not* be used.) Each vial should be visually inspected for discoloration (slightly straw-colored solution) and for the presence of particulate material. Highly colored solutions should not be used. Because ABBOKINASE contains no preservatives, it should not be reconstituted until immediately before using. Any unused portion of the reconstituted material should be discarded.

To minimize formation of filaments, avoid shaking the vial during reconstitution. Roll and tilt the vial to enhance reconstitution. The solution may be terminally filtered, e.g., through a 0.45 micron or smaller cellulose membrane filter. No other medication should be added to this solution.

Reconstituted ABBOKINASE is diluted with 0.9% Sodium Chloride Injection, USP or 5% Dextrose Injection, USP, prior to intravenous infusion. (See Table I, **Dose Preparation-Pulmonary Embolism.**)

Administration

Administer ABBOKINASE (urokinase for injection) by means of a constant infusion pump that is capable of delivering a total volume of 195 mL. The following table may be used as an aid in the preparation of ABBOKINASE (urokinase for injection) for administration.

[See table above]

A priming dose of 2,000 IU/lb (4,400 IU/kg) of ABBOKINASE is given as the ABBOKINASE-0.9% Sodium Chloride Injection or 5% Dextrose Injection admixture at a rate of 90 mL/hour over a period of 10 minutes. This is followed by a continuous infusion of 2,000 IU/lb/hr (4,400 IU/kg/hr) of ABBOKINASE at a rate of 15 mL/hour for 12 hours. Since some ABBOKINASE admixture will remain in the tubing at the end of an infusion pump delivery cycle, the following flush procedure should be performed to insure that the total dose of ABBOKINASE is administered. A solution of 0.9% Sodium Chloride Injection or 5% Dextrose Injection approximately equal in amount to the volume of the tubing in the infusion set should be administered via the pump to flush the ABBOKINASE admixture from the entire length of the infusion set. The pump should be set to administer the flush solution at the continuous infusion rate of 15 mL/hour.

Anticoagulation After Terminating Urokinase Treatment

At the end of urokinase therapy, treatment with heparin by continuous intravenous infusion is recommended to prevent recurrent thrombosis. Heparin treatment, without a loading dose, should not begin until the thrombin time has decreased to *less than twice* the normal control value (approximately 3 to 4 hours after completion of the infusion). See manufacturer's prescribing information for proper use of heparin. This should then be followed by oral anticoagulants in the conventional manner.

B. Lysis of Coronary Artery Thrombi:[9]

Preparation

Reconstitute three (3) 250,000 IU vials of ABBOKINASE by aseptically adding 5 mL of Sterile Water for Injection, USP,

Continued on next page

Abbokinase—Cont.

to each vial. (It is important that ABBOKINASE be reconstituted *only* with Sterile Water for Injection, USP, *without* preservatives. Bacteriostatic Water for Injection should *not* be used.) Each vial should be visually inspected for discoloration (slightly straw-colored solution) and for the presence of particulate material. Highly colored solutions should not be used. Because ABBOKINASE contains no preservatives, it should not be reconstituted until immediately before using. Any unused portion of the reconstituted material should be discarded.

To minimize formation of filaments, avoid shaking the vial during reconstitution. Roll and tilt the vial to enhance reconstitution. The solution may be terminally filtered, e.g., through a 0.45 micron or smaller cellulose membrane filter. Add the contents of the three (3) reconstituted ABBOKINASE vials to 500 mL of 5% Dextrose Injection, USP. The resulting solution admixture will have a concentration of approximately 1500 IU per mL. No other medication should be added to the solution.

The admixture should be administered immediately as described under Administration. Any solution remaining after administration should be discarded.

NOTE: Adsorption of drug from dilute protein solutions to various materials has been reported in the literature. Therefore, the directions for Preparation and Administration must be followed to assure that significant drug loss does not occur.

Administration

Prior to the infusion of ABBOKINASE, a bolus dose of heparin ranging from 2500 to 10,000 units should be administered intravenously. Prior heparin administration should be considered when calculating the heparin dose for this procedure. Following the bolus dose of heparin, the prepared ABBOKINASE solution should be infused into the occluded artery at a rate of 4 mL per minute (6000 IU per minute) for periods up to 2 hours. In a clinical study, the average total dose of ABBOKINASE utilized for lysis of coronary artery thrombi was 500,000 IU.[9]

To determine response to ABBOKINASE therapy, periodic angiography during the infusion is recommended. It is suggested that the angiography be repeated at approximately 15 minute intervals. ABBOKINASE therapy should be continued until the artery is maximally opened, usually 15 to 30 minutes after the initial opening. Following the infusion, coagulation parameters should be determined. It is advisable to continue heparin therapy after the artery is opened by ABBOKINASE.

When ABBOKINASE was administered selectively into thrombosed coronary arteries via coronary catheter within 6 hours following onset of symptoms of acute transmural myocardial infarction, 60% of the occlusions were opened.[9]

HOW SUPPLIED

ABBOKINASE (urokinase for injection) is supplied as a sterile lyophilized preparation (NDC 0074-6109-05). Each vial contains 250,000 IU urokinase activity, 25 mg mannitol, 250 mg Albumin (Human), and 50 mg sodium chloride. Store ABBOKINASE powder at 2° to 8°C.

REFERENCES

1. Sherry S, et al. Thrombolytic therapy in thrombosis: A National Institutes of Health consensus development conference. *Ann Intern Med.* 1980;93:141–144.
2. Bang NU. Physiology and biochemistry of fibrinolysis. In: Bang NU, Beller FK, Deutsch E, Mammen EF, eds. *Thrombosis and Bleeding Disorders.* New York, NY: Academic Press; 1971:292–327.
3. McNicol GP. The fibrinolytic enzyme system. *Postgrad Med J.* August 1973;49 (suppl 5):10–12.
4. Sasahara AA, Hyers TM, Cole CM, et al. The urokinase pulmonary embolism trial. *Circulation.* 1973;47 (suppl 2):1–108.
5. Urokinase pulmonary embolism trial study group: Urokinase-streptokinase embolism trial. *JAMA.* 1974;229:1606–1613.
6. Sasahara AA, Bell WR, Simon TL, et al. The Phase II urokinase-streptokinase pulmonary embolism trial, *Thrombos Diathes Haemorrh* (Stuttg). 1975;33:464–476.
7. Bell WR. Thrombolytic therapy: A comparison between urokinase and streptokinase, *Sem Thromb Hemost.* 1975;2:1–13.
8. Fratantoni JC, Ness P, Simon TL. Thrombolytic therapy: Current status. *N Eng J Med.* 1975;293:1073–1078.
9. Tennant SN, Campbell WB, et al. Intracoronary thrombolysis in acute myocardial infarction: Comparison of the efficacy of urokinase to streptokinase. *Circulation.* 1984;69:756–760.

Revised March, 1998

Ref. 58-0360-R12

Abbott Laboratories
North Chicago, IL 60064, U.S.A.

ABBOKINASE® OPEN-CATH® ℞
(Urokinase for Catheter Clearance)

DESCRIPTION

Urokinase is an enzyme (protein) produced by the kidney, and found in the urine. There are two forms of urokinase differing in molecular weight but having similar clinical effects. Urokinase is a thrombolytic agent obtained from human kidney cells by tissue culture techniques and is primarily the low molecular weight form. It is supplied as a sterile lyophilized white powder. Following reconstitution ABBOKINASE OPEN-CATH solution is clear and essentially colorless.

Each mL of reconstituted ABBOKINASE OPEN-CATH solution contains 5000 IU of urokinase activity, 5 mg gelatin, 15 mg mannitol, 1.7 mg sodium chloride and 4.6 mg monobasic sodium phosphate anhydrous. The pH is adjusted with sodium hydroxide and/or hydrochloric acid prior to lyophilization.

CLINICAL PHARMACOLOGY

Urokinase acts on the endogenous fibrinolytic system. It converts plasminogen to the enzyme plasmin. Plasmin degrades fibrin clots as well as fibrinogen and other plasma proteins.

When used as directed for I.V. catheter clearance, only small amounts of urokinase may reach the circulation; therefore, therapeutic serum levels are not expected to be achieved. Nevertheless, one should be aware of the clinical pharmacology of urokinase.

Intravenous infusion of urokinase in doses recommended for lysis of pulmonary embolism is followed by increased fibrinolytic activity. This effect disappears within a few hours after discontinuation, but a decrease in plasma levels of fibrinogen and plasminogen and an increase in the amount of circulating fibrin (ogen) degradation products may persist for 12–24 hours.[1,2] There is a lack of correlation between embolus resolution and changes in coagulation and fibrinolytic assay results.

Information is incomplete about the pharmacokinetic properties in man. Urokinase administered by intravenous infusion is cleared rapidly by the liver. The serum half-life in man is 20 minutes or less. Patients with impaired liver function (e.g., cirrhosis) would be expected to show a prolongation in half-life. Small fractions of an administered dose are excreted in bile and urine.

INDICATIONS AND USAGE

ABBOKINASE OPEN-CATH (urokinase for catheter clearance) is indicated for the restoration of patency to intravenous catheters, including central venous catheters, obstructed by clotted blood or fibrin.[3,4,5]

CONTRAINDICATIONS

Because thrombolytic therapy increases the risk of bleeding, urokinase is contraindicated in the following situations:

— Active internal bleeding
— History of cerebrovascular accident
— Recent (within two months) intracranial or intraspinal surgery
— Recent trauma including cardiopulmonary resuscitation
— Intracranial neoplasm, arteriovenous malformation, or aneurysm
— Known bleeding diathesis
— Severe uncontrolled arterial hypertension

There have been no reports, however, which would suggest a contraindication for the use of urokinase for I.V. catheter clearance.

WARNINGS

Excessive pressure should be avoided when ABBOKINASE solution is injected into the catheter. Such force could cause rupture of the catheter or expulsion of the clot into the circulation. During attempts to determine catheter occlusion, vigorous suction should not be applied due to possible damage to the vascular wall or collapse of soft-wall catheters.

Catheters may be occluded by substances other than fibrin clots such as drug precipitates. ABBOKINASE solution is not effective in such cases and there is the possibility that the substances may be forced into the vascular system.

PRECAUTIONS

Carcinogenicity
Adequate data is not available on the long-term potential for carcinogenicity in animals or humans.

Pregnancy
Pregnancy Category B. Reproduction studies have been performed in mice and rats at doses up to 1,000 times the human therapeutic dose and have revealed no evidence of impaired fertility or harm to the fetus due to urokinase. There are, however, no adequate and well-controlled studies in pregnant women. Because animal reproduction studies are not always predictive of human response, this drug should be used during pregnancy only if clearly needed.

Nursing Mothers
It is not known whether this drug is excreted in human milk. Because many drugs are excreted in human milk, caution should be exercised when urokinase is administered to a nursing woman.

Pediatric Use
Safety and effectiveness in children have not been established.

ADVERSE REACTIONS

The following reactions have been associated with ABBOKINASE (urokinase for injection) in doses recommended for lysis of pulmonary embolism.

Bleeding
The type of bleeding associated with thrombolytic therapy can be placed into two broad categories:
— Superficial or surface bleeding, observed mainly at invaded or disturbed sites (e.g., venous cutdowns, arterial punctures, sites of recent surgical intervention, etc.).
— Internal bleeding, involving, e.g., the gastrointestinal tract, genitourinary tract, vagina, or intramuscular, retroperitoneal, or intracranial sites.

Several fatalities due to intracranial or retroperitoneal hemorrhage have occurred during thrombolytic therapy. Should serious bleeding occur, urokinase infusion should be discontinued and, if necessary, blood loss and reversal of the bleeding tendency can be effectively managed with whole blood (fresh blood preferable), packed red blood cells and cryoprecipitate or plasma. Dextran and hetastarch should not be used. Although the use of aminocaproic acid (ACA, AMICAR®) in humans as an antidote for urokinase has not been documented, it may be considered in an emergency situation.

Allergic Reactions
In vitro tests with urokinase, as well as intradermal tests in humans, gave no evidence of induced antibody formation. Relatively mild allergic type reactions, e.g., bronchospasm and skin rash, have been reported. When such reactions occur, they usually respond to conventional therapy. In addition, rare cases of anaphylaxis have been reported.

Miscellaneous
Fever and chills, including shaking chills (rigors), nausea and/or vomiting, transient hypotension or hypertension, dyspnea, tachycardia, cyanosis, back pain, hypoxemia, and acidosis have been reported together and separately. Rare cases of myocardial infarction have also been reported. A cause and effect relationship has not been established. Aspirin is not recommended for treatment of fever.

DOSAGE AND ADMINISTRATION

BECAUSE ABBOKINASE OPEN-CATH POWDER CONTAINS NO PRESERVATIVE, RECONSTITUTED SOLUTION SHOULD BE USED IMMEDIATELY AFTER RECONSTITUTION. DISCARD ANY UNUSED PORTION.

Preparation of Solution:
Univial:
1. Remove protective cap. Turn plunger-stopper a quarter turn and press to force diluent into lower chamber.
2. Roll and tilt to effect solution. Use only a clear, essentially colorless solution.
3. Sterilize top of stopper with a suitable germicide.
4. Insert needle through the center of stopper until tip is barely visible. Withdraw dose.

It is recommended that vigorous shaking be avoided during reconstitution; roll and tilt to enhance reconstitution.

Parenteral drug products should be inspected visually for particulate matter and discoloration prior to administration, whenever solution and container permit.

Administration:
When the following procedure is used to clear a central venous catheter, the patient should be instructed to exhale and hold his breath any time the catheter is not connected to I.V. tubing or a syringe. This is to prevent air from entering the open catheter.

Aseptically disconnect the I.V. tubing connection at the catheter hub and attach an empty 10 mL syringe. Determine occlusion of the catheter by gently attempting to aspirate blood from the catheter with the 10 mL syringe. If aspiration is not possible, remove the 10 mL syringe and attach a syringe filled with an amount of prepared ABBOKINASE OPEN-CATH solution equal to the internal volume of the catheter. Slowly and gently inject the ABBOKINASE solution into the catheter. Aseptically remove the syringe and connect a 5 mL syringe to the catheter. Wait at least 5 minutes before attempting to aspirate the drug and residual clot with the empty syringe. Repeat aspiration attempts every 5 minutes. If the catheter is not open within 30 minutes, the catheter may be capped allowing ABBOKINASE solution to remain in the catheter for an additional 30 to 60 minutes before again attempting to aspirate. A second injection of ABBOKINASE (urokinase for catheter clearance) may be necessary in resistant cases.

When patency is restored, aspirate 4 to 5 mL of blood to assure removal of all drug and residual clot. Remove the blood-filled syringe and replace it with a 10 mL syringe filled with 0.9% Sodium Chloride Injection, USP. The catheter should then be gently irrigated with this solution to as-

sure patency of the catheter. After the catheter has been irrigated, remove the 10 mL syringe and aseptically reconnect sterile I.V. tubing to the catheter hub.

HOW SUPPLIED

ABBOKINASE OPEN-CATH (urokinase for catheter clearance) is supplied as a sterile lyophilized preparation in single dose Univial® packages of 1 mL (**NDC** 0074-6111-01) and 1.8 mL (**NDC** 0074-6145-02). Store powder below 77°F (25°C). Avoid freezing.

REFERENCES

1. Bang NU. Physiology and biochemistry of fibrinolysis. In: Bang NU, Beller FK, Deutsch E, Mammen EF, eds. *Thrombosis and Bleeding Disorders*. New York, NY: Academic Press; 1971: 292-327.
2. McNicol GP. The fibrinolytic enzyme system. *Postgrad Med J*. August 1973; 49 (suppl 5):10-12.
3. Hurtubise MR, Bottino JC, Lawson M, et al. Restoring patency of occluded central venous catheters. *Arch Surg*. 1980; 115:212-213.
4. Glynn MFX, et al. Therapy for thrombotic occlusion of long-term intravenous alimentation catheters. *Journal of Parenteral and Enteral Nutrition*. 1980; 4:387-390.
5. Lawson M, Bottino JC, Hurtubise MR, et al. The use of urokinase to restore the patency of occluded central venous catheters. *Am J IV Ther and Clin Nutr*. 1982; 9:29-30,32.

Revised: Aug., 1994
Univial-Sterile two-compartment vial, Abbott.
Ref. 06-9128-R8-Rev. August, 1994
Abbott Laboratories
North Chicago, IL 60064

BIAXIN® Filmtab®   ℞
(clarithromycin tablets)

BIAXIN® Granules   ℞
(clarithromycin for oral suspension)

DESCRIPTION

Clarithromycin is a semi-synthetic macrolide antibiotic. Chemically, it is 6-0-methylerythromycin. The molecular formula is $C_{38}H_{69}NO_{13}$, and the molecular weight is 747.96. The structural formula is:

Clarithromycin is a white to off-white crystalline powder. It is soluble in acetone, slightly soluble in methanol, ethanol, and acetonitrile, and practically insoluble in water.

BIAXIN is available as tablets and granules for oral suspension.

Each yellow oval film-coated BIAXIN tablet contains 250 mg or 500 mg of clarithromycin and the following inactive ingredients: cellulosic polymers, croscarmellose sodium, D&C Yellow No. 10, FD&C Blue No. 1, magnesium stearate, povidone, propylene glycol, silicon dioxide, sorbic acid, sorbitan monooleate, stearic acid, talc, titanium dioxide, and vanillin. The 250-mg tablet also contains pregelatinized starch.

After constitution, each 5 mL of BIAXIN suspension contains 125 mg or 250 mg of clarithromycin. Each bottle of BIAXIN granules contains 1250 mg (50 mL size), 2500 mg (50 and 100 mL sizes) or 5000 mg (100 mL size) of clarithromycin and the following inactive ingredients: carbomer, castor oil, citric acid, hydroxypropyl methylcellulose phthalate, maltodextrin, potassium sorbate, povidone, silicon dioxide, sucrose, xanthan gum, titanium dioxide and fruit punch flavor.

CLINICAL PHARMACOLOGY

Pharmacokinetics:

Clarithromycin is rapidly absorbed from the gastrointestinal tract after oral administration. The absolute bioavailability of 250-mg clarithromycin tablets was approximately 50%. Food slightly delays both the onset of clarithromycin absorption and the formation of the antimicrobially active metabolite, 14-OH clarithromycin, but does not affect the extent of bioavailability. Therefore, BIAXIN tablets may be given without regard to food.

In fasting healthy human subjects, peak serum concentrations were attained within 2 hours after oral dosing. Steady-state peak serum clarithromycin concentrations were attained in 2 to 3 days and were approximately 1 µg/mL with

---

Clarithromycin Tissue Concentrations
2 hours after Dose (µg/mL)/(µg/g)

Treatment	N	antrum	fundus	N	mucus
Clarithromycin	5	10.48±2.01	20.81±7.64	4	4.15±7.74
Clarithromycin + Omeprazole	5	19.96±4.71	24.25±6.37	4	39.29±32.79

---

a 250-mg dose administered every 12 hours, 2 to 3 µg/mL with a 500-mg dose administered every 12 hours, and 3 to 4 µg/mL with a 500 mg dose administered every 8 hours. The elimination half-life of clarithromycin was about 3 to 4 hours with 250 mg administered every 12 hours but increased to 5 to 7 hours with 500 mg administered every 8 to 12 hours. The nonlinearity of clarithromycin pharmacokinetics is slight at the recommended doses of 250 mg and 500 mg administered every 8 to 12 hours. With a 250 mg every 12 hours dosing, the principal metabolite, 14-OH clarithromycin, attains a peak steady-state concentration of about 0.6 µg/mL and has an elimination half-life of 5 to 6 hours. With a 500 mg every 8 to 12 hours dosing, the peak steady-state concentration of 14-OH clarithromycin is slightly higher (up to 1 µg/mL), and its elimination half-life is about 7 to 9 hours. With any of these dosing regimens, the steady-state concentration of this metabolite is generally attained within 2 to 3 days.

After a 250-mg tablet every 12 hours, approximately 20% of the dose is excreted in the urine as clarithromycin, while after a 500-mg tablet every 12 hours, the urinary excretion of clarithromycin is somewhat greater, approximately 30%. In comparison, after an oral dose of 250 mg (125 mg/5 mL) suspension every 12 hours, approximately 40% is excreted in urine as clarithromycin. The renal clearance of clarithromycin is, however, relatively independent of the dose size and approximates the normal glomerular filtration rate. The major metabolite found in urine is 14-OH clarithromycin, which accounts for an additional 10% to 15% of the dose with either a 250-mg or a 500-mg tablet administered every 12 hours.

Steady-state concentrations of clarithromycin and 14-OH clarithromycin observed following administration of 500-mg doses of clarithromycin every 12 hours to adult patients with HIV infection were similar to those observed in healthy volunteers. In adult HIV-infected patients taking 500- or 1000-mg doses of clarithromycin every 12 hours, steady-state clarithromycin C_{max} values ranged from 2 to 4 µg/mL and 5 to 10 µg/mL, respectively.

The steady-state concentrations of clarithromycin in subjects with impaired hepatic function did not differ from those in normal subjects; however, the 14-OH clarithromycin concentrations were lower in the hepatically impaired subjects. The decreased formation of 14-OH clarithromycin was at least partially offset by an increase in renal clearance of clarithromycin in the subjects with impaired hepatic function when compared to healthy subjects.

The pharmacokinetics of clarithromycin was also altered in subjects with impaired renal function. (See **PRECAUTIONS** and **DOSAGE AND ADMINISTRATION**.)

Clarithromycin and the 14-OH clarithromycin metabolite distribute readily into body tissues and fluids. There are no data available on cerebrospinal fluid penetration. Because of high intracellular concentrations, tissue concentrations are higher than serum concentrations. Examples of tissue and serum concentrations are presented below.

CONCENTRATION
(after 250 mg q12h)

Tissue Type	Tissue (µg/g)	Serum (µg/mL)
Tonsil	1.6	0.8
Lung	8.8	1.7

When 250-mg doses of clarithromycin as BIAXIN suspension were administered to fasting healthy adult subjects, peak plasma concentrations were attained around 3 hours after dosing. Steady-state peak plasma concentrations were attained in 2 to 3 days and were approximately 2 µg/mL for clarithromycin and 0.7 µg/mL for 14-OH clarithromycin when 250-mg doses of the clarithromycin suspension were administered every 12 hours. Elimination half-life of clarithromycin (3 to 4 hours) and that of 14-OH clarithromycin (5 to 7 hours) were similar to those observed at steady state following administration of equivalent doses of BIAXIN tablets.

For adult patients, the bioavailability of 10 mL of the 125 mg/5 mL suspension or 10 mL of the 250-mg/5 mL suspension is similar to a 250-mg or 500-mg tablet, respectively.

In children requiring antibiotic therapy, administration of 7.5 mg/kg q12h doses of clarithromycin as the suspension generally resulted in steady-state peak plasma concentrations of 3 to 7 µg/mL for clarithromycin and 1 to 2 µg/mL for 14-OH clarithromycin.

In HIV-infected children taking 15 mg/kg every 12 hours, steady-state clarithromycin peak concentrations generally ranged from 6 to 15 µg/mL.

Clarithromycin penetrates into the middle ear fluid of children with secretory otitis media.

CONCENTRATION
(after 7.5 mg/kg q12h for 5 doses)

Analyte	Middle Ear Fluid (µg/mL)	Serum (µg/mL)
Clarithromycin	2.5	1.7
14-OH Clarithromycin	1.3	0.8

In adults given 250 mg clarithromycin as suspension (n=22), food appeared to decrease mean peak plasma clarithromycin concentrations from 1.2 (±0.4) µg/mL to 1.0 (± 0.4) µg/mL and the extent of absorption from 7.2 (± 2.5) hr•µg/mL to 6.5 (± 3.7) hr•µg/mL.

When children (n=10) were administered a single oral dose of 7.5 mg/kg suspension, food increased mean peak plasma clarithromycin concentration from 3.6 (± 1.5) µg/mL to 4.6 (± 2.8) µg/mL and the extent of absorption from 10.0 (± 5.5) hr•µg/mL to 14.2 (± 9.4) hr•µg/mL.

Clarithromycin 500 mg every 8 hours was given in combination with omeprazole 40 mg daily to healthy adult males. The plasma levels of clarithromycin and 14-hydroxy-clarithromycin were increased by the concomitant administration of omeprazole. For clarithromycin, the mean C_{max} was 10% greater, the mean C_{min} was 27% greater, and the mean AUC_{0-8} was 15% greater when clarithromycin was administered with omeprazole than when clarithromycin was administered alone. Similar results were seen for 14-hydroxy-clarithromycin, the mean C_{max} was 45% greater, the mean C_{min} was 57% greater, and the mean AUC_{0-8} was 45% greater. Clarithromycin concentrations in the gastric tissue and mucus were also increased by concomitant administration of omeprazole.

[See table at top of page]

For information on omeprazole, refer to the CLINICAL PHARMACOLOGY section of the PRILOSEC package insert.

For information on ranitidine bismuth citrate, refer to the CLINICAL PHARMACOLOGY section of the TRITEC package insert.

For information on lansoprazole or amoxicillin, refer to the CLINICAL PHARMACOLOGY section of their package inserts.

Microbiology:

Clarithromycin exerts its antibacterial action by binding to the 50S ribosomal subunit of susceptible microorganisms resulting in inhibition of protein synthesis.

Clarithromycin is active *in vitro* against a variety of aerobic and anaerobic gram-positive and gram-negative microorganisms as well as most *Mycobacterium avium* complex (MAC) microorganisms.

Additionally, the 14-OH clarithromycin metabolite also has clinically significant antimicrobial activity. The 14-OH clarithromycin is twice as active against *Haemophilus influenzae* microorganisms as the parent compound. However, for *Mycobacterium avium* complex (MAC) isolates the 14-OH metabolite is 4 to 7 times less active than clarithromycin. The clinical significance of this activity against *Mycobacterium avium* complex is unknown.

Clarithromycin has been shown to be active against most strains of the following microorganisms both *in vitro* and in clinical infections as described in the **INDICATIONS AND USAGE** section:

Aerobic Gram-positive microorganisms
Staphylococcus aureus
Streptococcus pneumoniae
Streptococcus pyogenes

Aerobic Gram-negative microorganisms
Haemophilus influenzae
Moraxella catarrhalis

Other microorganisms
Mycoplasma pneumoniae
Chlamydia pneumoniae (TWAR)

Mycobacteria
Mycobacterium avium complex (MAC) consisting of:
Mycobacterium avium
Mycobacterium intracellulare

Beta-lactamase production should have no effect on clarithromycin activity.

Continued on next page

Biaxin—Cont.

NOTE: Most strains of methicillin-resistant and oxacillin-resistant staphylococci are resistant to clarithromycin. Clarithromycin has been shown to be active against most strains of *Helicobacter pylori in vitro* and in clinical infections when combined with omeprazole, lansoprazole and amoxicillin, or ranitidine bismuth citrate as described in the **INDICATIONS AND USAGE** section.

Helicobacter

Helicobacter pylori

Some *Helicobacter pylori* isolates obtained from patients treated with clarithromycin plus omeprazole demonstrated an increase in clarithromycin MIC's over time, indicating decreasing susceptibility and increasing resistance. In the two U.S. clarithromycin plus omeprazole clinical trials, 104 patients had *H. pylori* isolated and clarithromycin MIC's determined pre-treatment. Of these, 4 patients had resistant strains, 2 patients had strains with intermediate susceptibility, and 98 patients had susceptible strains. Of the patients with susceptible *H. pylori* pre-treatment, 72 patients were eradicated of the *H. pylori* and 26 patients had *H. pylori* present post-treatment. Isolates from 25 of these 26 patients became resistant to clarithromycin. The six patients with resistant or intermediate *H. pylori* strains pre-treatment had resistant strains isolated post-treatment.

Emerging clarithromycin resistance was not assessed for the ranitidine bismuth citrate plus clarithromycin regimen because there were no patients that had *H. pylori* isolates with both pre-treatment and post-treatment susceptibility tests. No adequate data were collected during clinical trials or *in vitro* studies to indicate that ranitidine bismuth citrate can either decrease or increase emerging clarithromycin resistance.

The following *in vitro* data are available, **but their clinical significance is unknown.** Clarithromycin exhibits *in vitro* activity against most strains of the following microorganisms; however, the safety and effectiveness of clarithromycin in treating clinical infections due to these microorganisms have not been established in adequate and well-controlled clinical trials.

Aerobic Gram-positive microorganisms

Streptococcus agalactiae
Streptococci (Groups C, F, G)
Viridans group streptococci

Aerobic Gram-negative microorganisms

Bordetella pertussis
Legionella pneumophila
Pasteurella multocida

Anaerobic Gram-positive microorganisms

Clostridium perfringens
Peptococcus niger
Propionibacterium acnes

Anaerobic Gram-negative microorganisms

Prevotella melaninogenica (formerly *Bacteriodes melaninogenicus*)

Susceptibility Testing Excluding Mycobacteria and Helicobacter:

Dilution Techniques:

Quantitative methods are used to determine antimicrobial minimal inhibitory concentrations (MIC's). These MIC's provide estimates of the susceptibility of bacteria to antimicrobial compounds. The MIC's should be determined using a standardized procedure. Standardized procedures are based on a dilution method[1] (broth or agar) or equivalent with standardized inoculum concentrations and standardized concentrations of clarithromycin powder. The MIC values should be interpreted according to the following criteria:

MIC (µg/mL)	Interpretation
≤2.0	Susceptible (S)
4.0	Intermediate (I)
≥8.0	Resistant (R)

A report of "Susceptible" indicates that the pathogen is likely to be inhibited if the antimicrobial compound in the blood reaches the concentrations usually achievable.

A report of "Intermediate" indicates that the result should be considered equivocal, and, if the microorganism is not fully susceptible to alternative, clinically feasible drugs, the test should be repeated. This category implies possible clinical applicability in body sites where the drug is physiologically concentrated or in situations where high dosage of drug can be used. This category also provides a buffer zone which prevents small uncontrolled technical factors from causing major discrepancies in interpretation.

A report of "Resistant" indicates that the pathogen is not likely to be inhibited if the antimicrobial compound in the blood reaches the concentrations usually achievable; other therapy should be selected.

Standardized susceptibility test procedures require the use of laboratory control microorganisms to control the technical aspects of the laboratory procedures. Standard clarithromycin powder should provide the following MIC values:

Microorganism		MIC (µg/mL)
S. aureus	ATCC 29213	0.12 to 0.5

Diffusion Techniques:

Quantitative methods that require measurement of zone diameters also provide reproducible estimates of the susceptibility of bacteria to antimicrobial compounds. One such standardized procedure[2] requires the use of standardized inoculum concentrations. This procedure uses paper disks impregnated with 15-µg clarithromycin to test the susceptibility of microorganisms to clarithromycin.

Reports from the laboratory providing results of the standard single-disk susceptibility test with a 15-µg clarithromycin disk should be interpreted according to the following criteria:

Zone diameter (mm)	Interpretation
≥ 18	Susceptible (S)
14 to 17	Intermediate (I)
≤ 13	Resistant (R)

Interpretation should be as stated above for results using dilution techniques. Interpretation involves correlation of the diameter obtained in the disk test with the MIC for clarithromycin. However, standardized diffusion methods for routine *in vitro* susceptibility testing, using the 15-µg clarithromycin disk, do not measure the additive antimicrobial activity of the 14-OH metabolite and, thus, may underestimate the drug's potential activity against *Haemophilus influenzae*. *Haemophilus influenzae* isolates falling into the "Intermediate" category often respond to treatment.

As with standardized dilution techniques, diffusion methods require the use of laboratory control microorganisms that are used to control the technical aspects of the laboratory procedures. For the diffusion technique, the 15-µg clarithromycin disk should provide the following zone diameters in this laboratory test quality control strain:

Microorganism		Zone diameter (mm)
S. aureus	ATCC 25923	26 to 32

In vitro Activity of Clarithromycin against Mycobacteria:

Clarithromycin has demonstrated *in vitro* activity against *Mycobacterium avium* complex (MAC) microorganisms isolated from both AIDS and non-AIDS patients. While gene probe techniques may be used to distinguish *M. avium* species from *M. intracellulare*, many studies only reported results on *M. avium* complex (MAC) isolates.

Various *in vitro* methodologies employing broth or solid media at different pH's, with and without oleic acid-albumin-dextrose-catalase (OADC), have been used to determine clarithromycin MIC values for mycobacterial species. In general, MIC values decrease more than 16-fold as the pH of Middlebrook 7H12 broth media increases from 5.0 to 7.4. At pH 7.4, MIC values determined with Mueller-Hinton agar were 4- to 8-fold higher than those observed with Middlebrook 7H12 media. Utilization of oleic acid-albumin-dextrose-catalase (OADC) in these assays has been shown to further alter MIC values.

Clarithromycin activity against 80 MAC isolates from AIDS patients and 211 MAC isolates from non-AIDS patients was evaluated using a microdilution method with Middlebrook 7H9 broth. Results showed an MIC value of ≤ 4.0 µg/mL in 81% and 89% of the AIDS and non-AIDS MAC isolates, respectively. Twelve percent of the non-AIDS isolates had an MIC value ≤ 0.5 µg/mL. Clarithromycin was also shown to be active against phagocytized *M. avium* complex (MAC) in mouse and human macrophage cell cultures as well as in the beige mouse infection model.

Clarithromycin activity was evaluated against *Mycobacterium tuberculosis* microorganisms. In one study utilizing the agar dilution method with Middlebrook 7H10 media, 3 of 30 clinical isolates had an MIC of 2.5 µg/mL. Clarithromycin inhibited all isolates at > 10.0 µg/mL.

Susceptibility Testing for *Mycobacterium avium* Complex (MAC):

The disk diffusion and dilution techniques for susceptibility testing against gram-positive and gram-negative bacteria should not be used for determining clarithromycin MIC values against mycobacteria. *In vitro* susceptibility testing methods and diagnostic products currently available for determining minimum inhibitory concentration (MIC) values against *Mycobacterium avium* complex (MAC) organisms have not been standardized or validated. Clarithromycin MIC values will vary depending on the susceptibility testing method employed, composition and pH of the media, and the utilization of nutritional supplements. Breakpoints to determine whether clinical isolates of *M. avium* or *M. intracellulare* are susceptible or resistant to clarithromycin have not been established.

In vitro Activity of Clarithromycin against Helicobacter pylori:

Clarithromycin has demonstrated *in vitro* activity against *Helicobacter pylori* isolated from patients with duodenal ulcers. *In vitro* susceptibility testing methods (broth microdilution, agar dilution, E-test, and disk diffusion) and diagnostic products currently available for determining minimum inhibitory concentrations (MIC's) and zone sizes have not been standardized, validated, or approved for testing *H. pylori*. The clarithromycin MIC values and zone sizes will vary depending on the susceptibility testing methodology employed, media, growth additives, pH, inoculum concentration tested, growth phase, incubation atmosphere, and time.

Susceptibility Test for *Helicobacter pylori*:

In vitro susceptibility testing methods and diagnostic products currently available for determining minimum inhibitory concentrations (MIC's) and zone sizes have not been standardized, validated, or approved for testing *H. pylori* microorganisms. MIC values for *H. pylori* isolates collected during the two U.S. clinical trials evaluating clarithromycin plus omeprazole, were determined by broth microdilution MIC methodology[3]. Results obtained during the clarithromycin plus omeprazole clinical trials fell into a distinct bimodal distribution of susceptible and resistant clarithromycin MIC's.

If the broth microdilution MIC methodology published in Hachem, et. al.[3] is used and the following tentative breakpoints are employed, there should be reasonable correlation between MIC results and clinical and microbiological outcomes for patients treated with clarithromycin plus omeprazole.

MIC (µg/mL)	Interpretation
≤0.06	Susceptible (S)
0.12 to 2.0	Intermediate (I)
≥4	Resistant (R)

These breakpoints should not be used to interpret results obtained using alternative methods.

INDICATIONS AND USAGE

BIAXIN Filmtab tablets and BIAXIN Granules for oral suspension are indicated for the treatment of mild to moderate infections caused by susceptible strains of the designated microorganisms in the conditions listed below:

Adults:

Pharyngitis/Tonsillitis due to *Streptococcus pyogenes* (The usual drug of choice in the treatment and prevention of streptococcal infections and the prophylaxis of rheumatic fever is penicillin administered by either the intramuscular or the oral route. Clarithromycin is generally effective in the eradication of *S. pyogenes* from the nasopharynx; however, data establishing the efficacy of clarithromycin in the subsequent prevention of rheumatic fever are not available at present.)

Acute maxillary sinusitis due to *Haemophilus influenzae*, *Moraxella catarrhalis*, or *Streptococcus pneumoniae*

Acute bacterial exacerbation of chronic bronchitis due to *Haemophilus influenzae*, *Moraxella catarrhalis*, or *Streptococcus pneumoniae*

Pneumonia due to *Mycoplasma pneumoniae*, *Streptococcus pneumoniae*, or *Chlamydia pneumoniae* (TWAR)

Uncomplicated skin and skin structure infections due to *Staphylococcus aureus*, or *Streptococcus pyogenes* (Abscesses usually require surgical drainage.)

Disseminated mycobacterial infections due to *Mycobacterium avium*, or *Mycobacterium intracellulare*

BIAXIN (clarithromycin) Filmtab tablets in combination with PREVACID (lansoprazole) Delayed-Release Capsules and amoxicillin, as triple therapy, are indicated for the treatment of patients with *H. pylori* infection and duodenal ulcer disease (active or one-year history of duodenal ulcer) to eradicate *H. pylori*.

BIAXIN Filmtab tablets in combination with PRILOSEC (omeprazole) capsules or TRITEC (ranitidine bismuth citrate) tablets are also indicated for the treatment of patients with an active duodenal ulcer associated with *H. pylori* infection. However, regimens which contain clarithromycin as the single antimicrobial agent are more likely to be associated with the development of clarithromycin resistance among patients who fail therapy. Clarithromycin-containing regimens should not be used in patients with known or suspected clarithromycin resistant isolates because the efficacy of treatment is reduced in this setting.

In patients who fail therapy, susceptibility testing should be done if possible. If resistance to clarithromycin is demonstrated, a non-clarithromycin-containing therapy is recommended. (For information on development of resistance see **Microbiology** section.) The eradication of *H. pylori* has been demonstrated to reduce the risk of duodenal ulcer recurrence.

Children:

Pharyngitis/Tonsillitis due to *Streptococcus pyogenes*

Pneumonia due to *Mycoplasma pneumoniae*, *Streptococcus pneumoniae*, or *Chlamydia pneumoniae* (TWAR)

Acute maxillary sinusitis due to *Haemophilus influenzae*, *Moraxella catarrhalis*, or *Streptococcus pneumoniae*

Acute otitis media due to *Haemophilus influenzae, Moraxella catarrhalis,* or *Streptococcus pneumoniae*
NOTE: For information on otitis media, see **CLINICAL STUDIES: Otitis Media.**
Uncomplicated skin and skin structure infections due to *Staphylococcus aureus,* or *Streptococcus pyogenes* (Abscesses usually require surgical drainage.)
Disseminated mycobacterial infections due to *Mycobacterium avium,* or *Mycobacterium intracellulare*
Prophylaxis:
BIAXIN Filmtab tablets and BIAXIN Granules for oral suspension are indicated for the prevention of disseminated *Mycobacterium avium* complex (MAC) disease in patients with advanced HIV infection.

CONTRAINDICATIONS

Clarithromycin is contraindicated in patients with a known hypersensitivity to clarithromycin, erythromycin, or any of the macrolide antibiotics.
Concomitant administration of clarithromycin with cisapride, pimozide, or terfenadine is contraindicated. There have been post-marketing reports of drug interactions when clarithromycin and/or erythromycin are co-administered with cisapride, pimozide, or terfenadine resulting in cardiac arrhythmias (QT prolongation, ventricular tachycardia, ventricular fibrillation, and torsades de pointes) most likely due to inhibition of hepatic metabolism of these drugs by erythromycin and clarithromycin. Fatalities have been reported.
For information on omeprazole, refer to the CONTRAINDICATIONS section of the PRILOSEC package insert.
For information on ranitidine bismuth citrate, refer to the CONTRAINDICATIONS section of the TRITEC package insert.
For information on lansoprazole or amoxicillin, refer to the CONTRAINDICATIONS section of their package inserts.

WARNINGS

CLARITHROMYCIN SHOULD NOT BE USED IN PREGNANT WOMEN EXCEPT IN CLINICAL CIRCUMSTANCES WHERE NO ALTERNATIVE THERAPY IS APPROPRIATE. IF PREGNANCY OCCURS WHILE TAKING THIS DRUG, THE PATIENT SHOULD BE APPRISED OF THE POTENTIAL HAZARD TO THE FETUS. CLARITHROMYCIN HAS DEMONSTRATED ADVERSE EFFECTS OF PREGNANCY OUTCOME AND/OR EMBRYO-FETAL DEVELOPMENT IN MONKEYS, RATS, MICE, AND RABBITS AT DOSES THAT PRODUCED PLASMA LEVELS 2 TO 17 TIMES THE SERUM LEVELS ACHIEVED IN HUMANS TREATED AT THE MAXIMUM RECOMMENDED HUMAN DOSES. (See PRECAUTIONS - *Pregnancy*.)
Pseudomembranous colitis has been reported with nearly all antibacterial agents, including clarithromycin, and may range in severity from mild to life threatening. Therefore, it is important to consider this diagnosis in patients who present with diarrhea subsequent to the administration of antibacterial agents.
Treatment with antibacterial agents alters the normal flora of the colon and may permit overgrowth of clostridia. Studies indicate that a toxin produced by *Clostridium difficile* is a primary cause of "antibiotic-associated colitis."
After the diagnosis of pseudomembranous colitis has been established, therapeutic measures should be initiated. Mild cases of pseudomembranous colitis usually respond to discontinuation of the drug alone. In moderate to severe cases, consideration should be given to management with fluids and electrolytes, protein supplementation, and treatment with an antibacterial drug clinically effective against *Clostridium difficile* colitis.
For information on omeprazole, refer to the WARNINGS section of the PRILOSEC package insert.
For information on ranitidine bismuth citrate, refer to the WARNINGS section of the TRITEC package insert.
For information on lansoprazole or amoxicillin, refer to the WARNINGS section of their package inserts.

PRECAUTIONS

General: Clarithromycin is principally excreted via the liver and kidney. Clarithromycin may be administered without dosage adjustment to patients with hepatic impairment and normal renal function. However, in the presence of severe renal impairment with or without coexisting hepatic impairment, decreased dosage or prolonged dosing intervals may be appropriate.
Clarithromycin in combination with ranitidine bismuth citrate therapy is not recommended in patients with creatinine clearance less than 25 mL/min. (See **DOSAGE AND ADMINISTRATION**.)
Clarithromycin in combination with ranitidine bismuth citrate should not be used in patients with a history of acute porphyria.
For information on omeprazole, refer to the PRECAUTIONS section of the PRILOSEC package insert.
For information on ranitidine bismuth citrate, refer to the PRECAUTIONS section of the TRITEC package insert.
For information on lansoprazole or amoxicillin, refer to the PRECAUTIONS section of their package inserts.

Information to Patients: BIAXIN tablets and oral suspension can be taken with or without food and can be taken with milk. Do **NOT** refrigerate the suspension.
Drug Interactions: Clarithromycin use in patients who are receiving theophylline may be associated with an increase of serum theophylline concentrations. Monitoring of serum theophylline concentrations should be considered for patients receiving high doses of theophylline or with baseline concentrations in the upper therapeutic range. In two studies in which theophylline was administered with clarithromycin (a theophylline sustained-release formulation was dosed at either 6.5 mg/kg or 12 mg/kg together with 250 or 500 mg q12h clarithromycin), the steady-state levels of C_{max}, C_{min}, and the area under the serum concentration time curve (AUC) of theophylline increased about 20%.
Concomitant administration of single doses of clarithromycin and carbamazepine has been shown to result in increased plasma concentrations of carbamazepine. Blood level monitoring of carbamazepine may be considered.
When clarithromycin and terfenadine were coadministered, plasma concentrations of the active acid metabolite of terfenadine were threefold higher, on average, than the values observed when terfenadine was administered alone. The pharmacokinetics of clarithromycin and the 14-hydroxy-clarithromycin were not significantly affected by coadministration of terfenadine once clarithromycin reached steady-state conditions. Concomitant administration of clarithromycin with terfenadine is contraindicated. (See **CONTRAINDICATIONS**.)
Clarithromycin 500 mg every 8 hours was given in combination with omeprazole 40 mg daily to healthy adult subjects. The steady-state plasma concentrations of omeprazole were increased (C_{max}, AUC_{0-24}, and $T_{1/2}$ increases of 30%, 89%, and 34%, respectively), by the concomitant administration of clarithromycin. The mean 24-hour gastric pH value was 5.2 when omeprazole was administered alone and 5.7 when co-administered with clarithromycin.
Co-administration of clarithromycin with ranitidine bismuth citrate resulted in increased plasma ranitidine concentrations (57%), increased plasma bismuth trough concentrations (48%), and increased 14-hydroxy-clarithromycin plasma concentrations (31%). These effects are clinically insignificant.
Simultaneous oral administration of BIAXIN tablets and zidovudine to HIV-infected adult patients resulted in decreased steady-state zidovudine concentrations. When 500 mg of clarithromycin were administered twice daily, steady-state zidovudine AUC was reduced by a mean of 12% (n=4). Individual values ranged from a decrease of 34% to an increase of 14%. Based on limited data in 24 patients, when BIAXIN tablets were administered two to four hours prior to oral zidovudine, the steady-state zidovudine C_{max} was increased by approximately 2-fold, whereas the AUC was unaffected.
Simultaneous administration of BIAXIN tablets and didanosine to 12 HIV-infected adult patients resulted in no statistically significant change in didanosine pharmacokinetics.
Concomitant administration of fluconazole 200 mg daily and clarithromycin 500 mg twice daily to 21 healthy volunteers led to increases in the mean steady-state clarithromycin C_{min} and AUC of 33% and 18%, respectively. Steady-state concentrations of 14-OH clarithromycin were not significantly affected by concomitant administration of fluconazole.
Concomitant administration of clarithromycin and ritonavir (n=22) resulted in a 77% increase in clarithromycin AUC and a 100% decrease in the AUC of 14-OH clarithromycin. Clarithromycin may be administered without dosage adjustment to patients with normal renal function taking ritonavir. However, for patients with renal impairment, the following dosage adjustments should be considered. For patients with CL_{CR} 30 to 60 mL/min, the dose of clarithromycin should be 50%. For patients with CL_{CR} < 30 mL/min, the dose of clarithromycin should be decreased by 75%
Spontaneous reports in the post-marketing period suggest that concomitant administration of clarithromycin and oral anticoagulants may potentiate the effects of the oral anticoagulants. Prothrombin times should be carefully monitored while patients are receiving clarithromycin and oral anticoagulants simultaneously.
Elevated digoxin serum concentrations in patients receiving clarithromycin and digoxin concomitantly have also been reported in post-marketing surveillance. Some patients have shown clinical signs consistent with digoxin toxicity, including arrhythmias. Serum digoxin levels should be carefully monitored while patients are receiving digoxin and clarithromycin simultaneously.
The following drug interactions, other than increased serum concentrations of carbamazepine and active acid metabolite of terfenadine, have not been reported in clinical trials with clarithromycin; however, they have been observed with erythromycin products and/or with clarithromycin in post-marketing experience.

Concurrent use of erythromycin or clarithromycin and ergotamine or dihydroergotamine has been associated in some patients with acute ergot toxicity characterized by severe peripheral vasospasm and dysesthesia.
Erythromycin has been reported to decrease the clearance of triazolam and, thus, may increase the pharmacologic effect of triazolam. There have been post-marketing reports of drug interactions and CNS effects (e.g., somnolence and confusion) with the concomitant use of clarithromycin and triazolam.
There have been reports of an interaction between erythromycin and astemizole resulting in QT prolongation and torsades de pointes. Concomitant administration of erythromycin and astemizole is contraindicated. Because clarithromycin is also metabolized by cytochrome P450, concomitant administration of clarithromycin with astemizole is not recommended.
The use of erythromycin and clarithromycin in patients concurrently taking drugs metabolized by the cytochrome P450 system may be associated with elevations in serum levels of these other drugs. There have been reports of interactions of erythromycin and/or clarithromycin with carbamazepine, cyclosporine, tacrolimus, hexobarbital, phenytoin, alfentanil, disopyramide, lovastatin, bromocriptine, valproate, terfenadine, cisapride, pimozide, and astemizole. Serum concentrations of drugs metabolized by the cytochrome P450 system should be monitored closely in patients concurrently receiving these drugs.
Carcinogenesis, Mutagenesis, Impairment of Fertility:
The following *in vitro* mutagenicity tests have been conducted with clarithromycin:

Salmonella/Mammalian Microsomes Test
Bacterial Induced Mutation Frequency Test
In Vitro Chromosome Aberration Test
Rat Hepatocyte DNA Synthesis Assay
Mouse Lymphoma Assay
Mouse Dominant Lethal Study
Mouse Micronucleus Test

All tests had negative results except the *In Vitro* Chromosome Aberration Test which was weakly positive in one test and negative in another.
In addition, a Bacterial Reverse-Mutation Test (Ames Test) has been performed on clarithromycin metabolites with negative results.
Fertility and reproduction studies have shown that daily doses of up to 160 mg/kg/day (1.3 times the recommended maximum human dose based on mg/m^2) to male and female rats caused no adverse effects on the estrous cycle, fertility, parturition, or number and viability of offspring. Plasma levels in rats after 150 mg/kg/day were 2 times the human serum levels.
In the 150 mg/kg/day monkey studies, plasma levels were 3 times the human serum levels. When given orally at 150 mg/kg/day (2.4 times the recommended maximum human dose based on mg/m^2), clarithromycin was shown to produce embryonic loss in monkeys. This effect has been attributed to marked maternal toxicity of the drug at this high dose.
In rabbits, *in utero* fetal loss occurred at an intravenous dose of 33 mg/m^2, which is 17 times less than the maximum proposed human oral daily dose of 618 mg/m^2.
Long-term studies in animals have not been performed to evaluate the carcinogenic potential of clarithromycin.
Pregnancy: Teratogenic Effects. Pregnancy Category C.
Four teratogenicity studies in rats (three with oral doses and one with intravenous doses up to 160 mg/kg/day administered during the period of major organogenesis) and two in rabbits at oral doses up to 125 mg/kg/day (approximately 2 times the recommended maximum human dose based on mg/m^2) or intravenous doses of 30 mg/kg/day administered during gestation days 6 to 18 failed to demonstrate any teratogenicity from clarithromycin. Two additional oral studies in a different rat strain at similar doses and similar conditions demonstrated a low incidence of cardiovascular anomalies at doses of 150 mg/kg/day administered during gestation days 6 to 15. Plasma levels after 150 mg/kg/day were 2 times the human serum levels. Four studies in mice revealed a variable incidence of cleft palate following oral doses of 1000 mg/kg/day (2 and 4 times the recommended maximum human dose based on mg/m^2, respectively) during gestation days 6 to 15. Cleft palate was also seen at 500 mg/kg/day. The 1000 mg/kg/day exposure resulted in plasma levels 17 times the human serum levels. In monkeys, an oral dose of 70 mg/kg/day (an approximate equidose of the recommended maximum human dose based on mg/m^2) produced fetal growth retardation at plasma levels that were 2 times the human serum levels.
There are no adequate and well-controlled studies in pregnant women. Clarithromycin should be used during pregnancy only if the potential benefit justifies the potential risk to the fetus. (See **WARNINGS**.)
Nursing Mothers: It is not known whether clarithromycin is excreted in human milk. Because many drugs are excreted in human milk, caution should be exercised when

Continued on next page

Biaxin—Cont.

clarithromycin is administered to a nursing woman. It is known that clarithromycin is excreted in the milk of lactating animals and that other drugs of this class are excreted in human milk. Preweaned rats, exposed indirectly via consumption of milk from dams treated with 150 mg/kg/day for 3 weeks, were not adversely affected, despite data indicating higher drug levels in milk than in plasma.

Pediatric Use: Safety and effectiveness of clarithromycin in children under 6 months of age have not been established. The safety of clarithromycin has not been studied in MAC patients under the age of 20 months. Neonatal and juvenile animals tolerated clarithromycin in a manner similar to adult animals. Young animals were slightly more intolerant to acute overdosage and to subtle reductions in erythrocytes, platelets and leukocytes but were less sensitive to toxicity in the liver, kidney, thymus, and genitalia.

Geriatric Use: In a steady-state study in which healthy elderly subjects (age 65 to 81 years old) were given 500 mg every 12 hours, the maximum serum concentrations and area under the curves of clarithromycin and 14-OH clarithromycin were increased compared to those achieved in healthy young adults. These changes in pharmacokinetics parallel known age-related decreases in renal function. In clinical trials, elderly patients did not have an increased incidence of adverse events when compared to younger patients. Dosage adjustment should be considered in elderly patients with severe renal impairment.

ADVERSE REACTIONS

The majority of side effects observed in clinical trials were of a mild and transient nature. Fewer than 3% of adult patients without mycobacterial infections and fewer than 2% of pediatric patients without mycobacterial infections discontinued therapy because of drug-related side effects.

The most frequently reported events in adults were diarrhea (3%), nausea (3%), abnormal taste (3%), dyspepsia (2%), abdominal pain/discomfort (2%), and headache (2%). In pediatric patients, the most frequently reported events were diarrhea (6%), vomiting (6%), abdominal pain (3%), rash (3%), and headache (2%). Most of these events were described as mild or moderate in severity. Of the reported adverse events, only 1% was described as severe.

In pneumonia studies conducted in adults comparing clarithromycin to erythromycin base or erythromycin stearate, there were fewer adverse events involving the digestive system in clarithromycin-treated patients compared to erythromycin-treated patients (13% vs 32%; p<0.01). Twenty percent of erythromycin-treated patients discontinued therapy due to adverse events compared to 4% of clarithromycin-treated patients.

In two U.S. studies of acute otitis media comparing clarithromycin to amoxicillin/potassium clavulanate in pediatric patients, there were fewer adverse events involving the digestive system in clarithromycin-treated patients compared to amoxicillin/potassium clavulanate-treated patients (21% vs 40%, p<0.001). One-third as many clarithromycin-treated patients reported diarrhea as did amoxicillin/potassium clavulanate-treated patients.

Post-Marketing Experience:

Allergic reactions ranging from urticaria and mild skin eruptions to rare cases of anaphylaxis and Stevens-Johnson syndrome have occurred. Other spontaneously reported adverse events include glossitis, stomatitis, oral moniliasis, vomiting, tongue discoloration, and dizziness. There have been reports of tooth discoloration in patients treated with BIAXIN. Tooth discoloration is usually reversible with professional dental cleaning. There have been isolated reports of hearing loss, which is usually reversible, occurring chiefly in elderly women. Reports of alterations of the sense of smell, usually in conjunction with taste perversion have also been reported.

Transient CNS events including anxiety, behavioral changes, confusional states, depersonalization, disorientation, hallucinations, insomnia, nightmares, psychosis, tinnitus, and vertigo have been reported during post-marketing surveillance. Events usually resolve with discontinuation of the drug.

Hepatic dysfunction, including increased liver enzymes, and hepatocellular and/or cholestatic hepatitis, with or without jaundice, has been infrequently reported with clarithromycin. This hepatic dysfunction may be severe and is usually reversible. In very rare instances, hepatic failure with fatal outcome has been reported and generally has been associated with serious underlying diseases and/or concomitant medications.

Rarely, erythromycin and clarithromycin have been associated with ventricular arrhythmias, including ventricular tachycardia and torsades de pointes, in individuals with prolonged QT$_c$ intervals.

Changes in Laboratory Values: Changes in laboratory values with possible clinical significance were as follows:
Hepatic-elevated SGPT (ALT) < 1%; SGOT (AST) < 1%; GGT < 1%; alkaline phosphatase <1%; LDH < 1%; total bilirubin < 1%

Hematologic-decreased WBC < 1%; elevated prothrombin time 1%

Renal-elevated BUN 4%; elevated serum creatinine < 1% GGT, alkaline phosphatase, and prothrombin time data are from adult studies only.

DOSAGE AND ADMINISTRATION

BIAXIN® Filmtab® (clarithromycin tablets) and BIAXIN® Granules (clarithromycin for oral suspension) may be given with or without food.

ADULT DOSAGE GUIDELINES

Infection	Dosage (q12h)	Normal Duration (days)
Pharyngitis/Tonsillitis	250 mg	10
Acute maxillary sinusitis	500 mg	14
Acute exacerbation of chronic bronchitis due to:		
S. pneumoniae	250 mg	7 to 14
M. catarrhalis	250 mg	7 to 14
H. influenzae	500 mg	7 to 14
Pneumonia due to:		
S. pneumoniae	250 mg	7 to 14
M. pneumoniae	250 mg	7 to 14
Uncomplicated skin and skin structure	250 mg	7 to 14

Active Duodenal Ulcer Associated with *H. pylori* Infection (28 day therapy) Clarithromycin + Omeprazole

Days 1 to 14	Days 15 to 28
Clarithromycin 500 mg tablet t.i.d. plus Omeprazole 2 × 20 mg capsules q AM	Omeprazole 20 mg capsule q AM

For information on omeprazole, refer to the DOSAGE AND ADMINISTRATION section of the PRILOSEC package insert.

Active Duodenal Ulcer Associated with *H. pylori* Infection (28 day therapy) Clarithromycin + Ranitidine Bismuth Citrate

Days 1 to 14	Days 15 to 28
Clarithromycin 500 mg tablet t.i.d. plus Ranitidine Bismuth Citrate 400 mg tablet b.i.d.	Ranitidine Bismuth Citrate 400 mg tablet b.i.d.

BIAXIN and ranitidine bismuth citrate combination therapy is not recommended in patients with creatinine clearance less than 25 mL/min.

For information on ranitidine bismuth citrate, refer to the DOSAGE AND ADMINISTRATION section of the TRITEC package insert.

H. pylori Eradication to Reduce the Risk of Duodenal Ulcer Recurrence Triple therapy: BIAXIN/lansoprazole/amoxicillin The recommended adult oral dose is 500 mg BIAXIN, 30 mg lansoprazole, and 1 gram amoxicillin, all given twice daily (q12h) for 14 days. (See **INDICATIONS AND USAGE.**)

For information on lansoprazole or amoxicillin, refer to the DOSAGE AND ADMINISTRATION section of their package inserts.

Children-The usual recommended daily dosage is 15 mg/kg/day divided q12h for 10 days.

PEDIATRIC DOSAGE GUIDELINES

Based on Body Weight

Weight kg	lbs	Dosing Calculated on 7.5 mg/kg q12h Dose (q12h)	125 mg/5 mL	250 mg/5 mL
9	20	62.5 mg	2.5 mL q12h	1.25 mL q12h
17	37	125 mg	5 mL q12h	2.5 mL q12h
25	55	187.5 mg	7.5 mL q12h	3.75 mL q12h
33	73	250 mg	10 mL q12h	5 mL q12h

Total volume after constitution	Clarithromycin concentration after constitution	Clarithromycin contents per bottle	NDC
50 mL	125 mg/5 mL	1250 mg	0074-3163-50
100 mL	125 mg/5 mL	2500 mg	0074-3163-13
50 mL	250 mg/5 mL	2500 mg	0074-3188-50
100 mL	250 mg/5 mL	5000 mg	0074-3188-13

[See first table above]

Clarithromycin may be administered without dosage adjustment in the presence of hepatic impairment if there is normal renal function. However, in the presence of severe renal impairment (CR$_{CL}$ < 30 mL/min), with or without coexisting hepatic impairment, the dose should be halved or the dosing interval doubled.

Mycobacterial infections:

Prophylaxis: The recommended dose of BIAXIN for the prevention of disseminated *Mycobacterium avium* disease is 500 mg b.i.d. In children, the recommended dose is 7.5 mg/kg b.i.d. up to 500 mg b.i.d. No studies of clarithromycin for MAC prophylaxis have been performed in pediatric populations and the doses recommended for prophylaxis are derived from MAC treatment studies in children. Dosing recommendations for children are in the table above.

Treatment: Clarithromycin is recommended as the primary agent for the treatment of disseminated infection due to *Mycobacterium avium* complex. Clarithromycin should be used in combination with other antimycobacterial drugs that have shown *in vitro* activity against MAC, or clinical benefit in MAC treatment. (See **CLINICAL STUDIES.**) The recommended dose for mycobacterial infections in adults is 500 mg b.i.d. In children, the recommended dose is 7.5 mg/kg b.i.d. up to 500 mg b.i.d. Dosing recommendations for children are in the table above.

Clarithromycin therapy should continue for life if clinical and mycobacterial improvements are observed.

Constituting Instructions

The table below indicates the volume of water to be added when constituting:

Total volume after constitution	Clarithromycin concentration after constitution	Amount of water to be added*
50 mL	125 mg/5 mL	27 mL
100 mL	125 mg/5 mL	55 mL
50 mL	250 mg/5 mL	27 mL
100 mL	250 mg/5 mL	55 mL

* see instructions below.

Add half the volume of water to the bottle and shake vigorously. Add the remainder of water to the bottle and shake. Shake well before each use. Oversize bottle provides shake space. Keep tightly closed. Do not refrigerate. After mixing, store at 15° to 30°C (59° to 86°F) and use within 14 days.

HOW SUPPLIED

BIAXIN® Filmtab® (clarithromycin tablets) are supplied as yellow oval film-coated tablets imprinted (on one side) in blue with the Abbott logo and a two-letter Abbo-Code designation, KT for the 250 mg tablet and KL for the 500 mg tablet, in the following packaging sizes:

250 mg tablets:

Bottles of 60 (**NDC** 0074-3368-60) and ABBO-PAC unit dose strip packages of 100 (**NDC** 0074-3368-11).

500 mg tablets:

Bottles of 60 (**NDC** 0074-2586-60), ABBO-PAC unit dose strip packages of 100 (**NDC** 0074-2586-11), and BIAXIN 7-PAK® unit-of-use package of 14 tablets in individual blisters (**NDC** 0074-2586-41).

BIAXIN® Granules (clarithromycin for oral suspension) is supplied in the following strengths and sizes:

[See second table from top of page]

Store tablets and granules for oral suspension at controlled room temperature 15° to 30°C (59° to 86°F) in a well-closed container. Protect from light. Do not refrigerate BIAXIN suspension.

CLINICAL STUDIES
Mycobacterial Infections
Prophylaxis:

A randomized, double-blind study (561) compared clarithromycin 500 mg b.i.d. to placebo in patients with CDC-defined AIDS and CD$_4$ counts <100 cells/μL. This study accrued 682 patients from November 1992 to January 1994, with a median CD$_4$ cell count at study entry of 30 cells/μL. Median duration of clarithromycin was 10.6 months vs. 8.2 months for placebo. More patients in the placebo arm than the clarithromycin arm discontinued prematurely from the study (75.6% and 67.4%, respectively). However, if premature discontinuations due to MAC or death are excluded, approximately equal percentages of patients on each arm (54.8% on clarithromycin and 52.5% on placebo) discontinued study drug early for other reasons. The study was designed to evaluate the following endpoints:

1. MAC bacteremia, defined as at least one positive culture for *M. avium* complex bacteria from blood or another normally sterile site.
2. Survival.
3. Clinically significant disseminated MAC disease, defined as MAC bacteremia accompanied by signs or symptoms of serious MAC infection, including fever, night sweats, weight loss, anemia, or elevations in liver function tests.

MAC bacteremia:
In patients randomized to clarithromycin, the risk of MAC bacteremia was reduced by 69% compared to placebo. The difference between groups was statistically significant (p<0.001). On an intent-to-treat basis, the one-year cumulative incidence of MAC bacteremia was 5.0% for patients randomized to clarithromycin and 19.4% for patients randomized to placebo. While only 19 of the 341 patients randomized to clarithromycin developed MAC, 11 of these cases were resistant to clarithromycin. The patients with resistant MAC bacteremia had a median baseline CD$_4$ count of 10 cells/mm^3 (range 2 to 25 cells/mm^3). Information regarding the clinical course and response to treatment of the patients with resistant MAC bacteremia is limited. The 8 patients who received clarithromycin and developed susceptible MAC bacteremia had a median baseline CD$_4$ count of 25 cells/mm^3 (range 10 to 80 cells/mm^3). Comparatively, 53 of the 341 placebo patients developed MAC; none of these isolates were resistant to clarithromycin. The median baseline CD$_4$ count was 15 cells/mm^3 (range 2 to 130 cells/mm^3) for placebo patients that developed MAC.

Survival:
A statistically significant survival benefit was observed.

Survival
All Randomized Patients

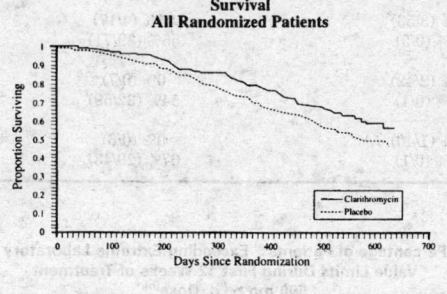

	Placebo Mortality	Clarithromycin Mortality	Reduction in Mortality on Clarithromycin
6 month	9.4%	6.5%	31%
12 month	29.7%	20.5%	31%
18 month	46.4%	37.5%	20%

Since the analysis at 18 months includes patients no longer receiving prophylaxis the survival benefit of clarithromycin may be underestimated.

Clinically significant disseminated MAC disease:
In association with the decreased incidence of bacteremia, patients in the group randomized to clarithromycin showed reductions in the signs and symptoms of disseminated MAC disease, including fever, night sweats, weight loss, and anemia.

Safety:
In AIDS patients treated with clarithromycin over long periods of time for prophylaxis against *M. avium*, it was often difficult to distinguish adverse events possibly associated with clarithromycin administration from underlying HIV disease or intercurrent illness. Median duration of treatment was 10.6 months for the clarithromycin group and 8.2 months for the placebo group.

Mean Reductions in Log CFU from Baseline (After 4 Weeks of Therapy)

500 mg b.i.d. (N=35)	1000 mg b.i.d. (N=32)	2000 mg b.i.d. (N=26)	Four Drug Regimen (N=24)
1.5	2.3	2.3	1.4

Resolution of Fever

b.i.d. dose (mg)	% ever afebrile	% afebrile ≥6 weeks
500	67%	23%
1000	67%	12%
2000	62%	22%

Resolution of Night Sweats

b.i.d. dose (mg)	% ever resolving	% resolving ≥6 weeks
500	85%	42%
1000	70%	33%
2000	72%	36%

Weight Gain >3%

b.i.d. dose (mg)	% ever gaining	% gaining ≥6 weeks
500	33%	14%
1000	26%	17%
2000	26%	12%

Hemoglobin Increase >1 gm

b.i.d. dose (mg)	% ever increasing	% increasing ≥6 weeks
500	58%	26%
1000	37%	6%
2000	62%	18%

Treatment-related* Adverse Event Incidence Rates (%) in Immunocompromised Adult Patients Receiving Prophylaxis Against *M. avium* Complex

Body System‡ Adverse Event	Clarithromycin (n=339) %	Placebo (n=339) %
Body as a Whole		
Abdominal pain	5.0%	3.5%
Headache	2.7%	0.9%
Digestive		
Diarrhea	7.7%	4.1%
Dyspepsia	3.8%	2.7%
Flatulence	2.4%	0.9%
Nausea	11.2%	7.1%
Vomiting	5.9%	3.2%
Skin & Appendages		
Rash	3.2%	3.5%
Special Senses		
Taste Perversion	8.0%	0.3%

* Includes those events possibly or probably related to study drug and excludes concurrent conditions.

‡ > 2% Adverse Event Incidence Rates for either treatment group.

Among these events, taste perversion was the only event that had significantly higher incidence in the clarithromycin-treated group compared to the placebo-treated group. Discontinuation due to adverse events was required in 18% of patients receiving clarithromycin compared to 17% of patients receiving placebo in this trial. Primary reasons for discontinuation in clarithromycin treated patients include headache, nausea, vomiting, depression and taste perversion.

Changes in Laboratory Values of Potential Clinical Importance:
In immunocompromised patients receiving prophylaxis against *M. avium*, evaluations of laboratory values were made by analyzing those values outside the seriously abnormal value (i.e., the extreme high or low limit) for the specified test.

Percentage of Patients(a) Exceeding Extreme Laboratory Value in Patients Receiving Prophylaxis Against *M. avium* Complex

		Clarithromycin 500 mg b.i.d.		Placebo	
Hemoglobin	< 8 g/dL	4/118	3%	5/103	5%
Platelet Count	< 50 × 10^9/L	11/249	4%	12/250	5%
WBC Count	<1 × 10^9/L	2/103	4%	0/95	0%
SGOT	>5 × ULN[b]	7/196	4%	5/208	2%
SGPT	>5 × ULN[b]	6/217	3%	4/232	2%
Alk. Phos.	>5 × ULN[b]	5/220	2%	5/218	2%

(a) Includes only patients with baseline values within the normal range or borderline high (hematology variables) and within the normal range or borderline low (chemistry variables).

(b) ULN = Upper Limit of Normal

Treatment:
Three randomized studies (500, 577, and 521) compared different dosages of clarithromycin in patients with CDC-de-

fined AIDS and CD$_4$ counts <100 cells/μL. These studies accrued patients from May 1991 to March 1992. Study 500 was randomized, double-blind; Study 577 was open-label compassionate use. Both studies used 500 and 1000 mg b.i.d. doses; Study 500 also had a 2000 mg b.i.d. group. Study 521 was a pediatric study at 3.75, 7.5, and 15 mg/kg b.i.d. Study 500 enrolled 154 adult patients, Study 577 enrolled 469 adult patients, and Study 521 enrolled 25 patients between the ages of 1 to 20. The majority of patients had CD$_4$ cell counts <50/μL at study entry. The studies were designed to evaluate the following end points:

1. Change in MAC bacteremia or blood cultures negative for *M. avium*.
2. Change in clinical signs and symptoms of MAC infection including one or more of the following: fever, night sweats, weight loss, diarrhea, splenomegaly, and hepatomegaly.

The results for the 500 study are described below. The 577 study results were similar to the results of the 500 study. Results with the 7.5 mg/kg b.i.d. dose in the pediatric study were comparable to those for the 500 mg b.i.d. regimen in the adult studies.

Study 069 compared the safety and efficacy of clarithromycin in combination with ethambutol versus clarithromycin in combination with ethambutol and clofazimine for the treatment of disseminated MAC (dMAC) infection[4]. This 24-week study enrolled 106 patients with AIDS and dMAC, with 55 patients randomized to receive clarithromycin and ethambutol, and 51 patients randomized to receive clarithromycin, ethambutol, and clofazimine. Baseline characteristics between study arms were similar with the exception of median CFU counts being at least 1 log higher in the clarithromycin, ethambutol, and clofazimine arm.

Compared to prior experience with clarithromycin monotherapy, the two-drug regimen of clarithromycin and ethambutol was well tolerated and extended the time to microbiologic relapse, largely through suppressing the emergence of clarithromycin resistant strains. However, the addition of clofazamine to the regimen added no additional microbiologic or clinical benefit. Tolerability of both multidrug regimens was comparable with the most common adverse events being gastrointestinal in nature. Patients receiving the clofazimine-containing regimen had reduced survival rates; however, their baseline mycobacterial colony counts were higher. The results of this trial support the addition of ethambutol to clarithromycin for the treatment of initial dMAC infections but do not support adding clofazimine as a third agent.

MAC bacteremia:
Decreases in MAC bacteremia or negative blood cultures were seen in the majority of patients in all dose groups. Mean reductions in colony forming units (CFU) are shown below. Included in the table are results from a separate study with a four drug regimen[5] (ciprofloxacin, ethambutol, rifampicin, and clofazimine). Since patient populations and study procedures may vary between these two studies, comparisons between the clarithromycin results and the combination therapy results should be interpreted cautiously.

[See table at top of page]

Although the 1000 mg and 2000 mg b.i.d. doses showed significantly better control of bacteremia during the first four weeks of therapy, no significant differences were seen beyond that point. The percent of patients whose blood was sterilized as shown by one or more negative cultures at any

Continued on next page

Biaxin—Cont.

time during acute therapy was 61% (30/49) for the 500 mg b.i.d. group and 59% (29/49) and 52% (25/48) for the 1000 and 2000 mg b.i.d. groups, respectively. The percent of patients who had 2 or more negative cultures during acute therapy that were sustained through study Day 84 was 25% (12/49) in both the 500 and 1000 mg b.i.d. groups and 8% (4/48) for the 2000 mg b.i.d. group. By Day 84, 23% (11/49), 37% (18/49), and 56% (27/48) of patients had died or discontinued from the study, and 14% (7/49), 12% (6/49), and 13% (6/48) of patients had relapsed in the 500, 1000, and 2000 mg b.i.d. dose groups, respectively. All of the isolates had an MIC < 8 µg/mL at pre-treatment. Relapse was almost always accompanied by an increase in MIC. The median time to first negative culture was 54, 41, and 29 days for the 500, 1000, and 2000 mg b.i.d. groups, respectively. The time to first decrease of at least 1 log in CFU count was significantly shorter with the 1000 and 2000 mg b.i.d. doses (median equal to 16 and 15 days, respectively) in comparison to the 500 mg b.i.d. group (median equal to 29 days). The median time to first positive culture or study discontinuation following the first negative culture was 43, 59 and 43 days for the 500, 1000, and 2000 mg b.i.d. groups, respectively.

Clinically significant disseminated MAC Disease:
Among patients experiencing night sweats prior to therapy, 84% showed resolution or improvement at some point during the 12 weeks of clarithromycin at 500 to 2000 mg b.i.d. doses. Similarly, 77% of patients reported resolution or improvement in fevers at some point. Response rates for clinical signs of MAC are given below:
[See second table at top of previous page]
The median duration of response, defined as improvement or resolution of clinical signs and symptoms, was 2 to 6 weeks.
Since the study was not designed to determine the benefit of monotherapy beyond 12 weeks, the duration of response may be underestimated for the 25 to 33% of patients who continued to show clinical response after 12 weeks.

Survival:
Median survival time from study entry (Study 500) was 249 days at the 500 mg b.i.d. dose compared to 215 days with the 1000 mg b.i.d. dose. However, during the first 12 weeks of therapy, there were 2 deaths in 53 patients in the 500 mg b.i.d. group versus 13 deaths in 51 patients in the 1000 mg b.i.d. group. The reason for this apparent mortality difference is not known. Survival in the two groups was similar beyond 12 weeks. The median survival times for these dosages were similar to recent historical controls with MAC when treated with combination therapies.[5]
Median survival time from study entry in Study 577 was 199 days for the 500 mg b.i.d. dose and 179 days for the 1000 mg b.i.d. dose. During the first four weeks of therapy, while patients were maintained on their originally assigned dose, there were 11 deaths in 255 patients taking 500 mg b.i.d. and 18 deaths in 214 patients taking 1000 mg b.i.d.

Safety:
The adverse event profiles showed that both the 500 and 1000 mg b.i.d. doses were well tolerated. The 2000 mg b.i.d. dose was poorly tolerated and resulted in a higher proportion of premature discontinuations.
In AIDS patients and other immunocompromised patients treated with the higher doses of clarithromycin over long periods of time for mycobacterial infections, it was often difficult to distinguish adverse events possibly associated with clarithromycin administration from underlying signs of HIV disease or intercurrent illness.
The following analyses summarize experience during the first 12 weeks of therapy with clarithromycin. Data are reported separately for Study 500 (randomized, double-blind) and Study 577 (open-label, compassionate use) and also combined. Adverse events were reported less frequently in Study 577, which may be due in part to differences in monitoring between the two studies. In adult patients receiving clarithromycin 500 mg b.i.d., the most frequently reported adverse events, considered possibly or probably related to study drug, with an incidence of 5% or greater, are listed below. Most of these events were mild to moderate in severity, although 5% (Study 500: 8%; Study 577: 4%) of patients receiving 500 mg b.i.d. and 5% (Study 500: 4%; Study 577: 6%) of patients receiving 1000 mg b.i.d. reported severe adverse events. Excluding those patients who discontinued therapy or died due to complications of their underlying non-mycobacterial disease, approximately 8% (Study 500: 15%; Study 577: 7%) of the patients who received 500 mg b.i.d. and 12% (Study 500: 14%; Study 577: 12%) of the patients who received 1000 mg b.i.d. discontinued therapy due to drug-related events during the first 12 weeks of therapy. Overall, the 500 and 1000 mg b.i.d. doses had similar adverse event profiles.

End-of-Treatment Ulcer Healing Rates
Percent of Patients Healed (n/N)

Study	Clarithromycin + Omeprazole	Omeprazole	Clarithromycin
U.S. Studies			
Study 100	94% (58/62)†	88% (60/68)	71% (49/69)
Study 067	88% (56/64)†	85% (55/65)	64% (44/69)
Non-U.S. Studies			
Study 058	99% (84/85)	95% (82/86)	N/A
Study 812b[1]	100% (64/64)	99% (71/72)	N/A

† p<0.05 for clarithromycin + omeprazole versus clarithromycin monotherapy.
[1] In Study 812b patients received omeprazole 40 mg daily for days 15 to 28.

H. pylori Eradication Rates (Per-Protocol Analysis) at 4 to 6 weeks
Percent of Patients Cured (n/N)

Study	Clarithromycin + Omeprazole	Omeprazole	Clarithromycin
U.S. Studies			
Study 100	64% (39/61)†‡	0% (0/59)	39% (17/44)
Study 067	74% (39/53)†‡	0% (0/54)	31% (13/42)
Non-U.S. Studies			
Study 058	74% (64/86)‡	1% (1/90)	N/A
Study 812b	83% (50/60)‡	1% (1/74)	N/A

† Statistically significantly higher than clarithromycin monotherapy (p<0.05).
‡ Statistically significantly higher than omeprazole monotherapy (p<0.05).

Ulcer Recurrence at 6 months by *H. pylori* Status at 4-6 Weeks

	H. pylori Negative	*H. pylori* Positive
U.S. Studies		
Study 100		
Clarithromycin + Omeprazole	6% (2/34)	56% (9/16)
Omeprazole	- (0/0)	71% (35/49)
Clarithromycin	12% (2/17)	32% (7/22)
Study 067		
Clarithromycin + Omeprazole	38% (11/29)	50% (6/12)
Omeprazole	- (0/0)	67% (31/46)
Clarithromycin	18% (2/11)	52% (14/27)
Non-U.S. Studies		
Study 058		
Clarithromycin + Omeprazole	6% (3/53)	24% (4/17)
Omeprazole	0% (0/3)	55% (39/71)
Study 812b*		
Clarithromycin + Omeprazole	5% (2/42)	0% (0/7)
Omeprazole	0% (0/1)	54% (32/59)
*12-month recurrence rates:		
Clarithromycin + Omeprazole	3% (1/40)	0% (0/6)
Omeprazole	0% (0/1)	67% (29/43)

Treatment-related* Adverse Event Incidence Rates (%) in Immunocompromised Adult Patients During the First 12 Weeks of Therapy with 500 mg b.i.d. Clarithromycin Dose

Adverse Event	Study 500 (n=53)	Study 577 (n=255)	Combined (n=308)
Abdominal Pain	7.5	2.4	3.2
Diarrhea	9.4	1.6	2.9
Flatulence	7.5	0.0	1.3
Headache	7.5	0.4	1.6
Nausea	28.3	9.0	12.3
Rash	9.4	2.0	3.2
Taste Perversion	18.9	0.4	3.6
Vomiting	24.5	3.9	7.5

* Includes those events possibly or probably related to study drug and excludes concurrent conditions.

A limited number of pediatric AIDS patients have been treated with clarithromycin suspension for mycobacterial infections. The most frequently reported adverse events, excluding those due to the patient's concurrent condition, were consistent with those observed in adult patients.

Changes in Laboratory Values:
In immunocompromised patients treated with clarithromycin for mycobacterial infections, evaluations of laboratory values were made by analyzing those values outside the seriously abnormal level (i.e., the extreme high or low limit) for the specified test.

Percentage of Patients[a] Exceeding Extreme Laboratory Value Limits During First 12 Weeks of Treatment 500 mg b.i.d. Dose[b]

		Study 500	Study 577	Combined
BUN	>50 mg/dL	0%	<1%	<1%
Platelet Count	<50 × 10⁹/L	0%	<1%	<1%
SGOT	>5 × ULN[c]	0%	3%	2%
SGPT	>5 × ULN[c]	0%	2%	1%
WBC	<1 × 10⁹/L	0%	1%	1%

(a) Includes only patients with baseline values within the normal range or borderline high (hematology variables) and within the normal range or borderline low (chemistry variables)
(b) Includes all values within the first 12 weeks for patients who start on 500 mg b.i.d.
(c) ULN = Upper Limit of Normal

Otitis Media
In a controlled clinical study of acute otitis media performed in the United States, where significant rates of beta-lactamase producing organisms were found, clarithromycin was compared to an oral cephalosporin. In this study, very strict evaluability criteria were used to determine clinical response. For the 223 patients who were evaluated for clinical efficacy, the clinical success rate (i.e., cure plus improvement) at the post-therapy visit was 88% for clarithromycin and 91% for the cephalosporin.
In a smaller number of patients, microbiologic determinations were made at the pre-treatment visit. The following presumptive bacterial eradication/clinical cure outcomes (i.e., clinical success) were obtained:

U.S. Acute Otitis Media Study
Clarithromycin vs. Oral Cephalosporin
EFFICACY RESULTS

PATHOGEN	OUTCOME
S. pneumoniae	clarithromycin success rate, 13/15 (87%), control 4/5
H. influenzae*	clarithromycin success rate, 10/14 (71%), control 3/4
M. catarrhalis	clarithromycin success rate, 4/5, control 1/1
S. pyogenes	clarithromycin success rate, 3/3, control 0/1
Overall	clarithromycin success rate, 30/37 (81%), control 8/11 (73%)

*None of the *H. influenzae* isolated pre-treatment was resistant to clarithromycin; 6% were resistant to the control agent.

Safety:
The incidence of adverse events in all patients treated, primarily diarrhea and vomiting, did not differ clinically or statistically for the two agents.
In two other controlled clinical trials of acute otitis media performed in the United States, where significant rates of beta-lactamase producing organisms were found, clarithromycin was compared to an oral antimicrobial agent that contained a specific beta-lactamase inhibitor. In these studies, very strict evaluability criteria were used to determine the clinical responses. In the 233 patients who were evaluated for clinical efficacy, the combined clinical success rate (i.e., cure and improvement) at the post-therapy visit was 91% for both clarithromycin and the control.
For the patients who had microbiologic determinations at the pre-treatment visit, the following presumptive bacterial eradication/clinical cure outcomes (i.e., clinical success) were obtained:

Two U.S. Acute Otitis Media Studies Clarithromycin vs. Antimicrobial/Beta-lactamase Inhibitor
EFFICACY RESULTS

PATHOGEN	OUTCOME
S. pneumoniae	clarithromycin success rate, 43/51 (84%), control 55/56 (98%)
H. influenzae*	clarithromycin success rate, 36/45 (80%), control 31/33 (94%)
M. catarrhalis	clarithromycin success rate, 9/10 (90%), control 6/6
S. pyogenes	clarithromycin success rate, 3/3, control 5/5
Overall	clarithromycin success rate, 91/109 (83%), control 97/100 (97%)

*Of the *H. influenzae* isolated pre-treatment, 3% were resistant to clarithromycin and 10% were resistant to the control agent.

Safety:
The incidence of adverse events in all patients treated, primarily diarrhea (15% vs. 38%) and diaper rash (3% vs. 11%) in young children, was clinically and statistically lower in the clarithromycin arm versus the control arm.

Duodenal Ulcer Associated with H. pylori Infection
Clarithromycin + Omeprazole Therapy
Four randomized, double-blind, multi-center studies (067, 100, 812b, and 058) evaluated clarithromycin 500 mg t.i.d. plus omeprazole 40 mg q.d. for 14 days, followed by omeprazole 20 mg q.d. (067, 100, and 058) or by omeprazole 40 mg q.d. (812b) for an additional 14 days in patients with active duodenal ulcer associated with *H. pylori*. Studies 067 and 100 were conducted in the U.S. and Canada and enrolled 242 and 256 patients, respectively. *H. pylori* infection and duodenal ulcer were confirmed in 219 patients in Study 067 and 228 patients in Study 100. These studies compared the combination regimen to omeprazole and clarithromycin monotherapies. Studies 812b and 058 were conducted in Europe and enrolled 154 and 215 patients, respectively. *H. pylori* infection and duodenal ulcer were confirmed in 148 patients in Study 812b and 208 patients in Study 058. These studies compared the combination regimen to omeprazole monotherapy. The results for the efficacy analyses for these studies are described below.
Duodenal Ulcer Healing:
The combination of clarithromycin and omeprazole was as effective as omeprazole alone for healing duodenal ulcer.
[See table at top of previous page]
Eradication of H. pylori Associated with Duodenal Ulcer:
The combination of clarithromycin and omeprazole was effective in eradicating *H. pylori*.
[See second table at top of previous page]
H. pylori eradication was defined as no positive test (culture or histology) at 4 weeks following the end of treatment, and

Adverse Events with an Incidence of 3% or Greater

Adverse Event	Clarithromycin + Omeprazole (N = 346) % of Patients	Omeprazole (N = 355) % of Patients	Clarithromycin (N = 166) % of Patients*
Taste Perversion	15%	1%	16%
Nausea	5%	1%	3%
Headache	5%	6%	9%
Diarrhea	4%	3%	7%
Vomiting	4%	<1%	1%
Abdominal Pain	3%	2%	1%
Infection	3%	4%	2%

*Studies 067 and 100, only

End-of-Treatment Ulcer Healing Rates*
Percent of Patients Healed†
[95% Confidence Interval]
(number of patients)

Study	Clarithromycin + Ranitidine Bismuth Citrate	Ranitidine Bismuth Citrate	Clarithromycin	Placebo
Study 305	75% [53%-90%] (n = 24)	73% [54%-88%] (n = 30)	70% [50%-86%] (n = 27)	56% [30%-80%] (n = 16)
Study 306	71%‡ [51%-87%] (n = 28)	79% [58%-93%] (n = 24)	53% [34%-72%] (n = 30)	21% [5%-51%] (n = 14)

* This analysis excludes dropouts and patients with major protocol violations.
† Ranitidine bismuth citrate alone has not been proven to be superior to ranitidine for duodenal ulcer healing.
‡ P<0.05 for clarithromycin + ranitidine bismuth citrate versus placebo.

H. pylori Eradication Rates*
Percent of Patients Cured
[95% Confidence Interval]
(number of patients)

Study	Clarithromycin + Ranitidine Bismuth Citrate	Ranitidine Bismuth Citrate	Clarithromycin	Placebo
Study 305	84%‡ [60%-97%] (n = 19)	0% [0%-14%] (n = 25)	25% [10%-47%] (n = 24)	0% [0%-21%] (n = 16)
Study 306	73%‡ [50%-89%] (n = 22)	0% [0%-15%] (n = 22)	25% [10%-47%] (n = 24)	0% [0%-23%] (n = 14)

**H. pylori* eradication was defined as no positive test (CLOtest™, culture, histology) at 4 weeks following the end of treatment. Patients must have had two tests performed and these must have been negative to be considered eradicated of *H. pylori*. The following patients were excluded: patients not infected with *H. pylori* prestudy, dropouts, patients with major protocol violations, patients with missing *H. pylori* tests, and patients that were not assessed for *H. pylori* eradication 4 weeks after the end of treatment because they were found to have an unhealed ulcer and were *H. pylori* negative at the end of treatment.
‡P<0.001 for clarithromycin + ranitidine bismuth citrate versus all other treatment groups.

Drug-Related Adverse Reactions During Treatment*

Adverse Reaction	TRITEC Tablets 800 mg + Clarithromycin 1,500 mg (n = 120)	Clarithromycin 1,500 mg (n = 120)	TRITEC Tablets 800 mg (n = 903)	Placebo (N = 469)
Gastrointestinal				
Diarrhea	8%	5%	2%	1%
Nausea & vomiting	3%	2%	<1%	1%
Constipation	0%	0%	1%	<1%
Neurological				
Headache	5%	<1%	1%	<1%
Dizziness	0%	2%	<1%	<1%
Miscellaneous				
Disturbance of taste	10%	11%	<1%	<1%
Sleep disorder	2%	<1%	<1%	<1%
Chest symptoms	2%	0%	0%	<1%
Skin				
Pruritus	3%	0%	<1%	0%
Urogenital				
Gynecological problems	3% (n = 34)	6% (n = 32)	<1% (n = 267)	0% (n = 159)

* Total daily dose.

two negative tests were required to be considered eradicated. In the per-protocol analysis, the following patients were excluded: dropouts, patients with major protocol violations, patients with missing *H. pylori* tests post-treatment, and patients that were not assessed for *H. pylori* eradica-

tion at 4 weeks after the end of treatment because they were found to have an unhealed ulcer at the end of treatment.

Continued on next page

Biaxin—Cont.

Ulcer recurrence at 6-months following the end of treatment was assessed for patients in whom ulcers were healed post-treatment.
[See third table at top of page 410]
Thus, in patients with duodenal ulcer associated with *H. pylori* infection, eradication of *H. pylori* reduced ulcer recurrence.
Safety:
The adverse event profiles for the four studies showed that the combination of clarithromycin 500 mg t.i.d. and omeprazole 40 mg q.d. for 14 days, followed by omeprazole 20 mg q.d. (067, 100, and 058) or 40 mg q.d. (812b) for an additional 14 days was well tolerated. Of the 346 patients who received the combination, 12 (3.5%) patients discontinued study drug due to adverse events.
Most of these events were mild to moderate in severity.
[See table at top of previous page]
Changes in Laboratory Values:
Changes in laboratory values with possible clinical significance in patients taking clarithromycin and omeprazole were as follows:
Hepatic-elevated direct bilirubin <1%; GGT <1%; SGOT (AST) <1%; SGPT (ALT) <1%.
Renal-elevated serum creatinine <1%.
For information on omeprazole, refer to the ADVERSE REACTIONS section of the PRILOSEC package insert.

Clarithromycin + Ranitidine Bismuth Citrate Therapy

BIAXIN alone and in combination with ranitidine bismuth citrate was evaluated in two U.S. double-blind, randomized, multicenter, placebo-controlled trials. Four-hundred and nine (409) patients were enrolled and 265 had *H. pylori* infection and active duodenal ulcer prestudy. Clarithromycin 500 mg t.i.d. for the first 2 weeks plus ranitidine bismuth citrate 400 mg b.i.d. for 4 weeks was found to have a significantly higher *H. pylori* eradication rate when compared to clarithromycin 500 mg t.i.d. for 2 weeks, ranitidine bismuth citrate 400 mg b.i.d. for 4 weeks, or placebo.
Duodenal Ulcer Healing at 4 Weeks (End of Treatment):
Ulcer healing rates for the two U.S. double-blind, randomized, multicenter, placebo-controlled trials are represented in the table below.
[See second table from top of previous page]
Eradication of H. pylori Associated with Active Duodenal Ulcer:
The combination of clarithromycin and ranitidine bismuth citrate was effective in eradicating *H. pylori*.
[See third table from top of previous page]
The relationship between *H. pylori* eradication and duodenal ulcer recurrence was assessed in a combined analysis of six U.S. randomized, double-blind, multicenter, placebo-controlled trials using ranitidine bismuth citrate with or without antibiotics. The results from approximately 650 U.S. patients showed that the risk of ulcer recurrence within 6 months of completing treatment was two times less likely in patients whose *H. pylori* infection was eradicated compared to patients in whom *H. pylori* infection was not eradicated.
Safety:
Placebo-controlled trials in patients with active duodenal ulcer in the United States included 240 patients given clarithromycin alone or in combination with ranitidine bismuth citrate, 903 patients given ranitidine bismuth citrate alone, and 469 patients given placebo.
Incidence of Drug-Related Adverse Reactions in Placebo-Controlled Clinical Trials:
The following table lists drug-related adverse reactions that occurred at a frequency of ≥1% among patients treated with ranitidine bismuth citrate who participated in U.S. placebo-controlled trials.
[See fourth table from top of previous page]
For information on ranitidine bismuth citrate, refer to the ADVERSE REACTIONS section of the TRITEC package insert.

Clarithromycin + Lansoprazole and Amoxicillin

H. pylori Eradication for Reducing the Risk of Duodenal Ulcer Recurrence:
Two U.S. randomized, double-blind clinical studies in patients with *H. pylori* and duodenal ulcer disease (defined as an active ulcer or history of an active ulcer within one year) evaluated the efficacy of clarithromycin in combination with lansoprazole and amoxicillin capsules as triple 14-day therapy for eradication of *H. pylori*. Based on the results of these studies, the safety and efficacy of the following eradication regimen were established:
Triple therapy: BIAXIN 500 mg b.i.d. + lansoprazole 30 mg b.i.d. + amoxicillin 1 gm b.i.d.
Treatment was for 14 days. *H. pylori* eradication was defined as two negative tests (culture and histology) at 4 to 6 weeks following the end of treatment.
The combination of BIAXIN plus lansoprazole and amoxicillin as triple therapy was effective in eradicating *H. pylori*. Eradication of *H. pylori* has been shown to reduce the risk of duodenal ulcer recurrence.
[See table below]
Safety:
In clinical trials using combination therapy with BIAXIN plus lansoprazole and amoxicillin, no adverse reactions peculiar to this drug combination have been observed. Adverse reactions that have occurred have been limited to those that have been previously reported with BIAXIN, lansoprazole, or amoxicillin.
Triple Therapy: Biaxin + lansoprazole + amoxicillin
The most frequently reported adverse events for patients who received triple therapy were diarrhea (7%), headache (6%), and taste perversion (5%). No treatment-emergent adverse events were observed at significantly higher rates with triple therapy than with any dual therapy regimen.

ANIMAL PHARMACOLOGY AND TOXICOLOGY

Clarithromycin is rapidly and well-absorbed with dose-linear kinetics, low protein binding, and a high volume of distribution. Plasma half-life ranged from 1 to 6 hours and was species dependent. High tissue concentrations were achieved, but negligible accumulation was observed. Fecal clearance predominated. Hepatotoxicity occurred in all species tested (i.e., in rats and monkeys at doses 2 times greater than and in dogs at doses comparable to the maximum human daily dose, based on mg/m²). Renal tubular degeneration (calculated on a mg/m² basis) occurred in rats at doses 2 times, in monkeys at doses 8 times, and in dogs at doses 12 times greater than the maximum human daily dose. Testicular atrophy (on a mg/m² basis) occurred in rats at doses 7 times, in dogs at doses 3 times, and in monkeys at doses 8 times greater than the maximum human daily dose. Corneal opacity (on a mg/m² basis) occurred in dogs at doses 12 times and in monkeys at doses 8 times greater than the maximum human daily dose. Lymphoid depletion (on a mg/m² basis) occurred in dogs at doses 3 times greater than and in monkeys at doses 2 times greater than the maximum human daily dose. These adverse events were absent during clinical trials.

REFERENCES

1. National Committee for Clinical Laboratory Standards, Methods for Dilution Antimicrobial Susceptibility Tests for Bacteria that Grow Aerobically - Fourth Edition. Approved Standard NCCLS Document M7-A4, Vol. 17, No. 2, NCCLS, Wayne, PA, January, 1997.
2. National Committee for Clinical Laboratory Standards, Performance Standards for Antimicrobial Disk Susceptibility Tests - Sixth Edition. Approved Standard NCCLS Document M2-A6, Vol. 17, No. 1, NCCLS, Wayne, PA, January, 1997.
3. Hachem, C. Y., J. E. Clarridge, R. Reddy, R. Flamm, D. G. Evans, S. K. Tanaka, and D. Y. Graham. Antimicrobial susceptibility testing of *Helicobacter pylori:* comparison of E-test, broth microdilution, and disk diffusion for ampicillin, clarithromycin, and metronidazole. *Diagnost. Microbiol. Infect. Dis.* 1996;24:37-41.
4. Chaisson RE, et al. Clarithromycin and Ethambutol with or without Clofazimine for the Treatment of Bacteremic *Mycobacterium avium* Complex Disease in Patients with HIV Infection. *AIDS*. 1997;11:311-317.
5. Kemper CA, et al. Treatment of *Mycobacterium avium* Complex Bacteremia in AIDS with a Four-Drug Oral Regimen. *Ann Intern Med.* 1992;116:466-472.

Filmtab - Film-sealed tablets, Abbott
Revised: October, 1997
Ref. 03-4821-R12

ABBOTT LABORATORIES
NORTH CHICAGO, IL 60064, U.S.A.
Shown in Product Identification Guide, page 303

H. pylori Eradication Rates-Triple Therapy Percent of Patients Cured [95% Confidence Interval] (number of patients)

Study	Triple Therapy (Evaluable Analysis)*	Triple Therapy (Intent-to-Treat Analysis)**
Study 131	92† [80.0–97.7] (n = 48)	86† [73.3–93.5] (n = 55)
Study 392	86‡ [75.7–93.6] (n = 66)	83‡ [72.0–90.8] (n = 70)

* Based on evaluable patients with confirmed duodenal ulcer (active or within one year) and *H. pylori* infection as baseline defined as at least two of three positive endoscopic tests from CLOtest (Delta West LTD., Bentley, Australia), histology and/or culture. Patients were included in the analysis if they completed the study. Additionally, if patients were dropped out of the study due to an adverse event related to the study drug, they were included as failures of therapy.
** Patients were included in the analysis if they had documented *H. pylori* infection at baseline as defined above and had a confirmed duodenal ulcer (active or within one year). All dropouts were included as failures of therapy.
† ($p<0.05$) versus BIAXIN/lansoprazole and lansoprazole/amoxicillin dual therapy.
‡ ($p<0.05$) versus BIAXIN/amoxicillin dual therapy.

CALCIJEX® ℞

CALCITRIOL INJECTION
1 mcg and 2 mcg/mL

DESCRIPTION

Calcijex® (calcitriol injection) is synthetically manufactured calcitriol and is available as a sterile, isotonic, clear, aqueous solution for intravenous injection. Calcijex is available in 1 mL ampuls. Each 1 mL contains calcitriol, 1 or 2 mcg; Polysorbate 20, 4 mg; sodium chloride 1.5 mg; sodium ascorbate 10 mg added; dibasic sodium phosphate, anhydrous 7.6 mg; monobasic sodium phosphate, monohydrate 1.8 mg; edetate disodium, dihydrate 1.1 mg added. pH 7.2 (6.5 to 8.0).
Calcitriol is a colorless, crystalline compound which occurs naturally in humans. It is soluble in organic solvents but relatively insoluble in water. Calcitriol is chemically designated (5Z,7E)-9, 10-secocholesta-5,7,10(19)-triene-1α,3β,25-triol and has the following structural formula:

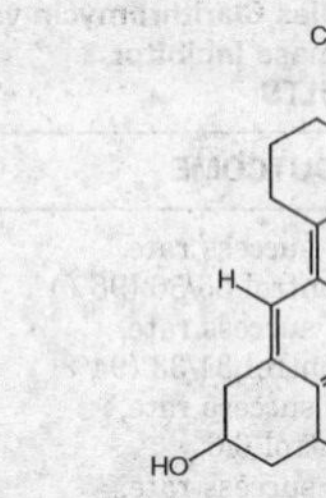

Molecular Formula: $C_{27}H_{44}O_3$
The other names frequently used for calcitriol are 1α,25-dihydroxycholecalciferol, 1α,25-dihydroxyvitamin D_3, 1,25-DHCC, 1,25$(OH)_2D_3$ and 1,25-diOHC.

CLINICAL PHARMACOLOGY

Calcitriol is the active form of vitamin D_3 (cholecalciferol). The natural or endogenous supply of vitamin D in man mainly depends on ultraviolet light for conversion of 7-dehydrocholesterol to vitamin D_3 in the skin. Vitamin D_3 must be metabolically activated in the liver and the kidney before it is fully active on its target tissues. The initial transformation is catalyzed by a vitamin D_3-25-hydroxylase enzyme present in the liver, and the product of this reaction is 25-$(OH)D_3$ (calcifediol). The latter undergoes hydroxylation in the mitochondria of kidney tissue, and this reaction is activated by the renal 25-hydroxyvitamin D_3-1-α-hydroxylase to produce 1,25-$(OH)_2D_3$ (calcitriol), the active form of vitamin D_3.
The known sites of action of calcitriol are intestine, bone, kidney and parathyroid gland. Calcitriol is the most active known form of vitamin D_3 in stimulating intestinal calcium transport. In acutely uremic rats, calcitriol has been shown to stimulate intestinal calcium absorption. In bone, calcitriol, in conjunction with parathyroid hormone, stimulates resorption of calcium; and in the kidney, calcitriol increases the tubular reabsorption of calcium. *In vitro* and *in vivo* studies have shown that calcitriol directly suppresses secretion and synthesis of PTH. A vitamin D-resistant state may exist in uremic patients because of the failure of the kidney to adequately convert precursors to the active compound, calcitriol.
Calcitriol when administered by bolus injection is rapidly available in the blood stream. Vitamin D metabolites are known to be transported in blood, bound to specific plasma proteins. The pharmacologic activity of an administered dose of calcitriol is about 3 to 5 days. Two metabolic pathways for calcitriol have been identified, conversion to 1,24,25-$(OH)_3D_3$ and to calcitroic acid.

INDICATIONS AND USAGE

Calcijex® (calcitriol injection) is indicated in the management of hypocalcemia in patients undergoing chronic renal

dialysis. It has been shown to significantly reduce elevated parathyroid hormone levels. Reduction of PTH has been shown to result in an improvement in renal osteodystrophy.

CONTRAINDICATIONS

Calcijex® (calcitriol injection) should not be given to patients with hypercalcemia or evidence of vitamin D toxicity.

WARNINGS

Since calcitriol is the most potent metabolite of vitamin D available, vitamin D and its derivatives should be withheld during treatment.

A non-aluminum phosphate-binding compound should be used to control serum phosphorus levels in patients undergoing dialysis.

Overdosage of any form of vitamin D is dangerous (see also OVERDOSAGE). Progressive hypercalcemia due to overdosage of vitamin D and its metabolites may be so severe as to require emergency attention. Chronic hypercalcemia can lead to generalized vascular calcification, nephrocalcinosis and other soft-tissue calcification. The serum calcium times phosphate (Ca x P) product should not be allowed to exceed 70. Radiographic evaluation of suspect anatomical regions may be useful in the early detection of this condition.

PRECAUTIONS

1. General

Excessive dosage of Calcijex® (calcitriol injection) induces hypercalcemia and in some instances hypercalciuria; therefore, early in treatment during dosage adjustment, serum calcium and phosphorus should be determined at least twice weekly. Should hypercalcemia develop, the drug should be discontinued immediately.

Calcijex should be given cautiously to patients on digitalis, because hypercalcemia in such patients may precipitate cardiac arrhythmias.

2. Information for the Patient

The patient and his or her parents should be informed about adherence to instructions about diet and calcium supplementation and avoidance of the use of unapproved non-prescription drugs, including magnesium-containing antacids. Patients should also be carefully informed about the symptoms of hypercalcemia (see ADVERSE REACTIONS).

3. Essential Laboratory Tests

Serum calcium, phosphorus, magnesium and alkaline phosphatase and 24-hour urinary calcium and phosphorus should be determined periodically. During the initial phase of the medication, serum calcium and phosphorus should be determined more frequently (twice weekly).

Adynamic bone disease may develop if PTH levels are suppressed to abnormal levels. If biopsy is not being done for other (diagnostic) reasons, PTH levels may be used to indicate the rate of bone turnover. If PTH levels fall below recommended target range (1.5 to 3 times the upper limit of normal), in patients treated with Calcijex, the Calcijex dose should be reduced or therapy discontinued. Discontinuation of Calcijex therapy may result in rebound effect, therefore, appropriate titration downward to a maintenance dose is recommended.

4. Drug Interactions

Magnesium-containing antacid and Calcijex should not be used concomitantly, because such use may lead to the development of hypermagnesemia.

5. Carcinogenesis, Mutagenesis, Impairment of Fertility

Long-term studies in animals have not been performed to evaluate the carcinogenic potential of Calcijex (calcitriol injection). There was no evidence of mutagenicity as studied by the Ames Method. No significant effects of calcitriol on fertility were reported using oral calcitriol.

6. Use in Pregnancy: *Pregnancy Category C:*

Calcitriol given orally has been reported to be teratogenic in rabbits when given in doses 4 and 15 times the dose recommended for human use.

All 15 fetuses in 3 litters at these doses showed external and skeletal abnormalities. However, none of the other 23 litters (156 fetuses) showed significant abnormalities compared with controls.

Teratology studies in rats showed no evidence of teratogenic potential. There are no adequate and well-controlled studies in pregnant women. Calcijex should be used during pregnancy only if the potential benefit justifies the potential risk to the fetus.

7. Nursing Mothers

It is not known whether this drug is excreted in human milk. Because many drugs are excreted in human milk and because of the potential for serious adverse reactions in nursing infants from calcitriol, a decision should be made whether to discontinue nursing or to discontinue the drug, taking into account the importance of the drug to the mother.

8. Pediatric Use

Safety and efficacy of Calcijex in pediatric patients have not been established.

ADVERSE REACTIONS

Adverse effects of Calcijex® (calcitriol injection) are, in general, similar to those encountered with excessive vitamin D intake. The early and late signs and symptoms of vitamin D intoxication associated with hypercalcemia include:

1. Early

Weakness, headache, somnolence, nausea, vomiting, dry mouth, constipation, muscle pain, bone pain and metallic taste.

2. Late

Polyuria, polydipsia, anorexia, weight loss, nocturia, conjunctivitis (calcific), pancreatitis, photophobia, rhinorrhea, pruritus, hyperthermia, decreased libido, elevated BUN, albuminuria, hypercholesterolemia, elevated SGOT and SGPT, ectopic calcification, hypertension, cardiac arrhythmias and, rarely, overt psychosis.

Occasional mild pain on injection has been observed.

OVERDOSAGE

Administration of Calcijex® (calcitriol injection) to patients in excess of their requirements can cause hypercalcemia, hypercalciuria and hyperphosphatemia. High intake of calcium and phosphate concomitant with Calcijex may lead to similar abnormalities.

1. Treatment of Hypercalcemia and Overdosage in Patients on Hemodialysis

General treatment of hypercalcemia (greater than 1 mg/dL above the upper limit of normal range) consists of immediate discontinuation of Calcijex therapy, institution of a low calcium diet and withdrawal of calcium supplements. Serum calcium levels should be determined daily until normocalcemia ensues. Hypercalcemia usually resolves in two to seven days. When serum calcium levels have returned to within normal limits, Calcijex therapy may be reinstituted at a dose 0.5 mcg less than prior therapy. Serum calcium levels should be obtained at least twice weekly after all dosage changes.

Persistent or markedly elevated serum calcium levels may be corrected by dialysis against a calcium-free dialysate.

2. Treatment of Accidental Overdosage of Calcitriol Injection

The treatment of acute accidental overdosage of Calcijex should consist of general supportive measures. Serial serum electrolyte determinations (especially calcium), rate of urinary calcium excretion and assessment of electrocardiographic abnormalities due to hypercalcemia should be obtained. Such monitoring is critical in patients receiving digitalis. Discontinuation of supplemental calcium and low calcium diet are also indicated in accidental overdosage. Due to the relatively short duration of the pharmacological action of calcitriol, further measures are probably unnecessary. Should, however, persistent and markedly elevated serum calcium levels occur, there are a variety of therapeutic alternatives which may be considered, depending on the patients' underlying condition. These include the use of drugs such as phosphates and corticosteroids as well as measures to induce an appropriate forced diuresis. The use of peritoneal dialysis against a calcium-free dialysate has also been reported.

DOSAGE AND ADMINISTRATION

The optimal dose of Calcijex® (calcitriol injection) must be carefully determined for each patient.

The effectiveness of Calcijex therapy is predicated on the assumption that each patient is receiving an adequate and appropriate daily intake of calcium. The RDA for calcium in adults is 800 mg. To ensure that each patient receives an adequate daily intake of calcium, the physician should either prescribe a calcium supplement or instruct the patient in proper dietary measures.

The recommended initial dose of Calcijex®, depending on the severity of the hypocalcemia and/or secondary hyperparathyroidism, is 1 mcg (0.02 mcg/kg) to 2 mcg administered three times weekly, approximately every other day. Doses as small as 0.5 mcg and as large as 4 mcg three times weekly have been used as an initial dose. If a satisfactory response is not observed, the dose may be increased by 0.5 to 1 mcg at two to four week intervals. During this titration period, serum calcium and phosphorus levels should be obtained at least twice weekly. If hypercalcemia or a serum calcium times phosphate product greater than 70 is noted, the drug should be immediately discontinued until these parameters are appropriate. Then, the Calcijex dose should be reinitiated at a lower dose. Doses may need to be reduced as the PTH levels decrease in response to the therapy. Thus, incremental dosing must be individualized and commensurate with PTH, serum calcium and phosphorus levels. The following is a suggested approach in dose titration:

PTH Levels	Calcijex Dose
the same or increasing	increase
decreasing by <30%	increase
decreasing by >30%, <60%	maintain
decreasing by >60%	decrease
one and one-half to three times the upper limit of normal	maintain

Parenteral drug products should be inspected visually for particulate matter and discoloration prior to administration, whenever solution and container permit.

Discard unused portion.

HOW SUPPLIED

Calcijex® (calcitriol injection) is supplied in 1 mL ampuls containing 1 mcg (List No. 1200) and 2 mcg (List No. 1210).

Protect from light.

Store at controlled room temperature 15° to 30°C (59° to 86°F).

Caution: Federal (USA) law prohibits dispensing without prescription.

06-9656-R8-Rev. Jun., 1997

ABBOTT LABORATORIES, NORTH CHICAGO, IL 60064, USA

CARTROL® ℞

[*kär ′trōl*]

(Carteolol Hydrochloride)

Filmtab® Tablets

DESCRIPTION

CARTROL (carteolol hydrochloride) is a synthetic, nonselective, beta-adrenergic receptor blocking agent with intrinsic sympathomimetic activity. It is chemically described as 5-[3-[(1,1-dimethylethyl)amino]-2-hydroxypropoxy]-3,4-dihydro-2(1H)-quinolinone monohydrochloride. The structural formula is:

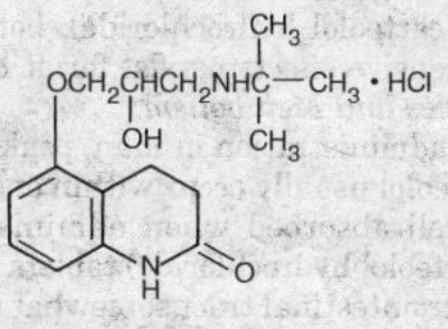

Carteolol hydrochloride is a stable, white crystalline powder which is soluble in water and slightly soluble in ethanol. The molecular weight is 328.84 and $C_{16}H_{24}N_2O_3{\cdot}HCl$ is the empirical formula.

CARTROL (carteolol hydrochloride) is available as tablets containing either 2.5 mg or 5 mg of carteolol hydrochloride for oral administration.

INACTIVE INGREDIENTS

2.5 mg Tablet: Cellulosic polymers, corn starch, iron oxide, lactose, magnesium stearate, microcrystalline cellulose, polyethylene glycol, propylene glycol, and titanium dioxide.

5 mg Tablet: Cellulosic polymers, corn starch, lactose, magnesium stearate, microcrystalline cellulose, polyethylene glycol, propylene glycol, and titanium dioxide.

CLINICAL PHARMACOLOGY

CARTROL (carteolol hydrochloride) is a long-acting, nonselective, beta-adrenergic receptor blocking agent with intrinsic sympathomimetic activity (ISA) and without significant membrane stabilizing (local anesthetic) activity.

Pharmacodynamics:

Carteolol specifically competes with beta-adrenergic receptor agonists for both $beta_1$-receptors located principally in cardiac muscle and $beta_2$-receptors located in the bronchial and vascular musculature, blocking the chronotropic, inotropic, and vasodilator responses to beta-adrenergic stimulation proportionately. Because of its partial agonist activity, however, carteolol does not reduce resting beta-agonist activity as much as beta-adrenergic blockers lacking this activity. Thus, in clinical trials in man, the decreases in resting pulse rate produced by carteolol (2–5 beats per minute in various studies) were less than those produced by beta-blockers (nadolol and propranolol) without ISA (10–12 beats per minute). There are also equivocal effects on renin secretion, in contrast to beta-blockers without ISA, which inhibit renin secretion.

In controlled clinical trials carteolol, at doses up to 20 mg as monotherapy or in combination with thiazide type diuretics, produced significantly greater reductions in blood pressure than did placebo, with the full effect seen between two and four weeks. The observed differences from placebo ranged from 3.1 to 6.7 mmHg for supine diastolic blood pressure. The antihypertensive effects of carteolol are smaller in

Continued on next page

Cartrol—Cont.

black populations but do not seem to be affected by age or sex. Doses of carteolol greater than 10 mg once a day did not produce greater reductions in blood pressure. In fact, doses of 20 mg and above appeared to produce blood pressure reductions less than those produced by 10 mg and below. When carteolol was compared to nadolol and propranolol, although the differences were not statistically significant in relatively small studies, carteolol at doses up to 20 mg produced supine diastolic blood pressure changes consistently 2 mmHg less than that produced by either nadolol or propranolol.

Although the mechanism of the antihypertensive effect of beta-adrenergic blocking agents has not been established, multiple factors are thought to contribute to the lowering of blood pressure, including diminished response to sympathetic nerve outflow from vasomotor centers in the brain, diminished release of renin from the kidneys, and decreased cardiac output. Carteolol does not have a consistent effect on renin and other agents with ISA have been shown to have less effect than other beta-blockers on resting cardiac output (although they cause the usual decrease in exercise cardiac output so that the difference is of uncertain clinical importance), so that the mechanism of its action is particularly uncertain.

Beta-blockade interferes with endogenous adrenergic bronchodilator activity and diminishes the response to exogenous bronchodilators. This is especially important in patients subject to bronchospasm.

Single intravenous doses of carteolol (0.5 mg, 1 mg, 2.5 mg and 5 mg) produced statistically, but not clinically, significant increases from baseline in AV node conduction time and RR and PR intervals.

CARTROL (carteolol hydrochloride) induced no significant alteration in total serum cholesterol and triglycerides.

Following discontinuation of carteolol treatment in man, pharmacologic activity (evaluated by blockade of the tachycardia induced by isoproterenol or postural changes) is present for 2 to 21 days (median 14 days) after the last dose of carteolol. Following administration of recommended doses of CARTROL (carteolol hydrochloride), both beta-blocking and antihypertensive effects persist for at least 24 hours.

Pharmacokinetics and Metabolism:

Following oral administration in man, peak plasma concentrations of carteolol usually occur within one to three hours. Carteolol is well absorbed when administered orally as CARTROL (carteolol hydrochloride) tablets. The presence of food in the gastrointestinal tract somewhat slows the rate of absorption, but the extent of absorption is not appreciably affected. Compared to intravenous administration, the absolute bioavailability of carteolol from CARTROL (carteolol hydrochloride) tablets is approximately 85%.

The plasma half-life of carteolol averages approximately six hours. Steady-state serum levels are achieved within one to two days after initiating therapeutic doses of carteolol in persons with normal renal function. Since approximately 50 to 70% of a carteolol dose is eliminated unchanged by the kidneys, the half-life is increased in patients with impaired renal function. Significant reductions in the rate of carteolol elimination (and prolongations of the half-life) occur in patients as creatinine clearance decreases. Therefore, a reduction in maintenance dose and/or prolongation in dosing interval is appropriate (see DOSAGE and ADMINISTRATION).

Carteolol is 23–30% bound to plasma proteins in humans. The major metabolites of carteolol are 8-hydroxycarteolol and the glucuronic acid conjugates of both carteolol and 8-hydroxycarteolol. In man, 8-hydroxycarteolol is an active metabolite with a half-life of approximately 8 to 12 hours and represents approximately 5% of the administered dose excreted in the urine.

INDICATIONS AND USAGE

CARTROL (carteolol hydrochloride) is indicated in the management of hypertension. It may be used alone or in combination with other antihypertensive agents, especially thiazide diuretics. Preliminary data indicate that carteolol does not have a favorable effect on arrhythmias.

CONTRAINDICATIONS

CARTROL (carteolol hydrochloride) is contraindicated in patients with: 1) bronchial asthma, 2) severe bradycardia, 3) greater than first degree heart block, 4) cardiogenic shock, and 5) clinically evident congestive heart failure (see WARNINGS).

WARNINGS

Congestive Heart Failure:

Sympathetic stimulation may be a vital component supporting circulatory function in patients with congestive heart failure, and impairing that support by beta-blockade may precipitate more severe decompensation. Although CARTROL (carteolol hydrochloride) should be avoided in clinically evident congestive heart failure, it can be used with caution, if necessary, in patients with a history of fail-

ure who are well-compensated and are receiving digitalis and diuretics. Beta-adrenergic blocking agents do not abolish the inotropic action of digitalis on heart muscle.

IN PATIENTS WITHOUT A HISTORY OF CONGESTIVE HEART FAILURE, the use of beta-blockers can, in some instances, lead to congestive heart failure. Therefore, at the first sign or symptom of cardiac decompensation, discontinuation of beta-blocker therapy should be considered. The patient should be closely observed and treatment should include a diuretic and/or digitalization as necessary.

Exacerbation of Angina Pectoris Upon Withdrawal:

In patients with angina pectoris, exacerbation of angina and, in some cases, myocardial infarction have been reported following abrupt discontinuation of therapy with some beta-blockers. Therefore such patients should be cautioned against interruption of therapy without a physician's advice. The long persistence of beta-adrenergic blockade following abrupt discontinuation of CARTROL (carteolol hydrochloride), however, might be expected to minimize the possibility of this complication. When discontinuation of CARTROL (carteolol hydrochloride) is planned, dosage should be tapered gradually, as it is with other beta-blockers. If exacerbation of angina occurs when CARTROL (carteolol hydrochloride) therapy is interrupted, it is advisable to reinstitute CARTROL (carteolol hydrochloride) or other beta-blocker therapy, at least temporarily, and to take other measures appropriate for the management of unstable angina pectoris.

PATIENTS WITHOUT CLINICALLY RECOGNIZED ANGINA PECTORIS should be carefully monitored after withdrawal of CARTROL (carteolol hydrochloride) therapy, since coronary artery disease may be unrecognized.

Nonallergic Bronchospasm (e.g., chronic bronchitis, emphysema):

Patients with bronchospastic disease generally should not receive beta-blocker therapy and carteolol is contraindicated in patients with bronchial asthma. If use of CARTROL (carteolol hydrochloride) is essential, it should be administered with caution since it may block bronchodilation produced by endogenous catecholamine stimulation of $beta_2$-receptors or diminish response to therapy with a beta-receptor agonist.

Major Surgery:

The necessity, or desirability, of withdrawal of beta-blocking therapy prior to major surgery is controversial. Because beta-blockade impairs the ability of the heart to respond to reflex stimuli and may increase risks of general anesthesia and surgical procedures resulting in protracted hypotension or low cardiac output, and difficulty in restarting or maintaining a heartbeat, it has been suggested that beta-blocker therapy should be withdrawn several days prior to surgery. It is also recognized, however, that increased sensitivity to catecholamines of patients recently withdrawn from beta-blocker therapy could increase certain risks. Given the persistence of the beta-blocking activity of CARTROL (carteolol hydrochloride), effective withdrawal would take several weeks and would ordinarily be impractical. When beta-blocker therapy is not discontinued, anesthetic agents that depress the myocardium should be avoided. In one study using intravenous carteolol during surgery, recovery from anesthesia was somewhat delayed in three patients who received carteolol near the end of anesthesia, and respiratory arrest occurred in one of these patients immediately following administration of intravenous carteolol.

In the event that CARTROL (carteolol hydrochloride) treatment is not discontinued before surgery, the anesthesiologist should be informed that the patient is receiving CARTROL (carteolol hydrochloride). The effects on the heart of beta-adrenergic blocking agents, such as CARTROL (carteolol hydrochloride), may be reversed by cautious administration of isoproterenol or dobutamine.

Diabetes Mellitus and Hypoglycemia:

Beta-adrenergic blockade may prevent the appearance of premonitory signs and symptoms (e.g., tachycardia and blood pressure changes) of acute hypoglycemia, and it inhibits glycogenolysis, a normal compensatory mechanism for hypoglycemia. This is especially important for patients with labile diabetes mellitus. Beta-blockade also reduces the release of insulin in response to hyperglycemia; therefore, it may be necessary to adjust the dose of antidiabetic agents used to treat hyperglycemia.

Thyrotoxicosis:

Beta-adrenergic blockade may mask certain clinical signs of hyperthyroidism such as tachycardia. Patients suspected of having thyrotoxicosis should be managed carefully to avoid abrupt withdrawal of beta-adrenergic blockade which might precipitate a thyroid storm.

PRECAUTIONS

General:

Impaired Renal Function:

CARTROL (carteolol hydrochloride) should be used with caution in patients with impaired renal function. Patients with impaired renal function clear carteolol at a reduced rate, and dosage should be reduced accordingly (see Dosage and Administration).

Beta-adrenoreceptor blockade can cause reduction in intraocular pressure. Therefore, CARTROL (carteolol hydrochloride) may interfere with glaucoma testing. Withdrawal may lead to a return of increased intraocular pressure.

Information for Patients:

Patients, especially those with evidence of coronary artery insufficiency, should be warned against interruption or discontinuation of CARTROL (carteolol hydrochloride) therapy without the physician's advice. Although cardiac failure rarely occurs in properly selected patients, patients being treated with beta-adrenergic blocking agents should be advised to consult the physician at the first sign or symptom of impending failure (i.e., fatigue with exertion, difficulty breathing, cough or unusually fast heartbeat).

Drug Interactions:

Catecholamine-depleting drugs (e.g., reserpine) may have an additive effect when given with beta-blocking agents. Therefore, patients treated with CARTROL (carteolol hydrochloride) plus a catecholamine-depleting agent must be observed carefully for evidence of hypotension and/or excessive bradycardia, which may produce syncope or postural hypotension.

Risk of Anaphylactic Reaction: While taking beta-blockers, patients with a history of severe anaphylactic reaction to a variety of allergens may be more reactive to repeated challenge, either accidental, diagnostic, or therapeutic. Such patients may be unresponsive to the usual doses of epinephrine used to treat allergic reaction.

Concurrent administration of *general anesthetics* and beta-blocking agents may result in exaggeration of the hypotension induced by general anesthetics (see WARNINGS, Major Surgery).

Blunting of the antihypertensive effect of beta-adrenoreceptor blocking agents by *non-steroidal anti-inflammatory drugs* has been reported. When using these agents concomitantly, patients should be observed carefully to confirm that the desired therapeutic effect has been obtained.

Literature reports suggest that *oral calcium antagonists* may be used in combination with beta-adrenergic blocking agents when heart function is normal, but should be avoided in patients with impaired cardiac function. Hypotension, AV conduction disturbances, and left ventricular failure have been reported in some patients receiving beta-adrenergic blocking agents when an oral calcium antagonist was added to the treatment regimen. Hypotension was more likely to occur if the calcium antagonist were a dihydropyridine derivative, e.g., nifedipine, while left ventricular failure and AV conduction disturbances were more likely to occur with either verapamil or diltiazem.

Intravenous calcium antagonists should be used with caution in patients receiving beta-adrenergic blocking agents. The concomitant use of beta-adrenergic blocking agents with digitalis and either diltiazem or verapamil may have additive effects in prolonging AV conduction time.

Concomitant use of oral antidiabetic agents or *insulin* with beta-blocking agents may be associated with hypoglycemia or possibly hyperglycemia. Dosage of the antidiabetic agent should be adjusted accordingly (see WARNINGS, Diabetes Mellitus and Hypoglycemia).

Carcinogenesis, Mutagenesis, Impairment of Fertility:

CARTROL (carteolol hydrochloride) did not produce carcinogenic effects at doses 280 times the maximum recommended human dose (10 mg/70 kg/day) in two-year oral rat and mouse studies.

Tests of mutagenicity, including the Ames Test, recombinant (rec)-assay, *in vivo* cytogenetics and dominant lethal assay demonstrated no evidence for mutagenic potential.

Fertility of male and female rats and male and female mice was unaffected by administration of CARTROL (carteolol hydrochloride) at dosages up to 150 mg/kg/day. This dosage is approximately 1052 times the maximum recommended human dose.

Pregnancy:

Teratogenic Effects: Pregnancy Category C. CARTROL (carteolol hydrochloride) increased resorptions and decreased fetal weights in rabbits and rats at maternally toxic doses approximately 1052 and 5264 times the maximum recommended human dose (10 mg/70 kg/day), respectively. A dose-related increase in wavy ribs was noted in the developing rat fetus when pregnant females received daily doses of approximately 212 times the maximum recommended human dose. No such effects were noted in pregnant mice subjected to up to 1052 times the maximum recommended human dose. There are no adequate and well-controlled studies in pregnant women. CARTROL (carteolol hydrochloride) should be used during pregnancy only if the potential benefit justifies the potential risk to the fetus.

Nursing Mothers:

Studies have not been conducted in lactating humans and, therefore, it is not known whether carteolol is excreted in human milk. Studies in lactating rats indicate that CARTROL (carteolol hydrochloride) is excreted in milk. Because many drugs are excreted in human milk, caution should be exercised when CARTROL (carteolol hydrochloride) is administered to a nursing woman.

Pediatric Use:
Safety and effectiveness in children have not been established.

ADVERSE REACTIONS

The prevalence of adverse reactions has been ascertained from clinical studies conducted primarily in the United States. All adverse experiences (events) reported during these studies were recorded as adverse reactions. The prevalence rates presented below are based on combined data from nineteen placebo-controlled studies of patients with hypertension, angina or dysrhythmias, using once-daily carteolol at doses up to 60 mg. Table 1 summarizes those adverse experiences reported for patients in these studies where the prevalence in the carteolol group is 1% or greater and exceeds the prevalence in the placebo group. Asthenia and muscle cramps were the only symptoms that were significantly more common in patients receiving carteolol than in patients receiving placebo. Patients in clinical trials were carefully selected to exclude those, such as patients with asthma or known bronchospasm, or congestive heart failure, who would be at high risk of experiencing beta-adrenergic blocker adverse effect (See WARNINGS and CONTRAINDICATIONS):

TABLE 1
Adverse Reactions During
Placebo-Controlled Studies

	Placebo (n=448) %	Carteolol (n=761) %
Body as a Whole		
†Asthenia	4.0	7.1*
Abdominal Pain	0.4	1.3
Back Pain	1.6	2.1
Chest Pain	1.8	2.2
Digestive System		
Diarrhea	2.0	2.1
Nausea	1.8	2.1
Metabolic/Nutritional Disorders		
Abnormal Lab Test	1.1	1.2
Peripheral Edema	1.1	1.7
Musculoskeletal System		
Arthralgia	1.1	1.2
Muscle Cramps	0.2	2.6*
Lower Extremity Pain	0.2	1.2
Nervous System		
Insomnia	0.7	1.7
Paresthesia	1.1	2.0
Respiratory System		
Nasal Congestion	0.9	1.1
Pharyngitis	0.9	1.1
Skin and Appendages		
Rash	1.1	1.3

† Includes weakness, tiredness, lassitude and fatigue.
* Statistically significant at p=0.05 level.

The adverse experiences were usually mild or moderate in intensity and transient, but sometimes were serious enough to interrupt treatment. The adverse reactions that were most bothersome, as judged by their being reported as reasons for discontinuation of therapy by at least 0.4% of the carteolol group are shown in Table 2.

TABLE 2
Discontinuations During
Placebo-Controlled Studies

	Placebo (n=448) %	Carteolol (n=761) %
Body as a Whole		
Asthenia	0.2	0.5
Headache	0.7	0.7
Chest Pain	0.2	0.4
Skin and Appendages		
Rash	0.0	0.4
Sweating	0.2	0.4
Digestive System		
Nausea	0.0	0.4
Overall Adverse Reactions	4.2	3.3

Additional adverse reactions have been reported, but these are, in general, not distinguishable from symptoms that might have occurred in the absence of exposure to carteolol. The following additional adverse reactions were reported by at least 1% of 1568 patients who received carteolol in controlled or open, short- or long-term clinical studies, or represent less common, but potentially important, reactions reported in clinical studies or marketing experience (these rarer reactions are shown in italics): *Body as a Whole:* fever, infection, injury, malaise, pain, neck pain, shoulder pain; *Cardiovascular System:* angina pectoris, arrhythmia, *heart failure,* palpitations, *second degree heart block,* vasodilation; *Digestive System:* acute hepatitis with jaundice, constipa-

tion, dyspepsia, flatulence, gastrointestinal disorder; *Metabolic/Nutritional Disorder:* gout; *Musculoskeletal System:* pain in extremity, joint disorder, arthritis; *Nervous System:* abnormal dreams, anxiety, depression, dizziness, nervousness, somnolence; *Respiratory System:* bronchitis, *bronchospasm,* cold symptoms, cough, dyspnea, flu symptoms, lung disorder, rhinitis, sinusitis, *wheezing; Skin and Appendages:* sweating; *Special Senses:* blurred vision, conjunctivitis, eye disorder, tinnitus; *Urogenital:* impotence, urinary frequency, urinary tract infection.

In studies of patients with hypertension or angina pectoris where carteolol and positive reference beta-adrenergic blocking agents [nadolol (n=82) and propranolol (n=50)] have been compared, the differences in prevalence rates between the carteolol group and the reference agent group were statistically significant (p≤0.05) for the adverse reactions listed in Table 3.

TABLE 3
Adverse Reactions During
Positive-Controlled Studies

	Reference Agents (n=132) %	Carteolol (n=135) %
Body as a Whole		
Chest Pain	5.3	0.7
Cardiovascular System		
Bradycardia	4.5	0.0
Digestive System		
Diarrhea	11.4	4.4
Nervous System		
Somnolence	0.8	7.4
Skin and Appendages		
Sweating	5.3	0.7

POTENTIAL ADVERSE REACTIONS

In addition, other adverse reactions not listed above have been reported with other beta-adrenergic blocking agents and should be considered potential adverse reactions of CARTROL (carteolol hydrochloride).
Body as a Whole:
Fever combined with aching and sore throat.
Cardiovascular System:
Intensification of AV block. (See *CONTRAINDICATIONS*).
Digestive System:
Mesenteric arterial thrombosis, ischemic colitis.
Hemic/Lymphatic System:
Agranurocytosis, thrombocytopenic and nonthrombocytopenic purpura.
Nervous System:
Reversible mental depression progressing to catatonia; an acute reversible syndrome characterized by disorientation to time and place, short-term memory loss, emotional lability, slightly clouded sensorium, and decreased performance on neuropsychometric testing.
Respiratory System: Laryngospasm, respiratory distress.
Skin and Appendages: Erythematous rash, reversible alopecia.
Urogenital System: Peyronie's disease.
The oculomucocutaneous syndrome associated with the beta-adrenergic blocking agent practolol has not been reported with carteolol.

OVERDOSAGE

No specific information on emergency treatment of overdosage in humans is available. The most common effects expected with overdosage of a beta-adrenergic blocking agent are bradycardia, bronchospasm, congestive heart failure and hypotension.
In case of overdosage, treatment with CARTROL (carteolol hydrochloride) should be discontinued and gastric lavage considered. The patient should be closely observed and vital signs carefully monitored. The prolonged effects of carteolol must be considered when determining the duration of corrective therapy. On the basis of the pharmacologic profile, the following additional measures should be considered as appropriate.
Symptomatic Bradycardia:
Administer atropine. If there is no response to vagal blockade, administer isoproterenol cautiously.
Bronchospasm:
Administer a beta₂-stimulating agent such as isoproterenol and/or a theophylline derivative.
Congestive Heart Failure:
Administer diuretics and digitalis glycosides as necessary.
Hypotension:
Administer vasopressors such as intravenous dopamine, epinephrine or norepinephrine bitartrate.

DOSAGE AND ADMINISTRATION

Dosage must be individualized. The initial dose of CARTROL (carteolol hydrochloride) is 2.5 mg given as a single daily oral dose either alone or added to diuretic therapy. If an adequate response is not achieved, the dose can be

gradually increased to 5 mg and 10 mg as single daily doses. Increasing the dose above 10 mg per day is unlikely to produce further substantial benefits and, in fact, may decrease the response. The usual maintenance dose of carteolol is 2.5 or 5 mg once daily.
Dosage Adjustment in Renal Impairment:
Carteolol is excreted principally by the kidneys. When administering CARTROL (carteolol hydrochloride) to patients with renal impairment, the dosage regimen should be adjusted individually by the physician. Guidelines for dose interval adjustment are shown below:

Creatinine Clearance (mL/min)	Dosage Interval (hours)
>60	24
20–60	48
<20	72

HOW SUPPLIED

CARTROL (carteolol hydrochloride) is supplied as:
2.5 mg gray tablets:
Bottles of 100 .... (NDC 0074-1664-13).
5 mg white tablets:
Bottles of 100 .... (NDC 0074-1665-13).
Recommended storage: Store under controlled room temperature, 59°–86°F (15°–30°C).
Revised: February, 1992
Ref. 01-2531-R3

CEFOL® Filmtab® Tablets ℞
[c 'full]
(B-Complex, Folic Acid, Vitamin E with 750 mg Vitamin C)

DESCRIPTION

Each oral tablet provides:
Ascorbic Acid (C) (as sodium ascorbate) .... 750 mg
Niacinamide .... 100 mg
Calcium Pantothenate .... 20 mg
Thiamine Mononitrate (B₁) .... 15 mg
Riboflavin (B₂) .... 10 mg
Pyridoxine Hydrochloride (B₆) .... 5 mg
Folic Acid .... 500 mcg
Cyanocobalamin (B₁₂) .... 6 mcg
Vitamin E (as dl-alpha tocopheryl acetate) .... 30 IU
Inactive Ingredients: Cellulosic polymers, colloidal silicon dioxide, corn starch, D&C Yellow No. 10, FD&C Blue No. 1, magnesium stearate, microcrystalline cellulose, polyethylene glycol, povidone, titanium dioxide, and vanillin.

CLINICAL PHARMACOLOGY

The vitamin components of Cefol are absorbed by the active transport process. All but Vitamin E are rapidly eliminated and not stored in the body. Vitamin E is stored in body tissues.

INDICATIONS AND USAGE

Indicated in non-pregnant* adults for treatment of Vitamin C deficiency states with associated deficient intake or increased need for Vitamin B-Complex, Folic Acid, and Vitamin E.

*Pregnancy may require greater Folic Acid intake.

CONTRAINDICATIONS

Rare hypersensitivity to Folic Acid.

WARNINGS

Folic Acid alone is improper treatment of pernicious anemia and other megaloblastic anemias where Vitamin B₁₂ is deficient.

PRECAUTIONS

Folic Acid above 0.1 mg daily may obscure pernicious anemia (hematologic remission may occur while neurological manifestations remain progressive).

ADVERSE REACTIONS

Allergic sensitization has been reported following oral and parenteral administration of Folic Acid.

DOSAGE

Usual adult dose is one tablet daily.

HOW SUPPLIED

Green tablets in bottles of 100.
Filmtab—Film-sealed tablets, Abbott.
Store below 77°F (25°C).
Ref. 03-2062-3/R24

Continued on next page

CYLERT® Ⓒ℞

[*cī 'lert*]
(PEMOLINE)

DESCRIPTION

CYLERT (pemoline) is a central nervous system stimulant. Pemoline is structurally dissimilar to the amphetamines and methylphenidate.
It is an oxazolidine compound and is chemically identified as 2-amino-5-phenyl-2-oxazolin-4-one. Pemoline has the following structural formula:

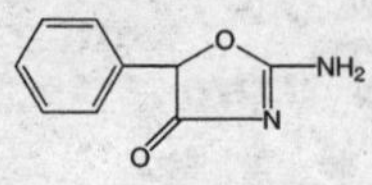

Pemoline is a white, tasteless, odorless powder, relatively insoluble (less than 1 mg/mL) in water, chloroform, ether, acetone, and benzene; its solubility in 95% ethyl alcohol is 2.2 mg/mL.
CYLERT (pemoline) is supplied as tablets containing 18.75 mg, 37.5 mg or 75 mg of pemoline for oral administration. CYLERT is also available as chewable tablets containing 37.5 mg of pemoline.

Inactive Ingredients

18.75 mg tablet: corn starch, gelatin, lactose, magnesium hydroxide, polyethylene glycol and talc.
37.5 mg tablet: corn starch, FD&C Yellow No. 6, gelatin, lactose, magnesium hydroxide, polyethylene glycol and talc.
37.5 mg chewable tablet: corn starch, FD&C Yellow No. 6, magnesium hydroxide, magnesium stearate, mannitol, polyethylene glycol, povidone, talc and artificial flavor.
75 mg tablet: corn starch, gelatin, iron oxide, lactose, magnesium hydroxide, polyethylene glycol and talc.

CLINICAL PHARMACOLOGY

CYLERT (pemoline) has a pharmacological activity similar to that of other known central nervous system stimulants; however, it has minimal sympathomimetic effects. Although studies indicate that pemoline may act in animals through dopaminergic mechanisms, the exact mechanism and site of action of the drug in man is not known.
There is neither specific evidence which clearly establishes the mechanism whereby CYLERT produces its mental and behavioral effects in children, nor conclusive evidence regarding how these effects relate to the condition of the central nervous system.
Pemoline is rapidly absorbed from the gastrointestinal tract. Approximately 50% is bound to plasma proteins. The serum half-life of pemoline is approximately 12 hours. Peak serum levels of the drug occur within 2 to 4 hours after ingestion of a single dose. Multiple dose studies in adults at several dose levels indicate that steady state is reached in approximately 2 to 3 days. In animals given radiolabeled pemoline, the drug was widely and uniformly distributed throughout the tissues, including the brain.
Pemoline is metabolized by the liver. Metabolites of pemoline include pemoline conjugate, pemoline dione, mandelic acid, and unidentified polar compounds. CYLERT is excreted primarily by the kidneys with approximately 50% excreted unchanged and only minor fractions present as metabolites.
CYLERT (pemoline) has a gradual onset of action. Using the recommended schedule of dosage titration, significant clinical benefit may not be evident until the third or fourth week of drug administration.

INDICATIONS AND USAGE

CYLERT (pemoline) is indicated in Attention Deficit Hyperactivity Disorder (ADHD). Because of its association with life threatening hepatic failure, CYLERT should not ordinarily be considered as first line therapy for ADHD (see **WARNINGS**).
CYLERT (pemoline) therapy should be part of a total treatment program which typically includes other remedial measures (psychological, educational, social) for a stabilizing effect in children with a behavioral syndrome characterized by the following group of developmentally inappropriate symptoms: moderate to severe distractibility, short attention span, hyperactivity, emotional lability, and impulsivity. The diagnosis of this syndrome should not be made with finality when these symptoms are only of comparatively recent origin. Nonlocalizing (soft) neurological signs, learning disability, and abnormal EEG may or may not be present, and a diagnosis of central nervous system dysfunction may or may not be warranted.

CONTRAINDICATIONS

CYLERT (pemoline) is contraindicated in patients with known hypersensitivity or idiosyncrasy to the drug. CYLERT should not be administered to patients with impaired hepatic function (see **ADVERSE REACTIONS**).

WARNINGS

> Because of its association with life threatening hepatic failure, CYLERT should not ordinarily be considered as first line drug therapy for ADHD (see **INDICATIONS AND USAGE**).
> Since CYLERT's marketing in 1975, 13 cases of acute hepatic failure have been reported to the FDA. While the absolute number of reported cases is not large, the rate of reporting ranges from 4 to 17 times the rate expected in the general population. This estimate may be conservative because of under reporting and because the long latency between initiation of CYLERT treatment and the occurrence of hepatic failure may limit recognition of the association. If only a portion of actual cases were recognized and reported, the risk could be substantially higher.
> Of the 13 cases reported as of May 1996, 11 resulted in death or liver transplantation, usually within four weeks of the onset of signs and symptoms of liver failure. The earliest onset of hepatic abnormalities occurred six months after initiation of CYLERT. Although some reports described dark urine and nonspecific prodromal symptoms (e.g., anorexia, malaise, and gastrointestinal symptoms), in other reports it was not clear if any prodromal symptoms preceded the onset of jaundice. It is also not clear if the recommended baseline and periodic liver function testing are predictive of these instances of acute liver failure. CYLERT should be discontinued if clinically significant hepatic dysfunction is observed during its use (see **PRECAUTIONS**).

Decrements in the predicted growth (i.e., weight gain and/or height) rate have been reported with the long-term use of stimulants in children. Therefore, patients requiring long-term therapy should be carefully monitored.

PRECAUTIONS

General:
Clinical experience suggests that in psychotic children, administration of CYLERT may exacerbate symptoms of behavior disturbance and thought disorder.
CYLERT should be administered with caution to patients with significantly impaired renal function.
Laboratory Tests:
Since CYLERT's market introduction, there have been reports of elevated liver enzymes associated with its use. Many of these patients had this increase detected several months after starting CYLERT. Most patients were asymptomatic, with the increase in liver enzymes returning to normal after CYLERT was discontinued. Liver function tests should be performed prior to and periodically during therapy with CYLERT. Treatment with CYLERT should be initiated only in individuals without liver disease and with normal baseline liver function tests.
The relationship, if any, between reversible elevations in liver function tests and the occurrence of life threatening hepatic failure in patients on long-term therapy with CYLERT is not known. Liver function testing may not predict the onset of acute liver failure. Nonetheless, CYLERT should be discontinued if clinically significant liver function test abnormalities are revealed at any time during therapy with this drug (see **WARNINGS**).
Drug Interactions:
The interaction of CYLERT (pemoline) with other drugs has not been studied in humans. Patients who are receiving CYLERT concurrently with other drugs, especially drugs with CNS activity, should be monitored carefully.
Decreased seizure threshold has been reported in patients receiving CYLERT concomitantly with *antiepileptic medications.*
Carcinogenesis:
Long-term studies have been conducted in rats with doses as high as 150 mg/kg/day for eighteen months. There was no significant difference in the incidence of any neoplasm between treated and control animals.
Mutagenesis:
Data are not available concerning long-term effects on mutagenicity in animals or humans.
Impairment of Fertility:
The results of studies in which rats were given 18.75 and 37.5 mg/kg/day indicated that pemoline did not affect fertility in males or females at those doses.
Pregnancy:
Teratogenic effects: Pregnancy Category B. Reproduction studies have been performed in rats and rabbits at doses of 18.75 and 37.5 mg/kg/day and have revealed no evidence of impaired fertility or harm to the fetus. There are, however, no adequate and well-controlled studies in pregnant women. Because animal reproduction studies are not always predictive of human response, this drug should be used during pregnancy only if clearly needed.
Nonteratogenic effects:
Studies in rats have shown an increased incidence of stillbirths and cannibalization when pemoline was administered at a dose of 37.5 mg/kg/day. Postnatal survival of offspring was reduced at doses of 18.75 and 37.5 mg/kg/day.
Nursing Mothers:
It is not known whether this drug is excreted in human milk. Because many drugs are excreted in human milk, caution should be exercised when CYLERT is administered to a nursing woman.
Pediatric Use:
Safety and effectiveness in children below the age of 6 years have not been established.
Long-term effects of CYLERT in children have not been established (see **WARNINGS**).
CNS stimulants, including pemoline, have been reported to precipitate motor and phonic tics and Tourette's syndrome. Therefore, clinical evaluation for tics and Tourette's syndrome in children and their families should precede use of stimulant medications.
Drug treatment is not indicated in all cases of ADHD and should be considered only in light of complete history and evaluation of the child. The decision to prescribe CYLERT (pemoline) should depend on the physician's assessment of the chronicity and severity of the child's symptoms and their appropriateness for his/her age. Prescription should not depend solely on the presence of one or more of the behavioral characteristics.

ADVERSE REACTIONS

The following are adverse reactions in decreasing order of severity within each category associated with CYLERT:
Hepatic: There have been reports of hepatic dysfunction, ranging from asymptomatic reversible increases in liver enzymes to hepatitis, jaundice and life-threatening hepatic failure, in patients taking CYLERT (see **PRECAUTIONS** and **WARNINGS**).
Hematopoietic: There have been isolated reports of aplastic anemia.
Central Nervous System: The following CNS effects have been reported with the use of CYLERT: convulsive seizures; literature reports indicate that CYLERT may precipitate attacks of Gilles de la Tourette syndrome; hallucinations; dyskinetic movements of the tongue, lips, face and extremities; abnormal oculomotor function including nystagmus and oculogyric crisis; mild depression; dizziness; increased irritability; headache; and drowsiness.
Insomnia is the most frequently reported side effect of CYLERT; it usually occurs early in therapy prior to an optimum therapeutic response. In the majority of cases it is transient in nature or responds to a reduction in dosage.
Gastrointestinal: Anorexia and weight loss may occur during the first weeks of therapy. In the majority of cases it is transient in nature; weight gain usually resumes within three to six months.
Nausea and stomach ache have also been reported.
Genitourinary: A case of elevated acid phosphatase in association with prostatic enlargement has been reported in a 63 year old male who was treated with CYLERT for sleepiness. The acid phosphatase normalized with discontinuation of CYLERT and was again elevated with rechallenge.
Miscellaneous: Suppression of growth has been reported with the long-term use of stimulants in children. (See **WARNINGS**.) Skin rash has been reported with CYLERT.
Mild adverse reactions appearing early during the course of treatment with CYLERT often remit with continuing therapy. If adverse reactions are of a significant or protracted nature, dosage should be reduced or the drug discontinued.

DRUG ABUSE AND DEPENDENCE

Controlled Substance: CYLERT is subject to control under DEA schedule IV.
Abuse: CYLERT failed to demonstrate a potential for self-administration in primates. However, the pharmacologic similarity of pemoline to other psychostimulants with known dependence liability suggests that psychological and/or physical dependence might also occur with CYLERT. There have been isolated reports of transient psychotic symptoms occurring in adults following the long-term misuse of excessive oral doses of pemoline. CYLERT should be given with caution to emotionally unstable patients who may increase the dosage on their own initiative.

OVERDOSAGE

Signs and symptoms of acute overdosage, resulting principally from overstimulation of the central nervous system and from excessive sympathomimetic effects, may include the following: vomiting, agitation, tremors, hyperreflexia, muscle twitching, convulsions (may be followed by coma), euphoria, confusion, hallucinations, delirium, sweating, flushing, headache, hyperpyrexia, tachycardia, hypertension and mydriasis. Consult with a Certified Poison Control Center regarding treatment for up to date guidance and advice. Treatment consists of appropriate supportive measures. The patient must be protected against self-injury and against external stimuli that would aggravate overstimulation already present. Gastric contents may be evacuated by gastric lavage. Other measures to detoxify the gut include administration of activated charcoal and a cathartic. Chlor-

promazine has been reported in the literature to be useful in decreasing CNS stimulation and sympathomimetic effects. Efficacy of peritoneal dialysis or extracorporeal hemodialysis for CYLERT overdosage has not been established.

DOSAGE AND ADMINISTRATION

CYLERT (pemoline) is administered as a single oral dose each morning. The recommended starting dose is 37.5 mg/day. This daily dose should be gradually increased by 18.75 mg at one week intervals until the desired clinical response is obtained. The effective daily dose for most patients will range from 56.25 to 75 mg. The maximum recommended daily dose of pemoline is 112.5 mg.

Clinical improvement with CYLERT is gradual. Using the recommended schedule of dosage titration, significant benefit may not be evident until the third or fourth week of drug administration.

Where possible, drug administration should be interrupted occasionally to determine if there is a recurrence of behavioral symptoms sufficient to require continued therapy.

HOW SUPPLIED

CYLERT (pemoline) is supplied as monogrammed, grooved tablets in three dosage strengths:

18.75 mg tablets (white) in bottles of 100 (**NDC** 0074-6025-13);

37.5 mg tablets (orange-colored) in bottles of 100 (**NDC** 0074-6057-13);

75 mg tablets (tan-colored) in bottles of 100 (**NDC** 0074-6073-13).

CYLERT (pemoline) Chewable is supplied as 37.5 mg monogrammed, grooved tablets (orange-colored) in bottles of 100 (**NDC** 0074-6088-13).

Recommended Storage: Store below 86°F (30°C).

Revised: December, 1996

Ref. 03-4735-R18

ABBOTT LABORATORIES

NORTH CHICAGO, IL 60064, U.S.A.

Shown in Product Identification Guide, page 303

DEPACON™ ℞
VALPROATE SODIUM INJECTION

BOX WARNING:

HEPATIC FAILURE RESULTING IN FATALITIES HAS OCCURRED IN PATIENTS RECEIVING VALPROIC ACID AND ITS DERIVATIVES. EXPERIENCE HAS INDICATED THAT CHILDREN UNDER THE AGE OF TWO YEARS ARE AT A CONSIDERABLY INCREASED RISK OF DEVELOPING FATAL HEPATOTOXICITY, ESPECIALLY THOSE ON MULTIPLE ANTICONVULSANTS, THOSE WITH CONGENITAL METABOLIC DISORDERS, THOSE WITH SEVERE SEIZURE DISORDERS ACCOMPANIED BY MENTAL RETARDATION, AND THOSE WITH ORGANIC BRAIN DISEASE. WHEN DEPACON IS USED IN THIS PATIENT GROUP, IT SHOULD BE USED WITH EXTREME CAUTION AND AS A SOLE AGENT. THE BENEFITS OF THERAPY SHOULD BE WEIGHED AGAINST THE RISKS. ABOVE THIS AGE GROUP, EXPERIENCE IN EPILEPSY HAS INDICATED THAT THE INCIDENCE OF FATAL HEPATOTOXICITY DECREASES CONSIDERABLY IN PROGRESSIVELY OLDER PATIENT GROUPS.

THESE INCIDENTS USUALLY HAVE OCCURRED DURING THE FIRST SIX MONTHS OF TREATMENT. SERIOUS OR FATAL HEPATOTOXICITY MAY BE PRECEDED BY NON-SPECIFIC SYMPTOMS SUCH AS MALAISE, WEAKNESS, LETHARGY, FACIAL EDEMA, ANOREXIA, AND VOMITING. IN PATIENTS WITH EPILEPSY, A LOSS OF SEIZURE CONTROL MAY ALSO OCCUR. PATIENTS SHOULD BE MONITORED CLOSELY FOR APPEARANCE OF THESE SYMPTOMS. LIVER FUNCTION TESTS SHOULD BE PERFORMED PRIOR TO THERAPY AND AT FREQUENT INTERVALS THEREAFTER, ESPECIALLY DURING THE FIRST SIX MONTHS.

TERATOGENICITY:

VALPROATE CAN PRODUCE TERATOGENIC EFFECTS SUCH AS NEURAL TUBE DEFECTS (E.G., SPINA BIFIDA), ACCORDINGLY, THE USE OF VALPROATE PRODUCTS IN WOMEN OF CHILDBEARING POTENTIAL REQUIRES THAT THE BENEFITS OF ITS USE BE WEIGHED AGAINST THE RISK OF INJURY TO THE FETUS.

DESCRIPTION

Valproate sodium is the sodium salt of valproic acid designated as sodium 2-propylpentanoate. Valproate sodium has the following structure:

[See chemical structure at top of next column]

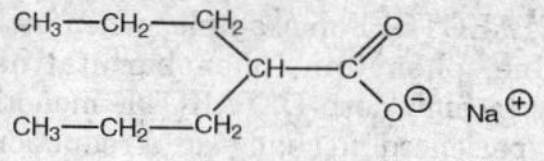

Valproate sodium has a molecular weight of 166.2. It occurs as an essentially white and odorless, crystalline, deliquescent powder.

DEPACON solution is available in 5 mL single-dose vials for intravenous injection. Each mL contains valproate sodium equivalent to 100 mg valproic acid, edetate disodium 0.40 mg, and water for injection to volume. The pH is adjusted to 7.6 with sodium hydroxide and/or hydrochloric acid. The solution is clear and colorless.

CLINICAL PHARMACOLOGY

DEPACON exists as the valproate ion in the blood. The mechanisms by which valproate exerts its therapeutic effects have not been established. It has been suggested that its activity in epilepsy is related to increased brain concentrations of gamma-aminobutyric acid (GABA).

Pharmacokinetics

Bioavailability

Equivalent doses of intravenous (IV) valproate and oral valproate products are expected to result in equivalent C_{max}, C_{min}, and total systemic exposure to the valproate ion. However, the rate of valproate ion absorption may vary with the formulation used. These differences should be of minor clinical importance under the steady state conditions achieved in chronic use in the treatment of epilepsy.

Administration of DEPAKOTE (divalproex sodium) tablets and IV valproate (given as a one hour infusion), 250 mg every 6 hours for 4 days to 18 healthy male volunteers resulted in equivalent AUC, C_{max}, C_{min} at steady state, as well as after the first dose. The T_{max} after IV DEPACON occurs at the end of the one hour infusion, while the T_{max} after oral dosing with DEPAKOTE occurs at approximately 4 hours. Because the kinetics of unbound valproate are linear, bioequivalence between DEPACON and DEPAKOTE up to the maximum recommended dose of 60 mg/kg/day can be assumed. The AUC and C_{max} resulting from administration of IV valproate 500 mg as a single one hour infusion and a single 500 mg dose of DEPAKENE syrup to 17 healthy male volunteers were also equivalent.

Patients maintained on valproic acid doses of 750 mg to 4250 mg daily (given in divided doses every 6 hours) as oral DEPAKOTE (divalproex sodium) alone (n=24) or with another stabilized antiepileptic drug [carbamazepine (n=15), phenytoin (n=11), or phenobarbital (n=1)], showed comparable plasma levels for valproic acid when switching from oral DEPAKOTE to IV valproate (1-hour infusion).

Distribution

Protein Binding:

The plasma protein binding of valproate is concentration dependent and the free fraction increases from approximately 10% at 40 μg/mL to 18.5% at 130 μg/mL. Protein binding of valproate is reduced in the elderly, in patients with chronic hepatic diseases, in patients with renal impairment, and in the presence of other drugs (e.g., aspirin). Conversely, valproate may displace certain protein-bound drugs (e.g., phenytoin, carbamazepine, warfarin, and tolbutamide). (See **PRECAUTIONS**, **Drug Interactions** for more detailed information on the pharmacokinetic interactions of valproate with other drugs.)

CNS Distribution:

Valproate concentrations in cerebrospinal fluid (CSF) approximate unbound concentrations in plasma (about 10% of total concentration).

Metabolism

Valproate is metabolized almost entirely by the liver. In adult patients on monotherapy, 30–50% of an administered dose appears in urine as a glucuronide conjugate. Mitochondrial β-oxidation is the other major metabolic pathway, typically accounting for over 40% of the dose. Usually, less than 15–20% of the dose is eliminated by other oxidative mechanisms. Less than 3% of an administered dose is excreted unchanged in urine.

The relationship between dose and total valproate concentration is nonlinear; concentration does not increase proportionally with the dose, but rather, increases to a lesser extent due to saturable plasma protein binding. The kinetics of unbound drug are linear.

Elimination

Mean plasma clearance and volume of distribution for total valproate are 0.56 L/hr/1.73 m^2 and 11 L/1.73 m^2, respectively. Mean terminal half-life for valproate monotherapy after a 60 minute intravenous infusion of 1000 mg was 16 ± 3.0 hours.

The estimates cited apply primarily to patients who are not taking drugs that affect hepatic metabolizing enzyme systems. For example, patients taking enzyme-inducing antiepileptic drugs (carbamazepine, phenytoin, and phenobarbital) will clear valproate more rapidly. Because of these changes in valproate clearance, monitoring of antiepileptic concentrations should be intensified whenever concomitant antiepileptics are introduced or withdrawn.

Special Populations

Effect of Age:

Neonates - Children within the first two months of life have a markedly decreased ability to eliminate valproate compared to older children and adults. This is a result of reduced clearance (perhaps due to delay in development of glucuronosyl transferase and other enzyme systems involved in valproate elimination) as well as increased volume of distribution (in part due to decreased plasma protein binding). For example, in one study, the half-life in children under 10 days ranged from 10 to 67 hours compared to a range of 7 to 13 hours in children greater than 2 months.

Children - Pediatric patients (i.e., between 3 months and 10 years) have 50% higher clearances expressed on weight (i.e., mL/min/kg) than do adults. Over the age of 10 years, children have pharmacokinetic parameters that approximate those of adults.

Elderly - The capacity of elderly patients (age range: 68 to 89 years) to eliminate valproate has been shown to be reduced compared to younger adults (age range: 22 to 26). Intrinsic clearance is reduced by 39%; the free fraction is increased by 44%. Accordingly, the initial dosage should be reduced in the elderly. (See **DOSAGE AND ADMINISTRATION**).

Effect of Gender:

There are no differences in the body surface area adjusted unbound clearance between males and females (4.8±0.17 and 4.7±0.07 L/hr per 1.73 m^2, respectively).

Effect of Race:

The effects of race on the kinetics of valproate have not been studied.

Effect of Disease:

Liver Disease - (See **BOXED WARNING**, **CONTRAINDICATIONS**, and **WARNINGS**). Liver disease impairs the capacity to eliminate valproate. In one study, the clearance of free valproate was decreased by 50% in 7 patients with cirrhosis and by 16% in 4 patients with acute hepatitis, compared with 6 healthy subjects. In that study, the half-life of valproate was increased from 12 to 18 hours. Liver disease is also associated with decreased albumin concentrations and larger unbound fractions (2 to 2.6 fold increase) of valproate. Accordingly, monitoring of total concentrations may be misleading since free concentrations may be substantially elevated in patients with hepatic disease whereas total concentrations may appear to be normal.

Renal Disease - A slight reduction (27%) in the unbound clearance of valproate has been reported in patients with renal failure (creatinine clearance < 10 mL/minute); however, hemodialysis typically reduces valproate concentrations by about 20%. Therefore, no dosage adjustment appears to be necessary in patients with renal failure. Protein binding in these patients is substantially reduced; thus, monitoring total concentrations may be misleading.

Plasma Levels and Clinical Effect

The relationship between plasma concentration and clinical response is not well documented. One contributing factor is the nonlinear, concentration dependent protein binding of valproate which affects the clearance of the drug. Thus, monitoring of total serum valproate cannot provide a reliable index of the bioactive valproate species.

For example, because the plasma protein binding of valproate is concentration dependent, the free fraction increases from approximately 10% at 40 μg/mL to 18.5% at 130 μg/mL. Higher than expected free fractions occur in the elderly, in hyperlipidemic patients, and in patients with hepatic and renal diseases.

Epilepsy:

The therapeutic range in epilepsy is commonly considered to be 50 to 100 μg/mL of total valproate, although some patients may be controlled with lower or higher plasma concentrations.

Equivalent doses of DEPACON and DEPAKOTE (divalproex sodium) yield equivalent plasma levels of the valproate ion (see **CLINICAL PHARMACOLOGY**, **Pharmacokinetics**).

Clinical Studies

The studies described in the following section were conducted with oral divalproex sodium products.

Epilepsy

The efficacy of DEPAKOTE (divalproex sodium) in reducing the incidence of complex partial seizures (CPS) that occur in isolation or in association with other seizure types was established in two controlled trials.

In one, multiclinic, placebo controlled study employing an add-on design (adjunctive therapy), 144 patients who continued to suffer eight or more CPS per 8 weeks during an 8 week period of monotherapy with doses of either carbamazepine or phenytoin sufficient to assure plasma concentrations within the "therapeutic range" were randomized to receive, in addition to their original antiepilepsy drug (AED), either DEPAKOTE or placebo. Randomized patients were to be followed for a total of 16 weeks. The following table presents the findings.

Continued on next page

Depacon—Cont.

Adjunctive Therapy Study
Median Incidence of CPS per 8 Weeks

Add-on Treatment	Number of Patients	Baseline Incidence	Experimental Incidence
DEPAKOTE	75	16.0	8.9*
Placebo	69	14.5	11.5

* Reduction from baseline statistically significantly greater for DEPAKOTE than placebo at p ≤ 0.05 level.

Figure 1 presents the proportion of patients (X axis) whose percentage reduction from baseline in complex partial seizure rates was at least as great as that indicated on the Y axis in the adjunctive therapy study. A positive percent reduction indicates an improvement (i.e., a decrease in seizure frequency), while a negative percent reduction indicates worsening. Thus, in a display of this type, the curve for an effective treatment is shifted to the left of the curve for placebo. This figure shows that the proportion of patients achieving any particular level of improvement was consistently higher for DEPAKOTE than for placebo. For example, 45% of patients treated with DEPAKOTE had a ≥ 50% reduction in complex partial seizure rate compared to 23% of patients treated with placebo.

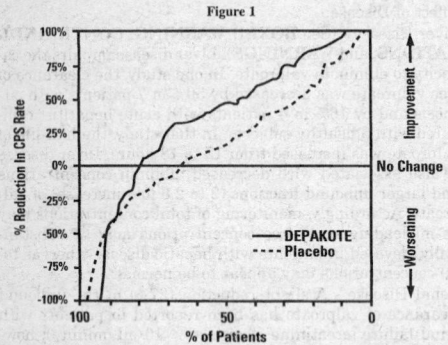

Figure 1

The second study assessed the capacity of DEPAKOTE to reduce the incidence of CPS when administered as the sole AED. The study compared the incidence of CPS among patients randomized to either a high or low dose treatment arm. Patients qualified for entry into the randomized comparison phase of this study only if 1) they continued to experience 2 or more CPS per 4 weeks during an 8 to 12 week long period of monotherapy with adequate doses of an AED (i.e., phenytoin, carbamazepine, phenobarbital, or primidone) and 2) they made a successful transition over a two week interval to DEPAKOTE. Patients entering the randomized phase were then brought to their assigned target dose, gradually tapered off their concomitant AED and followed for an interval as long as 22 weeks. Less than 50% of the patients randomized, however, completed the study. In patients converted to DEPAKOTE monotherapy, the mean total valproate concentrations during monotherapy were 71 and 123 µg/mL in the low dose and high dose groups, respectively.

The following table presents the findings for all patients randomized who had at least one post-randomization assessment.

Monotherapy Study
Median Incidence of CPS per 8 Weeks

Treatment	Number of Patients	Baseline Incidence	Randomized Phase Incidence
High dose DEPAKOTE	131	13.2	10.7*
Low dose DEPAKOTE	134	14.2	13.8

* Reduction from baseline statistically significantly greater for high dose than low dose at p ≤ 0.05 level.

Figure 2 presents the proportion of patients (X axis) whose percentage reduction from baseline in complex partial seizure rates was at least as great as that indicated on the Y axis in the monotherapy study. A positive percent reduction indicates an improvement (i.e., a decrease in seizure frequency), while a negative percent reduction indicates worsening. Thus, in a display of this type, the curve for a more effective treatment is shifted to the left of the curve for a less effective treatment. This figure shows that the proportion of patients achieving any particular level of reduction was consistently higher for high dose DEPAKOTE than for

low dose DEPAKOTE. For example, when switching from carbamazepine, phenytoin, phenobarbital or primidone monotherapy to high dose DEPAKOTE monotherapy, 63% of patients experienced no change or a reduction in complex partial seizure rates compared to 54% of patients receiving low dose DEPAKOTE.

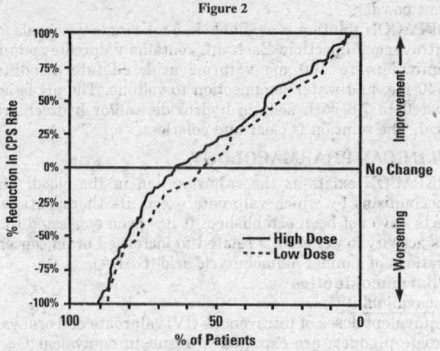

Figure 2

INDICATIONS AND USAGE

DEPACON is indicated as an intravenous alternative in patients for whom oral administration of valproate products is temporarily not feasible in the following conditions:
DEPACON is indicated as monotherapy and adjunctive therapy in the treatment of patients with complex partial seizures that occur either in isolation or in association with other types of seizures. DEPACON is also indicated for use as sole and adjunctive therapy in the treatment of patients with simple and complex absence seizures, and adjunctively in patients with multiple seizure types that include absence seizures.
Simple absence is defined as very brief clouding of the sensorium or loss of consciousness accompanied by certain generalized epileptic discharges without other detectable clinical signs. Complex absence is the term used when other signs are also present.
SEE **WARNINGS** FOR STATEMENT REGARDING FATAL HEPATIC DYSFUNCTION.

CONTRAINDICATIONS

VALPROATE SODIUM INJECTION SHOULD NOT BE ADMINISTERED TO PATIENTS WITH HEPATIC DISEASE OR SIGNIFICANT HEPATIC DYSFUNCTION.
Valproate sodium injection is contraindicated in patients with known hypersensitivity to the drug.

WARNINGS

Hepatic failure resulting in fatalities has occurred in patients receiving valproic acid. These incidents usually have occurred during the first six months of treatment. Serious or fatal hepatotoxicity may be preceded by non-specific symptoms such as malaise, weakness, lethargy, facial edema, anorexia, and vomiting. In patients with epilepsy, a loss of seizure control may also occur. Patients should be monitored closely for appearance of these symptoms. Liver function tests should be performed prior to therapy and at frequent intervals thereafter, especially during the first six months of valproate therapy. However, physicians should not rely totally on serum biochemistry since these tests may not be abnormal in all instances, but should also consider the results of careful interim medical history and physical examination.
Caution should be observed when administering valproate products to patients with a prior history of hepatic disease. Patients on multiple anticonvulsants, children, those with congenital metabolic disorders, those with severe seizure disorders accompanied by mental retardation, and those with organic brain disease may be at particular risk. Experience has indicated that children under the age of two years are at a considerably increased risk of developing fatal hepatotoxicity, especially those with the aforementioned conditions. When DEPACON is used in this patient group, it should be used with extreme caution and as a sole agent. The benefits of therapy should be weighed against the risks. Use of DEPACON has not been studied in children below the age of 2 years. Above this age group, experience with valproate products in epilepsy has indicated that the incidence of fatal hepatotoxicity decreases considerably in progressively older patient groups.
The drug should be discontinued immediately in the presence of significant hepatic dysfunction, suspected or apparent. In some cases, hepatic dysfunction has progressed in spite of discontinuation of drug.
The frequency of adverse effects (particularly elevated liver enzymes and thrombocytopenia [see **PRECAUTIONS**]) may be dose-related. In a clinical trial of DEPAKOTE as monotherapy in patients with epilepsy, 34/126 patients (27%) receiving approximately 50 mg/kg/day on average, had at least one value of platelets ≤ 75 × 10⁹/L. Approximately half of these patients had treatment discontinued,

with return of platelet counts to normal. In the remaining patients, platelet counts normalized with continued treatment. In this study, the probability of thrombocytopenia appeared to increase significantly at total valproate concentrations of ≥ 110 µg/mL (females) or ≥ 135 µg/mL (males). The therapeutic benefit which may accompany the higher doses should therefore be weighed against the possibility of a greater incidence of adverse effects.
A study was conducted to evaluate the effect of IV valproate in the prevention of post-traumatic seizures in patients with acute head injuries. Patients were randomly assigned to receive either IV valproate given for one week (followed by oral valproate products for either one or six months per random treatment assignment) or IV phenytoin given for one week (followed by placebo). In this study, the incidence of death was found to be higher in the two groups assigned to valproate treatment compared to the rate in those assigned to the IV phenytoin treatment group (13% vs 8.5%, respectively). Many of these patients were critically ill with multiple and/or severe injuries, and evaluation of the causes of death did not suggest any specific drug-related causation. Further, in the absence of a concurrent placebo control during the initial week of intravenous therapy, it is impossible to determine if the mortality rate in the patients treated with valproate was greater or less than that expected in a similar group not treated with valproate, or whether the rate seen in the IV phenytoin treated patients was lower than would be expected. Nonetheless, until further information is available, it seems prudent not to use DEPACON in patients with acute head trauma for the prophylaxis of post-traumatic seizures.
Usage In Pregnancy
ACCORDING TO PUBLISHED AND UNPUBLISHED REPORTS, VALPROIC ACID MAY PRODUCE TERATOGENIC EFFECTS IN THE OFFSPRING OF HUMAN FEMALES RECEIVING THE DRUG DURING PREGNANCY. THERE ARE MULTIPLE REPORTS IN THE CLINICAL LITERATURE WHICH INDICATE THAT THE USE OF ANTIEPILEPSY DRUGS DURING PREGNANCY RESULTS IN AN INCREASED INCIDENCE OF BIRTH DEFECTS IN THE OFFSPRING. ALTHOUGH DATA ARE MORE EXTENSIVE WITH RESPECT TO TRIMETHADIONE, PARAMETHADIONE, PHENYTOIN, AND PHENOBARBITAL, REPORTS INDICATE A POSSIBLE SIMILAR ASSOCIATION WITH THE USE OF OTHER ANTIEPILEPSY DRUGS. THEREFORE, ANTIEPILEPSY DRUGS SHOULD BE ADMINISTERED TO WOMEN OF CHILDBEARING POTENTIAL ONLY IF THEY ARE CLEARLY SHOWN TO BE ESSENTIAL IN THE MANAGEMENT OF THEIR SEIZURES.
THE INCIDENCE OF NEURAL TUBE DEFECTS IN THE FETUS MAY BE INCREASED IN MOTHERS RECEIVING VALPROATE DURING THE FIRST TRIMESTER OF PREGNANCY. THE CENTERS FOR DISEASE CONTROL (CDC) HAS ESTIMATED THE RISK OF VALPROIC ACID EXPOSED WOMEN HAVING CHILDREN WITH SPINA BIFIDA TO BE APPROXIMATELY 1 TO 2%.
OTHER CONGENITAL ANOMALIES (E.G., CRANIOFACIAL DEFECTS, CARDIOVASCULAR MALFORMATIONS AND ANOMALIES INVOLVING VARIOUS BODY SYSTEMS), COMPATIBLE AND INCOMPATIBLE WITH LIFE, HAVE BEEN REPORTED. SUFFICIENT DATA TO DETERMINE THE INCIDENCE OF THESE CONGENITAL ANOMALIES IS NOT AVAILABLE.
THE HIGHER INCIDENCE OF CONGENITAL ANOMALIES IN ANTIEPILEPSY DRUG-TREATED WOMEN WITH SEIZURE DISORDERS CANNOT BE REGARDED AS A CAUSE AND EFFECT RELATIONSHIP. THERE ARE INTRINSIC METHODOLOGIC PROBLEMS IN OBTAINING ADEQUATE DATA ON DRUG TERATOGENICITY IN HUMANS; GENETIC FACTORS OR THE EPILEPTIC CONDITION ITSELF, MAY BE MORE IMPORTANT THAN DRUG THERAPY IN CONTRIBUTING TO CONGENITAL ANOMALIES.
PATIENTS TAKING VALPROATE MAY DEVELOP CLOTTING ABNORMALITIES. A PATIENT WHO HAD LOW FIBRINOGEN WHEN TAKING MULTIPLE ANTICONVULSANTS INCLUDING VALPROATE GAVE BIRTH TO AN INFANT WITH AFIBRINOGENEMIA WHO SUBSEQUENTLY DIED OF HEMORRHAGE. IF VALPROATE IS USED IN PREGNANCY, THE CLOTTING PARAMETERS SHOULD BE MONITORED CAREFULLY.
HEPATIC FAILURE, RESULTING IN THE DEATH OF A NEWBORN AND OF AN INFANT, HAVE BEEN REPORTED FOLLOWING THE USE OF VALPROATE DURING PREGNANCY.
Animal studies have demonstrated valproate-induced teratogenicity. Increased frequencies of malformations, as well as intrauterine growth retardation and death, have been observed in mice, rats, rabbits, and monkeys following prenatal exposure to valproate. Malformations of the skeletal system are the most common structural abnormalities produced in experimental animals, but neural tube closure defects have been seen in mice exposed to maternal plasma valproate concentrations exceeding 230 µg/mL (2.3 times the upper limit of the human therapeutic range) during sus-

ceptible periods of embryonic development. Administration of an oral dose of 200 mg/kg/day or greater (50% of the maximum human daily dose or greater on a mg/m^2 basis) to pregnant rats during organogenesis produced malformations (skeletal, cardiac, and urogenital) and growth retardation in the offspring. These doses resulted in peak maternal plasma valproate levels of approximately 340 µg/mL or greater (3.4 times the upper limit of the human therapeutic range or greater). Behavioral deficits have been reported in the offspring of rats given a dose of 200 mg/kg/day throughout most of pregnancy. An oral dose of 350 mg/kg/day (2 times the maximum human daily dose on a mg/m^2 basis) produced skeletal and visceral malformations in rabbits exposed during organogenesis. Skeletal malformations, growth retardation, and death were observed in rhesus monkeys following administration of an oral dose of 200 mg/kg/day (equal to the maximum human daily dose on a mg/m^2 basis) during organogenesis. This dose resulted in peak maternal plasma valproate levels of approximately 280 µg/mL (2.8 times the upper limit of the human therapeutic range).

The prescribing physician will wish to weigh the benefits of therapy against the risks in treating or counseling women of childbearing potential. If this drug is used during pregnancy, or if the patient becomes pregnant while taking this drug, the patient should be apprised of the potential hazard to the fetus.

Antiepilepsy drugs should not be discontinued abruptly in patients in whom the drug is administered to prevent major seizures because of the strong possibility of precipitating status epilepticus with attendant hypoxia and threat to life. In individual cases where the severity and frequency of the seizure disorder are such that the removal of medication does not pose a serious threat to the patient, discontinuation of the drug may be considered prior to and during pregnancy, although it cannot be said with any confidence that even minor seizures do not pose some hazard to the developing embryo or fetus.

Tests to detect neural tube and other defects using current accepted procedures should be considered a part of routine prenatal care in childbearing women receiving valproate.

PRECAUTIONS

Hepatic Dysfunction

See **BOXED WARNING**, **CONTRAINDICATIONS** and **WARNINGS**.

General

Because of reports of thrombocytopenia (see **WARNINGS**), inhibition of the secondary phase of platelet aggregation, and abnormal coagulation parameters, (e.g., low fibrinogen), platelet counts and coagulation tests are recommended before initiating therapy and at periodic intervals. It is recommended that patients receiving DEPACON be monitored for platelet count and coagulation parameters prior to planned surgery. In a clinical trial of DEPAKOTE (divalproex sodium) as monotherapy in patients with epilepsy, 34/126 patients (27%) receiving approximately 50 mg/kg/day on average, had at least one value of platelets $\leq 75 \times 10^9$/L. Approximately half of these patients had treatment discontinued, with return of platelet counts to normal. In the remaining patients, platelet counts normalized with continued treatment. In this study, the probability of thrombocytopenia appeared to increase significantly at total valproate concentrations of $\geq$ 110 µg/mL (females) or $\geq$ 135 µg/mL (males). Evidence of hemorrhage, bruising, or a disorder of hemostasis/coagulation is an indication for reduction of the dosage or withdrawal of therapy.

Hyperammonemia with or without lethargy or coma has been reported and may be present in the absence of abnormal liver function tests. Asymptomatic elevations of ammonia are more common and when present require more frequent monitoring. If clinically significant symptoms occur, DEPACON therapy should be modified or discontinued.

Since DEPACON may interact with concurrently administered drugs which are capable of enzyme induction, periodic plasma concentration determinations of valproate and concomitant drugs are recommended during the early course of therapy. (See **PRECAUTIONS** - **Drug Interactions**.)

Valproate is partially eliminated in the urine as a keto-metabolite which may lead to a false interpretation of the urine ketone test.

There have been reports of altered thyroid function tests associated with valproate. The clinical significance of these is unknown.

Information for Patients

Since DEPACON may produce CNS depression, especially when combined with another CNS depressant (e.g., alcohol), patients should be advised not to engage in hazardous activities, such as driving an automobile or operating dangerous machinery, until it is known that they do not become drowsy from the drug.

Drug Interactions

Effects of Co-Administered Drugs on Valproate Clearance

Drugs that affect the level of expression of hepatic enzymes, particularly those that elevate levels of glucuronosyl transferases, may increase the clearance of valproate. For example, phenytoin, carbamazepine, and phenobarbital (or primidone) can double the clearance of valproate. Thus, patients on monotherapy will generally have longer half-lives and higher concentrations than patients receiving polytherapy with antiepilepsy drugs.

In contrast, drugs that are inhibitors of cytochrome P450 isozymes, e.g., antidepressants, may be expected to have little effect on valproate clearance because cytochrome P450 microsomal mediated oxidation is a relatively minor secondary metabolic pathway compared to glucuronidation and beta-oxidation.

Because of these changes in valproate clearance, monitoring of valproate and concomitant drug concentrations should be increased whenever enzyme inducing drugs are introduced or withdrawn.

The following list provides information about the potential for an influence of several commonly prescribed medications on valproate pharmacokinetics. The list is not exhaustive nor could it be, since new interactions are continuously being reported.

Drugs for which a potentially important interaction has been observed:

Aspirin - A study involving the co-administration of aspirin at antipyretic doses (11 to 16 mg/kg) with valproate to pediatric patients (n=6) revealed a decrease in protein binding and an inhibition of metabolism of valproate. Valproate free fraction was increased 4-fold in the presence of aspirin compared to valproate alone. The β-oxidation pathway consisting of 2-E-valproic acid, 3-OH-valproic acid, and 3-keto valproic acid was decreased from 25% of total metabolites excreted on valproate alone to 8.3% in the presence of aspirin. Caution should be observed if valproate and aspirin are to be co-administered.

Felbamate - A study involving the co-administration of 1200 mg/day of felbamate with valproate to patients with epilepsy (n=10) revealed an increase in mean valproate peak concentration by 35% (from 86 to 115 µg/mL) compared to valproate alone. Increasing the felbamate dose to 2400 mg/day increased the mean valproate peak concentration to 133 µg/mL (another 16% increase). A decrease in valproate dosage may be necessary when felbamate therapy is initiated.

Rifampin - A study involving the administration of a single dose of valproate (7 mg/kg) 36 hours after 5 nights of daily dosing with rifampin (600 mg) revealed a 40% increase in the oral clearance of valproate. Valproate dosage adjustment may be necessary when it is co-administered with rifampin.

Drugs for which either no interaction or a likely clinically unimportant interaction has been observed:

Antacids - A study involving the co-administration of valproate 500 mg with commonly administered antacids (Maalox, Trisogel, and Titralac - 160 mEq doses) did not reveal any effect on the extent of absorption of valproate.

Chlorpromazine - A study involving the administration of 100 to 300 mg/day of chlorpromazine to schizophrenic patients already receiving valproate (200 mg BID) revealed a 15% increase in trough plasma levels of valproate.

Haloperidol - A study involving the administration of 6 to 10 mg/day of haloperidol to schizophrenic patients already receiving valproate (200 mg BID) revealed no significant changes in valproate trough plasma levels.

Cimetidine and Ranitidine - Cimetidine and ranitidine do not affect the clearance of valproate.

Effects of Valproate on Other Drugs

Valproate has been found to be a weak inhibitor of some P450 isozymes, epoxide hydrase, and glucuronyl transferases.

The following list provides information about the potential for an influence of valproate co-administration on the pharmacokinetics or pharmacodynamics of several commonly prescribed medications. The list is not exhaustive, since new interactions are continuously being reported.

Drugs for which a potentially important valproate interaction has been observed:

Carbamazepine/carbamazepine-10,11-Epoxide - Serum levels of carbamazepine (CBZ) decreased 17% while that of carbamazepine-10,11-epoxide (CBZ-E) increased by 45% upon co-administration of valproate and CBZ to epileptic patients.

Clonazepam - The concomitant use of valproic acid and clonazepam may induce absence status in patients with a history of absence type seizures.

Diazepam - Valproate displaces diazepam from its plasma albumin binding sites and inhibits its metabolism. Co-administration of valproate (1500 mg daily) increased the free fraction of diazepam (10 mg) by 90% in healthy volunteers (n=6). Plasma clearance and volume of distribution for free diazepam were reduced by 25% and 20%, respectively, in the presence of valproate. The elimination half-life of diazepam remained unchanged upon addition of valproate.

Ethosuximide - Valproate inhibits the metabolism of ethosuximide. Administration of a single ethosuximide dose of 500 mg with valproate (800 to 1600 mg/day) to healthy volunteers (n=6) was accompanied by a 25% increase in elimination half-life of ethosuximide and a 15% decrease in its total clearance as compared to ethosuximide alone. Patients receiving valproate and ethosuximide, especially along with other anticonvulsants, should be monitored for alterations in serum concentrations of both drugs.

Lamotrigine - In a steady-state study involving 10 healthy volunteers, the elimination half-life of lamotrigine increased from 26 to 70 hours with valproate co-administration (a 165% increase). The dose of lamotrigine should be reduced when co-administered with valproate.

Phenobarbital - Valproate was found to inhibit the metabolism of phenobarbital. Co-administration of valproate (250 mg BID for 14 days) with phenobarbital to normal subjects (n=6) resulted in a 50% increase in half-life and a 30% decrease in plasma clearance of phenobarbital (60 mg single-dose). The fraction of phenobarbital dose excreted unchanged increased by 50% in presence of valproate.

There is evidence for severe CNS depression, with or without significant elevations of barbiturate or valproate serum concentrations. All patients receiving concomitant barbiturate therapy should be closely monitored for neurological toxicity. Serum barbiturate concentrations should be obtained, if possible, and the barbiturate dosage decreased, if appropriate.

Primidone, which is metabolized to a barbiturate, may be involved in a similar interaction with valproate.

Phenytoin - Valproate displaces phenytoin from its plasma albumin binding sites and inhibits its hepatic metabolism. Co-administration of valproate (400 mg TID) with phenytoin (250 mg) in normal volunteers (n=7) was associated with a 60% increase in the free fraction of phenytoin. Total plasma clearance and apparent volume of distribution of phenytoin increased 30% in the presence of valproate. Both the clearance and apparent volume of distribution of free phenytoin were reduced by 25%.

In patients with epilepsy, there have been reports of breakthrough seizures occurring with the combination of valproate and phenytoin. The dosage of phenytoin should be adjusted as required by the clinical situation.

Tolbutamide - From *in vitro* experiments, the unbound fraction of tolbutamide was increased from 20% to 50% when added to plasma samples taken from patients treated with valproate. The clinical relevance of this displacement is unknown.

Warfarin - In an *in vitro* study, valproate increased the unbound fraction of warfarin by up to 32.6%. The therapeutic relevance of this is unknown; however, coagulation tests should be monitored if valproate therapy is instituted in patients taking anticoagulants.

Zidovudine - In six patients who were seropositive for HIV, the clearance of zidovudine (100 mg q8h) was decreased by 38% after administration of valproate (250 or 500 mg q8h); the half-life of zidovudine was unaffected.

Drugs for which either no interaction or a likely clinically unimportant interaction has been observed:

Acetaminophen - Valproate had no effect on any of the pharmacokinetic parameters of acetaminophen when it was concurrently administered to three epileptic patients.

Amitriptyline/Nortriptyline - Administration of a single oral 50 mg dose of amitriptyline to 15 normal volunteers (10 males and 5 females) who received valproate (500 mg BID) resulted in a 21% decrease in plasma clearance of amitriptyline and a 34% decrease in the net clearance of nortriptyline.

Clozapine - In psychotic patients (n=11), no interaction was observed when valproate was co-administered with clozapine.

Lithium - Co-administration of valproate (500 mg BID) and lithium carbonate (300 mg TID) to normal male volunteers (n=16) had no effect on the steady-state kinetics of lithium.

Lorazepam - Concomitant administration of valproate (500 mg BID) and lorazepam (1 mg BID) in normal male volunteers (n=9) was accompanied by a 17% decrease in the plasma clearance of lorazepam.

Oral Contraceptive Steroids - Administration of a single-dose of ethinyloestradiol (50 µg)/levonorgestrel (250 µg) to 6 women on valproate (200 mg BID) therapy for 2 months did not reveal any pharmacokinetic interaction.

Carcinogenesis, Mutagenesis, Impairment of Fertility

Carcinogenesis

Valproic acid was administered orally to Sprague Dawley rats and ICR (HA/ICR) mice at doses of 80 and 170 mg/kg/day (approximately 10 to 50% of the maximum human daily dose on a mg/m^2 basis) for two years. A variety of neoplasms were observed in both species. The chief findings were a statistically significant increase in the incidence of subcutaneous fibrosarcomas in high dose male rats receiving valproic acid and a statistically significant dose-related trend for benign pulmonary adenomas in male mice receiving valproic acid. The significance of these findings for humans is unknown.

Mutagenesis

Valproate was not mutagenic in an *in vitro* bacterial assay (Ames test), did not produce dominant lethal effects in mice, and did not increase chromosome aberration frequency in

Continued on next page

Depacon—Cont.

an *in vivo* cytogenetic study in rats. Increased frequencies of sister chromatid exchange (SCE) have been reported in a study of epileptic children taking valproate, but this association was not observed in another study conducted in adults. There is some evidence that increased SCE frequencies may be associated with epilepsy. The biological significance of an increase in SCE frequency is not known.

Fertility

Chronic toxicity studies in juvenile and adult rats and dogs demonstrated reduced spermatogenesis and testicular atrophy at oral doses of 400 mg/kg/day or greater in rats (approximately equivalent to or greater than the maximum human daily dose on a mg/m^2 basis) and 150 mg/kg/day or greater in dogs (approximately 1.4 times the maximum human daily dose or greater on a mg/m^2 basis). Segment I fertility studies in rats have shown oral doses up to 350 mg/kg/day (approximately equal to the maximum human daily dose on a mg/m^2 basis) for 60 days to have no effect on fertility. THE EFFECT OF VALPROATE ON TESTICULAR DEVELOPMENT AND ON SPERM PRODUCTION AND FERTILITY IN HUMANS IS UNKNOWN.

Pregnancy

Pregnancy Category D: See **WARNINGS**.

Nursing Mothers

Valproate is excreted in breast milk. Concentrations in breast milk have been reported to be 1–10% of serum concentrations. It is not known what effect this would have on a nursing infant. Consideration should be given to discontinuing nursing when valproate is administered to a nursing woman.

Pediatric

Experience with oral valproate has indicated that children under the age of two years are at a considerably increased risk of developing fatal hepatotoxicity, especially those with the aforementioned conditions (see **BOXED WARNING**). The safety of DEPACON has not been studied in individuals below the age of 2 years. If a decision is made to use DEPACON in this age group, it should be used with extreme caution and as a sole agent. The benefits of therapy should be weighed against the risks. Above the age of 2 years, experience in epilepsy has indicated that the incidence of fatal hepatotoxicity decreases considerably in progressively older patient groups.

Younger children, especially those receiving enzyme-inducing drugs, will require larger maintenance doses to attain targeted total and unbound valproic acid concentrations.

The variability in free fraction limits the clinical usefulness of monitoring total serum valproic acid concentrations. Interpretation of valproic acid concentrations in children should include consideration of factors that affect hepatic metabolism and protein binding.

No unique safety concerns were identified in the 24 patients age 2 to 17 years who received DEPACON in clinical trials. The basic toxicology and pathologic manifestations of valproate sodium in neonatal (4-day old) and juvenile (14-day old) rats are similar to those seen in young adult rats. However, additional findings, including renal alterations in juvenile rats and renal alterations and retinal dysplasia in neonatal rats, have been reported. These findings occurred at 240 mg/kg/day, a dosage approximately equivalent to the human maximum recommended daily dose on a mg/m^2 basis. They were not seen at 90 mg/kg, or 40% of the maximum human daily dose on a mg/m^2 basis.

Geriatric Use

No unique safety concerns were identified in the 19 patients > 65 years of age receiving DEPACON in clinical trials.

ADVERSE REACTIONS

The adverse events that can result from DEPACON use include all of those associated with oral forms of valproate. The following describes experience specifically with DEPACON. DEPACON has been generally well tolerated in clinical trials involving 111 healthy adult male volunteers and 352 patients with epilepsy, given at doses of 125 to 6000 mg (total daily dose). A total of 2% of patients discontinued treatment with DEPACON due to adverse events. The most common adverse events leading to discontinuation were 2 cases each of nausea/vomiting and elevated amylase. Other adverse events leading to discontinuation were hallucinations, pneumonia, headache, injection site reaction, and abnormal gait. Dizziness and injection site pain were observed more frequently at a 100 mg/min infusion rate than at rates up to 33 mg/min. At a 200 mg/min rate, dizziness and taste perversion occurred more frequently than at a 100 mg/min rate. The maximum rate of infusion studied was 200 mg/min.

Adverse events reported by at least 0.5% of all subjects/patients in clinical trials of DEPACON are summarized in Table 1.

Table 1
Adverse Events Reported During Studies of DEPACON

Body System/Event	N = 463
Body as a Whole	
Chest Pain	1.7%
Headache	4.3%
Injection Site Inflammation	0.6%
Injection Site Pain	2.6%
Injection Site Reaction	2.4%
Pain (unspecified)	1.3%
Cardiovascular	
Vasodilation	0.9%
Dermatologic	
Sweating	0.9%
Digestive System	
Abdominal Pain	1.1%
Diarrhea	0.9%
Nausea	3.2%
Vomiting	1.3%
Nervous System	
Dizziness	5.2%
Euphoria	0.9%
Hypesthesia	0.6%
Nervousness	0.9%
Paresthesia	0.9%
Somnolence	1.7%
Tremor	0.6%
Respiratory	
Pharyngitis	0.6%
Special Senses	
Taste Perversion	1.9%

Epilepsy

Based on a placebo-controlled trial of adjunctive therapy for treatment of complex partial seizures, DEPAKOTE (divalproex sodium) was generally well tolerated with most adverse events rated as mild to moderate in severity. Intolerance was the primary reason for discontinuation in the DEPAKOTE-treated patients (6%), compared to 1% of placebo-treated patients.

Table 2 lists treatment-emergent adverse events which were reported by ≥ 5% of DEPAKOTE-treated patients and for which the incidence was greater than in the placebo group, in the placebo-controlled trial of adjunctive therapy for treatment of complex partial seizures. Since patients were also treated with other antiepilepsy drugs, it is not possible, in most cases, to determine whether the following adverse events can be ascribed to DEPAKOTE alone, or the combination of DEPAKOTE and other antiepilepsy drugs.

Table 2
Adverse Events Reported by ≥ 5% of Patients Treated with DEPAKOTE During Placebo-Controlled Trial of Adjunctive Therapy for Complex Partial Seizures

Body System/Event	Depakote (%) (n = 77)	Placebo (%) (n = 70)
Body as a Whole		
Headache	31	21
Asthenia	27	7
Fever	6	4
Gastrointestinal System		
Nausea	48	14
Vomiting	27	7
Abdominal Pain	23	6
Diarrhea	13	6
Anorexia	12	0
Dyspepsia	8	4
Constipation	5	1
Nervous System		
Somnolence	27	11
Tremor	25	6
Dizziness	25	13
Diplopia	16	9
Amblyopia/Blurred Vision	12	9
Ataxia	8	1
Nystagmus	8	1
Emotional Lability	6	4
Thinking Abnormal	6	0
Amnesia	5	1
Respiratory System		
Flu Syndrome	12	9
Infection	12	6
Bronchitis	5	1
Rhinitis	5	4
Other		
Alopecia	6	1
Weight Loss	6	0

Table 3 lists treatment-emergent adverse events which were reported by ≥ 5% of patients in the high dose DEPAKOTE group, and for which the incidence was greater

than in the low dose group, in a controlled trial of DEPAKOTE monotherapy treatment of complex partial seizures. Since patients were being titrated off another antiepilepsy drug during the first portion of the trial, it is not possible, in many cases, to determine whether the following adverse events can be ascribed to DEPAKOTE alone, or the combination of DEPAKOTE and other antiepilepsy drugs.

Table 3
Adverse Events Reported by ≥ 5% of Patients in the High Dose Group in the Controlled Trial of DEPAKOTE Monotherapy for Complex Partial Seizures[1]

Body System/Event	High Dose (%) (n = 131)	Low Dose (%) (n = 134)
Body as a Whole		
Asthenia	21	10
Digestive System		
Nausea	34	26
Diarrhea	23	19
Vomiting	23	15
Abdominal Pain	12	9
Anorexia	11	4
Dyspepsia	11	10
Hemic/Lymphatic System		
Thrombocytopenia	24	1
Ecchymosis	5	4
Metabolic/Nutritional		
Weight Gain	9	4
Peripheral Edema	8	3
Nervous System		
Tremor	57	19
Somnolence	30	18
Dizziness	18	13
Insomnia	15	9
Nervousness	11	7
Amnesia	7	4
Nystagmus	7	1
Depression	5	4
Respiratory System		
Infection	20	13
Pharyngitis	8	2
Dyspnea	5	1
Skin and Appendages		
Alopecia	24	13
Special Senses		
Amblyopia/Blurred Vision	8	4
Tinnitus	7	1

[1] Headache was the only adverse event that occurred in ≥ 5% of patients in the high dose group and at an equal or greater incidence in the low dose group.

The following additional adverse events were reported by greater than 1% but less than 5% of the 358 patients treated with DEPAKOTE in the controlled trials of complex partial seizures:

Body as a Whole: Back pain, chest pain, malaise.

Cardiovascular System: Tachycardia, hypertension, palpitation.

Digestive System: Increased appetite, flatulence, hematemesis, eructation, pancreatitis, periodontal abscess.

Hemic and Lymphatic System: Petechia.

Metabolic and Nutritional Disorders: SGOT increased, SGPT increased.

Musculoskeletal System: Myalgia, twitching, arthralgia, leg cramps, myasthenia.

Nervous System: Anxiety, confusion, abnormal gait, paresthesia, hypertonia, incoordination, abnormal dreams, personality disorder.

Respiratory System: Sinusitis, cough increased, pneumonia, epistaxis.

Skin and Appendages: Rash, pruritus, dry skin.

Special Senses: Taste perversion, abnormal vision, deafness, otitis media.

Urogenital System: Urinary incontinence, vaginitis, dysmenorrhea, amenorrhea, urinary frequency.

Other Patient Populations

Adverse events that have been reported with all dosage forms of valproate from epilepsy trials, spontaneous reports, and other sources are listed below by body system.

Gastrointestinal: The most commonly reported side effects at the initiation of therapy are nausea, vomiting, and indigestion. These effects are usually transient and rarely require discontinuation of therapy. Diarrhea, abdominal cramps, and constipation have been reported. Both anorexia with some weight loss and increased appetite with weight gain have also been reported. The administration of delayed-release divalproex sodium may result in reduction of gastrointestinal side effects in some patients using oral therapy.

CNS Effects: Sedative effects have occurred in patients receiving valproate alone but occur most often in patients receiving combination therapy. Sedation usually abates upon reduction of other antiepileptic medication. Tremor (may be

dose-related), hallucinations, ataxia, headache, nystagmus, diplopia, asterixis, "spots before eyes", dysarthria, dizziness, confusion, hypesthesia, vertigo, and incoordination. Rare cases of coma have occurred in patients receiving valproate alone or in conjunction with phenobarbital. In rare instances encephalopathy with fever has developed shortly after the introduction of valproate monotherapy without evidence of hepatic dysfunction or inappropriate plasma levels; all patients recovered after the drug was withdrawn.
Several reports have noted reversible cerebral atrophy and dementia in association with valproate therapy.
Dermatologic: Transient hair loss, skin rash, photosensitivity, generalized pruritus, erythema multiforme, and Stevens-Johnson syndrome. Rare cases of toxic epidermal necrolysis have been reported including a fatal case in a 6 month old infant taking valproate and several other concomitant medications. An additional case of toxic epidermal necrosis resulting in death was reported in a 35 year old patient with AIDS taking several concomitant medications and with a history of multiple cutaneous drug reactions.
Psychiatric: Emotional upset, depression, psychosis, aggression, hyperactivity, hostility, and behavioral deterioration.
Musculoskeletal: Weakness.
Hematologic: Thrombocytopenia and inhibition of the secondary phase of platelet aggregation may be reflected in altered bleeding time, petechiae, bruising, hematoma formation, epistaxis, and frank hemorrhage (see **PRECAUTIONS - General** and **Drug Interactions**). Relative lymphocytosis, macrocytosis, hypofibrinogenemia, leukopenia, eosinophilia, anemia including macrocytic with or without folate deficiency, bone marrow suppression, pancytopenia, aplastic anemia, and acute intermittent porphyria.
Hepatic: Minor elevations of transaminases (e.g., SGOT and SGPT) and LDH are frequent and appear to be dose-related. Occasionally, laboratory test results include increases in serum bilirubin and abnormal changes in other liver function tests. These results may reflect potentially serious hepatotoxicity (see **WARNINGS**).
Endocrine: Irregular menses, secondary amenorrhea, breast enlargement, galactorrhea, and parotid gland swelling. Abnormal thyroid function tests (see **PRECAUTIONS**).
There have been rare spontaneous reports of polycystic ovary disease. A cause and effect relationship has not been established.
Pancreatic: Acute pancreatitis including fatalities.
Metabolic: Hyperammonemia (see PRECAUTIONS), hyponatremia, and inappropriate ADH secretion.
There have been rare reports of Fanconi's syndrome occurring chiefly in children.
Decreased carnitine concentrations have been reported although the clinical relevance is undetermined.
Hyperglycinemia has occurred and was associated with a fatal outcome in a patient with preexistent nonketotic hyperglycinemia.
Genitourinary: Enuresis and urinary tract infection.
Special Senses: Hearing loss, either reversible or irreversible, has been reported; however, a cause and effect relationship has not been established. Ear pain has also been reported.
Other: Edema of the extremities, lupus erythematosus, bone pain, cough increased, pneumonia, otitis media, bradycardia, cutaneous vasculitis, and fever.

Mania

Although DEPACON has not been evaluated for safety and efficacy in the treatment of manic episodes associated with bipolar disorder, the following adverse events not listed above were reported by 1% or more of patients from two placebo-controlled clinical trials of DEPAKOTE (DIVALPROEX SODIUM) tablets.
Body as a Whole: Chills, neck pain, neck rigidity.
Cardiovascular System: Hypotension, postural hypotension.
Digestive System: Fecal incontinence, gastroenteritis, glossitis.
Musculoskeletal System: Arthrosis.
Nervous System: Agitation, catatonic reaction, hypokinesia, reflexes increased, tardive dyskinesia, vertigo.
Skin and Appendages: Furunculosis, maculopapular rash, seborrhea.
Special Senses: Conjunctivitis, dry eyes, eye pain.
Urogenital: Dysuria.

Migraine

Although DEPACON has not been evaluated for safety and efficacy in the prophylactic treatment of migraine headaches, the following adverse events not listed above were reported by 1% or more of patients from two placebo-controlled clinical trials of DEPAKOTE (DIVALPROEX SODIUM) tablets.
Body as a Whole: Face edema.
Digestive System: Dry mouth, stomatitis.
Urogenital System: Cystitis, metrorrhagia, and vaginal hemorrhage.

OVERDOSAGE

Overdosage with valproate may result in somnolence, heart block, and deep coma. Fatalities have been reported; however patients have recovered from valproate serum concentrations as high as 2120 μg/mL.
In overdose situations, the fraction of drug not bound to protein is high and hemodialysis or tandem hemodialysis plus hemoperfusion may result in significant removal of drug. General supportive measures should be applied with particular attention to the maintenance of adequate urinary output.
Naloxone has been reported to reverse the CNS depressant effects of valproate overdosage. Because naloxone could theoretically also reverse the antiepilepsy effects of valproate, it should be used with caution in patients with epilepsy.

DOSAGE AND ADMINISTRATION

DEPACON IS FOR INTRAVENOUS USE ONLY.
Use of DEPACON for periods of more than 14 days has not been studied. Patients should be switched to oral valproate products as soon as it is clinically feasible.
DEPACON should be administered as a 60 minute infusion (but not more than 20 mg/min) with the same frequency as the oral products, although plasma concentration monitoring and dosage adjustments may be necessary.

Initial Exposure to Valproate:

The following dosage recommendations were obtained from studies utilizing oral divalproex sodium products.
Complex Partial Seizures: For adults and children 10 years of age or older.
Monotherapy (Initial Therapy): DEPACON has not been systematically studied as initial therapy. Patients should initiate therapy at 10 to 15 mg/kg/day. The dosage should be increased by 5 to 10 mg/kg/week to achieve optimal clinical response. Ordinarily, optimal clinical response is achieved at daily doses below 60 mg/kg/day. If satisfactory clinical response has not been achieved, plasma levels should be measured to determine whether or not they are in the usually accepted therapeutic range (50 to 100 μg/mL). No recommendation regarding the safety of valproate for use at doses above 60 mg/kg/day can be made.
The probability of thrombocytopenia increases significantly at total trough valproate plasma concentrations above 110 μg/mL in females and 135 μg/mL in males. The benefit of improved seizure control with higher doses should be weighed against the possibility of a greater incidence of adverse reactions.
Conversion to Monotherapy: Patients should initiate therapy at 10 to 15 mg/kg/day. The dosage should be increased by 5 to 10 mg/kg/week to achieve optimal clinical response. Ordinarily, optimal clinical response is achieved at daily doses below 60 mg/kg/day. If satisfactory clinical response has not been achieved, plasma levels should be measured to determine whether or not they are in the usually accepted therapeutic range (50 - 100 μg/mL). No recommendation regarding the safety of valproate for use at doses above 60 mg/kg/day can be made. Concomitant antiepilepsy drug (AED) dosage can ordinarily be reduced by approximately 25% every 2 weeks. This reduction may be started at initiation of DEPACON therapy, or delayed by 1 to 2 weeks if there is a concern that seizures are likely to occur with a reduction. The speed and duration of withdrawal of the concomitant AED can be highly variable, and patients should be monitored closely during this period for increased seizure frequency.
Adjunctive Therapy: DEPACON may be added to the patient's regimen at a dosage of 10 to 15 mg/kg/day. The dosage may be increased by 5 to 10 mg/kg/week to achieve optimal clinical response. Ordinarily, optimal clinical response is achieved at daily doses below 60 mg/kg/day. If satisfactory clinical response has not been achieved, plasma levels should be measured to determine whether or not they are in the usually accepted therapeutic range (50 to 100 μg/mL). No recommendation regarding the safety of valproate for use at doses above 60 mg/kg/day can be made. If the total daily dose exceeds 250 mg, it should be given in divided doses.
In a study of adjunctive therapy for complex partial seizures in which patients were receiving either carbamazepine or phenytoin in addition to DEPAKOTE (divalproex sodium), no adjustment of carbamazepine or phenytoin dosage was needed (see **CLINICAL STUDIES**). However, since valproate may interact with these or other concurrently administered AEDs as well as other drugs (see **Drug Interactions**), periodic plasma concentration determinations of concomitant AEDs are recommended during the early course of therapy (see **PRECAUTIONS - Drug Interactions**).
Simple and Complex Absence Seizures: The recommended initial dose is 15 mg/kg/day, increasing at one week intervals by 5 to 10 mg/kg/day until seizures are controlled or side effects preclude further increases. The maximum recommended dosage is 60 mg/kg/day. If the total daily dose exceeds 250 mg, it should be given in divided doses.
A good correlation has not been established between daily dose, serum concentrations, and therapeutic effect. However, therapeutic valproate serum concentrations for most patients with absence seizures is considered to range from 50 to 100 μg/mL. Some patients may be controlled with lower or higher serum concentrations (see **CLINICAL PHARMACOLOGY**).
As the DEPACON dosage is titrated upward, blood concentrations of phenobarbital and/or phenytoin may be affected (see **PRECAUTIONS**).
Antiepilepsy drugs should not be abruptly discontinued in patients in whom the drug is administered to prevent major seizures because of the strong possibility of precipitating status epilepticus with attendant hypoxia and threat to life.

Replacement Therapy:

When switching from oral valproate products, the total daily dose of DEPACON should be equivalent to the total daily dose of the oral valproate product (see **CLINICAL PHARMACOLOGY**), and should be administered as a 60 minute infusion (but not more than 20 mg/min) with the same frequency as the oral products, although plasma concentration monitoring and dosage adjustments may be necessary. Patients receiving doses near the maximum recommended daily dose of 60 mg/kg/day, particularly those not receiving enzyme-inducing drugs, should be monitored more closely. If the total daily dose exceeds 250 mg, it should be given in a divided regimen. However, the equivalence shown between DEPACON and oral valproate products (DEPAKOTE) at steady state was only evaluated in an every 6 hour regimen. Whether, when DEPACON is given less frequently (i.e., twice or three times a day), trough levels fall below those that result from an oral dosage form given via the same regimen, is unknown. For this reason, when DEPACON is given twice or three times a day, close monitoring of trough plasma levels may be needed.

General Dosing Advice

Dosing in Elderly Patients - Due to a decrease in unbound clearance of valproate, the starting dose should be reduced; the ultimate therapeutic dose should be achieved on the basis of clinical response.
Dose-Related Adverse Events - The frequency of adverse effects (particularly elevated liver enzymes and thrombocytopenia) may be dose-related. The probability of thrombocytopenia appears to increase significantly at total valproate concentrations of ≥ 110 μg/mL (females) or ≥ 135 μg/mL (males) (see **PRECAUTIONS**). The benefit of improved therapeutic effect with higher doses should be weighed against the possibility of a greater incidence of adverse reactions.

Administration

Rapid infusion of DEPACON has been associated with an increase in adverse events. Infusion times of less than 60 minutes or rates of infusion > 20 mg/min have not been studied in patients with epilepsy (see **ADVERSE REACTIONS**).
DEPACON should be administered intravenously as a 60 minute infusion, as noted above. It should be diluted with at least 50 mL of a compatible diluent. Any unused portion of the vial contents should be discarded.
Parenteral drug products should be inspected visually for particulate matter and discoloration prior to administration whenever solution and container permit.

Compatibility and Stability

DEPACON was found to be physically compatible and chemically stable in the following parenteral solutions for at least 24 hours when stored in glass or polyvinyl chloride (PVC) bags at controlled room temperature 15–30°C (59–86°F).

- dextrose (5%) injection, USP
- sodium chloride (0.9%) injection, USP
- lactated ringer's injection, USP

HOW SUPPLIED

DEPACON (valproate sodium injection), equivalent to 100 mg of valproic acid per mL, is a clear, colorless solution in 5 mL single-dose vials, available in trays of 10 vials (**NDC** 0074-1564-10).
Recommended storage: Store vials at controlled room temperature 15–30°C (59–86°F). No preservatives have been added. Unused portion of container should be discarded.
Revised: January, 1998
Caution -- Federal (U.S.A.) law prohibits dispensing without a prescription.
Ref. 06-9798-R2-Rev. Jan., 1998
ABBOTT LABORATORIES
NORTH CHICAGO, IL 60064, U.S.A.

DEPAKENE® Capsules and Syrup ℞
[dep 'a-kāne]
(Valproic Acid)

WARNING:
HEPATIC FAILURE RESULTING IN FATALITIES HAS OCCURRED IN PATIENTS RECEIVING VALPROIC ACID. EXPERIENCE HAS INDICATED THAT CHILDREN UNDER THE AGE OF TWO YEARS ARE AT A CONSIDERABLY INCREASED RISK OF DEVELOPING FATAL HEPATOTOXICITY, ESPECIALLY

Continued on next page

Depakene—Cont.

THOSE ON MULTIPLE ANTICONVULSANTS, THOSE WITH CONGENITAL METABOLIC DISORDERS, THOSE WITH SEVERE SEIZURE DISORDERS ACCOMPANIED BY MENTAL RETARDATION, AND THOSE WITH ORGANIC BRAIN DISEASE. WHEN DEPAKENE PRODUCTS ARE USED IN THIS PATIENT GROUP, IT SHOULD BE USED WITH EXTREME CAUTION AND AS A SOLE AGENT. THE BENEFITS OF SEIZURE CONTROL SHOULD BE WEIGHED AGAINST THE RISKS. ABOVE THIS AGE GROUP, EXPERIENCE HAS INDICATED THAT THE INCIDENCE OF FATAL HEPATOTOXICITY DECREASES CONSIDERABLY IN PROGRESSIVELY OLDER PATIENT GROUPS.

THESE INCIDENTS USUALLY HAVE OCCURRED DURING THE FIRST SIX MONTHS OF TREATMENT. SERIOUS OR FATAL HEPATOTOXICITY MAY BE PRECEDED BY NON-SPECIFIC SYMPTOMS SUCH AS LOSS OF SEIZURE CONTROL, MALAISE, WEAKNESS, LETHARGY, FACIAL EDEMA, ANOREXIA, AND VOMITING. PATIENTS SHOULD BE MONITORED CLOSELY FOR APPEARANCE OF THESE SYMPTOMS. LIVER FUNCTION TESTS SHOULD BE PERFORMED PRIOR TO THERAPY AND AT FREQUENT INTERVALS THEREAFTER, ESPECIALLY DURING THE FIRST SIX MONTHS.

DESCRIPTION

DEPAKENE (valproic acid) is a carboxylic acid designated as 2-propylpentanoic acid. It is also known as dipropylacetic acid. Valproic acid has the following structure:

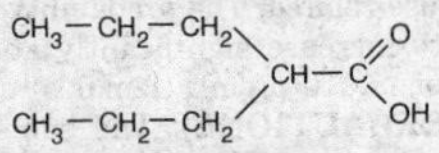

Valproic acid (pKa 4.8) has a molecular weight of 144 and occurs as a colorless liquid with a characteristic odor. It is slightly soluble in water (1.3 mg/mL) and very soluble in organic solvents.

DEPAKENE capsules and syrup are antiepileptics for oral administration. Each soft elastic capsule contains 250 mg valproic acid. The syrup contains the equivalent of 250 mg valproic acid per 5 mL as the sodium salt.

Inactive Ingredients

250 mg capsules: corn oil, FD&C Yellow No. 6, gelatin, glycerin, iron oxide, methylparaben, propylparaben, and titanium dioxide.

Syrup: FD&C Red No. 40, glycerin, methylparaben, propylparaben, sorbitol, sucrose, water, and natural and artificial flavors.

CLINICAL PHARMACOLOGY

Valproic acid is an antiepileptic agent which dissociates to the valproate ion in the gastrointestinal tract. The mechanism by which valproate exerts its antiepileptic effects has not been established. It has been suggested that its activity is related to increased brain levels of gamma-aminobutyric acid (GABA).

Valproic acid is rapidly absorbed after oral administration. Peak plasma concentrations of valproate ion are observed 1 to 4 hours after a single oral dose of valproic acid. A slight delay in absorption occurs when the drug is administered with meals, but this does not affect the total absorption.

Accordingly, administration of oral valproate products with food and substitution among the various DEPAKENE (valproic acid) and DEPAKOTE® (divalproex sodium) products should be without consequence. Nonetheless, any changes in dosage administration, or the addition or discontinuance of concomitant drugs should ordinarily be accompanied by close monitoring of clinical status and valproate plasma concentrations.

The plasma half-life of valproate is typically in the range of 6 to 16 hours. Half-lives in the lower part of the range are usually found in patients taking other antiepileptic drugs capable of enzyme induction.

Valproate is primarily metabolized in the liver. The major metabolic routes are glucuronidation, mitochrondrial beta oxidation, and microsomol oxidation. The major metabolites formed are the glucuronide conjugate, 2-propyl-3-keto-pentanoic acid, and 2-propyl-hydroxypentanoic acids. Other unsaturated metabolites have been reported. The major route of elimination of these metabolites is in the urine.

Patients on monotherapy will generally have longer half-lives and higher concentrations of valproate at a given dosage than patients receiving polytherapy. This is primarily due to enzyme induction caused by other antiepileptics, which results in enhanced clearance of valproate by glucuronidation and microsomal oxidation. Because of these changes in valproate clearance, monitoring of antiepileptic concentrations should be intensified whenever concomitant antiepileptics are introduced or withdrawn.

The therapeutic range is commonly considered to be 50 to 100 µg/mL of total valproate, although some patients may be controlled with lower or higher plasma concentrations.[4]

Valproate is highly bound (90%) to plasma proteins in the therapeutic range; however, protein binding is concentration-dependent and decreases at high valproate concentrations. The binding is variable among patients and may be affected by fatty acids or by highly bound drugs such as salicylate. Some clinicians favor monitoring free valproate concentrations, which may more accurately reflect CNS penetration of valproate. As yet, a consensus on the therapeutic range of free concentrations has not been established; however, monitoring total and free valproate may be informative when there are changes in clinical status, concomitant medication, or valproate dosage.

INDICATIONS AND USAGE

DEPAKENE (valproic acid) is indicated for use as sole and adjunctive therapy in the treatment of simple and complex absence seizures, and adjunctively in patients with multiple seizure types which include absence seizures.

Simple absence is defined as very brief clouding of the sensorium or loss of consciousness accompanied by certain generalized epileptic discharges without other detectable clinical signs. Complex absence is the term used when other signs are also present.

SEE WARNINGS FOR STATEMENT REGARDING FATAL HEPATIC DYSFUNCTION.

CONTRAINDICATIONS

VALPROIC ACID SHOULD NOT BE ADMINISTERED TO PATIENTS WITH HEPATIC DISEASE OR SIGNIFICANT DYSFUNCTION.

Valproic acid is contraindicated in patients with known hypersensitivity to the drug.

WARNINGS

Hepatic failure resulting in fatalities has occurred in patients receiving valproic acid. These incidents usually have occurred during the first six months of treatment. Serious or fatal hepatotoxicity may be preceded by nonspecific symptoms such as loss of seizure control, malaise, weakness, lethargy, facial edema, anorexia, and vomiting. Patients should be monitored closely for appearance of these symptoms. Liver function tests should be performed prior to therapy and at frequent intervals thereafter, especially during the first six months. However, physicians should not rely totally on serum biochemistry since these tests may not be abnormal in all instances, but should also consider the results of careful interim medical history and physical examination. Caution should be observed when administering DEPAKENE (valproic acid) to patients with a prior history of hepatic disease. Patients on multiple anticonvulsants, children, those with congenital metabolic disorders, those with severe seizure disorders accompanied by mental retardation, and those with organic brain disease may be at particular risk. Experience has indicated that children under the age of two years are at a considerably increased risk of developing fatal hepatotoxicity, especially those with the aforementioned conditions. When DEPAKENE products are used in this patient group, it should be used with extreme caution and as a sole agent. The benefits of seizure control should be weighed against the risks. Above this age group, experience has indicated that the incidence of fatal hepatotoxicity decreases considerably in progressively older patient groups.

The drug should be discontinued immediately in the presence of significant hepatic dysfunction, suspected or apparent. In some cases, hepatic dysfunction has progressed in spite of discontinuation of drug.

The frequency of adverse effects (particularly elevated liver enzymes) may be dose-related. The benefit of improved seizure control which may accompany the higher doses should be weighed against the possibility of a greater incidence of adverse effects.

Usage in Pregnancy: ACCORDING TO PUBLISHED AND UNPUBLISHED REPORTS, VALPROIC ACID MAY PRODUCE TERATOGENIC EFFECTS IN THE OFFSPRING OF HUMAN FEMALES RECEIVING THE DRUG DURING PREGNANCY.

THERE ARE MULTIPLE REPORTS IN THE CLINICAL LITERATURE WHICH INDICATE THAT THE USE OF ANTIEPILEPTIC DRUGS DURING PREGNANCY RESULTS IN AN INCREASED INCIDENCE OF BIRTH DEFECTS IN THE OFFSPRING. ALTHOUGH DATA ARE MORE EXTENSIVE WITH RESPECT TO TRIMETHADIONE, PARAMETHADIONE, PHENYTOIN, AND PHENOBARBITAL, REPORTS INDICATE A POSSIBLE SIMILAR ASSOCIATION WITH THE USE OF OTHER ANTIEPILEPTIC DRUGS. THEREFORE, ANTIEPILEPTIC DRUGS SHOULD BE ADMINISTERED TO WOMEN OF CHILDBEARING POTENTIAL ONLY IF THEY ARE CLEARLY SHOWN TO BE ESSENTIAL IN THE MANAGEMENT OF THEIR SEIZURES.

THE INCIDENCE OF NEURAL TUBE DEFECTS IN THE FETUS MAY BE INCREASED IN MOTHERS RECEIVING VALPROATE DURING THE FIRST TRIMESTER OF PREGNANCY. THE CENTERS FOR DISEASE CONTROL (CDC) HAS ESTIMATED THE RISK OF VALPROIC ACID EXPOSED WOMEN HAVING CHILDREN WITH SPINA BIFIDA TO BE APPROXIMATELY 1 to 2%.[1]

OTHER CONGENITAL ANOMALIES (EG, CRANIOFACIAL DEFECTS, CARDIOVASCULAR MALFORMATIONS AND ANOMALIES INVOLVING VARIOUS BODY SYSTEMS), COMPATIBLE AND INCOMPATIBLE WITH LIFE, HAVE BEEN REPORTED. SUFFICIENT DATA TO DETERMINE THE INCIDENCE OF THESE CONGENITAL ANOMALIES IS NOT AVAILABLE.

THE HIGHER INCIDENCE OF CONGENITAL ANOMALIES IN ANTIEPILEPTIC DRUG-TREATED WOMEN WITH SEIZURE DISORDERS CANNOT BE REGARDED AS A CAUSE AND EFFECT RELATIONSHIP. THERE ARE INTRINSIC METHODOLOGIC PROBLEMS IN OBTAINING ADEQUATE DATA ON DRUG TERATOGENICITY IN HUMANS; GENETIC FACTORS OR THE EPILEPTIC CONDITION ITSELF, MAY BE MORE IMPORTANT THAN DRUG THERAPY IN CONTRIBUTING TO CONGENITAL ANOMALIES.

PATIENTS TAKING VALPROATE MAY DEVELOP CLOTTING ABNORMALITIES. A PATIENT WHO HAD LOW FIBROGEN WHEN TAKING MULTIPLE ANTICONVULSANTS INCLUDING VALPROATE GAVE BIRTH TO AN INFANT WITH AFIBRINOGENEMIA WHO SUBSEQUENTLY DIED OF HEMORRHAGE. IF VALPROATE IS USED IN PREGNANCY, THE CLOTTING PARAMETERS SHOULD BE MONITORED CAREFULLY.

HEPATIC FAILURE, RESULTING IN THE DEATH OF A NEWBORN AND OF AN INFANT, HAVE BEEN REPORTED FOLLOWING THE USE OF VALPROATE DURING PREGNANCY.

ANIMAL STUDIES ALSO HAVE DEMONSTRATED VALPROATE INDUCED TERATOGENICITY. Studies in rats and human females demonstrated placental transfer of the drug. Doses greater than 65 mg/kg/day given to pregnant rats and mice produced skeletal abnormalities in the offspring, primarily involving ribs and vertebrae; doses greater than 150 mg/kg/day given to pregnant rabbits produced fetal resorptions and (primarily) soft-tissue abnormalities in the offspring. In rats a dose-related delay in the onset of parturition was noted. Postnatal growth and survival of the progeny were adversely affected, particularly when drug administration spanned the entire gestation and early lactation period.

Antiepileptic drugs should not be discontinued in patients in whom the drug is administered to prevent major seizures because of the strong possibility of precipitating status epilepticus with attendant hypoxia and threat to life. In individual cases where the severity and frequency of the seizure disorder are such that the removal of medication does not pose a serious threat to the patient, discontinuation of the drug may be considered prior to and during pregnancy, although it cannot be said with any confidence that even minor seizures do not pose some hazard to the developing embryo or fetus.

The prescribing physician will wish to weigh these considerations in treating or counseling epileptic women of childbearing potential.

Tests to detect neural tube and other defects using current accepted procedures should be considered a part of routine prenatal care in childbearing women receiving valproate.

PRECAUTIONS

Hepatic Dysfunction: See BOXED WARNING, CONTRAINDICATIONS, AND WARNINGS.

General: Because of reports of thrombocytopenia, inhibition of the secondary phase of platelet aggregation, and abnormal coagulation parameters (eg, low fibrinogen), platelet counts and coagulation tests are recommended before initiating therapy and at periodic intervals. It is recommended that patients receiving DEPAKENE (valproic acid) be monitored for platelet count and coagulation parameters prior to planned surgery. Evidence of hemorrhage, bruising, or a disorder of hemostasis/coagulation is an indication for reduction of the dosage or withdrawal of therapy.

Hyperammonemia with or without lethargy or coma has been reported and may be present in the absence of abnormal liver function tests. Asymptomatic elevations of ammonia are more common and when present require more frequent monitoring. If clinically significant symptoms occur, DEPAKENE therapy should be modified or discontinued.

Since valproate may interact with concurrently administered antiepileptic drugs, periodic plasma concentration determinations of concomitant antiepileptic drugs are recommended during the early course of therapy (see PRECAUTIONS—*Drug Interactions*).

Valproate is partially eliminated in the urine as a keto-metabolite which may lead to a false interpretation of the urine ketone test.

There have been reports of altered thyroid function tests associated with valproate. The clinical significance of these is unknown.

Information for Patients: Since DEPAKENE products may produce CNS depression, especially when combined with

another CNS depressant (eg, alcohol), patients should be advised not to engage in hazardous activities, such as driving an automobile or operating dangerous machinery, until it is known that they do not become drowsy from the drug.

Drug Interactions: Valproate may potentiate the action of CNS depressants (ie, alcohol, benzodiazepines, etc).

The concomitant administration of valproate with drugs that exhibit extensive protein binding (eg, aspirin, carbamazepine, dicumarol, and phenytoin) may result in alteration of serum drug concentrations.

There is evidence that valproate can cause an increase in serum phenobarbital concentrations by impairment of nonrenal clearance. This phenomenon can result in severe CNS depression. The combination of valproate and phenobarbital has also been reported to produce CNS depression without significant elevations of barbiturate or valproate serum concentrations. All patients receiving concomitant barbiturate therapy should be closely monitored for neurological toxicity. Serum barbiturate concentrations should be obtained, if possible, and the barbiturate dosage decreased, if appropriate.

Primidone is metabolized into a barbiturate and, therefore, may also be involved in a similar or identical interaction.

There have been reports of breakthrough seizures occurring with the combination of valproate and phenytoin. Most reports have noted a decrease in total plasma phenytoin concentration. However, increases in total phenytoin serum concentration have been reported. An initial fall with subsequent increase in total phenytoin concentrations has also been reported. In addition, a decrease in total serum phenytoin with an increase in the free vs. protein bound phenytoin concentrations has been reported. The dosage of phenytoin should be adjusted as required by the clinical situation.

The concomitant use of valproic acid and clonazepam may induce absence status in patients with a history of absence type seizures.

There is inconclusive evidence regarding the effects of valproate on serum ethosuximide concentrations. Patients receiving valproate and ethosuximide, especially along with other anticonvulsants, should be monitored for alterations in serum concentrations of both drugs.

Caution is recommended when valproate is used with drugs affecting coagulation (eg, aspirin, warfarin). See ADVERSE REACTIONS.

Evidence suggests that there is an association between the use of certain antiepileptics and failure of oral contraceptives. One explanation for this interaction is that enzyme-inducing antiepileptics effectively lower plasma concentrations of the relevant steroid hormones, resulting in unimpaired ovulation. However, other mechanisms, not related to enzyme induction may contribute to the failure of oral contraceptives. While valproate is not a significant enzyme inducer, and, therefore, would not be expected to decrease concentrations of steroid hormones, clinical data about the interaction of valproate with oral contraceptives is minimal.[2]

Carcinogenesis: Valproic acid was administered to Sprague Dawley rats and ICR (HA/ICR) mice at doses of 0, 80 and 170 mg/kg/day for two years. A variety of neoplasms were observed in both species. The chief findings were a statistically significant increase in the incidence of subcutaneous fibrosarcomas in high dose male rats receiving valproic acid and a statistically significant dose-related trend for benign pulmonary adenomas in male mice receiving valproic acid. The significance of these findings for man is unknown.

Mutagenesis: Studies of valproate have been performed using bacterial and mammalian systems. These studies have provided no evidence of a mutagenic potential for valproate.

Fertility: Chronic toxicity studies in juvenile and adult rats and dogs demonstrated reduced spermatogenesis and testicular atrophy at doses greater than 200 mg/kg/day in rats and greater than 90 mg/kg/day in dogs. Segment I fertility studies in rats have shown doses up to 350 mg/kg/day for 60 days to have no effect on fertility. THE EFFECT OF VALPROATE ON TESTICULAR DEVELOPMENT AND ON SPERM PRODUCTION AND FERTILITY IN HUMANS IS UNKNOWN.

Pregnancy: Pregnancy Category D: See WARNINGS.

Nursing Mothers: Valproate is excreted in breast milk. Concentrations in breast milk have been reported to be 1 to 10% of serum concentrations. It is not known what effect this would have on a nursing infant. Caution should be exercised when valproic acid is administered to a nursing woman.

ADVERSE REACTIONS

Since DEPAKENE (valproic acid) has usually been used with other antiepileptic drugs, it is not possible, in most cases, to determine whether the following adverse reactions can be ascribed to valproic acid alone, or the combination of drugs.

Gastrointestinal: The most commonly reported side effects at the initiation of therapy are nausea, vomiting, and indigestion. These effects are usually transient and rarely require discontinuation of therapy. Diarrhea, abdominal cramps, and constipation have been reported. Both anorexia with some weight loss and increased appetite with weight gain have also been reported. Some patients experiencing gastrointestinal side effects may benefit by converting therapy from DEPAKENE (valproic acid) to Depakote® (divalproex sodium).[3]

Weight (kg)	Weight (lb)	Total Daily Dose (mg)	Number of Capsules or Teaspoonfuls of Syrup: Dose 1	Dose 2	Dose 3
10—24.9	22— 54.9	250	0	0	1
25—39.9	55— 87.9	500	1	0	1
40—59.9	88—131.9	750	1	1	1
60—74.9	132—164.9	1,000	1	1	2
75—89.9	165—197.9	1,250	2	1	2

CNS Effects: Sedative effects have occurred in patients receiving valproate alone but occur most often in patients receiving combination therapy. Sedation usually abates upon reduction of other antiepileptic medication. Tremor (may be dose-related), hallucinations, ataxia, headache, nystagmus, diplopia, asterixis, "spots before eyes", dysarthria, dizziness, and incoordination. Rare cases of coma have been noted in patients receiving valproic acid alone or in conjunction with phenobarbital. In rare instances encephalopathy with fever has developed shortly after the introduction of valproate monotherapy without evidence of hepatic dysfunction or inappropriate plasma levels; all patients recovered after the drug was withdrawn.

Dermatologic: Transient hair loss, skin rash, photosensitivity, generalized pruritus, erythema multiforme, and Stevens-Johnson syndrome. A case of fatal epidermal necrolysis has been reported in a 6 month old infant taking valproate and several other concomitant medications.

Psychiatric: Emotional upset, depression, psychosis, aggression, hyperactivity and behavioral deterioration.

Musculoskeletal: Weakness.

Hematologic: Thrombocytopenia and inhibition of the secondary phase of platelet aggregation may be reflected in altered bleeding time, petechiae, bruising, hematoma formation and frank hemorrhage (see PRECAUTIONS—*General and Drug Interactions*). Relative lymphocytosis, macrocytosis, hypofibrinogenemia, leukopenia, eosinophilia, anemia including macrocytic with or without folate deficiency, bone marrow suppression, and acute intermittent porphyria.

Hepatic: Minor elevations of transaminases (eg, SGOT and SGPT) and LDH are frequent and appear to be dose-related. Occasionally, laboratory test results include increases in serum bilirubin and abnormal changes in other liver function tests. These results may reflect potentially serious hepatotoxicity. (See WARNINGS).

Endocrine: Irregular menses, secondary amenorrhea, breast enlargement, galactorrhea, and parotid gland swelling. Abnormal thyroid function tests (see PRECAUTIONS). There have been rare spontaneous reports of polycystic ovary disease. A cause and effect relationship has not been established.

Pancreatic: Acute pancreatitis, including fatalities.

Metabolic: Hyperammonemia (see PRECAUTIONS), hyponatremia, and inappropriate ADH secretion.

There have been rare reports of Fanconi's Syndrome occurring chiefly in children.

Decreased carnitine concentrations have been reported although the clinical relevance is undetermined.

Hyperglycinemia has occurred and was associated with a fatal outcome in a patient with preexistent nonketotic hyperglycinemia.

Genitourinary: Enuresis.

Special Senses: Hearing loss, either reversible or irreversible, has been reported; however, a cause and effect relationship has not been established.

Other: Edema of the extremities, lupus erythematosus, and fever.

OVERDOSAGE

Overdosage with valproate may result in somnolence, heart block, and deep coma. Fatalities have been reported.

Since valproic acid is absorbed very rapidly, the benefit of gastric lavage or emesis will vary with the time since ingestion. General supportive measures should be applied with particular attention to the maintenance of adequate urinary output.

Naloxone has been reported to reverse the CNS depressant effects of valproate overdosage. Because naloxone could theoretically also reverse the antiepileptic effects of valproate, it should be used with caution.

DOSAGE AND ADMINISTRATION

DEPAKENE (valproic acid) is administered orally. The recommended initial dose is 15 mg/kg/day, increasing at one week intervals by 5 to 10 mg/kg/day, until seizures are controlled or side effects preclude further increases. The maximum recommended dosage is 60 mg/kg/day. If the total daily dose exceeds 250 mg, it should be given in a divided regimen.

The following table is a guide for the initial daily dose of DEPAKENE (valproic acid) (15 mg/kg/day):

[See table above]

The frequency of adverse effects (particularly elevated liver enzymes) may be dose-related. The benefit of improved seizure control with higher doses should be weighed against the possibility of a greater incidence of adverse reactions.

A good correlation has not been established between daily dose, serum concentration and therapeutic effect. However, therapeutic valproate serum concentrations for most patients will range from 50 to 100 µg/mL. Some patients may be controlled with lower or higher serum concentrations (see CLINICAL PHARMACOLOGY).

As the DEPAKENE dosage is titrated upward, blood concentrations of phenobarbital and/or phenytoin may be affected. (See PRECAUTIONS).

Patients who experience G.I. irritation may benefit from administration of the drug with food or by slowly building up the dose from an initial low level.

THE CAPSULES SHOULD BE SWALLOWED WITHOUT CHEWING TO AVOID LOCAL IRRITATION OF THE MOUTH AND THROAT.

HOW SUPPLIED

DEPAKENE (valproic acid) is available as orange-colored soft gelatin capsules of 250 mg valproic acid, bearing the trademark DEPAKENE for product identification, in bottles of 100 capsules (**NDC** 0074-5681-13), and as a red syrup containing the equivalent of 250 mg valproic acid per 5 mL as the sodium salt in bottles of 16 ounces (**NDC** 0074-5682-16).

Store capsules at 59–77°F (15–25°C). Store syrup below 86°F (30°C).

REFERENCES

1. Centers for Disease Control, valproate: a new cause of birth defects—report from Italy and follow-up from France. *Morbidity and Mortality Weekly Report.* 1983;32(33):438–439.
2. Mattson, RH, et al. Use of oral contraceptives by women with epilepsy. *JAMA.* 1986;256(2):238–240.
3. Wilder, BJ, et al. Gastrointestinal tolerance of divalproex sodium. *Neurology.* 1983;33:808–811.
4. Hurst DL. Expanded therapeutic range of valproate. *Pediatr Neurol.* 1987;3:342–344.

Revised: January 1998

Caution—Federal (USA) Law prohibits dispensing without prescription.

Ref. 03-4840-R25

Shown in Product Identification Guide, page 303

DEPAKOTE® Sprinkle Capsules ℞

[*dəp' ā-coat*]

DIVALPROEX SODIUM

COATED PARTICLES IN CAPSULES

BOX WARNING:

HEPATIC FAILURE RESULTING IN FATALITIES HAS OCCURRED IN PATIENTS RECEIVING VALPROIC ACID AND ITS DERIVATIVES. EXPERIENCE HAS INDICATED THAT CHILDREN UNDER THE AGE OF TWO YEARS ARE AT A CONSIDERABLY INCREASED RISK OF DEVELOPING FATAL HEPATOTOXICITY, ESPECIALLY THOSE ON MULTIPLE ANTICONVULSANTS, THOSE WITH CONGENITAL METABOLIC DISORDERS, THOSE WITH SEVERE SEIZURE DISORDERS ACCOMPANIED BY MENTAL RETARDATION, AND THOSE WITH ORGANIC BRAIN DISEASE. WHEN DEPAKOTE IS USED IN THIS PATIENT GROUP, IT SHOULD BE USED WITH EXTREME CAUTION AND AS A SOLE AGENT. THE BENEFITS OF THERAPY SHOULD BE WEIGHED AGAINST THE RISKS. ABOVE THIS AGE GROUP, EXPERIENCE IN EPILEPSY HAS INDICATED THAT THE INCIDENCE OF FATAL HEPATOTOXICITY DECREASES CONSIDERABLY IN PROGRESSIVELY OLDER PATIENT GROUPS.

THESE INCIDENTS USUALLY HAVE OCCURRED DURING THE FIRST SIX MONTHS OF TREATMENT. SERIOUS OR FATAL HEPATOTOXICITY MAY BE PRECEDED BY NON-SPECIFIC SYMPTOMS SUCH

Continued on next page

Depakote Sprinkle—Cont.

AS MALAISE, WEAKNESS, LETHARGY, FACIAL EDEMA, ANOREXIA, AND VOMITING. IN PATIENTS WITH EPILEPSY, A LOSS OF SEIZURE CONTROL MAY ALSO OCCUR. PATIENTS SHOULD BE MONITORED CLOSELY FOR APPEARANCE OF THESE SYMPTOMS. LIVER FUNCTION TESTS SHOULD BE PERFORMED PRIOR TO THERAPY AND AT FREQUENT INTERVALS THEREAFTER, ESPECIALLY DURING THE FIRST SIX MONTHS.

TERATOGENICITY:
VALPROATE CAN PRODUCE TERATOGENIC EFFECTS SUCH AS NEURAL TUBE DEFECTS (E.G., SPINA BIFIDA), ACCORDINGLY, THE USE OF VALPROATE PRODUCTS IN WOMEN OF CHILDBEARING POTENTIAL REQUIRES THAT THE BENEFITS OF ITS USE BE WEIGHED AGAINST THE RISK OF INJURY TO THE FETUS.

DESCRIPTION

Divalproex sodium is a stable co-ordination compound comprised of sodium valproate and valproic acid in a 1:1 molar relationship and formed during the partial neutralization of valproic acid with 0.5 equivalent of sodium hydroxide. Chemically it is designated as sodium hydrogen bis (2-propyl pentanoate). Divalproex sodium has the following structure:

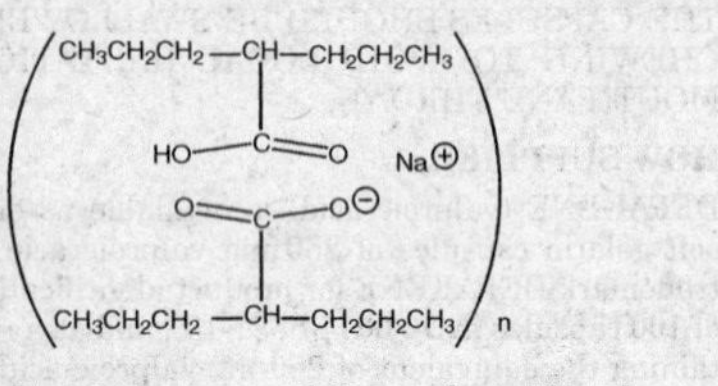
CH₃CH₂CH₂—CH—CH₂CH₂CH₃
HO—C=O
Na⊕
O=C—O⊖
CH₃CH₂CH₂—CH—CH₂CH₂CH₃
n

Divalproex sodium occurs as a white powder with a characteristic odor.

DEPAKOTE Sprinkle Capsules are for oral administration. DEPAKOTE Sprinkle Capsules contain specially coated particles of divalproex sodium equivalent to 125 mg of valproic acid in a hard gelatin capsule.

Inactive Ingredients

125 mg DEPAKOTE Sprinkle Capsules: cellulosic polymers, D&C Red No. 28, FD&C Blue No. 1, gelatin, iron oxide, magnesium stearate, silica gel, titanium dioxide, and triethyl citrate.

CLINICAL PHARMACOLOGY

Pharmacodynamics

Divalproex sodium dissociates to the valproate ion in the gastrointestinal tract. The mechanisms by which valproate exerts its therapeutic effects have not been established. It has been suggested that its activity in epilepsy is related to increased brain concentrations of gamma-aminobutyric acid (GABA).

Pharmacokinetics

Absorption/Bioavailability

Equivalent oral doses of DEPAKOTE (divalproex sodium) products and DEPAKENE (valproic acid) capsules deliver equivalent quantities of valproate ion systemically. Although the rate of valproate ion absorption may vary with the formulation administered (liquid, solid, or sprinkle), conditions of use (e.g., fasting or postprandial) and the method of administration (e.g., whether the contents of the capsule are sprinkled on food or the capsule is taken intact), these differences should be of minor clinical importance under the steady state conditions achieved in chronic use in the treatment of epilepsy.

However, it is possible that differences among the various valproate products in T_{max} and C_{max} could be important upon initiation of treatment. For example, in single dose studies, the effect of feeding had a greater influence on the rate of absorption of the tablet (increase in T_{max} from 4 to 8 hours) than on the absorption of the sprinkle capsules (increase in T_{max} from 3.3 to 4.8 hours).

While the absorption rate from the G.I. tract and fluctuation in valproate plasma concentrations vary with dosing regimen and formulation, the efficacy of valproate as an anticonvulsant in chronic use is unlikely to be affected. Experience employing dosing regimens from once-a-day to four-times-a-day, as well as studies in primate epilepsy models involving constant rate infusion, indicate that total daily systemic bioavailability (extent of absorption) is the primary determinant of seizure control and that differences in the ratios of plasma peak to trough concentrations between valproate formulations are inconsequential from a practical clinical standpoint.

Co-administration of oral valproate products with food and substitution among the various DEPAKOTE and DEPAKENE formulations should cause no clinical problems in the management of patients with epilepsy (see **DOSAGE AND ADMINISTRATION**). Nonetheless, any changes in dosage administration, or the addition or discontinuance of concomitant drugs should ordinarily be accompanied by close monitoring of clinical status and valproate plasma concentrations.

Distribution

Protein Binding:

The plasma protein binding of valproate is concentration dependent and the free fraction increases from approximately 10% at 40 µg/mL to 18.5% at 130 µg/mL. Protein binding of valproate is reduced in the elderly, in patients with chronic hepatic diseases, in patients with renal impairment, and in the presence of other drugs (e.g., aspirin). Conversely, valproate may displace certain protein-bound drugs (e.g., phenytoin, carbamazepine, warfarin, and tolbutamide). (See **PRECAUTIONS**, **Drug Interactions** for more detailed information on the pharmacokinetic interactions of valproate with other drugs.)

CNS Distribution:

Valproate concentrations in cerebrospinal fluid (CSF) approximate unbound concentrations in plasma (about 10% of total concentration).

Metabolism

Valproate is metabolized almost entirely by the liver. In adult patients on monotherapy, 30–50% of an administered dose appears in urine as a glucuronide conjugate. Mitochondrial β-oxidation is the other major metabolic pathway, typically accounting for over 40% of the dose. Usually, less than 15–20% of the dose is eliminated by other oxidative mechanisms. Less than 3% of an administered dose is excreted unchanged in urine.

The relationship between dose and total valproate concentration is nonlinear; concentration does not increase proportionally with the dose, but rather, increases to a lesser extent due to saturable plasma protein binding. The kinetics of unbound drug are linear.

Elimination

Mean plasma clearance and volume of distribution for total valproate are 0.56 L/hr/1.73 m^2 and 11 L/1.73 m^2, respectively. Mean plasma clearance and volume of distribution for free valproate are 4.6 L/hr/1.73 m^2 and 92 L/1.73 m^2. Mean terminal half-life for valproate monotherapy ranged from 9 to 16 hours following oral dosing regimens of 250 to 1000 mg.

The estimates cited apply primarily to patients who are not taking drugs that affect hepatic metabolizing enzyme systems. For example, patients taking enzyme-inducing antiepileptic drugs (carbamazepine, phenytoin, and phenobarbital) will clear valproate more rapidly. Because of these changes in valproate clearance, monitoring of antiepileptic concentrations should be intensified whenever concomitant antiepileptics are introduced or withdrawn.

Special Populations

Effect of Age:

Neonates - Children within the first two months of life have a markedly decreased ability to eliminate valproate compared to older children and adults. This is a result of reduced clearance (perhaps due to delay in development of glucuronosyltransferase and other enzyme systems involved in valproate elimination) as well as increased volume of distribution (in part due to decreased plasma protein binding). For example, in one study, the half-life in children under 10 days ranged from 10 to 67 hours compared to a range of 7 to 13 hours in children greater than 2 months.

Children - Pediatric patients (i.e., between 3 months and 10 years) have 50% higher clearances expressed on weight (i.e., mL/min/kg) than do adults. Over the age of 10 years, children have pharmacokinetic parameters that approximate those of adults.

Elderly - The capacity of elderly patients (age range: 68 to 89 years) to eliminate valproate has been shown to be reduced compared to younger adults (age range: 22 to 26). Intrinsic clearance is reduced by 39%; the free fraction is increased by 44%. Accordingly, the initial dosage should be reduced in the elderly. (See **DOSAGE AND ADMINISTRATION**).

Effect of Gender:

There are no differences in the body surface area adjusted unbound clearance between males and females (4.8±0.17 and 4.7±0.07 L/hr per 1.73 m^2, respectively).

Effect of Race:

The effects of race on the kinetics of valproate have not been studied.

Effect of Disease:

Liver Disease - (See **BOXED WARNING**, **CONTRAINDICATIONS**, and **WARNINGS**). Liver disease impairs the capacity to eliminate valproate. In one study, the clearance of free valproate was decreased by 50% in 7 patients with cirrhosis and by 16% in 4 patients with acute hepatitis, compared with 6 healthy subjects. In that study, the half-life of valproate was increased from 12 to 18 hours. Liver disease is also associated with decreased albumin concentrations and larger unbound fractions (2 to 2.6 fold increase) of valproate. Accordingly, monitoring of total concentrations may be misleading since free concentrations may be substantially elevated in patients with hepatic disease whereas total concentrations may appear to be normal.

Renal Disease - A slight reduction (27%) in the unbound clearance of valproate has been reported in patients with renal failure (creatinine clearance < 10 mL/minute); however, hemodialysis typically reduces valproate concentrations by about 20%. Therefore, no dosage adjustment appears to be necessary in patients with renal failure. Protein binding in these patients is substantially reduced; thus, monitoring total concentrations may be misleading.

Plasma Levels and Clinical Effect

The relationship between plasma concentration and clinical response is not well documented. One contributing factor is the nonlinear, concentration dependent protein binding of valproate which affects the clearance of the drug. Thus, monitoring of total serum valproate cannot provide a reliable index of the bioactive valproate species.

For example, because the plasma protein binding of valproate is concentration dependent, the free fraction increases from approximately 10% at 40 µg/mL to 18.5% at 130 µg/mL. Higher than expected free fractions occur in the elderly, in hyperlipidemic patients, and in patients with hepatic and renal diseases.

Epilepsy:

The therapeutic range in epilepsy is commonly considered to be 50 to 100 µg/mL of total valproate, although some patients may be controlled with lower or higher plasma concentrations.

CLINICAL STUDIES

Epilepsy

The efficacy of DEPAKOTE in reducing the incidence of complex partial seizures (CPS) that occur in isolation or in association with other seizure types was established in two controlled trials.

In one, a multiclinic, placebo controlled study employing an add-on design (adjunctive therapy), 144 patients who continued to suffer eight or more CPS per 8 weeks during an 8 week period of monotherapy with doses of either carbamazepine or phenytoin sufficient to assure plasma concentrations within the "therapeutic range" were randomized to receive, in addition to their original antiepilepsy drug (AED), either DEPAKOTE or placebo. Randomized patients were to be followed for a total of 16 weeks. The following table presents the findings.

Adjunctive Therapy Study
Median Incidence of CPS per 8 Weeks

Add-on Treatment	Number of Patients	Baseline Incidence	Experimental Incidence
DEPAKOTE	75	16.0	8.9*
Placebo	69	14.5	11.5

*Reduction from baseline statistically significantly greater for DEPAKOTE than placebo at p ≤0.05 level.

Figure 1 presents the proportion of patients (X axis) whose percentage reduction from baseline in complex partial seizure rates was at least as great as that indicated on the Y axis in the adjunctive therapy study. A positive percent reduction indicates an improvement (i.e., a decrease in seizure frequency), while a negative percent reduction indicates worsening. Thus, in a display of this type, the curve for an effective treatment is shifted to the left of the curve for placebo. This figure shows that the proportion of patients achieving any particular level of improvement was consistently higher for DEPAKOTE than for placebo. For example, 45% of patients treated with DEPAKOTE had a ≥50% reduction in complex partial seizure rate compared to 23% of patients treated with placebo.

Figure 1

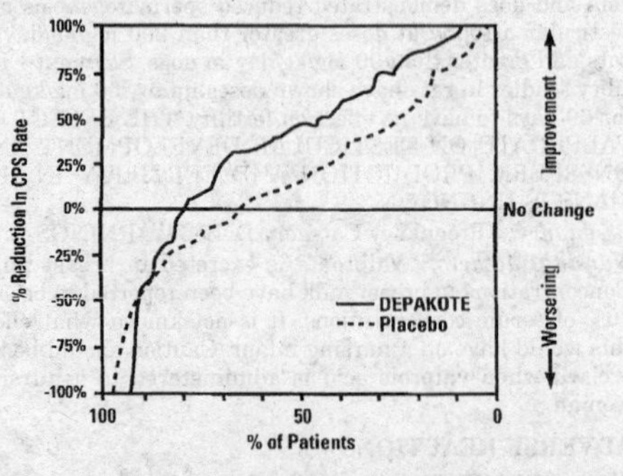
100%
75%
50%
25%
0%
-25%
-50%
-75%
-100%
% Reduction In CPS Rate
Improvement
No Change
Worsening
DEPAKOTE
Placebo
100
50
0
% of Patients

The second study assessed the capacity of DEPAKOTE to reduce the incidence of CPS when administered as the sole AED. The study compared the incidence of CPS among patients randomized to either a high or low dose treatment arm. Patients qualified for entry into the randomized comparison phase of this study only if 1) they continued to experience 2 or more CPS per 4 weeks during an 8 to 12 week long period of monotherapy with adequate doses of an

AED (i.e., phenytoin, carbamazepine, phenobarbital, or primidone) and 2) they made a successful transition over a two week interval to DEPAKOTE. Patients entering the randomized phase were then brought to their assigned target dose, gradually tapered off their concomitant AED and followed for an interval as long as 22 weeks. Less than 50% of the patients randomized, however, completed the study. In patients converted to DEPAKOTE monotherapy, the mean total valproate concentrations during monotherapy were 71 and 123 µg/mL in the low dose and high dose groups, respectively.

The following table presents the findings for all patients randomized who had at least one post-randomization assessment.

Monotherapy Study
Median Incidence of CPS per 8 Weeks

Treatment	Number of Patients	Baseline Incidence	Randomized Phase Incidence
High dose DEPAKOTE	131	13.2	10.7*
Low dose DEPAKOTE	134	14.2	13.8

* Reduction from baseline statistically significantly greater for high dose than low dose at p ≤0.05 level.

Figure 2 presents the proportion of patients (X axis) whose percentage reduction from baseline in complex partial seizure rates was at least as great as that indicated on the Y axis in the monotherapy study. A positive percent reduction indicates an improvement (i.e., a decrease in seizure frequency), while a negative percent reduction indicates worsening. Thus, in a display of this type, the curve for a more effective treatment is shifted to the left of the curve for a less effective treatment. This figure shows that the proportion of patients achieving any particular level of reduction was consistently higher for high dose DEPAKOTE than for low dose DEPAKOTE. For example, when switching from carbamazepine, phenytoin, phenobarbital or primidone monotherapy to high dose DEPAKOTE monotherapy, 63% of patients experienced no change or a reduction in complex partial seizure rates compared to 54% of patients receiving low dose DEPAKOTE.

Figure 2

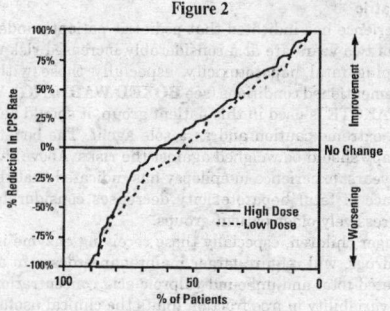

INDICATIONS AND USAGE

DEPAKOTE Sprinkle Capsules are indicated as monotherapy and adjunctive therapy in the treatment of patients with complex partial seizures that occur either in isolation or in association with other types of seizure. DEPAKOTE Sprinkle Capsules are also indicated for use as sole and adjunctive therapy in the treatment of simple and complex absence seizures, and adjunctively in patients with multiple seizure types that include absence seizures.

Simple absence is defined as very brief clouding of the sensorium or loss of consciousness accompanied by certain generalized epileptic discharges without other detectable clinical signs. Complex absence is the term used when other signs are also present.

SEE **WARNINGS** FOR STATEMENT REGARDING FATAL HEPATIC DYSFUNCTION.

CONTRAINDICATIONS

DIVALPROEX SODIUM SHOULD NOT BE ADMINISTERED TO PATIENTS WITH HEPATIC DISEASE OR SIGNIFICANT HEPATIC DYSFUNCTION.

Divalproex sodium is contraindicated in patients with known hypersensitivity to the drug.

WARNINGS

Hepatic failure resulting in fatalities has occurred in patients receiving valproic acid. These incidents usually have occurred during the first six months of treatment. Serious or fatal hepatotoxicity may be preceded by non-specific symptoms such as malaise, weakness, lethargy, facial edema, anorexia, and vomiting. In patients with epilepsy, a loss of seizure control may also occur. Patients should be monitored closely for appearance of these symptoms. Liver function tests should be performed prior to therapy and at

frequent intervals thereafter, especially during the first six months. However, physicians should not rely totally on serum biochemistry since these tests may not be abnormal in all instances, but should also consider the results of careful interim medical history and physical examination. Caution should be observed when administering DEPAKOTE products to patients with a prior history of hepatic disease. Patients on multiple anticonvulsants, children, those with congenital metabolic disorders, those with severe seizure disorders accompanied by mental retardation, and those with organic brain disease may be at particular risk. Experience has indicated that children under the age of two years are at a considerably increased risk of developing fatal hepatotoxicity, especially those with the aforementioned conditions. When DEPAKOTE is used in this patient group, it should be used with extreme caution and as a sole agent. The benefits of therapy should be weighed against the risks. Above this age group, experience in epilepsy has indicated that the incidence of fatal hepatotoxicity decreases considerably in progressively older patient groups.

The drug should be discontinued immediately in the presence of significant hepatic dysfunction, suspected or apparent. In some cases, hepatic dysfunction has progressed in spite of discontinuation of drug.

The frequency of adverse effects (particularly elevated liver enzymes and thrombocytopenia [see **PRECAUTIONS**]) may be dose-related. In a clinical trial of DEPAKOTE (divalproex sodium) as monotherapy in patients with epilepsy, 34/126 patients (27%) receiving approximately 50 mg/kg/day on average, had at least one value of platelets ≤75 x 10⁹/L. Approximately half of these patients had treatment discontinued, with return of platelet counts to normal. In the remaining patients, platelet counts normalized with continued treatment. In this study, the probability of thrombocytopenia appeared to increase significantly at total valproate concentrations of ≥110 µg/mL (females) or ≥135 µg/mL (males). The therapeutic benefit which may accompany the higher doses should therefore be weighed against the possibility of a greater incidence of adverse effects.

Usage In Pregnancy

ACCORDING TO PUBLISHED AND UNPUBLISHED REPORTS, VALPROIC ACID MAY PRODUCE TERATOGENIC EFFECTS IN THE OFFSPRING OF HUMAN FEMALES RECEIVING THE DRUG DURING PREGNANCY. THERE ARE MULTIPLE REPORTS IN THE CLINICAL LITERATURE WHICH INDICATE THAT THE USE OF ANTIEPILEPTIC DRUGS DURING PREGNANCY RESULTS IN AN INCREASED INCIDENCE OF BIRTH DEFECTS IN THE OFFSPRING. ALTHOUGH DATA ARE MORE EXTENSIVE WITH RESPECT TO TRIMETHADIONE, PARAMETHADIONE, PHENYTOIN, AND PHENOBARBITAL, REPORTS INDICATE A POSSIBLE SIMILAR ASSOCIATION WITH THE USE OF OTHER ANTIEPILEPTIC DRUGS.

THE INCIDENCE OF NEURAL TUBE DEFECTS IN THE FETUS MAY BE INCREASED IN MOTHERS RECEIVING VALPROATE DURING THE FIRST TRIMESTER OF PREGNANCY. THE CENTERS FOR DISEASE CONTROL (CDC) HAS ESTIMATED THE RISK OF VALPROIC ACID EXPOSED WOMEN HAVING CHILDREN WITH SPINA BIFIDA TO BE APPROXIMATELY 1 TO 2%.

OTHER CONGENITAL ANOMALIES (E.G., CRANIOFACIAL DEFECTS, CARDIOVASCULAR MALFORMATIONS AND ANOMALIES INVOLVING VARIOUS BODY SYSTEMS), COMPATIBLE AND INCOMPATIBLE WITH LIFE, HAVE BEEN REPORTED. SUFFICIENT DATA TO DETERMINE THE INCIDENCE OF THESE CONGENITAL ANOMALIES IS NOT AVAILABLE.

THE HIGHER INCIDENCE OF CONGENITAL ANOMALIES IN ANTIEPILEPTIC DRUG-TREATED WOMEN WITH SEIZURE DISORDERS CANNOT BE REGARDED AS A CAUSE AND EFFECT RELATIONSHIP. THERE ARE INTRINSIC METHODOLOGIC PROBLEMS IN OBTAINING ADEQUATE DATA ON DRUG TERATOGENICITY IN HUMANS; GENETIC FACTORS OR THE EPILEPTIC CONDITION ITSELF, MAY BE MORE IMPORTANT THAN DRUG THERAPY IN CONTRIBUTING TO CONGENITAL ANOMALIES.

PATIENTS TAKING VALPROATE MAY DEVELOP CLOTTING ABNORMALITIES. A PATIENT WHO HAD LOW FIBRINOGEN WHEN TAKING MULTIPLE ANTICONVULSANTS INCLUDING VALPROATE GAVE BIRTH TO AN INFANT WITH AFIBRINOGENEMIA WHO SUBSEQUENTLY DIED OF HEMORRHAGE. IF VALPROATE IS USED IN PREGNANCY, THE CLOTTING PARAMETERS SHOULD BE MONITORED CAREFULLY.

HEPATIC FAILURE, RESULTING IN THE DEATH OF A NEWBORN AND OF AN INFANT, HAVE BEEN REPORTED FOLLOWING THE USE OF VALPROATE DURING PREGNANCY.

Animal studies have demonstrated valproate-induced teratogenicity. Increased frequencies of malformations, as well as intrauterine growth retardation and death, have been observed in mice, rats, rabbits, and monkeys following prena-

tal exposure to valproate. Malformations of the skeletal system are the most common structural abnormalities produced in experimental animals, but neural tube closure defects have been seen in mice exposed to maternal plasma valproate concentrations exceeding 230 µg/mL (2.3 times the upper limit of the human therapeutic range) during susceptible periods of embryonic development. Administration of an oral dose of 200 mg/kg/day or greater (50% of the maximum human daily dose or greater on a mg/m² basis) to pregnant rats during organogenesis produced malformations (skeletal, cardiac, and urogenital) and growth retardation in the offspring. These doses resulted in peak maternal plasma valproate levels of approximately 340 µg/mL or greater (3.4 times the upper limit of the human therapeutic range or greater). Behavioral deficits have been reported in the offspring of rats given a dose of 200 mg/kg/day throughout most of pregnancy. An oral dose of 350 mg/kg/day (approximately 2 times the maximum human daily dose on a mg/m² basis) produced skeletal and visceral malformations in rabbits exposed during organogenesis. Skeletal malformations, growth retardation, and death were observed in rhesus monkeys following administration of an oral dose of 200 mg/kg/day (equal to the maximum human daily dose on a mg/m² basis) during organogenesis. This dose resulted in peak maternal plasma valproate levels of approximately 280 µg/mL (2.8 times the upper limit of the human therapeutic range).

The prescribing physician will wish to weigh the benefits of therapy against the risks in treating or counseling women of childbearing potential. If this drug is used during pregnancy, or if the patient becomes pregnant while taking this drug, the patient should be apprised of the potential hazard to the fetus.

Antiepileptic drugs should not be discontinued abruptly in patients in whom the drug is administered to prevent major seizures because of the strong possibility of precipitating status epilepticus with attendant hypoxia and threat to life. In individual cases where the severity and frequency of the seizure disorder are such that the removal of medication does not pose a serious threat to the patient, discontinuation of the drug may be considered prior to and during pregnancy, although it cannot be said with any confidence that even minor seizures do not pose some hazard to the developing embryo or fetus.

Tests to detect neural tube and other defects using current accepted procedures should be considered a part of routine prenatal care in childbearing women receiving valproate.

PRECAUTIONS
Hepatic Dysfunction
See **BOXED WARNING, CONTRAINDICATIONS** and **WARNINGS**.
General
Because of reports of thrombocytopenia (see **WARNINGS**), inhibition of the secondary phase of platelet aggregation, and abnormal coagulation parameters, (e.g., low fibrinogen), platelet counts and coagulation tests are recommended before initiating therapy and at periodic intervals. It is recommended that patients receiving DEPAKOTE be monitored for platelet count and coagulation parameters prior to planned surgery. In a clinical trial of DEPAKOTE as monotherapy in patients with epilepsy, 34/126 patients (27%) receiving approximately 50 mg/kg/day on average, had at least one value of platelets ≤75 x 10⁹/L. Approximately half of these patients had treatment discontinued, with return of platelet counts to normal. In the remaining patients, platelet counts normalized with continued treatment. In this study, the probability of thrombocytopenia appeared to increase significantly at total valproate concentrations of ≥110 µg/mL (females) or ≥135 µg/mL (males). Evidence of hemorrhage, bruising, or a disorder of hemostasis/coagulation is an indication for reduction of the dosage or withdrawal of therapy.

Hyperammonemia with or without lethargy or coma has been reported and may be present in the absence of abnormal liver function tests. Asymptomatic elevations of ammonia are more common and when present require more frequent monitoring. If clinically significant symptoms occur, DEPAKOTE therapy should be modified or discontinued.

Since DEPAKOTE may interact with concurrently administered drugs which are capable of enzyme induction, periodic plasma concentration determinations of valproate and concomitant drugs are recommended during the early course of therapy. (See **PRECAUTIONS - Drug Interactions.**)

Valproate is partially eliminated in the urine as a keto-metabolite which may lead to a false interpretation of the urine ketone test.

There have been reports of altered thyroid function tests associated with valproate. The clinical significance of these is unknown.

Information for Patients
Since DEPAKOTE products may produce CNS depression, especially when combined with another CNS depressant (e.g., alcohol), patients should be advised not to engage in

Continued on next page

Depakote Sprinkle—Cont.

hazardous activities, such as driving an automobile or operating dangerous machinery, until it is known that they do not become drowsy from the drug.

The specially coated particles in DEPAKOTE Sprinkle Capsules have been observed in the stool, but this occurrence has not been associated with clinically significant effects.

Drug Interactions

Effects of Co-Administered Drugs on Valproate Clearance

Drugs that affect the level of expression of hepatic enzymes, particularly those that elevate levels of glucuronosyltransferases, may increase the clearance of valproate. For example, phenytoin, carbamazepine, and phenobarbital (or primidone) can double the clearance of valproate. Thus, patients on monotherapy will generally have longer half-lives and higher concentrations than patients receiving polytherapy with antiepilepsy drugs.

In contrast, drugs that are inhibitors of cytochrome P450 isozymes, e.g., antidepressants, may be expected to have little effect on valproate clearance because cytochrome P450 microsomal mediated oxidation is a relatively minor secondary metabolic pathway compared to glucuronidation and beta-oxidation.

Because of these changes in valproate clearance, monitoring of valproate and concomitant drug concentrations should be increased whenever enzyme inducing drugs are introduced or withdrawn.

The following list provides information about the potential for an influence of several commonly prescribed medications on valproate pharmacokinetics. The list is not exhaustive nor could it be, since new interactions are continuously being reported.

Drugs for which a potentially important interaction has been observed:

Aspirin - A study involving the co-administration of aspirin at antipyretic doses (11 to 16 mg/kg) with valproate to pediatric patients (n=6) revealed a decrease in protein binding and an inhibition of metabolism of valproate. Valproate free fraction was increased 4-fold in the presence of aspirin compared to valproate alone. The β-oxidation pathway consisting of 2-E-valproic acid, 3-OH-valproic acid, and 3-keto valproic acid was decreased from 25% of total metabolites excreted on valproate alone to 8.3% in the presence of aspirin. Caution should be observed if valproate and aspirin are to be co-administered.

Felbamate - A study involving the co-administration of 1200 mg/day of felbamate with valproate to patients with epilepsy (n=10) revealed an increase in mean valproate peak concentration by 35% (from 86 to 115 μg/mL) compared to valproate alone. Increasing the felbamate dose to 2400 mg/day increased the mean valproate peak concentration to 133 μg/mL (another 16% increase). A decrease in valproate dosage may be necessary when felbamate therapy is initiated.

Rifampin - A study involving the administration of a single dose of valproate (7 mg/kg) 36 hours after 5 nights of daily dosing with rifampin (600 mg) revealed a 40% increase in the oral clearance of valproate. Valproate dosage adjustment may be necessary when it is co-administered with rifampin.

Drugs for which either no interaction or a likely clinically unimportant interaction has been observed:

Antacids - A study involving the co-administration of valproate 500 mg with commonly administered antacids (Maalox, Trisogel, and Titralac - 160 mEq doses) did not reveal any effect on the extent of absorption of valproate.

Chlorpromazine - A study involving the administration of 100 to 300 mg/day of chlorpromazine to schizophrenic patients already receiving valproate (200 mg BID) revealed a 15% increase in trough plasma levels of valproate.

Haloperidol - A study involving the administration of 6 to 10 mg/day of haloperidol to schizophrenic patients already receiving valproate (200 mg BID) revealed no significant changes in valproate trough plasma levels.

Cimetidine and Ranitidine - Cimetidine and ranitidine do not affect the clearance of valproate.

Effects of Valproate on Other Drugs

Valproate has been found to be a weak inhibitor of some P450 isozymes, epoxide hydrase, and glucuronosyltransferases.

The following list provides information about the potential for an influence of valproate co-administration on the pharmacokinetics or pharmacodynamics of several commonly prescribed medications. The list is not exhaustive, since new interactions are continuously being reported.

Drugs for which a potentially important valproate interaction has been observed:

Carbamazepine/carbamazepine-10,11-Epoxide - Serum levels of carbamazepine (CBZ) decreased 17% while that of carbamazepine-10,11-epoxide (CBZ-E) increased by 45% upon co-administration of valproate and CBZ to epileptic patients.

Clonazepam - The concomitant use of valproic acid and clonazepam may induce absence status in patients with a history of absence type seizures.

Diazepam - Valproate displaces diazepam from its plasma albumin binding sites and inhibits its metabolism. Co-administration of valproate (1500 mg daily) increased the free fraction of diazepam (10 mg) by 90% in healthy volunteers (n=6). Plasma clearance and volume of distribution for free diazepam were reduced by 25% and 20%, respectively, in the presence of valproate. The elimination half-life of diazepam remained unchanged upon addition of valproate.

Ethosuximide - Valproate inhibits the metabolism of ethosuximide. Administration of a single ethosuximide dose of 500 mg with valproate (800 to 1600 mg/day) to healthy volunteers (n=6) was accompanied by a 25% increase in elimination half-life of ethosuximide and a 15% decrease in its total clearance as compared to ethosuximide alone. Patients receiving valproate and ethosuximide, especially along with other anticonvulsants, should be monitored for alterations in serum concentrations of both drugs.

Lamotrigine - In a steady-state study involving 10 healthy volunteers, the elimination half-life of lamotrigine increased from 26 to 70 hours with valproate co-administration (a 165% increase). The dose of lamotrigine should be reduced when co-administered with valproate.

Phenobarbital - Valproate was found to inhibit the metabolism of phenobarbital. Co-administration of valproate (250 mg BID for 14 days) with phenobarbital to normal subjects (n=6) resulted in a 50% increase in half-life and a 30% decrease in plasma clearance of phenobarbital (60 mg single-dose). The fraction of phenobarbital dose excreted unchanged increased by 50% in presence of valproate.

There is evidence for severe CNS depression, with or without significant elevations of barbiturate or valproate serum concentrations. All patients receiving concomitant barbiturate therapy should be closely monitored for neurological toxicity. Serum barbiturate concentrations should be obtained, if possible, and the barbiturate dosage decreased, if appropriate.

Primidone, which is metabolized to a barbiturate, may be involved in a similar interaction with valproate.

Phenytoin - Valproate displaces phenytoin from its plasma albumin binding sites and inhibits its hepatic metabolism. Co-administration of valproate (400 mg TID) with phenytoin (250 mg) in normal volunteers (n=7) was associated with a 60% increase in the free fraction of phenytoin. Total plasma clearance and apparent volume of distribution of phenytoin increased 30% in the presence of valproate. Both the clearance and apparent volume of distribution of free phenytoin were reduced by 25%.

In patients with epilepsy, there have been reports of breakthrough seizures occurring with the combination of valproate and phenytoin. The dosage of phenytoin should be adjusted as required by the clinical situation.

Tolbutamide - From in vitro experiments, the unbound fraction of tolbutamide was increased from 20% to 50% when added to plasma samples taken from patients treated with valproate. The clinical relevance of this displacement is unknown.

Warfarin - In an in vitro study, valproate increased the unbound fraction of warfarin by up to 32.6%. The therapeutic relevance of this is unknown; however, coagulation tests should be monitored if DEPAKOTE therapy is instituted in patients taking anticoagulants.

Zidovudine - In six patients who were seropositive for HIV, the clearance of zidovudine (100 mg q8h) was decreased by 38% after administration of valproate (250 or 500 mg q8h); the half-life of zidovudine was unaffected.

Drugs for which either no interaction or a likely clinically unimportant interaction has been observed:

Acetaminophen - Valproate had no effect on any of the pharmacokinetic parameters of acetaminophen when it was concurrently administered to three epileptic patients.

Amitriptyline/Nortriptyline - Administration of a single oral 50 mg dose of amitriptyline to 15 normal volunteers (10 males and 5 females) who received valproate (500 mg BID) resulted in a 21% decrease in plasma clearance of amitriptyline and a 34% decrease in the net clearance of nortriptyline.

Clozapine - In psychotic patients (n=11), no interaction was observed when valproate was co-administered with clozapine.

Lithium - Co-administration of valproate (500 mg BID) and lithium carbonate (300 mg TID) to normal male volunteers (n=16) had no effect on the steady-state kinetics of lithium.

Lorazepam - Concomitant administration of valproate (500 mg BID) and lorazepam (1 mg BID) in normal male volunteers (n=9) was accompanied by a 17% decrease in the plasma clearance of lorazepam.

Oral Contraceptive Steroids - Administration of a single-dose of ethinyloestradiol (50 μg)/levonorgestrel (250 μg) to 6 women on valproate (200 mg BID) therapy for 2 months did not reveal any pharmacokinetic interaction.

Carcinogenesis, Mutagenesis, Impairment of Fertility

Carcinogenesis

Valproic acid was administered orally to Sprague Dawley rats and ICR (HA/ICR) mice at doses of 80 and 170 mg/kg/day (approximately 10 to 50% of the maximum human daily dose on a mg/m^2 basis) for two years. A variety of neoplasms were observed in both species. The chief findings were a statistically significant increase in the incidence of subcutaneous fibrosarcomas in high dose male rats receiving valproic acid and a statistically significant dose-related trend for benign pulmonary adenomas in male mice receiving valproic acid. The significance of these findings for humans is unknown.

Mutagenesis

Valproate was not mutagenic in an in vitro bacterial assay (Ames test), did not produce dominant lethal effects in mice, and did not increase chromosome aberration frequency in an in vivo cytogenetic study in rats. Increased frequencies of sister chromatid exchange (SCE) have been reported in a study of epileptic children taking valproate, but this association was not observed in another study conducted in adults. There is some evidence that increased SCE frequencies may be associated with epilepsy. The biological significance of increase in SCE frequency is not known.

Fertility

Chronic toxicity studies in juvenile and adult rats and dogs demonstrated reduced spermatogenesis and testicular atrophy at oral doses of 400 mg/kg/day or greater in rats (approximately equivalent to or greater than the maximum human daily dose on a mg/m^2 basis) and 150 mg/kg/day or greater in dogs (approximately 1.4 times the maximum human daily dose or greater on a mg/m^2 basis). Segment I fertility studies in rats have shown oral doses up to 350 mg/kg/day (approximately equal to the maximum human daily dose on a mg/m^2 basis) for 60 days to have no effect on fertility. THE EFFECT OF VALPROATE ON TESTICULAR DEVELOPMENT AND ON SPERM PRODUCTION AND FERTILITY IN HUMANS IS UNKNOWN.

Pregnancy

Pregnancy Category D: See **WARNINGS**.

Nursing Mothers

Valproate is excreted in breast milk. Concentrations in breast milk have been reported to be 1–10% of serum concentrations. It is not known what effect this would have on a nursing infant. Consideration should be given to discontinuing nursing when divalproex sodium is administered to a nursing woman.

Pediatric

Experience has indicated that pediatric patients under the age of two years are at a considerably increased risk of developing fatal hepatotoxicity, especially those with the aforementioned conditions (see **BOXED WARNING**). When DEPAKOTE is used in this patient group, it should be used with extreme caution and as a sole agent. The benefits of therapy should be weighed against the risks. Above the age of 2 years, experience in epilepsy has indicated that the incidence of fatal hepatotoxicity decreases considerably in progressively older patient groups.

Younger children, especially those receiving enzyme-inducing drugs, will require larger maintenance doses to attain targeted total and unbound valproic acid concentrations.

The variability in free fraction limits the clinical usefulness of monitoring total serum valproic acid concentrations. Interpretation of valproic acid concentrations in children should include consideration of factors that affect hepatic metabolism and protein binding.

The basic toxicology and pathologic manifestations of valproate sodium in neonatal (4-day old) and juvenile (14-day old) rats are similar to those seen in young adult rats. However, additional findings, including renal alterations in juvenile rats and renal alterations and retinal dysplasia in neonatal rats, have been reported. These findings occurred at 240 mg/kg/day, a dosage approximately equivalent to the human maximum recommended daily dose on a mg/m^2 basis. They were not seen at 90 mg/kg, or 40% of the maximum human daily dose on a mg/m^2 basis.

ADVERSE REACTIONS

Epilepsy

Based on a placebo-controlled trial of adjunctive therapy for treatment of complex partial seizures, DEPAKOTE was generally well tolerated with most adverse events rated as mild to moderate in severity. Intolerance was the primary reason for discontinuation in the DEPAKOTE-treated patients (6%), compared to 1% of placebo-treated patients.

Table 1 lists treatment-emergent adverse events which were reported by ≥5% of DEPAKOTE-treated patients and for which the incidence was greater than in the placebo group, in the placebo-controlled trial of adjunctive therapy for treatment of complex partial seizures. Since patients were also treated with other antiepilepsy drugs, it is not possible, in most cases, to determine whether the following adverse events can be ascribed to DEPAKOTE alone, or the combination of DEPAKOTE and other antiepilepsy drugs.

Table 1
Adverse Events Reported by ≥5% of Patients Treated with DEPAKOTE During Placebo-Controlled Trial of Adjunctive Therapy for Complex Partial Seizures

Body System/Event	Depakote (%) (n = 77)	Placebo (%) (n = 70)
Body as a Whole		
Headache	31	21
Asthenia	27	7
Fever	6	4
Gastrointestinal System		
Nausea	48	14
Vomiting	27	7
Abdominal Pain	23	6
Diarrhea	13	6
Anorexia	12	0
Dyspepsia	8	4
Constipation	5	1
Nervous System		
Somnolence	27	11
Tremor	25	6
Dizziness	25	13
Diplopia	16	9
Amblyopia/Blurred Vision	12	9
Ataxia	8	1
Nystagmus	8	1
Emotional Lability	6	4
Thinking Abnormal	6	0
Amnesia	5	1
Respiratory System		
Flu Syndrome	12	9
Infection	12	6
Bronchitis	5	1
Rhinitis	5	4
Other		
Alopecia	6	1
Weight Loss	6	0

Table 2 lists treatment-emergent adverse events which were reported by ≥ 5% of patients in the high dose DEPAKOTE group, and for which the incidence was greater than in the low dose group, in a controlled trial of DEPAKOTE monotherapy treatment of complex partial seizures. Since patients were being titrated off another antiepilepsy drug during the first portion of the trial, it is not possible, in many cases, to determine whether the following adverse events can be ascribed to DEPAKOTE alone, or the combination of DEPAKOTE and other antiepilepsy drugs.

Table 2
Adverse Events Reported by ≥5% of Patients in the High Dose Group in the Controlled Trial of DEPAKOTE Monotherapy for Complex Partial Seizures[1]

Body System/Event	High Dose (%) (n = 131)	Low Dose (%) (n = 134)
Body as a Whole		
Asthenia	21	10
Digestive System		
Nausea	34	26
Diarrhea	23	19
Vomiting	23	15
Abdominal Pain	12	9
Anorexia	11	4
Dyspepsia	11	10
Hemic/Lymphatic System		
Thrombocytopenia	24	1
Ecchymosis	5	4
Metabolic/Nutritional		
Weight Gain	9	4
Peripheral Edema	8	3
Nervous System		
Tremor	57	19
Somnolence	30	18
Dizziness	18	13
Insomnia	15	9
Nervousness	11	7
Amnesia	7	4
Nystagmus	7	1
Depression	5	4
Respiratory System		
Infection	20	13
Pharyngitis	8	2
Dyspnea	5	1
Skin and Appendages		
Alopecia	24	13
Special Senses		
Amblyopia/Blurred Vision	8	4
Tinnitus	7	1

[1] Headache was the only adverse event that occurred in ≥5% of patients in the high dose group and at an equal or greater incidence in the low dose group.

The following additional adverse events were reported by greater than 1% but less than 5% of the 358 patients treated with DEPAKOTE in the controlled trials of complex partial seizures:

Body as a Whole: Back pain, chest pain, malaise.
Cardiovascular System: Tachycardia, hypertension, palpitation.
Digestive System: Increased appetite, flatulence, hematemesis, eructation, pancreatitis, periodontal abscess.
Hemic and Lymphatic System: Petechia.
Metabolic and Nutritional Disorders: SGOT increased, SGPT increased.
Musculoskeletal System: Myalgia, twitching, arthralgia, leg cramps, myasthenia.
Nervous System: Anxiety, confusion, abnormal gait, paresthesia, hypertonia, incoordination, abnormal dreams, personality disorder.
Respiratory System: Sinusitis, cough increased, pneumonia, epistaxis.
Skin and Appendages: Rash, pruritus, dry skin.
Special Senses: Taste perversion, abnormal vision, deafness, otitis media.
Urogenital System: Urinary incontinence, vaginitis, dysmenorrhea, amenorrhea, urinary frequency.

Other Patient Populations
Adverse events that have been reported with all dosage forms of valproate from epilepsy trials, spontaneous reports, and other sources are listed below by body system.
Gastrointestinal: The most commonly reported side effects at the initiation of therapy are nausea, vomiting, and indigestion. These effects are usually transient and rarely require discontinuation of therapy. Diarrhea, abdominal cramps, and constipation have been reported. Both anorexia with some weight loss and increased appetite with weight gain have also been reported. The administration of delayed-release divalproex sodium may result in reduction of gastrointestinal side effects in some patients.
CNS Effects: Sedative effects have occurred in patients receiving valproate alone but occur most often in patients receiving combination therapy. Sedation usually abates upon reduction of other antiepileptic medication. Tremor (may be dose-related), hallucinations, ataxia, headache, nystagmus, diplopia, asterixis, "spots before eyes", dysarthria, dizziness, confusion, hypesthesia, vertigo, and incoordination. Rare cases of coma have occurred in patients receiving valproate alone or in conjunction with phenobarbital. In rare instances encephalopathy with fever has developed shortly after the introduction of valproate monotherapy without evidence of hepatic dysfunction or inappropriate plasma levels; all patients recovered after the drug was withdrawn.
Several reports have noted reversible cerebral atrophy and dementia in association with valproate therapy.
Dermatologic: Transient hair loss, skin rash, photosensitivity, generalized pruritus, erythema multiforme, and Stevens-Johnson syndrome. Rare cases of toxic epidermal necrolysis have been reported including a fatal case in a 6 month old infant taking valproate and several other concomitant medications. An additional case of toxic epidermal necrosis resulting in death was reported in a 35 year old patient with AIDS taking several concomitant medications and with a history of multiple cutaneous drug reactions.
Psychiatric: Emotional upset, depression, psychosis, aggression, hyperactivity, hostility, and behavioral deterioration.
Musculoskeletal: Weakness.
Hematologic: Thrombocytopenia and inhibition of the secondary phase of platelet aggregation may be reflected in altered bleeding time, petechia, bruising, hematoma formation, epistaxis, and frank hemorrhage (see **PRECAUTIONS - General** and **Drug Interactions**). Relative lymphocytosis, macrocytosis, hypofibrinogenemia, leukopenia, eosinophilia, anemia including macrocytic with or without folate deficiency, bone marrow suppression, pancytopenia, aplastic anemia, and acute intermittent porphyria.
Hepatic: Minor elevations of transaminases (eg, SGOT and SGPT) and LDH are frequent and appear to be dose-related. Occasionally, laboratory test results include increases in serum bilirubin and abnormal changes in other liver function tests. These results may reflect potentially serious hepatotoxicity (see **WARNINGS**).
Endocrine: Irregular menses, secondary amenorrhea, breast enlargement, galactorrhea, and parotid gland swelling. Abnormal thyroid function tests (see **PRECAUTIONS**).
There have been rare spontaneous reports of polycystic ovary disease. A cause and effect of relationship has not been established.
Pancreatic: Acute pancreatitis including fatalities.
Metabolic: Hyperammonemia (see **PRECAUTIONS**), hyponatremia, and inappropriate ADH secretion.
There have been rare reports of Fanconi's syndrome occurring chiefly in children.
Decreased carnitine concentrations have been reported although the clinical relevance is undetermined.

Hyperglycinemia has occurred and was associated with a fatal outcome in a patient with preexistent nonketotic hyperglycinemia.
Genitourinary: Enuresis and urinary tract infection.
Special Senses: Hearing loss, either reversible or irreversible, has been reported; however, a cause and effect relationship has not been established. Ear pain has also been reported.
Other: Edema of the extremities, lupus erythematosus, bone pain, cough increased, pneumonia, otitis media, bradycardia, cutaneous vasculitis, and fever.

Mania
Although DEPAKOTE Sprinkle Capsules have not been evaluated for safety and efficacy in the treatment of manic episodes associated with bipolar disorder, the following adverse events not listed above were reported by 1% or more of patients from two placebo-controlled clinical trials of DEPAKOTE tablets.
Body as a Whole: Chills, neck pain, neck rigidity.
Cardiovascular System: Hypotension, postural hypotension, vasodilation.
Digestive System: Fecal incontinence, gastroenteritis, glossitis.
Musculoskeletal System: Arthrosis.
Nervous System: Agitation, catatonic reaction, hypokinesia, reflexes increased, tardive dyskinesia, vertigo.
Skin and Appendages: Furunculosis, maculopapular rash, seborrhea.
Special Senses: Conjunctivitis, dry eyes, eye pain.
Urogenital System: Dysuria.

Migraine
Although DEPAKOTE Sprinkle Capsules have not been evaluated for safety and efficacy in the treatment of prophylaxis of migraine headaches, the following adverse events not listed above were reported by 1% or more of patients from two placebo-controlled clinical trials of DEPAKOTE tablets.
Body as a Whole: Face edema.
Digestive System: Dry mouth, stomatitis.
Urogenital System: Cystitis, metrorrhagia, and vaginal hemorrhage.

OVERDOSAGE
Overdosage with valproate may result in somnolence, heart block, and deep coma. Fatalities have been reported; however patients have recovered from valproate levels as high as 2120 μg/mL.
In overdose situations, the fraction of drug not bound to protein is high and hemodialysis or tandem hemodialysis plus hemoperfusion may result in significant removal of drug. The benefit of gastric lavage or emesis will vary with the time since ingestion. General supportive measures should be applied with particular attention to the maintenance of adequate urinary output.
Naloxone has been reported to reverse the CNS depressant effects of valproate overdosage. Because naloxone could theoretically also reverse the antiepileptic effects of valproate, it should be used with caution in patients with epilepsy.

DOSAGE AND ADMINISTRATION
Epilepsy
DEPAKOTE Sprinkle Capsules are administered orally. DEPAKOTE has been studied as monotherapy and adjunctive therapy in complex partial seizures, and in simple and complex absence seizures in adults and adolescents. As the DEPAKOTE dosage is titrated upward, concentrations of phenobarbital, carbamazepine, and/or phenytoin may be affected (see **PRECAUTIONS - Drug Interactions**).
Complex Partial Seizures: For adults and children 10 years of age or older.
Monotherapy (Initial Therapy): DEPAKOTE has not been systematically studied as initial therapy. Patients should initiate therapy at 10 to 15 mg/kg/day. The dosage should be increased by 5 to 10 mg/kg/week to achieve optimal clinical response. Ordinarily, optimal clinical response is achieved at daily doses below 60 mg/kg/day. If satisfactory clinical response has not been achieved, plasma levels should be measured to determine whether or not they are in the usually accepted therapeutic range (50 to 100 μg/mL). No recommendation regarding the safety of valproate for use at doses above 60 mg/kg/day can be made.
The probability of thrombocytopenia increases significantly at total trough valproate plasma concentrations above 110 μg/mL in females and 135 μg/mL in males. The benefit of improved seizure control with higher doses should be weighed against the possibility of a greater incidence of adverse reactions.
Conversion to Monotherapy: Patients should initiate therapy at 10 to 15 mg/kg/day. The dosage should be increased by 5 to 10 mg/kg/week to achieve optimal clinical response. Ordinarily, optimal clinical response is achieved at daily doses below 60 mg/kg/day. If satisfactory clinical response has not been achieved, plasma levels should be measured to determine whether or not they are in the usually accepted therapeutic range (50 - 100 μg/mL). No recommendation re-

Continued on next page

Depakote Sprinkle—Cont.

garding the safety of valproate for use at doses above 60 mg/kg/day can be made. Concomitant antiepilepsy drug (AED) dosage can ordinarily be reduced by approximately 25% every 2 weeks. This reduction may be started at initiation of DEPAKOTE therapy, or delayed by 1 to 2 weeks if there is a concern that seizures are likely to occur with a reduction. The speed and duration of withdrawal of the concomitant AED can be highly variable, and patients should be monitored closely during this period for increased seizure frequency.

Adjunctive Therapy: DEPAKOTE may be added to the patient's regimen at a dosage of 10 to 15 mg/kg/day. The dosage may be increased by 5 to 10 mg/kg/week to achieve optimal clinical response. Ordinarily, optimal clinical response is achieved at daily doses below 60 mg/kg/day. If satisfactory clinical response has not been achieved, plasma levels should be measured to determine whether or not they are in the usually accepted therapeutic range (50 to 100 µg/mL). No recommendation regarding the safety of valproate for use at doses above 60 mg/kg/day can be made. If the total daily dose exceeds 250 mg, it should be given in divided doses.

In a study of adjunctive therapy for complex partial seizures in which patients were receiving either carbamazepine or phenytoin in addition to DEPAKOTE, no adjustment of carbamazepine or phenytoin dosage was needed (see **CLINICAL STUDIES**). However, since valproate may interact with these or other concurrently administered AEDs as well as other drugs (see **Drug Interactions**), periodic plasma concentration determinations of concomitant AEDs are recommended during the early course of therapy (see **PRECAUTIONS - Drug Interactions**).

Simple and Complex Absence Seizures: The recommended initial dose is 15 mg/kg/day, increasing at one week intervals by 5 to 10 mg/kg/day until seizures are controlled or side effects preclude further increases. The maximum recommended dosage is 60 mg/kg/day. If the total daily dose exceeds 250 mg, it should be given in divided doses.

A good correlation has not been established between daily dose, serum concentrations, and therapeutic effect. However, therapeutic valproate serum concentrations for most patients with absence seizures is considered to range from 50 to 100 µg/mL. Some patients may be controlled with lower or higher serum concentrations (see **CLINICAL PHARMACOLOGY**).

As the DEPAKOTE dosage is titrated upward, blood concentrations of phenobarbital and/or phenytoin may be affected (see **PRECAUTIONS**).

Antiepilepsy drugs should not be abruptly discontinued in patients in whom the drug is administered to prevent major seizures because of the strong possibility of precipitating status epilepticus with attendant hypoxia and threat to life.

In epileptic patients previously receiving DEPAKENE (valproic acid) therapy, DEPAKOTE sprinkle capsules should be initiated at the same daily dose and dosing schedule. After the patient is stabilized on DEPAKOTE sprinkle capsules, a dosing schedule of two or three times a day may be elected in selected patients.

General Dosing Advice

Dosing in Elderly Patients - Due to a decrease in unbound clearance of valproate, the starting dose should be reduced; the ultimate therapeutic dose should be achieved on the basis of clinical response.

Dose-Related Adverse Events - The frequency of adverse effects (particularly elevated liver enzymes and thrombocytopenia) may be dose-related. The probability of thrombocytopenia appears to increase significantly at total valproate concentrations of ≥ 110 µg/mL (females) or ≥ 135 µg/mL (males) (see **PRECAUTIONS**). The benefit of improved therapeutic effect with higher doses should be weighed against the possibility of a greater incidence of adverse reactions.

G.I. Irritation - Patients who experience G.I. irritation may benefit from administration of the drug with food or by slowly building up the dose from an initial low level.

Administration of Sprinkle Capsules - DEPAKOTE Sprinkle Capsules may be swallowed whole or may be administered by carefully opening the capsule and sprinkling the entire contents on a small amount (teaspoonful) of soft food such as applesauce or pudding. The drug/food mixture should be swallowed immediately (avoid chewing) and not stored for future use. Each capsule is oversized to allow ease of opening.

HOW SUPPLIED

DEPAKOTE Sprinkle Capsules (divalproex sodium coated particles in capsules), 125 mg, are white opaque and blue, and are supplied in bottles of 100 (**NDC** 0074-6114-13) and Abbo-Pac® unit dose packages of 100 (**NDC** 0074-6114-11).

Recommended storage: Store capsules below 77°F (25°C).

Revised: January, 1998

Caution -- Federal (U.S.A.) Law prohibits dispensing without prescription.

Ref. 03-4842-R3

ABBOTT LABORATORIES
NORTH CHICAGO, IL 60064, U.S.A.

Shown in Product Identification Guide, page 303

DEPAKOTE® Tablets ℞

[dəp 'ā-coat]

DIVALPROEX SODIUM
DELAYED-RELEASE TABLETS

BOX WARNING:

HEPATIC FAILURE RESULTING IN FATALITIES HAS OCCURRED IN PATIENTS RECEIVING VALPROIC ACID AND ITS DERIVATIVES. EXPERIENCE HAS INDICATED THAT CHILDREN UNDER THE AGE OF TWO YEARS ARE AT A CONSIDERABLY INCREASED RISK OF DEVELOPING FATAL HEPATOTOXICITY, ESPECIALLY THOSE ON MULTIPLE ANTICONVULSANTS, THOSE WITH CONGENITAL METABOLIC DISORDERS, THOSE WITH SEVERE SEIZURE DISORDERS ACCOMPANIED BY MENTAL RETARDATION, AND THOSE WITH ORGANIC BRAIN DISEASE. WHEN DEPAKOTE IS USED IN THIS PATIENT GROUP, IT SHOULD BE USED WITH EXTREME CAUTION AND AS A SOLE AGENT. THE BENEFITS OF THERAPY SHOULD BE WEIGHED AGAINST THE RISKS. ABOVE THIS AGE GROUP, EXPERIENCE IN EPILEPSY HAS INDICATED THAT THE INCIDENCE OF FATAL HEPATOTOXICITY DECREASES CONSIDERABLY IN PROGRESSIVELY OLDER PATIENT GROUPS.

THESE INCIDENTS USUALLY HAVE OCCURRED DURING THE FIRST SIX MONTHS OF TREATMENT. SERIOUS OR FATAL HEPATOTOXICITY MAY BE PRECEDED BY NON-SPECIFIC SYMPTOMS SUCH AS MALAISE, WEAKNESS, LETHARGY, FACIAL EDEMA, ANOREXIA, AND VOMITING. IN PATIENTS WITH EPILEPSY, A LOSS OF SEIZURE CONTROL MAY ALSO OCCUR. PATIENTS SHOULD BE MONITORED CLOSELY FOR APPEARANCE OF THESE SYMPTOMS. LIVER FUNCTION TESTS SHOULD BE PERFORMED PRIOR TO THERAPY AND AT FREQUENT INTERVALS THEREAFTER, ESPECIALLY DURING THE FIRST SIX MONTHS.

TERATOGENICITY:

VALPROATE CAN PRODUCE TERATOGENIC EFFECTS SUCH AS NEURAL TUBE DEFECTS (E.G., SPINA BIFIDA), ACCORDINGLY, THE USE OF DEPAKOTE TABLETS IN WOMEN OF CHILDBEARING POTENTIAL REQUIRES THAT THE BENEFITS OF ITS USE BE WEIGHED AGAINST THE RISK OF INJURY TO THE FETUS. THIS IS ESPECIALLY IMPORTANT WHEN THE TREATMENT OF A SPONTANEOUSLY REVERSIBLE CONDITION NOT ORDINARILY ASSOCIATED WITH PERMANENT INJURY OR RISK OF DEATH (E.G., MIGRAINE) IS CONTEMPLATED. SEE WARNINGS, INFORMATION FOR PATIENTS.

AN INFORMATION SHEET DESCRIBING THE TERATOGENIC POTENTIAL OF VALPROATE IS AVAILABLE FOR PATIENTS.

DESCRIPTION

Divalproex sodium is a stable co-ordination compound comprised of sodium valproate and valproic acid in a 1:1 molar relationship and formed during the partial neutralization of valproic acid with 0.5 equivalent of sodium hydroxide. Chemically it is designated as sodium hydrogen bis(2-propylpentanoate). Divalproex sodium has the following structure:

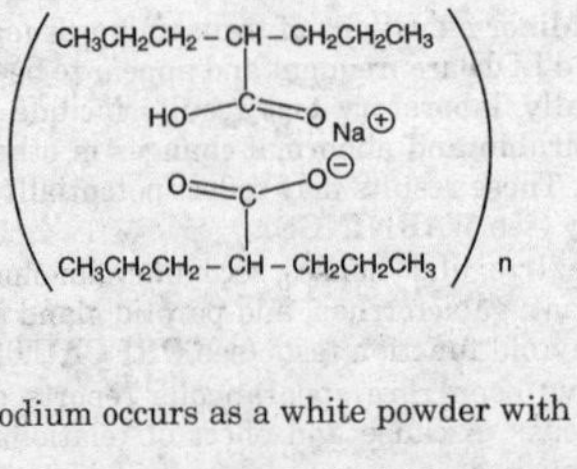
CH3CH2CH2 - CH - CH2CH2CH3
HO
Na⊕
O⊖
CH3CH2CH2 - CH - CH2CH2CH3
n

Divalproex sodium occurs as a white powder with a characteristic odor.

DEPAKOTE tablets are for oral administration.

DEPAKOTE tablets are supplied in three dosage strengths containing divalproex sodium equivalent to 125 mg, 250 mg, or 500 mg of valproic acid.

Inactive Ingredients

DEPAKOTE tablets: cellulosic polymers, diacetylated monoglycerides, povidone, pregelatinized starch (contains corn starch), silica gel, talc, titanium dioxide, and vanillin.

In addition, individual tablets contain:
125 mg tablets: FD&C Blue No. 1 and FD&C Red No. 40.
250 mg tablets: FD&C Yellow No. 6 and iron oxide.
500 mg tablets: D&C Red No. 30, FD&C Blue No. 2, and iron oxide.

CLINICAL PHARMACOLOGY

Pharmacodynamics

Divalproex sodium dissociates to the valproate ion in the gastrointestinal tract. The mechanisms by which valproate exerts its therapeutic effects have not been established. It has been suggested that its activity in epilepsy is related to increased brain concentrations of gamma-aminobutyric acid (GABA).

Pharmacokinetics

Absorption/Bioavailability

Equivalent oral doses of DEPAKOTE (divalproex sodium) products and DEPAKENE (valproic acid) capsules deliver equivalent quantities of valproate ion systemically. Although the rate of valproate ion absorption may vary with the formulation administered (liquid, solid, or sprinkle), conditions of use (e.g., fasting or postprandial) and the method of administration (e.g., whether the contents of the capsule are sprinkled on food or the capsule is taken intact), these differences should be of minor clinical importance under the steady state conditions achieved in chronic use in the treatment of epilepsy.

However, it is possible that differences among the various valproate products in T_{max} and C_{max} could be important upon initiation of treatment. For example, in single dose studies, the effect of feeding had a greater influence on the rate of absorption of the tablet (increase in T_{max} from 4 to 8 hours) than on the absorption of the sprinkle capsules (increase in T_{max} from 3.3 to 4.8 hours).

While the absorption rate from the G.I. tract and fluctuation in valproate plasma concentrations vary with dosing regimen and formulation, the efficacy of valproate as an anticonvulsant in chronic use is unlikely to be affected. Experience employing dosing regimens from once-a-day to four-times-a-day, as well as studies in primate epilepsy models involving constant rate infusion, indicate that total daily systemic bioavailability (extent of absorption) is the primary determinant of seizure control and that differences in the ratios of plasma peak to trough concentrations between valproate formulations are inconsequential from a practical clinical standpoint. Whether or not rate of absorption influences the efficacy of valproate as an antimanic or antimigraine agent is unknown.

Co-administration of oral valproate products with food and substitution among the various DEPAKOTE and DEPAKENE formulations should cause no clinical problems in the management of patients with epilepsy (see **DOSAGE AND ADMINISTRATION**). Nonetheless, any changes in dosage administration, or the addition or discontinuance of concomitant drugs should ordinarily be accompanied by close monitoring of clinical status and valproate plasma concentrations.

Distribution

Protein Binding:

The plasma protein binding of valproate is concentration dependent and the free fraction increases from approximately 10% at 40 µg/mL to 18.5% at 130 µg/mL. Protein binding of valproate is reduced in the elderly, in patients with chronic hepatic diseases, in patients with renal impairment, and in the presence of other drugs (e.g., aspirin). Conversely, valproate may displace certain protein-bound drugs (e.g., phenytoin, carbamazepine, warfarin, and tolbutamide). (See **PRECAUTIONS, Drug Interactions** for more detailed information on the pharmacokinetic interactions of valproate with other drugs.)

CNS Distribution:

Valproate concentrations in cerebrospinal fluid (CSF) approximate unbound concentrations in plasma (about 10% of total concentration).

Metabolism

Valproate is metabolized almost entirely by the liver. In adult patients on monotherapy, 30–50% of an administered dose appears in urine as a glucuronide conjugate. Mitochondrial β-oxidation is the other major metabolic pathway, typically accounting for over 40% of the dose. Usually, less than 15–20% of the dose is eliminated by other oxidative mechanisms. Less than 3% of an administered dose is excreted unchanged in urine.

The relationship between dose and total valproate concentration is nonlinear; concentration does not increase proportionally with the dose, but rather, increases to a lesser extent due to saturable plasma protein binding. The kinetics of unbound drug are linear.

Elimination

Mean plasma clearance and volume of distribution for total valproate are 0.56 L/hr/1.73 m^2 and 11 L/1.73 m^2, respectively. Mean plasma clearance and volume of distribution for free valproate are 4.6 L/hr/1.73 m^2 and 92 L/1.73 m^2. Mean terminal half-life for valproate monotherapy ranged from 9 to 16 hours following oral dosing regimens of 250 to 1000 mg.

The estimates cited apply primarily to patients who are not taking drugs that affect hepatic metabolizing enzyme systems. For example, patients taking enzyme-inducing antiepileptic drugs (carbamazepine, phenytoin, and phenobarbital) will clear valproate more rapidly. Because of these changes in valproate clearance, monitoring of antiepileptic concentrations should be intensified whenever concomitant antiepileptics are introduced or withdrawn.

Special Populations

Effect of Age:

Neonates - Children within the first two months of life have a markedly decreased ability to eliminate valproate compared to older children and adults. This is a result of reduced clearance (perhaps due to delay in development of glucuronosyltransferase and other enzyme systems involved in valproate elimination) as well as increased volume of distribution (in part due to decreased plasma protein binding). For example, in one study, the half-life in children under 10 days ranged from 10 to 67 hours compared to a range of 7 to 13 hours in children greater than 2 months.

Children - Pediatric patients (i.e., between 3 months and 10 years) have 50% higher clearances expressed on weight (i.e., mL/min/kg) than do adults. Over the age of 10 years, children have pharmacokinetic parameters that approximate those of adults.

Elderly - The capacity of elderly patients (age range: 68 to 89 years) to eliminate valproate has been shown to be reduced compared to younger adults (age range: 22 to 26). Intrinsic clearance is reduced by 39%; the free fraction is increased by 44%. Accordingly, the initial dosage should be reduced in the elderly. (See **DOSAGE AND ADMINISTRATION**).

Effect of Gender:

There are no differences in the body surface area adjusted unbound clearance between males and females (4.8±0.17 and 4.7±0.07 L/hr per 1.73 m², respectively).

Effect of Race:

The effects of race on the kinetics of valproate have not been studied.

Effect of Disease:

Liver Disease - (See **BOXED WARNING, CONTRAINDICATIONS**, and **WARNINGS**). Liver disease impairs the capacity to eliminate valproate. In one study, the clearance of free valproate was decreased by 50% in 7 patients with cirrhosis and by 16% in 4 patients with acute hepatitis, compared with 6 healthy subjects. In that study, the half-life of valproate was increased from 12 to 18 hours. Liver disease is also associated with decreased albumin concentrations and larger unbound fractions (2 to 2.6 fold increase) of valproate. Accordingly, monitoring of total concentrations may be misleading since free concentrations may be substantially elevated in patients with hepatic disease whereas total concentrations may appear to be normal.

Renal Disease - A slight reduction (27%) in the unbound clearance of valproate has been reported in patients with renal failure (creatinine clearance < 10 mL/minute); however, hemodialysis typically reduces valproate concentrations by about 20%. Therefore, no dosage adjustment appears to be necessary in patients with renal failure. Protein binding in these patients is substantially reduced; thus, monitoring total concentrations may be misleading.

Plasma Levels and Clinical Effect

The relationship between plasma concentration and clinical response is not well documented. One contributing factor is the nonlinear, concentration dependent protein binding of valproate which affects the clearance of the drug. Thus, monitoring of total serum valproate cannot provide a reliable index of the bioactive valproate species.

For example, because the plasma protein binding of valproate is concentration dependent, the free fraction increases from approximately 10% at 40 µg/mL to 18.5% at 130 µg/mL. Higher than expected free fractions occur in the elderly, in hyperlipidemic patients, and in patients with hepatic and renal diseases.

Epilepsy:

The therapeutic range in epilepsy is commonly considered to be 50 to 100 µg/mL of total valproate, although some patients may be controlled with lower or higher plasma concentrations.

Mania:

In placebo-controlled clinical trials of acute mania, patients were dosed to clinical response with trough plasma concentrations between 50 and 125 µg/mL (See **DOSAGE AND ADMINISTRATION**).

Clinical Trials

Mania

The effectiveness of DEPAKOTE for the treatment of acute mania was demonstrated in two 3-week, placebo controlled, parallel group studies.

(1) Study 1: The first study enrolled adult patients who met DSM-III-R criteria for Bipolar Disorder and who were hospitalized for acute mania. In addition, they had a history of failing to respond to or not tolerating previous lithium carbonate treatment. DEPAKOTE was initiated at a dose of 250 mg tid and adjusted to achieve serum valproate concentrations in a range of 50-100 µg/mL by day 7. Mean

DEPAKOTE doses for completers in this study were 1118, 1525, and 2402 mg/day at days 7, 14, and 21, respectively. Patients were assessed on the Young Mania Rating Scale (YMRS; score ranges from 0–60), an augmented Brief Psychiatric Rating Scale (BPRS-A), and the Global Assessment Scale (GAS). Baseline scores and change from baseline in the week 3 endpoint (last-observation-carry-forward) analysis were as follows:

Study 1
YMRS Total Score

Group	Baseline[1]	BL to Wk 3[2]	Difference[3]
Placebo	28.8	+0.2	
DEPAKOTE	28.5	−9.5	9.7

BPRS-A Total Score

Group	Baseline[1]	BL to Wk 3[2]	Difference[3]
Placebo	76.2	+1.8	
DEPAKOTE	76.4	−17.0	18.8

GAS Score

Group	Baseline[1]	BL to Wk 3[2]	Difference[3]
Placebo	31.8	0.0	
DEPAKOTE	30.3	+18.1	18.1

[1] Mean score at baseline
[2] Change from baseline to week 3 (LOCF)
[3] Difference in change from baseline to week 3 endpoint (LOCF) between DEPAKOTE and placebo

DEPAKOTE was statistically significantly superior to placebo on all three measures of outcome.

(2) Study 2: The second study enrolled adult patients who met Research Diagnostic Criteria for manic disorder and who were hospitalized for acute mania. DEPAKOTE was initiated at a dose of 250 mg tid and adjusted within a dose range of 750–2500 mg/day to achieve serum valproate concentrations in a range of 40-150 µg/mL. Mean DEPAKOTE doses for completers in this study were 1116, 1683, and 2006 mg/day at days 7, 14, and 21, respectively. Study 2 also included a lithium group for which lithium doses for completers were 1312, 1869, and 1984 mg/day at days 7, 14, and 21, respectively. Patients were assessed on the Manic Rating Scale (MRS; score ranges from 11–63), and the primary outcome measures were the total MRS score, and scores for two subscales of the MRS, i.e., the Manic Syndrome Scale (MSS) and the Behavior and Ideation Scale (BIS). Baseline scores and change from baseline in the week 3 endpoint (last-observation-carry-forward) analysis were as follows:

Study 2
MRS Total Score

Group	Baseline[1]	BL to Day 21[2]	Difference[3]
Placebo	38.9	−4.4	
Lithium	37.9	−10.5	6.1
DEPAKOTE	38.1	−9.5	5.1

MSS Total Score

Group	Baseline[1]	BL to Day 21[2]	Difference[3]
Placebo	18.9	−2.5	
Lithium	18.5	−6.2	3.7
DEPAKOTE	18.9	−6.0	3.5

BIS Total Score

Group	Baseline[1]	BL to Day 21[2]	Difference[3]
Placebo	16.4	−1.4	
Lithium	16.0	−3.8	2.4
DEPAKOTE	15.7	−3.2	1.8

[1] Mean score at baseline
[2] Change from baseline to day 21 (LOCF)
[3] Difference in change from baseline to day 21 endpoint (LOCF) between DEPAKOTE and placebo and lithium and placebo

DEPAKOTE was statistically significantly superior to placebo on all three measures of outcome. An exploratory analysis for age and gender effects on outcome did not suggest any differential responsiveness on the basis of age or gender.

A comparison of the percentage of patients showing ≥ 30% reduction in the symptom score from baseline in each treatment group, separated by study, is shown in Figure 1.
[See figure at top of next column]

Migraine

The results of two multicenter, randomized, double-blind, placebo-controlled clinical trials established the effectiveness of DEPAKOTE in the prophylactic treatment of migraine headache.

Both studies employed essentially identical designs and recruited patients with a history of migraine with or without aura (of at least 6 months in duration) who were experienc-

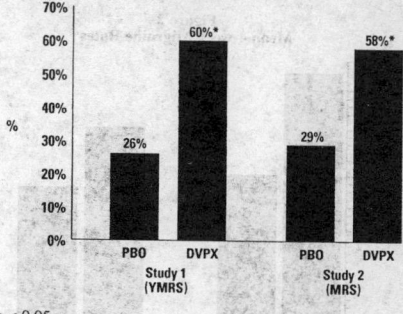

Figure 1
Percentage of Patients Achieving ≥ 30% Reduction in Symptom Score From Baseline

* p < 0.05
PBO = placebo, DVPX = DEPAKOTE

ing at least 2 migraine headaches a month during the 3 months prior to enrollment. Patients with cluster headaches were excluded. Women of childbearing potential were excluded entirely from one study, but were permitted in the other if they were deemed to be practicing an effective method of contraception.

In each study following a 4-week single-blind placebo baseline period, patients were randomized, under double blind conditions, to DEPAKOTE or placebo for a 12-week treatment phase, comprised of a 4-week dose titration period followed by an 8-week maintenance period. Treatment outcome was assessed on the basis of 4-week migraine headache rates during the treatment phase.

In the first study, a total of 107 patients (24 M, 83 F), ranging in age from 26 to 73 were randomized 2:1, DEPAKOTE to placebo. Ninety patients completed the 8-week maintenance period. Drug dose titration, using 250 mg tablets, was individualized at the investigator's discretion. Adjustments were guided by actual/sham trough total serum valproate levels in order to maintain the study blind. In patients on DEPAKOTE doses ranged from 500 to 2500 mg a day. Doses over 500 mg were given in three divided doses (TID). The mean dose during the treatment phase was 1087 mg/day resulting in a mean trough total valproate level of 72.5 µg/mL, with a range of 31 to 133 µg/mL.

The mean 4-week migraine headache rate during the treatment phase was 5.7 in the placebo group compared to 3.5 in the DEPAKOTE group (see Figure 2). These rates were significantly different.

In the second study, a total of 176 patients (19 males and 157 females), ranging in age from 17 to 76 years, were randomized equally to one of three DEPAKOTE dose groups (500, 1000, or 1500 mg/day) or placebo. The treatments were given in two divided doses (BID). One hundred thirty-seven patients completed the 8-week maintenance period. Efficacy was to be determined by a comparison of the 4-week migraine headache rate in the combined 1000/1500 mg/day group and placebo group.

The initial dose was 250 mg daily. The regimen was advanced by 250 mg every 4 days (8 days for 500 mg/day group), until the randomized dose was achieved. The mean trough total valproate levels during the treatment phase were 39.6, 62.5, and 72.5 µg/mL in the DEPAKOTE 500, 1000, and 1500 mg/day groups, respectively.

The mean 4-week migraine headache rates during the treatment phase, adjusted for differences in baseline rates, were 4.5 in the placebo group, compared to 3.3, 3.0, and 3.3 in the DEPAKOTE 500, 1000, and 1500 mg/day groups, respectively, based on intent-to-treat results (see Figure 2). Migraine headache rates in the combined DEPAKOTE 1000/1500 mg group were significantly lower than in the placebo group.

[See figure 2 at top of next column]

Epilepsy

The efficacy of DEPAKOTE in reducing the incidence of complex partial seizures (CPS) that occur in isolation or in association with other seizure types was established in two controlled trials.

In one, a multiclinic, placebo controlled study employing an add-on design, (adjunctive therapy) 144 patients who continued to suffer eight or more CPS per 8 weeks during an 8 week period of monotherapy with doses of either carbamazepine or phenytoin sufficient to assure plasma concentrations within the "therapeutic range" were randomized to receive, in addition to their original antiepilepsy drug (AED), either DEPAKOTE or placebo. Randomized patients were to be followed for a total of 16 weeks. The following table presents the findings.

Continued on next page

Depakote—Cont.

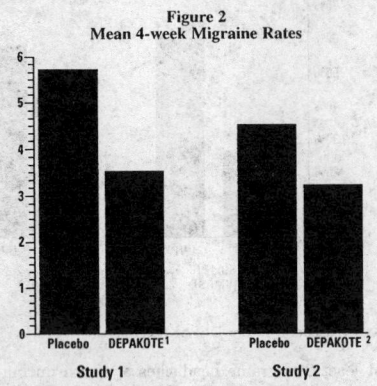

Figure 2
Mean 4-week Migraine Rates

[1] Mean dose of DEPAKOTE was 1087 mg/day.
[2] Dose of DEPAKOTE was 500 or 1000 mg/day.

Adjunctive Therapy Study
Median Incidence of CPS per 8 Weeks

Add-on Treatment	Number of Patients	Baseline Incidence	Experimental Incidence
DEPAKOTE	75	16.0	8.9*
Placebo	69	14.5	11.5

*Reduction from baseline statistically significantly greater for DEPAKOTE than placebo at p ≤ 0.05 level.

Figure 3 presents the proportion of patients (X axis) whose percentage reduction from baseline in complex partial seizure rates was at least as great as that indicated on the Y axis in the adjunctive therapy study. A positive percent reduction indicates an improvement (i.e., a decrease in seizure frequency), while a negative percent reduction indicates worsening. Thus, in a display of this type, the curve for an effective treatment is shifted to the left of the curve for placebo. This figure shows that the proportion of patients achieving any particular level of improvement was consistently higher for DEPAKOTE than for placebo. For example, 45% of patients treated with DEPAKOTE had a ≥ 50% reduction in complex partial seizure rate compared to 23% of patients treated with placebo.

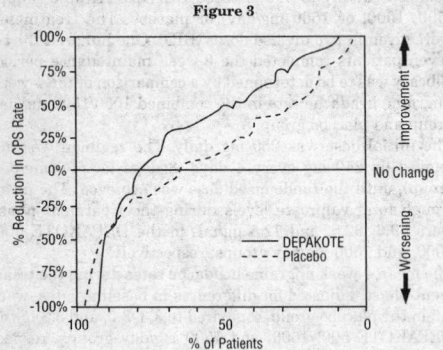

Figure 3

The second study assessed the capacity of DEPAKOTE to reduce the incidence of CPS when administered as the sole AED. The study compared the incidence of CPS among patients randomized to either a high or low dose treatment arm. Patients qualified for entry into the randomized comparison phase of this study only if 1) they continued to experience 2 or more CPS per 4 weeks during an 8 to 12 week long period of monotherapy with adequate doses of an AED (i.e., phenytoin, carbamazepine, phenobarbital, or primidone) and 2) they made a successful transition over a two week interval to DEPAKOTE. Patients entering the randomized phase were then brought to their assigned target dose, gradually tapered off their concomitant AED and followed for an interval as long as 22 weeks. Less than 50% of the patients randomized, however, completed the study. In patients converted to DEPAKOTE monotherapy, the mean total valproate concentrations during monotherapy were 71 and 123 μg/mL in the low dose and high dose groups, respectively.
The following table presents the findings for all patients randomized who had at least one post-randomization assessment.

Monotherapy Study
Median Incidence of CPS per 8 Weeks

Treatment	Number of Patients	Baseline Incidence	Randomized Phase Incidence
High dose DEPAKOTE	131	13.2	10.7*
Low dose DEPAKOTE	134	14.2	13.8

*Reduction from baseline statistically significantly greater for high dose than low dose at p ≤ 0.05 level.

Figure 4 presents the proportion of patients (X axis) whose percentage reduction from baseline in complex partial seizure rates was at least as great as that indicated on the Y axis in the monotherapy study. A positive percent reduction indicates an improvement (i.e., a decrease in seizure frequency), while a negative percent reduction indicates worsening. Thus, in a display of this type, the curve for a more effective treatment is shifted to the left of the curve for a less effective treatment. This figure shows that the proportion of patients achieving any particular level of reduction was consistently higher for high dose DEPAKOTE than for low dose DEPAKOTE. For example, when switching from carbamazepine, phenytoin, phenobarbital or primidone monotherapy to high dose DEPAKOTE monotherapy, 63% of patients experienced no change or a reduction in complex partial seizure rates compared to 54% of patients receiving low dose DEPAKOTE.

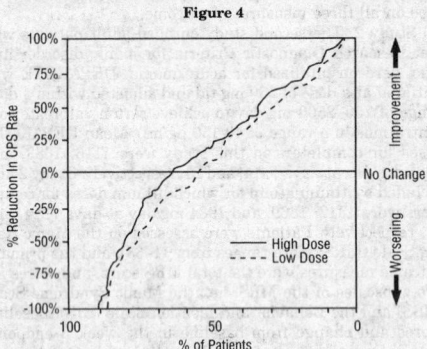

Figure 4

INDICATIONS AND USAGE
Mania
DEPAKOTE (divalproex sodium) is indicated for the treatment of the manic episodes associated with bipolar disorder. A manic episode is a distinct period of abnormally and persistently elevated, expansive, or irritable mood. Typical symptoms of mania include pressure of speech, motor hyperactivity, reduced need for sleep, flight of ideas, grandiosity, poor judgement, aggressiveness, and possible hostility. The efficacy of DEPAKOTE was established in 3-week trials with patients meeting DSM-III-R criteria for bipolar disorder who were hospitalized for acute mania (See **Clinical Trials** under **CLINICAL PHARMACOLOGY**).
The safety and effectiveness of DEPAKOTE for long-term use in mania, i.e., more than 3 weeks, has not been systematically evaluated in controlled clinical trials. Therefore, physicians who elect to use DEPAKOTE for extended periods should continually reevaluate the long-term usefulness of the drug for the individual patient.
Epilepsy
DEPAKOTE (divalproex sodium) is indicated as monotherapy and adjunctive therapy in the treatment of patients with complex partial seizures that occur either in isolation or in association with other types of seizures. DEPAKOTE (divalproex sodium) is also indicated for use as sole and adjunctive therapy in the treatment of simple and complex absence seizures, and adjunctively in patients with multiple seizure types that include absence seizures.
Simple absence is defined as very brief clouding of the sensorium or loss of consciousness accompanied by certain generalized epileptic discharges without other detectable clinical signs. Complex absence is the term used when other signs are also present.
Migraine
DEPAKOTE is indicated for prophylaxis of migraine headaches. There is no evidence that DEPAKOTE is useful in the acute treatment of migraine headaches. Because valproic acid may be a hazard to the fetus, DEPAKOTE should be considered for women of childbearing potential only after this risk has been thoroughly discussed with the patient and weighed against the potential benefits of treatment (see **WARNINGS - Usage In Pregnancy**, **PRECAUTIONS - Information for Patients**).
SEE **WARNINGS** FOR STATEMENT REGARDING FATAL HEPATIC DYSFUNCTION.

CONTRAINDICATIONS
DIVALPROEX SODIUM SHOULD NOT BE ADMINISTERED TO PATIENTS WITH HEPATIC DISEASE OR SIGNIFICANT HEPATIC DYSFUNCTION.
Divalproex sodium is contraindicated in patients with known hypersensitivity to the drug.

WARNINGS
Hepatic failure resulting in fatalities has occurred in patients receiving valproic acid. These incidents usually have occurred during the first six months of treatment. Serious or fatal hepatotoxicity may be preceded by non-specific symptoms such as malaise, weakness, lethargy, facial edema, anorexia, and vomiting. In patients with epilepsy, a loss of seizure control may also occur. Patients should be monitored closely for appearance of these symptoms. Liver function tests should be performed prior to therapy and at frequent intervals thereafter, especially during the first six months. However, physicians should not rely totally on serum biochemistry since these tests may not be abnormal in all instances, but should also consider the results of careful interim medical history and physical examination. Caution should be observed when administering DEPAKOTE products to patients with a prior history of hepatic disease. Patients on multiple anticonvulsants, children, those with congenital metabolic disorders, those with severe seizure disorders accompanied by mental retardation, and those with organic brain disease may be at particular risk. Experience has indicated that children under the age of two years are at a considerably increased risk of developing fatal hepatotoxicity, especially those with the aforementioned conditions. When DEPAKOTE is used in this patient group, it should be used with extreme caution and as a sole agent. The benefits of therapy should be weighed against the risks. Above this age group, experience in epilepsy has indicated that the incidence of fatal hepatotoxicity decreases considerably in progressively older patient groups.
The drug should be discontinued immediately in the presence of significant hepatic dysfunction, suspected or apparent. In some cases, hepatic dysfunction has progressed in spite of discontinuation of drug.
The frequency of adverse effects (particularly elevated liver enzymes and thrombocytopenia [see **PRECAUTIONS**]) may be dose-related. In a clinical trial of DEPAKOTE as monotherapy in patients with epilepsy, 34/126 patients (27%) receiving approximately 50 mg/kg/day on average, had at least one value of platelets ≤ 75 × 10⁹/L. Approximately half of these patients had treatment discontinued, with return of platelet counts to normal. In the remaining patients, platelet counts normalized with continued treatment. In this study, the probability of thrombocytopenia appeared to increase significantly at total valproate concentrations of ≥ 110 μg/mL (females) or ≥ 135 μg/mL (males). The therapeutic benefit which may accompany the higher doses should therefore be weighed against the possibility of a greater incidence of adverse effects.
Usage In Pregnancy
ACCORDING TO PUBLISHED AND UNPUBLISHED REPORTS, VALPROIC ACID MAY PRODUCE TERATOGENIC EFFECTS IN THE OFFSPRING OF HUMAN FEMALES RECEIVING THE DRUG DURING PREGNANCY. THERE ARE MULTIPLE REPORTS IN THE CLINICAL LITERATURE WHICH INDICATE THAT THE USE OF ANTIEPILEPTIC DRUGS DURING PREGNANCY RESULTS IN AN INCREASED INCIDENCE OF BIRTH DEFECTS IN THE OFFSPRING. ALTHOUGH DATA ARE MORE EXTENSIVE WITH RESPECT TO TRIMETHADIONE, PARAMETHADIONE, PHENYTOIN, AND PHENOBARBITAL, REPORTS INDICATE A POSSIBLE SIMILAR ASSOCIATION WITH THE USE OF OTHER ANTIEPILEPTIC DRUGS.
THE INCIDENCE OF NEURAL TUBE DEFECTS IN THE FETUS MAY BE INCREASED IN MOTHERS RECEIVING VALPROATE DURING THE FIRST TRIMESTER OF PREGNANCY. THE CENTERS FOR DISEASE CONTROL (CDC) HAS ESTIMATED THE RISK OF VALPROIC ACID EXPOSED WOMEN HAVING CHILDREN WITH SPINA BIFIDA TO BE APPROXIMATELY 1 TO 2%.
OTHER CONGENITAL ANOMALIES (EG, CRANIOFACIAL DEFECTS, CARDIOVASCULAR MALFORMATIONS AND ANOMALIES INVOLVING VARIOUS BODY SYSTEMS), COMPATIBLE AND INCOMPATIBLE WITH LIFE, HAVE BEEN REPORTED. SUFFICIENT DATA TO DETERMINE THE INCIDENCE OF THESE CONGENITAL ANOMALIES IS NOT AVAILABLE.
THE HIGHER INCIDENCE OF CONGENITAL ANOMALIES IN ANTIEPILEPTIC DRUG-TREATED WOMEN WITH SEIZURE DISORDERS CANNOT BE REGARDED AS A CAUSE AND EFFECT RELATIONSHIP. THERE ARE INTRINSIC METHODOLOGIC PROBLEMS IN OBTAINING ADEQUATE DATA ON DRUG TERATOGENICITY IN HUMANS; GENETIC FACTORS OR THE EPILEPTIC CONDITION ITSELF, MAY BE MORE IMPORTANT THAN DRUG THERAPY IN CONTRIBUTING TO CONGENITAL ANOMALIES.

PATIENTS TAKING VALPROATE MAY DEVELOP CLOTTING ABNORMALITIES. A PATIENT WHO HAD LOW FIBRINOGEN WHEN TAKING MULTIPLE ANTICONVULSANTS INCLUDING VALPROATE GAVE BIRTH TO AN INFANT WITH AFIBRINOGENEMIA WHO SUBSEQUENTLY DIED OF HEMORRHAGE. IF VALPROATE IS USED IN PREGNANCY, THE CLOTTING PARAMETERS SHOULD BE MONITORED CAREFULLY.

HEPATIC FAILURE, RESULTING IN THE DEATH OF A NEWBORN AND OF AN INFANT, HAVE BEEN REPORTED FOLLOWING THE USE OF VALPROATE DURING PREGNANCY.

Animal studies have demonstrated valproate-induced teratogenicity. Increased frequencies of malformations, as well as intrauterine growth retardation and death, have been observed in mice, rats, rabbits, and monkeys following prenatal exposure to valproate. Malformations of the skeletal system are the most common structural abnormalities produced in experimental animals, but neural tube closure defects have been seen in mice exposed to maternal plasma valproate concentrations exceeding 230 μg/mL (2.3 times the upper limit of the human therapeutic range) during susceptible periods of embryonic development. Administration of an oral dose of 200 mg/kg/day or greater (50% of the maximum human daily dose or greater on a mg/m² basis) to pregnant rats during organogenesis produced malformations (skeletal, cardiac, and urogenital) and growth retardation in the offspring. These doses resulted in peak maternal plasma valproate levels of approximately 340 μg/mL or greater (3.4 times the upper limit of the human therapeutic range or greater). Behavioral deficits have been reported in the offspring of rats given a dose of 200 mg/kg/day throughout most of pregnancy. An oral dose of 350 mg/kg/day (approximately 2 times the maximum human daily dose on a mg/m² basis) produced skeletal and visceral malformations in rabbits exposed during organogenesis. Skeletal malformations, growth retardation, and death were observed in rhesus monkeys following administration of an oral dose of 200 mg/kg/day (equal to the maximum human daily dose on a mg/m² basis) during organogenesis. This dose resulted in peak maternal plasma valproate levels of approximately 280 μg/mL (2.8 times the upper limit of the human therapeutic range).

The prescribing physician will wish to weigh the benefits of therapy against the risks in treating or counseling women of childbearing potential. If this drug is used during pregnancy, or if the patient becomes pregnant while taking this drug, the patient should be apprised of the potential hazard to the fetus.

Antiepileptic drugs should not be discontinued abruptly in patients in whom the drug is administered to prevent major seizures because of the strong possibility of precipitating status epilepticus with attendant hypoxia and threat to life. In individual cases where the severity and frequency of the seizure disorder are such that the removal of medication does not pose a serious threat to the patient, discontinuation of the drug may be considered prior to and during pregnancy, although it cannot be said with any confidence that even minor seizures do not pose some hazard to the developing embryo or fetus.

Tests to detect neural tube and other defects using current accepted procedures should be considered a part of routine prenatal care in childbearing women receiving valproate.

PRECAUTIONS
Hepatic Dysfunction
See **BOXED WARNING, CONTRAINDICATIONS** and **WARNINGS.**
General
Because of reports of thrombocytopenia (see **WARNINGS**), inhibition of the secondary phase of platelet aggregation, and abnormal coagulation parameters, (e.g., low fibrinogen), platelet counts and coagulation tests are recommended before initiating therapy and at periodic intervals. It is recommended that patients receiving DEPAKOTE be monitored for platelet count and coagulation parameters prior to planned surgery. In a clinical trial of DEPAKOTE as monotherapy in patients with epilepsy, 34/126 patients (27%) receiving approximately 50 mg/kg/day on average, had at least one value of platelets ≤ 75 × 10⁹/L. Approximately half of these patients had treatment discontinued, with return of platelet counts to normal. In the remaining patients, platelet counts normalized with continued treatment. In this study, the probability of thrombocytopenia appeared to increase significantly at total valproate concentrations of ≥ 110 μg/mL (females) or ≥ 135 μg/mL (males). Evidence of hemorrhage, bruising, or a disorder of hemostasis/coagulation is an indication for reduction of the dosage or withdrawal of therapy.

Hyperammonemia with or without lethargy or coma has been reported and may be present in the absence of abnormal liver function tests. Asymptomatic elevations of ammonia are more common and when present require more frequent monitoring. If clinically significant symptoms occur, DEPAKOTE therapy should be modified or discontinued.

Since DEPAKOTE may interact with concurrently administered drugs which are capable of enzyme induction, periodic plasma concentration determinations of valproate and concomitant drugs are recommended during the early course of therapy. (See **PRECAUTIONS-Drug Interactions**.)

Valproate is partially eliminated in the urine as a keto-metabolite which may lead to a false interpretation of the urine ketone test.

There have been reports of altered thyroid function tests associated with valproate. The clinical significance of these is unknown.

Suicidal ideation may be a manifestation of certain psychiatric disorders, and may persist until significant remission of symptoms occurs. Close supervision of high risk patients should accompany initial drug therapy.

Information for Patients
Since DEPAKOTE products may produce CNS depression, especially when combined with another CNS depressant (eg, alcohol), patients should be advised not to engage in hazardous activities, such as driving an automobile or operating dangerous machinery, until it is known that they do not become drowsy from the drug.

Migraine Patients: Since DEPAKOTE has been associated with certain types of birth defects, female patients of child-bearing age considering the use of DEPAKOTE for the prevention of migraine should be advised to read the **Patient Information Leaflet**, which appears as the last section of the labeling.

Drug Interactions
Effects of Co-Administered Drugs on Valproate Clearance
Drugs that affect the level of expression of hepatic enzymes, particularly those that elevate levels of glucuronosyltransferases, may increase the clearance of valproate. For example, phenytoin, carbamazepine, and phenobarbital (or primidone) can double the clearance of valproate. Thus, patients on monotherapy will generally have longer half-lives and higher concentrations than patients receiving polytherapy with antiepilepsy drugs.

In contrast, drugs that are inhibitors of cytochrome P450 isozymes, e.g., antidepressants, may be expected to have little effect on valproate clearance because cytochrome P450 microsomal mediated oxidation is a relatively minor secondary metabolic pathway compared to glucuronidation and beta-oxidation.

Because of these changes in valproate clearance, monitoring of valproate and concomitant drug concentrations should be increased whenever enzyme inducing drugs are introduced or withdrawn.

The following list provides information about the potential for an influence of several commonly prescribed medications on valproate pharmacokinetics. The list is not exhaustive nor could it be, since new interactions are continuously being reported.

Drugs for which a potentially important interaction has been observed:
Aspirin - A study involving the co-administration of aspirin at antipyretic doses (11 to 16 mg/kg) with valproate to pediatric patients (n=6) revealed a decrease in protein binding and an inhibition of metabolism of valproate. Valproate free fraction was increased 4-fold in the presence of aspirin compared to valproate alone. The β-oxidation pathway consisting of 2-E-valproic acid, 3-OH-valproic acid, and 3-keto valproic acid was decreased from 25% of total metabolites excreted on valproate alone to 8.3% in the presence of aspirin. Caution should be observed if valproate and aspirin are to be co-administered.

Felbamate - A study involving the co-administration of 1200 mg/day of felbamate with valproate to patients with epilepsy (n=10) revealed an increase in mean valproate peak concentration by 35% (from 86 to 115 μg/mL) compared to valproate alone. Increasing the felbamate dose to 2400 mg/day increased the mean valproate peak concentration to 133 μg/mL (another 16% increase). A decrease in valproate dosage may be necessary when felbamate therapy is initiated.

Rifampin - A study involving the administration of a single dose of valproate (7 mg/kg) 36 hours after 5 nights of daily dosing with rifampin (600 mg) revealed a 40% increase in the oral clearance of valproate. Valproate dosage adjustment may be necessary when it is co-administered with rifampin.

Drugs for which either no interaction or a likely clinically unimportant interaction has been observed:
Antacids - A study involving the co-administration of valproate 500 mg with commonly administered antacids (Maalox, Trisogel, and Titralac - 160 mEq doses) did not reveal any effect on the extent of absorption of valproate.

Chlorpromazine - A study involving the administration of 100 to 300 mg/day of chlorpromazine to schizophrenic patients already receiving valproate (200 mg BID) revealed a 15% increase in trough plasma levels of valproate.

Haloperidol - A study involving the administration of 6 to 10 mg/day of haloperidol to schizophrenic patients already receiving valproate (200 mg BID) revealed no significant changes in valproate trough plasma levels.

Cimetidine and Ranitidine - Cimetidine and ranitidine do not affect the clearance of valproate.

Effects of Valproate on Other Drugs
Valproate has been found to be a weak inhibitor of some P450 isozymes, epoxide hydrase, and glucuronosyltransferases.

The following list provides information about the potential for an influence of valproate co-administration on the pharmacokinetics or pharmacodynamics of several commonly prescribed medications. The list is not exhaustive, since new interactions are continuously being reported.

Drugs for which a potentially important valproate interaction has been observed:
Carbamazepine/carbamazepine-10,11-Epoxide - Serum levels of carbamazepine (CBZ) decreased 17% while that of carbamazepine-10,11-epoxide (CBZ-E) increased by 45% upon co-administration of valproate and CBZ to epileptic patients.

Clonazepam - The concomitant use of valproic acid and clonazepam may induce absence status in patients with a history of absence type seizures.

Diazepam - Valproate displaces diazepam from its plasma albumin binding sites and inhibits its metabolism. Co-administration of valproate (1500 mg daily) increased the free fraction of diazepam (10 mg) by 90% in healthy volunteers (n=6). Plasma clearance and volume of distribution for free diazepam were reduced by 25% and 20%, respectively, in the presence of valproate. The elimination half-life of diazepam remained unchanged upon addition of valproate.

Ethosuximide - Valproate inhibits the metabolism of ethosuximide. Administration of a single ethosuximide dose of 500 mg with valproate (800 to 1600 mg/day) to healthy volunteers (n=6) was accompanied by a 25% increase in elimination half-life of ethosuximide and a 15% decrease in its total clearance as compared to ethosuximide alone. Patients receiving valproate and ethosuximide, especially along with other anticonvulsants, should be monitored for alterations in serum concentrations of both drugs.

Lamotrigine - In a steady-state study involving 10 healthy volunteers, the elimination half-life of lamotrigine increased from 26 to 70 hours with valproate co-administration (a 165% increase). The dose of lamotrigine should be reduced when co-administered with valproate.

Phenobarbital - Valproate was found to inhibit the metabolism of phenobarbital. Co-administration of valproate (250 mg BID for 14 days) with phenobarbital to normal subjects (n=6) resulted in a 50% increase in half-life and a 30% decrease in plasma clearance of phenobarbital (60 mg single-dose). The fraction of phenobarbital dose excreted unchanged increased by 50% in presence of valproate.

There is evidence for severe CNS depression, with or without significant elevations of barbiturate or valproate serum concentrations. All patients receiving concomitant barbiturate therapy should be closely monitored for neurological toxicity. Serum barbiturate concentrations should be obtained, if possible, and the barbiturate dosage decreased, if appropriate.

Primidone, which is metabolized to a barbiturate, may be involved in a similar interaction with valproate.

Phenytoin - Valproate displaces phenytoin from its plasma albumin binding sites and inhibits its hepatic metabolism. Co-administration of valproate (400 mg TID) with phenytoin (250 mg) in normal volunteers (n=7) was associated with a 60% increase in the free fraction of phenytoin. Total plasma clearance and apparent volume of distribution of phenytoin increased 30% in the presence of valproate. Both the clearance and apparent volume of distribution of free phenytoin were reduced by 25%.

In patients with epilepsy, there have been reports of breakthrough seizures occurring with the combination of valproate and phenytoin. The dosage of phenytoin should be adjusted as required by the clinical situation.

Tolbutamide - From in vitro experiments, the unbound fraction of tolbutamide was increased from 20% to 50% when added to plasma samples taken from patients treated with valproate. The clinical relevance of this displacement is unknown.

Warfarin - In an in vitro study, valproate increased the unbound fraction of warfarin by up to 32.6%. The therapeutic relevance of this is unknown; however, coagulation tests should be monitored if DEPAKOTE therapy is instituted in patients taking anticoagulants.

Zidovudine - In six patients who were seropositive for HIV, the clearance of zidovudine (100 mg q8h) was decreased by 38% after administration of valproate (250 or 500 mg q8h); the half-life of zidovudine was unaffected.

Drugs for which either no interaction or a likely clinically unimportant interaction has been observed:
Acetaminophen - Valproate had no effect on any of the pharmacokinetic parameters of acetaminophen when it was concurrently administered to three epileptic patients.

Amitriptyline/Nortriptyline - Administration of a single oral 50 mg dose of amitriptyline to 15 normal volunteers (10 males and 5 females) who received valproate (500 mg BID)

Continued on next page

Depakote—Cont.

resulted in a 21% decrease in plasma clearance of amitriptyline and a 34% decrease in the net clearance of nortriptyline.

Clozapine - In psychotic patients (n=11), no interaction was observed when valproate was co-administered with clozapine.

Lithium - Co-administration of valproate (500 mg BID) and lithium carbonate (300 mg TID) to normal male volunteers (n=16) had no effect on the steady-state kinetics of lithium.

Lorazepam - Concomitant administration of valproate (500 mg BID) and lorazepam (1 mg BID) in normal male volunteers (n=9) was accompanied by a 17% decrease in the plasma clearance of lorazepam.

Oral Contraceptive Steroids - Administration of a single-dose of ethinyloestradiol (50 μg/levonorgestrel (250 μg) to 6 women on valproate (200 mg BID) therapy for 2 months did not reveal any pharmacokinetic interaction.

Carcinogenesis, Mutagenesis, Impairment of Fertility

Carcinogenesis

Valproic acid was administered orally to Sprague Dawley rats and ICR (HA/ICR) mice at doses of 80 and 170 mg/kg/day (approximately 10 to 50% of the maximum human daily dose on a mg/m^2 basis) for two years. A variety of neoplasms were observed in both species. The chief findings were a statistically significant increase in the incidence of subcutaneous fibrosarcomas in high dose male rats receiving valproic acid and a statistically significant dose-related trend for benign pulmonary adenomas in male mice receiving valproic acid. The significance of these findings for humans is unknown.

Mutagenesis

Valproate was not mutagenic in an *in vitro* bacterial assay (Ames test), did not produce dominant lethal effects in mice, and did not increase chromosome aberration frequency in an *in vivo* cytogenetic study in rats. Increased frequencies of sister chromatid exchange (SCE) have been reported in a study of epileptic children taking valproate, but this association was not observed in another study conducted in adults. There is some evidence that increased SCE frequencies may be associated with epilepsy. The biological significance of increase in SCE frequency is not known.

Fertility

Chronic toxicity studies in juvenile and adult rats and dogs demonstrated reduced spermatogenesis and testicular atrophy at oral doses of 400 mg/kg/day or greater in rats (approximately equivalent to or greater than the maximum human daily dose on a mg/m^2 basis) and 150 mg/kg/day or greater in dogs (approximately 1.4 times the maximum human daily dose or greater on a mg/m^2 basis). Segment I fertility studies in rats have shown doses up to 350 mg/kg/day (approximately equal to the maximum human daily dose on a mg/m^2 basis) for 60 days to have no effect on fertility. THE EFFECT OF VALPROATE ON TESTICULAR DEVELOPMENT AND ON SPERM PRODUCTION AND FERTILITY IN HUMANS IS UNKNOWN.

Pregnancy

Pregnancy Category D: See **WARNINGS**.

Nursing Mothers

Valproate is excreted in breast milk. Concentrations in breast milk have been reported to be 1-10% of serum concentrations. It is not known what effect this would have on a nursing infant. Consideration should be given to discontinuing nursing when divalproex sodium is administered to a nursing woman.

Pediatric

Experience has indicated that pediatric patients under the age of two years are at a considerably increased risk of developing fatal hepatotoxicity, especially those with the aforementioned conditions (see **BOXED WARNING**). When DEPAKOTE is used in this patient group, it should be used with extreme caution and as a sole agent. The benefits of therapy should be weighed against the risks. Above the age of 2 years, experience in epilepsy has indicated that the incidence of fatal hepatotoxicity decreases considerably in progressively older patient groups.

Younger children, especially those receiving enzyme-inducing drugs, will require larger maintenance doses to attain targeted total and unbound valproic acid concentrations.

The variability in free fraction limits the clinical usefulness of monitoring total serum valproic acid concentrations. Interpretation of valproic acid concentrations in children should include consideration of factors that affect hepatic metabolism and protein binding.

The safety and effectiveness of DEPAKOTE for the treatment of acute mania has not been studied in individuals below the age of 18 years.

The safety and effectiveness of DEPAKOTE for the prophylaxis of migraines has not been studied in individuals below the age of 16 years.

The basic toxicology and pathologic manifestations of valproate sodium in neonatal (4-day old) and juvenile (14-day old) rats are similar to those seen in young adult rats. However, additional findings, including renal alterations in ju-

venile rats and renal alterations and retinal dysplasia in neonatal rats, have been reported. These findings occurred at 240 mg/kg/day, a dosage approximately equivalent to the human maximum recommended daily dose on a mg/m^2 basis. They were not seen at 90 mg/kg, or 40% of the maximum human daily dose on a mg/m^2 basis.

Geriatric

No patients above the age of 65 years were enrolled in double-blind prospective clinical trials of mania associated with bipolar illness. In a case review study of 583 patients, 72 patients (12%) were greater than 65 years of age. A higher percentage of patients above 65 years of age reported accidental injury, infection, pain, somnolence, and tremor. Discontinuation of valproate was occasionally associated with the latter two events. It is not clear whether these events indicate additional risk or whether they result from preexisting medical illness and concomitant medication use among these patients.

There is insufficient information available to discern the safety and effectiveness of DEPAKOTE for the prophylaxis of migraines in patients over 65.

ADVERSE REACTIONS

Mania

The incidence of treatment-emergent events has been ascertained based on combined data from two placebo-controlled clinical trials of DEPAKOTE in the treatment of manic episodes associated with bipolar disorder. The adverse events were usually mild or moderate in intensity, but sometimes were serious enough to interrupt treatment. In clinical trials, the rates of premature termination due to intolerance were not statistically different between placebo, DEPAKOTE, and lithium carbonate. A total of 4%, 8% and 11% of patients discontinued therapy due to intolerance in the placebo, DEPAKOTE, and lithium carbonate groups, respectively.

Table 1 summarizes those adverse events reported for patients in these trials where the incidence rate in the DEPAKOTE-treated group was greater than 5% and greater than the placebo incidence, or where the incidence in the DEPAKOTE-treated group was statistically significantly greater than the placebo group. Vomiting was the only event that was reported by significantly ($p \leq 0.05$) more patients receiving DEPAKOTE compared to placebo.

Table 1

Adverse Events Reported by > 5% of DEPAKOTE-Treated Patients During Placebo-Controlled Trials of Acute Mania[1]

Adverse Event	DEPAKOTE (n=89)	Placebo (n=97)
Nausea	22%	15%
Somnolence	19%	12%
Dizziness	12%	4%
Vomiting	12%	3%
Asthenia	10%	7%
Abdominal pain	9%	8%
Dyspepsia	9%	8%
Rash	6%	3%

[1] The following adverse events occurred at an equal or greater incidence for placebo than for DEPAKOTE: back pain, headache, constipation, diarrhea, tremor, and pharyngitis.

The following additional adverse events were reported by greater than 1% but not more than 5% of the 89 divalproex sodium-treated patients in controlled clinical trials:

Body as a Whole: Chest pain, chills, chills and fever, fever, neck pain, neck rigidity.

Cardiovascular System: Hypertension, hypotension, palpitations, postural hypotension, tachycardia, vasodilation.

Digestive System: Anorexia, fecal incontinence, flatulence, gastroenteritis, glossitis, periodontal abscess.

Hemic and Lymphatic System: Ecchymosis.

Metabolic and Nutritional Disorders: Edema, peripheral edema.

Musculoskeletal System: Arthralgia, arthrosis, leg cramps, twitching.

Nervous System: Abnormal dreams, abnormal gait, agitation, ataxia, catatonic reaction, confusion, depression, diplopia, dysarthria, hallucinations, hypertonia, hypokinesia, insomnia, paresthesia, reflexes increased, tardive dyskinesia, thinking abnormalities, vertigo.

Respiratory System: Dyspnea, rhinitis.

Skin and Appendages: Alopecia, discoid lupus erythematosis, dry skin, furunculosis, maculopapular rash, seborrhea.

Special Senses: Amblyopia, conjunctivitis, deafness, dry eyes, ear pain, eye pain, tinnitus.

Urogenital System: Dysmenorrhea, dysuria, urinary incontinence.

Migraine

Based on two placebo-controlled clinical trials and their long term extension, DEPAKOTE was generally well tolerated with most adverse events rated as mild to moderate in severity. Of the 202 patients exposed to DEPAKOTE in the

placebo-controlled trials, 17% discontinued for intolerance. This is compared to a rate of 5% for the 81 placebo patients. Including the long term extension study, the adverse events reported as the primary reason for discontinuation by ≥1% of 248 DEPAKOTE-treated patients were alopecia (6%), nausea and/or vomiting (5%), weight gain (2%), tremor (2%), somnolence (1%), elevated SGOT and/or SGPT (1%), and depression (1%).

Table 2 includes those adverse events reported for patients in the placebo-controlled trials where the incidence rate in the DEPAKOTE-treated group was greater than 5% and was greater than that for placebo patients.

Table 2

Adverse Events Reported by >5% of DEPAKOTE-Treated Patients During Migraine Placebo-Controlled Trials with a Greater Incidence Than Patients Taking Placebo[1]

Body System Event	Depakote (N = 202)	Placebo (N = 81)
Gastrointestinal System		
Nausea	31%	10%
Dyspepsia	13%	9%
Diarrhea	12%	7%
Vomiting	11%	1%
Abdominal Pain	9%	4%
Increased appetite	6%	4%
Nervous System		
Asthenia	20%	9%
Somnolence	17%	5%
Dizziness	12%	6%
Tremor	9%	0%
Other		
Weight gain	8%	2%
Back pain	8%	6%
Alopecia	7%	1%

[1] The following adverse events occurred in at least 5% of DEPAKOTE-treated patients and at an equal or greater incidence for placebo than for DEPAKOTE: flu syndrome and pharyngitis.

The following additional adverse events were reported by greater than 1% but not more than 5% of the 202 divalproex sodium-treated patients in the controlled clinical trials:

Body as a Whole: Chest pain, chills, face edema, fever and malaise.

Cardiovascular System: Vasodilatation.

Digestive System: Anorexia, constipation, dry mouth, flatulence, gastrointestinal disorder (unspecified), and stomatitis.

Hemic and Lymphatic System: Ecchymosis.

Metabolic and Nutritional Disorders: Peripheral edema, SGOT increase, and SGPT increase.

Musculoskeletal System: Leg cramps and myalgia.

Nervous System: Abnormal dreams, amnesia, confusion, depression, emotional lability, insomnia, nervousness, paresthesia, speech disorder, thinking abnormalities, and vertigo.

Respiratory System: Cough increased, dyspnea, rhinitis, and sinusitis.

Skin and Appendages: Pruritus and rash.

Special Senses: Conjunctivitis, ear disorder, taste perversion, and tinnitus.

Urogenital System: Cystitis, metrorrhagia, and vaginal hemorrhage.

Epilepsy

Based on a placebo-controlled trial of adjunctive therapy for treatment of complex partial seizures, DEPAKOTE was generally well tolerated with most adverse events rated as mild to moderate in severity. Intolerance was the primary reason for discontinuation in the DEPAKOTE-treated patients (6%), compared to 1% of placebo-treated patients.

Table 3 lists treatment-emergent adverse events which were reported by ≥ 5% of DEPAKOTE-treated patients and for which the incidence was greater than in the placebo group, in the placebo-controlled trial of adjunctive therapy for treatment of complex partial seizures. Since patients were also treated with other antiepilepsy drugs, it is not possible, in most cases, to determine whether the following adverse events can be ascribed to DEPAKOTE alone, or the combination of DEPAKOTE and other antiepilepsy drugs.

Table 3

Adverse Events Reported by ≥5% of Patients Treated with DEPAKOTE During Placebo-Controlled Trial of Adjunctive Therapy for Complex Partial Seizures

Body System/Event	Depakote (%) (n = 77)	Placebo (%) (n = 70)
Body as a Whole		
Headache	31	21
Asthenia	27	7
Fever	6	4

Gastrointestinal System		
Nausea	48	14
Vomiting	27	7
Abdominal Pain	23	6
Diarrhea	13	6
Anorexia	12	0
Dyspepsia	8	4
Constipation	5	1
Nervous System		
Somnolence	27	11
Tremor	25	6
Dizziness	25	13
Diplopia	16	9
Amblyopia/Blurred Vision	12	9
Ataxia	8	1
Nystagmus	8	1
Emotional Lability	6	4
Thinking Abnormal	6	0
Amnesia	5	1
Respiratory System		
Flu Syndrome	12	9
Infection	12	6
Bronchitis	5	1
Rhinitis	5	4
Other		
Alopecia	6	1
Weight Loss	6	0

Table 4 lists treatment-emergent adverse events which were reported by ≥5% of patients in the high dose DEPAKOTE group, and for which the incidence was greater than in the low dose group, in a controlled trial of DEPAKOTE monotherapy treatment of complex partial seizures. Since patients were being titrated off another antiepilepsy drug during the first portion of the trial, it is not possible, in many cases, to determine whether the following adverse events can be ascribed to DEPAKOTE alone, or the combination of DEPAKOTE and other antiepilepsy drugs.

Table 4
Adverse Events Reported by ≥5% of Patients in the High Dose Group in the Controlled Trial of DEPAKOTE Monotherapy for Complex Partial Seizures[1]

Body System/Event	High Dose (%) (n = 131)	Low Dose (%) (n = 134)
Body as a Whole		
Asthenia	21	10
Digestive System		
Nausea	34	26
Diarrhea	23	19
Vomiting	23	15
Abdominal Pain	12	9
Anorexia	11	4
Dyspepsia	11	10
Hemic/Lymphatic System		
Thrombocytopenia	24	1
Ecchymosis	5	4
Metabolic/Nutritional		
Weight Gain	9	4
Peripheral Edema	8	3
Nervous System		
Tremor	57	19
Somnolence	30	18
Dizziness	18	13
Insomnia	15	9
Nervousness	11	7
Amnesia	7	4
Nystagmus	7	1
Depression	5	4
Respiratory System		
Infection	20	13
Pharyngitis	8	2
Dyspnea	5	1
Skin and Appendages		
Alopecia	24	13
Special Senses		
Amblyopia/Blurred Vision	8	4
Tinnitus	7	1

[1] Headache was the only adverse event that occurred in ≥5% of patients in the high dose group and at an equal or greater incidence in the low dose group.

The following additional adverse events were reported by greater than 1% but less than 5% of the 358 patients treated with DEPAKOTE in the controlled trials of complex partial seizures:

Body as a Whole: Back pain, chest pain, malaise.

Cardiovascular System: Tachycardia, hypertension, palpitation.

Digestive System: Increased appetite, flatulence, hematemesis, eructation, pancreatitis, periodontal abscess.

Hemic and Lymphatic System: Petechia.

Metabolic and Nutritional Disorders: SGOT increased, SGPT increased.

Musculoskeletal System: Myalgia, twitching, arthralgia, leg cramps, myasthenia.

Nervous System: Anxiety, confusion, abnormal gait, paresthesia, hypertonia, incoordination, abnormal dreams, personality disorder.

Respiratory System: Sinusitis, cough increased, pneumonia, epistaxis.

Skin and Appendages: Rash, pruritus, dry skin.

Special Senses: Taste perversion, abnormal vision, deafness, otitis media.

Urogenital System: Urinary incontinence, vaginitis, dysmenorrhea, amenorrhea, urinary frequency.

Other Patient Populations

Adverse events that have been reported with all dosage forms of valproate from epilepsy trials, spontaneous reports, and other sources are listed below by body system.

Gastrointestinal: The most commonly reported side effects at the initiation of therapy are nausea, vomiting, and indigestion. These effects are usually transient and rarely require discontinuation of therapy. Diarrhea, abdominal cramps, and constipation have been reported. Both anorexia with some weight loss and increased appetite with weight gain have also been reported. The administration of delayed-release divalproex sodium may result in reduction of gastrointestinal side effects in some patients.

CNS Effects: Sedative effects have occurred in patients receiving valproate alone but occur most often in patients receiving combination therapy. Sedation usually abates upon reduction of other antiepileptic medication. Tremor (may be dose-related), hallucinations, ataxia, headache, nystagmus, diplopia, asterixis, "spots before eyes", dysarthria, dizziness, confusion, hypesthesia, vertigo, and incoordination. Rare cases of coma have occurred in patients receiving valproate alone or in conjunction with phenobarbital. In rare instances encephalopathy with fever has developed shortly after the introduction of valproate monotherapy without evidence of hepatic dysfunction or inappropriate plasma levels; all patients recovered after the drug was withdrawn. Several reports have noted reversible cerebral atrophy and dementia in association with valproate therapy.

Dermatologic: Transient hair loss, skin rash, photosensitivity, generalized pruritus, erythema multiforme, and Stevens-Johnson syndrome. Rare cases of toxic epidermal necrolysis have been reported including a fatal case in a 6 month old infant taking valproate and several other concomitant medications. An additional case of toxic epidermal necrosis resulting in death was reported in a 35 year old patient with AIDS taking several concomitant medications and had with a history of multiple cutaneous drug reactions.

Psychiatric: Emotional upset, depression, psychosis, aggression, hyperactivity, hostility, and behavioral deterioration.

Musculoskeletal: Weakness.

Hematologic: Thrombocytopenia and inhibition of the secondary phase of platelet aggregation may be reflected in altered bleeding time, petechiae, bruising, hematoma formation, epistaxis, and frank hemorrhage (see **PRECAUTIONS - General** and **Drug Interactions**). Relative lymphocytosis, macrocytosis, hypofibrinogenemia, leukopenia, eosinophilia, anemia including macrocytic with or without folate deficiency, bone marrow suppression, pancytopenia, aplastic anemia, and acute intermittent porphyria.

Hepatic: Minor elevations of transaminases (eg, SGOT and SGPT) and LDH are frequent and appear to be dose-related. Occasionally, laboratory test results include increases in serum bilirubin and abnormal changes in other liver function tests. These results may reflect potentially serious hepatotoxicity (see **WARNINGS**).

Endocrine: Irregular menses, secondary amenorrhea, breast enlargement, galactorrhea, and parotid gland swelling. Abnormal thyroid function tests (see **PRECAUTIONS**).

There have been rare spontaneous reports of polycystic ovary disease. A cause and effect relationship has not been established.

Pancreatic: Acute pancreatitis including fatalities.

Metabolic: Hyperammonemia (see **PRECAUTIONS**), hyponatremia, and inappropriate ADH secretion.

There have been rare reports of Fanconi's syndrome occurring chiefly in children.

Decreased carnitine concentrations have been reported although the clinical relevance is undetermined.

Hyperglycinemia has occurred and was associated with a fatal outcome in a patient with preexistent nonketotic hyperglycinemia.

Genitourinary: Enuresis and urinary tract infection.

Special Senses: Hearing loss, either reversible or irreversible, has been reported; however, a cause and effect relationship has not been established. Ear pain has also been reported.

Other: Edema of the extremities, lupus erythematosus, bone pain, cough increased, pneumonia, otitis media, bradycardia, cutaneous vasculitis, and fever.

OVERDOSAGE

Overdosage with valproate may result in somnolence, heart block, and deep coma. Fatalities have been reported; however patients have recovered from valproate levels as high as 2120 µg/mL.

In overdose situations, the fraction of drug not bound to protein is high and hemodialysis or tandem hemodialysis plus hemoperfusion may result in significant removal of drug. The benefit of gastric lavage or emesis will vary with the time since ingestion. General supportive measures should be applied with particular attention to the maintenance of adequate urinary output.

Naloxone has been reported to reverse the CNS depressant effects of valproate overdosage. Because naloxone could theoretically also reverse the antiepileptic effects of valproate, it should be used with caution in patients with epilepsy.

DOSAGE AND ADMINISTRATION
Mania

DEPAKOTE tablets are administered orally. The recommended initial dose is 750 mg daily in divided doses. The dose should be increased as rapidly as possible to achieve the lowest therapeutic dose which produces the desired clinical effect or the desired range of plasma concentrations. In placebo-controlled clinical trials of acute mania, patients were dosed to a clinical response with a trough plasma concentration between 50 and 125 µg/mL. Maximum concentrations were generally achieved within 14 days. The maximum recommended dosage is 60 mg/kg/day.

There is no body of evidence available from controlled trials to guide a clinician in the longer term management of a patient who improves during DEPAKOTE treatment of an acute manic episode. While it is generally agreed that pharmacological treatment beyond an acute response in mania is desirable, both for maintenance of the initial response and for prevention of new manic episodes, there are no systematically obtained data to support the benefits of DEPAKOTE in such longer-term treatment. Although there are no efficacy data that specifically address longer-term antimanic treatment with DEPAKOTE, the safety of DEPAKOTE in long-term use is supported by data from record reviews involving approximately 360 patients treated with DEPAKOTE for greater than 3 months.

Epilepsy

DEPAKOTE tablets are administered orally. DEPAKOTE has been studied as monotherapy and adjunctive therapy in complex partial seizures, and in simple and complex absence seizures in adults and adolescents. As the DEPAKOTE dosage is titrated upward, concentrations of phenobarbital, carbamazepine, and/or phenytoin may be affected (see **PRECAUTIONS- Drug Interactions**).

Complex Partial Seizures: For adults and children 10 years of age or older.

Monotherapy (Initial Therapy): DEPAKOTE has not been systematically studied as initial therapy. Patients should initiate therapy at 10 to 15 mg/kg/day. The dosage should be increased by 5 to 10 mg/kg/week to achieve optimal clinical response. Ordinarily, optimal clinical response is achieved at daily doses below 60 mg/kg/day. If satisfactory clinical response has not been achieved, plasma levels should be measured to determine whether or not they are in the usually accepted therapeutic range (50 to 100 µg/mL). No recommendation regarding the safety of valproate for use at doses above 60 mg/kg/day can be made.

The probability of thrombocytopenia increases significantly at total trough valproate plasma concentrations above 110 µg/mL in females and 135 µg/mL in males. The benefit of improved seizure control with higher doses should be weighed against the possibility of a greater incidence of adverse reactions.

Conversion to Monotherapy: Patients should initiate therapy at 10 to 15 mg/kg/day. The dosage should be increased by 5 to 10 mg/kg/week to achieve optimal clinical response. Ordinarily, optimal clinical response is achieved at daily doses below 60 mg/kg/day. If satisfactory clinical response has not been achieved, plasma levels should be measured to determine whether or not they are in the usually accepted therapeutic range (50 - 100 µg/mL). No recommendation regarding the safety of valproate for use at doses above 60 mg/kg/day can be made. Concomitant antiepilepsy drug (AED) dosage can ordinarily be reduced by approximately 25% every 2 weeks. This reduction may be started at initiation of DEPAKOTE therapy, or delayed by 1 to 2 weeks if there is a concern that seizures are likely to occur with a reduction. The speed and duration of withdrawal of the concomitant AED can be highly variable, and patients should be monitored closely during this period for increased seizure frequency.

Adjunctive Therapy: DEPAKOTE may be added to the patient's regimen at a dosage of 10 to 15 mg/kg/day. The dosage may be increased by 5 to 10 mg/kg/week to achieve optimal clinical response. Ordinarily, optimal clinical response is achieved at daily doses below 60 mg/kg/day. If satisfactory clinical response has not been achieved, plasma levels should be measured to determine whether or not they are in the usually accepted therapeutic range (50 to 100 µg/mL). No recommendation regarding the safety of valproate for use at doses above 60 mg/kg/day can be made. If the total daily dose exceeds 250 mg, it should be given in divided doses.

Continued on next page

Depakote—Cont.

In a study of adjunctive therapy for complex partial seizures in which patients were receiving either carbamazepine or phenytoin in addition to DEPAKOTE, no adjustment of carbamazepine or phenytoin dosage was needed (see **CLINICAL STUDIES**). However, since valproate may interact with these or other concurrently administered AEDs as well as other drugs (see **Drug Interactions**), periodic plasma concentration determinations of concomitant AEDs are recommended during the early course of therapy (see **PRECAUTIONS - Drug Interactions**).

Simple and Complex Absence Seizures: The recommended initial dose is 15 mg/kg/day, increasing at one week intervals by 5 to 10 mg/kg/day until seizures are controlled or side effects preclude further increases. The maximum recommended dosage is 60 mg/kg/day. If the total daily dose exceeds 250 mg, it should be given in divided doses.

A good correlation has not been established between daily dose, serum concentrations, and therapeutic effect. However, therapeutic valproate serum concentrations for most patients with absence seizures is considered to range from 50 to 100 µg/mL. Some patients may be controlled with lower or higher serum concentrations (see **CLINICAL PHARMACOLOGY**).

As the DEPAKOTE dosage is titrated upward, blood concentrations of phenobarbital and/or phenytoin may be affected (see **PRECAUTIONS**).

Antiepilepsy drugs should not be abruptly discontinued in patients in whom the drug is administered to prevent major seizures because of the strong possibility of precipitating status epilepticus with attendant hypoxia and threat to life.

In epileptic patients previously receiving DEPAKENE (valproic acid) therapy, DEPAKOTE tablets should be initiated at the same daily dose and dosing schedule. After the patient is stabilized on DEPAKOTE tablets, a dosing schedule of two or three times a day may be elected in selected patients.

Migraine

DEPAKOTE tablets are administered orally. The recommended starting dose is 250 mg twice daily. Some patients may benefit from doses up to 1000 mg/day. In the clinical trials, there was no evidence that higher doses led to greater efficacy.

General Dosing Advice

Dosing in Elderly Patients - Due to a decrease in unbound clearance of valproate, the starting dose should be reduced; the ultimate therapeutic dose should be achieved on the basis of clinical response.

Dose-Related Adverse Events - The frequency of adverse effects (particularly elevated liver enzymes and thrombocytopenia) may be dose-related. The probability of thrombocytopenia appears to increase significantly at total valproate concentrations of ≥ 110 µg/mL (females) or ≥ 135 µg/mL (males) (see **PRECAUTIONS**). The benefit of improved therapeutic effect with higher doses should be weighed against the possibility of a greater incidence of adverse reactions. G.I. Irritation - Patients who experience G.I. irritation may benefit from administration of the drug with food or by slowly building up the dose from an initial low level.

HOW SUPPLIED

DEPAKOTE tablets (divalproex sodium delayed-release tablets) are supplied as:

125 mg salmon pink-colored tablets:
Bottles of 100 .... (**NDC** 0074-6212-13)
Abbo-Pac® unit dose packages of
100 .... (**NDC** 0074-6212-11).
250 mg peach-colored tablets:
Bottles of 100 .... (**NDC** 0074-6214-13)
Bottles of 500 .... (**NDC** 0074-6214-53)
Abbo-Pac® unit dose packages of
100 .... (**NDC** 0074-6214-11).
500 mg lavender-colored tablets:
Bottles of 100 .... (**NDC** 0074-6215-13)
Bottles of 500 .... (**NDC** 0074-6215-53)
Abbo-Pac® unit dose packages of
100 .... (**NDC** 0074-6215-11).

Recommended storage: Store tablets below 86°F (30°C).

Caution -- Federal (U.S.A.) Law prohibits dispensing without prescription.

Patient Information Leaflet

Important Information for Women Who Could Become Pregnant About the Use of Depakote® (divalproex sodium) Tablets for Migraine

Please read this leaflet carefully before you take Depakote® (divalproex sodium) tablets. This leaflet provides a summary of important information about taking Depakote for migraine to women who could become pregnant. Depakote is also prescribed for uses other than those discussed in this leaflet. If you have any questions or concerns, or want more information about Depakote, contact your doctor or pharmacist.

Information For Women Who Could Become Pregnant

Depakote is used to prevent or reduce the number of migraines you experience. Depakote can be obtained only by prescription from your doctor. The decision to use Depakote for the prevention of migraine is one that you and your doctor should make together, taking into account your individual needs and medical condition.

Before using Depakote, women who can become pregnant should consider the fact that **Depakote has been associated with birth defects, in particular, with spina bifida and other defects related to failure of the spinal canal to close normally. Although the incidence is unknown in migraine patients treated with Depakote, approximately 1 to 2% of children born to women with epilepsy taking Depakote in the first 12 weeks of pregnancy had these defects (based on data from the Centers for Disease Control, a U.S. agency based in Atlanta). The incidence in the general population is 0.1 to 0.2%.**

Information For Women Who Are Planning to Get Pregnant

- Women taking Depakote for the prevention of migraine who are planning to get pregnant should discuss with their doctor temporarily stopping Depakote, before and during their pregnancy.

Information For Women Who Become Pregnant While Taking Depakote

- If you become pregnant while taking Depakote for the prevention of migraine, you should contact your doctor immediately.

Other Important Information About Depakote Tablets

- Depakote tablets should be taken exactly as it is prescribed by your doctor to get the most benefits from Depakote and reduce the risk of side effects.
- If you have taken more than the prescribed dose of Depakote, contact your hospital emergency room or local poison center immediately.
- This medication was prescribed for your particular condition. Do not use it for another condition or give the drug to others.

Facts About Birth Defects

It is important to know that birth defects may occur even in children of individuals not taking any medications or without any additional risk factors.

Facts About Migraine

About 23 million Americans suffer from migraine headaches. About 75% of migraine sufferers are women. A migraine is described as a throbbing headache that gets worse with activity. Migraine may also include nausea and/or vomiting as well as sensitivity to light and sound. Migraine usually happens about once a month, but some people may have them as often as once or twice a week. Often, the symptoms from a migraine can cause people to miss work or school. If you have frequent migraines, or if acute treatment is not working for you, your doctor may prescribe a preventative therapy. Preventative (prophylactic) treatment is used to prevent attacks and reduce the frequency and severity of headache events.

This summary provides important information about the use of Depakote for migraine to women who could become pregnant. If you would like more information about the other potential risks and benefits of Depakote, ask your doctor or pharmacist to let you read the professional labeling and then discuss it with them. If you have any questions or concerns about taking Depakote, you should discuss them with your doctor.

Revised: January, 1998
Ref. 03-4841-R5
ABBOTT LABORATORIES
NORTH CHICAGO, IL 60064, U.S.A.

Shown in Product Identification Guide, page 303

DESOXYN® Ⓒ℞

(methamphetamine hydrochloride)
Gradumet® Tablets

METHAMPHETAMINE HAS A HIGH POTENTIAL FOR ABUSE. IT SHOULD THUS BE TRIED ONLY IN WEIGHT REDUCTION PROGRAMS FOR PATIENTS IN WHOM ALTERNATIVE THERAPY HAS BEEN INEFFECTIVE. ADMINISTRATION OF METHAMPHETAMINE FOR PROLONGED PERIODS OF TIME IN OBESITY MAY LEAD TO DRUG DEPENDENCE AND MUST BE AVOIDED. PARTICULAR ATTENTION SHOULD BE PAID TO THE POSSIBILITY OF SUBJECTS OBTAINING METHAMPHETAMINE FOR NON-THERAPEUTIC USE OR DISTRIBUTION TO OTHERS, AND THE DRUG SHOULD BE PRESCRIBED OR DISPENSED SPARINGLY.

DESCRIPTION

Methamphetamine hydrochloride, chemically known as (S)-N, α-dimethylbenzeneethanamine hydrochloride, is a member of the amphetamine group of sympathomimetic amines.

It has the following structural formula:

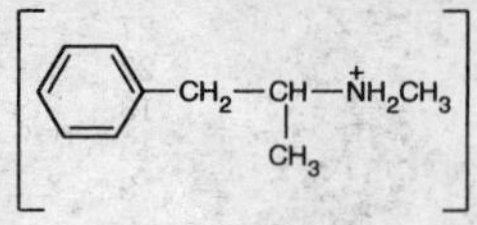

DESOXYN Gradumet sustained-release tablets are available containing 5 mg, 10 mg or 15 mg of methamphetamine hydrochloride for oral administration. The Gradumet is an inert, porous, plastic matrix, which is impregnated with methamphetamine hydrochloride. The drug is leached slowly from the Gradumet as it passes through the gastrointestinal tract. The expended matrix is not absorbed and is excreted in the stool.

Inactive Ingredients: 5 mg Gradumet tablet: magnesium stearate, methyl acrylate-methyl methacrylate copolymer, povidone and talc.

10 mg Gradumet tablet: FD&C Yellow No. 6 (sunset yellow), magnesium stearate, methyl acrylate-methyl methacrylate copolymer, povidone and talc.

15 mg Gradumet tablet: FD&C Yellow No. 5 (tartrazine), magnesium stearate, methyl acrylate-methyl methacrylate copolymer, povidone and talc.

CLINICAL PHARMACOLOGY

Methamphetamine is a sympathomimetic amine with CNS stimulant activity. Peripheral actions include elevation of systolic and diastolic blood pressures and weak bronchodilator and respiratory stimulant action. Drugs of this class used in obesity are commonly known as "anorectics" or "anorexigenics." It has not been established, however, that the action of such drugs in treating obesity is primarily one of appetite suppression. Other central nervous system actions, or metabolic effects, may be involved, for example.

Adult obese subjects instructed in dietary management and treated with "anorectic" drugs, lose more weight on the average than those treated with placebo and diet, as determined in relatively short-term clinical trials.

The magnitude of increased weight loss of drug-treated patients over placebo-treated patients is only a fraction of a pound a week. The rate of weight loss is greatest in the first weeks of therapy for both drug and placebo subjects and tends to decrease in succeeding weeks. The origins of the increased weight loss due to the various possible drug effects are not established. The amount of weight loss associated with the use of an "anorectic" drug varies from trial to trial, and the increased weight loss appears to be related in part to variables other than the drug prescribed, such as the physician-investigator, the population treated, and the diet prescribed. Studies do not permit conclusions as to the relative importance of the drug and non-drug factors on weight loss.

The natural history of obesity is measured in years, whereas the studies cited are restricted to a few weeks duration; thus, the total impact of drug-induced weight loss over that of diet alone must be considered clinically limited.

The mechanism of action involved in producing the beneficial behavioral changes seen in hyperkinetic children receiving methamphetamine is unknown.

In humans, methamphetamine is rapidly absorbed from the gastrointestinal tract. The primary site of metabolism is in the liver by aromatic hydroxylation, N-dealkylation and deamination. At least seven metabolites have been identified in the urine. The biological half-life has been reported in the range of 4 to 5 hours. Excretion occurs primarily in the urine and is dependent on urine pH. Alkaline urine will significantly increase the drug half-life. Approximately 62% of an oral dose is eliminated in the urine within the first 24 hours with about one-third as intact drug and the remainder as metabolites.

INDICATIONS AND USAGE

Attention Deficit Disorder with Hyperactivity —DESOXYN Gradumet tablets are indicated as an integral part of a total treatment program which typically includes other remedial measures (psychological, educational, social) for a stabilizing effect in children over 6 years of age with a behavioral syndrome characterized by the following group of developmentally inappropriate symptoms: moderate to severe distractibility, short attention span, hyperactivity, emotional lability, and impulsivity. The diagnosis of this syndrome should not be made with finality when these symptoms are only of comparatively recent origin. Nonlocalizing (soft) neurological signs, learning disability, and abnormal EEG may or may not be present, and a diagnosis of central nervous system dysfunction may or may not be warranted.

Exogenous Obesity —as a short-term (i.e., a few weeks) adjunct in a regimen of weight reduction based on caloric restriction, for patients in whom obesity is refractory to alternative therapy, e.g., repeated diets, group programs, and other drugs. The limited usefulness of DESOXYN Gradumet tablets (see **CLINICAL PHARMACOLOGY**) should be weighed against possible risks inherent in use of the drug, such as those described below.

CONTRAINDICATIONS

DESOXYN Gradumet tablets are contraindicated during or within 14 days following the administration of monoamine oxidase inhibitors; hypertensive crises may result. It is also contraindicated in patients with glaucoma, advanced arteriosclerosis, symptomatic cardiovascular disease, moderate to severe hypertension, hyperthyroidism or known hypersensitivity or idiosyncrasy to sympathomimetic amines. Methamphetamine should not be given to patients who are in an agitated state or who have a history of drug abuse.

WARNINGS

Tolerance to the anorectic effect usually develops within a few weeks. When this occurs, the recommended dose should not be exceeded in an attempt to increase the effect; rather, the drug should be discontinued (see **DRUG ABUSE AND DEPENDENCE**).

Decrements in the predicted growth (i.e., weight gain and/or height) rate have been reported with the long-term use of stimulants in children. Therefore, patients requiring long-term therapy should be carefully monitored.

Usage in Nursing Mothers: Amphetamines are excreted in human milk. Mothers taking amphetamines should be advised to refrain from nursing.

PRECAUTIONS

General: DESOXYN (methamphetamine hydrochloride) Gradumet tablets should be used with caution in patients with even mild hypertension.

Methamphetamine should not be used to combat fatigue or to replace rest in normal persons.

Prescribing and dispensing of methamphetamine should be limited to the smallest amount that is feasible at one time in order to minimize the possibility of overdosage.

The 15 mg dosage strength of DESOXYN Gradumet tablets contains FD&C Yellow No. 5 (tartrazine) which may cause allergic-type reactions (including bronchial asthma) in certain susceptible individuals. Although the overall incidence of FD&C Yellow No. 5 (tartrazine) sensitivity in the general population is low, it is frequently seen in patients who also have aspirin hypersensitivity.

Information for Patients: The patient should be informed that methamphetamine may impair the ability to engage in potentially hazardous activities, such as, operating machinery or driving a motor vehicle.

The patient should be cautioned not to increase dosage, except on advice of the physician.

Drug Interactions: Insulin requirements in diabetes mellitus may be altered in association with the use of methamphetamine and the concomitant dietary regimen.

Methamphetamine may decrease the hypotensive effect of *guanethidine.*

DESOXYN should not be used concurrently with *monoamine oxidase inhibitors* (see **CONTRAINDICATIONS**).

Concurrent administration of *tricyclic antidepressants* and indirect-acting sympathomimetic amines such as amphetamines, should be closely supervised and dosage carefully adjusted.

Phenothiazines are reported in the literature to antagonize the CNS stimulant action of the amphetamines.

Drug/Laboratory Test Interactions: Literature reports suggest that amphetamines may be associated with significant elevation of plasma corticosteroids. This should be considered if determination of plasma corticosteroid levels is desired in a person receiving amphetamines.

Carcinogensis, Mutagenesis, Impairment of Fertility: Data are not available on long-term potential for carcinogenicity, mutagenicity, or impairment of fertility.

Pregnancy: Teratogenic effects: Pregnancy Category C. Methamphetamine has been shown to have teratogenic and embryocidal effects in mammals given high multiples of the human dose. There are no adequate and well-controlled studies in pregnant women. DESOXYN Gradumet tablets should not be used during pregnancy unless the potential benefit justifies the potential risk to the fetus.

Nonteratogenic effects: Infants born to mothers dependent on amphetamines have an increased risk of premature delivery and low birth weight. Also, these infants may experience symptoms of withdrawal as demonstrated by dysphoria, including agitation and significant lassitude.

Nursing Mothers: See **WARNINGS**.

Pediatric Use: Safety and effectiveness for use as an anorectic agent in children below the age of 12 years have not been established.

Long-term effects of methamphetamine in children have not been established (see **WARNINGS**).

Drug treatment is not indicated in all cases of the behavioral syndrome characterized by moderate to severe distractibility, short attention span, hyperactivity, emotional lability and impulsivity. It should be considered only in light of the complete history and evaluation of the child. The decision to prescribe DESOXYN Gradumet tablets should depend on the physician's assessment of the chronicity and severity of the child's symptoms and their appropriateness for his/her age. Prescription should not depend solely on the presence of one or more of the behavioral characteristics.

When these symptoms are associated with acute stress reactions, treatment with DESOXYN Gradumet tablets is usually not indicated.

Clinical experience suggests that in psychotic children, administration of DESOXYN Gradumet tablets may exacerbate symptoms of behavior disturbance and thought disorder.

Amphetamines have been reported to exacerbate motor and phonic tics and Tourette's syndrome. Therefore, clinical evaluation for tics and Tourette's syndrome in children and their families should precede use of stimulant medications.

ADVERSE REACTIONS

The following are adverse reactions in decreasing order of severity within each category that have been reported:

Cardiovascular: Elevation of blood pressure, tachycardia and palpitation.

Central Nervous System: Psychotic episodes have been rarely reported at recommended doses. Dizziness, dysphoria, overstimulation, euphoria, insomnia, tremor, restlessness and headache. Exacerbation of motor and phonic tics and Tourette's syndrome.

Gastrointestinal: Diarrhea, constipation, dryness of mouth, unpleasant taste and other gastrointestinal disturbances.

Hypersensitivity: Urticaria.

Endocrine: Impotence and changes in libido.

Miscellaneous: Suppression of growth has been reported with the long-term use of stimulants in children (see **WARNINGS**).

DRUG ABUSE AND DEPENDENCE

Controlled Substance: DESOXYN Gradumet tablets are subject to control under DEA schedule II.

Abuse: Methamphetamine has been extensively abused. Tolerance, extreme psychological dependence, and severe social disability have occurred. There are reports of patients who have increased the dosage to many times that recommended. Abrupt cessation following prolonged high dosage administration results in extreme fatigue and mental depression; changes are also noted on the sleep EEG. Manifestations of chronic intoxication with methamphetamine include severe dermatoses, marked insomnia, irritability, hyperactivity, and personality changes. The most severe manifestation of chronic intoxication is psychosis often clinically indistinguishable from schizophrenia.

OVERDOSAGE

Manifestations of acute overdosage with methamphetamine include restlessness, tremor, hyperreflexia, rapid respiration, confusion, assaultiveness, hallucinations, panic states, hyperpyrexia, and rhabdomyolysis. Fatigue and depression usually follow the central stimulation. Cardiovascular effects include arrhythmias, hypertension or hypotension, and circulatory collapse. Gastrointestinal symptoms include nausea, vomiting, diarrhea, and abdominal cramps. Fatal poisoning usually terminates in convulsions and coma.

Consult with a Certified Poison Control Center regarding treatment for up to date guidance and advice. Management of acute methamphetamine intoxication is largely symptomatic and includes gastric evacuation, administration of activated charcoal, and sedation. Experience with hemodialysis or peritoneal dialysis is inadequate to permit recommendations in this regard.

Acidification of urine increases methamphetamine excretion, but is believed to increase risk of acute renal failure if myoglobinuria is present. Intravenous phentolamine (Regitine®) has been suggested for possible acute, severe hypertension, if this complicates methamphetamine overdosage. Usually a gradual drop in blood pressure will result when sufficient sedation has been achieved. Chlorpromazine has been reported to be useful in decreasing CNS stimulation and sympathomimetic effects.

Since the Gradumet tablet releases methamphetamine gradually, therapy should be directed at reversing the effects of the ingested drug and at supporting the patient until symptoms subside. Saline cathartics are useful for hastening the evacuation of the tablets that have not already released medication.

DOSAGE AND ADMINISTRATION

DESOXYN Gradumet tablets are given orally.

Methamphetamine should be administered at the lowest effective dosage, and dosage should be individually adjusted. Late evening medication should be avoided because of the resulting insomnia.

Attention Deficit Disorder with Hyperactivity:

For treatment of children 6 years or older with a behavioral syndrome characterized by moderate to severe distractibility, short attention span, hyperactivity, emotional lability and impulsivity: an initial dose of 5 mg DESOXYN once or twice a day is recommended. Daily dosage may be raised in increments of 5 mg at weekly intervals until optimum clinical response is achieved. The usual effective dose is 20 to 25 mg daily. The total daily dose may be given once daily using the Gradumet tablet. The Gradumet form should not be utilized for initiation of dosage nor until the titrated daily dosage is equal to or greater than the dosage provided in a Gradumet tablet.

Where possible, drug administration should be interrupted occasionally to determine if there is a recurrence of behavioral symptoms sufficient to require continued therapy.

For Obesity: one Gradumet tablet, 10 or 15 mg, once a day in the morning. Treatment should not exceed a few weeks in duration. Methamphetamine is not recommended for use as an anorectic agent in children under 12 years of age.

HOW SUPPLIED

DESOXYN (methamphetamine hydrochloride) Gradumet tablets are supplied as follows:

5 mg, white, in bottles of 100 (**NDC** 0074-6941-04); 10 mg, orange, in bottles of 100 (**NDC** 0074-6948-08); and 15 mg, yellow, in bottles of 100 (**NDC** 0074-6959-07).

® GRADUMET—Long-release dose form, Abbott.

Recommended Storage: Store below 86°F (30°C).

Revised: December, 1995

Ref. 03-4654-R3

Shown in Product Identification Guide, page 303

ENDURON® ℞

[en 'de-ron]

(methyclothiazide tablets, USP)

DESCRIPTION

Methyclothiazide is a member of the benzothiadiazine (thiazide) class of drugs. It is an analogue of hydrochlorothiazide and occurs as a white to practically white crystalline powder which is basically odorless. Methyclothiazide is very slightly soluble in water and chloroform, and slightly soluble in alcohol. Chemically, methyclothiazide is represented as 6-chloro-3- (chloromethyl) -3,4-dihydro-2-methyl-2H-1,2,4-benzothiadiazine-7-sulfonamide 1,1-dioxide. The structural formula is:

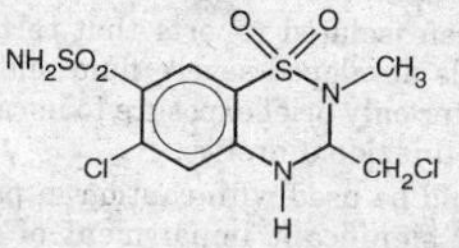

Clinically, ENDURON (methyclothiazide) is an oral diuretic-antihypertensive agent. ENDURON tablets are available in two dosage strengths containing 2.5 mg and 5 mg of methyclothiazide.

Inactive Ingredients

2.5 mg tablets: corn starch, FD&C Yellow No. 6, lactose, magnesium stearate and talc.

5 mg tablets: corn starch, D&C Red No. 36, lactose, magnesium stearate and talc.

CLINICAL PHARMACOLOGY

The diuretic and saluretic effects of methyclothiazide result from a drug-induced inhibition of the renal tubular reabsorption of electrolytes. The excretion of sodium and chloride is greatly enhanced. Potassium excretion is also enhanced to a variable degree, as it is with the other thiazides. Although urinary excretion of bicarbonate is increased slightly, there is usually no significant change in urinary pH. Methyclothiazide has a per mg natriuretic activity approximately 100 times that of the prototype thiazide, chlorothiazide. At maximal therapeutic dosages, all thiazides are approximately equal in their diuretic/natriuretic effects. There is significant natriuresis and diuresis within two hours after administration of a single dose of methyclothiazide. These effects reach a peak in about six hours and persist for 24 hours following oral administration of a single dose.

Like other benzothiadiazines, methyclothiazide also has antihypertensive properties, and may be used for this purpose either alone or to enhance the antihypertensive action of other drugs. The mechanism by which the benzothiadiazines, including methyclothiazide, produce a reduction of elevated blood pressure is not known. However, sodium depletion appears to be involved.

Methyclothiazide is rapidly absorbed and slowly eliminated by the kidneys as intact drug but primarily as an inactive metabolite. Additional information on the pharmacokinetics is not known at this time.

INDICATIONS AND USAGE

ENDURON (methyclothiazide) is indicated in the management of hypertension either as the sole therapeutic agent or to enhance the effect of other antihypertensive drugs in the more severe forms of hypertension.

ENDURON tablets are indicated as adjunctive therapy in edema associated with congestive heart failure, hepatic cirrhosis, and corticosteroid and estrogen therapy.

Continued on next page

Enduron—Cont.

ENDURON tablets have also been found useful in edema due to various forms of renal dysfunction such as the nephrotic syndrome, acute glomerulonephritis, and chronic renal failure.

Usage in Pregnancy: The routine use of diuretics in an otherwise healthy pregnant woman is inappropriate and exposes mother and fetus to unnecessary hazard. Diuretics do not prevent development of toxemia of pregnancy, and there is no satisfactory evidence that they are useful in the treatment of developed toxemia.

Edema during pregnancy may arise from pathological causes or from the physiological and mechanical consequences of pregnancy. Thiazides are indicated in pregnancy when edema is due to pathological causes, just as they are in the absence of pregnancy (see PRECAUTIONS—Pregnancy). Dependent edema in pregnancy, resulting from restriction of venous return by the expanded uterus, is properly treated through elevation of the lower extremities and use of support hose; use of diuretics to lower intravascular volume in this case is illogical and unnecessary. There is hypervolemia during normal pregnancy that is harmful to neither the fetus nor the mother (in the absence of cardiovascular disease), but that is associated with edema, including generalized edema, in the majority of pregnant women. If this edema produces discomfort, increased recumbency will often provide relief. In rare instances, this edema may cause extreme discomfort that is not relieved by rest. In these cases, a short course of diuretics may provide relief and may be appropriate.

CONTRAINDICATIONS

Methyclothiazide is contraindicated in patients with anuria and in patients with a history of hypersensitivity to this compound or other sulfonamide-derived drugs.

WARNINGS

Methyclothiazide shares with other thiazides the propensity to deplete potassium reserves to an unpredictable degree. There have been isolated reports that certain nonedematous individuals developed severe fluid and electrolyte derangements after only brief exposure to normal doses of thiazide and non-thiazide diuretics.

Thiazides should be used with caution in patients with renal disease or significant impairment of renal function, since azotemia may be precipitated and cumulative drug effects may occur.

Thiazides should be used with caution in patients with impaired hepatic function or progressive liver disease, since minor alterations of fluid and electrolyte balance may precipitate hepatic coma.

Sensitivity reactions may occur in patients with a history of allergy or bronchial asthma.

The possibility of exacerbation or activation of systemic lupus erythematosus has been reported.

Hyperuricemia may occur or frank gout may be precipitated in certain patients receiving thiazide therapy.

PRECAUTIONS

Laboratory Tests: Initial and periodic determinations of serum electrolytes should be performed at appropriate intervals for the purpose of detecting possible electrolyte imbalances such as hyponatremia, hypochloremic alkalosis, and hypokalemia. Serum and urine electrolyte determinations are particularly important when a patient is vomiting excessively or receiving parenteral fluids.

General: All patients should be observed for clinical signs of electrolyte imbalances such as dryness of mouth, thirst, weakness, lethargy, drowsiness, restlessness, muscle pains or cramps, muscular fatigue, hypotension, oliguria, tachycardia, and gastrointestinal disturbances such as nausea and vomiting.

Hypokalemia may develop, especially with brisk diuresis, when severe cirrhosis is present, during concomitant use of corticosteroids or ACTH, or after prolonged therapy.

Interference with adequate oral electrolyte intake will also contribute to hypokalemia. Hypokalemia may be avoided or treated by use of potassium supplements or foods with a high potassium content.

Any chloride deficit is generally mild and usually does not require specific treatment except under extraordinary circumstances (as in liver disease or renal disease). Dilutional hyponatremia may occur in edematous patients in hot weather; appropriate therapy is water restriction rather than administration of salt, except in rare instances when the hyponatremia is life threatening. In actual salt depletion, appropriate replacement is the therapy of choice.

Latent diabetes mellitus may become manifest during thiazide administration.

The antihypertensive effects of the drug may be enhanced in the postsympathectomy patient.

If progressive renal impairment becomes evident as indicated by a rising nonprotein nitrogen or blood urea nitro-

gen, a careful reappraisal of therapy is necessary with consideration given to withholding or discontinuing diuretic therapy.

Thiazides may decrease urinary calcium excretion. Thiazides may cause intermittent and slight elevation of serum calcium in the absence of known disorders of calcium metabolism. Marked hypercalcemia may be evidence of hidden hyperparathyroidism. Thiazides should be discontinued before carrying out tests for parathyroid function.

Thiazides may cause increased concentrations of total serum cholesterol, total triglycerides, and low-density lipoproteins in some patients. Use thiazides with caution in patients with moderate or high cholesterol concentrations and in patients with elevated triglyceride levels.

Information for Patients: Patients should inform their doctor if they have: 1) had an allergic reaction to methyclothiazide or other diuretics 2) asthma 3) kidney disease 4) liver disease 5) gout 6) systemic lupus erythematosus, or 7) been taking other drugs such as cortisone, digitalis, lithium carbonate, or drugs for diabetes.

The physician should inform patients of possible side effects and caution the patient to report any of the following symptoms of electrolyte imbalance: dryness of mouth, thirst, weakness, tiredness, drowsiness, restlessness, muscle pains or cramps, nausea, vomiting or increased heart rate.

The physician should advise the patient to take this medication every day as directed. Physicians should also caution patients that drinking alcohol can increase the chance of dizziness.

Drug Interactions: Hypokalemia can sensitize or exaggerate the response of the heart to the toxic effects of *digitalis* (e.g., increased ventricular irritability).

Hypokalemia may develop during concomitant use of *steroids* or *ACTH.*

Insulin requirements in diabetic patients may be increased, decreased, or unchanged.

Thiazides may decrease arterial responsiveness to *norepinephrine.* This diminution is not sufficient to preclude effectiveness of the pressor agent for therapeutic use.

Thiazide drugs may increase the responsiveness to *tubocurarine.*

Lithium renal clearance is reduced by thiazides, increasing the risk of lithium toxicity.

Thiazides may add to or potentiate the action of *other antihypertensive drugs.* Potentiation occurs with ganglionic or peripheral adrenergic blocking drugs.

Drug/Laboratory Test Interactions: Thiazides may decrease serum PBI levels without signs of thyroid disturbance.

Thiazides should be discontinued before carrying out tests for parathyroid function.

Carcinogenesis, Mutagenesis, Impairment of Fertility: No data are available concerning the potential for carcinogenicity or mutagenicity in animals or humans. Methyclothiazide did not impair fertility in rats receiving up to 4 mg/kg/day (at least 20 times the maximum recommended human dose of 10 mg, assuming patient weight equal to or greater than 50 kg).

Pregnancy—Teratogenic Effects: Pregnancy Category B. Reproduction studies performed in rats and rabbits at doses up to 4 mg/kg/day have revealed no evidence of harm to the fetus due to methyclothiazide. There are, however, no adequate and well-controlled studies in pregnant women. Because animal reproduction studies are not always predictive of human response, this drug should be used during pregnancy only if clearly needed.

Nonteratogenic Effects: Thiazides cross the placental barrier and appear in cord blood. The use of thiazides in pregnant women requires that the anticipated benefit be weighed against possible hazards to the fetus. These hazards include fetal or neonatal jaundice, thrombocytopenia and possible other adverse reactions that have occurred in the adult.

Nursing Mothers: Thiazides are excreted in breast milk. Because of the potential for serious adverse reactions in nursing infants, a decision should be made whether to discontinue nursing or to discontinue the drug taking into account the importance of the drug to the mother.

Pediatric Use: Safety and effectiveness in children have not been established.

ADVERSE REACTIONS

Adverse reactions are usually reversible upon reduction of dosage or discontinuation of ENDURON tablets. Whenever adverse reactions are moderate or severe, it may be necessary to discontinue the drug.

The following adverse reactions have been observed, but there has not been enough systematic collection of data to support an estimate of their frequency. Consequently the reactions are categorized by organ system and are listed in decreasing order of severity and not frequency.

Body as a Whole: Headache, cramping, weakness.

Cardiovascular System: Orthostatic hypotension (may be potentiated by alcohol, barbiturates, or narcotics).

Digestive System: Pancreatitis, jaundice (intrahepatic cholestatic), sialadenitis, vomiting, diarrhea, nausea, gastric irritation, constipation, anorexia.

Hemic and Lymphatic System: Aplastic anemia, hemolytic anemia, agranulocytosis, leukopenia, thrombocytopenia.

Hypersensitivity Reactions: Anaphylactic reactions, necrotizing angiitis (vasculitis, cutaneous vasculitis), Stevens-Johnson syndrome, respiratory distress including pneumonitis and pulmonary edema, fever, purpura, urticaria, rash, photosensitivity.

Metabolic and Nutritional Disorders: Hyperglycemia, hyperuricemia, electrolyte imbalance (see PRECAUTIONS section), hypercalcemia.

Nervous System: Vertigo, dizziness, paresthesias, muscle spasms, restlessness.

Special Senses: Transient blurred vision, xanthopsia.

Urogenital System: Glycosuria.

OVERDOSAGE

Symptoms of overdosage include electrolyte imbalance and signs of potassium deficiency such as confusion, dizziness, muscular weakness, and gastrointestinal disturbances. General supportive measures including replacement of fluids and electrolytes may be indicated in treatment of overdosage.

DOSAGE AND ADMINISTRATION

ENDURON (methyclothiazide) is administered orally. Therapy should be individualized according to patient response. This therapy should be titrated to gain maximal therapeutic response as well as the minimal dose possible to maintain that therapeutic response.

For edematous conditions: The usual adult dose ranges from 2.5 to 10 mg once daily. Maximum effective single dose is 10 mg; larger single doses do not accomplish greater diuresis, and are not recommended.

For the treatment of hypertension: The usual adult dose ranges from 2.5 to 5 mg once daily.

If control of blood pressure is not satisfactory after 8 to 12 weeks of therapy with 5 mg once daily, another antihypertensive drug should be added. Increasing the dosage of methyclothiazide will usually not result in further lowering of blood pressure.

Methyclothiazide may be either employed alone for mild to moderate hypertension or concurrently with other antihypertensive drugs in the management of more severe forms of hypertension. Combined therapy may provide adequate control of hypertension with lower dosage of the component drugs and fewer or less severe side effects. An enhanced response frequently follows its concurrent administration with Harmonyl® (deserpidine) so that dosage of both drugs may be reduced.

When other antihypertensive agents are to be added to the regimen, this should be accomplished gradually. Ganglionic blocking agents should be given at only half the usual dose since their effect is potentiated by pretreatment with ENDURON tablets.

HOW SUPPLIED

ENDURON (methyclothiazide tablets, USP) is provided in two dosage sizes as monogrammed, grooved, square-shaped tablets:

2.5 mg, orange-colored:
    bottles of 100 (**NDC** 0074-6827-01),
    bottles of 1000 (**NDC** 0074-6827-02).
5 mg, salmon-colored:
    bottles of 100 (**NDC** 0074-6812-01),
    bottles of 1000 (**NDC** 0074-6812-02),
    bottles of 5000 (**NDC** 0074-6812-03),
    Abbo-Pac® unit dose packages of 100
    (**NDC** 0074-6812-10).

Dispense in a USP tight container.
Recommended storage: Store below 86°F (30°C).
Revised: October, 1991
Ref. 03-4404-R9

ERY-PED®   ℞
[erē ' ped]
(ERYTHROMYCIN ETHYLSUCCINATE, USP)

DESCRIPTION

Erythromycin is produced by a strain of *Saccharopolyspora erythraea* (formerly *Streptomyces erythraeus*) and belongs to the macrolide group of antibiotics. It is basic and readily forms salts with acids. The base, the stearate salt, and the esters are poorly soluble in water. Erythromycin ethylsuccinate is an ester of erythromycin suitable for oral administration. Erythromycin ethylsuccinate is known chemically as erythromycin 2'-(ethyl succinate). The molecular formula is $C_{43}H_{75}NO_{16}$ and the molecular weight is 862.06. The structural formula is:
[See chemical structure at top of next column]
EryPed 200 and EryPed Drops (erythromycin ethylsuccinate for oral suspension) when reconstituted with water,

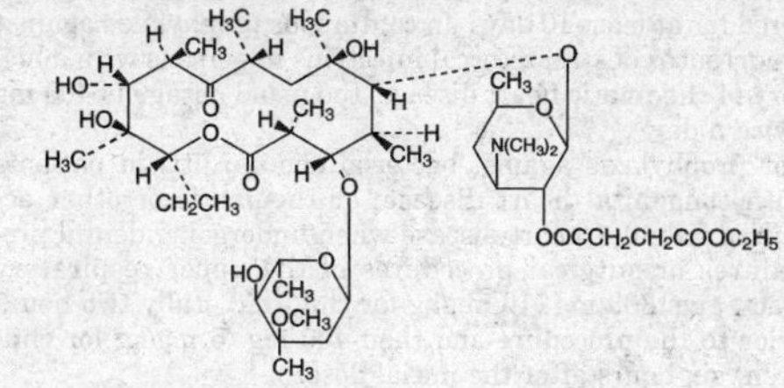

forms a suspension containing erythromycin ethylsuccinate equivalent to 200 mg erythromycin per 5 mL (teaspoonful) or 100 mg per 2.5 mL (dropperful) with an appealing fruit flavor. EryPed 400 when reconstituted with water, forms a suspension containing erythromycin ethylsuccinate equivalent to 400 mg of erythromycin per 5 mL (teaspoonful) with an appealing banana flavor.
Fruit-flavored EryPed Chewable tablets are easily ingested and are particularly acceptable for the administration of antibiotic medication to young children who are unable to swallow regular tablets or in whom persuasion of a pleasant taste insures cooperation.
Each chewable tablet contains erythromycin ethylsuccinate equivalent to 200 mg of erythromycin and is scored for division into half-dose (100 mg) portions.
These products are intended primarily for pediatric use but can also be used in adults.

Inactive Ingredients:
EryPed 200, EryPed 400 and EryPed Drops: Caramel, polysorbate, sodium citrate, sucrose, xanthan gum and artificial flavors.
EryPed Chewable Tablets: Citric acid, confectioner's sugar (contains corn starch), magnesium aluminum silicate, magnesium stearate, sodium carboxymethylcellulose, sodium citrate and artificial flavor.

CLINICAL PHARMACOLOGY

Orally administered erythromycin ethylsuccinate suspension is readily and reliably absorbed under both fasting and nonfasting conditions.
Erythromycin diffuses readily into most body fluids. Only low concentrations are normally achieved in the spinal fluid, but passage of the drug across the blood-brain barrier increases in meningitis. In the presence of normal hepatic function, erythromycin is concentrated in the liver and excreted in the bile; the effect of hepatic dysfunction on excretion of erythromycin by the liver into the bile is not known. Less than 5 percent of the orally administered dose of erythromycin is excreted in active form in the urine.
Erythromycin crosses the placental barrier, but fetal plasma levels are low. The drug is excreted in human milk.

Microbiology:
Erythromycin acts by inhibition of protein synthesis by binding 50 *S* ribosomal subunits of susceptible organisms. It does not affect nucleic acid synthesis. Antagonism has been demonstrated *in vitro* between erythromycin and clindamycin, lincomycin, and chloramphenicol.
Many strains of *Haemophilus influenzae* are resistant to erythromycin alone but are susceptible to erythromycin and sulfonamides used concomitantly.
Staphylococci resistant to erythromycin may emerge during a course of therapy.
Erythromycin has been shown to be active against most strains of the following microorganisms, both *in vitro* and in clinical infections as described in the **INDICATIONS AND USAGE** section.

Gram-positive Organisms:
Corynebacterium diphtheriae
Corynebacterium minutissimum
Listeria monocytogenes
Staphylococcus aureus (resistant organisms may emerge during treatment)
Streptococcus pneumoniae
Streptococcus pyogenes

Gram-negative Organisms:
Bordetella pertussis
Legionella pneumophila
Neisseria gonorrhoeae

Other Microorganisms:
Chlamydia trachomatis
Entamoeba histolytica
Mycoplasma pneumoniae
Treponema pallidum
Ureaplasma urealyticum

The following *in vitro* data are available, **but their clinical significance is unknown.**
Erythromycin exhibits *in vitro* minimal inhibitory concentrations (MIC's) of 0.5 µg/mL or less against most (≥ 90%) strains of the following microorganisms; however, the safety and effectiveness of erythromycin in treating clinical infections due to these microorganisms have not been established in adequate and well-controlled clinical trials.

Gram-positive Organisms:
Viridans group streptococci

Gram-negative Organisms:
Moraxella catarrhalis

Susceptibility Tests:

Dilution Techniques:
Quantitative methods are used to determine antimicrobial minimum inhibitory concentrations (MIC's). These MIC's provide estimates of the susceptibility of bacteria to antimicrobial compounds. The MIC's should be determined using a standardized procedure. Standardized procedures are based on a dilution method[1] (broth or agar) or equivalent with standardized inoculum concentrations and standardized concentrations of erythromycin powder. The MIC values should be interpreted according to the following criteria:

MIC (µg/mL)	Interpretation
≤0.5	Susceptible (S)
1–4	Intermediate (I)
≥8	Resistant (R)

A report of "Susceptible" indicates that the pathogen is likely to be inhibited if the antimicrobial compound in the blood reaches the concentrations usually achievable. A report of "Intermediate" indicates that the result should be considered equivocal, and, if the microorganism is not fully susceptible to alternative, clinically feasible drugs, the test should be repeated. This category implies possible clinical applicability in body sites where the drug is physiologically concentrated or in situations where high dosage of drug can be used. This category also provides a buffer zone which prevents small uncontrolled technical factors from causing major discrepancies in interpretation. A report of "Resistant" indicates that the pathogen is not likely to be inhibited if the antimicrobial compound in the blood reaches the concentrations usually achievable; other therapy should be selected.
Standardized susceptibility test procedures require the use of laboratory control microorganisms to control the technical aspects of the laboratory procedures. Standard erythromycin powder should provide the following MIC values:

Microorganism	MIC (µg/mL)
S. aureus ATCC 29213	0.12-0.5
*E. faecalis*ATCC 22912	1–4

Diffusion Techniques:
Quantitative methods that require measurement of zone diameters also provide reproducible estimates of the susceptibility of bacteria to antimicrobial compounds. One such standardized procedure[2] requires the use of standardized inoculum concentrations. This procedure uses paper disks impregnated with 15-µg erythromycin to test the susceptibility of microorganisms to erythromycin.
Reports from the laboratory providing results of the standard single-disk susceptibility test with a 15-µg erythromycin disk should be interpreted according to the following criteria:

Zone Diameter (mm)	Interpretation
≥23	Susceptible (S)
14–22	Intermediate (I)
≤13	Resistant (R)

Interpretation should be as stated above for results using dilution techniques. Interpretation involves correlation of the diameter obtained in the disk test with the MIC for erythromycin.
As with standardized dilution techniques, diffusion methods require the use of laboratory control microorganisms that are used to control the technical aspects of the laboratory procedures. For the diffusion technique, the 15-µg erythromycin disk should provide the following zone diameters in these laboratory test quality control strains:

Microorganism	Zone Diameter (mm)
*S. aureus*ATCC 25923	22–30

INDICATIONS AND USAGE

Ery-Ped is indicated in the treatment of infections caused by susceptible strains of the designated organisms in the diseases listed below:
Upper respiratory tract infections of mild to moderate degree caused by *Streptococcus pyogenes, Streptococcus pneumoniae*, or *Haemophilus influenzae* (when used concomitantly with adequate doses of sulfonamides, since many strains of *H. influenzae* are not susceptible to the erythromycin concentrations ordinarily achieved). (See appropriate sulfonamide labeling for prescribing information.)
Lower-respiratory tract infections of mild to moderate severity caused by *Streptococcus pneumoniae* or *Streptococcus pyogenes*.
Listeriosis caused by *Listeria monocytogenes*.
Pertussis (whooping cough) caused by *Bordetella pertussis*. Erythromycin is effective in eliminating the organism from the nasopharynx of infected individuals rendering them noninfectious. Some clinical studies suggest that erythromycin may be helpful in the prophylaxis of pertussis in exposed susceptible individuals.
Respiratory tract infections due to *Mycoplasma pneumoniae*.
Skin and skin structure infections of mild to moderate severity caused by *Streptococcus pyogenes* or *Staphylococcus aureus* (resistant staphylococci may emerge during treatment).
Diphtheria: Infections due to *Corynebacterium diphtheriae*, as an adjunct to antitoxin, to prevent establishment of carriers and to eradicate the organism in carriers.
Erythrasma: In the treatment of infections due to *Corynebacterium minutissimum*.
Intestinal amebiasis caused by *Entamoeba histolytica* (oral erythromycins only). Extraenteric amebiasis requires treatment with other agents.
Acute pelvic inflammatory disease caused by *Neisseria gonorrhoeae*: As an alternative drug in treatment of acute pelvic inflammatory disease caused by *N. gonorrhoeae* in female patients with a history of sensitivity to penicillin. Patients should have a serologic test for syphilis before receiving erythromycin as treatment of gonorrhea and a follow-up serologic test for syphilis after 3 months.
Syphilis caused by *Treponema pallidum*: Erythromycin is an alternate choice of treatment for primary syphilis in penicillin-allergic patients. In primary syphilis, spinal fluid examinations should be done before treatment and as part of follow-up after therapy.
Erythromycins are indicated for the treatment of the following infections caused by *Chlamydia trachomatis*: conjunctivitis of the newborn, pneumonia of infancy, and urogenital infections during pregnancy. When tetracyclines are contraindicated or not tolerated, erythromycin is indicated for the treatment of uncomplicated urethral, endocervical, or rectal infections in adults due to *Chlamydia trachomatis*.
When tetracyclines are contraindicated or not tolerated, erythromycin is indicated for the treatment of nongonococcal urethritis caused by *Ureaplasma urealyticum*.
Legionnaires' Disease caused by *Legionella pneumophila*. Although no controlled clinical efficacy studies have been conducted, *in vitro* and limited preliminary clinical data suggest that erythromycin may be effective in treating Legionnaires' Disease.

Prophylaxis:
Prevention of Initial Attacks of Rheumatic Fever: Penicillin is considered by the American Heart Association to be the drug of choice in the prevention of initial attacks of rheumatic fever (treatment of *Streptococcus pyogenes* infections of the upper respiratory tract, e.g., tonsillitis or pharyngitis). Erythromycin is indicated for the treatment of penicillin-allergic patients.[3] The therapeutic dose should be administered for 10 days.
Prevention of Recurrent Attacks of Rheumatic Fever: Penicillin or sulfonamides are considered by the American Heart Association to be the drugs of choice in the prevention of recurrent attacks of rheumatic fever. In patients who are allergic to penicillin and sulfonamides, oral erythromycin is recommended by the American Heart Association in the long-term prophylaxis of streptococcal pharyngitis (for the prevention of recurrent attacks of rheumatic fever).[3]
Prevention of Bacterial Endocarditis: Although no controlled clinical efficacy trials have been conducted, oral erythromycin has been recommended by the American Heart Association for prevention of bacterial endocarditis in penicillin-allergic patients with prosthetic cardiac valves, most congenital cardiac malformations, surgically constructed systemic pulmonary shunts, rheumatic or other acquired valvular dysfunction, idiopathic hypertrophic subaortic stenosis (IHSS), previous history of bacterial endocarditis or mitral valve prolapse with insufficiency when they undergo dental procedures or surgical procedures of the upper respiratory tract.[4]

CONTRAINDICATIONS

Erythromycin is contraindicated in patients with known hypersensitivity to this antibiotic.
Erythromycin is contraindicated in patients taking terfenadine, astemizole, or cisapride. (See **PRECAUTIONS** - *Drug Interactions*.)

WARNINGS

There have been reports of hepatic dysfunction, including increased liver enzymes, and hepatocellular and/or cholestatic hepatitis, with or without jaundice, occurring in patients receiving oral erythromycin products.

Continued on next page

Ery-Ped—Cont.

There have been reports suggesting that erythromycin does not reach the fetus in adequate concentration to prevent congenital syphilis. Infants born to women treated during pregnancy with oral erythromycin for early syphilis should be treated with an appropriate penicillin regimen.

Pseudomembranous colitis has been reported with nearly all antibacterial agents, including erythromycin, and may range in severity from mild to life threatening. Therefore, it is important to consider this diagnosis in patients who present with diarrhea subsequent to the administration of antibacterial agents.

Treatment with antibacterial agents alters the normal flora of the colon and may permit overgrowth of clostridia. Studies indicate that a toxin produced by *Clostridium difficile* is a primary cause of "antibiotic-associated colitis".

After the diagnosis of pseudomembranous colitis has been established, therapeutic measures should be initiated. Mild cases of pseudomembranous colitis usually respond to discontinuation of the drug alone. In moderate to severe cases, consideration should be given to management with fluids and electrolytes, protein supplementation, and treatment with an antibacterial drug clinically effective against *Clostridium difficile* colitis.

Rhabdomyolysis with or without renal impairment has been reported in seriously ill patients receiving erythromycin concomitantly with lovastatin. Therefore, patients receiving concomitant lovastatin and erythromycin should be carefully monitored for creatine kinase (CK) and serum transaminase levels. (See package insert for lovastatin.)

PRECAUTIONS

General: Since erythromycin is principally excreted by the liver, caution should be exercised when erythromycin is administered to patients with impaired hepatic function. (See **CLINICAL PHARMACOLOGY** and **WARNINGS** sections.)

There have been reports that erythromycin may aggravate the weakness of patients with myasthenia gravis.

Prolonged or repeated use of erythromycin may result in an overgrowth of nonsusceptible bacteria or fungi. If superinfection occurs, erythromycin should be discontinued and appropriate therapy instituted.

When indicated, incision and drainage or other surgical procedures should be performed in conjunction with antibiotic therapy.

Drug Interactions: Erythromycin use in patients who are receiving high doses of theophylline may be associated with an increase in serum theophylline levels and potential theophylline toxicity. In case of theophylline toxicity and/or elevated serum theophylline levels, the dose of theophylline should be reduced while the patient is receiving concomitant erythromycin therapy.

Concomitant administration of erythromycin and digoxin has been reported to result in elevated digoxin serum levels.

There have been reports of increased anticoagulant effects when erythromycin and oral anticoagulants were used concomitantly. Increased anticoagulation effects due to interactions of erythromycin with various oral anticoagulants may be more pronounced in the elderly.

Concurrent use of erythromycin and ergotamine or dihydroergotamine has been associated in some patients with acute ergot toxicity characterized by severe peripheral vasospasm and dysesthesia.

Erythromycin has been reported to decrease the clearance of triazolam and midazolam and, thus, may increase the pharmacologic effect of these benzodiazepines.

The use of erythromycin in patients concurrently taking drugs metabolized by the cytochrome P450 system may be associated with elevations in serum levels of these other drugs. There have been reports of interactions of erythromycin with carbamazepine, cyclosporine, tacrolimus, hexobarbital, phenytoin, alfentanil, cisapride, disopyramide, lovastatin, bromocriptine, valproate, terfenadine, and astemizole. Serum concentrations of drugs metabolized by the cytochrome P450 system should be monitored closely in patients concurrently receiving erythromycin.

Erythromycin has been reported to significantly alter the metabolism of the nonsedating antihistamines terfenadine and astemizole when taken concomitantly. Rare cases of serious cardiovascular adverse events, including electrocardiographic QT/QT_c interval prolongation, cardiac arrest, torsades de pointes, and other ventricular arrhythmias have been observed. (See **CONTRAINDICATIONS**.) In addition, deaths have been reported rarely with concomitant administration of terfenadine and erythromycin.

There have been post-marketing reports of drug interactions when erythromycin was coadministered with cisapride, resulting in QT prolongation, cardiac arrhythmias, ventricular tachycardia, ventricular fibrillation, and torsades de pointes most likely due to the inhibition of hepatic metabolism of cisapride by erythromycin. Fatalities have been reported. (See **CONTRAINDICATIONS**.)

Drug/Laboratory Test Interactions: Erythromycin interferes with the fluorometric determination of urinary catecholamines.

Carcinogenesis, Mutagenesis, Impairment of Fertility: Long-term (2-year) oral studies in rats with erythromycin ethylsuccinate and erythromycin base did not provide evidence of tumorigenicity. Mutagenicity studies have not been conducted. There was no apparent effect on male or female fertility in rats fed erythromycin (base) at levels up to 0.25% of diet.

Pregnancy: Teratogenic Effects. Pregnancy Category B: There is no evidence of teratogenicity or any other adverse effect on reproduction in female rats fed erythromycin base (up to 0.25% of diet) prior to and during mating, during gestation, and through weaning of two successive litters. There are, however, no adequate and well-controlled studies in pregnant women. Because animal reproduction studies are not always predictive of human response, this drug should be used during pregnancy only if clearly needed.

Labor and Delivery: The effect of erythromycin on labor and delivery is unknown.

Nursing Mothers: Erythromycin is excreted in human milk. Caution should be exercised when erythromycin is administered to a nursing woman.

Pediatric Use: See **INDICATIONS AND USAGE** and **DOSAGE AND ADMINISTRATION** sections.

ADVERSE REACTIONS

The most frequent side effects of oral erythromycin preparations are gastrointestinal and are dose-related. They include nausea, vomiting, abdominal pain, diarrhea and anorexia. Symptoms of hepatitis, hepatic dysfunction and/or abnormal liver function test results may occur. (See **WARNINGS** section.)

Onset of pseudomembranous colitis symptoms may occur during or after antibacterial treatment. (See **WARNINGS**.)

Rarely, erythromycin has been associated with the production of ventricular arrhythmias, including ventricular tachycardia and torsades de pointes, in individuals with prolonged QT intervals.

Allergic reactions ranging from urticaria to anaphylaxis have occurred. Skin reactions ranging from mild eruptions to erythema multiforme, Stevens-Johnson syndrome, and toxic epidermal necrolysis have been reported rarely.

There have been isolated reports of reversible hearing loss occurring chiefly in patients with renal insufficiency and in patients receiving high doses of erythromycin.

OVERDOSAGE

In case of overdosage, erythromycin should be discontinued. Overdosage should be handled with the prompt elimination of unabsorbed drug and all other appropriate measures should be instituted.

Erythromycin is not removed by peritoneal dialysis or hemodialysis.

DOSAGE AND ADMINISTRATION

EryPed (erythromycin ethylsuccinate) oral suspensions and chewable tablets may be administered without regard to meals.

Children: Age, weight, and severity of the infection are important factors in determining the proper dosage. In mild to moderate infections, the usual dosage of erythromycin ethylsuccinate for children is 30 to 50 mg/kg/day in equally divided doses every 6 hours. For more severe infections this dosage may be doubled. If twice-a-day dosage is desired, one-half of the total daily dose may be given every 12 hours. Doses may also be given three times daily by administering one-third of the total daily dose every 8 hours.

The following dosage schedule is suggested for mild to moderate infections:

Body Weight	Total Daily Dose
Under 10 lbs	30–50 mg/kg/day 15–25 mg/lb/day
10 to 15 lbs	200 mg
16 to 25 lbs	400 mg
26 to 50 lbs	800 mg
51 to 100 lbs	1200 mg
over 100 lbs	1600 mg

Adults: 400 mg erythromycin ethylsuccinate every 6 hours is the usual dose. Dosage may be increased up to 4 g per day according to the severity of the infection. If twice-a-day dosage is desired, one-half of the total daily dose may be given every 12 hours. Doses may also be given three times daily by administering one-third of the total daily dose every 8 hours.

For adult dosage calculation, use a ratio of 400 mg of erythromycin activity as the ethylsuccinate to 250 mg of erythromycin activity as the stearate, base or estolate.

In the treatment of streptococcal infections, a therapeutic dosage of erythromycin ethylsuccinate should be administered for at least 10 days. In continuous prophylaxis against recurrences of streptococcal infections in persons with a history of rheumatic heart disease, the usual dosage is 400 mg twice a day.

For prophylaxis against bacterial endocarditis in patients with congenital heart disease, or rheumatic or other acquired valvular heart disease when undergoing dental procedures or surgical procedures of the upper respiratory tract, give 800 mg (10 mg/kg for children) orally two hours prior to the procedure and then 400 mg (5 mg/kg for children) six hours after the initial dose.

For treatment of urethritis due to *C. trachomatis* or *U. urealyticum:* 800 mg three times a day for 7 days.

For treatment of primary syphilis: Adults: 48 to 64 g given in divided doses over a period of 10 to 15 days.

For intestinal amebiasis: Adults: 400 mg four times daily for 10 to 14 days. Children: 30 to 50 mg/kg/day in divided doses for 10 to 14 days.

For use in pertussis: Although optimal dosage and duration have not been established, doses of erythromycin utilized in reported clinical studies were 40 to 50 mg/kg/day, given in divided doses for 5 to 14 days.

For treatment of Legionnaires' Disease: Although optimal doses have not been established, doses utilized in reported clinical data were 1.6 to 4 g daily in divided doses.

For the EryPed 200 unit dose, reconstitute with 2.9 mL of water. For the EryPed 400 unit dose, reconstitute with 2.7 mL of water.

HOW SUPPLIED

EryPed 200 (erythromycin ethylsuccinate for oral suspension, USP) is supplied in bottles of 100 mL (**NDC** 0074-6302-13), 200 mL (**NDC** 0074-6302-53), and 5 mL unit dose ABBO-PAC® packages of 100 bottles (**NDC** 0074-6302-05).

EryPed 400 (erythromycin ethylsuccinate for oral suspension, USP) is supplied in bottles of 60 mL (**NDC** 0074-6305-60), 100 mL (**NDC** 0074-6305-13), 200 mL (**NDC** 0074-6305-53), and 5 mL unit dose ABBO-PAC packages of 100 bottles (**NDC** 0074-6305-05).

EryPed Drops (erythromycin ethylsuccinate for oral suspension) is supplied in 50 mL bottles (**NDC** 0074-6303-50).

EryPed Chewable (erythromycin ethylsuccinate tablets, USP) are fruit-flavored wafers containing activity equivalent to 200 mg of erythromycin and are available in packages of 40 (**NDC** 0074-6314-40). Each wafer is individually sealed in a blister package.

Recommended storage: Store EryPed Chewable below 86°F (30°C). Store EryPed 200, EryPed 400, and EryPed Drops, prior to mixing, below 86°F (30°C). After reconstitution, EryPed 200, EryPed 400, and EryPed Drops must be stored at or below 77°F (25°C) and used within 35 days; refrigeration is not required.

REFERENCES

1. National Committee for Clinical Laboratory Standards, *Method for Dilution Antimicrobial Susceptibility Tests for Bacteria that Grow Aerobically,* Third Edition. Approved Standard NCCLS Document M7-A3, Vol. 13, No. 25. NCCLS, Villanova, PA, December 1993.
2. National Committee for Clinical Laboratory Standards, *Performance Standards for Antimicrobial Disk Susceptibility Tests,* Fifth Edition. Approved Standard NCCLS Document M2-A5, Vol. 13, No. 24. NCCLS, Villanova, PA, December 1993.
3. Committee on Rheumatic Fever, Endocarditis, and Kawasaki Disease of the Council on Cardiovascular Disease in the Young, the American Heart Association: Prevention of Rheumatic Fever. *Circulation.* 78(4):1082-1086, October 1988.
4. Dajani, Adnan., M.D., et al.: Prevention of Bacterial Endocarditis Recommendations by the American Heart Association. *JAMA.* 264(22):2919-2922, December 12, 1990.

Ref. 03-4831-R9

Revised: December, 1998

ABBOTT LABORATORIES

NORTH CHICAGO, IL 60064, U.S.A.

Shown in Product Identification Guide, page 303

ERY-TAB® ℞

[*ērē 'tab*]

(erythromycin delayed-release tablets, USP)

Enteric-Coated

DESCRIPTION

Erythromycin is produced by a strain of *Streptomyces erythraeus* and belongs to the macrolide group of antibiotics. It is basic and readily forms salts with acids. The base is white to off-white crystals or powder slightly soluble in water, soluble in alcohol, in chloroform, and in ether. ERY-TAB (erythromycin delayed-release tablets) is specially enteric-coated to protect the contents from the inactivating effects of gastric acidity and to permit efficient absorption of the antibiotic in the small intestine.

ERY-TAB is available in three dosage strengths, each tablet containing either 250 mg, 333 mg, or 500 mg of erythromycin as the free base.

Inactive Ingredients: 250 mg tablet: cellulosic polymers, corn starch, diacetylated monoglycerides, D&C red No. 30, iron oxide, magnesium hydroxide, magnesium stearate, sodium starch glycolate, titanium dioxide and vanillin.

333 mg tablet: cellulosic polymers, diacetylated monoglycerides, FD&C blue No. 1, magnesium stearate, microcrystalline cellulose, povidone, sodium citrate, soybean derivatives, talc, titanium dioxide and vanillin.

500 mg tablet: cellulosic polymers, diacetylated monoglycerides, FD&C red No. 40, iron oxide, magnesium stearate, microcrystalline cellulose, povidone, sodium citrate, soybean derivatives, talc, titanium dioxide and vanillin.

ACTIONS

The mode of action of erythromycin is inhibition of protein synthesis without affecting nucleic acid synthesis. Resistance to erythromycin of some strains of *Hemophilus influenzae* and staphylococci has been demonstrated. Culture and susceptibility testing should be done. If the Kirby-Bauer method of disc susceptibility is used, a 15 mcg erythromycin disc should give a zone diameter of at least 18 mm when tested against an erythromycin susceptible organism. Bioavailability data are available from Abbott Laboratories, Dept. 355.

ERY-TAB is well absorbed and may be given without regard to meals.

After absorption, erythromycin diffuses readily into most body fluids. In the absence of meningeal inflammation, low concentrations are normally achieved in the spinal fluid but passage of the drug across the blood-brain barrier increases in meningitis. In the presence of normal hepatic function, erythromycin is concentrated in the liver and excreted in the bile; the effect of hepatic dysfunction on excretion of erythromycin by the liver into the bile is not known. After oral administration, less than 5 percent of the activity of the administered dose can be recovered in the urine.

Erythromycin crosses the placental barrier but fetal plasma levels are low.

INDICATIONS

Streptococcus pyogenes (Group A beta hemolytic streptococcus): For upper and lower respiratory tract, skin, and soft tissue infections of mild to moderate severity.

Injectable benzathine penicillin G is considered by the American Heart Association to be the drug of choice in the treatment and prevention of streptococcal pharyngitis and in long-term prophylaxis of rheumatic fever.

When oral medication is preferred for treatment of the above conditions, penicillin G, V, or erythromycin are alternate drugs of choice.

When oral medication is given, the importance of strict adherence by the patient to the prescribed dosage regimen must be stressed. A therapeutic dose should be administered for at least 10 days.

Alpha-hemolytic streptococci (viridans group): Although no controlled clinical efficacy trials have been conducted, oral erythromycin has been suggested by the American Heart Association and American Dental Association for use in a regimen for prophylaxis against bacterial endocarditis in patients hypersensitive to penicillin who have congenital heart disease, or rheumatic or other acquired valvular heart disease when they undergo dental procedures and surgical procedures of the upper respiratory tract.[1] Erythromycin is not suitable prior to genitourinary or gastrointestinal tract surgery. NOTE: When selecting antibiotics for the prevention of bacterial endocarditis the physician or dentist should read the full joint statement of the American Heart Association and the American Dental Association.[1]

Staphylococcus aureus: For acute infections of skin and soft tissue of mild to moderate severity. Resistant organisms may emerge during treatment.

Streptococcus pneumoniae (Diplococcus pneumoniae): For upper respiratory tract infections (e.g., otitis media, pharyngitis) and lower respiratory tract infection (e.g., pneumonia) of mild to moderate degree.

Mycoplasma pneumoniae (Eaton agent, PPLO): For respiratory infections due to this organism.

Hemophilus influenzae: For upper respiratory tract infections of mild to moderate severity when used concomitantly with adequate doses of sulfonamides. Not all strains of this organism are susceptible at the erythromycin concentrations ordinarily achieved (see appropriate sulfonamide labeling for prescribing information).

Chlamydia trachomatis: Erythromycin is indicated for treatment of the following infections caused by *Chlamydia trachomatis:* conjunctivitis of the newborn, pneumonia of infancy and urogenital infections during pregnancy. When tetracyclines are contraindicated or not tolerated, erythromycin is indicated for the treatment of uncomplicated urethral, endocervical, or rectal infections in adults due to *Chlamydia trachomatis.*[2]

Treponema pallidum: Erythromycin is an alternate choice of treatment for primary syphilis in patients allergic to the penicillins. In treatment of primary syphilis, spinal fluid examinations should be done before treatment and as part of follow-up after therapy.

Corynebacterium diphtheriae and C. minutissimum: As an adjunct to antitoxin, to prevent establishment of carriers, and to eradicate the organism in carriers.

In the treatment of erythrasma.

Entamoeba histolytica: In the treatment of intestinal amebiasis only. Extra-enteric amebiasis requires treatment with other agents.

Listeria monocytogenes: Infections due to this organism.

Neisseria gonorrhoeae: Erythrocin® Lactobionate-I.V. (erythromycin lactobionate for injection, USP) in conjunction with erythromycin base orally, as an alternative drug in treatment of acute pelvic inflammatory disease caused by *N. gonorrhoeae* in female patients with a history of sensitivity to penicillin. Before treatment of gonorrhea, patients who are suspected of also having syphilis should have a microscopic examination for *T. pallidum* (by immunofluorescence or darkfield) before receiving erythromycin, and monthly serologic tests for a minimum of 4 months.

Bordetella pertussis: Erythromycin is effective in eliminating the organism from the nasopharynx of infected individuals, rendering them non-infectious. Some clinical studies suggest that erythromycin may be helpful in the prophylaxis of pertussis in exposed susceptible individuals.

Legionnaires' Disease: Although no controlled clinical efficacy studies have been conducted, *in vitro* and limited preliminary clinical data suggest that erythromycin can be effective in treating Legionnaires' Disease.

CONTRAINDICATIONS

Erythromycin is contraindicated in patients with known hypersensitivity to this antibiotic.

WARNINGS

There have been reports of hepatic dysfunction with or without jaundice, occurring in patients receiving oral erythromycin products.

PRECAUTIONS

General: Erythromycin is principally excreted by the liver. Caution should be exercised when erythromycin is administered to patients with impaired hepatic function. (See "Clinical Pharmacology" and "Warnings" sections).

Prolonged or repeated use of erythromycin may result in an overgrowth of nonsusceptible bacteria or fungi. If superinfection occurs, erythromycin should be discontinued and appropriate therapy instituted.

When indicated, incision and drainage or other surgical procedures should be performed in conjunction with antibiotic therapy.

Laboratory Tests: Erythromycin interferes with the fluorometric determination of urinary catecholamines.

Drug Interactions: Erythromycin use in patients who are receiving high doses of theophylline may be associated with an increase in serum theophylline levels and potential theophylline toxicity. In case of theophylline toxicity and/or elevated serum theophylline levels, the dose of theophylline should be reduced while the patient is receiving concomitant erythromycin therapy.

Concomitant administration of erythromycin and digoxin has been reported to result in elevated digoxin serum levels. There have been reports of increased anticoagulant effects when erythromycin and oral anticoagulants were used concomitantly.

Concurrent use of erythromycin and ergotamine or dihydroergotamine has been associated in some patients with acute ergot toxicity characterized by severe peripheral vasospasm and dysesthesia.

Erythromycin has been reported to decrease the clearance of triazolam and thus may increase the pharmacologic effect of triazolam.

The use of erythromycin in patients concurrently taking drugs metabolized by the cytochrome P450 system may be associated with elevations in serum erythromycin with carbamazepine, cyclosporine, hexobarbital and phenytoin. Serum concentrations of drugs metabolized by the cytochrome P450 system should be monitored closely in patients concurrently receiving erythromycin.

Troleandomycin significantly alters the metabolism of terfenadine when taken concomitantly; therefore, observe caution when erythromycin and terfenadine are used concurrently.

Patients receiving concomitant lovastatin and erythromycin should be carefully monitored; cases of rhabdomyolysis have been reported in seriously ill patients.

Carcinogenesis, Mutagenesis, Impairment of Fertility: Long-term (2-year) oral studies conducted in rats with erythromycin base did not provide evidence of tumorigenicity. Mutagenicity studies have not been conducted. There was no apparent effect on male or female fertility in rats fed erythromycin (base) at levels up to 0.25 percent of diet.

Pregnancy: Pregnancy Category B: There is no evidence of teratogenicity or any other adverse effect on reproduction in female rats fed erythromycin base (up to 0.25 percent of diet) prior to and during mating, during gestation, and through weaning of two successive litters. There are, however, no adequate and well-controlled studies in pregnant women. Because animal reproduction studies are not always predictive of human response, this drug should be used during pregnancy only if clearly needed. Erythromycin has been reported to cross the placental barrier in humans, but fetal plasma levels are generally low.

Labor and Delivery: The effect of erythromycin on labor and delivery is unknown.

Nursing Mothers: Erythromycin is excreted in breast milk, therefore, caution should be exercised when erythromycin is administered to a nursing woman.

Pediatric Use: See "Indications and Usage" and "Dosage and Administration" sections.

ADVERSE REACTIONS

The most frequent side effects of oral erythromycin preparations are gastrointestinal and are dose-related. They include nausea, vomiting, abdominal pain, diarrhea and anorexia. Symptoms of hepatic dysfunction and/or abnormal liver function test results may occur (see "Warnings" section). Pseudomembranous colitis has been rarely reported in association with erythromycin therapy.

There have been isolated reports of transient central nervous system side effects including confusion, hallucinations, seizures, and vertigo; however, a cause and effect relationship has not been established.

Occasional case reports of cardiac arrhythmias such as ventricular tachycardia have been documented in patients receiving erythromycin therapy. There have been isolated reports of other cardiovascular symptoms such as chest pain, dizziness, and palpitations; however, a cause and effect relationship has not been established.

Allergic reactions ranging from urticaria and mild skin eruptions to anaphylaxis have occurred.

There have been isolated reports of reversible hearing loss occurring chiefly in patients with renal insufficiency and in patients receiving high doses of erythromycin.

OVERDOSAGE

In case of overdosage, erythromycin should be discontinued. Overdosage should be handled with the prompt elimination of unabsorbed drug and all other appropriate measures. Erythromycin is not removed by peritoneal dialysis or hemodialysis.

DOSAGE AND ADMINISTRATION

ERY-TAB (erythromycin delayed-release tablets) is well absorbed and may be given without regard to meals.

Adults: The usual dose is 250 mg four times daily in equally spaced doses. The 333 mg tablet is recommended if dosage is desired every 8 hours. If twice-a-day dosage is desired, the recommended dose is 500 mg every 12 hours.

Dosage may be increased up to 4 or more grams per day according to the severity of the infection. Twice-a-day dosing is not recommended when doses larger than 1 gram daily are administered.

Children: Age, weight, and severity of the infection are important factors in determining the proper dosage. 30 to 50 mg/kg/day, in divided doses, is the usual dose. For more severe infections, this dose may be doubled.

In the treatment of streptococcal infections, a therapeutic dosage of erythromycin should be administered for at least 10 days. In continuous prophylaxis of streptococcal infections in persons with a history of rheumatic heart disease, the dose is 250 mg twice a day.

For prophylaxis against bacterial endocarditis[1] in patients with congenital heart disease, or rheumatic or other acquired valvular heart disease when undergoing dental procedures or surgical procedures of the upper respiratory tract, give 1 g (20 mg/kg for children) orally $1\frac{1}{2}$ to 2 hours before the procedure, and then, 500 mg (10 mg/kg in children) orally every 6 hours for 8 doses.

For conjunctivitis of the newborn caused by *Chlamydia trachomatis:* Oral erythromycin suspension 50 mg/kg/day in 4 divided doses for at least 2 weeks.[2]

For pneumonia of infancy caused by *Chlamydia trachomatis:* Although the optimal duration of therapy has not been established, the recommended therapy is oral erythromycin suspension 50 mg/kg/day in 4 divided doses for at least 3 weeks.[2]

For urogenital infections during pregnancy due to *Chlamydia trachomatis:* Although the optimal dose and duration of therapy have not been established, the suggested treatment is erythromycin 500 mg, by mouth, 4 times a day for at least 7 days. For women who cannot tolerate this regimen, a decreased dose of 250 mg, by mouth, 4 times a day should be used for at least 14 days.[2]

For adults with uncomplicated urethral, endocervical, or rectal infections caused by *Chlamydia trachomatis* in whom tetracyclines are contraindicated or not tolerated: 500 mg, by mouth, 4 times a day for at least 7 days.[2]

For treatment of primary syphilis: 30 to 40 grams given in divided doses over a period of 10 to 15 days.

Continued on next page

Ery-Tab—Cont.

For treatment of acute pelvic inflammatory disease caused by *N. gonorrhoeae:* After initial treatment with Erythrocin® Lactobionate-I.V. (erythromycin lactobionate for injection, USP) 500 mg every 6 hours for 3 days, the oral dosage recommendation is 250 mg every 6 hours for 7 days.

For dysenteric amebiasis: 250 mg four times daily for 10 to 14 days, for adults; 30 to 50 mg/kg/day in divided doses for 10 to 14 days, for children.

For use in pertussis: Although optimal dosage and duration have not been established, doses of erythromycin utilized in reported clinical studies were 40 to 50 mg/kg/day, given in divided doses for 5 to 14 days.

For treatment of Legionnaires' Disease: Although optimal doses have not been established, doses utilized in reported clinical data were 1 to 4 grams erythromycin base daily in divided doses.

HOW SUPPLIED

ERY-TAB (erythromycin delayed-release tablets, USP), 250 mg, is supplied as pink tablets in bottles of 100 (**NDC** 0074-6304-13), bottles of 500 (**NDC** 0074-6304-53), and Abbo-Pac® unit dose packages of 100 (**NDC** 0074-6304-11).
ERY-TAB, 333 mg, is supplied as white tablets in bottles of 100 (**NDC** 0074-6320-13), bottles of 500 (**NDC** 0074-6320-53), and Abbo-Pac® unit dose packages of 100 (**NDC** 0074-6320-11).
ERY-TAB, 500 mg, is supplied as pink tablets in bottles of 100 (**NDC** 0074-6321-13) and Abbo-Pac® unit dose packages of 100 (**NDC** 0074-6321-11).
Recommended Storage: Store below 86°F (30°C).

REFERENCES

1. American Heart Association, 1977. Prevention of bacterial endocarditis, Circulation 56: 139A-143A.
2. CDC Sexually Transmitted Diseases Treatment Guidelines 1982.

333 mg and 500 mg tablets—U.S. Pat. No. 4,340,582.
Revised: August 1991
Ref. 01-2526-R6
Shown in Product Identification Guide, page 303

E.E.S.®   Rx
[ē-ē-s]
(ERYTHROMYCIN ETHYLSUCCINATE)

DESCRIPTION

Erythromycin is produced by a strain of *Saccharopolyspora erythraea* (formerly *Streptomyces erythraeus*) and belongs to the macrolide group of antibiotics. It is basic and readily forms salts with acids. The base, the stearate salt, and the esters are poorly soluble in water. Erythromycin ethylsuccinate is an ester of erythromycin suitable for oral administration. Erythromycin ethylsuccinate is known chemically as erythromycin 2′-(ethylsuccinate). The molecular formula is $C_{43}H_{75}NO_{16}$ and the molecular weight is 862.06. The structural formula is:

E.E.S. Granules are intended for reconstitution with water. Each 5-mL teaspoonful of reconstituted cherry-flavored suspension contains erythromycin ethylsuccinate equivalent to 200 mg of erythromycin.
The pleasant tasting, fruit-flavored liquids are supplied ready for oral administration.
E.E.S. 200 Liquid: Each 5-mL teaspoonful of fruit-flavored suspension contains erythromycin ethylsuccinate equivalent to 200 mg of erythromycin.
E.E.S. 400 Liquid: Each 5-mL teaspoonful of orange-flavored suspension contains erythromycin ethylsuccinate equivalent to 400 mg of erythromycin.
Granules and ready-made suspensions are intended primarily for pediatric use but can also be used in adults.
E.E.S. 400® Filmtab® Tablets: Each tablet contains erythromycin ethylsuccinate equivalent to 400 mg of erythromycin.
The Filmtab® tablets are intended primarily for adults or older children.

Inactive Ingredients:

E.E.S. 200 Liquid: FD&C Red No. 40, methylparaben, polysorbate 60, propylparaben, sodium citrate, sucrose, water, xanthan gum and natural and artificial flavors.
E.E.S. 400 Liquid: D&C Yellow No. 10, FD&C Yellow No. 6, methylparaben, polysorbate 60, propylparaben, sodium citrate, sucrose, water, xanthan gum and natural and artificial flavors.
E.E.S. Granules: Citric acid, FD&C Red No. 3, magnesium aluminum silicate, sodium carboxymethylcellulose, sodium citrate, sucrose and artificial flavor.
E.E.S. 400 Filmtab Tablets: Cellulosic polymers, confectioner's sugar (contains corn starch), corn starch, D&C Red No. 30, D&C Yellow No. 10, FD&C Red No. 40, magnesium stearate, polacrilin potassium, polyethylene glycol, propylene glycol, sodium citrate, sorbic acid, and titanium dioxide.

CLINICAL PHARMACOLOGY

Orally administered erythromycin ethylsuccinate suspensions and Filmtab tablets are readily and reliably absorbed. Comparable serum levels of erythromycin are achieved in the fasting and nonfasting states.
Erythromycin diffuses readily into most body fluids. Only low concentrations are normally achieved in the spinal fluid, but passage of the drug across the blood-brain barrier increases in meningitis. In the presence of normal hepatic function, erythromycin is concentrated in the liver and excreted in the bile; the effect of hepatic dysfunction on excretion of erythromycin by the liver into the bile is not known. Less than 5 percent of the orally administered dose of erythromycin is excreted in active form in the urine.
Erythromycin crosses the placental barrier, but fetal plasma levels are low. The drug is excreted in human milk.
Microbiology:
Erythromycin acts by inhibition of protein synthesis by binding 50 S ribosomal subunits of susceptible organisms. It does not affect nucleic acid synthesis. Antagonism has been demonstrated *in vitro* between erythromycin and clindamycin, lincomycin, and chloramphenicol.
Many strains of *Haemophilus influenzae* are resistant to erythromycin alone but are susceptible to erythromycin and sulfonamides used concomitantly.
Staphylocci resistant to erythromycin may emerge during a course of therapy.
Erythromycin has been shown to be active against most strains of the following microorganisms, both *in vitro* and in clinical infections as described in the **INDICATIONS AND USAGE** section.
Gram-positive Organisms:
   Corynebacterium diphtheriae
   Corynebacterium minutissimum
   Listeria monocytogenes
   Staphylococcus aureus (resistant organisms may emerge during treatment)
   Streptococcus pneumoniae
   Streptococcus pyogenes
Gram-negative Organisms:
   Bordetella pertussis
   Legionella pneumophila
   Neisseria gonorrhoeae
Other Microorganisms:
   Chlamydia trachomatis
   Entamoeba histolytica
   Mycoplasma pneumoniae
   Treponema pallidum
   Ureaplasma urealyticum
The following *in vitro* data are available, **but their clinical significance is unknown.**
Erythromycin exhibits *in vitro* minimal inhibitory concentrations (MIC's) of 0.5 μg/mL or less against most (≥90%) strains of the following microorganisms; however, the safety and effectiveness of erythromycin in treating clinical infections due to these microorganisms have not been established in adequate and well controlled clinical trials.
Gram-positive Organisms:
   Viridans group streptococci
Gram-negative Organisms:
   Moraxella catarrhalis
Susceptibility Tests:
Dilution Techniques:
Quantitative methods are used to determine antimicrobial minimum inhibitory concentrations (MIC's). These MIC's provide estimates of the susceptibility of bacteria to antimicrobial compounds. The MIC's should be determined using a standardized procedure. Standardized procedures are based on a dilution method[1] (broth or agar) or equivalent with standardized inoculum concentrations and standardized concentrations of erythromycin powder. The MIC values should be interpreted according to the following criteria:

MIC (μg/mL)	Interpretation
≤0.5	Susceptible (S)
1–4	Intermediate (I)
≥8	Resistant (R)

A report of "Susceptible" indicates that the pathogen is likely to be inhibited if the antimicrobial compound in the blood reaches the concentrations usually achievable. A report of "Intermediate" indicates that the result should be considered equivocal, and, if the microorganism is not fully susceptible to alternative, clinically feasible drugs, the test should be repeated. This category implies possible clinical applicability in body sites where the drug is physiologically concentrated or in situations where high dosage of drug can be used. This category also provides a buffer zone which prevents small uncontrolled technical factors from causing major discrepancies in interpretation. A report of "Resistant" indicates that the pathogen is not likely to be inhibited if the antimicrobial compound in the blood reaches the concentrations usually achievable; other therapy should be selected.
Standardized susceptibility test procedures require the use of laboratory control microorganisms to control the technical aspects of the laboratory procedures. Standard erythromycin powder should provide the following MIC values:

Microorganism	MIC (μg/mL)
S. aureus ATCC 25923	0.12–0.5
E. faecalis ATC 29212	1–4

Diffusion Techniques:
Quantitative methods that require measurement of zone diameters also provide reproducible estimates of the susceptibility of bacteria to antimicrobial compounds. One such standardized procedure[2] requires the use of standardized inoculum concentrations. This procedure uses paper disks impregnated with 15-μg erythromycin to test the susceptibility of microorganisms to erythromycin.
Reports from the laboratory providing results of the standard single-disk susceptibility test with a 15-μg erythromycin disk should be interpreted according to the following criteria:

Zone Diameter (mm)	Interpretation
≥23	Susceptible (S)
14–22	Intermediate (I)
≤13	Resistant (R)

Interpretation should be as stated above for results using dilution techniques. Interpretation involves correlation of the diameter obtained in the disk test with the MIC for erythromycin.
As with standardized dilution techniques, diffusion methods require the use of laboratory control microorganisms that are used to control the technical aspects of the laboratory procedures. For the diffusion technique, the 15-μg erythromycin disk should provide the following zone diameters in these laboratory test quality control strains:

Microorganism	Zone Diameter (mm)
S. aureus ATCC 25923	22–30

INDICATIONS AND USAGE

E.E.S. is indicated in the treatment of infections caused by susceptible strains of the designated organisms in the diseases listed below:
Upper respiratory tract infections of mild to moderate degree caused by *Streptococcus pyogenes, Streptococcus pneumoniae,* or *Haemophilus influenzae* (when used concomitantly with adequate doses of sulfonamides, since many strains of *H. influenzae* are not susceptible to the erythromycin concentrations ordinarily achieved). (See appropriate sulfonamide labeling for prescribing information.)
Lower-respiratory tract infections of mild to moderate severity caused by *Streptococcus pneumoniae* or *Streptococcus pyogenes.*
Listeriosis caused by *Listeria monocytogenes.*
Pertussis (whooping cough) caused by *Bordetella pertussis.* Erythromycin is effective in eliminating the organism from the nasopharynx of infected individuals rendering them noninfectious. Some clinical studies suggest that erythromycin may be helpful in the prophylaxis of pertussis in exposed susceptible individuals.
Respiratory tract infections due to *Mycoplasma pneumoniae.*
Skin and skin structure infections of mild to moderate severity caused by *Streptococcus pyogenes* or *Staphylococcus aureus* (resistant staphylococci may emerge during treatment).
Diphtheria: Infections due to *Corynebacterium diphtheriae,* as an adjunct to antitoxin, to prevent establishment of carriers and to eradicate the organism in carriers.
Erythrasma: In the treatment of infections due to *Corynebacterium minutissimum.*
Intestinal amebiasis caused by *Entamoeba histolytica* (oral erythromycins only). Extraenteric amebiasis requires treatment with other agents.

Acute pelvic inflammatory disease caused by *Neisseria gonorrhoeae*: As an alternative drug in treatment of acute pelvic inflammatory disease caused by *N. gonorrhoeae* in female patients with a history of sensitivity to penicillin. Patients should have a serologic test for syphilis before receiving erythromycin as treatment of gonorrhea and a follow-up serologic test for syphilis after 3 months.

Syphilis caused by *Treponema pallidum*: Erythromycin is an alternate choice of treatment for primary syphilis in patients allergic to the penicillins. In treatment of primary syphilis, spinal fluid examinations should be done before treatment and as part of follow-up after therapy.

Erythromycins are indicated for the treatment of the following infections caused by *Chlamydia trachomatis*: conjunctivitis of the newborn, pneumonia of infancy, and urogenital infections during pregnancy. When tetracyclines are contraindicated or not tolerated, erythromycin is indicated for the treatment of uncomplicated urethral, endocervical, or rectal infections in adults due to *Chlamydia trachomatis*.

When tetracyclines are contraindicated or not tolerated, erythromycin is indicated for the treatment of nongonococcal urethritis caused by *Ureaplasma urealyticum*.

Legionnaires' Disease caused by *Legionella pneumophila*. Although no controlled clinical efficacy studies have been conducted, *in vitro* and limited preliminary clinical data suggest that erythromycin may be effective in treating Legionnaires' Disease.

Prophylaxis:

Prevention of Initial Attacks of Rheumatic Fever: Penicillin is considered by the American Heart Association to be the drug of choice in the prevention of initial attacks of rheumatic fever (treatment of *Streptococcus pyogenes* infections of the upper respiratory tract, e.g., tonsillitis or pharyngitis). Erythromycin is indicated for the treatment of penicillin-allergic patients.[3] The therapeutic dose should be administered for 10 days.

Prevention of Recurrent Attacks of Rheumatic Fever: Penicillin or sulfonamides are considered by the American Heart Association to be the drugs of choice in the prevention of recurrent attacks of rheumatic fever. In patients who are allergic to penicillin and sulfonamides, oral erythromycin is recommended by the American Heart Association in the long-term prophylaxis of streptococcal pharyngitis (for the prevention of recurrent attacks of rheumatic fever).[3]

Prevention of Bacterial Endocarditis: Although no controlled clinical efficacy trials have been conducted, oral erythromycin has been recommended by the American Heart Association for prevention of bacterial endocarditis in penicillin-allergic patients with prosthetic cardiac valves, most congenital cardiac malformations, surgically constructed systemic pulmonary shunts, rheumatic or other acquired valvular dysfunction, idiopathic hypertrophic subaortic stenosis (IHSS), previous history of bacterial endocarditis or mitral valve prolapse with insufficiency when they undergo dental procedures or surgical procedures of the upper respiratory tract.[4]

CONTRAINDICATIONS

Erythromycin is contraindicated in patients with known hypersensitivity to this antibiotic.

Erythromycin is contraindicated in patients taking terfenadine, astemizole, or cisapride. (See **PRECAUTIONS** - *Drug Interactions*.)

WARNINGS

There have been reports of hepatic dysfunction, including increased liver enzymes, and hepatocellular and/or cholestatic hepatitis, with or without jaundice, occurring in patients receiving oral erythromycin products.

There have been reports suggesting that erythromycin does not reach the fetus in adequate concentration to prevent congenital syphilis. Infants born to women treated during pregnancy with oral erythromycin for early syphilis should be treated with an appropriate penicillin regimen.

Pseudomembranous colitis has been reported with nearly all antibacterial agents, including erythromycin, and may range in severity from mild to life threatening. Therefore, it is important to consider this diagnosis in patients who present with diarrhea subsequent to the administration of antibacterial agents.

Treatment with antibacterial agents alters the normal flora of the colon and may permit overgrowth of clostridia. Studies indicate that a toxin produced by *Clostridium difficile* is a primary cause of "antibiotic-associated colitis."

After the diagnosis of pseudomembranous colitis has been established, therapeutic measures should be initiated. Mild cases of pseudomembranous colitis usually respond to discontinuation of the drug alone. In moderate to severe cases, consideration should be given to management with fluids and electrolytes, protein supplementation, and treatment with an antibacterial drug clinically effective against *Clostridium difficile* colitis.

Rhabdomyolysis with or without renal impairment has been reported in seriously ill patients receiving erythromycin concomitantly with lovastatin. Therefore, patients receiving concomitant lovastatin and erythromycin should be carefully monitored for creatine kinase (CK) and serum transaminase levels. (See package insert for lovastatin.)

PRECAUTIONS

General: Since erythromycin is principally excreted by the liver, caution should be exercised when erythromycin is administered to patients with impaired hepatic function. (See **CLINICAL PHARMACOLOGY** and **WARNINGS** sections.)

There have been reports that erythromycin may aggravate the weakness of patients with myasthenia gravis.

Prolonged or repeated use of erythromycin may result in an overgrowth of nonsusceptible bacteria or fungi. If superinfection occurs, erythromycin should be discontinued and appropriate therapy instituted.

When indicated, incision and drainage or other surgical procedures should be performed in conjunction with antibiotic therapy.

Drug Interactions: Erythromycin use in patients who are receiving high doses of theophylline may be associated with an increase in serum theophylline levels and potential theophylline toxicity. In case of theophylline toxicity and/or elevated serum theophylline levels, the dose of theophylline should be reduced while the patient is receiving concomitant erythromycin therapy.

Concomitant administration of erythromycin and digoxin has been reported to result in elevated digoxin serum levels. There have been reports of increased anticoagulant effects when erythromycin and oral anticoagulants were used concomitantly. Increased anticoagulation effects due to interactions of erythromycin with various oral anticoagulants may be more pronounced in the elderly.

Concurrent use of erythromycin and ergotamine or dihydroergotamine has been associated in some patients with acute ergot toxicity characterized by severe peripheral vasospasm and dysesthesia.

Erythromycin has been reported to decrease the clearance of triazolam and midazolam and, thus, may increase the pharmacologic effect of these benzodiazepines.

The use of erythromycin in patients concurrently taking drugs metabolized by the cytochrome P450 system may be associated with elevations in serum levels of these other drugs. There have been reports of interactions of erythromycin with carbamazepine, cyclosporine, tacrolimus, hexobarbital, phenytoin, alfentanil, cisapride, disopyramide, lovastatin, bromocriptine, valproate, terfenadine, and astemizole. Serum concentrations of drugs metabolized by the cytochrome P450 system should be monitored closely in patients concurrently receiving erythromycin.

Erythromycin has been reported to significantly alter the metabolism of the nonsedating antihistamines terfenadine and astemizole when taken concomitantly. Rare cases of serious cardiovascular adverse events, including electrocardiographic QT/QT$_c$ interval prolongation, cardiac arrest, torsades de pointes, and other ventricular arrhythmias have been observed. (See **CONTRAINDICATIONS**.) In addition, deaths have been reported rarely with concomitant administration of terfenadine and erythromycin.

There have been post-marketing reports of drug interactions when erythromycin is coadministered with cisapride, resulting in QT prolongation, cardiac arrhythmias, ventricular tachycardia, ventricular fibrillation, and torsades de pointes, most likely due to inhibition of hepatic metabolism of cisapride by erythromycin. Fatalities have been reported. (See **CONTRAINDICATIONS**.)

Drug/Laboratory Test Interactions: Erythromycin interferes with the fluorometric determination of urinary catecholamines.

Carcinogenesis, Mutagenesis, Impairment of Fertility: Long-term (2-year) oral studies in rats with erythromycin ethylsuccinate and erythromycin base did not provide evidence of tumorigenicity. Mutagenicity studies have not been conducted. There was no apparent effect on male or female fertility in rats fed erythromycin (base) at levels up to 0.25% of diet.

Pregnancy: Teratogenic Effects. Pregnancy Category B: There is no evidence of teratogenicity or any other adverse effect on reproduction in female rats fed erythromycin base (up to 0.25% of diet) prior to and during mating, during gestation, and through weaning of two successive litters. There are, however, no adequate and well-controlled studies in pregnant women. Because animal reproduction studies are not always predictive of human response, this drug should be used during pregnancy only if clearly needed.

Labor and Delivery: The effect of erythromycin on labor and delivery is unknown.

Nursing Mothers: Erythromycin is excreted in human milk. Caution should be exercised when erythromycin is administered to a nursing woman.

Pediatric Use: See **INDICATIONS AND USAGE** and **DOSAGE AND ADMINISTRATION** sections.

ADVERSE REACTIONS

The most frequent side effects of oral erythromycin preparations are gastrointestinal and are dose-related. They include nausea, vomiting, abdominal pain, diarrhea and ano-rexia. Symptoms of hepatitis, hepatic dysfunction and/or abnormal liver function test results may occur. (See **WARNINGS**.)

Onset of pseudomembranous colitis symptoms may occur during or after antibiotic treatment. (See **WARNINGS**.)

Rarely, erythromycin has been associated with the production of ventricular arrhythmias, including ventricular tachycardia and torsades de pointes, in individuals with prolonged QT intervals.

Allergic reactions ranging from urticaria to anaphylaxis have occurred. Skin reactions ranging from mild eruptions to erythema multiforme, Stevens-Johnson syndrome, and toxic epidermal necrolysis have been reported rarely.

There have been isolated reports of reversible hearing loss occurring chiefly in patients with renal insufficiency and in patients receiving high doses of erythromycin.

OVERDOSAGE

In case of overdosage, erythromycin should be discontinued. Overdosage should be handled with the prompt elimination of unabsorbed drug and all other appropriate measures should be instituted.

Erythromycin is not removed by peritoneal dialysis or hemodialysis.

DOSAGE AND ADMINISTRATION

Erythromycin ethylsuccinate suspensions and Filmtab tablets may be administered without regard to meals.

Children: Age, weight, and severity of the infection are important factors in determining the proper dosage. In mild to moderate infections the usual dosage of erythromycin ethylsuccinate for children is 30 to 50 mg/kg/day in equally divided doses every 6 hours. For more severe infections this dosage may be doubled. If twice-a-day dosage is desired, one-half of the total daily dose may be given every 12 hours. Doses may also be given three times daily by administering one-third of the total daily dose every 8 hours.

The following dosage schedule is suggested for mild to moderate infections:

Body Weight	Total Daily Dose
Under 10 lbs	30–50 mg/kg/day 15–25 mg/kg/q 12 h
10 to 15 lbs	200 mg
16 to 25 lbs	400 mg
26 to 50 lbs	800 mg
51 to 100 lbs	1200 mg
over 100 lbs	1600 mg

Adults: 400 mg erythromycin ethylsuccinate every 6 hours is the usual dose. Dosage may be increased up to 4 g per day according to the severity of the infection. If twice-a-day dosage is desired, one-half of the total daily dose may be given every 12 hours. Doses may also be given three times daily by administering one-third of the total daily dose every 8 hours.

For adult dosage calculation, use a ratio of 400 mg of erythromycin activity as the ethylsuccinate to 250 mg of erythromycin activity as the stearate, base or estolate.

In the treatment of streptococcal infections, a therapeutic dosage of erythromycin ethylsuccinate should be administered for at least 10 days. In continuous prophylaxis against recurrences of streptococcal infections in persons with a history of rheumatic heart disease, the usual dosage is 400 mg twice a day.

For prophylaxis against bacterial endocarditis in patients with congenital heart disease, or rheumatic or other acquired valvular heart disease when undergoing dental procedures or surgical procedures of the upper respiratory tract, give 800 mg (10 mg/kg for children) orally 2 hours prior to the procedure and then 400 mg (5 mg/kg for children) six hours after the initial dose.

For treatment of urethritis due to *C. trachomatis* or *U. urealyticum*: 800 mg three times a day for 7 days.

For treatment of primary syphilis: Adults: 48 to 64 g given in divided doses over a period of 10 to 15 days.

For intestinal amebiasis: Adults: 400 mg four times daily for 10 to 14 days. Children: 30 to 50 mg/kg/day in divided doses for 10 to 14 days.

For use in pertussis: Although optimal dosage and duration have not been established, doses of erythromycin utilized in reported clinical studies were 40 to 50 mg/kg/day, given in divided doses for 5 to 14 days.

For treatment of Legionnaires' Disease: Although optimal doses have not been established, doses utilized in reported clinical data were those recommended above (1.6 to 4 g daily in divided doses).

Continued on next page

E.E.S.—Cont.

HOW SUPPLIED

E.E.S. 200 LIQUID (erythromycin ethylsuccinate oral suspension, USP) is supplied in 1 pint bottles (**NDC** 0074-6306-16) and in packages of six l00-mL bottles (**NDC** 0074-6306-13).

E.E.S. 400® LIQUID (erythromycin ethylsuccinate oral suspension, USP) is supplied in 1 pint bottles (**NDC** 0074-6373-16) and in packages of six l00-mL bottles (**NDC** 0074-6373-13).

Both liquid products require refrigeration to preserve taste until dispensed. Refrigeration by patient is not required if used within 14 days.

E.E.S. GRANULES (erythromycin ethylsuccinate for oral suspension, USP) is supplied in l00-mL (**NDC** 0074-6369-02) and 200-mL (**NDC** 0074-6369-10) size bottles.

E.E.S. 400 Filmtab tablets (erythromycin ethylsuccinate tablets, USP) 400 mg, are supplied as pink tablets imprinted with the Abbott logo, , and two letter Abbo-Code designation, EE, in bottles of 100 (**NDC** 0074-5729-13), 500 (**NDC** 0074-5729-53) and 1000 (**NDC** 0074-5729-19) and in ABBO-PAC unit dose strip packages of 100 (**NDC** 0074-5729-11).

Recommended storage: Store tablets below 86°F (30°C). Store granules, prior to mixing, below 86°F (30°C). After mixing, refrigerate and use within 10 days.

REFERENCES

1. National Committee for Clinical Laboratory Standards, *Methods for Dilution Antimicrobial Susceptibility Tests for Bacteria that Grow Aerobically*, Third Edition. Approved Standard NCCLS Document M7-A3, Vol. 13, No. 25. NCCLS, Villanova, PA, December 1993.
2. National Committee for Clinical Laboratory Standards, *Performance Standards for Antimicrobial Disk Susceptibility Tests*, Fifth Edition. Approved Standard NCCLS Document M2-A5, Vol. 13, No. 24. NCCLS, Villanova, PA, December 1993.
3. Committee on Rheumatic Fever, Endocarditis, and Kawasaki Disease of the Council on Cardiovascular Disease in the Young, the American Heart Association: Prevention of Rheumatic Fever. *Circulation*. 78(4): 1082-1086, October 1988.
4. Dajani, Adnan., M.D., et al.: Prevention of Bacterial Endocarditis Recommendations by the American Heart Association. *JAMA*. 264(22): 2919-2922, December 1990.

Filmtab—Film-sealed tablets, Abbott.
Ref. 03-4800-R19
Revised: May, 1997
ABBOTT LABORATORIES
NORTH CHICAGO, IL 60064, U.S.A.

Shown in Product Identification Guide, page 303

ERYTHROCIN® STEARATE ℞

[*e-ry 'thrō-sin*]
(erythromycin stearate tablets, USP)
Filmtab® Tablets

DESCRIPTION

Erythromycin is produced by a strain of *Streptomyces erythraeus* and belongs to the macrolide group of antibiotics. It is basic and readily forms salts with acids. The base, the stearate salt, and the esters are poorly soluble in water, and are suitable for oral administration.

ERYTHROCIN STEARATE Filmtab tablets (erythromycin stearate tablets, USP) contain the stearate salt of the antibiotic in a unique film coating.

Inactive Ingredients: 250 mg tablet: Cellulosic polymers, corn starch, D&C Red No. 7, polacrilin potassium, polyethylene glycol, povidone, propylene glycol, sodium carboxymethylcellulose, sodium citrate, sorbic acid, sorbitan monooleate and titanium dioxide.

500 mg tablet: Cellulosic polymers, corn starch, FD&C Red No. 3, magnesium hydroxide, polacrilin potassium, povidone, propylene glycol, sorbitan monooleate, titanium dioxide and vanillin.

ACTIONS

Microbiology

Biochemical tests demonstrate that erythromycin inhibits protein synthesis of the pathogen without directly affecting nucleic acid synthesis. Antagonism has been demonstrated between clindamycin and erythromycin.

NOTE: Many strains of *Hemophilus influenzae* are resistant to erythromycin alone, but are susceptible to erythromycin and sulfonamides together. Staphylococci resistant to erythromycin may emerge during a course of erythromycin therapy. Culture and susceptibility testing should be performed.

Disc Susceptibility Tests:

Quantitative methods that require measurement of zone diameters give the most precise estimates of antibiotic susceptibility. One recommended procedure (21 CFR section 460.1) uses erythromycin class discs for testing susceptibility; interpretations correlate zone diameters of this disc test with MIC values for erythromycin. With this procedure, a report from the laboratory of "susceptible" indicates that the infecting organism is likely to respond to therapy. A report of "resistant" indicates that the infective organism is not likely to respond to therapy. A report of "intermediate susceptibility" suggests that the organism would be susceptible if higher doses were used.

Clinical Pharmacology

Erythromycin binds to the 50 S ribosomal subunits of susceptible bacteria and suppresses protein synthesis.

Orally administered ERYTHROCIN STEARATE tablets are readily and reliably absorbed. Optimal serum levels of erythromycin are reached when the drug is taken in the fasting state or immediately before meals.

Erythromycin diffuses readily into most body fluids. Only low concentrations are normally achieved in the spinal fluid, but passage of the drug across the blood-brain barrier increases in meningitis. In the presence of normal hepatic function, erythromycin is concentrated in the liver and excreted in the bile; the effect of hepatic dysfunction on excretion of erythromycin by the liver into the bile is not known. Less than 5 percent of the orally administered dose of erythromycin is excreted in active form in the urine.

Erythromycin crosses the placental barrier and is excreted in breast milk.

INDICATIONS

Streptococcus pyogenes (Group A beta hemolytic streptococcus): Upper and lower respiratory tract, skin, and soft tissue infections of mild to moderate severity.

Injectable benzathine penicillin G is considered by the American Heart Association to be the drug of choice in the treatment and prevention of streptococcal pharyngitis and in long-term prophylaxis of rheumatic fever.

When oral medication is preferred for treatment of the above conditions, penicillin G, V, or erythromycin are alternate drugs of choice.

When oral medication is given, the importance of strict adherence by the patient to the prescribed dosage regimen must be stressed. A therapeutic dose should be administered for at least 10 days.

Alpha-hemolytic streptococci (viridans group):

Although no controlled clinical efficacy trials have been conducted, oral erythromycin has been suggested by the American Heart Association and American Dental Association for use in a regimen for prophylaxis against bacterial endocarditis in patients hypersensitive to penicillin who have congenital heart disease, or rheumatic or other acquired valvular heart disease when they undergo dental procedures and surgical procedures of the upper respiratory tract.[1] Erythromycin is not suitable prior to genitourinary or gastrointestinal tract surgery. NOTE: When selecting antibiotics for the prevention of bacterial endocarditis the physician or dentist should read the full joint statement of the American Heart Association and the American Dental Association.[1]

Staphylococcus aureus: Acute infections of skin and soft tissue of mild to moderate severity. Resistant organisms may emerge during treatment.

Streptococcus pneumoniae (Diplococcus pneumoniae): Upper respiratory tract infections (e.g., otitis media, pharyngitis) and lower respiratory tract infections (e.g., pneumonia) of mild to moderate degree.

Mycoplasma pneumoniae (Eaton agent, PPLO): For respiratory infections due to this organism.

Hemophilus influenzae: For upper respiratory tract infections of mild to moderate severity when used concomitantly with adequate doses of sulfonamides. (See sulfonamide labeling for appropriate prescribing information.) The concomitant use of the sulfonamides is necessary since not all strains of *Hemophilus influenzae* are susceptible to erythromycin at the concentrations of the antibiotic achieved with usual therapeutic doses.

Chlamydia trachomatis: Erythromycin is indicated for treatment of the following infections caused by *Chlamydia trachomatis:* conjunctivitis of the newborn, pneumonia of infancy and urogenital infections during pregnancy. When tetracyclines are contraindicated or not tolerated, erythromycin is indicated for the treatment of uncomplicated urethral, endocervical, or rectal infections in adults due to *Chlamydia trachomatis.*[2]

Treponema pallidum: Erythromycin is an alternate choice of treatment for primary syphilis in patients allergic to the penicillins. In treatment of primary syphilis, spinal fluid examinations should be done before treatment and as part of follow-up after therapy.

Corynebacterium diphtheriae: As an adjunct to antitoxin, to prevent establishment of carriers, and to eradicate the organism in carriers.

Corynebacterium minutissimum: For the treatment of erythrasma.

Entamoeba histolytica: In the treatment of intestinal amebiasis only. Extra-enteric amebiasis requires treatment with other agents.

Listeria monocytogenes: Infections due to this organism.

Neisseria gonorrhoeae: Erythrocin Lactobionate-I.V. (erythromycin lactobionate for injection) in conjunction with erythromycin stearate orally, as an alternative drug in treatment of acute pelvic inflammatory disease caused by *N. gonorrhoeae* in female patients with a history of sensitivity to penicillin. Before treatment of gonorrhea, patients who are suspected of also having syphilis should have a microscopic examination for *T. pallidum* (by immunofluorescence or darkfield) before receiving erythromycin, and monthly serologic tests for a minimum of 4 months.

Bordetella pertussis: Erythromycin is effective in eliminating the organism from the nasopharynx of infected individuals, rendering them non-infectious. Some clinical studies suggest that erythromycin may be helpful in the prophylaxis of pertussis in exposed susceptible individuals.

Legionnaires' Disease: Although no controlled clinical efficacy studies have been conducted, *in vitro* and limited preliminary clinical data suggest that erythromycin may be effective in treating Legionnaires' Disease.

CONTRAINDICATIONS

Erythromycin is contraindicated in patients with known hypersensitivity to this antibiotic.

WARNINGS

There have been reports of hepatic dysfunction with or without jaundice, occurring in patients receiving oral erythromycin products.

PRECAUTIONS

General: Erythromycin is principally excreted by the liver. Caution should be exercised when erythromycin is administered to patients with impaired hepatic function. (See "Clinical Pharmacology" and "Warnings" sections.)

Prolonged or repeated use of erythromycin may result in an overgrowth of nonsusceptible bacteria or fungi. If superinfection occurs, erythromycin should be discontinued and appropriate therapy instituted.

When indicated, incision and drainage or other surgical procedures should be performed in conjunction with antibiotic therapy.

Laboratory Tests: Erythromycin interferes with the fluorometric determination of urinary catecholamines.

Drug Interactions: Erythromycin use in patients who are receiving high doses of theophylline may be associated with an increase in serum theophylline levels and potential theophylline toxicity. In case of theophylline toxicity and/or elevated serum theophylline levels, the dose of theophylline should be reduced while the patient is receiving concomitant erythromycin therapy.

Concomitant administration of erythromycin and digoxin has been reported to result in elevated digoxin serum levels.

There have been reports of increased anticoagulant effects when erythromycin and oral anticoagulants were used concomitantly.

Concurrent use of erythromycin and ergotamine or dihydroergotamine has been associated in some patients with acute ergot toxicity characterized by severe peripheral vasospasm and dysesthesia.

Erythromycin has been reported to decrease the clearance of triazolam and thus may increase the pharmacologic effect of triazolam.

The use of erythromycin in patients concurrently taking drugs metabolized by the cytochrome P450 system may be associated with elevations in serum erythromycin with carbamazepine, cyclosporine, hexobarbital and phenytoin. Serum concentrations of drugs metabolized by the cytochrome P450 system should be monitored closely in patients concurrently receiving erythromycin.

Troleandomycin significantly alters the metabolism of terfenadine when taken concomitantly; therefore, observe caution when erythromycin and terfenadine are used concurrently.

Patients receiving concomitant lovastatin and erythromycin should be carefully monitored; cases of rhabdomyolysis have been reported in seriously ill patients.

Carcinogenesis, Mutagenesis, Impairment of Fertility: Long-term (2-year) oral studies conducted in rats with erythromycin base did not provide evidence of tumorigenicity. Mutagenicity studies have not been conducted. There was no apparent effect on male or female fertility in rats fed erythromycin (base) at levels up to 0.25 percent of diet.

Pregnancy: Pregnancy Category B: There is no evidence of teratogenicity or any other adverse effect on reproduction in female rats fed erythromycin base (up to 0.25 percent of diet) prior to and during mating, during gestation, and through weaning of two successive litters. There are, however, no adequate and well-controlled studies in pregnant women. Because animal reproduction studies are not always predictive of human response, this drug should be used during pregnancy only if clearly needed. Erythromycin has been reported to cross the placental barrier in humans, but fetal plasma levels are generally low.

Labor and Delivery: The effect of erythromycin on labor and delivery is unknown.

Nursing Mothers: Erythromycin is excreted in breast milk, therefore, caution should be exercised when erythromycin is administered to a nursing woman.

Pediatric Use: See "Indications and Usage" and "Dosage and Administration" sections.

ADVERSE REACTIONS

The most frequent side effects of oral erythromycin preparations are gastrointestinal and are dose-related. They include nausea, vomiting, abdominal pain, diarrhea and anorexia. Symptoms of hepatic dysfunction and/or abnormal liver function test results may occur (see "Warnings" section). Pseudomembranous colitis has been rarely reported in association with erythromycin therapy.

There have been isolated reports of transient central nervous system side effects including confusion, hallucinations, seizures, and vertigo; however, a cause and effect relationship has not been established.

Occasional case reports of cardiac arrhythmias such as ventricular tachycardia have been documented in patients receiving erythromycin therapy. There have been isolated reports of other cardiovascular symptoms such as chest pain, dizziness, and palpitations; however, a cause and effect relationship has not been established.

Allergic reactions ranging from urticaria and mild skin eruptions to anaphylaxis have occurred.

There have been isolated reports of reversible hearing loss occurring chiefly in patients with renal insufficiency and in patients receiving high doses of erythromycin.

OVERDOSAGE

In case of overdosage, erythromycin should be discontinued. Overdosage should be handled with the prompt elimination of unabsorbed drug and all other appropriate measures.

Erythromycin is not removed by peritoneal dialysis or hemodialysis.

DOSAGE AND ADMINISTRATION

Optimal serum levels of erythromycin are reached when ERYTHROCIN STEARATE (erythromycin stearate) is taken in the fasting state or immediately before meals.

Adults: The usual dosage is 250 mg every 6 hours; or 500 mg every 12 hours, taken in the fasting state or immediately before meals. Up to 4 g per day may be administered, depending upon the severity of the infection.

Children: Age, weight, and severity of the infection are important factors in determining the proper dosage. For the treatment of mild to moderate infections, the usual dosage is 30 to 50 mg/kg/day in 3 or 4 divided doses. When dosage is desired on a twice-a-day schedule, one-half of the total daily dose may be taken every 12 hours in the fasting state or immediately before meals. For the treatment of more severe infections the total daily dose may be doubled.

In the treatment of streptococcal infections, a therapeutic dosage of erythromycin should be administered for at least 10 days. In continuous prophylaxis of streptococcal infections in persons with a history of rheumatic heart disease, the dose is 250 mg twice a day.

For prophylaxis against bacterial endocarditis[1] in patients with congenital heart disease, or rheumatic or other acquired valvular heart disease when undergoing dental procedures or surgical procedures of the upper respiratory tract, give 1 g (20 mg/kg for children) orally 1½ to 2 hours before the procedure, and then, 500 mg (10 mg/kg for children) orally every 6 hours for 8 doses.

For conjunctivitis of the newborn caused by *Chlamydia trachomatis:* Oral erythromycin suspension 50 mg/kg/day in 4 divided doses for at least 2 weeks.[2]

For pneumonia of infancy caused by *Chlamydia trachomatis.* Although the optimal duration of therapy has not been established, the recommended therapy is oral erythromycin suspension 50 mg/kg/day in 4 divided doses for at least 3 weeks.[2]

For urogenital infections during pregnancy due to *Chlamydia trachomatis:* Although the optimal dose and duration of therapy have not been established, the suggested treatment is erythromycin 500 mg, by mouth, 4 times a day on an empty stomach for at least 7 days. For women who cannot tolerate this regimen, a decreased dose of 250 mg, by mouth, 4 times a day should be used for at least 14 days.[2]

For adults with uncomplicated urethral, endocervical, or rectal infections caused by *Chlamydia trachomatis* in whom tetracyclines are contraindicated or not tolerated: 500 mg, by mouth, 4 times a day for at least 7 days.[2]

For treatment of primary syphilis: 30 to 40 g given in divided doses over a period of 10 to 15 days.

For treatment of acute pelvic inflammatory disease caused by *N. gonorrhoeae:* 500 mg Erythrocin Lactobionate-I.V. (erythromycin lactobionate for injection) every 6 hours for 3 days, followed by 250 mg ERYTHROCIN STEARATE every 6 hours for 7 days.

For intestinal amebiasis: Adults: 250 mg four times daily for 10 to 14 days. Children: 30 to 50 mg/kg/day in divided doses for 10 to 14 days.

For use in pertussis: Although optimal dosage and duration have not been established, doses of erythromycin utilized in reported clinical studies were 40 to 50 mg/kg/day, given in divided doses for 5 to 14 days.

For treatment of Legionnaires' Disease: Although optimal doses have not been established, doses utilized in reported clinical data were 1 to 4 g daily in divided doses.

HOW SUPPLIED

ERYTHROCIN STEARATE Filmtab Tablets (erythromycin stearate tablets, USP) are supplied as:

ERYTHROCIN STEARATE Filmtab, 250 mg
Bottles of 100 .... (**NDC** 0074-6346-20)
Bottles of 500 .... (**NDC** 0074-6346-53)
Bottles of 1000 .... (**NDC** 0074-6346-19)
ABBO-PAC® unit dose strip packages of
100 tablets .... (**NDC** 0074-6346-38)

ERYTHROCIN STEARATE Filmtab, 500 mg
Bottles of 100 .... (**NDC** 0074-6316-13)
Recommended storage: Store below 86°F (30°C).

REFERENCES

1. American Heart Association. 1977. Prevention of bacterial endocarditis. Circulation 56: 139A-143A.
2. CDC Sexually Transmitted Diseases Treatment Guidelines 1982.

FILMTAB—Film-sealed tablets, Abbott
Ref. 01-2538-R13

Shown in Product Identification Guide, page 303

ERYTHROMYCIN Base Filmtab®   ℞
[*e-ri-thrō-mī 'sin*]
(erythromycin tablets, USP)

DESCRIPTION

Erythromycin is produced by a strain of *Streptomyces erythraeus* and belongs to the macrolide group of antibiotics. It is basic and readily forms salts with acids. The base, the stearate salt, and the esters are poorly soluble in water, and are suitable for oral administration.

ERYTHROMYCIN Base Filmtab tablets contain erythromycin, USP, in a unique, nonenteric film coating.

Inactive Ingredients: 250 mg tablet: Cellulosic polymers, corn starch, D&C Red No. 30, iron oxide, magnesium hydroxide, magnesium stearate, polyethylene glycol, propylene glycol, sodium starch glycolate, sorbic acid, sorbitan monooleate and titanium dioxide.

500 mg tablet: Cellulosic polymers, corn starch, D&C Red No. 30, magnesium hydroxide, magnesium stearate, microcrystalline cellulose, polyethylene glycol, propylene glycol, sodium starch glycolate, sorbic acid, sorbitan monooleate and titanium dioxide.

ACTIONS

Microbiology: Biochemical tests demonstrate that erythromycin inhibits protein synthesis of the pathogen without directly affecting nucleic acid synthesis. Antagonism has been demonstrated between clindamycin and erythromycin.

NOTE: Many strains of *Hemophilus influenzae* are resistant to erythromycin alone, but are susceptible to erythromycin and sulfonamides together. Staphylococci resistant to erythromycin may emerge during a course of erythromycin therapy. Culture and susceptibility testing should be performed.

Disc Susceptibility Tests: Quantitative methods that require measurement of zone diameters give the most precise estimates of antibiotic susceptibility. One recommended procedure (21 CFR section 460.1) uses erythromycin class discs for testing susceptibility; interpretations correlate zone diameters of this disc test with MIC values for erythromycin. With this procedure, a report from the laboratory of "susceptible" indicates that the infecting organism is likely to respond to therapy. A report of "resistant" indicates that the infective organism is not likely to respond to therapy. A report of "intermediate susceptibility" suggests that the organism would be susceptible if higher doses were used.

Clinical Pharmacology: Erythromycin binds to the 50 S ribosomal subunits of susceptible bacteria and suppresses protein synthesis.

Orally administered erythromycin is readily absorbed by most patients, especially on an empty stomach, but patient variation is observed. Due to its formulation and nonenteric coating, this erythromycin tablet gives reliable blood levels in the average subject; however, the levels may vary with the individual.

Erythromycin diffuses readily into most body fluids. Only low concentrations are normally achieved in the spinal fluid, but passage of the drug across the blood-brain barrier increases in meningitis. In the presence of normal hepatic function, erythromycin is concentrated in the liver and excreted in the bile; the effect of hepatic dysfunction on excretion of erythromycin by the liver into the bile is not known. Less than 5 percent of the orally administered dose of erythromycin is excreted in active form in the urine.

Erythromycin crosses the placental barrier and is excreted in breast milk.

INDICATIONS

Streptococcus pyogenes (Group A beta-hemolytic streptococcus): Upper and lower respiratory tract, skin, and soft tissue infections of mild to moderate severity.

Injectable benzathine penicillin G is considered by the American Heart Association to be the drug of choice in the treatment and prevention of streptococcal pharyngitis and in long-term prophylaxis of rheumatic fever.

When oral medication is preferred for treatment of the above conditions, penicillin G, V, or erythromycin are alternate drugs of choice.

When oral medication is given, the importance of strict adherence by the patient to the prescribed dosage regimen must be stressed. A therapeutic dose should be administered for at least 10 days.

Alpha-hemolytic streptococci (viridans group): Although no controlled clinical efficacy trials have been conducted, oral erythromycin has been suggested by the American Heart Association and American Dental Association for use in a regimen for prophylaxis against bacterial endocarditis in patients hypersensitive to penicillin who have congenital heart disease, or rheumatic or other acquired valvular heart disease when they undergo dental procedures and surgical procedures of the upper respiratory tract.[1] Erythromycin is not suitable prior to genitourinary or gastrointestinal tract surgery. NOTE: When selecting antibiotics for the prevention of bacterial endocarditis the physician or dentist should read the full joint statement of the American Heart Association and the American Dental Association.[1]

Staphylococcus aureus: Acute infections of skin and soft tissue of mild to moderate severity. Resistant organisms may emerge during treatment.

Streptococcus pneumoniae (Diplococcus pneumoniae): Upper respiratory tract infections (e.g., otitis media, pharyngitis) and lower respiratory tract infections (e.g., pneumonia) of mild to moderate degree.

Mycoplasma pneumoniae (Eaton agent, PPLO): For respiratory infections due to this organism.

Hemophilus influenzae: For upper respiratory tract infections of mild to moderate severity when used concomitantly with adequate doses of sulfonamides. (See sulfonamide labeling for appropriate prescribing information). The concomitant use of the sulfonamides is necessary since not all strains of *Hemophilus influenzae* are susceptible to erythromycin at the concentrations of the antibiotic achieved with usual therapeutic doses.

Chlamydia trachomatis: Erythromycin is indicated for treatment of the following infections caused by *Chlamydia trachomatis:* conjunctivitis of the newborn, pneumonia of infancy and urogenital infections during pregnancy. When tetracyclines are contraindicated or not tolerated, erythromycin is indicated for the treatment of uncomplicated urethral, endocervical, or rectal infections in adults due to *Chlamydia trachomatis.*[2]

Treponema pallidum: Erythromycin is an alternate choice of treatment for primary syphilis in patients allergic to the penicillins. In treatment of primary syphilis, spinal fluid examinations should be done before treatment and as part of follow-up after therapy.

Corynebacterium diphtheriae: As an adjunct to antitoxin, to prevent establishment of carriers, and to eradicate the organism in carriers.

Corynebacterium minutissimum: For the treatment of erythrasma.

Entamoeba histolytica: In the treatment of intestinal amebiasis only. Extra-enteric amebiasis requires treatment with other agents.

Listeria monocytogenes: Infections due to this organism.

Neisseria gonorrhoeae: Erythrocin® Lactobionate-I.V. (erythromycin lactobionate for injection) in conjunction with erythromycin base orally, as an alternative drug in treatment of acute pelvic inflammatory disease caused by *N. gonorrhoeae* in female patients with a history of sensitivity to penicillin. Before treatment of gonorrhea, patients who are suspected of also having syphilis should have a microscopic examination for *T. pallidum* (by immunofluorescence or darkfield) before receiving erythromycin, and monthly serologic tests for a minimum of 4 months.

Bordetella pertussis: Erythromycin is effective in eliminating the organism from the nasopharynx of infected individuals, rendering them non-infectious. Some clinical studies suggest that erythromycin may be helpful in the prophylaxis of pertussis in exposed susceptible individuals.

Legionnaires' Disease: Although no controlled clinical efficacy studies have been conducted, *in vitro* and limited preliminary clinical data suggest that erythromycin may be effective in treating Legionnaires' Disease.

CONTRAINDICATIONS

Erythromycin is contraindicated in patients with known hypersensitivity to this antibiotic.

Continued on next page

Erythromycin Base Filmtab—Cont.

WARNINGS

There have been reports of hepatic dysfunction with or without jaundice, occurring in patients receiving oral erythromycin products.

PRECAUTIONS

General: Erythromycin is principally excreted by the liver. Caution should be exercised when erythromycin is administered to patients with impaired hepatic function. (See "Clinical Pharmacology" and "Warnings" sections).

Prolonged or repeated use of erythromycin may result in an overgrowth of nonsusceptible bacteria or fungi. If superinfection occurs, erythromycin should be discontinued and appropriate therapy instituted.

When indicated, incision and drainage or other surgical procedures should be performed in conjunction with antibiotic therapy.

Laboratory Tests: Erythromycin interferes with the fluorometric determination of urinary catecholamines.

Drug Interactions: Erythromycin use in patients who are receiving high doses of theophylline may be associated with an increase in serum theophylline levels and potential theophylline toxicity. In case of theophylline toxicity and/or elevated serum theophylline levels, the dose of theophylline should be reduced while the patient is receiving concomitant erythromycin therapy.

Concomitant administration of erythromycin and digoxin has been reported to result in elevated digoxin serum levels.

There have been reports of increased anticoagulant effects when erythromycin and oral anticoagulants were used concomitantly.

Concurrent use of erythromycin and ergotamine or dihydroergotamine has been associated in some patients with acute ergot toxicity characterized by severe peripheral vasospasm and dysethesia.

Erythromycin has been reported to decrease the clearance of triazolam and thus may increase the pharmacologic effect of triazolam.

The use of erythromycin in patients concurrently taking drugs metabolized by the cytochrome P450 system may be associated with elevations in serum erythromycin with carbamazepine, cyclosporine, hexobarbital and phenytoin. Serum concentrations of drugs metabolized by the cytochrome P450 system should be monitored closely in patients concurrently receiving erythromycin.

Troleandomycin significantly alters the metabolism of terfenadine when taken concomitantly; therefore, observe caution when erythromycin and terfenadine are used concurrently.

Patients receiving concomitant lovastatin and erythromycin should be carefully monitored; cases of rhabdomyolysis have been reported in seriously ill patients.

Carcinogenesis, Mutagenesis, Impairment of Fertility: Long-term (2-year) oral studies conducted in rats with erythromycin base did not provide evidence of tumorigenicity. Mutagenicity studies have not been conducted. There was no apparent effect on male or female fertility in rats fed erythromycin (base) at levels up to 0.25 percent of diet.

Pregnancy: Pregnancy Category B: There is no evidence of teratogenicity or any other adverse effect on reproduction in female rats fed erythromycin base (up to 0.25 percent of diet) prior to and during mating, during gestation, and through weaning of two successive litters. There are, however, no adequate and well-controlled studies in pregnant women. Because animal reproduction studies are not always predictive of human response, this drug should be used during pregnancy only if clearly needed. Erythromycin has been reported to cross the placental barrier in humans, but fetal plasma levels are generally low.

Labor and Delivery: The effect of erythromycin on labor and delivery is unknown.

Nursing Mothers: Erythromycin is excreted in breast milk, therefore, caution should be exercised when erythromycin is administered to a nursing woman.

Pediatric Use: See "Indications and Usage" and "Dosage and Administration" sections.

ADVERSE REACTIONS

The most frequent side effects of oral erythromycin preparations are gastrointestinal and are dose-related. They include nausea, vomiting, abdominal pain, diarrhea and anorexia. Symptoms of hepatic dysfunction and/or abnormal liver function test results may occur (see "Warnings" section). Pseudomembranous colitis has been rarely reported in association with erythromycin therapy.

There have been isolated reports of transient central nervous system side effects including confusion, hallucinations, seizures, and vertigo; however, a cause and effect relationship has not been established.

Occasional case reports of cardiac arrhythmias such as ventricular tachycardia have been documented in patients receiving erythromycin therapy. There have been isolated reports of other cardiovascular symptoms such as chest pain, dizziness, and palpitations; however a cause and effect relationship has not been established.

Allergic reactions ranging from urticaria and mild skin eruptions to anaphylaxis have occurred.

There have been isolated reports of reversible hearing loss occurring chiefly in patients with renal insufficiency and in patients receiving high doses of erythromycin.

OVERDOSAGE

In case of overdosage, erythromycin should be discontinued. Overdosage should be handled with the prompt elimination of unabsorbed drug and all other appropriate measures.

Erythromycin is not removed by peritoneal dialysis or hemodialysis.

DOSAGE AND ADMINISTRATION

Optimum blood levels are obtained when doses are given on an empty stomach.

Adults: 250 mg every 6 hours is the usual dose; or 500 mg every 12 hours one hour before meals. Dosage may be increased up to 4 g per day according to the severity of the infection.

Children: Age, weight, and severity of the infection are important factors in determining the proper dosage. 30 to 50 mg/kg/day, in divided doses, is the usual dose. For more severe infections this dose may be doubled. If dosage is desired on a twice-a-day schedule, one-half of the total daily dose may be given every 12 hours, one hour before meals.

For treatment of streptococcal infections: a therapeutic dosage should be administered for at least 10 days. In continuous prophylaxis of streptococcal infections in persons with rheumatic heart disease history, the dose is 250 mg twice a day.

For prophylaxis against bacterial endocarditis[1] in patients with congenital heart disease, or rheumatic or other acquired valvular heart disease when undergoing dental procedures or surgical procedures of the upper respiratory tract, give 1 g (20 mg/kg for children) orally $1^1/_2$ to 2 hours before the procedure, and then, 500 mg (10 mg/kg for children) orally every 6 hours for 8 doses.

For conjunctivitis of the newborn caused by *Chlamydia trachomatis:* Oral erythromycin suspension 50 mg/kg/day in 4 divided doses for at least 2 weeks.[2]

For pneumonia of infancy caused by *Chlamydia trachomatis:* Although the optimal duration of therapy has not been established, the recommended therapy is oral erythromycin suspension 50 mg/kg/day in 4 divided doses for at least 3 weeks.[2]

For urogenital infections during pregnancy due to *Chlamydia trachomatis:* Although the optimal dose and duration of therapy have not been established, the suggested treatment is erythromycin 500 mg, by mouth, 4 times a day on an empty stomach for at least 7 days. For women who cannot tolerate this regimen, a decreased dose of 250 mg, by mouth, 4 times a day should be used for at least 14 days.[2]

For adults with uncomplicated urethral, endocervical, or rectal infections caused by *Chlamydia trachomatis* in whom tetracyclines are contraindicated or not tolerated: 500 mg, by mouth, 4 times a day for at least 7 days.[2]

For treatment of primary syphilis: 30 to 40 g given in divided doses over a period of 10 to 15 days.

For treatment of acute pelvic inflammatory disease caused by *N. gonorrhoeae:* 500 mg Erythrocin® Lactobionate-I.V. (erythromycin lactobionate for injection) every 6 hours for 3 days, followed by 250 mg erythromycin base every 6 hours for 7 days.

For intestinal amebiasis: Adults: 250 mg four times daily for 10 to 14 days. Children: 30 to 50 mg/kg/day in divided doses for 10 to 14 days.

For use in pertussis: Although optimal dosage and duration have not been established, doses of erythromycin utilized in reported clinical studies were 40 to 50 mg/kg/day, given in divided doses for 5 to 14 days.

For treatment of Legionnaires' Disease: Although optimal doses have not been established, doses utilized in reported clinical data were 1 to 4 g daily in divided doses.

HOW SUPPLIED

ERYTHROMYCIN Base Filmtab tablets (erythromycin tablets, USP) are supplied as pink, capsule-shaped tablets in two dosage strengths:

250 mg tablets:
Bottles of 100 .... (**NDC** 0074-6326-13);
Bottles of 500 .... (**NDC** 0074-6326-53);
ABBO-PAC® unit dose strip packages of
100 tablets .... (**NDC** 0074-6326-11).
500 mg tablets:
Bottles of 100 .... (**NDC** 0074-6227-13).
Recommended storage: Store below 86°F (30°C).

REFERENCES

1. American Heart Association. 1977. Prevention of bacterial endocarditis. Circulation. 56: 139A-143A.
2. CDC Sexually Transmitted Diseases Treatment Guidelines 1982.

FILMTAB—Film-sealed tablets, Abbott.

Revised: October, 1991
Ref. 01-2541-R3

ERYTHROMYCIN DELAYED-RELEASE CAPSULES, USP ℞

DESCRIPTION

Erythromycin Delayed-release Capsules contain enteric-coated pellets of erythromycin base for oral administration. Erythromycin is produced by a strain of *Streptomyces erythraeus* and belongs to the macrolide group of antibiotics. It is basic and readily forms salts with acids, but it is the base which is microbiologically active. Each Erythromycin Delayed-release Capsule contains 250 milligrams of erythromycin base.

Inactive Ingredients: Cellulosic polymers, citrate ester, D&C Red No. 30, D&C Yellow No. 10, magnesium stearate and povidone. The capsule shell contains FD&C Blue No. 1, FD&C Red No. 3, gelatin, and titanium dioxide.

Erythromycin base is (3R*, 4S*, 5S*, 6R*, 7R*, 9R*, 11R*, 12R*, 13S*, 14R*)-4-[(2,6-Dideoxy-3-C-methyl-3-0-methyl-α-L-*ribo*-hexopyranosyl)oxy]-14-ethyl-7,12,13-trihydroxy-3,5,7,9,11,13-hexamethyl-6-[[3,4,6-trideoxy-3-(dimethylamino)-β-D-*xylo*-hexopyranosyl]oxy]oxacyclotetradecane-2,10-dione. The structural formula is:

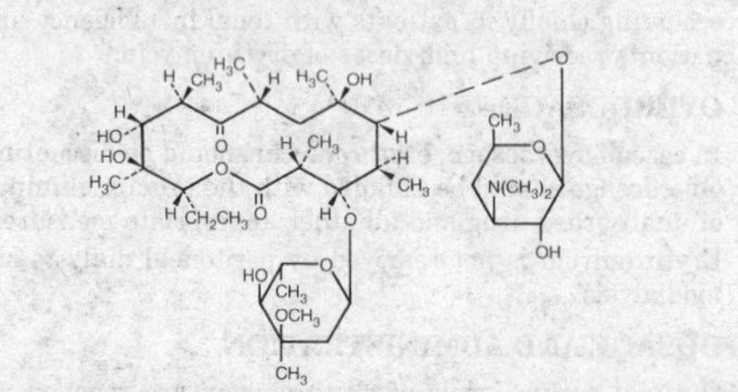

$C_{37}H_{67}NO_{13}$ MW 734

CLINICAL PHARMACOLOGY

Orally administered erythromycin base and its salts are readily absorbed in the microbiologically active form. Interindividual variations in the absorption of erythromycin are, however, observed, and some patients do not achieve acceptable serum levels. Erythromycin is largely bound to plasma proteins, and the freely dissociating bound fraction after administration of erythromycin base represents 90% of the total erythromycin absorbed. After absorption, erythromycin diffuses readily into most body fluids. In the absence of meningeal inflammation, low concentrations are normally achieved in the spinal fluid, but the passage of the drug across the blood-brain barrier increases in meningitis.

Erythromycin is excreted in breast milk. The drug crosses the placental barrier but plasma levels are low.

In the presence of normal hepatic function, erythromycin is concentrated in the liver and is excreted in the bile; the effect of hepatic dysfunction on biliary excretion of erythromycin is not known. After oral administration, less than 5% of the administered dose can be recovered in the active form in the urine.

The enteric coating of pellets in Erythromycin Delayed-release Capsules protects the erythromycin base from inactivation by gastric acidity. Because of their small size and enteric coating, the pellets readily pass intact from the stomach to the small intestine and dissolve efficiently to allow absorption of erythromycin in a uniform manner. After administration of a single dose of a 250 mg Erythromycin Delayed-release Capsule, peak serum levels in the range of 1.13 to 1.68 mcg/mL are attained in approximately 3 hours and decline to 0.30-0.42 mcg/mL in 6 hours. Optimal conditions for stability in the presence of gastric secretion and for complete absorption are attained when Erythromycin Delayed-release Capsules are taken on an empty stomach.

Microbiology:

Erythromycin acts by inhibition of protein synthesis by binding 50 S ribosomal subunits of susceptible organisms. It does not affect nucleic acid synthesis. Antagonism has been demonstrated between clindamycin and erythromycin. Resistance to erythromycin of many strains of *Haemophilus influenzae* and some strains of staphylococci has been demonstrated. Specimens should be obtained for culture and susceptibility testing.

Erythromycin is usually active against the following organisms *in vitro* and in clinical infections:

Streptococcus pyogenes
Alpha-hemolytic streptococci (viridans group)
Staphylococcus aureus (Resistant organisms may emerge during treatment.)
Streptococcus pneumoniae
Mycoplasma pneumoniae (Eaton's Agent)
Haemophilus influenzae (Many strains are resistant to erythromycin alone, but are susceptible to erythromycin and sulfonamides together.)

Treponema pallidum
Corynebacterium diphtheriae
Corynebacterium minutissimum
Entamoeba histolytica
Listeria monocytogenes
Neisseria gonorrhoeae
Bordetella pertussis
Legionella pneumophila (agent of Legionnaires' disease)

Susceptibility Testing

Quantitative methods that require measurement of zone diameters give the most precise estimates of antibiotic susceptibility. One such standardized single-disc procedure has been recommended for use with discs to test susceptibility to erythromycin.[1] Interpretation involves correlation of the zone diameters obtained in the disc test with minimal inhibitory concentration (MIC) values for erythromycin.

Reports from the laboratory giving results of the standardized single-disc susceptibility test using a 15 mcg erythromycin disc should be interpreted according to the following criteria:

Susceptible organisms produce zones of 18 mm or greater, indicating that the tested organism is likely to respond to therapy.

Resistant organisms produce zones of 13 mm or less, indicating that other therapy should be selected.

Organisms of intermediate susceptibility produce zones of 14 to 17 mm. The "intermediate" category provides a "buffer zone" which should prevent small, uncontrolled technical factors from causing major discrepancies in interpretations; thus, when a zone diameter falls within the "intermediate" range, the results may be considered equivocal. If alternative drugs are not available, confirmation by dilution tests may be indicated.

A bacterial isolate may be considered susceptible if the MIC value[2] (minimal inhibitory concentration) for erythromycin is not more than 2 mcg/mL. Organisms are considered resistant if the MIC is 8 mcg/mL or higher.

INDICATIONS AND USAGE

Erythromycin Delayed-release Capsules are indicated in adults and children for treatment of the following conditions:

Upper respiratory tract infections of mild to moderate degree caused by *Streptococcus pyogenes* (Group A beta-hemolytic streptococci); *Streptococcus pneumoniae (Diplococcus pneumoniae); Haemophilus influenzae* (when used concomitantly with adequate doses of sulfonamides, since many strains of *H. influenzae* are not susceptible to the erythromycin concentrations ordinarily achieved). (See appropriate sulfonamide labeling for prescribing information.)

Lower respiratory tract infections of mild to moderate severity caused by *Streptococcus pyogenes* (Group A beta-hemolytic streptococci); *Streptococcus pneumoniae (Diplococcus pneumoniae).*

Respiratory tract infections due to *Mycoplasma pneumoniae* (Eaton's agent).

Pertussis (whooping cough) caused by *Bordetella pertussis.* Erythromycin is effective in eliminating the organism from the nasopharynx of infected individuals, rendering them noninfectious. Some clinical studies suggest that erythromycin may be helpful in the prophylaxis of pertussis in exposed susceptible individuals.

Diphtheria—As an adjunct to antitoxin in infections due to *Corynebacterium diphtheriae,* to prevent establishment of carriers and to eradicate the organism in carriers.

Erythrasma—In the treatment of infections due to *Corynebacterium minutissimum.*

Intestinal amebiasis caused by *Entamoeba histolytica* (oral erythromycins only). Extraenteric amebiasis requires treatment with other agents.

Infections due to *Listeria monocytogenes.*

Skin and soft tissue infections of mild to moderate severity caused by *Streptococcus pyogenes* and *Staphylococcus aureus* (resistant staphylococci may emerge during treatment).

Primary syphilis caused by *Treponema pallidum.* Erythromycin (oral forms only) is an alternate choice of treatment for primary syphilis in patients allergic to the penicillins. In treatment of primary syphilis, spinal fluid should be examined before treatment and as part of the follow-up after therapy. The use of erythromycin for the treatment of *in utero* syphilis is not recommended. (See "CLINICAL PHARMACOLOGY" section.)

Erythromycins are indicated for treatment of the following infections caused by *Chlamydia trachomatis:* conjunctivitis of the newborn, pneumonia of infancy, and urogenital infections during pregnancy. When tetracyclines are contraindicated or not tolerated, erythromycin is indicated for the treatment of uncomplicated urethral, endocervical, or rectal infections in adults due to *Chlamydia trachomatis.*[3]

Legionnaires' Disease caused by *Legionella pneumophila.* Although no controlled clinical efficacy studies have been conducted, *in vitro* and limited preliminary clinical data suggest that erythromycin may be effective in treating Legionnaires' Disease.

Therapy with erythromycin should be monitored by bacteriological studies and by clinical response. (See "CLINICAL PHARMACOLOGY—Microbiology" section.)

Injectable benzathine penicillin G is considered by the American Heart Association to be the drug of choice in the treatment and prevention of streptococcal pharyngitis and in long-term prophylaxis of rheumatic fever. When oral medication is preferred for treatment of the above conditions, penicillin G, V or erythromycin are alternate drugs of choice.

Although no controlled clinical efficacy trials have been conducted, erythromycin has been suggested by the American Heart Association and the American Dental Association for use in a regimen for prophylaxis against bacterial endocarditis in patients allergic to penicillin who have congenital and/or rheumatic or other acquired valvular heart disease when they undergo dental procedures and surgical procedures of the upper respiratory tract.[3] (Erythromycin is not suitable prior to genitourinary surgery where the organisms likely to lead to bacteremia are gram-negative bacilli or the enterococcal group of streptococci.)

NOTE: When selecting antibiotics for the prevention of bacterial endocarditis the physician or dentist should read the full joint 1984 statement of the American Heart Association and the American Dental Association.[3]

CONTRAINDICATION

Erythromycin is contraindicated in patients with known hypersensitivity to this antibiotic.

WARNINGS

There have been a few reports of hepatic dysfunction, with or without jaundice, occurring in patients receiving oral erythromycin products.

PRECAUTIONS

General: Erythromycin is principally excreted by the liver. Caution should be exercised when erythromycin is administered to patients with impaired hepatic function. (See "Clinical Pharmacology" and "Warnings" sections).

Prolonged or repeated use of erythromycin may result in an overgrowth of nonsusceptible bacteria or fungi. If superinfection occurs, erythromycin should be discontinued and appropriate therapy instituted.

When indicated, incision and drainage or other surgical procedures should be performed in conjunction with antibiotic therapy.

Laboratory Tests: Erythromycin interferes with the fluorometric determination of urinary catecholamines.

Drug Interactions: Erythromycin use in patients who are receiving high doses of theophylline may be associated with an increase in serum theophylline levels and potential theophylline toxicity. In case of theophylline toxicity and/or elevated serum theophylline levels, the dose of theophylline should be reduced while the patient is receiving concomitant erythromycin therapy.

Concomitant administration of erythromycin and digoxin has been reported to result in elevated digoxin serum levels.

There have been reports of increased anticoagulant effects when erythromycin and oral anticoagulants were used concomitantly.

Concurrent use of erythromycin and ergotamine or dihydroergotamine has been associated in some patients with acute ergot toxicity characterized by severe peripheral vasospasm and dysesthesia.

Erythromycin has been reported to decrease the clearance of triazolam and thus may increase the pharmacologic effect of triazolam.

The use of erythromycin in patients concurrently taking drugs metabolized by the cytochrome P450 system may be associated with elevations in serum erythromycin with carbamazepine, cyclosporine, hexobarbital and phenytoin. Serum concentrations of drugs metabolized by the cytochrome P450 system should be monitored closely in patients concurrently receiving erythromycin.

Troleandomycin significantly alters the metabolism of terfenadine when taken concomitantly; therefore, observe caution when erythromycin and terfenadine are used concurrently.

Patients receiving concomitant lovastatin and erythromycin should be carefully monitored; cases of rhabdomyolysis have been reported in seriously ill patients.

Carcinogenesis, Mutagenesis, Impairment of Fertility: Long-term (2-year) oral studies conducted in rats with erythromycin base did not provide evidence of tumorigenicity. Mutagenicity studies have not been conducted. There was no apparent effect on male or female fertility in rats fed erythromycin (base) at levels up to 0.25 percent of diet.

Pregnancy: Pregnancy Category B: There is no evidence of teratogenicity or any other adverse effect on reproduction in female rats fed erythromycin base (up to 0.25 percent of diet) prior to and during mating, during gestation, and through weaning of two successive litters. There are, however, no adequate and well-controlled studies in pregnant women. Because animal reproduction studies are not always predictive of human response, this drug should be used during pregnancy only if clearly needed. Erythromycin has been reported to cross the placental barrier in humans, but fetal plasma levels are generally low.

Labor and Delivery: The effect of erythromycin on labor and delivery is unknown.

Nursing Mothers: Erythromycin is excreted in breast milk, therefore, caution should be exercised when erythromycin is administered to a nursing woman.

Pediatric Use: See "Indications and Usage" and "Dosage and Administration" sections.

ADVERSE REACTIONS

The most frequent side effects of oral erythromycin preparations are gastrointestinal and are dose-related. They include nausea, vomiting, abdominal pain, diarrhea and anorexia. Symptoms of hepatic dysfunction and/or abnormal liver function test results may occur (see "Warnings" section). Pseudomembranous colitis has been rarely reported in association with erythromycin therapy.

There have been isolated reports of transient central nervous system side effects including confusion, hallucinations, seizures, and vertigo; however, a cause and effect relationship has not been established.

Occasional case reports of cardiac arrhythmias such as ventricular tachycardia have been documented in patients receiving erythromycin therapy. There have been isolated reports of other cardiovascular symptoms such as chest pain, dizziness, and palpitations; however, a cause and effect relationship has not been established.

Allergic reactions ranging from urticaria and mild skin eruptions to anaphylaxis have occurred.

There have been isolated reports of reversible hearing loss occurring chiefly in patients with renal insufficiency and in patients receiving high doses of erythromycin.

OVERDOSAGE

In case of overdosage, erythromycin should be discontinued. Overdosage should be handled with the prompt elimination of unabsorbed drug and all other appropriate measures.

Erythromycin is not removed by peritoneal dialysis or hemodialysis.

DOSAGE AND ADMINISTRATION

Administration of a dose of Erythromycin Delayed-release Capsules in the presence of food lowers the blood levels of systemically available erythromycin. Although the blood levels obtained upon administration of enteric-coated erythromycin products in the presence of food are still above minimum inhibitory concentrations (MICs) of most organisms for which erythromycin is indicated, optimum blood levels are obtained on a fasting stomach (administration at least $^1/_2$ hour and preferably two hours before or after a meal).

Adults: The usual dose is 250 mg every 6 hours taken one hour before meals. If twice-a-day dosage is desired, the recommended dose is 500 mg every 12 hours. Dosage may be increased up to 4 grams per day, according to the severity of infection. Twice-a-day dosing is not recommended when doses larger than 1 gram daily are administered.

Children: Age, weight, and severity of the infection are important factors in determining the proper dosage. The usual dosage is 30 to 50 mg/kg/day, in divided doses. For the treatment of more severe infections this dosage may be doubled.

Streptococcal infections: A therapeutic dosage of oral erythromycin should be administered for at least ten days. For continuous prophylaxis against recurrences of streptococcal infections in persons with a history of rheumatic heart disease, the dose is 250 mg twice a day.

For the prevention of bacterial endocarditis in penicillin-allergic patients with valvular heart disease who are to undergo dental procedures or surgical procedures of the upper respiratory tract, the adult dose is 1 gram orally (20 mg/kg for children) one hour prior to the procedure and then 500 mg (10 mg/kg for children) orally 6 hours later.[3] (See "INDICATIONS AND USAGE" section.)

Primary syphilis: 30 to 40 g given in divided doses over a period of 10 to 15 days.

Intestinal amebiasis: 250 mg every 6 hours for 10 to 14 days for adults; 30 to 50 mg/kg/day in divided doses for 10 to 14 days for children.

Legionnaires' disease: Although optimal doses have not been established, doses utilized in reported clinical data were those recommended above (1 to 4 g daily in divided doses).

Urogenital infections during pregnancy due to *Chlamydia trachomatis:* Although the optimal dose and duration of therapy have not been established, the suggested treatment is 500 mg by mouth four times a day on an empty stomach for at least 7 days. For women who cannot tolerate this regimen, a decreased dose of 250 mg by mouth four times a day should be used for at least 14 days.[4]

For adults with uncomplicated urethral, endocervical, or rectal infections caused by *Chlamydia trachomatis,* when tetracycline is contraindicated or not tolerated, 500 mg of erythromycin by mouth four times a day for at least 7 days.[4]

Continued on next page

Erythromycin Delayed-Rel.—Cont.

Pertussis: Although optimum dosage and duration of therapy have not been established, doses of erythromycin utilized in reported clinical studies were 40 to 50 mg/kg/day, given in divided doses for 5 to 14 days.

HOW SUPPLIED

Erythromycin Delayed-release Capsules, USP, are clear and opaque maroon capsules with pink and yellow particles containing 250 mg of erythromycin supplied in bottles of 100 (NDC 0074-6301-13) and 500 (NDC 0074-6301-53).
Storage Conditions: Protect from moisture and excessive heat. **Store below 86°F (30°C).**

REFERENCES

1. Approved Standard ASM-2 "Performance Standards for Antimicrobial Disc Susceptibility Test." National Committee for Clinical Laboratory Standards, 771 East Lancaster Avenue, Villanova, PA 19085.
2. Ericson, H.M., Sherris, J.C.: "Antibiotic Sensitivity Testing Report of an International Collaborative Study." *Acta Pathologica et Microbiologica Scandinavica*, Section B, Supp. 217, 1971.
3. American Heart Assoc. and American Dental Assoc. "Prevention of Bacterial Endocarditis," *Circulation:* Vol. 70, No. 6, December, 1984, 1123A-1127A.
4. CDC Sexually Transmitted Diseases Treatment Guidelines 1982.

Revised: September, 1991
Ref. 01-2563-R4

Shown in Product Identification Guide, page 303

FERO–FOLIC–500® Filmtab® Tablets   ℞
[fe 'ro fo-lic]
Controlled-Release Iron with Folic Acid and Vitamin C

IBERET–FOLIC–500® Filmtab®   ℞
Tablets
Controlled-Release Iron with Vitamin C, and B-Complex including Folic Acid

> **WARNING:** Accidental overdose of iron-containing products is a leading cause of fatal poisoning in children under 6. Keep this product out of reach of children. In case of accidental overdose, call doctor or poison control center immediately.

DESCRIPTION

FERO-FOLIC-500 Filmtab tablets are a hematinic for oral administration containing iron in the Gradumet controlled-release vehicle; Vitamin C for enhancement of iron absorption; and folic acid. Each tablet provides 525 mg of ferrous sulfate (equivalent to 105 mg of elemental iron), 800 mcg of folic acid and 500 mg of ascorbic acid present as sodium ascorbate.

Inactive Ingredients: Castor oil, cellulosic polymers, D&C Red No. 30, magnesium stearate, methyl acrylate-methyl methacrylate copolymer, pregelatinized starch (contains corn starch), polyethylene glycol, povidone, propylene glycol, talc, titanium dioxide and vanillin.

IBERET-FOLIC-500 tablets are a hematinic for oral administration containing iron in the Gradumet® controlled-release vehicle; vitamin C for enhancement of iron absorption; and the B-Complex vitamins including folic acid.

Each Filmtab tablet provides:

*Ferrous Sulfate	525 mg
(equivalent to 105 mg of elemental iron)	
Ascorbic Acid (present as	
sodium ascorbate) (C)	500 mg
Niacinamide	30 mg
Calcium Pantothenate	10 mg
Thiamine Mononitrate (B_1)	6 mg
Riboflavin (B_2)	6 mg
Pyridoxine Hydrochloride (B_6)	5 mg
Folic Acid	800 mcg
Cyanocobalamin (B_{12})	25 mcg

*In controlled-release form (Gradumet)
Filmtab®-Film—Film-sealed tablets, Abbott

Inactive Ingredients: Castor oil, cellulosic polymers, corn starch, D&C Red No. 7, FD&C Blue No. 1, FD&C Blue No. 2, magnesium stearate, methyl acrylate-methyl methacrylate copolymer, polyethylene glycol, povidone, propylene glycol, stearic acid, talc, titanium dioxide and vanillin.

Controlled-release of iron from the Gradumet protects against gastric side effects. The Gradumet is an inert, porous, plastic matrix impregnated with ferrous sulfate. Iron is leached from the Gradumet as it passes through the gastrointestinal tract, and the expended matrix is excreted harmlessly in the stool. Controlled-release iron is particularly helpful in patients who have demonstrated intolerance to oral iron preparations.

CLINICAL PHARMACOLOGY

Oral iron is absorbed most efficiently when administered between meals. Conventional iron preparations frequently cause gastric irritation when taken on an empty stomach. Studies with iron in the Gradumet have indicated that relatively little of the iron is released in the stomach, gastric intolerance is seldom encountered, and hematologic response ranks with that obtained from plain ferrous sulfate. Iron is found in the body principally as hemoglobin. Storage in the form of ferritin occurs in the liver, spleen, and bone marrow. Concentrations of plasma iron and the total iron-binding capacity of plasma vary greatly in different physiological conditions and disease states.

Large amounts of ascorbic acid administered orally with ferrous sulfate have been shown to enhance iron absorption. Apparently this is due to the ability of ascorbic acid to prevent the oxidation of ferrous iron to the less effectively absorbed ferric form.

Folic acid and iron are absorbed in the proximal small intestine, particularly the duodenum. Folic acid is absorbed maximally and rapidly at this site, and iron is absorbed in a descending gradient from the duodenum distally.

After absorption folic acid is rapidly converted into its metabolically active forms. Approximately two-thirds is bound to plasma protein. Half of the folic acid stored in the body is found in the liver. Folic acid is also concentrated in spinal fluid.

Except for the folates ingested in liver, yeast, and egg yolk, the percentage of absorption of food folates averages about 10%.

The B-complex vitamins in IBERET-FOLIC-500 are absorbed by the active transport process. B-complex vitamins are rapidly eliminated and therefore are not stored in the body. Calcium pantothenate is absorbed readily from the gastrointestinal tract and distributed to all body tissues.

INDICATIONS AND USAGE

FERO-FOLIC-500 is indicated for the treatment of iron deficiency and prevention of concomitant folic acid deficiency in non-pregnant adults. FERO-FOLIC-500 is also indicated in pregnancy for the prevention and treatment of iron deficiency and to supply a maintenance dosage of folic acid.

IBERET-FOLIC-500 is indicated in non-pregnant adults for the treatment of iron deficiency and prevention of concomitant folic acid deficiency with an associated deficient intake or increased need for the B-complex vitamins. IBERET-FOLIC-500 is also indicated in pregnancy for the prevention and treatment of iron deficiency with a concomitant deficient intake or increased need for the B-complex vitamins (including folic acid).

CONTRAINDICATIONS

FERO-FOLIC-500 and IBERET-FOLIC-500 are contraindicated in patients with pernicious anemia.
FERO-FOLIC-500 and IBERET-FOLIC-500 are also contraindicated in the rare instance of hypersensitivity to folic acid.

WARNINGS

Folic acid alone is improper therapy in the treatment of pernicious anemia and other megaloblastic anemias where vitamin B_{12} is deficient. See **boxed WARNING** regarding overdose in children.

PRECAUTIONS

Where anemia exists, its nature should be established and underlying causes determined.
FERO-FOLIC-500 and IBERET-FOLIC-500 contain 800 mcg of folic acid per tablet. Folic acid especially in doses above 0.1 mg daily may obscure pernicious anemia, in that hematologic remission may occur while neurological manifestations remain progresssive. Concomitant parenteral therapy with vitamin B_{12} may be necessary in patients with deficiency of vitamin B_{12}. Pernicious anemia is rare in women of childbearing age, and the likelihood of its occurrence along with pregnancy is reduced by the impairment of fertility associated with vitamin B_{12} deficiency.

Laboratory Tests: In older patients and those with conditions tending to lead to vitamin B_{12} depletion, serum B_{12} levels should be regularly assessed during treatment with FERO-FOLIC-500 or IBERET-FOLIC-500.

Drug Interactions: Absorption of iron is inhibited by *magnesium trisilicate* and *antacids containing carbonates.*
Ferrous sulfate may interfere with the absorption of *tetracyclines.*
The antiparkinsonism effects of *levodopa* may be reversed by pyridoxine.
Iron absorption is inhibited by the ingestion of eggs or milk.

Carcinogenesis: Adequate data are not available on long-term potential for carcinogenesis in animals or humans.

Pregnancy: Pregnancy Category A. Studies in pregnant women have not shown that FERO-FOLIC-500 or IBERET-FOLIC-500 increase the risk of fetal abnormalities if administered during pregnancy. If either of these drugs is used during pregnancy, the possibility of fetal harm appears remote. Because studies cannot rule out the possibility of harm, however, FERO-FOLIC-500 or IBERET-FOLIC-500 should be used during pregnancy only if clearly needed.

Nursing Mothers: Folic acid, ascorbic acid, and B-complex vitamins are excreted in breast milk.

ADVERSE REACTIONS

The likelihood of gastric intolerance to iron in the controlled-release Gradumet vehicle is remote. If such should occur, the tablet may be taken after a meal. Allergic sensitization has been reported following both oral and parenteral administration of folic acid.

OVERDOSAGE

Signs of serious toxicity may be delayed because the iron is in a controlled-release dose form. Increased capillary permeability, reduced plasma volume, increased cardiac output, and sudden cardiovascular collapse may occur in acute iron intoxication. In overdosage, efforts should be made to hasten the elimination of the Gradumet tablets ingested. An emetic should be administered as soon as possible, followed by gastric lavage if indicated. Immediately following emesis, a large dose of a saline cathartic should be used to speed passage through the intestinal tract. X-ray examination may then be considered to determine the position and number of Gradumet tablets remaining in the gastrointestinal tract.

DOSAGE AND ADMINISTRATION

Adults, including Pregnant Females: The recommended dose is one Fero-Folic-500 or one Iberet-Folic-500 tablet daily on an empty stomach.

HOW SUPPLIED

FERO-FOLIC-500 red Filmtab tablets, imprinted with the Abbott logo Ⓐ and Abbo-Code identification letters AJ, are supplied in packages of 30 tablets (NDC 0074-7079-30) each containing 5 child-resistant blisters of 6 tablets.

IBERET-FOLIC-500 red Filmtab tablets, imprinted with the Abbott logo Ⓐ and Abbo-Code identification letters AK, are supplied in packaes of 30 tablets (NDC 0074-7125-30) each containing 5 child-resistant blisters of 6 tablets.

FILMTAB—Film-sealed tablets, Abbott.
GRADUMET—Controlled-release dose form, Abbott.

Recommended Storage: Store below 77°F (25°C). Protect from light to avoid tablet color changes.
Ref. 13-1743-8/R1 and 13-1746-7/R1

FERO–GRAD–500® Filmtab® tablets   OTC
[fe 'ro-grad]
High Potency Dietary Supplement
CONTROLLED-RELEASE IRON, plus Vitamin C
Well-tolerated once-daily iron supplement

> **WARNING:** Accidental overdose of iron-containing products is a leading cause of poisoning in children under 6. Keep this product out of reach of children. In case of accidental overdose, call doctor or poison control center immediately.

DESCRIPTION

Each Fero-Grad-500 tablet provides the equivalent of 105 mg of elemental iron (525 mg of ferrous sulfate) in a unique controlled-release vehicle, the Gradumet® and 500 mg of vitamin C (as sodium ascorbate).
Ingredients: Ferrous sulfate, sodium ascorbate, povidone, methyl acrylate-methyl methacrylate copolymer, polyethylene glycol, hydroxypropyl methylcellulose, pregelatinized starch (contains corn starch), talc, D & C Red No. 7, titanium dioxide, hydroxypropyl cellulose, magnesium stearate, ethylcellulose, propylene glycol, castor oil and vanillin.

DOSAGE AND ADMINISTRATION

Usual Adult Dose: One tablet daily, or as directed by the physician.
TO OPEN CHILD-RESISTANT BLISTER PACKAGE:
1. Tear from bottom edge on perforations at START TEAR arrows.
2. Fold back and peel paper from corner marked PEEL.
3. Push tablet through foil.

HOW SUPPLIED

Fero-Grad-500 is supplied as red tablets in reclosable cartons of 30 tablets (5 child-resistant blister packages of 6 tablets) list no. 0074-7238-30. Do not accept if blister unit has been opened or seal has been broken. The ingredients of these products are listed in one or more of the Medicare designated compendia.
Recommended storage: Store below 77°F (25°C). Protect from light to avoid tablet color changes.
Ref. 13-1745-8/R1

GABITRIL™ Filmtab® ℞

[*găb-ĭ-trĭll*]
(tiagabine hydrochloride)
Tablets

DESCRIPTION

GABITRIL (tiagabine HCl) is an antiepilepsy drug available as 4 mg, 12 mg, 16 mg, and 20 mg tablets for oral administration. Its chemical name is (-)-(R)-1-[4,4-Bis(3-methyl-2-thienyl)-3-butenyl]nipecotic acid hydrochloride, its molecular formula is $C_{20}H_{25}NO_2S_2$ HCl, and its molecular weight is 412.0. Tiagabine HCl is a white to off-white, odorless, crystalline powder. It is insoluble in heptane, sparingly soluble in water, and soluble in aqueous base. The structural formula is:

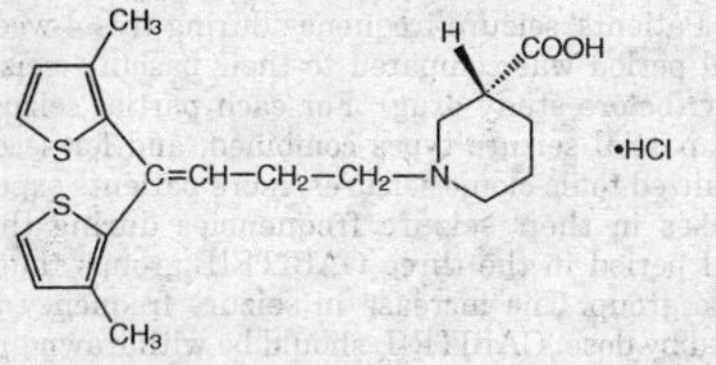

Inactive Ingredients

GABITRIL tablets contain the following inactive ingredients: Ascorbic acid, colloidal silicon dioxide, crospovidone, hydrogenated vegetable oil wax, hydroxypropyl cellulose, hydroxypropyl methylcellulose, lactose, magnesium stearate, microcrystalline cellulose, pregelatinized starch, stearic acid, and titanium dioxide.

In addition, individual tablets contain:

4 mg tablets: D&C Yellow No. 10.
12 mg tablets: D&C Yellow No. 10 and FD&C Blue No. 1.
16 mg tablets: FD&C Blue No. 2.
20 mg tablets: D&C Red No. 30.

CLINICAL PHARMACOLOGY

Mechanism of Action

The precise mechanism by which tiagabine exerts its antiseizure effect is unknown, although it is believed to be related to its ability, documented in *in vitro* experiments, to enhance the activity of gamma aminobutyric acid (GABA), the major inhibitory neurotransmitter in the central nervous system. These experiments have shown that tiagabine binds to recognition sites associated with the GABA uptake carrier. It is thought that, by this action, tiagabine blocks GABA uptake into presynaptic neurons, permitting more GABA to be available for receptor binding on the surfaces of post-synaptic cells. Inhibition of GABA uptake has been shown for synaptosomes, neuronal cell cultures, and glial cell cultures. In rat-derived hippocampal slices, tiagabine has been shown to prolong GABA-mediated inhibitory post-synaptic potentials. Tiagabine increases the amount of GABA available in the extracellular space of the globus pallidus, ventral palladum, and substantia nigra in rats at the ED_{50} and ED_{85} doses for inhibition of pentylenetetrazol (PTZ)-induced tonic seizures. This suggests that tiagabine prevents the propagation of neural impulses that contribute to seizures by a GABA-ergic action.

Tiagabine has shown efficacy in several animal models of seizures. It is effective against the tonic phase of subcutaneous PTZ-induced seizures in mice and rats, seizures induced by the proconvulsant DMCM in mice, audiogenic seizures in genetically epilepsy-prone rats (GEPR), and amygdala-kindled seizures in rats. Tiagabine has little efficacy against maximal electroshock seizures in rats and is only partially effective against subcutaneous PTZ-induced clonic seizures in mice, picrotoxin-induced tonic seizures in the mouse, bicuculline-induced seizures in the rat, and photic seizures in photosensitive baboons. Tiagabine produces a biphasic dose-response curve against PTZ- and DMCM-induced convulsions, with attenuated effectiveness at higher doses.

Based on *in vitro* binding studies, tiagabine does not significantly inhibit the uptake of dopamine, norepinephrine, serotonin, glutamate, or choline and shows little or no binding to dopamine D1 and D2, muscarinic, serotonin $5HT_{1A}$, $5HT_2$, and $5HT_3$, beta-1 and 2 adrenergic, alpha-1 and alpha-2 adrenergic, histamine H2 and H3, adenosine A_1 and A_2, opiate µ and K_1, NMDA glutamate, and $GABA_A$ receptors at 100 µM. It also lacks significant affinity for sodium or calcium channels. Tiagabine binds to histamine H1, serotonin $5HT_{1B}$, benzodiazepine, and chloride channel receptors at concentrations 20 to 400 times those inhibiting the uptake of GABA.

PHARMACOKINETICS

Tiagabine is well absorbed, with food slowing absorption rate but not altering the extent of absorption. Although its elimination half-life is 7 to 9 hours in normal volunteers, it is only 4 to 7 hours in patients receiving hepatic enzyme-inducing drugs (carbamazepine, phenytoin, primidone, and phenobarbital). In clinical trials, most patients were induced.

Table 1
Median Reduction and Median Percent Reduction from Baseline in 4-Week Seizure Rates in Study 1

		Placebo (N=91)	GABITRIL 16 mg/day (N=61)	GABITRIL 32 mg/day (N=87)	GABITRIL 56 mg/day (N=56)	Combined 32 + 56 mg/day (N=143)
Complex Partial	Median Reduction	0.6	0.8	2.2*	2.9*	2.6*
	Median % Reduction†	9%	13%	25%	32%	29%
All Partial	Median Reduction	0.2	1.2	2.7*	3.5*	2.9*
	Median % Reduction†	3%	12%	24%	36%	27%

* $p < 0.05$
† Statistical significance was not assessed for median % reduction.

Absorption and Distribution: Absorption of tiagabine is rapid, with peak plasma concentrations occurring at approximately 45 minutes following an oral dose in the fasting state. Tiagabine is nearly completely absorbed (>95%), with an absolute oral bioavailability of about 90%. A high fat meal decreases the rate (mean T_{max} was prolonged to 2.5 hours, and mean C_{max} was reduced by about 40%) but not the extent (AUC) of tiagabine absorption. In all clinical trials, tiagabine was given with meals.

The pharmacokinetics of tiagabine are linear over the single dose range of 2 to 24 mg. Following multiple dosing, steady state is achieved within 2 days.

Tiagabine is 96% bound to human plasma proteins, mainly to serum albumin and α1-acid glycoprotein over the concentration range of 10 ng/mL to 10,000 ng/mL. While the relationship between tiagabine plasma concentrations and clinical response is not currently understood, trough plasma concentrations observed in controlled clinical trials at doses from 30 to 56 mg/day ranged from <1 ng/mL to 234 ng/mL.

Metabolism and Elimination: Although the metabolism of tiagabine has not been fully elucidated, *in vivo* and *in vitro* studies suggest that at least two metabolic pathways for tiagabine have been identified in humans: 1) thiophene ring oxidation leading to the formation of 5-oxo-tiagabine; and 2) glucuronidation. The 5-oxo-tiagabine metabolite does not contribute to the pharmacologic activity of tiagabine.

Based on *in vitro* data, tiagabine is likely to be metabolized primarily by the 3A isoform subfamily of hepatic cytochrome P450 (CYP 3A), although contributions to the metabolism of tiagabine from CYP 1A2, CYP 2D6 or CYP 2C19 have not been excluded.

Approximately 2% of an oral dose of tiagabine is excreted unchanged, with 25% and 63% of the remaining dose excreted into the urine and feces, respectively, primarily as metabolites, at least 2 of which have not been identified. The mean systemic plasma clearance is 109 mL/min (CV = 23%) and the average elimination half-life for tiagabine in healthy subjects ranged from 7 to 9 hours. The elimination half-life decreased by 50 to 65% in hepatic enzyme-induced patients with epilepsy compared to uninduced patients with epilepsy.

A diurnal effect on the pharmacokinetics of tiagabine was observed. Mean steady-state C_{min} values were 40% lower in the evening than in the morning. Tiagabine steady-state AUC values were also found to be 15% lower following the evening tiagabine dose compared to the AUC following the morning dose.

SPECIAL POPULATIONS

Renal Insufficiency: The pharmacokinetics of total and unbound tiagabine were similar in subjects with normal renal function (creatinine clearance >80 mL/min) and in subjects with mild (creatinine clearance 40 to 80 mL/min), moderate (creatinine clearance 20 to 39 mL/min), or severe (creatinine clearance 5 to 19 mL/min) renal impairment. The pharmacokinetics of total and unbound tiagabine were also unaffected in subjects with renal failure requiring hemodialysis.

Hepatic Insufficiency: In patients with moderate hepatic impairment (Child-Pugh Class B), clearance of unbound tiagabine was reduced by about 60%. Patients with impaired liver function may require reduced initial and maintenance doses of tiagabine and/or longer dosing intervals compared to patients with normal hepatic function (see **PRECAUTIONS**).

Geriatric: The pharmacokinetic profile of tiagabine was similar in healthy elderly and healthy young adults.

Pediatric: Tiagabine has not been investigated in adequate and well-controlled clinical trials in patients below the age of 12. The apparent clearance and volume of distribution of tiagabine per unit body surface area or per kg were fairly similar in 25 children (age: 3 to 10 years) and in adults taking enzyme-inducing antiepilepsy drugs ([AEDs] e.g., carbamazepine or phenytoin). In children who were taking a non-inducing AED (e.g., valproate), the clearance of tiagabine based upon body weight and body surface area was 2 and 1.5-fold higher, respectively, than in uninduced adults with epilepsy.

Gender, Race and Cigarette Smoking: No specific pharmacokinetic studies were conducted to investigate the effect of gender, race and cigarette smoking on the disposition of tiagabine. Retrospective pharmacokinetic analyses, however, suggest that there is no clinically important difference between the clearance of tiagabine in males and females, when adjusted for body weight. Population pharmacokinetic analyses indicated that tiagabine clearance values were not significantly different in Caucasian (N=463), Black (N=23), or Hispanic (N=17) patients with epilepsy, and that tiagabine clearance values were not significantly affected by tobacco use.

Interactions with other Antiepilepsy Drugs: The clearance of tiagabine is affected by the co-administration of hepatic enzyme-inducing antiepilepsy drugs. Tiagabine is eliminated more rapidly in patients who have been taking hepatic enzyme-inducing drugs, e.g. carbamazepine, phenytoin, primidone and phenobarbital than in patients not receiving such treatment (see **PRECAUTIONS, Drug Interactions.**).

Interactions with Other Drugs: See **PRECAUTIONS, Drug Interactions.**

CLINICAL STUDIES

The effectiveness of GABITRIL as adjunctive therapy (added to other antiepilepsy drugs) was examined in three multi-center, double-blind, placebo-controlled, parallel-group, clinical trials in 769 patients with refractory partial seizures who were taking at least one hepatic enzyme-inducing antiepilepsy drug (AED), and two placebo-controlled cross-over studies in 90 patients. In the parallel-group trials, patients had a history of at least six complex partial seizures (Study 1 and Study 2, U.S. studies), or six partial seizures of any type (Study 3, European study), occurring alone or in combination with any other seizure type within the 8-week period preceding the first study visit in spite of receiving one or more AEDs at therapeutic concentrations. In the first two studies, the primary protocol-specified outcome measure was the median reduction from baseline in the 4-week complex partial seizure (CPS) rates during treatment. In the third study, the protocol-specified primary outcome measure was the proportion of patients achieving a 50% or greater reduction from baseline in the 4-week seizure rate of all partial seizures during treatment. The results given below include data for complex partial seizures and all partial seizures for the intent-to-treat population (all patients who received at least one dose of treatment and at least one seizure evaluation) in each study.

Study 1 was a double-blind, placebo-controlled, parallel-group trial comparing GABITRIL 16 mg/day, GABITRIL 32 mg/day, GABITRIL 56 mg/day, and placebo. Study drug was given as a four times a day regimen. After a prospective Baseline Phase of 12 weeks, patients were randomized to one of the four treatment groups described above. The 16-week Treatment Phase consisted of a 4-week Titration Period, followed by a 12-week Fixed-Dose Period, during which concomitant AED doses were held constant. The primary outcome was assessed for the combined 32 and 56 mg/day groups compared to placebo.

Study 2 was a double-blind, placebo-controlled, parallel-group trial consisting of an 8-week Baseline Phase and a 12-week Treatment Phase, the first 4 weeks of which constituted a Titration Period and the last 8 weeks a Fixed-Dose Period. This study compared GABITRIL 16 mg BID and 8 mg QID to placebo. The protocol-specified primary outcome measure was assessed separately for each group treated with GABITRIL.

The following tables display the results of the analyses of these two trials.

[See table 1 above]
[See table 2 at bottom of next page]

Continued on next page

Gabitril—Cont.

Figures 1 to 4 present the proportion of patients (X-axis) whose percent reduction from baseline in the all partial seizure rate was at least as great as that indicated on the Y axis in the three placebo-controlled adjunctive studies (Studies 1, 2, and 3). A positive value on the Y axis indicates an improvement from baseline (i.e., a decrease in seizure rate), while a negative value indicates a worsening from baseline (i.e., an increase in seizure rate). Thus, in a display of this type, the curve for an effective treatment is shifted to the left of the curve for placebo.

Figure 1 indicates that the proportion of patients achieving any particular level of reduction in seizure rate was consistently higher for the combined GABITRIL 32 mg and 56 mg groups compared to the placebo group in Study 1. For example, Figure 1 indicates that approximately 24% of patients treated with GABITRIL experienced a 50% or greater reduction, compared to 4% in the placebo group.

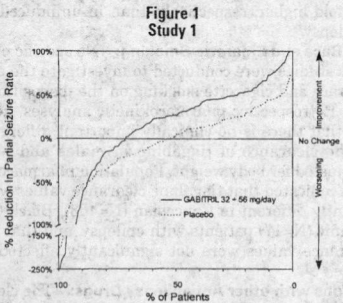

Figure 1
Study 1

Figure 2 also displays the results for Study 1, which was a dose-response study, by treatment group. Figure 2 indicates a dose-response relationship across the three GABITRIL groups. The proportion of patients achieving any particular level of reduction in all partial seizure rates was consistently higher as the dose of GABITRIL was increased. For example, Figure 2 indicates that approximately 4% of patients in the placebo group experienced a 50% or greater reduction in all partial seizure rate, compared to approximately 10% of the GABITRIL 16 mg/day group, 21% of the GABITRIL 32 mg/day group, and 30% of the GABITRIL 56 mg/day group.

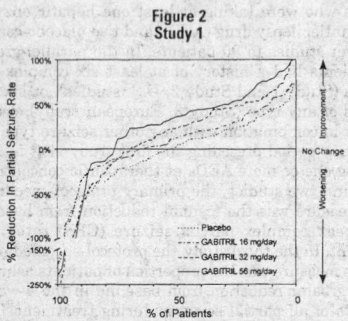

Figure 2
Study 1

Figure 3 indicates that the proportion of patients achieving any particular level of reduction in partial seizure rate was consistently greater in patients taking GABITRIL than in those taking placebo in Study 2. (Study 2 compared placebo to GABITRIL 32 mg/day; one of the GABITRIL groups received 8 mg QID, while the other GABITRIL group received 16 mg BID). For example, Figure 3 indicates that approximately 7% of patients in the placebo group experienced a 50% or greater reduction in their partial seizure rate, compared to approximately 23% of patients in the GABITRIL 8 mg QID group and 28% of patients in the GABITRIL 16 mg BID group.

[See figure 3 at top of next column]

Study 3 was a double-blind, placebo-controlled, parallel-group trial that compared GABITRIL 10 mg TID (N=77) with placebo (N=77). In this trial, patients were followed prospectively during a 12-week Baseline Phase and then randomized to receive study drug during an 18-week Treatment Phase. During the first 6 weeks of treatment (Titration Period), patients were titrated to 30 mg/day, after which they were maintained on this dose during the 12-week Fixed-Dose Period. The protocol-specified primary outcome measure (proportion of patients who achieved at least a 50% reduction from baseline in partial seizure rate) did not reach statistical significance. However, analyses of the median reduction from baseline in 4-week partial seizure rate (the analyses presented above for Study 1 and Study 2)

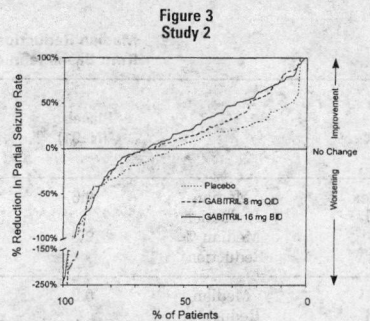

Figure 3
Study 2

were performed and showed a statistically significant improvement compared to placebo in all partial and complex partial seizure rates (Table 3):

[See table 3 below]

Figure 4 indicates that the proportion of patients achieving any particular level of reduction in seizure activity was consistently higher in those taking GABITRIL than those taking placebo in Study 3. For example, Figure 4 indicates that approximately 5% of patients in the placebo group experienced a 50% or greater reduction in their partial seizure rate compared to approximately 10% of patients in the GABITRIL group.

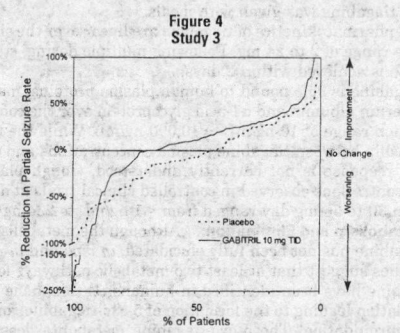

Figure 4
Study 3

The two other placebo-controlled trials that examined the effectiveness of GABITRIL were small cross-over trials (N=46 and 44). Both trials included an open Screening Phase during which patients were titrated to an optimal dose and then treated with this dose for an additional 4 weeks. After this Open Phase, patients were randomized to one of two blinded treatment sequences (GABITRIL followed by placebo or placebo followed by GABITRIL). The Double-Blind Phase consisted of two Treatment Periods, each lasting 7 weeks (with a 3 week washout between periods). The outcome measures were median with-in patient differences between placebo and GABITRIL Treatment Periods in 4-week complex partial and all partial seizure rates. The reductions in seizure rates were statistically significant in both studies.

INDICATIONS AND USAGE

GABITRIL (tiagabine hydrochloride) is indicated as adjunctive therapy in adults and children 12 years and older in the treatment of partial seizures.

CONTRAINDICATIONS

GABITRIL is contraindicated in patients who have demonstrated hypersensitivity to the drug or its ingredients.

WARNINGS

Withdrawal Seizures: As a rule, antiepilepsy drugs should not be abruptly discontinued because of the possibility of increasing seizure frequency. In a placebo-controlled, double-blind, dose-response study (Study 1 described in **CLINICAL STUDIES**) designed, in part, to investigate the capacity of GABITRIL to induce withdrawal seizures, study drug was tapered over a 4-week period after 16 weeks of treatment. Patients' seizure frequency during this 4-week withdrawal period was compared to their baseline seizure frequency (before study drug). For each partial seizure type, for all partial seizure types combined, and for secondarily generalized tonic-clonic seizures, more patients experienced increases in their seizure frequencies during the withdrawal period in the three GABITRIL groups than in the placebo group. The increase in seizure frequency was not affected by dose. GABITRIL should be withdrawn gradually to minimize the potential of increased seizure frequency, unless safety concerns require a more rapid withdrawal.

Cognitive/Neuropsychiatric Adverse Events: Adverse events most often associated with the use of GABITRIL were related to the central nervous system. The most significant of these can be classified into 2 general categories: 1) impaired concentration, speech or language problems, and confusion (effects on thought processes); and 2) somnolence and fatigue (effects on level of consciousness). The majority of these events were mild to moderate. In controlled clinical trials, these events led to discontinuation of treatment with GABITRIL in 6% (31 of 494) of patients compared to 2% (5 of 275) of the placebo-treated patients. A total of 1.6% (8 of 494) of the GABITRIL treated patients in the controlled trials were hospitalized secondary to the occurrence of these events compared to 0% of the placebo treated patients. Some of these events were dose related and usually began during initial titration.

Patients with a history of spike and wave discharges on EEG have been reported to have exacerbations of their EEG abnormalities associated with these cognitive/neuropsychiatric events. This raises the possibility that these clinical events may, in some cases, be a manifestation of underlying seizure activity (see **PRECAUTIONS, EEG**). In the documented cases of spike and wave discharges on EEG with cognitive/neuropsychiatric events, patients usually continued tiagabine, but required dosage adjustment.

Status Epilepticus: In the three double-blind, placebo-controlled, parallel-group studies (Studies 1, 2, and 3), the incidence of any type of status epilepticus (simple, complex, or generalized tonic-clonic) in patients receiving GABITRIL was 0.8% (4 of 494 patients) versus 0.7% (2 of 275 patients) receiving placebo. Among the patients treated with GABITRIL across all epilepsy studies (controlled and uncontrolled), 5% had some form of status epilepticus. Of the 5%,

Table 2
Median Reduction and Median Percent Reduction from Baseline in 4-Week Seizure Rates in Study 2

		Placebo (N=107)	GABITRIL 16 mg BID (N=106)	GABITRIL 8 mg QID (N=104)
Complex Partial	Median Reduction	0.3	1.6	1.3*
	Median % Reduction†	4%	22%	15%
All Partial	Median Reduction	0.5	1.6	1.3
	Median % Reduction†	5%	19%	13%

* p < 0.027, necessary for statistical significance due to multiple comparisons.
† Statistical significance was not assessed for median % reduction.

Table 3
Median Reduction and Median Percent Reduction from Baseline in 4-Week Seizure Rates in Study 3

		Placebo (N=77)	GABITRIL 30 mg/day (N=77)
Complex Partial‡	Median Reduction	-0.1	1.3*
	Median % Reduction†	-1%	14%
All Partial	Median Reduction	-0.5	1.1*
	Median % Reduction†	-7%	11%

* p < 0.05
† Statistical significance was not assessed for median % reduction.
‡ N=72 and 75 for placebo and GABITRIL, respectively.

57% of patients experienced complex partial status epilepticus. A critical risk factor for status epilepticus was the presence of a previous history; 33% of patients with a history of status epilepticus had recurrence during GABITRIL treatment. Because adequate information about the incidence of status epilepticus in a similar population of patients with epilepsy who have not received treatment with GABITRIL is not available, it is impossible to state whether or not treatment with GABITRIL is associated with a higher or lower rate of status epilepticus than would be expected to occur in a similar population not treated with GABITRIL.

Sudden Unexpected Death In Epilepsy (SUDEP): There have been as many as 10 cases of sudden unexpected deaths during the clinical development of tiagabine among 2531 patients with epilepsy (3831 patient-years of exposure). This represents an estimated incidence of 0.0026 deaths per patient-year. This rate is within the range of estimates for the incidence of sudden and unexpected deaths in patients with epilepsy not receiving GABITRIL (ranging from 0.0005 for the general population with epilepsy, 0.003 to 0.004 for clinical trial populations similar to that in the clinical development program for GABITRIL, to 0.005 for patients with refractory epilepsy). The estimated SUDEP rates in patients receiving GABITRIL are also similar to those observed in patients receiving other antiepilepsy drugs, chemically unrelated to GABITRIL, that underwent clinical testing in similar populations at about the same time. This evidence suggests that the SUDEP rates reflect population rates, not a drug effect.

PRECAUTIONS
General
Use in Non-Induced Patients: Virtually all experience with GABITRIL has been obtained in patients receiving at least one concomitant enzyme-inducing antiepilepsy drug (AED). Use in non-induced patients (e.g., patients receiving valproate monotherapy) may require lower doses or a slower dose titration of GABITRIL for clinical response. Patients taking a combination of inducing and non-inducing drugs (e.g., carbamazepine and valproate) should be considered to be induced.

Generalized Weakness: Moderately severe to incapacitating generalized weakness has been reported following administration of GABITRIL in 28 of 2531 (approximately 1%) patients with epilepsy. The weakness resolved in all cases after a reduction in dose or discontinuation of GABITRIL.

Binding in the Eye and Other Melanin-Containing Tissues: When dogs received a single dose of radiolabeled tiagabine, there was evidence of residual binding in the retina and uvea after 3 weeks (the latest time point measured). Although not directly measured, melanin binding is suggested. The ability of available tests to detect potentially adverse consequences, if any, of the binding of tiagabine to melanin-containing tissue is unknown and there was no systematic monitoring for relevant ophthalmological changes during the clinical development of GABITRIL. However, long term (up to one year) toxicological studies of tiagabine in dogs showed no treatment-related ophthalmoscopic changes and macro- and microscopic examinations of the eye were unremarkable. Accordingly, although there are no specific recommendations for periodic ophthalmologic monitoring, prescribers should be aware of the possibility of long-term ophthalmologic effects.

Use in Hepatically-Impaired Patients: Because the clearance of tiagabine is reduced in patients with liver disease, dosage reduction may be necessary in these patients.

Serious Rash: Four patients treated with tiagabine during the product's premarketing clinical testing developed what were considered to be serious rashes. In two patients, the rash was described as maculopapular; in one it was described as vesiculobullous; and in the 4th case, a diagnosis of Stevens Johnson Syndrome was made. In none of the 4 cases is it certain that tiagabine was the primary, or even a contributory, cause of the rash. Nevertheless, drug associated rash can, if extensive and serious, cause irreversible morbidity, even death.

Information for Patients: Patients should be instructed to take GABITRIL only as prescribed.

Patients should be advised that GABITRIL may cause dizziness, somnolence, and other symptoms and signs of CNS depression. Accordingly, they should be advised neither to drive nor to operate other complex machinery until they have gained sufficient experience on GABITRIL to gauge whether or not it affects their mental and/or motor performance adversely. Because of the possible additive depressive effects, caution should also be used when patients are taking other CNS depressants in combination with GABITRIL.

Because teratogenic effects were seen in the offspring of rats exposed to maternally toxic doses of tiagabine and because experience in humans is limited, patients should be advised to notify their physicians if they become pregnant or intend to become pregnant during therapy.

Because of the possibility that tiagabine may be excreted in breast milk, patients should be advised to notify those providing care to themselves and their children if they intend to breast-feed or are breast-feeding an infant.

Laboratory Tests
Therapeutic Monitoring of Plasma Concentrations of Tiagabine: A therapeutic range for tiagabine plasma concentrations has not been established. In controlled trials, trough plasma concentrations observed among patients randomized to doses of tiagabine that were statistically significantly more effective than placebo ranged from <1 ng/mL to 234 ng/mL (median, 10th and 90th percentiles are 23.7 ng/mL, 5.4 ng/mL, and 69.8 ng/mL, respectively). Because of the potential for pharmacokinetic interactions between GABITRIL and drugs that induce or inhibit hepatic metabolizing enzymes, it may be useful to obtain plasma levels of tiagabine before and after changes are made in the therapeutic regimen.

Clinical Chemistry and Hematology: During the development of GABITRIL, no systematic abnormalities on routine laboratory testing were noted. Therefore, no specific guidance is offered regarding routine monitoring; the practitioner retains responsibility for determining how best to monitor the patient in his/her care.

EEG: Patients with a history of spike and wave discharges on EEG have been reported to have exacerbations of their EEG abnormalities associated with cognitive/neuropsychiatric events. This raises the possibility that these clinical events may, in some cases, be a manifestation of underlying seizure activity (see **WARNINGS, Cognitive/Neuropsychiatric Adverse Events**). In the documented cases of spike and wave discharges on EEG with cognitive/neuropsychiatric events, patients usually continued tiagabine, but required dosage adjustment.

Drug Interactions
In evaluating the potential for interactions among co-administered antiepilepsy drugs (AEDs), whether or not an AED induces or does not induce metabolic enzymes is an important consideration. Phenytoin, phenobarbital and carbamazepine are generally classified as enzyme inducers; valproate and gabapentin are not. GABITRIL is considered to be a non-enzyme inducing AED.

The drug interaction data described in this section were obtained from studies involving either healthy subjects or patients with epilepsy.

Effects of GABITRIL on other Antiepilepsy Drugs (AEDs):
Phenytoin: Tiagabine had no effect on the steady-state plasma concentrations of phenytoin in patients with epilepsy.

Carbamazepine: Tiagabine had no effect on the steady-state plasma concentrations of carbamazepine or its epoxide metabolite in patients with epilepsy.

Valproate: Tiagabine causes a slight decrease (about 10%) in steady-state valproate concentrations.

Phenobarbital or Primidone: No formal pharmacokinetic studies have been performed examining the addition of tiagabine to regimens containing phenobarbital or primidone. The addition of tiagabine in a limited number of patients in three well-controlled studies caused no systematic changes in phenobarbital or primidone concentrations when compared to placebo.

Effects of other Antiepilepsy Drugs (AEDs) on GABITRIL:
Carbamazepine: Population pharmacokinetic analyses indicate that tiagabine clearance is 60% greater in patients taking carbamazepine with or without other enzyme-inducing AEDs.

Phenytoin: Population pharmacokinetic analyses indicate that tiagabine clearance is 60% greater in patients taking phenytoin with or without other enzyme-inducing AEDs.

Phenobarbital (Primidone): Population pharmacokinetic analyses indicate that tiagabine clearance is 60% greater in patients taking phenobarbital (primidone) with or without other enzyme-inducing AEDs.

Valproate: The addition of tiagabine to patients taking valproate chronically had no effect on tiagabine pharmacokinetics, but valproate significantly decreased tiagabine binding in vitro from 96.3 to 94.8%, which resulted in an increase of approximately 40% in the free tiagabine concentration. The clinical relevance of this in vitro finding is unknown.

Interaction of GABITRIL with Other Drugs:
Cimetidine: Co-administration of cimetidine (800 mg/day) to patients taking tiagabine chronically had no effect on tiagabine pharmacokinetics.

Theophylline: A single 10 mg dose of tiagabine did not affect the pharmacokinetics of theophylline at steady state.

Warfarin: No significant differences were observed in the steady-state pharmacokinetics of R-warfarin or S-warfarin with the addition of tiagabine given as a single dose. Prothrombin times were not affected by tiagabine.

Digoxin: Concomitant administration of tiagabine did not affect the steady-state pharmacokinetics of digoxin or the mean daily trough serum level of digoxin.

Ethanol or Triazolam: No significant differences were observed in the pharmacokinetics of triazolam (0.125 mg) and tiagabine (10 mg) when given together as a single dose. The pharmacokinetics of ethanol were not affected by multiple-dose administration of tiagabine. Tiagabine has shown no clinically important potentiation of the pharmacodynamic effects of triazolam or alcohol. Because of the possible addi-

tive effects of drugs that may depress the nervous system, ethanol or triazolam should be used cautiously in combination with tiagabine.

Oral Contraceptives: Multiple dose administration of tiagabine (8 mg/day monotherapy) did not alter the pharmacokinetics of oral contraceptives in healthy women of child-bearing age.

Antipyrine: Antipyrine pharmacokinetics were not significantly different before and after tiagabine multiple-dose regimens. This indicates that tiagabine does not cause induction or inhibition of the hepatic microsomal enzyme systems responsible for the metabolism of antipyrine.

Carcinogenesis: In rats, a study of the potential carcinogenicity associated with tiagabine HCl administration showed that 200 mg/kg/day (plasma exposure [AUC] 36 to 100 times that at the maximum recommended human dosage [MRHD] of 56 mg/day) for 2 years resulted in small, but statistically significant increases in the incidences of hepatocellular adenomas in females and Leydig cell tumors of the testis in males. The significance of these findings relative to the use of GABITRIL in humans is unknown. The no effect dosage for induction of tumors in this study was 100 mg/kg/day (17 to 50 times the exposure at the MRHD). No statistically significant increases in tumor formation were noted in mice at dosages up to 250 mg/kg/day (20 times the MRHD on a mg/m^2 basis).

Mutagenesis: Tiagabine produced an increase in structural chromosome aberration frequency in human lymphocytes in vitro in the absence of metabolic activation. No increase in chromosomal aberration frequencies was demonstrated in this assay in the presence of metabolic activation. No evidence of genetic toxicity was found in the in vitro bacterial gene mutation assays, the in vitro HGPRT forward mutation assay in Chinese hamster lung cells, the in vivo mouse micronucleus test, or an unscheduled DNA synthesis assay.

Impairment of Fertility: Studies of male and female rats administered dosages of tiagabine HCl prior to and during mating, gestation, and lactation have shown no impairment of fertility at doses up to 100 mg/kg/day. This dose represents approximately 16 times the maximum recommended human dose (MRHD) of 56 mg/day, based on body surface area (mg/m^2). Lowered maternal weight gain and decreased viability and growth in the rat pups were found at 100 mg/kg, but not at 20 mg/kg/day (3 times the MRHD on a mg/m^2 basis).

Pregnancy: Pregnancy Category C: Tiagabine has been shown to have adverse effects on embryo-fetal development, including teratogenic effects, when administered to pregnant rats and rabbits at doses greater than the human therapeutic dose.

An increased incidence of malformed fetuses (various craniofacial, appendicular, and visceral defects) and decreased fetal weights were observed following oral administration of 100 mg/kg/day to pregnant rats during the period of organogenesis. This dose is approximately 16 times the maximum recommended human dose (MRHD) of 56 mg/day, based on body surface area (mg/m^2). Maternal toxicity (transient weight loss/reduced maternal weight gain during gestation) was associated with this dose, but there is no evidence to suggest that the teratogenic effects were secondary to the maternal effects. No adverse maternal or embryofetal effects were seen at a dose of 20 mg/kg/day (3 times the MRHD on a mg/m^2 basis).

Decreased maternal weight gain, increased resorption of embryos and increased incidences of fetal variations, but not malformations, were observed when pregnant rabbits were given 25 mg/kg/day (8 times the MRHD on a mg/m^2 basis) during organogenesis. The no effect level for maternal and embryo-fetal toxicity in rabbits was 5 mg/kg/day (equivalent to the MRHD on a mg/m^2 basis).

When female rats were given tiagabine 100 mg/kg/day during late gestation and throughout parturition and lactation, decreased maternal weight gain during gestation, an increase in stillbirths, and decreased postnatal offspring viability and growth were found. There are no adequate and well-controlled studies in pregnant women. Tiagabine should be used during pregnancy only if clearly needed.

Use in Nursing Mothers: Studies in rats have shown that tiagabine HCl and/or its metabolites are excreted in the milk of that species. Levels of excretion of tiagabine and/or its metabolites in human milk have not been determined and effects on the nursing infant are unknown. GABITRIL should be used in women who are nursing only if the benefits clearly outweigh the risks.

Pediatric Use: Safety and effectiveness in pediatric patients below the age of 12 have not been established. The pharmacokinetics of tiagabine were evaluated in pediatric patients age 3 to 10 years (see **CLINICAL PHARMACOLOGY** - Pediatric).

Geriatric Use: Because few patients over the age of 65 (approximately 20) were exposed to GABITRIL during its clinical evaluation, no specific statements about the safety or effectiveness of GABITRIL in this age group could be made.

Continued on next page

Gabitril—Cont.

ADVERSE REACTIONS

The most commonly observed adverse events in placebo-controlled, parallel-group, add-on epilepsy trials associated with the use of GABITRIL in combination with other antiepilepsy drugs not seen at an equivalent frequency among placebo-treated patients were dizziness/light-headedness, asthenia/lack of energy, somnolence, nausea, nervousness/irritability, tremor, abdominal pain, and thinking abnormal/difficulty with concentration or attention.

Approximately 21% of the 2531 patients who received GABITRIL in clinical trials of epilepsy discontinued treatment because of an adverse event. The adverse events most commonly associated with discontinuation were dizziness (1.7%), somnolence (1.6%), depression (1.3%), confusion (1.1%), and asthenia (1.1%).

In Studies 1 and 2 (U.S. studies), the double-blind, placebo-controlled, parallel-group, add-on studies, the proportion of patients who discontinued treatment because of adverse events was 11% for the group treated with GABITRIL and 6% for the placebo group. The most common adverse events considered the primary reason for discontinuation were confusion (1.2%), somnolence (1.0%), and ataxia (1.0%).

Adverse Event Incidence in Controlled Clinical Trials: Table 4 lists treatment-emergent signs and symptoms that occurred in at least 1% of patients treated with GABITRIL for epilepsy participating in parallel-group, placebo-controlled trials and were numerically more common in the GABITRIL group. In these studies, either GABITRIL or placebo was added to the patient's current antiepilepsy drug therapy. Adverse events were usually mild or moderate in intensity. The prescriber should be aware that these figures, obtained when GABITRIL was added to concurrent antiepilepsy drug therapy, cannot be used to predict the frequency of adverse events in the course of usual medical practice when patient characteristics and other factors may differ from those prevailing during clinical studies. Similarly, the cited frequencies cannot be directly compared with figures obtained from other clinical investigations involving different treatments, uses, or investigators. An inspection of these frequencies, however, does provide the prescribing physician with one basis to estimate the relative contribution of drug and non-drug factors to the adverse event incidences in the population studied.

[See table 4 below]

Other events reported by 1% or more of patients treated with GABITRIL but equally or more frequent in the placebo group were: accidental injury, chest pain, constipation, flu syndrome, rhinitis, anorexia, back pain, dry mouth, flatulence, ecchymosis, twitching, fever, amblyopia, conjunctivitis, urinary tract infection, urinary frequency, infection, dyspepsia, gastroenteritis, nausea and vomiting, myalgia, diplopia, headache, anxiety, acne, sinusitis, and incoordination. Study 1 was a dose-response study including doses of 32 mg and 56 mg. Table 5 shows adverse events reported at a rate of ≥ 5% in at least one GABITRIL group and more frequent than in the placebo group. Among these events, tremor, difficulty with concentration/attention, and perhaps asthenia exhibited a positive relationship to dose.

[See table 5 at top of next page]

The effects of GABITRIL in relation to those of placebo on the incidence of adverse events and the types of adverse events reported were independent of age, weight, and gender. Because only 10% of patients were non-Caucasian in parallel-group, placebo-controlled trials, there is insufficient data to support a statement regarding the distribution of adverse experience reports by race.

Other Adverse Events Observed During All Clinical Trials: GABITRIL has been administered to 2531 patients during all phase 2/3 clinical trials, only some of which were placebo-controlled. During these trials, all adverse events were recorded by the clinical investigators using terminology of their own choosing. To provide a meaningful estimate of the proportion of individuals having adverse events, similar types of events were grouped into a smaller number of standardized categories using modified COSTART dictionary terminology. These categories are used in the listing below. The frequencies presented represent the proportion of the 2531 patients exposed to GABITRIL who experienced events of the type cited on at least one occasion while receiving GABITRIL. All reported events are included except those already listed above, events seen only three times or fewer (unless potentially important), events very unlikely to be drug-related, and those too general to be informative. Events are included without regard to determination of a causal relationship to tiagabine.

Events are further classified within body system categories and enumerated in order of decreasing frequency using the following definitions: frequent adverse events are defined as those occurring in at least 1/100 patients; infrequent adverse events are those occurring in 1/100 to 1/1000 patients; rare events are those occurring in fewer than 1/1000 patients.

Body as a Whole: *Frequent:* Allergic reaction, chest pain, chills, cyst, neck pain, and malaise. *Infrequent:* Abscess, cellulitis, facial edema, halitosis, hernia, neck rigidity, neoplasm, pelvic pain, photosensitivity reaction, sepsis, sudden death, and suicide attempt.

Cardiovascular System: *Frequent:* Hypertension, palpitation, syncope, and tachycardia. *Infrequent:* Angina pectoris, cerebral ischemia, electrocardiogram abnormal, hemorrhage, hypotension, myocardial infarct, pallor, peripheral vascular disorder, phlebitis, postural hypotension, and thrombophlebitis.

Digestive System: *Frequent:* Gingivitis and stomatitis. *Infrequent:* Abnormal stools, cholecystitis, cholelithiasis, dysphagia, eructation, esophagitis, fecal incontinence, gastritis, gastrointestinal hemorrhage, glossitis, gum hyperplasia, hepatomegaly, increased salivation, liver function tests abnormal, melena, periodontal abscess, rectal hemorrhage, thirst, tooth caries, and ulcerative stomatitis.

Endocrine System: *Infrequent:* Goiter and hypothyroidism.

Hemic and Lymphatic System: *Frequent:* Lymphadenopathy. *Infrequent:* Anemia, erythrocytes abnormal, leukopenia, petechia, and thrombocytopenia.

Metabolic and Nutritional: *Frequent:* Edema, peripheral edema, weight gain, and weight loss. *Infrequent:* Dehydration, hypercholesteremia, hyperglycemia, hyperlipemia, hypoglycemia, hypokalemia, and hyponatremia.

Musculoskeletal System: *Frequent:* Arthralgia. *Infrequent:* Arthritis, arthrosis, bursitis, generalized spasm, and tendinous contracture.

Nervous System: *Frequent:* Depersonalization, dysarthria, euphoria, hallucination, hyperkinesia, hypertonia, hypesthesia, hypokinesia, hypotonia, migraine, myoclonus, paranoid reaction, personality disorder, reflexes decreased, stupor, twitching, and vertigo. *Infrequent:* Abnormal dreams, apathy, choreoathetosis, circumoral paresthesia, CNS neoplasm, coma, delusions, dry mouth, dystonia, encephalopathy, hemiplegia, leg cramps, libido increased, libido decreased, movement disorder, neuritis, neurosis, paralysis, peripheral neuritis, psychosis, reflexes increased, and urinary retention.

Respiratory System: *Frequent:* Bronchitis, dyspnea, epistaxis, and pneumonia. *Infrequent:* Apnea, asthma, hemoptysis, hiccups, hyperventilation, laryngitis, respiratory disorder, and voice alteration.

Skin and Appendages: *Frequent:* Alopecia, dry skin, and sweating. *Infrequent:* Contact dermatitis, eczema, exfoliative dermatitis, furunculosis, herpes simplex, herpes zoster, hirsutism, maculopapular rash, psoriasis, skin benign neoplasm, skin carcinoma, skin discolorations, skin nodules, skin ulcer, subcutaneous nodule, urticaria, and vesiculobullous rash.

Special Senses: *Frequent:* Abnormal vision, ear pain, otitis media, and tinnitus. *Infrequent:* Blepharitis, blindness, deafness, eye pain, hyperacusis, keratoconjunctivitis, otitis externa, parosmia, photophobia, taste loss, taste perversion, and visual field defect.

Urogenital System: *Frequent:* Dysmenorrhea, dysuria, metrorrhagia, urinary incontinence, and vaginitis. *Infrequent:* Abortion, amenorrhea, breast enlargement, breast pain, cystitis, fibrocystic breast, hematuria, impotence, kidney failure, menorrhagia, nocturia, papanicolaou smear suspicious, polyuria, pyelonephritis, salpingitis, urethritis, urinary urgency, and vaginal hemorrhage.

DRUG ABUSE AND DEPENDENCE

The abuse and dependence potential of GABITRIL have not been evaluated in human studies.

OVERDOSAGE

Human Overdose Experience: Human experience of acute overdose with GABITRIL is limited. Eleven patients in clinical trials took single doses of GABITRIL up to 800 mg. All patients fully recovered, usually within one day. The most common symptoms reported after overdose included somnolence, impaired consciousness, agitation, confusion, speech difficulty, hostility, depression, weakness, and myoclonus. One patient who ingested a single dose of 400 mg experienced generalized tonic-clonic status epilepticus, which responded to intravenous phenobarbital.

Eleven individuals (including five children <7 years old) not in tiagabine clinical trials accidentally ingested tiagabine in single doses up to 20 mg. These individuals were asymptomatic in six cases. Symptoms exhibited in at least one of the

Table 4
Treatment-Emergent Adverse Event[1] Incidence in Parallel-Group, Placebo-Controlled, Add-On Trials (events in at least 1% of patients treated with GABITRIL and numerically more frequent than in the placebo group)

Body System/ COSTART	GABITRIL N=494 %	Placebo N=275 %
Body as a Whole		
Abdominal Pain	7	3
Pain (unspecified)	5	3
Cardiovascular		
Vasodilation	2	1
Digestive		
Nausea	11	9
Diarrhea	7	3
Vomiting	7	4
Increased Appetite	2	0
Mouth Ulceration	1	0
Musculoskeletal		
Myasthenia	1	0
Nervous System		
Dizziness	27	15
Asthenia	20	14
Somnolence	18	15
Nervousness	10	3
Tremor	9	3
Difficulty With Concentration/Attention*	6	2
Insomnia	6	4
Ataxia	5	3
Confusion	5	3
Speech Disorder	4	2
Difficulty With Memory*	4	3
Paresthesia	4	2
Depression	3	1
Emotional Lability	3	2
Abnormal Gait	3	2
Hostility	2	1
Nystagmus	2	3
Language Problems*	2	0
Agitation	1	0
Respiratory System		
Pharyngitis	7	4
Cough Increased	4	3
Skin and Appendages		
Rash	5	4
Pruritus	2	0

[1]Patients in these add-on studies were receiving one to three concomitant enzyme-inducing antiepilepsy drugs in addition to GABITRIL or placebo. Patients may have reported multiple adverse experiences; thus, patients may be included in more than one category.

* COSTART term substituted with a more clinically descriptive term.

Table 5
Treatment-Emergent Adverse Event Incidence in Study 1†
(events in at least 5% of patients treated with GABITRIL 32 or 56 mg
and numerically more frequent than in the placebo group)

Body System/ COSTART Term	GABITRIL 56 mg (N=57) %	GABITRIL 32 mg (N=88) %	Placebo (N=91) %
Body as a Whole			
Accidental Injury	21	15	20
Infection	19	10	12
Flu Syndrome	9	6	3
Pain	7	2	3
Abdominal Pain	5	7	4
Digestive System			
Diarrhea	2	10	6
Hemic and Lymphatic System			
Ecchymosis	0	6	1
Musculoskeletal System			
Myalgia	5	2	3
Nervous System			
Dizziness	28	31	12
Asthenia	23	18	15
Tremor	21	14	1
Somnolence	19	21	17
Nervousness	14	11	6
Difficulty With Concentration/Attention*	14	7	3
Ataxia	9	6	6
Depression	7	1	0
Insomnia	5	6	3
Abnormal Gait	5	5	3
Hostility	5	5	2
Respiratory System			
Pharyngitis	7	8	6
Special Senses			
Amblyopia	4	9	8
Urogenital System			
Urinary Tract Infection	5	0	2

† Patients in this study were receiving one to three concomitant enzyme-inducing antiepilepsy drugs in addition to GABITRIL or placebo. Patients may have reported multiple adverse experiences; thus, patients may be included in more than one category.
* COSTART term substituted with a more clinically descriptive term.

Table 6
Typical Dosing Titration Regimen for Patients Taking Enzyme-Inducing AEDs

	Initiation and Titration Schedule	Total Daily Dose
Week 1	Initiate at 4 mg once daily	4 mg/day
Week 2	Increase total daily dose by 4 mg	8 mg/day (in two divided doses)
Week 3	Increase total daily dose by 4 mg	12 mg/day (in three divided doses)
Week 4	Increase total daily dose by 4 mg	16 mg/day (in two to four divided doses)
Week 5	Increase total daily dose by 4 to 8 mg	20 to 24 mg/day (in two to four divided doses)
Week 6	Increase total daily dose by 4 to 8 mg	24 to 32 mg/day (in two to four divided doses)
Usual Adult Maintenance Dose:	32 to 56 mg/day in two to four divided doses	

other five individuals included ataxia, confusion, somnolence, impaired consciousness, impaired speech, agitation, lethargy, drowsiness, and myoclonus. One individual experienced a tonic-clonic seizure but was taking other agents which may be associated with seizures. All individuals recovered, usually within one day.
Management of Overdose: There is no specific antidote for overdose with GABITRIL. If indicated, elimination of unabsorbed drug should be achieved by emesis or gastric lavage; usual precautions should be observed to maintain the airway. General supportive care of the patient is indicated including monitoring of vital signs and observation of clinical status of the patient. Since tiagabine is mostly metabolized by the liver and is highly protein bound, dialysis is unlikely to be beneficial. A Certified Poison Control Center should be consulted for up to date information on the management of overdose with GABITRIL.

DOSAGE AND ADMINISTRATION
GABITRIL (tiagabine HCl) is recommended as adjunctive therapy in patients 12 years and older.
GABITRIL is given orally and should be taken with food. Adequate and controlled clinical studies with GABITRIL were conducted in patients taking enzyme-inducing AEDs

(e.g., phenytoin, carbamazepine, and barbiturates). Patients taking only non-enzyme-inducing AEDs (e.g., valproate, gabapentin, and lamotrigine) may require lower doses or a slower titration of GABITRIL for clinical response.
Adults and Adolescents 12 Years or Older: In adolescents 12 to 18 years old, GABITRIL should be initiated at 4 mg once daily. Modification of concomitant antiepilepsy drugs is not necessary, unless clinically indicated. The total daily dose of GABITRIL may be increased by 4 mg at the beginning of Week 2. Thereafter, the total daily dose may be increased by 4 to 8 mg at weekly intervals until clinical response is achieved or up to 32 mg/day. The total daily dose should be given in divided doses two to four times daily. Doses above 32 mg/day have been tolerated in a small number of adolescent patients for a relatively short duration.
In adults, GABITRIL should be initiated at 4 mg once daily. Modification of concomitant antiepilepsy drugs is not necessary, unless clinically indicated. The total daily dose of GABITRIL may be increased by 4 to 8 mg at weekly intervals until clinical response is achieved or, up to 56 mg/day. The total daily dose should be given in divided doses two to four times daily. Doses above 56 mg/day have not been systematically evaluated in adequate well-controlled trials.

Experience is limited in patients taking total daily doses above 32 mg/day using twice daily dosing. A typical dosing titration regimen for patients taking enzyme-inducing AEDs is provided in Table 6.
[See table 6 at left]

HOW SUPPLIED
GABITRIL Filmtab tablets are available in four dosage strengths.
4 mg yellow, round tablets, debossed with 🄰 on one side and the Abbo-Code FK on the opposite side, are available in bottles of 100 (**NDC** 0074-3904-13), and Abbo-Pac packages of 100 (**NDC** 0074-3904-11).
12 mg green, ovaloid tablets, debossed with 🄰 on one side and the Abbo-Code FL on the opposite side, are available in bottles of 100 (**NDC** 0074-3910-13), and Abbo-Pac packages of 100 (**NDC** 0074-3910-11).
16 mg blue, ovaloid tablets, debossed with 🄰 on one side and the Abbo-Code FM on the opposite side, are available in bottles of 100 (**NDC** 0074-3960-13), and Abbo-Pac packages of 100 (**NDC** 0074-3960-11).
20 mg pink, ovaloid tablets, debossed with 🄰 on one side and the Abbo-Code FN on the opposite side, are available in bottles of 100 (**NDC** 0074-3982-13), and Abbo-Pac packages of 100 (**NDC** 0074-3982-11).
Recommended Storage: Store tablets at controlled room temperature, between 20–25°C (68–77°F). See USP. Protect from light and moisture.

ANIMAL TOXICOLOGY
In repeat dose toxicology studies, dogs receiving daily oral doses of 5 mg/kg/day or greater experienced unexpected CNS effects throughout the study. These effects occurred acutely and included marked sedation and apparent visual impairment which was characterized by a lack of awareness of objects, failure to fix on and follow moving objects, and absence of a blink reaction. Plasma exposures (AUCs) at 5 mg/kg/day were equal to those in humans receiving the maximum recommended daily human dose of 56 mg/day. The effects were reversible upon cessation of treatment and were not associated with any observed structural abnormality. The implications of these findings for humans are unknown.

Filmtab® - Film-sealed tablets, Abbott

Revised: February, 1998

Ref.: 03-4834-R3

ABBOTT LABORATORIES 612-015-7822 **MASTER**
NORTH CHICAGO, IL 60064, U.S.A.
Shown in Product Identification Guide, page 303

HYTRIN® ℞
(terazosin hydrochloride)
Capsules

DESCRIPTION
HYTRIN (terazosin hydrochloride), an alpha-1-selective adrenoceptor blocking agent, is a quinazoline derivative represented by the following chemical name and structural formula:
(RS)-Piperazine, 1-(4-amino-6,7-dimethoxy-2-quinazolinyl)-4-[(tetra-hydro-2-furanyl)carbonyl]-, monohydrochloride, dihydrate.

Terazosin hydrochloride is a white, crystalline substance, freely soluble in water and isotonic saline and has a molecular weight of 459.93. HYTRIN capsules (terazosin hydrochloride capsules) for oral ingestion are supplied in four dosage strengths containing terazosin hydrochloride equivalent to 1 mg, 2 mg, 5 mg, or 10 mg of terazosin.
Inactive Ingredients:
1 mg capsules: gelatin, glycerin, iron oxide, methylparaben, mineral oil, polyethylene glycol, povidone, propylparaben, titanium dioxide, and vanillin.
2 mg capsules: D&C yellow No. 10, gelatin, glycerin, methylparaben, mineral oil, polyethylene glycol, povidone, propylparaben, titanium dioxide, and vanillin.
5 mg capsules: D&C red No. 28, FD&C red No. 40, gelatin, glycerin, methylparaben, mineral oil, polyethylene glycol, povidone, propylparaben, titanium dioxide, and vanillin.

Continued on next page

Hytrin—Cont.

10 mg capsules: FD&C blue No. 1, gelatin, glycerin, methylparaben, mineral oil, polyethylene glycol, povidone, propylparaben, titanium dioxide, and vanillin.

CLINICAL PHARMACOLOGY
Pharmacodynamics:
A. Benign Prostatic Hyperplasia (BPH)

The symptoms associated with BPH are related to bladder outlet obstruction, which is comprised of two underlying components: a static component and a dynamic component. The static component is a consequence of an increase in prostate size. Over time, the prostate will continue to enlarge. However, clinical studies have demonstrated that the size of the prostate does not correlate with the severity of BPH symptoms or the degree of urinary obstruction. The dynamic component is a function of an increase in smooth muscle tone in the prostate and bladder neck, leading to constriction of the bladder outlet. Smooth muscle tone is mediated by sympathetic nervous stimulation of alpha-1 adrenoceptors, which are abundant in the prostate, prostatic capsule and bladder neck. The reduction in symptoms and improvement in urine flow rates following administration of terazosin is related to relaxation of smooth muscle produced by blockade of alpha-1 adrenoceptors in the bladder neck and prostate. Because there are relatively few alpha-1 adrenoceptors in the bladder body, terazosin is able to reduce the bladder outlet obstruction without affecting bladder contractility.

Terazosin has been studied in 1222 men with symptomatic BPH. In three placebo-controlled studies, symptom evaluation and uroflowmetric measurements were performed approximately 24 hours following dosing. Symptoms were quantified using the Boyarsky Index. The questionnaire evaluated both obstructive (hesitancy, intermittency, terminal dribbling, impairment of size and force of stream, sensation of incomplete bladder emptying) and irritative (nocturia, daytime frequency, urgency, dysuria) symptoms by rating each of the 9 symptoms from 0–3, for a total score of 27 points. Results from these studies indicated that terazosin statistically significantly improved symptoms and peak urine flow rates over placebo as follows:

	Symptom Score (Range 0-27)		Peak Flow Rate (mL/sec)	
N	Mean Baseline	Mean Change (%)	N Mean Baseline	Mean Change (%)
Study 1 (10 mg)[a]				
Titration to fixed dose (12 wks)				
Placebo	55 9.7	−2.3 (24)	54 10.1	+1.0 (10)
Terazosin	54 10.1	−4.5 (45)*	52 8.8	+3.0 (34)*
Study 2 (2, 5, 10, 20 mg)[b]				
Titration to response (24 wks)				
Placebo	89 12.5	−3.8 (30)	88 8.8	+1.4 (16)
Terazosin	85 12.2	−5.3 (43)*	84 8.4	+2.9 (35)*
Study 3 (1, 2, 5, 10 mg)[c]				
Titration to response (24 wks)				
Placebo	74 10.4	−1.1 (11)	74 8.8	+1.2 (14)
Terazosin	73 10.9	−4.6 (42)*	73 8.6	+2.6 (30)*

[a] Highest dose 10 mg shown.
[b] 23% of patients on 10 mg, 41% of patients on 20 mg.
[c] 67% of patients on 10 mg.
* Significantly (p ≤ 0.05) more improvement than placebo.

In all three studies, both symptom scores and peak urine flow rates showed statistically significant improvement from baseline in patients treated with terazosin from week 2 (or the first clinic visit) and throughout the study duration.

Analysis of the effect of terazosin on individual urinary symptoms demonstrated that compared to placebo, terazosin significantly improved the symptoms of hesitancy, intermittency, impairment in size and force of urinary stream, sensation of incomplete emptying, terminal dribbling, daytime frequency and nocturia.

Global assessments of overall urinary function and symptoms were also performed by investigators who were blinded to patient treatment assignment. In studies 1 and 3, patients treated with terazosin had a significantly (p ≤ 0.001) greater overall improvement compared to placebo treated patients.

In a short term study (Study 1), patients were randomized to either 2, 5 or 10 mg of terazosin or placebo. Patients randomized to the 10 mg group achieved a statistically significant response in both symptoms and peak flow rate compared to placebo (Figure 1).
[See figure at top of next column]

In a long-term, open-label, non-placebo controlled clinical trial, 181 men were followed for 2 years and 58 of these men were followed for 30 months. The effect of terazosin on uri-

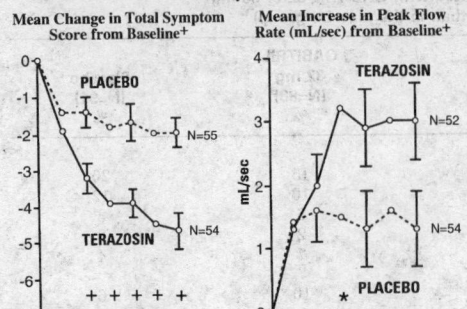

Figure 1
Study 1

Mean Change in Total Symptom Score from Baseline+

Mean Increase in Peak Flow Rate (mL/sec) from Baseline+

+ for baseline values see above table
* p ≤ 0.05, compared to placebo group

nary symptom scores and peak flow rates was maintained throughout the study duration (Figures 2 and 3):

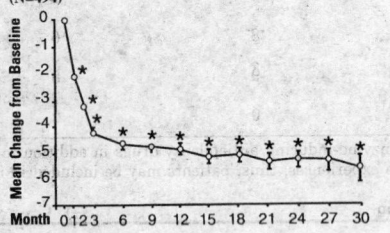

Figure 2
Mean Change in Total Symptom Score from Baseline
Long-Term, Open-Label, Non-Placebo Controlled Study
(N=494)

* p ≤ 0.05 vs. baseline
mean baseline = 10.7

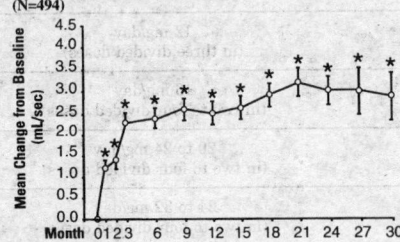

Figure 3
Mean Change in Peak Flow Rate from Baseline
Long-Term, Open-Label, Non-Placebo Controlled Study
(N=494)

* p ≤ 0.05 vs. baseline
mean baseline = 9.9

In this long-term trial, both symptom scores and peak urinary flow rates showed statistically significant improvement suggesting a relaxation of smooth muscle cells. Although blockade of alpha-1 adrenoceptors also lowers blood pressure in hypertensive patients with increased peripheral vascular resistance, terazosin treatment of normotensive men with BPH did not result in a clinically significant blood pressure lowering effect:

Mean Changes in Blood Pressure from Baseline to Final Visit in all Double-Blind, Placebo-Controlled Studies

	Group	Normotensive Patients DBP ≤90 mm Hg		Hypertensive Patients DBP >90 mm Hg	
		N	Mean Change	N	Mean Change
SBP	Placebo	293	−0.1	45	−5.8
(mm Hg)	Terazosin	519	−3.3*	65	−14.4*
DBP	Placebo	293	+0.4	45	−7.1
(mm Hg)	Terazosin	519	−2.2*	65	−15.1*

* p ≤ 0.05 vs. placebo

B. Hypertension

In animals, terazosin causes a decrease in blood pressure by decreasing total peripheral vascular resistance. The vasodilatory hypotensive action of terazosin appears to be produced mainly by blockade of alpha-1 adrenoceptors. Terazosin decreases blood pressure gradually within 15 minutes following oral administration.

Patients in clinical trials of terazosin were administered once daily (the great majority) and twice daily regimens with total doses usually in the range of 5–20 mg/day, and had mild (about 77%, diastolic pressure 95–105 mmHg) or moderate (23%, diastolic pressure 105–115 mmHg) hypertension. Because terazosin, like all alpha antagonists, can cause unusually large falls in blood pressure after the first dose or first few doses, the initial dose was 1 mg in virtually all trials, with subsequent titration to a specified fixed dose or titration to some specified blood pressure end point (usually a supine diastolic pressure of 90 mmHg).

Blood pressure responses were measured at the end of the dosing interval (usually 24 hours) and effects were shown to persist throughout the interval, with the usual supine responses 5–10 mmHg systolic and 3.5–8 mmHg diastolic greater than placebo. The responses in the standing position tended to be somewhat larger, by 1–3 mmHg, although this was not true in all studies. The magnitude of the blood pressure responses was similar to prazosin and less than hydrochlorothiazide (in a single study of hypertensive patients). In measurements 24 hours after dosing, heart rate was unchanged.

Limited measurements of peak response (2–3 hours after dosing) during chronic terazosin administration indicate that it is greater than about twice the trough (24 hour) response, suggesting some attenuation of response at 24 hours, presumably due to a fall in blood terazosin concentrations at the end of the dose interval. This explanation is not established with certainty, however, and is not consistent with the similarity of blood pressure response to once daily and twice daily dosing and with the absence of an observed dose-response relationship over a range of 5–20 mg, i.e., if blood concentrations had fallen to the point of providing less than full effect at 24 hours, a shorter dosing interval or larger dose should have led to increased response.

Further dose response and dose duration studies are being carried out. Blood pressure should be measured at the end of the dose interval; if response is not satisfactory, patients may be tried on a larger dose or twice daily dosing regimen. The latter should also be considered if possibly blood pressure-related side effects, such as dizziness, palpitations, or orthostatic complaints, are seen within a few hours after dosing.

The greater blood pressure effect associated with peak plasma concentrations (first few hours after dosing) appears somewhat more position-dependent (greater in the erect position) than the effect of terazosin at 24 hours and in the erect position there is also a 6–10 beat per minute increase in heart rate in the first few hours after dosing. During the first 3 hours after dosing 12.5% of patients had a systolic pressure fall of 30 mmHg or more from supine to standing, or standing systolic pressure below 90 mmHg with a fall of at least 20 mmHg, compared to 4% of a placebo group.

There was a tendency for patients to gain weight during terazosin therapy. In placebo-controlled monotherapy trials, male and female patients receiving terazosin gained a mean of 1.7 and 2.2 pounds respectively, compared to losses of 0.2 and 1.2 pounds respectively in the placebo group. Both differences were statistically significant.

During controlled clinical trials, patients receiving terazosin monotherapy had a small but statistically significant decrease (a 3% fall) compared to placebo in total cholesterol and the combined low-density and very-low-density lipoprotein fractions. No significant changes were observed in high-density lipoprotein fraction and triglycerides compared to placebo.

Analysis of clinical laboratory data following administration of terazosin suggested the possibility of hemodilution based on decreases in hematocrit, hemoglobin, white blood cells, total protein and albumin. Decreases in hematocrit and total protein have been observed with alpha-blockade and are attributed to hemodilution.

Pharmacokinetics:

Terazosin hydrochloride administered as HYTRIN capsules is essentially completely absorbed in man. Administration of capsules immediately after meals had a minimal effect on the extent of absorption. The time to reach peak plasma concentration however, was delayed by about 40 minutes. Terazosin has been shown to undergo minimal hepatic first-pass metabolism and nearly all of the circulating dose is in the form of parent drug. The plasma levels peak about one hour after dosing, and then decline with a half-life of approximately 12 hours. In a study that evaluated the effect of age on terazosin pharmacokinetics, the mean plasma half-lives were 14.0 and 11.4 hours for the age group ≥ 70 years and the age group of 20–39 years, respectively. After oral

administration the plasma clearance was decreased by 31.7% in patients 70 years of age or older compared to that in patients 20–39 years of age.

The drug is 90–94% bound to plasma proteins and binding is constant over the clinically observed concentration range. Approximately 10% of an orally administered dose is excreted as parent drug in the urine and approximately 20% is excreted in the feces. The remainder is eliminated as metabolites. Impaired renal function had no significant effect on the elimination of terazosin, and dosage adjustment of terazosin to compensate for the drug removal during hemodialysis (approximately 10%) does not appear to be necessary. Overall, approximately 40% of the administered dose is excreted in the urine and approximately 60% in the feces. The disposition of the compound in animals is qualitatively similar to that in man.

INDICATIONS AND USAGE

HYTRIN (terazosin hydrochloride) is indicated for the treatment of symptomatic benign prostatic hyperplasia (BPH). There is a rapid response, with approximately 70% of patients experiencing an increase in urinary flow and improvement in symptoms of BPH when treated with HYTRIN. The long-term effects of HYTRIN on the incidence of surgery, acute urinary obstruction or other complications of BPH are yet to be determined.

HYTRIN is also indicated for the treatment of hypertension. It can be used alone or in combination with other antihypertensive agents such as diuretics or beta-adrenergic blocking agents.

CONTRAINDICATIONS

HYTRIN capsules are contraindicated in patients known to be hypersensitive to terazosin hydrochloride.

WARNINGS

Syncope and "First-dose" Effect:

HYTRIN capsules, like other alpha-adrenergic blocking agents, can cause marked lowering of blood pressure, especially postural hypotension, and syncope in association with the first dose or first few days of therapy. A similar effect can be anticipated if therapy is interrupted for several days and then restarted. Syncope has also been reported with other alpha-adrenergic blocking agents in association with rapid dosage increases or the introduction of another antihypertensive drug. Syncope is believed to be due to an excessive postural hypotensive effect, although occasionally the syncopal episode has been preceded by a bout of severe supraventricular tachycardia with heart rates of 120–160 beats per minute. Additionally, the possibility of the contribution of hemodilution to the symptoms of postural hypotension should be considered. To decrease the likelihood of syncope or excessive hypotension, treatment should always be initiated with a 1 mg dose of terazosin, given at bedtime. The 2 mg, 5 mg and 10 mg capsules are not indicated as initial therapy. Dosage should then be increased slowly, according to recommendations in the Dosage and Administration section and additional antihypertensive agents should be added with caution. The patient should be cautioned to avoid situations, such as driving or hazardous tasks, where injury could result should syncope occur during initiation of therapy.

In early investigational studies, where increasing single doses up to 7.5 mg were given at 3 day intervals, tolerance to the first dose phenomenon did not necessarily develop and the "first-dose" effect could be observed at all doses. Syncopal episodes occurred in 3 of the 14 subjects given terazosin at doses of 2.5, 5 and 7.5 mg, which are higher than the recommended initial dose; in addition, severe orthostatic hypotension (blood pressure falling to 50/0 mmHg) was seen in two others and dizziness, tachycardia, and lightheadedness occurred in most subjects. These adverse effects all occurred within 90 minutes of dosing.

In three placebo-controlled BPH studies 1, 2, and 3 (see CLINICAL PHARMACOLOGY), the incidence of postural hypotension in the terazosin treated patients was 5.1%, 5.2%, and 3.7% respectively.

In multiple dose clinical trials involving nearly 2000 hypertensive patients treated with terazosin, syncope was reported in about 1% of patients. Syncope was not necessarily associated only with the first dose.

If syncope occurs, the patient should be placed in a recumbent position and treated supportively as necessary. There is evidence that the orthostatic effect of terazosin is greater, even in chronic use, shortly after dosing. The risk of the events is greatest during the initial seven days of treatment, but continues at all time intervals.

Priapism:

Rarely, (probably less than once in every several thousand patients) terazosin and other α_1-antagonists have been associated with priapism (painful penile erection, sustained for hours and unrelieved by sexual intercourse or masturbation). Two or three dozen cases have been reported. Because this condition can lead to permanent impotence if not promptly treated, patients must be advised about the seriousness of the condition (see **PRECAUTIONS: Information for Patients**).

PRECAUTIONS

General:

Prostatic Cancer

Carcinoma of the prostate and BPH cause many of the same symptoms. These two diseases frequently co-exist. Therefore, patients thought to have BPH should be examined prior to starting HYTRIN therapy to rule out the presence of carcinoma of the prostate.

Orthostatic Hypotension

While syncope is the most severe orthostatic effect of terazosin (see Warnings), other symptoms of lowered blood pressure, such as dizziness, lightheadedness and palpitations, were more common and occurred in some 28% of patients in clinical trials of hypertension. In BPH clinical trials, 21% of the patients experienced one or more of the following: dizziness, hypotension, postural hypotension, syncope, and vertigo. Patients with occupations in which such events represent potential problems should be treated with particular caution.

Information for Patients (see Patient Package Insert):

Patients should be made aware of the possibility of syncopal and orthostatic symptoms, especially at the initiation of therapy, and to avoid driving or hazardous tasks for 12 hours after the first dose, after a dosage increase and after interruption of therapy when treatment is resumed. They should be cautioned to avoid situations where injury could result should syncope occur during initiation of terazosin therapy. They should also be advised of the need to sit or lie down when symptoms of lowered blood pressure occur, although these symptoms are not always orthostatic, and to be careful when rising from a sitting or lying position. If dizziness, lightheadedness, or palpitations are bothersome they should be reported to the physician, so that dose adjustment can be considered.

Patients should also be told that drowsiness or somnolence can occur with terazosin, requiring caution in people who must drive or operate heavy machinery.

Patients should be advised about the possibility of priapism as a result of treatment with HYTRIN and other similar medications. Patients should know that this reaction to HYTRIN is extremely rare, but that if it is not brought to immediate medical attention, it can lead to permanent erectile dysfunction (impotence).

Laboratory Tests:

Small but statistically significant decreases in hematocrit, hemoglobin, white blood cells, total protein and albumin were observed in controlled clinical trials. These laboratory findings suggested the possibility of hemodilution. Treatment with terazosin for up to 24 months had no significant effect on prostate specific antigen (PSA) levels.

Drug Interactions:

In controlled trials, terazosin has been added to diuretics, and several beta-adrenergic blockers; no unexpected interactions were observed. Terazosin has also been used in patients on a variety of concomitant therapies; while these were not formal interaction studies, no interactions were observed. Terazosin has been used concomitantly in at least 50 patients on the following drugs or drug classes: 1) analgesic/anti-inflammatory (e.g., acetaminophen, aspirin, codeine, ibuprofen, indomethacin); 2) antibiotics (e.g., erythromycin, trimethoprim and sulfamethoxazole); 3) anti cholinergic/sympathomimetics (e.g., phenylephrine hydrochloride, phenylpropanolamine hydrochloride, pseudoephedrine hydrochloride); 4) antigout (e.g., allopurinol); 5) antihistamines (e.g., chlorpheniramine); 6) cardiovascular agents (e.g., atenolol, hydrochlorothiazide, methyclothiazide, propranolol); 7) corticosteroids; 8) gastrointestinal agents (e.g., antacids); 9) hypoglycemics; 10) sedatives and tranquilizers (e.g., diazepam).

Use with Other Drugs:

In a study (n=24) where terazosin and verapamil were administered concomitantly, terazosin's mean AUC_{0-24} increased 11% after the first verapamil dose and after 3 weeks of verapamil treatment it increased by 24% with associated increases in C_{max}(25%) and C_{min} (32%) means. Terazosin mean T_{max} decreased from 1.3 hours to 0.8 hours after 3 weeks of verapamil treatment. Statistically significant differences were not found in the verapamil level with and without terazosin. In a study (n=6) where terazosin and captopril were administered concomitantly, plasma disposition of captopril was not influenced by concomitant administration of terazosin and terazosin maximum plasma concentrations increased linearly with dose at steady-state after administration of terazosin plus captopril (see Dosage and Administration).

Carcinogenesis, Mutagenesis, Impairment of Fertility:

Terazosin was devoid of mutagenic potential when evaluated *in vivo* and *in vitro* (the Ames test, *in vivo* cytogenetics, the dominant lethal test in mice, *in vivo* Chinese hamster chromosome aberration test and V79 forward mutation assay).

Terazosin, administered in the feed to rats at doses of 8, 40, and 250 mg/kg/day (70, 350, and 2100 mg/M²/day), for two years, was associated with a statistically significant increase in benign adrenal medullary tumors of male rats exposed to the 250 mg/kg dose. This dose is 175 times the maximum recommended human dose of 20 mg (12 mg/M²). Female rats were unaffected. Terazosin was not oncogenic in mice when administered in feed for 2 years at a maximum tolerated dose of 32 mg/kg/day (110 mg/M²; 9 times the maximum recommended human dose). The absence of mutagenicity in a battery of tests, of tumorigenicity of any cell type in the mouse carcinogenicity assay, of increased total tumor incidence in either species, and of proliferative adrenal lesions in female rats, suggests a male rat species-specific event. Numerous other diverse pharmaceutical and chemical compounds have also been associated with benign adrenal medullary tumors in male rats without supporting evidence for carcinogenicity in man.

The effect of terazosin on fertility was assessed in a standard fertility/reproductive performance study in which male and female rats were administered oral doses of 8, 30 and 120 mg/kg/day. Four of 20 male rats given 30 mg/kg (240 mg/M²; 20 times the maximum recommended human dose) and five of 19 male rats given 120 mg/kg (960 mg/M²; 80 times the maximum recommended human dose) failed to sire a litter. Testicular weights and morphology were unaffected by treatment. Vaginal smears at 30 and 120 mg/kg/day, however, appeared to contain less sperm than smears from control matings and good correlation was reported between sperm count and subsequent pregnancy. Oral administration of terazosin for one or two years elicited a statistically significant increase in the incidence of testicular atrophy in rats exposed to 40 and 250 mg/kg/day (29 and 175 times the maximum recommended human dose), but not in rats exposed to 8 mg/kg/day (> 6 times the maximum recommended human dose). Testicular atrophy was also observed in dogs dosed with 300 mg/kg/day (> 500 times the maximum recommended human dose) for three months but not after one year when dosed with 20 mg/kg/day (38 times the maximum recommended human dose). This lesion has also been seen with Minipress®, another (marketed) selective-alpha-1 blocking agent.

Pregnancy:

Teratogenic effects: Pregnancy Category C. Terazosin was not teratogenic in either rats or rabbits when administered at oral doses up to 280 and 60 times, respectively, the maximum recommended human dose. Fetal resorptions occurred in rats dosed with 480 mg/kg/day, approximately 280 times the maximum recommended human dose. Increased fetal resorptions, decreased fetal weight and an increased number of supernumerary ribs were observed in offspring of rabbits dosed with 60 times the maximum recommended human dose. These findings (in both species) were most likely secondary to maternal toxicity. There are no adequate and well-controlled studies in pregnant women and the safety of terazosin in pregnancy has not been established. HYTRIN is not recommended during pregnancy unless the potential benefit justifies the potential risk to the mother and fetus.

Nonteratogenic effects: In a peri- and post-natal development study in rats, significantly more pups died in the group dosed with 120 mg/kg/day (> 75 times the maximum recommended human dose) than in the control group during the three-week postpartum period.

Nursing Mothers:

It is not known whether terazosin is excreted in breast milk. Because many drugs are excreted in breast milk, caution should be exercised when terazosin is administered to a nursing woman.

Pediatric Use:

Safety and effectiveness in children have not been determined.

ADVERSE REACTIONS

Benign Prostatic Hyperplasia

The incidence of treatment-emergent adverse events has been ascertained from clinical trials conducted worldwide. All adverse events reported during these trials were recorded as adverse reactions. The incidence rates presented below are based on combined data from six placebo-controlled trials involving once-a-day administration of terazosin at doses ranging from 1 to 20 mg. Table 1 summarizes those adverse events reported for patients in these trials when the incidence rate in the terazosin group was at least 1% and was greater than that for the placebo group, or where the reaction is of clinical interest. Asthenia, postural hypotension, dizziness, somnolence, nasal congestion/rhinitis, and impotence were the only events that were significantly (p ≤ 0.05) more common in patients receiving terazosin than in patients receiving placebo. The incidence of urinary tract infection was significantly lower in the patients receiving terazosin than in patients receiving placebo. An analysis of the incidence rate of hypotensive adverse events (see PRECAUTIONS) adjusted for the length of drug treatment has shown that the risk of the events is greatest during the initial seven days of treatment, but continues at all time intervals.

Continued on next page

Hytrin—Cont.

TABLE 1
ADVERSE REACTIONS DURING
PLACEBO-CONTROLLED TRIALS
BENIGN PROSTATIC HYPERPLASIA

Body System	Terazosin (N=636)	Placebo (N=360)
BODY AS A WHOLE		
† Asthenia	7.4%*	3.3%
Flu Syndrome	2.4%	1.7%
Headache	4.9%	5.8%
CARDIOVASCULAR SYSTEM		
Hypotension	0.6%	0.6%
Palpitations	0.9%	1.1%
Postural Hypotension	3.9%*	0.8%
Syncope	0.6%	0.0%
DIGESTIVE SYSTEM		
Nausea	1.7%	1.1%
METABOLIC AND NUTRITIONAL DISORDERS		
Peripheral Edema	0.9%	0.3%
Weight Gain	0.5%	0.0%
NERVOUS SYSTEM		
Dizziness	9.1%*	4.2%
Somnolence	3.6%*	1.9%
Vertigo	1.4%	0.3%
RESPIRATORY SYSTEM		
Dyspnea	1.7%	0.8%
Nasal Congestion/Rhinitis	1.9%*	0.0%
SPECIAL SENSES		
Blurred Vision/Amblyopia	1.3%	0.6%
UROGENITAL SYSTEM		
Impotence	1.6%*	0.6%
Urinary Tract Infection	1.3%	3.9%*

† Includes weakness, tiredness, lassitude and fatigue.
* p ≤ 0.05 comparison between groups.

Additional adverse events have been reported, but these are, in general, not distinguishable from symptoms that might have occurred in the absence of exposure to terazosin. The safety profile of patients treated in the long-term open-label study was similar to that observed in the controlled studies.

The adverse events were usually transient and mild or moderate in intensity, but sometimes were serious enough to interrupt treatment. In the placebo-controlled clinical trials, the rates of premature termination due to adverse events were not statistically different between the placebo and terazosin groups. The adverse events that were bothersome, as judged by their being reported as reasons for discontinuation of therapy by at least 0.5% of the terazosin group and being reported more often than in the placebo group, are shown in Table 2.

TABLE 2
DISCONTINUATION DURING
PLACEBO-CONTROLLED TRIALS
BENIGN PROSTATIC HYPERPLASIA

Body System	Terazosin (N=636)	Placebo (N=360)
BODY AS A WHOLE		
Fever	0.5%	0.0%
Headache	1.1%	0.8%
CARDIOVASCULAR SYSTEM		
Postural Hypotension	0.5%	0.0%
Syncope	0.5%	0.0%
DIGESTIVE SYSTEM		
Nausea	0.5%	0.3%
NERVOUS SYSTEM		
Dizziness	2.0%	1.1%
Vertigo	0.5%	0.0%
RESPIRATORY SYSTEM		
Dyspnea	0.5%	0.3%
SPECIAL SENSES		
Blurred Vision/Amblyopia	0.6%	0.0%
UROGENITAL SYSTEM		
Urinary Tract Infection	0.5%	0.3%

Hypertension

The prevalence of adverse reactions has been ascertained from clinical trials conducted primarily in the United States. All adverse experiences (events) reported during these trials were recorded as adverse reactions. The prevalence rates presented below are based on combined data from fourteen placebo-controlled trials involving once-a-day administration of terazosin, as monotherapy or in combination with other antihypertensive agents, at doses ranging from 1 to 40 mg. Table 3 summarizes those adverse experiences reported for patients in these trials where the prevalence rate in the terazosin group was at least 5%, where the prevalence rate for the terazosin group was at least 2% and was greater than the prevalence rate for the placebo group, or where the reaction is of particular interest. Asthenia, blurred vision, dizziness, nasal congestion, nausea, peripheral edema, palpitations and somnolence were the only symptoms that were significantly (p < 0.05) more common in patients receiving terazosin than in patients receiving placebo. Similar adverse reaction rates were observed in placebo-controlled monotherapy trials.

TABLE 3
ADVERSE REACTIONS DURING
PLACEBO-CONTROLLED TRIALS
HYPERTENSION

Body System	Terazosin (N=859)	Placebo (N=506)
BODY AS A WHOLE		
† Asthenia	11.3%*	4.3%
Back Pain	2.4%	1.2%
Headache	16.2%	15.8%
CARDIOVASCULAR SYSTEM		
Palpitations	4.3%*	1.2%
Postural Hypotension	1.3%	0.4%
Tachycardia	1.9%	1.2%
DIGESTIVE SYSTEM		
Nausea	4.4%*	1.4%
METABOLIC AND NUTRITIONAL DISORDERS		
Edema	0.9%	0.6%
Peripheral Edema	5.5%*	2.4%
Weight Gain	0.5%	0.2%
MUSCULOSKELETAL SYSTEM		
Pain-Extremities	3.5%	3.0%
NERVOUS SYSTEM		
Depression	0.3%	0.2%
Dizziness	19.3%*	7.5%
Libido Decreased	0.6%	0.2%
Nervousness	2.3%	1.8%
Paresthesia	2.9%	1.4%
Somnolence	5.4%*	2.6%
RESPIRATORY SYSTEM		
Dyspnea	3.1%	2.4%
Nasal Congestion	5.9%*	3.4%
Sinusitis	2.6%	1.4%
SPECIAL SENSES		
Blurred Vision	1.6%*	0.0%
UROGENITAL SYSTEM		
Impotence	1.2%	1.4%

† Includes weakness, tiredness, lassitude and fatigue.
* Statistically significant at p=0.05 level.

Additional adverse reactions have been reported, but these are, in general, not distinguishable from symptoms that might have occurred in the absence of exposure to terazosin. The following additional adverse reactions were reported by at least 1% of 1987 patients who received terazosin in controlled or open, short- or long-term clinical trials or have been reported during marketing experience: *Body as a Whole:* chest pain, facial edema, fever, abdominal pain, neck pain, shoulder pain; *Cardiovascular System:* arrhythmia, vasodilation; *Digestive System:* constipation, diarrhea, dry mouth, dyspepsia, flatulence, vomiting; *Metabolic/Nutritional Disorders:* gout; *Musculoskeletal System:* arthralgia, arthritis, joint disorder, myalgia; *Nervous System:* anxiety, insomnia; *Respiratory System:* bronchitis, cold symptoms, epistaxis, flu symptoms, increased cough, pharyngitis, rhinitis; *Skin and Appendages:* pruritus, rash, sweating; *Special Senses:* abnormal vision, conjunctivitis, tinnitus; *Urogenital System:* urinary frequency, urinary incontinence primarily reported in postmenopausal women, urinary tract infection.

Post-marketing experience indicates that in rare instances patients may develop allergic reactions, including anaphylaxis, following administration of terazosin hydrochloride. There have been reports of priapism during post-marketing surveillance.

The adverse reactions were usually mild or moderate in intensity but sometimes were serious enough to interrupt treatment. The adverse reactions that were most bothersome, as judged by their being reported as reasons for discontinuation of therapy by at least 0.5% of the terazosin group and being reported more often than in the placebo group, are shown in Table 4.

TABLE 4
DISCONTINUATIONS DURING
PLACEBO-CONTROLLED TRIALS
HYPERTENSION

Body System	Terazosin (N=859)	Placebo (N=506)
BODY AS A WHOLE		
Asthenia	1.6%	0.0%
Headache	1.3%	1.0%
CARDIOVASCULAR SYSTEM		
Palpitations	1.4%	0.2%
Postural Hypotension	0.5%	0.0%
Syncope	0.5%	0.2%
Tachycardia	0.6%	0.0%
DIGESTIVE SYSTEM		
Nausea	0.8%	0.0%
METABOLIC AND NUTRITIONAL DISORDERS		
Peripheral Edema	0.6%	0.0%
NERVOUS SYSTEM		
Dizziness	3.1%	0.4%
Paresthesia	0.8%	0.2%
Somnolence	0.6%	0.2%
RESPIRATORY SYSTEM		
Dyspnea	0.9%	0.6%
Nasal Congestion	0.6%	0.0%
SPECIAL SENSES		
Blurred Vision	0.6%	0.0%

OVERDOSAGE

Should overdosage of HYTRIN lead to hypotension, support of the cardiovascular system is of first importance. Restoration of blood pressure and normalization of heart rate may be accomplished by keeping the patient in the supine position. If this measure is inadequate, shock should first be treated with volume expanders. If necessary, vasopressors should then be used and renal function should be monitored and supported as needed. Laboratory data indicate that terazosin is 90–94% protein bound; therefore, dialysis may not be of benefit.

DOSAGE AND ADMINISTRATION

If HYTRIN administration is discontinued for several days, therapy should be reinstituted using the initial dosing regimen.

Benign Prostatic Hyperplasia:

Initial Dose:

1 mg at bedtime is the starting dose for all patients, and this dose should not be exceeded as an initial dose. Patients should be closely followed during initial administration in order to minimize the risk of severe hypotensive response.

Subsequent Doses:

The dose should be increased in a stepwise fashion to 2 mg, 5 mg, or 10 mg once daily to achieve the desired improvement of symptoms and/or flow rates. Doses of 10 mg once daily are generally required for the clinical response. Therefore, treatment with 10 mg for a minimum of 4–6 weeks may be required to assess whether a beneficial response has been achieved. Some patients may not achieve a clinical response despite appropriate titration. Although some additional patients responded at a 20 mg daily dose, there was an insufficient number of patients studied to draw definitive conclusions about this dose. There are insufficient data to support the use of higher doses for those patients who show inadequate or no response to 20 mg daily. **If terazosin administration is discontinued for several days or longer, therapy should be reinstituted using the initial dosing regimen.**

Use with Other Drugs:

Caution should be observed when HYTRIN is administered concomitantly with other antihypertensive agents, especially the calcium channel blocker verapamil, to avoid the possibility of developing significant hypotension. When using HYTRIN and other antihypertensive agents concomitantly, dosage reduction and retitration of either agent may be necessary (see Precautions).

Hypertension:
The dose of HYTRIN and the dose interval (12 or 24 hours) should be adjusted according to the patient's individual blood pressure response. The following is a guide to its administration:
Initial Dose:
1 mg at bedtime is the starting dose for all patients, and this dose should not be exceeded. This initial dosing regimen should be strictly observed to minimize the potential for severe hypotensive effects.
Subsequent Doses:
The dose may be slowly increased to achieve the desired blood pressure response. The usual recommended dose range is 1 mg to 5 mg administered once a day; however, some patients may benefit from doses as high as 20 mg per day. Doses over 20 mg do not appear to provide further blood pressure effect and doses over 40 mg have not been studied. Blood pressure should be monitored at the end of the dosing interval to be sure control is maintained throughout the interval. It may also be helpful to measure blood pressure 2–3 hours after dosing to see if the maximum and minimum responses are similar, and to evaluate symptoms such as dizziness or palpitations which can result from excessive hypotensive response. If response is substantially diminished at 24 hours an increased dose or use of a twice daily regimen can be considered. **If terazosin administration is discontinued for several days or longer, therapy should be reinstituted using the initial dosing regimen.** In clinical trials, except for the initial dose, the dose was given in the morning.
Use With Other Drugs: (see above)

HOW SUPPLIED

HYTRIN capsules (terazosin hydrochloride capsules) are available in four dosage strengths:
1 mg grey capsules (imprinted with [Abbott logo] and the Abbo-Code HH):
Bottles of 100 .... (**NDC** 0074-3805-13),
Abbo-Pac® unit dose strip packages
of 100 capsules .... (**NDC** 0074-3805-11).
2 mg yellow capsules (imprinted with [Abbott logo] and the Abbo-Code HY):
Bottles of 100 .... (**NDC** 0074-3806-13),
Abbo-Pac® unit dose strip packages
of 100 capsules .... (**NDC** 0074-3806-11).
5 mg red capsules (imprinted with [Abbott logo] and the Abbo-Code HK):
Bottles of 100 .... (**NDC** 0074-3807-13),
Abbo-Pac® unit dose strip packages
of 100 capsules .... (**NDC** 0074-3807-11).
10 mg blue capsules (imprinted with [Abbott logo] and the Abbo-Code HN):
Bottles of 100 .... (**NDC** 0074-3808-13),
Abbo-Pac® unit dose strip packages
of 100 capsules .... (**NDC** 0074-3808-11).
Recommended storage: Store at controlled room temperature between 20–25°C (68–77°F). See USP. Protect from light and moisture.
Revised: October, 1996
Ref. 03-4655-R3-Rev. Oct., 1996
ABBOTT LABORATORIES
NORTH CHICAGO, IL 60064, U.S.A
Shown in Product Identification Guide, page 303

IBERET®–500 Filmtab® tablets OTC

[ī 'be-ret]
High Potency Dietary Supplement
CONTROLLED-RELEASE IRON,
plus B-Complex & Vitamin C
Well-tolerated once-daily iron, B-complex and vitamin C supplement.

DESCRIPTION

> **WARNING:** Accidental overdose of iron-containing products is a leading cause of fatal poisoning in children under 6. Keep this product out of reach of children. In case of accidental overdose, call doctor or poison control center immediately.

Each Iberet-500 Filmtab tablet contains 525 mg of ferrous sulfate (equivalent to 105 mg of elemental iron) in the Gradumet® controlled-release vehicle. To enhance iron absorption, 500 mg of vitamin C has been added to each Iberet-500 Filmtab.
Each tablet provides:

*Ferrous Sulfate (equivalent to 105 mg of elemental iron)	525 mg
Vitamin C (as sodium ascorbate)	500 mg
Niacinamide	30 mg
Calcium Pantothenate	10 mg
Vitamin B_1 (Thiamine Mononitrate)	6 mg
Vitamin B_2 (Riboflavin)	6 mg
Vitamin B_6 (Pyridoxine Hydrochloride)	5 mg
Vitamin B_{12} (Cyanocobalamin)	25 mcg

*In Gradumet® controlled-release dose form.
Ingredients:
Ferrous sulfate, sodium ascorbate, methyl acrylate-methyl methacrylate copolymer, polyethylene glycol, hydroxypropyl methylcellulose, niacinamide, povidone, talc, calcium pantothenate, stearic acid, thiamine mononitrate, riboflavin,titanium dioxide, pyridoxine hydrochloride, FD&C Red No. 40, hyroxypropyl cellulose, ethylcellulose, magnesium stearate, propylene glycol, castor oil, FD&C Yellow No. 6, vanillin and cyanocobalamin (in corn starch).

DOSAGE AND ADMINISTRATION

Usual Adult Dose: One tablet daily, or as directed by the physician.
TO OPEN CHILD-RESISTANT BLISTER PACKAGE:
1. Tear from bottom edge on perforations at START TEAR arrows.
2. Fold back and peel paper from corner marked PEEL.
3. Push tablet through foil.

HOW SUPPLIED

Iberet-500 is supplied as red, oval shaped tablets in reclosable cartons of 30 tablets (5 child-resistant blister packages of 6 tablets), list no. 0074-7235-30. Do not accept if blister unit has been opened or seal has been broken.
Recommended storage: Store below 77°F (25°C). Protect from light to avoid tablet color changes.
Ref. 13-1744-4/R1

IBERET–FOLIC–500® Filmtab® Tablets ℞

Controlled-Release Iron with Vitamin C, and B-Complex including Folic Acid

See combined listing under FERO-FOLIC-500.

IBERET®–500 LIQUID OTC

[ī 'bê-rêt]
Hematinic Supplying Iron, Vitamin C and Vitamin B-Complex

IBERET®–LIQUID

Hematinic Supplying Iron, Vitamin C and Vitamin B-Complex

DESCRIPTION

Iberet-500 Liquid and Iberet-Liquid are hematinic preparations of ferrous sulfate, B-complex vitamins and ascorbic acid. Each teaspoonful (5 mL) of Iberet-500 Liquid provides:

Elemental Iron (as Ferrous Sulfate)	26.25 mg
Vitamin C (Ascorbic Acid)	125 mg
Niacinamide	7.5 mg
Dexpanthenol	2.5 mg
VitaminB_1 (Thiamine Hydrochloride)	1.5 mg
Vitamin B_2 (Riboflavin)	1.5 mg
Vitamin B_6 (Pyridoxine Hydrochloride)	1.25 mg
Vitamin B_{12} (Cyanocobalamin)	6.25 mcg

Iberet-500 liquid has a citrus-flavored vehicle.
Iberet-Liquid has a raspberry-mint flavored vehicle; Iberet-Liquid has a smaller amount of ascorbic acid: 37.5 mg per teaspoonful. Riboflavin 5′ phosphate sodium is the source of Vitamin B_2 in Iberet Liquid.
Inactive Ingredients:
Iberet-Liquid: Alcohol 1%, methylparaben, propylparaben, sorbitol, water, natural and artificial flavors.
Iberet-500 Liquid: Glycerin, methylparaben, propylene glycol, propylparaben, sodium bicarbonate, sorbitol, sucrose, water and artificial flavor.

INDICATIONS

Iberet-500 Liquid: For conditions in which iron deficiency occurs concomitantly with deficient intake or increased need for the B-complex vitamins.
Iberet-Liquid: For conditions in which iron deficiency and vitamin C deficiency occur concomitantly with deficient intake or increased need for the B-complex vitamins.

WARNING

Close tightly and keep out of reach of children. Contains iron, which can be harmful or fatal to children in large doses. In case of accidental overdose, seek professional assistance or contact a Poison Control Center immediately.

DOSAGE AND ADMINISTRATION

Iberet-500 Liquid: **Usual dosage: Adults, including pregnant females and children 4 years of age and older**—2 teaspoonfuls (10 mL) twice daily, after meals;
Children 1–3 years of age—1 teaspoonful (5 mL) twice daily, after meals. Otherwise as directed by the physician.
Iberet-Liquid: **Usual dosage: Adults, including pregnant females and children 4 years of age and older**—2 teaspoonfuls (10 mL) three times daily, after meals;
Children 1–3 years of age—1 teaspoonful (5 mL) three times daily, after meals. Otherwise as directed by the physician.

HOW SUPPLIED

Iberet-500 Liquid (**NDC** 0074-8422-02) and Iberet-Liquid (**NDC** 0074-7173-01) are supplied in 8 fl oz (236 mL) bottles. Bottle caps are child-resistant and provided with a tamper-evident band. Do not accept if printed band is broken or missing.
Recommended storage: Protect from temperatures above 77°F (25°C). Dispense in amber bottle only.
Ref. 02-7610-4/R23 and 02-7611-4/R20

K–LOR™ 20 mEq. ℞

[k 'lor]
(Potassium Chloride for Oral Solution, USP)

DESCRIPTION

Natural fruit-flavored K-LOR (potassium chloride for oral solution, USP) is an oral potassium supplement offered in individual packets as a powder for reconstitution. Each packet of K-LOR 20 mEq powder contains potassium 20 mEq and chloride 20 mEq provided by potassium chloride 1.5 g.
K-LOR powder is an electrolyte replenisher. The chemical name is potassium chloride, and the structural formula is KCl. Potassium chloride, USP, occurs as a white, granular powder or as colorless crystals. It is odorless and has a saline taste. Its solutions are neutral to litmus. It is freely soluble in water and insoluble in alcohol.
Inactive Ingredients: FD&C Yellow No. 6, maltodextrin (contains corn derivative), malic acid, saccharin, silica gel and natural flavoring.

CLINICAL PHARMACOLOGY

Potassium ion is the principal intracellular cation of most body tissues. Potassium ions participate in a number of essential physiological processes including the maintenance of intracellular tonicity, the transmission of nerve impulses, the contraction of cardiac, skeletal and smooth muscle, and the maintenance of normal renal function.
The intracellular concentration of potassium is approximately 150 to 160 mEq per liter. The normal adult plasma concentration is 3.5 to 5 mEq per liter. An active ion transport system maintains this gradient across the plasma membrane.
Potassium is a normal dietary constituent and under steady state conditions the amount of potassium absorbed from the gastrointestinal tract is equal to the amount excreted in the urine. The usual dietary intake of potassium is 50 to 100 mEq per day.
Potassium depletion will occur whenever the rate of potassium loss through renal excretion and/or loss from the gastrointestinal tract exceeds the rate of potassium intake. Such depletion usually develops as a consequence of therapy with diuretics, primary or secondary hyperaldosteronism, diabetic ketoacidosis, or inadequate replacement of potassium in patients on prolonged parenteral nutrition. Depletion can develop rapidly with severe diarrhea, especially if associated with vomiting. Potassium depletion due to these causes is usually accompanied by a concomitant loss of chloride and is manifested by hypokalemia and metabolic alkalosis. Potassium depletion may produce weakness, fatigue, disturbances of cardiac rhythm (primarily ectopic beats), prominent U-waves in the electrocardiogram, and, in advanced cases, flaccid paralysis and/or impaired ability to concentrate urine.
If potassium depletion associated with metabolic alkalosis cannot be managed by correcting the fundamental cause of the deficiency, e.g., where the patient requires long term diuretic therapy, supplemental potassium in the form of high potassium food or potassium chloride may restore normal potassium levels.
In rare circumstances, (e.g., patients with renal tubular acidosis), potassium depletion may be associated with metabolic acidosis and hyperchloremia. In such patients potassium replacement should be accomplished with potassium salts other than the chloride, such as potassium bicarbonate, potassium citrate, potassium acetate, or potassium gluconate.

INDICATIONS AND USAGE

1. For the treatment of patients with hypokalemia with or without metabolic alkalosis, in digitalis intoxication, and in patients with hypokalemic familial periodic paralysis. If hypokalemia is the result of diuretic therapy, consideration should be given to the use of a lower dose of diuretic, which may be sufficient without leading to hypokalemia.
2. For the prevention of hypokalemia in patients who would be at particular risk if hypokalemia were to develop, e.g., digitalized patients or patients with significant cardiac arrhythmias.

The use of potassium salts in patients receiving diuretics for uncomplicated essential hypertension is often unnecessary when such patients have a normal dietary pattern, and

Continued on next page

K-Lor—Cont.

when low doses of the diuretic are used. Serum potassium should be checked periodically, however, and, if hypokalemia occurs, dietary supplementation with potassium-containing foods may be adequate to control milder cases. In more severe cases, and if dose adjustment of the diuretic is ineffective or unwarranted, supplementation with potassium salts may be indicated.

CONTRAINDICATIONS

Potassium supplements are contraindicated in patients with hyperkalemia since a further increase in serum potassium concentration in such patients can produce cardiac arrest. Hyperkalemia may complicate any of the following conditions: chronic renal failure, systemic acidosis such as diabetic acidosis, acute dehydration, extensive tissue breakdown as in severe burns, adrenal insufficiency, or the administration of a potassium-sparing diuretic, e.g., spironolactone, triamterene, or amiloride (see OVERDOSAGE).
K-LOR (potassium chloride for oral solution) is contraindicated in patients with known hypersensitivity to any ingredient in this product.

WARNINGS

Hyperkalemia (See OVERDOSAGE)
In patients with impaired mechanisms for excreting potassium, the administration of potassium salts can produce hyperkalemia and cardiac arrest. This occurs most commonly in patients given potassium intravenously, but may also occur in patients given potassium orally. Potentially fatal hyperkalemia can develop rapidly and can be asymptomatic. The use of potassium salts in patients with chronic renal disease, or any other condition which impairs potassium excretion, requires particularly careful monitoring of the serum potassium concentration and appropriate dosage adjustment.
Interaction with Potassium-Sparing Diuretics
Hypokalemia should not be treated by the concomitant administration of potassium salts and a potassium-sparing diuretic, e.g., spironolactone, triamterene, or amiloride, since the simultaneous administration of these agents can produce severe hyperkalemia.
Interaction with Angiotensin Converting Enzyme Inhibitors
Angiotensin converting enzyme (ACE) inhibitors (e.g., captopril, enalapril) will produce some potassium retention by inhibiting aldosterone production. Potassium supplements should be given to patients receiving ACE inhibitors only with close monitoring
Metabolic Acidosis
Hypokalemia in patients with metabolic acidosis should be treated with an alkalinizing potassium salt such as potassium bicarbonate, potassium citrate, potassium acetate or potassium gluconate.

PRECAUTIONS

General: The diagnosis of potassium depletion is ordinarily made by demonstrating hypokalemia in a patient with a clinical history suggesting some cause for potassium depletion. In interpreting the serum potassium level, the physician should bear in mind that acute alkalosis *per se* can produce hypokalemia in the absence of a deficit in total body potassium, while acute acidosis *per se* can increase the serum potassium concentration to within the normal range even in the presence of a reduced total body potassium. The treatment of potassium depletion, particularly in the presence of cardiac disease, renal disease, or acidosis, requires careful attention to acid-base balance and appropriate monitoring of serum electrolytes, the electrocardiogram, and the clinical status of the patient.
Information for Patients: Physicians should consider reminding the patient of the following:
To dilute each packet of powder in 1/2 glassful of water or other liquid and take each dose after a meal.
To take this medicine following the frequency and amount prescribed by the physician. This is especially important if the patient is also taking diuretics and/or digitalis preparations.
Laboratory Tests: When blood is drawn for analysis of plasma potassium it is important to recognize that artifactual elevations can occur after improper venipuncture technique or as a result of *in vitro* hemolysis of the sample.
Drug Interactions: Potassium-sparing diuretics, angiotensin converting enzyme inhibitors (see WARNINGS).
Carcinogenesis, Mutagenesis, Impairment of Fertility: Carcinogenicity, mutagenicity and fertility studies in animals have not been performed. Potassium is a normal dietary constituent.
Pregnancy Category C: Animal reproduction studies have not been conducted with K-LOR powder. It is unlikely that potassium supplementation that does not lead to hyperkalemia would have an adverse effect on the fetus or would affect reproductive capacity.
Nursing Mothers: The normal potassium ion content of human milk is about 13 mEq per liter. Since oral potassium becomes part of the body potassium pool, as long as body potassium is not excessive, the contribution of potassium chloride supplementation should have little or no effect on the level in human milk.
Pediatric Use: Safety and effectiveness in children have not been established.

ADVERSE REACTIONS

One of the most severe adverse effects is hyperkalemia (see CONTRAINDICATIONS, WARNINGS and OVERDOSAGE).
The most common adverse reactions to oral potassium salts are nausea, vomiting, flatulence, abdominal pain/discomfort, and diarrhea. These symptoms are due to irritation of the gastrointestinal tract and are best managed by diluting the preparation further, taking the dose with meals, or reducing the amount taken at one time.
Skin rash has been reported rarely.

OVERDOSAGE

The administration of oral potassium salts to persons with normal excretory mechanisms for potassium rarely causes serious hyperkalemia. However, if excretory mechanisms are impaired or if intravenous administration is too rapid, potentially fatal hyperkalemia can result (see CONTRAINDICATIONS and WARNINGS). It is important to recognize that hyperkalemia is usually asymptomatic and may be manifested only by an increased serum potassium concentration (6.5–8.0 mEq/L) and characteristic electrocardiographic changes (peaking of T-waves, loss of P-waves, depression of S-T segments, and prolongation of the QT intervals). Late manifestations include muscle paralysis and cardiovascular collapse from cardiac arrest (9–12 mEq/L).
Treatment measures for hyperkalemia include the following:

1. Elimination of foods and medications containing potassium and of any agents with potassium-sparing properties;
2. Intravenous administration of 300 to 500 ml/hr of 10% dextrose solution containing 10–20 units of crystalline insulin per 1,000 ml;
3. Correction of acidosis, if present, with intravenous sodium bicarbonate;
4. Use of exchange resins, hemodialysis, or peritoneal dialysis.

In treating hyperkalemia, it should be recalled that in patients who have been stabilized on digitalis, lowering the serum potassium concentration too rapidly can produce digitalis toxicity.

DOSAGE AND ADMINISTRATION

The usual dietary potassium intake by the average adult is 50 to 100 mEq per day. Potassium depletion sufficient to cause hypokalemia usually requires the loss of 200 or more mEq of potassium from the total body store.
Dosage must be adjusted to the individual needs of each patient. The dose for the prevention of hypokalemia is typically in the range of 20 mEq per day. Doses of 40–100 mEq per day or more are used for the treatment of potassium depletion. Dosage should be divided if more than 20 mEq per day is given such that no more than 20 mEq is given in a single dose. The dose should be taken after a meal.
K-LOR 20 mEq powder provides 20 mEq of potassium chloride.
Each 20 mEq (one K-LOR mEq packet) of potassium should be dissolved in at least 4 oz (approximately 1/2 glassful) cold water or juice. This preparation, like other potassium supplements, must be properly diluted to avoid the possibility of gastrointestinal irritation.

HOW SUPPLIED

K-LOR 20 mEq (Potassium Chloride for Oral Solution, USP) is supplied in cartons of 30 packets (**NDC** 0074-3611-01), and in cartons of 100 packets (**NDC** 0074-3611-02). Each packet contains potassium, 20 mEq, and chloride, 20 mEq, provided by potassium chloride, 1.5 g.
Recommended storage: Store below 86°F (30°C).
Caution: Federal (U.S.A.) law prohibits dispensing without prescription.
TM—Trademark
Revised: June, 1994
Ref. 13-1379-5/R25

K-Tab® ℞
[*k 'tâb*]
(Potassium Chloride Extended-Release Tablets, USP)

DESCRIPTION

K-TAB (potassium chloride extended-release tablets) is a solid oral dosage form of potassium chloride containing 750 mg of potassium chloride, USP, equivalent to 10 mEq of potassium in a film-coated (not enteric-coated), wax matrix tablet. This formulation is intended to slow the release of potassium so that the likelihood of a high localized concentration of potassium chloride within the gastrointestinal tract is reduced. The expended inert, porous, wax/polymer matrix is not absorbed and may be excreted intact in the stool.
K-TAB tablets are an electrolyte replenisher. The chemical name is potassium chloride, and the structural formula is KCl. Potassium chloride, USP, occurs as a white, granular powder or as colorless crystals. It is odorless and has a saline taste. Its solutions are neutral to litmus. It is freely soluble in water and insoluble in alcohol.
Inactive Ingredients
Castor oil, cellulosic polymers, colloidal silicon dioxide, D&C Yellow No. 10, magnesium stearate, paraffin, polyvinyl acetate, titanium dioxide, vanillin and vitamin E.

CLINICAL PHARMACOLOGY

Potassium ion is the principal intracellular cation of most body tissues. Potassium ions participate in a number of essential physiological processes including the maintenance of intracellular tonicity, the transmission of nerve impulses, the contraction of cardiac, skeletal, and smooth muscle, and the maintenance of normal renal function.
The intracellular concentration of potassium is approximately 150 to 160 mEq per liter. The normal adult plasma concentration is 3.5 to 5 mEq per liter. An active ion transport system maintains this gradient across the plasma membrane.
Potassium is a normal dietary constituent and under steady state conditions the amount of potassium absorbed from the gastrointestinal tract is equal to the amount excreted in the urine. The usual dietary intake of potassium is 50 to 100 mEq per day.
Potassium depletion will occur whenever the rate of potassium loss through renal excretion and/or loss from the gastrointestinal tract exceeds the rate of potassium intake. Such depletion usually develops as a consequence of therapy with diuretics, primary or secondary hyperaldosteronism, diabetic ketoacidosis, or inadequate replacement of potassium in patients on prolonged parenteral nutrition. Depletion can develop rapidly with severe diarrhea, especially if associated with vomiting. Potassium depletion due to these causes is usually accompanied by a concomitant loss of chloride and is manifested by hypokalemia and metabolic alkalosis. Potassium depletion may produce weakness, fatigue, disturbances of cardiac rhythm (primarily ectopic beats), prominent U-waves in the electrocardiogram, and, in advanced cases, flaccid paralysis and/or impaired ability to concentrate urine.
If potassium depletion associated with metabolic alkalosis cannot be managed by correcting the fundamental cause of the deficiency, e.g., where the patient requires long term diuretic therapy, supplemental potassium in the form of high potassium food or potassium chloride may restore normal potassium levels.
In rare circumstances, (e.g., patients with renal tubular acidosis) potassium depletion may be associated with metabolic acidosis and hyperchloremia. In such patients potassium replacement should be accomplished with potassium salts other than the chloride, such as potassium bicarbonate, potassium citrate, potassium acetate, or potassium gluconate.

INDICATIONS AND USAGE

BECAUSE OF REPORTS OF INTESTINAL AND GASTRIC ULCERATION AND BLEEDING WITH CONTROLLED-RELEASE POTASSIUM CHLORIDE PREPARATIONS, THESE DRUGS SHOULD BE RESERVED FOR THOSE PATIENTS WHO CANNOT TOLERATE OR REFUSE TO TAKE LIQUID OR EFFERVESCENT POTASSIUM PREPARATIONS, OR FOR PATIENTS WITH WHOM THERE IS A PROBLEM OF COMPLIANCE WITH THESE PREPARATIONS.

1. For the treatment of patients with hypokalemia with or without metabolic alkalosis, in digitalis intoxication, and in patients with hypokalemic familial periodic paralysis. If hypokalemia is the result of diuretic therapy, consideration should be given to the use of a lower dose of diuretic, which may be sufficient without leading to hypokalemia.
2. For the prevention of hypokalemia in patients who would be at particular risk if hypokalemia were to develop, e.g., digitalized patients or patients with significant cardiac arrhythmias.

The use of potassium salts in patients receiving diuretics for uncomplicated essential hypertension is often unnecessary when such patients have a normal dietary pattern, and when low doses of the diuretic are used. Serum potassium should be checked periodically, however, and, if hypokalemia occurs, dietary supplementation with potassium-containing foods may be adequate to control milder cases. In more severe cases and if dose adjustment of the diuretic is ineffective or unwarranted supplementation with potassium salts may be indicated.

CONTRAINDICATIONS

Potassium supplements are contraindicated in patients with hyperkalemia since a further increase in serum potassium concentration in such patients can produce cardiac arrest. Hyperkalemia may complicate any of the following

conditions: chronic renal failure, systemic acidosis such as diabetic acidosis, acute dehydration, extensive tissue breakdown as in severe burns, adrenal insufficiency, or the administration of potassium-sparing diuretic, e.g., spironolactone, triamterene, or amiloride (see OVERDOSAGE).

K-TAB tablets are contraindicated in patients with known hypersensitivity to any ingredient in this product.

Controlled-release formulations of potassium chloride have produced esophageal ulceration in certain cardiac patients with esophageal compression due to an enlarged left atrium. Potassium supplementation, when indicated in such patients, should be given as a liquid preparation.

All solid oral dosage forms of potassium chloride are contraindicated in any patient in whom there is structural, pathological, e.g., diabetic gastroparesis, or pharmacologic (use of anticholinergic agents or other agents with anticholinergic properties at sufficient doses to exert anticholinergic effects) cause for arrest or delay in tablet passage through the gastrointestinal tract.

WARNINGS

Hyperkalemia (see OVERDOSAGE)

In patients with impaired mechanisms for excreting potassium, the administration of potassium salts can produce hyperkalemia and cardiac arrest. This occurs most commonly in patients given potassium intravenously, but may also occur in patients given potassium orally. Potentially fatal hyperkalemia can develop rapidly and can be asymptomatic. The use of potassium salts in patients with chronic renal disease, or any other condition which impairs potassium excretion, requires particularly careful monitoring of the serum potassium concentration and appropriate dosage adjustment.

Interaction with Potassium-Sparing Diuretics

Hypokalemia should not be treated by the concomitant administration of potassium salts and a potassium-sparing diuretic, e.g., spironolactone, triamterene, or amiloride, since the simultaneous administration of these agents can produce severe hyperkalemia.

Interaction with Angiotensin Converting Enzyme Inhibitors

Angiotensin converting enzyme (ACE) inhibitors (e.g., captopril, enalapril) will produce some potassium retention by inhibiting aldosterone production. Potassium supplements should be given to patients receiving ACE inhibitors only with close monitoring.

Gastrointestinal Lesions

Solid oral dosage forms of potassium chloride can produce ulcerative and/or stenotic lesions of the gastrointestinal tract. Based on spontaneous adverse reaction reports, enteric-coated preparations of potassium chloride are associated with an increased frequency of small bowel lesions (40-50 per 100,000 patient years) compared to sustained-release wax matrix formulations (less than one per 100,000 patient years). Because of the lack of extensive marketing experience with microencapsulated products, a comparison between such products and wax matrix or enteric-coated products is not available. K-TAB tablets consist of a wax matrix formulated to provide a controlled rate of release potassium chloride and thus to minimize the possibility of a high local concentration of potassium near the gastrointestinal wall.

Prospective trials have been conducted in normal human volunteers in which the upper gastrointestinal tract was evaluated by endoscopic inspection before and after one week of solid oral potassium chloride therapy. The ability of this model to predict events occuring in usual clinical practice is unknown. Trials which approximated usual clinical practice did not reveal any clear differences between the wax matrix and microencapsulated dosage forms. In contrast, there was a higher incidence of gastric and duodenal lesions in subjects receiving a high dose of a wax matrix controlled-release formulation under conditions which did not resemble usual or recommended clinical practice, i.e., 96 mEq per day in divided doses of potassium chloride administered, to fasted patients in the presence of an anticholinergic drug to delay gastric emptying. The upper gastrointestinal lesions observed by endoscopy were asymptomatic and were not accompanied by evidence of bleeding (hemoccult testing). The relevance of these findings to the usual conditions, i.e., nonfasting, no anticholinergic agent, and smaller doses, under which controlled-release potassium chloride products are used is uncertain. Epidemiologic studies have not identified an elevated risk, compared to microencapsulated products, for upper gastrointestinal lesions in patients receiving wax matrix formulations. K-TAB tablets should be discontinued immediately and the possibility of ulceration, obstruction or perforation considered if severe vomiting, abdominal pain, distention, or gastrointestinal bleeding occurs.

Metabolic Acidosis

Hypokalemia in patients with metabolic acidosis should be treated with an alkalinizing potassium salt such as potassium bicarbonate, potassium citrate, potassium acetate, or potassium gluconate.

PRECAUTIONS

General: The diagnosis of potassium depletion is ordinarily made by demonstrating hypokalemia in a patient with a clinical history suggesting some cause for potassium depletion. In interpreting the serum potassium level, the physician should bear in mind that acute alkalosis *per se* can produce hypokalemia in the absence of a deficit in total body potassium, while acute acidosis *per se* can increase the serum potassium concentration to within the normal range even in the presence of a reduced total body potassium. The treatment of potassium depletion, particularly in the presence of cardiac disease, renal disease, or acidosis, requires careful attention to acid-base balance and appropriate monitoring of serum electrolytes, the electrocardiogram, and the clinical status of the patient.

Information for Patients: Physicians should consider reminding the patient of the following:

To take each dose with meals and with a full glass of water or other liquid.

To take this medicine following the frequency and amount prescribed by the physician. This is especially important if the patient is also taking diuretics and/or digitalis preparations.

To check with the physician if there is trouble swallowing tablets or if the tablets seem to stick in the throat.

To check with the physician at once if tarry stools or other evidence of gastrointestinal bleeding is noticed.

To take each dose without crushing, chewing or sucking the tablets.

Laboratory Tests: When blood is drawn for analysis of plasma potassium it is important to recognize that artifactual elevations can occur after improper venipuncture technique or as a result of *in vitro* hemolysis of the sample.

Drug Interactions: Potassium-sparing diuretics, angiotensin converting enzyme inhibitors (see WARNINGS).

Carcinogenesis, Mutagenesis, Impairment of Fertility: Carcinogenicity, mutagenicity and fertility studies in animals have not been performed. Potassium is a normal dietary constituent.

Pregnancy Category C: Animal reproduction studies have not been conducted with K-TAB tablets. It is unlikely that potassium supplementation that does not lead to hyperkalemia would have an adverse effect on the fetus or would affect reproductive capacity.

Nursing Mothers: The normal potassium ion content of human milk is about 13 mEq per liter. Since oral potassium becomes part of the body potassium pool, as long as body potassium is not excessive, the contribution of potassium chloride supplementation should have little or no effect on the level in human milk.

Pediatric Use: Safety and effectiveness in children have not been established.

ADVERSE REACTIONS

One of the most severe adverse effects is hyperkalemia (see CONTRAINDICATIONS, WARNINGS, and OVERDOSAGE). There also have been reports of upper and lower gastrointestinal conditions including obstruction, bleeding, ulceration, and perforation (see CONTRAINDICATIONS and WARNINGS).

The most common adverse reactions to oral potassium salts are nausea, vomiting, flatulence, abdominal pain/discomfort, and diarrhea. These symptoms are due to irritation of the gastrointestinal tract and are best managed by taking the dose with meals, or reducing the amount taken at one time.

Skin rash has been reported rarely.

OVERDOSAGE

The administration of oral potassium salts to persons with normal excretory mechanisms for potassium rarely causes serious hyperkalemia. However, if excretory mechanisms are impaired or if intravenous administration is too rapid, potentially fatal hyperkalemia can result (see CONTRAINDICATIONS and WARNINGS). It is important to recognize that hyperkalemia is usually asymptomatic and may be manifested only by an increased serum potassium concentration (6.5-8.0 mEq/L) and characteristic electrocardiographic changes (peaking of T-waves, loss P-waves, depression of S-T segments, and prolongation of QT intervals). Late manifestations include muscle paralysis and cardiovascular collapse from cardiac arrest (9-12 mEq/L).

Treatment measures for hyperkalemia include the following:

1. Elimination of foods and medications containing potassium and of any agents with potassium-sparing properties;
2. Intravenous administration of 300 to 500 mL/hr of 10% dextrose solution containing 10-20 units of crystalline insulin per 1,000 mL;
3. Correction of acidosis, if present, with intravenous sodium bicarbonate;
4. Use of exchange resins, hemodialysis, or peritoneal dialysis.

In treating hyperkalemia, it should be recalled that in patients who have been stabilized on digitalis, lowering the serum potassium concentration too rapidly can produce digitalis toxicity.

DOSAGE AND ADMINISTRATION

The usual dietary potassium intake by the average adult is 50 to 100 mEq per day. Potassium depletion sufficient to cause hypokalemia usually requires the loss of 200 or more mEq of potassium from the total body store.

Dosage must be adjusted to the individual needs of each patient. The dose for the prevention of hypokalemia is typically in the range of 20 mEq per day. Doses of 40-100 mEq per day or more are used for the treatment of potassium depletion. Dosage should be divided if more than 20 mEq per day is given such that no more than 20 mEq is given in a single dose.

K-TAB tablets provide 10 mEq of potassium chloride.

K-TAB tablets should be taken with meals and with a glass of water or other liquid. This product should not be taken on an empty stomach because of its potential for gastric irritation (see WARNINGS).

NOTE: K-TAB tablets are to be swallowed whole without crushing, chewing or sucking the tablets.

HOW SUPPLIED

K-TAB (potassium chloride extended-release tablets, USP) contains 750 mg of potassium chloride (equivalent to 10 mEq). K-TAB tablets are provided as yellow, ovaloid, extended-release Filmtab® tablets in bottles of 100 (**NDC** 0074-7804-13), 1000 (**NDC** 0074-7804-19) and 5000 (**NDC** 0074-7804-59) and in ABBO-PAC® unit dose packages of 100 (**NDC** 0074-7804-11).

Recommended storage: Store below 86°F (30°C).

CAUTION: Federal (USA) law prohibits dispensing without prescription.

Revised: September, 1991

Filmtab—Film-sealed tablets, Abbott

Ref. 03-4415-R14 – Rev. September, 1991

Shown in Product Identification Guide, page 303

NEMBUTAL® SODIUM CAPSULES C-II ℞

[*nêm-bū-tal sō-dī-um*]

(pentobarbital sodium capsules, USP)

WARNING—MAY BE HABIT FORMING

DESCRIPTION

The barbiturates are nonselective central nervous system depressants which are primarily used as sedative hypnotics. The barbiturates and their sodium salts are subject to control under the Federal Controlled Substances Act (See "Drug Abuse and Dependence" section).

Barbiturates are substituted pyrimidine derivatives in which the basic structure common to these drugs is barbituric acid, a substance which has no central nervous system (CNS) activity. CNS activity is obtained by substituting alkyl, alkenyl, or aryl groups on the pyrimidine ring. Nembutal (pentobarbital sodium) is chemically represented by sodium 5-ethyl-5-(1-methylbutyl) barbiturate.

The structural formula for pentobarbitol sodium is:

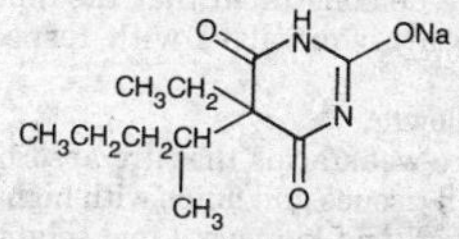

The sodium salt of pentobarbital occurs as a white, slightly bitter powder which is freely soluble in water and alcohol but practically insoluble in benzene and ether. Nembutal Sodium capsules for oral administration contain either 50 mg or 100 mg of pentobarbital sodium.

Inactive Ingredients: 50 mg Capsule: FD&C Blue No. 1, FD&C Red No. 3, FD&C Yellow No. 6, gelatin, lactose, magnesium stearate, polacrilin potassium and potassium chloride.

100 mg Capsule: colloidal silicon dioxide, corn starch, FD&C Blue No. 1, FD&C Red No. 3, FD&C Yellow No. 5 (tartrazine), FD&C Yellow No. 6, gelatin, magnesium stearate and potassium chloride.

CLINICAL PHARMACOLOGY

Barbiturates are capable of producing all levels of CNS mood alteration from excitation to mild sedation, to hypnosis, and deep coma. Overdosage can produce death. In high enough therapeutic doses, barbiturates induce anesthesia.

Barbiturates depress the sensory cortex, decrease motor activity, alter cerebellar function, and produce drowsiness, sedation, and hypnosis.

Barbiturate-induced sleep differs from physiological sleep. Sleep laboratory studies have demonstrated that barbiturates reduce the amount of time spent in the rapid eye movement (REM) phase of sleep or dreaming stage. Also, Stages III and IV sleep are decreased. Following abrupt ces-

Continued on next page

Nembutal Sodium Capsules—Cont.

sation of barbiturates used regularly, patients may experience markedly increased dreaming, nightmares, and/or insomnia. Therefore, withdrawal of a single therapeutic dose over 5 or 6 days has been recommended to lessen the REM rebound and disturbed sleep which contribute to drug withdrawal syndrome (for example, decrease the dose from 3 to 2 doses a day for 1 week).

In studies, secobarbital sodium and pentobarbital sodium have been found to lose most of their effectiveness for both inducing and maintaining sleep by the end of 2 weeks of continued drug administration at fixed doses. The short-, intermediate-, and, to a lesser degree, long-acting barbiturates have been widely prescribed for treating insomnia. Although the clinical literature abounds with claims that the short-acting barbiturates are superior for producing sleep while the intermediate-acting compounds are more effective in maintaining sleep, controlled studies have failed to demonstrate these differential effects. Therefore, as sleep medications, the barbiturates are of limited value beyond short-term use.

Barbiturates have little analgesic action at subanesthetic doses. Rather, in subanesthetic doses these drugs may increase the reaction to painful stimuli. All barbiturates exhibit anticonvulsant activity in anesthetic doses. However, of the drugs in this class, only phenobarbital, mephobarbital, and metharbital have been clinically demonstrated to be effective as oral anticonvulsants in subhypnotic doses.

Barbiturates are respiratory depressants. The degree of respiratory depression is dependent upon dose. With hypnotic doses, respiratory depression produced by barbiturates is similar to that which occurs during physiologic sleep with slight decrease in blood pressure and heart rate.

Studies in laboratory animals have shown that barbiturates cause reduction in the tone and contractility of the uterus, ureters, and urinary bladder. However, concentrations of the drugs required to produce this effect in humans are not reached with sedative-hypnotic doses.

Barbiturates do not impair normal hepatic function, but have been shown to induce liver microsomal enzymes, thus increasing and/or altering the metabolism of barbiturates and other drugs. (See "Precautions—*Drug Interactions*" section).

Pharmacokinetics: Barbiturates are absorbed in varying degrees following oral, rectal, or parenteral administration. The salts are more rapidly absorbed than are the acids. The rate of absorption is increased if the sodium salt is ingested as a dilute solution or taken on an empty stomach.

The onset of action for oral or rectal administration varies from 20 to 60 minutes.

Duration of action, which is related to the rate at which the barbiturates are redistributed throughout the body, varies among persons and in the same person from time to time. In Table 1, the barbiturates are classified according to their duration of action. This classification should not be used to predict the exact duration of effect, but the grouping of drugs should be used as a guide in the selection of barbiturates.

No studies have demonstrated that the different routes of administration are equivalent with respect to bioavailability.

[See Table 1 below]

Barbiturates are weak acids that are absorbed and rapidly distributed to all tissues and fluids with high concentrations in the brain, liver, and kidneys. Lipid solubility of the barbiturates is the dominant factor in their distribution within the body. The more lipid soluble the barbiturate, the more rapidly it penetrates all tissues of the body. Barbiturates are bound to plasma and tissue proteins to a varying degree with the degree of binding increasing directly as a function of lipid solubility.

Phenobarbital has the lowest lipid solubility, lowest plasma binding, lowest brain protein binding, the longest delay in onset of activity, and the longest duration of action. At the opposite extreme is secobarbital which has the highest lipid solubility, plasma protein binding, brain protein binding, the shortest delay in onset of activity, and the shortest duration of action. Butabarbital is classified as an intermediate barbiturate.

The plasma half-life for pentobarbital in adults is 15 to 50 hours and appears to be dose dependent.

Barbiturates are metabolized primarily by the hepatic microsomal enzyme system, and the metabolic products are excreted in the urine, and less commonly, in the feces. Approximately 25 to 50 percent of a dose of aprobarbital or phenobarbital is eliminated unchanged in the urine, whereas the amount of other barbiturates excreted unchanged in the urine is negligible. The excretion of unmetabolized barbiturate is one feature that distinguishes the long-acting category from those belonging to other categories which are almost entirely metabolized. The inactive metabolites of the barbiturates are excreted as conjugates of glucuronic acid.

INDICATIONS AND USAGE

Oral:
a. Sedatives.
b. Hypnotics, for the short-term treatment of insomnia, since they appear to lose their effectiveness for sleep induction and sleep maintenance after 2 weeks (See "Clinical Pharmacology" section).
c. Preanesthetics.

CONTRAINDICATIONS

Barbiturates are contraindicated in patients with known barbiturate sensitivity. Barbiturates are also contraindicated in patients with a history of manifest or latent porphyria.

WARNINGS

1. *Habit forming:* Barbiturates may be habit forming. Tolerance, psychological and physical dependence may occur with continued use. (See "Drug Abuse and Dependence" and "Pharmacokinetics" sections). Patients who have psychological dependence on barbiturates may increase the dosage or decrease the dosage interval without consulting a physician and may subsequently develop a physical dependence on barbiturates. To minimize the possibility of overdosage or the development of dependence, the prescribing and dispensing of sedative-hypnotic barbiturates should be limited to the amount required for the interval until the next appointment. Abrupt cessation after prolonged use in the dependent person may result in withdrawal symptoms, including delirium, convulsions, and possibly death. Barbiturates should be withdrawn gradually from any patient known to be taking excessive dosage over long periods of time. (See "Drug Abuse and Dependence" section).

2. *Acute or chronic pain:* Caution should be exercised when barbiturates are administered to patients with acute or chronic pain, because paradoxical excitement could be induced or important symptoms could be masked. However, the use of barbiturates as sedatives in the postoperative surgical period and as adjuncts to cancer chemotherapy is well established.

3. *Use in pregnancy:* Barbiturates can cause fetal damage when administered to a pregnant woman. Retrospective, case-controlled studies have suggested a connection between the maternal consumption of barbiturates and a higher than expected incidence of fetal abnormalities. Following oral or parenteral administration, barbiturates readily cross the placental barrier and are distributed throughout fetal tissues with highest concentrations found in the placenta, fetal liver, and brain.
Withdrawal symptoms occur in infants born to mothers who receive barbiturates throughout the last trimester of pregnancy. (See "Drug Abuse and Dependence" section). If this drug is used during pregnancy, or if the patient becomes pregnant while taking this drug, the patient should be apprised of the potential hazard to the fetus.

4. *Synergistic effects:* The concomitant use of alcohol or other CNS depressants may produce additive CNS depressant effects.

PRECAUTIONS

General: Barbiturates may be habit forming. Tolerance and psychological and physical dependence may occur with continuing use. (See "Drug Abuse and Dependence" section). Barbiturates should be administered with caution, if at all, to patients who are mentally depressed, have suicidal tendencies, or a history of drug abuse.

Elderly or debilitated patients may react to barbiturates with marked excitement, depression, and confusion. In some persons, barbiturates repeatedly produce excitement rather than depression.

In patients with hepatic damage, barbiturates should be administered with caution and initially in reduced doses. Barbiturates should not be administered to patients showing the premonitory signs of hepatic coma.

The 100 mg dosage strength of Nembutal Sodium capsules contains FD&C Yellow No. 5 (tartrazine) which may cause allergic-type reactions (including bronchial asthma) in certain susceptible individuals. Although the overall incidence of FD&C Yellow No. 5 (tartrazine) sensitivity in the general population is low, it is frequently seen in patients who also have aspirin hypersensitivity.

Information for the patient: Practitioners should give the following information and instructions to patients receiving barbiturates.

1. The use of barbiturates carries with it an associated risk of psychological and/or physical dependence. The patient should be warned against increasing the dose of the drug without consulting a physician.

2. Barbiturates may impair mental and/or physical abilities required for the performance of potentially hazardous tasks (e.g., driving, operating machinery, etc.).

3. Alcohol should not be consumed while taking barbiturates. Concurrent use of the barbiturates with other CNS depressants (e.g., alcohol, narcotics, tranquilizers, and antihistamines) may result in additional CNS depressant effects.

Laboratory tests: Prolonged therapy with barbiturates should be accompanied by periodic laboratory evaluation of organ systems, including hematopoietic, renal, and hepatic systems. (See "Precautions—General" and "Adverse Reactions" sections).

Drug interactions: Most reports of clinically significant drug interactions occurring with the barbiturates have involved phenobarbital. However, the application of these data to other barbiturates appears valid and warrants serial blood level determinations of the relevant drugs when there are multiple therapies.

1. *Anticoagulants:* Phenobarbital lowers the plasma levels of dicumarol (name previously used: bishydroxycoumarin) and causes a decrease in anticoagulant activity as measured by the prothrombin time. Barbiturates can induce hepatic microsomal enzymes resulting in increased metabolism and decreased anticoagulant response of oral anticoagulants (e.g., warfarin, acenocoumarol, dicumarol and phenprocoumon). Patients stabilized on anticoagulant therapy may require dosage adjustments if barbiturates are added to or withdrawn from their dosage regimen.

2. *Corticosteroids:* Barbiturates appear to enhance the metabolism of exogenous corticosteroids probably through the induction of hepatic microsomal enzymes. Patients stabilized on corticosteroid therapy may require dosage adjustments if barbiturates are added to or withdrawn from their dosage regimen.

3. *Griseofulvin:* Phenobarbital appears to interfere with the absorption of orally administered griseofulvin, thus decreasing its blood level. The effect of the resultant decreased blood levels of griseofulvin on therapeutic response has not been established. However, it would be preferable to avoid concomitant administration of these drugs.

4. *Doxycycline:* Phenobarbital has been shown to shorten the half-life of doxycycline for as long as 2 weeks after barbiturate therapy is discontinued.
This mechanism is probably through the induction of hepatic microsomal enzymes that metabolize the antibiotic. If phenobarbital and doxycycline are administered concurrently, the clinical response to doxycycline should be monitored closely.

5. *Phenytoin, sodium valproate, valproic acid:* The effect of barbiturates on the metabolism of phenytoin appears to be variable. Some investigators report an accelerating effect, while others report no effect. Because the effect of barbiturates on the metabolism of phenytoin is not predictable, phenytoin and barbiturate blood levels should be monitored more frequently if these drugs are given concurrently. Sodium valproate and valproic acid appear to decrease barbiturate metabolism; therefore, barbiturate blood levels should be monitored and appropriate dosage adjustments made as indicated.

6. *Central nervous system depressants:* The concomitant use of other central nervous system depressants, including other sedatives or hypnotics, antihistamines, tranquilizers, or alcohol, may produce additive depressant effects.

7. *Monoamine oxidase inhibitors (MAOI):* MAOI prolong the effects of barbiturates probably because metabolism of the barbiturate is inhibited.

8. *Estradiol, estrone, progesterone and other steroidal hormones:* Pretreatment with or concurrent administration of phenobarbital may decrease the effect of estradiol by increasing its metabolism. There have been reports of pa-

Table 1.—*Classification, Onset, and Duration of Action of Commonly used Barbiturates Taken Orally*

Classification	Onset of action	Duration of action
Long-acting Phenobarbital.	1 hour or longer	10 to 12 hours

Intermediate
    Amobarbital
    Butabarbital.
	$^3/_4$ to 1 hour	6 to 8 hours

Short-acting
    Pentobarbital
    Secobarbital.
	10 to 15 minutes	3 to 4 hours

tients treated with antiepileptic drugs (e.g., phenobarbital) who became pregnant while taking oral contraceptives. An alternate contraceptive method might be suggested to women taking phenobarbital.

Carcinogenesis: 1. Animal data. Phenobarbital sodium is carcinogenic in mice and rats after lifetime administration. In mice, it produced benign and malignant liver cell tumors. In rats, benign liver cell tumors were observed very late in life.

2. Human data. In a 29-year epidemiological study of 9,136 patients who were treated on an anticonvulsant protocol that included phenobarbital, results indicated a higher than normal incidence of hepatic carcinoma. Previously, some of these patients were treated with thorotrast, a drug that is known to produce hepatic carcinomas. Thus, this study did not provide sufficient evidence that phenobarbital sodium is carcinogenic in humans.

Data from one retrospective study of 235 children in which the types of barbiturates are not identified suggested an association between exposure to barbiturates prenatally and an increased incidence of brain tumor. (Gold, E., et al., "Increased Risk of Brain Tumors in Children Exposed to Barbiturates," Journal of National Cancer Institute, 61:1031–1034, 1978).

Pregnancy: 1. Teratogenic effects. Pregnancy Category D—See "Warnings—Use in Pregnancy" section.

2. *Nonteratogenic effects.* Reports of infants suffering from long-term barbiturate exposure in utero included the acute withdrawal syndrome of seizures and hyperirritability from birth to a delayed onset of up to 14 days. (See "Drug Abuse and Dependence" section).

Labor and delivery: Hypnotic doses of these barbiturates do not appear to significantly impair uterine activity during labor. Full anesthetic doses of barbiturates decrease the force and frequency of uterine contractions. Administration of sedative-hypnotic barbiturates to the mother during labor may result in respiratory depression in the newborn. Premature infants are particularly susceptible to the depressant effects of barbiturates. If barbiturates are used during labor and delivery, resuscitation equipment should be available.

Data are currently not available to evaluate the effect of these barbiturates when forceps delivery or other intervention is necessary. Also, data are not available to determine the effect of these barbiturates on the later growth, development, and functional maturation of the child.

Nursing mothers: Caution should be exercised when a barbiturate is administered to a nursing woman since small amounts of barbiturates are excreted in the milk.

ADVERSE REACTIONS

The following adverse reactions and their incidence were compiled from surveillance of thousands of hospitalized patients. Because such patients may be less aware of certain of the milder adverse effects of barbiturates, the incidence of these reactions may be somewhat higher in fully ambulatory patients.

More than 1 in 100 patients. The most common adverse reaction estimated to occur at a rate of 1 to 3 patients per 100 is: *Nervous System:* Somnolence.

Less than 1 in 100 patients. Adverse reactions estimated to occur at a rate of less than 1 in 100 patients listed below, grouped by organ system, and by decreasing order of occurrence are:

Nervous system: Agitation, confusion, hyperkinesia, ataxia, CNS depression, nightmares, nervousness, psychiatric disturbance, hallucinations, insomnia, anxiety, dizziness, thinking abnormality.

Respiratory system: Hypoventilation, apnea.

Cardiovascular system: Bradycardia, hypotension, syncope.

Digestive system: Nausea, vomiting, constipation.

Other reported reactions: Headache, injection site reactions, hypersensitivity reactions (angioedema, skin rashes, exfoliative dermatitis), fever, liver damage, megaloblastic anemia following chronic phenobarbital use.

DRUG ABUSE AND DEPENDENCE

Pentobarbital sodium capsules are subject to control by the Federal Controlled Substances Act under DEA schedule II.

Barbiturates may be habit forming. Tolerance, psychological dependence, and physical dependence may occur especially following prolonged use of high doses of barbiturates. Daily administration in excess of 400 milligrams (mg) of pentobarbital or secobarbital for approximately 90 days is likely to produce some degree of physical dependence. A dosage of from 600 to 800 mg taken for at least 35 days is sufficient to produce withdrawal seizures. The average daily dose for the barbiturate addict is usually about 1.5 grams. As tolerance to barbiturates develops, the amount needed to maintain the same level of intoxication increases; tolerance to a fatal dosage, however, does not increase more than two-fold. As this occurs, the margin between an intoxicating dosage and fatal dosage becomes smaller.

Symptoms of acute intoxication with barbiturates include unsteady gait, slurred speech, and sustained nystagmus.

Table 2.—*Concentration of Barbiturate in the Blood Versus Degree of CNS Depression*

Blood barbiturate level in ppm (μg/ml)

Barbiturate	Onset/duration	Degree of depression in nontolerant persons* 1	2	3	4	5
Pentobarbital	Fast/short	≤2	0.5 to 3	10 to 15	12 to 25	15 to 40
Secobarbital	Fast/short	≤2	0.5 to 5	10 to 15	15 to 25	15 to 40
Amobarbital	Intermediate/ intermediate	≤3	2 to 10	30 to 40	30 to 60	40 to 80
Butabarbital	Intermediate/ intermediate	≤5	3 to 25	40 to 60	50 to 80	60 to 100
Phenobarbital	Slow/long	≤10	5 to 40	50 to 80	70 to 120	100 to 200

* Categories of degree of depression in nontolerant persons:
1. Under the influence and appreciably impaired for purposes of driving a motor vehicle or performing tasks requiring alertness and unimpaired judgment and reaction time.
2. Sedated, therapeutic range, calm, relaxed, and easily aroused.
3. Comatose, difficult to arouse, significant depression of respiration.
4. Compatible with death in aged or ill persons or in presence of obstructed airway, other toxic agents, or exposure to cold.
5. Usual lethal level, the upper end of the range includes those who received some supportive treatment.

Mental signs of chronic intoxication include confusion, poor judgment, irritability, insomnia, and somatic complaints.

Symptoms of barbiturate dependence are similar to those of chronic alcoholism. If an individual appears to be intoxicated with alcohol to a degree that is radically disproportionate to the amount of alcohol in his or her blood the use of barbiturates should be suspected. The lethal dose of a barbiturate is far less if alcohol is also ingested.

The symptoms of barbiturate withdrawal can be severe and may cause death. Minor withdrawal symptoms may appear 8 to 12 hours after the last dose of a barbiturate. These symptoms usually appear in the following order: anxiety, muscle twitching, tremor of hands and fingers, progressive weakness, dizziness, distortion in visual perception, nausea, vomiting, insomnia, and orthostatic hypotension. Major withdrawal symptoms (convulsions and delirium) may occur within 16 hours and last up to 5 days after abrupt cessation of these drugs. Intensity of withdrawal symptoms gradually declines over a period of approximately 15 days. Individuals susceptible to barbiturate abuse and dependence include alcoholics and opiate abusers, as well as other sedative-hypnotic and amphetamine abusers.

Drug dependence to barbiturates arises from repeated administration of a barbiturate or agent with barbiturate-like effect on a continuous basis, generally in amounts exceeding therapeutic dose levels. The characteristics of drug dependence to barbiturates include: (a) a strong desire or need to continue taking the drug; (b) a tendency to increase the dose; (c) a psychic dependence on the effects of the drug related to subjective and individual appreciation of those effects; and (d) a physical dependence on the effects of the drug requiring its presence for maintenance of homeostasis and resulting in a definite, characteristic, and self-limited abstinence syndrome when the drug is withdrawn.

Treatment of barbiturate dependence consists of cautious and gradual withdrawal of the drug. Barbiturate-dependent patients can be withdrawn by using a number of different withdrawal regimens. In all cases withdrawal takes an extended period of time. One method involves substituting a 30 mg dose of phenobarbital for each 100 to 200 mg dose of barbiturate that the patient has been taking. The total daily amount of phenobarbital is then administered in 3 to 4 divided doses, not to exceed 600 mg daily. Should signs of withdrawal occur on the first day of treatment, a loading dose of 100 to 200 mg of phenobarbital may be administered IM in addition to the oral dose. After stabilization on phenobarbital, the total daily dose is decreased by 30 mg a day as long as withdrawal is proceeding smoothly. A modification of this regimen involves initiating treatment at the patient's regular dosage level and decreasing the daily dosage by 10 percent if tolerated by the patient.

Infants physically dependent on barbiturates may be given phenobarbital 3 to 10 mg/kg/day. After withdrawal symptoms (hyperactivity, disturbed sleep, tremors, hyperreflexia) are relieved, the dosage of phenobarbital should be gradually decreased and completely withdrawn over a 2 week period.

OVERDOSAGE

The toxic dose of barbiturates varies considerably. In general, an oral dose of 1 gram of most barbiturates produces serious poisoning in an adult. Death commonly occurs after 2 to 10 grams of ingested barbiturate. Barbiturate intoxication may be confused with alcoholism, bromide intoxication, and with various neurological disorders.

Acute overdosage with barbiturates is manifested by CNS and respiratory depression which may progress to Cheyne-Stokes respiration, areflexia, constriction of the pupils to a slight degree (though in severe poisoning they may show paralytic dilation), oliguria, tachycardia, hypotension, lowered body temperature, and coma. Typical shock syndrome (apnea, circulatory collapse, respiratory arrest, and death) may occur.

In extreme overdose, all electrical activity in the brain may cease, in which case a "flat" EEG normally equated with clinical death cannot be accepted. This effect is fully reversible unless hypoxic damage occurs. Consideration should be given to the possibility of barbiturate intoxication even in situations that appear to involve trauma.

Complications such as pneumonia, pulmonary edema, cardiac arrhythmias, congestive heart failure, and renal failure may occur. Uremia may increase CNS sensitivity to barbiturates. Differential diagnosis should include hypoglycemia, head trauma, cerebrovascular accidents, convulsive states, and diabetic coma. Blood levels from acute overdosage for some barbiturates are listed in Table 2.

[See table above]

Treatment of overdosage is mainly supportive and consists of the following:

1. Maintenance of an adequate airway, with assisted respiration and oxygen administration as necessary.
2. Monitoring of vital signs and fluid balance.
3. If the patient is conscious and has not lost the gag reflex, emesis may be induced with ipecac. Care should be taken to prevent pulmonary aspiration of vomitus. After completion of vomiting, 30 grams activated charcoal in a glass of water may be administered.
4. If emesis is contraindicated, gastric lavage may be performed with a cuffed endotracheal tube in place with the patient in the face down position. Activated charcoal may be left in the emptied stomach and a saline cathartic administered.
5. Fluid therapy and other standard treatment for shock, if needed.
6. If renal function is normal, forced diuresis may aid in the elimination of the barbiturate. Alkalinization of the urine increases renal excretion of some barbiturates, especially phenobarbital, also aprobarbital, and mephobarbital (which is metabolized to phenobarbital).
7. Although not recommended as a routine procedure, hemodialysis may be used in severe barbiturate intoxications or if the patient is anuric or in shock.
8. Patient should be rolled from side to side every 30 minutes.
9. Antibiotics should be given if pneumonia is suspected.
10. Appropriate nursing care to prevent hypostatic pneumonia, decubiti, aspiration, and other complications of patients with altered states of consciousness.

DOSAGE AND ADMINISTRATION

Adults: The usual hypnotic dose consists of 100 mg at bedtime.

Children: The preoperative dose is 2 to 6 mg/kg/24 hours (maximum 100 mg), depending on age, weight, and the desired degree of sedation.

The proper hypnotic dose for children must be judged on the basis of individual age and weight.

Dosages of barbiturates must be individualized with full knowledge of their particular characteristics and recommended rate of administration. Factors of consideration are the patient's age, weight, and condition.

Special patient population: Dosage should be reduced in the elderly or debilitated because these patients may be more sensitive to barbiturates. Dosage should be reduced for patients with impaired renal function or hepatic disease.

HOW SUPPLIED

NEMBUTAL Sodium Capsules (pentobarbital sodium capsules, USP) are supplied as follows:

50 mg transparent and orange-colored capsules (imprinted with ⊐ and the Abbo-Code CF) in bottles of 100 (**NDC** 0074-3150-11)

Continued on next page

Nembutal Sodium Capsules—Cont.

100 mg yellow capsules (imprinted with [logo] and the Abbo-Code CH) in bottles of 100 (**NDC** 0074-3114-01), and in the Abbo-Pac® unit dose packages of 100 (**NDC** 0074-3114-21).
Recommended Storage: Store below 86°F (30°C).
Revised: September, 1997
Ref. 03-4785-R11

Shown in Product Identification Guide, page 303

NEMBUTAL® SODIUM SOLUTION ℂ ℞

PENTOBARBITAL SODIUM INJECTION, USP
WARNING—MAY BE HABIT FORMING
Ampuls—Vials
DO NOT USE IF MATERIAL HAS PRECIPITATED

DESCRIPTION

The barbiturates are nonselective central nervous system depressants which are primarily used as sedative hypnotics and also anticonvulsants in subhypnotic doses. The barbiturates and their sodium salts are subject to control under the Federal Controlled Substances Act (See "Drug Abuse and Dependence" section).
The sodium salts of amobarbital, pentobarbital, phenobarbital, and secobarbital are available as sterile parenteral solutions.
Barbiturates are substituted pyrimidine derivatives in which the basic structure common to these drugs is barbituric acid, a substance which has no central nervous system (CNS) activity. CNS activity is obtained by substituting alkyl, alkenyl, or aryl groups on the pyrimidine ring.
NEMBUTAL Sodium Solution (pentobarbital sodium injection) is a sterile solution for intravenous or intramuscular injection. Each ml contains pentobarbital sodium 50 mg, in a vehicle of propylene glycol, 40%, alcohol, 10% and water for injection, to volume. The pH is adjusted to approximately 9.5 with hydrochloric acid and/or sodium hydroxide.
NEMBUTAL Sodium is a short-acting barbiturate, chemically designated as sodium 5-ethyl-5-(1-methylbutyl) barbiturate. The structural formula for pentobarbital sodium is:

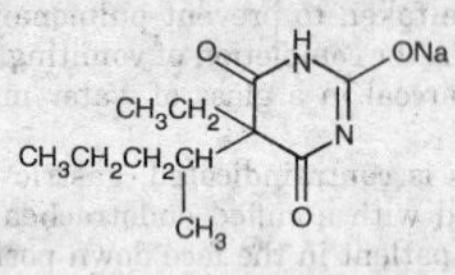

The sodium salt occurs as a white, slightly bitter powder which is freely soluble in water and alcohol but practically insoluble in benzene and ether.

CLINICAL PHARMACOLOGY

Barbiturates are capable of producing all levels of CNS mood alteration from excitation to mild sedation, to hypnosis, and deep coma. Overdosage can produce death. In high enough therapeutic doses, barbiturates induce anesthesia.
Barbiturates depress the sensory cortex, decrease motor activity, alter cerebellar function, and produce drowsiness, sedation, and hypnosis.
Barbiturate-induced sleep differs from physiological sleep. Sleep laboratory studies have demonstrated that barbiturates reduce the amount of time spent in the rapid eye movement (REM) phase of sleep or dreaming stage. Also, Stages III and IV sleep are decreased. Following abrupt cessation of barbiturates used regularly, patients may experience markedly increased dreaming, nightmares, and/or insomnia. Therefore, withdrawal of a single therapeutic dose over 5 or 6 days has been recommended to lessen the REM rebound and disturbed sleep which contribute to drug withdrawal syndrome (for example, decrease the dose from 3 to 2 doses a day for 1 week).
In studies, secobarbital sodium and pentobarbital sodium have been found to lose most of their effectiveness for both inducing and maintaining sleep by the end of 2 weeks of continued drug administration at fixed doses. The short-, intermediate-, and, to a lesser degree, long-acting barbiturates have been widely prescribed for treating insomnia. Although the clinical literature abounds with claims that the short-acting barbiturates are superior for producing sleep while the intermediate-acting compounds are more effective in maintaining sleep, controlled studies have failed to demonstrate these differential effects. Therefore, as sleep medications, the barbiturates are of limited value beyond short-term use.
Barbiturates have little analgesic action at subanesthetic doses. Rather, in subanesthetic doses these drugs may increase the reaction to painful stimuli. All barbiturates exhibit anticonvulsant activity in anesthetic doses. However, of the drugs in this class, only phenobarbital, mephobarbital, and metharbital have been clinically demonstrated to be effective as oral anticonvulsants in subhypnotic doses.
Barbiturates are respiratory depressants. The degree of respiratory depression is dependent upon dose. With hypnotic doses, respiratory depression produced by barbiturates is similar to that which occurs during physiologic sleep with slight decrease in blood pressure and heart rate.
Studies in laboratory animals have shown that barbiturates cause reduction in the tone and contractility of the uterus, ureters, and urinary bladder. However, concentrations of the drugs required to produce this effect in humans are not reached with sedative-hypnotic doses.
Barbiturates do not impair normal hepatic function, but have been shown to induce liver microsomal enzymes, thus increasing and/or altering the metabolism of barbiturates and other drugs. (See "Precautions—*Drug Interactions*" section).

Pharmacokinetics:
Barbiturates are absorbed in varying degrees following oral, rectal, or parenteral administration. The salts are more rapidly absorbed than are the acids.
The onset of action for oral or rectal administration varies from 20 to 60 minutes. For IM administration, the onset of action is slightly faster. Following IV administration, the onset of action ranges from almost immediately for pentobarbital sodium to 5 minutes for phenobarbital sodium. Maximal CNS depression may not occur until 15 minutes or more after IV administration for phenobarbital sodium.
Duration of action, which is related to the rate at which the barbiturates are redistributed throughout the body, varies among persons and in the same person from time to time.
No studies have demonstrated that the different routes of administration are equivalent with respect to bioavailability.
Barbiturates are weak acids that are absorbed and rapidly distributed to all tissues and fluids with high concentrations in the brain, liver, and kidneys. Lipid solubility of the barbiturates is the dominant factor in their distribution within the body. The more lipid soluble the barbiturate, the more rapidly it penetrates all tissues of the body. Barbiturates are bound to plasma and tissue proteins to a varying degree with the degree of binding increasing directly as a function of lipid solubility.
Phenobarbital has the lowest lipid solubility, lowest plasma binding, lowest brain protein binding, the longest delay in onset of activity, and the longest duration of action. At the opposite extreme is secobarbital which has the highest lipid solubility, plasma protein binding, brain protein binding, the shortest delay in onset of activity, and the shortest duration of action. Butabarbital is classified as an intermediate barbiturate.
The plasma half-life for pentobarbital in adults is 15 to 50 hours and appears to be dose dependent.
Barbiturates are metabolized primarily by the hepatic microsomal enzyme system, and the metabolic products are excreted in the urine, and less commonly, in the feces. Approximately 25 to 50 percent of a dose of aprobarbital or phenobarbital is eliminated unchanged in the urine, whereas the amount of other barbiturates excreted unchanged in the urine is negligible. The excretion of unmetabolized barbiturate is one feature that distinguishes the long-acting category from those belonging to other categories which are almost entirely metabolized. The inactive metabolites of the barbiturates are excreted as conjugates of glucuronic acid.

INDICATIONS AND USAGE

Parenteral:
a. Sedatives.
b. Hypnotics, for the short-term treatment of insomnia, since they appear to lose their effectiveness for sleep induction and sleep maintenance after 2 weeks (See "Clinical Pharmacology" section).
c. Preanesthetics.
d. Anticonvulsant, in anesthetic doses, in the emergency control of certain acute convulsive episodes, e.g., those associated with status epilepticus, cholera, eclampsia, meningitis, tetanus, and toxic reactions to strychnine or local anesthetics.

CONTRAINDICATIONS

Barbiturates are contraindicated in patients with known barbiturate sensitivity. Barbiturates are also contraindicated in patients with a history of manifest or latent porphyria.

WARNINGS

1. *Habit forming:* Barbiturates may be habit forming. Tolerance, psychological and physical dependence may occur with continued use. (See "Drug Abuse and Dependence" and "Pharmacokinetics" sections). Patients who have psychological dependence on barbiturates may increase the dosage or decrease the dosage interval without consulting a physician and may subsequently develop a physical dependence on barbiturates. To minimize the possibility of overdosage or the development of dependence, the prescribing and dispensing of sedative-hypnotic barbiturates should be limited to the amount required for the interval until the next appointment. Abrupt cessation after prolonged use in the dependent person may result in withdrawal symptoms, including delirium, convulsions, and possibly death. Barbiturates should be withdrawn gradually from any patient known to be taking excessive dosage over long periods of time. (See "Drug Abuse and Dependence" section).
2. *IV administration:* Too rapid administration may cause respiratory depression, apnea, laryngospasm, or vasodilation with fall in blood pressure.
3. *Acute or chronic pain:* Caution should be exercised when barbiturates are administered to patients with acute or chronic pain, because paradoxical excitement could be induced or important symptoms could be masked. However, the use of barbiturates as sedatives in the postoperative surgical period and as adjuncts to cancer chemotherapy is well established.
4. *Use in pregnancy:* Barbiturates can cause fetal damage when administered to a pregnant woman. Retrospective, case-controlled studies have suggested a connection between the maternal consumption of barbiturates and a higher than expected incidence of fetal abnormalities. Following oral or parenteral administration, barbiturates readily cross the placental barrier and are distributed throughout fetal tissues with highest concentrations found in the placenta, fetal liver, and brain. Fetal blood levels approach maternal blood levels following parenteral administration.
Withdrawal symptoms occur in infants born to mothers who receive barbiturates throughout the last trimester of pregnancy. (See "Drug Abuse and Dependence" section). If this drug is used during pregnancy, or if the patient becomes pregnant while taking this drug, the patient should be apprised of the potential hazard to the fetus.
5. *Synergistic effects:* The concomitant use of alcohol or other CNS depressants may produce additive CNS depressant effects.

PRECAUTIONS

General:
Barbiturates may be habit forming. Tolerance and psychological and physical dependence may occur with continuing use. (See "Drug Abuse and Dependence" section). Barbiturates should be administered with caution, if at all, to patients who are mentally depressed, have suicidal tendencies, or a history of drug abuse.
Elderly or debilitated patients may react to barbiturates with marked excitement, depression, and confusion. In some persons, barbiturates repeatedly produce excitement rather than depression.
In patients with hepatic damage, barbiturates should be administered with caution and initially in reduced doses. Barbiturates should not be administered to patients showing the premonitory signs of hepatic coma.
Parenteral solutions of barbiturates are highly alkaline. Therefore, extreme care should be taken to avoid perivascular extravasation or intra-arterial injection. Extravascular injection may cause local tissue damage with subsequent necrosis; consequences of intra-arterial injection may vary from transient pain to gangrene of the limb. Any complaint of pain in the limb warrants stopping the injection.

Information for the patient:
Practitioners should give the following information and instructions to patients receiving barbiturates.
1. The use of barbiturates carries with it an associated risk of psychological and/or physical dependence. The patient should be warned against increasing the dose of the drug without consulting a physician.
2. Barbiturates may impair mental and/or physical abilities required for the performance of potentially hazardous tasks (e.g., driving, operating machinery, etc.).
3. Alcohol should not be consumed while taking barbiturates. Concurrent use of the barbiturates with other CNS depressants (e.g., alcohol, narcotics, tranquilizers, and antihistamines) may result in additional CNS depressant effects.

Laboratory tests:
Prolonged therapy with barbiturates should be accompanied by periodic laboratory evaluation of organ systems, including hematopoietic, renal, and hepatic systems. (See "Precautions-*General*" and "Adverse Reactions" sections).

Drug interactions:
Most reports of clinically significant drug interactions occurring with the barbiturates have involved phenobarbital. However, the application of these data to other barbiturates appears valid and warrants serial blood level determinations of the relevant drugs when there are multiple therapies.
1. *Anticoagulants:* Phenobarbital lowers the plasma levels of dicumarol (name previously used: bishydroxycoumarin) and causes a decrease in anticoagulant activity as measured by the prothrombin time. Barbiturates can induce hepatic microsomal enzymes resulting in increased metabolism and decreased anticoagulant response of oral anticoagulants (e.g., warfarin, acenocoumarol, dicumarol, and phenprocoumon). Patients stabilized on anticoagu-

lant therapy may require dosage adjustments if barbiturates are added to or withdrawn from their dosage regimen.

2. *Corticosteroids:* Barbiturates appear to enhance the metabolism of exogenous corticosteroids probably through the induction of hepatic microsomal enzymes. Patients stabilized on corticosteroid therapy may require dosage adjustments if barbiturates are added to or withdrawn from their dosage regimen.
3. *Griseofulvin:* Phenobarbital appears to interfere with the absorption of orally administered griseofulvin, thus decreasing its blood level. The effect of the resultant decreased blood levels of griseofulvin on therapeutic response has not been established. However, it would be preferable to avoid concomitant administration of these drugs.
4. *Doxycycline:* Phenobarbital has been shown to shorten the half-life of doxycycline for as long as 2 weeks after barbiturate therapy is discontinued.

This mechanism is probably through the induction of hepatic microsomal enzymes that metabolize the antibiotic. If phenobarbital and doxycycline are administered concurrently, the clinical response to doxycycline should be monitored closely.

5. *Phenytoin, sodium valproate, valproic acid:* The effect of barbiturates on the metabolism of phenytoin appears to be variable. Some investigators report an accelerating effect, while others report no effect. Because the effect of barbiturates on the metabolism of phenytoin is not predictable, phenytoin and barbiturate blood levels should be monitored more frequently if these drugs are given concurrently. Sodium valproate and valproic acid appear to decrease barbiturate metabolism; therefore, barbiturate blood levels should be monitored and appropriate dosage adjustments made as indicated.
6. *Central nervous system depressants:* The concomitant use of other central nervous system depressants, including other sedatives or hypnotics, antihistamines, tranquilizers, or alcohol, may produce additive depressant effects.
7. *Monoamine oxidase inhibitors (MAOI):* MAOI prolong the effects of barbiturates probably because metabolism of the barbiturate is inhibited.
8. *Estradiol, estrone, progesterone and other steroidal hormones:* Pretreatment with or concurrent administration of phenobarbital may decrease the effect of estradiol by increasing its metabolism. There have been reports of patients treated with antiepileptic drugs (e.g., phenobarbital) who became pregnant while taking oral contraceptives. An alternate contraceptive method might be suggested to women taking phenobarbital.

Carcinogenesis:

1. *Animal data.* Phenobarbital sodium is carcinogenic in mice and rats after lifetime administration. In mice, it produced benign and malignant liver cell tumors. In rats, benign liver cell tumors were observed very late in life.
2. *Human data.* In a 29-year epidemiological study of 9,136 patients who were treated on an anticonvulsant protocol that included phenobarbital, results indicated a higher than normal incidence of hepatic carcinoma. Previously, some of these patients were treated with thorotrast, a drug that is known to produce hepatic carcinomas. Thus, this study did not provide sufficient evidence that phenobarbital sodium is carcinogenic in humans.

Data from one retrospective study of 235 children in which the types of barbiturates are not identified suggested an association between exposure to barbiturates prenatally and an increased incidence of brain tumor. (Gold, E., et al., "Increased Risk of Brain Tumors in Children Exposed to Barbiturates," Journal of National Cancer Institute, 61:1031-1034, 1978).

Pregnancy:

1. *Teratogenic effects.* Pregnancy Category D—See "Warnings—Use in Pregnancy" section.
2. *Nonteratogenic effects.* Reports of infants suffering from long-term barbiturate exposure *in utero* included the acute withdrawal syndrome of seizures and hyperirritability from birth to a delayed onset of up to 14 days. (See "Drug Abuse and Dependence" section).

Labor and delivery:

Hypnotic doses of these barbiturates do not appear to significantly impair uterine activity during labor. Full anesthetic doses of barbiturates decrease the force and frequency of uterine contractions. Administration of sedative-hypnotic barbiturates to the mother during labor may result in respiratory depression in the newborn. Premature infants are particularly susceptible to the depressant effects of barbiturates. If barbiturates are used during labor and delivery, resuscitation equipment should be available.

Data are currently not available to evaluate the effect of these barbiturates when forceps delivery or other intervention is necessary. Also, data are not available to determine the effect of these barbiturates on the later growth, development, and functional maturation of the child.

Nursing mothers:

Caution should be exercised when a barbiturate is administered to a nursing woman since small amounts of barbiturates are excreted in the milk.

Table 1.— *Concentration of Barbiturate in the Blood Versus Degree of CNS Depression*

		Blood barbiturate level in ppm (μg/ml)				
		Degree of depression in nontolerant persons*				
Barbiturate	Onset/ duration	1	2	3	4	5
Pentobarbital	Fast/short	≤2	0.5 to 3	10 to 15	12 to 25	15 to 40
Secobarbital	Fast/short	≤2	0.5 to 5	10 to 15	15 to 25	15 to 40
Amobarbital	Intermediate/ intermediate	≤3	2 to 10	30 to 40	30 to 60	40 to 80
Butabarbital	Intermediate/ intermediate	≤5	3 to 25	40 to 60	50 to 80	60 to 100
Phenobarbital	Slow/long	≤10	5 to 40	50 to 80	70 to 120	100 to 200

* Categories of degree of depression in nontolerant persons:
1. Under the influence and appreciably impaired for purposes of driving a motor vehicle or performing tasks requiring alertness and unimpaired judgment and reaction time.
2. Sedated, therapeutic range, calm, relaxed, and easily aroused.
3. Comatose, difficult to arouse, significant depression of respiration.
4. Compatible with death in aged or ill persons or in presence of obstructed airway, other toxic agents, or exposure to cold.
5. Usual lethal level, the upper end of the range includes those who received some supportive treatment.

ADVERSE REACTIONS

The following adverse reactions and their incidence were compiled from surveillance of thousands of hospitalized patients. Because such patients may be less aware of certain of the milder adverse effects of barbiturates, the incidence of these reactions may be somewhat higher in fully ambulatory patients.

More than 1 in 100 patients. The most common adverse reaction estimated to occur at a rate of 1 to 3 patients per 100 is: *Nervous System:* Somnolence.

Less than 1 in 100 patients. Adverse reactions estimated to occur at a rate of less than 1 in 100 patients listed below, grouped by organ system, and by decreasing order of occurrence are:

Nervous system: Agitation, confusion, hyperkinesia, ataxia, CNS depression, nightmares, nervousness, psychiatric disturbance, hallucinations, insomnia, anxiety, dizziness, thinking abnormality.

Respiratory system: Hypoventilation, apnea.

Cardiovascular system: Bradycardia, hypotension, syncope.

Digestive system: Nausea, vomiting, constipation.

Other reported reactions: Headache, injection site reactions, hypersensitivity reactions (angioedema, skin rashes, exfoliative dermatitis), fever, liver damage, megaloblastic anemia following chronic phenobarbital use.

DRUG ABUSE AND DEPENDENCE

Pentobarbital sodium injection is subject to control by the Federal Controlled Substances Act under DEA schedule II. Barbiturates may be habit forming. Tolerance, psychological dependence, and physical dependence may occur especially following prolonged use of high doses of barbiturates. Daily administration in excess of 400 milligrams (mg) of pentobarbital or secobarbital for approximately 90 days is likely to produce some degree of physical dependence. A dosage of from 600 to 800 mg taken for at least 35 days is sufficient to produce withdrawal seizures. The average daily dose for the barbiturate addict is usually about 1.5 grams. As tolerance to barbiturates develops, the amount needed to maintain the same level of intoxication increases; tolerance to a fatal dosage, however, does not increase more than two-fold. As this occurs, the margin between an intoxicating dosage and fatal dosage becomes smaller.

Symptoms of acute intoxication with barbiturates include unsteady gait, slurred speech, and sustained nystagmus. Mental signs of chronic intoxication include confusion, poor judgment, irritability, insomnia, and somatic complaints.

Symptoms of barbiturate dependence are similar to those of chronic alcoholism. If an individual appears to be intoxicated with alcohol to a degree that is radically disproportionate to the amount of alcohol in his or her blood the use of barbiturates should be suspected. The lethal dose of a barbiturate is far less if alcohol is also ingested.

The symptoms of barbiturate withdrawal can be severe and may cause death. Minor withdrawal symptoms may appear 8 to 12 hours after the last dose of a barbiturate. These symptoms usually appear in the following order: anxiety, muscle twitching, tremor of hands and fingers, progressive weakness, dizziness, distortion in visual perception, nausea, vomiting, insomnia, and orthostatic hypotension. Major withdrawal symptoms (convulsions and delirium) may occur within 16 hours and last up to 5 days after abrupt cessation of these drugs. Intensity of withdrawal symptoms gradually declines over a period of approximately 15 days. Individuals susceptible to barbiturate abuse and dependence include alcoholics and opiate abusers, as well as other sedative-hypnotic and amphetamine abusers.

Drug dependence to barbiturates arises from repeated administration of a barbiturate or agent with barbiturate-like effect on a continuous basis, generally in amounts exceeding therapeutic dose levels. The characteristics of drug dependence to barbiturates include: (a) a strong desire or need to continue taking the drug; (b) a tendency to increase the dose; (c) a psychic dependence on the effects of the drug related to subjective and individual appreciation of those effects; and (d) a physical dependence on the effects of the drug requiring its presence for maintenance of homeostasis and resulting in a definite, characteristic, and self-limited abstinence syndrome when the drug is withdrawn.

Treatment of barbiturate dependence consists of cautious and gradual withdrawal of the drug. Barbiturate-dependent patients can be withdrawn by using a number of different withdrawal regimens. In all cases withdrawal takes an extended period of time. One method involves substituting a 30 mg dose of phenobarbital for each 100 to 200 mg dose of barbiturate that the patient has been taking. The total daily amount of phenobarbital is then administered in 3 to 4 divided doses, not to exceed 600 mg daily. Should signs of withdrawal occur on the first day of treatment, a loading dose of 100 to 200 mg of phenobarbital may be administered IM in addition to the oral dose. After stabilization on phenobarbital, the total daily dose is decreased by 30 mg a day as long as withdrawal is proceeding smoothly. A modification of this regimen involves initiating treatment at the patient's regular dosage level and decreasing the daily dosage by 10 percent if tolerated by the patient.

Infants physically dependent on barbiturates may be given phenobarbital 3 to 10 mg/kg/day. After withdrawal symptoms (hyperactivity, disturbed sleep, tremors, hyperreflexia) are relieved, the dosage of phenobarbital should be gradually decreased and completely withdrawn over a 2-week period.

OVERDOSAGE

The toxic dose of barbiturates varies considerably. In general, an oral dose of 1 gram of most barbiturates produces serious poisoning in an adult. Death commonly occurs after 2 to 10 grams of ingested barbiturate. Barbiturate intoxication may be confused with alcoholism, bromide intoxication, and with various neurological disorders.

Acute overdosage with barbiturates is manifested by CNS and respiratory depression which may progress to Cheyne-Stokes respiration, areflexia, constriction of the pupils to a slight degree (though in severe poisoning they may show paralytic dilation), oliguria, tachycardia, hypotension, lowered body temperature, and coma. Typical shock syndrome (apnea, circulatory collapse, respiratory arrest, and death) may occur.

In extreme overdose, all electrical activity in the brain may cease, in which case a "flat" EEG normally equated with clinical death cannot be accepted. This effect is fully reversible unless hypoxic damage occurs. Consideration should be given to the possibility of barbiturate intoxication even in situations that appear to involve trauma.

Complications such as pneumonia, pulmonary edema, cardiac arrhythmias, congestive heart failure, and renal failure may occur. Uremia may increase CNS sensitivity to barbiturates. Differential diagnosis should include hypoglycemia, head trauma, cerebrovascular accidents, convulsive states, and diabetic coma. Blood levels from acute overdosage for some barbiturates are listed in Table 1.

[See table above]

Treatment of overdosage is mainly supportive and consists of the following:

1. Maintenance of an adequate airway, with assisted respiration and oxygen administration as necessary.
2. Monitoring of vital signs and fluid balance.
3. Fluid therapy and other standard treatment for shock, if needed.
4. If renal function is normal, forced diuresis may aid in the elimination of the barbiturate. Alkalinization of the urine

Continued on next page

Nembutal Sodium Solution—Cont.

increases renal excretion of some barbiturates, especially phenobarbital, also aprobarbital and mephobarbital (which is metabolized to phenobarbital).

5. Although not recommended as a routine procedure, hemodialysis may be used in severe barbiturate intoxications or if the patient is anuric or in shock.
6. Patient should be rolled from side to side every 30 minutes.
7. Antibiotics should be given if pneumonia is suspected.
8. Appropriate nursing care to prevent hypostatic pneumonia, decubiti, aspiration, and other complications of patients with altered states of consciousness.

DOSAGE AND ADMINISTRATION

Dosages of barbiturates must be individualized with full knowledge of their particular characteristics and recommended rate of administration. Factors of consideration are the patient's age, weight, and condition. Parenteral routes should be used only when oral administration is impossible or impractical.

Intramuscular Administration: IM injection of the sodium salts of barbiturates should be made deeply into a large muscle, and a volume of 5 ml should not be exceeded at any one site because of possible tissue irritation. After IM injection of a hypnotic dose, the patient's vital signs should be monitored. The usual adult dosage of NEMBUTAL Sodium Solution is 150 to 200 mg as a single IM injection; the recommended pediatric dosage ranges from 2 to 6 mg/kg as a single IM injection not to exceed 100 mg.

Intravenous Administration: NEMBUTAL Sodium Solution should not be admixed with any other medication or solution. IV injection is restricted to conditions in which other routes are not feasible, either because the patient is unconscious (as in cerebral hemorrhage, eclampsia, or status epilepticus), or because the patient resists (as in delirium), or because prompt action is imperative. Slow IV injection is essential, and patients should be carefully observed during administration. This requires that blood pressure, respiration, and cardiac function be maintained, vital signs be recorded, and equipment for resuscitation and artificial ventilation be available. The rate of IV injection should not exceed 50 mg/min for pentobarbital sodium.

There is no average intravenous dose of NEMBUTAL Sodium Solution (pentobarbital sodium injection) that can be relied on to produce similar effects in different patients. The possibility of overdose and respiratory depression is remote when the drug is injected slowly in fractional doses.

A commonly used initial dose for the 70 kg adult is 100 mg. Proportional reduction in dosage should be made for pediatric or debilitated patients. At least one minute is necessary to determine the full effect of intravenous pentobarbital. If necessary, additional small increments of the drug may be given up to a total of from 200 to 500 mg for normal adults.

Anticonvulsant use: In convulsive states, dosage of NEMBUTAL Sodium Solution should be kept to a minimum to avoid compounding the depression which may follow convulsions. The injection must be made slowly with due regard to the time required for the drug to penetrate the blood-brain barrier.

Special patient population: Dosage should be reduced in the elderly or debilitated because these patients may be more sensitive to barbiturates. Dosage should be reduced for patients with impaired renal function or hepatic disease.

Inspection: Parenteral drug products should be inspected visually for particulate matter and discoloration prior to administration, whenever solution containers permit. Solutions for injection showing evidence of precipitation should not be used.

HOW SUPPLIED

NEMBUTAL Sodium Solution (pentobarbital sodium injection, USP) is available in the following sizes: 20-ml multiple-dose vial, 1 g per vial (**NDC** 0074-3778-04); and 50-ml multiple-dose vial, 2.5 g per vial (**NDC** 0074-3778-05).

Each ml contains:

Pentobarbital Sodium, derivative of barbituric acid	50 mg
Warning - May be habit forming.	
Propylene glycol	40% v/v
Alcohol	10%
Water for Injection	qs

(pH adjusted to approximately 9.5 with hydrochloric acid and/or sodium hydroxide.)

Exposure of pharmaceutical products to heat should be minimized. Avoid excessive heat. Protect from freezing. It is recommended that the product be stored at room temperature-86°F (30°C); however, brief exposure up to 104° F (40°C) does not adversely affect the product.

Revised: February, 1998
Ref. 03-4715-R7

ABBOTT LABORATORIES
NORTH CHICAGO, IL 60064, U.S.A.

NEMBUTAL® SODIUM SUPPOSITORIES

CIII ℞

[*nêm-bū 'tal*]

(PENTOBARBITAL SODIUM SUPPOSITORIES)

WARNING: MAY BE HABIT FORMING

DESCRIPTION

The barbiturates are nonselective central nervous system depressants which are primarily used as sedative hypnotics. The barbiturates and their sodium salts are subject to control under the Federal Controlled Substances Act (See "Drug Abuse and Dependence" section).

Barbiturates are substituted pyrimidine derivatives in which the basic structure common to these drugs is barbituric acid, a substance which has no central nervous system (CNS) activity. CNS activity is obtained by substituting alkyl, alkenyl, or aryl groups on the pyrimidine ring. Nembutal (pentobarbital sodium) is chemically represented by sodium 5-ethyl-5-(1-methylbutyl) barbiturate.

The structural formula for pentobarbital sodium is:

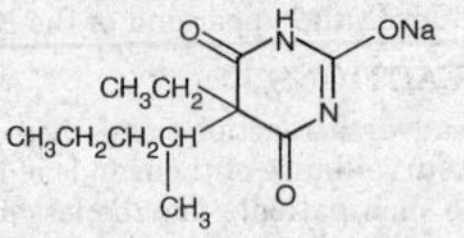

The sodium salt of pentobarbital occurs as a white, slightly bitter powder which is freely soluble in water and alcohol but practically insoluble in benzene and ether. Each rectal suppository contains either 30 mg, 60 mg, 120 mg, or 200 mg of pentobarbital sodium.

Inactive Ingredients: Semi-synthetic glycerides.

CLINICAL PHARMACOLOGY

Barbiturates are capable of producing all levels of CNS mood alteration from excitation to mild sedation, to hypnosis, and deep coma. Overdosage can produce death. In high enough therapeutic doses, barbiturates induce anesthesia. Barbiturates depress the sensory cortex, decrease motor activity, alter cerebellar function, and produce drowsiness, sedation, and hypnosis.

Barbiturate-induced sleep differs from physiological sleep. Sleep laboratory studies have demonstrated that barbiturates reduce the amount of time spent in the rapid eye movement (REM) phase of sleep or dreaming stage. Also, Stages III and IV sleep are decreased. Following abrupt cessation of barbiturates used regularly, patients may experience markedly increased dreaming, nightmares, and/or insomnia. Therefore, withdrawal of a single therapeutic dose over 5 or 6 days has been recommended to lessen the REM rebound and disturbed sleep which contribute to drug withdrawal syndrome (for example, decrease the dose from 3 to 2 doses a day for 1 week).

In studies, secobarbital sodium and pentobarbital sodium have been found to lose most of their effectiveness for both inducing and maintaining sleep by the end of 2 weeks of continued drug administration at fixed doses. The short-, intermediate-, and, to a lesser degree, long-acting barbiturates have been widely prescribed for treating insomnia. Although the clinical literature abounds with claims that the short-acting barbiturates are superior for producing sleep while the intermediate-acting compounds are more effective in maintaining sleep, controlled studies have failed to demonstrate these differential effects. Therefore, as sleep medications, the barbiturates are of limited value beyond short-term use.

Barbiturates have little analgesic action at subanesthetic doses. Rather, in subanesthetic doses these drugs may increase the reaction to painful stimuli. All barbiturates exhibit anticonvulsant activity in anesthetic doses. However, of the drugs in this class, only phenobarbital, mephobarbital, and metharbital have been clinically demonstrated to be effective as oral anticonvulsants in subhypnotic doses.

Barbiturates are respiratory depressants. The degree of respiratory depression is dependent upon dose. With hypnotic doses, respiratory depression produced by barbiturates is similar to that which occurs during physiologic sleep with slight decrease in blood pressure and heart rate.

Studies in laboratory animals have shown that barbiturates cause reduction in the tone and contractility of the uterus, ureters, and urinary bladder. However, concentrations of the drugs required to produce this effect in humans are not reached with sedative-hypnotic doses.

Barbiturates do not impair normal hepatic function, but have been shown to induce liver microsomal enzymes, thus increasing and/or altering the metabolism of barbiturates and other drugs. (See "Precautions—*Drug Interactions*" section).

Pharmacokinetics: Barbiturates are absorbed in varying degrees following oral, rectal, or parenteral administration. The onset of action for oral or rectal administration varies from 20 to 60 minutes.

Duration of action, which is related to the rate at which the barbiturates are redistributed throughout the body, varies among persons and in the same person from time to time. No studies have demonstrated that the different routes of administration are equivalent with respect to bioavailability.

Barbiturates are weak acids that are absorbed and rapidly distributed to all tissues and fluids with high concentrations in the brain, liver, and kidneys. Lipid solubility of the barbiturates is the dominant factor in their distribution within the body. The more lipid soluble the barbiturate, the more rapidly it penetrates all tissues of the body. Barbiturates are bound to plasma and tissue proteins to a varying degree with the degree of binding increasing directly as a function of lipid solubility.

Phenobarbital has the lowest lipid solubility, lowest plasma binding, lowest brain protein binding, the longest delay in onset of activity, and the longest duration of action. At the opposite extreme is secobarbital which has the highest lipid solubility, plasma protein binding, brain protein binding, the shortest delay in onset of activity, and the shortest duration of action. Butabarbital is classified as an intermediate barbiturate.

The plasma half-life for phentobarbital in adults is 15 to 50 hours and appears to be dose dependent.

Barbiturates are metabolized primarily by the hepatic microsomal enzyme system, and the metabolic products are excreted in the urine, and less commonly, in the feces. Approximately 25 to 50 percent of a dose of aprobarbital or phenobarbital is eliminated unchanged in the urine, whereas the amount of other barbiturates excreted unchanged in the urine is negligible. The excretion of unmetabolized barbiturate is one feature that distinguishes the long-acting category from those belonging to other categories which are almost entirely metabolized. The inactive metabolites of the barbiturates are excreted as conjugates of glucuronic acid.

INDICATIONS AND USAGE

Rectal: Barbiturates administered rectally are absorbed from the colon and are used when oral or parenteral administration may be undesirable.

1. Sedative.
2. Hypnotic, for the short-term treatment of insomnia, since they appear to lose their effectiveness for sleep induction and sleep maintenance after 2 weeks (See "Clinical Pharmacology" section).

CONTRAINDICATIONS

Barbiturates are contraindicated in patients with known barbiturate sensitivity. Barbiturates are also contraindicated in patients with a history of manifest or latent porphyria.

WARNINGS

1. *Habit forming:* Barbiturates may be habit forming. Tolerance, psychological and physical dependence may occur with continued use. (See "Drug Abuse and Dependence" and "Pharmacokinetics" sections). Patients who have psychological dependence on barbiturates may increase the dosage or decrease the dosage interval without consulting a physician and may subsequently develop a physical dependence on barbiturates. To minimize the possibility of overdosage or the development of dependence, the prescribing and dispensing of sedative-hypnotic barbiturates should be limited to the amount required for the interval until the next appointment. Abrupt cessation after prolonged use in the dependent person may result in withdrawal symptoms, including delirium, convulsions, and possibly death. Barbiturates should be withdrawn gradually from any patient known to be taking excessive dosage over long periods of time. (See "Drug Abuse and Dependence" section).

2. *Acute or chronic pain:* Caution should be exercised when barbiturates are administered to patients with acute or chronic pain, because paradoxical excitement could be induced or important symptoms could be masked. However, the use of barbiturates as sedatives in the postoperative surgical period and as adjuncts to cancer chemotherapy is well established.

3. *Use in pregnancy:* Barbiturates can cause fetal damage when administered to a pregnant woman. Retrospective, case-controlled studies have suggested a connection between the maternal consumption of barbiturates and a higher than expected incidence of fetal abnormalities. Following oral or parenteral administration, barbiturates readily cross the placental barrier and are distributed throughout fetal tissues with highest concentrations found in the placenta, fetal liver, and brain. It is presumed that this effect will also be seen following rectal administration. Withdrawal symptoms occur in infants born to mothers who receive barbiturates throughout the last trimester of pregnancy. (See "Drug Abuse and Dependence" section). If this drug is used during pregnancy, or if the patient becomes pregnant while taking this drug, the patient should be apprised of the potential hazard to the fetus.

4. *Synergistic effects:* The concomitant use of alcohol or other CNS depressants may produce additive CNS depressant effects.

PRECAUTIONS

General: Barbiturates may be habit forming. Tolerance and psychological and physical dependence may occur with continuing use. (See "Drug Abuse and Dependence" section). Barbiturates should be administered with caution, if at all, to patients who are mentally depressed, have suicidal tendencies, or a history of drug abuse.

Elderly or debilitated patients may react to barbiturates with marked excitement, depression, and confusion. In some persons, barbiturates repeatedly produce excitement rather than depression.

In patients with hepatic damage, barbiturates should be administered with caution and initially in reduced doses. Barbiturates should not be administered to patients showing the premonitory signs of hepatic coma.

Information for the patient: Practitioners should give the following information and instructions to patients receiving barbiturates.

1. The use of barbiturates carries with it an associated risk of psychological and/or physical dependence. The patient should be warned against increasing the dose of the drug without consulting a physician.
2. Barbiturates may impair mental and/or physical abilities required for the performance of potentially hazardous tasks (e.g., driving, operating machinery, etc.)
3. Alcohol should not be consumed while taking barbiturates. Concurrent use of the barbiturates with other CNS depressants (e.g., alcohol, narcotics, tranquilizers, and antihistamines) may result in additional CNS depressant effects.

Laboratory tests: Prolonged therapy with barbiturates should be accompanied by periodic laboratory evaluation of organ systems, including hematopoietic, renal, and hepatic systems. (See "Precautions — *General* " and "Adverse Reactions" sections).

Drug interactions: Most reports of clinically significant drug interactions occurring with the barbiturates have involved phenobarbital. However, the application of these data to other barbiturates appears valid and warrants serial blood level determinations of the relevant drugs when there are multiple therapies.

1. *Anticoagulants:* Phenobarbital lowers the plasma levels of dicumarol (name previously used: bishydroxycoumarin) and causes a decrease in anticoagulant activity as measured by the prothrombin time. Barbiturates can induce hepatic microsomal enzymes resulting in increased metabolism and decreased anticoagulant response of oral anticoagulants (e.g., warfarin, acenocoumarol, dicumarol, and phenprocoumon). Patients stabilized on anticoagulant therapy may require dosage adjustments if barbiturates are added to or withdrawn from their dosage regimen.
2. *Corticosteroids:* Barbiturates appear to enhance the metabolism of exogenous corticosteroids probably through the induction of hepatic microsomal enzymes. Patients stabilized on corticosteroid therapy may require dosage adjustments if barbiturates are added to or withdrawn from their dosage regimen.
3. *Griseofulvin:* Phenobarbital appears to interfere with the absorption of orally administered griseofulvin, thus decreasing its blood level. The effect of the resultant decreased blood levels of griseofulvin on therapeutic response has not been established. However, it would be preferable to avoid concomitant administration of these drugs.
4. *Doxycycline:* Phenobarbital has been shown to shorten the half-life of doxycycline for as long as 2 weeks after barbiturate therapy is discontinued.
   This mechanism is probably through the induction of hepatic microsomal enzymes that metabolize the antibiotic. If phenobarbital and doxycycline are administered concurrently, the clinical response to doxycycline should be monitored closely.
5. *Phenytoin, sodium valproate, valproic acid:* The effect of barbiturates on the metabolism of phenytoin appears to be variable. Some investigators report an accelerating effect, while others report no effect. Because the effect of barbiturates on the metabolism of phenytoin is not predictable, phenytoin and barbiturate blood levels should be monitored more frequently if these drugs are given concurrently. Sodium valproate and valproic acid appear to decrease barbiturate metabolism; therefore, barbiturate blood levels should be monitored and appropriate dosage adjustments made as indicated.
6. *Central nervous system depressants:* The concomitant use of other central nervous system depressants, including other sedatives or hypnotics, antihistamines, tranquilizers, or alcohol, may produce additive depressant effects.
7. *Monoamine oxidase inhibitors (MAOI):* MAOI prolong the effects of barbiturates probably because metabolism of the barbiturate is inhibited.
8. *Estradiol, estrone, progesterone and other steroidal hormones:* Pretreatment with or concurrent administration of phenobarbital may decrease the effect of estradiol by increasing its metabolism. There have been reports of patients treated with antiepileptic drugs (e.g., phenobarbital) who became pregnant while taking oral contraceptives. An alternate contraceptive method might be suggested to women taking phenobarbital.

Table 1.—*Concentration of Barbiturate in the Blood Versus Degree of CNS Depression*

Barbiturate	Onset/ duration	Blood barbiturate level in ppm (µg/ml) — Degree of depression in nontolerant persons* 1	2	3	4	5
Pentobarbital	Fast/short	≤2	0.5 to 3	10 to 15	12 to 25	15 to 40
Secobarbital	Fast/short	≤2	0.5 to 5	10 to 15	15 to 25	15 to 40
Amobarbital	Intermediate/ intermediate	≤3	2 to 10	30 to 40	30 to 60	40 to 80
Butabarbital	Intermediate/ intermediate	≤5	3 to 25	40 to 60	50 to 80	60 to 100
Phenobarbital	Slow/long	≤10	5 to 40	50 to 80	70 to 120	100 to 200

* Categories of degree of depression in nontolerant persons:
1. Under the influence and appreciably impaired for purposes of driving a motor vehicle or performing tasks requiring alertness and unimpaired judgment and reaction time.
2. Sedated, therapeutic range, calm, relaxed, and easily aroused.
3. Comatose, difficult to arouse, significant depression of respiration.
4. Compatible with death in aged or ill persons or in presence of obstructed airway, other toxic agents, or exposure to cold.
5. Usual lethal level, the upper end of the range includes those who received some supportive treatment.

Carcinogenesis:

1. Animal data. Phenobarbital sodium is carcinogenic in mice and rats after lifetime administration. In mice, it produced benign and malignant liver cell tumors. In rats, benign liver cell tumors were observed very late in life.
2. Human data. In a 29-year epidemiological study of 9,136 patients who were treated on an anticonvulsant protocol that included phenobarbital, results indicated a higher than normal incidence of hepatic carcinoma. Previously, some of these patients were treated with thorotrast, a drug that is known to produce hepatic carcinomas. Thus, this study did not provide sufficient evidence that phenobarbital sodium is carcinogenic in humans.

Data from one retrospective study of 235 children in which the types of barbiturates are not identified suggested an association between exposure to barbiturates prenatally and an increased incidence of brain tumor. (Gold, E., et al., "Increased Risk of Brain Tumors in Children Exposed to Barbiturates," Journal of National Cancer Institute, 61:1031–1034, 1978).

Pregnancy: *1. Teratogenic effects.* Pregnancy Category D — See "Warnings — Use in Pregnancy" section.

2. Nonteratogenic effects. Reports of infants suffering from long-term barbiturate exposure in utero included the acute withdrawal syndrome of seizures and hyperirritability from birth to a delayed onset of up to 14 days. (See "Drug Abuse and Dependence" section).

Labor and delivery: Hypnotic doses of these barbiturates do not appear to significantly impair uterine activity during labor. Full anesthetic doses of barbiturates decrease the force and frequency of uterine contractions. Administration of sedative-hypnotic barbiturates to the mother during labor may result in respiratory depression in the newborn. Premature infants are particularly susceptible to the depressant effects of barbiturates. If barbiturates are used during labor and delivery, resuscitation equipment should be available.

Data are currently not available to evaluate the effect of these barbiturates when forceps delivery or other intervention is necessary. Also, data are not available to determine the effect of these barbiturates on the later growth, development, and functional maturation of the child.

Nursing mothers: Caution should be exercised when a barbiturate is administered to a nursing woman since small amounts of barbiturates are excreted in the milk.

ADVERSE REACTIONS

The following adverse reactions and their incidence were compiled from surveillance of thousands of hospitalized patients. Because such patients may be less aware of certain of the milder adverse effects of barbiturates, the incidence of these reactions may be somewhat higher in fully ambulatory patients.

More than 1 in 100 patients. The most common adverse reaction estimated to occur at a rate of 1 to 3 patients per 100 is: *Nervous System:* Somnolence.

Less than 1 in 100 patients. Adverse reactions estimated to occur at a rate of less than 1 in 100 patients listed below, grouped by organ system, and by decreasing order of occurrence are:

Nervous system: Agitation, confusion, hyperkinesia, ataxia, CNS depression, nightmares, nervousness, psychiatric disturbance, hallucinations, insomnia, anxiety, dizziness, thinking abnormality.

Respiratory system: Hypoventilation, apnea.

Cardiovascular system: Bradycardia, hypotension, syncope.

Digestive system: Nausea, vomiting, constipation.

Other reported reactions: Headache, injection site reactions, hypersensitivity reactions (angioedema, skin rashes, exfoliative dermatitis), fever, liver damage, megaloblastic anemia following chronic phenobarbital use.

DRUG ABUSE AND DEPENDENCE

Pentobarbital sodium suppositories are subject to control by the Federal Controlled Substances Act under DEA schedule III.

Barbiturates may be habit forming. Tolerance, psychological dependence, and physical dependence may occur especially following prolonged use of high doses of barbiturates. Daily administration in excess of 400 milligrams (mg) of pentobarbital or secobarbital for approximately 90 days is likely to produce some degree of physical dependence. A dosage of from 600 to 800 mg taken for at least 35 days is sufficient to produce withdrawal seizures. The average daily dose for the barbiturate addict is usually about 1.5 grams. As tolerance to barbiturates develops, the amount needed to maintain the same level of intoxication increases; tolerance to a fatal dosage, however, does not increase more than two-fold. As this occurs, the margin between an intoxicating dosage and fatal dosage becomes smaller.

Symptoms of acute intoxication with barbiturates include unsteady gait, slurred speech, and sustained nystagmus. Mental signs of chronic intoxication include confusion, poor judgment, irritability, insomnia, and somatic complaints.

Symptoms of barbiturate dependence are similar to those of chronic alcoholism. If an individual appears to be intoxicated with alcohol to a degree that is radically disproportionate to the amount of alcohol in his or her blood the use of barbiturates should be suspected. The lethal dose of a barbiturate is far less if alcohol is also ingested.

The symptoms of barbiturate withdrawal can be severe and may cause death. Minor withdrawal symptoms may appear 8 to 12 hours after the last dose of a barbiturate. These symptoms usually appear in the following order: anxiety, muscle twitching, tremor of hands and fingers, progressive weakness, dizziness, distortion in visual perception, nausea, vomiting, insomnia, and orthostatic hypotension. Major withdrawal symptoms (convulsions and delirium) may occur within 16 hours and last up to 5 days after abrupt cessation of these drugs. Intensity of withdrawal symptoms gradually declines over a period of approximately 15 days. Individuals susceptible to barbiturate abuse and dependence include alcoholics and opiate abusers, as well as other sedative-hypnotic and amphetamine abusers.

Drug dependence to barbiturates arises from repeated administration of a barbiturate or agent with barbiturate-like effect on a continuous basis, generally in amounts exceeding therapeutic dose levels. The characteristics of drug dependence to barbiturates include: (a) a strong desire or need to continue taking the drug; (b) a tendency to increase the dose; (c) a psychic dependence on the effects of the drug related to subjective and individual appreciation of those effects; and (d) a physical dependence on the effects of the drug requiring its presence for maintenance of homeostasis and resulting in a definite, characteristic, and self-limited abstinence syndrome when the drug is withdrawn.

Treatment of barbiturate dependence consists of cautious and gradual withdrawal of the drug. Barbiturate-dependent patients can be withdrawn by using a number of different withdrawal regimens. In all cases withdrawal takes an extended period of time. One method involves substituting a 30 mg dose of phenobarbital for each 100 to 200 mg dose of barbiturate that the patient has been taking. The total daily amount of phenobarbital is then administered in 3 to 4 divided doses, not to exceed 600 mg daily. Should signs of withdrawal occur on the first day of treatment, a loading dose of 100 to 200 mg of phenobarbital may be administered

Continued on next page

Nembutal Suppositories—Cont.

IM in addition to the oral dose. After stabilization on phenobarbital, the total daily dose is decreased by 30 mg a day as long as withdrawal is proceeding smoothly. A modification of this regimen involves initiating treatment at the patient's regular dosage level and decreasing the daily dosage by 10 percent if tolerated by the patient.

Infants physically dependent on barbiturates may be given phenobarbital 3 to 10 mg/kg/day. After withdrawal symptoms (hyperactivity, disturbed sleep, tremors, hyperreflexia) are relieved, the dosage of phenobarbital should be gradually decreased and completely withdrawn over a 2 week period.

OVERDOSAGE

The toxic dose of barbiturates varies considerably. In general, an oral dose of 1 gram of most barbiturates produces serious poisoning in an adult. Death commonly occurs after 2 to 10 grams of ingested barbiturate. Barbiturate intoxication may be confused with alcoholism, bromide intoxication, and with various neurological disorders.

Acute overdosage with barbiturates is manifested by CNS and respiratory depression which may progress to Cheyne-Stokes respiration, areflexia, constriction of the pupils to a slight degree (though in severe poisoning they may show paralytic dilation), oliguria, tachycardia, hypotension, lowered body temperature, and coma. Typical shock syndrome (apnea, circulatory collapse, respiratory arrest, and death) may occur.

In extreme overdose, all electrical activity in the brain may cease, in which case a "flat" EEG normally equated with clinical death cannot be accepted. This effect is fully reversible unless hypoxic damage occurs. Consideration should be given to the possibility of barbiturate intoxication even in situations that appear to involve trauma.

Complications such as pneumonia, pulmonary edema, cardiac arrhythmias, congestive heart failure, and renal failure may occur. Uremia may increase CNS sensitivity to barbiturates. Differential diagnosis should include hypoglycemia, head trauma, cerebrovascular accidents, convulsive states, and diabetic coma. Blood levels from acute overdosage for some barbiturates are listed in Table 1.

[See table at top of previous page]

Treatment of overdosage is mainly supportive and consists of the following:

1. Maintenance of an adequate airway, with assisted respiration and oxygen administration as necessary.
2. Monitoring of vital signs and fluid balance.
3. Fluid therapy and other standard treatment for shock, if needed.
4. If renal function is normal, forced diuresis may aid in the elimination of the barbiturate. Alkalinization of the urine increases renal excretion of some barbiturates, especially phenobarbital, also aprobarbital, and mephobarbital (which is metabolized to phenobarbital).
5. Although not recommended as a routine procedure, hemodialysis may be used in severe barbiturate intoxications or if the patient is anuric or in shock.
6. Patient should be rolled from side to side every 30 minutes.
7. Antibiotics should be given if pneumonia is suspected.
8. Appropriate nursing care to prevent hypostatic pneumonia, decubiti, aspiration, and other complications of patients with altered states of consciousness.

DOSAGE AND ADMINISTRATION

Typical hypnotic doses for adults and children are given below. These are intended only as a guide, and administration should be adjusted to the individual needs of each patient. For sedation, in children 5–14 years and in adults, reduce dose appropriately.

Adults (average to above average weight)— one 120 mg or one 200 mg suppository.

Children —

12–14 years (80–110 lbs)	one 60 mg or one 120 mg suppository
5–12 years (40–80 lbs)	one 60 mg suppository
1–4 years (20–40 lbs)	one 30 mg or one 60 mg suppository
2 months–1 year (10–20 lbs)	one 30 mg suppository

Suppositories should not be divided.

Dosages of barbiturates must be individualized with full knowledge of their particular characteristics and recommended rate of administration. Factors of consideration are the patient's age, weight, and condition.

Special patient population: Dosage should be reduced in the elderly or debilitated because these patients may be more sensitive to barbiturates. Dosage should be reduced for patients with impaired renal function or hepatic disease.

HOW SUPPLIED

NEMBUTAL Sodium Suppositories (pentobarbital sodium suppositories) are available as suppositories containing pentobarbital sodium in the amount of 30 mg (**NDC** 0074-3272-01); 60 mg (**NDC** 0074-3148-01); 120 mg (**NDC** 0074-3145-01) and 200 mg (**NDC** 0074-3164-01). Supplied in boxes of 12 suppositories.

Store in a refrigerator (36°–46°F).

Revised: June, 1994

Ref. 03-4514-R13

NORVIR™ ℞

(ritonavir capsules)
(ritonavir oral solution)

WARNING
CO-ADMINISTRATION OF NORVIR WITH CERTAIN NONSEDATING ANTIHISTAMINES, SEDATIVE HYPNOTICS, ANTIARRHYTHMICS, OR ERGOT ALKALOID PREPARATIONS MAY RESULT IN POTENTIALLY SERIOUS AND/OR LIFE-THREATENING ADVERSE EVENTS DUE TO POSSIBLE EFFECTS OF NORVIR ON THE HEPATIC METABOLISM OF CERTAIN DRUGS. SEE **CONTRAINDICATIONS** AND **PRECAUTIONS** SECTIONS.

DESCRIPTION

NORVIR (ritonavir) is an inhibitor of HIV protease with activity against the Human Immunodeficiency Virus (HIV).

Ritonavir is chemically designated as 10-Hydroxy-2-methyl-5-(1-methylethyl)-1-[2-(1-methylethyl)-4-thiazolyl]-3,6-dioxo-8,11-bis(phenylmethyl)-2,4,7,12-tetraazatridecan-13-oic acid, 5-thiazolylmethyl ester, [5S-(5R*,8R*,10R*,11R*)]. Its molecular formula is $C_{37}H_{48}N_6O_5S_2$, and its molecular weight is 720.95. Ritonavir has the following structural formula:

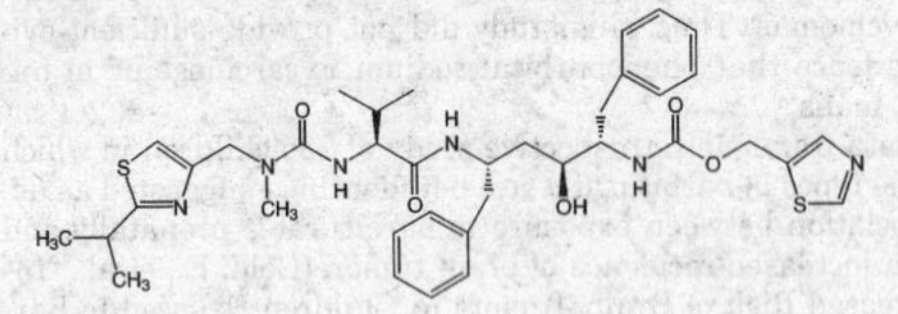

Ritonavir is a white-to-light-tan powder. Ritonavir has a bitter metallic taste. It is freely soluble in methanol and ethanol, soluble in isopropanol and practically insoluble in water.

NORVIR capsules are available for oral administration in a strength of 100 mg ritonavir with the following inactive ingredients: Caprylic/capric triglycerides, polyoxyl 35 castor oil, citric acid, gelatin, ethanol, polyglycolyzed glycerides, polysorbate 80, and propylene glycol.

NORVIR oral solution is available for oral administration as 80 mg/mL of ritonavir in a peppermint and caramel flavored vehicle. Each 8-ounce bottle contains 19.2 grams of ritonavir. NORVIR oral solution also contains ethanol, water, polyoxyl 35 castor oil, propylene glycol, anhydrous citric acid to adjust pH, saccharin sodium, peppermint oil, creamy caramel flavoring, and FD&C Yellow No. 6.

CLINICAL PHARMACOLOGY

Microbiology

Mechanism of action: Ritonavir is a peptidomimetic inhibitor of both the HIV-1 and HIV-2 proteases. Inhibition of HIV protease renders the enzyme incapable of processing the *gag-pol* polyprotein precursor which leads to production of non-infectious immature HIV particles.

Antiviral activity *in vitro*: The activity of ritonavir was assessed *in vitro* in acutely infected lymphoblastoid cell lines and in peripheral blood lymphocytes. The concentration of drug that inhibits 50% (EC_{50}) of viral replication ranged from 3.8 to 153 nM depending upon the HIV-1 isolate and the cells employed. The average EC_{50} for low passage clinical isolates was 22 nM (n=13). In MT_4 cells, ritonavir demonstrated additive effects against HIV-1 in combination with either zidovudine (ZDV) or didanosine (ddI). Studies which measured cytotoxicity of ritonavir on several cell lines showed that >20 µM was required to inhibit cellular growth by 50% resulting in an *in vitro* therapeutic index of at least 1000.

Resistance: HIV-1 isolates with reduced susceptibility to ritonavir have been selected *in vitro*. Genotypic analysis of these isolates showed mutations in the HIV protease gene at amino acid positions 84 (Ile to Val), 82 (Val to Phe), 71 (Ala to Val), and 46 (Met to Ile). Phenotypic (n=18) and genotypic (n=44) changes in HIV isolates from selected patients treated with ritonavir were monitored in phase I/II trials over a period of 3 to 32 weeks. Mutations associated with the HIV viral protease in isolates obtained from 41 patients appeared to occur in a stepwise and ordered fashion; in sequence, these mutations were position 82 (Val to Ala/Phe), 54 (Ile to Val), 71 (Ala to Val/Thr), and 36 (Ile to Leu), followed by combinations of mutations at an additional 5 specific amino acid positions. Of 18 patients for which both phenotypic and genotypic analysis were performed on free virus isolated from plasma, 12 showed reduced susceptibility to ritonavir *in vitro*. All 18 patients possessed one or more mutations in the viral protease gene. The 82 mutation appeared to be necessary but not sufficient to confer phenotypic resistance. Phenotypic resistance was defined as a ≥5-fold decrease in viral sensitivity *in vitro* from baseline. The clinical relevance of phenotypic and genotypic changes associated with ritonavir therapy has not been established.

Cross-resistance to other antiretrovirals: The potential for HIV cross-resistance between protease inhibitors has not been fully explored. Therefore, it is unknown what effect ritonavir therapy will have on the activity of concordantly or subsequently administered protease inhibitors. Serial HIV isolates obtained from six patients during ritonavir therapy showed a decrease in ritonavir susceptibility *in vitro* but did not demonstrate a concordant decrease in susceptibility to saquinavir *in vitro* when compared to matched baseline isolates. However, isolates from two of these patients demonstrated decreased susceptibility to indinavir *in vitro* (8-fold). Isolates from 5 patients were also tested for cross-resistance to VX-478 and nelfinavir; isolates from 2 patients had a decrease in susceptibility to nelfinavir (12-14-fold), and none to VX-478. Cross-resistance between ritonavir and reverse transcriptase inhibitors is unlikely because of the different enzyme targets involved. One ZDV-resistant HIV isolate tested *in vitro* retained full susceptibility to ritonavir.

Pharmacokinetics

The pharmacokinetics of ritonavir have been studied in healthy volunteers and HIV-infected patients (CD_4 ≥ 50 cells/µL). See Table 1 for ritonavir pharmacokinetic characteristics.

The absolute bioavailability of ritonavir has not been determined. After a 600 mg dose of oral solution, peak concentrations of ritonavir were achieved approximately 2 hours and 4 hours after dosing under fasting and non-fasting (514 KCal; 9% fat, 12% protein, and 79% carbohydrate) conditions, respectively. When the oral solution was given under non-fasting conditions, peak ritonavir concentrations decreased 23% and the extent of absorption decreased 7% relative to fasting conditions. Dilution of the oral solution, within one hour of administration, with 240 mL of chocolate milk, Advera® or Ensure® did not significantly affect the extent and rate of ritonavir absorption. After a single 600 mg dose under non-fasting conditions, in two separate studies, the capsule (n=21) and oral solution (n=18) formulations yielded mean ± SD areas under the plasma concentration-time curve (AUCs) of 129.5 ± 47.1 and 129.0 ± 39.3 µg•h/mL, respectively. Relative to fasting conditions, the extent of absorption of ritonavir from the capsule formulation was 15% higher when administered with a meal (771 KCal; 46% fat, 18% protein, and 37% carbohydrate).

Nearly all of the plasma radioactivity after a single oral 600 mg dose of ^{14}C-ritonavir oral solution (n=5) was attributed to unchanged ritonavir. Five ritonavir metabolites have been identified in human urine and feces. The isopropylthiazole oxidation metabolite (M-2) is the major metabolite and has antiviral activity similar to that of parent drug; however, the concentrations of this metabolite in plasma are low. Studies utilizing human liver microsomes have demonstrated that cytochrome P450 3A (CYP3A) is the major isoform involved in ritonavir metabolism, although CYP2D6 also contributes to the formation of M-2.

In a study of five subjects receiving a 600 mg dose of ^{14}C-ritonavir oral solution, 11.3 ± 2.8% of the dose was excreted into the urine, with 3.5 ± 1.8% of the dose excreted as unchanged parent drug. In that study, 86.4 ± 2.9% of the dose was excreted in the feces with 33.8 ± 10.8% of the dose excreted as unchanged parent drug. Upon multiple dosing, ritonavir accumulation is less than predicted from a single dose possibly due to a time and dose-related increase in clearance.

Table 1
Ritonavir Pharmacokinetic Characteristics

Parameter	n	Values (Mean ± SD)
C_{max} SS†	10	11.2 ± 3.6 µg/mL
C_{trough} SS†	10	3.7 ± 2.6 µg/mL
V_β/F‡	91	0.41 ± 0.25 L/kg
$t_{1/2}$		3 – 5 h
CL/F/SS†	10	8.8 ± 3.2 L/h
CL/F‡	91	4.6 ± 1.6 L/h
CL_R	62	<0.1 L/h
RBC/Plasma Ratio		0.14
Percent Bound*		98 to 99%

† SS = steady state; patients taking ritonavir 600 mg q12h.
‡ Single ritonavir 600 mg dose.
* Primarily bound to human serum albumin and alpha-1

acid glycoprotein over the ritonavir concentration range of 0.01 to 30 μg/mL.

The pharmacokinetic profile of ritonavir in pediatric patients below the age of 2 years has not been established. Steady-state pharmacokinetics were evaluated in 37 HIV-infected patients ages 2 to 14 years receiving doses ranging from 250 mg/m² b.i.d. to 400 mg/m² b.i.d. Across dose groups, ritonavir steady-state oral clearance (CL/F/m²) was approximately 1.5 times faster in pediatric patients than in adult subjects. Ritonavir concentrations obtained after 350 to 400 mg/m² twice daily in pediatric patients were comparable to those obtained in adults receiving 600 mg (approximately 330 mg/m²) twice daily.

Special Populations:

Gender, Race and Age: No age-related pharmacokinetic differences have been observed in adult patients (18 to 63 years). Ritonavir pharmacokinetics have not been studied in older patients. A study of ritonavir pharmacokinetics in healthy males and females showed no statistically significant differences in the pharmacokinetics of ritonavir. Pharmacokinetic differences due to race have not been identified.

Renal Insufficiency: Ritonavir pharmacokinetics have not been studied in patients with renal insufficiency, however since renal clearance is negligible, a decrease in total body clearance is not expected in patients with renal insufficiency.

Hepatic Insufficiency: Ritonavir pharmacokinetics have not been studied in subjects with hepatic insufficiency (see **PRECAUTIONS**).

Drug-Drug Interactions: Table 2 summarizes the effects on AUC and C_{max}, with 95% confidence intervals (95 CI), of co-administration of ritonavir with a variety of drugs. For information about clinical recommendations see **PRECAUTIONS-Drug Interactions**.

[See table above]

INDICATIONS AND USAGE

NORVIR is indicated in combination with other antiretroviral agents or as monotherapy for the treatment of HIV-infection. For patients with advanced HIV disease, this indication is based on the results from a study that showed a reduction in both mortality and AIDS-defining clinical events for patients who received NORVIR. Median duration of follow-up in this study was 6 months. The clinical benefit from NORVIR therapy for longer periods of treatment is unknown.

For patients with less advanced disease, this indication is based on changes in surrogate markers in studies evaluating patients who received NORVIR alone or in combination with other antiretroviral agents (see **Description of Clinical Studies**).

Description of Clinical Studies

The activity of NORVIR as monotherapy or in combination with nucleoside analogues has been evaluated in 1446 patients enrolled in two double-blind, randomized trials. NORVIR therapy in combination with zidovudine and zalcitabine was also evaluated in an open-label, non-comparative study of 32 patients. The clinical studies reported here were all conducted using ritonavir oral solution.

Advanced Patients with Prior Antiretroviral Therapy

Study 247 was a randomized, double-blind trial conducted in HIV-infected patients with at least nine months of prior antiretroviral therapy and baseline CD_4 cell counts ≤ 100 cells/μL. NORVIR 600 mg b.i.d. or placebo was added to each patient's baseline antiretroviral therapy regimen, which could have consisted of up to two approved antiretroviral agents. The study accrued 1090 patients, with mean baseline CD_4 cell count at study entry of 32 cells/μL. Median duration of follow-up was 6 months.

The six month cumulative incidence of clinical disease progression or death was 17% for patients randomized to NORVIR compared to 34% for patients randomized to placebo. This difference in rates was statistically significant (see Figure 1).

Figure 1
Time to Disease Progression or Death in Study 247

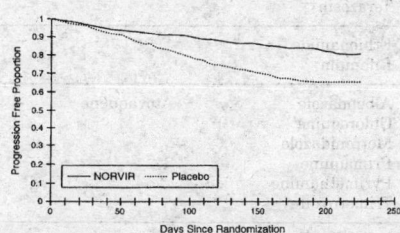

The six-month cumulative mortality was 5.8% for patients randomized to NORVIR and 10.1% for patients randomized to placebo. This difference in rates was statistically significant.

In addition, analyses of mean CD_4 cell count changes from baseline over the first 16 weeks of study for the first 211

patients enrolled (mean baseline CD_4 cell count = 29 cells/μL) showed that NORVIR was associated with larger increases in CD_4 cell counts than was placebo (see Figure 2).

Figure 2
Mean CD₄ Count Changes (cells/μL) From Baseline In Study 247

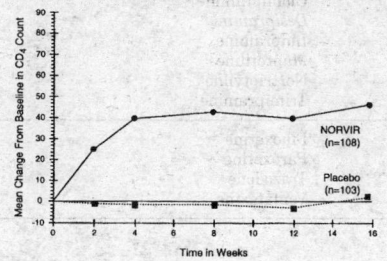

Figure 3 summarizes the mean changes from baseline in log HIV RNA levels for Study 247.

Figure 3
Mean Change From Baseline in Log HIV RNA Levels in Study 247

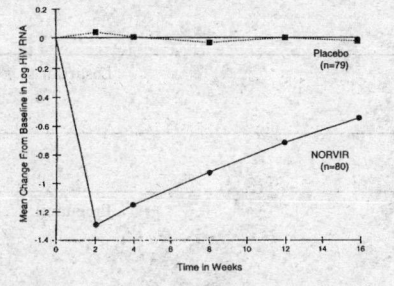

Patients Without Prior Antiretroviral Therapy

In ongoing Study 245, 356 antiretroviral-naive HIV-infected patients (mean baseline CD_4 = 364 cells/μL) were randomized to receive either NORVIR 600 mg b.i.d., zidovudine 200 mg t.i.d., or a combination of these drugs. In analyses of average CD_4 cell count changes from baseline over the first 16 weeks of study, both NORVIR monotherapy and combination therapy produced greater mean increases in CD_4 cell count than did zidovudine monotherapy (see Figure 4). The

CD_4 cell count increases for NORVIR monotherapy were larger than the increases for combination therapy.

Figure 4
Mean CD₄ Count Changes (cells/μL) From Baseline In Study 245

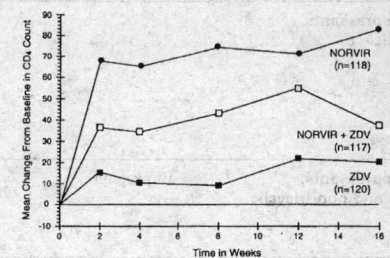

Figure 5 summarizes the mean changes from baseline in log HIV RNA levels for Study 245.

Figure 5
Mean Change From Baseline in Log HIV RNA Levels in Study 245

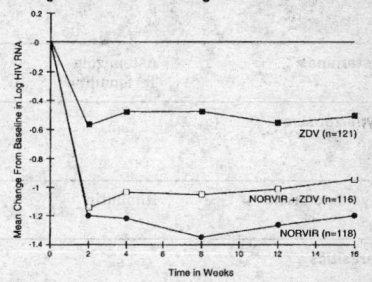

Combination Therapy with NORVIR, Zidovudine, and Zalcitabine in Antiretroviral-Naive Patients

In Study 208, an open-label uncontrolled trial, 32 antiretroviral-naive HIV-infected patients initially received NORVIR 600 mg b.i.d. monotherapy. Zidovudine 200 mg t.i.d. and zalcitabine 0.75 mg t.i.d. were added after 14 days of NORVIR monotherapy. Results of combination therapy for the first 20 weeks of this study show median increases in CD_4 cell

Table 2
Effects on AUC and C_max of Co-administration of Ritonavir With Other Drugs

Drug	Ritonavir Dosage	n	AUC % (95 CI)	C_{max} % (95 CI)
Effect on Ritonavir				
Clarithromycin 500 mg q12h 4 days	200 mg q8h 4 days	22	↑ 12% (2, 23%)	↑ 15% (2, 28%)
Didanosine 200 mg q12h 4 days	600 mg q12h 4 days	12	↔	↔
Fluconazole 400 mg day 1, 200 mg daily 4 days	200 mg q6h 4 days	8	↑ 12% (5, 20%)	↑ 15% (7, 22%)
Fluoxetine 30 mg q12h 8 days	600 mg single dose	16	↑ 19% (7, 34%)	↔
Rifampin 600 mg or 300 mg daily 10 days[2]	500 mg q12h 20 days	7,9*	↓ 35% (7, 55%)	↓ 25% (-5, 46%)
Zidovudine 200 mg q8h 4 days	300 mg q6h 4 days	10	↔	↔

Drug	Ritonavir Dosage	n	AUC % (95 CI)	C_{max} % (95 CI)
Effect on Co-administered Drug				
Alprazolam 1 mg single dose	500 mg q12h 10 days	12	↓ 12% (-5, 30%)	↓ 16% (5, 27%)
Clarithromycin 500 mg q12h 4 days	200 mg q8h 4 days	22	↑ 77% (56, 103%)	↑ 31% (15, 51%)
14-OH clarithromycin metabolite			↓ 100%	↓ 99%
Desipramine 100 mg single dose	500 mg q12h 12 days	14	↑ 145% (103, 211%)	↑ 22% (12, 35%)
2-OH desipramine metabolite			↓ 15% (3, 26%)	↓ 67% (62, 72%)
Didanosine 200 mg q12h 4 days	600 mg q12h 4 days	12	↓ 13% (0, 23%)	↓ 16% (5, 26%)
Ethinyl estradiol 50 μg single dose	500 mg q12h 16 days	23	↓ 40% (31, 49%)	↓ 32% (24, 39%)
Rifabutin 150 mg daily 16 days	500 mg q12h 10 days	5,11*	↑ 4-fold (2.8, 6.1X)	↑ 2.5-fold (1.9, 3.4X)
25-O-desacetyl rifabutin metabolite			↑ 35-fold (25, 78X)	↑ 16-fold (14, 20X)
Saquinavir 400 mg bid steady state[3]	400 mg bid steady state	7	↑ 17-fold (9, 31X)	↑ 14-fold (7, 28X)
Sulfamethoxazole 800 mg single dose[1]	500 mg q12h 12 days	15	↓ 20% (16, 23%)	↔
Theophylline 3 mg/kg q8h 15 days	500 mg q12h 10 days	13,11*	↓ 43% (42, 45%)	↓ 32% (29, 34%)
Trimethoprim 160 mg single dose[1]	500 mg q12h 12 days	15	↓ 20% (3, 43%)	↔
Zidovudine 200 mg q8h 4 days	300 mg q6h 4 days	9	↓ 25% (15, 34%)	↓ 27% (4, 45%)

[1] Sulfamethoxazole and trimethoprim taken as single combination tablet.
[2] Preliminary Data.
[3] Comparison to a standard saquinavir 600 mg t.i.d. regimen (n = 114).
↑ Indicates increase.
↓ Indicates decrease.
↔ Indicates no change.
* Parallel group design; entries are subjects receiving combination and control regimens, respectively.

Continued on next page

Norvir—Cont.

counts from baseline levels of 83 to 106 cells/μL over the treatment period. Mean decreases from baseline in HIV RNA particle levels ranged from 1.69 to 1.92 logs.

CONTRAINDICATIONS

NORVIR is contraindicated in patients with known hypersensitivity to ritonavir or any of its ingredients.

Ritonavir is expected to produce large increases in the plasma concentrations of the following drugs: amiodarone, astemizole, bepridil, bupropion, cisapride, clozapine, dihydroergotamine, encainide, ergotamine, flecainide, meperidine, pimozide, piroxicam, propafenone, propoxyphene, quinidine, rifabutin, and terfenadine. These agents have recognized risks of arrhythmias, hematologic abnormalities, seizures, or other potentially serious adverse effects. Additionally, postmarketing reports of co-administration of ritonavir with ergotamine or dihydroergotamine has been associated with acute ergot toxicity characterized by peripheral vasospasm and ischemia of the extremities. **These drugs should not be co-administered with ritonavir.**

Ritonavir co-administration is also expected to produce large increases in these highly metabolized sedatives and hypnotics: clorazepate, diazepam, estazolam, flurazepam, midazolam, triazolam, and zolpidem. **Due to the potential for extreme sedation and respiratory depression from these agents, these drugs should not be co-administered with ritonavir.**

WARNINGS

Allergic reactions including urticaria, mild skin eruptions, bronchospasm, and angioedema have been reported. Rare cases of anaphylaxis and Stevens-Johnson syndrome have also been reported.

Hepatic transaminase elevations exceeding five times the upper limit of normal, clinical hepatitis, and jaundice have occurred in patients receiving NORVIR alone or in combination with other antiretroviral drugs (see Table 5). There may be an increased risk for transaminase elevations in patients with underlying hepatitis B or C. Therefore, caution should be exercised when administering NORVIR to patients with pre-existing liver diseases, liver enzyme abnormalities, or hepatitis.

Table 3
Predicted Effects on Drugs Co-administered with Ritonavir. Contraindicated Medications are Listed in Column 1
(see PRECAUTIONS, Drug Interactions for Clinical Pharmacology Study Results)

Drug Category	Representative Drugs by Theoretical Prediction of Interaction Category					
	Contraindicated Medications	Large[1] ↑ AUC[2]	Moderate[1] ↑ AUC[2]	Moderate[1] ↑ or ↓ AUC[2]	Unknown	Possible ↓ AUC[2]
Analgesics, narcotic	Meperidine Propoxyphene	Alfentanil Fentanyl Methadone	Hydrocodone Oxycodone Tramadol		Levamethadyl (LAAM)	Codeine Hydromorphone Morphine
Analgesics, nonsteroidal	Piroxicam		Diclofenac Flurbiprofen Ibuprofen Indomethacin		Nabumetone Sulindac	Ketoprofen Ketorlac Naproxen
Antiarrhythmics	Amiodarone Encainide Flecainide Propafenone Quinidine	Lidocaine	Disopyramide Mexiletine		Tocainide†† Digoxin	
Antiasthmatic						Theophylline*
Antibiotics, macrolide		Erythromycin	Clarithromycin*			
Anticoagulant			R-warfarin	S-warfarin		
Anticonvulsants		Carbamazepine	Clonazepam Ethosuximide	Phenytoin	Phenobarbital	Divalproex Lamotrigine
Antidepressants, tricyclic			Amitriptyline Clomipramine Desipramine* Imipramine Maprotiline Nortriptyline Trimipramine		Doxepin††	
Antidepressants, SSRIs and non-tricyclic	Bupropion	Nefazodone Sertraline	Fluoxetine Paroxetine Trazodone Venlafaxine		Fluvoxamine	
Antidiarrheal						Diphenoxylate Loperamide
Antiemetics, Prokinetics	Cisapride		Dronabinol Ondansetron		Prochlorperazine†† Promethazine††	Metoclopramide
Antifungal agents		Itraconazole Ketoconazole Miconazole				
Antihistamines	Astemizole Terfenadine	Loratadine				
Antihypertensives				Losartan	Doxazosin†† Prazosin†† Terazosin††	
Antimycobacterials	Rifabutin				Ethionamide Rifampin	
Antiparasitics		Quinine		Proguanil	Albendazole Chloroquine Metronidazole Primaquine Pyrimethamine Trimetrexate	Atovaquone
Antiulcer agents				Lansoprazole Omeprazole		
β-blockers			Metoprolol Penbutolol Pindolol Timolol	Propranolol	Betaxolol††	

Table 3 (continued)
Predicted Effects on Drugs Co-administered with Ritonavir. Contraindicated Medications are Listed in Column 1
(see PRECAUTIONS, Drug Interactions for Clinical Pharmacology Study Results)

Calcium channel blockers	Bepridil	Amlodipine Diltiazem Felodipine Isradipine Nicardipine Nifedipine Nimodipine Nisoldipine Nitrendipine Verapamil				
Cancer chemotherapeutic agents		Tamoxifen	Etoposide Paclitaxel Vinblastine Vincristine	Cyclophosphamide† Ifosfamide†	Daunorubicin†† Doxorubicin††	
Ergot alkaloids and derivatives	Dihydroergotamine Ergotamine	Bromocriptine			Ergonavine†† Methylergonavine†† Methysergide††	
Hemorheologic agent					Pentoxifylline	
HIV antivirals		Indinavir *Saquinavir**			Nevirapine††	
Hypoglycemics				Glimepiride Glipizide Glyburide Tolbutamide		
Hypolipidemics		Fluvastatin Lovastatin Simvastatin	Pravastatin		Gemfibrozil	Clofibrate
Immunosuppressants		Cyclosporine Tacrolimus				
Neuroleptics	Clozapine Pimozide		Chlorpromazine Haloperidol Perphenazine Risperidone Thioridazine			
Sedative/hypnotics	Clorazepate Diazepam Estazolam Flurazepam Midazolam Triazolam Zolpidem					Lorazepam Oxazepam Propofol Temazepam
Steroids		Dexamethasone	Prednisone			*Ethinyl estradiol**
Stimulants			Dexfenfluramine Methamphetamine		Methylphenidate	

[1]   Large = > 3X; Moderate = 1.5–3X.
[2]   AUC = area under the plasma concentration-time curve, a measure of drug exposure.
†   An increase in the AUC of cyclophosphamide and ifosfamide, both activated by CYP, may correspond to a decrease in the AUC of the active metabolite(s) and a possible decrease in efficacy of these drugs.
††   A possible increase in concentrations is more likely when combined with ritonavir.
*   Clinical drug interaction study has been performed (see Table 2).

There have been postmarketing reports of hepatic dysfunction, including some fatalities. These have generally occurred in patients taking multiple concomitant medications and/or with advanced AIDS. A definitive causal relationship has not been established.

New onset diabetes mellitus, exacerbation of pre-existing diabetes mellitus, and hyperglycemia have been reported during post marketing surveillance in HIV-infected patients receiving protease inhibitor therapy. Some patients required either initiation or dose adjustments of insulin or oral hypoglycemic agents for treatment of these events. In some cases, diabetic ketoacidosis has occurred. In those patients who discontinued protease inhibitor therapy, hyperglycemia persisted in some cases. Because these events have been reported voluntarily during clinical practice, estimates of frequency cannot be made and a causal relationship between protease inhibitor therapy and these events has not been established.

PRECAUTIONS
General
Ritonavir is principally metabolized by the liver. Therefore, caution should be exercised when administering this drug to patients with impaired hepatic function (see **WARNINGS**).
Resistance/Cross-resistance
The potential for HIV cross-resistance between protease inhibitors has not been fully explored. Therefore, it is unknown what effect ritonavir therapy will have on the activity of subsequent protease inhibitors (see **Microbiology**).

Hemophilia
There have been reports of increased bleeding, including spontaneous skin hematomas and hemarthrosis, in patients with hemophilia type A and B treated with protease inhibitors. In some patients additional factor VIII was given. In more than half of the reported cases, treatment with protease inhibitors was continued or reintroduced. A causal relationship has not been established.
Information For Patients
Patients should be informed that NORVIR is not a cure for HIV infection and that they may continue to acquire illnesses associated with advanced HIV infection, including opportunistic infections.

Patients should be told that the long-term effects of NORVIR are unknown at this time. They should be informed that NORVIR therapy has not been shown to reduce the risk of transmitting HIV to others through sexual contact or blood contamination.

Patients should be advised to take NORVIR with food, if possible.

Patients should be informed to take NORVIR every day as prescribed. Patients should not alter the dose or discontinue NORVIR without consulting their doctor. If a dose is missed, patients should take the next dose as soon as possible. However, if a dose is skipped, the patient should not double the next dose.

Since NORVIR interacts with some drugs when taken together, patients should be advised to report to their doctor the use of any other medications, including prescription and nonprescription drugs.

Laboratory Tests
Ritonavir has been associated with alterations in triglycerides, cholesterol, SGOT, SGPT, GGT, CPK, and uric acid. Appropriate laboratory testing should be performed prior to initiating NORVIR therapy and at periodic intervals or if any clinical signs or symptoms occur during therapy. For comprehensive information concerning laboratory test alterations associated with nucleoside analogues, physicians should refer to the complete product information for each of these drugs.
Drug Interactions
Effects on ritonavir
Agents which increase CYP3A activity (e.g., phenobarbital, carbamazepine, dexamethasone, phenytoin, rifampin, and rifabutin) are expected to increase the clearance of ritonavir resulting in decreased ritonavir plasma concentrations. Tobacco use is associated with an 18% decrease in the AUC of ritonavir.
Effects on co-administered drugs
Ritonavir can produce large increases in plasma concentrations of certain highly metabolized drugs. Ritonavir has a high affinity for several cytochrome P450 (CYP) isoforms with the following rank order: CYP3A > CYP2D6 > CYP2C9, CYP2C19 >> CYP2A6, CYP1A2, CYP2E1. There is some evidence that ritonavir may increase the activity of glucuronosyltransferases; thus, loss of therapeutic effects from directly glucuronidated agents during ritonavir therapy may signify the need for dosage alteration of these agents.

Continued on next page

Norvir—Cont.

Clinical drug interaction studies with ritonavir and some commonly administered drugs have been conducted. Drugs that may need dose adjustment based on information from these studies are listed below in alphabetical order. Drugs that are predicted to be affected by co-administration with ritonavir are listed in Table 3.

Clarithromycin: The mean increase in the AUC of clarithromycin in the presence of ritonavir was 77%. Clarithromycin may be administered without dosage adjustment to patients with normal renal function. However, for patients with renal impairment the following dosage adjustments should be considered. For patients with CL_{CR} 30 to 60 mL/min the dose of clarithromycin should be reduced by 50%. For patients with CL_{CR} < 30 mL/min the dose of clarithromycin should be decreased by 75%.

Desipramine: Co-administration of ritonavir resulted in a 145% mean increase in the AUC of desipramine. Dosage reduction of desipramine should be considered in patients taking the combination.

Didanosine: The AUC of didanosine was decreased by 13% when co-administered with ritonavir. Didanosine may be administered without dosage adjustment to patients taking ritonavir; however, dosing of the two drugs should be separated by 2.5 hours to avoid formulation incompatibility.

Disulfiram/Metronidazole: Ritonavir formulations contain alcohol, which can produce reactions when co-administered with disulfiram or other drugs that produce disulfiram-like reactions (e.g., metronidazole).

Oral Contraceptives: The mean AUC of ethinyl estradiol, a component in oral contraceptives, was reduced 40% during concomitant dosing with ritonavir 500 mg q12h; dosage increase or alternate contraceptive measures should be considered.

Saquinavir: Ritonavir extensively inhibits the metabolism of saquinavir resulting in greatly increased saquinavir plasma concentrations. Following approximately 4 weeks of a combination regimen of saquinavir (400 or 600 mg b.i.d.) and ritonavir (400 or 600 mg b.i.d.) in HIV-infected patients, saquinavir AUC values were at least 17-fold greater than historical AUC values from patients who received saquinavir 600 mg t.i.d. without ritonavir. When used in combination therapy for up to 24 weeks, doses greater than 400 mg b.i.d. of either ritonavir or saquinavir were associated with an increase in adverse events. Plasma exposures achieved with Invirase® (saquinavir mesylate) (400 mg b.i.d.) and ritonavir (400 mg b.i.d.) are similar to those achieved with Fortovase™ (saquinavir) (400 mg b.i.d.) and ritonavir (400 mg b.i.d.).

Theophylline: The average AUC of theophylline was reduced by 43% when co-administered with ritonavir. Increased dosage of theophylline may be required.

A systematic review of over 200 medications prescribed to HIV-infected patients was performed to identify potential drug interactions with ritonavir. Table 3 summarizes some commonly prescribed drugs, categorized by the predicted magnitude of interaction that could result if co-administered with ritonavir. Drugs that are specifically contraindicated due to the expected magnitude of interaction and potential for serious adverse events are in the first column of Table 3. This table lists the predicted magnitude of drug interaction based on what is known about the metabolism for each medication. The actual magnitude of interaction could be larger or smaller than that listed; therefore, it is advised that concomitant use of any of these agents with ritonavir should be accompanied by therapeutic drug concentration monitoring and/or increased monitoring of therapeutic and adverse effects, especially for agents with narrow therapeutic margins (e.g., oral anticoagulants, immunosuppressants). Large dosage reductions (>50% reduction) may be required for those agents extensively metabolized by CYP3A.

[See table at bottom of page 466 and on previous page]

Post-Marketing Experience with Drugs Listed in Table 3

Cardiac and neurologic events have been reported when ritonavir has been co-administered with disopyramide, mexiletine, nefazodone, or fluoxetine. The possibility of drug interaction cannot be excluded.

Carcinogenesis and Mutagenesis

Long-term carcinogenicity studies of ritonavir in animal systems have not been completed. However, ritonavir was not mutagenic or clastogenic in a battery of *in vitro* and *in vivo* assays including bacterial reverse mutation (Ames) using *S. typhimurium* and *E. coli*, mouse lymphoma, mouse micronucleus, and chromosome aberrations in human lymphocytes.

Pregnancy, Fertility, and Reproduction

Pregnancy Category B: Ritonavir produced no effects on fertility in rats at drug exposures approximately 40% (male) and 60% (female) of that achieved with the proposed therapeutic dose. Higher dosages were not feasible due to hepatic toxicity.

Table 4
Percentage of Patients with Treatment-Emergent[1] Adverse Events of Moderate or Severe Intensity Occurring in ≥ 2% of Patients Receiving NORVIR

Adverse Events	Study 245 Naive Patients NORVIR + ZDV n = 116	NORVIR n = 117	ZDV n = 119	Study 247 Advanced Patients NORVIR n = 541	Placebo n = 547
Body as a Whole					
Abdominal Pain	4.3	3.4	4.2	7.0	3.1
Asthenia	27.6	9.4	10.1	14.2	5.3
Fever	1.7	0.9	1.7	4.4	2.2
Headache	7.8	5.1	7.6	6.3	4.0
Malaise	4.3	1.7	3.4	0.7	0.2
Cardiovascular					
Vasodilation	2.6	1.7	0.8	1.3	0.0
Digestive					
Anorexia	7.8	0.9	3.4	6.1	2.0
Constipation	2.6	0.0	0.8	1.0	0.4
Diarrhea	21.6	12.8	0.0	18.3	6.1
Dyspepsia	1.7	0.0	1.7	4.8	0.7
Flatulence	2.6	0.9	0.8	0.9	0.6
Local Throat Irritation	1.7	1.7	0.8	2.6	0.2
Nausea	46.6	23.1	24.4	26.2	5.7
Vomiting	22.4	12.8	12.6	15.2	2.6
Metabolic and Nutritional					
Creatine Phosphokinase					
Increased	1.7	3.4	3.4	0.9	0.2
Hyperlipidemia	1.7	1.7	0.0	4.1	0.0
Musculoskeletal					
Myalgia	1.7	1.7	0.8	2.2	0.9
Nervous					
Circumoral Paresthesia	5.2	2.6	0.0	5.9	0.2
Dizziness	5.2	2.6	1.7	3.3	1.1
Insomnia	3.4	2.6	0.8	1.3	0.6
Paresthesia	5.2	2.6	0.0	2.0	0.2
Peripheral Paresthesia	0.0	6.0	0.0	5.0	0.7
Somnolence	2.6	2.6	0.0	2.0	0.2
Thinking Abnormal	2.6	0.0	0.8	0.7	0.2
Respiratory					
Pharyngitis	0.9	2.6	0.0	0.4	0.4
Skin and Appendages					
Rash	0.9	0.0	0.8	2.6	0.9
Sweating	3.4	2.6	1.7	1.3	0.6
Special Senses					
Taste Perversion	15.5	10.3	7.6	5.4	1.7

[1] Includes those adverse events at least possibly related to study drug or of unknown relationship and excludes concurrent HIV conditions.

No treatment-related malformations were observed when ritonavir was administered to pregnant rats or rabbits. Developmental toxicity observed in rats (early resorptions, decreased fetal body weight and ossification delays and developmental variations) occurred at a maternally toxic dosage at an exposure equivalent to approximately 30% of that achieved with the proposed therapeutic dose. A slight increase in the incidence of cryptorchidism was also noted in rats at an exposure approximately 22% of that achieved with the proposed therapeutic dose.

Developmental toxicity observed in rabbits (resorptions, decreased litter size and decreased fetal weights) also occurred at a maternally toxic dosage equivalent to 1.8 times the proposed therapeutic dose based on a body surface area conversion factor.

There are, however, no adequate and well-controlled studies in pregnant women. Because animal reproduction studies are not always predictive of human response, this drug should be used during pregnancy only if clearly needed.

Nursing Mothers: It is not known whether this drug is excreted in human milk. Because many drugs are excreted in human milk, caution should be exercised when ritonavir is administered to a nursing woman. However, the U.S. Public Health Service Centers for Disease Control and Prevention advises HIV-infected women not to breast-feed to avoid postnatal transmission of HIV to a child who may not be infected.

Pediatric Use

The safety and pharmacokinetic profile of ritonavir in pediatric patients below the age of 2 years have not been established. In HIV-infected patients age 2 to 16 years, the adverse event profile seen during a clinical trial and postmarketing experience was similar to that for adult patients. The evaluation of the antiviral activity of ritonavir in pediatric patients in clinical trials is ongoing.

ADVERSE REACTIONS

The safety of NORVIR alone and in combination with nucleoside analogues was studied in 1140 patients. Table 4 lists treatment-emergent adverse events (at least possibly related and of at least moderate intensity) that occurred in 2% or greater of patients receiving NORVIR alone or in combination with nucleosides in Study 245 or Study 247. At the time of this safety assessment, the median duration of treatment in Study 245 and Study 247 was 3.7 and 2.4 months, respectively. However, safety data was collected on patients for greater than 6 months of treatment. The most frequently reported clinical adverse events, other than asthenia, among patients receiving NORVIR were gastrointestinal and neurological disturbances including nausea, diarrhea, vomiting, anorexia, abdominal pain, taste perversion, and circumoral and peripheral paresthesias. Similar adverse event profiles were reported in patients receiving ritonavir in other trials.

[See table 4 above]

Adverse events occurring in less than 2% of patients receiving NORVIR in all phase II/phase III studies and considered at least possibly related or of unknown relationship to treatment and of at least moderate intensity are listed below by body system.

Body as a Whole: Abdomen enlarged, accidental injury, allergic reaction, back pain, cachexia, chest pain, chills, facial edema, facial pain, flu syndrome, hormone level altered, hypothermia, kidney pain, neck pain, neck rigidity, pain (unspecified), substernal chest pain, and photosensitivity reaction.

Cardiovascular System: Hemorrhage, hypotension, migraine, palpitation, peripheral vascular disorder, postural hypotension, syncope, and tachycardia.

Digestive System: Abnormal stools, bloody diarrhea, cheilitis, cholangitis, colitis, dry mouth, dysphagia, eructation, esophagitis, gastritis, gastroenteritis, gastrointestinal disorder, gastrointestinal hemorrhage, gingivitis, hepatitis, hepatomegaly, ileitis, liver damage, liver function tests abnormal, mouth ulcer, oral moniliasis, pancreatitis, periodontal abscess, rectal disorder, tenesmus, and thirst.

Endocrine System: Diabetes mellitus.

Hemic and Lymphatic System: Anemia, ecchymosis, leukopenia, lymphadenopathy, lymphocytosis, and thrombocytopenia.

Metabolic and Nutritional Disorders: Avitaminosis, dehydration, edema, glycosuria, gout, hyper cholesteremia, peripheral edema, and weight loss.

Musculoskeletal System: Arthralgia, arthrosis, joint disorder, muscle cramps, muscle weakness, myositis, and twitching.

Nervous System: Abnormal dreams, abnormal gait, agitation, amnesia, anxiety, aphasia, ataxia, confusion, convulsion, depression, diplopia, emotional lability, euphoria, grand mal convulsion, hallucinations, hyperesthesia, incoordination, libido decreased, nervousness, neuralgia, neu-

Table 5
Percentage of Patients, by Study and Treatment Group, with Marked Chemistry and Hematology Laboratory Value Abnormalities

Variable	Limit	Study 245 Naive Patients NORVIR + ZDV	NORVIR	ZDV	Study 247 Advanced Patients NORVIR	Placebo
CHEMISTRY	HIGH					
Glucose	(>250 mg/dL)	2.0	-	0.9	0.4	1.1
Uric Acid	(>12 mg/dL)	-	-	-	3.6	0.2
Creatinine	(>3.6 mg/dL)	-	-	-	0.2	0.2
Potassium	(>6.0 mEq/L)	-	-	-	0.4	0.2
Chloride	(>122 mEq/L)	-	0.9	-	-	-
Total Bilirubin	(>3.6 mg/dL)	-	-	-	1.2	0.2
Alkaline Phosphatase	(>550 IU/L)	-	0.9	-	1.4	1.7
SGOT (AST)	(>180 IU/L)	2.9	6.5	1.7	3.8	4.3
SGPT (ALT)	(>215 IU/L)	3.9	5.6	2.6	6.1	2.6
GGT	(>300 IU/L)	2.0	2.8	0.9	14.7	6.7
LDH	(>1170 IU/L)	-	-	-	1.0	0.2
Triglycerides	(>1500 mg/dL)	1.0	2.8	-	10.1	0.2
Triglycerides Fasting	(>1500 mg/dL)	2.1	1.4	-	7.9	0.4
CPK	(>1000 IU/L)	7.0	7.5	7.1	8.6	4.5
Amylase	(>2 × ULN[1])	-	0.9	-	0.2	-
CHEMISTRY	LOW					
Albumin	(<2.0 g/dL)	-	-	-	0.2	0.6
Sodium	(<123 mEq/L)	-	-	-	0.2	-
Potassium	(<3.0 mEq/L)	-	0.9	-	2.0	1.1
Chloride	(<84 mEq/L)	-	0.9	-	-	0.4
Magnesium	(<1.0 mEq/L)	-	-	-	0.4	0.4
Calcium	(<6.9 mEq/L)	-	-	-	1.2	0.9
HEMATOLOGY	LOW					
Hemoglobin	(<8.0 g/dL)	-	-	-	2.8	2.4
Hematocrit	(<30%)	2.0	-	-	11.7	16.0
RBC	(<3.0 × 10^12/L)	1.0	-	1.7	14.9	19.7
WBC	(<2.5 × 10^9/L)	-	-	3.5	25.1	51.4
Platelet Count	(<20 × 10^9/L)	-	-	-	0.4	0.6
Neutrophils	(≤0.5 × 10^9/L)	-	-	-	4.0	6.9
HEMATOLOGY	HIGH					
WBC	(>25 × 10^9/L)	-	-	-	1.6	0.7
Neutrophils	(>20 × 10^9/L)	-	-	-	1.8	0.9
Eosinophils	(>1.0 × 10^9/L)	-	1.9	0.9	1.8	2.6
Prothrombin Time	(>1.5 × ULN[1])	1.0	-	-	1.0	1.3

[1] ULN = upper limit of the normal range.
- Indicates no events reported.

Pediatric Dosage Guidelines[1]

Body Surface Area* (m²)	Twice Daily Dose 250 mg/m²	Twice Daily Dose 300 mg/m²	Twice Daily Dose 350 mg/m²	Twice Daily Dose 400 mg/m²
0.25	0.8 mL (62.5 mg)	0.9 mL (75 mg)	1.1 mL (87.5 mg)	1.25 mL (100 mg)
0.50	1.6 mL (125 mg)	1.9 mL (150 mg)	2.2 mL (175 mg)	2.5 mL (200 mg)
1.0	3.1 mL (250 mg)	3.75 mL (300 mg)	4.4 mL (350 mg)	5 mL (400 mg)
1.25	3.9 mL (312.5 mg)	4.7 mL (375 mg)	5.5 mL (437.5 mg)	6.25 mL (500 mg)
1.50	4.7 mL (375 mg)	5.6 mL (450 mg)	6.6 mL (525 mg)	7.5 mL (600 mg)

* Body surface area can be calculated with the following equation:

$$BSA \ (m^2) = \sqrt{\frac{Ht \ (cm) \times Wt \ (kg)}{3600}}$$

ropathy, paralysis, peripheral neuropathy, peripheral sensory neuropathy, personality disorder, tremor, urinary retention, and vertigo.
Respiratory System: Asthma, dyspnea, epistaxis, hiccup, hypoventilation, increased cough, interstitial pneumonia, lung disorder, and rhinitis.
Skin and Appendages: Acne, contact dermatitis, dry skin, eczema, folliculitis, maculopapular rash, molluscum contagiosum, pruritus, psoriasis, seborrhea, urticaria, and vesiculobullous rash.
Special Senses: Abnormal electro-oculogram, abnormal electroretinogram, abnormal vision, amblyopia/blurred vision, blepharitis, ear pain, eye pain, hearing impairment, increased cerumen, iritis, parosmia, photophobia, taste loss, tinnitus, uveitis, and visual field defect.
Urogenital System: Dysuria, hematuria, impotence, kidney calculus, kidney failure, nocturia, penis disorder, polyuria, pyelonephritis, urethritis, and urinary frequency.
Post-Marketing Experience:
There have been postmarketing reports of seizure. Cause and effect relationship has not been established.
Dehydration, usually associated with gastrointestinal symptoms, and sometimes resulting in hypotension, syncope, or renal insufficiency has been reported. Syncope, orthostatic hypotension, and renal insufficiency have also been reported without known dehydration.
Laboratory Abnormalities
Table 5 shows the percentage of patients who developed marked laboratory abnormalities.
[See table 5 above]

OVERDOSAGE
Acute Overdosage
Human Overdose Experience: Human experience of acute overdose with NORVIR is limited. One patient in clinical trials took NORVIR 1500 mg/day for two days. The patient reported paresthesias which resolved after the dose was decreased. A post-marketing case of renal failure with eosinophilia has been reported with ritonavir overdose.
The approximate lethal dose was found to be greater than 20 times the related human dose in rats and 10 times the related human dose in mice.
Management of Overdosage
Treatment of overdose with NORVIR consists of general supportive measures including monitoring of vital signs and observation of the clinical status of the patient. There is no specific antidote for overdose with NORVIR. If indicated, elimination of unabsorbed drug should be achieved by emesis or gastric lavage; usual precautions should be observed to maintain the airway. Administration of activated charcoal may also be used to aid in removal of unabsorbed drug. Since ritonavir is extensively metabolized by the liver and is highly protein bound, dialysis is unlikely to be beneficial in significant removal of the drug. A Certified Poison Control Center should be consulted for up-to-date information on the management of overdose with NORVIR.

DOSAGE AND ADMINISTRATION
NORVIR is administered orally. It is recommended that NORVIR be taken with meals if possible. Patients may improve the taste of NORVIR oral solution by mixing with

chocolate milk, Ensure®, or Advera® within one hour of dosing. The effects of antacids on the absorption of ritonavir have not been studied.
Adults
The recommended dosage of ritonavir is 600 mg twice daily by mouth. Use of a dose titration schedule may help to reduce treatment-emergent adverse events while maintaining appropriate ritonavir plasma levels. Ritonavir should be started at no less than 300 mg twice daily and increased by 100 mg twice daily increments up to 600 mg twice daily.
Pediatric Patients
Ritonavir should be used in combination with other antiretroviral agents (see General Dosing Guidelines). The recommended dosage of ritonavir is 400 mg/m² twice daily by mouth and should not exceed 600 mg twice daily. Ritonavir should be started at 250 mg/m² and increased at 2 to 3 day intervals by 50 mg/m² twice daily. If patients do not tolerate 400 mg/m² twice daily due to adverse events, the highest tolerated dose should be used for maintenance therapy in combination with other antiretroviral agent. When possible, dose should be administered using a calibrated dosing syringe.
[See second table at left]
General Dosing Guidelines
Patients should be aware that frequently observed adverse events, such as mild to moderate gastrointestinal disturbances and paraesthesias, may diminish as therapy is continued. In addition, patients initiating combination regimens with NORVIR and nucleosides may improve gastrointestinal tolerance by initiating NORVIR alone and subsequently adding nucleosides before completing two weeks of NORVIR monotherapy.

HOW SUPPLIED
NORVIR (ritonavir capsules) are white capsules imprinted with the corporate logo ⊇ , 100 mg, and the Abbo-Code PI. NORVIR is available as 100 mg capsules in the following package size:
Packages of 2 bottles of 84 capsules each . (**NDC** 0074-9492-02).
Recommended storage: Store capsules in the refrigerator between 36-46°F (2-8°C). Protect from light.
NORVIR (ritonavir oral solution) is an orange-colored liquid, supplied in amber-colored, multi-dose bottles containing 600 mg ritonavir per 7.5 mL marked dosage cup (80 mg/mL) in the following size:
240 mL bottles .... (**NDC** 0074-1940-63).
Recommended storage: Store NORVIR oral solution in the refrigerator between 36-46°F (2-8°C) until it is dispensed. Refrigeration of NORVIR oral solution by the patient is recommended, but not required if used within 30 days and stored below 77°F (25°C). Product should be stored and dispensed in the original container. Avoid exposure to excessive heat. Keep cap tightly closed.

REFERENCES
1. Sewester CS. Calculations. In: Drug Facts and Comparisons, St. Louis, MO: J.B. Lippincott Co; January 1997: xix.
Revised: December, 1997
TM - Trademark
Caution-Federal (U.S.A.) Law prohibits dispensing without prescription.
Ref. 03-4838-R6
Shown in Product Identification Guide, page 303

PANHEMATIN®   ℞
[pan-hē 'ma-tin]
HEMIN FOR INJECTION
For I.V. Use Only

> PANHEMATIN (hemin for injection) should only be used by physicians experienced in the management of porphyrias in hospitals where the recommended clinical and laboratory diagnostic and monitoring techniques are available.
> PANHEMATIN therapy should be considered after an appropriate period of alternate therapy (i.e., 400 g glucose/day for 1 to 2 days). (See "WARNINGS", "PRECAUTIONS" and "DOSAGE AND ADMINISTRATION" sections.)

DESCRIPTION
PANHEMATIN (hemin for injection) is an enzyme inhibitor derived from processed red blood cells. Hemin for injection was known previously as hematin. The term hematin has been used to describe the chemical reaction product of hemin and sodium carbonate solution. Hemin is an iron containing metalloporphyrin. Chemically hemin is represented as chloro [7,12-diethenyl-3,8,13,17-tetramethyl-21H,23H-porphine-2,18-dipropanoato (2-)-N[21],N[22], N[23], N[24]] iron.

Continued on next page

Panhematin—Cont.

The structural formula for hemin is:

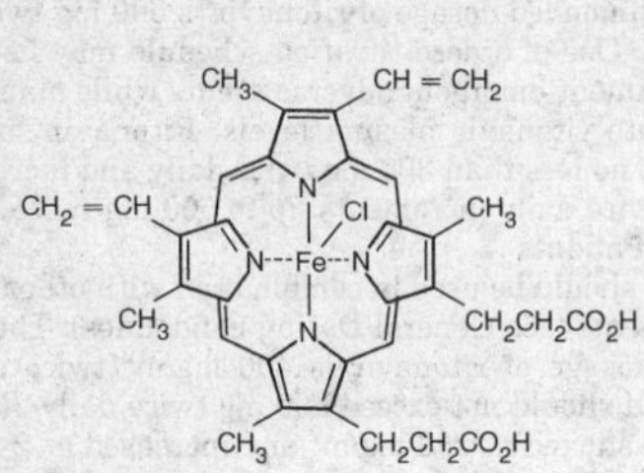

Panhematin is a sterile, lyophilized powder suitable for intravenous administration after reconstitution. Each dispensing vial of Panhematin contains the equivalent of 313 mg hemin, 215 mg sodium carbonate and 300 mg of sorbitol. The pH may have been adjusted with hydrochloric acid; the product contains no preservatives. When mixed as directed with Sterile Water for Injection, USP, each 43 ml provides the equivalent of approximately 301 mg hematin (7 mg/ml).

CLINICAL PHARMACOLOGY

Heme acts to limit the hepatic and/or marrow synthesis of porphyrin. This action is likely due to the inhibition of δ-aminolevulinic acid synthetase, the enzyme which limits the rate of the porphyrin/heme biosynthetic pathway. The exact mechanism by which hematin produces symptomatic improvement in patients with acute episodes of the hepatic porphyrias has not been elucidated.[1,9]

Following intravenous administration of hematin in non-jaundiced human patients, an increase in fecal urobilinogen can be observed which is roughly proportional to the amount of hematin administered. This suggests an entero-hepatic pathway as at least one route of elimination. Bilirubin metabolites are also excreted in the urine following hematin injections.[2]

Panhematin (hemin for injection) therapy for the acute porphyrias is not curative. After discontinuation of Panhematin treatment, symptoms generally return although in some cases remission is prolonged. Some neurological symptoms have improved weeks to months after therapy although little or no response was noted at the time of treatment.

Other aspects of human pharmacokinetics have not been defined.

INDICATIONS AND USAGE

Panhematin (hemin for injection) is indicated for the amelioration of recurrent attacks of acute intermittent porphyria temporally related to the menstrual cycle in susceptible women.

Manifestations such as pain, hypertension, tachycardia, abnormal mental status and mild to progressive neurologic signs may be controlled in selected patients with this disorder.

Similar findings have been reported in other patients with acute intermittent porphyria, porphyria variegata and hereditary coproporphyria. Panhematin is not indicated in porphyria cutanea tarda.

CONTRAINDICATIONS

Hemin for injection is contraindicated in patients with known hypersensitivity to this drug.

WARNINGS

PANHEMATIN (hemin for injection) is made from human blood. Products made from human blood may contain infectious agents, such as viruses, that can cause disease. The risk that such products will transmit an infectious agent has been reduced by screening blood donors for prior exposure to certain viruses, by testing for the presence of certain current virus infections, and by inactivating certain viruses. Despite these measures, such products can still potentially transmit disease. There is also the possibility that unknown infectious agents may be present in such products. ALL infections thought by a physician possibly to have been transmitted by this product should be reported by the physician or other healthcare provider to Abbott Laboratories, (800) 633-9110. The physician should discuss the risks and benefits of this product with the patient.

Panhematin therapy is intended to limit the rate of porphyria/heme biosynthesis possibly by inhibiting the enzyme δ-aminolevulinic acid synthetase. For this reason, drugs such as estrogens, barbituric acid derivatives and steroid metabolites which increase the activity of δ-aminolevulinic acid synthetase should be avoided.

Also, because Panhematin has exhibited transient, mild anticoagulant effects during clinical studies, concurrent anticoagulant therapy should be avoided.[9] The extent and duration of the hypocoagulable state induced by Panhematin has not been established.

PRECAUTIONS

General: Clinical benefit from Panhematin depends on prompt administration. Attacks of porphyria may progress to a point where irreversible neuronal damage has occurred. Panhematin therapy is intended to prevent an attack from reaching the critical stage of neuronal degeneration. Panhematin is not effective in repairing neuronal damage.[9]

Recommended dosage guidelines should be strictly followed. Reversible renal shutdown has been observed in a case where an excessive hematin dose (12.2 mg/kg) was administered in a single infusion. Oliguria and increased nitrogen retention occurred although the patient remained asymptomatic.[4] No worsening of renal function has been seen with administration of recommended dosages of hematin.[9]

A large arm vein or a central venous catheter should be utilized for the administration of hemin for injection to avoid the possibility of phlebitis.

Since reconstituted Panhematin is not transparent, any undissolved particulate matter is difficult to see when inspected visually. Therefore, terminal filtration through a sterile 0.45 micron or smaller filter is recommended.

Tests for Diagnosis and Monitoring of Therapy: Before Panhematin therapy is begun, the presence of acute porphyria must be diagnosed using the following criteria:[9]

a. Presence of clinical symptoms.
b. Positive Watson-Schwartz or Hoesch test. (A negative Watson-Schwartz or Hoesch test indicates a porphyric attack is highly unlikely. When in doubt quantitative measures of δ-aminolevulinic acid and porphobilinogen in serum or urine may aid in diagnosis.)

Urinary concentrations of the following compounds may be *monitored* during Panhematin therapy. Drug effect will be demonstrated by a decrease in one or more of the following compounds:[3–6]

ALA-δ-aminolevulinic acid
UPG-uroporphyrinogen
PBG-porphobilinogen
coproporphyrin

Carcinogenesis, Mutagenesis, Impairment of Fertility: No data are available on potential for carcinogenicity, mutagenicity or impairment of fertility in animals or humans.

Pregnancy: Teratogenic effects: Pregnancy Category C. Animal reproduction studies have not been conducted with hematin. It is also not known whether hematin can cause fetal harm when administered to a pregnant woman or can affect reproduction capacity. For this reason hemin for injection should not be given to a pregnant woman unless the expected benefits are sufficiently important to the health and welfare of the patient to outweigh the unknown hazard to the fetus.

Nursing Mothers: It is not known whether this drug is excreted in human milk. Because many drugs are excreted in human milk, caution should be exercised when hemin for injection is administered to a nursing woman.

Pediatric Use: Safety and effectiveness in pediatric patients under 16 years of age have not been established.

ADVERSE REACTIONS

Reversible renal shutdown has occurred with administration of excessive doses (See "PRECAUTIONS" section).

Phlebitis with or without leucocytosis and with or without mild pyrexia has occurred after administration of hematin through small arm veins.

There has been one report in the literature[8] of coagulopathy occurring in a patient receiving hematin therapy. This patient exhibited prolonged prothrombin time and partial thromboplastin time, thrombocytopenia, mild hypofibrinogenemia, mild elevation of fibrin split products and a 10% fall in hematocrit.

OVERDOSAGE

Reversible renal shutdown has been observed in a case where an excessive hematin dose (12.2 mg/kg) was administered in a single infusion. Treatment of this case consisted of ethacrynic acid and mannitol.[7]

DOSAGE AND ADMINISTRATION

Before administering hemin for injection, an appropriate period of alternate therapy (i.e., 400 g glucose/day for 1 to 2 days) must be considered. If improvement is unsatisfactory for the treatment of acute attacks of porphyria, an intravenous infusion of Panhematin containing a dose of 1 to 4 mg/kg/day of hematin should be given over a period of 10 to 15 minutes for 3 to 14 days based on the clinical signs. In more severe cases this dose may be repeated no earlier than every 12 hours. No more than 6 mg/kg of hematin should be given in any 24-hour period.

After reconstitution each mL of Panhematin contains the equivalent of approximately 7 mg of hematin. The drug may be administered directly from the vial.

Dosage Calculation Table

1 mg hematin equivalent	= 0.14 mL Panhematin
2 mg hematin equivalent	= 0.28 mL Panhematin
3 mg hematin equivalent	= 0.42 mL Panhematin
4 mg hematin equivalent	= 0.56 mL Panhematin

Since reconstituted Panhematin is not transparent, any undissolved particulate matter is difficult to see when inspected visually. Therefore, terminal filtration through a sterile 0.45 micron or smaller filter is recommended.

Preparation of Solution: Reconstitute Panhematin by aseptically adding 43 mL of Sterile Water for Injection, USP, to the dispensing vial. Immediately after adding diluent, the product should be shaken well for a period of 2 to 3 minutes to aid dissolution. **NOTE: Because Panhematin contains no preservative and because Panhematin undergoes rapid chemical decomposition in solution, it should not be reconstituted until immediately before use. After the first withdrawal from the vial, any solution remaining must be discarded.**

No drug or chemical agent should be added to a Panhematin fluid admixture unless its effect on the chemical and physical stability has first been determined.

HOW SUPPLIED

Panhematin (hemin for injection) is supplied as a sterile, lyophilized black powder in single dose dispensing vials (**NDC** 0074-2000-43). When mixed as directed with Sterile Water for Injection, USP, each 43 mL provides the equivalent of approximately 301 mg hematin (7 mg/mL). Store lyophilized powder in refrigerator (2–8°C) until time of use.

REFERENCES

1. Bickers, D., Treatment of the Porphyrias: Mechanisms of Action, *J Invest Dermatol* 77(1):107–113, 1981.
2. Watson, C. J., Hematin and Porphyria, editorial, *N Engl J Med* 293(12):605–607, September 18, 1975.
3. Lamon, J. M., Hematin Therapy for Acute Porphyria, *Medicine* 58(3):252–269, 1979.
4. Dhar, G. J., et al., Effects of Hematin in Hepatic Porphyria, *Ann Intern Med* 83:20–30, 1975.
5. Watson, C. J., et al., Use of Hematin in the Acute Attack of the "Inducible" Hepatic Porphyrias, *Adv Intern Med* 23:265–286, 1978.
6. McColl, K. E., et al., Treatment with Haematin in Acute Hepatic Porphyria, *Q J Med,* New Series L (198):161–174, Spring, 1981.
7. Dhar, G. J., et al., Transitory Renal Failure Following Rapid Administration of a Relatively Large Amount of Hematin in a Patient with Acute Intermittent Porphyria in Clinical Remission, *Acta Med Scand* 203:437–443, 1978.
8. Morris, D. L., et al., Coagulopathy Associated with Hematin Treatment for Acute Intermittent Porphyria, *Ann Intern Med* 95:700–701, 1981.
9. Pierach, C. A., Hematin Therapy for the Porphyric Attack, *Semin Liver Dis* 2(2):125–131, May, 1982.

Revised: July, 1997
Ref. 06-9681-R5

PCE® ℞

[*p-c-ē*]
(erythromycin particles in tablets)
Dispertab® Tablets

DESCRIPTION

PCE (erythromycin particles in tablets) is an antibacterial product containing specially coated erythromycin base particles for oral administration. The coating protects the antibiotic from the inactivating effects of gastric acidity and permits efficient absorption of the antibiotic in the small intestine. PCE is available in two strengths containing either 333 mg or 500 mg of erythromycin base. PCE 500 mg tablets contain no synthetic dyes or artificial colors.

Erythromycin is produced by a strain of *Saccharopolyspora erythraea* (formerly *Streptomyces erythraeus*) and belongs to the macrolide group of antibiotics. It is basic and readily forms salts with acids. Erythromycin is a white to off-white powder, slightly soluble in water, and soluble in alcohol, chloroform, and ether. Erythromycin is known chemically as (3R*, 4S*, 5S*, 6R*, 7R*, 9R*, 11R*, 12R*, 13S*, 14R*)-4-[(2,6-dideoxy-3-C-methyl-3-O-methyl-α-L-*ribo*-hexopyranosyl)oxy]-14-ethyl-7,12,13-trihydroxy-3,5,7,9,11,13-hexamethyl-6-[[3,4,6-trideoxy-3-(dimethylamino)-β-D-*xylo*-hexopyranosyl]oxy]oxacyclotetradecane-2,10-dione. The molecular formula is $C_{37}H_{67}NO_{13}$, and the molecular weight is 733.94. The structural formula is:

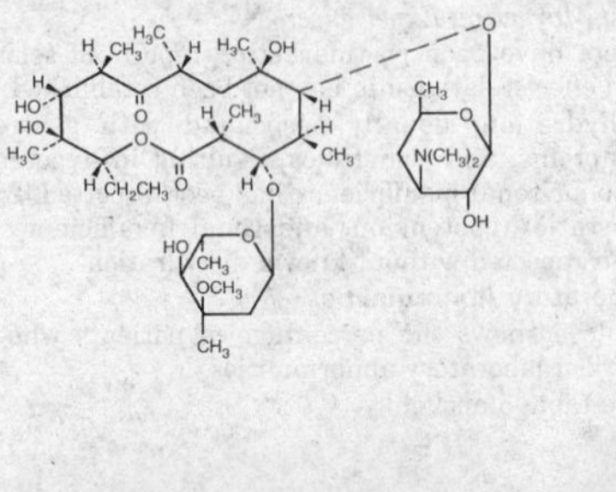

Inactive Ingredients:

PCE 333 mg tablets: Cellulosic polymers, citrate ester, colloidal silicon dioxide, D&C Red No. 30, hydrogenated vegetable oil wax, lactose, magnesium stearate, microcrystalline cellulose, povidone, propylene glycol, sodium starch glycolate, stearic acid and vanillin.

PCE 500 mg tablets: Cellulosic polymers, citrate ester, colloidal silicon dioxide, crospovidone, hydrogenated vegetable oil wax, iron oxide, microcrystalline cellulose, polyethylene glycol, povidone, propylene glycol, stearic acid, talc, titanium dioxide and vanillin.

CLINICAL PHARMACOLOGY

Orally administered erythromycin base and its salts are readily absorbed in the microbiologically active form. Interindividual variations in the absorption of erythromycin are, however, observed, and some patients do not achieve optimal serum levels. Erythromycin is largely bound to plasma proteins. After absorption, erythromycin diffuses readily into most body fluids. In the absence of meningeal inflammation, low concentrations are normally achieved in the spinal fluid but the passage of the drug across the blood-brain barrier increases in meningitis. Erythromycin crosses the placental barrier, but fetal plasma levels are low. The drug is excreted in human milk. Erythromycin is not removed by peritoneal dialysis or hemodialysis.

In the presence of normal hepatic function, erythromycin is concentrated in the liver and is excreted in the bile; the effect of hepatic dysfunction on biliary excretion of erythromycin is not known. After oral administration, less than 5% of the administered dose can be recovered in the active form in the urine.

The erythromycin particles in PCE tablets are coated with a polymer whose dissolution is pH dependent. This coating allows for minimal release of erythromycin in acidic environments, e.g. stomach. This delivery system is designed for optimal drug release and absorption in the small intestine. In multiple-dose, steady-state studies, PCE tablets have demonstrated rapid and generally adequate drug delivery in both fasting and nonfasting conditions. However, the presence of food results in lower blood levels, and optimal blood levels are obtained when PCE tablets are given in the fasting state (at least 1/2 hour and preferably 2 hours before meals). Bioavailability data are available from Abbott Laboratories, Dept. 422.

Microbiology:

Erythromycin acts by inhibition of protein synthesis by binding 50 S ribosomal subunits of susceptible organisms. It does not affect nucleic acid synthesis. Antagonism has been demonstrated *in vitro* between erythromycin and clindamycin, lincomycin, and chloramphenicol.

Many strains of *Haemophilus influenzae* are resistant to erythromycin alone, but are susceptible to erythromycin and sulfonamides used concomitantly.

Staphylococci resistant to erythromycin may emerge during a course of erythromycin therapy.

Erythromycin has been shown to be active against most strains of the following microorganisms, both *in vitro* and in clinical infections as described in the **INDICATIONS AND USAGE** section.

Gram-positive organisms:

Corynebacterium diphtheriae
Corynebacterium minutissimum
Listeria monocytogenes
Staphylococcus aureus (resistant organisms may emerge during treatment)
Streptococcus pneumoniae
Streptococcus pyogenes

Gram-negative organisms:

Bordetella pertussis
Legionella pneumophila
Neisseria gonorrhoeae

Other microorganisms:

Chlamydia trachomatis
Entamoeba histolytica
Mycoplasma pneumoniae
Treponema pallidum
Ureaplasma urealyticum

The following *in vitro* data are available, **but their clinical significance is unknown.**

Erythromycin exhibits *in vitro* minimal inhibitory concentrations (MIC's) of 0.5 µg/mL or less against most ($\geq 90\%$) strains of the following microorganisms; however, the safety and effectiveness of erythromycin in treating clinical infections due to these microorganisms have not been established in adequate and well-controlled clinical trials.

Gram-positive organisms:

Viridans group streptococci

Gram-negative organisms:

Moraxella catarrhalis
Susceptibility Tests:

Dilution Techniques:

Quantitative methods are used to determine antimicrobial minimum inhibitory concentrations (MIC's). These MIC's provide estimates of the susceptibility of bacteria to antimi-

crobial compounds. The MIC's should be determined using a standardized procedure. Standardized procedures are based on a dilution method[1] (broth or agar) or equivalent with standardized inoculum concentrations and standardized concentrations of erythromycin powder. The MIC values should be interpreted according to the following criteria:

MIC (µg/mL)	Interpretation
≤0.5	Susceptible (S)
1–4	Intermediate (I)
≥8	Resistant (R)

A report of "Susceptible" indicates that the pathogen is likely to be inhibited if the antimicrobial compound in the blood reaches the concentrations usually achievable. A report of "Intermediate" indicates that the result should be considered equivocal, and, if the microorganism is not fully susceptible to alternative, clinically feasible drugs, the test should be repeated. This category implies possible clinical applicability in body sites where the drug is physiologically concentrated or in situations where high dosage of drug can be used. This category also provides a buffer zone which prevents small uncontrolled technical factors from causing major discrepancies in interpretation. A report of "Resistant" indicates that the pathogen is not likely to be inhibited if the antimicrobial compound in the blood reaches the concentrations usually achievable; other therapy should be selected.

Standardized susceptibility test procedures require the use of laboratory control microorganisms to control the technical aspects of the laboratory procedures. Standard erythromycin powder should provide the following MIC values:

Microorganism	MIC (µg/mL)
S. aureus ATCC 29213	0.12–0.5
E. faecalis ATCC 29212	1–4

Diffusion Techniques:

Quantitative methods that require measurement of zone diameters also provide reproducible estimates of the susceptibility of bacteria to antimicrobial compounds. One such standardized procedure[2] requires the use of standardized inoculum concentrations. This procedure uses paper disks impregnated with 15-µg erythromycin to test the susceptibility of microorganisms to erythromycin.

Reports from the laboratory providing results of the standard single-disk susceptibility test with a 15-µg erythromycin disk should be interpreted according to the following criteria:

Zone Diameter (mm)	Interpretation
≥23	Susceptible (S)
14–22	Intermediate (I)
≤13	Resistant (R)

Interpretation should be as stated above for results using dilution techniques. Interpretation involves correlation of the diameter obtained in the disk test with the MIC for erythromycin.

As with standardized dilution techniques, diffusion methods require the use of laboratory control microorganisms that are used to control the technical aspects of the laboratory procedures. For the diffusion technique, the 15-µg erythromycin disk should provide the following zone diameters in these laboratory test quality control strains:

Microorganism	Zone Diameter (mm)
S. aureus ATCC 25923	22–30

INDICATIONS AND USAGE

PCE tablets are indicated in the treatment of infections caused by susceptible strains of the designated microorganisms in the diseases listed below:

Upper respiratory tract infections of mild to moderate degree caused by *Streptococcus pyogenes*; *Streptococcus pneumoniae*; *Haemophilus influenzae* (when used concomitantly with adequate doses of sulfonamides, since many strains of *H. influenzae* are not susceptible to the erythromycin concentrations ordinarily achieved). (See appropriate sulfonamide labeling for prescribing information.)

Lower respiratory tract infections of mild to moderate severity caused by *Streptococcus pyogenes* or *Streptococcus pneumoniae.*

Listeriosis caused by *Listeria monocytogenes.*

Respiratory tract infections due to *Mycoplasma pneumoniae.*

Skin and skin structure infections of mild to moderate severity caused by *Streptococcus pyogenes* or *Staphylococcus aureus* (resistant staphylococci may emerge during treatment).

Pertussis (whooping cough) caused by *Bordetella pertussis.* Erythromycin is effective in eliminating the organism from the nasopharynx of infected individuals, rendering them noninfectious. Some clinical studies suggest that erythromycin may be helpful in the prophylaxis of pertussis in exposed susceptible individuals.

Diphtheria: Infections due to *Corynebacterium diphtheriae,* as an adjunct to antitoxin, to prevent establishment of carriers and to eradicate the organism in carriers.

Erythrasma—In the treatment of infections due to *Corynebacterium minutissimum.*

Intestinal amebiasis caused by *Entamoeba histolytica* (oral erythromycins only). Extraenteric amebiasis requires treatment with other agents.

Acute pelvic inflammatory disease caused by *Neisseria gonorrhoeae:* Erythrocin® Lactobionate-I.V. (erythromycin lactobionate for injection, USP) followed by erythromycin base orally, as an alternative drug in treatment of acute pelvic inflammatory disease caused by *N. gonorrhoeae* in female patients with a history of sensitivity to penicillin. Patients should have a serologic test for syphilis before receiving erythromycin as treatment of gonorrhea and a follow-up serologic test for syphilis after 3 months.

Erythromycins are indicated for treatment of the following infections caused by *Chlamydia trachomatis*: conjunctivitis of the newborn, pneumonia of infancy, and urogenital infections during pregnancy. When tetracyclines are contraindicated or not tolerated, erythromycin is indicated for the treatment of uncomplicated urethral, endocervical, or rectal infections in adults due to *Chlamydia trachomatis.*

When tetracyclines are contraindicated or not tolerated, erythromycin is indicated for the treatment of nongonococcal urethritis caused by *Ureaplasma urealyticum.*

Primary syphilis caused by *Treponema pallidum.* Erythromycin (oral forms only) is an alternative choice of treatment for primary syphilis in patients allergic to the penicillins. In treatment of primary syphilis, spinal fluid should be examined before treatment and as part of the follow-up after therapy.

Legionnaires' Disease caused by *Legionella pneumophila.* Although no controlled clinical efficacy studies have been conducted, *in vitro* and limited preliminary clinical data suggest that erythromycin may be effective in treating Legionnaires' Disease.

Prophylaxis

Prevention of Initial Attacks of Rheumatic Fever—Penicillin is considered by the American Heart Association to be the drug of choice in the prevention of initial attacks of rheumatic fever (treatment of *Streptococcus pyogenes* infections of the upper respiratory tract e.g., tonsillitis, or pharyngitis).[3] Erythromycin is indicated for the treatment of penicillin-allergic patients. The therapeutic dose should be administered for ten days.

Prevention of Recurrent Attacks of Rheumatic Fever—Penicillin or sulfonamides are considered by the American Heart Association to be the drugs of choice in the prevention of recurrent attacks of rheumatic fever. In patients who are allergic to penicillin and sulfonamides, oral erythromycin is recommended by the American Heart Association in the long-term prophylaxis of streptococcal pharyngitis (for the prevention of recurrent attacks of rheumatic fever).[3]

Prevention of Bacterial Endocarditis—Although no controlled clinical efficacy trials have been conducted, oral erythromycin has been recommended by the American Heart Association for prevention of bacterial endocarditis in penicillin-allergic patients with prosthetic cardiac valves, most congenital cardiac malformations, surgically constructed systemic pulmonary shunts, rheumatic or other acquired valvular dysfunction, idiopathic hypertrophic subaortic stenosis (IHSS), previous history of bacterial endocarditis or mitral valve prolapse with insufficiency when they undergo dental procedures or surgical procedures of the upper respiratory tract.[4]

CONTRAINDICATIONS

Erythromycin is contraindicated in patients with known hypersensitivity to this antibiotic.

Erythromycin is contraindicated in patients taking terfenadine, astemizole, or cisapride. (See **PRECAUTIONS**-*Drug Interactions.*)

WARNINGS

There have been reports of hepatic dysfunction, including increased liver enzymes, and hepatocellular and/or cholestatic hepatitis, with or without jaundice, occurring in patients receiving oral erythromycin products.

There have been reports suggesting that erythromycin does not reach the fetus in adequate concentration to prevent congenital syphilis. Infants born to women treated during pregnancy with oral erythromycin for early syphilis should be treated with an appropriate penicillin regimen.

Rhabdomyolysis with or without renal impairment has been reported in seriously ill patients receiving erythromycin concomitantly with lovastatin. Therefore, patients receiving

Continued on next page

PCE—Cont.

concomitant lovastatin and erythromycin should be carefully monitored for creatine kinase (CK) and serum transaminase levels. (See package insert for lovastatin.)

Pseudomembranous colitis has been reported with nearly all antibacterial agents, including erythromycin, and may range in severity from mild to life threatening. Therefore, it is important to consider this diagnosis in patients who present with diarrhea subsequent to the administration of antibacterial agents.

Treatment with antibacterial agents alters the normal flora of the colon and may permit overgrowth of clostridia. Studies indicate that a toxin produced by *Clostridium difficile* is a primary cause of "antibiotic-associated colitis".

After the diagnosis of pseudomembranous colitis has been established, therapeutic measures should be initiated. Mild cases of pseudomembranous colitis usually respond to discontinuation of the drug alone. In moderate to severe cases, consideration should be given to management with fluids and electrolytes, protein supplementation, and treatment with an antibacterial drug clinically effective against *Clostridium difficile* colitis.

PRECAUTIONS

General: Since erythromycin is principally excreted by the liver, caution should be exercised when erythromycin is administered to patients with impaired hepatic function. (See **CLINICAL PHARMACOLOGY** and **WARNINGS**.)

There have been reports that erythromycin may aggravate the weakness of patients with myasthenia gravis.

Prolonged or repeated use of erythromycin may result in an overgrowth of nonsusceptible bacteria or fungi. If superinfection occurs, erythromycin should be discontinued and appropriate therapy instituted.

When indicated, incision and drainage or other surgical procedures should be performed in conjunction with antibiotic therapy.

Drug Interactions: Erythromycin use in patients who are receiving high doses of theophylline may be associated with an increase in serum theophylline levels and potential theophylline toxicity. In case of theophylline toxicity and/or elevated serum theophylline levels, the dose of theophylline should be reduced while the patient is receiving concomitant erythromycin therapy.

Concomitant administration of erythromycin and digoxin has been reported to result in elevated digoxin serum levels.

There have been reports of increased anticoagulant effects when erythromycin and oral anticoagulants were used concomitantly. Increased anticoagulation effects due to interactions of erythromycin with oral anticoagulants may be more pronounced in the elderly.

Concurrent use of erythromycin and ergotamine or dihydroergotamine has been associated in some patients with acute ergot toxicity characterized by severe peripheral vasospasm and dysesthesia.

Erythromycin has been reported to decrease the clearance of triazolam and midazolam and, thus, may increase the pharmacologic effect of these benzodiazepines.

The use of erythromycin in patients concurrently taking drugs metabolized by the cytochrome P450 system may be associated with elevations in serum levels of these other drugs. There have been reports of interactions of erythromycin with carbamazepine, cyclosporine, tacrolimus, hexobarbital, phenytoin, alfentanil, cisapride, disopyramide, lovastatin, bromocriptine, valproate, terfenadine, and astemizole. Serum concentrations of drugs metabolized by the cytochrome P450 system should be monitored closely in patients concurrently receiving erythromycin.

Erythromycin has been reported to significantly alter the metabolism of the nonsedating antihistamines terfenadine and astemizole when taken concomitantly. Rare cases of serious cardiovascular adverse events, including electrocardiographic QT/QT_c interval prolongation, cardiac arrest, torsades de pointes, and other ventricular arrhythmias, have been observed. (See **CONTRAINDICATIONS**.) In addition, deaths have been reported rarely with concomitant administration of terfenadine and erythromycin.

There have been post-marketing reports of drug interactions when erythromycin was coadministered with cisapride, resulting in QT prolongation, cardiac arrhythmias, ventricular tachycardia, ventricular fibrillation, and torsades de pointes, most likely due to the inhibition of hepatic metabolism of cisapride by erythromycin. Fatalities have been reported. (See **CONTRAINDICATIONS**).

Drug/Laboratory Test interactions: Erythromycin interferes with the fluorometric determination of urinary catecholamines.

Carcinogenesis, Mutagenesis, Impairment of Fertility: Long-term (2-year) oral studies conducted in rats with erythromycin base did not provide evidence of tumorigenicity. Mutagenicity studies have not been conducted. There was no apparent effect on male or female fertility in rats fed erythromycin (base) at levels up to 0.25 percent of diet.

Pregnancy: Teratogenic effects. Pregnancy Category B: There is no evidence of teratogenicity or any other adverse effect on reproduction in female rats fed erythromycin base (up to 0.25 percent of diet) prior to and during mating, during gestation, and through weaning of two successive litters. There are, however, no adequate and well-controlled studies in pregnant women. Because animal reproduction studies are not always predictive of human response, this drug should be used during pregnancy only if clearly needed.

Labor and Delivery: The effect of erythromycin on labor and delivery is unknown.

Nursing Mothers: Erythromycin is excreted in human milk. Caution should be exercised when erythromycin is administered to a nursing woman.

Pediatric Use: See **INDICATIONS AND USAGE** and **DOSAGE AND ADMINISTRATION**.

ADVERSE REACTIONS

The most frequent side effects of oral erythromycin preparations are gastrointestinal and are dose-related. They include nausea, vomiting, abdominal pain, diarrhea and anorexia. Symptoms of hepatitis, hepatic dysfunction and/or abnormal liver function test results may occur. (See **WARNINGS**.)

Onset of pseudomembranous colitis symptoms may occur during or after antibacterial treatment. (See **WARNINGS**.)

Rarely, erythromycin has been associated with the production of ventricular arrhythmias, including ventricular tachycardia and torsades de pointes, in individuals with prolonged QT interval.

Allergic reactions ranging from urticaria to anaphylaxis have occurred. Skin reactions ranging from mild eruptions to erythema multiforme, Stevens-Johnson syndrome, and toxic epidermal necrolysis have been reported rarely.

There have been isolated reports of reversible hearing loss occurring chiefly in patients with renal insufficiency and in patients receiving high doses of erythromycin.

OVERDOSAGE

In case of overdosage, erythromycin should be discontinued. Overdosage should be handled with the prompt elimination of unabsorbed drug and all other appropriate measures should be instituted.

Erythromycin is not removed by peritoneal dialysis or hemodialysis.

DOSAGE AND ADMINISTRATION

In most patients, PCE tablets are well absorbed and may be dosed orally without regard to meals. However, optimal blood levels are obtained when either PCE 333 mg or PCE 500 mg tablets are given in the fasting state (at least 1/2 hour and preferably 2 hours before meals).

Adults: The usual dosage of PCE is one 333 mg tablet every 8 hours or one 500 mg tablet every 12 hours. Dosage may be increased up to 4 g per day according to the severity of the infection. However, twice-a-day dosing is not recommended when doses larger than 1 g daily are administered.

Children: Age, weight, and severity of the infection are important factors in determining the proper dosage. The usual dosage is 30 to 50 mg/kg/day, in equally divided doses. For more severe infections this dosage may be doubled but should not exceed 4 g per day.

In the treatment of streptococcal infections of the upper respiratory tract (e.g., tonsillitis or pharyngitis), the therapeutic dosage of erythromycin should be administered for at least ten days.

The American Heart Association suggests a dosage of 250 mg of erythromycin orally, twice a day in long-term prophylaxis of streptococcal upper respiratory tract infections for the prevention of recurring attacks of rheumatic fever in patients allergic to penicillin and sulfonamides.[3]

In prophylaxis against bacterial endocarditis (See **INDICATIONS AND USAGE**) the oral regimen for penicillin allergic patients is erythromycin 1 gram, 1 hour before the procedure followed by 500 mg six hours later.[4]

Conjunctivitis of the newborn caused by *Chlamydia trachomatis*: Oral erythromycin suspension 50 mg/kg/day in 4 divided doses for at least 2 weeks.[3]

Pneumonia of infancy caused by *Chlamydia trachomatis*: Although the optimal duration of therapy has not been established, the recommended therapy is oral erythromycin suspension 50 mg/kg/day in 4 divided doses for at least 3 weeks.

Urogenital infections during pregnancy due to *Chlamydia trachomatis*: Although the optimal dose and duration of therapy have not been established, the suggested treatment is 500 mg of erythromycin by mouth four times a day or two erythromycin 333 mg tablets orally every 8 hours on an empty stomach for at least 7 days. For women who cannot tolerate this regimen, a decreased dose of one erythromycin 500 mg tablet orally every 12 hours, one 333 mg tablet orally every 8 hours or 250 mg by mouth four times a day should be used for at least 14 days.[5]

For adults with uncomplicated urethral, endocervical, or rectal infections caused by *Chlamydia trachomatis*, when tetracycline is contraindicated or not tolerated: 500 mg of erythromycin by mouth four times a day or two 333 mg tablets orally every 8 hours for at least 7 days.[5]

For patients with nongonococcal urethritis caused by *Ureaplasma urealyticum* when tetracycline is contraindicated or not tolerated: 500 mg of erythromycin by mouth four times a day or two 333 mg tablets orally every 8 hours for at least seven days.[5]

Primary syphilis: 30 to 40 g given in divided doses over a period of 10 to 15 days.

Acute pelvic inflammatory disease caused by *N. gonorrhoeae*: 500 mg Erythrocin Lactobionate-I.V. (erythromycin lactobionate for injection, USP) every 6 hours for 3 days, followed by 500 mg of erythromycin base orally every 12 hours, or 333 mg of erythromycin base orally every 8 hours for 7 days.

Intestinal amebiasis: Adults: 500 mg every 12 hours, 333 mg every 8 hours or 250 mg every 6 hours for 10 to 14 days. Children: 30 to 50 mg/kg/day in divided doses for 10 to 14 days.

Pertussis: Although optimal dosage and duration have not been established, doses of erythromycin utilized in reported clinical studies were 40 to 50 mg/kg/day, given in divided doses for 5 to 14 days.

Legionnaires' Disease: Although optimal dosage has not been established, doses utilized in reported clinical data were 1 to 4 g daily in divided doses.

HOW SUPPLIED

PCE (erythromycin particles in tablets) is supplied as unscored, ovaloid, Dispertab® tablets in the following strengths and packages.

333 mg, pink-speckled white (imprinted with and PCE):
Bottles of 60 .... (**NDC** 0074-6290-60).

500 mg, white (imprinted with and EK):
Bottles of 100 .... (**NDC** 0074-3389-13).

Recommended Storage: Store below 86°F (30°C).

REFERENCES

1. National Committee for Clinical Laboratory Standards. *Methods for Dilution Antimicrobial Susceptibility Tests for Bacteria that Grow Aerobically*, Third Edition. Approved Standard NCCLS Document M7-A3, Vol. 13, No. 25 NCCLS, Villanova, PA, December 1993.
2. National Committee for Clinical Laboratory Standards, *Performance Standards for Antimicrobial Disk Susceptibility Tests*, Fifth Edition. Approved Standard NCCLS Document M2-A5, Vol. 13, No. 24 NCCLS, Villanova, PA, December 1993.
3. Committee on Rheumatic Fever, Endocarditis, and Kawasaki Disease of the Council on Cardiovascular Disease in the Young, the American Heart Association: Prevention of Rheumatic Fever. *Circulation*. 78(4):1082-1086, October 1988.
4. Dajani, Adnan S.,M.D., et al.: Prevention of Bacterial Endocarditis Recommendations by the American Heart Association. *JAMA*. 264(22):2919-2922, December 1990.
5. Data on file, Abbott Laboratories.

Ref. 03-4802-R6
Revised: May, 1997
PCE 333 mg: U.S. Pat. No. 4,874,614.
PCE 500 mg: U.S. Pat. No. 4,874,614 and 5,009,897.

ABBOTT LABORATORIES
NORTH CHICAGO, IL 60064, U.S.A.

Shown in Product Identification Guide, page 303

PLACIDYL® CIV ℞
ETHCHLORVYNOL CAPSULES, USP
Oral hypnotic

DESCRIPTION

PLACIDYL (ethchlorvynol) is a tertiary carbinol. It is chemically designated as 1-chloro-3-ethyl-1-penten-4-yl-3-ol. Ethchlorvynol occurs as a liquid which is immiscible with water and miscible with most organic solvents. It has the following structural formula:

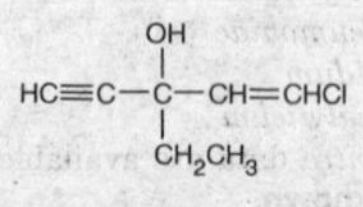

OH
HC≡C—C—CH=CHCl
CH2CH3

PLACIDYL is an oral hypnotic available as dark red capsules containing either 200 mg or 500 mg, or green capsules containing 750 mg of ethchlorvynol.

Each capsule contains the following inactive ingredients: gelatin, glycerin, iron oxide, methylparaben, polyethylene glycol, propylparaben, sorbitol and titanium dioxide. The 200 mg and 500 mg capsules also contain FD&C Red No. 40. The 750 mg capsule also contains FD&C Blue No. 1, FD&C Yellow No. 5 (tartrazine) and FD&C Yellow No. 6.

WARNING: Manufactured with carbon tetrachloride, a substance which harms public health and environment by destroying ozone in the upper atmosphere.

CLINICAL PHARMACOLOGY

The usual hypnotic dose of PLACIDYL induces sleep within 15 minutes to one hour. The duration of the hypnotic effect is about five hours. The mechanism of action is unknown.

PLACIDYL is rapidly absorbed from the gastrointestinal tract with peak plasma concentrations usually occurring within two hours after a single oral fasting dose. Plasma concentrations required for hypnotic effects are unknown. The plasma half-life ($t^{1}/_{2}$, β) of the parent compound is approximately ten to twenty hours. Studies with ^{14}C-PLACIDYL have demonstrated that within 24 hours, 33% of a single 500 mg dose is excreted in the urine mostly as metabolites. The major plasma and urinary metabolite is the secondary alcohol of PLACIDYL. The free and conjugated forms of this metabolite in the urine account for about 40% of the dose. Other minor metabolites have been identified as the primary alcohol and a secondary alcohol with an altered acetylene group. Studies with ^{14}C-PLACIDYL in animals indicate that the parent compound and its metabolites undergo extensive enterohepatic recirculation.

Distribution studies indicate that there is extensive tissue localization of ethchlorvynol, particularly in adipose tissue. Ethchlorvynol and/or its metabolites have also been detected in liver, kidneys, spleen, brain, bile and cerebrospinal fluid.

INDICATIONS AND USAGE

PLACIDYL is indicated as short-term hypnotic therapy for periods up to one week in duration for the management of insomnia. If retreatment becomes necessary, after drug-free intervals of one or more weeks, it should only be undertaken upon further evaluation of the patient.

CONTRAINDICATIONS

PLACIDYL is contraindicated in patients with known hypersensitivity to the drug and in patients with porphyria.

WARNINGS

PLACIDYL SHOULD BE ADMINISTERED WITH CAUTION TO MENTALLY DEPRESSED PATIENTS WITH OR WITHOUT SUICIDAL TENDENCIES. IT SHOULD ALSO BE ADMINISTERED WITH CAUTION TO THOSE WHO HAVE A PSYCHOLOGICAL POTENTIAL FOR DRUG DEPENDENCE. THE LEAST AMOUNT OF DRUG THAT IS FEASIBLE SHOULD BE PRESCRIBED FOR THESE PATIENTS.

Psychological and Physical Dependence

PROLONGED USE OF PLACIDYL MAY RESULT IN TOLERANCE AND PSYCHOLOGICAL AND PHYSICAL DEPENDENCE. PROLONGED ADMINISTRATION OF THE DRUG IS NOT RECOMMENDED. (See "Drug Abuse and Dependence" section.)

PRECAUTIONS

General: Elderly or debilitated patients should receive the smallest effective amount of PLACIDYL (ethchlorvynol).

Caution should be exercised when treating patients with impaired hepatic or renal function.

Patients who exhibit unpredictable behavior, or paradoxical restlessness or excitement in response to barbiturates or alcohol may react in this manner to PLACIDYL.

PLACIDYL should not be used for the management of insomnia in the presence of pain unless insomnia persists after pain is controlled with analgesics.

The 750 mg dosage strength of PLACIDYL contains FD&C Yellow No. 5 (tartrazine) which may cause allergic-type reactions (including bronchial asthma) in certain susceptible individuals. Although the overall incidence of FD&C Yellow No. 5 (tartrazine) sensitivity in the general population is low, it is frequently seen in patients who also have aspirin hypersensitivity.

Information for Patients: The use of ethchlorvynol carries with it an associated risk of psychological and/or physical dependence. The patient should be warned against increasing the dose of the drug without consulting a physician.

Patients should be advised that, for the duration of the effect of PLACIDYL, mental and/or physical abilities required for the performance of potentially hazardous tasks such as the operation of dangerous machinery including motor vehicles, may be impaired.

Patients should be cautioned to avoid the concomitant use of PLACIDYL with alcohol, barbiturates, other CNS depressants, or MAO inhibitors.

Drug Interactions: The concomitant use of PLACIDYL with alcohol, barbiturates, other CNS depressants, or MAO inhibitors may produce exaggerated depressant effects.

Ethchlorvynol may cause a decreased prothrombin time response to coumarin anticoagulants; therefore, the dosage of these drugs may require adjustment when therapy with ethchlorvynol is initiated and after it is discontinued.

Transient delirium has been reported with the concomitant use of PLACIDYL and amitriptyline; therefore, PLACIDYL should be administered with caution to patients receiving tricyclic antidepressants.

Carcinogenesis: A study in mice receiving oral doses of PLACIDYL up to 7 times the maximum human daily dose for 22 to 24 months produced equivocal results. When compared to controls, a statistically significant increase in total lung tumors was found in female mice given the high dose of PLACIDYL. However, the 48% incidence is not substantially higher than the high value (39%) reported for the historical laboratory controls.

No evidence of carcinogenic potential was observed in rats given PLACIDYL at 5 to 15 times the maximum human daily dose for up to 2 years.

Usage During Pregnancy: 1. Teratogenic—Pregnancy Category C. Ethchlorvynol has been associated with a higher percentage of stillbirths and a lower survival rate of progeny among rats given 40 mg/kg/day. There are no adequate and well-controlled studies in pregnant women. Therefore, ethchlorvynol is not recommended for use during the first and second trimesters of pregnancy. Ethchlorvynol should be used during pregnancy only if the potential benefit justifies the potential risk to the fetus.

2. Non-teratogenic—Clinical experience has indicated that ethchlorvynol taken during the third trimester of pregnancy may produce CNS depression and transient withdrawal symptoms in the newborn. These symptoms resemble congenital narcotic withdrawal symptoms (See "Drug Abuse and Dependence" section).

Nursing Mothers: It is not known whether this drug is excreted in breast milk. Because many drugs are excreted in human milk and because of the potential for serious adverse reactions in nursing infants from PLACIDYL, a decision should be made whether to discontinue nursing or to discontinue the drug, taking into account the importance of the drug to the mother.

Pediatric Use: PLACIDYL is not recommended for use in children since its safety and effectiveness in the pediatric age group has not been determined.

ADVERSE REACTIONS

Adverse effects in decreasing order of severity within each of the following categories are:

Hypersensitivity: cholestatic jaundice, urticaria and rash.

Hematologic: thrombocytopenia—one case of fatal immune thrombocytopenia due to ethchlorvynol has been reported.

Gastrointestinal: vomiting, gastric upset, nausea and aftertaste.

Neurologic: dizziness and facial numbness.

Miscellaneous: blurred vision, hypotension and mild "hangover".

The following idiosyncratic responses have been reported occasionally: syncope without marked hypotension, profound muscular weakness, hysteria, marked excitement, prolonged hypnosis and mild stimulation.

Transient ataxia, and giddiness have occurred in patients in whom absorption of the drug is especially rapid. These effects can sometimes be controlled by giving PLACIDYL with food.

(See "Drug Abuse and Dependence" section for the signs and symptoms of chronic intoxication).

DRUG ABUSE AND DEPENDENCE

PLACIDYL is subject to control by the Federal Controlled Substances Act under DEA schedule IV.

Abuse: Pulmonary edema of rapid onset has resulted from the I.V. abuse of PLACIDYL (ethchlorvynol).

Dependence: Signs and symptoms of intoxication have been reported with the prolonged use of doses as low as 1 g/day. Signs and symptoms of chronic intoxication may include incoordination, tremors, ataxia, confusion, slurred speech, hyperreflexia, diplopia, and generalized muscle weakness. Toxic amblyopia, scotoma, nystagmus, and peripheral neuropathy have also been reported with prolonged use of ethchlorvynol; these symptoms are usually reversible.

Severe withdrawal symptoms similar to those seen during barbiturate and alcohol withdrawal have been reported following abrupt discontinuance of prolonged use of PLACIDYL. These symptoms may appear as late as nine days after sudden withdrawal of the drug. Signs and symptoms of PLACIDYL withdrawal may include convulsions, delirium, hallucinations, schizoid reaction, perceptual distortions, memory loss, ataxia, insomnia, slurring of speech, unusual anxiety, irritability, agitation, and tremors. Other signs and symptoms may include anorexia, nausea, vomiting, weakness, dizziness, sweating, muscle twitching, and weight loss.

Management of a patient who manifests withdrawal symptoms from PLACIDYL involves readministration of the drug to approximately the same level of chronic intoxication which existed before the abrupt discontinuance. (Phenobarbital may be substituted for PLACIDYL.) A gradual, stepwise reduction of dosage may then be made over a period of days or weeks. A phenothiazine compound may be used in addition to this regimen for those patients who exhibit psychotic symptoms during the withdrawal period. The patient undergoing withdrawal from PLACIDYL must be hospitalized or closely observed, and given general supportive care as indicated.

In one report an infant born to a mother who received 500 mg PLACIDYL at bedtime daily throughout the third trimester, exhibited withdrawal symptoms on the second day of life. The symptoms included episodic jitteriness, hyperactivity, restlessness, irritability, disturbed sleep and hunger. The neonate responded to a single oral dose of phenobarbital(3 mg/kg). The withdrawal symptoms gradually decreased and completely disappeared by the tenth day of life.

OVERDOSAGE

Acute intoxication is characterized by prolonged deep coma, severe respiratory depression, hypothermia, hypotension, and relative bradycardia. Nystagmus and pancytopenia resulting from acute PLACIDYL overdose have been reported.

Although death has occurred following the ingestion of 6 g of PLACIDYL, there have been reports of patients who have survived overdoses of 50 g and more with intensive care. Fatal blood concentrations usually range from 20 to 50 μg/mL.[1] Because large amounts of ethchlorvynol are taken up by adipose tissue, the blood concentration is an unreliable indicator of the magnitude of overdose.

Management of acute PLACIDYL intoxication is similar to that of acute barbiturate intoxication.[2] Gastric evacuation should be performed immediately. (In the unconscious patient, gastric lavage should be preceded by tracheal intubation with a cuffed tube.) Supportive care (assisted ventilation, frequent and careful monitoring of vital signs, control of blood pressure) is essential. Emphasis should be placed on pulmonary care and monitoring of blood gases. Hemoperfusion utilizing the Amberlite column technique has been reported in the literature to be the most effective method in the management of acute PLACIDYL overdose.[3] In addition, hemodialysis and peritoneal dialysis have each been reported to be of some value. (Aqueous and oil dialysates have been used. Forced diuresis with maintenance of a high urinary output has also been reported of some value.) (See "Drug Abuse and Dependence" section for the signs and symptoms of chronic intoxication.)

DOSAGE AND ADMINISTRATION

The usual adult hypnotic dose of PLACIDYL (ethchlorvynol) is 500 mg taken orally at bedtime. A dose of 750 mg may be required for patients whose sleep response to a 500 mg capsule is inadequate, or for patients being changed from barbiturates or other nonbarbiturate hypnotics. Up to 1000 mg may be given as a single bedtime dose when insomnia is unusually severe. A single supplemental dose of 200 mg may be given to reinstitute sleep in patients who may awaken after the original bedtime dose of 500 or 750 mg.

For patients whose insomnia is characterized only by untimely awakening during the early morning hours, a single dose of 200 mg taken upon awakening may be adequate for relief.

The smallest effective dose of PLACIDYL should be given to elderly or debilitated patients.

PLACIDYL should not be prescribed for periods exceeding one week. (See "Drug Abuse and Dependence" section.)

HOW SUPPLIED

PLACIDYL (ethchlorvynol capsules, USP) is supplied as:

200 mg red capsules imprinted with the , Abbott corporate logo:

Bottles of 100 .... (**NDC** 0074-6661-08)

500 mg red capsules imprinted with the trademark PLACIDYL and 500:

Bottles of 100 .... (**NDC** 0074-6685-15)

ABBO-PAC® unit dose strip

packages of 100 .... (**NDC** 0074-6685-10)

750 mg green capsules imprinted with the trademark PLACIDYL and 750:

Bottles of 100 .... (**NDC** 0074-6630-01)

Recommended storage: 59°–77° F (15°–25° C).

REFERENCES

1. AMA Dept. of Drugs. *AMA Drug Evaluations,* Massachusetts: Publishing Sciences Group, Inc., 1980.
2. Khantzian, E. J., McKenna, G. J., Acute Toxic and Withdrawal Reactions Associated with Drug Use and Abuse, *Annals of Internal Medicine,* 90:361–372, 1979.
3. Lynn, R.I., et al., Resin Hemoperfusion for Treatment of Ethchlorvynol Overdose, *Annals of Internal Medicine,* 91: 549–553, 1979.

Revised: October, 1994

Ref. 03-4566-R12

Shown in Product Identification Guide, page 303

PROSOM™ Ⓒ℞

(estazolam tablets)

DESCRIPTION

ProSom (estazolam), a triazolobenzodiazepine derivative, is an oral hypnotic agent. Estazolam occurs as a fine, white, odorless powder that is soluble in alcohol and practically insoluble in water. The chemical name for estazolam is 8-chloro-6-phenyl-4H-s-triazolo[4,3-α] [1,4]benzodiazepine.

Continued on next page

Prosom—Cont.

The empirical formula is $C_{16}H_{11}ClN_4$. The structural formula is represented as follows:

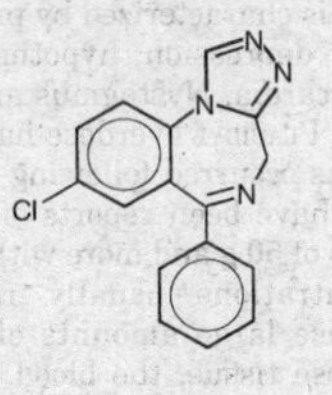

ProSom tablets are scored and contain either 1 mg or 2 mg of estazolam.
Inactive Ingredients: 1 mg tablets: corn starch, lactose, and stearic acid.
2 mg tablets: corn starch, iron oxide, lactose, and stearic acid.

CLINICAL PHARMACOLOGY

Pharmacokinetics: ProSom tablets have been found to be equivalent in absorption to an orally administered solution of estazolam. Independent of concentration, estazolam in plasma is 93% protein bound.
In healthy subjects who received up to three times the recommended dose of ProSom, peak estazolam plasma concentrations occurred within two hours after dosing (range 0.5 to 6.0 hours) and were proportional to the administered dose, suggesting linear pharmacokinetics over the dosage range tested.
The range of estimates for the mean elimination half-life of estazolam varied from 10 to 24 hours. The clearance of benzodiazepines is accelerated in smokers compared to nonsmokers, and there is evidence that this occurs with estazolam. This decrease in half-life, presumably due to enzyme induction by smoking, is consistent with other drugs with similar hepatic clearance characteristics. In all subjects and at all doses, the mean elimination half-life appeared to be independent of the dose.
In a small study (N=8) using various doses in older subjects (59 to 68 years), peak estazolam concentrations were found to be similar to those observed in younger subjects with a mean elimination half-life of 18.4 hours (range 13.5 to 34.6 hours).
Estazolam is extensively metabolized, and the metabolites are excreted primarily in the urine. Less than 5% of a 2 mg dose of estazolam is excreted unchanged in the urine, with only 4% of the dose appearing in the feces. 4′-hydroxy estazolam is the major metabolite in plasma, with concentrations approaching 12% of those of the parent eight hours after administration. While it and the lesser metabolite, 1-oxo-estazolam, have some pharmacologic activity, their low potencies and low concentrations preclude any significant contribution to the hypnotic effect of ProSom.
Postulated relationship between elimination rate of benzodiazepine hypnotics and their profile of common untoward effects: The type and duration of hypnotic effects and the profile of unwanted effects during administration of benzodiazepine drugs may be influenced by the biologic half-life of administered drug and any active metabolites formed. If half-lives are long, drug or metabolites may accumulate during periods of nightly administration and may be associated with impairments of cognitive and/or motor performance during waking hours; the possibility of interaction with other psychoactive drugs or alcohol will be increased. In contrast, if half-lives are short, drug and metabolites will be cleared before the next dose is ingested, and carry-over effects related to excessive sedation or CNS depression should be minimal or absent. However, during nightly use for an extended period, pharmacodynamic tolerance or adaptation to some effects of benzodiazepine hypnotics may develop. If the drug has a short elimination half-life, it is possible that a relative deficiency of the drug or its active metabolites (ie, in relationship to the receptor site) may occur at some point in the interval between each night's use. This sequence of events may account for two clinical findings reported to occur after several weeks of nightly use of rapidly eliminated benzodiazepine hypnotics, namely, increased wakefulness during the last third of the night and increased daytime anxiety in selected patients.
Controlled Trials Supporting Efficacy: In three 7-night, double-blind, parallel-group trials comparing estazolam 1 mg and/or 2 mg with placebo in adult outpatients with chronic insomnia, estazolam 2 mg was consistently superior to placebo in subjective measures of sleep induction (latency) and sleep maintenance (duration, number of awakenings, depth and quality of sleep); estazolam 1 mg was similarly superior to placebo on all measures of sleep maintenance, however, it significantly improved sleep induction in only one of two studies. In a similarly designed trial comparing estazolam 0.5 mg and 1 mg with placebo in geriatric outpatients with chronic insomnia, only the 1 mg estazolam dose was consistently superior to placebo in sleep induction (latency) and in only one measure of sleep maintenance (ie, duration of sleep).
In a single-night, double-blind, parallel-group trial comparing estazolam 2 mg and placebo in patients admitted for elective surgery and requiring sleep medications, estazolam was superior to placebo in subjective measures of sleep induction and maintenance.
In a 12-week, double-blind, parallel-group trial including a comparison of estazolam 2 mg and placebo in adult outpatients with chronic insomnia, estazolam was superior to placebo in subjective measures of sleep induction (latency) and maintenance (duration, number of awakenings, total wake time during sleep) at week 2, but produced consistent improvement over 12 weeks only for sleep duration and total wake time during sleep. Following withdrawal at week 12, rebound insomnia was seen at the first withdrawal week, but there was no difference between drug and placebo by the second withdrawal week in all parameters except latency, for which normalization did not occur until the fourth withdrawal week.
Adult outpatients with chronic insomnia were evaluated in a sleep laboratory trial comparing four doses of estazolam (0.25, 0.50, 1.0 and 2.0 mg) and placebo, each administered for 2 nights in a crossover design. The higher estazolam doses were superior to placebo in most EEG measures of sleep induction and maintenance, especially at the 2 mg dose, but only for sleep duration in subjective measures of sleep.

INDICATIONS AND USAGE

ProSom (estazolam) is indicated for the short-term management of insomnia characterized by difficulty in falling asleep, frequent nocturnal awakenings, and/or early morning awakenings. Both outpatient studies and a sleep laboratory study have shown that ProSom administered at bedtime improved sleep induction and sleep maintenance (see CLINICAL PHARMACOLOGY).
Because insomnia is often transient and intermittent, the prolonged administration of ProSom is generally neither necessary nor recommended. Since insomnia may be a symptom of several other disorders, the possibility that the complaint may be related to a condition for which there is a more specific treatment should be considered.
There is evidence to support the ability of ProSom to enhance the duration and quality of sleep for intervals up to 12 weeks (see CLINICAL PHARMACOLOGY).

CONTRAINDICATIONS

Benzodiazepines may cause fetal damage when administered during pregnancy. An increased risk of congenital malformations associated with the use of diazepam and chlordiazepoxide during the first trimester of pregnancy has been suggested in several studies. Transplacental distribution has resulted in neonatal CNS depression and also withdrawal phenomena following the ingestion of therapeutic doses of a benzodiazepine hypnotic during the last weeks of pregnancy.
ProSom is contraindicated in pregnant women. If there is a likelihood of the patient becoming pregnant while receiving ProSom she should be warned of the potential risk to the fetus and instructed to discontinue the drug prior to becoming pregnant. The possibility that a woman of childbearing potential is pregnant at the time of institution of therapy should be considered.

WARNINGS

ProSom, like other benzodiazepines, has CNS depressant effects. For this reason, patients should be cautioned against engaging in hazardous occupations requiring complete mental alertness, such as operating machinery or driving a motor vehicle, after ingesting the drug, including potential impairment of the performance of such activities that may occur the day following ingestion of ProSom. Patients should also be cautioned about possible combined effects with alcohol and other CNS depressant drugs.
As with all benzodiazepines, amnesia, paradoxical reactions (eg, excitement, agitation, etc.), and other adverse behavioral effects may occur unpredictably.
There have been reports of withdrawal signs and symptoms of the type associated with withdrawal from CNS depressant drugs following the rapid decrease or the abrupt discontinuation of benzodiazepines (see DRUG ABUSE AND DEPENDENCE).

PRECAUTIONS

General: Impaired motor and/or cognitive performance attributable to the accumulation of benzodiazepines and their active metabolites following several days of repeated use at their recommended doses is a concern in certain vulnerable patients (eg, those especially sensitive to the effects of benzodiazepines or those with a reduced capacity to metabolize and eliminate them) (see DOSAGE AND ADMINISTRATION).
Elderly or debilitated patients and those with impaired renal or hepatic function should be cautioned about these risks and advised to monitor themselves for signs of excessive sedation or impaired conditions.
ProSom appears to cause dose-related respiratory depression that is ordinarily not clinically relevant at recommended doses in patients with normal respiratory function. However, patients with compromised respiratory function may be at risk and should be monitored appropriately. As a class, benzodiazepines have the capacity to depress respiratory drive; there are insufficient data available, however, to characterize their relative potency in depressing respiratory drive at clinically recommended doses.
As with other benzodiazepines, ProSom should be administered with caution to patients exhibiting signs or symptoms of depression. Suicidal tendencies may be present in such patients and protective measures may be required. Intentional overdosage is more common in this group of patients; therefore, the least amount of drug that is feasible should be prescribed for the patient at any one time.
Information for Patients: To assure the safe and effective use of ProSom, the following information and instructions should be given to patients:

1. Inform your physician about any alcohol consumption and medicine you are taking now, including drugs you may buy without a prescription. Alcohol should not be used during treatment with hypnotics.
2. Inform your physician if you are planning to become pregnant, if you are pregnant, or if you become pregnant while you are taking this medicine.
3. You should not take this medicine if you are nursing, as the drug may be excreted in breast milk.
4. Until you experience the way this medicine affects you, do not drive a car, operate potentially dangerous machinery, or engage in hazardous occupations requiring complete mental alertness after taking this medicine.
5. Since benzodiazepines may produce psychological and physical dependence, you should not increase the dose before consulting your physician. In addition, since the abrupt discontinuation of ProSom may be associated with temporary sleep disturbances, you should consult your physician before abruptly discontinuing doses of 2 mg per night or more.

Laboratory Tests: Laboratory tests are not ordinarily required in otherwise healthy patients. When treatment with ProSom is protracted, periodic blood counts, urinalyses, and blood chemistry analyses are advisable.
Drug Interactions: If ProSom is given concomitantly with other drugs acting on the central nervous system, careful consideration should be given to the pharmacology of all agents. The action of the benzodiazepines may be potentiated by anticonvulsants, antihistamines, alcohol, barbiturates, monoamine oxidase inhibitors, narcotics, phenothiazines, psychotropic medications, or other drugs that produce CNS depression. Smokers have an increased clearance of benzodiazepines as compared to nonsmokers; this was seen in studies with estazolam (see CLINICAL PHARMACOLOGY).
Carcinogenesis, Mutagenesis, Impairment of Fertility: Two-year carcinogenicity studies were conducted in mice and rats at dietary doses of 0.8, 3, and 10 mg/kg/day and 0.5, 2, and 10 mg/kg/day, respectively. Evidence of tumorigenicity was not observed in either study. Incidence of hyperplastic liver nodules increased in female mice given the mid- and high-dose levels. The significance of such nodules in mice is not known at this time.
In vitro and *in vivo* mutagenicity tests including the Ames test, DNA repair in *B. subtilis*, *in vivo* cytogenetics in mice and rats, and the dominant lethal test in mice did not show a mutagenic potential for estazolam.
Fertility in male and female rats was not affected by doses up to 30 times the usual recommended human dose.
Pregnancy:

1. Teratogenic Effects: Pregnancy Category X (see CONTRAINDICATIONS).
2. Nonteratogenic Effects: The child born of a mother taking benzodiazepines may be at some risk for withdrawal symptoms during the postnatal period. Neonatal flaccidity has been reported in an infant born of a mother who received benzodiazepines during pregnancy.

Labor and Delivery: ProSom has no established use in labor or delivery.
Nursing Mothers: Human studies have not been conducted; however, studies in lactating rats indicate that estazolam and/or its metabolites are secreted in the milk. The use of ProSom in nursing mothers is not recommended.
Pediatric Use: Safety and effectiveness in pediatric patients below the age of 18 have not been established.
Geriatric Use: Approximately 18% of individuals participating in the premarketing clinical trials of ProSom were 60 years of age or older. Overall, the adverse event profile did not differ substantively from that observed in younger individuals. Care should be exercised when prescribing benzodiazepines to small or debilitated elderly patients (see DOSAGE AND ADMINISTRATION).

ADVERSE REACTIONS

Commonly Observed: The most commonly observed adverse events associated with the use of ProSom, not seen at

an equivalent incidence among placebo-treated patients were somnolence, hypokinesia, dizziness, and abnormal coordination.

Associated with Discontinuation of Treatment: Approximately 3% of 1277 patients who received ProSom in US premarketing clinical trials discontinued treatment because of an adverse clinical event. The only event commonly associated with discontinuation, accounting for 1.3% of the total, was somnolence.

Incidence in Controlled Clinical Trials: The table below enumerates adverse events that occurred at an incidence of 1% or greater among patients with insomnia who received ProSom in 7-night, placebo-controlled trials. Events reported by investigators were classified into standard dictionary (COSTART) terms to establish event frequencies. Event frequencies reported were not corrected for the occurrence of these events at baseline. The frequencies were obtained from data pooled across six studies: ProSom, N=685; placebo, N=433. The prescriber should be aware that these figures cannot be used to predict the incidence of side effects in the course of usual medical practice in which patient characteristics and other factors differ from those that prevailed in these six clinical trials. Similarly, the cited frequencies cannot be compared with figures obtained from other clinical investigators involving related drug products and uses, since each group of drug trials was conducted under a different set of conditions. However, the cited figures provide the physician with a basis of estimating the relative contribution of drug and nondrug factors to the incidence of side effects in the population studied.

INCIDENCE OF ADVERSE EXPERIENCES IN PLACEBO-CONTROLLED CLINICAL TRIALS
(Percentage of Patients Reporting)

Body System/ Adverse Event*	ProSom (N=685)	Placebo (N=433)
Body as a Whole		
Headache	16	27
Asthenia	11	8
Malaise	5	5
Low extremity pain	3	2
Back pain	2	2
Body pain	2	2
Abdominal pain	1	2
Chest pain	1	1
Digestive System		
Nausea	4	5
Dyspepsia	2	2
Musculoskeletal System		
Stiffness	1	–
Nervous System		
Somnolence	42	27
Hypokinesia	8	4
Nervousness	8	11
Dizziness	7	3
Coordination abnormal	4	1
Hangover	3	2
Confusion	2	–
Depression	2	3
Dream abnormal	2	2
Thinking abnormal	2	1
Respiratory System		
Cold symptoms	3	5
Pharyngitis	1	2
Skin and Appendages		
Pruritus	1	–

*Events reported by at least 1% of ProSom patients.

Other Adverse Events:
During clinical trials conducted by Abbott, some of which were not placebo-controlled, ProSom was administered to approximately 1300 patients. Untoward events associated with this exposure were recorded by clinical investigators using terminology of their own choosing. To provide a meaningful estimate of the proportion of individuals experiencing adverse events, similar types of untoward events must be grouped into a smaller number of standardized event categories. In the tabulations that follow, a standard COSTART dictionary terminology has been used to classify reported adverse events. The frequencies presented, therefore, represent the proportion of the 1277 individuals exposed to ProSom who experienced an event of the type cited on at least one occasion while receiving ProSom. All reported events are included except those already listed in the previous table, those COSTART terms too general to be informative, and those events where a drug cause was remote. Events are further classified within body system categories and enumerated in order of decreasing frequency using the following definitions: frequent adverse events are defined as those occurring on one or more occasions in at least 1/100 patients; infrequent adverse events are those occurring in 1/100 to 1/1000 patients; rare events are those occurring in less than 1/1000 patients. It is important to emphasize that, although the events reported did occur during treatment with ProSom, they were not necessarily caused by it.

Body as a Whole—Infrequent: allergic reaction, chills, fever, neck pain, upper extremity pain; Rare: edema, jaw pain, swollen breast.

Cardiovascular System—Infrequent: flushing, palpitation; Rare: arrhythmia, syncope.

Digestive System— Frequent: constipation, dry mouth; Infrequent: decreased appetite, flatulence, gastritis, increased appetite, vomiting; Rare: enterocolitis, melena, ulceration of the mouth.

Endocrine System—Rare: thyroid nodule.

Hematologic and Lymphatic System—Rare: leukopenia, purpura, swollen lymph nodes.

Metabolic/Nutritional Disorders—Infrequent: thirst; Rare: increased SGOT, weight gain, weight loss.

Musculoskeletal System— Infrequent: arthritis, muscle spasm, myalgia; Rare: arthralgia.

Nervous System—Frequent: anxiety; Infrequent: agitation, amnesia, apathy, emotional lability, euphoria, hostility, paresthesia, seizure, sleep disorder, stupor, twitch; Rare: ataxia, circumoral paresthesia, decreased libido, decreased reflexes, hallucinations, neuritis, nystagmus, tremor.

Minor changes in EEG patterns, usually low-voltage fast activity, have been observed in patients during ProSom therapy or withdrawal and are of no known clinical significance.

Respiratory System— Infrequent: asthma, cough, dyspnea, rhinitis, sinusitis; Rare: epistaxis, hyperventilation, laryngitis.

Skin and Appendages—Infrequent: rash, sweating, urticaria; Rare: acne, dry skin.

Special Senses—Infrequent: abnormal vision, ear pain, eye irritation, eye pain, eye swelling, perverse taste, photophobia, tinnitus; Rare: decreased hearing, diplopia, scotomata.

Urogenital System—Infrequent: frequent urination, menstrual cramps, urinary hesitancy, urinary urgency, vaginal discharge/itching; Rare: hematuria, nocturia, oliguria, penile discharge, urinary incontinence.

Postintroduction Reports— Voluntary reports of non-US postmarketing experience with estazolam have included rare occurrences of photosensitivity, Stevens-Johnson syndrome, and agranulocytosis. Because of the uncontrolled nature of these spontaneous reports, a causal relationship to estazolam treatment has not been determined.

DRUG ABUSE AND DEPENDENCE

Controlled Substance: ProSom tablets are a controlled substance in Schedule IV.

Abuse and Dependence: Withdrawal symptoms similar to those noted with sedatives/hypnotics and alcohol have occurred following the abrupt discontinuation of drugs in the benzodiazepine class. The symptoms can range from mild dysphoria and insomnia to a major syndrome that may include abdominal and muscle cramps, vomiting, sweating, tremors, and convulsions.

Although withdrawal symptoms are more commonly noted after the discontinuation of higher than therapeutic doses of benzodiazepines, a proportion of patients taking benzodiazepines chronically at therapeutic doses may become physically dependent on them. Available data, however, cannot provide a reliable estimate of the incidence of dependency or the relationship of the dependency to dose and duration of treatment. There is some evidence to suggest that gradual reduction of dosage will attenuate or eliminate some withdrawal phenomena. In most instances, withdrawal phenomena are relatively mild and transient; however, life-threatening events (eg, seizures, delirium, etc.) have been reported.

Gradual withdrawal is the preferred course for any patient taking benzodiazepines for a prolonged period. Patients with a history of seizures, regardless of their concomitant antiseizure drug therapy, should not be withdrawn abruptly from benzodiazepines.

Individuals with a history of addiction to or abuse of drugs or alcohol should be under careful surveillance when receiving benzodiazepines because of the risk of habituation and dependence to such patients.

OVERDOSAGE

As with other benzodiazepines, experience with ProSom indicates that manifestations of overdosage include somnolence, respiratory depression, confusion, impaired coordination, slurred speech, and ultimately, coma. Patients have recovered from overdosage as high as 40 mg. As in the management of intentional overdose with any drug, the possibility should be considered that multiple agents may have been taken.

Gastric evacuation, either by the induction of emesis, lavage, or both, should be performed immediately. Maintenance of adequate ventilation is essential. General supportive care, including frequent monitoring of the vital signs and close observation of the patient, is indicated. Fluids should be administered intravenously to maintain blood pressure and encourage diuresis. The value of dialysis in treatment of benzodiazepine overdose has not been determined. The physician may wish to consider contacting a Poison Control Center for up-to-date information on the management of hypnotic drug product overdose.

Flumazenil, a specific benzodiazepine receptor antagonist, is indicated for the complete or partial reversal of the sedative effects of benzodiazepines and may be used in situations when an overdose with a benzodiazepine is known or suspected. Prior to the administration of flumazenil, necessary measures should be instituted to secure airway, ventilation, and intravenous access. Flumazenil is intended as an adjunct to, not as a substitute for, proper management of benzodiazepine overdose. Patients treated with flumazenil should be monitored for resedation, respiratory depression, and other residual benzodiazepine effects for an appropriate period after treatment. **The prescriber should be aware of a risk of seizure in association with flumazenil treatment, particularly in long-term benzodiazepine users and in cyclic antidepressant overdose.** The complete flumazenil package insert including CONTRAINDICATIONS, WARNINGS, and PRECAUTIONS should be consulted prior to use.

DOSAGE AND ADMINISTRATION

The recommended initial dose for adults is 1 mg at bedtime; however, some patients may need a 2 mg dose. In healthy elderly patients, 1 mg is also the appropriate starting dose, but increases should be initiated with particular care. In small or debilitated older patients, a starting dose of 0.5 mg, while only marginally effective in the overall elderly population, should be considered.

HOW SUPPLIED

ProSom tablets are scored tablets supplied as:
ProSom Tablets 1 mg (white)
Bottles of 100 .... (**NDC** 0074-3735-13)
ProSom Tablets 2 mg (coral-colored)
Bottles of 100 .... (**NDC** 0074-3736-13)
Recommended storage: Store below 86°F (30°C).
Revised: March, 1997
Ref. 03-4728-R6
ABBOTT LABORATORIES
NORTH CHICAGO, IL 60064, U.S.A.
Shown in Product Identification Guide, page 303

TRANXENE® Ⓒ ℞

[tran' zēen]
T-TAB® Tablets
CLORAZEPATE DIPOTASSIUM
TRANXENE®-SD™
& TRANXENE®-SD™ HALF STRENGTH
CLORAZEPATE DIPOTASSIUM SINGLE DOSE TABLETS

DESCRIPTION

Chemically, TRANXENE is a benzodiazepine. The empirical formula is $C_{16}H_{11}ClK_2N_2O_4$; the molecular weight is 408.92; and the structural formula may be represented as follows:

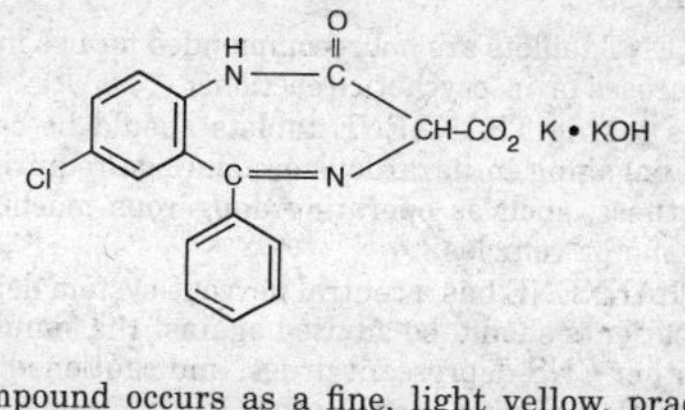

The compound occurs as a fine, light yellow, practically odorless powder. It is insoluble in the common organic solvents, but very soluble in water. Aqueous solutions are unstable, clear, light yellow, and alkaline.

TRANXENE T-TAB tablets contain either 3.75 mg, 7.5 mg or 15 mg of clorazepate dipotassium for oral administration. TRANXENE- SD and TRANXENE-SD HALF STRENGTH tablets contain 22.5 mg and 11.25 mg of clorazepate dipotassium respectively. TRANXENE-SD and TRANXENE-SD HALF STRENGTH tablets gradually release clorazepate and are designed for once-a-day administration in patients already stabilized on TRANXENE T-TAB tablets.

Inactive ingredients for TRANXENE T-TAB® Tablets: Colloidal silicon dioxide, FD&C Blue No. 2 (3.75 mg only), FD&C Yellow No. 6 (7.5 mg only), FD&C Red No. 3 (15 mg only), magnesium oxide, magnesium stearate, microcrystalline cellulose, potassium carbonate, potassium chloride, and talc. Inactive ingredients for TRANXENE-SD and TRANXENE-SD HALF STRENGTH Tablets: Castor oil wax, FD&C Blue No. 2 (SD Half Strength, 11.25 mg only), iron oxide (SD, 22.5 mg only), lactose, magnesium oxide, magnesium stearate, potassium carbonate, potassium chloride, and talc.

CLINICAL PHARMACOLOGY

Pharmacologically, clorazepate dipotassium has the characteristics of the benzodiazepines. It has depressant effects on

Continued on next page

Tranxene—Cont.

the central nervous system. The primary metabolite, nordiazepam, quickly appears in the blood stream. The serum half-life is about 2 days. The drug is metabolized in the liver and excreted primarily in the urine.

Studies in healthy men have shown that clorazenate dipotassium has depressant effects on the central nervous system. Prolonged administration of single daily doses as high as 120 mg was without toxic effects. Abrupt cessation of high doses was followed in some patients by nervousness, insomnia, irritability, diarrhea, muscle aches, or memory impairment.

Since orally administered clorazepate dipotassium is rapidly decarboxylated to form nordiazepam, there is essentially no circulating parent drug. Nordiazepam, the primary metabolite, quickly appears in the blood and is eliminated from the plasma with an apparent half-life of about 40 to 50 hours. Plasma levels of nordiazepam increase proportionally with TRANXENE dose and show moderate accumulation with repeated administration. The protein binding of nordiazepam in plasma is high (97-98%).

Within 10 days after oral administration of a 15 mg (50μCi) dose of ^{14}C-TRANXENE to two volunteers, 62–67% of the radioactivity was excreted in the urine and 15–19% was eliminated in the feces. Both subjects were still excreting measurable amounts of radioactivity in the urine (about 1% of the ^{14}C-dose) on day ten.

Nordiazepam is further metabolized by hydroxylation. The major urinary metabolite is conjugated oxazepam (3-hydroxynordiazepam), and smaller amounts of conjugated p-hydroxynordiazepam and nordiazepam are also found in the urine.

INDICATIONS AND USAGE

TRANXENE is indicated for the management of anxiety disorders or for the short-term relief of the symptoms of anxiety. Anxiety or tension associated with the stress of everyday life usually does not require treatment with an anxiolytic.

TRANXENE tablets are indicated as adjunctive therapy in the management of partial seizures.

The effectiveness of TRANXENE tablets in long-term management of anxiety, that is, more than 4 months, has not been assessed by systematic clinical studies. Long-term studies in epileptic patients, however, have shown continued therapeutic activity. The physician should reassess periodically the usefulness of the drug for the individual patient.

TRANXENE tablets are indicated for the symptomatic relief of acute alcohol withdrawal.

CONTRAINDICATIONS

TRANXENE tablets are contraindicated in patients with a known hypersensitivity to the drug and in those with acute narrow angle glaucoma.

WARNINGS

TRANXENE tablets are not recommended for use in depressive neuroses or in psychotic reactions.

Patients taking TRANXENE tablets should be cautioned against engaging in hazardous occupations requiring mental alertness, such as operating dangerous machinery including motor vehicles.

Since TRANXENE has a central nervous system depressant effect, patients should be advised against the simultaneous use of other CNS-depressant drugs, and cautioned that the effects of alcohol may be increased.

Because of the lack of sufficient clinical experience, TRANXENE tablets are not recommended for use in patients less than 9 years of age.

Physical and Psychological Dependence:
Withdrawal symptoms (similar in character to those noted with barbiturates and alcohol) have occurred following abrupt discontinuance of clorazepate. Withdrawal symptoms associated with the abrupt discontinuation of benzodiazepines have included convulsions, delirium, tremor, abdominal and muscle cramps, vomiting, sweating, nervousness, insomnia, irritability, diarrhea, and memory impairment. The more severe withdrawal symptoms have usually been limited to those patients who had received excessive doses over an extended period of time. Generally milder withdrawal symptoms have been reported following abrupt discontinuance of benzodiazepines taken continuously at therapeutic levels for several months. Consequently, after extended therapy, abrupt discontinuation of clorazepate should generally be avoided and a gradual dosage tapering schedule followed.

Caution should be observed in patients who are considered to have a psychological potential for drug dependence.

Evidence of drug dependence has been observed in dogs and rabbits which was characterized by convulsive seizures when the drug was abruptly withdrawn or the dose was reduced; the syndrome in dogs could be abolished by administration of clorazepate.

Usage in Pregnancy: **An increased risk of congenital malformations associated with the use of minor tranquilizers (chlordiazepoxide, diazepam, and meprobamate) during the first trimester of pregnancy has been suggested in several studies. Clorazepate dipotassium, a benzodiazepine derivative, has not been studied adequately to determine whether it, too, may be associated with an increased risk of fetal abnormality. Because use of these drugs is rarely a matter of urgency, their use during this period should almost always be avoided. The possibility that a woman of childbearing potential may be pregnant at the time of institution of therapy should be considered. Patients should be advised that if they become pregnant during therapy or intend to become pregnant they should communicate with their physician about the desirability of discontinuing the drug.**

Usage during Lactation:
TRANXENE tablets should not be given to nursing mothers since it has been reported that nordiazepam is excreted in human breast milk.

PRECAUTIONS

In those patients in which a degree of depression accompanies the anxiety, suicidal tendencies may be present and protective measures may be required. The least amount of drug that is feasible should be available to the patient.

Patients taking TRANXENE tablets for prolonged periods should have blood counts and liver function tests periodically. The usual precautions in treating patients with impaired renal or hepatic function should also be observed.

In elderly or debilitated patients, the initial dose should be small, and increments should be made gradually, in accordance with the response of the patient, to preclude ataxia or excessive sedation.

Information for Patients:
To assure the safe and effective use of benzodiazepines, patients should be informed that, since benzodiazepines may produce psychological and physical dependence, it is essential that they consult with their physician before either increasing the dose or abruptly discontinuing this drug.

Pediatric Use: See **WARNINGS**.

ADVERSE REACTIONS

The side effect most frequently reported was drowsiness. Less commonly reported (in descending order of occurrence) were: dizziness, various gastrointestinal complaints, nervousness, blurred vision, dry mouth, headache, and mental confusion. Other side effects included insomnia, transient skin rashes, fatigue, ataxia, genitourinary complaints, irritability, diplopia, depression, tremor, and slurred speech.

There have been reports of abnormal liver and kidney function tests and of decrease in hematocrit.

Decrease in systolic blood pressure has been observed.

DOSAGE AND ADMINISTRATION

For the symptomatic relief of anxiety:
TRANXENE T-TAB® tablets are administered orally in divided doses. The usual daily dose is 30 mg. The dose should be adjusted gradually within the range of 15 to 60 mg daily in accordance with the response of the patient. In elderly or debilitated patients it is advisable to initiate treatment at a daily dose of 7.5 to 15 mg.

TRANXENE tablets may also be administered in a single dose daily at bedtime; the recommended initial dose is 15 mg. After the initial dose, the response of the patient may require adjustment of subsequent dosage. Lower doses may be indicated in the elderly patient. Drowsiness may occur at the initiation of treatment and with dosage increment.

TRANXENE-SD (22.5 mg) tablets may be administered as a single dose every 24 hours. This tablet is intended as an alternate dosage form for the convenience of patients stabilized on a dose of 7.5 mg tablets three times a day. TRANXENE-SD tablets should not be used to initiate therapy.

TRANXENE-SD HALF STRENGTH (11.25 mg) tablets may be administered as a single dose every 24 hours. This tablet is intended as an alternate dosage form for the convenience of patients stabilized on a dose of 3.75 mg tablets three times a day. TRANXENE-SD HALF STRENGTH should not be used to initiate therapy.

For the symptomatic relief of acute alcohol withdrawal:
The following dosage schedule is recommended:

1st 24 hours (Day 1)	30 mg initially; followed by 30 to 60 mg in divided doses
2nd 24 hours (Day 2)	45 to 90 mg in divided doses
3rd 24 hours (Day 3)	22.5 to 45 mg in divided doses
Day 4	15 to 30 mg in divided doses

Thereafter, gradually reduce the daily dose to 7.5 to 15 mg. Discontinue drug therapy as soon as patient's condition is stable.

The maximum recommended total daily dose is 90 mg. Avoid excessive reductions in the total amount of drug administered on successive days.

As an Adjunct to Antiepileptic Drugs:
In order to minimize drowsiness, the recommended initial dosages and dosage increments should not be exceeded.

Adults: The maximum recommended initial dose in patients over 12 years old is 7.5 mg three times a day. Dosage should be increased by no more than 7.5 mg every week and should not exceed 90 mg/day.

Children (9-12 years): The maximum recommended initial dose is 7.5 mg two times a day. Dosage should be increased by no more than 7.5 mg every week and should not exceed 60 mg/day.

DRUG INTERACTIONS

If TRANXENE is to be combined with other drugs acting on the central nervous system, careful consideration should be given to the pharmacology of the agents to be employed. Animal experience indicates that clorazepate dipotassium prolongs the sleeping time after hexobarbital or after ethyl alcohol, increases the inhibitory effects of chlorpromazine, but does not exhibit monoamine oxidase inhibition. Clinical studies have shown increased sedation with concurrent hypnotic medications. The actions of the benzodiazepines may be potentiated by barbiturates, narcotics, phenothiazines, monoamine oxidase inhibitors or other antidepressants.

If TRANXENE tablets are used to treat anxiety associated with somatic disease states, careful attention must be paid to possible drug interaction with concomitant medication.

In bioavailability studies with normal subjects, the concurrent administration of antacids at therapeutic levels did not significantly influence the bioavailability of TRANXENE tablets.

OVERDOSAGE

Overdosage is usually manifested by varying degrees of CNS depression ranging from slight sedation to coma. As in the management of overdosage with any drug, it should be borne in mind that multiple agents may have been taken. The treatment of overdosage should consist of the general measures employed in the management of overdosage of any CNS depressant. Gastric evacuation either by the induction of emesis, lavage, or both, should be performed immediately. General supportive care, including frequent monitoring of the vital signs and close observation of the patient, is indicated. Hypotension, though rarely reported, may occur with large overdoses. In such cases the use of agents such as Levophed® Bitartrate (norepinephrine bitartrate injection, USP) or Aramine® Injection (metaraminol bitartrate injection, USP) should be considered.

While reports indicate that individuals have survived overdoses of clorazepate dipotassium as high as 450 to 675 mg, these doses are not necessarily an accurate indication of the amount of drug absorbed since the time interval between ingestion and the institution of treatment was not always known. Sedation in varying degrees was the most common physiological manifestation of clorazepate dipotassium overdosage. Deep coma when it occurred was usually associated with the ingestion of other drugs in addition to clorazepate dipotassium.

Flumazenil, a specific benzodiazepine receptor antagonist, is indicated for the complete or partial reversal of the sedative effects of benzodiazepines and may be used in situations when an overdose with a benzodiazepine is known or suspected. Prior to the administration of flumazenil, necessary measures should be instituted to secure airway, ventilation, and intravenous access. Flumazenil is intended as an adjunct to, not as a substitute for, proper management of benzodiazepine overdose. Patients treated with flumazenil should be monitored for resedation, respiratory depression, and other residual benzodiazepine effects for an appropriate period after treatment. **The prescriber should be aware of a risk of seizure in association with flumazenil treatment, particularly in long-term benzodiazepine users and in cyclic antidepressant overdose.** The complete flumazenil package insert including CONTRAINDICATIONS, WARNINGS, and PRECAUTIONS should be consulted prior to use.

ANIMAL PHARMACOLOGY AND TOXICOLOGY

Studies in rats and monkeys have shown a substantial difference between doses producing tranquilizing, sedative and toxic effects. In rats, conditioned avoidance response was inhibited at an oral dose of 10 mg/kg; sedation was induced at 32 mg/kg; the LD$_{50}$ was 1320 mg/kg. In monkeys aggressive behavior was reduced at an oral dose of 0.25 mg/kg; sedation (ataxia) was induced at 7.5 mg/kg; the LD$_{50}$ could not be determined because of the emetic effect of large doses, but the LD$_{50}$ exceeds 1600 mg/kg.

Twenty-four dogs were given clorazepate dipotassium orally in a 22-month toxicity study; doses up to 75 mg/kg were given. Drug-related changes occurred in the liver; weight

was increased and cholestasis with minimal hepatocellular damage was found, but lobular architecture remained well preserved.

Eighteen rhesus monkeys were given oral doses of clorazepate dipotassium from 3 to 36 mg/kg daily for 52 weeks. All treated animals remained similar to control animals. Although total leucocyte count remained within normal limits it tended to fall in the female animals on the highest doses. Examination of all organs revealed no alterations attributable to clorazepate dipotassium. There was no damage to liver function or structure.

Reproduction Studies: Standard fertility, reproduction, and teratology studies were conducted in rats and rabbits. Oral doses in rats up to 150 mg/kg and in rabbits up to 15 mg/kg produced no abnormalities in the fetuses. TRANXENE did not alter the fertility indices or reproductive capacity of adult animals. As expected, the sedative effect of high doses interfered with care of the young by their mothers (*see Usage in Pregnancy*).

HOW SUPPLIED

TRANXENE® 3.75 mg, scored T-TAB® tablets are supplied as blue-colored tablets bearing the Abbott logo, the distinctive T shape and a two-letter Abbo-Code designation, TL:

Bottles of 100 .... (**NDC** 0074-4389-13).
Bottles of 500 .... (**NDC** 0074-4389-53).
ABBO-PAC® unit dose packages:
100 .... (**NDC** 0074-4389-11).

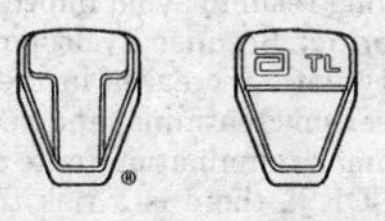

7.5 mg, scored T-TAB® tablets are supplied as peach-colored tablets bearing the Abbott logo, the distinctive T shape and a two-letter Abbo-Code designation, TM:

Bottles of 100 .... (**NDC** 0074-4390-13).
Bottles of 500 .... (**NDC** 0074-4390-53).
ABBO-PAC® unit dose packages:
100 .... (**NDC** 0074-4390-11).

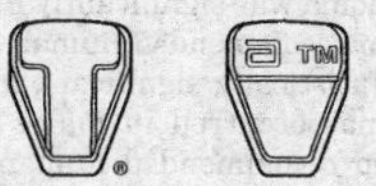

15 mg, scored T-TAB® tablets are supplied as lavender-colored tablets bearing the Abbott logo, the distinctive T shape and a two-letter Abbo-Code designation, TN:

Bottles of 100 .... (**NDC** 0074-4391-13).
Bottles of 500 .... (**NDC** 0074-4391-53).
ABBO-PAC® unit dose packages:
100 .... (**NDC** 0074-4391-11).

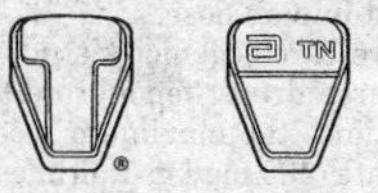

TRANXENE®-SD™ 22.5 mg, single dose tablets are supplied as tan-colored tablets bearing the Abbott logo and a two-letter Abbo-Code designation, TY:

Bottles of 100 .... (**NDC** 0074-2997-13).

TRANXENE®-SD™ HALF STRENGTH 11.25 mg, single dose tablets are supplied as blue-colored tablets bearing the Abbott logo and a two-letter Abbo-Code designation, TX:

Bottles of 100 .... (**NDC** 0074-2699-13).

T-TAB, tablet appearance and shape are trademarks of Abbott Laboratories.

Recommended storage: Store below 77°F (25°C)
U.S. Design Pat. No. D–300,879
Ref. 03-4833-R14

Shown in Product Identification Guide, page 303

Revised: December, 1997

TRICOR™ ℞
[trī cŏr]
(fenofibrate capsules), micronized

DESCRIPTION

TRICOR™ (fenofibrate capsules), micronized, is a lipid regulating agent available as capsules for oral administration. Each capsule contains 67 mg of micronized fenofibrate. Each capsule also contains lactose, NF; pregelatinized starch, NF; sodium lauryl sulfate, NF; crospovidone, NF; and magnesium stearate, NF. The chemical name for fenofibrate is 2-[4-(4-chlorobenzoyl) phenoxy]-2-methyl-propanoic acid, 1-methylethyl ester with the following structural formula:

[See chemical structure at top of next column]

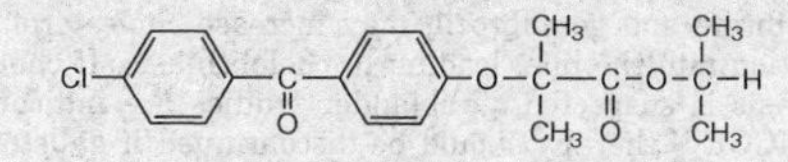

The empirical formula is $C_{20}H_{21}O_4Cl$ and the molecular weight is 360.83; fenofibrate is insoluble in water. The melting point is 79-82°C. Fenofibrate is a white solid which is stable under ordinary conditions.

CLINICAL PHARMACOLOGY

The effects of fenofibrate on serum triglycerides were studied in two randomized, double-blind clinical trials[1]. 147 hypertriglyceridemic patients (Types IV and V) were treated for eight weeks under protocols that differed only in that one entered patients with baseline triglyceride (TG) levels of 500 to 1500 mg/dL, and the other TG levels of 350 to 500 mg/dL. In patients with hypertriglyceridemia and normal cholesterolemia with or without hyperchylomicronemia (Type IV/V hyperlipidemia), treatment with fenofibrate at dosages equivalent to 3 capsules of 67 mg TRICOR™ per day decreased primarily very low density lipoprotein (VLDL) triglycerides and VLDL cholesterol. Treatment of patients with Type IV hyperlipoproteinemia and elevated triglycerides often results in an increase of low density lipoprotein (LDL) cholesterol.

The mechanism of action of TRICOR™ has not been clearly established in man. Fenofibric acid, the active metabolite of fenofibrate, lowers plasma triglycerides apparently by inhibiting triglyceride synthesis, resulting in a reduction of VLDL released into the circulation, and also by stimulating the catabolism of triglyceride-rich lipoprotein (i.e., VLDL). Fenofibrate also reduces serum uric acid levels in hyperuricemic and normal individuals by increasing the urinary excretion of uric acid.

Pharmacokinetics/Metabolism

Clinical experience has been obtained with two different formulations of fenofibrate: a "micronized" and "non-micronized" formulation. Comparisons of blood levels following oral administration of both formulations in healthy volunteers demonstrate that a single capsule containing 67 mg of the "micronized" formulation is bioequivalent to 100 mg of the "non-micronized" formulation.

Absorption

The absolute bioavailability of fenofibrate cannot be determined as the compound is virtually insoluble in aqueous media suitable for injection. However, fenofibrate is well absorbed from the gastrointestinal tract. Following oral administration in healthy volunteers, approximately 60% of a single dose of radiolabelled fenofibrate appeared in urine, primarily as fenofibric acid and its glucuronate conjugate, and 25% was excreted in the feces. Peak plasma levels of fenofibric acid occur within 6 to 8 hours after administration.

The absorption of fenofibrate is increased when administered with food. With micronized fenofibrate, the absorption is increased by approximately 35% under fed as compared to fasting conditions.

Distribution

In healthy volunteers, steady-state plasma levels of fenofibric acid were shown to be achieved within 5 days of dosing with single oral doses equivalent to 67 mg TRICOR™ and did not demonstrate accumulation across time following multiple dose administration. Serum protein binding was approximately 99% in normal and hyperlipidemic subjects.

Metabolism

Following oral administration, fenofibrate is rapidly hydrolyzed by esterases to the active metabolite, fenofibric acid; no unchanged fenofibrate is detected in plasma.

Fenofibric acid is primarily conjugated with glucuronic acid and then excreted in urine. A small amount of fenofibric acid is reduced at the carbonyl moiety to a benzhydrol metabolite which is, in turn, conjugated with glucuronic acid and excreted in urine.

Excretion

After absorption, fenofibrate is mainly excreted in the urine in the form of metabolites, primarily fenofibric acid and fenofibric acid glucuronide. After administration of radiolabelled fenofibrate, approximately 60% of the dose appeared in the urine and 25% was excreted in the feces.

The compound is eliminated with a half-life of 20 hours, allowing once daily administration in a clinical setting.

Special populations

Geriatrics

In elderly volunteers 77 – 87 years of age, the oral clearance of fenofibric acid following a single oral dose of fenofibrate was 1.2 L/h, which compares to 1.1 L/h in young adults. This indicates that a similar dosage regimen can be used in the elderly, without increasing accumulation of the drug or metabolites.

Pediatrics

No data are available. TRICOR™ is not indicated for use in the pediatric population.

Gender

No pharmacokinetic difference between male and female has been observed for fenofibrate.

Race

The influence of race on the pharmacokinetics of fenofibrate has not been studied but, as fenofibrate is not metabolized by enzymes known for exhibiting inter-ethnic variability, inter-ethnic pharmacokinetic differences are very unlikely.

Renal insufficiency

In a study in patients with severe renal impairment (creatinine clearance < 50 mL/min), the rate of clearance of fenofibric acid was greatly reduced, and the compound accumulated during chronic dosage. However, in patients having moderate renal impairment (creatinine clearance of 50 to 90 mL/min), the oral clearance and the oral volume of distribution of fenofibric acid are increased compared to healthy adults (2.1 L/h and 95 L versus 1.1 L/h and 30 L, respectively). Therefore, the dosage of TRICOR™ should be minimized in patients who have severe renal impairment, while no modification of dosage is required in patients having moderate renal impairment.

Hepatic insufficiency

No pharmacokinetic study has been conducted in patients having hepatic insufficiency.

Drug-drug interactions

Potentiation of coumarin-type anticoagulants has been observed with prolongation of the prothrombin time.

Bile acid sequestrants have been shown to bind other drugs given concurrently. Therefore, fenofibrate should be taken at least 1 hour before or 4–6 hours after a bile acid binding resin to avoid impeding its absorption. (See WARNINGS and PRECAUTIONS.)

INDICATIONS AND USAGE

TRICOR™ (fenofibrate capsules), micronized, is indicated as adjunctive therapy to diet for treatment of adult patients with very high elevations of serum triglyceride levels (Types IV and V hyperlipidemia) who are at risk of pancreatitis and who do not respond adequately to a determined dietary effort to control them. Patients who present such risk typically have serum triglycerides over 2000 mg/dL and have elevations of VLDL-cholesterol as well as fasting chylomicrons (Type V hyperlipidemia). Subjects who consistently have total serum or plasma triglycerides below 1000 mg/dL are unlikely to present a risk of pancreatitis. Improving glycemic control in diabetic patients showing fasting chylomicronemia will usually reduce fasting triglycerides and eliminate chylomicronemia thereby obviating the need for pharmacologic intervention. TRICOR™ therapy may be considered for those subjects with triglyceride elevations between 1000 and 2000 mg/dL who have a history of pancreatitis or of recurrent abdominal pain typical of pancreatitis. It is recognized that some Type IV patients with triglycerides under 1000 mg/dL may, through dietary or alcoholic indiscretion, convert to a Type V pattern with massive triglyceride elevations accompanying fasting chylomicronemia, but the influence of TRICOR™ therapy on the risk of pancreatitis in such situations has not been adequately studied. Drug therapy is not indicated for patients with Type I hyperlipoproteinemia, who have elevations of chylomicrons and plasma triglycerides, but who have normal levels of very low density lipoprotein (VLDL). Inspection of plasma refrigerated for 14 hours is helpful in distinguishing Types I, IV and V hyperlipoproteinemia[2].

The initial treatment for dyslipidemia is dietary therapy specific for the type of lipoprotein abnormality. Excess body weight and excess alcoholic intake may be important factors in hypertriglyceridemia and should be addressed prior to any drug therapy. Physical exercise can be an important ancillary measure. Diseases contributory to hyperlipidemia, such as hypothyroidism or diabetes mellitus should be looked for and adequately treated. Estrogen therapy, like thiazide diuretics and beta-blockers, is sometimes associated with massive rises in plasma triglycerides, especially in subjects with familial hypertriglyceridemia. In such cases, discontinuation of the specific etiologic agent may obviate the need for specific drug therapy of hypertriglyceridemia.

The use of drugs should be considered only when reasonable attempts have been made to obtain satisfactory results with non-drug methods. If the decision is made to use drugs, the patient should be instructed that this does not reduce the importance of adhering to diet.

Because the benefit/risk ratio of TRICOR™ has not been established in clinical trials of primary or secondary prevention to reduce the risk of developing coronary heart disease, TRICOR™ is not indicated for such use. (See WARNINGS and PRECAUTIONS.)

CONTRAINDICATIONS

1. Hepatic or severe renal dysfunction, including primary biliary cirrhosis, and patients with unexplained persistent liver function abnormality.
2. Preexisting gallbladder disease (see WARNINGS).
3. Hypersensitivity to fenofibrate.

WARNINGS

1. Because of chemical, pharmacological, and clinical similarities between TRICOR™ (fenofibrate capsules), mi-

Continued on next page

Tricor—Cont.

cronized, Atromid-S (clofibrate), and Lopid (gemfibrozil), the adverse findings in 4 large randomized, placebo-controlled clinical studies with these other fibrate drugs may also apply to TRICOR™. In the first of those studies, the Coronary Drug Project, 1000 subjects with previous myocardial infarction were treated for 5 years with clofibrate. There was no difference in mortality between the clofibrate-treated subjects and 3000 placebo-treated subjects, but twice as many clofibrate-treated subjects developed cholelithiasis and cholecystitis requiring surgery. In a study, conducted by the World Health Organization (WHO), 5000 subjects without known coronary heart disease were treated with clofibrate for 5 years and followed 1 year beyond. There was a statistically significant, 44% higher age-adjusted total mortality in the clofibrate-treated than in a comparable placebo-treated control group during the trial period. The excess mortality was due to a 33% increase in non-cardiovascular causes, including malignancy, post-cholecystectomy complications, and pancreatitis. The higher risk of clofibrate-treated subjects for gallbladder disease was confirmed.

During the 5 year primary prevention component of the Helsinki Heart Study involving 4081 middle-aged males treated with either gemfibrozil or placebo, and the 3.5 year open extension, total mortality was 22% higher in the original gemfibrozil randomization group (p=0.19, 95% confidence interval for relative risk G:P=0.91-1.64). Cancer deaths trended higher in the gemfibrozil group (p=0.11), while cancers (excluding basal cell carcinoma) were diagnosed in 2.5% of patients in both treatment groups. Because of the more limited size of the Helsinki Heart Study, the relative risk of death from any cause did not differ statistically from the relative risk of 1.29 clofibrate/placebo observed at the 9 year follow-up of the WHO study. Similarly, the numerical excess of gallbladder surgeries in the gemfibrozil group (0.9% vs. 0.5% with placebo) did not differ statistically from the excess observed in the clofibrate group compared to placebo in the WHO study.

The secondary prevention component of the Helsinki Heart Study involved 628 middle-aged males excluded from the primary prevention study because of known or suspected coronary heart disease and treated with either gemfibrozil or placebo for 5 years. Cardiac deaths trended higher in the gemfibrozil group (17/311 vs. 8/317 placebo patients, p=0.06, hazard ratio 2.2, 95% confidence interval for hazard ratio = 0.94-5.05). Gallbladder surgery was more frequent in the gemfibrozil group (1.9% vs. 0.3%, p=0.07), as was appendectomy (6 cases on gemfibrozil vs. 0 on placebo, p=0.029).

2. **Liver Function:** Fenofibrate use at doses equivalent to 2 to 3 capsules of 67 mg TRICOR™ per day is associated with significant increases in serum transaminases [AST (SGOT) or ALT (SGPT)]. Increases to > 3 times the upper limit of normal occurred in 6.3% of patients taking fenofibrate at doses equivalent to 2 to 3 capsules of 67 mg TRICOR™ per day in controlled multiple-dose trials lasting 8–24 weeks.

Patients with AST or ALT > 3x the Upper Normal Limits in Controlled Clinical Trials vs Fenofibrate*

	N	# Events	Events Rate
Control	336	4	1.2%
Fenofibrate	442	28	6.3%

*Dosages equivalent to 2 to 3 capsules of 67 mg TRICOR™ per day

When transaminase determinations were followed either after discontinuation of treatment or during continued treatment, a return to normal limits was usually observed. However, the transaminase determinations remained above normal limits in 2 of the 28 patients (7.1%) at the end of follow-up off treatment. Fenofibrate hepatotoxicity appears to be dose-related. In an 8-week dose-ranging study, the incidence of ALT or AST elevations to at least three times the upper limit of normal was 13% in patients receiving dosages equivalent to 2 to 3 capsules of 67 mg TRICOR™ per day and was 0% in those receiving dosages equivalent to one or ½ capsule per day, or placebo. Hepatocellular, chronic active and cholestatic hepatitis associated with fenofibrate therapy have been reported after exposures of weeks to several years. In extremely rare cases, cirrhosis has been reported in association with chronic active hepatitis.

Regular periodic monitoring of liver function, including serum ALT (SGPT) should be performed for the duration of therapy with TRICOR™, and therapy discontinued if enzyme levels persist above three times the normal limit.

3. **Cholelithiasis:** A gallstone prevalence substudy of 450 Helsinki Heart Study participants showed a trend toward a greater prevalence of gallstones during the study within the gemfibrozil treatment group. Fenofibrate, like clofibrate and gemfibrozil, may increase cholesterol excretion into the bile, leading to cholelithiasis. If cholelithiasis is suspected, gallbladder studies are indicated. TRICOR™ therapy should be discontinued if gallstones are found.

4. **Concomitant Oral Anticoagulants:** Caution should be exercised when anticoagulants are given in conjunction with TRICOR™ because of the potentiation of coumarin-type anticoagulants in prolonging the prothrombin time. The dosage of the anticoagulant should be reduced to maintain the prothrombin time at the desired level to prevent bleeding complications. Frequent prothrombin determinations are advisable until it has been definitely determined that the prothrombin level has stabilized.

5. Concomitant therapy with TRICOR™ and HMG-CoA reductase inhibitors (such as lovastatin, pravastatin, and simvastatin). No data exists on this combined therapy. The association of the chemically and pharmacologically related similar compound gemfibrozil and Mevacor® (lovastatin) has been associated with rhabdomyolysis, markedly elevated creatine kinase (CK) levels and myoglobinuria, leading in a high proportion of cases to acute renal failure.

In virtually all patients who have had an unsatisfactory lipid response to either drug alone, any potential lipid benefit of combined therapy with HMG CoA reductase inhibitors and TRICOR™ does not outweigh the risks of severe myopathy, rhabdomyolysis, and acute renal failure. The use of fibrates alone, including TRICOR™, may occasionally be associated with myositis, myopathy, or rhabdomyolysis. Patients receiving TRICOR™ and complaining of muscle pain, tenderness, or weakness should have prompt medical evaluation for myopathy, including serum creatine kinase level determination. If myopathy/myositis is suspected or diagnosed, TRICOR™ therapy should be stopped.

6. The effect of TRICOR™ on coronary heart disease morbidity and mortality and non-cardiovascular mortality has not been established. TRICOR™ should be administered only to those patients described under INDICATIONS AND USAGE. If a significant reduction in fasting chylomicronemia does not occur, TRICOR™ should be discontinued.

PRECAUTIONS

1. **Initial therapy:** Laboratory studies should be done to ascertain that the lipid levels are consistently abnormal before instituting TRICOR™ therapy. Every attempt should be made to control serum lipids with appropriate diet, exercise, weight loss in obese patients, and control of any medical problems such as diabetes mellitus and hypothyroidism that are contributing to the lipid abnormalities. Medications known to exacerbate hypertriglyceridemia (beta-blockers, thiazides, estrogens) should be discontinued or changed if possible prior to consideration of triglyceride-lowering drug therapy.

2. **Continued therapy:** Periodic determination of serum lipids should be obtained during initial therapy in order to establish the lowest effective dose of TRICOR™. Therapy should be withdrawn in patients who do not have an adequate response after two months of treatment with the maximum recommended dose of 3 capsules per day (201 mg).

3. **Pancreatitis** has been reported in patients taking fenofibrate, gemfibrozil, and clofibrate. This occurrence may represent a failure of efficacy or a secondary phenomenon through biliary tract stone or sludge formation and obstruction of the common bile duct.

4. **Hypersensitivity Reactions:** Acute hypersensitivity reactions including severe skin rashes requiring patient hospitalization and treatment with steroids have occurred very rarely during treatment with fenofibrate. Urticaria was seen in 1.25 vs 0%, and rash in 2.82 vs 1.23% of fenofibrate and placebo patients respectively in controlled trials.

5. **Hematologic Changes:** Mild to moderate hemoglobin, hematocrit, and white blood cell decreases have been observed in patients following initiation of fenofibrate therapy. However, these levels stabilize during long-term administration. Extremely rare spontaneous reports of thrombocytopenia and agranulocytosis have been received during post-marketing surveillance outside of the U.S. Periodic blood counts are recommended during the first 12 months of TRICOR™ administration.

6. **Skeletal muscle:** The use of fibrates alone, including TRICOR™ may occasionally be associated with myositis. Treatment with drugs of the fibrate class has been associated on rare occasions with rhabdomyolysis, usually in patients with impaired renal function. Myopathy should be considered in any patient with diffuse myalgias, muscle tenderness or weakness, and/or marked elevations of creatinine phosphokinase levels.

Patients should be advised to report promptly unexplained muscle pain, tenderness or weakness, particularly if accompanied by malaise or fever. CPK levels should be assessed in patients reporting these symptoms, and fenofibrate therapy should be discontinued if markedly elevated CPK levels occur or myopathy is diagnosed.

7. **Drug Interactions:**
(A) **Oral Anticoagulants:** CAUTION SHOULD BE EXERCISED WHEN ANTICOAGULANTS ARE GIVEN IN CONJUNCTION WITH TRICOR™. THE DOSAGE OF THE ANTICOAGULANTS SHOULD BE REDUCED TO MAINTAIN THE PROTHROMBIN TIME AT THE DESIRED LEVEL TO PREVENT BLEEDING COMPLICATIONS. FREQUENT PROTHROMBIN DETERMINATIONS ARE ADVISABLE UNTIL IT HAS BEEN DEFINITELY DETERMINED THAT THE PROTHROMBIN LEVEL HAS STABILIZED.

(B) **HMG-CoA reductase inhibitors:** Rhabdomyolysis has occurred when lovastatin was administered in combined therapy with gemfibrozil, a compound of the fibrate class related to fenofibrate. In most patients who have had an unsatisfactory lipid response to either drug alone, any possible benefit of combined therapy with an HMG-CoA reductase inhibitor and TRICOR™ is not outweighed by the risks of severe myopathy, rhabdomyolysis, and acute renal failure. There is no assurance that periodic monitoring of creatine kinase will prevent the occurrence of severe myopathy and kidney damage.

(C) **Resins:** Since bile acid sequestrants may bind other drugs given concurrently, patients should take TRICOR™ at least 1 hour before or 4–6 hours after a bile acid binding resin to avoid impeding its absorption.

(D) **Cyclosporine:** Because cyclosporine can produce nephrotoxicity with decreases in creatinine clearance and rises in serum creatinine, and because renal excretion is the primary elimination route of fibrate drugs including TRICOR™, there is a risk that an interaction will lead to deterioration. The benefits and risks of using TRICOR™ with immunosuppressants and other potentially nephrotoxic agents should be carefully considered, and the lowest effective dose employed.

8. **Carcinogenesis, Mutagenesis, Impairment of Fertility:** In a 24-month study in rats (10, 45, and 200 mg/kg; 0.3, 1, and 6 times the maximum recommended human dose on the basis of mg/meter² of surface area), the incidence of liver carcinoma was significantly increased at 6 times the maximum recommended human dose in males and females. A statistically significant increase in pancreatic carcinomas occurred in males at 1 and 6 times the maximum recommended human dose; there were also increases in pancreatic adenomas and benign testicular interstitial cell tumors at 6 times the maximum recommended human dose in males. In a second 24-month study in a different strain of rats (doses of 10 and 60 mg/kg; 0.3 and 2 times the maximum recommended human dose based on mg/meter² surface area), there were significant increases in the incidence of pancreatic acinar adenomas in both sexes and increases in interstitial cell tumors of the testes at 2 times the maximum recommended human dose.

A comparative carcinogenicity study was done in rats comparing three drugs: fenofibrate (10 and 70 mg/kg; 0.3 and 1.6 times the maximum recommended human dose), clofibrate (400 mg/kg; 1.6 times the human dose), and gemfibrozil (250 mg/kg; 1.7 times the human dose) (multiples based on mg/meter² surface area). Pancreatic acinar adenomas were increased in males and females on fenofibrate; hepatocellular carcinoma and pancreatic acinar adenomas were increased in males and hepatic neoplastic nodules in females treated with clofibrate; hepatic neoplastic nodules were increased in males and females treated with gemfibrozil while testicular interstitial cell tumors were increased in males on all three drugs.

In a 21-month study in mice at doses of 10, 45, and 200 mg/kg (approximately 0.2, 0.7 and 3 times the maximum recommended human dose on the basis of mg/meter² surface area), there were statistically significant increases in liver carcinoma at 3 times the maximum recommended human dose in both males and females. In a second 18-month study at the same doses, there was a significant increase in liver carcinoma in male mice and liver adenoma in female mice at 3 times the maximum recommended human dose.

Electron microscopy studies have demonstrated peroxisomal proliferation following fenofibrate administration to the rat. An adequate study to test for peroxisome proliferation in humans has not been done, but changes in peroxisome morphology and numbers have been observed in humans after treatment with other members of the fibrate class when liver biopsies were compared before and after treatment in the same individual.

Fenofibrate has been demonstrated to be devoid of mutagenic potential in the following tests: Ames, mouse lymphoma, chromosomal aberration and unscheduled DNA synthesis.

9. **Pregnancy Category C:** Fenofibrate has been shown to be embryocidal and teratogenic in rats when given in doses 7 to 10 times the maximum recommended human

dose and embryocidal in rabbits when given at 9 times the maximum recommended human dose (on the basis of mg/meter² surface area). There are no adequate and well-controlled studies in pregnant women. Fenofibrate should be used during pregnancy only if the potential benefit justifies the potential risk to the fetus.

Administration of 9 times the maximum recommended human dose of fenofibrate to female rats before and throughout gestation caused 100% of dams to delay delivery and resulted in a 60% increase in post-implantation loss, a decrease in litter size, a decrease in birth weight, a 40% survival of pups at birth, a 4% survival of pups as neonates, and a 0% survival of pups to weaning, and an increase in spina bifida.

Administration of 10 times the maximum recommended human dose to female rats on days 6–15 of gestation caused an increase in gross, visceral and skeletal findings in fetuses (domed head/hunched shoulders/rounded body/abnormal chest, kyphosis, stunted fetuses, elongated sternal ribs, malformed sternebrae, extra foramen in palatine, misshapen vertebrae, supernumerary ribs).

Administration of 7 times the maximum recommended human dose to female rats from day 15 of gestation through weaning caused a delay in delivery, a 40% decrease in live births, a 75% decrease in neonatal survival, and decreases in pup weight, at birth as well as on days 4 and 21 post-partum.

Administration of 9 and 18 times the maximum recommended human dose to female rabbits caused abortions in 10% of dams at 9 times and 25% of dams at 18 times the maximum recommended human dose and death of 7% of fetuses at 18 times the maximum recommended human dose.

10. **Nursing mothers:** Fenofibrate should not be used in nursing mothers. Because of the potential for tumorigenicity seen in animal studies, a decision should be made whether to discontinue nursing or to discontinue the drug.

11. **Use in Children:** Safety and efficacy in children have not been established.

ADVERSE REACTIONS

CLINICAL: Adverse events reported by 1% or more of patients treated with fenofibrate during the six month and the eight week double-blind, placebo-controlled trials in the U.S.[1,3] are listed in the table below. Adverse events led to discontinuation of treatment in 6% of patients treated with fenofibrate and in 2% treated with placebo. Skin rashes were the most frequent events, causing discontinuation of fenofibrate treatment in 2% of patients in double-blind trials.

BODY SYSTEM Adverse Event	Fenofibrate* (N=191)	PLACEBO (N=183)
BODY AS A WHOLE		
Asthenia/Fatigue	5%	3%
Infections	18%	15%
Flu Syndrome	5%	2%
Localized/Misc. Pain	8%	7%
Headache	5%	4%
CARDIOVASCULAR		
Arrhythmia	1%	1%
DIGESTIVE		
Dyspepsia	5%	7%
Eructation	1%	0%
Flatulence	3%	2%
Nausea/Vomiting	4%	3%
Abdominal Pain	3%	3%
Constipation	3%	2%
Diarrhea	3%	7%
MUSCULOSKELETAL		
Arthralgia	3%	4%
NERVOUS		
Decreased Libido	2%	1%
Paresthesia	1%	2%
Increased Appetite	1%	1%
Dizziness	2%	1%
Insomnia	1%	1%
RESPIRATORY		
Cough	1%	1%
Rhinitis	4%	3%
Sinusitis	1%	1%
SKIN & APPENDAGES		
Pruritis	3%	1%
Rash	6%	2%
SPECIAL SENSES		
Earache	1%	1%
Eye Floaters	1%	0%
Blurred Vision	1%	1%
Conjunctivitis	1%	2%
Eye Irritation	2%	1%

UROGENITAL

Polyuria	1%	1%
Vaginitis	1%	1%

*Dosage equivalent to 67 mg TRICOR™ t.i.d.

Additional clinical adverse events reported by fewer than 1% of patients in the U.S. double-blind studies, those reported in other clinical trials, and spontaneously reported in post-marketing surveillance outside the U.S. are listed below, categorized by causality.

PROBABLY CAUSALLY RELATED: Digestive: hepatitis, cholelithiasis, cholecystitis, hepatomegaly; Musculoskeletal: myalgia, myasthenia, rhabdomyolysis; Skin and appendages: photosensitivity, eczema; Respiratory: allergic pulmonary alveolitis.

CAUSAL RELATIONSHIP NOT ESTABLISHED: Body as a whole: facial edema, weight decrease, fever, epistaxis; Cardiovascular: peripheral edema, angina, palpitations, tachycardia, migraine; Digestive: hematemesis, pancreatitis; Respiratory: congestion; Nervous: dry mouth, vertigo, anxiety, sleep disorders, confusion; Skin and appendages: lupuslike syndrome, ichthyosis, telangiectasis, alopecia; Special senses: amblyopia, tinnitus; Urogenital: decreased male fertility, renal lithiasis.

LABORATORY: In the two U.S. placebo controlled studies, serum transaminase determinations (SGPT and/or SGOT) were increased to over three times the upper normal limit in 8 to 10% of patients taking fenofibrate at doses equivalent to three capsules of 67 mg TRICOR™ per day. (See WARNINGS). Other changes that occurred more frequently during fenofibrate treatment compared to placebo included increases in creatinine and blood urea, and decreases in hemoglobin and uric acid.

Additional laboratory findings that have been reported during fenofibrate treatment that are probably causally related include: anemia, leukopenia, eosinophilia, thrombocytopenia, and increased creatinine phosphokinase.

OVERDOSAGE

Because fenofibrate is highy bound to plasma proteins, hemodialysis should not be considered. While there has been no reported case of overdosage, symptomatic supportive measures should be taken should it occur.

DOSAGE AND ADMINISTRATION

Patients should be placed on an appropriate triglyceride-lowering diet before receiving TRICOR™, and should continue this diet during treatment with TRICOR™. TRICOR™ should be given with meals, thereby optimizing the bioavailability of the medication. The initial dose is usually 67 mg per day, depending on the physician's assessment of the patient's risk for pancreatitis (see INDICATIONS AND USAGE). Dosage should be individualized according to patient response, and should be increased sequentially if necessary following repeat serum triglyceride estimations at 4 to 8 week intervals. The maximum dose is 3 capsules per day (201 mg).

Treatment with TRICOR™ should be initiated at a dose of 67 mg/day in patients having impaired renal function, and increased only after evaluation of the effects on renal function and triglyceride levels at this dose. In the elderly, the initial dose should likewise be limited to 67 mg/day.

HOW SUPPLIED

TRICOR™ (fenofibrate capsules), micronized, is available as yellow, opaque, hard gelatin capsules. Each capsule contains 67 mg of micronized fenofibrate. Each capsule is printed with the corporate logo ⊇ and the Abbo-Code "FR". TRICOR™ is available in bottles of 90 (NDC 0074-4342-90).

STORAGE

Store at controlled room temperature, 15-30°C (59-86°F). Keep out of the reach of children. Protect from moisture.
Manufactured for Abbott Laboratories, North Chicago, IL 60064, U.S.A.
by Laboratoires Fournier, S.A., 21300 Chenôve, France
Made in France.
CAUTION—Federal law prohibits dispensing without prescription.

REFERENCES

1. GOLDBERG AC, et al. Fenofibrate for the Treatment of Type IV and V Hyperlipoproteinemias: A Double-Blind, Placebo-Controlled Multicenter US Study. *Clinical Therapeutics*, 11, pp. 69-83, 1989.
2. NIKKILA EA. Familial Lipoprotein Lipase Deficiency and Related Disorders of Chylomicron Metabolism. In Stanbury J.B., et al. (eds.): *The Metabolic Basis of Inherited Disease*, 5th edition, McGraw-Hill, 1983, Chap. 30, pp. 622-642.
3. BROWN WV, et al. Effects of Fenofibrate on Plasma Lipids: Double-Blind, Multicenter Study In Patients with Type IIA or IIB Hyperlipidemia. *Arteriosclerosis*. 6, pp. 670-678, 1986.

Revised: February, 1998
Ref.: 03-4844-R1

ABBOTT LABORATORIES 802-030-3280 **MASTER**
NORTH CHICAGO, IL 60064, U.S.A.
Shown in Product Identification Guide, page 303

ZEMPLAR™ ℞
[zĕm 'plăr]
Paricalcitol Injection
Fliptop Vial

DESCRIPTION

Zemplar™ (paricalcitol injection) is a synthetically manufactured vitamin D analog. It is available as a sterile, clear, colorless, aqueous solution for intravenous injection. Each mL contains paricalcitol, 5 mcg; propylene glycol, 30% (v/v); and alcohol, 20% (v/v).

Paricalcitol is a white powder chemically designated as 19-nor-1α,3β,25-trihydroxy-9,10-secoergosta-5(Z),7(E),22(E)-triene and has the following structural formula:

Molecular formula is $C_{27}H_{44}O_3$.
Molecular weight is 416.65.

CLINICAL PHARMACOLOGY

Mechanism of Action

Paricalcitol is a synthetic vitamin D analog. Vitamin D and paricalcitol have been shown to reduce parathyroid hormone (PTH) levels.

Pharmacokinetics

Distribution

The pharmacokinetics of paricalcitol have been studied in patients with chronic renal failure (CRF) requiring hemodialysis. Zemplar™ is administered as an intravenous bolus injection. Within two hours after administering doses ranging from 0.04 to 0.24 mcg/kg, concentrations of paricalcitol decreased rapidly; thereafter, concentrations of paricalcitol declined log-linearly with a mean half-life of about 15 hours. No accumulation of paricalcitol was observed with multiple dosing.

Elimination

In healthy subjects, plasma radioactivity after a single 0.16 mcg/kg intravenous bolus dose of ³H-paricalcitol (n=4) was attributed to parent drug. Paricalcitol was eliminated primarily by hepatobiliary excretion, as 74% of the radioactive dose was recovered in feces and only 16% was found in urine.

Metabolism

Several unknown metabolites were detected in both the urine and feces, with no detectable paricalcitol in the urine. These metabolites have not been characterized and have not been identified. Together, these metabolites contributed 51% of the urinary radioactivity and 59% of the fecal radioactivity. *In vitro* plasma protein binding of paricalcitol was extensive (>99.9%) and nonsaturable over the concentration range of 1 to 100 ng/mL.
[See table at top of next page]

Laboratory Tests

In placebo-controlled studies, paricalcitol reduced serum total alkaline phosphatase levels.

Special Populations

Paricalcitol pharmacokinetics have not been investigated in special populations (geriatric, pediatric, hepatic insufficiency), or for drug-drug interactions. Pharmacokinetics were not gender-dependent.

Clinical Studies

In three 12-week, placebo-controlled, phase 3 studies in chronic renal failure patients on dialysis, the dose of Zemplar™ was started at 0.04 mcg/kg 3 times per week. The dose was increased by 0.04 mcg/kg every 2 weeks until intact parathyroid hormone (iPTH) levels were decreased at least 30% from baseline or a fifth escalation brought the dose to 0.24 mcg/kg, or iPTH fell to less than 100 pg/mL, or the Ca x P product was greater than 75 within any 2 week period, or serum calcium became greater than 11.5 mg/dL at any time.

Patients treated with Zemplar™ achieved a mean iPTH reduction of 30% within 6 weeks. In these studies, there was no significant difference in the incidence of hypercalcemia or hyperphosphatemia between Zemplar™ and placebo-treated patients. The results from these studies are as follows:
[See second table at top of next page]

Continued on next page

Zemplar—Cont.

INDICATIONS AND USAGE

Zemplar™ is indicated for the prevention and treatment of secondary hyperparathyroidism associated with chronic renal failure. Studies in patients with chronic renal failure show that Zemplar™ suppresses PTH levels with no significant difference in the incidence of hypercalcemia or hyperphosphatemia when compared to placebo. However, the serum phosphorus, calcium and calcium x phosphorus product (Ca x P) may increase when Zemplar™ is administered.

CONTRAINDICATIONS

Zemplar™ should not be given to patients with evidence of vitamin D toxicity, hypercalcemia, or hypersensitivity to any ingredient in this product (see **PRECAUTIONS, General**).

WARNINGS

Acute overdose of Zemplar™ may cause hypercalcemia, and require emergency attention. During dose adjustment, serum calcium and phosphorus levels should be monitored closely (e.g., twice weekly). If clinically significant hypercalcemia develops, the dose should be reduced or interrupted. Chronic administration of Zemplar™ may place patients at risk of hypercalcemia, elevated Ca x P product, and metastatic calcification. Signs and symptoms of vitamin D intoxication associated with hypercalcemia include:

Early
Weakness, headache, somnolence, nausea, vomiting, dry mouth, constipation, muscle pain, bone pain, and metallic taste.

Late
Anorexia, weight loss, conjunctivitis (calcific), pancreatitis, photophobia, rhinorrhea, pruritus, hyperthermia, decreased libido, elevated BUN, hypercholesterolemia, elevated AST and ALT, ectopic calcification, hypertension, cardiac arrhythmias, somnolence, death, and, rarely, overt psychosis.

Treatment of patients with clinically significant hypercalcemia consists of immediate dose reduction or interruption of Zemplar™ therapy and includes a low calcium diet, withdrawal of calcium supplements, patient mobilization, attention to fluid and electrolyte imbalances, assessment of electrocardiographic abnormalities (critical in patients receiving digitalis), and hemodialysis or peritoneal dialysis against a calcium-free dialysate, as warranted. Serum calcium levels should be monitored frequently until normocalcemia ensues.

Phosphate or vitamin D-related compounds should not be taken concomitantly with Zemplar™.

PRECAUTIONS

General: Digitalis toxicity is potentiated by hypercalcemia of any cause, so caution should be applied when digitalis compounds are prescribed concomitantly with Zemplar™. Adynamic bone lesions may develop if PTH levels are suppressed to abnormal levels.

Information for the Patient: The patient should be instructed that, to ensure effectiveness of Zemplar™ therapy, it is important to adhere to a dietary regimen of calcium supplementation and phosphorus restriction. Appropriate types of phosphate-binding compounds may be needed to control serum phosphorus levels in patients with chronic renal failure (CRF), but excessive use of aluminum containing compounds should be avoided. Patients should also be carefully informed about the symptoms of elevated calcium.

Essential Laboratory Tests: During the initial phase of medication, serum calcium and phosphorus should be determined frequently (e.g., twice weekly). Once dosage has been established, serum calcium and phosphorus should be measured at least monthly. Measurements of serum or plasma PTH are recommended every 3 months. An intact PTH (iPTH) assay is recommended for reliable detection of biologically active PTH in patients with CRF. During dose adjustment of Zemplar™, laboratory tests may be required more frequently.

Drug Interactions: Specific interaction studies were not performed. Digitalis toxicity is potentiated by hypercalcemia of any cause, so caution should be applied when digitalis compounds are prescribed concomitantly with Zemplar™.

Carcinogenesis, Mutagenesis, Impairment of Fertility: Long-term studies in animals to evaluate the carcinogenic potential of paricalcitol have not been completed. Paricalcitol did not exhibit genetic toxicity *in vitro* with or without metabolic activation in the microbial mutagenesis assay (Ames Assay), mouse lymphoma mutagenesis assay (L5178Y), or a human lymphocyte cell chromosomal aberration assay. There was also no evidence of genetic toxicity in an *in vivo* mouse micronucleus assay. Zemplar™ had no effect on fertility (male or female) in rats at intravenous doses up to 20 mcg/kg/dose [equivalent to 13 times the highest recommended human dose (0.24 mcg/kg) based on surface area, mg/m^2].

Pregnancy: *Pregnancy Category C.* Paricalcitol has been shown to cause minimal decreases in fetal viability (5%)

when administered daily to rabbits at a dose 0.5 times the 0.24 mcg/kg human dose (based on surface area, mg/m^2) and when administered to rats at a dose 2 times the 0.24 mcg/kg human dose (based on plasma levels of exposure). At the highest dose tested (20 mcg/kg 3 times per week in rats, 13 times the 0.24 mcg/kg human dose based on surface area), there was a significant increase of the mortality of newborn rats at doses that were maternally toxic (hypercalcemia). No other effects on offspring development were observed. Paricalcitol was not teratogenic at the doses tested.

There are no adequate and well-controlled studies in pregnant women. Zemplar™ should be used during pregnancy only if the potential benefit justifies the potential risk to the fetus.

Nursing Mothers: It is not known whether paricalcitol is excreted in human milk. Because many drugs are excreted in human milk, caution should be exercised when Zemplar™ is administered to a nursing woman.

Pediatric Use: Safety and efficacy of Zemplar™ in pediatric patients have not been established.

Geriatric Use: Of the 40 patients receiving Zemplar™ in the three phase 3 placebo-controlled CRF studies, 10 patients were 65 years or over. In these studies, no overall differences in efficacy or safety were observed between patients 65 years or older and younger patients.

ADVERSE REACTIONS

Zemplar™ has been evaluated for safety in clinical studies in 270 CRF patients. In four, placebo-controlled, double-blind, multicenter studies, discontinuation of therapy due to any adverse event occurred in 6.5% of patients treated with Zemplar™ (dosage titrated as tolerated, see **CLINICAL PHARMACOLOGY, Clinical Studies**) and 2.0% of 51 patients treated with placebo for one to three months. Adverse events occurring with greater frequency in the Zemplar™ group at a frequency of 2% or greater, regardless of causality, are presented in the following table:
[See third table above]

OVERDOSAGE

Overdosage of Zemplar™ may lead to hypercalcemia (see **WARNINGS**).

DOSAGE AND ADMINISTRATION

The currently accepted target range for iPTH levels in CRF patients is no more than 1.5 to 3 times the non-uremic upper limit of normal.

Paricalcitol Pharmacokinetic Characteristics in CRF Patients (0.24 mcg/kg dose)

Parameter	n	Values (Mean ± SD)
C_{max} (5 min. after bolus)	6	1850 ± 664 (pg/mL)
$AUC_{0-\infty}$	5	27382 ± 8230 (pg•hr/mL)
CL	5	0.72 ± 0.24 (L/hr)
V_{ss}	5	6 ± 2 (L)

	Group (No. of Pts.)	Baseline Mean (Range)	Mean (SE) Change From Baseline to Final Evaluation
PTH (pg/mL)	Zemplar™ (n=40)	783 (291 – 2076)	−379 (43.7)
	placebo (n=38)	745 (320 – 1671)	−69.6 (44.8)
Alkaline Phosphatase (U/L)	Zemplar™ (n=31)	150 (40 – 600)	−41.5 (10.6)
	placebo (n=34)	169 (56 – 911)	+2.6 (10.1)
Calcium (mg/dL)	Zemplar™ (n=40)	9.3 (7.2 – 10.4)	+0.47 (0.1)
	placebo (n=38)	9.1 (7.8 – 10.7)	+0.02 (0.1)
Phosphorus (mg/dL)	Zemplar™ (n=40)	5.8 (3.7 – 10.2)	+0.47 (0.3)
	placebo (n=38)	6.0 (2.8 – 8.8)	−0.47 (0.3)
Calcium x Phosphorus Product	Zemplar™ (n=40)	54 (32 – 106)	+7.9 (2.2)
	placebo (n=38)	54 (26 – 77)	−3.9 (2.3)

Adverse Event Incidence Rates for All Treated Patients In All Placebo-Controlled Studies

Adverse Event	Zemplar™ (n=62) number of events, %	Placebo (n=51) number of events, %
Overall	71	78
Body as a Whole		
Chills	5	0
Feeling unwell	3	0
Fever	5	2
Flu	5	4
Sepsis	5	2
Cardiovascular System		
Palpitation	3	0
Digestive System		
Dry mouth	3	2
Gastrointestinal bleeding	5	2
Nausea	13	8
Vomiting	8	4
Metabolic and Nutritional Disorders		
Edema	7	
Nervous System		
Light-headedness	5	2
Respiratory System		
Pneumonia	5	0

A patient who reported the same medical term more than once was counted only once for that medical term.

List No.	Volume/Container	Concentration	Total Content
1658	1 mL/Fliptop Vial	5 mcg/mL	5 mcg
1658	2 mL/Fliptop Vial	5 mcg/mL	10 mcg

The recommended initial dose of Zemplar™ is 0.04 mcg/kg to 0.1 mcg/kg (2.8–7 mcg) administered as a bolus dose no more frequently than every other day at any time during dialysis. Doses as high as 0.24 mcg/kg (16.8 mcg) have been safely administered.

If a satisfactory response is not observed, the dose may be increased by 2 to 4 mcg at 2- to 4-week intervals. During any dose adjustment period, serum calcium and phosphorus levels should be monitored more frequently, and if an elevated calcium level or a Ca x P product greater than 75 is noted, the drug dosage should be immediately reduced or interrupted until these parameters are normalized. Then, Zemplar™ should be reinitiated at a lower dose. Doses may need to be decreased as the PTH levels decrease in response to therapy. Thus, incremental dosing must be individualized.

The following table is a suggested approach in dose titration:

Suggested Dosing Guidelines	
PTH Level	Zemplar™ Dose
the same or increasing	increase
decreasing by <30%	increase
decreasing by >30%, <60%	maintain
decreasing by >60%	decrease
one and one-half to three times upper limit of normal	maintain

Parenteral drug products should be inspected visually for particulate matter and discoloration prior to administration whenever solution and container permit.
Discard unused portion.

HOW SUPPLIED

Zemplar™ (paricalcitol injection) 5 mcg/mL is supplied as 1 and 2 mL single-dose Fliptop Vials.
[See fourth table on previous page]
Store at 25°C (77°F). Excursions permitted to 15°–30°C (59°–86°F).
Rx only
U.S. patents: 5,246,925; 5,587,497
©Abbott 1998   Reference 06-9998-R1-Rev. April, 1998
ABBOTT LABORATORIES, NORTH CHICAGO, IL 60064, USA

ZYFLO™ FILMTAB®
(zileuton tablets)   Rx

DESCRIPTION

Zileuton is an orally active inhibitor of 5-lipoxygenase, the enzyme that catalyzes the formation of leukotrienes from arachidonic acid. Zileuton has the chemical name (±)-1-(1-Benzo[b]thien-2-ylethyl)-l-hydroxyurea and the following chemical structure:

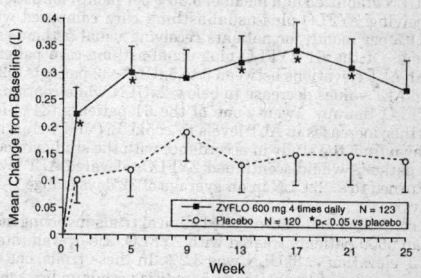

Zileuton has the molecular formula $C_{11}H_{12}N_2O_2S$ and a molecular weight of 236.29. It is a racemic mixture (50:50) of R(+) and S(-) enantiomers. Zileuton is a practically odorless, white, crystalline powder that is soluble in methanol and ethanol, slightly soluble in acetonitrile, and practically insoluble in water and hexane. The melting point ranges from 144.2°C to 145.2°C. ZYFLO tablets for oral administration is supplied in one dosage strength containing 600 mg of zileuton.
Inactive Ingredients: crospovidone, hydroxypropyl cellulose, hydroxypropyl methylcellulose, magnesium stearate, microcrystalline cellulose, pregelatinized starch, propylene glycol, sodium starch glycolate, talc, and titanium dioxide.

CLINICAL PHARMACOLOGY
Mechanism of Action:
Zileuton is a specific inhibitor of 5-lipoxygenase and thus inhibits leukotriene (LTB_4, LTC_4, LTD_4, and LTE_4) formation. Both the R(+) and S(-) enantiomers are pharmacologically active as 5-lipoxygenase inhibitors in in vitro systems. Leukotrienes are substances that induce numerous biological effects including augmentation of neutrophil and eosinophil migration, neutrophil and monocyte aggregation, leukocyte adhesion, increased capillary permeability, and smooth muscle contraction. These effects contribute to in-flammation, edema, mucus secretion, and bronchoconstriction in the airways of asthmatic patients. Sulfido-peptide leukotrienes (LTC_4, LTD_4, LTE_4, also known as the slow-releasing substances of anaphylaxis) and LTB4, a chemoattractant for neutrophils and eosinophils, can be measured in a number of biological fluids including bronchoalveolar lavage fluid (BALF) from asthmatic patients.

Zileuton is an orally active inhibitor of ex vivo LTB_4 formation in several species, including dogs, monkeys, rats, sheep, and rabbits. Zileuton inhibits arachidonic acid-induced ear edema in mice, neutrophil migration in mice in response to polyacrylamide gel, and eosinophil migration into the lungs of antigen-challenged sheep. Zileuton inhibits leukotriene-dependent smooth muscle contractions in vitro in guinea pig and human airways. The compound inhibits leukotriene-dependent bronchospasm in antigen and arachidonic acid-challenged guinea pigs. In antigen-challenged sheep, zileuton inhibits late-phase bronchoconstriction and airway hyperreactivity. In humans, pretreatment with zileuton attenuated bronchoconstriction caused by cold air challenge in patients with asthma.

PHARMACOKINETICS

Zileuton is rapidly absorbed upon oral administration with a mean time to peak plasma concentration (T_{max}) of 1.7 hours and a mean peak level (C_{max}) of 4.98 µg/mL. The absolute bioavailability of ZYFLO is unknown. Systemic exposure (mean AUC) following 600 mg ZYFLO administration is 19.2 µg.hr/mL. Plasma concentrations of zileuton are proportional to dose, and steady-state levels are predictable from single-dose pharmacokinetic data. Administration of ZYFLO with food resulted in a small but statistically significant increase (27%) in zileuton C_{max} without significant changes in the extent of absorption (AUC) or T_{max}. Therefore, ZYFLO can be administered with or without food (see **DOSAGE AND ADMINISTRATION**).

The apparent volume of distribution (V/F) of zileuton is approximately 1.2 L/kg. Zileuton is 93% bound to plasma proteins, primarily to albumin, with minor binding to αl-acid glycoprotein.

Elimination of zileuton is predominantly via metabolism with a mean terminal half-life of 2.5 hours. Apparent oral clearance of zileuton is 7.0 mL/min/kg. ZYFLO activity is primarily due to the parent drug. Studies with radiolabeled drug demonstrated that orally administered zileuton is well absorbed into the systemic circulation with 94.5% and 2.2% of the radiolabeled dose recovered in urine and feces, respectively. Several zileuton metabolites have been identified in human plasma and urine. These include two diastereomeric O-glucuronide conjugates (major metabolites) and an N-dehydroxylated metabolite of zileuton. The urinary excretion of the inactive N-dehydroxylated metabolite and unchanged zileuton each accounted for less than 0.5% of the dose. In vitro studies utilizing human liver microsomes have shown that zileuton and its N-dehydroxylated metabolite can be oxidatively metabolized by the cytochrome P450 isoenzymes 1A2, 2C9 and 3A4 (CYP1A2, CYP2C9 and CYP3A4).

Special populations:

Effect of age: Zileuton pharmacokinetics were similar in healthy elderly subjects (>65 years) compared to healthy younger adults (18 to 40 years).

Effect of gender: Across several studies, no significant gender effects were observed on the pharmacokinetics of zileuton.

Renal insufficiency: The pharmacokinetics of zileuton were similar in healthy subjects and in subjects with mild, moderate, and severe renal insufficiency. In subjects with renal failure requiring hemodialysis, zileuton pharmacokinetics were not altered by hemodialysis and a very small percentage of the administered zileuton dose (<0.5%) was removed by hemodialysis. Hence, dosing adjustment in patients with renal dysfunction or undergoing hemodialysis is not necessary.

Hepatic insufficiency: ZYFLO is contraindicated in patients with active liver disease (see **CONTRAINDICATIONS** and **PRECAUTIONS, Hepatic**).

CLINICAL STUDIES

Two double-blind, parallel, placebo-controlled, multi-center studies have established the efficacy of ZYFLO in the treatment of asthma. Three hundred seventy-three (373) patients were enrolled in the 6-month, double-blind phase of Study 1, and 401 patients were enrolled in the 3-month double-blind phase of Study 2. In these studies, the patients were mild-to-moderate asthmatics who had a mean baseline FEV_1 of approximately 2.3 liters and who used inhaled beta-agonists as needed, the mean being approximately 6 puffs of albuterol per day from a metered-dose inhaler. In each study, patients were randomized to receive either ZYFLO 400 mg four times daily, ZYFLO 600 mg four times daily, or placebo. Only the ZYFLO 600 mg four times daily dosage regimen was shown to be efficacious by demonstrating statistically significant improvement across several parameters.

Efficacy endpoints measured in Study 1 are shown in Table 1 below as mean change from baseline to the end of the study (six months). Statistically significant differences from placebo at the p<0.05 level are indicated by an asterisk(*). Similar results were observed after three months in Study 2.

Table 1
MEAN CHANGE FROM BASELINE TO END OF STUDY
(Six-Month Study)

	ZYFLO 600 mg	
Efficacy Endpoint	4 times/day	Placebo
Trough FEV_1 (L)	0.27	0.14
AM PEFE (L/min)	30.60*	5.04
PM PEFR (L/min)	24.59*	7.98
β-Agonist Use (puffs/day)	-1.77*	-0.22
Daily Symptom Score (0-3 Scale)	-0.49*	-0.28
Nocturnal Symptom Score (0-3 Scale)	-0.29*	-0.04

Figure 1 shows the mean effect of ZYLO versus placebo for the primary efficacy variable, trough FEV_1, over the course of Study 1.

Figure 1
Mean Change From Baseline in Trough FEV_1 (L)

[Graph: Mean Change from Baseline (L) on y-axis (0 to 0.4) vs Week on x-axis (0 to 25). Legend: ZYFLO 600 mg 4 times daily N = 123; Placebo N = 120; *p< 0.05 vs placebo]

Of all the patients in Study 1 and Study 2, 7.0% of those administered ZYFLO 600 mg four times daily required systemic corticosteroid therapy for exacerbation of asthma, whereas 18.7% of the placebo group required corticosteroid treatment. This difference was statistically significant.

In these trials, there was a statistically significant improvement from baseline in FEV_1, which occurred 2 hours after initial administration of ZYFLO. This mean increase was approximately 0.10 L greater than that in placebo-treated patients.

These studies evaluated patients receiving as-needed inhaled beta-agonist as their only asthma therapy. In this patient population, post-hoc analyses suggested that individuals with lower FEV_1 values at baseline showed a greater improvement.

The role of ZYFLO in the management of patients with more severe asthma, patients receiving anti-asthma therapy other than as-needed, inhaled beta-agonists, or patients receiving it as an oral or inhaled corticosteroid-sparing agent remains to be fully characterized.

INDICATIONS AND USAGE

ZYFLO is indicated for the prophylaxis and chronic treatment of asthma in adults and children 12 years of age and older.

CONTRAINDICATIONS

ZYFLO tablets are contraindicated in patients with:
- Active liver disease or transaminase elevations greater than or equal to three times the upper limit of normal (≥3xULN) (see **PRECAUTIONS, Hepatic**).
- Hypersensitivity to zileuton or any of its inactive ingredients.

WARNINGS

ZYFLO is not indicated for use in the reversal of bronchospasm in acute asthma attacks, including status asthmaticus. Therapy with ZYFLO can be continued during acute exacerbations of asthma.

Co-administration of ZYFLO and theophylline results in, on average, an approximate doubling of serum theophylline concentrations. Theophylline dosage in these patients should be reduced and serum theophylline concentrations monitored closely (see **PRECAUTIONS, Drug Interactions**).

Co-administration of ZYFLO and warfarin results in a clinically significant increase in prothrombin time (PT). Patients on oral warfarin therapy and ZYFLO should have their prothrombin times monitored closely and anticoagulant dose adjusted accordingly (see **PRECAUTIONS, Drug Interactions**).

Continued on next page

Zyflo—Cont.

Co-administration of ZYFLO and propranolol results in doubling of propranolol AUC and consequent increased beta-blocker activity. Patients on ZYFLO and propranolol should be closely monitored and the dose of the propranolol reduced as necessary (see **PRECAUTIONS**, **Drug Interactions**).

PRECAUTIONS

Hepatic: Elevations of one or more liver function tests may occur during ZYFLO therapy. These laboratory abnormalities may progress, remain unchanged, or resolve with continued therapy. In a few cases, initial transaminase elevations were first noted after discontinuing treatment, usually within 2 weeks. The ALT (SGPT) test is considered the most sensitive indicator of liver injury. In placebo-controlled clinical trials, the frequency of ALT elevations greater than or equal to three times the upper limit of normal (3xULN) was 1.9% for ZYFLO-treated patients, compared with 0.2% for placebo-treated patients.

In a long-term safety surveillance study, 2458 patients received ZYFLO in addition to their usual asthma care and 489 received their usual asthma care. In patients treated for up to 12 months with ZYFLO in addition to their usual asthma care, 4.6% developed an ALT of at least 3xULN, compared with 1.1% of patients receiving only their usual asthma care. Sixty-one percent of these elevations occurred during the first two months of ZYFLO therapy. After two months of treatment, the rate of new ALT elevations ≥ 3xULN stabilized at a mean of 0.30% per month for patients receiving ZYFLO-plus-usual-asthma care compared with 0.11% per month for patients receiving usual asthma care alone. Of the 61 ZYFLO-plus-usual-asthma-care patients with ALT elevations between 3 to 5xULN, 32 patients (52%) had ALT values decrease to below 2xULN while continuing ZYFLO therapy. Twenty-one of the 61 patients (34%) had further increases in ALT levels to ≥ 5xULN and were withdrawn from the study in accordance with the study protocol. In patients who discontinued ZYFLO, elevated ALT levels returned to < 2xULN in an average of 32 days (range 1–111 days).

In controlled and uncontrolled clinical trials involving more than 5000 patients treated with ZYFLO, the overall rate of ALT elevation ≥ 3xULN was 3.2%. In these trials, one patient developed symptomatic hepatitis with jaundice, which resolved upon discontinuation of therapy. An additional 3 patients with transaminase elevations developed mild hyperbilirubinemia that was less than three times the upper limit of normal. There was no evidence of hypersensitivity or other alternative etiologies for these findings. In subset analyses, females over the age of 65 appeared to be at an increased risk for ALT elevations. Patients with pre-existing transaminase elevations may also be at an increased risk for ALT elevations (see **CONTRAINDICATIONS**).

It is recommended that hepatic transaminases be evaluated at initiation of, and during therapy with, ZYFLO. Serum ALT should be monitored before treatment begins, once-a-month for the first 3 months, every two to three months for the remainder of the first year, and periodically thereafter for patients receiving long-term ZYFLO therapy. If clinical signs and/or symptoms of liver dysfunction (e.g., right upper quadrant pain, nausea, fatigue, lethargy, pruritus, jaundice, or "flu-like" symptoms) develop or transaminase elevations greater than 5 times the ULN occur, ZYFLO should be discontinued and transaminase levels followed until normal.

Since treatment with ZYFLO may result in increased hepatic transaminases, ZYFLO should be used with caution in patients who consume substantial quantities of alcohol and/or have a past history of liver disease.

Information for Patients: Patients should be told that:

- ZYFLO is indicated for the chronic treatment of asthma and should be taken regularly as prescribed, even during symptom-free periods.
- ZYFLO is not a bronchodilator and should not be used to treat acute episodes of asthma.
- When taking ZYFLO, they should not decrease the dose or stop taking any other antiasthma medications unless instructed by a physician.
- While using ZYFLO, medical attention should be sought if short-acting bronchodilators are needed more often than usual, or if more than the maximum number of inhalations of short-acting bronchodilator treatment prescribed for a 24-hour period are needed.
- The most serious side effect of ZYFLO is elevation of liver enzyme tests and that, while taking ZYFLO, they must return for liver enzyme test monitoring on a regular basis.
- If they experience signs and/or symptoms of liver dysfunction (e.g., right upper quadrant pain, nausea, fatigue, lethargy, pruritus, jaundice, or "flu-like" symptoms), they should contact their physician immediately.
- ZYFLO can interact with other drugs and that, while taking ZYFLO, they should consult their doctor before starting or stopping any prescription or non-prescription medicines.

A patient leaflet is included as part of this labeling.

Drug Interactions: In a drug-interaction study in 16 healthy volunteers, co-administration of multiple doses of zileuton (800 mg every 12 hours) and theophylline (200 mg every 6 hours) for 5 days resulted in a significant decrease (approximately 50%) in steady-state clearance of theophylline, an approximate doubling of theophylline AUC, and an increase in theophylline C_{max} (by 73%). The elimination half-life of theophylline was increased by 24%. Also, during co-administration, theophylline-related adverse events were observed more frequently than after theophylline alone. Upon initiation of ZYFLO in patients receiving theophylline, the theophylline dosage should be reduced by approximately one-half and plasma theophylline concentrations monitored. Similarly, when initiating therapy with theophylline in a patient receiving ZYFLO, the maintenance dose and/or dosing interval of theophylline should be adjusted accordingly and guided by serum theophylline determinations (see **WARNINGS**).

Concomitant administration of multiple doses of ZYFLO (600 mg every 6 hours) and warfarin (fixed daily dose obtained by titration in each subject) to 30 healthy male volunteers resulted in a 15% decrease in R-warfarin clearance and an increase in AUC of 22%. The pharmacokinetics of S-warfarin were not affected. These pharmacokinetic changes were accompanied by a clinically significant increase in prothrombin times. Monitoring of prothrombin time, or other suitable coagulation tests, with the appropriate dose titration of warfarin is recommended in patients receiving concomitant ZYFLO and warfarin therapy (see **WARNINGS**).

Co-administration of ZYFLO and propranolol results in a significant increase in propranolol concentrations. Administration of a single 80-mg dose of propranolol in 16 healthy male volunteers who received ZYFLO 600 mg every 6 hours for 5 days resulted in a 42% decrease in propranolol clearance. This resulted in an increase in propranolol C_{max}, AUC, and elimination half-life by 52%, 104%, and 25%, respectively. There was an increase in β-blockade and decrease in heart rate associated with the co-administration of these drugs. Patients on ZYFLO and propranolol should be closely monitored and the dose of propranolol reduced as necessary (see **WARNINGS**). No formal drug-drug interaction studies between ZYFLO and other beta-adrenergic blocking agents (i.e., β-blockers) have been conducted. It is reasonable to employ appropriate clinical monitoring when these drugs are co-administered with ZYFLO.

In a drug interaction study in 16 healthy volunteers, co-administration of multiple doses of terfenadine (60 mg every 12 hours) and ZYFLO (600 mg every 6 hours) for 7 days resulted in a decrease in clearance of terfenadine by 22% leading to a statistically significant increase in mean AUC and C_{max} of terfenadine of approximately 35%. This increase in terfenadine plasma concentration in the presence of ZYFLO was not associated with a significant prolongation of the QTc interval. Although there was no cardiac effect in this small number of healthy volunteers, given the high inter-individual pharmacokinetic variability of terfenadine, co-administration of ZYFLO and terfenadine is not recommended.

Drug-drug interaction studies conducted in healthy volunteers between ZYFLO and prednisone and ethinyl estradiol (oral contraceptive), drugs known to be metabolized by the P450 3A4 (CYP3A4) isoenzyme, have shown no significant interaction. However, no formal drug-drug interaction studies between ZYFLO and dihydropyridine, calcium channel blockers, cyclosporine, cisapride, and astemizole, also metabolized by CYP3A4, have been conducted. It is reasonable to employ appropriate clinical monitoring when these drugs are co-administered with ZYFLO.

Drug-drug interaction studies in healthy volunteers have been conducted with ZYFLO and digoxin, phenytoin, sulfasalazine, and naproxen. There was no significant interaction between ZYFLO and any of these drugs.

Carcinogenesis, Mutagenesis, Impairment of Fertility: In 2-year carcinogenicity studies, increases in the incidence of liver, kidney, and vascular tumors in female mice and a trend towards an increase in the incidence of liver tumors in male mice were observed at 450 mg/kg/day (providing approximately 4 times [females] or 7 times [males] the systemic exposure [AUC] achieved at the maximum recommended human daily oral dose). No increase in the incidence of tumors was observed at 150 mg/kg/day (providing approximately 2 times the systemic exposure [AUC] achieved at the maximum recommended human daily oral dose). In rats, an increase in the incidence of kidney tumors was observed in both sexes at 170 mg/kg/day (providing approximately 6 times [males] or 14 times [females] the systemic exposure [AUC] achieved at the maximum recommended human daily oral dose). No increased incidence of kidney tumors was seen at 80 mg/kg/day (providing approximately 4 times [males] or 6 times [females] the systemic exposure [AUC] achieved at the maximum recommended human daily oral dose). Although a dose-related increased incidence of benign Leydig cell tumors was observed, Leydig cell tumorigenesis was prevented by supplementing male rats with testosterone.

Zileuton was negative in genotoxicity studies including bacterial reverse mutation (Ames) using *S. typhimurium* and *E. coli*, chromosome aberration in human lymphocytes, *in vitro* unscheduled DNA synthesis (UDS), in rat hepatocytes with or without zileuton pretreatment and in mouse and rat kidney cells with zileuton pretreatment, and mouse micronucleus assays. However, a dose-related increase in DNA adduct formation was reported in kidneys and livers of female mice treated with zileuton. Although some evidence of DNA damage was observed in a UDS assay in hepatocytes isolated from Aroclor-1254 treated rats, no such finding was noticed in hepatocytes isolated from monkeys, where the metabolic profile of zileuton is more similar to that of humans.

In reproductive performance/fertility studies, zileuton produced no effects on fertility in rats at oral doses up to 300 mg/kg/day (providing approximately 8 times [male rats] and 18 times [female rats] the systemic exposure [AUC] achieved at the maximum recommended human daily oral dose). Comparative systemic exposure (AUC) is based on measurements in male rats or nonpregnant female rats at similar dosages. However, reduction in fetal implants was observed at oral doses of 150 mg/kg/day and higher (providing approximately 9 times the systemic exposure [AUC] achieved at the maximum recommended human daily oral dose). Increases in gestation length, prolongation of estrous cycle, and increases in stillbirths were observed at oral doses of 70 mg/kg/day and higher (providing approximately 4 times the systemic exposure (AUC) achieved at the maximum recommended human daily oral dose). In a perinatal/postnatal study in rats, reduced pup survival and growth were noted at an oral dose of 300 mg/kg/day (providing approximately 18 times the systemic exposure [AUC] achieved at the maximum recommended human daily oral dose).

Pregnancy: Pregnancy Category C: Developmental studies indicated adverse effects (reduced body weight and increased skeletal variations) in rats at an oral dose of 300 mg/kg/day (providing approximately 18 times the systemic exposure [AUC] achieved at the maximum recommended human daily oral dose). Comparative systemic exposure [AUC] is based on measurements in nonpregnant female rats at a similar dosage. Zileuton and/or its metabolites cross the placental barrier of rats. Three of 118 (2.5%) rabbit fetuses had cleft palates at an oral dose of 150 mg/kg/day (equivalent to the maximum recommended human daily oral dose on a mg/m² basis). There are no adequate and well-controlled studies in pregnant women. ZYFLO should be used during pregnancy only if the potential benefit justifies the potential risk to the fetus.

Nursing Mothers: Zileuton and/or its metabolites are excreted in rat milk. It is not known if zileuton is excreted in human milk. Because many drugs are excreted in human milk, and because of the potential for tumorigenicity shown for ZYFLO in animal studies, a decision should be made whether to discontinue nursing or to discontinue the drug, taking into account the importance of the drug to the mother.

Pediatric Use: The safety and effectiveness of ZYFLO in pediatric patients under 12 years of age have not been established.

ADVERSE REACTIONS

Clinical Studies: A total of 5542 patients have been exposed to zileuton in clinical trials, 2252 of them for greater than 6 months and 742 for greater than 1 year.

Adverse events most frequently occurring (frequency ≥3%) in ZYFLO-treated patients and at a frequency greater than placebo-treated patients are summarized in Table 2.

TABLE 2
Proportion of Patients Experiencing Adverse Events in Placebo-Controlled Studies in Asthma

BODY SYSTEM/Event	ZYFLO 600 mg 4 times daily % Occurrence (N=475)	Placebo % Occurrence (N=491)
BODY AS A WHOLE		
Headache	24.6	24.0
Pain (unspecified)	7.8	5.3
Abdominal Pain	4.6	2.4
Asthenia	3.8	2.4
Accidental Injury	3.4	2.0
DIGESTIVE SYSTEM		
Dyspepsia	8.2*	2.9
Nausea	5.5	3.7
MUSCULOSKELETAL		
Myalgia	3.2	2.9

* p ≤ 0.05 vs placebo

Less common adverse events occurring at a frequency of greater than 1% and more commonly in ZYFLO-treated patients included: arthralgia, chest pain, conjunctivitis, constipation, dizziness, fever, flatulence, hypertonia, insomnia, lymphadenopathy, malaise, neck pain/rigidity, nervousness, pruritus, somnolence, urinary tract infection, vaginitis, and vomiting.

The frequency of discontinuation from the asthma clinical studies due to any adverse event was comparable between ZYFLO (9.7%) and placebo-treated (8.4%) groups.

In placebo-controlled clinical trials, the frequency of ALT elevations ≥3xULN was 1.9% for ZYFLO-treated patients, compared with 0.2% for placebo-treated patients. In controlled and uncontrolled trials, one patient developed symptomatic hepatitis with jaundice, which resolved upon discontinuation of therapy. An additional 3 patients with transaminase elevations developed mild hyperbilirubinemia that was less than three times the upper limit of normal. There was no evidence of hypersensitivity or other alternative etiologies for these findings. ZYFLO is contraindicated in patients with active liver disease or transaminase elevations greater than or equal to 3xULN (see **CONTRA-INDICATIONS**). It is recommended that hepatic transaminases be evaluated at initiation of and during therapy with ZYFLO (see **PRECAUTIONS**, **Hepatic**).
Occurrences of low white blood cell count (≤ 2.8 x 10^9/L) were observed in 1.0% of 1,678 patients taking ZYFLO and 0.6% of 1,056 patients taking placebo in placebo-controlled studies. These findings were transient and the majority of cases returned toward normal or baseline with continued ZYFLO dosing. All remaining cases returned toward normal or baseline after discontinuation of ZYFLO. Similar findings were also noted in a long-term safety surveillance study of 2458 patients treated with ZYFLO plus usual asthma care versus 489 patients treated only with usual asthma care for up to one year. The clinical significance of these observations is not known.
In the long-term safety surveillance trial of ZYFLO plus usual asthma care versus usual asthma care alone, a similar adverse event profile was seen as in other clinical trials.

OVERDOSAGE

Human experience of acute overdose with zileuton is limited. A patient in a clinical trial took between 6.6 and 9.0 grams of zileuton in a single dose. Vomiting was induced and the patient recovered without sequelae. Zileuton is not removed by dialysis. Should an overdose occur, the patient should be treated symptomatically and supportive measures instituted as required. If indicated, elimination of unabsorbed drug should be achieved by emesis or gastric lavage; usual precautions should be observed to maintain the airway. A Certified Poison Control Center should be consulted for up-to-date information on management of overdose with ZYFLO.
The oral minimum lethal doses in mice and rats were 500-4000 and 300-1000 mg/kg in various preparations, respectively (providing greater than 3 and 9 times the systemic exposure [AUC] achieved at the maximum recommended human daily oral dose, respectively). No deaths occurred, but nephritis was reported in dogs at an oral dose of 1000 mg/kg (providing in excess of 12 times the systemic exposure [AUC] achieved at the maximum recommended human daily oral dose).

DOSAGE AND ADMINISTRATION

The recommended dosage of ZYFLO for the symptomatic treatment of patients with asthma is one 600-mg tablet four times a day for a total daily dose of 2400 mg. For ease of administration, ZYFLO may be taken with meals and at bedtime. Hepatic transaminases should be evaluated prior to initiation of ZYFLO and periodically during treatment (see **PRECAUTIONS**, **Hepatic**).

HOW SUPPLIED

ZYFLO Filmtab Tablets are available as 1 dosage strength: 600-mg white ovaloid tablets with single bisect, debossed on bisect side with Abbott logo and ZL (Abbo-Code), and 600 on the opposite side:
High-density polyethylene
bottles of 120 .... (**NDC** 0074-8036-22)
Recommended storage: Store tablets at controlled room temperature between 20°-25°C, (68°-77°F). See USP. Protect from light.
TM - Trademark
Filmtab - Film-sealed tablets, Abbott
Revised January, 1997
Ref. 03-4743-R2-Rev. January, 1997
ABBOTT LABORATORIES
NORTH CHICAGO, IL 60064, U.S.A
Shown in Product Identification Guide, page 303

Medication Guide
Zyflo™ Filmtab® Tablets
Generic Name: zileuton

Please read this leaflet carefully before you start taking Zyflo™ Filmtab® tablets. Also, read it each time you get your Zyflo prescription refilled.
This leaflet provides important information about taking Zyflo. It is not meant to take the place of your doctor's specific instructions. Talk to your doctor if you have any questions about Zyflo. Your doctor or pharmacist can also provide you with additional information about Zyflo.

What is the most important information I should know about Zyflo?
The most important things to remember are to take all your doses of Zyflo every day and to make sure that you return to your doctor's office for scheduled liver enzyme tests.
You should also know that you should seek medical help immediately if you need more "puffs" of your bronchodilator inhaler than normal or if you use the maximum number of "puffs" prescribed for one 24-hour period. These could be a sign of worsening asthma which means that your asthma therapy may need to be changed.

What is Zyflo?
Zyflo, which contains the active ingredient zileuton, blocks the formation of certain chemicals (leukotrienes) that may contribute to your asthma symptoms.

Who should not take Zyflo?
You should not take Zyflo if you:
- have active liver disease or have liver enzymes that are elevated.
- have ever had an allergic reaction to this medicine.

Your doctor will determine if it is safe for you to take Zyflo.

What should I tell my doctor before I take the first dose of Zyflo?
You should tell your doctor if you:
- have ever had liver disease, hepatitis, jaundice (yellow eyes or skin), or dark urine.
- drink alcohol.
- are taking any prescription or nonprescription medicines. Your doctor may adjust the doses of some of your other medicines while you are taking Zyflo.
- if you are taking theophylline for your asthma, the blood-thinning medication warfarin, or the blood-pressure medication propranolol. Your doctor may need to change the doses of these drugs.
- are pregnant, planning to become pregnant, or are breast-feeding.

How should I take Zyflo?
- Zyflo is taken four times a day with or without food. It may be easier to remember to take Zyflo if you make it part of your daily routine such as with meals and at bedtime.
- For Zyflo to help control your asthma symptoms, it must be taken every day as prescribed by your doctor. Zyflo WILL NOT relieve an asthma attack that has already started. While taking Zyflo, it is important to keep taking your other asthma medicines as directed and to follow all of your doctor's instructions.
- Even if you have no asthma symptoms, do not decrease the dose of Zyflo or stop taking the medicine without talking to your doctor first. Feeling good is a sign that the medicine is working.
- When you take your dose of Zyflo, the tablets may be swallowed whole or split in half to make them easier to swallow.

What should I avoid while taking Zyflo?
- Because Zyflo may affect how other medications work, always talk to your doctor before you start or stop taking any medicines while taking Zyflo. This includes all prescription and nonprescription medicines.
- Never take a larger dose of Zyflo or take it more often than your doctor has prescribed.
- It is also important for you to know that it may take several days or a few weeks to get the full benefit from Zyflo and that you should not stop taking it if you do not feel better right away.

What are the possible side effects of Zyflo?
All medicines, including Zyflo, cause side effects in some people. Some of the most common side effects are abdominal pain, upset stomach, and nausea. You should tell your doctor if you experience any new or unusual symptoms while taking Zyflo.
One side effect that occurs in a small number of patients is an increased release of substances from the liver called "enzymes." Liver enzymes can be measured by a simple blood test. It is important that your doctor makes sure that your liver enzymes do not become too high and that it is safe for you to continue taking Zyflo. To insure your safety, your doctor will do this blood test before you first start taking Zyflo and repeat it on a regular basis while you are taking the medicine.
Usually, even if your liver enzymes are increased, you will not notice any symptoms. However, some symptoms of increased liver enzymes are feeling more tired than normal, "flu-like" symptoms, itching, yellow skin and/or yellow color in the whites of the eyes, or urine that is darker than normal.
If you notice these or any other symptoms that you think may be caused by Zyflo, call your doctor immediately. Once the medicine is stopped, these symptoms usually go away.
Even if you do not have any of these symptoms, you should continue to see your doctor for regular check-ups and liver enzyme tests.

Where should I keep my supply of Zyflo?
Keep Zyflo and all medicines out of the reach of children. In case of an accidental overdose, call your doctor or a Poison Control Center immediately.
Protect Zyflo from light and replace the child-resistant cap each time after use. Store Zyflo between 68° – 77°F (20° – 25°C).
If you would like more information about Zyflo, ask your doctor or pharmacist. If you have any questions or concerns about taking Zyflo, discuss them with your doctor.
Filmtab - Film-sealed tablets, Abbott
TM - Trademark
Revised December, 1996
Ref. 03-4700-R1-Rev. December, 1996
ABBOTT LABORATORIES
NORTH CHICAGO, IL 60064, U.S.A.

Advanced Nutritional Technology®, Inc.

6988 SIERRA CT.
DUBLIN, CA 94568

Direct Inquiries to:
(925) 828–2128
FAX: (925) 828–6848

NUTR-E-SOL® OTC

(Water Soluble Natural Vitamin E For Maximum Absorption)

FORMULATIONS

400 I.U. Natural Vitamin E per tablespoon

PHYSIOLOGICAL CONSIDERATIONS

Advanced Nutritional Technology's Nutr-E-Sol is a high potency water soluble natural vitamin E designed for fast absorption.
Nutr-E-Sol contains a unique form of vitamin E (d-α-tocopheryl polyethylene glycol 1000 succinate or TPGS) that is absorbed directly through the intestinal wall without the use of bile for emulsification. Nutr-E-Sol is useful in raising vitamin E blood levels in diseases such as Cystic Fibrosis, Crohn's Disease, Short Bowel Syndrome, Biliary Cirrhosis and Cholestasis, where vitamin E blood levels are low.
Nutr-E-Sol may be taken alone or mixed with drinks. This product is tasteless and sugar-free for better compliance with the young and diabetic.
Studies indicate that Nutr-E-Sol's form of Vitamin E is absorbed better than other water-soluble vitamin E supplements, dry vitamin E supplements and emulsified forms of vitamin E.

DOSAGE

Liquid—One to three tablespoons per day.

HOW SUPPLIED

	SIZE	NDC #
Nutr-E-Sol®	8 oz.	62617-515-10
	16 oz.	62617-515-20

SUPER EPA® OTC

(Eicosapentaenoic Acid and Docosahexaenoic Acid)

FORMULATION

Each softgel contains the following omega-3 fatty acid potency.
SuperEPA 2000
1000 mg
SuperEPA 1200
720 mg
SuperEPA 1000
350 mg
All strengths are cholesterol free! No Vitamin A & D or sodium are added and each product is free of toxic metals.

PHYSIOLOGICAL CONSIDERATIONS

Advanced Nutritional Technology introduces the latest development in omega-3 fatty acid therapy. All of our highly concentrated fish oils are now in their natural triglyceride form. Compared with the commonly used ethyl ester form, the natural triglyceride form is better absorbed by the body. Moreover, natural triglyceride is more stable than the free fatty acid form occasionally used—guaranteeing a product that is not rancid with peroxides.
Taken for its cardiovascular benefits, SuperEPA fish oil concentrate in its natural triglyceride form provides more omega-3 fatty acids per milligram of fish body oil in each capsule than our previous formula. Available in three strengths, you can choose the potency that best meets your dietary needs.
SuperEPA 2000 contains the highest concentration of triglyceride fish oil concentrate at 1,250 mg, providing 80% pure omega-3 fatty acids (or 1000 mg) in one capsule. At a

Continued on next page

Super EPA—Cont.

dosage of only one or two capsules daily, this strength is the most convenient and promotes better compliance with users.

DOSAGE
SuperEPA 2000
One to two softgels daily, taken with meals.
SuperEPA 1200
One to three softgels daily, taken with meals.
SuperEPA 1000
One to six softgels daily, taken with meals

HOW SUPPLIED

	SIZE	NDC #
SuperEPA® 2000	90's	62617-050-03
SuperEPA® 1200	90's	62617-045-03
SuperEPA® 1000	90's	62617-040-03

Agouron Pharmaceuticals, Inc.
**10350 NORTH TORREY PINES ROAD
LA JOLLA, CA 92037-1020**

Direct Inquiries to:
Customer Communications
(888) VIRACEPT
FAX: (619) 678-8266
Medical Emergency Contact:
Medical Affairs
(888) VIRACEPT
FAX: (619) 678-8245

VIRACEPT® ℞
[vī 'ră-cĕpt]
nelfinavir mesylate
TABLETS AND ORAL POWDER

VIRACEPT is indicated for the treatment of HIV infection when antiretroviral therapy is warranted. This indication is based on surrogate marker changes in patients who received VIRACEPT in combination with nucleoside analogues or alone for up to 24 weeks. At present, there are no results from controlled trials evaluating the effect of therapy with VIRACEPT on clinical progression of HIV infection, such as survival or the incidence of opportunistic infections.

DESCRIPTION
VIRACEPT® (nelfinavir mesylate) is an inhibitor of the human immunodeficiency virus (HIV) protease. VIRACEPT Tablets are available for oral administration as a light blue, capsule-shaped tablet in a 250 mg strength (as nelfinavir free base). Each tablet also contains the following inactive ingredients: calcium silicate, crospovidon, magnesium stearate, and FD&C blue #2 powder. VIRACEPT Oral Powder is available for oral administration in a 50 mg/g strength (as nelfinavir free base) in bottles. The oral powder also contains the following inactive ingredients: microcrystalline cellulose, maltodextrin, dibasic potassium phosphate, crospovidone, hydroxypropyl methylcellulose, aspartame, sucrose palmitate, and natural and artificial flavor. The chemical name for nelfinavir mesylate is [3S-[2(2S*, 3S*), 3α,4aβ,8aβ]]-N-(1,1-dimethylethyl)decahydro-2-[2-hydroxy-3-[(3-hydroxy-2-methylbenzoyl)amino]-4-(phenylthio)butyl]-3-isoquinolinecarboxamide mono-methanesulfonate (salt) and the molecular weight is 663.90 (567.79 as the free base). Nelfinavir mesylate has the following structural formula:

Nelfinavir mesylate is a white to off-white amorphous powder, slightly soluble in water at pH ≤4 and freely soluble in methanol, ethanol, isopropanol and propylene glycol.

MICROBIOLOGY
Mechanism of Action: Nelfinavir is an inhibitor of the HIV-1 protease. Inhibition of the viral protease prevents cleavage of the gag-pol polyprotein resulting in the production of immature, non-infectious virus.
Antiviral Activity In Vitro: The antiviral activity of nelfinavir *in vitro* has been demonstrated in both acute and/or

Table 1
Effect of Nelfinavir on Coadministered Drug Plasma AUC and C$_{max}$

Coadministered Drug	Nelfinavir Dose	N	Coadministered Drug	
			AUC (95%CI)	C$_{max}$ (95%CI)
Lamivudine 150 mg Single Dose	750 mg q8h × 7–10 days	11	↑10% (1–20%)	↑31% (5–62%)
Stavudine 30–40 mg bid × 56 days	750 mg tid × 56 days	8	↔	↔
Zidovudine 200 mg Single Dose	750 mg q8h × 7–10 days	11	↓35% (28–41%)	↓31% (8–49%)
Indinavir 800 mg Single Dose	750 mg q8h × 7 days	6	↑51% (25–83%)	↔
Ritonavir 500 mg Single Dose	750 mg q8h × 5 doses	10	↔	↔
Saquinavir 1200 mg Single Dose*	750 mg tid × 4 days	14	↑392% (271–553%)	↑179% (105–280%)
Ethinyl estradiol 35 μg qd × 15 days	750 mg q8h × 7 days	12	↓47% (41–63%)	↓28% (14–39%)
Norethindrone 0.4 mg qd × 15 days	750 mg q8h × 7 days	12	↓18% (12–27%)	↔
Rifabutin 300 mg qd × 8 days	750 mg q8h × 7–8 days	10	↑207% (151–276%)	↑146% (112–186%)
Terfenadine 60 mg Single Dose	750 mg q8h × 7 days	12	Terfenadine plasma concentrations were transiently measurable when coadministered with VIRACEPT**	

↑ Indicates increase
↓ Indicates decrease
↔Indicates no change
* Using an experimental (soft-gelatin capsule) formulation of saquinavir 1200 mg
**Terfenadine and VIRACEPT should not be coadministered (see WARNINGS)

Table 2
Effect of Coadministered Drug on Nelfinavir Plasma AUC and C$_{max}$

Coadministered Drug	Nelfinavir Dose	N	Nelfinavir	
			AUC (95%CI)	C$_{max}$ (95%CI)
Didanosine 200 mg Single Dose	750 mg Single Dose	9	↔	↔
Zidovudine 200 mg + Lamivudine 150 mg Single Dose	750 mg q8h × 7–10 days	11	↔	↔
Indinavir 800 mg q8h × 7 days	750 mg Single Dose	6	↑83% (34–150%)	↑31% (13–52%)
Ritonavir 500 mg q8h × 3 doses	750 mg Single Dose	10	↑152% (86–242%)	↑44% (25–67%)
Saquinavir 1200 mg tid × 4 days*	750 mg Single Dose	14	↑18% (5–33%)	↔
Ketoconazole 400 mg qd ×7 days	500 mg q8h × 5–6 days	12	↑35% (21–49%)	↑25% (8–44%)
Rifabutin 300 mg qd × 8 days	750 mg q8h × 7–8 days	10	↓32% (10–48%)	↓25% (6–38%)
Rifampin 600 mg qd × 7 days	750 mg q8h × 5–6 days	12	↓82% (77–86%)	↓76% (67–83%)

↑ Indicates increase
↓ Indicates decrease
↔Indicates no change
* Using an experimental (soft-gelatin capsule) formulation of saquinavir 1200 mg

chronic HIV infections in lymphoblastoid cell lines, peripheral blood lymphocytes and monocytes/macrophages. Nelfinavir was found to be active against several laboratory strains of HIV-1 and several clinical isolates of HIV-1 and the HIV-2 strain ROD. The EC$_{95}$ (95% effective concentration) of nelfinavir ranged from 7 to 196 nM. In combination with reverse transcriptase inhibitors, nelfinavir demonstrated additive (didanosine or stavudine) to synergistic (zidovudine, lamivudine or zalcitabine) antiviral activity *in vitro* without enhanced cytotoxicity. Drug combination studies with protease inhibitors (ritonavir, saquinavir or indinavir) showed variable results ranging from antagonistic to synergistic. The clinical relevance of these *in vitro* findings is not known.
Drug Resistance: HIV-1 isolates with reduced susceptibility to nelfinavir have been selected *in vitro*. HIV isolates from selected patients treated with nelfinavir alone or in

combination with reverse transcriptase inhibitors were monitored for phenotypic (n=19) and genotypic (n=55) changes in phase I/II trials over a period of 2 to 52 weeks. One or more virus protease mutations at amino acid positions 30, 35, 36, 46, 71, 77 and 88 were detected in >10% of patients with evaluable isolates. Of 19 patients for which both phenotypic and genotypic analyses were performed on clinical isolates, 9 showed reduced susceptibility (5- to 93-fold) to nelfinavir *in vitro*. All 9 patients possessed one or more mutations in the virus protease gene. Amino acid position 30 appeared to be the most frequent mutation site. Phenotypic resistance was defined as a ≥5-fold decrease in viral sensitivity (EC$_{90}$) *in vitro* compared to baseline. The incidence of the D30N mutation in the virus protease of randomly selected patients receiving nelfinavir monotherapy (n=64) or nelfinavir in combination with zidovudine and lamivudine (n=49) at 12 to 16 weeks of therapy was 56% and 6%, respectively. However, the sample size includes pa-

tients with non-amplifiable virus at 12 to 16 weeks of therapy. The clinical relevance of phenotypic and genotypic changes associated with nelfinavir therapy has not been established.

Cross-resistance: HIV isolates obtained from 5 patients during nelfinavir therapy showed a 5- to 93-fold decrease in nelfinavir susceptibility *in vitro* when compared to matched baseline isolates, but did not demonstrate a concordant decrease in susceptibility to indinavir, ritonavir, saquinavir or 141W94, *in vitro*. Conversely, following ritonavir therapy, 6 of 7 clinical isolates with decreased ritonavir susceptibility (8- to 113-fold) *in vitro* compared to baseline also exhibited decreased susceptibility to nelfinavir *in vitro* (5- to 40-fold). An HIV isolate obtained from a patient receiving saquinavir therapy showed decreased susceptibility to saquinavir (7-fold), but did not demonstrate a concordant decrease in susceptibility to nelfinavir *in vitro*. Cross-resistance between nelfinavir and reverse transcriptase inhibitors is unlikely because different enzyme targets are involved. One zidovudine-resistant HIV-1 isolate and one pyridinone-resistant HIV-1 isolate tested *in vitro* retained susceptibility to nelfinavir. Because the potential for HIV cross-resistance between nelfinavir and other protease inhibitors has not been fully explored, it is unknown what effect nelfinavir therapy will have on the activity of coadministered or subsequently administered protease inhibitors.

CLINICAL PHARMACOLOGY

Pharmacokinetics

The pharmacokinetic properties of nelfinavir were evaluated in healthy volunteers and HIV-infected patients; no substantial differences were observed between the two groups.

Absorption: After single and multiple oral doses of 500 to 750 mg (two to three 250 mg tablets) with food, peak nelfinavir plasma concentrations were typically achieved in 2 to 4 hours. After multiple dosing with 750 mg three times daily (TID) for 28 days (steady-state), peak plasma concentrations (C_{max}) averaged 3–4 μg/mL and plasma concentrations prior to the morning dose (trough) were 1–3 μg/mL (trough sample collection times averaged 11 hours after the previous evening dose). A greater than dose-proportional increase in nelfinavir plasma concentrations was observed after single doses; however, this was not observed after multiple dosing.

Effect of Food on Oral Absorption: Maximum plasma concentrations and area under the plasma concentration-time curve (AUC) were 2- to 3-fold higher under fed conditions compared to fasting. The effect of food on nelfinavir absorption was evaluated in two studies (n=14, total). The meals evaluated contained 517 to 759 Kcal, with 153 to 313 Kcal derived from fat.

Distribution: The apparent volume of distribution following oral administration of nelfinavir was 2–7 L/kg. Nelfinavir in serum is extensively protein-bound (>98%).

Metabolism: Unchanged nelfinavir comprised 82–86% of the total plasma radioactivity after a single oral 750 mg dose of ^{14}C-nelfinavir. *In vitro*, multiple cytochrome P-450 isoforms including CYP3A are responsible for metabolism of nelfinavir. One major and several minor oxidative metabolites were found in plasma. The major oxidative metabolite has *in vitro* antiviral activity comparable to the parent drug.

Elimination: The terminal half-life in plasma was typically 3.5 to 5 hours. The majority (87%) of an oral 750 mg dose containing ^{14}C-nelfinavir was recovered in the feces; fecal radioactivity consisted of numerous oxidative metabolites (78%) and unchanged nelfinavir (22%). Only 1–2% of the dose was recovered in urine, of which unchanged nelfinavir was the major component.

Special Populations

Hepatic or Renal Insufficiency: The pharmacokinetics of nelfinavir have not been studied in patients with hepatic or renal insufficiency; however, less than 2% of nelfinavir is excreted in the urine, so the impact of renal impairment on nelfinavir elimination should be minimal.

Gender and Race: No significant pharmacokinetic differences have been detected between males and females. Pharmacokinetic differences due to race have not been evaluated.

Pediatrics: see PRECAUTIONS: Pediatric Use

Drug Interactions (also see PRECAUTIONS, Drug Interactions)

The potential ability of nelfinavir to inhibit the major human cytochrome P450 isoforms (CYP3A, CYP2C19, CYP2D6, CYP2C9, CYP1A2 and CYP2E1) has been investigated *in vitro*. Only CYP3A was inhibited at concentrations in the therapeutic range.

Specific drug interaction studies were performed with nelfinavir and a number of drugs. Tables 1 and 2 summarize the effects of coadministration of nelfinavir on the geometric mean AUC and C_{max}.

[See table 1 at top of previous page]

[See table 2 on previous page]

For information regarding clinical recommendations, see PRECAUTIONS, Drug Interactions.

INDICATIONS AND USAGE

VIRACEPT is indicated for the treatment of HIV infection when antiretroviral therapy is warranted. This indication is based on surrogate marker changes in patients who received VIRACEPT in combination with nucleoside analogues or alone for up to 24 weeks. At present, there are no results from controlled trials evaluating the effect of therapy with VIRACEPT on clinical progression of HIV infection, such as survival or the incidence of opportunistic infections.

Description of Studies

In the clinical studies described below, an experimental branched DNA signal amplification assay was used to estimate the level of circulating HIV RNA in plasma. Using this assay, values below an estimated 1,200 copies/mL could not be reliably quantified and were set to 1,200 copies/mL in all analyses. The units reported, copies/mL, may not represent actual viral copies on an absolute scale. Consequently, HIV RNA results summarized below should not be directly compared to results from other trials utilizing different HIV RNA assays.

Study 511: VIRACEPT + zidovudine + lamivudine versus zidovudine + lamivudine

Study 511 was a double-blind, randomized, placebo controlled trial comparing treatment with zidovudine and lamivudine plus 2 doses of VIRACEPT to zidovudine and lamivudine alone in 297 antiretroviral naive HIV-1 infected patients (median age 35 [range 21 to 63], 89% male and 78% Caucasian). Mean baseline CD4 cell count was 288 cells/mm^3 and mean baseline plasma HIV RNA was 153,044 copies/mL (mean of log_{10} baseline plasma HIV RNA was 4.86). Mean changes in plasma HIV RNA and CD4 cell count are summarized in Figures 1 and 2, respectively.

Figure 1

Study 511: Mean Log_{10} Change From Baseline in Plasma HIV RNA

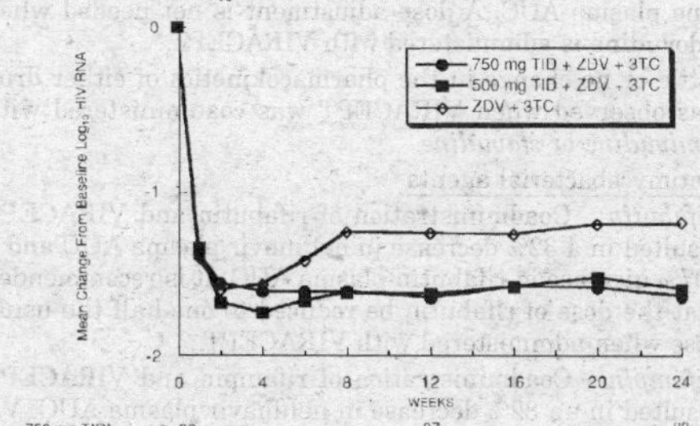
750 mg TID + ZDV + 3TC
500 mg TID + ZDV + 3TC
ZDV + 3TC
Mean Change From Baseline Log_{10} HIV RNA
0
-1
-2
0 4 8 12 16 20 24
WEEKS
750 mg TID* n=99 87 83
500 mg TID* n=97 81 79
Placebo* n=101 89 84
*All arms contain ZDV-3TC

At 24 weeks of therapy, 59, 73 and 30 patients randomized to receive VIRACEPT 500 mg TID plus zidovudine and lamivudine,VIRACEPT 750 mg TID plus zidovudine and lamivudine, or zidovudine and lamivudine, respectively, had plasma HIV RNA assigned a value of 1,200 copies/mL. The clinical significance of changes in plasma HIV RNA has not been established.

Figure 2

Study 511: Mean Change From Baseline in CD4 Cell Counts

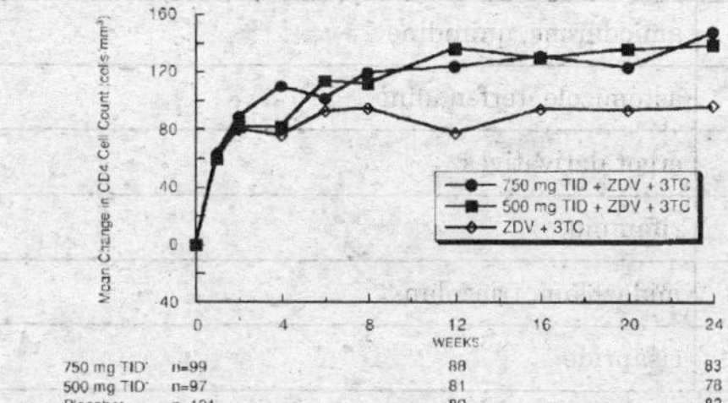
750 mg TID + ZDV + 3TC
500 mg TID + ZDV + 3TC
ZDV + 3TC
Mean Change in CD4 Cell Count (cells/mm³)
160
120
80
40
0
-40
0 4 8 12 16 20 24
WEEKS
750 mg TID* n=99 88 83
500 mg TID* n=97 81 78
Placebo* n=101 89 82
*All arms contain ZDV+3TC

Study 506: VIRACEPT + stavudine versus stavudine

Study 506 is an ongoing double-blind, randomized, placebo controlled trial comparing treatment with 2 doses of VIRACEPT + stavudine and stavudine monotherapy in 308 HIV-1 infected patients (median age 37 [range 21 to 69], 89% male and 75% Caucasian). Sixty-one out of 308 (20%) patients were antiretroviral naive; the remaining patients were experienced (mean duration of antiretroviral therapy 32 months). The mean baseline CD4 cell count for all patients was 279 cells/mm^3 and the mean baseline plasma HIV RNA was 141,369 copies/mL (mean of log_{10} baseline plasma HIV RNA was 4.86). Mean changes in plasma HIV RNA and CD4 cell count are summarized in Figures 3 and 4, respectively. The study allowed for treatment changes in the three study arms based on surrogate marker response or toxicity. By 24 weeks 43, 2 and 4 patients remaining on this study in the stavudine, stavudine plus VIRACEPT 500 mg TID, and stavudine plus VIRACEPT 750 mg TID arms, respectively, had altered initial therapy based primarily on their surrogate marker response. For patients receiving stavudine monotherapy, alteration of therapy was primarily the addition of nelfinavir. Figures 3 and 4 represent surrogate marker changes by original randomization group, without regard to treatment modification.

Figure 3

Study 506: Mean Log_{10} Change From Baseline in Plasma HIV RNA

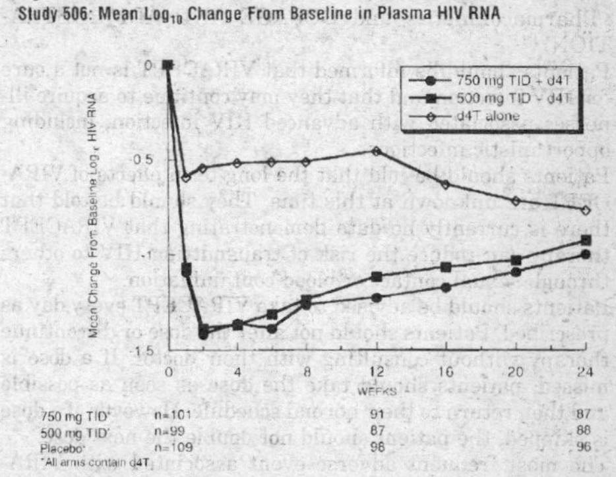
750 mg TID + d4T
500 mg TID + d4T
d4T alone
Mean Change From Baseline Log_{10} HIV RNA
0
0.5
-1
-1.5
0 4 8 12 16 20 24
WEEKS
750 mg TID* n=101 91 87
500 mg TID* n=99 87 88
Placebo* n=109 98 96
*All arms contain d4T

At 24 weeks of therapy, 24, 22 and 13 patients randomized to receive VIRACEPT 500 mg TID plus stavudine, VIRACEPT 750 mg TID plus stavudine, or stavudine alone, respectively, had plasma HIV RNA levels assigned a value of 1,200 copies/mL. The clinical significance of changes in plasma HIV RNA has not been established.

Figure 4

Study 506: Mean Change From Baseline in CD4 Cell Counts

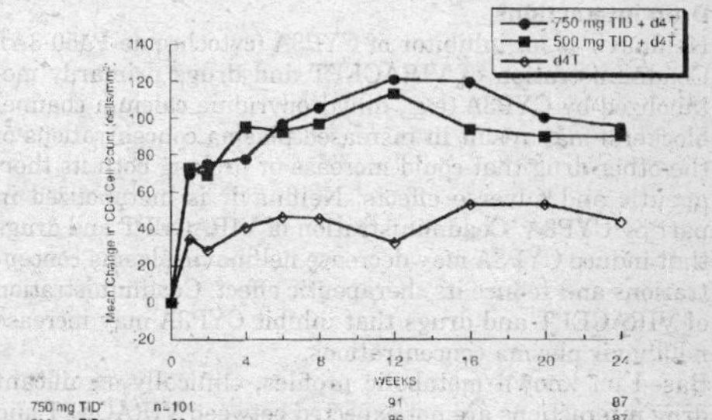
750 mg TID + d4T
500 mg TID + d4T
d4T
Mean Change in CD4 Cell Count (cells/mm³)
140
120
100
80
60
40
20
0
-20
0 4 8 12 16 20 24
WEEKS
750 mg TID* n=101 91 87
500 mg TID* n=99 86 87
Placebo* n=109 98 95
*All arms contain d4T

CONTRAINDICATIONS

VIRACEPT is contraindicated in patients with clinically significant hypersensitivity to any of its components.

WARNING

Patients with Phenylketonuria: VIRACEPT Oral Powder contains 11.2 mg phenylalanine per gram of powder.

VIRACEPT should not be administered concurrently with terfenadine, astemizole, cisapride, triazolam, midazolam, ergot derivatives, amiodarone or quinidine because VIRACEPT may effect the hepatic metabolism of these drugs and create the potential for serious and/or life-threatening adverse events. (see PRECAUTIONS, Drug Interactions).

New onset diabetes mellitus, exacerbation of pre-existing diabetes mellitus and hyperglycemia have been reported during post-marketing surveillance in HIV-infected patients receiving protease inhibitor therapy. Some patients required either initiation or dose adjustments of insulin or oral hypoglycemic agents for treatment of these events. In some cases diabetic ketoacidosis has occurred. In those patients who discontinued protease inhibitor therapy, hyperglycemia persisted in some cases. Because these events have been reported voluntarily during clinical practice, estimates of frequency cannot be made and a causal relationship between protease inhibitor therapy and these events has not been established.

PRECAUTIONS

General

Nelfinavir is principally metabolized by the liver. Therefore, caution should be exercised when administering this drug to patients with hepatic impairment.

Resistance/Cross Resistance: Because the potential for HIV cross resistance between protease inhibitors has not been fully explored, it is unknown what effect nelfinavir therapy will have on the activity of subsequently administered protease inhibitors. (See MICROBIOLOGY)

Hemophilia

There have been reports of increased bleeding, including spontaneous skin hematomas and hemarthrosis, in patients with hemophilia type A and B treated with protease inhibitors. In some patients, additional factor VIII was given. In more than half of the reported cases, treatment with protease inhibitors was continued or reintroduced. A causal relationship has not been established.

Continued on next page

Viracept—Cont.

Information For Patients

For optimal absorption, patients should be advised to take VIRACEPT with food (See CLINICAL PHARMACOLOGY: Pharmacokinetics and DOSAGE AND ADMINISTRATION).

Patients should be informed that VIRACEPT is not a cure for HIV infection and that they may continue to acquire illnesses associated with advanced HIV infection, including opportunistic infections.

Patients should be told that the long-term effects of VIRACEPT are unknown at this time. They should be told that there is currently no data demonstrating that VIRACEPT therapy can reduce the risk of transmitting HIV to others through sexual contact or blood contamination.

Patients should be advised to take VIRACEPT every day as prescribed. Patients should not alter the dose or discontinue therapy without consulting with their doctor. If a dose is missed, patients should take the dose as soon as possible and then return to their normal schedule. However, if a dose is skipped, the patient should not double the next dose.

The most frequent adverse event associated with VIRACEPT is diarrhea, which can usually be controlled with nonprescription drugs, such as loperamide, which slow gastrointestinal motility.

VIRACEPT may interact with some drugs, therefore, patients should be advised to report to their doctor the use of any other prescription or non-prescription medication.

Patients receiving oral contraceptives should be instructed that alternate or additional contraceptive measures should be used during therapy with VIRACEPT.

Drug Interactions

Nelfinavir is an inhibitor of CYP3A (cytochrome P450 3A). Coadministration of VIRACEPT and drugs primarily metabolized by CYP3A (e.g., dihydropyridine calcium channel blockers) may result in increased plasma concentrations of the other drug that could increase or prolong both its therapeutic and adverse effects. Nelfinavir is metabolized in part by CYP3A. Coadministration of VIRACEPT and drugs that induce CYP3A may decrease nelfinavir plasma concentrations and reduce its therapeutic effect. Coadministration of VIRACEPT and drugs that inhibit CYP3A may increase nelfinavir plasma concentrations.

Based on known metabolic profiles, clinically significant drug interactions are not expected between VIRACEPT and dapsone, trimethoprim/sulfamethoxazole, clarithromycin, azithromycin, erythromycin, itraconazole or fluconazole.

[See table below]

Antihistamines

Terfenadine: Administration of terfenadine with VIRACEPT resulted in the appearance of unchanged terfenadine in plasma; therefore, VIRACEPT should not be administered concurrently with terfenadine because of the potential for serious and/or life-threatening cardiac arrhythmias. Because a similar interaction is likely, VIRACEPT should also not be administered concurrently with *astemizole*.

Anti-HIV protease inhibitors

Indinavir: Coadministration of indinavir with VIRACEPT resulted in an 83% increase in nelfinavir plasma AUC and a 51% increase in indinavir plasma AUC. Currently, there are no safety and efficacy data available from the use of this combination.

Ritonavir: Coadministration of ritonavir with VIRACEPT resulted in a 152% increase in nelfinavir plasma AUC and very little change in ritonavir plasma AUC. Currently, there are no safety and efficacy data available from the use of this combination.

Saquinavir: Coadministration of saquinavir (using an experimental soft-gelatin capsule formulation of saquinavir 1200 mg) with VIRACEPT resulted in an 18% increase in nelfinavir plasma AUC and a 4-fold increase in saquinavir plasma AUC. If used in combination with saquinavir hard gelatin capsules at the recommended dose of 600 mg tid, no dose adjustments are needed. Currently, there are no safety and efficacy data available from the use of this combination.

Antifungal agents

Ketoconazole: Coadministration of ketoconazole with VIRACEPT resulted in a 35% increase in nelfinavir plasma AUC. This change was not considered clinically significant and no dose adjustment is needed when ketoconazole and VIRACEPT are coadministered.

Anti-HIV reverse transcriptase inhibitors

Didanosine: It is recommended that didanosine be administered on an empty stomach; therefore, nelfinavir should be administered (with food) one hour after or more than two hours before didanosine.

Zidovudine: Coadministration of zidovudine and lamivudine with VIRACEPT resulted in a 35% decrease in zidovudine plasma AUC. A dose adjustment is not needed when zidovudine is administered with VIRACEPT.

Little or no change in the pharmacokinetics of either drug was observed when VIRACEPT was coadministered with *lamivudine* or *stavudine*.

Antimycobacterial agents

Rifabutin: Coadministration of rifabutin and VIRACEPT resulted in a 32% decrease in nelfinavir plasma AUC and a 207% increase in rifabutin plasma AUC. It is recommended that the dose of rifabutin be reduced to one-half the usual dose when administered with VIRACEPT.

Rifampin: Coadministration of rifampin and VIRACEPT resulted in an 82% decrease in nelfinavir plasma AUC. VIRACEPT and rifampin should not be coadministered.

Oral Contraceptives

Ethinyl estradiol and *norethindrone:* Coadministration of VIRACEPT with OVCON-35 resulted in a 47% decrease in ethinyl estradiol and an 18% decrease in norethindrone plasma concentrations. Alternate or additional contraceptive measures should be used during therapy with VIRACEPT.

Carcinogenesis and Mutagenesis

Carcinogenicity studies in animals have not yet been completed. Nelfinavir was not, however, mutagenic or clastogenic in a battery of *in vitro* and *in vivo* tests including microbial mutagenesis (Ames), mouse lymphoma, chromosome aberrations in human lymphocytes, and an *in vivo* rat micronucleus assay.

Pregnancy, Fertility and Reproduction—Pregnancy Category B

Comparisons of systemic exposure are based on the steady-state area under the plasma concentration time curve (AUC) observed in humans receiving the recommended therapeutic dose. Nelfinavir produced no effects on either male or female mating and fertility or embryo survival in rat studies at exposures comparable to human therapeutic exposure. There were also no effects on fetal development or maternal toxicity when nelfinavir was administered to pregnant rats at systemic exposures comparable to human exposure. Administration of nelfinavir to pregnant rabbits resulted in no fetal development effects up to a dose at which a slight decrease in maternal body weight was observed; however, even at the highest dose evaluated, systemic exposure in rabbits was significantly lower than human exposure. Additional studies in rats indicated that exposure to nelfinavir in females from mid-pregnancy through lactation had no effect on the survival, growth, and development of the offspring through to weaning. Subsequent reproductive performance of these offspring was also not affected by maternal exposure to nelfinavir. However, there are no adequate and well-controlled studies in pregnant women. Because animal reproduction studies are not always predictive of human response, VIRACEPT should be used during pregnancy only if clearly needed.

Nursing Mothers

The US Public Health Service Centers for Disease Control and Prevention advises HIV-infected women not to breast-feed to avoid postnatal transmission of HIV to a child who may not yet be infected. Studies in lactating rats have demonstrated that nelfinavir is excreted in milk. It is not known whether nelfinavir is excreted in human milk.

Pediatric Use

Nelfinavir was studied in one open-label, uncontrolled trial in 38 pediatric patients ranging in age from 2 to 13 years. In order to achieve plasma concentrations in pediatric patients which approximate those observed in adults, the recommended pediatric dose is 20–30 mg/kg given three times daily with a meal or snack, not to exceed 750 mg three times a day. (See DOSAGE AND ADMINISTRATION)

A similar adverse event profile was seen during the pediatric clinical trial as in adult patients. The evaluation of the antiviral activity of nelfinavir in pediatric patients is ongoing.

The safety, effectiveness and pharmacokinetics of nelfinavir have not been evaluated in pediatric patients below the age of 2 years.

ADVERSE REACTIONS

The safety of VIRACEPT was studied in over 1500 patients who received drug either alone or in combination with nucleoside analogues (d4T or ZDV/3TC). The majority of adverse events were of mild intensity. The most frequently reported adverse event among patients receiving VIRACEPT was diarrhea, which was generally of mild to moderate intensity.

Drug-related clinical adverse experiences of moderate or severe intensity in ≥2% of patients treated with VIRACEPT coadministered with ZDV plus 3TC (Study 511) or in combination with d4T (Study 506) for up to 24 weeks are presented in Table 3.

[See table 3 at top of next page]

Adverse events occurring in less than 2% of patients receiving VIRACEPT in all phase II/III clinical trials and considered at least possibly related or of unknown relationship to treatment and of at least moderate severity are listed below.

Body as a Whole: accidental injury, allergic reaction, back pain, fever, headache, malaise, and pain.

Digestive System: anorexia, dyspepsia, epigastric pain, gastrointestinal bleeding, hepatitis, mouth ulceration, pancreatitis and vomiting.

Hemic/Lymphatic System: anemia, leukopenia and thrombocytopenia.

Metabolic/Nutritional System: increases in alkaline phosphate, amylase, creatine phosphokinase, lactic dehydrogenase, SGOT, SGPT and gamma glutamyl transpeptidase; hyperlipemia, hyperuricemia, hyperglycemia, hypoglycemia, dehydration, and liver function tests abnormal.

Musculoskeletal System: arthralgia, arthritis, cramps, myalgia, myasthenia and myopathy.

Drugs That Should Not Be Coadministered With VIRACEPT

Drug Class	Drugs Within Class Not to Be Coadministered With VIRACEPT
Antiarrhythmics	amiodarone, quinidine
Antihistamines	astemizole, terfenadine
Antimigrane	ergot derivatives
Antimycobacterial agents	rifampin
Benzodiazepines	midazolam, triazolam
GI motility agents	cisapride

Drugs Which Require a Dose Reduction When Coadministered With VIRACEPT

Drug Class	Drugs Within Class Which Require Dose Reduction
Antimycobacterial agents	rifabutin

Other Potentially Clinically Significant Drug Interactions With VIRACEPT*

Anticonvulsants: carbamazepine, phenobarbital, phenytoin	May decrease nelfinavir plasma concentrations**
Anti-HIV protease inhibitors: indinavir, ritonavir	May increase nelfinavir plasma concentrations
Oral contraceptives: ethinyl estradiol, norethindrone	Plasma concentrations may be decreased by VIRACEPT

* This table is not all inclusive
**VIRACEPT may not be effective due to decreased nelfinavir plasma concentrations in patients taking these agents concomitantly

Table 3
Percentage of Patients with Treatment-Emergent[1] Adverse Events of Moderate or Severe Intensity Reported in ≥2% of Patients

Adverse Events	Study 511 Naive Patients			Study 506 Experienced Patients		
	Placebo + ZDV/3TC (n=101)	500 mg TID VIRACEPT +ZDV/3TC (n=97)	750 mg TID VIRACEPT +ZDV/3TC (n=100)	Placebo + d4T (n=109)	500 mg TID VIRACEPT +d4T (n=98)	750 mg TID VIRACEPT +d4T (n=101)
Body as a Whole						
Abdominal Pain	1%	0	0	3%	2%	4%
Asthenia	2%	1%	1%	4%	3%	1%
Digestive System						
Diarrhea	3%	14%	20%	10%	28%	32%
Nausea	4%	3%	7%	1%	3%	2%
Flatulence	0	5%	2%	4%	8%	3%
Skin/Appendages						
Rash	1%	1%	3%	0	4%	3%

[1] Includes those adverse events at least possibly related to study drug or of unknown relationship and excludes concurrent HIV conditions

Table 4
Percentage of Patients by Treatment Group With Marked Laboratory Abnormalities[1] in >2% of Patients

	Study 511 Naive Patients			Study 506 Experienced Patients		
	Placebo + ZDV/3TC (n=101)	500 mg TID VIRACEPT +ZDV/3TC (n=97)	750 mg TID VIRACEPT +ZDV/3TC (n=100)	Placebo + d4T (n=109)	500 mg TID VIRACEPT +d4T (n=98)	750 mg TID VIRACEPT +d4T (n=101)
Hematology						
Hemoglobin	6%	3%	2%	0	0	0
Neutrophils	4%	3%	5%	1%	1%	4%
Lymphocytes	1%	6%	1%	1%	1%	0
Chemistry						
ALT (SGPT)	6%	1%	1%	1%	3%	2%
AST (SGOT)	4%	1%	0	0	3%	3%
Creatine Kinase	7%	2%	2%	4%	5%	6%

[1] Marked laboratory abnormalities are defined as a shift from Grade 0 at baseline to at least Grade 3 or from Grade 1 to Grade 4

Table 5
Pediatric Dose to be Administered Three Times Daily

Body Weight Kg	Lbs.	Number of Level 1 gm Scoops	Number of Level Teaspoons	Number of Tablets
7 to <8.5	15.5 to <18.5	4	1	—
8.5 to <10.5	18.5 to <23	5	1¼	—
10.5 to <12	23 to <26.5	6	1½	—
12 to <14	26.5 to <31	7	1¾	—
14 to <16	31 to <35	8	2	—
16 to <18	35 to <39.5	9	2¼	—
18 to <23	39.5 to <50.5	10	2½	2
≥23	≥50.5	15	3¾	3

Nervous System: anxiety, depression, dizziness, emotional lability, hyperkinesia, insomnia, migraine, paresthesia, seizures, sleep disorder, somnolence and suicide ideation.
Respiratory System: dyspnea, pharyngitis, rhinitis, and sinusitis.
Skin/Appendages: dermatitis, folliculitis, fungal dermatitis, maculopapular rash, pruritus, sweating, and urticaria.
Special Senses: acute iritis and eye disorder.
Urogenital System: kidney calculus, sexual dysfunction and urine abnormality.

Laboratory Abnormalities
Few patients experienced significant laboratory abnormalities while receiving VIRACEPT. The percentage of patients with marked laboratory abnormalities in Studies 511 and 506 are presented in Table 4. Marked laboratory abnormal-

ities are defined as a Grade 3 or 4 abnormality in a patient with a normal baseline value or a Grade 4 abnormality in a patient with a Grade 1 abnormality at baseline.
[See table 4 above]

OVERDOSAGE
Human experience of acute overdose with VIRACEPT is limited. There is no specific antidote for overdose with VIRACEPT. If indicated, elimination of unabsorbed drug should be achieved by emesis or gastric lavage. Administration of activated charcoal may also be used to aid removal of unabsorbed drug. Since nelfinavir is highly protein bound, dialysis is unlikely to significantly remove drug from blood.

DOSAGE AND ADMINISTRATION
Adults: The recommended dose is 750 mg (three 250 mg tablets) three times daily. VIRACEPT should be taken with a meal or light snack. Antiviral activity is enhanced when VIRACEPT is administered in combination with nucleoside analogues. Therefore, it is recommended that VIRACEPT be used in combination with nucleoside analogues.
Pediatric patients (2–13 years): The recommended oral dose of VIRACEPT for pediatric patients 2 to 13 years of age is 20–30 mg/kg per dose, three times daily with a meal or a light snack. For children unable to take tablets, VIRACEPT Oral Powder may be administered. The oral powder may be mixed with a small amount of water, milk, formula, soy formula, soy milk or dietary supplements; once mixed, the entire contents must be consumed in order to obtain the full dose. The recommended use period for storage of the product in these media is 6 hours. Acidic food or juice (e.g., orange juice, apple juice or apple sauce) are not recommended to be used in combination with VIRACEPT, because the combination may result in a bitter taste. VIRACEPT Oral Powder should not be reconstituted with water in its original container. The recommended pediatric dose of VIRACEPT to be administered three times daily is described in Table 5:
[See table 5 below]

HOW SUPPLIED
VIRACEPT (nelfinavir mesylate) Tablets, 250 mg are light blue, capsule-shaped tablets engraved with "VIRACEPT" on one side and "250 mg" on the other.
Available as:
NDC 63010-010-27, bottle containing 270 tablets
VIRACEPT (nelfinavir mesylate) Oral Powder, 50 mg/g is an off-white powder containing 50 mg (as nelfinavir free base) in each level scoopful (1 gram).
Available as:
NDC 63010-011–90, multiple use bottle containing 144 grams of powder with scoop.
VIRACEPT Tablets and Oral Powder should be stored at 15° to 30°C (59° to 86°F).
Issued 10/29/97
VIRACEPT is a registered trademark of Agouron Pharmaceuticals, Inc.
Shown in Product Identification Guide, page 303

Alcon Laboratories, Inc.
and its affiliates
CORPORATE HEADQUARTERS
6201 SOUTH FREEWAY
FORT WORTH, TX 76134

Direct Inquiries to:
Ophthalmic/Vision Care: (800) 451-3937
(Pharmaceuticals/Lens Care)
Surgical: (800) 862-5266
(Instrumentation/Surgical Meds)
Systems: (800) 289-1991
(Medical Management Information Systems)
6201 South Freeway
Fort Worth, TX 76134
(817) 293-0450

OPHTHALMIC PRODUCTS

For information on Alcon ophthalmic products, consult the PDR For Ophthalmology. See a complete listing of products in the Manufacturers' Index section of this book. For information, literature, samples or service items contact Alcon at the phone numbers listed above.

BETOPTIC® ℞
(betaxolol hydrochloride)
0.5% as base
Sterile Ophthalmic Solution

DESCRIPTION
BETOPTIC® Sterile Ophthalmic Solution contains betaxolol hydrochloride, a cardioselective beta-adrenergic receptor blocking agent, in a sterile isotonic solution. Betaxolol hydrochloride is a white, crystalline powder, soluble in water, with a molecular weight of 343.89.
Chemical Name:
(±)-1-[p-[2-(Cyclopropylmethoxy)ethyl]phenoxy]-3-(isopropylamino)-2-propanol hydrochloride.
Each mL of BETOPTIC Ophthalmic Solution (0.5%) contains: Active: 5.6 mg betaxolol hydrochloride equivalent to betaxolol base 5 mg. Preservative: Benzalkonium Chloride

Continued on next page

Betoptic—Cont.

0.01%. Inactives: Edetate Disodium, Sodium Chloride, Hydrochloric Acid and/or Sodium Hydroxide (to adjust pH), and Purified Water.

CLINICAL PHARMACOLOGY

Betaxolol HCl, a cardioselective (beta-1-adrenergic) receptor blocking agent, does not have significant membrane-stabilizing (local anesthetic) activity and is devoid of intrinsic sympathomimetic action. Orally administered beta-adrenergic blocking agents reduce cardiac output in healthy subjects and patients with heart disease. In patients with severe impairment of myocardial function, beta-adrenergic receptor antagonists may inhibit the sympathetic stimulatory effect necessary to maintain adequate cardiac function. When instilled in the eye, BETOPTIC Ophthalmic Solution has the action of reducing elevated as well as normal intraocular pressure, whether or not accompanied by glaucoma. Ophthalmic betaxolol has minimal effect on pulmonary and cardiovascular parameters.

Ophthalmic betaxolol (one drop in each eye) was compared to timolol and placebo in a three-way crossover study challenging nine patients with reactive airway disease who were selected on the basis of having at least a 15% reduction in the forced expiratory volume in one second (FEV_1) after administration of ophthalmic timolol. Betaxolol HCl had no significant effect on pulmonary function as measured by FEV_1, Forced Vital Capacity (FVC) and FEV_1/VC. Additionally, the action of isoproterenol, a beta stimulant, administered at the end of the study was not inhibited by ophthalmic betaxolol. In contrast, ophthalmic timolol significantly decreased these pulmonary functions.

[See table above]

No evidence of cardiovascular beta-adrenergic blockade during exercise was observed with betaxolol in a double-masked, three-way crossover study in 24 normal subjects comparing ophthalmic betaxolol, timolol and placebo for effect on blood pressure and heart rate. Mean arterial blood pressure was not affected by any treatment; however, ophthalmic timolol produced a significant decrease in the mean heart rate.

[See table below]

CLINICAL STUDIES

Optic nerve head damage and visual field loss are the result of a sustained elevated intraocular pressure and poor ocular perfusion. BETOPTIC Ophthalmic Solution has the action of reducing elevated as well as normal intraocular pressure, and the mechanism of ocular hypotensive action appears to be a reduction of aqueous production as demonstrated by tonography and aqueous fluorophotometry. The onset of action with BETOPTIC Ophthalmic Solution can generally be noted within 30 minutes and the maximal effect can usually be detected 2 hours after topical administration. A single dose provides a 12-hour reduction in intraocular pressure. Clinical observation of glaucoma patients treated with BETOPTIC Ophthalmic Solution for up to three years shows that the intraocular pressure lowering effect is well maintained.

Clinical studies show that topical BETOPTIC Ophthalmic Solution reduces mean intraocular pressure 25% from baseline. In trials using 22 mmHg as a generally accepted index of intraocular pressure control, BETOPTIC Ophthalmic Solution was effective in more than 94% of the population studied, of which 73% were treated with the beta blocker alone. In controlled, double-masked studies, the magnitude and duration of the ocular hypotensive effect of BETOPTIC Ophthalmic Solution and ophthalmic timolol solution were clinically equivalent.

	FEV$_1$ —Percent Change from Baseline[1]		
	Means		
	Betaxolol 1.0%[a]	Timolol 0.5%	Placebo
Baseline	1.6	1.4	1.4
60 Minutes	2.3	−25.7*	5.8
120 Minutes	1.6	−27.4*	7.5
240 Minutes	−6.4	−26.9*	6.9
Isoproterenol[b]	36.1	−12.4*	42.8

[1] Schoene, R. B. et al., Am. J. Ophthal. 97:86, 1984.
[a] Twice the clinical concentration.
[b] Inhaled at 240 minutes; measurement at 270 minutes.
* Timolol statistically different from betaxolol and placebo (p<0.05).

BETOPTIC Ophthalmic Solution has also been used successfully in glaucoma patients who have undergone a laser trabeculoplasty and have needed additional long-term ocular hypotensive therapy.

BETOPTIC Ophthalmic Solution has been well tolerated in glaucoma patients wearing hard or soft contact lenses and in aphakic patients.

BETOPTIC Ophthalmic Solution does not produce miosis or accommodative spasm which are frequently seen with miotic agents. The blurred vision and night blindness often associated with standard miotic therapy are not associated with BETOPTIC Ophthalmic Solution. Thus, patients with central lenticular opacities avoid the visual impairment caused by a constricted pupil.

INDICATIONS AND USAGE

BETOPTIC Ophthalmic Solution has been shown to be effective in lowering intraocular pressure and is indicated in the treatment of ocular hypertension and chronic open-angle glaucoma. It may be used alone or in combination with other anti-glaucoma drugs.

In clinical studies BETOPTIC® was safely used to lower intraocular pressure in 47 patients with both glaucoma and reactive airway disease who were followed for a mean period of 15 months. However, caution should be used in treating patients with severe reactive airway disease or a history of asthma.

CONTRAINDICATIONS

Hypersensitivity to any component of is product. BETOPTIC Ophthalmic Solution is contraindicated in patients with sinus bradycardia, greater than a first degree atrioventricular block, cardiogenic shock, or patients with overt cardiac failure.

WARNING

Topically applied beta-adrenergic blocking agents may be absorbed systemically. The same adverse reactions found with systemic administration of beta-adrenergic blocking agents may occur with topical administration. For example, severe respiratory reactions and cardiac reactions, including death due to bronchospasm in patients with asthma, and rarely death in association with cardiac failure, have been reported with topical application of beta-adrenergic blocking agents.

BETOPTIC Ophthalmic Solution has been shown to have a minor effect on heart rate and blood pressure in clinical studies. Caution should be used in treating patients with a history of cardiac failure or heart block. Treatment with BETOPTIC Ophthalmic Solution should be discontinued at the first signs of cardiac failure.

PRECAUTIONS

General: Information for Patients. Do not touch dropper tip to any surface as this may contaminate the solution.

Diabetes Mellitus. Beta-adrenergic blocking agents should be administered with caution in patients subject to spontaneous hypoglycemia or to diabetic patients (especially those with labile diabetes) who are receiving insulin or oral hypoglycemic agents. Beta-adrenergic receptor blocking agents may mask the signs and symptoms of acute hypoglycemia.

Thyrotoxicosis. Beta-adrenergic blocking agents may mask certain clinical signs (e.g., tachycardia) of hyperthyroidism. Patients suspected of developing thyrotoxicosis should be managed carefully to avoid abrupt withdrawal of beta-adrenergic blocking agents, which might precipitate a thyroid storm.

Muscle Weakness. Beta-adrenergic blockade has been reported to potentiate muscle weakness consistent with certain myasthenic symptoms (e.g., diplopia, ptosis, and generalized weakness).

Major Surgery. Consideration should be given to the gradual withdrawal of beta-adrenergic blocking agents prior to general anesthesia because of the reduced ability of the heart to respond to beta-adrenergically mediated sympathetic reflex stimuli.

Pulmonary. Caution should be exercised in the treatment of glaucoma patients with excessive restriction of pulmonary function. There have been reports of asthmatic attacks and pulmonary distress during betaxolol treatment. Although rechallenges of some such patients with ophthalmic betaxolol has not adversely affected pulmonary function test results, the possibility of adverse pulmonary effects in patients sensitive to beta blockers cannot be ruled out.

Risk from Anaphylactic Reaction: While taking beta-blockers, patients with a history of atopy or a history of severe anaphylactic reaction to a variety of allergens may be more reactive to repeated accidental, diagnostic, or therapeutic challenge with such allergens. Such patients may be unresponsive to the usual doses of epinephrine used to treat anaphylactic reactions.

Drug Interactions: Patients who are receiving a beta-adrenergic blocking agent orally and BETOPTIC Ophthalmic Solution should be observed for a potential additive effect either on the intraocular pressure or on the known systemic effects of beta blockade.

Close observation of the patient is recommended when a beta blocker is administered to patients receiving catecholamine-depleting drugs such as reserpine, because of possible additive effects and the production of hypotension and/or bradycardia.

Betaxolol is an adrenergic blocking agent; therefore, caution should be exercised in patients using concomitant adrenergic psychotropic drugs.

Ocular: In patients with angle-closure glaucoma, the immediate treatment objective is to reopen the angle by constriction of the pupil with a miotic agent. Betaxolol has little or no effect on the pupil. When BETOPTIC Ophthalmic Solution is used to reduce elevated intraocular pressure in angle-closure glaucoma, it should be used with a miotic and not alone.

Carcinogenesis, Mutagenesis, Impairment of Fertility: Lifetime studies with betaxolol HCl have been completed in mice at oral doses of 6, 20 or 60 mg/kg/day and in rats at 3, 12 or 48 mg/kg/day; betaxolol HCl demonstrated no carcinogenic effect. Higher dose levels were not tested.

In a variety of in vitro and in vivo bacterial and mammalian cell assays, betaxolol HCl was nonmutagenic.

Pregnancy: Pregnancy Category C. Reproduction, teratology, and peri- and postnatal studies have been conducted with orally administered betaxolol HCl in rats and rabbits. There was evidence of drug related postimplantation loss in rabbits and rats at dose levels above 12 mg/kg and 128 mg/kg, respectively. Betaxolol HCl was not shown to be teratogenic, however, and there were no other adverse effects on reproduction at subtoxic dose levels. There are no adequate and well-controlled studies in pregnant women. BETOPTIC

	Mean Heart Rates[1]		
	TREATMENT		
Bruce Stress Exercise Test			
Minutes	Betaxolol 1%[a]	Timolol 0.5%	Placebo
0	79.2	79.3	81.2
2	130.2	126.0	130.4
4	133.4	128.0*	134.3
6	136.4	129.2*	137.9
8	139.8	131.8*	139.4
10	140.8	131.8*	141.3

[1] Atkins, J. M. et al., Am. J. Oph. 99:173–175, Feb., 1985.
[a] Twice the clinical concentration.
* Mean pulse rate significantly lower for timolol than betaxolol or placebo (p<0.05).

Ophthalmic Solution should be used during pregnancy only if the potential benefit justifies the potential risk to the fetus.

Nursing Mothers: It is not known whether betaxolol HCl is excreted in human milk. Because many drugs are excreted in human milk, caution should be exercised when BETOPTIC Ophthalmic Solution is administered to nursing women.

Pediatric Use: Safety and effectiveness in pediatric patients have not been established.

ADVERSE REACTIONS

The following adverse reactions have been reported in clinical trials with BETOPTIC Ophthalmic Solution.

Ocular: Discomfort of short duration was experienced by one in four patients, but none discontinued therapy; occasional tearing has been reported. Rare instances of decreased corneal sensitivity, erythema, itching sensation, corneal punctate staining, keratitis, anisocoria, edema, and photophobia have been reported.

Additional medical events reported with other formulations of betaxolol include blurred vision, foreign body sensation, dryness of the eyes, inflammation, discharge, ocular pain, decreased visual acuity, and crusty lashes.

Systemic: Systemic reactions following administration of BETOPTIC Ophthalmic Solution 0.5% or BETOPTIC S Ophthalmic Suspension 0.25% have been rarely reported. These include:

Cardiovascular: Bradycardia, heart block and congestive failure.

Pulmonary: Pulmonary distress characterized by dyspnea, bronchospasm, thickened bronchial secretions, asthma and respiratory failure.

Central Nervous System: Insomnia, dizziness, vertigo, headaches, depression, lethargy, and increase in signs and symptoms of myasthenia gravis.

Other: Hives, toxic epidermal necrolysis, hair loss and glossitis.

OVERDOSAGE

No information is available on overdosage of humans. The oral LD_{50} of the drug ranged from 350–920 mg/kg in mice and 860–1050 mg/kg in rats. The symptoms which might be expected with an overdose of a systemically administered beta-1-adrenergic receptor blocker agent are bradycardia, hypotension and acute cardiac failure. A topical overdose of BETOPTIC Ophthalmic Solution may be flushed from the eye(s) with warm tap water.

DOSAGE AND ADMINISTRATION

The recommended dose is one to two drops of BETOPTIC Ophthalmic Solution in the affected eye(s) twice daily. In some patients, the intraocular pressure lowering responses to BETOPTIC Ophthalmic Solution may require a few weeks to stabilize. As with any new medication, careful monitoring of patients is advised.

If the intraocular pressure of the patient is not adequately controlled on this regimen, concomitant therapy with pilocarpine and other miotics, and/or epinephrine and/or carbonic anhydrase inhibitors can be instituted.

HOW SUPPLIED

BETOPTIC Ophthalmic Solution is a sterile, isotonic, aqueous solution of betaxolol hydrochloride. Supplied as follows: 2.5, 5, 10 and 15 mL in plastic ophthalmic DROP-TAINER® dispensers.

2.5 mL: **NDC** 0065-0245-20
5 mL: **NDC** 0065-0245-05
10 mL: **NDC** 0065-0245-10
15 mL: **NDC** 0065-0245-15

STORAGE

Store at room temperature.
Rx Only
U.S. Patents Nos. 4,252,984; 4,311,708; 4,342,783

BETOPTIC® S   ℞
(betaxolol HCl)
0.25% as base
Sterile Ophthalmic Suspension

DESCRIPTION

BETOPTIC S Ophthalmic Suspension 0.25% contains betaxolol hydrochloride, a cardioselective beta-adrenergic receptor blocking agent, in a sterile resin suspension formulation. Betaxolol hydrochloride is a white, crystalline powder, with a molecular weight of 343.89.
Chemical Name:
  (±)-1-[p-[2-(cyclopropylmethoxy)ethyl]
  phenoxy]-3-(isopropylamino)-2-propanol hydrochloride.
Each mL of BETOPTIC S Ophthalmic Suspension contains:
Active: betaxolol HCl 2.8 mg equivalent to 2.5 mg of betaxolol base. **Preservative:** benzalkonium chloride 0.01%. **Inactive:** Mannitol, Poly(Styrene-Divinyl Benzene) sulfonic acid, Carbomer 934P, edetate disodium, hydrochloric acid or sodium hydroxide (to adjust pH) and purified water.

CLINICAL PHARMACOLOGY

Betaxolol HCl, a cardioselective (beta-1-adrenergic) receptor blocking agent, does not have significant membrane-stabilizing (local anesthetic) activity and is devoid of intrinsic sympathomimetic action. Orally administered beta-adrenergic blocking agents reduce cardiac output in healthy subjects and patients with heart disease. In patients with severe impairment of myocardial function, beta-adrenergic receptor antagonists may inhibit the sympathetic stimulatory effect necessary to maintain adequate cardiac function. When instilled in the eye, BETOPTIC S Ophthalmic Suspension 0.25% has the action of reducing elevated intraocular pressure, whether or not accompanied by glaucoma. Ophthalmic betaxolol has minimal effect on pulmonary and cardiovascular parameters.

Elevated IOP presents a major risk factor in glaucomatous field loss. The higher the level of IOP, the greater the likelihood of optic nerve damage and visual field loss. Betaxolol has the action of reducing elevated as well as normal intraocular pressure and the mechanism of ocular hypotensive action appears to be a reduction of aqueous production as demonstrated by tonography and aqueous fluorophotometry. The onset of action with betaxolol can generally be noted within 30 minutes and the maximal effect can usually be detected 2 hours after topical administration. A single dose provides a 12-hour reduction in intraocular pressure. In controlled, double-masked studies, the magnitude and duration of the ocular hypotensive effect of BETOPTIC S Ophthalmic Suspension 0.25% and BETOPTIC Ophthalmic Solution 0.5% were clinically equivalent. BETOPTIC S Suspension was significantly more comfortable than BETOPTIC Solution.

Ophthalmic betaxolol solution at 1% (one drop in each eye) was compared to placebo in a crossover study challenging nine patients with reactive airway disease. Betaxolol HCl had no significant effect on pulmonary function as measured by FEV_1, Forced Vital Capacity (FVC), FEV_1/FVC and was not significantly different from placebo. The action of isoproterenol, a beta stimulant, administered at the end of the study was not inhibited by ophthalmic betaxolol.

No evidence of cardiovascular beta adrenergic-blockade during exercise was observed with betaxolol in a double-masked, crossover study in 24 normal subjects comparing ophthalmic betaxolol and placebo for effects on blood pressure and heart rate.

INDICATIONS AND USAGE

BETOPTIC S Ophthalmic Suspension 0.25% has been shown to be effective in lowering intraocular pressure and may be used in patients with chronic open-angle glaucoma and ocular hypertension. It may be used alone or in combination with other intraocular pressure lowering medications.

CONTRAINDICATIONS

Hypersensitivity to any component of this product. BETOPTIC S Ophthalmic Suspension 0.25% is contraindicated in patients with sinus bradycardia, greater than a first degree atrioventricular block, cardiogenic shock, or patients with overt cardiac failure.

WARNING

Topically applied beta-adrenergic blocking agents may be absorbed systemically. The same adverse reactions found with systemic administration of beta-adrenergic blocking agents may occur with topical administration. For example, severe respiratory reactions and cardiac reactions, including death due to bronchospasm in patients with asthma, and rarely death in association with cardiac failure, have been reported with topical application of beta-adrenergic blocking agents.

BETOPTIC S Ophthalmic Suspension 0.25% has been shown to have a minor effect on heart rate and blood pressure in clinical studies. Caution should be used in treating patients with a history of cardiac failure or heart block. Treatment with BETOPTIC S Ophthalmic Suspension 0.25% should be discontinued at the first signs of cardiac failure.

PRECAUTIONS

General:

Diabetes Mellitus. Beta-adrenergic blocking agents should be administered with caution in patients subject to spontaneous hypoglycemia or to diabetic patients (especially those with labile diabetes) who are receiving insulin or oral hypoglycemic agents. Beta-adrenergic receptor blocking agents may mask the signs and symptoms of acute hypoglycemia.

Thyrotoxicosis. Beta-adrenergic blocking agents may mask certain clinical signs (e.g., tachycardia) of hyperthyroidism. Patients suspected of developing thyrotoxicosis should be managed carefully to avoid abrupt withdrawal of beta-adrenergic blocking agents, which might precipitate a thyroid storm.

Muscle Weakness. Beta-adrenergic blockade has been reported to potentiate muscle weakness consistent with certain myasthenic symptoms (e.g., diplopia, ptosis and generalized weakness).

Major Surgery. Consideration should be given to the gradual withdrawal of beta-adrenergic blocking agents prior to general anesthesia because of the reduced ability of the heart to respond to beta-adrenergically mediated sympathetic reflex stimuli.

Pulmonary. Caution should be exercised in the treatment of glaucoma patients with excessive restriction of pulmonary function. There have been reports of asthmatic attacks and pulmonary distress during betaxolol treatment. Although rechallenges of some such patients with ophthalmic betaxolol has not adversely affected pulmonary function test results, the possibility of adverse pulmonary effects in patients sensitive to beta blockers cannot be ruled out.

Information for Patients: Do not touch dropper tip to any surface, as this may contaminate the contents. Do not use with contact lenses in eyes.

Drug Interactions: Patients who are receiving a beta-adrenergic blocking agent orally and BETOPTIC S Ophthalmic Suspension 0.25% should be observed for a potential additive effect either on the intraocular pressure or on the known systemic effects of beta blockade.

Close observation of the patient is recommended when a beta blocker is administered to patients receiving catecholamine-depleting drugs such as reserpine, because of possible additive effects and the production of hypotension and/or bradycardia.

Betaxolol is an adrenergic blocking agent; therefore, caution should be exercised in patients using concomitant adrenergic psychotropic drugs.

Risk from anaphylactic reaction: While taking beta-blockers, patients with a history of atopy or a history of severe anaphylactic reaction to a variety of allergens may be more reactive to repeated accidental, diagnostic, or therapeutic challenge with such allergens. Such patients may be unresponsive to the usual doses of epinephrine used to treat anaphylactic reactions.

Ocular: In patients with angle-closure glaucoma, the immediate treatment objective is to reopen the angle by constriction of the pupil with a miotic agent. Betaxolol has little or no effect on the pupil. When BETOPTIC S Ophthalmic Suspension 0.25% is used to reduce elevated intraocular pressure in angle-closure glaucoma, it should be used with a miotic and not alone.

Carcinogenesis, Mutagenesis, Impairment of Fertility: Lifetime studies with betaxolol HCl have been completed in mice at oral doses of 6, 20 or 60 mg/kg/day and in rats at 3, 12 or 48 mg/kg/day; betaxolol HCl demonstrated no carcinogenic effect. Higher dose levels were not tested.

In a variety of *in vitro* and *in vivo* bacterial and mammalian cell assays, betaxolol HCl was nonmutagenic.

Pregnancy: Pregnancy Category C. Reproduction, teratology, and peri- and postnatal studies have been conducted with orally administered betaxolol HCl in rats and rabbits. There was evidence of drug related postimplantation loss in rabbits and rats at dose levels above 12 mg/kg and 128 mg/kg, respectively. Betaxolol HCl was not shown to be teratogenic, however, and there were no other adverse effects on reproduction at subtoxic dose levels. There are no adequate and well-controlled studies in pregnant women. BETOPTIC S should be used during pregnancy only if the potential benefit justifies the potential risk to the fetus.

Nursing Mothers: It is not known whether betaxolol HCl is excreted in human milk. Because many drugs are excreted in human milk, caution should be exercised when BETOPTIC S Ophthalmic Suspension 0.25% is administered to nursing women.

Pediatric Use: Safety and effectiveness in pediatric patients not have been established.

ADVERSE REACTIONS

Ocular: In clinical trials, the most frequent event associated with the use of BETOPTIC S Ophthalmic Suspension 0.25% has been transient ocular discomfort. The following other conditions have been reported in small numbers of patients: blurred vision, corneal punctate keratitis, foreign body sensation, photophobia, tearing, itching, dryness of eyes, erythema, inflammation, discharge, ocular pain, decreased visual acuity and crusty lashes.

Additional medical events reported with other formulations of betaxolol include allergic reactions, decreased corneal sensitivity, corneal punctate staining which may appear in dendritic formations, edema and anisocoria.

Systemic: Systemic reactions following administration of BETOPTIC S Ophthalmic Suspension 0.25% or BETOPTIC Ophthalmic Solution 0.5% have been rarely reported. These include:

Cardiovascular: Bradycardia, heart block and congestive failure.

Pulmonary: Pulmonary distress characterized by dyspnea, bronchospasm, thickened bronchial secretions, asthma and respiratory failure.

Central Nervous System: Insomnia, dizziness, vertigo, headaches, depression, lethargy, and increase in signs and symptoms of myasthenia gravis.

Continued on next page

Betoptic S—Cont.

Other: Hives, toxic epidermal necrolysis, hair loss, and glossitis. Perversions of taste and smell have been reported.

OVERDOSAGE

No information is available on overdosage of humans. The oral LD50 of the drug ranged from 350–920 mg/kg in mice and 860–1050 mg/kg in rats. The symptoms which might be expected with an overdose of a systemically administered beta-1-adrenergic receptor blocking agent are bradycardia, hypotension and acute cardiac failure.

A topical overdose of BETOPTIC S Ophthalmic Suspension 0.25% may be flushed from the eye(s) with warm tap water.

DOSAGE AND ADMINISTRATION

The recommended dose is one to two drops of BETOPTIC S Ophthalmic Suspension 0.25% in the affected eye(s) twice daily. In some patients, the intraocular pressure lowering responses to BETOPTIC S may require a few weeks to stabilize. As with any new medication, careful monitoring of patients is advised.

If the intraocular pressure of the patient is not adequately controlled on this regimen, concomitant therapy with pilocarpine and other miotics, and/or epinephrine and/or carbonic anhydrase inhibitors can be instituted.

HOW SUPPLIED

BETOPTIC S Ophthalmic Suspension 0.25% is supplied as follows: 2.5, 5, 10 and 15 mL in plastic ophthalmic DROP-TAINER® dispensers.

2.5 mL: **NDC 0065-0246-20**
5 mL: **NDC 0065-0246-05**
10 mL: **NDC 0065-0246-10**
15 mL: **NDC 0065-0246-15**

STORAGE

Store upright at room temperature. Shake well before using.

Rx Only.

U.S. Patents Nos. 4,252,984; 4,311,708; 4,342,783; 4,911,920.

BION® TEARS
Lubricant Eye Drops   OTC

DESCRIPTION

BION® TEARS are specially designed to be physiologically compatible with the surface of the eye and to treat dry eye symptoms by replacing needed tear components. BION® TEARS advanced formula contains:

The unique DUASORB® polymeric system which combines with natural tears to soothe sensitive dry spots.

A special lubricating vehicle designed to match the electrolyte balance of sodium, potassium, calcium, magnesium, zinc and bicarbonate found in natural tears.

No preservatives or decongestants that may cause irritation or limit use. BION® TEARS may be used as often as necessary to provide relief.

BION® TEARS special formula requires special packaging. Airtight foil pouches are used to maintain the delicate balance of ingredients until the product is ready for use in the eye. **To ensure optimal effectiveness once the pouch is opened, the containers inside the pouch must be used within four days (96 hours).**

PLEASE READ THESE WARNINGS PRIOR TO USING BION® TEARS LUBRICANT EYE DROPS AND KEEP THIS INSERT FOR FUTURE REFERENCE.

WARNINGS

If you experience eye pain, changes in vision, continued redness or irritation of the eye, or if the condition worsens or persists for more than 72 hours, discontinue use and consult a doctor.

If solution changes color or becomes cloudy, do not use.

To avoid contamination, do not touch tip of container to any surface. Do not reuse. Once opened, discard. Keep this and all drugs out of the reach of children. In case of accidental ingestion, seek professional assistance or contact a Poison Control Center immediately.

HOW SUPPLIED

BION® TEARS Lubricant Eye Drops are supplied in boxes of 28 0.015 fl. oz. single-use containers.
Product Code 0065-0419-28

CILOXAN®   ℞
(Ciprofloxacin HCl)
0.3% as base
Sterile Ophthalmic Solution and Ointment

DESCRIPTION

CILOXAN® (Ciprofloxacin HCl) Ophthalmic Solution and Ointment are synthetic, sterile, multiple dose, antimicrobial for topical ophthalmic use. Ciprofloxacin is a fluoroquinolone antibacterial active against a broad spectrum of gram-positive and gram-negative ocular pathogens. It is available as the monohydrochloride monohydrate salt of 1-cyclopropyl-6-fluoro-1,4-dihydro-4-oxo-7-(1-piperazinyl)-3-quinoline-carboxylic acid. It is a faint to light yellow crystalline powder with a molecular weight of 385.8. Its empirical formula is $C_{17}H_{18}FN_3O_3 \cdot HCl \cdot H_2O$.

Ciprofloxacin differs from other quinolones in that it has a fluorine atom at the 6-position, a piperazine moiety at the 7-position, and a cyclopropyl ring at the 1-position.

Each mL of CILOXAN Ophthalmic Solution contains: **Active:** Ciprofloxacin HCl 3.5 mg equivalent to 3 mg base. **Preservative:** Benzalkonium Chloride 0.006%. **Inactive:** Sodium Acetate, Acetic Acid, Mannitol 4.6%, Edetate Disodium 0.05%, Hydrochloric Acid and/or Sodium Hydroxide (to adjust pH) and Purified Water. The pH is approximately 4.5 and the osmolality is approximately 300 mOsm.

Each gram of CILOXAN Ophthalmic Ointment contains: **Active:** Ciprofloxacin HCl 3.33 mg equivalent to 3 mg base. **Inactives:** Mineral Oil, White Petrolatum.

CLINICAL PHARMACOLOGY

Systemic Absorption: A systemic absorption study was performed in which CILOXAN Ophthalmic Solution was administerd in each eye every two hours while awake for two days followed by every four hours while awake for an additional 5 days. The maximum reported plasma concentration of ciprofloxacin was less than 5 ng/mL. The mean concentration was usually less than 2.5 ng/mL. Ointment mean concentration levels have not been determined but are expected to be similar.

Microbiology: Ciprofloxacin has in vitro activity against a wide range of gram-negative and gram-positive organisms. The bactericidal action of ciprofloxacin results from interference with the enzyme DNA gyrase which is needed for the synthesis of bacterial DNA.

Ciprofloxacin has been shown to be active against most strains of the following organisms both in vitro and in clinical infections. (See INDICATIONS AND USAGE section).

Gram-Positive:
Staphylococcus aureus (including methicillin-susceptible and methicillin-resistant strains)
Staphylococcus epidermidis
Streptococcus pneumoniae
Streptococcus (Viridans Group)

Gram-Negative:
Haemophilus influenzae
Pseudomonas aeruginosa
Serratia marcescens

Ciprofloxacin has been shown to be active in vitro against most strains of the following organisms, however, the clinical significance of these data is unknown:

Gram-Positive:
Bacillus species
Corynebacterium species
Enterococcus faecalis (Many strains are only moderately susceptible)
Staphylococcus haemolyticus
Staphylococcus hominis
Staphylococcus saprophyticus
Streptococcus pyogenes

Gram-Negative:
Acinetobacter caloacetius subsp anitratus
Aeromonas caviae
Aeromonas hydrophilia
Brucella melitensis
Campylobacter coli
Campylobacter jejuni
Citrobacter diversus
Citrobacter freundii
Edwardsiella tarda
Enterobacter aerogenes
Enterobacter cloacae
Eschricia coli
Haemophilius ducreyl
Haemophilius parainfluenzae
Klebsiella pneumoniae
Klebsiella oxytoca
Legionella pneumophila
Moraxella (Branhamella) catarrhalis
Morganella morganii
Neisseria gonorrhea
Neisseria meningitidis
Pasteurella multocida
Proteus mirabilis
Proteus vulgaris
Providencia rettgeri
Providencia stuartii
Salmonella enteritidis
Salmonella typhi
Shigella sonnei
Shigella flexneri
Vibrio cholerae
Vibrio parahaemolyticus
Vibrio vulnificus
Yersinia enterocolitica

Other Organisms:
Chlamydia trachomatis (only moderately susceptible) and Mycobacterium tuberculosis (only moderately susceptible). Most strains of Pseudomonas cepacia and Burkholderia cepacia and some strains of Pseudomonas maltophilia and Stenotrophomonas maltophilia are resistant to ciprofloxacin as are most anaerobic bacteria, including Bacteroides fragilis and Clostridium difficile.

The minimal bactericidal concentration (MBC) generally does not exceed the minimal inhibitory concentration (MIC) by more than a factor of 2. Resistance to ciprofloxacin in vitro usually develops slowly (multiple-step mutation).

Ciprofloxacin does not cross-react with other antimicrobial agents such as beta-lactams or aminoglycosides; therefore, organisms resistant to these drugs may be susceptible to ciprofloxacin. Organisms resistant to ciprofloxacin may be susceptible to beta-lactams or aminoglycosides.

Clinical Studies:
Following therapy with CILOXAN Ophthalmic Solution, 76% of the patients with corneal ulcers and positive bacterial cultures were clinically cured and complete re-epithelialization occurred in about 92% of the ulcers.

In 3 and 7 day multicenter trials, 52% of the patients with conjunctivitis and positive conjunctival cultures were clinically cured and 70–80% had all causative pathogens eradicated by the end of treatment. Following therapy with CILOXAN Ointment 75% of the patients with signs and symptoms of bacterial conjunctivitis and positive conjunctival cultures were clinically cured and approximately 80% had presumed pathogens eradicated by the end of treatment (day 7).

INDICATIONS AND USAGE

CILOXAN Ophthalmic Solution and CILOXAN Ophthalmic Ointment are indicated for the treatment of infections caused by susceptible strains of the designated microorganisms in the conditions listed below:

Conjunctivitis — Solution and Ointment:
Haemophilus influenzae
Staphylococcus aureus
Staphylococcus epidermidis
Streptococcus pneumoniae
Streptococcus (Viridans Group)

Corneal Ulcers — Solution only:
Pseudomonas aeruginosa
Serratia marcescens*
Staphylococcus aureus
Staphylococcus epidermidis
Streptococcus pneumoniae
Streptococcus (Viridans Group)*

*Efficacy for these organisms was studied in fewer than 10 infections.

CONTRAINDICATIONS

A history of hypersensitivity to ciprofloxacin or any other component of the medication is a contraindication to its use. A history of hypersensitivity to other quinolones may also contraindicate the use of ciprofloxacin.

WARNINGS

NOT FOR INJECTION INTO THE EYE.

Serious and occasionally fatal hypersensitivity (anaphylactic) reactions, some following the first dose, have been reported in patients receiving systemic quinolone therapy. Some reactions were accompanied by cardiovascular collapse, loss of consciousness, tingling, pharyngeal or facial edema, dyspnea, urticaria, and itching. Only a few patients had a history of hypersensitivity reactions. Serious anaphylactic reactions require immediate emergency treatment with epinephrine and other resuscitation measures, including oxygen, intravenous fluids, intravenous antihistamines, corticosteroids, pressor amines and airway management, as clinically indicated.

PRECAUTIONS

General: As with other antibacterial preparations, prolonged use of ciprofloxacin may result in overgrowth of non-susceptible organisms, including fungi. If superinfection occurs, appropriate therapy should be initiated. Whenever clinical judgment dictates, the patient should be examined with the aid of magnification, such as slit lamp biomicroscopy and, where appropriate, fluorescein staining.

Ciprofloxacin should be discontinued at the first appearance of a skin rash or any other sign of hypersensitivity reaction. Ophthalmic ointments may retard corneal healing and cause visual blurring. Patients should be advised not to wear contact lenses if they have signs and symptoms of bacterial conjunctivitis.

In clinical studies of patients with bacterial corneal ulcer, a white crystalline precipitate located in the superficial portion of the corneal defect was observed in 35 (16.6%) of 210 patients. The onset of the precipitate was within 24 hours to 7 days after starting therapy. In one patient, the precipitate was immediately irrigated out upon its appearance. In 17 patients, resolution of the precipitate was seen in 1 to 8 days (seven within the first 24–72 hours), in five patients,

resolution was noted in 10–13 days. In nine patients, exact resolution days were unavailable; however, at follow-up examinations, 18–44 days after onset of the event, complete resolution of the precipitate was noted. In three patients, outcome information was unavailable. The precipitate did not preclude continued use of ciprofloxacin, nor did it adversely affect the clinical course of the ulcer or visual outcome. (SEE ADVERSE REACTIONS).

Information for patients: Do not touch tip of any surface, as this may contaminate the product.

Drug Interactions: Specific drug interaction studies have not been conducted with ophthalmic ciprofloxacin. However, the systemic administration of some quinolones has been shown to elevate plasma concentrations of theophylline, interfere with the metabolism of caffeine, enhance the effects of the oral anticoagulant, warfarin, and its derivatives and has been associated with transient elevations in serum creatinine in patients receiving cyclosporine concomitantly.

Carcinogenesis, Mutagenesis, Impairment of Fertility: Eight in vitro mutagenicity tests have been conducted with ciprofloxacin and the test results are listed below:

Salmonella/Microsome Test (Negative)
E. coli DNA Repair Assay (Negative)
Mouse Lymphoma Cell Forward Mutation Assay (Positive)
Chinese Hamster V79 Cell HGPRT Test (Negative)
Syrian Hamster Embryo Cell Transformation Assay (Negative)
Saccharomyces cerevisiae Point Mutation Assay (Negative)
Saccharomyces cerevisiae Mitotic Crossover and Gene Conversion Assay (Negative)
Rat Hepatocyte DNA Repair Assay (Positive)

Thus, two of the eight tests were positive, but the results of the following three in vivo test systems gave negative results:

Rat Hepatocyte DNA Repair Assay
Micronucleus Test (Mice)
Dominant Lethal Test (Mice)

Long term carcinogenicity studies in mice and rats have been completed. After daily oral dosing for up to two years, there is no evidence that ciprofloxacin had any carcinogenic or tumorigenic effects in these species.

Pregnancy—Pregnancy Category C: Reproduction studies have been performed in rats and mice at doses up to six times the usual daily human oral dose and have revealed no evidence of impaired fertility or harm to the fetus due to ciprofloxacin. In rabbits, as with most antimicrobial agents, ciprofloxacin (30 and 100 mg/kg orally) produced gastrointestinal disturbances resulting in maternal weight loss and an increased incidence of abortion. No teratogenicity was observed at either dose. After intravenous administration, at doses up to 20 mg/kg, no maternal toxicity was produced and no embryotoxicity or teratogenicity was observed. There are no adequate and well controlled studies in pregnant women. CILOXAN® should be used during pregnancy only if the potential benefit justifies the potential risk to the fetus.

Nursing Mothers: It is not known whether topically applied ciprofloxacin is excreted in human milk; however, it is known that orally administered ciprofloxacin is excreted in the milk of lactating rats and oral ciprofloxacin has been reported in human breast milk after a single 500 mg dose. Caution should be exercised when CILOXAN is administered to a nursing mother.

Pediatric Use: Safety and effectiveness in pediatric patients below the age of 1 year (solution) and 2 years (ointment) have not been established.

Although ciprofloxacin and other quinolones cause arthropathy in immature Beagle dogs after oral administration, topical ocular administration of ciprofloxacin to immature animals did not cause any arthropathy and there is no evidence that the ophthalmic dosage form has any effect on the weight bearing joints.

ADVERSE REACTIONS

The most frequently reported drug related adverse reaction was local burning or discomfort. In corneal ulcer studies with frequent administration of the drug, white crystalline precipitates were seen in approximately 17% (solution) and 13% (ointment) of patients (SEE PRECAUTIONS). Other reactions occurring in less than 10% of patients included lid margin crusting, crystals/scales, foreign body sensation, itching, conjunctival hyperemia and a bad taste following instillation. Additional events occurring in less than 1% of patients included corneal staining, keratopathy/keratitis, allergic reactions, lid edema, tearing, photophobia, corneal infiltrates, nausea and decreased vision, blurred vision, dry eye, epitheliopathy, eye pain, irritation and dermatitis.

OVERDOSAGE

A topical overdose of CILOXAN Opthalmic Solution may be flushed from the (eye(s) with warm tap water.

DOSAGE AND ADMINISTRATION

Bacterial Conjunctivitis: Solution: The recommended dosage regimen for the treatment of bacterial conjunctivitis is one or two drops of CILOXAN Ophthalmic Solution instilled into the conjunctival sac(s) every two hours while awake for two days and one or two drops every four hours while awake for the next five days. Ointment: Apply a ½" ribbon into the conjunctival sac three times a day on the first two days, then apply a ½" ribbon two times a day for the next five days.

Corneal Ulcers: The recommended dosage regimen for the treatment of corneal ulcers is two drops of the Solution into the affected eye every 15 minutes for the first six hours and then two drops into the affected eye every 30 minutes for the remainder of the first day. On the second day, instill two drops in the affected eye hourly. On the third through the fourteenth day, place two drops in the affected eye every four hours. Treatment may be continued after 14 days if corneal re-epithelialization has not occurred.

HOW SUPPLIED

As a sterile ophthalmic solution in 2.5 mL (NDC 0065-0656-25) and 5 mL (NDC 0065-0656-05) in plastic DROP-TAINER® dispensers. Sterile ophthalmic ointment in 3.5 g ophthalmic tube (NDC 0065-0654-35).

STORAGE

Solution: Store at 2° to 30°C (36° to 86°F). Protect from light.

Ointment: Store at 36°F to 77°F (2°C to 25°C)

ANIMAL PHARMACOLOGY

Ciprofloxacin and related drugs have been shown to cause arthropathy in immature animals of most species tested following oral administration. However, a one-month topical ocular study using immature Beagle dogs did not demonstrate any articular lesions.

Rx Only

U.S. Patent No. 4,670,444
ALCON LABORATORIES, INC.
FORT WORTH, TEXAS 76134 USA

NAPHCON® A — OTC

Eye Drops
Relieves Itching & Redness

Temporary relief of the minor eye symptoms of itching and redness caused by ragweed, pollen, grass, animal hair, and dander.

DESCRIPTION

Active: Pheniramine Maleate 0.3%, Naphazoline Hydrochloride 0.025%. **Preservative:** Benzalkonium Chloride 0.01%. **Inactive:** Sodium Chloride, Boric Acid, Sodium Borate, Edetate Disodium 0.01%, Sodium Hydroxide and/or Hydrochloric Acid (to adjust pH), Purified Water. The sterile ophthalmic solution has a pH of about 6 and a tonicity of about 270 mOsm/Kg.

DIRECTIONS

Instill 1 or 2 drops in the affected eye(s) up to 4 times daily.

WARNINGS

To avoid contamination, do not touch tip of container to any surface. Replace cap after using.

If solution changes color or becomes cloudy, do not use.

If you experience eye pain, changes in vision, continued redness or irritation of the eye, or if the condition worsens, or persists for more than 72 hours, discontinue use and consult a physician. Overuse of this product may produce increased redness of the eye.

If you are sensitive to any ingredient in this product, do not use. Do not use use this product if you have heart disease, high blood pressure, difficulty in urination due to enlargement of the prostate gland or narrow angle glaucoma unless directed by a physician.

Accidental oral ingestion in infants and children may lead to coma and marked reduction in body temperature. Before using in children under 6 years of age, consult your physician.

Keep this and all drugs out of reach of children. In case of accidental ingestion, seek professional assistance or contact a Poison Control Center immediately.

Remove contact lenses before using.

Store at 36°–80°F (2°–27°C).

Protect from light.

Use before the expiration date marked on the carton or bottle.

Keep this and all drugs out of reach of children.

PATANOL® — ℞

(olopatadine hydrochloride ophthalmic solution) 0.1%

DESCRIPTION

PATANOL® (olopatadine hydrochloride ophthalmic solution) 0.1% is a sterile ophthalmic solution containing olopatadine, a relatively selective H_1-receptor antagonist and inhibitor of histamine release from the mast cell for topical administration to the eyes. Olopatadine hydrochloride is a white, crystalline, water-soluble powder with a molecular weight of 373.88.

Chemical Name: 11-[(Z)-3-(Dimethylamino)propylidene]-6-11-dihydrodibenz[b,e] oxepin-2-acetic acid hydrochloride

Each mL of PATANOL contains: **Active:** 1.11 mg olopatadine hydrochloride equivalent to 1 mg olopatadine. **Preservative:** benzalkonium chloride 0.01%. **Inactives:** dibasic sodium phosphate; sodium chloride; hydrochloric acid/sodium hydroxide (adjust pH); and purified water.

It has a pH of approximately 7 and an osmolality of approximately 300 mOsm/kg. DM-00

CLINICAL PHARMACOLOGY

Olopatadine is an inhibitor of the release of histamine from the mast cell and a relatively selective histamine H_1-antagonist that inhibits the *in vivo* and *in vitro* type 1 immediate hypersensitivity reaction. Olopatadine is devoid of effects on alpha-adrenergic, dopamine, muscarinic type 1 and 2, and serotonin receptors.

Following topical ocular administration in man, olopatadine was shown to have low systemic exposure. Two studies in normal volunteers (totaling 24 subjects) dosed bilaterally with olopatadine 0.15% ophthalmic solution once every 12 hours for 2 weeks demonstrated plasma concentrations to be generally below the quantitation limit of the assay (<0.5 ng/mL). Samples in which olopatadine was quantifiable were typically found within 2 hours of dosing and ranged from 0.5 to 1.3 ng/mL. The half-life in plasma was approximately 3 hours, and elimination was predominantly through renal excretion. Approximately 60–70% of the dose was recovered in the urine as parent drug. Two metabolites, the mono-desmethyl and the N-oxide, were detected at low concentrations in the urine.

Results from conjunctival antigen challenge studies demonstrated that PATANOL, when subjects were challenged with antigen both initially and up to 8 hours after dosing, was significantly more effective than its vehicle in preventing ocular itching associated with allergic conjunctivitis.

INDICATIONS AND USAGE

PATANOL (olopatadine hydrochloride ophthalmic solution) 0.1% is indicated for the temporary prevention of itching of the eye due to allergic conjunctivitis.

CONTRAINDICATIONS

PATANOL is contraindicated in persons with a known hypersensitivity to olopatadine hydrochloride or any components of PATANOL.

WARNINGS

PATANOL is for topical use only and not for injection or oral use.

PRECAUTIONS

Information for Patients To prevent contaminating the dropper tip and solution, care should be taken not to touch the eyelids or surrounding areas with the dropper tip of the bottle. Keep bottle tightly closed when not in use.

Patients should be advised not to wear a contact lens if their eye is red. PATANOL should not be used to treat contact lens related irritation. The preservative in PATANOL, benzalkonium chloride, may be absorbed by soft contact lenses. Patients who wear soft contact lenses and **whose eyes are not red**, should be instructed to wait at least ten minutes after instilling PATANOL before they insert their contact lenses.

Carcinogenesis, Mutagenesis, Impairment of Fertility: Olopatadine administered orally was not carcinogenic in mice and rats in doses up to 500 mg/kg/day and 200 mg/kg/day, respectively. Based on a 40 µl drop size, these doses were 78,125 and 31,250 times higher than the maximum recommended ocular human dose (MROHD). No mutagenic potential was observed when olopatadine was tested in an *in vitro* bacterial reverse mutation (Ames) test, an *in vitro* mammalian chromosome aberration assay or an *in vivo* mouse micronucleus test. Olopatadine administered to male and female rats at oral doses of 62,500 times MROHD level resulted in a slight decrease in the fertility index and reduced implantation rate; no effects on reproductive function were observed at doses of 7,800 times the maximum recommended ocular human use level.

Pregnancy: Pregnancy Category C. Olopatadine was found not to be teratogenic in rats and rabbits. However, rats treated at 600 mg/kg/day, or 93,750 times the MROHD and rabbits treated at 400 mg/kg/day, or 62,500 times the MROHD, during organogenesis showed a decrease in live fetuses. There are, however, no adequate and well controlled studies in pregnant women. Because animal studies are not always predictive of human responses, this drug should be used in pregnant women only if the potential benefit to the mother justifies the potential risk to the embryo or fetus.

Nursing Mothers: Olopatadine has been identified in the milk of nursing rats following oral administration. It is not known whether topical ocular administration could result in

Continued on next page

Patanol—Cont.

sufficient systemic absorption to produce detectable quantities in the human breast milk. Nevertheless, caution should be exercised when PATANOL is administered to a nursing mother.

Pediatric Use: Safety and effectiveness in pediatric patients below the age of 3 years have not been established.

ADVERSE REACTIONS

Headaches were reported at an incidence of 7%. The following adverse experiences were reported in less than 5% of patients: Asthenia, burning or stinging, cold syndrome, dry eye, foreign body sensation, hyperemia, keratitis, lid edema, pharyngitis, pruritus, rhinitis, sinusitis, and taste perversion. Some of these events were similar to the underlying disease being studied.

DOSAGE AND ADMINISTRATION

The recommended dose is one to two drops in each affected eye two times per day at an interval of 6 to 8 hours.

HOW SUPPLIED

PATANOL (olopatadine hydrochloride ophthalmic solution) 0.1% is supplied as follows: 5 mL in plastic DROP-TAINER® dispenser.

5 mL: NDC 0065-0271-05

Storage:

Store at 39°F to 86°F (4°C to 30°C)

U.S. Patents Nos. 4,871,865; 4,923,892; 5,116,863; 5,641,805.

Rx Only.

TEARS NATURALE® II — OTC
Lubricant Eye Drops
TEARS NATURALE FREE®
Lubricant Eye Drops

DESCRIPTION

TEARS NATURALE II is the only lubricant eye drop preserved with safe, nonsensitizing POLYQUAD 0.001%. *In vitro* studies have shown that POLYQUAD substantially avoids the damaging effects of epithelial cell toxicity possible with other tear substitute preservatives and allows epithelial cell growth. POLYQUAD has been shown to be 99% reaction-free in normal subjects and 97% reaction-free in subjects known to be preservative sensitive. TEARS NATURALE FREE is a preservative-free version of TEARS NATURALE II.

With their unique mucin like polymeric formulation, and with their natural pH, low viscosity, and isotonicity, TEARS NATURALE II and TEARS NATURALE FREE provide dry eye patients with comfort and prompt relief of dry eye symptoms.

Sterile-For Topical Eye Use Only

INGREDIENTS

TEARS NATURALE II: Each mL contains: **Active:** DUASORB®, a water soluble polymeric system containing Dextran 70 0.1% and Hydroxypropyl Methylcellulose 2910 0.3%.

Preservative: POLYQUAD® (Polyquaternium-1) 0.001%. **Inactive:** Sodium Borate, Potassium Chloride, Sodium Chloride, Purified Water. May contain Hydrochloric Acid and/or Sodium Hydroxide to adjust pH.

TEARS NATURALE FREE: Each mL contains:

Active: DUASORB®, a water soluble polymeric system containing Dextran 70 0.1% and Hydroxypropyl Methylcellulose 2910 0.3%.

Inactives: Sodium Borate, Potassium Chloride, Sodium Chloride, Purified Water. May contain Hydrochloric Acid and/or Sodium Hydroxide to adjust pH.

INDICATIONS

For the temporary relief of burning and irritation due to dryness of the eye and for use as a protectant against further irritation. For temporary relief of discomfort due to minor irritations of the eye or to exposure to wind or sun.

WARNINGS

Remove contact lenses before using. If you experience eye pain, changes in vision, continued redness or irritation of the eye, or if the condition worsens or persists for more than 72 hours, discontinue use and consult a doctor.

If solution changes color or becomes cloudy, do not use.

To avoid contamination, do not touch tip of container to any surface. Replace cap after using. Keep this and all drugs out of the reach of children. In case of accidental ingestion, seek professional assistance or contact a Poison Control Center immediately.

DIRECTIONS

TEARS NATURALE II: Instill 1 or 2 drops in the affected eye(s) as needed. TEARS NATURALE FREE: Completely TWIST off tab: do NOT pull. Instill 1 or 2 drops in the affected eye(s) as needed. To close, press tab down over container tip and twist. Reclosed vial may leak under pressure. **DISCARD CONTAINER 12 HOURS AFTER OPENING.**

HOW SUPPLIED

TEARS NATURALE II Lubricant Eye Drops are supplied in 15 mL and 30 mL plastic DROP-TAINER® bottles.

15 mL NDC 0065-0418-15
30 mL NDC 0065-0418-30

TEARS NATURALE FREE Lubricant Eye Drops are supplied in boxes of 32 0.03 fl. oz. re-closable containers.

NDC 0065-0416-32

STORAGE

Store at room temperature.

TOBRADEX® — ℞
(tobramycin and dexamethasone ophthalmic suspension and ointment)
Sterile

DESCRIPTION

TOBRADEX® (tobramycin and dexamethasone) ophthalmic suspension and ointment are sterile, multiple dose antibiotic and steroid combinations for topical ophthalmic use.

Tobramycin

Chemical name:

O -3-Amino-3-deoxy-α-D-glucopyranosyl-(1→4)-*O* -[2,6-diamino-2,3,6-trideoxy-α-D-*ribo* -hexopyranosyl-(1→6)]-2-deoxy-L-streptamine

Dexamethasone

Chemical Name:

9-Fluoro-11β,17,21-trihydroxy-16α-methylpregna-1,4-diene-3,20-dione

Each mL of TOBRADEX® Suspension contains: Active: Tobramycin 0.3% (3 mg) and Dexamethasone 0.1% (1 mg). Preservative: Benzalkonium Chloride 0.01%. Inactives: Tyloxapol, Edetate Disodium, Sodium Chloride, Hydroxyethyl Cellulose, Sodium Sulfate, Sulfuric Acid and/or Sodium Hydroxide (to adjust pH) and Purified Water.

Each gram of TOBRADEX® Ointment contains: Actives: Tobramycin 0.3% (3 mg) and Dexamethasone 0.1% (1 mg). Preservative: Chlorobutanol 0.5%. Inactives: Mineral Oil and White Petrolatum.

CLINICAL PHARMACOLOGY

Corticoids suppress the inflammatory response to a variety of agents and they probably delay or slow healing. Since corticoids may inhibit the body's defense mechanism against infection, a concomitant antimicrobial drug may be used when this inhibition is considered to be clinically significant. Dexamethasone is a potent corticoid.

The antibiotic component in the combination (tobramycin) is included to provide action against susceptible organisms. *In vitro* studies have demonstrated that tobramycin is active against susceptible strains of the following microorganisms:

Staphylococci, including *S. aureus* and *S. epidermidis* (coagulase-positive and coagulase-negative), including penicillin-resistant strains.

Streptococci, including some of the Group A-beta-hemolytic species, some nonhemolytic species, and some *Streptococcus pneumoniae.*

Pseudomonas aeruginosa, Escherichia coli, Klebsiella pneumoniae, Enterobacter aerogenes, Proteus mirabilis, Morganella morganii, most *Proteus vulgaris* strains, *Haemophilus influenzae* and *H. aegyptius, Moraxella lacunata, Acinetobacter calcoaceticus* and some *Neisseria* species.

Bacterial susceptibility studies demonstrate that in some cases microorganisms resistant to gentamicin remain susceptible to tobramycin.

No data are available on the extent of systemic absorption from TOBRADEX® Ophthalmic Suspension or Ointment; however, it is known that some systemic absorption can occur with ocularly applied drugs. If the maximum dose of TOBRADEX Ophthalmic Suspension is given for the first 48 hours (two drops in each eye every 2 hours) and complete systemic absorption occurs, which is highly unlikely, the daily dose of dexamethasone would be 2.4 mg. The usual physiologic replacement dose is 0.75 mg daily. If TOBRADEX Ophthalmic Suspension is given after the first 48 hours as two drops in each eye every 4 hours, the administered dose of dexamethasone would be 1.2 mg daily. The administered dose for TOBRADEX Ophthalmic Ointment in both eyes four times daily would be 0.4 mg of dexamethasone daily.

INDICATIONS AND USAGE

TOBRADEX® Ophthalmic Suspension and Ointment are indicated for steroid-responsive inflammatory ocular conditions for which a corticosteroid is indicated and where superficial bacterial ocular infection or a risk of bacterial ocular infection exists.

Ocular steroids are indicated in inflammatory conditions of the palpebral and bulbar conjunctiva, cornea and anterior segment of the globe where the inherent risk of steroid use in certain infective conjunctivitides is accepted to obtain a diminution in edema and inflammation. They are also indicated in chronic anterior uveitis and corneal injury from chemical, radiation or thermal burns, or penetration of foreign bodies.

The use of a combination drug with an anti-infective component is indicated where the risk of superficial ocular infection is high or where there is an expectation that potentially dangerous numbers of bacteria will be present in the eye.

The particular anti-infective drug in this product is active against the following common bacterial eye pathogens:

Staphylococci, including *S. aureus* and *S. epidermidis* (coagulase-positive and coagulase-negative), including penicillin-resistant strains.

Streptococci, including some of the Group A-beta-hemolytic species, some nonhemolytic species, and some *Streptococcus pneumoniae.*

Pseudomonas aeruginosa, Escherichia coli, Klebsiella pneumoniae, Enterobacter aerogenes, Proteus mirabilis, Morganella morganii, most *Proteus vulgaris* strains, *Haemophilus influenzae* and *H. aegyptius, Moraxella lacunata, Acinetobacter calcoaceticus* and some *Neisseria* species.

CONTRAINDICATIONS

Epithelial herpes simplex keratitis (dendritic keratitis), vaccinia, varicella, and many other viral diseases of the cornea and conjunctiva. Mycobacterial infection of the eye. Fungal diseases of ocular structures. Hypersensitivity to a component of the medication.

WARNINGS

NOT FOR INJECTION INTO THE EYE. Sensitivity to topically applied aminoglycosides may occur in some patients. If a sensitivity reaction does occur, discontinue use.

Prolonged use of steroids may result in glaucoma, with damage to the optic nerve, defects in visual acuity and fields of vision, and posterior subcapsular cataract formation. Intraocular pressure should be routinely monitored even though it may be difficult in children and uncooperative patients. Prolonged use may suppress the host response and thus increase the hazard of secondary ocular infections. In those diseases causing thinning of the cornea or sclera, perforations have been known to occur with the use of topical steroids. In acute purulent conditions of the eye, steroids may mask infection or enhance existing infection.

PRECAUTIONS

General. The possibility of fungal infections of the cornea should be considered after long-term steroid dosing. As with other antibiotic preparations, prolonged use may result in overgrowth of nonsusceptible organisms, including fungi. If superinfection occurs, appropriate therapy should be initiated. When multiple prescriptions are required, or whenever clinical judgement dictates, the patient should be examined with the aid of magnification, such as slit lamp biomicroscopy and, where appropriate, fluorescein staining.

Cross-sensitivity to other aminoglycoside antibiotics may occur; if hypersensitivity develops with this product, discontinue use and institute appropriate therapy.

Information for Patients: Do not touch dropper or tube tip to any surface, as this may contaminate the contents.

Carcinogenesis, Mutagenesis, Impairment of Fertility. No studies have been conducted to evaluate the carcinogenic or mutagenic potential. No impairment of fertility was noted in studies of subcutaneous tobramycin in rats at doses of 50 and 100 mg/kg/day.

Pregnancy Category C. Corticosteroids have been found to be teratogenic in animal studies. Ocular administration of 0.1% dexamethasone resulted in 15.6% and 32.3% incidence of fetal anomalies in two groups of pregnant rabbits. Fetal growth retardation and increased mortality rates have been observed in rats with chronic dexamethasone therapy. Reproduction studies have been performed in rats and rabbits with tobramycin at doses up to 100 mg/ kg/day parenterally and have revealed no evidence of impaired fertility or harm to the fetus. There are no adequate and well-controlled studies in pregnant women. TOBRADEX® Ophthalmic Suspension and Ointment should be used during pregnancy only if the potential benefit justifies the potential risk to the fetus.

Nursing Mothers.

Systemically administered corticosteroids appear in human milk and could suppress growth, interfere with endogenous corticosteroid production, or cause other untoward effects. It is not known whether topical administration of corticosteroids could result in sufficient systemic absorption to produce detectable quantities in human milk. Because many drugs are excreted in human milk, caution should be exercised when TOBRADEX® Ophthalmic Suspension or ointment is administered to a nursing woman.

Pediatric Use. Safety and effectiveness in pediatric patients have not been established.

ADVERSE REACTIONS

Adverse reactions have occurred with steroid/anti-infective combination drugs which can be attributed to the steroid

component, the anti-infective component, or the combination. Exact incidence figures are not available. The most frequent adverse reactions to topical ocular tobramycin (TOBREX) are hypersensitivity and localized ocular toxicity, including lid itching and swelling, and conjunctival erythema. These reactions occur in less than 4% of patients. Similar reactions may occur with the topical use of other aminoglycoside antibiotics. Other adverse reactions have not been reported; however, if topical ocular tobramycin is administered concomitantly with systemic aminoglycoside antibiotics, care should be taken to monitor the total serum concentration. The reactions due to the steroid component are: elevation of intraocular pressure (IOP) with possible development of glaucoma, and infrequent optic nerve damage; posterior subcapsular cataract formation; and delayed wound healing.

Secondary Infection. The development of secondary infection has occurred after use of combinations containing steroids and antimicrobials. Fungal infections of the cornea are particularly prone to develop coincidentally with long-term applications of steroids. The possibility of fungal invasion must be considered in any persistent corneal ulceration where steroid treatment has been used. Secondary bacterial ocular infection following suppression of host responses also occurs.

OVERDOSAGE

Clinically apparent signs and symptoms of an overdose of TOBRADEX Ophthalmic Ointment (punctate keratitis, erythema, increased lacrimation, edema and lid itching) may be similar to adverse reaction effects seen in some patients.

DOSAGE AND ADMINISTRATION

Apply a small amount (approximately 1/2 inch ribbon) into the conjunctival sac(s) up to three or four times daily.
Suspension: One or two drops instilled into the conjunctival sac(s) every four to six hours. During the initial 24 to 48 hours, the dosage may be increased to one or two drops every two (2) hours. Frequency should be decreased gradually as warranted by improvement in clinical signs. Care should be taken not to discontinue therapy prematurely. **Ointment.** Apply a small amount (approximately $^1/_2$ inch ribbon) into the conjunctival sac(s) up to three or four times daily.
How to apply TOBRADEX Ophthalmic Ointment:
1. Tilt your head back.
2. Place a finger on your cheek just under your eye and gently pull down until a "V" pocket is formed between your eyeball and your lower lid.
3. Place a small amount (about 1/2 inch) of TOBRADEX Ophthalmic Ointment in the "V" pocket. Do not let the tip of the tube touch your eye.
4. Look downward before closing your eye.
Not more than 20 mL or 8 g should be prescribed initially and the prescription should not be refilled without further evaluation as outlined in PRECAUTIONS above.

HOW SUPPLIED

Sterile ophthalmic suspension in 2.5 mL (NDC 0065-0647-25), 5 mL (NDC 0065-0647-05) and 10 mL (NDC 0065-0647-10) DROP-TAINER® dispensers. Sterile ophthalmic ointment in 3.5 g ophthalmic tube (NDC 0065-0648-35).

STORAGE

Store at 8° to 27°C (46° to 80°F).
Store suspension upright and shake well before using.
Rx Only.
U.S. Patent No. 5,149,694

Allergan, Inc.
2525 DUPONT DRIVE
P.O. BOX 19534
IRVINE, CA 92623-9534

Direct Inquiries to:
(714) 246-4500

OPHTHALMIC PRODUCTS

For information on Allergan, Inc., prescription, OTC, and ophthalmic products, consult the Physicians' Desk Reference for Ophthalmology. For literature, service items, or sample material, contact Allergan directly. See a complete listing of products in the Manufacturers' Index section of this book.

ACULAR®   ℞
(ketorolac tromethamine ophthalmic solution) 0.5% Sterile

PRODUCT OVERVIEW

ACULAR® (ketorolac tromethamine ophthalmic solution) 0.5% is the only topical NSAID indicated for the temporary

relief of ocular itching due to seasonal allergic conjunctivitis. ACULAR® is also indicated for the treatment of postoperative inflammation in patients who have undergone cataract extraction.
ACULAR® relieves the ocular itch associated with seasonal allergic conjunctivitis and inflammation following cataract surgery due in part to its ability to inhibit prostaglandin biosynthesis.
In two double-masked, paired studies (N=241), ACULAR® Solution was found to be superior to placebo in relieving the ocular itch of seasonal allergic conjunctivitis.[1]
Two controlled clinical studies showed that patients treated for two weeks with ACULAR® ophthalmic solution were less likely to have measurable signs of inflammation (cell and flare) than patients treated with its vehicle.
ACULAR® Solution is also proven safe in clinical trials, and avoids steroid-like side effects (e.g., no significant effect upon IOP).[1] There is no significant ocular toxicity reported in clinical studies to date with ACULAR®.
The most frequently reported adverse events have been transient stinging and burning on instillation (approximately 40%). Caution should be used in patients with sensitivities to other NSAIDs.
ACULAR® Solution is available in 3 mL, 5 mL and 10 mL plastic bottles with a controlled-dropper tip.
Please see full prescribing information included.
1. Data on file, Syntex (U.S.A.) Inc.
ACULAR®, a registered trademark of Syntex (U.S.A.) Inc., is manufactured and distributed by Allergan, Inc. under license from its developer, Syntex (U.S.A.) Inc., Palo Alto, CA.
ACULAR® is marketed by Allergan, Inc.

PRESCRIBING INFORMATION

ACULAR®   ℞
(ketorolac tromethamine ophthalmic solution) 0.5% Sterile

DESCRIPTION

ACULAR® (ketorolac tromethamine ophthalmic solution) is a member of the pyrrolo-pyrrole group of nonsteroidal anti-inflammatory drugs (NSAIDs) for ophthalmic use. Its chemical name is $(\pm)$-5-benzoyl-2,3-dihydro-1H-pyrrolizine-1-carboxylic acid compound with 2-amino-2-(hydroxymethyl)-1,3-propanediol (1:1).
ACULAR® is supplied as a sterile isotonic aqueous 0.5% solution, with a pH of 7.4. ACULAR® is a racemic mixture of R-(+)- and S-(-)- ketorolac tromethamine. Ketorolac tromethamine may exist in three crystal forms. All forms are equally soluble in water. The pKa of ketorolac is 3.5. This white to off-white crystalline substance discolors on prolonged exposure to light. The molecular weight of ketorolac tromethamine is 376.41. Each mL of ACULAR® ophthalmic solution contains: Active: ketorolac tromethamine 0.5%. Preservative: benzalkonium chloride 0.01%. Inactives: edetate disodium 0.1%; octoxynol 40; sodium chloride; hydrochloric acid and/or sodium hydroxide to adjust the pH; and purified water. The osmolality of ACULAR® is 290 mOsmol/kg.

ANIMAL PHARMACOLOGY

Ketorolac tromethamine prevented the development of increased intraocular pressure induced in rabbits with topically applied arachidonic acid. Ketorolac did not inhibit rabbit lens aldose reductase *in vitro*.
Ketorolac tromethamine ophthalmic solution did not enhance the spread of ocular infections induced in rabbits with *Candida albicans*, *Herpes simplex* virus type one, or *Pseudomonas aeruginosa*.

CLINICAL PHARMACOLOGY

Ketorolac tromethamine is nonsteroidal anti-inflammatory drug which, when administered systemically, has demonstrated analgesic, anti-inflammatory, and anti-pyretic activity. The mechanism of its action is thought to be due, in part, to its ability to inhibit prostaglandin biosynthesis. Ketorolac tromethamine given systemically does not cause pupil constriction.
Prostaglandins have been shown in many animal models to be mediators of certain kinds of intraocular inflammation. In studies performed in animal eyes, prostaglandins have been shown to produce disruption of the blood-aqueous humor barrier, vasodilation, increased vascular permeability, leukocytosis, and increased intraocular pressure. Prostaglandins also appear to play a role in the miotic response produced during ocular surgery by constricting the iris sphincter independently of cholinergic mechanisms.
Two drops (0.1 mL) of 0.5% ACULAR® ophthalmic solution instilled into the eyes of patients 12 hours and 1 hour prior to cataract extraction achieved measurable levels in 8 of 9 patients' eyes (mean ketorolac concentration 95 ng/mL aqueous humor, range 40 to 170 ng/mL). Ocular administration of ketorolac tromethamine reduces prostaglandin E_2 (PGE$_2$) levels in aqueous humor. The mean concentration of PGE$_2$ was 80 pg/mL in the aqueous humor of eyes receiving vehicle and 28 pg/mL in the eyes receiving ACULAR® 0.5% ophthalmic solution.

One drop (0.05 mL) of 0.5% ACULAR® ophthalmic solution was instilled into one eye and one drop of vehicle into the other eye TID in 26 normal subjects. Only 5 of 26 subjects had a detectable amount of ketorolac in their plasma (range 10.7 to 22.5 ng/mL) at Day 10 during topical ocular treatment. When ketorolac tromethamine 10 mg is administered systemically every 6 hours, peak plasma levels at steady state are around 960 ng/mL.
Two controlled clinical studies showed that ACULAR® ophthalmic solution was significantly more effective than its vehicle in relieving ocular itching caused by seasonal allergic conjunctivitis.
Two controlled clinical studies showed that patients treated for two weeks with ACULAR® ophthalmic solution were less likely to have measurable signs of inflammation (cell and flare) than patients treated with its vehicle.
Results from clinical studies indicate that ACULAR® has no significant effect upon intraocular pressure; however, changes in intraocular pressure may occur following cataract surgery.
ACULAR® ophthalmic solution has been safely administered in conjunction with other ophthalmic medications such as antibiotics, beta blockers, carbonic anhydrase inhibitors, cycloplegics, and mydriatics.

INDICATIONS AND USAGE

ACULAR® ophthalmic solution is indicated for the temporary relief of ocular itching due to seasonal allergic conjunctivitis. ACULAR® is also indicated for the treatment of postoperative inflammation in patients who have undergone cataract extraction.

CONTRAINDICATIONS

ACULAR® ophthalmic solution is contraindicated in patients with previously demonstrated hypersensitivity to any of the ingredients in the formulation.

WARNINGS

There is the potential for cross-sensitivity to acetylsalicylic acid, phenylacetic acid derivatives, and other nonsteroidal anti-inflammatory agents. Therefore, caution should be used when treating individuals who have previously exhibited sensitivities to these drugs.
With some nonsteroidal anti-inflammatory drugs, there exists the potential for increased bleeding time due to interference with thrombocyte aggregation. There have been reports that ocularly applied nonsteroidal anti-inflammatory drugs may cause increased bleeding of ocular tissues (including hyphemas) in conjunction with ocular surgery.

PRECAUTIONS

General: It is recommended that ACULAR® ophthalmic solution be used with caution in patients with known bleeding tendencies or who are receiving other medications which may prolong bleeding time.
Information for Patients: ACULAR® should not be administered while wearing contact lenses.
Carcinogenesis, Mutagenesis, and Impairment of Fertility: An 18-month study in mice at oral doses of ketorolac tromethamine equal to the parenteral MRHD (Maximum Recommended Human Dose) and a 24-month study in rats at oral doses 2.5 times the parenteral MRHD, showed no evidence of tumorigenicity.
Ketorolac tromethamine was not mutagenic in Ames test, unscheduled DNA synthesis and repair, and in forward mutation assays. Ketorolac did not cause chromosome breakage in the *in vivo* mouse micronucleus assay. At 1590 ug/mL (approximately 1000 times the average human plasma levels) and at higher concentrations, ketorolac tromethamine increased the incidence of chromosomal aberrations in Chinese hamster ovarian cells.
Impairment of fertility did not occur in male or female rats at oral doses of 9 mg/kg and 16 mg/kg respectively.
Pregnancy:
Pregnancy Category C. Reproduction studies have been performed in rabbits, using daily oral doses at 3.6 mg/kg and in rats at 10 mg/kg during organogenesis. Results of these studies did not reveal evidence of teratogenicity to the fetus. Oral doses of ketorolac tromethamine at 1.5 mg/kg, which was half of the human oral exposure, administered after gestation day 17 caused dystocia and higher pup mortality in rats. There are no adequate and well-controlled studies in pregnant women. Ketorolac tromethamine should be used during pregnancy only if the potential benefit justifies the potential risk to the fetus.
Nonteratogenic Effects: Because of the known effects of prostaglandin-inhibiting drugs on the fetal cardiovascular system (closure of the ductus arteriosus), the use of ACULAR® ophthalmic solution during late pregnancy should be avoided.
Nursing Mothers: Caution should be exercised when ACULAR® is administered to a nursing woman.
Pediatric Use: Safety and efficacy in pediatric patients below the age of 12 have not been established.

Continued on next page

Acular—Cont.

ADVERSE REACTIONS

In controlled clinical studies, the most frequent adverse events reported with the use of ACULAR® ophthalmic solution have been transient stinging and burning on instillation. These events were reported by up to 40% of patients treated with ACULAR® ophthalmic solution. In all development studies conducted, other adverse events occurring less than 5% of the time during treatment with ACULAR® included ocular irritation, allergic reactions, superficial ocular infections, and superficial keratitis.
Other adverse events reported rarely with the use of ACULAR® ophthalmic solution include: eye dryness, corneal infiltrates, corneal ulcer, and visual disturbance (blurry vision).

DOSAGE AND ADMINISTRATION

The recommended dose of ACULAR® ophthalmic solution is one drop (0.25 mg) four times a day for relief of ocular itching due to seasonal allergic conjunctivitis.
For the treatment of postoperative inflammation in patients who have undergone cataract extraction, one drop of ACULAR® ophthalmic solution should be applied to the affected eye(s) four times daily beginning 24 hours after cataract surgery and continuing through the first 2 weeks of the postoperative period.

HOW SUPPLIED

ACULAR® (ketorolac tromethamine ophthalmic solution) is available for topical ophthalmic administration as a 0.5% sterile solution, and is supplied in white opaque plastic bottles with a controlled dropper tip in the following sizes:
3 mL —NDC 0023-2181-03
5 mL —NDC 0023-2181-05
10 mL—NDC 0023-2181-10
Store at controlled room temperature 15–30°C (59–86°F) with protection from light.
Rx only
U.S. Patent Nos. 4,089,969; 4,454,151; 5,110,493
ACULAR®, a registered trademark of Syntex (U.S.A.) Inc., is manufactured and distributed by Allergan, Inc. under license from its developer, Syntex (U.S.A.) Inc., Palo Alto, California, U.S.A.

ALLERGAN

©1997 Allergan, Inc.
Irvine, CA 92612

ACULAR® PF ℞
(ketorolac tromethamine ophthalmic solution) 0.5% Preservative-Free

DESCRIPTION

ACULAR® PF (ketorolac tromethamine ophthalmic solution) Preservative-Free is a member of the pyrrolo-pyrrole group of nonsteroidal anti-inflammatory drugs (NSAIDs) for ophthalmic use. Ketorolac tromethamine's chemical name is (±)-5-benzoyl-2,3-dihydro-1H pyrrolizine-1-carboxylic acid compound with 2-amino-2-(hydroxymethyl)-1,3-propanediol (1:1).
ACULAR® PF is a racemic mixture of R-(+) and S-(-)-ketorolac tromethamine. Ketorolac tromethamine may exist in three crystal forms. All forms are equally soluble in water. The pKa of ketorolac is 3.5. This white to off-white crystalline substance discolors on prolonged exposure to light. The molecular weight of ketorolac tromethamine is 376.41. The osmolality of ACULAR® PF is 290 mOsmol/kg. Each ml of ACULAR® PF contains: Active ingredient: ketorolac tromethamine 0.5%. Inactives: sodium chloride; hydrochloric acid and/or sodium hydroxide to adjust the pH to 7.4; and purified water.

CLINICAL PHARMACOLOGY

Ketorolac tromethamine is a nonsteroidal anti-inflammatory drug which, when administered systemically, has demonstrated analgesic, anti-inflammatory, and anti-pyretic activity. The mechanism of its action is thought to be due to its ability to inhibit prostaglandin biosynthesis. Ketorolac tromethamine given systemically does not cause pupil constriction.
One drop (0.05 mL) of ketorolac tromethamine (preserved) was instilled into one eye and one drop of vehicle into the other eye TID in 26 normal subjects. Only 5 of 26 subjects had a detectable amount of ketorolac in their plasma (range 10.7 to 22.5 ng/mL) at day 10 during topical ocular treatment. When ketorolac tromethamine 10 mg is administered systemically every 6 hours, peak plasma levels at steady state are around 960 ng/mL.
In two double-masked, multi-centered, parallel-group studies, 340 patients who had undergone incisional refractive surgery received ACULAR® PF or its vehicle QID for up to 3 days. Significant differences favored ACULAR® PF for the treatment of ocular pain and photophobia.
Results from clinical studies indicate that ketorolac tromethamine has no significant effect upon intraocular pressure.

INDICATIONS AND USAGE

ACULAR® PF ophthalmic solution is indicated for the reduction of ocular pain and photophobia following incisional refractive surgery.

CONTRAINDICATIONS

ACULAR® PF is contraindicated in patients with previously demonstrated hypersensitivity to any of the ingredients in the formulation.

WARNINGS

There is the potential for cross-sensitivity to acetylsalicylic acid, phenylacetic acid derivatives, and other nonsteroidal anti-inflammatory agents. Therefore, caution should be used when treating individuals who have previously exhibited sensitivities to these drugs.
With some nonsteroidal anti-inflammatory drugs, there exists the potential for increased bleeding time due to interference with thrombocyte aggregation. There have been reports that ocularly applied nonsteroidal anti-inflammatory drugs may cause increased bleeding of ocular tissues (including hyphemas) in conjunction with ocular surgery.

PRECAUTIONS

General: It is recommended that ACULAR® PF be used with caution in surgical patients with known bleeding tendencies or who are receiving other medications which may prolong bleeding time.
Wound healing may be delayed with the use of ACULAR® PF.
Information for Patients: ACULAR® PF should not be administered while wearing contact lenses.
The solution from one individual single-use vial is to be used immediately after opening for administration to one or both eyes, and the remaining contents should be discarded immediately after administration. To avoid contamination, do not touch tip of unit-dose vial to eye or any other surface.
Carcinogenesis, Mutagenesis, and Impairment of Fertility: An 18-month study in mice at oral doses of ketorolac tromethamine equal to the parenteral MRHD (Maximum Recommended Human Dose) and a 24-month study in rats at oral doses 2.5 times the parenteral MRHD, showed no evidence of tumorigenicity.
Ketorolac tromethamine was not mutagenic in the Ames test, unscheduled DNA synthesis and repair, and forward mutation assays. Ketorolac did not cause chromosome breakage in the *in vivo* mouse micronucleus assay. At 1590 µg/mL (approximately 1000 times the average human plasma levels) and at higher concentrations, ketorolac tromethamine increased the incidence of chromosomal aberrations in Chinese hamster ovarian cells.
Impairment of fertility did not occur in male or female rats at oral doses of 9 mg/kg and 16 mg/kg, respectively.
Pregnancy: Teratogenic Effects: Pregnancy Category C: Reproduction studies have been performed in rabbits, using daily oral doses at 3.6 mg/kg and in rats at 10 mg/kg during organogenesis. Results of these studies did not reveal evidence of teratogenicity to the fetus. Oral doses of ketorolac tromethamine at 1.5 mg/kg, which was half of the human oral exposure, administered after gestation day 17 caused dystocia and higher pup mortality in rats. There are no adequate and well-controlled studies in pregnant women. Ketorolac tromethamine should be used during pregnancy only if the potential benefit justifies the potential risk to the fetus.
Nonteratogenic Effects: Because of the known effects of prostaglandin-inhibiting drugs on the fetal cardiovascular system (closure of the ductus arteriosus), the use of ACULAR® PF during late pregnancy should be avoided.
Nursing Mothers: Caution should be exercised when ACULAR® PF is administered to a nursing woman.
Pediatric Use: Safety and efficacy in pediatric patients below the age of 12 years have not been established.

ADVERSE REACTIONS

The most frequent adverse events reported with the use of ketorolac tromethamine ophthalmic solutions have been transient stinging and burning on instillation. These events were reported by approximately 20% of patients participating in clinical trials.
Other adverse events occurring 1%–10% of the time during treatment with ketorolac tromethamine ophthalmic solutions included ocular irritation, allergic reactions, superficial ocular infections, superficial keratitis, ocular inflammation, corneal edema, and iritis.
Other adverse events reported rarely with the use of ketorolac tromethamine ophthalmic solutions include: eye dryness, corneal infiltrates, corneal ulcer, visual disturbance (blurry vision), and headaches.

DOSAGE AND ADMINISTRATION

The recommended dose of ACULAR® PF Preservative-Free is one drop (0.25 mg) four times a day in the operated eye as needed for pain and photophobia for up to 3 days after incisional refractive surgery.

HOW SUPPLIED

ACULAR® PF (ketorolac tromethamine ophthalmic solution) 0.5% Preservative-Free is available as a sterile solution supplied in single-use vials as follows: ACULAR® PF 12 Single-Use Vials 0.4 mL each - NDC 0023-9055-04. Store ACULAR® PF between 15°C–30°C (59°F–86°F) with protection from light.
Rx only
U.S. Patent Nos. 4,089,969; 4,454,151; 5,110,493
ALLERGAN ©1997 Allergan, Irvine, CA 92612, U.S.A.
ACULAR® is a registered trademark of SYNTEX (U.S.A.) Inc. ACULAR® PF is manufactured and distributed by ALLERGAN under license from its developer, SYNTEX (U.S.A.) Inc., Palo Alto, California, U.S.A. November 1997

ALPHAGAN® ℞
(brimonidine tartrate ophthalmic solution) 0.2%

DESCRIPTION

ALPHAGAN® (brimonidine tartrate ophthalmic solution) 0.2% is a relatively selective alpha-2 adrenergic agonist for ophthalmic use. The chemical name of brimonidine tartrate is 5-bromo-6-(2-imidazolidinylideneamino) quinoxaline L-tartrate. It is an off-white, pale yellow to pale pink powder. In solution, ALPHAGAN® has a clear, greenish-yellow color. It has a molecular weight of 442.24 as the tartrate salt and is water soluble (34 mg/mL). The molecular formula is $C_{11}H_{10}BrN_5 \cdot C_4H_6O_6$.
ALPHAGAN® (brimonidine tartrate ophthalmic solution) 0.2% is a sterile ophthalmic solution. Each mL of ALPHAGAN® Solution contains:
ACTIVE: brimonidine tartrate 2 mg (equivalent to 1.32 mg as brimonidine free base).
PRESERVATIVE: benzalkonium chloride (0.05 mg)
INACTIVES: polyvinyl alcohol; sodium chloride; sodium citrate; citric acid; and purified water. Hydrochloric acid and/or sodium hydroxide may be added to adjust pH (6.3–6.5).

CLINICAL PHARMACOLOGY

Mechanism of Action
ALPHAGAN® is an alpha adrenergic receptor agonist. It has a peak ocular hypotensive effect occurring at two hours post-dosing. Fluorophotometric studies in animals and humans suggest that brimonidine tartrate has a dual mechanism of action by reducing aqueous humor production and increasing uveoscleral outflow.
Pharmacokinetics
After ocular administration of a 0.2% solution, plasma concentrations peaked within 1 to 4 hours and declined with a systemic half-life of approximately 3 hours.
In humans, systemic metabolism of brimonidine is extensive. It is metabolized primarily by the liver. Urinary excretion is the major route of elimination of the drug and its metabolites. Approximately 87% of an orally-administered radioactive dose was eliminated within 120 hours, with 74% found in the urine.
Clinical Studies
Elevated IOP presents a major risk factor in glaucomatous field loss. The higher the level of IOP, the greater the likelihood of optic nerve damage and visual field loss. ALPHAGAN® has the action of lowering intraocular pressure with minimal effect on cardiovascular and pulmonary parameters.
In comparative clinical studies with timolol 0.5%, lasting up to one year, the IOP lowering effect of ALPHAGAN® was approximately 4–6 mm Hg compared with approximately 6 mm Hg for timolol. In these studies, both patient groups were dosed BID, however, due to the duration of action of ALPHAGAN®, it is recommended that ALPHAGAN® be dosed TID. Eight percent of the subjects were discontinued from studies due to inadequately controlled intraocular pressure, which in 30% of these patients occurred during the first month of therapy. Approximately 20% were discontinued due to adverse experiences.

INDICATIONS AND USAGE

ALPHAGAN® is indicated for lowering intraocular pressure in patients with open-angle glaucoma or ocular hypertension. The IOP lowering efficacy of ALPHAGAN® Ophthalmic Solution diminishes over time in some patients. This loss of effect appears with a variable time of onset in each patient and should be closely monitored.

CONTRAINDICATIONS

ALPHAGAN® is contraindicated in patients with hypersensitivity to brimonidine tartrate or any component of this medication. It is also contraindicated in patients receiving monoamine oxidase (MAO) inhibitor therapy.

PRECAUTIONS

General: Although ALPHAGAN® had minimal effect on blood pressure of patients in clinical studies, caution should be exercised in treating patients with severe cardiovascular disease.

ALPHAGAN® has not been studied in patients with hepatic or renal impairment; caution should be used in treating such patients.

ALPHAGAN® should be used with caution in patients with depression, cerebral or coronary insufficiency, Raynaud's phenomenon, orthostatic hypotension or thromboangitis obliterans.

During the studies there was a loss of effect in some patients. The IOP-lowering efficacy observed with ALPHAGAN® Ophthalmic Solution during the first month of therapy may not always reflect the long-term level of IOP reduction. Patients prescribed IOP-lowering medication should be routinely monitored for IOP.

Information for Patients: The preservative in ALPHAGAN®, benzalkonium chloride, may be absorbed by soft contact lenses. Patients wearing soft contact lenses should be instructed to wait at least 15 minutes after instilling ALPHAGAN® to insert soft contact lenses.

As with other drugs in this class, ALPHAGAN® may cause fatigue and/or drowsiness in some patients. Patients who engage in hazardous activities should be cautioned of the potential for a decrease in mental alertness.

Drug Interactions: Although specific drug interaction studies have not been conducted with ALPHAGAN®, the possibility of an additive or potentiating effect with CNS depressants (alcohol, barbiturates, opiates, sedatives, or anesthetics) should be considered. ALPHAGAN® did not have significant effects on pulse and blood pressure in clinical studies. However, since alpha-agonists, as a class, may reduce pulse and blood pressure, caution in using concomitant drugs such as beta-blockers (ophthalmic and systemic), antihypertensives and/or cardiac glycosides is advised.

Tricyclic antidepressants have been reported to blunt the hypotensive effect of systemic clonidine. It is not known whether the concurrent use of these agents with ALPHAGAN® can lead to an interference in IOP lowering effect. No data on the level of circulating catecholamines after ALPHAGAN® is instilled are available. Caution, however, is advised in patients taking tricyclic antidepressants which can affect the metabolism and uptake of circulating amines.

Carcinogenesis, mutagenesis, impairment of fertility: No compound-related carcinogenic effects were observed in 21 month and 2 year studies in mice and rats given oral doses of 2.5 mg/kg/day (as the free base) and 1.0 mg/kg/day, respectively (~77 and 118 times, respectively, the human plasma drug concentration following the recommended ophthalmic dose).

ALPHAGAN® was not mutagenic or cytogenic in a series of *in vitro* and *in vivo* studies including the Ames test, host-mediated assay, chromosomal aberration assay in Chinese Hamster Ovary (CHO) cells, cytogenic studies in mice and dominant lethal assay.

Pregnancy: Teratogenic Effects: Pregnancy Category B. Reproduction studies performed in rats with oral doses of 0.66 mg base/kg revealed no evidence of impaired fertility or harm to the fetus due to ALPHAGAN®. Dosing at this level produced 100 times the plasma drug concentration level seen in humans following multiple ophthalmic doses.

There are no studies of ALPHAGAN® in pregnant women, however in animal studies, brimonidine crossed the placenta and entered into the fetal circulation to a limited extent. ALPHAGAN® should be used during pregnancy only if the potential benefit to the mother justifies the potential risk to the fetus.

Nursing Mothers: It is not known whether ALPHAGAN® is excreted in human milk, although in animal studies, brimonidine tartrate has been shown to be excreted in breast milk. A decision should be made whether to discontinue nursing or to discontinue the drug, taking into account the importance of the drug to the mother.

Pediatric Use: Safety and effectiveness in pediatric patients have not been established. Symptoms of bradycardia, hypotension, hypothermia, hypotoria, and apnea have been reported (rarely) in neonates receiving brimonidine.

ADVERSE REACTIONS

Adverse events occurring in approximately 10–30% of the subjects, in descending order of incidence, included oral dryness, ocular hyperemia, burning and stinging, headache, blurring, foreign body sensation, fatigue/drowsiness, conjunctival follicles, ocular allergic reactions, and ocular pruritus.

Events occurring in approximately 3–9% of the subjects, in descending order included corneal staining/erosion, photophobia, eyelid erythema, ocular ache/pain, ocular dryness, tearing, upper respiratory symptoms, eyelid edema, conjunctival edema, dizziness, blepharitis, ocular irritation, gastrointestinal symptoms, asthenia, conjunctival blanching, abnormal vision and muscular pain.

The following adverse reactions were reported in less than 3% of the patients: lid crusting, conjunctival hemorrhage, abnormal taste, insomnia, conjunctival discharge, depression, hypertension, anxiety, palpitations, nasal dryness and syncope.

OVERDOSAGE

No information is available on overdosage in humans. Treatment of an oral overdose includes supportive and symptomatic therapy; a patent airway should be maintained.

DOSAGE AND ADMINISTRATION

The recommended dose is one drop of ALPHAGAN® in the affected eye(s) three times daily, approximately 8 hours apart.

HOW SUPPLIED

ALPHAGAN® (brimonidine tartrate ophthalmic solution) 0.2% is supplied sterile in white opaque plastic dropper bottles as follows:

5 mL   NDC 0023-8665-05
10 mL NDC 0023-8665-10
15 mL NDC 0023-8665-15

NOTE: Store at or below 25° C (77° F).

Rx only

ALLERGAN

© January 1998 Allergan, Inc., Irvine, CA 92612
70830/11C

AZELEX®
(azelaic acid cream) 20%
For Dermatologic Use Only
Not for Ophthalmic Use

℞

DESCRIPTION

AZELEX® (azelaic acid cream) 20% contains azelaic acid, a naturally occurring saturated dicarboxylic acid.

Structural Formula: $HOOC-(CH_2)_7-COOH$. Chemical Name: 1,7-heptanedicarboxylic acid. Empirical Formula: $C_9H_{16}O_4$. Molecular Weight: 188.22.

Active Ingredient: Each gram of AZELEX® contains azelaic acid .... 0.2 gm (20% w/w).

Inactive Ingredients: cetearyl octanoate, glycerin, glyceryl stearate and cetearyl alcohol and cetyl palmitate and cocoglycerides, PEG-5 glyceryl stearate, propylene glycol and purified water. Benzoic acid is present as a preservative.

CLINICAL PHARMACOLOGY

The exact mechanism of action of azelaic acid is not known. The following *in vitro* data are available, but their clinical significance is unknown. Azelaic acid has been shown to possess antimicrobial activity against *Propionibacterium acnes* and *Staphylococcus epidermidis.* The antimicrobial action may be attributable to inhibition of microbial cellular protein synthesis.

A normalization of keratinization leading to an anticomedonal effect of azelaic acid may also contribute to its clinical activity. Electron microscopic and immunohistochemical evaluation of skin biopsies from human subjects treated with AZELEX® demonstrated a reduction in the thickness of the stratum corneum, a reduction in number and size of keratohyalin granules, and a reduction in the amount and distribution of filaggrin (a protein component of keratohyalin) in epidermal layers. This is suggestive of the ability to decrease microcomedo formation.

Pharmacokinetics: Following a single application of AZELEX® to human skin *in vitro,* azelaic acid penetrates into the stratum corneum (approximately 3 to 5% of the applied dose) and other viable skin layers (up to 10% of the dose is found in the epidermis and dermis). Negligible cutaneous metabolism occurs after topical application. Approximately 4% of the topically applied azelaic acid is systemically absorbed. Azelaic acid is mainly excreted unchanged in the urine but undergoes some β-oxidation to shorter chain dicarboxylic acids. The observed half-lives in healthy subjects are approximately 45 minutes after oral dosing and 12 hours after topical dosing, indicating percutaneous absorption rate-limited kinetics.

Azelaic acid is a dietary constituent (whole grain cereals and animal products), and can be formed endogenously from longer-chain dicarboxylic acids, metabolism of oleic acid, and ω-oxidation of monocarboxylic acids. Endogenous plasma concentration (20 to 80 ng/mL) and daily urinary excretion (4 to 28 mg) of azelaic acid are highly dependent on dietary intake. After topical treatment with AZELEX® in humans, plasma concentration and urinary excretion of azelaic acid are not significantly different from baseline levels.

INDICATIONS AND USAGE

AZELEX® is indicated for the topical treatment of mild-to-moderate inflammatory acne vulgaris.

CONTRAINDICATIONS

AZELEX® is contraindicated in individuals who have shown hypersensitivity to any of its components.

WARNINGS

AZELEX® is for dermatologic use only and not for ophthalmic use.

There have been isolated reports of hypopigmentation after use of azelaic acid. Since azelaic acid has not been well studied in patients with dark complexions, these patients should be monitored for early signs of hypopigmentation.

PRECAUTIONS

General: If sensitivity or severe irritation develop with the use of AZELEX®, treatment should be discontinued and appropriate therapy instituted.

Information for patients: Patients should be told: 1. To use AZELEX® for the full prescribed treatment period. 2. To avoid the use of occlusive dressings or wrappings. 3. To keep AZELEX® away from the mouth, eyes and other mucous membranes. If it does come in contact with the eyes, they should wash their eyes with large amounts of water and consult a physician if eye irritation persists. 4. If they have dark complexions, to report abnormal changes in skin color to their physician. 5. Due in part to the low pH of azelaic acid, temporary skin irritation (pruritus, burning, or stinging) may occur when AZELEX® is applied to broken or inflamed skin, usually at the start of treatment. However, this irritation commonly subsides if treatment is continued. If it continues, AZELEX® should be applied only once-a-day, or the treatment should be stopped until these effects have subsided. If troublesome irritation persists, use should be discontinued, and patients should consult their physician. (See **ADVERSE REACTIONS**.)

Carcinogenesis, mutagenesis, impairment of fertility: Azelaic acid is a human dietary component of a simple molecular structure that does not suggest carcinogenic potential, and it does not belong to a class of drugs for which there is a concern about carcinogenicity. Therefore, animal studies to evaluate carcinogenic potential with AZELEX® Cream were not deemed necessary. In a battery of tests (Ames assay, HGPRT test in Chinese hamster ovary cells, human lymphocyte test, dominant lethal assay in mice), azelaic acid was found to be nonmutagenic. Animal studies have shown no adverse effects on fertility.

Pregnancy: Teratogenic Effects: Pregnancy Category B. Embryotoxic effects were observed in Segment I and Segment II oral studies with rats receiving 2500 mg/kg/day of azelaic acid. Similar effects were observed in Segment II studies in rabbits given 150 to 500 mg/kg/day and in monkeys given 500 mg/kg/day. The doses at which these effects were noted were all within toxic dose ranges for the dams. No teratogenic effects were observed. There are, however, no adequate and well-controlled studies in pregnant women. Because animal reproduction studies are not always predictive of human response, this drug should be used during pregnancy only if clearly needed.

Nursing Mothers: Equilibrium dialysis was used to assess human milk partitioning *in vitro.* At an azelaic acid concentration of 25 μg/mL, the milk/plasma distribution coefficient was 0.7 and the milk/buffer distribution was 1.0, indicating that passage of drug into maternal milk may occur. Since less than 4% of a topically applied dose is systemically absorbed, the uptake of azelaic acid into maternal milk is not expected to cause a significant change from baseline azelaic acid levels in the milk. However, caution should be exercised when AZELEX® is administered to a nursing mother.

Pediatric Use: Safety and effectiveness in pediatric patients under 12 years of age have not been established.

ADVERSE REACTIONS

During U.S. clinical trials with AZELEX®, adverse reactions were generally mild and transient in nature. The most common adverse reactions occurring in approximately 1–5% of patients were pruritus, burning, stinging and tingling. Other adverse reactions such as erythema, dryness, rash, peeling, irritation, dermatitis, and contact dermatitis were reported in less than 1% of subjects. There is the potential for experiencing allergic reactions with use of AZELEX®.

In patients using azelaic acid formulations, the following additional adverse experiences have been reported rarely: worsening of asthma, vitiligo depigmentation, small depigmented spots, hypertrichosis, reddening (signs of keratosis pilaris), and exacerbation of recurrent herpes labialis.

DOSAGE AND ADMINISTRATION

After the skin is thoroughly washed and patted dry, a thin film of AZELEX® should be gently but thoroughly massaged into the affected areas twice daily, in the morning and evening. The hands should be washed following application. The duration of use of AZELEX® can vary from person to person and depends on the severity of the acne. Improvement of the condition occurs in the majority of patients with inflammatory lesions within four weeks.

HOW SUPPLIED

AZELEX® is supplied in collapsible tubes in a 30 gm size:
30 g—NDC 0023-8694-30.

Continued on next page

Azelex—Cont.

Note: Protect from freezing. Store between 15°–30°C (59°–86°F).
Rx only
Distributed under license; U.S. Patent No. 4,386,104.
April 1997
Distributed by
ALLERGAN
Irvine, California 92612, U.S.A.
© 1997 Allergan, Inc.
Made in Germany

BLEPHAMIDE® ℞

(sulfacetamide sodium and prednisolone acetate ophthalmic ointment USP)
10%/0.2% sterile

DESCRIPTION

BLEPHAMIDE® (sulfacetamide sodium and prednisolone acetate ophthalmic ointment USP) is a sterile topical ophthalmic ointment combining an antibacterial and a corticosteroid.

Contains: Actives: sulfacetamide sodium 10% and prednisolone acetate 0.2%. Inactives: phenylmercuric acetate (0.0008%); mineral oil; white petrolatum; and petrolatum (and) lanolin alcohol.

Chemical Names: Sulfacetamide sodium: N-sulfanilylacetamide monosodium salt monohydrate.
Prednisolone acetate: 11β, 17, 21-trihydroxypregna-1,4-diene-3, 20-dione, 21-acetate.

CLINICAL PHARMACOLOGY

Corticosteroids suppress the inflammatory response to a variety of agents and they probably delay or slow healing. Since corticosteroids may inhibit the body's defense mechanism against infection, a concomitant antibacterial drug may be used when this inhibition is considered to be clinically significant in a particular case.

When a decision to administer both a corticosteroid and an antibacterial is made, the administration of such drugs in combination has the advantage of greater patient compliance and convenience, with the added assurance that the appropriate dosage of both drugs is administered, plus assured compatibility of ingredients when both types of drugs are in the same formulation and, particularly, that the correct volume of drug is delivered and retained.

The relative potency of corticosteroids depends on the molecular structure, concentration and release from the vehicle.

Microbiology: Sulfacetamide exerts a bacteriostatic effect against susceptible bacteria by restricting the synthesis of folic acid required for growth through competition with p-amino benzoic acid.

Some strains of these bacteria may be resistant to sulfacetamide or resistant strains may emerge *in vivo.*

The anti-infective component in BLEPHAMIDE® ointment is included to provide action against specific organisms susceptible to it. Sulfacetamide sodium is active *in vitro* against susceptible strains of the following microorganisms: *Escherichia coli, Staphylococcus aureus, Streptococcus pneumoniae, Streptococcus* (viridans group), *Haemophilus influenzae, Klebsiella* species, and *Enterobacter* species.

This product does not provide adequate coverage against: *Neisseria* species, *Pseudomonas* species, and *Serratia marcescens* (see **INDICATIONS AND USAGE**).

INDICATIONS AND USAGE

BLEPHAMIDE® ophthalmic ointment is indicated for steroid-responsive inflammatory ocular conditions for which a corticosteroid is indicated and where superficial bacterial ocular infection or a risk of bacterial ocular infection exists.

Ocular corticosteroids are indicated in inflammatory conditions of the palpebral and bulbar conjunctiva, cornea, and anterior segment of the globe where the inherent risk of corticosteroid use in certain infective conjunctivitides is accepted to obtain diminution in edema and inflammation. They are also indicated in chronic anterior uveitis and corneal injury from chemical, radiation or thermal burns or penetration of foreign bodies.

The use of a combination drug with an anti-infective component is indicated where the risk of superficial ocular infection is high or where there is an expectation that potentially dangerous numbers of bacteria will be present in the eye.

The particular antibacterial drug in this product is active against the following common bacterial eye pathogens: *Escherichia coli, Staphylococcus aureus, Streptococcus pneumoniae, Streptococcus* (viridans group), *Haemophilus influenzae, Klebsiella* species, and *Enterobacter* species.

The product does not provide adequate coverage against: *Neisseria* species, *Pseudomonas* species, and *Serratia marcescens.*

A significant percentage of staphylococcal isolates are completely resistant to sulfa drugs.

CONTRAINDICATIONS

BLEPHAMIDE® ophthalmic ointment is contraindicated in most viral diseases of the cornea and conjunctiva including epithelial herpes simplex keratitis (dendritic keratitis), vaccinia, and varicella, and also in mycobacterial infection of the eye and fungal diseases of ocular structures.

This product is also contraindicated in individuals with known or suspected hypersensitivity to any of the ingredients of this preparation, to other sulfonamides and to other corticosteroids. See **WARNINGS**. (Hypersensitivity to the antimicrobial component occurs at a higher rate than for other components).

WARNINGS

NOT FOR INJECTION INTO THE EYE.

Prolonged use of corticosteroids may result in ocular hypertension/glaucoma with damage to the optic nerve, defects in visual acuity and fields of vision, and in posterior subcapsular cataract formation.

Acute anterior uveitis may occur in susceptible individuals, primarily Blacks.

Prolonged use of BLEPHAMIDE® ophthalmic ointment may suppress the host response and thus increase the hazard of secondary ocular infections. In those diseases causing thinning of the cornea or sclera, perforation has been known to occur with the use of topical corticosteroids. In acute purulent conditions of the eye, corticosteroids may mask infection or enhance existing infection.

If the product is used for 10 days or longer, intraocular pressure should be routinely monitored even though it may be difficult in children and uncooperative patients. Corticosteroids should be used with caution in the presence of glaucoma. Intraocular pressure should be checked frequently.

A significant percentage of staphylococcal isolates are completely resistant to sulfonamides.

The use of steroids after cataract surgery may delay healing and increase the incidence of filtering blebs.

The use of ocular corticosteroids may prolong the course and may exacerbate the severity of many viral infections of the eye (including herpes simplex). Employment of corticosteroid medication in the treatment of herpes simplex requires great caution.

Topical steroids are not effective in mustard gas keratitis and Sjogren's keratoconjunctivitis.

Fatalities have occurred, although rarely, due to severe reactions to sulfonamides including Stevens-Johnson syndrome, toxic epidermal necrolysis, fulminant hepatic necrosis, agranulocytosis, aplastic anemia and other blood dyscrasias. Sensitization may recur when a sulfonamide is readministered, irrespective of the route of administration.

If signs of hypersensitivity or other serious reactions occur, discontinue use of this preparation. Cross-sensitivity among corticosteroids has been demonstrated (see **ADVERSE REACTIONS**).

PRECAUTIONS

General: The initial prescription and renewal of the medication order beyond 8 g of ointment should be made by a physician only after examination of the patient with the aid of magnification, such as slit lamp biomicroscopy and, where appropriate, fluorescein staining. If signs and symptoms fail to improve after two days, the patient should be re-evaluated. The possibility of fungal infections of the cornea should be considered after prolonged corticosteroid dosing. Use with caution in patients with severe dry eye. Fungal cultures should be taken when appropriate.

The p-amino benzoic acid present in purulent exudates competes with sulfonamides and can reduce their effectiveness. Ophthalmic ointments may retard corneal healing.

Information for Patients: If inflammation or pain persists longer than 48 hours or becomes aggravated, the patient should be advised to discontinue use of the medication and consult a physician (see **WARNINGS**).

This product is sterile when packaged. To prevent contamination, care should be taken to avoid touching the tube tip to eyelids or to any other surface. The use of this tube by more than one person may spread infection. Keep tube tightly closed when not in use. Keep out of the reach of children.

Laboratory Tests: Eyelid cultures and tests to determine the susceptibility of organisms to sulfacetamide may be indicated if signs and symptoms persist or recur in spite of the recommended course of treatment with BLEPHAMIDE® ophthalmic ointment.

Drug Interactions: BLEPHAMIDE® ophthalmic ointment is incompatible with silver preparations. Local anesthetics related to p-amino benzoic acid may antagonize the action of the sulfonamides.

Carcinogenesis, Mutagenesis, Impairment of Fertility: Prednisolone has been reported to be noncarcinogenic. Long-term animal studies for carcinogenic potential have not been performed with sulfacetamide.

One author detected chromosomal nondisjunction in the yeast *Saccharomyces cerevisiae* following application of sulfacetamide sodium. The significance of this finding to topical ophthalmic use of sulfacetamide sodium in the human is unknown.

Mutagenic studies with prednisolone have been negative. Studies on reproduction and fertility have not been performed with sulfacetamide. A long-term chronic toxicity study in dogs showed that high oral doses of prednisolone prevented estrus. A decrease in fertility was seen in male and female rats that were mated following oral dosing with another glucocorticosteroid.

Pregnancy: Teratogenic Effects: Pregnancy Category C. Animal reproduction studies have not been conducted with sulfacetamide sodium. Prednisolone has been shown to be teratogenic in rabbits, hamsters, and mice. In mice, prednisolone has been shown to be teratogenic when given in doses 1 to 10 times the human ocular dose. Dexamethasone, hydrocortisone and prednisolone were ocularly applied to both eyes of pregnant mice five times per day on days 10 through 13 of gestation. A significant increase in the incidence of cleft palate was observed in the fetuses of the treated mice. There are no adequate well-controlled studies in pregnant women dosed with corticosteroids.

Kernicterus may be precipitated in infants by sulfonamides being given systemically during the third trimester of pregnancy. It is not known whether sulfacetamide sodium can cause fetal harm when administered to a pregnant woman or whether it can affect reproductive capacity.

BLEPHAMIDE® ophthalmic ointment should be used during pregnancy only if the potential benefit justifies the potential risk to the fetus.

Nursing Mothers: It is not known whether topical administration of corticosteroids could result in sufficient systemic absorption to produce detectable quantities in human milk. Systemically administered corticosteroids appear in human milk and could suppress growth, interfere with endogenous corticosteroid production, or cause other untoward effects. Systemically administered sulfonamides are capable of producing kernicterus in infants of lactating women. Because of the potential for serious adverse reactions in nursing infants from sulfacetamide sodium and prednisolone acetate ophthalmic ointments, a decision should be made whether to discontinue nursing or to discontinue the medication.

Pediatric Use: Safety and effectiveness in children below the age of six have not been established.

ADVERSE REACTIONS

Adverse reactions have occurred with corticosteroid/antibacterial combination drugs which can be attributed to the corticosteroid component, the antibacterial component, or the combination. Exact incidence figures are not available since no denominator of treated patients is available.

Reactions occurring most often from the presence of the antibacterial ingredient are allergic sensitizations. Fatalities have occurred, although rarely, due to severe reactions to sulfonamides including Stevens-Johnson syndrome, toxic epidermal necrolysis, fulminant hepatic necrosis, agranulocytosis, aplastic anemia, and other blood dyscrasias (See **WARNINGS**).

Sulfacetamide sodium may cause local irritation.

The reactions due to the corticosteroid component in decreasing order of frequency are: elevation of intraocular pressure (IOP) with possible development of glaucoma and infrequent optic nerve damage, posterior subcapsular cataract formation, and delayed wound healing.

Although systemic effects are extremely uncommon, there have been rare occurrences of systemic hypercorticoidism after use of topical steroids.

Corticosteroid-containing preparations can also cause acute anterior uveitis or perforation of the globe. Mydriasis, loss of accommodation and ptosis have occasionally been reported following local use of corticosteroids.

Secondary Infection: The development of secondary infection has occurred after use of combinations containing corticosteroids and antibacterials. Fungal and viral infections of the cornea are particularly prone to develop coincidentally with long-term applications of corticosteroid. The possibility of fungal invasion must be considered in any persistent corneal ulceration where corticosteroid treatment has been used.

Secondary bacterial ocular infection following suppression of host responses also occurs.

DOSAGE AND ADMINISTRATION

A small amount, approximately $^1/_2$ inch ribbon of ointment, should be applied in the conjunctival sac three or four times daily and once or twice at night.

Not more than 8 g should be prescribed initially.

The dosing of BLEPHAMIDE® ophthalmic ointment may be reduced, but care should be taken not to discontinue therapy prematurely. In chronic conditions, withdrawal of treatment should be carried out by gradually decreasing the frequency of application.

If signs and symptoms fail to improve after two days, the patient should be re-evaluated (see **PRECAUTIONS**).

HOW SUPPLIED

BLEPHAMIDE® (sulfacetamide sodium and prednisolone acetate ophthalmic ointment USP) 10%/0.2% is supplied sterile in 3.5 gram ointment tubes:

NDC 0023-0313-04.

Note: Store away from heat.

Rx only

BLEPHAMIDE®
(sulfacetamide sodium-prednisolone acetate)

℞

LIQUIFILM®
sterile ophthalmic suspension

DESCRIPTION

BLEPHAMIDE® LIQUIFILM® sterile ophthalmic suspension is a topical anti-inflammatory/anti-infective combination product for ophthalmic use.

Chemical Names:

Sulfacetamide sodium: N-Sulfanilylacetamide monosodium salt monohydrate.

Prednisolone acetate: 11β, 17, 21-Trihydroxypregna-1, 4-diene-3, 20-dione 21-acetate.

Contains:

Actives: sulfacetamide sodium 10.0%, prednisolone acetate (microfine suspension) 0.2%; Preservative: benzalkonium chloride: Inactives: LIQUIFILM® (polyvinyl alcohol) 1.4%; polysorbate 80; edetate disodium; sodium phosphate, dibasic; potassium phosphate, monobasic; sodium thiosulfate; hydrochloric acid and/or sodium hydroxide to adjust the pH; and purified water.

CLINICAL PHARMACOLOGY

Corticosteroids suppress the inflammatory response to a variety of agents and they probably delay or slow healing. Since corticosteroids may inhibit the body's defense mechanism against infection, a concomitant antimicrobial drug may be used when this inhibition is considered to be clinically significant in a particular case.

The anti-infective component in BLEPHAMIDE® is included to provide action against specific organisms susceptible to it. Sulfacetamide sodium is considered active against the following microorganisms: *Escherichia coli, Staphylococcus aureus, Streptococcus pneumoniae, Streptococcus* (viridans group), *Pseudomonas species, Haemophilus influenzae, Klebsiella* species, and *Enterobacter* species.

When a decision to administer both a corticosteroid and an antimicrobial is made, the administration of such drugs in combination has the advantage of greater patient compliance and convenience, with the added assurance that the appropriate dosage of both drugs is administered. When both types of drugs are in the same formulation, compatibility of ingredients is assured and the correct volume of drug is delivered and retained. The relative potency of corticosteroids depends on the molecular structure, concentration, and release from the vehicle.

INDICATIONS AND USAGE

A steroid/anti-infective combination is indicated for steroid-responsive inflammatory ocular conditions for which a corticosteroid is indicated and where bacterial infection or a risk of bacterial ocular infection exists.

Ocular steroids are indicated in inflammatory conditions of the palpebral and bulbar conjunctiva, cornea, and anterior segment of the globe where the inherent risk of steroid use in certain infective conjunctivitides is accepted to obtain a diminution in edema and inflammation. They are also indicated in chronic anterior uveitis and corneal injury from chemical, radiation, or thermal burns or penetration of foreign bodies.

The use of a combination drug with an anti-infective component is indicated where the risk of infection is high or where there is an expectation that potentially dangerous numbers of bacteria will be present in the eye.

The particular anti-infective drug in this product is active against the following common bacterial eye pathogens: *Escherichia coli, Staphylococcus aureus, Streptococcus pneumoniae, Streptococcus* (viridans group), *Pseudomonas* species, *Haemophilus influenzae, Klebsiella* species, and *Enterobacter* species. This product does not provide adequate coverage against *Neisseria* species and *Serratia marcescens.*

CONTRAINDICATIONS

BLEPHAMIDE® ophthalmic suspension is contraindicated in most viral diseases of the cornea and conjunctiva including epithelial herpes simplex keratitis (dendritic keratitis), vaccinia, and varicella, and also in mycobacterial infection of the eye and fungal diseases of ocular structures.

This product is also contraindicated in individuals with known or suspected hypersensitivity to any of the ingredients of this preparation, to other sulfonamides and to other corticosteroids. See **WARNINGS.** (Hypersensitivity to the antimicrobial component occurs at a higher rate than for other components.)

WARNINGS

NOT FOR INJECTION INTO THE EYE.

Prolonged use of corticosteroids may result in ocular hypertension/glaucoma with damage to the optic nerve, defects in visual acuity and fields of vision, and in posterior subcapsular cataract formation.

Acute anterior uveitis may occur in susceptible individuals, primarily Blacks.

Prolonged use of BLEPHAMIDE® ophthalmic suspension may suppress the host response and thus increase the hazard of secondary ocular infections. In those diseases causing thinning of the cornea or sclera, perforation has been known to occur with the use of topical corticosteroids. In acute purulent conditions of the eye, corticosteroids may mask infection or enhance existing infection.

If the product is used for 10 days or longer, intraocular pressure should be routinely monitored even though it may be difficult in children and uncooperative patients. Corticosteroids should be used with caution in the presence of glaucoma. Intraocular pressure should be checked frequently.

A significant percentage of staphylococcal isolates are completely resistant to sulfonamides.

The use of steroids after cataract surgery may delay healing and increase the incidence of filtering blebs.

The use of ocular corticosteroids may prolong the course and may exacerbate the severity of many viral infections of the eye (including herpes simplex). Employment of corticosteroid medication in the treatment of herpes simplex requires great caution.

Topical steroids are not effective in mustard gas keratitis and Sjogren's keratoconjunctivitis.

Fatalities have occurred, although rarely, due to severe reactions to sulfonamides including Stevens-Johnson syndrome, toxic epidermal necrolysis, fulminant hepatic necrosis, agranulocytosis, aplastic anemia and other blood dyscrasias. Sensitization may recur when a sulfonamide is readministered, irrespective of the route of administration.

If signs of hypersensitivity or other serious reactions occur, discontinue use of this preparation. Cross-sensitivity among corticosteroids has been demonstrated (see **ADVERSE REACTIONS**).

PRECAUTIONS

General: The initial prescription and renewal of the medication order beyond 20 milliliters of the suspension should be made by a physician only after examination of the patient with the aid of magnification, such as slit lamp biomicroscopy and, where appropriate, fluorescein staining. If signs and symptoms fail to improve after two days, the patient should be re-evaluated.

The possibility of fungal infections of the cornea should be considered after prolonged corticosteroid dosing. Use with caution in patients with severe dry eye. Fungal cultures should be taken when appropriate.

The p-amino benzoic acid present in purulent exudates competes with sulfonamides and can reduce their effectiveness.

Information for Patients: If inflammation or pain persists longer than 48 hours or becomes aggravated, the patient should be advised to discontinue use of the medication and consult a physician (see **WARNINGS**).

This product is sterile when packaged. To prevent contamination, care should be taken to avoid touching the applicator tip to eyelids or to any other surface. The use of this bottle by more than one person may spread infection. Keep bottle tightly closed when not in use. Keep out of the reach of children.

Laboratory Tests: Eyelid cultures and tests to determine the susceptibility of organisms to sulfacetamide may be indicated if signs and symptoms persist or recur in spite of the recommended course of treatment with BLEPHAMIDE® ophthalmic suspension.

Drug Interactions: BLEPHAMIDE® ophthalmic suspension is incompatible with silver preparations. Local anesthetics related to p-amino benzoic acid may antagonize the action of the sulfonamides.

Carcinogenesis, Mutagenesis, Impairment of Fertility: Prednisolone has been reported to be noncarcinogenic. Long-term animal studies for carcinogenic potential have not been performed with sulfacetamide.

One author detected chromosomal nondisjunction in the yeast *Saccharomyces cerevisiae* following application of sulfacetamide sodium. The significance of this finding to topical ophthalmic use of sulfacetamide sodium in the human is unknown.

Mutagenic studies with prednisolone have been negative. Studies on reproduction and fertility have not been performed with sulfacetamide. A long-term chronic toxicity study in dogs showed that high oral doses of prednisolone prevented estrus. A decrease in fertility was seen in male and female rats that were mated following oral dosing with another glucocorticosteroid.

Pregnancy: Teratogenic Effects: Pregnancy Category C. Animal reproduction studies have not been conducted with sulfacetamide sodium. Prednisolone has been shown to be teratogenic in rabbits, hamsters, and mice. In mice, prednisolone has been shown to be teratogenic when given in

doses 1 to 10 times the human ocular dose. Dexamethasone, hydrocortisone and prednisolone were ocularly applied to both eyes of pregnant mice five times per day on days 10 through 13 of gestation. A significant increase in the incidence of cleft palate was observed in the fetuses of the treated mice. There are no adequate well-controlled studies in pregnant women dosed with corticosteroids.

Kernicterus may be precipitated in infants by sulfonamides being given systemically during the third trimester of pregnancy. It is not known whether sulfacetamide sodium can cause fetal harm when administered to a pregnant woman or whether it can affect reproductive capacity.

BLEPHAMIDE® ophthalmic suspension should be used during pregnancy only if the potential benefit justifies the potential risk to the fetus.

Nursing Mothers: It is not known whether topical administration of corticosteroids could result in sufficient systemic absorption to produce detectable quantities in human milk. Systemically administered corticosteroids appear in human milk and could suppress growth, interfere with endogenous corticosteroid production, or cause other untoward effects. Systemically administered sulfonamides are capable of producing kernicterus in infants of lactating women. Because of the potential for serious adverse reactions in nursing infants from sulfacetamide sodium and prednisolone acetate ophthalmic suspensions, a decision should be made whether to discontinue nursing or to discontinue the medication.

Pediatric Use: Safety and effectiveness in pediatric patients below the age of six have not been established.

ADVERSE REACTIONS

Adverse reactions have occurred with corticosteroid/antibacterial combination drugs which can be attributed to the corticosteroid component, the antibacterial component, or the combination. Exact incidence figures are not available since no denominator of treated patients is available.

Reactions occurring most often from the presence of the anti-bacterial ingredient are allergic sensitizations. Fatalities have occurred, although rarely, due to severe reactions to sulfonamides including Stevens-Johnson syndrome, toxic epidermal necrolysis, fulminant hepatic necrosis, agranulocytosis, aplastic anemia, and other blood dyscrasias (See **WARNINGS**).

Sulfacetamide sodium may cause local irritation.

The reactions due to the corticosteroid component in decreasing order of frequency are: elevation of intraocular pressure (IOP) with possible development of glaucoma and infrequent optic nerve damage, posterior subcapsular cataract formation, and delayed wound healing.

Although systemic effects are extremely uncommon, there have been rare occurrences of systemic hypercorticoidism after use of topical steroids.

Corticosteroid-containing preparations can also cause acute anterior uveitis or perforation of the globe. Mydriasis, loss of accommodation and ptosis have occasionally been reported following local use of corticosteroids.

Secondary Infection: The development of secondary infection has occurred after use of combinations containing corticosteroids and antibacterials. Fungal and viral infections of the cornea are particularly prone to develop coincidentally with long-term applications of corticosteroid. The possibility of fungal invasion must be considered in any persistent corneal ulceration where corticosteroid treatment has been used.

Secondary bacterial ocular infection following suppression of host responses also occurs.

DOSAGE AND ADMINISTRATION

Optimal dosage is 1 drop two to four times daily, depending upon the severity of the condition.

In general, during early or acute stages of blepharitis, BLEPHAMIDE® LIQUIFILM® sterile ophthalmic suspension produces results most rapidly—and most efficiently—with instillation directly into the eye, with the excess spread on the lid (Method I). When the condition is confined to the lid, however, BLEPHAMIDE® may be applied directly to the site of the lesions (Method II).

METHOD I: In the Eye and On the Lid.

1. Wash hands carefully. Tilt head back and drop **1 drop** into the eye.

2. Close the eye and spread the excess medication present after closing the eye on the full length of the upper and lower lids.

3. Do not wipe any of the medication off the lids. It will dry completely in 4 or 5 minutes to a clear film that remains on the lids for several hours—it cannot be seen by others, nor will it interfere with vision.

4. The medication should be washed off the lids once or twice daily. **However, it should be reapplied after each washing.**

METHOD II: On the Lid.

1. Wash hands carefully. Tilt the head back and with **eye closed** drop 1 drop onto the lid—preferably at the corner of the eye close to the nose.

Continued on next page

Blephamide—Cont.

2. Spread the medication over the full length of the upper and lower lids.
3. Do not wipe away any medication—it will dry in 4 to 5 minutes to a clear, invisible film which will remain on the lids for several hours.
4. The medication should be washed off the lids once or twice a day. **However, it should be reapplied after each washing.**

Not more than 20 milliliters should be prescribed initially and the prescription should not be refilled without further evaluation as outlined in PRECAUTIONS above.

HOW SUPPLIED

BLEPHAMIDE® LIQUIFILM® is supplied in plastic dropper bottles in the following sizes:
5 mL—NDC 11980-022-05 10 mL—NDC 11980-022-10
Note: Protect from freezing. **Shake well before using.**
Caution: Rx only

BOTOX® ℞
(Botulinum Toxin Type A) Purified Neurotoxin Complex

DESCRIPTION

BOTOX® (Botulinum Toxin Type A) Purified Neurotoxin Complex is a sterile, vacuum-dried form of purified botulinum toxin type A, produced from a culture of the Hall strain of *Clostridium botulinum* grown in a medium containing N-Z amine and yeast extract. It is purified from the culture solution by a series of acid precipitations to a crystalline complex consisting of the active high molecular weight toxin protein and an associated hemagglutinin protein. The crystalline complex is re-dissolved in a solution containing saline and albumin and sterile filtered (0.2 microns) prior to vacuum-drying. **BOTOX®** is to be reconstituted with sterile non-preserved saline prior to intramuscular injection.

Each vial of **BOTOX®** contains 100 units (U) of *Clostridium botulinum* toxin type A, 0.5 milligrams of albumin (human), and 0.9 milligrams of sodium chloride in a sterile, vacuum-dried form without a preservative. One unit (U) corresponds to the calculated median lethal intraperitoneal dose (LD/50) in mice of the reconstituted **BOTOX®** injected.

CLINICAL PHARMACOLOGY

BOTOX® (Botulinum Toxin Type A) Purified Neurotoxin Complex blocks neuromuscular conduction by binding to receptor sites on motor nerve terminals, entering the nerve terminals, and inhibiting the release of acetylcholine. When injected intramuscularly at therapeutic doses, **BOTOX®** produces a localized chemical denervation muscle paralysis. When the muscle is chemically denervated, it atrophies and may develop extrajunctional acetylcholine receptors. There is evidence that the nerve can sprout and reinnervate the muscle, with the weakness thus being reversible.

The paralytic effect on muscles injected with **BOTOX®** Purified Neurotoxin Complex is useful in reducing the excessive, abnormal contractions associated with blepharospasm. When used for the treatment of strabismus, it is postulated that the administration of **BOTOX®** affects muscle pairs by inducing an atrophic lengthening of the injected muscle and a corresponding shortening of the muscle's antagonist. Following peri-ocular injection of **BOTOX®**, distant muscles show electrophysiologic changes but no clinical weakness or other clinical change for a period of several weeks or months, parallel to the duration of local clinical paralysis.

In one study, botulinum toxin was evaluated in 27 patients with essential blepharospasm. Twenty-six of the patients had previously undergone drug treatment utilizing benztropine mesylate, clonazepam and/or baclofen without adequate clinical results. Three of these patients then underwent muscle stripping surgery still without an adequate outcome. One patient of the 27 was previously untreated. Upon using botulinum toxin, 25 of the 27 patients reported improvement within 48 hours. One of the other patients was later controlled with a higher dosage. The remaining patient reported only mild improvement but remained functionally impaired.

In another study, 12 patients with blepharospasm were evaluated in a double-blind, placebo-controlled study. All patients receiving botulinum toxin (n=8) were improved compared with no improvements in the placebo group (n=4). The mean dystonia score improved by 72%, the self-assessment score rating improved by 61%, and a videotape evaluation rating improved by 39%. The effects of the treatment lasted a mean of 12.5 weeks.

One thousand six hundred eighty-four patients with blepharospasm evaluated in an open trial showed clinical improvement lasting an average of 12.5 weeks prior to the need for re-treatment.

Six hundred seventy-seven patients with strabismus treated with one or more injections of **BOTOX®** Purified Neurotoxin Complex were evaluated in an open trial. Fifty-five percent of these patients were improved to an alignment of 10 prism diopters or less when evaluated six months or more following injection. These results are consistent with results from additional open label trials which were conducted for this indication.

INDICATIONS AND USAGE

BOTOX® (Botulinum Toxin Type A) Purified Neurotoxin Complex is indicated for the treatment of strabismus and blepharospasm associated with dystonia, including benign essential blepharospasm or VII nerve disorders in patients 12 years of age and above.

The efficacy of **BOTOX®** Purified Neurotoxin Complex in deviations over 50 prism diopters, in restrictive strabismus, in Duane's syndrome with lateral rectus weakness, and in secondary strabismus caused by prior surgical over-recession of the antagonist is doubtful, or multiple injections over time may be required. **BOTOX®** is ineffective in chronic paralytic strabismus except to reduce antagonist contracture in conjunction with surgical repair.

Presence of antibodies to botulinum toxin type A may reduce the effectiveness of **BOTOX®** Purified Neurotoxin Complex therapy. In clinical studies, reduction in effectiveness due to antibody production has occurred in one patient with blepharospasm receiving three doses of **BOTOX®** over a six week period totalling 92 U, and in several patients with torticollis who received multiple doses experimentally, totalling over 300 U in a one-month period. For this reason, the dose of **BOTOX®** for strabismus and blepharospasm should be kept as low as possible, in any case below 200 U in a one month period.

CONTRAINDICATIONS

BOTOX® (Botulinum Toxin Type A) Purified Neurotoxin Complex is contraindicated in individuals with known hypersensitivity to any ingredient in the formulation.

WARNINGS

The recommended dosages and frequencies of administration for **BOTOX®** Purified Neurotoxin Complex should not be exceeded. There have not been any reported instances of systemic toxicity resulting from accidental injection or oral ingestion of **BOTOX®**. Should accidental injection or oral ingestion occur, the person should be medically supervised for several days on an office or outpatient basis for signs or symptoms of systemic weakness or muscle paralysis. The entire contents of a vial is below the estimated dose for systemic toxicity in humans weighing 6 kg. or greater.

In the event of overdosage or injection into the wrong muscle, additional information may be obtained by contacting Allergan, Inc. at (800) 433-8871.

The effect of botulinum toxin may be potentiated by aminoglycoside antibiotics or any other drugs that interfere with neuromuscular transmission. Caution should be exercised when **BOTOX®** is used in patients taking any of these drugs.

PRECAUTIONS

General: The safe and effective use of **BOTOX®** (Botulinum Toxin Type A) Purified Neurotoxin Complex depends upon proper storage of the product, selection of the correct dose, and proper reconstitution and administration techniques. Physicians administering **BOTOX®** must understand the relevant neuromuscular and orbital anatomy and any alterations to the anatomy due to prior surgical procedures, and standard electromyographic techniques.

As with all biologic products, epinephrine and other precautions as necessary should be available should an anaphylactic reaction occur.

During the administration of **BOTOX®** Purified Neurotoxin Complex for the treatment of strabismus, retrobulbar hemorrhages sufficient to compromise retinal circulation have occurred from needle penetrations into the orbit. It is recommended that appropriate instruments to decompress the orbit be accessible. Ocular (globe) penetrations by needles have also occurred. An ophthalmoscope to diagnose this condition should be available.

Reduced blinking from **BOTOX®** Purified Neurotoxin Complex injection of the orbicularis muscle can lead to corneal exposure, persistent epithelial defect and corneal ulceration, especially in patients with VII nerve disorders. One case of corneal perforation in an aphakic eye requiring corneal grafting has occurred because of this effect. Careful testing of corneal sensation in eyes previously operated upon, avoidance of injection into the lower lid area to avoid ectropion, and vigorous treatment of any epithelial defect should be employed. This may require protective drops, ointment, therapeutic soft contact lenses, or closure of the eye by patching or other means.

Information for Patients: Patients with blepharospasm may have been extremely sedentary for a long time. Sedentary patients should be cautioned to resume activity slowly and carefully following the administration of **BOTOX®** Purified Neurotoxin Complex.

Drug Interactions: The effect of botulinum toxin may be potentiated by aminoglycoside antibiotics or any other drugs that interfere with neuromuscular transmission. Caution should be exercised when **BOTOX®** Purified Neurotoxin Complex is used in patients taking any of these drugs. (See **Warnings**).

Pregnancy: ***Pregnancy Category C:*** Animal reproduction studies have not been conducted with **BOTOX®** Purified Neurotoxin Complex. It is also not known whether **BOTOX®** can cause fetal harm when administered to a pregnant woman or can affect reproduction capacity. **BOTOX®** should be administered to pregnant women only if clearly needed.

Carcinogenesis, Mutagenesis, Impairment of Fertility: Long term studies in animals have not been performed to evaluate carcinogenic potential of **BOTOX®** Purified Neurotoxin Complex.

Nursing Mothers: It is not known whether this drug is excreted in human milk. Because many drugs are excreted in human milk, caution should be exercised when **BOTOX®** Purified Neurotoxin Complex is administered to a nursing woman.

Pediatric Use: Safety and effectiveness in children below the age of 12 have not been established.

ADVERSE REACTIONS

There have been reports of seven cases of diffuse skin rash and two cases of local swelling of the eyelid skin lasting for several days following eyelid injection.

Strabismus: Inducing paralysis in one or more extraocular muscles may produce spatial disorientation, double vision, or past-pointing. Covering the affected eye may alleviate these symptoms. Extraocular muscles adjacent to the injection site are often affected, causing ptosis or vertical deviation, especially with higher doses of **BOTOX®** (Botulinum Toxin Type A) Purified Neurotoxin Complex. The incidence rates of these side effects in 2058 adults who received 3650 injections for horizontal strabismus are listed below:

Ptosis	15.7%
Vertical deviation	16.9%

The incidence of ptosis was much less after inferior rectus injection (0.9%) and much greater after superior rectus injection (37.7%).

The incidence rates of these side effects persisting for over six months in an enlarged series of 5587 injections of horizontal muscles in 3104 patients are listed below:

Ptosis lasting over 180 days	0.3%
Vertical deviation greater than 2 prism diopters lasting over 180 days	2.1%

In these patients, the injection procedure itself caused nine scleral perforations. A vitreous hemorrhage occurred and later cleared in one case. No retinal detachment or visual loss occurred in any case. Sixteen retrobulbar hemorrhages occurred. Decompression of the orbit after five minutes was done to restore retinal circulation in one case. No eye lost vision from retrobulbar hemorrhage. Five eyes had pupillary change consistent with ciliary ganglion damage (Adies pupil).

Blepharospasm: In 1684 patients who received 4258 treatments (involving multiple injections) for blepharospasm, the incidence rates of adverse reactions per treated eye are listed below:

Ptosis	11.0%
Irritation/Tearing (includes dry eye, lagophthalmos, and photophobia)	10.0%

Ectropion, keratitis, diplopia and entropion were reported rarely (incidence less than 1%)

Ecchymosis occurs easily in the soft eyelid tissues. This can be prevented by applying pressure at the injection site immediately after the injection.

In two cases of VII nerve disorder (one case of an aphakic eye) reduced blinking from **BOTOX®** Purified Neurotoxin Complex injection of the orbicularis muscle led to serious corneal exposure, persistent epithelial defect and corneal ulceration. Perforation requiring corneal grafting occurred in one case, an aphakic eye. Avoidance of injection into the lower lid area to avoid ectropion may reduce this hazard. Vigorous treatment of any corneal epithelial defect should be employed. This may require protective drops, ointment, therapeutic soft contact lenses, or closure of the eye by patching or other means.

Two patients previously incapacitated by blepharospasm experienced cardiac collapse attributed to over-exertion within three weeks following **BOTOX®** therapy. Sedentary patients should be cautioned to resume activity slowly and carefully following the administration of **BOTOX®**.

OVERDOSAGE

In the event of overdosage or injection into the wrong muscle, additional information may be obtained by contacting Allergan, Inc. at (800) 433-8871.

DOSAGE AND ADMINISTRATION

Strabismus: **BOTOX®** (Botulinum Toxin Type A) Purified Neurotoxin Complex is intended for injection into extraocular muscles utilizing the electrical activity recorded from the tip of the injection needle as a guide to placement within the target muscle. Injection without surgical exposure or electromyographic guidance should not be attempted. Physicians should be familiar with electromyographic technique.

An injection of **BOTOX®** Purified Neurotoxin Complex is prepared by drawing into a sterile 1.0 mL tuberculin syringe an amount of the properly diluted toxin (see Dilution Table) slightly greater than the intended dose. Air bubbles in the syringe barrel are expelled and the syringe is attached to the electromyographic injection needle, preferably a 1.5 inch, 27 gauge needle. Injection volume in excess of the intended dose is expelled through the needle into an appropriate waste container to assure patency of the needle and to confirm that there is no syringe-needle leakage. A new, sterile needle and syringe should be used to enter the vial on each occasion for dilution or removal of **BOTOX®**.

To prepare the eye for **BOTOX®** Purified Neurotoxin Complex injection, it is recommended that several drops of a local anesthetic and an ocular decongestant be given several minutes prior to injection.

Note: The volume of **BOTOX®** injected for treatment of strabismus should be between 0.05 mL to 0.15 mL per muscle.

Strabismus dosage: The initial listed doses of the diluted **BOTOX®** Purified Neurotoxin Complex (see Dilution Table below) typically create paralysis of injected muscles beginning one to two days after injection and increasing in intensity during the first week. The paralysis lasts for 2–6 weeks and gradually resolves over a similar time period. Overcorrections lasting over 6 months have been rare. About one half of patients will require subsequent doses because of inadequate paralytic response of the muscle to the initial dose, or because of mechanical factors such as large deviations or restrictions, or because of the lack of binocular motor fusion to stabilize the alignment.

I. Initial doses in units (abbreviated as U). Use the lower listed doses for treatment of small deviations. Use the larger doses only for large deviations.
A. For vertical muscles, and for horizontal strabismus of less than 20 prism diopters: 1.25 U to 2.5 U in any one muscle.
B. For horizontal strabismus of 20 prism diopters to 50 prism diopters: 2.5 U to 5.0 U in any one muscle.
C. For persistent VI nerve palsy of one month or longer duration: 1.25 U to 2.5 U in the medial rectus muscle.
II. Subsequent doses for residual or recurrent strabismus.
A. It is recommended that patients be re-examined 7–14 days after each injection to assess the effect of that dose.
B. Patients experiencing adequate paralysis of the target muscle that require subsequent injections should receive a dose comparable to the initial dose.
C. Subsequent doses for patients experiencing incomplete paralysis of the target muscle may be increased up to twice the size of the previously administered dose.
D. Subsequent injections should not be administered until the effects of the previous dose have dissipated as evidenced by substantial function in the injected and adjacent muscles.
E. The maximum recommended dose as a single injection for any one muscle is 25 U.

Blepharospasm: For blepharospasm, diluted **BOTOX®** Purified Neurotoxin Complex (see Dilution Table) is injected using a sterile, 27–30 gauge needle without electromyographic guidance. 1.25 U to 2.5 U (0.05 mL to 0.1 mL volume at each site) injected into the medial and lateral pretarsal orbicularis oculi of the upper lid and into the lateral pre-tarsal orbicularis oculi of the lower lid is the initial recommended dose. In general, the initial effect of the injections is seen within three days and reaches a peak at one to two weeks post-treatment. Each treatment lasts approximately three months, following which the procedure can be repeated indefinitely. At repeat treatment sessions, the dose may be increased up to two-fold if the response from the initial treatment is considered insufficient—usually defined as an effect that does not last longer than two months. However there appears to be little benefit obtainable from injecting more than 5.0 U per site. Some tolerance may be found when **BOTOX®** is used in treating blepharospasm if treatments are given any more frequently than every three months, and it is rare to have the effect be permanent.

The cumulative dose of **BOTOX®** Purified Neurotoxin Complex in a 30-day period should not exceed 200 U.

DILUTION TECHNIQUE

To reconstitute vacuum-dried **BOTOX®** (Botulinum Toxin Type A) Purified Neurotoxin Complex, use sterile normal saline **without** a preservative; 0.9% Sodium Chloride Injection is the recommended diluent. Draw up the proper amount of diluent in the appropriate size syringe. Since **BOTOX®** is denatured by bubbling or similar violent agitation, inject the diluent into the vial gently. Discard the vial if a vacuum does not pull the diluent into the vial. Record the date and time of reconstitution on the space on the label. **BOTOX®** should be administered within 4 hours after reconstitution.

During this time period, reconstituted **BOTOX®** Purified Neurotoxin Complex should be stored in a refrigerator (2° to 8°C). Reconstituted **BOTOX®** should be clear, colorless and free of particulate matter. Parenteral drug products should be inspected visually for particulate matter and discoloration prior to administration and whenever the solution and the container permit. The use of one vial for more than one patient is not recommended because the product and diluent do not contain a preservative.

Dilution Table

Diluent Added (0.9% Sodium Chloride Injection)	Resulting dose in Units per 0.1 mL
1.0 mL	10.0 U
2.0 mL	5.0 U
4.0 mL	2.5 U
8.0 mL	1.25 U

Note: These dilutions are calculated for an injection volume of 0.1 mL. A decrease or increase in the **BOTOX®** Purified Neurotoxin Complex dose is also possible by administering a smaller or larger injection volume—from 0.05 mL (50% decrease in dose) to 0.15 mL (50% increase in dose).

HOW SUPPLIED

Each vial contains 100 U of vacuum-dried *Clostridium botulinum* toxin type A. NDC 0023-1145-01.

Rx only

STORAGE

Store the vacuum-dried product in a freezer at or below −5°C. Administer **BOTOX®** (Botulinum Toxin Type A) Purified Neurotoxin Complex within four hours after the vial is removed from the freezer and reconstituted. During these four hours, reconstituted **BOTOX®** should be stored in a refrigerator (2° to 8°C). Reconstituted **BOTOX®** should be clear, colorless and free of particulate matter.

All vials, including expired vials, or equipment used with the drug should be disposed of carefully as is done with all medical waste.

ELIMITE® Cream (permethrin) 5% *

℞

DESCRIPTION

ELIMITE® (permethrin) 5% Cream is a topical scabicidal agent for the treatment of infestation with *Sarcoptes scabiei* (scabies). It is available in an off-white, vanishing cream base. ELIMITE® Cream is for topical use only.

Chemical Name: The permethrin used is an approximate 1:3 mixture of the cis and trans isomers of the pyrethroid (±)-3-phenoxybenzyl 3-(2,2-dichlorovinyl)-2,2-dimethylcyclopropanecarboxylate. Permethrin has a molecular formula of $C_{21}H_{20}Cl_2O_3$ and a molecular weight of 391.29. It is a yellow to light orange-brown, low melting solid or viscous liquid.

Active Ingredient: Each gram contains permethrin 50 mg (5%).

Inactive Ingredients: Butylated hydroxytoluene, carbomer 934P, fractionated coconut oil, glycerin, glyceryl monostearate, isopropyl myristate, lanolin alcohols, mineral oil, polyoxyethylene cetyl ethers, purified water, and sodium hydroxide. Formaldehyde 1 mg (0.1%) is added as a preservative.

CLINICAL PHARMACOLOGY

Permethrin, a pyrethroid, is active against a broad range of pests including lice, ticks, fleas, mites, and other arthropods. It acts on the nerve cell membrane to disrupt the sodium channel current by which the polarization of the membrane is regulated. Delayed repolarization and paralysis of the pests are the consequences of this disturbance. Permethrin is rapidly metabolized by ester hydrolysis to inactive metabolites which are excreted primarily in the urine. Although the amount of permethrin absorbed after a single application of the 5% cream has not been determined precisely, data from studies with ^{14}C-labeled permethrin and absorption studies of the cream applied to patients with moderate to severe scabies indicate it is 2% or less of the amount applied.

INDICATIONS AND USAGE

ELIMITE® (permethrin) 5% Cream is indicated for the treatment of infestation with *Sarcoptes scabiei* (scabies).

CONTRAINDICATIONS

ELIMITE® is contraindicated in patients with known hypersensitivity to any of its components, to any synthetic pyrethroid or pyrethrin.

WARNINGS

If hypersensitivity to ELIMITE® occurs, discontinue use.

PRECAUTIONS

General: Scabies infestation is often accompanied by pruritus, edema and erythema. Treatment with ELIMITE® may temporarily exacerbate these conditions.

Information for patients: Patients with scabies should be advised that itching, mild burning and/or stinging may occur after application of ELIMITE®. In clinical trials approximately 75% of patients treated with ELIMITE® who continued to manifest pruritus at 2 weeks had cessation by 4 weeks. If irritation persists, they should consult their physician. ELIMITE® may be very mildly irritating to the eyes. Patients should be advised to avoid contact with eyes during application and to flush with water immediately if ELIMITE® gets in the eyes.

Carcinogenesis, mutagenesis, impairment of fertility: Six carcinogenicity bioassays were evaluated with permethrin, three each in rats and mice. No tumorigenicity was seen in the rat studies. However, species-specific increases in pulmonary adenomas, a common benign tumor of mice of high spontaneous background incidence, were seen in the three mouse studies. In one of these studies there was an increased incidence of pulmonary alveolar-cell carcinomas and benign liver adenomas only in female mice when permethrin was given in their food at a concentration of 5000 ppm. Mutagenicity assays, which give useful correlative data for interpreting results from carcinogenicity bioassays in rodents, were negative. Permethrin showed no evidence of mutagenic potential in a battery of *in vitro* and *in vivo* genetic toxicity studies.

Permethrin did not have any adverse effect on reproductive function at a dose of 180 mg/kg/day orally in a three-generation rat study.

Pregnancy: *teratogenic effects:* Pregnancy Category B: Reproduction studies have been performed in mice, rats, and rabbits (200 to 400 mg/kg/day orally) and have revealed no evidence of impaired fertility or harm to the fetus due to permethrin. There are, however, no adequate and well-controlled studies in pregnant women. Because animal reproduction studies are not always predictive of human response, this drug should be used during pregnancy only if clearly needed.

Nursing mothers: It is not known whether this drug is excreted in human milk. Because many drugs are excreted in human milk and because of the evidence for tumorigenic potential of permethrin in animal studies, consideration should be given to discontinuing nursing temporarily or withholding the drug while the mother is nursing.

Pediatric use: ELIMITE® is safe and effective in pediatric patients two months of age and older. Safety and effectiveness in infants less than two months of age have not been established.

ADVERSE REACTIONS

In clinical trials, generally mild and transient burning and stinging followed application with ELIMITE® in 10% of patients and was associated with the severity of infestation. Pruritus was reported in 7% of patients at various times post-application. Erythema, numbness, tingling, and rash were reported in 1 to 2% or less of patients (see PRECAUTIONS: General).

OVERDOSAGE

No instance of accidental ingestion of ELIMITE® has been reported. If ingested, gastric lavage and general supportive measures should be employed.

DOSAGE AND ADMINISTRATION

Adults and children: Thoroughly massage ELIMITE® into the skin from the head to the soles of the feet. Scabies rarely infests the scalp of adults, although the hairline, neck, temple, and forehead may be infested in infants and geriatric patients. Usually 30 grams is sufficient for an average adult. The cream should be removed by washing (shower or bath) after 8 to 14 hours. Infants should be treated on the scalp, temple and forehead. ONE APPLICATION IS GENERALLY CURATIVE.

Patients may experience persistent pruritus after treatment. This is rarely a sign of treatment failure and is not an indication for retreatment. Demonstrable living mites after 14 days indicate that retreatment is necessary.

HOW SUPPLIED

ELIMITE® (permethrin) 5% (wt./wt.) Cream is supplied in tubes in the following size: 60 g NDC 0023-7915-60.

Note: Store at 15° to 25°C (59° to 77°F).

Rx only

Manufactured for:
Allergan, Inc.
Irvine, CA 92612, U.S.A.
by Catalytica Pharmaceuticals, Inc.
Research Triangle Park, NC 27709
© 1998 Allergan, Inc.

ERYGEL®

℞

[ār 'ē-jel]
(Erythromycin
Topical Gel USP) 2%

Active Ingredient: erythromycin, USP ...... 2% (20 mg/g)
Inactive Ingredients: alcohol 92% and hydroxypropyl cellulose

Continued on next page

Erygel—Cont.

HOW SUPPLIED

ERYGEL® (erythromycin) 2% Topical Gel is supplied in plastic tubes in the following sizes: 30 g—NDC 0023-4312-30. 60 g—NDC 0023-4312-60.

Note: FLAMMABLE. Keep away from heat and flame. Keep tube tightly closed. Store at room temperature.
© 1996 Allergan, Inc.

ERYMAX® ℞
(Erythromycin Topical Solution USP) 2%

Active Ingredient: erythromycin .... 2% (20 mg/mL).
Inactive Ingredients: SD Alcohol 40-2 with tertiary butyl alcohol and brucine sulfate (66%), propylene glycol, and citric acid.

HOW SUPPLIED

In a 2 fl oz plastic bottle with optional Dab-O-Matic applicator and a 4 fl oz plastic bottle:
  2 fl oz (59 mL)—NDC 0023-0540-02
  4 fl oz (118 mL)—NDC 0023-0540-04
© 1995 Allergan, Inc.

EXSEL® Lotion/Shampoo ℞
(Selenium Sulfide Lotion, USP) 2.5%

Active Ingredient: selenium sulfide .... 2.5% (w/v) in aqueous suspension.
Inactive Ingredients: edetate disodium; bentonite; sodium dodecylbenzene sulfonate; sodium C14-16 olefin sulfonate; glyceryl ricinoleate; dimethicone copolyol; titanium dioxide; citric acid monohydrate; sodium phosphate monobasic, monohydrate; fragrance; and purified water.

HOW SUPPLIED

EXSEL® is available in a 4 fl oz plastic bottle—NDC 0023-0817-99
© 1995 Allergan, Inc.

FLUONID® ℞
(fluocinolone acetonide) 0.01%
Topical Solution

Active Ingredient: fluocinolone acetonide 0.01%
Active Ingredient: propylene glycol and citric acid

HOW SUPPLIED

Topical Solution 0.01%—60 mL plastic squeeze bottles.
  60 mL NDC 0023-0878-60
© 1995 Allergan, Inc.

FLUOROPLEX® ℞
(fluorouracil)
1% Topical Cream
and
1% Topical Solution

PRODUCT OVERVIEW
KEY FACTS

Effective treatment for multiple Actinic Keratoses sites.
Provides effective treatment for both clinical and subclinical lesions.
FLUOROPLEX® Cream does not contain irritating parabens or propylene glycol.

MAJOR USES

Multiple actinic keratoses.

SAFETY INFORMATION

Contraindicated in persons hypersensitive to fluorouracil or its listed ingredients.
Contraindicated in pregnancy.
Prolonged exposure to sunlight or other forms of ultraviolet irradiation may increase intensity of reaction.
Adequate long-term studies in animals to evaluate carcinogenic potential have not been conducted with fluorouracil.

PRESCRIBING INFORMATION

FLUOROPLEX® ℞
(fluorouracil)
1% Topical Cream
and
1% Topical Solution

DESCRIPTION

FLUOROPLEX® (fluorouracil) 1% Topical Cream and 1% Topical Solution are antineoplastic/antimetabolite products for dermatological use. Fluorouracil has the empirical formula $C_4H_3FN_2O_2$ and a molecular weight of 130.08. It is sparingly soluble in water and slightly soluble in alcohol. The pH is approximately 8.5 for FLUOROPLEX® Topical Cream and 9.2 for FLUOROPLEX® Topical Solution.

Chemical Name:
2,4(1*H*, 3*H*)-Pyrimidinedione, 5-fluoro-.
FLUOROPLEX® 1% Topical Cream contains:
Active Ingredient: fluorouracil .... 1.0%.
Inactive Ingredients: benzyl alcohol, emulsifying wax, mineral oil, isopropyl myristate, sodium hydroxide and purified water.
FLUOROPLEX® 1% Topical Solution contains:
Active Ingredient: fluorouracil 1.0%
Inactive Ingredients: propylene glycol, sodium hydroxide and/or hydrochloric acid to adjust the pH, and purified water.

CLINICAL PHARMACOLOGY

There is evidence that fluorouracil (or its metabolites) blocks the methylation reaction of deoxyuridylic acid to thymidylic acid. In this fashion, fluorouracil interferes with the synthesis of deoxyribonucleic acid (DNA) and to a lesser extent inhibits the formation of ribonucleic acid (RNA).

INDICATIONS AND USAGE

FLUOROPLEX® is indicated for the topical treatment of multiple actinic (solar) keratoses.

CONTRAINDICATIONS

Fluorouracil is contraindicated in women who are or may become pregnant. These products should not be used by patients who are allergic to any of their components.

WARNINGS

There exists the potential for a delayed hypersensitivity reaction to fluorouracil. Patch testing to prove hypersensitivity may be inconclusive.[1]
If an occlusive dressing is used, there may be an increase in the incidence of inflammatory reactions in the adjacent normal skin.
The patient should avoid prolonged exposure to sunlight or other forms of ultraviolet irradiation during treatment with FLUOROPLEX®, as the intensity of the reaction may be increased.

PRECAUTIONS

General: There is a possibility of increased absorption through ulcerated or inflamed skin.
Information for patients: The medication should be applied with care near the eyes, nose and mouth. Excessive reaction in these areas may occur due to irritation from accumulation of drug. If FLUOROPLEX® is applied with the fingers, the hands should be washed immediately afterward.
The reaction to FLUOROPLEX® in treated areas may be unsightly during therapy, and, in some cases, for several weeks following cessation of therapy.
Laboratory Tests: To rule out the presence of a frank neoplasm, a biopsy should be made of those areas failing to respond to treatment or recurring after treatment.
Carcinogenesis, mutagenesis, impairment of fertility: Adequate long-term studies in animals to evaluate carcinogenic potential have not been conducted with fluorouracil. In three *in vitro* cell transformation assays, fluorouracil produced morphological transformation of cells. Morphological transformation was also produced in one of these *in vitro* assays by a metabolite of fluorouracil and the transformed cells produced malignant tumors when injected into immunosuppressed syngeneic mice. Fluorouracil has been shown to exert mutagenic activity in the yeast cells, **Bacillus subtilis,** and **Drosophila** assays. In addition, fluorouracil has produced chromosome damage at concentrations of 1.0 and 2.0 mcg/mL in an *in vitro* hamster fibroblast assay and increases in micronuclei formation in the bone marrow of mice at intraperitoneal doses within the human therapeutic dose range of 12–15 mg/kg/day. Patients receiving cumulative doses of 0.24–1.0 g of fluorouracil parenterally have shown an increase in numerical and structural chromosome aberrations in peripheral blood lymphocytes. Fluorouracil has been shown to impair fertility after parenteral administration in rats. In mice, single-dose intravenous and intraperitoneal injections of fluorouracil have been reported to kill differentiated spermatogonia and spermatocytes at a dose of 500 mg/kg and produce abnormalities in spermatids at 50 mg/kg.
Fluorouracil was negative in the dominant lethal mutation assay performed in mice.
Pregnancy: Teratogenic effects: Pregnancy Category X:
Fluorouracil may cause fetal harm when administered to a pregnant woman. Fluorouracil administered parenterally has been shown to be teratogenic in mice, rats and hamsters, and embryolethal in monkeys. Fluorouracil is contraindicated in women who are or may become pregnant. If this drug is used during pregnancy, or if the patient becomes pregnant while taking this drug, the patient should be apprised of the potential hazard to the fetus.
Nursing mothers: It is not known whether this drug is excreted in human milk. Because many drugs are excreted in human milk, and because there is some systemic absorption of fluorouracil after topical administration (see **PRECAUTIONS: General**), mothers should not nurse their infants while receiving this drug.
Pediatric use: Safety and effectiveness in pediatric patients have not been established.

ADVERSE REACTIONS

Pain, pruritus, burning, irritation, inflammation, allergic contact dermatitis and telangiectasia have been reported. Occasionally, hyperpigmentation and scarring have also been reported.

OVERDOSAGE

Ordinarily, overdosage will not cause acute problems. If FLUOROPLEX® accidentally comes in contact with the eye(s), flush the eye(s) with water or normal saline. If FLUOROPLEX® is accidentally ingested, induce emesis and gastric lavage. Administer symptomatic and supportive care as needed.

DOSAGE AND ADMINISTRATION

The patient should be instructed to apply sufficient medication to cover the entire face or other affected areas.
Apply medication twice daily with non-metallic applicator or fingertips and wash hands afterwards. A treatment period of 2–6 weeks is usually required.
Increasing the frequency of application and a longer period of administration with FLUOROPLEX® may be required on areas other than the head and neck.
When FLUOROPLEX® is applied to keratotic skin, a response occurs with the following sequence: erythema, usually followed by scaling, tenderness, erosion, ulceration, necrosis and re-epithelization. When the inflammatory reaction reaches the erosion, ulceration and necrosis stages, the use of the drug should be terminated. Responses may sometimes occur in areas which appear clinically normal. These may be sites of subclinical actinic (solar) keratosis which the medication is affecting.

HOW SUPPLIED

FLUOROPLEX® (fluorouracil) 1% Topical Cream is available in 30 g tubes (NDC 0023-0812-30).
FLUOROPLEX® (fluorouracil) 1% Topical Solution is available in 30 mL plastic dropper bottles (NDC 0023-0810-30).
Note: Avoid freezing. Store at 15°–30°C (59°–86 °F) in tight containers.

Rx only

REFERENCE

1. Epstein E. Testing for 5-fluorouracil allergy: patch and intradermal tests. *Contact Dermatitis* 1984; 10:311.
© 1995 Allergan, Inc.

GRIS-PEG® ℞
(griseofulvin ultramicrosize)
Tablets, USP
125 mg; 250 mg

DESCRIPTION

GRIS-PEG® Tablets contain ultramicrosize crystals of griseofulvin, an antibiotic derived from a species of *Penicillium*.
Each GRIS-PEG® Tablet contains:
Active Ingredient: griseofulvin ultramicrosize ..... 125 mg
Inactive Ingredients: colloidal silicon dioxide, lactose, magnesium stearate; methylcellulose; methylparaben; polyethylene glycol 400 and 8000, polyvinylpyrrolidone; and titanium dioxide.
or
Active Ingredient: griseofulvin ultramicrosize ..... 250 mg
Inactive Ingredients: colloidal silicon dioxide; magnesium stearate; methylcellulose; methylparaben; polyethylene glycol 400 and 8000; povidone; sodium lauryl sulfate; and titanium dioxide.

ACTION

Microbiology—Griseofulvin is fungistatic with *in vitro* activity against various species of *Microsporum, Epidermophyton* and *Trichophyton*. It has no effect on bacteria or other genera of fungi.
Human Pharmacology—Following oral administration, griseofulvin is deposited in the keratin precursor cells and has a greater affinity for diseased tissue. The drug is tightly bound to the new keratin which becomes highly resistant to fungal invasions.
The efficiency of gastrointestinal absorption of ultramicrocrystalline griseofulvin is approximately one and one-half times that of the conventional microsize griseofulvin. This factor permits the oral intake of two-thirds as much ultramicrocrystalline griseofulvin as the microsize form. However, there is currently no evidence that this lower dose confers any significant clinical differences with regard to safety and/or efficacy.

INDICATIONS

GRIS-PEG® (griseofulvin ultramicrosize) is indicated for the treatment of the following ringworm infections; tinea corporis (ringworm of the body), tinea pedis (athlete's foot), tinea cruris (ringworm of the groin and thigh), tinea barbae (barber's itch), tinea capitis (ringworm of the scalp), and tinea unguium (onychomycosis, ringworm of the nails), when caused by one or more of the following genera of fungi: *Trichophyton rubrum, Trichophyton tonsurans, Trichophyton mentagrophytes, Trichophyton interdigitalis, Trichophyton verrucosum, Trichophyton megnini, Trichophyton gallinae, Trichophyton crateriform, Trichophyton sulphureum, Trichophyton schoenleini, Microsporum audouini, Microsporum canis, Microsporum gypseum* and *Epidermophyton floccosum.* Note: Prior to therapy, the type of fungi responsible for the infection should be identified. The use of the drug is not justified in minor or trivial infections which will respond to topical agents alone. Griseofulvin is *not* effective in the following: bacterial infections, candidiasis (moniliasis), histoplasmosis, actinomycosis, sporotrichosis, chromoblastomycosis, coccidioidomycosis, North American blastomycosis, cryptococcosis (torulosis), tinea versicolor and nocardiosis.

CONTRAINDICATIONS

Two cases of conjoined twins have been reported since 1977 in patients taking griseofulvin during the first trimester of pregnancy. Griseofulvin should not be prescribed to pregnant patients. If the patient becomes pregnant while taking this drug, the patient should be apprised of the potential hazard to the fetus.

This drug is contraindicated in patients with porphyria or hepatocellular failure and in individuals with a history of hypersensitivity to griseofulvin.

WARNINGS

Prophylactic Usage —Safety and efficacy of griseofulvin for prophylaxis of fungal infections have not been established.

Animal Toxicology —Chronic feeding of griseofulvin, at levels ranging from 0.5%–2.5% of the diet resulted in the development of liver tumors in several strains of mice, particularly in males. Smaller particle sizes result in an enhanced effect. Lower oral dosage levels have not been tested. Subcutaneous administration of relatively small doses of griseofulvin once a week during the first three weeks of life has also been reported to induce hepatomata in mice. Thyroid tumors, mostly adenomas but some carcinomas, have been reported in male rats receiving griseofulvin at levels of 2.0%, 1.0% and 0.2% of the diet, and in female rats receiving the two higher dose levels. Although studies in other animal species have not yielded evidence of tumorigenicity, these studies were not of adequate design to form a basis for conclusion in this regard. In subacute toxicity studies, orally administered griseofulvin produced hepatocellular necrosis in mice, but this has not been seen in other species. Disturbances in porphyrin metabolism have been reported in griseofulvin-treated laboratory animals. Griseofulvin has been reported to have a colchicine-like effect on mitosis and cocarcinogenicity with methylcholanthrene in cutaneous tumor induction in laboratory animals.

Usage in Pregnancy —See CONTRAINDICATIONS section.

Animal Reproduction Studies —It has been reported in the literature that griseofulvin was found to be embryotoxic and teratogenic on oral administration to pregnant rats. Pups with abnormalities have been reported in the litters of a few bitches treated with griseofulvin. Suppression of spermatogenesis has been reported to occur in rats, but investigation in man failed to confirm this.

PRECAUTIONS

Patients on prolonged therapy with any potent medication should be under close observation. Periodic monitoring of organ system function, including renal, hepatic and hematopoietic, should be done. Since griseofulvin is derived from species of *Penicillium,* the possibility of cross-sensitivity with penicillin exists; however, known penicillin-sensitive patients have been treated without difficulty. Since a photosensitivity reaction is occasionally associated with griseofulvin therapy, patients should be warned to avoid exposure to intense natural or artificial sunlight. Lupus erythematosus or lupus-like syndromes have been reported in patients receiving griseofulvin. Griseofulvin decreases the activity of warfarin-type anticoagulants so that patients receiving these drugs concomitantly may require dosage adjustment of the anticoagulant during and after griseofulvin therapy. Barbiturates usually depress griseofulvin activity and concomitant administration may require a dosage adjustment of the antifungal agent. There have been reports in the literature of possible interactions between griseofulvin and oral contraceptives. The effect of alcohol may be potentiated by griseofulvin, producing such effects as tachycardia and flush.

ADVERSE REACTIONS

When adverse reactions occur, they are most commonly of the hypersensitivity type such as skin rashes, urticaria, erythema multiforme-like drug reactions, and rarely, angioneurotic edema, and may necessitate withdrawal of therapy and appropriate countermeasures. Paresthesias of the hands and feet have been reported rarely after extended therapy. Other side effects reported occasionally are oral thrush, nausea, vomiting, epigastric distress, diarrhea, headache, fatigue, dizziness, insomnia, mental confusion, and impairment of performance of routine activities. Proteinuria and leukopenia have been reported rarely. Administration of the drug should be discontinued if granulocytopenia occurs. When rare, serious reactions occur with griseofulvin, they are usually associated with high dosages, long periods of therapy, or both.

DOSAGE AND ADMINISTRATION

Accurate diagnosis of the infecting organism is essential. Identification should be made either by direct microscopic examination of a mounting of infected tissue in a solution of potassium hydroxide or by culture on an appropriate medium. Medication must be continued until the infecting organism is completely eradicated as indicated by appropriate clinical or laboratory examination. Representative treatment periods are tinea capitis, 4 to 6 weeks; tinea corporis, 2 to 4 weeks; tinea pedis, 4 to 8 weeks; tinea unguium—depending on rate of growth—fingernails, at least 4 months; toenails, at least 6 months.

General measures in regard to hygiene should be observed to control sources of infection or reinfection. Concomitant use of appropriate topical agents is usually required, particularly in treatment of tinea pedis. In some forms of athlete's foot, yeasts and bacteria may be involved as well as fungi. Griseofulvin will not eradicate the bacterial or monilial infection.

Adults: Daily administration of 375 mg (as a single dose or in divided doses) will give a satisfactory response in most patients with tinea corporis, tinea cruris, and tinea capitis. For those fungal infections more difficult to eradicate, such as tinea pedis and tinea unguium, a divided dose of 750 mg is recommended.

Pediatric Use: Approximately 3.3 mg per pound of body weight per day of ultramicrosize griseofulvin is an effective dose for most pediatric patients. On this basis, the following dosage schedule is suggested: Children weighing 35–60 pounds—125 mg to 187.5 mg daily. Children weighing over 60 pounds—187.5 mg to 375 mg daily. Children and infants 2 years of age and younger—dosage has not been established.

Clinical experience with griseofulvin in children with tinea capitis indicates that a single daily dose is effective. Clinical relapse will occur if the medication is not continued until the infecting organism is eradicated.

HOW SUPPLIED

GRIS-PEG® (griseofulvin ultramicrosize) Tablets, 125 mg, white, scored, elliptical-shaped, embossed "GRIS-PEG" on one side and "125" on the other. GRIS-PEG® (griseofulvin ultramicrosize) Tablets, 250 mg, white, scored, capsule-shaped, embossed "GRIS-PEG" on one side and "250" on the other. The 125 mg strength is available in bottles of 100 (NDC 0023-0763-04). The 250 mg strength is available in bottles of 100, and 500 (NDC 0023-0773-04, and NDC 0023-0773-50 respectively). Both strengths are film-coated.

Rx only

STORAGE

Store GRIS-PEG® tablets at controlled room temperature 15°–30°C (59°–86°F) in tight, light-resistant containers.

Manufactured for ALLERGAN
Irvine, CA 92612, U.S.A.
by SANDOZ PHARMACEUTICALS CORPORATION
© 1996 Allergan, Inc.

MAXIFLOR® ℞
(diflorasone diacetate)
Cream, USP, 0.05%
Ointment, USP, 0.05%

DESCRIPTION

MAXIFLOR® Cream Contains:

Active Ingredient: 0.5 mg diflorasone diacetate, USP, in an emulsified and hydrophilic cream base.

Inactive Ingredients: Propylene glycol, stearic acid, polysorbate 60, sorbitan monostearate and monooleate, sorbic acid, citric acid and water. The corticosteroid is formulated as a solution in the vehicle using 15 percent propylene glycol to optimize drug delivery.

MAXIFLOR® Ointment Contains:

Active Ingredient: 0.5 mg diflorasone diacetate, USP, in an emollient, occlusive base. *Inactive Ingredients:* Polyoxypropylene 15-stearyl ether, stearic acid, lanolin alcohol and white petrolatum.

HOW SUPPLIED

MAXIFLOR® (diflorasone diacetate) Cream, USP, 0.05% is available in collapsible tubes in the following sizes:
30 gram NDC 0023-0766-30
60 gram NDC 0023-0766-60

MAXIFLOR® (diflorasone diacetate) Ointment, USP, 0.05% is available in collapsible tubes in the following sizes:
30 gram NDC 0023-0770-30
60 gram NDC 0023-0770-60

Manufactured for ALLERGAN
Irvine, California 92715, USA
by Pharmacia & Upjohn Company
Kalamazoo, Michigan 49001
© 1996 Allergan, Inc.

NAFTIN® ℞
(naftifine hydrochloride) 1%
Cream

DESCRIPTION

NAFTIN® Cream, 1% contains the synthetic, broad-spectrum, antifungal agent naftifine hydrochloride.

NAFTIN® Cream, 1% is for topical use only.

Chemical Name: (E)-N-Cinnamyl-N-methyl-1-naphthalenemethyl-amine hydrochloride. Naftifine hydrochloride has an empirical formula of $C_{21}H_{21}N \cdot HCl$ and a molecular weight of 323.86.

Active Ingredient: Naftifine hydrochloride 1%

Inactive Ingredients: benzyl alcohol, cetyl alcohol, cetyl esters wax, isopropyl myristate, polysorbate 60, purified water, sodium hydroxide, sorbitan monostearate, and stearyl alcohol. Hydrochloric acid may be added to adjust pH.

CLINICAL PHARMACOLOGY

Naftifine hydrochloride is a synthetic allylamine derivative. The following *in vitro* data are available, but their clinical significance is unknown. Naftifine hydrochloride has been shown to exhibit fungicidal activity *in vitro* against a broad spectrum of organisms including *Trichophyton rubrum, Trichophyton mentagrophytes, Trichophyton tonsurans, Epidermophyton floccosum, Microsporum canis, Microsporum audouini,* and *Microsporum gypseum;* and fungistatic activity against *Candida* species, including *Candida albicans.* NAFTIN® Cream, 1% has only been shown to be clinically effective against the disease entities listed in the INDICATIONS AND USAGE section.

Although the exact mechanism of action against fungi is not known, naftifine hydrochloride appears to interfere with sterol biosynthesis by inhibiting the enzyme squalene 2,3-epoxidase. This inhibition of enzyme activity results in decreased amounts of sterols, especially ergosterol, and a corresponding accumulation of squalene in the cells.

Pharmacokinetics: *In vitro* and *in vivo* bioavailability studies have demonstrated that naftifine penetrates the stratum corneum in sufficient concentration to inhibit the growth of dermatophytes.

Following a single topical application of 1% naftifine cream to the skin of healthy subjects, systemic absorption of naftifine was approximately 6% of the applied dose. Naftifine and/or its metabolites are excreted via the urine and feces with a half-life of approximately two to three days.

INDICATIONS AND USAGE

NAFTIN® Cream, 1% is indicated for topical application in the treatment of tinea pedis, tinea cruris and tinea corporis caused by the organisms *Tricophyton rubrum, Tricophyton mentagrophytes,* and *Epidermophyton floccosum.*

CONTRAINDICATIONS

NAFTIN® Cream, 1% is contraindicated in individuals who have shown hypersensitivity to any of its components.

WARNING

NAFTIN® Cream, 1% is for topical use only and not for ophthalmic use.

PRECAUTIONS

General: NAFTIN® Cream, 1% is for external use only. If irritation or sensitivity develops with the use of NAFTIN® Cream 1%, treatment should be discontinued and appropriate therapy instituted. Diagnosis of the disease should be confirmed either by direct microscopic examination of a mounting of infected tissue in a solution of potassium hydroxide or by culture on an appropriate medium.

Information for patients: The patient should be told to:

1. Avoid the use of occlusive dressings or wrappings unless otherwise directed by the physician.
2. Keep NAFTIN® Cream, 1% away from the eyes, nose, mouth and other mucous membranes.

Carcinogenesis, mutagenesis, impairment of fertility: Long-term animal studies to evaluate the carcinogenic potential of NAFTIN® Cream, 1% have not been performed. *In vitro* and animal studies have not demonstrated any mutagenic effect or effect on fertility.

Pregnancy: Teratogenic Effects: Pregnancy Category B: Reproduction studies have been performed in rats and rabbits (via oral administration) at doses 150 times or more the

Continued on next page

Naftin—Cont.

topical human dose and have revealed no significant evidence of impaired fertility or harm to the fetus due to naftifine. There are, however, no adequate and well-controlled studies in pregnant women. Because animal reproduction studies are not always predictive of human response, this drug should be used during pregnancy only if clearly needed.

Nursing mothers: It is not known whether this drug is excreted in human milk. Because many drugs are excreted in human milk, caution should be exercised when NAFTIN® Cream, 1% is administered to a nursing woman.

Pediatric use: Safety and effectiveness in pediatric patients have not been established.

ADVERSE REACTIONS

During clinical trials with NAFTIN® Cream 1%, the incidence of adverse reactions was as follows: burning/stinging (6%), dryness (3%), erythema (2%), itching (2%), local irritation (2%).

DOSAGE AND ADMINISTRATION

A sufficient quantity of NAFTIN® Cream, 1% should be gently massaged into the affected and surrounding skin areas once a day. The hands should be washed after application.

If no clinical improvement is seen after four weeks of treatment with NAFTIN® Cream, 1% the patient should be reevaluated.

HOW SUPPLIED

NAFTIN® (naftifine hydrochloride) 1% Cream is supplied in collapsible tubes in the following sizes:
15 g-NDC-0023-4126-15
30 g-NDC-0023-4126-30
60 g-NDC-0023-4126-60
Note: Store below 30°C (86°F).
Rx only
©1996 Allergan, Inc.

NAFTIN®   ℞
(naftifine hydrochloride) 1%
Gel

DESCRIPTION

NAFTIN® Gel, 1% contains the synthetic, broad-spectrum, antifungal agent naftifine hydrochloride.
NAFTIN® Gel, 1% is for topical use only.
Chemical Name: (E)-N-Cinnamyl-N-methyl-1-naphthalene-methylamine hydrochloride. Naftifine hydrochloride has an empirical formula of $C_{21}H_{21}N \cdot HCl$ and a molecular weight of 323.86.
Contains:
Active Ingredient: Naftifine hydrochloride 1%
Inactive Ingredients: polysorbate 80, carbomer 934P, diisopropanolamine, edetate disodium, alcohol (52% v/v), and purified water.

CLINICAL PHARMACOLOGY

Naftifine hydrochloride is a synthetic allylamine derivative. The following *in vitro* data are available but their clinical significance is unknown. Naftifine hydrochloride has been shown to exhibit fungicidal activity *in vitro* against a broad spectrum of organisms including *Trichophyton rubrum, Trichophyton mentagrophytes, Trichophyton tonsurans, Epidermophyton floccosum,* and *Microsporum canis, Microsporum audouini,* and *Microsporum gypseum;* and fungistatic activity against *Candida* species including *Candida albicans.* NAFTIN® Gel, 1% has only been shown to be clinically effective against the disease entities listed in the INDICATIONS AND USAGE section.

Although the exact mechanism of action against fungi is not known, naftifine hydrochloride appears to interfere with sterol biosynthesis by inhibiting the enzyme squalene 2,3-epoxidase. This inhibition of enzyme activity results in decreased amounts of sterols, especially ergosterol, and a corresponding accumulation of squalene in the cells.

Pharmacokinetics: *In vitro* and *in vivo* bioavailability studies have demonstrated that naftifine penetrates the stratum corneum in sufficient concentration to inhibit the growth of dermatophytes.

Following single topical application of ^{3}H-labeled naftifine gel 1% to the skin of healthy subjects, up to 4.2% of the applied dose was absorbed. Naftifine and/or its metabolites are excreted via the urine and feces with a half-life of approximately two to three days.

INDICATION AND USAGE

NAFTIN® Gel, 1% is indicated for the topical treatment of tinea pedis, tinea cruris and tinea corporis caused by the organisms *Trichophyton rubrum, Trichophyton mentagro-*

phytes, Trichophyton tonsurans* and *Epidermophyton floccosum.**

*Efficacy for this organism in this organ system was studied in fewer than 10 infections.

CONTRAINDICATIONS

NAFTIN® Gel, 1% is contraindicated in individuals who have shown hypersensitivity to any of its components.

WARNINGS

NAFTIN® Gel, 1% is for topical use only and not for ophthalmic use.

PRECAUTIONS

General: NAFTIN® Gel, 1% is for external use only. If irritation or sensitivity develop with the use of NAFTIN® Gel, 1%, treatment should be discontinued and appropriate therapy instituted. Diagnosis of the disease should be confirmed either by direct microscopic examination of a mounting of infected tissue in a solution of potassium hydroxide or by culture on an appropriate medium.

Information for patients:
The patient should be told to:
1. Avoid the use of occlusive dressings or wrappings unless otherwise directed by the physician.
2. Keep NAFTIN® Gel, 1% away from the eyes, nose, mouth and other mucous membranes.

Carcinogenesis, mutagenesis, impairment of fertility: Long-term studies to evaluate the carcinogenic potential of NAFTIN® Gel, 1% have not been performed. *In vitro* and animal studies have not demonstrated any mutagenic effect or effect on fertility.

Pregnancy: Teratogenic Effects: Pregnancy Category B: Reproduction studies have been performed in rats and rabbits (via oral administration) at doses 150 times or more than the topical human dose and have revealed no evidence of impaired fertility or harm to the fetus due to naftifine. There are, however, no adequate and well-controlled studies in pregnant women. Because animal reproduction studies are not always predictive of human response, this drug should be used during pregnancy only if clearly needed.

Nursing mothers: It is not known whether this drug is excreted in human milk. Because many drugs are excreted in human milk, caution should be exercised when NAFTIN® Gel, 1% is administered to a nursing woman.

Pediatric use: Safety and effectiveness in pediatric patients have not been established.

ADVERSE REACTIONS

During clinical trials with NAFTIN® Gel, 1%, the incidence of adverse reactions was as follows: burning/stinging (5.0%), itching (1.0%), erythema (0.5%), rash (0.5%), skin tenderness (0.5%).

DOSAGE AND ADMINISTRATION

A sufficient quantity of NAFTIN® Gel, 1% should be gently massaged into the affected and surrounding skin areas twice a day, in the morning and evening. The hands should be washed after application.

If no clinical improvement is seen after four weeks of treatment with NAFTIN® Gel, 1%, the patient should be reevaluated.

HOW SUPPLIED

NAFTIN® (naftifine hydrochloride) is supplied in collapsible tubes in the following sizes:
20 g-NDC-0023-4770-20
40 g-NDC-0023-4770-40
60 g-NDC-0023-4770-60
Note: Store at room temperature.
Rx only
© 1996 Allergan, Inc.

OCUFLOX®   ℞
(ofloxacin ophthalmic solution)
0.3% sterile

DESCRIPTION

OCUFLOX® (ofloxacin ophthalmic solution) 0.3% is a sterile ophthalmic solution. It is a fluorinated carboxyquinolone anti-infective for topical ophthalmic use.
Structural Formula:

ofloxacin

$C_{18}H_{20}FN_3O_4$ Mol Wt 361.37

Chemical Name: (±)-9-Fluoro-2,3-dihydro-3-methyl-10-(4-methyl-1-piperazinyl)-7-oxo-7H-pyrido[1,2,3-de]-1,4 benzoxazine-6-carboxylic acid.

Contains:
Active: ofloxacin 0.3% (3 mg/mL);
Preservative: benzalkonium chloride (0.005%);
Inactives: sodium chloride and purified water. May also contain hydrochloric acid and/or sodium hydroxide to adjust pH.

OCUFLOX® solution is unbuffered and formulated with a pH of 6.4 (range—6.0 to 6.8). It has an osmolality of 300 mOsm/kg. Ofloxacin is a fluorinated 4-quinolone which differs from other fluorinated 4-quinolones in that there is a six member (pyridobenzoxazine) ring from positions 1 to 8 of the basic ring structure.

CLINICAL PHARMACOLOGY

Pharmacokinetics: Serum, urine and tear concentrations of ofloxacin were measured in 30 healthy women at various time points during a ten-day course of treatment with OCUFLOX® solution. The mean serum ofloxacin concentration ranged from 0.4 ng/mL to 1.9 ng/mL. Maximum ofloxacin concentration increased from 1.1 ng/mL on day one to 1.9 ng/mL on day 11 after QID dosing for $10^1/_2$ days. Maximum serum ofloxacin concentrations after ten days of topical ophthalmic dosing were more than 1000 times lower than those reported after standard oral doses of ofloxacin.

Tear ofloxacin concentrations ranged from 5.7 to 31 µg/g during the 40 minute period following the last dose on day 11. Mean tear concentration measured four hours after topical ophthalmic dosing was 9.2 µg/g.

Corneal tissue concentrations of 4.4 µg/mL were observed four hours after beginning topical ocular application of two drops of OCUFLOX® every 30 minutes. Ofloxacin was excreted in the urine primarily unmodified.

Microbiology: Ofloxacin has in vitro activity against a broad range of gram-positive and gram-negative aerobic and anaerobic bacteria. Ofloxacin is bactericidal at concentrations equal to or slightly greater than inhibitory concentrations. Ofloxacin is thought to exert a bactericidal effect on susceptible bacterial cells by inhibiting DNA gyrase, an essential bacterial enzyme which is a critical catalyst in the duplication, transcription, and repair of bacterial DNA.

Cross-resistance has been observed between ofloxacin and other fluoroquinolones. There is generally no cross-resistance between ofloxacin and other classes of antibacterial agents such as beta-lactams or aminoglycosides.

Ofloxacin has been shown to be active against most strains of the following organisms both in vitro and clinically, in conjunctival and/or corneal ulcer infections as described in the **INDICATIONS AND USAGE** section.

AEROBES, GRAM-POSITIVE:
Staphylococcus aureus
Staphylococcus epidermidis
Streptococcus pneumoniae
AEROBES, GRAM-NEGATIVE:
Enterobacter cloacae
Haemophilus influenzae
Proteus mirabilis
Pseudomonas aeruginosa
Serratia marcescens*
ANAEROBIC SPECIES:
Propionibacterium acnes
*Efficacy for this organism was studied in fewer than 10 infections.

The safety and effectiveness of OCUFLOX® in treating ophthalmologic infections due to the following organisms have not been established in adequate and well-controlled clinical trials. OCUFLOX® has been shown to be active in vitro against most strains of these organisms but the clinical significance in ophthalmologic infections is unknown.

AEROBES, GRAM-POSITIVE:
Enterococcus faecalis
Listeria monocytogenes
Staphylococcus capitis
Staphylococcus hominus
Staphylococcus simulans
Streptococcus pyogenes
AEROBES, GRAM-NEGATIVE:
Acinetobacter calcoaceticus var. *anitratus*
Acinetobacter calcoaceticus var. *lwoffii*
Citrobacter diversus
Citrobacter freundii
Enterobacter aerogenes
Enterobacter agglomerans
Escherichia coli
Haemophilus parainfluenzae
Klebsiella oxytoca
Klebsiella pneumoniae
Moraxella (Branhamella) catarrhalis
Moraxella lacunata
Morganella morganii
Neisseria gonorrhoeae
Pseudomonas acidovorans
Pseudomonas fluorescens
Shigella sonnei
OTHER:
Chlamydia trachomatis

Clinical Studies:

Conjunctivitis: In a randomized, double-masked, multicenter clinical trial, OCUFLOX® solution was superior to its vehicle after 2 days of treatment in patients with conjunctivitis and positive conjunctival cultures. Clinical outcomes for the trial demonstrated a clinical improvement rate of 86% (54/63) for the ofloxacin treated group versus 72% (48/67) for the placebo treated group after 2 days of therapy. Microbiological outcomes for the same clinical trial demonstrated an eradication rate for causative pathogens of 65% (41/63) for the ofloxacin treated group versus 25% (17/67) for the vehicle treated group after 2 days of therapy. Please note that microbiologic eradication does not always correlate with clinical outcome in anti-infective trials.

Corneal Ulcers: In a randomized, double-masked, multicenter trial of 140 subjects with positive cultures, OCUFLOX® treated subjects had an overall clinical success rate (complete re-epithelialization and no progression of the infiltrate for two consecutive visits) of 82% (61/74) compared to 80% (53/66) for the fortified antibiotic group, consisting of 1.5% tobramycin and 10% cefazolin solutions. The median time to clinical success was 11 days for the ofloxacin treated group and 10 days for the fortified treatment group.

INDICATIONS AND USAGE

OCUFLOX® solution is indicated for the treatment of infections caused by susceptible strains of the following bacteria in the conditions listed below:

CONJUNCTIVITIS:

Gram-positive bacteria:
Staphylococcus aureus
Staphylococcus epidermidis
Streptococcus pneumoniae

Gram-negative bacteria:
Enterobacter cloacae
Haemophilus influenzae
Proteus mirabilis
Pseudomonas aeruginosa

CORNEAL ULCERS:

Gram-positive bacteria:
Staphylococcus aureus
Staphylococcus epidermidis
Streptococcus pneumoniae

Gram-negative bacteria:
Pseudomonas aeruginosa
*Serratia marcescens**

Anaerobic species:
Propionibacterium acnes

*Efficacy for this organism was studied in fewer than 10 infections.

CONTRAINDICATIONS

OCUFLOX® solution is contraindicated in patients with a history of hypersensitivity to ofloxacin, to other quinolones, or to any of the components in this medication.

WARNINGS

NOT FOR INJECTION.

OCUFLOX® solution should not be injected subconjunctivally, nor should it be introduced directly into the anterior chamber of the eye.

Serious and occasionally fatal hypersensitivity (anaphylactic) reactions, some following the first dose, have been reported in patients receiving systemic quinolones, including ofloxacin. Some reactions were accompanied by cardiovascular collapse, loss of consciousness, angioedema (including laryngeal, pharyngeal or facial edema), airway obstruction, dyspnea, urticaria, and itching. A rare occurrence of Stevens-Johnson syndrome, which progressed to toxic epidermal necrolysis, has been reported in a patient who was receiving topical ophthalmic ofloxacin. If an allergic reaction to ofloxacin occurs, discontinue the drug. Serious acute hypersensitivity reactions may require immediate emergency treatment. Oxygen and airway management, including intubation should be administered as clinically indicated.

PRECAUTIONS

General: As with other anti-infectives, prolonged use may result in overgrowth of nonsusceptible organisms, including fungi. If superinfection occurs, discontinue use and institute alternative therapy. Whenever clinical judgment dictates, the patient should be examined with the aid of magnification, such as slit lamp biomicroscopy and, where appropriate, fluorescein staining. Ofloxacin should be discontinued at the first appearance of a skin rash or any other sign of hypersensitivity reaction.

The systemic administration of quinolones, including ofloxacin, has led to lesions or erosions of the cartilage in weight-bearing joints and other signs of arthropathy in immature animals of various species. Ofloxacin, administered systemically at 10 mg/kg/day in young dogs (equivalent to 110 times the maximum recommended daily *adult ophthalmic* dose) has been associated with these types of effects.

Information for Patients: Avoid contaminating the applicator tip with material from the eye, fingers, or other source. Systemic quinolones, including ofloxacin, have been associated with hypersensitivity reactions, even following a single dose. Discontinue use immediately and contact your physician at the first sign of a rash or allergic reaction.

Drug Interactions: Specific drug interaction studies have not been conducted with OCUFLOX® ophthalmic solution. However, the systemic administration of some quinolones has been shown to elevate plasma concentrations of theophylline, interfere with the metabolism of caffeine, and enhance the effects of the oral anticoagulant warfarin and its derivatives, and has been associated with transient elevations in serum creatinine in patients receiving cyclosporine concomitantly.

Carcinogenesis, Mutagenesis, Impairment of Fertility: Long term studies to determine the carcinogenic potential of ofloxacin have not been conducted.

Ofloxacin was not mutagenic in the Ames test, in vitro and in vivo cytogenic assay, sister chromatid exchange assay (Chinese hamster and human cell lines), unscheduled DNA synthesis (UDS) assay using human fibroblasts, the dominant lethal assay, or mouse micronucleus assay. Ofloxacin was positive in the UDS test using rat hepatocyte, and in the mouse lymphoma assay.

In fertility studies in rats, ofloxacin did not affect male or female fertility or morphological or reproductive performance at oral dosing up to 360 mg/kg/day (equivalent to 4000 times the maximum recommended daily ophthalmic dose).

Pregnancy: Teratogenic Effects. Pregnancy Category C: Ofloxacin has been shown to have embryocidal effect in rats and in rabbits when given in doses of 810 mg/kg/day (equivalent to 9000 times the maximum recommended daily ophthalmic dose) and 160 mg/kg/day (equivalent to 1800 times the maximum recommended daily ophthalmic dose). These dosages resulted in decreased fetal body weight and increased fetal mortality in rats and rabbits, respectively. Minor fetal skeletal variations were reported in rats receiving doses of 810 mg/kg/day. Ofloxacin has not been shown to be teratogenic at doses as high as 810 mg/kg/day and 160 mg/kg/day when administered to pregnant rats and rabbits, respectively.

Nonteratogenic Effects: Additional studies in rats with doses up to 360 mg/kg/day during late gestation showed no adverse effect on late fetal development, labor, delivery, lactation, neonatal viability, or growth of the newborn.

There are, however, no adequate and well-controlled studies in pregnant women. OCUFLOX® solution should be used during pregnancy only if the potential benefit justifies the potential risk to the fetus.

Nursing Mothers: In nursing women a single 200 mg oral dose resulted in concentrations of ofloxacin in milk which were similar to those found in plasma. It is not known whether ofloxacin is excreted in human milk following topical ophthalmic administration. Because of the potential for serious adverse reactions from ofloxacin in nursing infants, a decision should be made whether to discontinue nursing or to discontinue the drug, taking into account the importance of the drug to the mother.

Pediatric Use: Safety and effectiveness in infants below the age of one year have not been established.

Quinolones, including ofloxacin, have been shown to cause arthropathy in immature animals after oral administration; however, topical ocular administration of ofloxacin to immature animals has not shown any arthropathy. There is no evidence that the ophthalmic dosage form of ofloxacin has any effect on weight bearing joints.

ADVERSE REACTIONS

Ophthalmic Use: The most frequently reported drug-related adverse reaction was transient ocular burning or discomfort. Other reported reactions include stinging, redness, itching, chemical conjunctivitis/keratitis, periocular/facial edema, foreign body sensation, photophobia, blurred vision, tearing, dryness, and eye pain. Rare reports of dizziness have been received.

DOSAGE AND ADMINISTRATION

The recommended dosage regimen for the treatment of **bacterial conjunctivitis** is:

Days 1 and 2
Instill one to two drops every two to four hours in the affected eye(s).

Days 3 through 7
Instill one to two drops four times daily.

The recommended dosage regimen for the treatment of **bacterial corneal ulcer** is:

Days 1 and 2
Instill one to two drops into the affected eye every 30 minutes, while awake. Awaken at approximately four and six hours after retiring and instill one to two drops.

Days 3 through 7 to 9
Instill one to two drops hourly, while awake.

Days 7 to 9 through treatment completion
Instill one to two drops, four times daily.

HOW SUPPLIED

OCUFLOX® (ofloxacin ophthalmic solution) 0.3% is supplied sterile in plastic dropper bottles of the following sizes:
1 mL—NDC 11980–779–01
5 mL—NDC 11980–779–05
10 mL—NDC 11980–779–10

Note: Store at 15–25°C (59–77°F)

Caution: Rx only

May 1996

Allergan America, Hormigueros, Puerto Rico 00660

Licensed from: Daiichi Pharmaceutical Co., Ltd., Tokyo, Japan and Santen Pharmaceutical Co., Ltd., Osaka, Japan

U.S. PAT. NOS. 4,382,892; 4,551,456

©1996 Allergan, Inc. 70829 10B

Shown in Product Identification Guide, page 303

OPTICROM® ℞

(cromolyn sodium ophthalmic solution, USP) 4%
Sterile

Prescribing Information

DESCRIPTION

OPTICROM® (cromolyn sodium ophthalmic solution, USP) 4% is a clear, colorless, sterile solution intended for topical ophthalmic use.

Cromolyn sodium is represented by the following structural formula:

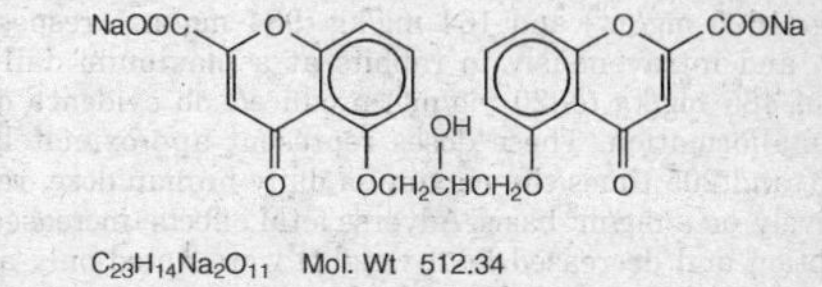
NaOOC
O
COONa
O
OH
O
OCH2CHCH2O
O

$C_{23}H_{14}Na_2O_{11}$ Mol. Wt 512.34

Chemical Name: Disodium 5-5′ - [(2-hydroxy trimethylene) dioxy] bis [4-oxo-4*H*-1-benzopyran-2-carboxylate].

Pharmacologic Category: Mast cell stabilizer

Each mL contains: **Active:** Cromolyn sodium 40 mg (4%); **Preservative:** Benzalkonium chloride 0.01%; **Inactives:** Edetate disodium 0.1% and purified water. It has a pH of 4.0 to 7.0.

CLINICAL PHARMACOLOGY

In vitro and *in vivo* animal studies have shown that cromolyn sodium inhibits the degranulation of sensitized mast cells which occurs after exposure to specific antigens. Cromolyn sodium acts by inhibiting the release of histamine and SRS-A (slow-reacting substance of anaphylaxis) from the mast cell.

Another activity demonstrated *in vitro* is the capacity of cromolyn sodium to inhibit the degranulation of non-sensitized rat mast cells by phospholipase A and the subsequent release of chemical mediators. Another study showed that cromolyn sodium did not inhibit the enzymatic activity of released phospholipase A on its specific substrate.

Cromolyn sodium has no intrinsic vasoconstrictor, antihistamine, or anti-inflammatory activity.

Cromolyn sodium is poorly absorbed. When multiple doses of cromolyn sodium ophthalmic solution are instilled into normal rabbit eyes, less than 0.07% of the administered dose of cromolyn sodium is absorbed into the systemic circulation (presumably by way of the eye, nasal passages, buccal cavity, and gastro intestinal tract). Trace amounts (less than 0.01%) of the cromolyn sodium dose penetrate into the aqueous humor and clearance from this chamber is virtually complete within 24 hours after treatment is stopped.

In normal volunteers, analysis of drug excretion indicates that approximately 0.03% of cromolyn sodium is absorbed following administration to the eye.

INDICATIONS AND USAGE

OPTICROM® is indicated in the treatment of vernal keratoconjunctivitis, vernal conjunctivitis, and vernal keratitis.

CONTRAINDICATIONS

OPTICROM® is contraindicated in those patients who have shown hypersensitivity to cromolyn sodium or to any of the other ingredients.

PRECAUTIONS

General: Patients may experience a transient stinging or burning sensation following application of OPTICROM.® The recommended frequency of administration should not be exceeded (see **DOSAGE AND ADMINISTRATION**).

Information for Patients: Patients should be advised to follow the patient instructions listed on the Information for Patients sheet.

Continued on next page

Opticrom—Cont.

Users of contact lenses should refrain from wearing lenses while exhibiting the signs and symptoms of vernal keratoconjunctivitis, vernal conjunctivitis, or vernal keratitis. Do not wear contact lenses during treatment with OPTICROM.®

Carcinogenesis, Mutagenesis, and Impairment of Fertility: Long term studies of cromolyn sodium in mice (12 months intraperitoneal administration at doses up to 150 mg/kg three days per week), hamsters (intraperitoneal administration at doses up to 52.6 mg/kg three days per week for 15 weeks followed by 17.5 mg/kg three days per week for 37 weeks), and rats (18 months subcutaneous administration at doses up to 75 mg/kg six days per week) showed no neoplastic effects. The average daily maximum dose levels administered in these studies were 192.9 mg/m^2 for mice, 47.2 mg/m^2 for hamsters and 385.8 mg/m^2 for rats. These doses correspond to approximately 6.8, 1.7, and 14 times the maximum daily human dose of 28 mg/m^2.

Cromolyn sodium showed no mutagenic potential in the Ames *Salmonella*/microsome plate assays, mitotic gene conversion in *Saccharomyces cerevisiae* and in an *in vitro* cytogenetic study in human peripheral lymphocytes.

No evidence of impaired fertility was shown in laboratory reproduction studies conducted subcutaneously in rats at the highest doses tested, 175 mg/kg/day (1050 mg/m^2) in males and 100 mg/kg/day (600 mg/m^2) in females. These doses are approximately 37 and 21 times the maximum daily human dose, respectively, based on mg/m^2.

Pregnancy

Teratogenic Effects: Pregnancy Category B. Reproduction studies with cromolyn sodium administered subcutaneously to pregnant mice and rats at maximum daily doses of 540 mg/kg (1620 mg/m^2) and 164 mg/kg (984 mg/m^2), respectively, and intravenously to rabbits at a maximum daily dose of 485 mg/kg (5820 mg/m^2) produced no evidence of fetal malformation. These doses represent approximately 57, 35, and 205 times the maximum daily human dose, respectively, on a mg/m^2 basis. Adverse fetal effects (increased resorption and decreased fetal weight) were noted only at the very high parenteral doses that produced maternal toxicity. There are, however, no adequate and well-controlled studies in pregnant women. Because animal reproduction studies are not always predictive of human response, this drug should be used during pregnancy only if clearly needed.

Nursing Mothers: It is not known whether this drug is excreted in human milk. Because many drugs are excreted in human milk, caution should be exercised when OPTICROM® is administered to a nursing woman.

Pediatric Use: Safety and effectiveness in children below the age of 4 years have not been established.

ADVERSE REACTIONS

The most frequently reported adverse reaction attributed to the use of OPTICROM®, on the basis of reoccurrence following readministration, is transient ocular stinging or burning upon instillation.

The following adverse reactions have been reported as infrequent events. It is unclear whether they are attributed to the drug:

Conjunctival injection; watery eyes; itchy eyes; dryness around the eye; puffy eyes; eye irritation; and styes.

Immediate hypersensitivity reactions have been reported rarely and include dyspnea, edema, and rash.

DOSAGE AND ADMINISTRATION

The dose is 1–2 drops in each eye 4–6 times a day at regular intervals. One drop contains approximately 1.6 mg cromolyn sodium.

Patients should be advised that the effect of OPTICROM® therapy is dependent upon its administration at regular intervals, as directed.

Symptomatic response to therapy (decreased itching, tearing, redness, and discharge) is usually evident within a few days, but longer treatment for up to six weeks is sometimes required. Once symptomatic improvement has been established, therapy should be continued for as long as needed to sustain improvement. If required, corticosteroids may be used concomitantly with OPTICROM.®

HOW SUPPLIED

OPTICROM® (cromolyn sodium ophthalmic solution, USP) 4% is supplied as 10 mL of solution in an opaque polyethylene eye drop bottle.

10 mL **NDC** 0023-6422-10

Store at Controlled Room Temperature 20–25°C (68–77°F). Protect from light - store in original carton. Keep tightly closed and out of the reach of children.

Rx only

ALLERGAN

©1998 Allergan, Inc., Irvine, CA 92612 U.S.A.

OPTICROM® is a registered trademark under exclusive license from Fisons plc.

Revised February 1998

IN-F9541
70568 US 10D RX9419

PENECORT® ℞
(hydrocortisone)
Cream, USP, 1%
Topical Solution 1%

PENECORT® Cream contains:
Active Ingredient: hydrocortisone, USP 1%
Inactive Ingredients: benzyl alcohol; petrolatum; stearyl alcohol; propylene glycol; isopropyl myristate; polyoxyl 40 stearate; carbomer 934; sodium lauryl sulfate; edetate disodium; sodium hydroxide to adjust the pH; and purified water.

PENECORT® Topical Solution contains:
Active Ingredient: hydrocortisone, USP 1%
Inactive Ingredients: SD Alcohol 40–2 with tertiary butyl alcohol and brucine sulfate (57%); propylene glycol; benzyl alcohol; and purified water.

HOW SUPPLIED

PENECORT® (hydrocortisone):
Cream, USP, 1%—30 g collapsible tubes: NDC 0023-0510-30
Topical Solution 1%—30 mL and 60 mL plastic bottles:
30 mL NDC 0023-0889-30; 60 mL NDC 0023-0889-60

Note: Store at controlled room temperature 15°–30°C (59°–86°F). Store away from heat. Protect from freezing.

Rx only

© 1995 Allergan, Inc.

POLYTRIM® ℞
(TRIMETHOPRIM AND POLYMYXIN B SULFATE OPHTHALMIC SOLUTION) Sterile

DESCRIPTION

Polytrim® (trimethoprim and polymyxin B sulfate ophthalmic solution) is a sterile antimicrobial solution for topical ophthalmic use. It has pH of 4.0 to 6.2 and osmolarity of 270 to 310 mOsm/kg.

Chemical Names: Trimethoprim, 2,4-Diamino-5-(3,4,5-trimethoxybenzyl)pyrimidine is a white, odorless, crystalline powder with a molecular weight of 678.72.

Polymyxin B sulfate is the sulfate salt of polymyxin B_1 and B_2 which are produced by the growth of *Bacillus polymyxa* (Prazmowski) Migula (Fam. Bacillaceae). It has a potency of not less than 6,000 polymyxin B units per mg, calculated on an anhydrous basis.

Contains: Actives: trimethoprim 1 mg/mL, polymyxin B sulfate 10,000 units/mL. Preservative: benzalkonium chloride 0.04 mg/mL. Inactives: sodium chloride, sulfuric acid and purified water. May also contain sodium hydroxide for pH adjustment.

CLINICAL PHARMACOLOGY

Trimethoprim is a synthetic antibacterial drug active against a wide variety of aerobic gram-positive and gram-negative ophthalmic pathogens. Trimethoprim blocks the production of tetrahydrofolic acid from dihydrofolic acid by binding to and reversibly inhibiting the enzyme dihydrofolate reductase. This binding is stronger for the bacterial enzyme than for the corresponding mammalian enzyme and therefore selectively interferes with bacterial biosynthesis of nucleic acids and proteins.

Polymyxin B, a cyclic lipopeptide antibiotic, is bactericidal for a variety of gram-negative organisms, especially *Pseudomonas aeruginosa*. It increases the permeability of the bacterial cell membrane by interacting with the phospholipid components of the membrane.

Blood samples were obtained from 11 human volunteers at 20 minutes, 1 hour and 3 hours following instillation in the eye of 2 drops of ophthalmic solution containing 1 mg trimethoprim and 10,000 units polymyxin B per mL. Peak serum concentrations were approximately 0.03 µg/mL trimethoprim and 1 unit/mL polymyxin B.

Microbiology: *In vitro* studies have demonstrated that the anti-infective components of Polytrim are active against the following bacterial pathogens that are capable of causing external infections of the eye:

Trimethoprim: *Staphylococcus aureus* and *Staphylococcus epidermidis, Streptococcus pyogenes, Streptococcus faecalis, Streptococcus pneumoniae, Haemophilus influenzae, Haemophilus aegyptius, Escherichia coli, Klebsiella pneumoniae, Proteus mirabilis* (indole-negative), *Proteus vulgaris* (indole-positive), *Enterobacter aerogenes,* and *Serratia marcescens.*

Polymyxin B: *Pseudomonas aeruginosa, Escherichia coli, Klebsiella pneumoniae, Enterobacter aerogenes* and *Haemophilus influenzae.*

INDICATIONS AND USAGE

Polytrim Ophthalmic Solution is indicated in the treatment of surface ocular bacterial infections, including acute bacterial conjunctivitis, and blepharoconjunctivitis, caused by susceptible strains of the following microorganisms: *Staphylococcus aureus, Staphylococcus epidermidis, Streptococcus pneumoniae, Streptococcus viridans, Haemophilus influenzae* and *Pseudomonas aeruginosa.**

*Efficacy for this organism in this organ system was studied in fewer than 10 infections.

CONTRAINDICATIONS

Polytrim Ophthalmic Solution is contraindicated in patients with known hypersensitivity to any of its components.

WARNINGS

NOT FOR INJECTION INTO THE EYE. If a sensitivity reaction to Polytrim occurs, discontinue use. Polytrim Ophthalmic Solution is not indicated for the prophylaxis or treatment of ophthalmia neonatorum.

PRECAUTIONS

General: As with other antimicrobial preparations, prolonged use may result in overgrowth of nonsusceptible organisms, including fungi. If superinfection occurs, appropriate therapy should be initiated.

Information for Patients: Avoid contaminating the applicator tip with material from the eye, fingers, or other source. This precaution is necessary if the sterility of the drops is to be maintained.

If redness, irritation, swelling or pain persists or increases, discontinue use immediately and contact your physician. Unless deemed medically necessary, patients should be advised not to wear contact lenses if they have signs and symptoms of ocular bacterial infections.

Carcinogenesis, Mutagenesis, Impairment of Fertility:

Carcinogenesis: Long-term studies in animals to evaluate carcinogenic potential have not been conducted with polymyxin B sulfate or trimethoprim.

Mutagenesis: Trimethoprim was demonstrated to be non-mutagenic in the Ames assay. In studies at two laboratories no chromosomal damage was detected in cultured Chinese hamster ovary cells at concentrations approximately 500 times human plasma levels after oral administration; at concentrations approximately 1000 times human plasma levels after oral administration in these same cells a low level of chromosomal damage was induced at one of the laboratories. Studies to evaluate mutagenic potential have not been conducted with polymyxin B sulfate.

Impairment of Fertility: Polymyxin B sulfate has been reported to impair the motility of equine sperm, but its effects on male or female fertility are unknown.

No adverse effects on fertility or general reproductive performance were observed in rats given trimethoprim in oral dosages as high as 70 mg/kg/day for males and 14 mg/kg/day for females.

Pregnancy: ***Teratogenic Effects:*** Pregnancy Category C. Animal reproduction studies have not been conducted with polymyxin B sulfate. It is not known whether polymyxin B sulfate can cause fetal harm when administered to a pregnant woman or can affect reproduction capacity.

Trimethoprim has been shown to be teratogenic in the rat when given in oral doses 40 times the human dose. In some rabbit studies, the overall increase in fetal loss (dead and resorbed and malformed conceptuses) was associated with oral doses 6 times the human therapeutic dose.

While there are no large well-controlled studies on the use of trimethoprim in pregnant women, Brumfitt and Pursell, in a retrospective study, reported the outcome of 186 pregnancies during which the mother received either placebo or oral trimethoprim in combination with sulfamethoxazole. The incidence of congenital abnormalities was 4.5% (3 of 66) in those who received placebo and 3.3% (4 of 120) in those receiving trimethoprim and sulfamethoxazole. There were no abnormalities in the 10 children whose mothers received the drug during the first trimester. In a separate survey, Brumfitt and Pursell also found no congenital abnormalities in 35 children whose mothers had received oral trimethoprim and sulfamethoxazole at the time of conception or shortly thereafter.

Because trimethoprim may interfere with folic acid metabolism, trimethoprim should be used during pregnancy only if the potential benefit justifies the potential risk to the fetus.

Nonteratogenic Effects: The oral administration of trimethoprim to rats at a dose of 70 mg/kg/day commencing with the last third of gestation and continuing through parturition and lactation caused no deleterious effects on gestation or pup growth and survival.

Nursing mothers: It is not known whether this drug is excreted in human milk. Because many drugs are excreted in human milk, caution should be exercised when Polytrim Ophthalmic Solution is administered to a nursing woman.

Pediatric Use: Safety and effectiveness in children below the age of 2 months have not been established (see WARNINGS).

ADVERSE REACTIONS

The most frequent adverse reaction to Polytrim Ophthalmic Solution is local irritation consisting of increased redness, burning, stinging, and/or itching. This may occur on instillation, within 48 hours, or at any time with extended use. There are also multiple reports of hypersensitivity reactions consisting of lid edema, itching, increased redness, tearing, and/or circumocular rash. Photosensitivity has been reported in patients taking oral trimethoprim.

DOSAGE AND ADMINISTRATION

Adults: In mild to moderate infections, instill one drop in the affected eye(s) every three hours (maximum of 6 doses per day) for a period of 7 to 10 days.

HOW SUPPLIED

A sterile ophthalmic solution, each mL contains trimethoprim 1 mg and polymyxin B sulfate 10,000 units in a plastic dropper bottle of 10 mL (NDC 0023-7824-10). 5 mL (NDC 0023-7824-05)

Note: Store at 15°–25°C (59°–77°F) and protect from light.

Rx only

TAZORAC® ℞

[*tăz ō răc*]

(tazarotene topical gel) 0.05%
(tazarotene topical gel) 0.1%

FOR DERMATOLOGIC USE ONLY
NOT FOR OPHTHALMIC USE

DESCRIPTION

TAZORAC® is a translucent, aqueous gel and contains the compound tazarotene, a member of the acetylenic class of retinoids. It is for topical dermatologic use only. The active ingredient is represented by the following structural formula:

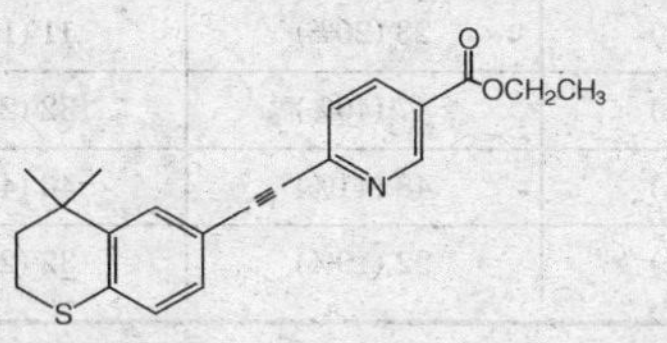

TAZAROTENE

$C_{21}H_{21}NO_2S$

Molecular Weight: **351.46**

Chemical Name: ethyl 6-[2-(4,4-dimethylthiochroman-6-yl)-ethynyl] nicotinate

Contains:

Active: Tazarotene .... 0.05% or 0.1% (w/w)

Preservative: Benzyl alcohol .... 1.0% (w/w)

Inactives: Ascorbic acid, butylated hydroxyanisole, butylated hydroxytoluene, carbomer 934P, edetate disodium, hexylene glycol, purified water, poloxamer 407, polyethylene glycol 400, polysorbate 40, and tromethamine.

CLINICAL PHARMACOLOGY

Tazarotene is a retinoid prodrug which is converted to its active form, the cognate carboxylic acid of tazarotene (AGN 190299), by rapid deesterification in most biological systems. AGN 190299 binds to all three members of the retinoic acid receptor (RAR) family: RARα, RARβ, and RARγ, but shows relative selectivity for RARβ, and RARγ and may modify gene expression. The clinical significance of these findings is unknown.

Psoriasis: The mechanism of tazarotene action in psoriasis is not defined. Topical tazarotene blocks induction of mouse epidermal ornithine decarboxylase (ODC) activity, which is associated with cell proliferation and hyperplasia. In cell culture and *in vitro* models of skin, tazarotene suppresses expression of MRP8, a marker of inflammation present in the epidermis of psoriasis subjects at high levels. In human keratinocyte cultures, it inhibits cornified envelope formation, whose build-up is an element of the psoriatic scale. The clinical significance of these findings is unknown.

Acne: The mechanism of tazarotene action in acne is not defined. Tazarotene inhibited corneocyte accumulation in rhino mouse skin and cross-linked envelope formation in cultured human keratinocytes. The clinical significance of these findings is unknown.

Pharmacokinetics:

Following topical application, tazarotene undergoes esterase hydrolysis to form its active metabolite, AGN 190299. Little parent compound could be detected in the plasma. AGN 190299 was highly bound to plasma proteins (>99%). Tazarotene and AGN 190299 were metabolized to sulfoxides, sulfones and other polar metabolites which were eliminated through urinary and fecal pathways. The half-life of AGN 190299 following topical application of tazarotene was similar in normal and psoriatic subjects, approximately 18 hours.

Plaque Elevation, Scaling and Erythema in Two Controlled Clinical Trials for Psoriasis

		TAZORAC® 0.05% Gel				TAZORAC® 0.1% Gel				Vehicle Gel			
		Trunk/Arm/ Leg lesions		Knee/Elbow lesions		Trunk/Arm/ Leg lesions		Knee/Elbow lesions		Trunk/Arm/ Leg lesions		Knee/Elbow lesions	
		N=108	N=111	N=108	N=111	N=108	N=112	N=108	N=112	N=108	N=113	N=108	N=113
Plaque elevation	B*	2.5	2.6	2.6	2.6	2.5	2.6	2.6	2.6	2.4	2.6	2.6	2.6
	C-12*	-1.4	-1.3	-1.3	-1.1	-1.4	-1.4	-1.5	-1.3	-0.8	-0.7	-0.7	-0.6
	C-24*	-1.2		-1.1		-1.1		-1.0		-0.9		-0.7	
Scaling	B*	2.4	2.5	2.5	2.6	2.4	2.6	2.5	2.7	2.4	2.6	2.5	2.7
	C-12*	-1.1	-1.1	-1.1	-0.9	-1.3	-1.3	-1.2	-1.2	-0.7	-0.7	-0.6	-0.6
	C-24*	-0.9		-0.8		-1.0		-0.8		-0.8		-0.7	
Erythema	B*	2.4	2.7	2.2	2.5	2.4	2.8	2.3	2.5	2.3	2.7	2.2	2.5
	C-12*	-1.0	-0.8	-0.9	-0.8	-1.0	-1.1	-1.0	-0.8	-0.6	-0.5	-0.5	-0.5
	C-24*	-1.1		-0.7		-0.9		-0.8		-0.7		-0.6	

Plaque elevation, scaling and erythema scored on a 0-4 scale with 0=none, 1=mild, 2=moderate, 3=severe and 4=very severe.

*B=Mean Baseline Severity: C-12=Mean Change from Baseline at end of 12 weeks of therapy: C-24=Mean Change from Baseline at week 24 (12 weeks after the end of therapy).

The human *in vivo* studies described below were conducted with tazarotene gel applied topically at approximately 2 mg/cm^2 and left on the skin for 10 to 12 hours. Both the peak plasma concentration (Cmax) and area under the plasma concentration time curve (AUC) refer to the active metabolite only.

Two single, topical dose studies were conducted using ^{14}C-tazarotene gel. Systemic absorption, as determined from radioactivity in the excreta, was less than 1% of the applied dose (without occlusion) in six psoriatic patients and approximately 5% of the applied dose (under occlusion) in six healthy subjects. One non-radiolabeled single-dose study comparing the 0.05% gel to the 0.1% gel in healthy subjects indicated that the Cmax and AUC were 40% higher for the 0.1% gel.

After 7 days of topical dosing with measured doses of tazarotene 0.1% gel on 20% of the total body surface without occlusion in 24 healthy subjects, the Cmax was 0.72 ± 0.58 ng/mL (mean ± SD) occurring 9 hours after the last dose, and the AUC_{0-24hr} was 10.1 ± 7.2 ng·hr/mL. Systemic absorption was 0.91 ± 0.67% of the applied dose.

In a 14-day study in five psoriatic patients, measured doses of tazarotene 0.1% gel were applied daily by nursing staff to involved skin without occlusion (8 to 18% of total body surface area; mean ± SD: 13 ± 5%). The Cmax was 12.0 ± 7.6 ng/mL occurring 6 hours after the final dose, and the AUC_{0-24hr} was 105 ± 55 ng·hr/mL. Systemic absorption was 14.8 ± 7.6% of the applied dose. Extrapolation of these results to represent dosing on 20% of total body surface yielded estimates of Cmax of 18.9 ± 10.6 ng/mL and AUC_{0-24hr} of 172 ± 88 ng·hr/mL.

An *in vitro* percutaneous absorption study, using radiolabeled drug and freshly excised human skin or human cadaver skin, indicated that approximately 4 to 5% of the applied dose was in the stratum corneum (tazarotene: AGN 190299 = 5:1) and 2 to 4% was in the viable epidermis-dermis layer (tazarotene: AGN 190299 = 2:1) 24 hours after topical application of the gel.

Clinical Studies:

Psoriasis:

In two large vehicle-controlled clinical studies, tazarotene 0.05% and 0.1% gels applied once daily for 12 weeks were significantly more effective than vehicle in reducing the severity of the clinical signs of stable plaque psoriasis covering up to 20% of body surface area. In one of the studies, patients were followed up for an additional 12 weeks following cessation of therapy with TAZORAC®. Mean baseline scores and changes from baseline (reductions) after treatment in these two studies are shown in the following table:

[See table above]

[See first table at top of next page]

The 0.1% gel was more effective than the 0.05% gel, but the 0.05% gel was associated with less local irritation than the 0.1% gel (see ADVERSE REACTIONS section).

Acne:

In two large vehicle-controlled studies, tazarotene 0.1% gel applied once daily was significantly more effective than vehicle in the treatment of facial acne vulgaris of mild to moderate severity. Percent reductions in lesion counts after treatment for 12 weeks in these two studies are shown in the following table:

[See second table at top of next page]

[See third table at top of next page]

INDICATIONS AND USAGE

TAZORAC® (tazarotene topical gel) 0.05% and 0.1% are indicated for the topical treatment of patients with stable plaque psoriasis of up to 20% body surface area involvement.

TAZORAC® (tazarotene topical gel) 0.1% is also indicated for the topical treatment of patients with facial acne vulgaris of mild to moderate severity.

The efficacy of TAZORAC® in the treatment of acne previously treated with other retinoids or resistant to oral antibiotics has not been established.

CONTRAINDICATIONS

Retinoids may cause fetal harm when administered to a pregnant woman.

In rats, tazarotene 0.05%, administered **topically** during gestation days 6 through 17 at 0.25 mg/kg/day (1.5 mg/m^2/day) resulted in reduced fetal body weights and reduced skeletal ossification. Rabbits dosed **topically** with 0.25 mg/kg/day (2.75 mg/m^2 total body surface area/day) tazarotene during gestation days 6 through 18 were noted with single incidences of known retinoid malformations, including spina bifida, hydrocephaly, and heart anomalies. As with other retinoids, when tazarotene was given **orally** to experimental animals, developmental delays were seen in rats, and teratogenic effects and post-implantation fetal loss were seen in rats and rabbits at doses producing 0.7 and 13 times, respectively, the systemic exposure (AUC_{0-24hr}) in human psoriasis patients, when extrapolated for **topical** treatment of 20% of body surface area. THUS, SYSTEMIC EXPOSURE IN TOPICALLY TREATED PSORIASIS PATIENTS (FOR USE ON UP TO 20% OF BODY SURFACE AREA) COULD BE IN THE SAME ORDER OF MAGNITUDE AS IN THESE ORALLY TREATED ANIMALS.

Systemic exposure anticipated in the treatment of facial acne may be less, due to a more limited area of application.

Six women inadvertently exposed to TAZORAC® during pregnancy in clinical trials have subsequently delivered healthy babies. As the exact timing and extent of exposure in relation to the gestation time are not certain, the significance of these findings is not known.

TAZORAC® is contraindicated in women who are or may become pregnant. If this drug is used during pregnancy, or if the patient becomes pregnant while taking this drug, treatment should be discontinued and the patient apprised of the potential hazard to the fetus. Women of childbearing potential should be warned of the potential risk and use adequate birth-control measures when TAZORAC® is used. The possibility that a woman of childbearing potential is pregnant at the time of institution of therapy should be considered. A negative result for pregnancy test having a sensitivity down to at least 50 mIU/mL for human chorionic gonadotropin (hCG) should be obtained within 2 weeks prior to TAZORAC® therapy, which should begin during a normal menstrual period.

TAZORAC® is contraindicated in individuals who have shown hypersensitivity to any of its components.

WARNINGS

Pregnancy Category X: See CONTRAINDICATIONS section. Women of childbearing potential should be warned of the potential risk and use adequate birth-control measures when TAZORAC® is used. The possibility that a woman of childbearing potential is pregnant at the time of institution of therapy should be considered. A negative result for pregnancy test having a sensitivity down to at least 50 mIU/mL for hCG should be obtained within 2 weeks prior to TAZORAC® therapy, which should begin during a normal menstrual period.

PRECAUTIONS

General: TAZORAC® should only be applied to the affected areas. For external use only. Avoid contact with

Continued on next page

Tazorac—Cont.

eyes, eyelids, and mouth. If contact with eyes occurs, rinse thoroughly with water. The safety of use over more than 20% of body surface area has not been established in psoriasis or acne.

Retinoids should not be used on eczematous skin, as they may cause severe irritation.

Because of heightened burning susceptibility, exposure to sunlight (including sunlamps) should be avoided unless deemed medically necessary, and in such cases, exposure should be minimized during the use of TAZORAC®. Patients must be warned to use sunscreens (minimum SPF of 15) and protective clothing when using TAZORAC®. Patients with sunburn should be advised not to use TAZORAC® until fully recovered. Patients who may have considerable sun exposure due to their occupation and those patients with inherent sensitivity to sunlight should exercise particular caution when using TAZORAC® and ensure that the precautions outlined in the Information for Patients subsection are observed.

TAZORAC® should be administered with caution if the patient is also taking drugs known to be photosensitizers (e.g., thiazides, tetracyclines, fluoroquinolones, phenothiazines, sulfonamides) because of the increased possibility of augmented photosensitivity.

If pruritus, burning, skin redness or peeling is excessive, the medication should be discontinued until the integrity of the skin is restored.

Weather extremes, such as wind or cold, may be more irritating to patients using TAZORAC®.

Information for Patients: See attached Patient Package Insert.

Drug Interactions: Concomitant dermatologic medications and cosmetics that have a strong drying effect should be avoided. It is also advisable to "rest" a patient's skin until the effects of such preparations subside before use of TAZORAC® is begun.

Carcinogenesis, mutagenesis, impairment of fertility: Long-term studies of tazarotene following oral administration of 0.025, 0.050, and 0.125 mg/kg/day to rats showed no indications of increased carcinogenic risks. However, in other rat studies, oral doses twice that of the highest dose in the rat carcinogenicity study produced an AUC_{0-24hr} that was less (0.7 times) than that in topically treated psoriatic patients extrapolated for treatment of 20% of body surface area. In evaluation of photocarcinogenicity, median time to onset of tumors was decreased and the number of tumors increased in hairless mice following chronic topical dosing with intercurrent exposure to ultraviolet radiation at tazarotene concentrations of 0.001%, 0.005%, and 0.01% for up to 40 weeks.

A long-term topical application study in mice terminated at 88 weeks showed that dose levels of 0.05, 0.125, 0.25 and 1.0 mg/kg/day (reduced to 0.5 mg/kg/day for males after 41 weeks due to severe dermal irritation) revealed no apparent carcinogenic effects when compared to vehicle control animals; untreated control animals were not completely evaluated. The AUC_{0-12hr}'s for these doses were 82.7, 137, 183, 136 (males at 1.0/0.5 mg/kg) and 344 ng·hr/mL (females at 1.0 mg/kg), respectively. The mean AUC_{0-24hr} for psoriatic patients was 172 ng·hr/mL, extrapolated for 20% total body surface area.

Tazarotene was found to be non-mutagenic in the Ames assay and did not produce structural chromosomal aberrations in a human lymphocyte assay. Tazarotene was also non-mutagenic in the CHO/HPRT mammalian cell forward gene mutation assay and was non-clastogenic in the *in vivo* mouse micronucleus test.

No impairment of fertility occurred in rats when male animals were treated for 70 days prior to mating and female animals were treated for 14 days prior to mating and continuing through gestation and lactation with topical doses of TAZORAC® gel of up to 0.125 mg/kg/day (0.738 mg/m²/day).

Reproductive capabilities of F1 animals, including F2 survival and development, were not affected by topical administration of TAZORAC® gel to female F0 parental rats from gestation day 16 through lactation day 20 at the maximum tolerated dose of 0.125 mg/kg/day (0.738 mg/m²/day).

Pregnancy: Teratogenic Effects: Pregnancy Category X: See CONTRAINDICATIONS section. Women of childbearing potential should use adequate birth-control measures when TAZORAC® is used. The possibility that a woman of childbearing potential is pregnant at the time of institution of therapy should be considered. A negative result for pregnancy test having a sensitivity down to at least 50 mIU/mL for hCG should be obtained within 2 weeks prior to TAZORAC® therapy, which should begin during a normal menstrual period.

Nursing Mothers: After single topical doses of ^{14}C-tazarotene to the skin of lactating rats, secretion of radioactivity was detected in milk, suggesting that there would be transfer of drug-related material to the offspring via milk. It is not known whether this drug is excreted in human milk.

Global improvement over baseline at the end of 12 weeks of treatment in these two studies is shown in the following table:

	TAZORAC® 0.05% Gel		TAZORAC® 0.1% Gel		Vehicle Gel	
	N=81	N=93	N=79	N=69	N=84	N=91
100% improvement	2 (2%)	1 (1%)	0	0	1 (1%)	0
≥75% improvement	23 (28%)	17 (18%)	30 (38%)	17 (25%)	10 (12%)	9 (10%)
≥50% improvement	42 (52%)	39 (42%)	51 (65%)	36 (52%)	28 (33%)	21 (23%)
1-49% improvement	21 (26%)	32 (34%)	18 (23%)	23 (33%)	27 (32%)	32 (35%)
No change or worse	18 (22%)	22 (24%)	10 (13%)	10 (14%)	29 (35%)	38 (42%)

Reduction in Lesion Counts after 12 Weeks of Treatment in Two Controlled Clinical Trials for Acne

	TAZORAC® 0.1% Gel		Vehicle Gel	
	N=150	N=149	N=148	N=149
Noninflammatory lesions	55%	43%	35%	27%
Inflammatory lesions	42%	47%	30%	28%
Total lesions	52%	45%	33%	27%

Global improvement over baseline at the end of 12 weeks of treatment in these two studies is shown in the following table:

	TAZORAC® 0.1% Gel		Vehicle Gel	
	N=105	N=117	N=117	N=110
100% improvement	1 (1%)	0	0	0
≥75% improvement	40 (38%)	21 (18%)	23 (20%)	11 (10%)
≥50% improvement	71 (68%)	56 (48%)	47 (40%)	32 (29%)
1-49% improvement	23 (22%)	49 (42%)	48 (41%)	46 (42%)
No change or worse	11 (10%)	12 (10%)	22 (19%)	32 (29%)

Caution should be exercised when tazarotene is administered to a nursing woman.

Pediatric Use: The safety and efficacy of tazarotene have not been established in pediatric patients under the age of 12 years.

ADVERSE REACTIONS

Psoriasis:

The most frequent adverse events reported with TAZORAC® 0.05% and 0.1% gels were limited to the skin. Those occurring in 10 to 30% of patients, in descending order, included pruritus, burning/stinging, erythema, worsening of psoriasis, irritation, and skin pain. Events occurring in 1 to 10% of patients included rash, desquamation, irritant contact dermatitis, skin inflammation, fissuring, bleeding and dry skin. Increases in "psoriasis worsening" and "sun-induced erythema" were noted in some patients over the 4th to 12th months as compared to the first three months of a 1 year study. In general, the incidence of adverse events with TAZORAC® 0.05% gel was 2 to 5% lower than that seen with TAZORAC® 0.1% gel.

Acne:

The most frequent adverse events reported with TAZORAC® 0.1% gel were limited to the skin. Those events occurring in 10 to 30% of patients, in descending order, included desquamation, burning/stinging, dry skin, erythema and pruritus. Events occurring in 1 to 10% of patients included irritation, skin pain, fissuring, localized edema and skin discoloration.

In human dermal safety studies, tazarotene 0.05% and 0.1% gels did not induce contact sensitization, phototoxicity or photoallergy.

OVERDOSAGE

Excessive topical use of TAZORAC® may lead to marked redness, peeling, or discomfort (see PRECAUTIONS).

TAZORAC® is not for oral use. Oral ingestion of the drug may lead to the same adverse effects as those associated with excessive oral intake of Vitamin A (hypervitaminosis A) or other retinoids. If oral ingestion occurs, the patient should be monitored, and appropriate supportive measures should be administered as necessary.

DOSAGE AND ADMINISTRATION

General: Application may cause a transitory feeling of burning or stinging. If irritation is excessive, application should be discontinued.

For psoriasis: Apply TAZORAC® once a day, in the evening, to psoriatic lesions, using enough (2 mg/cm²) to cover only the lesion with a thin film to no more than 20% of body surface area. If a bath or shower is taken prior to application, the skin should be dry before applying the gel. Because unaffected skin may be more susceptible to irritation, application of tazarotene to these areas should be carefully avoided. TAZORAC® was investigated for up to 12 months during clinical trials for psoriasis.

For acne: Cleanse the face gently. After the skin is dry, apply a thin film of TAZORAC® (2 mg/cm²) once a day, in the evening, to the skin where acne lesions appear. Use enough to cover the entire affected area. TAZORAC® was investigated for up to 12 weeks during clinical trials for acne.

HOW SUPPLIED

TAZORAC® (tazarotene topical gel) is available in concentrations of 0.05% and 0.1%. It comes in collapsible aluminum tubes, in 30 gm and 100 gm sizes.

	TAZORAC® Gel 0.05%	TAZORAC® Gel 0.1%
30 mg	NDC 0023-8335-03	NDC 0023-0042-03
100 mg	NDC 0023-8335-10	NDC 0023-0042-10

NOTE: TAZORAC® gel should be stored at 25°C (77°F): excursion permitted to 15–30°C (59–86°F).

Rx only

ALLERGAN
Irvine, California 92612, USA
©1997 Allergan, Inc.

September 1997

For information on over-the-counter drugs, consult **PDR For Nonprescription Drugs**.

Alpha Therapeutic Corporation
5555 VALLEY BLVD.
LOS ANGELES, CA 90032

Direct Inquiries to:
(213) 225-2221
(800) 421-0008
FAX: (213) 227-7027

For Medical Information Contact:
In Emergencies:
Clyde McAuley, M.D., Medical Director
(213) 227-7419
After Hours Emergency Orders:
(800) 421-0008

ALBUTEIN® 5%   ℞
Albumin (Human), USP, 5% Solution

10 bottles per case.
250mL bottle & IV set   NDC 49669-5211-1
500mL bottle & IV set   NDC 49669-5211-2

ALBUTEIN® 25%   ℞
Albumin (Human), USP, 25% Solution

10 bottles per case.
50mL bottle & IV set   NDC 49669-5213-2
100mL bottle & IV set   NDC 49669-5213-3

ALPHANATE®   ℞
Antihemophilic Factor, (Human)
Solvent Detergent/Heat Treated

DESCRIPTION
Alphanate® Antihemophilic Factor (Human) Solvent Detergent/Heat Treated is a highly purified Factor VIII product for the treatment of Hemophilia A and acquired Factor VIII deficiency. It is intended for intravenous administration. The product is purified by column chromatography and utilizes a solvent detergent treatment for viral inactivation.

HOW SUPPLIED
The product is available in the following potencies:

Factor VIII Activity	Diluent	NDC Number
250 i.u.	5 mL	49669-4600-01
500 i.u.	5 mL	49669-4600-01
1000 i.u.	10 mL	49669-4600-02
1500 i.u.	10 mL	49669-4600-02

Each carton contains a single dose vial of concentrate, sterile water for injection, a double ended transfer needle and microaggregate filter, and a package insert with full prescribing information. 12 vials per case.

AlphaNine®-SD   ℞
Coagulation Factor IX (Human)
Solvent Detergent Treated/Virus Filtered

AlphaNine®-SD, Coagulation Factor IX (Human) is available in 250, 500, 1000, 1250, and 1500 assay ranges with 10 mL diluent. For intravenous administration only. Each carton and single dose vial is labeled with Factor IX dose contained; carton contains sterile diluent, transfer needle, and microaggregate filter. 12 vials per case. ASSAY RANGE 0-2000 F IX Units/Vial NDC 49669-3600-02

PROFILNINE® SD   ℞
Factor IX Complex
Solvent Detergent Treated

DESCRIPTION
Profilnine® SD, Factor IX Complex, Solvent Detergent Treated is a lyophilized concentrate containing factors II, IX, and X plus low levels of factor VII. The product is available in single dose vials of Factor IX for the treatment of Hemophilia B (Factor IX deficiency).

HOW SUPPLIED
The product is available in the following potencies:

Factor IX Activity	Diluent	NDC Number
500 i.u.	5 mL	49669-3200-02
1000 i.u.	10 mL	49669-3200-03
1500 i.u.	10 mL	49669-3200-03

Each individual carton contains a single dose vial of Factor IX, sterile water for injection, transfer needle, microaggregate filter, and a package insert with full prescribing information. 12 vials per case.

VENOGLOBULIN®–S 5% Solution   ℞
Immune Globulin Intravenous (Human)
SOLVENT DETERGENT TREATED

Venoglobulin®-S 5% Solution, Solvent Detergent Treated is a sterile, highly purified solution of intact, unmodified human immunoglobulin G intended for intravenous use. IgG is isolated from large pools of human plasma using the Cohn-Oncley cold alcohol fractionation process, followed by polyethylene glycol fractionation and ion exchange chromatography. The manufacturing process includes treatment with a mixture of tri-n-butyl phosphate (TNBP) and polysorbate 80.

The process used to produce Venoglobulin®-S inactivates and/or partitions up to 13 cumulative logs of Human Immunodeficiency Virus Type 1 (HIV-1) based on in vitro studies. Additional solvent-detergent treatment further removes greater than 10 logs of HIV-1 and greater than 6 logs of HIV-2 as demonstrated in vitro, thereby providing an extra measure of safety.

Venoglobulin®-S contains all IgG antibody activities present in the donor population. The distribution of IgG subclasses corresponds to that of normal human plasma. Gamma globulin is isolated without additional chemical or enzymatic modification and the Fc portion of the molecule is maintained functionally intact. Typically IgG purity exceeds 99%.

The composition of Venoglobulin®-S is as follows:

Component	Quantity/mL
Human immunoglobulin G	50 mg
D-sorbitol	50 mg
Albumin (Human)	<1.3 mg
Polyethylene glycol	<100 mcg
Polysorbate 80	<100 mcg
Tri-n-butyl phosphate	< 10 mcg

This formulation contains no preservatives. The pH of the solution ranges from 5.2 to 5.8. The osmolarity is approximately 300 mOsm/L.

HOW SUPPLIED

Vial size	Grams of IgG	NDC Number
50 mL	2.5 g	49669-1612-1
100 mL	5.0 g	49669-1613-1
200 mL	10.0 g	49669-1614-1

All sizes are packaged with a sterile I.V. administration set. 10 vials per case. Store at or below 25°C or 77°F. Do not freeze.

VENOGLOBULIN®-S 10% Solution   ℞
Immune Globulin Intravenous (Human)
SOLVENT DETERGENT TREATED

DESCRIPTION
Venoglobulin®-S 10% Solution, Solvent Detergent Treated is a sterile, highly purified solution of intact, unmodified human immunoglobulin G intended for intravenous use. IgG is isolated from large pools of human plasma using the Cohn-Oncley cold alcohol fractionation process, followed by polyethylene glycol fractionation and ion exchange chromatography. The manufacturing process also includes a solvent detergent viral inactivation step.

The composition of Venoglobulin®-S 10% is as follows:

Component	Quantity/mL	
Human immunoglobulin G	100	mg
D-sorbitol	50	mg
Albumin (Human)	≤2.6	mg
Polyethylene glycol	≤200	mcg
Polysorbate 80	≤200	mcg
Tri-n-butyl phosphate	≤20	mcg

This formulation contains no preservatives. The pH of the solution ranges from 5.2 to 5.8. The osmolarity is approximately 330 mOsm/L.

HOW SUPPLIED

Vial size	Grams of IgG	NDC Number
50 mL	5.0 g	49669-1622-1
100 mL	10.0 g	49669-1623-1
200 mL	20.0 g	49669-1624-1

All sizes are packaged with a sterile IV administration set. 10 vials per case. Store at or below 25°C (77°F). Do not freeze. Warm to room temperature before infusion.

Alpharma™
U.S. Pharmaceuticals Division
Makers of Barre and NMC Products
7205 WINDSOR BLVD.
BALTIMORE, MD 21244

For General Inquiries Contact:
Customer Service
(800) 638–9096

LINDANE LOTION USP, 1%   ℞

DESCRIPTION
Lindane Lotion USP, 1% is an ectoparasiticide and ovicide effective against Sarcoptes scabiei (scabies). In addition to the active ingredient, lindane, it contains glycerol monostearate, cetyl alcohol, stearic acid, trolamine, carrageenan, 2-amino-2-methyl-1-propanol, methylparaben, butylparaben, perfume and water to form a non-greasy lotion. Lindane, which is the highly purified gamma isomer of 1, 2, 3, 4, 5, 6, hexachlorocyclohexane, has the following structural formula:

$C_6H_6Cl_6$ 290.83

CLINICAL PHARMACOLOGY
Lindane exerts its parasiticidal action by being directly absorbed into the parasites and their ova. Feldmann and Maibach[1] reported approximately 10% absorption of a lindane acetone solution applied to the forearm and left in place for 24 hours. Dale, et al[2], reported a blood level of 290 ng/mL associated with convulsions following the accidental ingestion of a lindane-containing product. Ginsburg[3] found a mean peak blood level of 28 ng/mL 6 hours after total body application of lindane lotion to scabietic infants and children. The half-life was determined to be 18 hours.

INDICATIONS AND USAGE
Because post-treatment pruritus is common and may lead to misuse, lindane lotion is indicated only for the treatment of patients infested with Sarcoptes scabiei (scabies) who have either failed to respond to adequate doses, or are intolerant of, other approved therapies. Reinfestation should be considered carefully before attributing the posttreatment presence of ectoparasites to a failure of response to adequate doses of other approved therapies.

CONTRAINDICATIONS
Lindane lotion is contraindicated for premature neonates because their skin may be more permeable than full term infants and their liver enzymes may not be sufficiently developed. It is also contraindicated for patients with Norwegian (crusted) scabies due to possible increased absorption. It is also contraindicated for patients with known seizure disorders and for individuals with a known sensitivity to the product or any of its components.

WARNINGS
LINDANE PENETRATES HUMAN SKIN AND HAS THE POTENTIAL FOR CNS TOXICITY (SEE CLINICAL PHARMACOLOGY SECTION). LINDANE LOTION SHOULD BE USED ACCORDING TO RECOMMENDED DOSAGE (SEE DIRECTIONS FOR USE) ESPECIALLY ON INFANTS, PREGNANT WOMEN AND NURSING MOTHERS. ANIMAL STUDIES INDICATE THAT POTENTIAL TOXIC EFFECTS OF TOPICALLY APPLIED LINDANE ARE GREATER IN THE YOUNG. SEIZURES AND, IN RARE INSTANCES, DEATHS HAVE BEEN REPORTED AFTER EXCESS DOSAGE, OVER-EXPOSURE, FREQUENT REAPPLICATIONS, AND ACCIDENTAL AND INTENTIONAL INGESTION OF LINDANE. THESE INSTANCES OF PATIENT MISUSE HAVE BEEN ASSOCIATED WITH LACK OF PATIENT UNDERSTANDING ON DIRECTIONS OF USE, PRESCRIBING OR DISPENSING EXCESSIVE QUANTITIES, AND IMPROPER REAP-

Continued on next page

Lindane Lotion—Cont.

PLICATIONS. IN EXCEEDINGLY RARE CASES SEIZURES HAVE BEEN REPORTED WHEN USED ACCORDING TO DIRECTIONS. NO RESIDUAL EFFECTS HAVE BEEN DEMONSTRATED, THEREFORE, THIS PRODUCT SHOULD NOT BE USED TO WARD OFF A POSSIBLE INFESTATION. If accidental ingestion occurs, prompt gastric lavage is indicated. Because oils may enhance absorption, saline rather than oily cathartics should be used. Central nervous excitation can be controlled by the administration of pentobarbital, phenobarbital or diazepam.

PRECAUTIONS

General: Care should be taken to avoid contact with the eyes. If such contact occurs, eyes should be immediately flushed with water. If irritation or sensitization occurs, the patient should be advised to consult a physician.

Geriatric: Dosage may have to be reduced due to the possibility of increased absorption through elderly skin.

Information for Patients: Patients must be instructed on the proper use of the medication, especially as to amount applied and duration of use. Patients Directions for Use must accompany the product.

Laboratory Tests: No laboratory tests are needed for the proper use of this medication.

Drug Interactions: Oils may enhance absorption, therefore, simultaneous use of creams, ointments or oils should be avoided.

Carcinogenesis: Although no studies have been conducted with lindane lotion, numerous long-term feeding studies have been conducted in mice and rats to evaluate the carcinogenic potential of the technical grade of hexachlorocyclohexane (BHC) as well as the alpha, beta, gamma (lindane) and delta isomers. Both oral and topical applications have been evaluated. Nagasaki[4], Goto[5] and Hanada[6] found varying amounts of benign and malignant hepatomas associated with BHC and the alpha, delta and epsilon isomers. None reported a carcinogenic potential for lindane. Tumors were found only in the animals which had received the alpha isomer. Weisse and Herbst[7] also evaluated the carcinogenic potential of lindane in mice but could find no evidence of lindane carcinogenicity. The National Cancer Institute[8] also found no evidence of carcinogenicity.

Thorpe and Walker[9] compared beta BHC with lindane, dieldrin, DDT and hexabarbital in mice. Despite the unusually high incidence of tumors in the control group, they concluded that 600 ppm of lindane was associated with a significant increase in the incidence of hepatoma and thus, considered it a tumorigen.

Orr[10] and Kashyap, et al[11], evaluated the carcinogenic potential in mice of topically applied BHC. In neither study was there any evidence of a tumorigenic or carcinogenic potential associated with topical application of BHC.

Mutagenicity tests have been used as predictive information about the carcinogenicity of various chemical compounds. Numerous types of mutagenicity tests have been performed with lindane. The results of these tests do not indicate that lindane is mutagenic.

Pregnancy: *Teratogenic Effects*-Pregnancy Category B. Reproduction, including multigeneration, studies have been performed in mice, rats, rabbits, pigs, and dogs at doses up to 10 times the human dose and have revealed no evidence of impaired fertility or harm to the fetus due to orally administered lindane. There are, however, no adequate and well-controlled studies in pregnant women. Because animal reproduction studies are not always predictive of human response, the recommended dosage should not be exceeded on pregnant women. They should be treated no more than twice during a pregnancy.

Nursing Mothers: Lindane is secreted in human milk in low concentrations. Studies conducted in the United States as well as in Europe and South America found levels of lindane in human milk ranging from 0 to 113 ppb, as the result of ingestion of foods which had been treated with lindane. There appeared to be no difference in concentrations between country and urban dwellers. Although the levels of lindane found in blood after topical application with lindane lotion make it unlikely that amounts of lindane sufficient to cause serious adverse reactions will be excreted in the milk of nursing mothers who have used lindane lotion, if there is any concern, an alternate method of feeding may be used for 4 days.

Pediatric Use: Refer to the CONTRAINDICATIONS and WARNINGS sections.

ADVERSE REACTIONS

Lindane has been reported to cause central nervous stimulation ranging from dizziness to convulsions. Cases of convulsions have been reported in connection with lindane lotion therapy. However, these incidents were almost always associated with accidental oral ingestion or misuse of the product. In exceedingly rare cases, seizures have been reported when used according to directions. Eczematous eruptions due to irritation from this product have also been reported. Incidence of these adverse reactions is relatively infrequent, occurring in less than 1 in 100,000 patients.

DRUG ABUSE AND DEPENDENCE

Lindane lotion is not subject to abuse, nor is there any dependence on the drug.

OVERDOSAGE

Overdosage or oral ingestion of lindane lotion can cause central nervous system excitation and, if taken in sufficient quantities, convulsions may occur. If accidental ingestion occurs, prompt gastric lavage should be instituted. However, since oils favor absorption, saline cathartics for intestinal evacuation should be given rather than oil laxatives. If central nervous system manifestations occur, they can be antagonized by the administration of pentobarbital, phenobarbital or diazepam.

DOSAGE AND ADMINISTRATION

CAUTION: USE ONLY AS DIRECTED. DO NOT EXCEED RECOMMENDED DOSAGE.

No residual effects have been demonstrated, therefore, this product should not be used to ward off a possible infestation. However, sexual contacts should be treated simultaneously.

NOTE: PLEASE READ CAREFULLY.

DIRECTIONS FOR USE:

WARNING:

THIS PRODUCT CAN BE POISONOUS IF MISUSED. CHILDREN MUST NOT BE ALLOWED TO APPLY THIS DRUG WITHOUT DIRECT ADULT SUPERVISION. USE LOTION FOR SCABIES ONLY. APPLY ONLY ONCE. USE ONLY ENOUGH TO COVER THE BODY IN A THIN LAYER. 1 OUNCE (HALF OF A 2 OUNCE CONTAINER) SHOULD BE ALL THAT IS NEEDED FOR CHILDREN UNDER 6 YEARS OF AGE; 1 TO 2 OUNCES FOR OLDER CHILDREN AND ADULTS. DO NOT LEAVE ON FOR MORE THAN 12 HOURS. DO NOT INGEST. KEEP AWAY FROM MOUTH AND EYES. COVER INFANTS' HANDS AND FEET DURING TREATMENT TO PREVENT SUCKING AND LICKING OF LOTION. DO NOT USE IF OPEN WOUNDS, CUTS OR SORES ARE PRESENT, UNLESS DIRECTED BY YOUR PHYSICIAN.

(LOTION: SHAKE WELL)

1. APPLY THIS PREPARATION TO DRY SKIN IN A THIN LAYER AND RUB IN THOROUGHLY.
2. TRIM NAILS AND APPLY UNDER NAILS WITH TOOTHBRUSH (THROW AWAY TOOTHBRUSH AFTER USE).
3. IF A WARM BATH IS TAKEN BEFORE APPLICATION, ALLOW THE SKIN TO DRY AND COOL COMPLETELY BEFORE APPLYING THE MEDICATION.
4. A TOTAL BODY APPLICATION SHOULD BE MADE FROM THE NECK DOWN, INCLUDING SOLES OF FEET, UNLESS OTHERWISE DIRECTED BY YOUR PHYSICIAN.
5. THE LOTION SHOULD BE LEFT ON FOR 8 TO 12 HOURS (USUALLY OVERNIGHT) AND THEN REMOVED BY THOROUGH WASHING (BATH OR SHOWER).
6. AVOID UNNECESSARY CONTACT WITH YOUR SKIN IF YOU ARE APPLYING TO ANOTHER PERSON. IF TREATING MORE THAN ONE PERSON, PERSON APPLYING LOTION (ESPECIALLY PREGNANT OR NURSING WOMEN) SHOULD WEAR RUBBER GLOVES.
7. ALL RECENTLY WORN CLOTHING, UNDERWEAR AND PAJAMAS, AND USED SHEETS, PILLOW CASES, AND TOWELS SHOULD BE WASHED IN VERY HOT WATER OR DRY-CLEANED.

AFTER ONE APPLICATION, ITCHING WILL CONTINUE FOR SEVERAL WEEKS. THIS IS NORMAL AND DOES NOT REQUIRE REAPPLICATION.

IF YOU HAVE ANY QUESTIONS OR CONCERNS ABOUT YOUR CONDITION OR USE OF THE LOTION, CONTACT YOUR PHYSICIAN.

HOW SUPPLIED

Lindane Lotion USP, 1% in patient-size 2 fl oz (59 mL), pharmacy-size only pint (473 mL) and pharmacy-size only gallon (3785 mL) bottles.

SHAKE WELL BEFORE USING.

Store at controlled room temperature 15°–30°C (59°–86°F).

Dispense in a tight, light-resistant container as defined in the USP, with a child-resistant closure.

CAUTION: Federal law prohibits dispensing without prescription.

REFERENCES

1. Feldmann, R.J. and Maiback, H.I., *Toxicol. Applied. Pharmacol.*, 28:126, 1974.
2. Dale, W.E., Curly, A. and Cueto, C. *Life Sci* 5:47, 1966.
3. Ginsburg, C.M., et al., *J. Pediatr.* 91:6 998–1000, 1977.
4. Nagasaki, T., Tomii, S., Mega, T., Marugami, M. and lto. N. *Gann* (Cancer) 63(3):393, 1972.
5. Goto, M., Hattori, M., Miyagawa, T. and Enomoto, M., *Chemosphere* 6:279, 1972.
6. Hanada, M., Yatani, C., Miyaji, T., *Gann* 64:511, 1973.
7. Weisse, I., and Herbst, M., *Toxicol.* 7:233, 1977.
8. Technical Report Series, NCI-CG-TR-14, *HEW PUBLICATIONS,* No. (NIH) 77–814.
9. Thorpe, E., and Walker, A.I.T., *Food Cosmetic Toxicol.* 11:433, 1973.
10. Orr, J.W., *Nature* 162:189, 1948.
11. Kashyap, S.K. et. al., *J. Environ, Sci. Health* 14:305–318, 1979.

Manufactured by
Barre-National Inc.
Baltimore, MD 21244
an ALPHARMA USPD Company

FORM NO. 0570-02 Rev. 4/96 B1

PHARMACIST—DETACH AND GIVE TO PATIENT

LINDANE LOTION USP 1%
DIRECTIONS FOR USE

WARNING:

THIS PRODUCT CAN BE POISONOUS IF MISUSED. CHILDREN MUST NOT BE ALLOWED TO APPLY THIS DRUG WITHOUT DIRECT ADULT SUPERVISION. USE LOTION FOR SCABIES ONLY. APPLY ONLY ONCE. USE ONLY ENOUGH TO COVER THE BODY IN A THIN LAYER. 1 OUNCE (HALF OF A 2 OUNCE CONTAINER) SHOULD BE ALL THAT IS NEEDED FOR CHILDREN UNDER 6 YEARS OF AGE; 1 TO 2 OUNCES FOR OLDER CHILDREN AND ADULTS. DO NOT LEAVE ON FOR MORE THAN 12 HOURS. DO NOT INGEST. KEEP AWAY FROM MOUTH AND EYES. COVER INFANTS' HANDS AND FEET DURING TREATMENT TO PREVENT SUCKING AND LICKING OF LOTION. DO NOT USE IF OPEN WOUNDS, CUTS OR SORES ARE PRESENT, UNLESS DIRECTED BY YOUR PHYSICIAN.

(Lotion: Shake Well)

1. Apply this preparation to dry skin in a thin layer and rub in thoroughly.
2. Trim nails and apply under nails with toothbrush (throw away toothbrush after use).
3. If a warm bath is taken before application, allow the skin to dry and cool completely before applying the medication.
4. A total body application should be made from the neck down, including soles of feet, unless otherwise directed by your physician.
5. The lotion should be left on for 8 to 12 hours (usually overnight) and then removed by thorough washing (bath or shower).
6. If applying lotion to another person, wear rubber gloves, especially if you are pregnant or a nursing mother.
7. All recently worn clothing, underwear and pajamas, and used sheets, pillow cases, and towels should be washed in very hot water or dry-cleaned.

After one application, itching will continue for several weeks. This is normal and does not require reapplication.

If you have any questions or concerns about your condition or use of the lotion, contact your physician.

0570-02

LINDANE SHAMPOO, USP 1% ℞

DESCRIPTION

Lindane Shampoo, USP 1% is an ectoparasiticide and ovicide effective against *Pediculosis capitis* (head lice), *Pediculosis pubis* (crab lice) and their ova. In addition to the active ingredient, lindane, it contains trolamine lauryl sulfate, polysorbate 60, acetone and water to form a cosmetically pleasant shampoo. The pH may be adjusted with Citric Acid and/or Trolamine. Lindane, which is the highly purified gamma isomer of 1, 2, 3, 4, 5, 6, hexachlorocyclohexane, has the following structural formula:

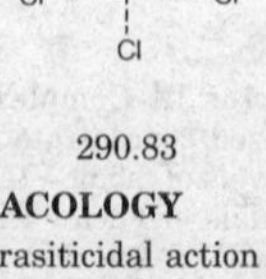

$C_6H_6Cl_6$ 290.83

CLINICAL PHARMACOLOGY

Lindane exerts its parasiticidal action by being directly absorbed into the parasites and their ova. Dale, et al[1], reported a blood level of 290 ng/mL associated with convulsions following the accidental ingestion of a lindane-containing product. Analysis of blood taken from subjects before and after the use of lindane shampoo showed a mean peak blood level of only 3 ng/mL which appeared at six hours and disappeared at eight hours after the shampoo was applied.

INDICATIONS AND USAGE

Because post-treatment pruritus is common and may lead to misuse, lindane shampoo is indicated only for the treat-

ment of patients with pediculosis capitis (head lice) and pediculosis pubis (crab lice) who have either failed to respond to adequate doses, or are intolerant of, other approved therapies. Reinfestation should be considered carefully before attributing the posttreatment presence of ectoparasites to a failure of response to adequate doses of other approved therapies.

CONTRAINDICATIONS

Lindane shampoo is contraindicated for premature neonates because their skin may be more permeable than full term infants and their liver enzymes may not be sufficiently developed. It is also contraindicated for patients with known seizure disorders and for individuals with a known sensitivity to the product or any of its components.

WARNINGS

LINDANE PENETRATES HUMAN SKIN AND HAS THE POTENTIAL FOR CNS TOXICITY (SEE CLINICAL PHARMACOLOGY SECTION). LINDANE SHAMPOO SHOULD BE USED ACCORDING TO RECOMMENDED DOSAGE (SEE DIRECTIONS FOR USE) ESPECIALLY ON INFANTS, PREGNANT WOMEN AND NURSING MOTHERS. ANIMAL STUDIES INDICATE THAT POTENTIAL TOXIC EFFECTS OF TOPICALLY APPLIED LINDANE ARE GREATER IN THE YOUNG. SEIZURES AND, IN RARE INSTANCES, DEATHS HAVE BEEN REPORTED AFTER EXCESS DOSAGE, OVER-EXPOSURE, FREQUENT REAPPLICATIONS, AND ACCIDENTAL AND INTENTIONAL INGESTION OF LINDANE. THESE INSTANCES OF PATIENT MISUSE HAVE BEEN ASSOCIATED WITH LACK OF PATIENT UNDERSTANDING OF DIRECTIONS FOR USE, PRESCRIBING OR DISPENSING EXCESSIVE QUANTITIES, AND IMPROPER REAPPLICATIONS. IN EXCEEDINGLY RARE CASES SEIZURES HAVE BEEN REPORTED WHEN USED ACCORDING TO DIRECTIONS. NO RESIDUAL EFFECTS OF LINDANE TREATMENT HAVE BEEN DEMONSTRATED, THEREFORE, THIS PRODUCT SHOULD NOT BE USED TO WARD OFF A POSSIBLE INFESTATION.

If accidental ingestion occurs, prompt gastric lavage is indicated. Because oils may enhance absorption, saline rather than oily cathartics should be used. Central nervous excitation can be controlled by the administration of pentobarbital, phenobarbital or diazepam.

PRECAUTIONS

General: Care should be taken to avoid contact with the eyes. If such contact occurs, eyes should be immediately flushed with water. If irritation or sensitization occurs, the patient should be advised to consult a physician.

Information for Patients: Patients must be instructed on the proper use of the medication, especially as to amount applied and duration of use. Patients Directions for Use must accompany the product.

Laboratory Tests: No laboratory tests are needed for the proper use of this medication.

Drug Interactions: Oils may enhance absorption, therefore, avoid using oil treatments, or oil based hair dressings or conditioners immediately before and after applying lindane shampoo.

Carcinogenesis: Although no studies have been conducted with lindane shampoo, numerous long-term feeding studies have been conducted in mice and rats to evaluate the carcinogenic potential of the technical grade of hexachlorocyclohexane (BHC) as well as the alpha, beta, gamma (lindane) and delta isomers. Both oral and topical applications have been evaluated. Nagasaki[2], Goto[3] and Hanada[4] found varying amounts of benign and malignant hepatomas associated with BHC and the alpha, delta and epsilon isomers. None reported a carcinogenic potential for lindane. Tumors were found only in the animals which had received the alpha isomer. Weisse and Herbst[5] also evaluated the carcinogenic potential of lindane in mice but could find no evidence of lindane carcinogenicity. The National Cancer Institute[6] had also found no evidence of carcinogenicity.

Thorpe and Walker[7] compared beta BHC with lindane, dieldrin, DDT and hexabarbital in mice. Despite the unusually high incidence of tumors in the control group, they concluded that 600 ppm of lindane was associated with a significant increase in the incidence of hepatoma and thus, considered it a tumorigen.

Orr[8] and Kashyap, et al[9] evaluated the carcinogenic potential in mice of topically applied BHC. In neither study was there any evidence of a tumorigenic or carcinogenic potential associated with topical application of BHC.

Mutagenicity tests have been used as predictive information about the carcinogenicity of various chemical compounds. Numerous types of mutagenicity tests have been performed with lindane. The results of these tests do not indicate that lindane is mutagenic.

Pregnancy: *Teratogenic Effects*—Pregnancy Category B. Reproduction, including multigeneration, studies have been performed in mice, rats, rabbits, pigs, and dogs at doses up to 10 times the human dose and have revealed no evidence of impaired fertility or harm to the fetus due to orally administered lindane. There are, however, no adequate and well-controlled studies in pregnant women. Because animal reproduction studies are not always predictive of human response, the recommended dosage should not be exceeded on pregnant women. They should be treated no more than twice during a pregnancy.

Nursing Mothers: Lindane is secreted in human milk in low concentrations. Studies conducted in the United States as well as in Europe and South America found levels of lindane in human milk ranging from 0 to 113 ppb, as the result of ingestion of foods which had been treated with lindane. There appeared to be no difference in concentrations between country and urban dwellers. Although the levels of lindane found in blood after topical application with lindane shampoo make it unlikely that amounts of lindane sufficient to cause serious adverse reactions will be excreted in the milk of nursing mothers who have used lindane shampoo, if there is any concern, an alternate method of feeding may be used for 4 days.

Pediatric Use: Refer to the CONTRAINDICATIONS and WARNINGS sections.

ADVERSE REACTIONS

Lindane has been reported to cause central nervous stimulation ranging from dizziness to convulsions. Cases of convulsions have been reported in connection with lindane shampoo therapy. However, these incidents were almost always associated with accidental oral ingestion or misuse of the product. In exceedingly rare cases, seizures have been reported when used according to directions. Eczematous eruptions due to irritation from this product have also been reported. Incidence of these adverse reactions is relatively infrequent, occurring in less than 1 in 100,000 patients.

DRUG ABUSE AND DEPENDENCE

Lindane shampoo is not subject to abuse, nor is there any dependence on the drug.

OVERDOSAGE

Overdosage or oral ingestion of lindane shampoo can cause central nervous system excitation and, if taken in sufficient quantities, convulsions may occur.

If accidental ingestion occurs, prompt gastric lavage should be instituted. However, since oils favor absorption, saline cathartics for intestinal evacuation should be given rather than oil laxatives. If central nervous system manifestations occur, they can be antagonized by the administration of pentobarbital, phenobarbital or diazepam.

DOSAGE AND ADMINISTRATION

CAUTION: USE ONLY AS DIRECTED. DO NOT EXCEED RECOMMENDED DOSAGE.

No residual effects of lindane shampoo treatment have been demonstrated, therefore, this product should not be used to ward off a possible infestation. However, sexual contacts should be treated simultaneously.

NOTE: PLEASE READ CAREFULLY.
DIRECTIONS FOR USE
WARNING:

THIS PRODUCT CAN BE POISONOUS IF MISUSED. CHILDREN MUST NOT BE ALLOWED TO APPLY THIS DRUG WITHOUT DIRECT ADULT SUPERVISION. USE SHAMPOO FOR HEAD AND PUBIC LICE ONLY. DO NOT USE FOR SCABIES. USE ONLY IN AMOUNTS DIRECTED BELOW. IN NO CASE SHOULD MORE THAN 2 OUNCES BE USED BY ONE PERSON IN ONE APPLICATION. DO NOT INGEST. KEEP AWAY FROM MOUTH AND EYES. DO NOT USE IF OPEN WOUNDS, CUTS OR SORES ARE PRESENT ON SCALP OR GROIN, UNLESS DIRECTED BY YOUR PHYSICIAN.
AVOID USING OIL TREATMENTS, OIL BASED HAIR DRESSINGS OR CONDITIONERS IMMEDIATELY BEFORE AND AFTER APPLYING LINDANE SHAMPOO.
(SHAKE WELL)

1. BEFORE APPLYING LINDANE SHAMPOO, USE REGULAR SHAMPOO (WITHOUT CONDITIONERS), RINSE AND COMPLETELY DRY HAIR.
2. USE 1 OUNCE (HALF OF A 2 OUNCE BOTTLE) FOR SHORT HAIR; 1.5 OUNCES (THREE-QUARTERS OF A 2 OUNCE BOTTLE) FOR MEDIUM LENGTH HAIR; AND FULL 2 OUNCE BOTTLE FOR LONG HAIR.
3. APPLY SHAMPOO DIRECTLY TO DRY HAIR WITHOUT ADDING WATER. WORK THOROUGHLY INTO THE HAIR AND ALLOW TO REMAIN IN PLACE FOR 4 MINUTES ONLY.
4. AFTER 4 MINUTES, ADD SMALL QUANTITIES OF WATER TO HAIR UNTIL A GOOD LATHER FORMS.
5. IMMEDIATELY RINSE ALL LATHER AWAY. AVOID UNNECESSARY CONTACT OF LATHER WITH OTHER BODY SURFACES.
6. TOWEL BRISKLY AND REMOVE NITS WITH NIT COMB OR TWEEZERS.
7. AVOID UNNECESSARY CONTACT WITH YOUR SKIN IF YOU ARE APPLYING SHAMPOO TO ANOTHER PERSON. IF TREATING MORE THAN ONE PERSON, PERSON APPLYING SHAMPOO (ESPECIALLY PREGNANT AND/OR NURSING WOMEN) SHOULD WEAR RUBBER GLOVES.
RE-TREATMENT IS USUALLY NOT NECESSARY, BUT PRESENCE OF LIVING LICE IN HAIR 7 DAYS AFTER TREATMENT INDICATES THAT RE-TREATMENT MAY BE NECESSARY. DO NOT RETREAT WITHOUT THE ADVICE OF A PHYSICIAN.

HOW SUPPLIED

Lindane Shampoo, USP 1% in patient-size 2 fl oz (59 mL), pharmacy-size only pint (473 mL) and pharmacy-size only gallon (3785 mL) bottles.
SHAKE WELL BEFORE USING.
Store at controlled room temperature 15°–30°C (59°–86°F). Dispense in a tight, light-resistant container as defined in the USP, with a child-resistant closure.
CAUTION: Federal law prohibits dispensing without prescription.

REFERENCES

1. Dale, W.E., Curly, A. and Cueto, C. *Life Sci* 5:47, 1966.
2. Nagasaki, T., Tomii, S., Mega, T., Marugami, M. and Ito, N. *Gann* (Cancer) 63(3):373, 1972.
3. Goto, M., Hattori, M., Miyagawa, T. and Enomoto, M., *Chemosphere* 6:279, 1972.
4. Hanada, M., Yatani, C., Miyaji, T., *Gann* 64:511, 1973.
5. Weisse, I., and Herbst, M., *Toxicol.* 7:233, 1977.
6. Technical Report Series, NCl-CG-TR-14, *HEW PUBLICATIONS*, No. (NIH) 77–814.
7. Thorpe, E., and Walker, A.I.T., *Food Cosmetic Toxicol.* 11: 433, 1973.
8. Orr, J.W., *Nature* 162:189, 1948.
9. Kashyap, S.K. et al, *J. Environ. Sci. Health* 14:305–318, 1979.

Manufactured by
Barre-National Inc.
Baltimore, MD 21244
an ALPHARMA USPD Company

FORM NO. 0572-02   Rev. 4/96 B1

PHARMACIST — DETACH AND GIVE TO PATIENT

LINDANE SHAMPOO, USP 1%
A SHAMPOO
FOR THE TREATMENT OF HEAD OR PUBIC LICE
CAUTION: USE ONLY AS DIRECTED. DO NOT EXCEED RECOMMENDED DOSE.
NOTE: PLEASE READ CAREFULLY.
DIRECTIONS FOR USE:
WARNING:

THIS PRODUCT CAN BE POISONOUS IF MISUSED. CHILDREN MUST NOT BE ALLOWED TO APPLY THIS DRUG WITHOUT DIRECT ADULT SUPERVISION. USE SHAMPOO FOR HEAD AND PUBIC LICE ONLY. DO NOT USE FOR SCABIES. USE ONLY IN AMOUNTS DIRECTED BELOW. IN NO CASE SHOULD MORE THAN 2 OUNCES BE USED BY ONE PERSON IN ONE APPLICATION. DO NOT INGEST. KEEP AWAY FROM MOUTH AND EYES. DO NOT USE IF OPEN WOUNDS, CUTS OR SORES ARE PRESENT ON SCALP OR GROIN, UNLESS DIRECTED BY YOUR PHYSICIAN.
AVOID USING OIL TREATMENTS, OIL BASED HAIR DRESSINGS OR CONDITIONERS IMMEDIATELY BEFORE AND AFTER APPLYING LINDANE SHAMPOO.
(SHAKE WELL)

1. BEFORE APPLYING LINDANE SHAMPOO, USE REGULAR SHAMPOO (WITHOUT CONDITIONERS), RINSE AND COMPLETELY DRY HAIR.
2. USE 1 OUNCE (HALF OF A 2 OUNCE BOTTLE) FOR SHORT HAIR; 1.5 OUNCES (THREE-QUARTERS OF A 2 OUNCE BOTTLE) FOR MEDIUM LENGTH HAIR; AND FULL 2 OUNCE BOTTLE FOR LONG HAIR.
3. APPLY SHAMPOO DIRECTLY TO DRY HAIR WITHOUT ADDING WATER. WORK THOROUGHLY INTO THE HAIR AND ALLOW TO REMAIN IN PLACE FOR 4 MINUTES ONLY.
4. AFTER 4 MINUTES, ADD SMALL QUANTITIES OF WATER TO HAIR UNTIL A GOOD LATHER FORMS.
5. IMMEDIATELY RINSE ALL LATHER AWAY. AVOID UNNECESSARY CONTACT OF LATHER WITH OTHER BODY SURFACES.
6. TOWEL BRISKLY AND REMOVE NITS WITH NIT COMB OR TWEEZERS.
7. AVOID UNNECESSARY CONTACT WITH YOUR SKIN IF YOU ARE APPLYING SHAMPOO TO ANOTHER PERSON. IF TREATING MORE THAN ONE PERSON, PERSON APPLYING SHAMPOO (ESPECIALLY PREGNANT AND/OR NURSING WOMEN) SHOULD WEAR RUBBER GLOVES.
RE-TREATMENT IS USUALLY NOT NECESSARY, BUT PRESENCE OF LIVING LICE IN HAIR 7 DAYS AFTER TREATMENT INDICATES THAT RE-TREATMENT MAY BE NECESSARY. DO NOT RE-TREAT WITHOUT THE ADVICE OF A PHYSICIAN.

Alra Laboratories, Inc.
3850 CLEARVIEW CT.
GURNEE, IL 60031

Direct Inquiries to:
Professional Services
(847) 244-9440
(800) 248-ALRA
FAX: (847) 244-9464

CHOLAC
[kō 'lac]
Ŗ
CONSTILAC
[kŏn 'stil-ac]
Ŗ
Lactulose Solution, USP

Each 15 mL syrup contains:
10 g lactulose (and less than 1.6 g galactose, less than 1.2 g lactose, 0.1 g or less of fructose); plus water and coloring. Sodium hydroxide used to adjust pH.

HOW SUPPLIED
1 fl. oz. bottle (30 mL) (unit-dose)
    100 bottles/carton   NDC #51641-225-61
8 fl. oz. bottle (240 mL)   NDC #51641-224-68
16 fl oz. bottle (480 mL)   NDC #51641-225-76
32 fl. oz. bottle (960 mL)   NDC #51641-224-82
64 fl. oz. bottle (1920 mL)   NDC #51641-225-94
1 gal. (3785 mL)   NDC #51641-225-97

ERYZOLE Granules for Suspension
Ŗ
erythromycin ethylsuccinate and sulfisoxazole acetyl for oral suspension USP

When reconstituted each 5mL of suspension contains: Erythromycin Ethylsuccinate equivalent to 200mg erythromycin and Sulfisoxazole Acetyl equivalent to 600mg sulfisoxazole.

HOW SUPPLIED
Eryzole suspension is available for teaspoon dosage in bottles of,
100 mL (NDC 51641-111-64)
150 mL (NDC 51641-111-66)
200 mL (NDC 51641-111-68)
in the form of granules to be reconstituted with water.

GELPIRIN TABLETS
OTC

Each tablet contains:
    Acetaminophen .... 125 mg.
    Aspirin .... 240 mg.
    Caffeine .... 32 mg.
Along with two buffering agents

HOW SUPPLIED
Bottle of 100 (NDC 51641-711-01)
Bottle of 1000 (NDC 51641-711-10)

GELPIRIN-M TABLETS (FILM COATED)
OTC

Each tablet contains:
    Aspirin .... 250 mg.
    Acetaminophen .... 250 mg.
    Caffeine .... 65 mg.
Along with two buffering agents

HOW SUPPLIED
Bottle of 30 (NDC 51641-717-30)
Bottle of 60 (NDC 51641-717-60)
Bottle of 125 (NDC 51641-717-01)

Gen–XENE®
Ⓒ Ŗ
[jen 'zēn]
Clorazepate Dipotassium Tablets

Gen–XENE Tablets are available in 3.75 mg, 7.5 mg or 15 mg strengths for oral administration.

HOW SUPPLIED
3.75 mg gray, scored tablets debossed with ALRA and GX:
Unit dose packages of 100: NDC 51641-242-11
Bottles of 30 NDC 51641-242-03
Bottles of 100 NDC 51641-242-01
Bottles of 500 NDC 51641-242-05

7.5 mg yellow, scored tablets debossed with ALRA and GT:
Unit dose packages of 100: NDC 51641-243-11
Bottles of 30 NDC 51641-243-03
Bottles of 100 NDC 51641-243-01
Bottles of 500 NDC 51641-243-05

15 mg green, scored tablets debossed with ALRA and GN:
Unit dose packages of 100: NDC 51641-244-11
Bottles of 30 NDC 51641-244-03
Bottles of 100 NDC 51641-244-01
Bottles of 500 NDC 51641-244-05

IBU–TAB
Ibuprofen Tablets, USP

Ibuprofen Tablets are available in 200, 400, 600 and 800 mg strengths for oral administration.

HOW SUPPLIED
IBU-TAB OTC
Ibuprofen Tablets, 200 mg (orange) film-coated, round tablets. Debossed 'ALRA' on one side and 215 on the other.
Bottles of 30   NDC 51641-215-03
Bottles of 60   NDC 51641-215-60
Bottles of 100   NDC 51641-215-01
Bottles of 250   NDC 51641-215-25
IBU-TAB Ŗ
Ibuprofen Tablets, 400 mg (orange) film-coated, round tablets. Debossed 'ALRA' on one side and IF 400 on the other.
Bottles of 100   NDC 51641-214-01
Bottles of 500   NDC 51641-214-05
Bottles of 1000   NDC 51641-214-10
Unit-dose packages of 100   NDC 51641-214-11
Ibuprofen Tablets, 600 mg (orange) film-coated, oval tablets. Debossed 'ALRA' on one side and IF 600 on the other.
Bottles of 100   NDC 51641-213-01
Bottles of 500   NDC 51641-213-05
Bottles of 1000   NDC 51641-213-10
Unit-dose packages of 100   NDC 51641-213-11
Ibuprofen Tablets, 800 mg (light peach) film-coated, oval tablets. Debossed 'ALRA' on one side and IF 800 on the other.
Bottles of 100   NDC 51641-212-01
Bottles of 500   NDC 51641-212-05
Bottles of 1000   NDC 51641-212-10
Unit-dose packages of 100   NDC 51641-212-11

K+ 8
Ŗ
Potassium Chloride Extended-release Tablets, USP

Each K+ 8 tablet contains:
    Potassium Chloride, USP .... 8 mEq (600 mg)
    Equivalent to 8 mEq (312 mg) of potassium and 8 mEq (288 mg) of chloride)

HOW SUPPLIED
8 mEq (600 mg) yellow, coated, round tablets debossed ALRA on one side and K+8 on the other side:
Bottles of 100 (NDC 51641-175-01)
Bottles of 500 (NDC 51641-175-05)
8 mEq (600 mg) white, coated, round tablets debossed ALRA on one side and K+8 on the other side:
Bottles of 100 (NDC 51641-275-01)
Bottles of 500 (NDC 51641-275-05)

K + 10
Ŗ
Potassium Chloride Extended-release Tablets, USP

Each K + 10 tablet contains:
    Potassium Chloride, USP .... 10 mEq (750 mg)
    [Equivalent to 10 mEq (390 mg) of potassium and 10 mEq (360 mg) of chloride]

HOW SUPPLIED
10 mEq (750 mg) yellow, coated, capsule shaped tablets debossed ALRA on one side and K+10 on the other side.
Bottles of 100 (NDC 51641-177-01)
Bottles of 500 (NDC 51641-177-05)
Bottles of 1000 (NDC 51641-177-10)
Unit dose (100) in strips (NDC 51641-177-11)
10 mEq (750 mg) white, coated, capsule shaped tablets debossed ALRA on one side and K+10 on the other side.
Bottles of 100 (NDC 51641-277-01)
Bottles of 500 (NDC 51641-277-05)
Bottles of 1000 (NDC 51641-277-10)

K + CARE ET 25 mEq
Ŗ
Potassium Bicarbonate Effervescent Tablets For Oral Solution, USP

Each tablet contains .... 25 mEq of Potassium
    (From 2.5 Gm. of Potassium Bicarbonate)

HOW SUPPLIED
Carton of 30 (NDC 51641-135-03) Orange flavor
Carton of 30 (NDC 51641-125-03) Lime flavor
Carton of 100 (NDC 51641-135-01) Orange flavor
Carton of 100 (NDC 51641-125-01) Lime flavor

LIQUID VITAMINS, Geriatrics
SILVER STRENGTH
OTC
FEMALE—GERIATRIC
MULTI-VIT/MULTI-MIN LIQUID

Contains:
Vitamin A, E, C, B_1, B_2, B_6, B_{12}, D_2, Biotin, Pantothenic Acid, Niacin, Iodine, Iron, Zinc, Manganese, Chromium and Molybdenum

HOW SUPPLIED
Bottle of 8oz (NDC 51641-771-68)
Bottle of 16oz (NDC 51641-771-76)

SILVER STRENGTH
OTC
MALE—GERIATRIC
MULTI-VIT/MULTI-MIN LIQUID

Contains:
Vitamin A, E, C, B_1, B_2, B_6, B_{12}, D_2, Biotin, Pantothenic Acid, Niacin, Iodine, Iron, Zinc, Manganese, Chromium and Molybdenum

HOW SUPPLIED
Bottle of 8oz (NDC 51641-770-68)
Bottle of 16oz (NDC 51641-770-76)

LIQUID VITAMINS, Pediatrics

INFANT FORMULA
Ŗ
MULTI-VIT/FLUORIDE
DROPS 0.25 mg

Contains:
    Vitamin A, D, E, C, B_1, B_2, B_6, B_{12}, Niacin & Fluoride.

HOW SUPPLIED
Bottle of 50mL (NDC 51641-727-50)
Bottle of 120mL (NDC 51641-727-64)

INFANT FORMULA
Ŗ
MULTI-VIT/FLUORIDE
DROPS 0.50 mg
Contains:
    Vitamin A, D, E, C, B_1, B_2, B_6, B_{12}, Niacin & Fluoride.

HOW SUPPLIED
Bottle of 50mL (NDC 51641-730-50)
Bottle of 120mL (NDC 51641-730-64)

INFANT FORMULA
Ŗ
TRI-VIT/FLUORIDE DROPS 0.25 mg
Contains:
    Vitamin A, D, C, and Fluoride.

HOW SUPPLIED
Bottle of 50mL (NDC 51641-724-50)
Bottle of 120mL (NDC 51641-724-64)

INFANT FORMULA
Ŗ
TRI-VIT/FLUORIDE DROPS 0.50 mg
Contains:
    Vitamin A, D, C, and Fluoride.

HOW SUPPLIED
Bottle of 50mL (NDC 51641-725-50)
Bottle of 120mL (NDC 51641-725-64)

ALZA Pharmaceuticals,
**A division of ALZA Corporation
950 PAGE MILL ROAD
P.O. BOX 10950
PALO ALTO, CA 94303-0802**

Direct Inquiries to:
Customer Service
(800) 227-9953
FAX: (415) 962-4212

For Medical Information or Medical Emergencies Contact:
Medical Communications
(800) 634-8977
FAX: (415) 962-2488

Medical Communications (for Ethyol)
(800) 506-4959
FAX: (415) 962-2488

BICITRA® ℞

[bye"si-trah]

**Brand of sodium citrate and
citric acid oral solution, USP**

DESCRIPTION

BICITRA® is a stable and pleasant-tasting oral systemic alkalizer solution containing sodium citrate and citric acid in a sugar-free base. It is a nonparticulate neutralizing buffer. BICITRA® contains in each teaspoonful (5 mL):
SODIUM CITRATE Dihydrate 500 mg (0.34 Molar)
CITRIC ACID Monohydrate 334 mg (0.32 Molar)
Each mL contains 1 mEq sodium ion and is equivalent to 1 mEq bicarbonate (HCO_3). BICITRA® also contains butylparaben, flavoring, maltitol, and sodium saccharin.

CLINICAL PHARMACOLOGY

Sodium citrate is absorbed and metabolized to sodium bicarbonate, thus acting as a systemic alkalizer. The effects are essentially those of chlorides before absorption and those of bicarbonates subsequently. Oxidization is virtually complete so that less than 5% of sodium citrate is excreted in the urine unchanged.

INDICATIONS AND USAGE

Bicitra® is an effective alkalinizing agent. It is useful in those conditions where long-term maintenance of an alkaline urine is desirable, and is of value in the alleviation of chronic metabolic acidosis, such as results from chronic renal insufficiency or the syndrome of renal tubular acidosis, especially when the administration of potassium salts is undesirable or contraindicated. BICITRA® is also useful for buffering and neutralizing gastric hydrochloric acid quickly and effectively.
BICITRA® is concentrated, and when administered after meals and before bedtime, allows one to maintain an alkaline urinary pH around the clock, usually without the necessity of a 2 A.M. dose. BICITRA® alkalinizes the urine without producing a systemic alkalosis in the recommended dosage. BICITRA® is highly palatable, pleasant tasting, and tolerable, even when administered for long periods. BICITRA® is sugar-free.

CONTRAINDICATIONS

Patients on sodium-restricted diets or with severe renal impairment. In certain situations, potassium citrate, as contained in POLYCITRA®-K, may be preferable.

PRECAUTIONS

Should be used with caution by patients with low urinary output unless under the supervision of a physician. BICITRA® should not be administered concurrently with aluminum-based antacids. Patients should be directed to dilute adequately with water, and preferably, to take each dose after meals to avoid saline laxative effect. Sodium salts should be used cautiously in patients with cardiac failure, hypertension, impaired renal function, peripheral and pulmonary edema, and toxemia of pregnancy. Periodic examinations and determinations of serum electrolytes, particularly serum bicarbonate level, should be carried out in those patients with renal disease in order to avoid these complications.

ADVERSE REACTIONS

BICITRA® is generally well tolerated, without any unpleasant side effects, when given in recommended doses to patients with normal renal function and urinary output. However, as with any alkalinizing agent, caution must be used in certain patients with abnormal renal mechanisms to avoid development of alkalosis, especially in the presence of hypocalcemia.

OVERDOSAGE

Overdosage with sodium salts may cause diarrhea, nausea, vomiting, hypernoia, and convulsions.

DOSAGE AND ADMINISTRATION

BICITRA® should be taken diluted in water, followed by additional water, if desired. Palatability is enhanced if chilled before taking.
For Systemic Alkalization:
Usual Adult Dose: 2 to 6 teaspoonfuls (10 to 30 mL), diluted in 1 to 3 ounces of water, after meals and at bedtime, or as directed by a physician.
Usual Pediatric Dose: 1 to 3 teaspoonfuls (5 to 15 mL), diluted in 1 to 3 ounces of water, after meals and at bedtime, or as directed by a physician. For children under two years of age, use is based on consultation with a physician.
As a neutralizing buffer: 3 teaspoonfuls (15 mL), diluted with 15 mL water, taken as a single dose, or as directed by a physician.

HOW SUPPLIED

BICITRA® is a grape flavored citrate solution supplied as:
16 fl. oz. (473 mL)
  (NDC 17314-9330-1);
30 mL Unit Dose
  (NDC 17314-9330-5);

15 mL Unit Dose
  (NDC 17314-9330-4).
Keep tightly closed and protect from excessive heat or freezing.
Rx only
©1998 Baker Norton
Pharmaceuticals, Inc.
BICITRA® is a registered
trademark of Baker Norton
Pharmaceuticals, Inc.
under license to
ALZA Corporation
Distributed by:
ALZA Corporation
Mountain View, CA 94043
Mfd. by:
  Draxis Pharma Inc.
  Kirkland, Quebec H9H 4J4
  Canada
ALZA Pharmaceuticals
A division of ALZA Corp.
Mountain View, CA 94043
1001721   Rev 9804
REV9804   (212001)

DITROPAN® ℞

**(oxybutynin chloride)
Tablets and Syrup**

DESCRIPTION

Each scored biconvex, engraved blue DITROPAN® Tablet contains 5 mg of oxybutynin chloride. Each 5 mL of DITROPAN® Syrup contains 5 mg of oxybutynin chloride. Chemically, oxybutynin chloride is d,l (racemic) 4-diethylamino-2-butynyl phenylcyclohexylglycolate hydrochloride. The empirical formula of oxybutynin chloride is $C_{22}H_{31}NO_3 \cdot HCl$. The structural formula appears below:

Oxybutynin chloride is a white crystalline solid with a molecular weight of 393.9. It is readily soluble in water and acids, but relatively insoluble in alkalis.
DITROPAN® Tablets
Also contains: calcium stearate, FD&C Blue #1 Lake, lactose, and microcrystalline cellulose.
DITROPAN® Syrup
Also contains: citric acid, FD&C Green #3, glycerin, methylparaben, flavor, sodium citrate, sorbitol, sucrose, and water.
DITROPAN® Tablets and Syrup are for oral administration.
Therapeutic Category: Antispasmodic, anticholinergic.

CLINICAL PHARMACOLOGY

DITROPAN® (oxybutynin chloride) exerts direct antispasmodic effect on smooth muscle and inhibits the muscarinic action of acetylcholine on smooth muscle. DITROPAN exhibits only one fifth of the anticholinergic activity of atropine on the rabbit detrusor muscle, but four to ten times the antispasmodic activity. No blocking effects occur at skeletal neuromuscular junctions or autonomic ganglia (antinicotinic effects).
DITROPAN relaxes bladder smooth muscle. In patients with conditions characterized by involuntary bladder contractions, cystometric studies have demonstrated that DITROPAN increases bladder (vesical) capacity, diminishes the frequency of uninhibited contractions of the detrusor muscle, and delays the initial desire to void. DITROPAN thus decreases urgency and the frequency of both incontinent episodes and voluntary urination.
DITROPAN was well tolerated in patients administered the drug in controlled studies of 30 days' duration and in uncontrolled studies in which some of the patients received the drug for 2 years. Pharmacokinetic information is not currently available.

INDICATIONS AND USAGE

DITROPAN is indicated for the relief of symptoms of bladder instability associated with voiding in patients with uninhibited neurogenic or reflex neurogenic bladder (ie, urgency, frequency, urinary leakage, urge incontinence, dysuria).

CONTRAINDICATIONS

DITROPAN® (oxybutynin chloride) is contraindicated in patients with untreated angle closure glaucoma and in patients with untreated narrow anterior chamber angles since anticholinergic drugs may aggravate these conditions.

It is also contraindicated in partial or complete obstruction of the gastrointestinal tract, paralytic ileus, intestinal atony of the elderly or debilitated patient, megacolon, toxic megacolon complicating ulcerative colitis, severe colitis, and myasthenia gravis. It is contraindicated in patients with obstructive uropathy and in patients with unstable cardiovascular status in acute hemorrhage.
DITROPAN is contraindicated in patients who have demonstrated hypersensitivity to the product.

WARNINGS

DITROPAN® (oxybutynin chloride), when administered in the presence of high environmental temperature, can cause heat prostration (fever and heat stroke due to decreased sweating).
Diarrhea may be an early symptom of incomplete intestinal obstruction, especially in patients with ileostomy or colostomy. In this instance treatment with DITROPAN would be inappropriate and possibly harmful.
DITROPAN may produce drowsiness or blurred vision. The patient should be cautioned regarding activities requiring mental alertness such as operating a motor vehicle or other machinery or performing hazardous work while taking this drug.
Alcohol or other sedative drugs may enhance the drowsiness caused by DITROPAN.

PRECAUTIONS

DITROPAN® (oxybutynin chloride) should be used with caution in the elderly and in all patients with autonomic neuropathy, hepatic or renal disease. DITROPAN may aggravate the symptoms of hyperthyroidism, coronary heart disease, congestive heart failure, cardiac arrhythmias, hiatal hernia, tachycardia, hypertension, and prostatic hypertrophy. Administration of DITROPAN® (oxybutynin chloride) to patients with ulcerative colitis may suppress intestinal motility to the point of producing a paralytic ileus and precipitate or aggravate toxic megacolon, a serious complication of the disease.
Carcinogenesis, Mutagenesis, Impairment of Fertility. A 24-month study in rats at dosages up to approximately 400 times the recommended human dosage showed no evidence of carcinogenicity.
DITROPAN showed no increase of mutagenic activity when tested in *Schizosaccharomyces pompholiciformis*, *Saccharomyces cerevisiae* and *Salmonella typhimurium* test systems. Reproduction studies in the hamster, rabbit, rat, and mouse have shown no definite evidence of impaired fertility.
Pregnancy. Category B. Reproduction studies in the hamster, rabbit, rat, and mouse have shown no definite evidence of impaired fertility or harm to the animal fetus. The safety of DITROPAN administered to women who are or who may become pregnant has not been established. Therefore, DITROPAN should not be given to pregnant women unless, in the judgment of the physician, the probable clinical benefits outweigh the possible hazards.
Nursing Mothers. It is not known whether this drug is excreted in human milk. Because many drugs are excreted in human milk, caution should be exercised when DITROPAN is administered to a nursing woman.
Pediatric Use. The safety and efficacy of DITROPAN administration have been demonstrated for pediatric patients 5 years of age and older (see DOSAGE AND ADMINISTRATION). However, as there is insufficient clinical data for pediatric populations under age 5, DITROPAN is not recommended for this age group.

ADVERSE REACTIONS

Following administration of DITROPAN® (oxybutynin chloride), the symptoms that can be associated with the use of other anticholinergic drugs may occur:
Cardiovascular: Palpitations, tachycardia, vasodilation
Dermatologic: Decreased sweating, rash
Gastrointestinal/Genitourinary: Constipation, decreased gastrointestinal motility, dry mouth, nausea, urinary hesitance and retention
Nervous System: Asthenia, dizziness, drowsiness, hallucinations, insomnia, restlessness
Ophthalmic: Amblyopia, cycloplegia, decreased lacrimation, mydriasis
Other: Impotence, suppression of lactation

OVERDOSAGE

The symptoms of overdosage with DITROPAN® (oxybutynin chloride) may be any of those seen with other anticholinergic agents. Symptoms may include signs of central nervous system excitation (eg, restlessness, tremor, irritability, convulsions, delirium, hallucinations), flushing, fever, nausea, vomiting, tachycardia, hypotension or hypertension, respiratory failure, paralysis, and coma.
In the event of an overdose or exaggerated response, treatment should be symptomatic and supportive. Maintain respiration and induce emesis or perform gastric lavage (emesis is contraindicated in precomatose, convulsive, or psychotic state). Activated charcoal may be administered as

Continued on next page

Ditropan—Cont.

well as a cathartic. Physostigmine may be considered to reverse symptoms of anticholinergic intoxication. Hyperpyrexia may be treated symptomatically with ice bags or other cold applications and alcohol sponges.

DOSAGE AND ADMINISTRATION

Tablets

Adults: The usual dose is one 5-mg tablet two to three times a day. The maximum recommended dose is one 5-mg tablet four times a day.

Pediatric patients over 5 years of age: The usual dose is one 5-mg tablet two times a day. The maximum recommended dose is one 5-mg tablet three times a day.

Syrup

Adults: The usual dose is one teaspoon (5 mg/5 mL) syrup two to three times a day. The maximum recommended dose is one teaspoon (5 mg/5 mL) syrup four times a day.

Pediatric patients over 5 years of age: The usual dose is one teaspoon (5 mg/5 mL) two times a day. The maximum recommended dose is one teaspoon (5 mg/5 mL) three times a day.

HOW SUPPLIED

DITROPAN® (oxybutynin chloride) Tablets are supplied in bottles of 100 tablets (NDC 17314-9200-1) and 1000 tablets (NDC 17314-9200-2) and in Unit Dose Identification Paks of 100 tablets (NDC 17314-9200-3).

Blue scored tablets (5 mg) are engraved with DITROPAN on one side with 92 and 00, separated by a horizontal score, on the other side.

DITROPAN® Syrup (5 mg/5 mL) is supplied in bottles of 16 fluid ounces (473 mL) (NDC 17314-9201-4).

Pharmacist: Dispense in tight, light-resistant container as defined in the USP.

Store at controlled room temperature (59–86°F).

Rx ONLY

Manufactured by Hoechst Marion Roussel, Inc., Kansas City, MO 64137

Distributed by ALZE Corporation, Mountain View, CA 94043   50016519
                                                             Edition: 01/98

ELMIRON®-100 mg   ℞
(pentosan polysulfate sodium)
Capsules

DESCRIPTION

Pentosan polysulfate sodium is a semi-synthetically produced heparin-like macromolecular carbohydrate derivative which chemically and structurally resembles glycosaminoglycans. It is a white odorless powder, slightly hygroscopic and soluble in water to 50% at pH 6. It has a molecular weight of 4000 to 6000 Dalton with the following structural formula:

ELMIRON® is supplied in white opaque hard gelatin capsules containing 100 mg pentosan polysulfate sodium, microcrystalline cellulose, and magnesium stearate. It is formulated for oral use.

CLINICAL PHARMACOLOGY

GENERAL: Pentosan polysulfate sodium is a low molecular weight heparin-like compound. It has anticoagulant and fibrinolytic effects. The mechanism of action of pentosan polysulfate sodium in interstitial cystitis is not known.

PHARMACOKINETICS:

Absorption: In preliminary clinical studies with different doses of radio labeled pentosan polysulfate sodium, absorption was approximately 3% of the administered dose (n=3).

Distribution: Preclinical studies with parenterally administered radio labeled pentosan polysulfate sodium showed distribution to the uroepithelium of the genitourinary tract with lesser amounts found in the liver, spleen, lung, skin, periosteum, and bone marrow. Erythrocyte penetration is low in animals.

Metabolism: Preliminary literature studies of metabolism in 5 healthy volunteers with radio labeled drug suggest that 68% of the dose, at about 1 hour after IV administration, undergoes partial desulfation in the liver and spleen. In an-

other study of 3 healthy volunteers, partial depolymerization occurs in the kidney. Both the desulfation and depolymerization can be saturated with continued dosing.

Excretion: In preliminary clinical studies in 8 healthy male volunteers, the elimination half-life of pentosan polysulfate sodium had a mean value at 24 hours after IV injection of 40 mg.

The elimination half-life in urine following orally administered radio labeled pentosan polysulfate sodium was determined to be 4.8 hours for the unchanged drug.

In preliminary human studies in 3 healthy male volunteers, after single doses of radio labeled drug, urinary excretion averaged 3.5% of the administered dose. After multiple doses of pentosan polysulfate sodium, urine excretion of radioactivity averaged 11% of the administered dose.

Further analyses of the urinary fraction obtained after repeated dosing showed that about 3% of the dose may be unchanged pentosan polysulfate sodium.

Special Populations: Dose adjustments in geriatric patients and in patients with hepatic or renal impairment were not studied.

PHARMACODYNAMICS:

The mechanism by which pentosan polysulfate sodium achieves its effects in patients is unknown. In preliminary clinical models, pentosan polysulfate sodium adhered to the bladder wall mucosal membrane. The drug may act as a buffer to control cell permeability preventing irritating solutes in the urine from reaching the cells.

Food effects: The effect of food on absorption of pentosan polysulfate sodium is now known. In clinical trials, ELMIRON® was administered with water 1 hour before or 2 hours after meals.

Drug-Drug Interactions:
Not studied.

CLINICAL TRIALS

ELMIRON® was evaluated in two clinical trials for the relief of pain in patients with chronic interstitial cystitis (IC). All patients met the NIH definition of IC based upon the results of cystoscopy, cytology, and biopsy. One blinded, randomized, placebo controlled study evaluated 151 patients (145 women, 5 men, 1 unknown) with a mean age of 44 years (range 18 to 81). Approximately equal numbers of patients received either placebo or ELMIRON® 100 mg three times a day for 3 months. Clinical improvement in bladder pain was based upon the patient's own assessment. In this study, 28/74 (38%) of patients who received ELMIRON® and 13/74 (18%) of patients who received placebo, showed greater than 50% improvement in bladder pain (p=0.005).

A second clinical trial, the physician's usage study, was a prospectively designed retrospective analysis of 2499 patients who received ELMIRON® 300 mg a day without blinding. Of the 2499 patients, 2220 were women, 254 were men, and 25 were of unknown sex. The patients had a mean age of 47 years and 23% were over 60 years of age. By 3 months, 1307 (52%) of the patients had dropped out or were ineligible for analysis, overall, 1192 (48%) received ELMIRON® for 3 months; 892 (36%) received ELMIRON® for 6 months; and 598 (24%) received ELMIRON® for one year. Patients had unblinded evaluations every 3 months for the patient's rating of overall change in pain in comparison to baseline and for the difference calculated in "pain/discomfort" scores. At baseline, pain/discomfort scores for the original 2499 patients were severe or unbearable in 60%, moderate in 33% and mild or none in 7% of patients. The extent of the patients' pain improvement is shown in Table 1.

Table 1:
Pain Scores in Reference to Baseline in Open Label Physician's Usage Study (N=2499)[1]

Efficacy Parameter	3 months[2]	6 months[2]
Patient Rating of Overall Change in Pain (Recollection of difference between current pain and baseline pain)[2]	N=1161 Median=3 Mean=3.44 CI: (3.37, 3.51)	N=724 Median=4 Mean=3.91 CI: (3.83, 3.99)
Change in Pain/ Discomfort Score (Calculated difference in scores at the time point and baseline)[4].	N=1440 Median=1 Mean=0.51 CI: (0.45, 0.57)	N=904 Median=1 Mean=0.66 CI: (0.61, 0.71)

[1] Trial not designed to detect onset of pain relief.
[2] CI=95% confidence interval.
[3] 6-point-scale: 1 = worse, 2 = no better,
  3 = slightly improved, 4 = moderately
  improved, 5 = greatly improved,
  6=symptom gone.

[4] 3-point scale:
  1=none or mild,
  2=moderate,
  3=severe or unbearable.

At 3 months, 722/2499 (29%) of the patients originally in the study had pain scores that improved by one or two categories. By 6 months, in the 892 patients who continued taking ELMIRON®, an additional 116/2499 (5%) of patients had improved pain scores. After 6 months, the percent of patients who reported the first onset of pain relief was less than 1.5% of patients who originally entered in the study (see Table 2).

Table 2:
Number (%) of Patients with New Relief of Pain/Discomfort in the Open-Label Physician's Usage Study (N=2499)

	at 3 months[2] (n=1192)	at 6 months[3] (n=892)
Considering only the patients who continued treatment	722/1192 (61%)	116/892 (13%)
Considering all the patients originally enrolled in the study	722/2499 (29%)	116/2499 (5%)

[1] First-time improvement in pain/discomfort score by 1 or 2 categories.
[2] Number (%) of patients with improvement of pain/discomfort score at 3 months when compared to baseline.
[2] Number (%) of patients without pain/ discomfort improvement at 3 months who had improvement at 6 months.

INDICATIONS AND USAGE

ELMIRON® (pentosan polysulfate sodium) is indicated for the relief of bladder pain or discomfort associated with interstitial cystitis.

CONTRAINDICATIONS

ELMIRON® (pentosan polysulfate sodium) is contraindicated in patients with known hypersensitivity to the drug, structurally related compounds, or excipients.

WARNINGS

None.

PRECAUTIONS

GENERAL:

ELMIRON® (pentosan polysulfate sodium) is a weak anticoagulant (1/15 the activity of heparin). Bleeding complications of ecchymosis, epistaxis, and gum hemorrhage have been reported (see **ADVERSE REACTIONS**). Patients undergoing invasive procedures or having signs/symptoms of underlying coagulopathy or other increased risk of bleeding (due to other therapies such as coumarin anticoagulants, heparin, t-PA streptokinase, or high dose aspirin) should be evaluated for hemorrhage. Patients with diseases such as aneurysms, thrombocytopenia, hemophilia, gastrointestinal ulcerations, polyps, or diverticula should be carefully evaluated before starting ELMIRON®.

A similar product that was given subcutaneously, sublingually, or intramuscularly (and not initially metabolized by the liver) is associated with delayed immunoallergic thrombocytopenia with symptoms of thrombosis and hemorrhage. Caution should be exercised when using ELMIRON® in patients who have a history of heparin induced thrombocytopenia.

Hepatic Insufficiency: Pentosan polysulfate sodium is desulfated by both the liver and the spleen. The extent to which hepatic insufficiency or splenic disorders may increase the bioavailability of the parent or active metabolites of pentosan polysulfate sodium is not known. Caution should be exercised when using ELMIRON® in these patients.

Mildly (<2.5 × normal) elevated transaminase, alkaline phosphatase, γ-glutamyl transpeptidase, and lactic dehydrogenase occurred in 1.2% of patients. The increases usually appeared 3 to 12 months after the start of ELMIRON® therapy, and were not associated with jaundice or other clinical signs or symptoms. These abnormalities are usually transient, may remain essentially unchanged, or may rarely progress with continued use. Increases in PTT and PT (<1% for both) or thrombocytopenia (0.2%) were noted.

Alopecia is associated with pentosan polysulfate and with heparin products. In clinical trials of ELMIRON®, alopecia could begin within the first 4 weeks of treatment. Ninety-seven percent (97%) of the cases of alopecia reported were alopecia areata, limited to a single area on the scalp.

INFORMATION FOR PATIENTS:

Patients should take the drug as prescribed, in the dosage prescribed, and no more frequently than prescribed. Patients should be reminded that ELMIRON® has a weak anticoagulant effect. This effect may increase bleeding times.

LABORATORY TEST FINDINGS:

Pentosan polysulfate sodium did not affect prothrombin time (PT) or partial thromboplastin time (PTT) up to 1200 mg per day in 24 healthy male subjects treated for 8 days. Pentosan polysulfate sodium also inhibits the generation of factor Xa in plasma and inhibits thrombin-induced platelet aggregation in human platelet rich plasma ex vivo. (See **PRECAUTIONS**-Hepatic Insufficiency Section for additional information).

CARCINOGENICITY, MUTAGENESIS, IMPAIRMENT OF FERTILITY:

Long term studies in animals have not been performed to evaluate the carcinogenic potential of ELMIRON®. Pentosan polysulfate sodium was not clastogenic or mutagenic when tested in the mouse micronucleus test or the Ames test (*S. typhimurium*). The effect of pentosan polysulfate sodium on spermatogenesis has not been investigated.

PREGNANCY CATEGORY B:

Reproduction studies have been performed in mice and rats with intravenous daily doses of 15 mg/kg, and in rabbits with 7.5 mg/kg. These doses are 0.42 and 0.14 times the daily oral human doses of ELMIRON® when normalized to body surface area. These studies did not reveal evidence of impaired fertility or harm to the fetus from ELMIRON®. Direct in vitro bathing of cultured mouse embryos with pentosan polysulfate sodium (PPS) at a concentration of 1 mg/mL may cause reversible limb bud abnormalities. Adequate and well controlled studies have not been performed in pregnant women. Because animal studies are not always predictive of human response, this drug should be used in pregnancy only if clearly needed.

NURSING MOTHERS:

It is not known whether this drug is excreted in human milk. Because many drugs are excreted in human milk, caution should be exercised when ELMIRON® is administered to a nursing woman.

PEDIATRIC USE:

Safety and effectiveness in pediatric patients below the age of 16 years have not been established.

ADVERSE REACTIONS

ELMIRON® was evaluated in clinical trials in a total of 2627 patients (2343 women, 262 men, 22 unknown) with a mean age of 47 [range 18 to 88 with 581 (22%) over 60 years of age]. Of the 2627 patients, 128 patients were in a 3 month trial and the remaining 2499 patients were in a long term, unblinded trial.

Deaths occurred in 6/2627 (0.2%) patients who received the drug over a period of 3 to 75 months. The deaths appear to be related to other concurrent illnesses or procedures, except in one patient for whom the cause was not known.

Serious adverse events occurred in 33/2627 (1.3%) patients. Two patients had severe abdominal pain or diarrhea and dehydration that required hospitalization. Because there was not a control group of patients with interstitial cystitis who were concurrently evaluated, it is difficult to determine which events are associated with ELMIRON® and which events are associated with concurrent illness, medicine, or other factors.

Adverse Experience In Placebo-Controlled Clinical Trials of ELMIRON® 100 mg Three Times a Day for 3 Months

Body System/ Adverse Experience	Elmiron® n=128	Placebo n=130
CNS		
Overall Number of Patients*	3	5
Insomnia	1	0
Headache	1	3
Severe Emotional Lability/Depression	2	1
Nystagmus/Dizziness	1	1
Hyperkinesia	1	1
GI		
Overall Number of Patients*	7	7
Nausea	3	3
Diarrhea	3	6
Dyspepsia	1	0
Jaundice	0	1
Vomiting	0	2
Skin/Allergic		
Overall Number of Patients*	2	4
Rash	0	2
Pruritus	0	2
Lacrimation	1	1
Rhinitis	1	1
Increased Sweating	1	0
Other		
Overall Number of Patients*	1	3
Amenorrhea	0	1
Arthralgia	0	1
Vaginitis	1	1
Total Events	17	27
Total Number of Patients Reporting Adverse Events	13	19

* Within a body system, the individual events do not sum to equal overall number of patients because a patient may have more than one event.

The adverse events described below were reported in an unblinded clinical trial of 2499 interstitial cystitis patients treated with ELMIRON®. Of the original 2499 patients, 1192 (48%) received ELMIRON® for 3 months; 892 (36%) received ELMIRON® for 6 months; and 598 (24%) received ELMIRON® for one year, 355 (14%) received ELMIRON® for 2 years, and 145 (6%) for 4 years.

FREQUENCY (1 to 4%): Alopecia (4%), diarrhea (4%), nausea (4%), headache (3%), rash (3%), dyspepsia (2%), abdominal pain (2%), liver function abnormalities (1%), dizziness (1%).

FREQUENCY (≤1%):

Digestive: Vomiting, mouth ulcer, colitis, esophagitis, gastritis, flatulence, constipation, anorexia, gum hemorrhage.

Hematologic: Anemia, ecchymosis, increased prothrombin time, increased partial thromboplastin time, leukopenia, thrombocytopenia.

Hypersensitive Reactions: Allergic reaction, photosensitivity.

Respiratory System: Pharyngitis, rhinitis, epistaxis, dyspnea.

Skin and Appendages: Pruritus, urticaria.

Special Senses: Conjunctivitis, tinnitus, optic neuritis, amblyopia, retinal hemorrhage.

OVERDOSAGE

Overdose has not been reported. Based upon the pharmacodynamics of the drug, toxicity is likely to be reflected as anticoagulation, bleeding, thrombocytopenia, liver function abnormalities, and gastric distress. (See **CLINICAL PHARMACOLOGY** and **PRECAUTIONS** sections). In the event of acute overdose, the patient should be given gastric lavage if possible, carefully observed and given symptomatic and supportive treatment.

DOSAGE AND ADMINISTRATION

The recommended dose of ELMIRON® is 300 mg/day taken as one 100 mg capsule orally three times daily. The capsules should be taken with water at least 1 hour before meals or 2 hours after meals.

Patients receiving ELMIRON® should be reassessed after 3 months. If improvement has not occurred and if limiting adverse events are not present, ELMIRON® may be continued for another 3 months.

The clinical value and risks of continued treatment in patients whose pain has not improved by 6 months is not known.

HOW SUPPLIED

ELMIRON® is supplied in white opaque hard gelatin capsules imprinted "BNP7600" containing 100 mg pentosan polysulfate sodium. Supplied in bottles of 100 capsules. NDC NUMBER 17314-9300-1

STORAGE

Store at controlled room temperature 15°–30°C (59°–86°F).

CAUTION: Federal (USA) law prohibits dispensing without prescription.

ELMIRON® is a Registered Trademark of Baker Norton Pharmaceuticals, Inc. under license to ALZA Corporation.
©1998 Baker Norton Pharmaceuticals, Inc.

ALZA Pharmaceuticals
A division of ALZA Corp.
Mountain View, CA 94043
Manufactured by:
Baker Norton Pharmaceuticals, Inc.
Miami, FL 33178
Distributed by
ALZA Corporation
Mountain View, CA 94043
1001719   REV 9801
Patent #5, 180, 715

Shown in Product Identification Guide, page 303

ETHYOL®   ℞
[*a-thī-ol*]
(amifostine) for Injection

DESCRIPTION

ETHYOL (amifostine) is an organic thiophosphate cytoprotective agent known chemically as ethanethiol, 2-[(3-aminopropyl)amino]-, dihydrogen phosphate (ester) and has the following structural formula:

$$H_2N(CH_2)_3NH(CH_2)_2S\text{-}PO_3H_2$$

Amifostine is a white crystalline powder which is freely soluble in water. Its empirical formula is $C_5H_{15}N_2O_3PS$ and it has a molecular weight of 214.22.

ETHYOL is the trihydrate form of amifostine and is supplied as a sterile lyophilized powder requiring reconstitution for intravenous infusion. Each single-use 10 mL vial contains 500 mg of amifostine on the anhydrous basis.

CLINICAL PHARMACOLOGY

ETHYOL is a prodrug that is dephosphorylated by alkaline phosphatase in tissues to a pharmacologically active free thiol metabolite that can reduce the toxic effects of cisplatin. The ability to differentially protect normal tissues is attributed to the higher capillary alkaline phosphatase activity, higher pH and better vascularity of normal tissues relative to tumor tissue, which results in a more rapid generation of the active thiol metabolite as well as a higher rate constant for uptake. The higher concentration of free thiol in normal tissues is available to bind to, and thereby detoxify, reactive metabolites of cisplatin; and also can act as a scavenger of free radicals that may be generated in tissues exposed to cisplatin. Several preclinical studies in mice and rats have demonstrated that pretreatment with ETHYOL results in protection from nephrotoxicity following administration of single and multiple doses of cisplatin.

Pharmacokinetics: Clinical pharmacokinetic studies show that ETHYOL is rapidly cleared from the plasma with a distribution half-life of <1 minute and an elimination half-life of approximately 8 minutes. Less than 10% of ETHYOL remains in the plasma 6 minutes after drug administration. ETHYOL is rapidly metabolized to an active free thiol metabolite. A disulfide metabolite is produced subsequently and is less active than the free thiol. After a 10-second bolus dose of 150 mg/m² of ETHYOL, renal excretion of the parent drug and its two metabolites was low during the hour following drug administration, averaging 0.69%, 2.64% and 2.22% of the administered dose for the parent, thiol and disulfide, respectively. Measurable levels of the free thiol metabolite have been found in bone marrow cells 5–8 minutes after intravenous infusion of amifostine. Pretreatment with dexamethasone or metoclopramide has no effect on ETHYOL pharmacokinetics.

Clinical Studies: A randomized controlled trial compared six cycles of cyclophosphamide 1000 mg/m², and cisplatin 100 mg/m² with or without amifostine pretreatment at 910 mg/m², in two successive cohorts of 121 patients with advanced ovarian cancer. In both cohorts, after multiple cycles of chemotherapy, pretreatment with ETHYOL significantly reduced the cumulative renal toxicity associated with cisplatin as assessed by the proportion of patients who had ≥40% decrease in creatinine clearance from pretreatment values, protracted elevations in serum creatinine (>1.5 mg/dL), or severe hypomagnesemia. Subgroup analyses suggested that the effect of ETHYOL was present in patients who had received nephrotoxic antibiotics, or who had preexisting diabetes or hypertension (and thus may have been at increased risk for significant nephrotoxicity), as well as in patients who lacked these risks. Selected analyses of the effects of ETHYOL in reducing the cumulative renal toxicity of cisplatin in the randomized ovarian cancer study are provided in TABLES 1 and 2, below.

TABLE 1
Proportion of Patients with ≥40% Reduction in Calculated Creatinine Clearance*

	Amifostine + CP	CP	p-value 2-sided
All Patients	16/122 (13%)	36/120 (30%)	0.001
First Cohort	10/63	20/58	0.018
Second Cohort	6/59	16/62	0.026

*Creatinine clearance values were calculated using the Cockcroft-Gault formula. *Nephron* 1976; 16:31–41.

[See table 2 at top of next page]

In the randomized ovarian cancer study, ETHYOL had no detectable effect on the antitumor efficacy of cisplatin-cyclophosphamide chemotherapy. Objective response rates (including pathologically confirmed complete remission rates), time to progression, and survival duration were all similar

Continued on next page

Ethyol—Cont.

in the amifostine and control study groups. The table below summarizes the principal efficacy findings of the randomized ovarian cancer study.

[See table 3 below]

A Phase II trial of Ethyol, 740–910 mg/m², and cisplatin, 120 mg/m², administered on day 1 and vinblastine, 5mg/m², administered on days 1, 8, 15 and 22 of each monthly cycle was conducted in 25 patients with Stage IV non-small cell lung cancer. This regimen was repeated until disease progression or unacceptable toxicity occurred, or a maximum of six cycles had been administered. Among 13 patients who received 4 or more cycles of this intensive cisplatin regimen, 1 had a ≥40% reduction in creatinine clearance. These results are consistent with the randomized ovarian cancer trial.

Sixteen of the 25 patients treated demonstrated a partial response to chemotherapy. With a median follow-up of 19 months, the median survival was 17 months. At one year, 64% of the patients were alive. These results indicate that ETHYOL may not adversely affect the efficacy of this chemotherapy for non-small cell lung cancer.

INDICATIONS AND USAGE

ETHYOL (amifostine) is indicated to reduce the cumulative renal toxicity associated with repeated administration of cisplatin in patients with advanced ovarian cancer or non-small cell lung cancer. In these settings, the clinical data do not suggest that the effectiveness of cisplatin based chemotherapy regimens is altered by ETHYOL. There are at present only limited data on the effects of ETHYOL on the efficacy of chemotherapy in other settings; therefore ETHYOL should not be administered to patients in other settings where chemotherapy can produce a significant survival benefit or cure (e.g., certain malignancies of germ cell origin), except in the context of a clinical study.

CONTRAINDICATIONS

ETHYOL is contraindicated in patients with known sensitivity to aminothiol compounds.

WARNINGS

1. Effectiveness of the Cytotoxic Regimen
Limited data are currently available regarding the preservation of antitumor efficacy when amifostine is administered prior to cisplatin therapy in settings other than advanced ovarian cancer or non-small cell lung cancer. Although some animal data suggest interference is possible, in most tumor models the antitumor effects of chemotherapy are not altered by amifostine. The possibility of interference with the efficacy of cancer treatment would be of particular concern in those settings where chemotherapy can produce a significant survival benefit or cure. ETHYOL should therefore not be used in patients receiving chemotherapy for other malignancies in which chemotherapy can produce a significant survival benefit or cure (e.g. certain malignancies of germ cell origin), except in the context of a clinical study.

2. Hypotension
Patients who are hypotensive or in a state of dehydration should not receive ETHYOL. Patients receiving antihypertensive therapy that cannot be stopped for 24 hours preceding ETHYOL treatment also should not receive ETHYOL. Patients should be adequately hydrated prior to ETHYOL infusion and kept in a supine position during the infusion. Blood pressure should be monitored every 5 minutes during the infusion. It is important that the duration of the infusion be 15 minutes, as administration of ETHYOL as a longer infusion is associated with a higher incidence of side effects. If hypotension requiring interruption of therapy occurs, patients should be placed in the Trendelenburg position and be given an infusion of normal saline using a separate i.v. line. Guidelines for interrupting and restarting ETHYOL infusion if a decrease in systolic blood pressure should occur are provided in the DOSAGE AND ADMINISTRATION section.

3. Nausea and Vomiting
Antiemetic medication should be administered prior to and in conjunction with ETHYOL (see DOSAGE and ADMINISTRATION). When ETHYOL is administered with highly emetogenic chemotherapy, the fluid balance of the patient should be carefully monitored.

4. Hypocalcemia
Serum calcium levels should be monitored in patients at risk of hypocalcemia, such as those with nephrotic syndrome or patients receiving multiple doses of Ethyol. If necessary, calcium supplements can be administered.

PRECAUTIONS

GENERAL
Patients should be adequately hydrated prior to the infusion and blood pressure should be monitored during the infusion. ETHYOL (amifostine) should be administered as a 15-minute infusion (See DOSAGE and ADMINISTRATION).

The safety of ETHYOL administration has not been established in elderly patients, or patients with preexisting cardiovascular or cerebrovascular conditions such as ischemic heart disease, arrhythmias, congestive heart failure, or history of stroke or transient ischemic attacks. ETHYOL should be used with particular care in these and other patients in whom the common ETHYOL adverse effects of nausea/vomiting and hypotension may be more likely to have serious consequences.

Drug Interactions
There are no known drug interactions with ETHYOL. However, special consideration should be given to the administration of ETHYOL in patients receiving antihypertensive medications or other drugs that could potentiate hypotension.

Carcinogenesis, Mutagenesis and Impairment of Fertility
No long-term animal studies have been performed to evaluate the carcinogenic potential of ETHYOL. ETHYOL was negative in the Ames test and in the mouse micronucleus test. The free thiol metabolite, however, was positive in the Ames test with S9 microsomal fraction in the TA1535 *Salmonella typhimurium* strain and at the TK locus in the mouse L5178Y cell assay. The metabolite was negative in the mouse micronucleus test and negative for clastogenicity in human lymphocytes.

Pregnancy
Pregnancy Category C. ETHYOL has been shown to be embryotoxic in rabbits at doses of 50 mg/kg, approximately sixty percent of the recommended dose in humans on a body surface area basis. There are no adequate and well-controlled studies in pregnant women. ETHYOL should be used during pregnancy only if the potential benefit justifies the potential risk to the fetus.

Nursing Mothers
No information is available on the excretion of ETHYOL or its metabolites into human milk. Because many drugs are excreted in human milk and because of the potential for adverse reactions in nursing infants, it is recommended that breast feeding be discontinued if the mother is treated with ETHYOL.

Pediatric Use
The safety and effectiveness in pediatric patients have not been established.

ADVERSE REACTIONS

ETHYOL produced a transient reduction in blood pressure in 62% of patients treated. The mean time of onset was 14 minutes into the 15-minute period of ETHYOL infusion, and the mean duration was 6 minutes. In some cases, the infusion had to be prematurely terminated due to a more pronounced drop in systolic blood pressure. In general, the blood pressure returned to normal within 5–15 minutes. Fewer than 3% of patients discontinued ETHYOL due to blood pressure reductions. Short term, reversible loss of consciousness has been reported rarely. Blood pressure reductions by ETHYOL administration have not been reported to cause long-term CNS, cardiovascular or renal sequelae, but clinical studies performed to date have not evaluated the safety of ETHYOL in elderly patients or patients with pre-existing cardiovascular or cerebrovascular conditions.

Hypotension that requires interruption of the ETHYOL Infusion should be treated with fluid infusion and postural management of the patient (supine or Trendelenburg position). If the blood pressure returns to normal within 5 minutes and the patient is asymptomatic, the infusion may be restarted, so that the full dose of ETHYOL can be administered.

Nausea and/or vomiting occur frequently after amifostine infusion and may be severe. In the ovarian cancer randomized study, the incidence of severe nausea/vomiting on day 1 of cyclophosphamide-cisplatin chemotherapy was 10% in patients who did not receive ETHYOL, and 19% in patients who did receive ETHYOL. Other effects which have been described during or following ETHYOL infusion are flushing/feeling of warmth, chills/feeling of coldness, dizziness, somnolence, hiccups and sneezing. These effects have not generally precluded the completion of chemotherapy.

Decrease in serum calcium concentrations is a known pharmacological effect of ETHYOL. At the recommended doses, clinically significant hypocalcemia has occurred rarely (<1%) (see WARNINGS).

Allergic reactions, ranging from mild skin rashes to rigors, have occurred rarely (<1%). There has been no reported occurrence of anaphylaxis with ETHYOL.

OVERDOSAGE

In clinical trials, the maximum single dose of ETHYOL was 1300 mg/m². No information is available on single doses higher than this in adults. In the setting of a clinical trial, children have received single ETHYOL doses of up to 2700 mg/m². At the higher doses, anxiety and reversible urinary retention occurred. Administration of ETHYOL at 2 and 4 hours after the initial dose has not led to increased nausea and vomiting or hypotension. The most likely symptom of overdosage is hypotension, which should be managed by infusion of normal saline and other supportive measures, as clinically indicated.

DOSAGE AND ADMINISTRATION

In adults, the recommended starting dose of ETHYOL is 910 mg/m² administered once daily as a 15-minute i.v. infusion, starting 30 minutes prior to chemotherapy.

The 15-minute infusion is better tolerated than more extended infusions. Further reductions in infusion times have not been systematically investigated.

The infusion of ETHYOL should be interrupted if the systolic blood pressure decreases significantly from the baseline value as listed in the guideline below:

TABLE 2
NCI Toxicity Grades of Serum Magnesium Levels for Each Patient's Last Cycle of Therapy

NCI-CTC Grade: (mEq/L)	0 >1.4	1 ≤1.4->1.1	2 ≤1.1->0.8	3 ≤0.8->0.5	4 ≤0.5	p-value*
All Patients						
Amifostine +CP	92	13	3	0	0	0.001
CP	73	18	7	5	1	
First Cohort						
Amifostine +CP	49	10	3	0	0	0.017
CP	35	8	6	3	1	
Second Cohort						
Amifostine +CP	43	3	0	0	0	0.012
CP	38	10	1	2	0	

* Based on 2-sided Mantel-Haenszel Chi-Square statistic.

TABLE 3

	ETHYOL +CP	CP
Complete pathologic tumor response rate	21.3%	15.8%
Time to progression (months)		
Median (± 95% Cl)	15.8 (13.2, 25.1)	18.1 (12.5, 20.4)
Mean (± Std error)	19.8 (±1.04)	19.1 (±1.58)
Hazard ratio (95% Confidence Interval)	.98 (.64, 1.4)	
Survival (months)		
Median (± 95% Cl)	31.3 (28.3, 38.2)	31.8 (26.3, 39.8)
Mean (± Std error)	33.7 (±2.03)	34.3 (±2.04)
Hazard ratio (95% Confidence Interval)	.97 (.69, 1.32)	

Guideline for Interrupting ETHYOL Infusion Due to Decrease in Systolic Blood Pressure

	Baseline Systolic Blood Pressure (mm Hg)				
	<100	100–119	120–139	140–179	≥180
Decrease in systolic blood pressure during infusion of ETHYOL (mm Hg)	20	25	30	40	50

If the blood pressure returns to normal within 5 minutes and the patient is asymptomatic, the infusion may be restarted so that the full dose of ETHYOL may be administered. If the full dose of ETHYOL cannot be administered, the dose of ETHYOL for subsequent cycles should be 740 mg/m².

Only limited experience is available for the usage of ETHYOL in children or elderly patients (more than 70 years of age).

It is recommended that antiemetic medication, including dexamethasone 20 mg i.v. and a serotonin 5HT₃ receptor antagonist, be administered prior to and in conjunction with ETHYOL. Additional antiemetics may be required based on the chemotherapy drugs administered.

Reconstitution

ETHYOL (amifostine) for Injection is supplied as a sterile lyophilized powder requiring reconstitution for intravenous infusion. Each single-use vial contains 500 mg of amifostine on the anhydrous basis.

Prior to intravenous injection, Ethyol is reconstituted with 9.7 mL of sterile 0.9% Sodium Chloride Injection, USP. The reconstituted solution (500 mg amifostine/10 mL) is chemically stable for up to 5 hours at room temperature (approximately 25°C) or up to 24 hours under refrigeration (2°C to 8°C).

ETHYOL prepared in polyvinylchloride (PVC) bags at concentrations ranging from 5 mg/mL to 40 mg/mL is chemically stable for up to 5 hours when stored at room temperature (approximately 25°C) or up to 24 hours when stored under refrigeration (2°C to 8°C).

CAUTION: Parenteral products should be inspected visually for particulate matter and discoloration prior to administration whenever solution and container permit. Do not use if cloudiness or precipitate is observed.

Incompatibilities

The compatibility of amifostine with solutions other than 0.9% Sodium Chloride for Injection, or Sodium Chloride solutions with other additives, has not been examined. The use of other solutions is not recommended.

HOW SUPPLIED

ETHYOL (amifostine) for Injection is supplied as a sterile lyophilized powder in 10 mL single-use vials (NDC 17314-7253-1). Each single-use vial contains 500 mg of amifostine on the anhydrous basis. The vials are available packaged as follows:

3 pack—3 vials per carton (NDC 17314-7253-3)

Store the lyophilized dosage form at Controlled Room Temperature 20°–25°C (68°–77°F) [see USP].

CAUTION: Federal (U.S.A.) law prohibits dispensing without prescription.

U.S. Patents 5,424,471; 5,591,731

Manufactured by:
USB Pharma B.V.
6545 CG Nijmegen
The Netherlands

Marketed by:
Alza Pharmaceuticals
A division of Alza Corporation
Palo Alto,
California 94303

And:
U.S. Bioscience, Inc.
West Conshohocken,
Pennsylvania 19428
1-800-506-4959
©1995, U.S. Bioscience, Inc.
Revision Date 12/97   N-LB2022 PB
Shown in Product Identification Guide, page 303

MYCELEX®
(clotrimazole) TROCHE
FOR TOPICAL ORAL ADMINISTRATION

℞

DESCRIPTION

Each Mycelex® Troche contains 10mg clotrimazole [1–(o-chloro-α,α-diphenylbenzyl) imidazole], a synthetic antifungal agent, for topical use in the mouth.

Structural Formula:

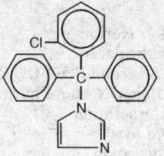

Chemical Formula:
$C_{22}H_{17}ClN_2$

The troche dosage from is a large, slowly dissolving tablet (lozenge) containing 10 mg of clotrimazole dispersed in dextrose, microcrystalline cellulose, povidone, and magnesium stearate.

CLINICAL PHARMACOLOGY

Clotrimazole is a broad-spectrum antifungal agent that inhibits the growth of pathogenic yeasts by altering the permeability of cell membranes. The action of clotrimazole is fungistatic at concentrations of drug up to 20 mcg/mL and may be fungicidal *in vitro* against *Candida albicans* and other species of the genus *Candida* at higher concentrations. No single-step or multiple-step resistance to clotrimazole has developed during successive passages of *Candida albicans* in the laboratory; however, individual organism tolerance has been observed during successive passages in the laboratory. Such *in vitro* tolerance has resolved once the organism has been removed from the antifungal environment.

After oral administration of a 10 mg clotrimazole troche to healthy volunteers, concentrations sufficient to inhibit most species of *Candida* persist in saliva for up to three hours following the approximately 30 minutes needed for a troche to dissolve. The long term persistence of drug in salvia appears to be related to the slow release of clotrimazole from the oral mucosa to which the drug is apparently bound. Repetitive dosing at three hour intervals maintains salivary levels above the minimum inhibitory concentrations of most strains of *Candida;* however, the relationship between *in vitro* susceptibility of pathogenic fungi to clotrimazole and prophylaxis or cure of infections in humans has not been established.

In another study, the mean serum concentrations were 4.98 ± 3.7 and 3.23 ± 1.4 nanograms/mL of clotrimazole at 30 and 60 minutes, respectively, after administration as a troche.

INDICATIONS AND USAGE

Mycelex® Troches are indicated for the local treatment of oropharyngeal candidiasis. The diagnosis should be confirmed by a KOH smear and/or culture prior to treatment. Mycelex® Troches are also indicated prophylactically to reduce the incidence of oropharyngeal candidasis in patients immunocompromised by conditions that include chemotherapy, radiotherapy, or steroid therapy utilized in the treatment of leukemia, solid tumors, or renal transplantation. There are no data from adequate and well-controlled trials to establish the safety and efficacy of this product for prophylactic use in patients immuncompromised by etiologies other than those listed in the previous sentence (See DOSAGE AND ADMINISTRATION.)

CONTRAINDICATIONS

Mycelex® Troches are contra-indicated in patients who are hypersensitive to any of its components.

WARNINGS

Mycelex® Troches are not indicated for the treatment of systemic mycoses including systemic candidiasis.

PRECAUTIONS

Abnormal liver function tests have been reported in patients treated with clotrimazole troches; elevated SGOT levels were reported in about 15% of patients in the clinical trials. In most cases the elevations were minimal and it was often impossible to distinguish effects of clotrimazole from those of other therapy and the underly disease (malignancy in most cases). Periodic assessment of hepatic function is advisable particularly in patients with pre-existing hepatic impairment.

Since patients must be instructed to allow each troche to dissolve slowly in the mouth in order to achieve maximum effect of the medication, they must be of such an age and physical and/or mental condition to comprehend such instructions.

Carcinogenesis: An 18 month dosing study with clo-trimazole in rats has not revealed any carcinogenic effect.

Usage in Pregnancy: Pregnancy Category C: Clotrimazole has been shown to be embryotoxic in rats and mice when given in doses 100 times the adult human dose (in mg/kg), possibly secondary to maternal toxicity. The drug was not teratogenic in mice, rabbits, and rats when given in doses up to 200, 180, and 100 times the human dose.

Clotrimazole given orally to mice from nine weeks before mating through weaning at a dose 120 times the human dose was associated with impairment of mating, decreased number of viable young, and decreased survival to weaning. No effects were observed at 60 times the human dose. When the drug was given to rats during a similar time period at 50 times the human dose, there was a slight decrease in the number of pups per litter and decreased pup viability.

There are no adequate and well controlled studies in pregnant women. Clotrimazole troches should be used during pregnancy only if the potential benefit justifies the potential risk to the fetus.

PEDIATRIC USE Safety and effectiveness of clotrimazole in children below the age of 3 years have not been established; therefore, its use in such patients is not recommended.

The safety and efficacy of the prophylactic use of clotrimazole troches in children have not been established.

ADVERSE REACTIONS

Abnormal liver function tests have been reported in patients treated with clotrimazole troches; elevated SGOT levels were reported in about 15% of patients in the clinical trials (See Precautions section).

Nausea, vomiting, unpleasant mouth sensations and pruritus have also been reported with the use of the troche.

OVERDOSAGE

No data available.

DRUG ABUSE AND DEPENDENCE

No data available.

DOSAGE AND ADMINISTRATION

Mycelex® Troches are administered only as a lozenge that must be slowly dissolved in the mouth. The recommended dose is one troche five times a day for fourteen consecutive days. Only limited data are available on the safety and effectiveness of the clotrimazole troche after prolonged administration; therefore, therapy should be limited to short term use, if possible.

For prophylaxis to reduce the incidence of orophar-yngeal candidasis in patients immunocompromised by conditions that include chemotherapy, radio-therapy, or steroid therapy utilized in the treatment of leukemia, solid tumors, or renal transplantation, the recommended dose is one troche three times daily for the duration of chemotherapy or until steroids are reduced to maintenance levels.

HOW SUPPLIED

Mycelex® Troches, white discoid, uncoated tablets are supplied in bottles of 70 and 140. Mycelex Troches are also available for insti-tutional use in foil packages of 70 tablets. Each tablet will be identified with the following: Mycelex 10.

Store below 86°F (30°C).
Avoid freezing.
Manufactured by Bayer Corporation
West Haven, CT 06516

Distributed by ALZA Pharmaceuticals
A Division of ALZA Corporation
Mountain View, CA 94043
PD100797   11/97   BAY 5097
©1997 Bayer Corporation   7973
Shown in Product Identification Guide, page 303

POLYCITRA® SYRUP   ℞
POLYCITRA®-LC   ℞
[polly "si-trah]
(tricitrates oral solution)

DESCRIPTION

Syrup POLYCITRA® and POLYCITRA®-LC are stable and pleasant-tasting oral systemic alkalizers containing potassium citrate, sodium citrate, and citric acid. Syrup POLYCITRA® is a sugar-base preparation. POLYCITRA®-LC is a sugar-free solution, to be used by patients who desire a low-carbohydrate diet. Both products are non-alcoholic and contain identical amounts of active ingredients.

COMPOSITION

Syrup POLYCITRA® or POLYCITRA®-LC contains in each teaspoonful (5 mL):

POTASSIUM CITRATE Monohydrate	550 mg
SODIUM CITRATE Dihydrate	500 mg
CITRIC ACID Monohydrate	334 mg

Each mL contains 1 mEq potassium ion and 1 mEq sodium ion and is equivalent to 2 mEq bicarbonate (HCO_3).

ACTIONS

Potassium citrate and sodium citrate are absorbed and metabolized to potassium bicarbonate and sodium bicarbonate, thus acting as systemic alkalizers. The effects are essentially those of chlorides before absorption and those of bicar-

Continued on next page

Polycitra/Polycitra-LC—Cont.

bonates subsequently. Oxidation is virtually complete so that less than 5% of the citrates are excreted in the urine unchanged.

INDICATIONS AND ADVANTAGES

Syrup POLYCITRA® and POLYCITRA®-LC are effective alkalinizing agents useful in those conditions where long-term maintenance of an alkaline urine is desirable, such as in patients with uric acid and cystine calculi of the urinary tract. In addition, they are valuable adjuvants when administered with uricosuric agents in gout therapy, since urates tend to crystallize out of an acid urine. They are also effective in correcting the acidosis of certain renal tubular disorders. Syrup POLYCITRA® and POLYCITRA®-LC are highly concentrated, and when administered after meals and before bedtime, allow one to maintain an alkaline urine pH around the clock, usually without the necessity of a 2 A.M. dose. Syrup POLYCITRA® and POLYCITRA®-LC alkalinize the urine without producing a systemic alkalosis in recommended dosage. They are highly palatable, pleasant tasting and tolerable, even when administered for long periods. Potassium citrate and sodium citrate do not neutralize the gastric juice or disturb digestion.

CONTRAINDICATIONS

Severe renal impairment with oliguria or azotemia, untreated Addison's disease, or severe myocardial damage. In certain situations, when patients are on a sodium-restricted diet, the use of potassium citrate, as contained in POLYCITRA®-K may be preferable; or when patients are on a potassium-restricted diet the use of sodium citrate, as contained in BICITRA®, may be preferable.

PRECAUTIONS AND WARNINGS

Should be used with caution by patients with low urinary output or reduced glomerular filtration rates unless under the supervision of a physician. Aluminum-based antacids should be avoided in these patients. Patients should be directed to dilute adequately with water, and preferably, to take each dose after meals, to minimize the possibility of gastrointestinal injury associated with oral ingestion of potassium salt preparations and to avoid saline laxative effect. Sodium salts should be used cautiously in patients with cardiac failure, hypertension, peripheral and pulmonary edema, and toxemia of pregnancy.

Concurrent administration of potassium-containing medication, potassium-sparing diuretics, angiotensin-converting enzyme (ACE) inhibitors, or cardiac glycosides may lead to toxicity. Periodic examination and determinations of serum electrolytes, particularly serum bicarbonate level should be carried out in those patients with renal disease in order to avoid these complications.

ADVERSE REACTIONS

Syrup POLYCITRA® and POLYCITRA®-LC are generally well tolerated without any unpleasant side effects when given in recommended doses to patients with normal renal function and urinary output. However, as with any alkalinizing agent, caution must be used in certain patients with abnormal renal mechanisms to avoid development of hyperkalemia or alkalosis, especially in the presence of hypocalcemia. Potassium intoxication causes listlessness, weakness, mental confusion, and tingling of extremities.

DOSAGE AND ADMINISTRATION

Syrup POLYCITRA® and POLYCITRA®-LC should be taken diluted in water, followed by additional water, if desired. Palatability is enhanced if chilled before taking.
Usual Adult Dose: 3 to 6 teaspoonfuls (15 to 30 mL), diluted in water, four times a day, after meals and at bedtime, or as directed by physician.
Usual Pediatric Dose: 1 to 3 teaspoonfuls (5 to 15 mL), diluted in water, four times a day, after meals and at bedtime, or as directed by physician.
Usual Dosage Range: 2 to 3 teaspoonfuls (10 to 15 mL), diluted with water, taken four times a day, will usually maintain a urine pH of 6.5–7.4. 3 to 4 teaspoonfuls (15 to 20 mL), diluted with water, taken four times a day, will usually maintain a urine pH of 7.0–7.6 throughout most of the 24 hours, without unpleasant side effects. To check urine pH, HYDRION Paper (pH 6.0–8.0) or NITRAZINE Paper (pH 4.5–7.5) are available and easy to use.

OVERDOSAGE

Overdosage with sodium salts may cause diarrhea, nausea, vomiting, hypernoia, and convulsions. Overdosage with potassium salts may cause hyperkalemia and alkalosis, especially in the presence of renal disease.

HOW SUPPLIED

POLYCITRA®-Syrup
  16 fl. oz. (473 mL)
    (NDC 17314-9322-1)
POLYCITRA®-LC
  16 fl. oz. (473 mL)
    (NDC 17314-9323-1)

Keep tightly closed and protect from excessive heat and freezing.
Rx only
©1998Baker Norton
Pharmaceuticals, Inc.
POLYCITRA® and POLYCITRA®-LC are Registered Trademarks of Baker Norton Pharmaceuticals, Inc. under license to ALZA Corporation.
Distributed by:
ALZA Corporation
Mountain View, CA 94043
Manufactured by:
Draxis Pharma Inc.
Kirkland, Quebec H9H 4J4
Canada
MADE IN CANADA
ALZA Pharmaceuticals
A division of ALZA Corp.
Mountain View, CA 94043
1001739   REV9804
(212011)

POLYCITRA–K CRYSTALS® ℞

[polly "si-trah- kăy]
(Potassium Citrate and Citric Acid for Oral Solution)

DESCRIPTION

POLYCITRA–K CRYSTALS® is a pleasant-tasting oral systemic alkalizer containing potassium citrate and citric acid in a sugar-free base.

COMPOSITION

POLYCITRA-K CRYSTALS® (potassium citrate and citric acid for oral solution)—each unit dose packet contains:
POTASSIUM CITRATE
  Monohydrate   3300 mg
CITRIC ACID
  Monohydrate   1002 mg
Each unit dose packet, when reconstituted, supplies the same amount of active ingredients as is contained in 15 mL (one tablespoonful) POLYCITRA®-K Oral Solution and provides 30 mEq potassium ion and is equivalent to 30 mEq bicarbonate (HCO_3).

ACTIONS

Potassium citrate is absorbed and metabolized to potassium bicarbonate, thus acting as a systemic alkalizer. The effects are essentially those of chlorides before absorption and those of bicarbonates subsequently. Oxidation is virtually complete so that less than 5% of the potassium citrate is excreted in the urine unchanged.

INDICATIONS AND USAGE

POLYCITRA-K CRYSTALS® is an effective alkalinizing agent useful in those conditions where long-term maintenance of an alkaline urine is desirable, such as in patients with uric acid and cystine calculi of the urinary tract, especially when the administration of sodium salts is undesirable or contraindicated. In addition, it is a valuable adjuvant when administered with uricosuric agents in gout therapy, since urates tend to crystallize out of an acid urine. It is also effective in correcting the acidosis of certain renal tubular disorders where the administration of potassium citrate may be preferable. POLYCITRA-K CRYSTALS® is highly concentrated, and when administered after meals and before bedtime, allows one to maintain an alkaline urinary pH around the clock, usually without the necessity of a 2 A.M. dose. POLYCITRA-K CRYSTALS® alkalinizes the urine without producing a systemic alkalosis in recommended dosage. It is highly palatable, pleasant tasting, and tolerable, even when administered for long periods. Potassium citrate does not neutralize the gastric juice or disturb digestion.

CONTRAINDICATIONS

Severe renal impairment with oliguria or azotemia, untreated Addison's disease, adynamia episodica hereditaria, acute dehydration, heat cramps, anuria, severe myocardial damage, and hyperkalemia from any cause.

WARNING

Large doses may cause hyperkalemia and alkalosis, especially in the presence of renal disease. Concurrent administration of potassium-containing medication, potassium-sparing diuretics, angiotensin-converting enzyme (ACE) inhibitors, or cardiac glycosides may lead to toxicity.

PRECAUTIONS

Should be used with caution by patients with low urinary output unless under the supervision of a physician. As with all liquids containing a high concentration of potassium, patients should be directed to dilute adequately with water to minimize the possibility of gastrointestinal injury associated with the oral ingestion of concentrated potassium salt preparations; and preferably, to take each dose after meals to avoid saline laxative effect.

ADVERSE REACTIONS

POLYCITRA-K CRYSTALS® is generally well tolerated without any unpleasant side effects when given in recommended doses to patients with normal renal function and urinary output. However, as with any alkalinizing agent, caution must be used in certain patients with abnormal renal mechanisms to avoid development of hyperkalemia or alkalosis. Potassium intoxication causes listlessness, weakness, mental confusion, tingling of extremities, and other symptoms associated with a high concentration of potassium in the serum. Periodic determinations of serum electrolytes should be carried out in those patients with renal disease in order to avoid these complications. Hyperkalemia may exhibit the following electrocardiographic abnormalities: Disappearance of the P wave, widening and slurring of QRS complex, changes of the S-T segment, tall peaked T waves, etc.

OVERDOSAGE

The administration of oral potassium salts to persons with normal excretory mechanisms for potassium rarely causes serious hyperkalemia. However, if excretory mechanisms are impaired, hyperkalemia can result (see Contraindications and Warnings). Hyperkalemia, when detected, must be treated immediately because lethal levels can be reached in a few hours.

TREATMENT OF HYPERKALEMIA

Should hyperkalemia occur, treatment measures include the following: (1) Elimination of foods or medications containing potassium. (2) The intravenous administration of 300 to 500 mL/hr of dextrose solution (10 to 25%), containing 10 units of insulin /20 gm dextrose. (3) The use of exchange resins, hemodialysis, or peritoneal dialysis. In treating hyperkalemia, it should be recalled that in patients who have been stabilized on digitalis, too rapid a lowering of the plasma potassium concentration can produce digitalis toxicity.

DOSAGE AND ADMINISTRATION

POLYCITRA-K CRYSTALS® should be taken mixed in cool water or juice according to directions, followed by additional water or juice, if desired.
Usual Adult Dose: POLYCITRA-K CRYSTALS®—Contents of 1 packet reconstituted with at least 6 ounces of cool water or juice, after meals and at bedtime, or as directed by physician.
Usual Pediatric Dose: POLYCITRA-K CRYSTALS® is not recommended for pediatric use. Dosage can be more easily regulated using POLYCITRA®-K Oral Solution.
Usual Dosage Range: Contents of 1 packet POLYCITRA-K CRYSTALS®, reconstituted as directed and taken four times a day, will usually maintain a urinary pH of 6.5–7.4. To check urinary pH, HYDRION Paper (pH 6.0–8.0) or NITRAZINE Paper (pH 4.5–7.5) are available and easy to use.

HOW SUPPLIED

POLYCITRA-K CRYSTALS®
—Unit Dose Packets, 100/box (NDC 17314–9320–1).
Protect from excessive heat or freezing.
Rx only
©1998 Baker Norton
Pharmaceuticals, Inc.
POLYCITRA-K Crystals® is a
registered Trademark of
Baker Norton Pharmaceuticals, Inc.
under license to ALZA Corporation
POLYCITRA-K Crystals® is
Distributed by
ALZA Corporation
Mountain view, CA 94043
Manufactured by
Zenith Goldline
Pharmaceuticals, Inc.
Miami, FL 33137
ALZA Pharmaceuticals
A division of
ALZA Corp.
Mountain View, CA 94043
1001734   REV9802

POLYCITRA®–K ORAL SOLUTION ℞

[polly" si-trah-kăy]
Potassium Citrate and Citric Acid Oral Solution, USP

DESCRIPTION

POLYCITRA®-K is a stable and pleasant-tasting oral systemic alkalizer containing potassium citrate and citric acid in a sugar-free non-alcoholic base.

COMPOSITION

POLYCITRA®–K Oral Solution (potassium citrate and citric acid oral solution, USP) contains in each teaspoonful (5 mL):

POTASSIUM CITRATE
Monohydrate   1100 mg
CITRIC ACID
Monohydrate   334 mg

Each mL contains 2 mEq potassium ion and is equivalent to 2 mEq bicarbonate (HCO_3).

ACTIONS

Potassium citrate is absorbed and metabolized to potassium bicarbonate, thus acting as a systemic alkalizer. The effects are essentially those of chlorides before absorption and those of bicarbonates subsequently. Oxidation is virtually complete so that less than 5% of the potassium citrate is excreted in the urine unchanged.

INDICATIONS AND USAGE

POLYCITRA®-K Oral Solution is an effective alkalinizing agent useful in those conditions where long-term mainte-nance of an alkaline urine is desirable, such as in patients with uric acid and cystine calculi of the urinary tract, espe-cially when the administration of sodium salts is undesir-able or contraindicated. In addition, it is a valuable adju-vant when administered with uricosuric agents in gout therapy, since urates tend to crystallize out of an acid urine. It is also effective in correcting the acidosis of certain renal tubular disorders where the administered of potassium ci-trate may be preferable. POLYCITRA®-K Oral Solution is highly concentrated, and when administered after meals and before bedtime, allows one to maintain an alkaline uri-nary pH around the clock, usually without the necessity of a 2 A.M. dose. POLYCITRA®-K Oral Solution alkalinizes the urine without producing a systemic alkalosis in recom-mended dosage. It is highly palatable, pleasant tasting, and tolerable, even when administered for long periods. Potas-sium citrate does not neutralize the gastric juice or disturb digestion.

CONTRAINDICATIONS

Severe renal impairment with oliguria or azotemia, un-treated Addison's disease, adynamia episodica hereditaria, acute dehydration, heat cramps, anuria, severe myocardial damage, and hyperkalemia from any cause.

WARNING

Large doses may cause hyperkalemia and alkalosis, espe-cially in the presence of renal disease. Concurrent adminis-tration of potassium-containing medication, potassium-sparing diuretics, angiotensin-converting enzyme (ACE) in-hibitors, or cardiac glycosides may lead to toxicity.

PRECAUTIONS

Should be used with caution by patients with low urinary output unless under the supervision of a physician. As with all liquids containing a high concentration of potassium, pa-tients should be directed to dilute adequately with water to minimize the possibility of gastrointestinal injury associ-ated with the oral ingestion of concentrated potassium salt preparations; and preferably, to take each dose after meals to avoid saline laxative effect.

ADVERSE REACTIONS

POLYCITRA®-K Oral Solution is generally well tolerated without any unpleasant side effects when given in recom-mended doses to patients with normal renal function and urinary output. However, as with any alkalinizing agent, caution must be used in certain patients with abnormal re-nal mechanisms to avoid development of hyperkalemia or alkalosis. Potassium intoxication causes listlessness, weak-ness, mental confusion, tingling of extremities, and other symptoms associated with a high concentration of potas-sium in the serum. Periodic determinations of serum elec-trolytes should be carried out in those patients with renal disease in order to avoid these complications. Hyperkalemia may exhibit the following electrocardiographic abnormali-ties: Disappearance of the P wave, widening and slurring of QRS complex, changes of the S-T segment, tall peaked T waves, etc.

OVERDOSAGE

The administration of oral potassium salts to persons with normal excretory mechanisms for potassium rarely causes serious hyperkalemia. However, if excretory mechanisms are impaired, hyperkalemia can result (see Contraindica-tions and Warnings). Hyperkalemia, when detected, must be treated immediately because lethal levels can be reached in a few hours.

TREATMENT OF HYPERKALEMIA

Should hyperkalemia occur, treatment measures include the following: (1) Elimination of foods or medications con-taining potassium. (2) The intravenous administration of 300 to 500 mL/hr of dextrose solution (10 to 25%), contain-ing 10 units of insulin /20 gm dextrose. (3) The use of ex-change resins, hemodialysis, or peritoneal dialysis. In treat-ing hyperkalemia, it should be recalled that in patients who have been stabilized on digitalis, too rapid a lowering of the plasma potassium concentration can produce digitalis toxic-ity.

DOSAGE AND ADMINISTRATION

POLYCITRA®-K Oral Solution should be taken diluted in water according to directions, followed by additional water, if desired. Palatability is enhanced if chilled before taking.
Usual Adult Dose: POLYCITRA®-K Oral Solution—3 to 6 teaspoonfuls (15 to 30 mL), diluted with 1 glass of water, after meals and at bedtime, or as directed by physician.
Usual Pediatric Dose: POLYCITRA®-K Oral Solution—1 to 3 teaspoonfuls (5 to 15 mL), diluted with 1/2 glass of wa-ter, after meals and at bedtime, or as directed by a physi-cian.
Usual Dosage Range: 2 to 3 teaspoonfuls (10 to 15 mL) POLYCITRA®-K Oral Solution, diluted with a glassful of water, taken four times a day, will usually maintain a uri-nary pH of 6.5–7.4. 3 to 4 teaspoonfuls (15 to 20 mL) POLY-CITRA®-K Oral Solution, diluted with a glassful of water, taken four time a day, will usually maintain a urinary pH of 7.0–7.6 throughout most of the 24 hours without unpleasant side effects. To check urinary pH, HYDRION Paper (pH 6.0–8.0) or NITRAZINE Paper (pH 4.5–7.5) are available and easy to use.

HOW SUPPLIED
POLYCITRA®–K ORAL SOLUTION
—16 fl. oz. (473 mL).
(NDC 17314-9321-1).
Keep tightly closed and protect from excessive heat or freez-ing.
Rx only
©1998 Baker Norton Pharmaceuticals, Inc.
POLYCITRA®-K is a Registered Trademark of Baker Nor-ton Pharmaceuticals, Inc. under license to ALZA Corpora-tion.

Distributed by:
  ALZA Corporation
  Mountain View, CA 94043

Manufactured by:
  Draxis Pharma Inc.
  Kirkland, Quebec H9H 4J4
  Canada
MADE IN CANADA
ALZA Pharmaceuticals
A division of ALZA Corp.
Mountain View, CA 94043
1001729   REV 9804
(212021)

TESTODERM® TTS
[tes-tō-derm]
Testosterone Transdermal System
5 mg/day
TESTODERM®
Testosterone Transdermal System
4 or 6 mg/day
TESTODERM® WITH ADHESIVE
Testosterone Transdermal System
6 mg/day

CONTROLLED DELIVERY
FOR ONCE-DAILY APPLICATION

DESCRIPTION
TESTODERM® TTS, TESTODERM®, and TESTODERM® WITH ADHESIVE Testosterone Transdermal Systems (re-ferred to collectively as the TESTODERM® products) are designed to release controlled amounts of testosterone, the primary circulating endogenous androgen, continuously upon application to the arm, back or upper buttocks (TESTODERM® TTS) or scrotal skin (TESTODERM®, and TESTODERM® WITH ADHESIVE). The TESTODERM® products are described below.
[See table below]
The active component of each of the systems is testosterone. Testosterone USP is a white or creamy-white crystalline powder or crystals chemically described as 17-beta hy-droxyandrost-4-en-3-one. The remaining components of the systems are pharmacologically inactive.
[See chemical structure at top of next column]

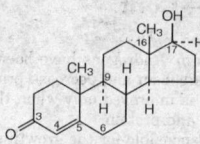

Testosterone
$C_{19}H_{28}O_2$ MW 288.43

TESTODERM® TTS is composed of the following layers: a flexible backing of transparent polyester/ethylene-vinyl ac-etate copolymer film, a drug reservoir of testosterone USP and 1.2 mL alcohol USP gelled with hydroxypropyl cellu-lose, and an ethylene-vinyl acetate copolymer membrane coated with a layer of polyisobutylene adhesive formulation that controls the rate of release of testosterone from the sys-tem. A protective liner of silicone-coated polyester covers the adhesive surface. The liner must be removed before appli-cation.

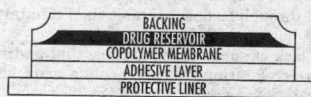

TESTODERM® TTS is composed of two layers. a soft flexi-ble backing of polyester and a testosterone-containing film of ethylene-vinyl acetate copolymer that contacts the skin surface and modulates the availability of the steroid. A pro-tective liner of fluorocarbon diacrylate or silicone-coated polyester covers the drug film. The liner must be removed before application.

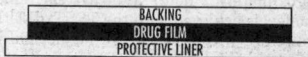

TESTODERM® WITH ADHESIVE is composed of three layers: a soft flexible backing of polyester and a testoste-rone-containing film of ethylene-vinyl acetate copolymer. The surface of the drug film is partially covered by the third layer: thin and narrow adhesive stripes composed of poly-isobutylene and colloidal silicon dioxide. A protective liner of fluorocarbon diacrylate-coated polyester covers the adhesive stripes and te adhesive-free area of the drug film. The liner must be removed before application.

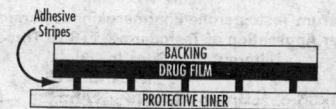

CLINICAL PHARMACOLOGY
Testosterone
The TESTOSDERM® products deliver physiologic amounts of testosterone, the primary endogenous androgenic hor-mone. Endogenous testosterone serum concentrations in normal males follow a circadian pattern. Daily morning ap-plication of any of the TESTODERM® products results in a serum testosterone profile that approximates the natural endogenous pattern of normal men.
General Androgen Effects
Endogenous androgens, including testosterone and dihydro-testosterone (DHT), are responsible for the normal growth and development of the male sex organs and for mainte-nance of secondary sex characteristics. These effects include the growth and maturation of prostate, seminal vesicles, pe-nis, and scrotum; the development of male hair distribution, such as facial, pubic, chest, and axillary hair; laryngeal en-largement, vocal chord thickening, alterations in body mus-culature, and fat distribution. DHT is necessary for the nor-mal development of secondary sex characteristics.
Male hypogonadism results from insufficient secretion of testosterone and is characterized by low serum testosterone concentrations. Symptoms associated with male hypogonad-ism include impotence and decreased sexual desire, fatigue and loss of energy, mood depression, and regression of sec-ondary sexual characteristics.
Drugs in the androgen class also cause retention of nitro-gen, sodium, potassium, phosphorus, and decreased urinary

Continued on next page

Product	Dose (mg/day)	Size (cm²)	Application Site
Testoderm® TTS	5	60	Arm, Back, Upper Buttocks
Testoderm®*	6	60	Scrotum
Testoderm®*	4	40	Scrotum
Testoderm® with Adhesive	6	60	Scrotum

* The composition of the two sizes per unit area is identical.

Testoderm—Cont.

excretion of calcium. Androgens have been reported to increase protein anabolism and decrease protein catabolism. Nitrogen balance is improved only when there is sufficient intake of calories and protein.

Androgens are responsible for the growth spurt of adolescence and for the eventual termination of linear growth brought about by fusion of the epiphyseal growth centers. In children, exogenous androgens accelerate linear growth rates but may cause a disproportionate advancement in bone maturation. Use over long periods may result in fusion of the epiphyseal growth centers and termination of the growth process. Androgens have been reported to stimulate the production of red blood cells by enhancing the production of erythropoietin.

During exogenous administration of androgens, endogenous testosterone release may be inhibited through feedback inhibition of pituitary luteinizing hormone (LH). At large doses of exogenous androgens, spermatogenesis may also be suppressed through feedback inhibition of pituitary follicle-stimulating hormone (FSH).

There is a lack of substantial evidence that androgens are effective in accelerating fracture healing or in shortening post-surgical convalescence.

Pharmacokinetics

Absorption

Daily morning application of any of the TESTODERM® products approximates the natural endogenous pattern of serum testosterone of normal males. Following application, testosterone is continuously absorbed during the 24-hour dosing period. The serum testosterone concentrations rise to a maximum at 2 to 4 hours and return toward baseline within approximately 2 hours after system removal. The testosterone levels achieved with the TESTODERM® products generally are within the range for normal men. Patients vary in their ability to absorb testosterone transdermally (see **Clinical Studies**).

TESTODERM® TTS

For TESTODERM® TTS three skin sites (arm, back, and upper buttocks), representing recommended application sites, are interchangeable based on equivalent testosterone $AUC_{(0\text{-}27)}$ (area under serum concentration curve) values. The estimated mean pharmacokinetic parameters after Testoderm® TTS application to various skin sites are presented in Table 1.

Table 1
Mean Serum Testosterone Pharmacokinetic Parameters after Application of Testoderm® TTS to Three Different Skin Sites (n=13)

PARAMETERS	TREATMENTS Upper Buttocks	Arm	Back
C_{max} (ng/dL)	482	462	499
*T_{max} (h)	3.9	4.0	3.9
AUC (ng•h/dL)	9,560	8,651	8,988

*Median value

In clinical trials, 94% of patients on TESTODERM® TTS treatment achieved maximum and average serum testosterone concentrations (C_{max} and C_{avg}, respectively) within the normal range; the average C_{max} and C_{avg} serum testosterone concentrations were 531 ng/dL and 366 ng/dL, respectively. Within-subject coefficient of variation in testosterone C_{avg} for subjects on TESTODERM® TTS therapy was 17%. The typical steady state serum testosterone concentration pattern achieved with a nominal testosterone dose of 5 mg/day from TESTODERM® TTS is shown in Figure 1.

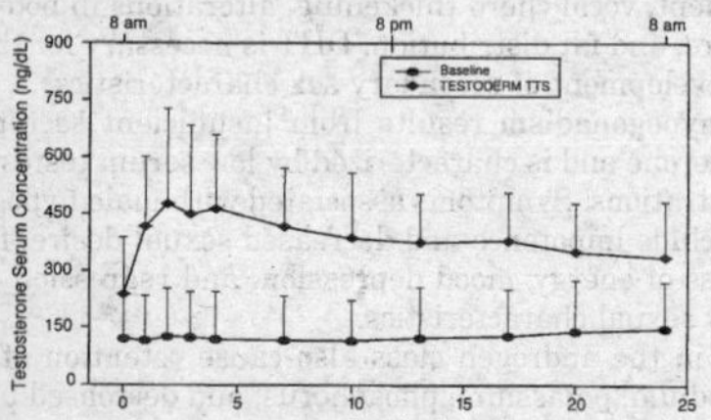

Figure 1. *Serum concentrations of testosterone (mean ± SD) during pretreatment baseline or while wearing a TESTODERM® TTS system on the upper buttocks (n=32). Systems were applied at 0 hours (8 AM) and removed 24 hours later.*

Normal range serum testosterone concentrations are reached during the first day of dosing.

There is no accumulation of testosterone following repeated application of TESTODERM® TTS.

Two TESTODERM® TTS systems deliver a testosterone dose which is twice that delivered by a single system.

There is no first-pass skin metabolism of testosterone to DHT when applied to arm, back or upper buttocks skin sites as recommended.

TESTODERM®

Scrotal skin is at least five times more permeable to testosterone than other skin sites. TESTODERM® or TESTODERM® WITH ADHESIVE will not produce adequate serum testosterone concentrations if applied to non-scrotal skin.

Hypogonadal men using TESTODERM® therapy have trough serum testosterone concentrations that are about 15% of peak levels. Serum levels reach a plateau at 3 to 4 weeks.

TESTODERM® WITH ADHESIVE

Data from a pharmacokinetic trial in 50 normal male subjects show that TESTODERM® WITH ADHESIVE applied to scrotal skin is equivalent to TETODERM ® with respect to rate (C_{max}) and extent (AUC) of testosterone delivery.

Distribution

Circulating testosterone is chiefly bound in the serum to sex hormone-binding globulin (SHBG) and albumin. The albumin-bound fraction of testosterone easily dissociates from albumin and is presumed to be bioactive. The portion of testosterone bound to SHBG is not considered biologically active. The amount of SHBG in the serum and the total testosterone level will determine the distribution of bioactive and nonbioactive androgen. SHBG-binding capacity is high in prepubertal children, declines during puberty and adulthood, and increases again during the later decades of life.

Metabolism

There is considerable variation in the half-life of testosterone as reported in the literature, ranging from 10 to 100 minutes. Testosterone is a substrate for conversion to an active metabolite, dihydrotestosterone (DHT). Testosterone is metabolized to various 17-keto steroids through two different pathways, and the major active metabolites are estradiol and DHT. Concentrations of estrodiol in normal men are 1.0 to 5.0 ng/dL. DHT concentrations in normal male serum are 30 to 85 ng/dL. DHT binds with greater affinity to SHBG than does testosterone. In many tissues the activity of testosterone appears to depend on reduction to DHT, which binds to cytosol receptor proteins. The steroid-receptor complex is transported to the nucleus where it initiates transcription and cellular changes related to androgen action. In reproductive tissues, DHT is further metabolized to 3-alpha and 3-beta androstanediol.

Composite results of all studies with TESTODERM® show elevated DHT concentrations and a change in the ratio of testosterone to DHT (T/DHT) during treatment. The range in this ratio was 0.7–12.5, as compared with a ratio of 3.6–15.2 in normal untreated men. The long-term effects of the change in this ratio are not known.

The T/DHT ratio during TESTODERM® TTS treatment was not statistically significantly different from placebo treatment.

Excretion

About 90% of a dose of testosterone given intramuscularly is excreted in the urine as glucuronic and sulfuric acid conjugates of testosterone and its metabolites; about 6% of a dose is excreted in the feces, mostly in the unconjugated form. Inactivation of testosterone occurs primarily in the liver.

Special Populations

Geriatric

In clinical trials with TESTODERM® TTS, C_{avg} testosterone concentrations were not different between men aged 65 and older and younger adult males.

Race

There is insufficient information available from trials with the TESTODERM® products to compare testosterone pharmacokinetics in different racial groups.

Renal Insufficiency

There is no experience with the use of the TESTODERM® products in patients with renal insufficiency.

Hepatic Insufficiency

There is no experience with the use of the TESTODERM® products in patients with hepatic insufficiency.

Drug-Drug Insufficiency

See PRECAUTIONS: Drug Interactions.

Clinical Studies

TESTODERM® TTS

Of 32 hypogonadal men receiving daily application of a single TESTODERM® TTS system, 94% achieved normal serum concentrations of testosterone as determined by C_{max} and C_{avg} (200-1000 ng/dL). Mean free testosterone, estrodiol, and dihydrotestosterone concentrations were also in the normal range aftr application of TESTODERM® TTS.

TESTODERM® and TESTODERM® WITH ADHESIVE

After at least 3 weeks of TESTODERM® therapy when steadt-state is obtained, 30 hypogonadal men treated with 6 mg/day systems for 22 hours daily achieved mean maximum serum testosterone concentrations of 593 ng/dL at 2 to 4 hours post application. Sixty percent of the patients achieved individual maximal testosterone concentrations >500 ng/dL. The mean 24 hour steady-state AUC (area under the curve) value was 9132 ng/dL. The mean DHT serum concentrations ranged from 134 to 162 ng/dL. Normal levels of testosterone have been maintained in patients who have worn the systems for up to six years. DHT levels also remain stable. The increase in serum testosterone concentration is proportional to the size of the system.

The variability of total testosterone concentrations among patients receiving TESTODERM® treatment was 35% to 49%. The coefficient of variation of total testosterone concentrations within individual patients was 30% to 41%. This variability is comparable to the values reported in the literature for both normal and hypogonadal men.

In two 12-week clinical studies in 72 hypogonadal men, TESTODERM® therapy produced positive effects on mood and sexual behavior. By five weeks, 45 patients not previously treated with TESTODERM® showed statistically significant increases in sexual activity. Compared to baseline, mean sexual events per week increased for sexual intercourse (0.3 to 0.8, orgasm (0.4 to 1.2), waking erections (1.0 to 3.5), and spontaneous erections (0.4 to 2.8).

Changes in nonfasting serum lipid concentrations were observed during TESTODERM® therapy. By three months total cholesterol and high-density lipoprotein cholesterol decreased on average of 8% and 13%, respectively. High density lipoprotein cholesterol remained stable thereafter. Total cholesterol continued to decrease through two years. At the end of two years, the total cholesterol/high-density lipoprotein cholesterol ratio was not different from pretreatment values.

Estradiol levels increased to the normal range with treatment. Sporadic elevations of estradiol above the normal range for men were observed in 3 of 72 patients and these were not associated with feminizing side effects.

INDICATIONS AND USAGE

The TESTODERM® products are indicated for replacement therapy in males for conditions associated with a deficiency or absence of endogenous testosterone:

1. Primary hypogonadism (congenital or acquired) – testicular failure due to cryptorchidism, bilateral torsion, orchitis, vanishing testis syndrome, orchidectomy, Klinefelter's syndrome, chemotherapy, or toxic damage from alcohol or heave metals. These men usually have low serum testosterone levels and gonadropins (FSH, LH) above the normal range.
2. Hypogonadotropic hypogonadism (congenital or acquired)—idiopathic gonodotropin or LHRH deficiency or pituitary-hypothalamic injury from tumors, trauma, or radiation. These men have low testosterone serum levels but have gonadotropins in the normal or low range.

The TESTODERM® products have not been evaluated clinically in males under 18 years of age.

CONTRAINDICATIONS

Androgens are contraindicated in men with carcinoma of the breast or known or suspected carcinoma of the prostate.

The TESTODERM® products are not indicated for use in women, have not been evaluated in women, and must not be used in women. Testosterone may cause fetal harm.

The TESTODERM® products should not be used in patients with known hypersensitivity to any components of the respective systems, e.g., ethanol (alcohol USP is a component of TESTODERM® TTS).

WARNINGS

1. Prolonged use of high doses of orally active 17-alpha-alkyl androgens (e.g., methyltestosterone) has been associated with serious hepatic adverse effects (peliosis hepatis, hepatic neoplasms, cholestatic hepatitis, and jaundice). Peliosis hepatis can be a life-threatening or fatal complication. Long-term therapy with testosterone enanthate, which elevates blood levesl for prolonged periods, has produced multiple hepatic adenomos. Testosterone is not known to produce these adverse effects.
2. Geriatric patients treated with androgens may be at an increased risk for the development of prostatic hyperplasia and prostatic carcinoma.
3. Geriatric patients and other patients with clinical or demographic characteristics that are recognized to be associated with an increased risk of prostate cancer should be evaluated for the presence of prostate cancer prior to initiation of testosterone replacement therapy. In men receiving testosterone replacement therapy, surveillance for prostate cancer should be consistent with current practices for eugonadal men (see **PRECAUTIONS:** Carcinogenesis, Mutagenesis, Impairment of Fertility and Laboratory Tests).
4. Edema with or without congestive heart failure may be a serious complication in patients with preexisting cardiac, renal, or hepatic disease. In addition to discontinuation of the drug, diuretic therapy may be required.
5. Gynecomastia frequently develops and occasionally persists in patients being treated for hypogonadism.
6. There are literature reports that the treatment of hypogonadal men with testosterone esters may potentiate sleep apena in some patients,[1,2] especially those with risk factors such as obesity or chronic lung diseases.[3,4,5]

PRECAUTIONS

General

The physician should instruct patients to report any of the following:

- Too frequent or persistent erections of the penis.
- Any nausea, vomiting, changes in skin color, or ankle swelling.
- Breathing disturbances, including those associated with sleep.

Virilization of female partners has been reported with use of a topical testosterone solution.

Percutaneous creams leave as much as 90 mg residual testosterone on the skin. The results from one study indicated that, after removal of a TESTODERM® system, the potential for transfer of testosterone to a sexual partner was 6 µg, 1/45th the daily endogenous testosterone production by the female body. TESTODERM® TTS, unlike TESTODERM® and TESTODERM® WITH ADHESIVE, has an occlusive backing that prevents the partner from coming in contact with the active material in the system. If a TESTODERM® TTS system is inadvertently transferred to a female partner, it should be removed immediately and the contacted skin washed. Changes in body hair distribution or significant increase in acne of the female partner should be brought to the attention of a physician.

Information for Patients

An information brochure containing instructions for the use of TESTODERM® TTS is available. A separate instruction booklet is available for TESTODERM® and TESTODERM® WITH ADHESIVE. These booklets contain important information and instructions on how to properly use and dispose of the TESTODERM® products. Patients should be encouraged to ask questions of the physician and pharmacist.

Advise patients of the following:

- TESTODERM® TTS should not be aplied to the scrotum.
- TESTODERM® and TESTODERM® WITH ADHESIVE are designed for application to scrotal skin only.
- The TESTODERM® products should be applied once daily to dry, clean skin. If the TESTODERM® product has come off after it has been worn for more than 12 hours and it cannot be reapplied, the patient may wait until the next routine application time to apply a new system.

Laboratory Tests

1. Hemoglobin and hematocrit levels should be checked periodically (to detect polycythemia) in patients on long-term androgen therapy.
2. Liver function, prostatic specific antigen, cholesterol, and high-density lipoprotein should be checked periodically.
3. To ensure proper dosing, serum testosterone concentrations may be measured (see **DOSAGE AND ADMINISTRATION**).

Drug Interactions

Anticoagulants: C-17 substituted derivatives of testosterone, such as methandrostenolone, have been reported to decrease the anticoagulant requirements of patients receiving oral anticoagulants. Patients receiving oral anticoagulant therapy require close monitoring, especially when androgens are started or stopped.

Oxyphenbutazone: Concurrent administration of oxyphenbutazone and androgens may result in elevated serum levels of oxyphenbutazone.

Insulin: In diebetic patients, the metabolic effects of androgens may decrease blood glucose and, therefore, insulin requirements.

Propranolol: In a published pharmacokinetic study of an injectable testosterone product, administration of testosterone cypionate led to an increased clearance of propranolol in the majority of men tested.[6]

Corticosteroids: The concurrent administration of testosterone with ACTH or corticosteroids may enhance edema formation; thus these drugs should be administered cautiously, particularly in patients with cardiac or hepatic disease.[7]

Drug/Laboratory Test Interactions

Androgens may decrease levels of thyroxin-binding globulin, resulting in decreased total T_4 serum levels and increased resin uptake of T_3 and T_4. Free thyroid hormone levels remain unchanged, however, and there is no clinical evidence of thyroid dysfunction.

Carcinogenesis, Mutagenesis, Impairment of Fertility Animal Data: Testosterone has been tested by subcutaneous injection and implantation in mice and rats. In mice, the implant induced cervical-uterine tumors, which metastasized in some cases. There is suggestive evidence that injection of testosterone into some strains of female mice increases their susceptibility to hepatoma. Testosterone is also known to increase the number of tumors and decrease the degree of differentiation of chemically induced carcinomas of the liver in rats.

Human Data: There are rare reports of hepatocellular carcinoma in patients receiving long-term therapy with androgens in high doses. Withdrawal of the drugs did not lead to regression of the tumors in all cases.

Geriatric patients treated with androgens may be at an increased risk for the development of prostatic hyperplasia and prostatic carcinoma.

Geriatric patients and other patients with clinical or demographic characteristics that are recognized to be associated with an increased risk of prostate cancer should be evaluated for the presence of prostate cancer prior to initiation of testosterone replacement therapy.

In men receiving testosterone replacement therapy, surveillance for prostate cancer should be consistent with current practices for eugonadal men.

Pregnancy Category X (see* Contraindications*). Teratogenic Effects: The TESTODERM® products are not indicated for women and must not be used in women.

Nursing Mothers: The TESTODERM® products are not indicated for women and must not be used in women.

Pediatric Use: Safety and efficacy of the TESTODERM® products in pediatric patients has not been established.

ADVERSE REACTIONS

Adverse events are reported in this section by product. Adverse events reported during use of a given product may occur in patients who are treated with any TESTODERM® product.

Adverse Events with TESTODERM® TTS

In clinical studies of 457 participants (116 hypogonadal males and 341 healthy adult males) treated for up to 6 weeks with TESTODERM® TTS, the most commonly reported adverse events were application site reactions of transient itching (12%) and moderate or severe erythema (3%).

Table 2
Adverse events reported in clinical trials in males (n=457) receiving TESTODERM® TTS by 1% or more of users.

Event	Percent of Patients
Itching (ASR)*	12
Headache	5
Erythema† (ASR)*	3
Myalgia	2
Accidental injury	2
Pruritus	2
Pain	2
Asthenia	1
Flu syndrome	1
Libido increased	1
Burning sensation (ASR)*	1
Rash	1

* ASR = Application Site Reaction
† Moderate or severe

Adverse events reported by less than 1% of TESTODERM® TTS users in clinical trials that were of probable or unknown relationship to drug were: *Body as a Whole:* abdominal pain, back pain, infection; *Cardiovascular System:* congestive heart failure, hypertension, tachycardia; *Digestive System:* diarrhea, nausea; *Metabolic and Nutritional System:* hyperglycemia, hyperlipemia, hyponatremia; *Musculoskeletal System:* arthralgia; *Nervous System:* nervousness, depression, dizziness, dry mouth, insomnia, decreased libido, personality disorder, CNS stimulation; *Respiratory System:* bronchitis; *Skin System:* application site reactions – papules/pustules, edema, vesicles, pain, other—, acne, alopecia, hirsutism; *Urogenital System:* abnormal ejaculation, breast pain, dysuria, urinary tract infection, and impaired urination.

Topical Reactions

Of 457 study participants, 3 men (1%) discontinued prematurely because of application site reactions.

There were no clinically significant differences in skin tolerability in younger (<65 years old) and older (≥ 65 years old) subjects.

A contact sensitization rate of 0.5% for TESTODERM® TTS was observed in a 6-week study of 233 normal male volunteers.

In one study with 14 days of daily use, 42% of patients reported 3 or more detachments of their TESTODERM® TTS; of these detachments, 33% occurred during exercise.

Adverse Events with TESTODERM®

In clinical studies of 104 patients treated with TESTODERM®, the most common adverse effects reported were local effects. In US clinical trials, most of the 72 patients filling out a daily questionnaire reported scrotal itching, discomfort, or irritation at some time during therapy. Of all the daily questionnaire responses, 7% reported itching, 4% discomfort, and 2% irritation. All topical reactions decreased with duration of use.

The following adverse effects (greater than 1%) were reported in association with TESTODERM® therapy in 104 patients using the product for up to three years. These effects are listed in decreasing frequency of occurrence with the percentages of patients reporting the effect in parentheses: Gynecomastia (5%), acne (4%), prostatitis/urinary tract infection (4%), breast tenderness (3%), stroke (2%). For this same patient population, the following adverse effects were reported by 1% of users: memory loss, pupillary dilation, abnormal liver enzymes, scrotal cellulitis, deep vein phlebitis, benign prostatic hyperplasia, rectal mucosal lesion over prostate, hematuria/bladder cancer, papilloma on scrotum, and congestive heart failure.

See **CLINICAL PHARMACOLOCY**, Clinical Studies, regarding effects on serum lipids.

Adverse Events with TESTODERM® WITH ADHESIVE

In a pharmacokinetic study in 50 normal men, skin assessment scores following a single 24-hour application of TESTODERM® WITH ADHESIVE to scrotal skin were similar to those for TESTODERM®. Other adverse events reported during the study were headache (6%), dizziness (6%), back pain, pain, nausea, and pustular rash (1% each).

General Adverse Events with Androgen Replacement Therapy

Skin and Appendages: Hirsutism, male pattern baldness, seborrhea, and acne.

Endocrine and Urogenital: Gynecomastia and excessive frequency and duration of penile erections. Oligospermia may occur at high doses)see **CLINICAL PHARMACOLOGY**),

Fluid and Electrolyte Disturbances: Retention of sodium, chloride, water, potassium, calcium, and inorganic phosphates.

Gastrointestinal: Nausea, cholestatic jaundice, alterations in liver function tests. Rare instances of hepatocellular neoplasms and peliosis hepatis have occurred (see **WARNINGS**).

Hematologic: Suppression of clotting factors II, V, VII, and X, bleeding in patients on concomitant anticoagulant therapy, and polycythemia.

Nervous System: Increased or decreased libido, headache, anxiety, depression, and generalized paresthesia.

Metabolic: Increased serum cholesterol.

Miscellaneous: Rarely, anaphylactoid reactions.

DRUG ABUSE AND DEPENDENCE

The TESTODERM® products contain a Schedule III controlled substance as defined by the Anabolic Steroids Control Act.

TESTODERM® TTS is designed for application to arm, back or upper buttocks skin.

TESTODERM® and TESTODERM® WITH ADHESIVE are designed for application to scrotal skin only. Because scrotal skin is at least five times more permeable to testosterone than other skin sites, TESTODERM® or TESTODERM® WITH ADHESIVE will not produce adequate serum testosterone concentrations if applied to non-scrotal skin.

Ingestion of testosterone, or the contents of any of the TESTODERM® products will not result in clinically significant serum testosterone concentrations due to extensive first-pass metabolism. In addition, an intramuscular injection of testosterone from any of the TESTODERM® products will not produce adequate serum testosterone levels due to its short half-life (about 10 minutes).

OVERDOSAGE

There is one report of acute overdosage by injection of testosterone enanthate: testosterone levels of up to 11,400 ng/dL were implicated in a cerebrovascular accident.

DOSAGE AND ADMINISTRATION

TESTODERM® TTS

One system is applied at about the same time each day. The adhesive side of the TESTODERM® TTS system should be placed on a clean, dry area of skin on the arm, back or upper buttocks immediately upon removal from the protective pouch. DO NOT APPLY TO THE SCROTUM. The area selected should not be oily, damaged, or irritated. The system should be pressed firmly in place with the palm of the hand for about 10 seconds, making sure there is good contact, especially around the edges. In the event that a system should fall off, the same system may be reapplied. If the system comes off after it has been worn for more than 12 hours and it cannot be reapplied, a new system may be applied at the next routine application time. In either case, the daily treatment schedule should be continued. The TESTODERM® TTS system should be worn approximately 24 hours and then replaced. To ensure proper dosing, serum testosterone concentration may be measured 2–4 hours after an application of TESTODERM® TTS. If the serum testosterone concentrations are low, the dosing regimen may be increased to 2 systems. Because of variability in analytical values among diagnostic laboratories, all testosterone measurements should be performed at the same laboratory.

TESTODERM® and TESTODERM® WITH ADHESIVE

Patients should start therapy with a 6 mg/day system of either TESTODERM® and TESTODERM® WITH ADHESIVE applied daily; if the scrotal area cannot accommodate a 6 mg/day system, a 4 mg/day TESTODERM® system should be used. One TESTODERM® or TESTODERM® WITH ADHESIVE system should be placed on clean, dry, scrotal skin. Scrotal hair should be dry-shaved for optimal skin contact. Chemical depilatories should not be used (see Patient Information). TESTODERM® or TESTODERM® WITH ADHESIVE should be worn 22–24 hours.

After 3–4 weeks of daily system use, blood should be drawn 2–4 hours after system application for determination of serum total testosterone. Because of variability in analyti-

Continued on next page

Testoderm—Cont.

cal values among diagnostic laboratories, this laboratory work and later analyses for assessing the effect of the TESTODERM® and TESTODERM® WITH ADHESIVE therapy should be performed at the same laboratory.

If patients have not achieved desired results by the end of 6–8 weeks of treatment with any of the TESTODERM® products, another form of testosterone replacement therapy should be considered.

HOW SUPPLIED

TESTODERM® TTS, TESTODERM®, and TESTODERM® WITH ADHESIVE testosterone transdermal systems contain a Schedule III controlled substance as defined by the Anabolic Steroids Control Act.

TESTODERM® TTS

TESTODERM® TTS systems are supplied as individually pouched systems, 30 per carton. TESTODERM® TTS 5 mg/day (Testosterone Transdermal System) – each 60 cm² system contains 328 mg trestoterone USP for nominal dose of 5 mg/day.

Carton of 30 TESTODERM® TTS 5 mg/day systems
.... NDC 17314-4717-3

TESTODERM® and TESTODERM® WITH ADHESIVE

TESTODERM® and TESTODERM® WITH ADHESIVE systems are supplied as individually pouched systems, 30 per carton.

TESTODERM® 4 mg/day (Testosterone Transdermal System) – each 40 cm² system contains 10 mg testosterone USP for naminal delivery of 4 mg for one day.

Carton of 30 TESTODERM® 4 mg/day systems
.... NDC 17314-4608-3

TESTODERM® WITH ADHESIVE

6 mg/day (Testosterone Transdermal System) – each 60 cm² system contains 15 mg testosterone USP for nominal delivery of 6 mg for one day.

Carton of 30 TESTODERM® 6 mg/day systems
.... NDC 17314-4609-3

Carton of 30 TESTODERM® WITH ADHESIVE 6 mg/day systems
.... NDC 17314-2836-3

Storage

TESTODERM® TTS

Store at controlled room temperature below 25°C (77°F).

TESTODERM® and TESTODERM® WITH ADHESIVE

Store at room temperature 15–30°C (59–86°F).

Disposal

TESTODERM® products should be discarded in household trash in a manner that prevents accidental application or ingestion by children or pets.

REFERENCES

1. Matsumoto AM, Sandblom RE, Schoene RB et al. *Testosterone replacement in hypogonadal men: Effects on obstructive sleep apnoea, respiratory drives, and sleep.* Clin Endocrinol (1985) 22: 713–721.
2. Schneider BK, Pickett CK, Zwillich CW et al. *Influence of testosterone on breathing during sleep.* J Appl Physiol (1986) 61: 618–623.
3. Matsumoto AM. *Hormonal therapy of male hypogonadism.* Endocrinol Metab Clin North Am. (1994) 23: 857–875.
4. Bardin CW, Swerdloff RS, Santen RJ. *Androgens: Risks and benefits.* J Clin Endocinol Metab (1991) 73: 4–7.
5. Nieschlag E, Wang CCL. *Guidelines for the use of androgens in men.* Geneva: World Health Organization (1992); 1–16.
6. Walle T, Walle UK, Mathur RS et al. *Propranolol metabolism in normal subjects: Association with sex steroid hormones.* Curr Pharmacol Ther (1994) 56:127–132.
7. Physicians' Generic Rx: The Complete Drug Reference. (1996); II-1972

Caution: Federal law prohibits dispensing with prescription.

Manufactured by ALZA Corporations, Palo Alto, CA 94304, USA.

**ALZA PHARMACEUTICALS
A DIVISION OF ALZA CORPORATION
Edition: 01/98**

00071210

Shown in Product Identification Guide, page 304

PROGESTASERT EDUCATIONAL MATERIAL

All progestasert educational materials are complimentary.

Booklets—Brochures

A. Patient Information Leaflet
   (English and Spanish)
B. Clinical Evidence Brochure
C. Demonstration Kit

Videos—Audiotapes—Slides

A. Progestasert® System Insertion Technique
   Videocassette
B. Patient Audiocassette Tape
C. Instructional Slide Program

American Lecithin Company
**115 HURLEY ROAD, UNIT 2B
OXFORD, CT 06478**

Direct Inquiries to:
Randall E. Zigmont
(203) 262-7100
Fax: (203) 262-7101

**For Medical Emergencies Contact:
In Emergencies:**
Randall E. Zigmont
(203) 262-7100
Fax: (203) 262-7101

PHOSCHOL®   OTC
[fos 'kol]
**Phosphatidylcholine (highly purified lecithin)
Softgels and Concentrate**

DESCRIPTION

PhosChol 900 contains 900 mg of pure phosphatidylcholine in each softgel.

PhosChol Concentrate contains 3000 mg of pure phosphatidylcholine in each teaspoonful.

ACTION & USES

Choline circulating in the blood after PC ingestion is taken up into all cells of the body. The brain has a unique way of ensuring that its nerve cells will receive adequate supplies of circulating choline.

A special protein molecule within the brain's capillaries traps the circulating choline, and then transports it across the blood-brain barrier, into the brain. Once in the brain, choline is incorporated into the brain's own PC, which is an essential and major part of neuronal membranes. Circulating choline transported into the brain has an additional very important function for a special group of nerve cells that make a biochemical, acetylcholine, which is released into synapses as a neurotransmitter. It provides the essential precursor used to synthesize acetylcholine. Moreover, when nerve cells are active, firing frequently and releasing large quantities of acetylcholine, their ability to make adequate amounts of the neurotransmitter requires that they receive adequate amounts of choline from the blood stream. In the absence of adequate choline, the ability of nerve cells to transmit messages to other cells across synapses is impaired and neuronal cell membranes can be depleted of PC causing cell damage. In contrast, when supplemental choline is provided, these messages can be amplified and membrane structure maintained.

PhosChol® brand of highly purified lecithin has been carefully developed to contain the highest concentration of phosphatidylcholine commercially available and can provide for the highest blood choline levels.

Figure 1.
LEVELS OF CHOLINE IN HUMAN PLASMA AFTER THE ADMINISTRATION OF 3, 6, 9, AND 18 GRAM DOSES OF PHOSCHOL

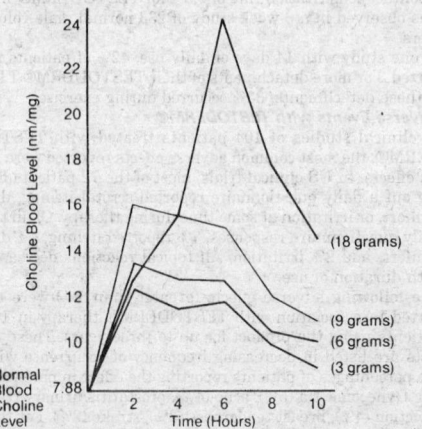

(One 9-gram dose at baseline, one 9-gram dose at 4 hours)

ADMINISTRATION

PhosChol® nutritional supplements may be recommended for two purposes:

To guard against low blood choline levels, and to restore blood choline levels in patients suffering from selected brain disorders. Amounts of PC sufficient to increase blood choline levels would help support normal cellular membrane composition and repair; they would also provide sufficient precursor choline for the maintenance of acetylcholine biosynthesis. Taken according to these schedules, dietary supplements of PC are an aid to good health, and protect against low choline stores.

To increase blood choline by 50%, patients should take 3 grams of PhosChol before meals by noon. To double blood choline levels, patients should take 9 grams of PhosChol before meals by noon. If ingestion before meals causes intestinal distress, it is recommended that PhosChol be taken either with meals or immediately thereafter.

ADVERSE REACTIONS

No major side effects have been reported in connection with consumption of large quantities of phosphatidylcholine or commercially available (less pure) lecithin.

Minor side effects may be seen such as increased salivation, nausea and upset stomach.

HOW SUPPLIED

Two strengths as clear, amber colored, one-piece sealed softgels.

PhosChol 900 contains 900 mg of pure phosphatidylcholine in each softgel and is available in bottles of 30, 100 and 300 softgels. Ten softgels a day provide 9 grams of phosphatidylcholine.

PhosChol 565 contains 565 mg of pure phosphatidylcholine and is available in bottles of 100.

One strength as a liquid concentrate.

PhosChol Concentrate contains 3000 mg of pure phosphatidylcholine in each teaspoonful and is available in 8 oz., and 16 oz. bottles. Three teaspoonsful a day provide 9 grams of phosphatidylcholine.

American Red Cross
**NATIONAL HEADQUARTERS
BIOMEDICAL SERVICES
1616 FORT MYER DRIVE, 17th FLOOR
ARLINGTON, VA 22209-3100**

Direct Inquiries to:
Professional Services Department
800-293-5023
FAX: 703-312-8742
Customer Service Department
800-446-8883
FAX: 703-312-8746

ALBUMARC® 5%   ℞
ALBUMIN (HUMAN), USP, 5% SOLUTION

6 bottles per case
250mL bottle   52769-450-25
500mL bottle   52769-450-50

ALBUMARC® 25%   ℞
ALBUMIN (HUMAN), USP, 25% SOLUTION

10 bottles per case
50mL bottle   52769-451-05
100mL bottle   52769-451-10

MONARC-M™   ℞
**ANTIHEMOPHILIC FACTOR (HUMAN)
Method M
Monoclonal Purified**

This product is derived from blood collected from volunteer donors by the American Red Cross Blood Services. The cost of processing, testing and packaging was paid by the American Red Cross Blood Services.

DESCRIPTION

MONARC-M™, Antihemophilic Factor (Human), Method M Monoclonal Purified, is a sterile, nonpyrogenic, dried preparation of antihemophilic factor (Factor VIII, Factor VIII:C, AHF) in concentrated form with a specific activity range of 2 to 15 AHF International Units/mg of total protein. When reconstituted with the appropriate volume of diluent, it contains approximately 12.5 mg/mL Albumin (Human), 1.5 mg/mL polyethylene glycol (3350), 0.055 M histidine and 0.030 M glycine as stabilizing agents. In the absence of the added Albumin (Human), the specific activity is approximately 2,000 AHF International Units/mg of protein. It also contains, per AHF International Unit, not more than 0.1 ng mouse protein, 18 ng organic solvent tri-n-butyl phosphate and 50 ng detergent (Triton X-100). **See CLINICAL PHARMACOLOGY.**

MONARC–M™ is prepared by the Method M process from pooled human plasma by immunoaffinity chromatography utilizing a murine monoclonal antibody to Factor VIII:C, followed by an ion exchange chromatography step for further purification. Method M also includes an organic solvent [tri(n-butyl) phosphate] and detergent (Triton X-100) virus inactivation step designed to reduce the risk of transmission of hepatitis and other viral diseases. However, no procedure has been shown to be totally effective in removing viral infectivity from coagulation factor products.

Each bottle of MONARC–M™ is labeled with the AHF activity expressed in International Units per bottle, which is referenced to the WHO International Standard.

MONARC–M™ is to be administered only intravenously.

HOW SUPPLIED

MONARC–M™, is available as single dose bottles. Each bottle is labeled with the potency in International Units, and is packaged together with 10 mL of Sterile Water for Injection, USP, a double-ended needle, and a filter needle.
NDC 52769-460-01

Manufactured for:
+ American Red Cross
Biomedical Services
Arlington, VA 22209, USA

Manufactured by:
Baxter Healthcare Corporation
Hyland Division
Glendale, CA 91203 USA
U.S. License No. 140
June, 1998

POLYGAM® S/D
IMMUNE GLOBULIN INTRAVENOUS
SOLVENT/DETERGENT TREATED
(HUMAN)   R

This product is derived from blood collected from volunteer donors by the American Red Cross Blood Services. The cost of processing, testing and packaging was paid by the American Red Cross Blood Services.

DESCRIPTION

Immune Globulin Intravenous (Human) [IGIV], Polygam® S/D, is a solvent/detergent treated, sterile, freeze-dried preparation of highly purified immunoglobulin G (IgG) derived from large pools of human plasma. The product is manufactured by the Cohn-Oncley cold ethanol fractionation process followed by ultrafiltration and ion exchange chromatography. The manufacturing process includes treatment with an organic solvent/detergent mixture,[1,2] composed of tri-n-butyl phosphate, octoxynol 9 and polysorbate 80.[3] The Polygam® S/D manufacturing process provides a significant viral reduction in *in vitro* studies.[3] These reductions are achieved through a combination of process chemistry, partitioning and/or inactivation during cold ethanol fractionation and the solvent/detergent treatment.[3]

When reconstituted with the total volume of diluent (Sterile Water for Injection, USP) supplied, this preparation contains approximately 50 mg of protein per mL (5%), of which at least 90% is gamma globulin. The product, reconstituted to 5%, contains a physiological concentration of sodium chloride (approximately 8.5 mg/mL) and has a pH of 6.8 ± 0.4. Stabilizing agents and additional components are present in the following maximum amounts for a 5% solution: 3 mg/mL Albumin (Human), 22.5 mg/mL glycine, 20 mg/mL glucose, 2 mg/mL polyethylene glycol (PEG), 1 μg/mL tri(n-butyl) phosphate, 1μg/mL octoxynol 9, and 100 μg/mL polysorbate 80. If it is necessary to prepare a 10% (100 mg/mL) solution for infusion, half the volume of diluent should be added as described in the **DOSAGE AND ADMINISTRATION** section. In this case, the stabilizing agents and other components will be present at double the concentrations given for the 5% solution.

The manufacturing process for Immune Globulin Intravenous (Human), Polygam® S/D, isolates IgG without additional chemical or enzymatic modification and the Fc portion is maintained intact. Immune Globulin Intravenous (Human), Polygam® S/D, contains all of the IgG antibody activities which are present in the donor population. On the average, the distribution of IgG subclasses present in this product is similar to that in normal plasma.[3] Immune Globulin Intravenous (Human), Polygam® S/D, contains only trace amounts of IgA (<3.7 μg/mL in a 5% solution). IgM is also present in trace amounts.

Immune Globulin Intravenous (Human), Polygam® S/D, contains no preservative.

HOW SUPPLIED

Immune Globulin Intravenous (Human), Polygam® S/D, is supplied in 2.5 g, 5 g or 10 g single use bottles. Each bottle of Immune Globulin Intravenous (Human), Polygam® S/D, is furnished with a suitable volume of Sterile Water for Injection, USP, a transfer device and an administration set which contains an integral airway and a 15 micron filter.

2.5g   NDC 52769-471-72
5g   NDC 52769-471-75
10g   NDC 52769-471-80

Manufactured for:
+ American Red Cross
Biomedical Services
Arlington, VA 22209, USA

Manufactured by:
Baxter Healthcare Corporation
Hyland Division
Glendale, CA 91203 USA
U.S. License No. 140
June, 1998

Panglobulin™   R
IMMUNE GLOBULIN INTRAVENOUS (HUMAN)

CAUTION: US Federal law prohibits dispensing without prescription.

DESCRIPTION

Immune globulin Intravenous (Human), Panglobulin™, is a sterile, highly purified polyvalent antibody product containing in concentrated form all the IgG antibodies which regularly occur in the donor population (1). The fractionation process by which IGIV is prepared from plasma includes several filtration steps which are carried out in the presence of filter aids. Four of these steps were validated for virus elimination. The cumulative LRFs (log_{10} of reduction factors) were 15.5 for HIV (human immunodeficiency virus), 16.0 for PRV (pseudorabies virus), 9.3 for SFV (Semliki Forest virus), 12.4 for Sindbis virus, and 14.1 for BEV (bovine entero-virus).

Panglobulin™ (IGIV) is made suitable for intravenous use by treatment at acid pH in the presence of trace amounts of pepsin (2,3). Treatment with pepsin at pH4 rapidly inactivates enveloped viruses. LRFs were ≥6.1 for HIV, ≥5.3 for PRV, ≥4.4 for BVDV (bovine viral diarrhea virus), and ≥6.8 for SFV. PRV and the two model viruses for HCV (hepatitis C virus), BVDV and SFV, were all inactivated within 1/10, and HIV within 1/2 of the total incubation time used during production of Immune Globulin Intravenous (Human) Panglobulin™. Overall viral clearance by either elimination and/or inactivation during the manufacturing process has been documented to be ≥21 for HIV, ≥19 for PRV, ≥15 for SFV, and ≥14 for BEV (expressed as LRF).

The preparation contains at least 96% of IgG and after reconstitution with a neutral unbuffered diluent has a pH of 6.6 ± 0.2. Most of the immunoglobulins are monomeric (7 S) IgG; the remainder consists of dimeric IgG and a small amount of polymeric IgG, traces of IgA and IgM and immunoglobulin fragments (4). The distribution of the IgG subclasses corresponds to that of normal serum (5,6,7,8). Final container lyophilized units are prepared so as to contain 1, 3, 6, or 12 g protein with 1.67 g sucrose and less than 20 mg NaCl per gram of protein. The lyophilized preparation is devoid of any preservatives and may be reconstituted with sterile water, 5% dextrose or 0.9% saline to a solution with protein concentrations ranging from 3% to 12%.

HOW SUPPLIED

Immune Globulin Intravenous (Human), Panglobulin™, is available as a white lyophilized powder in 6 and 12 g size vials. The only diluents which may be used to reconstitute the product are sterile (0.9%) Sodium Chloride Injection USP, 5% Dextrose, or Sterile Water.
Panglobulin™ (IGIV) is available in individual vial packages.
1 g
3 g
6 g
• Individual vial package   NDC 52769-270-76
12 g
• Individual vial package   NDC 52769-270-82

REFERENCES

1. Gardi A: Quality control in the production of an immunoglobulin for intravenous use. Blut 48:337-344, 1984.
2. Römer J. Morgenthaler JJ, Scherz R, et al: Characterization of various immunoglobulin-preparations for intravenous application.
I. Protein composition and antibody content. Vox Sang 42: 62-73, 1982.
3. Römer J, Späth PJ, Skvaril F, et al: Characterization of various immunoglobulin preparations for intravenous application. II. Complement activation and binding to Staphylococcus protein A. Vox Sang 42:74-80, 1982.
4. Römer J, Späth PJ: Molecular composition of immunoglobulin preparations and its relation to complement activation, in Nydegger UE (ed): Immunohemotherapy: A Guide to Immunoglobulin Prophylaxis and Therapy. London, Academic Press, 1981. p 123.
5. Skvaril F, Roth-Wicky B, and Barandun S: IgG subclasses in human-g-globulin preparations for intravenous use and their reactivity with Staphylococcus protein A. Vox Sang 38: 147, 1980.
6. Skvaril F: Qualitative and quantitative aspects of IgG subclasses in i.v. immunoglobulin preparations, in Nydegger UE (ed): Immunohemotherapy: A Guide to Immunoglobulin Prophylaxis and Therapy. London, Academic Press, 1981, p 113.
7. Skvaril F, and Barandun S: In vitro characterization of immunoglobulins for intravenous use, in Alving BM, Finlayson JS (eds): Immunoglobulins: Characteristics and Uses of Intravenous Preparations, DHHS Publication No. (FDA)-80-9005. US Government Printing Office, 1980, pp 201-206.
8. Burckhardt JJ, Gardi A, Oxelius V, et al: Immunoglobulin G subclass distribution in three human intravenous immunoglobulin preparations. Vox Sang 57:10-14, 1989.

Manufactured For:
American Red Cross
Biomedical Services
Arlington, Va. 22209, USA

Manufactured By:
Central Laboratory
Blood Transfusion Service
Swiss Red Cross
Wankdorfstrasse 10, 3000 Berne 22
Switzerland
US License No. 647
June, 1998

Amgen
AMGEN INC.
ONE AMGEN CENTER DRIVE
THOUSAND OAKS, CA 91320-1789

Direct Inquiries to:
Customer Services Department
(800) 282-6436
FAX: (800) 292-6436

For Medical Information Contact:
Professional Services Department
(800) 772-6436
FAX: 805-376-8550
In Emergencies:
(800) 772-6436
After Hours and Weekends:
(800) 772-6436

Sales and Ordering:
Customer Services Department
(800) 282-6436
FAX: (800) 292-6436

EPOGEN®   R
EPOETIN ALFA
RECOMBINANT
For Injection

DESCRIPTION

Erythropoietin is a glycoprotein which stimulates red blood cell production. It is produced in the kidney and stimulates the division and differentiation of committed erythroid progenitors in the bone marrow. EPOGEN® (Epoetin alfa), a 165 amino acid glycoprotein manufactured by recombinant DNA technology, has the same biological effects as endogenous erythropoietin.[1] It has a molecular weight of 30,400 daltons and is produced by mammalian cells into which the human erythropoietin gene has been introduced. The product contains the identical amino acid sequence of isolated natural erythropoietin.

EPOGEN® is formulated as a sterile, colorless liquid in an isotonic sodium chloride/sodium citrate buffered solution for intravenous (IV) or subcutaneous (SC) administration.

Single-dose, Preservative-free Vial: Each 1 mL of solution contains 2000, 3000, 4000 or 10,000 Units of Epoetin alfa, 2.5 mg Albumin (Human), 5.8 mg sodium citrate, 5.8 mg sodium chloride, and 0.06 mg citric acid in Water for Injection, USP (pH 6.9 ± 0.3). This formulation contains no preservative.

Multidose, Preserved Vial: 2 mL (20,000 Units, 10,000 Units/mL). Each 1 mL of solution contains 10,000 Units of Epoetin alfa, 2.5 mg Albumin (Human), 1.3 mg sodium citrate, 8.2 mg sodium chloride, 0.11 mg citric acid, and 1% benzyl alcohol as preservative in Water for Injection, USP (pH 6.1 ± 0.3).

Multidose, Preserved Vial: 1 mL (20,000 Units/mL). Each 1 mL of solution contains 20,000 Units of Epoetin alfa, 2.5 mg

Continued on next page

Epogen—Cont.

Albumin (Human), 1.3 mg sodium citrate, 8.2 mg sodium chloride, 0.11 mg citric acid, and 1% benzyl alcohol as preservative in Water for Injection, USP (pH 6.1 ± 0.3).

CLINICAL PHARMACOLOGY

Chronic Renal Failure Patients

Endogenous production of erythropoietin is normally regulated by the level of tissue oxygenation. Hypoxia and anemia generally increase the production of erythropoietin, which in turn stimulates erythropoiesis.[2] In normal subjects, plasma erythropoietin levels range from 0.01 to 0.03 Units/mL and increase up to 100- to 1000-fold during hypoxia or anemia.[2,3] In contrast, in patients with chronic renal failure (CRF), production of erythropoietin is impaired, and this erythropoietin deficiency is the primary cause of their anemia.[3,4]

Chronic renal failure is the clinical situation in which there is a progressive and usually irreversible decline in kidney function. Such patients may manifest the sequelae of renal dysfunction, including anemia, but do not necessarily require regular dialysis. Patients with end-stage renal disease (ESRD) are those patients with CRF who require regular dialysis or kidney transplantation for survival.

EPOGEN® has been shown to stimulate erythropoiesis in anemic patients with CRF, including both patients on dialysis and those who do not require regular dialysis.[4–13] The first evidence of a response to the three times weekly (TIW) administration of EPOGEN® is an increase in the reticulocyte count within 10 days, followed by increases in the red cell count, hemoglobin, and hematocrit, usually within 2 to 6 weeks.[4,5] Because of the length of time required for erythropoiesis—several days for erythroid progenitors to mature and be released into the circulation—a clinically significant increase in hematocrit is usually not observed in less than 2 weeks and may require up to 6 weeks in some patients. Once the hematocrit reaches the suggested target range (30% to 36%), that level can be sustained by EPOGEN® therapy in the absence of iron deficiency and concurrent illnesses.

The rate of hematocrit increase varies between patients and is dependent upon the dose of EPOGEN®, within a therapeutic range of approximately 50 to 300 Units/kg TIW.[4] A greater biologic response is not observed at doses exceeding 300 Units/kg TIW.[6] Other factors affecting the rate and extent of response include availability of iron stores, the baseline hematocrit, and the presence of concurrent medical problems.

Zidovudine-treated HIV-infected Patients

Responsiveness to EPOGEN® in HIV-infected patients is dependent upon the endogenous serum erythropoietin level prior to treatment. Patients with endogenous serum erythropoietin levels ≤500 mUnits/mL, and who are receiving a dose of zidovudine ≤4200 mg/week, may respond to EPOGEN® therapy. Patients with endogenous serum erythropoietin levels >500 mUnits/mL do not appear to respond to EPOGEN® therapy. In a series of four clinical trials involving 255 patients, 60% to 80% of HIV-infected patients treated with zidovudine had endogenous serum erythropoietin levels ≤500 mUnits/mL.

Response to EPOGEN® in zidovudine-treated HIV-infected patients is manifested by reduced transfusion requirements and increased hematocrit.

Cancer Patients on Chemotherapy

Anemia in cancer patients may be related to the disease itself or the effect of concomitantly administered chemotherapeutic agents. EPOGEN® has been shown to increase hematocrit and decrease transfusion requirements after the first month of therapy (months 2 and 3), in anemic cancer patients undergoing chemotherapy.

A series of clinical trials enrolled 131 anemic cancer patients who were receiving cyclic cisplatin- or non cisplatin-containing chemotherapy. Endogenous baseline serum erythropoietin levels varied among patients in these trials with approximately 75% (n=83/110) having endogeneous serum erythropoietin levels ≤132 mUnits/mL, and approximately 4% (n=4/110) of patients having endogenous serum erythropoietin levels >500 mUnits/mL. In general, patients with lower baseline serum erythropoietin levels responded more vigorously to EPOGEN® than patients with higher baseline erythropoietin levels. Although no specific serum erythropoietin level can be stipulated above which patients would be unlikely to respond to EPOGEN® therapy, treatment of patients with grossly elevated serum erythropoietin levels (eg, >200 mUnits/mL) is not recommended.

Pharmacokinetics

Intravenously administered EPOGEN® is eliminated at a rate consistent with first order kinetics with a circulating half-life ranging from approximately 4 to 13 hours in patients with CRF. Within the therapeutic dose range, detectable levels of plasma erythropoietin are maintained for at least 24 hours.[7] After SC administration of EPOGEN® to patients with CRF, peak serum levels are achieved within 5 to 24 hours after administration and decline slowly thereafter. There is no apparent difference in half-life between patients not on dialysis whose serum creatinine levels were greater than 3, and patients maintained on dialysis.

In normal volunteers, the half-life of IV administered EPOGEN® is approximately 20% shorter than the half-life in CRF patients. The pharmacokinetics of EPOGEN® have not been studied in HIV-infected patients.

INDICATIONS AND USAGE

Treatment of Anemia of Chronic Renal Failure Patients

EPOGEN® is indicated for the treatment of anemia associated with CRF, including patients on dialysis (ESRD) and patients not on dialysis. EPOGEN® is indicated to elevate or maintain the red blood cell level (as manifested by the hematocrit or hemoglobin determinations) and to decrease the need for transfusions in these patients.

Non-dialysis patients with symptomatic anemia considered for therapy should have a hematocrit less than 30%.

EPOGEN® is not intended for patients who require immediate correction of severe anemia. EPOGEN® may obviate the need for maintenance transfusions but is not a substitute for emergency transfusion.

Prior to initiation of therapy, the patient's iron stores should be evaluated. Transferrin saturation should be at least 20% and ferritin at least 100 ng/mL. Blood pressure should be adequately controlled prior to initiation of EPOGEN® therapy, and must be closely monitored and controlled during therapy.

EPOGEN® should be administered under the guidance of a qualified physician (see DOSAGE AND ADMINISTRATION).

Treatment of Anemia in Zidovudine-treated HIV-infected Patients

EPOGEN® is indicated for the treatment of anemia related to therapy with zidovudine in HIV-infected patients. EPOGEN® is indicated to elevate or maintain the red blood cell level (as manifested by the hematocrit or hemoglobin determinations) and to decrease the need for transfusions in these patients. EPOGEN® is not indicated for the treatment of anemia in HIV-infected patients due to other factors such as iron or folate deficiencies, hemolysis or gastrointestinal bleeding, which should be managed appropriately.

EPOGEN®, at a dose of 100 Units/kg TIW, is effective in decreasing the transfusion requirement and increasing the red blood cell level of anemic, HIV-infected patients treated with zidovudine, when the endogenous serum erythropoietin level is ≤500 mUnits/mL and when patients are receiving a dose of zidovudine ≤4200 mg/week.

Treatment of Anemia in Cancer Patients on Chemotherapy

EPOGEN® is indicated for the treatment of anemia in patients with non-myeloid malignancies where anemia is due to the effect of concomitantly administered chemotherapy. EPOGEN® is indicated to decrease the need for transfusions in patients who will be receiving concomitant chemotherapy for a minimum of 2 months. EPOGEN® is not indicated for the treatment of anemia in cancer patients due to other factors such as iron or folate deficiencies, hemolysis or gastrointestinal bleeding which should be managed appropriately.

Reduction of Allogeneic Blood Transfusion in Surgery Patients

EPOGEN® is indicated for the treatment of anemic patients (hemoglobin >10 to ≤ 13 g/dL) scheduled to undergo elective, noncardiac, nonvascular surgery to reduce the need for allogeneic blood transfusions.[14–16] EPOGEN® is indicated for patients at high risk for perioperative transfusions with significant, anticipated blood loss. EPOGEN® is not indicated for anemic patients who are willing to donate autologous blood. The safety of the perioperative use of EPOGEN® has been studied only in patients who are receiving anticoagulant prophylaxis.

CLINICAL EXPERIENCE: RESPONSE TO EPOGEN®

Chronic Renal Failure Patients

Response to EPOGEN® was consistent across all studies. In the presence of adequate iron stores (see IRON EVALUATION), the time to reach the target hematocrit is a function of the baseline hematocrit and the rate of hematocrit rise. The rate of increase in hematocrit is dependent upon the dose of EPOGEN® administered and individual patient variation. In clinical trials at starting doses of 50 to 150 Units/kg TIW, patients responded with an average rate of hematocrit rise of:

STARTING DOSE (TIW IV)	HEMATOCRIT INCREASE POINTS/DAY	POINTS/2 WEEKS
50 Units/kg	0.11	1.5
100 Units/kg	0.18	2.5
150 Units/kg	0.25	3.5

Over this dose range, approximately 95% of all patients responded with a clinically significant increase in hematocrit, and by the end of approximately 2 months of therapy virtually all patients were transfusion-independent. Changes in the quality of life of patients treated with EPOGEN® were assessed as part of a Phase 3 clinical trial.[5,8] Once the target hematocrit (32% to 38%) was achieved, statistically significant improvements were demonstrated for most quality of life parameters measured, including energy and activity level, functional ability, sleep and eating behavior, health status, satisfaction with health, sex life, well-being, psychological effect, life satisfaction, and happiness. Patients also reported improvement in their disease symptoms. They showed a statistically significant increase in exercise capacity (VO_2 max), energy, and strength with a significant reduction in aching, dizziness, anxiety, shortness of breath, muscle weakness, and leg cramps.[8,17]

Patients on Dialysis

Thirteen clinical studies were conducted, involving IV administration to a total of 1010 anemic patients on dialysis for 986 patient-years of EPOGEN® therapy. In the three largest of these clinical trials, the median maintenance dose necessary to maintain the hematocrit between 30% to 36% was approximately 75 Units/kg TIW. In the US multicenter Phase 3 study, approximately 65% of the patients required doses of 100 Units/kg TIW, or less, to maintain their hematocrit at approximately 35%. Almost 10% of patients required a dose of 25 Units/kg, or less, and approximately 10% required a dose of more than 200 Units/kg TIW to maintain their hematocrit at this level.

A multicenter unit dose study was also conducted in 119 patients receiving peritoneal dialysis who self-administered EPOGEN® subcutaneously for approximately 109 patient-years of experience. Patients responded to EPOGEN® administered SC in a manner similar to patients receiving IV administration.[18]

Patients with CRF Not Requiring Dialysis

Four clinical trials were conducted in patients with CRF not on dialysis involving 181 patients treated with EPOGEN® for approximately 67 patient-years of experience. These patients responded to EPOGEN® therapy in a manner similar to that observed in patietns on dialysis. Patients with CRF not on dialysis demonstrated a dose-dependent and sustained increase in hematocrit when EPOGEN® was administered by either an IV or SC route, with similar rates of rise of hematocrit when EPOGEN® was administered by either route. Moreover, EPOGEN® doses of 75 to 150 Units/kg per week have been shown to maintain hematocrits of 36% to 38% for up to 6 months. Correcting the anemia of progressive renal failure will allow patients to remain active even though their renal function continues to decrease.[19–21]

Zidovudine-treated HIV-infected Patients

EPOGEN® has been studied in four placebo-controlled trials enrolling 297 anemic (hematocrit < 30%) HIV-infected (AIDS) patients receiving concomitant therapy with zidovudine (all patients were treated with Epoetin alfa manufactured by Amgen Inc.). In the subgroup of patients (89/125 EPOGEN® and 88/130 placebo) with prestudy endogenous serum erythropoietin levels ≤ 500 mUnits/mL, EPOGEN® reduced the mean cumulative number of units of blood transfused per patient by approximately 40% as compared to the placebo group.[22] Among those patients who required transfusions at baseline, 43% of patients treated with EPOGEN® versus 18% of placebo-treated patients were transfusion-independent during the second and third months of therapy. EPOGEN® therapy also resulted in significant increases in hematocrit in comparison to placebo. When examining the results according to the weekly dose of zidovudine received during month 3 of therapy, there was a statistically significant ($p < 0.003$) reduction in transfusion requirements in patients treated with EPOGEN® ($n = 51$) compared to placebo treated patients ($n = 54$) whose mean weekly zidovudine dose was ≤ 4200 mg/week.[22]

Approximately 17% of the patients with endogenous serum erythropoietin levels ≤ 500 mUnits/mL receiving EPOGEN® in doses from 100 to 200 Units/kg TIW achieved a hematocrit of 38% without administration of transfusions or significant reduction in zidovudine dose. In the subgroup of patients whose prestudy endogenous serum erythropoietin levels were > 500 mUnits/mL, EPOGEN® therapy did not reduce transfusion requirements or increase hematocrit, compared to the corresponding responses in placebo-treated patients. In a six month open-label EPOGEN® study, patients responded with decreased transfusion requirements and sustained increases in hematocrit and hemoglobin with doses of EPOGEN® up to 300 Units/kg TIW.[21–23]

Responsiveness to EPOGEN® therapy may be blunted by intercurrent infectious/inflammatory episodes and by an increase in zidovudine dosage. Consequently, the dose of EPOGEN® must be titrated based on these factors to maintain the desired erythropoietic response.

Cancer Patients on Chemotherapy

EPOGEN® has been studied in a series of placebo-controlled, double-blind trials in a total of 131 anemic cancer patients. Within this group, 72 patients were treated with concomitant non cisplatin-containing chemotherapy regimens and 59 patients were treated with concomitant cisplatin-containing chemotherapy regimens. Patients were randomized to EPOGEN® 150 Units/kg or placebo subcutaneously TIW for 12 weeks.

EPOGEN® therapy was associated with a significantly ($p < 0.008$) greater hematocrit response than in the corresponding placebo-treated patients (see table).[22]

HEMATOCRIT (%):
MEAN CHANGE FROM BASELINE TO FINAL VALUE*

STUDY	*EPOGEN®*	*PLACEBO*
Chemotherapy	7.6	1.3
Cisplatin	6.9	0.6

* Significantly higher in EPOGEN® patients than in placebo patients ($p<0.008$)

In the two types of chemotherapy studies (utilizing an EPOGEN® dose of 150 Units/kg TIW), the mean number of units of blood transfused per patient after the first month of therapy was significantly ($p < 0.02$) lower in patients treated with EPOGEN® (0.71 units in months 2, 3) than in corresponding placebo-treated patients (1.84 units in months 2, 3). Moreover, the proportion of patients transfused during months 2 and 3 of therapy combined was significantly ($p < 0.03$) lower in the patients treated with EPOGEN® than in the corresponding placebo-treated patients (22% vs 43%).[22]
Comparable intensity of chemotherapy in the EPOGEN® and placebo groups in the chemotherapy trials was suggested by a similar area under the neutrophil time curve in patients treated with EPOGEN® and placebo-treated patients as well as by a similar proportion of patients in groups treated with EPOGEN® and placebo-treated groups whose absolute neutrophil counts fell below 1000 cells/µL. Available evidence suggests that patients with lymphoid and solid cancers respond equivalently to EPOGEN® therapy, and that patients with or without tumor infiltration of the bone marrow respond equivalently to EPOGEN® therapy.

Surgery Patients

EPOGEN® has been studied in a placebo-controlled, double-blind trial enrolling 316 patients scheduled for major, elective orthopedic hip or knee surgery who were expected to require ≥ 2 units of blood and who were not able or willing to participate in an autologous blood donation program. Based on previous studies which demonstrated that pretreatment hemoglobin is a predictor of risk of receiving transfusion,[16,24] patients were stratified into one of three groups based on their pretreatment hemoglobin [≤ 10 (n = 2), > 10 to ≤ 13 (n = 96), and > 13 to ≤ 15 g/dL (n = 218)] and then randomly assigned to receive 300 Units/kg EPOGEN®, 100 Units/kg EPOGEN® or placebo by SC injection for 10 days before surgery, on the day of surgery, and for four days after surgery.[14] All patients received oral iron and a low-dose post-operative warfarin regimen.[14]
Treatment with EPOGEN® 300 Units/kg significantly ($p = 0.024$) reduced the risk of allogeneic transfusion in patients with a pretreatment hemoglobin of > 10 to ≤ 13 g/dL; 5/31 (16%) of EPOGEN® 300 Units/kg, 6/26 (23%) of EPOGEN® 100 Units/kg, and 13/29 (45%) of placebo-treated patients were transfused.[14] There was no significant difference in the number of patients transfused between EPOGEN® (9% 300 Units/kg, 6% 100 Units/kg) and placebo (13%) in the > 13 to ≤ 15 g/dL hemoglobin stratum. There were too few patients in the ≤ 10 g/dL group to determine if EPOGEN® is useful in this hemoglobin strata. In the > 10 to ≤ 13 g/dL pretreatment stratum, the mean number of units transfused per EPOGEN® treated patient (0.45 units blood for 300 Units/kg, 0.42 units blood for 100 Units/kg) was less than the mean transfused per placebo-treated patient (1.14 units) (overall $p = 0.028$). In addition, mean hemoglobin, hematocrit and reticulocyte counts increased significantly during the presurgery period in patients treated with EPOGEN®.[14]
EPOGEN® was also studied in an open-label, parallel-group trial enrolling 145 subjects with a pretreatment hemoglobin level of ≥ 10 to ≤ 13 g/dL who were scheduled for major orthopedic hip or knee surgery and who were not participating in an autologous program.[15] Subjects were randomly assigned to receive one of two SC dosing regimens of EPOGEN® (600 Units/kg once weekly for three weeks prior to surgery and on the day of surgery, or 300 Units/kg once daily for 10 days prior to surgery, on the day of surgery and for 4 days after surgery). All subjects received oral iron and appropriate pharmacologic anticoagulation therapy.
From pretreatment to presurgery, the mean increase in hemoglobin in the 600 Units/kg weekly group (1.44 g/dL) was greater than observed in the 300 Units/kg daily group.[15] The mean increase in absolute reticulocyte count was smaller in the weekly group ($0.11 \times 10^6/mm^3$) compared to the daily group ($0.17 \times 10^6/mm^3$). Mean hemoglobin levels were similar for the two treatment groups throughout the postsurgical period.
The erythropoietic response observed in both treatment groups resulted in similar transfusion rates [11/69 (16%) in the 600 Units/kg weekly group and 14/71 (20%) in the 300 Units/kg daily group].[15] The mean number of units transfused per subject was approximately 0.3 units in both treatment groups.

CONTRAINDICATIONS

EPOGEN® is contraindicated in patients with:

1. Uncontrolled hypertension.
2. Known hypersensitivity to mammalian cell-derived products.
3. Known hypersensitivity to Albumin (Human).

WARNINGS

Pediatric Use

The multidose preserved formulation contains benzyl alcohol. Benzyl alcohol has been reported to be associated with an increased incidence of neurological and other complications in premature infants which are sometimes fatal. The safety and effectiveness of Epoetin alfa in pediatric patients have not been established.

Thrombotic Events and Increased Mortality

A randomized, prospective trial of 1265 hemodialysis patients with clinically evident cardiac disease (ischemic heart disease or congestive heart failure) was conducted in which patients were assigned to EPOGEN® treatment targeted to a maintenance hematocrit of either 42 ± 3% or 30 ± 3%. Increased mortality was observed in 634 patients randomized to a target hematocrit of 42% [221 deaths (35% mortality)] compared to 631 patients targeted to remain at a hematocrit of 30% [185 deaths (29% mortality)]. The reason for the increased mortality observed in these studies is unknown, however the incidence of non-fatal myocardial infarctions (3.1% vs 2.3%), vascular access thromboses (39% vs 29%), and all other thrombotic events (22% vs 18%) were also higher in the group randomized to achieve a hematocrit of 42%.
Increased mortality was also observed in a randomized placebo-controlled study of EPOGEN® in patients who did not have CRF who were undergoing coronary artery bypass surgery (7 deaths in 126 patients randomized to EPOGEN® versus no deaths among 56 patients receiving placebo). Four of these deaths occurred during the period of study drug administration and all 4 deaths were associated with thrombotic events. While the extent of the population affected is unknown, in patients at risk for thrombosis, the anticipated benefits of EPOGEN® treatment should be weighed against the potential for increased risks associated with therapy.

Chronic Renal Failure Patients

Hypertension: Patients with uncontrolled hypertension should not be treated with EPOGEN®; blood pressure should be controlled adequately before initiation of therapy. Up to 80% of patients with CRF have a history of hypertension.[25] Although there does not appear to be any direct pressor effects of EPOGEN®, blood pressure may rise during EPOGEN® therapy. During the early phase of treatment when the hematocrit is increasing, approximately 25% of patients on dialysis may require initiation of, or increases in, antihypertensive therapy. Hypertensive encephalopathy and seizures have been observed in patients with CRF treated with EPOGEN®.
Special care should be taken to closely monitor and agressively control blood pressure in patients treated with EPOGEN®. Patients should be advised as to the importance of compliance with antihypertensive therapy and dietary restrictions. If blood pressure is difficult to control by initiation of appropriate measures, the hematocrit may be reduced by decreasing or withholding the dose of EPOGEN®. A clinically significant decrease in hematocrit may not be observed for several weeks.
It is recommended that the dose of EPOGEN® be decreased if the hematocrit increase exceeds 4 points in any 2-week period, because of the possible association of excessive rate of rise of hematocrit with an exacerbation of hypertension. In CRF patients on hemodialysis with clinically evident ischemic heart disease or congestive heart failure, the hematocrit should be managed carefully, not to exceed 36% (SEE THROMBOTIC EVENTS).
Seizures: Seizures have occurred in patients with CRF participating in EPOGEN® clinical trials.
In patients on dialysis, there was a higher incidence of seizures during the first 90 days of therapy (occurring in approximately 2.5% of patients) as compared with later timepoints.
Given the potential for an increased risk of seizures during the first 90 days of therapy, blood pressure and the presence of premonitory neurologic symptoms should be monitored closely. Patients should be cautioned to avoid potentially hazardous activities such as driving or operating heavy machinery during this period.
While the relationship between seizures and the rate of rise of hematocrit is uncertain, it is recommended that the dose of EPOGEN® be decreased if the hematocrit increase exceeds 4 points in any 2-week period.
Thrombotic Events: During hemodialysis, patients treated with EPOGEN® may require increased anticoagulation with heparin to prevent clotting of the artificial kidney (see ADVERSE REACTIONS for more information about thrombotic events).
Other thrombotic events (eg, myocardial infarction, cerebrovascular accident, transient ischemic attack) have occurred in clinical trials at an annualized rate of less than 0.04 events per patient per year of EPOGEN® therapy. These trials were conducted in patients with CRF (whether on dialysis or not) in whom the target hematocrit was 32% to 40%. However, the risk of thrombotic events, including vascular access thrombosis, was significantly increased in patients with ischemic heart disease or congestive heart failure receiving EPOGEN® therapy with the goal of reaching a normal hematocrit (42%) as compared to a target hematocrit of 30%. Patients with pre-existing cardiovascular disease should be monitored closely.

Zidovudine-treated HIV-infected Patients

In contrast to CRF patients, EPOGEN® therapy has not been linked to exacerbation of hypertension, seizures, and thrombotic events in HIV-infected patients.

PRECAUTIONS

The parenteral administration of any biologic product should be attended by appropriate precautions in case allergic or other untoward reactions occur (see CONTRAINDICATIONS). In clinical trials, while transient rashes were occasionally observed concurrently with EPOGEN® therapy, no serious allergic or anaphylactic reactions were reported (see ADVERSE REACTIONS for more information regarding allergic reactions).
The safety and efficacy of EPOGEN® therapy have not been established in patients with a known history of a seizure disorder or underlying hematologic disease (eg, sickle cell anemia, myelodysplastic syndromes, or hypercoagulable disorders).
In some female patients, menses have resumed following EPOGEN® therapy; the possibility of pregnancy should be discussed and the need for contraception evaluated.

Hematology

Exacerbation of porphyria has been observed rarely in patients with CRF treated with EPOGEN®. However, EPOGEN® has not caused increased urinary excretion of porphyrin metabolites in normal volunteers, even in the presence of a rapid erythropoietic response. Nevertheless, EPOGEN® should be used with caution in patients with known porphyria.
In preclinical studies in dogs and rats, but not in monkeys, EPOGEN® therapy was associated with subclinical bone marrow fibrosis. Bone marrow fibrosis is a known complication of CRF in humans and may be related to secondary hyperparathyroidism or unknown factors. The incidence of bone marrow fibrosis was not increased in a study of patients on dialysis who were treated with EPOGEN® for 12 to 19 months, compared to the incidence of bone marrow fibrosis in a matched group of patients who had not been treated with EPOGEN®.
Hematocrit in CRF patients should be measured twice a week, zidovudine-treated HIV-infected and cancer patients should have hematocrit measured once a week until hematocrit has been stabilized, and measured periodically thereafter.

Delayed or Diminished Response

If the patient fails to respond or to maintain a response to doses within the recommended dosing range, the following etiologies should be considered and evaluated:

1. Iron deficiency: Virtually all patients will eventually require supplemental iron therapy (see IRON EVALUATION).
2. Underlying infectious, inflammatory, or malignant processes.
3. Occult blood loss.
4. Underlying hematologic diseases (ie, thalassemia, refractory anemia, or other myelodysplastic disorders).
5. Vitamin deficiencies: Folic acid or vitamin B12.
6. Hemolysis.
7. Aluminum intoxication.
8. Osteitis fibrosa cystica.

Iron Evlauation

During EPOGEN® therapy, absolute or functional iron deficiency may develop. Functional iron deficiency, with normal ferritin levels but low transferrin saturation, is presumably due to the inability to mobilize iron stores rapidly enough to support increased erythropoiesis. Transferrin saturation should be at least 20% and ferritin should be at least 100 ng/mL.
Prior to and during EPOGEN® therapy, the patient's iron status, including transferrin saturation (serum iron divided by iron binding capacity) and serium ferritin, should be evaluated. Virtually all patients will eventually require supplemental iron to increase or maintain transferrin saturation to levels which will adequately support erythropoiesis stimulated by EPOGEN®. All surgery patients being treated with EPOGEN® should receive adequate iron supplementation throughout the course of therapy in order to support erythropoiesis and avoid depletion of iron stores.

Drug Interaction

No evidence of interaction of EPOGEN® with other drugs was observed in the course of clinical trials.

Continued on next page

Epogen—Cont.

Carcinogenesis, Mutagenesis, and Impairment of Fertility
Carcinogenic potential of EPOGEN® has not been evaluated. EPOGEN® does not induce bacterial gene mutation (Ames Test), chromosomal aberrations in mammalian cells, micronuclei in mice, or gene mutation at the HGPRT locus. In female rats treated IV with EPOGEN®, there was a trend for slightly increased fetal wastage at doses of 100 and 500 Units/kg.

Pregnancy Category C
EPOGEN® has been shown to have adverse effects in rats when given in doses 5 times the human dose. There are no adequate and well-controlled studies in pregnant women. EPOGEN® should be used during pregnancy only if potential benefit justifies the potential risk to the fetus.

In studies of female rats, there were decreases in body weight gain, delays in appearance of abdominal hair, delayed eyelid opening, delayed ossification, and decreases in the number of caudal vertebrae in the F1 fetuses of the 500 Units/kg group. In female rats treated IV, there was a trend for slightly increased fetal wastage at dosages of 100 and 500 Units/kg. EPOGEN® has not shown any adverse effect at doses as high as 500 Units/kg in pregnant rabbits (from day 6 to 18 of gestation).

Nursing Mothers
Postnatal observations of the live offspring (F1 generation) of female rats treated with EPOGEN® during gestation and lactation revealed no effect of EPOGEN® at doses of up to 500 Units/kg. There were, however, decreases in body weight gain, delays in appearance of abdominal hair, eyelid opening, and decreases in the number of caudal vertebrae in the F1 fetuses of the 500 Units/kg group. There were no EPOGEN®-related effects on the F2 generation fetuses.

It is not known whether EPOGEN® is excreted in human milk. Because many drugs are excreted in human milk, caution should be exercised when EPOGEN® is administered to a nursing woman.

Pediatric Use
The safety and effectiveness of EPOGEN® in pediatric patients have not been established (see WARNINGS).

Chronic Renal Failure Patients

Patients with CRF Not Requiring Dialysis
Blood pressure and hematocrit should be monitored no less frequently than for patients maintained on dialysis. Renal function and fluid and electrolyte balance should be closely monitored, as an improved sense of well-being may obscure the need to initiate dialysis in some patients.

Hematology: Sufficient time should be allowed to determine a patient's responsiveness to a dosage of EPOGEN® before adjusting the dose. Because of the time required for erythropoiesis and the red cell half-life, an interval of 2 to 6 weeks may occur between the time of a dose adjustment (initiation, increase, decrease, or discontinuation) and a significant change in hematocrit.

In order to avoid reaching the suggested target hematocrit too rapidly, or exceeding the suggested target range (hematocrit of 30% to 36%), the guidelines for dose and frequency of dose adjustments (see DOSAGE AND ADMINISTRATION) should be followed.

For patients who respond to EPOGEN® with a rapid increase in hematocrit (eg, more than 4 points in any 2-week period), the dose of EPOGEN® should be reduced because of the possible association of excessive rate of rise of hematocrit with an exacerbation of hypertension.

The elevated bleeding time characteristic of CRF decreases toward normal after correction of anemia in patients treated with EPOGEN®. Reduction of bleeding time also occurs after correction of anemia by transfusion.

Laboratory Monitoring: The hematocrit should be determined twice a week until it has stabilized in the suggested target range and the maintenance dose has been established. After any dose adjustment, the hematocrit should also be determined twice weekly for at least 2 to 6 weeks until it has been determined that the hematocrit has stabilized in response to the dose change. The hematocrit should then be monitored at regular intervals.

A complete blood count with differential and platelet count should be performed regularly. During clinical trials, modest increases were seen in platelets and white blood cell counts. While these changes were statistically significant, they were not clinically significant and the values remained within normal ranges.

In patients with CRF, serum chemistry values [including blood urea nitrogen (BUN), uric acid, creatinine, phosphorus, and potassium] should be monitored regularly. During clinical trials in patients on dialysis, modest increases were seen in BUN, creatinine, phosphorus, and potassium. In some patients with CRF not on dialysis, treated with EPOGEN®, modest increases in serum uric acid and phosphorus were observed. While changes were statistically significant, the values remained within the ranges normally seen in patients with CRF.

Diet: As the hematocrit increases and patients experience an improved sense of well-being and quality of life, the importance of compliance with dietary and dialysis prescriptions should be reinforced. In particular, hyperkalemia is not uncommon in patients with CRF. In US studies in patients on dialysis, hyperkalemia has occurred at an annualized rate of approximately 0.11 episodes per patient-year of EPOGEN® therapy, often in association with poor compliance to medication, diet, and/or dialysis.

Dialysis Management: Therapy with EPOGEN® results in an increase in hematocrit and a decrease in plasma volume which could affect dialysis efficiency. In studies to date, the resulting increase in hematocrit did not appear to adversely affect dialyzer function[9,10] or the efficiency of high flux hemodialysis.[11] During hemodialysis, patients treated with EPOGEN® may require increased anticoagulation with heparin to prevent clotting of the artificial kidney.

Patients who are marginally dialyzed may require adjustments in their dialysis prescription. As with all patients on dialysis, the serum chemistry values (including BUN, creatinine, phosphorus, and potassium) in patients treated with EPOGEN® should be monitored regularly to assure the adequacy of the dialysis prescription.

Information for Patients: In those situations in which the physician determines that a home dialysis patient can safely and effectively self-administer EPOGEN®, the patient should be instructed as to the proper dosage and administration. Home dialysis patients should be referred to the full "Information for Home Dialysis Patients" insert; it is not a disclosure of all possible effects. Patients should be informed of the signs and symptoms of allergic drug reaction and advised of appropriate actions. If home use is prescribed for a home dialysis patient, the patient should be thoroughly instructed in the importance of proper disposal and cautioned against the reuse of needles, syringes, or drug product. A puncture-resistant container for the disposal of used syringes and needles should be available to the patient. The full container should be disposed of according to the directions provided by the physician.

Renal Function: In patients with CRF not on dialysis, renal function and fluid and electrolyte balance should be closely monitored, as an improved sense of well-being may obscure the need to initiate dialysis in some patients. In patients with CRF not on dialysis, placebo-controlled studies of progression of renal dysfunction over periods of greater than one year have not been completed. In shorter term trials in patients with CRF not on dialysis, changes in creatinine and creatinine clearance were not significantly different in patients treated with EPOGEN®, compared with placebo-treated patients. Analysis of the slope of 1/serum creatinine versus time plots in these patients indicates no significant change in the slope after the initiation of EPOGEN® therapy.

Zidovudine-treated HIV-infected Patients
Hypertension: Exacerbation of hypertension has not been observed in zidovudine-treated HIV-infected patients treated with EPOGEN®. However, EPOGEN® should be withheld in these patients if pre-existing hypertension is uncontrolled, and should not be started until blood pressure is controlled. In double-blind studies, a single seizure has been experienced by a patient treated with EPOGEN®.[22]

Cancer Patients on Chemotherapy
Hypertension: Hypertension, associated with a significant increase in hematocrit, has been noted rarely in patients treated with EPOGEN®. Nevertheless, blood pressure in patients treated with EPOGEN® should be monitored carefully, particularly in patients with an underlying history of hypertension or cardiovascular disease.

Seizures: In double-blind, placebo-controlled trials, 3.2% (n=2/63) of patients treated with EPOGEN® and 2.9% (n=2/68) of placebo-treated patients had seizures. Seizures in 1.6% (n=1/63) of patients treated with EPOGEN® occurred in the context of a significant increase in blood pressure and hematocrit from baseline values. However, both patients treated with EPOGEN® also had underlying CNS pathology which may have been related to seizure activity.

Thrombotic Events: In double-blind, placebo-controlled trials, 3.2% (n=2/63) of patients treated with EPOGEN® and 11.8% (n=8/68) of placebo-treated patients had thrombotic events (eg, pulmonary embolism, cerebrovascular accident).

Growth Factor Potential: EPOGEN® is a growth factor that primarily stimulates red cell production. However, the possibility that EPOGEN® can act as a growth factor for any tumor type, particularly myeloid malignancies, cannot be excluded.

Surgery patients
Thrombotic/Vascular Events: In perioperative clinical trials with orthopedic patients, the overall incidence of thrombotic/vascular events was similar in Epoetin alfa and placebo-treated patients who had a pretreatment hemoglobin of >10 to ≤13 g/dL. In patients with a hemoglobin of >13 g/dL treated with 300 Units/kg of Epoetin alfa, the possibility that EPOGEN® treatment may be associated with an increased risk of postoperative thrombotic/vascular events cannot be excluded.[14–16]

In one study in which Epoetin alfa was administered in the perioperative period to patients undergoing coronary artery bypass graft surgery, there were seven deaths in the group treated with Epoetin alfa (n=126) and no deaths in the placebo-treated group (n=56). Among the seven deaths in the patients treated with Epoetin alfa, four were at the time of therapy (between study day 2 and 8). The four deaths at the time of therapy (3%) were associated with thrombotic/vascular events. A causative role of Epoetin alfa cannot be excluded (see WARNINGS).

Hypertension: Blood pressure may rise in the perioperative period in patients being treated with EPOGEN®. Therefore, blood pressure should be monitored carefully.

ADVERSE REACTIONS

Chronic Renal Failure Patients
EPOGEN® is generally well-tolerated. The adverse events reported are frequent sequelae of CRF and are not necessarily attributable to EPOGEN® therapy. In double-blind, placebo-controlled studies involving over 300 patients with CRF, the events reported in greater than 5% of patients treated with EPOGEN® during the blinded phase were:

PERCENT OF PATIENTS REPORTING EVENT

Event	Patients Treated with EPOGEN® (n = 200)	Placebo-Treated Patients (n =135)
Hypertension	24%	19%
Headache	16%	12%
Arthralgias	11%	6%
Nausea	11%	9%
Edema	9%	10%
Fatigue	9%	14%
Diarrhea	9%	6%
Vomiting	8%	5%
Chest Pain	7%	9%
Skin Reaction, Administration Site	7%	12%
Asthenia	7%	12%
Dizziness	7%	13%
Clotted Access	7%	2%

Significant adverse events of concern in patients with CRF treated in double-blind, placebo-controlled trials occurred in the following percent of patients during the blinded phase of the studies:

Seizure	1.1%	1.1%
CVA/TIA	0.4%	0.6%
MI	0.4%	1.1%
Death	0%	1.7%

In the US EPOGEN® studies in patients on dialysis (over 567 patients), the incidence (number of events per patient-year) of the most frequently reported adverse events were hypertension (0.75), headache (0.40), tachycardia (0.31), nausea/vomiting (0.26), clotted vascular access (0.25), shortness of breath (0.14), hyperkalemia (0.11), and diarrhea (0.11). Other reported events occurred at a rate of less than 0.10 events per patient per year.

Events reported to have occurred within several hours of administration of EPOGEN® were rare, mild, and transient, and included injection site stinging in dialysis patients and flu-like symptoms such as arthralgias and myalgias.

In all studies analyzed to date, EPOGEN® administration was generally well-tolerated, irrespective of the route of administration.

Hypertension: Increases in blood pressure have been reported in clinical trials, often during the first 90 days of therapy. On occasion, hypertensive encephalopathy and seizures have been observed in patients with CRF treated with EPOGEN®. When data from all patients in the US Phase 3 multicenter trial were analyzed, there was an apparent trend of more reports of hypertensive adverse events in patients on dialysis with a faster rate of rise of hematocrit (greater than 4 hematocrit points in any 2–week period). However, in a double-blind, placebo-controlled trial, hypertensive adverse events were not reported at an increased rate in the group treated with EPOGEN® (150 Units/kg TIW) relative to the placebo group.

Seizures: There have been 47 seizures in 1010 patients on dialysis treated with EPOGEN® in clinical trials, with an exposure of 986 patient-years for a rate of approximately 0.048 events per patient-year. However, there appeared to be a higher rate of seizures during the first 90 days of therapy (occurring in approximately 2.5% of patients) when compared to subsequent 90–day periods. The baseline incidence of seizures in the untreated dialysis population is difficult to determine; it appears to be in the range of 5% to 10% per patient-year.[26–28]

Thrombotic Events: In clinical trials where the maintenance hematocrit was 35 ± 3% on EPOGEN®, clotting of the vascular access (A-V shunt) has occurred at an annualized rate of about 0.25 events per patient-year, and other thrombotic events (eg, myocardial infarction, cerebral vascular accident, transient ischemic attack, and pulmonary

PRODUCT INFORMATION

embolism) occurred at a rate of 0.04 events per patient-year. In a separate study of 1111 untreated dialysis patients, clotting of the vascular access occurred at a rate of 0.50 events per patient-year. However, in CRF patients on hemodialysis who also had clinically evident ischemic heart disease or congestive heart failure, the risk of A-V shunt thrombosis was higher (39% vs 29%, p <0.001), and myocardial infarctions, vascular ischemic events, and venous thrombosis were increased, in patients targeted to a hematocrit of 42 ± 3% compared to those maintained at 30 ± 3% (see WARNINGS).

In patients treated with commercial EPOGEN®, there have been rare reports of serious or unusual thrombo-embolic events including migratory thrombophlebitis, microvascular thrombosis, pulmonary embolus, and thrombosis of the retinal artery, and temporal and renal veins. A causal relationship has not been established.

Allergic Reactions: There have been no reports of serious allergic reactions or anaphylaxis associated with EPOGEN® administration during clinical trials. Skin rashes and urticaria have been observed rarely and when reported have generally been mild and transient in nature.

There have been rare reports of potentially serious allergic reactions including urticaria with associated respiratory symptoms or circumoral edema, or urticaria alone. Most reactions occurred in situations where a causal relationship could not be established. Symptoms recurred with rechallenge in a few instances, suggesting that allergic reactivity may occasionally be associated with EPOGEN® therapy. There has been no evidence for development of antibodies to erythropoietin in patients tested to date, including those receiving EPOGEN® for over 4 years. Nevertheless, if an anaphylactoid reaction occurs, EPOGEN® should be immediately discontinued and appropriate therapy initiated.

Zidovudine-treated HIV-infected Patients

Adverse events reported in clinical trials with EPOGEN® in zidovudine-treated HIV-infected patients were consistent with the progression of HIV infection. In double-blind, placebo-controlled studies of three-months duration involving approximately 300 zidovudine-treated HIV-infected patients, adverse events with an incidence of ≥ 10% in either patients treated with EPOGEN® or placebo-treated patients were:

PERCENT OF PATIENTS REPORTING EVENT

Event	Patients Treated with EPOGEN® (n = 144)	Placebo-Treated Patients (n = 153)
Pyrexia	38%	29%
Fatigue	25%	31%
Headache	19%	14%
Cough	18%	14%
Diarrhea	16%	18%
Rash	16%	8%
Congestion, Respiratory	15%	10%
Nausea	15%	12%
Shortness of Breath	14%	13%
Asthenia	11%	14%
Skin Reaction, Medication Site	10%	7%
Dizziness	9%	10%

There were no statistically significant differences between treatment groups in the incidence of the above events. In the 297 patients studied, EPOGEN® was not associated with significant increses in opportunistic infections or mortality.[22] In 71 patients from this group treated with EPOGEN® at 150 Units/kg TIW, serum p24 antigen levels did not appear to increase.[23] Preliminary data showed no enhancement of HIV replication in infected cell lines in vitro.[22] Peripheral white blood cell and platelet counts are unchanged following EPOGEN® therapy.

Allergic Reactions: Two zidovudine-treated HIV-infected patients had urticarial reactions within 48 hours of their first exposure to study medication. One patient was treated with EPOGEN® and one was treated with placebo (EPOGEN® vehicle alone). Both patients had positive immediate skin tests against their study medication with a negative saline control. The basis for this apparent pre-existing hypersitivity to components of the EPOGEN® formulation is unknown, but may be related to HIV-induced immunosuppression or prior exposure to blood products.

Seizures: In double-blind and open-label trials of EPOGEN® in zidovudine-treated HIV-infected patients, 10 patients have experienced seizures.[22] In general, these seizures appear to be related to underlying pathology, such as meningitis or cerebral neoplasms, not EPOGEN® therapy.

Cancer Patients on Chemotherapy

Adverse experiences reported in clinical trials with EPOGEN® in cancer patients were consistent with the underlying disease state. In double-blind, placebo-controlled studies of up to 3 months duration involving 131 cancer patients, adverse effects with an incidence > 10% in either patients treated with EPOGEN® or placebo-treated patients were as indicated below:

PERCENT OF PATIENTS REPORTING EVENT

Event	Patients Treated with EPOGEN® 300 U/kg (n = 112)[a]	Patients Treated with EPOGEN® 100 U/kg (n = 101)[a]	Placebo-treated Patients (n = 103)[a]	Patients Treated with EPOGEN® 600 U/kg (n = 73)[b]	Patients Treated with EPOGEN® 300 U/kg (n = 72)[b]
Pyrexia	51%	50%	60%	47%	42%
Nausea	48%	43%	45%	45%	58%
Constipation	43%	42%	43%	51%	53%
Skin reaction, Medication site	25%	19%	22%	26%	29%
Vomiting	22%	12%	14%	21%	29%
Skin Pain	18%	18%	17%	5%	4%
Pruritus	16%	16%	14%	14%	22%
Insomnia	13%	16%	13%	21%	18%
Headache	13%	11%	9%	10%	19%
Dizziness	12%	9%	12%	11%	21%
Urinary Tract Infection	12%	3%	11%	11%	8%
Hypertension	10%	11%	10%	5%	10%
Diarrhea	10%	7%	12%	10%	6%
Deep Venous Thrombosis	10%	3%	5%	0%[c]	0%[c]
Dyspepsia	9%	11%	6%	7%	8%
Anxiety	7%	2%	11%	11%	4%
Edema	6%	11%	8%	11%	7%

[a] Study including patients undergoing orthopedic surgery treated with EPOGEN® or placebo for 15 days
[b] Study including patients undergoing orthopedic surgery treated with EPOGEN® 600 Units/kg weekly × 4 or 300 Units/kg daily × 15
[c] Determined by clinical symptoms

Although some statistically significant differences between patients being treated with EPOGEN®- and placebo-treated patients were noted, the overall safety profile of EPOGEN® appeared to be consistent with the disease process of advanced cancer. During double-blind and subsequent open-label therapy in which patients (n = 72 for total exposure to EPOGEN®) were treated for up to 32 weeks with doses as high as 927 Units/kg, the adverse experience profile of EPOGEN® was consistent with the progression of advanced cancer.

Based on comparable survival data and on the percentage of patients treated with EPOGEN® and placebo-treated patients who discontinued therapy due to death, disease progression, or adverse experiences (22% and 13%, respectively; p = 0.25), the clinical outcome in patients treated with EPOGEN® and placebo-treated patients appeared to be similar. Available data from animal tumor models and measurement of proliferation of solid tumor cells from clinical biopsy specimens in response to EPOGEN® suggest that EPOGEN® does not potentiate tumor growth. Nevertheless, as a growth factor, the possibility that EPOGEN® may potentiate growth of some tumors, particularly myeloid tumors, cannot be excluded. A randomized controlled Phase 4 study is currently ongoing to further evaluate this issue. The mean peripheral white blood cell count was unchanged following EPOGEN® therapy compared to the corresponding value in the placebo-treated group.

Surgery Patients

Adverse events with an incidence of ≥ 10% are shown in the following table:
[See table at top of page]

PERCENT OF PATIENTS REPORTING EVENT

Event	Patients Treated with EPOGEN® (n = 63)	Placebo-Treated Patients (n = 68)
Pyrexia	29%[a]	19%
Diarrhea	21%[a]	7%
Nausea	17%[b]	32%
Vomiting	17%	15%
Edema	17%[c]	1%
Asthenia	13%	16%
Fatigue	13%	15%
Shortness of Breath	13%	9%
Parasthesia	11%	6%
Upper Respiratory Infection	11%	4%
Dizziness	5%	12%
Trunk Pain	3%[d]	16%

[a] p=0.041,
[b] p=0.069,
[c] p=0.0016,
[d] p=0.017

Thrombotic/Vascular Events: In three double-blind, placebo-controlled orthopedic surgery studies, the rate of deep venous thrombosis (DVT) was similar among Epoetin alfa and placebo-treated patients in the recommended population of patients with a pretreatment hemoglobin of > 10 to ≤ 13 g/dL.[14,16,24] However, in 2 of 3 orthopedic surgery studies the overall rate (all pretreatment hemoglobin groups combined) of DVTs detected by postoperative ultrasonography and/or surveillance venography was higher in the group treated with Epoetin alfa than in the placebo-treated group (11% vs 6%). This finding was attributable to the difference in DVT rates observed in the subgroup of patients with pretreatment hemoglobin > 13 g/dL. However, the incidence of DVTs was within the range of that reported in the literature for orthopedic surgery patients.

In the orthopedic surgery study of patients with pretreatment hemoglobin of > 10 to ≤ 13 g/dL which compared two dosing regimens (600 Units/kg weekly × 4 and 300 Units/kg daily × 15), 4 subjects in the 600 Units/kg weekly EPOGEN® group (5%) and no subjects in the 300 Units/kg daily group had a thrombotic vascular event during the study period.[15]

In a study examining the use of Epoetin alfa in 182 patients scheduled for coronary artery bypass graft surgery 23% of patients treated with Epoetin alfa and 29% treated with placebo experienced thrombotic/vascular events. There were 4 deaths among the Epoetin alfa-treated patients that were associated with a thrombotic/vascular event. A causative role of Epoetin alfa cannot be excluded (see WARNINGS).

OVERDOSAGE

The maximum amount of EPOGEN® that can be safely administered in single or multiple doses has not been determined. Doses of up to 1500 Units/kg TIW for 3 to 4 weeks have been administered without any direct toxic effects of EPOGEN® itself.[6] Therapy with EPOGEN® can result in polycythemia if the hematocrit is not carefully monitored and the dose appropriately adjusted. If the suggested target range is exceeded, EPOGEN® may be temporarily withheld until the hematocrit returns to the suggested target range; EPOGEN® therapy may then be resumed using a lower dose (see DOSAGE AND ADMINISTRATION). If polycythemia is of concern, phlebotomy may be indicated to decrease the hematocrit.

DOSAGE AND ADMINISTRATION

Chronic Renal Failure Patients

Starting doses of EPOGEN® over the range of 50 to 100 Units/kg TIW have been shown to be safe and effective in increasing hematocrit and eliminating transfusion dependency in patients with CRF (see CLINICAL EXPERIENCE). The dose of EPOGEN® should be reduced as the hematocrit approaches 36% or increases by more than 4 points in any 2-week period. The dosage of EPOGEN® must be individualized to maintain the hematocrit within the suggested target range. At the physician's discretion, the suggested target hematocrit range may be expanded to achieve maximal patient benefit.

Continued on next page

Epogen—Cont.

EPOGEN® may be given either as an IV or SC injection. In patients on hemodialysis, EPOGEN® usually has been administered as an IV bolus TIW. While the administration of EPOGEN® is independent of the dialysis procedure, EPOGEN® may be administered into the venous line at the end of the dialysis procedure to obviate the need for additional venous access. In patients with CRF not on dialysis, EPOGEN® may be given either as an IV or SC injection.
Patients who have been judged competent by their physicians to self-administer EPOGEN® without medical or other supervision may give themselves either an IV or SC injection. The table below provides general therapeutic guidelines for patients with CRF:

Starting Dose:	50 to 100 Units/kg TIW; IV or SC
Reduce Dose When:	1. Hct. approaches 36% or, 2. Hct. increases > 4 points in any 2-week period
Increase Dose If:	Hct. does not increase by 5 to 6 points after 8 weeks of therapy, and hct. is below suggested target range
Maintenance Dose:	Individually titrate
Suggested Target Hct. Range:	30% to 36%

During therapy, hematological parameters should be monitored regularly (see LABORATORY MONITORING).

Pre-therapy Iron Evaluation: Prior to and during EPOGEN® therapy, the patient's iron stores, including transferrin saturation (serum iron divided by iron binding capacity) and serum ferritin, should be evaluated. Transferrin saturation should be at least 20%, and ferritin should be at least 100 ng/mL. Virtually all patients will eventually require supplemental iron to increase or maintain transferrin saturation to levels that will adequately support erythropoiesis stimulated by EPOGEN®.

Dose Adjustment: Following EPOGEN® therapy, a period of time is required for erythroid progenitors to mature and be released into circulation resulting in an eventual increase in hematocrit. Additionally, red blood cell survival time affects hematocrit and may vary due to uremia. As a result, the time required to elicit a clinically significant change in hematocrit (increase or decrease) following any dose adjustment may be 2 to 6 weeks.
Dose adjustment should not be made more frequently than once a month, unless clinically indicated. After any dose adjustment, the hematocrit should be determined twice weekly for at least 2 to 6 weeks (see LABORATORY MONITORING).

- If the hematocrit is increasing and approaching 36%, the dose should be reduced to maintain the suggested target hematocrit range. If the reduced dose does not stop the rise in hematocrit, and it exceeds 36%, doses should be temporarily withheld until the hematocrit begins to decrease, at which point therapy should be reinitiated at a lower dose.
- At any time, if the hematocrit increases by more than 4 points in a 2-week period, the dose should be immediately decreased. After the dose reduction, the hematocrit should be monitored twice weekly for 2 to 6 weeks, and further dose adjustments should be made as outlined in MAINTENANCE DOSE.
- If a hematocrit increase of 5 to 6 points is not achieved after an 8-week period and iron stores are adequate (see DELAYED OR DIMINISHED RESPONSE), the dose of EPOGEN® may be incrementally increased. Further increases may be made at 4 to 6 week intervals until the desired response is attained.

Maintenance Dose: The maintenance dose must be individualized for each patient on dialysis. In the US Phase 3 multicenter trial in patients on hemodialysis, the median maintenance dose was 75 Units/kg TIW, with a range from 12.5 to 525 Units/kg TIW. Almost 10% of the patients required a dose of 25 Units/kg, or less, and approximately 10% of the patients required more than 200 Units/kg TIW to maintain their hematocrit in the suggested target range.
If the hematocrit remains below, or falls below, the suggested target range, iron stores should be re-evaluated. If the transferrin saturation is less than 20%, supplemental iron should be administered. If the transferrin saturation is greater than 20%, the dose of EPOGEN® may be increased. Such dose increases should not be made more frequently than once a month, unless clinically indicated, as the response time of the hematocrit to a dose increase can be 2 to 6 weeks. Hematocrit should be measured twice weekly for 2 to 6 weeks following dose increases. In patients with CRF not on dialysis, the maintenance dose must also be individualized. EPOGEN® doses of 75 to 150 Units/kg per week have been shown to maintain hematocrits of 36% to 38% for up to 6 months.

Delayed or Diminished Response: Over 95% of patients with CRF responded with clinically significant increases in hematocrit, and virtually all patients were transfusion-independent within approximately 2 months of initiation of EPOGEN® therapy.
If a patient fails to respond or maintain a response, other etiologies should be considered and evaluated as clinically indicated (see PRECAUTIONS for discussion of delayed or diminshed response).

Zidovudine-treated HIV-infected Patients

Prior to beginning EPOGEN®, it is recommended that the endogenous serum erythropoietin level be determined (prior to transfusion). Available evidence suggests that patients receiving zidovudine with endogenous serum erythropoietin levels > 500 mUnits/mL are unlikely to respond to therapy with EPOGEN®.

Starting Dose: For patients with serum erythropoietin levels ≤ 500 mUnits/mL who are receiving a dose of zidovudine ≤ 4200 mg/week, the recommended starting dose of EPOGEN® is 100 Units/kg as an IV or SC injection TIW for 8 weeks.

Increase Dose: During the dose adjustment phase of therapy, the hematocrit should be monitored weekly. If the response is not satisfactory in terms of reducing transfusion requirements or increasing hematocrit after 8 weeks of therapy, the dose of EPOGEN® can be increased by 50 to 100 Units/kg TIW. Response should be evaluated every 4 to 8 weeks thereafter and the dose adjusted accordingly by 50 to 100 Units/kg increments TIW. If patients have not responded satisfactorily to an EPOGEN® dose of 300 Units/kg TIW, it is unlikely that they will respond to higher doses of EPOGEN®.

Maintenance Dose: After attainment of the desired response (ie, reduced transfusion requirements or increased hematocrit), the dose of EPOGEN® should be titrated to maintain the response based on factors such as variations in zidovudine dose and the presence of intercurrent infectious or inflammatory episodes. If the hematocrit exceeds 40%, the dose should be discontinued until the hematocrit drops to 36%. The dose should be reduced by 25% when treatment is resumed and then titrated to maintain the desired hematocrit.

Cancer Patients on Chemotherapy

Baseline endogenous serum erythropoietin levels varied among patients in these trials with approximately 75% (n = 83/110) having endogenous serum erythropoietin levels < 132 mUnits/mL, and approximately 4% (n = 4/110) of patients having endogenous serum erythropoietin levels > 500 mUnits/mL. In general, patients with lower baseline serum erythropoietin levels responded more vigorously to EPOGEN® than patients with higher erythropoietin levels. Although no specific serum erythropoietin level can be stipulated above which patients would be unlikely to respond to EPOGEN® therapy, treatment of patients with grossly elevated serum erythropoietin levels (eg, > 200 mUnits/mL) is not recommended. The hematocrit should be monitored on a weekly basis in patients receiving EPOGEN® therapy until hematocrit becomes stable.

Starting Dose: The recommended starting dose of EPOGEN® is 150 Units/ kg SC TIW.

Dose Adjustment: If the response is not satisfactory in terms of reducing transfusion requirements or increasing hematocrit after 8 weeks of therapy, the dose of EPOGEN® can be increased up to 300 Units/kg TIW. If patients have not responded satisfactorily to an EPOGEN® dose of 300 Units/kg TIW, it is unlikely that they will respond to higher doses of EPOGEN®. If the hematocrit exceeds 40%, the dose of EPOGEN® should be withheld until the hematocrit falls to 36%. The dose of EPOGEN® should be reduced by 25% when treatment is resumed and titrated to maintain the desired hematocrit. If the initial dose of EPOGEN® includes a very rapid hematocrit response (eg, an increase of more than 4 percentage points in any 2-week period), the dose of EPOGEN® should be reduced.

Surgery Patients

Prior to initiating treatment with EPOGEN® a hemoglobin should be obtained to establish that it is > 10 to ≤ 13 g/dL.[14] The recommended dose of EPOGEN® is 300 Units/kg/day subcutaneously for 10 days before surgery, on the day of surgery, and for 4 days after surgery.
An alternate dose schedule is 600 Units/kg EPOGEN® subcutaneously in once weekly doses (21, 14, and 7 days before surgery) plus a fourth dose on the day of surgery.[15]
All patients should receive adequate iron supplementation. Iron supplementation should be initiated no later than the beginning of treatment with EPOGEN® and should continue throughout the course of therapy.

PREPARATION AND ADMINISTRATION OF EPOGEN®

1. Do not shake. It is not necessary to shake EPOGEN®. Prolonged vigorous shaking may denature any glycoprotein, rendering it biologically inactive.
2. Parenteral drug products should be inspected visually for particulate matter and discoloration prior to administration. Do not use any vials exhibiting particulate matter or discoloration.
3. Using aspetic techniques, attach a sterile needle to a sterile syringe. Remove the flip top from the vial containing EPOGEN®, and wipe the septum with a disinfectant. Insert the needle into the vial, and withdraw into the syringe an appropriate volume of solution.
4. **Single-dose** 1 mL vial contains no preservative. Use one dose per vial; do not re-enter the vial. Discard unused portions.
   Multidose 1 mL and 2 mL vials contain preservative. Store at 2° to 8°C after initial entry and between doses. Discard 21 days after initial entry.
5. Do not dilute or administer in conjunction with other drug solutions. However, at the time of SC administration, preservative-free EPOGEN® from single-use vials may be admixed in a syringe with bacteriostatic 0.9% sodium chloride injection, USP, with benzyl alcohol 0.9% (bacteriostatic saline) at a 1:1 ratio using aseptic technique. The benzyl alcohol in the bacteriostatic saline acts as a local anesthetic which may amerliorate SC injection site discomfort. Admixing is not necessary when using the multidose vials of EPOGEN® containing benzyl alcohol.

HOW SUPPLIED

EPOGEN®, containing Epoetin alfa, is available in the following packages:

1 mL **Single-dose, Preservative-free** Solution
2000 Units/mL (NDC 55513-126-10)
3000 Units/mL (NDC 55513-267-10)
4000 Units/mL (NDC 55513-148-10)
10,000 Units/mL (NDC 55513-144-10)
Supplied in cartons containing 10 single-dose vials.

2 mL **Multidose, Preserved** Solution
10,000 Units/mL (NDC 55513-283-10)

1 mL **Multidose, Preserved** Solution
20,000 Units/mL (NDC 55513-478-10)
Supplied in cartons containing 10 multidose vials.

STORAGE

Store at 2° to 8°C (36° to 46°F). Do not freeze or shake.

REFERENCES

1. Egrie JC, Strickland TW, Lane J, et al. Characterization and Biological Effects of Recombinant Human Erythropoietin. *Immunobiol.* 1986; 72:213–224.
2. Graber SE, Krantz SB. Erythropoietin and the Control of Red Cell Production. *Ann Rev Med.* 1978;29:51–66.
3. Eschbach JW, Adamson JW. Anemia of End-Stage Renal Disease (ESRD). *Kidney Intl.* 1985;28:1–5
4. Eschbach JW, Egrie JC, Downing MR, et al. Correction of the Anemia of End-Stage Renal Disease with Recombinant Human Erythropoietin. *NEJM.* 1987;316:73–78.
5. Eschbach JW, Abdulhadi MH, Browne JK, et al. Recombinant Human Erythropoietin in Anemic Patients with End-Stage Renal Disease. *Ann Intern Med.* 1989;111: 992–1000.
6. Eschbach JW, Egrie JC, Downing MR, et al. The Use of Recombinant Human Erythropoietin (r-HuEPO): Effect in End-Stage Renal Disease (ESRD). In: Friedman, Beyer, DeSanto, Giordano, eds. *Prevention of Chronic Uremia.* Philadelphia, PA: Field and Wood Inc; 1989: 148–155.
7. Egrie JC, Eschbach JW, McGuire T, Adamson JW, Pharmacokinetics of Recombinant Human Erythropoietin (r-HuEPO) Administered to Hemodialysis (HD) Patients. *Kidney Intl.* 1988;33:262.
8. Evans RW, Radar B, Manninen DL, et al. The Quality of Life of Hemodialysis Recipients Treated with Recombinant Human Erythropoietin. *JAMA.* 1990;263:825–830.
9. Paganini E, Garcia J, Ellis P, et al. Clinical Sequelae of Correction of Anemia with Recombinant Human Erythropoietin (r-HuEPO); Urea Kinetics, Dialyzer Function and Reuse. *Am J Kid Dis.* 1988;11:16.
10. Delano BG, Lundin AP, Golansky R, et al. Dialyzer Urea and Creatinine Clearances Not Significantly Changed in r-HuEPO Treated Maintenance Hemodialysis (MD) Patients. *Kidney Intl.* 1988;33:219.
11. Stivelman J, Van Wyck D, Ogden D. Use of Recombinant Erythropoietin (r-HuEPO) with High Flux Dialysis (HFD) Does Not Worsen Azotemia or Shorten Access Survival. *Kidney Intl.* 1988;33:239.
12. Lim VS, DeGowin RL, Zavala D, et al. Recombinant Human Erythropoietin Treatment in Pre-Dialysis Patients: A Double-Blind Placebo Controlled Trial. *Ann Int. Med.* 1989;110:108–114.
13. Stone WJ, Graber SE, Krantz SB, et al. Treatment of the Anemia of Pre-Dialysis Patients with Recombinant Human Erythropoietin: A Randomized, Placebo-Controlled Trial. *Am J Med Sci.* 1988;296:171–179.
14. deAndrade JR and Jove M. Baseline Hemoglobin as a Predictor of Risk of Transfusion and Response to Epoetin alfa in Orthopedic Surgery Patients. *Am. J. of Orthoped.* 1996;25 (8):533–542.
15. Goldberg MA and McCutchen JW. A Safety and Efficacy Comparison Study of Two Dosing Regimens of Epoetin alfa in Patients Undergoing Major Orthopedic Surgery. *Am. J. of Orthoped.* 1996;25 (8):544–552.
16. Faris PM and Ritter MA. The Effects of Recombinant Human Erythropoietin on Perioperative Transfusion

Requirements in Patients Having a Major Orthopedic Operation. *J. Bone and Joint Surgery.* 1996; 78-A:62-72.

17. Lundin AP, Akerman MJH, Chesler RM, et al. Exercise in Hemodialysis Patients after Treatment with Recombinant Human Erythropoietin. *Nephron.* 1991;58:315-319.

18. Amgen Inc., data on file.

19. Eschbach JW, Kelly MR, Galey NR, et al. Treatment of the Anemia of Progressive Renal Failure with Recombinant Human Erythropoietin. *NEJM.* 1989;321:158-163.

20. The US Recombinant Human Erythropoietin Predialysis Study Group. Double-Blind, Placebo-Controlled Study of the Therapeutic Use of Recombinant Human Erythropoietin for Anemia Associated with Chronic Renal Failure in Predialysis Patients. *Am J Kid Dis.* 1991;18(1):50-59.

21. Danna RP, Rudnick SA, Abels RI. Erythropoietin Therapy for the Anemia Associated with AIDS and AIDS Therapy and Cancer. In: MB Garnick, ed. *Erythropoietin in Clinical Applications—An International Perspective.* New York, NY: Marcel Dekker; 1990:301-324.

22. Ortho Biologics, Inc., data on file.

23. Fischl M, Galpin JE, Levine JD, et al. Recombinant Human Erythropoietin for Patients with AIDS Treated with Zidovudine. *NEJM.* 1990;322:1488-1493.

24. Laupacis A. Effectiveness of Perioperative Recombinant Human Erythropoietin in Elective Hip Replacement. *Lancet.* 1993;341:1228-1232.

25. Kerr DN. Chronic Renal Failure. In: Beeson PB, McDermott W, Wyngaarden JB, eds. Cecil *Textbook of Medicine.* Philadelphia, PA: W.B. Saunders; 1979:1351-1367.

26. Raskin NH, Fishman RA. Neurologic Disorders in Renal Failure (First of Two Parts). *NEJM.* 1976;294:143-148.

27. Raskin NH and Fishman RA. Neurologic Disorder in Renal Failure (Second of Two parts). *NEJM.* 1976;294:204-210.

28. Messing RO, Simon RP. Seizures as a Manifestation of Systemic Disease. *Neurologic Clinics.* 1986;4:563-584.

AMGEN®

Manufactured by:
Amgen Inc.
1840 DeHavilland Drive
Thousand Oaks, CA
91320-1789
Issue Date: 12/23/96

EPOGEN®(Epoetin alfa)
Information for Home Dialysis Patients

AMGEN®
EPOGEN®
(RECOMBINANT EPOETIN ALFA)

What is EPOGEN® and how does it work?

EPOGEN® is a copy of human erythropoietin, a hormone produced primarily by healthy kidneys. EPOGEN® replaces the erythropoietin that the failed kidneys can no longer produce, and signals the bone marrow to make the oxygen-carrying red blood cells once again. EPOGEN® is produced in mammalian cells that have been genetically altered by the addition of gene for the natural substance erythropoietin.

How should I take EPOGEN®?

In those situations where your doctor has determined that you, as a home dialysis patient, can self-administer EPOGEN®, you will receive instruction on how much EPOGEN® to use, how to inject it, how often you should inject it, and how you should dispose of the unused portions of each vial.

You will be instructed to monitor your blood pressure carefully everyday and to report any changes outside of the guidelines that your doctor has given you. When the number of red blood cells increases, your blood pressure can also increase, so your doctor may prescribe some new or additional blood pressure medication. Be sure to follow your doctor's orders. You may also be instructed to have certain laboratory tests, such as additional hematocrit or iron level measurements, done more frequently. You may be asked to report these tests to your doctor or dialysis center. Also, your doctor may prescribe additional iron for you to take. Be sure to comply with your doctor's orders.

Continue to check your access, as your doctor or nurse has shown you, to make sure it is working. Be sure to let your health care professional know right away if there is a problem.

Allergy to EPOGEN®

Patients occasionally experience redness, swelling, or itching at the site of injection of EPOGEN®. This may indicate an allergy to the components of EPOGEN®, or it may indicate a local reaction. If you have a local reaction, consult your doctor. A potentially more serious reaction would be a generalized allergy to EPOGEN®, which could cause a rash over the whole body, shortness of breath, wheezing, reduction in blood pressure, fast pulse, or sweating. Severe cases of generalized allergy may be life-threatening. If you think you are having a generalized allergic reaction, stop taking EPOGEN® and notify a doctor or emergency medical personnel imediately.

How will I know if EPOGEN® is working?

The effectiveness of EPOGEN® is measured by the increase in hematocrit (the amount of red blood cells in the blood) that results from EPOGEN® therapy. The rise in hematocrit is not immediate. It usually takes about 2 to 6 weeks before the hematocrit starts to rise. The amount of time it takes, and the dose of EPOGEN® that is needed to make the hematocrit increase, varies from patient to patient.

What is the most important information I should know about EPOGEN® and CHRONIC RENAL FAILURE?

EPOGEN® has been prescribed for you by your doctor because you:
1. Have anemia due to your kidney disease.
2. Are able to dialyze at home.
3. Have been determined to be able to administer EPOGEN® without direct medical or other supervision.

A lack of energy or feeling of tiredness is the major symptom of anemia. Additional symptoms include shortness of breath, chest pain, and feeling cold all the time. The reason for these symptoms is that there is a lack of red blood cells. Red blood cells carry oxygen, which is important for all of the body's functions. When there are fewer red blood cells, the body does not get all the oxygen it needs.

Kidneys remove toxins from the blood; they also measure the amount of oxygen in the blood. If there is not enough oxygen, the kidneys will produce a hormone called erythropoietin. Erythropoietin is released into the bloodstream and travels to the bone marrow where red blood cells are made. Erythropoietin signals the bone marrow to make more oxygen-carrying red blood cells.

As the kidneys fail, they stop cleansing toxins from your body. They also make less erythropoietin than they should. Therefore, the bone marrow does not receive a strong-enough signal to make the oxygen-carrying red blood cells. Fewer red blood cells are produced so the muscles, brain, and other parts of the body do not get the oxygen they need to function properly.

Most patients treated with EPOGEN® no longer need blood transfusions. However, certain medical conditions, or unexpected blood loss, may result in the need for a transfusion.

What do I need to know if I am giving myself EPOGEN® injections?

When you receive your EPOGEN® from the dialysis center, doctor's office or home dialysis supplier, always check to see that:
1. The name EPOGEN® appears on the carton and vial label.
2. You will be able to use EPOGEN® before the expiration date stamped on the package.

The EPOGEN® solution in the vial should always be clear and colorless. Do not use EPOGEN® if the contents of the vial appear discolored or cloudy, or if the vial appears to contain lumps, flakes, or particles. In addition, if the vial has been shaken vigorously, the solution may appear to be frothy and should not be used. Therefore, care should be taken not to shake the EPOGEN® vial vigorously before use.

Single Use Vials–S

If you have been prescribed EPOGEN® vials for single use, your vial will have a capital "S" with a number next to it identifying the concentration of EPOGEN® in the vial, printed in a colored dot on the front left side of the label (for example, "S2" identifies a single use vial with 2000 Units/mL). Single use means the vial cannot be used more than once, and any unused portion of the vial should be discarded as directed by your doctor or dialysis center.

Multidose Use Vials–M

If you have been prescribed EPOGEN® Multidose vials, your vial will have a capital "M" with a number under it identifying the concentration of EPOGEN® in the vial, printed in a colored dot on the front left side of the label (for example, "M10" identifies a Multidose vial with 10,000 Units/mL). Multidose EPOGEN® can be used to inject multiple doses as prescribed by your doctor, and may be stored in the refrigerator (but not the freezing compartment) between doses for up to 21 days. Follow your doctor's or dialysis center's instructions on what to do with the used vials.

How should I store EPOGEN®?

EPOGEN® should be stored in the refrigerator, but not in the freezing compartment. Do not let the vial freeze and do not leave it in direct sunlight. Do not use a vial of EPOGEN® that has been frozen or after the expiration date that is stamped on the label. If you have any questions about the safety of a vial of EPOGEN® that has been subjected to temperature extremes, be sure to check with your dialysis unit staff.

Always use the correct syringe

Your doctor has instructed you on how to give yourself the correct dosage of EPOGEN®. This dosage will usually be measured in Units per milliliter or CCs. It is important to use a syringe that is marked in tenths of milliliters (for example, 0.2 mL or CC). Failure to use the proper syringe can lead to a mistake in dosage, and you may receive too much or too little EPOGEN®. Too little EPOGEN® may not be effective in increasing your hematocrit, and too much EPOGEN® may lead to a hematocrit that is too high. Only use disposable syringes and needles as they do not require sterilization; they should be used once and disposed of as instructed by your doctor.

IMPORTANT: TO HELP AVOID CONTAMINATION AND POSSIBLE INFECTION, FOLLOW THESE INSTRUCTIONS EXACTLY.

PREPARING THE DOSE

1. Wash your hands thoroughly with soap and water before preparing the medication.

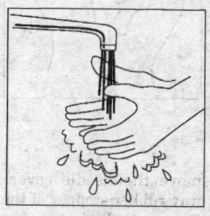

2. Check the date on the EPOGEN® vial to be sure that the drug has not expired.

3. Remove the vial of EPOGEN® from the refrigerator and allow it to reach room temperature. Unless you are using a Multidose vial, each EPOGEN® vial is designed to be used only once. It is not necessary to shake EPOGEN®. Prolonged vigorous shaking may damage the product. Assemble the other supplies you will need for your injection.

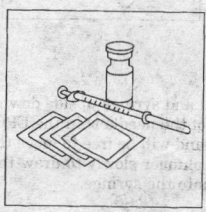

4. Hemodialysis patients should wipe off the venous port of the hemodialysis tubing with an antiseptic swab. Peritoneal dialysis patients should cleanse the skin with an antiseptic swab where the injection is to be made.

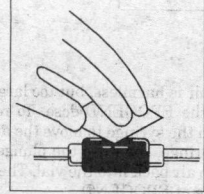 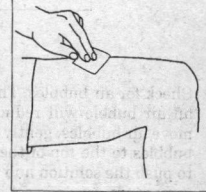

5. Flip off the red protective cap but do not remove the gray rubber stopper. Wipe the top of the gray rubber stopper with an antiseptic swab.

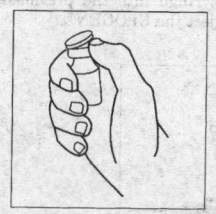 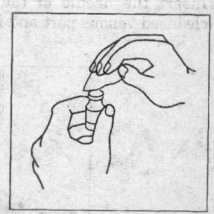

Continued on next page

Epogen—Cont.

6. Using a syringe and needle designed for subcutaneous injection, draw air into the syringe by pulling back on the plunger. The amount of air should be equal to your EPOGEN® dose.

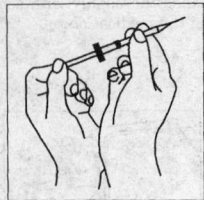

7. Carefully remove the needle cover. Put the needle through the gray rubber stopper of the EPOGEN® vial.
8. Push the plunger in to discharge air into the vial. The air injected into the vial will allow EPOGEN® to be easily withdrawn into the syringe.

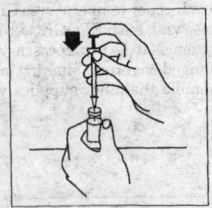

9. Turn the vial and syringe upside down in one hand. Be sure the tip of the needle is in the EPOGEN® solution. Your other hand will be free to move the plunger. Draw back on the plunger slowly to draw the correct dose of EPOGEN® into the syringe.

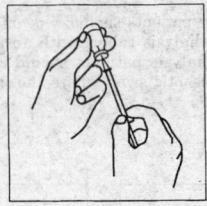

10. Check for air bubbles. The air is harmless, but too large an air bubble will reduce the EPOGEN® dose. To remove air bubbles, gently tap the syringe to move the air bubbles to the top of the syringe, then use the plunger to push the solution and the air back into the vial. Then remeasure your correct dose of EPOGEN®.
11. Double check your dose. Remove the needle from the vial. Do not lay the syringe down or allow the needle to touch anything.

INJECTING THE DOSE
Patients on home hemodialysis using the intravenous injection route:
1. Insert the needle of the syringe into the previously cleansed venous port and inject the EPOGEN®.

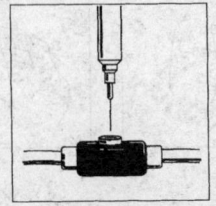

2. Remove the syringe and dispose of the whole unit. **Use the disposable syringe only once.** Dispose of syringes and needles as directed by your doctor, by following these simple steps:
   - Place all used needles and syringes in a hard plastic container with a screw-on-cap, or a metal container with a plastic lid, such as a coffee can properly labeled as to content. If a metal container is used, cut a small hole in the plastic lid and tape the lid to the metal container. If a hard-plastic container is used, always screw the cap on tightly after each use. When the container is full, tape around the cap or lid, and dispose of according to your doctor's instructions.
   - Do not use glass or clear plastic containers, or any container that will be recycled or returned to a store.
   - Always store the container out of the reach of children.
   - Please check with your doctor, nurse, or pharmacist for other suggestions. There may be special state and local laws that they will discuss with you.

Patients on home peritoneal dialysis or home hemodialysis using the subcutaneous route:
1. With one hand, stabilize the previously cleansed skin by spreading it or by pinching up a large area with your free hand.

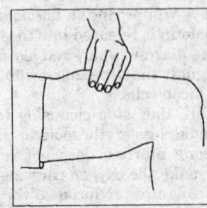

2. Hold the syringe with the other hand, as you would a pencil. Double check that the correct amount of EPOGEN® is in the syringe. Insert the needle straight into the skin (90 degree angle). Pull the plunger back slightly. If blood comes into the syringe, do not inject EPOGEN®, as the needle has entered a blood vessel; withdraw the syringe and inject at a different site. Inject the EPOGEN® by pushing the plunger all the way down.

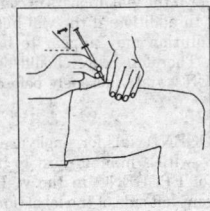 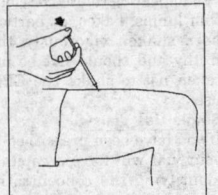

3. Hold an antiseptic swab near the needle and pull the needle straight out of the skin. Press the antiseptic swab over the injection site for several seconds.
4. **Use the disposable syringe only once.** Dispose of syringes and needles as directed by your doctor, by following these simple steps:
   - Place all used needles and syringes in a hard plastic container with a screw-on-cap, or a metal container with a plastic lid, such as a coffee can properly labeled as to content. If a metal container is used, cut a small hole in the plastic lid and tape the lid to the metal container. If a hard-plastic container is used, always screw the cap on tightly after each use. When the container is full, taper around the cap or lid, and dispose of according to your doctor's instructions.
   - Do not use glass or clear plastic containers, or any container that will be recycled or returned to a store.
   - Always store the container out of the reach of children.
   - Please check with your doctor, nurse, or pharmacist for other suggestions. There may be special state and local laws that they will discuss with you.
5. Always change the site for each injection as directed. Occasionally a problem may develop at the injection site. If you notice a lump, swelling, or bruising that doesn't go away, contact your doctor. You may wish to record the site just used so that you can keep track.
[See figure at top of next column]

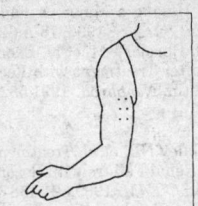 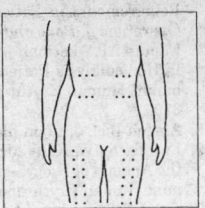

USAGE IN PREGNANCY
If you are pregnant or nursing a baby, consult your doctor before using EPOGEN®.

IMPORTANT NOTES
Since you are a home dialysis patient and your doctor allows you to self-administer EPOGEN®, please note the following:
1. Always follow the instructions of your doctor concerning the dosage and administration of EPOGEN®. Do not change the dose or instructions for administration of EPOGEN® without consulting your doctor.
2. Your doctor will tell you what to do if you miss a dose of EPOGEN®. Always keep a spare syringe and needle on hand.
3. Always consult your doctor if you notice anything unusual about your condition or your use of EPOGEN®.

AMGEN®
Manufactured by:
Amgen Inc.
1840 DeHavilland Drive
Thousand Oaks, CA
91320-1789

Issue Date: 11/14/96 US EPO PI Copy Rev
©1996, 1997 Amgen Inc. All Rights Reserved.
P30035D   25M/1-97
Shown in Product Identification Guide, page 304

INFERGEN®   ℞
(Interferon alfacon-1)

DESCRIPTION
Interferon alfacon-1 is a recombinant non-naturally occurring type-I interferon. The 166-amino acid sequence of Interferon alfacon-1 was derived by scanning the sequences of several natural interferon alpha subtypes and assigning the most frequently observed amino acid in each corresponding position.[1] Four additional amino acid changes were made to facilitate the molecular construction, and a corresponding synthetic DNA sequence was constructed using chemical synthesis methodology. Interferon alfacon-1 differs from interferon alfa-2 at 20/166 amino acids (88% homology), and comparison with interferon-beta shows identity at over 30% of the amino acid positions, a greater similarity than any natural interferon alpha subtype. Interferon alfacon-1 is produced in *Escherichia coli (E coli)* cells that have been genetically altered by insertion of a synthetically constructed sequence that codes for Interferon alfacon-1. Prior to final purification, Interferon alfacon-1 is allowed to oxidize to its native state, and its final purity is achieved by sequential passage over a series of chromatography columns. This protein has a molecular weight of 19,434 daltons. Infergen® is the Amgen Inc. trademark for Interferon alfacon-1.

Infergen is a sterile, clear, colorless, preservative-free liquid formulated with 100 mM sodium chloride and 25 mM sodium phosphate at pH 7.0 ± 0.2. The product is available in single-use vials containing 9 mcg and 15 mcg Interferon alfacon-1 at a fill volume of 0.3 mL and 0.5 mL, respectively. Infergen vials contain 0.03 mg/mL of Interferon alfacon-1, 5.9 mg/mL sodium chloride, and 3.8 mg/mL sodium phosphate in Water for Injection, USP. Infergen is to be administered undiluted by subcutaneous (SC) injection.

Formulation, filling, and packaging operations for Infergen are performed by Amgen Puerto Rico, a wholly-owned subsidiary of Amgen Inc.

CLINICAL PHARMACOLOGY
General
Interferons are a family of naturally occurring, small protein molecules with molecular weights of 15,000 to 21,000 daltons that are produced and secreted by cells in response to viral infections or to various synthetic and biological inducers. Two major classes of interferons have been identified (ie, type-I and type-II). Type-I interferons include a family of more than 25 interferon alphas as well as interferon beta and interferon omega. While all alpha interferons have similar biological effects, not all the activities are

shared by each alpha interferon and, in many cases, the extent of activity varies substantially for each interferon subtype.

All type-I interferons share common biological activities generated by binding of interferon to the cell-surface receptor, leading to the production of several interferon-stimulated gene products. Type-I interferons induce pleiotropic biologic responses which include antiviral, antiproliferative and immunomodulatory effects, regulation of cell surface major histocompatibility antigen (HLA class I and class II) expression and regulation of cytokine expression. Examples of interferon-stimulated gene products include 2′5′ oligoadenylate synthetase (2′5′ OAS) and β-2 microglobulin.

The antiviral, antiproliferative, NK cell activation, and gene-induction activities of Infergen have been compared with other recombinant alfa interferons in *in vitro* assays and have demonstrated similar ranges of activity. Infergen exhibited at least five times higher specific activity *in vitro* than Interferon alfa-2a and Interferon alfa-2b.[2] Comparison of Infergen with a WHO international potency standard for recombinant interferon alfa (83/514) revealed that the specific activity of Infergen in both an *in vitro* antiviral cytopathic effect assay and an antiproliferative assay was 1×10^9 units/mg. However, correlation between *in vitro* activity and clinical activity of any interferon is unknown.

Pharmacokinetics and Pharmacodynamics

The pharmacokinetic properties of Infergen have not been evaluated in patients with chronic hepatitis C. Pharmacokinetic profiles were evaluated in normal, healthy volunteer subjects after SC injection of 1, 3, or 9 mcg Interferon alfacon-1. Plasma levels of Infergen after SC administration of any dose were too low to be detected by either ELISA or by inhibition of viral cytopathic effect. However, analysis of Infergen-induced cellular products (induction of 2′5′ OAS and β-2 microglobulin) after treatment in these subjects revealed a statistically significant, dose-related increase in the area under the curve (AUC) for the levels of 2′5′ OAS or β-2 microglobulin induced over time ($p < 0.001$ for all comparisons). Concentrations of 2′5′ OAS were maximal at 24 hours after dosing, while serum levels of β-2 microglobulin appeared to reach a maximum 24 to 36 hours after dosing. The dose-response relationships observed for 2′5′ OAS and β-2 microglobulin were indicative of biological activity after SC administration of 1 to 9 mcg Infergen.

Preclinical Experience

All interferons have been shown to be highly species specific. Antiviral activity of Infergen was observed in the rhesus monkey LLC cell line and golden Syrian hamster BHK cell line. Antiviral activity of Infergen in the golden Syrian hamster was confirmed further *in vivo*.[3] Pharmacokinetic studies of Infergen in golden Syrian hamsters and rhesus monkeys demonstrated rapid absorption following SC injection. Peak serum concentrations of Infergen were observed at 1 hour and 4 hours in golden Syrian hamsters and in rhesus monkeys, respectively. Subcutaneous bioavailability was high in both species, averaging 99% in golden Syrian hamsters and 83% to 104% in rhesus monkeys. Clearance of Infergen, averaging 1.99 mL/minute/kg in golden Syrian hamsters and 0.71 to 0.92 mL/minute/kg in rhesus monkeys, was due predominantly to catabolism and excretion by the kidneys. The terminal half-life of Infergen following SC dosing was 1.3 hours in golden Syrian hamsters and 3.4 hours in rhesus monkeys. Upon 7-day multiple SC dosing, no accumulation of serum levels was observed in golden Syrian hamsters.

In preclinical toxicology studies in golden Syrian hamsters and rhesus monkeys, administration of Infergen at doses of up to 100 mcg/kg/day was associated with decreased body weight, decreased food consumption, and bone marrow suppression. High-dose chronic exposure at doses of 10 to 100 mcg/kg/day (50- to 500-fold higher than the maximum clinical dose given daily) in rhesus monkeys was not tolerated for greater than 1 month, due to the development of vascular leak syndrome.

Reproductive toxicity studies in pregnant rhesus monkeys and golden Syrian hamsters demonstrated an increase in fetal loss in hamsters treated with Infergen at doses of greater than 150 mcg/kg/day, and in rhesus monkeys at doses of 3 and 10 mcg/kg/day. The Infergen toxicity profile described is consistent with the known toxicity profile of other alfa interferons.[4]

CLINICAL EXPERIENCE: RESPONSE TO INFERGEN

Infergen was studied in an open-label dose escalation study using 3, 6, 9, 12, or 15 mcg administered three times per week (TIW) to patients with compensated liver disease secondary to chronic hepatitis C virus (HCV) infection. The 15 mcg dose was the maximal tolerated dose. All doses demonstrated an acceptable safety profile and preliminary evidence of efficacy.

The efficacy of 3 and 9 mcg doses of Infergen in the treatment of chronic HCV infection was examined in a randomized, double-blind clinical trial involving 704 patients previously untreated with alfa interferon. Patients were 18 years or older, had compensated liver disease, tested positive for HCV RNA, and had elevated serum alanine aminotransferase (ALT) concentrations averaging > 1.5 times the upper limit of normal. Staging of chronic liver disease was confirmed by a liver biopsy taken within 1 year prior to enrollment. Other causes of chronic liver disease were ruled out prior to randomization. Notable exclusion criteria were decompensated liver disease, thyroid abnormality, or history of depression.

Efficacy of Infergen therapy was assessed on an intent to treat basis and was determined by measurement of serum ALT concentrations at the end of therapy (24 weeks) and following 24 weeks of observation after the end of treatment. Serum HCV RNA was also assessed using a quantitative reverse transcriptase polymerase chain reaction (RT-PCR) assay with a lower limit of sensitivity of 100 copies/mL. Liver histology was assessed by comparing the histology activity index (HAI) score[5] of a pretreatment biopsy specimen with the HAI score from a specimen obtained 24 weeks after cessation of interferon therapy.

Patients enrolled in the study were randomized to one of three treatment groups: Infergen at a dose of 3 mcg (n = 232), Infergen at a dose of 9 mcg (n = 232), or Interferon alfa-2b recombinant [IFN α-2b, Intron® A (Intron® is a registered trademark of the Schering Corporation)] at a dose of 3 million international units (IU) (approximately 15 mcg) (n = 240). All patients were scheduled to receive their respective interferons SC TIW for 24 weeks (end of treatment). Following treatment, patients were observed for an additional 24 weeks to assess durability of ALT normalization (end of post-treatment observation). In all patients, a complete response was defined as a decrease in serum ALT concentration to at or below the upper limit of normal (48 U/L) at the end of the post-treatment observation period, even if ALT normalization had not been observed at the end of treatment. Complete response was dependent on two consecutive normal serum ALT values determined 4 weeks apart. Reduction of HCV RNA to < 100 copies/mL was measured as a secondary efficacy endpoint (two consecutive measurements).

Sustained response rates by ALT normalization and HCV RNA reductions to below detectable limits are included in Table 1. Among the Infergen treatment groups in this study, the 9 mcg dosage arm demonstrated a similar efficacy profile when compared to the IFN α-2b dosage arm. The 3 mcg Infergen dosage arm had lesser efficacy; 3% of patients receiving 3 mcg Infergen had sustained reductions in their ALT concentrations to within the normal range and 3% had sustained reductions in HCV RNA to below detectable limits.

[See table above]

Table 1. Rates (95% CI[a]) of ALT Normalization and HCV RNA Reductions to Below Detectable Limits

	End of 24-week Treatment		End of Observation (Sustained Response Rate)	
	Infergen 9 mcg	IFN α-2b 3 Million IU[b]	Infergen 9 mcg	IFN α-2b 3 Million IU[b]
Normalized ALT	39% (33%, 46%)	35% (29%, 41%)	17% (12%, 22%)	17% (13%, 22%)
HCV RNA Negative	33% (27%, 39%)	25% (19%, 31%)	9% (6%,14%)	8% (5%, 13%)

[a]CI = Confidence Interval.
[b]3 million IU IFN α-2b is equivalent to approximately 15 mcg IFN α-2b.

In this study, liver biopsies were taken at baseline and at the end of post-treatment observation. Similar improvement in liver histology, assessed by HAI score,[5] was observed in the 9 mcg Infergen (68%), 3 mcg Infergen (63%), and IFN α-2b (65%) dosage arms.

Subsequent treatment with 15 mcg of Infergen was evaluated in an open-label clinical trial in 107 patients who had failed initial therapy with either 9 mcg Infergen or 3 million IU (approximately 15 mcg) IFN α-2b. Of these patients, 74/107 had failed to normalize ALT concentrations during either the initial treatment period or the post-treatment observation period, while 33/107 achieved a normal ALT concentration during initial treatment, but experienced relapse (return of abnormal ALT concentration) during post-treatment observation. Patients were assessed for normalization of ALT (ALT response rate) and HCV RNA reduction to < 100 copies/mL (HCV response rate) at the end of 24 weeks of observation. Response rates (expressed as fraction of patients, percentage of patients, and 95% confidence interval of percentage) are presented for all patients and two subsets of patients: patients who had relapsed following initial therapy and patients who had never normalized following initial therapy.

Overall 16/107 [15% (9–23% CI)] patients had a sustained ALT response. Of patients who had relapsed following initial therapy 10/33 [30% (16–49% CI)] had a sustained ALT response and 6/74 [8% (3–17% CI)] who never normalized their ALT concentration had a sustained ALT response. Overall 10/107 [9% (5–17% CI)] patients had a sustained HCV response (< 100 copies/mL). Of patients who had relapsed following initial therapy 8/32 [25% (11–43% CI)] had a sustained HCV response and 2/75 [3% (0–9% CI)] who never had a reduction in HCV RNA to < 100 copies/mL had a sustained HCV response.

Serum antibody levels were measured in all patients using both an Infergen-binding radioimmunoassay and an IFN α-2b-binding ELISA. A patient was considered to have developed binding antibodies if, using serum samples from two consecutive time points, a positive response was detected in either assay. The number of patients developing positive binding antibody responses in either assay was similar in the 9 mcg Infergen (11%) and 3 million IU IFN α-2b groups (15%). The titer of neutralizing antibodies to interferon was not measured. Sustained ALT response rates in patients treated with Infergen who developed binding antibodies (4/25) were similar to sustained ALT response rates in patients who did not develop detectable antibody titers (40/195). The most frequently observed time to first antibody response was week 16 of interferon treatment. Following cessation of interferon therapy, the number of patients with a positive antibody response declined during post-treatment observation.

INDICATIONS AND USAGE

Infergen is indicated for the treatment of chronic HCV infection in patients 18 years of age or older with compensated liver disease who have anti-HCV serum antibodies and/or the presence of HCV RNA. Other causes of hepatitis, such as viral hepatitis B or auto-immune hepatitis should be ruled out prior to initiation of therapy with Infergen. In some patients with chronic HCV infection, Infergen normalizes serum ALT concentrations, reduces serum HCV RNA concentrations to undetectable quantities (< 100 copies/mL), and improves liver histology.

CONTRAINDICATIONS

Infergen is contraindicated in patients with known hypersensitivity to alpha interferons, to *E coli*-derived products, or to any component of the product.

WARNINGS

Treatment with Infergen should be administered under the guidance of a qualified physician, and may lead to moderate-to-severe adverse experiences requiring dose reduction, temporary dose cessation, or discontinuation of further therapy.

Withdrawal from study for adverse events occurred in 7% of patients treated with 9 mcg Infergen (including 4% due to psychiatric events).

SEVERE PSYCHIATRIC ADVERSE EVENTS MAY MANIFEST IN PATIENTS RECEIVING THERAPY WITH INTERFERON, INCLUDING INFERGEN. DEPRESSION, SUICIDAL IDEATION, AND SUICIDE ATTEMPT MAY OCCUR. The incidence of psychiatric events of suicidal ideation was small (1%) for patients treated with 9 mcg Infergen compared to the overall incidence (55%) of psychiatric events. Infergen should be used with caution in patients who report a history of depression and physicians should monitor all patients for evidence of depression. Physicians should inform patients of the possible development of depression prior to initiation of Infergen therapy, and patients should report any sign or symptom of depression immediately. Other prominent psychiatric adverse events may also occur, including nervousness, anxiety, emotional lability, abnormal thinking, agitation, or apathy (see PRECAUTIONS).

INFERGEN SHOULD BE ADMINISTERED WITH CAUTION TO PATIENTS WITH PRE-EXISTING CARDIAC DISEASE. Hypertension and supraventricular arrhythmias, chest pain and myocardial infarction have been associated with interferon therapies.[6]

No studies with Infergen have been conducted in patients with decompensated hepatic disease. Patients with decompensated hepatic disease should not be treated with Infergen, and patients who develop symptoms of hepatic decompensation, such as jaundice, ascites, coagulopathy, or decreased serum albumin, should halt further interferon therapy.

PRECAUTIONS

General

Since the use of type-I interferons has been associated with depression, Infergen therapy should not be used in patients

Continued on next page

Infergen—Cont.

with a history of severe psychiatric disorders and should be discontinued in patients developing severe depression, suicidal ideation, or other severe psychiatric disorders (see WARNINGS).

Infergen should be used with caution in patients with a history of cardiac disease. Hypertension (5%), tachycardia (4%), and palpitation (3%) were the most common cardiovascular adverse events reported for 9 mcg Infergen therapy, with 1% of patients reporting tachyarrhythmias which were dose-limiting (see WARNINGS).

Infergen should be used cautiously in patients with abnormally low peripheral blood cell counts or who are receiving agents that are known to cause myelosuppression. Leukopenia, particularly granulocytopenia, may be severe in patients treated with alpha interferons, including Infergen, and may necessitate dose reduction or temporary dose cessation. Thrombocytopenia is a common, but less severe, event often associated with alpha interferon therapy. Therapy should be withheld if the absolute neutrophil count (ANC) is $< 500 \times 10^6$/L or if the platelet count is $< 50 \times 10^9$/L. Transplantation patients, or other chronically immunosuppressed patients, should receive Infergen therapy with caution.

Serious acute hypersensitivity reactions have been reported in rare instances following treatment with alpha interferons. If hypersensitivity reactions occur (eg, urticaria, angioedema, bronchoconstriction, anaphylaxis), the drug should be discontinued immediately and appropriate medical treatment instituted.

Infergen should be administered with caution to patients with a history of endocrine disorders. Abnormal thyroid stimulating hormone (TSH) and free thyroxine (T_4) level with hypothyroidism occurred in 4% of patients administered 9 mcg Infergen, and thyroid supplements were required in approximately two thirds of those patients.

Ophthalmologic disorders have been reported with treatment with alpha interferons. Investigators using alpha interferons have reported the occurrence of retinal hemorrhages, cotton wool spots, and retinal artery or vein obstruction in rare instances. Any patient complaining of loss of visual acuity or visual field should have an eye examination. Because these ocular events may occur in conjunction with other disease states, a visual exam prior to initiation of interferon therapy is recommended in patients with diabetes mellitus or hypertension.

Exacerbation of autoimmune disease has been reported in patients receiving type-I interferon therapy. Infergen should not be used in patients with autoimmune hepatitis and be used with caution in patients with other autoimmune disorders.

While fever may be related to the flu-like symptoms reported in patients treated with Infergen, when fever occurs, other possible causes of persistent fever should be ruled out.

Information for Patients

If home use is determined to be desirable by the physician, instructions on appropriate use should be given by a health care professional. The patient must be instructed as to the proper dosage and administration. Information included in the full "Information for Patients" leaflet (provided separately) should be fully reviewed with the patient; it is not a disclosure of all, or possible, adverse effects. The most common adverse reactions occurring with Infergen therapy are flu-like symptoms including fatigue, fever, rigors, headache, arthralgia, myalgia, and increased sweating. Non-narcotic analgesics and bedtime administration of Infergen may be used to prevent or lessen some of these symptoms. Additionally, patients must be thoroughly instructed in the importance of proper disposal procedures and cautioned against the reuse of needles, syringes, or re-entry of the drug product. A puncture-resistant container for the disposal of used syringes and needles should be used by the patient and should be disposed of according to the directions provided by the health care provider.

Laboratory Tests

Laboratory tests are recommended for all patients on Infergen therapy, prior to beginning treatment (baseline), 2 weeks after initiation of therapy, and periodically thereafter during the 24 weeks of therapy at the discretion of the physician. Following completion of Infergen therapy, any abnormal test values should be monitored periodically. The entrance criteria that were used for the clinical study of Infergen may be considered as a guideline to acceptable baseline values for initiation of treatment:

- Platelet count $\geq 75 \times 10^9$/L
- Hemoglobin concentration ≥ 100 g/L
- ANC $\geq 1500 \times 10^6$/L
- Serum creatinine concentration < 180 μmol/L (< 2.0 mg/dL) or creatinine clearance > 0.83 mL/second (> 50 mL/minute)
- Serum albumin concentration ≥ 25 g/L
- Bilirubin within normal limits
- TSH and T_4 within normal limits

Table 2. Patient Incidence of Adverse Events in Phase 3 Clinical Trials Regardless of Attribution[a]

Body System	Preferred Term	Initial Treatment[b] Infergen 9 mcg (n = 231)	IFN α-2b 3 Million IU (n = 236)	Subsequent Treatment[b] Infergen 15 mcg (n = 165)
		% of Patients		% of Patients
APPLICATION SITE				
	Injection Site Erythema	23	15	17
	Injection Site Pain	9	3	8
	Injection Site Ecchymosis	6	7	5
BODY AS A WHOLE				
	Body Pain	54	45	39
	Influenza-like Symptoms[c]	15	11	8
	Hot Flushes	13	7	7
	Pain Chest–Non-cardiac	13	14	5
	Malaise	11	10	2
	Asthenia	9	11	10
	Edema Peripheral	9	8	4
	Access Pain	8	9	1
	Allergic Reaction	7	5	3
	Weight Decrease	5	7	5
CARDIOVASCULAR				
	Hypertension	5	3	2
	Palpitation	3	6	5
CNS/PNS				
	Insomnia	39	30	24
	Dizziness	22	25	18
	Paresthesia	13	10	9
	Amnesia	10	6	2
	Hypoesthesia	10	8	8
	Hypertonia	7	10	6
	Confusion	4	6	4
	Somnolence	4	8	5
ENDOCRINE DISORDERS				
	Thyroid Test Abnormal	9	5	4
FLU-LIKE SYMPTOMS				
	Headache	82	83	78
	Fatigue	69	67	65
	Fever	61	45	58
	Myalgia	58	56	51
	Rigors	57	45	62
	Arthralgia	51	45	43
	Sweating Increased	12	11	13
GASTRO-INTESTINAL				
	Abdominal Pain	41	40	24
	Nausea	40	36	30
	Diarrhea	29	24	24
	Anorexia	24	17	21
	Dyspepsia	21	18	12
	Vomiting	12	11	13
	Constipation	9	6	5
	Flatulence	8	9	6
	Tooth Ache	7	7	3
	Hemorrhoids	6	3	1
	Saliva Decreased	6	7	4
HEARING-VESTIBULAR				
	Tinnitus	6	4	4
	Earache	5	7	5
	Otitis	2	5	1
HEMATOLOGIC				
	Granulocytopenia	23	25	42
	Thrombocytopenia	19	16	18
	Leukopenia	15	13	19
	Ecchymosis	6	4	4
	Lymphadenopathy	6	8	4
	Lymphocytosis	5	7	11
	PT Increased	3	5	1
LIVER AND BILIARY				
	Liver Tender	5	3	5
	Hepatomegaly	3	5	5
METABOLIC-NUTRITION				
	Hypertriglyceridemia	6	7	5
MUSCULO-SKELETAL				
	Back Pain	42	37	29
	Limb Pain	26	25	13
	Neck Pain	14	13	8
	Skeletal Pain	14	14	10
	Musculo-Skeletal Disorder	4	4	7
PSYCHIATRIC DISORDER				
	Nervousness	31	29	16
	Depression	26	25	18
	Anxiety	19	18	10
	Emotional Lability	12	11	6
	Thinking Abnormal	8	12	10
	Agitation	6	6	4
	Libido Decreased	5	5	5

Continued on next page

Table 2. (continued) Patient Incidence of Adverse Events in Phase 3 Clinical Trials Regardless of Attribution[a]

Body System	Preferred Term	Initial Treatment[b] Infergen 9 mcg (n = 231)	Initial Treatment[b] IFN α-2b 3 Million IU (n = 236)	Subsequent Treatment[b] Infergen 15 mcg (n = 165)
		% of Patients	% of Patients	% of Patients
REPRODUCTIVE-FEMALE				
	Dysmenorrhea	9	9	2
	Vaginitis	8	2	5
	Menstrual Disorder	6	5	2
	Moniliasis Genital	2	6	2
	Pain Breast	0	5	2
RESISTANCE MECHANISM				
	Infection	3	5	2
RESPIRATORY				
	Pharyngitis	34	31	17
	Infection Upper Respiratory	31	34	16
	Cough	22	17	12
	Sinusitis	17	22	12
	Rhinitis	13	16	7
	Respiratory Tract Congestion	12	7	5
	Upper Respiratory Tract Congestion	10	14	7
	Epistaxis	8	12	6
	Dyspnea	7	12	8
	Bronchitis	6	6	2
SKIN AND APPENDAGES				
	Alopecia	14	25	10
	Pruritus	14	14	11
	Rash	13	15	13
	Erythema	6	6	6
	Skin Dry	6	5	2
	Wound	4	7	3
SPECIAL SENSES				
	Taste Perversion	3	6	3
VISION DISORDERS				
	Conjunctivitis	8	8	4
	Eye Pain	5	6	4
	Vision Abnormal	3	5	5

[a] Only events that occurred at a frequency of ≥5% in any treatment group are included. Patients can appear more than once in Table 2. Because the two studies were conducted at different times with nonidentical patient groups, the adverse events profile for the subsequent treatment study is not directly comparable to the initial treatment study.
[b] Adverse events reported in patients during treatment or post-treatment observation in the pivotal initial treatment and subsequent treatment studies are listed regardless of attribution to treatment.
[c] Influenza-like Symptoms; presumed viral etiology.

Neutropenia, thrombocytopenia, hypertriglyceridemia, and thyroid disorders have been reported with administration of Infergen (see ADVERSE REACTIONS). Therefore, these laboratory parameters should be monitored closely.

Drug Interactions
No formal drug interaction studies have been conducted with Infergen. Infergen should be used cautiously in patients who are receiving agents that are known to cause myelosuppression or with agents known to be metabolized via the cytochrome P-450 pathway.[7] Patients taking drugs that are metabolized by this pathway should be monitored closely for changes in the therapeutic and/or toxic levels of concomitant drugs.

Carcinogenesis, Mutagenesis, Impairment of Fertility
Carcinogenesis: No carcinogenicity data for Infergen are available in animals or humans.
Mutagenesis: Infergen was not mutagenic when tested in several *in vitro* assays, including the Ames bacterial mutagenicity assay and an *in vitro* cytogenetic assay in human lymphocytes, either in the presence or absence of metabolic activation.
Impairment of Fertility: Infergen at doses as high as 100 mcg/kg did not selectively affect reproductive performance or the development of the offspring when administered SC to male and female golden Syrian hamsters for 70 and 14 days before mating, respectively, and then through mating and to day 7 of pregnancy.

Pregnancy Category C
Infergen has been shown to have embryolethal or abortifacient effects in golden Syrian hamsters when given at 135 times the human dose and in cynomolgus and rhesus monkeys when given at 9 to 81 times (based on body surface area) the human dose. There are no adequate and well-controlled studies in pregnant women. Infergen should not be used during pregnancy. If a woman becomes pregnant or plans to become pregnant while taking Infergen, she should be informed of the potential hazards to the fetus. Males and females treated with Infergen should be advised to use effective contraception.

Nursing Mothers
It is not known whether Infergen is excreted in human milk. Because many drugs are excreted in human milk, caution should be exercised if Infergen is administered to a nursing woman. The effect on the nursing neonate of orally ingested Infergen in breast milk has not been evaluated.

Pediatric Use
The safety and effectiveness of Infergen have not been established in patients below the age of 18 years. Infergen therapy is not recommended in pediatric patients.

ADVERSE REACTIONS
Adverse experiences that were reported, regardless of attribution to treatment, in at least 5% of the patients in the 9 mcg Infergen or 3 million IU IFN α-2b groups of the pivotal study are presented in Table 2, listed in decreasing order by the 9 mcg Infergen group. The incidence of adverse events is expressed based on the number of patients experiencing each event at least once during treatment or post-treatment of the study.
Most adverse events were mild-to-moderate in severity and abated with cessation of therapy. Flu-like symptoms (ie, headache, fatigue, fever, rigors, myalgia, sweating increased, and arthralgia) were the most frequently reported treatment-related adverse reactions. Most were short-lived and could be treated symptomatically.
Depression, usually mild-to-moderate in severity, was reported in 26% of patients who received 9 mcg Infergen and was the most common adverse event resulting in study drug discontinuation.
In patients who had tolerated previous interferon therapy and failed to normalize ALT concentration or who had achieved normalization of ALT concentration during the treatment period but who relapsed during the post-treatment observation period, further treatment with 15 mcg TIW of Infergen for 24 weeks was generally tolerated (see Table 2). The higher dose of Infergen used in these patients was associated with a greater incidence of leukopenia and granulocytopenia, and one or more dose reductions for all causes were required in 33% of patients. Patients who do not tolerate initial standard interferon therapy should not receive therapy with 15 mcg TIW of Infergen.
[See table 2 at top of previous page and above]

Laboratory Values
The following laboratory variables were found to be affected by therapy with Infergen in the 231 patients who received treatment with 9 mcg Infergen.

Hemoglobin and Hematocrit: Treatment with Infergen was associated with gradual decreases in mean values for hemoglobin and hematocrit, which were 4% and 5% below baseline at the end of treatment. Decreases from baseline of 20% or more in hemoglobin or hematocrit were seen in 1% of patients or less.
White Blood Cells: Infergen treatment was associated with decreases in mean values for both total white blood cell (WBC) count and ANC within the first 2 weeks of treatment. By the end of treatment, mean decreases from baseline of 19% for WBCs and 23% for ANC were observed. These effects reversed during the post-treatment observation period. In two Infergen-treated patients in the phase 3 trial, decreases in ANC to levels below 500×10^6 cells/L were seen. In both cases, the ANC returned to clinically acceptable levels with reduction of the dose of Infergen, and these transient decreases in neutrophils were not associated with infections.
Platelets: Infergen treatment was associated with alterations in platelet count. Decreases in mean platelet count of 16% compared to baseline were seen by the end of treatment. These decreases were reversed during the post-treatment observation period. Values below normal were common during treatment with 3% of patients developing values less than 50×10^9 cells/L, usually necessitating dose reduction.
Triglycerides: Mean values for serum triglyceride increased shortly after the start of administration of Infergen, with increases of 41%, compared with baseline, at the end of the treatment period. Seven percent of the patients developed values which were at least three times above pretreatment levels during treatment. This effect was promptly reversed after discontinuation of treatment.
Thyroid Function: Infergen treatment was associated with biochemical changes consistent with hypothyroidism including increases in TSH and decreases in T_4 mean values. Increases in TSH to greater than 7 mU/L were seen in 10% of 9 mcg Infergen-treated patients either during the treatment period or the 24-week post-treatment observation period. Thyroid supplements were instituted in approximately one third of these patients.
Laboratory Values for Subsequent Treatment: From a database of 165 patients receiving treatment with 15 mcg of Infergen after failing initial interferon therapy, similar changes in the laboratory variables as outlined above were observed. However, mean decreases from baseline of 23% for WBCs and 27% for ANC were observed, which was greater than during initial treatment. Reductions in WBCs and ANC resulted in alteration of doses in 11 patients (7%). Two patients experienced reversible reductions in ANC to < 500 $\times 10^6$ cells/L, which were not associated with infectious complications. No patients discontinued as a result of hematologic toxicity.

OVERDOSAGE
In Infergen trials, the maximum overdose reported was a dose of 150 mcg Infergen administered SC in a patient enrolled in a phase 1 advanced malignancy trial. The patient received 10 times the prescribed dosage for 3 days. The patient experienced a mild increase in anorexia, chills, fever, and myalgia. Increases in ALT (15 to 127 IU/L), aspartate transaminase (AST) (15 to 164 IU/L), and lactic dehydrogenase (LDH) (183 to 281 IU/L) were reported. These laboratory values returned to normal or to the patient's baseline values within 30 days.

DOSAGE AND ADMINISTRATION
The recommended dose of Infergen for treatment of chronic HCV infection is 9 mcg TIW administered SC as a single injection for 24 weeks. At least 48 hours should elapse between doses of Infergen.
Patients who tolerated previous interferon therapy and did not respond or relapsed following its discontinuation may be subsequently treated with 15 mcg of Infergen TIW for 6 months. Patients should not be treated with 15 mcg of Infergen TIW if they have not received, or have not tolerated, an initial course of interferon therapy.
There are significant differences in specific activities among interferons. Health care providers should be aware that changes in interferon brand may require adjustments of dosage and/or change in route of administration. Patients should be warned not to change brands of interferon without medical consultation. Patients should also be instructed by their physician not to reduce the dosage of Infergen prior to medical consultation.

Dose Reduction
For patients who experience a severe adverse reaction on Infergen, dosage should be withheld temporarily. If the adverse reaction does not become tolerable, therapy should be discontinued. Dose reduction to 7.5 mcg may be necessary following an intolerable adverse event. In the pivotal study, 11% of patients (26/231) who initially received Infergen at a dose of 9 mcg (0.3 mL) were dose-reduced to 7.5 mcg (0.25 mL).
If adverse reactions continue to occur at the reduced dosage, the physician may discontinue treatment or reduce dosage further. However, decreased efficacy may result from continued treatment at dosages below 7.5 mcg.

Continued on next page

Infergen—Cont.

During subsequent treatment with 15 mcg of Infergen, 33% of patients required dose reductions in 3 mcg increments.

Administration of Infergen

If home use is determined to be desirable by the physician, instructions on appropriate use should be given by a health care professional. After administration of Infergen, it is essential to follow the procedure for proper disposal of syringes and needles. See "Information For Patients" leaflet for detailed instructions provided separately.

Storage

Infergen should be stored in the refrigerator at 2° to 8°C (36° to 46°F). Do not freeze. Avoid vigorous shaking. Just prior to injection, Infergen may be allowed to reach room temperature.

Parenteral drug products should be inspected visually for particulate matter and discoloration prior to administration; if particulates or discoloration are observed, the container should not be used.

HOW SUPPLIED

Infergen: Use only one dose per vial; do not re-enter the vial. Discard unused portions. Do not save unused drug for later administration.

Single-dose, preservative-free vials containing 9 mcg (0.3 mL) of Interferon alfacon-1 are available in dispensing packs of six vials (NDC 55513-554-06).

Single-dose, preservative-free vials containing 15 mcg (0.5 mL) of Interferon alfacon-1 are available in dispensing packs of six vials (NDC 55513-562-06).

Infergen should be stored at 2° to 8°C (36° to 46°F). Do not freeze. Avoid vigorous shaking.

REFERENCES

1. Alton K, Stabinsky Y, Richards R, et al. Production, characterization and biological effects of recombinant DNA derived human IFN-α and IFN-γ analogs. In: De Maeyer E, Schellekens H, eds. *The Biology of the Interferon System 1983.* Elsevier Science Publishers: Amsterdam. 1983;119–128.
2. Blatt LM, Davis J, Klein SB, Taylor MW. The biologic activity and molecular characterization of a novel synthetic interferon-alpha species, consensus interferon. *J Interferon Cytokine Res.*1996;16:489–499.
3. Fish EN, Banerjee K, Levine HL, Stebbing N. Antiherpetic effects of a human alpha inteferon analog, IFN-alpha Con_1, in hamsters. *Antimicrob Agents Chemother.* 1986;30:52–56.
4. Trown PW, Willis RJ, Kamm JJ. The preclinical development of Roferon®-A. *Cancer.* 1986;57:1648–1656.
5. Knodell RG, Ishak KG, Black WC, et al. Formulation and application of a numerical scoring system for assessing histological activity in asymptomatic chronic active hepatitis. *Hepatology.* 1981;1:431–435.
6. Vial T, Descotes J. Clinical toxicity of interferons. *Drug Safety.* 1994; 10:115–150
7. Horsmans Y, Brenard R, Geubel AP. Short report: interferon-α decreases ^{14}C-aminopyrine breath test values in patients with chronic hepatitis C. *Aliment Pharmacol Ther.* 1994;8:353–355.

This product and its use are covered by the following US Patent Nos.: 4,695,623; 5,372,808; 5,541,293.

Manufactured by:
Amgen Inc.
One Amgen Center Drive
Thousand Oaks, CA
91320–1789

Issue Date: October 1997
P80080 200M/10–97

Shown in Product Identification Guide, page 304

NEUPOGEN® ℞
(Filgrastim)

DESCRIPTION

Filgrastim is a human granulocyte colony stimulating factor (G-CSF), produced by recombinant DNA technology. NEUPOGEN® is the Amgen Inc. trademark for Filgrastim, which has been selected as the name for recombinant methionyl human granulocyte colony stimulating factor (r-metHuG-CSF).

NEUPOGEN is a 175 amino acid protein manufactured by recombinant DNA technology.[1] NEUPOGEN is produced by *Escherichia coli (E coli)* bacteria into which has been inserted the human granulocyte colony stimulating factor gene. NEUPOGEN has a molecular weight of 18,800 daltons. The protein has an amino acid sequence that is identical to the natural sequence predicted from human DNA sequence analysis, except for the addition of an N-terminal methionine necessary for expression in *E coli*. Because NEUPOGEN is produced in *E coli*, the product is nonglycosylated and thus differs from G-CSF isolated from a human cell.

NEUPOGEN is a sterile, clear, colorless, preservative-free liquid for parenteral administration. Each single-use vial of NEUPOGEN contains 300 mcg/mL of Filgrastim at a specific activity of $1.0 \pm 0.6 \times 10^8$ U/mg, (as measured by a cell mitogenesis assay). The product is formulated in a 10 mM sodium acetate buffer at pH 4.0, containing 5% sorbitol, and 0.004% Tween® 80. The quantitative composition (per mL) of NEUPOGEN is:

Filgrastim	300 mcg
Acetate	0.59 mg
Sorbitol	50.0 mg
Tween® 80	0.004%
Sodium	0.035 mg
Water for Injection USP q.s. ad	1.0 mL

CLINICAL PHARMACOLOGY

Colony Stimulating Factors

Colony stimulating factors are glycoproteins which act on hematopoietic cells by binding to specific cell surface receptors and stimulating proliferation, differentiation commitment, and some end-cell functional activation.

Endogenous G-CSF is a lineage specific colony stimulating factor which is produced by monocytes, fibroblasts, and endothelial cells. G-CSF regulates the production of neutrophils within the bone marrow and affects neutrophil progenitor proliferation,[2,3] differentiation,[2,4] and selected end-cell functional activation (including enhanced phagocytic ability,[5] priming of the cellular metabolism associated with respiratory burst,[6] antibody dependent killing,[7] and the increased expression of some functions associated with cell surface antigens[8]). G-CSF is not species specific and has been shown to have minimal direct *in vivo* or *in vitro* effects on the production of hematopoietic cell types other than the neutrophil lineage.

Preclinical Experience

Filgrastim was administered to monkeys, dogs, hamsters, rats, and mice as part of a preclinical toxicology program which included single-dose acute, repeated-dose subacute, subchronic, and chronic studies. Single-dose administration of Filgrastim by the oral, intravenous (IV), subcutaneous (SC), or intraperitoneal (IP) routes resulted in no significant toxicity in mice, rats, hamsters, or monkeys. Although no deaths were observed in mice, rats, or monkeys at dose levels up to 3450 mcg/kg or in hamsters using single doses up to approximately 860 mcg/kg, deaths were observed in a subchronic (13-week) study in monkeys. In this study, evidence of neurological symptoms was seen in monkeys treated with doses of Filgrastim greater than 1150 mcg/kg/day for up to 18 days. Deaths were seen in five of the eight treated animals and were associated with 15- to 28-fold increases in peripheral leukocyte counts, and neutrophil-infiltrated hemorrhagic foci were seen in both the cerebrum and cerebellum. In contrast, no monkeys died following 13 weeks of daily IV administration of Filgrastim at a dose level of 115 mcg/kg. In an ensuing 52-week study, one 115 mcg/kg dose female monkey died after 18 weeks of daily IV administration of Filgrastim. Death was attributed to cardiopulmonary insufficiency.

In subacute, repeated-dose studies, changes observed were attributable to the expected pharmacological actions of Filgrastim (i.e., dose-dependent increases in white cell counts, increased circulating segmented neutrophils, and increased myeloid:erythroid ratio in bone marrow). In all species, histopathologic examination of the liver and spleen revealed evidence of ongoing extramedullary granulopoiesis; increased spleen weights were seen in all species and appeared to be dose-related. A dose-dependent increase in serum alkaline phosphatase was observed in rats, and may reflect increased activity of osteoblasts and osteoclasts. Changes in serum chemistry values were reversible following discontinuation of treatment.

In rats treated at doses of 1150 mcg/kg/day for 4 weeks (5 of 32 animals) and for 13 weeks at doses of 100 mcg/kg/day (4 of 32 animals) and 500 mcg/kg/day (6 of 32 animals), articular swelling of the hind legs was observed. Some degree of hind leg dysfunction was also observed; however, symptoms reversed following cessation of dosing. In rats, osteoclasis and osteoanagenesis were found in the femur, humerus, coccyx, and hind legs (where they were accompanied by synovitis) after IV treatment for 4 weeks (115 to 1150 mcg/kg/day), and in the sternum after IV treatment for 13 weeks (115 to 575 mcg/kg/day). These effects reversed to normal within 4 to 5 weeks following cessation of treatment.

In the 52-week chronic, repeated-dose studies performed in rats (IP injection up to 57.5 mcg/kg/day), and cynomolgus monkeys (IV injection of up to 115 mcg/kg/day), changes observed were similar to those noted in the subacute studies. Expected pharmacological actions of Filgrastim included dose-dependent increases in white cell counts, increased circulating segmented neutrophils and alkaline phosphatase levels, and increased myeloid:erythroid ratios in the bone marrow. Decreases in platelet counts were also noted in primates. In no animals tested were hemorrhagic complications observed. Rats displayed dose-related swelling of the hind limb, accompanied by some degree of hind limb dysfunction; osteopathy was noted microscopically. Enlarged spleens (both species) and livers (monkeys), reflective of ongoing extramedullary granulopoiesis, as well as myeloid hyperplasia of the bone marrow, were observed in a dose-dependent manner.

Pharmacologic Effects of NEUPOGEN

In phase 1 studies involving 96 patients with various nonmyeloid malignancies, NEUPOGEN administration resulted in a dose-dependent increase in circulating neutrophil counts over the dose range of 1 to 70 mcg/kg/day.[9–11] This increase in neutrophil counts was observed whether NEUPOGEN was administered IV (1 to 70 mcg/kg twice daily),[9] SC (1 to 3 mcg/kg once daily),[11] or by continuous SC infusion (3 to 11 mcg/kg/day).[10] With discontinuation of NEUPOGEN therapy, neutrophil counts returned to baseline, in most cases within 4 days. Isolated neutrophils displayed normal phagocytic (measured by zymosan-stimulated chemoluminescence) and chemotactic [measured by migration under agarose using N-formyl-methionyl-leucyl-phenylalanine (fMLP) as the chemotaxin] activity *in vitro*.

The absolute monocyte count was reported to increase in a dose-dependent manner in most patients receiving NEUPOGEN, however, the percentage of monocytes in the differential count remained within the normal range. In all studies to date, absolute counts of both eosinophils and basophils did not change and were within the normal range following administration of NEUPOGEN. Increases in lymphocyte counts following NEUPOGEN administration have been reported in some normal subjects and cancer patients.

White blood cell (WBC) differentials obtained during clinical trials have demonstrated a shift towards earlier granulocyte progenitor cells (left shift), including the appearance of promyelocytes and myeloblasts, usually during neutrophil recovery following the chemotherapy-induced nadir. In addition, Dohle bodies, increased granulocyte granulation, as well as hypersegmented neutrophils have been observed. Such changes were transient, and were not associated with clinical sequelae nor were they necessarily associated with infection.

Pharmacokinetics

Absorption and clearance of NEUPOGEN follows first-order pharmacokinetic modeling without apparent concentration dependence. A positive linear correlation occurred between the parenteral dose and both the serum concentration and area under the concentration-time curves. Continuous IV infusion of 20 mcg/kg of NEUPOGEN over 24 hours resulted in mean and median serum concentrations of approximately 48 and 56 ng/mL, respectively. Subcutaneous administration of 3.45 mcg/kg and 11.5 mcg/kg resulted in maximum serum concentrations of 4 and 49 ng/mL, respectively, within 2 to 8 hours. The volume of distribution averaged 150 mL/kg in both normal subjects and cancer patients. The elimination half-life, in both normal subjects and cancer patients, was approximately 3.5 hours. Clearance rates of NEUPOGEN were approximately 0.5 to 0.7 mL/minute/kg. Single parenteral doses or daily IV doses, over a 14-day period, resulted in comparable half-lives. The half-lives were similar for IV administration (231 minutes, following doses of 34.5 mcg/kg) and for SC administration (210 minutes, following NEUPOGEN doses of 3.45 mcg/kg). Continuous 24-hour IV infusions of 20 mcg/kg over an 11- to 20-day period produced steady-state serum concentrations of NEUPOGEN with no evidence of drug accumulation over the time period investigated.

CLINICAL EXPERIENCE

Cancer Patients Receiving Myelosuppressive Chemotherapy

NEUPOGEN has been shown to be safe and effective in accelerating the recovery of neutrophil counts following a variety of chemotherapy regimens. In a phase 3 clinical trial in small cell lung cancer, patients received SC administration of NEUPOGEN (4 to 8 mcg/kg/day, days 4 to 17) or placebo. In this study, the benefits of NEUPOGEN therapy were shown to be prevention of infection as manifested by febrile neutropenia, decreased hospitalization, and decreased IV antibiotic usage. No difference in survival or disease progression was demonstrated.

In the phase 3, randomized, double-blind, placebo-controlled trial conducted in patients with small cell lung cancer, patients were randomized to receive NEUPOGEN (n = 99) or placebo (n = 111) starting on day 4, after receiving standard dose chemotherapy with cyclophosphamide, doxorubicin, and etoposide. A total of 210 patients were evaluated for efficacy and 207 evaluated for safety. Treatment with NEUPOGEN resulted in a clinically and statistically significant reduction in the incidence of infection, as manifested by febrile neutropenia; the incidence of at least one infection over all cycles of chemotherapy was 76% (84/111) for placebo-treated patients, versus 40% (40/99) for NEUPOGEN-treated patients ($p < 0.001$). The following secondary analyses were also performed. The requirements for in-patient hospitalization and antibiotic use were also significantly decreased during the first cycle of chemotherapy; incidence of hospitalization was 69% (77/111) for placebo-treated patients in cycle one, versus 52% (51/99) for NEUPOGEN-treated patients ($p = 0.032$). The incidence of IV antibiotic usage was 60% (67/111) for placebo-treated patients in cycle one, versus 38% (38/99) for NEUPOGEN-

treated patients (p = 0.003). The incidence, severity, and duration of severe neutropenia [absolute neutrophil count (ANC) $< 500/mm^3$] following chemotherapy were all significantly reduced. The incidence of severe neutropenia in cycle one was 84% (83/99) for patients receiving NEUPOGEN versus 96% (106/110) for patients receiving placebo (p = 0.004). Over all cycles, patients randomized to NEUPOGEN had a 57% (286/500 cycles) rate of severe neutropenia versus 77% (416/543 cycles) for patients randomized to placebo. The median duration of severe neutropenia in cycle one was reduced from 6 days (range 0 to 10 days) for patients receiving placebo to 2 days (range 0 to 9 days) for patients receiving NEUPOGEN ($p < 0.001$). The mean duration of neutropenia in cycle one was 5.64 ± 2.27 days for patients receiving placebo versus 2.44 ± 1.90 days for patients receiving NEUPOGEN. Over all cycles, the median duration of neutropenia was 3 days for patients randomized to placebo versus 1 day for patients randomized to NEUPOGEN. The median severity of neutropenia (as measured by ANC nadir) was $72/mm^3$ (range $0/mm^3$ to $7912/mm^3$) in cycle one for patients receiving NEUPOGEN versus $38/mm^3$ (range $0/mm^3$ to $9520/mm^3$) for patients receiving placebo (p = 0.012). The mean severity of neutropenia in cycle one was $496/mm^3 \pm 1382/mm^3$ for patients receiving NEUPOGEN versus $204/mm^3 \pm 953/mm^3$ for patients receiving placebo. Over all cycles, the ANC nadir for patients randomized to NEUPOGEN was $403/mm^3$, versus $161/mm^3$ for patients randomized to placebo. Administration of NEUPOGEN resulted in an earlier ANC nadir following chemotherapy than was experienced by patients receiving placebo (day 10 vs day 12). NEUPOGEN was well tolerated when given SC daily at doses of 4 to 8 mcg/kg for up to 14 consecutive days following each cycle of chemotherapy (see ADVERSE REACTIONS).

Several other phase 1/2 studies, which did not directly measure the incidence of infection, but which did measure increases in neutrophils, support the efficacy of NEUPOGEN. The regimens are presented to provide some background on the clinical experience with NEUPOGEN. No claim regarding the safety or efficacy of the chemotherapy regimens is made. The effects of NEUPOGEN on tumor growth or on the anti-tumor activity of the chemotherapy were not assessed. The doses of NEUPOGEN used in these studies are considerably greater than those found to be effective in the phase 3 study described above. Such phase 1/2 studies are summarized in the following table.

[See table above]

Type of Malignancy	Regimen	Chemotherapy Dose	No. Pts.	Trial Phase	NEUPOGEN Daily Dosage[a]
Small Cell Lung Cancer	Cyclophosphamide	$1 g/m^2/day$	210	3	4-8 mc/kg SC days 4–17
	Doxorubicin	$50 mg/m^2/day$			
	Etoposide	$120 mg/m^2/day \times 3$ q 21 days			
Small Cell Lung Cancer[11]	Ifosfamide	$5 g/m^2/day$	12	1/2	5.75–46 mcg/kg IV days 4–17
	Doxorubicin	$50 mg/m^2/day$			
	Etoposide	$120 mg/m^2/day \times 3$			
	Mesna	$8 g/m^2/day$ q 21 days			
Urothelial Cancer[12]	Methotrexate	$30 mg/m^2/day \times 2$	40	1/2	3.45-69 mcg/kg IV days 4–11
	Vinblastine	$3 mg/m^2/day \times 2$			
	Doxorubicin	$30 mg/m^2/day$			
	Cisplatin	$70 mg/m^2/day$ q 28 days			
Various Non-Myeloid Malignancies[13]	Cyclophosphamide	$2.5 g/m^2/day \times 2$	18	1/2	23-69 mcg/kg[b] IV days 8–28
	Etoposide	$500 mg/m^2/day \times 3$			
	Cisplatin	$50 mg/m^2/day \times 3$ q 28 days			
Breast/Ovarian Cancer[14]	Doxorubicin[c]	$75 mg/m^2$ $100 mg/m^2$ $125 mg/m^2$ $150 mg/m^2$ q 14 days	21	2	11.5 mcg/kg IV days 2–9 5.75 mcg/kg IV days 10–12
Neuroblastoma	Cyclophosphamide	$150 mg/m^2 \times 7$	12	2	5.45–17.25 mcg/kg SC days 6–19
	Doxorubicin	$35 mg/m^2$			
	Cisplatin	$90 mg/m^2$ q 28 days (cycles 1,3,5)[d]			

[a] NEUPOGEN doses were those that accelerated neutrophil production. Doses which provided no additional acceleration beyond that achieved at the next lower dose are not reported.
[b] Lowest dose(s) tested in the study.
[c] Patients received doxorubicin at either 75, 100, 125, or 150 mg/m^2.
[d] Cycles 2,6 = cyclophosphamide $150 mg/m^2 \times 7$ and etoposide $280 mg/m^2 \times 3$. Cycle 4 = cisplatin $90 mg/m^2 \times 1$ and etoposide $280 mg/m^2 \times 3$.

Patients With Acute Myeloid Leukemia Receiving Induction or Consolidation Chemotherapy

In a randomized, double-blind, placebo-controlled, multicenter, phase 3 clinical trial, 521 patients (median age 54, range 16 to 89 years) were treated for de novo acute myeloid leukemia (AML). Following a standard induction chemotherapy regimen comprising daunorubicin, cytosine arabinoside, and etoposide[17] (DAV 3+7+5), patients received either NEUPOGEN at 5 mcg/kg/day or placebo, SC, from 24 hours after the last dose of chemotherapy until neutrophil recovery (ANC $1000/mm^3$ for 3 consecutive days or $10,000/mm^3$ for 1 day) or for a maximum of 35 days.

Treatment with NEUPOGEN significantly reduced the median time to ANC recovery and the median duration of fever, antibiotic use, and hospitalization following induction chemotherapy. In the NEUPOGEN-treated group, the median time from initiation of chemotherapy to ANC recovery (ANC $\geq 500/mm^3$) was 20 days (vs 25 days in the control group, p = 0.0001), the median duration of fever was reduced by 1.5 days (p = 0.009), and there were statistically significant reductions in the durations of IV antibiotic use and hospitalization. During consolidation therapy (DAV 2+5+5), patients treated with NEUPOGEN also experienced significant reductions in the incidence of severe neutropenia, time to neutrophil recovery, the incidence and duration of fever, and in the durations of IV antibiotic use and hospitalization. Patients treated with a further course of standard (DAV 2+5+5) or high-dose cytosine arabinoside consolidation also experienced significant reductions in the duration of neutropenia.

There were no statistically significant differences between NEUPOGEN and placebo groups in complete remission rate (69% NEUPOGEN vs 68% placebo, p = 0.77), disease-free survival [median 342 days NEUPOGEN (n = 178), 322 days placebo (n = 177), p = 0.99], time to progression of all randomized patients (median 165 days NEUPOGEN, 186 days placebo, p = 0.87), or overall survival (median 380 days NEUPOGEN, 425 days placebo, p = 0.83).

Cancer Patients Receiving Bone Marrow Transplant

In two separate randomized, controlled trials, patients with Hodgkin's disease (HD) and non-Hodgkin's lymphoma (NHL) were treated with myeloablative chemotherapy and autologous bone marrow transplantation (ABMT). In one study (n = 54), NEUPOGEN was administered at doses of 10 or 30 mcg/kg/day; a third treatment group in this study received no NEUPOGEN. A statistically significant reduction in the median number of days of severe neutropenia (ANC $< 500/mm^3$) occurred in the NEUPOGEN-treated group versus the control group [23 days in the control group, 11 days in the 10 mcg/kg/day group, and 14 days in the 30 mcg/kg/day group, (11 days in the combined treatment groups, p = 0.004)]. In the second study (n = 44, 43 patients evaluable), NEUPOGEN was administered at doses of 10 or 20 mcg/kg/day; a third treatment group in this study received no NEUPOGEN. A statistically significant reduction in the median number of days of severe neutropenia occurred in the NEUPOGEN-treated group versus the control group (21.5 days in the control group and 10 days in both treatment groups, $p < 0.001$). The number of days of febrile neutropenia was also reduced significantly in this study [13.5 days in the control group, 5 days in the 10 mcg/kg/day group, and 5.5 days in the 20 mcg/kg/day group, (5 days in the combined treatment groups, $p < 0.0001$)]. Reductions in the number of days of hospitalization and antibiotic use were also seen, although these reductions were not statistically significant. There were no effects on red blood cell or platelet levels.

In a randomized, placebo-controlled trial, 70 patients with myeloid and nonmyeloid malignancies were treated with myeloablative therapy and allogeneic bone marrow transplant followed by 300 $mcg/m^2/day$ of a Filgrastim product. A statistically significant reduction in the median number of days of severe neutropenia occurred in the treated group versus the control group (19 days in the control group and 15 days in the treatment group, $p < 0.001$) and time to recovery of ANC to $\geq 500/mm^3$ (21 days in the control group and 16 days in the treatment group, $p < 0.001$).

In three nonrandomized studies (n = 119), patients received ABMT and treatment with NEUPOGEN. One study (n = 45) involved patients with breast cancer and malignant melanoma. A second study (n = 39) involved patients with HD. The third study (n = 35) involved patients with NHL, acute lymphoblastic leukemia (ALL), and germ cell tumor. In these studies, the recovery of the ANC to $\geq 500/mm^3$ ranged from a median of 11.5 to 13 days.

None of the conditioning regimens used in the ABMT studies included radiation therapy.

While these studies were not designed to compare survival, this information was collected and evaluated. The overall survival and disease progression of patients receiving NEUPOGEN in these studies were similar to those observed in the respective control groups and to historical data.

Peripheral Blood Progenitor Cell Collection and Therapy in Cancer Patients

All patients in the Amgen-sponsored trials received a similar mobilization/collection regimen: NEUPOGEN was administered for 6 to 7 days, with an apheresis procedure on days 5, 6, and 7 (except for a limited number of patients receiving apheresis on days 4, 6, and 8). In a non-Amgen-sponsored study, patients underwent mobilization to a target number of mononuclear cells (MNC), with apheresis starting on day 5. There are no data on the mobilization of peripheral blood progenitor cells (PBPC) after days 4 to 5 that are not confounded by leukapheresis.

Mobilization: Mobilization of PBPC was studied in 50 heavily pretreated patients (median number of prior cycles = 9.5) with NHL, HD, or ALL (Amgen study 1). CFU-GM was used as the marker for engraftable PBPC. The median CFU-GM level on each day of mobilization was determined from the data available (CFU-GM assays were not obtained on all patients on each day of mobilization). These data are presented below.

The data from Amgen study 1 were supported by data from Amgen study 2 in which 22 pretreated breast cancer patients (median number of prior cycles = 3) were studied. Both the CFU-GM and $CD34^+$ cells reached a maximum on day 5 at > 10-fold over baseline and then remained elevated with leukapheresis.

[See table at top of next page]

In three studies of patients with prior exposure to chemotherapy, the median CFU-GM yield in the leukapheresis product ranged from 20.9 to 32.7×10^4/kg body weight (n = 105). In two of these studies where $CD34^+$ yields in the leukapheresis product were also determined, the median $CD34^+$ yields were 3.11 and 2.80×10^6/kg, respectively (n = 56). In an additional study of 18 chemotherapy-naive patients, the median CFU-GM yield was 123.4×10^4/kg.

Engraftment: Engraftment following NEUPOGEN-mobilized PBPC is summarized for 101 patients in the table below. In all studies, a Cox regression model showed that the total number of CFU-GM and/or $CD34^+$ cells collected was a significant predictor of time to platelet recovery.

In a randomized unblinded study of patients with HD or NHL undergoing myeloablative chemotherapy (Amgen study 3), 27 patients received NEUPOGEN-mobilized PBPC followed by NEUPOGEN and 31 patients received ABMT followed by NEUPOGEN. Patients randomized to the NEUPOGEN-mobilized PBPC group compared to the ABMT group had significantly fewer days of platelet transfusions (median 6 vs 10 days), a significantly shorter time to a sustained platelet count $> 20,000/mm^3$ (median 16 vs 23 days), a significantly shorter time to recovery of a sustained ANC $\geq 500/mm^3$ (median 11 vs 14 days), significantly fewer days of red blood cell transfusions (median 2 vs 3 days) and a significantly shorter duration of posttransplant hospitalization.

Continued on next page

Neupogen—Cont.

[See table at bottom of page]

Three of the 101 patients (3%) did not achieve the criteria for engraftment as defined by a platelet count $\geq 20,000/$ mm^3 by day 28. In clinical trials of NEUPOGEN for the mobilization of PBPC, NEUPOGEN was administered to patients at 5 to 24 mcg/kg/day after reinfusion of the collected cells until a sustainable ANC ($\geq 500/mm^3$) was reached. The rate of engraftment of these cells in the absence of NEUPOGEN posttransplantation has not been studied.

Patients With Severe Chronic Neutropenia

Severe Chronic Neutropenia (SCN) (idiopathic, cyclic, and congenital) is characterized by a selective decrease in the number of circulating neutrophils and an enhanced susceptibility to bacterial infections.

The daily administration of NEUPOGEN has been shown to be safe and effective in causing a sustained increase in the neutrophil count and a decrease in infectious morbidity in children and adults with the clinical syndrome of SCN.[15] In the phase 3 trial, summarized in the following table, daily treatment with NEUPOGEN resulted in significant beneficial changes in the incidence and duration of infection, fever, antibiotic use, and oropharyngeal ulcers. In this trial, 120 patients with a median age of 12 years (range 1 to 76 years) were treated.

[See table at bottom of next page]

The incidence for each of these five clinical parameters was lower in the NEUPOGEN arm compared to the control arm for cohorts in each of the three major diagnostic categories. All three diagnostic groups showed favorable trends in favor of treatment. An analysis of variance showed no significant interaction between treatment and diagnosis, suggesting that efficacy did not differ substantially in the different diseases. Although NEUPOGEN substantially reduced neutropenia in all patient groups, in patients with cyclic neutropenia, cycling persisted but the period of neutropenia was shortened to 1 day.

As a result of the lower incidence and duration of infections, there was also a lower number of episodes of hospitalization [28 hospitalizations in 62 patients in the treated group vs 44 hospitalizations in 60 patients in the control group over a 4-month period (p = 0.0034)]. Patients treated with NEUPOGEN also reported a lower number of episodes of diarrhea, nausea, fatigue, and sore throat.

In the phase 3 trial, untreated patients had a median ANC of $210/mm^3$ (range 0 to $1550/mm^3$). NEUPOGEN therapy was adjusted to maintain the median ANC between 1500 and $10,000/mm^3$. Overall, the response to NEUPOGEN was observed in 1 to 2 weeks. The median ANC after 5 months of NEUPOGEN therapy for all patients was $7460/mm^3$ (range 30 to $30,880/mm^3$). NEUPOGEN dosing requirements were generally higher for patients with congenital neutropenia (2.3 to 40 mcg/kg/day) than for patients with idiopathic (0.6 to 11.5 mcg/kg/day) or cyclic (0.5 to 6 mcg/kg/day) neutropenia.

INDICATIONS AND USAGE

Cancer Patients Receiving Myelosuppressive Chemotherapy

NEUPOGEN is indicated to decrease the incidence of infection, as manifested by febrile neutropenia, in patients with nonmyeloid malignancies receiving myelosuppressive anticancer drugs associated with a significant incidence of severe neutropenia with fever (see CLINICAL EXPERIENCE). A complete blood count (CBC) and platelet count should be obtained prior to chemotherapy, and twice per week (see LABORATORY MONITORING) during NEUPOGEN therapy to avoid leukocytosis and to monitor the neutrophil count. In phase 3 clinical studies, NEUPOGEN therapy was discontinued when the ANC was $\geq 10,000/mm^3$ after the expected chemotherapy-induced nadir.

Patients With Acute Myeloid Leukemia Receiving Induction or Consolidation Chemotherapy

NEUPOGEN is indicated for reducing the time to neutrophil recovery and the duration of fever, following induction or consolidation chemotherapy treatment of adults with AML.

Progenitor Cell Levels in Peripheral Blood by Mobilization Day

	Overall Study 1 CFU-GM/mL		Study 2 CFU-GM/mL		Study 2 CD34+ ($\times 10^4$/mL)	
	No. Samples	Median (25%–75%)	No. Samples	Median (25%–75%)	No. Samples	Median (25%–75%)
Day 1	11	18 (13–62)	20	42 (15–151)	20	0.13 (0.02–0.66)
Day 2	7	22 (3–61)	n/a	n/a	n/a	n/a
Day 3	10	138 (39–364)	n/a	n/a	n/a	n/a
Day 4	18	365 (158–864)	18	576 (108–1819)	17	2.11 (0.58–3.93)
Day 5	36	781 (391–1608)	21	960 (72–1677)	22	3.16 (1.08–6.11)
Day 6	46	505 (199–1397)	22	756 (70–3486)	22	2.67 (1.09–4.40)
Day 7	37	333 (111–938)	22	597 (118–2009)	21	2.64 (0.78–4.22)
Day 8	15	383 (94–815)	12	51 (10–746)	12	1.61 (0.38–4.31)

n/a = not available

Cancer Patients Receiving Bone Marrow Transplant

NEUPOGEN is indicated to reduce the duration of neutropenia and neutropenia-related clinical sequelae, e.g., febrile neutropenia, in patients with nonmyeloid malignancies undergoing myeloablative chemotherapy followed by marrow transplantation (see CLINICAL EXPERIENCE). It is recommended that CBCs and platelet counts be obtained at a minimum of three times per week (see LABORATORY MONITORING) following marrow infusion to monitor the recovery of marrow reconstitution.

Patients Undergoing Peripheral Blood Progenitor Cell Collection and Therapy

NEUPOGEN is indicated for the mobilization of hematopoietic progenitor cells into the peripheral blood for collection by leukapheresis. Mobilization allows for the collection of increased numbers of progenitor cells capable of engraftment compared with collection by leukapheresis without mobilization or bone marrow harvest. After myeloablative chemotherapy, the transplantation of an increased number of progenitor cells can lead to more rapid engraftment, which may result in a decreased need for supportive care (see CLINICAL EXPERIENCE).

Patients With Severe Chronic Neutropenia

NEUPOGEN is indicated for chronic administration to reduce the incidence and duration of sequelae of neutropenia (e.g., fever, infections, oropharyngeal ulcers) in symptomatic patients with congenital neutropenia, cyclic neutropenia, or idiopathic neutropenia (see CLINICAL EXPERIENCE). It is essential that serial CBCs with differential and platelet counts, and an evaluation of bone marrow morphology and karyotype be performed prior to initiation of NEUPOGEN therapy. The use of NEUPOGEN prior to confirmation of SCN may impair diagnostic efforts and may thus impair or delay evaluation and treatment of an underlying condition, other than SCN, causing the neutropenia.

CONTRAINDICATIONS

NEUPOGEN is contraindicated in patients with known hypersensitivity to E coli-derived proteins, Filgrastim, or any component of the product.

WARNINGS

Allergic-type reactions occurring on initial or subsequent treatment have been reported in < 1 in 4000 patients treated with NEUPOGEN. These have generally been characterized by systemic symptoms involving at least two body systems, most often skin (rash, urticaria, facial edema), respiratory (wheezing, dyspnea), and cardiovascular (hypoten-

sion, tachycardia). Some reactions occurred on initial exposure. Reactions tended to occur within the first 30 minutes after administration and appeared to occur more frequently in patients receiving NEUPOGEN IV. Rapid resolution of symptoms occurred in most cases after administration of antihistamines, steroids, bronchodilators, and/or epinephrine. Symptoms recurred in more than half the patients who were rechallenged.

Patients With Severe Chronic Neutropenia

The safety and efficacy of NEUPOGEN in the treatment of neutropenia due to other hematopoietic disorders (e.g., myelodysplastic disorders or myeloid leukemia) have not been established. Care should be taken to confirm the diagnosis of SCN before initiating NEUPOGEN therapy.

While 9 of 325 patients developed myelodysplasia or myeloid leukemia while receiving NEUPOGEN during clinical trials, AML or abnormal cytogenetics have been reported to occur in the natural history of SCN without cytokine therapy.[16] Abnormal cytogenetics have been associated with the eventual development of myeloid leukemia. The effect of NEUPOGEN on the development of abnormal cytogenetics and the effect of continued NEUPOGEN administration in patients with abnormal cytogenetics are unknown. If a patient with SCN develops abnormal cytogenetics, the risks and benefits of continuing NEUPOGEN should be carefully considered (see ADVERSE REACTIONS).

PRECAUTIONS

General

Simultaneous Use With Chemotherapy and Radiation Therapy

The safety and efficacy of NEUPOGEN given simultaneously with cytotoxic chemotherapy have not been established. Because of the potential sensitivity of rapidly dividing myeloid cells to cytotoxic chemotherapy, do not use NEUPOGEN in the period 24 hours before through 24 hours after the administration of cytotoxic chemotherapy (see DOSAGE AND ADMINISTRATION).

The efficacy of NEUPOGEN has not been evaluated in patients receiving chemotherapy associated with delayed myelosuppression (e.g., nitrosoureas) or with mitomycin C or with myelosuppressive doses of anti-metabolites such as 5-fluorouracil.

The safety and efficacy of NEUPOGEN have not been evaluated in patients receiving concurrent radiation therapy. Simultaneous use of NEUPOGEN with chemotherapy and radiation therapy should be avoided.

Potential Effect on Malignant Cells

NEUPOGEN is a growth factor that primarily stimulates neutrophils. However, the possibility that NEUPOGEN can act as a growth factor for any tumor type cannot be excluded. In a randomized study evaluating the effects of NEUPOGEN versus placebo in patients undergoing remission induction for AML, there was no significant difference in remission rate, disease-free or overall survival (see CLINICAL EXPERIENCE).

The safety of NEUPOGEN in chronic myeloid leukemia (CML) and myelodysplasia (MDS) has not been established. When NEUPOGEN is used to mobilize PBPC, tumor cells may be released from the marrow and subsequently collected in the leukapheresis product. The effect of reinfusion of tumor cells has not been well-studied, and the limited data available are inconclusive.

Leukocytosis

Cancer Patients Receiving Myelosuppressive Chemotherapy

White blood cell counts of $100,000/mm^3$ or greater were observed in approximately 2% of patients receiving NEUPO-

	Amgen-sponsored Study 1 N=13	Amgen-sponsored Study 2 N=22	Amgen-sponsored Study 3 N=27	Non-Amgen-sponsored Study N=39
Median PBPC/kg Collected:				
MNC	9.5×10^8	9.5×10^8	8.1×10^8	10.3×10^8
CD34+	n/a	3.1×10^6	2.8×10^6	6.2×10^6
CFU-GM	63.9×10^4	25.3×10^4	32.6×10^4	n/a
Days to ANC $\geq 500/mm^3$:				
Median	9	10	11	10
Range	8–10	8–15	9–38	7–40
Days to Plt. $\geq 20,000/mm^3$:				
Median	10	12.5	16	15.5
Range	7–16	10–30	8–52	7–63

n/a = not available.

GEN at doses above 5 mcg/kg/day. There were no reports of adverse events associated with this degree of leukocytosis. In order to avoid the potential complications of excessive leukocytosis, a CBC is recommended twice per week during NEUPOGEN therapy (see LABORATORY MONITORING).

Premature Discontinuation of NEUPOGEN Therapy

Cancer Patients Receiving Myelosuppressive Chemotherapy

A transient increase in neutrophil counts is typically seen 1 to 2 days after initiation of NEUPOGEN therapy. However, for a sustained therapeutic response, NEUPOGEN therapy should be continued following chemotherapy until the post nadir ANC reaches 10,000/mm^3. Therefore, the premature discontinuation of NEUPOGEN therapy, prior to the time of recovery from the expected neutrophil nadir, is generally not recommended (see DOSAGE AND ADMINISTRATION).

Other

In studies of NEUPOGEN administration following chemotherapy, most reported side effects were consistent with those usually seen as a result of cytotoxic chemotherapy (see ADVERSE REACTIONS). Because of the potential of receiving higher doses of chemotherapy (i.e., full doses on the prescribed schedule), the patient may be at greater risk of thrombocytopenia, anemia, and nonhematologic consequences of increased chemotherapy doses (please refer to the prescribing information of the specific chemotherapy agents used). Regular monitoring of the hematocrit and platelet count is recommended. Furthermore, care should be exercised in the administration of NEUPOGEN in conjunction with other drugs known to lower the platelet count. In septic patients receiving NEUPOGEN, the physician should be alert to the theoretical possibility of adult respiratory distress syndrome, due to the possible influx of neutrophils at the site of inflammation.

There have been rare reports (< 1 in 7000 patients) of cutaneous vasculitis in patients treated with NEUPOGEN. In most cases, the severity of cutaneous vasculitis was moderate or severe. Most of the reports involved patients with SCN receiving long-term NEUPOGEN therapy. Symptoms of vasculitis generally developed simultaneously with an increase in the ANC and abated when the ANC decreased. Many patients were able to continue NEUPOGEN at a reduced dose.

Information for Patients

In those situations in which the physician determines that the patient can safely and effectively self-administer NEUPOGEN, the patient should be instructed as to the proper dosage and administration. Patients should be referred to the "Information for Patients" labeling included with the Package Insert in each dispensing carton of NEUPOGEN. This patient information, however, is not intended to be a disclosure of all known or possible effects. If home use is prescribed, patients should be thoroughly instructed in the importance of proper disposal and cautioned against the reuse of needles, syringes, or drug product. A puncture-resistant container for the disposal of used syringes and needles should be available to the patient. The full container should be disposed of according to the directions provided by the physician.

Laboratory Monitoring

Cancer Patients Receiving Myelosuppressive Chemotherapy

A CBC and platelet count should be obtained prior to chemotherapy, and at regular intervals (twice per week) during NEUPOGEN therapy. Following cytotoxic chemotherapy, the neutrophil nadir occurred earlier during cycles when NEUPOGEN was administered, and WBC differentials demonstrated a left shift, including the appearance of promyelocytes and myeloblasts. In addition, the duration of severe neutropenia was reduced, and was followed by an accelerated recovery in the neutrophil counts. Therefore, regular monitoring of WBC counts, particularly at the time of the recovery from the postchemotherapy nadir, is recommended in order to avoid excessive leukocytosis.

Cancer Patients Receiving Bone Marrow Transplant

Frequent CBCs and platelet counts are recommended (at least three times per week) following marrow transplantation.

Event	% of Blinded Cycles with Events	
	NEUPOGEN N=384 Patient Cycles	Placebo N=257 Patient Cycles
Nausea/Vomiting	57	64
Skeletal Pain	22	11
Alopecia	18	27
Diarrhea	14	23
Neutropenic Fever	13	35
Mucositis	12	20
Fever	12	11
Fatigue	11	16
Anorexia	9	11
Dyspnea	9	11
Headache	7	9
Cough	6	8
Skin Rash	6	9
Chest Pain	5	6
Generalized Weakness	4	7
Sore Throat	4	9
Stomatitis	5	10
Constipation	5	10
Pain (Unspecified)	2	7

Patients With Severe Chronic Neutropenia

During the initial 4 weeks of NEUPOGEN therapy and during the 2 weeks following any dose adjustment, a CBC with differential and platelet count should be performed twice weekly. Once a patient is clinically stable, a CBC with differential and platelet count should be performed monthly. In clinical trials, the following laboratory results were observed.

— Cyclic fluctuations in the neutrophil counts were frequently observed in patients with congenital or idiopathic neutropenia after initiation of NEUPOGEN therapy.

— Platelet counts were generally at the upper limits of normal prior to NEUPOGEN therapy. With NEUPOGEN therapy, platelet counts decreased but usually remained within normal limits (see ADVERSE REACTIONS).

— Early myeloid forms were noted in peripheral blood in most patients, including the appearance of metamyelocytes and myelocytes. Promyelocytes and myeloblasts were noted in some patients.

— Relative increases were occasionally noted in the number of circulating eosinophils and basophils. No consistent increases were observed with NEUPOGEN therapy.

— As in other trials, increases were observed in serum uric acid, lactic dehydrogenase, and serum alkaline phosphatase.

Drug Interaction

Drug interactions between NEUPOGEN and other drugs have not been fully evaluated. Drugs which may potentiate the release of neutrophils, such as lithium, should be used with caution.

Carcinogenesis, Mutagenesis, Impairment of Fertility

The carcinogenic potential of NEUPOGEN has not been studied. NEUPOGEN failed to induce bacterial gene mutations in either the presence or absence of a drug metabolizing enzyme system. NEUPOGEN had no observed effect on the fertility of male or female rats, or on gestation at doses up to 500 mcg/kg.

Pregnancy Category C

NEUPOGEN has been shown to have adverse effects in pregnant rabbits when given in doses 2 to 10 times the human dose. There are no adequate and well-controlled studies in pregnant women. NEUPOGEN should be used during pregnancy only if the potential benefit justifies the potential risk to the fetus.

In rabbits, increased abortion and embryolethality were observed in animals treated with NEUPOGEN at 80 mcg/kg/day. NEUPOGEN administered to pregnant rabbits at doses of 80 mcg/kg/day during the period of organogenesis was associated with increased fetal resorption, genitourinary bleeding, developmental abnormalities, decreased body weight, live births, and food consumption. External abnormalities were not observed in the fetuses of dams treated at 80 mcg/kg/day. Reproductive studies in pregnant rats have shown that NEUPOGEN was not associated with lethal, teratogenic, or behavioral effects on fetuses when administered by daily IV injection during the period of organogenesis at dose levels up to 575 mcg/kg/day.

In Segment III studies in rats, offspring of dams treated at > 20 mcg/kg/day exhibited a delay in external differentiation (detachment of auricles and descent of testes) and slight growth retardation, possibly due to lower body weight of females during rearing and nursing. Offspring of dams treated at 100 mcg/kg/day exhibited decreased body weights at birth, and a slightly reduced 4-day survival rate.

Nursing Mothers

It is not known whether NEUPOGEN is excreted in human milk. Because many drugs are excreted in human milk, caution should be exercised if NEUPOGEN is administered to a nursing woman.

Pediatric Use

Serious long-term risks associated with daily administration of NEUPOGEN have not been identified in pediatric patients (ages 4 months to 17 years) with SCN. Limited data from patients who were followed in the phase 3 study for 1.5 years did not suggest alterations in growth and development, sexual maturation, or endocrine function.

The safety and efficacy in neonates and patients with autoimmune neutropenia of infancy have not been established. In the cancer setting, 12 pediatric patients with neuroblastoma have received up to 6 cycles of cyclophosphamide, cisplatin, doxorubicin, and etoposide chemotherapy concurrently with NEUPOGEN; in this population, NEUPOGEN was well tolerated. There was one report of palpable splenomegaly associated with NEUPOGEN therapy, however, the only consistently reported adverse event was musculoskeletal pain, which is no different from the experience in the adult population.

ADVERSE REACTIONS

Cancer Patients Receiving Myelosuppressive Chemotherapy

In clinical trials involving over 350 patients receiving NEUPOGEN following nonmyeloablative cytotoxic chemotherapy, most adverse experiences were the sequelae of the underlying malignancy or cytotoxic chemotherapy. In all phase 2 and 3 trials, medullary bone pain, reported in 24% of patients, was the only consistently observed adverse reaction attributed to NEUPOGEN therapy. This bone pain was generally reported to be of mild-to-moderate severity, and could be controlled in most patients with non-narcotic analgesics; infrequently, bone pain was severe enough to require narcotic analgesics. Bone pain was reported more frequently in patients treated with higher doses (20 to 100 mcg/kg/day) administered IV, and less frequently in patients treated with lower SC doses of NEUPOGEN (3 to 10 mcg/kg/day).

In the randomized, double-blind, placebo-controlled trial of NEUPOGEN therapy following combination chemotherapy in patients (n = 207) with small cell lung cancer, the following adverse events were reported during blinded cycles of study medication (placebo or NEUPOGEN at 4 to 8 mcg/kg/day). Events are reported as exposure adjusted since patients remained on double-blind NEUPOGEN a median of 3 cycles versus 1 cycle for placebo.

[See table above]

In this study, there were no serious, life-threatening, or fatal adverse reactions attributed to NEUPOGEN therapy. Specifically, there were no reports of flu-like symptoms, pleuritis, pericarditis, or other major systemic reactions to NEUPOGEN.

Overall Significant Changes in Clinical Endpoints
Median Incidence^a (events) or Duration (days) per 28-day Period

	Control Patients^b	NEUPOGEN-treated Patients	p-value
Incidence of Infection	0.50	0.20	<0.001
Incidence of Fever	0.25	0.20	<0.001
Duration of Fever	0.63	0.20	0.005
Incidence of Oropharyngeal Ulcers	0.26	0.00	<0.001
Incidence of Antibiotic Use	0.49	0.20	<0.001

a Incidence values were calculated for each patient, and are defined as the total number of events experienced divided by the number of 28-day periods of exposure (on-study). Median incidence values were then reported for each patient group.
b Control patients were observed for a 4-month period.

Continued on next page

Neupogen—Cont.

Spontaneously reversible elevations in uric acid, lactate dehydrogenase, and alkaline phosphatase occurred in 27% to 58% of 98 patients receiving blinded NEUPOGEN therapy following cytotoxic chemotherapy; increases were generally mild to moderate. Transient decreases in blood pressure (< 90/60 mmHg), which did not require clinical treatment, were reported in 7 of 176 patients in phase 3 clinical studies following administration of NEUPOGEN. Cardiac events (myocardial infarctions, arrhythmias) have been reported in 11 of 375 cancer patients receiving NEUPOGEN in clinical studies; the relationship to NEUPOGEN therapy is unknown. No evidence of interaction of NEUPOGEN with other drugs was observed in the course of clinical trials (see PRECAUTIONS).

There has been no evidence for the development of antibodies or of a blunted or diminished response to NEUPOGEN in treated patients, including those receiving NEUPOGEN daily for almost 2 years.

Patients With Acute Myeloid Leukemia

In a randomized phase 3 clinical trial, 259 patients received NEUPOGEN and 262 patients received placebo postchemotherapy. Overall, the frequency of all reported adverse events was similar in both the NEUPOGEN and placebo groups (83% vs 82% in Induction 1, 61% vs 64% in Consolidation 1). Adverse events reported more frequently in the NEUPOGEN-treated group included: petechiae (17% vs 14%), epistaxis (9% vs 5%), and transfusion reactions (10% vs 5%). There were no significant differences in the frequency of these events.

There were a similar number of deaths in each treatment group during induction (25 NEUPOGEN vs 27 placebo). The primary causes of death included infection (9 vs 18), persistent leukemia (7 vs 5), and hemorrhage (6 vs 3). Of the hemorrhagic deaths, five cerebral hemorrhages were reported in the NEUPOGEN group and one in the placebo group. Other serious nonfatal hemorrhagic events were reported in the respiratory tract (4 vs 1), skin (4 vs 4), gastrointestinal tract (2 vs 2), urinary tract (1 vs 1), ocular (1 vs 0), and other nonspecific sites (2 vs 1). While 19 (7%) patients in the NEUPOGEN group and five (2%) patients in the placebo group experienced severe or fatal hemorrhagic events, overall, hemorrhagic adverse events were reported at a similar frequency in both groups (40% vs 38%). The time to transfusion-independent platelet recovery and the number of days of platelet transfusions were similar in both groups.

Cancer Patients Receiving Bone Marrow Transplant

In clinical trials, the reported adverse effects were those typically seen in patients receiving intensive chemotherapy followed by bone marrow transplant (BMT). The most common events reported in both control and treatment groups included stomatitis, nausea, and vomiting, generally of mild-to-moderate severity and were considered unrelated to NEUPOGEN. In the randomized studies of BMT involving 167 patients who received study drug, the following events occurred more frequently in patients treated with Filgrastim than in controls: nausea (10% vs 4%), vomiting (7% vs 3%), hypertension (4% vs 0%), rash (12% vs 10%), and peritonitis (2% vs 0%). None of these events were reported by the Investigator to be related to NEUPOGEN. One event of erythema nodosum was reported moderate in severity and possibly related to NEUPOGEN.

Generally, adverse events observed in nonrandomized studies were similar to those seen in randomized studies, occurred in a minority of patients, and were of mild-to-moderate severity. In one study (n = 45), three serious adverse events reported by the Investigator were considered possibly related to NEUPOGEN. These included two events of renal insufficiency and one event of capillary leak syndrome. The relationship of these events to NEUPOGEN remains unclear since they occurred in patients with culture-proven infection with clinical sepsis who were receiving potentially nephrotoxic antibacterial and antifungal therapy.

Cancer Patients Undergoing Peripheral Blood Progenitor Cell Collection and Therapy

In clinical trials, 126 patients received NEUPOGEN for PBPC mobilization. In this setting, NEUPOGEN was generally well tolerated. Adverse events related to NEUPOGEN consisted primarily of mild-to-moderate musculoskeletal symptoms, reported in 44% of patients. These symptoms were predominantly events of medullary bone pain (33%). Headache was reported related to NEUPOGEN in 7% of patients. Transient increases in alkaline phosphatase related

to NEUPOGEN were reported in 21% of the patients who had serum chemistries measured; most were mild-to-moderate. All patients had increases in neutrophil counts during mobilization, consistent with the biological effects of NEUPOGEN. Two patients had a WBC count > 100,000/mm^3. No sequelae were associated with any grade of leukocytosis.

Sixty-five percent of patients had mild-to-moderate anemia and 97% of patients had decreases in platelet counts; five patients (out of 126) had decreased platelet counts to < 50,000/mm^3. Anemia and thrombocytopenia have been reported to be related to leukapheresis; however, the possibility that NEUPOGEN mobilization may contribute to anemia or thrombocytopenia has not been ruled out.

Patients with Severe Chronic Neutropenia

Mild-to-moderate bone pain was reported in approximately 33% of patients in clinical trials. This symptom was readily controlled with non-narcotic analgesics. Generalized musculoskeletal pain was also noted in higher frequency in patients treated with NEUPOGEN. Palpable splenomegaly was observed in approximately 30% of patients. Abdominal or flank pain was seen infrequently and thrombocytopenia (< 50,000/mm^3) was noted in 12% of patients with palpable spleens. Fewer than 3% of all patients underwent splenectomy, and most of these had a prestudy history of splenomegaly. Fewer than 6% of patients had thrombocytopenia (< 50,000/mm^3) during NEUPOGEN therapy, most of whom had a pre-existing history of thrombocytopenia. In most cases, thrombocytopenia was managed by NEUPOGEN dose reduction or interruption. An additional 5% of patients had platelet counts between 50,000 to 100,000/mm^3. There were no associated serious hemorrhagic sequelae in these patients. Epistaxis was noted in 15% of patients treated with NEUPOGEN, but was associated with thrombocytopenia in 2% of patients. Anemia was reported in approximately 10% of patients, but in most cases appeared to be related to frequent diagnostic phlebotomy, chronic illness, or concomitant medications. In clinical trials, myelodysplasia or myeloid leukemia was reported to have developed during NEUPOGEN therapy in approximately 3% of patients (9 of 325) (see WARNINGS). Twelve patients from a subset of 102 who had normal cytogenetic evaluations at baseline were subsequently found to have abnormalities, including monosomy 7, on routine repeat evaluation conducted after 18 to 52 months of NEUPOGEN therapy. It is unknown whether the development of these findings is related to chronic daily NEUPOGEN administration or reflects the natural history of SCN. Other adverse events infrequently observed and possibly related to NEUPOGEN therapy were: injection site reaction, rash, hepatomegaly, arthralgia, osteoporosis, cutaneous vasculitis, hematuria/proteinuria, alopecia, and exacerbation of some pre-existing skin disorders (e.g., psoriasis).

OVERDOSAGE

In cancer patients receiving NEUPOGEN as an adjunct to myelosuppressive chemotherapy, it is recommended, to avoid the potential risks of excessive leukocytosis, that NEUPOGEN therapy be discontinued if the ANC surpasses 10,000/mm^3 after the chemotherapy-induced ANC nadir has occurred. Doses of NEUPOGEN that increase the ANC beyond 10,000/mm^3 may not result in any additional clinical benefit.

The maximum tolerated dose of NEUPOGEN has not been determined. Efficacy was demonstrated at doses of 4 to 8 mcg/kg/day in the phase 3 study of nonmyeloablative chemotherapy. Patients in the BMT studies received up to 138 mcg/kg/day without toxic effects, although there was a flattening of the dose response curve above daily doses of greater than 10 mcg/kg/day.

In NEUPOGEN clinical trials of cancer patients receiving myelosuppressive chemotherapy, WBC counts > 100,000/mm^3 have been reported in less than 5% of patients, but were not associated with any reported adverse clinical effects.

In cancer patients receiving myelosuppressive chemotherapy, discontinuation of NEUPOGEN therapy usually results in a 50% decrease in circulating neutrophils within 1 to 2 days, with a return to pretreatment levels in 1 to 7 days.

DOSAGE AND ADMINISTRATION

Cancer Patients Receiving Myelosuppressive Chemotherapy

The recommended starting dose of NEUPOGEN is 5 mcg/kg/day, administered as a single daily injection by SC bolus

injection, by short IV infusion (15 to 30 minutes), or by continuous SC or continuous IV infusion. A CBC and platelet count should be obtained before instituting NEUPOGEN therapy, and monitored twice weekly during therapy. Doses may be increased in increments of 5 mcg/kg for each chemotherapy cycle, according to the duration and severity of the ANC nadir.

NEUPOGEN should be administered no earlier than 24 hours after the administration of cytotoxic chemotherapy. NEUPOGEN should not be administered in the period 24 hours before the administration of chemotherapy (see PRECAUTIONS). NEUPOGEN should be administered daily for up to 2 weeks, until the ANC has reached 10,000/mm^3 following the expected chemotherapy-induced neutrophil nadir. The duration of NEUPOGEN therapy needed to attenuate chemotherapy-induced neutropenia may be dependent on the myelosuppressive potential of the chemotherapy regimen employed. NEUPOGEN therapy should be discontinued if the ANC surpasses 10,000/mm^3 after the expected chemotherapy-induced neutrophil nadir (see PRECAUTIONS). In phase 3 trials, efficacy was observed at doses of 4 to 8 mcg/kg/day.

Cancer Patients Receiving Bone Marrow Transplant

The recommended dose of NEUPOGEN following BMT is 10 mcg/kg/day given as an IV infusion of 4 or 24 hours, or as a continuous 24-hour SC infusion. For patients receiving BMT, the first dose of NEUPOGEN should be administered at least 24 hours after cytotoxic chemotherapy and at least 24 hours after bone marrow infusion.

During the period of neutrophil recovery, the daily dose of NEUPOGEN should be titrated against the neutrophil response as follows:
[See table below]

Peripheral Blood Progenitor Cell Collection and Therapy in Cancer Patients

The recommended dose of NEUPOGEN for the mobilization of PBPC is 10 mcg/kg/day SC, either as a bolus or a continuous infusion. It is recommended that NEUPOGEN be given for at least 4 days before the first leukapheresis procedure and continued until the last leukapheresis. Although the optimal duration of NEUPOGEN administration and leukapheresis schedule have not been established, administration of NEUPOGEN for 6 to 7 days with leukaphereses on days 5, 6, and 7 was found to be safe and effective (see CLINICAL EXPERIENCE for schedules used in clinical trials). Neutrophil counts should be monitored after 4 days of NEUPOGEN, and NEUPOGEN dose modification should be considered for those patients who develop a WBC count > 100,000/mm^3.

In all clinical trials of NEUPOGEN for the mobilization of PBPC, NEUPOGEN was also administered after reinfusion of the collected cells (see CLINICAL EXPERIENCE).

Patients With Severe Chronic Neutropenia

NEUPOGEN should be administered to those patients in whom a diagnosis of congenital, cyclic, or idiopathic neutropenia has been definitively confirmed. Other diseases associated with neutropenia should be ruled out.

Starting Dose:
Congenital Neutropenia: The recommended daily starting dose is 6 mcg/kg BID SC every day.
Idiopathic or Cyclic Neutropenia: The recommended daily starting dose is 5 mcg/kg as a single injection SC every day.
Dose Adjustments:
Chronic daily administration is required to maintain clinical benefit. Absolute neutrophil count should not be used as the sole indication of efficacy. The dose should be individually adjusted based on the patient's clinical course as well as ANC. In the phase 3 study, the target ANC was 1500/mm^3 to 10,000/mm^3. However, patients may experience clinical benefit with ANCs below this target range. The dose should be reduced if the ANC is persistently greater than 10,000/mm^3.

Dilution

If required, NEUPOGEN may be diluted in 5% dextrose. NEUPOGEN diluted to concentrations between 5 and 15 mcg/mL should be protected from adsorption to plastic materials by the addition of Albumin (Human) to a final concentration of 2 mg/mL. When diluted in 5% dextrose or 5% dextrose plus Albumin (Human), NEUPOGEN is compatible with glass bottles, PVC and polyolefin IV bags, and polypropylene syringes.

Dilution of NEUPOGEN to a final concentration of less than 5 mcg/mL is not recommended at any time. **Do not dilute with saline at any time; product may precipitate.**

Storage

NEUPOGEN should be stored in the refrigerator at 2° to 8°C (36° to 46°F). Avoid shaking. Prior to injection, NEUPOGEN may be allowed to reach room temperature for a maximum of 24 hours. Any vial left at room temperature for greater than 24 hours should be discarded. Parenteral drug products should be inspected visually for particulate matter and discoloration prior to administration, whenever solution and container permit; if particulates or discoloration are observed, the container should not be used.

HOW SUPPLIED

NEUPOGEN: Use only one dose per vial; do not re-enter the vial. Discard unused portions. Do not save unused drug for later administration.

Absolute Neutrophil Count	NEUPOGEN Dose Adjustment
When ANC > 1000/mm^3 for 3 consecutive days then:	Reduce to 5 mcg/kg/day[a]
If ANC remains > 1000/mm^3 for 3 more consecutive days then:	Discontinue NEUPOGEN
If ANC decreases to < 1000/mm^3	Resume at 5 mcg/kg/day

[a] If ANC decreases to < 1000/mm^3 at any time during the 5 mcg/kg/day administration, NEUPOGEN should be increased to 10 mcg/kg/day, and the above steps should then be followed.

Single-dose, preservative-free vials containing 300 mcg (1 mL) of Filgrastim (300 mcg/mL). Dispensing packs of 10 (NDC 55513-530-10).
Single-dose, preservative-free vials containing 480 mcg (1.6 mL) of Filgrastim (300 mcg/mL). Dispensing packs of 10 (NDC 55513-546-10).

NEUPOGEN should be stored at 2° to 8° C (36° to 46° F). Avoid shaking.

REFERENCES

1. Zsebo KM, Cohen AM, Murdock DC, et al. Recombinant human granulocyte colony-stimulating factor: Molecular and biological characterization. *Immunobiol.* 1986;172:175–184.
2. Welte K, Bonilla MA, Gillio AP, et al. Recombinant human G-CSF: Effects on hematopoiesis in normal and cyclophosphamide treated primates. *J Exp Med.* 1987;165:941–948.
3. Duhrsen U, Villeval JL, Boyd J, et al. Effects of recombinant human granulocyte colony-stimulating factor on hematopoietic progenitor cells in cancer patients. *Blood.* 1988;72:2074–2081.
4. Souza LM, Boone TC, Gabrilove J, et al. Recombinant human granulocyte colony-stimulating factor: Effects on normal and leukemic myeloid cells. *Science.* 1986;232:61–65.
5. Weisbart RH, Kacena A, Schuh A, and Golde DW. GM-CSF induces human neutrophil IgA-mediated phagocytosis by an IgA Fc receptor activation mechanism. *Nature.* 1988;332:647–648.
6. Kitagawa S, Yuo A, Souza LM, Saito M, Miura Y, and Takaku F. Recombinant human granulocyte colony-stimulating factor enhances superoxide release in human granulocytes stimulated by chemotactic peptide. *Biochem Biophys Res Commun.* 1987;144:1143.
7. Glaspy JA, Baldwin GC, Robertson PA, et al. Therapy for neutropenia in hairy cell leukemia with recombinant human granulocyte colony-stimulating factor. *Ann Int Med.* 1988;109:789–795.8.
8. Yuo A, Kitagawa S, Ohsaka A, et al. Recombinant human granulocyte colony-stimulating factor as an activator of human granulocytes: Potentiation of responses triggered by receptor-mediated agonists and stimulation of C3bi receptor expression and adherance. *Blood.* 1989;74:2144–2149.
9. Gabrilove JL, Jakubowski A, Fain K, et al. Phase I study of granulocyte colony-stimulating factor in patients with transitional cell carcinoma of the urothelium. *J Clin Invest.* 1988;82:1454–1461.
10. Morstyn G, Souza L, Keech J, et al. Effect of granulocyte colony-stimulating factor on neutropenia induced by cytotoxic chemotherapy. *Lancet.* 1988;1:667–672.
11. Bronchud MH, Scarffe JH, Thatcher N, et al. Phase I/II study of recombinant human granulocyte colony-stimulating factor in patients receiving intensive chemotherapy for small cell lung cancer. *Br J Cancer.* 1987;56:809–813.
12. Gabrilove JL, Jakubowski A, Scher H, et al. Effect of granulocyte colony-stimulating factor on neutropenia and associated morbidity due to chemotherapy for transitional cell carcinoma of the urothelium. *N Engl J Med.* 1988;318:1414–1422.
13. Neidhart J, Mangalik A, Kohler W, et al. Granulocyte colony-stimulating factor stimulates recovery of granulocytes in patients receiving dose-intensive chemotherapy without bone-marrow transplantation. *J Clin Oncol.* 1989;7:1685–1691.
14. Bronchud MH, Howell A, Crowther D, et al. The use of granulocyte colony-stimulating factor to increase the intensity of treatment with doxorubicin in patients with advanced breast and ovarian cancer. *Br J Cancer.* 1989;60:121–128.
15. Dale DC, Bonilla MA, Davis MW, et al. A randomized controlled phase III trial of recombinant human granulocyte colony-stimulating factor (Filgrastim) for treatment of severe chronic neutropenia. *Blood.* 1993;81:2496–2502.
16. Schroeder TM and Kurth R. Spontaneous chromosomal breakage and high incidence of leukemia in inherited disease. *Blood.* 1971;37:96–112.
17. Heil G, Hoelzer D, Sanz MA, et al. A randomized, double-blind, placebo-controlled, phase III study of Filgrastim in remission induction and consolidation therapy for adults with de novo Acute Myeloid Leukemia. *Blood.* 1997;90:4710–4718.

This product and its use are covered by the following US Patent Nos.: 4,810,643; 4,999,291; 5,528,823; 5,580,755.

AMGEN®

Manufactured by:
Amgen Inc.
One Amgen Center Drive
Thousand Oaks, CA
91320-1789

©1991-1998 Amgen Inc.
All rights reserved.

Issue Date: 04/2/98

NEUPOGEN®
(FILGRASTIM)
Information for People Taking NEUPOGEN®

What is NEUPOGEN® and how does it work?

Colony stimulating factors (CSFs) are substances naturally produced by the body. They stimulate the growth of different types of cells found in the blood and the immune system. One type of CSF is called Granulocyte Colony Stimulating Factor or G-CSF. NEUPOGEN® brand of Filgrastim is a form of G-CSF. NEUPOGEN increases the production of infection-fighting white blood cells called neutrophils (**nu**-tro-fils).

If your physician has recommended chemotherapy, please refer to the section titled *NEUPOGEN for People Receiving Chemotherapy.* If your physician has recommended a bone marrow transplant (BMT), please refer to the section titled *NEUPOGEN for People Undergoing Bone Marrow Transplant (BMT).* If your physician has recommended a peripheral blood progenitor cell transplant (PBPCT), please refer to the section titled *NEUPOGEN for People Undergoing Peripheral Blood Progenitor Cell Transplant (PBPCT).* If your physician has recommended NEUPOGEN for the treatment of severe chronic neutropenia, please refer to the section titled *NEUPOGEN for People with Severe Chronic Neutropenia (SCN).*

How should I take NEUPOGEN?

NEUPOGEN can be given by a health care professional as an injection under the skin or into a vein by IV infusion. Some people may self-inject NEUPOGEN at home. If you are able to give it to yourself, it is important that you know how much NEUPOGEN to use, how to inject it, and how often to inject. Whether you receive NEUPOGEN at your doctor's office, a clinic, a hospital, or at home, it must be taken exactly as directed by your doctor to have the most beneficial effect.

What are the possible side effects of NEUPOGEN?

NEUPOGEN is generally well tolerated. Side effects from NEUPOGEN are not experienced by everyone. Some people experience discomfort usually described as aching in the bones and muscles. If this occurs, it can usually be relieved with a non-aspirin pain reliever, such as acetaminophen. Possible effects you may experience when receiving NEUPOGEN following a bone marrow transplant (BMT) include nausea, vomiting, hypertension, and rash. You should ask your doctor or nurse about ways to relieve any discomfort you may experience.

Allergy to NEUPOGEN

Patients occasionally experience redness, swelling, or itching at the site of injection of NEUPOGEN. This may indicate an allergy to the components of NEUPOGEN, or it may indicate a local reaction. If you suspect an allergy or a local reaction, consult your physician. A potentially more serious reaction, however, would be a generalized allergy to NEUPOGEN, which could cause a rash over the whole body, shortness of breath, wheezing, reduction in blood pressure, fast pulse, or sweating. Severe cases of generalized allergy, although very rare, may be life-threatening. If you think you are having a generalized allergic reaction, stop taking NEUPOGEN and notify a physician or emergency medical personnel immediately.

How will I know if NEUPOGEN is working?

To make sure NEUPOGEN is working for you, your doctor may require you to have blood tests to check your white blood cell count routinely while you are taking NEUPOGEN.

It is important to note that taking NEUPOGEN will reduce your risk of infection, but will not eliminate the risk entirely. In some people, an infection could still occur during the short period when neutrophil levels are low. You must take extreme care to minimize the risk of infection, which could possibly require you to go to the hospital. Therefore, it is important to recognize and be alert for some of the common signs of infection, such as a sore throat; fever; chills; rash; diarrhea; or redness, swelling, or pain around a wound or sore. If you experience one of these symptoms tell your doctor or nurse immediately.

NEUPOGEN for People Receiving Chemotherapy

What is the most important information I should know about NEUPOGEN and chemotherapy?

As your doctor has explained, the drugs used in chemotherapy may help destroy rapidly growing cells like cancer cells. Unfortunately, these anti-cancer medications also destroy some normal cells in addition to cancer cells. As a result, infection-fighting white blood cells (neutrophils) may also be destroyed while a person is receiving chemotherapy treatments.

These white blood cells, specifically neutrophils, are very important because they fight infection. They are produced inside your bones, in the bone marrow, and are part of your body's defense against invading bacteria. Because you need neutrophils to fight infection, a person with only a few neutrophils is at particular risk for developing a serious infection. When the number of neutrophils in the blood falls too low, the condition is called neutropenia (nu-tro-**peen**-ee-ah).

If you are taking NEUPOGEN because your doctor has advised you to receive chemotherapy, you will usually be given your first dose a day after your last dose of chemotherapy in each cycle. NEUPOGEN helps to speed the recovery of white blood cells (neutrophils), reduces the chance of serious infection, and helps keep you out of the hospital. NEUPOGEN is not a treatment for cancer. It works only to help protect against infection, during the time when you are at risk following chemotherapy.

You should not receive NEUPOGEN in the period 24 hours before through 24 hours after receiving your chemotherapy. You will need to have laboratory tests done twice a week so your doctor can monitor your white blood cell count.

NEUPOGEN for People Undergoing Bone Marrow Transplant (BMT)

What is the most important information I should know about NEUPOGEN and bone marrow transplant (BMT)?

If your doctor had advised you to undergo a bone marrow transplant*, NEUPOGEN may be given after chemotherapy and after bone marrow has been put into your body, to help restore and maintain your white blood cell count and prevent infection. Your doctor will routinely check your white blood cell count to see if the number of neutrophils is increasing as expected, and to change the dose of NEUPOGEN, if needed.

**The information and consent for the bone marrow transplant procedure will be provided to you separately.*

NEUPOGEN for People Undergoing Peripheral Blood Progenitor Cell Transplant (PBPCT)

What is the most important information I should know about NEUPOGEN and peripheral blood progenitor cell transplant (PBPCT)?

As an alternative to bone marrow transplant, your doctor may advise you to undergo a peripheral blood progenitor cell transplant (PBPCT). You will be given NEUPOGEN injections for several days in a row. NEUPOGEN will increase the number of progenitor cells circulating in your blood. Progenitor cells are immature cells in your bone marrow that will eventually develop into blood cells. The progenitor cells circulating in your blood will be removed using a procedure called apheresis (ay-fuh-**ree**-sis). The cells collected will be frozen, stored, and returned to your bloodstream (transplanted) after you have had your chemotherapy treatment. The transplanted cells will help to restore your blood counts after chemotherapy. The transplanted cells may also help to reduce the risk of infection, the number of blood and platelet transfusions you need, and the length of your hospital stay.

NEUPOGEN for People with Severe Chronic Neutropenia (SCN)

What is the most important information I should know about NEUPOGEN and severe chronic neutropenia?

Severe chronic neutropenia is a disease which results in a deficiency of infection-fighting white blood cells called neutrophils (**nu**-tro-fils). When the number of these infection-fighting cells is too low, a person becomes more likely to develop a fever and/or serious infection.

NEUPOGEN works by increasing the number of neutrophils in the blood and by preventing them from decreasing to dangerously low levels. It helps to make and keep the right number of neutrophils, and to reduce your chances of a serious infection. People with severe chronic neutropenia are required to take NEUPOGEN for a long period of time.

What do I need to know if I am giving myself NEUPOGEN injections?

When you receive your NEUPOGEN from the doctor or pharmacist, always check to see that the name NEUPOGEN is on the carton and vial. Use NEUPOGEN before the expiration date stamped on the package.

How should I store NEUPOGEN?

NEUPOGEN should be stored in your refrigerator, but not in the freezer. If the vial is accidentally frozen, allow it to thaw in your refrigerator before administering your next dose. However, if the vial is frozen a second time, do not use it and contact your doctor or nurse for further instructions. You can leave your NEUPOGEN out at room temperature for up to 24 hours. Do not leave your NEUPOGEN in direct sunlight. If you have any questions about storage, contact your doctor or nurse for further instructions.

How should I take NEUPOGEN?

NEUPOGEN is given as an injection under the skin. It is important to take your NEUPOGEN every day.

Always use the correct syringe

Your doctor or nurse has instructed you on how to give yourself the correct dosage of NEUPOGEN. This dosage will usually be measured in milliliters. It is important to use a syringe that is marked in tenths of milliliters, or mL's (for example, 0.2 mL). Your doctor or nurse may refer to mL's as cc's. Failure to use the proper syringe can lead to a mistake in dosage, and you may receive too much or too little NEUPOGEN. Too little NEUPOGEN may not be effective in reducing your risk of infections, and too much NEUPOGEN may lead to neutrophil levels that are too high.

Continued on next page

Neupogen—Cont.

How do I give myself an injection?
Step-by-step guide to subcutaneous self-injection

Step 1: Setting up for self-injection

You should find a comfortable, well-lit working place and self-inject at the same time each day. Remove the vial of NEUPOGEN from the refrigerator, check the date on the NEUPOGEN vial to be sure that the drug has not expired, and allow it to reach room temperature. Each NEUPOGEN vial is designed to be used only once; do not re-enter the vial. DO NOT SHAKE THE VIAL VIGOROUSLY. If the medication has particles or is discolored, do not use it, and check with a health professional.

1. Assemble the other supplies you will need for your injection.
2. Clean your work area.
3. Assemble supplies—vial, sterile disposable syringe, alcohol swabs, puncture-proof disposal container.
4. Wash your hands thoroughly with soap and water before preparing the medication.

Step 2: Selecting and preparing the injection site

5. Find the site for injection.
   a. Back of the upper arms (if someone is giving you the injection)
   b. Abdomen, except for the naval and waist
   c. Upper thighs

Alternate the injection site each time you inject to avoid soreness at any one site.

6. Clean the injection site with an alcohol swab. Use circular motions from the inside to the outside. Keep the used alcohol swab nearby.

Step 3: Preparing the dose and injecting the medication

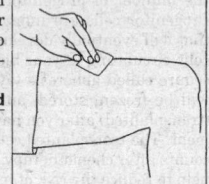

7. Remove the colored cap from the vial, exposing the rubber stopper.

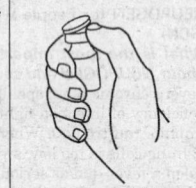

8. Clean the rubber stopper with a fresh alcohol swab, then cover the stopper with the swab.
9. Remove the syringe from its packagi the sterile covering is open, dispose of that syringe in the puncture-proof disposal container).

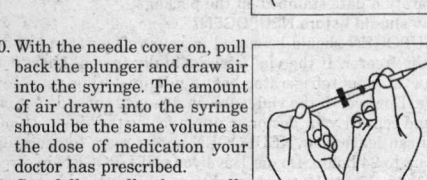

10. With the needle cover on, pull back the plunger and draw air into the syringe. The amount of air drawn into the syringe should be the same volume as the dose of medication your doctor has prescribed.
11. Carefully pull the needle cover straight off.
12. While keeping the vial on a flat surface, insert the needle straight through the rubber stopper.

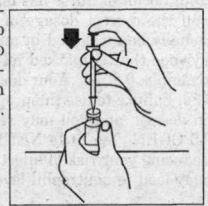

13. Push the plunger of the syringe down and inject air into the vial. The air injected into the vial will allow NEUPOGEN to be easily withdrawn from the vial into the syringe.

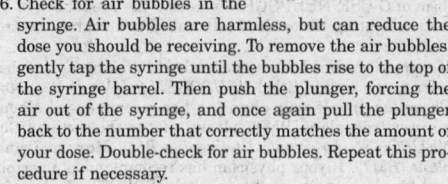

14. Keeping the needle in the vial, turn the vial upside down and make sure that the needle is in the liquid medication.
15. Slowly pull back on the plunger and let the medication enter the syringe, filling up to the dose your doctor prescribed.
16. Check for air bubbles in the syringe. Air bubbles are harmless, but can reduce the dose you should be receiving. To remove the air bubbles, gently tap the syringe until the bubbles rise to the top of the syringe barrel. Then push the plunger, forcing the air out of the syringe, and once again pull the plunger back to the number that correctly matches the amount of your dose. Double-check for air bubbles. Repeat this procedure if necessary.
17. Double-check to make sure you have drawn up the correct dose.
18. Take the needle out of the vial and hold the syringe in the hand that you will use to inject yourself. Do not lay the syringe down or allow the needle to touch anything.

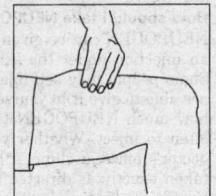

19. Use the other hand to pinch a fold of skin at the previously prepared injection site.

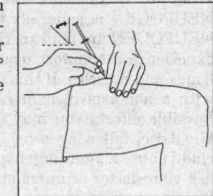

20. Hold the syringe the way you would hold a pencil and insert the needle either straight up and down (90° angle) or at a slight angle (45°) to the skin.

21. After the needle is in, let go of the skin. Pull plunger back slightly. If blood appears, do not inject NEUPOGEN, because the needle has entered a blood vessel. Withdraw the syringe and inject it in a different place. Repeat this procedure checking for blood.
22. If no blood appears, slowly push down on the plunger all the way, until all the medication is gone from the syringe.
23. As you pull the needle out of the skin, place the alcohol swab over the injection site, then press for several seconds.
24. Use the disposable syringe only once to ensure sterility of the syringe and needle, and to ensure accuracy of the dose. Dispose of syringes and needles as directed by your physician, or by following these simple steps:

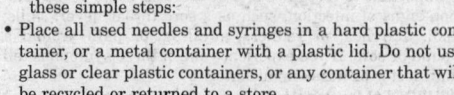

- Place all used needles and syringes in a hard plastic container, or a metal container with a plastic lid. Do not use glass or clear plastic containers, or any container that will be recycled or returned to a store.
- Properly label the container to indicate its contents. If a metal container such as a coffee can with a plastic lid is used, cut a small hole in the plastic lid and tape the lid onto the metal container. When the container is full, cover the hole and dispose of the container according to your doctor's or nurse's instructions.
- If an opaque (do not use clear plastic), hard plastic container with a screw-on cap is used, always screw the cap on tightly after each use. When the container is full, tape around the cap or lid and dispose of the container according to your doctor's or nurse's instructions.
- Please check with your doctor, nurse, or pharmacist for other suggestions for disposal. There may be special state and local laws that they will discuss with you.
- Always store the container out of the reach of children.

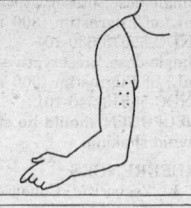

25. Always change the site for each injection as directed by your doctor. Occasionally a problem may develop at the injection site. If you notice a lump, swelling, or bruising that doesn't go away, contact your physician.

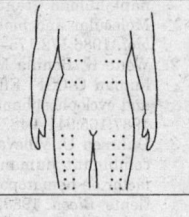

26. Try to take your NEUPOGEN at the same time each day. If you miss your dose by more than a few hours, contact your doctor or nurse.
27. NEUPOGEN should be stored in the refrigerator at 36° to 46°F (2° to 8°C), but not in the freezer. For instructions on how to transport NEUPOGEN, contact your doctor, nurse, or pharmacist.

For further information about self-injection, please call your doctor or nurse.

Usage in Pregnancy
If you are pregnant or nursing a baby, consult your physician before using NEUPOGEN.

Important Notes
If your doctor allows you to self-administer NEUPOGEN, please note the following:

1. Always follow your doctor's or nurse's instruction concerning the dosage and administration of NEUPOGEN. Do not change the dose or method of administration of NEUPOGEN without consulting your physician.
2. Your doctor will tell you what to do if you miss a dose of NEUPOGEN. Always keep a spare syringe and needle on hand.
3. If you develop a fever or symptoms of infection, contact your doctor.
4. Consult your doctor if you notice anything unusual about your condition or your use of NEUPOGEN.

AMGEN®
Manufactured by:
Amgen Inc.
One Amgen Center Drive
Thousand Oaks, CA
91320-1789
Issue Date: 12/20/96
©1996, 1997, 1998 Amgen Inc. All Rights Reserved.
P40047H 50M/Rev. 4-98

Shown in Product Identification Guide, page 304

Apothecon
A Bristol-Myers Squibb Company
P.O. BOX 4500
PRINCETON, NJ 08543-4500

For Medical Information Contact:
Generally:
Bristol-Myers Squibb Drug Information Department
P.O. Box 4500
Princeton, NJ 08543-4500
(800) 321-1335
Adverse Drug Experiences
and Product Defects Reporting call
between 8:30 am-4:30 pm EST:
(609) 818-3737
Sales and Ordering:
Orders for Apothecon Products may be placed by:
1. Calling toll-free between 8:30 am-6:00 pm EST:
   (800) 631-5244
2. Mailing your purchase orders to:
   Apothecon
   Attn: Customer Service Department
   P.O. Box 5250
   Princeton, NJ 08543-5250
3. Faxing your purchase orders to:
   Customer Service Department
   (800) 523-2965

For listing of standard, purified, and human insulins, see Novo Nordisk Pharmaceuticals Inc.

UNILOG®
(Tablet and Capsule Identification Code)
ALPHABETICAL INDEX

AL 1.0 G	**Alprazolam Tablets**, 1 mg
AL G2	**Alprazolam Tablets**, 2 mg
INV 211	**Amantadine Hydrochloride Capsules, USP** 100 mg
BMS 37	**Amoxicillin Tablets, USP (Chewable)** 125 mg
BMS 38	**Amoxicillin Tablets, USP (Chewable)** 250 mg
INV 259	**Atenolol Tablets** 25 mg
INV 256	**Atenolol Tablets** 50 mg
INV 257	**Atenolol Tablets** 100 mg
BMS 5040	**Atenolol Tablets** 50 mg
BMS 5240	**Atenolol Tablets** 100 mg
INV 208	**Benztropine Mesylate Tablets, USP** 0.5 mg
INV 209	**Benztropine Mesylate Tablets, USP** 1 mg
INV 210	**Benztropine Mesylate Tablets, USP** 2 mg
AP 8818	**Buspirone HCl Tablets** 5 mg
AP 8819	**Buspirone HCl Tablets** 10 mg
Bristol 7271	**Cefadroxil Tablets, USP** 500 mg
AP 7045	**Captopril Tablets, USP** 12.5 mg
AP 7046	**Captopril Tablets, USP** 25 mg
AP 7047	**Captopril Tablets, USP** 50 mg
AP 7048	**Captopril Tablets, USP** 100 mg
AP 7491	**Cefaclor Capsules** 250 mg
AP 7494	**Cefaclor Capsules** 500 mg
7375	**Cephalexin Capsules USP** 250 mg
7376	**Cephalexin Capsules USP** 500 mg
Squibb 181	**Cephalexin Capsules USP** 250 mg
Squibb 239	**Cephalexin Capsules USP** 500 mg
832 2L	**Cimetidine Tablets, USP** 200 mg
832 3L	**Cimetidine Tablets, USP** 300 mg
LEK CT4	**Cimetidine Tablets, USP** 400 mg
832 8L	**Cimetidine Tablets, USP** 800 mg
INV 321	**Clomipramine HCl Capsules** 25 mg
INV 322	**Clomipramine HCl Capsules** 50 mg
INV 323	**Clomipramine HCl Capsules** 75 mg
INV 353	**Clonazepam Tablets** .5 mg
INV 354	**Clonazepam Tablets** 1 mg
INV 355	**Clonazepam Tablets** 2 mg
Squibb W028	**Cloxacillin Sodium Capsules USP** 250 mg
Squibb W038	**Cloxacillin Sodium Capsules USP** 500 mg
7936	**Cloxacillin Sodium Capsules USP** 250 mg
7496	**Cloxacillin Sodium Capsules USP** 500 mg
INV 252	**Cyclobenzaprine Hydrochloride Tablets, USP** 10 mg
MJ775	**Desyrel Tablets** (Trazodone Hydrochloride Tablets) 50 mg
MJ776	**Desyrel Tablets** (Trazodone Hydrochloride Tablets) 100 mg
MJ778	**Desyrel Dividose Tablets** (Trazodone Hydrochloride Tablets) 150 mg
MJ796	**Desyrel Dividose Tablets** (Trazodone Hydrochloride Tablets) 300 mg
W048	**Dicloxacillin Sodium Capsules USP** 250 mg
W058	**Dicloxacillin Sodium Capsules USP** 500 mg
BMS 52 50	**Diltiazem Hydrochloride** 30 mg
BMS 55 50	**Diltiazem Hydrochloride** 60 mg
BMS 57 70	**Diltiazem Hydrochloride** 90 mg
BMS 58 50	**Diltiazem Hydrochloride** 120 mg
AP 0837	**Doxycycline Hyclate Capsules USP** 50 mg
AP 0814	**Doxycycline Hyclate Capsules USP** 100 mg
AP 812	**Doxycycline Hyclate Tablets USP** 100 mg
7892	**Dynapen Capsules** (Dicloxacillin Sodium Capsules USP) 125 mg
W048	**Dynapen Capsules** (Dicloxacillin Sodium Capsules USP) 250 mg
W058	**Dynapen Capsules** (Dicloxacillin Sodium Capsules USP) 500 mg
AP 025	**Estradiol Tablets** .5 mg
AP 026	**Estradiol Tablets** 1.0 mg
AP 027	**Estradiol Tablets** 2.0 mg
INV 359	**Etodolac Capsules** 200 mg
INV 360	**Etodolac Capsules** 300 mg
INV 350	**Etodolac Capsules** 400 mg
Squibb 429	**Florinef Tablets** Fludrocortisone Acetate Tablets USP) 0.1 mg
INV 320	**Gemfibrozil Tablets, USP** 600 mg
INV 291	**Glipizide Tablets, USP** 5 mg
INV 292	**Glipizide Tablets, USP** 10 mg
INV 250	**Hydroxychloroquine Sulfate Tablets, USP** 200 mg

INV 246	**Indapamide Tablets, USP** 1.25 mg
INV 247	**Indapamide Tablets, USP** 2.5 mg
Bristol 3506	**Kantrex Capsules** (Kanamycin Sulfate Capsules) 500 mg
BL 770	**Klotrix Tablets** (Potassium Chloride Tablets) 10 mEq
531 MD	**Methylphenidate HCl Tablets**, 5 mg
530 MD	**Methylphenidate HCl Tablets**, 10 mg
562 MD	**Methylphenidate HCl Tablets**, 20 mg ER
532 MD	**Methylphenidate HCl Tablets**, 20 mg
INV 351	**Methylprednisolone Tablets** 4 mg
INV 263	**Metoclopramide Tablets, USP** 5 mg
INV 264	**Metoclopramide Tablets, USP** 10 mg
BMS W921	**Metoprolol Tartrate Tablets, USP** 50 mg
BMS W933	**Metoprolol Tartrate Tablets, USP** 100 mg
Squibb 580	**Mycostatin Oral Tablets** (Nystatin Tablets USP) 500,000 u.
AP 2461	**Nadolol Tablets, USP** 20 mg
AP 2462	**Nadolol Tablets, USP** 40 mg
AP 2463	**Nadolol Tablets, USP** 80 mg
AP 2464	**Nadolol Tablets, USP** 120 mg
AP 2465	**Nadolol Tablets, USP** 160 mg
BL NI	**Naldecon Tablets**
INV 286	**Naproxen Sodium Tablets, USP** 275 mg
INV 287	**Naproxen Sodium Tablets, USP** 550 mg
PPP 606	**Naturetin Tablets** (Bendroflumethiazide Tablets USP) 5 mg
PPP 618	**Naturetin Tablets** (Bendroflumethazide Tablets USP) 10 mg
Squibb 611	**Niacin Tablets USP** 50 mg
Squibb 612	**Niacin Tablets USP** 100 mg
Squibb 537	**Niacin Tablets USP** 500 mg
P5 G	**Pindolol Tablets, USP** 5 mg
P10 G	**Pindolol Tablets, USP** 10 mg
O26 G	**Piroxicam Capsules, USP** 10 mg
O27 G	**Piroxicam Capsules, USP** 20 mg
AP 6910	**Potassium Chloride Extended Release Tablets** 10 meq
Bristol 7992	**Principen Capsules** (Ampicillin Capsules USP) 250 mg
Bristol 7993	**Principen Capsules** (Ampicillin Capsules USP) 500 mg
INV 275	**Prochlorperazine Maleate Tablets, USP** 5 mg
INV 276	**Prochlorperazine Maleate Tablets, USP** 10 mg
PPP 863	**Prolixin Tablets** (Fluphenazine Hydrochloride Tablets USP) 1 mg
PPP 864	**Prolixin Tablets** (Fluphenazine Hydrochloride Tablets USP) 2.5 mg
PPP 877	**Prolixin Tablets** (Fluphenazine Hydrochloride Tablets USP) 5 mg
PPP 956	**Prolixin Tablets** (Fluphenazine Hydrochloride Tablets USP) 10 mg
PPP 758	**Pronestyl Capsules** (Procainamide Hydrochloride Capsules USP) 250 mg
PPP 756	**Pronestyl Capsules** (Procainamide Hydrochloride Capsules USP) 375 mg
PPP 757	**Pronestyl Capsules** (Procainamide Hydrochloride Capsules USP) 500 mg
PPP 431	**Pronestyl Tablets** (Procainamide Hydrochloride Tablets USP) 250 mg
PPP 434	**Pronestyl Tablets** (Procainamide Hydrochloride Tablets USP) 375 mg
PPP 438	**Pronestyl Tablets** (Procainamide Hydrochloride Tablets USP) 500 mg
PPP 775	**Pronestyl-SR Tablets** (Procainamide Hydrochloride Tablets USP) 500 mg
APO 025	**Ranitidine Tablets**, 150 mg
APO 26	**Ranitidine Tablets**, 300 mg
AP 908	**Selegiline Tablets**, 5 mg
PPP 769	**Rauzide Tablets** (Rauwolfia Serpentina with Bendroflumethiazide Tablets) 50 mg - 4 mg

138	**SMZ/TMP Tablets** (Sulfamethoxazole and Trimethoprim Tablets USP) 400 mg - 80 mg
171	**SMZ/TMP Tablets** (Sulfamethoxazole and Trimethoprim Tablets USP) 800 mg - 160 mg
Squibb 655	**Sumycin Capsules** (Tetracycline Hydrochloride Capsules USP) 250 mg
Squibb 763	**Sumycin Capsules** (Tetracycline Hydrochloride Capsules USP) 500 mg
Squibb 663	**Sumycin Tablets** (Tetracycline Hydrochloride Tablets USP) 250 mg
Squibb 603	**Sumycin Tablets** (Tetracycline Hydrochloride Tablets USP) 500 mg
Squibb 535	**Theragran Hematinic Tablets**
AP 778	**Trazodone Hydrochloride Tablets**, 150 mg
Bristol 7278	**Trimox Capsules** (Amoxicillin Capsules USP) 250 mg
Bristol 7279	**Trimox Capsules** (Amoxicillin Capsules USP) 500 mg
MJ 543	**Vasodilan Tablets** (Isoxsuprine Hydrochloride) 10 mg
MJ 544	**Vasodilan Tablets** (Isoxsuprine Hydrochloride) 20 mg
BL V1	**Veetids Tablets** (Penicillin V Potassium Tablets, USP) 250 mg
BL V2	**Veetids Tablets** (Penicillin v Potassium Tablets, USP) 500 mg
Squibb 113	**Velosef '250' Capsules** (Cephradine Capsules USP) 250 mg
Squibb 114	**Velosef '500' Capsules** (Cephradine Capsules USP) 500 mg

---

DESYREL® Tablets
[*des 'ē-rel*]
(trazodone HCl Tablets, USP)

℞

DESCRIPTION

DESYREL (trazodone hydrochloride) is an antidepressant chemically unrelated to tricyclic, tetracyclic, or other known antidepressant agents. Trazodone hydrochloride is a triazolopyridine derivative designated as 2-[3-[4-(3-chlorophenyl)-1-piperazinyl] propyl]-1,2,4-triazolo[4, 3-a]pyridin-3(2H)-one hydrochloride. It is a white odorless crystalline powder which is freely soluble in water. Its molecular weight is 408.3. The empirical formula is $C_{19}H_{22}ClN_5O\cdot HCl$ and the structural formula is represented as follows:

DESYREL is supplied for oral administration in 50 mg, 100 mg, 150 mg and 300 mg tablets.

DESYREL Tablets, 50 mg, contain the following inactive ingredients: dibasic calcium phosphate, castor oil, microcrystalline cellulose, ethylcellulose, FD&C Yellow No. 6 (aluminum lake), lactose, magnesium stearate, povidone, sodium starch glycolate, and starch (corn).

DESYREL Tablets, 100 mg, contain the following inactive ingredients: dibasic calcium phosphate, castor oil, microcrystalline cellulose, ethylcellulose, lactose, magnesium stearate, povidone, sodium starch glycolate, and starch (corn).

DESYREL Tablets, 150 mg, contain the following inactive ingredients: microcrystalline cellulose, FD&C Yellow No. 6 (aluminum lake), magnesium stearate, pregelatinized starch, and stearic acid.

DESYREL Tablets, 300 mg, contain the following inactive ingredients: microcrystalline cellulose, yellow ferric oxide, magnesium stearate, sodium starch glycolate, pregelatinized starch, and stearic acid.

CLINICAL PHARMACOLOGY

The mechanism of DESYREL's antidepressant action in man is not fully understood. In animals, DESYREL selectively inhibits serotonin uptake by brain synaptosomes and potentiates the behavioral changes induced by the serotonin precursor, 5-hydroxytryptophan. Cardiac conduction effects of DESYREL in the anesthetized dog are qualitatively dissimilar and quantitatively less pronounced than those seen with tricyclic antidepressants. DESYREL is not a monoamine oxidase inhibitor and, unlike amphetamine-type drugs, does not stimulate the central nervous system.

Continued on next page

Desyrel—Cont.

In man, DESYREL is well absorbed after oral administration without selective localization in any tissue. When DESYREL is taken shortly after ingestion of food, there may be an increase in the amount of drug absorbed, a decrease in maximum concentration, and a lengthening in the time to maximum concentration. Peak plasma levels occur approximately one hour after dosing when DESYREL is taken on an empty stomach or two hours after dosing when taken with food. Elimination of DESYREL is biphasic, consisting of an initial phase (half-life 3–6 hours) followed by a slower phase (half-life 5–9 hours), and is unaffected by the presence or absence of food. Since the clearance of DESYREL from the body is sufficiently variable, in some patients DESYREL may accumulate in the plasma.

For those patients who responded to DESYREL, one-third of the inpatients and one-half of the outpatients had a significant therapeutic response by the end of the first week of treatment. Three-fourths of all responders demonstrated a significant therapeutic effect by the end of the second week. One-fourth of responders required 2–4 weeks for a significant therapeutic response.

INDICATIONS AND USAGE

DESYREL is indicated for the treatment of depression. The efficacy of DESYREL has been demonstrated in both inpatient and outpatient settings and for depressed patients with and without prominent anxiety. The depressive illness of patients studied corresponds to the Major Depressive Episode criteria of the American Psychiatric Association's Diagnostic and Statistical Manual, III.[a]

Major Depressive Episode implies a prominent and relatively persistent (nearly every day for at least two weeks) depressed or dysphoric mood that usually interferes with daily functioning, and includes at least four of the following eight symptoms: change in appetite, change in sleep, psychomotor agitation or retardation, loss of interest in usual activities or decrease in sexual drive, increased fatigability, feelings of guilt or worthlessness, slowed thinking or impaired concentration, and suicidal ideation or attempts.

CONTRAINDICATIONS

DESYREL is contraindicated in patients hypersensitive to DESYREL.

WARNINGS

TRAZODONE HAS BEEN ASSOCIATED WITH THE OCCURRENCE OF PRIAPISM. IN MANY OF THE CASES REPORTED, SURGICAL INTERVENTION WAS REQUIRED AND, IN SOME OF THESE CASES, PERMANENT IMPAIRMENT OF ERECTILE FUNCTION OR IMPOTENCE RESULTED. MALE PATIENTS WITH PROLONGED OR INAPPROPRIATE ERECTIONS SHOULD IMMEDIATELY DISCONTINUE THE DRUG AND CONSULT THEIR PHYSICIAN.

The detumescence of priapism and drug-induced penile erections has been accomplished by both pharmacologic, e.g., the intracavernosal injection of alpha-adrenergic stimulants such as epinephrine and norepinephrine, as well as surgical procedures.[b-g] Any pharmacologic or surgical procedure utilized in the treatment of priapism should be performed under the supervision of a urologist or a physician familiar with the procedure and should not be initiated without urologic consultation if the priapism has persisted for more than 24 hours.

DESYREL (trazodone hydrochloride) is not recommended for use during the initial recovery phase of myocardial infarction.

Caution should be used when administering DESYREL to patients with cardiac disease, and such patients should be closely monitored, since antidepressant drugs (including DESYREL) have been associated with the occurrence of cardiac arrhythmias. Recent clinical studies in patients with pre-existing cardiac disease indicate that DESYREL may be arrhythmogenic in some patients in that population. Arrhythmias identified include isolated PVCs, ventricular couplets, and in two patients short episodes (3–4 beats) of ventricular tachycardia.

PRECAUTIONS

General

The possibility of suicide in seriously depressed patients is inherent in the illness and may persist until significant remission occurs. Therefore, prescriptions should be written for the smallest number of tablets consistent with good patient management.

Hypotension, including orthostatic hypotension and syncope, has been reported to occur in patients receiving DESYREL. Concomitant administration of antihypertensive therapy with DESYREL may require a reduction in the dose of the antihypertensive drug.

Little is known about the interaction between DESYREL and general anesthetics; therefore, prior to elective surgery, DESYREL should be discontinued for as long as clinically feasible.

As with all antidepressants, the use of DESYREL should be based on the consideration of the physician that the expected benefits of therapy outweigh potential risk factors.

Information for Patients

Because priapism has been reported to occur in patients receiving DESYREL, patients with prolonged or inappropriate penile erection should immediately discontinue the drug and consult with the physician (see **WARNINGS**).

Antidepressants may impair the mental and/or physical ability required for the performance of potentially hazardous tasks, such as operating an automobile or machinery; the patient should be cautioned accordingly.

DESYREL may enhance the response to alcohol, barbiturates, and other CNS depressants.

DESYREL should be given shortly after a meal or light snack. Within any individual patient, total drug absorption may be up to 20% higher when the drug is taken with food rather than on an empty stomach. The risk of dizziness/lightheadedness may increase under fasting conditions.

Laboratory Tests

Occasional low white blood cell and neutrophil counts have been noted in patients receiving DESYREL. These were not considered clinically significant and did not necessitate discontinuation of the drug; however, the drug should be discontinued in any patient whose white blood cell count or absolute neutrophil count falls below normal levels. White blood cell and differential counts are recommended for patients who develop fever and sore throat (or other signs of infection) during therapy.

Drug Interactions

Increased serum digoxin or phenytoin levels have been reported to occur in patients receiving DESYREL concurrently with either of those two drugs.

It is not known whether interactions will occur between monoamine oxidase (MAO) inhibitors and DESYREL. Due to the absence of clinical experience, if MAO inhibitors are discontinued shortly before or are to be given concomitantly with DESYREL, therapy should be initiated cautiously with gradual increase in dosage until optimum response is achieved.

Therapeutic Interactions

Concurrent administration with electroshock therapy should be avoided because of the absence of experience in this area.

There have been reports of increased and decreased prothrombin time occurring in warfarinized patients who take DESYREL.

Carcinogenesis, Mutagenesis, Impairment of Fertility

No drug- or dose-related occurrence of carcinogenesis was evident in rats receiving DESYREL in daily oral doses up to 300 mg/kg for 18 months.

Pregnancy Category C

DESYREL has been shown to cause increased fetal resorption and other adverse effects on the fetus in two studies using the rat when given at dose levels approximately 30–50 times the proposed maximum human dose. There was also an increase in congenital anomalies in one of three rabbit studies at approximately 15–50 times the maximum human dose. There are no adequate and well-controlled studies in pregnant women. DESYREL should be used during pregnancy only if the potential benefit justifies the potential risk to the fetus.

Nursing Mothers

DESYREL and/or its metabolites have been found in the milk of lactating rats, suggesting that the drug may be secreted in human milk. Caution should be exercised when DESYREL is administered to a nursing woman.

	Treatment-Emergent Symptom Incidence			
	Inpatients		Outpatients	
	D	P	D	P
Number of Patients	142	95	157	158
% of Patients Reporting				
Allergic				
Skin Condition/Edema	2.8	1.1	7.0	1.3
Autonomic				
Blurred Vision	6.3	4.2	14.7	3.8
Constipation	7.0	4.2	7.6	5.7
Dry Mouth	14.8	8.4	33.8	20.3
Cardiovascular				
Hypertension	2.1	1.1	1.3	*
Hypotension	7.0	1.1	3.8	0.0
Shortness of Breath	*	1.1	1.3	0.0
Syncope	2.8	2.1	4.5	1.3
Tachycardia/Palpitations	0.0	0.0	7.0	7.0
CNS				
Anger/Hostility	3.5	6.3	1.3	2.5
Confusion	4.9	0.0	5.7	7.6
Decreased Concentration	2.8	2.1	1.3	0.0
Disorientation	2.1	0.0	*	0.0
Dizziness/Lightheadedness	19.7	5.3	28.0	15.2
Drowsiness	23.9	6.3	40.8	19.6
Excitement	1.4	1.1	5.1	5.7
Fatigue	11.3	4.2	5.7	2.5
Headache	9.9	5.3	19.8	15.8
Insomnia	9.9	10.5	6.4	12.0
Impaired Memory	1.4	0.0	*	*
Nervousness	14.8	10.5	6.4	8.2
Gastrointestinal				
Abdominal/Gastric Disorder	3.5	4.2	5.7	4.4
Bad Taste in Mouth	1.4	0.0	0.0	0.0
Diarrhea	0.0	1.1	4.5	1.9
Nausea/Vomiting	9.9	1.1	12.7	9.5
Musculoskeletal				
Musculoskeletal Aches/Pains	5.6	3.2	5.1	2.5
Neurological				
Incoordination	4.9	0.0	1.9	0.0
Paresthesia	1.4	0.0	0.0	*
Tremors	2.8	1.1	5.1	3.8
Sexual Function				
Decreased Libido	*	1.1	1.3	*
Other				
Decreased Appetite	3.5	5.3	0.0	*
Eyes Red/Tired/Itching	2.8	0.0	0.0	0.0
Head Full-Heavy	2.8	0.0	0.0	0.0
Malaise	2.8	0.0	0.0	0.0
Nasal/Sinus Congestion	2.8	0.0	5.7	3.2
Nightmares/Vivid Dreams	*	1.1	5.1	5.7
Sweating/Clamminess	1.4	1.1	*	*
Tinnitus	1.4	0.0	0.0	*
Weight Gain	1.4	0.0	4.5	1.9
Weight Loss	*	3.2	5.7	2.5

*Incidence less than 1%.

D = DESYREL   P = Placebo

Pediatric Use
Safety and effectiveness in children below the age of 18 have not been established.

ADVERSE REACTIONS

Because the frequency of adverse drug effects is affected by diverse factors (eg, drug dose, method of detection, physician judgment, disease under treatment, etc.), a single meaningful estimate of adverse event incidence is difficult to obtain. This problem is illustrated by the variation in adverse event incidence observed and reported from the inpatients and outpatients treated with DESYREL. It is impossible to determine precisely what accounts for the differences observed.

Clinical Trial Reports
The table below is presented solely to indicate the relative frequency of adverse events reported in representative controlled clinical studies conducted to evaluate the safety and efficacy of DESYREL® (trazodone hydrochloride).
The figures cited cannot be used to predict precisely the incidence of untoward events in the course of usual medical practice where patient characteristics and other factors often differ from those which prevailed in the clinical trials. These incidence figures, also, cannot be compared with those obtained from other clinical studies involving related drug products and placebo as each group of drug trials is conducted under a different set of conditions.
[See table at bottom of previous page]
Occasional sinus bradycardia has occurred in long-term studies.
In addition to the relatively common (ie, greater than 1%) untoward events enumerated above, the following adverse events have been reported to occur in association with the use of DESYREL® (trazodone hydrochloride) in the controlled clinical studies: akathisia, allergic reaction, anemia, chest pain, delayed urine flow, early menses, flatulence, hallucinations/delusions, hematuria, hypersalivation, hypomania, impaired speech, impotence, increased appetite, increased libido, increased urinary frequency, missed periods, muscle twitches, numbness, and retrograde ejaculation.

Postintroduction Reports:
Although the following adverse reactions have been reported in DESYREL users, the causal association has neither been confirmed nor refuted.
Voluntary reports received since market introduction include the following: abnormal dreams, agitation, alopecia, anxiety, aphasia, apnea, ataxia, breast enlargement or engorgement, cardiospams, cerebrovascular accident, chills, cholestatis, clitorism, congestive heart failure, diplopia, edema, extrapyramidal symptoms, grand mal seizures, hallucinations, hemolytic anemia, hirsutism, hyperbilirubinema, increased amylase, increased salivation, insomnia, leukocytosis, leukonychia, jaundice, lactation, liver enzyme alterations, methemoglobinemia, nausea/vomiting (most frequently), paresthesia, paranoid reaction, priapism (see **WARNINGS** and **PRECAUTIONS, Information for Patients;** some patients have required surgical intervention), pruritus, psoriasis, psychosis, rash, stupor, inappropriate ADH syndrome, tardive dyskinesia, unexplained death, urinary incontinence, urinary retention, urticaria, vasodilation, vertigo, and weakness.
Cardiovascular system effects which have been reported include the following: conduction block, orthostatic hypotension and syncope, palpitations, bradycardia, atrial fibrillation, myocardial infarction, cardiac arrest, arrhythmia, and ventricular ectopic activity, including ventricular tachycardia (see **WARNINGS**).

OVERDOSE

Animal Oral LD_{50}
The oral LD_{50} of the drug is 610 mg/kg in mice, 486 mg/kg in rats, and 560 mg/kg in rabbits.

Signs and Symptoms
Death from overdose has occurred in patients ingesting DESYREL (trazodone hydrochloride) and other drugs concurrently (namely, alcohol; alcohol + chloral hydrate + diazepam; amobarbital; chlordiazepoxide; or meprobamate).
The most severe reactions reported to have occurred with overdose of DESYREL alone have been priapism, respiratory arrest, seizures, and EKG changes. The reactions reported most frequently have been drowsiness and vomiting. Overdosage may cause an increase in incidence or severity of any of the reported adverse reactions (see **ADVERSE REACTIONS**).

Treatment
There is no specific antidote for DESYREL. Treatment should be symptomatic and supportive in the case of hypotension or excessive sedation. Any patient suspected of having taken an overdose should have the stomach emptied by gastric lavage. Forced diuresis may be useful in facilitating elimination of the drug.

DOSAGE AND ADMINISTRATION

The dosage should be initiated at a low level and increased gradually, noting the clinical response and any evidence of intolerance. Occurrence of drowsiness may require the administration of a major portion of the daily dose at bedtime or a reduction of dosage. DESYREL should be taken shortly after a meal or light snack. Symptomatic relief may be seen during the first week, with optimal antidepressant effects typically evident within two weeks. Twenty-five percent of those who respond to DESYREL require more than two weeks (up to four weeks) of drug administration.

Usual Adult Dosage
An initial dose of 150 mg/day in divided doses is suggested. The dose may be increased by 50 mg/day every three to four days. The maximum dose for outpatients usually should not exceed 400 mg/day in divided doses. Inpatients (i.e., more severely depressed patients) may be given up to but not in excess of 600 mg/day in divided doses.

Maintenance
Dosage during prolonged maintenance therapy should be kept at the lowest effective level. Once an adequate response has been achieved, dosage may be gradually reduced, with subsequent adjustment depending on therapeutic response.
Although there has been no systematic evaluation of the efficacy of DESYREL beyond six weeks, it is generally recommended that a course of antidepressant drug treatment should be continued for several months.

HOW SUPPLIED

DESYREL® (trazodone hydrochloride tablets, USP)
Tablets, **50 mg**—round, orange/scored, film-sealed (debossed with **DESYREL** and **MJ 775**)

NDC 0087-0775-41	Bottles of 100
NDC 0087-0775-43	Bottles of 1000
NDC 0087-0775-42	Cartons of 100 Unit Doses

Tablets, **100 mg**—round, white/scored, film-sealed (debossed with **DESYREL** and **MJ 776**)

NDC 0087-0776-41	Bottles of 100
NDC 0087-0776-43	Bottles of 1000
NDC 0087-0776-42	Cartons of 100 Unit Doses

Tablets, **150 mg**—orange, in the Dividose® tablet design (debossed with **MJ** and **778** on front; **50, 50, 50** on reverse)

NDC 0087-0778-43	Bottles of 100
NDC 0087-0778-44	Bottles of 500

Tablets, **300 mg**—yellow, in the Dividose® tablet design (debossed with **MJ** and **796** on front; **100, 100, 100** on reverse)

NDC 0087-0796-41	Bottles of 100

U.S. Patent Nos. 4,215,104
4,258,027

Storage
Store at room temperature. Protect from temperatures above 104°F (40°C). Dispense in tight, light-resistant container (USP).

Caution: Federal law prohibits dispensing without prescription.

REFERENCES

a. Williams JBW, Ed: Diagnostic and Statistical Manual of Mental Disorders-III, American Psychiatric Association, May, 1980.
b. Lue TF, Physiology of erection and pathophysiology of impotence. In: Wash PC, Retik AB, Stamey TA, Vaughan ED, eds. Campbell's Urology. Sixth edition. Philadelphia: W.B. Saunders; 1992: 722–725.
c. Goldstein I, Krane RJ, Diagnosis and therapy of erectile dysfunction. In: Wash PC, Retik AB, Stamey TA, Vaughan ED, eds. Campbell's Urology. Sixth edition. Philadelphia: W.B. Saunders: 1992: 3071–3072.
d. Yealy DM, Hogya PT: Priapism. Emerg Med Clin North Am. 1988; 6:509–520.
e. Banos JE, Bosch F, Farre M, Drug-induced priapism. Its aetiology, incidence and treatment. Med Toxicol Adverse Drug Exp. 1989; 4:46–58.
f. O'Brien WM, O'Connor KP, Lynch JH. Priapism: current concepts. Ann Emerg Med. 1989: 980–983.
g. Bardin ED, Krieger JN. Pharmacological priapism: comparison of trazodone- and papaverine-associated cases. Int Urol Nephrol. 1990; 22:147–152.

Des18207

FLORINEF® ACETATE ℞
Fludrocortisone Acetate Tablets USP

DESCRIPTION

Florinef Acetate (Fludrocortisone Acetate Tablets USP) contains fludrocortisone acetate, a synthetic adrenocortical steroid possessing very potent mineralocorticoid properties and high glucocorticoid activity; it is used only for its mineralocorticoid effects. The chemical name for fludrocortisone acetate is 9-fluoro-11β, 17, 21-trihydroxypregn-4-ene-3,20-dione 21-acetate; its graphic formula is:
[See chemical structure at top of next column]
Florinef Acetate is available for oral administration as scored tablets providing 0.1 mg fludrocortisone acetate per tablet. Inactive ingredients: calcium phosphate, color additive (D&C Red No. 27), corn starch, lactose, magnesium stearate, sodium benzoate, and talc.

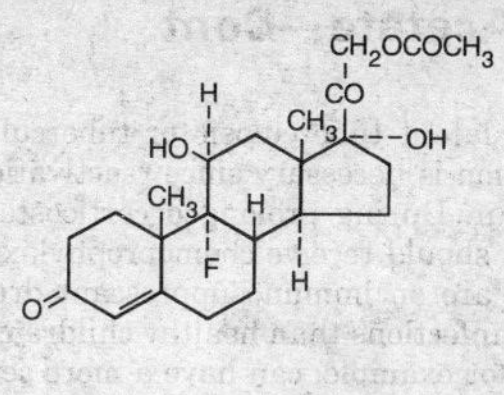

$C_{23}H_{31}FO_6$ MW422.49

CLINICAL PHARMACOLOGY

Corticosteroids are thought to act, at least in part, by controlling the rate of synthesis of proteins. Although there are a number of instances in which the synthesis of specific proteins is known to be induced by corticosteroids, the links between the initial actions of the hormones and the final metabolic effects have not been completely elucidated.
The physiologic action of fludrocortisone acetate is similar to that of hydrocortisone. However, the effects of fludrocortisone acetate, particularly on electrolyte balance, but also on carbohydrate metabolism, are considerably heightened and prolonged. Mineralocorticoids act on the distal tubules of the kidney to enhance the reabsorption of sodium ions from the tubular fluid into the plasma; they increase the urinary excretion of both potassium and hydrogen ions. The consequence of these three primary effects together with similar actions on cation transport in other tissues appear to account for the entire spectrum of physiological activities that are characteristic of mineralocorticoids. In small oral doses, fludrocortisone acetate produces marked sodium retention and increased urinary potassium excretion. It also causes a rise in blood pressure, apparently because of these effects on electrolyte levels.
In larger doses, fludrocortisone acetate inhibits endogenous adrenal cortical secretion, thymic activity, and pituitary corticotropin excretion; promotes the deposition of liver glycogen; and, unless protein intake is adequate, induces negative nitrogen balance.
The approximate plasma half-life of fludrocortisone (fluorohydrocortisone) is 3.5 hours or more and the biological half-life is 18 to 36 hours.

INDICATIONS AND USAGE

Florinef Acetate is indicated as partial replacement therapy for primary and secondary adrenocortical insufficiency in Addison's disease and for the treatment of salt-losing adrenogenital syndrome.

CONTRAINDICATIONS

Corticosteroids are contraindicated in patients with systemic fungal infections and in those with a history of possible or known hypersensitivity to these agents.

WARNINGS

BECAUSE OF ITS MARKED EFFECT ON SODIUM RETENTION, THE USE OF FLUDROCORTISONE ACETATE IN THE TREATMENT OF CONDITIONS OTHER THAN THOSE INDICATED HEREIN IS NOT ADVISED.
Corticosteroids may mask some signs of infection, and new infections may appear during their use. There may be decreased resistance and inability to localize infection when corticosteroids are used. If an infection occurs during fludrocortisone acetate therapy, it should be promptly controlled by suitable antimicrobial therapy.
Prolonged use of corticosteroids may produce posterior subcapsular cataracts, glaucoma with possible damage to the optic nerves, and may enhance the establishment of secondary ocular infections due to fungi or viruses.
Average and large doses of hydrocortisone or cortisone can cause elevation of blood pressure, salt and water retention, and increased excretion of potassium. These effects are less likely to occur with the synthetic derivatives except when used in large doses. However, since fludrocortisone acetate is a potent mineralocorticoid, both the dosage and salt intake should be carefully monitored in order to avoid the development of hypertension, edema, or weight gain. **Periodic checking of serum electrolyte levels is advisable during prolonged therapy; dietary salt restriction and potassium supplementation may be necessary.** All corticosteroids increase calcium excretion.
Patients should not be vaccinated against smallpox while on corticosteroid therapy. Other immunization procedures should not be undertaken in patients who are on corticosteroids, especially on high dose, because of possible hazards of neurological complications and a lack of antibody response.
The use of Florinef Acetate (Fludrocortisone Acetate Tablets USP) in patients with active tuberculosis should be restricted to those cases of fulminating or disseminated tuberculosis in which the corticosteroid is used for the management of the disease in conjunction with an appropriate antituberculous regimen. If corticosteroids are indicated in

Continued on next page

Florinef Acetate—Cont.

patients with latent tuberculosis or tuberculin reactivity, close observation is necessary since reactivation of the disease may occur. During prolonged corticosteroid therapy these patients should receive chemoprophylaxis.

Children who are on immunosuppressant drugs are more susceptible to infections than healthy children. Chicken pox and measles, for example, can have a more serious or even fatal course in children on immunosuppressant corticosteroids. In such children, or in adults who have not had these diseases, particular care should be taken to avoid exposure. If exposed, therapy with varicella zoster immune globulin (VZIG) or pooled intravenous immunoglobulin (IVIG), as appropriate, may be indicated. If chicken pox develops, treatment with antiviral agents may be considered.

PRECAUTIONS

General

Adverse reactions to corticosteroids may be produced by too rapid withdrawal or by continued use of large doses.

To avoid drug-induced adrenal insufficiency, supportive dosage may be required in times of stress (such as trauma, surgery, or severe illness) both during treatment with fludrocortisone acetate and for a year afterwards.

There is an enhanced corticosteroid effect in patients with hypothyroidism and in those with cirrhosis.

Corticosteroids should be used cautiously in patients with ocular herpes simplex because of possible corneal perforation.

The lowest possible dose of corticosteroid should be used to control the condition being treated. A gradual reduction in dosage should be made when possible.

Psychic derangement may appear when corticosteroids are used. These may range from euphoria, insomnia, mood swings, personality changes, and severe depression to frank psychotic manifestations. Existing emotional instability or psychotic tendencies may also be aggravated by corticosteroids.

Aspirin should be used cautiously in conjunction with corticosteroids in patients with hypoprothrombinemia.

Corticosteroids should be used with caution in patients with nonspecific ulcerative colitis if there is a probability of impending perforation, abscess, or other pyogenic infection. Corticosteroids should also be used cautiously in patients with diverticulitis, fresh intestinal anastomoses, active or latent peptic ulcer, renal insufficiency, hypertension, osteoporosis, and myasthenia gravis.

Information for Patients

The physician should advise the patient to report any medical history of heart disease, high blood pressure, or kidney or liver disease and to report current use of any medicines to determine if these medicines might interact adversely with fludrocortisone acetate (see **Drug Interactions**).

Patients who are on immunosuppressant doses of corticosteroids should be warned to avoid exposure to chicken pox or measles and, if exposed, to obtain medical advice.

The patient's understanding of his steroid-dependent status and increased dosage requirement under widely variable conditions of stress is vital. Advise the patient to carry medical identification indicating his dependence on steroid medication and, if necessary, instruct him to carry an adequate supply of medication for use in emergencies.

Stress to the patient the importance of regular follow-up visits to check his progress and the need to promptly notify the physician of dizziness, severe or continuing headaches, swelling of feet or lower legs, or unusual weight gain.

Advise the patient to use the medicine only as directed, to take a missed dose as soon as possible, unless it is almost time for the next dose, and not to double the next dose.

Inform the patient to keep this medication and all drugs out of the reach of children.

Laboratory Tests

Patients should be monitored regularly for blood pressure determinations and serum electrolyte determinations (see **WARNINGS**).

Drug Interactions

When administered concurrently, the following drugs may interact with adrenal corticosteroids.

Amphotericin B or potassium-depleting diuretics (benzothiadiazines and related drugs, ethacrynic acid and furosemide)—enhanced hypokalemia. Check serum potassium levels at frequent intervals; use potassium supplements if necessary (see **WARNINGS**).

Digitalis glycosides—enhanced possibility of arrhythmias or digitalis toxicity associated with hypokalemia. Monitor serum potassium levels; use potassium supplements if necessary.

Oral anticoagulants—decreased prothrombin time response. Monitor prothrombin levels and adjust anticoagulant dosage accordingly.

Antidiabetic drugs (oral agents and insulin)—diminished antidiabetic effect. Monitor for symptoms of hyperglycemia; adjust dosage of antidiabetic drug upward if necessary.

Aspirin—increased ulcerogenic effect; decreased pharmacologic effect of aspirin. Rarely salicylate toxicity may occur in patients who discontinue steroids after concurrent high-dose aspirin therapy. Monitor salicylate levels or the therapeutic effect for which aspirin is given; adjust salicylate dosage accordingly if effect is altered (see **PRECAUTIONS, General**).

Barbiturates, phenytoin, or rifampin—increased metabolic clearance of fludrocortisone acetate because of the induction of hepatic enzymes. Observe the patient for possible diminished effect of steroid and increase the steroid dosage accordingly.

Anabolic steroids (particularly C-17 alkylated androgens such as oxymetholone, methandrostenolone, norethandrolone, and similar compounds)—enhanced tendency toward edema. Use caution when giving these drugs together, especially in patients with hepatic or cardiac disease.

Vaccines—neurological complications and lack of antibody response (see **WARNINGS**).

Estrogen—increased levels of corticosteroid-binding globulin, thereby increasing the bound (inactive) fraction; this effect is at least balanced by decreased metabolism of corticosteroids. When estrogen therapy is initiated, a reduction in corticosteroid dosage may be required, and increased amounts may be required when estrogen is terminated.

Drug/Laboratory Test Interactions

Corticosteroids may affect the nitrobluetetrazolium test for bacterial infection and produce false-negative results.

Carcinogenesis, Mutagenesis, Impairment of Fertility

Adequate studies have not been performed in animals to determine whether fludrocortisone acetate has carcinogenic or mutagenic activity or whether it affects fertility in males or females.

Pregnancy. Category C.

Adequate animal reproduction studies have not been conducted with fludrocortisone acetate. However, many corticosteroids have been shown to be teratogenic in laboratory animals at low doses. Teratogenicity of these agents in man has not been demonstrated. It is not known whether fludrocortisone acetate can cause fetal harm when administered to a pregnant woman or can affect reproduction capacity. Fludrocortisone acetate should be given to a pregnant woman only if clearly needed.

Pregnancy. Nonteratogenic Effects.

Infants born of mothers who have received substantial doses of fludrocortisone acetate during pregnancy should be carefully observed for signs of hypoadrenalism.

Maternal treatment with corticosteroids should be carefully documented in the infant's medical records to assist in follow up.

Nursing Mothers

Corticosteroids are found in the breast milk of lactating women receiving systemic therapy with these agents. Caution should be exercised when fludrocortisone acetate is administered to a nursing woman.

Pediatric Use

Safety and effectiveness in children have not been established.

Growth and development of infants and children on prolonged corticosteroid therapy should be carefully observed.

ADVERSE REACTIONS

Most adverse reactions are caused by the drug's mineralocorticoid activity (retention of sodium and water) and include hypertension, edema, cardiac enlargement, congestive heart failure, potassium loss, and hypokalemic alkalosis.

When fludrocortisone is used in the small dosages recommended, the glucocorticoid side effects often seen with cortisone and its derivatives are not usually a problem; however the following untoward effects should be kept in mind, particularly when fludrocortisone is used over a prolonged period of time or in conjunction with cortisone or a similar glucocorticoid.

Musculoskeletal—muscle weakness, steroid myopathy, loss of muscle mass, osteoporosis, vertebral compression fractures, aseptic necrosis of femoral and humeral heads, pathologic fracture of long bones, and spontaneous fractures.

Gastrointestinal—peptic ulcer with possible perforation and hemorrhage, pancreatitis, abdominal distention, and ulcerative esophagitis.

Dermatologic—impaired wound healing, thin fragile skin, bruising, petechiae and ecchymoses, facial erythema, increased sweating, subcutaneous fat atrophy, purpura, striae, hyperpigmentation of the skin and nails, hirsutism, acneiform eruptions, and hives reactions to skin tests may be suppressed.

Neurological—convulsions, increased intracranial pressure with papilledema (pseudotumor cerebri) usually after treatment, vertigo, headache, and severe mental disturbances.

Endocrine—menstrual irregularities, development of the cushingoid state; suppression of growth in children; secondary adrenocortical and pituitary unresponsiveness, particularly in times of stress (e.g., trauma, surgery, or illness); decreased carbohydrate tolerance; manifestations of latent diabetes mellitus; and increased requirements for insulin or oral hypoglycemic agents in diabetics.

Ophthalmic—posterior subcapsular cataracts, increased intraocular pressure, glaucoma, and exophthalmos.

Metabolic—hyperglycemia, glycosuria, and negative nitrogen balance due to protein catabolism.

Allergic Reactions—allergic skin rash, maculopapular rash, and urticaria.

Other adverse reactions that may occur following the administration of a corticosteroid are necrotizing angiitis, thrombophlebitis, aggravation or masking of infections, insomnia, syncopal episodes, and anaphylactoid reactions.

OVERDOSAGE

Development of hypertension, edema, hypokalemia, excessive increase in weight, and increase in heart size are signs of overdosage of fludrocortisone acetate. When these are noted, administration of the drug should be discontinued, after which the symptoms will usually subside within several days; subsequent treatment with fludrocortisone acetate should be with a reduced dose. Muscular weakness may develop due to excessive potassium loss and can be treated by administering a potassium supplement. Regular monitoring of blood pressure and serum electrolytes can help to prevent overdosage (see **WARNINGS**).

DOSAGE AND ADMINISTRATION

Dosage depends on the severity of the disease and the response of the patient. Patients should be continually monitored for signs that indicate dosage adjustment is necessary, such as remissions or exacerbations of the disease and stress (surgery, infection, trauma) (see **WARNINGS** and **PRECAUTIONS, General**).

Addison's Disease

In Addison's disease, the combination of Florinef Acetate (Fludrocortisone Acetate Tablets USP) with a glucocorticoid such as hydrocortisone or cortisone provides substitution therapy approximating normal adrenal activity with minimal risks of unwanted effects.

The usual dose is 0.1 mg of Florinef Acetate daily, although dosage ranging from 0.1 mg three times a week to 0.2 mg daily has been employed. In the event transient hypertension develops as a consequence of therapy, the dose should be reduced to 0.05 mg daily. Florinef Acetate is preferably administered in conjunction with cortisone (10 mg to 37.5 mg daily in divided doses) or hydrocortisone (10 mg to 30 mg daily in divided doses).

Salt-Losing Adrenogenital Syndrome

The recommended dosage for treating the salt-losing adrenogenital syndrome is 0.1 mg to 0.2 mg of Florinef Acetate daily.

HOW SUPPLIED

Florinef Acetate Tablets (Fludrocortisone Acetate Tablets USP), 0.1 mg/tablet: light pink, round, biconvex, scored tablets in bottles of 100 (NDC 0003-0429-50); identification no. **429.**

Storage

Store at room temperature; avoid excessive heat.

CAUTION: Federal law prohibits dispensing without prescription.

Apothecon®
A Bristol-Myers Squibb Co.
Princeton, NJ 08540

P3345-01 Revised January 1996 P3345-01

NYDRAZID® INJECTION ℞

Isoniazid Injection USP

WARNING

Severe and sometimes fatal hepatitis associated with isoniazid therapy has been reported and may occur or may develop even after many months of treatment. The risk of developing hepatitis is age related. Approximate case rates by age are: less than 1 per 1,000 for persons under 20 years of age, 3 per 1,000 for persons in the 20–34 year age group, 12 per 1,000 for persons in the 35–49 year age group, 23 per 1,000 for persons in the 50–64 year age group, and 8 per 1,000 for persons over 65 years of age. The risk of hepatitis is increased with daily consumption of alcohol. Precise data to provide a fatality rate for isoniazid-related hepatitis is not available; however, in a U.S. Public Health Service Surveillance Study of 13,838 persons taking isoniazid, there were 8 deaths among 174 cases of hepatitis.

Therefore, patients given isoniazid should be carefully monitored and interviewed at monthly intervals. For persons 35 and older, in addition to monthly symptom reviews, hepatic enzymes (specifically, AST and ALT (formerly SGOT and SGPT, respectively)) should be measured prior to starting isoniazid therapy and periodically throughout treatment. Isoniazid-associated hepatitis usually occurs during the first three months of treatment. Usually, enzyme levels return to normal despite continuance of drug, but in some cases progressive liver dysfunction occurs. Other factors associated with an increased risk of hepatitis include daily use of alcohol, chronic liver disease and injection drug use. A re-

port suggests an increased risk of fatal hepatitis associated with isoniazid among women, particularly black and Hispanic women. The risk may also be increased during the post partum period. More careful monitoring should be considered in these groups, possibly including more frequent laboratory monitoring. If abnormalities of liver function exceed three to five times the upper limit of normal, discontinuation of isoniazid should be strongly considered. Liver function tests are not a substitute for a clinical evaluation at monthly intervals or for the prompt assessment of signs or symptoms of adverse reactions occurring between regularly scheduled evaluations. Patients should be instructed to immediately report signs or symptoms consistent with liver damage or other adverse effects. These include any of the following: unexplained anorexia, nausea, vomiting, dark urine, icterus, rash, persistent paresthesias of the hands and feet, persistent fatigue, weakness or fever of greater than 3 days duration and/or abdominal tenderness, especially right upper quadrant discomfort. If these symptoms appear or if signs suggestive of hepatic damage are detected, isoniazid should be discontinued promptly, since continued use of the drug in these cases has been reported to cause a more severe form of liver damage.
Patients with tuberculosis who have hepatitis attributed to isoniazid should be given appropriate treatment with alternative drugs. If isoniazid must be reinstituted, it should be reinstituted only after symptoms and laboratory abnormalities have cleared. The drug should be restarted in very small and gradually increasing doses and should be withdrawn immediately if there is any indication of recurrent liver involvement.
Preventive treatment should be deferred in persons with acute hepatic diseases.

DESCRIPTION

Isoniazid is the hydrazide of isonicotinic acid. Nydrazid Injection (Isoniazid Injection) provides 100 mg isoniazid per ml with 0.25% chlorobutanol (chloral derivative) as a preservative; the pH has been adjusted to 6.0 to 7.0 with sodium hydroxide or hydrochloric acid. At the time of manufacture, the air in the container is replaced by nitrogen.
Isoniazid is chemically known as isonicotinyl hydrazine or isonicotinic acid hydrazide. It has an empirical formula of $C_6H_7N_3O$ and a molecular weight of 137.14. It has the following structure:

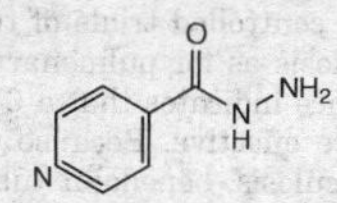

Isoniazid is odorless, and occurs as a colorless or white crystalline powder or as white crystals. It is freely soluble in water, sparingly soluble in alcohol, and slightly soluble in chloroform and in ether. Isoniazid is slowly affected by exposure to air and light.

CLINICAL PHARMACOLOGY

Isoniazid acts against actively growing tubercle bacilli.
Within one to two hours after oral administration, isoniazid produces peak blood levels which decline to 50 percent or less within six hours. It diffuses readily into all body fluids (cerebrospinal, pleural, and ascitic), tissues, organs, and excreta (saliva, sputum, and feces). The drug also passes through the placental barrier and into milk in concentrations comparable to those in the plasma. From 50 to 70 percent of a dose of isoniazid is excreted in the urine in 24 hours.
Isoniazid is metabolized primarily by acetylation and dehydrazination. The rate of acetylation is genetically determined. Approximately 50 percent of Blacks and Caucasians are "slow acetylators" and the rest are "rapid acetylators"; the majority of Eskimos and Orientals are "rapid acetylators."
The rate of acetylation does not significantly alter the effectiveness of isoniazid therapy when dosage is administered daily. However, slow acetylation may lead to higher blood levels of the drug and thus an increase in toxic reactions.
Pyridoxine (B_6) deficiency is sometimes observed in adults with high doses of isoniazid and is considered probably due to its competition with pyridoxal phosphate for the enzyme apotryptophanase.

Mechanism of Action

Isoniazid inhibits the synthesis of mycoloic acids, an essential component of the bacterial cell wall. At therapeutic levels isoniazid is bacteriocidal against actively growing intracellular and extracellular *Mycobacterium tuberculosis* organisms.

Isoniazid resistant *Mycobacterium tuberculosis* bacilli develop rapidly when isoniazid monotherapy is administered.

Microbiology:

Two standardized *in vitro* susceptibility methods are available for testing isoniazid against *Mycobacterium tuberculosis* organisms. The agar proportion method (CDC or NCCLS M24-P) utilizes middlebrook 7H10 medium impregnated with isoniazid at two final concentrations, 0.2 and 1.0 mcg/mL. MIC_{99} values are calculated by comparing the quantity of organisms growing in the medium containing drug to the control cultures. Mycobacterial growth in the presence of drug ≥ 1% of the control indicates resistance.
The radiometric broth method employs the BACTEC 460 machine to compare the growth index from untreated control cultures to cultures grown in the presence of 0.2 and 1.0 mcg/mL of isoniazid. Strict adherence to the manufacturer's instructions for sample processing and data interpretation is required for this assay.
Mycobacterium tuberculosis isolates with an MIC_{99} ≤ 0.2 mcg/mL are considered to be susceptible to isoniazid. Susceptibility test results obtained by the two different methods discussed above cannot be compared unless equivalent drug concentrations are evaluated.
The clinical relevance of *in vitro* susceptibility for mycobacterium species other than *M. tuberculosis* using either the BACTEC or the proportion method has not been determined.

INDICATIONS AND USAGE

Nydrazid Injection (Isoniazid Injection) is recommended for all forms of tuberculosis in which organisms are susceptible. However, active tuberculosis must be treated with multiple concomitant antituberculosis medications to prevent the emergence of drug resistance. Single-drug treatment of active tuberculosis with isoniazid, or any other medication, is inadequate therapy.
Intramuscular administration is intended for use whenever administration by the oral route is not possible.
Isoniazid is recommended as preventive therapy for the following groups, regardless of age. (Note: the criterion for a positive reaction to a skin test (in millimeters of induration) for each group is given in parenthesis):

1. Persons with human immunodeficiency virus (HIV) infection (≥ 5 mm) and persons with risk factors for HIV infection whose HIV infection status is unknown but who are suspected of having HIV infection.
   Preventive therapy may be considered for HIV infected persons who are tuberculin-negative but belong to groups in which the prevalence of tuberculosis infection is high. Candidates for preventive therapy who have HIV infection should have a minimum of 12 months of therapy.
2. Close contacts of persons with newly diagnosed infectious tuberculosis (≥ 5 mm). In addition, tuberculin-negative (< 5 mm) children and adolescents who have been close contacts of infectious persons within the past 3 months are candidates for preventive therapy until a repeat tuberculin skin test is done 12 weeks after contact with the infectious source. If the repeat skin test is positive (> 5 mm), therapy should be continued.
3. Recent converters, as indicated by a tuberculin skin test (≥ 10 mm increase within a 2-year period for those < 35 years old; ≥ 15 mm increase for those ≥ 35 years of age). All infants and children younger than 4 years of age with a > 10 mm skin test are included in this category.
4. Persons with abnormal chest radiographs that show fibrotic lesions likely to represent old healed tuberculosis (≥ 5mm). Candidates for preventive therapy who have fibrotic pulmonary lesions consistent with healed tuberculosis or who have pulmonary silicosis should have 12 months of isoniazid or 4 months of isoniazid and rifampin, concomitantly.
5. Intravenous drug users known to be HIV-seronegative (> 10 mm).
6. Persons with the following medical conditions that have been reported to increase the risk of tuberculosis (≥ 10 mm); silicosis; diabetes mellitus; prolonged therapy with adrenocorticosteroids; immunosuppressive therapy; some hematologic and reticulendothelial disease; such as leukemia or Hodgkin's disease; end-stage renal disease; clinical situations associated with substantial rapid weight loss or chronic undernutrition (including: intestinal bypass surgery for obesity, the postgastrectomy state (with or without weight loss), chronic peptic ulcer disease, chronic malabsorption syndromes, and carcinomas of the oropharynx and upper gastrointestinal tract that prevent adequate nutritional intake). Candidates for preventive therapy who have fibrotic pulmonary lesions consistent with healed tuberculosis or who have pulmonary silicosis should have 12 months of isoniazid or 4 months of isoniazid and rifampin, concomitantly.

Additionally, in the absence of any of the above risk factors, persons under the age of 35 with a tuberculin skin test reaction of 10 mm or more are also appropriate candidates for preventive therapy if they are a member of any of the following high-incidence groups:

1. Foreign-born persons from high-prevalence countries who never received BCG vaccine.
2. Medically underserved low-income populations, including high-risk racial or ethnic minority populations, especially blacks, Hispanics, and Native Americans,
2. Residents of facilities for long-term care (e.g., correctional institutions, nursing homes, and mental institutions).

Children who are less than 4 years old are candidates for isoniazid preventive therapy if they have > 10 mm induration from a PPD Mantoux tuberculin skin test.
Finally, persons under the age of 35 who a) have none of the above risk factors (1–6); b) belong to none of the high-incidence groups; and c) have a tuberculin skin test reaction of 15 mm or more, are appropriate candidates for preventive therapy.
The risk of hepatitis must be weighed against the risk of tuberculosis in positive tuberculin reactors over the age of 35. However, the use of isoniazid is recommended for those with the additional risk factors listed above (1–6) and on an individual basis in situations where there is likelihood of serious consequences to contacts who may become infected.

CONTRAINDICATIONS

Isoniazid is contraindicated in patients who develop severe hypersensitivity reactions, including drug-induced hepatitis; previous isoniazid-associated hepatic injury; severe adverse reactions to isoniazid such as drug fever, chills, arthritis; and acute liver disease of any etiology.

WARNINGS

See the boxed warning.

PRECAUTIONS

General

General drugs should be stopped and an evaluation made at the first sign of a hypersensitivity reaction. If isoniazid therapy must be reinstituted, the drug should be given only after symptoms have cleared. The drug should be restarted in very small and gradually increasing doses and should be withdrawn immediately if there is any indication of recurrent hypersensitivity reaction.
Use of isoniazid should be carefully monitored in the following:

1. Daily users of alcohol. Daily ingestion of alcohol may be associated with a higher incidence of + isoniazid hepatitis.
2. Patients with active chronic liver disease or severe renal dysfunction.
3. Age >35.
4. Concurrent use of any chronically administered medication.
5. History of previous discontinuation of isoniazid.
6. Existence of peripheral neuropathy or conditions predisposing to neuropathy.
7. Pregnancy.
8. Injection drug use.
9. Women belonging to minority groups, particularly in the postpartum period.
10. HIV seropositive patients.

Periodic ophthalmologic examinations during isoniazid therapy are recommended when visual symptoms occur.

Laboratory Tests

Because there is a higher frequency of isoniazid associated hepatitis among certain patient groups, including Age > 35, daily users of alcohol, chronic liver disease, injection drug use and women belonging to minority groups, particularly in the post-partum period, transaminase measurements should be obtained prior to starting and monthly during preventative therapy, or more frequently as needed. If any of the values exceed three to five times the upper limit of normal, isoniazid should be temporarily discontinued and consideration given to restarting therapy.

DRUG INTERACTIONS:

Food: Isoniazid should not be administered with food. Studies have shown that the bioavailability of isoniazid is reduced significantly when administered with food.
Acetaminophen: A report of severe acetaminophen toxicity was reported in a patient receiving Isoniazid. It is believed that the toxicity may have resulted from a previously unrecognized interaction between isoniazid and acetaminophen and a molecular basis for this interaction has been proposed. However, current evidence suggests that isoniazid does induce P-450IIE1, a mixed-function oxidase enzyme that appears to generate the toxic metabolites, in the liver. Furthermore it has been proposed that isoniazid resulted in induction of P-450IIE1 in the patients liver which, in turn, resulted in a greater proportion of the ingested acetaminophen being converted to the toxic metabolites. Studies have demonstrated that pretreatment with isoniazid potentiates acetaminophen hepatotoxicity in rats[1,2].
Carbamazepine: Isoniazid is known to slow the metabolism of carbamazepine and increase its serum levels. Carbamazepine levels should be determined prior to concurrent administration with isoniazid, signs and symptoms of carbamazepine toxicity should be monitored closely, and appropriate dosage adjustment of the anticonvulsant should be made[3].
Ketoconazole: Potential interaction of Ketoconazole and isoniazid may exist. When Ketoconazole is given in combina-

Continued on next page

Nydrazid—Cont.

tion with isoniazid and rifampin the AUC of Ketoconazole is decreased by as much as 88% after 5 months of concurrent Isoniazid and Rifampin therapy[4].

Phenytoin: Isoniazid may increase serum levels of phenytoin. To avoid phenytoin intoxication, appropriate adjustment of the anticonvulsant should be made[5,6].

Theophylline: A recent study has shown that concomitant administration of isoniazid and theophylline may cause elevated plasma levels of theophylline, and in some instances a slight decrease in the elimination of isoniazid. Since the therapeutic range of theophylline is narrow, theophylline serum levels should be monitored closely, and appropriate dosage adjustments of theophylline should be made[7].

Valproate: A recent case study has shown a possible increase in the plasma level of valproate when co-administered with isoniazid. Plasma valproate concentration should be monitored when isoniazid and valproate are co-administered, and appropriate dosage adjustments of valproate should be made[5].

Carcinogenesis and Mutagenesis

Isoniazid has been shown to induce pulmonary tumors in a number of strains of mice. Isoniazid has not been shown to be carcinogenic in humans. (Note: a diagnosis of mesothelioma in a child with prenatal exposure to isoniazid and no other apparent risk factors has been reported). Isoniazid has been found to be weakly mutagenic in strains TA 100 and TA 1535 of *Salmonella typhimurium* (Ames assay) without metalbolic activation.

Pregnancy

Teratogenic Effects: Pregnancy Category C: Isoniazid has been shown to have an embryocidal effect in rats and rabbits when given orally during pregnancy. Isoniazid was not teratogenic in reproduction studies in mice, rats, and rabbits. There are no adequate and well-controlled studies in pregnant women. Isoniazid should be used as a treatment for active tuberculosis during pregnancy brcause the benefit justifies the potential risk to the fetus. The benefit of preventive therapy also should be weighed against a possible risk to the fetus. Preventive therapy generally should be started after delivery to prevent putting the fetus at risk of exposure; the low levels of isoniazid in breast milk do not threaten the neonate.

Since isoniazid is known to cross the placental barrier, neonates of isoniazid-treated mothers should be carefully observed for any evidence of adverse effects.

Nonteratogenic Effects: Since isoniazid is known to cross the placental barrier, neonates of isoniazid-treated mothers should be carefully observed for any evidence of adverse effects.

Nursing Mothers

The small concentrations of isoniazid in breast milk do not produce toxicity in the nursing newborn; therefore, breast feeding should not be discouraged. However, because levels of isoniazid are so low in breast milk, they can not be relied upon for prophylaxis or therapy of nursing infants.

ADVERSE REACTIONS

The most frequent reactions are those affecting the nervous system and the liver.

Nervous system: Peripheral neuropathy is the most common toxic effect. It is dose related, occurs most often in the malnourished and in those predisposed to neuritis (e.g., alcoholics and diabetics), and is usually preceded by paresthesias of the feet and hands. The incidence is higher in "slow acetylators."

Other neurotoxic effects which are uncommon with conventional doses are convulsions, toxic encephalopathy, optic neuritis and atrophy, memory impairment, and toxic psychosis.

Gastrointestinal: Nausea, vomiting, and epigastric distress.

Hepatic: See boxed warning. Elevated serum transaminases (SGOT; SGPT), bilirubinemia, bilirubinuria, jaundice, and occasionally severe and sometimes fatal hepatitis. The common prodromal symptoms of hepatitis are anorexia, nausea, vomiting, fatigue, malaise, and weakness. Mild hepatic dysfunction, evidenced by mild and transient elevation of serum transaminase levels occurs in 10 to 20 percent of patients taking isoniazid. The abnormality usually appears in the first 1 to 3 months of treatment but can occur at any time during therapy. In most instances, enzyme levels return to normal, and generally, there is no necessity to discontinue medication during the period of mild serum transaminase elevation. In occasional instances, progressive liver damage occurs, with accompanying symptoms. If the SGOT value exceeds three to five times the upper limit of normal, discontinuation of the isoniazid should be strongly considered. The frequency of progressive liver damage increases with age. It is rare in persons under 20, but occurs in up to 2.3 percent of those over 50 years of age.

Hematologic: Agranulocytosis; hemolytic, sideroblastic, or aplastic anemia; thrombocytopenia; and eosinophilia.

Hypersensitivity: Fever, skin eruptions (morbilliform, maculopapular, purpuric, or exfoliative), lymphadenopathy, and vasculitis.

Metabolic and endocrine: Pyridoxine deficiency, pellagra, hyperglycemia, metabolic acidosis, and gynecomastia.

Miscellaneous: Rheumatic syndrome and systemic lupus erythematosus-like syndrome. Local irritation has been observed at the site of intramuscular injection.

OVERDOSAGE

Signs and Symptoms

Isoniazid overdosage produces signs and symptoms within 30 minutes to three hours after ingestion. Nausea, vomiting, dizziness, slurring of speech, blurring of vision, and visual hallucinations (including bright colors and strange designs) are among the early manifestations. With marked overdosage, respiratory distress and CNS depression, progressing rapidly from stupor to profound coma, are to be expected, along with severe, intractable seizures. Severe metabolic acidosis, acetonuria, and hyperglycemia are typical laboratory findings.

Treatment

Untreated or inadequately treated cases of gross isoniazid overdosage, 80 mg/kg-150mg/kg, can cause neurotoxicity[6] and terminate fatally, but good response has been reported in most patients brought under adequate treatment within the first few hours after drug ingestion.

For the Asymptomatic Patient: Absorption of drugs from the GI tract may be decreased by giving activated charcoal. Gastric emptying should also be employed in the asymptomatic patient. Safeguard the patient's airway when employing these procedures. Patients who acutely ingest > 80 mg/kg should be treated with intravenous pyridoxine on a gram per gram basis equal to the isoniazid dose. If an unknown amount of isoniazid is ingested, consider an initial dose of 5 grms of pyridoxine given over *30 to 60 minutes* in adults, or 80 mg/kg of pyridoxine in children.

For the Symptomatic Patient: Ensure adequate ventilation, support cardiac output, and protect the airway while treating seizures and attempting to limit absorption. If the dose of isoniazid is known, the patient should be treated initially with a slow intravenous bolus of pyridoxine, over 3 to 5 minutes, on a gram per gram basis, equal to the isoniazid dose. If the quantity of isoniazid ingestion is unknown, then consider an initial intravenous bolus of pyridoxine of 5 grams in the adult or 80 mg/kg in the child. If seizures continue, the dosage of pyridoxine may be repeated. It would be rare that more than 10 grams of pyridoxine would need to be given. the maximum safe dose of pyridoxine in isoniazid intoxication is not known. If the patient does not respond to pyridoxine, diazepam may be administered. Phenytoin should be used cautiously, because isoniazid inteferes with the metabolism of phenytoin.

General: Obtain blood samples for immediate determination of gases, electrolytes, BUN, glucose, etc.; type and cross-match blood in preparation for possible hemodialysis.

Rapid control of metabolic acidosis: Patients with this degree of INH intoxication are likely to have hypoventilation. The administration of sodium bicarbonate under these circumstances can cause exacerbation of hypercarbia. Ventilation must be monitored carefully, by measuring blood carbon dioxide levels, and supported mechanically, if there is respiratory insufficiency.

Dialysis: Both peritoneal and hemodialysis have been used in the management of isoniazid overdosage. These procedures are probably not required if control of seizures and acidosis is achieved with pyridoxine, diazepam and bicarbonate.

Along with measures based on initial and repeated determination of blood gases and other laboratory tests as needed, utilize meticulous respiratory and other intensive care to protect against hypoxia, hypotension, aspiration pneumonitis, etc.

DOSAGE AND ADMINISTRATION (SEE ALSO INDICATIONS)

NOTE: For preventive therapy of tuberculous infection and treatment of tuberculosis, it is recommended that physicians be familiar with the following publications: (1) the recommendations of the Advisory Council for the Elimination of Tuberculosis, published in the MMWR: vol 42; RR-4, 1993 and (2) Treatment of Tuberculosis and Tuberculosis Infection in Adults and Children, American Journal of Respiratory and Critical Care Medicine: vol 149; 1359–1374, 1994.

For Treatment of Tuberculosis

Drug susceptibility testing should be performed on the organism initially isolated from all patients with newly diagnosed tuberculosis. If the bacilli becomes resistant, therapy must be changed to agents to which the bacilli are susceptible.

USUAL PARENTERAL DOSAGE (DEPENDING ON THE REGIMEN USED)

Adults: 5 mg/kg up to 300 mg daily in a single dose; or 15 mg/kg up to 900 mg/day, two or three times/week.

Children: 10–15 mg/kg up to 300 mg daily in a single dose; or 20–40 mg/kg up to 900 mg/day, two or three times/week.

Patients with Pulmonary Tuberculosis Without HIV Infection

There are 3 regimen options for the initial treatment of tuberculosis in children and adults:

Option 1: Daily isoniazid, rifampin, and pyrazinamide for 8 weeks followed by 16 weeks of isoniazid and rifampin daily or 2–3 times weekly. Ethambutol or streptomycin should be added to the initial regimen until sensitivity to isoniazid and rifampin is demonstrated. The addition of a fourth drug is optional if the relative prevalence of isoniazid-resistant *Mycobacterium tuberculosis* isolates in the community is less than or equal to four percent.

Option 2: Daily isoniazid, rifampin, pyrazinamide and streptomycin or ethambutol for 2 weeks followed by twice weekly administration of the same drugs for 6 weeks, subsequently twice weekly isoniazid and rifampin for 16 weeks.

Option 3: Three times weekly with isoniazid, rifampin, pyrazinamide and ethambutol or streptomycin for 6 months.

*All regimens given twice weekly or 3 times weekly should be administered by directly observed therapy (see also *Directly Observed Therapy*).

The above treatment guidelines apply only when the disease is caused by organisms that are susceptible to the standard antituberculous agents. Because of the impact of resistance to isoniazid and rifampin on the response to therapy, it is essential that physicians initiating therapy for tuberculosis be familiar with the prevalence of drug resistance in their communities. It is suggested that ethambutol not be used in children whose vital acuity cannot be monitored.

Patients with Pulmonary Tuberculosis and HIV Infection

The response of the immunologically impaired host to treatment may not be satisfactory as that of a person with normal host responsiveness. For this reason, therapeutic decisions for the impaired host must be individualized. Since patients co-infected with HIV may have problems with malabsorption, screening of antimycobacterial drug levels, especially in patients with advanced HIV disease, may be necessary to prevent the emergence of MDRTB.

Patients with Extra Pulmonary Tuberculosis

The basic principles that underlie the treatment of pulmonary tuberculosis also apply to Extra pulmonary forms of the disease. Although there have not been the same kinds of carefully conducted controlled trials of treatment of Extra pulmonary tuberculosis as for pulmonary disease, increasing clinical experience indicates that a 6 to 9 month short-course regimens are effective. Because of the insufficient data, miliary tuberculosis, bone/joint tuberculosis, and tuberculosis meningitis in infants and children should receive 12 month therapy.

Bacteriologic evaluation of Extra pulmonary tuberculosis may be limited by the relative inaccessibility of the sites of disease. Thus, response to treatment often must be judged on the basis of clinical and radiographic findings.

The use of adjunctive therapies such as surgery and corticosteroids is more commonly required in Extra pulmonary tuberculosis than in pulmonary disease. Surgery may be necessary to obtain specimens for diagnosis and to treat such processes as constrictive pericarditis and spinal cord compression form Pott's Disease. Corticosteroids have been shown to be of benefit in preventing cardiac constriction form tuberculous pericarditis and in decreasing the neurologic sequaelae of all stages of tuberculosis meningitis, expecially when administered early in the course of the disease.

Pregnant Women with Tuberculosis

The options listed above must be adjusted for the pregnant patient. Streptomycin interferes with in utero development of the ear and may cause congenital deafness. Routine use of pyrazinamide is also not recommended in pregnancy because of inadequate teratogenicity data. The intial treatment regimen should consist of isoniazid and rifampin. Ethambutol should be include unless primary isoniazid resistance is unlikely (isoniazid resistance rate documented to be less than 4%).

Treatment of Patients with Multi-Drug Resistant Tuberculosis (MDRTB)

Multiple-drug resistant tuberculosis (i.e., resistance to at least isoniazid and rifampin) presents difficult treatment problems. Treatment must be individualized and based on susceptibility studies. In such cases, consultation with an expert in tuberculosis is recommended.

Directly Observed Therapy (DOT)

A major cause of drug-resistant tuberculosis is patient noncompliance with treatment. The use of DOT can help assure patient compliance with drug therapy. DOT is the observation of the patient by a health care provider or other responsible person as the patient ingests anti-tuberculosis medications. DOT can be achieved with daily, twice weekly or thrice weekly regimens, and is recommended for all patients.

For Preventive Therapy of Tuberculosis

Before isoniazid preventive therapy is initiated, bacteriologically positive or radiographically progressive tuberculosis must be excluded. Appropriate evaluations should be performed in Extra pulmonary tuberculosis is suspected.

Adults over 30 Kg: 300 mg per day in a single dose.

Infants and Children: 10 mg/kg (up to 300 mg daily) in a single dose.

In situations where adherence with daily preventative therapy cannot be assured, 20–30 mg/kg (not to exceed 900 mg) twice weekly under the direct observation of a health care worker at the time of administration[8].

Continuous administration of isoniazid for a sufficient period of time is an essential part of the regimen because relapse rates are higher if chemotherapy is stopped prematurely. In the treatment of tuberculosis, resistant organisms may multiply and the emergence during the treatment may necessitate a change in the regimen.

For following patient compliance: the Potts-Cozart test[9], a simple colorimetric[6] method of checking for isoniazid in the urine, is a useful tool for assuring patient compliance, which is essential for effective tuberculosis control. Additionally, isoniazid test strips are also available to check patient compliance.

Concomitant administration of pyridoxine (B_6) is recommended in the malnourished and in those predisposed to neuropathy (e.g., alcoholics and diabetics).

HOW SUPPLIED

Nydrazid Injection (Isoniazid Injection USP) is available for intramuscular use in 10 mL vials providing 100 mg isoniazid per mL (NDC 0003-0643-50).

Storage

Store at controlled room temperature 15°–30°C (59°–86°F). Protect from light.

Nydrazid Injection may crystallize at low temperatures. If this occurs, warm the vial to room temperature before use to redissolve the crystals.

REFERENCES

1. Murphy, R. *et al: Annuals of Internal Medicine*; 1990: November 15; volume 113:799–800.
2. Burke, R.F., *et al: Res Commun Chem Pathol Pharmacol*, 1990; July; vol. 69; 115–118.
3. Fleenor, M.F., *et al: Chest* (United States) *Letter*,; 1991: June;99 (6):1554.
4. Baciewicz, A.M. and Baciewicz, Jr. F.A.,: Arch Int Med 1993, September; volume 153; 1970–1971.
5. Jonville, A.P., *et al: European Journal of Clinical Pharmacol (Germany)*, 1991:40 (2) p198.
6. American Thoracic Society/Centers for disease Control: Treatment of Tuberculosis and Tuberculosis Infection in Adults and Children. Amer. J. Respir Crit Care Med. 1994; 149: p1359–1374.
7. Hoglund P., *et al:European Journal of Respir Dis* (Denmark) 1987: February; 70 (2) p110–116.
8. Committee on Infectious Diseases American Academy of Pediatrics: 1994, Red Book: Report of the Committee on Infectious Diseases; 23 edition; p487.
9. Schraufnagel, DE;*Testing for Isoniazid;Chest* (United States) 1990, August: 98 (2) p314–316.

CAUTION: Federal law prohibits dispensing without prescription.

APOTHECON®
A Bristol-Myers Squibb Company
Princeton, NJ 08540 USA

J4-491A

STADOL® ℞

[stā 'dŏl]
(butorphanol tartrate injection, USP)

Full prescribing information for the above product appears under Bristol-Myers Squibb Company.

Arco Pharmaceuticals, Inc.
105 ORVILLE DRIVE
BOHEMIA, NY 11716

Direct Inquiries to:
Professional Service Department
(516) 567-9500

ARCO-LASE® OTC
(broad pH spectrum digestant)

COMPOSITION

Each soft, mint flavored tablet contains Trizyme*, 38 mg., and Lipase, 25 mg.
*Contains the following standardized enzymes: amylolytic 30 mg.; proteolytic 6 mg.; cellulolytic 2 mg.

ACTION AND USES

Indicated for most gastrointestinal disorders due to poor digestion. Flatulence, gas and bloating, dyspepsia, distention, fullness, heartburn, or in any condition where normal digestion is impaired by digestive insufficiencies. Arcolase provides the highest standardized enzymatic activity, plus the protective action of the widest pH range. Thus it is effective throughout the entire G.I. tract. Requiring no enteric coating, there is assurance of a positive breakdown of its factors. This is advantageous, because quite often patients with digestive disorders cannot digest their food properly, let alone hard, or enteric coated capsules or tablets.

SIDE EFFECTS
None.

ADMINISTRATION AND DOSAGE

One tablet with or immediately following meals. Tablet may be swallowed or chewed.

SUPPLIED

Bottles of 50's. NDC 275-4040.

ARCO–LASE® PLUS ℞

COMPOSITION

Same as Arco-Lase, plus the addition of Hyoscyamine sulfate 0.10 mg., atropine sulfate 0.02 mg. and phenobarbital $^1/_8$ gr. (Warning: may be habit forming.)

ACTION AND USES

Gastrointestinal disturbances, such as cramps, bloating, spasms, diarrhea, nausea, vomiting and peptic ulcer. The enzymes correct the digestive insufficiencies.
The antispasmodic and phenobarbital contribute to the symptomatic relief of hypermotility and nervous tension, which usually accompanies functional disturbances of the bowel.

ADMINISTRATION AND DOSAGE

One tablet following meals.

SIDE EFFECTS

May cause rapid pulse, dryness of mouth and blurred vision.

CONTRAINDICATIONS

This product is contraindicated in the presence of glaucoma or prostatic hypertrophy.

SUPPLIED

Bottles of 50's. NDC 275-45-45.

LITERATURE AVAILABLE
Yes.

MEGA-B® OTC
(super potency vitamin B complex, sugar & starch free)

COMPOSITION

Each Mega-B Tablet contains the following Mega Vitamins:

B_1 (Thiamine Mononitrate)	100 mg.
B_2 (Riboflavin)	100 mg.
B_6 (Pyridoxine Hydrochloride)	100 mg.
B_{12} (Cyanocobalamin)	100 mcg.
Choline Bitartrate	100 mg.
Inositol	100 mg.
Niacinamide	100 mg.
Folic Acid	100 mcg.
Pantothenic Acid	100 mg.
d-Biotin	100 mcg.
Para-Aminobenzoic Acid (PABA)	100 mg.

In a base of yeast to provide the identified and unidentified B-Complex Factors.

ADVANTAGES

Each Mega-B capsule-shaped tablet provides the highest vitamin B complex available in a single dose.
Mega-B was designed for those patients who require truly Mega vitamin potencies with the convenience of minimum dosage.

INDICATIONS

Mega-B is indicated in conditions characterized by depletions or increased demand of the water-soluble B-complex vitamins. It may be useful in the nutritional management of patients during prolonged convalescence associated with major surgery. It is also indicated for stress conditions, as an adjunct to antibiotics and diuretic therapy, pre and post operative cases, liver conditions, gastrointestinal disorders interfering with intake or absorption of water-soluble vitamins, prolonged or wasting diseases, diabetes, burns, fractures, severe infections, and some psychological disorders.

WARNING

NOT INTENDED FOR TREATMENT OF PERNICIOUS ANEMIA, OR OTHER PRIMARY OR SECONDARY ANEMIAS.

DOSAGE

Usual dosage is one Mega-B tablet daily, or varied, depending on clinical needs.

SUPPLIED

Yellow capsule shaped tablets in bottles of 30, 100 and 500.

MEGADOSE™ OTC
(multiple mega-vitamin formula with minerals, sugar and starch free)

COMPOSITION

Vitamin A	25,000	USP Units
Vitamin D	1,000	USP Units
Vitamin C w/Rose Hips	250	mg.
Vitamin E	100	IU
Folic Acid	400	mcg.
Vitamin B_1	80	mg.
Vitamin B_2	80	mg.
Niacinamide	80	mg.
Vitamin B_6	80	mg.
Vitamin B_{12}	80	mcg.
Biotin	80	mcg.
Pantothenic Acid	80	mg.
Choline Bitartrate	80	mg.
Inositol	80	mg.
Para-Aminobenzoic Acid	80	mg.
Rutin	30	mg.
Citrus Bioflavonoids	30	mg.
Betaine Hydrochloride	30	mg.
Glutamic Acid	30	mg.
Hesperidin Complex	5	mg.
Iodine (from Kelp)	0.15	mg.
Calcium Gluconate*	50	mg.
Zinc Gluconate*	25	mg.
Potassium Gluconate*	10	mg.
Ferrous Gluconate*	10	mg.
Magnesium Gluconate*	7	mg.
Manganese Gluconate*	6	mg.
Copper Gluconate*	0.5	mg.

*Natural mineral chelates in a base containing natural ingredients.

DOSAGE
One tablet daily.

SUPPLIED

Capsule shaped tablets in bottles of 30, 100 and 250.

For information on over-the-counter drugs,
consult **PDR For Nonprescription Drugs.**

Astra Merck Inc.

See Astra Pharmaceuticals, L.P.

Astra Pharmaceuticals, L.P.

725 CHESTERBROOK BOULEVARD
WAYNE, PA 19087-5677

For Medical Information,
Adverse Drug Experiences,
and Customer Service
Contact: (800) 236-9933

ALBUTEROL SULFATE, USP ℞

Solution for Inhalation 0.5%*
Arm-a-Med®*
(*Potency expressed as albuterol)

DESCRIPTION

Albuterol Sulfate Solution for Inhalation contains albuterol sulfate, USP, the racemic form of albuterol and a relatively selective beta$_2$-adrenergic bronchodilator (see **CLINICAL PHARMACOLOGY** section below). Albuterol sulfate has the chemical name α[1]-[(*tert*-Butylamino) methyl]-4-hydroxy-*m*-xylene-α,α′-diol sulfate (2:1) (salt), and the following chemical structure:

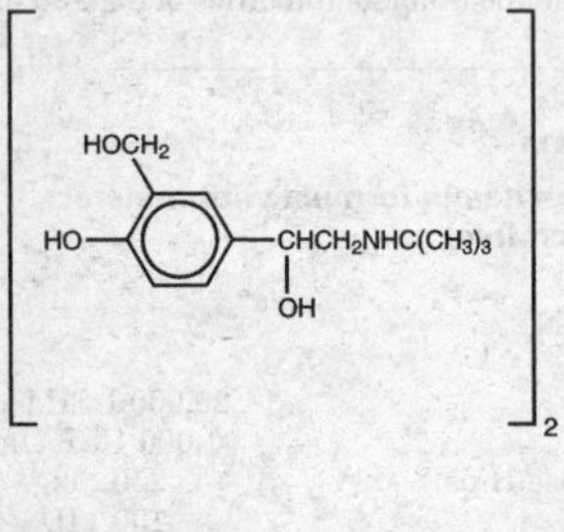

Albuterol sulfate has a molecular weight of 576.7 and the empirical formula $(C_{13}H_{21}NO_3)_2 \bullet H_2SO_4$. Albuterol sulfate is a white crystalline powder, soluble in water and slightly soluble in ethanol.

The World Health Organization's recommended name for albuterol base is salbutamol.

Albuterol Sulfate Solution for Inhalation 0.5% is in concentrated form. Dilute 0.5 mL of the solution to 3 mL with sterile normal saline solution prior to administration.

Each mL of Albuterol Sulfate Solution for Inhalation 0.5% contains 5 mg of albuterol (as 6.0 mg of albuterol sulfate) in an aqueous solution containing benzalkonium chloride; sulfuric acid is used to adjust the pH between 3 and 5. Albuterol Sulfate Solution for Inhalation 0.5% contains no sulfiting agents. It is supplied in 20 mL bottles.

Albuterol Sulfate Solution for Inhalation is a clear, colorless to light yellow solution.

CLINICAL PHARMACOLOGY

The prime action of beta-adrenergic drugs is to stimulate adenyl cyclase, the enzyme which catalyzes the formation of cyclic-3′, 5′-adenosine monophosphate (cyclic AMP) from adenosine triphosphate (ATP). The cyclic AMP thus formed mediates the cellular responses. *In vitro* studies and *in vivo* pharmacologic studies have demonstrated that albuterol has a preferential effect on beta$_2$-adrenergic receptors compared with isoproterenol. While it is recognized that beta$_2$-adrenergic receptors are the predominant receptors in bronchial smooth muscle, recent data indicate that 10% to 50% of the beta receptors in the human heart may be beta$_2$ receptors. The precise function of these receptors, however, is not yet established. Albuterol has been shown in most controlled clinical trials to have more effect on the respiratory tract, in the form of bronchial smooth muscle relaxation, than isoproterenol at comparable doses while producing fewer cardiovascular effects. Controlled clinical studies and other clinical experience have shown that inhaled albuterol, like other beta-adrenergic agonist drugs, can produce a significant cardiovascular effect in some patients, as measured by pulse rate, blood pressure, symptoms, and/or ECG changes.

Albuterol is longer acting than isoproterenol in most patients by any route of administration because it is not a substrate for the cellular uptake processes for catecholamines nor for catechol-*O*-methyl transferase.

Studies in asthmatic patients have shown that less than 20% of a single alubterol dose was absorbed following either IPPB or nebulizer administration; the remaining amount was recovered from the nebulizer and apparatus and expired air. Most of the absorbed dose was recovered in the urine 24 hours after drug administration. Following a 3.0 mg dose of nebulized albuterol, the maximum albuterol plasma level at 0.5 hour was 2.1 ng/mL (range 1.4 to 3.2 ng/mL). There was a significant dose-related response in FEV$_1$ and peak flow rate (PFR). It has been demonstrated that following oral administration of 4 mg albuterol, the elimination half-life was 5 to 6 hours.

Animal studies show that albuterol does not pass the blood-brain barrier. Recent studies in laboratory animals (minipigs, rodents, and dogs) recorded the occurrence of cardiac arrhythmias and sudden death (with histologic evidence of myocardial necrosis) when beta-agonists and methylxanthines were administered concurrently. The significance of these findings when applied to humans is currently unknown.

In controlled clinical trials, most patients exhibited an onset of improvement in pulmonary function within 5 minutes as determined by FEV$_1$. FEV$_1$ measurements also showed that the maximum average improvement in pulmonary function usually occurred at approximately 1 hour following inhalation of 2.5 mg of albuterol by compressor-nebulizer, and remained close to peak for 2 hours. Clinically significant improvement in pulmonary function (defined as maintenance of a 15% or more increase in FEV$_1$ over baseline values) continued for 3 to 4 hours in most patients and in some patients continued up to 6 hours.

In repetitive dose studies, continued effectiveness was demonstrated throughout the 3-month period of treatment in some patients.

INDICATIONS AND USAGE

Albuterol Sulfate Solution for Inhalation is indicated for the relief of bronchospasm in patients with reversible obstructive airway disease and acute attacks of bronchospasm.

CONTRAINDICATIONS

Albuterol Sulfate Solution for Inhalation is contraindicated in patients with a history of hypersensitivity to any of its components.

WARNINGS

As with other inhaled beta-adrenergic agonists, Albuterol Sulfate Solution for Inhalation can produce paradoxical bronchospasm, which can be life threatening. If it occurs, the preparation should be discontinued immediately and alternative therapy instituted.

Fatalities have been reported in association with excessive use of inhaled sympathomimetic drugs and with the home use of sympathomimetic nebulizers. It is, therefore, essential that the physician instruct the patient in the need for further evaluation if his/her asthma becomes worse. In individual patients, any beta$_2$-adrenergic agonist, including albuterol inhalation solution and solution for inhalation, may have a clinically significant cardiac effect.

Immediate hypersensitivity reactions may occur after administration of albuterol as demonstrated by rare cases of urticaria, angioedema, rash, bronchospasm, and oropharyngeal edema.

PRECAUTIONS

General: Albuterol, as with all sympathomimetic amines, should be used with caution in patients with cardiovascular disorders, especially coronary insufficiency, cardiac arrhythmias and hypertension, in patients with convulsive disorders, hyperthyroidism or diabetes mellitus, and in patients who are unusually responsive to sympathomimetic amines.

Large doses of intravenous albuterol have been reported to aggravate preexisting diabetes mellitus and ketoacidosis. Additionally, beta-agonists, including albuterol, when given intravenously may cause a decrease in serum potassium, possibly through intracellular shunting. The decrease is usually transient, not requiring supplementation. The relevance of these observations to the use of Albuterol Sulfate Solution for Inhalation is unknown.

To avoid contaminating the multi-dose bottle of Albuterol Sulfate Solution for Inhalation, proper aseptic technique should be used when withdrawing and delivering the dose into the nebulizer.

Information for Patients: The action of Albuterol Sulfate Solution for Inhalation may last up to 6 hours and therefore it should not be used more frequently than recommended. Do not increase the dose or frequency of medication without medical consultation. If symptoms get worse, medical consultation should be sought promptly. While taking Albuterol Sulfate Solution for Inhalation, other anti-asthma medicines should not be used unless prescribed.

Drug stability and safety of Albuterol Sulfate Solution for Inhalation when mixed with other drugs in a nebulizer have not been established.

See illustrated **"Patient's Instructions for Use."**

Drug Interactions: Other sympathomimetic aerosol bronchodilators or epinephrine should not be used concomitantly with albuterol.

Albuterol should be administered with extreme caution to patients being treated with monoamine oxidase inhibitors or tricyclic antidepressants, since the action of albuterol on the vascular system may be potentiated.

Beta-receptor blocking agents and albuterol inhibit the effect of each other.

Since albuterol may lower serum potassium, care should be taken in patients also using other drugs which lower serum potassium as the effects may be additive.

Carcinogenesis, Mutagenesis, and Impairment of Fertility: Albuterol sulfate, like other agents in its class, caused a significant dose-related increase in the incidence of benign leiomyomas of the mesovarium in a 2-year study in the rat, at oral doses corresponding to 10, 50, and 250 times the maximum human nebulizer dose. In another study, this effect was blocked by the coadministration of propranolol. The relevance of these findings to humans is not known. An 18-month study in mice and a lifetime study in hamsters revealed no evidence of tumorigenicity. Studies with albuterol revealed no evidence of mutagenesis. Reproduction studies in rats revealed no evidence of impaired fertility.

Teratogenic Effects—Pregnancy Category C: Albuterol has been shown to be teratogenic in mice when given subcutaneously in doses corresponding to the human nebulization dose. There are no adequate and well-controlled studies in pregnant women. Albuterol should be used during pregnancy only if the potential benefit justifies the potential risk to the fetus. A reproduction study in CD-1 mice with albuterol (0.025, 0.25, and 2.5 mg/kg subcutaneously, corresponding to 0.1, 1, and 12.5 times the maximum human nebulization dose, respectively) showed cleft palate formation in 5 of 111 (4.5%) fetuses at 0.25 mg/kg and in 10 of 108 (9.3%) fetuses at 2.5 mg/kg. None were observed at 0.025 mg/kg. Cleft palate also occurred in 22 of 72 (30.5%) fetuses treated with 2.5 mg/kg isoproterenol (positive control). A reproduction study in Stride Dutch rabbits revealed cranioschisis in 7 of 19 (37%) fetuses at 50 mg/kg, corresponding to 250 times the maximum human nebulization dose. During marketing, various congenital anomalies, including cleft palate and limb defects, have been reported in the offspring of patients being treated with albuterol. Some of the mothers were taking multiple medications during their pregnancies. Because no consistent pattern of defects can be discerned, a relationship between albuterol use and congenital anomalies cannot be established.

Labor and Delivery: Oral albuterol has been shown to delay preterm labor in some reports. There are presently no well-controlled studies which demonstrate that it will stop preterm labor or prevent labor at term. Therefore, cautious use of Albuterol Sulfate Solution for Inhalation is required in pregnant patients when given for relief of bronchospasm so as to avoid interference with uterine contractility.

Nursing Mothers: It is not known whether this drug is excreted in human milk. Because of the potential for tumorigenicity shown for alubterol in some animal studies, a decision should be made whether to discontinue nursing or to discontinue the drug, taking into account the importance of the drug to the mother.

Pediatric Use: Safety and effectiveness of albuterol inhalation solution and solution for inhalation in children below the age of 12 years have not been established.

ADVERSE REACTIONS

The results of clinical trials with Albuterol Sulfate Solution for Inhalation in 135 patients showed the following side effects which were considered probably or possibly drug related:

Central Nervous System: tremors (20%), dizziness (7%), nervousness (4%), headache (3%), insomnia (1%).
Gastrointestinal: nausea (4%), dyspepsia (1%).
Ear, Nose, and Throat: pharyngitis (<1%), nasal congestion (1%).
Cardiovascular: tachycardia (1%), hypertension (1%).
Respiratory: bronchospasm (8%), cough (4%), bronchitis (4%), wheezing (1%).

No clinically relevant laboratory abnormalities related to Albuterol Sulfate Solution for Inhalation administration were determined in these studies.

In comparing the adverse reactions reported for patients treated with Albuterol Sulfate Solution for Inhalation with those of patients treated with isoproterenol during clinical trials of 3 months, the following moderate to severe reactions, as judged by the investigators, were reported. This table does not include mild reactions.

Percent Incidence of Moderate to Severe Adverse Reactions

Reaction	Albuterol N=65	Isoproterenol N=65
Central Nervous System		
Tremors	10.7%	13.8%
Headache	3.1%	1.5%
Insomnia	3.1%	1.5%

Cardiovascular		
Hypertension	3.1%	3.1%
Arrhythmias	0%	3.0%
*Palpitation	0%	22.0%
Respiratory		
†Bronchospasm	15.4%	18.0%
Cough	3.1%	5.0%
Bronchitis	1.5%	5.0%
Wheeze	1.5%	1.5%
Sputum Increase	1.5%	1.5%
Dyspnea	1.5%	1.5%
Gastrointestinal		
Nausea	3.1%	0%
Dyspepsia	1.5%	0%
Systemic		
Malaise	1.5%	0%

* The finding of no arrhythmias and no palpitations after albuterol administration in this clinical study should not be interpreted as indicating that these adverse effects cannot occur after the administration of inhaled albuterol.

† In most cases of bronchospasm, this term was generally used to describe exacerbations in the underlying pulmonary disease.

Rare cases of urticaria, angioedema, rash, bronchospasm, and oropharyngeal edema have been reported after the use of inhaled albuterol.

OVERDOSAGE

Manifestations of overdosage may include anginal pain, hypertension, hypokalemia, and exaggeration of the pharmacological effects listed in **ADVERSE REACTIONS**.
The oral LD$_{50}$ in rats and mice was greater than 2,000 mg/kg. The inhalational LD$_{50}$ could not be determined.
There is insufficient evidence to determine if dialysis is beneficial for overdosage of Albuterol Sulfate Solution for Inhalation.

DOSAGE AND ADMINISTRATION

The usual dosage for adults and children 12 years and older is 2.5 mg of albuterol administered 3 to 4 times daily by nebulization. More frequent administration or higher doses are not recommended. To administer 2.5 mg of albuterol, dilute 0.5 mL of the 0.5% solution for inhalation to a total volume of 3 mL with sterile normal saline solution and administer by nebulization. The flow rate is regulated to suit the particular nebulizer so that the Albuterol Sulfate Solution for Inhalation will be delivered over approximately 5 to 15 minutes.
Drug stability and safety of Albuterol Sulfate Solution for Inhalation when mixed with other drugs in a nebulizer have not been established.
The use of Albuterol Sulfate Solution for Inhalation can be continued as medically indicated to control recurring bouts of bronchospasm. During treatment, most patients gain optimum benefit from regular use of the nebulizer solution.
If a previously effective dosage regimen fails to provide the usual relief, medical advice should be sought immediately, as this is often a sign of seriously worsening asthma which would require reassessment of therapy.

HOW SUPPLIED

Albuterol Sulfate Solution for Inhalation 0.5% is a clear, colorless to light yellow solution, and is supplied in amber glass bottles of 20 mL fill (NDC 0186-1490-01) with accompanying calibrated dropper; boxes of one.
Store between 2° and 25°C (36° and 77°F).

PATIENT'S INSTRUCTIONS FOR USE

Albuterol Sulfate, USP
Solution for Inhalation 0.5%*
*Potency expressed as albuterol
Note: The Albuterol Sulfate Solution contained in the 20 mL multiple-dose bottle is concentrated and must be diluted.
Read complete instructions carefully before using.
1. Draw 0.5 mL of Albuterol Sulfate Solution into the specially marked dropper that comes with each multi-dose bottle (Figure 1).

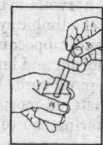

Figure 1

2. Squeeze the solution into the nebulizer reservoir through the appropriate opening (Figure 2).

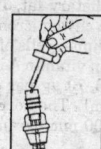

Figure 2

3. Add 2.5 mL of diluting fluid–sterile normal saline solution (as your physician has directed).
4. Gently swirl the nebulizer to mix the contents and connect it with the mouthpiece or face mask (Figure 3).

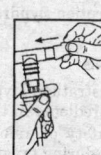

Figure 3

5. Connect the nebulizer to the compressor.
6. Sit in a comfortable, upright position; place the mouthpiece in your mouth (Figure 4) (or put on the face mask); and turn the compressor on.

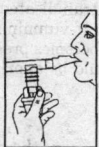

Figure 4

7. Breathe as calmly, deeply, and evenly as possible until no more mist is formed in the nebulizer chamber (about 5-15 minutes). At this point, the treatment is finished.
8. Clean the nebulizer (see manufacturer's instructions).

Note: Use only as directed by your physician. More frequent administration or higher doses are not recommended.
Drug stability and safety of Albuterol Sulfate Solution for Inhalation when mixed with other drugs in a nebulizer have not been established.
Store Albuterol Sulfate Solution for Inhalation 0.5%* between 2° and 25°C (36° and 77°F).
Manufactured by:
Warrick Pharmaceuticals Corporation
Reno, NV 89506 USA
Manufactured for:
Astra USA, Inc., Westborough, MA 01581
Illustrations Copyright© 1993 by
Astra USA, Inc., Westborough, MA 01581
Copyright© 1994, 1995, 1996, Warrick
Pharmaceuticals Corporation, Reno, NV
89506 USA. All rights reserved.
000539R02
Rev. 3/96
B-17954130

AQUASOL A®
Vitamin A Capsules, USP   ℞

DESCRIPTION

Each Vitamin A capsule, 15 mg for oral administration, contains the equivalent in activity to 15 mg of retinol or 50,000 USP Vitamin A Units. Each Vitamin A capsule, 7.5 mg, for oral administration, contains the equivalent of 7.5 mg retinol or 25,000 USP Vitamin A Units.
One USP unit is equal to 0.3 mcg of retinol or 0.6 mcg of beta-carotene. One molecule of beta-carotene yields 2 molecules of retinol, which is known as provitamin A.
Vitamin A synthetic (palmitate) is a clear, yellow to light-amber, oily liquid that has only a slight odor. It is a preisomerized vitamin A palmitate of synthetic origin. It is miscible with ether and with chloroform and is slightly soluble in alcohol.
Ordinarily fat-soluble, the vitamin A in this product has been water solubilized by special processing* to enable better absorption and utilization particularly in conditions in which absorption or utilization of fats and fat-soluble substances is impaired. The capsules also contain ethyl vanillin, FD&C Red #40, gelatin, glycerin, methylparaben, polysorbate 80, and propylparaben.

* Oil-soluble Vitamin A alcohol, water solubilized with polysorbate 80.

The structural formula of Vitamin A, retinol, is as follows:

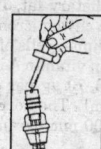

CLINICAL PHARMACOLOGY

Beta-carotene, retinol, and retinal have effective and reliable vitamin A activity. Retinal and retinol are in chemical equilibrium in the body and have equivalent antixerophthalmic activity. Retinal combines with the rod pigment, opsin, in the retina to form rhodopsin, necessary for visual dark adaptation. Vitamin A prevents retardation of growth and preserves the epithelial cells integrity. Normal adult liver storage is sufficient to satisfy two years requirements of vitamin A.
Vitamin A is readily absorbed from the gastrointestinal tract, where the biosynthesis of vitamin A from beta-carotene takes place. Vitamin A absorption requires bile salts, pancreatic lipase, and dietary fat. It is transported in the blood to the liver by the chylomicron fraction of the lymph. Vitamin A is stored in Kupffer cells of the liver mainly as the palmitate. Normal serum vitamin A is 80–300 USP units per 100 mL (plasma range is 30–70 mcg per dL) and for carotenoids 270 to 753 USP units per 100 mL. The normal adult liver contains approximately 100 to 300 micrograms per gram, mostly as retinol palmitate.

INDICATIONS AND USAGE

Vitamin A capsules are effective for the treatment of vitamin A deficiency.

CONTRAINDICATIONS

Vitamin A is contraindicated in hypervitaminosis A; malabsorption syndrome; or when there is sensitivity to any of the ingredients of this preparation.
Usage in Pregnancy: Safety of amounts exceeding 6,000 USP units of vitamin A daily during pregnancy has not been established at this time. The use of vitamin A in excess of the recommended dietary allowance may cause fetal harm when administered to a pregnant woman.
Animal reproduction studies have shown fetal abnormalities associated with overdosage in several species. Malformations of the central nervous system, the eye, the palate, and the urogenital tract are recorded.
Vitamin A in excess of the recommended dietary allowance is contraindicated in women who are or may become pregnant. If vitamin A is used during pregnancy, or if the patient becomes pregnant while taking vitamin A, the patient should be apprised of the potential hazard to the fetus.

WARNINGS

Avoid overdosage. Keep out of the reach of children.

PRECAUTIONS

General: Protect from light. Prolonged daily administration over 25,000 USP units of vitamin A should be under close supervision. Blood level assays are not a direct measure of liver storage. Liver storage should be adequate before discontinuing therapy. Single vitamin A deficiency is rare. Multiple vitamin deficiency is expected in any dietary deficiency.
Drug Interactions: Women on oral contraceptives have shown a significant increase in plasma vitamin A levels.
Carcinogenesis: There are no studies that show that administration of vitamin A will cause or prevent cancer.
Pregnancy Category X: See CONTRAINDICATIONS section.
Nursing Mothers: The U.S. Recommended Daily Allowance (RDA) of vitamin A (5,000 USP units) is recommended for nursing mothers.

ADVERSE REACTIONS

See OVERDOSAGE section.

OVERDOSAGE

The following amounts have been found to be toxic orally. Toxicity manifestations depended on the age, dosage size, and duration of administration.
Acute Toxicity —single dose (25,000 USP units/kg body weight)
  Infant: 350,000 USP units
  Adult: Over 2 million USP units
Chronic Toxicity —(4,000 USP units/kg body weight for 6 to 15 months)
  Infants 3 to 6 months old: 18,500 USP units (water dispersed)/day for one to three months.
  Adults: 1 million USP units daily for three days; 50,000 USP units daily for longer than 18 months: 500,000 USP units daily for two months.
Hypervitaminosis A Syndrome:
1. *General manifestations:*
  Fatigue, malaise, lethargy, abdominal discomfort, anorexia, and vomiting.

Continued on next page

Aquasol A—Cont.

2. *Specific manifestations:*
   a. Skeletal: slow growth, hard tender cortical thickening over the radius and the tibia, migratory arthralgia, and premature closure of the epiphysis.
   b. Central Nervous System: irritability, headache, and increased intracranial pressure as manifested by bulging fontanels, papilledema, and exophthalmos.
   c. Dermatologic: fissures of the lips, drying and cracking of the skin, alopecia, scaling, massive desquamation, and increased pigmentation.
   d. Systemic: hypomenorrhea, hepatosplenomegaly, jaundice, leukopenia, vitamin A plasma level over 1,200 USP units/100 mL.

The treatment of hypervitaminosis A consists of immediate withdrawal of the vitamin along with symptomatic and supportive treatment.

DOSAGE AND ADMINISTRATION
Adults and Children Over 8 years of age:
100,000 USP units daily for three days followed by 50,000 USP units daily for two weeks.

Follow-up therapy with an oral therapeutic multivitamin preparation, containing 10,000 to 20,000 USP units vitamin A for persons over 8 years old is recommended daily for two months. In malabsorption, the parenteral route must be used for an equivalent preparation.

Poor dietary habits should be corrected and an abundant and well-balanced dietary intake should be prescribed.

HOW SUPPLIED
Aquasol A capsules (vitamin A capsules USP) are available as:

NDC 0186-4301-00; 15 mg retinol (50,000 USP Units), Bottles of 100.

NDC 0186-4291-00; 7.5 mg retinol (25,000 USP Units), Bottles of 100.

These products are dark red, soft gelatin capsules.

Store at controlled room temperature, 15°–30°C (59°–86°F). Protect from light. Dispense in a tight, light-resistant container as defined in the USP.

These products are manufactured for Astra USA, Inc., by R.P. Scherer Corp., Clearwater, FL 33518.

Caution: Federal law prohibits dispensing without prescription.

021678R30   8/93 (30)

AQUASOL A®
Parenteral   ℞
water-miscible vitamin A Palmitate

50,000 USP Units

(15 mg retinol)/mL

with 0.5% chlorobutanol as preservative; 12% polysorbate 80, 0.1% citric acid, 0.03% butylated hydroxyanisole, 0.03% butylated hydroxytoluene; and sodium hydroxide to adjust pH.

THIS IS A STERILE PRODUCT FOR INTRAMUSCULAR INJECTION

DESCRIPTION
AQUASOL A PARENTERAL (water-miscible vitamin A Palmitate) provides 50,000 USP Units of vitamin A per mL as retinol ($C_{20}H_{30}O$) in the form of vitamin A palmitate, a light yellow to amber oil. The structural formula of retinol is:

Ordinarily oil-soluble, the vitamin A in this product has been water solubilized by special processing* and is available in a water solution for intramuscular injection.

One USP Unit is equivalent to one international unit (IU) and to 0.3 mcg of retinol or 0.6 mcg of beta-carotene.

CLINICAL PHARMACOLOGY
Beta-carotene, retinol, and retinal have effective and reliable vitamin A activity. Retinal and retinol are in chemical equilibrium in the body and have equivalent antixerophthalmic activity. Retinal combines with the rod pigment, opsin, in the retina to form rhodopsin, necessary for visual dark adaptation. Vitamin A prevents retardation of growth and preserves the epithelial cells' integrity. Normal adult liver storage is sufficient to satisfy two years' requirements of vitamin A.

---

*Oil-soluble vitamin A water solubilized with polysorbate 80.

Vitamin A is readily absorbed from the gastrointestinal tract, where the biosynthesis of vitamin A from beta-carotene takes place. Vitamin A absorption requires bile salts, pancreatic lipase, and dietary fat. It is transported in the blood to the liver by the chylomicron fraction of the lymph. Vitamin A is stored in Kupffer cells of the liver mainly as the palmitate. Normal serum vitamin A is 80–300 Units per 100 mL (plasma range is 30–70 μg per dl) and for carotenoids 270–753 Units per 100 mL. The normal adult liver contains approximately 100 to 300 micrograms per gram, mostly as retinol palmitate.

INDICATIONS
Vitamin A injection is effective for the treatment of vitamin A deficiency.

The parenteral administration is indicated when the oral administration is not feasible as in anorexia, nausea, vomiting, pre- and post-operative conditions, or it is not available as in the "Malabsorption Syndrome" with accompanying steatorrhea.

CONTRAINDICATIONS
The intravenous administration. Hypervitaminosis A. Sensitivity to any of the ingredients in this preparation.

Use in Pregnancy: Safety of amounts exceeding 6,000 Units of vitamin A daily during pregnancy has not been established at this time. The use of vitamin A in excess of the recommended dietary allowance may cause fetal harm when administered to a pregnant woman. Animal reproduction studies have shown fetal abnormalities associated with overdosage in several species. Malformations of the central nervous system, the eye, the palate, and the urogenital tract are recorded. Vitamin A in excess of the recommended dietary allowance is contraindicated in women who are or may become pregnant. If vitamin A is used during pregnancy, or if the patient becomes pregnant while taking vitamin A, the patient should be apprised of the potential hazard to the fetus.

WARNINGS
Avoid overdosage. Keep out of the reach of children.

PRECAUTIONS
General: Protect from light. Prolonged daily dose administration over 25,000 Units vitamin A should be under close supervision. Blood level assays are not a direct measure of liver storage. Liver storage should be adequate before discontinuing therapy. Single vitamin A deficiency is rare. Multiple vitamin deficiency is expected in any dietary deficiency.

Drug Interactions: Women on oral contraceptives have shown a significant increase in plasma vitamin A levels.

Carcinogenesis: There are no studies that show that administration of vitamin A will cause or prevent cancer.

Pregnancy Category X:
See CONTRAINDICATIONS section.

Nursing Mothers: The U.S. Recommended Daily Allowance (RDA) of vitamin A (5,000 Units) is recommended for nursing mothers.

ADVERSE REACTIONS
See OVERDOSAGE section. Anaphylactic shock and death have been reported using the intravenous route. Allergic reactions have been reported rarely with administration of Aquasol A Parenteral including one case of an anaphylactoid type reaction.

OVERDOSAGE
The following amounts have been found to be toxic orally. Toxicity manifestations depend on the age, dosage, size, and duration of administration.
Acute toxicity—single dose (25,000 Units/kg body weight)
   Infant: 350,000 Units
   Adult: Over 2 million Units
Chronic toxicity (4,000 Units/kg body weight for 6 to 15 months)
   Infants 3 to 6 months old: 18,500 Units (water dispersed)/day for one to three months.
   Adult: 1 million Units daily for three days; 50,000 Units daily for longer than 18 months; 500,000 Units daily for two months.

Hypervitaminosis A Syndrome:
1. *General manifestations:*
   Fatigue, malaise, lethargy, abdominal discomfort, anorexia, and vomiting.
2. *Specific manifestations:*
   a. Skeletal: slow growth, hard tender cortical thickening over the radius and tibia, migratory arthralgia and premature closure of the epiphysis.
   b. Central Nervous System: irritability, headache, and increased intracranial pressure as manifested by bulging fontanels, papilledema, and exophthalmos.
   c. Dermatologic: fissures of the lips, drying and cracking of the skin, alopecia, scaling, massive desquamation, and increased pigmentation.

d. Systemic: hypomenorrhea, hepatosplenomegaly, jaundice, leukopenia, vitamin A plasma level over 1,200 Units/100 mL.
The treatment of hypervitaminosis A consists of immediate withdrawal of the vitamin along with symptomatic and supportive treatment.

DOSAGE AND ADMINISTRATION
For intramuscular use.
I. Adults
   100,000 Units daily for three days followed by 50,000 daily for two weeks.
II. Children 1 to 8 years old
   17,500 to 35,000 Units daily for 10 days.
III. Infants
   7,500 to 15,000 Units daily for 10 days.
Follow-up therapy with an oral therapeutic multi-vitamin preparation, containing 10,000 to 20,000 Units vitamin A for persons over 8 years old and 5,000 to 10,000 Units for infants and children, is recommended daily for two months. In malabsorption, the parenteral route must be used for an equivalent preparation.

Poor dietary habits should be corrected and an abundant and well-balanced dietary intake should be prescribed.

HOW SUPPLIED
Aquasol A Parenteral (water-miscible vitamin A Palmitate) is available as: NDC 0186-4239-62; 50,000 USP Units (15 mg retinol/mL); 2 mL single-dose vial, box of 10.
Store at 2°–8°C (36°–46°F). Do not freeze.
Caution: Federal law prohibits dispensing without prescription.
Manufactured by:
Centeon L.L.C., Kankakee, IL 60901

Manufactured for:
Astra USA, Inc., Westborough, MA 01581
021646R01   Rev. 6/96

ASTRAMORPH/PF™   ℞
[ăs '-trā-mŏrf '']
(morphine sulfate Injection, USP) Preservative-Free

DESCRIPTION
Morphine is the most important alkaloid of opium and is a phenanthrene derivative. It is available as the sulfate, having the following structural formula:

7,8-Didehydro-4,5-epoxy-17-methyl-(5α,6α)-morphinan-3,6-diol sulfate (2:1) (salt), pentahydrate
Preservative-free Astramorph/PF (morphine sulfate Injection, USP) is a sterile, pyrogen-free, isobaric solution free of antioxidants, preservatives or other potentially neurotoxic additives, and is intended for intravenous, epidural or intrathecal administration as a narcotic analgesic. Each milliliter contains morphine sulfate 0.5 mg or 1 mg (Warning: May Be Habit Forming) and sodium chloride 9 mg in Water for Injection. pH may be adjusted with hydrochloric acid to 2.5–6.5. Containers are sealed under nitrogen. Each container is intended for SINGLE USE ONLY. Discard any unused portion. DO NOT AUTOCLAVE.

CLINICAL PHARMACOLOGY
Morphine exerts its primary effects on the central nervous system and organs containing smooth muscle. Pharmacologic effects include analgesia, drowsiness, alteration in mood (euphoria), reduction in body temperature (at low doses), dose-related depression of respiration, interference with adrenocortical response to stress (at high doses), reduction in peripheral resistance with little or no effect on cardiac index and miosis.

Morphine, as other opioids, acts as an agonist interacting with stereo-specific and saturable binding sites/receptors in the brain, spinal cord and other tissues. These sites have been classified as μ receptors and are widely distributed throughout the central nervous system being present in highest concentration in the limbic system (frontal and temporal cortex, amygdala and hippocampus), thalamus, striatum, hypothalamus, midbrain and laminae I, II, IV and V of the dorsal horn in the spinal cord. It has been postulated that exogenously administered morphine exerts its analgesic effect, in part, by altering the central release of neurotransmitter from afferent nerves sensitive to noxious stimuli. Peripheral threshold or responsiveness to noxious stimuli is unaffected leaving monosynaptic reflexes such as the patellar or the Achilles tendon reflex intact.

Autonomic reflexes are not affected by epidural or intrathecal morphine, however morphine exerts spasmogenic effects on the gastrointestinal tract that result in decreased peristaltic activity.

Central nervous system effects of intravenously administered morphine sulfate are influenced by ability to cross the blood-brain barrier.

The delay in the onset of analgesia following epidural or intrathecal injection may be attributed to its relatively poor lipid solubility (i.e., an oil/water partition coefficient of 1.42), and its slow access to the receptor sites. The hydrophilic character of morphine may also explain its retention in the CNS and its slow release into the systemic circulation, resulting in a prolonged effect.

Nausea and vomiting may be prominent and are thought to be the result of central stimulation of the chemoreceptor trigger zone. Histamine release is common; allergic manifestations of urticaria and, rarely, anaphylaxis may occur. Bronchoconstriction may occur either as an idiosyncratic reaction or from large dosages.

Approximately one-third of intravenous morphine is bound to plasma proteins. Free morphine is rapidly redistributed in parenchymatous tissues. The major metabolic pathway is through conjugation with glucuronic acid in the liver. Elimination half-life is approximately 1.5 to 2 hours in healthy volunteers. For intravenously administered morphine, 90% is excreted in the urine within 24 hours and traces are detectable in urine up to 48 hours. About 7–10% of administered morphine eventually appears in the feces as conjugated morphine.

Peak serum levels following epidural or intrathecal administration of Astramorph/PF are reached within 30 minutes in most subjects and decline to very low levels during the next 2 to 4 hours. The onset of action occurs in 15 to 60 minutes following epidural administration or intrathecal administration; analgesia may last up to 24 hours. Due to this extended duration of action, sustained pain relief can be provided with lower daily doses (by these two routes) than are usually required with intravenous or intramuscular morphine administration.

INDICATIONS AND USAGE

Preservative-free Astramorph/PF is a systemic narcotic analgesic for administration by the intravenous, epidural or intrathecal routes. It is used for the management of pain not responsive to non-narcotic analgesics. Morphine sulfate, administered epidurally or intrathecally, provides pain relief for extended periods without attendant loss of motor, sensory or sympathetic function.

CONTRAINDICATIONS

Astramorph/PF is contraindicated in those medical conditions which would preclude the administration of opioids by the intravenous route—allergy to morphine or other opiates, acute bronchial asthma, upper airway obstruction.

Administration of morphine by the epidural or intrathecal route is contraindicated in the presence of infection at the injection site, anticoagulant therapy, bleeding diathesis, parenterally administered corticosteroids within a two week period or other concomitant drug therapy or medical condition which would contraindicate the technique of epidural or intrathecal analgesia.

WARNINGS

Astramorph/PF administration should be limited to use by those familiar with the management of respiratory depression, and in the case of epidural or intrathecal administration, familiar with the techniques and patient management problems associated with epidural or intrathecal drug administration. Because epidural administration has been associated with lessened potential for immediate or late adverse effects than intrathecal administration, the epidural route should be used whenever possible. Rapid intravenous administration may result in chest wall rigidity.

FACILITIES WHERE ASTRAMORPH/PF IS ADMINISTERED MUST BE EQUIPPED WITH RESUSCITATIVE EQUIPMENT, OXYGEN, NALOXONE INJECTION, AND OTHER RESUSCITATIVE DRUGS. WHEN THE EPIDURAL OR INTRATHECAL ROUTE OF ADMINISTRATION IS EMPLOYED, PATIENTS MUST BE OBSERVED IN A FULLY EQUIPPED AND STAFFED ENVIRONMENT FOR AT LEAST 24 HOURS.

SEVERE RESPIRATORY DEPRESSION UP TO 24 HOURS FOLLOWING EPIDURAL OR INTRATHECAL ADMINISTRATION HAS BEEN REPORTED.

Morphine sulfate may be habit forming. (See DRUG ABUSE AND DEPENDENCE section.)

PRECAUTIONS

General: Preservative-free Astramorph/PF (morphine sulfate Injection, USP) should be administered with extreme caution in aged or debilitated patients, in the presence of increased intracranial/intraocular pressure and in patients with head injury. Pupillary changes (miosis) may obscure the course of intracranial pathology. Care is urged in patients who have a decreased respiratory reserve (e.g., emphysema, severe obesity, kyphoscoliosis).

Seizures may result from high doses. Patients with known seizure disorders should be carefully observed for evidence of morphine-induced seizure activity.

It is recommended that administration of Astramorph/PF by the epidural or intrathecal routes be limited to the lumbar area. Intrathecal use has been associated with a higher incidence of respiratory depression than epidural use.

Smooth muscle hypertonicity may result in biliary colic, difficulty in urination and possible urinary retention requiring catheterization. Consideration should be given to risks inherent in urethral catheterization, e.g., sepsis, when epidural or intrathecal administration is considered, especially in the perioperative period.

Elimination half-life may be prolonged in patients with reduced metabolic rates and with hepatic or renal dysfunction. Hence, care should be exercised in administering morphine in these conditions, particularly with repeated dosing. Patients with reduced circulating blood volume, impaired myocardial function or on sympatholytic drugs should be observed carefully for orthostatic hypotension, particularly in transport.

Patients with chronic obstructive pulmonary disease and patients with acute asthmatic attack may develop acute respiratory failure with administration of morphine. Use in these patients should be reserved for those whose conditions require endotracheal intubation and respiratory support or control of ventilation.

Drug Interactions: Depressant effects of morphine are potentiated by either concomitant administration or in the presence of other CNS depressants such as alcohol, sedatives, antihistaminics or psychotropic drugs (e.g., MAO inhibitors, phenothiazines, butyrophenones and tricyclic antidepressants). Premedication or intra-anesthetic use of neuroleptics with morphine may increase the risk of respiratory depression.

Carcinogenesis, Mutagenesis, Impairment of Fertility: Studies of morphine sulfate in animals to evaluate the carcinogenic and mutagenic potential or the effect on fertility have not been conducted.

Pregnancy: *Teratogenic effects—Pregnancy Category C* Animal reproduction studies have not been conducted with morphine sulfate. It is also not known whether morphine sulfate can cause fetal harm when administered to a pregnant woman or can affect reproductive capacity. Morphine sulfate should be given to a pregnant woman only if clearly needed.

Nonteratogenic effects—Infants born from mothers who have been taking morphine chronically may exhibit withdrawal symptoms.

Labor and Delivery: *Intravenous* morphine readily passes into the fetal circulation and may result in respiratory depression in the neonate. Naloxone and resuscitative equipment should be available for reversal of narcotic-induced respiratory depression in the neonate. In addition, intravenous morphine may reduce the strength, duration and frequency of uterine contraction resulting in prolonged labor. *Epidurally and intrathecally* administered morphine readily passes into the fetal circulation and may result in respiratory depression of the neonate. Controlled clinical studies have shown that *epidural* administration has little or no effect on the relief of labor pain.

However, studies have suggested that in most cases 0.2 to 1 mg of morphine *intrathecally* provides adequate pain relief with little effect on the duration of first stage labor. The second stage labor, though, may be prolonged if the parturient is not encouraged to bear down. A continuous intravenous infusion of naloxone, 0.6 mg/hr, for 24 hours after intrathecal injection may be employed to reduce the incidence of potential side effects.

Nursing Mothers: Morphine is excreted in maternal milk. Effect on the nursing infant is not known.

Pediatric Use: Safety and effectiveness in children have not been established.

ADVERSE REACTIONS

The most serious side effect is respiratory depression. Because of delay in maximum CNS effect with intravenously administered drug (30 min), rapid administration may result in overdosing. Bolus administration by the epidural or intrathecal route may result in early respiratory depression due to direct venous redistribution of morphine to the respiratory centers in the brain. Late (up to 24 hours) onset of acute respiratory depression has been reported with administration by the epidural or intrathecal route and is believed to be the result of rostral spread. Reports of respiratory depression following intrathecal administration have been more frequent, but the dosage used in most of these cases has been considerably higher than that recommended. This depression may be severe and could require intervention (see WARNINGS and OVERDOSAGE sections). Even without clinical evidence of ventilatory inadequacy, a diminished CO_2 ventilation response may be noted for up to 22 hours following epidural or intrathecal administration.

While low doses of intravenously administered morphine have little effect on cardiovascular stability, high doses are excitatory, resulting from sympathetic hyperactivity and in-

crease in circulating catecholamines. Excitation of the central nervous system resulting in convulsions may accompany high doses of morphine given intravenously. Dysphoric reactions may occur and toxic psychoses have been reported.

Epidural or intrathecal administration is accompanied by a high incidence of pruritus which is dose related but not confined to site of administration. Nausea and vomiting are frequently seen in patients following morphine administration. Urinary retention which may persist for 10–20 hours following single epidural or intrathecal administration has been reported in approximately 90% of males. Incidence is somewhat lower in females. Patients may require catheterization (see PRECAUTIONS). Pruritus, nausea/vomiting and urinary retention frequently can be alleviated by the intravenous administration of low doses of naloxone (0.2 mg).

Tolerance and dependence to chronically administered morphine, by whatever route, is known to occur (see DRUG ABUSE AND DEPENDENCE section).

Miscellaneous side effects include constipation, headache, anxiety, depression of cough reflex, interference with thermal regulation and oliguria. Evidence of histamine release such as urticaria, wheals and/or local tissue irritation may occur.

In general, side effects are amenable to reversal by narcotic antagonists. **NALOXONE HYDROCHLORIDE INJECTION AND RESUSCITATIVE EQUIPMENT SHOULD BE IMMEDIATELY AVAILABLE FOR ADMINISTRATION IN CASE OF LIFE THREATENING OR INTOLERABLE SIDE EFFECTS.**

DRUG ABUSE AND DEPENDENCE

Controlled Substance: Morphine sulfate Injection is a Schedule II substance under the Drug Enforcement Administration classification.

Abuse: Morphine has recognized abuse and dependence potential.

Dependence: Cerebral and spinal receptors may develop tolerance/dependence independently, as a function of local dosage. Care must be taken to avert withdrawal in those patients who have been maintained on parenteral/oral narcotics when epidural or intrathecal administration is considered. Withdrawal may occur following chronic epidural or intrathecal administration, as well as the development of tolerance to morphine by these routes. (See NONTERATOGENIC EFFECTS under Pregnancy).

OVERDOSAGE

Overdosage is characterized by respiratory depression with or without concomitant CNS depression. Since respiratory arrest may result either through direct depression of the respiratory center or as the result of hypoxia, primary attention should be given to the establishment of adequate respiratory exchange through provision of a patent airway and institution of assisted or controlled ventilation. The narcotic antagonist, naloxone hydrochloride, is a specific antidote. Naloxone hydrochloride (see package insert for full prescribing information) should be administered intravenously, simultaneously with respiratory resuscitation. *As the duration of effect of naloxone is considerably shorter than that of epidural or intrathecal morphine, repeated administration may be necessary.* Patients should be closely observed for evidence of renarcotization. *Note: Respiratory depression may be delayed in onset up to 24 hours following epidural or intrathecal administration.* In painful conditions, reversal of narcotic effect may result in acute onset of pain and release of catecholamines. Careful administration of naloxone may permit reversal of side effects without affecting analgesia. Parenteral administration of narcotics in patients receiving epidural or intrathecal morphine may result in overdosage.

DOSAGE AND ADMINISTRATION

Preservative-free Astramorph/PF (morphine sulfate Injection, USP) is intended for intravenous, epidural or intrathecal administration.

Intravenous Administration

Dosage—The initial dose of morphine sulfate should be 2 mg to 10 mg/70 kg of body weight. Patients under the age of 18; no information available.

Epidural Administration

ASTRAMORPH/PF SHOULD BE ADMINISTERED EPIDURALLY ONLY BY PHYSICIANS EXPERIENCED IN THE TECHNIQUES OF EPIDURAL ADMINISTRATION AND WHO ARE THOROUGHLY FAMILIAR WITH THE LABELING. IT SHOULD BE ADMINISTERED ONLY IN SETTINGS WHERE ADEQUATE PATIENT MONITORING IS POSSIBLE. RESUSCITATIVE EQUIPMENT AND A SPECIFIC ANTAGONIST (NALOXONE HYDROCHLORIDE INJECTION) SHOULD BE IMMEDIATELY AVAILABLE FOR THE MANAGEMENT OF RESPIRATORY DEPRESSION AS WELL AS COMPLICATIONS WHICH MIGHT RESULT FROM INADVERTENT INTRATHECAL OR INTRAVASCULAR INJECTION. (NOTE: INTRATHECAL DOSAGE IS USUALLY $^1/_{10}$ THAT OF EPIDURAL

Continued on next page

Astramorph/PF—Cont.

DOSAGE.) PATIENT MONITORING SHOULD BE CONTINUED FOR AT LEAST 24 HOURS AFTER EACH DOSE, SINCE DELAYED RESPIRATORY DEPRESSION MAY OCCUR.
Proper placement of a needle or catheter in the epidural space should be verified before Astramorph/PF is injected. Acceptable techniques for verifying proper placement include: a) aspiration to check for absence of blood or cerebrospinal fluid, or b) administration of 5 mL (3 mL in obstetric patients) of UNPRESERVED 1.5% Lidocaine and Epinephrine (1:200,000) Injection and then observe the patient for lack of tachycardia (this indicates that vascular injection has *not* been made) and lack of sudden onset of segmental anesthesia (this indicates that intrathecal injection has *not* been made).
Epidural Adult Dosage—Initial injection of 5 mg in the lumbar region may provide satisfactory pain relief for up to 24 hours. If adequate pain relief is not achieved within one hour, careful administration of incremental doses of 1 to 2 mg at intervals sufficient to assess effectiveness may be given. No more than 10 mg/24 hr should be administered.
Thoracic administration has been shown to dramatically increase the incidence of early and late respiratory depression even at doses of 1 to 2 mg.
For continuous infusion an initial dose of 2 to 4 mg/24 hours is recommended. Further doses of 1 to 2 mg may be given if pain relief is not achieved initially.
Aged or debilitated patients-Administer with extreme caution (see PRECAUTIONS section). Doses of less than 5 mg may provide satisfactory pain relief for up to 24 hours.
Epidural Pediatric Use—No information on use in pediatric patients is available.
Intrathecal Administration

NOTE: INTRATHECAL DOSAGE IS USUALLY 1/10 THAT OF EPIDURAL DOSAGE.

ASTRAMORPH/PF SHOULD BE ADMINISTERED INTRATHECALLY ONLY BY PHYSICIANS EXPERIENCED IN THE TECHNIQUES OF INTRATHECAL ADMINISTRATION AND WHO ARE THOROUGHLY FAMILIAR WITH THE LABELING. IT SHOULD BE ADMINISTERED ONLY IN SETTINGS WHERE ADEQUATE PATIENT MONITORING IS POSSIBLE. RESUSCITATIVE EQUIPMENT AND A SPECIFIC ANTAGONIST (NALOXONE HYDROCHLORIDE INJECTION) SHOULD BE IMMEDIATELY AVAILABLE FOR THE MANAGEMENT OF RESPIRATORY DEPRESSION AS WELL AS COMPLICATIONS WHICH MIGHT RESULT FROM INADVERTENT INTRAVASCULAR INJECTION. **PATIENT MONITORING SHOULD BE CONTINUED FOR AT LEAST 24 HOURS AFTER EACH DOSE, SINCE DELAYED RESPIRATORY DEPRESSION MAY OCCUR. RESPIRATORY DEPRESSION (BOTH EARLY AND LATE ONSET) HAS OCCURRED MORE FREQUENTLY FOLLOWING INTRATHECAL ADMINISTRATION.**
Intrathecal Adult Dosage—A single injection of 0.2 to 1 mg may provide satisfactory pain relief for up to 24 hours. **(CAUTION: THIS IS ONLY 0.4 TO 2 ML OF THE 0.5 MG/ML POTENCY OR 0.2 to 1 ML OF THE 1 MG/ML POTENCY OF ASTRAMORPH/PF.) DO NOT INJECT INTRATHECALLY MORE THAN 2 ML OF THE 0.5 MG/ML POTENCY OR 1 ML OF THE 1 MG/ML POTENCY. USE IN THE LUMBAR AREA ONLY IS RECOMMENDED.** Repeated intrathecal injections of Astramorph/PF are not recommended. A constant intravenous infusion of naloxone hydrochloride, 0.6 mg/hr, for 24 hours after intrathecal injection may be used to reduce the incidence of potential side effects.
Aged or debilitated patients-Administer with extreme caution (see PRECAUTIONS section). A lower dosage is usually satisfactory.
Repeat Dosage—If pain recurs, alternative routes of administration should be considered, since experience with repeated doses of morphine by the intrathecal route is limited.
Intrathecal Pediatric Use—No information on use in pediatric patients is available.
Parenteral drug products should be inspected for particulate matter and discoloration prior to administration, whenever solution and container permit.

HOW SUPPLIED
The following strengths and container types of Astramorph/PF are available:

0.5 mg/mL

NDC 0186-1159-03	2 mL (1 mg) Ampule, Boxes of 10
NDC 0186-1150-02	10 mL (5 mg) Ampule, Boxes of 5
NDC 0186-1152-12	10 mL (5 mg) Single Dose Vial, Boxes of 5 Astra E-Z OFF® vial closure

1 mg/mL

NDC 0186-1160-03	2 mL (2 mg) Ampule, Boxes of 10
NDC 0186-1151-02	10 mL (10 mg) Ampule, Boxes of 5
NDC 0186-1153-12	10 mL (10 mg) Single Dose Vial, Boxes of 5 Astra E-Z OFF® vial closure

Storage
Protect from light. Store in carton at controlled room temperature, 15° to 30° C (59° to 86°F) until ready to use. Astramorph/PF contains no preservative. DISCARD ANY UNUSED PORTION. DO NOT AUTOCLAVE. Do not use the injection if darker than pale yellow or if discolored in any other way, or if it contains a precipitate.
Caution: Federal law prohibits dispensing without prescription.
021865R04 Rev. 5/97

ATACAND® ℞
(CANDESARTAN CILEXETIL)
TABLETS

USE IN PREGNANCY
When used in pregnancy during the second and third trimesters, drugs that act directly on the renin-angiotensin system can cause injury and even death to the developing fetus. When pregnancy is detected, ATACAND should be discontinued as soon as possible. See WARNINGS, *Fetal/Neonatal and Mortality.*

DESCRIPTION

ATACAND* (candesartan cilexetil), a prodrug, is hydrolyzed to candesartan during absorption from the gastrointestinal tract. Candesartan is a selective AT_1 subtype angiotensin II receptor antagonist.
Candesartan cilexetil, a nonpeptide, is chemically described as (±)-1-[[(cyclohexyloxy)carbonyl]oxy]ethyl 2-ethoxy-1-[[2'-(1H-tetrazol-5-yl)[1,1'-biphenyl]-4-yl]methyl]-1H-benzimidazole-7-carboxylate.
Its empirical formula is $C_{33}H_{34}N_6O_6$ and its structural formula is:

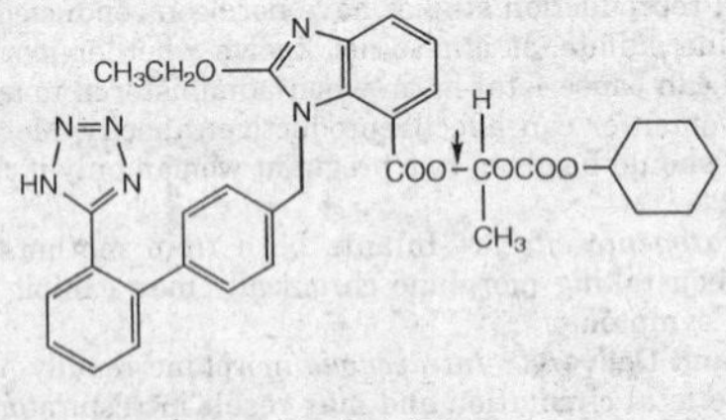

↓ site of ester hydrolysis

Candesartan cilexetil is a white to off-white powder with a molecular weight of 610.67. It is practically insoluble in water and sparingly soluble in methanol. Candesartan cilexetil is a racemic mixture containing one chiral center at the cyclohexyloxycarbonyloxy ethyl ester group. Following oral administration, candesartan cilexetil undergoes hydrolysis at the ester link to form the active drug, candesartan, which is achiral.
ATACAND is available for oral use as tablets containing either 4 mg, 8 mg, 16 mg, or 32 mg of candesartan cilexetil and the following inactive ingredients: hydroxypropyl cellulose, polyethylene glycol, lactose, corn starch, carboxymethylcellulose calcium, and magnesium stearate. Ferric oxide (reddish brown) is added to the 8-mg, 16-mg, and 32-mg tablets as a colorant.

* Registered Trademark of Astra AB
COPYRIGHT © ASTRA Pharmaceuticals, L.P. 1998
All rights reserved

CLINICAL PHARMACOLOGY

Mechanism of Action
Angiotensin II is formed from angiotensin I in a reaction catalyzed by angiotensin converting enzyme (ACE, kininase II). Angiotensin II is the principal pressor agent of the renin-angiotensin system, with effects that include vasoconstriction, stimulation of synthesis and release of aldosterone, cardiac stimulation, and renal reabsorption of sodium. Candesartan blocks the vasoconstrictor and aldosterone-secreting effects of angiotensin II by selectively blocking the binding of angiotensin II to the AT_1 receptor in many tissues, such as vascular smooth muscle and the adrenal gland. Its action is, therefore, independent of the pathways for angiotensin II synthesis.
There is also an AT_2 receptor found in many tissues, but AT_2 is not known to be associated with cardiovascular homeostasis. Candesartan has much greater affinity (>10,000-fold) for the AT_1 receptor than for the AT_2 receptor.
Blockade of the renin-angiotensin system with ACE inhibitors, which inhibit the biosynthesis of angiotensin II from angiotensin I, is widely used in the treatment of hypertension. ACE inhibitors also inhibit the degradation of bradykinin, a reaction also catalyzed by ACE. Because candesartan does not inhibit ACE (kininase II), it does not affect the response to bradykinin. Whether this difference has clinical relevance is not yet known. Candesartan does not bind to or block other hormone receptors or ion channels known to be important in cardiovascular regulation.
Blockage of the angiotensin II receptor inhibits the negative regulatory feedback of angiotensin II on renin secretion, but the resulting increased plasma renin activity and angiotensin II circulating levels do not overcome the effect of candesartan on blood pressure.
Pharmacokinetics
General
Candesartan cilexetil is rapidly and completely bioactivated by ester hydrolysis during absorption from the gastrointestinal tract to candesartan, a selective AT_1 subtype angiotensin II receptor antagonist. Candesartan is mainly excreted unchanged in urine and feces (via bile). It undergoes minor hepatic metabolism by O-deethylation to an inactive metabolite. The elimination half-life of candesartan is approximately 9 hours. After single and repeated administration, the pharmacokinetics of candesartan are linear for oral doses up to 32 mg of candesartan cilexetil. Candesartan and its inactive metabolite do not accumulate in serum upon repeated once daily dosing.
Following administration of candesartan cilexetil, the absolute bioavailability of candesartan was estimated to be 15%. After tablet ingestion, the peak serum concentration (C_{max}) is reached after 3–4 hours. Food with a high-fat content does not affect the bioavailability of candesartan after candesartan cilexetil administration.
Metabolism and Excretion
Total plasma clearance of candesartan is 0.37 mL/min/kg, with a renal clearance of 0.19 mL/min/kg. When candesartan is administered orally, about 26% of the dose is excreted unchanged in urine. Following an oral dose of ^{14}C-labeled candesartan cilexetil, approximately 33% of radioactivity is recovered in urine and approximately 67% in feces. Following an intravenous dose of ^{14}C-labeled candesartan, approximately 59% of radioactivity is recovered in urine and approximately 36% in feces. Biliary excretion contributes to the elimination of candesartan.
Distribution
The volume of distribution of candesartan is 0.13 L/kg. Candesartan is highly bound to plasma proteins (>99%) and does not penetrate red blood cells. The protein binding is constant at candesartan plasma concentrations well above the range achieved with recommended doses. In rats, it has been demonstrated that candesartan crosses the blood-brain barrier poorly, if at all. It has also been demonstrated in rats that candesartan passes across the placental barrier and is distributed in the fetus.
Special Populations
Pediatric: The pharmacokinetics of candesartan cilexetil have not been investigated in patients <18 years of age.
Geriatric and Gender: The pharmacokinetics of candesartan have been studied in the elderly (≥65 years) and in both sexes. The plasma concentration of candesartan was higher in the elderly (C_{max} was approximately 50% higher, and AUC was approximately 80% higher) compared to younger subjects administered the same dose. The pharmacokinetics of candesartan were linear in the elderly, and candesartan and its inactive metabolite did not accumulate in the serum of these subjects upon repeated, once-daily administration. No initial dosage adjustment is necessary. (See DOSAGE AND ADMINISTRATION.) There is no difference in the pharmacokinetics of candesartan between male and female subjects.
Renal Insufficiency: In hypertensive patients with renal insufficiency, serum concentrations of candesartan were elevated. After repeated dosing, the AUC and C_{max} were approximately doubled in patients with severe renal impairment (creatinine clearance <30 mL/min/1.73m^2) compared to patients with normal kidney function. The pharmacokinetics of candesartan in hypertensive patients undergoing hemodialysis are similar to those in hypertensive patients with severe renal impairment. Candesartan cannot be removed by hemodialysis. No initial dosage adjustment is necessary in patients with renal insufficiency. (See DOSAGE AND ADMINISTRATION.)
Hepatic Insufficiency: No differences in the pharmacokinetics of candesartan were observed in patients with mild to moderate chronic liver disease. The pharmacokinetics after candesartan cilexetil administration have not been investigated in patients with severe hepatic insufficiency. No initial dosage adjustment is necessary in patients with mild hepatic disease. (See DOSAGE AND ADMINISTRATION.)
Drug Interactions: *(See* **PRECAUTIONS**, *Drug Interactions.)*
Pharmacodynamics
Candesartan inhibits the pressor effects of angiotensin II infusion in a dose-dependent manner. After one week of once-daily dosing of 8-mg candesartan cilexetil, the pressor effect was inhibited by approximately 90% at peak with approximately 50% inhibition persisting for 24 hours.

Plasma concentrations of angiotensin I, angiotensin II and plasma renin activity (PRA), increased in a dose-dependent manner after single and repeated administration of candesartan cilexetil to healthy subjects and hypertensive patients. ACE activity was not altered in healthy subjects after repeated candesartan cilexetil administration. The once-daily administration of up to 16 mg of candesartan cilexetil the healthy subjects did not influence plasma aldosterone concentrations, but a decrease in the plasma concentration of aldosterone was observed when 32 mg of candesartan cilexetil was administered to hypertensive patients. In spite of the effect of candesartan cilexetil on aldosterone secretion, very little effect on serum potassium was observed.

In multiple-dose studies with hypertensive patients, there were no clinically significant changes in metabolic function including serum levels of cholesterol, triglycerides, glucose, or uric acid. In a 12-week study of 161 patients with non-insulin-dependent (type II) diabetes mellitus and hypertension, there was no change in the level of HbA$_{1c}$.

Clinical Trials

The antihypertensive effects of ATACAND were examined in 14 placebo-controlled trials of 4- to 12-weeks duration, primarily at daily doses of 2 to 32 mg per day in patients with baseline diastolic blood pressures of 95–114 mmHg. Most of the trials were of candesartan cilexetil as a single agent, but it was also studied as add-on to hydrochlorothiazide and amlodipine. These studies included a total of 2350 patients randomized to one of several doses of candesartan cilexetil and 1027 to placebo. Except for a study in diabetics, all studies showed significant effects, generally dose related, of 2–32 mg on trough (24 hour) systolic and diastolic pressures compared to placebo, with doses of 8–32 mg giving effects of about 8–12/4–8 mmHg. There were no exaggerated first dose effects in these patients. Most of the antihypertensive effect was seen within 2 weeks of initial dosing, and the full effect in 4 weeks. With once-daily dosing, blood pressure effect was maintained over 24 hours, with trough to peak ratios of blood pressure effect generally over 80%. Candesartan cilexetil had an additional blood pressure lowering effect when added to hydrochlorothiazide.

The antihypertensive effect was similar in men and women and in patients older and younger than 65. Candesartan was effective in reducing blood pressure regardless of race, although the effect was somewhat less in blacks (usually a low-renin population). This has been generally true for angiotensin II antagonists and ACE inhibitors.

In long-term studies of up to 1 year, the antihypertensive effectiveness of candesartan cilexetil was maintained, and there was no rebound after abrupt withdrawal.

There were no changes in the heart rate of patients treated with candesartan cilexetil in controlled trials.

INDICATIONS AND USAGE

ATACAND is indicated for the treatment of hypertension. It may be used alone or in combination with other antihypertensive agents.

CONTRAINDICATIONS

ATACAND is contraindicated in patients who are hypersensitive to any component of this product.

WARNINGS

Fetal/Neonatal Morbidity and Mortality

Drugs that act directly on the renin-angiotensin system can cause fetal and neonatal morbidity and death when administered to pregnant women. Several dozen cases have been reported in the world literature in patients who were taking angiotensin converting enzyme inhibitors. When pregnancy is detected, ATACAND should be discontinued as soon as possible.

The use of drugs that act directly on the renin-angiotensin system during the second and third trimesters of pregnancy has been associated with fetal and neonatal injury, including hypotension, neonatal skull hypoplasia, anuria, reversible or irreversible renal failure, and death. Oligohydramnios has also been reported, presumably resulting from decreased fetal function; oligohydramnios in this setting has been associated with fetal limb contractures, craniofacial deformation, and hypoplastic lung development. Prematurity, intrauterine growth retardation, and patent ductus arteriosus have also been reported, although it is not clear whether these occurrences were due to exposure to the drug.

These adverse effects do not appear to have resulted from intrauterine drug exposure that has been limited to the first trimester. Mothers whose embryos and fetuses are exposed to an angiotensin II receptor antagonist only during the first trimester should be so informed. Nonetheless, when patients become pregnant, physicians should have the patient discontinue the use of ATACAND as soon as possible. Rarely (probably less often than once in every thousand pregnancies), no alternative to a drug acting on the renin-angiotensin system will be found. In these rare cases, the mothers should be apprised of the potential hazards to their fetuses, and serial ultrasound examinations should be performed to assess the intra-amniotic environment.

If oligohydramnios is observed, ATACAND should be discontinued unless it is considered life-saving for the mother. Contraction stress testing (CST), a nonstress test (NST), or biophysical profiling (BPP) may be appropriate, depending upon the week of pregnancy. Patients and physicians should be aware, however, that oligohydramnios may not appear until after the fetus has sustained irreversible injury.

Infants with histories of in utero exposure to an angiotensin II receptor antagonist should be closely observed for hypotension, oliguria, and hyperkalemia. If oliguria occurs, attention should be directed toward support of blood pressure and renal perfusion. Exchange transfusion or dialysis may be required as means of reversing hypotension and/or substituting for disordered renal function.

There is no clinical experience with the use of ATACAND in pregnant women. Oral doses $\geq$ 10-mg candesartan cilexetil/kg/day administered to pregnant rats during late gestation and continued through lactation were associated with reduced survival and an increased incidence of hydronephrosis in the offspring. The 10-mg/kg/day dose in rats is approximately 2.8 times the maximum recommended daily human dose (MRHD) of 32 mg on a mg/m^2 basis (comparison assumes human body weight of 50 kg). Candesartan cilexetil given to pregnant rabbits at an oral dose of 3 mg/kg/day (approximately 1.7 times the MRHD on a mg/m^2 basis) caused maternal toxicity (decreased body weight and death) but, in surviving dams, had no adverse effects on fetal survival, fetal weight or on external, visceral or skeletal development. No maternal toxicity or adverse effects on fetal development were observed when oral doses up to 1000-mg candesartan cilexetil/kg/day (approximately 138 times the MRHD on a mg/m^2 basis) were administered to pregnant mice.

Hypotension in Volume- and Salt-Depleted Patients

In patients with an activated renin-angiotensin system, such as volume- and/or salt-depleted patients (e.g., those being treated with diuretics), symptomatic hypotension may occur. These conditions should be corrected prior to administration of ATACAND, or the treatment should start under close medical supervision (see DOSAGE AND ADMINISTRATION).

If hypotension occurs, the patients should be placed in the supine position and, if necessary, given an intravenous infusion of normal saline. A transient hypotensive response is not a contraindication to further treatment which usually can be continued without difficulty once the blood pressure has stabilized.

PRECAUTIONS

General

Impaired Renal Function: As a consequence of inhibiting the renin-angiotensin-aldosterone system, changes in renal function may be anticipated in susceptible individuals treated with ATACAND. In patients whose renal function may depend upon the activity of the renin-angiotensin-aldosterone system (e.g. patients with severe congestive heart failure), treatment with angiotensin converting enzyme inhibitors and angiotensin receptor antagonists has been associated with oliguria and/or progressive azotemia and (rarely) with acute renal failure and/or death. Similar results may be anticipated in patients treated with ATACAND. (See CLINICAL PHARMACOLOGY, Special Populations.)

In studies of ACE inhibitors in patients with unilateral or bilateral renal artery stenosis, increases in serum creatinine or blood urea nitrogen (BUN) have been reported. There has been no long-term use of ATACAND in patients with unilateral or bilateral renal artery stenosis, but similar results may be expected.

Information for Patients

Pregnancy: Female patients of childbearing age should be told about the consequences of second and third trimester exposure to drugs that act on the renin-angiotensin system, and they should also be told that these consequences do not appear to have resulted from intrauterine drug exposure that has been limited to the first trimester. These patients should be asked to report pregnancies to their physicians as soon as possible.

Drug Interactions

No significant drug interactions have been reported in studies of candesartan cilexetil given with other drugs such as glyburide, nifedipine, digoxin, warfarin, hydrochlorothiazide and oral contraceptives in healthy volunteers. Because candesartan is not metabolized by the cytochrome P450 system and has no effects on P450 enzymes, interactions with drugs that inhibit, or are metabolized by, those enzymes would not be expected.

Carcinogenesis, Mutagenesis, Impairment of Fertility

There was no evidence of carcinogenicity when candesartan cilexetil was orally administered to mice and rats for up to 104 weeks at doses up to 300 and 1000 mg/kg/day, respectively. Rats received the drug by gavage; whereas, mice received the drug by dietary administration. These (maximal-ly-tolerated) doses of candesartan cilexetil provided systemic exposures to candesartan (AUCs) that were, in mice, approximately 7 times and, in rats, more than 70 times the exposure in man at the maximum recommended daily human dose (32 mg).

Candesartan cilexetil was not genotoxic in the microbial mutagenesis and mammalian cell mutagenesis assays and in the in vivo chromosomal aberration and rat unscheduled DNA synthesis assays. In addition, candesartan was not genotoxic in the microbial mutagenesis, mammalian cell mutagenesis, and in vitro and in vivo chromosome aberration assays.

Fertility and reproductive performance were not affected in studies with male and female rats given oral doses of up to 300 mg/kg/day (83-times the maximum daily human dose of 32 mg on a body surface area basis).

Pregnancy

Pregnancy Categories C (first trimester) and D (second and third trimesters). See WARNINGS, Fetal/Neonatal Morbidity and Mortality.

Nursing Mothers

It is not known whether candesartan is excreted in human milk, but candesartan has been shown to be present in rat milk. Because of the potential for adverse effects on the nursing infant, a decision should be made whether to discontinue nursing or discontinue the drug, taking into account the importance of the drug to the mother.

Pediatric Use

Safety and effectiveness in pediatric patients have not been established.

Geriatric Use

Of the total number of subjects in clinical studies of ATACAND, 21% were 65 and over, while 3% were 75 and over. No overall differences in safety or effectiveness were observed between these subjects and younger subjects, and other reported clinical experience has not identified differences in responses between the elderly and younger patients, but greater sensitivity of some older individuals cannot be ruled out. In a placebo-controlled trial of about 200 elderly hypertensive patients (ages 65 to 87 years), administration of candesartan cilexetil was well tolerated and lowered blood pressure by about 12/6 mmHg more than placebo.

ADVERSE REACTIONS

ATACAND has been evaluated for safety in more than 3600 patients/subjects, including more than 3200 patients treated for hypertension. About 600 of these patients were studied for at least 6 months and about 200 for more than at least 1 year. In general, treatment with ATACAND was well-tolerated. The overall incidence of adverse events reported with ATACAND was similar to placebo.

The rate of withdrawals due to adverse events in all trials in patients (7510 total) was 3.3% (i.e., 108 of 3260) of patients treated with candesartan cilexetil as monotherapy and 3.5% (i.e., 39 of 1106) of patients treated with placebo. In placebo controlled trials, discontinuation of therapy due to clinical adverse events occurred in 2.4% (i.e., 57 of 2350) of patients treated with ATACAND and 3.4% (i.e., 35 of 1027) of patients treated with placebo.

The most common reasons for discontinuation of therapy with ATACAND were headache (0.6%) and dizziness (0.3%). The adverse events that occurred in placebo-controlled clinical trials in at least 1% of patients treated with ATACAND and at a higher incidence in candesartan cilexetil (n=2350) than placebo (n=1027) patients included back pain (3% vs. 2%), dizziness (4% vs. 3%), upper respiratory tract infection (6% vs. 4%), pharyngitis (2% vs. 1%), and rhinitis (2% vs. 1%).

The following adverse experiences occurred in placebo-controlled clinical trials at a more than 1% rate but at about the same or greater incidence in patients receiving placebo compared to candesartan cilexetil: fatigue, peripheral edema, chest pain, headache, bronchitis, coughing, sinusitis, nausea, abdominal pain, diarrhea, vomiting, arthralgia, albuminuria.

Other potentially important adverse events that have been reported, whether or not attributed to treatment, with an incidence of 0.5% or greater from the more than 3200 patients worldwide treated with ATACAND are listed below. It cannot be determined whether these events were causally related to ATACAND. **Body as a Whole:** asthenia, fever; **Central and Peripheral Nervous System:** paraesthesia, vertigo; **Gastrointestinal System Disorder:** dyspepsia, gastroenteritis; **Heart Rate and Rhythm Disorders:** tachycardia, palpitation; **Metabolic and Nutritional Disorders:** creatine phosphokinase increased, hyperglycemia, hypertriglyceridemia, hyperuricemia; **Musculoskeletal System Disorders:** myalgia; **Platelet/Bleeding Clotting Disorders:** epistaxis; **Psychiatric Disorders:** anxiety, depression, somnolence; **Respiratory System Disorders:** dyspnea; **Skin and Appendages Disorders:** rash, sweating increased; **Urinary System Disorders:** hematuria.

Continued on next page

Atacand—Cont.

Other reported events seen less frequently included angina pectoris, myocardial infarction, and angioedema.

Adverse events occurred at about the same rates in men and women, older and younger patients, and black and nonblack patients.

Laboratory Test Findings

In controlled clinical trials, clinically important changes in standard laboratory parameters were rarely associated with the administration of ATACAND.

Creatinine, Blood Urea Nitrogen: Minor increases in blood urea nitrogen (BUN) and serum creatinine were observed infrequently.

Hyperuricemia: Hyperuricemia was rarely found (19 or 0.6% of 3260 patients treated with candesartan cilexetil and 5 or 0.5% of 1106 patients treated with placebo).

Hemoglobin and Hematocrit: Small decreases in hemoglobin and hematocrit (mean decreases of approximately 0.2 grams/dL and 0.5 volume percent, respectively), were observed in patients treated with ATACAND alone but were rarely of clinical importance. Anemia, leukopenia and thrombocytopenia were associated with withdrawal of one patient each from clinical trials.

Potassium: A small increase (mean increase of 0.1 mEq/L) was observed in patients treated with ATACAND alone but was rarely of clinical importance. One patient from a congestive heart failure trial was withdrawn for hyperkalemia (serum potassium = 7.5 mEq/L). This patient was also receiving spironolactone.

Liver Function Tests: Elevations of liver enzymes and/or serum bilirubin were observed infrequently. Five patients assigned to candesartan cilexetil in clinical trials were withdrawn because of abnormal liver chemistries. All had elevated transaminases. Two had mildly elevated total bilirubin, but one on these patients was diagnosed with Hepatitis A.

OVERDOSAGE

No lethality was observed in acute toxicity studies in mice, rats, and dogs given single oral doses of up to 2000 mg/kg of candesartan cilexetil. In mice given single oral doses of the primary metabolite, candesartan, the minimum lethal dose was greater than 1000 mg/kg but less than 2000 mg/kg.

Limited data are available in regard to overdosage in humans. In one recorded case of an intentional overdose, a 43 year old female patient (Body Mass Index of 31 kg/m²) ingested an estimated 160 mg of candesartan cilexetil, in conjunction with multiple other pharmaceutical agents (ibuprofen, naproxen sodium, diphenhydramine hydrochloride, and ketoprofen). Gastric lavage was performed; the patient was monitored in hospital for several days and was discharged without sequelae.

Candesartan cannot be removed by hemodialysis.

Treatment: To obtain up-to-date information about the treatment of overdosage, consult your Regional Poison-Control Center. Telephone numbers of certified poison-control centers are listed in the *Physicians' Desk Reference (PDR)*. In managing overdose, consider the possibilities of multiple-drug overdoses, drug-drug interactions, and altered pharmacokinetics in your patient.

The most likely manifestation of overdosage with ATACAND would be hypotension, dizziness, and, tachycardia; bradycardia could occur from parasympathetic (vagal) stimulation. If symptomatic hypotension should occur, supportive treatement should be instituted.

DOSAGE AND ADMINISTRATION

Dosage must be individualized. Blood pressure response is dose related over the range of 2–32 mg. The usual recommended starting dose of ATACAND is 16 mg once daily when it is used as monotherapy in patients who are not volume depleted. ATACAND can be administered once or twice daily with total daily doses ranging from 8 mg to 32 mg. Larger doses do not appear to have a greater effect, and there is relatively little experience with such doses. Most of the antihypertensive effect is present within 2 weeks, and maximal blood pressure reduction is generally obtained within 4 to 6 weeks of ATACAND treatment.

No initial dosage adjustment is necessary for elderly patients, for patients with mildly impaired renal function, or for patients with mildly impaired hepatic function (see CLINICAL PHARMACOLOGY, *Special Populations*). For patients with possible depletion of intravascular volume (e.g., patients treated with diuretics, particularly those with impaired renal function), ATACAND should be initiated under close medical supervision and consideration should be given to administration of a lower dose (see WARNINGS, *Hypotension in Volume- and Salt-Depleted Patients*).

ATACAND may be administered with or without food.

If blood pressure is not controlled by ATACAND alone, a diuretic may be added. ATACAND may be administered with other antihypertensive agents.

HOW SUPPLIED

No. 3782—Tablets ATACAND, 4 mg, are white to off-white, circular/biconvex shaped, non–film-coated tablets, coded ACF on one side and 004 on the other. They are supplied as follows:
NDC 61113-004-31 unit of use bottles of 30
No. 3780—Tablets ATACAND, 8 mg, are light pink, circular/biconvex shaped, non–film-coated tablets, coded ACG on one side and 008 on the other. They are supplied as follows:
NDC 61113-008-31 unit of use bottles of 30
No. 3781—Tablets ATACAND, 16 mg, are pink, circular/biconvex shaped, non–film-coated tablets, coded ACH on one side and 016 on the other. They are supplied as follows:
NDC 61113-016-31 unit of use bottles of 30
NDC 61113-016-28 unit dose of packages of 100
No. 3791—Tablets ATACAND, 32 mg, are pink, circular/biconvex shaped, non–film-coated tablets, coded ACL on one side and 032 on the other. They are supplied as follows:
NDC 61113-032-31 unit of use bottles of 30
NDC 61113-032-28 unit dose of packages of 100

Storage

Store at 25°C (77°F); excursions permitted to 15–30°C (59–86°F) [see USP Controlled Room Temperature]. Keep container tightly closed.

Distributed by:
Astra Pharmaceuticals, L.P.
Wayne, PA 19087, USA
Packaged by:
Merck & Co., Inc., West Point, PA 19486, USA
Manufactured under the license from Takeda Chemical Industries, Ltd.
by: Astra AB, S-151 85 Södertälje, Sweden.
Issued June 1998   9119501

Shown in Product Identification Guide, page 304

ATROPINE SULFATE INJECTION, USP   ℞

[ā 'trow-peen]
0.1 mg/mL
Adult Strength

(For details of indications, dosage and administration, precautions, and adverse reactions, see circular in package.)

HOW SUPPLIED

Prefilled Syringes:
5 mL (0.5 mg) NDC 0186-0648-01
with a 21 G 15/16″ Needle
10 mL (1 mg) NDC 0186-0649-01
with a 21 G 15/16″ Needle
Solution should be stored at controlled room temperature 15°–30°C (59°–86°F).
Caution: Federal law prohibits dispensing without prescription.
021880R04   Rev. 9/95

BRETYLIUM TOSYLATE INJECTION   ℞

For Intramuscular or Intravenous Use.

(For details of indications, dosage and administration, precautions, and adverse reactions, see circular in package.)

HOW SUPPLIED

NDC 0186-1131-04, 10 mL single dose vial, box of 1
NDC 0186-0663-01, 10 mL syringe, 21 G 15/16″ Needle, box of 1
Each unit contains 500 mg bretylium tosylate in Water for Injection, USP. The pH is adjusted when necessary, with hydrochloric acid and/or sodium hydroxide. Sterile, non-pyrogenic.
021810R05   Rev. 1/97

CALCITONIN-SALMON INJECTION, SYNTHETIC   ℞

DESCRIPTION

Calcitonin is a polypeptide hormone secreted by the parafollicular cells of the thyroid gland in mammals and by the ultimobranchial gland of birds and fish.

Calcitonin-salmon injection, synthetic is a synthetic polypeptide of 32 amino acids in the same linear sequence that is found in calcitonin of salmon origin. This is shown by the following graphic formula:

```
H—Cys—Ser—Asn—Leu—Ser—Thr—Cys Val—Leu—Gly—Lys—Leu—Ser—Gln—Glu—Leu—
    1    2    3    4    5    6    7    8    9   10   11   12   13   14   15   16

His—Lys—Leu—Gln—Thr—Tyr—Pro—Arg—Thr—Asn—Thr—Gly—Ser—Gly—Thr—Pro—NH₂
 17   18   19   20   21   22   23   24   25   26   27   28   29   30   31   32
```

It is provided in sterile solution for subcutaneous or intramuscular injection. Each milliliter contains 200 I.U. calcitonin-salmon; 5 mg phenol (as preservative); with sodium chloride, sodium acetate, glacial acetic acid, and sodium hydroxide to adjust tonicity and pH between 3.9 and 4.5. Filled under nitrogen.

The activity of calcitonin-salmon is stated in International Units based on bioassay in comparison with the International Reference Preparation of calcitonin-salmon for Bioassay, distributed by the National Institute for Biological Standards and Control, Holly Hill, London.

HOW SUPPLIED

Calcitonin-salmon injection, synthetic is available as:
NDC 0186-1608-13; 2 mL multiple dose vial containing 200 I.U. per mL, Box of 1
Store in refrigerator, between 2°-8°C (36°-46°F).
Caution: Federal law prohibits dispensing without prescription.
021713R02   Rev. 2/97

10% CALCIUM CHLORIDE   ℞

[cal 'cium chlor 'ide]
Injection, USP
1 gram (100 mg/mL)
27.3 mg (1.4 mEq) Ca⁺⁺/mL
2.04 mOsm/mL (calc.)
A HYPERTONIC SOLUTION FOR INTRAVENOUS INJECTION

Caution: This solution must not be injected intramuscularly or subcutaneously.

(For details of indications, dosage and administration, precautions, and adverse reactions, see circular in package.)

HOW SUPPLIED

10% Calcium Chloride Injection, USP is supplied as follows:
NDC 0186-1166-04 10 mL single dose vials in packages of 25
NDC 0186-0651-01 10 mL prefilled syringes with 21 G 15/16″ Needle
The solution should be stored at controlled room temperature 15°–30°C (59°–86°F).
021710R04   Rev. 7/96

COCAINE HYDROCHLORIDE   Ⓒ
Topical Solution

DESCRIPTION

Each mL contains 40 mg or 100 mg cocaine HCl (Warning: May be habit forming), benzoic acid, citric acid, FD&C green #3 dye, D&C yellow #10 dye. An aqueous solution.

NOT FOR INJECTION OR OPHTHALMIC USE

NOTE (for Glass Bottle): Do not steam autoclave.
Cocaine Hydrochloride USP is a crystalline, granular, or powder substance having a saline, slightly bitter taste that numbs tongue and lips. Cocaine Hydrochloride is a local anesthetic.

CLINICAL PHARMACOLOGY

Cocaine blocks the initiation or conduction of the nerve impulse following local application, thereby effecting local anesthetic action.

Cocaine is absorbed from all sites of application, including mucous membranes and the gastrointestinal mucosa. Cocaine is degraded by plasma esterases, with the half-life in the plasma being approximately one hour.

INDICATIONS AND USAGE

Cocaine Hydrochloride Topical Solution is indicated for the introduction of local (topical) anesthesia of accessible mucous membranes of the oral, laryngeal and nasal cavities.

CONTRAINDICATIONS

Cocaine Hydrochloride is contraindicated in patients with a known history of hypersensitivity to the drug or to the components of the topical solution.

WARNINGS

RESUSCITATIVE EQUIPMENT AND DRUGS SHOULD BE IMMEDIATELY AVAILABLE WHEN ANY LOCAL ANESTHETIC IS USED.

Carcinogenesis, Mutagenesis: Long-term studies to determine the carcinogenic and mutagenic potential of cocaine are not available.

Pregnancy: Teratogenic Effects —*Pregnancy Category C:* Animal reproduction studies have not been conducted with cocaine. It is also not known whether cocaine can cause fetal harm when administered to a pregnant woman or can affect reproduction capacity. Cocaine should be given to a pregnant woman only if needed.

PRECAUTIONS

The safety and effectiveness of Cocaine Hydrochloride Topical Solution depends on proper dosage, correct technique, adequate precautions, and readiness for emergencies. Standard textbooks should be consulted for specific techniques and precautions for various anesthetic procedures.

The lowest dosage that results in effective anesthesia should be used to avoid high plasma levels and serious adverse effects. Debilitated, elderly patients, acutely ill patients, and children should be given reduced doses commensurate with their age and physical status.

Cocaine Hydrochloride Topical Solution should be used with caution in patients with severely traumatized mucosa and sepsis in the region of the proposed application. Use with caution in persons with known drug sensitivities.

ADVERSE REACTIONS

Adverse reactions may be due to high plasma levels as a result of excessive and rapid absorption of the drug. Reactions are systemic in nature and involve the central nervous system and/or the cardiovascular system. A small number of reactions may result from hypersensitivity, idiosyncrasy or diminished tolerance on the part of the patient.

CNS reactions are excitatory and/or depressant and may be characterized by nervousness, restlessness and excitement. Tremors and eventually clonicotonic convulsions may result. Emesis may occur. Central stimulation is followed by depression, with death resulting from respiratory failure.

Small doses of cocaine slow the heart rate, but after moderate doses, the rate is increased due to central sympathetic stimulation.

Cocaine is pyrogenic, augmenting heat production in stimulating muscular activity and causing vasoconstriction which decreases heat loss. Cocaine is known to interfere with the uptake of norepinephrine by adrenergic nerve terminals, producing sensitization to catecholamines, causing vasoconstriction and mydriasis.

Cocaine causes sloughing of the corneal epithelium, causing clouding, pitting, and occasionally ulceration of the cornea. The drug is not meant for ophthalmic use.

OVERDOSAGE

The fatal dose of cocaine has been approximated at 1.2 g, although severe toxic effects have been reported from doses as low as 20 mg.

Symptoms: The symptoms of cocaine poisoning are referable to the CNS, namely the patient becomes excited, restless, garrulous, anxious and confused. Enhanced reflexes, headache, rapid pulse, irregular respiration, chills, rise in body temperature, mydriasis, exophthalmos, nausea, vomiting and abdominal pain are noticed. In severe overdoses, delirium, Cheyne-Stokes respiration, convulsions, unconsciousness, and death from respiratory arrest result. Acute poisoning by cocaine is rapid in developing.

Treatment: The specific treatment of acute cocaine poisoning is the intravenous administration of a short-acting barbiturate or diazepam. Artificial respiration may be necessary. It is important to limit absorption of the drug. If entrance of the drug into circulation can be checked, and respiratory exchange maintained, the prognosis is favorable since cocaine is eliminated fairly rapidly.

DOSAGE AND ADMINISTRATION

The dosage varies and depends upon the area to be anesthetized, vascularity of the tissues, individual tolerance, and the technique of anesthesia. The lowest dosage needed to provide effective anesthesia should be administered. Dosages should be reduced for children and for elderly and debilitated patients. Cocaine Hydrochloride Topical Solution can be administered by means of cotton applicators or packs, instilled into a cavity, or as a spray.

HOW SUPPLIED

4% Cocaine Hydrochloride Topical Solution

NDC 0186-1790-78	4 mL Bottle Box of 1
NDC 0186-1791-13	10 mL Multiple Dose Bottle Box of 1

10% Cocaine Hydrochloride Topical Solution

NDC 0186-1792-78	4 mL Bottle Box of 1
NDC 0186-1793-13	10 mL Multiple Dose Bottle Box of 1

Store at controlled room temperature 15°–30°C (59°–86°F).

Caution: Federal law prohibits dispensing without prescription.

021661R04 Rev. 1/97

50% DEXTROSE Injection, USP ℞

[dex 'trose]

Concentrated Dextrose
For Intravenous Administration

NOTE: This solution is hypertonic—see WARNINGS and PRECAUTIONS

(For details of indications, dosage and administration, precautions, and adverse reactions, see circular in package.)

HOW SUPPLIED

50% Dextrose Injection, USP is supplied as follows:
50 mL Prefilled Syringe with 19 G $^{15}/_{16}''$ needle, NDC 0186-0654-01

The solution should be stored at controlled room temperature 15°–30°C (59°–86°F).

021857R07 Rev. 7/96

DOBUTAMINE INJECTION, USP ℞

[dō-bū-tă-mən]

(For details of indications, dosage and administration, precautions, and adverse reactions, see circular in package.)

DESCRIPTION

Dobutamine Injection, USP is 1,2-benzenediol, 4-[2-[[3-(4-hydroxyphenyl)-1-methylpropyl]amino]ethyl]-, hydrochloride, (±)-. It is a synthetic catecholamine.

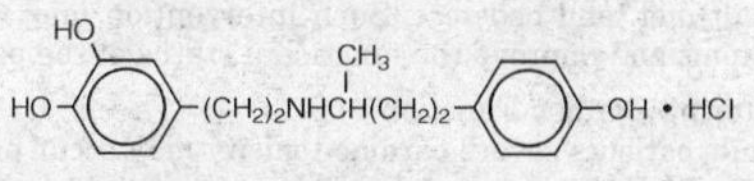

Molecular Formula: $C_{18}H_{23}NO_3 \cdot HCl$
Molecular Weight: 337.85

The clinical formulation is supplied in a sterile form for intravenous use only. Each mL contains 12.5 mg (41.5 μmol) dobutamine, 0.24 mg sodium metabisulfite (added during manufacture), and water for injection, q.s. Hydrochloric acid and/or sodium hydroxide may have been added during manufacture to adjust the pH.

HOW SUPPLIED

NDC 0186-1931-01, 20 mL single dose vial containing 250 mg dobutamine (as the hydrochloride), box of 1.

Store at controlled room temperature, 15° to 30°C (59° to 86°F).

021648R05 Rev. 4/98

DOPAMINE HYDROCHLORIDE Injection, USP ℞

[dó-pa-mean]

(For details of indications, dosage and administration, precautions, and adverse reactions, see circular in package.)

HOW SUPPLIED

Dopamine HCl 200 mg is supplied in the following form:
Additive Syringe 5 mL (40 mg/mL) NDC 0186-0638-01
Dopamine HCl 400 mg is supplied in the following forms:
Additive Syringe 5 mL (80 mg/mL) NDC 0186-0641-01
10 mL (40 mg/mL) NDC 0186-0639-01
Dopamine HCl 800 mg is supplied in the following form:
Additive Syringe 5 mL (160 mg/mL) NDC 0186-0642-01

Packages are color coded according to the total dosage content; 200 mg coded blue/white, 400 mg coded green/white and 800 mg coded yellow/white.

Store at controlled room temperature 15°–30°C (59°–86°F). Avoid contact with alkalies (including sodium bicarbonate), oxidizing agents, or iron salts.

NOTE: Do not use the injection if it is darker than slightly yellow or discolored in any other way.

WARNING: NOT FOR DIRECT INTRAVENOUS INJECTION. MUST BE DILUTED BEFORE USE.

Caution: Federal (USA) law prohibits dispensing without prescription.

021861R09 Rev. 11/97

DOXORUBICIN HYDROCHLORIDE INJECTION, USP ℞
DOXORUBICIN HYDROCHLORIDE FOR INJECTION, USP

FOR INTRAVENOUS USE ONLY.

WARNING

1. Severe local tissue necrosis will occur if there is extravasation during administration (see DOSAGE AND ADMINISTRATION). Doxorubicin must not be given by the intramuscular or subcutaneous route.
2. Myocardial toxicity manifested in its most severe form by potentially fatal congestive heart failure may occur either during therapy or months to years after termination of therapy. The probability of developing impaired myocardial function based on a combined index of signs, symptoms and decline in left ventricular ejection fraction (LVEF) is estimated to be 1 to 2% at a total cumulative dose of 300 mg/m^2 of doxorubicin, 3 to 5% at a dose of 400 mg/m^2, 5 to 8% at 450 mg/m^2 and 6 to 20% at 500 mg/m^2. Data on file are available at Pharmacia Adria. The risk of developing CHF increases rapidly with increasing total cumulative doses of doxorubicin in excess of 450 mg/m^2. This toxicity may occur at lower cumulative doses in patients with prior mediastinal irradiation or on concurrent cyclophosphamide therapy or with pre-existing heart disease.
3. Dosage should be reduced in patients with impaired hepatic function.
4. Severe myelosuppression may occur.
5. Doxorubicin should be administered only under the supervision of a physician who is experienced in the use of cancer chemotherapeutic agents.

DESCRIPTION

Doxorubicin is a cytotoxic anthracycline antibiotic isolated from cultures of *Streptomyces peucetius* var. *caesius*.

Doxorubicin consists of a naphthacenequinone nucleus linked through a glycosidic bond at ring atom 7 to an amino sugar, daunosamine.

Chemically, doxorubicin hydrochloride is: 5,12-Naphthacenedione, 10-[(3-amino-2,3,6-trideoxy-α-L-*lyxo*-hexopyranosyl)oxy]-7,8,9,10-tetrahydro-6,8,11-trihydroxy-8-(hydroxylacetyl)-1-methoxy-, hydrochloride (8S-*cis*)-. The structural formula is as follows:

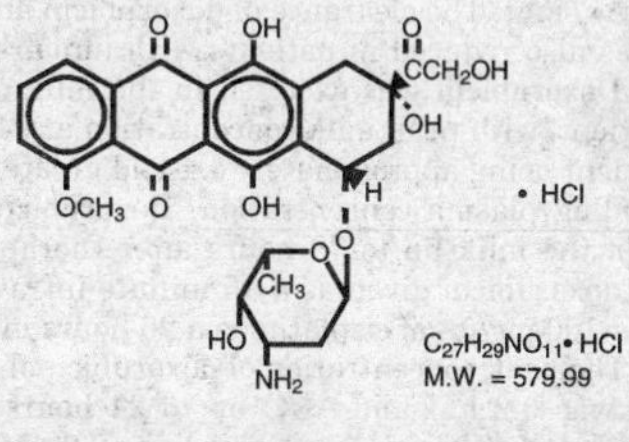
$C_{27}H_{29}NO_{11} \cdot HCl$
M.W. = 579.99

Doxorubicin binds to nucleic acids, presumably by specific intercalation of the planar anthracycline nucleus with the DNA double helix. The anthracycline ring is lipophilic, but the saturated end of the ring system contains abundant hydroxyl groups adjacent to the amino sugar, producing a hydrophilic center. The molecule is amphoteric, containing acidic functions in the ring phenolic groups and a basic function in the sugar amino group. It binds to cell membranes as well as plasma proteins.

Doxorubicin Hydrochloride Injection, USP is a sterile parenteral, isotonic solution for intravenous use only, containing no preservative, available in 10 mg (5 mL), 20 mg (10 mL) and 50 mg (25 mL) single dose vials and 2 mg/mL (100 mL) multidose vials. Each mL contains 2 mg doxorubicin hydrochloride and the following inactive ingredients: sodium chloride 9 mg and water for injection q.s. Hydrochloric acid is used to adjust pH to a target pH of 3.0.

Doxorubicin Hydrochloride for Injection, USP, a sterile red lyophilized powder for intravenous use only, is available in 10 mg, 20 mg and 50 mg single dose vials. Each single dose vial contains 10, 20 or 50 mg doxorubicin hydrochloride and 50 mg, 100 mg or 250 mg lactose monohydrate respectively, as a sterile red lyophilized powder.

CLINICAL PHARMACOLOGY

The cytotoxic effect of doxorubicin on malignant cells and its toxic effects on various organs are thought to be related to nucleotide base intercalation and cell membrane lipid binding activities of doxorubicin. Intercalation inhibits nucleotide replication and action of DNA and RNA polymerases. The interaction of doxorubicin with topoisomerase II to form DNA-cleavable complexes appears to be an important mechanism of doxorubicin cytocidal activity. Doxorubicin cellular membrane binding may effect a variety of cellular functions. Enzymatic electron reduction of doxorubicin by a variety of oxidases, reductases and dehydrogenases generate highly reactive species including the hydroxyl free radical OH•. Free radical formation has been implicated in doxorubicin cardiotoxicity by means of Cu (II) and Fe (III) reduction at the cellular level.

Animal studies have shown activity in a spectrum of experimental tumors, immunosuppression, carcinogenic properties in rodents, induction of a variety of toxic effects, including delayed and progressive cardiac toxicity, myelosuppression in all species and atrophy to testes in rats and dogs.

Pharmacokinetic studies, determined in patients with various types of tumors undergoing either single or multi-agent therapy have shown that doxorubicin follows a multiphasic disposition after intravenous injection. The initial distributive half-life of approximately 5.0 minutes suggests rapid tissue uptake of doxorubicin, while its slow elimination from tissues is reflected by a terminal half-life of 20 to 48 hours. Steady-state distribution volumes exceed 20 to 30 L/kg and are indicative of extensive drug uptake into tissues. Plasma clearance is in the range of 8 to 20 mL/min/kg

Continued on next page

Doxorubicin Hydrochloride—Cont.

and is predominately by metabolism and biliary excretion. Approximately 40% of the dose appears in the bile in 5 days, while only 5 to 12% of the drug and its metabolites appear in the urine during the same time period. Binding of doxorubicin and its major metabolite, doxorubicinol to plasma proteins is about 74 to 76% and is independent of plasma concentration of doxorubicin up to $2 \mu M$. Enzymatic reduction at the 7 position and cleavage of the daunosamine sugar yields aglycones which are accompanied by free radical formation, the local production of which may contribute to the cardiotoxic activity of doxorubicin. Disposition of doxorubicinol (DOX-OL) in patients is formation rate limited. The terminal half-life of DOX-OL is similar to doxorubicin. The relative exposure of DOX-OL, compared to doxorubicin ranges between 0.4 to 0.6. In urine, < 3% of the dose was recovered as DOX-OL over 7 days. The literature contains no information regarding gender related differences in the pharmacokinetics of doxorubicin and doxorubicinol.

In four patients, dose-independent pharmacokinetics have been shown for doxorubicin in the dose range of 30 to 70 mg/m^2. Systemic clearance of doxorubicin is significantly reduced in obese women with ideal body weight greater than 130%. There was a significant reduction in clearance without any change in volume of distribution in obese patients when compared with normal patients with less than 115% ideal body weight. The clearance of doxorubicin and doxorubicinol was also reduced in patients with impaired hepatic function. Doxorubicin was excreted in the milk of one lactating patient, with peak milk concentration at 24 hours after treatment being approximately 4.4-fold greater than the corresponding plasma concentration. Doxorubicin was detectable in the milk up to 72 hours after therapy with 70 mg/m^2 of doxorubicin given as a 15 minute intravenous infusion and 100 mg/m^2 of cisplatin as a 26 hours intravenous infusion. The peak concentration of doxorubicinol in milk at 24 hours was 0.2 μM and AUC up to 24 hours was 16.5 $\mu M.hr$ while the AUC for doxorubicin was 9.9 $\mu M.hr$. Doxorubicin does not cross the blood brain barrier.

INDICATIONS AND USAGE

Injectable doxorubicin hydrochloride has been used successfully to produce regression in disseminated neoplastic conditions such as acute lymphoblastic leukemia, acute myeloblastic leukemia, Wilms' tumor, neuroblastoma, soft tissue and bone sarcomas, breast carcinoma, ovarian carcinoma, transitional cell bladder carcinoma, thyroid carcinoma, gastric carcinoma, Hodgkin's disease, malignant lymphoma and bronchogenic carcinoma in which the small cell histologic type is the most responsive compared to other cell types.

CONTRAINDICATIONS

Doxorubicin therapy should not be started in patients who have marked myelosuppression induced by previous treatment with other antitumor agents or by radiotherapy. Doxorubicin treatment is contraindicated in patients who received previous treatment with complete cumulative doses of doxorubicin, daunorubicin, idarubicin and/or other anthracyclines and anthracenes.

WARNINGS

Special attention must be given to the cardiotoxicity induced by doxorubicin. Irreversible myocardial toxicity, manifested in its most severe form by life-threatening and potentially fatal congestive heart failure, may occur either during therapy or months to years after termination of therapy. The probability of developing impaired myocardial function, based on a combined index of signs, symptoms and decline in left ventricular ejection fraction (LVEF) is estimated to be 1 to 2% at a total cumulative dose of 300 mg/m^2 of doxorubicin, 3 to 5% at a dose of 400 mg/m^2, 5 to 8% at a dose of 450 mg/m^2 and 6 to 20% at a dose of 500 mg/m^2 given in a schedule of a bolus injection once every 3 weeks (data on file at Pharmacia Adria). In a retrospective review by Von Hoff et al, the probability of developing congestive heart failure was reported to be 5/168 (3%) at a cumulative dose of 430 mg/m^2 of doxorubicin, 8/110 (7%) at 575 mg/m^2 and 3/14 (21%) at 728 mg/m^2. The cumulative incidence of CHF was 2.2%. In a prospective study of doxorubicin in combination with cyclophosphamide, fluorouracil and/or vincristine in patients with breast cancer or small cell lung cancer, the cumulative incidence of congestive heart failure was 5 to 6%. The probability of CHF at various cumulative doses of doxorubicin was 1.5% at 300 mg/m^2, 4.9% at 400 mg/m^2, 7.7% at 450 mg/m^2 and 20.5% at 500 mg/m^2.

Cardiotoxicity may occur at lower doses in patients with prior mediastinal irradiation, concurrent cyclophosphamide therapy and advanced age. Data also suggest that pre-existing heart disease is a cofactor for increased risk of doxorubicin cardiotoxicity. In such cases, cardiac toxicity may occur at doses lower than the respective recommended cumulative dose of doxorubicin. Studies have suggested that concomitant administration of doxorubicin and calcium channel entry blockers may increase the risk of doxorubicin

cardiotoxicity. The total dose of doxorubicin administered to the individual patient should also take into account previous or concomitant therapy with related compounds such as daunorubicin, idarubicin and mitoxantrone. Cardiomyopathy and/or congestive heart failure may be encountered several months or years after discontinuation of doxorubicin therapy.

The risk of congestive heart failure and other acute manifestations of doxorubicin cardiotoxicity in children may be as much or lower than in adults. Children appear to be at particular risk for developing delayed cardiac toxicity in that doxorubicin induced cardiomyopathy impairs myocardial growth as children mature, subsequently leading to possible development of congestive heart failure during early adulthood. As many as 40% of children may have subclinical cardiac dysfunction and 5 to 10% of children may develop congestive heart failure on a long term follow-up. This late cardiac toxicity may be related to the dose of doxorubicin. The longer the length of follow-up the greater the increase in the detection rate.

Treatment of doxorubicin induced congestive heart failure includes the use of digitalis, diuretics, after load reducers such as angiotensin I converting enzyme (ACE) inhibitors, low salt diet, and bed rest. Such intervention may relieve symptoms and improve the functional status of the patient.

Monitoring Cardiac Function

In adult patients severe cardiac toxicity may occur precipitously without antecedent ECG changes. Cardiomyopathy induced by anthracyclines is usually associated with very characteristic histopathologic changes on an endomyocardial biopsy (EM biopsy), and a decrease of left ventricular ejection fraction (LVEF), as measured by multi-gated radionuclide angiography (MUGA scans) and/or echocardiogram (ECHO), from pretreatment baseline values. However, it has not been demonstrated that monitoring of the ejection fraction will predict when individual patients are approaching their maximally tolerated cumulative dose of doxorubicin. Cardiac function should be carefully monitored during treatment to minimize the risk of cardiac toxicity. A baseline cardiac evaluation with an ECG, LVEF, and/or an echocardiogram (ECHO) is recommended especially in patients with risk factors for increased cardiac toxicity (pre-existing heart disease, mediastinal irradiation, or concurrent cyclophosphamide therapy). Subsequent evaluations should be obtained at a cumulative dose of doxorubicin of at least 400 mg/m^2 and periodically thereafter during the course of therapy. Children are at increased risk for developing delayed cardiotoxicity following doxorubicin administration and therefore a follow-up cardiac evaluation is recommended periodically to monitor for this delayed cardiotoxicity.

In adults, a 10% decline in LVEF to below the lower limit of normal or an absolute LVEF of 45%, or a 20% decline in LVEF at any level is indicative of deterioration in cardiac function. In children, deterioration in cardiac function during or after the completion of therapy with doxorubicin is indicated by a drop in fractional shortening (FS) by an absolute value of ≥10 percentile units or below 29%, and a decline in LVEF of 10 percentile units or an LVEF below 55%. In general, if test results indicate deterioration in cardiac function associated with doxorubicin, the benefit of continued therapy should be carefully evaluated against the risk of producing irreversible cardiac damage.

Acute life-threatening arrhythmias have been reported to occur during or within a few hours after doxorubicin hydrochloride administration.

There is a high incidence of bone marrow depression, primarily of leukocytes, requiring careful hematologic monitoring. With the recommended dose schedule, leukopenia is usually transient, reaching its nadir at 10 to 14 days after treatment with recovery usually occurring by the 21st day. White blood cell counts as low as 1000/mm^3 are to be expected during treatment with appropriate doses of doxorubicin. Red blood cell and platelet levels should also be monitored since they may also be depressed. Hematologic toxicity may require dose reduction or suspension or delay of doxorubicin therapy. Persistent severe myelosuppression may result in superinfection or hemorrhage.

Doxorubicin may potentiate the toxicity of other anticancer therapies. Exacerbation of cyclophosphamide induced hemorrhagic cystitis and enhancement of the hepatotoxicity of 6-mercaptopurine have been reported. Radiation induced toxicity to the myocardium, mucosae, skin and liver have been reported to be increased by the administration of doxorubicin.

Since metabolism and excretion of doxorubicin occurs predominantly by the hepatobiliary route, toxicity to recommended doses of doxorubicin can be enhanced by hepatic impairment; therefore, prior to the individual dosing, evaluation of hepatic function is recommended using conventional clinical laboratory tests, such as SGOT, SGPT, alkaline phosphatase and bilirubin. (See DOSAGE AND ADMINISTRATION.)

Necrotizing colitis manifested by typhlitis (cecal inflammation), bloody stools and severe and sometimes fatal infections have been associated with a combination of doxorubicin given by i.v. push daily for 3 days and cytarabine given by continuous infusion daily for 7 or more days.

On intravenous administration of doxorubicin, extravasation may occur with or without an accompanying stinging or burning sensation, even if blood returns well on aspiration of the infusion needle (see DOSAGE AND ADMINISTRATION). If any signs or symptoms of extravasation have occurred, the injection or infusion should be immediately terminated and restarted in another vein.

Pregnancy Category D: Safe use of doxorubicin in pregnancy has not been established. Doxorubicin is embryotoxic and teratogenic in rats and embryotoxic and abortifacient in rabbits. There are no adequate and well-controlled studies in pregnant women. If doxorubicin is to be used during pregnancy, or if the patient becomes pregnant during therapy, the patient should be apprised of the potential hazard to the fetus. Women of childbearing age should be advised to avoid becoming pregnant.

PRECAUTIONS

General: Doxorubicin is not an anti-microbial agent.

Information for Patients: Doxorubicin imparts a red coloration to the urine for 1 to 2 days after administration, and patients should be advised to expect this during active therapy.

Drug Interactions: Literature contain the following drug interactions with doxorubicin in humans: cyclosporine (Sandimmune) may induce coma and/or seizures, phenobarbital increases the elimination of doxorubicin, phenytoin levels may be decreased by doxorubicin, streptozocin (Zanosar) may inhibit the hepatic metabolism, and administration of live vaccines to immunosuppressed patients, including those undergoing cytotoxic chemotherapy, may be hazardous. Information on other potential drug interactions may be found in the literature.

Laboratory Tests: Initial treatment with doxorubicin requires observation of the patient and periodic monitoring of complete blood counts, hepatic function test, and radionuclide left ventricular ejection fraction (see WARNINGS section).

Like other cytotoxic drugs, doxorubicin may induce "tumor lysis syndrome" and hyperuricemia in patients with rapidly growing tumors. Appropriate supportive and pharmacologic measures may prevent or alleviate this complication.

Carcinogenesis, Mutagenesis, Impairment of Fertility: Formal long-term carcinogenicity studies have not been conducted with doxorubicin. Doxorubicin and related compounds have been shown to have mutagenic and carcinogenic properties when tested in experimental models (including bacterial systems, mammalian cells in culture, and female Sprague-Dawley rats).

The possible adverse effect on fertility in males and females in humans or experimental animals have not been adequately evaluated. Testicular atrophy was observed in rats and dogs.

A variant of chemotherapy-related acute non-lymphocytic leukemia has been reported to occur infrequently a few years after multiple drug treatment of some neoplasms, which sometimes included doxorubicin. The exact role of doxorubicin has not been elucidated.

Pregnancy Category D: (see WARNINGS section).

Nursing Mothers: Because of the potential for serious adverse reactions in nursing infants from doxorubicin, mothers should be advised to discontinue nursing during doxorubicin therapy.

ADVERSE REACTIONS

Dose limiting toxicities of therapy are myelosuppression and cardiotoxicity. Other reactions reported are:

Cardiotoxicity—(see WARNINGS section).

Cutaneous—Reversible and complete alopecia occurs in most cases. Hyperpigmentation of nailbeds and dermal crease, primarily in children, and onycholysis have been reported in a few cases. Recall of skin reaction due to prior radiotherapy has occurred with doxorubicin administration.

Gastrointestinal—Acute nausea and vomiting occurs frequently and may be severe. This may be alleviated by antiemetic therapy. Mucositis (stomatitis and esophagitis) may occur 5 to 10 days after administration. The effect may be severe leading to ulceration and represents a site of origin for severe infections. The dosage regimen consisting of administration of doxorubicin on three consecutive days results in the greater incidence and severity of mucositis. Ulceration and necrosis of the colon, especially the cecum, may occur leading to bleeding or severe infections which can be fatal. This reaction has been reported in patients with acute non-lymphocytic leukemia treated with a 3-day course of doxorubicin combined with cytarabine. Anorexia and diarrhea have been occasionally reported.

Vascular—Phlebosclerosis has been reported especially when small veins are used or a single vein is used for repeated administration. Facial flushing may occur if the injection is given too rapidly.

Local—Severe cellulitis, vesication and tissue necrosis will occur if extravasation of doxorubicin occurs during administration. Erythematous streaking along the vein proximal to the site of the injection has been reported. (See DOSAGE AND ADMINISTRATION.)

Hematologic—The occurrence of secondary acute myeloid leukemia with or without a preleukemic phase has been reported rarely in patients concurrently treated with doxorubicin in association with DNA-damaging antineoplastic agents. Such cases could have a short (1–3 years) latency period.
Hypersensitivity—Fever, chills and urticaria have been reported occasionally. Anaphylaxis may occur. A case of apparent cross sensitivity to lincomycin has been reported.
Other—Conjunctivitis and lacrimation occur rarely.

OVERDOSAGE

Acute overdosage with doxorubicin enhances the toxic effects of mucositis, leukopenia and thrombocytopenia. Treatment of acute overdosage consists of treatment of the severely myelosuppressed patient with hospitalization, antimicrobials, platelet transfusions and symptomatic treatment of mucositis. Use of hemopoietic growth factor (G-CSF, GM-CSF) may be considered.
The 200 mg vial is packaged as a multiple dose vial and caution should be exercised to prevent inadvertent overdosage.
Cumulative dosage with doxorubicin increases the risk of cardiomyopathy and resultant congestive heart failure (see WARNINGS section). Treatment consists of vigorous management of congestive heart failure with digitalis preparations, diuretics, and after-load reducers such as ACE inhibitors.

DOSAGE AND ADMINISTRATION

Care in the administration of doxorubicin hydrochloride will reduce the chance of perivenous infiltration (see WARNINGS). It may also decrease the chance of local reactions such as urticaria and erythematous streaking. On intravenous administration of doxorubicin, extravasation may occur with or without an accompanying burning or stinging sensation, even if blood returns well on aspiration of the infusion needle. If any signs or symptoms of extravasation have occurred, the injection or infusion should be immediately terminated and restarted in another vein. If extravasation is suspected, intermittent application of ice to the site for 15 min. q.i.d. × 3 days may be useful. The benefit of local administration of drugs has not been clearly established. Because of the progressive nature of extravasation reactions, close observation and plastic surgery consultation is recommended. Blistering, ulceration and/or persistent pain are indications for wide excision surgery, followed by split-thickness skin grafting[1].
The most commonly used dosage schedule is 60 to 75 mg/m^2 as a single intravenous injection administered at 21 day intervals. The lower dose should be given to patients with inadequate marrow reserves due to old age, or prior therapy, or neoplastic marrow infiltration. Doxorubicin has been used concurrently with other approved chemotherapeutic agents. Evidence is available that in some types of neoplastic disease combination chemotherapy is superior to single agents. The benefits and risks of such therapy continue to be elucidated. When used in combination with other chemotherapy drugs, the most commonly used dosage of doxorubicin is 40 to 60 mg/m^2 given as a single intravenous injection every 21 to 28 days. Doxorubicin dosage must be reduced in case of hyperbilirubinemia as follows:

Plasma bilirubin concentration (mg/dL)	Dosage reduction (%)
1.2–3.0	50
3.1–5.0	75

Reconstitution Directions: Doxorubicin Hydrochloride for Injection, 10 mg, 20 mg and 50 mg vials should be reconstituted with 5 mL, 10 mL and 25 mL, respectively, of Sodium Chloride Injection 0.9% to give a final concentration of 2 mg/mL of doxorubicin hydrochloride. An appropriate volume of air should be withdrawn from the vial during reconstitution to avoid excessive pressure buildup. Bacteriostatic diluents are not recommended.
After adding the diluent, the vial should be shaken and the contents allowed to dissolve. The reconstituted solution is stable for 7 days at room temperature and under normal room light (100 foot-candles) and 15 days under refrigeration (2°C to 8°C). It should be protected from exposure to sunlight. Discard any unused solution from the 10 mg, 20 mg and 50 mg single dose vials.
It is recommended that doxorubicin be slowly administered into the tubing of a freely running intravenous infusion of Sodium Chloride Injection, USP or 5% Dextrose Injection, USP. The tubing should be attached to a Butterfly® needle inserted preferably into a large vein. If possible, avoid veins over joints or in extremities with compromised venous or lymphatic drainage. The rate of administration is dependent on the size of the vein, and the dosage. However, the dose should be administered in not less than 3 to 5 minutes. Local erythematous streaking along the vein as well as facial flushing may be indicative of too rapid an administration. A burning or stinging sensation may be indicative of perivenous infiltration and the infusion should be immediately terminated and restarted in another vein. Perivenous infiltration may occur painlessly. Doxorubicin should not be mixed with heparin or fluorouracil since it has been reported that these drugs are incompatible to the extent that a precipitate may form. Until specific compatibility data are available, it is not recommended that doxorubicin be mixed with other drugs.
Parenteral drug products should be inspected visually for particulate matter and discoloration prior to administration, whenever solution and container permit.
Handling and Disposal: Skin reactions associated with doxorubicin have been reported. Skin accidently exposed to doxorubicin should be rinsed copiously with soap and warm water, and if the eyes are involved, standard irrigation techniques should be used immediately. The use of goggles, gloves, and protective gowns is recommended during preparation and administration of the drug.
Procedures for proper handling and disposal of anti-cancer drugs should be considered. Several guidelines on this subject have been published [2–8].
There is no general agreement that all the procedures recommended in the guidelines are necessary or appropriate.

HOW SUPPLIED

Doxorubicin Hydrochloride Injection, USP
SINGLE DOSE VIALS:
Sterile single use only, contains no preservatives.
NDC 0186-1532-31, 10 mg vial, 2 mg/mL, 5 mL, single vial packs.
NDC 0186-1532-41, 20 mg vial, 2 mg/mL, 10 mL, single vial packs.
NDC 0186-1532-61, 50 mg vial, 2 mg/mL, 25 mL, single vial packs.
Store under refrigeration 2°C to 8°C (36°F to 46°F). Protect from light.
Retain in carton until time of use. Discard unused portion.
MULTIDOSE VIAL:
Sterile multidose vial, contains no preservatives.
NDC 0186-1532-81, 200 mg vial, 2 mg/mL, 100 mL, multidose vial, single vial packs.
Store under refrigeration, 2°C to 8°C (36°F to 46°F). Protect from light.
Retain in carton until contents are used.
Doxorubicin Hydrochloride for Injection, USP is available as follows:
NDC 0186-1533-28 (Product No. 1530-13), 10 mg, single dose vial, box of 5.
NDC 0186-1535-28 (Product No. 1575-12), 20 mg, single dose vial, box of 5.
NDC 0186-1534-28 (Product No. 1531-01), 50 mg, single dose vial, box of 1.
Store at controlled room temperature, 15°C to 30°C (59°F to 86°F). Protect from light.
Retain in carton until time of use. Contains no preservative. Discard unused portion.

RECONSTITUTED SOLUTION STABILITY

After adding the diluent, the vial should be shaken and the contents allowed to dissolve. The reconstituted solution is stable for 7 days at room temperature and under normal room light (100 foot-candles) and 15 days under refrigeration (2°C to 8°C). It should be protected from exposure to sunlight. Discard any unused solution from the 10 mg, 20 mg and 50 mg single dose vials.
Caution: Federal law prohibits dispensing without prescription.

REFERENCES

1. Rudolph R, Larson DL: Etiology and Treatment of Chemotherapeutic Agent Extravasation Injuries: A Review. J Clin Oncol 5: 1116-1126, 1987.
2. Recommendations for the Safe Handling of Parenteral Antineoplastic Drugs. NIH Publication No. 83-2621. For sale by the Superintendent of Documents, US Government Printing Office, Washington, DC 20402.
3. AMA Council Report, Guidelines for Handling Parenteral Antineoplastics, JAMA. 1985; 253 (11): 1590-1592.
4. National Study Commission on Cytotoxic Exposure - Recommendations for Handling Cytotoxic Agents. Available from Louis P. Jeffrey, Sc.D., Chairman, National Study Commission on Cytotoxic Exposure, Massachusetts College of Pharmacy and Allied Health Sciences, 179 Longwood Avenue, Boston, Massachusetts 02115.
5. Clinical Oncological Society of Australia. Guidelines and Recommendations for Safe Handling of Antineoplastic Agents. Med J Australia. 1983; 1: 426-428.
6. Jones RB, et al: Safe Handling of Chemotherapeutic Agents: A Report from the Mount Sinai Medical Center. Ca-A Cancer Journal for Clinicians. 1983; (Sept/Oct) 258-263.
7. American Society of Hospital Pharmacists Technical Assistance Bulletin on Handling Cytotoxic and Hazardous Drugs. Am J Hosp Pharm. 1990; 47: 1033-1049.
8. OSHA Work-Practice Guidelines for Personnel Dealing with Cytotoxic (Antineoplastic) Drugs. Am J Hosp Pharm. 1986; 43: 1193-1204.

MANUFACTURED FOR:
Astra USA, Inc., Westborough, MA 01581
MANUFACTURED BY:
PHARMACHEMIE B.V.
Haarlem, The Netherlands
021794R05 93.144.129–B
DATE:
November 1996

DURANEST® ℞

[dur 'a-nest]
(etidocaine hydrochloride)
Injections for infiltration and nerve block

DESCRIPTION

Duranest (etidocaine HCl) Injections are sterile aqueous solutions that contain a local anesthetic agent and are administered parenterally by injection. See INDICATIONS AND USAGE for specific uses. The specific quantitative composition of each available solution is shown in Table 1.
Duranest Injections contain etidocaine HCl, which is chemically designated as butanamide, N-(2,6-dimethylphenyl)-2-(ethylpropylamine)-, monohydrochloride and has the following structural formula:

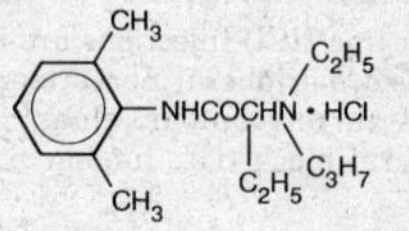

Epinephrine is (-)-3, 4-Dihydroxy-α-[(methylamino) methyl] benzyl alcohol and has the following structural formula:

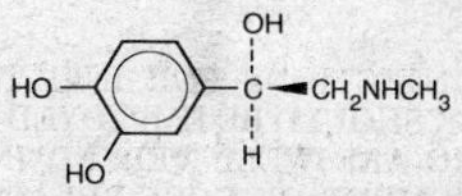

The pK$_a$ of etidocaine (7.74) is similar to that of lidocaine (7.86). However, etidocaine possesses a greater degree of lipid solubility and protein binding capacity than does lidocaine. Duranest Injections are sterile and, except for the 1.5% concentration, are available with or without epinephrine 1:200,000. Single dose containers of Duranest Injection without epinephrine may be reautoclaved if necessary.
See Table 1 for composition of available injections.
[See table at top of next page]

CLINICAL PHARMACOLOGY

Mechanism of Action: Etidocaine stabilizes the neuronal membrane by inhibiting the ionic fluxes required for the initiation and conduction of impulses, thereby effecting local anesthetic action.
Onset and Duration of Action: *In vivo* animal studies have shown that etidocaine has a rapid onset (3–5 minutes) and a prolonged duration of action (5–10 hours). Based on comparative clinical studies of lidocaine and etidocaine, the anesthetic properties of etidocaine in man may be characterized as follows: Initial onset of sensory analgesia and motor blockade is rapid (usually 3–5 minutes) and similar to that produced by lidocaine. Duration of sensory analgesia is 1.5 to 2 times longer than that of lidocaine by the peridural route. The difference in analgesic duration between etidocaine and lidocaine may be even greater following peripheral nerve blockade than following central neural block. Duration of analgesia in excess of 9 hours is not infrequent when etidocaine is used for peripheral nerve blocks such as brachial plexus blockade. Etidocaine produces a profound degree of motor blockade and abdominal muscle relaxation when used for peridural analgesia.
Hemodynamics: Excessive blood levels may cause changes in cardiac output, total peripheral resistance, and mean arterial pressure. With central neural blockade these changes may be attributable to block of autonomic fibers, a direct depressant effect of the local anesthetic agent on various components of the cardiovascular system, and/or the beta-adrenergic receptor stimulating action of epinephrine when present. The net effect is normally a modest hypotension when the recommended dosages are not exceeded.
Pharmacokinetics and Metabolism: Information derived from diverse formulations, concentrations and usages reveals that etidocaine is completely absorbed following parenteral administration, its rate of absorption depending, for example, upon such factors as the site of administration and the presence or absence of a vasconstrictor agent. Except for intravenous administration, the highest blood levels are obtained following intercostal nerve block and the lowest after subcutaneous administration.

Continued on next page

Duranest—Cont.

The plasma binding of etidocaine is dependent on drug concentration, and the fraction bound decreases with increasing concentration. At 0.5–1.0 μg/mL, 95% is bound to plasma protein.
Etidocaine crosses the blood-brain and placental barriers, presumably by passive diffusion.
Etidocaine is metabolized rapidly by the liver, and metabolites and unchanged drug are excreted by the kidney. Biotransformation includes oxidative N-dealkylation, ring hydroxylation, cleavage of the amide linkage, and conjugation. To date, approximately 20 metabolites of etidocaine have been found in the urine. The percent of dose excreted as unchanged drug is less than 10%.
The mean elimination half-life of etidocaine following a bolus intravenous injection is about 2.5 hours. Because of the rapid rate at which etidocaine is metabolized, any condition that affects liver function may alter etidocaine kinetics. Renal dysfunction may not affect etidocaine kinetics but may increase the accumulation of metabolites.
Factors such as acidosis and the concomitant use of CNS stimulants and depressants affect the CNS levels of etidocaine required to produce overt systemic effects. In the rhesus monkey, arterial blood levels of 4.5 μg/mL have been shown to be threshold for convulsive activity.

INDICATIONS AND USAGE

Duranest (etidocaine HCl) Injections are indicated for infiltration anesthesia, peripheral nerve blocks (e.g., brachial plexus, intercostal, retrobulbar, ulnar, inferior alveolar), and central neural block (i.e., lumbar or caudal epidural blocks).

CONTRAINDICATIONS

Etidocaine is contraindicated in patients with a known history of hypersensitivity to local anesthetics of the amide type.

WARNINGS

DURANEST INJECTIONS FOR INFILTRATION AND NERVE BLOCK SHOULD BE EMPLOYED ONLY BY CLINICIANS WHO ARE WELL VERSED IN DIAGNOSIS AND MANAGEMENT OF DOSE-RELATED TOXICITY AND OTHER ACUTE EMERGENCIES THAT MIGHT ARISE FROM THE BLOCK TO BE EMPLOYED AND THEN ONLY AFTER ENSURING THE *IMMEDIATE* AVAILABILITY OF OXYGEN, OTHER RESUSCITATIVE DRUGS, CARDIOPULMONARY EQUIPMENT, AND THE PERSONNEL NEEDED FOR PROPER MANAGEMENT OF TOXIC REACTIONS AND RELATED EMERGENCIES (see also ADVERSE REACTIONS and PRECAUTIONS). DELAY IN PROPER MANAGEMENT OF DOSE-RELATED TOXICITY, UNDERVENTILATION FROM ANY CAUSE AND/OR ALTERED SENSITIVITY MAY LEAD TO THE DEVELOPMENT OF ACIDOSIS, CARDIAC ARREST, AND POSSIBLY DEATH.
To avoid intravascular injection, aspiration should be performed before the local anesthetic solution is injected. The needle must be repositioned until no return of blood can be elicited by aspiration. Note, however, that the absence of blood in the syringe does not guarantee that intravascular injection has been avoided.
Local anesthetic solutions containing antimicrobial preservatives (e.g., methylparaben) should not be used for epidural anesthesia because the safety of these agents has not been established with regard to intrathecal injection, either intentional or accidental.
Vasopressor agents administered for the treatment of hypotension related to caudal or other epidural blocks should not be used in the presence of ergot-type oxytocic drugs, since severe persistent hypertension and even rupture of cerebral blood vessels may occur.
Duranest with epinephrine solutions contain sodium metabisulfite, a sulfite that may cause allergic-type reactions including anaphylactic symptoms and life-threatening or less severe asthmatic episodes in certain susceptible people. The overall prevalence of sulfite sensitivity in the general population is unknown and probably low. Sulfite sensitivity is seen more frequently in asthmatic than in nonasthmatic people.

PRECAUTIONS

General: The safety and effectiveness of etidocaine depend on proper dosage, correct technique, adequate precautions, and readiness for emergencies. Standard textbooks should be consulted for specific techniques and precautions for various regional anesthetic procedures. Resuscitative equipment, oxygen, and other resuscitative drugs should be available for immediate use. (See WARNINGS and ADVERSE REACTIONS.) The lowest dosage that results in effective anesthesia should be used to avoid high plasma levels and serious adverse effects. Syringe aspirations should also be performed before and during each supplemental injection when using indwelling catheter techniques. During the administration of epidural anesthesia, it is recommended that a test dose be administered initially and that the patient be monitored for central nervous system toxicity and cardiovascular toxicity, as well as for signs of unintended intrathecal administration, before proceeding. When clinical conditions permit, consideration should be given to employing local anesthetic solutions that contain epinephrine for the test dose because circulatory changes compatible with epinephrine may also serve as a warning sign of unintended intravascular injection. An intravascular injection is still possible even if aspirations for blood are negative. Repeated doses of etidocaine may cause significant increases in blood levels with each repeated dose because of slow accumulation of the drug or its metabolites. Tolerance to elevated blood levels varies with the status of the patient. Debilitated, elderly patients, acutely ill patients, and children should be given reduced doses commensurate with their age and physical condition.
Etidocaine should also be used with caution in patients with severe shock or heart block.
Lumbar and caudal epidural anesthesia should be used with extreme caution in persons with the following conditions: existing neurological disease, spinal deformities, septicemia, and severe hypertension.
Local anesthetic solutions containing a vasoconstrictor should be used cautiously and in carefully circumscribed quantities in areas of the body supplied by end arteries or having otherwise compromised blood supply. Patients with peripheral vascular disease and those with hypertensive vascular disease may exhibit exaggerated vasoconstrictor response. Ischemic injury or necrosis may result. Preparations containing a vasoconstrictor should be used with caution in patients during or following the administration of potent general anesthetic agents, since cardiac arrhythmias may occur under such conditions.
Careful and constant monitoring of cardiovascular and respiratory (adequacy of ventilation) vital signs and the patient's state of consciousness should be accomplished after each local anesthetic injection. It should be kept in mind at such times that restlessness, anxiety, tinnitus, dizziness, blurred vision, tremors, depression or drowsiness may be early warning signs of central nervous system toxicity.
Since amide-type local anesthetics are metabolized by the liver, Duranest Injections should be used with caution in patients with hepatic disease.
Patients with severe hepatic disease, because of their inability to metabolize local anesthetics normally, are at greater risk of developing toxic plasma concentrations.
Duranest Injection should also be used with caution in patients with impaired cardiovascular function since they may be less able to compensate for functional changes associated with the prolongation of A-V conduction produced by these drugs.
Many drugs used during the conduct of anesthesia are considered potential triggering agents for familial malignant hyperthermia. Since it is not known whether amide-type local anesthetics may trigger this reaction and since the need for supplemental general anesthesia cannot be predicted in advance, it is suggested that a standard protocol for the management of malignant hyperthermia should be available. Early unexplained signs of tachycardia, tachypnea, labile blood pressure and metabolic acidosis may precede temperature elevation. Successful outcome is dependent on early diagnosis, prompt discontinuance of the suspect triggering agent(s) and institution of treatment, including oxygen therapy, indicated supportive measures and dantrolene (consult dantrolene sodium intravenous package insert before using).
Etidocaine should be used with caution in persons with known drug sensitivities. Patients allergic to para-aminobenzoic acid derivatives (procaine, tetracaine, benzocaine, etc.) have not shown cross sensitivity to etidocaine.
Use in the Head and Neck Area: Small doses of local anesthetics injected into the head and neck area, including retrobulbar, dental and stellate ganglion blocks, may produce adverse reactions similar to systemic toxicity seen with unintentional intravascular injections of larger doses. The injection procedures require the utmost care. Confusion, convulsions, respiratory depression and/or respiratory arrest, and cardiovascular stimulation or depression have been reported. These reactions may be due to intra-arterial injection of the local anesthetic with retrograde flow to the cerebral circulation. They may also be due to puncture of the dural sheath of the optic nerve during retrobulbar block with diffusion of any local anesthetic along the subdural space to the midbrain. Patients receiving these blocks should have their circulation and respiration monitored and be constantly observed. Resuscitative equipment and personnel for treating adverse reactions should be immediately available. Dosage recommendations should not be exceeded. (See DOSAGE AND ADMINISTRATION.)
Use in Ophthalmic Surgery: When local anesthetic injections are employed for retrobulbar block, lack of corneal sensation should not be relied upon to determine whether or not the patient is ready for surgery. This is because complete lack of corneal sensation usually precedes clinically acceptable external ocular muscle akinesia.
Use in Dentistry: Because of the long duration of anesthesia, when Duranest 1.5% with epinephrine is used for dental injections, patients should be cautioned about the possibility of inadvertent trauma to tongue, lips and buccal mucosa and advised not to chew solid foods or test the anesthetized area by biting or probing.
Information for Patients: When appropriate, patients should be informed in advance that they may experience temporary loss of sensation and motor activity, usually in the lower half of the body, following proper administration of epidural anesthesia.
Clinically Significant Drug Interactions: The administration of local anesthetic solutions containing epinephrine or norepinephrine to patients receiving monoamine oxidase inhibitors, tricyclic antidepressants or phenothiazines may produce severe, prolonged hypotension or hypertension. Concurrent use of these agents should generally be avoided. In situations when concurrent therapy is necessary, careful patient monitoring is essential.
Concurrent administration of vasopressor drugs (for the treatment of hypotension related to epidural blocks) and ergot-type oxytocic drugs may cause severe, persistent hypertension or cerebrovascular accidents.
Drug Laboratory Test Interactions: The intramuscular injection of etidocaine may result in an increase in creatine phosphokinase levels. Thus, the use of this enzyme determination, without isoenzyme separation, as a diagnostic test for the presence of acute myocardial infarction may be compromised by the intramuscular injection of etidocaine.
Carcinogenesis, Mutagenesis, Impairment of Fertility: Studies of etidocaine in animals to evaluate the carcinogenic and mutagenic potential have not been conducted. Studies in rats at 1.7 times the maximum recommended human dose have revealed no impairment of fertility.
Use in Pregnancy: Teratogenic Effects. Pregnancy Category B. Reproduction studies have been performed in rats and rabbits at doses up to 1.7 times the human dose and have revealed no evidence of harm to the fetus caused by etidocaine. There are, however, no adequate and well-controlled studies in pregnant women. Animal reproduction studies are not always predictive of human response. General consideration should be given to this fact before administering etidocaine to women of childbearing potential, especially during early pregnancy when maximum organogenesis takes place.
Labor and Delivery: Local anesthetics rapidly cross the placenta and when used for epidural, paracervical, pudendal or caudal block anesthesia, can cause varying degrees of maternal, fetal and neonatal toxicity. (See CLINICAL PHARMACOLOGY—Pharmacokinetics.) The incidence and degree of toxicity depend upon the procedure performed, the type and amount of drug used, and the technique of drug administration. Adverse reactions in the parturient, fetus and neonate involve alterations of the central nervous system, peripheral vascular tone and cardiac function.
Maternal hypotension has resulted from regional anesthesia. Local anesthetics produce vasodilation by blocking sympathetic nerves. Elevating the patient's legs and positioning her on her left side will help prevent decreases in blood pressure. The fetal heart rate also should be monitored continuously and electronic fetal monitoring is highly advisable.
Epidural anesthesia may alter the forces of parturition through changes in uterine contractility or maternal expul-

Table 1. Composition of Available Injections

Product Identification			Formula		
Duranest (etidocaine HCl) Concentration % (mg/mL)	Epinephrine Dilution (as the bitartrate) (mg/mL)	pH	Sodium chloride (mg/mL)	Single Dose Vials/ Dental Cartridge Sodium metabisulfite (mg/mL)	Citric acid (mg/mL)
1.0 (10)	None	4.0–5.0	7.1	None	—
1.0 (10)	1:200,000 (0.005 mg/mL)	3.0–4.5	7.1	0.5	0.2
1.5 (15)	1:200,000 (0.005 mg/mL)	3.0–4.5	6.2	0.5	0.2

NOTE: pH of all solutions adjusted with sodium hydroxide and/or hydrochloric acid. Duranest dental cartridges are only available as 1.5% solution with epinephrine 1:200,000. Filled under nitrogen.

sive efforts. Because Duranest Injection may produce profound motor block, it is not recommended for epidural anesthesia in normal delivery. Duranest Injection is, however, recommended for epidural anesthesia when caesarean section is to be performed.

The use of some local anesthetic drug products during labor and delivery may be followed by diminished muscle strength and tone for the first day or two of life. The long-term significance of these observations is unknown.

Fetal bradycardia may occur in 20 to 30 percent of patients receiving paracervical nerve block anesthesia with the amide-type local anesthetics and may be associated with fetal acidosis. Fetal heart rate should always be monitored during paracervical anesthesia. The physician should weigh the possible advantages against risks when considering paracervical block in prematurity, toxemia of pregnancy, and fetal distress. Careful adherence to recommended dosage is of the utmost importance in obstetrical paracervical block. Failure to achieve adequate analgesia with recommended doses should arouse suspicion of intravascular or fetal intracranial injection. Cases compatible with unintended fetal intracranial injection of local anesthetic solution have been reported following intended paracervical or pudendal block or both. Babies so affected present with unexplained neonatal depression at birth, which correlates with high local anesthetic serum levels, and often manifest seizures within six hours. Prompt use of supportive measures combined with forced urinary excretion of the local anesthetic has been used successfully to manage this complication. Case reports of maternal convulsions and cardiovascular collapse following use of some local anesthetics for paracervical block in early pregnancy (as anesthesia for elective abortion) suggest that systemic absorption under these circumstances may be rapid. There are inadequate data in support of safe and effective use of etidocaine for obstetrical or non-obstetrical paracervical block, therefore, such use is not recommended.

Nursing Mothers: It is not known whether this drug is excreted in human milk. Because many drugs are excreted in human milk, caution should be exercised when etidocaine is administered to a nursing woman.

Pediatric Use: No information is currently available on appropriate pediatric doses.

ADVERSE REACTIONS

Systemic: Adverse experiences following the administration of etidocaine are similar in nature to those observed with other amide local anesthetic agents. These adverse experiences are, in general, dose-related and may result from high plasma levels caused by excessive dosage, rapid absorption or unintended intravascular injection, or may result from a hypersensitivity, idiosyncrasy or diminished tolerance on the part of the patient. Serious adverse experiences are generally systemic in nature. The following types are those most commonly reported:

Central Nervous System: CNS manifestations are excitatory and/or depressant and may be characterized by lightheadedness, nervousness, apprehension, euphoria, confusion, dizziness, drowsiness, tinnitus, blurred or double vision, vomiting, sensations of heat, cold or numbness, twitching, tremors, convulsions, unconsciousness, respiratory depression and arrest. The excitatory manifestations may be very brief or may not occur at all, in which case the first manifestation of toxicity may be drowsiness merging into unconsciousness and respiratory arrest.

Drowsiness following the administration of etidocaine is usually an early sign of a high blood level of the drug and may occur as a consequence of rapid absorption.

Cardiovascular System: Cardiovascular manifestations are usually depressant and are characterized by bradycardia, hypotension, and cardiovascular collapse, which may lead to cardiac arrest.

Allergic: Allergic reactions are characterized by cutaneous lesions, urticaria, edema or anaphylactoid reactions. Allergic reactions may occur as a result of sensitivity either to local anesthetic agents or to the methylparaben used as a preservative in multiple dose vials. The detection of sensitivity by skin testing is of doubtful value.

Neurologic: The incidences of adverse reactions associated with the use of local anesthetics may be related to the total dose of local anesthetic administered and are also dependent upon the particular drug used, the route of administration and the physical status of the patient.

In the practice of caudal or lumbar epidural block, occasional unintentional penetration of the subarachnoid space by the catheter may occur. Subsequent adverse effects may depend partially on the amount of drug administered subdurally. These may include spinal block of varying magnitude (including total spinal block), hypotension secondary to spinal block, loss of bladder and bowel control, and loss of perineal sensation and sexual function. Persistent motor, sensory and/or autonomic (sphincter control) deficit of some lower spinal segments with slow recovery (several months) or incomplete recovery have been reported in rare instances when caudal or lumbar epidural block has been attempted. Backache and headache have also been noted following use of these anesthetic procedures.

Table 2. Dosage Recommendations

PROCEDURE	Duranest HCl with epinephrine 1:200,000 Conc. (%)	Vol. (mL)	Total Dose (mg)	PROCEDURE	Duranest HCl with epinephrine 1:200,000 Conc. (%)	Vol. (mL)	Total Dose (mg)
Peripheral Nerve Block Central Neural Block Lumbar Peridural	1.0	5–40	50–400	Caudal	1.0	10–30	100–300
				Retrobulbar	1.0 or 1.5	2–4	20–60
				Maxillary Infiltration and/or inferior Alveolar Nerve Block	1.5	1–5	15–75
Intra-abdominal or Pelvic Surgery Lower Limb Surgery Caesarean Section	1.0 or 1.5	10–30 10–20	100–300 150–300				

HOW SUPPLIED

Dosage Form and Volume	Duranest Injection Concentration	Epinephrine Dilution (as the bitartrate)	pH	NDC Number
Single Dose Vials* 30 mL	1.0%	None	4.0–5.0	0186-0820-01
	1.0%	1:200,000	3.0–4.5	0186-0825-01
20 mL	1.5%	1:200,000	3.0–4.5	0186-0836-03
Dental Cartridge** 1.8 mL	1.5%	1:200,000	3.0–4.5	0186-0840-14

Solutions containing epinephrine should be protected from light.
*Store at controlled room temperature 15°–30°C (59°–86°F).
**Store at room temperature, approx. 25°C (77°F).

There have been reported cases of permanent injury to extraocular muscles requiring surgical repair following retrobulbar administration.

Other: There have been rare reports of TRISMUS in patients who have received Duranest (etidocaine HCl) for dental anesthesia. Onset of symptoms occurs within hours or days upon resolution of blockade. No correlation has been demonstrated with dosage, administration technique or dental procedure. In most patients, symptoms resolved within days to weeks, although some reports have suggested that symptoms were present for many months. Symptomatic treatment with analgesics, moist heat and physiotherapy was helpful in some cases.

OVERDOSAGE

Acute emergencies from local anesthetics are generally related to high plasma levels encountered during therapeutic use of local anesthetics or to unintended subarachnoid injection of local anesthetic solution (see ADVERSE REACTIONS, WARNINGS, and PRECAUTIONS).

Management of Local Anesthetic Emergencies: The first consideration is prevention, best accomplished by careful and constant monitoring of cardiovascular and respiratory vital signs and the patient's state of consciousness after each local anesthetic injection. At the first sign of change, oxygen should be administered.

The first step in the management of convulsions, as well as underventilation or apnea due to unintentional subarachnoid injection of drug solution, consists of immediate attention to the maintenance of a patent airway and assisted or controlled ventilation with oxygen and a delivery system capable of permitting immediate positive airway pressure by mask. Immediately after the institution of these ventilatory measures, the adequacy of the circulation should be evaluated, keeping in mind that drugs used to treat convulsions sometimes depress the circulation when administered intravenously. Should convulsions persist despite adequate respiratory support, and if the status of the circulation permits, small increments of an ultra-short acting barbiturate (such as thiopental or thiamylal) or a benzodiazepine (such as diazepam) may be administered intravenously. The clinician should be familiar, prior to use of local anesthetics, with these anticonvulsant drugs. Supportive treatment of circulatory depression may require administration of intravenous fluids and, when appropriate, a vasopressor as directed by the clinical situation (e.g., ephedrine).

If not treated immediately, both convulsions and cardiovascular depression can result in hypoxia, acidosis, bradycardia, arrhythmias and cardiac arrest. Underventilation or apnea due to unintentional subarachnoid injection of local anesthetic solution may produce these same signs and also lead to cardiac arrest if ventilatory support is not instituted. If cardiac arrest should occur, standard cardiopulmonary resuscitative measures should be instituted.

Endotracheal intubation, employing drugs and techniques familiar to the clinician, may be indicated, after initial administration of oxygen by mask, if difficulty is encountered in the maintenance of a patent airway or if prolonged ventilatory support (assisted or controlled) is indicated.

Dialysis is of negligible value in the treatment of acute overdosage with etidocaine.

The intravenous LD_{50} of etidocaine HCl in female mice is 7.6 (6.6–8.5) mg/kg and the subcutaneous LD_{50} is 112 (96–166) mg/kg.

DOSAGE AND ADMINISTRATION

As with all local anesthetic agents, the dose of Duranest (etidocaine HCl) Injection to be employed will depend upon the area to be anesthetized, the vascularity of the tissues, the number of neuronal segments to be blocked, the type of regional anesthetic technique, and the physical condition and tolerance of the individual patient.

The maximum dose to be employed as a single injection should be determined on the basis of the status of the patient and the type of regional anesthetic technique to be performed. Although single injections of 450 mg have been employed for regional anesthesia without adverse effects, at present it is strongly recommended that the maximal dose as a single injection should not exceed 400 mg (approximately 8.0 mg/kg or 3.6 mg/lb based on a 50 kg person) with epinephrine 1:200,000 and 300 mg (approximately 6 mg/kg or 2.7 mg/lb based on a 50 kg person) without epinephrine. Because etidocaine has been shown to disappear quite rapidly from blood, toxicity is influenced by rapidity of administration, and therefore, slow injection in vascular areas is highly recommended. Incremental doses of Duranest Injection may be repeated at 2–3 hour intervals.

Caudal and Lumbar Epidural Block: As a precaution against the adverse experiences sometimes observed following unintentional penetration of the subarachnoid space, a test dose of 2–5 mL should be administered at least 5 minutes prior to injecting the total volume required for a lumbar or caudal epidural block. The test dose should be repeated if the patient is moved in a manner that may have displaced the catheter. Epinephrine, if contained in the test dose (10–15 μg have been suggested), may serve as a warning of unintentional intravascular injection. If injected into a blood vessel, this amount of epinephrine is likely to produce a transient "epinephrine response" within 45 seconds, consisting of an increase in heart rate and systolic blood pressure, circumoral pallor, palpitations and nervousness in the unsedated patient. The sedated patient may exhibit only a pulse rate increase of 20 or more beats per minute for 15 or more seconds. Patients on beta-blockers may not manifest changes in heart rate, but blood pressure monitoring can detect an evanescent rise in systolic blood pressure. Ad-

Continued on next page

Duranest—Cont.

equate time should be allowed for onset of anesthesia after administration of each test dose. The rapid injection of a large volume of Duranest Injection through the catheter should be avoided, and when feasible, fractional doses should be administered.
In the event of the known injection of a large volume of local anesthetic solution into the subarachnoid space, after suitable resuscitation, and if the catheter is in place, consider attempting the recovery of drug by draining a moderate amount of cerebrospinal fluid (such as 10 mL) through the epidural catheter.
Use in Dentistry: When used for local anesthesia in dental procedures the dosage of Duranest (etidocaine HCl) Injection depends on the physical status of the patient, the area of the oral cavity to be anesthetized, the vascularity of the oral tissues, and the technique of anesthesia. The least volume of solution that results in effective local anesthesia should be administered. For specific techniques and procedures of local anesthesia in the oral cavity, refer to standard textbooks.
Dosage requirements should be determined on an individual basis. In maxillary infiltration and/or inferior alveolar nerve block, initial dosages of 1.0–5.0 mL ($^1/_2$–$2^1/_2$ cartridges) of Duranest Injection 1.5% with epinephrine 1:200,000 are usually effective.
Aspiration is recommended since it reduces the possibility of intravascular injection, thereby keeping the incidence of side effects and anesthetic failures to a minimum.
The following dosage recommendations are intended as guides for the use of Duranest Injection in the average adult patient. As indicated previously, the dosage should be reduced for elderly or debilitated patients or patients with severe renal disease.
NOTE:
Parenteral drug products should be inspected visually for particulate matter and discoloration prior to administration whenever the solution and container permit. The Injection is not to be used if its color is pinkish or darker than slightly yellow or if it contains a precipitate.
[See table 2 at top of previous page]

HOW SUPPLIED

[See second table from top on previous page]
021842R31 Rev. 3/97

DYCLONE® (dyclonine HCl) ℞
0.5% and 1% Topical Solutions, USP
[dié-clone]

DESCRIPTION

Dyclone (dyclonine HCl) 0.5% and 1% Topical Solutions contain a local anesthetic agent and are administered topically. See INDICATIONS for specific uses.
Dyclone 0.5% and 1% Topical Solutions contain dyclonine HCl, which is chemically designated as 4'-butoxy-3-piperidinopropiophenone HCl. Dyclonine HCl is a white crystalline powder that is sparingly soluble in water and has the following structural formula:

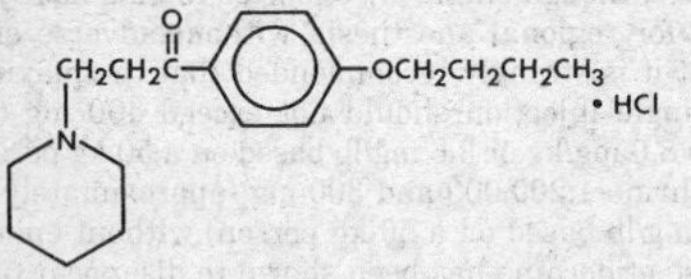

COMPOSITION OF DYCLONE 0.5% AND 1% TOPICAL SOLUTIONS

Each mL of Dyclone 0.5% Solution contains dyclonine HCl, 5 mg.
Each mL of Dyclone 1% Solution contains dyclonine HCl, 10 mg.
Both solutions also contain chlorbutanol hydrous and sodium chloride, and the pH is adjusted to 3.0–5.0 by means of hydrochloric acid.

CLINICAL PHARMACOLOGY

Dyclone Topical Solutions effect surface anesthesia when applied topically to mucous membranes. Effective anesthesia varies with different patients, but usually occurs from 2 to 10 minutes after application and persists for approximately 30 minutes.

INDICATIONS AND USAGE

Dyclone Topical Solutions are indicated for anesthetizing accessible mucous membranes (e.g., the mouth, pharynx, larynx, trachea, esophagus, and urethra) prior to various endoscopic procedures.
Dyclone 0.5% Topical Solution may also be used to block the gag reflex, to relieve the pain of oral ulcers or stomatitis and to relieve pain associated with ano-genital lesions.

CONTRAINDICATIONS

Dyclonine is contraindicated in patients known to be hypersensitive (allergic) to the local anesthetic or to other components of Dyclone Topical Solutions.

WARNINGS

IN ORDER TO MANAGE POSSIBLE ADVERSE REACTIONS, RESUSCITATIVE EQUIPMENT, OXYGEN AND OTHER RESUSCITATIVE DRUGS SHOULD BE IMMEDIATELY AVAILABLE WHENEVER LOCAL ANESTHETIC AGENTS, SUCH AS DYCLONINE, ARE ADMINISTERED TO MUCOUS MEMBRANES.
Dyclone Topical Solutions should not be injected into tissue or used in the eyes because of highly irritant properties.
Dyclone Topical Solutions should be used with extreme caution in the presence of sepsis or severely traumatized mucosa in the area of application since under such conditions there is the potential for rapid systemic absorption.

PRECAUTIONS

General: The safety and effectiveness of dyclonine depend on proper dosage, correct technique, adequate precautions, and readiness for emergencies (See WARNINGS and ADVERSE REACTIONS). The lowest dosage that results in effective anesthesia should be used to avoid high plasma levels and serious adverse effects. Repeated doses of dyclonine may cause significant increases in blood levels with each repeated dose because of slow accumulation of the drug or its metabolites. Tolerance to elevated blood levels varies with the status of the patient. Debilitated, elderly patients, acutely ill patients, and children should be given reduced doses commensurate with their age, weight and physical condition. Dyclonine should also be used with caution in patients with severe shock or heart block.
Dyclone Topical Solutions should be used with caution in persons with known drug sensitivities.
Information for Patients: When topical anesthetics are used in the mouth or throat, the patient should be aware that the production of topical anesthesia may impair swallowing and thus enhance the danger of aspiration. For this reason, food should not be ingested for 60 minutes following use of local anesthetic preparations in the mouth or throat area. This is particularly important in children because of their frequency of eating.
Numbness of the tongue or buccal mucosa may increase the danger of biting trauma. When Dyclone 0.5% Topical Solution is used to relieve the pain of oral ulcers or stomatitis which interferes with eating, patients should be warned about the risk of biting trauma before they accept this treatment; caution should be exercised in selecting food and eating. Following other uses in the mouth and throat area, food and/or chewing gum should not be used while the area is anesthetized.
Drug/Laboratory Test Interactions: Dyclone Topical Solutions should not be used in cystoscopic procedures following intravenous pyelography because an iodine precipitate occurs which interferes with visualization.
Carcinogenesis, Mutagenesis, Impairment of Fertility: Studies of dyclonine in animals to evaluate the carcinogenic and mutagenic potential or the effect on fertility have not been conducted.
Use in Pregnancy: Teratogenic Effects:
Pregnancy Category C. Animal reproduction studies have not been conducted with dyclonine. It is also not known whether dyclonine can cause fetal harm when administered to a pregnant woman or can affect reproduction capacity. General consideration should be given to this fact before administering dyclonine to women of childbearing potential, especially during early pregnancy when maximum organogenesis takes place.
Nursing Mothers: It is not known whether this drug is excreted in human milk. Because many drugs are excreted in human milk, caution should be exercised when dyclonine is administered to a nursing woman.
Pediatric Use: Safety and effectiveness in children under the age of 12 have not been established.

ADVERSE REACTIONS

Adverse experiences following the administration of dyclonine are similar in nature to those observed with other local anesthetic agents. These adverse experiences are, in general, dose-related and may result from high plasma levels caused by excessive dosage or rapid absorption, or may result from a hypersensitivity, idiosyncrasy or diminished tolerance on the part of the patient. Serious adverse experiences are generally systemic in nature. The following types are those most commonly reported:
Central Nervous System: CNS manifestations are excitatory and/or depressant and may be characterized by lightheadedness, nervousness, apprehension, euphoria, confusion, dizziness, drowsiness, tinnitus, blurred or double vision, vomiting, sensations of heat, cold or numbness, twitching, tremors, convulsions, unconsciousness, respiratory depression and arrest. The excitatory manifestations may be very brief or may not occur at all, in which case the first manifestation of toxicity may be drowsiness merging into unconsciousness and respiratory arrest.
Drowsiness following the administration of dyclonine is usually an early sign of a high blood level of the drug and may occur as a consequence of rapid absorption.
Cardiovascular System: Cardiovascular manifestations are usually depressant and are characterized by bradycardia, hypotension, and cardiovascular collapse, which may lead to cardiac arrest.
Allergic: Allergic reactions are characterized by cutaneous lesions, urticaria, edema or anaphylactoid reactions. Allergic reactions may occur as a result of sensitivity either to the local anesthetic agent or to the other ingredients used in this formulation. Allergic reactions, if they occur, should be managed by conventional means. The detection of sensitivity by skin testing is of doubtful value. Local reactions include irritation, stinging, urethritis with and without bleeding.

OVERDOSAGE

Acute emergencies from local anesthetics are generally related to high plasma levels encountered during therapeutic use of local anesthetics. (See ADVERSE REACTIONS, WARNINGS, and PRECAUTIONS).
Management of Local Anesthetic Emergencies: The first consideration is prevention, best accomplished by careful and constant monitoring of cardiovascular and respiratory vital signs and the patient's state of consciousness after each local anesthetic administration.
The first step in the management of convulsions consists of immediate attention to the maintenance of a patent airway and assisted or controlled ventilation with oxygen and a delivery system capable of permitting immediate positive airway pressure by mask. Immediately after the institution of these ventilatory measures, the adequacy of the circulation should be evaluated, keeping in mind that drugs used to treat convulsions sometimes depress the circulation when administered intravenously. Should convulsions persist despite adequate respiratory support, and if the status of the circulation permits, small increments of an ultra-short acting barbiturate (such as thiopental or thiamylal) or a benzodiazepine (such as diazepam) may be administered intravenously. The clinician should be familiar, prior to use of local anesthetics, with these anticonvulsant drugs. Supportive treatment of circulatory depression may require administration of intravenous fluids and, when appropriate, a vasopressor as directed by the clinical situation (e.g., ephedrine).
If not treated immediately, both convulsions and cardiovascular depression can result in hypoxia, acidosis, bradycardia, arrhythmias and cardiac arrest. If cardiac arrest should occur, standard cardiopulmonary resuscitative measures should be instituted.
The median lethal dose (LD_{50}) of dyclonine HCl administered orally to female rats is 176 mg/kg and 90 mg/kg in female mice. Intraperitoneally the LD_{50} in female rats is 31 mg/kg and 43 mg/kg in female mice.

DOSAGE AND ADMINISTRATION

As with all local anesthetics, the dosage varies and depends upon the area to be anesthetized, vascularity of the tissues, individual tolerance and the technique of anesthesia. The lowest dosage needed to provide effective anesthesia should be administered.
A maximum dose of 30 mL of 1% Dyclone Topical Solution (300 mg of dyclonine HCl) may be used, although satisfactory anesthesia is usually produced within the range of 4 to 20 mL. For specific techniques and procedures refer to standard textbooks.
Although as much as 300 mg of dyclonine HCl (as a 1% solution) have been tolerated, this dosage as a 0.5% solution has not been administered primarily because satisfactory anesthesia in endoscopic procedures can usually be produced by lesser amounts. For specific techniques for endoscopic procedures refer to standard textbooks.

PROCTOLOGY

Apply pledgets of cotton or sponges moistened with the Dyclone 0.5% Solution to postoperative wounds for the relief of discomfort and pain.

GYNECOLOGY

Apply Dyclone 0.5% Solution as wet compresses or as a spray to relieve the discomfort of episiotomy or perineorrhaphy wounds.

ONCOLOGY-RADIOLOGY

Apply Dyclone 0.5% Solution as a rinse or swab to inflamed or ulcerated mucous membrane of the mouth caused by antineoplastic chemotherapy or radiation therapy. In lesions of the esophagus, 5–15 mL of the anesthetic may be swallowed to relieve pain and allow more comfortable deglutition.

OTORHINOLARYNGOLOGY

To suppress the gag reflex and to facilitate examination of the posterior pharynx or larynx, apply Dyclone 0.5% Solution as a spray or gargle.

Dyclone 0.5% Solution may be applied as a rinse or swab to relieve the discomfort of aphthous stomatitis, herpetic stomatitis, or other painful oral lesions.

DENTISTRY

Dyclone 0.5% Topical Solution is useful to suppress the gag reflex in the positioning of x-ray films, making prosthetic impressions, and doing surgical procedures in the molar areas. It is also useful as a preinjection mucous membrane anesthetic or applied to the gums prior to scaling (prophylaxis). The anesthetic can be applied as a mouthwash or gargle and the excess spit out.

HOW SUPPLIED

Sterile, in one fluid ounce bottles, DYCLONE 0.5% TOPICAL SOLUTION (NDC 0186-3001-67) and DYCLONE 1% TOPICAL SOLUTION (NDC 0186-3002-67). Keep tightly closed. Store at controlled room temperature: 15°–30°C (59°–86°F). Avoid excessive heat (temperatures above 40°C (104°F). Subject to damage by freezing.

021859R03 Rev. 11/97

EMLA® Anesthetic Disc ℞

(lidocaine 2.5% and prilocaine 2.5% cream)
Topical Adhesive System

EMLA® CREAM ℞

(lidocaine 2.5% and prilocaine 2.5%)

DESCRIPTION

EMLA Cream (lidocaine 2.5% and prilocaine 2.5%) is an emulsion in which the oil phase is a eutectic mixture of lidocaine and prilocaine in a ratio of 1:1 by weight. This eutectic mixture has a melting point below room temperature and therefore both local anesthetics exist as a liquid oil rather than as crystals. It is packaged in 5 gram and 30 gram tubes. It is also packaged in the Anesthetic Disc, which is a single-dose unit of EMLA contained within an occlusive dressing. The Anesthetic Disc is composed of a laminate backing, an absorbent cellulose disc, and an adhesive tape ring. The disc contains 1 gram of EMLA emulsion, the active contact surface being approximately 10 cm^2. The surface area of the entire anesthetic disc is approximately 40 cm^2.

Lidocaine is chemically designated as acetamide, 2-(diethylamino)-N-(2,6-dimethylphenyl), has an octanol:water partition ratio of 43 at pH 7.4, and has the following structure:

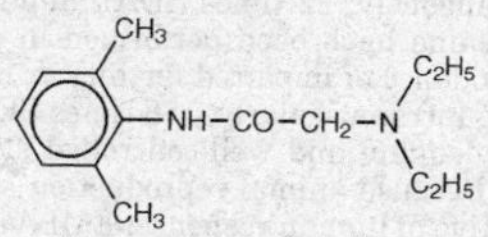

$C_{14}H_{22}N_2O$ M.W. 234.3

Prilocaine is chemically designated as propanamide, N-(2-methylphenyl)-2-(propylamino), has an octanol:water partition ratio of 25 at pH 7.4, and has the following structure:

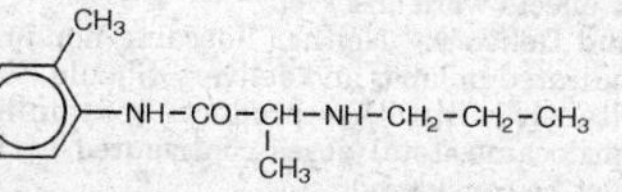

$C_{13}H_{20}N_2O$ M.W. 220.3

Each gram of EMLA contains lidocaine 25 mg, prilocaine 25 mg, polyoxethylene fatty acid esters (as emulsifiers), carboxypolymethylene (as a thickening agent), sodium hydroxide to adjust to a pH approximating 9, and purified water to 1 gram. EMLA contains no preservative, however it passes the USP antimicrobial effectiveness test due to the pH. The specific gravity of EMLA Cream is 1.00.

CLINICAL PHARMACOLOGY

Mechanism of Action: EMLA (lidocaine 2.5% and prilocaine 2.5%), applied to intact skin under occlusive dressing, provides dermal analgesia by the release of lidocaine and prilocaine from the cream into the epidermal and dermal layers of the skin and by the accumulation of lidocaine and prilocaine in the vicinity of dermal pain receptors and nerve endings. Lidocaine and prilocaine are amide-type local anesthetic agents. Both lidocaine and prilocaine stabilize neuronal membranes by inhibiting the ionic fluxes required for the initiation and conduction of impulses, thereby effecting local anesthetic action.

The onset, depth and duration of dermal analgesia provided by EMLA depends primarily on the duration of application. To provide sufficient analgesia for clinical procedures such as intravenous catheter placement and venipuncture, EMLA should be applied under an occlusive dressing for at least 1 hour. To provide dermal analgesia for clinical procedures such as split skin graft harvesting, EMLA should be applied under occlusive dressing for at least 2 hours. Satisfactory dermal analgesia is achieved 1 hour after application, reaches maximum at 2 to 3 hours, and persists for 1 to 2 hours after removal.

TABLE 1
Absorption of Lidocaine and Prilocaine from EMLA Cream: Normal Volunteers (N=16)

EMLA (g)	Area (cm^2)	Time on (hrs)	Drug Content (mg)	Absorbed (mg)	Cmax (μg/mL)	Tmax (hr)
60	400	3	lidocaine 1500	54	0.12	4
			prilocaine 1500	92	0.07	4
60	400	24*	lidocaine 1500	243	0.28	10
			prilocaine 1500	503	0.14	10

*Maximum recommended duration of exposure is 4 hours.

Dermal application of EMLA may cause a transient, local blanching followed by a transient, local redness or erythema.

Pharmacokinetics: EMLA is a eutectic mixture of lidocaine 2.5% and prilocaine 2.5% formulated as an oil in water emulsion. In this eutectic mixture, both anesthetics are liquid at room temperature (see DESCRIPTION) and the penetration and subsequent systemic absorption of both prilocaine and lidocaine are enhanced over that which would be seen if each component in crystalline form was applied separately as a 2.5% topical cream.

The amount of lidocaine and prilocaine systemically absorbed from EMLA is directly related to both the duration of application and to the area over which it is applied. In two pharmacokinetic studies, 60 g of EMLA Cream (1.5 g lidocaine and 1.5 g prilocaine) was applied to 400 cm^2 of intact skin on the lateral thigh and then covered by an occlusive dressing. The subjects were then randomized such that one-half of the subjects had the occlusive dressing and residual cream removed after 3 hours, while the remainder left the dressing in place for 24 hours. The results from these studies are summarized below.

[See table above]

When 60 g of EMLA Cream was applied over 400 cm^2 for 24 hours, peak blood levels of lidocaine are approximately 1/20 the systemic toxic level. Likewise, the maximum prilocaine level is about 1/36 the toxic level. In a pharmacokinetic study, EMLA Cream was applied to penile skin in 20 adult male patients in doses ranging from 0.5 g to 3.3 g for 15 minutes. Plasma concentrations of lidocaine and prilocaine following EMLA Cream application in this study were consistently low (2.5–16 ng/mL for lidocaine and 2.5–7 ng/mL for prilocaine). The application of EMLA to broken or inflamed skin, or to 2,000 cm^2 or more of skin where more of both anesthetics are absorbed, could result in higher plasma levels that could, in susceptible individuals, produce a systemic pharmacologic response. When each drug is administered intravenously, the steady-state volume of distribution is 1.1 to 2.1 L/kg (mean 1.5, ±0.3 SD, n=13) for lidocaine and is 0.7 to 4.4 L/kg (mean 2.6, ±1.3 SD, n=13) for prilocaine. The larger distribution volume for prilocaine produces the lower plasma concentrations of prilocaine observed when equal amounts of prilocaine and lidocaine are administered. At concentrations produced by application of EMLA, lidocaine is approximately 70% bound to plasma proteins, primarily alpha-1-acid glycoprotein. At much higher plasma concentrations (1 to 4 μg/mL of free base) the plasma protein binding of lidocaine is concentration dependent. Prilocaine is 55% bound to plasma proteins. Both lidocaine and prilocaine cross the placental and blood brain barrier, presumably by passive diffusion.

It is not known if lidocaine or prilocaine are metabolized in the skin. Lidocaine is metabolized rapidly by the liver to a number of metabolites including monoethylglycinexylidide (MEGX) and glycinexylidide (GX), both of which have pharmacologic activity similar to, but less potent than that of lidocaine. The metabolite, 2,6-xylidine, has unknown pharmacologic activity but is carcinogenic in rats (see Carcinogenesis subsection of PRECAUTIONS). Following intravenous administration, MEGX and GX concentrations in serum range from 11 to 36% and from 5 to 11% of lidocaine concentrations, respectively. Prilocaine is metabolized in both the liver and kidneys by amidases to various metabolites including *ortho*-toluidine and N-n-propylalanine. It is not metabolized by plasma esterases. The *ortho*-toluidine metabolite has been shown to be carcinogenic in several animal models (see Carcinogenesis subsection of PRECAUTIONS). In addition, *ortho*-toluidine can produce methemoglobinemia following systemic doses of prilocaine approximating 8 mg/kg (see ADVERSE REACTIONS). Very young patients, patients with glucose-6-phosphate deficiencies and patients taking oxidizing drugs such as antimalarials and sulfonamides are more susceptible to methemoglobinemia (see Methemoglobinemia subsection of PRECAUTIONS).

The half-life of lidocaine elimination from the plasma following IV administration is approximately 65 to 150 minutes (mean 110, ±24 SD, n=13). This half-life may be increased in cardiac or hepatic dysfunction. More than 98% of an absorbed dose of lidocaine can be recovered in the urine as metabolites or parent drug. The systemic clearance is 10 to 20 mL/min/kg (mean 13, ± 3 SD, n=13). The elimination half-life of prilocaine is approximately 10 to 150 minutes (mean 70, ±48 SD, n=13). The systemic clearance is 18 to 64 mL/min/kg (mean 38, ±15 SD, n=13). Prilocaine's half-life also may be increased in hepatic or renal dysfunction since both of these organs are involved in prilocaine metabolism.

CLINICAL STUDIES

EMLA Cream application in adults prior to IV cannulation or venipuncture was studied in 200 patients in four clinical studies in Europe. Application for at least 1 hour provided significantly more dermal analgesia than placebo cream or ethyl chloride. EMLA Cream was comparable to subcutaneous lidocaine, but was less efficacious than intradermal lidocaine. Most patients found EMLA Cream treatment preferable to lidocaine infiltration or ethyl chloride spray.

EMLA Cream was compared with 0.5% lidocaine infiltration prior to skin graft harvesting in one open label study in 80 adult patients in England. Application of EMLA Cream for 2 to 5 hours provided dermal analgesia comparable to lidocaine infiltration.

EMLA Cream application in children was studied in seven non-US studies (320 patients) and one US study (100 patients). In controlled studies, application of EMLA Cream for at least 1 hour with or without presurgical medication prior to needle insertion provided significantly more pain reduction than placebo. In children under the age of seven years, EMLA Cream was less effective than in older children or adults.

EMLA Cream was compared with placebo in the laser treatment of facial port-wine stains in 72 pediatric patients (ages 5–16). EMLA Cream was effective in providing pain relief during laser treatment.

EMLA Cream alone was compared to EMLA Cream followed by lidocaine infiltration and lidocaine infiltration alone prior to cryotherapy for the removal of male genital warts. The data from 121 patients demonstrated that EMLA Cream was not effective as a sole anesthetic agent in managing the pain from the surgical procedure. The administration of EMLA Cream prior to lidocaine infiltration provided significant relief of discomfort associated with local anesthetic infiltration and thus was effective in the overall reduction of pain from the procedure only when used in conjunction with local anesthetic infiltration of lidocaine.

Local dermal effects associated with EMLA Cream application in these studies on intact skin included paleness, redness and edema and were transient in nature (see ADVERSE REACTIONS).

Individualization of Dose: The dose of EMLA which provides effective analgesia depends on the duration of the application over the treated area.

All pharmacokinetic and clinical studies employed a thick layer of EMLA Cream (1–2 g/10 cm^2). The duration of application prior to venipuncture was 1 hour. The duration of application prior to taking split thickness skin grafts was 2 hours. Although a thinner application may be efficacious, such has not been studied and may result in less complete analgesia or a shorter duration of adequate analgesia.

The systemic absorption of lidocaine and prilocaine is a side effect of the desired local effect. The amount of drug absorbed depends on surface area and duration of application. The systemic blood levels depend on the amount absorbed and patient size (weight) and rate of systemic drug elimination. Long duration of application, large treatment area, small patients, or impaired elimination may result in high blood levels. The systemic blood levels are typically a small fraction (1/20 to 1/36) of the blood levels which produce toxicity. Table 2 which follows gives maximum recommended doses and application areas for infants and children.

[See table at top of next page]

An IV antiarrhythmic dose of lidocaine is 1 mg/kg (70 mg/70 kg) and gives a blood level of about 1 μg/mL. Toxicity would be expected at blood levels above 5 μg/mL. Smaller areas of treatment are recommended in a debilitated patient, a small child or a patient with impaired elimination. Decreasing the duration of application is likely to decrease the analgesic effect.

Continued on next page

Emla—Cont.

INDICATIONS AND USAGE

EMLA (a eutectic mixture of lidocaine 2.5% and prilocaine 2.5%) is indicated as a topical anesthetic for use on **normal intact skin** for local analgesia.

EMLA is not recommended for use on mucous membranes because limited studies show much greater absorption of lidocaine and prilocaine than through intact skin. Safe dosing recommendations for use on mucous membranes cannot be made because it has not been studied adequately.

EMLA is not recommended in any clinical situation in which penetration or migration beyond the tympanic membrane into the middle ear is possible because of the ototoxic effects observed in animal studies (see WARNINGS).

CONTRAINDICATIONS

EMLA (lidocaine 2.5% and prilocaine 2.5%) is contraindicated in patients with a known history of sensitivity to local anesthetics of the amide type or to any other component of the product.

WARNINGS

Application of EMLA to larger areas or for longer times than those recommended could result in sufficient absorption of lidocaine and prilocaine resulting in serious adverse effects (see Individualization of Dose).

Studies in laboratory animals (guinea pigs) have shown that EMLA has an ototoxic effect when instilled into the middle ear. In these same studies, animals exposed to EMLA Cream in the external auditory canal only, showed no abnormality. EMLA should not be used in any clinical situation in which its penetration or migration beyond the tympanic membrane into the middle ear is possible.

Methemoglobinemia: EMLA should not be used in those rare patients with congenital or idiopathic methemoglobinemia and in infants under the age of twelve months who are receiving treatment with methemoglobin-inducing agents. Very young patients or patients with glucose-6-phosphate deficiencies are more susceptible to methemoglobinemia.

Patients taking drugs associated with drug-induced methemoglobinemia such as sulfonamides, acetaminophen, acetanilid, aniline dyes, benzocaine, chloroquine, dapsone, naphthalene, nitrates and nitrites, nitrofurantoin, nitroglycerin, nitroprusside, pamaquine, para-aminosalicylic acid, phenacetin, phenobarbital, phenytoin, primaquine, quinine, are also at greater risk for developing methemoglobinemia.

There have been reports of significant methemoglobinemia (20–30%) in infants and children following excessive applications of EMLA Cream. These cases involved the use of large doses, larger than recommended areas of application, or infants under the age of 3 months who did not have fully mature enzyme systems. Most patients recovered spontaneously after removal of the cream. Treatment with IV methylene blue may be effective if required.

Physicians are cautioned to make sure that parents or other caregivers understand the need for careful application of EMLA, to ensure that the doses and areas of application recommended in Table 2 are not exceeded (especially in children under the age of 3 months) and to limit the period of application to the minimum required to achieve the desired anesthesia.

PRECAUTIONS

General: Repeated doses of EMLA may increase blood levels of lidocaine and prilocaine. EMLA should be used with caution in patients who may be more sensitive to the systemic effects of lidocaine and prilocaine including acutely ill, debilitated, or elderly patients.

EMLA coming in contact with the eye should be avoided because animal studies have demonstrated severe eye irritation. Also the loss of protective reflexes can permit corneal irritation and potential abrasion. Absorption of EMLA in conjunctival tissues has not been determined. If eye contact occurs, immediately wash out the eye with water or saline and protect the eye until sensation returns.

Patients allergic to para-aminobenzoic acid derivatives (procaine, tetracaine, benzocaine, etc.) have not shown cross sensitivity to lidocaine and/or prilocaine, however, EMLA should be used with caution in patients with a history of drug sensitivities, especially if the etiologic agent is uncertain.

Patients with severe hepatic disease, because of their inability to metabolize local anesthetics normally, are at greater risk of developing toxic plasma concentrations of lidocaine and prilocaine.

Lidocaine and prilocaine have been shown to inhibit viral and bacterial growth. The effect of EMLA on **intradermal** injections of **live** vaccines has not been determined.

Information for Patients: When EMLA is used, the patient should be aware that the production of dermal analgesia may be accompanied by the block of all sensations in the treated skin. For this reason, the patient should avoid inadvertent trauma to the treated area by scratching, rubbing, or exposure to extreme hot or cold temperatures until complete sensation has returned.

TABLE 2
EMLA MAXIMUM RECOMMENDED DOSE AND APPLICATION AREA BY AGE AND WEIGHT*
For Infants and Children Based on Application to Intact Skin

Age and Body Weight Requirements	Maximum Total Dose of EMLA	Maximum Application Area**
1 to 3 months or <5 kg	1 g	10 cm^2
4 to 12 months and >5 kg	2 g	20 cm^2
1 to 6 years and >10 kg	10 g	100 cm^2
7 to 12 years and >20 kg	20 g	200 cm^2

Please note: If a patient greater than 3 months old does not meet the minimum weight requirement, the maximum total dose of EMLA should be restricted to that which corresponds to the patient's **weight.**

* These are broad guidelines for avoiding systemic toxicity in applying EMLA to patients with normal intact skin and with normal renal and hepatic function.

**For more individualized calculation of how much lidocaine and prilocaine may be absorbed, physicians can use the following estimates of lidocaine and prilocaine absorption for children and adults:
The estimated mean (±SD) absorption of lidocaine is 0.045 (±0.016) mg/cm^2/hr.
The estimated mean (±SD) absorption of prilocaine is 0.077 (±0.036) mg/cm^2/hr.

Drug Interactions: EMLA should be used with caution in patients receiving Class I antiarrhythmic drugs (such as tocainide and mexiletine) since the toxic effects are additive and potentially synergistic.

Prilocaine may contribute to the formation of methemoglobin in patients treated with other drugs known to cause this condition (see Methemoglobinemia subsection of WARNINGS).

Carcinogenesis, Mutagenesis, Impairment of Fertility:
Carcinogenesis: Metabolites of both lidocaine and prilocaine have been shown to be carcinogenic in laboratory animals. In the animal studies reported below, doses or blood levels are compared to the Single Dermal Administration (SDA) of 60 g of EMLA Cream to 400 cm^2 for 3 hours to a small person (50 kg). The typical application of EMLA Cream for one or two treatments for venipuncture sites (2.5 or 5 g) would be 1/24 or 1/12 of that dose in an adult or about the same mg/kg dose in an infant. The typical application of EMLA Anesthetic Disc for one or two treatments for venipuncture sites (1 or 2 g) would be 1/60 or 1/30 of that dose in an adult or about half the mg/kg dose in an infant.

A two-year oral toxicity study of 2,6-xylidine, a metabolite of lidocaine, has shown that in both male and female rats 2,6-xylidine in daily doses of 900 mg/m^2 (60 times SDA) resulted in carcinomas and adenomas of the nasal cavity. With daily doses of 300 mg/m^2 (20 times SDA), the increase in incidence of nasal carcinomas and/or adenomas in each sex of the rat were not statistically greater than the control group. In the low dose (90 mg/m^2; 6 times SDA) and control groups, no nasal tumors were observed. A rhabdomyosarcoma, a rare tumor, was observed in the nasal cavity of both male and female rats at the high dose of 900 mg/m^2. In addition, the compound caused subcutaneous fibromas and/or fibrosarcomas in both male and female rats and neoplastic nodules of the liver in the female rats with a significantly positive trend test; pairwise comparisons using Fisher's Exact Test showed significance only at the high dose of 900 mg/m^2. The animal study was conducted at oral doses of 15, 50, and 150 mg/kg/day. The dosages have been converted to mg/m^2 for the SDA calculations above.

Chronic oral toxicity studies of *ortho*-toluidine, a metabolite of prilocaine, in mice (900 to 14,400 mg/m^2; 60 to 960 times SDA) and rats (900 to 4,800 mg/m^2; 60 to 320 times SDA) have shown that *ortho*-toluidine is a carcinogen in both species. The tumors included hepatocarcinomas/adenomas in female mice, multiple occurrences of hemangiosarcomas/hemangiomas in both sexes of mice, sarcomas of multiple organs, transitional-cell carcinomas/papillomas of urinary bladder in both sexes of rats, subcutaneous fibromas/fibrosarcomas and mesotheliomas in male rats, and mammary gland fibroadenomas/adenomas in female rats. The lowest dose tested (900 mg/m^2; 60 times SDA) was carcinogenic in both species. Thus the no-effect dose must be less than 60 times SDA. The animal studies were conducted at 150 to 2,400 mg/kg in mice and at 150 to 800 mg/kg in rats. The dosages have been converted to mg/m^2 for the SDA calculations above.

Mutagenesis: The mutagenic potential of lidocaine HCl has been tested in the Ames Salmonella/mammalian microsome test and by analysis of structural chromosome aberrations in human lymphocytes *in vitro,* and by the mouse micronucleus test *in vivo*. There was no indication in these three tests of any mutagenic effects.

The mutagenicity of 2,6-xylidine, a metabolite of lidocaine, has been studied in different tests with mixed results. The compound was found to be weakly mutagenic in the Ames test only under metabolic activation conditions. In addition, 2,6-xylidine was observed to be mutagenic at the thymidine kinase locus, with or without activation, and induced chromosome aberrations and sister chromatid exchanges at con-

centrations at which the drug precipitated out of the solution (1.2 mg/mL). No evidence of genotoxicity was found in the *in vivo* assays measuring unscheduled DNA synthesis in rat hepatocytes, chromosome damage in polychromatic erythrocytes or preferential killing of DNA repair-deficient bacteria in liver, lung, kidney, testes and blood extracts from mice. However, covalent binding studies of DNA from liver and ethmoid turbinates in rats indicate that 2,6-xylidine may be genotoxic under certain conditions *in vivo*.

Ortho-toluidine, a metabolite of prilocaine, (0.5 µg/mL) showed positive results in *Escherichia coli* DNA repair and phage-induction assays. Urine concentrates from rats treated with *ortho*-toluidine (300 mg/kg orally; 300 times SDA) were mutagenic for *Salmonella typhimurium* with metabolic activation. Several other tests on *ortho*-toluidine, including reverse mutations in five different *Salmonella typhimurium* strains with or without metabolic activation and with single strand breaks in DNA of V79 Chinese hamster cells, were negative.

Impairment of Fertility: See Use in Pregnancy.

Use in Pregnancy: Teratogenic Effects: Pregnancy Category B.

Reproduction studies with lidocaine have been performed in rats and have revealed no evidence of harm to the fetus (30 mg/kg subcutaneously; 22 times SDA). Reproduction studies with prilocaine have been performed in rats and have revealed no evidence of impaired fertility or harm to the fetus (300 mg/kg intramuscularly; 188 times SDA). There are, however, no adequate and well-controlled studies in pregnant women. Because animal reproduction studies are not always predictive of human response, EMLA should be used during pregnancy only if clearly needed.

Reproduction studies have been performed in rats receiving subcutaneous administration of an aqueous mixture containing lidocaine HCl and prilocaine HCl at 1:1 (w/w). At 40 mg/kg each, a dose equivalent to 29 times SDA lidocaine and 25 times SDA prilocaine, no teratogenic, embryotoxic or fetotoxic effects were observed.

Labor and Delivery: Neither lidocaine nor prilocaine are contraindicated in labor and delivery. Should EMLA be used concomitantly with other products containing lidocaine and/or prilocaine, total doses contributed by all formulations must be considered.

Nursing Mothers: Lidocaine, and probably prilocaine, are excreted in human milk. Therefore, caution should be exercised when EMLA is administered to a nursing mother since the milk:plasma ratio of lidocaine is 0.4 and is not determined for prilocaine.

Pediatric Use: Controlled studies of EMLA Cream in children under the age of seven years have shown less overall benefit than in older children or adults. These results illustrate the importance of emotional and psychological support of younger children undergoing medical or surgical procedures.

EMLA should be used with care in patients with conditions or therapy associated with methemoglobinemia (see Methemoglobinemia subsection of WARNINGS).

When using EMLA in young children, especially infants under the age of 3 months, care must be taken to insure that the caregiver understands the need to limit the dose and area of application, and to prevent accidental ingestion (see DOSAGE AND ADMINISTRATION and Methemoglobinemia).

Due to the potential risk of methemoglobinemia and the lack of proven efficacy, EMLA Cream is not recommended for use prior to circumcision in pediatric patients.

In children above the age of one month weighing less than 20 kg, the area and duration of application should be limited (see TABLE 2 in Individualization of Dose).

ADVERSE REACTIONS

Localized Reactions: During or immediately after treatment with EMLA, the skin at the site of treatment may develop erythema or edema or may be the locus of abnormal

sensation. Rare cases of hyperpigmentation following the use of EMLA Cream have been reported. The relationship to EMLA Cream or the underlying procedure has not been established. In clinical studies involving over 1,300 EMLA Cream-treated subjects, one or more such local reactions were noted in 56% of patients, and were generally mild and transient, resolving spontaneously within 1 or 2 hours. There were no serious reactions which were ascribed to EMLA Cream.

In patients treated with EMLA Cream, local effects observed in the trials included: paleness (pallor or blanching) 37%, redness (erythema) 30%, alterations in temperature sensations 7%, edema 6%, itching 2% and rash, less than 1%.

Allergic Reactions: Allergic and anaphylactoid reactions associated with lidocaine or prilocaine can occur. They are characterized by urticaria, angioedema, bronchospasm, and shock. If they occur they should be managed by conventional means. The detection of sensitivity by skin testing is of doubtful value.

Systemic (Dose Related) Reactions: Systemic adverse reactions following appropriate use of EMLA are unlikely due to the small dose absorbed (see Pharmacokinetics subsection of CLINICAL PHARMACOLOGY). Systemic adverse effects of lidocaine and/or prilocaine are similar in nature to those observed with other amide local anesthetic agents including CNS excitation and/or depression (light-headedness, nervousness, apprehension, euphoria, confusion, dizziness, drowsiness, tinnitus, blurred or double vision, vomiting, sensations of heat, cold or numbness, twitching, tremors, convulsions, unconsciousness, respiratory depression and arrest). Excitatory CNS reactions may be brief or not occur at all, in which case the first manifestation may be drowsiness merging into unconsciousness. Cardiovascular manifestations may include bradycardia, hypotension and cardiovascular collapse leading to arrest.

OVERDOSAGE

Peak blood levels following a 60 g application to 400 cm^2 for 3 hours are 0.05 to 0.16 $\mu g/mL$ for lidocaine and 0.02 to 0.10 $\mu g/mL$ for prilocaine. Toxic levels of lidocaine (>5 $\mu g/mL$) and/or prilocaine (>6 $\mu g/mL$) cause decreases in cardiac output, total peripheral resistance and mean arterial pressure. These changes may be attributable to direct depressant effects of these local anesthetic agents on the cardiovascular system. In the absence of massive topical overdose or oral ingestion, evaluation should include evaluation of other etiologies for the clinical effects or overdosage from other sources of lidocaine, prilocaine or other local anesthetics. Consult the package inserts for parenteral Xylocaine (lidocaine HCl) or Citanest (prilocaine HCl) for further information for the management of overdose.

DOSAGE AND ADMINISTRATION

Adult Patients

EMLA Cream and Anesthetic Disc

A thick layer of EMLA Cream is applied to intact skin and covered with an occlusive dressing, or alternatively, an EMLA Anesthetic Disc is applied to intact skin:

Minor Dermal Procedures: For minor procedures such as intravenous cannulation and venipuncture, apply 2.5 grams of EMLA Cream (1/2 the 5 g tube) over 20 to 25 cm^2 of skin surface, or 1 EMLA Anesthetic Disc (1g over 10 cm^2) for at least 1 hour. In controlled clinical trials using EMLA Cream, two sites were usually prepared in case there was a technical problem with cannulation or venipuncture at the first site.

EMLA Cream

A thick layer of EMLA Cream is applied to intact skin and covered with an occlusive dressing:

Major Dermal Procedures: For more painful dermatological procedures involving a larger skin area such as split thickness skin graft harvesting, apply 2 grams of EMLA Cream per 10 cm^2 of skin and allow to remain in contact with the skin for at least 2 hours.

Adult Male Genital Skin: As an adjunct prior to local anesthetic infiltration, apply a thick layer of EMLA Cream (1 g/10 cm^2) to the skin surface for 15 minutes. Local anesthetic infiltration should be performed immediately after removal of EMLA Cream.

Dermal analgesia can be expected to increase for up to 3 hours under occlusive dressing and persist for 1 to 2 hours after removal of the cream. The amount of lidocaine and prilocaine absorbed during the period of application can be estimated from the information in Table 2, ** footnote, in Individualization of Dose.

Pediatric Patients

The following are the maximum recommended doses and areas of application for EMLA based on a child's age and weight:

[See table above]

Please note: If a patient greater than 3 months old does not meet the minimum weight requirement, the maximum total dose of EMLA should be restricted to that which corresponds to the patient's **weight**.

Age and Body Weight Requirements	Maximum Total Dose of EMLA	Maximum Application Area
1 to 3 months or < 5 kg	1 g	10 cm^2
4 to 12 months and > 5 kg	2 g	20 cm^2
1 to 6 years and > 10 kg	10 g	100 cm^2
7 to 12 years and > 20 kg	20 g	200 cm^2

Practitioners should carefully instruct caregivers to avoid application of excessive amounts of EMLA (see Precautions).

When applying EMLA to the skin of young children, care must be taken to maintain careful observation of the child to prevent accidental ingestion of EMLA, the occlusive dressing, or the anesthetic disc. A secondary protective covering to prevent inadvertent disruption of the application site may be useful.

EMLA should not be used in infants under the age of one month nor in infants under the age of twelve months who are receiving treatment with methemoglobin-inducing agents (see Methemoglobinemia subsection of WARNINGS).

When EMLA (lidocaine 2.5% and prilocaine 2.5%) is used concomitantly with other products containing local anesthetic agents, the amount absorbed from all formulations must be considered (see Individualization of Dose.) The amount absorbed in the case of EMLA is determined by the area over which it is applied and the duration of application under occlusion (see Table 2, ** footnote, in Individualization of Dose).

Although the incidence of systemic adverse reactions with EMLA is very low, caution should be exercised, particularly when applying it over large areas and leaving it on for longer than 2 hours. The incidence of systemic adverse reactions can be expected to be directly proportional to the area and time of exposure (see Individualization of Dose).

HOW SUPPLIED

EMLA Cream is available as the following:
NDC 0186-1515-01   5 gram tube,   box of 1, contains 2 Tegaderm® dressings (6 cm × 7 cm)
NDC 0186-1515-03   5 gram tube,   box of 5, contains 12 Tegaderm® dressings (6 cm × 7 cm)
NDC 0186-1516-01   30 gram tube,   box of 1
EMLA Anesthetic Disc is available in the following:
NDC 0186-1512-70   1 gram Anesthetic Disc,   box of 2
NDC 0186-1512-71   1 gram Anesthetic Disc,   box of 10
NOT FOR OPHTHALMIC USE.
KEEP CONTAINER TIGHTLY CLOSED AT ALL TIMES WHEN NOT IN USE.
Store at controlled room temperature 15°–30°C (59°–86°F).
EMLA Anesthetic Disc manufactured by:
Astra Pharmaceutical Production, AB
Södertälje, Sweden
EMLA Cream manufactured by:
Astra USA, Inc., Westborough, MA 01581

INSTRUCTIONS FOR APPLICATION

EMLA®
Anesthetic Disc
(lidocaine 2.5% and prilocaine 2.5% cream)
Topical Adhesive System

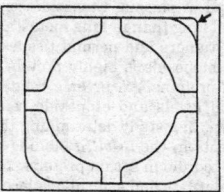

1. Make sure that the area to be anesthetized is clean and dry. Take hold of the aluminum flap at the corner of the Anesthetic disc and bend it backwards. Next, take hold of the corner of the beige-colored Anesthetic Disc layer.

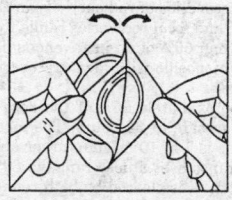

2. Pull the two layers apart, separating the adhesive surface from the protective liner, as shown. Make sure that you do not touch the white, round disc, which contains EMLA.

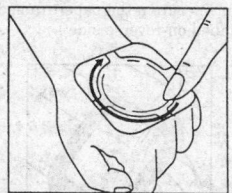

3. Press firmly around the *edges* of the Anesthetic Disc to ensure good adhesion to the skin. **Do not press on the center of the Anesthetic Disc.** This may cause EMLA to spread under the adhesive.

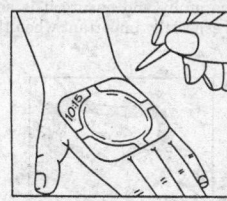

4. The time of application may be easily marked along the border of the Anesthetic Disc. (A ballpoint pen may be used for this purpose.)
EMLA Anesthetic Disc must be applied at least **one hour** before the start of a procedure.
PRECAUTIONS
   1. Do not apply near eyes or on open wounds.
   2. Do not use in children under one month of age.
   3. Keep out of reach of children.
Manufactured by: Astra Pharmaceutical Production, AB
Södertälje, Sweden
Manufactured for:
Astra USA, Inc., Westborough, MA 01581
021792R02   Iss. 5/98

INSTRUCTIONS FOR APPLICATION

EMLA®
CREAM (lidocaine 2.5% and prilocaine 2.5%)

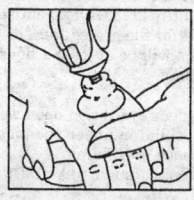

1. In adults, apply 2.5 g of cream (1/2 the 5 g tube) per 20 to 25 cm^2 (approx. 2 in. by 2 in.) of skin in a thick layer at the site of the procedure. For pediatric patients, apply ONLY as prescribed by your physician. If your child is below the age of 3 months or small for their age, please inform your doctor before applying EMLA, which can be harmful, if applied over too much skin at one time in young children.
If your child becomes very dizzy, excessively sleepy, or develops duskiness of the face or lips after applying EMLA, remove the cream and contact your physician at once.

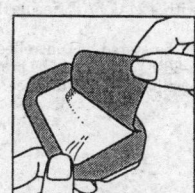

2. Take an occlusive dressing (provided with the 5 g tubes only) and remove the center cut-out piece.

Continued on next page

Emla—Cont.

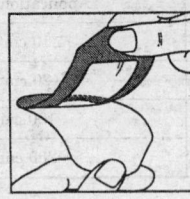

3. Peel the paper liner from the paper framed dressing. (Instructions continued on reverse side.)

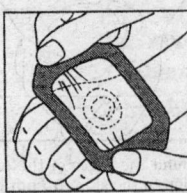

4. Cover the EMLA® Cream so that you get a thick layer underneath. Do not spread out the cream. Smooth down the dressing edges carefully and ensure it is secure to avoid leakage. (This is especially important when the patient is a child.)

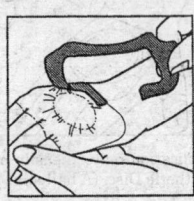

5. Remove the paper frame. The time of application can easily be marked directly on the occlusive dressing. EMLA® must be applied at least 1 hour before the start of a routine procedure and for 2 hours before the start of a painful procedure.

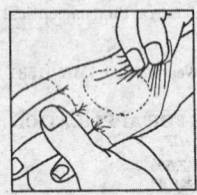

6. Remove the occlusive dressing, wipe off the EMLA® Cream, clean the entire area with an antiseptic solution and prepare the patient for the procedure. The duration of effective skin anesthesia will be at least 1 hour after removal of the occlusive dressing.

PRECAUTIONS

   1. Do not apply near eyes or on open wounds.
   2. Do not use in children under one month of age.
   3. Keep out of reach of children.

Astra USA, Inc., Westborough, MA 01581
021700R02   Iss. 5/98
Shown in Product Identification Guide, page 304

EPINEPHRINE Injection, USP   ℞
[ep-ē-nef'-rin]
1:10,000 (0.1 mg/mL) Adult Strength

(For details of indications, dosage and administration, precautions, and adverse reactions, see circular in package.)

HOW SUPPLIED

Epinephrine Injection, USP, 1:10,000, is supplied in: 10 mL prefilled syringes with a 21 G $^{15}/_{16}$" Needle (NDC 0186-0653-01).

The solution should be stored at controlled room temperature 15°–30°C (59°–86°F) and should be protected from light by storage in the original carton until use.
021687R02   Rev. 7/96

ETOPOSIDE   ℞
INJECTION

WARNINGS
Etoposide should be administered under the supervision of a qualified physician experienced in the use of cancer chemotherapeutic agents. Severe myelosuppression with resulting infection or bleeding may occur.

DESCRIPTION

Etoposide (also commonly known as VP-16) is a semisynthetic derivative of podophyllotoxin used in the treatment of certain neoplastic diseases. It is 4'-demethylepipodophyllotoxin 9-[4,6-0-(R) ethylidene-β-D-glucopyranoside]. It is very soluble in methanol and chloroform, slightly soluble in ethanol, and sparingly soluble in water and ether. It is made more miscible with water by means of organic solvents. It has a molecular weight of 588.58 and a molecular formula of $C_{29}H_{32}O_{13}$.

Etoposide injection is available for intravenous use as 20 mg/mL (100 mg/5 mL) sterile solution in 5 mL multiple dose vials. The pH of the clear yellow solution is 3 to 4. Each mL contains 20 mg etoposide, 2 mg citric acid, 30 mg benzyl alcohol, 80 mg polysorbate 80, 650 mg polyethylene glycol 300, and 30.5 percent (v/v) alcohol. The structural formula is:

CLINICAL PHARMACOLOGY

Etoposide has been shown to cause metaphase arrest in chick fibroblasts. Its main effect, however, appears to be at the G_2 portion of the cell cycle in mammalian cells. Two different dose-dependent responses are seen. At high concentrations (10 µg/mL or more), lysis of cells entering mitosis is observed. At low concentrations (0.3 to 10 µg/mL), cells are inhibited from entering prophase. It does not interfere with microtubular assembly. The predominant macromolecular effect of etoposide appears to be DNA synthesis inhibition.
Pharmacokinetics: On intravenous administration, the disposition of etoposide is best described as a biphasic process with a distribution half-life of about 1.5 hours and terminal elimination half-life ranging from 4 to 11 hours. Total body clearance values range from 33 to 48 mL/min or 16 to 36 mL/min/m² and, like the terminal elimination half-life, are independent of dose over a range 100 to 600 mg/m². Over the same dose range, the areas under the plasma concentration vs. time curves (AUC) and the maximum plasma concentration (C_{max}) values increase linearly with dose. Etoposide does not accumulate in the plasma following daily administration of 100 mg/m² for 4 to 5 days.

The mean volumes of distribution at steady state fall in the range of 18 to 29 liters or 7 to 17 L/m². Etoposide enters the CSF poorly. Although it is detectable in CSF and intracerebral tumors, the concentrations are lower than in extracerebral tumors and in plasma. Etoposide concentrations are higher in normal lung than in lung metastases and are similar in primary tumors and normal tissues of the myometrium. *In vitro*, etoposide is highly protein bound (97%) to human plasma proteins. An inverse relationship between plasma albumin levels and etoposide renal clearance is found in children. In a study determining the effect of other therapeutic agents in the *in vitro* binding of carbon-14 labeled etoposide to human serum proteins, only phenylbutazone, sodium salicylate and aspirin displaced protein-bound etoposide at concentrations achieved *in vivo*[1].

Etoposide binding ratio correlates directly with serum albumin in patients with cancer and in normal volunteers. The unbound fraction of etoposide significantly correlated with bilirubin in a population of cancer patients[2, 3].

After intravenous administration of ³H-etoposide (70 to 290 mg/m²), mean recoveries of radioactivity in the urine range from 42 to 67%, and fecal recoveries range from 0 to 16% of the dose. Less than 50% of an intravenous dose is excreted in the urine as etoposide with mean recoveries of 8 to 35% within 24 hours.

In children, approximately 55% of the dose is excreted in the urine as etoposide in 24 hours. The mean renal clearance of etoposide is 7 to 10 mL/min/m² or about 35% of the total body clearance over a dose range of 80 to 600 mg/m². Etoposide, therefore, is cleared by both renal and nonrenal processes, i.e., metabolism and biliary excretion. The effect of renal disease on plasma etoposide clearance is not known. Biliary excretion appears to be a minor route of etoposide elimination. Only 6% or less of an intravenous dose is recovered in the bile as etoposide. Metabolism accounts for most of the nonrenal clearance of etoposide. The major urinary metabolite of etoposide in adults and children is the hydroxy acid [4'-demethylepipodophyllic acid-9-[4,6-O-(R)-ethylidene-β-D-glucopyranoside)], formed by opening of the lactone ring. It is also present in human plasma, presumably as the trans isomer. Glucuronide and/or sulfate conjugates of etoposide are excreted in human urine and represent 5 to 22% of the dose.

After intravenous infusion, the C_{max} and AUC values exhibit marked intra- and inter-subject variability.

In adults, the total body clearance of etoposide is correlated with creatinine clearance, serum albumin concentration, and nonrenal clearance. In children, elevated serum SGPT levels are associated with reduced drug total body clearance. Prior use of cisplatin may also result in a decrease of etoposide total body clearance in children.

INDICATIONS AND USAGE

Etoposide Injection is indicated in the management of the following neoplasms:
Refractory Testicular Tumors: In combination therapy with other approved chemotherapeutic agents in patients with refractory testicular tumors who have already received appropriate surgical, chemotherapeutic, and radiotherapeutic therapy.
Small Cell Lung Cancer: Etoposide injection and/or capsules in combination with other approved chemotherapeutic agents as first line treatment in patients with small cell lung cancer.

CONTRAINDICATIONS

Etoposide Injection is contraindicated in patients who have demonstrated a previous hypersensitivity to it.

WARNINGS

Patients being treated with etoposide must be frequently observed for myelosuppression both during and after therapy. Dose-limiting bone marrow suppression is the most significant toxicity associated with etoposide therapy. Therefore, the following studies should be obtained at the start of therapy and prior to each subsequent dose of etoposide: platelet count, hemoglobin, white blood cell count, and differential. The occurrence of a platelet count below 50,000/mm³ or an absolute neutrophil count below 500/mm³ is an indication to withhold further therapy until the blood counts have sufficiently recovered.

Physicians should be aware of the possible occurrence of an anaphylactic reaction manifested by chills, fever, tachycardia, bronchospasm, dyspnea, and hypotension. (See **"ADVERSE REACTIONS"** section). Treatment is symptomatic. The infusion should be terminated immediately, followed by the administration of pressor agents, corticosteroids, antihistamines, or volume expanders at the discretion of the physician.

Etoposide injection should be given only by slow intravenous infusion (usually over a 30 to 60 minute period) since hypotension has been reported as a possible side effect of rapid intravenous injection.

Pregnancy: Pregnancy "Category D". Etoposide can cause fetal harm when administered to pregnant women. Etoposide has been shown to be teratogenic in mice and rats. There are no adequate and well-controlled studies in pregnant women. If this drug is used during pregnancy, or if the patient becomes pregnant while receiving this drug, the patient should be apprised of the potential hazard to the fetus. Women of childbearing potential should be advised to avoid becoming pregnant.

Etoposide is teratogenic and embryocidal in rats and mice at doses of 1 to 3% of the recommended clinical dose based on body surface area.

In a teratology study in SPF rats, etoposide was administered intravenously at doses of 0.13, 0.4, 1.2, and 3.6 mg/kg/day on days 6 to 15 of gestation. Etoposide caused dose-related maternal toxicity, embryotoxicity, and teratogenicity at dose levels of 0.4 mg/kg/day and higher. Embryonic resorptions were 90 and 100% at the 2 highest dosages. At 0.4 and 1.2 mg/kg, fetal weights were decreased and fetal abnormalities including decreased weight, major skeletal abnormalities, exencephaly, encephalocele, and anophthalmia occurred. Even at the lowest dose tested, 0.13 mg/kg, a significant increase in retarded ossification was observed.

Etoposide administered as a single intraperitoneal, injection in Swiss-Albino mice at dosages of 1, 1.5 and 2 mg/kg on days 6, 7, or 8 of gestation caused dose-related embryotoxicity, cranial abnormalities, and major skeletal malformations.

PRECAUTIONS

General: In all instances where the use of etoposide is considered for chemotherapy, the physician must evaluate the need and usefulness of the drug against the risk of adverse reactions. Most such adverse reactions are reversible if detected early. If severe reactions occur, the drug should be reduced in dosage or discontinued and appropriate correc-

tive measures should be taken according to the clinical judgement of the physician. Reinstitution of etoposide therapy should be carried out with caution, and with adequate consideration of the further need for the drug and alertness as to possible recurrence of toxicity.

Laboratory Tests: Periodic complete blood counts should be done during the course of etoposide treatment. They should be performed prior to therapy and at appropriate intervals during and after therapy. At least one determination should be done prior to each dose of etoposide.

Carcinogenesis, Mutagenesis, Impairment of Fertility: Carcinogenicity tests with etoposide have not been conducted in laboratory animals. Etoposide should be considered a potential carcinogen in humans. The occurence of acute leukemia with a preleukemic phase has been reported rarely in patients treated with etoposide in association with other antineo-plastic agents.

The mutagenic and genotoxic potential of etoposide has been established in mammalian cells. Etoposide caused aberrations in chromosome number and structure in embryonic murine cells and human hematopoietic cells; gene mutations in Chinese hamster ovary cells; and DNA damage by strand breakage and DNA-protein cross-links in mouse leukemia cells. Etoposide also caused a dose-related increase in sister chromatid exchanges in Chinese hamster ovary cells. Treatment of Swiss-Albino mice with 1.5 mg/kg IP of etoposide on day 7 of gestation increased the incidence of intrauterine death and fetal malformations as well as significantly decreased the average fetal body weight. Maternal weight gain was not affected.

Treatment of pregnant SPF rats with 1.2 mg/kg/day IV of etoposide for 10 days led to a prenatal mortality of 92%, and 50% of the implanting fetuses were abnormal.

Pregnancy: Pregnancy "Category D" (See **"WARNINGS"** section).

Nursing Mothers: It is not known whether this drug is excreted in human milk. Because many drugs are excreted in human milk and because of the potential for serious adverse reactions in nursing infants from etoposide, a decision should be made whether to discontinue nursing or to discontinue the drug, taking into account the importance of the drug to the mother.

Pediatric Use: Safety and effectiveness in pediatric patients have not been established.

Etoposide Injection contains polysorbate 80. In premature infants, a life-threatening syndrome consisting of liver and renal failure, pulmonary deterioration, thrombocytopenia, and ascites has been associated with an injectable vitamin E product containing polysorbate 80.

ADVERSE REACTIONS

The following data on adverse reactions are based on both oral and intravenous administration of etoposide as a single agent, using several different dose schedules for treatment of a wide variety of malignancies.

Hematologic Toxicity: Myelosuppression is dose related and dose limiting, with granulocyte nadirs occurring 7 to 14 days after drug administration and platelet nadirs occurring 9 to 16 days after drug administration. Bone marrow recovery is usually complete by day 20, and no cumulative toxicity has been reported.

The occurrence of acute leukemia with or without a preleukemic phase has been reported rarely in patients treated with etoposide in association with other antineoplastic agents.

Gastrointestinal Toxicity: Nausea and vomiting are the major gastrointestinal toxicities. The severity of such nausea and vomiting is generally mild to moderate with treatment discontinuation required in 1% of patients. Nausea and vomiting can usually be controlled with standard antiemetic therapy. Gastrointestinal toxicities are slightly more frequent after oral administration than after intravenous infusion.

Hypotension: Transient hypotension following rapid intravenous administration has been reported in 1% to 2% of patients. It has not been associated with cardiac toxicity or electrocardiographic changes. No delayed hypotension has been noted. To prevent this rare occurrence, it is recommended that etoposide be administered by slow intravenous infusion over a 30 to 60 minute period. If hypotension occurs, it usually responds to cessation of the infusion and administration of fluids or other supportive therapy as appropriate. When restarting the infusion, a slower administration rate should be used.

Allergic Reactions: Anaphylactic-like reactions characterized by chills, fever, tachycardia, bronchospasm, dyspnea, and/or hypotension have been reported to occur in 0.7% to 2% of patients receiving intravenous etoposide and in less than 1% of the patients treated with the oral capsules. These reactions have usually responded promptly to the cessation of the infusion and administration of pressor agents, corticosteroids, antihistamines or volume expanders as appropriate; however, the reactions can be fatal. Hypertension and/or flushing have also been reported. Blood pressure usually normalizes within a few hours after cessation of the infusion. Anaphylactic-like reactions have occurred during the initial infusion of etoposide.

Facial/tongue swelling, coughing, diaphoresis, cyanosis, tightness in throat, laryngospasm, back pain, and/or loss of consciousness have sometimes occurred in association with the above reactions. In addition, an apparent hypersensitivity, associated apnea has been reported rarely.

Rash, urticaria, and/or pruritis have infrequently been reported at recommended doses. At investigational doses, a generalized pruritic erythymatous maculopapular rash, consistent with perivasculitis, has been reported.

Alopecia: Reversible alopecia, sometimes progressing to total baldness was observed in up to 66% of patients.

Other Toxicities: The following adverse reactions have been infrequently reported: aftertaste, fever, pigmentation, abdominal pain, constipation, dysphagia, transient cortical blindness, optical neuritis and a single report of radiation recall dermatitis.

Hepatic toxicity, generally in patients receiving higher doses of the drug than those recommended, has been reported with etoposide. Metabolic acidosis also has been reported in patients receiving these higher doses.

The incidence of adverse reactions in the table that follows are derived from multiple data bases from studies in 2,081 patients when etoposide was used either orally or by injection as a single agent.

ADVERSE DRUG EFFECT	PERCENT RANGE OF REPORTED INCIDENCE
Hematologic Toxicity	
Leukopenia (less than 1,000 WBC/mm³)	3-17
Leukopenia (less than 4,000 WBC/mm³)	60-91
Thrombocytopenia (less than 50,000 platelets/mm³)	1-20
Thrombocytopenia (less than 100,000 platelets/mm³)	22-41
Anemia	0-33
Gastrointestinal Toxicity	
Nausea and vomiting	31-43
Abdominal pain	0-2
Anorexia	10-13
Diarrhea	1-13
Stomatitis	1-6
Hepatic	0-3
Alopecia	8-66
Peripheral neurotoxicity	1-2
Hypotension	1-2
Allergic reactions	1-2

OVERDOSAGE

No proven antidotes have been established for etoposide overdosage.

DOSAGE AND ADMINISTRATION

Note: Plastic devices made of acrylic or ABS (a polymer composed of acrylonitrile, butadiene, and styrene) have been reported to crack and leak when used with undiluted Etoposide Injection.

The usual dose of Etoposide Injection in testicular cancer in combination with other approved chemotherapeutic agents ranges from 50 to 100 mg/m²/day on days 1 through 5 to 100 mg/m²/ day on days 1, 3, and 5.

In small cell lung cancer, the Etoposide Injection dose in combination with other approved chemotherapeutic drugs ranges from 35 mg/m²/day for 4 days to 50 mg/m²/day for 5 days.

Chemotherapy courses are repeated at 3- to 4-week intervals after adequate recovery from any toxicity.

The dosage should be modified to take into account the myelosuppressive effects of other drugs in the combination or the effects of prior X-ray therapy or chemotherapy which may have compromised bone marrow reserve.

Administration Precautions: As with other potentially toxic compounds, caution should be exercised in handling and preparing the solution of etoposide. Skin reactions associated with accidental exposure to etoposide may occur. The use of gloves is recommended. If etoposide solution contacts the skin or mucosa, immediately wash the skin or mucosa thoroughly with soap and water.

Preparation for Intravenous Administration: Etoposide Injection must be diluted prior to use with either dextrose injection 5% or sodium chloride injection 0.9%, to give a final concentration of 0.2 mg/mL to 0.4 mg/mL. If solutions are prepared at concentrations above 0.4 mg/mL, precipitation may occur. Hypotension following rapid intravenous administration has been reported, hence, it is recommended that the etoposide solution is administered over a 30 to 60 minute period. A longer duration of administration may be used if the volume of fluid to be infused is a concern. **Etoposide should not be given by rapid intravenous injection.**

Parenteral drug products should be inspected visually for particulate matter and discoloration (see **"DESCRIPTION"** section) prior to administration whenever solution and container permit.

Stability: Unopened vials of Etoposide Injection are stable for 24 months at room temperature 15°C–30°C (59°F–86°F). Vials diluted as recommended to a concentration of 0.2 mg/mL or 0.4 mg/mL are stable for 96 and 24 hours, respectively, at room temperature 15°C–30°C (59°F–86°F) under normal room fluorescent light in both glass and plastic containers.

Procedures for proper handling and disposal of anticancer drugs should be considered. Several guidelines on this subject have been published[4-10]. There is no general agreement that all of the procedures recommended in the guidelines are necessary or appropriate.

HOW SUPPLIED

Etoposide Injection is supplied as a sterile, clear, yellow solution, in a 5 mL multi-dose vial.
NDC 0186-1571-31, 100 mg (20 mg/mL).
Store at controlled room temperature 15°C–30°C (59°F–86°F).

Caution: Federal law prohibits dispensing without prescription.

REFERENCES

1. Gaver RC, Deeb G. The effect of other drugs on the in vitro binding of ¹⁴C-etoposide to human serum proteins. Proc Am Assoc Cancer Res 1989;30:A2132.
2. Stewart CF, Pieper JA, Arbuck SG, Evans WE. Altered protein binding of etoposide in patients with cancer. Clin Pharmacol Ther 1989;45:49–55.
3. Stewart CF, Arbuck SG, Fleming RA, Evans WE. Prospective evaluation of a model for predicting etoposide plasma protein binding in cancer patients. Proc Am Assoc Cancer Res 1989;30:A958.
4. Recommendations for the Safe Handling of Parenteral Antineoplastic Drugs. NIH Publication No. 83–2621. For sale by the Superintendent of Documents, US Government Printing Office, Washington, DC 20402.
5. AMA Council Report. Guidelines for Handling Parenteral Antineoplastics. JAMA 1985 March 15.
6. National Study Commissions on Cytotoxic Exposure-Recommendations for Handling Cytotoxic Agents. Available from Louis P. Jeffrey, Sc.D., Chairman, National Study Commission on Cytotoxic Exposure, Massachusetts College of Pharmacy and Allied Health Sciences, 179 Longwood Avenue, Boston, Massachusetts 02115.
7. Clinical Oncological Society of Australia. Guidelines and Recommendations for Safe Handling of Antineoplastic Agents. Med J Australia 1983; 1:426–428.
8. Jones RB, et al: Safe handling of chemotherapeutic agents: A report from the Mount Sinai Medical Center. CA-A Cancer Journal for Clinicians 1983;Sept/Oct:258–263.
9. American Society of Hospital Pharmacists Technical Assistance Bulletin on Handling Cytotoxic and Hazardous Drugs. Am J Hosp Pharm 1990; 47:1033–1049.
10. OSHA Work-Practice Guidelines for Personnel Dealing with Cytotoxic (Antineoplastic) Drugs. Am J Hosp Pharm 1986;43:1193–1204.

MANUFACTURED BY
PHARMACHEMIE B.V.
Haarlem, The Netherlands
MANUFACTURED FOR
Astra USA, Inc., Westborough, MA 01581
021796R01   Iss. 6/95

FENTANYL CITRATE* and DROPERIDOL INJECTION Ⓒ
*WARNING: May be habit forming.
FOR INTRAVENOUS OR INTRAMUSCULAR USE ONLY.

The two components of Fentanyl Citrate and Droperidol Injection, fentanyl citrate and droperidol, have different pharmacologic actions. Before administering Fentanyl Citrate and Droperidol Injection, the user should become familiar with the special properties of each drug, particularly the widely differing durations of action.

(For details of indications, dosage and administration, precautions, and adverse reactions, see circular in package.)

HOW SUPPLIED

Each mL of Fentanyl Citrate and Droperidol Injection contains fentanyl citrate (WARNING: May be habit forming) equivalent to 0.05 mg (50 mcg) of fentanyl base, droperidol 2.5 mg and lactic acid to adjust pH and is available in the following dosage forms:

Ampules
NDC 0186-1230-03, 2 mL ampule, packages of 10

Continued on next page

Fentanyl Citrate—Cont.

Vials
NDC 0186-1232-13, 2 mL single dose vial, packages of 10 (FOR INTRAVENOUS USE BY HOSPITAL PERSONNEL SPECIFICALLY TRAINED IN THE USE OF OPIOID ANALGESICS.)
Protect from light. Store at controlled room temperature 15°–30°C (59°–86°F).
Caution: Federal law prohibits dispensing without prescription.
021881R03   Rev. 12/94

FOSCAVIR® (foscarnet sodium) Injection   ℞

WARNING
RENAL IMPAIRMENT IS THE MAJOR TOXICITY OF FOSCAVIR. FREQUENT MONITORING OF SERUM CREATININE, WITH DOSE ADJUSTMENT FOR CHANGES IN RENAL FUNCTION, AND ADEQUATE HYDRATION WITH ADMINISTRATION OF FOSCAVIR, IS IMPERATIVE. (See ADMINISTRATION section; Hydration.)
SEIZURES, RELATED TO ALTERATIONS IN PLASMA MINERALS AND ELECTROLYTES, HAVE BEEN ASSOCIATED WITH FOSCAVIR TREATMENT. THEREFORE, PATIENTS MUST BE CAREFULLY MONITORED FOR SUCH CHANGES AND THEIR POTENTIAL SEQUELAE. MINERAL AND ELECTROLYTE SUPPLEMENTATION MAY BE REQUIRED.
FOSCAVIR IS INDICATED FOR USE ONLY IN IMMUNOCOMPROMISED PATIENTS WITH CMV RETINITIS AND MUCOCUTANEOUS ACYCLOVIR-RESISTANT HSV INFECTIONS. (See INDICATIONS section.)

DESCRIPTION
FOSCAVIR is the brand name for foscarnet sodium. The chemical name of foscarnet sodium is phosphonoformic acid, trisodium salt. Foscarnet sodium is a white, crystalline powder containing 6 equivalents of water of hydration with an empirical formula of $Na_3CO_5P \cdot 6 H_2O$ and a molecular weight of 300.1. The structural formula is:

$$3\ Na+\ \begin{bmatrix} O \\ \| \\ O-P-C-O^- \\ \| \quad \| \\ O^- \quad O \end{bmatrix} \cdot 6\ H_2O$$

FOSCAVIR has the potential to chelate divalent metal ions, such as calcium and magnesium, to form stable coordination compounds. FOSCAVIR INJECTION is a sterile, isotonic aqueous solution for intravenous administration only. The solution is clear and colorless. Each milliliter of FOSCAVIR contains 24 mg of foscarnet sodium hexahydrate in Water for Injection, USP. Hydrochloric acid and/or sodium hydroxide may have been added to adjust the pH of the solution to 7.4. FOSCAVIR INJECTION contains no preservatives.

VIROLOGY
Mechanism of Action: FOSCAVIR is an organic analogue of inorganic pyrophosphate that inhibits replication of herpesviruses *in vitro* including cytomegalovirus (CMV) and herpes simplex virus types 1 and 2 (HSV-1 and HSV-2).
FOSCAVIR exerts its antiviral activity by a selective inhibition at the pyrophosphate binding site on virus-specific DNA polymerases at concentrations that do not affect cellular DNA polymerases. FOSCAVIR does not require activation (phosphorylation) by thymidine kinase or other kinases and therefore is active *in vitro* against HSV TK deficient mutants and CMV UL97 mutants. Thus, HSV strains resistant to acyclovir or CMV strains resistant to ganciclovir may be sensitive to FOSCAVIR. However, acyclovir or ganciclovir resistant mutants with alterations in the viral DNA polymerase may be resistant to FOSCAVIR and may not re-

spond to therapy with FOSCAVIR. The combination of FOSCAVIR and ganciclovir has been shown to have enhanced activity *in vitro*.

Antiviral Activity *in vitro* and *in vivo*: The quantitative relationship between the *in vitro* susceptibility of human cytomegalovirus (CMV) or herpes simplex virus 1 and 2 (HSV-1 and HSV-2) to FOSCAVIR and clinical response to therapy has not been established and virus sensitivity testing has not been standardized. Sensitivity test results, expressed as the concentration of drug required to inhibit by 50% the growth of virus in cell culture (IC_{50}), vary greatly depending on the assay method used, cell type employed and the laboratory performing the test. A number of sensitive viruses and their IC_{50} values are listed below (Table 1).

TABLE 1
FOSCARNET Inhibition of virus multiplication in cell culture

Virus	IC_{50} (μM)
CMV	50–800*
HSV-1, HSV-2	10–130
Ganciclovir resistant CMV	190
HSV-TK negative mutant	67
HSV-DNA polymerase mutants	5–443

* Mean = 269 μM

Statistically significant decreases in positive CMV cultures from blood and urine have been demonstrated in two studies (FOS-03 and ACTG-015/915) of patients treated with FOSCAVIR. Although median time to progression of CMV retinitis was increased in patients treated with FOSCAVIR, reductions in positive blood or urine cultures have not been shown to correlate with clinical efficacy in individual patients.

TABLE 2
BLOOD AND URINE CULTURE RESULTS FROM CMV RETINITIS PATIENTS*

Blood	+CMV	−CMV
Baseline	27	34
End of Induction**	1	60

Urine	+CMV	−CMV
Baseline	52	6
End of Induction**	21	37

* A total of 77 patients was treated with FOSCAVIR in two clinical trials (FOS-03 and ACTG-015/915). Not all patients had blood or urine cultures done and some patients had results from both cultures.

** (60 mg/kg FOSCAVIR TID for 2–3 weeks).

Resistance: Strains of both HSV and CMV that are resistant to FOSCAVIR can be readily selected *in vitro* by passage of wild type virus in the presence of increasing concentrations of the drug. All FOSCAVIR resistant mutants are known to be generated through mutation in the viral DNA polymerase gene. CMV strains with double mutations conferring resistance to both FOSCAVIR and ganciclovir have been isolated from patients with AIDS. The possibility of viral resistance should be considered in patients who show poor clinical response or experience persistent viral excretion during therapy.

CLINICAL PHARMACOLOGY
Pharmacokinetics: The pharmacokinetics of foscarnet have been determined after administration as an intermittent intravenous infusion during induction therapy in AIDS patients with CMV retinitis. Observed plasma foscarnet concentrations in four studies (FOS-01, ACTG-015, FP48PK, FP49PK) are summarized in Table 3:

TABLE 3
Foscarnet Pharmacokinetic Characteristics*

Parameter	60 mg/kg Q8h	90 mg/kg Q12h
C_{max} at steady-state (μM)	589 ± 192 (24)	623 ± 132 (19)
C_{trough} at steady-state (μM)	114 ± 91 (24)	63 ± 57 (17)
Volume of distribution (L/kg)	0.41 ± 0.13 (12)	0.52 ± 0.20 (18)
Plasma half-life (hr)	4.0 ± 2.0 (24)	3.3 ± 1.4 (18)
Systemic clearance (L/hr)	6.2 ± 2.1 (24)	7.1 ± 2.7 (18)
Renal clearance (L/hr)	5.6 ± 1.9 (5)	6.4 ± 2.5 (13)
CSF:plasma ratio	0.69 ± 0.19 (9)†	0.66 ± 0.11 (5)‡

* Values expressed as mean ± S.D. (number of subjects studied) for each parameter
† 50 mg/kg Q8h for 28 days, samples taken 3 hrs after end of 1 hr infusion (Astra Report 815-04 AC025-1)
‡ 90 mg/kg Q12h for 28 days, samples taken 1 hr after end of 2 hr infusion (Hengge et al., 1993)

Distribution: *In vitro* studies have shown that 14–17% of foscarnet is protein bound at plasma drug concentrations of 1–1000 μM.
The foscarnet terminal half-life determined by urinary excretion was 87.5 ± 41.8 hours, possibly due to release of foscarnet from bone. Postmortem data on several patients in European clinical trials provide evidence that foscarnet does accumulate in bone in humans; however, the extent to which this occurs has not been determined. In animal studies (mice), 40% of an intravenous dose of FOSCAVIR was deposited in bone in young animals and 7% was deposited in adult animals.
Special Populations:
Adults with Impaired Renal Function—The pharmacokinetic properties of foscarnet have been determined in a small group of adult subjects with normal and impaired renal function, as summarized in Table 4:
[See table 4 below]
Total systemic clearance (CL) of foscarnet decreased and half-life increased with diminishing renal function (as expressed by creatinine clearance). Based on these observations, it is necessary to modify the dosage of foscarnet in patients with renal impairment (see DOSAGE AND ADMINISTRATION).

CLINICAL TRIALS
CMV Retinitis: A prospective, randomized, controlled clinical trial (FOS-03) was conducted in 24 patients with AIDS and CMV retinitis comparing treatment with FOSCAVIR to no treatment. Patients received induction treatment of FOSCAVIR, 60 mg/kg every 8 hours for 3 weeks, followed by maintenance treatment with 90 mg/kg/day until retinitis progression (appearance of a new lesion or advancement of the border of a posterior lesion greater than 750 microns in diameter). All diagnoses and determinations of retinitis progression were made from masked reading of retinal photographs. The 13 patients randomized to treatment with FOSCAVIR had a significant delay in progression of CMV retinitis compared to untreated controls. Median times to retinitis progression from study entry were 93 days (range 21– >364) and 22 days (range 7–42), respectively.
In another prospective clinical trial of CMV retinitis in patients with AIDS (ACTG-915), 33 patients were treated with two to three weeks of FOSCAVIR induction (60 mg/kg TID) and then randomized to either 90 mg/kg/day or 120 mg/kg/day maintenance therapy. The median times from study entry to retinitis progression were not significantly different between the treatment groups, 96 (range 14– >176) days and 140 (range 16– >233) days, respectively.
In study ACTG 129/FGCRT SOCA study 107 patients with newly diagnosed CMV retinitis were randomized to treatment with FOSCAVIR (induction: 60 mg/kg TID for 2 weeks; maintenance: 90 mg/kg QD) and 127 were randomized to treatment with ganciclovir (induction: 5 mg/kg BID; maintenance: 5 mg/kg QD). The median time to progression on the two drugs was similar (Fos=59 and Gcv=56 days).
Relapsed CMV Retinitis: The CMV Retinitis Retreatment Trial (ACTG 228/SOCA CRRT) was a randomized, open-label comparison of FOSCAVIR or ganciclovir monotherapy to the combination of both drugs for the treatment of persistently active or relapsed CMV retinitis in patients with AIDS. Subjects were randomized to one of the three treatments: FOSCAVIR 90 mg/kg BID induction followed by 120 mg/kg QD maintenance (Fos); ganciclovir 5 mg/kg BID induction followed by 10 mg/kg QD maintenance (Gcv); or the combination of the two drugs, consisting of continuation of the subject's current therapy and induction dosing of the other drug (as above), followed by maintenance with

TABLE 4
Pharmacokinetic Parameters (mean ± S.D.) After a Single 60 mg/kg Dose of FOSCAVIR in 4 Groups* of Adults with Varying Degrees of Renal Function

Parameter	Group 1 (N=6)	Group 2 (N=6)	Group 3 (N=6)	Group 4 (N=4)
Creatinine clearance (mL/min)	108 ± 16	68 ± 8	34 ± 9	20 ± 4
Foscarnet CL (mL/min/kg)	2.13 ± 0.71	1.33 ± 0.43	0.46 ± 0.14	0.43 ± 0.26
Foscarnet half-life (hr)	1.93 ± 0.12	3.35 ± 0.87	13.0 ± 4.05	25.3 ± 18.7

* Group 1 patients had normal renal function defined as a creatinine clearance (CrCl) of >80 mL/min, Group 2 CrCl was 50–80 mL/min, Group 3 CrCl was 25–49 mL/min and Group 4 CrCl was 10–24 mL/min.

FOSCAVIR 90 mg/kg QD plus ganciclovir 5 mg/kg QD (Cmb). Assessment of retinitis progression was performed by masked evaluation of retinal photographs. The median times to retinitis progression or death were 39 days for the FOSCAVIR group, 61 days for the ganciclovir group and 105 days for the combination group. For the alternative endpoint of retinitis progression (censoring on death), the median times were 39 days for the FOSCAVIR group, 61 days for the ganciclovir group and 132 days for the combination group. Due to censoring on death, the latter analysis may overestimate the treatment effect. Treatment modifications due to toxicity were more common in the combination group than in the FOSCAVIR or ganciclovir monotherapy groups (see ADVERSE REACTIONS section).

Mucocutaneous Acyclovir-Resistant HSV Infections: In a controlled trial, patients with AIDS and mucocutaneous, acyclovir-resistant HSV infection were randomized to either FOSCAVIR (N=8) at a dose of 40 mg/kg TID or vidarabine (N=6) at a dose of 15 mg/kg per day. Eleven patients were nonrandomly assigned to receive treatment with FOSCAVIR because of prior intolerance to vidarabine. Lesions in the eight patients randomized to FOSCAVIR healed after 11 to 25 days; seven of the 11 patients non-randomly treated with FOSCAVIR healed their lesions in 10 to 30 days. Vidarabine was discontinued because of intolerance (N=4) or poor therapeutic response (N=2). In a second trial, forty AIDS patients and three bone marrow transplant recipients with mucocutaneous, acyclovir-resistant HSV infections were randomized to receive FOSCAVIR at a dose of either 40 mg/kg BID or 40 mg/kg TID. Fifteen of the 43 patients had healing of their lesions in 11 to 72 days with no difference in response between the two treatment groups.

INDICATIONS

CMV Retinitis: FOSCAVIR is indicated for the treatment of CMV retinitis in patients with acquired immunodeficiency syndrome (AIDS). Combination therapy with FOSCAVIR and ganciclovir is indicated for patients who have relapsed after monotherapy with either drug. SAFETY AND EFFICACY OF FOSCAVIR HAVE NOT BEEN ESTABLISHED FOR TREATMENT OF OTHER CMV INFECTIONS (e.g., PNEUMONITIS, GASTROENTERITIS); CONGENITAL OR NEONATAL CMV DISEASE; OR NON-IMMUNOCOMPROMISED INDIVIDUALS.

Mucocutaneous Acyclovir-Resistant HSV Infections: FOSCAVIR is indicated for the treatment of acyclovir-resistant mucocutaneous HSV infections in immunocompromised patients. SAFETY AND EFFICACY OF FOSCAVIR HAVE NOT BEEN ESTABLISHED FOR TREATMENT OF OTHER HSV INFECTIONS (e.g., RETINITIS, ENCEPHALITIS); CONGENITAL OR NEONATAL HSV DISEASE; OR HSV IN NON-IMMUNOCOMPROMISED INDIVIDUALS.

CONTRAINDICATIONS

FOSCAVIR is contraindicated in patients with clinically significant hypersensitivity to foscarnet sodium.

WARNINGS

Renal Impairment: THE MAJOR TOXICITY OF FOSCAVIR IS RENAL IMPAIRMENT (see ADVERSE REACTIONS section). Renal impairment is most likely to become clinically evident during the second week of induction therapy, but may occur at any time during FOSCAVIR treatment. Renal function should be monitored carefully during both induction and maintenance therapy (see PATIENT MONITORING section). Elevations in serum creatinine are usually, but not always, reversible following discontinuation or dose adjustment of FOSCAVIR. Safety and efficacy data for patients with baseline serum creatinine levels greater than 2.8 mg/dL or measured 24-hour creatinine clearances <50 mL/min are limited.

BECAUSE OF FOSCAVIR'S POTENTIAL TO CAUSE RENAL IMPAIRMENT, DOSE ADJUSTMENT BASED ON SERUM CREATININE IS NECESSARY. Hydration may reduce the risk of nephrotoxicity. It is recommended that 750–1000 mL of normal saline or 5% dextrose solution should be given prior to the first infusion of FOSCAVIR to establish diuresis. With subsequent infusions, 750–1000 mL of hydration fluid should be given with 90-120 mg/kg of FOSCAVIR, and 500 mL with 40–60 mg/kg of FOSCAVIR. Hydration fluid may need to be decreased if clinically warranted.

After the first dose, the hydration fluid should be administered concurrently with each infusion of FOSCAVIR.

Mineral and Electrolyte Abnormalities: FOSCAVIR has been associated with changes in serum electrolytes including hypocalcemia, hypophosphatemia, hyperphosphatemia, hypomagnesemia, and hypokalemia (see ADVERSE REACTIONS section). FOSCAVIR may also be associated with a dose-related decrease in ionized serum calcium which may not be reflected in total serum calcium. This effect is likely to be related to chelation of divalent metal ions such as calcium by foscarnet. Patients should be advised to report symptoms of low ionized calcium such as perioral tingling, numbness in the extremities and paresthesias. Particular caution and careful management of serum electrolytes is advised in patients with altered calcium or other electrolyte levels before treatment and especially in those with neurologic or cardiac abnormalities and those receiving other drugs known to influence minerals and electrolytes (see PATIENT MONITORING and Drug Interactions sections). Physicians should be prepared to treat these abnormalities and their sequalae such as tetany, seizures or cardiac disturbances. The rate of FOSCAVIR infusion may also affect the decrease in ionized calcium. **Therefore, an infusion pump must be used for administration to prevent rapid intravenous infusion (see DOSAGE AND ADMINISTRATION section).** Slowing the infusion rate may decrease or prevent symptoms.

Seizures: Seizures related to mineral and electrolyte abnormalities have been associated with FOSCAVIR treatment (see WARNING section; Mineral and Electrolyte Abnormalities). Several cases of seizures were associated with death. Risk factors associated with seizures included impaired baseline renal function, low total serum calcium, and underlying CNS conditions.

PRECAUTIONS

General: Care must be taken to infuse solutions containing FOSCAVIR only into veins with adequate blood flow to permit rapid dilution and distribution to avoid local irritation (see DOSAGE AND ADMINISTRATION). Local irritation and ulcerations of penile epithelium have been reported in male patients receiving FOSCAVIR, possibly related to the presence of drug in the urine. One case of vulvovaginal ulcerations in a female receiving FOSCAVIR has been reported. Adequate hydration with close attention to personal hygiene may minimize the occurrence of such events.

Hemopoietic System: Anemia has been reported in 33% of patients receiving FOSCAVIR in controlled studies. Granulocytopenia has been reported in 17% of patients receiving FOSCAVIR in controlled studies; however, only 1% (2/189) were terminated from these studies because of neutropenia.

Information for Patients:

CMV Retinitis—Patients should be advised that FOSCAVIR is not a cure for CMV retinitis, and that they may continue to experience progression of retinitis during or following treatment. They should be advised to have regular ophthalmologic examinations.

Mucocutaneous Acyclovir-Resistant HSV Infections—Patients should be advised that FOSCAVIR is not a cure for HSV infections. While complete healing is possible, relapse occurs in most patients. Because relapse may be due to acyclovir-sensitive HSV, sensitivity testing of the viral isolate is advised. In addition, repeated treatment with FOSCAVIR has led to the development of resistance associated with poorer response. In the case of poor therapeutic response, sensitivity testing of the viral isolate also is advised.

General—Patients should be informed that the major toxicities of foscarnet are renal impairment, electrolyte disturbances, and seizures, and that dose modifications and possibly discontinuation may be required. The importance of close monitoring while on therapy must be emphasized. Patients should be advised of the importance of reporting to their physicians symptoms of perioral tingling, numbness in the extremities or paresthesias during or after infusion as possible symptoms of electrolyte abnormalities. Should such symptoms occur, the infusion of FOSCAVIR should be stopped, appropriate laboratory samples for assessment of electrolyte concentrations obtained, and a physician consulted before resuming treatment. The rate of infusion must be no more than 1 mg/kg/minute. The potential for renal impairment may be minimized by accompanying FOSCAVIR administration with hydration adequate to establish and maintain a diuresis during dosing.

Drug Interactions: A possible drug interaction of FOSCAVIR and intravenous pentamidine has been described. Concomitant treatment of four patients in the United Kingdom with FOSCAVIR and intravenous pentamidine may have caused hypocalcemia; one patient died with severe hypocalcemia. Toxicity associated with concomitant use of aerosolized pentamidine has not been reported.

Because of foscarnet's tendency to cause renal impairment, the use of FOSCAVIR should be avoided in combination with potentially nephrotoxic drugs such as aminoglycosides, amphotericin B and intravenous pentamidine (see above) unless the potential benefits outweigh the risks to the patient.

Abnormal renal function has been reported in connection with the use of FOSCAVIR in combination with ritonavir and/or saquinavir.

Since FOSCAVIR decreases serum concentrations of ionized calcium, concurrent treatment with other drugs known to influence serum calcium concentrations should be used with particular caution.

Ganciclovir—The pharmacokinetics of foscarnet and ganciclovir were not altered in 13 patients receiving either concomitant therapy or daily alternating therapy for maintenance of CMV disease.

Carcinogenesis, Mutagenesis, Impairment of Fertility: Carcinogenicity studies were conducted in rats and mice at oral doses of 500 mg/kg/day and 250 mg/kg/day. Oral bioavailability in unfasted rodents is < 20%. No evidence of oncogenicity was reported at plasma drug levels equal to 1/3 and 1/5, respectively, of those in humans (at the maximum recommended human daily dose) as measured by the area-under-the-time/concentration curve (AUC).

FOSCAVIR showed genotoxic effects in the BALB/3T3 *in vitro* transformation assay at concentrations greater than 0.5 mcg/mL and an increased frequency of chromosome aberrations in the sister chromatid exchange assay at 1000 mcg/mL. A high dose of foscarnet (350 mg/kg) caused an increase in micronucleated polychromatic erythrocytes *in vivo* in mice at doses that produced exposures (area under curve) comparable to that anticipated clinically.

Pregnancy: Teratogenic Effect:

Pregnancy, Category C: FOSCAVIR did not adversely affect fertility and general reproductive performance in rats. The results of peri- and post-natal studies in rats were also negative. However, these studies used exposures that are inadequate to define the potential for impairment of fertility at human drug exposure levels.

Daily subcutaneous doses up to 75 mg/kg administered to female rats prior to and during mating, during gestation, and 21 days post-partum caused a slight increase (< 5%) in the number of skeletal anomalies compared with the control group. Daily subcutaneous doses up to 75 mg/kg administered to rabbits and 150 mg/kg administered to rats during gestation caused an increase in the frequency of skeletal anomalies/variations. On the basis of estimated drug exposure (as measured by AUC), the 150 mg/kg dose in rats and 75 mg/kg dose in rabbits were approximately one-eighth (rat) and one-third (rabbit) the estimated maximal daily human exposure. These studies are inadequate to define the potential teratogenicity at levels to which women will be exposed.

There are no adequate and well controlled studies in pregnant women. Because animal reproductive studies are not always predictive of human response, FOSCAVIR should be used during pregnancy only if clearly needed.

Nursing Mothers: It is not known whether FOSCAVIR is excreted in human milk; however, in lactating rats administered 75 mg/kg, FOSCAVIR was excreted in maternal milk at concentrations three times higher than peak maternal blood concentrations.

Pediatric Use: The safety and effectiveness of FOSCAVIR in pediatric patients have not been established. FOSCAVIR is deposited in teeth and bone and deposition is greater in young and growing animals. FOSCAVIR has been demonstrated to adversely affect development of tooth enamel in mice and rats. The effects of this deposition on skeletal development have not been studied. Since deposition in human bone has also been shown to occur, it is likely that it does so to a greater degree in developing bone in pediatric patients. Administration to pediatric patients should be undertaken only after careful evaluation and only if the potential benefits for treatment outweigh the risks.

Use in the Elderly: No studies of the efficacy or safety of FOSCAVIR in persons over age 65 have been conducted. Since these individuals frequently have reduced glomerular filtration, particular attention should be paid to assessing renal function before and during FOSCAVIR administration (see DOSAGE AND ADMINISTRATION).

ADVERSE REACTIONS

THE MAJOR TOXICITY OF FOSCAVIR IS RENAL IMPAIRMENT (see WARNINGS section). Approximately 33% of 189 patients with AIDS and CMV retinitis who received FOSCAVIR (60 mg/kg TID), without adequate hydration, developed significant impairment of renal function (serum creatinine ≥ 2.0 mg/dL). The incidence of renal impairment in subsequent clinical trials in which 1000 mL of normal saline or 5% dextrose solution was given with each infusion of FOSCAVIR was 12% (34/280).

FOSCAVIR has been associated with changes in serum electrolytes including hypocalcemia (15–30%), hypophosphatemia (8–26%) and hyperphosphatemia (6%), hypomagnesemia (15–30%), and hypokalemia (16–48%) (see WARNINGS section). The higher percentages were derived from those patients receiving hydration.

FOSCAVIR treatment was associated with seizures in 18/189 (10%) AIDS patients in the initial five controlled studies (see WARNINGS section). Risk factors associated with seizures included impaired baseline renal function, low total serum calcium, and underlying CNS conditions predisposing the patient to seizures. The rate of seizures did not increase with duration of treatment. Three cases were associated with overdoses of FOSCAVIR (see OVERDOSAGE section).

In five controlled U.S. clinical trials the most frequently reported adverse events in patients with AIDS and CMV retinitis are shown in Table 5. These figures were calculated without reference to drug relationship or severity.

TABLE 5—Adverse Events Reported in Five Controlled US Clinical Trials

	n = 189		n = 189
Fever	65%	**Abnormal Renal Function**	27%
Nausea	47%	**Vomiting**	26%

Continued on next page

Foscavir—Cont.

Anemia	33%	**Headache**	26%
Diarrhea	30%	**Seizures**	10%

From the same controlled studies, adverse events categorized by investigator as "severe" are shown in Table 6. Although death was specifically attributed to FOSCAVIR in only one case, other complications of FOSCAVIR (i.e., renal impairment, electrolyte abnormalities, and seizures) may have contributed to patient deaths (see WARNINGS section).

TABLE 6—Severe Adverse Events

	n = 189
Death	14%
Abnormal Renal Function	14%
Marrow Suppression	10%
Anemia	9%
Seizures	7%

From the five initial U.S. controlled trials of FOSCAVIR, the following list of adverse events has been compiled regardless of causal relationship to FOSCAVIR. Evaluation of these reports was difficult because of the diverse manifestations of the underlying disease and because most patients received numerous concomitant medications.

Incidence 5% or Greater

Body as a Whole: fever, fatigue, rigors, asthenia, malaise, pain, infection, sepsis, death

Central and Peripheral Nervous System: headache, paresthesia, dizziness, involuntary muscle contractions, hypoesthesia, neuropathy, seizures including grand mal seizures (see WARNINGS)

Gastrointestinal System: anorexia, nausea, diarrhea, vomiting, abdominal pain

Hematologic: anemia, granulocytopenia, leukopenia (see PRECAUTIONS)

Metabolic and Nutritional: mineral and electrolyte imbalances (see WARNINGS) including hypokalemia, hypocalcemia, hypomagnesemia, hypophosphatemia, hyperphosphatemia

Psychiatric: depression, confusion, anxiety

Respiratory System: coughing, dyspnea

Skin and Appendages: rash, increased sweating

Urinary: alterations in renal function including increased serum creatinine, decreased creatinine clearance, and abnormal renal function (see WARNINGS)

Special Senses: vision abnormalities

Incidence between 1% and 5%

Application Site: injection site pain, injection site inflammation

Body as a Whole: back pain, chest pain, edema, influenza-like symptoms, bacterial infections, moniliasis, fungal infections, abscess

Cardiovascular: hypertension, palpitations, ECG abnormalities including sinus tachycardia, first degree AV block and non-specific ST-T segment changes, hypotension, flushing, cerebrovascular disorder (see WARNINGS)

Central and Peripheral Nervous System: tremor, ataxia, dementia, stupor, generalized spasms, sensory disturbances, meningitis, aphasia, abnormal coordination, leg cramps, EEG abnormalities (see WARNINGS)

Gastrointestinal: constipation, dysphagia, dyspepsia, rectal hemorrhage, dry mouth, melena, flatulence, ulcerative stomatitis, pancreatitis

Hematologic: thrombocytopenia, platelet abnormalities, thrombosis, white blood cell abnormalities, lymphadenopathy

Liver and Biliary: abnormal A-G ratio, abnormal hepatic function, increased SGPT, increased SGOT

Metabolic and Nutritional: hyponatremia, decreased weight, increased alkaline phosphatase, increased LDH, increased BUN, acidosis, cachexia, thirst, hypercalcemia (see WARNINGS)

Musculo-Skeletal: arthralgia, myalgia

Neoplasms: lymphoma-like disorder, sarcoma

Psychiatric: insomnia, somnolence, nervousness, amnesia, agitation, aggressive reaction, hallucination

Respiratory System: pneumonia, sinusitis, pharyngitis, rhinitis, respiratory disorders, respiratory insufficiency, pulmonary infiltration, stridor, pneumothorax, hemoptysis, bronchospasm

Skin and Appendages: pruritus, skin ulceration, seborrhea, erythematous rash, maculo-papular rash, skin discoloration

Special Senses: taste perversions, eye abnormalities, eye pain, conjunctivitis

Urinary System: albuminuria, dysuria, polyuria, urethral disorder, urinary retention, urinary tract infections, acute renal failure, nocturia, facial edema

Selected adverse events occurring at a rate of less than 1% in the five initial U.S. controlled clinical trials of FOSCAVIR include: syndrome of inappropriate antidiuretic hormone secretion, pancytopenia, hematuria, dehydration, hypoproteinemia, increases in amylase and creatinine phosphokinase, cardiac arrest, coma, and other cardiovascular and neurologic complications.

Selected adverse event data from the Foscarnet vs. Ganciclovir CMV Retinitis Trial (FGCRT), performed by the Studies of the Ocular Complications of AIDS (SOCA) Research Group, are shown in Table 7 (see CLINICAL TRIALS section).

[See table 7 below]

Selected adverse events from ACTG Study 228 (CRRT) comparing combination therapy with FOSCAVIR or ganciclovir monotherapy are shown in Table 8. The most common reason for a treatment change in patients assigned to either FOSCAVIR or ganciclovir was retinitis progression. The most frequent reason for a treatment change in the combination treatment group was toxicity.

[See table 8 at bottom of next page]

Adverse events that have been reported in post-marketing surveillance include: ventricular arrhythmia, prolongation of QT interval, diabetes insipidus (usually nephrogenic), and muscle disorders including myopathy, myositis, muscle weakness and rare cases of rhabdomyolysis. Cases of vesiculobullous eruptions including erythema multiforme, toxic epidermal necrolysis, and Stevens-Johnson Syndrome have been reported. In most cases, patients were taking other medications that have been associated with toxic epidermal necrolysis or Stevens-Johnson Syndrome.

OVERDOSAGE

In controlled clinical trials performed in the United States, overdosage with FOSCAVIR was reported in 10 out of 189 patients. All 10 patients experienced adverse events and all except one made a complete recovery. One patient died after receiving a total daily dose of 12.5 g for three days instead of the intended 10.9 g. The patient suffered a grand mal seizure and became comatose. Three days later the patient expired with the cause of death listed as respiratory/cardiac arrest. The other nine patients received doses ranging from 1.14 times to 8 times their recommended doses with an average of 4 times their recommended doses. Overall, three patients had seizures, three patients had renal function impairment, four patients had paresthesias either in limbs or periorally, and five patients had documented electrolyte disturbances primarily involving calcium and phosphate.

The pattern of adverse events associated with overdose in post-marketing surveillance is consistent with the symptoms previously observed during foscarnet therapy.

There is no specific antidote for FOSCAVIR overdose. Hemodialysis and hydration may be of benefit in reducing drug plasma levels in patients who receive an overdosage of FOSCAVIR, but the effectiveness of these interventions has not been evaluated. The patient should be observed for signs and symptoms of renal impairment and electrolyte imbalance. Medical treatment should be instituted if clinically warranted.

DOSAGE AND ADMINISTRATION

CAUTION—DO NOT ADMINISTER FOSCAVIR BY RAPID OR BOLUS INTRAVENOUS INJECTION. THE TOXICITY OF FOSCAVIR MAY BE INCREASED AS A RESULT OF EXCESSIVE PLASMA LEVELS. CARE SHOULD BE TAKEN TO AVOID UNINTENTIONAL OVERDOSE BY CAREFULLY CONTROLLING THE RATE OF INFUSION. THEREFORE, AN INFUSION PUMP MUST BE USED. IN SPITE OF THE USE OF AN INFUSION PUMP, OVERDOSES HAVE OCCURRED.

ADMINISTRATION

FOSCAVIR is administered by controlled intravenous infusion, either by using a central venous line or by using a peripheral vein. The standard 24 mg/mL solution may be used with or without dilution when using a central venous catheter for infusion. When a peripheral vein catheter is used, the 24 mg/mL solution **must** be diluted to 12 mg/mL with 5% dextrose in water or with a normal saline solution prior to administration to avoid local irritation of peripheral veins. Since the dose of FOSCAVIR is calculated on the basis of body weight, it may be desirable to remove and discard any unneeded quantity from the bottle before starting with the infusion to avoid overdosage. Dilutions and/or removals of excess quantities should be accomplished under aseptic conditions. Solutions thus prepared should be used within 24 hours of first entry into a sealed bottle. *To reduce the risk of nephrotoxicity, creatinine clearance (mL/min/kg) should be calculated even if serum creatinine is within the normal range, and doses should be adjusted accordingly.*

Hydration: Hydration may reduce the risk of nephrotoxicity. It is recommended that 750–1000 mL of normal saline or 5% dextrose solution should be given prior to the first infusion of FOSCAVIR to establish diuresis. With subsequent infusions, 750–1000 mL of hydration fluid should be given with 90–120 mg/kg of FOSCAVIR, and 500 mL with 40–60 mg/kg of FOSCAVIR. Hydration fluid may need to be decreased if clinically warranted.

After the first dose, the hydration fluid should be administered concurrently with each infusion of FOSCAVIR.

Compatibility With Other Solutions/Drugs: Other drugs and supplements can be administered to a patient receiving FOSCAVIR. However, care must be taken to ensure that FOSCAVIR is only administered with normal saline or 5% dextrose solution and that no other drug or supplement is administered concurrently via the same catheter. Foscarnet has been reported to be chemically incompatible with 30% dextrose, amphotericin B, and solutions containing calcium such as Ringer's lactate and TPN. Physical incompatibility with other IV drugs has also been reported including acyclovir sodium, ganciclovir, trimetrexate glucuronate, pentamidine isethionate, vancomycin, trimethoprim/sulfamethoxazole, diazepam, midazolam, digoxin, phenytoin, leucovorin, and prochlorperazine. Because of foscarnet's chelating properties, a precipitate can potentially occur when divalent cations are administered concurrently in the same catheter.

Parenteral drug products must be inspected visually for particulate matter and discoloration prior to administration whenever the solution and container permit. Solutions that are discolored or contain particulate matter should not be used.

Accidental Exposure: Accidental skin and eye contact with foscarnet sodium solution may cause local irritation and burning sensation. If accidental contact occurs, the exposed area should be flushed with water.

DOSAGE

THE RECOMMENDED DOSAGE, FREQUENCY, OR INFUSION RATES SHOULD NOT BE EXCEEDED. ALL DOSES MUST BE INDIVIDUALIZED FOR PATIENTS' RENAL FUNCTION.

Induction Treatment: The recommended initial dose of FOSCAVIR for patients with normal renal function is:

- For CMV retinitis patients, either 90 mg/kg (1-1/2 to 2 hour infusion) every twelve hours or 60 mg/kg (minimum one hour infusion) every eight hours over 2-3 weeks depending on clinical response.
- For acyclovir-resistant HSV patients, 40 mg/kg (minimum one hour infusion) either every 8 or 12 hours for 2-3 weeks or until healed.

An infusion pump must be used to control the rate of infusion. Adequate hydration is recommended to establish a diuresis (see Hydration for recommendation), both prior to and during treatment to minimize renal toxicity (see WARNINGS), provided there are no clinical contraindications.

Maintenance Treatment: Following induction treatment the recommended maintenance dose of FOSCAVIR for CMV retinitis is 90 mg/kg/day to 120 mg/kg/day (individualized for renal function) given as an intravenous infusion over 2 hours. Because the superiority of the 120 mg/kg/day has not been established in controlled trials, and given the likely relationship of higher plasma foscarnet levels to toxicity, it is

TABLE 7—FGCRT: SELECTED ADVERSE EVENTS*

EVENT	GANCICLOVIR No. of Events	GANCICLOVIR No. of Patients	GANCICLOVIR Rates§	FOSCARNET No. of Events	FOSCARNET No. of Patients	FOSCARNET Rates§
Absolute neutrophil count decreasing to <0.50 × 10^9 per liter	63	41	1.30	31	17	0.72
Serum creatinine increasing to >260 μmol per liter (>2.9 mg/dL)	6	4	0.12	13	9	0.30
Seizure‡	21	13	0.37	19	13	0.37
Catheterization-related infection	49	27	1.26	51	28	1.46
Hospitalization	209	91	4.74	202	75	5.03

* Values for the treatment groups refer only to patients who completed at least one follow-up visit—i.e., 113 to 119 patients in the ganciclovir group and 93 to 100 in the foscarnet group. "Events" denotes all events observed and "patients" the number of patients with one or more of the indicated events.

‡ Final frozen SOCA I database dated October 1991.

§ Per person-year at risk

recommended that most patients be started on maintenance treatment with a dose of 90 mg/kg/day. Escalation to 120 mg/kg/day may be considered should early reinduction be required because of retinitis progression. Some patients who show excellent tolerance to FOSCAVIR may benefit from initiation of maintenance treatment at 120 mg/kg/day earlier in their treatment.

An infusion pump must be used to control the rate of infusion with all doses. Again, hydration to establish diuresis both prior to and during treatment is recommended to minimize renal toxicity, provided there are no clinical contraindications (see WARNINGS).

Patients who experience progression of retinitis while receiving FOSCAVIR maintenance therapy may be retreated with the induction and maintenance regimens given above or with a combination of FOSCAVIR and ganciclovir (see CLINICAL TRIALS section). **Because of physical incompatibility, FOSCAVIR and ganciclovir must NOT be mixed.**
Use in Patients with Abnormal Renal Function: FOSCAVIR should be used with caution in patients with abnormal renal function because reduced plasma clearance of foscarnet will result in elevated plasma levels (see CLINICAL PHARMACOLOGY). In addition, FOSCAVIR has the potential to further impair renal function (see WARNINGS). Safety and efficacy data for patients with baseline serum creatinine levels greater than 2.8 mg/dL or measured 24-hour creatinine clearances < 50 mL/min are limited.

Renal function must be monitored carefully at baseline and during induction and maintenance therapy with appropriate dose adjustments for FOSCAVIR as outlined below (see Dose Adjustment and PATIENT MONITORING). During FOSCAVIR therapy if creatinine clearance falls below the limits of the dosing nomograms (0.4 mL/min/kg), FOSCAVIR should be discontinued, the patient hydrated, and monitored daily until resolution of renal impairment is ensured.

Dose Adjustment: FOSCAVIR dosing must be individualized according to the patient's renal function status. Refer to Table 9 below for recommended doses and adjust the dose as indicated. Even patients with serum creatinine in the normal range may require dose adjustment; therefore, the dose should be calculated at baseline and frequently thereafter. To use this dosing guide, actual 24-hour creatinine clearance (mL/min) must be divided by body weight (kg), or the estimated creatinine clearance in mL/min/kg can be calculated from serum creatinine (mg/dL) using the following formula (modified Cockcroft and Gault equation):

For males:

$$\frac{140 - age}{serum\ creatinine \times 72} \quad (\times\ 0.85\ for\ females) = mL/min/kg$$

[See table 9 above]

PATIENT MONITORING

The majority of patients will experience some decrease in renal function due to FOSCAVIR administration. Therefore it is recommended that creatinine clearance, either measured or estimated using the modified Cockcroft and Gault equation based on serum creatinine, be determined at baseline, 2–3 times per week during induction therapy and at least every one to two weeks during maintenance therapy, with FOSCAVIR dose adjusted accordingly (see Dose Adjustment). More frequent monitoring may be required for some patients. It is also recommended that a 24-hour creatinine clearance be determined at baseline and periodically

thereafter to ensure correct dosing (assuming verification of an adequate collection using creatinine index). FOSCAVIR should be discontinued if creatinine clearance drops below 0.4 mL/min/kg.

Due to FOSCAVIR's propensity to chelate divalent metal ions and alter levels of serum electrolytes, patients must be monitored closely for such changes. It is recommended that a schedule similar to that recommended for serum creatinine (see above) be used to monitor serum calcium, magnesium, potassium and phosphorus. Particular caution is advised in patients with decreased total serum calcium or other electrolyte levels before treatment, as well as in patients with neurologic or cardiac abnormalities, and in patients receiving other drugs known to influence serum calcium levels. Any clinically significant metabolic changes should be corrected. Also, patients who experience mild (e.g., perioral numbness or paresthesias) or severe (e.g., seizures) symptoms of electrolyte abnormalities should have serum electrolyte and mineral levels assessed as close in time to the event as possible.

Careful monitoring and appropriate management of electrolytes, calcium, magnesium and creatinine are of particular importance in patients with conditions that may predispose them to seizures (see WARNINGS).

HOW SUPPLIED

FOSCAVIR (foscarnet sodium) INJECTION, 24 mg/mL for intravenous infusion, is supplied in glass bottles as follows:
NDC 0186-1906-01   500 mL bottles,   cases of 12
NDC 0186-1905-01   250 mL bottles,   cases of 12

TABLE 9
FOSCAVIR DOSING GUIDE
INDUCTION

CrCl (mL/min/kg)	HSV: Equivalent to		CMV: Equivalent to	
	80 mg/kg/day total (40 mg/kg Q12h)	120 mg/kg/day total (40 mg/kg Q8h)	180 mg/kg/day total (60 mg/kg Q8h)	(90 mg/kg Q12h)
>1.4	40 Q12h	40 Q8h	60 Q8h	90 Q12h
>1.0–1.4	30 Q12h	30 Q8h	45 Q8h	70 Q12h
>0.8–1.0	20 Q12h	**35 Q12h**	**50 Q12h**	50 Q12h
>0.6–0.8	**35 Q24h**	25 Q12h	**40 Q12h**	**80 Q24h**
>0.5–0.6	**25 Q24h**	40 Q24h	60 Q24h	**60 Q24h**
≥0.4–0.5	**20 Q24h**	35 Q24h	50 Q24h	**50 Q24h**
<0.4	Not Recommended	Not Recommended	Not Recommended	Not Recommended

MAINTENANCE

CrCl (mL/min/kg)	CMV: Equivalent to	
	90 mg/kg/day (once daily)	120 mg/kg/day (once daily)
>1.4	90 Q24h	120 Q24h
>1.0–1.4	70 Q24h	90 Q24h
>0.8–1.0	50 Q24h	65 Q24h
>0.6–0.8	**80 Q48h**	**105 Q48h**
>0.5–0.6	**60 Q48h**	**80 Q48h**
≥0.4–0.5	**50 Q48h**	**65 Q48h**
<0.4	Not Recommended	Not Recommended

> means "greater than"; ≥ means "greater than or equal to"; < means "less than"

FOSCAVIR INJECTION should be stored at controlled room temperature, 15°–30°C (59°–86°F), and should be protected from excessive heat (above 40°C) and from freezing. FOSCAVIR INJECTION should be used only if the bottle and seal are intact, a vacuum is present, and the solution is clear and colorless.
Caution: Federal law prohibits dispensing without prescription.
Manufactured by:
Abbott Laboratories, North Chicago, IL 60064
Manufactured for:
Astra USA, Inc., Westborough, MA 01581
000571R07   Rev. 2/98

FUROSEMIDE INJECTION, USP   ℞
[fū "rō 'sĕ-mīde]
10 mg/mL

PROTECT FROM LIGHT · DO NOT USE IF THE SOLUTION IS DISCOLORED · STORE AT CONTROLLED ROOM TEMPERATURE
WARNING: Furosemide is a potent diuretic which, if given in excessive amounts, can lead to a profound diuresis with water and electrolyte depletion. Therefore, careful medical supervision is required, and the dose and dose schedule have to be adjusted to each patient's needs.
(See under DOSAGE AND ADMINISTRATION.)
(For details of indications, dosage, and administration, precautions, and adverse reactions, see circular in package.)

HOW SUPPLIED

Furosemide Injection, USP, 10 mg/mL is supplied in the following forms:
Single Dose Vials
2 mL   (20 mg),   25 per package,   NDC 0186-1114-13
4 mL   (40 mg),   25 per package,   NDC 0186-1115-13
8 mL   (80 mg),   25 per package,   NDC 0186-1116-12
10 mL (100 mg),   25 per package,   NDC 0186-1117-12
Prefilled Syringes supplied with 21 gauge × $^{15}/_{16}$" needle
4 mL   (40 mg),   Boxes of 10,   NDC 0186-0635-01
10 mL (100 mg), Boxes of 10,   NDC 0186-0636-01
Store in carton to protect from light.
To insure patient safety, this needle should be handled with care and should be destroyed and discarded if damaged in any manner. If cannula is bent, no attempt should be made to straighten.
To prevent needle-stick injuries, needles should not be recapped, purposely bent, or broken by hand.
All solutions should be stored at controlled room temperature 15°–30°C (59°–86°F) and should be protected from light. Do not use if the solution is discolored.
021877R13   Rev. 11/97

HYDROMORPHONE HCl INJECTION   ℞

(For details of indications, dosages and administration, precautions, and adverse reactions, see circular in package.)

TABLE 8
CRRT: Selected Adverse Events

	Foscavir N=88			Ganciclovir N=93			Combination N=93		
	No. Events	No. Pts.†	Rate‡	No. Events	No. Pts.†	Rate‡	No. Events	No. Pts.†	Rate‡
Anemia (Hgb <70 g/L)	11	7	0.20	9	7	0.14	19	15	0.33
Neutropenia§									
ANC <0.75 × 10⁹ cells/L	86	32	1.53	95	41	1.51	107	51	1.91
ANC <0.50 × 10⁹ cells/L	50	25	0.91	49	28	0.80	50	28	0.85
Thrombocytopenia									
Platelets <50 × 10⁹/L	28	14	0.50	19	8	0.43	40	15	0.56
Platelets <20 × 10⁹/L	1	1	0.01	6	2	0.05	7	6	0.18
Nephrotoxicity									
Creatinine >260 μmol/L (>2.9 mg/dL)	9	7	0.15	10	7	0.17	11	10	0.20
Seizures	6	6	0.17	7	6	0.15	10	5	0.18
Hospitalizations	86	53	1.86	111	59	2.36	118	64	2.36

† Pts. = patients with event;
‡ Rate = events/person/year;
§ ANC = absolute neutrophil count

Hydromorphone HCl—Cont.

HOW SUPPLIED

NDC 0186-1309-01   2 mg/mL - 20 mL multiple dose vials
Storage: Store at 15°–30°C (59°–86°F). Protect from light.
021888R01   11/91 (1)

LEUCOVORIN CALCIUM TABLETS, USP ℞
5 mg and 25 mg

DESCRIPTION

Leucovorin Calcium Tablets contain either 5 mg or 25 mg of leucovorin as the calcium salt of N-[4-[[(2-amino-5-formyl-1,4,5,6,7,8-hexahydro-4-oxo-6-pteridinyl)-methyl]amino]benzoyl]-L-glutamic acid. This is equivalent to 5.40 mg or 27.01 mg of anhydrous leucovorin calcium.
Leucovorin is a water soluble form of reduced folate in the folate group; it is useful as an antidote to drugs which act as folic acid antagonists. These tablets are intended for oral administration only. The structural formula of leucovorin calcium (which normally exists as a hydrate, 8% to 15% water) is:

$C_{20}H_{21}CaN_7O_7$ 511.51

Each tablet for oral administration contains leucovorin calcium, equivalent to 5 mg or 25 mg of leucovorin. The inactive ingredients are lactose monohydrate, potato starch, povidone, magnesium stearate and colloidal silicon dioxide.

CLINICAL PHARMACOLOGY

Leucovorin is a racemic mixture of the diastereoisomers of the 5-formyl derivative of tetrahydrofolic acid. The biologically active component of the mixture is the (-)-L-isomer, known as *Citrovorum factor*, or (-)-folinic acid. Leucovorin does **not** require reduction by the enzyme dihydrofolate reductase in order to participate in reactions utilizing folates as a source of "one-carbon" moieties. Following oral administration, leucovorin is rapidly absorbed and enters the general body pool of *reduced folates*. The increase in plasma and serum folate activity (determined microbiologically with *Lactobacillus casei*) seen after oral administration of leucovorin is predominantly due to 5-methyltetrahydrofolate.
Twenty normal men were given a single, oral 15 mg dose (7.5 mg/m²) of leucovorin calcium and serum folate concentrations were assayed with L casei. Mean values observed (± one standard error) were:
a) Time to peak serum folate concentration:
1.72 ± 0.08 hrs.,
b) Peak serum folate concentration achieved:
268 ± 18 ng/mL,
c) Serum folate half-disappearance time: 3.5 hours.
Oral tablets yielded areas under the serum folate concentration-time curves (AUC's) that were 12% greater than equal amounts of leucovorin given intramuscularly and equal to the same amounts given intravenously.
Oral absorption of leucovorin is saturable at doses above 25 mg. The apparent bioavailability of leucovorin was 97% for 25 mg, 75% for 50 mg and 37% for 100 mg.

INDICATIONS AND USAGE

Leucovorin Calcium Tablets are indicated to diminish the toxicity and counteract the effects of impaired methotrexate elimination and of inadvertent overdosages of folic acid antagonists.

CONTRAINDICATIONS

Leucovorin is improper therapy for pernicious anemia and other megaloblastic anemias secondary to the lack of vitamin B_{12}. A hematologic remission may occur while neurological manifestations continue to progress.

WARNINGS

In the treatment of accidental overdosage of folic acid antagonists, leucovorin should be administered as promptly as possible. As the time interval between antifolate administration (e.g., methotrexate) and leucovorin rescue increases, leucovorin's effectiveness in counteracting hematologic toxicity decreases.
Monitoring of the serum methotrexate concentration is essential in determining the optimal dose and duration of treatment with leucovorin.
Delayed methotrexate excretion may be caused by a third space fluid accumulation (i.e., ascites, pleural effusion), renal insufficiency, or inadequate hydration. Under such circumstances, higher doses of leucovorin or prolonged administration may be indicated. Doses higher than those recommended for oral use must be given intravenously.
Leucovorin may enhance the toxicity of fluorouracil. Deaths from severe enterocolitis, diarrhea, and dehydration have

been reported in elderly patients receiving weekly leucovorin and fluorouracil[1]. Concomitant granulocytopenia and fever were present in some but not all of the patients.
The concomitant use of leucovorin with trimethoprim-sulfamethoxazole for the acute treatment of *Pneumocystis carinii* pneumonia in patients with HIV infection was associated with increased rates of treatment failure and morbidity in a placebo-controlled study.

PRECAUTIONS

General: Parenteral administration of leucovorin is preferable to oral dosing if there is a possibility that the patient may vomit or not absorb the leucovorin. Leucovorin has no effect on other established toxicities of methotrexate such as the nephrotoxicity resulting from drug and/or metabolite precipitation in the kidney.
Drug Interactions: Folic acid in large amounts may counteract the antiepileptic effect of phenobarbital, phenytoin and primidone, and increase the frequency of seizures in susceptible children.
Preliminary animal and human studies have shown that small quantities of systemically administered leucovorin enter the CSF primarily as 5-methyltetrahydrofolate and, in humans, remain 1 to 3 orders of magnitude lower than the usual methotrexate concentration following intrathecal administration. However, high doses of leucovorin may reduce the efficacy of intrathecally administered methotrexate.
Leucovorin may enhance the toxicity of fluorouracil (see WARNINGS).
Pregnancy: *Teratogenic Effects*—Pregnancy Category C. Animal reproduction studies have not been conducted with leucovorin. It is also not known whether leucovorin can cause fetal harm when administered to a pregnant woman or can affect reproduction capacity. Leucovorin should be given to a pregnant woman only if clearly needed.
Nursing Mothers: It is not known whether this drug is excreted in human milk. Because many drugs are excreted in human milk, caution should be exercised when leucovorin is administered to a nursing mother.
Pediatric Use: See "Drug Interactions" subsection.

ADVERSE REACTIONS

Allergic sensitization, including anaphylactoid reactions and urticaria, has been reported following the administration of both oral and parenteral leucovorin.

OVERDOSAGE

Excessive amounts of leucovorin may nullify the chemotherapeutic effect of folic acid antagonists.

DOSAGE AND ADMINISTRATION

Leucovorin Calcium Tablets are intended for oral administration. Because absorption is saturable, oral administration of doses greater than 25 mg is not recommended.
Impaired Methotrexate Elimination or Inadvertent Overdosage: Leucovorin rescue should begin as soon as possible after an inadvertent overdosage and within 24 hours of methotrexate administration when there is delayed excretion (see WARNINGS). Leucovorin 15 mg (10 mg/m²) should be administered IM, IV, or PO every 6 hours until the serum methotrexate level is less than 10⁻⁸M. In the presence of gastrointestinal toxicity, nausea or vomiting, leucovorin should be administered parenterally.
Serum creatinine and methotrexate levels should be determined at 24 hour intervals. If the 24 hour serum creatinine has increased 50% over baseline or if the 24 hour methotrexate level is greater than 5×10^{-6}M or the 48 hour level is greater than 9×10^{-7}M, the dose of leucovorin should be increased to 150 mg (100 mg/m²) IV every 3 hours until the methotrexate level is less than 10⁻⁸M. Doses greater than 25 mg should be given parenterally (see CLINICAL PHARMACOLOGY).
Hydration (3L/d) and urinary alkalinization with sodium bicarbonate should be employed concomitantly. The bicarbonate dose should be adjusted to maintain the urine pH at 7.0 or greater.
The recommended dose of leucovorin to counteract hematologic toxicity from folic acid antagonists with less affinity for mammalian dihydrofolate reductase than methotrexate (i.e., trimethoprim, pyrimethamine) is substantially less and 5 to 15 mg of leucovorin per day has been recommended by some investigators.
Patients who experience delayed early methotrexate elimination are likely to develop reversible non-oliguric renal failure. In addition to appropriate leucovorin therapy, these patients require continuing hydration and urinary alkalinization, and close monitoring of fluid and electrolyte status, until the serum methotrexate level has fallen to below 0.05 micromolar and the renal failure has resolved.
Some patients will have abnormalities in methotrexate elimination or renal function following methotrexate administration, which are significant but less severe. These abnormalities may or may not be associated with significant clinical toxicity. If significant clinical toxicity is observed, leucovorin rescue should be extended for an additional 24 hours (total of 14 doses over 84 hours) in subsequent courses of therapy. The possibility that the patient is taking

other medications which interact with methotrexate (e.g., medications which may interfere with methotrexate elimination or binding to serum albumin) should always be reconsidered when laboratory abnormalities or clinical toxicities are observed.

HOW SUPPLIED

Leucovorin Calcium Tablets equivalent to 5 mg of leucovorin are round, yellowish-white, scored tablets, identified with PCH on one side and RES above the score and 5 below the score on the other side, available in packages of 50 tablets (10 strips of 5 tablets), NDC 0186-1601-78, and in containers with respectively 30 or 100 tablets, NDC 0186-1601-30 or NDC 0186-1601-05.
Leucovorin Calcium Tablets equivalent to 25 mg of leucovorin are round, yellowish-white, scored tablets, identified with PCH on one side and RES above the score and 25 below the score on the other side, available in packages of 10 tablets (2 strips of 5 tablets), NDC 0186-1603-78, and in a container with 25 tablets, NDC 0186-1603-25.
Store between 15° to 25°C (59° to 77°F) [see USP].

REFERENCES

1. Grem JL, Shoemaker DD, Petrelli NJ, Douglass HO Jr. Severe and fatal toxic effects observed in treatment with high- and low-dose leucovorin plus 5-fluorouracil for colorectal carcinoma. *Cancer Treat Rep* 1987;71:1122.
2. Link MP, Goorin AM, Miser AW, et al. The effect of adjuvant chemotherapy on relapse-free survival patients with osteosarcoma of the extremity. *N Engl J Med* 1986; 314: 1600–1606.

Manufactured by:
Pharmachemie B.V., Haarlem, Holland

Manufactured for:
Astra USA, Inc., Westborough, MA 01581
001601R00   Iss. 8/97

LEXXEL® ℞
(ENALAPRIL MALEATE-FELODIPINE ER) TABLETS

USE IN PREGNANCY

When used in pregnancy during the second and third trimesters, ACE inhibitors can cause injury and even death to the developing fetus. When pregnancy is detected, LEXXEL should be discontinued as soon as possible. See WARNINGS, *Fetal/Neonatal Morbidity and Mortality*.

DESCRIPTION

LEXXEL* (Enalapril Maleate-Felodipine ER) is a combination product, consisting of an outer layer of enalapril maleate surrounding a core tablet of an extended-release felodipine formulation.
Enalapril maleate is the maleate salt of enalapril, the ethyl ester of a long-acting angiotensin converting enzyme inhibitor, enalaprilat. Enalapril maleate is chemically described as (S)-1-[N-[1-(ethoxycarbonyl)-3-phenylpropyl]-L-alanyl]-L-proline, (Z)-2-butenedioate salt (1:1). Its empirical formula is $C_{20}H_{28}N_2O_5 \cdot C_4H_4O_4$, and its structural formula is:

Enalapril maleate is a white to off-white, crystalline powder with a molecular weight of 492.53. It is sparingly soluble in water, soluble in ethanol, and freely soluble in methanol.
Felodipine, a calcium channel blocker, is a dihydropyridine derivative that is chemically described as ± ethyl methyl 4-(2,3-dichlorophenyl)-1,4-dihydro-2,6-dimethyl-3,5-pyridinedicarboxylate. Its empirical formula is $C_{18}H_{19}Cl_2NO_4$ and its structural formula is:

Felodipine is a slightly yellowish, crystalline powder with a molecular weight of 384.26. It is insoluble in water and is freely soluble in dichloromethane and ethanol. Felodipine is a racemic mixture; however, *S*-felodipine is the more biologically active enantiomer.

LEXXEL is available for oral use as tablets containing 5 mg of enalapril maleate, and 5 mg of felodipine as an extended-release formulation. Inactive ingredients include: propyl gallate, polyoxyl 40 hydrogenated castor oil, cellulose compounds, lactose, aluminum silicate, sodium stearyl fumarate, carnauba wax, and black iron oxide. The tablets are imprinted with an ink of synthetic black iron oxide which contains pharmaceutical glaze in SD-45, n-butyl alcohol, propylene glycol, isopropyl alcohol, methyl alcohol, and ammonium hydroxide.

*Registered trademark of Astra Pharmaceuticals, L.P.

CLINICAL PHARMACOLOGY

Mechanism of Action

The two components of LEXXEL have complementary antihypertensive actions. **Enalapril** is a pro-drug; following oral administration, it is bioactivated by hydrolysis of the ethyl ester to enalaprilat, which is the active angiotensin converting enzyme (ACE) inhibitor. Enalaprilat inhibits angiotensin-converting enzyme in humans and animals. ACE is a peptidyl dipeptidase that catalyzes the conversion of angiotensin I to the vasoconstrictor substance, angiotensin II. Angiotensin II also stimulates aldosterone secretion by the adrenal cortex. The beneficial effects of enalapril in hypertension appear to result primarily from suppression of the renin-angiotensin-aldosterone system.

Inhibition of ACE results in decreased plasma angiotensin II, which leads to decreased vasopressor activity, and to decreased aldosterone secretion. Although the latter decrease is small, it results in small increases of serum potassium. In hypertensive patients treated with enalapril maleate alone for up to 48 weeks, mean increases in serum potassium of approximately 0.2 mEq/L were observed. In patients treated with enalapril maleate plus a thiazide diuretic, there was essentially no change in serum potassium. (See PRECAUTIONS.) Removal of angiotensin II negative feedback on renin secretion leads to increased plasma renin activity.

ACE is identical to kininase, an enzyme that degrades bradykinin. Whether increased levels of bradykinin, a potent vasodepressor peptide, play a role in the therapeutic effects of enalapril maleate remains to be elucidated.

While the mechanism through which enalapril lowers blood pressure is believed to be primarily suppression of the renin-angiotensin-aldosterone system, enalapril is antihypertensive even in patients with low-renin hypertension. Although enalapril was antihypertensive in all races studied, black hypertensive patients (usually a low-renin hypertensive population) had a smaller average response to enalapril monotherapy than non-black patients.

Felodipine is a dihydropyridine calcium channel blocker that reduces the influx of Ca^{++} by an effect on the voltage dependent L-channels in vascular smooth muscle and cultured rabbit atrial cells, and blocks potassium-induced contracture of the rat portal vein.

Pharmacologic studies show that the effects of felodipine on contractile processes are selective, with greater effects on vascular smooth muscle than cardiac muscle. Negative inotropic effects can be detected *in vitro*, but such effects have not been seen in intact animals.

The consequences of vasodilation produced by felodipine include a modest, short-lived reflex increase in heart rate. A mild diuretic effect is seen in several animal species and man, but most of the effects of felodipine are accounted for by its effects on peripheral vascular resistance.

Pharmacokinetics and Metabolism

Concomitant administration of enalapril and felodipine as an extended-release formulation has little effect on the bioavailability of either compound. The rate and extent of absorption of enalapril from LEXXEL is not significantly different from that of enalapril in VASOTEC** (Enalapril Maleate). The rate and extent of absorption of felodipine from LEXXEL has not been directly compared to the extended-release formulation of felodipine in PLENDIL*** (Felodipine).

Following oral administration of LEXXEL, peak concentrations of enalapril occur within about one hour. Enalapril is hydrolyzed to enalaprilat, which is a more potent angiotensin converting enzyme inhibitor than enalapril. Peak serum concentrations of enalaprilat occur about three hours after an oral dose of LEXXEL. Based on urinary recovery, the extent of absorption of enalapril is approximately 60 percent.

**Registered trademark of Merck & Co., Inc.

***Registered trademark of Astra AB

Peak concentrations of the isomers of felodipine are generally seen at 3–6 hours after administration of LEXXEL. Following oral administration, felodipine is almost completely absorbed and undergoes extensive first-pass metabolism; the systemic bioavailability of felodipine ER is approximately 20 percent.

When LEXXEL is taken with food (a substantial meal of 650 kcal or greater), some of the pharmacokinetics of its components are changed. Although the $AUC_{(0-48\ hr)}$ of felodipine is not changed, the peak concentration of its isomers is almost doubled, and the trough concentration is approximately halved. The bioavailability of enalapril, as measured by total urinary recovery of enalaprilat, is slightly reduced. As with other dihydropyridine calcium channel blockers, the bioavailability of felodipine was increased when taken with grapefruit juice, compared to when taken with water or orange juice.

The systemic plasma clearance of felodipine in young healthy subjects is about 0.8 L/min, and the apparent volume of distribution is 10 L/kg. Approximately 99 percent of felodipine is bound to plasma proteins.

Following administration of ^{14}C-labeled intravenous or immediate-release oral felodipine in man, about 70 percent of the dose of radioactivity was recovered in urine and 10 percent in the feces. A negligible amount of intact felodipine was recovered in the urine and feces (<0.5%). Six metabolites, which account for 23 percent of the oral dose, have been identified; none has significant vasodilating activity. Following oral administration of the immediate-release formulation, the plasma levels of felodipine declined polyexponentially with a mean terminal half-life of 11 to 16 hours.

Excretion of enalaprilat and enalapril is primarily renal. Approximately 94 percent of the dose is recovered in the urine and feces as enalaprilat or enalapril. The principal components in urine are enalaprilat, accounting for about 40 percent of the dose, and intact enalapril. There is no evidence of metabolites of enalapril, other than enalaprilat. The serum concentration profile of enalaprilat exhibits a prolonged terminal phase, apparently representing a small fraction of the administered dose that has been bound to ACE. The amount bound does not increase with dose, indicating a saturable site of binding. The effective half-life for accumulation of enalaprilat following multiple doses of enalapril maleate is 11 hours.

The disposition of enalapril and enalaprilat in patients with renal insufficiency is similar to that in patients with normal renal function until the glomerular filtration rate is reduced to 30 mL/min or less. With glomerular filtration rate ≤30 mL/min, peak and trough enalaprilat levels increase, time to peak concentration increases, and time to steady state may be delayed. The effective half-life of enalaprilat following multiple doses of enalapril maleate is prolonged at this level of renal insufficiency. Enalaprilat is dialyzable at a rate of 62 mL/min.

Plasma concentrations of felodipine, after a single dose and at steady state, increase with age. Mean clearance of felodipine in elderly hypertensives (mean age 74) was only 45 percent of that for young volunteers (mean age 26). At steady state, the mean AUC for young patients was 39 percent of that for the elderly. Data for intermediate age ranges suggest that the AUCs fall between the extremes of the young and the elderly.

In patients with hepatic disease, the clearance of felodipine was reduced to about 60 percent of that seen in normal young volunteers.

Blood Brain Barrier and Blood Placental Barrier: Animal studies have shown that felodipine crosses the blood brain barrier. The plasma to brain concentration ratio of felodipine is about 20:1. Felodipine crosses the placenta. Fetal plasma levels of felodipine are similar to maternal plasma levels. Studies in dogs indicate that enalapril crosses the blood brain barrier poorly, if at all; enalaprilat does not enter the brain. Multiple doses of enalapril maleate in rats do not result in accumulation in any tissues. Milk of lactating rats contains radioactivity following administration of ^{14}C enalapril maleate. Radioactivity was found to cross the placenta following administration of labeled drug to pregnant hamsters.

Pharmacodynamics

Administration of **enalapril** maleate to patients with hypertension of severity ranging from mild to severe results in a reduction of both supine and standing blood pressure, usually with no orthostatic component. Symptomatic postural hypotension is infrequent with enalapril alone, although it might be anticipated in volume-depleted patients. (See WARNINGS.) In most patients studied, after oral administration of a single dose of enalapril, onset of antihypertensive activity was seen at one hour, with peak reduction of blood pressure achieved by 4 to 6 hours. At recommended doses, antihypertensive effects have been maintained for at least 24 hours. In some patients the effects may diminish toward the end of the dosing interval.

In most patients, achievement of optimal blood pressure reduction may require several weeks of therapy. The antihypertensive effects of enalapril have continued during long-term therapy. Abrupt withdrawal of enalapril has not been associated with a rapid increase in blood pressure. In hemodynamic studies in patients with essential hypertension, blood pressure reduction was accompanied by a reduction in peripheral arterial resistance with an increase in cardiac output and little or no change in heart rate. Following administration of enalapril maleate, there is an increase in renal blood flow; glomerular filtration rate is usually unchanged. The effects appear to be similar in patients with renovascular hypertension.

In a clinical pharmacology study, indomethacin or sulindac was administered to hypertensive patients receiving enalapril. In this study there was no evidence of a blunting of the antihypertensive action of enalapril.

The effect of **felodipine** on blood pressure is principally a consequence of a dose-related decrease in peripheral vascular resistance. Blood pressure response following administration of felodipine ER to hypertensive patients is correlated with dose and plasma concentrations of felodipine. A reduction in blood pressure generally occurs within 2 to 5 hours. During chronic administration, substantial blood pressure control lasts for 24 hours, with trough reductions in diastolic blood pressure approximately 40–50 percent of peak reductions. A reflex increase in heart rate frequently occurs during the first week of therapy; this increase attenuates over time. Heart rate increases of 5–10 beats per minute may be seen during chronic dosing. The increase is inhibited by beta-blocking agents.

Felodipine has no significant effect on cardiac conduction (P-R, P-Q, and H-V intervals). In clinical trials in hypertensive patients without clinical evidence of left ventricular dysfunction, no symptoms suggestive of a negative inotropic effect were noted; however, none would be expected in this population.

In an 8-week, fixed-dose, parallel-group, double-blind study, 707 hypertensive patients were randomized among all possible combinations of enalapril (0, 5, or 20 mg), and extended-release felodipine (0, 2.5, 5, or 10 mg), both taken once daily. Each of the non-placebo combinations was significantly more effective than placebo in reducing seated systolic and diastolic blood pressure at peak (three to five hours after dosing) and trough (24 hours after dosing). Enalapril and felodipine contributed additively to the effect, so that each active-active combination was significantly more effective than either of its component monotherapies. Most of the drug effect seen at peak was still present at trough. The efficacy of combination therapy relative to monotherapy was not significantly affected by race, sex, or age.

During chronic dosing with LEXXEL, the maximum reduction in blood pressure is generally achieved after one to two weeks. The antihypertensive effects of LEXXEL have continued during chronic therapy for at least one year.

INDICATIONS AND USAGE

LEXXEL is indicated for the treatment of hypertension.

This fixed combination drug is not indicated for the initial therapy of hypertension. (See DOSAGE AND ADMINISTRATION.)

In using LEXXEL, consideration should be given to the fact that another angiotensin converting enzyme inhibitor, captopril, has caused agranulocytosis, particularly in patients with renal impairment or collagen vascular disease, and that available data are insufficient to show that enalapril (a component of LEXXEL) does not have a similar risk. (See WARNINGS, *Neutropenia/Agranulocytosis.*)

In considering use of LEXXEL, it should be noted that black patients receiving ACE inhibitors have been reported to have a higher incidence of angioedema compared to non-blacks. (See WARNINGS, *Angioedema.*)

CONTRAINDICATIONS

LEXXEL is contraindicated in patients who are hypersensitive to any component of this product. Because of the enalapril component, LEXXEL is contraindicated in patients with a history of angioedema related to previous treatment with an angiotensin converting enzyme inhibitor.

WARNINGS

Anaphylactoid and Possibly Related Reactions: Presumably because angiotensin-converting enzyme inhibitors affect the metabolism of eicosanoids and polypeptides, including endogenous bradykinin, patients receiving ACE inhibitors (including LEXXEL) may be subject to a variety of adverse reactions, some of them serious.

Angioedema: Angioedema of the face, extremities, lips, tongue, glottis and/or larynx has been reported in patients treated with angiotensin converting enzyme inhibitors, including enalapril. This may occur at any time during treatment. In such cases LEXXEL should be promptly discontinued, and appropriate therapy and monitoring should be provided until complete and sustained resolution of signs and symptoms has occurred. In instances where swelling has been confined to the face and lips the condition has generally resolved without treatment, although antihistamines have been useful in relieving symptoms. Angioedema associated with laryngeal edema may be fatal. **Where there is involvement of the tongue, glottis or larynx, likely to cause**

Continued on next page

Lexxel—Cont.

airway obstruction, appropriate therapy, e.g., subcutaneous epinephrine solution 1:1000 (0.3 mL to 0.5 mL) and/or measures necessary to ensure a patent airway, should be promptly provided. (See ADVERSE REACTIONS.)

Patients with a history of angioedema unrelated to ACE inhibitor therapy may be at increased risk of angioedema while receiving an ACE inhibitor (see also INDICATIONS AND USAGE and CONTRAINDICATIONS.)

Anaphylactoid Reactions During Desensitization: Two patients undergoing desensitizing treatment with hymenoptera venom while receiving ACE inhibitors sustained life-threatening anaphylactoid reactions. In the same patients, these reactions were avoided when ACE inhibitors were temporarily withheld, but they reappeared upon inadvertent rechallenge.

Anaphylactoid Reactions During Membrane Exposure: Anaphylactoid reactions have been reported in patients dialyzed with high-flux membranes and treated concomitantly with an ACE inhibitor. Anaphylactoid reactions have also been reported in patients undergoing low-density lipoprotein apheresis with dextran sulfate absorption.

Hypotension: LEXXEL can occasionally cause symptomatic hypotension.

Excessive hypotension is rare in uncomplicated hypertensive patients treated with enalapril alone. Patients at risk for excessive hypotension, sometimes associated with oliguria and/or progressive azotemia, and rarely with acute renal failure and/or death, include those with the following conditions or characteristics: heart failure, hyponatremia, high dose diuretic therapy, recent intensive diuresis or increase in diuretic dose, renal dialysis, or severe volume and/or salt depletion of any etiology. It may be advisable to eliminate the diuretic (except in patients with heart failure), reduce the diuretic dose or increase salt intake cautiously before initiating therapy with enalapril maleate in patients at risk for excessive hypotension who are able to tolerate such adjustments. (See PRECAUTIONS, *Drug Interactions* and ADVERSE REACTIONS.) In patients at risk for excessive hypotension, therapy should be started under very close medical supervision and such patients should be followed closely for the first 2 weeks of treatment and whenever the dose of enalapril and/or diuretic is increased. Similar considerations may apply to patients with ischemic heart or cerebrovascular disease, in whom an excessive fall in blood pressure could result in a myocardial infarction or cerebrovascular accident.

If excessive hypotension occurs, the patient should be placed in the supine position and, if necessary, receive an intravenous infusion of normal saline. A transient hypotensive response is not a contraindication to further doses of enalapril maleate, which usually can be given without difficulty once the blood pressure has stabilized. If symptomatic hypotension develops, a dose reduction or discontinuation of enalapril or diuretic may be necessary.

Felodipine, like other calcium channel blockers, may occasionally precipitate significant hypotension, and rarely syncope. It may lead to reflex tachycardia which in susceptible individuals may precipitate angina pectoris. (See ADVERSE REACTIONS.)

Neutropenia/Agranulocytosis: Another angiotensin converting enzyme inhibitor, captopril, has been shown to cause agranulocytosis and bone marrow depression, rarely in uncomplicated patients but more frequently in patients with renal impairment, especially if they also have a collagen vascular disease. Available data from clinical trials of enalapril are insufficient to show that enalapril does not cause agranulocytosis at similar rates. Marketing experience has revealed several cases of neutropenia or agranulocytosis in which a causal relationship to enalapril cannot be excluded. Periodic monitoring of white blood cell counts in patients with collagen vascular disease and renal disease should be considered.

Hepatic Failure: Rarely, ACE inhibitors have been associated with a syndrome that starts with cholestatic jaundice and progresses to fulminant hepatic necrosis and (sometimes) death. The mechanism of this syndrome is not understood. Patients receiving ACE inhibitors who develop jaundice or marked elevations of hepatic enzymes should discontinue the ACE inhibitor and receive appropriate medical follow-up.

Fetal/Neonatal Morbidity and Mortality: ACE inhibitors can cause fetal and neonatal morbidity and death when administered to pregnant women. Several dozen cases have been reported in the world literature. When pregnancy is detected, LEXXEL should be discontinued as soon as possible.

The use of ACE inhibitors during the second and third trimesters of pregnancy has been associated with fetal and neonatal injury, including hypotension, neonatal skull hypoplasia, anuria, reversible or irreversible renal failure, and death. Oligohydramnios has also been reported, presumably resulting from decreased fetal renal function; oligohydramnios in this setting has been associated with fetal limb con-

tractures, craniofacial deformation, and hypoplastic lung development. Prematurity, intrauterine growth retardation, and patent ductus arteriosus have also been reported, although it is not clear whether these occurrences were due to the ACE-inhibitor exposure.

These adverse effects do not appear to have resulted from intrauterine ACE-inhibitor exposure that has been limited to the first trimester. Mothers whose embryos and fetuses are exposed to ACE inhibitors only during the first trimester should be so informed. Nonetheless, when patients become pregnant, physicians should make every effort to discontinue the use of LEXXEL as soon as possible.

Rarely (probably less than once in every thousand pregnancies), no alternative to ACE inhibitors will be found. In these rare cases, the mothers should be apprised of the potential hazards to their fetuses, and serial ultrasound examinations should be performed to assess the intra-amniotic environment.

If oligohydramnios is observed, LEXXEL should be discontinued unless it is considered lifesaving for the mother. Contraction stress testing (CST), a non-stress test (NST), or biophysical profiling (BPP) may be appropriate, depending upon the week of pregnancy. Patients and physicians should be aware, however, that oligohydramnios may not appear until after the fetus has sustained irreversible injury.

Infants with histories of *in utero* exposure to ACE inhibitors should be closely observed for hypotension, oliguria, and hyperkalemia. If oliguria occurs, attention should be directed toward support of blood pressure and renal perfusion. Exchange transfusion or dialysis may be required as means of reversing hypotension and/or substituting for disordered renal function. Enalapril, which crosses the placenta, has been removed from neonatal circulation by peritoneal dialysis with some clinical benefit, and theoretically may be removed by exchange transfusion, although there is no experience with the latter procedure.

No teratogenic effects of enalapril were seen in studies of pregnant rats and rabbits. On a body surface area basis, the doses used were 57 times and 12 times, respectively, the maximum recommended human daily dose (MRHDD).

In rats administered the combination of enalapril and felodipine (enalapril [E]=1.9-felodipine [F]=2.5 mg/kg/day), an increased incidence of fetuses with dilated renal pelvis/ureter was observed. However, there was no evidence of this effect in the offspring postweaning. In mice, with doses of E=23, F=30 mg/kg/day or greater, there was an increased incidence of both early and late *in utero* deaths. Other than a transient and slight decrease in body weight gain in the first generation offspring, there were no adverse effects in offspring with regard to sexual maturation, behavioral development, fertility or fecundity.

Enalapril-felodipine given to pregnant mice (enalapril 20.8, felodipine 27 mg/kg/day) and rats (enalapril =17.3, felodipine =22.5 mg/kg/day) produced plasma levels (C_{max} and AUC values) of enalapril/enalaprilat that were 76 to 418-fold greater and plasma levels of felodipine that were 151 to 433-fold greater than those expected in humans (non-pregnant) at the dose to be used in humans.

PRECAUTIONS

General

Impaired Renal Function: As a consequence of inhibiting the renin-angiotensin-aldosterone system, changes in renal function may be anticipated in susceptible individuals treated with enalapril. In patients with severe heart failure whose renal function may depend on the activity of the renin-angiotensin-aldosterone system, treatment with angiotensin converting enzyme inhibitors, including enalapril, may be associated with oliguria and/or progressive azotemia and rarely with acute renal failure and/or death.

In clinical studies in hypertensive patients with unilateral or bilateral renal artery stenosis, increases in blood urea nitrogen and serum creatinine were observed in 20 percent of patients treated with enalapril. These increases were almost always reversible upon discontinuation of enalapril and/or diuretic therapy. In such patients, renal function should be monitored during the first few weeks of therapy. Some enalapril-treated patients with hypertension or heart failure, with no apparent pre-existing renal vascular disease, have developed increases in blood urea and serum creatinine, usually minor and transient, especially when enalapril has been given concomitantly with a diuretic. This is more likely to occur in patients with pre-existing renal impairment. Dosage reduction of enalapril or discontinuation of the diuretic may be required.

Evaluation of the hypertensive patient should always include assessment of renal function.

Hyperkalemia: Elevated serum potassium (greater than 5.7 mEq/L) was observed in approximately one percent of hypertensive patients in clinical trials treated with enalapril alone. In most cases these were isolated values which resolved despite continued therapy. Hyperkalemia was a cause of discontinuation of therapy in 0.28 percent of hypertensive patients. In clinical trials in heart failure, hyperkalemia was observed in 3.8 percent of patients but was not a cause for discontinuation.

Risk factors for the development of hyperkalemia include renal insufficiency, diabetes mellitus, and the concomitant use of potassium-sparing diuretics, potassium supplements and/or potassium-containing salt substitutes, which should be used cautiously, if at all, with enalapril. (See *Drug Interactions*.)

Elderly Patients or Patients with Impaired Liver Function: Patients over 65 years of age or patients with impaired liver function may have elevated plasma concentrations of felodipine. (See DOSAGE AND ADMINISTRATION.)

Cough: Presumably due to the inhibition of the degradation of endogenous bradykinin, persistent nonproductive cough has been reported with all ACE inhibitors, always resolving after discontinuation of therapy. ACE inhibitor-induced cough should be considered in the diagnosis of cough.

Surgery/Anesthesia: In patients undergoing major surgery or during anesthesia with agents that produce hypotension, enalapril may block angiotensin II formation secondary to compensatory renin release. If hypotension occurs and is considered to be due to this mechanism, it can be corrected by volume expansion.

Peripheral Edema: Peripheral edema, generally mild and not associated with generalized fluid retention, was the most common adverse event in the felodipine clinical trials. The incidence of peripheral edema was both dose and age dependent. This adverse event generally occurs within 2–3 weeks of the initiation of treatment.

Information for Patients

Patients should be instructed to take LEXXEL whole and not to divide, crush or chew the tablet.

All patients should be advised to consult their physician if they experience any of the following conditions:

Angioedema: Angioedema, including laryngeal edema, may occur at any time during treatment with angiotensin converting enzyme inhibitors, including enalapril. Patients should be so advised and told to report immediately any signs or symptoms suggesting angioedema (swelling of face, extremities, eyes, lips, tongue, difficulty in swallowing or breathing) and to take no more drug until they have consulted with the prescribing physician.

Hypotension: Patients should be cautioned to report light headedness especially during the first few days of therapy. If actual syncope occurs, the patients should be told to discontinue LEXXEL until they have consulted with the prescribing physician. All patients should be cautioned that excessive perspiration and dehydration may lead to an excessive fall in blood pressure because of reduction in fluid volume. Other causes of volume depletion, such as vomiting or diarrhea, may also lead to a fall in blood pressure; patients should be advised to consult with the physician.

Hyperkalemia: Patients should be told not to use salt substitutes containing potassium without consulting their physician.

Neutropenia: Patients should be told to report promptly any indication of infection (e.g., sore throat, fever) which may be a sign of neutropenia.

Pregnancy: Female patients of childbearing age should be told about the consequences of second- and third-trimester exposure to ACE inhibitors, and they should also be told that these consequences do not appear to have resulted from intrauterine ACE-inhibitor exposure that has been limited to the first trimester. These patients should be asked to report pregnancies to their physicians as soon as possible.

Gingival Hyperplasia: Patients should be told that mild gingival hyperplasia (gum swelling) has been reported. Good dental hygiene decreases its incidence and severity.

Note: As with many other drugs, certain advice to patients being treated with LEXXEL is warranted. This information is intended to aid in the safe and effective use of this medication. It is not disclosure of all possible adverse or intended effects.

Drug Interactions

Hypotension—Patients on Diuretic Therapy: Patients on diuretics, and especially those in whom diuretic therapy was recently instituted, may occasionally experience an excessive reduction of blood pressure after initiation of therapy with enalapril. The possibility of hypotensive effects with enalapril can be minimized by either discontinuing the diuretic or increasing the salt intake prior to initiation of treatment with enalapril. If it is necessary to continue the diuretic, provide close medical supervision after the initial dose for at least two hours and until blood pressure has stabilized for at least an additional hour. (See WARNINGS and DOSAGE AND ADMINISTRATION.)

Agents Causing Renin Release: The antihypertensive effect of enalapril is augmented by antihypertensive agents that cause renin release (e.g., diuretics).

Agents Increasing Serum Potassium: Enalapril attenuates potassium loss caused by thiazide-type diuretics. Potassium-sparing diuretics (e.g., spironolactone, triamterene, or amiloride), potassium supplements, or potassium-containing salt substitutes may lead to significant increases in serum potassium. Therefore, if concomitant use of these

agents is indicated because of demonstrated hypokalemia, they should be used with caution and with frequent monitoring of serum potassium.

Lithium: Lithium toxicity has been reported in patients receiving lithium concomitantly with drugs which cause elimination of sodium, including ACE inhibitors. A few cases of lithium toxicity have been reported in patients receiving concomitant enalapril and lithium and were reversible upon discontinuation of both drugs. It is recommended that serum lithium levels be monitored frequently if enalapril is administered concomitantly with lithium.

Beta-Blocking Agents: Enalapril has been used concomitantly with beta adrenergic-blocking agents without evidence of clinically significant adverse interactions.

A pharmacokinetic study of felodipine in conjunction with metoprolol demonstrated no significant effects on the pharmacokinetics of felodipine. The AUC and C_{max} of metoprolol, however, were increased approximately 31 and 38 percent, respectively. In controlled clinical trials, however, beta blockers including metoprolol were concurrently administered with felodipine and were well tolerated.

Cimetidine: In healthy subjects, pharmacokinetic studies showed an approximately 50 percent increase in the area under the plasma concentration time curve (AUC) as well as the C_{max} of felodipine when given concomitantly with cimetidine. It is anticipated that a clinically significant interaction may occur in some hypertensive patients.

Digoxin: Enalapril has been used concomitantly with digoxin without evidence of clinically significant adverse interactions.

When given concomitantly with felodipine ER, the pharmacokinetics of digoxin in patients with heart failure were not significantly altered.

Anticonvulsants: In a pharmacokinetic study, maximum plasma concentrations of felodipine were considerably lower in epileptic patients on long-term anticonvulsant therapy (e.g., phenytoin, carbamazepine, or phenobarbital) than in healthy volunteers. In such patients, the mean area under the felodipine plasma concentration-time curve was also reduced to approximately 6 percent of that observed in healthy volunteers. Since a clinically significant interaction may be anticipated, alternative antihypertensive therapy should be considered in these patients.

Other Concomitant Therapy: In healthy subjects, there were no clinically significant interactions when felodipine was given concomitantly with indomethacin or spironolactone.

Enalapril has been used concomitantly with methyldopa, nitrates, hydralazine, and prazosin without evidence of clinically significant adverse interactions.

Carcinogenesis, Mutagenesis, Impairment of Fertility

No long-term carcinogenicity tests have been performed with the combination. Enalapril-felodipine was not mutagenic with or without metabolic activation *in vitro* in the Ames microbial mutation assay, the V-79 mammalian cell forward mutation assay, the alkaline elution assay with rat hepatocytes or the CHO mammalian cell cytogenetics assay. An *in vivo* mouse bone marrow cytogenetics assay was also negative.

In rats given enalapril-felodipine, there was no effect on fertility in males at doses up to 6.9/9 mg/kg/day, and in females at doses up to 17.3/22.5 mg/kg/day.

There was no evidence of a tumorigenic effect when enalapril was administered for 106 weeks to male and female rats at doses up to 90 mg/kg/day or for 94 weeks to male and female mice at doses up to 90 and 180 mg/kg/day, respectively. These doses are 26 times (in rats and female mice) and 13 times (in male mice) the maximum recommended human daily dose (MRHDD) when compared on a body surface area basis.

Neither enalapril maleate nor the active diacid was mutagenic in the Ames microbial mutagen test with or without metabolic activation. Enalapril was also negative in the following genotoxicity studies: rec-assay, reverse mutation assay with *E. coli*, sister chromatid exchange with cultured mammalian cells, and the micronucleus test with mice, as well as in an *in vivo* cytogenic study using mouse bone marrow.

There were no adverse effects on reproductive performance of male and female rats treated with up to 90 mg/kg/day of enalapril (26 times the MRHDD when compared on a body surface area basis).

In a 2-year carcinogenicity study in rats fed felodipine at doses of 7.7, 23.1 or 69.3 mg/kg/day (up to 28 times† the maximum recommended human dose on a mg/m² basis), a dose-related increase in the incidence of benign interstitial cell tumors of the testes (Leydig cell tumors) was observed in treated male rats. These tumors were not observed in a similar study in mice at doses up to 138.6 mg/kg/day (28 times† the maximum recommended human dose on a mg/m² basis). Felodipine, at the doses employed in the 2-year rat study, has been shown to lower testicular testosterone and to produce a corresponding increase in serum luteinizing hormone in rats. The Leydig cell tumor development is possibly secondary to these hormonal effects which have not been observed in man.

†Based on patient weight of 50 kg.

Percent of Patients with Adverse Events in the Double-Blind Trial
(Percent discontinuation shown in parentheses)

Body System Adverse Event	Enalapril[a] Felodipine ER[b] N=319	Enalapril[a] N=133	Felodipine ER[b] N=176	Placebo N=79
Body as a Whole				
Edema/Swelling	4.1(0.3)	2.3(0.0)	10.8(1.7)	1.3(0.0)
Asthenia/Fatigue	1.9(0.0)	2.3(0.8)	0.6(0.6)	3.8(0.0)
Nervous/Psychiatric				
Headache	10.3(0.6)	3.8(0.0)	10.2(1.1)	7.6(1.3)
Dizziness	4.4(0.3)	1.5(0.0)	2.8(0.6)	0.0(0.0)
Respiratory				
Cough	2.2(0.6)	2.3(0.0)	0.6(0.0)	0.0(0.0)
Skin				
Flushing	1.6(0.3)	0.0(0.0)	2.3(1.1)	0.0(0.0)

[a]Combination of dose of 5 and 20 mg daily
[b]Combination of dose 2.5, 5 and 10 mg daily

In this same rat study, a dose-related increase in the incidence of focal squamous cell hyperplasia, compared to control, was observed in the esophageal groove of male and female rats in all dose groups. No other drug-related esophageal or gastric pathology was observed in the rats or with chronic administration in mice and dogs. The latter species, like man, has no anatomical structure comparable to the esophageal groove.

Felodipine was not carcinogenic when fed to mice at doses of up to 138.6 mg/kg/day (28 times† the maximum recommended human dose on a mg/m² basis) for periods of up to 80 weeks in males and 99 weeks in females.

Felodipine did not display any mutagenic activity *in vitro* in the Ames microbial mutagenicity test or in the mouse lymphoma forward mutation assay. No clastogenic potential was seen *in vivo* in the mouse micronucleus test at oral doses up to 2500 mg/kg (506 times† the maximum recommended human dose on a mg/m² basis) or *in vitro* in a human lymphocyte chromosome aberration assay.

A fertility study in which male and female rats were administered doses of 3.8, 9.6, or 26.9 mg/kg/day showed no significant effect of felodipine on reproductive performance.

Pregnancy

Pregnancy Categories C (first trimester) *and D* (second and third trimesters). See WARNINGS, *Fetal/Neonatal Morbidity and Mortality.*

Teratogenic Effects: Studies in pregnant rabbits administered doses of felodipine 0.46, 1.2, 2.3, and 4.6 mg/kg/day (from 0.4 to 4 times† the maximum recommended human dose on a mg/m² basis) showed digital anomalies consisting of reduction in size and degree of ossification of the terminal phalanges in the fetuses. The frequency and severity of the changes appeared dose-related and were noted even at the lowest dose. These changes have been shown to occur with other members of the dihydropyridine class and are possibly a result of compromised uterine blood flow. Similar fetal anomalies were not observed in rats given felodipine.

In a teratology study in cynomolgus monkeys, no reduction in the size of the terminal phalanges was observed, but an abnormal position of the distal phalanges was noted in about 40 percent of the fetuses.

Nonteratogenic Effects: A prolongation of parturition with difficult labor and an increased frequency of fetal and early postnatal deaths were observed in rats administered felodipine doses of 9.6 mg/kg/day (4 times† the maximum human dose on a mg/m² basis) and above.

Significant enlargement of the mammary glands, in excess of the normal enlargement for pregnant rabbits, was found with doses greater than or equal to 1.2 mg/kg/day (equal to the maximum human dose on a mg/m² basis). This effect occurred only in pregnant rabbits and regressed during lactation. Similar changes in the mammary glands were not observed in rats or monkeys.

There are no adequate and well-controlled studies with felodipine in pregnant women. If felodipine is used during pregnancy, or if the patient becomes pregnant while taking this drug, she should be apprised of the potential hazard to the fetus, possible digital anomalies of the infant, and the potential effects of felodipine on labor and delivery, and on the mammary glands of pregnant females.

†Based on patient weight of 50 kg

Nursing Mothers

Enalapril and enalaprilat are detected in human breast milk. It is not known whether felodipine administered as monotherapy is secreted in human milk; studies of the combination of enalapril and felodipine in rats indicate that felodipine concentrates in milk to a level almost ten-fold that found in plasma. Because of the potential for serious adverse reactions from enalapril and felodipine in the infant, a decision should be made either to discontinue nursing or to discontinue the drug, taking into account the importance of the drug to the mother. Therefore, caution should be exercised when LEXXEL is given to a nursing mother.

Pediatric Use

Safety and effectiveness in pediatric patients have not been established.

ADVERSE REACTIONS

In a factorial study, combinations of enalapril at doses of 0, 5, and 20 mg and felodipine ER at doses of 0, 2.5, 5, and 10 mg were evaluated for safety in more than 700 patients with hypertension. In addition more than 500 patients received various combinations of enalapril (5 or 10 mg) and felodipine ER (2.5, 5, or 10 mg) with or without hydrochlorothiazide (12.5 mg) in an open-labeled study up to 52 weeks (mean 33 weeks). Adverse events were similar to those described with the individual components.

In general, treatment with enalapril maleate-felodipine ER was well tolerated and adverse events were mild and transient in nature. In the placebo-controlled, double-blind trial, discontinuation of therapy due to adverse events considered related (possibly, probably or definitely) occurred in 2.8 percent vs 1.3 percent of patients treated with the combination or placebo, respectively. The most frequently observed clinical adverse events considered related to treatment with the combination were headache, edema or swelling, and dizziness.

Clinical adverse events considered related (possibly, probably, or definitely) to treatment with enalapril-felodipine ER that occurred with an incidence of one percent or greater with the combination during the placebo-controlled, double-blind trial are compared to individual components and placebo in the table below:

[See table above]

Other clinical adverse events considered related (possibly, probably, or definitely) to treatment with enalapril-felodipine ER that occurred with an incidence of less than one percent in the placebo-controlled, double-blind trial are listed below. These events are listed in order of decreasing frequency within each category. ***Body as a Whole:*** Syncope, facial edema, orthostatic effects, chest pain; ***Cardiovascular:*** Palpitation, hypotension, bradycardia, premature ventricular contraction, increased blood pressure; ***Digestive:*** Dry mouth, constipation, dyspepsia, flatulence, acid regurgitation, vomiting, diarrhea, nausea, anal/rectal pain; ***Metabolic:*** Gout; ***Musculoskeletal:*** Neck pain, joint swelling; ***Nervous/Psychiatric:*** Insomnia, nervousness, somnolence, ataxia, agitation, paresthesia, tremor; ***Respiratory:*** Dyspnea, respiratory congestion, pharyngeal discomfort, dry throat; ***Skin:*** Rash, angioedema, pruritus, alopecia, dry skin; ***Special Senses:*** Increased intraocular pressure; ***Urogenital:*** Impotence, hot flashes.

Other infrequently reported adverse events were seen in clinical trials with enalapril-felodipine ER (causal relationship unknown). These included: ***Body as a Whole:*** Abdominal pain, fever; ***Digestive:*** Dental pain; ***Metabolic:*** Increased ALT and AST, hyperglycemia; ***Musculoskeletal:*** Back pain, myalgia, foot pain, knee pain, shoulder pain, tendinitis; ***Respiratory:*** Upper respiratory infection, sinusitis, pharyngitis, bronchitis, nasal congestion, influenza, sinus disorder; ***Special Senses:*** Conjunctivitis; ***Urogenital:*** Proteinuria, pyuria, urinary tract infection.

Enalapril Maleate

Other adverse events that have been reported with enalapril, without regard to causality, are listed (in decreasing severity) below:

Angioedema: Angioedema has been reported in patients receiving enalapril maleate, with an incidence higher in black than in non-black patients. Angioedema associated with laryngeal edema may be fatal. If angioedema of the

Continued on next page

Lexxel—Cont.

face, extremities, lips, tongue, glottis and/or larynx occurs, treatment with LEXXEL should be discontinued and appropriate therapy instituted immediately. (See WARNINGS.)
Body as a Whole: Anaphylactoid reactions (see WARNINGS, *Anaphylactoid and Possibly Related Reactions*); ***Cardiovascular:*** Cardiac arrest, myocardial infarction or cerebrovascular accident, possibly secondary to excessive hypotension in high risk patients (see WARNINGS, *Hypotension*), orthostatic hypotension, pulmonary embolism and infarction, pulmonary edema, rhythm disturbances including atrial tachycardia and bradycardia, atrial fibrillation, angina pectoris; ***Digestive:*** Ileus, pancreatitis, hepatic failure, hepatitis (hepatocellular [proven on rechallenge] or cholestatic jaundice) (see WARNINGS, *Hepatic Failure*), melena, anorexia, glossitis, stomatitis; ***Endocrine:*** Gynecomastia; ***Hematologic:*** Rare cases of neutropenia, thrombocytopenia and bone marrow depression; ***Musculoskeletal:*** Muscle cramps; ***Nervous/Psychiatric:*** Depression, confusion, peripheral neuropathy (e.g. paresthesia, dysesthesia), vertigo; ***Respiratory:*** Bronchospasm, rhinorrhea, sore throat and hoarseness, asthma, pneumonia, pulmonary infiltrates; ***Skin:*** Exfoliative dermatitis, toxic epidermal necrolysis, Stevens-Johnson syndrome, pemphigus, herpes zoster, erythema multiforme, urticaria, diaphoresis, photosensitivity; ***Special Senses:*** Blurred vision, taste alteration, anosmia, tinnitus, dry eyes, tearing; ***Urogenital:*** Renal failure, oliguria, renal dysfunction (see PRECAUTIONS), flank pain, gynecomastia. ***Miscellaneous:*** A symptom complex has been reported which may include a positive ANA, an elevated erythrocyte sedimentation rate, arthralgia/arthritis, myalgia/myositis, fever, serositis, vasculitis, leukocytosis, eosinophilia, photosensitivity rash and other dermatologic manifestations; ***Fetal/Neonatal Morbidity and Mortality:*** See WARNINGS, *Fetal/Neonatal Morbidity and Mortality.*

Felodipine as an Extended-Release Formulation
Other adverse events that have been reported with felodipine ER, without regard to causality, are listed (in decreasing severity) below:
Body as a Whole: Flu-like illness; ***Cardiovascular:*** Myocardial infarction, angina pectoris, arrhythmia, tachycardia, premature beats; ***Digestive:*** Gingival hyperplasia; ***Hematologic:*** Anemia; ***Musculoskeletal:*** Arthralgia, leg pain, muscle cramps, arm pain, hip pain; ***Nervous/Psychiatric:*** Depression, anxiety disorders, irritability, decreased libido; ***Respiratory:*** Upper respiratory infection, rhinorrhea, sneezing, pharyngitis, influenza, epistaxis, respiratory infection; ***Skin:*** Contusion, erythema, urticaria; ***Special Senses:*** Visual disturbances; ***Urogenital:*** Urinary frequency, urinary urgency, dysuria, polyuria.

Laboratory Test Findings
In controlled clinical trials with enalapril-felodipine ER, clinically important changes in standard laboratory parameters associated with administration of LEXXEL were rare. No changes peculiar to the combination treatment were observed.
Serum Electrolytes: See PRECAUTIONS.
Creatinine: Minor reversible increases in serum creatinine were observed in patients treated with LEXXEL. Increases in creatinine are more likely to occur in patients with renal insufficiency or those pretreated with a diuretic and based on experience with other ACE inhibitors, would be expected to be especially likely in patients with renal artery stenosis (see PRECAUTIONS).
Other: Minor reversible increases or decreases in serum potassium were infrequently observed in patients treated with LEXXEL; rarely were these measurements outside the normal range.

OVERDOSAGE

Limited data are available in regard to enalapril overdosage in humans. In a suicide attempt, one patient took 150 mg felodipine together with 15 tablets each of atenolol and spironolactone and 20 tablets of nitrazepam. The patient's blood pressure and heart rate were normal on admission to hospital; he subsequently recovered without significant sequelae.
Human overdoses with any combination of enalapril and felodipine ER have not been reported.
Single oral doses of enalapril above 1000 mg/kg and ≥1775 mg/kg were associated with lethality in mice and rats, respectively. Oral doses of felodipine at 240 mg/kg and 264 mg/kg in male and female mice, respectively, and 2390 mg/kg and 2250 mg/kg in male and female rats, respectively, caused significant lethality.
In interaction studies on the acute oral toxicity of the combination in mice, pretreatment with felodipine (50 mg/kg) for one hour led to an increase in mortality at doses of enalapril maleate that exceeded 1000 mg/kg. Significant lethality with felodipine was not increased by pretreatment of mice for one hour with 100 mg/kg of enalapril maleate.
Treatment: To obtain up-to-date information about the treatment of overdose, consult your Regional Poison-Control Center. Telephone numbers of certified poison-control centers are listed in the *Physicians' Desk Reference (PDR)*. In managing overdose, consider the possibilities of multiple-drug overdoses, drug-drug interactions, and unusual drug kinetics in your patient.
The most likely effect of overdose with LEXXEL is vasodilation, with consequent hypotension and tachycardia. Repletion of central fluid volume (Trendelenburg positioning, infusion of crystalloids) may be sufficient therapy, but pressor agents (norepinephrine or high-dose dopamine) may be required.
Enalaprilat may be removed from general circulation by hemodialysis at a rate of 62 mL/min and has been removed from neonatal circulation by peritoneal dialysis. It has not been established whether felodipine can be removed from the circulation by hemodialysis.

DOSAGE AND ADMINSTRATION

LEXXEL is an effective treatment for hypertension. This fixed combination drug is not indicated for initial therapy of hypertension.
The recommended initial dose of enalapril maleate for hypertension in patients not receiving diuretics is 5 mg once a day. The usual dosage range of enalapril maleate for hypertension is 10–40 mg per day administered in a single dose or two divided doses. In some patients treated once daily with enalapril, the antihypertensive effect may diminish toward the end of the dosing interval. In such patients, an increase in dosage or twice daily administration should be considered. The recommended initial dose of felodipine ER is 5 mg once a day with a usual dosage range of 2.5 mg-10 mg once a day. In elderly or hepatically impaired patients, the recommended initial dose of felodipine is 2.5 mg. When LEXXEL is taken with food, the peak concentration of felodipine is almost doubled, and the trough (24-hour) concentration is approximately halved (see CLINICAL PHARMACOLOGY, *Pharmacokinetics and Metabolism*).
In clinical trials of enalapril-felodipine ER combination therapy using enalapril doses of 5–20 mg and felodipine ER doses of 2.5–10 mg once daily, the antihypertensive effects increased with increasing doses of each component in all patient groups.
The hazards (see WARNINGS and ADVERSE REACTIONS) of enalapril are generally independent of dose; those of felodipine are a mixture of dose-dependent phenomena (primarily peripheral edema) and dose-independent phenomena, the former much more common than the latter. Therapy with any combination of enalapril and felodipine will thus be associated with both sets of dose-independent hazards.
Rarely, the dose-independent hazards associated with enalapril or felodipine are serious. To minimize dose-independent hazards, it is usually appropriate to begin therapy with LEXXEL only after a patient has failed to achieve the desired antihypertensive effect with one or the other monotherapy.
Replacement Therapy: Although the felodipine component of LEXXEL has not been shown to be bioequivalent to the available extended-release felodipine (PLENDIL), patients receiving enalapril and felodipine from separate tablets once a day may instead wish to receive the tablets of LEXXEL containing the same component doses.
Therapy Guided By Clinical Effect: A patient whose blood pressure is not adequately controlled with felodipine or enalapril monotherapy may be switched to combination therapy with LEXXEL, initially one tablet daily. If blood pressure control is inadequate after a week or two, the dose may be increased to two tablets daily. If control remains unsatisfactory, consider addition of a thiazide diuretic.
Use in Patients with Metabolic Impairments: Regimens of therapy with LEXXEL need not be adjusted for renal function as long as the patient's creatinine clearance is >30 mL/min/1.73m^2 (serum creatinine roughly ≤3 mg/dL or 265 µmol/L). In patients with more severe renal impairment, the recommended initial dose of enalapril is 2.5 mg.
LEXXEL should regularly be taken either without food or with a light meal (see CLINICAL PHARMACOLOGY, *Pharmacokinetics and Metabolism*). LEXXEL should be swallowed whole and not divided, crushed or chewed.

HOW SUPPLIED

No. 3661—Tablets LEXXEL, 5-5 are white, round/biconvex-shaped, film-coated tablets, coded LEXXEL 1, 5-5 on one side and no markings on the other. Each tablet contains 5 mg of enalapril maleate and 5 mg of felodipine as an extended-release formulation. They are supplied as follows:
NDC 61113-001-31 unit of use bottles of 30 (with desiccants)
NDC 61113-001-68 bottles of 100 (with desiccants)
NDC 61113-001-28 unit dose packages of 100.
Storage:
Store at 25°C (77°F); excursions permitted between 15°C and 30°C (59°F and 86°F) [See USP Controlled Room Temperature]. Keep container tightly closed. Protect from moisture and light. Dispense in a tight container, if product package is subdivided.
Distributed by:
Astra Pharmaceuticals, L.P.
Wayne, PA 19087, USA
Manufactured by: MERCK & CO., INC.,
West Point, PA 19486, USA
Issued March 1998 7989602
©1998 Astra Merck Inc. All rights reserved.
Shown in Product Identification Guide, page 304

MAGNESIUM SULFATE INJECTION, USP ℞

(For details of indications, dosages and administration, precautions, and adverse reactions, see circular in package.)

HOW SUPPLIED

[See table below]
No preservative added. Unused portion of container should be discarded. Use only if solution is clear, and seal intact.
021874R02 Rev. 7/96

MANNITOL Injection, USP 25% ℞

[man-ĭ-tall]

(For details of indications, dosage and administration, precautions, and adverse reactions, see circular in package.)

HOW SUPPLIED

Mannitol Injection, USP 25% is a sterile solution supplied in single dose containers as follows:
NDC 0186-1168-04: 50 mL vials, 25 vials per package
NDC 0186-0652-01: 50 mL syringes, 10 syringes per package
Caution: Federal law prohibits dispensing without prescription.
Store at controlled room temperature 15°–30°C (59°–86°F).
NOTE: Crystals may form in mannitol solutions especially if solutions are chilled. See PRECAUTIONS to dissolve the crystals.
021855R04 Rev. 7/96

MEPERIDINE HCl INJECTION, USP Ⓒ

WARNING: May be habit forming.
(For details of indications, dosage and administration, precautions, and adverse reactions, see circular in package.)

HOW SUPPLIED

Meperidine Hydrochloride Injection, USP is available as:
Multiple Dose Vials

NDC 0186-1283-01	100 mg/mL,	20 mL vial, box of 1
NDC 0186-1284-01	50 mg/mL,	30 mL vial, box of 1

Store at controlled room temperature 15°–30°C (59°–86°F).
021889R04 7/92 (4)

MORPHINE SULFATE (Immediate Release) Ⓒ
Concentrated Oral Solution

(WARNING: May be habit forming.)
(For details of indications, dosage and administration, precautions, and adverse reactions, see circular in package.)

MAGNESIUM SULFATE INJECTION, USP

NDC No. 0186-	Magnesium Sulfate Heptahydrate Concentration	Container Type	Fill Volume	Magnesium per mL	Sulfate per mL
1203-04	10%	Vial	20 mL	9.9 mg	38.9 mg
1204-04	10%	Vial	50 mL	9.9 mg	38.9 mg
1209-04	50%	Vial	2 mL	49.3 mg	194.7 mg
1210-04	50%	Vial	10 mL	49.3 mg	194.7 mg
1211-04	50%	Vial	20 mL	49.3 mg	194.7 mg
0684-01	50%	Additive Syringe	5 mL	49.3 mg	194.7 mg
0685-01	50%	Additive Syringe	10 mL	49.3 mg	194.7 mg

DESCRIPTION

Each mL of Morphine Sulfate (Immediate Release) Concentrated Oral Solution contains:

Morphine Sulfate .... 20 mg
(WARNING: May be habit forming.)

Chemically, Morphine Sulfate is Morphinan-3,6-diol, 7,8-didehydro-4,5-epoxy-17-methyl-, (5α,6α)-, sulfate (2:1)(salt), pentahydrate, which can be represented by the following structural formula:

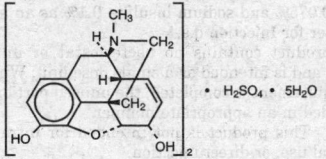

Morphine Sulfate acts as a narcotic analgesic.

HOW SUPPLIED

Morphine Sulfate (Immediate Release) Concentrated Oral Solution is available as follows:

NDC 0186-1123-85, 20 mg/mL, 120 mL bottle with calibrated dropper (box of one).

DEA Order Form Required.

Caution: Federal law prohibits dispensing without prescription.

021702R01   Rev. 6/97

MORPHINE SULFATE
Immediate Release Oral Solution

(WARNING: May be habit forming.)

DESCRIPTION

Each 5 mL of Morphine Sulfate Immediate Release Oral Solution contains:

Morphine Sulfate .... 10 mg
(WARNING: May be habit forming.)

Chemically, Morphine Sulfate is Morphinan-3,6-diol, 7,8-didehydro-4,5-epoxy-17-methyl-, (5α,6α)-, sulfate (2:1) (salt), pentahydrate, which can be represented by the following structural formula:

Morphine Sulfate acts as a narcotic analgesic.

HOW SUPPLIED

Morphine Sulfate Immediate Release Oral Solution is available as follows:

NDC 0186-1124-95, 10 mg/5 mL, 500 mL Bottle

DEA Order Form Required.

Caution: Federal law prohibits dispensing without prescription.

021694R01   Iss. 8/97

MORPHINE SULFATE INJECTION, USP

DESCRIPTION

Morphine Sulfate Injection, USP is a sterile product intended for subcutaneous, intramuscular, or intravenous injection.

In the 2 mL size vials and ampules, each mL of solution contains 8 mg (1/8 gr.), 10 mg (1/6 gr.) or 15 mg (1/4 gr.) morphine sulfate (Warning-May be habit forming) in Water for Injection, USP, with not more than 5 mg chlorobutanol and 1 mg edetate disodium. Sulfuric acid is present to adjust pH between 2.5–6.5. The 2 mL size containers have a 1 mL fill to permit mixing with other compatible medications immediately prior to use. Filled under nitrogen.

In multiple dose vial form, each mL of solution contains 15 mg (1/4 gr.) morphine sulfate (Warning-May be habit forming) in Water for Injection, USP, with not more than 5 mg chlorobutanol and 1 mg sodium bisulfite. The pH of this solution is between 2.5–6.5. Filled under nitrogen.

Morphine is one of the naturally occurring phenanthrene alkaloids of opium derived from the opium poppy. It is classified pharmacologically as a narcotic analgesic.

Morphine sulfate may be designated chemically as 7,8-Didehydro-4,5 α-epoxy-17-methylmorphinan-3,6 α-diol sulfate (2:1) (salt) pentahydrate, with the following structural formula:

Morphine sulfate occurs as white, feathery, silky crystals, cubical masses of crystals, or white crystalline powder; it is soluble in water and slightly soluble in alcohol.

CLINICAL PHARMACOLOGY

Like other narcotic analgesics, morphine exerts its principal pharmacological effects on the central nervous system and gastrointestinal tract, its primary actions of therapeutic value are analgesia and sedation. The analgesic effects of morphine are due to its central action; however, the precise sites of action have not been determined and the mechanisms involved appear to be quite complex. Morphine appears to increase the patient's tolerance for pain and to decrease the perception of suffering, although the presence of the pain itself may still be recognized.

In addition to analgesia, alterations in mood, including euphoria and dysphoria, drowsiness, and mental clouding commonly occur. Morphine depresses various respiratory centers, depresses the cough reflex, and constricts the pupils. Morphine may cause nausea and vomiting by stimulating the chemoreceptor trigger zone (CTZ); however, it also depresses the vomiting center, so that subsequent doses are unlikely to produce vomiting. Nausea and vomiting are significantly more common in ambulatory than in recumbent patients.

Morphine increases the tone and decreases the propulsive contractions of the smooth muscle of the gastrointestinal tract. The resultant prolongation in gastrointestinal transit time is responsible for the constipating effect of morphine. Because morphine may increase biliary tract pressure, some patients with biliary colic may experience worsening rather than relief of pain.

While morphine generally increases the tone of urinary tract smooth muscle, the net effect tends to be variable, in some cases producing urinary urgency. In others, difficulty in urination. Morphine has been reported to cause antidiuretic hormone (ADH) to be released, thereby reducing urine output.

In therapeutic dosage, morphine does not usually exert major effects on the cardiovascular system. However, some patients exhibit a propensity to develop orthostatic hypotension and fainting. Rapid intravenous injection is more likely to precipitate a fall in blood pressure than are intramuscular or subcutaneous injections.

Narcotic analgesics cause histamine release, which appears to be responsible for wheals or urticaria sometimes seen at the site of injection. Histamine release may also produce dilation of cutaneous blood vessels, with resultant flushing of the face and neck, pruritus, and sweating.

Morphine is well absorbed after intramuscular and subcutaneous injection. It is relatively ineffective orally, reportedly because of extensive "first-pass" biotransformation by the intestinal mucosa and the liver. The major pathway of morphine metabolism is conjugation with glucuronic acid. Morphine 3-glucuronide as well as some free morphine are excreted in the urine, over 90% of the total excretion occurring in the first 24 hours. Some conjugated morphine appears in the bile and about 7 to 10% of an administered dose is excreted via the feces. The elimination half-life of morphine administered by various parenteral routes has been reported to be in the range of 2.1 to about 2.6 hours.

Peak analgesia occurs within fifty to ninety minutes following subcutaneous injection, thirty to sixty minutes after intramuscular injection, and twenty minutes after intravenous injection. The duration of analgesia is usually three to six hours.

INDICATIONS AND USAGE

Morphine Sulfate Injection, USP is indicated for the relief of severe pain in adults, infants, and children. It is effective in the control of postoperative pain in addition to relieving preoperative apprehension.

CONTRAINDICATIONS

Morphine is contraindicated in patients with a known hypersensitivity to the drug. Narcotic analgesics, including morphine, are contraindicated in premature infants or during labor when delivery of a premature infant is anticipated.

WARNINGS

General: The multiple dose vial of morphine sulfate contains sodium bisulfite, a sulfite that may cause allergic-type reactions including anaphylactic symptoms and life-threatening or less severe asthmatic episodes in certain susceptible people. The overall prevalence of sulfite sensitivity in the general population is unknown and probably low. Sulfite sensitivity is seen more frequently in asthmatic than in nonasthmatic people.

Head Injury and Increased Intracranial Pressure: The respiratory-depressant effects of morphine and its capacity to elevate cerebrospinal fluid pressure may be markedly exaggerated in the presence of head injury, other intracranial lesions, or a preexisting increase in intracranial pressure. Furthermore, narcotics produce adverse reactions which may obscure the clinical course of patients with head injuries. In such patients, morphine must be used with extreme caution and only if its use is deemed essential.

Asthma and Other Respiratory Conditions: Morphine should be used with extreme caution in patients having an acute asthmatic attack, patients with chronic obstructive pulmonary disease or cor pulmonale, patients having a substantially decreased respiratory reserve, and patients with preexisting respiratory depression, hypoxia or hypercapnia. In such patients, even usual therapeutic doses of narcotics may decrease respiratory drive while simultaneously increasing airway resistance to the point of apnea.

Intravenous Use: If necessary morphine may be given intravenously, but the injection should be given very slowly. Rapid intravenous injection of narcotic analgesics, including morphine, increases the incidence of adverse reactions; severe respiratory depression, apnea, hypotension, peripheral circulatory collapse, cardiac arrest, as well as anaphylactoid reactions, have occurred. Morphine should not be administered intravenously unless a narcotic antagonist and the facilities for resuscitation and assisted or controlled respiration are immediately available. When morphine is given parenterally, especially intravenously, the patient should be lying down.

Hypotensive Effect: The administration of morphine may result in severe hypotension in an individual whose ability to maintain his blood pressure has already been compromised by a depleted blood volume or concurrent administration of drugs such as the phenothiazines or certain anesthetics.

Morphine may produce orthostatic hypotension in ambulatory patients.

PRECAUTIONS

General: Narcotic analgesics, including morphine, should be administered with caution and the initial dose reduced in patients with acute abdominal conditions, convulsive disorders, significant hepatic or renal impairment, fever, hypothyroidism, Addison's disease, ulcerative colitis, prostatic hypertrophy, in patients with recent gastrointestinal urinary tract surgery, and in the very young or elderly or debilitated patients.

Caution must be used when injecting any opioid subcutaneously or intramuscularly into chilled areas or in patients with hypotension or shock, since impaired perfusion may prevent complete absorption; if repeated injections are administered, an excessive amount may be suddenly absorbed if normal circulation is reestablished.

Information for Patients: Morphine may impair the mental and/or physical abilities required for the performance of potentially hazardous tasks, such as driving a vehicle or operating machinery. The concomitant use of alcohol or other central nervous system depressants, including sedatives, hypnotics, tranquilizers, phenothiazines, and antihistamines, may have an additive effect. Morphine, like other narcotic analgesics, may produce orthostatic hypotension in ambulatory patients. Patients should be cautioned accordingly.

Drug Interactions: Morphine should be administered cautiously and in reduced dosage to avoid additive effects when other central nervous system depressants, including other narcotic analgesics, general anesthetics, phenothiazines, tricyclic antidepressants, tranquilizers, and alcohol, are given concomitantly.

Virtually all drug interactions involving MAO inhibitors and narcotic analgesics have been reported with meperidine, which is contraindicated in such patients. In patients receiving MAO inhibitors, therefore, before initiating therapy with other narcotic analgesics, including morphine, an initial small test dose is advisable to allow observation of excessive narcotic effects of MAOI interaction.

Drug/Laboratory Test Interactions: Because narcotic analgesics may increase biliary tract pressure, with resultant increases in plasma amylase or lipase levels, determination of these enzyme levels may be unreliable for 24 hours after a narcotic analgesic has been given.

Carcinogenesis, Mutagenesis, Impairment of Fertility: Long-term animal studies have not been performed to assess the carcinogenic potential of morphine, nor are there any other animal or human data available concerning carcinogenesis, mutagenesis, or impairment of fertility with this drug.

Continued on next page

Morphine Sulfate—Cont.

PREGNANCY

Teratogenic Effects—Pregnancy Category C: Morphine has been reported to be teratogenic in mice when administered in single subcutaneous doses over 2000 times the human therapeutic dose. The authors noted that the effects produced resembled hypoxia-induced malformations. In another study, morphine was reported to be teratogenic in golden hamsters at a minimal teratogenic dose of 35 mg/kg, over 230 times the usual therapeutic dose in humans. There are no adequate and well-controlled studies in pregnant women. Morphine should be used in pregnancy only if the potential benefit justifies the potential risk to the fetus.

Nonteratogenic Effects: Dependence has been reported in newborns whose mothers took opiates regularly during pregnancy. Withdrawal signs include irritability, excessive crying, tremors, hyperreflexia, fever, vomiting, and diarrhea. Signs usually appear during the first few days of life.

Labor and Delivery: Narcotic analgesics cross the placental barrier. The closer to delivery and the larger the dose used, the greater the possibility of respiratory depression in the newborn. Narcotic analgesics should be avoided during labor if delivery of a premature infant is anticipated. If the mother has received narcotic analgesics during labor, newborn infants should be observed closely for signs of respiratory depression. Resuscitation may be required (see OVERDOSAGE). The effect of morphine, if any, on the later growth, development, and functional maturation of the child is unknown.

Clinical studies have failed to demonstrate any effect of morphine on the uterus itself or on the pattern of contractions during labor. However, therapeutic doses of morphine have been reported to somewhat increase the duration of labor. The mechanism involved and the clinical significance of this observation, if any, are unknown.

Nursing Mothers: Caution should be exercised when morphine is administered to a nursing woman. Some studies, but not others, have reported detectable amounts of morphine in breast milk. The levels are probably not clinically significant after usual therapeutic dosage. The possibility of clinically important amounts being excreted in breast milk in individuals abusing morphine should be considered.

Pediatric Use: Narcotic analgesics, including morphine, should not be used in premature infants (see CONTRAINDICATIONS). Narcotics are reported to cross the immature blood-brain barrier to a greater extent, thereby producing disproportionate respiratory depression. Narcotic analgesics should be administered to infants and small children only with great caution and in carefully monitored dosage. Safety and effectiveness of morphine in newborn infants have not been established.

ADVERSE REACTIONS

The major hazards of morphine, as with other narcotic analgesics, are respiratory depression and, to a lesser degree, circulatory depression; respiratory arrest, shock, and cardiac arrest have occurred, particularly with overdosage or rapid intravenous administration. Rarely, anaphylactoid reactions have been reported when morphine or other phenanthrene alkaloids of opium are administered intravenously.

The most frequently observed reactions include sedation, light-headedness, dizziness, nausea, vomiting, and sweating. These effects seem to be more prominent in ambulatory patients and in those who are not experiencing severe pain. In such individuals, lower doses are advisable. Some adverse reactions in ambulatory patients may be alleviated if the patient lies down.

Other adverse reactions include:

Central Nervous System—Euphoria, dysphoria, weakness, headache, agitation, tremor, uncoordinated muscle movements, transient hallucinations and disorientation, visual disturbances.

Gastrointestinal—Constipation, biliary tract spasm. Patients with chronic ulcerative colitis may experience increased colonic motility; in patients with acute ulcerative colitis, toxic dilation has been reported.

Cardiovascular—Tachycardia, bradycardia, palpitation, faintness, syncope, and orthostatic hypotension.

Genitourinary—Oliguria and urinary retention; an antidiuretic effect has been reported.

Allergic—Allergic reactions to opiates occur infrequently; pruritus, urticaria, and other skin rashes are most common. Rarely, anaphylactoid reactions have been reported following intravenous administration.

Other—Opiate-induced histamine release may be responsible for the flushing of the face, sweating, and pruritus often seen with these drugs. Wheals and urticaria at the site of injection are probably related to histamine release. Local tissue irritation, pain, and induration have been reported following repeated subcutaneous injection.

DRUG ABUSE AND DEPENDENCE

Controlled Substance: Morphine Sulfate Injection, USP is a Schedule II Controlled Substance.

Abuse: Morphine is known to be a subject of abuse. Opiates produce relaxation, indifference to pain and stress, lethargy and euphoria. Patients who receive narcotics regularly for more than a few days may exhibit mild symptoms, which may not be recognized as withdrawal, upon discontinuation of therapy. However, the overwhelming majority of patients who receive opiates for medical reasons do not develop drug-seeking behavior or compulsive drug use. Personality characteristics play a major role in determining which patients are likely to abuse drugs. Morphine must be administered only under close supervision to patients with a history of drug abuse or dependence.

Dependence: Psychological dependence, physical dependence, and tolerance are known to occur with morphine. The severity of the abstinence syndrome is related to the degree of dependence, the abruptness of withdrawal, and the drug used. If abstinence syndrome is precipitated by administration of a narcotic antagonist, symptoms appear within a few minutes and are maximal within thirty minutes. Administration of a narcotic antagonist as a means of detecting dependence is not usually recommended.

Withdrawal symptoms in patients dependent on morphine begin shortly before the time of the next scheduled dose, reach a peak at 36 to 72 hours after the last dose, then slowly subside over a period of 7 to 10 days. Symptoms include yawning, sweating, lacrimation, rhinorrhea, a restless tossing sleep, dilated pupils, gooseflesh, irritability, tremor, nausea, vomiting, and diarrhea. Treatment of the abstinence syndrome is primarily symptomatic and supportive, including maintenance of proper fluid and electrolyte balance.

OVERDOSAGE

Symptoms: Serious overdose with morphine is characterized by respiratory depression (a decrease in respiratory rate and/or tidal volume, Cheyne-Stokes respiration, cyanosis), extreme somnolence progressing to stupor or coma, skeletal muscle flaccidity, cold and clammy skin, and sometimes bradycardia and hypotension. The triad of coma, pinpoint pupils, and respiratory depression is strongly suggestive of opiate poisoning. In severe overdosage, particularly by the intravenous route, apnea, circulatory collapse, cardiac arrest, and death may occur.

It is difficult to determine with opiates what constitutes a standard toxic or lethal dose. Parenteral doses of morphine in excess of 30 mg are likely to produce serious toxic effects in the normal adult. Infants and children are believed to be relatively more sensitive to opiates on a body-weight basis. Elderly patients are also comparatively intolerant to opiates.

Treatment: Primary attention should be given to the reestablishment of adequate respiratory exchange through provision of a patent airway and institution of assisted or controlled ventilation. The narcotic antagonists, naloxone hydrochloride and levallorphan tartrate, are specific antidotes against respiratory depression which may result from overdosage or unusual sensitivity to narcotics. Therefore, an appropriate dose of one of these antagonists should be administered, preferably by the intravenous route, simultaneously with efforts at respiratory resuscitation.

An antagonist should only be administered in the presence of clinically significant respiratory or cardiovascular depression induced by a narcotic. Oxygen, intravenous fluids, vasopressors, and other supportive measures should be employed as indicated.

NOTE: In an individual physically dependent on narcotics, the administration of the usual dose of a narcotic antagonist will precipitate an acute withdrawal syndrome. The severity of this syndrome will depend on the degree of physical dependence and the dose of the antagonist administered. The use of narcotic antagonists in such individuals should be avoided if possible. If a narcotic antagonist must be used to treat serious respiratory depression in the physically dependent patient, the antagonist should be administered with extreme care and only one-tenth to one-fifth the usual initial dose administered.

DOSAGE AND ADMINISTRATION

Parenteral drug products should be inspected visually for particulate matter and discoloration prior to administration, whenever solution and container permit. Do not use the injection if darker than pale yellow or if discolored in any other way, or if it contains a precipitate.

Morphine Sulfate Injection has been reported to be chemically or physically incompatible with a variety of other injectable medications. Before diluting with any intravenous solution or combining with any other medication, consult specialized references. Do not use if there is any indication of precipitation or other signs of incompatibility.

Adults: The usual initial dose is 10 mg subcutaneously or intramuscularly. The usual adult dosage range is 5 to 20 mg, every four hours, as needed. For more rapid effect, intravenous administration may be indicated (see WARNINGS, Intravenous Use). The usual intravenous dose is 4 to 10 mg, administered very slowly.

Infants and Children: Do not use in premature infants (see CONTRAINDICATIONS). Safety and effectiveness in newborn infants have not been established.

Infants and children may receive 0.1 to 0.2 mg/kg per dose subcutaneously. A single pediatric dose should not exceed 15 mg.

HOW SUPPLIED

Morphine Sulfate Injection, USP is available in the following dosage strengths:

NDC 0186-1139-13 10 mg (1/6 gr.)/mL 2 mL (1 mL fill) Vial Boxes of 25

NDC 0186-1158-02 15 mg (1/4 gr.)/mL 20 mL Multiple Dose Vial Box of 1

021869R06 Rev. 7/97

MORPHINE SULFATE INJECTION, USP Ⓒ

WARNING—MAY BE HABIT FORMING.
FOR INTRAVENOUS USE AFTER DILUTION.
NOT FOR EPIDURAL OR INTRATHECAL USE.

(For details of indications, dosage and administration, precautions, and adverse reactions, see circular in package.)

DESCRIPTION

Morphine is a tertiary nitrogen base containing a phenanthrene nucleus; it has two hydroxyl groups, one phenolic and the other alcoholic (secondary). The sulfate salt occurs as white, feathery, silky crystals, cubical masses of crystals, or white, crystalline powder.

The chemical name of morphine sulfate is 7,8-didehydro-4,5α-epoxy-17-methylmorphinan-3,6α-diol sulfate (2:1) (salt), pentahydrate.

The molecular formula is $(C_{17}H_{19}NO_3)_2 \cdot H_2SO_4 \cdot 5H_2O$, and the structural formula is as follows:

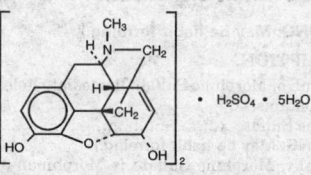

Morphine Sulfate Injection, USP, 25 mg/mL, 20 mL is a sterile solution of morphine sulfate for intravenous infusion after dilution.

Each mL contains: Morphine sulfate 25 mg, edetate disodium 0.075% and sodium bisulfite 0.1% as an antioxidant, in Water for Injection q.s.

This product contains no bacteriostat or antimicrobial agents and is intended as a single dose unit. When the dosing requirement is completed, the unused portion should be discarded in an appropriate manner.

NOTE: This product is not intended for intrathecal use, epidural use, or direct injection.

HOW SUPPLIED

Morphine Sulfate Injection, USP, 25 mg/mL is available in a single dose vial as follows:
NDC 0186-1135-51, 25 mg/mL, 20 mL vial, (box of one)
Store at controlled room temperature 15°–30°C (59°–86°F).
PROTECT FROM LIGHT.
CAUTION: Federal law prohibits dispensing without prescription.
021643R00 Iss. 9/94

MORPHINE SULFATE INJECTION, USP Ⓒ

WARNING—MAY BE HABIT FORMING.
For Intravenous Infusion Only.
Not For Epidural Or Intrathecal Use.

(For details of indications, dosage and administration, precautions, and adverse reactions, see circular in package.)

DESCRIPTION

Morphine is a tertiary nitrogen base containing a phenanthrene nucleus; it has two hydroxyl groups, one phenolic and the other alcoholic (secondary). The sulfate salt occurs as white, feathery, silky crystals, cubical masses of crystals or white, crystalline powder.

The chemical name of morphine sulfate is 7,8-didehydro-4,5α-epoxy-17-methylmorphinan-3,6α-diol sulfate (2:1) (salt), pentahydrate.

The empirical formula is $(C_{17}H_{19}NO_3)_2 \cdot H_2SO_4 \cdot 5H_2O$ and the structure is as follows:

[See chemical structure at top of next column]

Morphine Sulfate Injection, USP, is a sterile solution of 1 mg/mL or 2 mg/mL morphine sulfate pentahydrate in Water for Injection, USP. The 1 mg/mL and 2 mg/mL solutions contain Sodium Chloride 7.6 mg; with citric acid, anhydrous 0.4 mg and sodium citrate, dihydrate 0.2 mg added as buf-

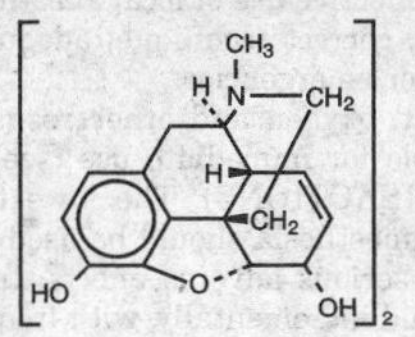

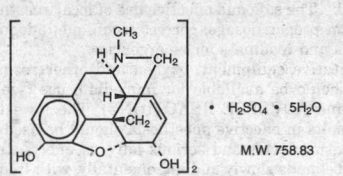

• H_2SO_4 • $5H_2O$

M.W. 758.83

fers. Sodium metabisulfite 0.9 mg is added as an antioxidant. May contain additional citric acid and sodium citrate for pH adjustment.

The solutions contain no bacteriostat or antimicrobial agents and are intended only as single dose units for slow intravenous use by infusion pump. When the dosing requirement is completed, the unused portion should be discarded in an appropriate manner.

HOW SUPPLIED

Morphine Sulfate Injection, USP, is available in single-dose vials as follows:
NDC 0186-1120-81 1 mg/mL, 60 mL vial (box of one)
Store at controlled room temperature 15°–30°C (59°–86°F).
PROTECT FROM LIGHT.
NOTE: Morphine sulfate solutions may darken with age.
CAUTION: Federal law prohibits dispensing without prescription.
021691R01 Rev. 3/97

M.V.I.®-12 ℞

Multi-Vitamin Infusion
For dilution in intravenous infusions only.

(For details of indications, dosage and administration, precautions, and adverse reactions, see circular in package.)

After M.V.I.-12 is diluted in an intravenous infusion, the resulting solution is ready for immediate use. Some of the vitamins in this product, particularly A and D and riboflavin, are light sensitive, and exposure to light should be minimized.
Store at 2°–8°C (36°–46°F).

HOW SUPPLIED

M.V.I.-12—NDC 0186-1199-31 Boxes of 25 and cartons of 100. Each box contains two vials—Vial 1 (5 mL) and Vial 2 (5 mL), both vials to be used for a single dose.
M.V.I.-12 Multi-Dose (PHARMACY BULK PACKAGE)–NDC 0186-1199-10 Boxes of 20 vials, 50 mL each (10 Vial 1 and 10 Vial 2). Mix contents of Vial 1 with Vial 2 to provide ten single doses.
M.V.I.-12 UNIT VIAL—NDC 0186-1199-35 Boxes of 25 two-chambered 10 mL vials.
Caution: Federal law prohibits dispensing without prescription.
Manufactured by:
Centeon L.L.C.
Kankakee, Illinois 60901
Manufactured for:
Astra USA, Inc.
Westborough, MA 01581
021644R02 Rev. 10/97

M.V.I.® PEDIATRIC ℞

Multi-Vitamins for Infusion
For dilution in intravenous infusions only.

(For details of indications, dosage and administration, precautions, and adverse reactions, see circular in package.)

DISCARD ANY UNUSED PORTION.
Parenteral drug products should be inspected visually for particulate matter and discoloration prior to administration, whenever solution and container permit.
After M.V.I. Pediatric is reconstituted it should be immediately diluted into the intravenous solution. The resulting solution should be administered immediately. Some of the vitamins in this product, particularly vitamins A and D and riboflavin, are light-sensitive and exposure to light should be minimized.

HOW SUPPLIED

M.V.I Pediatric is available as:
NDC 0186-1839-35, Single Dose Vial, Boxes of 25.
NDC 0186-1839-25, Single-use, multiple dose vials (PHARMACY BULK PACKAGE), Boxes of 5.
Store at controlled room temperature, 15°–30°C (59°–86°F).
Caution: Federal law prohibits dispensing without prescription.
Manufactured by:
Centeon L.L.C. Kankakee, Illinois 60901
Manufactured for:
Astra USA, Inc. Westborough, MA 01581
021645R02 Rev. 10/97

NALBUPHINE HCl INJECTION ℞

(For details of indications, dosage and administration, precautions, and adverse reactions, see circular in package.)

HOW SUPPLIED

Nalbuphine HCl Injection for intramuscular, subcutaneous or intravenous use is available in the following dosage forms:
Vials
10 mg/mL, 10 mL vial (box of 1), NDC 0186-1262-12
20 mg/mL, 10 mL vial (box of 1), NDC 0186-1266-12
Store at controlled room temperature 15°–30°C (59°–86°F).
Protect from light.
021886R05 Rev. 6/97

NAROPIN™ ℞

[nă-rōpin]
(ropivacaine HCl Injection)

DESCRIPTION

Naropin™ (ropivacaine HCl Injection) is a member of the amino amide class of local anesthetics. Naropin injections are sterile, isotonic solutions that contain the enantiomerically pure drug substance, sodium chloride for isotonicity and Water for Injection. Sodium hydroxide and/or hydrochloric acid may be used for pH adjustment. These solutions are administered parenterally.
Naropin contains ropivacaine HCl which is chemically described as S-(-)-1-propyl-2′,6′-pipecoloxylidide hydrochloride monohydrate. The drug substance is a white crystalline powder, with a chemical formula of $C_{17}H_{26}N_2O{\cdot}HCl{\cdot}H_2O$, molecular weight of 328.89 and the following structural formula:

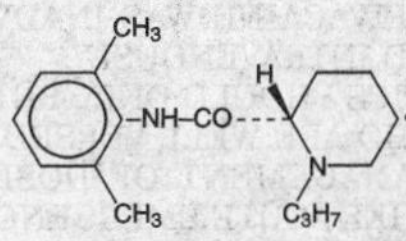

• HCl • H_2O

At 25°C ropivacaine HCl has a solubility of 53.8 mg/mL in water, a distribution ratio between n-octanol and phosphate buffer at pH 7.4 of 141 and a pKa of 8.07 in 0.1 M KCl solution. The pKa of ropivacaine is approximately the same as bupivacaine (8.1) and is similar to that of mepivacaine (7.7). However, ropivacaine has an intermediate degree of lipid solubility compared to bupivacaine and mepivacaine.
Naropin is preservative free and is available in single dose containers in 2.0, 5.0, 7.5 and 10.0 mg/mL concentrations. The specific gravity of Naropin solutions range from 1.002 to 1.005 at 25°C.

CLINICAL PHARMACOLOGY

Mechanism of Action: Ropivacaine is a member of the amino amide class of local anesthetics and is supplied as the pure S-(-)-enantiomer. Local anesthetics block the generation and the conduction of nerve impulses, presumably by increasing the threshold for electrical excitation in the nerve, by slowing the propagation of the nerve impulse, and by reducing the rate of rise of the action potential. In general, the progression of anesthesia is related to the diameter, myelination and conduction velocity of affected nerve fibers. Clinically, the order of loss of nerve function is as follows: (1) pain, (2) temperature, (3) touch, (4) proprioception, and (5) skeletal muscle tone.

PHARMACOKINETICS

Absorption: The systemic concentration of ropivacaine is dependent on the total dose and concentration of drug administered, the route of administration, the patient's hemodynamic/circulatory condition and the vascularity of the administration site.
From the epidural space, ropivacaine shows complete and biphasic absorption. The half-lives of the two phases, (mean ± SD) are 14 ± 7 minutes and 4.2 ± 0.9 h, respectively. The slow absorption is the rate limiting factor in the elimination of ropivacaine which explains why the terminal half-life is longer after epidural than after intravenous administration. Ropivacaine shows dose-proportionality up to the highest intravenous dose studied, 80 mg, corresponding to a mean ± SD peak plasma concentration of 1.9 ±0.3 μg/mL.
Distribution: After intravascular infusion, ropivacaine has a steady state volume of distribution of 41 ± 7 liters. Ropivacaine is 94% protein bound, mainly to α_1-acid glycoprotein. An increase in total plasma concentrations during continuous epidural infusion has been observed, related to a postoperative increase of α_1-acid glycoprotein. Variations in unbound, i.e. pharmacologically active, concentrations have been less than in total plasma concentration. Ropivacaine readily crosses the placenta and equilibrium in regard to unbound concentration will be rapidly reached (see PRECAUTIONS, Labor and Delivery).
Metabolism: Ropivacaine is extensively metabolized in the liver, predominantly by aromatic hydroxylation mediated by cytochrome P4501A to 3-hydroxy ropivacaine. Approximately 37% of the total dose is excreted in the urine as both free and conjugated 3-hydroxy ropivacaine. Low concentrations of 3-hydroxy ropivacaine have been found in the plasma. Urinary excretion of the 4-hydroxy and both the 3-hydroxy and 4-hydroxy N-dealkylated metabolites accounts for less than 3% of dose. An additional metabolite, 2-hydroxy-methyl-ropivacaine, has been identified but not quantified in the urine. Both 3-hydroxy and 4-hydroxy ropivacaine have a local anesthetic activity in animal models less than that of ropivacaine. There is no evidence of *in vivo* racemization in urine of S-(-)-ropivacaine to R-(+)-ropivacaine.
Elimination: The kidney is the main excretory organ for most local anesthetic metabolites. In total, 86% of the ropivacaine dose is excreted in the urine after intravenous administration of which only 1% relates to unchanged drug. Ropivacaine has a mean ± SD total plasma clearance of 387 ± 107 mL/min, an unbound plasma clearance of 7.2 ± 1.6 L/min, and a renal clearance of 1 mL/min. The mean ± SD terminal half-life is 1.8 ± 0.7 h after intravascular administration and 4.2 ± 1.0 h after epidural administration (see Absorption).
Pharmacodynamics: Studies in humans have demonstrated that, unlike most other local anesthetics, the presence of epinephrine has no major effect on either the time of onset or the duration of action of ropivacaine. Likewise, addition of epinephrine to ropivacaine has no effect on limiting systemic absorption of ropivacaine.
Systemic absorption of local anesthetics can produce effects on the central nervous and cardiovascular systems. At blood concentrations achieved with therapeutic doses, changes in cardiac conduction, excitability, refractoriness, contractility, and peripheral vascular resistance are minimal. However, toxic blood concentrations depress cardiac conduction and excitability, which may lead to atrioventricular block, ventricular arrhythmias and to cardiac arrest, sometimes resulting in fatalities. In addition, myocardial contractility is depressed and peripheral vasodilation occurs, leading to decreased cardiac output and arterial blood pressure.
Following systemic absorption, local anesthetics can produce central nervous system stimulation, depression or both. Apparent central stimulation is usually manifested as restlessness, tremors and shivering, progressing to convulsions, followed by depression and coma, progressing ultimately to respiratory arrest. However, the local anesthetics have a primary depressant effect on the medulla and on higher centers. The depressed stage may occur without a prior excited stage.
In two clinical pharmacology studies (total n=24) ropivacaine and bupivacaine were infused (10 mg/min) in human volunteers until the appearance of CNS symptoms, e.g., visual or hearing disturbances, perioral numbness, tingling and others. Similar symptoms were seen with both drugs. In one study, the mean ± SD maximum tolerated intravenous dose of ropivacaine infused (124 ± 38 mg) was significantly higher than that of bupivacaine (99 ± 30 mg) while in the other study the doses were not different (115 ± 29 mg of ropivacaine and 103 ± 30 mg of bupivacaine). In the latter study, the number of subjects reporting each symptom was similar for both drugs with the exception of muscle twitching which was reported by more subjects with bupivacaine than ropivacaine at comparable intravenous doses. At the end of the infusion, ropivacaine in both studies caused significantly less depression of cardiac conductivity (less QRS widening) than bupivacaine. Ropivacaine and bupivacaine caused evidence of depression of cardiac contractility, but there were no changes in cardiac output.
In nonclinical pharmacology studies comparing ropivacaine and bupivacaine in several animal species, the cardiac toxicity of ropivacaine was less than that of bupivacaine, although both were considerably more toxic than lidocaine. Arrhythmogenic and cardiodepressant effects were seen in animals at significantly higher doses of ropivacaine than bupivacaine. The incidence of successful resuscitation was not significantly different between the ropivacaine and bupivacaine groups.
Clinical Trials: Ropivacaine was studied as a local anesthetic both for surgical anesthesia and for acute pain management. (See DOSAGE AND ADMINISTRATION.)
The onset, depth and duration of sensory block are, in general, similar to bupivacaine. However, the depth and duration of motor block, in general, are less than that with bupivacaine.

Continued on next page

Naropin—Cont.

Epidural Administration In Surgery—There were 25 clinical studies performed in 900 patients to evaluate Naropin epidural injection for general surgery. Naropin was used in doses ranging from 75 to 250 mg. In doses of 100-200 mg, the median (1st-3rd quartile) onset time to achieve a T10 sensory block was 10 (5-13) minutes and the median (1st-3rd quartile) duration at the T10 level was 4 (3-5) hours. (See DOSAGE AND ADMINISTRATION.)
Higher doses produced a more profound block with a greater duration of effect.
Epidural Administration In Cesarean Section—There were 8 studies performed in 218 patients to evaluate Naropin for cesarean section. 5 mg/mL (0.5%) Naropin was used in doses up to 150 mg. Median onset measured at T6 ranged from 11 to 26 minutes. Median duration of sensory block at T6 ranged from 1.7 to 3.2 h, and duration of motor block ranged from 1.4 to 2.9 h. Naropin provided adequate muscle relaxation for surgery in all cases.
Epidural Administration In Labor And Delivery—There were 10 double-blind clinical studies performed to evaluate Naropin versus bupivacaine for epidural block for management of labor pain (Naropin, n=258; bupivacaine, n=231). When administered in doses up to 278 mg as intermittent injections or as a continuous infusion, Naropin produced adequate pain relief.
A prospective meta-analysis on 6 of these studies provided detailed evaluation of the delivered newborns and showed no difference in clinical outcomes compared to bupivacaine. There were significantly fewer instrumental deliveries in mothers receiving ropivacaine as compared to bupivacaine.

LABOR AND DELIVERY META-ANALYSIS: MODE OF DELIVERY

Delivery Mode	Naropin n=199		Bupivacaine n=188	
	n	%	n	%
Spontaneous Vertex	116	58	92	49
Vacuum Extractor	26		33	
		}27*		}40
Forceps	28		42	
Cesarean Section	29	15	21	11

* p=0.004 versus bupivacaine

Epidural Administration In Postoperative Pain Management—There were 8 clinical studies performed in 382 patients to evaluate Naropin for postoperative pain management after upper and lower abdominal surgery and after orthopedic surgery. The studies utilized intravascular morphine via PCA as a rescue medication and as an efficacy variable. Epidural anesthesia with Naropin was used intraoperatively for each of these procedures prior to initiation of postoperative Naropin. The incidence and intensity of the motor block were dependent on the dose rate of Naropin and the site of injection. Cumulative doses of up to 770 mg of ropivacaine were administered over 24 hours (intraoperative block plus postoperative continuous infusion). The overall quality of pain relief, as judged by the patients, in the ropivacaine groups was rated as good or excellent (73% to 100%). The frequency of motor block was greatest at 4 hours and decreased during the infusion period in all groups. At least 80% of patients in the upper and lower abdominal studies and 42% in the orthopedic studies had no motor block at the end of the 21-hour infusion period. Sensory block was also dose rate-dependent and a decrease in spread was observed during the infusion period. Clinical studies with 2 mg/mL (0.2%) Naropin have demonstrated that infusion rates of 6–10 mL (12–20 mg) per hour provide adequate analgesia with only slight and non-progressive motor block in cases of moderate to severe postoperative pain. In these studies, this technique resulted in a significant reduction in patients' morphine rescue dose-requirement. Clinical experience supports the use of Naropin epidural infusions for up to 24 hours.
Epidural infusion of Naropin has, in some cases, been associated with transient increases in temperature to > 38.5°C. This occurred more frequently at doses >16 mg/h.
Peripheral Nerve Block—Naropin, 5 mg/mL, (0.5%), was evaluated for its ability to provide anesthesia for surgery using the techniques of Peripheral Nerve Block. There were 13 studies performed including a series of 4 pharmacodynamic and pharmacokinetic studies performed on minor nerve blocks. From these, 235 Naropin treated patients were evaluable for efficacy. Naropin was used in doses up to 275 mg. When used for brachial plexus block, onset depended on technique used. Supraclavicular blocks were consistently more successful than axillary blocks. The median onset of sensory block (anesthesia) produced by ropivacaine 0.5% via axillary block ranged from 10 minutes (medial brachial cutaneous nerve) to 45 minutes (musculocutaneous nerve). Median duration ranged from 3.7 hours (medial brachial cutaneous nerve) to 8.7 hours (ulnar nerve). The 5 mg/mL (0.5%) Naropin solution gave success rates from 56% to 86% for axillary blocks, compared with 92% for supraclavicular blocks.
Local Infiltration—There were 7 clinical studies performed to evaluate the local infiltration of Naropin to produce anesthesia for surgery and analgesia in postoperative pain management. In these studies, 297 patients who received Naropin in doses up to 200 mg were evaluable for efficacy. With infiltration of 100–200 mg Naropin, the time to first request for analgesic was 2–6 hours. When compared to placebo, Naropin produced lower pain scores and a reduction of analgesic consumption.

INDICATIONS AND USAGE

Naropin is indicated for the production of local or regional anesthesia for surgery, for postoperative pain management and for obstetrical procedures.

Surgical Anesthesia:	epidural block for surgery including cesarean section; major nerve block; local infiltration
Acute Pain Management:	epidural continuous infusion or intermittent bolus e.g., postoperative or labor; local infiltration

Standard current textbooks should be consulted to determine the accepted procedures and techniques for the administration of local anesthetic agents.

CONTRAINDICATIONS

Naropin is contraindicated in patients with a known hypersensitivity to Naropin or to any local anesthetic agent of the amide type.

WARNINGS

FOR CESAREAN SECTION, THE 5 MG/ML (0.5%) NAROPIN SOLUTION IN DOSES UP TO 150 MG IS RECOMMENDED. AS WITH ALL LOCAL ANESTHETICS, NAROPIN SHOULD BE ADMINISTERED IN INCREMENTAL DOSES. SINCE NAROPIN SHOULD NOT BE INJECTED RAPIDLY IN LARGE DOSES, IT IS NOT RECOMMENDED FOR EMERGENCY SITUATIONS, WHERE A FAST ONSET OF SURGICAL ANESTHESIA IS NECESSARY. HISTORICALLY, PREGNANT PATIENTS WERE REPORTED TO HAVE A HIGH RISK FOR CARDIAC ARRHYTHMIAS, CARDIAC/ CIRCULATORY ARREST AND DEATH WHEN BUPIVACAINE WAS INADVERTENTLY RAPIDLY INJECTED INTRAVENOUSLY.
LOCAL ANESTHETICS SHOULD ONLY BE EMPLOYED BY CLINICIANS WHO ARE WELL VERSED IN THE DIAGNOSIS AND MANAGEMENT OF DOSE RELATED TOXICITY AND OTHER ACUTE EMERGENCIES WHICH MIGHT ARISE FROM THE BLOCK TO BE EMPLOYED, AND THEN ONLY AFTER INSURING THE **IMMEDIATE (WITHOUT DELAY)** AVAILABILITY OF OXYGEN, OTHER RESUSCITATIVE DRUGS, CARDIOPULMONARY RESUSCITATIVE EQUIPMENT, AND THE PERSONNEL RESOURCES NEEDED FOR PROPER MANAGEMENT OF TOXIC REACTIONS AND RELATED EMERGENCIES (See also ADVERSE REACTIONS and PRECAUTIONS). DELAY IN PROPER MANAGEMENT OF DOSE RELATED TOXICITY, UNDERVENTILATION FROM ANY CAUSE AND/OR ALTERED SENSITIVITY MAY LEAD TO THE DEVELOPMENT OF ACIDOSIS, CARDIAC ARREST AND, POSSIBLY, DEATH.
SOLUTIONS OF NAROPIN SHOULD NOT BE USED FOR THE PRODUCTION OF OBSTETRICAL PARACERVICAL BLOCK ANESTHESIA, RETROBULBAR BLOCK OR SPINAL ANESTHESIA (SUBARACHNOID BLOCK) DUE TO INSUFFICIENT DATA TO SUPPORT SUCH USE. INTRAVENOUS REGIONAL ANESTHESIA (BIER BLOCK) SHOULD NOT BE PERFORMED DUE TO A LACK OF CLINICAL EXPERIENCE AND THE RISK OF ATTAINING TOXIC BLOOD LEVELS OF NAROPIN.
It is essential that aspiration for blood, or cerebrospinal fluid (where applicable), be done prior to injecting any local anesthetic, both the original dose and all subsequent doses, to avoid intravascular or subarachnoid injection. However, a negative aspiration does *not* ensure against an intravascular or subarachnoid injection.
A well-known risk of epidural anesthesia may be an unintentional subarachnoid injection of local anesthetic. Two clinical studies have been performed to verify the safety of Naropin at a volume of 3 mL injected into the subarachnoid space since this dose represents an incremental epidural volume that could be unintentionally injected. The 15 and 22.5 mg doses injected resulted in sensory levels as high as T5 and T4, respectively. Sensory analgesia started in the sacral dermatomes in 2-3 minutes, extended to the T10 level in 10–13 minutes and lasted for approximately 2 hours. The results of these two clinical studies showed that a 3 mL dose did not produce any serious adverse events when spinal anesthesia blockade was achieved.
Naropin should be used with caution in patients receiving other local anesthetics or agents structurally related to amide-type local anesthetics, since the toxic effects of these drugs are additive.

PRECAUTIONS

General: The safe and effective use of local anesthetics depends on proper dosage, correct technique, adequate precautions and readiness for emergencies.
Resuscitative equipment, oxygen and other resuscitative drugs should be available for immediate use (see WARNINGS and ADVERSE REACTIONS). The lowest dosage that results in effective anesthesia should be used to avoid high plasma levels and serious adverse effects. Injections should be made slowly and incrementally, with frequent aspirations before and during the injection to avoid intravascular injection. When a continuous catheter technique is used, syringe aspirations should also be performed before and during each supplemental injection. During the administration of epidural anesthesia, it is recommended that a test dose of a local anesthetic with a fast onset be administered initially and that the patient be monitored for central nervous system and cardiovascular toxicity, as well as for signs of unintended intrathecal administration before proceeding. When clinical conditions permit, consideration should be given to employing local anesthetic solutions which contain epinephrine for the test dose because circulatory changes compatible with epinephrine may also serve as a warning sign of unintended intravascular injection. An intravascular injection is still possible even if aspirations for blood are negative. Administration of higher than recommended doses of Naropin to achieve greater motor blockade or increased duration of sensory blockade may negate the advantages of Naropin's favorable cardiovascular depression profile in the event that an inadvertent intravascular injection occurs.
Injection of repeated doses of local anesthetics may cause significant increases in plasma levels with each repeated dose due to slow accumulation of the drug or its metabolites or to slow metabolic degradation. Tolerance to elevated blood levels varies with the physical condition of the patient. Debilitated, elderly patients, and acutely ill patients and children should be given reduced doses commensurate with their age and physical condition. Local anesthetics should also be used with caution in patients with hypotension, hypovolemia or heart block.
Careful and constant monitoring of cardiovascular and respiratory vital signs (adequacy of ventilation) and the patient's state of consciousness should be performed after each local anesthetic injection. It should be kept in mind at such times that restlessness, anxiety, incoherent speech, lightheadedness, numbness and tingling of the mouth and lips, metallic taste, tinnitus, dizziness, blurred vision, tremors, twitching, depression, or drowsiness may be early warning signs of central nervous system toxicity.
Because amide-type local anesthetics such as Naropin are metabolized by the liver, these drugs, especially repeat doses, should be used cautiously in patients with hepatic disease. Patients with severe hepatic disease, because of their inability to metabolize local anesthetics normally, are at a greater risk of developing toxic plasma concentrations. Local anesthetics should also be used with caution in patients with impaired cardiovascular function because they may be less able to compensate for functional changes associated with the prolongation of A-V conduction produced by these drugs.
Many drugs used during the conduct of anesthesia are considered potential triggering agents for malignant hyperthermia. Amide-type local anesthetics are not known to trigger this reaction. However, since the need for supplemental general anesthesia cannot be predicted in advance, it is suggested that a standard protocol for management should be available.
Epidural Anesthesia: During epidural administration, Naropin should be administered in incremental doses of 3 to 5 mL with sufficient time between doses to detect toxic manifestations of unintentional intravascular or intrathecal injection. Syringe aspirations should also be performed before and during each supplemental injection in continuous (intermittent) catheter techniques. An intravascular injection is still possible even if aspirations for blood are negative. During the administration of epidural anesthesia, it is recommended that a test dose be administered initially and the effects monitored before the full dose is given. When clinical conditions permit, the test dose should contain epinephrine (10 to 15 μg have been suggested) to serve as a warning of unintentional intravascular injection. If injected into a blood vessel, this amount of epinephrine is likely to produce a transient "epinephrine response" within 45 seconds, consisting of an increase in heart rate and systolic blood pressure, circumoral pallor, palpitations and nervousness in the unsedated patient. The sedated patient may exhibit only a pulse rate increase of 20 or more beats per minute for 15 or more seconds. Therefore, following the test dose, the heart should be continuously monitored for a heart rate increase. Patients on beta-blockers may not manifest changes in heart rate, but blood pressure monitoring can detect a rise in systolic blood pressure. A test dose of a short-acting amide anesthetic such as 30 to 40 mg of lidocaine is recommended to detect an unintentional intrathecal administration. This will be manifested within a few minutes by

signs of spinal block (e.g., decreased sensation of the buttocks, paresis of the legs, or, in the sedated patient, absent knee jerk). An intravascular or subarachnoid injection is still possible even if results of the test dose are negative. The test dose itself may produce a systemic toxic reaction, high spinal or epinephrine-induced cardiovascular effects.

Use in Head and Neck Area: Small doses of local anesthetics injected into the head and neck area may produce adverse reactions similar to systemic toxicity seen with unintentional intravascular injections of larger doses. The injection procedures require the utmost care. Confusion, convulsions, respiratory depression, and/or respiratory arrest, and cardiovascular stimulation or depression have been reported. These reactions may be due to intraarterial injection of the local anesthetic with retrograde flow to the cerebral circulation. Patients receiving these blocks should have their circulation and respiration monitored and be constantly observed. Resuscitative equipment and personnel for treating adverse reactions should be immediately available. Dosage recommendations should not be exceeded (see DOSAGE AND ADMINISTRATION).

Use in Ophthalmic Surgery: The use of Naropin in retrobulbar blocks for ophthalmic surgery has not been studied. Until appropriate experience is gained, the use of Naropin for such surgery is not recommended.

Information for Patients: When appropriate, patients should be informed in advance that they may experience temporary loss of sensation and motor activity in the anesthetized part of the body following proper administration of lumbar epidural anesthesia. Also, when appropriate, the physician should discuss other information including adverse reactions in the Naropin package insert.

Clinically Significant Drug-Drug Interactions: Naropin should be used with caution in patients receiving other local anesthetics or agents structurally related to amide-type local anesthetics, since the toxic effects of these drugs are additive.

In vitro studies indicate that cytochrome P4501A is involved in the formation of 3-hydroxy ropivacaine, the major metabolite. Thus agents likely to be administered concomitantly with Naropin, which are metabolized by this isozyme family may potentially interact with Naropin. Such interaction might be a possibility with drugs known to be metabolized by P4501A2 via competitive inhibition such as theophylline, imipramine and with potent inhibitors such as fluvoxamine and verapamil.

Carcinogenesis, Mutagenesis, Impairment of Fertility: Long term studies in animals of most local anesthetics, including Naropin, to evaluate the carcinogenic potential have not been conducted.

Weak mutagenic activity was seen in the mouse lymphoma test. Mutagenicity was not noted in the other assays, demonstrating that the weak signs of *in vitro* activity in the mouse lymphoma test were not manifest under diverse *in vivo* conditions.

Studies performed with ropivacaine in rats did not demonstrate an effect on fertility or general reproductive performance over two generations.

Pregnancy Category B: Teratogenicity studies in rats and rabbits did not show evidence of any adverse effects on organogenesis or early fetal development in rats or rabbits. The doses used were approximately equal to 5 and 2.5 times, respectively, the maximum recommended human dose (250 mg) based on body weight. There were no treatment related effects on late fetal development, parturition, lactation, neonatal viability or growth of the offspring in 2 perinatal and postnatal studies in rats, at dose levels up to approximately 5 times the maximum recommended human dose based on body weight. In another study with a higher dose, 23 mg/kg, an increased pup loss was seen during the first 3 days postpartum, which was considered secondary to impaired maternal care due to maternal toxicity.

There are no adequate and well-controlled studies in pregnant women of the effects of Naropin on the developing fetus. Naropin should be used during pregnancy only if clearly needed. This does not preclude the use of Naropin after fetal organogenesis is completed or for obstetrical anesthesia or analgesia. (See Labor and Delivery).

Labor and Delivery: Local anesthetics, including Naropin, rapidly cross the placenta, and when used for epidural block can cause varying degrees of maternal, fetal and neonatal toxicity (see CLINICAL PHARMACOLOGY, PHARMACOKINETICS). The incidence and degree of toxicity depend upon the procedure performed, the type and amount of drug used, and the technique of drug administration. Adverse reactions in the parturient, fetus and neonate involve alterations of the central nervous system, peripheral vascular tone and cardiac function.

Maternal hypotension has resulted from regional anesthesia with Naropin for obstetrical pain relief. Local anesthetics produce vasodilation by blocking sympathetic nerves. Elevating the patient's legs and positioning her on her left side will help prevent decreases in blood pressure. The fetal heart rate also should be monitored continuously, and electronic fetal monitoring is highly advisable.

Table 2. Common Events (Epidural Administration)

Adverse Reaction	Naropin 5 mg/mL total N=256		Naropin 7.5 mg/mL total N=297		Naropin 10 mg/mL total N=207		Bupivacaine 5 mg/mL total N=236		Bupivacaine 7.5 mg/mL total N=174	
	N	(%)	N	(%)	N	(%)	N	(%)	N	(%)
hypotension	99	(38.7)	146	(49.2)	113	(54.6)	91	(38.6)	89	(51.1)
nausea	34	(13.3)	68	(22.9)			41	(17.4)	36	(20.7)
bradycardia	29	(11.3)	58	(19.5)	40	(19.3)	32	(13.6)	25	(14.4)
back pain	18	(7.0)	23	(7.7)	34	(16.4)	21	(8.9)	23	(13.2)
vomiting	18	(7.0)	33	(11.1)	23	(11.1)	19	(8.1)	14	(8.0)
headache	12	(4.7)	20	(6.7)	16	(7.7)	13	(5.5)	9	(5.2)
fever	8	(3.1)	5	(1.7)	18	(8.7)	11	(4.7)		
chills	6	(2.3)	7	(2.4)	6	(2.9)	4	(1.7)	3	(1.7)
urinary retention	5	(2.0)	8	(2.7)	10	(4.8)	10	(4.2)		
paresthesia	5	(2.0)	10	(3.4)	5	(2.4)	7	(3.0)		
pruritus			14	(4.7)	3	(1.4)			7	(4.0)

Epidural anesthesia has been reported to prolong the second stage of labor by removing the parturient's reflex urge to bear down or by interfering with motor function. Spontaneous vertex delivery occurred more frequently in patients receiving Naropin than in those receiving bupivacaine.

Nursing Mothers: Some local anesthetic drugs are excreted in human milk and caution should be exercised when they are administered to a nursing woman. The excretion of ropivacaine or its metabolites in human milk has not been studied. Based on the milk/plasma concentration ratio in rats, the estimated daily dose to a pup will be about 4% of the dose given to the mother. Assuming that the milk/plasma concentration in humans is of the same order, the total Naropin dose to which the baby is exposed by breast feeding is far lower than by exposure in utero in pregnant women at term (see PRECAUTIONS).

Pediatric Use: No special studies were conducted in pediatrics. Until further experience is gained in children younger than 12 years, administration of Naropin in this age group is not recommended.

ADVERSE REACTIONS

Reactions to Naropin are characteristic of those associated with other amide-type local anesthetics. A major cause of adverse reactions to this group of drugs may be associated with excessive plasma levels, which may be due to overdosage, unintentional intravascular injection or slow metabolic degradation.

The reported adverse events are derived from controlled clinical trials in the U.S. and other countries. The reference drug was usually bupivacaine. The studies were conducted using a variety of premedications, sedatives, and surgical procedures of varying length. Most adverse events reported were mild and transient, and may reflect the surgical procedures, patient characteristics (including disease) and/or medications administered.

Of the 3558 patients enrolled in the clinical trials, 2404 were exposed to Naropin. Each patient was counted once for each type of adverse event.

Incidence >5%

hypotension, fetal bradycardia, nausea, bradycardia, vomiting, paresthesia, back pain

Incidence 1-5%

fever, headache, pain, postoperative complications, urinary retention, dizziness, pruritus, rigors, anemia, hypertension, tachycardia, anxiety, oliguria, hypoesthesia, chest pain, fetal disorders including tachycardia and fetal distress, and neonatal disorders including jaundice, tachypnea, fever, respiratory disorder and vomiting

A comparison has been made between Naropin and bupivacaine for events with a frequency of 1% or greater. Tables 1a and 1b show adverse events (number and percentage) in patients exposed to *similar doses* in double-blind controlled clinical trials. In the trials, Naropin was administered as an epidural anesthetic/analgesic for surgery, labor, or cesarean section. In addition, patients that received Naropin for peripheral nerve block or local infiltration are included.

Table 1a.
Adverse Events Reported in ≥1% of Adult Patients Receiving Regional Or Local Anesthesia (Surgery, Labor, Cesarean Section, Peripheral Nerve Block and Local Infiltration)

Adverse Reaction	Naropin total N = 742		Bupivacaine total N = 737	
	N	(%)	N	(%)
hypotension	237	(31.9)	225	(30.5)
nausea	92	(12.4)	96	(13.0)
paresthesia	51	(6.9)	44	(6.0)
vomiting	48	(6.5)	38	(5.2)
back pain	36	(4.9)	47	(6.4)
pain	39	(5.3)	40	(5.4)
bradycardia	32	(4.3)	38	(5.2)
headache	23	(3.1)	26	(3.5)
fever	25	(3.4)	20	(2.7)
chills	16	(2.2)	14	(1.9)
dizziness	18	(2.4)	10	(1.4)
pruritus	16	(2.2)	11	(1.5)
urinary retention	10	(1.3)	12	(1.6)
hypoesthesia	8	(1.1)	10	(1.4)

Table 1b.
Adverse Events Reported in ≥1% of Fetuses or Neonates of Mothers Who Received Regional Anesthesia (Cesarean Section and Labor Studies)

Adverse Reaction	Naropin total N = 337		Bupivacaine total N = 317	
	N	(%)	N	(%)
fetal bradycardia	58	(17.2)	53	(16.7)
neonatal jaundice	12	(3.6)	12	(3.8)
neonatal tachypnea	8	(2.4)	11	(3.5)
fetal tachycardia	7	(2.1)	8	(2.5)
neonatal fever	6	(1.8)	8	(2.5)
fetal distress	4	(1.2)	8	(2.5)
neonatal respiratory distress	5	(1.5)	4	(1.3)
neonatal vomiting	5	(1.5)	1	(0.3)

Incidence <1%

The following list includes all adverse and intercurrent events which were recorded in more than one patient, but occurred at an overall rate of less than one percent, and were considered clinically relevant.

Application Site Reactions - injection site pain

Cardiovascular System- vasovagal reaction, syncope, postural hypotension, non-specific ECG abnormalities

Female Reproductive - poor progression of labor, uterine atony

Gastrointestinal System - fecal incontinence, tenesmus

General and Other Disorders - hypothermia, malaise, asthenia, accident and/or injury

Hearing and Vestibular - tinnitus, hearing abnormalities

Heart Rate and Rhythm - extrasystoles, non-specific arrhythmias, atrial fibrillation

Liver and Biliary System - jaundice

Metabolic Disorders - hypokalemia, hypomagnesemia

Musculoskeletal System - myalgia, cramps

Myo/Endo/Pericardium - ST segment changes, myocardial infarction

Nervous System - tremor, Horner's syndrome, paresis, dyskinesia, neuropathy, vertigo, coma, convulsion, hypokinesia, hypotonia, ptosis, stupor

Psychiatric Disorders - agitation, confusion, somnolence, nervousness, amnesia, hallucination, emotional lability, insomnia, nightmares

Respiratory System - dyspnea, bronchospasm, coughing

Skin Disorders - rash, urticaria

Urinary System Disorders - urinary incontinence, urinary tract infection, micturition disorder

Vascular - deep vein thrombosis, phlebitis, pulmonary embolism

Vision - vision abnormalities

For the indication epidural anesthesia for surgery, the 15 most common adverse events were compared between different concentrations of Naropin and bupivacaine. Table 2 is based on data from trials in the U.S. and other countries where Naropin was administered as an epidural anesthetic for surgery.

[See table 2 above]

Continued on next page

Naropin—Cont.

Using data from the same studies, the number (%) of patients experiencing hypotension is displayed by patient age, drug and concentration in Table 4. In Table 3, the adverse events for Naropin are broken down by gender.

Table 3.
Most Common Adverse Events by Gender (Epidural Administration)
Total N: Females = 405, Males = 355

Adverse Reaction	Female N	Female (%)	Male N	Male (%)
hypotension	220	(54.3)	138	(38.9)
nausea	119	(29.4)	23	(6.5)
bradycardia	65	(16.0)	56	(15.8)
vomiting	59	(14.6)	8	(2.3)
back pain	41	(10.1)	23	(6.5)
headache	33	(8.1)	17	(4.8)
chills	18	(4.4)	5	(1.4)
fever	16	(4.0)	3	(0.8)
pruritus	16	(4.0)	1	(0.3)
pain	12	(3.0)	4	(1.1)
urinary retention	11	(2.7)	7	(2.0)
dizziness	9	(2.2)	4	(1.1)
hypoesthesia	8	(2.0)	2	(0.6)
paresthesia	8	(2.0)	10	(2.8)

[See table 4 below]

Systemic Reactions: The most commonly encountered acute adverse experiences that demand immediate countermeasures are related to the central nervous system and the cardiovascular system. These adverse experiences are generally dose-related and due to high plasma levels which may result from overdosage, rapid absorption from the injection site, diminished tolerance or from unintentional intravascular injection of the local anesthetic solution. In addition to systemic dose-related toxicity, unintentional subarachnoid injection of drug during the intended performance of lumbar epidural block or nerve blocks near the vertebral column (especially in the head and neck region) may result in underventilation or apnea ("Total or High Spinal"). Also, hypotension due to loss of sympathetic tone and respiratory paralysis or underventilation due to cephalad extension of the motor level of anesthesia may occur. This may lead to secondary cardiac arrest if untreated. Factors influencing plasma protein binding, such as acidosis, systemic diseases that alter protein production or competition with other drugs for protein binding sites, may diminish individual tolerance.

Central Nervous System Reactions: These are characterized by excitation and/or depression. Restlessness, anxiety, dizziness, tinnitus, blurred vision or tremors may occur, possibly proceeding to convulsions. However, excitement may be transient or absent, with depression being the first manifestation of an adverse reaction. This may quickly be followed by drowsiness merging into unconsciousness and respiratory arrest. Other central nervous system effects may be nausea, vomiting, chills, and constriction of the pupils.

The incidence of convulsions associated with the use of local anesthetics varies with the route of administration and the total dose administered. In a survey of studies of epidural anesthesia, overt toxicity progressing to convulsions occurred in approximately 0.1 percent of local anesthetic administrations.

Cardiovascular System Reactions: High doses or unintentional intravascular injection may lead to high plasma levels and related depression of the myocardium, decreased cardiac output, heart block, hypotension, bradycardia, ventricular arrhythmias, including ventricular tachycardia and ventricular fibrillation, and possibly cardiac arrest. (See WARNINGS, PRECAUTIONS, and OVERDOSAGE sections.)

Allergic Reactions: Allergic type reactions are rare and may occur as a result of sensitivity to the local anesthetic (see WARNINGS). These reactions are characterized by signs such as urticaria, pruritus, erythema, angioneurotic edema (including laryngeal edema), tachycardia, sneezing, nausea, vomiting, dizziness, syncope, excessive sweating, elevated temperature, and possibly, anaphylactoid symptomatology (including severe hypotension). Cross sensitivity among members of the amide-type local anesthetic group has been reported. The usefulness of screening for sensitivity has not been definitively established.

Neurologic Reactions: The incidence of adverse neurologic reactions associated with the use of local anesthetics may be related to the total dose and concentration of local anesthetic administered and are also dependent upon the particular drug used, the route of administration and the physical status of the patient. Many of these observations may be related to local anesthetic techniques, with or without a contribution from the drug.

During lumbar epidural block, occasional unintentional penetration of the subarachnoid space by the catheter or needle may occur. Subsequent adverse effects may depend partially on the amount of drug administered intrathecally and the physiological and physical effects of a dural puncture. These observations may include spinal block of varying magnitude (including high or total spinal block), hypotension secondary to spinal block, urinary retention, loss of bladder and bowel control (fecal and urinary incontinence), and loss of perineal sensation and sexual function. Signs and symptoms of subarachnoid block typically start within 2-3 minutes of injection. Doses of 15 and 22.5 mg of Naropin resulted in sensory levels as high as T5 and T4, respectively. Sensory analgesia started in the sacral dermatomes in 2-3 minutes and extended to the T10 level in 10-13 minutes and lasted for approximately 2 hours. Other neurological effects following unintentional subarachnoid administration during epidural anesthesia may include persistent anesthesia, paresthesia, weakness, paralysis of the lower extremities and loss of sphincter control, all of which may have slow, incomplete or no recovery. Headache, septic meningitis, meningismus, slowing of labor, increased incidence of forceps delivery, or cranial nerve palsies due to traction on nerves from loss of cerebrospinal fluid have been reported (see DOSAGE AND ADMINISTRATION discussion of Lumbar Epidural Block). A high spinal is characterized by paralysis of the arms, loss of consciousness, respiratory paralysis and bradycardia.

OVERDOSAGE

Acute emergencies from local anesthetics are generally related to high plasma levels encountered during therapeutic use of local anesthetics or to unintended subarachnoid or intravascular injection of local anesthetic solution. (See ADVERSE REACTIONS, WARNINGS, and PRECAUTIONS.)

Management of Local Anesthetic Emergencies: The practitioner should be familiar with standard contemporary textbooks that address the management of local anesthetic emergencies. No specific information is available on the treatment of overdosage with Naropin; treatment should be symptomatic and supportive. Therapy with Naropin should be discontinued.

The first consideration is prevention, best accomplished by incremental injection of Naropin, careful and constant monitoring of cardiovascular and respiratory vital signs and the patient's state of consciousness after each local anesthetic injection and during continuous infusion. At the first sign of change, oxygen should be administered.

The first step in the management of systemic toxic reactions, as well as underventilation or apnea due to unintentional subarachnoid injection of drug solution, consists of immediate attention to the establishment and maintenance of a patent airway and effective assisted or controlled ventilation with 100% oxygen with a delivery system capable of permitting immediate positive airway pressure by mask. This may prevent convulsions if they have not already occurred.

If necessary, use drugs to control convulsions. Intravenous barbiturates, anticonvulsant agents, or muscle relaxants should only be administered by those familiar with their use. Immediately after the institution of these ventilatory measures, the adequacy of the circulation should be evaluated. Supportive treatment of circulatory depression may require administration of intravenous fluids, and, when appropriate, a vasopressor dictated by the clinical situation (such as ephedrine or epinephrine to enhance myocardial contractile force).

The mean dosages of ropivacaine producing seizures, after intravenous infusion in dogs, nonpregnant and pregnant sheep were 4.9, 6.1 and 5.9 mg/kg, respectively. These doses were associated with peak arterial total plasma concentrations of 11.4, 4.3 and 5.0 µg/mL, respectively. In rats, the LD_{50} is 9.9 and 12 mg/kg by the intravenous route for males and females respectively.

In human volunteers given intravenous Naropin, the mean maximum tolerated total and free arterial plasma concentrations were 4.3 and 0.6 µg/mL respectively, at which time moderate CNS symptoms (muscle twitching) were noted.

Clinical data from patients experiencing local anesthetic induced convulsions demonstrated rapid development of hypoxia, hypercarbia and acidosis within a minute of the onset of convulsions. These observations suggest that oxygen consumption and carbon dioxide production are greatly increased during local anesthetic convulsions and emphasize the importance of immediate and effective ventilation with oxygen which may avoid cardiac arrest.

If difficulty is encountered in the maintenance of a patent airway or if prolonged ventilatory support (assisted or controlled) is indicated, endotracheal intubation, employing drugs and techniques familiar to the clinician, may be indicated after initial administration of oxygen by mask.

The supine position is dangerous in pregnant women at term because of aorta-caval compression by the gravid uterus. Therefore, during treatment of systemic toxicity, maternal hypotension or fetal bradycardia following regional block, the parturient should be maintained in the left lateral decubitus position if possible, or manual displacement of the uterus off the great vessels should be accomplished. Resuscitation of obstetrical patients may take longer than resuscitation of non-pregnant patients and closed-chest cardiac compression may be ineffective. Rapid delivery of the fetus may improve the response to resuscitative efforts.

DOSAGE AND ADMINISTRATION

The rapid injection of a large volume of local anesthetic solution should be avoided and fractional (incremental) doses should always be used. The smallest dose and concentration required to produce the desired result should be administered.

The dose of any local anesthetic administered varies with the anesthetic procedure, the area to be anesthetized, the vascularity of the tissues, the number of neuronal segments to be blocked, the depth of anesthesia and degree of muscle relaxation required, the duration of anesthesia desired, individual tolerance, and the physical condition of the patient. Patients in poor general condition due to aging or other compromising factors such as partial or complete heart conduction block, advanced liver disease or severe renal dysfunction require special attention although regional anesthesia is frequently indicated in these patients. To reduce the risk of potentially serious adverse reactions, attempts should be made to optimize the patient's condition before major blocks are performed, and the dosage should be adjusted accordingly.

Use an adequate test dose (3-5 mL of a short acting local anesthetic solution containing epinephrine) prior to induction of complete block. This test dose should be repeated if the patient is moved in such a fashion as to have displaced the epidural catheter. Allow adequate time for onset of anesthesia following administration of each test dose.

Parenteral drug products should be inspected visually for particulate matter and discoloration prior to administration, whenever solution and container permit. Solutions which are discolored or which contain particulate matter should not be administered. For specific techniques and procedures, refer to standard contemporary textbooks.

[See table at top of next page]

The doses in the table are those considered to be necessary to produce a successful block and should be regarded as guidelines for use in adults. Individual variations in onset and duration occur. The figures reflect the expected average dose range needed. For other local anesthetic techniques standard current textbooks should be consulted.

When prolonged blocks are used, either through continuous infusion or through repeated bolus administration, the risks of reaching a toxic plasma concentration or inducing local neural injury must be considered. Experience to date indicates that a cumulative dose of up to 770 mg Naropin administered over 24 hours is well tolerated in adults when used for postoperative pain management.

For treatment of postoperative pain, the following technique can be recommended: If regional anesthesia was not used intraoperatively, then an epidural block with Naropin is induced via an epidural catheter. Analgesia is maintained with an infusion of Naropin, 2 mg/mL (0.2%). Clinical studies have demonstrated that infusion rates of 6-10 mL (12-20 mg), per hour provide adequate analgesia with only slight and nonprogressive motor block in cases of moderate to severe postoperative pain. If patients require additional pain relief, higher infusion rates of up to 14 mL (28 mg) per hour may be used. With this technique a significant reduction in the need for opioids was demonstrated. Clinical experience supports the use of Naropin epidural infusions for up to 24 hours.

HOW SUPPLIED

Naropin™ Astra E-Z Off® Single Dose Vials:

Table 4.
Effects of Age on Hypotension (Epidural Administration)
Total N: Naropin = 760, bupivacaine = 410

	Naropin						Bupivacaine			
AGE	5 mg/mL		7.5 mg/mL		10 mg/mL		5 mg/mL		7.5 mg/mL	
	N	(%)	N	(%)	N	(%)	N	(%)	N	(%)
<65	68	(32.2)	99	(43.2)	87	(51.5)	64	(33.5)	73	(48.3)
≥65	31	(68.9)	47	(69.1)	26	(68.4)	27	(60.0)	16	(69.6)

Dosage Recommendations

	Conc. mg/mL	(%)	Volume mL	Dose mg	Onset min	Duration hours
SURGICAL ANESTHESIA						
Lumbar Epidural	5.0	(0.5%)	15–30	75–150	15–30	2–4
Administration	7.5	(0.75%)	15–25	113–188	10–20	3–5
Surgery	10.0	(1.0%)	15–20	150–200	10–20	4–6
Lumbar Epidural Administration	5.0	(0.5%)	20–30	100–150	15–25	2–4
Cesarean Section						
Thoracic Epidural Administration	5.0	(0.5%)	5–15	25–75	10–20	n/a[1]
To establish block for postoperative pain relief						
Major Nerve Block	5.0	(0.5%)	35–50	175–250	15–30	5–8
(e.g. brachial plexus block)						
Field Block	5.0	(0.5%)	1–40	5–200	1–15	2–6
(e.g. minor nerve blocks and infiltration)						
LABOR PAIN MANAGEMENT						
Lumbar Epidural Administration						
Initial Dose	2.0	(0.2%)	10–20	20–40	10–15	0.5–1.5
Continuous infusion[2]	2.0	(0.2%)	6–14 mL/h	12–28 mg/h	n/a[1]	n/a[1]
Incremental injections (top-up)[2]	2.0	(0.2%)	10–15 mL/h	20–30 mg/h	n/a[1]	n/a[1]
POSTOPERATIVE PAIN MANAGEMENT						
Lumbar Epidural Administration						
Continuous infusion[3]	2.0	(0.2%)	6–10 mL/h	12–20 mg/h	n/a[1]	n/a[1]
Thoracic Epidural Administration	2.0	(0.2%)	4–8 mL/h	8–16 mg/h	n/a[1]	n/a[1]
Continuous infusion[3]						
Infiltration	2.0	(0.2%)	1–100	2–200	1–5	2–6
(e.g. minor nerve block)	5.0	(0.5%)	1–40	5–200	1–5	2–6

1 = Not Applicable

2 = Median dose of 21 mg per hour was administered by continuous infusion or by incremental injections (top-ups) over a median delivery time of 5.5 hours.

3 = Cumulative doses up to 770 mg of Naropin over 24 hours for postoperative pain management have been well tolerated in adults.

7.5 mg/mL	10 mL	NDC 0186-0867-41	
10.0 mg/mL	10 mL	NDC 0186-0868-41	
Naropin™ Single Dose Vials:			
2.0 mg/mL	20 mL	NDC 0186-0859-51	
5.0 mg/mL	30 mL	NDC 0186-0863-61	
7.5 mg/mL	20 mL	NDC 0186-0867-51	
10.0 mg/mL	20 mL	NDC 0186-0868-51	
Naropin™ Single Dose Ampules:			
2.0 mg/mL	20 mL	NDC 0186-0859-52	
5.0 mg/mL	30 mL	NDC 0186-0863-62	
7.5 mg/mL	20 mL	NDC 0186-0867-52	
10.0 mg/mL	20 mL	NDC 0186-0868-52	
Naropin™ Single Dose Infusion Bottles:			
2.0 mg/mL	100 mL	NDC 0186-0859-81	
2.0 mg/mL	200 mL	NDC 0186-0859-91	
Naropin™ Sterile-Pak® Single Dose Vials:			
2.0 mg/mL	20 mL	Product Code 0859-59	
5.0 mg/mL	30 mL	Product Code 0863-69	
7.5 mg/mL	20 mL	Product Code 0867-59	
10.0 mg/mL	20 mL	Product Code 0868-59	

The solubility of ropivacaine is limited at pH above 6. Thus care must be taken as precipitation may occur if Naropin is mixed with alkaline solutions.

Disinfecting agents containing heavy metals, which cause release of respective ions (mercury, zinc, copper, etc.) should not be used for skin or mucous membrane disinfection since they have been related to incidents of swelling and edema. When chemical disinfection of the container surface is desired, either isopropyl alcohol (91%) or ethyl alcohol (70%) is recommended. It is recommended that chemical disinfection be accomplished by wiping the ampule or vial stopper thoroughly with cotton or gauze that has been moistened with the recommended alcohol just prior to use. When a container is required to have a sterile outside, a Sterile-Pak should be chosen. Glass containers may, as an alternative, be autoclaved once. Stability has been demonstrated using a targeted F_0 of 7 minutes at 121°C.

Solutions should be stored at controlled room temperature 20° - 25°C (68° - 77°F) [see USP].

These products are intended for single use and are free from preservatives. Any solution remaining from an opened container should be discarded promptly. In addition, continuous infusion bottles should not be left in place for more than 24 hours.

Caution: Federal law prohibits dispensing without prescription.

021683R00   Iss. 9/96

Shown in Product Identification Guide, page 304

NESACAINE® ℞
(chloroprocaine HCl Injection, USP)
[nes' a-caine]

NESACAINE®-MPF
(chloroprocaine HCl Injection, USP)
For Infiltration and Nerve Block.

DESCRIPTION

Nesacaine and Nesacaine-MPF Injections are sterile non pyrogenic local anesthetics. The active ingredient in Nesacaine and Nesacaine-MPF Injections is chloroprocaine HCl (benzoic acid, 4-amino-2-chloro-2-(diethylamino) ethyl ester, monohydrochloride), which is represented by the following structural formula:

$$NH_2-C_6H_3(Cl)-COOCH_2CH_2N(C_2H_5)_2 \cdot HCl$$

[See table 1 below]

The solutions are adjusted to pH 2.7–4.0 by means of sodium hydroxide and/or hydrochloric acid. Filled under nitrogen.

Nesacaine and Nesacaine-MPF Injections should not be resterilized by autoclaving.

CLINICAL PHARMACOLOGY

Chloroprocaine, like other local anesthetics, blocks the generation and the conduction of nerve impulses, presumably by increasing the threshold for electrical excitation in the nerve, by slowing the propagation of the nerve impulse and by reducing the rate of rise of the action potential. In general, the progression of anesthesia is related to the diameter, myelination and conduction velocity of affected nerve fibers. Clinically, the order of loss of nerve function is as follows: (1) pain, (2) temperature, (3) touch, (4) proprioception, and (5) skeletal muscle tone.

Systemic absorption of local anesthetics produces effects on the cardiovascular and central nervous systems. At blood concentrations achieved with normal therapeutic doses, changes in cardiac conduction, excitability, refractoriness, contractility, and peripheral vascular resistance are minimal. However, toxic blood concentrations depress cardiac conduction and excitability, which may lead to atrioventricular block and ultimately to cardiac arrest. In addition, with toxic blood concentrations myocardial contractility may be depressed and peripheral vasodilation may occur, leading to decreased cardiac output and arterial blood pressure.

Following systemic absorption, toxic blood concentrations of local anesthetics can produce central nervous system stimulation, depression, or both. Apparent central stimulation may be manifested as restlessness, tremors and shivering, which may progress to convulsions. Depression and coma may occur, possibly progressing ultimately to respiratory arrest. However, the local anesthetics have a primary depressant effect on the medulla and on higher centers. The depressed stage may occur without a prior stage of central nervous system stimulation.

PHARMACOKINETICS

The rate of systemic absorption of local anesthetic drugs is dependent upon the total dose and concentration of drug administered, the route of administration, the vascularity of the administration site, and the presence or absence of epinephrine in the anesthetic injection. Epinephrine usually reduces the rate of absorption and plasma concentration of local anesthetics and is sometimes added to local anesthetic injections in order to prolong the duration of action. The onset of action with chloroprocaine is rapid (usually within 6 to 12 minutes), and the duration of anesthesia, depending upon the amount used and the route of administration, may be up to 60 minutes.

Local anesthetics appear to cross the placenta by passive diffusion. However, the rate and degree of diffusion varies considerably among the different drugs as governed by: (1) the degree of plasma protein binding, (2) the degree of ionization, and (3) the degree of lipid solubility. Fetal/maternal ratios of local anesthetics appear to be inversely related to the degree of plasma protein binding, since only the free, unbound drug is available for placental transfer. Thus, drugs with the highest protein binding capacity may have the lowest fetal/maternal ratios. The extent of placental transfer is also determined by the degree of ionization and lipid solubility of the drug. Lipid soluble, nonionized drugs readily enter the fetal blood from the maternal circulation. Depending upon the route of administration, local anesthetics are distributed to some extent to all body tissues, with high concentrations found in highly perfused organs such as the liver, lungs, heart, and brain.

Various pharmacokinetic parameters of the local anesthetics can be significantly altered by the presence of hepatic or renal disease, addition of epinephrine, factors affecting urinary pH, renal blood flow, the route of administration, and the age of the patient. The *in vitro* plasma half-life of chloroprocaine in adults is 21 ± 2 seconds for males and 25 ± 1 seconds for females. The *in vitro* plasma half-life in neonates is 43 ± 2 seconds.

Chloroprocaine is rapidly metabolized in plasma by hydrolysis of the ester linkage by pseudocholinesterase. The hydrolysis of chloroprocaine results in the production of β-diethylaminoethanol and 2-chloro-4-aminobenzoic acid, which inhibits the action of the sulfonamides (see PRECAUTIONS).

The kidney is the main excretory organ for most local anesthetics and their metabolites. Urinary excretion is affected by urinary perfusion and factors affecting urinary pH.

INDICATIONS AND USAGE

Nesacaine 1% and 2% Injections, in multidose vials with methylparaben as preservative, are indicated for the production of local anesthesia by infiltration and peripheral nerve block. They are not to be used for lumbar or caudal epidural anesthesia.

Nesacaine-MPF 2% and 3% Injections, in single dose vials without preservative and without EDTA, are indicated for

Continued on next page

Table 1: Composition of Available Injections

Product Identification	Chloroprocaine HCl	Sodium Chloride	Disodium EDTA dihydrate	Methylparaben
Nesacaine 1%	10	6.7	0.111	1
Nesacaine 2%	20	4.7	0.111	1
Nesacaine-MPF 2%	20	4.7	—	—
Nesacaine-MPF 3%	30	3.3	—	—

(Formula (mg/mL))

Nesacaine/Nesacaine-MPF—Cont.

the production of local anesthesia by infiltration, peripheral and central nerve block, including lumbar and caudal epidural blocks.
Nesacaine and Nesacaine-MPF Injections are not to be used for subarachnoid administration.

CONTRAINDICATIONS

Nesacaine and Nesacaine-MPF Injections are contraindicated in patients hypersensitive (allergic) to drugs of the PABA ester group.
Lumbar and caudal epidural anesthesia should be used with extreme caution in persons with the following conditions: existing neurological disease, spinal deformities, septicemia, and severe hypertension.

WARNINGS

LOCAL ANESTHETICS SHOULD ONLY BE EMPLOYED BY CLINICIANS WHO ARE WELL VERSED IN DIAGNOSIS AND MANAGEMENT OF DOSE RELATED TOXICITY AND OTHER ACUTE EMERGENCIES WHICH MIGHT ARISE FROM THE BLOCK TO BE EMPLOYED, AND THEN ONLY AFTER ENSURING THE *IMMEDIATE* AVAILABILITY OF OXYGEN, OTHER RESUSCITATIVE DRUGS, CARDIOPULMONARY RESUSCITATIVE EQUIPMENT, AND THE PERSONNEL RESOURCES NEEDED FOR PROPER MANAGEMENT OF TOXIC REACTIONS AND RELATED EMERGENCIES (see also ADVERSE REACTIONS and PRECAUTIONS). DELAY IN PROPER MANAGEMENT OF DOSE RELATED TOXICITY, UNDERVENTILATION FROM ANY CAUSE AND/OR ALTERED SENSITIVITY MAY LEAD TO THE DEVELOPMENT OF ACIDOSIS, CARDIAC ARREST AND, POSSIBLY, DEATH. NESCAINE (chloroprocaine HCl Injection, USP) contains methylparaben and should not be used for lumbar or caudal epidural anesthesia because safety of this antimicrobial preservative has not been established with regard to intrathecal injection, either intentional or unintentional. NESACAINE-MPF Injection contains no preservative; discard unused injection remaining in vial after initial use.
Vasopressors should not be used in the presence of ergot type oxytocic drugs, since a severe persistent hypertension may occur.
To avoid intravascular injection, aspiration should be performed before the anesthetic solution is injected. The needle must be repositioned until no blood return can be elicited. However, the absence of blood in the syringe does not guarantee that intravascular injection has been avoided.
Mixtures of local anesthetics are sometimes employed to compensate for the slower onset of one drug and the shorter duration of action of the second drug. Experiments in primates suggest that toxicity is probably additive when mixtures of local anesthetics are employed, but some experiments in rodents suggest synergism. Caution regarding toxic equivalence should be exercised when mixtures of local anesthetics are employed.

PRECAUTIONS

General: The safety and effective use of chloroprocaine depend on proper dosage, correct technique, adequate precautions and readiness for emergencies. Resuscitative equipment, oxygen and other resuscitative drugs should be available for immediate use. (See WARNINGS and ADVERSE REACTIONS.) The lowest dosage that results in effective anesthesia should be used to avoid high plasma levels and serious adverse effects. Injections should be made slowly, with frequent aspirations before and during the injection to avoid intravascular injection. Syringe aspirations should also be performed before and during each supplemental injection in continuous (intermittent) catheter techniques. During the administration of epidural anesthesia, it is recommended that a test dose be administered (3 mL of 3% or 5 mL of 2% Nesacaine-MPF Injection) initially and that the patient be monitored for central nervous system toxicity and cardiovascular toxicity, as well as for signs of unintended intrathecal administration, before proceeding. When clinical conditions permit, consideration should be given to employing a chloroprocaine solution that contains epinephrine for the test dose because circulatory changes characteristic of epinephrine may also serve as a warning sign of unintended intravascular injection. An intravascular injection is still possible even if aspirations for blood are negative. With the use of continuous catheter techniques, it is recommended that a fraction of each supplemental dose be administered as a test dose in order to verify proper location of the catheter.
Injection of repeated doses of local anesthetics may cause significant increases in plasma levels with each repeated dose due to slow accumulation of the drug or its metabolites. Tolerance to elevated blood levels varies with the physical condition of the patient. Debilitated, elderly patients, acutely ill patients, and children should be given reduced doses commensurate with their age and physical status. Local anesthetics should also be used with caution in patients with hypotension or heart block.
Careful and constant monitoring of cardiovascular and respiratory (adequacy of ventilation) vital signs and the patient's state of consciousness should be accomplished after each local anesthetic injection. It should be kept in mind at such times that restlessness, anxiety, tinnitus, dizziness, blurred vision, tremors, depression or drowsiness may be early warning signs of central nervous system toxicity.
Local anesthetic injections containing a vasoconstrictor should be used cautiously and in carefully circumscribed quantities in areas of the body supplied by end arteries or having otherwise compromised blood supply. Patients with peripheral vascular disease and those with hypertensive vascular disease may exhibit exaggerated vasoconstrictor response. Ischemic injury or necrosis may result.
Since ester-type local anesthetics are hydrolyzed by plasma cholinesterase produced by the liver, chloroprocaine should be used cautiously in patients with hepatic disease.
Local anesthetics should also be used with caution in patients with impaired cardiovascular function since they may be less able to compensate for functional changes associated with the prolongation of A-V conduction produced by these drugs.
Use in Ophthalmic Surgery—When local anesthetic injections are employed for retrobulbar block, lack of corneal sensation should not be relied upon to determine whether or not the patient is ready for surgery. This is because complete lack of corneal sensation usually precedes clinically acceptable external ocular muscle akinesia.
Information for Patients: When appropriate, patients should be informed in advance that they may experience temporary loss of sensation and motor activity, usually in the lower half of the body, following proper administration of epidural anesthesia.
Clinically Significant Drug Interactions: The administration of local anesthetic solutions containing epinephrine or norepinephrine to patients receiving monoamine oxidase inhibitors, tricyclic antidepressants or phenothiazines may produce severe, prolonged hypotension or hypertension. Concurrent use of these agents should generally be avoided. In situation when concurrent therapy is necessary, careful patient monitoring is essential.
Concurrent administration of vasopressor drugs (for the treatment of hypotension related to obstetric blocks) and ergot-type oxytocic drugs may cause severe, persistent hypertension or cerebrovascular accidents.
The para-aminobenzoic acid metabolite of chloroprocaine inhibits the action of sulfonamides. Therefore, chloroprocaine should not be used in any condition in which a sulfonamide drug is being employed.
Carcinogenesis, Mutagenesis, and Impairment of Fertility: Long-term studies in animals to evaluate carcinogenic potential and reproduction studies to evaluate mutagenesis or impairment of fertility have not been conducted with chloroprocaine.
Pregnancy: Category C: Animal reproduction studies have not been conducted with chloroprocaine. It is also not known whether chloroprocaine can cause fetal harm when administered to a pregnant woman or can affect reproduction capacity. Chloroprocaine should be given to a pregnant woman only if clearly needed. This does not preclude the use of chloroprocaine at term for the production of obstetrical anesthesia.
Labor and Delivery: Local anesthetics rapidly cross the placenta, and when used for epidural, paracervical, pudendal or caudal block anesthesia, can cause varying degrees of maternal, fetal and neonatal toxicity. (See CLINICAL PHARMACOLOGY and PHARMACOKINETICS.)
The incidence and degree of toxicity depend upon the procedure performed, the type and amount of drug used, and the technique of drug administration. Adverse reactions in the parturient, fetus and neonate involve alterations of the central nervous system, peripheral vascular tone and cardiac function.
Maternal hypotension has resulted from regional anesthesia. Local anesthetics produce vasodilation by blocking sympathetic nerves. Elevating the patient's legs and positioning her on her left side will help prevent decreases in blood pressure. The fetal heart rate also should be monitored continuously, and electronic fetal monitoring is highly advisable.
Epidural, paracervical, or pudendal anesthesia may alter the forces of parturition through changes in uterine contractility or maternal expulsive efforts. In one study, paracervical block anesthesia was associated with a decrease in the mean duration of first stage labor and facilitation of cervical dilation. However, epidural anesthesia has also been reported to prolong the second stage of labor by removing the parturient's reflex urge to bear down or by interfering with motor function. The use of obstetrical anesthesia may increase the need for forceps assistance.
The use of some local anesthetic drug products during labor and delivery may be followed by diminished muscle strength and tone for the first day or two of life. The long-term significance of these observations is unknown.
Careful adherence to recommended dosage is of the utmost importance in obstetrical paracervical block. Failure to achieve adequate analgesia with recommended doses should arouse suspicion of intravascular or fetal intracranial injection. Cases compatible with unintended fetal intracranial injection of local anesthetic injection have been reported following intended paracervical or pudendal block or both. Babies so affected present with unexplained neonatal depression at birth which correlates with high local anesthetic serum levels and usually manifest seizures within six hours. Prompt use of supportive measures combined with forced urinary excretion of the local anesthetic has been used successfully to manage this complication.
Case reports of maternal convulsions and cardiovascular collapse following use of some local anesthetics for paracervical block in early pregnancy (as anesthesia for elective abortion) suggest that systemic absorption under these circumstances may be rapid. The recommended maximum dose of each drug should not be exceeded. Injection should be made slowly and with frequent aspiration. Allow a 5-minute interval between sides.
There are no data concerning use of chloroprocaine for obstetrical paracervical block when toxemia of pregnancy is present or when fetal distress or prematurity is anticipated in advance of the block; such use is, therefore, not recommended.
The following information should be considered by clinicians who select chloroprocaine for obstetrical paracevical block anesthesia:

1. Fetal bradycardia (generally a heart rate of less than 120 per minute for more than 2 minutes) has been noted by electronic monitoring in about 5 to 10 percent of the cases (various studies) where initial total doses of 120 mg to 400 mg of chloroprocaine were employed. The incidence of bradycardia, within this dose range, might not be dose related.
2. Fetal acidosis has not been demonstrated by blood gas monitoring around the time of bradycardia or afterwards. These data are limited and generally restricted to non-toxemic cases where fetal distress or prematurity was not anticipated in advance of the block.
3. No intact chloroprocaine and only trace quantities of a hydrolysis product, 2-chloro-4-aminobenzoic acid, have been demonstrated in umbilical cord arterial or venous plasma following properly administered paracervical block with chloroprocaine.
4. The role of drug factors and non-drug factors associated with fetal bradycardia following paracervical block are unexplained at this time.

Nursing Mothers: It is not known whether this drug is excreted in human milk. Because many drugs are excreted in human milk, caution should be exercised when chloroprocaine is administered to a nursing woman.
Pediatric Use: Guidelines for the administration of Nesacaine and Nesacaine-MPF Injections to children are presented in DOSAGE AND ADMINISTRATION.

ADVERSE REACTIONS

Systemic: The most commonly encountered acute adverse experiences that demand immediate countermeasures are related to the central nervous system and the cardiovascular system. These adverse experiences are generally dose related and may result from rapid absorption from the injection site, diminished tolerance, or from unintentional intravascular injection of the local anesthetic solution. In addition to systemic dose-related toxicity, unintentional subarachnoid injection of drug during the intended performance of caudal or lumbar epidural block or nerve blocks near the vertebral column (especially in the head and neck region) may result in underventilation or apnea ("Total Spinal"). Factors influencing plasma protein binding, such as acidosis, systemic diseases that alter protein production, or competition of other drugs for protein binding sites, may diminish individual tolerance. Plasma cholinesterase deficiency may also account for diminished tolerance to ester type local anesthetics.
Central Nervous System Reactions: These are characterized by excitation and/or depression. Restlessness, anxiety, dizziness, tinnitus, blurred vision or tremors may occur, possibly proceeding to convulsions. However, excitement may be transient or absent, with depression being the first manifestation of an adverse reaction. This may quickly be followed by drowsiness merging into unconsciousness and respiratory arrest.
The incidence of convulsions associated with the use of local anesthetics varies with the procedure used and the total dose administered. In a survey of studies of epidural anesthesia, overt toxicity progressing to convulsions occurred in approximately 0.1 percent of local anesthetic administrations.
Cardiovascular System Reactions: High doses, or unintended intravascular injection, may lead to high plasma levels and related depression of the myocardium, hypotension, bradycardia, ventricular arrhythmias, and, possibly, cardiac arrest.
Allergic: Allergic type reactions are rare and may occur as a result of sensitivity to the local anesthetic or to other formulation ingredients, such as the antimicrobial preserva-

tive methylparaben, contained in multiple dose vials. These reactions are characterized by signs such as urticaria, pruritis, erythema, angioneurotic edema (including laryngeal edema), tachycardia, sneezing, nausea, vomiting, dizziness, syncope, excessive sweating, elevated temperature, and possibly, anaphylactoid type symptomatology (including severe hypotension). Cross sensitivity among members of the ester-type local anesthetic group has been reported. The usefulness of screening for sensitivity has not been definitely established.

Neurologic: In the practice of caudal or lumbar epidural block, occasional unintentional penetration of the subarachnoid space by the catheter may occur (see PRECAUTIONS). Subsequent adverse observations may depend partially on the amount of drug administered intrathecally. These observations may include spinal block of varying magnitude (including total spinal block), hypotension secondary to spinal block, loss of bladder and bowel control, and loss of perineal sensation and sexual function. Arachnoiditis, persistent motor, sensory and/or autonomic (sphincter control) deficit of some lower spinal segments with slow recovery (several months) or incomplete recovery have been reported in rare instances. (See DOSAGE AND ADMINISTRATION discussion of Caudal and Lumbar Epidural Block.) Backache and headache have also been noted following lumbar epidural or caudal block.

OVERDOSAGE

Acute emergencies from local anesthetics are generally related to high plasma levels encountered during therapeutic use of local anesthetics or to unintended subarachnoid injection of local anesthetic solution (see ADVERSE REACTIONS, WARNINGS and PRECAUTIONS).

In mice, the intravenous LD_{50} of chloroprocaine HCl is 97 mg/kg and the subcutaneous LD_{50} of chloroprocaine HCl is 950 mg/kg.

Management of Local Anesthetic Emergencies: The first consideration is prevention, best accomplished by careful and constant monitoring of cardiovascular and respiratory vital signs and the patient's state of consciousness after each local anesthetic injection. At the first sign of change, oxygen should be administered.

The first step in the management of convulsions, as well as underventilation or apnea due to unintentional subarachnoid injection of drug solution, consists of immediate attention to the maintenance of a patent airway and assisted or controlled ventilation with oxygen and a delivery system capable of permitting immediate positive airway pressure by mask. Immediately after the institution of these ventilatory measures, the adequacy of the circulation should be evaluated, keeping in mind that drugs used to treat convulsions sometimes depress the circulation when administered intravenously. Should convulsions persist despite adequate respiratory support, and if the status of the circulation permits, small increments of an ultra-short acting barbiturate (such as thiopental or thiamylal) or a benzodiazepine (such as diazepam) may be administered intravenously; the clinician should be familiar, prior to the use of anesthetics, with these anticonvulsant drugs. Supportive treatment of circulatory depression may require administration of intravenous fluids and, when appropriate, a vasopressor dictated by the clinical situation (such as ephedrine to enhance myocardial contractile force).

If not treated immediately, both convulsions and cardiovascular depression can result in hypoxia, acidosis, bradycardia, arrhythmias and cardiac arrest. Underventilation or apnea due to unintentional subarachnoid injection of local anesthetic solution may produce these same signs and also lead to cardiac arrest if ventilatory support is not instituted. If cardiac arrest should occur, standard cardiopulmonary resuscitative measures should be instituted. Recovery has been reported after prolonged resuscitative efforts.

Endotracheal intubation, employing drugs and techniques familiar to the clinician, may be indicated, after initial administration of oxygen by mask, if difficulty is encountered in the maintenance of a patent airway or if prolonged ventilatory support (assisted or controlled) is indicated.

DOSAGE AND ADMINISTRATION

Chloroprocaine may be administered as a single injection or continuously through an indwelling catheter. As with all local anesthetics, the dose administered varies with the anesthetic procedure, the vascularity of the tissues, the depth of anesthesia and degree of muscle relaxation required, the duration of anesthesia desired, and the physical condition of the patient. The smallest dose and concentration required to produce the desired result should be used. Dosage should be reduced for children, elderly and debilitated patients and patients with cardiac and/or liver disease. The maximum single recommended doses of chloroprocaine in adults are: without epinephrine, 11 mg/kg, not to exceed a maximum total dose of 800 mg; with epinephrine (1:200,000), 14 mg/kg, not to exceed a maximum total dose of 1000 mg. For specific techniques and procedures, refer to standard textbooks.

Caudal and Lumbar Epidural Block: In order to guard against adverse experiences sometimes noted following unintended penetration of the subarachnoid space, the following procedure modifications are recommended:

Anesthetic Procedure	Solution Concentration %	Volume (mL)	Total Dose (mg)
Mandibular	2	2–3	40–60
Infraorbital	2	0.5–1	10–20
Brachial plexus	2	30–40	600–800
Digital (without epinephrine)	1	3–4	30–40
Pudendal	2	10 each side	400
Paracervical (see also PRECAUTIONS)	1	3 per each of 4 sites	up to 120

1. Use an adequate test dose (3 mL of Nesacaine-MPF 3% Injection or 5 mL of Nesacaine-MPF 2% Injection) prior to induction of complete block. This test dose should be repeated if the patient is moved in such a fashion as to have displaced the epidural catheter. Allow adequate time for onset of anesthesia following administration of each test dose.
2. Avoid the rapid injection of a large volume of local anesthetic injection through the catheter. Consider fractional doses, when feasible.
3. In the event of the known injection of a large volume of local anesthetic injection into the subarachnoid space, after suitable resuscitation and if the catheter is in place, consider attempting the recovery of drug by draining a moderate amount of cerebrospinal fluid (such as 10 mL) through the epidural catheter.

As a guide for some routine procedures, suggested doses are given below:

1. Infiltration and Peripheral Nerve Block: NESACAINE or NESACAINE-MPF (chloroprocaine HCl Injection, USP) [See table above]
2. Caudal and Lumbar Epidural Block: NESACAINE-MPF INJECTION. For caudal anesthesia, the initial dose is 15 to 25 mL of a 2% or 3% solution. Repeated doses may be given at 40 to 60 minute intervals.
   For lumbar epidural anesthesia, 2 to 2.5 mL per segment of a 2% or 3% solution can be used. The usual total volume of Nesacaine-MPF Injection is from 15 to 25 mL. Repeated doses 2 to 6 mL less than the original dose may be given at 40 to 50 minute intervals.

The above dosages are recommended as a guide for use in the average adult. Maximum dosages of all local anesthetics must be individualized after evaluating the size and physical condition of the patient and the rate of systemic absorption from a particular injection site.

Pediatric Dosage: It is difficult to recommend a maximum dose of any drug for children, since this varies as a function of age and weight. For children over 3 years of age who have a normal lean body mass and normal body development, the maximum dose is determined by the child's age and weight and should not exceed 11 mg/kg (5 mg/lb). For example, in a child of 5 years weighing 50 lbs (23 kg), the dose of chloroprocaine HCl without epinephrine would be 250 mg. Concentrations of 0.5–1.0% are suggested for infiltration and 1.0–1.5% for nerve block. In order to guard against systemic toxicity, the lowest effective concentration and lowest effective dose should be used at all times. Some of the lower concentrations for use in infants and smaller children are not available in pre-packaged containers; it will be necessary to dilute available concentrations with the amount of 0.9% sodium chloride injection necessary to obtain the required final concentration of chloroprocaine injection.

Preparation of Epinephrine Injections—To prepare a 1:200,000 epinephrine-chloroprocaine HCl injection, add 0.1 mL of a 1 to 1000 Epinephrine Injection USP to 20 mL of Nesacaine-MPF Injection.

Chloroprocaine is incompatible with caustic alkalis and their carbonates, soaps, silver salts, iodine and iodides.

Parenteral drug products should be inspected visually for particulate matter and discoloration prior to administration, whenever injection and container permit. As with other anesthetics having a free aromatic amino group, Nesacaine and Nesacaine-MPF Injections are slightly photosensitive and may become discolored after prolonged exposure to light. It is recommended that these vials be stored in the original outer containers, protected from direct sunlight. Discolored injection should not be administered. If exposed to low temperatures, Nesacaine and Nesacaine-MPF Injections may deposit crystals of chloroprocaine HCl which will redissolve with shaking when returned to room temperature. The product should not be used if it contains undissolved (e.g., particulate) material.

HOW SUPPLIED

NESACAINE (chloroprocaine HCl Injection, USP) with preservatives is supplied as follows:

1% solution (NDC 0186-0971-66) in 30 mL multiple dose vials

2% solution (NDC 0186-0972-66) in 30 mL multiple dose vials

NESACAINE-MPF (chloroprocaine HCl Injection, USP) without preservatives and without EDTA is supplied as follows:

2% solution (NDC 0186-0991-66) in 20 mL single dose vials

3% solution (NDC 0186-0992-66) in 20 mL single dose vials

Keep from freezing. Protect from light. Store at controlled room temperature 15°–30°C (59°–86°F).

021849R11 Rev. 2/97

PANCURONIUM BROMIDE INJECTION ℞

THIS DRUG SHOULD BE ADMINISTERED BY ADEQUATELY TRAINED INDIVIDUALS FAMILIAR WITH ITS ACTIONS, CHARACTERISTICS, AND HAZARDS.

(For details of indications, dosage and administration, precautions, and adverse reactions, see circular in package.)

HOW SUPPLIED

Pancuronium Bromide Injection is packaged in the following forms:

Vials, 1 mg/mL
NDC 0186-1322-12, 10 mL size—boxes of 5,
Flip-Off vial closure

Vials, 2 mg/mL
NDC 0186-1331-13, 2 mL size—boxes of 10,
Astra E-Z OFF® vial closure
NDC 0186-1334-03, 2 mL size—boxes of 10,
Flip-Off vial closure
NDC 0186-1332-13, 5 mL size—boxes of 10,
Astra E-Z OFF® vial closure
NDC 0186-1335-03, 5 mL size—boxes of 10,
Flip-Off vial closure

Syringes, 2 mg/mL
NDC 0186-1333-23, 2 mL size—boxes of 10, 22 G, $1^1/_4$″ needle
NDC 0186-1336-23, 2 mL size—boxes of 10, Luer Hub Only
NDC 0186-0676-01, 5 mL size—box of 1, 21 G, $^{15}/_{16}$″ needle
NDC 0186-0692-01, 5 mL size—box of 1, Luer Hub Only

STORAGE

Both concentrations of Pancuronium Bromide Injection will maintain full clinical potency for six months if kept at a room temperature of 18°-22°C (65°-72°F); or for 18 months when refrigerated at 2°-8°C (36°-46°F).

Caution: Federal law prohibits dispensing without prescription.

021887R06 Rev. 7/96

TABLETS
PLENDIL® ℞
(FELODIPINE)
EXTENDED-RELEASE TABLETS

DESCRIPTION

PLENDIL* (Felodipine) is a calcium antagonist (calcium channel blocker). Felodipine is a dihydropyridine derivative that is chemically described as ± ethyl methyl 4-(2,3-dichlorophenyl)-1,4-dihydro-2,6-dimethyl-3,5-pyridinedicarboxylate. Its empirical formula is $C_{18}H_{19}Cl_2NO_4$ and its structural formula is:

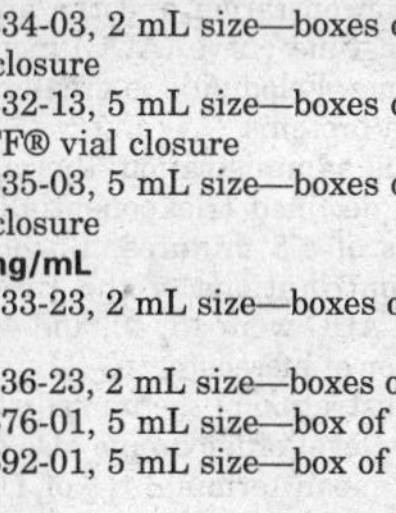

Felodipine is a slightly yellowish, crystalline powder with a molecular weight of 384.26. It is insoluble in water and is freely soluble in dichloromethane and ethanol. Felodipine is a racemic mixture.

Continued on next page

Plendil—Cont.

Tablets PLENDIL provide extended release of felodipine. They are available as tablets containing 2.5 mg, 5 mg, or 10 mg of felodipine for oral administration. In addition to the active ingredient felodipine, the tablets contain the following inactive ingredients: Tablets PLENDIL 2.5 mg — hydroxypropyl cellulose, lactose, FD&C Blue 2, sodium stearyl fumarate, titanium dioxide, yellow iron oxide and other ingredients. Tablets PLENDIL 5 mg and 10 mg — cellulose, red and yellow oxide, lactose, polyethylene glycol, sodium stearyl fumarate, titanium dioxide and other ingredients.

---

*Registered trademark of Astra AB

CLINICAL PHARMACOLOGY

Mechanism of Action

Felodipine is a member of the dihydropyridine class of calcium channel antagonists (calcium channel blockers). It reversibly competes with nitrendipine and/or other calcium channel blockers for dihydropyridine binding sites, blocks voltage-dependent Ca^{++} currents in vascular smooth muscle and cultured rabbit atrial cells, and blocks potassium-induced contracture of the rat portal vein.

In vitro studies show that the effects of felodipine on contractile processes are selective, with greater effects on vascular smooth muscle than cardiac muscle. Negative inotropic effects can be detected in vitro, but such effects have not been seen in intact animals.

The effect of felodipine on blood pressure is principally a consequence of a dose-related decrease of peripheral vascular resistance in man, with a modest reflex increase in heart rate (see Cardiovascular Effects). With the exception of a mild diuretic effect seen in several animal species and man, the effects of felodipine are accounted for by its effects on peripheral vascular resistance.

Pharmacokinetics and Metabolism

Following oral administration, felodipine is almost completely absorbed and undergoes extensive first-pass metabolism. The systemic bioavailability of PLENDIL is approximately 20 percent. Mean peak concentrations following the administration of PLENDIL are reached in 2.5 to 5 hours. Both peak plasma concentration and the area under the plasma concentration time curve (AUC) increase linearly with doses up to 20 mg. Felodipine is greater than 99 percent bound to plasma proteins.

Following intravenous administration, the plasma concentration of felodipine declined triexponentially with mean disposition half-lives of 4.8 minutes, 1.5 hours, and 9.1 hours. The mean contributions of the three individual phases to the overall AUC were 15, 40, and 45 percent, respectively, in the order of increasing $t_{1/2}$.

Following oral administration of the immediate-release formulation, the plasma level of felodipine also declined polyexponentially with a mean terminal $t_{1/2}$ of 11 to 16 hours. The mean peak and trough steady-state plasma concentrations achieved after 10 mg of the immediate-release formulation given once a day to normal volunteers, were 20 and 0.5 nmol/L, respectively. The trough plasma concentration of felodipine in most individuals was substantially below the concentration needed to effect a half-maximal decline in blood pressure (EC_{50}) [4–6 nmol/L for felodipine], thus precluding once a day dosing with the immediate-release formulation.

Following administration of a 10-mg dose of PLENDIL, the extended-release formulation, to young, healthy volunteers, mean peak and trough steady-state plasma concentrations of felodipine were 7 and 2 nmol/L, respectively. Corresponding values in hypertensive patients (mean age 64) after a 20-mg dose of PLENDIL were 23 and 7 nmol/L. Since the EC_{50} for felodipine is 4 to 6 nmol/L, a 5 to 10-mg dose of PLENDIL in some patients, and a 20-mg dose in others, would be expected to provide an antihypertensive effect that persists for 24 hours (see Cardiovascular Effects below and DOSAGE AND ADMINISTRATION).

The systemic plasma clearance of felodipine in young healthy subjects is about 0.8 L/min, and the apparent volume of distribution is about 10 L/kg.

Following an oral or intravenous dose of ^{14}C-labeled felodipine in man, about 70 percent of the dose of radioactivity was recovered in urine and 10 percent in the feces. A negligible amount of intact felodipine is recovered in the urine and feces (< 0.5%). Six metabolites, which account for 23 percent of the oral dose, have been identified; none has significant vasodilating activity.

Following administration of PLENDIL to hypertensive patients, mean peak plasma concentrations at steady state are about 20 percent higher than after a single dose. Blood pressure response is correlated with plasma concentrations of felodipine.

The bioavailability of PLENDIL is influenced by the presence of food. When administered either with a high fat or carbohydrate diet, C_{max} is increased by approximately 60 percent. AUC is unchanged. When PLENDIL was administered after a light meal (orange juice, toast, and cereal),

however, there is no effect on felodipine's pharmacokinetics. The bioavailability of felodipine was increased approximately two-fold when taken with grapefruit juice. Orange juice does not appear to modify the kinetics of PLENDIL. A similar finding has been seen with other dihydropyridine calcium antagonists, but to a lesser extent than that seen with felodipine.

Age Effects: Plasma concentrations of felodipine, after a single dose and at steady state, increase with age. Mean clearance of felodipine in elderly hypertensives (mean age 74) was only 45 percent of that of young volunteers (mean age 26). At steady state mean AUC for young patients was 39 percent of that for the elderly. Data for intermediate age ranges suggest that the AUCs fall between the extremes of the young and the elderly.

Hepatic Dysfunction: In patients with hepatic disease, the clearance of felodipine was reduced to about 60 percent of that seen in normal young volunteers.

Renal impairment does not alter the plasma concentration profile of felodipine; although higher concentrations of the metabolites are present in the plasma due to decreased urinary excretion, these are inactive.

Animal studies have demonstrated that felodipine crosses the blood-brain barrier and the placenta.

Cardiovascular Effects

Following administration of PLENDIL, a reduction in blood pressure generally occurs within 2 to 5 hours. During chronic administration, substantial blood pressure control lasts for 24 hours, with trough reductions in diastolic blood pressure approximately 40–50 percent of peak reductions. The antihypertensive effect is dose-dependent and correlates with the plasma concentration of felodipine.

A reflex increase in heart rate frequently occurs during the first week of therapy; this increase attenuates over time. Heart rate increases of 5–10 beats per minute may be seen during chronic dosing. The increase is inhibited by beta-blocking agents.

The P-R interval of the ECG is not affected by felodipine when administered alone or in combination with a beta-blocking agent. Felodipine alone or in combination with a beta-blocking agent has been shown, in clinical and electrophysiologic studies, to have no significant effect on cardiac conduction (P-R, P-Q, and H-V intervals).

In clinical trials in hypertensive patients without clinical evidence of left ventricular dysfunction, no symptoms suggestive of a negative inotropic effect were noted; however, none would be expected in this population (see PRECAUTIONS).

Renal/Endocrine Effects

Renal vascular resistance is decreased by felodipine while glomerular filtration rate remains unchanged. Mild diuresis, natriuresis, and kaliuresis have been observed during the first week of therapy. No significant effects on serum electrolytes were observed during short- and long-term therapy.

In clinical trials in patients with hypertension, increases in plasma noradrenaline levels have been observed.

Clinical Studies

Felodipine produces dose-related decreases in systolic and diastolic blood pressure as demonstrated in six placebo-controlled, dose response studies using either immediate-release or extended-release dosage forms. These studies enrolled over 800 patients on active treatment, at total daily doses ranging from 2.5 to 20 mg. In those studies felodipine was administered either as monotherapy or was added to beta blockers. The results of the two studies with PLENDIL given once daily as monotherapy are shown in the table below:

MEAN REDUCTIONS IN BLOOD PRESSURE (mmHg)*
Systolic/Diastolic

Dose	N	Mean Peak Response	Mean Trough Response	Trough/Peak Ratios (%s)
		Study 1 (8 weeks)		
2.5 mg	68	9.4/4.7	2.7/2.5	29/53
5 mg	69	9.5/6.3	2.4/3.7	25/59
10 mg	67	18.0/10.8	10.0/6.0	56/56
		Study 2 (4 weeks)		
10 mg	50	5.3/7.2	1.5/3.2	33/40**
20 mg	50	11.3/10.2	4.5/3.2	43/34**

*Placebo response subtracted
**Different number of patients available for peak and trough measurements

INDICATIONS AND USAGE

PLENDIL is indicated for the treatment of hypertension. PLENDIL may be used alone or concomitantly with other antihypertensive agents.

CONTRAINDICATIONS

PLENDIL is contraindicated in patients who are hypersensitive to this product.

PRECAUTIONS

General

Hypotension: Felodipine, like other calcium antagonists, may occasionally precipitate significant hypotension and, rarely, syncope. It may lead to reflex tachycardia which in susceptible individuals may precipitate angina pectoris. (See ADVERSE REACTIONS.)

Heart Failure: Although acute hemodynamic studies in a small number of patients with NYHA Class II or III heart failure treated with felodipine have not demonstrated negative inotropic effects, safety in patients with heart failure has not been established. Caution, therefore, should be exercised when using PLENDIL in patients with heart failure or compromised ventricular function, particularly in combination with a beta blocker.

Elderly Patients or Patients with Impaired Liver Function: Patients over 65 years of age or patients with impaired liver function may have elevated plasma concentrations of felodipine and may respond to lower doses of PLENDIL; therefore, a starting dose of 2.5 mg once a day is recommended. These patients should have their blood pressure monitored closely during dosage adjustment of PLENDIL. (See CLINICAL PHARMACOLOGY and DOSAGE AND ADMINISTRATION.)

Peripheral Edema: Peripheral edema, generally mild and not associated with generalized fluid retention, was the most common adverse event in the clinical trials. The incidence of peripheral edema was both dose- and age- dependent. Frequency of peripheral edema ranged from about 10 percent in patients under 50 years of age taking 5 mg daily to about 30 percent in those over 60 years of age taking 20 mg daily. This adverse effect generally occurs within 2–3 weeks of the initiation of treatment.

Information for Patients

Patients should be instructed to take PLENDIL whole and not to crush or chew the tablets. They should be told that mild gingival hyperplasia (gum swelling) has been reported. Good dental hygiene decreases its incidence and severity.

NOTE: As with many other drugs, certain advice to patients being treated with PLENDIL is warranted. This information is intended to aid in the safe and effective use of this medication. It is not a disclosure of all possible adverse or intended effects.

Drug Interactions

Beta-Blocking Agents: A pharmacokinetic study of felodipine in conjunction with metoprolol demonstrated no significant effects on the pharmacokinetics of felodipine. The AUC and C_{max} of metoprolol, however, were increased approximately 31 and 38 percent, respectively. In controlled clinical trials, however, beta blockers including metoprolol were concurrently administered with felodipine and were well tolerated.

Cimetidine: In healthy subjects pharmacokinetic studies showed an approximately 50 percent increase in the area under the plasma concentration time curve (AUC) as well as the C_{max} of felodipine when given concomitantly with cimetidine. It is anticipated that a clinically significant interaction may occur in some hypertensive patients. Therefore, it is recommended that low doses of PLENDIL be used when given concomitantly with cimetidine.

Digoxin: When given concomitantly with PLENDIL the pharmacokinetics of digoxin in patients with heart failure were not significantly altered.

Anticonvulsants: In a pharmacokinetic study, maximum plasma concentrations of felodipine were considerably lower in epileptic patients on long-term anticonvulsant therapy (e.g., phenytoin, carbamazepine, or phenobarbital) than in healthy volunteers. In such patients, the mean area under the felodipine plasma concentration-time curve was also reduced to approximately six percent of that observed in healthy volunteers. Since a clinically significant interaction may be anticipated, alternative antihypertensive therapy should be considered in these patients.

Other Concomitant Therapy: In healthy subjects there were no clinically significant interactions when felodipine was given concomitantly with indomethacin or spironolactone.

Interaction with Food: See CLINICAL PHARMACOLOGY, Pharmacokinetics and Metabolism.

Carcinogenesis, Mutagenesis, Impairment of Fertility

In a 2-year carcinogenicity study in rats fed felodipine at doses of 7.7, 23.1 or 69.3 mg/kg/day (up to 28 times** the maximum recommended human dose on a mg/m² basis), a dose-related increase in the incidence of benign interstitial cell tumors of the testes (Leydig cell tumors) was observed in treated male rats. These tumors were not observed in a similar study in mice at doses up to 138.6 mg/kg/day (28 times** the maximum recommended human dose on a mg/m² basis). Felodipine, at the doses employed in the 2-year rat study, has been shown to lower testicular testos-

terone and to produce a corresponding increase in serum luteinizing hormone in rats. The Leydig cell tumor development is possibly secondary to these hormonal effects which have not been observed in man.
In this same rat study a dose-related increase in the incidence of focal squamous cell hyperplasia compared to control was observed in the esophageal groove of male and female rats in all dose groups. No other drug-related esophageal or gastric pathology was observed in the rats or with chronic administration in mice and dogs. The latter species, like man, has no anatomical structure comparable to the esophageal groove.
Felodipine was not carcinogenic when fed to mice at doses of up to 138.6 mg/kg/day (28 times** the maximum recommended human dose on a mg/m^2 basis) for periods of up to 80 weeks in males and 99 weeks in females.
Felodipine did not display any mutagenic activity *in vitro* in the Ames microbial mutagenicity test or in the mouse lymphoma forward mutation assay. No clastogenic potential was seen *in vivo* in the mouse micronucleus test at oral doses up to 2500 mg/kg (506 times** the maximum recommended human dose on a mg/m^2 basis) or *in vitro* in a human lymphocyte chromosome aberration assay.
A fertility study in which male and female rats were administered doses of 3.8, 9.6 or 26.9 mg/kg/day showed no significant effect of felodipine on reproductive performance.
Pregnancy
Pregnancy Category C
Teratogenic Effects: Studies in pregnant rabbits administered doses of 0.46, 1.2, 2.3, and 4.6 mg/kg/day (from 0.4 to 4 times** the maximum recommended human dose on a mg/m^2 basis) showed digital anomalies consisting of reduction in size and degree of ossification of the terminal phalanges in the fetuses. The frequency and severity of the changes appeared dose-related and were noted even at the lowest dose. These changes have been shown to occur with other members of the dihydropyridine class and are possibly a result of compromised uterine blood flow. Similar fetal anomalies were not observed in rats given felodipine.
In a teratology study in cynomolgus monkeys, no reduction in the size of the terminal phalanges was observed, but an abnormal position of the distal phalanges was noted in about 40 percent of the fetuses.
Nonteratogenic Effects: A prolongation of parturition with difficult labor and an increased frequency of fetal and early postnatal deaths were observed in rats administered doses of 9.6 mg/kg/day (4 times** the maximum human dose on a mg/m^2 basis) and above.
Significant enlargement of the mammary glands, in excess of the normal enlargement for pregnant rabbits, was found with doses greater than or equal to 1.2 mg/kg/day (equal to the maximum human dose on a mg/m^2 basis). This effect occurred only in pregnant rabbits and regressed during lactation. Similar changes in the mammary glands were not observed in rats or monkeys.
There are no adequate and well-controlled studies in pregnant women. If felodipine is used during pregnancy, or if the patient becomes pregnant while taking this drug, she should be apprised of the potential hazard to the fetus, possible digital anomalies of the infant, and the potential effects of felodipine on labor and delivery, and on the mammary glands of pregnant females.
Nursing Mothers
It is not known whether this drug is secreted in human milk and because of the potential for serious adverse reactions from felodipine in the infant, a decision should be made whether to discontinue nursing or to discontinue the drug, taking into account the importance of the drug to the mother.
Pediatric Use
Safety and effectiveness in pediatric patients have not been established.

**Based on patient weight of 50 kg

ADVERSE REACTIONS

In controlled studies in the United States and overseas, approximately 3000 patients were treated with felodipine as either the extended-release or the immediate-release formulation.
The most common clinical adverse events reported with PLENDIL administered as monotherapy at the recommended dosage range of 2.5 mg to 10 mg once a day were peripheral edema and headache. Peripheral edema was generally mild, but it was age- and dose- related and resulted in discontinuation of therapy in about 3 percent of the enrolled patients. Discontinuation of therapy due to any clinical adverse event occurred in about 6 percent of the patients receiving PLENDIL, principally for peripheral edema, headache, or flushing.
Adverse events that occurred with an incidence of 1.5 percent or greater at any of the recommended doses of 2.5 mg to 10 mg once a day (PLENDIL, N = 861; Placebo, N = 334), without regard to causality, are compared to placebo and are listed by dose in the table below. These events are reported from controlled clinical trials with patients who were randomized to a fixed dose of PLENDIL or titrated from an initial dose of 2.5 mg or 5 mg once a day. A dose of 20 mg once a day has been evaluated in some clinical studies. Although the antihypertensive effect of PLENDIL is increased at 20 mg once a day, there is a disproportionate increase in adverse events, especially those associated with vasodilatory effects (see DOSAGE and ADMINISTRATION).
[See table above]

Percent of Patients with Adverse Events in Controlled Trials* of PLENDIL (N=861) as Monotherapy without Regard to Causality
(Incidence of discontinuations shown in parentheses)

Body System Adverse Events	Placebo N=334	2.5 mg N=255	5 mg N=581	10 mg N=408
Body as a Whole				
Peripheral Edema	3.3 (0.0)	2.0 (0.0)	8.8 (2.2)	17.4 (2.5)
Asthenia	3.3 (0.0)	3.9 (0.0)	3.3 (0.0)	2.2 (0.0)
Warm Sensation	0.0 (0.0)	0.0 (0.0)	0.9 (0.2)	1.5 (0.0)
Cardiovascular				
Palpitation	2.4 (0.0)	0.4 (0.0)	1.4 (0.3)	2.5 (0.5)
Digestive				
Nausea	1.5 (0.9)	1.2 (0.0)	1.7 (0.3)	1.0 (0.7)
Dyspepsia	1.2 (0.0)	3.9 (0.0)	0.7 (0.0)	0.5 (0.0)
Constipation	0.9 (0.0)	1.2 (0.0)	0.3 (0.0)	1.5 (0.2)
Nervous				
Headache	10.2 (0.9)	10.6 (0.4)	11.0 (1.7)	14.7 (2.0)
Dizziness	2.7 (0.3)	2.7 (0.0)	3.6 (0.5)	3.7 (0.5)
Paresthesia	1.5 (0.3)	1.6 (0.0)	1.2 (0.0)	1.2 (0.2)
Respiratory				
Upper Respiratory Infection	1.8 (0.0)	3.9 (0.0)	1.9 (0.0)	0.7 (0.0)
Cough	0.3 (0.0)	0.8 (0.0)	1.2 (0.0)	1.7 (0.0)
Rhinorrhea	0.0 (0.0)	1.6 (0.0)	0.2 (0.0)	0.2 (0.0)
Sneezing	0.0 (0.0)	1.6 (0.0)	0.0 (0.0)	0.0 (0.0)
Skin				
Rash	0.9 (0.0)	2.0 (0.0)	0.2 (0.0)	0.2 (0.0)
Flushing	0.9 (0.3)	3.9 (0.0)	5.3 (0.7)	6.9 (1.2)

* Patients in titration studies may have been exposed to more than one dose level of PLENDIL.

Adverse events that occurred in 0.5 up to 1.5 percent of patients who received PLENDIL in all controlled clinical trials at the recommended dosage range of 2.5 mg to 10 mg once a day, and serious adverse events that occurred at a lower rate, or events reported during marketing experience (those lower rate events are in italics) are listed below. These events are listed in order of decreasing severity within each category, and the relationship of these events to administration of PLENDIL is uncertain: ***Body as a Whole:*** Chest pain, facial edema, flu-like illness; ***Cardiovascular:*** *Myocardial infarction, hypotension, syncope, angina pectoris, arrhythmia,* tachycardia, premature beats; ***Digestive:*** Abdominal pain, diarrhea, vomiting, dry mouth, flatulence, acid regurgitation; ***Endocrine:*** Gynecomastia; ***Hematologic:*** *Anemia;* ***Metabolic:*** ALT (SGPT) increased; ***Musculoskeletal:*** Arthralgia, back pain, leg pain, foot pain, muscle cramps, myalgia, arm pain, knee pain, hip pain; ***Nervous/Psychiatric:*** Insomnia, depression, anxiety disorders, irritability, nervousness, somnolence, decreased libido; ***Respiratory:*** Dyspnea, pharyngitis, bronchitis, influenza, sinusitis, epistaxis, respiratory infection; ***Skin:*** Contusion, erythema, urticaria; ***Special Senses:*** Visual disturbances; ***Urogenital:*** Impotence, urinary frequency, urinary urgency, dysuria, polyuria.
Gingival Hyperplasia: Gingival hyperplasia, usually mild, occurred in <0.5 percent of patients in controlled studies. This condition may be avoided or may regress with improved dental hygiene. (See PRECAUTIONS, *Information for Patients.*)
Clinical Laboratory Test Findings
Serum Electrolytes: No significant effects on serum electrolytes were observed during short- and long-term therapy (see CLINICAL PHARMACOLOGY, *Renal/Endocrine Effects*).
Serum Glucose: No significant effects on fasting serum glucose were observed in patients treated with PLENDIL in the U.S. controlled study.
Liver Enzymes: One of two episodes of elevated serum transaminases decreased once drug was discontinued in clinical studies; no follow-up was available for the other patient.

OVERDOSAGE

Oral doses of 240 mg/kg and 264 mg/kg in male and female mice, respectively, and 2390 mg/kg and 2250 mg/kg in male and female rats, respectively, caused significant lethality.
In a suicide attempt, one patient took 150 mg felodipine together with 15 tablets each of atenolol and spironolactone and 20 tablets of nitrazepam. The patient's blood pressure and heart rate were normal on admission to hospital; he subsequently recovered without significant sequelae.
Overdosage might be expected to cause excessive peripheral vasodilation with marked hypotension and possibly bradycardia.
If severe hypotension occurs, symptomatic treatment should be instituted. The patient should be placed supine with the legs elevated. The administration of intravenous fluids may be useful to treat hypotension due to overdosage with calcium antagonists. In case of accompanying bradycardia, atropine (0.5–1 mg) should be administered intravenously. Sympathomimetic drugs may also be given if the physician feels they are warranted.
It has not been established whether felodipine can be removed from the circulation by hemodialysis.
To obtain up-to-date information about the treatment of overdose, consult your Regional Poison-Control Center. Telephone numbers of certified poison-control centers are listed in the *Physicians' Desk Reference (PDR)*. In managing overdose, consider the possibilities of multiple-drug overdoses, drug-drug interactions, and unusual drug kinetics in your patient.

DOSAGE AND ADMINISTRATION

The recommended starting dose is 5 mg once a day. Depending on the patient's response, the dosage can be decreased to 2.5 mg or increased to 10 mg once a day. These adjustments should occur generally at intervals of not less than 2 weeks. The recommended dosage range is 2.5–10 mg once daily. In clinical trials, doses above 10 mg daily showed an increased blood pressure response but a large increase in the rate of peripheral edema and other vasodilatory adverse events (see ADVERSE REACTIONS). Modification of the recommended dosage is usually not required in patients with renal impairment.
PLENDIL should regularly be taken either without food or with a light meal (see CLINICAL PHARMACOLOGY, *Pharmacokinetics and Metabolism*). PLENDIL should be swallowed whole and not crushed or chewed.
Use in the Elderly or Patients with Impaired Liver Function: Patients over 65 years of age, or patients with impaired liver function, may develop higher plasma concentrations of felodipine; therefore, a starting dose of 2.5 mg once a day is recommended. Dosage may be adjusted as described above. (See PRECAUTIONS.)

HOW SUPPLIED

No. 3584—Tablets PLENDIL, 2.5 mg, are sage green, round convex tablets, with code 450 on one side and PLENDIL on the other. They are supplied as follows:
NDC 61113-450-28 unit dose packages of 100
NDC 61113-450-58 unit of use bottles of 100
NDC 61113-450-31 unit of use bottles of 30.
No. 3585—Tablets PLENDIL, 5 mg, are light red-brown, round convex tablets, with code 451 on one side and PLENDIL on the other. They are supplied as follows:
NDC 61113-451-28 unit dose packages of 100
(6505-01-350-0354, 5 mg individually sealed 100's)
NDC 61113-451-58 unit of use bottles of 100
(6505-01-350-0356, 5 mg 100's)
NDC 61113-451-31 unit of use bottles of 30
(6505-01-350-0352, 5 mg 30's).

Continued on next page

Plendil—Cont.

No. 3586—Tablets PLENDIL, 10 mg, are red-brown, round convex tablets, with code 452 on one side and PLENDIL on the other. They are supplied as follows:

NDC 61113-452-28 unit dose packages of 100
(6505-01-350-0353, 10 mg individually sealed 100's)
NDC 61113-452-58 unit of use bottles of 100
(6505-01-350-0355, 10 mg 100's)
NDC 61113-452-31 unit of use bottles of 30
(6505-01-350-0357, 10 mg 30's)

Storage:
Store below 30°C (86°F). Keep container tightly closed. Protect from light.
Distributed by:
Astra Pharmaceuticals, L.P.
Wayne, PA 19087, USA
Manufactured by: MERCK & CO., INC.,
West Point, PA 19486, USA
Issued January 1998   7909010
© 1998 Astra Pharmaceuticals, L.P. All rights reserved.
Shown in Product Identification Guide, page 304

POLOCAINE®   ℞
[pō '-lō-caine ″]
(Mepivacaine Hydrochloride Injection, USP)

POLOCAINE®-MPF
(Mepivacaine Hydrochloride Injection, USP)
THESE SOLUTIONS ARE NOT INTENDED FOR SPINAL ANESTHESIA OR DENTAL USE

(For details of indications, dosage and administration, precautions, and adverse reactions, see circular in package.)

HOW SUPPLIED

POLOCAINE-MPF (Mepivacaine HCl Injection, USP) without preservatives is available as follows:
1% Single-dose vials of 30 mL (NDC 0186-0412-01)
1.5% Single-dose vials of 30 mL (NDC 0186-0418-01)
2% Single-dose vials of 20 mL (NDC 0186-0422-01)
POLOCAINE (Mepivacaine HCl Injection, USP) with preservatives is available as follows:
1% Multiple-dose vials of 50 mL (NDC 0186-0410-01)
2% Multiple-dose vials of 50 mL (NDC 0186-0420-01)
Unused portions of solutions not containing preservatives should be discarded.
Store at controlled room temperature 15°–30°C (59°–86°F).
021668R00   Iss. 1/92

PRILOSEC®   ℞
(OMEPRAZOLE)
DELAYED-RELEASE CAPSULES

DESCRIPTION

The active ingredient in PRILOSEC* (Omeprazole) Delayed-Release Capsules is a substituted benzimidazole, 5-methoxy-2-[[(4-methoxy-3, 5-dimethyl-2-pyridinyl) methyl] sulfinyl]-1H-benzimidazole, a compound that inhibits gastric acid secretion. Its empirical formula is $C_{17}H_{19}N_3O_3S$, with a molecular weight of 345.42. The structural formula is:

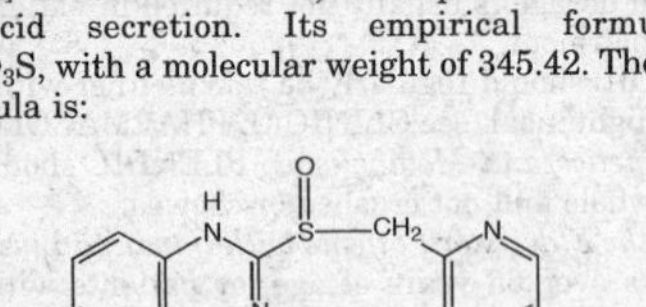

Omeprazole is a white to off-white crystalline powder which melts with decomposition at about 155°C. It is a weak base, freely soluble in ethanol and methanol, and slightly soluble in acetone and isopropanol and very slightly soluble in water. The stability of omeprazole is a function of pH; it is rapidly degraded in acid media, but has acceptable stability under alkaline conditions.
PRILOSEC is supplied as delayed-release capsules for oral administration. Each delayed-release capsule contains either 10 mg, 20 mg or 40 mg of omeprazole in the form of enteric-coated granules with the following inactive ingredients: cellulose, disodium hydrogen phosphate, hydroxypropyl cellulose, hydroxypropyl methylcellulose, lactose, mannitol, sodium lauryl sulfate and other ingredients. The capsule shells have the following inactive ingredients: gelatin-NF, FD&C blue #1, FD&C Red #40, D&C Red #28, titanium dioxide, synthetic black iron oxide, isopropanol, butyl alcohol, FD&C Blue #2, D&C Red #7 Calcium Lake, and, in addition, the 10 mg and 40 mg capsule shells also contain D&C Yellow #10.
*Registered trademark of Astra AB.

CLINICAL PHARMACOLOGY

Pharmacokinetics and Metabolism: Omeprazole
PRILOSEC Delayed-Release Capsules contain an enteric-coated granule formulation of omeprazole (because omeprazole is acid-labile), so that absorption of omeprazole begins only after the granules leave the stomach. Absorption is rapid, with peak plasma levels of omeprazole occurring within 0.5 to 3.5 hours. Peak plasma concentrations of omeprazole and AUC are approximately proportional to doses up to 40 mg, but because of a saturable first-pass effect, a greater than linear response in peak plasma concentration and AUC occurs with doses greater than 40 mg. Absolute bioavailability (compared to intravenous administration) is about 30–40% at doses of 20–40 mg, due in large part to presystemic metabolism. In healthy subjects the plasma half-life is 0.5 to 1 hour, and the total body clearance is 500–600 mL/min. Protein binding is approximately 95%.
The bioavailability of omeprazole increases slightly upon repeated administration of PRILOSEC Delayed-Release Capsules.
Following single dose oral administration of a buffered solution of omeprazole, little if any unchanged drug was excreted in urine. The majority of the dose (about 77%) was eliminated in urine as at least six metabolites. Two were identified as hydroxyomeprazole and the corresponding carboxylic acid. The remainder of the dose was recoverable in feces. This implies a significant biliary excretion of the metabolites of omeprazole. Three metabolites have been identified in plasma — the sulfide and sulfone derivatives of omeprazole, and hydroxyomeprazole. These metabolites have very little or no antisecretory activity.
In patients with chronic hepatic disease, the bioavailability increased to approximately 100% compared to an I.V. dose, reflecting decreased first-pass effect, and the plasma half-life of the drug increased to nearly 3 hours compared to the half-life in normals of 0.5–1 hour. Plasma clearance averaged 70mL/min, compared to a value of 500–600 mL/min in normal subjects.
In patients with chronic renal impairment, whose creatinine clearance ranged between 10 and 62 mL/min/1.73 m², the disposition of omeprazole was very similar to that in healthy volunteers, although there was a slight increase in bioavailability. Because urinary excretion is a primary route of excretion of omeprazole metabolites, their elimination slowed in proportion to the decreased creatinine clearance.
The elimination rate of omeprazole was somewhat decreased in the elderly, and bioavailability was increased. Omeprazole was 76% bioavailable when a single 40 mg oral dose of omeprazole (buffered solution) was administered to healthy elderly volunteers, versus 58% in young volunteers given the same dose. Nearly 70% of the dose was recovered in urine as metabolites of omeprazole and no unchanged drug was detected. The plasma clearance of omeprazole was 250 mL/min (about half that of young volunteers) and its plasma half-life averaged one hour, about twice that of young healthy volunteers.
In pharmacokinetic studies of single 20 mg omeprazole doses, an increase in AUC of approximately four-fold was noted in Asian subjects compared to Caucasians. Dose adjustment, particularly where maintenance of healing of erosive esophagitis is indicated, for the hepatically impaired and Asian subjects should be considered.
Pharmacokinetics: Combination Therapy with Clarithromycin
Omeprazole 40 mg daily was given in combination with clarithromycin 500 mg every 8 hours to healthy adult male subjects. The steady state plasma concentrations of omeprazole were increased (C_{max}, AUC_{0-24}, and $T_{1/2}$ increases of 30%, 89% and 34% respectively) by the concomitant administration of clarithromycin. The observed increases in omeprazole plasma concentration were associated with the following pharmacological effects. The mean 24-hour gastric pH value was 5.2 when omeprazole was administered alone and 5.7 when co-administered with clarithromycin.
The plasma levels of clarithromycin and 14-hydroxy-clarithromycin were increased by the concomitant administration of omeprazole. For clarithromycin, the mean C_{max} was 10% greater, the mean C_{min} was 27% greater, and the mean AUC_{0-8} was 15% greater when clarithromycin was administered with omeprazole than when clarithromycin was administered alone. Similar results were seen for 14-hydroxy-clarithromycin, the mean C_{max} was 45% greater, the mean C_{min} was 57% greater, and the mean AUC_{0-8} was 45% greater. Clarithromycin concentrations in the gastric tissue and mucus were also increased by concomitant administration of omeprazole.

Clarithromycin Tissue Concentrations
2 hours after Dose[1]

Tissue	Clarithromycin	Clarithromycin + Omeprazole
Antrum	10.48 ± 2.01 (n = 5)	19.96 ± 4.71 (n = 5)
Fundus	20.81 ± 7.64 (n = 5)	24.25 ± 6.37 (n = 5)
Mucus	4.15 ± 7.74 (n = 4)	39.29 ± 32.79 (n = 4)

[1] Mean ± SD (μg/g)

For information on clarithromycin pharmacokinetics and microbiology, consult the clarithromycin package insert, CLINICAL PHARMACOLOGY section.
Pharmacodynamics
Mechanism of Action
Omeprazole belongs to a new class of antisecretory compounds, the substituted benzimidazoles, that do not exhibit anticholinergic or H_2 histamine antagonistic properties, but that suppress gastric acid secretion by specific inhibition of the H^+/K^+ ATPase enzyme system at the secretory surface of the gastric parietal cell. Because this enzyme system is regarded as the acid (proton) pump within the gastric mucosa, omeprazole has been characterized as a gastric acid-pump inhibitor, in that it blocks the final step of acid production. This effect is dose-related and leads to inhibition of both basal and stimulated acid secretion irrespective of the stimulus. Animal studies indicate that after rapid disappearance from plasma, omeprazole can be found within the gastric mucosa for a day or more.
Antisecretory Activity
After oral administration, the onset of the antisecretory effect of omeprazole occurs within one hour, with the maximum effect occurring within two hours. Inhibition of secretion is about 50% of maximum at 24 hours and the duration of inhibition lasts up to 72 hours. The antisecretory effect thus lasts far longer than would be expected from the very short (less than one hour) plasma half-life, apparently due to prolonged binding to the parietal H^+/K^+ ATPase enzyme. When the drug is discontinued, secretory activity returns gradually, over 3 to 5 days. The inhibitory effect of omeprazole on acid secretion increases with repeated once-daily dosing, reaching a plateau after four days.
Results from numerous studies of the antisecretory effect of multiple doses of 20 mg and 40 mg of omeprazole in normal volunteers and patients are shown below. The "max" value represents determinations at a time of maximum effect (2–6 hours after dosing), while "min" values are those 24 hours after the last dose of omeprazole.

Range of Mean Values from Multiple Studies
of the Mean Antisecretory Effects of Omeprazole
After Multiple Daily Dosing

Parameter	Omeprazole 20 mg		Omeprazole 40 mg	
% Decrease in	Max	Min	Max	Min
Basal Acid Output	78*	58-80	94*	80-93
% Decrease in Peak Acid Output	79*	50-59	88*	62-68
% Decrease in 24-hr. Intragastric Acidity		80-97		92-94

*Single Studies

Single daily oral doses of omeprazole ranging from a dose of 10 mg to 40 mg have produced 100% inhibition of 24-hour intragastric acidity in some patients.
Enterochromaffin-like (ECL) Cell Effects
In 24-month carcinogenicity studies in rats, a dose-related significant increase in gastric carcinoid tumors and ECL cell hyperplasia was observed in both male and female animals (see PRECAUTIONS, *Carcinogenesis, Mutagenesis, Impairment of Fertility*). Carcinoid tumors have also been observed in rats subjected to fundectomy or long-term treatment with other proton pump inhibitors or high doses of H_2-receptor antagonists.
Human gastric biopsy specimens have been obtained from more than 3000 patients treated with omeprazole in long-term clinical trials. The incidence of ECL cell hyperplasia in these studies increased with time; however, no case of ECL cell carcinoids, dysplasia, or neoplasia has been found in these patients. (See also CLINICAL PHARMACOLOGY, *Pathological Hypersecretory Conditions*.)
Serum Gastrin Effects
In studies involving more than 200 patients, serum gastrin levels increased during the first 1 to 2 weeks of once-daily administration of therapeutic doses of omeprazole in parallel with inhibition of acid secretion. No further increase in serum gastrin occurred with continued treatment. In comparison with histamine H_2-receptor antagonists, the median increases produced by 20 mg doses of omeprazole were higher (1.3 to 3.6 fold vs. 1.1 to 1.8 fold increase). Gastrin values returned to pretreatment levels, usually within 1 to 2 weeks after discontinuation of therapy.
Other Effects
Systemic effects of omeprazole in the CNS, cardiovascular and respiratory systems have not been found to date. Omeprazole, given in oral doses of 30 or 40 mg for 2 to 4 weeks, had no effect on thyroid function, carbohydrate metabolism, or circulating levels of parathyroid hormone, cortisol, estradiol, testosterone, prolactin, cholecystokinin or secretin. No effect on gastric emptying of the solid and liquid components of a test meal was demonstrated after a single dose of

omeprazole 90 mg. In healthy subjects, a single I.V. dose of omeprazole (0.35 mg/kg) had no effect on intrinsic factor secretion. No systematic dose-dependent effect has been observed on basal or stimulated pepsin output in humans. However, when intragastric pH is maintained at 4.0 or above, basal pepsin output is low, and pepsin activity is decreased.

As do other agents that elevate intragastric pH, omeprazole administered for 14 days in healthy subjects produced a significant increase in the intragastric concentrations of viable bacteria. The pattern of the bacterial species was unchanged from that commonly found in saliva. All changes resolved within three days of stopping treatment.

Clinical Studies
Duodenal Ulcer Disease
Active Duodenal Ulcer: In a multicenter, double-blind, placebo-controlled study of 147 patients with endoscopically documented duodenal ulcer, the percentage of patients healed (per protocol) at 2 and 4 weeks was significantly higher with PRILOSEC 20 mg once a day than with placebo ($p \leq 0.01$).

Treatment of Active Duodenal Ulcer
% of Patients Healed

	PRILOSEC 20 mg a.m. (n = 99)	Placebo a.m. (n = 48)
Week 2	*41	13
Week 4	*75	27

*($p \leq 0.01$)

Complete daytime and nighttime pain relief occurred significantly faster ($p \leq 0.01$) in patients treated with PRILOSEC 20 mg than in patients treated with placebo. At the end of the study, significantly more patients who had received PRILOSEC had complete relief of daytime pain ($p \leq 0.05$) and nighttime pain ($p \leq 0.01$).

In a multicenter, double-blind study of 293 patients with endoscopically documented duodenal ulcer, the percentage of patients healed (per protocol) at 4 weeks was significantly higher with PRILOSEC 20 mg once a day than with ranitidine 150 mg b.i.d. ($p < 0.01$).

Treatment of Active Duodenal Ulcer
% of Patients Healed

	PRILOSEC 20 mg a.m. (n = 145)	Ranitidine 150 mg b.i.d. (n = 148)
Week 2	42	34
Week 4	*82	63

*($p < 0.01$)

Healing occurred significantly faster in patients treated with PRILOSEC than in those treated with ranitidine 150 mg b.i.d. ($p < 0.01$).

In a foreign multinational randomized, double-blind study of 105 patients with endoscopically documented duodenal ulcer, 20 mg and 40 mg of PRILOSEC were compared to 150 mg b.i.d. of ranitidine at 2, 4 and 8 weeks. At 2 and 4 weeks both doses of PRILOSEC were statistically superior (per protocol) to ranitidine, but 40 mg was not superior to 20 mg of PRILOSEC, and at 8 weeks there was no significant difference between any of the active drugs.

Treatment of Active Duodenal Ulcer
% of Patients Healed

	PRILOSEC 20 mg (n = 34)	PRILOSEC 40 mg (n = 36)	Ranitidine 150 mg b.i.d. (n = 35)
Week 2	*83	*83	53
Week 4	*97	*100	82
Week 8	100	100	94

*($p \leq 0.01$)

Duodenal Ulcer Recurrence
Four randomized double blind clinical studies in patients with *H. pylori* infection and active duodenal ulcer disease compared omeprazole plus clarithromycin to omeprazole. Two of these studies, one in the U.S. and Canada, included a clarithromycin alone arm. The dose regimen in the two multicenter U.S. studies (n=498) was PRILOSEC 40 mg q.d. plus clarithromycin 500 mg t.i.d. for 14 days followed by PRILOSEC 20 mg q.d. for 14 days; PRILOSEC 40 mg q.d. for 14 days followed by PRILOSEC 20 mg q.d. for 14 days; clarithromycin 500 mg t.i.d. for 14 days. Two foreign studies (n=369) compared PRILOSEC and clarithromycin to PRILOSEC, and did not include a clarithromycin alone arm. The dose regimen was the same as that used in the U.S. studies except for one study (M92-812b) where PRILOSEC 40 mg q.d. was used throughout the 28 day treatment period. Endpoints studied were: eradication of *H. pylori*, duodenal ulcer healing and recurrence. *H. pylori* status was determined by histology and another bacteriological test. For a given patient, *H. pylori* was considered eradicated if at least one of these tests was negative, and none was positive.

The combination of omeprazole and clarithromycin was effective in eradicating *H. pylori*.

H. pylori Eradication Rates
% of Patients Cured† [95% Confidence Interval]

	PRILOSEC + Clarithromycin	PRILOSEC	Clarithromycin
U.S. Studies			
Study M93-067	*74 [61, 85] (n = 58)	0 [0, 6] (n = 55)	34 [20, 50] (n = 44)
Study M93-100	*64 [51, 76] (n = 64)	0 [0, 6] (n = 62)	38 [24, 53] (n = 48)
Non U.S. Studies			
Study M92-812b	*83 [72, 91] (n = 69)	1 [0, 7] (n = 75)	N/A
Study M93-058	*74 [64, 83] (n = 93)	4 [1, 10] (n = 96)	N/A

† Evaluable patients with confirmed duodenal ulcer and *H. pylori* infection at baseline who are healed at week 4, and for whom results were available for the 4-6 week post-treatment visit are included in this analysis.
*($p \leq 0.01$) versus PRILOSEC or clarithromycin

Ulcer healing was not significantly different when clarithromycin was added to omeprazole therapy compared to omeprazole therapy alone.
The combination of omeprazole and clarithromycin was effective in eradicating *H. pylori* and reduced duodenal ulcer recurrence.

Duodenal Ulcer Recurrence Rates by
H. pylori Eradication Status
% of Patients with Ulcer Recurrence

	H. pylori eradicated#	*H. pylori* not eradicated#
U.S. Studies†		
6 months post-treatment		
Study M93-067	*35 (n = 49)	60 (n = 88)
Study M93-100	* 8 (n = 53)	60 (n = 106)
Non U.S. Studies‡		
6 months post-treatment		
Study M92-812b	* 5 (n = 43)	46 (n = 78)
Study M93-058	* 6 (n = 53)	43 (n = 107)
12 months post-treatment		
Study M92-812b	* 5 (n = 39)	68 (n = 71)

#*H. pylori* eradication status assessed at same timepoint as ulcer recurrence
†Combined results for PRILOSEC + clarithromycin, PRILOSEC, and clarithromycin treatment arms
‡Combined results for PRILOSEC + clarithromycin and PRILOSEC treatment arms
*($p \leq 0.01$) versus proportion with duodenal ulcer recurrence who were not *H. pylori* eradicated

Gastric Ulcer
In a U.S. multicenter, double-blind, study of omeprazole 40 mg once a day, 20 mg once a day, and placebo in 520 patients with endoscopically diagnosed gastric ulcer, the following results were obtained.

Treatment of Gastric Ulcer
% of Patients Healed
(All Patients Treated)

	PRILOSEC 20 mg q.d. (n = 202)	PRILOSEC 40 mg q.d. (n = 214)	Placebo (n = 104)
Week 4	47.5**	55.6**	30.8
Week 8	74.8**	82.7**,†	48.1

**($p < 0.01$) PRILOSEC 40 mg or 20 mg versus placebo
†($p < 0.05$) PRILOSEC 40 mg versus 20 mg

For the stratified groups of patients with ulcer size less than or equal to 1 cm, no difference in healing rates between 40 mg and 20 mg was detected at either 4 or 8 weeks. For patients with ulcer size greater than 1 cm, 40 mg was significantly more effective than 20 mg at 8 weeks.

In a foreign, multinational, double-blind study of 602 patients with endoscopically diagnosed gastric ulcer, omeprazole 40 mg once a day, 20 mg once a day, and ranitidine 150 mg twice a day were evaluated.

Treatment of Gastric Ulcer
% of Patients Healed
(All Patients Treated)

	PRILOSEC 20 mg q.d. (n = 200)	PRILOSEC 40 mg q.d. (n = 187)	Ranitidine 150 mg b.i.d. (n = 199)
Week 4	63.5	78.1**,††	56.3
Week 8	81.5	91.4**,††	78.4

**($p < 0.01$) PRILOSEC 40 mg versus ranitidine
††($p < 0.01$) PRILOSEC 40 mg versus 20 mg

Gastroesophageal Reflux Disease (GERD)
Symptomatic GERD
A placebo controlled study was conducted in Scandinavia to compare the efficacy of omeprazole 20 mg or 10 mg once daily for up to 4 weeks in the treatment of heartburn and other symptoms in GERD patients without erosive esophagitis. Results are shown below.

% Successful Symptomatic Outcome[a]

	PRILOSEC 20 mg a.m.	PRILOSEC 10 mg a.m.	Placebo a.m.
All patients	46*,† (n = 205)	31† (n = 199)	13 (n = 105)
Patients with confirmed GERD	56*,† (n = 115)	36† (n = 109)	14 (n = 59)

[a] Defined as complete resolution of heartburn
*($p < 0.005$) versus 10 mg
†($p < 0.005$) versus placebo

Erosive Esophagitis
In a U.S. multicenter double-blind placebo controlled study of 20 mg or 40 mg of PRILOSEC Delayed-Release Capsules in patients with symptoms of GERD and endoscopically diagnosed erosive esophagitis of grade 2 or above, the percentage healing rates (per protocol) were as follows:

Week	20 mg PRILOSEC (n = 83)	40 mg PRILOSEC (n = 87)	Placebo (n = 43)
4	39**	45**	7
8	74**	75**	14

**($p < 0.01$) PRILOSEC versus placebo.

In this study, the 40 mg dose was not superior to the 20 mg dose of PRILOSEC in the percentage healing rate. Other controlled clinical trials have also shown that PRILOSEC is effective in severe GERD. In comparisons with histamine H_2-receptor antagonists in patients with erosive esophagitis, grade 2 or above, PRILOSEC in a dose of 20 mg was significantly more effective than the active controls. Complete daytime and nighttime heartburn relief occurred significantly faster ($p < 0.01$) in patients treated with PRILOSEC than in those taking placebo or histamine H_2-receptor antagonists.

In this and five other controlled GERD studies, significantly more patients taking 20 mg omeprazole (84%) reported complete relief of GERD symptoms than patients receiving placebo (12%).
Long Term Maintenance Treatment of Erosive Esophagitis
In a U.S. double-blind, randomized, multicenter, placebo controlled study, two dose regimens of PRILOSEC were studied in patients with endoscopically confirmed healed esophagitis. Results to determine maintenance of healing of erosive esophagitis are shown below.

Life Table Analysis

	PRILOSEC 20 mg q.d. (n = 138)	PRILOSEC 20 mg 3 days per week (n = 137)	Placebo (n = 131)
Percent in endoscopic remission at 6 months	*70	34	11

*($p < 0.01$) PRILOSEC 20 mg q.d. versus PRILOSEC 20 mg 3 consecutive days per week or placebo.

In an international multicenter double-blind study, PRILOSEC 20 mg daily and 10 mg daily were compared to ranitidine 150 mg twice daily in patients with endoscopically confirmed healed esophagitis. The table below provides the results of this study for maintenance of healing of erosive esophagitis.

Life Table Analysis

	PRILOSEC 20 mg q.d. (n = 131)	PRILOSEC 10 mg q.d. (n = 133)	Ranitidine 150 mg b.i.d. (n = 128)
Percent in endoscopic remission at 12 months	*77	‡58	46

Continued on next page

Prilosec—Cont.

*(p = 0.01) PRILOSEC 20 mg q.d. versus PRILOSEC 10 mg q.d. or Ranitidine.
‡(p = 0.03) PRILOSEC 10 mg q.d. versus Ranitidine.

In patients who initially had grades 3 or 4 erosive esophagitis, for maintenance after healing 20 mg daily of PRILOSEC was effective, while 10 mg did not demonstrate effectiveness.

Pathological Hypersecretory Conditions
In open studies of 136 patients with pathological hypersecretory conditions, such as Zollinger-Ellison (ZE) syndrome with or without multiple endocrine adenomas, PRILOSEC Delayed-Release Capsules significantly inhibited gastric acid secretion and controlled associated symptoms of diarrhea, anorexia, and pain. Doses ranging from 20 mg every other day to 360 mg per day maintained basal acid secretion below 10 mEq/hr in patients without prior gastric surgery, and below 5 mEq/hr in patients with prior gastric surgery. Initial doses were titrated to the individual patient need, and adjustments were necessary with time in some patients (see DOSAGE AND ADMINISTRATION). PRILOSEC was well tolerated at these high dose levels for prolonged periods (> 5 years in some patients). In most ZE patients, serum gastrin levels were not modified by PRILOSEC. However, in some patients serum gastrin increased to levels greater than those present prior to initiation of omeprazole therapy. At least 11 patients with ZE syndrome on long-term treatment with PRILOSEC developed gastric carcinoids. These findings are believed to be a manifestation of the underlying condition, which is known to be associated with such tumors, rather than the result of the administration of PRILOSEC. (See ADVERSE REACTIONS.)

INDICATIONS AND USAGE
Duodenal Ulcer
PRILOSEC Delayed-Release Capsules are indicated for short-term treatment of active duodenal ulcer. Most patients heal within four weeks. Some patients may require an additional four weeks of therapy.

PRILOSEC Delayed-Release Capsules, in combination with clarithromycin, are also indicated for treatment of patients with *H. pylori* infection and active duodenal ulcer to eradicate *H. pylori*. Eradication of *H. pylori* has been shown to reduce the risk of duodenal ulcer recurrence (see CLINICAL PHARMACOLOGY, *Clinical Studies* and DOSAGE AND ADMINISTRATION).

In patients who fail therapy, susceptibility testing should be done. If resistance to clarithromycin is demonstrated or susceptibility testing is not possible, alternative antimicrobial therapy should be instituted. (See the clarithromycin package insert, MICROBIOLOGY section.)

Gastric Ulcer
PRILOSEC Delayed-Release Capsules are indicated for short-term treatment (4–8 weeks) of active benign gastric ulcer. (See CLINICAL PHARMACOLOGY, *Clinical Studies*, *Gastric Ulcer*.)

Treatment of Gastroesophageal Reflux Disease (GERD)
Symptomatic GERD
PRILOSEC Delayed-Release Capsules are indicated for the treatment of heartburn and other symptoms associated with GERD.

Erosive Esophagitis
PRILOSEC Delayed-Release Capsules are indicated for the short-term treatment (4–8 weeks) of erosive esophagitis which has been diagnosed by endoscopy.
(See CLINICAL PHARMACOLOGY, *Clinical Studies*.)
The efficacy of PRILOSEC used for longer than 8 weeks in these patients has not been established. In the rare instance of a patient not responding to 8 weeks of treatment, it may be helpful to give up to an additional 4 weeks of treatment. If there is recurrence of erosive esophagitis or GERD symptoms (e.g. heartburn), additional 4–8 week courses of omeprazole may be considered.

Maintenance of Healing of Erosive Esophagitis
PRILOSEC Delayed-Release Capsules are indicated to maintain healing of erosive esophagitis.
Controlled studies do not extend beyond 12 months.

Pathological Hypersecretory Conditions
PRILOSEC Delayed-Release Capsules are indicated for the long-term treatment of pathological hypersecretory conditions (e.g., Zollinger-Ellison syndrome, multiple endocrine adenomas and systemic mastocytosis).

CONTRAINDICATIONS
Omeprazole
PRILOSEC Delayed-Release Capsules are contraindicated in patients with known hypersensitivity to any component of the formulation.
Clarithromycin
Clarithromycin is contraindicated in patients with a known hypersensitivity to any macrolide antibiotic.
Concomitant administration of clarithromycin with cisapride, pimozide, or terfenadine is contraindicated. There have been post-marketing reports of drug interactions when clarithromycin and/or erythromycin are co-administered

with cisapride, pimozide, or terfenadine resulting in cardiac arrhythmias (QT prolongation, ventricular tachycardia, ventricular fibrillation, and torsades de pointes) most likely due to inhibition of hepatic metabolism of these drugs by erythromycin and clarithromycin. Fatalities have been reported. (Please refer to full prescribing information for clarithromycin before prescribing.)

WARNING:
Clarithromycin
CLARITHROMYCIN SHOULD NOT BE USED IN PREGNANT WOMEN EXCEPT IN CLINICAL CIRCUMSTANCES WHERE NO ALTERNATIVE THERAPY IS APPROPRIATE. IF PREGNANCY OCCURS WHILE TAKING CLARITHROMYCIN, THE PATIENT SHOULD BE APPRISED OF THE POTENTIAL HAZARD TO THE FETUS. (See WARNINGS in prescribing information for clarithromycin.)

PRECAUTIONS
General
Symptomatic response to therapy with omeprazole does not preclude the presence of gastric malignancy.
Atrophic gastritis has been noted occasionally in gastric corpus biopsies from patients treated long-term with omeprazole.
Information for Patients
PRILOSEC Delayed-Release Capsules should be taken before eating. Patients should be cautioned that the PRILOSEC Delayed-Release Capsule should not be opened, chewed or crushed, and should be swallowed whole.
Drug Interactions
Other
Omeprazole can prolong the elimination of diazepam, warfarin and phenytoin, drugs that are metabolized by oxidation in the liver. Although in normal subjects no interaction with theophylline or propranolol was found, there have been clinical reports of interaction with other drugs metabolized via the cytochrome P-450 system (e.g., cyclosporine, disulfiram, benzodiazepines). Patients should be monitored to determine if it is necessary to adjust the dosage of these drugs when taken concomitantly with PRILOSEC.
Because of its profound and long lasting inhibition of gastric acid secretion, it is theoretically possible that omeprazole may interfere with absorption of drugs where gastric pH is an important determinant of their bioavailability (e.g., ketoconazole, ampicillin esters, and iron salts). In the clinical trials, antacids were used concomitantly with the administration of PRILOSEC.
Combination Therapy with Clarithromycin
Co-administration of omeprazole and clarithromycin may result in increases in plasma levels of omeprazole, clarithromycin, and 14-hydroxy-clarithromycin. (See also CLINICAL PHARMACOLOGY, *Pharmacokinetics: Combination Therapy with Clarithromycin.*)
Concomitant administration of clarithromycin with cisapride, pimozide, or terfenadine is contraindicated.
There have been reports of an interaction between erythromycin and astemizole resulting in QT prolongation and torsades de pointes. Concomitant administration of erythromycin and astemizole is contraindicated. Because clarithromycin is also metabolized by cytochrome P450, concomitant administration of clarithromycin with astemizole is not recommended. (See also CONTRAINDICATIONS, *Clarithromycin*, above. Please refer to full prescribing information for clarithromycin before prescribing.)
Carcinogenesis, Mutagenesis, Impairment of Fertility
In two 24-month carcinogenicity studies in rats, omeprazole at daily doses of 1.7, 3.4,13.8, 44.0 and 140.8 mg/kg/day (approximately 4 to 352 times the human dose, based on a patient weight of 50 kg and a human dose of 20 mg) produced gastric ECL cell carcinoids in a dose-related manner in both male and female rats; the incidence of this effect was markedly higher in female rats, which had higher blood levels of omeprazole. Gastric carcinoids seldom occur in the untreated rat. In addition, ECL cell hyperplasia was present in all treated groups of both sexes. In one of these studies, female rats were treated with 13.8 mg omeprazole/kg/day (approximately 35 times the human dose) for one year, then followed for an additional year without the drug. No carcinoids were seen in these rats. An increased incidence of treatment-related ECL cell hyperplasia was observed at the end of one year (94% treated vs 10% controls). By the second year the difference between treated and control rats was much smaller (46% vs 26%) but still showed more hyperplasia in the treated group. An unusual primary malignant tumor in the stomach was seen in one rat (2%). No similar tumor was seen in male or female rats treated for two years. For this strain of rat no similar tumor has been noted historically, but a finding involving only one tumor is difficult to interpret. A 78-week mouse carcinogenicity study of omeprazole did not show increased tumor occurrence, but the study was not conclusive.
Omeprazole was not mutagenic in an *in vitro* Ames *Salmonella typhimurium* assay, an *in vitro* mouse lymphoma cell assay and an *in vivo* rat liver DNA damage assay. A mouse micronucleus test at 625 and 6250 times the human dose gave a borderline result, as did an *in vivo* bone marrow

chromosome aberration test. A second mouse micronucleus study at 2000 times the human dose, but with different (suboptimal) sampling times, was negative.
In a rat fertility and general reproductive performance test, omeprazole in a dose range of 13.8 to 138.0 mg/kg/day (approximately 35 to 345 times the human dose) was not toxic or deleterious to the reproductive performance of parental animals.
Pregnancy
Omeprazole
Pregnancy Category C
Teratology studies conducted in pregnant rats at doses up to 138 mg/kg/day (approximately 345 times the human dose) and in pregnant rabbits at doses up to 69 mg/kg/day (approximately 172 times the human dose) did not disclose any evidence for a teratogenic potential of omeprazole.
In rabbits, omeprazole in a dose range of 6.9 to 69.1 mg/kg/day (approximately 17 to 172 times the human dose) produced dose-related increases in embryo-lethality, fetal resorptions and pregnancy disruptions. In rats, dose-related embryo/fetal toxicity and postnatal developmental toxicity were observed in offspring resulting from parents treated with omeprazole 13.8 to 138.0 mg/kg/day (approximately 35 to 345 times the human dose). There are no adequate or well-controlled studies in pregnant women. Sporadic reports have been received of congenital abnormalities occurring in infants born to women who have received omeprazole during pregnancy. Omeprazole should be used during pregnancy only if the potential benefit justifies the potential risk to the fetus.
Clarithromycin
Pregnancy Category C. See WARNINGS (above) and full prescribing information for clarithromycin before using in pregnant women.
Nursing Mothers
It is not known whether omeprazole is excreted in human milk. In rats, omeprazole administration during late gestation and lactation at doses of 13.8 to 138 mg/kg/day (35 to 345 times the human dose) resulted in decreased weight gain in pups. Because many drugs are excreted in human milk, because of the potential for serious adverse reactions in nursing infants from omeprazole, and because of the potential for tumorigenicity shown for omeprazole in rat carcinogenicity studies, a decision should be made whether to discontinue nursing or to discontinue the drug, taking into account the importance of the drug to the mother.
Pediatric Use
Safety and effectiveness in children have not been established.

ADVERSE REACTIONS
PRILOSEC Delayed-Release Capsules were generally well tolerated during domestic and international clinical trials in 3096 patients.
In the U.S. clinical trial population of 465 patients (including duodenal ulcer, Zollinger-Ellison syndrome and resistant ulcer patients), the following adverse experiences were reported to occur in 1% or more of patients on therapy with PRILOSEC. Numbers in parentheses indicate percentages of the adverse experiences considered by investigators as possibly, probably or definitely related to the drug:

	Omeprazole (n = 465)	Placebo (n = 64)	Ranitidine (n = 195)
Headache	6.9 (2.4)	6.3	7.7 (2.6)
Diarrhea	3.0 (1.9)	3.1 (1.6)	2.1 (0.5)
Abdominal Pain	2.4 (0.4)	3.1	2.1
Nausea	2.2 (0.9)	3.1	4.1 (0.5)
URI	1.9	1.6	2.6
Dizziness	1.5 (0.6)	0.0	2.6 (1.0)
Vomiting	1.5 (0.4)	4.7	1.5 (0.5)
Rash	1.5 (1.1)	0.0	0.0
Constipation	1.1 (0.9)	0.0	0.0
Cough	1.1	0.0	1.5
Asthenia	1.1 (0.2)	1.6 (1.6)	1.5 (1.0)
Back Pain	1.1	0.0	0.5

The following adverse reactions which occurred in 1% or more of omeprazole-treated patients have been reported in international double-blind, and open-label, clinical trials in which 2,631 patients and subjects received omeprazole.

	Incidence of Adverse Experiences ≥ 1% Causal Relationship not Assessed	
	Omeprazole (n = 2631)	Placebo (n = 120)
Body as a Whole, *site unspecified*		
Abdominal pain	5.2	3.3
Asthenia	1.3	0.8
Digestive System		
Constipation	1.5	0.8
Diarrhea	3.7	2.5
Flatulence	2.7	5.8
Nausea	4.0	6.7
Vomiting	3.2	10.0

Acid regurgitation	1.9	3.3
Nervous System/Psychiatric		
Headache	2.9	2.5

Additional adverse experiences occurring in < 1% of patients or subjects in domestic and/or international trials, or occurring since the drug was marketed, are shown below within each body system. In many instances, the relationship to PRILOSEC was unclear.

Body As a Whole: Fever, pain, fatigue, malaise, abdominal swelling

Cardiovascular: Chest pain or angina, tachycardia, bradycardia, palpitation, elevated blood pressure, peripheral edema

Gastrointestinal: Pancreatitis (some fatal), anorexia, irritable colon, flatulence, fecal discoloration, esophageal candidiasis, mucosal atrophy of the tongue, dry mouth. During treatment with omeprazole, gastric fundic gland polyps have been noted rarely. These polyps are benign and appear to be reversible when treatment is discontinued.

Gastro-duodenal carcinoids have been reported in patients with ZE syndrome on long-term treatment with PRILOSEC. This finding is believed to be a manifestation of the underlying condition, which is known to be associated with such tumors.

Hepatic: Mild and, rarely, marked elevations of liver function tests [ALT (SGPT), AST (SGOT), γ-glutamyl transpeptidase, alkaline phosphatase, and bilirubin (jaundice)]. In rare instances, overt liver disease has occurred, including hepatocellular, cholestatic, or mixed hepatitis, liver necrosis (some fatal), hepatic failure (some fatal), and hepatic encephalopathy.

Metabolic/Nutritional: Hyponatremia, hypoglycemia, weight gain

Musculoskeletal: Muscle cramps, myalgia, muscle weakness, joint pain, leg pain

Nervous System/Psychiatric: Psychic disturbances including depression, aggression, hallucinations, confusion, insomnia, nervousness, tremors, apathy, somnolence, anxiety, dream abnormalities; vertigo; paresthesia; hemifacial dysesthesia

Respiratory: Epistaxis, pharyngeal pain

Skin: Rash and, very rarely, cases of severe generalized skin reactions including toxic epidermal necrolysis (TEN; some fatal), Stevens-Johnson syndrome, and erythema multiforme (some severe); skin inflammation, urticaria, angioedema, pruritus, alopecia, dry skin, hyperhidrosis

Special Senses: Tinnitus, taste perversion

Urogenital: Interstitial nephritis (some with positive rechallenge), urinary tract infection, microscopic pyuria, urinary frequency, elevated serum creatinine, proteinuria, hematuria, glycosuria, testicular pain, gynecomastia

Hematologic: Rare instances of pancytopenia, agranulocytosis (some fatal), thrombocytopenia, neutropenia, anemia, leucocytosis, and hemolytic anemia have been reported.

The incidence of clinical adverse experiences in patients greater than 65 years of age was similar to that in patients 65 years of age or less.

Combination Therapy with Clarithromycin

In clinical trials using combination therapy with PRILOSEC and clarithromycin, no adverse experiences peculiar to this drug combination have been observed. Adverse experiences that have occurred have been limited to those that have been previously reported with omeprazole or clarithromycin.

Adverse experiences observed in controlled clinical trials using combination therapy with PRILOSEC and clarithromycin (n=346) which differed from those previously described for omeprazole alone were: Taste perversion (15%), tongue discoloration (2%), rhinitis (2%), pharyngitis (1%) and flu syndrome (1%).

For more information on clarithromycin, refer to the clarithromycin package insert, ADVERSE REACTIONS section.

OVERDOSAGE

Rare reports have been received of overdosage with omeprazole. Doses ranged from 320 mg to 900 mg (16–45 times the usual recommended clinical dose). Manifestations were variable, but included confusion, drowsiness, blurred vision, tachycardia, nausea, diaphoresis, flushing, headache, and dry mouth. Symptoms were transient, and no serious clinical outcome has been reported. No specific antidote for omeprazole overdosage is known. Omeprazole is extensively protein bound and is, therefore, not readily dialyzable. In the event of overdosage, treatment should be symptomatic and supportive.

Lethal doses of omeprazole after single oral administration are about 1500 mg/kg in mice and greater than 4000 mg/kg in rats, and about 100 mg/kg in mice and greater than 40 mg/kg in rats given single intravenous injections. Animals given these doses showed sedation, ptosis, convulsions, and decreased activity, body temperature, and respiratory rate and increased depth of respiration.

DOSAGE AND ADMINISTRATION

Duodenal Ulcer

Short-Term Treatment of Active Duodenal Ulcer: The recommended adult oral dose of PRILOSEC is 20 mg once daily. Most patients heal within four weeks. Some patients may require an additional four weeks of therapy. (See INDICATIONS AND USAGE.)

Reduction of the Risk of Duodenal Ulcer Recurrence: Combination Therapy with Clarithromycin

Days 1-14:	Days 15-28:
PRILOSEC 40 mg q.d. (in the morning) plus clarithromycin 500 mg t.i.d.	PRILOSEC 20 mg q.d.

Please refer to clarithromycin full prescribing information for CONTRAINDICATIONS and WARNING, and for information regarding dosing in elderly and renally impaired patients (PRECAUTIONS: *General*, PRECAUTIONS: *Geriatric Use* and PRECAUTIONS: *Drug Interactions*).

Gastric Ulcer

The recommended adult oral dose is 40 mg once a day for 4-8 weeks. (See CLINICAL PHARMACOLOGY, *Clinical Studies, Gastric Ulcer*, and INDICATIONS AND USAGE, *Gastric Ulcer*.)

Gastroesophageal Reflux Disease (GERD)

The recommended adult oral dose for the treatment of patients with symptomatic GERD and no esophageal lesions is 20 mg daily for up to 4 weeks. The recommended adult oral dose for the treatment of patients with erosive esophagitis and accompanying symptoms due to GERD is 20 mg daily for 4 to 8 weeks. (See INDICATIONS AND USAGE.)

Maintenance of Healing of Erosive Esophagitis

The recommended adult oral dose is 20 mg daily. (See CLINICAL PHARMACOLOGY, *Clinical Studies*.)

Pathological Hypersecretory Conditions

The dosage of PRILOSEC in patients with pathological hypersecretory conditions varies with the individual patient. The recommended adult oral starting dose is 60 mg once a day. Doses should be adjusted to individual patient needs and should continue for as long as clinically indicated. Doses up to 120 mg t.i.d. have been administered. Daily dosages of greater than 80 mg should be administered in divided doses. Some patients with Zollinger-Ellison syndrome have been treated continuously with PRILOSEC for more than 5 years.

No dosage adjustment is necessary for patients with renal impairment, hepatic dysfunction or for the elderly.

PRILOSEC Delayed-Release Capsules should be taken before eating. In the clinical trials, antacids were used concomitantly with PRILOSEC.

Patients should be cautioned that the PRILOSEC Delayed-Release Capsule should not be opened, chewed or crushed, and should be swallowed whole.

HOW SUPPLIED

No. 3426 - PRILOSEC Delayed-Release Capsules, 10 mg, are opaque, hard gelatin, apricot and amethyst colored capsules, coded 606 on cap and PRILOSEC 10 on the body. They are supplied as follows:

NDC 61113-606-31 unit of use bottles of 30

NDC 61113-606-68 bottles of 100

NDC 61113-606-28 unit dose packages of 100.

No. 3440 - PRILOSEC Delayed-Release Capsules, 20 mg, are opaque, hard gelatin, amethyst colored capsules, coded 742 on cap and PRILOSEC 20 on body. They are supplied as follows:

NDC 61113-742-31 unit of use bottles of 30

(6505-01-314-2716, 20 mg 30's)

NDC 61113-742-28 unit dose package of 100

(6505-01-314-2717, 20 mg individually sealed 100's)

NDC 61113-742-82 bottles of 1000.

No. 3428–PRILOSEC Delayed-Release Capsules, 40 mg, are opaque, hard gelatin, apricot and amethyst colored capsules, coded 743 on cap and PRILOSEC 40 on the body. They are supplied as follows:

NDC 61113-743-31 unit of use bottles of 30

NDC 61113-743-68 bottles of 100

NDC 61113-743-28 unit dose packages of 100

NDC 61113-743-82 bottles of 1000.

Storage

Store PRILOSEC Delayed-Release Capsules in a tight container protected from light and moisture. Store between 15°C and 30°C (59°F and 86°F).

Distributed by:

ASTRA Pharmaceuticals, L.P.

Wayne, PA 19087, USA

Manufactured by:

MERCK & CO., INC.,

West Point, PA 19486, USA

© 1998 Astra Pharmaceuticals, L.P. All rights reserved.

Issued September 1997   7910927

Shown in Product Identification Guide, page 304

PULMICORT TURBUHALER® 200 mcg ℞

[pull' mĭ-cört]

(budesonide inhalation powder)

For Oral Inhalation Only.

DESCRIPTION

Budesonide, the active component of PULMICORT TURBUHALER 200 mcg, is a corticosteroid designated chemically as (RS)-11β, 16α, 17,21-Tetrahydroxypregna-1,4-diene-3,20-dione cyclic 16,17-acetal with butyraldehyde. Budesonide is provided as a mixture of two epimers (22R and 22S). The empirical formula of budesonide is $C_{25}H_{34}O_6$ and its molecular weight is 430.5. Its structural formula is:

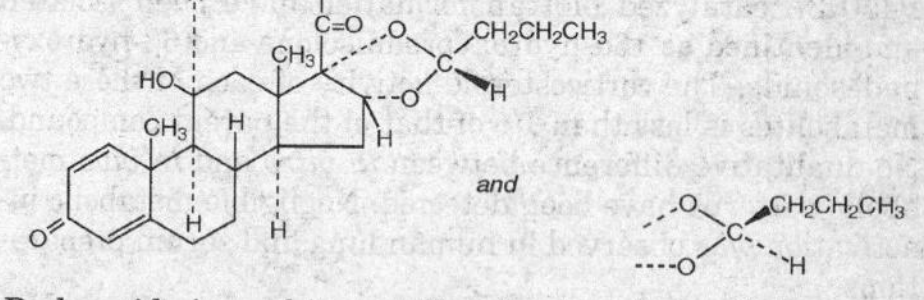

Budesonide is a white to off-white, tasteless, odorless powder that is practically insoluble in water and in heptane, sparingly soluble in ethanol, and freely soluble in chloroform. Its partition coefficient between octanol and water at pH 7.4 is 1.6×10^3.

PULMICORT TURBUHALER is an inhalation-driven multi-dose dry powder inhaler which contains only micronized budesonide. Each actuation of PULMICORT TURBUHALER provides 200 mcg budesonide per metered dose, which delivers approximately 160 mcg budesonide from the mouthpiece (based on *in vitro* testing at 60 L/min for 2 sec). The amount of drug delivered to the lung will depend on patient factors such as inspiratory flow (see Patient's Instructions for Use). In adult patients with asthma (mean FEV$_1$ 2.9 L [0.8 - 5.1 L]) mean peak inspiratory flow (PIF) through PULMICORT TURBUHALER was 78 (40-111) L/min. Similar results (mean PIF 82 [43-125] L/min) were obtained in asthmatic children (6 to 15 years, mean FEV$_1$ 2.1 L [0.9 - 5.4 L]).

CLINICAL PHARMACOLOGY

Budesonide is an anti-inflammatory corticosteroid that exhibits potent glucocorticoid activity and weak mineralocorticoid activity. In standard *in vitro* and animal models, budesonide has approximately a 200-fold higher affinity for the glucocorticoid receptor and a 1000-fold higher topical anti-inflammatory potency than cortisol (rat croton oil ear edema assay). As a measure of systemic activity, budesonide is 40 times more potent than cortisol when administered subcutaneously and 25 times more potent when administered orally in the rat thymus involution assay.

The precise mechanism of corticosteroid actions on inflammation in asthma is not known. Corticosteroids have been shown to have a wide range of inhibitory activities against multiple cell types (e.g., mast cells, eosinophils, neutrophils, macrophages, and lymphocytes) and mediators (e.g., histamine, eicosanoids, leukotrienes, and cytokines) involved in allergic and non-allergic-mediated inflammation. These anti-inflammatory actions of corticosteroids may contribute to their efficacy in asthma.

Studies in asthmatic patients have shown a favorable ratio between topical anti-inflammatory activity and systemic corticosteroid effects over a wide range of doses from PULMICORT TURBUHALER. This is explained by a combination of a relatively high local anti-inflammatory effect, extensive first pass hepatic degradation of orally absorbed drug (85–95%), and the low potency of formed metabolites (see below).

Pharmacokinetics: The activity of PULMICORT TURBUHALER is due to the parent drug, budesonide. In glucocorticoid receptor affinity studies, the 22R form was two times as active as the 22S epimer. *In vitro* studies indicated that the two forms of budesonide do not interconvert. The 22R form was preferentially cleared by the liver with systemic clearance of 1.4 L/min vs. 1.0 L/min for the 22S form. The terminal half-life, 2 to 3 hours, was the same for both epimers and was independent of dose. In asthmatic patients, budesonide showed a linear increase in AUC and C_{max} with increasing dose after both a single dose and repeated dosing from PULMICORT TURBUHALER.

Absorption: After oral administration of budesonide, peak plasma concentration was achieved in about 1 to 2 hours and the absolute systemic availability was 6–13%. In contrast, most of budesonide delivered to the lungs is systemically absorbed. In healthy subjects, 34% of the metered dose was deposited in the lungs (as assessed by plasma concentration method) with an absolute systemic availability of 39% of the metered dose. Pharmacokinetics of budesonide do not differ significantly in healthy volunteers and asthmatic patients. Peak plasma concentrations of budesonide occurred within 30 minutes of inhalation from PULMICORT TURBUHALER.

Continued on next page

Pulmicort—Cont.

Distribution: The volume of distribution of budesonide was approximately 3 L/kg. It was 85–90% bound to plasma proteins. Protein binding was constant over the concentration range (1–100 nmol/L) achieved with, and exceeding, recommended doses of PULMICORT TURBUHALER. Budesonide showed little or no binding to corticosteroid binding globulin. Budesonide rapidly equilibrated with red blood cells in a concentration independent manner with a blood/plasma ratio of about 0.8.

Metabolism: *In vitro* studies with human liver homogenates have shown that budesonide is rapidly and extensively metabolized. Two major metabolites formed via cytochrome P450 3A catalyzed biotransformation have been isolated and identified as 16α-hydroxyprednisolone and 6β-hydroxybudesonide. The corticosteroid activity of each of these two metabolites is less than 1% of that of the parent compound. No qualitative difference between *in vitro* and *in vivo* metabolic patterns have been detected. Negligible metabolic inactivation was observed in human lung and serum preparations.

Excretion: Budesonide was excreted in urine and feces in the form of metabolites. Approximately 60% of an intravenous radiolabelled dose was recovered in the urine. No unchanged budesonide was detected in the urine.

Special Populations: No pharmacokinetic differences have been identified due to race, gender or advanced age.

Pediatric: Following intravenous dosing in pediatric patients age 10–14 years, plasma half-life was shorter than in adults (1.5 hrs vs 2.0 hrs in adults). In the same population following inhalation of budesonide via a pressurized metered-dose inhaler, absolute systemic availability was similar to that in adults.

Hepatic Insufficiency: Reduced liver function may affect the elimination of corticosteroids. The pharmacokinetics of budesonide were affected by compromised liver function as evidenced by a doubled systemic availability after oral ingestion. The intravenous pharmacokinetics of budesonide were, however, similar in cirrhotic patients and in healthy subjects.

Drug-drug Interactions: Ketoconazole, a potent inhibitor of cytochrome P450 3A, the main metabolic enzyme for corticosteroids, increased plasma levels of orally ingested budesonide. At recommended doses, cimetidine had a slight but clinically insignificant effect on the pharmacokinetics of oral budesonide.

Pharmacodynamics: To confirm that systemic absorption is not a significant factor in the clinical efficacy of inhaled budesonide, a clinical study in patients with asthma was performed comparing 400 mcg budesonide administered via a pressurized metered dose inhaler with a tube spacer to 1400 mcg of oral budesonide and placebo. The study demonstrated the efficacy of inhaled budesonide but not orally ingested budesonide despite comparable systemic levels. Thus, the therapeutic effect of conventional doses of orally inhaled budesonide are largely explained by its direct action on the respiratory tract.

Generally, PULMICORT TURBUHALER has a relatively rapid onset of action for an inhaled corticosteroid. Improvement in asthma control following inhalation of PULMICORT TURBUHALER can occur within 24 hours of beginning treatment although maximum benefit may not be achieved for 1 to 2 weeks, or longer.

PULMICORT TURBUHALER has been shown to decrease airway reactivity to various challenge models, including histamine, methacholine, sodium metabisulfite, and adenosine monophosphate in hyperreactive patients. The clinical relevance of these models is not certain.

Pretreatment with PULMICORT TURBUHALER 1600 mcg daily (800 mcg twice daily) for 2 weeks reduced the acute (early-phase reaction) and delayed (late-phase reaction) decrease in FEV_1 following inhaled allergen challenge.

The effects of PULMICORT TURBUHALER on the hypothalamic-pituitary-adrenal (HPA) axis were studied in 905 adults and 404 pediatric patients with asthma. For most patients, the ability to increase cortisol production in response to stress, as assessed by cosyntropin (ACTH) stimulation test, remained intact with PULMICORT TURBUHALER treatment at recommended doses. For adult patients treated with 100, 200, 400, or 800 mcg twice daily for 12 weeks, 4%, 2%, 6%, and 13% respectively, had an abnormal stimulated cortisol response (peak cortisol <14.5 mcg/dL assessed by liquid chromatography following short-cosyntropin test) as compared to 8% of patients treated with placebo. Similar results were obtained in pediatric patients. In another study in adults, doses of 400, 800 and 1600 mcg budesonide twice daily via PULMICORT TURBUHALER for 6 weeks were examined; 1600 mcg twice daily (twice the maximum recommended dose) resulted in a 27% reduction in stimulated cortisol (6-hour ACTH infusion) while 10 mg prednisone resulted in a 35% reduction. In this study, no patient on PULMICORT TURBUHALER at doses of 400 and 800 mcg twice daily met the criterion for an abnormal stimulated cortisol response (peak cortisol <14.5 mcg/dL assessed by liquid chromatography) following ACTH infusion. An open-label, long-term follow-up of 1133 patients for up to 52 weeks confirmed the minimal effect on the HPA axis (both basal and stimulated plasma cortisol) of PULMICORT TURBUHALER when administered at recommended doses. In patients who had previously been oral steroid-dependent, use of PULMICORT TURBUHALER in recommended doses was associated with higher stimulated cortisol response compared to baseline following 1 year of therapy.

The administration of budesonide via PULMICORT TURBUHALER in doses up to 800 mcg/day (mean daily dose 445 mcg/day) or via a pressurized metered-dose inhaler in doses up to 1200 mcg/day (mean daily dose 620 mcg/day) to 216 pediatric patients (age 3 to 11 years) for 2 to 6 years had no significant effect on statural growth compared with non-corticosteroid therapy in 62 matched control patients. However, the long-term effect of PULMICORT TURBUHALER on growth is not fully known.

CLINICAL TRIALS

The therapeutic efficacy of PULMICORT TURBUHALER has been evaluated in controlled clinical trials involving more than 1300 patients (6 years and older) with asthma of varying disease duration (<1 year to >20 years) and severity.

Double-blind, parallel, placebo-controlled clinical trials of 12 weeks duration and longer have shown that, compared with placebo, PULMICORT TURBUHALER significantly improved lung function (measured by PEF and FEV_1), significantly decreased morning and evening symptoms of asthma, and significantly reduced the need for as needed inhaled β_2-agonist use at doses of 400 mcg to 1600 mcg per day (200 mcg to 800 mcg twice daily) in adults and 400 mcg to 800 mcg per day (200 mcg to 400 mcg twice daily) in pediatric patients 6 years of age and older.

Improved lung function (morning PEF) was observed within 24 hours of initiating treatment in both adult and pediatric patients 6 years of age and older, although maximum benefit was not achieved for 1 to 2 weeks, or longer, after starting treatment. Improved lung function was maintained throughout the 12 weeks of the double-blind portion of the trials.

Patients Not Receiving Corticosteroid Therapy: In a 12-week clinical trial in 273 patients with mild to moderate asthma (mean baseline FEV_1 2.27 L) who were not well controlled by bronchodilators alone, PULMICORT TURBUHALER was evaluated at doses of 200 mcg twice daily and 400 mcg twice daily versus placebo. The FEV_1 results from this trial are shown in the figure below. Pulmonary function improved significantly on both doses of PULMICORT TURBUHALER compared with placebo.

A 12-Week Trial in Patients Not on Corticosteroid Therapy Prior to Study Entry

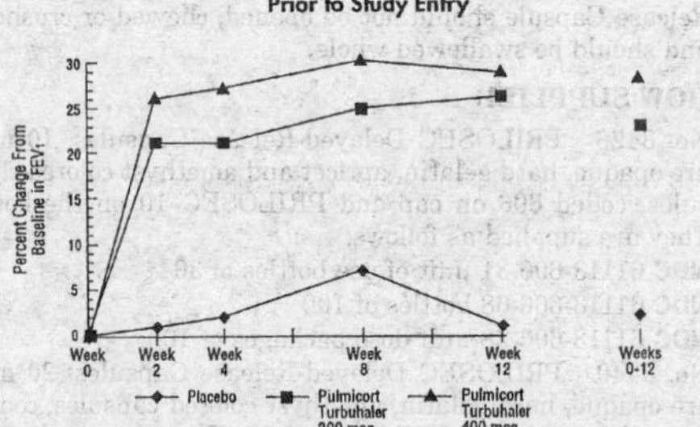

In a 12-month controlled trial in 75 patients not previously receiving corticosteroids, PULMICORT TURBUHALER at 200 mcg twice daily resulted in improved lung function (measured by PEF) and reduced bronchial hyperreactivity compared to placebo.

Patients Previously Maintained on Inhaled Corticosteroids: The safety and efficacy of PULMICORT TURBUHALER was also evaluated in adult and pediatric patients (age 6 to 18 years) previously maintained on inhaled corticosteroids (adults: N = 473, mean baseline FEV_1 2.04 L, baseline doses of beclomethasone dipropionate 126–1008 mcg/day; pediatrics: N = 404, mean baseline FEV_1 2.09 L, baseline doses of beclomethasone dipropionate 126–672 mcg/day or triamcinolone acetonide 300–1800 mcg/day). The FEV_1 results of these two trials, both 12 weeks in duration, are presented in the following figures. Pulmonary function improved significantly with all doses of PULMICORT TURBUHALER compared to placebo in both trials.

[See figures at top of next column]

Patients Previously Maintained on Oral Corticosteroids: In a clinical trial in 159 severe asthmatic patients requiring chronic oral prednisone therapy (mean baseline prednisone dose 19.3 mg/day) PULMICORT TURBUHALER at doses of 400 mcg twice daily and 800 mcg twice daily was compared to placebo over a 20-week period. Approximately two-thirds (68% on 400 mcg twice daily and 64% on 800 mcg twice daily) of PULMICORT TURBUHALER-treated patients were able to achieve sustained (at least 2 weeks) oral corticosteroid cessation (compared with 8% of placebo-treated patients) and improved asthma control. The average oral corticosteroid dose was reduced by 83% on 400 mcg twice daily and 79% on 800 mcg twice daily for PULMICORT TURBUHALER-treated patients vs. 27% for placebo. Additionally, 58 out of 64 patients (91%) who completely eliminated oral corticosteroids during the double-blind phase of the trial remained off oral corticosteroids for an additional 12 months while receiving PULMICORT TURBUHALER.

Adult Patients Previously Maintained on Inhaled Corticosteroids

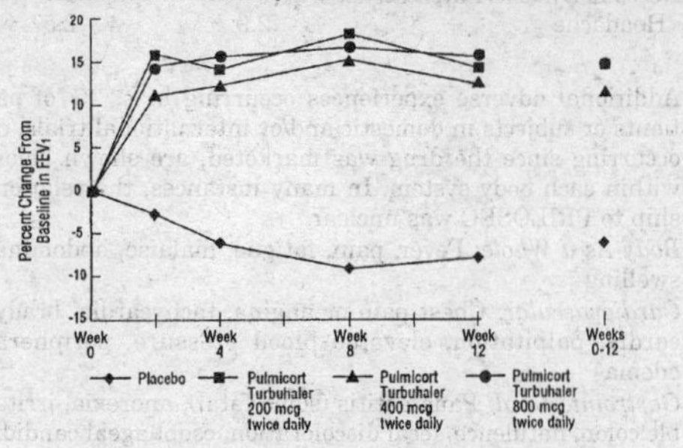

Pediatric Patients Age 6 to 18 Years Previously Maintained on Inhaled Corticosteroids

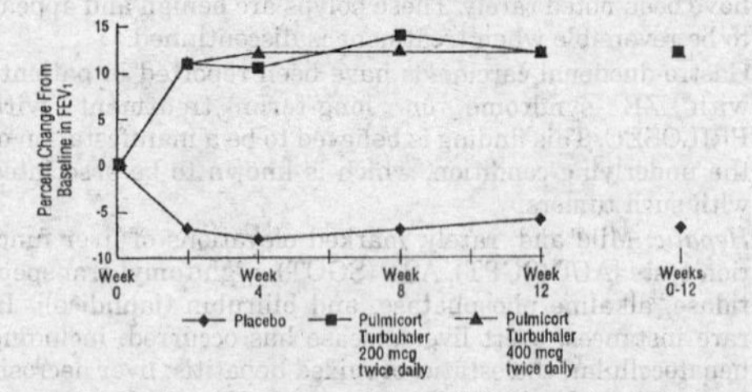

INDICATIONS AND USAGE

PULMICORT TURBUHALER is indicated for the maintenance treatment of asthma as prophylactic therapy in adult and pediatric patients six years of age or older. It is also indicated for patients requiring oral corticosteroid therapy for asthma. Many of those patients may be able to reduce or eliminate their requirement for oral corticosteroids over time.

PULMICORT TURBUHALER is NOT indicated for the relief of acute bronchospasm.

CONTRAINDICATIONS

PULMICORT TURBUHALER is contraindicated in the primary treatment of status asthmaticus or other acute episodes of asthma where intensive measures are required. Hypersensitivity to budesonide contraindicates the use of PULMICORT TURBUHALER.

WARNINGS

Particular care is needed for patients who are transferred from systemically active corticosteroids to PULMICORT TURBUHALER because deaths due to adrenal insufficiency have occurred in asthmatic patients during and after transfer from systemic corticosteroids to less systemically available inhaled corticosteroids. After withdrawal from systemic corticosteroids, a number of months are required for recovery of HPA function. Patients who have been previously maintained on 20 mg or more per day of prednisone (or its equivalent) may be most susceptible, particularly when their systemic corticosteroids have been almost completely withdrawn. During this period of HPA suppression, patients may exhibit signs and symptoms of adrenal insufficiency when exposed to trauma, surgery, or infection (particularly gastroenteritis) or other conditions associated with severe electrolyte loss. Although PULMICORT TURBUHALER may provide control of asthma symptoms during these episodes, in recommended doses it supplies less than normal physiological amounts of glucocorticoid systemically and does NOT provide the mineralocorticoid activity that is necessary for coping with these emergencies.

During periods of stress or a severe asthma attack, patients who have been withdrawn from systemic corticosteroids should be instructed to resume oral corticosteroids (in large doses) immediately and to contact their physicians for further instruction. These patients should also be instructed to carry a medical identification card indicating that they may need supplementary systemic corticosteroids during periods of stress or a severe asthma attack.

Transfer of patients from systemic corticosteroid therapy to PULMICORT TURBUHALER may unmask allergic conditions previously suppressed by the systemic corticosteroid therapy, e.g., rhinitis, conjunctivitis, and eczema (See Dosage and Administration).

Patients who are on drugs which suppress the immune system are more susceptible to infection than healthy individuals. Chicken pox and measles, for example, can have a more serious or even fatal course in susceptible pediatric patients or adults on immunosuppressant doses of corticosteroids. In pediatric or adult patients who have not had these diseases, particular care should be taken to avoid exposure. How the dose, route and duration of corticosteroid administration affects the risk of developing a disseminated infection is not known. The contribution of the underlying disease and/or prior corticosteroid treatment to the risk is also not known. If exposed, therapy with varicella zoster immune globulin (VZIG) or pooled intravenous immunoglobulin (IVIG), as appropriate, may be indicated. If exposed to measles, prophylaxis with pooled intramuscular immunoglobulin (IG) may be indicated. (See the respective package insert for complete VZIG and IG prescribing information.) If chicken pox develops, treatment with antiviral agents may be considered.

PULMICORT TURBUHALER is not a bronchodilator and is not indicated for rapid relief of bronchospasm or other acute episodes of asthma.

As with other inhaled asthma medications, bronchospasm, with an immediate increase in wheezing, may occur after dosing. If bronchospasm occurs following dosing with PULMICORT TURBUHALER, it should be treated immediately with a fast-acting inhaled bronchodilator. Treatment with PULMICORT TURBUHALER should be discontinued and alternate therapy instituted.

Patients should be instructed to contact their physician immediately when episodes of asthma not responsive to their usual doses of bronchodilators occur during treatment with PULMICORT TURBUHALER. During such episodes, patients may require therapy with oral corticosteroids.

PRECAUTIONS

General: During withdrawal from oral corticosteroids, some patients may experience symptoms of systemically active corticosteroid withdrawal, e.g., joint and/or muscular pain, lassitude, and depression, despite maintenance or even improvement of respiratory function.

PULMICORT TURBUHALER will often permit control of asthma symptoms with less suppression of HPA function than therapeutically equivalent oral doses of prednisone. Since budesonide is absorbed into the circulation and can be systemically active at higher doses, the full beneficial effects of PULMICORT TURBUHALER in minimizing HPA dysfunction may be expected only when recommended dosages are not exceeded and individual patients are titrated to the lowest effective dose. Since individual sensitivity to effects on cortisol production exists, physicians should consider this information when prescribing PULMICORT TURBUHALER.

Because of the possibility of systemic absorption of inhaled corticosteroids, patients treated with these drugs should be observed carefully for any evidence of systemic corticosteroid effects. Particular care should be taken in observing patients postoperatively or during periods of stress for evidence of inadequate adrenal response.

It is possible that systemic corticosteroid effects such as hypercorticism and adrenal suppression may appear in a small number of patients, particularly at higher doses. If such changes occur, PULMICORT TURBUHALER should be reduced slowly, consistent with accepted procedures for management of asthma symptoms and for tapering of systemic steroids.

A reduction of growth velocity in children or teenagers may occur as a result of inadequate control of chronic diseases such as asthma or from use of corticosteroids for treatment. Physicians should closely follow the growth of adolescents taking corticosteroids by any route and weigh the benefits of corticosteroid therapy and asthma control against the possibility of growth suppression if an adolescent's growth appears slowed.

Although patients in clinical trials have received PULMICORT TURBUHALER on a continuous basis for periods of 1 to 2 years, the long-term local and systemic effects of PULMICORT TURBUHALER in human subjects are not completely known. In particular, the effects resulting from chronic use of PULMICORT TURBUHALER on developmental or immunological processes in the mouth, pharynx, trachea, and lung are unknown.

In clinical trials with PULMICORT TURBUHALER, localized infections with Candida albicans occurred in the mouth and pharynx in some patients. If oropharyngeal candidiasis develops, it should be treated with appropriate local or systemic (i.e., oral) antifungal therapy while still continuing with PULMICORT TURBUHALER therapy, but at times therapy with PULMICORT TURBUHALER may need to be temporarily interrupted under close medical supervision.

Inhaled corticosteroids should be used with caution, if at all, in patients with active or quiescent tuberculosis infection of the respiratory tract, untreated systemic fungal, bacterial, viral or parasitic infections; or ocular herpes simplex.

Rare instances of glaucoma, increased intraocular pressure, and cataracts have been reported following the inhaled administration of corticosteroids.

Information for Patients: For proper use of PULMICORT TURBUHALER and to attain maximum improvement, the patient should read and follow the accompanying Patient's Instructions for Use carefully. In addition, patients being treated with PULMICORT TURBUHALER should receive the following information and instructions. This information is intended to aid the patient in the safe and effective use of the medication. It is not a disclosure of all possible adverse or intended effects.

- Patients should take the medication as directed and use PULMICORT TURBUHALER at regular intervals twice daily since its effectiveness depends on regular use. The patient should not alter the prescribed dosage unless advised to do so by the physician.
- PULMICORT TURBUHALER is not a bronchodilator and is not intended to treat acute or life-threatening episodes of asthma.
- PULMICORT TURBUHALER must be in the upright position (mouthpiece on top) during loading in order to provide the correct dose. PULMICORT TURBUHALER must be primed when the unit is used for the very first time. To prime the unit, hold the unit in an upright position and turn the brown grip fully to the right, then fully to the left until it clicks. Repeat. The unit is now primed and ready to load the first dose by turning the grip fully to the right and fully to the left until it clicks.

  On subsequent uses, it is not necessary to prime the unit. However, it must be loaded in the upright position immediately prior to use. Turn the brown grip fully to the right, then fully to the left until it clicks. During inhalation, PULMICORT TURBUHALER must be held in the upright (mouthpiece up) or horizontal position. Do not shake the inhaler. Place the mouthpiece between lips and inhale forcefully and deeply. The powder is then delivered to the lungs.
- Patients should not exhale through PULMICORT TURBUHALER.
- Due to the small volume of powder, the patient may not taste or sense the presence of any medication entering the lungs when inhaling from TURBUHALER. This lack of "sensation" does not indicate that the patient is not receiving benefit from PULMICORT TURBUHALER.
- Rinsing the mouth with water without swallowing after each dosing may decrease the risk of the development of oral candidiasis.
- When there are 20 doses remaining in PULMICORT TURBUHALER, a red mark will appear in the indicator window.
- PULMICORT TURBUHALER should not be used with a spacer.
- The mouthpiece should not be bitten or chewed.
- The cover should be replaced securely after each opening.
- Keep PULMICORT TURBUHALER clean and dry at all times.
- Improvement in asthma control following inhalation of PULMICORT TURBUHALER can occur within 24 hours of beginning treatment although maximum benefit may not be achieved for 1 to 2 weeks, or longer. If symptoms do not improve in that time frame, or if the condition worsens, the patient should be instructed to contact the physician.
- Patients should be warned to avoid exposure to chicken pox or measles and if they are exposed, to consult their physicians without delay.
- For proper use of PULMICORT TURBUHALER and to attain maximum improvement, the patient should read and follow the accompanying Patient's Instructions for Use.

Drug Interactions: In clinical studies, concurrent administration of budesonide and other drugs commonly used in the treatment of asthma has not resulted in an increased frequency of adverse events. Ketoconazole, a potent inhibitor of cytochrome P450 3A, may increase plasma levels of budesonide during concomitant dosing. The clinical significance of concomitant administration of ketoconazole with PULMICORT TURBUHALER is not known, but caution may be warranted.

Carcinogenesis, Mutagenesis, Impairment of Fertility: Long-term studies were conducted in mice and rats using oral administration to evaluate the carcinogenic potential of budesonide.

There was no evidence of a carcinogenic effect when budesonide was administered orally for 91 weeks to mice at doses up to 200 mcg/kg/day (approximately $^1/_2$ the maximum recommended human daily inhalation dose on a mcg/m^2 basis).

In a 104-week carcinogenicity study in Sprague-Dawley rats, a statistically significant increase in the incidence of gliomas was observed in male rats receiving oral doses of 50 mcg/kg/day (approximately $^1/_4$ the maximum recommended human daily inhalation dose on a mcg/m^2 basis); no such changes were seen in male rats receiving oral doses of 10 and 25 mcg/kg/day (approximately $^1/_{20}$ and $^1/_8$ the maximum recommended human daily inhalation dose on a mcg/m^2 basis) or in female rats at oral doses up to 50 mcg/kg/day (approximately ¼ the maximum recommended human daily inhalation dose on a mcg/m^2 basis).

Two additional 104-week carcinogenicity studies have been performed with oral budesonide at doses of 50 mcg/kg/day (approximately $^1/_4$ the maximum recommended human daily inhalation dose on a mcg/m^2 basis) in male Sprague-Dawley and Fischer rats. These studies did not demonstrate an increased glioma incidence in budesonide-treated animals as compared with concurrent controls or reference corticosteroid-treated groups (prednisolone and triamcinolone acetonide). Compared with concurrent controls, a statistically significant increase in the incidence of hepatocellular tumors was observed in all three steroid groups (budesonide, prednisolone, triamcinolone acetonide) in these studies.

The mutagenic potential of budesonide was evaluated in six different test systems; Ames Salmonella/microsome plate test, mouse micronucleus test, mouse lymphoma test, chromosome aberration test in human lymphocytes, sex-linked recessive lethal test in Drosophila melanogaster, and DNA repair analysis in rat hepatocyte culture. Budesonide was not mutagenic or clastogenic in any of these tests.

The effect of subcutaneous budesonide on fertility and general reproductive performance was studied in rats. At 20 mcg/kg/day (approximately $^1/_{10}$ the maximum recommended human daily inhalation dose on a mcg/m^2 basis), decreases in maternal body weight gain, prenatal viability, and viability of the young at birth and during lactation were observed. No such effects were noted at 5 mcg/kg (approximately $^1/_{40}$ the maximum recommended human daily inhalation dose on a mcg/m^2 basis).

Pregnancy: Teratogenic Effects: Pregnancy Category C: As with other glucocorticoids, budesonide produced fetal loss, decreased pup weight and skeletal abnormalities at subcutaneous doses of 25 mcg/kg/day (approximately $^1/_4$ the maximum recommended human daily inhalation dose on a mcg/m^2 basis) in rabbits and 500 mcg/kg/day (approximately $2^1/_2$ times the maximum recommended human daily inhalation dose on a mcg/m^2 basis) in rats.

No teratogenic or embryocidal effects were observed in rats when budesonide was administered by inhalation at doses of 100 to 250 mcg/kg/day (approximately $^1/_2$ to $1^1/_4$ times the maximum recommended human daily inhalation dose on a mcg/m^2 basis).

There are no adequate and well-controlled studies in pregnant women. Budesonide should be used during pregnancy only if the potential benefit justifies the potential risk to the fetus.

Experience with oral corticosteroids since their introduction in pharmacologic as opposed to physiologic doses suggests that rodents are more prone to teratogenic effects from corticosteroids than humans.

Nonterotogenic Effects: Hypoadrenalism may occur in infants born of mothers receiving corticosteroids during pregnancy. Such infants should be carefully observed.

Nursing Mothers: Corticosteroids are secreted in human milk. Because of the potential for adverse reactions in nursing infants from any corticosteroid, a decision should be made whether to discontinue nursing or discontinue the drug, taking into account the importance of the drug to the mother. Actual data for budesonide are lacking.

Pediatric Use: Safety and effectiveness of PULMICORT TURBUHALER in pediatric patients below 6 years of age have not been established.

In pediatric asthma patients the frequency of adverse events observed with PULMICORT TURBUHALER was similar between the 6- to 12-year age group (N = 172) compared with the 13- to 17-year age group (N = 124).

Oral corticosteroids have been shown to cause growth suppression in pediatric and adolescent patients, particularly with higher doses over extended periods. If a pediatric or adolescent patient on any corticosteroid appears to have growth suppression, the possibility that they are particularly sensitive to this effect of corticosteroids should be considered (see PRECAUTIONS).

Geriatric Use: One hundred patients 65 years or older were included in the US and non-US controlled clinical trials of PULMICORT TURBUHALER. There were no differences in the safety and efficacy of the drug compared to those seen in younger patients.

ADVERSE REACTIONS

The following adverse reactions were reported in patients treated with PULMICORT TURBUHALER.

The incidence of common adverse events is based upon double-blind, placebo-controlled US clinical trials in which 1,116 adult and pediatric patients age 6–70 years (472 females and 644 males) were treated with PULMICORT TURBUHALER (200 to 800 mcg twice daily for 12 to 20 weeks) or placebo.

Continued on next page

Pulmicort—Cont.

The following table shows the incidence of adverse events in patients previously receiving bronchodilators and/or inhaled corticosteroids in US controlled clinical trials. This population included 232 male and 62 female pediatric patients (age 6 to 17 years) and 332 male and 331 female adult patients (age 18 years and greater).

[See table below]

The table above includes all events (whether considered drug-related or non drug-related by the investigators) that occurred at a rate of ≥3% in any one PULMICORT TURBUHALER group and were more common than in the placebo group. In considering these data, the increased average duration of exposure for PULMICORT TURBUHALER patients should be taken into account.

The following other adverse events occurred in these clinical trials using PULMICORT TURBUHALER with an incidence of 1 to 3% and were more common on PULMICORT TURBUHALER than on placebo.

Body As A Whole: neck pain
Cardiovascular: syncope
Digestive: abdominal pain, dry mouth, vomiting
Metabolic and Nutritional: weight gain
Musculoskeletal: fracture, myalgia
Nervous: hypertonia, migraine
Platelet, Bleeding and Clotting: ecchymosis
Psychiatric: insomnia
Resistance Mechanisms: infection
Special Senses: taste perversion

In a 20-week trial in adult asthmatics who previously required oral corticosteroids, the effects of PULMICORT TURBUHALER 400 mcg twice daily (N=53) and 800 mcg twice daily (N=53) were compared with placebo (N=53) on the frequency of reported adverse events. Adverse events, whether considered drug-related or non drug-related by the investigators, reported in more than five patients in the PULMICORT TURBUHALER group and which occurred more frequently with PULMICORT TURBUHALER than placebo are shown below (% PULMICORT TURBUHALER and % placebo). In considering these data, the increased average duration of exposure for PULMICORT TURBUHALER patients (78 days for PULMICORT TURBUHALER vs. 41 days for placebo) should be taken into account.

Body As A Whole: asthenia (9% and 2%)
headache (12% and 2%)
pain (10% and 2%)
Digestive: dyspepsia (8% and 0%)
nausea (6% and 0%)
oral candidiasis (10% and 0%)
Musculoskeletal: arthralgia (6% and 0%)
Respiratory: cough increased (6% and 2%)
respiratory infection (32% and 13%)
rhinitis (6% and 2%)
sinusitis (16% and 11%)

Pediatric Studies: In a 12-week placebo-controlled trial in 404 pediatric patients 6 to 18 years of age previously maintained on inhaled corticosteroids, the frequency of adverse events for each age category (6 to 12 years, 13 to 18 years) was comparable for PULMICORT TURBUHALER (at 100, 200 and 400 mcg twice daily) and placebo. There were no

clinically relevant differences in the pattern or severity of adverse events in children compared with those reported in adults.

Adverse Event Reports From Other Sources: Rare adverse events reported in the published literature or from marketing experience include: immediate and delayed hypersensitivity reactions including rash, contact dermatitis, urticaria, angioedema and bronchospasm; symptoms of hypocorticism and hypercorticism; psychiatric symptoms including depression, aggressive reactions, irritability, anxiety and psychosis.

OVERDOSAGE

The potential for acute toxic effects following overdose of PULMICORT TURBUHALER is low. If used at excessive doses for prolonged periods, systemic corticosteroid effects such as hypercorticism may occur (see PRECAUTIONS). PULMICORT TURBUHALER at twice the highest recommended dose (3200 mcg daily) administered for 6 weeks caused a significant reduction (27%) in the plasma cortisol response to a 6-hour infusion of ACTH compared with placebo (+1%). The corresponding effect of 10 mg prednisone daily was a 35% reduction in the plasma cortisol response to ACTH.

The minimal inhalation lethal dose in mice was 100 mg/kg (approximately 250 times the maximum recommended human daily inhalation dose on a mcg/m^2 basis). There were no deaths following the administration of an inhalation dose of 68 mg/kg in rats (approximately 345 times the maximum recommended human daily inhalation dose on a mcg/m^2 basis). The minimal oral lethal dose was 200 mg/kg in mice and less than 100 mg/kg in rats (approximately 500 times the maximum recommended human daily inhalation dose based on a mcg/m^2 basis).

DOSAGE AND ADMINISTRATION

PULMICORT TURBUHALER should be administered by the orally inhaled route in asthmatic patients age 6 years and older. Individual patients will experience a variable onset and degree of symptom relief. Generally, PULMICORT TURBUHALER has a relatively rapid onset of action for an inhaled corticosteroid. Improvement in asthma control following inhaled administration of PULMICORT TURBUHALER can occur within 24 hours of initiation of treatment, although maximum benefit may not be achieved for 1 to 2 weeks, or longer. The safety and efficacy of PULMICORT TURBUHALER when administered in excess of recommended doses have not been established.

The recommended starting dose and the highest recommended dose of PULMICORT TURBUHALER, based on prior asthma therapy, are listed in the following table.

[See table at top of next page]

Patients Maintained on Chronic Oral Corticosteroids: Initially, PULMICORT TURBUHALER should be used concurrently with the patient's usual maintenance dose of systemic corticosteroid. After approximately one week, gradual withdrawal of the systemic corticosteroid is started by reducing the daily or alternate daily dose. The next reduction is made after an interval of one or two weeks, depending on the response of the patient. Generally, these decrements should not exceed 2.5 mg of prednisone or its equivalent. A slow rate of withdrawal is strongly recommended. During reduction of oral corticosteroids, patients should be care-

fully monitored for asthma instability, including objective measures of airway function, and for adrenal insufficiency (see WARNINGS). During withdrawal, some patients may experience symptoms of systemic corticosteroid withdrawal, e.g., joint and/or muscular pain, lassitude and depression, despite maintenance or even improvement in pulmonary function. Such patients should be encouraged to continue with PULMICORT TURBUHALER but should be monitored for objective signs of adrenal insufficiency. If evidence of adrenal insufficiency occurs, the systemic corticosteroid doses should be increased temporarily and thereafter withdrawal should continue more slowly. During periods of stress or a severe asthma attack, transfer patients may require supplementary treatment with systemic corticosteroids.

NOTE: In all patients it is desirable to titrate to the lowest effective dose once asthma stability is achieved.

Patients should be instructed to prime PULMICORT TURBUHALER prior to its initial use, and instructed to inhale deeply and forcefully each time the unit is used. Rinsing the mouth after inhalation is also recommended.

Directions for Use: Illustrated Patient's Instructions for Use accompany each package of PULMICORT TURBUHALER.

HOW SUPPLIED

PULMICORT TURBUHALER consists of a number of assembled plastic details, the main parts being the dosing mechanism, the storage unit for drug substance and the mouthpiece. The inhaler is protected by a white outer tubular cover screwed onto the inhaler. The body of the inhaler is white and the turning grip is brown. The following wording is printed on the grip in raised lettering, "Pulmicort™ 200 mcg." TURBUHALER cannot be refilled and should be discarded when empty.

PULMICORT TURBUHALER is available as 200 mcg/dose, 200 doses.

Store at controlled room temperature 20°C to 25°C (68°F to 77°F) [see USP].

PATIENT'S INSTRUCTIONS FOR USE

Please read this leaflet carefully before you start to take your medicine. It provides a summary of information on your medicine.

FOR FURTHER INFORMATION ASK YOUR DOCTOR OR PHARMACIST.

WHAT YOU SHOULD KNOW ABOUT PULMICORT TURBUHALER®

Your doctor has prescribed Pulmicort Turbuhaler 200 mcg. It contains a medication called budesonide, which is a synthetic corticosteroid. Corticosteroids are natural substances found in the body that help fight inflammation. They are used to treat asthma because they reduce the swelling and irritation in the walls of the small air passages in the lungs and ease breathing problems. When inhaled regularly, corticosteroids also help to prevent attacks of asthma.

Pulmicort Turbuhaler treats the inflammation—the "quiet part" of asthma that you cannot hear, see, or feel. When inflammation is left untreated, your asthma symptoms and attacks can increase. Pulmicort Turbuhaler works to prevent and reduce your asthma symptoms and attacks.

IMPORTANT POINTS TO REMEMBER ABOUT PULMICORT TURBUHALER

1. MAKE SURE that this medicine is suitable for you (see "BEFORE USING YOUR PULMICORT TURBUHALER" below).

2. It is important that you inhale each dose as your doctor has advised.

3. Use your Turbuhaler as directed by your doctor. **DO NOT STOP TREATMENT OR REDUCE YOUR DOSE EVEN IF YOU FEEL BETTER,** unless told to do so by your doctor.

4. DO NOT inhale more doses or use your Turbuhaler more often than instructed by your doctor.

5. This medicine is **NOT** intended to provide rapid relief of your breathing difficulties during an asthma attack. It must be taken at regular intervals as recommended by your doctor, and not as an emergency measure.

6. Your doctor may prescribe additional medication (such as bronchodilators) for emergency relief if an acute asthma attack occurs. Please contact your doctor if:

→ an asthma attack does not respond to the additional medication,

→ you require more of the additional medication than usual.

7. If you also use another medicine by inhalation, you should consult your doctor for instructions on when to use it in relation to using your Pulmicort Turbuhaler.

BEFORE USING YOUR PULMICORT TURBUHALER TELL YOUR DOCTOR BEFORE STARTING TO TAKE THIS MEDICINE:

→ if you are pregnant (or intending to become pregnant),
→ if you are breast-feeding a baby,
→ if you are allergic to budesonide or any other orally inhaled corticosteroid.

Adverse Events with ≥ 3% Incidence reported by Patients on PULMICORT TURBUHALER

Adverse Event	Placebo N=284 %	PULMICORT TURBUHALER 200 mcg twice daily N=286 %	PULMICORT TURBUHALER 400 mcg twice daily N=289 %	PULMICORT TURBUHALER 800 mcg twice daily N=98 %
Respiratory System				
Respiratory infection	17	20	24	19
Pharyngitis	9	10	9	5
Sinusitis	7	11	7	2
Voice alteration	0	1	2	6
Body As A Whole				
Headache	7	14	13	14
Flu syndrome	6	6	6	14
Pain	2	5	5	5
Back pain	1	2	3	6
Fever	2	2	4	0
Digestive System				
Oral candidiasis	2	2	4	4
Dyspepsia	2	1	2	4
Gastroenteritis	1	1	2	3
Nausea	2	2	1	3
Average Duration of Exposure (days)	59	79	80	80

	Previous Therapy	Recommended Starting Dose	Highest Recommended Dose
Adults:	Bronchodilators alone	200 to 400 mcg twice daily	400 mcg twice daily
	Inhaled Corticosteroids	200 to 400 mcg twice daily	800 mcg twice daily
	Oral Corticosteroids	400 to 800 mcg twice daily	800 mcg twice daily
Children:	Bronchodilators alone	200 mcg twice daily	400 mcg twice daily
	Inhaled Corticosteroids	200 mcg twice daily	400 mcg twice daily
	Oral Corticosteroids	The highest recommended dose in children is 400 mcg twice daily	

In some circumstances, this medicine may not be suitable and your doctor may wish to give you a different medicine. Make sure that your doctor knows what other medicines you are taking.

USING YOUR PULMICORT TURBUHALER
→ Follow the instructions shown on the other side. If you have any problems, tell your doctor or pharmacist.
→ It is important that you inhale each dose as directed by your doctor. The pharmacy label will usually tell you what dose to take and how often. If it doesn't, or you are not sure, ask your doctor or pharmacist.

DOSAGE
→ Use as directed by your doctor.
→ It is **VERY IMPORTANT** that you follow your doctor's instructions as to how many inhalations to take and how often to use your Pulmicort Turbuhaler.
→ **DO NOT** inhale more doses or use your Pulmicort Turbuhaler more often than your doctor advises.
→ It may take 1 to 2 weeks or longer before you feel maximum improvement, so **IT IS VERY IMPORTANT THAT YOU USE PULMICORT TURBUHALER REGULARLY. DO NOT STOP TREATMENT OR REDUCE YOUR DOSE EVEN IF YOU ARE FEELING BETTER,** unless told to do so by your doctor.
→ If you miss a dose, just take your regularly scheduled next dose when it is due. **DO NOT DOUBLE** the dose.

HOW TO USE YOUR PULMICORT TURBUHALER®
Read the complete instructions carefully and use only as directed.

BEFORE YOU USE A NEW PULMICORT TURBUHALER
Before you use a new Pulmicort Turbuhaler for the first time, you should prime it. To do this, turn the cover and lift off. Hold Pulmicort Turbuhaler upright (with mouthpiece up), then twist the brown grip fully to the right and back again to the left. Repeat. Now you are ready to use it. **You do not have to prime it any other time after this, even if you put it aside for a prolonged period of time.**

FOLLOW THE INSTRUCTIONS BELOW:

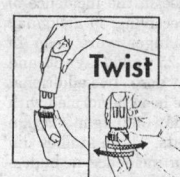

1. LOADING A DOSE
→ Twist the cover and lift off.
→ In order to provide the correct dose, Pulmicort Turbuhaler <u>must</u> be held in the

upright position (mouthpiece up) whenever a dose of medication is being loaded.
→ Twist the brown grip fully to the right as far as it will go. Twist it back again fully to the left.

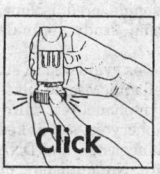

→ You will hear a click.
→ Turn your head away from the inhaler and breathe out. **Do not blow or exhale into the inhaler. Do not shake the inhaler after loading it.**

2. INHALING THE DOSE
→ When you are inhaling, Pulmicort Turbuhaler <u>must</u> be held in the upright (mouthpiece up) or horizontal position.

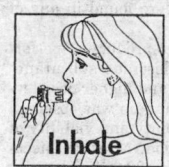

→ Place the mouthpiece between your lips and inhale deeply and forcefully.
→ If more than one dose is required, just repeat the steps above.
→ **When you are finished, place the cover back on** the inhaler and twist shut. **Rinse your mouth with water. Do not swallow.**
→ **Keep your Pulmicort Turbuhaler clean and dry at all times.**

STORING YOUR PULMICORT TURBUHALER
→ After each use, place the white cover back on and twist it firmly into place.
→ Keep Pulmicort Turbuhaler in a dry place at controlled room temperature, 68° to 77°F (20° to 25°C).

→ Keep your Pulmicort Turbuhaler out of the **reach of young children.**
→ **DO NOT** use after the date shown on the body of your Turbuhaler.

HOW TO KNOW WHEN YOUR PULMICORT TURBUHALER IS EMPTY
THERE ARE 200 DOSES IN EACH PULMICORT TURBUHALER.
Your Pulmicort Turbuhaler has a convenient dose indicator window just below the mouthpiece.

→ **When a red mark appears at the top of the window, there are 20 doses of medicine remaining.** Now is the time to get your next Pulmicort Turbuhaler.

→ **When the red mark reaches the bottom of the window, your inhaler is empty. Discard it.** (You may still hear a sound if you shake it—this sound is not the medicine. This sound is produced by the drying agent inside Turbuhaler.)
→ **Do not immerse it in water to find out if it is empty. Simply check your dose indicator window.**

FURTHER INFORMATION ABOUT PULMICORT TURBUHALER
→ Pulmicort Turbuhaler delivers your medicine as a very fine powder **that you may not taste, smell, or feel.** By following the instructions for use in this leaflet, you can be confident that you have received the correct dose.
→ Pulmicort Turbuhaler should not be used with a spacer.
→ Pulmicort Turbuhaler contains only budesonide and does not contain any inactive ingredients.
→ Pulmicort Turbuhaler is specially designed to deliver only one dose at a time, no matter how often you click the brown grip. If you accidentally blow into your inhaler after loading a dose, simply follow the instructions for loading a new dose.

This leaflet does not contain the complete information about your medicine. If you have any questions, or are not sure about something, then you should ask your doctor or pharmacist.
You may want to read this leaflet again. Please DO NOT THROW IT AWAY until you have finished your medicine.
REMEMBER: This medicine has been prescribed for you by your doctor. DO NOT give this medicine to anyone else.
USE THIS PRODUCT AS DIRECTED, UNLESS INSTRUCTED TO DO OTHERWISE BY YOUR DOCTOR.
If you have further questions about the use of
Pulmicort Turbuhaler, call:
1-800-343-4777

000641R01   Rev. 10/97
Shown in Product Identification Guide, page 304

RHINOCORT® Nasal Inhaler   ℞
(budesonide)
For Intranasal Use Only. Shake Well Before Use.

DESCRIPTION
Budesonide, the active component of Rhinocort® Nasal Inhaler, is an anti-inflammatory glucocorticosteroid. It is designated chemically as (RS)-11β,16α,17,21-Tetrahydroxypregna-1,4-diene-3,20-dione cyclic 16,17-acetal with butyraldehyde. Budesonide is provided as a mixture of two epimers (22R and 22S). The empirical formula of budesonide is $C_{25}H_{34}O_6$ and its molecular weight is 430.5. Its structural formula is:

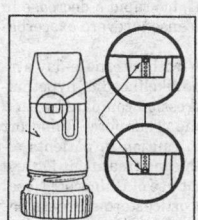

Budesonide is a white to off-white odorless powder that is practically insoluble in water and in heptane, sparingly sol-

uble in ethanol, and freely soluble in chloroform. Its partition coefficient between octanol and water at pH 7.4 is 1.6×10^3.
Rhinocort Nasal Inhaler is a metered-dose pressurized aerosol unit containing a suspension of micronized budesonide in a mixture of propellants, (dichlorodifluoromethane, trichloromonofluoromethane, and dichlorotetrafluoroethane) and sorbitan trioleate.
Each actuation releases 50 μg budesonide from the valve and delivers approximately 32 μg budesonide from the nasal adapter (dose to patient). Throughout the package insert 32 μg per actuation is used to calculate the dose administered. One canister provides at least 200 metered doses.

CLINICAL PHARMACOLOGY
Budesonide is a glucocorticosteroid having a potent glucocorticoid and weak mineralocorticoid activity. In standard *in vitro* and animal models, budesonide has an approximately 200 fold higher affinity for the glucocorticoid receptor and a 1000 fold higher topical anti-inflammatory potency than cortisol (rat croton oil ear edema assay). As a measure of systemic activity, budesonide is 40 times more potent than cortisol when administered subcutaneously and 25 times more potent when administered orally in the rat thymus involution assay.
The precise mechanism of glucocorticosteroid actions on allergic and nonallergic rhinitis is not known. Glucocorticosteroids have been shown to have a wide range of inhibitory activities against multiple cell types (e.g., mast cells, eosinophils, neutrophils, macrophages and lymphocytes) and mediators (e.g., histamine, eicosanoids, leukotrienes and cytokines) involved in allergic and nonallergic/irritant-mediated inflammation.
Corticoids affect the delayed (6 hour) response to an allergen challenge more than the histamine-associated immediate response (20 minute). The clinical significance of these findings is unknown.
Pharmacokinetics: The pharmacokinetics of budesonide have been studied following nasal, oral and intravenous administration. Pharmacokinetic studies were performed with doses higher than those used clinically because at clinical doses the resulting plasma levels are below the limits of detection.
The results are as follows:
[See table at top of next page]
Only about 20% of an intranasal dose from the Rhinocort Nasal Inhaler reaches the systemic circulation.
While budesonide is well absorbed from the GI tract, the oral bioavailability of budesonide is low (~10%) primarily due to extensive first pass metabolism in the liver. After reaching the systemic circulation, plasma levels decline in a log linear manner with an apparent elimination half-life of approximately 2 hours.
Budesonide has a volume of distibution of approximately 200 L and is 88% protein bound in the plasma. Budesonide is a mixture of two epimers, 22R and 22S. In glucocorticoid receptor affinity studies, the 22R form is two times as active as the 22S epimer. It is also preferentially cleared by the liver with an apparent systemic clearance of 1.4 +/− 0.3 L/min., vs. 1.0 +/− 0.2 L/min. for the 22S form. *In vitro* studies indicate that the two forms of budesonide do not interconvert.
Budesonide is rapidly and extensively metabolized in man by the liver. *In vitro* studies looking at sites of metabolism showed negligible metabolism in skin, lung, and serum. After intranasal administration of a radiolabeled dose, $^2/_3$ of the radioactivity was found in the urine and the remainder in the feces by 96 hours. The primary metabolites of budesonide in the urine following IV administration are 16α-hydroxyprednisolone (24%) and 6β-hydroxybudesonide (5%). An additional 34% of the radioactivity recovered in the urine were conjugates. No unchanged budesonide was found in the urine. These results regarding the metabolic fate of budesonide parallel results obtained in *in vitro* metabolic studies using human liver homogenates.
In vitro studies of the binding of the two primary metabolites to the glucocorticoid receptor indicate that they have less than 1% of the affinity for the receptor as the parent compound budesonide.
Pharmacodynamics: The effect of Rhinocort Nasal Inhaler at a dosage of two sprays in each nostril morning and evening (total daily dose of 256 μg) on hypothalamic-pituitary-adrenal (HPA) axis function has been evaluated in 275 adults and 61 children following short-term use (<2 months) and in 113 adults and 116 children following longer use (6–48 months). Early morning plasma cortisol and the short cosyntropin stimulation test (30–60 minutes) were the most commonly performed assessments of HPA function.
Twenty-four hour urinary cortisol levels were determined in 50 adults (short term) and 96 children (long term). There were no statistically significant changes from baseline measurements in early morning plasma cortisol or 24-hour urinary cortisol excretion or in response to cosyntropin.

Continued on next page

Rhinocort—Cont.

In a crossover trial using single doses of 200, 400 and 800 μg of an aqueous formulation of budesonide administered intranasally at 10 P.M., a dose-dependent decrease in urinary cortisol excretion was found between 10 P.M. and 8 A.M. the following morning. The same study has not been performed with Rhinocort Nasal Inhaler. However, in a study using the Rhinocort Nasal Inhaler administered at 10 P.M., doses four (1024 μg) and eight (2048 μg) times higher than the recommended daily dose (256 μg) were followed by a significant decrease in plasma cortisol levels at 8 A.M. the following morning (17% and 22%, respectively).
A 3 week clinical study in seasonal rhinitis, comparing Rhinocort Nasal Inhaler and orally ingested budesonide with placebo in 98 patients with allergic rhinitis due to birch pollen, demonstrated that the therapeutic effect of budesonide can be attributed to the topical effects of budesonide. Intranasally, 128 μg of budesonide applied twice daily (55 μg systemically absorbed/day) provided clinically and statistically significant evidence of efficacy, whereas 250 μg of budesonide ingested twice a day as a capsule (65 μg systemically absorbed/day) was no different from placebo in reducing nasal symptoms.

Clinical Trials: The prophylactic and therapeutic efficacy of Rhinocort Nasal Inhaler has been evaluated in 20 controlled clinical trials of seasonal or perennial rhinitis. The number of patients treated with budesonide in these studies was 50 male and 33 female patients ages 6 to 12 years old, 77 males and 62 females ages 13 to 18 years old, 185 males and 246 females ages 19 to 64 and 1 male and 2 females over 64. The patients were predominantly caucasian.
Double-blind clinical trials of two to four weeks duration have shown that, compared with placebo, Rhinocort Nasal Inhaler 128 μg b.i.d. (two sprays in each nostril morning and evening) or 256 μg q.d. (four sprays in each nostril in the morning) provides statistically significant relief of nasal symptoms such as blockage, rhinorrhea, itching, and sneezing in adults and children with seasonal allergic rhinitis or perennial allergic rhinitis. Similar improvement has also been demonstrated in adults with nonallergic perennial rhinitis.
The therapeutic effect of Rhinocort Nasal Inhaler compared with placebo has been demonstrated by rhinoscopic examinations in children and adults with seasonal or perennial allergic rhinitis and adults with nonallergic perennial rhinitis. Biopsies of the nasal mucosa of 50 adult patients after 12 months of treatment and of 10 patients after 3–5 years of therapy showed no histopathological evidence of adverse effects. The clinical significance of either of these findings is unknown.

Individualization of Dosage: It is recommended that the starting dose for all adults be 256 μg daily, as either two sprays in each nostril twice per day, morning and evening, or as four sprays in each nostril once a day in the morning. The effect should be assessed 3–7 days after initiating treatment and then periodically until the patient's symptoms are stable. If adequate relief of symptoms is not achieved after 3 weeks of treatment, then Rhinocort Nasal Inhaler should be discontinued.
In patients who do achieve a good result it is desirable, once the maximum benefit seems to have been achieved, to titrate an individual patient to the minimum effective dose. Because of the generally short duration of therapy for seasonal allergic rhinitis, it is usually not necessary to do this. In patients with perennial allergic rhinitis, once adequate relief has been obtained the dose should be gradually decreased every 2–4 weeks as long as the desired clinical effect is maintained. If symptoms return, the dose may briefly be increased to the patient's starting dose and then returned to the dose the patient was on before symptoms reoccurred.
As with other aerosolized nasal glucocorticosteroids, the vehicle used to deliver the glucocorticosteroid may cause symptoms that are difficult to distinguish from the patient's rhinitis symptoms. The corticoid may suppress symptoms caused by the vehicle at higher doses but as the dose is decreased symptoms from the vehicle may emerge. If a patient needs chronic treatment and the daily dose cannot be decreased from the starting dose, it may be advisable to try alternative therapy.

INDICATIONS AND USAGE

Rhinocort Nasal Inhaler is indicated for the management of symptoms of seasonal or perennial allergic rhinitis in adults and children and nonallergic perennial rhinitis in adults.
Rhinocort Nasal Inhaler is not recommended for treatment of nonallergic rhinitis in children because adequate numbers of such children have not been studied.

CONTRAINDICATIONS

Hypersensitivity to any of the ingredients of this preparation contraindicates its use.

WARNINGS

The replacement of a systemic glucocorticosteroid with a topical glucocorticosteroid can be accompanied by signs of adrenal insufficiency, and in addition some patients may experience symptoms of withdrawal, e.g., joint and/or muscular pain, lassitude and depression. Patients previously treated for prolonged periods with systemic glucocorticosteroids and transferred to topical glucocorticosteroids should be carefully monitored for acute adrenal insufficiency in response to stress. In those patients who have asthma or other clinical conditions requiring long-term systemic glucocorticosteroid treatment, too rapid a decrease in systemic glucocorticosteroids may cause a severe exacerbation of their symptoms.
The use of Rhinocort Nasal Inhaler with alternate-day systemic prednisone could increase the likelihood of hypothalamic-pituitary-adrenal (HPA) suppression compared with a therapeutic dose of either one alone. Therefore, Rhinocort Nasal Inhaler should be used with caution in patients already receiving alternate-day prednisone treatment for any disease. In addition, the concomitant use of Rhinocort Nasal Inhaler with other inhaled glucocorticosteroids could increase the risk of signs or symptoms of hypercorticism and/or suppression of the HPA-axis.
Patients who are on drugs which suppress the immune system are more susceptible to infections than healthy individuals. Chicken pox and measles, for example, can have a more serious or even fatal course in non-immune children or adults on immunosuppressant doses of corticosteroids. In such children or adults, who have not had these diseases, particular care should be taken to avoid exposure. How the dose, route and duration of corticosteroid administration affects the risk of developing a disseminated infection is not known. The contribution of the underlying disease and/or prior corticosteroid treatment to the risk is also not known. If exposed to chicken pox, prophylaxis with varicella zoster immune globulin (VZIG) may be indicated. If exposed to measles, prophylaxis with pooled intramuscular immunoglobulin (IG) may be indicated. (See the respective package insert for complete VZIG and IG prescribing information). If chicken pox develops, treatment with antiviral agents may be considered.

Route of Administration		Mean* [range]				
		T_{max} (hr)	C_{max}** (nmol/L)	Systemic Availability***	V_D (L)	Clearance (L/min)
Nasal Inhaler	(N=9)	0.6 [0.3–2]	0.52 [0.24–0.88]	21 [16–27]	—	—
Oral Capsule	(N=11)	1.0 [0.5–2]	0.33 [0.19–0.50]	12 [8–20]	—	—
I.V.	(N=11)	—	—	100	201 [102–275]	1.2 [0.8–1.5]

* mean of the two epimers
** dose normalized to a 256 μg dose
*** % of delivered dose

PRECAUTIONS

General: Rarely, immediate hypersensitivity reactions or contact dermatitis may occur after the intranasal administration of budesonide. Rare instances of wheezing, nasal septum perforation and increased intraocular pressure have been reported following the intranasal application of aerosolized glucocorticosteroids.
Like other glucocorticosteroids, budesonide is absorbed into the circulation. Use of excessive doses of glucocorticosteroids may lead to signs or symptoms of hypercorticism, suppression of HPA function and/or suppression of growth in children or teenagers. In short term studies of the acute effect of inhaled budesonide 256 μg/day on lower leg growth (knemometry), it like other inhaled and intramuscular corticoids which have been studied showed a decrease in the rate of lower leg growth. The clinical significance of this finding is not known. In two one-year studies in 92 children taking recommended doses of Rhinocort Nasal Inhaler, height and skeletal stature were consistent with chronological age. Physicians should closely follow the growth of children taking corticoids, by any route, and weigh the benefits of corticoid therapy against the possibility of growth suppression if a child's growth appears slowed.
Although systemic effects have been minimal with recommended doses of Rhinocort Nasal Inhaler, this potential risk increases with larger doses. Therefore, larger than recommended doses of Rhinocort Nasal Inhaler should be avoided. When used at larger doses, systemic glucocorticosteroid effects such as hypercorticism and adrenal suppression may appear. If such changes occur, the dosage of Rhinocort Nasal Inhaler should be discontinued slowly, consistent with accepted procedures for discontinuing oral glucocorticosteroid therapy.
In clinical studies with budesonide administered intranasally, the development of localized infections of the nose and pharynx with Candida albicans has occurred only rarely. When such an infection develops, it may require treatment with appropriate local therapy and discontinuation of treatment with Rhinocort Nasal Inhaler. Patients using Rhinocort Nasal Inhaler over several months or longer should be examined periodically for evidence of Candida infection or other signs of adverse effects on the nasal mucosa.
Rhinocort Nasal Inhaler should be used with caution, if at all, in patients with active or quiescent tuberculous infections, untreated fungal, bacterial, or systemic viral infections, or ocular herpes simplex.
Because of the inhibitory effect of glucocorticosteroids on wound healing, patients who have experienced recent nasal septal ulcers, nasal surgery, or nasal trauma should not use a nasal glucocorticosteroid until healing has occurred.

Information for Patients: Patients being treated with Rhinocort Nasal Inhaler should receive the following information and instructions.
Patients should use Rhinocort Nasal Inhaler as prescribed. A decrease in symptoms may occur as soon as 24 hours after starting glucocorticosteroid therapy and generally can be expected to occur within a few days of initiating therapy in allergic rhinitis. The patient should contact the physician if symptoms do not improve by three weeks, or if the condition worsens. Nasal irritation and/or burning after use of the spray occur only rarely with this product. The patient should contact the physician if they occur repeatedly.
Patients who are on corticosteroids should be warned to avoid exposure to chicken pox or measles. Patients should also be advised that if they are exposed, they should consult their physician without delay.
For the proper use of this unit and to attain maximum improvement, the patient should read and follow the accompanying patient instructions carefully.

Carcinogenesis, Mutagenesis, Impairment of Fertility: Long-term studies were conducted in mice and rats using oral administration to evaluate the carcinogenic potential of budesonide.
There was no evidence of a carcinogenic effect when budesonide was administered orally for 91 weeks to mice at doses up to 200 μg/kg/day (600 μg/m^2/day).
In a 104-week carcinogenicity study in Sprague-Dawley rats (41), a statistically significant increase in the incidence of gliomas was observed in male rats receiving 50 μg/kg/day (300 μg/m^2/day) orally; no such changes were seen in male rats receiving doses of 10 and 25 μg/kg/day (60 and 150 μg/m^2/day) or in female rats at any dose. Two additional 104-week carcinogenicity studies have been performed with oral budesonide at doses of 50 μg/kg/day (300 μg/m^2/day) in male Sprague-Dawley and Fischer rats. These studies did not demonstrate an increased glioma incidence in budesonide treated animals as compared with concurrent controls or reference glucocorticosteroid treated groups (prednisolone and triamcinolone acetonide).
Compared with concurrent control male Sprague-Dawley rats there was a statistically significant increase in the incidence of hepatocellular tumors. This finding was confirmed in all three steroid groups (budesonide, prednisolone, triamcinolone acetonide) in the second study in male Sprague-Dawley rats.
The mutagenic potential of budesonide was evaluated in six different test systems; Ames Salmonella/microsome plate test, mouse micronucleus test, mouse lymphoma test, chromosome aberration test in human lymphocytes, sex-linked recessive lethal test in Drosophila melanogaster, and DNA repair analysis in rat hepatocyte culture. No mutagenic or clastogenic properties of budesonide were found in any of the tests.
The effect upon fertility and general reproductive performance was studied in rats given budesonide subcutaneously. At 20 μg/kg/day (120 μg/m^2/day) and higher dose levels, a decrease in maternal body-weight gain was observed along with a decrease in prenatal viability and viability of the young at birth and during lactation. No such effects were noted at the dose level 5 μg/kg/day (30 μg/m^2/day).

Pregnancy: Teratogenic Effects: Pregnancy Category C: As with other glucocorticoids budesonide has been shown to be teratogenic and embryocidal in rabbits and rats when given subcutaneously in doses exceeding 5 and 100 μg/kg/day (59 and 600 μg/m^2/day), respectively. In these studies budesonide at 25 μg/kg/day (295 μg/m^2/day) given to rabbits and 500 μg/kg/day (3000 μg/m^2/day) given to rats was found to produce fetal loss, decreased pup weights and skeletal abnormalities. No teratogenic or embryocidal effects have been seen in rats when budesonide was administered by inhalation at doses of 100–250 μg/kg/day (600–1500 μg/m^2/day, approximately 27–68 times the human recommended starting dose based on μg/kg/day or 4–10 times the human dose based on μg/m^2/day).

There are no adequate and well-controlled studies in pregnant women. Budesonide should be used during pregnancy only if the potential benefit justifies the potential risk to the fetus. Experience with oral glucocorticosteroids since their introduction in pharmacologic, as opposed to physiologic, doses suggests that rodents are more prone to teratogenic effects from glucocorticosteroids than humans. In addition, because there is a natural increase in glucocorticosteroid production during pregnancy, most women will require a lower exogenous glucocorticosteroid dose and many will not need glucocorticosteroid treatment during pregnancy.

Nonteratogenic Effects: Hypoadrenalism may occur in infants born of mothers receiving glucocorticosteroids during pregnancy. Such infants should be carefully observed.

Nursing Mothers: It is not known whether budesonide is excreted in human milk. Because other glucocorticosteroids are excreted in human milk, caution should be exercised when Rhinocort Nasal Inhaler is administered to nursing women.

Pediatric Use: Safety and effectiveness in children below 6 years of age have not been established. Oral glucocorticosteroids have been shown to cause growth suppression in children and teenagers with extended use. If a child or teenager on any glucocorticosteroid appears to have growth suppression, the possibility that they are particularly sensitive to this effect of glucocorticosteroids should be considered (see PRECAUTIONS).

ADVERSE REACTIONS

Adverse reaction information is derived from blinded-controlled clinical trials (see Clinical Trials), open label studies and marketing experience. In the description below, rates of rare events are derived principally from marketing experience and publications, and accurate estimates of incidence are not possible.

The incidence of common adverse reactions is based upon controlled clinical trials in 606 patients [101 girls and 145 boys (<19 years of age) and 203 female and 157 male adults] treated with Rhinocort Nasal Inhaler 128 μg twice daily over 2–4 weeks. The most common adverse reactions were symptoms of irritation of the nasal mucous membranes. All common adverse reactions were reported with approximately the same frequency by placebo patients suggesting the possibility that the vehicle or the rhinitis itself was responsible for the symptoms. Sneezing after use of the inhaler occurred in 2% of Rhinocort treated patients and in 11% of patients using the placebo.

Systemic glucocorticosteroid side-effects were not reported during controlled clinical studies with Rhinocort Nasal Inhaler. If recommended doses are exceeded, however, or if individuals are particularly sensitive, symptoms of hypercorticism, i.e., Cushing's syndrome, could occur.

Incidence Greater than 1% (Based on controlled clinical trials):

Respiratory: nasal irritation*, pharyngitis*, cough increased*, epistaxis*.

Digestive: dry mouth, dyspepsia.

*incidence 3 to 9%; incidence of unmarked reactions 1 to 3%.

Incidence Less than 1% (Based on controlled clinical trials):

Respiratory: dyspnea, moniliasis, hoarseness, wheezing, nasal pain.

Special Senses: reduced sense of smell, bad taste.

Digestive: nausea.

Skin and Appendages: facial edema, rash, pruritus, herpes simplex.

Nervous System: nervousness.

Musculoskeletal: myalgia, arthralgia.

Adverse Event Reports from Other Sources: Rare adverse events reports in the published literature or from marketing experience include: immediate and delayed hypersensitivity reactions including rash, contact dermatitis, urticaria, angioedema, and bronchospasm; nasal septal disorders including atrophy, necrosis and/or perforation; symptoms of hypocorticism and hypercorticism; alopecia; psychiatric symptoms including depression, aggressive reactions, irritability, anxiety and psychosis.

OVERDOSAGE

Acute overdosage with this dosage form is unlikely since one canister of Rhinocort Nasal Inhaler only contains approximately 12.7 mg of budesonide. Chronic overdosage may result in signs/symptoms of hyerpcorticism (see WARNINGS and PRECAUTIONS).

DOSAGE AND ADMINISTRATION

Adults and children 6 years of age and older: The recommended starting dose is 256 μg daily, given as either two sprays in each nostril morning and evening or as four sprays in each nostril in the morning.

A decrease in symptoms may occur as soon as 24 hours after onset of treatment with Rhinocort Nasal Inhaler but generally it takes 3–7 days to reach maximum benefit.

If no improvement has been obtained by the third week of treatment with Rhinocort Nasal Inhaler, treatment should be discontinued.

After the desired clinical effect has been obtained, the maintenance dose should be reduced to the smallest amount necessary for control of symptoms (see Individualization of Dosage, CLINICAL PHARMACOLOGY section).

If glucocorticosteroids are discontinued when they still are needed, symptoms may not recur for several days.

At recommended doses, Rhinocort's therapeutic effects are localized to the nose, therefore, concomitant treatment may be necessary to counteract allergic eye symptoms. Doses exceeding 256 μg daily (4 sprays/nostril) are not recommended. Rhinocort Nasal Inhaler is not recommended for children below 6 years of age or for children with nonallergic perennial rhinitis because adequate numbers of these children have not been studied.

Directions for Use: Illustrated Patient's Instructions for Use accompany each package of Rhinocort Nasal Inhaler.

HOW SUPPLIED

Rhinocort Nasal Inhaler is supplied in a 7.0 g canister containing 200 metered doses provided with a metering valve and nasal adapter together with Patient's Instructions for Use. Each actuation delivers approximately 32 μg of micronized budesonide from the nasal adapter to the patient.

Caution: Federal (USA) law prohibits dispensing without prescription.

Rhinocort Nasal Inhaler should be stored between 15°C (59°F) and 30°C (86°F) with the valve up. Shake well before use.

Each inhaler with actuator is packaged in an aluminum foil pouch to protect the product from moisture. After opening the aluminum pouch, the product should be used within 6 months and storage in an area of high humidity should be avoided.

Contents under pressure. Do not puncture. Do not use or store near heat or open flame. Exposure to temperatures above 50°C (120°F) may cause the canister to explode. Never throw the container into fire or an incinerator. Keep out of reach of children.

Note: The indented statement below is required by the Federal government's Clean Air Act for all products containing or manufactured with chlorofluorocarbons (CFCs).

> **WARNING:** Contains trichloromonofluoromethane, dichlorotetrafluoroethane, and dichlorodifluoromethane, substances which harm public health and environment by destroying ozone in the upper atmosphere.

A notice similar to the above WARNING has been placed in the patient information leaflet of this product pursuant to EPA regulations.

Patient's Instructions For Use

Use a pair of scissors to cut the pouch open. Read the information before using Rhinocort Nasal Inhaler.
Follow the directions carefully.

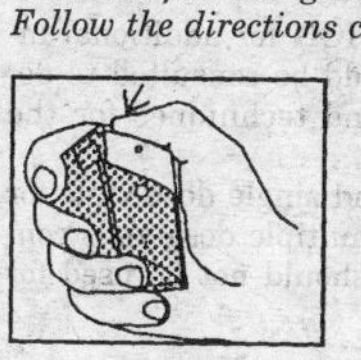

1. Blow your nose. Open the nasal inhaler by pressing on the arrow and rotating until it clicks into the locked position. Shake the canister thoroughly before using.

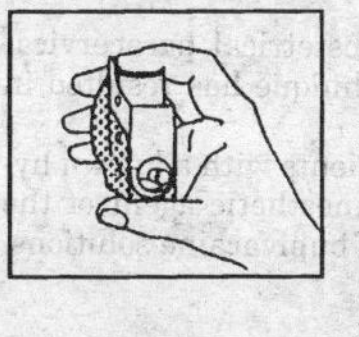

2. Place your thumb on the bottom of the unit (on the grid) while placing your index finger on the top of the canister. Wrap your fingers securely around the back. Press straight down on the canister to deliver a dose. Spray into the air 4 times before using for the first time.

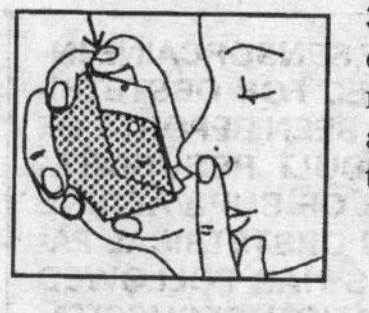

3. Close one nostril and insert the end of the inhaler tube into the other nostril. Hold your breath and deliver a dose. For optimum results, shake the canister between sprays.

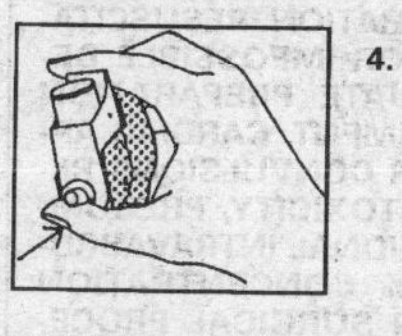

4. Rotate the unit closed for storage.

5. If Rhinocort is unused for 8 weeks, spray into the air 4 times before reuse.

WARNING: Contains trichloromonofluoromethane, dichlorotetrafluoroethane, and dichlorodifluoromethane, substances which harm the environment by destroying ozone in the upper atmosphere. Your physician has determined that this product is likely to help your personal health. USE THIS PRODUCT AS DIRECTED, UNLESS INSTRUCTED TO DO OTHERWISE BY YOUR PHYSICIAN. If you have any questions about alternatives, consult with your physician.

N.B.

Follow your doctor's directions and do not use Rhinocort Nasal Inhaler more often than prescribed. Contact your doctor if you find the effect strongly reduced.

Rhinocort Nasal Inhaler does not give immediate relief. Generally it will take a few days to achieve full effect. It is therefore very important that Rhinocort is used regularly.

Rhinocort Nasal Inhaler should be used within 6 months after the aluminum pouch has been opened. After opening the pouch, avoid storage in areas of high humidity.

Cleaning: Remove the aerosol container and wash the plastic parts regularly in warm-not hot-water with addition of mild detergent if necessary. Allow the plastic parts to dry completely and then replace the container.

Contents under pressure. Do not puncture or throw container into incinerator. Using or storing near open flame or heating above 120°F (50°C) may cause container to burst.

Manufactured for: Astra USA, Inc., Westborough, MA 01581

001053R03 Rev. 5/98

Shown in Product Identification Guide, page 304

SENSORCAINE® ℞

[*sén-sor-caine*]

(bupivacaine HCl Injection, USP)

SENSORCAINE®–MPF

(bupivacaine HCl Injection, USP)

SENSORCAINE® with Epinephrine

(bupivacaine HCl and epinephrine Injection, USP)

1:200,000 (as bitartrate)

SENSORCAINE®–MPF with Epinephrine

(bupivacaine HCl and epinephrine Injection, USP)

1:200,000 (as bitartrate)

DESCRIPTION

Sensorcaine® (bupivacaine HCl) injections are sterile isotonic solutions that contain a local anesthetic agent with and without epinephrine (as bitartrate) 1:200,000 and are administered parenterally by injection. See INDICATIONS AND USAGE for specific uses. Solutions of bupivacaine HCl may be autoclaved if they do not contain epinephrine.

Sensorcaine® injections contain bupivacaine HCl which is chemically designated as 2-piperidinecarboxamide, 1-butyl-N-(2,6-dimethylphenyl)-, monohydrochloride, monohydrate and has the following structure:

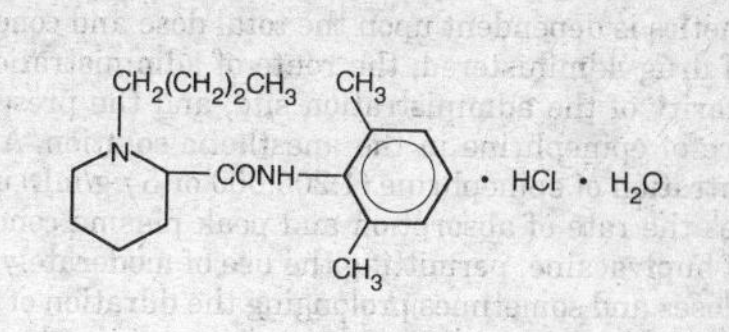

Epinephrine is (-)-3,4-Dihydroxy-α [(methylamino)methyl] benzyl alcohol. It has the following structural formula:

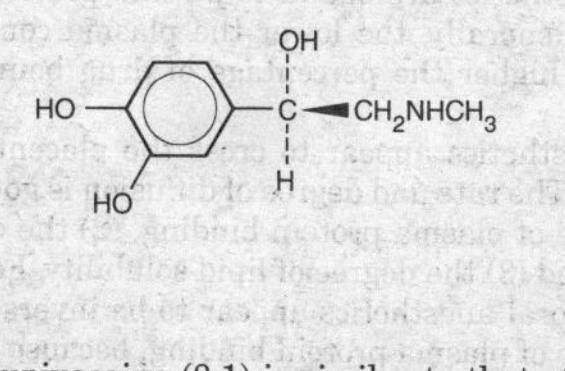

The pK_a of bupivacaine (8.1) is similar to that of lidocaine (7.86). However, bupivacaine possesses a greater degree of lipid solubility and is protein bound to a greater extent than lidocaine.

Bupivacaine is related chemically and pharmacologically to the aminoacyl local anesthetics. It is a homologue of mepivacaine and is chemically related to lidocaine. All three of these anesthetics contain an amide linkage between the aromatic nucleus and the amino or piperidine group. They differ in this respect from the procaine-type local anesthetics, which have an ester linkage.

Dosage forms listed as Sensorcaine-MPF indicates single dose solutions that are Methyl Paraben Free (MPF).

Sensorcaine-MPF is a sterile isotonic solution containing sodium chloride. Sensorcaine in multiple dose vials, each mL

Continued on next page

Sensorcaine/Sensorcaine-MPF—Cont

also contains 1 mg methylparaben as antiseptic preservative. The pH of these solutions is adjusted to between 4.0 and 6.5 with sodium hydroxide and/or hydrochloric acid. Sensorcaine-MPF with Epinephrine 1:200,000 (as bitartrate) is a sterile isotonic solution containing sodium chloride. Each mL contains bupivacaine hydrochloride and 0.005 mg epinephrine, with 0.5 mg sodium metabisulfite as an antioxidant and 0.2 mg citric acid (anhydrous) as stabilizer. Sensorcaine with Epinephrine 1:200,000 (as bitartrate) in multiple dose vials, each mL also contains 1 mg methylparaben as antiseptic preservative. The pH of these solutions is adjusted to between 3.3 to 5.5 with sodium hydroxide and/or hydrochloric acid. Filled under nitrogen.

Note: The user should have an appreciation and awareness of the formulations and their intended uses. (See DOSAGE AND ADMINISTRATION.)

CLINICAL PHARMACOLOGY

Local anesthetics block the generation and the conduction of nerve impulses, presumably by increasing the threshold for electrical excitation in the nerve, by slowing the propagation of the nerve impulse, and by reducing the rate of rise of the action potential. In general, the progression of anesthesia is related to the diameter, myelination and conduction velocity of affected nerve fibers. Clinically, the order of loss of nerve function is as follows: (1) pain, (2) temperature, (3) touch, (4) proprioception, and (5) skeletal muscle tone.

Systemic absorption of local anesthetics produces effects on the cardiovascular and central nervous systems. At blood concentrations achieved with therapeutic doses, changes in cardiac conduction, excitability, refractoriness, contractility, and peripheral vascular resistance are minimal. However, toxic blood concentrations depress cardiac conduction and excitability, which may lead to atrioventricular block, ventricular arrhythmias and to cardiac arrest, sometimes resulting in fatalities. In addition, myocardial contractility is depressed and peripheral vasodilation occurs, leading to decreased cardiac output and arterial blood pressure. Recent clinical reports and animal research suggest that these cardiovascular changes are more likely to occur after unintended intravascular injection of bupivacaine. Therefore, incremental dosing is necessary.

Following systemic absorption, local anesthetics can produce central nervous system stimulation, depression or both. Apparent central stimulation is usually manifested as restlessness, tremors and shivering, progressing to convulsions, followed by depression and coma, progressing ultimately to respiratory arrest. However, the local anesthetics have a primary depressant effect on the medulla and on higher centers. The depressed stage may occur without a prior excited stage.

Pharmacokinetics: The rate of systemic absorption of local anesthetics is dependent upon the total dose and concentration of drug administered, the route of administration, the vascularity of the administration site, and the presence or absence of epinephrine in the anesthetic solution. A dilute concentration of epinephrine (1:200,000 or 5 µg/mL) usually reduces the rate of absorption and peak plasma concentration of bupivacaine, permitting the use of moderately larger total doses and sometimes prolonging the duration of action. The onset of action with bupivacaine is rapid and anesthesia is long-lasting. The duration of anesthesia is significantly longer with bupivacaine than with any other commonly used local anesthetic. It has also been noted that there is a period of analgesia that persists after the return of sensation, during which time the need for potent analgesics is reduced.

Local anesthetics are bound to plasma proteins in varying degrees. Generally, the lower the plasma concentration of drug, the higher the percentage of drug bound to plasma proteins.

Local anesthetics appear to cross the placenta by passive diffusion. The rate and degree of diffusion is governed by: (1) the degree of plasma protein binding, (2) the degree of ionization, and (3) the degree of lipid solubility. Fetal/maternal ratios of local anesthetics appear to be inversely related to the degree of plasma protein binding, because only the free, unbound drug is available for placental transfer. Bupivacaine, with a high protein binding capacity (95%), has a low fetal/maternal ratio (0.2–0.4). The extent of placental transfer is also determined by the degree of ionization and lipid solubility of the drug. Lipid soluble, nonionized drugs readily enter the fetal blood from the maternal circulation. Depending upon the route of administration, local anesthetics are distributed to some extent to all body tissues, with high concentrations found in highly perfused organs such as the liver, lungs, heart, and brain.

Pharmacokinetic studies on the plasma profile of bupivacaine after direct intravenous injection suggest a three-compartment open model. The first compartment is represented by the rapid intravascular distribution of the drug. The second compartment represents the equilibration of the drug throughout the highly perfused organs such as the brain, myocardium, lungs, kidneys, and liver. The third compartment represents an equilibration of the drug with poorly perfused tissues, such as muscle and fat. The elimination of drug from tissue depends largely upon the ability of binding sites in the circulation to carry it to the liver where it is metabolized.

After injection of Sensorcaine for caudal, epidural or peripheral nerve block in man, peak levels of bupivacaine in the blood are reached in 30 to 45 minutes, followed by a decline to insignificant levels during the next 3 to 6 hours.

Various pharmacokinetic parameters of the local anesthetics can be significantly altered by the presence of hepatic or renal disease, addition of epinephrine, factors affecting urinary pH, renal blood flow, the route of drug administration, and the age of the patient. The half-life of bupivacaine in adults is 3.5 ± 2.0 hours and in neonates 8.1 hours.

Amide-type local anesthetics such as bupivacaine are metabolized primarily in the liver via conjugation with glucuronic acid.

Patients with hepatic disease, especially those with severe hepatic disease, may be more susceptible to the potential toxicities of the amide-type local anesthetics. The major metabolite of bupivacaine is 2,6-pipecoloxylidine.

The kidney is the main excretory organ for most local anesthetics and their metabolites. Urinary excretion is affected by renal perfusion and factors affecting urinary pH. Only 5% of bupivacaine is excreted unchanged in the urine.

When administered in recommended doses and concentrations, Sensorcaine does not ordinarily produce irritation or tissue damage and does not cause methemoglobinemia.

INDICATIONS AND USAGE

Sensorcaine is indicated for the production of local or regional anesthesia or analgesia for surgery, for oral surgery procedures, for diagnostic and therapeutic procedures, and for obstetrical procedures. Only the 0.25% and 0.5% concentrations are indicated for obstetrical anesthesia. (See WARNINGS.)

Experience with non-obstetrical surgical procedures in pregnant patients is not sufficient to recommend use of the 0.75% concentration in these patients. Sensorcaine is not recommended for intravenous regional anesthesia (Bier Block). (See WARNINGS.)

The routes of administration and indicated Sensorcaine concentrations are:

local infiltration	0.25%
peripheral nerve block	0.25%, 0.5%
retrobulbar block	0.75%
sympathetic block	0.25%
lumbar epidural	0.25%, 0.5% and 0.75% (non-obstetrical)
caudal	0.25%, 0.5%

epidural test dose (see PRECAUTIONS)
(See DOSAGE AND ADMINISTRATION for additional information.) Standard textbooks should be consulted to determine the accepted procedures and techniques for the administration of Sensorcaine.

Use only the single dose ampules and single dose vials for caudal or epidural anesthesia; the multiple dose vials contain a preservative and, therefore, should not be used for these procedures.

CONTRAINDICATIONS

Sensorcaine is contraindicated in obstetrical paracervical block anesthesia. Its use by this technique has resulted in fetal bradycardia and death.

Sensorcaine is contraindicated in patients with a known hypersensitivity to it or to any local anesthetic agent of the amide type or to other components of bupivacaine solutions.

WARNINGS

THE 0.75% CONCENTRATION OF SENSORCAINE INJECTION IS NOT RECOMMENDED FOR OBSTETRICAL ANESTHESIA. THERE HAVE BEEN REPORTS OF CARDIAC ARREST WITH DIFFICULT RESUSCITATION OR DEATH DURING USE OF BUPIVACAINE FOR EPIDURAL ANESTHESIA IN OBSTETRICAL PATIENTS. IN MOST CASES, THIS HAS FOLLOWED USE OF THE 0.75% CONCENTRATION. RESUSCITATION HAS BEEN DIFFICULT OR IMPOSSIBLE DESPITE APPARENTLY ADEQUATE PREPARATION AND APPROPRIATE MANAGEMENT. CARDIAC ARREST HAS OCCURRED AFTER CONVULSIONS RESULTING FROM SYSTEMIC TOXICITY, PRESUMABLY FOLLOWING UNINTENTIONAL INTRAVASCULAR INJECTION. THE 0.75% CONCENTRATION SHOULD BE RESERVED FOR SURGICAL PROCEDURES WHERE A HIGH DEGREE OF MUSCLE RELAXATION AND PROLONGED EFFECT ARE NECESSARY.

LOCAL ANESTHETICS SHOULD ONLY BE EMPLOYED BY CLINICIANS WHO ARE WELL VERSED IN DIAGNOSIS AND MANAGEMENT OF DOSE-RELATED TOXICITY AND OTHER ACUTE EMERGENCIES WHICH MIGHT ARISE FROM THE BLOCK TO BE EMPLOYED, AND THEN ONLY AFTER INSURING THE *IMMEDIATE* AVAILABILITY OF OXYGEN, OTHER RESUSCITATIVE DRUGS, CARDIOPULMONARY RESUSCITATIVE EQUIPMENT, AND THE PERSONNEL RESOURCES NEEDED FOR PROPER MANAGEMENT OF TOXIC REACTIONS AND RELATED EMERGENCIES. (See also ADVERSE REACTIONS, PRECAUTIONS, and OVERDOSAGE.) DELAY IN PROPER MANAGEMENT OF DOSE-RELATED TOXICITY, UNDERVENTILATION FROM ANY CAUSE AND /OR ALTERED SENSITIVITY MAY LEAD TO THE DEVELOPMENT OF ACIDOSIS, CARDIAC ARREST AND, POSSIBLY, DEATH. Local anesthetic solutions containing antimicrobial preservatives, i.e., those supplied in multiple dose vials, should not be used for epidural or caudal anesthesia because safety has not been established with regard to intrathecal injection, either intentional or unintentional, of such preservatives.

It is essential that aspiration for blood or cerebrospinal fluid (where applicable) be done prior to injecting any local anesthetic, both the original dose and all subsequent doses, to avoid intravascular or subarachnoid injection. However, a negative aspiration does *not* ensure against an intravascular or subarachnoid injection.

Bupivacaine and Epinephrine Injection or other vasopressors should not be used concomitantly with ergot-type oxytocic drugs, because a severe persistent hypertension may occur. Likewise, solutions of bupivacaine containing a vasoconstrictor, such as epinephrine, should be used with extreme caution in patients receiving monoamine oxidase (MAO) inhibitors or antidepressants of the triptyline or imipramine types, because severe prolonged hypertension may result.

Until further experience is gained in children younger than 12 years, administration of bupivacaine in this age group is not recommended.

Reports of cardiac arrest and death have occurred with the use of bupivacaine for intravenous regional anesthesia (Bier Block). Information on safe dosages or techniques of administration of this product are lacking; therefore, bupivacaine is not recommended for use by this technique.

Prior use of chloroprocaine may interfere with subsequent use of bupivacaine. Because of this, and because safety of intercurrent use of bupivacaine and chloroprocaine has not been established, such use is not recommended.

Sensorcaine with epinephrine solutions contain sodium metabisulfite, a sulfite that may cause allergic-type reactions including anaphylactic symptoms and life-threatening or less severe asthmatic episodes in certain susceptible people. The overall prevalence of sulfite sensitivity in the general population is unknown and probably low. Sulfite sensitivity is seen more frequently in asthmatic than in non-asthmatic people.

PRECAUTIONS

General: The safety and effectiveness of local anesthetics depend on proper dosage, correct technique, adequate precautions and readiness for emergencies. Resuscitative equipment, oxygen, and other resuscitative drugs should be available for immediate use. (See WARNINGS, ADVERSE REACTIONS, and OVERDOSAGE.) During major regional nerve blocks, the patient should have I.V. fluids running via an indwelling catheter to assure a functioning intravenous pathway. The lowest dosage of local anesthetic that results in effective anesthesia should be used to avoid high plasma levels and serious adverse effects. The rapid injection of a large volume of local anesthetic solution should be avoided and fractional (incremental) doses should be used when feasible.

Epidural Anesthesia: During epidural administration of bupivacaine, concentrated solutions (0.5–0.75%) should be administered in incremental doses of 3 to 5 mL with sufficient time between doses to detect toxic manifestations of unintentional intravascular or intrathecal injection. Syringe aspirations should also be performed before and during each supplemental injection in continuous (intermittent) catheter techniques. An intravascular injection is still possible even if aspirations for blood are negative.

During the administration of epidural anesthesia, it is recommended that a test dose be administered initially and the effects monitored before the full dose is given. When using a "continuous" catheter technique, test doses should be given prior to both the original and all reinforcing doses, because plastic tubing in the epidural space can migrate into a blood vessel or through the dura. When clinical conditions permit, the test dose should contain epinephrine (10 to 15 µg have been suggested) to serve as a warning of unintentional intravascular injection. If injected into a blood vessel, this amount of epinephrine is likely to produce a transient "epinephrine response" within 45 seconds, consisting of an increase in heart rate and systolic blood pressure, circumoral pallor, palpitations and nervousness in the unsedated patient. The sedated patient may exhibit only a pulse rate increase of 20 or more beats per minute for 15 or more seconds. Therefore, following the test dose, the heart rate should be monitored for a heart rate increase. Patients on beta-blockers may not manifest changes in heart rate, but blood pressure monitoring can detect an evanescent rise in systolic blood pressure. The test dose should also contain 10

to 15 mg of Sensorcaine or an equivalent dose of a short-acting amide anesthetic such as 30 to 40 mg of lidocaine, to detect an unintentional intrathecal administration. This will be manifested within a few minutes by signs of spinal block (e.g., decreased sensation of the buttocks, paresis of the legs, or, in the sedated patient, absent knee jerk). An intravascular or subarachnoid injection is still possible even if results of the test dose are negative. The test dose itself may produce a systemic toxic reaction, high spinal or epinephrine-induced cardiovascular effects.

Injection of repeated doses of local anesthetics may cause significant increases in plasma levels with each repeated dose due to slow accumulation of the drug or its metabolites or to slow metabolic degradation. Tolerance to elevated blood levels varies with the physical condition of the patient. Debilitated, elderly patients, acutely ill patients and children should be given reduced doses commensurate with their age and physical condition. Local anesthetics should also be used with caution in patients with hypotension or heart block.

Careful and constant monitoring of cardiovascular and respiratory vital signs (adequacy of ventilation) and the patient's state of consciousness should be performed after each local anesthetic injection. It should be kept in mind at such times that restlessness, anxiety, incoherent speech, light-headedness, numbness and tingling of the mouth and lips, metallic taste, tinnitus, dizziness, blurred vision, tremors, twitching, depression, or drowsiness may be early warning signs of central nervous system toxicity.

Local anesthetic solutions containing a vasoconstrictor should be used cautiously and in carefully restricted quantities in areas of the body supplied by end arteries or having otherwise compromised blood supply such as digits, nose, external ear, penis, etc. Patients with hypertensive vascular disease may exhibit exaggerated vasoconstrictor response. Ischemic injury or necrosis may result.

Because amide-type local anesthetics such as bupivacaine are metabolized by the liver, these drugs, especially repeat doses, should be used cautiously in patients with hepatic disease. Patients with severe hepatic disease, because of their inability to metabolize local anesthetics normally, are at a greater risk of developing toxic plasma concentrations. Local anesthetics should also be used with caution in patients with impaired cardiovascular function because they may be less able to compensate for functional changes associated with the prolongation of A-V conduction produced by these drugs.

Serious dose-related cardiac arrhythmias may occur if preparations containing a vasoconstrictor such as epinephrine are employed in patients during or following the administration of potent inhalation anesthetics. In deciding whether to use these products concurrently in the same patient, the combined action of both agents upon the myocardium, the concentration and volume of vasoconstrictor used, and the time since injection, when applicable, should be taken into account.

Many drugs used during the conduct of anesthesia are considered potential triggering agents for familial malignant hyperthermia. Because it is not known whether amide-type local anesthetics may trigger this reaction and because the need for supplemental general anesthesia cannot be predicted in advance, it is suggested that a standard protocol for management should be available. Early unexplained signs of tachycardia, tachypnea, labile blood pressure and metabolic acidosis may precede temperature elevation. Successful outcome is dependent on early diagnosis, prompt discontinuance of the suspect triggering agent(s) and prompt treatment, including oxygen therapy, dantrolene (consult dantrolene sodium intravenous package insert before using) and other supportive measures.

Use in Head and Neck Area: Small doses of local anesthetics injected into the head and neck area, including retrobulbar, dental and stellate ganglion blocks, may produce adverse reactions similar to systemic toxicity seen with unintentional intravascular injections of larger doses. The injection procedures require the utmost care. Confusion, convulsions, respiratory depression and/or respiratory arrest, and cardiovascular stimulation or depression have been reported. These reactions may be due to intraarterial injection of the local anesthetic with retrograde flow to the cerebral circulation. They also may be due to puncture of the dural sheath of the optic nerve during retrobulbar block with diffusion of any local anesthetic along the subdural space to the midbrain. Patients receiving these blocks should have their circulation and respiration monitored and be constantly observed. Resuscitative equipment and personnel for treating adverse reactions should be immediately available. Dosage recommendations should not be exceeded (See DOSAGE AND ADMINISTRATION).

Use in Ophthalmic Surgery: Clinicians who perform retrobulbar blocks should be aware that there have been reports of respiratory arrest following local anesthetic injection. Prior to retrobulbar block, as with all other regional procedures, the immediate availability of equipment, drugs, and personnel to manage respiratory arrest or depression, convulsions, and cardiac stimulation or depression should be

assured (see also WARNINGS and *Use in Head and Neck Area*, above). As with other anesthetic procedures, patients should be constantly monitored following ophthalmic blocks for signs of these adverse reactions, which may occur following relatively low total doses. A concentration of 0.75% bupivacaine is indicated for retrobulbar block; however, this concentration is not indicated for any other peripheral nerve block, including the facial nerve and not indicated for local infiltration, including the conjunctiva (see INDICATIONS and PRECAUTIONS, *General*). Mixing Sensorcaine (bupivacaine HCl) with other local anesthetics is not recommended because of insufficient data on the clinical use of such mixtures.

When Sensorcaine 0.75% is used for retrobulbar block, complete corneal anesthesia usually precedes onset of clinically acceptable external ocular muscle akinesia. Therefore, presence of akinesia rather than anesthesia alone should determine readiness of the patient for surgery.

Information for Patients: When appropriate, patients should be informed in advance that they may experience temporary loss of sensation and motor activity, usually in the lower half of the body following proper administration of caudal or lumbar epidural anesthesia. Also, when appropriate, the physician should discuss other information including adverse reactions in the Sensorcaine package insert.

Clinically Significant Drug Interactions: The administration of local anesthetic solutions containing epinephrine or norepinephrine to patients receiving monoamine oxidase inhibitors or tricyclic antidepressants may produce severe, prolonged hypertension. Concurrent use of these agents should generally be avoided. In situations in which concurrent therapy is necessary, careful patient monitoring is essential.

Concurrent administration of vasopressor drugs and of ergot-type oxytocic drugs may cause severe, persistent hypertension or cerebrovascular accidents.

Phenothiazines and butyrophenones may reduce or reverse the pressor effect of epinephrine.

Carcinogenesis, Mutagenesis, and Impairment of Fertility: Long-term studies in animals of most local anesthetics, including bupivacaine, to evaluate the carcinogenic potential have not been conducted. Mutagenic potential or the effect on fertility has not been determined. There is no evidence from human data that bupivacaine may be carcinogenic or mutagenic or that it impairs fertility.

Pregnancy Category C: Decreased pup survival in rats and embryocidal effect in rabbits have been observed when bupivacaine HCl was administered to these species in doses comparable to nine and five times, respectively, the maximum recommended daily human dose (400 mg). There are no adequate and well-controlled studies in pregnant women of the effect of bupivacaine on the developing fetus. Sensorcaine should be used during pregnancy only if the potential benefit justifies the potential risk to the fetus. This does not exclude the use of Sensorcaine (0.25% and 0.5% concentrations) at term for obstetrical anesthesia or analgesia. (See *Labor and Delivery*.)

Labor and Delivery: See Box WARNINGS regarding obstetrical use in 0.75% concentration.

Sensorcaine is contraindicated in obstetrical paracervical block anesthesia.

Local anesthetics rapidly cross the placenta, and when used for epidural, caudal or pudendal block anesthesia, can cause varying degrees of maternal, fetal and neonatal toxicity. (See *Pharmacokinetics* in CLINICAL PHARMACOLOGY.) The incidence and degree of toxicity depend upon the procedure performed, the type and amount of drug used, and the technique of drug administration. Adverse reactions in the parturient, fetus and neonate involve alterations of the central nervous system, peripheral vascular tone and cardiac function.

Maternal hypotension has resulted from regional anesthesia. Local anesthetics produce vasodilation by blocking sympathetic nerves. Elevating the patient's legs and positioning her on her left side will help prevent decreases in blood pressure. The fetal heart rate also should be monitored continuously, and electronic fetal monitoring is highly advisable.

Epidural, caudal, or pudendal anesthesia may alter the forces of parturition through changes in uterine contractility or maternal expulsive efforts. Epidural anesthesia has been reported to prolong the second stage of labor by removing the parturient's reflex urge to bear down or by interfering with motor function. The use of obstetrical anesthesia may increase the need for forceps assistance.

The use of some local anesthetic drug products during labor and delivery may be followed by diminished muscle strength and tone for the first day or two of life. This has not been reported with Sensorcaine.

It is extremely important to avoid aortocaval compression by the gravid uterus during administration of regional block to parturients. To do this, the patient must be maintained in the left lateral decubitus position or a blanket roll or sandbag may be placed beneath the right hip and the gravid uterus displaced to the left.

Nursing Mothers: It is not known whether local anesthetic drugs are excreted in human milk. Because many drugs are excreted in human milk, caution should be exercised when local anesthetics are administered to a nursing mother.

Pediatric Use: Until further experience is gained in children younger than 12 years, administration of Sensorcaine (bupivacaine HCl) Injection in this age group is not recommended.

ADVERSE REACTIONS

Reactions to bupivacaine are characteristic of those associated with other amide-type local anesthetics. A major cause of adverse reactions to this group of drugs may be associated with its excessive plasma levels, which may be due to overdosage, unintentional intravascular injection or slow metabolic degradation.

Systemic: The most commonly encountered acute adverse experiences that demand immediate countermeasures are related to the central nervous system and the cardiovascular system. These adverse experiences are generally dose related and due to high plasma levels which may result from overdosage, rapid absorption from the injection site, diminished tolerance or from unintentional intravascular injection of the local anesthetic solution. In addition to systemic dose-related toxicity, unintentional subarachnoid injection of drug during the intended performance of caudal or lumbar epidural block or nerve blocks near the vertebral column (especially in the head and neck region) may result in underventilation or apnea ("Total or High Spinal"). Also, hypotension due to loss of sympathetic tone and respiratory paralysis or underventilation due to cephalad extension of the motor level of anesthesia may occur. This may lead to secondary cardiac arrest if untreated. Factors influencing plasma protein binding, such as acidosis, systemic diseases that alter protein production or competition with other drugs for protein binding sites, may diminish individual tolerance.

Central Nervous System Reactions: These are characterized by excitation and/or depression. Restlessness, anxiety, dizziness, tinnitus, blurred vision or tremors may occur, possibly proceeding to convulsions. However, excitement may be transient or absent, with depression being the first manifestation of an adverse reaction. This may quickly be followed by drowsiness merging into unconsciousness and respiratory arrest. Other central nervous system effects may be nausea, vomiting, chills, and constriction of the pupils.

The incidence of convulsions associated with the use of local anesthetics varies with the procedure used and the total dose administered. In a survey of studies of epidural anesthesia, overt toxicity progressing to convulsions occurred in approximately 0.1 percent of local anesthetic administrations.

Cardiovascular System Reactions: High doses or unintentional intravascular injection may lead to high plasma levels and related depression of the myocardium, decreased cardiac output, heart block, hypotension, bradycardia, ventricular arrhythmias, including ventricular tachycardia and ventricular fibrillation, and cardiac arrest. (See WARNINGS, PRECAUTIONS, and OVERDOSAGE sections.)

Allergic: Allergic type reactions are rare and may occur as a result of sensitivity to the local anesthetic or to other formulation ingredients, such as the antimicrobial preservative methylparaben contained in multiple dose vials or sulfites in epinephrine-containing solutions (see WARNINGS). These reactions are characterized by signs such as urticaria, pruritus, erythema, angioneurotic edema (including laryngeal edema), tachycardia, sneezing, nausea, vomiting, dizziness, syncope, excessive sweating, elevated temperature, and possibly, anaphylactoid symptomatology (including severe hypotension). Cross sensitivity among members of the amide-type local anesthetic group has been reported. The usefulness of screening for sensitivity has not been definitely established.

Neurologic: The incidence of adverse neurologic reactions associated with the use of local anesthetics may be related to the total dose of local anesthetic administered and are also dependent upon the particular drug used, the route of administration and the physical status of the patient. Many of these effects may be related to local anesthetic techniques, with or without a contribution from the drug.

In the practice of caudal or lumbar epidural block, occasional unintentional penetration of the subarachnoid space by the catheter or needle may occur. Subsequent adverse effects may depend partially on the amount of drug administered intrathecally and the physiological and physical effects of a dural puncture. A high spinal is characterized by paralysis of the legs, loss of consciousness, respiratory paralysis and bradycardia.

Neurologic effects following unintentional subarachnoid administration during epidural or caudal anesthesia may include spinal block by varying magnitude (including high or total spinal block); hypotension secondary to spinal block; urinary retention; fecal and urinary incontinence; loss of

Continued on next page

Sensorcaine/Sensorcaine-MPF—Cont

perineal sensation and sexual function; persistent anesthesia, paresthesia, weakness, paralysis of the lower extremities and loss of sphincter control, all of which may have slow, incomplete or no recovery; headache; backache; septic meningitis; meningismus; slowing of labor; increased incidence of forceps delivery; or cranial nerve palsies due to traction on nerves from loss of cerebrospinal fluid.

OVERDOSAGE

Acute emergencies from local anesthetics are generally related to high plasma levels encountered during therapeutic use of local anesthetics or to unintended subarachnoid injection of local anesthetic solution. (See ADVERSE REACTIONS, WARNINGS, and PRECAUTIONS.)

Management of Local Anesthetic Emergencies: The first consideration is prevention, best accomplished by careful and constant monitoring of cardiovascular and respiratory vital signs and the patient's state of consciousness after each local anesthetic injection. At the first sign of change, oxygen should be administered.

The first step in the management of systemic toxic reactions, as well as underventilation or apnea due to unintentional subarachnoid injection of drug solution, consists of ***immediate*** *attention to the establishment and maintenance of a patent airway and effective assisted or controlled ventilation with 100% oxygen with a delivery system capable of permitting immediate positive airway pressure by mask.* This may prevent convulsions if they have not already occurred.

If necessary, use drugs to control the convulsions. A 50 to 100 mg bolus I.V. injection of succinylcholine will paralyze the patient without depressing the central nervous or cardiovascular systems and facilitate ventilation. A bolus I.V. dose of 5 to 10 mg of diazepam or 50 to 100 mg of thiopental will permit ventilation and counteract central nervous system stimulation, but these drugs also depress the central nervous system, respiratory and cardiac function, add to postictal depression, and may result in apnea. Intravenous barbiturates, anticonvulsant agents, or muscle relaxants should only be administered by those familiar with their use. Immediately after the institution of these ventilatory measures, the adequacy of the circulation should be evaluated. Supportive treatment of circulatory depression may require administration of intravenous fluids, and, when appropriate, a vasopressor dictated by the clinical situation (such as ephedrine or epinephrine to enhance myocardial contractile force).

If difficulty is encountered in the maintenance of a patent airway or if prolonged ventilatory support (assisted or controlled) is indicated, endotracheal intubation, employing drugs and techniques familiar to the clinician, may be indicated after initial administration of oxygen by mask.

Recent clinical data from patients experiencing local anesthetic induced convulsions demonstrated rapid development of hypoxia, hypercarbia, and acidosis with bupivacaine within a minute of the onset of convulsions. These observations suggest that oxygen consumption and carbon dioxide production are greatly increased during local anesthetic convulsions and emphasize the importance of immediate and effective ventilation with oxygen which may avoid cardiac arrest.

If not treated immediately, convulsions with simultaneous hypoxia, hypercarbia and acidosis, plus myocardial depression from the direct effects of the local anesthetic may result in cardiac arrhythmias, bradycardia, asystole, ventricular fibrillation, or cardiac arrest. Respiratory abnormalities, including apnea, may occur. Underventilation or apnea due to unintentional subarachnoid injection of local anesthetic solution may produce these same signs and also lead to cardiac arrest if ventilatory support is not instituted. *If cardiac arrest should occur, a successful outcome may require prolonged resuscitative efforts.*

The supine position is dangerous in pregnant women at term because of aortocaval compression by the gravid uterus. Therefore, during treatment of systemic toxicity, maternal hypotension or fetal bradycardia following regional block, the parturient should be maintained in the left lateral decubitus position if possible, or manual displacement of the uterus off the great vessels be accomplished.

The mean seizure dosage of bupivacaine in rhesus monkeys was found to be 4.4 mg/kg with mean arterial plasma concentration of 4.5 mcg/mL. The intravenous and subcutaneous LD_{50} in mice is 6 to 8 mg/kg and 38 to 54 mg/kg respectively.

DOSAGE AND ADMINISTRATION

The dose of any local anesthetic administered varies with the anesthetic procedure, the area to be anesthetized, the vascularity of the tissues, the number of neuronal segments to be blocked, the depth of anesthesia and degree of muscle relaxation required, the duration of anesthesia desired, individual tolerance, and the physical condition of the patient. The smallest dose and concentration required to produce the desired result should be administered. Dosages of Sensorcaine should be reduced for young, elderly and debilitated patients and patients with cardiac and/or liver disease. The rapid injection of a large volume of local anesthetic solution should be avoided and fractional (incremental) doses should be used when feasible.

TABLE 1. DOSAGE RECOMMENDATIONS—SENSORCAINE (bupivacaine HCl) INJECTIONS

Type of Block	Conc.	Each Dose (mL)	(mg)	Motor Block[1]
Local Infiltration	0.25%[4]	up to max.	up to max.	—
Epidural	0.75%[2,4]	10–20	75–150	complete
	0.5%[4]	10–20	50–100	moderate to complete
	0.25%[4]	10–20	25–50	partial to moderate
Caudal	0.5%[4]	15–30	75–150	moderate to complete
	0.25%[4]	15–30	37.5–75	moderate
Peripheral Nerves	0.5%[4]	5 to max.	25 to max.	moderate to complete
	0.25%[4]	5 to max.	12.5 to max.	moderate to complete
Retrobulbar[3]	0.75%[4]	2–4	15–30	complete
Sympathetic	0.25%	20–50	50–125	—
Epidural[3]Test Dose	0.5% w/epi	2–3	10–15 (See PRECAUTIONS)	—

[1]With continuous (intermittent) techniques, repeat doses increase the degree of motor block. The first repeat dose of 0.5% may produce complete motor block. Intercostal nerve block with 0.25% may also produce complete motor block for intra-abdominal surgery.
[2]For single dose use, not for intermittent (catheter) epidural technique. Not for obstetric anesthesia.
[3]See PRECAUTIONS.
[4]Solutions with or without epinephrine.

Sensorcaine-MPF (methylparaben free) is available in the following forms:

Single Dose Ampules:	
5 mL	0.5% with epinephrine 1:200,000
30 mL	0.25%, 0.5% and 0.75% without epinephrine
	0.5% and 0.75% with epinephrine 1:200,000
Single Dose Vials:	
10 mL with Astra E-Z Off® vial closure;	0.25%, 0.5% and 0.75% without epinephrine
	0.25%, 0.5% and 0.75% with epinephrine 1:200,000
30 mL	0.25%, 0.5% and 0.75% without epinephrine
	0.25%, 0.5% and 0.75% with epinephrine 1:200,000

Sensorcaine is available in the following forms:

Multiple Dose Vials:	
50 mL	0.25% and 0.5% without epinephrine
	0.25% and 0.5% with epinephrine 1:200,000

For specific techniques and procedures, refer to standard textbooks.

In recommended doses, Sensorcaine produces complete sensory block, but the effect on motor function differs among the three concentrations.

0.25%—when used for caudal, epidural, or peripheral nerve block, produces incomplete motor block. Should be used for operations in which muscle relaxation is not important, or when another means of providing muscle relaxation is used concurrently. Onset of action may be slower than with the 0.5% or 0.75% solutions.

0.5%—provides motor blockade for caudal, epidural, or nerve block, but muscle relaxation may be inadequate for operations in which complete muscle relaxation is essential.

0.75%—produces complete motor block. Most useful for epidural block in abdominal operations requiring complete muscle relaxation, and for retrobulbar anesthesia. Not for obstetrical anesthesia.

The duration of anesthesia with Sensorcaine is such that for most indications, a single dose is sufficient.

Maximum dosage limit must be individualized in each case after evaluating the size and physical status of the patient, as well as the usual rate of systemic absorption from a particular injection site. Most experience to date is with single doses of Sensorcaine up to 225 mg with epinephrine 1:200,000 and 175 mg without epinephrine; more or less drug may be used depending on individualization of each case.

These doses may be repeated up to once every three hours. In clinical studies to date, total daily doses up to 400 mg have been reported. Until further experience is gained, this dose should not be exceeded in 24 hours. The duration of anesthetic effect may be prolonged by the addition of epinephrine.

The dosages in Table 1 have generally proved satisfactory and are recommended as a guide for use in the average adult. These dosages should be reduced for young, elderly or debilitated patients. Until further experience is gained Sensorcaine is not recommended for children younger than 12 years. Sensorcaine is contraindicated for obstetrical paracervical blocks, and is not recommended for intravenous regional anesthesia (Bier Block).

Use in Epidural Anesthesia: During epidural administration of Sensorcaine, 0.5% and 0.75% solutions should be administered in incremental doses of 3 mL to 5 mL with sufficient time between doses to detect toxic manifestations of unintentional intravascular or intrathecal injection. In obstetrics, only the 0.5% and 0.25% concentrations should be used; incremental doses of 3 mL to 5 mL of the 0.5% solution not exceeding 50 mg to 100 mg at any dosing interval are recommended. Repeat doses should be preceded by a test dose containing epinephrine if not contraindicated. Use only the single dose ampules and single dose vials for caudal or epidural anesthesia; the multiple dose vials contain a preservative and therefore should not be used for these procedures.

Test dose for Caudal and Lumbar Epidural Blocks: See PRECAUTIONS.

Unused portions of solutions in single dose containers should be discarded, since this product form contains no preservatives.

[See table 1 above]

NOTE: Parenteral drug products should be inspected visually for particulate matter and discoloration prior to administration whenever the solution and container permit. The Injection is not to be used if its color is pinkish or darker than slightly yellow or if it contains a precipitate.

HOW SUPPLIED

SOLUTIONS OF SENSORCAINE (BUPIVACAINE HYDROCHLORIDE) SHOULD NOT BE USED FOR THE PRODUCTION OF SPINAL ANESTHESIA (SUBARACHNOID BLOCK) BECAUSE OF INSUFFICIENT DATA TO SUPPORT SUCH USE.

[See second table above]

Disinfecting agents containing heavy metals, which cause release of respective ions (mercury, zinc, copper, etc.), should not be used for skin or mucous membrane disinfection since they have been related to incidents of swelling and edema. When chemical disinfection of the container surface is desired, either isopropyl alcohol (91%) or ethyl alcohol (70%) is recommended. It is recommended that chemical disinfection be accomplished by wiping the ampule or vial stopper thoroughly with cotton or gauze that has been moistened with the recommended alcohol just prior to use.

Solutions should be stored at controlled room temperature 15° to 30°C (59°–86°F).

Solutions containing epinephrine should be protected from light.

Caution: Federal law prohibits dispensing without prescription.

021680R03 Rev. 3/97

Shown in Product Identification Guide, page 304

SENSORCAINE®-MPF SPINAL INJECTION ℞

[sén-sor-caine]

(bupivacaine HCl in dextrose Injection, USP)

bupivacaine HCl 0.75% in dextrose 8.25% Injection

Sterile Hyperbaric Solution for Spinal Anesthesia

(For details of indications, dosage and administration, precautions, and adverse reactions, see circular in package.)

HOW SUPPLIED

NDC 0186-1026-03 2 mL ampule (15 mg bupivacaine HCl with 165 mg dextrose), boxes of 10.
Store at controlled room temperature, between 15°C and 30°C (59°F and 86°F).

021868R04   Rev. 5/97

SODIUM BICARBONATE INJECTION, USP ℞

[so '-dēum by-car '-bōw-nāte]

FOR CORRECTION OF METABOLIC ACIDOSIS AND OTHER CONDITIONS REQUIRING SYSTEMIC ALKALINIZATION.
(For details of indications, dosage and administration, precautions, and adverse reactions, see circular in package.)

HOW SUPPLIED

Sodium Bicarbonate Injection, USP is supplied in the following dosage forms:
[See table below]

021701R06   8/95

STREPTASE® ℞

(Streptokinase)

DESCRIPTION

Streptase®, Streptokinase, is a sterile, purified preparation of a bacterial protein elaborated by group C β-hemolytic streptococci. It is supplied as a lyophilized white powder containing 25 mg cross-linked gelatin polypeptides, 25 mg sodium L-glutamate, sodium hydroxide to adjust pH, and 100 mg Albumin (Human) per vial or infusion bottle as stabilizers. The preparation contains no preservatives and is intended for intravenous and intracoronary administration.

CLINICAL PHARMACOLOGY

Streptase, Streptokinase, acts with plasminogen to produce an "activator complex" that converts plasminogen to the proteolytic enzyme plasmin. The $t^1/_2$ of the activator complex is about 23 minutes; the complex is inactivated, in part, by antistreptococcal antibodies. The mechanism by which dissociated streptokinase is eliminated is clearance by sites in the liver; however, no metabolites of streptokinase have been identified. Plasmin degrades fibrin clots as well as fibrinogen and other plasma proteins. Plasmin is inactivated by circulating inhibitors, such as α-2-plasmin inhibitor or α-2-macroglobulin. These inhibitors are rapidly consumed at high doses of streptokinase.

Intravenous infusion of Streptokinase is followed by increased fibrinolytic activity, which decreases plasma fibrinogen levels for 24 to 36 hours. The decrease in plasma fibrinogen is associated with decreases in plasma and blood viscosity and red blood cell aggregation. The hyperfibrinolytic effect disappears within a few hours after discontinuation, but a prolonged thrombin time may persist for up to 24 hours due to the decrease in plasma levels of fibrinogen and an increase in the amount of circulating fibrin(ogen) degradation products (FDP). Depending upon the dosage and duration of infusion of Streptokinase, the thrombin time will decrease to less than two times the normal control value within 4 hours, and return to normal by 24 hours.

Intravenous administration has been shown to reduce blood pressure and total peripheral resistance with a corresponding reduction in cardiac afterload. These expected responses were not studied with the intracoronary administration of Streptase, Streptokinase. The quantitative benefit has not been evaluated.

Variable amounts of circulating antistreptokinase antibody are present in individuals as a result of recent streptococcal infections. The recommended dosage schedule usually obviates the need for antibody titration.

Two very large, randomized, placebo-controlled studies[1,2] involving almost 30,000 patients have demonstrated that a 60-minute intravenous infusion of 1,500,000 IU of Streptokinase significantly reduces mortality following a myocardial infarction. One of these studies also evaluated concomitant oral administration of low dose aspirin (160 mg/d over one month).

In the GISSI study the reduction in mortality was time dependent. There was a 47% reduction in mortality among patients treated within one hour of the onset of chest pain, a 23% reduction among patients treated within three hours, and a 17% reduction among patients treated between three and six hours. There was also a reduction in mortality in patients treated between six and twelve hours from the onset of symptoms, but the reduction was not statistically significant.

In the ISIS-2 study the reduction in mortality was also time dependent. If Streptokinase and aspirin were administered within the first hour after symptom onset, the reduction in mortality was 44%. The reduction in the odds of death in patients treated within four hours was 53% for the combination of Streptokinase and aspirin, and 35% for Streptokinase alone. However, the reduction was still significant when treatment was started 5–24 hours after symptom onset: 33% for the combined therapy and 17% for Streptokinase alone. Overall, in the 0–24 hour time period there was a 42% reduction in the odds of death with combined treatment (Streptokinase and aspirin) versus placebo (2p<0.00001) and a 25% reduction in the odds of death with Streptokinase alone versus placebo (2p<0.00001).

One of eight smaller studies using a similar dosing schedule showed a statistically significant reduction in mortality. When all of these studies were pooled, the overall decrease in mortality was approximately 23%. Results from pooling several studies using different dosages with long term infusion corroborate these observations.

In addition, studies measuring left ventricular ejection fraction (LVEF) at discharge showed the mean LVEFs were 3–6 percentage points higher in the Streptokinase group than in the control group. This difference was statistically significant in some of the studies[3,4]. Furthermore, some studies reported greater improvement in LVEF among patients treated within three hours than in patients treated later. Results from a randomized controlled trial in over 11,000 patients show that, following treatment with IV Streptokinase, there is a reduction in the number of patients with clinical congestive heart failure during the 14–21 day in-hospital period. Clinical congestive heart failure occurred in 12.8% of Streptokinase-treated patients compared with 15% of the control patients (p=0.001)[1].

The rate of reocclusion of the infarct-related vessel has been reported to be approximately 15–20%. The rate of reocclusion depends on dosage, additional anticoagulant therapy and residual stenosis. When the reinfarctions were evaluated in studies involving 8800 Streptokinase-treated patients, the overall rate was 3.8% (range 2–15%). In over 8500 control patients, the rate of reinfarction was 2.4%. However, the ISIS-2 study showed that an increase in reinfarction was avoided when Streptokinase was combined with low dose aspirin. The rate of reinfarction in the combination group was 1.8% vs 1.9% in the group given aspirin alone.

Streptase, Streptokinase, administered by the intracoronary route has resulted in thrombolysis usually within one hour, and ensuing reperfusion results in improvement of cardiac function and reduction of mortality[5,6]. LVEF was increased in patients treated with Streptokinase when compared to patients treated with conventional therapy. When the initial LVEF was low, the Streptokinase-treated patients showed greater improvement than did the controls. Spontaneous reperfusion is known to occur and has been observed with angiography at various time points after infarction. Data from one study show that 73% of Streptokinase-treated patients and 47% of the placebo-allocated patients reperfused during hospitalization.

Studies with thrombolytic therapy for pulmonary embolism show no significant difference in lung perfusion scan between the thrombolysis group and the heparin group at one-year follow-up. However, measurements of pulmonary capillary blood volumes and diffusing capacities at two weeks and one year after therapy indicate that a more complete resolution of thrombotic obstruction and normalization of pulmonary physiology was achieved with thrombolytic therapy, thus preventing the long term sequelae of pulmonary hypertension and pulmonary failure[7].

The long term benefit of Streptase, Streptokinase, therapy for deep vein thrombosis (DVT) has been evaluated veno-

graphically[8]. The combined results of five randomized studies show no residual thrombotic material in 60-75% of patients treated with Streptokinase versus only 10% of those treated with heparin. Thrombolytic therapy also preserves venous valve function in a majority of cases, thus avoiding the pathologic venous changes that produce the clinical post-phlebitic syndrome which occurs in 90% of the DVT patients treated with heparin.

There is a time-related decrease in effectiveness when Streptase, Streptokinase, is used in the management of peripheral arterial thromboembolism. When administered three to ten days after onset of obstruction, rates of clearance of 50–75% were reported.

INDICATIONS AND USAGE

Acute Evolving Transmural Myocardial Infarction: Streptase, Streptokinase, is indicated for use in the management of acute myocardial infarction (AMI) in adults, for the lysis of intracoronary thrombi, the improvement of ventricular function, and the reduction of mortality associated with AMI, when administered by either the intravenous or the intracoronary route, as well as for the reduction of infarct size and congestive heart failure associated with AMI when administered by the intravenous route. Earlier administration of Streptokinase is correlated with greater clinical benefit. (See CLINICAL PHARMACOLOGY.)

Pulmonary Embolism: Streptase, Streptokinase, is indicated for the lysis of objectively diagnosed (angiography or lung scan) pulmonary emboli, involving obstruction of blood flow to a lobe or multiple segments, with or without unstable hemodynamics.

Deep Vein Thrombosis: Streptase, Streptokinase, is indicated for the lysis of objectively diagnosed (preferably ascending venography), acute, extensive thrombi of the deep veins such as those involving the popliteal and more proximal vessels.

Arterial Thrombosis or Embolism: Streptase, Streptokinase, is indicated for the lysis of acute arterial thrombi and emboli. Streptokinase is not indicated for arterial emboli originating from the left side of the heart due to the risk of new embolic phenomena such as cerebral embolism.

Occlusion of Arteriovenous Cannulae: Streptase, Streptokinase, is indicated as an alternative to surgical revision for clearing totally or partially occluded arteriovenous cannulae when acceptable flow cannot be achieved.

CONTRAINDICATIONS

Because thrombolytic therapy increases the risk of bleeding, Streptase, Streptokinase, is contraindicated in the following situations:

- active internal bleeding
- recent (within 2 months) cerebrovascular accident, intracranial or intraspinal surgery (see WARNINGS)
- intracranial neoplasm
- severe uncontrolled hypertension

Streptokinase should not be administered to patients having experienced severe allergic reaction to the product.

WARNINGS

Bleeding: Following intravenous high-dose brief-duration Streptokinase therapy in acute myocardial infarction, severe bleeding complications requiring transfusion are extremely rare (0.3–0.5%), and combined therapy with low dose aspirin does not appear to increase the risk of major bleeding. The addition of aspirin to Streptokinase may cause a slight increase in the risk of minor bleeding (3.1% without aspirin vs. 3.9% with)[2].

Streptokinase will cause lysis of hemostatic fibrin deposits such as those occurring at sites of needle punctures, particularly when infused over several hours, and bleeding may occur from such sites. In order to minimize the risk of bleeding during treatment with Streptokinase, venipunctures and physical handling of the patient should be performed carefully and as infrequently as possible, and intramuscular injections must be avoided.

Should an arterial puncture be necessary during intravenous therapy, upper extremity vessels are preferable. Pressure should be applied for at least 30 minutes, a pressure dressing applied, and the puncture site checked frequently for evidence of bleeding.

In the following conditions the risks of therapy may be increased and should be weighed against the anticipated benefits.

- Recent (within 10 days) major surgery, obstetrical delivery, organ biopsy, previous puncture of noncompressible vessels

Continued on next page

SODIUM BICARBONATE

NDC No. 0186-	Dosage Form	Conc. %	mg/mL (NaHCO₃)	mEq/mL (Na+)	mEq/mL (HCO₃)	mEq/Container size (mL)	mOsm
0650-01	Syringe	8.4	84	1.0	1.0	50/50	2/mL
0656-01	Syringe/Pediatric	8.4	84	1.0	1.0	10/10	2/mL
0647-01	Syringe	7.5	75	0.9	0.9	44.6/50	1.79/mL
0646-01	Syringe/Infant	4.2	42	0.5	0.5	5/10	1/mL
0645-01	Syringe/Infant	4.2	42	0.5	0.5	2.5/5	1/mL

Solutions should be stored at controlled room temperature 15°–30°C (59°–86°F).

Streptase—Cont.

- Recent (within 10 days) serious gastrointestinal bleeding
- Recent (within 10 days) trauma including cardiopulmonary resuscitation
- Hypertension: systolic BP >180 mm Hg and/or diastolic BP >110 mm Hg
- High likelihood of left heart thrombus, e.g., mitral stenosis with atrial fibrillation
- Subacute bacterial endocarditis
- Hemostatic defects including those secondary to severe hepatic or renal disease
- Pregnancy
- Age >75 years
- Cerebrovascular disease
- Diabetic hemorrhagic retinopathy
- Septic thrombophlebitis or occluded AV cannula at seriously infected site
- Any other condition in which bleeding constitutes a significant hazard or would be particularly difficult to manage because of its location.

Should serious spontaneous bleeding (not controllable by local pressure) occur, the infusion of Streptase, Streptokinase, should be terminated immediately and treatment instituted as described under ADVERSE REACTIONS.

Bleeding into the pericardium, sometimes associated with myocardial rupture, has been seen in individual cases and has resulted in fatalities.

Arrhythmias: Rapid lysis of coronary thrombi has been shown to cause reperfusion atrial or ventricular dysrhythmias requiring immediate treatment. Careful monitoring for arrhythmia is recommended during and immediately following administration of Streptase, Streptokinase, for acute myocardial infarction. Occasionally, tachycardia and bradycardia have been observed.

Hypotension: Hypotension, sometimes severe, not secondary to bleeding or anaphylaxis has been observed during intravenous Streptase, Streptokinase, infusion in 1% to 10% of patients. Patients should be monitored closely and, should symptomatic or alarming hypotension occur, appropriate treatment should be administered. This treatment may include a decrease in the intravenous Streptokinase infusion rate. Smaller hypotensive effects are common and have not required treatment.

Cholesterol Embolism: Cholesterol embolism has been reported rarely in patients treated with all types of thrombolytic agents; the true incidence is unknown. This serious condition, which can be lethal, is also associated with invasive vascular procedures (e.g., cardiac catheterization, angiography, vascular surgery) and/or anticoagulant therapy. Clinical features of cholesterol embolism may include livedo reticularis, "purple toe" syndrome, acute renal failure, gangrenous digits, hypertension, pancreatitis, myocardial infarction, cerebral infarction, spinal cord infarction, retinal artery occlusion, bowel infarction, and rhabdomyolysis.

Other: Non-cardiogenic pulmonary edema has been reported rarely in patients treated with Streptase, Streptokinase. The risk of this appears greatest in patients who have large myocardial infarctions and are undergoing thrombolytic therapy by the intracoronary route.

Rarely, polyneuropathy has been temporally related to the use of Streptase, Streptokinase, with some cases described as Guillain Barré Syndrome.

Should pulmonary embolism or recurrent pulmonary embolism occur during Streptase, Streptokinase, therapy, the originally planned course of treatment should be completed in an attempt to lyse the embolus. While pulmonary embolism may occasionally occur during Streptokinase treatment, the incidence is no greater than when patients are treated with heparin alone. In addition to pulmonary embolism, embolization to other sites during Streptase treatment, has been observed.

PRECAUTIONS

General: There have been rare cases where Streptase, Streptokinase, has been administered for suspected AMI subsequently diagnosed as pancreatitis. Fatalities have occurred under these circumstances.

Repeated Administration — Because of the increased likelihood of resistance due to antistreptokinase antibody, Streptase, Streptokinase, may not be effective if administered between five days and twelve months of prior Streptokinase or Anistreplase administration, or streptococcal infections, such as streptococcal pharyngitis, acute rheumatic fever, or acute glomerulonephritis secondary to a streptococcal infection.

Laboratory Tests

Intravenous or Intracoronary Infusion for Myocardial Infarction — Intravenous administration of Streptase, Streptokinase, will cause marked decreases in plasminogen and fibrinogen and increases in thrombin time (TT), activated partial thromboplastin time (APTT), and prothrombin time (PT), which usually normalize within 12–24 hours. These changes may also occur in some patients with intracoronary administration of Streptokinase.

Intravenous Infusion for Other Indications — Before commencing thrombolytic therapy, it is desirable to obtain an activated partial thromboplastin time (APTT), a prothrombin time (PT), a thrombin time (TT), or fibrinogen levels, and a hematocrit and platelet count. If heparin has been given, it should be discontinued and the TT or APTT should be less than twice the normal control value before thrombolytic therapy is started.

During the infusion, decreases in plasminogen and fibrinogen levels and an increase in the level of FDP (the latter two causing a prolongation in the clotting times of coagulation tests) will generally confirm the existence of a lytic state. Therefore, lytic therapy can be confirmed by performing the TT, APTT, PT, or fibrinogen levels approximately 4 hours after initiation of therapy. If heparin is to be (re)instituted following the Streptase, Streptokinase, infusion, the TT or APTT should be less than twice the normal control value (see manufacturer's prescribing information for proper use of heparin).

Drug Interactions: The interaction of Streptase, Streptokinase, with other drugs has not been well studied.

Use of Anticoagulants and Antiplatelet Agents — Streptase, Streptokinase, alone or in combination with antiplatelet agents and anticoagulants, may cause bleeding complications. Therefore, careful monitoring is advised. In the treatment of acute MI, aspirin, when not otherwise contraindicated, should be administered with Streptokinase (see below).

Anticoagulation and Antiplatelets After Treatment for Myocardial Infarction — In the treatment of acute myocardial infarction, the use of aspirin has been shown to reduce the incidence of reinfarction and stroke. The addition of aspirin to Streptokinase causes a minimal increase in the risk of minor bleeding (3.9% vs. 3.1%), but does not appear to increase the incidence of major bleeding (see ADVERSE REACTIONS)[2]. The use of anticoagulants following administration of Streptokinase increases the risk of bleeding, but has not yet been shown to be of unequivocal clinical benefit. Therefore, whereas the use of aspirin is recommended unless otherwise contraindicated, the use of anticoagulants should be decided by the treating physician.

Anticoagulation After IV Treatment for Other Indications — Continuous intravenous infusion of heparin, without a loading dose, has been recommended following termination of Streptase, Streptokinase, infusion for treatment of pulmonary embolism or deep vein thrombosis to prevent rethrombosis. The effect of Streptokinase on thrombin time (TT) and activated partial thromboplastin time (APTT) will usually diminish within 3 to 4 hours after Streptokinase therapy, and heparin therapy without a loading dose can be initiated when the TT or the APTT is less than twice the normal control value.

Pregnancy

Pregnancy Category C — Animal reproduction studies have not been conducted with Streptase, Streptokinase. It is also not known whether Streptokinase can cause fetal harm when administered to a pregnant woman or can affect reproduction capacity. Streptokinase should be given to a pregnant woman only if clearly needed.

Pediatric Use: Controlled clinical studies have not been conducted in children to determine safety and efficacy in the pediatric population. The evidence of clinical benefits and risks is solely based on anecdotal reports in patients ranging in age from <1 month to 16 years. The largest number of patient reports have pertained to the use of streptokinase in arterial occlusions. For arterial occlusions the most frequently used loading dose was 1000 IU/kg; fewer numbers of patients received 3000 IU/kg. Loading dose durations have typically ranged from 5 minutes to 30 minutes. Continuous infusion doses were frequently 1000 IU/kg/hr; fewer were at 1500 IU/kg/hr. Infusions were maintained for ≤ 12 hours in approximately half of the published cases; a smaller proportion were between 12 hours and 24 hours. Reported adverse events associated with the use of streptokinase in the pediatric population are similar in nature to those associated with its use in adults. Rates of all bleeding complications have been variable, and as high as 50% at catheter sites in some studies. Occasionally bleeding has required transfusion. Careful monitoring of patient status is necessary.

ADVERSE REACTIONS

The following adverse reactions have been associated with intravenous therapy and may also occur with intracoronary artery infusion:

Bleeding: The reported incidence of bleeding (major or minor) has varied widely depending on the indication, dose, route and duration of administration, and concomitant therapy.

Minor bleeding can be anticipated mainly at invaded or disturbed sites. If such bleeding occurs, local measures should be taken to control the bleeding.

Severe internal bleeding involving gastrointestinal (including hepatic bleeding), genitourinary, retroperitoneal, or intracerebral sites has occurred and has resulted in fatalities. In the treatment of acute myocardial infarction with intravenous Streptokinase, the GISSI and ISIS-2 studies reported a rate of major bleeding (requiring transfusion) of 0.3–0.5%. However, rates as high as 16% have been reported in studies which required administration of anticoagulants and invasive procedures.

Major bleed rates are difficult to determine for other dosages and patient populations because of the different dosing and intervals of infusions. The rates reported appear to be within the ranges reported for intravenous administration in acute myocardial infarction.

Should uncontrollable bleeding occur, Streptokinase infusion should be terminated immediately, rather than slowing the rate of administration of or reducing the dose of Streptokinase. If necessary, bleeding can be reversed and blood loss effectively managed with appropriate replacement therapy. Although the use of aminocaproic acid in humans as an antidote for Streptokinase has not been documented, it may be considered in an emergency situation.

Allergic Reactions: Fever and shivering, occurring in 1–4% of patients[1,2], are the most commonly reported allergic reactions with intravenous use of Streptase, Streptokinase, in acute myocardial infarction. Anaphylactic and anaphylactoid reactions ranging in severity from minor breathing difficulty to bronchospasm, periorbital swelling or angioneurotic edema have been observed rarely. Other milder allergic effects such as urticaria, itching, flushing, nausea, headache and musculoskeletal pain have also been observed, as have delayed hypersensitivity reactions such as vasculitis and interstitial nephritis. Anaphylactic shock is very rare, having been reported in 0–0.1% of patients[1,2,4]. Mild or moderate allergic reactions may be managed with concomitant antihistamine and/or corticosteroid therapy. Severe allergic reactions require immediate discontinuation of Streptase, Streptokinase, with adrenergic, antihistamine, and/or corticosteroid agents administered intravenously as required.

Respiratory: There have been reports of respiratory depression in patients receiving Streptokinase. In some cases, it was not possible to determine whether the respiratory depression was associated with Streptokinase or was a symptom of the underlying process. If respiratory depression is associated with Streptokinase, the occurrence is believed to be rare.

Other Adverse Reactions: Transient elevations of serum transaminases have been observed. The source of these enzyme rises and their clinical significance is not fully understood.

There have been reports in the literature of cases of back pain associated with the use of Streptokinase. In most cases the pain developed during Streptokinase intravenous infusion and ceased within minutes of discontinuation of the infusion.

DOSAGE AND ADMINISTRATION

Acute Evolving Transmural Myocardial Infarction: Administer Streptokinase as soon as possible after onset of symptoms. The greatest benefit in mortality reduction was observed when Streptokinase was administered within four hours, but statistically significant benefit has been reported up to 24 hours (see CLINICAL PHARMACOLOGY).

Route	Total Dose	Dosage/Duration
Intravenous infusion	1,500,000 IU	1,500,000 IU within 60 min.
Intracoronary infusion	140,000 IU	20,000 IU by bolus followed by 2,000 IU/min. for 60 min.

Pulmonary Embolism, Deep Vein Thrombosis, Arterial Thrombosis or Embolism: Streptase, Streptokinase, treatment should be instituted as soon as possible after onset of the thrombotic event, preferably within 7 days. Any delay in instituting lytic therapy to evaluate the effect of heparin therapy decreases the potential for optimal efficacy. Since human exposure to streptococci is common, antibodies to Streptokinase are prevalent. Thus, a loading dose of Streptokinase sufficient to neutralize these antibodies is required. A dose of 250,000 IU of Streptokinase infused into a peripheral vein over 30 minutes has been found appropriate in over 90% of patients. Furthermore, if the thrombin time or any other parameter of lysis after 4 hours of therapy is not significantly different from the normal control level, discontinue Streptokinase because excessive resistance is present.

Indication	Loading Dose	IV Infusion Dosage/Duration
Pulmonary Embolism	250,000 IU/30 min.	100,000 IU/hr for 24 hr (72 hrs if concurrent DVT is suspected).
Deep Vein Thrombosis	250,000 IU/30 min.	100,000 IU/hr for 72 hr
Arterial Thrombosis or Embolism	250,000 IU/30 min.	100,000 IU/hr for 24–72 hr

TABLE 1
SUGGESTED DILUTIONS AND INFUSION RATES

Dosage	Vial Size (IU)	Total Solution Volume	Infusion Rate
1. Acute Myocardial Infarction			
A. Intravenous Infusion	1,500,000	45 mL	Infuse 45 mL within 60 min.
B. Intracoronary Infusion	250,000	125 mL	
1. 20,000 IU bolus			1. Loading Dose of 10 mL
2. 2,000 IU/minute for 60 minutes			2. Then 60 mL/hour
II. Pulmonary Embolism, Deep Vein Thrombosis, Arterial Thrombosis or Embolism			
Intravenous Infusion			
A. 1. 250,000 IU loading dose over 30 minutes	1,500,000	90 mL	1. Infuse 30 mL/hour for 30 minutes
2. 100,000 IU/hour maintenance dose			2. Infuse 6 mL per hour
B. SAME	1,500,000 infusion bottle	45 mL	1. 15 mL/hour for 30 minutes
			2. Infuse 3 mL per hour

Arteriovenous Cannulae Occlusion: Before using Streptase, Streptokinase, an attempt should be made to clear the cannula by careful syringe technique, using heparinized saline solution. If adequate flow is not reestablished, Streptokinase may be employed. Allow the effect of any pretreatment anticoagulants to diminish. Instill 250,000 IU Streptokinase in 2 mL of solution into each occluded limb of the cannula slowly. Clamp off cannula limb(s) for 2 hours. Observe the patient closely for possible adverse effects. After treatment, aspirate contents of infused cannula limb(s), flush with saline, reconnect cannula.

Pediatric Patients: Specific dosage and administration recommendations cannot be made based on the limited data available. However, published experience generally supports loading and continuous infusion doses administered on a weight-adjusted basis. See Precautions, Pediatric Use.

Reconstitution and Dilution: The protein nature and lyophilized form of Streptase, Streptokinase, require careful reconstitution and dilution. Slight flocculation (described as thin translucent fibers) of reconstituted Streptokinase occurred occasionally during clinical trials but did not interfere with the safe use of the solution. The following reconstitution and dilution procedures are recommended:

Vials and Infusion Bottles

1. Slowly add 5 mL Sodium Chloride Injection, USP or 5% Dextrose Injection, USP to the Streptase, Streptokinase, vial, directing the diluent at the side of the vacuum-packed vial rather than into the drug powder.
2. Roll and tilt the vial gently to reconstitute. Avoid shaking. (Shaking may cause foaming.) (If necessary, total volume may be increased to a maximum of 500 mL in glass or 50 mL in plastic containers, and the infusion pump rate in Table 1 should be adjusted accordingly.) To facilitate setting the infusion pump rate, a total volume of 45 mL, or a multiple thereof, is recommended.
3. Withdraw the entire reconstituted contents of the vial; slowly and carefully dilute further to a total volume as recommended in Table 1. Avoid shaking and agitation on dilution.
4. When diluting the 1,500,000 IU infusion bottle (50 mL), slowly add 5 mL Sodium Chloride Injection, USP, or 5% Dextrose Injection, USP, directing it at the side of the bottle rather than into the drug powder. Roll and tilt the bottle gently to reconstitute. Avoid shaking as it may cause foaming. Add an additional 40 mL of diluent to the bottle, avoiding shaking and agitation. (Total volume = 45 mL). Administer by infusion pump at the rate indicated in Table 1.
5. Parenteral drug products should be inspected visually for particulate matter and discoloration prior to administration. (The Albumin (Human) may impart a slightly yellow color to the solution.)
6. The reconstituted solution can be filtered through a 0.8 μm or larger pore size filter.
7. Because Streptase, Streptokinase, contains no preservatives, it should be reconstituted immediately before use. The solution may be used for direct intravenous administration within eight hours following reconstitution if stored at 2–8°C (36–46°F).
8. Do not add other medication to the container of Streptase, Streptokinase.
9. Unused reconstituted drug should be discarded.
[See table above]

For Use In Arteriovenous Cannulae: Slowly reconstitute the contents of 250,000 IU Streptase, Streptokinase, vacuum-packed vial with 2 mL Sodium Chloride Injection, USP or 5% Dextrose Injection, USP.

HOW SUPPLIED

Streptase, Streptokinase, is supplied as a lyophilized white powder in 50 mL infusion bottles (1,500,000 IU) or in 6.5 mL vials with a color-coded label corresponding to the amount of purified Streptokinase in each vial as follows:

green	250,000 IU	NDC 0186-1770-01	box of 1
blue	750,000 IU	NDC 0186-1771-01	box of 1
red	1,500,000 IU	NDC 0186-1773-01	box of 1 (vials)
red	1,500,000 IU	NDC 0186-1774-01	box of 1 (infusion bottles)

Store unopened vials at controlled room temperature (15–30°C or 59–86°F).

REFERENCES

1. GISSI: Effectiveness of intravenous thrombolytic treatment in acute myocardial infarction. Lancet I: 397-402, 1986.
2. ISIS-2 Collaborative Group: Randomized trial of streptokinase, oral aspirin, both, or neither among 17,187 cases of suspected acute myocardial infarction: ISIS-2. Lancet II:349-360, 1988.
3. White, H., Norris, R., Brown, M., et al: Effect of intravenous streptokinase on left ventricular function and early survival after acute myocardial infarction. N Engl J Med 317: 850-5, 1987.
4. The I.S.A.M. Study Group: A prospective trial of intravenous streptokinase in acute myocardial infarction (I.S.A.M.). N Engl J Med 314: 1465-1471, 1986.
5. Anderson, J., Marshall, H., Bray, B., et al: A randomized trial of intracoronary streptokinase in the treatment of acute myocardial infarction. N Engl J Med 308: 1312-8, 1983.
6. Kennedy, J., Ritchie, J., Davis, K., Fritz, J.: Western Washington randomized trial of intracoronary streptokinase in acute myocardial infarction. N Engl J Med 309: 1477-82, 1983.
7. Sharma, G., Burleson, V., Sasahara, A.: Effect of thrombolytic therapy on pulmonary-capillary blood volume in patients with pulmonary embolism. N Engl J Med 303: 842-5, 1980.
8. Arnesen, H., Heilo, A., Jakobsen, E., et al: A prospective study of streptokinase and heparin in the treatment of venous thrombosis. Acta Med Scand 203: 457-463, 1978.

Manufactured by Hoechst Marion Roussel Deutschland GmbH in Marburg/Lahn, Germany US License No. 1232
Distributed by Astra USA, Inc., Westborough, MA 01581
021596R10 (Revised 10/97)

TOBRAMYCIN SULFATE INJECTION, USP ℞

For Intravenous or Intramuscular Use.

> **WARNINGS**
> Patients treated with tobramycin sulfate injection and other aminoglycosides should be under close clinical observation, because these drugs have an inherent potential for causing ototoxicity and nephrotoxicity.
> Neurotoxicity, manifested as both auditory and vestibular ototoxicity, can occur. The auditory changes are irreversible, are usually bilateral, and may be partial or total. Eighth-nerve impairment and nephrotoxicity may develop, primarily in patients having preexisting renal damage and in those with normal renal function to whom aminoglycosides are administered for longer periods or in higher doses than those recommended. Other manifestations of neurotoxicity may include numbness, skin tingling, muscle twitching, and convulsions. The risk of aminoglycoside-induced hearing loss increases with the degree of exposure to either high peak or high trough serum concentrations. Patients who develop cochlear damage may not have symptoms during therapy to warn them of eighth-nerve toxicity, and partial or total irreversible bilateral deafness may continue to develop after the drug has been discontinued.
> Rarely, nephrotoxicity may not become apparent until the first few days after cessation of therapy. Aminoglycoside-induced nephrotoxicity usually is reversible.
> Renal and eighth-nerve function should be closely monitored in patients with known or suspected renal impairment and also in those whose renal function is initially normal but who develop signs of renal dysfunction during therapy. Peak and trough serum concentrations of aminoglycosides should be monitored periodically during therapy to assure adequate levels and to avoid potentially toxic levels. Prolonged serum concentrations above 12 μg/mL should be avoided. Rising trough levels

(above 2 μg/mL) may indicate tissue accumulation. Such accumulation, excessive peak concentrations, advanced age, and cumulative dose may contribute to ototoxicity and nephrotoxicity (see PRECAUTIONS). Urine should be examined for decreased specific gravity and increased excretion of protein, cells, and casts. Blood urea nitrogen, serum creatinine, and creatinine clearance should be measured periodically. When feasible, it is recommended that serial audiograms be obtained in patients old enough to be tested, particularly high-risk patients. Evidence of impairment of renal, vestibular, or auditory function requires discontinuation of the drug or dosage adjustment.
> Tobramycin should be used with caution in premature and neonatal infants because of their renal immaturity and the resulting prolongation of serum half-life of the drug.
> Concurrent and sequential use of other neurotoxic and/or nephrotoxic antibiotics, particularly other aminoglycosides (e.g., amikacin, streptomycin, neomycin, kanamycin, gentamicin, and paromomycin), cephaloridine, viomycin, polymyxin B, colistin, cisplatin, and vancomycin, should be avoided. Other factors that may increase patient risk are advanced age and dehydration. Aminoglycosides should not be given concurrently with potent diuretics, such as ethacrynic acid and furosemide. Some diuretics themselves cause ototoxicity, and intravenously administered diuretics enhance aminoglycoside toxicity by altering antibiotic concentrations in serum and tissue.
> Aminoglycosides can cause fetal harm when administered to a pregnant woman (see PRECAUTIONS).

For further information see PRECAUTIONS in full prescribing information.
(For details of indications, dosage and administration, precautions, and adverse reactions, see circular in package.)

DESCRIPTION

Tobramycin sulfate, a water-soluble antibiotic of the aminoglycoside group, is derived from the actinomycete *Streptomyces tenebrarius*. Tobramycin sulfate injection, is a clear and colorless sterile aqueous solution for parenteral administration.

Tobramycin sulfate is O-3-amino-3-deoxy-α-D-glucopyranosyl-(1→4)-O-[2,6-diamino-2,3,6-trideoxy-α-D-*ribo*-hexopyranosyl-(1→6)]-2-deoxy-L-streptamine, sulfate (2:5) (salt) and has the chemical formula ($C_{18}H_{37}N_5O_9$)$_2$·5H_2SO_4. The molecular weight is 1,425.45. The structural formula for tobramycin is as follows:

Each mL contains 40 mg tobramycin, 5 mg phenol as a preservative, 3.2 mg sodium bisulfite, 0.1 mg edetate disodium, and Water for Injection. Sulfuric acid and, if necessary, sodium hydroxide have been added to adjust the pH to 3.0–6.5. Filled under nitrogen.

HOW SUPPLIED

Tobramycin Sulfate Injection, USP is available in the following forms:

Multiple Dose Vials
NDC 0186-1783-04 80 mg*/2 mL, (40 mg*/mL) 2 mL vial—box of 25
NDC 0186-1784-01 40 mg*/mL, 30 mL—box of 1
*equivalent to tobramycin
Store at controlled room temperature 15°–30°C (59°–86°F).
021832R09 Rev. 6/98

TABLETS

TONOCARD® ℞
(TOCAINIDE HCl)

> **WARNINGS**
> *Blood Dyscrasias:* Agranulocytosis, bone marrow depression, leukopenia, neutropenia, aplastic/hypoplastic anemia, thrombocytopenia and sequelae such as septicemia and septic shock have been reported in patients receiving TONOCARD. Most of these patients received TONOCARD within the recommended dosage range.

Continued on next page

Tonocard—Cont.

Fatalities have occurred (with approximately 25 percent mortality in reported agranulocytosis cases). Since most of these events have been noted during the first 12 weeks of therapy, it is recommended that complete blood counts, including white cell, differential and platelet counts be performed, optimally, at weekly intervals for the first three months of therapy; and frequently thereafter. Complete blood counts should be performed promptly if the patient develops any signs of infection (such as fever, chills, sore throat, or stomatitis), bruising, or bleeding. If any of these hematologic disorders is identified, TONOCARD should be discontinued and appropriate treatment should be instituted if necessary. Blood counts usually return to normal within one month of discontinuation. Caution should be used in patients with pre-existing marrow failure or cytopenia of any type. (See ADVERSE REACTIONS.)

Pulmonary Fibrosis: Pulmonary fibrosis, interstitial pneumonitis, fibrosing alveolitis, pulmonary edema, and pneumonia have been reported in patients receiving TONOCARD. Many of these events occurred in patients who were seriously ill. Fatalities have been reported. The experiences are usually characterized by bilateral infiltrates on x-ray and are frequently associated with dyspnea and cough. Fever may or may not be present. Patients should be instructed to promptly report the development of any pulmonary symptoms such as exertional dyspnea, cough or wheezing. Chest x-rays are advisable at that time. If these pulmonary disorders develop, TONOCARD should be discontinued. (See ADVERSE REACTIONS.)

DESCRIPTION

TONOCARD* (Tocainide HCl) is a primary amine analog of lidocaine with antiarrhythmic properties useful in the treatment of ventricular arrhythmias. The chemical name for tocainide hydrochloride is 2-amino-*N*-(2,6-dimethylphenyl) propanamide hydrochloride. Its empirical formula is $C_{11}H_{16}N_2O \bullet HCl$, with a molecular weight of 228.72. The structural formula is:

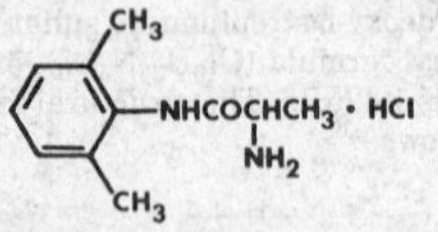

Tocainide hydrochloride is a white crystalline powder with a bitter taste and is freely soluble in water. It is supplied as 400 mg and 600 mg tablets for oral administration. Each tablet contains the following inactive ingredients: hydroxypropyl methylcellulose, iron oxide, magnesium stearate, methylcellulose, polyethylene glycol, and titanium dioxide.

*Registered trademark of Astra Pharmaceuticals, L.P.

CLINICAL PHARMACOLOGY

Action

Tocainide, like lidocaine, produces dose dependent decreases in sodium and potassium conductance, thereby decreasing the excitability of myocardial cells. In experimental animal models, the dose-related depression of sodium current is more pronounced in ischemic tissue than in normal tissue.

Electrophysiology

Tocainide is a Class I antiarrhythmic compound with electrophysiologic properties in man similar to those of lidocaine, but dissimilar from quinidine, procainamide, and disopyramide.

In studies of isolated dog Purkinje fibers, tocainide in concentrations of 1–50 mcg/mL had no significant effect on resting membrane potential, but reduced the amplitude and rate of depolarization (dv/dt) of the action potential. Tocainide decreased the effective refractory period (ERP) to a lesser extent than the action potential duration (APD) resulting in an increase in the ERP/APD ratio.

In patients with cardiac disease, TONOCARD produced no clinically significant changes in sinus nodal function, effective refractory periods, or intracardiac conduction times when studied under electrophysiologic testing procedures.

Tocainide, like lidocaine, characteristically does not prolong ventricular depolarization (QRS duration) or repolarization (QT intervals) as measured by electrocardiography. Theoretically, therefore, TONOCARD may be useful in the treatment of ventricular arrhythmias associated with a prolonged QT interval.

Patients who respond to lidocaine also respond to TONOCARD in a majority of cases. Failure to respond to lidocaine usually predicts failure to respond to TONOCARD, but there are exceptions to this.

In a controlled comparison with quinidine, 600 mg b.i.d. of TONOCARD produced a mean reduction of 42 percent in PVC count, compared to a 54 percent reduction by quinidine 300 mg every 6 hours. Among all patients entered into the study, about one-fifth of tocainide recipients and one-third of quinidine recipients had 75 percent or greater reductions in PVC count or had elimination of ventricular tachycardia.

Pharmacokinetics

Following oral administration of tocainide, peak plasma concentrations occur within 0.5 to 2 hours. The average plasma half-life in patients is approximately 15 hours. Although the effective plasma concentration may vary from patient to patient, the usual therapeutic plasma range (as defined by 50–80 percent PVC suppression) is 4–10 mcg/mL (18–45 micromole/L), expressed as tocainide hydrochloride. Tocainide is approximately 10 percent bound to plasma protein.

In contrast to lidocaine, tocainide undergoes negligible first pass hepatic degradation. Following oral administration, the bioavailability of TONOCARD approaches 100 percent. The extent of its bioavailability is unaffected by food. Tocainide has no cardioactive metabolites. Approximately 40 percent of the administered dose of tocainide is excreted unchanged in the urine. Acidification of the urine has not been shown to significantly alter tocainide excretion in the urine, but alkalinization of the urine results in a significant decrease in the percent of tocainide excreted unchanged in the urine. Animal data indicate that tocainide crosses the blood-brain barrier; however, it has less lipid solubility than lidocaine.

Hemodynamics

Cardiac catheterization studies in man utilizing intravenous tocainide infusions (0.5–0.75 mg/kg/min over 15 min) have shown that tocainide usually produces a small degree of depression of parameters of left ventricular function, such as left ventricular dP/dt, and left ventricular end diastolic pressure. There were usually no changes in cardiac output or clinical evidence of increasing congestive heart failure in the well-compensated patients studied. Small but statistically significant increases in aortic and pulmonary arterial pressures have been consistently observed and are probably related to small increases in vascular resistance. When used concomitantly with a beta-blocking drug, tocainide further reduced cardiac index and left ventricular dP/dt and further increased pulmonary wedge pressure.

No clinically significant changes in heart rate, blood pressure, or signs of myocardial depression were observed in a study of 72 post-myocardial infarction patients receiving long-term therapy with oral TONOCARD at usual doses (400 mg q8h). When tocainide was administered orally at a dose of 120 mg/kg to anesthetized dogs (14 times the initial maximum dose recommended for humans), a negative inotropic effect was observed: the rate of change of left ventricular pressure decreased by up to 29 percent of control at 3 hours after administration. This effect was not observed at lower doses (60 mg/kg). Tocainide has been used safely in patients with acute myocardial infarction and various degrees of congestive heart failure. It has, however, a small negative inotropic effect and can increase peripheral resistance slightly. It therefore should be used cautiously in patients with known heart failure, particularly if a beta blocker is given as well. (See PRECAUTIONS.)

INDICATIONS AND USAGE

TONOCARD is indicated for the treatment of documented ventricular arrhythmias, such as sustained ventricular tachycardia, that, in the judgment of the physician, are life-threatening. Because of the proarrhythmic effects of TONOCARD, as well as its potential for other serious adverse effects, (see WARNINGS), its use to treat lesser arrhythmias is not recommended. Treatment of patients with asymptomatic ventricular premature contractions should be avoided. Initiation of treatment with TONOCARD, as with other antiarrhythmic agents used to treat life-threatening arrhythmias, should be carried out in the hospital. It is essential that each patient given TONOCARD be evaluated electrocardiographically and clinically prior to, and during, therapy with TONOCARD to determine whether the response to TONOCARD supports continued treatment.

Antiarrhythmic drugs have not been shown to enhance survival in patients with ventricular arrhythmias.

CONTRAINDICATIONS

Patients who are hypersensitive to this product or to local anesthetics of the amide type.

Patients with second or third degree atrioventricular block in the absence of an artificial ventricular pacemaker.

WARNINGS

Mortality: **In the National Heart, Lung and Blood Institute's Cardiac Arrhythmia Suppression Trial (CAST), a long-term, multi-center, randomized, double-blind study in patients with asymptomatic non-life-threatening ventricular arrhythmias who had a myocardial infarction more than six days but less than two years previously, an excessive mortality or non-fatal cardiac arrest rate (7.7%) was seen in patients treated with encainide or flecainide compared with that seen in patients assigned to carefully matched placebo-treated groups (3.0%). The average duration of treatment with encainide or flecainide in this study was ten months. The applicability of the CAST results to other populations (e.g., those without recent myocardial infarction) is uncertain. Considering the known proarrhythmic properties of TONOCARD (Tocainide HCl) and the lack of evidence of improved survival for any antiarrhythmic drug in patients without life-threatening arrhythmias, the use of TONOCARD as well as other antiarrhythmic agents should be reserved for patients with life-threatening ventricular arrhythmias.**

Acceleration of Ventricular Rate: Acceleration of ventricular rate occurs infrequently when antiarrhythmics are administered to patients with atrial flutter or fibrillation (see ADVERSE REACTIONS).

PRECAUTIONS

General

In patients with known heart failure or minimal cardiac reserve, TONOCARD should be used with caution because of the potential for aggravating the degree of heart failure. Caution should be used in the institution or continuation of antiarrhythmic therapy in the presence of signs of increasing depression of cardiac conductivity.

In patients with severe liver or kidney disease, the rate of drug elimination may be significantly decreased (see DOSAGE AND ADMINISTRATION).

Since antiarrhythmic drugs may be ineffective in patients with hypokalemia, the possibility of a potassium deficit should be explored and, if present, the deficit should be corrected.

Like all other oral antiarrhythmics, TONOCARD has been reported to increase arrhythmias in some patients (see ADVERSE REACTIONS).

Information for Patients

Patients should be instructed to promptly report the development of bruising or bleeding; any signs of infections such as fever, chills, sore throat, or soreness and ulcers in the mouth; any pulmonary symptoms, such as exertional dyspnea, cough, or wheezing; rash.

Laboratory Tests

As with other antiarrhythmics, abnormal liver function tests, particularly in the early stages of therapy, have been reported. Periodic monitoring of liver function should be considered. Hepatitis and jaundice have been reported in some patients.

Drug Interactions

Tocainide and lidocaine are pharmacodynamically similar. The concomitant use of these two agents may cause an increased incidence of adverse reactions, including central nervous system adverse reactions such as seizure.

Specific interaction studies with cimetidine, digoxin, metoprolol and warfarin have been conducted, no clinically significant interaction was seen with cimetidine, digoxin or warfarin; but tocainide and metoprolol had additive effects on wedge pressure and cardiac index. TONOCARD has also been used in open studies with digitalis, beta-blocking agents, other antiarrhythmic agents, anticoagulants, and diuretics, without evidence of clinically significant interactions. Nevertheless, caution should be exercised in the use of multiple drug therapy.

TONOCARD is equally effective in digitalized and nondigitalized patients. In 17 patients with refractory ventricular arrhythmias on concomitant therapy, serum digoxin levels (1.1 ± 0.4 ng/mL) remained in the expected normal range (0.5–2.5 ng/mL) during tocainide administration.

Carcinogenesis, Mutagenesis, Impairment of Fertility

The carcinogenic potential of tocainide was studied in mice using oral doses up to 300 mg/kg/day (about 6 times the maximum recommended human dose) for up to 94 weeks in males and 102 weeks in females and in rats at doses up to 200 mg/kg/day for 24 months. Tocainide did not affect the type or incidence of neoplasia in the two studies.

Tocainide did not show any mutagenic potential when evaluated *in vivo* in the micronucleus test using mice at oral doses up to 187.5 mg/kg/day (about 7 times the usual human dose). Also, no mutagenic activity was seen *in vitro* in the Ames microbial mutagen test or in the mouse lymphoma forward mutation assay.

Reproduction and fertility studies in rats showed no adverse effects on male or female fertility at oral doses up to 200 mg/kg/day (about 8 times the usual human dose).

Pregnancy

Pregnancy Category C. In a teratogenicity study in rabbits, tocainide was administered orally at doses of 25, 50,

and 100 mg/kg/day (about 1 to 4 times the usual human dose). No evidence of a drug-related teratogenic effect was noted; however, these doses were maternotoxic and produced a dose-related increase in abortions and stillbirths. In a teratogenicity study in rats, an oral dose of 300 mg/kg/day (about 12 times the usual human dose) showed no evidence of treatment-related fetal malformations, but maternotoxicity and an increase in fetal resorptions were noted. An oral dose of 30 mg/kg/day (about twice the usual human dose) did not produce any adverse effects.

In reproduction studies in rats at maternotoxic oral doses of 200 and 300 mg/kg/day (about 8 and 12 times the usual human dose, respectively), dystocia, and delayed parturition occurred which was accompanied by an increase in stillbirths and decreased survival in offspring during the first week postpartum. Growth and viability of surviving offspring were not affected for the remainder of the lactation period.

There are no adequate and well-controlled studies in pregnant women. TONOCARD should be used during pregnancy only if the potential benefit justifies the potential risk to the fetus.

Nursing Mothers

It is not known whether tocainide is secreted in human milk. Because many drugs are secreted in human milk and because of the potential for serious adverse reactions in nursing infants from TONOCARD, a decision should be made whether to discontinue nursing or to discontinue the drug, taking into account the importance of the drug to the mother.

Pediatric Use

Safety and effectiveness in children have not been established.

ADVERSE REACTIONS

TONOCARD commonly produces minor, transient, nervous system and gastrointestinal adverse reactions, but is otherwise generally well tolerated. TONOCARD has been evaluated in both short-term (n = 1,358) and long-term (n = 262) controlled studies as well as a compassionate use program. Dosages were lower in most of the controlled studies (1200 mg/day) and higher in the compassionate use program (1800 mg and more). In long-term (2–6 months) controlled studies, the most frequent adverse reactions were dizziness/vertigo (15.3 percent), nausea (14.5 percent), paresthesia (9.2 percent), and tremor (8.4 percent). These reactions were generally mild, transient, dose-related and reversible with a reduction in dosage, by taking the drug with food, or by therapy discontinuation. Tremor, when present, may be useful as a clinical indicator that the maximum dose is being approached. Adverse reactions leading to therapy discontinuation occurred in 21 percent of patients in long-term controlled trials and were usually related to the nervous system or digestive system.

Adverse reactions occurring in greater than one percent of patients from the short-term and long-term controlled studies appear in the following table:

| | Percent of Patients Controlled Studies | |
	Short-term (n = 1,358)	Long-term (n = 262)
BODY AS A WHOLE		
Tiredness/drowsiness/ fatigue/lethargy/ lassitude/sleepiness	1.6	0.8
Hot/cold feelings	0.5	1.5
CARDIOVASCULAR		
Hypotension	3.4	2.7
Bradycardia	1.8	0.4
Palpitations	1.8	0.4
Chest pain	1.6	0.4
Conduction disorders	1.5	0.0
Left ventricular failure	1.4	0.0
DIGESTIVE		
Nausea	15.2	14.5
Vomiting	8.3	4.6
Anorexia	1.2	1.9
Diarrhea/loose stools	0.0	3.8
NERVOUS SYSTEM/PSYCHIATRIC		
Dizziness/vertigo	8.0	15.3
Paresthesia	3.5	9.2
Tremor	2.9	8.4
Confusion/disorientation/ hallucinations	2.1	2.7
Headache	2.1	4.6
Nervousness	1.5	0.4
Altered mood/awareness	1.5	3.4
Incoordination/ unsteadiness/walking disturbances	1.2	0.0
Anxiety	1.1	1.5
Ataxia	0.2	3.0
SKIN		
Diaphoresis	5.1	2.3
Rash/skin lesion	0.4	8.4
SPECIAL SENSES		
Blurred vision/visual disturbances	1.3	1.5
Tinnitus/hearing loss	0.4	1.5
Nystagmus	0.0	1.1

An additional group of about 2,000 patients has been treated in a program allowing for the use of TONOCARD under compassionate use circumstances. These patients were seriously ill with the large majority on multiple drug therapy, and comparatively high doses of TONOCARD were used. Fifty-four percent of the patients continued in the program for one year or longer, and 12 percent were treated for longer than three years, with the longest duration of therapy being nine years. Adverse reactions leading to therapy discontinuation occurred in 12 percent of patients (usually central nervous system effects or rash). A tabulation of adverse reactions occurring in one percent or more of patients follows:

	Percent of Patients Compassionate Use (n = 1,927)
CARDIOVASCULAR	
Increased ventricular arrhythmias/ PVCs	10.9
CHF/progression of CHF	4.0
Tachycardia	3.2
Hypotension	1.8
Conduction disorders	1.3
Bradycardia	1.0
DIGESTIVE	
Nausea	24.6
Anorexia	11.3
Vomiting	9.0
Diarrhea/loose stools	6.8
MUSCULOSKELETAL	
Arthritis/arthralgia	4.7
Myalgia	1.7
NERVOUS SYSTEM/PSYCHIATRIC	
Dizziness/vertigo	25.3
Tremor	21.6
Nervousness	11.5
Confusion/disorientation/ hallucinations	11.2
Altered mood/awareness	11.0
Ataxia	10.8
Paresthesia	9.2
SKIN	
Rash/skin lesion	12.2
Diaphoresis	8.3
Lupus	1.6
SPECIAL SENSES	
Blurred vision/vision disturbances	10.0
Nystagmus	1.1

Adverse reactions occurring in less than one percent of patients in either the controlled studies or the compassionate use program or since the drug was marketed are as follows:

Body as a Whole: Septicemia; septic shock; syncope; vaso-vagal episodes; edema; fever; chills; cinchonism; asthenia; malaise.

Cardiovascular: Ventricular fibrillation; extension of acute myocardial infarction; cardiogenic shock; pulmonary embolism; angina; AV block; hypertension; claudication; increased QRS duration; pleurisy/pericarditis; prolonged QT interval; right bundle branch block; cardiomegaly; sinus arrest; vasculitis; orthostatic hypotension; cold extremities.

Digestive: Hepatitis, jaundice (see PRECAUTIONS); abnormal liver function tests; pancreatitis; abdominal pain/discomfort; constipation; dysphagia; gastrointestinal symptoms (including dyspepsia); stomatitis; dry mouth; thirst.

Hematologic: Agranulocytosis; bone marrow depression; aplastic/hypoplastic anemia; hemolytic anemia; anemia; leukopenia; neutropenia; thrombocytopenia; eosinophilia.

Metabolic and Immune: Hypersensitivity Reaction (including some of the following symptoms or signs: rash, fever, joint pains, abnormal liver function tests, eosinophilia); increased ANA.

Musculoskeletal: Muscle cramps; muscle twitching/spasm; neck pain; pain radiating from neck; pressure on shoulder.

Nervous System/Psychiatric: Coma; convulsions/seizures; myasthenia gravis; depression; psychosis; psychic disturbances; agitation; decreased mental acuity; dysarthria; impaired memory; increased stuttering/slurred speech; insomnia/sleeping disturbances; local anesthesia; dream abnormalities.

Respiratory: Respiratory arrest; pulmonary edema; pulmonary fibrosis; fibrosing alveolitis; pneumonia; interstitial pneumonitis; dyspnea; hiccough; yawning.

Skin: Stevens-Johnson syndrome; exfoliative dermatitis; erythema multiforme; urticaria; alopecia; pruritus; pallor/flushed face.

Special Senses: Diplopia; earache; taste perversion/smell perversion.

Urogenital: Urinary retention; polyuria/increased diuresis.

Agranulocytosis, bone marrow depression, leukopenia, neutropenia, aplastic/hypoplastic anemia, and thrombocytopenia have been reported (0.18 percent) in patients receiving TONOCARD in controlled trials and the compassionate use program. Most of these events have been noted during the first 12 weeks of therapy. (See Box WARNINGS.)

Pulmonary fibrosis, interstitial pneumonitis, fibrosing alveolitis, pulmonary edema, and pneumonia, have been reported in patients receiving TONOCARD. The incidence of pulmonary fibrosis (including interstitial pneumonitis and fibrosing alveolitis) was 0.11 percent in controlled trials and the compassionate use program. These events usually occurred in seriously ill patients. Symptoms of these pulmonary disorders and/or x-ray changes usually occurred following 3–18 weeks of therapy. Fatalities have been reported. (See Box WARNINGS.)

A number of disorders, in which a causal relationship with TONOCARD has not been established, have been reported in seriously ill patients. These include: renal failure, renal dysfunction, myocardial infarction, cerebrovascular accidents and transient ischemic attacks. These disorders may be related to the patient's underlying condition.

DRUG ABUSE AND DEPENDENCE

Drug withdrawal after chronic treatment has not shown any indication of psychological or physical dependence.

OVERDOSAGE

The initial and most important signs and symptoms of overdosage would be expected to be related to the central nervous system. Other adverse reactions, such as gastrointestinal disturbances, may follow. (See ADVERSE REACTIONS.)

Should convulsions or cardiopulmonary depression or arrest develop, the patency of the airway and adequacy of ventilation must be assured immediately. Should convulsions persist despite ventilatory therapy with oxygen, small increments of anticonvulsive agents may be given intravenously. Examples of such agents include a benzodiazepine (e.g., diazepam), an ultrashort-acting barbiturate (e.g., thiopental or thiamylal), or a short-acting barbiturate (e.g., pentobarbital or secobarbital).

The oral LD_{50} of tocainide was calculated to be about 800 mg/kg in mice, 1000 mg/kg in rats, and 230 mg/kg in guinea pigs; deaths were usually preceded by convulsions.

Studies in normal individuals to date indicate that tocainide has a hemodialysis clearance approximately equivalent to its renal clearance.

DOSAGE AND ADMINISTRATION

The dosage of TONOCARD must be individualized on the basis of antiarrhythmic response and tolerance, both of which are dose-related. Clinical and electrocardiographic evaluation (including Holter monitoring if necessary for evaluation) are needed to determine whether the desired antiarrhythmic response has been obtained and to guide titration and dose adjustment. Adverse effects appearing shortly after dosing, for example, suggest a need for dividing the dose further with a shorter dose-interval. Loss of arrhythmia control prior to the next dose suggests use of a shorter dose interval and/or a dose increase. Absence of a clear response suggests reconsideration of therapy.

The recommended initial dosage is 400 mg every 8 hours. The usual adult dosage is between 1200 and 1800 mg/day in a three dose daily divided regimen. Doses beyond 2400 mg per day have been administered infrequently. Patients who tolerate the t.i.d. regimen may be tried on a twice daily regimen with careful monitoring.

Some patients, particularly those with renal or hepatic impairment, may be adequately treated with less than 1200 mg/day.

HOW SUPPLIED

No. 3409—Tablets TONOCARD, 400 mg, are oval, yellow, scored, film-coated tablets, coded 707 on one side and TONOCARD on the other side. They are supplied as follows:
NDC 61113-707-68 bottles of 100
(6505-01-203-6240, 400 mg 100's)
NDC 61113-707-28 unit dose packages of 100.

Continued on next page

Tonocard—Cont.

No. 3410—Tablets TONOCARD, 600 mg, are oblong, yellow, scored, film-coated tablets, coded 709 on one side and TONOCARD on the other side. They are supplied as follows:
NDC 61113-709-68 bottles of 100
(6505-01-206-0273, 600 mg 100's)
NDC 61113-709-28 unit dose packages of 100.
Storage
Store below 40°C (104°F), preferably between 15°C and 30°C (59°F and 86°F). Store in a well-closed container.
Distributed by:
Astra Pharmaceuticals, L.P.
Wayne, PA 19087, USA
Manufactured by: MERCK & CO., INC.,
West Point, PA 19486, USA
Issued July 1995   7911313
©1998 Astra Pharmaceuticals, L.P. All rights reserved.
Shown in Product Identification Guide, page 304

TOPROL-XL® TABLETS   ℞
(metoprolol succinate)
Extended Release Tablets
Tablets: 50 mg, 100 mg, and 200 mg

DESCRIPTION

Toprol-XL, metoprolol succinate, is a beta$_1$-selective (cardioselective) adrenoceptor blocking agent, for oral administration, available as extended release tablets. Toprol-XL has been formulated to provide a controlled and predictable release of metoprolol for once daily administration. The tablets comprise a multiple unit system containing metoprolol succinate in a multitude of controlled release pellets. Each pellet acts as a separate drug delivery unit and is designed to deliver metoprolol continuously over the dosage interval. The tablets contain 47.5 mg, 95 mg and 190 mg of metoprolol succinate equivalent to 50, 100 and 200 mg of metoprolol tartrate, USP, respectively. Its chemical name is (±)1-(isopropylamino)-3-[p-(2-methoxyethyl)phenoxy]-2-propanol succinate (2:1) (salt). Its structural formula is:

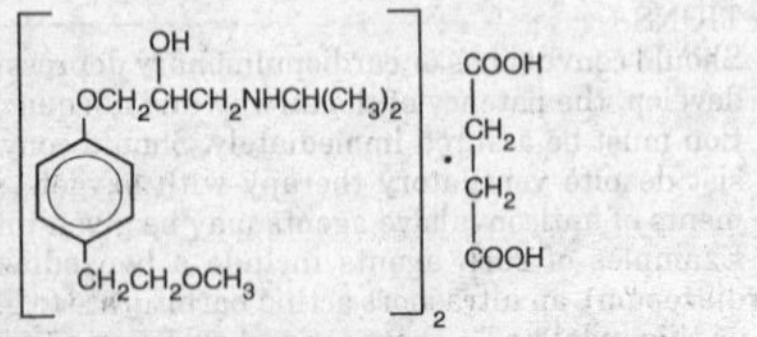

Metoprolol succinate is a white crystalline powder with a molecular weight of 652.8. It is freely soluble in water; soluble in methanol; sparingly soluble in ethanol; slightly soluble in dichloromethane and 2-propanol; practically insoluble in ethyl-acetate, acetone, diethylether and heptane. Inactive ingredients: silicon dioxide, cellulose compounds, sodium stearyl fumarate, polyethylene glycol, titanium dioxide, paraffin.

CLINICAL PHARMACOLOGY

Metoprolol is a beta$_1$-selective (cardioselective) adrenergic receptor blocking agent. This preferential effect is not absolute, however, and at higher plasma concentrations, metoprolol also inhibits beta$_2$-adrenoreceptors, chiefly located in the bronchial and vascular musculature. Metoprolol has no intrinsic sympathomimetic activity, and membrane-stabilizing activity is detectable only at plasma concentrations much greater than required for beta-blockade. Animal and human experiments indicate that metoprolol slows the sinus rate and decreases AV nodal conduction.
Clinical pharmacology studies have confirmed the beta-blocking activity of metoprolol in man, as shown by (1) reduction in heart rate and cardiac output at rest and upon exercise, (2) reduction of systolic blood pressure upon exercise, (3) inhibition of isoproterenol-induced tachycardia, and (4) reduction of reflex orthostatic tachycardia.
The relative beta$_1$-selectivity of metoprolol has been confirmed by the following: (1) In normal subjects, metoprolol is unable to reverse the beta$_2$-mediated vasodilating effects of epinephrine. This contrasts with the effect of nonselective beta-blockers, which completely reverse the vasodilating effects of epinephrine. (2) In asthmatic patients, metoprolol reduces FEV$_1$ and FVC significantly less than a nonselective beta-blocker, propranolol, at equivalent beta$_1$-receptor blocking doses.
In five controlled studies in normal healthy subjects, the same daily doses of Toprol-XL and immediate release metoprolol were compared in terms of the extent and duration of beta$_1$-blockade produced. Both formulations were given in a dose range equivalent to 100–400 mg of immediate release metoprolol per day. In these studies, Toprol-XL was administered once a day and immediate release metoprolol was administered once to four times a day. A sixth controlled study compared the beta$_1$-blocking effects of a 50 mg daily dose of the two formulations. In each study, beta$_1$-blockade was expressed as the percent change from baseline, in exercise heart rate following standardized submaximal exercise tolerance tests at steady state. Toprol-XL administered once a day, and immediate release metoprolol administered once to four times a day, provided comparable total beta$_1$-blockade over 24 hours (area under the beta$_1$-blockade versus time curve) in the dose range 100–400 mg. At a dosage of 50 mg once daily, Toprol-XL produced significantly higher total beta$_1$-blockade over 24 hours than immediate release metoprolol. For Toprol-XL, the percent reduction in exercise heart rate was relatively stable throughout the entire dosage interval and the level of beta$_1$-blockade increased with increasing doses from 50 to 300 mg daily. The effects at peak/ trough (i.e. at 24 hours post dosing) were; 14/9, 16/10, 24/14, 27/22 and 27/20% reduction in exercise heart rate for doses of 50, 100, 200, 300 and 400 mg Toprol-XL once a day, respectively. In contrast to Toprol-XL immediate release metoprolol given at a dose of 50–100 mg once a day, produced a significantly larger peak effect on exercise tachycardia, but the effect was not evident at 24 hours. To match the peak to trough ratio obtained with Toprol-XL over the dosing range of 200 to 400 mg, a t.i.d. to q.i.d. divided dosing regimen was required for immediate release metoprolol.
The relationship between plasma metoprolol levels and reduction in exercise heart rate is independent of the pharmaceutical formulation. Using the E$_{max}$ model, the maximal beta$_1$-blocking effect has been estimated to produce a 28.3% reduction in exercise heart rate. Beta$_1$-blocking effects in the range of 30–80% of the maximal effect (corresponding to approximately 8–23% reduction in exercise heart rate) are expected to occur at metoprolol plasma concentrations ranging from 30–540 nmol/L. The concentration-effect curve begins reaching a plateau between 200–300 nmol/L, and higher plasma levels produce little additional beta$_1$-blocking effect. The relative beta$_1$-selectivity of metoprolol diminishes and blockade of beta$_2$-adrenoceptors increases at higher plasma concentrations.
Although beta-adrenergic receptor blockade is useful in the treatment of angina and hypertension, there are situations in which sympathetic stimulation is vital. In patients with severely damaged hearts, adequate ventricular function may depend on sympathetic drive. In the presence of AV block, beta-blockade may prevent the necessary facilitating effect of sympathetic activity on conduction. Beta$_2$-adrenergic blockade results in passive bronchial constriction by interfering with endogenous adrenergic bronchodilator activity in patients subject to bronchospasm and may also interfere with exogenous bronchodilators in such patients.
Hypertension: The mechanism of the antihypertensive effects of beta-blocking agents has not been elucidated. However, several possible mechanisms have been proposed: (1) competitive antagonism of catecholamines at peripheral (especially cardiac) adrenergic neuron sites, leading to decreased cardiac output; (2) a central effect leading to reduced sympathetic outflow to the periphery; and (3) suppression of renin activity.
In controlled clinical studies, an immediate release dosage form of metoprolol has been shown to be an effective antihypertensive agent when used alone or as concomitant therapy with thiazide-type diuretics at dosages of 100–450 mg daily. Toprol-XL, in dosages of 100 to 400 mg once daily, has been shown to possess comparable β$_1$-blockade as conventional metoprolol tablets administered two to four times daily. In addition, Toprol-XL administered at a dose of 50 mg once daily has been shown to lower blood pressure 24-hours post-dosing in placebo controlled studies. In controlled, comparative, clinical studies, immediate release metoprolol appeared comparable as an antihypertensive agent to propranolol, methyldopa, and thiazide-type diuretics, and affected both supine and standing blood pressure. Because of variable plasma levels attained with a given dose and lack of a consistent relationship of antihypertensive activity to drug plasma concentration, selection of proper dosage requires individual titration.
Angina Pectoris: By blocking catecholamine-induced increases in heart rate, in velocity and extent of myocardial contraction, and in blood pressure, metoprolol reduces the oxygen requirements of the heart at any given level of effort, thus making it useful in the long-term management of angina pectoris. However, in patients with heart failure, beta-adrenergic blockade may increase oxygen requirements by increasing left ventricular fiber length and end-diastolic pressure.
In controlled clinical trials, an immediate release formulation of metoprolol has been shown to be an effective anti-anginal agent, reducing the number of angina attacks and increasing exercise tolerance. The dosage used in these studies ranged from 100 to 400 mg daily. Toprol-XL, in dosages of 100 to 400 mg once daily, has been shown to possess comparable β$_1$-blockade as conventional metoprolol tablets administered two to four times daily.
Pharmacokinetics: In man, absorption of metoprolol is rapid and complete. Plasma levels following oral administration of conventional metoprolol tablets, however, approximate 50% of levels following intravenous administration, indicating about 50% first-pass metabolism. Metoprolol crosses the blood-brain barrier and has been reported in the CSF in a concentration 78% of the simultaneous plasma concentration.
Plasma levels achieved are highly variable after oral administration. Only a small fraction of the drug (about 12%) is bound to human serum albumin. Elimination is mainly by biotransformation in the liver, and the plasma half-life ranges from approximately 3 to 7 hours. Less than 5% of an oral dose of metoprolol is recovered unchanged in the urine; the rest is excreted by the kidneys as metabolites that appear to have no clinical significance. Following intravenous administration of metoprolol, the urinary recovery of unchanged drug is approximately 10%. The systemic availability and half-life of metoprolol in patients with renal failure do not differ to a clinically significant degree from those in normal subjects. Consequently, no reduction in dosage is usually needed in patients with chronic renal failure.
In comparison to conventional metoprolol, the plasma metoprolol levels following administration of Toprol-XL are characterized by lower peaks, longer time to peak and significantly lower peak to trough variation. The peak plasma levels following once daily administration of Toprol-XL average one-fourth to one-half the peak plasma levels obtained following a corresponding dose of conventional metoprolol, administered once daily or in divided doses. At steady state the average bioavailability of metoprolol following administration of Toprol- XL, across the dosage range of 50 to 400 mg once daily, was 77% relative to the corresponding single or divided doses of conventional metoprolol. Nevertheless, over the 24 hour dosing interval, β$_1$-blockade is comparable and dose-related (see CLINICAL PHARMACOLOGY). The bioavailability of metoprolol shows a dose-related, although not directly proportional increase with dose and is not significantly affected by food following Toprol-XL administration.

INDICATIONS AND USAGE
Hypertension: Toprol-XL tablets are indicated for the treatment of hypertension. They may be used alone or in combination with other antihypertensive agents.
Angina Pectoris: Toprol-XL tablets are indicated in the long-term treatment of angina pectoris.

CONTRAINDICATIONS
Hypertension and Angina: Toprol-XL is contraindicated in sinus bradycardia, heart block greater than first degree, cardiogenic shock, and overt cardiac failure (see WARNINGS).

WARNINGS
Hypertension and Angina
Cardiac Failure—Sympathetic stimulation is a vital component supporting circulatory function in congestive heart failure, and beta-blockade carries the potential hazard of further depressing myocardial contractility and precipitating more severe failure. In hypertensive and angina patients who have congestive heart failure controlled by digitalis and diuretics, Toprol-XL should be administered cautiously. Both digitalis and Toprol-XL slow AV conduction.
In Patients Without a History of Cardiac Failure—Continued depression of the myocardium with beta-blocking agents over a period of time can, in some cases, lead to cardiac failure. At the first sign or symptom of impending cardiac failure, patients should be fully digitalized and/or given a diuretic. The response should be observed closely. If cardiac failure continues, despite adequate digitalization and diuretic therapy, Toprol-XL should be withdrawn.

> *Ischemic Heart Disease:* Following abrupt cessation of therapy with certain beta-blocking agents, exacerbations of angina pectoris and, in some cases, myocardial infarction have occurred. When discontinuing chronically administered Toprol-XL, particularly in patients with ischemic heart disease, the dosage should be gradually reduced over a period of 1–2 weeks and the patient should be carefully monitored. If angina markedly worsens or acute coronary insufficiency develops, Toprol-XL administration should be reinstated promptly, at least temporarily, and other measures appropriate for the management of unstable angina should be taken. Patients should be warned against interruption or discontinuation of therapy without the physician's advice. Because coronary artery disease is common and may be unrecognized, it may be prudent not to discontinue Toprol-XL therapy abruptly even in patients treated only for hypertension.

Bronchospastic Diseases—PATIENTS WITH BRONCHOSPASTIC DISEASES SHOULD, IN GENERAL, NOT RECEIVE BETA-BLOCKERS. Because of its relative beta$_1$-selectivity, however, Toprol-XL may be used with caution in patients with bronchospastic disease who do not respond to, or cannot tolerate, other antihypertensive treatment. Since beta$_1$-selectivity is not absolute, a beta$_2$-stimulating agent

should be administered concomitantly, and the lowest possible dose of Toprol-XL should be used (see DOSAGE AND ADMINISTRATION).

Major Surgery—The necessity or desirability of withdrawing beta-blocking therapy prior to major surgery is controversial; the impaired ability of the heart to respond to reflex adrenergic stimuli may augment the risks of general anesthesia and surgical procedures.

Toprol-XL like other beta-blockers, is a competitive inhibitor of beta-receptor agonists, and its effects can be reversed by administration of such agents, e.g., dobutamine or isoproterenol. However, such patients may be subject to protracted severe hypotension. Difficulty in restarting and maintaining the heart beat has also been reported with beta-blockers.

Diabetes and Hypoglycemia—Toprol-XL should be used with caution in diabetic patients if a beta-blocking agent is required. Beta-blockers may mask tachycardia occurring with hypoglycemia, but other manifestations such as dizziness and sweating may not be significantly affected.

Thyrotoxicosis—Beta-adrenergic blockade may mask certain clinical signs (e.g., tachycardia) of hyperthyroidism. Patients suspected of developing thyrotoxicosis should be managed carefully to avoid abrupt withdrawal of beta-blockade, which might precipitate a thyroid storm.

PRECAUTIONS

General: Toprol-XL should be used with caution in patients with impaired hepatic function.

Information for Patients: Patients should be advised to take Toprol-XL regularly and continuously, as directed, preferably with or immediately following meals. If a dose should be missed, the patient should take only the next scheduled dose (without doubling it). Patients should not discontinue Toprol-XL without consulting the physician.

Patients should be advised (1) to avoid operating automobiles and machinery or engaging in other tasks requiring alertness until the patient's response to therapy with Toprol- XL has been determined; (2) to contact the physician if any difficulty in breathing occurs; (3) to inform the physician or dentist before any type of surgery that he or she is taking Toprol-XL.

Laboratory Tests: Clinical laboratory findings may include elevated levels of serum transaminase, alkaline phosphatase, and lactate dehydrogenase.

Drug Interactions: Catecholamine-depleting drugs (e.g., reserpine) may have an additive effect when given with beta-blocking agents. Patients treated with Toprol-XL plus a catecholamine depletor should therefore be closely observed for evidence of hypotension or marked bradycardia, which may produce vertigo, syncope, or postural hypotension.

Carcinogenesis, Mutagenesis, Impairment of Fertility: Long-term studies in animals have been conducted to evaluate the carcinogenic potential of metoprolol tartrate. In 2-year studies in rats at three oral dosage levels of up to 800 mg/kg/day, there was no increase in the development of spontaneously occurring benign or malignant neoplasms of any type. The only histologic changes that appeared to be drug related were an increased incidence of generally mild focal accumulation of foamy macrophages in pulmonary alveoli and a slight increase in biliary hyperplasia. In a 21-month study in Swiss albino mice at three oral dosage levels of up to 750 mg/kg/day, benign lung tumors (small adenomas) occurred more frequently in female mice receiving the highest dose than in untreated control animals. There was no increase in malignant or total (benign plus malignant) lung tumors, nor in the overall incidence of tumors or malignant tumors. This 21-month study was repeated in CD-1 mice, and no statistically or biologically significant differences were observed between treated and control mice of either sex for any type of tumor.

All mutagenicity tests performed on metoprolol tartrate (a dominant lethal study in mice, chromosome studies in somatic cells, a Salmonella/mammalian-microsome mutagenicity test, and a nucleus anomaly test in somatic interphase nuclei) and metoprolol succinate (a Salmonella/mammalian-microsome mutagenicity test) were negative.

No evidence of impaired fertility due to metoprolol tartrate was observed in a study performed in rats at doses up to 55.5 times the maximum daily human dose of 450 mg.

Pregnancy Category C: Metoprolol tartrate has been shown to increase post-implantation loss and decrease neonatal survival in rats at doses up to 55.5 times the maximum daily human dose of 450 mg. Distribution studies in mice confirm exposure of the fetus when metoprolol tartrate is administered to the pregnant animal. These studies have revealed no evidence of impaired fertility or teratogenicity. There are no adequate and well-controlled studies in pregnant women. Because animal reproduction studies are not always predictive of human response, this drug should be used during pregnancy only if clearly needed.

Nursing Mothers: Metoprolol is excreted in breast milk in very small quantities. An infant consuming 1 liter of breast milk daily would receive a dose of less than 1 mg of the drug. Caution should be exercised when Toprol-XL is administered to a nursing woman.

Pediatric Use: Safety and effectiveness in pediatric patients have not been established.

Risk of Anaphylactic Reactions: While taking beta-blockers, patients with a history of severe anaphylactic reactions to a variety of allergens may be more reactive to repeated challenge, either accidental, diagnostic or therapeutic. Such patients may be unresponsive to the usual doses of epinephrine used to treat allergic reaction.

ADVERSE REACTIONS

Hypertension and Angina: Most adverse effects have been mild and transient. The following adverse reactions have been reported for metoprolol tartrate.

Central Nervous System—Tiredness and dizziness have occurred in about 10 of 100 patients. Depression has been reported in about 5 of 100 patients. Mental confusion and short-term memory loss have been reported. Headache, somnolence, nightmares, and insomnia have also been reported.

Cardiovascular—Shortness of breath and bradycardia have occurred in approximately 3 of 100 patients. Cold extremities; arterial insufficiency, usually of the Raynaud type; palpitations; congestive heart failure; peripheral edema; syncope; chest pain; and hypotension have been reported in about 1 of 100 patients (see CONTRAINDICATIONS, WARNINGS and PRECAUTIONS).

Respiratory—Wheezing (bronchospasm) and dyspnea have been reported in about 1 of 100 patients (see WARNINGS).

Gastrointestinal—Diarrhea has occurred in about 5 of 100 patients. Nausea, dry mouth, gastric pain, constipation, flatulence, digestive tract disorders and heartburn have been reported in about 1 of 100 patients.

Hypersensitive Reactions—Pruritus or rash have occurred in about 5 of 100 patients. Worsening of psoriasis has also been reported.

Miscellaneous—Peyronie's disease has been reported in fewer than 1 of 100,000 patients. Musculoskeletal pain, blurred vision, decreased libido and tinnitus have also been reported.

There have been rare reports of reversible alopecia, agranulocytosis, and dry eyes. Discontinuation of the drug should be considered if any such reaction is not otherwise explicable. The oculomucocutaneous syndrome associated with the beta-blocker practolol has not been reported with metoprolol.

Potential Adverse Reactions: A variety of adverse reactions not listed above have been reported with other beta-adrenergic blocking agents and should be considered potential adverse reactions to Toprol-XL.

Central Nervous System—Reversible mental depression progressing to catatonia; an acute reversible syndrome characterized by disorientation for time and place, short-term memory loss, emotional lability, slightly clouded sensorium, and decreased performance on neuropsychometrics.

Cardiovascular—Intensification of AV block (see CONTRAINDICATIONS).

Hematologic—Agranulocytosis, nonthrombocytopenic purpura, thrombocytopenic purpura.

Hypersensitive Reactions—Fever combined with aching and sore throat, laryngospasm, and respiratory distress.

OVERDOSAGE

Acute Toxicity: There have been a few reports of overdosage with Toprol-XL and no specific overdosage information was obtained with this drug, with the exception of animal toxicology data. However, since Toprol-XL (metoprolol succinate salt) contains the same active moiety, metoprolol, as conventional metoprolol tablets (metoprolol tartrate salt), the recommendations on overdosage for metoprolol conventional tablets are applicable to Toprol-XL.

Signs and Symptoms: Potential signs and symptoms associated with overdosage with metoprolol are bradycardia, hypotension, bronchospasm, and cardiac failure.

Treatment: There is no specific antidote.

In general, patients with acute or recent myocardial infarction may be more hemodynamically unstable than other patients and should be treated accordingly. On the basis of the pharmacologic actions of metoprolol tartrate, the following general measures should be employed.

Elimination of the Drug—Gastric lavage should be performed.

Bradycardia—Atropine should be administered. If there is no response to vagal blockade, isoproterenol should be administered cautiously.

Hypotension—A vasopressor should be administered, e.g., levarterenol or dopamine.

Bronchospasm—A beta$_2$-stimulating agent and/or a theophylline derivative should be administered.

Cardiac Failure—A digitalis glycoside and diuretics should be administered. In shock resulting from inadequate cardiac contractility, administration of dobutamine, isoproterenol or glucagon may be considered.

DOSAGE AND ADMINISTRATION

Toprol-XL is an extended release tablet intended for once-a-day administration. When switching from immediate release metoprolol tablet to Toprol-XL, the same total daily dose of Toprol-XL should be used.

As with immediate release metoprolol, dosages of Toprol-XL should be individualized and titration may be needed in some patients.

Toprol-XL tablets are scored and can be divided; however, the whole or half tablet should be swallowed whole and not chewed or crushed.

Hypertension: The usual initial dosage is 50 to 100 mg daily in a single dose, whether used alone or added to a diuretic. The dosage may be increased at weekly (or longer) intervals until optimum blood pressure reduction is achieved. In general, the maximum effect of any given dosage level will be apparent after 1 week of therapy. Dosages above 400 mg per day have not been studied.

Angina Pectoris: The dosage of Toprol-XL should be individualized. The usual initial dosage is 100 mg daily, given in a single dose. The dosage may be gradually increased at weekly intervals until optimum clinical response has been obtained or there is a pronounced slowing of the heart rate. Dosages above 400 mg per day have not been studied. If treatment is to be discontinued, the dosage should be reduced gradually over a period of 1–2 weeks (see WARNINGS).

HOW SUPPLIED

Tablets 50 mg:
Contain 47.5 mg of metoprolol succinate equivalent to 50 mg of metoprolol tartrate, USP
Are white, biconvex, round, film-coated
Engraved A/mo on one side and scored on the other
Bottles of 100 NDC 0186-1090-05

Tablets 100 mg:
Contain 95 mg of metoprolol succinate equivalent to 100 mg of metoprolol tartrate, USP
Are white, biconvex, round, film-coated
Engraved A/ms on one side and scored on the other
Bottles of 100 NDC 0186-1092-05

Tablets 200 mg:
Contain 190 mg of metoprolol succinate equivalent to 200 mg of metoprolol tartrate, USP
Are white, biconvex, oval, film-coated
Engraved A/my and scored on one side
Bottles of 100 NDC 0186-1094-05

Store at controlled room temperature 15°-30°C (59°–86°F).

Manufactured by:
Astra Pharmaceutical Production, AB
Södertälje, Sweden
Manufactured for:
Astra USA, Inc., Westborough, MA 01581
021671R37 Rev. 4/98

Shown in Product Identification Guide, page 304

XYLOCAINE® (lidocaine HCl Injection, USP) ℞
[*zī 'lo-caine*]
XYLOCAINE®
(lidocaine HCl and epinephrine Injection, USP)
For Infiltration and Nerve Block

DESCRIPTION

Xylocaine (lidocaine HCl) Injections are sterile, non pyrogenic, aqueous solutions that contain a local anesthetic agent with or without epinephrine and are administered parenterally by injection. See INDICATIONS for specific uses.

Xylocaine solutions contain lidocaine HCl, which is chemically designated as acetamide, 2-(diethylamino)-N-(2,6-dimethylphenyl)-, monohydrochloride and has the molecular wt. 270.8. Lidocaine HCl ($C_{14}H_{22}N_2O{\bullet}HCl$) has the following structural formula:

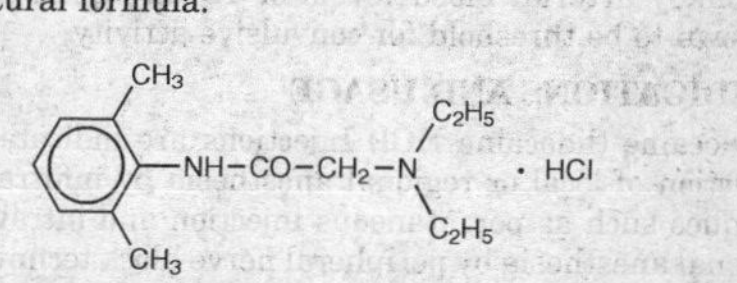

Epinephrine is (-) -3, 4-Dihydroxy-α-[(methylamino) methyl] benzyl alcohol and has the molecular wt. 183.21. Epinephrine ($C_9H_{13}NO_3$) has the following structural formula:

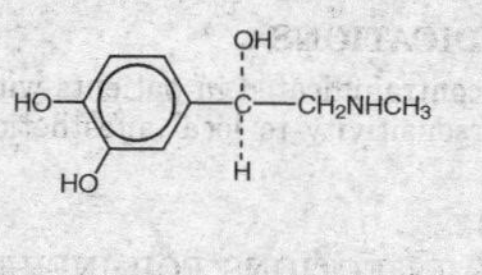

Continued on next page

Xylocaine—Cont.

Dosage forms listed as Xylocaine-MPF indicate single dose solutions that are Methyl Paraben Free (MPF).

Xylocaine MPF is a sterile, non pyrogenic, isotonic solution containing sodium chloride. Xylocaine in multiple dose vials, each mL also contains 1 mg methylparaben as antiseptic preservative. The pH of these solutions is adjusted to approximately 6.5 (5.0–7.0) with sodium hydroxide and/or hydrochloric acid.

Xylocaine MPF with Epinephrine is a sterile, non pyrogenic, isotonic solution containing sodium chloride. Each mL contains lidocaine hydrochloride and epinephrine, with 0.5 mg sodium metabisulfite as an antioxidant and 0.2 mg citric acid as a stabilizer. Xylocaine with Epinephrine in multiple dose vials, each mL also contains 1 mg methylparaben as antiseptic preservative. The pH of these solutions is adjusted to approximately 4.5 (3.3–5.5) with sodium hydroxide and/or hydrochloric acid. Filled under nitrogen.

CLINICAL PHARMACOLOGY

Mechanism of Action: Lidocaine stabilizes the neuronal membrane by inhibiting the ionic fluxes required for the initiation and conduction of impulses thereby effecting local anesthetic action.

Hemodynamics: Excessive blood levels may cause changes in cardiac output, total peripheral resistance, and mean arterial pressure. With central neural blockade these changes may be attributable to block of autonomic fibers, a direct depressant effect of the local anesthetic agent on various components of the cardiovascular system, and/or the beta-adrenergic receptor stimulating action of epinephrine when present. The net effect is normally a modest hypotension when the recommended dosages are not exceeded.

Pharmacokinetics and Metabolism: Information derived from diverse formulations, concentrations and usages reveals that lidocaine is completely absorbed following parenteral administration, its rate of absorption depending, for example, upon various factors such as the site of administration and the presence or absence of a vasoconstrictor agent. Except for intravascular administration, the highest blood levels are obtained following intercostal nerve block and the lowest after subcutaneous administration.

The plasma binding of lidocaine is dependent on drug concentration, and the fraction bound decreases with increasing concentration. At concentrations of 1 to 4 μg of free base per mL 60 to 80 percent of lidocaine is protein bound. Binding is also dependent on the plasma concentration of the alpha-1-acid glycoprotein.

Lidocaine crosses the blood-brain and placental barriers, presumably by passive diffusion.

Lidocaine is metabolized rapidly by the liver, and metabolites and unchanged drug are excreted by the kidneys. Biotransformation includes oxidative N-dealkylation, ring hydroxylation, cleavage of the amide linkage, and conjugation. N-dealkylation, a major pathway of biotransformation, yields the metabolites monoethylglycinexylidide and glycinexylidide. The pharmacological/toxicological actions of these metabolites are similar to, but less potent than, those of lidocaine. Approximately 90% of lidocaine administered is excreted in the form of various metabolites, and less than 10% is excreted unchanged. The primary metabolite in urine is a conjugate of 4-hydroxy-2,6-dimethylaniline.

The elimination half-life of lidocaine following an intravenous bolus injection is typically 1.5 to 2.0 hours. Because of the rapid rate at which lidocaine is metabolized, any condition that affects liver function may alter lidocaine kinetics. The half-life may be prolonged two-fold or more in patients with liver dysfunction. Renal dysfunction does not affect lidocaine kinetics but may increase the accumulation of metabolites.

Factors such as acidosis and the use of CNS stimulants and depressants affect the CNS levels of lidocaine required to produce overt systemic effects. Objective adverse manifestations become increasingly apparent with increasing venous plasma levels about 6.0 μg free base per mL. In the rhesus monkey arterial blood levels of 18–21 μg/mL have been shown to be threshold for convulsive activity.

INDICATIONS AND USAGE

Xylocaine (lidocaine HCl) Injections are indicated for production of local or regional anesthesia by infiltration techniques such as percutaneous injection and intravenous regional anesthesia by peripheral nerve block techniques such as brachial plexus and intercostal and by central neural techniques such as lumbar and caudal epidural blocks, when the accepted procedures for these techniques as described in standard textbooks are observed.

CONTRAINDICATIONS

Lidocaine is contraindicated in patients with a known history of hypersensitivity to local anesthetics of the amide type.

WARNINGS

XYLOCAINE INJECTIONS FOR INFILTRATION AND NERVE BLOCK SHOULD BE EMPLOYED ONLY BY CLINICIANS WHO ARE WELL VERSED IN DIAGNOSIS AND MANAGEMENT OF DOSE-RELATED TOXICITY AND OTHER ACUTE EMERGENCIES THAT MIGHT ARISE FROM THE BLOCK TO BE EMPLOYED AND THEN ONLY AFTER ENSURING THE *IMMEDIATE* AVAILABILITY OF OXYGEN, OTHER RESUSCITATIVE DRUGS, CARDIOPULMONARY EQUIPMENT AND THE PERSONNEL NEEDED FOR PROPER MANAGEMENT OF TOXIC REACTIONS AND RELATED EMERGENCIES. (See also ADVERSE REACTIONS and PRECAUTIONS.) DELAY IN PROPER MANAGEMENT OF DOSE-RELATED TOXICITY, UNDERVENTILATION FROM ANY CAUSE AND/OR ALTERED SENSITIVITY MAY LEAD TO THE DEVELOPMENT OF ACIDOSIS, CARDIAC ARREST AND, POSSIBLY, DEATH.

To avoid intravascular injection, aspiration should be performed before the local anesthetic solution is injected. The needle must be repositioned until no return of blood can be elicited by aspiration. Note, however, that the absence of blood in the syringe does not guarantee that intravascular injection has been avoided.

Local anesthetic solutions containing antimicrobial preservatives, (e.g., methylparaben) should not be used for epidural or spinal anesthesia because the safety of these agents has not been established with regard to intrathecal injection, either intentional or accidental.

Xylocaine with epinephrine solutions contain sodium metabisulfite, a sulfite that may cause allergic-type reactions including anaphylactic symptoms and life-threatening or less severe asthmatic episodes in certain susceptible people. The overall prevalence of sulfite sensitivity in the general population is unknown and probably low. Sulfite sensitivity is seen more frequently in asthmatic than in non-asthmatic people.

PRECAUTIONS

General: The safety and effectiveness of lidocaine depend on proper dosage, correct technique, adequate precautions, and readiness for emergencies. Standard textbooks should be consulted for specific techniques and precautions for various regional anesthetic procedures.

Resuscitative equipment, oxygen, and other resuscitative drugs should be available for immediate use. (See WARNINGS and ADVERSE REACTIONS.) The lowest dosage that results in effective anesthesia should be used to avoid high plasma levels and serious adverse effects. Syringe aspirations should also be performed before and during each supplemental injection when using indwelling catheter techniques. During the administration of epidural anesthesia, it is recommended that a test dose be administered initially and that the patient be monitored for central nervous system toxicity and cardiovascular toxicity, as well as for signs of unintended intrathecal administration, before proceeding. When clinical conditions permit, consideration should be given to employing local anesthetic solutions that contain epinephrine for the test dose because circulatory changes compatible with epinephrine may also serve as a warning sign of unintended intravascular injection. An intravascular injection is still possible even if aspirations for blood are negative. Repeated doses of lidocaine may cause significant increases in blood levels with each repeated dose because of slow accumulation of the drug or its metabolites. Tolerance to elevated blood levels varies with the status of the patient. Debilitated, elderly patients, acutely ill patients, and children should be given reduced doses commensurate with their age and physical condition. Lidocaine should also be used with caution in patients with severe shock or heart block.

Lumbar and caudal epidural anesthesia should be used with extreme caution in persons with the following conditions: existing neurological disease, spinal deformities, septicemia and severe hypertension.

Local anesthetic solutions containing a vasoconstrictor should be used cautiously and in carefully circumscribed quantities in areas of the body supplied by end arteries or having otherwise compromised blood supply. Patients with peripheral vascular disease and those with hypertensive vascular disease may exhibit exaggerated vasoconstrictor response. Ischemic injury or necrosis may result. Preparations containing a vasoconstrictor should be used with caution in patients during or following the administration of potent general anesthetic agents, since cardiac arrhythmias may occur under such conditions.

Careful and constant monitoring of cardiovascular and respiratory (adequacy of ventilation) vital signs and the patient's state of consciousness should be accomplished after each local anesthetic injection. It should be kept in mind at such times that restlessness, anxiety, tinnitus, dizziness, blurred vision, tremors, depression or drowsiness may be early warning signs of central nervous system toxicity.

Since amide-type local anesthetics are metabolized by the liver, Xylocaine injection should be used with caution in patients with hepatic disease. Patients with severe hepatic disease, because of their inability to metabolize local anesthetics normally, are at greater risk of developing toxic plasma concentrations. Xylocaine Injection should also be used with caution in patients with impaired cardiovascular function since they may be less able to compensate for functional changes associated with the prolongation of A-V conduction produced by these drugs.

Many drugs used during the conduct of anesthesia are considered potential triggering agents for familial malignant hyperthermia. Since it is not known whether amide-type local anesthetics may trigger this reaction and since the need for supplemental general anesthesia cannot be predicted in advance, it is suggested that a standard protocol for the management of malignant hyperthermia should be available. Early unexplained signs of tachycardia, tachypnea, labile blood pressure and metabolic acidosis may precede temperature elevation. Successful outcome is dependent on early diagnosis, prompt discontinuance of the suspect triggering agent(s) and institution of treatment, including oxygen therapy, indicated supportive measures and dantrolene (consult dantrolene sodium intravenous package insert before using).

Proper tourniquet technique, as described in publications and standard textbooks, is essential in the performance of intravenous regional anesthesia. Solutions containing epinephrine or other vasoconstrictors should not be used for this technique.

Lidocaine should be used with caution in persons with known drug sensitivities. Patients allergic to para-aminobenzoic acid derivatives (procaine, tetracaine, benzocaine, etc.) have not shown cross sensitivity to lidocaine.

Use in the Head and Neck Area: Small doses of local anesthetics injected into the head and neck area, including retrobulbar, dental and stellate ganglion blocks, may produce adverse reactions similar to systemic toxicity seen with unintentional intravascular injections of larger doses. Confusion, convulsions, respiratory depression and/or respiratory arrest, and cardiovascular stimulation or depression have been reported. These reactions may be due to intra-arterial injection of the local anesthetic with retrograde flow to the cerebral circulation. Patients receiving these blocks should have their circulation and respiration monitored and be constantly observed. Resuscitative equipment and personnel for treating adverse reactions should be immediately available. Dosage recommendations should not be exceeded. (See DOSAGE and ADMINISTRATION.)

Information for Patients: When appropriate, patients should be informed in advance that they may experience temporary loss of sensation and motor activity, usually in the lower half of the body, following proper administration of epidural anesthesia.

Clinically Significant Drug Interactions: The administration of local anesthetic solutions containing epinephrine or norepinephrine to patients receiving monoamine oxidase inhibitors or tricyclic antidepressants may produce severe, prolonged hypertension.

Phenothiazines and butyrophenones may reduce or reverse the pressor effect of epinephrine.

Concurrent use of these agents should generally be avoided. In situations when concurrent therapy is necessary, careful patient monitoring is essential.

Concurrent administration of vasopressor drugs (for the treatment of hypotension related to obstetric blocks) and ergot-type oxytocic drugs may cause severe, persistent hypertension or cerebrovascular accidents.

Drug/Laboratory Test Interactions: The intramuscular injection of lidocaine may result in an increase in creatine phosphokinase levels. Thus, the use of this enzyme determination, without isoenzyme separation, as a diagnostic test for the presence of acute myocardial infarction may be compromised by the intramuscular injection of lidocaine.

Carcinogenesis, Mutagenesis, Impairment of Fertility: Studies of lidocaine in animals to evaluate the carcinogenic and mutagenic potential or the effect on fertility have not been conducted.

Pregnancy: *Teratogenic Effects*—Pregnancy Category B. Reproduction studies have been performed in rats at doses up to 6.6 times the human dose and have revealed no evidence of harm to the fetus caused by lidocaine. There are, however, no adequate and well-controlled studies in pregnant women. Animal reproduction studies are not always predictive of human response. General consideration should be given to this fact before administering lidocaine to women of childbearing potential, especially during early pregnancy when maximum organogenesis takes place.

Labor and Delivery: Local anesthetics rapidly cross the placenta and when used for epidural, paracervical, pudendal or caudal block anesthesia, can cause varying degrees of maternal, fetal and neonatal toxicity. (see CLINICAL PHARMACOLOGY, Pharmacokinetics.) The potential for toxicity depends upon the procedure performed, the type and amount of drug used, and the technique of drug administration. Adverse reactions in the parturient, fetus and neonate involve alterations of the central nervous system, peripheral vascular tone and cardiac function.

Maternal hypotension has resulted from regional anesthesia. Local anesthetics produce vasodilation by blocking sympathetic nerves. Elevating the patient's legs and positioning her on her left side will help prevent decreases in blood pressure.

The fetal heart rate also should be monitored continuously, and electronic fetal monitoring is highly advisable.

Epidural, spinal, paracervical, or pudendal anesthesia may alter the forces of parturition through changes in uterine contractility or maternal expulsive efforts. In one study, paracervical block anesthesia was associated with a decrease in the mean duration of first stage labor and facilitation of cervical dilation. However, spinal and epidural anesthesia have also been reported to prolong the second stage of labor by removing the parturient's reflex urge to bear down or by interfering with motor function. The use of obstetrical anesthesia may increase the need for forceps assistance.

The use of some local anesthetic drug products during labor and delivery may be followed by diminished muscle strength and tone for the first day or two of life. The long-term significance of these observations is unknown. Fetal bradycardia may occur in 20 to 30 percent of patients receiving paracervical nerve block anesthesia with the amide-type local anesthetics and may be associated with fetal acidosis. Fetal heart rate should always be monitored during paracervical anesthesia. The physician should weigh the possible advantages against risks when considering a paracervical block in prematurity, toxemia of pregnancy, and fetal distress. Careful adherence to recommended dosage is of the utmost importance in obstetrical paracervical block. Failure to achieve adequate analgesia with recommended doses should arouse suspicion of intravascular or fetal intracranial injection. Cases compatible with unintended fetal intracranial injection of local anesthetic solution have been reported following intended paracervical or pudendal block or both. Babies so affected present with unexplained neonatal depression at birth, which correlates with high local anesthetic serum levels, and often manifest seizures within six hours. Prompt use of supportive measures combined with forced urinary excretion of the local anesthetic has been used successfully to manage this complication.

Case reports of maternal convulsions and cardiovascular collapse following use of some local anesthetics for paracervical block in early pregnancy (as anesthesia for elective abortion) suggest that systemic absorption under these circumstances may be rapid. The recommended maximum dose of each drug should not be exceeded. Injection should be made slowly and with frequent aspiration. Allow a 5-minute interval between sides.

Nursing Mothers: It is not known whether this drug is excreted in human milk. Because many drugs are excreted in human milk, caution should be exercised when lidocaine is administered to a nursing woman.

Pediatric Use: Dosages in children should be reduced, commensurate with age, body weight and physical condition. See DOSAGE AND ADMINISTRATION.

ADVERSE REACTIONS

Systemic: Adverse experiences following the administration of lidocaine are similar in nature to those observed with other amide local anesthetic agents. These adverse experiences are, in general, dose-related and may result from high plasma levels caused by excessive dosage, rapid absorption or inadvertent intravascular injection, or may result from a hypersensitivity, idiosyncrasy or diminished tolerance on the part of the patient. Serious adverse experiences are generally systemic in nature. The following types are those most commonly reported:

Central Nervous System: CNS manifestations are excitatory and/or depressant and may be characterized by lightheadedness, nervousness, apprehension, euphoria, confusion, dizziness, drowsiness, tinnitus, blurred or double vision, vomiting, sensations of heat, cold or numbness, twitching, tremors, convulsions, unconsciousness, respiratory depression and arrest. The excitatory manifestations may be very brief or may not occur at all, in which case the first manifestation of toxicity may be drowsiness merging into unconsciousness and respiratory arrest.

Drowsiness following the administration of lidocaine is usually an early sign of a high blood level of the drug and may occur as a consequence of rapid absorption.

Cardiovascular System: Cardiovascular manifestations are usually depressant and are characterized by bradycardia, hypotension, and cardiovascular collapse, which may lead to cardiac arrest.

Allergic: Allergic reactions are characterized by cutaneous lesions, urticaria, edema or anaphylactoid reactions. Allergic reactions may occur as a result of sensitivity either to local anesthetic agents or to the methylparaben used as a preservative in the multiple dose vials. Allergic reactions as a result of sensitivity to lidocaine are extremely rare and, if they occur, should be managed by conventional means. The detection of sensitivity by skin testing is of doubtful value.

Neurologic: The incidences of adverse reactions associated with the use of local anesthetics may be related to the total dose of local anesthetic administered and are also dependent upon the particular drug used, the route of administration and the physical status of the patient. In a prospective review of 10,440 patients who received lidocaine for spinal anesthesia, the incidences of adverse reactions were reported to be about 3 percent each for positional headaches, hypotension and backache; 2 percent for shivering; and less than 1 percent each for peripheral nerve symptoms, nausea, respiratory inadequacy and double vision. Many of these observations may be related to local anesthetic techniques, with or without a contribution from the local anesthetic.

In the practice of caudal or lumbar epidural block, occasional unintentional penetration of the subarachnoid space by the catheter may occur. Subsequent adverse effects may depend partially on the amount of drug administered subdurally. These may include spinal block of varying magnitude (including total spinal block), hypotension secondary to spinal block, loss of bladder and bowel control, and loss of perineal sensation and sexual function. Persistent motor, sensory and/or autonomic (sphincter control) deficit of some lower spinal segments with slow recovery (several months) or incomplete recovery have been reported in rare instances when caudal or lumbar epidural block has been attempted. Backache and headache have also been noted following use of these anesthetic procedures.

There have been reported cases of permanent injury to extraocular muscles requiring surgical repair following retrobulbar administration.

OVERDOSAGE

Acute emergencies from local anesthetics are generally related to high plasma levels encountered during therapeutic use of local anesthetics or to unintended subarachnoid injection of local anesthetic solution (see ADVERSE REACTIONS, WARNINGS, and PRECAUTIONS).

Management of Local Anesthetic Emergencies: The first consideration is prevention, best accomplished by careful and constant monitoring of cardiovascular and respiratory vital signs and the patient's state of consciousness after each local anesthetic injection. At the first sign of change, oxygen should be administered.

The first step in the management of convulsions, as well as underventilation or apnea due to unintended subarachnoid injection of drug solution, consists of immediate attention to the maintenance of a patent airway and assisted or controlled ventilation with oxygen and a delivery system capable of permitting immediate positive airway pressure by mask. Immediately after the institution of these ventilatory measures, the adequacy of the circulation should be evaluated, keeping in mind that drugs used to treat convulsions sometimes depress the circulation when administered intravenously. Should convulsions persist despite adequate respiratory support, and if the status of the circulation permits, small increments of an ultra-short acting barbiturate (such as thiopental or thiamylal) or a benzodiazepine (such as diazepam) may be administered intravenously. The clinician should be familiar, prior to the use of local anesthetics, with these anticonvulsant drugs. Supportive treatment of circulatory depression may require administration of intravenous fluids and, when appropriate, a vasopressor as directed by the clinical situation (e.g., ephedrine).

If not treated immediately, both convulsions and cardiovascular depression can result in hypoxia, acidosis, bradycardia, arrhythmias and cardiac arrest. Underventilation or apnea due to unintentional subarachnoid injection of local anesthetic solution may produce these same signs and also lead to cardiac arrest if ventilatory support is not instituted. If cardiac arrest should occur, standard cardiopulmonary resuscitative measures should be instituted.

Endotracheal intubation, employing drugs and techniques familiar to the clinician, may be indicated, after initial administration of oxygen by mask, if difficulty is encountered in the maintenance of a patent airway or if prolonged ventilatory support (assisted or controlled) is indicated.

Dialysis is of negligible value in the treatment of acute overdosage with lidocaine.

The oral LD_{50} of lidocaine HCl in non-fasted female rats is 459 (346–773) mg/kg (as the salt) and 214 (159–324) mg/kg (as the salt) in fasted female rats.

DOSAGE AND ADMINISTRATION

Table 1 (Recommended Dosages) summarizes the recommended volumes and concentrations of Xylocaine Injection for various types of anesthetic procedures. The dosages suggested in this table are for normal healthy adults and refer to the use of epinephrine-free solutions. When larger volumes are required, only solutions containing epinephrine should be used except in those cases where vasopressor drugs may be contraindicated.

These recommended doses serve only as a guide to the amount of anesthetic required for most routine procedures. The actual volumes and concentrations to be used depend on a number of factors such as type and extent of surgical procedure, depth of anesthesia and degree of muscular relaxation required, duration of anesthesia required, and the physical condition of the patient. In all cases the lowest concentration and smallest dose that will produce the desired result should be given. Dosages should be reduced for children and for the elderly and debilitated patients and patients with cardiac and/or liver disease.

The onset of anesthesia, the duration of anesthesia and the degree of muscular relaxation are proportional to the volume and concentration (i.e., total dose) of local anesthetic used. Thus, an increase in volume and concentration of Xylocaine Injection will decrease the onset of anesthesia, prolong the duration of anesthesia, provide a greater degree of muscular relaxation and increase the segmental spread of anesthesia. However, increasing the volume and concentration of Xylocaine Injection may result in a more profound fall in blood pressure when used in epidural anesthesia. Although the incidence of side effects with lidocaine is quite low, caution should be exercised when employing large volumes and concentrations, since the incidence of side effects is directly proportional to the total dose of local anesthetic agent injected.

For intravenous regional anesthesia, only the 50 mL single dose vial containing Xylocaine (lidocaine HCl) 0.5% Injection should be used.

Epidural Anesthesia

For epidural anesthesia, only the following dosage forms of Xylocaine Injection are recommended:

1% without epinephrine	10 mL Polyamp DuoFit™
1% without epinephrine	20 mL Polyamp DuoFit™
1% without epinephrine	30 mL single dose solutions
1% with epinephrine 1:200,000	30 mL single dose solutions
1.5% without epinephrine	10 mL Polyamp DuoFit™
1.5% without epinephrine	20 mL Polyamp DuoFit™
1.5% without epinephrine	20 mL ampules, 20 mL single dose solutions
1.5% with epinephrine 1:200,000	30 mL ampules, 30 mL single dose solutions
2% without epinephrine	10 mL Polyamp DuoFit™
2% without epinephrine	10 mL ampules, 10 mL single dose solutions
2% with epinephrine 1:200,000	20 mL ampules, 20 mL single dose solutions

Although these solutions are intended specifically for epidural anesthesia, they may also be used for infiltration and peripheral nerve block, provided they are employed as single dose units. These solutions contain no bacteriostatic agent.

In epidural anesthesia, the dosage varies with the number of dermatomes to be anesthetized (generally 2–3 mL of the indicated concentration per dermatome).

Caudal and Lumbar Epidural Block: As a precaution against the adverse experience sometimes observed following unintentional penetration of the subarachnoid space, a test dose such as 2–3 mL of 1.5% lidocaine should be administered at least 5 minutes prior to injecting the total volume required for a lumbar or caudal epidural block. The test dose should be repeated if the patient is moved in a manner that may have displaced the catheter. Epinephrine, if contained in the test dose, (10–15 μg have been suggested), may serve as a warning of unintentional intravascular injection. If injected into a blood vessel, this amount of epinephrine is likely to produce a transient "epinephrine response" within 45 seconds, consisting of an increase in heart rate and systolic blood pressure, circumoral pallor, palpitations and nervousness in the unsedated patient. The sedated patient may exhibit only a pulse rate increase of 20 or more beats per minute for 15 or more seconds. Patients on beta blockers may not manifest changes in heart rate, but blood pressure monitoring can detect an evanescent rise in systolic blood pressure. Adequate time should be allowed for onset of anesthesia after administration of each test dose. The rapid injection of a large volume of Xylocaine Injection through the catheter should be avoided, and, when feasible, fractional doses should be administered.

In the event of the known injection of a large volume of local anesthetic solution into the subarachnoid space, after suitable resuscitation and if the catheter is in place, consider attempting the recovery of drug by draining a moderate amount of cerebrospinal fluid (such as 10 mL) through the epidural catheter.

MAXIMUM RECOMMENDED DOSAGES

Adults

For normal healthy adults, the individual maximum recommended dose of lidocaine HCl with epinephrine should not exceed 7 mg/kg (3.5 mg/lb) of body weight, and in general it is recommended that the maximum total dose not exceed 500 mg. When used without epinephrine the maximum in-

Continued on next page

Xylocaine—Cont.

dividual dose should not exceed 4.5 mg/kg (2 mg/lb) of body weight, and in general it is recommended that the maximum total dose does not exceed 300 mg. For continuous epidural or caudal anesthesia, the maximum recommended dosage should not be administered at intervals of less than 90 minutes. When continuous lumbar or caudal epidural anesthesia is used for non-obstetrical procedures, more drug may be administered if required to produce adequate anesthesia.

The maximum recommended dose per 90 minute period of lidocaine hydrochloride for paracervical block in obstetrical patients and non-obstetrical patients is 200 mg total. One half of the total dose is usually administered to each side. Inject slowly, five minutes between sides. (See also discussion of paracervical block in PRECAUTIONS.)

For intravenous regional anesthesia, the dose administered should not exceed 4 mg/kg in adults.

Children

It is difficult to recommend a maximum dose of any drug for children, since this varies as a function of age and weight. For children over 3 years of age who have a normal lean body mass and normal body development, the maximum dose is determined by the child's age and weight. For example, in a child of 5 years weighing 50 lbs the dose of lidocaine HCl should not exceed 75–100 mg (1.5–2 mg/lb). The use of even more dilute solutions (i.e., 0.25–0.5%) and total dosages not to exceed 3 mg/kg (1.4 mg/lb) are recommended for induction of intravenous regional anesthesia in children.

In order to guard against systemic toxicity, the lowest effective concentration and lowest effective dose should be used at all times. In some cases it will be necessary to dilute available concentrations with 0.9% sodium chloride injection in order to obtain the required final concentration.

NOTE: Parenteral drug products should be inspected visually for particulate matter and discoloration prior to administration whenever the solution and container permit. The injection is not to be used if its color is pinkish or darker than slightly yellow or if it contains a precipitate.

Table 1. Recommended Dosages

Procedure	Xylocaine (lidocaine hydrochloride) Injection (without epinephrine)		
	Conc (%)	Vol (mL)	Total Dose (mg)
Infiltration			
Percutaneous	0.5 or 1	1–60	5–300
Intravenous regional	0.5	10–60	50–300
Peripheral Nerve Blocks, e.g.			
Brachial	1.5	15–20	225–300
Dental	2	1–5	20–100
Intercostal	1	3	30
Paravertebral	1	3–5	30–50
Pudendal (each side)	1	10	100
Paracervical			
Obstetrical analgesia (each side)	1	10	100
Sympathetic Nerve Blocks, e.g.			
Cervical (stellate ganglion)	1	5	50
Lumbar	1	5–10	50–100
Central Neural Blocks			
Epidural*			
Thoracic	1	20–30	200–300
Lumbar			
Analgesia	1	25–30	250–300
Anesthesia	1.5	15–20	225–300
	2	10–15	200–300
Caudal			
Obstetrical analgesia	1	20–30	200–300
Surgical anesthesia	1.5	15–20	225–300

* Dose determined by number of dermatomes to be anesthetized (2–3 mL/dermatome).

THE ABOVE SUGGESTED CONCENTRATIONS AND VOLUMES SERVE ONLY AS A GUIDE. OTHER VOLUMES AND CONCENTRATIONS MAY BE USED PROVIDED THE TOTAL MAXIMUM RECOMMENDED DOSE IS NOT EXCEEDED.

STERILIZATION, STORAGE AND TECHNICAL PROCEDURES

Disinfecting agents containing heavy metals, which cause release of respective ions (mercury, zinc, copper, etc.) should not be used for skin or mucous membrane disinfection as they have been related to incidents of swelling and edema. When chemical disinfection of multi-dose vials is desired, either isopropyl alcohol (91%) or ethyl alcohol (70%) is recommended. Many commercially available brands of rubbing alcohol, as well as solutions of ethyl alcohol not of U.S.P. grade, contain denaturants which are injurious to rubber and therefore are not to be used.

Dosage forms listed as Xylocaine-MPF indicate single dose solutions that are Methyl Paraben Free (MPF).

[See table at bottom of page]

All solutions should be stored at room temperature, approximately 25°C (77°F).

Protect from light.

002201R00   Iss. 6/98

Shown in Product Identification Guide, page 305

XYLOCAINE® ℞
[zī 'lo-caine]
(lidocaine HCl Injection, USP)
For Ventricular Arrhythmias

(For details of indications, dosage and administration, precautions, and adverse reactions, see circular in package.)

DESCRIPTION

Xylocaine (lidocaine HCl Injection, USP) is a sterile non pyrogenic solution of an antiarrhythmic agent administered intravenously by either direct injection or continuous infusion.

Xylocaine Injections are composed of aqueous solutions of lidocaine hydrochloride. Lidocaine HCl ($C_{14}H_{22}N_2O \cdot HCl$) is chemically designated acetamide, 2-(diethylamino)-N-(2,6 dimethylphenyl)-, monohydrochloride.

HOW SUPPLIED

For direct intravenous injection, Xylocaine (lidocaine HCl Injection, USP) without preservatives is supplied in the following dosage forms:

NDC 0186-0615-01	50 mg	5 mL Prefilled Syringe with a 21G 15/16″ Needle
NDC 0186-0611-01	100 mg	5 mL Prefilled Syringe with a 21G 15/16″ Needle
NDC 0186-0232-03	100 mg	5 mL Ampule

For preparing solutions for intravenous infusions, Xylocaine (lidocaine HCl Injection, USP) without sodium chloride or preservatives is supplied in the following dosage forms:

NDC 0186-0166-01	1 gram	25 mL Single Use Vial without transfer unit
NDC 0186-0169-01	2 grams	50 mL Single Use Vial without transfer unit
NDC 0186-0167-01	1 gram	25 mL Single Use Vial with presterilized transfer unit
NDC 0186-0168-01	2 grams	50 mL Single Use Vial with presterilized transfer unit

Solutions should be stored at controlled room temperature 15°–30°C (59°–86°F).

021679R03   Rev. 6/97

4% XYLOCAINE®-MPF (lidocaine HCl) ℞
[zī 'lo-caine]
Sterile Solution

(For details of indications, dosage and administration, precautions, and adverse reactions, see circular in package.)

DESCRIPTION

4% Xylocaine-MPF (lidocaine HCl) Sterile Solution (Methylparaben Free) contains a local anesthetic agent and is administered topically or by injection. See INDICATIONS for specific uses.

4% Xylocaine-MPF Sterile Solution contains lidocaine HCl, which is chemically designated as acetamide, 2-(diethylamino)-N-(2,6-dimethylphenyl)-mono-hydrochloride.

4% Xylocaine-MPF Sterile Solution in 5 mL ampules may be autoclaved repeatedly if necessary.

Composition of 4% Xylocaine-MPF Sterile Solution Each mL contains lidocaine HCl, 40.0 mg, and sodium hydroxide and/or hydrochloric acid to adjust pH to 5.0–7.0. A sterile, aqueous solution.

HOW SUPPLIED

4% Xylocaine-MPF (lidocaine HCl) Sterile Solution, 5 mL ampule (NDC 0186-0235-03) and 5 mL prefilled sterile disposable syringe packaged in a presterilized kit containing a laryngotracheal cannula (NDC 0186-0235-72).

Store at controlled room temperature: 15°–30°C (59°–86°F).

021562R09   Rev. 2/97

4% XYLOCAINE® (lidocaine HCl) ℞
[zī 'lo-caine]
TOPICAL SOLUTION

(For details of indications, dosage and administration, precautions, and adverse reactions, see circular in package.)

DESCRIPTION

Xylocaine (lidocaine HCl) 4% Topical Solution contains a local anesthetic agent and is administered topically. See INDICATIONS for specific uses.

Xylocaine 4% Topical Solution contains lidocaine HCl, which is chemically designated as acetamide, 2-(diethylamino)-N-(2, 6-dimethylphenyl)-, monohydrochloride.

The 50 mL screw-cap bottle should not be autoclaved, because the closure employed cannot withstand autoclaving temperatures and pressures. Composition of Xylocaine (lidocaine HCl) 4% Topical Solution: Each mL contains lidocaine HCl, 40 mg, methylparaben, and sodium hydroxide and/or hydrochloric acid to adjust pH to 6.0 – 7.0. An aqueous solution. NOT FOR INJECTION.

HOW SUPPLIED

Xylocaine (lidocaine HCl) 4% Topical Solution 50 mL screw-cap bottle, cartoned (NDC 0186-0320-01). NOT FOR INJECTION.

Store at controlled room temperature 15°-30°C (59°-86°F).

021708R00   Rev. 4/97

1.5% XYLOCAINE®-MPF ℞
with Dextrose 7.5% Injection
(lidocaine HCl and dextrose anhydrous Injection)
For Spinal Anesthesia in Obstetrics.

(For details of indications, dosage and administration, precautions, and adverse reactions, see circular in package.)

HOW SUPPLIED

Xylocaine (lidocaine HCl) Concentration	Epinephrine Dilution (if present)	Xylocaine-MPF													Xylocaine		
		Ampules (mL)					Polyamp DuoFit™ (mL)		Single Dose Vial (mL)						Multiple Dose Vial (mL)		
		2	5	10	20	30	10	20	2	5	10	20	30	50	10	20	50
0.5%														X			X
0.5%	1:200,000																X
1%		X	X			X	X	X	X	X	X				X	X	X
1%	1:100,000														X	X	X
1%	1:200,000					X				X	X						
1.5%					X		X	X	X	X							
1.5%	1:200,000		X			X				X	X						
2%		X		X			X	X	X	X	X				X	X	X
2%	1:100,000														X	X	X
2%	1:200,000				X				X	X	X						

HOW SUPPLIED

Xylocaine-MPF 1.5% with Dextrose 7.5% Injection (lidocaine HCl and dextrose anhydrous Injection), NDC 0186-0212-03, is supplied in 2 mL ampules in packages of 10. Store at controlled room temperature 15°–30°C (59°–86°F).

021836R09   Rev. 9/97

5% XYLOCAINE®-MPF
With Glucose 7.5% Injection   ℞
[zī 'lo-cain]
(lidocaine HCl and dextrose anhydrous Injection)

(For details of indications, dosage and administration, precautions, and adverse reactions, see circular in package.)

HOW SUPPLIED

Xylocaine-MPF 5% with Glucose 7.5% Injection (lidocaine HCl and dextrose anhydrous Injection), NDC 0186-0225-03, is supplied in 2 mL ampules in packages of 10. Store at controlled room temperature 15°–30°C (59°–86°F).

021564R14   Rev. 9/97

XYLOCAINE® 2% Jelly (lidocaine hydrochloride)   ℞
[zī 'lo-caine]

(For details of indications, dosage and administration, precautions, and adverse reactions, see circular in package.)

DESCRIPTION

Xylocaine (lidocaine HCl) 2% Jelly is a sterile aqueous product that contains a local anesthetic agent and is administered topically. (See INDICATIONS for specific uses.)
Xylocaine 2% Jelly contains lidocaine HCl which is chemically designated as acetamide, 2-(diethylamino)-N-(2,-6-dimethylphenyl)-, monohydrochloride.
Xylocaine 2% Jelly also contains hydroxypropylmethylcellulose, and the resulting mixture maximizes contact with mucosa and provides lubrication for instrumentation. The unused portion should be discarded after initial use.
Composition of Xylocaine 2% Jelly (30 mL and 5 mL tubes): Each mL contains 20 mg of lidocaine HCl. The formulation also contains methylparaben, propylparaben, hydroxypropylmethylcellulose, and sodium hydroxide and/or hydrochloric acid to adjust pH to 6.0–7.0.
Composition of Xylocaine 2% Jelly (10 mL and 20 mL syringes): Each mL contains 20 mg of lidocaine HCl. The formulation also contains hydroxypropylmethylcellulose, and sodium hydroxide and/or hydrochloric acid to adjust pH to 6.2–6.8.

HOW SUPPLIED

Xylocaine (lidocaine HCl) 2% Jelly is supplied in the listed dosage forms.
NDC 0186-0330-01, 30 mL aluminum tube, Box of 1.
A detachable applicator cone and a key for expressing the contents are included.
NDC 0186-0330-36 5 mL plastic tube, Box of 10
NDC 0186-0330-43 10 mL polypropylene syringe, Box of 10
NDC 0186-0330-53 20 mL polypropylene syringe, Box of 10
Store at controlled room temperature 20°–25°C (68°–77°F) [see USP].
Xylocaine Jelly Syringes are manufactured by Astra Production Liquid Products AB, Kariskoga, Sweden.

000807R03   Iss. 5/98

Shown in Product Identification Guide, page 305

5% XYLOCAINE® OINTMENT (lidocaine)   ℞
[zī 'lo-caine]

(For details of indications, dosage and administration, precautions, and adverse reactions, see circular in package.)

DESCRIPTION

Xylocaine (lidocaine) 5% Ointment contains a local anesthetic agent and is administered topically. See INDICATIONS for specific uses.
Xylocaine 5% Ointment contains lidocaine, which is chemically designated as acetamide, 2-(diethylamino)-N-(2,6-dimethylphenyl)-.
Composition of Xylocaine 5% Ointment:
Each gram of the plain and flavored ointments contains lidocaine, 50 mg, polyethylene glycol 540 blend, polyethylene glycol 3350 and propylene glycol. The flavored ointment contains sodium saccharin, peppermint oil and spearmint oil.

HOW SUPPLIED

Xylocaine (lidocaine) 5% Ointment (NDC 0186-0315-21) is available in 35 gm tubes.
Xylocaine (lidocaine) 5% Ointment Flavored for application within the oral cavity, is dispensed in 3.5 gram tubes, 10 tubes per carton (NDC 0186-0350-03), and in 35-gram jars (NDC 0186-0350-01).

KEEP CONTAINER TIGHTLY CLOSED AT ALL TIMES WHEN NOT IN USE.
Store at controlled room temperature 15°–30°C (59°–86°F).

021563R00   Rev. 5/97

XYLOCAINE ® 2.5% OINTMENT (lidocaine)   OTC
[zī 'lo-cain]

(See PDR For Nonprescription Drugs.)

10% XYLOCAINE® Oral Spray (lidocaine)   ℞
[zī 'lo-caine]
Flavored Topical Anesthetic Aerosol
For Use In The Oral Cavity

WARNING—CONTENTS UNDER PRESSURE

(For details of indications, dosage and administration, precautions, and adverse reactions, see circular in package.)

DESCRIPTION

Xylocaine (lidocaine) 10% Oral Spray contains a local anesthetic agent and is administered topically in the oral cavity. See INDICATIONS for specific uses.
Xylocaine 10% Oral Spray contains lidocaine, which is chemically designated as acetamide, 2-(diethylamino)-N-(2,6-dimethylphenyl)-.
Composition of Xylocaine (lidocaine) 10% Oral Spray:
Each actuation of the metered dose valve delivers a solution containing lidocaine, 10 mg, cetylpyridinium chloride, absolute alcohol, saccharin, flavor, and polyethylene glycol.
And as propellants: trichlorofluoromethane/dichlorodifluoromethane (65%/35%).

WARNING: Contains trichlorofluoromethane and dichlorodifluoromethane, substances which harm public health and environment by destroying ozone in the upper atmosphere.

HOW SUPPLIED

NDC 0186-0356-01:   A 26.8 mL aerosol container provides a total amount of 3.3 g (w/w) of the active ingredient lidocaine. Each actuation of the metered dose valve delivers 10 mg of lidocaine.
Contents under pressure. Do not puncture or incinerate container. Do not expose to heat or store at temperatures above 120°F. Avoid contact with the eyes. Inhalation and swallowing should be avoided.
Keep out of the reach of children.
Use only as directed; intentional misuse by deliberately concentrating and inhaling the contents can be harmful or fatal.
STORE AT CONTROLLED ROOM TEMPERATURE 15°–30°C (59°–86°F).
Manufactured by Armstrong Laboratories, Inc., West Roxbury, MA 02132.
Manufactured for Astra USA, Inc., Westborough, MA 01581
A flexible, disposable Cannula, 9035-05, is available in boxes of 50, to provide directed spray for easier access to oropharynx.

021731R31   11/93(31)

2% XYLOCAINE® Viscous   ℞
(lidocaine hydrochloride) Solution
[zī 'lo-caine]
A Topical Anesthetic for the Mucous
Membranes of the Mouth and Pharynx

(For details of indications, dosage and administration, precautions, and adverse reactions, see circular in package.)

DESCRIPTION

Xylocaine (lidocaine HCl) 2% Viscous Solution contains a local anesthetic agent and is administered topically. Xylocaine 2% Viscous Solution contains lidocaine HCl, which is chemically designated as acetamide, 2-(diethylamino)-N-(2,6-dimethylphenyl)-, monohydrochloride.
The molecular formula of lidocaine is $C_{14}H_{22}N_2O$. The molecular weight is 234.34.

HOW SUPPLIED

Xylocaine (lidocaine HCl) 2% Viscous Solution is available in 100 mL (NDC 0186-0360-01) and 450 mL (NDC 0186-0360-11) polyethylene squeeze bottles and in unit of use (adult dose) packages of 25 (20 mL) polyethylene bottles (NDC 0186-0361-78).
The solutions should be stored at controlled room temperature 15°–30°C (59°–86°F).

021899R02   4/94 (2)

Astra USA, Inc.
See Astra Pharmaceuticals, L.P.

Athena Neurosciences, Inc.
**800 GATEWAY BOULEVARD
SOUTH SAN FRANCISCO, CA 94080**

For Medical Information or To Report Adverse Events Contact:
888-NEURO-05
(888-63876-05)

ATAMET®   ℞
CARBIDOPA AND LEVODOPA TABLETS, USP

DESCRIPTION

When Carbidopa and Levodopa Tablets are to be given to patients who are being treated with levodopa, levodopa must be discontinued at least eight hours before therapy with this combination product is started. In order to reduce adverse reactions, it is necessary to individualize therapy. See the WARNINGS and DOSAGE AND ADMINISTRATION sections before initiating therapy.
Carbidopa, an inhibitor of aromatic amino acid decarboxylation, is a white, crystalline compound, slightly soluble in water. It is designated chemically as (−)-L-α-hydrazino-α-methyl-β-(3, 4-dihydroxybenzene) propanoic acid monohydrate, and has the following structural formula:

$C_{10}H_{14}N_2O_4 \cdot H_2O$ M.W. 244.25
Tablet content is expressed in terms of anhydrous carbidopa which has a molecular weight of 226.23.
Levodopa, an aromatic amino acid, is a white, crystalline compound, slightly soluble in water. It is designated chemically as (−)-L-α-amino-β-(3,4-dihydroxybenzene) propanoic acid, and has the following structural formula:

$C_9H_{11}NO_4$ M.W. 197.2
Carbidopa and Levodopa is supplied as tablets in two strengths:
Carbidopa and Levodopa Tablets 25 mg/100 mg, containing 25 mg of carbidopa and 100 mg of levodopa.
Carbidopa and Levodopa Tablets 25 mg/250 mg, containing 25 mg of carbidopa and 250 mg of levodopa.
Inactive ingredients are magnesium stearate, microcrystalline cellulose, pregelatinized starch, and corn starch. Carbidopa and Levodopa Tablets 25 mg/250 mg also contain FD&C Blue 2. Carbidopa and Levodopa Tablets 25 mg/100 mg contain D&C Yellow 10 and FD&C Yellow 6.

CLINICAL PHARMACOLOGY

Current evidence indicates that symptoms of Parkinson's disease are related to depletion of dopamine in the corpus striatum. Administration of dopamine is ineffective in the treatment of Parkinson's disease apparently because it does not cross the blood-brain barrier. However, levodopa, the metabolic precursor of dopamine, does cross the blood-brain barrier, and presumably is converted to dopamine in the basal ganglia. This is thought to be the mechanism whereby levodopa relieves symptoms of Parkinson's disease.
When levodopa is administered orally it is rapidly converted to dopamine in extracerebral tissues so that only a small portion of a given dose is transported unchanged to the central nervous system. For this reason, large doses of levodopa are required for adequate therapeutic effect and these may often be attended by nausea and other adverse reactions, some of which are attributable to dopamine formed in extracerebral tissues.
Since levodopa competes with certain amino acids, the absorption of levodopa may be impaired in some patients on a high protein diet.
Carbidopa inhibits decarboxylation of peripheral levodopa. It does not cross the blood-brain barrier and does not affect the metabolism of levodopa within the central nervous system.
Since its decarboxylase inhibiting activity is limited to extracerebral tissues, administration of carbidopa with levodopa makes more levodopa available for transport to the brain. In dogs, reduced formation of dopamine in extra-

Continued on next page

Atamet—Cont.

cerebral tissues, such as the heart, provides protection against the development of dopamine-induced cardiac arrhythmias. Clinical studies tend to support the hypothesis of a similar protective effect in humans although controlled data are too limited at the present time to draw firm conclusions.

Carbidopa reduces the amount of levodopa required by about 75 percent and, when administered with levodopa, increases both plasma levels and the plasma half-life of levodopa, and decreases plasma and urinary dopamine and homovanillic acid.

In clinical pharmacologic studies, simultaneous administration of carbidopa and levodopa produced greater urinary excretion of levodopa in proportion to the excretion of dopamine than administration of the two drugs at separate times.

Pyridoxine hydrochloride (vitamin B_6), in oral doses of 10 mg to 25 mg, may reverse the effects of levodopa by increasing the rate of aromatic amino acid decarboxylation. Carbidopa inhibits this action of pyridoxine.

INDICATIONS AND USAGE

Carbidopa and levodopa tablets are indicated in the treatment of the symptoms of idiopathic Parkinson's disease (paralysis agitans), postencephalitic parkinsonism, and symptomatic parkinsonism which may follow injury to the nervous system by carbon monoxide intoxication and manganese intoxication. This product is indicated in these conditions to permit the administration of lower doses of levodopa with reduced nausea and vomiting, with more rapid dosage titration, with a somewhat smoother response, and with supplemental pyridoxine (vitamin B_6).

The incidence of levodopa-induced nausea and vomiting is less with this combination product than with levodopa. In many patients this reduction in nausea and vomiting will permit more rapid dosage titration.

In some patients a somewhat smoother antiparkinsonian effect results from therapy with carbidopa and levodopa than with levodopa. However, patients with markedly irregular ("on-off") responses to levodopa have not been shown to benefit from carbidopa and levodopa therapy.

Since carbidopa prevents the reversal of levodopa effects caused by pyridoxine, carbidopa and levodopa can be given to patients receiving supplemental pyridoxine (vitamin B_6).

Although the administration of carbidopa permits control of parkinsonism and Parkinson's disease with much lower doses of levodopa, there is no conclusive evidence at present that this is beneficial other than in reducing nausea and vomiting, permitting more rapid titration, and providing a somewhat smoother response to levodopa. *Carbidopa does not decrease adverse reactions due to central effects of levodopa. By permitting more levodopa to reach the brain, particularly when nausea and vomiting is not a dose-limiting factor, certain adverse CNS effects, e.g., dyskinesias, may occur at lower dosages and sooner during therapy with carbidopa and levodopa than with levodopa.*

Certain patients who responded poorly to levodopa have improved when carbidopa and levodopa was substituted. This is most likely due to decreased peripheral decarboxylation of levodopa which results from administration of carbidopa rather than to a primary effect of carbidopa on the nervous system. Carbidopa has not been shown to enhance the intrinsic efficacy of levodopa in parkinsonian syndromes.

In considering whether to give this combination product to patients already on levodopa who have nausea and/or vomiting, the practitioner should be aware that, while many patients may be expected to improve, some do not. Since one cannot predict which patients are likely to improve, this can only be determined by a trial of therapy. It should be further noted that in controlled trials comparing carbidopa and levodopa with levodopa, about half of the patients with nausea and/or vomiting on levodopa improved spontaneously despite being retained on the same dose of levodopa during the controlled portion of the trial.

CONTRAINDICATIONS

Monoamine oxidase inhibitors and carbidopa and levodopa should not be given concomitantly. These inhibitors must be discontinued at least two weeks prior to initiating therapy with this combination product.

Carbidopa and levodopa is contraindicated in patients with known hypersensitivity to this drug, and in narrow angle glaucoma.

Because levodopa may activate a malignant melanoma, it should not be used in patients with suspicious, undiagnosed skin lesions or a history of melanoma.

WARNINGS

When patients are receiving levodopa, it must be discontinued at least eight hours before therapy with this combination product is started. Carbidopa and levodopa should be substituted at a dosage that will provide approximately 25

percent of the previous levodopa dosage (see DOSAGE AND ADMINISTRATION). Patients who are taking this combination product should be instructed not to take additional levodopa unless it is prescribed by the physician.

As with levodopa, the combination product may cause involuntary movements and mental disturbances. These reactions are thought to be due to increased brain dopamine following administration of levodopa. All patients should be observed carefully for the development of depression with concomitant suicidal tendencies. Patients with past or current psychoses should be treated with caution. *Because carbidopa permits more levodopa to reach the brain and, thus, more dopamine to be formed, dyskinesias may occur at lower dosages and sooner with carbidopa and levodopa than with levodopa.* The occurrence of dyskinesias may require dosage reduction.

Carbidopa and levodopa should be administered cautiously to patients with severe cardiovascular or pulmonary disease, bronchial asthma, renal, hepatic or endocrine disease. Care should be exercised in administering the combination product, as with levodopa, to patients with a history of myocardial infarction who have residual atrial, nodal, or ventricular arrhythmias. In such patients, cardiac function should be monitored with particular care during the period of initial dosage adjustment, in a facility with provisions for intensive cardiac care.

As with levodopa there is a possibility of upper gastrointestinal hemorrhage in patients with a history of peptic ulcer. A symptom complex resembling the neuroleptic malignant syndrome including muscular rigidity, elevated body temperature, mental changes, and increased serum creatine phosphokinase has been reported when antiparkinsonian agents were withdrawn abruptly. Therefore, patients should be observed carefully when the dosage of carbidopa and levodopa is reduced abruptly or discontinued, especially if the patient is receiving neuroleptics.

Usage in Pregnancy and Lactation: Although the effects of carbidopa and levodopa on human pregnancy and lactation are unknown, both levodopa and combinations of carbidopa and levodopa have caused visceral and skeletal malformations in rabbits. Use of carbidopa and levodopa in women of childbearing potential requires that the anticipated benefits of the drug be weighed against possible hazards to mother and child. This product should not be given to nursing mothers.

Usage in Children: The safety of carbidopa and levodopa tablets in patients under 18 years of age has not been established.

PRECAUTIONS

As with levodopa, periodic evaluations of hepatic, hematopoietic, cardiovascular, and renal function are recommended during extended therapy.

Patients with chronic wide angle glaucoma may be treated cautiously with carbidopa and levodopa provided the intraocular pressure is well controlled and the patient is monitored carefully for changes in intraocular pressure during therapy.

Laboratory Tests

Abnormalities in laboratory tests may include elevations of liver function tests such as alkaline phosphatase, SGOT (AST), SGPT (ALT), lactic dehydrogenase, and bilirubin. Abnormalities in protein-bound iodine, blood urea nitrogen and positive Coombs test have also been reported. Commonly, levels of blood urea nitrogen, creatinine, and uric acid are lower during administration of this combination product than with levodopa.

Carbidopa and levodopa may cause a false-positive reaction for urinary ketone bodies when a test tape is used for determination of ketonuria. This reaction will not be altered by boiling the urine specimen. False-negative tests may result with the use of glucose-oxidase methods of testing for glucosuria.

Drug Interactions

Caution should be exercised when the following drugs are administered concomitantly with carbidopa and levodopa.

Symptomatic postural hypotension can occur when carbidopa and levodopa is added to the treatment of a patient receiving antihypertensive drugs. Therefore, when carbidopa and levodopa therapy is started, dosage adjustment of the antihypertensive drug may be required. For patients receiving monoamine oxidase inhibitors, see CONTRAINDICATIONS.

There have been rare reports of adverse reactions, including hypertension and dyskinesia, resulting from the concomitant use of tricyclic antidepressants and carbidopa and levodopa.

Phenothiazines and butyrophenones may reduce the therapeutic effects of levodopa. In addition, the beneficial effects of levodopa in Parkinson's disease have been reported to be reversed by phenytoin and papaverine. Patients taking these drugs with carbidopa and levodopa should be carefully observed for loss of therapeutic response.

ADVERSE REACTIONS

The most common serious adverse reactions occurring with carbidopa and levodopa are choreiform, dystonic, and other

involuntary movements. Other serious adverse reactions are mental changes including paranoid ideation and psychotic episodes, depression with or without development of suicidal tendencies, and dementia. Convulsions also have occurred; however, a causal relationship with carbidopa and levodopa has not been established.

A common but less serious effect is nausea.

Less frequent adverse reactions are cardiac irregularities and/or palpitation, orthostatic hypotensive episodes, bradykinetic episodes (the "on-off" phenomenon), anorexia, vomiting, and dizziness.

Rarely, gastrointestinal bleeding, development of duodenal ulcer, hypertension, phlebitis, hemolytic and non-hemolytic anemia, thrombocytopenia, leukopenia, and agranulocytosis have occurred.

Laboratory tests which have been reported to be abnormal are alkaline phosphatase, SGOT (AST), SGPT (ALT), lactic dehydrogenase, bilirubin, blood urea nitrogen, protein-bound iodine, and Coombs test.

Other adverse reactions that have been reported with levodopa are:

Nervous System: ataxia, numbness, increased hand tremor, muscle twitching, muscle cramps, blepharospasm (which may be taken as an early sign of excess dosage, consideration of dosage reduction may be made at this time), trismus, activation of latent Horner's syndrome.

Psychiatric: confusion, sleepiness, insomnia, nightmares, hallucinations, delusions, agitation, anxiety, euphoria.

Gastrointestinal: dry mouth, bitter taste, sialorrhea, dysphagia, bruxism, hiccups, abdominal pain and distress, constipation, diarrhea, flatulence, burning sensation of tongue.

Metabolic: weight gain or loss, edema.

Integumentary: malignant melanoma (see also CONTRA-INDICATIONS), flushing, increased sweating, dark sweat, skin rash, loss of hair.

Genitourinary: urinary retention, urinary incontinence, dark urine, priapism.

Special Senses: diplopia, blurred vision, dilated pupils, oculogyric crises.

Miscellaneous: weakness, faintness, fatigue, headache, hoarseness, malaise, hot flashes, sense of stimulation, bizarre breathing patterns, neuroleptic malignant syndrome.

OVERDOSAGE

Management of acute overdosage with carbidopa and levodopa is basically the same as management of acute overdosage with levodopa; however, pyridoxine is not effective in reversing the actions of this product.

General supportive measures should be employed, along with immediate gastric lavage. Intravenous fluids should be administered judiciously and an adequate airway maintained. Electrocardiographic monitoring should be instituted and the patient carefully observed for the development of arrhythmias; if required, appropriate antiarrhythmic therapy should be given. The possibility that the patient may have taken other drugs as well as carbidopa and levopoda tablets should be taken into consideration. To date, no experience has been reported with dialysis; hence, its value in overdosage is not known.

DOSAGE AND ADMINISTRATION

The optimum daily dosage of carbidopa and levodopa must be determined by careful titration in each patient. Carbidopa and levodopa tablets are available in a 1:4 ratio of carbidopa to levodopa (25 mg/100 mg) as well as 1:10 ratio (25 mg/250 mg and 10 mg/100 mg). Tablets of the two ratios may be given separately or combined as needed to provide the optimum dosage.

Studies show that peripheral dopa decarboxylase is saturated by carbidopa at approximately 70 to 100 mg a day. Patients receiving less than this amount of carbidopa are more likely to experience nausea and vomiting.

Usual Initial Dosage

Dosage is best initiated with one tablet of carbidopa and levodopa 25 mg/100 mg three times a day. This dosage schedule provides 75 mg of carbidopa per day. Dosage may be increased by one tablet every day or every other day, as necessary, until a dosage of eight tablets of carbidopa and levodopa 25 mg/100 mg a day is reached.

If carbidopa and levodopa 10 mg/100 mg is used, dosage may be initiated with one tablet three or four times a day. However, this will not provide an adequate amount of carbidopa for many patients. Dosage may be increased by one tablet every day or every other day until a total of eight tablets (2 tablets q.i.d.) is reached.

How to Transfer Patients from Levodopa

Levodopa must be discontinued at least eight hours before starting this combination product. A daily dosage of carbidopa and levodopa should be chosen that will provide approximately 25 percent of the previous levodopa dosage. Patients who are taking less than 1500 mg of levodopa a day should be started on one tablet of carbidopa and levodopa 25 mg/100 mg three or four times a day. The suggested starting dosage for most patients taking more than 1500 mg of levodopa is one tablet of carbidopa and levodopa 25 mg/250 mg three or four times a day.

Maintenance

Therapy should be individualized and adjusted according to the desired therapeutic response. At least 70 to 100 mg of carbidopa per day should be provided. When a greater proportion of carbidopa is required, one 25 mg/100 mg tablet may be substituted for each 10 mg/100 mg tablet. When more levodopa is required, each 25 mg/250 mg tablet should be substituted for a 25 mg/100 mg tablet or a 10 mg/100 mg tablet. If necessary, the dosage of carbidopa and levodopa 25 mg/250 mg may be increased by one-half or one tablet every day or every other day to a maximum of eight tablets a day. Experience with total daily dosages of carbidopa greater than 200 mg is limited.

Because both therapeutic and adverse responses occur more rapidly with this combination product than with levodopa alone, patients should be monitored closely during the dose adjustment period. Specifically, involuntary movements will occur more rapidly with carbidopa and levodopa than with levodopa. The occurrence of involuntary movements may require dosage reduction. Blepharospasm may be a useful early sign of excess dosage in some patients.

Current evidence indicates that other standard drugs for Parkinson's disease (except levodopa) may be continued while carbidopa and levodopa is being administered, although their dosage may have to be adjusted.

If general anesthesia is required, carbidopa and levodopa may be continued as long as the patient is permitted to take fluids and medication by mouth. If therapy is interrupted temporarily, the usual daily dosage may be administered as soon as the patient is able to take oral medication.

HOW SUPPLIED

Carbidopa and Levodopa Tablets 25 mg/100 mg NDC 59075-585-10 are available in the following form:

Mottled yellow, round, scored tablets, engraved A-"585" on the scored side, and packaged in bottles of 100.

Carbidopa and Levodopa Tablets 25 mg/250 mg NDC 59075-587-10 are available in the following form:

Mottled blue, round, scored tablets, engraved A-"587" on the scored side, and packaged in bottles of 100.

Store at controlled room temperature 15°–30°C (59°–86°F). PROTECT FROM LIGHT.

Dispense in a tight, light-resistant container as defined in the USP, with a child-resistant closure (as required).

CAUTION: Federal law prohibits dispensing without prescription.

Rev. B 4/92

Manufactured by:
TEVA PHARMACEUTICAL IND. LTD.
Jerusalem, 91010, Israel
Distributed by:
ATHENA NEUROSCIENCES, Inc.
South San Francisco, CA 94080

Shown in Product Identification Guide, page 305

ATAPRYL™ ℞
[at-ă-pril]
SELEGILINE HYDROCHLORIDE TABLETS USP

DESCRIPTION

Selegiline hydrochloride is a levorotatory acetylenic derivative of phenethylamine. It is commonly referred to in the clinical and pharmacological literature as 1-deprenyl.

The chemical name is: (-)-(R)-*N*, α-dimethyl-*N*-2-propynylphenethylamine hydrochloride. It is a white to near white crystalline powder, freely soluble in water, chloroform, and methanol, and has a molecular weight of 223.75. The structural formula is as follows:

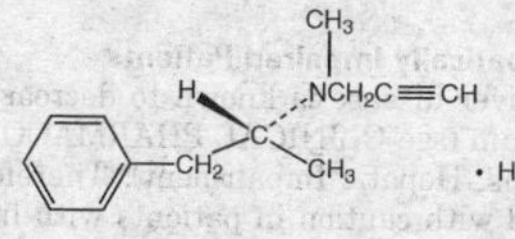

Molecular Formula: $C_{13}H_{17}N{\cdot}HCl$

Each tablet, for oral administration, contains 5 mg of selegiline hydrochloride. Inactive ingredients are lactose monohydrate, starch (corn), povidone, magnesium stearate and talc.

HOW SUPPLIED

Selegiline Hydrochloride Tablets USP are available containing 5 mg of selegiline hydrochloride. Each white to off white, round, unscored, flat face beveled edge, compressed tablet is engraved with **A** over **660** on one side and 5 on the reverse. They are available as:

NDC 59075-660-60 bottles of 60

Store at controlled room temperature, 15° to 30°C (59° to 86°F).

CAUTION: Federal (U.S.A.) law prohibits dispensing without prescription.

Manufactured by: Novopharm Limited
Toronto, Canada
M1B 2K9

Manufactured for: Athena Neurosciences Inc
South San Francisco, CA 94080
Issued Sept 1996
83520 Rev 00

Shown in Product Identification Guide, page 305

DIASTAT® Rectal Delivery System Ⓒ℞
[dī 'ă-stat]
(diazepam rectal gel)

DESCRIPTION

Diastat* rectal delivery system is a non-sterile diazepam gel provided in a prefilled, unit-dose, rectal delivery system. Diastat contains 5 mg/mL diazepam, propylene glycol, ethyl alcohol (10%), hydroxypropyl methylcellulose, sodium benzoate, benzyl alcohol (1.5%), benzoic acid and water. Diastat is clear to slightly yellow and has a pH between 6.5–7.2.

Diazepam, the active ingredient of Diastat, is a benzodiazepine anticonvulsant with the chemical name 7-chloro-1,3-dihydro-1-methyl-5-phenyl-2H-1,4-benzodiazepin-2-one. The structural formula is as follows:

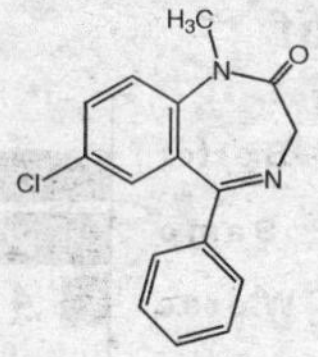

* Registered trademark of Athena Neurosciences, Inc.

CLINICAL PHARMACOLOGY

Mechanism of Action

Although the precise mechanism by which diazepam exerts its antiseizure effects is unknown, animal and *in vitro* studies suggest that diazepam acts to suppress seizures through an interaction with γ-aminobutyric acid (GABA) receptors of the A-type ($GABA_A$). GABA, the major inhibitory neurotransmitter in the central nervous system, acts at this receptor to open the membrane channel allowing chloride ions to flow into neurons. Entry of chloride ions causes an inhibitory potential that reduces the ability of neurons to depolarize to the threshold potential necessary to produce action potentials. Excessive depolarization of neurons is implicated in the generation and spread of seizures. It is believed that diazepam enhances the actions of GABA by causing GABA to bind more tightly to the $GABA_A$ receptor.

Pharmacokinetics

Pharmacokinetic information of diazepam following rectal administration was obtained from studies conducted in healthy adult subjects. No pharmacokinetic studies were conducted in pediatric patients. Therefore, information from the literature is used to define pharmacokinetic labeling in the pediatric population.

Diastat is well absorbed following rectal administration, reaching peak plasma concentrations in 1.5 hours. The absolute bioavailability of Diastat relative to Valium® injectable is 90%. The volume of distribution of Diastat is calculated to be approximately 1 L/kg. The mean elimination half-life of diazepam and desmethyldiazepam following administration of a 15 mg dose of Diastat was found to be about 46 hours (CV=43%) and 71 hours (CV=37%), respectively. Both diazepam and its major active metabolite desmethyldiazepam bind extensively to plasma proteins (95–98%).

[See figure 1 at top of next page]

Metabolism and Elimination: It has been reported in the literature that diazepam is extensively metabolized to one major active metabolite (desmethyldiazepam) and two minor active metabolites, 3-hydroxydiazepam (temazepam) and 3-hydroxy-N-diazepam (oxazepam) in plasma. At therapeutic doses, desmethyldiazepam is found in plasma at concentrations equivalent to those of diazepam while oxazepam and temazepam are not usually detectable. The metabolism of diazepam is primarily hepatic and involves demethylation (involving primarily CYP2C19 and CYP3A4) and 3-hydroxylation (involving primarily CYP3A4), followed by glucuronidation. The marked inter-individual variability in the clearance of diazepam reported in the literature is probably attributable to variability of CYP2C19 (which is known to exhibit genetic polymorphism; about 3–5% of Caucasians have little or no activity and are "poor metabolizers") and CYP3A4. No inhibition was demonstrated in the presence of inhibitors selective for CYP2A6, CYP2C9, CYP2D6, CYP2E1, or CYP1A2, indicating that these enzymes are not significantly involved in metabolism of diazepam.

Special Populations

Hepatic Impairment: No pharmacokinetic studies were conducted with Diastat in hepatically impaired subjects. Literature review indicates that following administration of 0.1 to 0.15 mg/kg of diazepam intravenously, the half-life of diazepam was prolonged by two to five-fold in subjects with alcoholic cirrhosis (n=24) compared to age-matched control subjects (n=37) with a corresponding decrease in clearance by half: however, the exact degree of hepatic impairment in these subjects was not characterized in this literature (see PRECAUTIONS section).

Renal Impairment: The pharmacokinetics of diazepam have not been studied in renally impaired subjects (see PRECAUTIONS section).

Pediatrics: No pharmacokinetic studies were conducted with Diastat in the pediatric population. However, literature review indicates that following IV administration (0.33 mg/kg), diazepam has a longer half-life in neonates (birth up to one month; approximately 50–95 hours) and infants (one month up to two years; about 40–50 hours), whereas it has a shorter half-life in children (two to 12 years; approximately 15–21 hours) and adolescents (12 to 16 years; about 18–20 years) (see PRECAUTIONS section).

Elderly: A study of single dose IV administration of diazepam (0.1 mg/kg) indicates that the elimination half-life of diazepam increases linearly with age, ranging from about 15 hours at 18 years (healthy young adults) to about 100 hours at 95 years (healthy elderly) with a corresponding decrease in clearance of free diazepam (see PRECAUTIONS and DOSAGE AND ADMINISTRATION sections).

Effect of Gender, Race, and Cigarette Smoking: No targeted pharmacokinetic studies have been conducted to evaluate the effect of gender, race, and cigarette smoking on the pharmacokinetics of diazepam. However, covariate analysis of a population of treated patients following administration of Diastat indicated that neither gender nor cigarette smoking had any effect on the pharmacokinetics of diazepam.

Clinical Studies

The effectiveness of Diastat has been established in two adequate and well-controlled clinical studies in children and adults exhibiting the seizure pattern described below under INDICATIONS.

A randomized, double-blind study compared sequential doses of Diastat and placebo in 91 patients (47 children, 44 adults) exhibiting the appropriate seizure profile. The first dose was given at the onset of an identified episode. Children were dosed again four hours after the first dose and were observed for a total of 12 hours. Adults were dosed at four and 12 hours after the first dose and were observed for a total of 24 hours. Primary outcomes for this study were seizure frequency during the period of observation and a global assessment that took into account the severity and nature of the seizures as well as their frequency.

The median seizure frequency for the Diastat treated group was zero seizures per hour, compared to a median seizure frequency of 0.3 seizures per hour for the placebo group, a difference that was statistically significant ($p < 0.0001$). All three categories of the global assessment (seizure frequency, seizure severity, and "overall") were also found to be statistically significant in favor of Diastat ($p < 0.0001$). The following histogram displays the results for the "overall" category of the global assessment.

[See figure 2 on next page]

Patients treated with Diastat experienced prolonged time-to-next-seizure compared to placebo ($p = 0.0002$) as shown in the following graph.

[See figure 3 on page 611]

In addition, 62% of patients treated with Diastat were seizure-free during the observation period compared to 20% of placebo patients.

Analysis of response by gender and age revealed no substantial differences between treatment in either of these subgroups. Analysis of response by race was considered unreliable, due to the small percentage of non-Caucasions.

A second double-blind study compared single doses of Diastat and placebo in 114 patients (53 children, 61 adults). The dose was given at the onset of the identified episode and patients were observed for a total of 12 hours. The primary outcome in this study was seizure frequency. The median seizure frequency for the Diastat-treated group was zero seizures per 12 hours, compared to a median seizure frequency of 2.0 seizures per 12 hours for the placebo group, a difference that was statistically significant ($p < 0.03$). Patients treated with Diastat experienced prolonged time-to-next-seizure compared to placebo ($p = 0.0072$) as shown in the following graph.

[See figure 4 on page 611]

In addition, 55% of patients treated with Diastat were seizure-free during the observation period compared to 34% of patients receiving placebo. Overall, caregivers judged Diastat to be more effective than placebo (p=0.018), based on a 10 centimeter visual analog scale. In addition, investigators also evaluated the effectiveness of Diastat and judged Diastat to be more effective than placebo ($p < 0.001$).

An analysis of response by gender revealed a statistically significant difference between treatments in females but not in males in this study, and the difference between the 2 genders in response to the treatments reached borderline sta-

Continued on next page

Diastat—Cont.

tistical significance. Analysis of response by race was considered unreliable, due to the small percentage of non-Caucasions.

INDICATIONS AND USAGE
Diastat is a gel formulation of diazepam intended for rectal administration in the management of selected, refractory, patients with epilepsy, on stable regimens of AEDs, who require intermittent use of diazepam to control bouts of increased seizure activity.

Evidence to support the use of Diastat was adduced in two controlled trials (see CLINICAL PHARMACOLOGY, CLINICAL STUDIES subsection) that enrolled patients with partial onset or generalized convulsive seizures who were identified jointly by their caregivers and physicians as suffering intermittent and periodic episodes of markedly increased seizure activity, sometimes heralded by non-convulsive symptoms, that for the individual patient were characteristic and were deemed by the prescriber to be of a kind for which a benzodiazepine would ordinarily be administered acutely. Although these clusters or bouts of seizures differed among patients, for any individual patient the clusters of seizure activity were not only stereotypic but were judged by those conducting and participating in these studies to be distinguishable from other seizures suffered by that patient. The conclusion that a patient experienced such unique episodes of seizure activity was based on historical information.

CONTRAINDICATIONS
Diastat is contraindicated in patients with a known hypersensitivity to diazepam. Diastat may be used in patients with open angle glaucoma who are receiving appropriate therapy but is contraindicated in acute narrow angle glaucoma.

WARNINGS
General
Diastat should only be administered by caregivers who in the opinion of the prescribing physician 1) are able to distinguish the distinct cluster of seizures (and/or the events presumed to herald their onset) from the patient's ordinary seizure activity, 2) have been instructed and judged to be competent to administer the treatment rectally, 3) understand explicitly which seizure manifestations may or may not be treated with Diastat, and 4) are able to monitor the clinical response and recognize when that response is such that immediate professional medical evaluation is required.
CNS Depression
Because Diastat produces CNS depression, patients receiving this drug who are otherwise capable and qualified to do so should be cautioned against engaging in hazardous occupations requiring mental alertness, such as operating machinery, driving a motor vehicle, or riding a bicycle until they have completely returned to their level of baseline functioning.

Although Diastat is indicated for use solely on an intermittent basis, the potential for a synergistic CNS-depressant effect when used simultaneously with alcohol or other CNS depressants must be considered by the prescribing physician, and appropriate recommendations made to the patient and/or caregiver.

Prolonged CNS depression has been observed in neonates treated with diazepam. Therefore, Diastat is not recommended for use in children under six months of age.
Pregnancy Risks
No clinical studies have been conducted with Diastat in pregnant women. Data from several sources raise concerns about the use of diazepam during pregnancy.
Animal Findings: Diazepam has been shown to be teratogenic in mice and hamsters when given orally at single doses of 100 mg/kg or greater (approximately eight times the maximum recommended human dose [MRHD=1 mg/kg/day] or greater on a mg/m^2 basis). Cleft palate and exencephaly are the most common and consistently reported malformations produced in these species by administration of high, maternally-toxic doses of diazepam during organogenesis. Rodent studies have indicated that prenatal exposure to diazepam doses similar to those used clinically can produce long-term changes in cellular immune responses, brain neurochemistry, and behavior.
General Concerns and Considerations About Anticonvulsants: Reports suggest an association between the use of anticonvulsant drugs by women with epilepsy and an elevated incidence of birth defects in children born to these women. Data are more extensive with respect to phenytoin and phenobarbital, but a smaller number of systematic or anecdotal reports suggest a possible similar association with the use of all known anticonvulsant drugs.

The reports suggesting an elevated incidence of birth defects in children of drug-treated epileptic women cannot be regarded as adequate to prove a definite cause and effect relationship. There are intrinsic methodologic problems in obtaining adequate data on drug teratogenicity in humans;

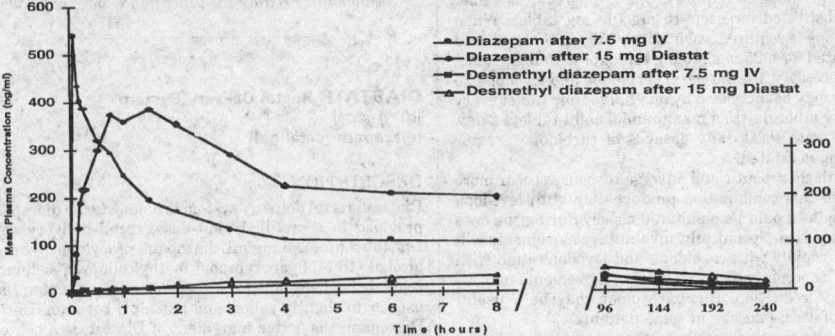

FIGURE 1: Plasma Concentrations of Diazepam and Dimethyldiazepam Following Diastat or IV Diazepam

- Diazepam after 7.5 mg IV
- Diazepam after 15 mg Diastat
- Desmethyl diazepam after 7.5 mg IV
- Desmethyl diazepam after 15 mg Diastat

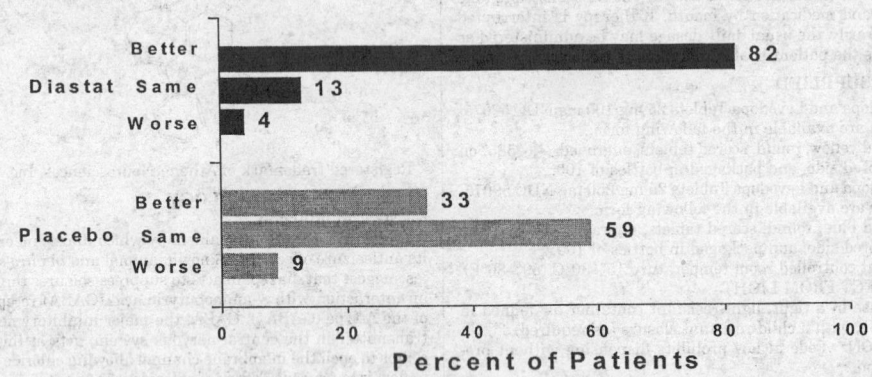

FIGURE 2: Caregiver Overall Global Assessment of the Efficacy of Diastat

Diastat — Better 82, Same 13, Worse 4
Placebo — Better 33, Same 59, Worse 9

Percent of Patients

the possibility also exists that other factors, e.g., genetic factors or the epileptic condition itself, may be more important than drug therapy in leading to birth defects. The great majority of mothers on anticonvulsant medication deliver normal infants. It is important to note that anticonvulsant drugs should not be discontinued in patients in whom the drug is administered to prevent seizures because of the strong possibility of precipitating *status epilepticus* with attendant hypoxia and threat to life. In individual cases where the severity and frequency of the seizure disorder are such that the removal of medication does not pose a serious threat to the patient, discontinuation of the drug may be considered prior to and during pregnancy, although it cannot be said with any confidence that even mild seizures do not pose some hazards to the developing embryo or fetus.
General Concerns About Benzodiazepines: An increased risk of congenital malformations associated with the use of benzodiazepine drugs has been suggested in several studies. There may also be non-teratogenic risks associated with the use of benzodiazepines during pregnancy. There have been reports of neonatal flaccidity, respiratory and feeding difficulties, and hypothermia in children born to mothers who have been receiving benzodiazepines late in pregnancy. In addition, children born to mothers receiving benzodiazepines on a regular basis late in pregnancy may be at some risk of experiencing withdrawal symptoms during the postnatal period.
Advice Regarding the Use of Diastat in Women of Childbearing Potential: In general, the use of Diastat in women of childbearing potential, and more specifically during known pregnancy, should be considered only when the clinical situation warrants the risk to the fetus.

The specific considerations addressed above regarding the use of anticonvulsants in epileptic women of childbearing potential should be weighed in treating or counseling these women.

Because of experience with other members of the benzodiazepine class, Diastat is assumed to be capable of causing an increased risk of congenital abnormalities when administered to a pregnant woman during the first trimester. The possibility that a woman of childbearing potential may be pregnant at the time of institution of therapy should be considered. If this drug is used during pregnancy, or if the patient becomes pregnant while taking this drug, the patient should be apprised of the potential hazard to the fetus. Patients should also be advised that if they become pregnant during therapy or intend to become pregnant they should communicate with their physician about the desirability of

discontinuing the drug.
Withdrawal Symptoms
Withdrawal symptoms of the barbiturate type have occurred after the discontinuation regular use of benzodiazepines (see DRUG ABUSE AND DEPENDENCE section).
Chronic Use
Diastat is not recommended for chronic, daily use as an anticonvulsant because of the potential for development of tolerance to diazepam. Chronic daily use of diazepam may increase the frequency and/or severity of tonic clonic seizures, requiring an increase in the dosage of standard anticonvulsant medication. In such cases, abrupt withdrawal of chronic diazepam may also be associated with a temporary increase in the frequency and/or severity of seizures.
Use in Patients with Petit Mal Status
Tonic *status epilepticus* has been precipitated in patients treated with IV diazepam for petit mal status or petit mal variant status.

PRECAUTIONS
Caution in Renally Impaired Patients
Metabolites of Diastat are excreted by the kidneys; to avoid their excess accumulation, caution should be exercised in the administration of the drug to patients with impaired renal function.
Caution in Hepatically Impaired Patients
Concomitant liver disease is known to decrease the clearance of diazepam (see CLINICAL PHARMACOLOGY, Special Populations, Hepatic Impairment). Therefore, Diastat should be used with caution in patients with liver disease.
Use in Pediatrics
The controlled trials demonstrating the effectiveness of Diastat included children two years of age and older. Clinical studies have not been conducted to establish the efficacy and safety of Diastat in children under two years of age.
Use in Patients with Compromised Respiratory Function
Diastat should be used with caution in patients with compromised respiratory function related to a concurrent disease process (e.g., asthma, pneumonia) or neurologic damage.
Use in Elderly
In elderly patients Diastat should be used with caution due to an increase in half-life with a corresponding decrease in the clearance of free diazepam. It is also recommended that the dosage be decreased to reduce the likelihood of ataxia or oversedation.
Information to be Communicated by the Prescriber to the Caregiver
Prescribers are strongly advised to take all reasonable steps to ensure that caregivers fully understand their role and ob-

ligations vis a vis the administration of Diastat to individuals in their care. Prescribers should routinely discuss the steps in the Patient/Caregiver Package Insert (see Patient/Caregiver Insert printed at the end of the product labeling and also included in the product carton). The successful and safe use of Diastat depends in large measure on the competence and performance of the caregiver.

Prescribers should advise caregivers that they expect to be informed immediately if a patient develops any new findings which are not typical of the patient's characteristic seizure episode.

Interference With Cognitive and Motor Performance: Because benzodiazepines have the potential to impair judgment, thinking, or motor skills, patients should be cautioned about operating hazardous machinery, including automobiles, until they are reasonably certain that Diastat therapy does not affect them adversely.

Pregnancy: Patients should be advised to notify their physician if they become pregnant or intend to become pregnant during therapy with Diastat (see WARNINGS section).

Nursing: Because diazepam and its metabolites may be present in human breast milk for prolonged periods of time after acute use of Diastat, patients should be advised not to breast-feed for an appropriate period of time after receiving treatment with Diastat.

Concomitant Medication

Although Diastat is indicated for use solely on an intermittent basis, the potential for a synergistic CNS-depressant effect when used simultaneously with alcohol or other CNS-depressants must be considered by the prescribing physician, and appropriate recommendations made to the patient and/or caregiver.

Drug Interactions

If Diastat is to be combined with other psychotropic agents or other CNS depressants, careful consideration should be given to the pharmacology of the agents to be employed—particularly with known compounds which may potentiate the action of diazepam, such as phenothiazines, narcotics, barbiturates, MAO inhibitors and other antidepressants. The clearance of diazepam and certain other benzodiazepines can be delayed in association with cimetidine administration. The clinical significance of this is unclear.

Valproate may potentiate the CNS-depressant effects of diazepam.

There have been no clinical studies or reports in literature to evaluate the interaction of rectally administered diazepam with other drugs. As with all drugs, the potential for interaction by a variety of mechanisms is a possibility.

Effect of Other Drugs On Diazepam Metabolism: *In vitro* studies using human liver preparations suggest that CYP2C19 and CYP3A4 are the principal isozymes involved in the initial oxidative metabolism of diazepam. Therefore, potential interactions may occur when diazepam is given concurrently with agents that affect CYP2C19 and CYP3A4 activity. Potential inhibitors of CYP2C19 (e.g., cimetidine, quinidine, and tranylcypromine) and CYP3A4 (e.g., ketoconazole, troleandomycin, and clotrimazole) could decrease the rate of diazepam elimination, while inducers of CYP2C19 (e.g., rifampin) and CYP3A4 (e.g., carbamazepine, phenytoin, dexamethasone and phenobarbital) could increase the rate of elimination of diazepam.

Effect of Diazepam On the Metabolism of Other Drugs: There are no reports as to which isozymes could be inhibited or induced by diazepam. But, based on the fact that diazepam is a substrate for CYP2C19 and CYP3A4, it is possible that diazepam may interfere with the metabolism of drugs which are substrates for CYP2C19, (e.g. omeprazole, propranolol, and imipramine) and CYP3A4 (e.g. cyclosporine, paclitaxel, terfenadine, theophylline, and warfarin) leading to a potential drug-drug interaction.

Carcinogenesis, Mutagenesis, Impairment of Fertility

The carcinogenic potential of rectal diazepam has not been evaluated. In studies in which mice and rats were administered diazepam in the diet at a dose of 75 mg/kg/day (approximately six and 12 times, respectively, the maximum recommended human dose [MRHD=1 mg/kg/day] on a mg/m² basis) for 80 and 104 weeks, respectively, an increased incidence of liver tumors was observed in males of both species.

The data currently available are inadequate to determine the mutagenic potential of diazepam.

Reproduction studies in rats showed decreases in the number of pregnancies and in the number of surviving offspring following administration of an oral dose of 100 mg/kg/day (approximately 16 times the MRHD on a mg/m² basis) prior to and during mating and throughout gestation and lactation. No adverse effects on fertility or offspring viability were noted at a dose of 80 mg/kg/day (approximately 13 times the MRHD on a mg/m² basis).

Pregnancy—Category D (see WARNINGS section.)

Labor and Delivery

In humans, measurable amounts of diazepam have been found in maternal and cord blood, indicating placental transfer of the drug. Until additional information is available, Diastat is not recommended for obstetrical use.

Nursing Mothers

Because diazepam and its metabolites may be present in human breast milk for prolonged periods of time after acute use of Diastat, patients should be advised not to breast-feed for an appropriate period of time after receiving treatment with Diastat.

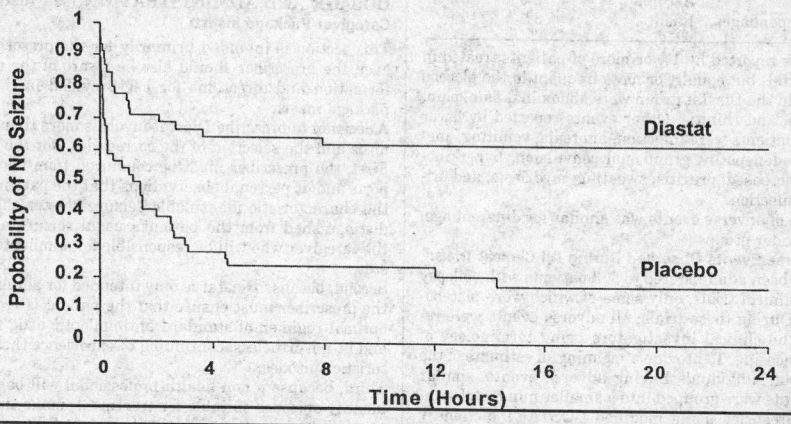

FIGURE 3: Kaplan-Meier Survival Analysis of Time-to-Next-Seizure - First Study

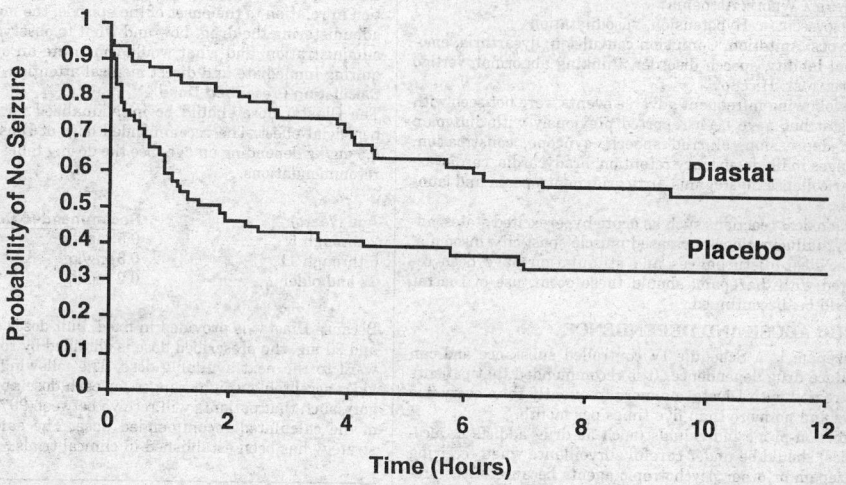

FIGURE 4: Kaplan-Meier Survival Analysis of Time-to-Next-Seizure - Second Study

ADVERSE REACTIONS

Diastat adverse event data were collected from double-blind, placebo-controlled studies and open-label studies. The majority of adverse events were mild to moderate in severity and transient in nature.

Two patients who received Diastat died seven to 15 weeks following treatment; neither of these deaths was deemed related to Diastat.

The most frequent adverse event reported to be related to Diastat in the two double-blind, placebo-controlled studies was somnolence (23%). Less frequent adverse events were dizziness, headache, pain, abdominal pain, nervousness, vasodilatation, diarrhea, ataxia, euphoria, incoordination, asthma, rhinitis, and rash, which occurred in approximately 2–5% of patients.

Approximately 1.4% of the 573 patients who received Diastat in clinical trials of epilepsy discontinued treatment because of an adverse event. The adverse event most frequently associated with discontinuation (occurring in three patients) was somnolence. Other adverse events most commonly associated with discontinuation and occurring in two patients were hypoventilation and rash. Adverse events occurring in one patient were asthenia, hyperkinesia, incoordination, vasodilatation and urticaria. These events were judged to be related to Diastat.

In the two domestic double-blind, placebo-controlled, parallel-group studies, the proportion of patients who discontinued treatment because of adverse events was 2% for the group treated with Diastat, versus 2% for the placebo group. In the Diastat group, the adverse events considered the primary reason for discontinuation were different in the two patients who discontinued treatment; one discontinued due to rash and one discontinued due to lethargy. The primary reason for discontinuation in the patients treated with placebo was lack of effect.

Adverse Event Incidence in Controlled Clinical Trials

Table 1 lists treatment-emergent signs and symptoms that occurred in >1% of patients enrolled in parallel-group, placebo-controlled trials and were numerically more common in the Diastat group. Adverse events were usually mild or moderate in intensity.

The prescriber should be aware that these figures, obtained when Diastat was added to concurrent antiepileptic drug therapy, cannot be used to predict the frequency of adverse events in the course of usual medical practice when patient characteristics and other factors may differ from those prevailing during clinical studies. Similarly, the cited frequencies cannot be directly compared with figures obtained from other clinical investigations involving different treatments, uses, or investigators. An inspection of these frequencies, however, does provide the prescribing physician with a basis to estimate the relative contribution of drug and non-drug factors to the adverse event incidences in the population studied.

TABLE 1: Treatment-Emergent Signs And Symptoms That Occurred In >1% Of Patients Enrolled In Parallel-Group, Placebo-Controlled Trials And Were Numerically More Common In The Diastat Group

Body System	COSTART Term	Diastat N = 101 %	Placebo N = 104 %
Body As A Whole	Headache	5%	4%
Cardiovascular	Vasodilatation	2%	0%
Digestive	Diarrhea	4%	<1%
Nervous	Ataxia	3%	<1%
	Dizziness	3%	2%
	Euphoria	3%	0%
	Incoordination	3%	0%
	Somnolence	23%	8%

Continued on next page

Diastat—Cont.

Respiratory	Asthma	2%	0%
Skin and Appendages	Rash	3%	0%

Other events reported by 1% or more of patients treated in controlled trials but equally or more frequent in the placebo group than in the Diastat group were abdominal pain, pain, nervousness, and rhinitis. Other events reported by fewer than 1% of patients were infection, anorexia, vomiting, anemia, lymphadenopathy, grand mal convulsion, hyperkinesia, cough increased, pruritis, sweating, mydriasis, and urinary tract infection.
The pattern of adverse events was similar for different age, race and gender groups.

Other Adverse Events Observed During All Clinical Trials: Diastat has been administered to 573 patients with epilepsy during all clinical trials, only some of which were placebo-controlled. During these trials, all adverse events were recorded by the clinical investigators using terminology of their own choosing. To provide a meaningful estimate of the proportion of individuals having adverse events, similar types of events were grouped into a smaller number of standardized categories using modified COSTART dictionary terminology. These categories are used in the listing below. All of the events listed below occurred in at least 1% of the 573 individuals exposed to Diastat. All reported events are included except those already listed above, events unlikely to be drug-related, and those too general to be informative. Events are included without regard to determination of a causal relationship to diazepam.

BODY AS A WHOLE: Asthenia
CARDIOVASCULAR: Hypotension, vasodilatation
NERVOUS: Agitation, Confusion convulsion, dysarthria, emotional lability, speech disorder, thinking abnormal, vertigo
RESPIRATORY: Hiccup

The following infrequent adverse events were not seen with Diastat but have been reported previously with diazepam use: depression, slurred speech, syncope, constipation, changes in libido, urinary retention, bradycardia, cardiovascular collapse, nystagmus, urticaria, neutropenia and jaundice.
Paradoxical reactions such as acute hyperexcited states, anxiety, hallucinations, increased muscle spasticity, insomnia, rage, sleep disturbances and stimulation have been reported with diazepam; should these occur, use of Diastat should be discontinued.

DRUG ABUSE AND DEPENDENCE

Diazepam is a Schedule IV controlled substance and can produce drug dependence. It is recommended that patients be treated with Diastat no more frequently than every five days and no more than five times per month.
Addiction-prone individuals (such as drug addicts or alcoholics) should be under careful surveillance when receiving diazepam or other psychotropic agents because of the predisposition of such patients to habituation and dependence.
Abrupt discontinuation of diazepam following chronic regular use has resulted in withdrawal symptoms, similar in character to those noted with barbiturates and alcohol (convulsions, tremor, abdominal and muscle cramps, vomiting and sweating). The more severe withdrawal symptoms have usually been limited to those patients who had received excessive doses over an extended period of time. Generally milder withdrawal symptoms (e.g., dysphoria and insomnia) have been reported following abrupt discontinuation of benzodiazepines taken continuously at therapeutic levels for several months.

OVERDOSAGE

Two patients in the clinical studies received more than twice the target dose; no adverse events were reported.
Previous reports of diazepam overdosage have shown that manifestations of diazepam overdosage include somnolence, confusion, coma, and diminished reflexes. Respiration, pulse and blood pressure should be monitored, as in all cases of drug overdosage, although, in general, these effects have been minimal. General supportive measures should be employed, along with intravenous fluids, and an adequate airway maintained. Hypotension may be combated by the use of levarterenol or metaraminol. Dialysis is of limited value.
Flumazenil, a specific benzodiazepine-receptor antagonist, is indicated for the complete or partial reversal of the sedative effects of benzodiazepines and may be used in situations when an overdose with a benzodiazepine is known or suspected. Prior to the administration of flumazenil, necessary measures should be instituted to secure airway, ventilation and intravenous access. Flumazenil is intended as an adjunct to, not as a substitute for, proper management of benzodiazepine overdose. Patients treated with flumazenil should be monitored for resedation, respiratory depression and other residual benzodiazepine effects for an appropriate period after treatment. **The prescriber should be aware of a risk of seizure in association with flumazenil treatment, particularly in long-term benzodiazepine users and in cyclic antidepressant overdose.** The complete flumazenil package insert, including CONTRAINDICATIONS, WARNINGS and PRECAUTIONS, should be consulted prior to use.

DOSAGE AND ADMINISTRATION (see Also Patient/Caregiver Package Insert)

This section is intended primarily for the prescriber; however, the prescriber should also be aware of the dosing information and directions for use provided in the patient package insert.
A decision to prescribe Diastat involves more than the diagnosis and the selection of the correct dose for the patient.
First, the prescriber must be convinced from historical reports and/or personal observations that the patient exhibits the characteristic identifiable seizure cluster that can be distinguished from the patient's usual seizure activity by the caregiver who will be responsible for administering Diastat.
Second, because Diastat is only intended for adjunctive use, the prescriber must ensure that the patient is receiving an optimal regimen of standard anti-epileptic drug treatment and is, nevertheless, continuing to experience these characteristic episodes.
Third, because a non-health professional will be obliged to identify episodes suitable for treatment, make the decision to administer treatment upon that identification, administer the drug, monitor the patient, and assess the adequacy of the response to treatment, a major component of the prescribing process involves the necessary instruction of this individual.
Fourth, the prescriber and caregiver must have a common understanding of what is and is not an episode of seizures that is appropriate for treatment, the timing of administration in relation to the onset of the episode, the mechanics of administering the drug, how and what to observe following administration, and what would constitute an outcome requiring immediate and direct medical attention.

Calculating Prescribed Dose
The Diastat dose should be individualized for maximum beneficial effect. The recommended dose of Diastat is 0.2–0.5 mg/kg depending on age. See the dosing table for specific recommendations.

Age (years)	Recommended Dose
2 through 5	0.5 mg/kg
6 through 11	0.3 mg/kg
12 and older	0.2 mg/kg

Because Diastat is provided in fixed, unit-doses of 5, 10, 15 and 20 mg, the prescribed dose is obtained by rounding upward to the next available dose. The following table provides acceptable weight ranges for each dose and age category, such that patients will receive between 90% and 180% of the calculated recommended dose. The safety of this strategy has been established in clinical trials.

2-5 Years 0.5 mg/kg		6-11 Years 0.3 mg/kg		12+ Years 0.2 mg/kg	
Weight (kg)	Dose (mg)	Weight (kg)	Dose (mg)	Weight (kg)	Dose (mg)
6 to 11	5	10 to 18	5	14 to 27	5
12 to 22	10	19 to 37	10	28 to 50	10
23 to 33	15	38 to 55	15	51 to 75	15
34 to 44	20	56 to 74	20	76 to 111	20

The rectal delivery system includes a plastic applicator with a flexible, molded tip available in two lengths, designated for convenience as Pediatric and Adult. The 2.5, 5.0, and 10.0 mg dosages are available with a 4.4 cm pediatric tip. The 10.0, 15.0, and 20.0 mg dosages are available with a 6.0 cm adult tip.
It is important to note that if a 15 mg dose is to be administered to a pediatric patient utilizing the plastic applicator with a pediatric tip, prescriptions must be written for 2 different twin packs, one for the 5 mg dosage and one for the 10 mg dosage (see HOW SUPPLIED section).
In elderly and debilitated patients, it is recommended that the dosage be adjusted downward to reduce the likelihood of ataxia or oversedation.
The prescribed dose of Diastat should be adjusted by the physician periodically to reflect changes in the patient's age or weight. It is recommended that dosage be reviewed at six month intervals.
A 2.5 mg dose is available for use as a supplemental dose. This dose may be prescribed at the discretion of the physician for patients who require more precise dose titration than is achieved using one of the four standard doses provided. The 2.5 mg dose may also be used as a partial replacement dose for patients who may expel a portion of the first dose.

Additional Dose
The prescriber may wish to prescribe a second dose of Diastat. A second dose, when required, may be given 4–12 hours after the first dose.

Treatment Frequency
It is recommended that Diastat be used to treat no more than five episodes per month and no more than one episode every five days.

HOW SUPPLIED

Diastat (diazepam rectal gel) rectal delivery system is a non-sterile diazepam gel provided in a prefilled, unit-dose, rectal delivery system. The rectal delivery system includes a plastic applicator with a flexible, molded tip available in two lengths, designated for convenience as Pediatric and Adult. Diastat is available in the following six presentations:

Dosage Strength	Rectal Tip Size	NDC Number
2.5 mg Twin Pack	Pediatric (4.4 cm)	NDC 59075-650-20
5.0 mg Twin Pack	Pediatric	NDC 59075-651-20
10.0 mg Twin Pack	Pediatric	NDC 59075-652-20
10.0 mg Twin Pack	Adult (6.0 cm)	NDC 59075-653-20
15.0 mg Twin Pack	Adult	NDC 59075-654-20
20.0 mg Twin Pack	Adult	NDC 59075-655-20

Each Twin Pack contains two Diastat rectal delivery systems, two packets of lubricating jelly, and Patient/Caregiver Package Insert.
Store at controlled room temperature 15–30°C (59–86°F).
CAUTION: Federal law prohibits dispensing without prescription.
CAUTION: Federal law prohibits the transfer of this drug to any person other than the patient for whom it was prescribed.
Distributed by:
ATHENA NEUROSCIENCES, INC.
South San Francisco, California 94080
Manufactured by:
DPT Laboratories, Inc.
San Antonio, Texas 78215

Diastat™ ADMINISTRATION INSTRUCTIONS Ⓒ
(diazepam rectal gel)

IMPORTANT
Read first before using
To the caregiver:
Please do not give DIASTAT® until:
1. you have thoroughly read these instructions,
2. reviewed administration steps with the doctor,
3. understand the directions.

Please do not administer DIASTAT until you feel comfortable with how to use DIASTAT. The doctor will tell you exactly when to use DIASTAT. When you use DIASTAT correctly and safely you will help bring seizures under control. Be sure to discuss every aspect of your role with the doctor. If you are not comfortable, then discuss your role with the doctor again.

To help the person with seizures:
- ✔You must be able to tell the difference between a cluster and ordinary seizures.
- ✔You must be comfortable and satisfied that you are able to give DIASTAT.
- ✔You need to agree with the doctor on the exact conditions when to treat with DIASTAT.
- ✔You must know how and for how long you should check the person after giving DIASTAT.

To know what responses to expect:
- ✔You need to know how soon seizures should stop or decrease in frequency after giving DIASTAT.
- ✔You need to know what you should do if the seizures do not stop or there is a change in the person's breathing, behavior or condition that alarms you.

If you have any questions or feel unsure about using the treatment, CALL THE DOCTOR before using DIASTAT.

Where can I find more information and support?
The two best places to go for information and support are:
ASAP™ (Appropriate Seizure Action Program) sponsored by Athena Neurosciences, Inc. You can reach ASAP by calling 1-888-801-ASAP (2727).
EFA (Epilepsy Foundation of America). You can reach EFA by calling 800-EFA-1000 or www.efa.org.

When to treat. *Based on the doctor's directions or prescription.*

Special considerations.
DIASTAT should be used with caution:
- In people with respiratory (breathing) difficulties (e.g., asthma or pneumonia)

- In the elderly
- In women of child bearing potential, pregnancy or nursing mothers

Discuss beforehand with the doctor any additional steps you may need to take if there is leakage of DIASTAT or a bowel movement.

Patient's DIASTAT dosage is: _____ **mg**

Patient's resting breathing rate _____ Patient's current weight _____

Check expiration date and always remove cap and seal pin before using.

TREATMENT 1

....

Important things to tell the doctor.

	Seizures Before DIASTAT		
Date	Time	Seizure Type	No. of Seizures

Seizures After DIASTAT		
Time	Seizure Type	No. of Seizures

Things to do after treatment with DIASTAT.

Stay with the person for 4 hours and make notes of the following:

- Changes in breathing rate _____
- Changes in color _____
- Confirm current weight is still the same as when DIASTAT was prescribed _____
- Possible side effects from treatment _____

TREATMENT 2

....

Important things to tell the doctor.

	Seizures Before DIASTAT		
Date	Time	Seizure Type	No. of Seizures

Seizures After DIASTAT		
Time	Seizure Type	No. of Seizures

Things to do after treatment with DIATSTAT.

- Changes in resting breathing rate _____
- Changes in color _____
- Confirm current weight is still the same as when DIASTAT was prescribed _____
- Possible side effects from treatment _____

Disposal

- Discard all used material in the garbage can.
- Do not reuse.
- Discard in a safe place away from children.

DIASTAT is a registered trademark of Athena Neurosciences, Inc.

HOW TO ADMINISTER Dia*stat*™ Ⓘⱽ (diazepam rectal gel)

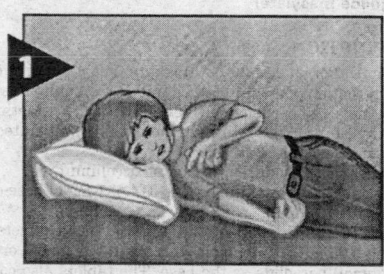

Put person on their side where they can't fall

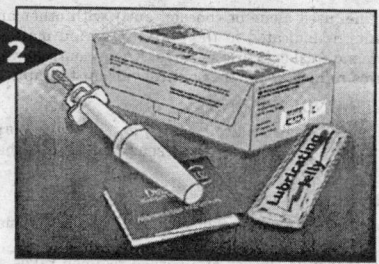

Get medicine

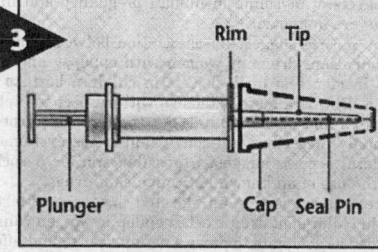

Get syringe

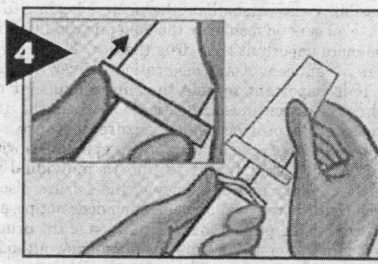

Push up with thumb and pull to remove protective cover from syringe

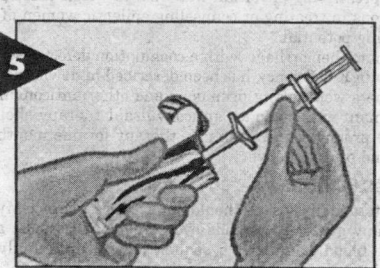

Lubricate rectal tip with lubricating jelly

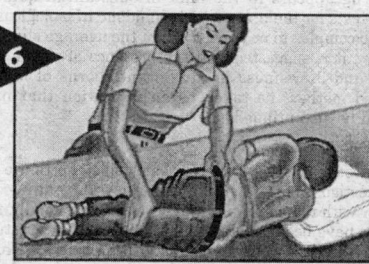

Turn person on side facing you

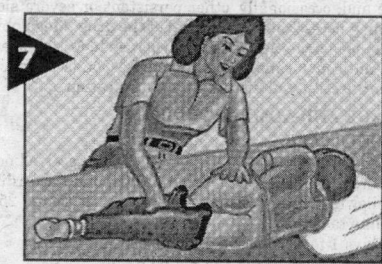

Bend upper leg forward to expose rectum

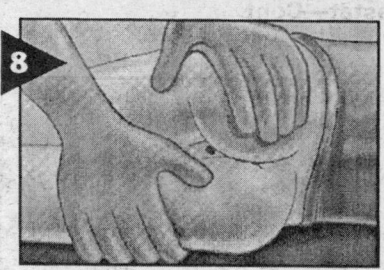

Separate buttocks to expose rectum

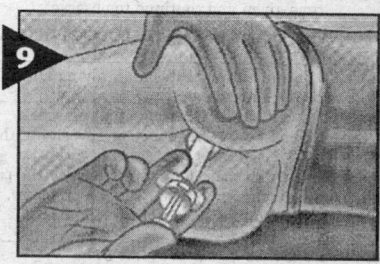

Gently insert syringe tip into rectum
Note: Rim should be snug against rectal opening.
SLOWLY COUNT OUT LOUD TO THREE...1...2...3

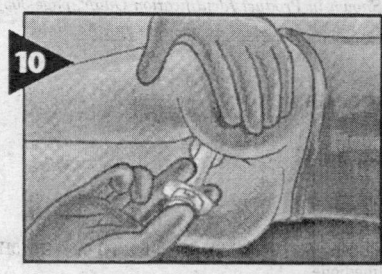

Slowly count to 3 while gently pushing plunger in until it stops

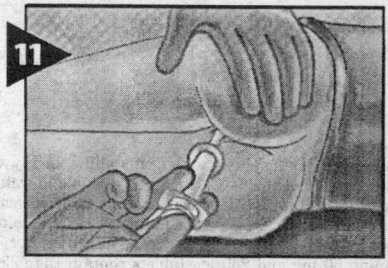

Slowly count to 3 before removing the syringe from rectum

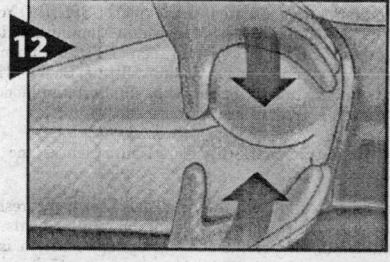

Slowly count to 3 while holding buttocks together to prevent leakage

Continued on next page

Diastat—Cont.

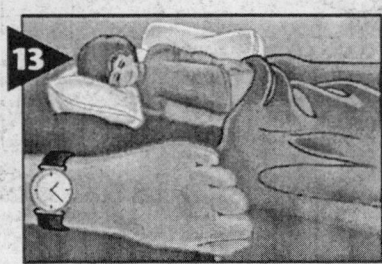

Keep person on side facing you, note
time given and continue to observe

CALL FOR HELP IF ANY OF THE FOLLOWING OCCUR

- Seizure(s) continues 15 minutes after giving DIASTAT or per the doctor's instructions.
- Seizure behavior is different from other episodes.
- You are alarmed by the frequency or severity of the seizure(s).
- You are alarmed by the color or breathing of the person.
- The person is having unusual or serious problems.

Local Emergency Number: **Doctor's Number:**

(please be sure to note if your area has 911)

Information for Emergency Squad: *Time DIASTAT given:*
_____ *Dose:*_____

DIASTAT is a registered trademark of Athena Neurosciences, Inc.
ASAP is a trademark of Athena Neurosciences, Inc.
© 1997 Athena Neurosciences, Inc.   Rev 11/97
Shown in Product Identification Guide, page 305

MYSOLINE® ℞
[mī 'sō-lēn]
(primidone)
Anticonvulsant

Rx Only

DESCRIPTION
Chemical name: 5-ethyldihydro-5-phenyl-4,6 (1H, 5H) pyrimidinedione.
Structural formula:

Mysoline* (primidone) is a white, crystalline, highly stable substance, M.P. 279–284°C. It is poorly soluble in water (60 mg per 100 mL at 37°C) and in most organic solvents. It possesses no acidic properties, in contrast to its barbiturate analog.
Mysoline 50 mg and 250 mg tablets contain the following inactive ingredients: Microcrystalline Cellulose, NF; Lactose, USP; Methylcellulose, USP; Sodium Starch Glycolate, NF; Talc, USP; Sodium Lauryl Sulfate, NF; Magnesium Stearate, NF; Water, USP, Purified.
Mysoline 250 mg tablets also contain Yellow Iron Oxide, NF.
Mysoline suspension contains these inactive ingredients: Ammonia Solution, Diluted; Citric Acid, USP; D&C Yellow No. 10; FD&C Yellow No. 6; Magnesium Aluminum Silicate; Methylparaben, NF; Propylparaben, NF; Saccharin Sodium, NF; Sodium Alginate; Sodium Citrate; Sodium Hypochlorite Solution, USP; Sorbic Acid, NF; Sorbitan Monolaurate; Water, USP, Purified; Flavors.

* Registered trademark of Athena Neurosciences, Inc.

ACTIONS
Mysoline raises electro- or chemoshock seizure thresholds or alters seizure patterns in experimental animals. The mechanism(s) of primidone's antiepileptic action is not known.
Primidone *per se* has anticonvulsant activity as do its two metabolites, phenobarbital and phenylethylmalonamide (PEMA). In addition to its anticonvulsant activity, PEMA potentiates the anticonvulsant activity of phenobarbital in experimental animals.

INDICATIONS
Mysoline, used alone or concomitantly with other anticonvulsants, is indicated in the control of grand mal, psychomotor, and focal epileptic seizures. It may control grand mal seizures refractory to other anticonvulsant therapy.

CONTRAINDICATIONS
Primidone is contraindicated in: 1) patients with porphyria and 2) patients who are hypersensitive to phenobarbital (see ACTIONS).

WARNINGS
The abrupt withdrawal of antiepileptic medication may precipitate status epilepticus.
The therapeutic efficacy of a dosage regimen takes several weeks before it can be assessed.
USAGE IN PREGNANCY
The effects of Mysoline in human pregnancy and nursing infants are unknown.
Recent reports suggest an association between the use of anticonvulsant drugs by women with epilepsy and an elevated incidence of birth defects in children born to these women. Data are more extensive with respect to diphenylhydantoin and phenobarbital, but these are also the most commonly prescribed anticonvulsants; less systematic or anecdotal reports suggest a possible similar association with the use of all known anticonvulsant drugs.
The reports suggesting an elevated incidence of birth defects in children of drug-treated epileptic women cannot be regarded as adequate to prove a definite cause-and-effect relationship. There are intrinsic methodologic problems in obtaining adequate data on drug teratogenicity in humans: the possibility also exists that other factors leading to birth defects, e.g., genetic factors or the epileptic condition itself, may be more important than drug therapy. The majority of mothers on anticonvulsant medication deliver normal infants. It is important to note that anticonvulsant drugs should not be discontinued in patients in whom the drug is administered to prevent major seizures because of the strong possibility of precipitating status epilepticus with attendant hypoxia and threat to life. In individual cases where the severity and frequency of the seizure disorders are such that the removal of medication does not pose a serious threat to the patient, discontinuation of the drug may be considered prior to and during pregnancy, although it cannot be said with any confidence that even minor seizures do not pose some hazard to the developing embryo or fetus. The prescribing physician will wish to weigh these considerations in treating or counseling epileptic women of childbearing potential.
Neonatal hemorrhage, with a coagulation defect resembling vitamin K deficiency, has been described in newborns whose mothers were taking primidone and other anticonvulsants. Pregnant women under anticonvulsant therapy should receive prophylactic vitamin K_1 therapy for one month prior to, and during, delivery.

PRECAUTIONS
The total daily dosage should not exceed 2 g. Since Mysoline therapy generally extends over prolonged periods, a complete blood count and a sequential multiple analysis-12 (SMA-12) test should be made every six months.
IN NURSING MOTHERS
There is evidence that in mothers treated with primidone, the drug appears in the milk in substantial quantities. Since tests for the presence of primidone in biological fluids are too complex to be carried out in the average clinical laboratory, it is suggested that the presence of undue somnolence and drowsiness in nursing newborns of Mysoline-treated mothers be taken as an indication that nursing should be discontinued.

ADVERSE REACTIONS
The most frequently occurring early side effects are ataxia and vertigo. These tend to disappear with continued therapy, or with reduction of initial dosage. Occasionally, the following have been reported: nausea, anorexia, vomiting, fatigue, hyperirritability, emotional disturbances, sexual impotency, diplopia, nystagmus, drowsiness, and morbilliform skin eruptions. Granulocytopenia, agranulocytosis, and red-cell hypoplasia and aplasia, have been reported rarely. These and, occasionally, other persistent or severe side effects may necessitate withdrawal of the drug. Megaloblastic anemia may occur as a rare idiosyncrasy to Mysoline and to other anticonvulsants. The anemia responds to folic acid without necessity of discontinuing medication.

DOSAGE AND ADMINISTRATION
ADULT DOSAGE
Patients 8 years of age and older who have received no previous treatment may be started on Mysoline according to the following regimen using either 50 mg or scored 250 mg Mysoline tablets.

    Days 1 to 3: 100 to 125 mg at bedtime
    Days 4 to 6: 100 to 125 mg b.i.d.
    Days 7 to 9: 100 to 125 mg t.i.d.
    Day 10 to maintenance: 250 mg t.i.d.

For most adults and children 8 years of age and over, the usual maintenance dosage is three to four 250 mg Mysoline tablets daily in divided doses (250 mg t.i.d. or q.i.d.). If required, an increase to five or six 250 mg tablets daily may be made but daily doses should not exceed 500 mg q.i.d.

INITIAL: ADULTS AND CHILDREN OVER 8

KEY: ·=50 mg tablet   •=250 mg tablet

DAY	1	2	3	4	5	6
AM				··		··
NOON						
PM	··	··	··	··	··	··

DAY	7	8	9	10	11	12
AM		··		•		
NOON	··	··	··	•	Adjust to
PM	··	··	··	•	Maintenance

Dosage should be individualized to provide maximum benefit. In some cases, serum blood level determinations of primidone may be necessary for optimal dosage adjustment. The clinically effective serum level for primidone is between 5 to 12 µg/mL.
IN PATIENTS ALREADY RECEIVING OTHER ANTICONVULSANTS
Mysoline should be started at 100 to 125 mg at bedtime and gradually increased to maintenance level as the other drug is gradually decreased. This regimen should be continued until satisfactory dosage level is achieved for the combination, or the other medication is completely withdrawn. When therapy with Mysoline alone is the objective, the transition from concomitant therapy should not be completed in less than two weeks.
PEDIATRIC DOSAGE
For children under 8 years of age, the following regimen may be used:

    Days 1 to 3:   50 mg at bedtime
    Days 4 to 6:   50 mg b.i.d.
    Days 7 to 9:   100 mg b.i.d.
    Day 10 to maintenance: 125 mg t.i.d. to 250 mg t.i.d.

For children under 8 years of age, the usual maintenance dosage is 125 to 250 mg three times daily or, 10 to 25 mg/kg/day in divided doses.

HOW SUPPLIED
MYSOLINE TABLETS
Each square-shaped, scored, yellow tablet, identified by "MYSOLINE 250" and an embossed M, contains 250 mg of primidone, in bottles of 100 (NDC 59075-691-10) and 1,000 (NDC 59075-691-11).
Also available in a unit-dose package of 100 (NDC 59075-691-81).
Each square-shaped, scored, white tablet, identified by "MYSOLINE 50 " and an embossed M, contains 50 mg of primidone, in bottles of 100 (NDC 59075-690-10) and 500 (NDC 59075-690-50).
The appearance of these tablets is a trademark of Athena Neurosciences, Inc.
MYSOLINE SUSPENSION
Each 5 mL (teaspoonful) contains 250 mg of primidone, in bottles of 8 fluid ounces (NDC 59075-692-50).

Store at room temperature, approximately 25° C (77° F).
Dispense in a tight, light-resistant container as defined in the U.S.P.
Distributed by:
Athena Neurosciences, Inc.
South San Francisco, CA 94080

Rev. 6/98

Shown in Product Identification Guide, page 305

PERMAX® ℞
[pĕr 'măks]
(pergolide mesylate)

DESCRIPTION
Permax® (Pergolide Mesylate) is an ergot derivative dopamine receptor agonist at both D_1 and D_2 receptor sites. Pergolide mesylate is chemically designated as 8β-[(Methylthio)methyl]-6-propylergoline monomethanesulfonate; the structural formula is as follows:
[See chemical structure at top of next column]
The formula weight of the base is 314.5; 1 mg of base corresponds to 3.18 µmol.
Permax is provided for oral administration in tablets containing 0.05 mg (0.159 µmol), 0.25 mg (0.795 µmol), or 1 mg (3.18 µmol) pergolide as the base. The tablets also contain croscarmellose sodium, iron oxide, lactose, magnesium stearate, and povidone. The 0.05-mg tablet also contains methionine, and the 0.25-mg tablet also contains F D & C Blue No. 2.

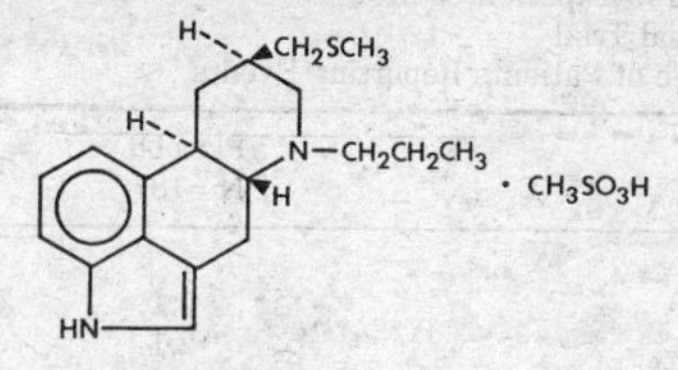

CLINICAL PHARMACOLOGY

Pharmacodynamic Information —Pergolide mesylate is a potent dopamine receptor agonist. Pergolide is 10 to 1,000 times more potent than bromocriptine on a milligram per milligram basis in various in vitro and in vivo test systems. Pergolide mesylate inhibits the secretion of prolactin in humans; it causes a transient rise in serum concentrations of growth hormone and a decrease in serum concentrations of luteinizing hormone. In Parkinson's disease, pergolide mesylate is believed to exert its therapeutic effect by directly stimulating postsynaptic dopamine receptors in the nigrostriatal system.

Pharmacokinetic Information (Absorption, Distribution, Metabolism, and Elimination) —Information on oral systemic bioavailability of pergolide mesylate is unavailable because of the lack of a sufficiently sensitive assay to detect the drug after the administration of a single dose. However, following oral administration of ^{14}C radiolabeled pergolide mesylate, approximately 55% of the administered radioactivity can be recovered from the urine and 5% from expired CO_2, suggesting that a significant fraction is absorbed. Nothing can be concluded about the extent of presystemic clearance, if any. Data on postabsorption distribution of pergolide are unavailable.

At least 10 metabolites have been detected, including N-despropylpergolide, pergolide sulfoxide, and pergolide sulfone. Pergolide sulfoxide and pergolide sulfone are dopamine agonists in animals. The other detected metabolites have not been identified, and it is not known whether any other metabolites are active pharmacologically.

The major route of excretion is the kidney.

Pergolide is approximately 90% bound to plasma proteins. This extent of protein binding may be important to consider when pergolide mesylate is coadministered with other drugs known to affect protein binding.

INDICATIONS AND USAGE

Permax is indicated as adjunctive treatment to levodopa/carbidopa in the management of the signs and symptoms of Parkinson's disease.

Evidence to support the efficacy of pergolide mesylate as an antiparkinsonian adjunct was obtained in a multicenter study enrolling 376 patients with mild to moderate Parkinson's disease who were intolerant to *l* -dopa/carbidopa as manifested by moderate to severe dyskinesia and/or on-off phenomena. On average, the patients evaluated had been on *l* -dopa/carbidopa for 3.9 years (range, 2 days to 16.8 years). The administration of pergolide mesylate permitted a 5% to 30% reduction in the daily dose of *l* -dopa. On average these patients treated with pergolide mesylate maintained an equivalent or better clinical status than they exhibited at baseline.

CONTRAINDICATIONS

Pergolide mesylate is contraindicated in patients who are hypersensitive to this drug or other ergot derivatives.

WARNINGS

Symptomatic Hypotension —In clinical trials, approximately 10% of patients taking pergolide mesylate with *l* -dopa versus 7% taking placebo with *l* -dopa experienced symptomatic orthostatic and/or sustained hypotension, especially during initial treatment. With gradual dosage titration, tolerance to the hypotension usually develops. It is therefore important to warn patients of the risk, to begin therapy with low doses, and to increase the dosage in carefully adjusted increments over a period of 3 to 4 weeks (*see* Dosage and Administration).

Hallucinosis —In controlled trials, pergolide mesylate with *l* -dopa caused hallucinosis in about 14% of patients as opposed to 3% taking placebo with *l* -dopa. This was of sufficient severity to cause discontinuation of treatment in about 3% of those enrolled; tolerance to this untoward effect was not observed.

Fatalities —In the placebo-controlled trial, 2 of 187 patients treated with placebo died as compared with 1 of 189 patients treated with pergolide mesylate. Of the 2,299 patients treated with pergolide mesylate in premarketing studies evaluated as of October 1988, 143 died while on the drug or shortly after discontinuing it. Because the patient population under evaluation was elderly, ill, and at high risk for death, it seems unlikely that pergolide mesylate played any role in these deaths, but the possibility that pergolide shortens survival of patients cannot be excluded with absolute certainty.

In particular, a case-by-case review of the clinical course of the patients who died failed to disclose any unique set of signs, symptoms, or laboratory results that would suggest that treatment with pergolide caused their deaths. Sixty-eight percent (68%) of the patients who died were 65 years of age or older. No death (other than a suicide) occurred within the first month of treatment; most of the patients who died had been on pergolide for years. A relative frequency of the causes of death by organ system are: Pulmonary failure/Pneumonia, 35%; Cardiovascular, 30%; Cancer, 11%; Unknown, 8.4%; Infection, 3.5%; Extrapyramidal syndrome, 3.5%; Stroke, 2.1%; Dysphagia, 2.1%; Injury, 1.4%; Suicide, 1.4%; Dehydration, 0.7%; Glomerulonephritis, 0.7%.

Serious Inflammation and Fibrosis —There have been rare reports of pleuritis, pleural effusion, pleural fibrosis, pericarditis, pericardial effusion or retroperitoneal fibrosis in patients taking pergolide. Some patients had experienced similar events while taking the ergot derivative bromocriptine. Pergolide should be used with caution in patients with a history of these conditions, particularly those patients who experienced the events while taking ergot derivatives. Patients with a history of such events should be carefully monitored clinically and with appropriate radiographic and laboratory studies while taking pergolide.

PRECAUTIONS

General —Caution should be exercised when administering pergolide mesylate to patients prone to cardiac dysrhythmias.

In a study comparing pergolide mesylate and placebo, patients taking pergolide mesylate were found to have significantly more episodes of atrial premature contractions (APCs) and sinus tachycardia.

The use of pergolide mesylate in patients on *l* -dopa may cause and/or exacerbate preexisting states of confusion and hallucinations (*see* Warnings) and preexisting dyskinesia. Also, the abrupt discontinuation of pergolide mesylate in patients receiving it chronically as an adjunct to *l*-dopa may precipitate the onset of hallucinations and confusion; these may occur within a span of several days. Discontinuation of pergolide should be undertaken gradually whenever possible, even if the patient is to remain on *l*-dopa.

A symptom complex resembling the neuroleptic malignant syndrome (NMS) (characterized by elevated temperature, muscular rigidity, altered consciousness, and autonomic instability), with no other obvious etiology, has been reported in association with rapid dose reduction, withdrawal of, or changes in antiparkinsonian therapy, including pergolide.

Information for Patients —Patients and their families should be informed of the common adverse consequences of the use of pergolide mesylate (*see* Adverse Reactions) and the risk of hypotension (*see* Warnings).

Patients should be advised to notify their physician if they become pregnant or intend to become pregnant during therapy.

Patients should be advised to notify their physician if they are breast feeding an infant.

Laboratory Tests —No specific laboratory tests are deemed essential for the management of patients on Permax. Periodic routine evaluation of all patients, however, is appropriate.

Drug Interactions —Dopamine antagonists, such as the neuroleptics (phenothiazines, butyrophenones, thioxanthines) or metoclopramide, ordinarily should not be administered concurrently with Permax (a dopamine agonist); these agents may diminish the effectiveness of Permax.

Because pergolide mesylate is approximately 90% bound to plasma proteins, caution should be exercised if pergolide mesylate is coadministered with other drugs known to affect protein binding.

Carcinogenesis, Mutagenesis, and Impairment of Fertility —A 2-year carcinogenicity study was conducted in mice using dietary levels of pergolide mesylate equivalent to oral doses of 0.6, 3.7, and 36.4 mg/kg/day in males and 0.6, 4.4, and 40.8 mg/kg/day in females. A 2-year study in rats was conducted using dietary levels equivalent to oral doses of 0.04, 0.18, and 0.88 mg/kg/day in males and 0.05, 0.28, and 1.42 mg/kg/day in females. The highest doses tested in the mice and rats were approximately 340 and 12 times the maximum human oral dose administered in controlled clinical trials (6 mg/day equivalent to 0.12 mg/kg/day).

A low incidence of uterine neoplasms occurred in both rats and mice. Endometrial adenomas and carcinomas were observed in rats. Endometrial sarcomas were observed in mice. The occurrence of these neoplasms is probably attributable to the high estrogen/progesterone ratio that would occur in rodents as a result of the prolactin-inhibiting action of pergolide mesylate. The endocrine mechanisms believed to be involved in the rodents are not present in humans. However, even though there is no known correlation between uterine malignancies occurring in pergolide-treated rodents and human risk, there are no human data to substantiate this conclusion.

Pergolide mesylate was evaluated for mutagenic potential in a battery of tests that included an Ames bacterial mutation assay, a DNA repair assay in cultured rat hepatocytes, an in vitro mammalian cell-point-mutation assay in cultured L5178Y cells, and a determination of chromosome alteration in bone marrow cells of Chinese hamsters. A weak mutagenic response was noted in the mammalian cell-point-mutation assay only after metabolic activation with rat liver microsomes. No mutagenic effects were obtained in the 2 other in vitro assays and in the vivo assay. The relevance of these findings in humans is unknown.

A fertility study in male and female mice showed that fertility was maintained at 0.6 and 1.7 mg/kg/day but decreased at 5.6 mg/kg/day. Prolactin has been reported to be involved in stimulating and maintaining progesterone levels required for implantation in mice, and, therefore, the impaired fertility at the high dose may have occurred because of depressed prolactin levels.

Usage in Pregnancy —Pregnancy Category B —Reproduction studies were conducted in mice at doses of 5, 16, and 45 mg/kg/day and in rabbits at doses of 2, 6, and 16 mg/kg/day. The highest doses tested in mice and rabbits were 375 and 133 times the 6 mg/day maximum human dose administered in controlled clinical trials. In these studies, there was no evidence of harm to the fetus due to pergolide mesylate. There are, however, no adequate and well-controlled studies in pregnant women. Among women who received pergolide mesylate for endocrine disorders in premarketing studies, there were 33 pregnancies that resulted in healthy babies and 6 pregnancies that resulted in congenital abnormalities (3 major, 3 minor); a causal relationship has not been established. Because human data are limited and because animal reproduction studies are not always predictive of human response, this drug should be used during pregnancy only if clearly needed.

Nursing Mothers —It is not known whether this drug is excreted in human milk. The pharmacologic action of pergolide mesylate suggests that it may interfere with lactation. Because many drugs are excreted in human milk and because of the potential for serious adverse reactions to pergolide mesylate in nursing infants, a decision should be made whether to discontinue nursing or to discontinue the drug, taking into account the importance of the drug to the mother.

Pediatric Use —Safety and effectiveness in pediatric patients have not been established.

ADVERSE REACTIONS

Commonly Observed —In premarketing clinical trials, the most commonly observed adverse events associated with use of pergolide mesylate which were not seen at an equivalent incidence among placebo-treated patients were: nervous system complaints, including dyskinesia, hallucinations, somnolence, insomnia; digestive complaints, including nausea, constipation, diarrhea, dyspepsia; and respiratory system complaints, including rhinitis.

Associated With Discontinuation of Treatment —Twenty-seven percent (27%) of approximately 1,200 patients receiving pergolide mesylate for treatment of Parkinson's disease in premarketing clinical trials in the US and Canada discontinued treatment due to adverse reactions. The events most commonly causing discontinuation were related to the nervous system (15.5%), primarily hallucinations (7.8%) and confusion (1.8%).

Fatalities —*See* Warnings.

Incidence in Controlled Clinical Trials —The table that follows enumerates adverse events that occurred at a frequency of 1% or more among patients taking pergolide mesylate who participated in the premarketing controlled clinical trials comparing pergolide mesylate with placebo. In a double-blind, controlled study of 6 months' duration, patients with Parkinson's disease were continued on *l* -dopa/carbidopa and were randomly assigned to receive either pergolide mesylate or placebo as additional therapy.

The prescriber should be aware that these figures cannot be used to predict the incidence of side effects in the course of usual medical practice where patient characteristics and other factors differ from those which prevailed in the clinical trials. Similarly, the cited frequencies cannot be compared with figures obtained from other clinical investigations involving different treatments, uses, and investigators. The cited figures, however, do provide the prescribing physician with some basis for estimating the relative contribution of drug and nondrug factors to the side-effect incidence rate in the population studied.

[See table at top of next page]

Events Observed During the Premarketing Evaluation of Permax— This section reports event frequencies evaluated as of October 1988 for adverse events occurring in a group of approximately 1,800 patients who took multiple doses of pergolide mesylate. The conditions and duration of exposure to pergolide mesylate varied greatly, involving well-controlled studies as well as experience in open and uncontrolled clinical settings. In the absence of appropriate controls in some of the studies, a causal relationship between these events and treatment with pergolide mesylate cannot be determined.

Continued on next page

Permax—Cont.

The following enumeration by organ system describes events in terms of their relative frequency of reporting in the data base. Events of major clinical importance are also described in the Warnings and Precautions sections.

The following definitions of frequency are used: frequent adverse events are defined as those occurring in at least 1/100 patients; infrequent adverse events are those occurring in 1/100 to 1/1,000 patients; rare events are those occurring in fewer than 1/1,000 patients.

Body as a Whole—*Frequent:* headache, asthenia, accidental injury, pain, abdominal pain, chest pain, back pain, flu syndrome, neck pain, fever; *Infrequent:* facial edema, chills, enlarged abdomen, malaise, neoplasm, hernia, pelvic pain, sepsis, cellulitis, moniliasis, abscess, jaw pain, hypothermia; *Rare:* acute abdominal syndrome, LE syndrome

Cardiovascular System—*Frequent:* postural hypotension, syncope, hypertension, palpitations, vasodilatations, congestive heart failure; *Infrequent:* myocardial infarction, tachycardia, heart arrest, abnormal electrocardiogram, angina pectoris, thrombophlebitis, bradycardia, ventricular extrasystoles, cerebrovascular accident, ventricular tachycardia, cerebral ischemia, atrial fibrillation, varicose vein, pulmonary embolus, AV block, shock; *Rare:* vasculitis, pulmonary hypertension, pericarditis, migraine, heart block, cerebral hemorrhage

Digestive System—*Frequent:* nausea, vomiting, dyspepsia, diarrhea, constipation, dry mouth, dysphagia; *Infrequent:* flatulence, abnormal liver function tests, increased appetite, salivary gland enlargement, thirst, gastroenteritis, gastritis, periodontal abscess, intestinal obstruction, nausea and vomiting, gingivitis, esophagitis, cholelithiasis, tooth caries, hepatitis, stomach ulcer, melena, hepatomegaly, hematemesis, eructation; *Rare:* sialadenitis, peptic ulcer, pancreatitis, jaundice, glossitis, fecal incontinence, duodenitis, colitis, cholecystitis, aphthous stomatitis, esophageal ulcer

Endocrine System—*Infrequent:* hypothyroidism, adenoma, diabetes mellitus, ADH inappropriate; *Rare:* endocrine disorder, thyroid adenoma

Hemic and Lymphatic System—*Frequent:* anemia; *Infrequent:* leukopenia, lymphadenopathy, leukocytosis, thrombocytopenia, petechia, megaloblastic anemia, cyanosis; *Rare:* purpura, lymphocytosis, eosinophilia, thrombocythemia, acute lymphoblastic leukemia, polycythemia, splenomegaly

Metabolic and Nutritional System—*Frequent:* peripheral edema, weight loss, weight gain; *Infrequent:* dehydration, hypokalemia, hypoglycemia, iron deficiency anemia, hyperglycemia, gout, hypercholesteremia; *Rare:* electrolyte imbalance, cachexia, acidosis, hyperuricemia

Musculoskeletal System—*Frequent:* twitching, myalgia, arthralgia; *Infrequent:* bone pain, tenosynovitis, myositis, bone sarcoma, arthritis; *Rare:* osteoporosis, muscle atrophy, osteomyelitis

Nervous System—*Frequent:* dyskinesia, dizziness, hallucinations, confusion, somnolence, insomnia, dystonia, paresthesia, depression, anxiety, tremor, akinesia, extrapyramidal syndrome, abnormal gait, abnormal dreams, incoordination, psychosis, personality disorder, nervousness, choreoathetosis, amnesia, paranoid reaction, abnormal thinking; *Infrequent:* akathisia, neuropathy, neuralgia, hypertonia, delusions, convulsion, libido increased, euphoria, emotional lability, libido decreased, vertigo, myoclonus, coma, apathy, paralysis, neurosis, hyperkinesia, ataxia, acute brain syndrome, torticollis, meningitis, manic reaction, hypokinesia, hostility, agitation, hypotonia; *Rare:* stupor, neuritis, intracranial hypertension, hemiplegia, facial paralysis, brain edema, myelitis, hallucinations and confusion after abrupt discontinuation

Respiratory System—*Frequent:* rhinitis, dyspnea, pneumonia, pharyngitis, cough increased; *Infrequent:* epistaxis, hiccup, sinusitis, bronchitis, voice alteration, hemoptysis, asthma, lung edema, pleural effusion, laryngitis, emphysema, apnea, hyperventilation; *Rare:* pneumothorax, lung fibrosis, larynx edema, hypoxia, hypoventilation, hemothorax, carcinoma of lung

Skin and Appendages System—*Frequent:* sweating, rash; *Infrequent:* skin discoloration, pruritus, acne, skin ulcer, alopecia, dry skin, skin carcinoma, seborrhea, hirsutism, herpes simplex, eczema, fungal dermatitis, herpes zoster; *Rare:* vesiculobullous rash, subcutaneous nodule, skin nodule, skin benign neoplasm, lichenoid dermatitis

Special Senses System—*Frequent:* abnormal vision, diplopia; *Infrequent:* otitis media, conjunctivitis, tinnitus, deafness, taste perversion, ear pain, eye pain, glaucoma, eye hemorrhage, photophobia, visual field defect; *Rare:* blindness, cataract, retinal detachment, retinal vascular disorder

Urogenital System—*Frequent:* urinary tract infection, urinary frequency, urinary incontinence, hematuria, dysmenorrhea; *Infrequent:* dysuria, breast pain, menorrhagia, impotence, cystitis, urinary retention, abortion, vaginal hemorrhage, vaginitis, priapism, kidney calculus, fibrocystic breast, lactation, uterine hemorrhage, urolithiasis, salpingitis, pyuria, metrorrhagia, menopause, kidney failure, breast carcinoma, cervical carcinoma; *Rare:* amenorrhea, bladder

Body System/ Adverse Event*	Pergolide Mesylate N = 189	Placebo N =187
Body as a Whole		
Pain	7.0	2.1
Abdominal pain	5.8	2.1
Injury, accident	5.8	7.0
Headache	5.3	6.4
Asthenia	4.2	4.8
Chest pain	3.7	2.1
Flu syndrome	3.2	2.1
Neck pain	2.7	1.6
Back pain	1.6	2.1
Surgical procedure	1.6	<1
Chills	1.1	0
Face edema	1.1	0
Infection	1.1	0
Cardiovascular		
Postural hypotension	9.0	7.0
Vasodilatation	3.2	<1
Palpitation	2.1	<1
Hypotension	2.1	<1
Syncope	2.1	1.1
Hypertension	1.6	1.1
Arrhythmia	1.1	<1
Myocardial infarction	1.1	<1
Digestive		
Nausea	24.3	12.8
Constipation	10.6	5.9
Diarrhea	6.4	2.7
Dyspepsia	6.4	2.1
Anorexia	4.8	2.7
Dry mouth	3.7	<1
Vomiting	2.7	1.6
Hemic and Lymphatic		
Anemia	1.1	<1
Metabolic and Nutritional		
Peripheral edema	7.4	4.3
Edema	1.6	0
Weight gain	1.6	0
Musculoskeletal		
Arthralgia	1.6	2.1
Bursitis	1.6	<1
Myalgia	1.1	<1
Twitching	1.1	0
Nervous System		
Dyskinesia	62.4	24.6
Dizziness	19.1	13.9
Hallucinations	13.8	3.2
Dystonia	11.6	8.0
Confusion	11.1	9.6
Somnolence	10.1	3.7
Insomnia	7.9	3.2
Anxiety	6.4	4.3
Tremor	4.2	7.5
Depression	3.2	5.4
Abnormal dreams	2.7	4.3
Personality disorder	2.1	<1
Psychosis	2.1	0
Abnormal gait	1.6	1.6
Akathisia	1.6	0
Extrapyramidal syndrome	1.6	1.1
Incoordination	1.6	<1
Paresthesia	1.6	3.2
Akinesia	1.1	1.1
Hypertonia	1.1	0
Neuralgia	1.1	<1
Speech disorder	1.1	1.6
Respiratory System		
Rhinitis	12.2	5.4
Dyspnea	4.8	1.1
Epistaxis	1.6	<1
Hiccup	1.1	0
Skin and Appendages		
Rash	3.2	2.1
Sweating	2.1	2.7
Special Senses		
Abnormal vision	5.8	5.4
Diplopia	2.1	0
Taste perversion	1.6	0
Eye disorder	1.1	0
Urogenital System		
Urinary frequency	2.7	6.4
Urinary tract infection	2.7	3.7
Hematuria	1.1	<1

Incidence of Treatment-Emergent Adverse Experiences in the Placebo-Controlled Clinical Trial
Percentage of Patients Reporting Events

* Events reported by at least 1% of patients receiving pergolide mesylate are included.

carcinoma, breast engorgement, epididymitis, hypogonadism, leukorrhea, nephrosis, pyelonephritis, urethral pain, uricaciduria, withdrawal bleeding

Postintroduction Reports—Voluntary reports of adverse events temporally associated with pergolide that have been received since market introduction and which may have no causal relationship with the drug, include the following: neuroleptic malignant syndrome.

OVERDOSAGE

There is no clinical experience with massive overdosage. The largest overdose involved a young hospitalized adult patient who was not being treated with pergolide mesylate but who intentionally took 60 mg of the drug. He experienced vomiting, hypotension, and agitation. Another patient receiving a daily dosage of 7 mg of pergolide mesylate unintentionally took 19 mg/day for 3 days, after which his vital signs were normal but he experienced severe hallucinations. Within 36 hours of resumption of the prescribed dosage level, the hallucinations stopped. One patient unintentionally took 14 mg/day for 23 days instead of her prescribed 1.4 mg/day dosage. She experienced severe involuntary movements and tingling in her arms and legs. Another patient who inadvertently received 7 mg instead of the prescribed 0.7 mg experienced palpitations, hypotension, and ventricular extrasystoles. The highest total daily dose (prescribed for several patients with refractory Parkinson's disease) has exceeded 30 mg.

Symptoms —Animal studies indicate that the manifestations of overdosage in man might include nausea, vomiting, convulsions, decreased blood pressure, and CNS stimulation. The oral median lethal doses in mice and rats were 54 and 15 mg/kg respectively.

Treatment —To obtain up-to-date information about the treatment of overdose, a good resource is your certified Regional Poison Control Center. Telephone numbers of certified poison control centers are listed in the *Physicians' Desk Reference (PDR).* In managing overdosage, consider the possibility of multiple drug overdoses, interaction among drugs, and unusual drug kinetics in your patient.

Management of overdosage may require supportive measures to maintain arterial blood pressure. Cardiac function should be monitored; an antiarrhythmic agent may be necessary. If signs of CNS stimulation are present, a phenothiazine or other butyrophenone neuroleptic agent may be indicated; the efficacy of such drugs in reversing the effects of overdose has not been assessed.

Protect the patient's airway and support ventilation and perfusion. Meticulously monitor and maintain, within acceptable limits, the patient's vital signs, blood gases, serum electrolytes, etc. Absorption of drugs from the gastrointestinal tract may be decreased by giving activated charcoal, which, in many cases, is more effective than emesis or lavage; consider charcoal instead of or in addition to gastric emptying. Repeated doses of charcoal over time may hasten elimination of some drugs that have been absorbed. Safeguard the patient's airway when employing gastric emptying or charcoal.

There is no experience with dialysis or hemoperfusion, and these procedures are unlikely to be of benefit.

DOSAGE AND ADMINISTRATION

Administration of Permax should be initiated with a daily dosage of 0.05 mg for the first 2 days. The dosage should then be gradually increased by 0.1 or 0.15 mg/day every third day over the next 12 days of therapy. The dosage may then be increased by 0.25 mg/day every third day until an optimal therapeutic dosage is achieved.

Permax is usually administered in divided doses 3 times per day. During dosage titration, the dosage of concurrent *l*-dopa/carbidopa may be cautiously decreased.

In clinical studies, the mean therapeutic daily dosage of Permax was 3 mg/day. The average concurrent daily dosage of *l*-dopa/carbidopa (expressed as *l*-dopa) was approximately 650 mg/day. The efficacy of Permax at doses above 5 mg/day has not been systematically evaluated.

HOW SUPPLIED

Tablets (scored):

0.05 mg, ivory, debossed with A615, (UC5336)—(RxPak* of 30) NDC 59075-615-30

0.25 mg, green, debossed with A625, (UC5337)—(RxPak of 100) NDC 59075-625-10

1 mg, pink, debossed with A630, (UC5338)—(RxPak of 100) NDC 59075-630-10

*All RxPaks (prescription packages, Lilly) have safety closures.

Store at controlled room temperature, 59° to 86°F (15° to 30°C).

CAUTION—Federal (USA) law prohibits dispensing without prescription.

Literature revised July 19, 1996

Manufactured by:
Eli Lilly & Co.
Indianapolis, IN 46285, USA
Distributed by:
Athena Neurosciences, Inc.
South San Francisco, CA 94080

Shown in Product Identification Guide, page 305

PV2276UCP

ZANAFLEX® ℞

[*zan̆-ă-flex*]
(tizanidine hydrochloride)
Tablets 4 mg

DESCRIPTION

ZANAFLEX* (tizanidine hydrochloride) is a centrally acting α_2-adrenergic agonist. Tizanidine HCl (tizanidine) is a white to off-white, fine crystalline powder, odorless or with a faint characteristic odor. Tizanidine is slightly soluble in water and methanol; solubility in water decreases as the pH increases. Its chemical name is 5-chloro-4-(2-imidazolin-2-ylamino)-2,1,3-benzothiodiazole hydrochloride. Tizanidine's molecular formula is $C_9H_8ClN_5S{\cdot}HCl$, its molecular weight is 290.2 and its structural formula is:

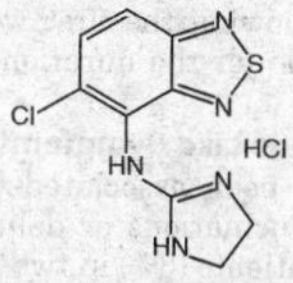

Zanaflex is supplied as 4 mg tablets for oral administration. Zanaflex tablets are composed of the active ingredient, tizanidine hydrochloride (4.576 mg equivalent to 4 mg tizanidine base), and the inactive ingredients, silicon dioxide colloidal, stearic acid, microcrystalline cellulose and anhydrous lactose.

* Registered trademark of Athena Neurosciences, Inc.

CLINICAL PHARMACOLOGY

Mechanism of Action

Tizanidine is an agonist at α_2-adrenergic receptor sites and presumably reduces spasticity by increasing presynaptic inhibition of motor neurons. In animal models, tizanidine has no direct effect on skeletal muscle fibers or the neuromuscular junction, and no major effect on monosynaptic spinal reflexes. The effects of tizanidine are greatest on polysynaptic pathways. The overall effect of these actions is thought to reduce facilitation of spinal motor neurons.

The imidazoline chemical structure of tizanidine is related to that of the anti-hypertensive drug clonidine and other α_2-adrenergic agonists. Pharmacological studies in animals show similarities between the two compounds, but tizanidine was found to have one-tenth to one-fiftieth (1/50) of the potency of clonidine in lowering blood pressure.

Pharmacokinetics

Following oral administration, tizanidine is essentially completely absorbed and has a half-life of approximately 2.5 hours (coefficient of variation [CV] = 33%). Following administration of tizanidine, peak plasma concentrations occurred at 1.5 hours (CV = 40%) after dosing. Food increases C_{max} by approximately one-third and shortens time to peak concentration by approximately 40 minutes, but the extent of tizanidine absorption is not affected. Tizanidine has linear pharmacokinetics over a dose of 1 to 20 mg. The absolute oral bioavailability of tizanidine is approximately 40% (CV = 24%), due to extensive first-pass metabolism in the liver; approximately 95% of an administered dose is metabolized. Tizanidine metabolites are not known to be active; their half-lives range from 20 to 40 hours. Tizanidine is widely distributed throughout the body; mean steady state volume of distribution is 2.4 L/kg (CV = 21%) following intravenous administration in healthy adult volunteers.

Following single and multiple oral dosing of ^{14}C-tizanidine, an average of 60% and 20% of total radioactivity was recovered in the urine and feces, respectively.

Tizanidine is approximately 30% bound to plasma proteins, independent of concentration over the therapeutic range.

Special Populations

Age Effects: No specific pharmacokinetic study was conducted to investigate age effects. Cross study comparison of pharmacokinetic data following single dose administration of 6 mg tizanidine showed that younger subjects cleared the drug four times faster than the elderly subjects. Tizanidine has not been evaluated in children (see PRECAUTIONS).

Hepatic Impairment: Pharmacokinetic differences due to hepatic impairment have not been studied (see WARNINGS).

Renal Impairment: Tizanidine clearance is reduced by more than 50% in elderly patients with renal insufficiency (creatinine clearance < 25 mL/min) compared to healthy elderly subjects; this would be expected to lead to a longer duration of clinical effect. Tizanidine should be used with caution in renally impaired patients (see PRECAUTIONS).

Gender Effects: No specific pharmacokinetic study was conducted to investigate gender effects. Retrospective analysis of pharmacokinetic data, however, following single and multiple dose administration of 4 mg tizanidine showed that gender had no effect on the pharmacokinetics of tizanidine.

Race Effects: Pharmacokinetic differences due to race have not been studied.

Drug Interactions-Oral Contraceptives: No specific pharmacokinetic study was conducted to investigate interaction between oral contraceptives and tizanidine. Retrospective analysis of population pharmacokinetic data following single and multiple dose administration of 4 mg tizanidine, however, showed that women concurrently taking oral contraceptives had 50% lower clearance of tizanidine compared to women not on oral contraceptives (see PRECAUTIONS).

CLINICAL STUDIES

Tizanidine's capacity to reduce increased muscle tone associated with spasticity was demonstrated in two adequate and well controlled studies in patients with multiple sclerosis or spinal cord injury.

In one study, patients with multiple sclerosis were randomized to receive single oral doses of drug or placebo. Patients and assessors were blind to treatment assignment and efforts were made to reduce the likelihood that assessors would become aware indirectly of treatment assignment (e.g., they did not provide direct care to patients and were prohibited from asking questions about side effects). In all, 140 patients received either placebo, 8 mg or 16 mg of tizanidine.

Response was assessed by physical examination; muscle tone was rated on a 5 point scale (Ashworth score), with a score of 0 used to describe normal muscle tone. A score of 1 indicated a slight spastic catch while a score of 2 indicated more marked muscle resistance. A score of 3 was used to describe considerable increase in tone, making passive movement difficult. A muscle immobilized by spasticity was given a score of 4. Spasm counts were also collected.

Assessments were made at 1, 2, 3 and 6 hours after treatment. A statistically significant reduction of the Ashworth score for Zanaflex compared to placebo was detected at 1, 2 and 3 hours after treatment. Figure 1 below shows a comparison of the mean change in muscle tone from baseline as measured by the Ashworth scale. The greatest reduction in muscle tone was 1 to 2 hours after treatment. By 6 hours after treatment, muscle tone in the 8 and 16 mg tizanidine groups was indistinguishable from muscle tone in placebo treated patients. Within a given patient, improvement in muscle tone was correlated with plasma concentration. Plasma concentrations were variable from patient to patient at a given dose. Although 16 mg produced a larger effect, adverse events including hypotension were more common and more severe than in the 8 mg group. There were no differences in the number of spasms occurring in each group.

FIGURE 1: Single Dose Study - Mean Change in Muscle Tone from Baseline as Measured by the Ashworth Scale +/- 95% Confidence Interval
(A Negative Ashworth Score Signifies an Improvement in Muscle Tone from Baseline)

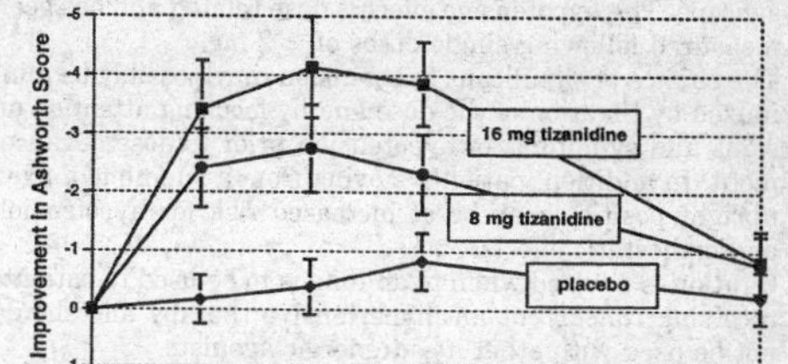

In a multiple dose study, 118 patients with spasticity secondary to spinal cord injury were randomized to either placebo or tizanidine. Steps similar to those taken in the first study were employed to ensure the integrity of blinding.

Patients were titrated over 3 weeks up to a maximum tolerated dose or 36 mg daily given in three unequal doses (e.g., 10 mg given in the morning and afternoon and 16 mg given at night). Patients were then maintained on their maximally tolerated dose for 4 additional weeks (i.e., maintenance phase). Throughout the maintenance phase, muscle tone was assessed on the Ashworth scale within a period of 2.5 hours following either the morning or afternoon dose. The number of daytime spasms was recorded daily by patients.

At endpoint (the protocol-specified time of outcome assessment), there was a statistically significant reduction in muscle tone and frequency of spasms in the tizanidine treated group compared to placebo. The reduction in muscle tone was not associated with a reduction in muscle strength (a desirable outcome) but also did not lead to any consistent advantage of tizanidine treated patients on measures of activities of daily living. Figure 2 below shows a comparison of the mean change in muscle tone from baseline as measured by the Ashworth scale.

[See figure at top of next column]

Continued on next page

Zanaflex—Cont.

FIGURE 2: Multiple Dose Study - Mean Change in Muscle Tone 0.5-2.5 Hours after Dosing as Measured by the Ashworth Scale +/- 95% Confidence Interval (A Negative Ashworth Score Signifies an Improvement in Muscle Tone from Baseline)

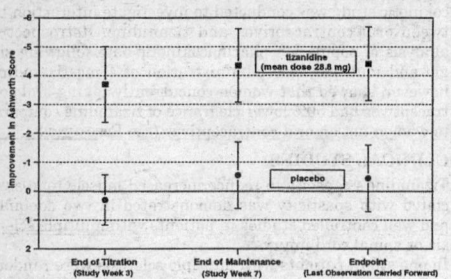

INDICATIONS AND USAGE

Tizanidine is a short-acting drug for the management of spasticity. Because of the short duration of effect, treatment with tizanidine should be reserved for those daily activities and times when relief of spasticity is most important (see DOSAGE AND ADMINISTRATION).

CONTRAINDICATIONS

Zanaflex is contraindicated in patients with known hypersensitivity to Zanaflex or its ingredients.

WARNINGS

Limited data base for chronic use of single doses above 8 mg and multiple doses above 24 mg per day

Clinical experience with long-term use of tizanidine at doses of 8 to 16 mg single doses or total daily doses of 24 to 36 mg (see DOSAGE AND ADMINISTRATION) is limited. Approximately 75 patients have been exposed to individual doses of 12 mg or more for at least one year or more and approximately 80 patients have been exposed to total daily doses of 30 to 36 mg/day for at least one year or more. There is essentially no long-term experience with single, daytime doses of 16 mg. Because long-term clinical study experience at high doses is limited, only those adverse events with a relatively high incidence are likely to have been identified (see WARNINGS, PRECAUTIONS and ADVERSE REACTIONS).

Hypotension

Tizanidine is an α_2-adrenergic agonist (like clonidine) and can produce hypotension. In a single dose study where blood pressure was monitored closely after dosing, two-thirds of patients treated with 8 mg of tizanidine had a 20% reduction in either the diastolic or systolic BP. The reduction was seen within 1 hour after dosing, peaked 2 to 3 hours after dosing and was associated, at times, with bradycardia, orthostatic hypotension, lightheadedness/dizziness and rarely syncope. The hypotensive effect is dose related and has been measured following single doses of $\geq$ 2 mg.

The chance of significant hypotension may possibly be minimized by titration of the dose and by focusing attention on signs and symptoms of hypotension prior to dose advancement. In addition, patients moving from a supine to a fixed upright position may be at increased risk for hypotension and orthostatic effects.

Caution is advised when tizanidine is to be used in patients receiving concurrent antihypertensive therapy and should not be used with other α_2-adrenergic agonists.

Risk of Liver Injury

Tizanidine occasionally causes liver injury, most often hepatocellular in type. In controlled clinical studies, approximately 5% of patients treated with tizanidine had elevations of liver function tests (ALT/SGPT, AST/SGOT) to greater than 3 times the upper limit of normal (or 2 times if baseline levels were elevated) compared to 0.4% in the control patients. Most cases resolved rapidly upon drug withdrawal with no reported residual problems. In occasional symptomatic cases, nausea, vomiting, anorexia and jaundice have been reported. In postmarketing experience, three deaths associated with liver failure have been reported in patients treated with tizanidine. In one case, a 49 year-old male developed jaundice and liver enlargement following 2 months of tizanidine treatment, primarily at 6 mg tid. A liver biopsy showed multilobular necrosis without eosinophilic infiltration. Treatment was discontinued and the patient died in hepatic coma 10 days later. There was no evidence of hepatitis B and C in this patient and other therapy included only oxezepam and ranitidine. There was thus no explanation, other than a reaction to tizanidine, to explain the liver injury. In the two other cases, patients were taking other drugs with known potential for liver toxicity. One patient, treated with tizanidine at a dose of 4 mg/day, was also on carbamazepine when he developed cholestatic jaundice after 2 months of treatment; this patient died with pneumonia about 20 days later. Another patient, treated with tizanidine for 11 days, was also treated with dantrolene for about 2 weeks prior to developing fatal fulminant hepatic failure.

Monitoring of aminotransferase levels is recommended during the first 6 months of treatment (e.g., baseline, 1, 3 and 6 months) and periodically thereafter, based on clinical status. Because of the potential toxic hepatic effect of tizanidine, the drug should be used only with extreme caution in patients with impaired hepatic function.

Sedation

In the multiple dose, controlled clinical studies, 48% of patients receiving any dose of tizanidine reported sedation as an adverse event. In 10% of these cases, the sedation was rated as severe compared to <1% in the placebo treated patients. Sedation may interfere with everyday activity.

The effect appears to be dose related. In a single dose study, 92% of the patients receiving 16 mg, when asked, reported that they were drowsy during the 6 hour study. This compares to 76% of the patients on 8 mg and 35% of the patients on placebo. Patients began noting this effect 30 minutes following dosing. The effect peaked 1.5 hours following dosing. Of the patients who received a single dose of 16 mg, 51% continued to report drowsiness 6 hours following dosing compared to 13% in the patients receiving placebo or 8 mg of tizanidine.

In the multiple dose studies, the prevalence of patients with sedation peaked following the first week of titration and then remained stable for the duration of the maintenance phase of the study.

Hallucinosis/Psychotic-Like Symptoms

Tizanidine use has been associated with hallucinations. Formed, visual hallucinations or delusions have been reported in 5 of 170 patients (3%) in two North American controlled clinical studies. These 5 cases occurred within the first 6 weeks. Most of the patients were aware that the events were unreal. One patient developed psychoses in association with the hallucinations. One patient among these 5 continued to have problems for at least 2 weeks following discontinuation of tizanidine.

PRECAUTIONS

Cardiovascular

Prolongation of the QT interval and bradycardia were noted in chronic toxicity studies in dogs at doses equal to the maximum human dose on a mg/m^2 basis. ECG evaluation was not performed in the controlled clinical studies. Reduction in pulse rate has been noted in association with decreases in blood pressure in the single dose controlled study (see WARNINGS).

Ophthalmic

Dose-related retinal degeneration and corneal opacities have been found in animal studies at doses equivalent to approximately the maximum recommended dose on a mg/m^2 basis. There have been no reports of corneal opacities or retinal degeneration in the clinical studies.

Use in Renally Impaired Patients

Tizanidine should be used with caution in patients with renal insufficiency (creatinine clearance < 25 mL/min), as clearance is reduced by more than 50%. In these patients, during titration, the individual doses should be reduced. If higher doses are required, individual doses rather than dosing frequency should be increased. These patients should be monitored closely for the onset or increase in severity of the common adverse events (dry mouth, somnolence, asthenia and dizziness) as indicators of potential overdose.

Use in Women Taking Oral Contraceptives

Tizanidine should be used with caution in women taking oral contraceptives, as clearance of tizanidine is reduced by approximately 50% in such patients. In these patients, during titration, the individual doses should be reduced.

Information for Patients

Patients should be advised of the limited clinical experience with tizanidine both in regard to duration of use and the higher doses required to reduce muscle tone (see WARNINGS).

Because of the possibility of tizanidine lowering blood pressure, patients should be warned about the risk of clinically significant orthostatic hypotension (see WARNINGS).

Because of the possibility of sedation, patients should be warned about performing activities requiring alertness, such as driving a vehicle or operating machinery (see WARNINGS). Patients should also be instructed that the sedation may be additive when Zanaflex is taken in conjunction with drugs (baclofen, benzodiazepines) or substances (e.g., alcohol) that act as CNS depressants.

Zanaflex should be used with caution where spasticity is utilized to sustain posture and balance in locomotion or whenever spasticity is utilized to obtain increased function.

Drug Interactions

In vitro studies of cytochrome P450 isoenzymes using human liver microsomes indicate that neither tizanidine nor the major metabolites are likely to affect the metabolism of other drugs metabolized by cytochrome P450 isoenzymes.

Acetaminophen: Tizanidine delayed the T$_{max}$ of acetaminophen by 16 minutes. Acetaminophen did not affect the pharmacokinetics of tizanidine.

Alcohol: Alcohol increased the AUC of tizanidine by approximately 20% while also increasing its C$_{max}$ by approximately

15%. This was associated with an increase in side effects of tizanidine. The CNS depressant effects of tizanidine and alcohol are additive.

Oral Contraceptives: No specific pharmacokinetic study was conducted to investigate interaction between oral contraceptives and tizanidine, but retrospective analysis of population pharmacokinetic data following single and multiple dose administration of 4 mg tizanidine showed that women concurrently taking oral contraceptives had 50% lower clearance of tizanidine than women not on oral contraceptives.

Carcinogenesis, Mutagenesis, Impairment of Fertility

No evidence for carcinogenicity was seen in two dietary studies in rodents. Tizanidine was administered to mice for 78 weeks at doses up to 16 mg/kg, which is equivalent to 2 times the maximum recommended human dose on a mg/m^2 basis. Tizanidine was also administered to rats for 104 weeks at doses up to 9 mg/kg, which is equivalent to 2.5 times the maximum recommended human dose on a mg/m^2 basis. There was no statistically significant increase in tumors in either species.

Tizanidine was not mutagenic or clastogenic in the following *in vitro* assays: the bacterial Ames test and the mammalian gene mutation test and chromosomal aberration test in Chinese hamster cells. It was also negative in the following *in vivo* assays: the bone marrow micronucleus test in mice, the bone marrow micronucleus and cytogenicity test in Chinese hamsters, the dominant lethal mutagenicity test in mice, and the unscheduled DNA synthesis (UDS) test in mice.

Tizanidine did not affect fertility in male rats at doses of 10 mg/kg, approximately 2.7 times the maximum recommended human dose on a mg/m^2 basis, and in females at doses of 3 mg/kg, approximately equal to the maximum recommended human dose on a mg/m^2 basis; fertility was reduced in males receiving 30 mg/kg (8 times the maximum recommended human dose on a mg/m^2 basis) and in females receiving 10 mg/kg (2.7 times the maximum recommended human dose on a mg/m^2 basis). At these doses, maternal behavioral effects and clinical signs were observed including marked sedation, weight loss, and ataxia.

Pregnancy

Pregnancy Category C: Reproduction studies performed in rats at a dose of 3 mg/kg, equal to the maximum recommended human dose on a mg/m^2 basis, and in rabbits at 30 mg/kg, 16 times the maximum recommended human dose on a mg/m^2 basis, did not show evidence of teratogenicity. Tizanidine at doses that are equal to and up to 8 times the maximum recommended human dose on a mg/m^2 basis increased gestation duration in rats. Prenatal and postnatal pup loss was increased and developmental retardation occurred. Postimplantation loss was increased in rabbits at doses of 1 mg/kg or greater, equal to or greater than 0.5 times the maximum recommended human dose on a mg/m^2 basis. Tizanidine has not been studied in pregnant women. Tizanidine should be given to pregnant women only if clearly needed.

Labor and Delivery

The effect of tizanidine on labor and delivery in humans is unknown.

Nursing Mothers

It is not known whether tizanidine is excreted in human milk, although as a lipid soluble drug, it might be expected to pass into breast milk.

Geriatric Use

Tizanidine should be used with caution in elderly patients because clearance is decreased four-fold.

Pediatric Use

There are no adequate and well-controlled studies to document the safety and efficacy of tizanidine in children.

ADVERSE REACTIONS

In multiple dose, placebo-controlled clinical studies, 264 patients were treated with tizanidine and 261 with placebo. Adverse events, including severe adverse events, were more frequently reported with tizanidine than with placebo.

Common Adverse Events Leading to Discontinuation

Forty-five of 264 (17%) patients receiving tizanidine and 13 of 261 (5%) patients receiving placebo in three multiple dose, placebo-controlled clinical studies discontinued treatment for adverse events. When patients withdrew from the study, they frequently had more than one reason for discontinuing. The adverse events most frequently leading to withdrawal of tizanidine treated patients in the controlled clinical studies were asthenia (weakness, fatigue and/or tiredness) (3%), somnolence (3%), dry mouth (3%), increased spasm or tone (2%) and dizziness (2%).

Most Frequent Adverse Clinical Events Seen in Association With the Use of Tizanidine

In multiple dose, placebo-controlled clinical studies involving 264 patients with spasticity, the most frequent adverse events were dry mouth, somnolence/sedation, asthenia (weakness, fatigue and/or tiredness), and dizziness. Three-quarters of the patients rated the events as mild to moderate and one-quarter of the patients rated the events as being severe. These events appeared to be dose related.

Adverse Events Reported in Controlled Studies

The events cited reflect experience gained under closely monitored conditions of clinical studies in a highly selected patient population. In actual clinical practice or in other clinical studies, these frequency estimates may not apply, as the conditions of use, reporting behavior, and the kinds of patients treated may differ. Table 1 lists treatment emergent signs and symptoms that were reported in greater than 2% of patients in three multiple dose, placebo-controlled studies who received tizanidine where the frequency in the tizanidine group was at least as common as in the placebo group. These events are not necessarily related to tizanidine treatment. For comparison purposes, the corresponding frequency of the event (per 100 patients) among placebo treated patients is also provided.

TABLE 1: Multiple Dose, Placebo-Controlled Studies - Frequent (> 2%) Adverse Events Reported for Which Zanaflex Incidence is Greater Than Placebo

Event	Placebo N = 261 %	Zanaflex N = 264 %
Dry mouth	10	49
Somnolence	10	48
Asthenia (weakness, fatigue and/or tiredness)	16	41
Dizziness	4	16
UTI	7	10
Infection	5	6
Constipation	1	4
Liver function tests abnormal	<1	3
Vomiting	0	3
Speech disorder	0	3
Amblyopia (blurred vision)	<1	3
Urinary frequency	2	3
Flu syndrome	2	3
SGPT/ALT increased	<1	3
Dyskinesia	0	3
Nervousness	<1	3
Pharyngitis	1	3
Rhinitis	2	3

In the single dose, placebo-controlled study involving 142 patients with spasticity, the patients were specifically asked if they had experienced any of the four most common adverse events: dry mouth, somnolence (drowsiness), asthenia (weakness, fatigue and/or tiredness), and dizziness. In addition, hypotension and bradycardia were observed. The occurrence of these adverse events are summarized in Table 2. Other events were, in general, reported at a rate of 2% or less.

TABLE 2: Single Dose, Placebo-Controlled Study - Common Adverse Events Reported

Event	Placebo N = 48 %	Zanaflex 8 mg N = 45 %	Zanaflex 16 mg N = 49 %
Somnolence	31	78	92
Dry mouth	35	76	88
Asthenia (weakness, fatigue and/or tiredness)	40	67	78
Dizziness	4	22	45
Hypotension	0	16	33
Bradycardia	0	2	10

Other Adverse Events Observed During the Evaluation of Tizanidine

Tizanidine was administered to 1187 patients in additional clinical studies where adverse event information was available. The conditions and duration of exposure varied greatly, and included (in overlapping categories) double-blind and open-label studies, uncontrolled and controlled studies, inpatient and outpatient studies, and titration studies. Untoward events associated with this exposure were recorded by clinical investigators using terminology of their own choosing. Consequently, it is not possible to provide a meaningful estimate of the proportion of individuals experiencing adverse events without first grouping similar types of untoward events into a smaller number of standardized event categories.

In the tabulations that follow, reported adverse events were classified using a standard COSTART-based dictionary terminology. The frequencies presented, therefore, represent the proportion of the 1187 patients exposed to tizanidine who experienced an event of the type cited on at least one occasion while receiving tizanidine. All reported events are included except those already listed in Table 1. If the COSTART term for an event was so general as to be uninformative, it was replaced with a more informative term. It is im-

portant to emphasize that, although the events reported occurred during treatment with tizanidine, they were not necessarily caused by it.

Events are further categorized by body system and listed in order of decreasing frequency according to the following definitions: frequent adverse events are those occurring on one or more occasions in at least 1/100 patients (only those not already listed in the tabulated results from placebo-controlled studies appear in this listing); infrequent adverse events are those occurring in 1/100 to 1/1000 patients.

Body as a Whole: Frequent: fever; *Infrequent:* allergic reaction, moniliasis, malaise, abscess, neck pain, sepsis, cellulitis, death, overdose; *Rare:* carcinoma, congenital anomaly, suicide attempt.

Cardiovascular System: Infrequent: vasodilatation, postural hypotension, syncope, migraine, arrhythmia; *Rare:* angina pectoris, coronary artery disorder, heart failure, myocardial infarct, phlebitis, pulmonary embolus, ventricular extrasystoles, ventricular tachycardia.

Digestive System: Frequent: abdomen pain, diarrhea, dyspepsia; *Infrequent:* dysphagia, cholelithiasis, fecal impaction, flatulence, gastrointestinal hemorrhage, hepatitis, melena; *Rare:* gastroenteritis, hematemesis, hepatoma, intestinal obstruction, liver damage.

Hemic and Lymphatic System: Infrequent: ecchymosis, hypercholesteremia, anemia, hyperlipemia, leukopenia, leukocytosis, sepsis; *Rare:* petechia, purpura, thrombocythemia, thrombocytopenia.

Metabolic and Nutritional System: Infrequent: edema, hypothyroidism, weight loss; *Rare:* adrenal cortex insufficiency, hyperglycemia, hypokalemia, hyponatremia, hypoproteinemia, respiratory acidosis.

Musculoskeletal System: Frequent: myasthenia, back pain; *Infrequent:* pathological fracture, arthralgia, arthritis, bursitis.

Nervous System: Frequent: depression, anxiety, paresthesia; *Infrequent:* tremor, emotional lability, convulsion, paralysis, thinking abnormal, vertigo, abnormal dreams, agitation, depersonalization, euphoria, migraine, stupor, dysautonomia, neuralgia; *Rare:* dementia, hemiplegia, neuropathy.

Respiratory System: Infrequent: sinusitis, pneumonia, bronchitis; *Rare:* asthma.

Skin and Appendages: Frequent: rash, sweating, skin ulcer; *Infrequent:* pruritus, dry skin, acne, alopecia, urticaria; *Rare:* exfoliative dermatitis, herpes simplex, herpes zoster, skin carcinoma.

Special Senses: Infrequent: ear pain, tinnitus, deafness, glaucoma, conjunctivitis, eye pain, optic neuritis, otitis media, retinal hemorrhage, visual field defect; *Rare:* iritis, keratitis, optic atrophy.

Urogenital System: Infrequent: urinary urgency, cystitis, menorrhagia, pyelonephritis, urinary retention, kidney calculus, uterine fibroids enlarged, vaginal moniliasis, vaginitis; *Rare:* albuminuria, glycosuria, hematuria, metrorrhagia.

DRUG ABUSE AND DEPENDENCE

Abuse potential was not evaluated in human studies. Rats were able to distinguish tizanidine from saline in a standard discrimination paradigm, after training, but failed to generalize the effects of morphine, cocaine, diazepam or phenobarbital to tizanidine. Monkeys were shown to self-administer tizanidine in a dose-dependent manner, and abrupt cessation of tizanidine produced transient signs of withdrawal at doses > 35 times the maximum recommended human dose on a mg/m² basis. These transient withdrawal signs (increased locomotion, body twitching, and aversive behavior toward the observer) were not reversed by naloxone administration.

OVERDOSAGE

One significant overdosage of tizanidine has been reported. Attempted suicide by a 46 year-old male with multiple sclerosis resulted in coma very shortly after the ingestion of one-hundred 4 mg tizanidine tablets. Pupils were not dilated and nystagmus was not present. The patient had marked respiratory depression with Cheyne-Stokes respiration. Gastric lavage and forced diuresis with furosemide and mannitol were instituted. The patient recovered several hours later without sequelae. Laboratory findings were normal.

Should overdosage occur, basic steps to ensure the adequacy of an airway and the monitoring of cardiovascular and respiratory systems should be undertaken. For the most recent information concerning the management of overdose, contact a poison control center.

DOSAGE AND ADMINISTRATION

A single oral dose of 8 mg of tizanidine reduces muscle tone in patients with spasticity for a period of several hours. The effect peaks at approximately 1 to 2 hours and dissipates between 3 to 6 hours. Effects are dose-related.

Although single doses of less than 8 mg have not been demonstrated to be effective in controlled clinical studies, the dose-related nature of tizanidine's common adverse events make it prudent to begin treatment with single oral doses of

4 mg. Increase the dose gradually (2 to 4 mg steps) to optimum effect (satisfactory reduction of muscle tone at a tolerated dose).

The dose can be repeated at 6 to 8 hour intervals, as needed, to a maximum of three doses in 24 hours. The total daily dose should not exceed 36 mg.

Experience with single doses exceeding 8 mg and daily doses exceeding 24 mg is limited. There is essentially no experience with repeated, single, daytime doses greater than 12 mg or total daily doses greater than 36 mg (see WARNINGS).

HOW SUPPLIED

Zanaflex® (tizanidine hydrochloride) is available as 4 mg white tablets, embossed with the Athena logo and "594" on one side and cross-scored on the other. The tablets are available in bottles of 150 (NDC 59075-594-15).

Store at 15-30°C (59-86°F). Dispense in containers with child resistant closure.

Caution: Federal law prohibits dispensing without prescription.

Manufactured by Sandoz Pharma, Ltd., Basle, Switzerland for

Athena Neurosciences, Inc., South San Francisco, California 94080

Rev. 3-3-98

Shown in Product Identification Guide, page 305

Axcan Pharma U.S. Inc.
3940 QUEBEC AVENUE NORTH
MINNEAPOLIS, MN 55427

Direct Inquiries to:
Medical Department
(612) 417-0684
FAX: (612) 417-9039
Medical Emergency Contact:
(800) 742-6706

URSO® ℞
[*ūr-so*]
Ursodiol Tablets 250 mg

DESCRIPTION

URSO® is a bile acid available as 250 mg film-coated tablets for oral administration.

URSO® is ursodiol (ursodeoxycholic acid), a naturally occurring bile acid found in small quantities in normal human bile and in larger quantities in the biles of certain species of bears. It is a bitter-tasting white powder consisting of crystalline particles freely soluble in ethanol and glacial acetic acid, slightly soluble in chloroform, sparingly soluble in ether, and practically insoluble in water. The chemical name of ursodiol is 3α,7β-dihydroxy-5β-cholan-24-oic ($C_{24}H_{40}O_4$). Ursodiol has a molecular weight of 392.56. Its structure is shown below.

Inactive ingredients: microcrystalline cellulose, povidone, sodium starch glycolate, magnesium stearate, ethylcellulose, dibutyl sebacate, carnauba wax, hydroxypropyl methylcellulose, PEG 3350, PEG 8000, cetyl alcohol, sodium lauryl sulfate and hydrogen peroxide.

CLINICAL PHARMACOLOGY

Ursodiol (UDCA) is normally present as a minor fraction of the total bile acids in humans (about 5%). Following oral administration, the majority of ursodiol is absorbed by passive diffusion and its absorption is incomplete. Once absorbed, ursodiol undergoes hepatic extraction to the extent of about 50% in the absence of liver disease. As the severity of liver disease increases, the extent of extraction decreases. In the liver, ursodiol is conjugated with glycine or taurine, then secreted into bile. These conjugates of ursodiol are absorbed in the small intestine by passive and active mechanisms. The conjugates can also be deconjugated in the ileum by intestinal enzymes, leading to the formation of free ursodiol that can be reabsorbed and reconjugated in the liver. Nonabsorbed ursodiol passes into the colon where it is mostly 7-dehydroxylated to lithocholic acid. Some ursodiol is epimerized to chenodiol (CDCA) via a 7-oxo intermediate.

Continued on next page

Urso—Cont.

Chenodiol also undergoes 7-dehydroxylation to form litho-cholic acid. These metabolites are poorly soluble and ex-creted in the feces. A small portion of lithocholic acid is re-absorbed, conjugated in the liver with glycine, or taurine and sulfated at the 3 position. The resulting sulfated litho-cholic acid conjugates are excreted in bile and then lost in feces.

Lithocholic acid, when administered chronically to animals, causes cholestatic liver injury that may lead to death from liver failure in certain species unable to form sulfate conju-gates. Ursodiol is 7-dehydroxylated more slowly than cheno-diol. For equimolar doses of ursodiol and chenodiol, steady state levels of lithocholic acid in biliary bile acids are lower during ursodiol administration than with chenodiol admin-istration. Humans and chimpanzees can sulfate lithocholic acid. Although liver injury has not been associated with ur-sodiol therapy, a reduced capacity to sulfate may exist in some individuals. Nonetheless, such a deficiency has not yet been clearly demonstrated and must be extremely rare, given the several thousand patient-years of clinical experi-ence with ursodiol.

In healthy subjects, at least 70% of ursodiol (unconjugated) is bound to plasma protein. No information is available on the binding of conjugated ursodiol to plasma protein in healthy subjects or primary biliary cirrhosis (PBC) patients. Its volume of distribution has not been determined, but is expected to be small since the drug is mostly distributed in the bile and small intestine. Ursodiol is excreted primarily in the feces. With treatment, urinary excretion increases, but remains less than 1% except in severe cholestatic liver disease.

During chronic administration of ursodiol, it becomes a ma-jor biliary and plasma bile acid. At a chronic dose of 13–15 mg/kg/day, ursodiol constitutes 30–50% of biliary and plasma bile acids.

CLINICAL STUDIES

A U.S., multicenter, randomized, double-blind, placebo-con-trolled study was conducted to evaluate the efficacy of ur-sodeoxycholic acid at a dose of 13–15 mg/kg/day, adminis-tered in 4 divided doses in 180 patients with PBC. Upon completion of the double-blind portion, all patients entered an open-label active treatment extension phase.

Treatment failure, the main efficacy end point measured during this study, was defined as death, need for liver trans-plantation, histologic progression by two stages or to cirrho-sis, development of varices, ascites or encephalopathy, marked worsening of fatigue or pruritus, inability to toler-ate the drug, doubling of serum bilirubin and voluntary withdrawal. After two years of double-blind treatment, the incidence of treatment failure was significantly reduced in the URSO® group (n=89) as compared to the placebo group (n=91). Time to treatment failure was also significantly de-layed in the URSO® treated group regardless of either his-tologic stage or baseline bilirubin levels (>1.8 or ≤1.8 mg/dl).

Using a definition of treatment failure which excluded dou-bling of serum bilirubin and voluntary withdrawal, time to treatment failure was significantly delayed in the URSO® group. In comparison with placebo, treatment with URSO® resulted in a significant improvement in the following serum hepatic biochemistries when compared to baseline: total bilirubin, SGOT, alkaline phosphatase and IgM.

A second study conducted in Canada randomized 222 PBC patients to ursodiol, 14 mg/kg/day or placebo, in a double-blind manner during a two-year period. At two years, a sta-tistically significant difference between the two treatments, in favor of ursodiol, was demonstrated in the following: re-duction in the proportion of patients exhibiting a more than 50% increase in serum bilirubin; median percent decrease in bilirubin, transaminases and alkaline phosphatase; inci-dence of treatment failure; and time to treatment failure. The definition of treatment failure included: discontinuing the study for any reason; a total serum bilirubin level greater than or equal to 1.5 mg/dl or increasing to a level equal to or greater than two times the baseline level; and the development of ascites or encephalopathy.

INDICATIONS AND USAGE

URSO® (ursodiol) tablets are indicated for the treatment of patients with primary biliary cirrhosis.

CONTRAINDICATIONS

Hypersensitivity or intolerance to ursodiol or any of the components of the formulation.

PRECAUTIONS

Patients with variceal bleeding, hepatic encephalopathy, ascites or in need of an urgent liver transplant, should re-ceive appropriate specific treatment.

Drug Interactions

Bile acid sequestering agents such as cholestyramine and colestipol may interfere with the action of URSO® by reduc-ing its absorption. Aluminum-based antacids have been shown to adsorb bile acids *in vitro* and may be expected to interfere with URSO® in the same manner as the bile acid sequestering agents. Estrogens, oral contraceptives, and clofibrate (and perhaps other lipid-lowering drugs) increase hepatic cholesterol secretion, and encourage cholesterol gallstone formation and hence may counteract the effective-ness of URSO®.

Carcinogenicity, Mutagenicity and Impairment of Fertility

In two 24-month oral carcinogenicity studies in mice, urso-diol at doses up to 1,000 mg/kg/day (3,000 mg/m²/day) was not tumorigenic. Based on body surface area, for a 50 kg person of average height (1.46 m² body surface area), this dose represents 5.4 times the recommended maximum clin-ical dose of 15 mg/kg/day (555 mg/m²/day).

In a two-year oral carcinogenicity study in Fischer 344 rats, ursodiol at doses up to 300 mg/kg/day (1,800 mg/m²/day, 3.2 times the recommended maximum human dose based on body surface area) was not tumorigenic.

In a life-span (126–138 weeks) oral carcinogenicity study, Sprague-Dawley rats were treated with doses of 33 to 300 mg/kg/day, 0.4 to 3.2 times the recommended maximum hu-man dose based on body surface area. Ursodiol produced a significantly (p≤0.5, Fisher's exact test) increased incidence of pheochromocytomas of the adrenal medulla in females of the highest dose group.

In 103-week oral carcinogenicity studies of lithocholic acid, a metabolite of ursodiol, doses up to 250 mg/kg/day in mice and 500 mg/kg/day in rats did not produce any tumors. In a 78-week rat study, intrarectal instillation of lithocholic acid (1 mg/kg/day) for 13 months did not produce colorectal tu-mors. A tumor-promoting effect was observed when it was administered after a single intrarectal dose of a known car-cinogen N-methyl-N'-nitro-N-nitrosoguanidine. On the other hand, in a 32-week rat study, ursodiol at a daily dose of 240 mg/kg (1,440 mg/m², 2.6 times the maximum recom-mended human dose based on body surface area) sup-pressed the colonic carcinogenic effect of another known car-cinogen azoxymethane.

Ursodiol was not genotoxic in the Ames test, the mouse lym-phoma cell (L5178Y, TK⁺/⁻) forward mutation test, the hu-man lymphocyte sister chromatid exchange test, the mouse spermatogenia chromosome aberration test, the Chinese hamster micronucleus test and the Chinese hamster bone marrow cell chromosome aberration test.

Ursodiol at oral doses of up to 2,700 mg/kg/day (16,200 mg/m²/day, 29 times the recommended maximum human dose based on body surface area) was found to have no effect on fertility and reproductive performance of male and female rats.

Pregnancy, Teratogenic Effects. Pregnancy Category B

Teratology studies have been performed in pregnant rats at oral doses up to 2,000 mg/kg/day (12,000 mg/m²/day, 22 times the recommended maximum human dose based on body surface area) and in pregnant rabbits at oral doses up to 300 mg/kg/day (3,600 mg/m²/day, 7 times the recom-mended maximum human dose based on body surface area) and have revealed no evidence of impaired fertility or harm to the fetus due to ursodiol.

There are no adequate or well-controlled studies in preg-nant women. Because animal reproduction studies are not always predictive of human response, this drug should be used during pregnancy only if clearly needed.

Nursing Mothers

It is not known whether ursodiol is excreted in human milk. Because many drugs are excreted in human milk, caution should be exercised when URSO® is administered to a nurs-ing mother.

Pediatric Use

The safety and effectiveness of URSO® in pediatric patients have not been established.

[See table below]

Note: Those AEs occurring at the same or higher incidence in the placebo as in the UDCA group have been deleted from this table (this includes diarrhea and thrombocytopenia at 12 months, nausea/vomiting, fever and other toxicity).

UDCA = Ursodeoxycholic acid = Ursodiol

Adverse events are reported regardless of attribution to the test medication.

OVERDOSE

Accidental or intentional overdosage with ursodiol has not been reported. The most severe manifestation of overdosage would likely consist of diarrhea which should be treated symptomatically.

Single oral doses of ursodiol at 10, 5 and 10 g/kg in mice, rats and dogs, respectively were not lethal. A single oral dose of ursodiol at 1.5 g/kg was lethal in hamsters. Symp-toms of acute toxicity were salivation and vomiting in dogs; and ataxia, dyspnea, ptosis, agonal convulsions and coma in hamsters.

DOSAGE AND ADMINISTRATION

The recommended adult dosage for URSO® in the treat-ment of PBC is 13–15 mg/kg/day administered in four di-vided doses with food.

HOW SUPPLIED

Each URSO® film-coated tablet, white, engraved with "URS785", contains 250 mg of ursodiol. Available in bottles of 100 tablets (NDC 0091-0785-01). Store at 20°C to 25°C (68°F to 77°F). Dispense in a tight container.

Caution: Federal law prohibits dispensing without a pre-scription.

Manufactured by:
GLOBAL PHARM INC.
North York, Ontario M3B 1Y5
Canada
for:
AXCAN PHARMA U.S. INC
3940 Quebec Avenue North
Minneapolis, MN 55427
USA
Distributed by:
SCHWARZ PHARMA
Milwaukee, WI 53201
USA
®Reg. TM of AXCAN PHARMA U.S. INC.
April 1998

Shown in Product Identification Guide, page 305

VIOKASE®   R

[*vī'ō-kās*]
Pancrelipase, USP
Tablets, Powder

DESCRIPTION

Viokase (pancrelipase, USP) is a pancreatic enzyme concen-trate of porcine origin containing standardized lipase, pro-tease, and amylase as well as other pancreatic enzymes. Viokase is available in tablet and powder dosage form for oral administration.

The enzyme potencies of the tablets and powder are:

	Each tablet	Each 0.7 g powder (1/4 teaspoonful)
Lipase, USP units	8,000	16,800
Protease, USP units	30,000	70,000
Amylase, USP units	30,000	70,000

Inactive Ingredients:
Tablets: Lactose, magnesium stearate, sodium chloride, stearic acid.
Powder: Lactose, sodium chloride.

ADVERSE EVENTS (AEs)

ADVERSE EVENTS	VISIT AT 12 MONTHS		VISIT AT 24 MONTHS	
	UDCA n (%)	Placebo n (%)	UDCA n (%)	Placebo n (%)
Diarrhea	—	—	1 (1.32)	—
Elevated creatinine	—	—	1 (1.32)	—
Elevated blood glucose	1 (1.18)	—	1 (1.32)	—
Leukopenia	—	—	2 (2.63)	—
Peptic ulcer	—	—	1 (1.32)	—
Skin rash	—	—	2 (2.63)	—

CLINICAL PHARMACOLOGY

The natural digestive enzymes in Viokase hydrolyze fats into fatty acids and glycerol, split protein into amino acids, and convert carbohydrates to dextrins and short chain sugars.

Under conditions of the USP test method (in vitro) Viokase has the following total digestive capacity:

	Each tablet	Each 0.7 g powder (1/4 teaspoonful)
Dietary fat, grams	28	59
Dietary protein, grams	30	70
Dietary starch, grams	30	70

Viokase Tablets are not enteric coated.
The digestive capacity of a pancreatic enzyme concentrate depends on the amount that passes through the stomach unchanged and is available at the site of action in the small intestine.

INDICATIONS

Viokase (Pancrelipase, USP) is indicated as a digestive aid in the treatment of exocrine pancreatic insufficiency as associated with but not limited to cystic fibrosis, chronic pancreatitis, pancreatectomy, or obstruction of the pancreas ducts.

CONTRAINDICATIONS

Do not use in patients hypersensitive to pork protein.

PRECAUTIONS

General: Individuals previously sensitized to trypsin, pancreatin or pancrelipase may have allergic manifestations.
Information for patients: Viokase should not be held in the mouth as the proteolytic action may cause irritation of the mucosa.
Avoid inhalation of the powder when administering Viokase.
Carcinogenesis, Mutagenesis, Impairment of fertility: Longterm studies in animals have not been performed to evaluate carcinogenic potential.
Pregnancy Category C: Animal reproduction studies have not been conducted with Viokase. It is also not known whether Viokase can cause fetal harm when administered to a pregnant woman or can affect reproduction capacity. Viokase should be given to a pregnant woman only if clearly needed.
Nursing Mothers: It is not known whether this drug is excreted in human milk. Because many drugs are excreted in human milk, caution should be exercised when Viokase is administered to a nursing mother.

ADVERSE REACTIONS

The dust or finely powdered pancreatic enzyme concentrate is irritating to the nasal mucosa and the respiratory tract. It has been documented that inhalation of the airborne powder can precipitate an asthma attack. The literature also contains several references to asthma due to inhalation in patients sensitized to pancreatic enzyme concentrates. Extremely high doses of exogenous pancreatic enzymes have been associated with hyperuricemia and hyperuricosuria. Overdosage of pancreatic enzyme concentrate may cause diarrhea or transient intestinal upset.

OVERDOSAGE

Acute toxicity determinations in animals have not been possible since the maximum dose that could be given orally produced no toxic reaction. In chronic feeding tests, rats developed swollen salivary glands. This is believed to be due to the proteolytic activity and the mucosal irritation caused by tissue digestion.
No acute toxic reactions have been reported.

DOSAGE AND ADMINISTRATION

Powder: Dosage for patients with cystic fibrosis – ¼ teaspoonful (0.7 grams) with meals. *Tablets:* Dosage for patients with cystic fibrosis or chronic pancreatitis – 1 to 3 tablets with meals or as directed by physician. As a digestive aid in patients with pancreatectomy or obstruction of pancreatic ducts – 1 to 2 tablets taken at 2 - hour intervals or as directed by physician.

HOW SUPPLIED

Tablets: Tan, round, compressed tablets engraved Viokase on one side and 9111 on the other side in bottles of 100 (NDC 0574-9111-63) and 500 (NDC 0574-9111-70). *Powder:* Tan powder in bottles of 8 oz. (227 grams) (NDC 0574-9115-25).
Store in tightly closed container in a dry place at a temperature not exceeding 25°C (77°F).
Dispense tablets and powder in tight container, preferably with a desiccant.

CLINICAL STUDIES

The effectiveness of Viokase as a digestive aid in the treatment of patients with exocrine pancreatic insufficiency has been documented in the literature as follows:
1. Regan PT, Malagelada J-R, DiMagno EP, Glanzman SL, Go VLW. Comparative effects of antacids, cimetidine and enteric coating on the therapeutic response to oral enzymes in severe pancreatic insufficiency. N. Engl. J. Med. 297: 854-8, 1977.
2. Graham DY. Enzyme replacement therapy of exocrine pancreatic insufficiency in man. N. Eng. J. Med. 296:1314-7, 1977.
CAUTION: Federal law prohibits dispensing without a prescription.
® = Registered trademark of Axcan Pharma U.S. Inc.
Manufactured for:
AXCAN PHARMA U.S. INC.
Minneapolis, MN 55427
Distributed by:
Paddock Laboratories, Inc.
Minneapolis, MN 55427
For product information please call 1-800-742-6706
92757   Rev. Sept. 1997   5310B
Shown in Product Identification Guide, page 305

Ayerst Laboratories Inc.
A Wyeth-Ayerst Company

See listing under Wyeth-Ayerst Laboratories for prescription products and Whitehall-Robins for nonprescription products.

Baxter Healthcare Corporation
Hyland Division
550 NORTH BRAND BLVD.
GLENDALE, CA 91203

Direct Inquiries to:
Product Management
(800) 423-2090

For Medical Information Contact:
In Emergencies:
Edward Gomperts, M.D.
Medical Director,
Baxter Healthcare Corporation:
(818) 956-3200

BUMINATE® 5% ℞
Albumin (Human), USP,
5% Solution

DESCRIPTION

Albumin (Human), 5% Solution, Buminate® 5% is a sterile, nonpyrogenic preparation of albumin in a single dosage form for intravenous administration. Each 100 mL contains 5 g of albumin and was prepared from human venous plasma using the Cohn cold ethanol fractionation process. It has been adjusted to physiological pH with sodium bicarbonate and/or sodium hydroxide and has been stabilized with 0.004 M sodium acetyltryptophanate and 0.004 M sodium caprylate. The sodium content is 145 ± 15 mEq/L. The solution contains no preservative and none of the coagulation factors found in fresh whole blood or plasma. Albumin (Human), 5% Solution, Buminate 5% is a transparent or slightly opalescent solution which may have a greenish tint or may vary from a pale straw to an amber color.
The likelihood of the presence of viable hepatitis viruses has been reduced by heating the product for 10 hours at 60°C. This procedure has been shown to be an effective method of inactivating hepatitis virus in albumin solutions even when those solutions were prepared from plasma known to be infective.[1–3]
Albumin (Human), 5% Solution, Buminate 5% contains no blood group isoagglutinins thereby permitting its administration without regard to the recipient's blood group.

HOW SUPPLIED

Albumin (Human), 5% Solution, Buminate 5% is supplied in 250 mL and 500 mL bottles.

BUMINATE® 25% ℞
Albumin (Human), USP,
25% Solution

DESCRIPTION

Albumin (Human), 25% Solution, Buminate® 25% is a sterile, nonpyrogenic preparation of albumin in a single dosage form for intravenous administration. Each 100 mL contains 25 g of albumin and was prepared from human venous plasma using the Cohn cold ethanol fractionation process. It has been adjusted to physiological pH with sodium bicarbonate and/or sodium hydroxide and stabilized with 0.02 M sodium acetyltryptophanate and 0.02 M sodium caprylate. The sodium content is 145 ± 15 mEq/L. This solution contains no preservative and none of the coagulation factors found in fresh whole blood or plasma. Albumin (Human), 25% Solution, Buminate 25% is a transparent or slightly opalescent solution which may have a greenish tint or may vary from a pale straw to an amber color.
The likelihood of the presence of viable hepatitis viruses has been minimized by heating the product for 10 hours at 60°C. This procedure has been shown to be an effective method of inactivating hepatitis virus in albumin solutions even when those solutions were prepared from plasma known to be infective.[1–3]

HOW SUPPLIED

Albumin (Human), 25% Solution, Buminate 25% is supplied in 20 mL, 50 mL and 100 mL bottles.

IMMUNE GLOBULIN INTRAVENOUS (HUMAN) ℞
GAMMAGARD® S/D
SOLVENT/DETERGENT TREATED

DESCRIPTION

Immune Globulin Intravenous (Human) [IGIV], Gammagard® S/D*, is a solvent/detergent treated, sterile, freeze-dried preparation of highly purified immunoglobulin G (IgG) derived from large pools of human plasma. The product is manufactured by the Cohn-Oncley cold ethanol fractionation process followed by ultrafiltration and ion exchange chromatography. The manufacturing process includes treatment with an organic solvent/detergent mixture,[1,2] composed of tri-n-butyl phosphate, octoxynol 9 and polysorbate 80.[3] The Gammagard® S/D manufacturing process provides a significant viral reduction in *in vitro* studies.[3] These studies, summarized in Table 1, demonstrate virus clearance during Gammagard® S/D manufacturing using infectious Human Immunodeficiency virus, Types 1 and 2 (HIV-1, HIV-2); Sindbis virus (SIN), a model virus for Hepatitis C virus; Pseudorabies virus (PRV), a model virus for lipid-enveloped DNA viruses such as Herpes; and Vesicular stomatitis virus (VSV), a model virus for lipid-enveloped RNA viruses.[3] These reductions are achieved through a combination of process chemistry, partitioning and/or inactivation during cold ethanol fractionation and the solvent/detergent treatment.[3]
[See table at top of next page]
When reconstituted with the total volume of diluent (Sterile Water for Injection, USP) supplied, this preparation contains approximately 50 mg of protein per mL (5%), of which at least 90% is gamma globulin. The product, reconstituted to 5%, contains a physiological concentration of sodium chloride (approximately 8.5 mg/mL) and has a pH of 6.8 ± 0.4. Stabilizing agents and additional components are present in the following maximum amounts for a 5% solution: 3 mg/mL Albumin (Human), 22.5 mg/mL glycine, 20 mg/mL glucose, 2 mg/mL polyethylene glycol (PEG), 1 μg/mL tri-n-butyl phosphate, 1 μg/mL octoxynol 9, and 100 μg/mL polysorbate 80. If it is necessary to prepare a 10% (100 mg/mL) solution for infusion, half the volume of diluent should be added, as described in the **DOSAGE AND ADMINISTRATION** section. In this case, the stabilizing agents and other components will be present at double the concentrations given for the 5% solution.
*Manufactured under U.S. Patent No. 4,439,421.
©Copyright 1986, 1987, 1988, 1989, 1990, 1994, 1995, 1997 Baxter Healthcare Corporation. All rights reserved.
The manufacturing process for Immune Globulin Intravenous (Human), Gammagard® S/D, isolates IgG without additional chemical or enzymatic modification, and the Fc portion is maintained intact. Immune Globulin Intravenous (Human), Gammagard® S/D, contains all of the IgG antibody activities which are present in the donor population. On the average, the distribution of IgG subclasses present in this product is similar to that of normal plasma.[3] Immune Globulin Intravenous (Human), Gammagard® S/D, contains only trace amounts of IgA (<3.7 μg/mL in a 5% solution). IgM is also present in trace amounts.
Immune Globulin Intravenous (Human), Gammagard® S/D, contains no preservative.

Continued on next page

Gammagard S/D—Cont.

CLINICAL PHARMACOLOGY

Immune Globulin Intravenous (Human), Gammagard® S/D, contains a broad spectrum of IgG antibodies against bacterial and viral agents that are capable of opsonization and neutralization of microbes and toxins.

Peak levels of IgG are reached immediately after infusion of Immune Globulin Intravenous (Human), Gammagard® S/D. It has been shown that, after infusion, exogenous IgG is distributed relatively rapidly between plasma and extravascular fluid until approximately half is partitioned in the extravascular space. Therefore a rapid initial drop in serum IgG levels is to be expected.[4]

As a class, IgG survives longer *in vivo* than other serum proteins.[4,5] Studies show that the half-life of Immune Globulin Intravenous (Human), Gammagard® S/D, is approximately 37.7 ± 15 days.[3] Previous studies reported IgG half-life values of 21 to 25 days.[4,5,6] The half-life of IgG can vary considerably from person to person, however. In particular, high concentrations of IgG and hypermetabolism associated with fever and infection have been seen to coincide with a shortened half-life of IgG.[4,5,6,7]

INDICATIONS AND USAGE

Primary Immunodeficiency Diseases

Immune Globulin Intravenous (Human), Gammagard® S/D, is indicated for the treatment of primary immunodeficient states, such as: congenital agammaglobulinemias, common variable immunodeficiency, Wiskott-Aldrich syndrome, and severe combined immunodeficiencies.[6,7] This indication was supported by a clinical trial of 17 patients with primary immunodeficiency who received a total of 341 infusions. Immune Globulin Intravenous (Human), Gammagard® S/D, is especially useful when high levels or rapid elevation of circulating IgG are desired or when intramuscular injections are contraindicated (e.g., small muscle mass).

B-cell Chronic Lymphocytic Leukemia (CLL)

Immune Globulin Intravenous (Human), Gammagard® S/D, is indicated for prevention of bacterial infections in patients with hypogammaglobulinemia and/or recurrent bacterial infections associated with B-cell Chronic Lymphocytic Leukemia (CLL). In a study of 81 patients, 41 of whom were treated with Immune Globulin Intravenous (Human), Gammagard®, bacterial infections were significantly reduced in the treatment group.[8,9] In this study, the placebo group had approximately twice as many bacterial infections as the IGIV group. The median time to first bacterial infection for the IGIV group was greater than 365 days. By contrast, the time to first bacterial infection in the placebo group was 192 days. The number of viral and fungal infections, which were for the most part minor, was not statistically different between the two groups.

Idiopathic Thrombocytopenic Purpura (ITP)

When a rapid rise in platelet count is needed to prevent and/or to control bleeding in a patient with Idiopathic Thrombocytopenic Purpura, the administration of Immune Globulin Intravenous (Human), Gammagard® S/D, should be considered.

The efficacy of Immune Globulin Intravenous (Human), Gammagard®, has been demonstrated in a clinical study involving 16 patients. Of these 16 patients, 13 had chronic ITP (11 adults, 2 children), and 3 patients had acute ITP (one adult, 2 children). All 16 patients (100%) demonstrated a clinically significant rise in platelet count to a level greater than 40,000/mm^3 following the administration of Immune Globulin Intravenous (Human), Gammagard®. Ten of the 16 patients (62.5%) exhibited a significant rise to greater than 80,000 platelets/mm^3. Of these 10 patients, 7 had chronic ITP (5 adults, 2 children), and 3 patients had acute ITP (one adult, 2 children).

The rise in platelet count to greater than 40,000/mm^3 occurred after a single 1 g/kg infusion of Gammagard® in 8 patients with chronic ITP (6 adults, 2 children), and in 2 patients with acute ITP (one adult, one child). A similar response was observed after two 1 g/kg infusions in 3 adult patients with chronic ITP, and one child with acute ITP. The remaining 2 adult patients with chronic ITP received more than two 1 g/kg infusions before achieving a platelet count greater than 40,000/mm^3. The rise in platelet count was generally rapid, occurring within 5 days. However, this rise was transient and not considered curative. Platelet count rises lasted 2 to 3 weeks, with a range of 12 days to 6 months. It should be noted that childhood ITP may resolve spontaneously without treatment.

CONTRAINDICATIONS

None known.

WARNINGS

Immune Globulin Intravenous (Human), Gammagard® S/D, should only be administered intravenously. Other routes of administration have not been evaluated.

Immediate anaphylactic and hypersensitivity reactions are a remote possibility. Epinephrine should be available for treatment of any acute anaphylactoid reactions.

Table 1
***In Vitro* Virus Clearance During Gammagard® S/D Manufacturing**

Process Step No.	Process Step Evaluated	Virus Clearance, log$_{10}$				
		HIV-1	HIV-2	SIN	PRV	VSV
1	Fraction I +II +III Wash to Fraction I +III Supernatant	8.2*	N.D.**	5.2*	N.D.**	N.D.**
2	Fraction I +III Supernatant to Fraction I +III Filtrate	8.2*	N.D.**	4.6*	N.D.**	N.D.**
3	Fraction I +III Filtrate to Fraction II Precipitate	8.1*	N.D.**	N.A.***	N.D.**	N.D.**
4	Treatment of Resuspended Fraction II Precipitate with Solvent/Detergent Mixture	8.4*	5.7*	5.1*	4.3*	6.0*

* Minimum log reduction due to detection limit of the assay.
** Not determined.
*** Not applicable. Sindbis virus co-precipitates with Fraction II proteins.

Immune Globulin Intravenous (Human), Gammagard® S/D, contains only trace amounts of IgA (<3.7 µg/mL in a 5% solution). Nonetheless, it should be given with caution to patients with antibodies to IgA or selective IgA deficiencies.[7,10]

PRECAUTIONS

There is clinical evidence of a possible association between Immune Globulin Intravenous (Human) (IGIV) administration and thrombotic events. The exact cause of this is unknown; therefore, caution should be exercised in the prescribing and infusion of IGIV in patients with a history of cardiovascular disease or thrombotic episodes.[12-17]

An aseptic meningitis syndrome (AMS) has been reported to occur infrequently in association with Immune Globulin Intravenous (Human) (IGIV) treatment. Discontinuation of IGIV treatment has resulted in remission of AMS within several days without sequelae. The syndrome usually begins within several hours to two days following IGIV treatment. It is characterized by symptoms and signs including severe headache, nuchal rigidity, drowsiness, fever, photophobia, painful eye movements, and nausea and vomiting. Cerebrospinal fluid (CSF) studies are frequently positive with pleocytosis up to several thousand cells per cu.mm., predominantly from the granulocytic series, and elevated protein levels up to several hundred mg/dL. Patients exhibiting such symptoms and signs should receive a thorough neurological examination, including CSF studies, to rule out other causes of meningitis. AMS may occur more frequently in association with high dose (2 g/kg) IGIV treatment.

Certain components used in the packaging of this product contain natural rubber latex.

Drug Interactions

See **DOSAGE AND ADMINISTRATION** Section.

Pregnancy Category C

Animal reproduction studies have not been conducted with Immune Globulin Intravenous (Human), Gammagard® S/D. It is also not known whether Immune Globulin Intravenous (Human), Gammagard® S/D, can cause fetal harm when administered to a pregnant woman or can affect reproduction capacity. Immune Globulin Intravenous (Human), Gammagard® S/D, should be given to a pregnant woman only if clearly needed.

ADVERSE REACTIONS

In general, reported adverse reactions to Immune Globulin Intravenous (Human) Gammagard®, in patients with either congenital or acquired immunodeficiencies are similar in kind and frequency. Various minor reactions, such as headache, fatigue, chills, backache, leg cramps, lightheadedness, fever, urticaria, flushing, slight elevation of blood pressure, nausea and vomiting may occasionally occur. Slowing or stopping the infusion usually allows the symptoms to disappear promptly.

Immediate anaphylactic and hypersensitivity reactions are a remote possibility. Epinephrine should be available for treatment of any acute anaphylactoid reaction. (See **WARNINGS.**)

Primary Immunodeficiency Diseases

Twenty-one adverse reactions occurred in 341 infusions (6%), when using Immune Globulin Intravenous (Human), Gammagard® (5% solution), in a clinical trial of 17 patients with primary immunodeficiency.[11] Of the 17 patients, 12 (71%) were adults, and 5 (29%) were children (16 years or younger).

In a cross-over study comparing Gammagard® and Gammagard® S/D (5% solutions) conducted in a small number (n=10) of primary immunodeficient patients, no unusual or unexpected adverse reactions were observed in the Gammagard® S/D group. The adverse reactions experienced in the Gammagard® S/D group were similar in frequency and nature to those observed in the control group consisting of patients receiving Gammagard®.

Gammagard®, reconstituted to a concentration of 10%, was administered intravenously at rates varying from 2–11 mL/kg/Hr. Systemic reactions occurred in 23 (10.5%) of 219 infusions. This compares with an adverse reaction incidence of 6% (only systemic reactions reported) for primary immunodeficient patients previously treated with a 5% solution at infusion rates varying between 2 and 8 mL/kg/Hr, as described above (also, see reference 11). Local pain or irritation was experienced during 35 (16%) of 219 infusions. Application of a warm compress to the infusion site alleviated local symptoms. These local reactions tended to be associated with hand vein infusions and their incidence may be reduced by infusions via the antecubital vein.

B-cell Chronic Lymphocytic Leukemia (CLL)

In the study of patients with B-cell Chronic Lymphocytic Leukemia, the incidence of adverse reactions associated with Gammagard® infusions was approximately 1.3% while that associated with placebo (normal saline) infusions was 0.6%.[9]

Idiopathic Thrombocytopenic Purpura (ITP)

During the clinical study of Gammagard® for the treatment of Idiopathic Thrombocytopenic Purpura, the only adverse reaction reported was headache which occurred in 12 of 16 patients (75%). Of these 12 patients, 11 had chronic ITP (9 adults, 2 children), and one child had acute ITP. Oral antihistamines and analgesics alleviated the symptoms and were used as pretreatment for those patients requiring additional IGIV therapy. The remaining 4 patients did not report any side effects and did not require pretreatment.

DOSAGE AND ADMINISTRATION

Primary Immunodeficiency Diseases

For patients with primary immunodeficiencies, monthly doses of at least 100 mg/kg are recommended. Initially, patients may receive 200–400 mg/kg. As there are significant differences in the half-life of IgG among patients with primary immunodeficiencies, the frequency and amount of immunoglobulin therapy may vary from patient to patient. The proper amount can be determined by monitoring clinical response. The minimum serum concentration of IgG necessary for protection has not been established.

B-cell Chronic Lymphocytic Leukemia (CLL)

For patients with hypogammaglobulinemia and/or recurrent bacterial infections due to B-cell Chronic Lymphocytic Leukemia, a dose of 400 mg/kg every 3 to 4 weeks is recommended.

Idiopathic Thrombocytopenic Purpura (ITP)

For patients with acute or chronic Idiopathic Thrombocytopenic Purpura, a dose of 1 g/kg is recommended. The need for additional doses can be determined by clinical response and platelet count. Up to three separate doses may be given on alternate days if required.

Reconstitution: Use Aseptic Technique

A. 5% Solution

1. **Note: Reconstitute immediately before use.**
2. If refrigerated, warm the Sterile Water for Injection, USP (diluent) and Immune Globulin Intravenous (Human), Gammagard® S/D (dried concentrate), to room temperature.
3. Remove caps from concentrate and diluent bottles to expose central portion of rubber stoppers.
4. Cleanse stoppers with germicidal solution.
5. Remove protective covering from the spike at one end of the transfer device (Fig. 1).
6. Place the diluent bottle on a flat surface and, while holding the bottle to prevent slipping, insert the spike of the transfer device **perpendicularly through the center** of the bottle stopper.

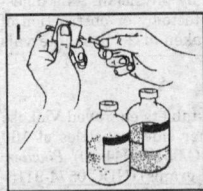

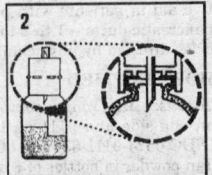

7. Press down firmly so that the transfer device fits snugly against the diluent bottle (Fig. 2). **Caution: Failure to use center of stopper may result in dislodging the stopper.**

8. Remove the protective covering from the other end of the transfer device. Hold diluent bottle to prevent slipping.
9. Hold concentrate bottle firmly and at an angle of approximately 45 degrees. Invert the diluent bottle with the transfer device at an angle complementary to the concentrate bottle (approximately 45 degrees) and firmly insert the transfer device into the concentrate bottle through the center of the rubber stopper (Fig. 3)
Note: Invert the diluent bottle with attached transfer device rapidly into the concentrate bottle in order to avoid loss of diluent.
Caution: Failure to use center of stopper may result in dislodging the stopper and loss of vacuum.
10. The diluent will flow into the concentrate bottle quickly. When diluent transfer is complete, remove empty diluent bottle and transfer device from concentrate bottle. Discard transfer device after single use.
11. Thoroughly wet the dried material by tilting or inverting and gently rotating the bottle (Fig. 4). **Do not shake. Avoid foaming.**
12. Repeat gentle rotation as long as undissolved product is observed.

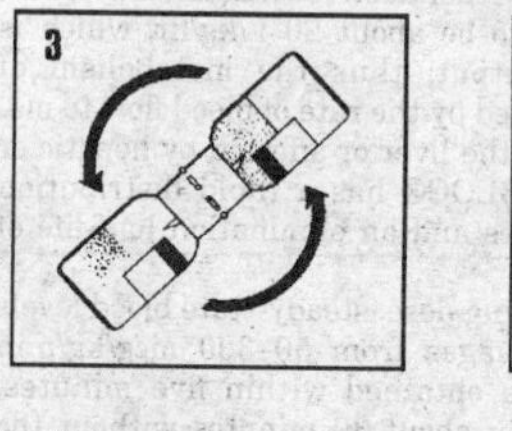

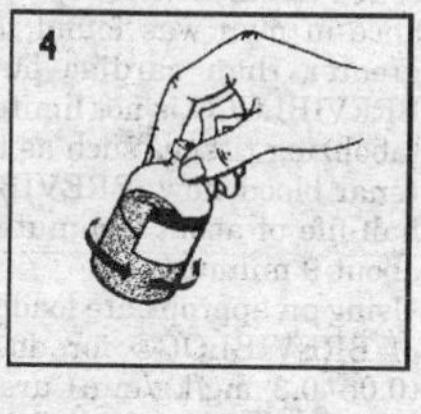

B. 10% Solution

Follow steps 1–4 as previously described in **A.**

5. To prepare a 10% solution, reconstitute with the appropriate volume of diluent as indicated in Table 2, which indicates the volume of diluent required for a 5% or 10% concentration. Using aseptic technique, draw the required volume of diluent into a sterile hypodermic syringe and needle. Discard the filled syringe.

Table 2
Required Diluent Volume

Concentration	2.5 g bottle	5 g bottle	10 g bottle
5%	50 mL	96 mL	192 mL
10%	25 mL	48 mL	96 mL

6. Using the residual diluent in the diluent vial, follow steps 5–12 as previously described in A.

Rate of Administration

It is recommended that initially a 5% solution be infused at a rate of 0.5 mL/kg/Hr. If infusion at this rate and concentration causes the patient no distress, the administration rate may be gradually increased to a maximum rate of 4 mL/kg/Hr. Patients who tolerate the 5% concentration at 4 mL/kg/Hr can be infused with the 10% concentration starting at 0.5 mL/kg/Hr. If no adverse effects occur, the rate can be increased gradually up to a maximum of 8 mL/kg/Hr.
It is recommended that antecubital veins be used especially for 10% solutions, if possible. This may reduce the likelihood of the patient experiencing discomfort at the infusion site (see **ADVERSE REACTIONS**).
A rate of administration which is too rapid may cause flushing and changes in pulse rate and blood pressure. Slowing or stopping the infusion usually allows the symptoms to disappear promptly.

Drug Interactions

Admixtures of Immune Globulin Intravenous (Human), Gammagard® S/D, with other drugs and intravenous solutions have not been evaluated. It is recommended that Immune Globulin Intravenous (Human), Gammagard® S/D, be administered separately from other drugs or medications which the patient may be receiving. The product should not be mixed with Immune Globulin Intravenous (Human) from other manufacturers.
Antibodies in immune globulin preparations may interfere with patient responses to live vaccines, such as those for measles, mumps, and rubella. The immunizing physician should be informed of recent therapy with Immune Globulin Intravenous (Human) so that appropriate precautions can be taken.

Administration

Immune Globulin Intravenous (Human), Gammagard® S/D, should be administered as soon after reconstitution as possible. Administration should begin not more than 2 hours after reconstitution.
The reconstituted material should be at room temperature during administration.
Parenteral drug products should be inspected visually for particulate matter and discoloration prior to administration, whenever solution and container permit. Do not use if particulate matter and/or discoloration is observed.
Follow directions for use which accompany the administration set provided. If another administration set is used, ensure that the set contains a similar filter.

HOW SUPPLIED

Immune Globulin Intravenous (Human), Gammagard® S/D, is supplied in 2.5 g, 5 g or 10 g single use bottles. Each bottle of Immune Globulin Intravenous (Human), Gammagard® S/D, is furnished with a suitable volume of Sterile Water for Injection, USP, a transfer device and an administration set which contains an integral airway and a 15 micron filter.

STORAGE

Immune Globulin Intravenous (Human), Gammagard® S/D, is to be stored at a temperature not to exceed 25°C (77°F). Freezing should be avoided to prevent the diluent bottle from breaking.

REFERENCES

1. Prince AM, Horowitz B, Brotman B: Sterilisation of hepatitis and HTLV-III viruses by exposure to tri(n-butyl) phosphate and sodium cholate. **Lancet** 1:706–710, 1986
2. Horowitz B, Wiebe ME, Lippin A, *et al*: Inactivation of viruses in labile blood derivatives: I. Disruption of lipid enveloped viruses by tri(n-butyl) phosphate detergent combinations. **Transfusion 25**:516–522, 1985
3. Unpublished data in the files of Baxter Healthcare Corporation.
4. Waldmann TA, Storber W: Metabolism of immunoglobulins. **Prog Allergy 13**: 1–110, 1969
5. Morell A, Riesen W: Structure, function and catabolism of immunoglobulins in **Immunohemotherapy.** Nydegger UE (ed), London, Academic Press, 1981, pp 17–26
6. Stiehm ER: Standard and special human immune serum globulins as therapeutic agents. **Pediatrics 63**: 301–319, 1979
7. Buckley RH: Immunoglobulin replacement therapy: Indications and contraindications for use and variable IgG levels achieved in **Immunoglobulins: Characteristics and Use of Intravenous Preparations.** Alving BM, Finlayson JS (eds), Washington, DC, U.S. Department of Health and Human Services, 1979, pp 3–8
8. Bunch C, Chapel HM, Rai K, *et al:* Intravenous Immune Globulin reduces bacterial infections in Chronic Lymphocytic Leukemia: A controlled randomized clinical trial. **Blood 70 Suppl 1**: 753, 1987
9. Cooperative Group for the Study of Immunoglobulin in Chronic Lymphocytic Leukemia: Intravenous immunoglobulin for the prevention of infection in Chronic Lymphocytic Leukemia: A randomized, controlled clinical trial. **N Eng J Med 319**: 902–907, 1988
10. Burks AW, Sampson HA, Buckley RH: Anaphylactic reactions after gammaglobulin administration in patients with hypogammaglobulinemia: Detection of IgE antibodies to IgA. **N Eng J Med 314**: 560–564, 1986
11. Ochs HD, Lee ML, Fischer SH, *et al*: Efficacy of a New Intravenous Immunoglobulin Preparation in Primary Immunodeficient Patients. **Clinical Therapeutics 9**:512–522, 1987
12. Reinhart WH, Berchtold PE. Effect of high-dose intravenous immunoglobulin therapy on blood rheology. **Lancet 339**: 662–664, 1992
13. Dalakas MC. High-dose intravenous immunoglobulin and serum viscosity: Risk of precipitating thromboembolic events. **Neurology 44**: 223–226, 1994
14. Harkness K, Howell SJL, Davies-Jones GAB. Encephalopathy associated with intravenous immunoglobulin treatment for Guillain-Barre syndrome. **Journal of Neurology 60**: 586–598, 1996
15. Woodruff RK, Grigg AP, Firkin FC, Smith IL. Fatal thrombotic events during treatment of autoimmune thrombocytopenia with intravenous immunoglobulin in elderly patients. **Lancet ii**: 217–18, 1986
16. Silbert PL, Knezevic WV, Bridge DT. Cerebral infarction complicating intravenous immunoglobulin therapy for polyneuritis cranialis. **Neurology 42**: 257–258, 1992
17. Duhem C, Dicato MA, Ries F. Side effects of intravenous immune globulins. **Clin Exp Immunol 97: (Suppl 1)**70–83, 1994

BIBLIOGRAPHY

Bussel JB, Kimberly RP, Inman RD, *et al:* Intravenous gammaglobulin treatment of chronic idiopathic thrombocytopenic purpura. **Blood 62**: 480–486, 1983

Baxter Healthcare Corporation
Hyland Division
Glendale, CA 91203 USA
U.S. License No. 140

HEMOFIL® M ℞
Antihemophilic Factor (Human)
Method M, Monoclonal Purified

DESCRIPTION

Antihemophilic Factor (Human), Hemofil® M, Method M, is a sterile, nonpyrogenic, dried preparation of antihemophilic factor (Factor VIII, Factor VIII:C, AHF) in concentrated form with a specific activity range of 2 to 15 AHF International Units/mg of total protein. When reconstituted with the appropriate volume of diluent, it contains approximately 12.5 mg/mL Albumin (Human), 1.5 mg/mL polyethylene glycol (3350), 0.055 M histidine and 0.030 M glycine as stabilizing agents. In the absence of the added Albumin (Human), the specific activity is approximately 2,000 AHF International Units/mg of protein. It also contains, per AHF International Unit, not more than 0.1 ng mouse protein, 18 ng organic solvent [tri-n-butyl phosphate] and 50 ng detergent (Triton X-100).
Hemofil® M is prepared by the Method M process from pooled human plasma by immuno affinity chromatography utilizing a murine monoclonal antibody to Factor VIII:C, followed by an ion exchange chromatography step for further purification. Source material may be provided by other US licensed manufacturers. Hemofil® M also includes an organic solvent [tri-n-butyl phosphate] and detergent (Triton X-100) virus inactivation step designed to reduce the risk of transmission of hepatitis and other viral diseases. However, no procedure has been shown to be totally effective in removing viral infectivity from coagulation factor products.
Each bottle of Hemofil® M is labeled with the AHF activity expressed in International Units per bottle, which is referenced to the WHO International Standard.
Hemofil® M is to be administered only intravenously.

HOW SUPPLIED

Hemofil® M is available as single dose bottles. Each bottle is labeled with the potency in International Units, and is packaged together with 10 mL of Sterile Water for Injection, USP, a double-ended needle, and a filter needle.

PROPLEX® T ℞
Factor IX Complex, Heat Treated

DESCRIPTION

Factor IX Complex, Heat Treated, Proplex® T, is a sterile product prepared from normal human plasma. It contains, in concentrated form, clotting Factors II (prothrombin), VII (proconvertin), IX (PTC, antihemophilic factor B), and X (Stuart-Prower factor). Other proteins are also present in minimal amounts. The product also contains a small amount of heparin, 1.5 units or less per mL of reconstituted material as a stabilizing agent. This amount does not affect the clinical usefulness of the complex in moderate dosage.
Factor IX Complex **must** be administered intravenously.
During the manufacturing process, this product was heated for 144 hours at 60°C.
This heating step was designed to reduce the risk of transmission of hepatitis and other viral infections. No procedure has been shown to be totally effective in removing viral infectivity from Factor IX Complex.

HOW SUPPLIED

Factor IX Complex, Proplex® T, is furnished with a suitable volume of Sterile Water for Injection, USP; a double-ended needle, and a filter needle.

RECOMBINATE™ ℞
Antihemophilic Factor
(Recombinant)

DESCRIPTION

Antihemophilic Factor (Recombinant), Recombinate™ is a glycoprotein synthesized by a genetically engineered Chinese Hamster Ovary (CHO) cell line. In culture the CHO cell line secretes recombinant antihemophilic factor (rAHF) into the cell culture medium. The rAHF is purified from the culture medium utilizing a series of chromatography columns. A key step in the purification process is an immunoaffinity chromatography methodology in which a purification matrix prepared by immobilization of a monoclonal antibody directed to Factor VIII is utilized to selectively isolate the rAHF in the medium. The synthesized rAHF produced by the CHO cells has the same biological effects as Antihemophilic Factor (Human) [AHF (Human)] and structurally has a similar combination of heterogeneous heavy and light chains as found in AHF (Human).
Recombinate™ is formulated as a sterile, nonpyrogenic, off-white to faint yellow, lyophilized powder preparation of concentrated recombinant AHF for intravenous injection and is available in single-dose bottles which contain nominally 250, 500 and 1000 International Units per bottle. When reconstituted with the appropriate volume of diluent, it contains the following stabilizers in maximum amounts: 12.5 mg/mL Albumin (Human), 0.20 mg/mL calcium, 1.5 mg/mL polyethylene glycol (3350), 180 mEq/L sodium, 55 mM his-

Continued on next page

Recombinate—Cont.

tidine, 1.5 µg/AHF International Unit (IU) polysorbate-80. Von Willebrand Factor (vWF) is co-expressed with the Antihemophilic Factor (Recombinant) and helps to stabilize it. The final product contains not more than 2 ng vWF/IU rAHF which will not have any clinically relevant effect in patients with von Willebrand's disease. The product contains no preservative.

Manufacturing of Recombinate™ is shared by Baxter Healthcare Corporation, Hyland Division and Genetics Institute, Inc. Genetics Institute produces Antihemophilic Factor Concentrate (Recombinant) (For Further Manufacturing Use) which is then formulated and packaged at Baxter Healthcare Corporation, Hyland Division.

Each bottle of Recombinate™ is labeled with the AHF activity expressed in IU per bottle. Biological potency is determined by an *in vitro* assay which is referenced to the World Health Organization (WHO) International Standard for Factor VIII:C Concentrate.

HOW SUPPLIED

Antihemophilic Factor (Recombinant), Recombinant™ is available in single-dose bottles which contain nominally 250, 500 and 1000 International Units per bottle. Recombinate™ is packaged with 10 mL of Sterile Water for Injection, USP, a double-ended needle, a filter needle, and a package insert.

Baxter Pharmaceutical Products Inc.

**110 ALLEN ROAD, PO BOX 804
LIBERTY CORNER, NJ 07938-0804**

Direct Inquiries to:
Professional Services Department
(800) ANA DRUG
(800) 262-3784

For Medical Information Contact:
In Emergencies:
Raul Trillo, MD
Director, Medical Services
(800) ANA-DRUG
(800) 262-3784

Sales and Ordering:
To place an order between 7:00 AM and 6:00 PM (central)
(800) 345-2700

ATRACURIUM BESYLATE ℞
[ătră-cŭr-ē-ŭm -bĕ-syl-āte]
Injection

This drug should be used only by adequately trained individuals familiar with its actions, characteristics, and hazards.

DESCRIPTION

Atracurium Besylate Injection is an intermediate-duration, nondepolarizing, skeletal muscle relaxant for intravenous administration. Atracurium besylate is designated as 2,2'-[1,5-pentanediylbis[oxy(3-oxo-3,1-propanediyl)]]bis[1-[(3,4-dimethoxyphenyl)methyl]-1,2,3,4-tetrahydro-6,7-dimethoxy-2-methylisoquinolinium] dibenzenesulfonate. It has a molecular weight of 1243.49, and its molecular formula is $C_{65}H_{82}N_2O_{18}S_2$. The structural formula is:

Atracurium besylate is a complex molecule containing four sites at which different stereochemical configurations can occur. The symmetry of the molecule, however, results in only ten, instead of sixteen, possible different isomers. The manufacture of atracurium besylate results in these isomers being produced in unequal amounts but with a consistent ratio. Those molecules in which the methyl group attached to the quarternary nitrogen projects on the opposite side to the adjacent substituted-benzyl moiety predominate by approximately 3:1.

Atracurium Besylate Injection is a sterile, non-pyrogenic aqueous solution for intravenous administration. Each mL contains 10 mg atracurium besylate. The pH is adjusted to 3.25–3.65 with benzenesulfonic acid. The multiple dose vial contains 0.9% benzyl alcohol added as a preservative. Atracurium Besylate Injection slowly loses potency with time at

the rate of approximately 6% per *year* under refrigeration (5°C). Atracurium Besylate Injection should be refrigerated at 2° to 8°C (36° to 46°F) to preserve potency. Rate of loss in potency increases to approximately 5% per *month* at 25°C (77°F). Upon removal from refrigeration to room temperature storage conditions (25°C/77°F), use Atracurium Besylate Injection within 14 days even if refrigerated.

HOW SUPPLIED

Atracurium Besylate Injection, 10 mg atracurium besylate in each mL.
5 mL *Single Dose* Vial (50 mg per vial) – Packaged in 10s (NDC 10019-002-05).
10 mL *Multiple Dose* Vial (100 mg per vial). Contains benzyl alcohol (see WARNINGS in full prescribing information). Packaged in 10s (NDC 10019-001-10).

ATROPINE ℞
[a 'troe-peen]
Sulfate Injection, USP
For IM, IV or SC Use

DESCRIPTION

Atropine Sulfate Injection, USP is a sterile solution of atropine sulfate in water for injection. Each mL contains Atropine Sulfate 0.4 mg or 1.0 mg; Sodium Chloride 9 mg; Benzyl Alcohol 9 mg; Water for injection qs; pH may be adjusted with H_2SO_4 if necessary. pH: 3.0–6.5.

Atropine Sulfate Injection, USP may be given intramuscularly, intravenously or subcutaneously.

Atropine is a white crystalline alkaloid which may be extracted from belladonna root or may be produced synthetically. It is used as atropine sulfate because this compound has much greater solubility.

Atropine sulfate is an anticholinergic drug. The empirical formula of atropine sulfate is $(C_{17}H_{23}NO_3)_2 \cdot H_2SO_4 \cdot H_2O$. The structural formula is:

HOW SUPPLIED

NDC Number	Atropine Sulfate per mL	Volume
10019-250-12	0.4 mg/mL	1 mL in a 2 mL vial
10019-251-12	1 mg/mL	1 mL in a 2 mL vial
10019-250-20	0.4 mg/mL	20 mL in a 20 mL vial

2 mL vials packaged 25 per shelf pack.
20 mL multiple dose vials packaged 10 per shelf pack.

BREVIBLOC® INJECTION ℞
[brĕv ə-blŏc]
(esmolol hydrochloride)
10 mL Ampul—2500 mg

**NOT FOR DIRECT INTRAVENOUS INJECTION.
AMPUL MUST BE DILUTED PRIOR TO ITS INFUSION - SEE DOSAGE AND ADMINISTRATION.**

10 mL Single Dose Vial—100 mg

DESCRIPTION

BREVIBLOC® (esmolol HCl) is a beta₁-selective (cardioselective) adrenergic receptor blocking agent with a very short duration of action (elimination half-life is approximately 9 minutes). Esmolol HCl is:
(±)-Methyl p-[2-hydroxy-3-(isopropylamino) propoxy] hydrocinnamate hydrochloride and has the following structure:

Esmolol HCl has the empirical formula $C_{16}H_{26}NO_4Cl$ and a molecular weight of 331.8. It has one asymmetric center and exists as an enantiomeric pair.

Esmolol HCl is a white to off-white crystalline powder. It is a relatively hydrophilic compound which is very soluble in water and freely soluble in alcohol. Its partition coefficient (octanol/water) at pH 7.0 is 0.42 compared to 17.0 for propranolol.

BREVIBLOC® INJECTION is a clear, colorless to light yellow, sterile, nonpyrogenic solution.

2500 mg, 10 mL Ampul—Each mL contains 250 mg esmolol HCl in 25% Propylene Glycol, USP, 25% Alcohol, USP and

Water for Injection, USP; buffered with 17.0 mg Sodium Acetate, USP, and 0.00715 mL Glacial Acetic Acid, USP. Sodium hydroxide and/or hydrochloric acid added, as necessary, to adjust pH to 3.5–5.5.

100 mg, 10 mL Single Dose Vial—Each mL contains 10 mg esmolol HCl and Water for Injection, USP; buffered with 2.8 mg Sodium Acetate, USP and 0.546 mg Glacial Acetic Acid, USP. Sodium hydroxide and/or hydrochloric acid added, as necessary to adjust pH to 4.5–5.5.

CLINICAL PHARMACOLOGY

BREVIBLOC® (esmolol HCl) is a beta₁-selective (cardioselective) adrenergic receptor blocking agent with rapid onset, a very short duration of action, and no significant intrinsic sympathomimetic or membrane stabilizing activity at therapeutic dosages. Its elimination half-life after intravenous infusion is approximately 9 minutes. BREVIBLOC® inhibits the beta₁ receptors located chiefly in cardiac muscle, but this preferential effect is not absolute and at higher doses it begins to inhibit beta₂ receptors located chiefly in the bronchial and vascular musculature.

Pharmacokinetics and Metabolism

BREVIBLOC® (esmolol HCl) is rapidly metabolized by hydrolysis of the ester linkage, chiefly by the esterases in the cytosol of red blood cells and not by plasma cholinesterases or red cell membrane acetylcholinesterase. Total body clearance in man was found to be about 20 L/kg/hr, which is greater than cardiac output; thus the metabolism of BREVIBLOC® is not limited by the rate of blood flow to metabolizing tissues such as the liver or affected by hepatic or renal blood flow. BREVIBLOC® has a rapid distribution half-life of about 2 minutes and an elimination half-life of about 9 minutes.

Using an appropriate loading dose, steady-state blood levels of BREVIBLOC® for dosages from 50–300 mcg/kg/min (0.05–0.3 mg/kg/min) are obtained within five minutes. (Steady-state is reached in about 30 minutes without the loading dose.) Steady-state blood levels of BREVIBLOC® increase linearly over this dosage range and elimination kinetics are dose-independent over this range. Steady-state blood levels are maintained during infusion but decrease rapidly after termination of the infusion. Because of its short half-life, blood levels of BREVIBLOC® can be rapidly altered by increasing or decreasing the infusion rate and rapidly eliminated by discontinuing the infusion.

Consistent with the high rate of blood-based metabolism of BREVIBLOC®, less than 2% of the drug is excreted unchanged in the urine. Within 24 hours of the end of infusion, approximately 73–88% of the dosage has been accounted for in the urine as the acid metabolite of BREVIBLOC®.

Metabolism of BREVIBLOC® results in the formation of the corresponding free acid and methanol. The acid metabolite has been shown in animals to have about 1/1500th the activity of esmolol and in normal volunteers its blood levels do not correspond to the level of beta blockade. The acid metabolite has an elimination half-life of about 3.7 hours and is excreted in the urine with a clearance approximately equivalent to the glomerular filtration rate. Excretion of the acid metabolite is significantly decreased in patients with renal disease, with the elimination half-life increased to about ten-fold that of normals, and plasma levels considerably elevated.

Methanol blood levels, monitored in subjects receiving BREVIBLOC® for up to 6 hours at 300 mcg/kg/min (0.3 mg/kg/min) and 24 hours at 150 mcg/kg/min (0.15 mg/kg/min), approximated endogenous levels and were less than 2% of levels usually associated with methanol toxicity.

BREVIBLOC® has been shown to be 55% bound to human plasma protein, while the acid metabolite is only 10% bound.

Pharmacodynamics

Clinical pharmacology studies in normal volunteers have confirmed the beta blocking activity of BREVIBLOC® (esmolol HCl), showing reduction in heart rate at rest and during exercise, and attenuation of isoproterenol-induced increases in heart rate. Blood levels of BREVIBLOC® have been shown to correlate with extent of beta blockade. After termination of infusion, substantial recovery from beta blockade is observed in 10–20 minutes.

In human electrophysiology studies, BREVIBLOC® produced effects typical of a beta blocker; a decrease in the heart rate, increase in sinus cycle length, prolongation of the sinus node recovery time, prolongation of the AH interval during normal sinus rhythm and during atrial pacing, and an increase in antegrade Wenckebach cycle length.

In patients undergoing radionuclide angiography, BREVIBLOC®, at dosages of 200 mcg/kg/min (0.2 mg/kg/min) produced reductions in heart rate, systolic blood pressure, rate pressure product, left and right ventricular ejection fraction and cardiac index at rest, which were similar in magnitude to those produced by intravenous propranolol (4 mg). During exercise, BREVIBLOC® produced reductions in heart rate, rate pressure product and cardiac index which were also similar to those produced by propranolol, but produced a significantly larger fall in systolic blood pressure. In patients undergoing cardiac catheterization,

the maximum therapeutic dose of 300 mcg/kg/min (0.3 mg/kg/min) of BREVIBLOC® produced similar effects and, in addition, there were small, clinically insignificant increases in the left ventricular end diastolic pressure and pulmonary capillary wedge pressure. At thirty minutes after the discontinuation of BREVIBLOC® infusion, all of the hemodynamic parameters had returned to pretreatment levels.

The relative cardioselectivity of BREVIBLOC® was demonstrated in 10 mildly asthmatic patients. Infusions of BREVIBLOC® [100, 200 and 300 mcg/kg/min (0.1, 0.2 and 0.3 mg/kg/min)] produced no significant increases in specific airway resistance compared to placebo. At 300 mcg/kg/min (0.3 mg/kg/min), BREVIBLOC® produced slightly enhanced bronchomotor sensitivity to dry air stimulus. These effects were not clinically significant, and BREVIBLOC® was well tolerated by all patients. Six of the patients also received intravenous propranolol, and at a dosage of 1 mg, two experienced significant, symptomatic bronchospasm requiring bronchodilator treatment. One other propranolol-treated patient also experienced dry air-induced bronchospasm. No adverse pulmonary effects were observed in patients with COPD who received therapeutic dosages of BREVIBLOC® for treatment of supraventricular tachycardia (51 patients) or in perioperative settings (32 patients).

Supraventricular Tachycardia
In two multicenter, randomized, double-blind, controlled comparisons of BREVIBLOC® (esmolol HCl) with placebo and propranolol, maintenance doses of 50 to 300 mcg/kg/min (0.05 to 0.3 mg/kg/min) of BREVIBLOC® were found to be more effective than placebo and about as effective as propranolol, 3–6 mg given by bolus injections, in the treatment of supraventricular tachycardia, principally atrial fibrillation and atrial flutter. The majority of these patients developed their arrhythmias postoperatively. About 60–70% of the patients treated with BREVIBLOC® had a desired therapeutic effect (either a 20% reduction in heart rate, a decrease in heart rate to less than 100 bpm, or, rarely, conversion to NSR) and about 95% of those who responded did so at a dosage of 200 mcg/kg/min (0.2 mg/kg/min) or less. The average effective dosage of BREVIBLOC® was approximately 100–115 mcg/kg/min (0.1–0.115 mg/kg/min) in the two studies. Other multicenter baseline-controlled studies gave essentially similar results. In the comparison with propranolol, about 50% of patients in both the BREVIBLOC® and propranolol groups were on concomitant digoxin. Response rates were slightly higher with both beta blockers in the digoxin-treated patients.

In all studies significant decreases of blood pressure occurred in 20–50% of patients, identified either as adverse reaction reports by investigators, or by observation of systolic pressure less than 90 mmHg or diastolic pressure less than 50 mmHg. The hypotension was symptomatic (mainly diaphoresis or dizziness) in about 12% of patients, and therapy was discontinued in about 11% of patients, about half of whom were symptomatic. In comparison to propranolol, hypotension was about three times as frequent with BREVIBLOC®, 53% vs. 17%. The hypotension was rapidly reversible with decreased infusion rate or after discontinuation of therapy with BREVIBLOC®. For both BREVIBLOC® and propranolol, hypotension was reported less frequently in patients receiving concomitant digoxin.

INDICATIONS AND USAGE
Supraventricular Tachycardia
BREVIBLOC® (esmolol HCl) is indicated for the rapid control of ventricular rate in patients with atrial fibrillation or atrial flutter in perioperative, postoperative, or other emergent circumstances where short term control of ventricular rate with a short-acting agent is desirable. BREVIBLOC® is also indicated in noncompensatory sinus tachycardia where, in the physician's judgment, the rapid heart rate requires specific intervention. BREVIBLOC® is not intended for use in chronic settings where transfer to another agent is anticipated.

Intraoperative and Postoperative Tachycardia and/or Hypertension
BREVIBLOC® (esmolol HCl) is indicated for the treatment of tachycardia and hypertension that occur during induction and tracheal intubation, during surgery, on emergence from anesthesia, and in the postoperative period, when in the physician's judgment such specific intervention is considered indicated.
Use of BREVIBLOC® to prevent such events is not recommended.

CONTRAINDICATIONS
BREVIBLOC® (esmolol HCl) is contraindicated in patients with sinus bradycardia, heart block greater than first degree, cardiogenic shock or overt heart failure (see WARNINGS).

WARNINGS
Hypotension: In clinical trials 20–50% of patients treated with BREVIBLOC® (esmolol HCl) have experienced hypotension, generally defined as systolic pressure less than 90 mmHg and/or diastolic pressure less than 50 mmHg. About 12% of the patients have been symptomatic (mainly diaphoresis or dizziness). Hypotension can occur at any dose but is

dose-related so that doses beyond 200 mcg/kg/min (0.2 mg/kg/min) are not recommended. Patients should be closely monitored, especially if pretreatment blood pressure is low. Decrease of dose or termination of infusion reverses hypotension, usually within 30 minutes.

Cardiac Failure: Sympathetic stimulation is necessary in supporting circulatory function in congestive heart failure, and beta blockade carries the potential hazard of further depressing myocardial contractility and precipitating more severe failure. Continued depression of the myocardium with beta blocking agents over a period of time can, in some cases, lead to cardiac failure. At the first sign or symptom of impending cardiac failure, BREVIBLOC® (esmolol HCl) should be withdrawn. Although withdrawal may be sufficient because of the short elimination half-life of BREVIBLOC®, specific treatment may also be considered (see OVERDOSAGE). The use of BREVIBLOC® for control of ventricular response in patients with supraventricular arrhythmias should be undertaken with caution when the patient is compromised hemodynamically or is taking other drugs that decrease any or all of the following: peripheral resistance, myocardial filling, myocardial contractility, or electrical impulse propagation in the myocardium. Despite the rapid onset and offset of the effects of BREVIBLOC®, several cases of death have been reported in complex clinical states where BREVIBLOC® was presumably being used to control ventricular rate.

Intraoperative and Postoperative Tachycardia and/or Hypertension: BREVIBLOC® (esmolol HCl) should not be used as the treatment for hypertension in patients in whom the increased blood pressure is primarily due to the vasoconstriction associated with hypothermia.

Bronchospastic Diseases: PATIENTS WITH BRONCHOSPASTIC DISEASES SHOULD, IN GENERAL, NOT RECEIVE BETA BLOCKERS. Because of its relative beta$_1$ selectivity and titratability, BREVIBLOC® (esmolol HCl) may be used with caution in patients with bronchospastic diseases. However, since beta$_1$ selectivity is not absolute, BREVIBLOC® should be carefully titrated to obtain the lowest possible effective dose. In the event of bronchospasm, the infusion should be terminated immediately; a beta$_2$ stimulating agent may be administered if conditions warrant but should be used with particular caution as patients already have rapid ventricular rates.

Diabetes Mellitus and Hypoglycemia: BREVIBLOC® (esmolol HCl) should be used with caution in diabetic patients requiring a beta blocking agent. Beta blockers may mask tachycardia occurring with hypoglycemia, but other manifestations such as dizziness and sweating may not be significantly affected.

PRECAUTIONS
General
Infusion concentrations of 20 mg/mL were associated with more serious venous irritation, including thrombophlebitis, than concentrations of 10 mg/mL. Extravasation of 20 mg/mL may lead to a serious local reaction and possible skin necrosis. Concentrations greater than 10 mg/mL or infusion into small veins or through a butterfly catheter should be avoided.

Because the acid metabolite of BREVIBLOC® is primarily excreted unchanged by the kidney, BREVIBLOC® (esmolol HCl) should be administered with caution to patients with impaired renal function. The elimination half-life of the acid metabolite was prolonged ten-fold and the plasma level was considerably elevated in patients with end-stage renal disease.

Care should be taken in the intravenous administration of BREVIBLOC® as sloughing of the skin and necrosis have been reported in association with infiltration and extravasation of intravenous infusions.

Drug Interactions
Catecholamine-depleting drugs, e.g., reserpine, may have an additive effect when given with beta blocking agents. Patients treated concurrently with BREVIBLOC® (esmolol HCl) and a catecholamine depletor should therefore be closely observed for evidence of hypotension or marked bradycardia, which may result in vertigo, syncope, or postural hypotension.

A study of interaction between BREVIBLOC® and warfarin showed that concomitant administration of BREVIBLOC® and warfarin does not alter warfarin plasma levels. BREVIBLOC® concentrations were equivocally higher when given with warfarin, but this is not likely to be clinically important.

When digoxin and BREVIBLOC® were concomitantly administered intravenously to normal volunteers, there was a 10–20% increase in digoxin blood levels at some time points. Digoxin did not affect BREVIBLOC® pharmacokinetics. When intravenous morphine and BREVIBLOC® were concomitantly administered in normal subjects, no effect on morphine blood levels was seen, but BREVIBLOC® steady-state blood levels were increased by 46% in the presence of morphine. No other pharmacokinetic parameters were changed.

The effect of BREVIBLOC® on the duration of succinylcholine-induced neuromuscular blockade was studied in patients undergoing surgery. The onset of neuromuscular blockade by succinylcholine was unaffected by BREVIBLOC®, but the duration of neuromuscular blockade was prolonged from 5 minutes to 8 minutes.

Although the interactions observed in these studies do not appear to be of major clinical importance, BREVIBLOC® should be titrated with caution in patients being treated concurrently with digoxin, morphine, succinylcholine or warfarin.

While taking beta blockers, patients with a history of severe anaphylactic reaction to a variety of allergens may be more reactive to repeated challenge, either accidental, diagnostic, or therapeutic. Such patients may be unresponsive to the usual doses of epinephrine used to treat allergic reaction.

Caution should be exercised when considering the use of BREVIBLOC® and verapamil in patients with depressed myocardial function. Fatal cardiac arrests have occurred in patients receiving both drugs. Additionally, BREVIBLOC® should not be used to control supraventricular tachycardia in the presence of agents which are vasoconstrictive and inotropic such as dopamine, epinephrine, and norepinephrine because of the danger of blocking cardiac contractility when systemic vascular resistance is high.

Carcinogenesis, Mutagenesis, Impairment of Fertility
Because of its short term usage no carcinogenicity, mutagenicity or reproductive performance studies have been conducted with BREVIBLOC® (esmolol HCl).

Pregnancy Category C
Teratogenicity studies in rats at intravenous dosages of BREVIBLOC® (esmolol HCl) up to 3000 mcg/kg/min (3 mg/kg/min) (ten times the maximum human maintenance dosage) for 30 minutes daily produced no evidence of maternal toxicity, embryotoxicity or teratogenicity, while a dosage of 10,000 mcg/kg/min (10 mg/kg/min) produced maternal toxicity and lethality. In rabbits, intravenous dosages up to 1000 mcg/kg/min (1 mg/kg/min) for 30 minutes daily produced no evidence of maternal toxicity, embryotoxicity or teratogenicity, while 2500 mcg/kg/min (2.5 mg/kg/min) produced minimal maternal toxicity and increased fetal resorptions.

Although there are no adequate and well-controlled studies in pregnant women, use of esmolol in the last trimester of pregnancy or during labor or delivery has been reported to cause fetal bradycardia, which continued after termination of drug infusion. BREVIBLOC® should be used during pregnancy only if the potential benefit justifies the potential risk to the fetus.

Nursing Mothers
It is not known whether BREVIBLOC® (esmolol HCl) is excreted in human milk; however, caution should be exercised when BREVIBLOC® is administered to a nursing woman.

Pediatric Use
The safety and effectiveness of BREVIBLOC® (esmolol HCl) in children have not been established.

ADVERSE REACTIONS
The following adverse reaction rates are based on use of BREVIBLOC® (esmolol HCl) in clinical trials involving 369 patients with supraventricular tachycardia and over 600 intraoperative and postoperative patients enrolled in clinical trials. Most adverse effects observed in controlled clinical trial settings have been mild and transient. The most important adverse effect has been hypotension (see WARNINGS). Deaths have been reported in post-marketing experience occurring during complex clinical states where BREVIBLOC® was presumably being used simply to control ventricular rate (see WARNINGS/Cardiac Failure).

Cardiovascular—Symptomatic hypotension (diaphoresis, dizziness) occurred in 12% of patients, and therapy was discontinued in about 11%, about half of whom were symptomatic. Asymptomatic hypotension occurred in about 25% of patients. Hypotension resolved during BREVIBLOC® (esmolol HCl) infusion in 63% of these patients and within 30 minutes after discontinuation of infusion in 80% of the remaining patients. Diaphoresis accompanied hypotension in 10% of patients. Peripheral ischemia occurred in approximately 1% of patients. Pallor, flushing, bradycardia (heart rate less than 50 beats per minute), chest pain, syncope, pulmonary edema and heart block have each been reported in less than 1% of patients. In two patients without supraventricular tachycardia but with serious coronary artery disease (post inferior myocardial infarction or unstable angina), severe bradycardia/sinus pause/asystole has developed, reversible in both cases with discontinuation of treatment.

Central Nervous System—Dizziness has occurred in 3% of patients; somnolence in 3%; confusion, headache, and agitation in about 2%; and fatigue in about 1% of patients. Paresthesia, asthenia, depression, abnormal thinking, anxiety, anorexia, and lightheadedness were reported in less than 1% of patients. Seizures were also reported in less than 1% of patients, with one death.

Continued on next page

Brevibloc—Cont.

Respiratory—Bronchospasm, wheezing, dyspnea, nasal congestion, rhonchi, and rales have each been reported in less than 1% of patients.

Gastrointestinal—Nausea was reported in 7% of patients. Vomiting has occurred in about 1% of patients. Dyspepsia, constipation, dry mouth, and abdominal discomfort have each occurred in less than 1% of patients. Taste perversion has also been reported.

Skin (Infusion Site)—Infusion site reactions including inflammation and induration were reported in about 8% of patients. Edema, erythema, skin discoloration, burning at the infusion site, thrombophlebitis, and local skin necrosis from extravasation have each occurred in less than 1% of patients.

Miscellaneous—Each of the following has been reported in less than 1% of patients: Urinary retention, speech disorder, abnormal vision, midscapular pain, rigors, and fever.

OVERDOSAGE

Acute Toxicity

Overdoses of BREVIBLOC® (esmolol HCl) can cause cardiac arrest. In addition, overdoses can produce bradycardia, hypotension, electromechanical dissociation and loss of consciousness. Cases of massive accidental overdoses of BREVIBLOC® have occurred due to dilution errors. Some of these overdoses have been fatal while others resulted in permanent disablility. Bolus doses in the range of 625 mg to 2.5 g (12.5–50 mg/kg) have been fatal. Patients have recovered completely from overdoses as high as 1.75 g given over one minute or doses of 7.5 g given over one hour for cardiovascular surgery. The patients who survived appear to be those whose circulation could be supported until the effects of BREVIBLOC® resolved.

Because of its approximately 9-minute elimination half-life, the first step in the management of toxicity should be to discontinue the BREVIBLOC® infusion. Then, based on the observed clinical effects, the following general measures should also be considered.

Bradycardia: Intravenous administration of atropine or another anticholinergic drug.

Bronchospasm: Intravenous administration of $beta_2$ stimulating agent and/or a theophylline derivative.

Cardiac Failure: Intravenous administration of a diuretic and/or digitalis glycoside. In shock resulting from inadequate cardiac contractility, intravenous administration of dopamine, dobutamine, isoproterenol, or amrinone may be considered.

Symptomatic Hypotension: Intravenous administration of fluids and/or pressor agents.

DOSAGE AND ADMINISTRATION

2500 mg AMPUL

THE 2500 mg AMPUL IS NOT FOR DIRECT INTRAVENOUS INJECTION. THIS DOSAGE FORM IS A CONCENTRATED, POTENT DRUG WHICH MUST BE DILUTED PRIOR TO ITS INFUSION. BREVIBLOC® SHOULD NOT BE ADMIXED WITH SODIUM BICARBONATE. BREVIBLOC® SHOULD NOT BE MIXED WITH OTHER DRUGS PRIOR TO DILUTION IN A SUITABLE INTRAVENOUS FLUID.

(See Compatibility Section below.)

Dilution: Aseptically prepare a 10 mg/mL infusion by adding two 2500 mg ampuls to a 500 mL container or one 2500 mg ampul to a 250 mL container of a compatible intravenous solution listed below. (Remove overage prior to dilution as appropriate.) This yields a final concentration of 10 mg/mL. The diluted solution is stable for at least 24 hours at room temperature. Note: Concentrations of BREVIBLOC® (esmolol HCl) greater than 10 mg/mL are likely to produce irritation on continued infusion (see PRECAUTIONS). BREVIBLOC® has, however, been well tolerated when administered via a central vein.

100 mg VIAL

This dosage form is prediluted to provide a ready-to-use 10 mg/mL concentration recommended for BREVIBLOC® intravenous administration. It may be used to administer the appropriate BREVIBLOC® (esmolol HCl) loading dosage infusions by hand-held syringe while the maintenance infusion is being prepared.

When using the 100 mg vial, a loading dose of 0.5 mg/kg/min for a 70 kg patient would be 3.5 mL.

Supraventricular Tachycardia

In the treatment of supraventricular tachycardia, responses to BREVIBLOC® (esmolol HCl) usually (over 95%) occur within the range of 50 to 200 mcg/kg/min (0.05 to 0.2 mg/kg/min). The average effective dosage is approximately 100 mcg/kg/min (0.1 mg/kg/min) although dosages as low as 25 mcg/kg/min (0.025 mg/kg/min) have been adequate in some patients. Dosages as high as 300 mcg/kg/min (0.3 mg/kg/min) have been used, but these provide little added effect and an increased rate of adverse effects, and are not recommended. Dosage of BREVIBLOC® in supraventricular tachycardia must be individualized by titration in which each step consists of a loading dosage followed by a maintenance dosage.

To initiate treatment of a patient with supraventricular tachycardia, administer a loading infusion of 500 mcg/kg/min (0.5 mg/kg/min) over one minute followed by a four-minute maintenance infusion of 50 mcg/kg/min (0.05 mg/kg/min). If an adequate therapeutic effect is observed over the five minutes of drug administration, maintain the maintenance infusion dosage with periodic adjustments up or down as needed. If an adequate therapeutic effect is not observed, the same loading dosage is repeated over one minute followed by an increased maintenance infusion rate of 100 mcg/kg/min (0.1 mg/kg/min).

Continue titration procedure as above, repeating the original loading infusion of 500 mcg/kg/min (0.5 mg/kg/min) over 1 minute, but increasing the maintenance infusion rate over the subsequent four minutes by 50 mcg/kg/min (0.05 mg/kg/min) increments. As the desired heart rate or blood pressure is approached, omit subsequent loading doses and titrate the maintenance dosage up or down to endpoint. Also, if desired, increase the interval between steps from 5 to 10 minutes.

Time (minutes)	Loading Dose (over 1 minute) mcg/kg/min	Loading Dose (over 1 minute) mg/kg/min	Maintenance Dose (over 4 minutes) mcg/kg/min	Maintenance Dose (over 4 minutes) mg/kg/min
0–1	500	0.5		
1–5			50	0.05
5–6	500	0.5		
6–10			100	0.1
10–11	500	0.5		
11–15			150	0.15
15–16	•	•		
16–20			*200	* 0.2
20–(24 hrs)			Maintenance dose titrated to heart rate or other clinical endpoint.	

* As the desired heart rate or endpoint is approached, the loading infusion may be omitted and the maintenance infusion titrated to 300 mcg/kg/min (0.3 mg/kg/min) or downward as appropriate. Maintenance dosages above 200 mcg/kg/min (0.2 mg/kg/min) have not been shown to have significantly increased benefits. The interval between titration steps may be increased.

This specific dosage regimen has not been studied intraoperatively and, because of the time required for titration, may not be optimal for intraoperative use.

The safety of dosages above 300 mcg/kg/min (0.3 mg/kg/min) has not been studied.

In the event of an adverse reaction, the dosage of BREVIBLOC® may be reduced or discontinued. If a local infusion site reaction develops, an alternate infusion site should be used and caution should be taken to prevent extravasation. The use of butterfly needles should be avoided.

Abrupt cessation of BREVIBLOC® in patients has not been reported to produce the withdrawal effects which may occur with abrupt withdrawal of beta blockers following chronic use in coronary artery disease (CAD) patients. However, caution should still be used in abruptly discontinuing infusions of BREVIBLOC® in CAD patients.

After achieving an adequate control of the heart rate and a stable clinical status in patients with supraventricular tachycardia, transition to alternative antiarrhythmic agents such as propranolol, digoxin, or verapamil, may be accomplished. A recommended guideline for such a transition is given below but the physician should carefully consider the labeling instructions for the alternative agent selected.

Alternative Agent	Dosage
Propranolol hydrochloride	10–20 mg q 4–6 hrs
Digoxin	0.125–0.5 mg q 6 hrs (p.o. or i.v.)
Verapamil	80 mg q 6 hrs

The dosage of BREVIBLOC® (esmolol HCl) should be reduced as follows:

1. Thirty minutes following the first dose of the alternative agent, reduce the infusion rate of BREVIBLOC® by one-half (50%).
2. Following the second dose of the alternative agent, monitor the patient's response and if satisfactory control is maintained for the first hour, discontinue BREVIBLOC®.

The use of infusions of BREVIBLOC® up to 24 hours has been well documented; in addition, limited data from 24–48 hrs (N=48) indicate that BREVIBLOC® is well tolerated up to 48 hours.

Intraoperative and Postoperative Tachycardia and/or Hypertension

In the intraoperative and postoperative settings it is not always advisable to slowly titrate the dose of BREVIBLOC® (esmolol HCl) to a therapeutic effect. Therefore, two dosing options are presented: immediate control dosing and a gradual control when the physician has time to titrate.

1. Immediate Control
   For intraoperative treatment of tachycardia and/or hypertension give an 80 mg (approximately 1 mg/kg) bolus dose over 30 seconds followed by a 150 mcg/kg/min infusion, if necessary. Adjust the infusion rate as required up to 300 mcg/kg/min to maintain desired heart rate and/or blood pressure.
2. Gradual Control
   For postoperative tachycardia and hypertension, the dosing schedule is the same as that used in supraventricular tachycardia. To initiate treatment, administer a loading dosage infusion of 500 mcg/kg/min of BREVIBLOC® for one minute followed by a four-minute maintenance infusion of 50 mcg/kg/min. If an adequate therapeutic effect is not observed within five minutes, repeat the same loading dosage and follow with a maintenance infusion increased to 100 mcg/kg/min (see above Supraventricular Tachycardia).
   Note: Higher dosages (250–300 mcg/kg/min) may be required for adequate control of blood pressure than those required for the treatment of atrial fibrillation, flutter and sinus tachycardia. One third of the postoperative hypertensive patients required these higher doses.

Compatibility with Commonly Use Intravenous Fluids

BREVIBLOC® INJECTION was tested for compatibility with ten commonly used intravenous fluids at a final concentration of 10 mg esmolol HCl per mL. BREVIBLOC® INJECTION was found to be compatible with the following solutions and was stable for at least 24 hours at controlled room temperature or under refrigeration:

- Dextrose (5%) Injection, USP
- Dextrose (5%) in Lactated Ringer's Injection
- Dextrose (5%) in Ringer's Injection
- Dextrose (5%) and Sodium Chloride (0.45%) Injection, USP
- Dextrose (5%) and Sodium Chloride (0.9%) Injection, USP
- Lactated Ringer's Injection, USP
- Potassium Chloride (40 mEq/liter) in Dextrose (5%) Injection, USP
- Sodium Chloride (0.45%) Injection, USP
- Sodium Chloride (0.9%) Injection, USP

BREVIBLOC® INJECTION was NOT compatible with Sodium Bicarbonate (5%) Injection, USP.

Note: Parenteral drug products should be inspected visually for particulate matter and discoloration prior to administration, whenever solution and container permit.

HOW SUPPLIED

NDC 10019-015-71, 100 mg—10 mL vial, Box of 20
NDC 10019-025-18, 2500 mg—10 mL ampul, Box of 10
STORE AT CONTROLLED ROOM TEMPERATURE (59°–86° F, 15°–30° C). Freezing does not adversely affect the product, but exposure to elevated temperatures should be avoided.

OHMEDA
THE BOC GROUP
Mfd. for: Ohmeda Pharmaceutical Products Division Inc
110 Allen Road PO Box 804 Liberty Corner NJ 07938 0804
Mfd. by: Faulding Puerto Rico, Inc. P.O. Box 471 Aguadilla, PR 00604
For Product Inquiry 1 800 ANA DRUG
400-277-02 Rev. 7-95

BUMETANIDE Injection, USP ℞

[bumĕ-tanide]

WARNING: Bumetanide is a potent diuretic which, if given in excessive amounts, can lead to a profound diuresis with water and electrolyte depletion. Therefore, careful medical supervision is required, and dose and dosage schedule have to be adjusted to the individual patient's needs. (See **DOSAGE AND ADMINISTRATION** in full prescribing information.)

DESCRIPTION

Bumetanide is a loop diuretic, available as 2 mL vials, 4 mL vials and 10 mL vials (0.25 mg/mL) for intravenous or intramuscular injection as a sterile solution.

Each mL contains: Bumetanide 0.25 mg, Sodium Chloride 8.5 mg and Ammonium Acetate 4.0 mg as buffers, Disodium Edetate 0.1 mg, Benzyl Alcohol 10 mg as preservative, Water for Injection q.s. pH adjusted with Sodium Hydroxide. pH 6.8–7.8

Chemically, bumetanide is 3-(butylamino)-4-phenoxy-5-sulfamoylbenzoic acid. It is a practically white powder, slightly soluble in water; soluble in alkaline solutions, having the following structural formula:

[See chemical structure at top of next column]

HOW SUPPLIED

Bumetanide Injection, USP 0.25 mg/mL is supplied in amber vials as follows:

NDC Number	Size
10019-506-02	2 mL
10019-506-45	4 mL
10019-506-10	10 mL Mutliple Dose Vial

Store at controlled room temperature 15°–30°C (59°–86°F).

COOH

CH$_3$(CH$_2$)$_3$HN— —SO$_2$NH$_2$

OC$_6$H$_5$

C$_{17}$H$_{20}$N$_2$O$_5$S   364.42

DILTIAZEM HYDROCHLORIDE INJECTION
0.5% (5 mg/mL)   ℞
[dĭl'tia-zem]

Rx only

DESCRIPTION

Diltiazem hydrochloride is a calcium ion influx inhibitor (slow channel blocker or calcium channel antagonist). Chemically, diltiazem hydrochloride is 1,5-benzothiazepin-4(5H)one,3-(acetyloxy)-5-[2-(dimethylamino)ethyl]-2,3-dihydro-2-(4-methoxyphenyl)-,monohydrochloride,(+)-cis-. The structural formula is:

The molecular formula is C$_{22}$H$_{26}$N$_2$O$_4$S•HCl

Diltiazem hydrochloride is a white to off-white crystalline powder with a bitter taste. It is soluble in water, methanol, and chloroform. It has a molecular weight of 450.99.

Diltiazem hydrochloride injection is a clear, colorless, sterile, nonpyrogenic solution. It has a pH range of 3.7 to 4.1.

Diltiazem hydrochloride injection is for direct intravenous bolus injection and continuous intravenous infusion.

Each mL contains: 5 mg diltiazem hydrochloride, 0.75 mg citric acid USP, 0.65 mg sodium citrate dihydrate USP, 71.4 mg sorbitol solution USP, and water for injection USP up to 1 mL. Sodium hydroxide and/or hydrochloric acid are used for pH adjustment.

HOW SUPPLIED

Diltiazem Hydrochloride Injection, 0.5% (5 mg/mL) is supplied:

5 mL vials in cartons of 6; NDC 10019-510-05
10 mL vials in cartons of 6; NDC 10019-510-10
SINGLE-USE CONTAINERS. DISCARD UNUSED PORTION.

DOBUTAMINE   ℞
[dō-bū-tă-mēn]
Hydrochloride Injection

DESCRIPTION

Dobutamine Hydrochloride Injection is (±)-4-[2-[[3-(p-Hydroxyphenyl)-1-methylpropyl]amino]ethyl]-pyrocatechol hydrochloride. It is a synthetic catecholamine.

Molecular Formula: C$_{18}$H$_{23}$NO$_3$·HCl
Molecular Weight: 337.85

The clinical formulation is supplied in a sterile form for intravenous use only. Each mL contains: Dobutamine hydrochloride, equivalent to 12.5 mg (41.5 μmol) dobutamine; Sodium Bisulfite 0.28 mg (added during manufacture), and water for injection q.s. Hydrochloric acid and/or sodium hydroxide may have been added during manufacture to adjust the pH (2.5–5.5).

HOW SUPPLIED

Dobutamine Hydrochloride Injection, 20 mL single dose vials containing the equivalent of 250 mg dobutamine per 20 mL; one vial per carton, in packs of 10. NDC 10019-181-20.

DURAMORPH®   ℞
[dŭră-morph]
PRESERVATIVE-FREE
(morphine sulfate injection, USP)
WARNING: May be habit forming

DESCRIPTION

Morphine is the most important alkaloid of opium and is a phenanthrene derivative. It is available as the sulfate salt, having the following structural formula:

•H$_2$SO$_4$•5H$_2$O

7,8-Didehydro-4,5-epoxy-17-methyl-(5α,6α)-morphinan-3,6-diol sulfate (2:1) (salt), pentahydrate

(C$_{17}$H$_{19}$NO$_3$)$_2$•H$_2$SO$_4$•5H$_2$O   Molecular weight is 758.83

Preservative-free DURAMORPH® (morphine sulfate injection, USP) is a sterile, nonpyrogenic, isobaric solution of morphine sulfate, free of antioxidants, preservatives or other potentially neurotoxic additives and is intended for intravenous, epidural or intrathecal administration as a narcotic analgesic. Each milliliter contains morphine sulfate 0.5 mg or 1 mg and sodium chloride 9 mg in Water for Injection. pH range is 2.5–6.5. Ampuls are sealed under nitrogen. Each 10 mL DOSETTE® ampul of DURAMORPH® is intended for **SINGLE USE ONLY**. *Discard any unused portion.* DO NOT HEAT-STERILIZE.

HOW SUPPLIED

Preservative-free DURAMORPH® (morphine sulfate injection, USP) is available in amber DOSETTE® ampuls for intravenous, epidural and intrathecal administration:

5 mg/10 mL (0.5 mg/mL) packaged in 10s (NDC 10019-006-73)

10 mg/10 mL (1 mg/1 mL) packaged in 10s (NDC 10019-007-73)

Duramorph® and DOSETTE® are registered trademarks of A.H. Robins Company.

ENLON®   ℞
[ĕn 'lon]
(edrophonium chloride injection, USP)

DESCRIPTION

Enlon® is a short and rapid-acting cholinergic drug. Chemically, edrophonium chloride is ethyl(m-hydroxyphenyl) dimethylammonium chloride and its structural formula is:

C$_2$H$_5$
HO— —N$^+$(CH$_3$)$_2$ Cl$^-$

Each mL contains, in a sterile solution, 10 mg edrophonium chloride compounded with 0.45% phenol as a preservative, and 0.2% sodium sulfite as an antioxidant, buffered with sodium citrate and citric acid, and pH adjusted to approximately 5.4.

Enlon® is intended for IV and IM use.

HOW SUPPLIED

ENLON® (edrophonium chloride injection, USP):
NDC 10019-873-15   15 mL vials

ENLON-PLUS®   ℞
[ĕn '-lon ' plus]
(edrophonium chloride, USP and atropine sulfate, USP) Injection

DESCRIPTION

Enlon-Plus® (edrophonium chloride, USP and atropine sulfate, USP) Injection, for intravenous use, is a sterile, nonpyrogenic, nondepolarizing neuromuscular relaxant antagonist. Enlon-Plus® is a combination drug containing a rapid acting acetylcholinesterase inhibitor, edrophonium chloride, and an anticholinergic, atropine sulfate. Chemically, edrophonium chloride is ethyl (m-hydroxyphenyl) dimethylammonium chloride; its structural formula is:

C$_2$H$_5$
HO— —N$^+$(CH$_3$)$_2$ Cl$^-$

Molecular Formula: C$_{10}$H$_{16}$ClNO
Molecular Weight: 201.70

Chemically, atropine sulfate is:
endo-(±)-alpha-(hydroxymethyl)-8-methyl-8-azabicyclo [3.2.1]oct-3-yl benzeneacetate sulfate (2:1) monohydrate. Its structural formula is:

CH$_3$
N
•H$_2$SO$_4$ • H$_2$O
OC—CH—
CH$_2$OH

Molecular Formula: (C$_{17}$H$_{23}$NO$_3$)$_2$.H$_2$SO$_4$.H$_2$O
Molecular Weight: 694.84

Enlon-Plus® contains in each mL of sterile solution:
5 mL Ampuls: 10 mg edrophonium chloride and 0.14 mg atropine sulfate compounded with 2.0 mg sodium sulfite as a preservative and buffered with sodium citrate and citric acid. The pH is adjusted in the range of 4.4–4.6.

15 mL Multidose Vials: 10 mg edrophonium chloride and 0.14 mg atropine sulfate compounded with 2.0 mg sodium sulfite and 4.5 mg phenol as a preservative and buffered with sodium citrate and citric acid. The pH is adjusted in the range of 4.4–4.6.

HOW SUPPLIED

Enlon-Plus® (edrophonium chloride, USP and atropine sulfate, USP) Injection should be stored between 15°–26°C (59°–78°F)

NDC 10019-180-05   5 mL ampuls, boxes of 10
NDC 10019-195-15   15 mL multidose vials

ÉTHRANE®   ℞
[ē 'thrān]
(enflurane, USP)
Liquid For Inhalation

CAUTION: Federal Law Prohibits Dispensing without Prescription.

DESCRIPTION

Éthrane® (enflurane, USP), a nonflammable liquid administered by vaporizing, is a general inhalation anesthetic drug. It is 2-chloro-1,1,2-trifluoroethyl difluoromethyl ether (CHF$_2$OCF$_2$CHFCl). The boiling point is 56.5° C at 760 mm Hg, and the vapor pressure (in mm Hg) is 175 at 20° C, 218 at 25° C, and 345 at 36° C. Vapor pressures can be calculated using the equation:

$$\log_{10}P_{vap}=A+\frac{B}{T}$$

A = 7.967
B = −1678.4
T = °C+ 273.16 (Kelvin)

The specific gravity (25°/25° C) is 1.517. The refractive index at 20° C is 1.3026–1.3030. The blood/gas coefficient is 1.91 at 37° C and the oil/gas coefficient is 98.5 at 37° C. Enflurane is a clear, colorless, stable liquid whose purity exceeds 99.9% (area percent by gas chromatography). No stabilizers are added as these have been found, through controlled laboratory tests, to be unnecessary even in the presence of ultraviolet light. Enflurane is stable to strong base, does not decompose in contact with soda lime (at normal operating temperatures), and does not react with aluminum, tin, brass, iron or copper. The partition coefficients of enflurane at 25° C are 74 in conductive rubber and 120 in polyvinyl chloride.

HOW SUPPLIED

Éthrane® (enflurane, USP) is packaged in 125 and 250 mL amber-colored bottles.
     125 mL—NDC 10019-350-50
     250 mL—NDC 10019-350-60
Storage: Store at room temperature 15°–30° C (59°–86° F). Enflurane contains no additives and has been demonstrated to be stable at room temperature for periods in excess of five years.

FENTANYL Citrate Injection, USP   ℞
[fĕn tăn-ill]
WARNING: May be habit forming.

DESCRIPTION

Fentanyl Citrate Injection is a sterile, non-pyrogenic solution for intravenous or intramuscular use as a potent narcotic analgesic. Each mL contains fentanyl citrate equivalent to 50 mcg (0.05 mg) fentanyl base (WARNING: May be habit forming) in Water for Injection. pH 4.0–7.5; sodium hydroxide and/or hydrochloric acid added, if needed, for pH adjustment. Contains no preservative.

Continued on next page

Fentanyl Citrate—Cont.

Fentanyl citrate is chemically identified as N-(1-phenethyl-4-piperidyl)propionanilide citrate (1:1) with the following structural formula:

$C_{32}H_{28}N_2O \cdot C_8H_8O_7$ MW 528.60

HOW SUPPLIED

Fentanyl Citrate Injection, USP, equivalent to 50 mcg (0.05 mg) fentanyl base per mL, is available as follows

2 mL DOSETTE® ampuls packaged in 10s (NDC 10019-038-67)

5 mL DOSETTE® ampuls packaged in 10s (NDC 10019-033-72)

For Intravenous Use by Hospital Personnel Specifically Trained in the Use of Narcotic Analgesics:

10 mL DOSETTE® ampuls packaged in 5s (NDC 10019-034-73)

20 mL DOSETTE® ampuls packaged in 5s (NDC 10019-035-74)

50 mL *SINGLE DOSE* vials packaged individually (NDC 10019-037-83)

DOSETTE® is a registered trademark of A.H. Robins Company.

FORANE®   ℞

[for 'ăn]

(isoflurane, USP)
Liquid For Inhalation

CAUTION:

Federal Law Prohibits Dispensing without Prescription.

DESCRIPTION

FORANE® (isoflurane, USP), a nonflammable liquid administered by vaporizing, is a general inhalation anesthetic drug. It is 1-chloro-2,2,2-trifluoroethyl difluoromethyl ether, and its structural formula is:

Some physical constants are:

Molecular weight	184.5
Boiling point at 760 mm Hg	48.5 °C (uncorr.)
Refractive index n_D^{20}	1.2990–1.3005
Specific gravity 25 °/25 °C	1.496
Vapor pressure in mm Hg** 20 °C	238
25 °C	295
30 °C	367
35 °C	450

**Equation for vapor pressure calculation:

$$\log_{10}P_{vap} = A + \frac{B}{T}$$ where: A = 8.056
B = −1664.58
T = °C + 273.16 (Kelvin)

Partition coefficients at 37 °C

Water/gas	0.61
Blood/gas	1.43
Oil/gas	90.8

Partition coefficients at 25 °C—rubber and plastic

Conductive rubber/gas	62.0
Butyl rubber/gas	75.0
Polyvinyl chloride/gas	110.0
Polyethylene/gas	~2.0
Polyurethane/gas	~1.4
Polyolefin/gas	~1.1
Butyl acetate/gas	~2.5
Purity by gas chromatography	>99.9%
Lower limit of flammability in oxygen or nitrous oxide at 9 joules/sec. and 23°C	None
Lower limit of flammability in oxygen or nitrous oxide at 900 joules/sec. and 23°C	Greater than useful concentration in anesthesia.

Isoflurane is a clear, colorless, stable liquid containing no additives or chemical stabilizers. Isoflurane has a mildly pungent, musty, ethereal odor. Samples stored in indirect sunlight in clear, colorless glass for five years, as well as samples directly exposed for 30 hours to a 2 amp, 115 volt, 60 cycle long wave U.V. light were unchanged in composition as determined by gas chromatography. Isoflurane in one normal sodium methoxide-methanol solution, a strong base, for over six months consumed essentially no alkali, indicative of strong base stability. Isoflurane does not decompose in the presence of soda lime (at normal operating temperatures), and does not attack aluminum, tin, brass, iron or copper.

HOW SUPPLIED

FORANE® (isoflurane, USP) is packaged in 100 mL and 250 mL amber-colored bottles.

100 mL – NDC 10019-360-40
250 mL – NDC 10019-360-60

FUROSEMIDE INJECTION, USP   ℞

[fūr-o-sĕmīde]

WARNING

Furosemide is a potent diuretic which, if given in excessive amounts, can lead to a profound diuresis with water and electrolyte depletion. Therefore, careful medical supervision is required and dose and dosage schedule have to be adjusted to individual patient's needs. (See DOSAGE AND ADMINISTRATION in full prescribing information.)

DESCRIPTION

Furosemide is a diuretic which is an anthranilic acid derivative, chemically known as 4-chloro-N-furfuryl-5-sulfamoylanthranilic acid. Furosemide is a white to off-white odorless crystalline powder. It is practically insoluble in water, sparingly soluble in alcohol, freely soluble in dilute alkali solutions and insoluble in dilute acids. The structural formula is as follows:

$C_{12}H_{11}ClN_2O_5S$ MW 330.74

Furosemide Injection, for intramuscular or slow intravenous use, is a sterile, non-pyrogenic solution of furosemide in Water for Injection prepared with the aid of sodium hydroxide. Each mL contains furosemide 10 mg and sodium chloride for isotonicity. pH adjusted to 8.0–9.3 with sodium hydroxide; hydrochloric acid used, if needed. The preparation contains no antimicrobial preservatives.

HOW SUPPLIED

Furosemide Injection, USP is available in the following:
10 mg/mL DOSETTE® Ampuls
40 mg/4 mL packaged in 25s (NDC 10019-010-76)
DOSETTE® is a registered trademark of A.H. Robins Company.

LIDOCAINE HCl Injection, USP   ℞

[lĭdō' caīne]

FOR INFILTRATION AND NERVE BLOCK

Do Not Use Solutions Containing Preservatives for Spinal or Epidural Anesthesia.

DESCRIPTION

Lidocaine Hydrochloride Injection is a sterile solution of Lidocaine Hydrochloride 1% or 2% in Water for Injection. Each mL of the available solutions of Lidocaine Hydrochloride Injection contains the ingredients listed in Table 1.
[See table below]
pH 5.0–7.0; sodium hydroxide and/or hydrochloric acid added, if needed, for pH adjustment.
Lidocaine hydrochloride is a local anesthetic that is administered parenterally by injection and is chemically designated as 2-(diethylamino)-N-(2,6-dimethylphenyl) acet-

amide monohydrochloride. The molecular weight is 270.80 and the molecular formula is $C_{14}H_{22}N_2O \cdot HCl$. The structural formula is:

Lidocaine Hydrochloride Injection is available with and without epinephrine. Lidocaine Hydrochloride Injection without epinephrine may be reautoclaved if necessary.

HOW SUPPLIED

Lidocaine Hydrochloride Injection, USP, with preservative, is available as:

1% (10 mg/mL)
30 mL Multiple Dose vials packaged in 25s (NDC 10019-017-56)
50 mL Multiple Dose vials packaged in 25s (NDC 10019-017-57)
2% (20 mg/mL)
30 mL Multiple Dose vials packaged in 25s (NDC 10019-019-56)
50 mL Multiple Dose vials packaged in 25s (NDC 10019-019-57)

MEPERIDINE   Ⓒ

[mĕ'pĕr-ĭdĭne]
Hydrochloride Injection, USP

WARNING: May be habit forming

DESCRIPTION

Meperidine hydrochloride is ethyl 1-methyl-4-phenylisonipecotate hydrochloride, a white, crystalline compound with a melting point of 186°–189° C. It has a slightly bitter taste and is readily soluble in water. Aqueous solutions may be boiled for short periods without decomposition.
In addition to the stated concentration of meperidine hydrochloride (see **HOW SUPPLIED**), each mL of the product in **TUBEX®** Sterile Cartridge-Needle Units contains sodium acetate buffer. The parenteral products are intended for intramuscular, subcutaneous or slow "slow intravenous" use.

HOW SUPPLIED

For Parenteral Use
Meperidine HCl Injection, USP, is available in **TUBEX®** Sterile Cartridge-Needle Units, boxes of 10 **TUBEX® TAMP-R-TEL®** tamper-resistant packages in the following dosage strengths:
25 mg per mL, NDC 10019-151-47, 1 mL fill in 2 mL size (22 gauge × 1-1/4 inch needle)
50 mg per mL, NDC 10019-152-47, 1 mL fill in 2 mL size (22 gauge × 1-1/4 inch needle)
75 mg per mL, NDC 10019-153-47, 1 mL fill in 2 mL size (22 gauge × 1-1/4 inch needle)
100 mg per mL, NDC 10019-154-47, 1 mL fill in 2 mL size (22 gauge × 1-1/4 inch needle)
Store at room temperature, 15°–25° C (59°–77° F).
TUBEX® and **TAMP-R-TEL®** are registered trademarks of Wyeth-Ayerst Laboratories.

MEPERIDINE   Ⓒ

[mĕ'pĕr-ĭdĭne]
Hydrochloride Injection, USP

WARNING: May be habit forming

DESCRIPTION

Meperidine Hydrochloride Injection, USP is a sterile solution for intramuscular, subcutaneous or slow intravenous use as a narcotic analgesic.
Each mL of the DOSETTE® vial contains meperidine hydrochloride 50 mg, sodium metabisulfite 1.5 mg and phenol 5 mg in Water for Injection. Buffered with acetic acid-sodium acetate. pH 3.5–6.0. Sealed under nitrogen.
Meperidine hydrochloride is ethyl 1-methyl-4-phenylisonipecotate hydrochloride, a white crystalline substance with a melting point of 186°–189°C. It is readily soluble in water and has a slightly bitter taste.
Its structural formula is as follows:

$C_{15}H_{21}NO_2 \cdot HCl$ MW 283.80

TABLE 1
Composition of Available Solutions

Product	Composition		
	Lidocaine HCl (mg/mL)	Sodium Chloride (mg/mL)	Methylparaben (mg/mL)
Lidocaine Hydrochloride Inection 1%, preserved	10	7	1
Lidocaine Hydrochloride Inection 2%, preserved	20	6	1

HOW SUPPLIED

Meperidine Hydrochloride Injection, USP is available as follows:

50 mg/mL, 1 mL DOSETTE® vials packaged in 25s (NDC 10019-152-44)

DOSETTE® is a registered trademark of A.H. Robins Company.

METOCLOPRAMIDE ℞
[mĕtō clō-pra-mide]
Injection, USP

DESCRIPTION

Metoclopramide Injection, USP is a clear, colorless, sterile solution with a pH of 2.5–6.5 for intravenous or intramuscular administration.

Each mL contains Metoclopramide 5 mg (present as the hydrochloride); Sodium Chloride 8.5 mg; Water for Injection qs; pH is adjusted with Hydrochloric Acid and/or Sodium Hydroxide if necessary. pH 2.5–6.5.

Metoclopramide hydrochloride is a white or practically white, crystalline, odorless or practically odorless powder. It is very soluble in water, freely soluble in alcohol, sparingly soluble in chloroform, practically insoluble in ether. Chemically, it is 4-amino-5-chloro-N-[2-(diethylamino)ethyl]-2-methoxy benzamide monohydrochloride monohydrate. Molecular weight, 354.3, with the following structural formula:

$$C_{14}H_{22}ClN_3O_2 \cdot HCl \cdot H_2O$$

HOW SUPPLIED

Metoclopramide Injection, USP, is supplied in 2 mL vials packaged 25 per shelf pack.

NDC Number	Metoclopramide Injection USP	Volume
10019-450-02	5 mg/mL	2 mL in a 2 mL vial

MORPHINE Sulfate Injection, USP Ⓒ
[mōre-phēne]
WARNING: May be habit forming
FOR SUBCUTANEOUS, INTRAMUSCULAR OR SLOW INTRAVENOUS ADMINISTRATION NOT FOR EPIDURAL OR INTRATHECAL ADMINISTRATION

DESCRIPTION
Chemistry
Morphine Sulfate Injection, USP is a sterile solution for subcutaneous, intramuscular or intravenous injection. Each mL contains morphine sulfate, either 5 mg, 10 mg or 15 mg, monobasic sodium phosphate, monohydrate 10 mg, dibasic sodium phosphate, anhydrous 2.8 mg, sodium formaldehyde sulfoxylate 3 mg and phenol 2.5 mg in Water for Injection; sulfuric acid added, if needed, for pH adjustment. The pH range is 2.5–6.5. Sealed under nitrogen.

Because of the presence and nature of the preservative and antioxidant, the product may have a characteristic odor.

Morphine is a phenanthrene-derivative opiate agonist. It is the principal alkaloid of opium and is considered to be the prototype of the opiate agonists.

Morphine sulfate occurs as white, feathery, silky crystals; cubical masses of crystals; or a white, crystalline powder. The drug contains five molecules of water of hydration and is soluble in water, having an aqueous solubility of approximately 62.5 mg/mL at 25°C, and slightly soluble in alcohol. The chemical name of morphine sulfate is 7,8-didehydro-4,5α-epoxy-17-methylmorphinan-3,6α-diol sulfate (2:1) (salt) pentahydrate, with the following structural formula:

$$(C_{17}H_{19}NO_3)_2 \cdot H_2SO_4 \cdot 5H_2O \qquad MW\ 758.83$$

HOW SUPPLIED
Morphine Sulfate Injection, USP is available in the following:
5 mg/mL
1 mL DOSETTE® vials packaged in 25s (NDC 10019-176-44)

NDC Number	Neostigmine Methylsulfate per mL	Volume
NDC 10019-271-02	1:2000 (0.5 mg/mL)	1 mL in a 2 mL Vial
NDC 10019-271-10	1:2000 (0.5 mg/mL)	10 mL in a 10 mL Vial
NDC 10019-270-10	1:1000 (1 mg/mL)	10 mL in a 10 mL Vial

10 mg/mL
1 mL DOSETTE® vials packaged in 25s (NDC 10019-178-44)
1 mL DOSETTE® ampules packaged in 25s (NDC 10019-178-68)
10 mL Multiple Dose amber vials packaged individually (NDC 10019-178-62)
15 mg/mL
20 mL Multiple Dose amber vials packaged individually (NDC 10019-179-63)
DOSETTE® is a registered trademark of A.H. Robins Company.

NALOXONE HCl Injection, USP ℞
[nă-lŏ xōne]

DESCRIPTION

Naloxone hydrochloride, a narcotic antagonist, is a synthetic congener of oxymorphone. In structure it differs from oxymorphone in that the methyl group on the nitrogen atom is replaced by an allyl group.

The structure for naloxone hydrochloride is as follows:

(-)-17-Allyl-4, 5α-epoxy-3,14-dihydroxymorphinan-6-one hydrochloride
$$C_{19}H_{21}NO_4 \cdot HCl \qquad MW\ 363.84$$

Naloxone hydrochloride occurs as a white to slightly off-white powder, and is soluble in water, in dilute acids, and in strong alkali; slightly soluble in alcohol; practically insoluble in ether and in chloroform.

Naloxone Hydrochloride Injection is a sterile solution intended for intramuscular, subcutaneous or intravenous use. Each mL contains naloxone hydrochloride 400 micrograms (0.4 mg), solium chloride 8.6 mg, methylparaben 1.8 mg and propylparaben 0.2 mg in Water for Injection, pH 3.0–4.5; hydrochloric acid and/or sodium hydroxide used, if needed, for pH adjustment. Sealed under nitrogen.

HOW SUPPLIED
Naloxone Hydrochloride Injection is available in the following package:
0.4 mg/mL
1 mL DOSETTE® ampuls packaged in 10s (NDC 10019-039-68)
DOSETTE® is a registered trademark of A.H. Robins Company.

NEOSTIGMINE ℞
[nē-ō-stĭg-mĕn]
Methylsulfate Injection, USP

DESCRIPTION

Neostigmine methylsulfate is the dimethylcarbamate of (m-hydroxyphenyl) trimethylammonium methylsulfate.
The chemical structure is:

Neostigmine methylsulfate, an anticholinesterase agent, is a bitter tasting, white crystalline powder and is very soluble in water and soluble in alcohol. Neostigmine Methylsulfate Injection is a sterile solution intended for intramuscular, subcutaneous or slow intravenous use. Each mL of the 1:1000 concentration contains neostigmine methylsulfate 1 mg, methylparaben 1.8 mg and propylparaben 0.2 mg in water for injection qs; pH adjusted with NaOH if necessary. pH: 5.0–6.5. Each mL of the 1:2000 concentration contains neostigmine methylsulfate 0.5 mg, methylparaben 1.8 mg, propylparaben 0.2 mg, water for injection qs; pH adjusted with NaOH if necessary. pH: 5.0–6.5.

HOW SUPPLIED
[See table above]
10 mL multiple dose and 1 mL vials packaged in 10 per shelf pack.

PANCURONIUM BROMIDE ℞
[pan 'cŭ-rō-nē-ŭm brō 'mīde]
Injection

This drug should be administered by adequately trained individuals familiar with its actions, characteristics, and hazards.

DESCRIPTION
Pancuronium bromide is a nondepolarizing, neuromuscular blocking agent chemically designated as the aminosteroid 2β, 16β-dipiperidino-5α-androstane-3α, 17-β diol diacetate dimethobromide. The structural formula is:

Each mL contains: pancuronium bromide 1 mg or 2 mg; sodium acetate, anhydrous, 2 mg; sodium chloride, 4 mg to make isotonic; benzyl alcohol 10 mg (as preservative); water for injection qs; pH is adjusted with acetic acid and/or sodium hydroxide if necessary. pH: 3.8–4.2

HOW SUPPLIED

NDC Number	Pancuronium Bromide	Volume
NDC 10019-281-02	2 mg/mL	2 mL in a 2 mL vial
NDC 10019-281-05	2 mg/mL	5 mL in a 5 mL vial
NDC 10019-280-10	1 mg/mL	10 mL in a 10 mL vial

2 mL vials packaged 25 per shelf pack.
5 mL multiple dose vials packaged 25 per shelf pack.
10 mL multiple dose vials packaged 10 per shelf pack.

PHENYLEPHRINE ℞
[phē-nyl-eph-rĭn]
Hydrochloride Injection, USP

WARNING: Physicians should completely familiarize themselves with the complete contents of the full prescribing information before prescribing Phenylephrine Hydrochloride Injection.

DESCRIPTION

Phenylephrine hydrochloride is a vasoconstrictor and pressor drug chemically related to epinephrine and ephedrine. Phenylephrine hydrochloride is a synthetic sympathomimetic agent in sterile form for parenteral injection. Chemically, phenylephrine hydrochloride is (-)-m-Hydroxy-α-[(methylamino)methyl]benzyl alcohol hydrochloride, and has the following structural formula:

Phenylephrine Hydrochloride Injection, USP is available as a 1% (10 mg/mL) 1 mL vial. Each mL contains: Phenylephrine Hydrochloride 10 mg; Sodium Chloride 3.5 mg; Sodium Citrate Dihydrate 4.56 mg; Citric Acid Monohydrate 1 mg; Sodium Metabisulfite not more than 2 mg; Water for Injection q.s. Air replaced with Nitrogen. pH adjusted with Sodium Hydroxide and/or Hydrochloric Acid if necessary. pH 3.0–6.5

HOW SUPPLIED
Phenylephrine Hydrochloride Injection, USP 1% (10 mg/mL) is supplied as follows:
NDC 10019-163-12   1 mL fill in 2 mL vial

Continued on next page

Phenylephrine Hydrochloride—Cont.

1 mL vials are packaged in shelf cartons of 25.
Store at controlled room temperature 15°-30°C (59°-86°F).
Protect from light. Keep covered in carton until time of use.

REVEX®
[Rē-vĕx]
(nalmefene hydrochloride injection)   ℞

DESCRIPTION

REVEX® (nalmefene hydrochloride injection), an opioid antagonist, is a 6-methylene analogue of naltrexone. The chemical structure is shown below:

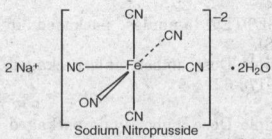

Molecular Formula: $C_{21}H_{25}NO_3 \cdot HCl$
Molecular Weight: 375.9, CAS # 58895-64-0
Chemical Name: 17-(Cyclopropylmethyl)-4,5α-epoxy-6-
                         methylenemorphinan-3,14-diol, hy-
                         drochloride salt.
Nalmefene hydrochloride is a white to off-white crystalline powder which is freely soluble in water up to 130 mg/mL and slightly soluble in chloroform up to 0.13 mg/mL, with a pK_a of 7.6.
REVEX® is available as a sterile solution for intravenous, intramuscular, and subcutaneous administration in two concentrations, containing 100 µg or 1.0 mg of nalmefene free base per mL. The 100 µg/mL concentration contains 110.8 µg of nalmefene hydrochloride and the 1.0 mg/mL concentration contains 1.108 mg of nalmefene hydrochloride per mL. Both concentrations contain 9.0 mg of sodium chloride per mL and the pH is adjusted to 3.9 with hydrochloric acid.
Concentrations and dosages of REVEX® are expressed as the free base equivalent of nalmefene.

HOW SUPPLIED

REVEX® (nalmefene hydrochloride injection) is available in the following presentations:
An ampul containing 1 mL of 100 µg/mL nalmefene base (Blue Label) Box of 10 (NDC 10019-315-21)
An ampul containing 2 mL of 1 mg/mL nalmefene base (Green Label) Box of 10 (NDC 10019-311-22)
A syringe containing 2 mL of 1 mg/mL nalmefene base (Green Label) (NDC 10019-311-32)
Syringe is supplied with 22 gauge × 1 1/4″ needle. See the REVEX® Syringe Carton for "Directions for Use of the Syringe".
Store at controlled room temperature.

SODIUM NITROPRUSSIDE   ℞
[sōdĭum nitrō′prussīde]
Injection

Sodium Nitroprusside Injection is not suitable for direct injection. The solution must be further diluted in 5% Dextrose Injection before infusion.
Sodium Nitroprusside Injection can cause precipitous decreases in blood pressure (see **DOSAGE AND ADMINISTRATION** in full prescribing information). In patients not properly monitored, these decreases can lead to irreversible ischemic injuries or death. Sodium nitroprusside should be used only when available equipment and personnel allow blood pressure to be continuously monitored.
Except when used briefly or at low (< 2 µg/kg/min) infusion rates, sodium nitroprusside gives rise to important quantities of cyanide ion, which can reach toxic, potentially lethal levels (see **WARNINGS** in full prescribing information). The usual dose rate is 0.5–10 µg/kg/min, but infusion at the maximum dose rate should never last more than 10 minutes. If blood pressure has not been adequately controlled after 10 minutes of infusion at the maximum rate, administration of sodium nitroprusside should be terminated immediately.
Although acid-base balance and venous oxygen concentration should be monitored and may indicate cyanide toxicity, these laboratory tests provide imperfect guidance.

The full prescribing information should be thoroughly reviewed before administration of Sodium Nitroprusside Injection.

DESCRIPTION

Sodium nitroprusside is disodium pentacyanonitrosylferrate (2-)dihydrate, an inorganic hypotensive agent whose structural formula is

$$2\,Na^+ \quad \left[\begin{array}{c} CN \\ NC - Fe - CN \\ ON \quad CN \end{array} \right]^{-2} \cdot 2H_2O$$

Sodium Nitroprusside

whose molecular formula is $Na_2[Fe(CN)_5NO] \cdot 2H_2O$, and whose molecular weight is 297.95. Dry sodium nitroprusside is a reddish-brown powder, soluble in water. In an aqueous solution infused intravenously, sodium nitroprusside is a rapid-acting vasodilator, active on both arteries and veins.
Sodium nitroprusside solution is rapidly degraded by trace contaminants, often with resulting color changes. (See **DOSAGE AND ADMINISTRATION** section of full prescribing information.) The solution is also sensitive to certain wavelengths of light, and it must be protected from light in clinical use.
Each 2 mL of Sodium Nitroprusside Injection contains the equivalent of 50 mg Sodium Nitroprusside Dihydrate in Sterile Water for Injection.

HOW SUPPLIED

Sodium Nitroprusside Injection is supplied as follows in amber-colored, single-dose 50 mg/2mL containers:
    NDC 10019-082-02   25 mg/mL vials packaged individually

SUFENTANIL CITRATE Injection, USP   Ⓒ
[sū′fĕn-tănĭl]
WARNING: May be habit forming.

DESCRIPTION

Sufentanil Citrate Injection, USP is a sterile, nonpyrogenic, aqueous solution for intravenous and epidural injection. Each mL contains sufentanil citrate equivalent to 50 mcg (0.05 mg) of sufentanil in Water for Injection. pH 3.5–6.0; citric acid added, if needed, for pH adjustment. Contains no preservative. Sufentanil Citrate is a potent opioid analgesic chemically designated as N-[4-(methoxymethyl)-1-[2-(2-thienyl)ethyl]-4-piperidinyl]-N-phenylpropanamide 2-hydroxy-1,2,3-propanetricarboxylate (1:1) with the following structural formula:

$C_{22}H_{30}N_2O_2S \cdot C_6H_8O_7$ MW 578.68

HOW SUPPLIED

Sufentanil Citrate Injection, USP, equivalent to 50 mcg (0.05 mg) sufentanil per mL, is available in the following:
    1 mL (50 mcg) DOSETTE® ampuls packaged in 10s (NDC 10019-050-43)
    2 mL (100 mcg) DOSETTE® ampuls packaged in 10s (NDC 10019-050-21)
    5 mL (250 mcg) DOSETTE® ampuls packaged in 10s (NDC 10019-050-06)
DOSETTE® is a registered trademark of A.H. Robins Company.

SUPRANE®   ℞
[sū′prān]
(desflurane, USP)
Volatile Liquid for Inhalation

DESCRIPTION

SUPRANE® (desflurane, USP), a nonflammable liquid administered via vaporizer, is a general inhalation anesthetic. It is (±)1,2,2,2-tetrafluoroethyl difluoromethyl ether:

Some physical constants are:

Molecular weight	168.04
Specific gravity (at 20°C/4°C)	1.465
Vapor pressure in mm Hg	669 mm Hg @ 20°C
	731 mm Hg @ 22°C
	757 mm Hg @ 22.8°C
	(boiling point; 1atm)
	764 mm Hg @ 23°C
	798 mm Hg @ 24°C
	869 mm Hg @ 26°C

Partition coefficients at 37°C:

Blood/Gas	0.424
Olive Oil/Gas	18.7
Brain/Gas	0.54

Mean Component/Gas Partition Coefficients:

Polypropylene (Y piece)	6.7
Polyethylene (circuit tube)	16.2
Latex rubber (bag)	19.3
Latex rubber (bellows)	10.4
Polyvinylchloride (endotracheal tube)	34.7

Desflurane is nonflammable as defined by the requirements of International Electrotechnical Commission 601-2-13. Desflurane is a colorless, volatile liquid below 22.8°C. Data indicate that desflurane is stable when stored under normal room lighting conditions according to instructions.
Desflurane is chemically stable. The only known degradation reaction is through prolonged direct contact with soda lime producing low levels of fluoroform (CHF_3). The amount of CHF_3 obtained is similar to that produced with MAC-equivalent doses of isoflurane. No discernible degradation occurs in the presence of strong acids.
Desflurane does not corrode stainless steel, brass, aluminum, anodized aluminum, nickel plated brass, copper, or beryllium.

CLINICAL PHARMACOLOGY

SUPRANE® (desflurane, USP) is a volatile liquid inhalation anesthetic minimally biotransformed in the liver in humans. Less than 0.02% of the SUPRANE® absorbed can be recovered as urinary metabolites (compared to 0.2% for isoflurane).
Minimum alveolar concentration (MAC) of desflurane in oxygen for a 25 year-old adult is 7.3%. The MAC of SUPRANE® (desflurane, USP) decreases with increasing age and with addition of depressants such as opioids or benzodiazepines. (See DOSAGE AND ADMINISTRATION for details).

Pharmacokinetics

Due to the volatile nature of desflurane in plasma samples, the washin-washout profile of desflurane was used as a surrogate of plasma pharmacokinetics. Eight healthy male volunteers first breathed 70% N_2O/30% O_2 for 30 minutes and then a mixture of SUPRANE® (desflurane, USP) 2.0%, isoflurane 0.4%, and halothane 0.2% for another 30 minutes. During this time, inspired and end-tidal concentrations (F_I and F_A) were measured. The F_A/F_I (washin) value at 30 minutes for desflurane was 0.91, compared to 1.00 for N_2O, 0.74 for isoflurane, and 0.58 for halothane (See Figure 1). The washin rates for halothane and isoflurane were similar to literature values. The washin was faster for desflurane than for isoflurane and halothane at all time points. The F_A/F_{AO} (washout) value at 5 minutes was 0.12 for desflurane, 0.22 for isoflurane, and 0.25 for halothane (See Figure 2). The washout for SUPRANE® was more rapid than that for isoflurane and halothane at all elimination time points. By 5 days, the F_A/F_{AO} for desflurane is 1/20th of that for halothane or isoflurane.

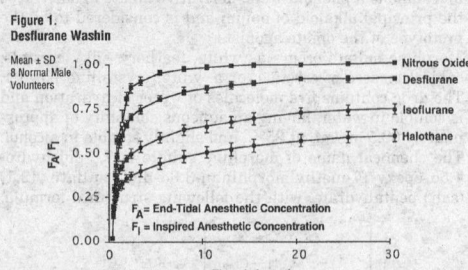

Figure 1.
Desflurane Washin

F_A = End-Tidal Anesthetic Concentration
F_I = Inspired Anesthetic Concentration

[See figure 2 at top of next column]

Pharmacodynamics

Changes in the clinical effects of SUPRANE® (desflurane, USP) rapidly follow changes in the inspired concentration. The duration of anesthesia and selected recovery measures for SUPRANE® are given in the following tables:
In 178 female outpatients undergoing laparoscopy, premedicated with fentanyl (1.5–2.0 µg/kg), anesthesia was initiated with propofol 2.5 mg/kg, desflurane/N_2O 60% in O_2 or desflurane/O_2 alone. Anesthesia was maintained with either propofol 1.5–9.0 mg/kg/hr, desflurane 2.6–8.4% in N_2O 60% in O_2, or desflurane 3.1–8.9% in O_2.

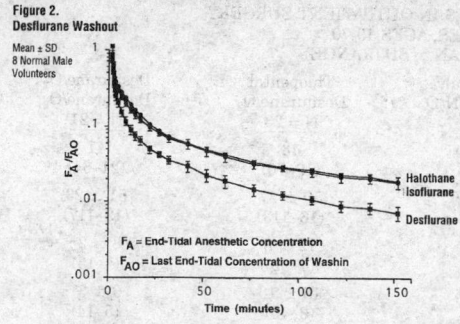

Figure 2.
Desflurane Washout

Mean ± SD
8 Normal Male
Volunteers

F_A = End-Tidal Anesthetic Concentration
F_{AO} = Last End-Tidal Concentration of Washin

	Propofol	Propofol	Desflurane/N$_2$O	Desflurane/O$_2$
Induction:	Propofol	Desflurane	Desflurane/N$_2$O	Desflurane/O$_2$
Maintenance:	Propofol/N$_2$O	Desflurane/N$_2$O		
Number of Pts:	N = 48	N = 44	N = 43	N = 43
Median age	30	26	29	30
	(20–43)	(21–47)	(21–42)	(20–40)
Anesthetic	49 ± 53	45 ± 35	44 ± 29	41 ± 26
Time	(8–336)	(11–178)	(14–149)	(19–126)
Time to open	7 ± 3	5 ± 2*	5 ± 2*	4 ± 2*
eyes	(2–19)	(2–10)	(2–12)	(1–11)
Time to state	9 ± 4	8 ± 3	7 ± 3*	7 ± 3*
name	(4–22)	(3–18)	(3–16)	(2–15)
Time to stand	80 ± 34	86 ± 55	81 ± 38	77 ± 38
	(40–200)	(30–320)	(35–190)	(35–200)
Time to walk	110 ± 6	122 ± 85	108 ± 59	108 ± 66
	(47–285)	(37–375)	(48–220)	(49–250)
Time to fit for	152 ± 75	157 ± 80	150 ± 66	155 ± 73
discharge	(66–375)	(73–385)	(68–310)	(69–325)

EMERGENCE AND RECOVERY AFTER OUTPATIENT LAPAROSCOPY
178 FEMALES, AGES 20-47
TIMES IN MINUTES: MEAN ± SD (RANGE)

*Differences were statistically significant (p < 0.05) by Dunnett's procedure comparing all treatments to the propofol-propofol/N$_2$O (induction and maintenance) group. Results for comparisons greater than one hour after anesthesia show no differences between groups and considerable variability within groups.

[See table above]
In 88 unpremedicated outpatients, anesthesia was initiated with thiopental 3–9 mg/kg or desflurane in O$_2$. Anesthesia was maintained with isoflurane 0.7–1.4% in N$_2$O 60%, desflurane 1.8–7.7% in N$_2$O 60%, or desflurane 4.4–11.9% in O$_2$.
[See first table at top of next page]
Recovery from anesthesia was assessed at 30, 60, and 90 minutes following 0.5 MAC desflurane (3%) or isoflurane (0.6%) in N$_2$O 60% using subjective and objective tests. At 30 minutes after anesthesia, only 43% of the isoflurane group were able to perform the psychometric tests compared to 76% in the desflurane group (p < 0.05).
[See second table on next page]
SUPRANE® (desflurane, USP) was studied in twelve volunteers receiving no other drugs. Hemodynamic effects during controlled ventilation (PaCO$_2$ 38mm Hg) were:
[See third table on next page]
When the same volunteers breathed spontaneously during desflurane anesthesia, systemic vascular resistance and mean arterial blood pressure decreased; cardiac index, heart rate, stroke volume, and central venous pressure (CVP) increased compared to values when the volunteers were conscious. Cardiac index, stroke volume, and CVP were greater during spontaneous ventilation than during controlled ventilation.
During spontaneous ventilation in the same volunteers, increasing the concentration of SUPRANE® (desflurane, USP) from 3% to 12% decreased tidal volume and increased arterial carbon dioxide tension and respiratory rate. The combination of N$_2$O 60% with a given concentration of desflurane gave results similar to those with desflurane alone. Respiratory depression produced by desflurane is similar to that produced by other potent inhalation agents.
The use of desflurane concentrations higher than 1.5 MAC may produce apnea.

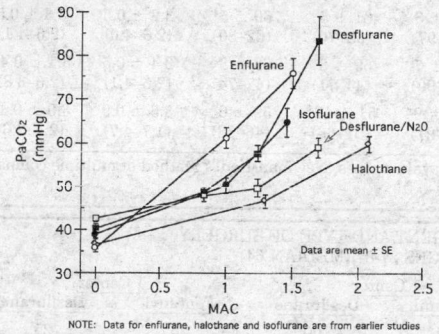

Figure 3. PaCO$_2$ During Spontaneous Ventilation in Unstimulated Volunteers

Data are mean ± SE

NOTE: Data for enflurane, halothane and isoflurane are from earlier studies.

CLINICAL TRIALS

SUPRANE® (desflurane, USP) was evaluated in 1,843 patients including ambulatory (N=1,061), cardiovascular (N=277), geriatric (N=103), neurosurgical (N=40), and pediatric (N=235) patients. Clinical experience with these patients and with 1,087 control patients in these studies not receiving desflurane are described below. Although desflurane can be used in adults for the inhalation induction of anesthesia via mask, it produces a high incidence of respiratory irritation (coughing, breathholding, apnea, increased secretions, laryngospasm). For incidence, see ADVERSE REACTIONS. Oxyhemoglobin saturation below 90% occurred in 6% of patients (from pooled data, N = 370 adults).

Ambulatory Surgery
SUPRANE® (desflurane, USP) plus N$_2$O was compared to isoflurane plus N$_2$O in multicenter studies (21 sites) of 792 ASA physical status I, II, or III patients aged 18–76 years (median 32).
Induction: Anesthetic induction begun with thiopental and continued with desflurane was associated with a 7% incidence of oxyhemoglobin saturation of 90% or less (from

pooled data, N = 307) compared with 5% in patients in whom anesthesia was induced with thiopental and isoflurane (from pooled data, N = 152).
Maintenance & Recovery: SUPRANE® (desflurane, USP) with or without N$_2$O or other anesthetics was generally well tolerated. There were no differences between desflurane and the other anesthetics studied in the times that patients were judged fit for discharge.
In one outpatient study, patients received a standardized anesthetic consisting of thiopental 4.2–4.4 mg/kg, fentanyl 3.5–4.0 µg/kg, vecuronium 0.05–0.07 mg/kg, and N$_2$O 60% in oxygen with either desflurane 3% or isoflurane 0.6%. Emergence times were significantly different; but times to sit up and discharge were not different (see Table).

RECOVERY PROFILES AFTER DESFLURANE 3% IN
N$_2$O 60% vs ISOFLURANE 0.6% IN N$_2$O 60% IN
OUTPATIENTS 16 MALES, 22 FEMALES, AGES 20-65
MEAN ± SD

	Isoflurane	Desflurane
Number	21	17
Anesthetic time (min)	127 ± 80	98 ± 55
Recovery time to:		
Follow commands (min)	11.1 ± 7.9	6.5 ± 2.3*
Sit up (min)	113 ± 27	95 ± 56
Fit for discharge (min)	231 ± 40	207 ± 54

* Difference was statistically significant from the isoflurane group (p < 0.05), unadjusted for multiple comparisons.

Cardiovascular Surgery
Desflurane was compared to isoflurane, sufentanil or fentanyl for the anesthetic management of coronary artery bypass graft (CABG), abdominal aortic aneurysm, peripheral vascular and carotid endarterectomy surgery in 7 studies at 15 centers involving a total of 558 patients. In all patients except the desflurane vs sufentanil study, the volatile anesthetics were supplemented with intravenous opioids, usually fentanyl. Blood pressure and heart rate were controlled by changes in concentration of the volatile anesthetics or opioids and cardiovascular drugs if necessary. Oxygen (100%) was the carrier gas in 253 of 277 desflurane cases (24 of 277 received N$_2$O/O$_2$).
[See fourth table on next page]
No differences were found in cardiovascular outcome (death, myocardial infarction, ventricular tachycardia or fibrillation, heart failure) among desflurane and the other anesthetics.
Induction: Desflurane should not be used as the sole agent for anesthetic induction in patients with coronary artery disease or any patients where increases in heart rate or blood pressure are undesirable. In the desflurane vs sufentanil study, anesthetic induction with desflurane without opioids was associated with new transient ischemia in 14 patients vs 0 in the sufentanil group. In the desflurane group, mean heart rate, arterial pressure, and pulmonary blood pressure increased and stroke volume decreased in contrast to no change in the sufentanil group. Cardiovascular drugs were used frequently in both groups: especially esmolol in the desflurane group (56% vs 0%) and phenylephrine in the sufentanil group (43% vs 27%). When 10 µg/kg of fentanyl was used to supplement induction of anesthesia at one other center, continuous 2-lead ECG analysis showed a low incidence of myocardial ischemia and no difference between desflurane and isoflurane. If desflurane is to be used

in patients with coronary artery disease, it should be used in combination with other medications for induction of anesthesia, preferably intravenous opioids and hypnotics.
Maintenance and Recovery: In studies where desflurane or isoflurane anesthesia was supplemented with fentanyl, there were no differences in hemodynamic variables or the incidence of myocardial ischemia in the patients anesthetized with desflurane compared to those anesthetized with isoflurane.
During the precardiopulmonary bypass period, in the desflurane vs sufentanil study where the desflurane patients received no intravenous opioids, more desflurane patients required cardiovascular adjuvants to control hemodynamics than the sufentanil patients. During this period, the incidence of ischemia detected by ECG or echocardiography was not statistically different between desflurane (18 of 99) and sufentanil (9 of 98) groups. However, the duration and severity of ECG-detected myocardial ischemia was significantly less in the desflurane group. The incidence of myocardial ischemia after cardiopulmonary bypass and in the ICU did not differ between groups.

Geriatric Surgery
SUPRANE® (desflurane, USP) plus N$_2$O was compared to isoflurane plus N$_2$O in a multicenter study (6 sites) of 203 ASA physical status II or III elderly patients, aged 57–91 years (median 71).
Induction: Most patients were premedicated with fentanyl (mean 2 µg/kg), preoxygenated, and received thiopental (mean 4.3 mg/kg IV) or thiamylal (mean 4 mg/kg IV) followed by succinylcholine (mean 1.4 mg/kg IV) for intubation.
Maintenance and Recovery: Heart rate and arterial blood pressure remained within 20% of preinduction baseline values during administration of SUPRANE® (desflurane, USP) 0.5–7.7% (average 3.6%) with 50–60% N$_2$O. Induction, maintenance, and recovery cardiovascular measurements did not differ from those during isoflurane/N$_2$O administration nor did the postoperative incidence of nausea and vomiting differ. The most common cardiovascular adverse event was hypotension occurring in 8% of the SUPRANE® patients and 6% of the isoflurane patients.

Neurosurgery
SUPRANE® (desflurane, USP) was studied in 38 patients aged 26–76 years (median 48 years), ASA physical status II or III undergoing neurosurgical procedures for intracranial lesions.
Induction: Induction consisted of standard neuroanesthetic techniques including hyperventilation and thiopental.
Maintenance: No change in cerebrospinal fluid pressure (CSFP) was observed in 8 patients who had intracranial tumors when the dose of desflurane was 0.5 MAC in N$_2$O 50%. In another study of 9 patients with intracranial tumors, 0.8 MAC desflurane/air/O$_2$ did not increase CSFP above postinduction baseline values. In a different study of 10 patients receiving 1.1 MAC desflurane/air/O$_2$, CSFP increased 7mm Hg (range 3–13 mm Hg increase, with final values of 11–26 mm Hg) above the predrug values.
All volatile anesthetics may increase intracranial pressure in patients with intracranial space occupying lesions. In such patients, desflurane should be administered at 0.8 MAC or less, and in conjunction with a barbiturate induction and hyperventilation (hypocapnia) in the period before cranial decompression. Appropriate attention must be paid to maintain cerebral perfusion pressure. The use of a lower

Continued on next page

Suprane—Cont.

dose of desflurane and the administration of a barbiturate and mannitol would be predicted to lessen the effect of desflurane on CSFP.

Under hypocapnic conditions ($PaCO_2$ 27 mm Hg) desflurane 1 and 1.5 MAC did not increase cerebral blood flow (CBF) in 9 patients undergoing craniotomies. CBF reactivity to increasing $PaCO_2$ from 27 to 35 mm Hg was also maintained at 1.25 MAC desflurane/air/O_2.

Pediatric Surgery
SUPRANE® (desflurane, USP) or halothane with or without N_2O was used to anesthetize 235 patients aged 2 weeks-12 years (median 2 years), ASA physical status I or II.

Induction: SUPRANE® (desflurane, USP) is not recommended for induction of general anesthesia in infants or children because of a high incidence of moderate to severe laryngospasm, coughing, breathholding, and secretions. The occurrence of oxyhemoglobin desaturation was 26%. For incidence, see ADVERSE REACTIONS.

Maintenance and Recovery: The concentration of SUPRANE® (desflurane, USP) required for maintenance of general anesthesia is age-dependent (see INDIVIDUALIZATION of DOSE). Changes in blood pressure during maintenance of and recovery from anesthesia with desflurane/N_2O/O_2 are similar to those observed with halothane/N_2O/O_2. Heart rate during maintenance of anesthesia is approximately 10 beats per minute faster with desflurane than with halothane. Patients were judged fit for discharge from post-anesthesia care units within one hour with both desflurane and halothane. There were no differences in the incidence of nausea and vomiting between patients receiving desflurane or halothane.

INDIVIDUALIZATION of DOSE

(Also see DOSAGE and ADMINISTRATION)
Preanesthetic Medication: Issues such as whether or not to premedicate and the choice of premedicant(s) must be individualized. In clinical studies, patients scheduled to be anesthetized with desflurane frequently received IV preanesthetic medication, such as opioid and/or benzodiazepine.

Induction: In adults, some premedicated with opioid, a frequent starting concentration was 3% desflurane, increased in 0.5–1.0% increments every 2 to 3 breaths. End-tidal concentrations of 4–11% SUPRANE® (desflurane, USP) with and without N_2O, produced desflurane within 2 to 4 minutes. When desflurane was tested as the primary anesthetic induction agent, the incidence of upper airway irritation (apnea, breathholding, laryngospasm, coughing and secretions) was high (see ADVERSE REACTIONS). During induction in adults, the overall incidence of oxyhemoglobin desaturation (SpO_2 < 90%) was 6%.

After induction in adults with an intravenous drug such as thiopental or propofol, desflurane can be started at approximately 0.5–1 MAC, whether the carrier gas is O_2 or N_2O/O_2.

Maintenance: Surgical levels of anesthesia in adults may be maintained with concentrations of 2.5–8.5% SUPRANE® (desflurane, USP) with or without the concomitant use of nitrous oxide. In children, surgical levels of anesthesia may be maintained with concentrations of 5.2–10% SUPRANE® with or without the concomitant use of nitrous oxide.

During the maintenance of anesthesia, increasing concentrations of SUPRANE® (desflurane, USP) produce dose-dependent decreases in blood pressure. Excessive decreases in blood pressure may be due to depth of anesthesia and in such instances may be corrected by decreasing the inspired concentration of SUPRANE®.

Concentrations of desflurane exceeding 1 MAC may increase heart rate. Thus with this drug, an increased heart rate may not serve reliably as a sign of inadequate anesthesia. SUPRANE® (desflurane, USP) decreases the doses of neuromuscular blocking agents required (see PRECAUTIONS, Drug Interactions).

INDICATIONS AND USAGE

SUPRANE® (desflurane, USP) is indicated as an inhalation agent for induction and/or maintenance of anesthesia for inpatient and outpatient surgery in adults (see PRECAUTIONS).

SUPRANE® (desflurane, USP) is not recommended for induction of anesthesia in pediatric patients because of a high incidence of moderate to severe upper airway adverse events (see WARNINGS). After induction of anesthesia with agents other than SUPRANE®, and tracheal intubation, SUPRANE® is indicated for maintenance of anesthesia in infants and children.

CONTRAINDICATIONS

SUPRANE® (desflurane, USP) should not be used in patients with a known or suspected genetic susceptibility to malignant hyperthermia.

Known sensitivity to SUPRANE® (desflurane, USP) or to other halogenated agents.

EMERGENCE AND RECOVERY TIMES IN OUTPATIENT SURGERY
46 MALES, 42 FEMALES, AGES 19-70
TIMES IN MINUTES: MEAN ± SD (RANGE)

Induction: Maintenance: Number of Pts:	Thiopental Isoflurane/N_2O N = 23	Thiopental Desflurane/N_2O N = 21	Thiopental Desflurane/O_2 N = 23	Desflurane/O_2 Desflurane/O_2 N = 21
Median age	43 (20–70)	40 (22–67)	43 (19–70)	41 (21–64)
Anesthetic Time	49 ± 23 (11–94)	50 ± 19 (16–80)	50 ± 27 (16–113)	51 ± 23 (19–117)
Time to open eyes	13 ± 7 (5–33)	9 ± 3* (4–16)	12 ± 8 (4–39)	8 ± 2* (4–13)
Time to state name	17 ± 10 (6–44)	11 ± 4* (6–19)	15 ± 10 (6–46)	9 ± 3* (5–14)
Time to walk	195 ± 67 (124–365)	176 ± 60 (101–315)	168 ± 34 (119–258)	181 ± 42 (92–252)
Time to fit for discharge	205 ± 53 (153–365)	202 ± 41 (144–315)	197 ± 35 (155–280)	194 ± 37 (134–288)

*Differences were statistically significant (p < 0.05) by Dunnett's procedure comparing all treatments to the thiopental-isoflurane/N_2O (induction and maintenance) group. Results for comparisons greater than one hour after anesthesia show no differences between groups and considerable variability within groups.

RECOVERY TESTS: PERCENT OF PREOPERATIVE BASELINE VALUES
16 MALES, 22 FEMALES, AGES 20-65
PERCENT: MEAN ± SD

Maintenance:	60 minutes After Anesthesia Desflurane/N_2O	Isoflurane/N_2O	90 minutes After Anesthesia Desflurane/N_2O	Isoflurane/N_2O
Confusion Δ	66±6	47±8	75±7*	56±8
Fatigue Δ	70±9*	33±6	89±12*	47±8
Drowsiness Δ	66±5*	36±8	76±7*	49±9
Clumsiness Δ	65±5	49±8	80±7*	57±9
Comfort Δ	59±7*	30±6	60±8*	31±7
DSST† score	74±4*	50±9	75±4*	55±7
Trieger Tests††	67±5	74±6	90±6	83±7

Δ Visual analog scale (values from 0-100; 100=baseline)
† DSST = Digit Symbol Substitution Test
†† Trieger Test = Dot Connecting Test
* Differences were statistically significant (p < 0.05) using a two-sample t-test

HEMODYNAMIC EFFECTS OF DESFLURANE DURING CONTROLLED VENTILATION
12 MALE VOLUNTEERS, AGES 16-26
MEAN ± SD (RANGE)

Total MAC Equivalent	End-Tidal % Des/O_2	End-Tidal %Des/N_2O	Heart Rate (beats/min) O_2	N_2O	Mean Arterial Pressure (mmHg) O_2	N_2O	Cardiac Index (L/min/m²) O_2	N_2O
0	0%/21%	0%/0%	69 ± 4 (63–76)	70 ± 6 (62–85)	85 ± 9 (74–102)	85 ± 9 (74–102)	3.7 ± 0.4 (3.0–4.2)	3.7 ± 0.4 (3.0–4.2)
0.8	6%/94%	3%/60%	73 ± 5 (67–80)	77 ± 8 (67–97)	61 ± 5* (55–70)	69 ± 5* (62–80)	3.2 ± 0.5 (2.6–4.0)	3.3 ± 0.5 (2.6–4.1)
1.2	9%/91%	6%/60%	80 ± 5* (72–84)	77 ± 7 (67–90)	59 ± 8* (44–71)	63 ± 8* (47–74)	3.4 ± 0.5 (2.6–4.1)	3.1 ± 0.4* (2.6–3.8)
1.7	12%/88%	9%/60%	94 ± 14* (78–109)	79 ± 9 (61–91)	51 ± 12* (31–66)	59 ± 6* (46–68)	3.5 ± 0.9 (1.7–4.7)	3.0 ± 0.4* (2.4–3.6)

*Differences were statistically significant (p<0.05) compared to awake values, Newman-Keul's method of multiple comparison.

CARDIOVASCULAR PATIENTS BY AGENT AND TYPE OF SURGERY
418 MALES, 140 FEMALES, AGES 27-87 (MEDIAN 64)

Type of Surgery	13 Centers Isoflurane	Desflurane	1 Center Sufentanil	Desflurane	1 Center Fentanyl	Desflurane
CABG	58	57	100	100	25	25
Abd Aorta	29	25	-	-	-	-
Periph Vasc	24	24	-	-	-	-
Carotid Art	45	46	-	-	-	-
Total	156	152	100	100	25	25

WARNINGS

Pediatric Use: SUPRANE® (desflurane, USP) is not recommended for induction of general anesthesia via mask in infants or children because of the high incidence of moderate to severe laryngospasm in 50% of patients, coughing 72%, breathholding 68%, increase in secretions 21% and oxyhemoglobin desaturation 26%.

SUPRANE® (desflurane, USP) should be administered only by persons trained in the administration of general anesthesia, using a vaporizer specifically designed and designated for use with desflurane. Facilities for maintenance of a patent airway, artificial ventilation, oxygen enrichment, and circulatory resuscitation must be immediately available. Hypotension and respiratory depression increase as anesthesia is deepened.

SUPRANE® (desflurane, USP) may present an increased risk in patients with a known sensitivity to halogenated anesthetic agents.

PRECAUTIONS

During the maintenance of anesthesia, increasing concentrations of SUPRANE® (desflurane, USP) produce dose-dependent decreases in blood pressure. Excessive decreases in blood pressure may be related to depth of anesthesia and in such instances may be corrected by decreasing the inspired concentration of SUPRANE®.

Concentrations of desflurane exceeding 1 MAC may increase heart rate. Thus an increased heart rate may not be a sign of inadequate anesthesia.

In patients with intracranial space occupying lesions, SUPRANE® (desflurane, USP) should be administered at 0.8

MAC or less, in conjunction with a barbiturate induction and hyperventilation (hypocapnia). Appropriate measures should be taken to maintain cerebral perfusion pressure (see CLINICAL STUDIES, Neurosurgery).

In patients with coronary artery disease, maintenance of normal hemodynamics is important to the avoidance of myocardial ischemia. Desflurane should not be used as the sole agent for anesthetic induction in patients with coronary artery disease or patients where increases in heart rate or blood pressure are undesirable. It should be used with other medications, preferably intravenous opioids and hypnotics (see CLINICAL STUDIES, Cardiovascular Surgery).

Inspired concentrations of SUPRANE® (desflurane, USP) greater than 12% have been safely administered to patients, particularly during induction of anesthesia. Such concentrations will proportionately dilute the concentration of oxygen; therefore, maintenance of an adequate concentration of oxygen may require a reduction of nitrous oxide or air if these gases are used concurrently.

The recovery from general anesthesia should be assessed carefully before patients are discharged from the post anesthesia care unit (PACU).

SUPRANE® (desflurane, USP), like some other inhalational anesthetics, can react with desiccated carbon dioxide (CO_2) absorbents to produce carbon monoxide which may result in elevated levels of carboxyhemoglobin in some patients. Case reports suggest that barium hydroxide lime and soda lime become desiccated when fresh gases are passed through the CO_2 absorber cannister at high flow rates over many hours or days. When a clinician suspects that CO_2 absorbent may be desiccated, it should be replaced before the administration of SUPRANE® (desflurane, USP).

As with other halogenated anesthetic agents, SUPRANE® (desflurane, USP) may cause sensitivity hepatitis in patients who have been sensitized by previous exposure to halogenated anesthetics (see CONTRAINDICATIONS).

Drug Interactions
No clinically significant adverse interactions with commonly used preanesthetic drugs, or drugs used during anesthesia (muscle relaxants, intravenous agents, and local anesthetic agents) were reported in clinical trials. The effect of desflurane on the disposition of other drugs has not been determined.

Like isoflurane, desflurane does not predispose to premature ventricular arrhythmias in the presence of exogenously infused epinephrine in swine.

BENZODIAZEPINES and OPIOIDS (MAC Reduction):
Benzodiazepines (midazolam 25–50 µg/kg) decrease the MAC of desflurane by 16% as do the opioids (fentanyl 3–6 µg/kg) by 50% (see DOSAGE AND ADMINISTRATION).

NEUROMUSCULAR BLOCKING AGENTS:
Anesthetic concentrations of desflurane at equilibrium (administered for 15 or more minutes before testing) reduced the ED_{95} of succinylcholine by approximately 30% and that of atracurium and pancuronium by approximately 50% compared to N_2O/opioid anesthesia. The effect of desflurane on duration of nondepolarizing neuromuscular blockade has not been studied.

DOSAGE OF MUSCLE RELAXANT CAUSING 95% DEPRESSION IN NEUROMUSCULAR BLOCKADE

Desflurane Concentration	Mean ED_{95} (µg/kg)		
	Pancuronium	Atracurium	Succinylcholine
0.65 MAC 60% N_2O/O_2	26	123	-
1.25 MAC 60% N_2O/O_2	18	91	-
1.25 MAC O_2	22	120	362

Dosage reduction of neuromuscular blocking agents during induction of anesthesia may result in delayed onset of conditions suitable for endotracheal intubation or inadequate muscle relaxation, because potentiation of neuromuscular blocking agents requires equilibration of muscle with the delivered partial pressure of desflurane.

Among nondepolarizing drugs, only pancuronium and atracurium interactions have been studied. In the absence of specific guidelines:
1. For endotracheal intubation, do not reduce the dose of nondepolarizing muscle relaxants or succinylcholine.
2. During maintenance of anesthesia, the dose of nondepolarizing muscle relaxants is likely to be reduced compared to that during N_2O/opioid anesthesia. Administration of supplemental doses of muscle relaxants should be guided by the response to nerve stimulation.

Malignant Hyperthermia: In susceptible individuals, potent inhalation anesthetic agents may trigger a skeletal muscle hypermetabolic state leading to high oxygen demand and the clinical syndrome known as malignant hyperthermia. In genetically susceptible pigs, desflurane induced malignant hyperthermia. The clinical syndrome is signalled by hypercapnia, and may include muscle rigidity, tachycardia, tachypnea, cyanosis, arrhythmias, and/or unstable blood pressure. Some of these nonspecific signs may also appear during light anesthesia: acute hypoxia, hypercapnia, and hypovolemia.

Treatment of malignant hyperthermia includes discontinuation of triggering agents, administration of intravenous dantrolene sodium, and application of supportive therapy. (Consult prescribing information for dantrolene sodium intravenous for additional information on patient management.) Renal failure may appear later, and urine flow should be monitored and sustained if possible.

Renal or Hepatic Insufficiency
Nine patients receiving SUPRANE® (desflurane, USP) (N=9) were compared to 9 patients receiving isoflurane, all with chronic renal insufficiency (serum creatinine 1.5–6.9 mg/dL). No differences in hematological or biochemical tests, including renal function evaluation, were seen between the two groups. Similarly, no differences were found in a comparison of patients receiving either SUPRANE® (desflurane, USP) (N=28) or isoflurane (N=30) undergoing renal transplant.

Eight patients receiving SUPRANE® (desflurane, USP) were compared to six patients receiving isoflurane, all with chronic hepatic disease (viral hepatitis, alcoholic hepatitis, or cirrhosis). No differences in hematological or biochemical tests, including hepatic enzymes and hepatic function evaluation, were seen.

Carcinogenesis, Mutagenesis, Impairment of Fertility
Animal carcinogenicity studies have not been performed with SUPRANE® (desflurane, USP). In vitro and in vivo genotoxicity studies did not demonstrate mutagenicity or chromosomal damage by SUPRANE®. Tests for genotoxicity included the Ames mutation assay, the metaphase analysis of human lymphocytes, and the mouse micronucleus assay. Fertility was not affected after 1 MAC-Hour per day exposure (cumulative 63 and 14 MAC-Hours for males and females, respectively). At higher doses, parental toxicity (mortalities and reduced weight gain) was observed which could affect fertility.

Teratogenic Effects: No teratogenic effect was observed at approximately 10 and 13 cumulative MAC-Hour exposures at 1 MAC-Hour per day during organogenesis in rats or rabbits. At higher doses increased incidences of post-implantation loss and maternal toxicity were observed. However, at 10 MAC-Hours cumulative exposure in rats, about 6% decrease in the weight of male pups was observed at preterm caesarean delivery.

Pregnancy Category B: There are no adequate and well-controlled studies in pregnant women. SUPRANE® (desflurane, USP) should be used during pregnancy only if the potential benefit justifies the potential risk to the fetus.

Rats exposed to desflurane at 1 MAC-hour per day from gestation day 15 to lactation day 21, did not show signs of dystocia. Body weight of pups delivered by these dams at birth and during lactation were comparable to that of control pups. No treatment related behavioral changes were reported in these pups during lactation.

Labor and Delivery: The safety of desflurane during labor or delivery has not been demonstrated.

Nursing Mothers: The concentrations of desflurane in milk are probably of no clinical importance 24 hours after anesthesia. Because of rapid washout, desflurane concentrations in milk are predicted to be below those found with other volatile potent anesthetics.

Geriatric Use: The average MAC for SUPRANE® (desflurane, USP) in a 70 year old patient is two-thirds the MAC for a 20 year old patient (see DOSAGE AND ADMINISTRATION).

Pediatric Use: SUPRANE® (desflurane, USP) is not recommended for induction of general anesthesia via mask in infants or children because of the high incidence of moderate to severe laryngospasm, coughing, breathholding and increase in secretions and oxyhemoglobin desaturation (see WARNINGS).

Neurosurgical Use: SUPRANE® (desflurane, USP) may produce a dose-dependent increase in cerebrospinal fluid pressure (CSFP) when administered to patients with intracranial space occupying lesions. Desflurane should be administered at 0.8 MAC or less, and in conjunction with a barbiturate induction and hyperventilation (hypocapnia) until cerebral decompression in patients with known or suspected increases in CSFP. Appropriate attention must be paid to maintain cerebral perfusion pressure (see CLINICAL STUDIES, Neurosurgery).

ADVERSE REACTIONS

Adverse event information is derived from controlled clinical trials, the majority of which were conducted in the United States. The studies were conducted using a variety of premedications, other anesthetics, and surgical procedures of varying length. Most adverse events reported were mild and transient, and may reflect the surgical procedures, patient characteristics (including disease) and/or medications administered.

Of the 1,843 patients exposed to SUPRANE® (desflurane, USP) in clinical trials, 370 adults and 152 children were induced with desflurane alone and 687 patients were maintained principally with desflurane. The frequencies given reflect the percent of patients with the event. Each patient was counted once for each type of adverse event. They are presented in alphabetical order according to body system.

PROBABLY CAUSALLY RELATED: Incidence greater than 1%.

Induction (use as a mask inhalation agent):

Adult patients (N=370):	Coughing 34%, breathholding 30%, apnea 15%, increased secretions*, laryngospasm*, oxyhemoglobin desaturation (SpO_2<90%)*, pharyngitis*.
Pediatric patients (N=152):	Coughing 72%, breathholding 68%, laryngospasm 50%, oxyhemoglobin desaturation (SpO_2<90%) 26%, increased secretions 21%, bronchospasm*. (See WARNINGS)

Maintenance or Recovery
Adult and pediatric patients (N=687):

Body as a Whole:	Headache.
Cardiovascular:	Bradycardia, hypertension, nodal arrhythmia, tachycardia.
Digestive:	Nausea 27%, vomiting 16%.
Nervous system:	Increased Salivation.
Respiratory:	Apnea*, breathholding, cough increased*, laryngospasm*, pharyngitis.
Special Senses:	Conjunctivitis (conjunctival hyperemia)

* Incidence of events: 3%–10%

PROBABLY CAUSALLY RELATED: Incidence less than 1% and reported in 3 or more patients, regardless of severity (N=1,843)

Cardiovascular:	Arrhythmia, bigeminy, abnormal electrocardiogram myocardial ischemia, vasodilation.
Nervous System:	Agitation, dizziness.
Respiratory:	Asthma, dyspnea, hypoxia.

CAUSAL RELATIONSHIP UNKNOWN: Incidence less than 1% and reported in 3 or more patients, regardless of severity (N=1,843)

Body as a Whole:	Fever.
Cardiovascular:	Hemorrhage, myocardial infarct.
Metabolic and Nutrition:	Increased creatinine phosphokinase.
Musculoskeletal System:	Myalgia.
Skin and Appendages:	Pruritis.

See PRECAUTIONS for information regarding pediatric use and malignant hyperthermia.

Laboratory Findings: Transient elevations in glucose and white blood cell count may occur as with use of other anesthetic agents.

DRUG ABUSE AND DEPENDENCE

The potential drug abuse liability, and dependence associated with SUPRANE® (desflurane, USP) have not been studied.

OVERDOSAGE

In the event of overdosage, or suspected overdosage, take the following actions: discontinue administration of SUPRANE® (desflurane, USP), maintain a patent airway, initiate assisted or controlled ventilation with oxygen, and maintain adequate cardiovascular function.

DOSAGE AND ADMINISTRATION

Deliver SUPRANE® (desflurane, USP) from a vaporizer specifically designed and designated for use with desflurane.

The administration of general anesthesia must be individualized based on the patient's response (see INDIVIDUALIZATION of DOSE). The following two tables provide mean relative potency based upon age and drug interaction studies in predominately ASA physical status I or II patients.

EFFECT OF AGE ON MAC OF DESFLURANE
MEAN ± SD (percent atmospheres)

Age	N	O_2 100%	N	N_2O 60%
2 weeks	6	9.2 ± 0.0	-	-
10 weeks	5	9.4 ± 0.4	-	-
9 months	4	10.0 ± 0.7	5	7.5 ± 0.8
2 years	3	9.1 ± 0.6	-	-
3 years	-	-	5	6.4 ± 0.4
4 years	4	8.6 ± 0.6	-	-
7 years	5	8.1 ± 0.6	-	-
25 years	4	7.3 ± 0.0	4	4.0 ± 0.3

Continued on next page

Suprane—Cont.

45 years	4	6.0 ± 0.3	6	2.8 ± 0.6	
70 years	6	5.2 ± 0.6	6	1.7 ± 0.4	

N = number of crossover pairs (using up-and-down method of quantal response)

Opioids or benzodiazepines decrease the amounts of SUPRANE® (desflurane, USP) required to produce anesthesia. The following table is based on studies of drug interaction (MAC reduction).

SUPRANE® (desflurane, USP) MAC WITH FENTANYL OR MIDAZOLAM
MEAN ± SD (percent reduction)

Dose	18-30 years	31-65 years
No fentanyl	6.4 ± 0.0	6.3 ± 0.4
3 µg/kg fentanyl	3.5 ± 1.9 (46%)	3.1 ± 0.6 (51%)
6 µg/kg fentanyl	3.0 ± 1.2 (53%)	2.3 ± 1.0 (64%)
No midazolam	6.9 ± 0.1	5.9 ± 0.6
25 µg/kg midazolam	-	4.9 ± 0.9 (16%)
50 µg/kg midazolam	-	4.9 ± 0.5 (17%)

SUPRANE® (desflurane, USP) decreases the doses of neuromuscular blocking agents required (see PRECAUTIONS, Drug Interactions).
During the maintenance of anesthesia with inflow rates of 2 L/min or more, the alveolar concentration of desflurane will usually be within 10% of the inspired concentration. (F_A/F_I, see Figure 1 in Pharmacokinetics section.)

HOW SUPPLIED
SUPRANE® (desflurane, USP), NDC 10019-641-24, is packaged in amber-colored bottles containing 240 mL desflurane.

SAFETY AND HANDLING
Occupational Caution: There is no specific work exposure limit established for SUPRANE® (desflurane, USP). However, the National Institute for Occupational Safety and Health Administration has recommended an 8-hr, time-weighted average limit of 2 ppm for halogenated anesthetic agents in general (0.5 ppm when coupled with exposure to N_2O).
The predicted effects of acute overexposure by inhalation of SUPRANE® (desflurane, USP) include headache, dizziness or (in extreme cases) unconsciousness.
There are no documented adverse effects of chronic exposure to halogenated anesthetic vapors (Waste Anesthetic Gases or WAGs) in the workplace. Although results of some epidemiological studies suggest a link between exposure to halogenated anesthetics and increased health problems (particularly spontaneous abortion), the relationship is not conclusive. Since exposure to WAGs is one possible factor in the findings for these studies, operating room personnel, and pregnant women in particular, should minimize exposure. Precautions include adequate general ventilation in the operating room, the use of a well-designated and well-maintained scavenging system, work practices to minimize leaks and spills while the anesthetic agent is in use, and routine equipment maintenance to minimize leaks.

STORAGE
Store at room temperature, 15°–30°C (59°–86°F). SUPRANE® (desflurane, USP) has been demonstrated to be stable for the period defined by the expiration dating on the label.

CAUTION
Federal Law Prohibits Dispensing without a Prescription.
OHMEDA
THE BOC GROUP
Manufactured By: Ohmeda Caribe Inc, Guayama, PR 00784
For: Ohmeda Pharmaceutical Products Division Inc, Liberty Corner NJ 07938
For Product Inquiry 1 800 ANA DRUG
400-447-04   Rev. 3-98

THIOPENTAL SODIUM ⓒ ℞
[thī-ō-pent-ăl sō-dē-ŭm]
For Injection, USP
WARNING: MAY BE HABIT FORMING

DESCRIPTION
Thiopental Sodium for Injection, USP is a thiobarbiturate, the sulfur analogue of sodium pentobarbital.
The drug is prepared as a sterile lyophilized powder and, after reconstitution with an appropriate diluent, is administered by the intravenous route.

Cat/Kit Number	Thiopental Sodium for Injection, USP	Diluent Volume	Reconstituted Concentration (%)	NDC Number
Syringe Kits[1]				
2580-0101	500 mg	20 mL	2.5	10019-258-96
Injection Kits[2]				
2530-0101	1 g	40 mL	2.5	10019-253-99
2540-0101	2.5 g	100 mL	2.5	10019-252-97
2550-0101	5 g	200 mL	2.5	10019-255-98

[1] Syringe Kits contain 1 vial of Thiopental Sodium for Injection, USP; 1 vial of 0.9% Sodium Chloride Injection, USP; 1 sterile syringe and needle.
[2] Injection Kits contain 1 vial of Thiopental Sodium for Injection, USP; 1 vial of Sterile Water for Injection, USP; sterile transfer spikes.

Thiopental Sodium, USP is chemically designated sodium 5-ethyl-5-(1-methylbutyl)-2-thiobarbiturate and has the following structural formula:

The drug is a yellowish, hygroscopic powder, stabilized with anhydrous sodium carbonate as a buffer (60 mg/g of Thiopental Sodium).

HOW SUPPLIED
Thiopental Sodium for Injection, USP, (Lyophilized) is available as follows:
[See table above]
Syringe Kits and Injection Kits are individually packaged.

EDUCATIONAL MATERIAL

Educational Resources
Baxter Pharmaceutical Products Inc offers a wide range of educational materials free of charge to physicians, nurse-anesthetists, post-anesthesia nurses and hospital pharmacists. They are available from Baxter PPI sales representatives or by writing to: Baxter Pharmaceutical Products Inc, 110 Allen Road, P.O. Box 804, Liberty Corner, NJ 07938-0804, or by calling (800) 262-3784.

Bayer Corporation
Pharmaceutical Division
400 MORGAN LANE
WEST HAVEN, CT 06516

For Medical Information Contact:
Director, Medical Services
(800) 468-0894
(203) 812-2000

ADALAT®   ℞
Capsules
(nifedipine)
For Oral Use

DESCRIPTION
ADALAT® (nifedipine) is an antianginal drug belonging to a class of pharmacological agents, the calcium channel blockers. Nifedipine is 3,5-pyridinedicarboxylic acid, 1,4-dihydro-2,6-dimethyl-4-(2-nitrophenyl)-, dimethyl ester, $C_{17}H_{18}N_2O_6$, and has the structural formula:

Nifedipine is a yellow crystalline substance, practically insoluble in water but soluble in ethanol. It has a molecular weight of 346.3. ADALAT® CAPSULES are formulated as soft gelatin capsules for oral administration each containing 10 mg or 20 mg of nifedipine.
Inert ingredients in the formulations are: glycerin; peppermint oil; polyethylene glycol 400; soft gelatin capsules (which contain FD&C Yellow No. 6, Red Ferric Oxide and other inert ingredients), and water. The 10 mg capsules also contain saccharin sodium.

CLINICAL PHARMACOLOGY
ADALAT® is a calcium ion influx inhibitor (slow channel blocker or calcium ion antagonist) and inhibits the transmembrane influx of calcium ions into cardiac muscle and smooth muscle. The contractile processes of cardiac muscle and vascular smooth muscle are dependent upon the movement of extracellular calcium ions into these cells through specific ion channels. ADALAT® selectively inhibits calcium ion influx across the cell membrane of cardiac muscle and vascular smooth muscle without changing serum calcium concentrations.

Mechanism of Action
The precise means by which this inhibition relieves angina has not been fully determined, but includes at least the following two mechanisms:

(1) Relaxation and Prevention of Coronary Artery Spasm
ADALAT® dilates the main coronary arteries and coronary arterioles, both in normal and ischemic regions, and is a potent inhibitor of coronary artery spasm, whether spontaneous or ergonovine-induced. This property increases myocardial oxygen delivery in patients with coronary artery spasm, and is responsible for the effectiveness of ADALAT® in vasospastic (Prinzmetal's or variant) angina. Whether this effect plays any role in classical angina is not clear, but studies of exercise tolerance have not shown an increase in the maximum exercise rate-pressure product, a widely accepted measure of oxygen utilization. This suggests that, in general, relief of spasm or dilation of coronary arteries is not an important factor in classical angina.

(2) Reduction of Oxygen Utilization
ADALAT® regularly reduces arterial pressure at rest and at a given level of exercise by dilating peripheral arterioles and reducing the total peripheral resistance (afterload) against which the heart works. This unloading of the heart reduces myocardial energy consumption and oxygen requirements and probably accounts for the effectiveness of ADALAT® in chronic stable angina.

Pharmacokinetics and Metabolism
ADALAT® is rapidly and fully absorbed after oral administration. The drug is detectable in serum 10 minutes after oral administration, and peak blood levels occur in approximately 30 minutes. Bioavailability is proportional to dose from 10 to 30 mg; half-life does not change significantly with dose. There is little difference in relative bioavailability when ADALAT® capsules are given orally and swallowed whole, bitten and swallowed, or bitten and held sublingually. However, biting through the capsule prior to swallowing does result in slightly earlier plasma concentrations (27 ng/mL 10 minutes after 10 mg) than if capsules are swallowed intact. It is highly bound by serum proteins. ADALAT® is extensively converted to inactive metabolites and approximately 80 percent of ADALAT® and metabolites are eliminated via the kidneys. The half-life of nifedipine in plasma is approximately two hours. Since hepatic biotransformation is the predominant route for the disposition of nifedipine, the pharmacokinetics may be altered in patients with chronic liver disease. Patients with hepatic impairment (liver cirrhosis) have a longer disposition half-life and higher bioavailability of nifedipine than healthy volunteers. The degree of serum protein binding of nifedipine is high (92–98%). Protein binding may be greatly reduced in patients with renal or hepatic impairment.

Hemodynamics
Like other slow channel blockers, ADALAT® exerts a negative inotropic effect on isolated myocardial tissue. This is rarely, if ever, seen in intact animals or man, probably because of reflex responses to its vasodilating effects. In man, ADALAT® causes decreased peripheral vascular resistance and a fall in systolic and diastolic pressure, usually modest (5–10mm Hg systolic), but sometimes larger. There is usually a small increase in heart rate, a reflex response to vasodilation. Measurements of cardiac function in patients with normal ventricular function have generally found a small increase in cardiac index without major effects on ejection fraction, left ventricular end diastolic pressure (LVEDP) or volume (LVEDV). In patients with impaired ventricular function, most acute studies have shown some increase in ejection fraction and reduction in left ventricular filling pressure.

Electrophysiologic Effects
Although like other members of its class, ADALAT® decreases sinoatrial node function and atrioventricular con-

duction in isolated myocardial preparations, such effects have not been seen in studies in intact animals or in man. In formal electrophysiologic studies, predominantly in patients with normal conduction system, ADALAT® has had no tendency to prolong atrioventricular conduction, prolong sinus node recovery time, or slow sinus rate.

INDICATIONS AND USAGE

I. Vasospastic Angina

ADALAT® (nifedipine) is indicated for the management of vasospastic angina confirmed by any of the following criteria: 1) classical pattern of angina at rest accompanied by ST segment elevation, 2) angina or coronary artery spasm provoked by ergonovine, or 3) angiographically demonstrated coronary artery spasm. In those patients who have had angiography, the presence of significant fixed obstructive disease is not incompatible with the diagnosis of vasospastic angina, provided that the above criteria are satisfied. ADALAT® may also be used where the clinical presentation suggests a possible vasospastic component but where vasospasm has not been confirmed, e.g., where pain has a variable threshold on exertion or when angina is refractory to nitrates and/or adequate doses of beta blockers.

II. Chronic Stable Angina
(Classical Effort-Associated Angina)

ADALAT® is indicated for the management of chronic stable angina (effort-associated angina) without evidence of vasospasm in patients who remain symptomatic despite adequate dose of beta blockers and/or organic nitrates or who cannot tolerate those agents.

In chronic stable angina (effort-associated angina) ADALAT® has been effective in controlled trials of up to eight weeks duration in reducing angina frequency and increasing exercise tolerance, but confirmation of sustained effectiveness and evaluation of long term safety in these patients are incomplete.

Controlled studies in small numbers of patients suggest concomitant use of ADALAT® and beta blocking agents may be beneficial in patients with chronic stable angina, but available information is not sufficient to predict with confidence the effects of concurrent treatment, especially in patients with compromised left ventricular function or cardiac conduction abnormalities. When introducing such concomitant therapy, care must be taken to monitor blood pressure closely since severe hypotension can occur from the combined effects of the drugs (See WARNINGS).

CONTRAINDICATIONS

Known hypersensitivity reaction to ADALAT®.

WARNINGS

Excessive Hypotension

Although in most patients, the hypotensive effect of ADALAT® CAPSULES is modest and well tolerated, occasional patients have had excessive and poorly tolerated hypotension. These responses have usually occurred during initial titration or at the time of subsequent upward dosage adjustment, and may be more likely in patients on concomitant beta blockers.

Although not approved for this purpose, ADALAT® CAPSULES and other immediate-release nifedipine capsules have been used (orally and sublingually) for acute reduction of blood pressure. Several well-documented reports describe profound hypotension, myocardial infarction, and death when immediate-release nifedipine capsules were used in this way. **ADALAT® CAPSULES should not be used for acute reduction of blood pressure.**

ADALAT® CAPSULES and other immediate-release nifedipine capsules have also been used for the long-term control of essential hypertension although no properly-controlled studies have been conducted to define an appropriate dose or dose interval for such treatment. **ADALAT® CAPSULES should not be used for the control of essential hypertension.**

Several well-controlled, randomized trials studied the use of immediate-release nifedipine capsules in patients who had just sustained myocardial infarctions. In none of these trials did immediate-release nifedipine appear to provide any benefit. In some of the trials, patients who received immediate-release nifedipine had significantly worse outcomes than patients who received placebo. **ADALAT® CAPSULES should not be administered for 1 week after myocardial infarction, and it should also be avoided in the setting of acute coronary syndrome (when infarction may be imminent).**

Severe hypotension and/or increased fluid volume requirements have been reported in patients receiving ADALAT® together with a beta blocking agent who underwent coronary artery bypass surgery using high dose fentanyl anesthesia. The interaction with high dose fentanyl appears to be due to the combination of ADALAT® and a beta blocker, but the possibility that it may occur with ADALAT® alone, with low doses of fentanyl, in other surgical procedures, or with other narcotic analgesics cannot be ruled out. In ADALAT® treated patients where surgery using high dose fentanyl anesthesia is contemplated, the physician should be aware of these potential problems and, if the patient's con-

dition permits, sufficient time (at least 36 hours) should be allowed for ADALAT® to be washed out of the body prior to surgery.

Increased Angina and/or Myocardial Infarction

Rarely, patients, particularly those who have severe obstructive coronary artery disease, have developed well documented increased frequency, duration and/or severity of angina or acute myocardial infarction on starting ADALAT® or at the time of dosage increase. The mechanism of this effect is not established.

Beta Blocker Withdrawal

Patients recently withdrawn from beta blockers may develop a withdrawal syndrome with increased angina, probably related to increased sensitivity to catecholamines. Initiation of ADALAT® treatment will not prevent this occurrence and might be expected to exacerbate it by provoking reflex catecholamine release. There have been occasional reports of increased angina in a setting of beta blocker withdrawal and ADALAT® initiation. It is important to taper beta blockers if possible, rather than stopping them abruptly before beginning ADALAT®.

Congestive Heart Failure

Rarely, patients (usually those receiving a beta blocker) have developed heart failure after beginning ADALAT®. Patients with tight aortic stenosis may be at greater risk for such an event since the unloading effect of ADALAT® would be expected to be of less benefit to these patients, owing to the fixed impedance to flow across the aortic valve.

PRECAUTIONS

General: Hypotension: Because ADALAT® decreases peripheral vascular resistance, careful monitoring of blood pressure during the initial administration and titration of ADALAT® is suggested. Close observation is especially recommended for patients already taking medications that are known to lower blood pressure (See WARNINGS).

Peripheral Edema: Mild to moderate peripheral edema, typically associated with arterial vasodilation and not due to left ventricular dysfunction, occurs in about one in ten patients treated with ADALAT® (nifedipine). This edema occurs primarily in the lower extremities and usually responds to diuretic therapy. With patients whose angina is complicated by congestive heart failure, care should be taken to differentiate this peripheral edema from the effects of increasing left ventricular dysfunction.

Laboratory Tests: Rare, usually transient, but occasionally significant elevations of enzymes such as alkaline phosphatase, CPK, LDH, SGOT, and SGPT have been noted. The relationship to ADALAT® therapy is uncertain in most cases, but probable in some. These laboratory abnormalities have rarely been associated with clinical symptoms, however, cholestasis with or without jaundice has been reported. Rare instances of allergic hepatitis have been reported.

ADALAT®, like other calcium channel blockers, decreases platelet aggregation *in vitro*. Limited clinical studies have demonstrated a moderate but statistically significant decrease in platelet aggregation and increase in bleeding time in some ADALAT® patients. This is thought to be a function of inhibition of calcium transport across the platelet membrane. No clinical significance for these findings has been demonstrated.

Positive direct Coombs test with/without hemolytic anemia has been reported.

Although ADALAT® has been used safely in patients with renal dysfunction and has been reported to exert a beneficial effect in certain cases, rare reversible elevations in BUN and serum creatinine have been reported in patients with pre-existing chronic renal insufficiency. The relationship to ADALAT® therapy is uncertain in most cases, but probable in some.

Drug Interactions: *Beta-adrenergic blocking agents:* (See INDICATIONS and WARNINGS). Experience in over 1400 patients in a non-comparative clinical trial has shown that concomitant administration of ADALAT® and beta blocking agents is usually well tolerated, but there have been occasional literature reports suggesting that the combination may increase the likelihood of congestive heart failure, severe hypotension or exacerbation of angina.

Long acting nitrates: ADALAT® may be safely co-administered with nitrates, but there have been no controlled studies to evaluate the antianginal effectiveness of this combination.

Digitalis: Since there have been isolated reports of patients with elevated digoxin levels, and there is a possible interaction between digoxin and nifedipine, it is recommended that digoxin levels be monitored when initiating, adjusting and discontinuing nifedipine to avoid possible over- or under-digitalization.

Coumarin anticoagulants: There have been rare reports of increased prothrombin time in patients taking coumarin anticoagulants to whom ADALAT® was administered. However, the relationship to ADALAT® therapy is uncertain.

Cimetidine: A study in six healthy volunteers has shown a significant increase in peak nifedipine plasma levels (80%) and area-under-the-curve (74%) after a one week course of

cimetidine at 1000 mg per day and nifedipine at 40 mg per day. Ranitidine produced smaller, non-significant increases. The effect may be mediated by the known inhibition of cimetidine on hepatic cytochrome P-450, the enzyme system probably responsible for the first-pass metabolism of nifedipine. If nifedipine therapy is initiated in a patient currently receiving cimetidine, cautious titration is advised.

Quinidine: There have been rare reports of an interaction between quinidine and nifedipine (with a decreased plasma level of quinidine).

Carcinogenesis, Mutagenesis, Impairment of Fertility: Nifedipine was administered orally to rats for two years and was not shown to be carcinogenic. When given to rats prior to mating, nifedipine caused reduced fertility at a dose approximately 30 times the maximum recommended human dose. *In vivo* mutagenicity studies were negative.

Pregnancy: Pregnancy Category C. In rodents, rabbits, and monkeys, nifedipine has been shown to have a variety of embryotoxic, placentoxic, and fetotoxic effects, including stunted fetuses (rats, mice, and rabbits), digital anomalies (rats and rabbits), rib deformities (mice), cleft palate (mice), small placentas and underdeveloped chorionic villi (monkeys), embryonic and fetal deaths (rats, mice, and rabbits), prolonged pregnancy (rats; not evaluated in other species), and decreased neonatal survival (rats; not evaluated in other species). On a mg/kg or mg/m² basis, some of the doses associated with these various effects are higher than the maximum recommended human dose and some are lower, but all are within one order of magnitude of it.

The digital anomalies seen in nifedipine-exposed rabbit pups are strikingly similar to those seen in pups exposed to phenytoin, and these are in turn similar to the phalangeal deformities that are the most common malformation seen in human children with *in utero* exposure to phenytoin.

There are no adequate and well controlled studies in pregnant women. ADALAT® should be used during pregnancy only if the potential benefit justifies the potential risk to the fetus.

Nursing Mothers: Nifedipine is excreted in human milk. Therefore, a decision should be made to discontinue nursing or to discontinue the drug, taking into account the importance of the drug to the mother.

ADVERSE REACTION

In multiple-dose U.S. and foreign controlled studies in which adverse reactions were reported spontaneously, adverse effects were frequent but generally not serious and rarely required discontinuation of therapy or dosage adjustment. Most were expected consequences of the vasodilator effects of ADALAT®.

Adverse Effect	ADALAT® (%) (N=226)	Placebo (%) (N=235)
Dizziness, lightheadedness, giddiness	27	15
Flushing, heat sensation	25	8
Headache	23	20
Weakness	12	10
Nausea, heartburn	11	8
Muscle cramps, tremor	8	3
Peripheral edema	7	1
Nervousness, mood changes	7	4
Palpitation	7	5
Dyspnea, cough, wheezing	6	3
Nasal congestion, sore throat	6	8

There is also a large uncontrolled experience in over 2100 patients in the United States. Most of the patients had vasospastic or resistant angina pectoris, and about half had concomitant treatment with beta-adrenergic blocking agents. The most common adverse events were:

Incidence Approximately 10%
Cardiovascular: peripheral edema
Central Nervous System: dizziness or lightheadedness
Gastrointestinal: nausea
Systemic: headache and flushing, weakness.

Incidence Approximately 5%
Cardiovascular: transient hypotension.

Incidence 2% or Less
Cardiovascular: palpitation
Respiratory: nasal and chest congestion, shortness of breath
Gastrointestinal: diarrhea, constipation, cramps, flatulence
Musculoskeletal: inflammation, joint stiffness, muscle cramps
Central Nervous System: shakiness, nervousness, jitteriness, sleep disturbances, blurred vision, difficulties in balance
Other: dermatitis, pruritus, urticaria, fever, sweating, chills, sexual difficulties.

Incidence Approximately 0.5%
Cardiovascular: syncope. Syncopal episodes occurred mostly with initial dose and/or increase of dosage.

Continued on next page

Adalat—Cont.

Incidence Less Than 0.5%

Hematologic: thrombocytopenia, anemia, leukopenia, purpura
Gastrointestinal: allergic hepatitis
Face and Throat: angioedema (mostly orpharyngeal edema with breathing difficulty in a few patients), gingival hyperplasia.
CNS: depression, paranoid syndrome
Musculoskeletal: myalgia
Special Senses: transient blindness at the peak of plasma level
Urogenital: nocturia, polyuria
Other: erythromelalgia, arthritis with ANA (+), gynecomastia, exfoliative dermatitis.

Several of these side effects appear to be dose related. Peripheral edema occurred in about one in 25 patients at doses less than 60 mg per day and in about one patient in eight at 120 mg per day or more. Transient hypotension, generally mild to moderate severity and seldom requiring discontinuation of therapy, occurred in one of 50 patients at less than 60 mg per day and in one of 20 patients at 120 mg per day or more. Very rarely, introduction of ADALAT® therapy was associated with an increase in anginal pain, possibly due to associated hypotension.

In addition, more serious adverse events were observed, not readily distinguishable from the natural history of the disease in these patients. It remains possible, however, that some or many of these events were drug related. Myocardial infarction occurred in about 4% of patients and congestive heart failure or pulmonary edema in about 2%. Ventricular arrhythmias or conduction disturbances each occurred in fewer than 0.5% of patients.

In a subgroup of over 1000 patients receiving ADALAT® with concomitant beta blocker therapy, the pattern and incidence of adverse experiences were not different from that of the entire group of ADALAT® (nifedipine) treated patients (See PRECAUTIONS).

In a subgroup of approximately 250 patients with a diagnosis of congestive heart failure as well as angina, dizziness or lightheadedness, peripheral edema, headache or flushing each occurred in one in eight patients. Hypotension occurred in about one in 20 patients. Syncope occurred in approximately one patient in 250. Myocardial infarction or symptoms of congestive heart failure each occurred in about one patient in 15. Atrial or ventricular dysrhythmias each occurred in about one patient in 150.

OVERDOSAGE

Experience with nifedipine overdosage is limited. Generally, overdosage with nifedipine leading to pronounced hypotension calls for active cardiovascular support including monitoring of cardiovascular and respiratory function, elevation of extremities, judicious use of calcium infusion, pressor agents and fluids. Clearance of nifedipine would be expected to be prolonged in patients with impaired liver function. Since nifedipine is highly protein bound, dialysis is not likely to be of any benefit; however, plasmapheresis may be beneficial.

DOSAGE AND ADMINISTRATION

The dosage of ADALAT® needed to suppress angina and that can be tolerated by the patient must be established by titration. Excessive doses can result in hypotension.

Therapy should be initiated with the 10 mg capsule. The starting dose is one 10 mg capsule, swallowed whole, 3 times/day. The usual effective dose range is 10–20 mg three times daily. Some patients, especially those with evidence of coronary artery spasm, respond only to higher doses, more frequent administration, or both. In such patients, doses of 20–30 mg three or four times daily may be effective. Doses above 120 mg daily are rarely necessary. More than 180 mg per day is not recommended.

In most cases, ADALAT® titration should proceed over a 7–14 day period so that the physician can assess the response to each dose level and monitor the blood pressure before proceeding to higher doses.

If symptoms so warrant, titration may proceed more rapidly provided that the patient is assessed frequently. Based on the patient's physical activity level, attack frequency, and sublingual nitroglycerin consumption, the dose of ADALAT® may be increased from 10 mg t.i.d. to 20 mg t.i.d. and then to 30 mg t.i.d. over a three-day period.

In hospitalized patients under close observation, the dose may be increased in 10 mg increments over four to six-hour periods as required to control pain and arrhythmias due to ischemia. A single dose should rarely exceed 30 mg.

No "rebound effect" has been observed upon discontinuation of ADALAT®. However, if discontinuation of ADALAT® is necessary, sound clinical practice suggests that the dosage should be decreased gradually with close physician supervision.

Co-Administration with Other Antianginal Drugs

Sublingual nitroglycerin may be taken as required for the control of acute manifestations of angina, particularly during ADALAT® titration. See **PRECAUTIONS, Drug Interactions,** for information on co-administration of ADALAT® with beta blockers or long acting nitrates.

HOW SUPPLIED

ADALAT® soft gelatin capsules are supplied in:

Bottles of 100:	10 mg (NDC 0026-8811-51) orange 20 mg (NDC 0026-8821-51) orange and light brown
Bottles of 300:	10 mg (NDC 0026-8811-18) orange 20 mg (NDC 0026-8821-18) orange and light brown
Unit dose packages of 100:	10 mg (NDC 0026-8811-48) orange 20 mg (NDC 0026-8821-48) orange and light brown

The capsules are identified as follows: 10 mg (Adalat 10), 20 mg (Adalat 20).

The capsules should be protected from light and moisture and stored at controlled room temperature 59° to 77°F (15° to 25°C). Dispense in tight, light resistant containers (USP).

Bayer Corporation
Pharmaceutical Division
400 Morgan Lane
West Haven, CT 06516

Encapsulated by
R.P. Scherer N.A., Clearwater, FL 33518

Caution: Federal (USA) law prohibits dispensing without prescription.

PD500034 3/96 BAY a 1040 6128

Shown in Product Identification Guide, page 305

ADALAT® CC ℞

(nifedipine)
Extended Release Tablets
For Oral Use

DESCRIPTION

ADALAT® CC is an extended release tablet dosage form of the calcium channel blocker nifedipine. Nifedipine is 3,5-pyridinedicarboxylic acid, 1,4-dihydro-2,6-dimethyl-4-(2-nitrophenyl)-dimethyl ester, $C_{17}H_{18}N_2O_6$, and has the structural formula:

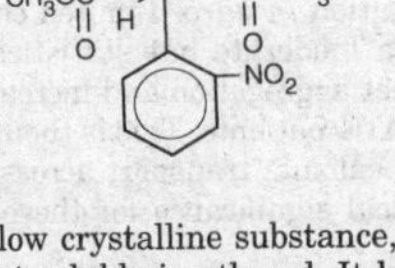

Nifedipine is a yellow crystalline substance, practically insoluble in water but soluble in ethanol. It has a molecular weight of 346.3. ADALAT CC tablets consist of an external coat and an internal core. Both contain nifedipine, the coat as a slow release formulation and the core as a fast release formulation. ADALAT CC tablets contain either 30, 60, or 90 mg of nifedipine for once-a-day oral administration.

Inert ingredients in the formulation are: hydroxypropylcellulose, lactose, corn starch, crospovidone, microcrystalline cellulose, silicon dioxide, and magnesium stearate. The inert ingredients in the film coating are: hydroxypropylmethylcellulose, polyethylene glycol, ferric oxide, and titanium dioxide.

CLINICAL PHARMACOLOGY

Nifedipine is a calcium ion influx inhibitor (slow-channel blocker or calcium ion antagonist) which inhibits the transmembrane influx of calcium ions into vascular smooth muscle and cardiac muscle. The contractile processes of vascular smooth muscle and cardiac muscle are dependent upon the movement of extracellular calcium ions into these cells through specific ion channels. Nifedipine selectively inhibits calcium ion influx across the cell membrane of vascular smooth muscle and cardiac muscle without altering serum calcium concentrations.

Mechanism of Action: The mechanism by which nifedipine reduces arterial blood pressure involves peripheral arterial vasodilatation and consequently, a reduction in peripheral vascular resistance. The increased peripheral vascular resistance that is an underlying cause of hypertension results from an increase in active tension in the vascular smooth muscle. Studies have demonstrated that the increase in active tension reflects an increase in cytosolic free calcium.

Nifedipine is a peripheral arterial vasodilator which acts directly on vascular smooth muscle. The binding of nifedipine to voltage-dependent and possibly receptor-operated channels in vascular smooth muscle results in an inhibition of calcium influx through these channels. Stores of intracellular calcium in vascular smooth muscle are limited and thus dependent upon the influx of extracellular calcium for contraction to occur. The reduction in calcium influx by nifedipine causes arterial vasodilation and decreased peripheral vascular resistance which results in reduced arterial blood pressure.

Pharmacokinetics and Metabolism: Nifedipine is completely absorbed after oral administration. The bioavailability of nifedipine as ADALAT CC relative to immediate release nifedipine is in the range of 84%–89%. After ingestion of ADALAT CC tablets under fasting conditions, plasma concentrations peak at about 2.5–5 hours with a second small peak or shoulder evident at approximately 6–12 hours post dose. The elimination half-life of nifedipine administered as ADALAT CC is approximately 7 hours in contrast to the known 2 hour elimination half-life of nifedipine administered as an immediate release capsule.

When ADALAT CC is administered as multiples of 30 mg tablets over a dose range of 30 mg to 90 mg, the area under the curve (AUC) is dose proportional; however, the peak plasma concentration for the 90 mg dose given as 3 × 30 mg is 29% greater than predicted from the 30 mg and 60 mg doses.

Two 30 mg ADALAT CC tablets may be interchanged with a 60 mg ADALAT CC tablet. Three 30 mg ADALAT CC tablets, however, result in substantially higher C_{max} values than those after a single 90 mg ADALAT CC tablet. Three 30 mg tablets should, therefore, not be considered interchangeable with a 90 mg tablet.

Once daily dosing of ADALAT CC under fasting conditions results in decreased fluctuations in the plasma concentration of nifedipine when compared to t.i.d. dosing with immediate release nifedipine capsules. The mean peak plasma concentration of nifedipine following a 90 mg ADALAT CC tablet, administered under fasting conditions, is approximately 115 ng/mL. When ADALAT CC is given immediately after a high fat meal in healthy volunteers, there is an average increase of 60% in the peak plasma nifedipine concentration, a prolongation in the time to peak concentration, but no significant change in the AUC. Plasma concentrations of nifedipine when ADALAT CC is taken after a fatty meal result in slightly lower peaks compared to the same daily dose of the immediate release formulation administered in three divided doses. This may be, in part, because ADALAT CC is less bioavailable than the immediate release formulation.

Nifedipine is extensively metabolized to highly water soluble, inactive metabolites accounting for 60% to 80% of the dose excreted in the urine. Only traces (less than 0.1% of the dose) of the unchanged form can be detected in the urine. The remainder is excreted in the feces in metabolized form, most likely as a result of biliary excretion.

No studies have been performed with ADALAT CC in patients with renal failure; however, significant alterations in the pharmacokinetics of nifedipine immediate release capsules have not been reported in patients undergoing hemodialysis or chronic ambulatory peritoneal dialysis. Since the absorption of nifedipine from ADALAT CC could be modified by renal disease, caution should be exercised in treating such patients.

Because hepatic biotransformation is the predominant route for the disposition of nifedipine, its pharmacokinetics may be altered in patients with chronic liver disease. ADALAT CC has not been studied in patients with hepatic disease; however, in patients with hepatic impairment (liver cirrhosis) nifedipine has a longer elimination half-life and higher bioavailability than in healthy volunteers.

The degree of protein binding of nifedipine is high (92%–98%). Protein binding may be greatly reduced in patients with renal or hepatic impairment.

After administration of ADALAT CC to healthy elderly men and women (age > 60 years), the mean C_{max} is 36% higher and the average plasma concentration is 70% greater than in younger patients.

Clinical Studies: ADALAT CC produced dose-related decreases in systolic and diastolic blood pressure as demonstrated in two double-blind, randomized, placebo-controlled trials in which over 350 patients were treated with ADALAT CC 30, 60 or 90mg once daily for 6 weeks. In the first study, ADALAT CC was given as monotherapy and in the second study, ADALAT CC was added to a beta-blocker in patients not controlled on a beta-blocker alone. The mean trough (24 hours post-dose) blood pressure results from these studies are shown below:

MEAN REDUCTIONS IN TROUGH SUPINE BLOOD PRESSURE (mmHg) SYSTOLIC/DIASTOLIC
STUDY 1

ADALAT CC DOSE	N	MEAN TROUGH REDUCTION*
30 MG	60	5.3/2.9
60 MG	57	8.0/4.1
90 MG	55	12.5/8.1

ADALAT CC DOSE	STUDY 2 N	MEAN TROUGH REDUCTION*
30 MG	58	7.6/3.8
60 MG	63	10.1/5.3
90 MG	62	10.2/5.8

*Placebo response subtracted.

The trough/peak ratios estimated from 24 hour blood pressure monitoring ranged from 41%–78% for diastolic and 46%–91% for systolic blood pressure.

Hemodynamics: Like other slow-channel blockers, nifedipine exerts a negative inotropic effect on isolated myocardial tissue. This is rarely, if ever, seen in intact animals or man, probably because of reflex responses to its vasodilating effects. In man, nifedipine decreases peripheral vascular resistance which leads to a fall in systolic and diastolic pressures, usually minimal in normotensive volunteers (less than 5–10 mm Hg systolic), but sometimes larger. With ADALAT CC, these decreases in blood pressure are not accompanied by any significant change in heart rate. Hemodynamic studies of the immediate release nifedipine formulation in patients with normal ventricular function have generally found a small increase in cardiac index without major effects on ejection fraction, left ventricular end-diastolic pressure (LVEDP) or volume (LVEDV). In patients with impaired ventricular function, most acute studies have shown some increase in ejection fraction and reduction in left ventricular filling pressure.

Electrophysiologic Effects: Although, like other members of its class, nifedipine causes a slight depression of sinoatrial node function and atrioventricular conduction in isolated myocardial preparations, such effects have not been seen in studies in intact animals or in man. In formal electrophysiologic studies, predominantly in patients with normal conduction systems, nifedipine administered as the immediate release capsule has had no tendency to prolong atrioventricular conduction or sinus node recovery time, or to slow sinus rate.

INDICATION AND USAGE

ADALAT CC is indicated for the treatment of hypertension. It may be used alone or in combination with other antihypertensive agents.

CONTRAINDICATIONS

Known hypersensitivity to nifedipine.

WARNINGS

Excessive Hypotension: Although in most patients the hypotensive effect of nifedipine is modest and well tolerated, occasional patients have had excessive and poorly tolerated hypotension. These responses have usually occurred during initial titration or at the time of subsequent upward dosage adjustment, and may be more likely in patients using concomitant beta-blockers.

Severe hypotension and/or increased fluid volume requirements have been reported in patients who received immediate release capsules together with a beta-blocking agent and who underwent coronary artery bypass surgery using high dose fentanyl anesthesia. The interaction with high dose fentanyl appears to be due to the combination of nifedipine and a beta-blocker, but the possibility that it may occur with nifedipine alone, with low doses of fentanyl, in other surgical procedures, or with other narcotic analgesics cannot be ruled out. In nifedipine-treated patients where surgery using high dose fentanyl anesthesia is contemplated, the physician should be aware of these potential problems and, if the patient's condition permits, sufficient time (at least 36 hours) should be allowed for nifedipine to be washed out of the body prior to surgery.

Increased Angina and/or Myocardial Infarction: Rarely, patients, particularly those who have severe obstructive coronary artery disease, have developed well documented increased frequency, duration and/or severity of angina or acute myocardial infarction upon starting nifedipine or at the time of dosage increase. The mechanism of this effect is not established.

Beta-Blocker Withdrawal: When discontinuing a beta-blocker it is important to taper its dose, if possible, rather than stopping abruptly before beginning nifedipine. Patients recently withdrawn from beta blockers may develop a withdrawal syndrome with increased angina, probably related to increased sensitivity to catecholamines. Initiation of nifedipine treatment will not prevent this occurrence and on occasion has been reported to increase it.

Congestive Heart Failure: Rarely, patients (usually while receiving a beta-blocker) have developed heart failure after beginning nifedipine. Patients with tight aortic stenosis may be at greater risk for such an event, as the unloading effect of nifedipine would be expected to be of less benefit to these patients, owing to their fixed impedance to flow across the aortic valve.

PRECAUTIONS

General—Hypotension: Because nifedipine decreases peripheral vascular resistance, careful monitoring of blood pressure during the initial administration and titration of ADALAT CC is suggested. Close observation is especially recommended for patients already taking medications that are known to lower blood pressure (See WARNINGS).

Peripheral Edema: Mild to moderate peripheral edema occurs in a dose-dependent manner with ADALAT CC. The placebo subtracted rate is approximately 8% at 30 mg, 12% at 60 mg and 19% at 90 mg daily. This edema is a localized phenomenon, thought to be associated with vasodilation of dependent arterioles and small blood vessels and not due to left ventricular dysfunction or generalized fluid retention. With patients whose hypertension is complicated by congestive heart failure, care should be taken to differentiate this peripheral edema from the effects of increasing left ventricular dysfunction.

Information for Patients: ADALAT CC is an extended release tablet and should be swallowed whole and taken on an empty stomach. It should not be administered with food. Do not chew, divide or crush tablets.

Laboratory Tests: Rare, usually transient, but occasionally significant elevations of enzymes such as alkaline phosphatase, CPK, LDH, SGOT, and SGPT have been noted. The relationship to nifedipine therapy is uncertain in most cases, but probable in some. These laboratory abnormalities have rarely been associated with clinical symptoms; however, cholestasis with or without jaundice has been reported. A small increase (<5%) in mean alkaline phosphatase was noted in patients treated with ADALAT CC. This was an isolated finding and it rarely resulted in values which fell outside the normal range. Rare instances of allergic hepatitis have been reported with nifedipine treatment. In controlled studies, ADALAT CC did not adversely affect serum uric acid, glucose, cholesterol or potassium.

Nifedipine, like other calcium channel blockers, decreases platelet aggregation *in vitro*. Limited clinical studies have demonstrated a moderate but statistically significant decrease in platelet aggregation and increase in bleeding time in some nifedipine patients. This is thought to be a function of inhibition of calcium transport across the platelet membrane. No clinical significance for these findings has been demonstrated.

Positive direct Coombs' test with or without hemolytic anemia has been reported but a causal relationship between nifedipine administration and positivity of this laboratory test, including hemolysis, could not be determined.

Although nifedipine has been used safely in patients with renal dysfunction and has been reported to exert a beneficial effect in certain cases, rare reversible elevations in BUN and serum creatinine have been reported in patients with pre-existing chronic renal insufficiency. The relationship to nifedipine therapy is uncertain in most cases but probable in some.

Drug Interactions: Beta-adrenergic blocking agents: (See WARNINGS).

ADALAT CC was well tolerated when administered in combination with a beta blocker in 187 hypertensive patients in a placebo-controlled clinical trial. However, there have been occasional literature reports suggesting that the combination of nifedipine and beta-adrenergic blocking drugs may increase the likelihood of congestive heart failure, severe hypotension, or exacerbation of angina in patients with cardiovascular disease.

Digitalis: Since there have been isolated reports of patients with elevated digoxin levels, and there is a possible interaction between digoxin and ADALAT CC, it is recommended that digoxin levels be monitored when initiating, adjusting, and discontinuing ADALAT CC to avoid possible over- or under-digitalization.

Coumarin Anticoagulants: There have been rare reports of increased prothrombin time in patients taking coumarin anticoagulants to whom nifedipine was administered. However, the relationship to nifedipine therapy is uncertain.

Quinidine: There have been rare reports of an interaction between quinidine and nifedipine (with a decreased plasma level of quinidine).

Cimetidine: Both the peak plasma level of nifedipine and the AUC may increase in the presence of cimetidine. Ranitidine produces smaller non-significant increases. This effect of cimetidine may be mediated by its known inhibition of hepatic cytochrome P-450, the enzyme system probably responsible for the first-pass metabolism of nifedipine. If nifedipine therapy is initiated in a patient currently receiving cimetidine, cautious titration is advised.

Carcinogenesis, Mutagenesis, Impairment of Fertility: Nifedipine was administered orally to rats for two years and was not shown to be carcinogenic. When given to rats prior to mating, nifedipine caused reduced fertility at a dose approximately 30 times the maximum recommended human dose. *In vivo* mutagenicity studies were negative.

Pregnancy: Pregnancy Category C. In rodents, rabbits and monkeys, nifedipine has been shown to have a variety of embryotoxic, placentotoxic and fetotoxic effects, including stunted fetuses (rats, mice and rabbits), digital anomalies (rats and rabbits), rib deformities (mice), cleft palate (mice), small placentas and underdeveloped chorionic villi (monkeys), embryonic and fetal deaths (rats, mice and rabbits), prolonged pregnancy (rats; not evaluated in other species), and decreased neonatal survival (rats; not evaluated in other species). On a mg/kg or mg/m^2 basis, some of the doses associated with these various effects are higher than the maximum recommended human dose and some are lower, but all are within an order of magnitude of it.

The digital anomalies seen in nifedipine-exposed rabbit pups are strikingly similar to those seen in pups exposed to phenytoin, and these are in turn similar to the phalangeal deformities that are the most common malformation seen in human children with *in utero* exposure to phenytoin.

There are no adequate and well-controlled studies in pregnant women. ADALAT CC should be used during pregnancy only if the potential benefit justifies the potential risk to the fetus.

Nursing Mothers: Nifedipine is excreted in human milk. Therefore, a decision should be made to discontinue nursing or to discontinue the drug, taking into account the importance of the drug to the mother.

ADVERSE EXPERIENCES

The incidence of adverse events during treatment with ADALAT CC in doses up to 90 mg daily were derived from multi-center placebo-controlled clinical trials in 370 hypertensive patients. Atenolol 50 mg once daily was used concomitantly in 187 of the 370 patients on ADALAT CC and in 64 of the 126 patients on placebo. All adverse events reported during ADALAT CC therapy were tabulated independently of their causal relationship to medication. The most common adverse event reported with ADALAT® CC was peripheral edema. This was dose related and the frequency was 18% on ADALAT CC 30 mg daily, 22% on ADALAT CC 60 mg daily and 29% on ADALAT CC 90 mg daily versus 10% on placebo.

Other common adverse events reported in the above placebo-controlled trials include:

Adverse Event	ADALAT CC (%) (n=370)	PLACEBO (%) (n=126)
Headache	19	13
Flushing/heat sensation	4	0
Dizziness	4	2
Fatigue/asthenia	4	4
Nausea	2	1
Constipation	1	0

Where the frequency of adverse events with ADALAT CC and placebo is similar, causal relationship cannot be established.

The following adverse events were reported with an incidence of 3% or less in daily doses up to 90 mg:

Body as a Whole/Systemic: chest pain, leg pain
Central Nervous System: paresthesia, vertigo
Dermatologic: rash
Gastrointestinal: constipation
Musculoskeletal: leg cramps
Respiratory: epistaxis, rhinitis
Urogenital: impotence, urinary frequency

Other adverse events reported with an incidence of less than 1.0% were:

Body as a Whole/Systemic: cellulitis, chills, facial edema, neck pain, pelvic pain, pain
Cardiovascular: atrial fibrillation, bradycardia, cardiac arrest, extrasystole, hypotension, palpitations, phlebitis, postural hypotension, tachycardia, cutaneous angiectases
Central Nervous System: anxiety, confusion, decreased libido, depression, hypertonia, insomnia, somnolence
Dermatologic: pruritus, sweating
Gastrointestinal: abdominal pain, diarrhea, dry mouth, dyspepsia, esophagitis, flatulence, gastrointestinal hemorrhage, vomiting
Hematologic: lymphadenopathy
Metabolic: gout, weight loss
Musculoskeletal: arthralgia, arthritis, myalgia
Respiratory: dyspnea, increased cough, rales, pharyngitis
Special Senses: abnormal vision, amblyopia, conjunctivitis, diplopia, tinnitus
Urogenital/Reproductive: kidney calculus, nocturia, breast engorgement

The following adverse events have been reported rarely in patients given nifedipine in other formulations: allergenic hepatitis, alopecia, anemia, arthritis with ANA (+), depression, erythromelalgia, exfoliative dermatitis, fever, gingival hyperplasia, gynecomastia, leukopenia, mood changes, muscle cramps, nervousness, paranoid syndrome, purpura, shakiness, sleep disturbances, syncope, taste perversion, thrombocytopenia, transient blindness at the peak plasma level, tremor and urticaria.

Continued on next page

Adalat CC—Cont.

OVERDOSAGE

Experience with nifedipine overdosage is limited. Generally, overdosage with nifedipine leading to pronounced hypotension calls for active cardiovascular support including monitoring of cardiovascular and respiratory function, elevation of extremities, judicious use of calcium infusion, pressor agents and fluids. Clearance of nifedipine would be expected to be prolonged in patients with impaired liver function. Since nifedipine is highly protein bound, dialysis is not likely to be of any benefit; however, plasmapheresis may be beneficial.

There has been one reported case of massive overdosage with tablets of another extended release formulation of nifedipine. The main effects of ingestion of approximately 4800 mg of nifedipine in a young man attempting suicide as a result of cocaine-induced depression was initial dizziness, palpitations, flushing, and nervousness. Within several hours of ingestion, nausea, vomiting, and generalized edema developed. No significant hypotension was apparent at presentation, 18 hours post ingestion. Blood chemistry abnormalities consisted of a mild, transient elevation of serum creatinine, and modest elevations of LDH and CPK, but normal SGOT. Vital signs remained stable, no electrocardiographic abnormalities were noted and renal function returned to normal within 24 to 48 hours with routine supportive measures alone. No prolonged sequelae were observed.

The effect of a single 900 mg ingestion of nifedipine capsules in a depressed anginal patient on tricyclic antidepressants was loss of consciousness within 30 minutes of ingestion, and profound hypotension, which responded to calcium infusion, pressor agents, and fluid replacement. A variety of ECG abnormalities were seen in this patient with a history of bundle branch block, including sinus bradycardia and varying degrees of AV block. These dictated the prophylactic placement of a temporary ventricular pacemaker, but otherwise resolved spontaneously. Significant hyperglycemia was seen initially in this patient, but plasma glucose levels rapidly normalized without further treatment.

A young hypertensive patient with advanced renal failure ingested 280 mg of nifedipine capsules at one time, with resulting marked hypotension responding to calcium infusion and fluids. No AV conduction abnormalities, arrhythmias, or pronounced changes in heart rate were noted, nor was there any further deterioration in renal function.

DOSAGE AND ADMINISTRATION

Dosage should be adjusted according to each patient's needs. It is recommended that ADALAT CC be administered orally once daily on an empty stomach. ADALAT CC is an extended release dosage form and tablets should be swallowed whole, not bitten or divided. In general, titration should proceed over a 7–14 day period starting with 30 mg once daily. Upward titration should be based on therapeutic efficacy and safety. The usual maintenance dose is 30 mg to 60 mg once daily. Titration to doses above 90 mg daily is not recommended.

If discontinuation of ADALAT CC is necessary, sound clinical practice suggests that the dosage should be decreased gradually with close physician supervision.

Care should be taken when dispensing ADALAT CC to assure that the extended release dosage form has been prescribed.

HOW SUPPLIED

ADALAT CC extended release tablets are supplied as 30 mg, 60 mg, and 90 mg round film coated tablets. The different strengths can be identified as follows:

Strength	Color	Markings
30 mg	Pink	30 on one side and ADALAT CC on the other side
60 mg	Salmon	60 on one side and ADALAT CC on the other side
90 mg	Dark Red	90 on one side and ADALAT CC on the other side

ADALAT® CC Tablets are supplied in:

	Strength	NDC Code
Bottles of 100	30 mg	0026-8841-51
	60 mg	0026-8851-51
	90 mg	0026-8861-51
Unit Dose	30 mg	0026-8841-48
Packages of 100	60 mg	0026-8851-48
	90 mg	0026-8861-48

The tablets should be protected from light and moisture and stored below 86°F (30°C). Dispense in tight, light-resistant containers.

Distributed by:
Bayer Corporation
Pharmaceutical Division
400 Morgan Lane
West Haven, CT 06516 USA

PZ500064 4/97
©1997 Bayer Corporation 7198
Shown in Product Identification Guide, page 305

BAYCOL™ ℞
(cerivastatin sodium tablets)

DESCRIPTION

Cerivastatin sodium is sodium [S-[R*,S*-(E)]]-7-[4-(4-fluorophenyl)-5-methoxymethyl)-2,6bis(1-methylethyl)-3-pyridinyl]-3,5-dihydroxy-6-heptenoate. The empirical formula for cerivastatin sodium is $C_{26}H_{33}FNO_5Na$ and its molecular weight is 481.5. It has the following chemical structure:

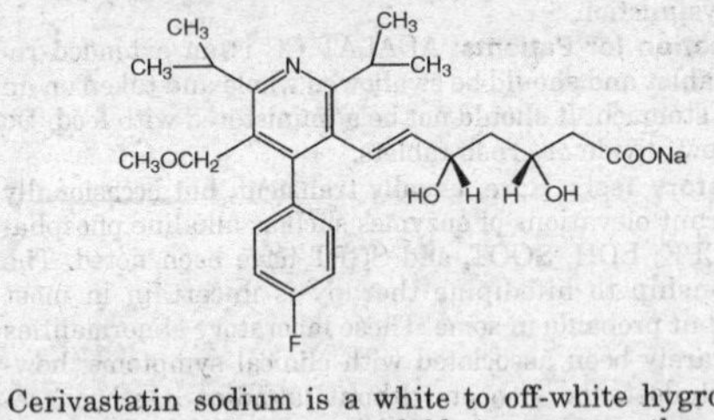

Cerivastatin sodium is a white to off-white hygroscopic amorphous powder that is soluble in water, methanol, and ethanol, and very slightly soluble in acetone.

Cerivastatin sodium is an entirely synthetic, enantiomerically pure inhibitor of 3-hydroxy-3-methylglutaryl-coenzyme A (HMG-CoA) reductase. HMG-CoA reductase catalyzes the conversion of HMG-CoA to mevalonate, which is an early and rate-limiting step in the biosynthesis of cholesterol.

BAYCOL™ (cerivastatin sodium tablets) is supplied as tablets containing 0.2 or 0.3 mg of cerivastatin sodium, for oral administration. Active ingredient: cerivastatin sodium. Inactive ingredients: mannitol, magnesium stearate, sodium hydroxide, crospovidone, povidone, iron oxide yellow, methylhydroxypropylcellulose, polyethylene glycol, and titanium dioxide.

CLINICAL PHARMACOLOGY

Cholesterol and triglycerides circulate as part of lipoprotein complexes throughout the bloodstream. These complexes can be separated via ultracentrifugation into high-density lipoprotein (HDL), intermediate-density lipoprotein (IDL), low-density lipoprotein (LDL) and very-low-density lipoprotein (VLDL) fractions. In the liver, cholesterol and triglycerides (TG) are synthesized, incorporated into VLDL, and released into the plasma for delivery to peripheral tissues. A variety of clinical studies have demonstrated that elevated levels of total cholesterol (total-C), LDL-C, and apolipoprotein B (apo-B, a membrane complex for LDL-C) promote human atherosclerosis. Similarly, decreased levels of HDL-C (and its transport complex, apolopoprotein A) are associated with the development of atherosclerosis. Epidemiologic investigations have established that cardiovascular morbidity and mortality vary directly with the level of total-C and LDL-C and inversely with the level of HDL-C. In patients with hypercholesterolemia, BAYCOL™ (cerivastatin sodium tablets) has been shown to reduce plasma total cholesterol, LDL-C, and apolipoprotein B. In addition, it also reduces plasma triglycerides and increases plasma HDL-C. The agent has no consistent effect on plasma Lp(a). The effect of BAYCOL™ on cardiovascular morbidity and mortality has not been determined.

Mechanism of Action: Cerivastatin is a competitive inhibitor of HMG-CoA reductase, which is responsible for the conversion of 3-hydroxy-3-methyl-glutaryl-coenzyme A (HMG-CoA) to mevalonate, a precursor of sterols, including cholesterol. The inhibition of cholesterol biosynthesis by cerivastatin reduces the level of cholesterol in hepatic cells, which stimulates the synthesis of LDL receptors, thereby increasing the uptake of cellular LDL particles. The end result of these biochemical processes is a reduction of the plasma cholesterol concentration.

Pharmacokinetics: Absorption

BAYCOL™ (cerivastatin sodium tablets) is administered orally in the active form. The mean absolute bioavailability of cerivastatin following a 0.2-mg tablet oral dose is 60% (range 39–101%). In general, the coefficient of variation (based on the inter-subject variability) for both systemic exposure (area under the curve, AUC) and C_{max} is in the 20% to 40% range. The bioavailability of cerivastatin sodium tablets is equivalent to that of a solution of cerivastatin sodium. No unchanged cerivastatin is excreted in feces. Cerivastatin exhibits linear kinetics over the dose range of 0.05 to 0.3 mg daily. Mean maximum concentrations (C_{max}) following evening cerivastatin tablet doses of 0.05, 0.1, 0.2, and 0.3 mg are 0.6, 1.3, 2.4, and 3.8 µg/L, respectively. AUC values are also dose-proportional over this dose range and the mean time to maximum concentration (t_{max}) is approximately 2.5 hours for all dose strengths. Following oral administration, the terminal elimination half-life ($t_{1/2}$) for cerivastatin is 2 to 3 hours. Steady-state plasma concentrations show no evidence of cerivastatin accumulation following administration of up to 0.40 mg daily.

Results from an overnight pharmacokinetic evaluation following single-dose administration of cerivastatin with the evening meal or 4 hours after the evening meal showed that administration of cerivastatin with the evening meal did not significantly alter either AUC or C_{max} compared to dosing the drug 4 hours after the evening meal. In patients given 0.2 mg cerivastatin sodium once daily for 4 weeks, either at mealtime or at bedtime, there were no differences in the lipid-lowering effects of cerivastatin. Both regimens of 0.2 mg once daily were slightly more efficacious than 0.1 mg twice daily.

Distribution: The volume of distribution (VD_{SS}) is calculated to be 0.3 L/kg. More than 99% of the circulating drug is bound to plasma proteins (80% to albumin). Binding is reversible and independent of drug concentration up to 100 mg/L.

Metabolism: Biotransformation pathways for cerivastatin in humans include the following: demethylation of the benzylic methyl ether to form M1 and hydroxylation of the methyl group in the 6′-isopropyl moiety to form M23. The combination of both reactions leads to formation of metabolite M24. The major circulating blood components are cerivastatin and the pharmacologically active M1 and M23 metabolites. The relative potencies of metabolites M1 and M23 are approximately 50% and 80% of the parent compound, respectively. Following a 0.3-mg dose of cerivastatin to 6 healthy volunteers, mean C_{max} values for cerivastatin, M1, and M23 were 3.0, 0.2, and 0.5 µg/L, respectively. Therefore, the cholesterol-lowering effect is due primarily to the parent compound, cerivastatin.

Excretion: Cerivastatin itself is not found in either urine or feces; M1, and M23 are the major metabolites excreted by these routes. Following an oral dose of 0.4 mg ^{14}C-cerivastatin to healthy volunteers, excretion of radioactivity is about 24% in the urine and 70% in the feces. The parent compound, cerivastatin, accounts for less than 2% of the total radioactivity excreted. The plasma clearance for cerivastatin in humans after intravenous dosing is 12 to 13 liters per hour.

SPECIAL POPULATIONS

Geriatric:	Plasma concentrations of cerivastatin are similar in healthy elderly male subjects (>65 years) and in young males (<40 years).
Gender:	Plasma concentrations of cerivastatin in females are slightly higher than in males (approximately 12% higher for C_{max} and 16% higher for AUC)
Pediatric:	Cerivastatin pharmacokinetics have not been studied in pediatric patients.
Race:	Cerivastatin pharmacokinetics were compared across studies in Caucasian, Japanese and Black subjects. No significant differences in AUC, C_{max}, t_{max} and $t_{1/2}$ were found.
Renal:	Steady-state plasma concentrations of cerivastatin are similar in healthy volunteers (Cl_{cr}>90 mL/min/1.73m²) and in patients with mild renal impairment (Cl_{cr} 61–90 mL/min/1.73m²). In patients with moderate (Cl_{cr} 31–60 mL/min/1.73m²) or severe (Cl_{cr}≤30 mL/min/1.73m²) renal impairment, AUC is up to 60% higher, C_{max} up to 23% higher, and $t_{1/2}$ up to 47% longer compared to subjects with normal renal function.
Hemodialysis:	While studies have not been conducted in patients with end-stage renal disease, hemodialysis is not expected to significantly enhance clearance of cerivastatin since the drug is extensively bound to plasma proteins.
Hepatic:	Cerivastatin has not been studied in patients with active liver disease (see CONTRAINDICATIONS). Caution should be exercised when BAYCOL™ (cerivastatin sodium tablets) is administered to patients with a history of liver disease or heavy alcohol ingestion (see WARNINGS).

Clinical Studies: BAYCOL™ (cerivastatin sodium tablets) has been studied in controlled trials in North America, Europe, Israel, and South Africa and has been shown to be effective in reducing plasma total cholesterol (Total-C) and LDL cholesterol (LDL-C) in heterozygous familial and non-familial forms of hypercholesterolemia and in mixed hyperlipidemia. Over 2,800 patients with Type IIa and IIb hypercholesterolemia were treated in trials of 4 to 104 weeks duration. In a 24-week, randomized, double-blind, placebo-controlled US trial in 934 patients with primary hypercholesterolemia, BAYCOL™ (cerivastatin sodium tablets) 0.05 to 0.3 mg once daily produced dose-related reductions in plasma LDL-C and Total-C. Significant reductions in mean total-C and LDL-C were evident after one week, peaked at four weeks, and were maintained for the duration

of the trial. Reductions in plasma triglycerides (TG) and increases in HDL-C were also observed. The results from this study in patients treated with the marketed doses of cerivastatin are summarized in Table 1.

Table 1
Response in Patients with Primary Hypercholesterolemia Mean Percent Change from Baseline after 24 Weeks

Dosage	n	Total-C	LDL-C	HDL-C	TG	Apo-B
Placebo	137*	+1.7	+1.8	+3.1	+1.1	+3.2
BAYCOL™						
0.2 mg qd**	143†	−17.4	−25.3	+10.4	−10.7	−18.7
0.3 mg qd**	135‡	−19.4	−28.2	+10.3	−12.7	−20.5

* 137 patients were evaluated for all parameters except LDL-C which had 136 patients
† 143 patients were evaluated for Total-C, HDL-C and TG. For LDL-C and Apo-B there were 140 and 141 patients evaluated, respectively.
‡ 135 patients were evaluated for all parameters except LDL-C which had 134 patients.
** qd = once daily

In a separate dose-scheduling study, BAYCOL™ (cerivastatin sodium tablets) was given as either a 0.2-mg dose once daily with dinner or at bedtime or as a 0.1-mg dose twice daily (morning and evening). Mean LDL-C reduction in response to BAYCOL dosed once with dinner or at bedtime was about 4% greater than the mean reduction in response to twice daily (divided) dosing ($p<0.05$).

INDICATIONS AND USAGE

Therapy with lipid-altering drugs should be a component of multiple risk factor intervention in those patients at significantly high risk for atherosclerotic vascular disease due to hypercholesterolemia. BAYCOL™ (cerivastatin sodium tablets) is indicated as an adjunct to diet for the reduction of elevated total and LDL cholesterol levels in patients with primary hypercholesterolemia and mixed dyslipidemia (Fredrickson Types IIa and IIb) when the response to dietary restriction of saturated fat and cholesterol and other non-pharmacological measures alone has been inadequate.

Before considering therapy with lipid-altering agents, secondary causes of hypercholesterolemia, e.g., poorly controlled diabetes mellitus, hypothyroidism, nephrotic syndrome, dysproteinemias, obstructive liver disease, other drug therapy, alcoholism, should be excluded and a lipid profile performed to measure Total-C, HDL-C, and triglycerides (TG). For patients with TG less than 400 mg/dL, LDL-C can be estimated using the following equation:

$$\text{LDL-C} = [\text{Total-C}] \text{ minus } [\text{HDL-C} + \text{TG}/5]$$

For TG levels > 400mg/dL, this equation is less accurate and LDL-C concentrations should be directly measured by preparative ultracentrifugation. In many hypertriglyceridemic patients, LDL-C may be low or normal despite elevated Total-C. In such cases, BAYCOL™ (cerivastatin sodium tablets) is not indicated.

Lipid determinations should be performed at intervals of no less than four weeks.

The National Cholesterol Education Program (NCEP) Treatment Guidelines are summarized in Table 2.

Table 2
National Cholesterol Education Program (NCEP) Treatment Guidelines
LDL-Cholesterol mg/dL (mmol/L)

Definite Atherosclerotic Disease*	Two or More Other Risk Factors**	Initiation Level***	Goal
NO	NO	≥190 (≥4.9)	<160 (<4.1)
NO	YES	≥160 (≥4.1)	<130 (<3.4)
YES	YES or NO	≥130 (≥3.4)	<100 (<2.6)

* Coronary heart disease or peripheral vascular disease (including symptomatic carotid artery disease).
** Other risk factors for coronary heart disease (CHD) include the following: age (males: ≥45 years; females: ≥55 years or premature menopause without estrogen replacement therapy); family history of premature CHD; current cigarette smoking; hypertension; confirmed HDL-C <35 mg/dL (<0.91mmol/L); and diabetes mellitus. Subtract one risk factor if HDL-C is ≥60mg/dL (≥1.6 mmol/L).
*** In CHD patients with LDL-C levels 100-129 mg/dL, the physician should exercise clinical judgment in deciding whether to initiate drug treatment.

At the time of hospitalization for an acute coronary event, consideration can be given to initiating drug therapy at discharge if the LDL-C level is ≥ 130 mg/dL (NCEP-ATP II).

Since the goal of treatment is to lower LDL-C, the NCEP recommends that LDL-C levels be used to initiate and assess treatment response. Only if LDL-C levels are not available, should the Total-C be used to monitor therapy.

Although BAYCOL may be useful to reduce elevated LDL-cholesterol levels in patients with combined hypercholesterolemia and hypertriglyceridemia where hypercholesterolemia is the major abnormality (Type IIb hyperlipoproteinemia), it has not been studied in conditions where the major abnormality is elevation of chylomicrons, VLDL, or IDL (i.e., hyperlipoproteinemia types I, III, IV, or V).[1]

CONTRAINDICATIONS

Active liver disease or unexplained persistent elevations of serum transaminases (see **WARNINGS**).

Pregnancy and lactation. Atherosclerosis is a chronic process, and the discontinuation of lipid-lowering drugs during pregnancy should have little impact on the outcome of long-term therapy of primary hypercholesterolemia. Moreover, cholesterol and other products of the cholesterol biosynthesis pathway are essential components for fetal development, including synthesis of steroids and cell membranes. Since HMG-CoA reductase inhibitors decrease cholesterol synthesis and possibly the synthesis of other biologically active substances derived from cholesterol, they may cause fetal harm when administered to pregnant women. Therefore, HMG-CoA reductase inhibitors are contraindicated during pregnancy and in nursing mothers. **Cerivastatin sodium should be administered to women of child-bearing age only when such patients are highly unlikely to conceive and have been informed of the potential hazards.** If the patient becomes pregnant while taking this drug, cerivastatin sodium should be discontinued and the patient should be apprised of the potential hazard to the fetus.

Hypersensitivity to any component of this medication.

WARNINGS

Liver Enzymes: HMG-CoA reductase inhibitors have been associated with biochemical abnormalities of liver function. Persistent increases of serum transaminase (ALT, AST) values to more than 3 times the upper limit of normal (occurring on two or more not necessarily sequential occasions) have been reported in less than 1.0% of patients treated with cerivastatin sodium in the US over an average period of 11 months. Most of these abnormalities occurred within the first 6 weeks of treatment, resolved after discontinuation of the drug, and were not associated with cholestasis. In most cases, these biochemical abnormalities were asymptomatic.

It is recommended that liver function tests be performed before the initiation of treatment, at 6 and 12 weeks after initiation of therapy or elevation in dose, and periodically thereafter e.g., semiannually. Patients who develop increased transaminase levels should be monitored with a second liver function evaluation to confirm the finding and be followed thereafter with frequent liver function tests until the abnormality(ies) return to normal. Should an increase in AST or ALT of three times the upper limit of normal or greater persist, withdrawal of cerivastatin sodium therapy is recommended.

Active liver disease or unexplained transaminase elevations are contraindications to the use of BAYCOL™ (cerivastatin sodium tablets) (see **CONTRAINDICATIONS**). Caution should be exercised when cerivastatin sodium is administered to patients with a history of liver disease or heavy alcohol ingestion (see **CLINICAL PHARMACOLOGY: Pharmacokinetics/Metabolism**). Such patients should be started at the low end of the recommended dosing range and closely monitored.

Skeletal Muscle: **Rare cases of rhabdomyolysis with acute renal failure secondary to myoglobinuria have been reported with other HMG-CoA reductase inhibitors.** Myopathy, defined as muscle aching or muscle weakness, associated with increases in plasma creatine kinase (CK) values to greater than 10 times the upper limit of normal, was rare (<0.2%) in U.S. cerivastatin clinical trials. Myopathy should be considered in any patient with diffuse myalgias, muscle tenderness or weakness, and/or marked elevation of CK. Patients should be advised to report promptly unexplained muscle pain, tenderness, or weakness, particularly if accompanied by malaise or fever. BAYCOL™ (cerivastatin sodium tablets) therapy should be discontinued if markedly elevated CK levels occur or myopathy is diagnosed or suspected. **BAYCOL™ (cerivastatin sodium tablets) should be temporarily withheld in any patient experiencing an acute or serious condition predisposing to the development of renal failure secondary to rhabdomyolysis, e.g., sepsis; hypotension; major surgery; trauma; severe metabolic, endocrine or electrolyte disorders; or uncontrolled epilepsy.**

The risk of myopathy during treatment with other HMG-CoA reductase inhibitors is increased with concurrent administration of cyclosporine, fibric acid derivatives, erythromycin, azole antifungals or lipid-lowering doses of niacin.

Uncomplicated myalgia has been observed infrequently in patients treated with cerivastatin sodium at rates that could not be distinguished from placebo.

The use of fibrates alone occasionally may be associated with myopathy. The combined use of HMG-CoA inhibitors and fibrates generally should be avoided.

PRECAUTIONS

General: Before instituting therapy with BAYCOL™ (cerivastatin sodium tablets), an attempt should be made to control hypercholesterolemia with appropriate diet, exercise, weight reduction in obese patients, and treatment of underlying medical problems (see INDICATIONS AND USAGE).

Cerivastatin sodium may elevate creatine kinase and transaminase levels (see ADVERSE REACTIONS). This should be considered in the differential diagnosis of chest pain in a patient on therapy with cerivastatin sodium.

Homozygous Familial Hypercholesterolemia: Cerivastatin sodium has not been evaluated in patients with rare homozygous familial hypercholesterolemia. HMG-CoA reductase inhibitors have been reported to be less effective in these patients because they lack functional LDL receptors.

Information for Patients: Patients should be advised to report promptly unexplained muscle pain, tenderness, or weakness, particularly if accompanied by malaise or fever.

Drug Interactions: Immunosuppressive Drugs, Fibric Acid Derivatives, Niacin (Nicotinic Acid), Erythromycin, Azole Antifungals: See WARNINGS: Skeletal Muscle.

ANTACID (Magnesium-Aluminum Hydroxide): Cerivastatin plasma concentrations were not affected by co-administration of antacid.

CIMETIDINE: Cerivastatin plasma concentrations were not affected by co-administration of cimetidine.

CHOLESTYRAMINE: The influence of the bile-acid-sequestering agent cholestyramine on the pharmacokinetics of cerivastatin sodium was evaluated in 12 healthy males in 2 separate randomized crossover studies. In the first study, concomitant administration of 0.2 mg cerivastatin sodium and 12 g cholestyramine resulted in decreases of more than 22% for AUC and 40% for C_{max} when compared to dosing cerivastatin sodium alone. However, in the second study, administration of 12 g cholestyramine 1 hour before the evening meal and 0.3 mg cerivastatin sodium approximately 4 hours after the same evening meal resulted in a decrease in the cerivastatin AUC of less than 8%, and a decrease in C_{max} of about 30% when compared to dosing cerivastatin sodium alone. Therefore, it would be expected that a dosing schedule of cerivastatin sodium given at bedtime and cholestyramine given before the evening meal would not result in a significant decrease in the clinical effect of cerivastatin sodium.

DIGOXIN: Plasma digoxin levels and digoxin clearance at steady-state were not affected by co-administration of 0.2 mg cerivastatin sodium. Cerivastatin plasma concentrations were also not affected by co-administration of digoxin.

WARFARIN: Co-administration of warfarin and cerivastatin to healthy volunteers did not result in any changes in prothrombin time or clotting factor VII when compared to co-administration of warfarin and placebo. The AUC and C_{max} of both the (R) and (S) isomers of warfarin were unaffected by concurrent dosing of 0.3 mg cerivastatin sodium. Co-administration of warfarin and cerivastatin did not alter the pharmacokinetics of cerivastatin sodium.

ERYTHROMYCIN: In hypercholesterolemic patients, steady-state cerivastatin AUC and C_{max} increased approximately 50% and 24% respectively after 10 days with co-administration of erythromycin, a known inhibitor of cytochrome P450 3A4.

OTHER CONCOMITANT THERAPY: Although specific interaction studies were not performed, in clinical studies, cerivastatin sodium was used concomitantly with angiotensin-converting enzyme (ACE) inhibitors, beta-blockers, calcium-channel blockers, diuretics, and nonsteroidal anti-inflammatory drugs (NSAIDs) without evidence of clinically significant adverse interactions.

Endocrine Function: HMG-CoA reductase inhibitors interfere with cholesterol synthesis and lower cholesterol levels and, as such, might theoretically blunt adrenal or gonadal steroid hormone production.

Clinical studies have shown that cerivastatin sodium has no adverse effect on sperm production and does not reduce basal plasma cortisol concentration, impair adrenal reserve or have an adverse effect on thyroid metabolism as assessed by TSH. Results of clinical trials with drugs in this class have been inconsistent with regard to drug effect on basal and reserve steroid levels. The effects of HMG-CoA reductase inhibitors on male fertility have not been studied in adequate numbers of male patients. The effects, if any, on the pituitary-gonadal axis in pre-menopausal women are unknown.

Patients treated with cerivastatin sodium who develop clinical evidence of endocrine dysfunction should be evaluated appropriately. Caution should be exercised if an HMG-CoA reductase inhibitor or other agent used to lower cholesterol levels is administered to patients also receiving other drugs that may decrease the levels or activity of endogenous steroid hormones, e.g., ketoconazole, spironolactone, or cimetidine.

CNS and other Toxicities: Chronic administration of cerivastatin to rodent and non-rodent species demonstrated the principal toxicologic targets and effects observed with other HMG-CoA reductase inhibitors: Hemorrhage and edema in multiple organs and tissues including CNS (dogs); cataracts

Continued on next page

Baycol—Cont.

(dogs); degeneration of muscle fibers (dogs, rats, and mice); hyperkeratosis in the nonglandular stomach (rats, and mice, this organ has no human equivalent); liver lesions (dogs, rats and mice).
CNS lesions were characterized by multifocal bleeding with fibrinoid degeneration of vessel walls in the plexus chorioideus of the brain stem and in the ciliary body of the eye at 0.1 mg/kg/day in the dog. This dose resulted in plasma levels of cerivastatin (C_{max}), that were about 23 times higher than the mean values in humans taking 0.3 mg/day. No CNS lesions were observed after chronic treatment with cerivastatin for up to two years in the mouse (C_{max} up to 7 times that of humans at 0.3 mg/day) and rat (C_{max} up to 2 times that of humans).

Carcinogenesis, Mutagenesis, Impairment of Fertility: A 2-year study was conducted in rats at average daily doses of cerivastatin of 0.007, 0.034, or 0.158 mg/kg. The high dosage level corresponded to plasma drug levels (AUC) of approximately 1–2 times the mean human plasma drug concentrations after a 0.3-mg oral dose. Tumor incidences of treated rats were comparable to controls in all treatment groups. In a 2-year carcinogenicity study in mice with average daily doses of cerivastatin of 0.4, 1.8, 9.1, or 55 mg/kg hepatocellular adenomas were significantly increased in male and female mice at ≥9.1 mg/kg and hepatocellular carcinomas were significantly increased in male mice at ≥1.8 mg/kg. These doses were in the range of human exposure (dose of 0.3 mg/day).
No evidence of genotoxicity was observed *in vitro* with or without metabolic activation in the following assays: microbial mutagen tests using mutant strains of *S. typhimurium* or *E. coli*, Chinese Hamster Ovary Forward Mutation Assay, Unscheduled DNA Synthesis in rat primary hepatocytes, chromosome aberrations in Chinese Hamster Ovary cells, and spindle inhibition in human lymphocytes. In addition, there was no evidence of genotoxicity *in vivo* in a mouse Micronucleus Test; there was equivocal evidence of mutagenicity in a mouse Dominant Lethal Test.
In a combined male and female rat fertility study, cerivastatin had no adverse effects on fertility or reproductive performance at doses up to 0.1 mg/kg/day, a dose that produced plasma drug levels (C_{max}) about 1–2 times higher than mean plasma drug levels for humans receiving 0.3 mg cerivastatin/day. At a dose of 0.3 mg/kg/day (plasma C_{max} 4–5 times the human level), the length of gestation was marginally prolonged, stillbirths were increased, and the survival rate up to day 4 postpartum was decreased. In the fetuses (F1), a marginal reduction in fetal weight and delay in bone development was observed. In the mating of the F1 generation, there was a reduced number of female rats that littered.
In the testicles of dogs treated chronically with cerivastatin at a dose of 0.008 mg/kg/day (approximately 2 fold the human exposure at doses of 0.3 mg based on C_{max}), atrophy, vacuolization of the germinal epithelium, spermatidic giant cells, and focal oligospermia were observed. In another 1-year study in dogs treated with 0.1 mg/kg/day (approximately 23 fold the human exposure at doses of 0.3 mg based on C_{max}), ejaculate volume was small and libido was decreased. Semen analysis revealed an increased number of morphologically altered spermatozoa indicating disturbances of epididymal sperm maturation that was reversible when drug administration was discontinued.

Pregnancy: Pregnancy Category X: (See CONTRAINDICATIONS): Cerivastatin caused a significant increase in incomplete ossification of the lumbar center of the vertebrae in rats at an oral dose of 0.72 mg/kg. Cerivastatin did not cause any anomalies or malformations in rabbits at oral doses up to 0.75 mg/kg. These doses resulted in plasma levels (C_{max}) 6–7 times the human exposure for rats and 3–4 times the human exposure for rabbits (human dose 0.3 mg). Cerivastatin crossed the placenta and was found in fetal liver, gastrointestinal tract, and kidneys when pregnant rats were given a single oral dose of 2 mg/kg.
Safety in pregnant women has not been established. Cerivastatin should be administered to women of child-bearing potential only when such patients are highly unlikely to conceive and have been informed of the potential hazards. Rare reports of congenital anomalies have been received following intrauterine exposure to other HMG-CoA reductase inhibitors. In a review of approximately 100 prospectively followed pregnancies in women exposed to simvastatin or lovastatin, the incidences of congenital anomalies, spontaneous abortions and fetal deaths/stillbirths did not exceed what would be expected in the general population. The number of cases is adequate only to exclude a three- to fourfold increase in congenital anomalies over the background incidence. In 89% of the prospectively followed pregnancies, drug treatment was initiated prior to pregnancy and was discontinued at some point in the first trimester when pregnancy was identified. As safety in pregnant women has not been established and there is no apparent benefit to therapy with BAYCOL™ during pregnancy (see CONTRAINDICATIONS), treatment should be immediately discontinued as soon as pregnancy is recognized. If a women becomes pregnant while taking cerivastatin, the drug should be discontinued and the patient advised again as to potential hazards to the fetus.

Nursing Mothers: Based on preclinical data, cerivastatin is present in breast milk in a 1.3:1 ratio (milk:plasma). Because of the potential for serious adverse reactions in nursing infants, nursing women should not take cerivastatin (see CONTRAINDICATIONS).

Pediatric Use: Safety and effectiveness in pediatric patients have not been established.

Geriatric Use: In clinical pharmacology studies, there were no clinically relevant effects of age on the pharmacokinetics of cerivastatin sodium.

Renal Insufficiency: Patients with significant renal impairment (Cl_{cr} ≤ 60 mL/min/1.73m²) have increased AUC (up to 60%) and C_{max} (up to 23%) and should be administered BAYCOL™ with caution.

Hepatic Insufficiency: Safety and effectiveness in hepatically impaired patients have not been established. Cerivastatin should be used with caution in patients who have a history of liver disease and/or consume substantial quantities of alcohol (see Contraindications and Warnings).

ADVERSE REACTIONS

In the U.S. placebo-controlled clinical studies, discontinuations due to adverse events occurred in 3% of cerivastatin sodium treated patients and in 3% of patients treated with placebo. Adverse reactions have usually been mild and transient. Cerivastatin sodium has been evaluated for adverse events in more than 3,000 patients and is generally well-tolerated.

Clinical Adverse Experiences: Adverse experiences occurring with a frequency ≥2% for marketed doses of cerivastatin sodium, regardless of causality assessment, in U.S. placebo-controlled clinical studies, are shown in the Table 3 below:

Table 3
Adverse Experiences Occurring In ≥2% of Patients In U.S. Placebo-Controlled Clinical Studies

Adverse Event	BAYCOL™ (n=552)	Placebo (n=247)
Body as a Whole		
Headache	11.8%	12.6%
Accidental Injury	7.1%	6.9%
Flu Syndrome	6.3%	8.1%
Back Pain	4.0%	6.1%
Abdominal Pain	3.4%	3.6%
Asthenia	3.4%	2.8%
Chest Pain	2.9%	2.8%
Leg Pain	2.0%	1.2%
Cardiovascular		
Peripheral Edema	2.0%	1.2%
Digestive		
Dyspepsia	5.6%	4.9%
Diarrhea	4.0%	3.6%
Flatulence	3.4%	3.6%
Nausea	2.7%	3.2%
Constipation	1.8%	2.0%
Surgery	1.4%	3.6%
Musculoskeletal		
Arthralgia	6.7%	4.5%
Myalgia	2.7%	1.2%
Nervous		
Dizziness	2.5%	3.6%
Insomnia	2.2%	1.2%
Respiratory		
Rhinitis	13.2%	12.1%
Pharyngitis	12.0%	17.0%
Sinusitis	6.9%	5.7%
Cough Increased	2.7%	2.0%
Skin and Appendages		
Rash	3.4%	5.7%
Urogenital		
Urinary Tract Infection	1.6%	2.4%

The following effects have been reported with drugs in this class.
Skeletal: myopathy, muscle cramps, rhabdomyolysis, arthralgias, myalgia.
Neurological: dysfunction of certain cranial nerves (including alteration of taste, impairment of extra-ocular movement, facial paresis), tremor, dizziness, memory loss, vertigo, paresthesia, peripheral neuropathy, peripheral nerve palsy, anxiety, insomnia, depression, psychic disturbances.
Hypersensitivity Reactions: An apparent hypersensitivity syndrome has been reported rarely that included one or more of the following features: anaphylaxis, angioedema, lupus erythematosus-like syndrome, polymyalgia rheumatica, dermatomyositis, vasculitis, purpura, thrombocytopenia, leukopenia, hemolytic anemia, positive ANA, ESR increase, eosinophilia, arthritis, arthralgia, urticaria, asthenia, photosensitivity, fever, chills, flushing, malaise, dyspnea, toxic epidermal necrolysis, erythema multiforme, including Stevens-Johnson syndrome.
Gastrointestinal: pancreatitis, hepatitis, including chronic active hepatitis, cholestatic jaundice, fatty change in liver, and, rarely, cirrhosis, fulminant hepatic necrosis, and hepatoma; anorexia, vomiting.
Skin: alopecia, pruritus. A variety of skin changes, e.g., nodules, discoloration, dryness of skin/mucous membranes, changes to hair/nails, have been reported.
Reproductive: gynecomastia, loss of libido, erectile dysfunction.
Eye: progression of cataracts (lens opacities), ophthalmoplegia.
Laboratory Abnormalities: elevated transaminases, alkaline phosphatase, γ-glutamyl transpeptidase, and bilirubin; thyroid function abnormalities.

Concomitant Therapy: In studies where cerivastatin sodium has been administered concomitantly with cholestyramine, no adverse reactions unique to this combination or in addition to those previously reported for this class of drugs were reported. Myopathy and rhabdomyolysis (with or without acute renal failure) have been reported when another HMG-CoA reductase inhibitor was used in combination with immunosuppressive drugs, fibric acid derivatives, erythromycin, azole antifungals or lipid-lowering doses of nicotinic acid. Concomitant therapy with HMG-CoA reductase inhibitors and these agents is generally not recommended (*See* WARNINGS: *Skeletal Muscle*).

OVERDOSAGE

The maximum single oral dose of cerivastatin sodium received by healthy volunteers and patients is 0.4 mg.
No specific recommendations concerning the treatment of an overdosage can be made. Should an overdose occur, it should be treated symptomatically and supportive measures should be undertaken as required.
Dialysis of cerivastatin sodium is not expected to significantly enhance clearance since the drug is extensively (99%) bound to plasma proteins.

DOSAGE AND ADMINISTRATION

The patient should be placed on a standard cholesterol-lowering diet before receiving cerivastatin sodium and should continue on this diet during treatment with cerivastatin sodium. (See NCEP Treatment Guidelines for details on dietary therapy).
The recommended starting dose is 0.3 mg once daily in the evening. Cerivastatin sodium may be taken with or without food. The recommended starting dose in patients with significant renal impairment (creatinine clearance ≤60 mL/min/1.73m²) is 0.2 mg once daily in the evening.
Since the maximal effect of cerivastatin sodium is seen within 4 weeks, lipid determinations should be performed at this time.

Concomitant Therapy: The lipid-lowering effects of LDL-C and Total-C are additive when cerivastatin sodium is combined with a bile-acid-binding resin. When co-administering cerivastatin sodium and a bile-acid-exchange resin, e.g., cholestyramine, cerivastatin sodium should be given at least 2 hours after the resin (*See also* ADVERSE REACTIONS: *Concomitant Therapy*).

Dosage in Patients with Renal Insufficiency: No dose adjustment is necessary for patients with mild renal dysfunction (Cl_{cr} 61–90 mL/min/1.73m²). For patients with moderate or severe renal dysfunction, a starting dose of 0.2 mg is recommended (see CLINICAL PHARMACOLOGY—Special Populations – Renal).

HOW SUPPLIED

BAYCOL™ (cerivastatin sodium tablets) is supplied as 0.2-mg and 0.3-mg tablets. The different tablet strengths can be identified as follows:

Strength	Color	Markings Front	Markings Back
0.2 mg	light yellow	283	200 MCG
0.3 mg	yellow brown	284	300 MCG

BAYCOL™ (cerivastatin sodium tablets) is supplied as follows:
Bottles of 100: 0.2 mg (NDC 0026-2883-51)
0.3 mg (NDC 0026-2884-51)
The tablets should be protected from moisture and stored below 77°F (25°C). Dispense in tight containers.

References:
[1]Classification of Hyperlipoproteinemias

Type	Lipoproteins Elevated	Lipid Elevations major	Lipid Elevations minor
I (rare)	chylomicrons	TG	↑→C
IIa	LDL	C	—
IIb	LDL, VLDL	C	TG
III (rare)	IDL	C/TG	—
IV	VLDL	TG	↑→C
V (rare)	chylomicrons, VLDL	TG	↑→C

C=cholesterol, TG=triglycerides, LDL=low-density lipoprotein, VLDL=very-low-density lipoprotein, IDL=intermediate-density lipoprotein.

Caution: Federal (USA) Law prohibits dispensing without a prescription.
Bayer Corporation
Pharmaceutical Division
400 Morgan Lane
West Haven, CT 06516 USA
Made in Germany
PZ500041 7/97 © 1997 Bayer Corporation 7422
Shown in Product Identification Guide, page 305

BILTRICIDE® Tablets ℞
(praziquantel)

DESCRIPTION
BILTRICIDE® (praziquantel) is a trematodicide provided in tablet form for the oral treatment of schistosome infections and infections due to liver fluke.
BILTRICIDE® (praziquantel) is 2-(cyclohexylcarbonyl)-1,2,3,6,7, 11b-hexahydro-4H-pyrazino [2, 1-a] isoquinolin-4-one with the molecular formula; $C_{19}H_{24}N_2O_2$. The structural formula is as follows:

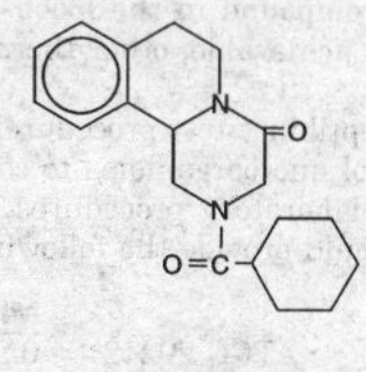

Praziquantel is a white to nearly white crystalline powder of bitter taste. The compound is stable under normal conditions and melts at 136–140°C with decomposition. The active substance is hygroscopic. Praziquantel is easily soluble in chloroform and dimethylsulfoxide, soluble in ethanol and very slightly soluble in water.
BILTRICIDE® tablets contain 600 mg of praziquantel. Inactive ingredients: corn starch, magnesium stearate, microcrystalline cellulose, povidone, sodium lauryl sulfate, polyethylene glycol, titanium dioxide and HPM cellulose.

CLINICAL PHARMACOLOGY
BILTRICIDE® induces a rapid contraction of schistosomes by a specific effect on the permeability of the cell membrane. The drug further causes vacuolization and disintegration of the schistosome tegument.
After oral administration BILTRICIDE® is rapidly absorbed (80%), subjected to a first pass effect, metabolized and eliminated by the kidneys. Maximal serum concentration is achieved 1–3 hours after dosing. The half-life of praziquantel in serum is 0.8–1.5 hours.

INDICATIONS AND USAGE
BILTRICIDE® is indicated for the treatment of infections due to: all species of schistosoma (e.g. *Schistosoma mekongi, Schistosoma japonicum, Schistosoma mansoni* and *Schistosoma hematobium),* and infections due to the liver flukes, *Clonorchis sinensis / Opisthorchis viverrini* (approval of this indication was based on studies in which the two species were not differentiated).

CONTRAINDICATIONS
BILTRICIDE® should not be given to patients who previously have shown hypersensitivity to the drug. Since parasite destruction within the eye may cause irreparable lesions, ocular cysticercosis should not be treated with this compound.

PRECAUTIONS
Information for the patient: Patients should be warned not to drive a car and not to operate machinery on the day of BILTRICIDE® treatment and the following day.
Minimal increases in liver enzymes have been reported in some patients.
When schistosomiasis or fluke infection is found to be associated with cerebral cysticercosis it is advised to hospitalize the patient for the duration of treatment.
Drug Interactions: No data are available regarding interaction of BILTRICIDE® with other drugs.
Mutagenesis, Carcinogenesis: Mutagenic effects in Salmonella tests found by one laboratory have not been confirmed in the same tested strain by other laboratories. Long term carcinogenicity studies in rats and golden hamsters did not reveal any carcinogenic effect.
Pregnancy Category B: Reproduction studies have been performed in rats and rabbits at doses up to 40 times the human dose and have revealed no evidence of impaired fertility or harm to the fetus due to BILTRICIDE®. There are, however, no adequate and well-controlled studies in pregnant women. An increase of the abortion rate was found in rats at three times the single human therapeutic dose. While animal reproduction studies are not always predictive of human response, this drug should be used during pregnancy only if clearly needed.
Nursing mothers: BILTRICIDE® appeared in the milk of nursing women at a concentration of about $^1/_4$ that of maternal serum. Women should not nurse on the day of BILTRICIDE® treatment and during the subsequent 72 hours.
Pediatric use: Safety in children under 4 years of age has not been established.

ADVERSE EFFECTS
In general BILTRICIDE® is very well tolerated. Side effects are usually mild and transient and do not require treatment. The following side effects were observed generally in order of severity: malaise, headache, dizziness, abdominal discomfort with or without nausea, rise in temperature and, rarely, urticaria. Such symptoms can, however, also result from the infection itself. Such side effects may be more frequent and/or serious in patients with a heavy worm burden. In patients with liver impairment caused by the infection, no adverse effects of BILTRICIDE® have occurred which would necessitate restriction in use.

OVERDOSAGE
In rats and mice the acute LD_{50} was about 2,500 mg/kg. No data are available in humans. In the event of overdose a fast-acting laxative should be given.

DOSAGE AND ADMINISTRATION
The dosage recommended for the treatment of schistosomiasis is: 3 × 20 mg/kg bodyweight as a one day treatment. The recommended dose for clonorchiasis and opisthorchiasis is: 3 × 25 mg/kg as a one day treatment. The tablets should be washed down unchewed with some liquid during meals. Keeping the tablets or segments thereof in the mouth can reveal a bitter taste which can promote gagging or vomiting. The interval between the individual doses should not be less than 4 and not more than 6 hours.

HOW SUPPLIED
BILTRICIDE® is supplied as a 600 mg white to orange tinged, filmcoated, oblong tablets with three scores. The tablet is coded with "BAYER" on one side and "LG" on the reverse side. When broken each of the four segments contain 150 mg of active ingredient so that the dosage can be easily adjusted to the patient's bodyweight.
Segments are broken off by pressing the score (notch) with thumbnails. If $^1/_4$ of a tablet is required, this is best achieved by breaking the segment from the outer end.
BILTRICIDE® is available in bottles of 6 tablets.

	Strength	NDC
Bottles of 6:	600 mg	0026-2521-06

Store below 86°F (30°C).
Bayer Corporation
Pharmaceutical Division
400 Morgan Lane
West Haven, CT 06516 USA
Made in Germany
Caution: Federal (USA) law prohibits dispensing without a prescription.
PD500021 10/96 EMBAY 8440 6788
© 1996 Bayer Corporation
Shown in Product Identification Guide, page 305

CIPRO® ℞
(ciprofloxacin hydrochloride)
TABLETS
CIPRO®
(ciprofloxacin) 5% and 10%
ORAL SUSPENSION

DESCRIPTION
CIPRO® (ciprofloxacin hydrochloride) Tablets and CIPRO® (ciprofloxacin) Oral Suspension are synthetic broad spectrum antimicrobial agents for oral administration. Ciprofloxacin hydrochloride, USP, a fluoroquinolone, is the monohydrochloride monohydrate salt of 1-cyclopropyl-6-fluoro-1,4-dihydro-4-oxo-7-(1-piperazinyl)-3-quinolinecarboxylic acid. It is a faintly yellowish to light yellow crystalline substance with a molecular weight of 385.8. Its empirical formula is $C_{17}H_{18}FN_3O_3 \bullet HCl \bullet H_2O$ and its chemical structure is as follows:

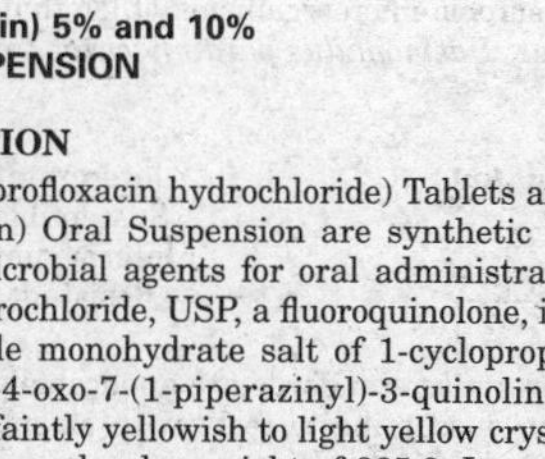

Ciprofloxacin is 1-cyclopropyl-6-fluoro-1, 4-dihydro-4-oxo-7-(1-piperazinyl)-3-quinolinecarboxylic acid. Its empirical formula is $C_{17}H_{18}FN_3O_3$ and its molecular weight is 331.4. It is a faintly yellowish to light yellow crystalline substance and its chemical structure is as follows:
[See chemical structure at top of next column]
Ciprofloxacin differs from other quinolones in that it has a fluorine atom at the 6-position, a piperazine moiety at the 7-position, and a cyclopropyl ring at the 1-position.

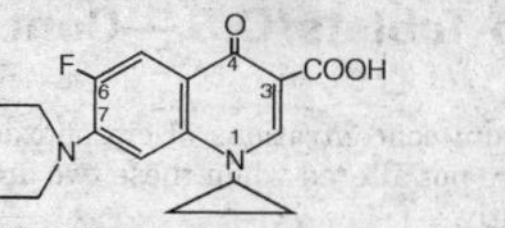

CIPRO® film-coated tablets are available in 100-mg, 250-mg, 500-mg and 750-mg (ciprofloxacin equivalent) strengths. The inactive ingredients are starch, microcrystalline cellulose, silicon dioxide, crospovidone, magnesium stearate, hydroxypropyl methylcellulose, titanium dioxide, polyethylene glycol and water.
Ciprofloxacin Oral Suspension is available in 5% (5 g ciprofloxacin in 100 mL) and 10% (10 g ciprofloxacin in 100 mL) strengths. Ciprofloxacin Oral Suspension is a white to slightly yellowish suspension with strawberry flavor which may contain yellow-orange droplets. It is composed of ciprofloxacin microcapsules and diluent which are mixed prior to dispensing (See instructions for USE/HANDLING). The components of the suspension have the following compositions:
Microcapsules - ciprofloxacin, polyvinylpyrrolidone, methacrylic acid copolymer, hydroxypropyl methylcellulose, magnesium stearate, and Polysorbate 20.
Diluent - medium-chain triglycerides, sucrose, lecithin, water, and strawberry flavor.

CLINICAL PHARMACOLOGY
Ciprofloxacin given as an oral tablet is rapidly and well absorbed from the gastrointestinal tract after oral administration. The absolute bioavailability is approximately 70% with no substantial loss by first pass metabolism. Ciprofloxacin maximum serum concentrations and area under the curve are shown in the chart for the 250-mg to 1000-mg dose range.

Dose (mg)	Maximum Serum Concentration (µg/mL)	Area Under Curve (AUC) (µg • hr/mL)
250	1.2	4.8
500	2.4	11.6
750	4.3	20.2
1000	5.4	30.8

Maximum serum concentrations are attained 1 to 2 hours after oral dosing. Mean concentrations 12 hours after dosing with 250, 500, or 750-mg are 0.1, 0.2, and 0.4 µg/mL, respectively. The serum elimination half-life in subjects with normal renal function is approximately 4 hours. Serum concentrations increase proportionately with doses up to 1000-mg. The serum elimination half-life in subjects with normal renal function is approximately 4 hours. Approximately 40 to 50% of an orally administered dose is excreted in the urine as unchanged drug. After a 250-mg oral dose, urine concentrations of ciprofloxacin usually exceed 200 mg/mL during the first two hours and are approximately 30 mg/mL at 8 to 12 hours after dosing. The urinary excretion of ciprofloxacin is virtually complete within 24 hours after dosing. The renal clearance of ciprofloxacin, which is approximately 300 mL/minute, exceeds the normal glomerular filtration rate of 120 mL/minute. Thus, active tubular secretion would seem to play a significant role in its elimination. Co-administration of probenecid with ciprofloxacin results in about a 50% reduction in the ciprofloxacin renal clearance and a 50% increase in its concentration in the systemic circulation. Although bile concentrations of ciprofloxacin are several fold higher than serum concentrations after oral dosing, only a small amount of the dose administered is recovered from the bile as unchanged drug. An additional 1 to 2% of the dose is recovered from the bile in the form of metabolites. Approximately 20 to 35% of an oral dose is recovered from the feces within 5 days after dosing. This may arise from either biliary clearance of transintestinal elimination. Four metabolites have been identified in human urine which together account for approximately 15% of an oral dose. The metabolites have antimicrobial activity, but are less active than unchanged ciprofloxacin.
With oral administration, a 500-mg dose, given as 10 mL of the 5% CIPRO® Suspension (containing 250-mg ciprofloxacin/5mL) is bioequivalent to the 500-mg tablet. A 10 mL volume of the 5% CIPRO® Suspension (containing 250-mg ciprofloxacin/5mL) is bioequivalent to a 5 mL volume of the 10% CIPRO® Suspension (containing 500-mg ciprofloxacin/5mL).
When CIPRO® Tablet is given concomitantly with food, there is a delay in the absorption of the drug, resulting in peak concentrations that occur closer to 2 hours after dosing rather than 1 hour whereas there is no delay observed when CIPRO® Suspension is given with food. The overall absorption of CIPRO® Tablet or CIPRO® Suspension, however, is not substantially affected. The pharmacokinetics of ciprofloxacin given as the suspension are also not afftected by food. Concurrent administration of antacids containing magnesium hydroxide or aluminum hydroxide may reduce the bioavailability of ciprofloxacin by as much as 90%. (See **PRECAUTIONS**.)

Continued on next page

Cipro Tablets/O.S.—Cont.

The serum concentrations of ciprofloxacin and metronidazole were not altered when these two drugs were given concomitantly.

Concomitant administration of ciprofloxacin with theophylline decreases the clearance of theophylline resulting in elevated serum theophylline levels and increased risk of a patient developing CNS or other adverse reactions. Ciprofloxacin also decreases caffeine clearance and inhibits the formation of paraxanthine after caffeine administration. (See **PRECAUTIONS**.)

In patients with reduced renal function, the half-life of ciprofloxacin is slightly prolonged. Dosage adjustments may be required. (See **DOSAGE AND ADMINISTRATION**.)

In preliminary studies in patients with stable chronic liver cirrhosis, no significant changes in ciprofloxacin pharmacokinetics have been observed. The kinetics of ciprofloxacin in patients with acute hepatic insufficiency, however, have not been fully elucidated.

The binding of ciprofloxacin to serum proteins is 20 to 40% which is not likely to be high enough to cause significant protein binding interactions with other drugs.

After oral administration, ciprofloxacin is widely distributed throughout the body. Tissue concentrations often exceed serum concentrations in both men and women, particularly in genital tissue including the prostate. Ciprofloxacin is present in active form in the saliva, nasal and bronchial secretions, mucosa of the sinuses, sputum, skin blister fluid, lymph, peritoneal fluid, bile, and prostatic secretions. Ciprofloxacin has also been detected in lung, skin, fat, muscle, cartilage, and bone. The drug diffuses into the cerebrospinal fluid (CSF); however, CSF concentrations are generally less than 10% of peak serum concentrations. Low levels of the drug have been detected in the aqueous and vitreous humors of the eye.

Microbiology: Ciprofloxacin has *in vitro* activity against a wide range of gram-negative and gram-positive organisms. The bactericidal action of ciprofloxacin results from interference with the enzyme DNA gyrase which is needed for the synthesis of bacterial DNA. Ciprofloxacin does not cross-react with other antimicrobial agents such as beta-lactams or aminoglycosides; therefore, organisms resistant to these drugs may be susceptible to ciprofloxacin. *In vitro* studies have shown that additive activity often results when ciprofloxacin is combined with other antimicrobial agents such as beta-lactams, aminoglycosides, clindamycin, or metronidazole. Synergy has been reported particularly with the combination of ciprofloxacin and a beta-lactam; antagonism is observed only rarely.

Ciprofloxacin has been shown to be active against most strains of the following microorganisms, both *in vitro* and in clinical infections as described in the **INDICATIONS AND USAGE** section of the package insert for CIPRO® (ciprofloxacin hydrochloride) Tablets and CIPRO® (ciprofloxacin) 5% and 10% Oral Suspension.

Aerobic gram-positive microorganisms

Enterococcus faecalis
   (Many strains are only moderately susceptible.)
Staphylococcus aureus (methicillin susceptible)
Staphylococcus epidermidis
Staphylococcus saprophyticus
Streptococcus pneumoniae
Streptococcus pyogenes

Aerobic gram-negative microorganisms

Campylobacter jejuni
Citrobacter diversus
Citrobacter freundii
Enterobacter cloacae
Escherichia coli
Haemophilus influenzae
Haemophilus parainfluenzae
Klebsiella pneumoniae
Moraxella catarrhalis
Morganella morganii
Neisseria gonorrhoeae
Proteus mirabilis
Proteus vulgaris
Providencia rettgeri
Providencia stuartii
Pseudomonas aeruginosa
Salmonella typhi
Serratia marcescens
Shigella boydii
Shigella dysenteriae
Shigella flexneri
Shigella sonnei

Ciprofloxacin has been shown to be active against most strains of the following microorganisms, both *in vitro* and in clinical infections as described in the **INDICATIONS AND USAGE** section of the package insert for CIPRO® I.V. (ciprofloxacin for intravenous infusion).

Aerobic gram-positive microorganisms

Enterococcus faecalis
   (Many strains are only moderately susceptible.)

Staphylococcus aureus (methicillin susceptible)
Staphylococcus epidermidis
Staphylococcus saprophyticus
Streptococcus pneumoniae
Streptococcus pyogenes

Aerobic gram-negative microorganisms

Citrobacter diversus
Citrobacter freundii
Enterobacter cloacae
Escherichia coli
Haemophilus influenzae
Haemophilus parainfluenzae
Klebsiella pneumoniae
Morganella morganii
Proteus mirabilis
Proteus vulgaris
Providencia rettgeri
Providencia stuartii
Pseudomonas aeruginosa
Serratia marcescens

The following *in vitro* data are available, **but their clinical significance is unknown.**

Ciprofloxacin exhibits *in vitro* minimum inhibitory concentrations (MICs) of 1 μg/mL or less against most (≥90%) strains of the following microorganisms; however, the safety and effectiveness of ciprofloxacin in treating clinical infections due to these microorganisms have not been established in adequate and well-controlled clinical trials.

Aerobic gram-positive microorganisms

Staphylococcus haemolyticus
Staphylococcus hominis

Aerobic gram-negative microorganisms

Acinetobacter lwoffi
Aeromonas hydrophila
Edwardsiella tarda
Enterobacter aerogenes
Klebsiella oxytoca
Legionella pneumophila
Pasteurella multocida
Salmonella enteritidis
Vibrio cholerae
Vibrio parahaemolyticus
Vibrio vulnificus
Yersinia enterocolitica

Most strains of *Burkholderia cepacia* and some strains of *Stenotrophomonas maltophilia* are resistant to ciprofloxacin as are most anaerobic bacteria, including *Bacteroides fragilis* and *Clostridium difficile*.

Ciprofloxacin is slightly less active when tested at acidic pH. The inoculum size has little effect when tested *in vitro*. The minimal bactericidal concentration (MBC) generally does not exceed the minimal inhibitory concentration (MIC) by more than a factor of 2. Resistance to ciprofloxacin *in vitro* develops slowly (multiple-step mutation).

Susceptibility Tests

Dilution Techniques: Quantitative methods are used to determine antimicrobial minimum inhibitory concentrations (MICs). These MICs provide estimates of the susceptibility of bacteria to antimicrobial compounds. The MICs should be determined using a standardized procedure. Standardized procedures are based on a dilution method[1] (broth or agar) or equivalent with standardized inoculum concentrations and standardized concentrations of ciprofloxacin powder. The MIC values should be interpreted according to the following criteria:

For testing aerobic microorganisms other than *Haemophilus influenzae*, *Haemophilus parainfluenzae*, and *Neisseria gonorrhoeae*[a]:

MIC (μg/mL)	Interpretation
≤ 1	Susceptible (S)
2	Intermediate (I)
≥ 4	Resistant (R)

[a] These interpretive standards are applicable only to broth microdilution susceptibility tests with streptococci using cation-adjusted Mueller-Hinton broth with 2–5% lysed horse blood.

For testing *Haemophilus influenzae* and *Haemophilus parainfluenzae*[b]:

MIC (μg/mL)	Interpretation
≤ 1	Susceptible (S)

[b] This interpretive standard is applicable only to broth microdilution susceptibility tests with *Haemophilus influenzae* and *Haemophilus parainfluenzae* using *Haemophilus* Test Medium[1].

The current absence of data on resistant strains precludes defining any results other than "Susceptible". Strains yielding MIC results suggestive of a "nonsusceptible" category should be submitted to a reference laboratory for further testing.

For testing *Neisseria gonorrhoeae*[c]:

MIC (μg/mL)	Interpretation
≤ 0.06	Susceptible (S)

[c] This interpretive standard is applicable only to agar dilution test with GC agar base and 1% defined growth supplement.

The current absence of data on resistant strains precludes defining any results other than "Susceptible". Strains yielding MIC results suggestive of a "nonsusceptible" category should be submitted to a reference laboratory for further testing.

A report of "Susceptible" indicates that the pathogen is likely to be inhibited if the antimicrobial compound in the blood reaches the concentrations usually achievable. A report of "Intermediate" indicates that the result should be considered equivocal, and, if the microorganism is not fully susceptible to alternative, clinically feasible drugs, the test should be repeated. This category implies possible clinical applicability in body sites where the drug is physiologically concentrated or in situations where high dosage of drug can be used. This category also provides a buffer zone which prevents small uncontrolled technical factors from causing major discrepancies in interpretation. A report of "Resistant" indicates that the pathogen is not likely to be inhibited if the antimicrobial compound in the blood reaches the concentrations usually achievable; other therapy should be selected.

Standardized susceptibility test procedures require the use of laboratory control microorganisms to control the technical aspects of the laboratory procedures. Standard ciprofloxacin powder should provide the following MIC values:

Organism		MIC (μg/mL)
E. faecalis	ATCC 29212	0.25 – 2.0
E. coli	ATCC 25922	0.004 – 0.015
H. influenzae[a]	ATCC 49247	0.004 – 0.03
N. gonorrhoeae[b]	ATCC 49226	0.001 – 0.008
P. aeruginosa	ATCC 27853	0.25 – 1.0
S. aureus	ATCC 29213	0.12 – 0.5

[a] This quality control range is applicable to only *H. influenzae* ATCC 49247 tested by a broth microdilution procedure using *Haemophilus* Test Medium (HTM)[1].

[b] This quality control range is applicable to only *N. gonorrhoeae* ATCC 49226 tested by an agar dilution procedure using GC agar base and 1% defined growth supplement.

Diffusion Techniques: Quantitative methods that require measurement of zone diameters also provide reproducible estimates of the susceptibility of bacteria to antimicrobial compounds. One such standardized procedure[2] requires the use of standardized inoculum concentrations. This procedure uses paper disks impregnated with 5-μg ciprofloxacin to test the susceptibility of microorganisms to ciprofloxacin. Reports from the laboratory providing results of the standard single-disk susceptibility test with a 5-μg ciprofloxacin disk should be interpreted according to the following criteria:

For testing aerobic microorganisms other than *Haemophilus influenzae*, *Haemophilus parainfluenzae*, and *Neisseria gonorrhoeae*[a]:

Zone Diameter (mm)	Interpretation
≥ 21	Susceptible (S)
16 – 20	Intermediate (I)
≤ 15	Resistant (R)

[a] These zone diameter standards are applicable only to tests performed for streptococci using Mueller-Hinton agar supplemented with 5% sheep blood incubated in 5% CO_2.

For testing *Haemophilus influenzae* and *Haemophilus parainfluenzae*[b]:

Zone Diameter (mm)	Interpretation
≥ 21	Susceptible (S)

[b] This zone diameter standard is applicable only to tests with *Haemophilus influenzae* and *Haemophilus parainfluenzae* using *Haemophilus* Test Medium (HTM)[2].

The current absence of data on resistant strains precludes defining any results other than "Susceptible". Strains yielding zone diameter results suggestive of a "nonsusceptible" category should be submitted to a reference laboratory for further testing.

For testing *Neisseria gonorrhoeae*[c]:

Zone Diameter (mm)	Interpretation
≥ 36	Susceptible (S)

[c] This zone diameter standard is applicable only to disk diffusion tests with GC agar base and 1% defined growth supplement.

The current absence of data on resistant strains precludes defining any results other than "Susceptible". Strains yielding zone diameter results suggestive of a "nonsusceptible" category should be submitted to a reference laboratory for further testing.

Interpretation should be as stated above for results using dilution techniques. Interpretation involves correlation of the diameter obtained in the disk test with the MIC for ciprofloxacin.

As with standardized dilution techniques, diffusion methods require the use of laboratory control microorganisms that are used to control the technical aspects of the laboratory procedures. For the diffusion technique, the 5-µg ciprofloxacin disk should provide the following zone diameters in these laboratory test quality control strains:

Organism		Zone Diameter (mm)
E. coli	ATCC 25922	30 – 40
H. influenzae[a]	ATCC 49247	34 – 42
N. gonorrhoeae[b]	ATCC 49226	48 – 58
P. aeruginosa	ATCC 27853	25 – 33
S. aureus	ATCC 25923	22 – 30

[a] These quality control limits are applicable to only *H. influenzae* ATCC 49247 testing using *Haemophilus Test Medium* (HTM)[2].
[b] These quality control limits are applicable only to tests conducted with *N. gonorrhoeae* ATCC 49226 performed by disk diffusion using GC agar base and 1% defined growth supplement.

INDICATIONS AND USAGE

CIPRO® is indicated for the treatment of infections caused by susceptible strains of the designated microorganisms in the conditions listed below. Please see **DOSAGE AND ADMINISTRATION** for specific recommendations.

Acute Sinusitis caused by *Haemophilus influenzae, Streptococcus pneumoniae,* or *Moraxella catarrhalis.*

Lower Respiratory Tract Infections caused by *Escherichia coli, Klebsiella pneumoniae, Enterobacter cloacae, Proteus mirabilis, Pseudomonas aeruginosa, Haemophilus influenzae, Haemophilus parainfluenzae,* or *Streptococcus pneumoniae.* Also, *Moraxella catarrhalis* for the treatment of acute exacerbations of chronic bronchitis.
NOTE: Although effective in clinical trials, ciprofloxacin is not a drug of first choice in the treatment of presumed or confirmed pneumonia secondary to *Streptococcus pneumoniae.*

Urinary Tract Infections caused by *Escherichia coli, Klebsiella pneumoniae, Enterobacter cloacae, Serratia marcescens, Proteus mirabilis, Providencia rettgeri, Morganella morganii, Citrobacter diversus, Citrobacter freundii, Pseudomonas aeruginosa, Staphylococcus epidermidis, Staphylococcus saprophyticus,* or *Enterococcus faecalis.*

Acute Uncomplicated Cystitis in females caused by *Escherichia coli* or *Staphylococcus saprophyticus.* (See **DOSAGE AND ADMINISTRATION.**)

Chronic Bacterial Prostatitis caused by *Escherichia coli* or *Proteus mirabilis.*

Complicated Intra-Abdominal Infections (used in combination with metronidazole) caused by *Escherichia coli, Pseudomonas aeruginosa, Proteus mirabilis, Klebsiella pneumoniae,* or *Bacteroides fragilis.* (See **DOSAGE AND ADMINISTRATION.**)

Skin and Skin Structure Infections caused by *Escherichia coli, Klebsiella pneumoniae, Enterobacter cloacae, Proteus mirabilis, Proteus vulgaris, Providencia stuartii, Morganella morganii, Citrobacter freundii, Pseudomonas aeruginosa, Staphylococcus aureus* (methicillin susceptible), *Staphylococcus epidermidis,* or *Streptococcus pyogenes.*

Bone and Joint Infections caused by *Enterobacter cloacae, Serratia marcescens,* or *Pseudomonas aeruginosa.*

Infectious Diarrhea caused by *Escherichia coli* (enterotoxigenic strains), *Campylobacter jejuni, Shigella boydii*, Shigella dysenteriae, Shigella flexneri* or *Shigella sonnei** when antibacterial therapy is indicated.

Typhoid Fever (Enteric Fever) caused by *Salmonella typhi.*
NOTE: The efficacy of ciprofloxacin in the eradication of the chronic typhoid carrier state has not been demonstrated.

Uncomplicated cervical and urethral gonorrhea due to *Neisseria gonorrhoeae.*

*Although treatment of infections due to this organism in this organ system demonstrated a clinically significant outcome, efficacy was studied in fewer than 10 patients.

If anaerobic organisms are suspected of contributing to the infection, appropriate therapy should be administered.
Appropriate culture and susceptibility tests should be performed before treatment in order to isolate and identify organisms causing infection and to determine their susceptibility to ciprofloxacin. Therapy with CIPRO® may be initiated before results of these tests are known; once results become available appropriate therapy should be continued.
As with other drugs, some strains of *Pseudomonas aeruginosa* may develop resistance fairly rapidly during treatment with ciprofloxacin. Culture and susceptibility testing performed periodically during therapy will provide information not only on the therapeutic effect of the antimicrobial agent but also on the possible emergence of bacterial resistance.

CONTRAINDICATIONS

CIPRO® (ciprofloxacin hydrochloride) is contraindicated in persons with a history of hypersensitivity to ciprofloxacin or any member of the quinolone class of antimicrobial agents.

WARNINGS

THE SAFETY AND EFFECTIVENESS OF CIPROFLOXACIN IN PEDIATRIC PATIENTS AND ADOLESCENTS (LESS THAN 18 YEARS OF AGE), PREGNANT WOMEN, AND LACTATING WOMEN HAVE NOT BEEN ESTABLISHED. (See **PRECAUTIONS: Pediatric Use, Pregnancy** and **Nursing Mothers** subsections.) The oral administration of ciprofloxacin caused lameness in immature dogs. Histopathological examination of the weight-bearing joints of these dogs revealed permanent lesions of the cartilage. Related quinolone-class drugs also produce erosions of cartilage of weight-bearing joints and other signs of arthropathy in immature animals of various species. (see **ANIMAL PHARMACOLOGY.**)

Convulsions, increased intracranial pressure, and toxic psychosis have been reported in patients receiving quinolones, including ciprofloxacin. Ciprofloxacin may also cause central nervous system (CNS) events including: dizziness, confusion, tremors, hallucinations, depression, and, rarely, suicidal thoughts or acts. These reactions may occur following the first dose. If these reactions occur in patients receiving ciprofloxacin, the drug should be discontinued and appropriate measures instituted. As with all quinolones, ciprofloxacin should be used with caution in patients with known or suspected CNS disorders that may predispose to seizures or lower the seizure threshold (e.g. severe cerebral arteriosclerosis, epilepsy), or in the presence of other risk factors that may predispose to seizures or lower the seizure threshold (e.g. certain drug therapy, renal dysfunction). See **PRECAUTIONS: General, Information for Patients, Drug Interactions** and **ADVERSE REACTIONS.**)

SERIOUS AND FATAL REACTIONS HAVE BEEN REPORTED IN PATIENTS RECEIVING CONCURRENT ADMINISTRATION OF CIPROFLOXACIN AND THEOPHYLLINE. These reactions have included cardiac arrest, seizure, status epilepticus, and respiratory failure. Although similar serious adverse effects have been reported in patients receiving theophylline alone, the possibility that these reactions may be potentiated by ciprofloxacin cannot be eliminated. If concomitant use cannot be avoided, serum levels of theophylline should be monitored and dosage adjustments made as appropriate.
Serious and occasionally fatal hypersensitivity (anaphylactic) reactions, some following the first dose, have been reported in patients receiving quinolone therapy. Some reactions were accompanied by cardiovascular collapse, loss of consciousness, tingling, pharyngeal or facial edema, dyspnea, urticaria, and itching. Only a few patients had a history of hypersensitivity reactions. Serious anaphylactic reactions require immediate emergency treatment with epinephrine. Oxygen, intravenous steroids, and airway management, including intubation, should be administered as indicated.
Severe hypersensitivity reactions characterized by rash, fever, eosinophilia, jaundice, and hepatic necrosis with fatal outcome have been rarely reported in patients receiving ciprofloxacin along with other drugs. The possibility that these reactions were related to ciprofloxacin cannot be excluded. Ciprofloxacin should be discontinued at the first appearance of a skin rash or any other sign of hypersensitivity.
Pseudomembranous colitis has been reported with nearly all antibacterial agents, including ciprofloxacin, and may range in severity from mild to life-threatening. Therefore, it is important to consider this diagnosis in patients who present with diarrhea subsequent to the administration of antibacterial agents.
Treatment with antibacterial agents alters the normal flora of the colon and may permit overgrowth of clostridia. Studies indicate that a toxin produced by *Clostridium difficile* is one primary cause of "antibiotic-associated colitis."
After the diagnosis of pseudomembranous colitis has been established, therapeutic measures should be initiated. Mild cases of pseudomembranous colitis usually respond to drug discontinuation alone. In moderate to severe cases, consideration should be given to management with fluids and electrolytes, protein supplementation, and treatment with an antibacterial drug clinically effective against *C. difficile* colitis.
Achilles and other tendon ruptures that required surgical repair or resulted in prolonged disability have been reported with ciprofloxacin and other quinolones. Ciprofloxacin should be discontinued if the patient experiences pain, inflammation, or rupture of a tendon.
Ciprofloxacin has not been shown to be effective in the treatment of syphilis. Antimicrobial agents used in high dose for short periods of time to treat gonorrhea may mask or delay the symptoms of incubating syphilis. All patients with gonorrhea should have a serologic test for syphilis at the time of diagnosis. Patients treated with ciprofloxacin should have a follow-up serologic test for syphilis after three months.

PRECAUTIONS

General: Crystals of ciprofloxacin have been observed rarely in the urine of human subjects but more frequently in the urine of laboratory animals, which is usually alkaline. (See **ANIMAL PHARMACOLOGY.**) Crystalluria related to ciprofloxacin has been reported only rarely in humans because human urine is usually acidic. Alkalinity of the urine should be avoided in patients receiving ciprofloxacin. Patients should be well hydrated to prevent the formation of highly concentrated urine.

Quinolones, including ciprofloxacin, may also cause central nervous system (CNS) events, including: nervousness, agitation, insomnia, anxiety, nightmares or paranoia. (See **WARNINGS, Information for Patients,** and **Drug Interactions.**)
Alteration of the dosage regimen is necessary for patients with impairment of renal function. (See **DOSAGE AND ADMINISTRATION.**)
Moderate to severe phototoxicity manifested as an exaggerated sunburn reaction has been observed in patients who are exposed to direct sunlight while receiving some members of the quinolone class of drugs. Excessive sunlight should be avoided. Therapy should be discontinued if phototoxicity occurs.
As with any potent drug, periodic assessment of organ system functions, including renal, hepatic, and hematopoietic function, is advisable during prolonged therapy.

Information for Patients:
Patients should be advised:
• that ciprofloxacin may be taken with or without meals. The preferred time of dosing is two hours after a meal. Patients should also be advised to drink fluids liberally and not take antacids containing magnesium, aluminum, or calcium, products containing iron, or multivitamins containing zinc. Ciprofloxacin should not be taken concurrently with milk or yogurt alone, since absorption of ciprofloxacin may be significantly reduced. Dietary calcium as part of a meal, however, does not significantly affect ciprofloxacin absorption.
• that ciprofloxacin may be associated with hypersensitivity reactions, even following a single dose, and to discontinue the drug at the first sign of a skin rash or other allergic reaction.
• to avoid excessive sunlight or artificial ultraviolet light while receiving ciprofloxacin and to discontinue therapy if phototoxicity occurs.
• to discontinue treatment; rest and refrain from exercise; and inform their physician if they experience pain, inflammation, or rupture of a tendon.
• that ciprofloxacin may cause dizziness and lightheadedness; therefore, patients should know how they react to this drug before they operate an automobile or machinery or engage in activities requiring mental alertness or coordination.
• that ciprofloxacin may increase the effects of theophylline and caffeine. There is a possibility of caffeine accumulation when products containing caffeine are consumed while taking quinolones.
• that convulsions have been reported in patients receiving quinolones, including ciprofloxacin, and to notify their physician before taking this drug if there is a history of this condition.

Drug Interactions: As with some other quinolones, concurrent administration of ciprofloxacin with theophylline may lead to elevated serum concentrations of theophylline and prolongation of its elimination half-life. This may result in increased risk of theophylline-related adverse reactions. (See **WARNINGS.**) If concomitant use cannot be avoided, serum levels of theophylline should be monitored and dosage adjustments made as appropriate.
Some quinolones, including ciprofloxacin, have also been shown to interfere with the metabolism of caffeine. This may lead to reduced clearance of caffeine and a prolongation of its serum half-life.
Concurrent administration of ciprofloxacin with antacids containing magnesium, aluminum, or calcium; with sucralfate or divalent and trivalent cations such as iron may substantially interfere with the absorption of ciprofloxacin, resulting in serum and urine levels considerably lower than desired. To a lesser extent this effect is demonstrated with zinc-containing multivitamins. (See **DOSAGE AND ADMINISTRATION** for concurrent administration of these agents with ciprofloxacin.)
Altered serum levels of phenytoin (increased and decreased) have been reported in patients receiving concomitant ciprofloxacin.
The concomitant administration of ciprofloxacin with the sulfonylurea glyburide has, on rare occasions, resulted in severe hypoglycemia.
Some quinolones, including ciprofloxacin, have been associated with transient elevations in serum creatinine in patients receiving cyclosporine concomitantly.
Quinolones have been reported to enhance the effects of the oral anticoagulant warfarin or its derivatives. When these products are administered concomitantly, prothrombin time or other suitable coagulation tests should be closely monitored.

Continued on next page

Cipro Tablets/O.S.—Cont.

DOSAGE GUIDELINES

Infection	Type or Severity	Unit Dose	Frequency	Usual Durations†
Acute Sinusitis	Mild/Moderate	500-mg	q 12 h	10 Days
Lower Respiratory Tract	Mild/Moderate	500-mg	q 12 h	7 to 14 Days
	Severe/Complicated	750-mg	q 12 h	7 to 14 Days
Urinary Tract	Acute Uncomplicated	100-mg	q 12 h	3 Days
	Mild/Moderate	250-mg	q 12 h	7 to 14 Days
	Severe/Complicated	500-mg	q 12 h	7 to 14 Days
Chronic Bacterial Prostatitis	Mild/Moderate	500-mg	q 12 h	28 Days
Intra-Abdominal*	Complicated	500-mg	q 12 h	7 to 14 Days
Skin and Skin Structure	Mild/Moderate	500-mg	q 12 h	7 to 14 Days
	Severe/Complicated	750-mg	q 12 h	7 to 14 Days
Bone and Joint	Mild/Moderate	500-mg	q 12 h	≥ 4 to 6 weeks
	Severe/Complicated	750-mg	q 12 h	≥ 4 to 6 weeks
Infectious Diarrhea	Mild/Moderate/Severe	500-mg	q 12 h	5 to 7 Days
Typhoid Fever	Mild/Moderate	500-mg	q 12 h	10 Days
Urethral and Cervical Gonococcal Infections	Uncomplicated	250-mg	single dose	single dose

* used in conjunction with metronidazole
† Generally ciprofloxacin should be continued for at least 2 days after the signs and symptoms of infection have disappeared.

Probenecid interferes with renal tubular secretion of ciprofloxacin and produces an increase in the level of ciprofloxacin in the serum. This should be considered if patients are receiving both drugs concomitantly.
As with other broad spectrum antimicrobial agents, prolonged use of ciprofloxacin may result in overgrowth of nonsusceptible organisms. Repeated evaluation of the patient's condition and microbial susceptibility testing is essential. If superinfection occurs during therapy, appropriate measures should be taken.

Carcinogenesis, Mutagenesis, Impairment of Fertility: Eight *in vitro* mutagenicity tests have been conducted with ciprofloxacin, and the test results are listed below:

- Salmonella/Microsome Test (Negative)
- *E. coli* DNA Repair Assay (Negative)
- Mouse Lymphoma Cell Forward Mutation Assay (Positive)
- Chinese Hamster V_{79} Cell HGPRT Test (Negative)
- Syrian Hamster Embryo Cell Transformation Assay (Negative)
- *Saccharomyces cerevisiae* Point Mutation Assay (Negative)
- *Saccharomyces cerevisiae* Mitotic Crossover and Gene Conversion Assay (Negative)
- Rat Hepatocyte DNA Repair Assay (Positive)

Thus, 2 of the 8 tests were positive, but results of the following 3 *in vivo* test systems gave negative results:

- Rat Hepatocyte DNA Repair Assay
- Micronucleus Test (Mice)
- Dominant Lethal Test (Mice)

Long-term carcinogenicity studies in mice and rats have been completed. After daily oral doses of 750 mg/kg (mice) and 250 mg/kg (rats) were administered for up to 2 years, there was no evidence that ciprofloxacin had any carcinogenic or tumorigenic effects in these species.
Results from photo co-carcinogenicity testing indicate that ciprofloxacin does not reduce the time to appearance of UV-induced skin tumors as compared to vehicle control. Hairless (Skh-1) mice were exposed to UVA light for 3.5 hours five times every two weeks for up to 78 weeks while concurrently being administered ciprofloxacin. The time to development of the first skin tumors was 50 weeks in mice treated concomitantly with UVA and ciprofloxacin (mouse dose approximately equal to maximum recommended human dose based upon mg/m^2), as opposed to 34 weeks when animals were treated with both UVA and vehicle. The times to development of skin tumors ranged from 16–32 weeks in mice treated concomitantly with UVA and other quinolones.[3]
In this model, mice treated with ciprofloxacin alone did not develop skin or systemic tumors. There are no data from similar models using pigmented mice and/or fully haired mice. The clinical significance of these findings to humans is unknown.
Fertility studies performed in rats at oral doses of ciprofloxacin up to 100 mg/kg (0.8 times the highest recommended human dose of 1200 mg based upon body surface area) revealed no evidence of impairment.

Pregnancy: Teratogenic Effects. Pregnancy Category C: Reproduction studies have been performed in rats and mice using oral doses up to 100 mg/kg (0.6 and 0.3 times the maximum daily human dose based upon body surface area, respectively) and have revealed no evidence of harm to the fetus due to ciprofloxacin. In rabbits, ciprofloxacin (30 and 100 mg/kg orally) produced gastrointestinal disturbances resulting in maternal weight loss and an increased incidence of abortion, but no teratogenicity was observed at either dose. After intravenous administration of doses up to 20 mg/kg, no maternal toxicity was produced in the rabbit, and no embryotoxicity or teratogenicity was observed. There are, however, no adequate and well-controlled studies in pregnant women. Ciprofloxacin should be used during pregnancy only if the potential benefit justifies the potential risk to the fetus. (See **WARNINGS**.)

Nursing Mothers: Ciprofloxacin is excreted in human milk. Because of the potential for serious adverse reactions in infants nursing from mothers taking ciprofloxacin, a decision should be made whether to discontinue nursing or to discontinue the drug, taking into account the importance of the drug to the mother.

Pediatric Use: Safety and effectiveness in pediatric patients and adolescents less than 18 years of age have not been established. Ciprofloxacin causes arthropathy in juvenile animals. (See **WARNINGS**.)
Short-term safety data from a single trial in pediatric cystic fibrosis patients are available. In a randomized, double-blind clinical trial for the treatment of acute pulmonary exacerbations in cystic fibrosis patients (ages 5–17 years), 67 patients received ciprofloxacin I.V. 10 mg/kg/dose q8h for one week followed by ciprofloxacin tablets 20 mg/kg/dose q12h to complete 10–21 days treatment and 62 patients received the combination of ceftazidime I.V. 50 mg/kg/dose q8h and tobramycin I.V. 3 mg/kg/dose q8h for a total of 10–21 days. Patients less than 5 years of age were not studied. Safety monitoring in the study included periodic range of motion examinations and gait assessments by treatment-blinded examiners. Patients were followed for an average of 23 days after completing treatment (range 0–93 days). This study was not designed to determine long term effects and the safety of repeated exposure to ciprofloxacin.
In the study, injection site reactions were more common in the ciprofloxacin group (24%) than in the comparison group (8%). Other adverse events were similar in nature and frequency between treatment arms. Musculoskeletal adverse events were reported in 22% of the patients in the ciprofloxacin group and 21% in the comparison group. Decreased range of motion was reported in 12% of the subjects in the ciprofloxacin group and 16% in the comparison group. Arthralgia was reported in 10% of the patients in the ciprofloxacin group and 11% in the comparison group. One of sixty-seven patients developed arthritis of the knee nine days after a ten day course of treatment with ciprofloxacin. Clinical symptoms resolved, but an MRI showed knee effusion without other abnormalities eight months after treatment. However, the relationship of this event to the patient's course of ciprofloxacin can not be definitively determined, particularly since patients with cystic fibrosis may develop arthralgias/arthritis as part of their underlying disease process.

ADVERSE REACTIONS

During clinical investigation with the tablet, 2,799 patients received 2,868 courses of the drug. Adverse events that were considered likely to be drug related occurred in 7.3% of patients treated, possibly related in 9.2% (total of 16.5% thought to be possibly or probably related to drug therapy), and remotely related in 3.0%. Ciprofloxacin was discontinued because of an adverse event in 3.5% of patients treated, primarily involving the gastrointestinal system (1.5%), skin (0.6%), and central nervous system (0.4%).
The most frequently reported events, drug related or not, were nausea (5.2%), diarrhea (2.3%), vomiting (2.0%), abdominal pain/discomfort (1.7%), headache (1.2%), restlessness (1.1%), and rash (1.1%).
Additional events that occurred in less than 1% of ciprofloxacin patients are listed below.

CARDIOVASCULAR: palpitation, atrial flutter, ventricular ectopy, syncope, hypertension, angina pectoris, myocardial infarction, cardiopulmonary arrest, cerebral thrombosis

CENTRAL NERVOUS SYSTEM: dizziness, lightheadedness, insomnia, nightmares, hallucinations, manic reaction, irritability, tremor, ataxia, convulsive seizures, lethargy, drowsiness, weakness, malaise, anorexia, phobia, depersonalization, depression, paresthesia (See above.) (See **PRECAUTIONS**.)

GASTROINTESTINAL: painful oral mucosa, oral candidiasis, dysphagia, intestinal perforation, gastrointestinal bleeding (See above.) Cholestatic jaundice has been reported.

MUSCULOSKELETAL: arthralgia or back pain, joint stiffness, achiness, neck or chest pain, flare up of gout

RENAL/UROGENITAL: interstitial nephritis, nephritis, renal failure, polyuria, urinary retention, urethral bleeding, vaginitis, acidosis

RESPIRATORY: dyspnea, epistaxis, laryngeal or pulmonary edema, hiccough, hemoptysis, bronchospasm, pulmonary embolism

SKIN/HYPERSENSITIVITY: pruritus, urticaria, photosensitivity, flushing, fever, chills, angioedema, edema of the face, neck, lips, conjunctivae or hands, cutaneous candidiasis, hyperpigmentation, erythema nodosum (See above.)

Allergic reactions ranging from urticaria to anaphylactic reactions have been reported. (See **WARNINGS**.)

SPECIAL SENSES: blurred vision, disturbed vision (change in color perception, overbrightness of lights), decreased visual acuity, diplopia, eye pain, tinnitus, hearing loss, bad taste

Most of the adverse events reported were described as only mild or moderate in severity, abated soon after the drug was discontinued, and required no treatment.
In several instances nausea, vomiting, tremor, irritability, or palpitation were judged by investigators to be related to elevated serum levels of theophylline possibly as a result of drug interaction with ciprofloxacin.
In domestic clinical trials involving 214 patients receiving a single 250–mg oral dose, approximately 5% of patients reported adverse experiences without reference to drug relationship. The most common adverse experiences were vaginitis (2%), headache (1%), and vaginal pruritus (1%). Additional reactions, occurring in 0.3%–1% of patients, were abdominal discomfort, lymphadenopathy, foot pain, dizziness, and breast pain. Less than 20% of these patients had laboratory values obtained, and these results were generally consistent with the pattern noted for multi-dose therapy.
In randomized, double-blind controlled clinical trials comparing ciprofloxacin tablets (500 mg BID) to cefuroxime axetil (250 mg – 500 mg BID) and to clarithromycin (500 mg BID) in patients with respiratory tract infections, ciprofloxacin demonstrated a CNS adverse event profile comparable to the control drugs.

Post-Marketing Adverse Events: Additional adverse events, regardless of relationship to drug, reported from worldwide marketing experience with quinolones, including ciprofloxacin, are:

BODY AS A WHOLE: change in serum phenytoin

CARDIOVASCULAR: postural hypotension, vasculitis

CENTRAL NERVOUS SYSTEM: agitation, confusion, delirium, dysphasia, myoclonus, nystagmus, toxic psychosis

GASTROINTESTINAL: constipation, dyspepsia, flatulence, hepatic necrosis, jaundice, pancreatitis, pseudomembranous colitis (The onset of pseudomembranous colitis symptoms may occur during or after antimicrobial treatment.)

HEMIC/LYMPHATIC: agranulocytosis, hemolytic anemia, methemoglobinemia, prolongation of prothrombin time

METABOLIC/NUTRITIONAL: elevation of serum triglycerides, cholesterol, blood glucose, serum potassium

MUSCULOSKELETAL: myalgia, possible exacerbation of myasthenia gravis, tendinitis/tendon rupture

RENAL/UROGENITAL: albuminuria, candiduria, renal calculi, vaginal candidasis

SKIN/HYPERSENSITIVITY: anaphylactic reactions, erythema multiforme/Stevens-Johnson syndrome, exfoliative dermatitis, toxic epidermal necrolysis

SPECIAL SENSES: anosmia, taste loss (See **PRECAUTIONS**.)

Adverse Laboratory Changes: Changes in laboratory parameters listed as adverse events without regard to drug relationship are listed below:

Hepatic—Elevations of ALT (SGPT) (1.9%), AST (SGOT) (1.7%), alkaline phosphatase (0.8%), LDH (0.4%), serum bilirubin (0.3%).

Hematologic—Eosinophilia (0.6%), leukopenia (0.4%), decreased blood platelets (0.1%), elevated blood platelets (0.1%), pancytopenia (0.1%).

Renal—Elevations of serum creatinine (1.1%), BUN (0.9%), CRYSTALLURIA, CYLINDRURIA, AND HEMATURIA HAVE BEEN REPORTED.

Other changes occurring in less than 0.1% of courses were: elevation of serum gammaglutamyl transferase, elevation of serum amylase, reduction in blood glucose, elevated uric acid, decrease in hemoglobin, anemia, bleeding diathesis, increase in blood monocytes, leukocytosis.

OVERDOSAGE

In the event of acute overdosage, the stomach should be emptied by inducing vomiting or by gastric lavage. The patient should be carefully observed and given supportive treatment. Adequate hydration must be maintained. Only a small amount of ciprofloxacin (<10%) is removed from the body after hemodialysis or peritoneal dialysis.

In mice, rats, rabbits and dogs, significant toxicity including tonic/clonic convulsions was observed at intravenous doses of ciprofloxacin between 125 and 300 mg/kg.

Single doses of ciprofloxacin were relatively non-toxic via the oral route of administration in mice, rats, and dogs. No deaths occurred within a 14-day post treatment observation period at the highest oral doses tested; up to 5000 mg/kg in either rodent species, or up to 2500 mg/kg in the dog. Clinical signs observed included hypoactivity and cyanosis in both rodent species and severe vomiting in dogs. In rabbits, significant mortality was seen at doses of ciprofloxacin >2500 mg/kg. Mortality was delayed in these animals, occurring 10–14 days after dosing.

DOSAGE AND ADMINISTRATION

The recommended adult dosage for acute sinusitis is 500-mg every 12 hours.

Lower respiratory tract infections may be treated with 500-mg every 12 hours. For more severe or complicated infections, a dosage of 750-mg may be given every 12 hours. Severe/complicated urinary tract infections or urinary tract infections caused by organisms not highly susceptible to ciprofloxacin may be treated with 500-mg every 12 hours. For other mild/moderate urinary infections, the usual adult dosage is 250-mg every 12 hours.

In acute uncomplicated cystitis in females, the usual dosage is 100-mg every 12 hours. For acute uncomplicated cystitis in females, 3 days of treatment is recommended while 7 to 14 days is suggested for other mild/moderate, severe or complicated urinary tract infections.

The recommended adult dosage for chronic bacterial prostatitis is 500-mg every 12 hours.

The recommended adult dosage for oral sequential therapy of complicated intra-abdominal infections is 500-mg every 12 hours. (To provide appropriate anaerobic activity, metronidazole should be given according to product labeling.) (See CIPRO® I.V. package insert.)

Skin and skin structure infections and bone and joint infections may be treated with 500-mg every 12 hours. For more severe or complicated infections, a dosage of 750-mg may be given every 12 hours.

The recommended adult dosage for infectious diarrhea or typhoid fever is 500-mg every 12 hours. For the treatment of uncomplicated urethral and cervical gonococcal infections, a single 250-mg dose is recommended.

See Instructions To The Pharmacist for Use/Handling of CIPRO® Oral Suspension.

[See table at top of previous page]

One teaspoonful (5 mL) of 5% ciprofloxacin oral suspension = 250-mg of ciprofloxacin.

One teaspoonful (5 mL) of 10% ciprofloxacin oral suspension = 500-mg of ciprofloxacin.

See Instructions for USE/HANDLING.

Dosage	Volume (mL) of Oral Suspension	
	5%	**10%**
250-mg	5 mL	2.5 mL
500-mg	10 mL	5 mL
750-mg	15 mL	7.5 mL

Complicated Intra-Abdominal Infections: Sequential therapy [parenteral to oral – 400-mg CIPRO I.V. q 12 h (plus I.V. metronidazole) → 500-mg CIPRO Tablets q 12 h (plus oral metronidazole)] can be instituted at the discretion of the physician.

The determination of dosage for any particular patient must take into consideration the severity and nature of the infec-

Men: Creatinine clearance (mL/min) = $\dfrac{\text{Weight (kg)} \times (140 - \text{age})}{72 \times \text{serum creatinine (mg/dL)}}$

Women: 0.85 × the value calculated for men

	Strength	NDC Code	Tablet Identification	
Bottles of 50:	750-mg	NDC 0026-8514-50	CIPRO	750
Bottles of 100:	250-mg	NDC 0026-8512-51	CIPRO	250
	500-mg	NDC 0026-8513-51	CIPRO	500
Unit Dose Package of 100:	250-mg	NDC 0026-8512-48	CIPRO	250
	500-mg	NDC 0026-8513-48	CIPRO	500
	750-mg	NDC 0026-8514-48	CIPRO	750
Cystitis Package of 6:	100-mg	NDC 0026-8511-06	CIPRO	100

Total volume after reconstitution	Ciprofloxacin contents after reconstitution	Ciprofloxacin contents per bottle	NDC Code
100 mL	250 mg/5 mL	5,000 mg	0026-8551-36
100 mL	500 mg/5 mL	10,000 mg	0026-8553-36

Drug Regimen	Clinical Response Resolution n (%)	Bacteriological Response By Organism (Eradication Rate) E. coli n (%)	S. saprophyticus n (%)
		STUDY 1	
CIPRO 100-mg BID × 3 days	82/94 (87)	64/70 (91)	8/8 (100)
CIPRO 250-mg BID × 7days	81/86 (94)	67/69 (97)	4/4 (100)
		STUDY 2	
CIPRO 100-mg BID × 3 days	134/141 (95)	117/123 (95)	8/8 (100)
Control (3 days)	128/133 (96)	103/105 (98)	10/10 (100)

tion, the susceptibility of the causative organism, the integrity of the patient's host-defense mechanisms, and the status of renal function and hepatic function.

The duration of treatment depends upon the severity of infection. Generally ciprofloxacin should be continued for at least 2 days after the signs and symptoms of infection have disappeared. The usual duration is 7 to 14 days; however, for severe and complicated infections more prolonged therapy may be required. Bone and joint infections may require treatment for 4 to 6 weeks or longer. Chronic Bacterial Prostatitis should be treated for 28 days. Infectious diarrhea may be treated for 5–7 days Typhoid fever should be treated for 10 days.

Concurrent Use With Antacids or Multivalent Cations: Concurrent administration of ciprofloxacin with sucralfate or divalent and trivalent cations such as iron or antacids containing magnesium, aluminum, or calcium may substantially interfere with the absorption of ciprofloxacin, resulting in serum and urine levels considerably lower than desired. Therefore, concurrent administration of these agents with ciprofloxacin should be avoided. However, usual dietary intake of calcium has not been shown to alter the bioavailability of ciprofloxacin. Single dose bioavailability studies have shown that antacids may be administered either 2 hours after or 6 hours before ciprofloxacin dosing without a significant decrease in bioavailability. Histamine H_2-receptor antagonists appear to have no significant effect on the bioavailability of ciprofloxacin.

Impaired Renal Function: Ciprofloxacin is eliminated primarily by renal excretion; however, the drug is also metabolized and partially cleared through the biliary system of the liver and through the intestine. These alternate pathways of drug elimination appear to compensate for the reduced renal excretion in patients with renal impairment. Nonetheless, some modification of dosage is recommended, particularly for patients with severe renal dysfunction. The following table provides dosage guidelines for use in patients with renal impairment; however, monitoring of serum drug levels provides the most reliable basis for dosage adjustment:

RECOMMENDED STARTING AND MAINTENANCE DOSES FOR PATIENTS WITH IMPAIRED RENAL FUNCTION

Creatinine Clearance (mL/min)	Dose
> 50	See Usual Dosage.
30 – 50	250 – 500 mg q 12 h
5 – 29	250 – 500 mg q 18 h
Patients on hemodialysis or Peritoneal dialysis	250 – 500 mg q 24 h (after dialysis)

When only the serum creatinine concentration is known, the following formula may be used to estimate creatinine clearance.

[See first table above]

The serum creatinine should represent a steady state of renal function.

In patients with severe infections and severe renal impairment, a unit dose of 750-mg may be administered at the intervals noted above; however, patients should be carefully monitored and the serum ciprofloxacin concentration should be measured periodically. Peak concentrations (1–2 hours after dosing) should generally range from 2 to 4 µg/mL.

For patients with changing renal function or for patients with renal impairment and hepatic insufficiency, measurement of serum concentrations of ciprofloxacin will provide additional guidance for adjusting dosage.

HOW SUPPLIED

CIPRO® (ciprofloxacin hydrochloride) Tablets are available as round, slightly yellowish film-coated tablets containing 100-mg or 250-mg ciprofloxacin. The 100-mg tablet is coded with the word "CIPRO" on one side and "100" on the reverse side. The 250-mg tablet is coded with the word "CIPRO" on one side and "250" on the reverse side. CIPRO® is also available as capsule shaped, slightly yellowish film-coated tablets containing 500-mg or 750-mg ciprofloxacin. The 500-mg tablet is coded with the word "CIPRO" on one side and "500" on the reverse side. The 750-mg tablet is coded with the word "CIPRO" on one side and "750" on the reverse side. CIPRO® 250-mg, 500-mg, and 750-mg are available in bottles of 50, 100, and Unit Dose packages of 100. The 100-mg strength, is available only as CIPRO® Cystitis pack containing 6 tablets for use only in female patients with acute uncomplicated cystitis.

[See second table above]

Store below 30°C (86°F).

CIPRO® Oral Suspension is supplied in 5% (5g ciprofloxacin in 100 mL) and 10% (10g ciprofloxacin in 100 mL) strengths. The drug product is composed of two components (microcapsules and diluent) which are mixed prior to dispensing. See Instructions To The Pharmacist For Use/Handling.

[See third table above]

Microcapsules and diluent should be stored below 25°C (77°F) and protected from freezing.

Reconstituted product may be stored below 30°C (86°F). Protect from freezing. A teaspoon is provided for the patient.

ANIMAL PHARMACOLOGY

Ciprofloxacin and other quinolones have been shown to cause arthropathy in immature animals of most species tested (See **WARNINGS**.) Damage of weight bearing joints was observed in juvenile dogs and rats. In young beagles, 100 mg/kg ciprofloxacin, given daily for 4 weeks, caused de-

Continued on next page

Cipro Tablets/O.S.—Cont.

generative articular changes of the knee joint. At 30 mg/kg, the effect on the joint was minimal. In a subsequent study in beagles, removal of weight bearing from the joint reduced the lesions but did not totally prevent them.

Crystalluria, sometimes associated with secondary nephropathy, occurs in laboratory animals dosed with ciprofloxacin. This is primarily related to the reduced solubility of ciprofloxacin under alkaline conditions, which predominate in the urine of test animals; in man, crystalluria is rare since human urine is typically acidic. In rhesus monkeys, crystalluria without nephropathy has been noted after single oral doses as low as 5 mg/kg. After 6 months of intravenous dosing at 10 mg/kg/day, no nephropathological changes were noted; however, nephropathy was observed after dosing at 20 mg/kg/day for the same duration.

In dogs, ciprofloxacin at 3 and 10 mg/kg by rapid IV injection (15 sec.) produces pronounced hypotensive effects. These effects are considered to be related to histamine release, since they are partially antagonized by pyrilamine, an antihistamine. In rhesus monkeys, rapid IV injection also produces hypotension but the effect in the species is inconsistent and less pronounced.

In mice, concomitant administration of nonsteroidal antiinflammatory drugs such as phenylbutazone and indomethacin with quinolones has been reported to enhance the CNS stimulatory effect of quinolones.

Ocular toxicity seen with some related drugs has not been observed in ciprofloxacin-treated animals.

CLINICAL STUDIES

Acute Sinusitis Studies

Ciprofloxacin tablets (500-mg BID) were evaluated for the treatment of acute sinusitis in two randomized, double-blind, controlled clinical trials conducted in the United States. Study 1 compared ciprofloxacin with cefuroxime axetil (250-mg BID) and enrolled 501 patients (400 of which were valid for the primary efficacy analysis). Study 2 compared ciprofloxacin with clarithromycin (500-mg BID) and enrolled 560 patients (418 of whom were valid for the primary efficacy analysis). The primary test of cure endpoint was a follow-up visit performed approximately 30 days after the completion of treatment with study medication. Clinical response data from these studies are summarized below:

Drug Regimen	Clinical Response Resolution at 30 Day Follow-up n(%)
STUDY 1	
CIPRO 500-mg BID × 10 days	152/197 (77)
Cefuroxime Axetil 250-mg BID × 10 days	145/203 (71)
STUDY 2	
CIPRO 500-mg BID × 10 days	168/212 (79)
Clarithromycin 500-mg BID × 14 days	169/206 (82)

In ciprofloxacin-treated patients enrolled in controlled and uncontrolled acute sinusitis studies, all of which included antral puncture, bacteriological eradication/presumed eradication was documented at the 30 day follow-up visit in 44 of 50 (88%) H. influenzae, 17 of 21 (80.9%) M. catarrhalis, and 42 of 51 (82.3%) S. pneumoniae. Patients infected with S. pneumoniae strains whose baseline susceptibilities were intermediate or resistant to ciprofloxacin had a lower success rate than patients infected with susceptible strains.

Uncomplicated Cystitis Studies

Efficacy: Two U.S. double-blind, controlled clinical studies of acute uncomplicated cystitis in women compared ciprofloxacin 100-mg BID for 3 days to ciprofloxacin 250-mg BID for 7 days or control drug. In these two studies, using strict evaluability criteria and microbiologic and clinical response criteria at the 5–9 day post-therapy follow-up, the following clinical resolution and bacterial eradication rates were obtained:

[See fourth table from top of previous page]

Instructions To The Pharmacist For Use/Handling Of CIPRO® Oral Suspension:

Preparation of the suspension:

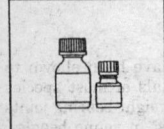

1. The small bottle contains the microcapsules, the large bottle contains the diluent.

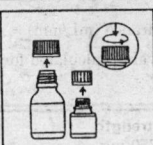

2. Open both bottles. Child-proof cap: Press down according to instructions on the cap while turning to the left.

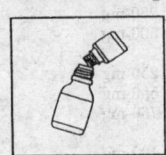

3. Pour the microcapsules completely into the large bottle of diluent. **Do not add water to the suspension.**

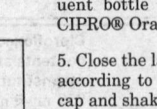

4. Remove the top layer of the diluent bottle label (to reveal the CIPRO® Oral Suspension label).

5. Close the large bottle completely according to the directions on the cap and shake vigorously for about 15 seconds. The suspension is ready for use.

Instructions To The Patient For Taking CIPRO® Oral Suspension:

Shake vigorously each time before use for approximately 15 seconds.

Swallow the prescribed amount of suspension. Do not chew the microcapsules. Reclose the bottle completely after use according to the instructions on the cap. The suspension is stable for 14 days when stored in a refrigerator or at room temperature (below 86°F). After treatment has been completed, any remaining suspension should not be reused.

REFERENCES

1. National Committee for Clinical Laboratory Standards, Methods for Dilution Antimicrobial Susceptibility Tests for Bacteria That Grow Aerobically-Fourth Edition. Approved Standard NCCLS Document M7-A4, Vol. 17, No. 2, NCCLS, Wayne, PA, January 1997. **2.** National Committee for Clinical Laboratory Standards. Performance Standards for Antimicrobial Disk Susceptibility Tests-Sixth Edition. Approved Standard NCCLS Document M2-A6, Vol. 17, No. 1, NCCLS, Wayne, PA, January, 1997. **3.** Report presented at the FDA's Anti-Infective Drug and Dermatological Drug Product's Advisory Committee meeting, March 31, 1993, Silver Spring, MD. Report available from FDA, CDER, Advisors and Consultants Staff, HFD-21, 1901 Chapman Avenue, Room 200, Rockville, MD 20852, USA

Bayer Corporation
Pharmaceutical Division
400 Morgan Lane
West Haven, CT 06516 USA

Rx only
CIPRO® (ciprofloxacin) 5% and 10% Oral Suspension made in Italy.
PD500087 7/98 Bay o 9867 5202-2-A-U.S.-6 ©1998 Bayer Corporation   8424
Shown in Product Identification Guide, page 305

CIPRO® HC OTIC   ℞
(ciprofloxacin hydrochloride and hydrocortisone otic suspension)

DESCRIPTION

CIPRO® HC OTIC (ciprofloxacin hydrochloride and hydrocortisone otic suspension) contains the synthetic broad spectrum antibacterial agent, ciprofloxacin hydrochloride, combined with the anti-inflammatory corticosteroid, hydrocortisone, in a preserved, nonsterile suspension for otic use. Each mL of CIPRO HC OTIC contains ciprofloxacin hydrochloride (equivalent to 2 mg ciprofloxacin), 10 mg hydrocortisone, and 9 mg benzyl alcohol as a preservative. The inactive ingredients are polyvinyl alcohol, sodium chloride, sodium acetate, glacial acetic acid, phospholipon 90HB (modified lecithin), polysorbate, and purified water. Sodium hydroxide or hydrochloric acid may be added for adjustment of pH.

Ciprofloxacin, a fluoroquinolone, is available as the monohydrochloride monohydrate salt of 1-cyclopropyl-6-fluoro-1,4-dihydro-4-oxo-7-(1-piperazinyl)-3-quinolinecarboxylic acid. Its empirical formula is $C_{17}H_{18}FN_3O_3 \cdot HCl \cdot H_2O$ and its chemical structure is as follows:

Hydrocortisone, pregn-4-ene-3, 20-dione, 11, 17, 21-trihydroxy-(11β)-, is an anti-inflammatory corticosteroid. Its empirical formula is $C_{21}H_{30}O_5$ and it chemical structure is:

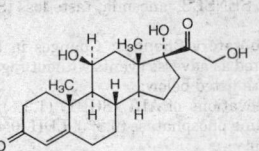

CLINICAL PHARMACOLOGY

The plasma concentrations of ciprofloxacin were not measured following three drops of otic suspension administration because the systemic exposure to ciprofloxacin is expected to be below the limit of quantitation of the assay (0.05 µg/mL).

Similarly, the predicted C_{max} of hydrocortisone is within the range of endogenous hydrocortisone concentration (0–150 ng/mL), and therefore can not be differentiated from the endogenous cortisol.

Preclinical studies have shown that CIPRO HC OTIC was not toxic to the guinea pig cochlea when administered intratympanically twice daily for 30 days and was only weakly irritating to rabbit skin upon repeated exposure.

Hydrocortisone has been added to aid in the resolution of the inflammatory response accompanying bacterial infection.

Microbiology

Ciprofloxacin has *in vitro* activity against a wide range of gram-positive and gram-negative microorganisms. The bactericidal action of ciprofloxacin results from interference with the enzyme, DNA gyrase, which is needed for the synthesis of bacterial DNA. Cross-resistance has been observed between ciprofloxacin and other fluoroquinolones. There is generally no cross-resistance between ciprofloxacin and other classes of antibacterial agents such as beta-lactams or aminoglycosides.

Ciprofloxacin has been shown to be active against most strains of the following microorganisms, both *in vitro* and in clinical infections of acute otitis externa as described in the **INDICATIONS AND USAGE** section:

Aerobic gram-positive microorganism
Staphylococcus aureus

Aerobic gram-negative microorganisms
Proteus mirabilis
Pseudomonas aeruginosa

INDICATIONS AND USAGE

CIPRO HC OTIC is indicated for the treatment of acute otitis externa in adult and pediatric patients, one year and older, due to susceptible strains of *Pseudomonas aeruginosa*, *Staphylococcus aureus*, and *Proteus mirabilis*.

CONTRAINDICATIONS

CIPRO HC OTIC is contraindicated in persons with a history of hypersensitivity to hydrocortisone, ciprofloxacin or any member of the quinolone class of antimicrobial agents. This nonsterile product should not be used if the tympanic membrane is perforated. Use of this product is contraindicated in viral infections of the external canal including varicella and herpes simplex infections.

WARNINGS

NOT FOR OPHTHALMIC USE. NOT FOR INJECTION.
CIPRO HC OTIC should be discontinued at the first appearance of a skin rash or any other sign of hypersensitivity. Serious and occasionally fatal hypersensitivity (anaphylactic) reactions, some following the first dose, have been reported in patients receiving systemic quinolones. Serious acute hypersensitivity reactions may require immediate emergency treatment.

PRECAUTIONS

GENERAL: As with other antibiotic preparations, use of this product may result in overgrowth of nonsusceptible organisms, including fungi. If the infection is not improved after one week of therapy, cultures should be obtained to guide further treatment.

Information for Patients:
If rash or allergic reaction occurs, discontinue use immediately and contact your physician.
Do not use in the eyes.
Avoid contaminating the dropper with material from the ear, fingers, or other sources.
Protect from light.
Shake well immediately before using.
Discard unused portion after therapy is completed.

Carcinogenesis, Mutagenesis, Impairment of Fertility:
Eight *in vitro* mutagenicity tests have been conducted with ciprofloxacin, and the test results are listed below:
Salmonella/Microsome Test (Negative)
E. coli DNA Repair Assay (Negative)
Mouse Lymphoma Cell Forward Mutation Assay (Positive)
Chinese Hamster V_{79} Cell HGPRT Test (Negative)

Syrian Hamster Embryo Cell Transformation Assay (Negative)
Saccharomyces cerevisiae Point Mutation Assay (Negative)
Saccharomyces cerevisiae Mitotic Crossover and Gene Conversion Assay (Negative)
Rat Hepatocyte DNA Repair Assay (Positive)

Thus, 2 of the 8 tests were positive, but results of the following 3 *in vivo* test systems gave negative results:

Rat Hepatocyte DNA Repair Assay
Micronucleus Test (Mice)
Dominant Lethal Test (Mice)

Long-term carcinogenicity studies in mice and rats have been completed for ciprofloxacin. After daily oral doses of 750 mg/kg (mice) and 250 mg/kg (rats) were administered for up to 2 years, there was no evidence that ciprofloxacin had any carcinogenic or tumorigenic effects in these species. No long term studies of CIPRO HC OTIC have been performed to evaluate carcinogenic potential.

Fertility studies performed in rats at oral doses of ciprofloxacin up to 100 mg/kg/day revealed no evidence of impairment. This would be over 1000 times the maximum recommended clinical dose of ototopical ciprofloxacin based upon body surface area, assuming total absorption of ciprofloxacin from the ear of a patient treated with CIPRO HC OTIC twice per day.

Long term studies have not been performed to evaluate the carcinogenic potential or the effect on fertility of topical hydrocortisone. Mutagenicity studies with hydrocortisone were negative.

Pregnancy: Teratogenic Effects. Pregnancy Category C: Reproduction studies have been performed in rats and mice using oral doses of up to 100 mg/kg and IV doses up to 30 mg/kg and have revealed no evidence of harm to the fetus as a result of ciprofloxacin. In rabbits, ciprofloxacin (30 and 100 mg/kg orally) produced gastrointestinal disturbances resulting in maternal weight loss and an increased incidence of abortion, but no teratogenicity was observed at either dose. After intravenous administration of doses up to 20 mg/kg, no maternal toxicity was produced in the rabbit, and no embryotoxicity or teratogenicity was observed.

Corticosteroids are generally teratogenic in laboratory animals when administered systemically at relatively low dosage levels. The more potent corticosteroids have been shown to be teratogenic after dermal application in laboratory animals.

Animal reproduction studies have not been conducted with CIPRO HC OTIC. No adequate and well controlled studies have been performed in pregnant women. Caution should be exercised when CIPRO HC OTIC is used by a pregnant woman.

Nursing Mothers: Ciprofloxacin is excreted in human milk with systemic use. It is not known whether ciprofloxacin is excreted in human milk following topical otic administration. Because of the potential for serious adverse reactions in nursing infants, a decision should be made whether to discontinue nursing or to discontinue the drug, taking into account the importance of the drug to the mother.

Pediatric Use: The safety and efficacy of CIPRO HC OTIC have been established in pediatric patients 2 years and older (131 patients) in adequate and well-controlled clinical trials. Although no data are available on patients less than age 2 years, there are no known safety concerns or differences in the disease process in this population which would preclude use of this product in patients one year and older. See **DOSAGE AND ADMINISTRATION.**

ADVERSE REACTIONS

In Phase 3 clinical trials, a total of 564 patients were treated with CIPRO HC OTIC. Adverse events with at least remote relationship to treatment included headache (1.2%) and pruritus (0.4%). The following treatment-related adverse events were each reported in a single patient: migraine, hypesthesia, paresthesia, fungal dermatitis, cough, rash, urticaria, and alopecia.

DOSAGE AND ADMINISTRATION

SHAKE WELL IMMEDIATELY BEFORE USING.

For children (age 1 year and older) and adults, 3 drops of the suspension should be instilled into the affected ear twice daily for seven days. The suspension should be warmed by holding the bottle in the hand for 1–2 minutes to avoid the dizziness which may result from the instillation of a cold solution into the ear canal. The patient should lie with the affected ear upward and then the drops should be instilled. This position should be maintained for 30–60 seconds to facilitate penetration of the drops into the ear. Repeat, if necessary, for the opposite ear. Discard unused portion after therapy is completed.

HOW SUPPLIED

CIPRO HC OTIC is supplied as a white to off-white opaque suspension in a 10 mL bottle with a dropper dispenser.
NDC Number 0026-8531-10
Store below 77°F (25°C). Avoid freezing. Protect from light.

Bayer Corporation
Pharmaceutical Division
400 Morgan Lane
West Haven, CT. 06516

Caution: Federal (USA) law prohibits dispensing without a prescription.

PZ500083 3/98 Bay o 9867 5202-2-A-U.S.-6

Shown in Product Identification Guide, page 305

CIPRO® I.V. ℞
(ciprofloxacin)
For Intravenous Infusion

DESCRIPTION

CIPRO® I.V. (ciprofloxacin) is a synthetic broad-spectrum antimicrobial agent for intravenous (I.V.) administration. Ciprofloxacin, a fluoroquinolone, is 1-cyclopropyl-6-fluoro-1,4-dihydro-4-oxo-7-(1-piperazinyl)-3-quinolinecarboxylic acid. Its empirical formula is $C_{17}H_{18}FN_3O_3$ and its chemical structure is:

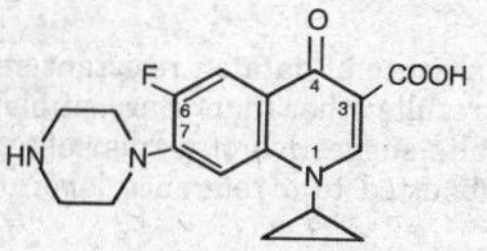

Ciprofloxacin is a faint to light yellow crystalline powder with a molecular weight of 331.4. It is soluble in dilute (0.1N) hydrochloric acid and is practically insoluble in water and ethanol. Ciprofloxacin differs from other quinolones in that it has a fluorine atom at the 6-position, a piperazine moiety at the 7-position, and a cyclopropyl ring at the 1-position. CIPRO® I.V. solutions are available as sterile 1.0% aqueous concentrates, which are intended for dilution prior to administration, and as 0.2% ready-for-use infusion solutions in 5% Dextrose Injection. All formulas contain lactic acid as a solubilizing agent and hydrochloric acid for pH adjustment. The pH range for the 1.0% aqueous concentrates in vials is 3.3 to 3.9. The pH range for the 0.2% ready-for-use infusion solutions is 3.5 to 4.6.

The plastic container is fabricated from a specially formulated polyvinyl chloride. Solutions in contact with the plastic container can leach out certain of its chemical components in very small amounts within the expiration period, e.g., di(2-ethylhexyl) phthalate (DEHP), up to 5 parts per million. The suitability of the plastic has been confirmed in tests in animals according to USP biological tests for plastic containers as well as by tissue culture toxicity studies.

CLINICAL PHARMACOLOGY

Following 60-minute intravenous infusions of 200 mg and 400 mg ciprofloxacin to normal volunteers, the mean maximum serum concentrations achieved were 2.1 and 4.6 μg/mL, respectively; the concentrations at 12 hours were 0.1 and 0.2 μg/mL, respectively.

Steady-state Ciprofloxacin Serum Concentrations (μg/mL) After 60-minute I.V. Infusions q 12 h.

	Time after starting the infusion					
Dose	**30 min**	**1 hr**	**3 hr**	**6 hr**	**8 hr**	**12 hr**
200 mg	1.7	2.1	0.6	0.3	0.2	0.1
400 mg	3.7	4.6	1.3	0.7	0.5	0.2

The pharmacokinetics of ciprofloxacin are linear over the dose range of 200 to 400 mg administered intravenously. The serum elimination half-life is approximately 5–6 hours and the total clearance is around 35 L/hr. Comparison of the pharmacokinetic parameters following the 1st and 5th I.V. dose on a q 12 h regimen indicates no evidence of drug accumulation.

The absolute bioavailability of oral ciprofloxacin is within a range of 70–80% with no substantial loss by first pass metabolism. An intravenous infusion of 400 mg ciprofloxacin given over 60 minutes every 12 hours has been shown to produce an area under the serum concentration time curve (AUC) equivalent to that produced by a 500-mg oral dose given every 12 hours. An intravenous infusion of 400 mg ciprofloxacin given over 60 minutes every 8 hours has been shown to produce an AUC at steady-state equivalent to that produced by a 750-mg oral dose given every 12 hours. A 400-mg I.V. dose results in a C_{max} similar to that observed with a 750-mg oral dose. An infusion of 200 mg ciprofloxacin given every 12 hours produces an AUC equivalent to that produced by a 250-mg oral dose given every 12 hours.

[See table at bottom of next page]

After intravenous administration, approximately 50% to 70% of the dose is excreted in the urine as unchanged drug. Following a 200-mg I.V. dose, concentrations in the urine usually exceed 200 μg/mL 0–2 hours after dosing and are generally greater than 15 μg/mL 8–12 hours after dosing. Following a 400-mg I.V. dose, urine concentrations generally exceed 400 μg/mL 0–2 hours after dosing and are usually greater than 30 μg/mL 8–12 hours after dosing. The renal clearance is approximately 22 L/hr. The urinary excretion of ciprofloxacin is virtually complete by 24 hours after dosing.

The serum concentrations of ciprofloxacin and metronidazole were not altered when these two drugs were given concomitantly.

Co-administration of probenecid with ciprofloxacin results in about a 50% reduction in the ciprofloxacin renal clearance and a 50% increase in its concentration in the systemic circulation. Although bile concentrations of ciprofloxacin are severalfold higher than serum concentrations after intravenous dosing, only a small amount of the administered dose (<1%) is recovered from the bile as unchanged drug. Approximately 15% of an I.V. dose is recovered from the feces within 5 days after dosing.

After I.V. administration, three metabolites of ciprofloxacin have been identified in human urine which together accounted for approximately 10% of the intravenous dose.

In patients with reduced renal function, the half-life of ciprofloxacin is slightly prolonged and dosage adjustments may be required. (See **DOSAGE AND ADMINISTRATION.**)

In preliminary studies in patients with stable chronic liver cirrhosis, no significant changes in ciprofloxacin pharmacokinetics have been observed. However, the kinetics of ciprofloxacin in patients with acute hepatic insufficiency have not been fully elucidated.

Following infusion of 400 mg I.V. ciprofloxacin every eight hours in combination with 50 mg/kg I.V. piperacillin sodium every 4 hours, mean serum ciprofloxacin concentrations were 3.02 μg/mL 1/2 hour and 1.18 μg/mL between 6–8 hours after the end of infusion.

The binding of ciprofloxacin to serum proteins is 20 to 40%. After intravenous administration, ciprofloxacin is present in saliva, nasal and bronchial secretions, sputum, skin blister fluid, lymph, peritoneal fluid, bile, and prostatic secretions. It has also been detected in the lung, skin, fat, muscle, cartilage, and bone. Although the drug diffuses into cerebrospinal fluid (CSF), CSF concentrations are generally less than 10% of peak serum concentrations. Levels of the drug in the aqueous and vitreous chambers of the eye are lower than in serum.

Microbiology: Ciprofloxacin has *in vitro* activity against a wide range of gram-negative and gram-positive microorganisms. The bactericidal action of ciprofloxacin results from interference with the enzyme DNA gyrase which is needed for the synthesis of bacterial DNA.

Ciprofloxacin has been shown to be active against most strains of the following microorganisms, both *in vitro* and in clinical infections as described in the **INDICATIONS AND USAGE** section of the package insert for CIPRO® I.V. (ciprofloxacin for intravenous infusion).

Aerobic gram-positive microorganisms
Enterococcus faecalis
(Many strains are only
moderately susceptible.)
Staphylococcus aureus
(methicillin susceptible)
Staphylococcus epidermidis
Staphylococcus saprophyticus
Streptococcus pneumoniae
Streptococcus pyogenes

Aerobic gram-negative microorganisms
Citrobacter diversus
Citrobacter freundii
Enterobacter cloacae
Escherichia coli
Haemophilus influenzae
Haemophilus parainfluenzae
Klebsiella pneumoniae
Morganella morganii
Proteus mirabilis
Proteus vulgaris
Providencia rettgeri
Providencia stuartii
Pseudomonas aeruginosa
Serratia marcescens

Ciprofloxacin has been shown to be active against most strains of the following microorganisms, both *in vitro* and in clinical infections as described in the **INDICATIONS AND USAGE** section of the package insert for CIPRO® (ciprofloxacin hydrochloride) Tablets.

Aerobic gram-positive microorganisms
Enterococcus faecalis
Many strains are only
moderately susceptible.)
Staphylococcus aureus
(methicillin susceptible)
Staphylococcus epidermidis
Staphylococcus saprophyticus

Continued on next page

Cipro I.V.—Cont.

Streptococcus pneumoniae
Streptococcus pyogenes

Aerobic gram-negative microorganisms
Campylobacter jejuni
Citrobacter diversus
Citrobacter freundii
Enterobacter cloacae
Escherichia coli
Haemophilus influenzae
Haemophilus parainfluenzae
Klebsiella pneumoniae
Moraxella catarrhalis
Morganella morganii
Neisseria gonorrhoeae
Proteus mirabilis
Proteus vulgaris
Providencia rettgeri
Providencia stuartii
Pseudomonas aeruginosa
Salmonella typhi
Serratia marcescens
Shigella boydii
Shigella dysenteriae
Shigella flexneri
Shigella sonnei

The following *in vitro* data are available, **but their clinical significance is unknown.**
Ciprofloxacin exhibits *in vitro* minimum inhibitory concentrations (MICs) of 1 μg/mL or less against most (≥ 90%) strains of the following microorganisms; however, the safety and effectiveness of ciprofloxacin in treating clinical infections due to these microorganisms have not been established in adequate and well-controlled clinical trials.

Aerobic gram-positive microorganisms
Staphylococcus haemolyticus
Staphylococcus hominis

Aerobic gram-negative microorganisms
Acinetobacter lwoffi
Aeromonas hydrophila
Edwardsiella tarda
Enterobacter aerogenes
Klebsiella oxytoca
Legionella pneumophila
Pasteurella multocida
Salmonella enteritidis
Vibrio cholerae
Vibrio parahaemolyticus
Vibrio vulnificus
Yersinia enterocolitica
Most strains of *Burkholderia cepacia* and some strains of *Stenotrophomonas maltophilia* are resistant to ciprofloxacin as are most anaerobic bacteria, including *Bacteroides fragilis* and *Clostridium difficile*.
Ciprofloxacin is slightly less active when tested at acidic pH. The inoculum size has little effect when tested *in vitro*. The minimum bactericidal concentration (MBC) generally does not exceed the minimum inhibitory concentration (MIC) by more than a factor of 2. Resistance to ciprofloxacin *in vitro* usually develops slowly (multiple-step mutation). Ciprofloxacin does not cross-react with other antimicrobial agents such as beta-lactams or aminoglycosides; therefore, organisms resistant to these drugs may be susceptible to ciprofloxacin.
In vitro studies have shown that additive activity often results when ciprofloxacin is combined with other antimicrobial agents such as beta-lactams, aminoglycosides, clindamycin, or metronidazole. Synergy has been reported particularly with the combination of ciprofloxacin and a beta-lactam; antagonism is observed only rarely.

Susceptibility Tests
Dilution Techniques: Quantitative methods are used to determine antimicrobial minimum inhibitory concentrations (MICs). These MICs provide estimates of the susceptibility of bacteria to antimicrobial compounds. The MICs should be determined using a standardized procedure. Standardized procedures are based on a dilution method[1] (broth or agar) or equivalent with standardized inoculum concentrations and standardized concentrations of ciprofloxacin powder. The MIC values should be interpreted according to the following criteria:

For testing aerobic microorganisms other than *Haemophilus influenzae*, *Haemophilus parainfluenzae*, and *Neisseria gonorrhoeae*[a]:

MIC (μg/mL)	Interpretation
≤ 1	Susceptible (S)
2	Intermediate (I)
≥ 4	Resistant (R)

[a] These interpretive standards are applicable only to broth microdilution susceptibility tests with streptococci using cation-adjusted Mueller-Hinton broth with 2–5% lysed horse blood.

For testing *Haemophilus influenzae* and *Haemophilus parainfluenzae*[b]:

MIC (μg/mL)	Interpretation
≤ 1	Susceptible (S)

[b] This interpretive standard is applicable only to broth microdilution susceptibility tests with *Haemophilus influenzae* and *Haemophilus parainfluenzae* using *Haemophilus* Test Medium[1].

The current absence of data on resistant strains precludes defining any results other than "Susceptible". Strains yielding MIC results suggestive of a "nonsusceptible" category should be submitted to a reference laboratory for further testing.
For testing *Neisseria gonorrhoeae*[c]:

MIC (μg/mL)	Interpretation
≤ 0.06	Susceptible (S)

[c] This interpretive standard is applicable only to agar dilution test with GC agar base and 1% defined growth supplement.

The current absence of data on resistant strains precludes defining any results other than "Susceptible". Strains yielding MIC results suggestive of a "nonsusceptible" category should be submitted to a reference laboratory for further testing.
A report of "Susceptible" indicates that the pathogen is likely to be inhibited if the antimicrobial compound in the blood reaches the concentrations usually achievable. A report of "Intermediate" indicates that the result should be considered equivocal, and, if the microorganism is not fully susceptible to alternative, clinically feasible drugs, the test should be repeated. This category implies possible clinical applicability in body sites where the drug is physiologically concentrated or in situations where high dosage of drug can be used. This category also provides a buffer zone which prevents small uncontrolled technical factors from causing major discrepancies in interpretation. A report of "Resistant" indicates that the pathogen is not likely to be inhibited if the antimicrobial compound in the blood reaches the concentrations usually achievable; other therapy should be selected.
Standardized susceptibility test procedures require the use of laboratory control microorganisms to control the technical aspects of the laboratory procedures. Standard ciprofloxacin powder should provide the following MIC values:

Organism		MIC (μg/mL)
E. faecalis	ATCC 29212	0.25 – 2.0
E. coli	ATCC 25922	0.004 – 0.015
H. influenzae[a]	ATCC 49247	0.004 – 0.03
N. gonorrhoeae[b]	ATCC 49226	0.001 – 0.008
P. aeruginosa	ATCC 27853	0.25 – 1.0
S. aureus	ATCC 29213	0.12 – 0.5

[a] This quality control range is applicable to only *H. influenzae* ATCC 49247 tested by a broth microdilution procedure using *Haemophilus* Test Medium (HTM)[1].
[b] This quality control range is applicable to only *N. gonorrhoeae* ATCC 49226 tested by an agar dilution procedure using GC agar base and 1% defined growth supplement.

Diffusion Techniques: Quantitative methods that require measurement of zone diameters also provide reproducible estimates of the susceptibility of bacteria to antimicrobial compounds. One such standardized procedure[2] requires the use of standardized inoculum concentrations. This procedure uses paper disks impregnated with 5-μg ciprofloxacin to test the susceptibility of microorganisms to ciprofloxacin. Reports from the laboratory providing results of the standard single-disk susceptibility test with a 5-μg ciprofloxacin disk should be interpreted according to the following criteria:
For testing aerobic microorganisms other than *Haemophilus influenzae*, *Haemophilus parainfluenzae*, and *Neisseria gonorrhoeae*[a]:

Zone Diameter (mm)	Interpretation
≥ 21	Susceptible (S)
16–20	Intermediate (I)
≤ 15	Resistant (R)

[a] These zone diameter standards are applicable only to tests performed for streptococci using Mueller-Hinton agar supplemented with 5% sheep blood incubated in 5% CO_2.

For testing *Haemophilus influenzae* and *Haemophilus parainfluenzae*[b]:

Zone Diameter (mm)	Interpretation
≥ 21	Susceptible (S)

[b] This zone diameter standard is applicable only to tests with *Haemophilus influenzae* and *Haemophilus parainfluenzae* using *Haemophilus* Test Medium (HTM)[2].

The current absence of data on resistant strains precludes defining any results other than "Susceptible". Strains yielding zone diameter results suggestive of a "nonsusceptible" category should be submitted to a reference laboratory for further testing.
For testing *Neisseria gonorrhoeae*[c]:

Zone Diameter (mm)	Interpretation
≥ 36	Susceptible (S)

[c] This zone diameter standard is applicable only to disk diffusion tests with GC agar base and 1% defined growth supplement.

The current absence of data on resistant strains precludes defining any results other than "Susceptible". Strains yielding zone diameter results suggestive of a "nonsusceptible" category should be submitted to a reference laboratory for further testing.
Interpretation should be as stated above for results using dilution techniques. Interpretation involves correlation of the diameter obtained in the disk test with the MIC for ciprofloxacin.
As with standardized dilution techniques, diffusion methods require the use of laboratory control microorganisms that are used to control the technical aspects of the laboratory procedures. For the diffusion technique, the 5-μg ciprofloxacin disk should provide the following zone diameters in these laboratory test quality control strains:

Organism		Zone Diameter (mm)
E. coli	ATCC 25922	30–40
H. influenzae[a]	ATCC 49247	34–42
N. gonorrhoeae[b]	ATCC 49226	48–58
P. aeruginosa	ATCC 27853	25–33
S. aureus	ATCC 25923	22–30

[a] These quality control limits are applicable to only *H. influenzae* ATCC 49247 testing using *Haemophilus* Test Medium (HTM)[2].
[b] These quality control limits are applicable only to tests conducted with *N. gonorrhoeae* ATCC 49226 performed by disk diffusion using GC agar base and 1% defined growth supplement.

INDICATIONS AND USAGE
CIPRO® I.V. is indicated for the treatment of infections caused by susceptible strains of the designated microorgan-

Steady-state Pharmacokinetic Parameter Following Multiple Oral and I.V. Doses				
Parameters	500 mg q12h, P.O.	400 mg q12h, I.V.	750 mg q12h, P.O.	400 mg q8h, I.V.
AUC (μg·hr/mL)	13.7[a]	12.7[a]	31.6[b]	32.9[c]
C_{max} (μg/mL)	2.97	4.56	3.59	4.07

[a] AUC_{0-12h}
[b] $AUC\ 24h = AUC_{0-12h} \times 2$
[c] $AUC\ 24h = AUC_{0-8h} \times 3$

Total	Ciprofloxacin/Piperacillin N = 233	Tobramycin/Piperacillin N = 237
Median Age (years)	47.0 (range 19–84)	50.0 (range 18–81)
Male	114 (48.9%)	117 (49.4%)
Female	119 (51.1%)	120 (50.6%)
Leukemia/Bone Marrow Transplant	165 (70.8%)	158 (66.7%)
Solid Tumor/Lymphoma	68 (29.2%)	79 (33.3%)
Median Duration of Neutropenia (days)	15.0 (range 1–61)	14.0 (range 1–89)

isms in the conditions listed below when the intravenous administration offers a route of administration advantageous to the patient. Please see **DOSAGE AND ADMINISTRATION** for specific recommendations.

Urinary Tract Infections caused by *Escherichia coli* (including cases with secondary bacteremia), *Klebsiella pneumoniae* subspecies *pneumoniae*, *Enterobacter cloacae*, *Serratia marcescens*, *Proteus mirabilis*, *Providencia rettgeri*, *Morganella morganii*, *Citrobacter diversus*, *Citrobacter freundii*, *Pseudomonas aeruginosa*, *Staphylococcus epidermidis*, *Staphylococcus saprophyticus*, or *Enterococcus faecalis*.

Lower Respiratory Infections caused by *Escherichia coli*, *Klebsiella pneumoniae* subspecies *pneumoniae*, *Enterobacter cloacae*, *Proteus mirabilis*, *Pseudomonas aeruginosa*, *Haemophilus influenzae*, *Haemophilus parainfluenzae*, or *Streptococcus pneumoniae*.

NOTE: Although effective in clinical trials, ciprofloxacin is not a drug of first choice in the treatment of presumed or confirmed pneumonia secondary to *Streptococcus pneumoniae*.

Nosocomial Pneumonia caused by *Haemophilus influenzae* or *Klebsiella pneumoniae*.

Skin and Skin Structure Infections caused by *Escherichia coli*, *Klebsiella pneumoniae* subspecies *pneumoniae*, *Enterobacter cloacae*, *Proteus mirabilis*, *Proteus vulgaris*, *Providencia stuartii*, *Morganella morganii*, *Citrobacter freundii*, *Pseudomonas aeruginosa*, *Staphylococcus aureus* (methicillin susceptible), *Staphylococcus epidermidis*, or *Streptococcus pyogenes*.

Bone and Joint Infections caused by *Enterobacter cloacae*, *Serratia marcescens*, or *Pseudomonas aeruginosa*.

Complicated Intra-Abdominal Infections (used in conjunction with metronidazole) caused by *Escherichia coli*, *Pseudomonas aeruginosa*, *Proteus mirabilis*, *Klebsiella pneumoniae*, or *Bacteroides fragilis*. (See **DOSAGE AND ADMINISTRATION**.)

Empirical Therapy for Febrile Neutropenic Patients in combination with piperacillin sodium. (See **DOSAGE AND ADMINISTRATION** and **CLINICAL STUDIES**.)

If anaerobic organisms are suspected of contributing to the infection, appropriate therapy should be administered.

Appropriate culture and susceptibility tests should be performed before treatment in order to isolate and identify organisms causing infection and to determine their susceptibility to ciprofloxacin. Therapy with CIPRO® I.V. may be initiated before the results of these tests are known; once results become available, appropriate therapy should be continued.

As with other drugs, some strains of *Pseudomonas aeruginosa* may develop resistance fairly rapidly during treatment with ciprofloxacin. Culture and susceptibility testing performed periodically during therapy will provide information not only on the therapeutic effect of the antimicrobial agent but also on the possible emergence of bacterial resistance.

CLINICAL STUDIES
EMPIRICAL THERAPY IN FEBRILE NEUTROPENIC PATIENTS
The safety and efficacy of ciprofloxacin, 400 mg I.V. q 8h, in combination with piperacillin sodium, 50 mg/kg I.V. q 4h, for the empirical therapy of febrile neutropenic patients were studied in one large pivotal multicenter, randomized trial and were compared to those of tobramycin, 2 mg/kg I.V. q 8h, in combination with piperacillin sodium, 50 mg/kg I.V. q 4h.

The demographics of the evaluable patients were as follows: [See table above]
Clinical response rates observed in this study were as follows: [See table below]

CONTRAINDICATIONS
CIPRO® I.V. (ciprofloxacin) is contraindicated in patients with a history of hypersensitivity to ciprofloxacin or any member of the quinolone class of antimicrobial agents.

WARNINGS
THE SAFETY AND EFFECTIVENESS OF CIPROFLOXACIN IN PEDIATRIC PATIENTS AND ADOLESCENTS (LESS THAN 18 YEARS OF AGE), PREGNANT WOMEN, AND LACTATING WOMEN HAVE NOT BEEN ESTABLISHED. (See **PRECAUTIONS: Pediatric Use, Pregnancy**, and **Nursing Mothers** subsections). Ciprofloxacin causes lameness in immature dogs. Histopathological examination of the weight-bearing joints of these dogs revealed permanent lesions of the cartilage. Related quinolone-class drugs also produce erosions of cartilage of weight-bearing joints and other signs of arthropathy in immature animals of various species. (See **ANIMAL PHARMACOLOGY**.)

Convulsions, increased intracranial pressure, and toxic psychosis have been reported in patients receiving quinolones, including ciprofloxacin. Ciprofloxacin may also cause central nervous system (CNS) events including: dizziness, confusion, tremors, hallucinations, depression, and, rarely, suicidal thoughts or acts. These reactions may occur following the first dose. If these reactions occur in patients receiving ciprofloxacin, the drug should be discontinued and appropriate measures instituted. As with all quinolones, ciprofloxacin should be used with caution in patients with known or suspected CNS disorders that may predispose to seizures or lower the seizure threshold (e.g. severe cerebral arteriosclerosis, epilepsy), or in the presence of other risk factors that may predispose to seizures or lower the seizure threshold (e.g. certain drug therapy, renal dysfunction). (See **PRECAUTIONS: General, Information for Patients, Drug Interactions** and **ADVERSE REACTIONS**.)

SERIOUS AND FATAL REACTIONS HAVE BEEN REPORTED IN PATIENTS RECEIVING CONCURRENT ADMINISTRATION OF INTRAVENOUS CIPROFLOXACIN AND THEOPHYLLINE. These reactions have included cardiac arrest, seizure, status epilepticus, and respiratory failure. Although similar serious adverse events have been reported in patients receiving theophylline alone, the possibility that these reactions may be potentiated by ciprofloxacin cannot be eliminated. If concomitant use cannot be avoided, serum levels of theophylline should be monitored and dosage adjustments made as appropriate.

Serious and occasionally fatal hypersensitivity (anaphylactic) reactions, some following the first dose, have been reported in patients receiving quinolone therapy. Some reactions were accompanied by cardiovascular collapse, loss of consciousness, tingling, pharyngeal or facial edema, dyspnea, urticaria, and itching. Only a few patients had a history of hypersensitivity reactions. Serious anaphylactic reactions require immediate emergency treatment with epinephrine and other resuscitation measures, including oxygen, intravenous fluids, intravenous antihistamines, corticosteroids, pressor amines, and airway management, as clinically indicated.

Severe hypersensitivity reactions characterized by rash, fever, eosinophilia, jaundice, and hepatic necrosis with fatal outcome have also been reported extremely rarely in patients receiving ciprofloxacin along with other drugs. The possibility that these reactions were related to ciprofloxacin cannot be excluded. Ciprofloxacin should be discontinued at the first appearance of a skin rash or any other sign of hypersensitivity.

Pseudomembranous colitis has been reported with nearly all antibacterial agents, including ciprofloxacin, and may range from mild to life-threatening. Therefore, it is important to consider this diagnosis in patients who present with diarrhea subsequent to the administration of antibacterial agents.

Treatment with antibacterial agents alters the normal flora of the colon and may permit overgrowth of clostridia. Studies indicate that a toxin produced by *Clostridium difficile* is one primary cause of "antibiotic associated colitis".

After the diagnosis of pseudomembranous colitis has been established, therapeutic measures should be initiated. Mild cases of pseudomembranous colitis usually respond to drug discontinuation alone. In moderate to severe cases, consideration should be given to management with fluids and electrolytes, protein supplementation and treatment with an antibacterial drug clinically effective against *C. difficile* colitis.

Achilles and other tendon ruptures that required surgical repair or resulted in prolonged disability have been reported with ciprofloxacin and other quinolones. Ciprofloxacin should be discontinued if the patient experiences pain, inflammation, or rupture of a tendon.

PRECAUTIONS
General: INTRAVENOUS CIPROFLOXACIN SHOULD BE ADMINISTERED BY SLOW INFUSION OVER A PERIOD OF 60 MINUTES. Local I.V. site reactions have been reported with the intravenous administration of ciprofloxacin. These reactions are more frequent if infusion time is 30 minutes or less or if small veins of the hand are used. (See **ADVERSE REACTIONS**.)

Quinolones, including ciprofloxacin, may also cause central nervous system (CNS) events, including nervousness, agitation, insomnia, anxiety, nightmares or paranoia. (See **WARNINGS, Information for Patients** and **Drug Interactions**.)

Crystals of ciprofloxacin have been observed rarely in the urine of human subjects but more frequently in the urine of laboratory animals, which is usually alkaline. (See **ANIMAL PHARMACOLOGY**.) Crystalluria related to ciprofloxacin has been reported only rarely in humans because human urine is usually acidic. Alkalinity of the urine should be avoided in patients receiving ciprofloxacin. Patients should be well hydrated to prevent the formation of highly concentrated urine.

Alteration of the dosage regimen is necessary for patients with impairment of renal function. (See **DOSAGE AND ADMINISTRATION**.)

Moderate to severe phototoxicity manifested as an exaggerated sunburn reaction has been observed in some patients who were exposed to direct sunlight while receiving some members of the quinolone class of drugs. Excessive sunlight should be avoided.

As with any potent drug, periodic assessment of organ system functions, including renal, hepatic, and hematopoietic, is advisable during prolonged therapy.

Information for Patients: Patients should be advised that ciprofloxacin may be associated with hypersensitivity reactions, even following a single dose, and to discontinue the drug at the first sign of a rash or other allergic reaction.

Ciprofloxacin may cause dizziness and lightheadedness; therefore, patients should know how they react to this drug before they operate an automobile or machinery or engage in activities requiring mental alertness or coordination.

Patients should be advised that ciprofloxacin may increase the effect of theophylline and caffeine. There is a possibility of caffeine accumulation when products containing caffeine are consumed while taking ciprofloxacin.

Patients should be advised to discontinue treatment; rest and refrain from exercise; and inform their physician if they experience pain, inflammation, or rupture of a tendon.

Patients should be advised that convulsions have been reported in patients taking quinolones, including ciprofloxacin, and to notify their physician before taking this drug if there is a history of this condition.

Drug Interactions: As with some other quinolones, concurrent administration of ciprofloxacin with theophylline may lead to elevated serum concentrations of theophylline and prolongation of its elimination half-life. This may result in increased risk of theophylline-related reactions. (See **WARNINGS**.) If concomitant use cannot be avoided, serum levels of theophylline should be monitored and dosage adjustments made as appropriate.

Some quinolones, including ciprofloxacin, have also been shown to interfere with the metabolism of caffeine. This may lead to reduced clearance of caffeine and prolongation of its serum half-life.

Outcomes	Ciprofloxacin/Piperacillin N = 233 Success (%)	Tobramycin/Piperacillin N = 237 Success (%)
Clinical Resolution of Initial Febrile Episode with No Modifications of Empirical Regimen*	63 (27.0%)	52 (21.9%)
Clinical Resolution of Initial Febrile Episode Including Patients with Modifications of Empirical Regimen	187 (80.3%)	185 (78.1%)
Overall Survival	224 (96.1%)	223 (94.1%)

* To be evaluated as a clinical resolution, patients had to have: (1) resolution of fever; (2) microbiological eradication of infection (if an infection was microbiologically documented); (3) resolution of signs/symptoms of infection; and (4) no modification of empirical antibiotic regimen.

Continued on next page

Cipro I.V.—Cont.

Some quinolones, including ciprofloxacin, have been associated with transient elevations in serum creatinine in patients receiving cyclosporine concomitantly.

Altered serum levels of phenytoin (increased and decreased) have been reported in patients receiving concomitant ciprofloxacin.

The concomitant administration of ciprofloxacin with the sulfonylurea glyburide has, in some patients, resulted in severe hypoglycemia. Fatalities have been reported.

Quinolones have been reported to enhance the effects of the oral anticoagulant warfarin or its derivatives. When these products are administered concomitantly, prothrombin time or other suitable coagulation tests should be closely monitored.

Probenecid interferes with renal tubular secretion of ciprofloxacin and produces an increase in the level of ciprofloxacin in the serum. This should be considered if patients are receiving both drugs concomitantly.

As with other broad-spectrum antimicrobial agents, prolonged use of ciprofloxacin may result in overgrowth of nonsusceptible organisms. Repeated evaluation of the patient's condition and microbial susceptibility testing are essential. If superinfection occurs during therapy, appropriate measures should be taken.

Carcinogenesis, Mutagenesis, Impairment of Fertility: Eight *in vitro* mutagenicity tests have been conducted with ciprofloxacin. Test results are listed below:

- Salmonella/Microsome Test (Negative)
- *E. coli* DNA Repair Assay (Negative)
- Mouse Lymphoma Cell Forward Mutation Assay (Positive)
- Chinese Hamster V_{79} Cell HGPRT Test (Negative)
- Syrian Hamster Embryo Cell Transformation Assay (Negative)
- *Saccharomyces cerevisiae* Point Mutation Assay (Negative)
- *Saccharomyces cerevisiae* Mitotic Crossover and Gene Conversion Assay (Negative)
- Rat Hepatocyte DNA Repair Assay (Positive)

Thus, two of the eight tests were positive, but results of the following three *in vivo* test systems gave negative results:

- Rat Hepatocyte DNA Repair Assay
- Micronucleus Test (Mice)
- Dominant Lethal Test (Mice)

Long-term carcinogenicity studies in mice and rats have been completed. After daily oral doses of 750 mg/kg (mice) and 250 mg/kg (rats) were administered for up to 2 years, there was no evidence that ciprofloxacin had any carcinogenic or tumorigenic effects in these species.

Results from photo co-carcinogenicity testing indicate that ciprofloxacin does not reduce the time to appearance of UV-induced skin tumors as compared to vehicle control. Hairless (Skh-1) mice were exposed to UVA light for 3.5 hours five times every two weeks for up to 78 weeks while concurrently being administered ciprofloxacin. The time to development of the first skin tumors was 50 weeks in mice treated concomitantly with UVA and ciprofloxacin (mouse dose approximately equal to maximum recommended human dose based upon mg/m^2), as opposed to 34 weeks when animals were treated with both UVA and vehicle. The times to development of skin tumors ranged from 16–32 weeks in mice treated concomitantly with UVA and other quinolones.[3]

In this model, mice treated with ciprofloxacin alone did not develop skin or systemic tumors. There are no data from similar models using pigmented mice and/or fully haired mice. The clinical significance of these findings to humans is unknown.

Fertility studies performed in rats at oral doses of ciprofloxacin up to 100 mg/kg (0.8 times the highest recommended human dose of 1200 mg based upon body surface area) revealed no evidence of impairment.

Pregnancy: Teratogenic Effects. Pregnancy Category C: Reproduction studies have been performed in rats and mice using oral doses of up to 100 mg/kg (0.8 and 0.4 times the maximum daily human dose based upon body surface area, respectively) and I.V. doses of up to 30 mg/kg (0.24 and 0.12 times the maximum daily human dose based upon body surface area, respectively) and have revealed no evidence of harm to the fetus due to ciprofloxacin. In rabbits, ciprofloxacin (30 and 100 mg/kg orally) produced gastrointestinal disturbances resulting in maternal weight loss and an increased incidence of abortion, but no teratogenicity was observed at either dose. After intravenous administration of doses up to 20 mg/kg, no maternal toxicity was produced in the rabbit, and no embryotoxicity or teratogenicity was observed. There are, however, no adequate and well-controlled studies in pregnant women. Ciprofloxacin should be used during pregnancy only if the potential benefit justifies the potential risk to the fetus. (See **WARNINGS**.)

Nursing Mothers: Ciprofloxacin is excreted in human milk. Because of the potential for serious adverse reactions in infants nursing from mothers taking ciprofloxacin, a decision should be made whether to discontinue nursing or to discontinue the drug, taking into account the importance of the drug to the mother.

DOSAGE GUIDELINES

Intravenous

Infection†	Type or Severity	Unit Dose	Frequency	Daily Dose
Urinary tract	Mild/Moderate	200 mg	q12h	400 mg
	Severe/Complicated	400 mg	q12h	800 mg
Lower Respiratory Tract	Mild/Moderate	400 mg	q12h	800 mg
	Severe/Complicated	400 mg	q8h	1200 mg
Nosocomial Pneumonia	Mild/Moderate/Severe	400 mg	q8h	1200 mg
Skin and Skin Structure	Mild/Moderate	400 mg	q12h	800 mg
	Severe/Complicated	400 mg	q8h	1200 mg
Bone and Joint	Mild/Moderate	400 mg	q12h	800 mg
	Severe/Complicated	400 mg	q8h	1200 mg
Intra-Abdominal*	Complicated	400 mg	q12h	800 mg
Empirical Therapy in Febrile Neutropenic Patients	Severe Ciprofloxacin	400 mg	q8h	1200 mg
	+ Piperacillin	50 mg/kg	q4h	Not to exceed 24 g/day

* used in conjunction with metronidazole. (See product labeling for prescribing information.)

† DUE TO THE DESIGNATED PATHOGENS (See **INDICATIONS AND USAGE**.)

Pediatric Use: Safety and effectiveness in pediatric patients and adolescents less than 18 years of age have not been established. Ciprofloxacin causes arthropathy in juvenile animals. (See **WARNINGS**.)

Short-term safety data from a single trial in pediatric cystic fibrosis patients are available. In a randomized, double-blind clinical trial for the treatment of acute pulmonary exacerbations in cystic fibrosis patients (ages 5–17 years), 67 patients received ciprofloxacin I.V. 10 mg/kg/dose q8h for one week followed by ciprofloxacin tablets 20 mg/kg/dose q12h to complete 10–21 days treatment and 62 patients received the combination of ceftazidime I.V. 50 mg/kg/dose q8h and tobramycin I.V. 3 mg/kg/dose q8h for a total of 10–21 days. Patients less than 5 years of age were not studied. Safety monitoring in the study included periodic range of motion examinations and gait assessments by treatment-blinded examiners. Patients were followed for an average of 23 days after completing treatment (range 0–93 days). This study was not designed to determine long term effects and the safety of repeated exposure to ciprofloxacin.

In the study, injection site reactions were more common in the ciprofloxacin group (24%) than in the comparison group (8%). Other adverse events were similar in nature and frequency between treatment arms. Musculoskeletal adverse events were reported in 22% of the patients in the ciprofloxacin group and 21% in the comparison group. Decreased range of motion was reported in 12% of the subjects in the ciprofloxacin group and 16% in the comparison group. Arthralgia was reported in 10% of the patients in the ciprofloxacin group and 11% in the comparison group. One of sixty-seven patients developed arthritis of the knee nine days after a ten day course of treatment with ciprofloxacin. Clinical symptoms resolved, but an MRI showed knee effusion without other abnormalities eight months after treatment. However, the relationship of this event to the patient's course of ciprofloxacin can not be definitively determined, particularly since patients with cystic fibrosis may develop arthralgias/arthritis as part of their underlying disease process.

ADVERSE REACTIONS

The most frequently reported events, without regard to drug relationship, among patients treated with intravenous ciprofloxacin were nausea, diarrhea, central nervous system disturbance, local I.V. site reactions, abnormalities of liver associated enzymes (hepatic enzymes), and eosinophilia. Headache, restlessness, and rash were also noted in greater than 1% of patients treated with the most common doses of ciprofloxacin.

Local I.V. site reactions have been reported with the intravenous administration of ciprofloxacin. These reactions are more frequent if the infusion time is 30 minutes or less. These may appear as local skin reactions which resolve rapidly upon completion of the infusion. Subsequent intravenous administration is not contraindicated unless the reactions recur or worsen.

Additional events, without regard to drug relationship or route of administration, that occurred in 1% or less of ciprofloxacin patients are listed below:

CARDIOVASCULAR: cardiovascular collapse, cardiopulmonary arrest, myocardial infarction, arrhythmia, tachycardia, palpitation, cerebral thrombosis, syncope, cardiac murmur, hypertension, hypotension, angina pectoris

CENTRAL NERVOUS SYSTEM: convulsive seizures, paranoia, toxic psychosis, depression, dysphasia, phobia, depersonalization, manic reaction, unresponsiveness, ataxia, confusion, hallucinations, dizziness, lightheadedness, paresthesia, anxiety, tremor, insomnia, nightmares, weakness, drowsiness, irritability, malaise, lethargy

GASTROINTESTINAL: ileus, jaundice, gastrointestinal bleeding, *C. difficile* associated diarrhea, pseudomembranous colitis, pancreatitis, hepatic necrosis, intestinal perforation, dyspepsia, epigastric or abdominal pain, vomiting, constipation, oral ulceration, oral candidiasis, mouth dryness, anorexia, dysphagia, flatulence

I.V. INFUSION SITE: thrombophlebitis, burning, pain, pruritus, paresthesia, erythema, swelling

MUSCULOSKELETAL: arthralgia, jaw, arm or back pain, joint stiffness, neck and chest pain, achiness, flare up of gout

RENAL/UROGENITAL: renal failure, interstitial nephritis, hemorrhagic cystitis, renal calculi, frequent urination, acidosis, urethral bleeding, polyuria, urinary retention, gynecomastia, candiduria, vaginitis. Crystalluria, cylindruria, hematuria, and albuminuria have also been reported.

RESPIRATORY: respiratory arrest, pulmonary embolism, dyspnea, pulmonary edema, respiratory distress, pleural effusion, hemoptysis, epistaxis, hiccough

SKIN/HYPERSENSITIVITY: anaphylactic reactions, erythema multiforme/Stevens-Johnson syndrome, exfoliative dermatitis, toxic epidermal necrolysis, vasculitis, angioedema, edema of the lips, face, neck, conjunctivae, hands or lower extremities, purpura, fever, chills, flushing, pruritus, urticaria, cutaneous candidiasis, vesicles, increased perspiration, hyperpigmentation, erythema nodosum, photosensitivity

Allergic reactions ranging from urticaria to anaphylactic reactions have been reported. (See **WARNINGS**.)

SPECIAL SENSES: decreased visual acuity, blurred vision, disturbed vision, (flashing lights, change in color perception, overbrightness of lights, diplopia), eye pain, anosmia, hearing loss, tinnitus, nystagmus, a bad taste

Also reported were agranulocytosis, prolongation of prothrombin time, and possible exacerbation of myasthenia gravis.

Many of these events were described as only mild or moderate in severity, abated soon after the drug was discontinued, and required no treatment.

In several instances, nausea, vomiting, tremor, irritability, or palpitation were judged by investigators to be related to elevated serum levels of theophylline possibly as a result of drug interaction with ciprofloxacin.

In randomized, double-blind controlled clinical trials comparing ciprofloxacin (I.V. and I.V. P.O. sequential) with intravenous beta-lactam control antibiotics, the CNS adverse event profile of ciprofloxacin was comparable to that of the control drugs.

Post-Marketing Adverse Events: Additional adverse events, regardless of relationship to drug, reported from worldwide marketing experience with quinolones, including ciprofloxacin, are:

BODY AS A WHOLE: change in serum phenytoin

CARDIOVASCULAR: postural hypotension, vasculitis

CENTRAL NERVOUS SYSTEM: agitation, confusion, delirium, dysphasia, myoclonus, nystagmus, toxic psychosis

Men: Creatinine clearance (mL/min) = $\dfrac{\text{Weight (kg)} \times (140 - \text{age})}{72 \times \text{serum creatinine (mg/dL)}}$

Women: 0.85 × the value calculated for men.

VIAL:

SIZE	STRENGTH	NDC NUMBER
20 mL	200 mg, 1%	0026-8562-20
40 mL	400 mg, 1%	0026-8564-64

FLEXIBLE CONTAINER: manufactured for Bayer Corporation by Abbott Laboratories, North Chicago, IL 60064.

SIZE	STRENGTH	NDC NUMBER
100 mL 5% dextrose	200 mg, 0.2%	0026-8552-36
200 mL 5% dextrose	400 mg, 0.2%	0026-8554-63

FLEXIBLE CONTAINER: manufactured for Bayer Corporation by Baxter Healthcare Corporation, Deerfield, IL 60015.

SIZE	STRENGTH	NDC NUMBER
100 mL 5% dextrose	200 mg, 0.2%	0026-8527-36
200 mL 5% dextrose	400 mg, 0.2%	0026-8527-63

GASTROINTESTINAL: constipation, dyspepsia, flatulence, hepatic necrosis, jaundice, pancreatitis, pseudomembranous colitis (The onset of pseudomembranous colitis symptoms may occur during or after antimicrobial treatment.)
HEMIC/LYMPHATIC: agranulocytosis, hemolytic anemia, methemoglobinemia, prolongation of prothrombin time
METABOLIC/NUTRITIONAL: elevation of serum triglycerides, cholesterol, blood glucose, serum potassium
MUSCULOSKELETAL: myalgia, possible exacerbation of myasthenia gravis, tendinitis/tendon rupture
RENAL/UROGENITAL: albuminuria, candiduria, renal calculi, vaginal candidiasis
SKIN/HYPERSENSITIVITY: anaphylactic reactions, erythema multiforme/Stevens-Johnson syndrome, exfoliative dermatitis, toxic epidermal necrolysis
SPECIAL SENSES: anosmia
(See **PRECAUTIONS**.)
Adverse Laboratory Changes: The most frequently reported changes in laboratory parameters with intravenous ciprofloxacin therapy, without regard to drug relationship are listed below:
Hepatic—elevations of AST (SGOT), ALT (SGPT), alkaline phosphatase, LDH, and serum bilirubin;
Hematologic—elevated eosinophil and platelet counts, decreased platelet counts, hemoglobin and/or hematocrit;
Renal—elevations of serum creatinine, BUN, and uric acid;
Other—elevations of serum creatinine, phosphokinase, serum theophylline (in patients receiving theophylline concomitantly), blood glucose, and triglycerides.

Other changes occurring infrequently were: decreased leukocyte count, elevated atypical lymphocyte count, immature WBCs, elevated serum calcium, elevation of serum gamma-glutamyl transpeptidase (γ GT), decreased BUN, decreased uric acid, decreased total serum protein, decreased serum albumin, decreased serum potassium, elevated serum potassium, elevated serum cholesterol.
Other changes occurring rarely during administration of ciprofloxacin were: elevation of serum amylase, decrease of blood glucose, pancytopenia, leukocytosis, elevated sedimentation rate, change in serum phenytoin, decreased prothrombin time, hemolytic anemia, and bleeding diathesis.

OVERDOSAGE
In the event of acute overdosage, the patient should be carefully observed and given supportive treatment. Adequate hydration must be maintained. Only a small amount of ciprofloxacin (<10%) is removed from the body after hemodialysis or peritoneal dialysis.
In mice, rats, rabbits and dogs, significant toxicity including tonic/clonic convulsions was observed at intravenous doses of ciprofloxacin between 125 and 300 mg/kg.

DOSAGE AND ADMINISTRATION
The recommended adult dosage for urinary tract infections of mild to moderate severity is 200 mg I.V. every 12 hours. For severe or complicated urinary tract infections, the recommended dosage is 400 mg I.V. every 12 hours.
The recommended adult dosage for lower respiratory tract infections, skin and skin structure infections, and bone and joint infections of mild to moderate severity is 400 mg I.V. every 12 hours.
For severe/complicated infections of the lower respiratory tract, skin and skin structure, and bone and joint, the recommended adult dosage is 400 mg I.V. every 8 hours.
The recommended adult dosage for mild, moderate, and severe nosocomial pneumonia is 400 mg I.V. every 8 hours.
Complicated Intra-Abdominal Infections: Sequential therapy [parenteral to oral—400 mg CIPRO® I.V. q 12 h (plus I.V. metronidazole) → 500 mg CIPRO® Tablets q 12 h (plus oral metronidazole)] can be instituted at the discretion of the physician. Metronidazole should be give according to product labeling to provide appropriate anaerobic coverage.
The recommended adult dosage for empirical therapy of febrile neutropenic patients is 400 mg I.V. every 8 hours in combination with piperacillin sodium 50 mg/kg I.V. q 4 hours, not to exceed 24 g/day (300 mg/kg/day), for 7–14 days.
The determination of dosage for any particular patient must take into consideration the severity and nature of the infection, the susceptibility of the causative microorganism, the integrity of the patient's host-defense mechanisms and the status of renal and hepatic function.
[See table at top of previous page]
CIPRO® I.V. should be administered by intravenous infusion over a period of 60 minutes.
Parenteral drug products should be inspected visually for particulate matter and discoloration prior to administration.
Ciprofloxacin hydrochloride (CIPRO® Tablets) for oral administration are available. Parenteral therapy may be changed to oral CIPRO® Tablets when the condition warrants, at the discretion of the physician. For complete dosage and administration information, see CIPRO® Tablets package insert.
Impaired Renal Function: The following table provides dosage guidelines for use in patients with renal impairment; however, monitoring of serum drug levels provides the most reliable basis for dosage adjustment.

RECOMMENDED STARTING AND MAINTENANCE DOSES FOR PATIENTS WITH IMPAIRED RENAL FUNCTION

Creatinine Clearance (mL/min)	Dosage
> 30	See usual dosage.
5–29	200–400 mg q 18–24 hr

When only the serum creatinine concentration is known, the following formula may be used to estimate creatinine clearance:
[See first table above]
The serum creatinine should represent a steady state of renal function.
For patients with changing renal function or for patients with renal impairment and hepatic insufficiency, measurement of serum concentrations of ciprofloxacin will provide additional guidance for adjusting dosage.
INTRAVENOUS ADMINISTRATION
CIPRO® I.V. should be administered by intravenous infusion over a period of 60 minutes. Slow infusion of a dilute solution into a large vein will minimize patient discomfort and reduce the risk of venous irritation.
Vials (Injection Concentrate): THIS PREPARATION MUST BE DILUTED BEFORE USE. The intravenous dose should be prepared by aseptically withdrawing the concentrate from the vial of CIPRO® I.V. This should be diluted with a suitable intravenous solution to a final concentration of 1–2 mg/mL. (See **COMPATIBILITY AND STABILITY**.) The resulting solution should be infused over a period of 60 minutes by direct infusion or through a Y-type intravenous infusion set which may already be in place.
If this method or the "piggyback" method of administration is used, it is advisable to discontinue temporarily the administration of any other solutions during the infusion of CIPRO® I.V.
Flexible Containers: CIPRO® I.V. is also available as a 0.2% premixed solution in 5% dextrose in flexible containers of 100 mL or 200 mL. The solutions in flexible containers may be infused as described above.
COMPATIBILITY AND STABILITY
Ciprofloxacin injection 1% (10 mg/mL), when diluted with the following intravenous solutions to concentrations of 0.5 to 2.0 mg/mL, is stable for up to 14 days at refrigerated or room temperature storage.
0.9% Sodium Chloride Injection, USP
5% Dextrose Injection, USP
Sterile Water for Injection
10% Dextrose for Injection
5% Dextrose and 0.225% Sodium Chloride for Injection
5% Dextrose and 0.45% Sodium Chloride for Injection
Lactated Ringer's for Injection

If CIPRO® I.V. is to be given concomitantly with another drug, each drug should be given separately in accordance with the recommended dosage and route of administration for each drug.

HOW SUPPLIED
CIPRO® I.V. (ciprofloxacin) is available as a clear, colorless to slightly yellowish solution. CIPRO® I.V. is available in 200 mg and 400 mg strengths. The concentrate is supplied in vials while the premixed solution is supplied in flexible containers as follows:
[See second table from top of page]
STORAGE
Vial: Store between 5–30°C (41–86°F).
Flexible Container: Store between 5–25°C (41–77°F). Protect from light, avoid excessive heat, protect from freezing.
CIPRO® I.V. (ciprofloxacin) is also available in a 120 mL Pharmacy Bulk Package.
Ciprofloxacin is also available as CIPRO® (ciprofloxacin HCl) Tablets 100, 250, 500, and 750 mg and CIPRO® (ciprofloxacin) 5% and 10% Oral Suspension.

ANIMAL PHARMACOLOGY
Ciprofloxacin and other quinolones have been shown to cause arthropathy in immature animals of most species tested. (See **WARNINGS**.) Damage of weight-bearing joints was observed in juvenile dogs and rats. In young beagles, 100 mg/kg ciprofloxacin given daily for 4 weeks caused degenerative articular changes of the knee joint. At 30 mg/kg, the effect on the joint was minimal. In a subsequent study in beagles, removal of weight-bearing from the joint reduced the lesions but did not totally prevent them.
Crystalluria, sometimes associated with secondary nephropathy, occurs in laboratory animals dosed with ciprofloxacin. This is primarily related to the reduced solubility of ciprofloxacin under alkaline conditions, which predominate in the urine of test animals; in man, crystalluria is rare since human urine is typically acidic. In rhesus monkeys, crystalluria without nephropathy has been noted after intravenous doses as low as 5 mg/kg. After 6 months of intravenous dosing at 10 mg/kg/day, no nephropathological changes were noted; however, nephropathy was observed after dosing at 20 mg/kg/day for the same duration.
In dogs, ciprofloxacin administered at 3 and 10 mg/kg by rapid intravenous injection (15 sec.) produces pronounced hypotensive effects. These effects are considered to be related to histamine release because they are partially antagonized by pyrilamine, an antihistamine. In rhesus monkeys, rapid intravenous injection also produces hypotension, but the effect in this species is inconsistent and less pronounced.
In mice, concomitant administration of nonsteroidal anti-inflammatory drugs, such as phenylbutazone and indomethacin, with quinolones has been reported to enhance the CNS stimulatory effect of quinolones.
Ocular toxicity, seen with some related drugs, has not been observed in ciprofloxacin-treated animals.

REFERENCES
1. National Committee for Clinical Laboratory Standards, Methods for Dilution Antimicrobial Susceptibility Tests for Bacteria That Grow Aerobically—Fourth Edition. Approved Standard NCCLS Document M7-A4, Vol. 17, No. 2, NCCLS, Wayne, PA, January, 1997. **2.** National Committee for Clinical Laboratory Standards, Performance Standards for Antimicrobial Disk Susceptibility Tests—Sixth Edition. Approved Standard NCCLS Document M2-A6, Vol. 17, No. 1, NCCLS, Wayne, PA, January, 1997. **3.** Report presented at the FDA's Anti-Infective Drug and Dermatological Drug Products Advisory Committee Meeting, March 31, 1993, Silver Spring, MD. Report available from FDA, CDER, Advisors and Consultants Staff, HFD-21, 1901 Chapman Avenue, Room 200, Rockville, MD 20852, USA.

Bayer Corporation
Pharmaceutical Division
400 Morgan Lane
West Haven, CT 06516 USA

Rx Only

PD500088 7/98 BAY q 3939 5202-4-A-U.S.-3 © 1998
Bayer Corporation 8418
06-9198

Shown in Product Identification Guide, page 305

CIPRO® I.V. ℞
(ciprofloxacin)
For Intravenous Infusion

PHARMACY BULK PACKAGE—NOT FOR DIRECT INFUSION

DESCRIPTION
The pharmacy bulk package is a single-entry container of a sterile preparation for parenteral use that contains many

Continued on next page

Cipro I.V. Pharm Bulk—Cont.

single doses. It contains ciprofloxacin as a 1% aqueous solution concentrate. The contents are intended for use in a pharmacy admixture program and are restricted to the preparation of admixtures for intravenous infusion.
CIPRO® I.V. (ciprofloxacin) is a synthetic broad-spectrum antimicrobial agent for intravenous (I.V.) administration.
Ciprofloxacin, a fluoroquinolone, is 1-cyclopropyl-6-fluoro-1,4-dihydro-4-oxo-7-(1-piperazinyl)-3-quinolinecarboxylic acid. Its empirical formula is $C_{17}H_{18}FN_3O_3$ and its chemical structure is:

Ciprofloxacin is a faint to light yellow crystalline powder with a molecular weight of 331.4. It is soluble in dilute (0.1N) hydrochloric acid and is practically insoluble in water and ethanol. Ciprofloxacin differs from other quinolones in that it has a fluorine atom at the 6-position, a piperazine moiety at the 7-position, and a cyclopropyl ring at the 1-position. CIPRO® I.V. solution is available as sterile 1.0% aqueous concentrate, which is intended for dilution prior to administration. Ciprofloxacin solution contains lactic acid as a solubilizing agent and hydrochloric acid for pH adjustment. The pH range for the 1.0% aqueous concentrate is 3.3 to 3.9.

CLINICAL PHARMACOLOGY

Following 60-minute intravenous infusions of 200 mg and 400 mg ciprofloxacin to normal volunteers, the mean maximum serum concentrations achieved were 2.1 and 4.6 µg/mL, respectively; the concentrations at 12 hours were 0.1 and 0.2 µg/mL, respectively.

Steady-state Ciprofloxacin Serum Concentrations (µg/mL)
After 60-minute I.V. Infusions q 12 h.

Dose	Time after starting the infusion					
	30 min	1hr	3 hr	6 hr	8 hr	12 hr
200 mg	1.7	2.1	0.6	0.3	0.2	0.1
400 mg	3.7	4.6	1.3	0.7	0.5	0.2

The pharmacokinetics of ciprofloxacin are linear over the dose range of 200 to 400 mg administered intravenously. The serum elimination half-life is approximately 5–6 hours and the total clearance is around 35 L/hr. Comparison of the pharmacokinetic parameters following the 1st and 5th I.V. dose on a q 12 h regimen indicates no evidence of drug accumulation.
The absolute bioavailability of oral ciprofloxacin is within a range of 70–80% with no substantial loss by first pass metabolism. An intravenous infusion of 400 mg ciprofloxacin given over 60 minutes every 12 hours has been shown to produce an area under the serum concentration time curve (AUC) equivalent to that produced by a 500-mg oral dose given every 12 hours. An intravenous infusion of 400 mg ciprofloxacin given over 60 minutes every 8 hours has been shown to produce an AUC at steady-state equivalent to that produced by a 750-mg oral dose given every 12 hours. A 400-mg I.V. dose results in a C_{max} similar to that observed with a 750-mg oral dose. An infusion of 200 mg ciprofloxacin given every 12 hours produces an AUC equivalent to that produced by a 250-mg oral dose given every 12 hours.
[See table below]
After intravenous administration, approximately 50% to 70% of the dose is excreted in the urine as unchanged drug. Following a 200-mg I.V. dose, concentrations in the urine usually exceed 200 µg/mL 0–2 hours after dosing and are generally greater than 15 µg/mL 8–12 hours after dosing. Following a 400-mg I.V. dose, urine concentrations generally exceed 400 µg/mL 0–2 hours after dosing and are usually greater than 30 µg/mL 8–12 hours after dosing. The renal clearance is approximately 22 L/hr. The urinary excretion of ciprofloxacin is virtually complete by 24 hours after dosing.
The serum concentrations of ciprofloxacin and metronidazole were not altered when these two drugs were given concomitantly.

Co-administration of probenecid with ciprofloxacin results in about a 50% reduction in the ciprofloxacin renal clearance and a 50% increase in its concentration in the systemic circulation. Although bile concentrations of ciprofloxacin are severalfold higher than serum concentrations after intravenous dosing, only a small amount of the administered dose (<1%) is recovered from the bile as unchanged drug. Approximately 15% of an I.V. dose is recovered from the feces within 5 days after dosing.
After I.V. administration, three metabolites of ciprofloxacin have been identified in human urine which together account for approximately 10% of the intravenous dose.
In patients with reduced renal function, the half-life of ciprofloxacin is slightly prolonged and dosage adjustments may be required. (See **DOSAGE AND ADMINISTRATION.**)
In preliminary studies in patients with stable chronic liver cirrhosis, no significant changes in ciprofloxacin pharmacokinetics have been observed. However, the kinetics of ciprofloxacin in patients with acute hepatic insufficiency have not been fully elucidated.
Following infusion of 400 mg I.V. ciprofloxacin every eight hours in combination with 50 mg/kg I.V. piperacillin sodium every 4 hours, mean serum ciprofloxacin concentrations were 3.02 µg/mL $^1/_2$ hour and 1.18 µg/mL between 6–8 hours after the end of infusion.
The binding of ciprofloxacin to serum proteins is 20 to 40%. After intravenous administration, ciprofloxacin is present in saliva, nasal and bronchial secretions, sputum, skin blister fluid, lymph, peritoneal fluid, bile, and prostatic secretions. It has also been detected in the lung, skin, fat, muscle, cartilage, and bone. Although the drug diffuses into cerebrospinal fluid (CSF), CSF concentrations are generally less than 10% of peak serum concentrations. Levels of the drug in the aqueous and vitreous chambers of the eye are lower than in serum.
Microbiology: Ciprofloxacin has *in vitro* activity against a wide range of gram-negative and gram-positive microorganisms. The bactericidal action of ciprofloxacin results from interference with the enzyme DNA gyrase which is needed for the synthesis of bacterial DNA.
Ciprofloxacin has been shown to be active against most strains of the following microorganisms, both *in vitro* and in clinical infections as described in the **INDICATIONS AND USAGE** section of the package insert for CIPRO® I.V. (ciprofloxacin for intravenous infusion).

Aerobic gram-positive microorganisms
Enterococcus faecalis
   (Many strains are only moderately susceptible.)
Staphylococcus aureus (methicillin susceptible)
Staphylococcus epidermidis
Staphylococcus saprophyticus
Streptococcus pneumoniae
Streptococcus pyogenes

Aerobic gram-negative microorganisms
Citrobacter diversus
Citrobacter freundii
Enterobacter cloacae
Escherichia coli
Haemophilus influenzae
Haemophilus parainfluenzae
Klebsiella pneumoniae
Morganella morganii
Proteus mirabilis
Proteus vulgaris
Providencia rettgeri
Providencia stuartii
Pseudomonas aeruginosa
Serratia marcescens
Ciprofloxacin has been shown to be active against most strains of the following microorganisms, both *in vitro* and in clinical infections as described in the **INDICATIONS AND USAGE** section of the package insert for CIPRO® (ciprofloxacin hydrochloride) Tablets.

Aerobic gram-positive microorganisms
Enterococcus faecalis
   (Many strains are only moderately susceptible.)
Staphylococcus aureus (methicillin susceptible)
Staphylococcus epidermidis
Staphylococcus saprophyticus
Streptococcus pneumoniae
Streptococcus pyogenes

Aerobic gram-negative microorganisms
Campylobacter jejuni
Citrobacter diversus
Citrobacter freundii
Enterobacter cloacae
Escherichia coli
Haemophilus influenzae
Haemophilus parainfluenzae
Klebsiella pneumoniae
Moraxella catarrhalis
Morganella morganii
Neisseria gonorrhoeae
Proteus mirabilis
Proteus vulgaris
Providencia rettgeri
Providencia stuartii
Pseudomonas aeruginosa
Salmonella typhi
Serratia marcescens
Shigella boydii
Shigella dysenteriae
Shigella flexneri
Shigella sonnei
The following *in vitro* data are available, **but their clinical significance is unknown.**
Ciprofloxacin exhibits *in vitro* minimum inhibitory concentrations (MICs) of 1 µg/mL or less against most (≥ 90%) strains of the following microorganisms; however, the safety and effectiveness of ciprofloxacin in treating clinical infections due to these microorganisms have not been established in adequate and well-controlled clinical trials.

Aerobic gram-positive microorganisms
Staphylococcus haemolyticus
Staphylococcus hominis

Aerobic gram-negative microorganisms
Acinetobacter lwoffi
Aeromonas hydrophila
Edwardsiella tarda
Enterobacter aerogenes
Klebsiella oxytoca
Legionella pneumophila
Pasteurella multocida
Salmonella enteritidis
Vibrio cholerae
Vibrio parahaemolyticus
Vibrio vulnificus
Yersinia enterocolitica
Most strains of *Burkholderia cepacia* and some strains of *Stenotrophomonas maltophilia* are resistant to ciprofloxacin as are most anaerobic bacteria, including *Bacteroides fragilis* and *Clostridium difficile*.
Ciprofloxacin is slightly less active when tested at acidic pH. The inoculum size has little effect when tested *in vitro*. The minimum bactericidal concentration (MBC) generally does not exceed the minimum inhibitory concentration (MIC) by more than a factor of 2. Resistance of ciprofloxacin *in vitro* usually develops slowly (multiple-step mutation).
Ciprofloxacin does not cross-react with other antimicrobial agents such as beta-lactams or aminoglycosides; therefore, organisms resistant to these drugs may be susceptible to ciprofloxacin.
In vitro studies have shown that additive activity often results when ciprofloxacin is combined with other antimicrobial agents such as beta-lactams, aminoglycosides, clindamycin, or metronidazole. Synergy has been reported particularly with the combination of ciprofloxacin and a beta-lactam; antagonism is observed only rarely.

Susceptibility Tests
Dilution Techniques: Quantitative methods are used to determine antimicrobial minimum inhibitory concentrations (MICs). These MICs provide estimates of the susceptibility of bacteria to antimicrobial compounds. The MICs should be determined using a standardized procedure. Standardized procedures are based on a dilution method[1] (broth or agar) or equivalent with standardized inoculum concentrations and standardized concentrations of ciprofloxacin powder. The MIC values should be interpreted according to the following criteria:
For testing aerobic microorganisms other than *Haemophilus influenzae*, *Haemophilus parainfluenzae*, and *Neisseria gonorrhoeae*[a]:

MIC (µg/mL)	Interpretation
≤1	Susceptible (S)
2	Intermediate (I)
≥4	Resistant (R)

[a] These interpretive standards are applicable only to broth microdilution susceptibility tests with streptococci using

Steady-state Pharmacokinetic Parameter
Following Multiple Oral and I.V. Doses

Parameters	500 mg q12h, P.O.	400 mg q12h, I.V.	750 mg q12h, P.O.	400 mg q8h, I.V.
AUC (µg·hr/mL)	13.7[a]	12.7[a]	31.6[b]	32.9[c]
C_{max} (µg/mL)	2.97	4.56	3.59	4.07

[a] $AUC_{0–12h}$
[b] $AUC\ 24h = AUC_{0–12h} \times 2$
[c] $AUC\ 24h = AUC_{0–8h} \times 3$

cation-adjusted Mueller-Hinton broth with 2–5% lysed horse blood.

For testing *Haemophilus influenzae* and *Haemophilus parainfluenzae*[b]:

MIC (μg/mL)	Interpretation
≤1	Susceptible (S)

[b] This interpretive standard is applicable only to broth microdilution susceptibility tests with *Haemophilus influenzae* and *Haemophilus parainfluenzae* using *Haemophilus* Test Medium[1].

The current absence of data on resistant strains precludes defining any results other than "Susceptible". Strains yielding MIC results suggestive of a "nonsusceptible" category should be submitted to a reference laboratory for further testing.

For testing *Neisseria gonorrhoeae*[c]:

MIC (μg/mL)	Interpretation
≤0.06	Susceptible (S)

[c] This interpretive standard is applicable only to agar dilution test with GC agar base and 1% defined growth supplement.

The current absence of data on resistant strains precludes defining any results other than "Susceptible". Strains yielding MIC results suggestive of a "nonsusceptible" category should be submitted to a reference laboratory for further testing.

A report of "Susceptible" indicates that the pathogen is likely to be inhibited if the antimicrobial compound in the blood reaches the concentrations usually achievable. A report of "Intermediate" indicates that the result should be considered equivocal, and, if the microorganism is not fully susceptible to alternative, clinically feasible drugs, the test should be repeated. This category implies possible clinical applicability in body sites where the drug is physiologically concentrated or in situations where high dosage of drug can be used. This category also provides a buffer zone which prevents small uncontrolled technical factors from causing major discrepancies in interpretation. A report of "Resistant" indicates that the pathogen is not likely to be inhibited if the antimicrobial compound in the blood reaches the concentrations usually achievable; other therapy should be selected.

Standardized susceptibility test procedures require the use of laboratory control microorganisms to control the technical aspects of the laboratory procedures. Standard ciprofloxacin powder should provide the following MIC values:

Organism		MIC (μg/mL)
E. faecalis	ATCC 29212	0.25 –2.0
E. coli	ATCC 25922	0.004–0.015
H. influenzae[a]	ATCC 49247	0.004–0.03
N. gonorrhoeae[b]	ATCC 49226	0.001–0.008
P. aeruginosa	ATCC 27853	0.25 –1.0
S. aureus	ATCC 29213	0.12 –0.5

[a] This quality control range is applicable to only *H. influenzae* ATCC 49247 tested by a broth microdilution procedure using *Haemophilus* Test Medium (HTM)[1].

[b] This quality control range is applicable to only *N. gonorrhoeae* ATCC 49226 tested by an agar dilution procedure using GC agar base and 1% defined growth supplement.

Diffusion Techniques: Quantitative methods that require measurement of zone diameters also provide reproducible estimates of the susceptibility of bacteria to antimicrobial compounds. One such standardized procedure[2] requires the use of standardized inoculum concentrations. This procedure uses paper disks impregnated with 5-μg ciprofloxacin to test the susceptibility of microorganisms to ciprofloxacin. Reports from the laboratory providing results of the standard single-disk susceptibility test with a 5-μg ciprofloxacin disk should be interpreted according to the following criteria:

For testing aerobic microorganisms other than *Haemophilus influenzae, Haemophilus parainfluenzae*, and *Neisseria gonorrhoeae*[a]:

Zone Diameter (mm)	Interpretation
≥21	Susceptible (S)
16–20	Intermediate (I)
≤ 15	Resistant (R)

[a] These zone diameter standards are applicable only to tests performed for streptococci using Mueller-Hinton agar supplemented with 5% sheep blood incubated in 5% CO_2.

For testing *Haemophilus influenzae* and *Haemophilus parainfluenzae*[b]:

Total	Ciprofloxacin/Piperacillin N = 233	Tobramycin/Piperacillin N = 237
Median Age (years)	47.0 (range 19–84)	50.0 (range 18–81)
Male	114 (48.9%)	117 (49.4%)
Female	119 (51.1%)	120 (50.6%)
Leukemia/Bone Marrow Transplant	165 (70.8%)	158 (66.7%)
Solid Tumor/Lymphoma	68 (29.2%)	79 (33.3%)
Median Duration of Neutropenia (days)	15.0 (range 1–61)	14.0 (range 1–89)

Zone Diameter (mm)	Interpretation
≥21	Susceptible (S)

[b] This zone diameter standard is applicable only to tests with *Haemophilus influenzae* and *Haemophilus parainfluenzae* using *Haemophilus* Test Medium (HTM)[2].

The current absence of data on resistant strains precludes defining any results other than "Susceptible". Strains yielding zone diameter results suggestive of a "nonsusceptible" category should be submitted to a reference laboratory for further testing.

For testing *Neisseria gonorrhoeae*[c]:

Zone Diameter (mm)	Interpretation
≥36	Susceptible (S)

[c] This zone diameter standard is applicable only to disk diffusion tests with GC agar base and 1% defined growth supplement.

The current absence of data on resistant strains precludes defining any results other than "Susceptible". Strains yielding zone diameter results suggestive of a "nonsusceptible" category should be submitted to a reference laboratory for further testing.

Interpretation should be as stated above for results using dilution techniques. Interpretation involves correlation of the diameter obtained in the disk test with the MIC for ciprofloxacin.

As with standardized dilution techniques, diffusion methods require the use of laboratory control microorganisms that are used to control the technical aspects of the laboratory procedures. For the diffusion technique, the 5-μg ciprofloxacin disk should provide the following zone diameters in these laboratory test quality control strains:

Organism		Zone Diameter (mm)
E. coli	ATCC 25922	30–40
H. influenzae[a]	ATCC 49247	34–42
N. gonorrhoeae[b]	ATCC 49226	48–58
P. aeruginosa	ATCC 27853	25–33
S. aureus	ATCC 25923	22–30

[a] These quality control limits are applicable to only *H. influenzae* ATCC 49247 testing using *Haemophilus* Test Medium (HTM)[2].

[b] These quality control limits are applicable only to tests conducted with *N. gonorrhoeae* ATCC 49226 performed by disk diffusion using GC agar base and 1% defined growth supplement.

INDICATIONS AND USAGE

CIPRO® I.V. is indicated for the treatment of infections caused by susceptible strains of the designated microorganisms in the conditions listed below when the intravenous administration offers a route of administration advantageous to the patient. Please see **DOSAGE AND ADMINISTRATION** for specific recommendations.

Urinary Tract Infections caused by *Escherichia coli* (including cases with secondary bacteremia), *Klebsiella pneumoniae* subspecies *pneumoniae, Enterobacter cloacae, Serratia marcescens, Proteus mirabilis, Providencia rettgeri, Morganella morganii, Citrobacter diversus, Citrobacter freundii, Pseudomonas aeruginosa, Staphylococcus epidermidis, Staphylococcus saprophyticus*, or *Enterococcus faecalis*.

Lower Respiratory Infections caused by *Escherichia coli, Klebsiella pneumoniae* subspecies *pneumoniae, Enterobacter cloacae, Proteus mirabilis, Pseudomonas aeruginosa, Haemophilus influenzae, Haemophilus parainfluenzae*, or *Streptococcus pneumoniae*.

NOTE: Although effective in clinical trials, ciprofloxacin is not a drug of first choice in the treatment of presumed or confirmed pneumonia secondary to *Streptococcus pneumoniae*.

Nosocomial Pneumonia caused by *Haemophilus influenzae* or *Klebsiella pneumoniae*.

Skin and Skin Structure Infections caused by *Escherichia coli, Klebsiella pneumoniae* subspecies *pneumoniae, Enterobacter cloacae, Proteus mirabilis, Proteus vulgaris, Providencia stuartii, Morganella morganii, Citrobacter freundii, Pseudomonas aeruginosa, Staphylococcus aureus* (methicillin susceptible), *Staphylococcus epidermidis*, or *Streptococcus pyogenes*.

Bone and Joint Infections caused by *Enterobacter cloacae, Serratia marcescens*, or *Pseudomonas aeruginosa*.

Complicated Intra-Abdominal Infections (used in conjunction with metronidazole) caused by *Escherichia coli, Pseudomonas aeruginosa, Proteus mirabilis, Klebsiella pneumoniae*, or *Bacteroides fragilis*. (See **DOSAGE AND ADMINISTRATION**.)

Empirical Therapy for Febrile Neutropenic Patients in combination with piperacillin sodium. (See **DOSAGE AND ADMINISTRATION** and **CLINICAL STUDIES**.)

If anaerobic organisms are suspected of contributing to the infection, appropriate therapy should be administered.

Appropriate culture and susceptibility tests should be performed before treatment in order to isolate and identify organisms causing infection and to determine their susceptibility to ciprofloxacin. Therapy with CIPRO® I.V. may be initiated before results of these tests are known; once results become available, appropriate therapy should be continued.

As with other drugs, some strains of *Pseudomonas aeruginosa* may develop resistance fairly rapidly during treatment with ciprofloxacin. Culture and susceptibility testing performed periodically during therapy will provide information not only on the therapeutic effect of the antimicrobial agent but also on the possible emergence of bacterial resistance.

CLINICAL STUDIES

EMPIRICAL THERAPY IN FEBRILE NEUTROPENIC PATIENTS

The safety and efficacy of ciprofloxacin, 400 mg I.V. q 8h, in combination with piperacillin sodium, 50 mg/kg I.V. q 4h, for the empirical therapy of febrile neutropenic patients were studied in one large pivotal multicenter, randomized trial and were compared to those of tobramycin, 2 mg/kg I.V. q 8h, in combination with piperacillin sodium, 50 mg/kg I.V. q 4h.

The demographics of the evaluable patients were as follows:
[See table above]

Clinical response rates observed in this study were as follows:
[See table at top of next page]

CONTRAINDICATIONS

CIPRO® I.V. (ciprofloxacin) is contraindicated in persons with a history of hypersensitivity to ciprofloxacin or any member of the quinolone class of antimicrobial agents.

WARNINGS

THE SAFETY AND EFFECTIVENESS OF CIPROFLOXACIN IN PEDIATRIC PATIENTS AND ADOLESCENTS (LESS THAN 18 YEARS OF AGE), PREGNANT WOMEN, AND LACTATING WOMEN HAVE NOT BEEN ESTABLISHED. (See **PRECAUTIONS: Pediatric Use, Pregnancy** and **Nursing Mothers** subsections.) Ciprofloxacin causes lameness in immature dogs. Histopathological examination of the weight-bearing joints of these dogs revealed permanent lesions of the cartilage. Related quinolone-class drugs also produce erosions of cartilage of weight-bearing joints and other signs of arthropathy in immature animals of various species. (See **ANIMAL PHARMACOLOGY**.)

Convulsions, increased intracranial pressure, and toxic psychosis have been reported in patients receiving quinolones, including ciprofloxacin. Ciprofloxacin may also cause central nervous system (CNS) events including: dizziness, confusion, tremors, hallucinations, depression, and, rarely, suicidal thoughts or acts. These reactions may occur following the first dose. If these reactions occur in patients receiving ciprofloxacin, the drug should be discontinued and appropriate measures instituted. As with all quinolones, ciprofloxacin should be used with caution in patients with known or suspected CNS disorders that may predispose to seizures or lower the seizure threshold (e.g. severe cerebral arteriosclerosis, epilepsy), or in the presence of other risk factors that may predispose to seizures or lower the seizure threshold (e.g. certain drug therapy, renal dysfunction). (See **PRECAUTIONS: General, Information for Patients, Drug Interactions** and **ADVERSE REACTIONS**.)

SERIOUS AND FATAL REACTIONS HAVE BEEN REPORTED IN PATIENTS RECEIVING CONCURRENT ADMINISTRATION

Continued on next page

Cipro I.V. Pharm Bulk—Cont.

OF INTRAVENOUS CIPROFLOXACIN AND THEOPHYLLINE. These reactions have included cardiac arrest, seizure, status epilepticus, and respiratory failure. Although similar serious adverse events have been reported in patients receiving theophylline alone, the possibility that these reactions may be potentiated by ciprofloxacin cannot be eliminated. If concomitant use cannot be avoided, serum levels of theophylline should be monitored and dosage adjustments made as appropriate.

Serious and occasionally fatal hypersensitivity (anaphylactic) reactions, some following the first dose, have been reported in patients receiving quinolone therapy. Some reactions were accompanied by cardiovascular collapse, loss of consciousness, tingling, pharyngeal or facial edema, dyspnea, urticaria, and itching. Only a few patients had a history of hypersensitivity reactions. Serious anaphylactic reactions require immediate emergency treatment with epinephrine and other resuscitation measures, including oxygen, intravenous fluids, intravenous antihistamines, corticosteroids, pressor amines, and airway management, as clinically indicated.

Severe hypersensitivity reactions characterized by rash, fever, eosinophilia, jaundice, and hepatic necrosis with fatal outcome have also been reported extremely rarely in patients receiving ciprofloxacin along with other drugs. The possibility that these reactions were related to ciprofloxacin cannot be excluded. Ciprofloxacin should be discontinued at the first appearance of a skin rash or any other sign of hypersensitivity.

Pseudomembranous colitis has been reported with nearly all antibacterial agents, including ciprofloxacin, and may range in severity from mild to life-threatening. Therefore, it is important to consider this diagnosis in patients who present with diarrhea subsequent to the administration of antibacterial agents.

Treatment with antibacterial agents alters the normal flora of the colon and may permit overgrowth of clostridia. Studies indicate that a toxin produced by *Clostridium difficile* is one primary cause of "antibiotic-associated colitis".

After the diagnosis of pseudomembranous colitis has been established, therapeutic measures should be initiated. Mild cases of pseudomembranous colitis usually respond to drug discontinuation alone. In moderate to severe cases, consideration should be given to management with fluids and electrolytes, protein supplementation and treatment with an antibacterial drug clinically effective against *C. difficile* colitis.

Achilles and other tendon ruptures that required surgical repair or resulted in prolonged disability have been reported with ciprofloxacin and other quinolones. Ciprofloxacin should be discontinued if the patient experiences pain, inflammation, or rupture of a tendon.

PRECAUTIONS

General: INTRAVENOUS CIPROFLOXACIN SHOULD BE ADMINISTERED BY SLOW INFUSION OVER A PERIOD OF 60 MINUTES. Local I.V. site reactions have been reported with the intravenous administration of ciprofloxacin. These reactions are more frequent if infusion time is 30 minutes or less or if small veins of the hand are used. (See **ADVERSE REACTIONS.**)

Quinolones, including ciprofloxacin, may also cause central nervous system (CNS) events, including nervousness, agitation, insomnia, anxiety, nightmares or paranoia. (See **WARNINGS, Information for Patients,** and **Drug Interactions.**)

Crystals of ciprofloxacin have been observed rarely in the urine of human subjects but more frequently in the urine of laboratory animals, which is usually alkaline. (See **ANIMAL PHARMACOLOGY.**) Crystalluria related to ciprofloxacin has been reported only rarely in humans because human urine is usually acidic. Alkalinity of the urine should be avoided in patients receiving ciprofloxacin. Patients should be well hydrated to prevent the formation of highly concentrated urine.

Alteration of the dosage regimen is necessary for patients with impairment of renal function. (See **DOSAGE AND ADMINISTRATION.**)

Moderate to severe phototoxicity manifested as an exaggerated sunburn reaction has been observed in some patients who were exposed to direct sunlight while receiving some members of the quinolone class of drugs. Excessive sunlight should be avoided.

As with any potent drug, periodic assessment of organ system functions, including renal, hepatic, and hematopoietic, is advisable during prolonged therapy.

Information For Patients: Patients should be advised that ciprofloxacin may be associated with hypersensitivity reactions, even following a single dose, and to discontinue the drug at the first sign of a skin rash or other allergic reaction.

Ciprofloxacin may cause dizziness and lightheadedness; therefore, patients should know how they react to this drug before they operate an automobile or machinery or engage in activities requiring mental alertness or coordination.

Outcomes	Ciprofloxacin/Piperacillin N = 233 Success (%)	Tobramycin/Piperacillin N = 237 Success (%)
Clinical Resolution of Initial Febrile Episode with No Modification of Empirical Regimen*	63 (27.0%)	52 (21.9%)
Clinical Resolution of Initial Febrile Episode Including Patients with Modifications of Empirical Regimen	187 (80.3%)	185 (78.1%)
Overall Survival	224 (96.1%)	223 (94.1%)

* To be evaluated as a clinical resolution, patients had to have: (1) resolution of fever; (2) microbiological eradication of infection (if an infection was microbiologically documented); (3) resolution of signs/symptoms of infection; and (4) no modification of empirical antibiotic regimen.

Patients should be advised that ciprofloxacin may increase the effects of theophylline and caffeine. There is a possibility of caffeine accumulation when products containing caffeine are consumed while taking ciprofloxacin.

Patients should be advised to discontinue treatment; rest and refrain from exercise; and inform their physician if they experience pain, inflammation, or rupture of a tendon.

Patients should be advised that convulsions have been reported in patients taking quinolones, including ciprofloxacin, and to notify their physician before taking this drug if there is a history of this condition.

Drug Interactions: As with some other quinolones, concurrent administration of ciprofloxacin with theophylline may lead to elevated serum concentrations of theophylline and prolongation of its elimination half-life. This may result in increased risk of theophylline-related adverse reactions. (See **WARNINGS.**) If concomitant use cannot be avoided, serum levels of theophylline should be monitored and dosage adjustments made as appropriate.

Some quinolones, including ciprofloxacin, have also been shown to interfere with the metabolism of caffeine. This may lead to reduced clearance of caffeine and prolongation of its serum half-life.

Some quinolones, including ciprofloxacin, have been associated with transient elevations in serum creatinine in patients receiving cyclosporine concomitantly.

Altered serum levels of phenytoin (increased and decreased) have been reported in patients receiving concomitant ciprofloxacin.

The concomitant administration of ciprofloxacin with the sulfonylurea glyburide has, in some patients, resulted in severe hypoglycemia. Fatalities have been reported.

Quinolones have been reported to enhance the effects of the oral anticoagulant warfarin or its derivatives. When these products are administered concomitantly, prothrombin time or other suitable coagulation tests should be closely monitored.

Probenecid interferes with renal tubular secretion of ciprofloxacin and produces an increase in the level of ciprofloxacin in the serum. This should be considered if patients are receiving both drugs concomitantly.

As with other broad-spectrum antimicrobial agents, prolonged use of ciprofloxacin may result in overgrowth of nonsusceptible organisms. Repeated evaluation of the patient's condition and microbial susceptibility testing are essential. If superinfection occurs during therapy, appropriate measures should be taken.

Carcinogenesis, Mutagenesis, Impairment of Fertility: Eight *in vitro* mutagenicity tests have been conducted with ciprofloxacin. Test results are listed below:

Salmonella/Microsome Test (Negative)

E. coli DNA Repair Assay (Negative)

Mouse Lymphoma Cell Forward Mutation Assay (Positive)

Chinese Hamster V_{79} Cell HGPRT Test (Negative)

Syrian Hamster Embryo Cell Transformation Assay (Negative)

Saccharomyces cerevisiae Point Mutation Assay (Negative)

Saccharomyces cerevisiae Mitotic Crossover and Gene Conversion Assay (Negative)

Rat Hepatocyte DNA Repair Assay (Positive)

Thus, two of the eight tests were positive, but results of the following three *in vivo* test systems gave negative results:

Rat Hepatocyte DNA Repair Assay

Micronucleus Test (Mice)

Dominant Lethal Test (Mice)

Long-term carcinogenicity studies in mice and rats have been completed. After daily oral doses of 750 mg/kg (mice) and 250 mg/kg (rats) were administered for up to 2 years, there was no evidence that ciprofloxacin had any carcinogenic or tumorigenic effects in these species.

Results from photo co-carcinogenicity testing indicate that ciprofloxacin does not reduce the time to appearance of UV-induced skin tumors as compared to vehicle control. Hairless (Skh-1) mice were exposed to UVA light for 3.5 hours five times every two weeks for up to 78 weeks while concurrently being administered ciprofloxacin. The time to devel-

opment of the first skin tumors was 50 weeks in mice treated concomitantly with UVA and ciprofloxacin (mouse dose approximately equal to maximum recommended human dose based upon mg/m^2), as opposed to 34 weeks when animals were treated with both UVA and vehicle. The times to development of skin tumors ranged from 16–32 weeks in mice treated concomitantly with UVA and other quinolones.[3]

In this model, mice treated with ciprofloxacin alone did not develop skin or systemic tumors. There are no data from similar models using pigmented mice and/or fully haired mice. The clinical significance of these findings to humans is unknown.

Fertility studies performed in rats at oral doses of ciprofloxacin up to 100 mg/kg (0.8 times the highest recommended human dose of 1200 mg based upon body surface area) revealed no evidence of impairment.

Pregnancy: Teratogenic Effects. Pregnancy Category C: Reproduction studies have been performed in rats and mice using oral doses of up to 100 mg/kg (0.8 and 0.4 times the maximum daily human dose based upon body surface area, respectively) and I.V. doses of up to 30 mg/kg (0.24 and 0.12 times the maximum daily human dose based upon body surface area, respectively) and have revealed no evidence of harm to the fetus due to ciprofloxacin. In rabbits, ciprofloxacin (30 and 100 mg/kg orally) produced gastrointestinal disturbances resulting in maternal weight loss and an increased incidence of abortion, but no teratogenicity was observed at either dose. After intravenous administration of doses up to 20 mg/kg, no maternal toxicity was produced in the rabbit, and no embryotoxicity or teratogenicity was observed. There are, however, no adequate and well-controlled studies in pregnant women. Ciprofloxacin should be used during pregnancy only if the potential benefit justifies the potential risk to the fetus. (See **WARNINGS.**)

Nursing Mothers: Ciprofloxacin is excreted in human milk. Because of the potential for serious adverse reactions in infants nursing from mothers taking ciprofloxacin, a decision should be made whether to discontinue nursing or to discontinue the drug, taking into account the importance of the drug to the mother.

Pediatric Use: Safety and effectiveness in pediatric patients and adolescents less than 18 years of age have not been established. Ciprofloxacin causes arthropathy in juvenile animals. (See **WARNINGS.**)

Short-term safety data from a single trial in pediatric cystic fibrosis patients are available. In a randomized, double-blind clinical trial for the treatment of acute pulmonary exacerbations in cystic fibrosis patients (ages 5–17 years), 67 patients received ciprofloxacin I.V. 10 mg/kg/dose q8h for one week followed by ciprofloxacin tablets 20 mg/kg/dose q12h to complete 10–21 days treatment and 62 patients received the combination of ceftazidime I.V. 50 mg/kg/dose q8h and tobramycin I.V. 3 mg/kg/dose q8h for a total of 10–21 days. Patients less than 5 years of age were not studied. Safety monitoring in the study included periodic range of motion examinations and gait assessments by treatment-blinded examiners. Patients were followed for an average of 23 days after completing treatment (range 0–93 days). This study was not designed to determine long term effects and the safety of repeated exposure to ciprofloxacin.

In the study, injection site reactions were more common in the ciprofloxacin group (24%) than in the comparison group (8%). Other adverse events were similar in nature and frequency between treatment arms. Musculoskeletal adverse events were reported in 22% of the patients in the ciprofloxacin group and 21% in the comparison group. Decreased range of motion was reported in 12% of the subjects in the ciprofloxacin group and 16% in the comparison group. Arthralgia was reported in 10% of the patients in the ciprofloxacin group and 11% in the comparison group. One of sixty-seven patients developed arthritis of the knee nine days after a ten day course of treatment with ciprofloxacin. Clinical symptoms resolved, but an MRI showed knee effusion without other abnormalities eight months after treatment. However, the relationship of this event to the patient's

course of ciprofloxacin can not be definitively determined, particularly since patients with cystic fibrosis may develop arthralgias/arthritis as part of their underlying disease process.

ADVERSE REACTIONS

The most frequently reported events, without regard to drug relationship, among patients treated with intravenous ciprofloxacin were nausea, diarrhea, central nervous system disturbance, local I.V. site reactions, abnormalities of liver associated enzymes (hepatic enzymes), and eosinophilia. Headache, restlessness, and rash were also noted in greater than 1% of patients treated with the most common doses of ciprofloxacin.

Local I.V. site reactions have been reported with the intravenous administration of ciprofloxacin. These reactions are more frequent if the infusion time is 30 minutes or less. These may appear as local skin reactions which resolve rapidly upon completion of the infusion. Subsequent intravenous administration is not contraindicated unless the reactions recur or worsen.

Additional events, without regard to drug relationship or route of administration, that occurred in 1% or less of ciprofloxacin patients are listed below:

CARDIOVASCULAR: cardiovascular collapse, cardiopulmonary arrest, myocardial infarction, arrhythmia, tachycardia, palpitation, cerebral thrombosis, syncope, cardiac murmur, hypertension, hypotension, angina pectoris

CENTRAL NERVOUS SYSTEM: convulsive seizures, paranoia, toxic psychosis, depression, dysphasia, phobia, depersonalization, manic reaction, unresponsiveness, ataxia, confusion, hallucinations, dizziness, lightheadedness, paresthesia, anxiety, tremor, insomnia, nightmares, weakness, drowsiness, irritability, malaise, lethargy

GASTROINTESTINAL: ileus, jaundice, gastrointestinal bleeding, C. difficile associated diarrhea, pseudomembranous colitis, pancreatitis, hepatic necrosis, intestinal perforation, dyspepsia, epigastric or abdominal pain, vomiting, constipation, oral ulceration, oral candidiasis, mouth dryness, anorexia, dysphagia, flatulence

I.V. INFUSION SITE: thrombophlebitis, burning, pain, pruritus, paresthesia, erythema, swelling

MUSCULOSKELETAL: arthralgia, jaw, arm or back pain, joint stiffness, neck and chest pain, achiness, flare up of gout

RENAL/UROGENITAL: renal failure, interstitial nephritis, hemorrhagic cystitis, renal calculi, frequent urination, acidosis, urethral bleeding, polyuria, urinary retention, gynecomastia, candiduria, vaginitis. Crystalluria, cylindruria, hematuria, and albuminuria have also been reported.

RESPIRATORY: respiratory arrest, pulmonary embolism, dyspnea, pulmonary edema, respiratory distress, pleural effusion, hemoptysis, epistaxis, hiccough

SKIN/HYPERSENSITIVITY: anaphylactic reactions, erythema multiforme/Stevens-Johnson syndrome, exfoliative dermatitis, toxic epidermal necrolysis, vasculitis, angioedema, edema of the lips, face, neck, conjunctivae, hands or lower extremities, purpura, fever, chills, flushing, pruritus, urticaria, cutaneous candidiasis, vesicles, increased perspiration, hyperpigmentation, erythema nodosum, photosensitivity

Allergic reactions ranging from urticaria to anaphylactic reactions have been reported. (See WARNINGS.)

SPECIAL SENSES: decreased visual acuity, blurred vision, disturbed vision (flashing lights, change in color perception, overbrightness of lights, diplopia), eye pain, anosmia, hearing loss, tinnitus, nystagmus, a bad taste

Also reported were agranulocytosis, prolongation of prothrombin time, and possible exacerbation of myasthenia gravis.

Many of these events were described as only mild or moderate in severity, abated soon after the drug was discontinued, and required no treatment.

In several instances, nausea, vomiting, tremor, irritability, or palpitation were judged by investigators to be related to elevated serum levels of theophylline possibly as a result of drug interaction with ciprofloxacin.

In randomized, double-blind controlled clinical trials comparing ciprofloxacin (I.V. and I.V. P.O. sequential) with intravenous beta-lactam control antibiotics, the CNS adverse event profile of ciprofloxacin was comparable to that of the control drugs.

Post-Marketing Adverse Events: Additional adverse events, regardless of relationship to drug, reported from worldwide marketing experience with quinolones, including ciprofloxacin, are:

BODY AS A WHOLE: change in serum phenytoin

CARDIOVASCULAR: postural hypotension, vasculitis

CENTRAL NERVOUS SYSTEM: agitation, confusion, delirium, dysphasia, myoclonus, nystagmus, toxic psychosis

GASTROINTESTINAL: constipation, dyspepsia, flatulence, hepatic necrosis, jaundice, pancreatitis, pseudo-

membranous colitis (The onset of pseudomembranous colitis symptoms may occur during or after antimicrobial treatment.)

HEMIC/LYMPHATIC: agranulocytosis, hemolytic anemia, methemoglobinemia, prolongation of prothrombin time

METABOLIC/NUTRITIONAL: elevation of serum triglycerides, cholesterol, blood glucose, serum potassium

MUSCULOSKELETAL: myalgia, possible exacerbation of myasthenia gravis, tendinitis/tendon rupture

RENAL/UROGENITAL: albuminuria, candiduria, renal calculi, vaginal candidiasis

SKIN/HYPERSENSITIVITY: anaphylactic reactions, erythema multiforme/Stevens-Johnson syndrome, exfoliative dermatitis, toxic epidermal necrolysis

SPECIAL SENSES: anosmia

(See PRECAUTIONS.)

Adverse Laboratory Changes: The most frequently reported changes in laboratory parameters with intravenous ciprofloxacin therapy, without regard to drug relationship are listed below:

Hepatic—elevations of AST (SGOT), ALT (SGPT), alkaline phosphatase, LDH, and serum bilirubin;

Hematologic—elevated eosinophil and platelet counts, decreased platelet counts, hemoglobin and/or hematocrit;

Renal—elevations of serum creatinine, BUN, and uric acid;

Other—elevations of serum creatinine, phosphokinase, serum theophylline (in patients receiving theophylline concomitantly), blood glucose, and triglycerides.

Other changes occurring infrequently were: decreased leukocyte count, elevated atypical lymphocyte count, immature WBCs, elevated serum calcium, elevation of serum gamma-glutamyl transpeptidase (γ GT), decreased BUN, decreased uric acid, decreased total serum protein, decreased serum albumin, decreased serum potassium, elevated serum potassium, elevated serum cholesterol.

Other changes occurring rarely during administration of ciprofloxacin were: elevation of serum amylase, decrease of blood glucose, pancytopenia, leukocytosis, elevated sedimentation rate, change in serum phenytoin, decreased prothrombin time, hemolytic anemia, and bleeding diathesis.

DOSAGE GUIDELINES
Intravenous

Infection†	Type or Severity	Unit Dose	Frequency	Daily Dose
Urinary tract	Mild/Moderate	200 mg	q12h	400 mg
	Severe/Complicated	400 mg	q12h	800 mg
Lower Respiratory Tract	Mild/Moderate	400 mg	q12h	800 mg
	Severe/Complicated	400 mg	q8h	1200 mg
Nosocomial Pneumonia	Mild/Moderate/Severe	400 mg	q8h	1200 mg
Skin and Skin Structure	Mild/Moderate	400 mg	q12h	800 mg
	Severe/Complicated	400 mg	q8h	1200 mg
Bone and Joint	Mild/Moderate	400 mg	q12h	800 mg
	Severe/Complicated	400 mg	q8h	1200 mg
Intra-Abdominal*	Complicated	400 mg	q12h	800 mg
Empirical Therapy in Febrile Neutropenic Patients	Severe Ciprofloxacin + Piperacillin	400 mg 50 mg/kg	q8h q4h	1200 mg Not to exceed 24 g/day

* used in conjunction with metronidazole. (See product labeling for prescribing information.)
† DUE TO THE DESIGNATED PATHOGENS (See INDICATIONS AND USAGE.)

Men: Creatinine clearance (mL/min) = $\dfrac{\text{Weight (kg)} \times (140 - \text{age})}{72 \times \text{serum creatinine (mg/dL)}}$

Women: $0.85 \times$ the value calculated for men.

CONTAINER	SIZE	STRENGTH	NDC NUMBER
Pharmacy Bulk Package:	120 mL	1200-mg, 1%	0026-8566-65

VIAL:	SIZE	STRENGTH	NDC NUMBER
	20 mL	200 mg, 1%	0026-8562-20
	40 mL	400 mg, 1%	0026-8564-64

FLEXIBLE CONTAINER: manufactured for Bayer Corporation by Abbott Laboratories, North Chicago, IL 60064.

	SIZE	STRENGTH	NDC NUMBER
	100 mL 5% dextrose	200 mg, 0.2%	0026-8552-36
	200 mL 5% dextrose	400 mg, 0.2%	0026-8554-63

FLEXIBLE CONTAINER: manufactured for Bayer Corporation by Baxter Healthcare Corporation, Deerfield, IL 60015.

	SIZE	STRENGTH	NDC NUMBER
	100 mL 5% dextrose	200 mg, 0.2%	0026-8527-36
	200 mL 5% dextrose	400 mg, 0.2%	0026-8527-63

OVERDOSAGE

In the event of acute overdosage, the patient should be carefully observed and given supportive treatment. Adequate hydration must be maintained. Only a small amount of ciprofloxacin (<10%) is removed from the body after hemodialysis or peritoneal dialysis.

In mice, rats, rabbits and dogs, significant toxicity including tonic/clonic convulsions was observed at intravenous doses of ciprofloxacin between 125 and 300 mg/kg.

DOSAGE AND ADMINISTRATION

The recommended adult dosage for urinary tract infections of mild to moderate severity is 200 mg I.V. every 12 hours. For severe or complicated urinary tract infections, the recommended dosage is 400 mg I.V. every 12 hours.

The recommended adult dosage for lower respiratory tract infections, skin and skin structure infections, and bone and joint infections of mild to moderate severity is 400 mg I.V. every 12 hours.

For severe/complicated infections of the lower respiratory tract, skin and skin structure, and bone and joint, the recommended adult dosage is 400 mg I.V. every 8 hours.

The recommended adult dosage for mild, moderate, and severe nosocomial pneumonia is 400 mg I.V. every 8 hours.

Complicated Intra-Abdominal Infections: Sequential therapy [parenteral to oral—400 mg CIPRO® I.V. q 12 h (plus I.V. metronidazole) → 500 mg CIPRO® Tablets q 12 h (plus oral metronidazole)] can be instituted at the discretion of the physician. Metronidazole should be given according to product labeling to provide appropriate anaerobic coverage. The recommended adult dosage for empirical therapy of febrile neutropenic patients is 400 mg I.V. every 8 hours in combination with piperacillin sodium 50 mg/kg I.V. q 4 hours, not to exceed 24 g/day (300 mg/kg/day), for 7–14 days.

The determination of dosage for any particular patient must take into consideration the severity and nature of the infection, the susceptibility of the causative microorganism, the integrity of the patient's host-defense mechanisms and the status of renal and hepatic function.

Continued on next page

Cipro I.V. Pharm Bulk—Cont.

[See first table at top of previous page]

After dilution CIPRO® I.V. should be administered by intravenous infusion over a period of 60 minutes.

Parenteral drug products should be inspected visually for particulate matter and discoloration prior to administration.

CIPRO® (ciprofloxacin hydrochloride) Tablets for oral administration are available. Parenteral therapy may be changed to oral CIPRO® Tablets when the condition warrants, at the discretion of the physician. For complete dosage and administration information, see CIPRO® Tablets package insert.

Impaired Renal Function: The following table provides dosage guidelines for use in patients with renal impairment; however, monitoring of serum drug levels provides the most reliable basis for dosage adjustment.

RECOMMENDED STARTING AND MAINTENANCE DOSES FOR PATIENTS WITH IMPAIRED RENAL FUNCTION

Creatinine Clearance (mL/min)	Dosage
>30	See usual dosage.
5–29	200–400 mg q 18–24 hr

When only the serum creatinine concentration is known, the following formula may be used to estimate creatinine clearance:

[See second table from top of previous page]

The serum creatinine should represent a steady state of renal function.

For patients with changing renal function or for patients with renal impairment and hepatic insufficiency, measurement of serum concentrations of ciprofloxacin will provide additional guidance for adjusting dosage.

INTRAVENOUS ADMINISTRATION

After dilution, CIPRO® I.V. should be administered by intravenous infusion over a period of 60 minutes. Slow infusion of a dilute solution into a large vein will minimize patient discomfort and reduce the risk of venous irritation.

PHARMACY BULK PACKAGE: The pharmacy bulk package is a single-entry container of a sterile preparation for parenteral use that contains many single doses. It contains ciprofloxacin as a 1% aqueous solution concentrate. The contents are intended for use in a pharmacy admixture program and are restricted to the preparation of admixtures for intravenous infusion. **THE CLOSURE SHALL BE PENETRATED ONLY ONE TIME** with a suitable sterile transfer set or dispensing device which allows measured dispensing of the contents.

The pharmacy bulk package is to be used only in a suitable work area such as laminar flow hood or an equivalent clean air or compounding area. **THIS PREPARATION MUST BE DILUTED BEFORE USE.** The intravenous dose should be prepared by aseptically withdrawing the CIPRO® I.V. concentrate from the pharmacy bulk package and diluting the appropriate volume with a suitable intravenous solution to a final concentration of 0.5–2 mg/mL. (See **COMPATIBILITY AND STABILITY.**) The resulting solution should be infused over a period of 60 minutes by direct infusion or through a Y-type intravenous set which may already be in place. If this method or the "piggyback" method of administration is used, it is advisable to discontinue the administration of any other intravenous solutions during the infusion of CIPRO® I.V.

COMPATIBILITY AND STABILITY

Ciprofloxacin injection 1% (10 mg/mL), when diluted with the following intravenous solutions to concentrations of 0.5 to 2.0 mg/mL, is stable for up to 14 days at refrigerated or room temperature storage.

- 0.9% Sodium Chloride Injection, USP
- 5% Dextrose Injection, USP
- Sterile Water for Injection
- 10% Dextrose for Injection
- 5% Dextrose and 0.225% Sodium Chloride for Injection
- 5% Dextrose and 0.45% Sodium Chloride for Injection
- Lactated Ringer's for Injection

If CIPRO® I.V. is to be given concomitantly with another drug, each drug should be given separately in accordance with the recommended dosage and route of administration for each drug.

HOW SUPPLIED

CIPRO® I.V. (ciprofloxacin) is available as a clear, colorless to slightly yellowish solution supplied in the pharmacy bulk package as follows:

[See third table from top of previous page]

STORAGE

Store between 5–30°C (41–86°F).

Protect from light, avoid excessive heat, protect from freezing.

CIPRO® I.V. (ciprofloxacin) is also available as follows:

[See fourth table from top of previous page]

Ciprofloxacin is also available as CIPRO® (ciprofloxacin HCl) Tablets 100, 250, 500, and 750 mg and as CIPRO® (ciprofloxacin) 5% and 10% Oral Suspension.

ANIMAL PHARMACOLOGY

Ciprofloxacin and other quinolones have been shown to cause arthropathy in immature animals of most species tested. (See **WARNINGS.**) Damage of weight-bearing joints was observed in juvenile dogs and rats. In young beagles, 100 mg/kg ciprofloxacin given daily for 4 weeks caused degenerative articular changes of the knee joint. At 30 mg/kg, the effect on the joint was minimal. In a subsequent study in beagles, removal of weight-bearing from the joint reduced the lesions but did not totally prevent them.

Crystalluria, sometimes associated with secondary nephropathy, occurs in laboratory animals dosed with ciprofloxacin. This is primarily related to the reduced solubility of ciprofloxacin under alkaline conditions, which predominate in the urine of test animals; in man, crystalluria is rare since human urine is typically acidic. In rhesus monkeys, crystalluria without nephropathy has been noted after intravenous doses as low as 5 mg/kg. After 6 months of intravenous dosing at 10 mg/kg/day, no nephropathological changes were noted; however, nephropathy was observed after dosing at 20 mg/kg/day for the same duration.

In dogs, ciprofloxacin administered at 3 and 10 mg/kg by rapid intravenous injection (15 sec.) produces pronounced hypotensive effects. These effects are considered to be related to histamine release because they are partially antagonized by pyrilamine, an antihistamine. In rhesus monkeys, rapid intravenous injection also produces hypotension, but the effect in this species is inconsistent and less pronounced.

In mice, concomitant administration of nonsteroidal anti-inflammatory drugs, such as phenylbutazone and indomethacin, with quinolones has been reported to enhance the CNS stimulatory effect of quinolones.

Ocular toxicity, seen with some related drugs, has not been observed in ciprofloxacin-treated animals.

REFERENCES

1. National Committee for Clinical Laboratory Standards, Methods for Dilution Antimicrobial Susceptibility Tests for Bacteria That Grow Aerobically—Fourth Edition. Approved Standard NCCLS Document M7-A4, Vol. 17, No. 2, NCCLS, Wayne, PA, January, 1997. **2.** National Committee for Clinical Laboratory Standards, Performance Standards for Antimicrobial Disk Susceptibility Tests—Sixth Edition. Approved Standard NCCLS Document M2-A6, Vol. 17, No. 1, NCCLS, Wayne, PA, January, 1997. **3.** Report presented at the FDA's Anti-Infective Drug and Dermatological Drug Products Advisory Committee Meeting, March 31, 1993, Silver Spring, MD. Report available from FDA, CDER, Advisors and Consultants Staff, HFD-21, 1901 Chapman Avenue, Room 200, Rockville, MD 20852, USA.

Bayer Corporation
Pharmaceutical Division
400 Morgan Lane
West Haven, CT 06516 USA

Rx Only

PD500113 7/98 BAY q 3939 5202-4-A-U.S.-4 ©1998 Bayer Corporation 8399

Shown in Product Identification Guide, page 305

DTIC-Dome® ℞
(dacarbazine)
Sterile

> **WARNING**
> It is recommended that DTIC-Dome (dacarbazine) be administered under the supervision of a qualified physician experienced in the use of cancer chemotherapeutic agents.
> 1. Hemopoietic depression is the most common toxicity with DTIC-Dome (See Warnings).
> 2. Hepatic necrosis has been reported (See Warnings).
> 3. Studies have demonstrated this agent to have a carcinogenic and teratogenic effect when used in animals.
> 4. In treatment of each patient, the physician must weigh carefully the possibility of achieving therapeutic benefit against the risk of toxicity.

DESCRIPTION

DTIC-Dome Sterile (dacarbazine) is a colorless to an ivory colored solid which is light sensitive. Each vial contains 100 mg of dacarbazine, or 200 mg of dacarbazine (the active ingredient), anhydrous citric acid and mannitol. DTIC-Dome is reconstituted and administered intravenously (pH 3–4). DTIC-Dome is an anticancer agent. Chemically, DTIC-Dome is 5-(3,3-dimethyl-l-triazeno)-imidazole-4-carboxamide (DTIC) with the following structural formula:

[See chemical structure at top of next column]

CLINICAL PHARMACOLOGY

After intravenous administration of DTIC-Dome, the volume of distribution exceeds total body water content sug-

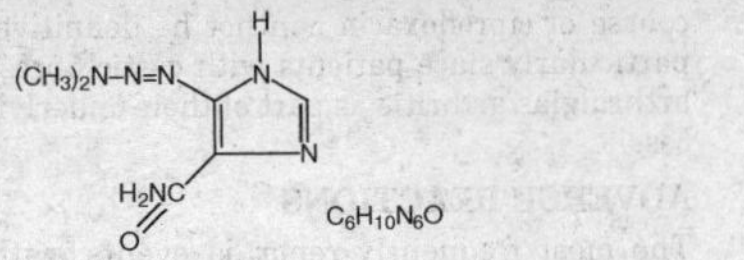
(CH3)2N–N=N
H2N
C6H10N6O

gesting localization in some body tissue, probably the liver. Its disappearance from the plasma is biphasic with initial half-life of 19 minutes and a terminal half-life of 5 hours.[1] In a patient with renal and hepatic dysfunctions, the half-lives were lengthened to 55 minutes and 7.2 hours.[1] The average cumulative excretion of unchanged DTIC in the urine is 40% of the injected dose in 6 hours.[1] DTIC is subject to renal tubular secretion rather than glomerular filtration. At therapeutic concentrations DTIC is not appreciably bound to human plasma protein.

In man, DTIC is extensively degraded. Besides unchanged DTIC, 5-aminoimidazole -4 carboxamide (AIC) is a major metabolite of DTIC excreted in the urine. AIC is not derived endogenously but from the injected DTIC, because the administration of radioactive DTIC labeled with ^{14}C in the imidazole portion of the molecule (DTIC-2-^{14}C) gives rise to AIC-2-^{14}C.[1]

Although the exact mechanism of action of DTIC-Dome is not known, three hypotheses have been offered:
1. inhibition of DNA synthesis by acting as a purine analog
2. action as an alkylating agent
3. interaction with SH groups

INDICATIONS AND USAGE

DTIC-Dome is indicated in the treatment of metastatic malignant melanoma. In addition, DTIC-Dome is also indicated for Hodgkin's disease as a secondary-line therapy when used in combination with other effective agents.

CONTRAINDICATIONS

DTIC-Dome is contraindicated in patients who have demonstrated a hypersensitivity to it in the past.

WARNINGS

Hemopoietic depression is the most common toxicity with DTIC-Dome and involves primarily the leukocytes and platelets, although, anemia may sometimes occur. Leukopenia and thrombocytopenia may be severe enough to cause death. The possible bone marrow depression requires careful monitoring of white blood cells, red blood cells, and platelet levels. Hemopoietic toxicity may warrant temporary suspension or cessation of therapy with DTIC-Dome.

Hepatic toxicity accompanied by hepatic vein thrombosis and hepatocellular necrosis resulting in death, has been reported. The incidence of such reactions has been low; approximately 0.01% of patients treated. This toxicity has been observed mostly when DTIC-Dome has been administered concomitantly with other anti-neoplastic drugs; however, it has also been reported in some patients treated with DTIC-Dome alone.

Anaphylaxis can occur following the administration of DTIC-Dome.

PRECAUTIONS

Hospitalization is not always necessary but adequate laboratory study capability must be available. Extravasation of the drug subcutaneously during intravenous administration may result in tissue damage and severe pain. Local pain, burning sensation, and irritation at the site of injection may be relieved by locally applied hot packs.

Carcinogenicity of DTIC was studied in rats and mice. Proliferative endocardial lesions, including fibrosarcomas and sarcomas were induced by DTIC in rats. In mice, administration of DTIC resulted in the induction of angiosarcomas of the spleen.

Pregnancy Category C. DTIC-Dome has been shown to be teratogenic in rats when given in doses 20 times the human daily dose on day 12 of gestation. DTIC when administered in 10 times the human daily dose to male rats (twice weekly for 9 weeks) did not affect the male libido, although female rats mated to male rats had higher incidence of resorptions than controls. In rabbits, DTIC daily dose 7 times the human daily dose given on Days 6–15 of gestation resulted in fetal skeletal anomalies. There are no adequate and well controlled studies in pregnant women. DTIC-Dome should be used during pregnancy only if the potential benefit justifies the potential risk to the fetus.

It is not known whether this drug is excreted in human milk. Because many drugs are excreted in human milk and because of the potential for tumorigenicity shown for DTIC-Dome in animal studies, a decision should be made whether to discontinue nursing or to discontinue the drug, taking into account the importance of the drug to the mother.

ADVERSE REACTIONS

Symptoms of anorexia, nausea, and vomiting are the most frequently noted of all toxic reactions. Over 90% of patients are affected with the initial few doses. The vomiting lasts 1–12 hours and is incompletely and unpredictably palliated with phenobarbital and/or prochlorperazine. Rarely, intrac-

table nausea and vomiting have necessitated discontinuance of therapy with DTIC-Dome. Rarely, DTIC-Dome has caused diarrhea. Some helpful suggestions include restricting the patient's oral intake of food for 4–6 hours prior to treatment. The rapid toleration of these symptoms suggests that a central nervous system mechanism may be involved, and usually these symptoms subside after the first 1 or 2 days.

There are a number of minor toxicities that are infrequently noted. Patients have experienced an influenza-like syndrome of fever to 39°C, myalgias and malaise. These symptoms occur usually after large single doses, may last for several days, and they may occur with successive treatments. Alopecia has been noted as has facial flushing and facial paresthesia. There have been few reports of significant liver or renal function test abnormalities in man. However, these abnormalities have been observed more frequently in animal studies.

Erythematous and urticarial rashes have been observed infrequently after administration of DTIC-Dome. Rarely, photosensitivity reactions may occur.

OVERDOSAGE

Give supportive treatment and monitor blood cell counts.

DOSAGE AND ADMINISTRATION

Malignant Melanoma: The recommended dosage is 2 to 4.5mg/kg/day for 10 days. Treatment may be repeated at 4 week intervals.[2]

An alternate recommended dosage is 250mg/square meter body surface/day I.V. for 5 days. Treatment may be repeated every 3 weeks.[3,4]

Hodgkin's Disease: The recommended dosage of DTIC-Dome in the treatment of Hodgkin's disease is 150mg/square meter body surface/day for 5 days, in combination with other effective drugs. Treatment may be repeated every 4 weeks.[5] An alternative recommended dosage is 375mg/square meter body surface on day 1, in combination with other effective drugs, to be repeated every 15 days.[6]

DTIC-Dome (dacarbazine) 100mg/vial and 200mg/vial are reconstituted with 9.9 mL and 19.7 mL, respectively, of Sterile Water for Injection, U.S.P. The resulting solution contains 10mg/mL of dacarbazine having a pH of 3.0 to 4.0. The calculated dose of the resulting solution is drawn into a syringe and administered *only* intravenously.

The reconstituted solution may be further diluted with 5% dextrose injection, U.S.P. or sodium chloride injection, U.S.P. and administered as an intravenous infusion.

After reconstitution and prior to use, the solution in the vial may be stored at 4°C for up to 72 hours or at normal room conditions (temperature and light) for up to 8 hours. If the reconstituted solution is further diluted in 5% dextrose, injection, U.S.P. or sodium chloride injection, U.S.P., the resulting solution may be stored at 4°C for up to 24 hours or at normal room conditions for up to 8 hours.

Procedures for proper handling and disposal of anticancer drugs should be considered. Several guidelines on this subject have been published.[7–12] There is no general agreement that all of the procedures recommended in the guidelines are necessary or appropriate.

HOW SUPPLIED

10 mL vials containing 100 mg or 20 mL vials containing 200 mg of DTIC-Dome as sterile dacarbazine in boxes of 12. Store in a refrigerator 2°C to 8°C (36°F to 46°F).

REFERENCES

1. Loo, T.J., *et al.:* Mechanism of action and pharmacology studies with DTIC (NSC-45388). Cancer Treatment Reports 60: 149–152, 1976.
2. Nathanson, L., *et al.:* Characteristics of prognosis and response to an imidazole carboxamide in malignant melanoma. Clinical Pharmacology and Therapeutics 12: 955–962, 1971.
3. Costanza, M.E., *et al.:* Therapy of malignant melanoma with an imidazole carboxamide and bischloroethyl nitrosourea. Cancer 30: 1457–1461, 1972.
4. Luce, J.K., *et al.:* Clinical trials with the antitumor agent 5-(3, 3-dimethyl-l-triazeno) imidazole-4-carboxamide (NSC-45388). Cancer Chemotherapy Reports 54: 119–124, 1970.
5. Bonadonna, G., *et al.:* Combined Chemotherapy (MOPP or ABVD)—radiotherapy approach in advanced Hodgkin's disease. Cancer Treatment Reports 61: 769–777, 1977.

6. Santoro, A., and Bonadonna, G.: Prolonged disease-free survival in MOPP-resistant Hodgkin's disease after treatment with adriamycin, bleomycin, vinblastine and dacarbazine (ABVD). Cancer Chemotherapy Pharmacol. 2: 101–105, 1979.
7. Recommendations for the Safe Handling of Parenteral Antineoplastic Drugs. NIH Publication No. 83-2621. For sale by the Superintendent of Documents, U.S. Government Printing Office, Washington, D.C. 20402.
8. AMA Council Report. Guidelines for Handling Parenteral Antineoplastics. JAMA, March 15, 1985.
9. National Study Commission on Cytotoxic Exposure—Recommendations for Handling Cytotoxic Agents. Available from Louis P. Jeffrey, Sc. D., Director of Pharmacy Services, Rhode Island Hospital, 593 Eddy Street, Providence, Rhode Island 02902.
10. Clinical Oncological Society of Australia: Guidelines and recommendations for safe handling of antineoplastic agents. Med. J. Australia 1: 426–428, 1983.
11. Jones, R.B., *et al.:* Safe handling of chemotherapeutic agents: A report from the Mount Sinai Medical Center. Ca-A Cancer Journal for Clinicians Sept./Oct. 258–263, 1983.
12. American Society of Hospital Pharmacists technical assistance bulletin on handling cytotoxic drugs in hospitals. Am. J. Hosp. Pharm. 42: 131–137, 1985.

Manufactured by:
Ben Venue Laboratories
Bedford, Ohio 44146
Distributed by:
Bayer Corporation
Pharmaceutical Division
400 Morgan Lane
West Haven, CT 06516 USA
PZ500002 2/95 ©1995 Bayer Corporation 5071

MEZLIN® ℞
Sterile mezlocillin sodium
for intravenous or intramuscular use.
BAYPEN®

DESCRIPTION

MEZLIN® (sterile mezlocillin sodium) is a semisynthetic broad spectrum penicillin antibiotic for parenteral administration. It is the monohydrate sodium salt of 6-[D-2 [3-(methyl-sulfonyl) -2- OXO- imidazolidine-1-carboxamido]-2-phenyl acetamido] penicillanic acid.

Structural Formula:

Empirical Formula:
$C_{21}H_{24}N_5O_8S_2Na \cdot H_2O$

MEZLIN® has a molecular weight of 579.6 and contains 42.6 mg (1.85 mEq) of sodium per one gram of mezlocillin activity. The dosage form is supplied as a sterile white to pale yellow crystalline powder, which is freely soluble in water. When reconstituted, solutions of MEZLIN® are clear and range from colorless to pale yellow with a pH of 4.5 to 8.0.

CLINICAL PHARMACOLOGY

Intravenous Administration. In healthy adult volunteers, mean serum levels of mezlocillin 5 minutes after a 5-minute intravenous injection of 1g, 2g, or 5g are 100, 253, or 411 mcg/mL, respectively. Serum levels, as noted below, lack dose proportionality:
[See table below]
Fifteen minutes after a 4g intravenous injection (2–5 min.), the concentration in serum is 254 mcg/mL; 1 hour and 4 hours later levels are 93 mcg/mL and 9.1 mcg/mL, respectively:
[See table at top of next page]
After an intravenous infusion (15 min.) of 3g, mean levels 15 minutes after dosing are 269 mcg/mL (170–280).

A 30-minute intravenous infusion of 3g produces mean peak concentrations of 263 mcg/mL; 1 hour and 4 hours later the concentrations are 57 mcg/mL and 4.4 mcg/mL, respectively:
[See table at bottom of next page]
Following intravenous infusion (2 hr.) of a 3g dose of mezlocillin every 4 hours for 7 days, mean peak serum concentrations are higher than 100 mcg/mL, and levels above 50 mcg/mL are maintained throughout dosing.

Intramuscular Administration. MEZLIN® is rapidly absorbed after intramuscular injection. In healthy volunteers, the mean peak serum concentration occurs approximately 45 minutes after a single dose of 1g and is about 15 mcg/mL. The oral administration of 1g probenecid before injection produces an increase in mezlocillin serum levels of about 50%. After repetitive intramuscular doses of 1g mezlocillin every 6 hours, peak levels in the serum generally range between 35 and 45 mcg/mL. The relationship between the pharmacokinetics of intramuscular and intravenous dosing has not yet been clearly established.

General. As with other penicillins, mezlocillin is excreted primarily by glomerular filtration and tubular secretion. The rate of elimination is dose dependent and related to the degree of renal functional impairment. In patients with normal renal function, approximately 55% of the administered dose is recovered from the urine within the first 6 hours after dosing. Two hours after an intravenous injection of 2g, concentrations of active drug in urine generally exceed 4000 mcg/mL. By 4–6 hours after injection, concentrations usually decline to a range of about 50 to 200 mcg/mL. The serum elimination half-life of mezlocillin after intravenous dosing is approximately 55 minutes.

In patients with reduced renal function, the half-life is only slightly prolonged. Dosage adjustments are usually not necessary except in patients with severe renal impairment. (See Dosage and Administration.) As with other penicillins, mezlocillin is metabolized only slightly; less than 10% of the drug excreted in the urine is in the form of the penicilloate or penilloate. The drug is readily removed from the serum by hemodialysis and, to a lesser extent, by peritoneal dialysis.

Up to 26% of a dose of mezlocillin is recovered from the bile of patients with normal liver function. Following intravenous doses of 2 to 5g, concentrations of active drug in bile generally range from 500 to 2500 mcg/mL. The biliary excretion of mezlocillin is reduced in patients with common bile duct obstruction.

Mezlocillin is not appreciably absorbed when given orally. Following parenteral administration, the apparent volume of distribution is approximately equal to the extracellular fluid volume. The drug is present in active form in the serum, urine, bile, peritoneal fluid, pleural fluid, bronchial and wound secretions, bone and other tissues. As with other penicillins, penetration into the cerebrospinal fluid (CSF) is generally poor, however higher CSF concentrations are obtained in the presence of meningeal inflammation.

Protein binding studies indicate that the degree of mezlocillin binding is low (16–42%) and depends upon testing methods and concentrations of drug studied.

Microbiology

Mezlocillin is a bactericidal antibiotic which acts by interfering with synthesis of cell wall components. It is active against a variety of gram-negative and gram-positive bacteria, including aerobic and anaerobic strains. Mezlocillin is usually active *in vitro* against most strains of the following organisms:

Gram-negative bacteria
Escherichia coli
Proteus mirabilis
Proteus vulgaris
Morganella morganii (formerly *P. morganii*)
Providencia rettgeri (formerly *Proteus rettgeri*)
Providencia stuartii
Citrobacter species*
Klebsiella species (including *K. pneumoniae*)
Enterobacter species
Shigella species*
Pseudomonas aeruginosa (and other species)
Haemophilus influenzae
Haemophilus parainfluenzae
Neisseria species

Continued on next page

MEZLOCILLIN SERUM LEVELS IN ADULTS (mcg/mL) 5 MIN. IV INJECTION											
DOSE	0	5 min.	10 min.	20 min.	30 min.	1 hr.	2 hr.	3 hr.	4 hr.	6 hr.	8 hr.
1g	**149** (132–185)	**100** (64–143)	**66** (47–87)	**50** (31–87)	**40** (22–83)	**18** (8–31)	**5.3** (3.3–7.7)	**2.5** (1.7–3.7)	**1.7** (0.7–2.8)	**0.5** (0–1.2)	**0.1** (0–0.2)
2g	**314** (207–362)	**253** (161–364)	**161** (113–214)	**117** (76–174)	**82** (55–112)	**56** (23–88)	**20** (7.5–32)	**11** (3.8–16)	**4.4** (1.6–8.7)	**1.5** (0.5–2.6)	**0.6** (0.1–1.4)
5g	**547** (268–854)	**411** (199–597)	**357** (246–456)	**250** (203–353)	**226** (190–333)	**131** (104–193)	**76** (59–104)	**31** (20–40)	**13** (6.4–17)	**4.6** (2.1–9.4)	**1.9** (1.1–3.6)

Mezlin—Cont.

MEZLOCILLIN SERUM LEVELS IN ADULTS (mcg/mL) 2–5 MIN. IV INJECTION

DOSE	0	15 min.	30 min.	45 min.	1 hr.	2 hr.	3 hr.	4 hr.	6 hr.
4g	—	**254** (155–400)	**163** (99–260)	**122** (78–215)	**93** (67–133)	**47** (22–96)	**20** (8–45)	**9.1** (6–13)	**8.4** (5–17)

Many strains of *Serratia, Salmonella**, and *Acinetobacter** are also susceptible.

Gram-positive bacteria

Staphylococcus aureus (non-penicillinase producing strains)
Beta-hemolytic *streptococci* (Groups A and B)
Streptococcus pneumoniae (formerly *Diplococcus Pneumoniae*)
Streptococcus faecalis (enterococcus)

Anaerobic Organisms

Peptococcus species
Peptostreptococcus species
Clostridium species*
Bacteroides species (including *B. fragilis* group)
Fusobacterium species*
Veillonella species*
Eubacterium species*

*Mezlocillin has been shown to be active *in vitro* against these organisms, however clinical efficacy has not yet been established.

Noteworthy is mezlocillin's broadened spectrum of *in vitro* activity against important pathogenic aerobic gram-negative bacteria, including strains of *Pseudomonas, Klebsiella, Enterobacter, Serratia, Proteus, Escherichia* and *Haemophilus,* as well as *Bacteroides* and other anaerobes; and its excellent inhibitory effect against gram-positive organisms including *Streptococcus faecalis* (enterococcus). It is inactive against penicillinase-producing strains of *Staphylococcus aureus.*

In vitro studies have shown that mezlocillin combined with an aminoglycoside (e.g., gentamicin, tobramycin, amikacin, sisomicin) acts synergistically against strains of *Streptococcus faecalis* and *Pseudomonas aeruginosa.* In some instances, this combination also acts synergistically *in vitro* against other gram-negative bacteria such as *Serratia, Klebsiella* and *Acinetobacter* species.

Mezlocillin is slightly more active when tested at alkaline pH and, as with other penicillins, has reduced activity when tested *in vitro* with increasing inoculum. The minimum bactericidal concentration (MBC) generally exceeds the minimum inhibitory concentration (MIC) by a factor of 2 or 3. Resistance to mezlocillin *in vitro* develops slowly (multiple step mutation). Some strains of *Pseudomonas aeruginosa* have developed resistance fairly rapidly. Mezlocillin is not stable in the presence of penicillinase and strains of *Staphylococcus aureus* resistant to penicillin are also resistant to mezlocillin.

Susceptibility Tests

Quantitative methods that require measurement of zone diameters give good estimates of bacterial susceptibility. One such procedure* has been recommended for use with discs to test susceptibility to antimicrobials. When the causative organism is tested by the Kirby-Bauer method of disc susceptibility, a 75 mcg mezlocillin disc should give a zone of 18 mm or greater to indicate susceptibility. Zone sizes of 14 mm or less indicate resistance. Zone sizes of 15 to 17 mm indicate intermediate susceptibility. Susceptible strains of *Haemophilus* and *Neisseria* species give zones of ≥29 mm, resistant strains ≤28 mm. With this procedure, a report from the laboratory of "Susceptible" indicates that the infecting organism is likely to respond to therapy. A report of "Resistant" indicates that the infecting organism is not likely to respond to therapy; other therapy should be selected. A report of "Intermediate Susceptibility" suggests that the organism may be susceptible if the infection is confined to tissues and fluids (e.g., urine), in which high antibiotic levels are attained. The mezlocillin disc should be used for testing susceptibility to mezlocillin. In certain conditions, it may be desirable to do additional susceptibility testing by broth or agar dilution techniques. Dilution methods, preferably the agar plate dilution procedure, are most accurate for susceptibility testing of obligate anaerobes. *Enterobacteriaceae, Pseudomonas* species and *Acinetobacter* species are considered susceptible if the MIC of mezlocillin is no greater than 64 mcg/mL and are considered resistant if the MIC is greater than 128 mcg/mL. *Haemophilus* species and *Neisseria* species are considered susceptible if the MIC of mezlocillin is less than or equal to 1 mcg/mL. Mezlocillin standard is available for broth or agar dilution studies.

*Bauer, A.W., Kirby, W.M., Sherris, J.C. and Turck, M.: Antibiotic Testing by a Standardized Single Disc Method, Am. J. Clin. Pathol., 45:493, 1966; Standardized Disc Susceptibility Test, FEDERAL REGISTER, 39:19182–19184, 1974.

INDICATIONS AND USAGE

MEZLIN® is indicated for the treatment of serious infections caused by susceptible strains of the designated microorganisms in the conditions listed below:

LOWER RESPIRATORY TRACT INFECTIONS including pneumonia and lung abscess caused by *Haemophilus influenzae, Klebsiella* species including *K. pneumoniae, Proteus mirabilis, Pseudomonas* species including *P. aeruginosa, E. coli,* and *Bacteroides* species including *B. fragilis.*

INTRA-ABDOMINAL INFECTIONS including acute cholecystitis, cholangitis, peritonitis, hepatic abscess and intra-abdominal abscess caused by susceptible *E. coli, Proteus mirabilis, Klebsiella* species, *Pseudomonas* species, *S. faecalis* (enterococcus), *Bacteroides* species, *Peptococcus* species, and *Peptostreptococcus* species.

URINARY TRACT INFECTIONS caused by susceptible *E. coli, Proteus mirabilis,* the indole positive *Proteus* species, *Morganella morganii; Klebsiella* species, *Enterobacter* species, *Serratia* species, *Pseudomonas* species, *S. faecalis* (enterococcus).

Uncomplicated gonorrhea due to susceptible *Neisseria gonorrhoeae.*

GYNECOLOGICAL INFECTIONS including endometritis, pelvic cellulitis, and pelvic inflammatory disease associated with susceptible *Neisseria gonorrhoeae, Peptococcus* species, *Peptostreptococcus* species, *Bacteroides* species, *E. coli, Proteus mirabilis, Klebsiella* species, and *Enterobacter* species.

SKIN AND SKIN STRUCTURE INFECTIONS caused by susceptible *S. faecalis* (enterococcus), *E. coli, Proteus mirabilis,* the indole positive *Proteus* species, *Proteus vulgaris,* and *Providencia rettgeri; Klebsiella* species, *Enterobacter* species, *Pseudomonas* species, *Peptococcus* species, and *Bacteroides* species.

SEPTICEMIA including bacteremia caused by susceptible *E. coli, Klebsiella* species, *Enterobacter* species, *Pseudomonas* species, *Bacteroides* species, and *Peptococcus* species.

Mezlocillin has also been shown to be effective for the treatment of infections caused by *Streptococcus* species including Group A Beta-hemolytic *Streptococcus* and *Streptococcus pneumoniae* (formerly *Diplococcus pneumoniae*) however, infections caused by these organisms are ordinarily treated with more narrow spectrum penicillins.

Appropriate culture and susceptibility tests should be performed before treatment in order to isolate and identify organisms causing infection and to determine their susceptibility to mezlocillin. Therapy with MEZLIN® may be initiated before results of these tests are known; once results become available, appropriate therapy should be continued.

Mezlocillin's broad spectrum of activity makes it particularly useful for treating mixed infections caused by susceptible strains of both gram-negative and gram-positive aerobic or anaerobic bacteria. It is not effective, however, against infections caused by penicillinase-producing *Staphylococcus aureus.*

In certain severe infections, when the causative organisms are unknown, MEZLIN® may be administered in conjunction with an aminoglycoside or a cephalosporin antibiotic as initial therapy. As soon as results of culture and susceptibility tests become available, antimicrobial therapy should be adjusted if indicated. Culture and sensitivity testing, performed periodically during therapy, will provide information on the therapeutic effect of the antimicrobial and will monitor for the possible emergence of bacterial resistance.

MEZLIN® has been used effectively in combination with an aminoglycoside antibiotic for the treatment of life-threatening infections caused by *Pseudomonas aeruginosa.* For the treatment of febrile episodes in immunosuppressed patients with granulocytopenia, MEZLIN® should be combined with an aminoglycoside or a cephalosporin antibiotic.

Prevention: The administration of MEZLIN® perioperatively (preoperatively, intraoperatively, and postoperatively) may reduce the incidence of infections in patients undergoing surgical procedures (e.g. vaginal hysterectomy and colorectal surgery) that may be classified as contaminated or potentially contaminated. Effective perioperative use for surgery depends on the time of administration. To achieve effective tissue levels, MEZLIN® should be given $^1/_2$ hour to $1^1/_2$ hours before surgery.

In patients undergoing Caesarean section, intraoperative (after clamping the umbilical cord) and postoperative use of MEZLIN® may reduce the incidence of certain postoperative infections. (See DOSAGE AND ADMINISTRATION section.)

For patients undergoing colorectal surgery, preoperative bowel preparation by mechanical cleansing as well as with a non-absorbable antibiotic (e.g. neomycin) is recommended.

If there are signs of infection, specimens for culture should be obtained for identification of the causative organism so that appropriate therapy may be instituted.

CONTRAINDICATIONS

MEZLIN® is contraindicated in patients with a history of hypersensitivity reactions to any of the penicillins.

WARNINGS

Serious and occasionally fatal hypersensitivity (anaphylactic) reactions have occurred in patients receiving a penicillin. These reactions are more apt to occur in individuals with a history of sensitivity to multiple allergens. There have been reports of individuals with a history of penicillin hypersensitivity reactions who have experienced severe hypersensitivity reactions when treated with cephalosporin. Before therapy with mezlocillin is instituted, careful inquiry should be made to determine whether the patient has had previous hypersensitivity reactions to penicillins, cephalosporins or other drugs. Antibiotics should be used with caution in any patient who has demonstrated some form of allergy, particularly to drugs.

If an allergic reaction occurs during therapy with mezlocillin, the drug should be discontinued. SERIOUS ANAPHYLACTOID REACTIONS REQUIRE IMMEDIATE EMERGENCY TREATMENT. EPINEPHRINE, OXYGEN, INTRAVENOUS STEROIDS, AND AIRWAY MANAGEMENT, INCLUDING INTUBATION, SHOULD BE PROVIDED AS INDICATED.

PRECAUTIONS

General

Although MEZLIN® shares with other penicillins the low potential for toxicity, as with any potent drug, periodic assessment of organ system functions, including renal, hepatic and hematopoietic, is advisable during prolonged therapy. MEZLIN® has been reported rarely to cause acute interstitial nephritis.

Bleeding manifestations have occurred in some patients receiving beta-lactam antibiotics. These reactions have been associated with abnormalities of coagulation tests, such as clotting time, platelet aggregation and prothrombin time and are more likely to occur in patients with renal impairment. Although MEZLIN® has rarely been associated with clinical bleeding, the possibility of this occurring should be kept in mind, particularly in patients with severe renal impairment receiving maximum doses of the drug.

MEZLIN® has only rarely been reported to cause hypokalemia; however, the possibility of this occurring should also be kept in mind, particularly when treating patients with fluid and electrolyte imbalance. Periodic monitoring of serum potassium may be advisable in patients receiving prolonged therapy.

MEZLIN® is a monosodium salt containing only 42.6 mg (1.85 mEq) of sodium per gram of mezlocillin. This should be considered when treating patients requiring restricted salt intake.

As with any penicillin, an allergic reaction, including anaphylaxis, may occur during MEZLIN® administration, particularly in a hypersensitive individual.

As with other antibiotics, prolonged use of MEZLIN® may result in overgrowth of non-susceptible organisms. If this occurs, appropriate measures should be taken.

MEZLIN®, along with other ureidopenicillins, has been reported in one study to prolong neuromuscular blockage of vecuronium. Caution is indicated when mezlocillin is used perioperatively.

Antimicrobials used in high doses for short periods to treat gonorrhea may mask or delay the symptoms of incubating syphilis. Therefore, prior to treatment, patients with gonorrhea should also be evaluated for syphilis. Specimens for dark field examination should be obtained from any suspected primary lesion and serologic tests should be performed. Patients treated with MEZLIN® should undergo follow-up serologic tests three months after therapy.

Interactions with Drugs and Laboratory Tests

As with other penicillins, the mixing of mezlocillin with an aminoglycoside in solutions for parenteral administration can result in substantial inactivation of the aminoglycoside.

Probenecid interferes with the renal tubular secretion of mezlocillin, thereby increasing serum concentrations and prolonging serum half-life of the antibiotic.

High urine concentrations of mezlocillin may produce false positive protein reactions (pseudoproteinuria) with the fol-

MEZLOCILLIN SERUM LEVELS IN ADULTS (mcg/mL) 30 MIN. IV INFUSION

DOSE	0	5 min.	15 min.	30 min.	45 min.	1 hr.	2 hr.	3 hr.	4 hr.	6 hr.	8 hr.
3g	**263** (87–489)	**170** (63–371)	**141** (75–301)	**109** (56–288)	**79** (41–135)	**57** (28–100)	**26** (14–55)	**12** (5.8–26)	**4.4** (2.2–6.5)	**1.6** (1.0–3.4)	**<1**

MEZLIN® DOSAGE GUIDE (ADULTS)

Condition	Daily Dosage Range	Usual Daily Dosage	Frequency and Route of Administration
Urinary tract infection (uncomplicated)	100–125 mg/kg	6–8g	1.5–2g every 6 hours IV or IM
Urinary tract infection (complicated)	150–200 mg/kg	12g	3g every 6 hours IV
Lower respiratory tract infection Intra-abdominal infection Gynecological infection Skin & skin structure infection Septicemia	225–300 mg/kg	16–18g	4g every 6 hours or 3g every 4 hours IV

MEZLIN® DOSAGE GUIDE FOR PATIENTS WITH IMPAIRED RENAL FUNCTION

Creatinine Clearance mL/min.	Urinary Tract Infection (Uncomplicated)	Urinary Tract Infection (Complicated)	Serious Systemic Infection
>30	Usual Recommended Dosage		
10–30	1.5g every 8 hours	1.5g every 6 hours	3g every 8 hours
<10	1.5g every 8 hours	1.5g every 8 hours	2g every 8 hours

MEZLIN® DOSAGE GUIDE (NEWBORNS)

BODY WEIGHT	AGE	
(gm)	≤7 DAYS	>7 DAYS
≤2000	75 mg/kg every 12 hours (150 mg/kg/day)	75 mg/kg every 8 hours (225 mg/kg/day)
>2000	75 mg/kg every 12 hours (150 mg/kg/day)	75 mg/kg every 6 hours (300 mg/kg/day)

STABILITY

INTRAVENOUS SOLUTION	Controlled Room Temperature	Refrigeration
Sterile Water for Injection, USP	48 hours	7 days
0.9% Sodium Chloride Injection, USP	48 hours	7 days
5% Dextrose Injection, USP	48 hours	7 days
5% Dextrose in 0.225% Sodium Chloride Injection, USP	72 hours	7 days
Lactated Ringer's Injection, USP	24 hours	7 days
5% Dextrose in Electrolyte #75 Injection	72 hours	7 days
5% Dextrose in 0.45% Sodium Chloride Injection, USP*	48 hours	48 hours
Ringer's Injection	24 hours	24 hours
10% Dextrose Injection	24 hours	24 hours
5% Fructose Injection	24 hours	24 hours

If precipitation should occur under refrigeration, the product should be warmed to 37°C for 20 minutes in a water bath and shaken well.

* This solution is stable from 10 mg/mL to 50 mg/mL under refrigeration.

lowing methods: sulfosalicylic acid and boiling test, acetic acid test, biuret reaction, and nitric acid test. The bromphenol blue (Multi-stix®) reagent strip test has been reported to be reliable.

Pregnancy Category B

Reproduction studies have been performed in rats and mice at doses up to 2 times the human dose, and have revealed no evidence of impaired fertility or harm to the fetus, due to MEZLIN®. There are however no adequate and well-controlled studies in pregnant women. Because animal reproductive studies are not always predictive of human response, this drug should be used during pregnancy only if clearly needed. Mezlocillin crosses the placenta and is found in low concentrations in cord blood and amniotic fluid.

Nursing Mothers

Mezlocillin is detected in low concentrations in the milk of nursing mothers, therefore caution should be exercised when MEZLIN® is administered to a nursing woman.

ADVERSE REACTIONS

As with other penicillins, the following adverse reactions may occur:

Hypersensitivity reactions: skin rash, pruritus, urticaria, drug fever, acute interstitial nephritis and anaphylactic reactions.

Gastrointestinal disturbances: abnormal taste sensation, nausea, vomiting and diarrhea. If diarrhea persists, pseudomembranous colitis should be considered.

Hemic and Lymphatic Systems: thrombocytopenia, leukopenia, neutropenia, eosinophilia, reduction of hemoglobin or hematocrit, and positive Coombs' test.

Abnormalities of hepatic and renal function tests: elevation of serum aspartate aminotransferase (SGOT), serum alanine aminotransferase (SGPT), serum alkaline phosphatase, serum bilirubin. Elevation of serum creatinine and/or BUN. Reduction in serum potassium.

Central nervous system: convulsive seizures or neuromuscular hyperirritability.

Local reactions: thrombophlebitis with intravenous administration, pain with intramuscular injection.

OVERDOSAGE

As with other penicillins, MEZLIN® in overdosage has the potential to cause neuromuscular hyperirritability or convulsive seizures. Hemodialysis, if necessary, will aid in the removal of drug from the blood.

DOSAGE AND ADMINISTRATION

MEZLIN® (sterile mezlocillin sodium) may be administered intravenously or intramuscularly. For serious infections, the intravenous route of administration should be used. Intramuscular doses should not exceed 2g per injection.

The recommended adult dosage for serious infections is 200–300 mg/kg per day given in 4 to 6 divided doses. The usual dose is 3g given every 4 hours (18g/day) or 4g given every 6 hours (16g/day). For life-threatening infections, up to 350 mg/kg per day may be administered, but the total daily dosage should ordinarily not exceed 24g.

[See first table above]

For patients with life-threatening infections, 4g may be administered every 4 hours (24g/day).

Dosage for any individual patient must take into consideration the site and severity of infection, the susceptibility of the organisms causing infection, and the status of the patient's host defense mechanism.

The duration of therapy depends upon the severity of infection. Generally, MEZLIN® should be continued for at least 2 days after the signs and symptoms of infection have disappeared. The usual duration is 7 to 10 days; however, in difficult and complicated infections, more prolonged therapy may be required. Antibiotic therapy for Group A Beta-hemolytic streptococcal infections should be maintained for at least 10 days to reduce the risk of rheumatic fever or glomerulonephritis.

In certain deep-seated infections, involving abscess formation, appropriate surgical drainage should be performed in conjunction with antimicrobial therapy.

For acute, uncomplicated gonococcal urethritis, the usual dose is 1–2g given once intravenously or by intramuscular injection. Probenecid 1g may be given orally at the time of dosing or up to $1/2$-hour before. (For full prescribing information, refer to probenecid package insert.)

Prevention

To prevent postoperative infection in contaminated or potentially contaminated surgery, the following doses are recommended:

4g IV given $1/2$ hour to $1^{1}/2$ hours prior to the start of surgery.

4g IV given 6 hours and 12 hours later.

Caesarean Section Patients.

The first dose of 4g is given intravenously as soon as the umbilical cord is clamped. The second and third doses of 4g should be given intravenously 4 and 8 hours, respectively, after the first dose.

Patients with Impaired Renal Function

The rate of elimination of mezlocillin is dose dependent and related to the degree of renal function impairment. After an intravenous dose of 3g, the serum half-life is approximately 1 hour in patients with creatinine clearances above 60 mL/min., 1.3 hr. in those with clearances of 30–59 mL/min., 1.6 hr. in those with clearances of 10–29 mL/min. and approximately 3.6 hr. in patients with clearances of less than 10 mL/min. Dosage adjustments of MEZLIN® are not required in patients with mild impairment of renal function. For patients with a creatinine clearance of ≤30 mL/min. (serum creatinine of approximately 3.0 mg% or greater), the following dosage guide may be used:

[See second table above]

For life-threatening infections, 3g may be given every 6 hours to patients with creatinine clearances between 10–30 mL/min. and 2g every 6 hours to those with clearances less than 10 mL/min.

For patients with serious systemic infection undergoing hemodialysis for renal failure, 3–4g may be administered after each dialysis and then every 12 hours. Patients undergoing peritoneal dialysis may receive 3g every 12 hours.

For patients with renal failure and hepatic insufficiency, measurement of serum levels of mezlocillin will provide additional guidance for adjusting dosage.

Intravenous Administration

MEZLIN® may be administered by intermittent infusion or by direct intravenous injection.

Infusion. Each gram of mezlocillin should be reconstituted by vigorous shaking with at least 9–10 mL of Sterile Water for Injection, 5% Dextrose Injection or 0.9% Sodium Chloride Injection. The dissolved drug should be further diluted to desired volume (50–100 mL) with an appropriate intravenous solution. (See Compatibility and Stability section.) The solution of reconstituted drug may then be administered over a period of 30 minutes by direct infusion, or through a Y-type intravenous infusion set which may already be in place. If this method or the "piggyback" method of administration is used, it is advisable to discontinue temporarily the administration of any other solutions during the infusion of MEZLIN®.

Injection. The reconstituted solution of MEZLIN® may also be injected directly into a vein or into intravenous tubing; when administered this way, the injection should be given slowly over a period of 3–5 minutes. To minimize venous irritation, the concentration of drug should not exceed 10%.

When MEZLIN® is given in combination with another antimicrobial, such as an aminoglycoside, each drug should be given separately in accordance with the recommended dosage and routes of administration for each drug.

Continued on next page

Mezlin—Cont.

Intramuscular Administration

Each gram of mezlocillin may be reconstituted by vigorous shaking with 3–4 mL of Sterile Water for Injection or with 3–4 mL of 0.5 or 1.0% Lidocaine Hydrochloride solution (without epinephrine). (For full prescribing information, refer to lidocaine package insert.) Intramuscular doses of MEZLIN® should not exceed 2g per injection.

As with all intramuscular preparations, MEZLIN® should be injected well within the body of a relatively large muscle, such as the upper outer quadrant of the buttock (i.e., gluteus maximus); aspiration will help avoid unintentional injection into a blood vessel. Slow injection (12–15 sec.) will minimize the discomfort associated with intramuscular administration.

Infants and Children

Only limited data are available on the safety and effectiveness of MEZLIN® in the treatment of infants and children with documented serious infection. In the event a child has an infection for which MEZLIN® may be judged particularly appropriate, the following dosage guide may be used: [See third table at top of previous page]

For infants beyond one month of age and children up to the age of 12 years, 50 mg/kg may be administered every 4 hours (300 mg/kg/day).

The drug may be infused intravenously over 30-minutes or be given by intramuscular injection.

COMPATIBILITY AND STABILITY

MEZLIN® at concentrations of 10 mg/mL and 100 mg/mL is stable (loss of potency less than 10%) in the following intravenous solutions for the time periods stated.
[See fourth table at top of previous page]

MEZLIN® at concentrations up to 250 mg/mL is stable for 24 hours at room temperature in the following diluents:

Sterile Water for Injection, USP

0.9% Sodium Chloride Injection, USP

0.5% and 1.0% Lidocaine Hydrochloride solution (without epinephrine)

MEZLIN® is stable for up to 28 days when frozen at −12°C at concentrations up to 100 mg/mL in the following diluents:

Sterile Water for Injection, USP

0.9% Sodium Chloride Injection, USP or 5% Dextrose Injection, USP

HOW SUPPLIED

MEZLIN® (sterile mezlocillin sodium) is a white to pale yellow crystalline powder supplied as listed below:

MEZLIN® is available in vials, infusion bottles, pharmacy bulk packages and ADD-Vantage® vials containing mezlocillin sodium equivalent to mezlocillin, as specified:

	NDC Number
1g Vial	0026-8211-10
2g Vial	0026-8212-30
2g Infusion Bottle	0026-8212-36
3g Vial	0026-8213-35
3g Infusion Bottle	0026-8213-36
3g ADD-Vantage® Vial	0026-8213-19
4g Vial	0026-8214-35
4g Infusion Bottle	0026-8214-36
4g ADD-Vantage® Vial	0026-8214-19
20g Pharmacy Bulk Package	0026-8220-31

Unreconstituted MEZLIN® should be stored at temperatures not exceeding 86°F (30°C). The powder as well as the reconstituted solution of drug may darken slightly, depending upon storage conditions, but potency is not affected.

Bayer Corporation
Pharmaceutical Division
400 Morgan Lane
West Haven, CT 06516 USA
Made in Germany
PD 100790   3/95   Bay f   1353   5202/A/US/Bayer
©1995 Bayer   Printed in USA   4998

MEZLIN®
Sterile mezlocillin sodium
BAYPEN®

℞

DESCRIPTION

A pharmacy bulk package is a container of a sterile preparation for parenteral use that contains many single doses. The contents are intended for use in a pharmacy admixture program and are restricted to the preparation of admixtures for intravenous infusion, or the filling of empty sterile syringes for intravenous injection for patients with individualized dosing requirements (see Dosage and Administration section).

MEZLIN® (sterile mezlocillin sodium) is a semisynthetic broad spectrum penicillin antibiotic for parenteral administration. It is the monohydrate sodium salt of 6-[D-2 [3-(methyl-sulfonyl) -2-OXO-imidazolidine -1- carboxamido] -2-phenyl acetamido] penicillanic acid.

Structural Formula:

Empirical Formula: $C_{21}H_{24}N_5O_8S_2Na \cdot H_2O$

MEZLIN® has a molecular weight of 579.6 and contains 42.6 mg (1.85 mEq) of sodium per one gram of mezlocillin activity. The dosage form is supplied as a sterile white to pale yellow crystalline powder, which is freely soluble in water. When reconstituted, solutions of MEZLIN® are clear and range from colorless to pale yellow with a pH of 4.5 to 8.0.

CLINICAL PHARMACOLOGY

Intravenous Administration. In healthy adult volunteers, mean serum levels of mezlocillin 5 minutes after a 5-minute intravenous injection of 1g, 2g, or 5g are 100, 253, or 411 mcg/mL, respectively. Serum levels, as noted below, lack dose proportionality:
[See table below]

Fifteen minutes after a 4g intravenous injection (2–5 min.), the concentration in serum is 254 mcg/mL; 1 hour and 4 hours later levels are 93 mcg/mL and 9.1 mcg/mL, respectively:
[See table at top of next page]

After an intravenous infusion (15 min.) of 3g, mean levels 15 minutes after dosing are 269 mcg/mL (170–280).

A 30-minute intravenous infusion of 3g produces mean peak concentrations of 263 mcg/mL; 1 hour and 4 hours later the concentrations are 57 mcg/mL and 4.4 mcg/mL, respectively:
[See table at bottom of next page]

Following intravenous infusion (2 hr.) of a 3g dose of mezlocillin every 4 hours for 7 days, mean peak serum concentrations are higher than 100 mcg/mL, and levels above 50 mcg/mL are maintained throughout dosing.

Intramuscular Administration. MEZLIN® is rapidly absorbed after intramuscular injection. In healthy volunteers, the mean peak serum concentration occurs approximately 45 minutes after a single dose of 1g and is about 15 mcg/mL. The oral administration of 1g probenecid before injection produces an increase in mezlocillin serum levels of about 50%. After repetitive intramuscular doses of 1g mezlocillin every 6 hours, peak levels in the serum generally range between 35 and 45 mcg/mL. The relationship between the pharmacokinetics of intramuscular and intravenous dosing has not yet been clearly established.

General. As with other penicillins, mezlocillin is excreted primarily by glomerular filtration and tubular secretion. The rate of elimination is dose dependent and related to the degree of renal functional impairment. In patients with normal renal function, approximately 55% of the administered dose is recovered from the urine within the first 6 hours after dosing. Two hours after an intravenous injection of 2g, concentrations of active drug in urine generally exceed 4000 mcg/mL. By 4–6 hours after injection, concentrations usually decline to a range of about 50 to 200 mcg/mL. The serum elimination half-life of mezlocillin after intravenous dosing is approximately 55 minutes.

In patients with reduced renal function, the half-life is only slightly prolonged. Dosage adjustments are usually not necessary except in patients with severe renal impairment. (See Dosage and Administration.) As with other penicillins, mezlocillin is metabolized only slightly; less than 10% of the drug excreted in the urine is in the form of the penicilloate

or penilloate. The drug is readily removed from the serum by hemodialysis and, to a lesser extent, by peritoneal dialysis.

Up to 26% of a dose of mezlocillin is recovered from the bile of patients with normal liver function. Following intravenous doses of 2g to 5g, concentrations of active drug in bile generally range from 500 to 2500 mcg/mL. The biliary excretion of mezlocillin is reduced in patients with common bile duct obstruction.

Mezlocillin is not appreciably absorbed when given orally. Following parenteral administration, the apparent volume of distribution is approximately equal to the extracellular fluid volume. The drug is present in active form in the serum, urine, bile, peritoneal fluid, pleural fluid, bronchial and wound secretions, bone and other tissues. As with other penicillins, penetration into the cerebrospinal fluid (CSF) is generally poor, however higher CSF concentrations are obtained in the presence of meningeal inflammation.

Protein binding studies indicate that the degree of mezlocillin binding is low (16–42%) and depends upon testing methods and concentrations of drug studied.

Microbiology

Mezlocillin is a bactericidal antibiotic which acts by interfering with synthesis of cell wall components. It is active against a variety of gram-negative and gram-positive bacteria, including aerobic and anaerobic strains. Mezlocillin is usually active *in vitro* against most strains of the following organisms:

Gram-negative bacteria
Escherichia coli
Proteus mirabilis
Proteus vulgaris
Morganella morganii (formerly *P. morganii*)
Providencia rettgeri (formerly *Proteus rettgeri*)
Providencia stuartii
Citrobacter species*
Klebsiella species (including *K. pneumoniae*)
Enterobacter species
Shigella species*
Pseudomonas aeruginosa (and other species)
Haemophilus influenzae
Haemophilus parainfluenzae
Neisseria species
Many strains of *Serratia, Salmonella*, and *Acinetobacter** are also susceptible.

Gram-positive bacteria
Staphylococcus aureus (non-penicillinase producing strains)
Beta-hemolytic *streptococci* (Groups A and B)
Streptococcus pneumoniae (formerly *Diplococcus pneumoniae*)
Streptococcus faecalis (enterococcus)

Anaerobic Organisms
Peptococcus species
Peptostreptococcus species
Clostridium species*
Bacteroides species (including *B. fragilis* group)
Fusobacterium species*
Veillonella species*
Eubacterium species*

*Mezlocillin has been shown to be active *in vitro* against these organisms, however clinical efficacy has not yet been established.

Noteworthy is mezlocillin's broadened spectrum of *in vitro* activity against important pathogenic aerobic gram-negative bacteria, including strains of *Pseudomonas, Klebsiella, Enterobacter, Serratia, Proteus, Escherichia* and *Haemophilus,* as well as *Bacteroides* and other anaerobes; and its excellent inhibitory effect against gram-positive organisms including *Streptococcus faecalis* (enterococcus). It is inactive against penicillinase-producing strains of *Staphylococcus aureus.*

In vitro studies have shown that mezlocillin combined with an aminoglycoside (e.g., gentamicin, tobramycin, amikacin, sisomicin) acts synergistically against strains of *Streptococcus faecalis* and *Pseudomonas aeruginosa.* In some instances, this combination also acts synergistically *in vitro* against other gram-negative bacteria such as *Serratia, Klebsiella* and *Acinetobacter* species.

Mezlocillin is slightly more active when tested at alkaline pH and, as with other penicillins, has reduced activity when tested *in vitro* with increasing inoculum. The minimum bactericidal concentration (MBC) generally exceeds the minimum inhibitory concentration (MIC) by a factor of 2 or 3. Resistance to mezlocillin *in vitro* develops slowly (multiple

MEZLOCILLIN SERUM LEVELS IN ADULTS (mcg/mL) 5 MIN. IV INJECTION

DOSE	0	5 min	10 min	20 min	30 min	1 hr	2 hr	3 hr	4 hr	6 hr	8 hr
1g	149 (132–185)	100 (64–143)	66 (47–87)	50 (31–87)	40 (22–83)	18 (8–31)	5.3 (3.3–7.7)	2.5 (1.7–3.7)	1.7 (0.7–2.8)	0.5 (0–1.2)	0.1 (0–0.2)
2g	314 (207–362)	253 (161–364)	161 (113–214)	117 (76–174)	82 (55–112)	56 (23–88)	20 (7.5–32)	11 (3.8–16)	4.4 (1.6–8.7)	1.5 (0.5–2.6)	0.6 (0.1–1.4)
5g	547 (268–854)	411 (199–597)	357 (246–456)	250 (203–353)	226 (190–333)	131 (104–193)	76 (59–104)	31 (20–40)	13 (6.4–17)	4.6 (2.1–9.4)	1.9 (1.1–3.6)

MEZLOCILLIN SERUM LEVELS IN ADULTS (mcg/mL) 2–5 MIN. IV INJECTION

DOSE	0	15 min	30 min	45 min	1 hr	2 hr	3 hr	4 hr	6 hr
4g	—	**254** (155–400)	**163** (99–260)	**122** (78–215)	**93** (67–133)	**47** (22–96)	**20** (8–45)	**9.1** (6–13)	**8.4** (5–17)

step mutation). Some strains of *Pseudomonas aeruginosa* have developed resistance fairly rapidly. Mezlocillin is not stable in the presence of penicillinase and strains of *Staphylococcus aureus* resistant to penicillin are also resistant to mezlocillin.

Susceptibility Tests

Quantitative methods that require measurement of zone diameters give good estimates of bacterial susceptibility. One such procedure* has been recommended for use with discs to test susceptibility to antimicrobials. When the causative organism is tested by the Kirby-Bauer method of disc susceptibility, a 75 mcg mezlocillin disc should give a zone of 18 mm or greater to indicate susceptibility. Zone sizes of 14 mm or less indicate resistance. Zone sizes of 15 to 17 mm indicate intermediate susceptibility. Susceptibile strains of *Haemophilus* and *Neisseria* species give zones of ≥29 mm, resistant strains ≤28 mm. With this procedure, a report from the laboratory of "Susceptibile" indicates that the infecting organism is likely to respond to therapy. A report of "Resistant" indicates that the infecting organism is not likely to respond to therapy; other therapy should be selected. A report of "Intermediate Susceptibility" suggests that the organism may be susceptible if the infection is confined to tissues and fluids (e.g., urine), in which high antibiotic levels are attained. The mezlocillin disc should be used for testing susceptibility to mezlocillin. In certain conditions, it may be desirable to do additional susceptibility testing by broth or agar dilution techniques. Dilution methods, preferably the agar plate dilution procedure, are most accurate for susceptibility testing of obligate anaerobes. *Enterobacteriaceae, Pseudomonas* species and *Acinetobacter* species are considered susceptible if the MIC of mezlocillin is no greater than 64 mcg/mL and are considered resistant if the MIC is greater than 128 mcg/mL. *Haemophilus* species and *Neisseria* species are considered susceptible if the MIC of mezlocillin is less than or equal to 1 mcg/mL. Mezlocillin standard is available for broth or agar dilution studies.

*Bauer, A.W., Kirby, W.M., Sherris, J.C., and Turck, M.: Antibiotic Testing by a Standardized Single Disc Method, Am. J. Clin. Pathol., 45:493, 1966; Standardized Disc Susceptibility Test, FEDERAL REGISTER, 39: 19182-19184, 1974.

INDICATIONS AND USAGE

MEZLIN® is indicated for the treatment of serious infections caused by susceptible strains of the designated microorganisms in the conditions listed below:

LOWER RESPIRATORY TRACT INFECTIONS including pneumonia and lung abscess caused by *Haemophilus influenzae, Klebsiella* species including *K. pneumoniae, Proteus mirabilis, Pseudomonas* species including *P. aeruginosa, E. coli,* and *Bacteroides* species including *B. fragilis.*

INTRA-ABDOMINAL INFECTIONS including acute cholecystitis, cholangitis, peritonitis, hepatic abscess and intra-abdominal abscess caused by susceptible *E. coli, Proteus mirabilis, Klebsiella* species, *Pseudomonas* species, *S. faecalis* (enterococcus), *Bacteroides* species, *Peptococcus* species, and *Peptostreptococcus* species.

URINARY TRACT INFECTIONS caused by susceptible *E. coli, Proteus mirabilis,* the indole positive *Proteus* species, *Morganella morganii; Klebsiella* species, *Enterobacter* species, *Serratia* species, *Pseudomonas* species, *S. faecalis* (enterococcus).

Uncomplicated gonorrhea due to susceptible *Neisseria gonorrhoeae.*

GYNECOLOGICAL INFECTIONS including endometritis, pelvic cellulitis, and pelvic inflammatory disease associated with susceptible *Neisseria gonorrhoeae, Peptococcus* species, *Peptostreptococcus* species, *Bacteroides* species, *E. coli, Proteus mirabilis, Klebsiella* species, and *Enterobacter* species.

SKIN AND SKIN STRUCTURE INFECTIONS caused by susceptible *S. faecalis* (enterococcus), *E. coli, Proteus mirabilis,* the indole positive *Proteus* species, *Proteus vulgaris,* and *Providencia rettgeri; Klebsiella* species, *Enterobacter* species, *Pseudomonas* species, *Peptococcus* species, and *Bacteroides* species.

SEPTICEMIA including bacteremia caused by susceptible *E. coli, Klebsiella* species, *Enterobacter* species, *Pseudomonas* species, *Bacteroides* species, and *Peptococcus* species.

Mezlocillin has also been shown to be effective for the treatment of infections caused by *Streptococcus* species including Group A Beta-hemolytic *Streptococcus* and *Streptococcus pneumoniae* (formerly *Diplococcus pneumoniae*) however, infections caused by these organisms are ordinarily treated with more narrow spectrum penicillins.

Appropriate culture and susceptibility tests should be performed before treatment in order to isolate and identify organisms causing infection and to determine their susceptibility to mezlocillin. Therapy with MEZLIN® may be initiated before results of these tests are known; once results become available, appropriate therapy should be continued.

Mezlocillin's broad spectrum of activity makes it particularly useful for treating mixed infections caused by susceptible strains of both gram-negative and gram-positive aerobic or anaerobic bacteria. It is not effective, however, against infections caused by penicillinase-producing *Staphylococcus aureus.*

In certain severe infections, when the causative organisms are unknown, MEZLIN® may be administered in conjunction with an aminoglycoside or a cephalosporin antibiotic as initial therapy. As soon as results of culture and susceptibility tests become available, antimicrobial therapy should be adjusted if indicated. Culture and sensitivity testing, performed periodically during therapy, will provide information on the therapeutic effect of the antimicrobial and will monitor for the possible emergence of bacterial resistance.

MEZLIN® has been used effectively in combination with an aminoglycoside antibiotic for the treatment of life-threatening infections caused by *Pseudomonas aeruginosa.* For the treatment of febrile episodes in immunosuppressed patients with granulocytopenia, MEZLIN® should be combined with an aminoglycoside or a cephalosporin antibiotic.

Prevention: The administration of MEZLIN® perioperatively (preoperatively, intraoperatively, and postoperatively) may reduce the incidence of infections in patients undergoing surgical procedures (e.g. vaginal hysterectomy and colorectal surgery) that may be classified as contaminated or potentially contaminated. Effective perioperative use for surgery depends on the time of administration. To achieve effective tissue levels, MEZLIN® should be given $^1/_2$ hour to $1^1/_2$ hours before surgery.

In patients undergoing Caesarean section, intraoperative (after clamping the umbilical cord) and postoperative use of MEZLIN® may reduce the incidence of certain postoperative infections. (See DOSAGE AND ADMINISTRATION section.)

For patients undergoing colorectal surgery, preoperative bowel preparation by mechanical cleansing as well as with a non-absorbable antibiotic (e.g. neomycin) is recommended. If there are signs of infection, specimens for culture should be obtained for identification of the causative organism so that appropriate therapy may be instituted.

CONTRAINDICATIONS

MEZLIN® is contraindicated in patients with a history of hypersensitivity reactions to any of the penicillins.

WARNINGS

Serious and occasionally fatal hypersensitivity (anaphylactic) reactions have occurred in patients receiving a penicillin. These reactions are more apt to occur in individuals with a history of sensitivity to multiple allergens. There have been reports of individuals with a history of penicillin hypersensitivity reactions who have experienced severe hypersensitivity reactions when treated with cephalosporin. Before therapy with mezlocillin is instituted, careful inquiry should be made to determine whether the patient has had previous hypersensitivity reactions to penicillins, cephalosporins or other drugs. Antibiotics should be used with caution in any patient who has demonstrated some form of allergy, particularly to drugs.

If an allergic reaction occurs during therapy with mezlocillin, the drug should be discontinued. SERIOUS ANAPHYLACTOID REACTIONS REQUIRE IMMEDIATE EMERGENCY TREATMENT. EPINEPHRINE, OXYGEN, INTRAVENOUS STEROIDS, AND AIRWAY MANAGEMENT, INCLUDING INTUBATION, SHOULD BE PROVIDED AS INDICATED.

PRECAUTIONS

General

Although MEZLIN® shares with other penicillins the low potential for toxicity, as with any other potent drug, periodic assessment of organ system functions, including renal, hepatic and hematopoietic, is advisable during prolonged therapy. MEZLIN® has been reported rarely to cause acute interstitial nephritis.

Bleeding manifestations have occurred in some patients receiving beta-lactam antibiotics. These reactions have been associated with abnormalities of coagulation tests, such as clotting time, platelet aggregation and prothrombin time and are more likely to occur in patients with renal impairment. Although MEZLIN® has rarely been associated with clinical bleeding, the possibility of this occurring should be kept in mind, particularly in patients with severe renal impairment receiving maximum doses of the drug.

MEZLIN® has only rarely been reported to cause hypokalemia; however, the possibility of this occurring should also be kept in mind, particularly when treating patients with fluid and electrolyte imbalance. Periodic monitoring of serum potassium may be advisable in patients receiving prolonged therapy.

MEZLIN® is a monosodium salt containing only 42.6 mg (1.85 mEq) of sodium per gram of mezlocillin. This should be considered when treating patients requiring restricted salt intake.

As with any penicillin, an allergic reaction, including anaphylaxis, may occur during MEZLIN® administration, particularly in a hypersensitive individual.

As with other antibiotics, prolonged use of MEZLIN® may result in overgrowth of non-susceptible organisms. If this occurs, appropriate measures should be taken.

MEZLIN®, along with other ureidopenicillins, has been reported in one study to prolong neuromuscular blockage of vecuronium. Caution is indicated when mezlocillin is used perioperatively.

Antimicrobials used in high doses for short periods to treat gonorrhea may mask or delay the symptoms of incubating syphilis. Therefore, prior to treatment, patients with gonorrhea should also be evaluated for syphilis. Specimens for dark field examination should be obtained from any suspected primary lesion and serologic tests should be performed. Patients treated with MEZLIN® should undergo follow-up serologic tests three months after therapy.

Interactions with Drugs and Laboratory Tests

As with other penicillins, the mixing of mezlocillin with an aminoglycoside in solutions for parenteral administration can result in substantial inactivation of the aminoglycoside.

Probenecid interferes with the renal tubular secretion of mezlocillin, thereby increasing serum concentrations and prolonging serum half-life of the antibiotic.

High urine concentrations of mezlocillin may produce false positive protein reactions (pseudoproteinuria) with the following methods: sulfosalicylic acid and boiling test, acetic acid test, biuret reaction, and nitric acid test. The bromphenol blue (Multi-stix®) reagent strip test has been reported to be reliable.

Pregnancy Category B

Reproduction studies have been performed in rats and mice at doses up to 2 times the human dose, and have revealed no evidence of impaired fertility or harm to the fetus, due to MEZLIN®. There are however no adequate and well-controlled studies in pregnant women. Because animal reproductive studies are not always predictive of human response, this drug should be used during pregnancy only if clearly needed. Mezlocillin crosses the placenta and is found in low concentrations in cord blood and amniotic fluid.

Nursing Mothers

Mezlocillin is detected in low concentrations in the milk of nursing mothers. Therefore caution should be exercised when MEZLIN® is administered to a nursing woman.

ADVERSE REACTIONS

As with other penicillins, the following adverse reactions may occur:

Hypersensitivity reactions: skin rash, pruritus, urticaria, drug fever, acute interstitial nephritis and anaphylactic reactions.

Gastrointestinal disturbances: abnormal taste sensation, nausea, vomiting and diarrhea. If diarrhea persists, pseudomembranous colitis should be considered.

Hematologic and Lymphatic Systems: thrombocytopenia, leukopenia, neutropenia, eosinophilia, reduction of hemoglobin or hematocrit, and positive Coombs' test.

Abnormalities of hepatic and renal function tests: elevation of serum aspartate aminotransferase (SGOT), serum alanine aminotransferase (SGPT), serum alkaline phosphatase, serum bilirubin. Elevation of serum creatinine and/or BUN. Reduction in serum potassium.

Continued on next page

MEZLOCILLIN SERUM LEVELS IN ADULTS (mcg/mL) 30 MIN. IV INFUSION

DOSE	0	5 min	15 min	30 min	45 min	1 hr	2 hr	3 hr	4 hr	6 hr	8 hr
3g	**263** (87–489)	**170** (63–371)	**141** (75–301)	**109** (56–288)	**79** (41–135)	**57** (28–100)	**26** (14–55)	**12** (5.8–26)	**4.4** (2.2–6.5)	**1.6** (1.0–3.4)	**<1**

Mezlin Bulk—Cont.

Central nervous system: convulsive seizures or neuromuscular hyperirritability.
Local reactions: thrombophlebitis with intravenous administration, pain with intramuscular injection.

OVERDOSAGE

As with other penicillins, MEZLIN® in overdosage has the potential to cause neuromuscular hyperirritability or convulsive seizures. Hemodialysis, if necessary, will aid in the removal of drug from the blood.

DOSAGE AND ADMINISTRATION

MEZLIN® (sterile mezlocillin sodium) may be administered intravenously or intramuscularly. For serious infections, the intravenous route of administration should be used. Intramuscular doses should not exceed 2g per injection.

The 20g pharmacy bulk package is intended for the preparation of solutions for intravenous use. When intramuscular administration is required, the MEZLIN® vial should be used.

The recommended adult dosage for serious infections is 200–300 mg/kg per day given in 4 to 6 divided doses. The usual dose is 3g given every 4 hours (18g/day) or 4g given every 6 hours (16g/day). For life-threatening infections, up to 350 mg/kg per day may be administered, but the total daily dosage should ordinarily not exceed 24g.
[See first table above]

For patients with life-threatening infections, 4g may be administered every 4 hours (24g/day).

Dosage for any individual patient must take into consideration the site and severity of infection, the susceptibility of the organisms causing infection, and the status of the patient's host defense mechanism.

The duration of therapy depends upon the severity of infection. Generally, MEZLIN® should be continued for at least 2 days after the signs and symptoms of infection have disappeared. The usual duration is 7 to 10 days; however, in difficult and complicated infections, more prolonged therapy may be required. Antibiotic therapy for Group A Beta-hemolytic streptococcal infections should be maintained for at least 10 days to reduce the risk of rheumatic fever or glomerulonephritis.

In certain deep-seated infections, involving abscess formation, appropriate surgical drainage should be performed in conjunction with antimicrobial therapy.

For acute, uncomplicated gonococcal urethritis, the usual dose is 1–2g given once intravenously or by intramuscular injection. Probenecid 1g may be given orally at the time of dosing or up to ½-hour before. (For full prescribing information, refer to probenecid package insert.)

Prevention

To prevent postoperative infection in contaminated or potentially contaminated surgery, the following doses are recommended:

4g IV given ½ hour to 1½ hours prior to the start of surgery.

4g IV given 6 hours and 12 hours later.

Caesarean Section Patients.

The first dose of 4g is given intravenously as soon as the umbilical cord is clamped. The second and third doses of 4g should be given intravenously 4 and 8 hours, respectively, after the first dose.

Patients with Impaired Renal Function

The rate of elimination of mezlocillin is dose dependent and related to the degree of renal function impairment. After an intravenous dose of 3g, the serum half-life is approximately 1 hour in patients with creatinine clearances above 60 mL/min., 1.3 hr. in those with clearances of 30–59 mL/min., 1.6 hr. in those with clearances of 10–29 mL/min. and approximately 3.6 hr. in patients with clearances of less than 10 mL/min. Dosage adjustments of MEZLIN® are not required in patients with mild impairment of renal function. For patients with a creatinine clearance of ≤30 mL/min. (serum creatinine of approximately 3.0 mg% or greater), the following dosage guide may be used:
[See second table above]

For life-threatening infections, 3g may be given every 6 hours to patients with creatinine clearances between 10–30 mL/min. and 2g every 6 hours to those with clearances less than 10 mL/min.

For patients with serious systemic infection undergoing hemodialysis for renal failure, 3–4g may be administered after each dialysis and then every 12 hours. Patients undergoing peritoneal dialysis may receive 3g every 12 hours.

For patients with renal failure and hepatic insufficiency, measurement of serum levels of mezlocillin will provide additional guidance for adjusting dosage.

Directions for Proper Use of 20 gram Pharmacy Bulk Package

A pharmacy bulk package is a container of a sterile preparation for parenteral use that contains many single doses. The contents are intended for use in a pharmacy admixture program and are restricted to the preparation of admixtures

for intravenous infusion, or the filling of empty sterile syringes for intravenous injection for patients with individualized dosing requirements.

THE CLOSURE SHALL BE PENETRATED ONLY ONE TIME AFTER RECONSTITUTION with a suitable sterile transfer set or dispensing device which allows measured dispensing of the contents. The pharmacy bulk package is to be used only in a suitable work area such as a laminar flow hood or an equivalent clean air compounding area.

Reconstitute by vigorous shaking with 186 mL of Sterile Water for Injection, 5% Dextrose Injection or 0.9% Sodium Chloride Injection resulting in a solution containing approximately 100 mg/mL which should be stored at controlled room temperature or under refrigeration. Within 8 hours of reconstitution, the desired dosages should be withdrawn and may be further diluted with an appropriate intravenous solution (see Compatability & Stability section).

Intravenous Administration

MEZLIN® may be administered intravenously by intermittent infusion or by direct intravenous injection.

Infusion. The dissolved drug should be further diluted to desired volume (50–100 mL) with an appropriate intravenous solution. (See Compatibility and Stability section.) The solution of reconstituted drug may then be administered over a period of 30 minutes by direct infusion, or through a Y-type intravenous infusion set which may already be in place. If this method or the "piggyback" method of administration is used, it is advisable to discontinue temporarily the administration of any other solutions during the infusion of MEZLIN®.

Injection. The reconstituted solution of MEZLIN® may also be injected directly into a vein or into intravenous tubing; when administered this way, the injection should be given slowly over a period of 3–5 minutes. To minimize venous irritation, the concentration of drug should not exceed 10%. When MEZLIN® is given in combination with another antimicrobial, such as an aminoglycoside, each drug should be given separately in accordance with the recommended dosage and routes of administration for each drug.

Intramuscular Administration

For intramuscular administration, please refer to the Dosage and Administration section of the MEZLIN® vial package insert.

Infants and Children

Only limited data are available on the safety and effectiveness of MEZLIN® in the treatment of infants and children with documented serious infection. In the event a child has an infection for which MEZLIN® may be judged particularly appropriate, the following dosage guide may be used:

MEZLIN® DOSAGE GUIDE (ADULTS)

Condition	Daily Dosage Range	Usual Daily Dosage	Frequency and Route of Administration
Urinary tract infection (uncomplicated)	100–125 mg/kg	6–8g	1.5–2g every 6 hours IV or IM
Urinary tract infection (complicated)	150–200 mg/kg	12g	3g every 6 hours IV
Lower respiratory tract infection Intra-abdominal infection Gynecological infection Skin & skin structure infection Septicemia	225–300 mg/kg	16–18g	4g every 6 hours or 3g every 4 hours IV

MEZLIN® DOSAGE GUIDE FOR PATIENTS WITH IMPAIRED RENAL FUNCTION

Creatinine Clearance mL/min.	Urinary Tract Infection (Uncomplicated)	Urinary Tract Infection (Complicated)	Serious Systemic Infection
>30	Usual Recommended Dosage		
10–30	1.5g every 8 hours	1.5g every 6 hours	3g every 8 hours
<10	1.5g every 8 hours	1.5g every 8 hours	2g every 8 hours

STABILITY

INTRAVENOUS SOLUTION	Controlled Room Temperature	Refrigeration
Sterile Water for Injection, USP	48 hours	7 days
0.9% Sodium Chloride Injection, USP	48 hours	7 days
5% Dextrose Injection, USP	48 hours	7 days
5% Dextrose in 0.225% Sodium Chloride Injection, USP	72 hours	7 days
Lactated Ringer's Injection, USP	72 hours	7 days
5% Dextrose in Electrolyte #75 Injection	72 hours	7 days
5% Dextrose in 0.45% Sodium Chloride Injection, USP*	48 hours	48 hours
Ringer's Injection	24 hours	24 hours
10% Dextrose Injection	24 hours	24 hours
5% Fructose Injection	24 hours	24 hours

If precipitation should occur under refrigeration, the product should be warmed to 37°C for 20 minutes in a water bath and shaken well.

*This solution is stable from 10 mg/mL to 50 mg/mL under refrigeration.

MEZLIN DOSAGE GUIDE (NEWBORNS)

BODY WEIGHT	AGE	
(gm)	≤7 DAYS	>7 DAYS
≤2000	75 mg/kg every 12 hours (150 mg/kg/day)	75 mg/kg every 8 hours (225 mg/kg/day)
>2000	75 mg/kg every 12 hours (150 mg/kg/day)	75 mg/kg every 6 hours (300 mg/kg/day)

For infants beyond one month of age and children up to the age of 12 years, 60 mg/kg may be administered every 4 hours (300 mg/kg/day).

The drug may be infused intravenously over 30-minutes or be given by intramuscular injection.

COMPATIBILITY AND STABILITY

MEZLIN® at concentrations of 10 mg/mL and 100 mg/mL is stable (loss of potency less than 10%) in the following intravenous solutions for the time periods stated (includes time retained in pharmacy bulk package after reconstitution):
[See third table from top of page]

MEZLIN® is stable for up to 28 days when frozen at −12°C at concentrations up to 100 mg/mL in the following diluents:

Sterile Water for Injection, USP
0.9% Sodium Chloride Injection, USP or 5% Dextrose Injection, USP

HOW SUPPLIED

MEZLIN® (sterile mezlocillin sodium) is a white to pale yellow crystalline powder supplied as listed below:
MEZLIN® is available in vials, infusion bottles, pharmacy bulk packages and ADD-Vantage® vials containing mezlocillin sodium equivalent to mezlocillin, as specified:

	NDC Number
1g Vial	0026-8211-10
2g Vial	0026-8212-30
2g Infusion Bottle	0026-8212-36
3g Vial	0026-8213-35
3g Infusion Bottle	0026-8213-36
3g ADD-Vantage® Vial	0026-8213-19
4g Vial	0026-8214-35
4g Infusion Bottle	0026-8214-36
4g ADD-Vantage® Vial	0026-8214-19
20g Pharmacy Bulk Package	0026-8220-31

Unreconstituted MEZLIN® should be stored at temperatures not exceeding 86°F (30°C). The powder as well as the reconstituted solution of drug may darken slightly, depending upon storage conditions, but potency is not affected.

Bayer Corporation
Pharmaceutical Division
400 Morgan Lane
West Haven, CT 06516 USA
PD100668 ©Bayer Corp. 9/88 BAY f 1353 5202/4/A/US/
Bayer

0626

MITHRACIN® ℞
(plicamycin)
FOR INTRAVENOUS USE

WARNING

IT IS RECOMMENDED THAT MITHRACIN (plicamycin) BE ADMINISTERED ONLY TO HOSPITALIZED PATIENTS BY OR UNDER THE SUPERVISION OF A QUALIFIED PHYSICIAN WHO IS EXPERIENCED IN THE USE OF CANCER CHEMOTHERAPEUTIC AGENTS, BECAUSE OF THE POSSIBILITY OF SEVERE REACTIONS. FACILITIES FOR THE DETERMINATION OF NECESSARY LABORATORY STUDIES MUST BE AVAILABLE.
SEVERE THROMBOCYTOPENIA, A HEMORRHAGIC TENDENCY AND EVEN DEATH MAY RESULT FROM THE USE OF MITHRACIN. ALTHOUGH SEVERE TOXICITY IS MORE APT TO OCCUR IN PATIENTS WHO HAVE FAR-ADVANCED DISEASE OR ARE OTHERWISE CONSIDERED POOR RISKS FOR THERAPY, SERIOUS TOXICITY MAY ALSO OCCASIONALLY OCCUR EVEN IN PATIENTS WHO ARE IN RELATIVELY GOOD CONDITION.
IN THE TREATMENT OF EACH PATIENT, THE PHYSICIAN MUST WEIGH CAREFULLY THE POSSIBILITY OF ACHIEVING THERAPEUTIC BENEFIT VERSUS THE RISK OF TOXICITY WHICH MAY OCCUR WITH MITHRACIN THERAPY. THE FOLLOWING DATA CONCERNING THE USE OF MITHRACIN IN THE TREATMENT OF TESTICULAR TUMORS, HYPERCALCEMIC AND/OR HYPERCALCIURIC CONDITIONS ASSOCIATED WITH VARIOUS ADVANCED MALIGNANCIES, SHOULD BE THOROUGHLY REVIEWED BEFORE ADMINISTERING THIS COMPOUND.

DESCRIPTION

Mithracin (plicamycin) is a yellow crystalline compound which is produced by a microorganism, *Streptomyces plicatus*. Mithracin is available in vials as a freeze-dried, sterile preparation for intravenous administration. Each vial contains 2500 mcg (2.5 mg) of Mithracin with 100 mg of mannitol and sufficient disodium phosphate to adjust to pH 7. After reconstitution with sterile water for injection, the solution has a pH of 7. The drug is unstable in acid solutions with a pH below 4.
Mithracin is an antineoplastic agent. It has an empirical formula of $C_{52}H_{76}O_{24}$. The following structural formula has been proposed for this compound.

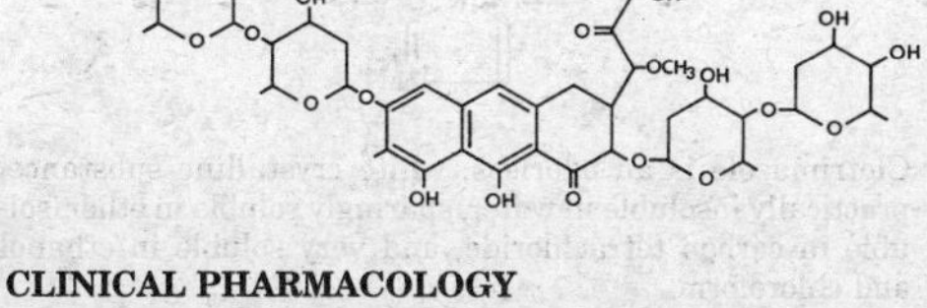

CLINICAL PHARMACOLOGY

Although the exact mechanism by which Mithracin causes tumor inhibition is not yet known, studies have indicated that this compound forms a complex with deoxyribonucleic acid (DNA) and inhibits cellular ribonucleic acid (RNA) and enzymic RNA synthesis. The binding of Mithracin to DNA in the presence of Mg^{++} (or other divalent cations) is responsible for the inhibition of DNA-dependent or DNA-directed RNA synthesis. This action presumably accounts for the biological properties of Mithracin.
Mithracin shows potent cytotoxicity against malignant cells of human origin (Hela cells) growing in tissue culture. Mithracin is lethal to Hela cells in 48 hours at concentrations as low as 0.5 micrograms per milliliter of tissue culture medium. Mithracin has shown significant anti-tumor activity against experimental leukemia in mice when administered intraperitoneally.
Plicamycin may lower serum calcium levels; the exact mechanism (or mechanisms) by which the drug exerts this effect is unknown. It appears that plicamycin may block the hypercalcemic action of pharmacologic doses of vitamin D. It has also been suggested that plicamycin may lower calcium serum levels by inhibiting the effect of parathyroid hormone upon osteoclasts. Plicamycin's inhibition of DNA-dependent RNA synthesis appears to render osteoclasts unable to fully respond to parathyroid hormone with the biosynthesis necessary for osteolysis. Decreases in serum phosphate levels and urinary calcium excretion accompany the lowering of serum calcium concentrations.
Radioautography studies[1] with ^{3}H-labeled plicamycin in C3H mice show that the greatest concentrations of the isotope are in the Kupffer cells of the liver and cells of the renal tubules. Plicamycin is rapidly cleared from the blood within the first 2 hours and excretion is also rapid. Sixty-seven percent of measured excretion occurs within 4 hours, 75% within 8 hours, and 90% is recovered in the first 24 hours after injection. There is no evidence of protein binding, nor is there any evidence of metabolism of the carbohydrate moiety of the drug to carbon dioxide and water with loss through respiration. Plicamycin crosses the blood-brain barrier; the concentration found in brain tissue is low but it persists longer than in other tissues. The experimental results in animals correlate closely with results achieved in man.[2]

INDICATIONS

Mithracin is a potent antineoplastic agent which has been shown to be useful in the treatment of carefully selected hospitalized patients with malignant tumors of the testis in whom successful treatment by surgery and/or radiation is impossible. Also, on the basis of limited clinical experience to date, it may be considered in the treatment of certain symptomatic patients with hypercalcemia and hypercalciuria associated with a variety of advanced neoplasms.
The use of Mithracin in other types of neoplastic disease is not recommended at the present time.

CONTRAINDICATIONS

Mithracin (plicamycin) is contraindicated in patients with thrombocytopenia, thrombocytopathy, coagulation disorder or an increased susceptibility to bleeding due to other causes. Mithracin should not be administered to any patient with impairment of bone marrow function.
Mithracin may cause fetal harm when administered to a pregnant woman. Mithracin is contraindicated in women who are or may become pregnant. If this drug is used during pregnancy, or if the patient becomes pregnant while taking this drug, the patient should be apprised of the potential hazard to the fetus.

PRECAUTIONS

General: Mithracin should be administered only to patients who are hospitalized and who can be observed carefully and frequently during and after therapy.
Severe thrombocytopenia, a hemorrhagic tendency and even death may result from the use of Mithracin. Although severe toxicity is more apt to occur in patients who have far-advanced disease or are otherwise considered poor risks for therapy, serious toxicity may also occasionally occur even in patients who are in relatively good condition.
Electrolyte imbalance, especially hypocalcemia, hypokalemia, and hypophosphatemia, should be corrected with appropriate electrolyte therapy prior to treatment with Mithracin.
Mithracin should be used with extreme caution in patients with significant impairment of renal or hepatic function.
Mithracin should not normally be administered to patients who are pregnant or to mothers who are breast feeding.
In the treatment of each patient, the physician must weigh carefully the possibility of achieving therapeutic benefit versus the risk of toxicity which may occur with Mithracin therapy.
Laboratory Tests: The following laboratory studies should be obtained frequently during therapy and for several days following the last dose: platelet count, prothrombin time, bleeding time. The occurrence of thrombocytopenia or a significant prolongation of prothrombin time or bleeding time is an indication for the termination of therapy.
Carcinogenesis, mutagenesis, impairment of fertility: No long-term studies in animals have been performed to evaluate the carcinogenic potential of Mithracin. Histologic evidence of inhibition of spermatogenesis was observed in a substantial number of male rats receiving doses of 0.6 mg/kg/day and above.
Pregnancy Category X: See "Contraindications" section.
Nursing Mothers: It is not known whether this drug is excreted in human milk. Because many drugs are excreted in human milk and because of the potential for serious adverse reactions in nursing infants from Mithracin, a decision should be made whether to discontinue nursing or to discontinue the drug, taking into account the importance of the drug to the mother.

ADVERSE REACTIONS

THE MOST IMPORTANT FORM OF TOXICITY ASSOCIATED WITH THE USE OF MITHRACIN CONSISTS OF A BLEEDING SYNDROME WHICH USUALLY BEGINS WITH AN EPISODE OF EPISTAXIS. This bleeding tendency may only consist of a single or several episodes of epistaxis and progress no further. However, in some cases, this hemorrhagic syndrome can start with an episode of hematemesis which may progress to more widespread hemorrhage in the gastrointestinal tract or to a more generalized bleeding tendency. This hemorrhagic diathesis is most likely due to abnormalities in multiple clotting factors.
A detailed analysis of the clinical data in 1,160 patients treated with Mithracin indicates that the hemorrhagic syndrome is dose related. With doses of 30 mcg/kg/day or less for 10 or fewer doses, the incidence of bleeding episodes has been 5.4% with an associated drug-related mortality rate of 1.6%. With doses greater than 30 mcg/kg/day and/or for more than 10 doses, a significantly larger number of bleeding episodes occurred (11.9%) and the associated drug-related mortality rate was also significantly higher (5.7%).
The most common side effects reported with the use of Mithracin consist of gastrointestinal symptoms: anorexia, nausea, vomiting, diarrhea, and stomatitis. Other less frequently reported side effects include fever, drowsiness, weakness, lethargy, malaise, headache, depression, phlebitis, facial flushing, and skin rash.
The following laboratory abnormalities have been reported during therapy with Mithracin and in most instances were reversible following cessation of treatment:
Hematologic Abnormalities: Depression of platelet count, white count, hemoglobin and prothrombin content; elevation of clotting time and bleeding time; abnormal clot retraction.
Thrombocytopenia may be rapid in onset and may occur at any time during therapy or within several days following the last dose. With the occurrence of severe thrombocytopenia, the infusion of platelet concentrates of platelet-rich plasma may be helpful in elevating the platelet count.
The occurrence of leukopenia with the use of Mithracin is relatively uncommon, occurring only in approximately 6% of patients.
It has been uncommon for abnormalities in clotting time or clot retraction to be demonstrated prior to the onset of an overt bleeding episode noted in some patients treated with Mithracin. Nevertheless, the performance of these tests periodically is recommended because in a few instances, an abnormality in one of these studies may have served as a warning to terminate therapy because of impending serious toxicity.
Abnormal Liver Function Tests: Increased levels of serum glutamic oxalacetic transaminase, serum glutamic pyruvic transaminase, lactic dehydrogenase, alkaline phosphatase, serum bilirubin, ornithine carbamyl transferase, isocitric dehydrogenase, and increased retention of bromsulphalein.
Abnormal Renal Function Tests: Increased blood urea nitrogen and serum creatinine; proteinuria.
Abnormalities in Electrolyte Concentrations: Depression of serum calcium, phosphorus, and potassium.

OVERDOSAGE

Generally, adverse effects following the use of Mithracin, especially the hemorrhagic syndrome, are dose related. Therefore, following administration of an overdose, patients can be expected to experience an exaggeration of the usual adverse effects. Close monitoring of the hematologic picture, including factors involved in the clotting mechanism, hepatic and renal functions, and serum electrolytes, is necessary. No specific antidote for Mithracin is known. Management of overdosage would include general supportive measures to sustain the patient through the period of toxicity.

DOSAGE AND ADMINISTRATION

The daily dose of Mithracin is based on the patient's body weight. If a patient has abnormal fluid retention such as edema, hydrothorax or ascites, the patient's ideal weight rather than actual body weight should be used to calculate the dose.
Treatment of Testicular Tumors: In the treatment of patients with testicular tumors the recommended daily dose of Mithracin (plicamycin) is 25 to 30 mcg (0.025–0.030 mg) per kilogram of body weight. Therapy should be continued for a period of 8 to 10 days unless significant side effects or tox-

Continued on next page

Mithracin—Cont.

icity occur during therapy. A course of therapy consisting of more than 10 daily doses is not recommended. Individual daily doses should not exceed 30 mcg (0.030 mg) per kilogram of body weight.

In those patients with responsive tumors, some degree of tumor regression is usually evident within 3 or 4 weeks following the initial course of therapy. If tumor masses remain unchanged following an initial course of therapy, additional courses of therapy at monthly intervals are warranted.

When a significant tumor regression is obtained, it is suggested that additional courses of therapy be given at monthly intervals until a complete regression of tumor masses is achieved or until definite tumor progression or new tumor masses occur in spite of continued courses of therapy.

Treatment of Hypercalcemia and Hypercalciuria: Reversal of hypercalcemia and hypercalciuria can usually be achieved with Mithracin at doses considerably lower than those recommended for use in the treatment of testicular tumors.

In hypercalcemia and hypercalciuria associated with advanced malignancy the recommended course of treatment with Mithracin is 25 mcg (0.025 mg) per kilogram of body weight per day for 3 or 4 days.

If the desired degree of reversal of hypercalcemia or hypercalciuria is not achieved with the initial course of therapy, additional courses of therapy may then be administered at intervals of one week or more to achieve the desired result or to maintain serum calcium and urinary calcium excretion at normal levels. It may be possible to maintain normal calcium balance with single, weekly doses or with a schedule of 2 or 3 doses per week.

NOTE: BECAUSE OF THE DRUG'S TOXICITY AND THE LIMITED CLINICAL EXPERIENCE TO DATE IN THESE INDICATIONS, THE FOLLOWING RECOMMENDATIONS SHOULD BE KEPT IN MIND BY THE PHYSICIAN.

1. CONSIDER CASES OF HYPERCALCEMIA AND HYPERCALCIURIA NOT RESPONSIVE TO CONVENTIONAL TREATMENT.
2. APPLY SAME CONTRAINDICATIONS AND PRECAUTIONARY MEASURES AS IN ANTITUMOR TREATMENT.
3. RENAL FUNCTION SHOULD BE CAREFULLY MONITORED BEFORE, DURING, AND AFTER TREATMENT.
4. BENEFITS OF USE DURING PREGNANCY OR IN WOMEN OF CHILDBEARING AGE SHOULD BE WEIGHED AGAINST POTENTIAL TOXICITY TO EMBRYO OR FETUS.

ADMINISTRATION

By IV administration only. The appropriate daily dose of Mithracin should be diluted in one liter of 5% Dextrose Injection, USP or Sodium Chloride Injection, USP and administered by slow intravenous infusion over a period of 4 to 6 hours. Rapid direct intravenous injection of Mithracin should be avoided as it may be associated with a higher incidence and greater severity of gastrointestinal side effects. Extravasation of solutions of Mithracin may cause local irritation and cellulitis at injection sites. Should thrombophlebitis or perivascular cellulitis occur, the infusion should be terminated and reinstituted at another site. The application of moderate heat to the site of extravasation may help to disperse the compound and minimize discomfort and local tissue irritation. The use of antiemetic compounds prior to and during treatment with Mithracin may be helpful in relieving nausea and vomiting.

Procedures for proper handling and disposal of anti-cancer drugs should be considered. Several guidelines on this subject have been published.[3-8] There is no general agreement that all of the procedures recommended in the guidelines are necessary or appropriate.

HOW SUPPLIED

Mithracin is available in vials as a freeze-dried preparation for intravenous administration. Each vial contains 2500 mcg (2.5 mg) of Mithracin with 100 mg of mannitol and sufficient disodium phosphate to adjust to pH 7. These vials should be stored at refrigerator temperatures between 2°C to 8°C (36°F to 46°F).

To reconstitute, add aseptically 4.9 mL of Sterile Water for Injection to the contents of the vial and shake to dissolve. Each mL of the resulting solution will then contain 500 mcg (0.5 mg) of Mithracin. NOTE: 1 mg (milligram)=1000 mcg (micrograms). AFTER REMOVAL OF THE APPROPRIATE DOSE, THE REMAINING UNUSED SOLUTION MUST BE DISCARDED, FRESH SOLUTIONS MUST BE PREPARED IN THE ABOVE MANNER EACH DAY OF THERAPY.

ANIMAL PHARMACOLOGY AND TOXICOLOGY

In mice the average intravenous LD_{50} of Mithracin is 2,000 mcg/kg of body weight. When administered orally, it is not toxic to mice even at doses 100 times greater than the intravenous LD_{50}. In rats the average intravenous LD_{50} of Mithracin is 1,700 mcg/kg of body weight. It is not toxic to rats when administered orally at doses 17 times greater than the intravenous LD_{50}. In dogs and monkeys Mithracin is essentially non-toxic when administered intravenously for 24 days at daily doses as high as 50 and 24 mcg/kg of body weight, respectively. However, at higher doses of 100 mcg/kg/day intravenously it is lethal to dogs and monkeys. Signs of toxicity in dogs and monkeys included anorexia, vomiting, listlessness, melena, anemia, lymphopenia, elevated alkaline phosphatase, serum glutamic oxalacetic transaminase, serum glutamic pyruvic transaminase values, hypochloremia, and azotemia. Dogs also showed marked thrombocytopenia, hyponatremia, hypokalemia, hypocalcemia, and decreased prothrombin consumption. Necropsy findings consisted of necrosis of lymphoid tissue and multiple generalized hemorrhages. Mithracin (plicamycin) was only mildly irritating when injected intramuscularly in rabbits and subcutaneously in guinea pigs. Histologic evidence of inhibition of spermatogenesis was observed in a substantial number of male rats receiving doses of 0.6 mg/kg/day and above. This preclinical finding of selective drug effect constituted the scientific rationale for clinical trials in testicular tumors.

CLINICAL REPORTS

Treatment of Patients with Inoperable Testicular Tumors: In a combined series of 305 patients with inoperable testicular tumors treated with Mithracin, 33 patients (10.8%) showed a complete disappearance of tumor masses and an additional 80 patients (26.2%) responded with significant partial regression of tumor masses. The longest duration of a continuing complete response is now over $8 \frac{1}{2}$ years. The therapeutic responses in this series of patients have been summarized by type of testicular tumor in the accompanying table.

[See table below]

Mithracin may be useful in the treatment of patients with testicular tumors which are resistant to other chemotherapeutic agents. Prior radiation therapy or prior chemotherapy did not alter the response rate with Mithracin. This suggests that there is no significant cross resistance between Mithracin and other chemotherapeutic agents.

Treatment of Patients with Hypercalcemia and Hypercalciuria: A limited number of patients with hypercalcemia (range: 12.0–25.8 mg%) and patients with hypercalciuria (range 215–492 mg/day) associated with malignant disease were treated with Mithracin. Hypercalcemia and hypercalciuria were promptly reversed in all patients. In some patients, the primary malignancy was of non-testicular origin.

REFERENCES

1. Kennedy, B.D., et al: Cancer Res. 27 :1534, 1967.
2. Ransohoff, J., et al: Cancer Chemother. Rep. 49 :51, 1965.

3. Recommendations for the Safe Handling of Parenteral Antineoplastic Drugs. NIH Publication No. 83-2621. For sale by the Superintendent of Documents, U.S. Government Printing Office, Washington, D.C. 20402.
4. AMA Council Report. Guidelines for Handling Parenteral Antineoplastics. JAMA, March 15, 1985.
5. National Study Commission on Cytotoxic Exposure—Recommendations for Handling Cytotoxic Agents. Available from Louis P. Jeffrey, Sc.D., Director of Pharmacy Services, Rhode Island Hospital, 593 Eddy Street, Providence, Rhode Island 02902.
6. Clinical Oncological Society of Australia: Guidelines and recommendations for safe handling of antineoplastic agents. Med J Australia 1 :426–428, 1983.
7. Jones, R.B., et al: Safe handling of chemotherapeutic agents: A report from the Mount Sinai Medical Center. Ca—A Cancer Journal for Clinicians, Sept./Oct. 258–263, 1983.
8. American Society of Hospital Pharmacists technical assistance bulletin on handling cytotoxic drugs in hospitals. Am J Hosp Pharm 42 :131–137, 1985.

Manufactured for
Bayer Corporation
Pharmaceutical Division
400 Morgan Lane
West Haven, CT 06516
by Ben Venue Laboratories
Bedford, Ohio 44146
PD100654—60-4178-81-4   Revised Feb. 1995

MYCELEX®-G 500 mg   ℞
brand of clotrimazole
Vaginal Tablets

PRODUCT OVERVIEW

KEY FACTS

Mycelex®-G 500 mg is an effective antifungal containing 500 mg of clotrimazole (the active ingredient). Clotrimazole is a broad spectrum antifungal which exhibits fungicidal activity *in vitro* against *Candida albicans* and other species of the genus *Candida*. No single-step or multiple-step resistance to clotrimazole has developed during successive passages of *Candida albicans*.

MAJOR USES

Mycelex®-G 500 mg has proved to be clinically effective for local treatment of vulvovaginal candidiasis when one day therapy is felt warranted. In the case of severe vulvovaginal candidiasis longer antimycotic therapy such as Mycelex®-G 100 mg tablets or Mycelex®-G Cream is recommended.

SAFETY INFORMATION

Mycelex®-G 500 Vaginal Tablets are contraindicated in women who have shown hypersensitivity to any components of the compound. If there is a lack of response to treatment with Mycelex®-G 500 mg, appropriate microbiological studies should be performed to confirm the diagnosis and rule out other pathogens before instituting another course of antimycotic therapy. There are, however, no adequate and well-controlled studies in pregnant women during the first trimester of pregnancy.

PRESCRIBING INFORMATION

MYCELEX®-G 500 mg   ℞
brand of clotrimazole
Vaginal Tablets

DESCRIPTION

Each Mycelex®-G 500 mg Vaginal Tablet contains 500 mg clotrimazole (the active ingredient) dispersed in lactose, microcrystalline cellulose, lactic acid, corn starch, crospovidone, calcium lactate, magnesium stearate, silicon dioxide and hydroxypropyl methylcellulose. Chemically, clotrimazole is [1-(o-Chloro-α, α-diphenylbenzyl) imidazole], a synthetic antifungal agent having the chemical formula $C_{22}H_{17}ClN_2$; a molecular weight of 344.84; and the following chemical structure:

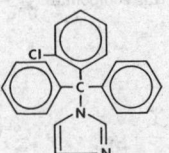

Clotrimazole is an odorless, white crystalline substance, practically insoluble in water, sparingly soluble in ether, soluble in carbon tetrachloride, and very soluble in ethanol and chloroform.

CLINICAL PHARMACOLOGY

Serum levels and levels in vaginal secretions of clotrimazole were measured in six healthy volunteers who had one 500

MITHRACIN
RESULTS IN 305 TESTICULAR TUMOR CASES BY TUMOR TYPE

TYPE OF TESTICULAR TUMOR	TOTAL	COMPLETE RESPONSE	PARTIAL RESPONSE	NO RESPONSE
EMBRYONAL CELL	173	26	42	105
TERATOMA	5	0	1	4
TERATOCARCINOMA	23	0	5	18
SEMINOMA	18	0	7	11
CHORIOCARCINOMA	13	1	6	6
MIXED TUMOR	73	6	19	48
TOTALS	305	33	80	192

mg vaginal tablet inserted. Although serum levels of clotrimazole were higher than those in other volunteers given 100 mg and 200 mg vaginal tablets these levels did not exceed 10 nanograms/mL. It has been estimated that three to ten percent of a vaginal dose of clotrimazole may be absorbed, but the drug rapidly and efficiently degrades to microbiologically inactive metabolites. The clotrimazole concentrations remaining in vaginal secretions were still in the mg/mL range for 48 hours and in two of the six subjects at 72 hours.

The findings of high clotrimazole concentrations in vaginal secretions for up to 72 hours and low concentrations in the serum suggest that nearly all the clotrimazole given in the 500 mg vaginal tablet remains in the vagina for 48 hours, and in some cases 72 hours, in fungicidal concentrations.

Clotrimazole is a broad-spectrum antifungal agent. It has been postulated that the compound affects the permeability characteristics of the membrane allowing the leakage of essential intracellular components with a consequent inhibition of the synthesis of such macromolecules as protein, lipid, DNA, and polysaccharides.

At concentrations as low as 2–5 µg/mL, clotrimazole exhibits fungicidal activity *in vitro* against *Candida albicans* and other species of the genus *Candida*.

No single-step or multiple-step resistance to clotrimazole has developed during successive passages of *Candida albicans*.

INDICATIONS

Mycelex-G 500 mg Vaginal Tablets are indicated for the local treatment of vulvovaginal candidiasis when one day therapy is felt warranted. In the case of severe vulvovaginitis due to candidiasis, longer antimycotic therapy is recommended. The diagnosis should be confirmed by KOH smears and/or cultures. Other pathogens commonly associated with vulvovaginitis, *Trichomonas* and *Gardnerella (Haemophilus) vaginalis,* should be ruled out by appropriate laboratory methods.

CONTRAINDICATIONS

Mycelex-G 500 mg Vaginal Tablets are contraindicated in women who have shown hypersensitivity to any components of the preparation.

WARNINGS

None.

PRECAUTIONS

If there is a lack of response to Mycelex-G 500 mg Vaginal Tablets, appropriate microbiological studies should be repeated to confirm the diagnosis and rule out other pathogens before instituting another course of antimycotic therapy.

CARCINOGENESIS

No long term studies in animals have been performed to evaluate the carcinogenic potential of Mycelex-G 500 mg Vaginal Tablets intravaginally. A long term study in rats (Wistar strains) where clotrimazole was administered orally provided no indication of carcinogenicity.

USAGE IN PREGNANCY

Pregnancy Category B: The disposition of ^{14}C-clotrimazole has been studied in humans and animals. Clotrimazole is poorly absorbed following intravaginal administration to humans, whereas it is rather well absorbed after oral administration.

In clinical trials, use of vaginally applied clotrimazole in pregnant women in their second and third trimesters has not been associated with ill effects. There are, however, no adequate and well-controlled studies in pregnant women during the first trimester of pregnancy.

Studies in pregnant rats given repeated intravaginal doses up to 100 mg/kg/day have revealed no evidence of harm to the fetus due to clotrimazole.

Repeated high oral doses of clotrimazole in rats and mice ranging from 50 to 120 mg/kg resulted in embryotoxicity (possibly secondary to maternal toxicity), impairment of mating, decreased litter size and number of viable young and decreased pup survival to weaning. However, clotrimazole was not teratogenic in mice, rabbits and rats at oral doses up to 200, 180 and 100 mg/kg, respectively. Oral absorption in the rat amounts to approximately 90% of the administered dose.

Because animal reproduction studies are not always predictive of human response, this drug should be used only if clearly indicated during the first trimester of pregnancy.

ADVERSE REACTIONS

Of 297 patients in double-blind studies with the 500 mg vaginal tablet, 3 of 149 patients treated with active drug and 3 of 148 patients treated with placebo reported complaints during therapy that were possibly drug related. In the active drug group, vomiting occurred in one patient, vaginal soreness with coitus in another, and complaints of vaginal irritation, itching, burning and dyspareunia in the third patient. In the placebo group, clitoral irritation occurred in one patient and dysuria, described as remotely related to drug, in the other. A third patient in the placebo group developed bacterial vaginitis which the investigator classed as possibly related to drug.

Eighteen (1.6%) of the 1116 patients treated with Mycelex-G in other formulations in double-blind studies reported complaints during therapy that were possibly drug-related. Mild burning occurred in six patients while other complaints such as skin rash, itching, vulval irritation, lower abdominal cramps and bloating, slight cramping, slight urinary frequency, and burning or irritation in the sexual partner, occurred rarely.

OVERDOSAGE

No data available.

DRUG ABUSE AND DEPENDENCE

Drug abuse and dependence with Mycelex-G 500 mg Vaginal Tablets has not been reported.

DOSAGE AND ADMINISTRATION

The recommended dose is one tablet inserted intravaginally one time only, preferably at bedtime. In the event of treatment failure, that is, persistence of signs and symptoms of vaginitis after five days, other pathogens commonly responsible for vaginitis should be ruled out before instituting another course of antimycotic therapy.

HOW SUPPLIED

Mycelex-G 500 mg Vaginal Tablets are white, bullet shaped, uncoated tablets, coded with Bayer on one side and 097 on the other, supplied as a single 500 mg tablet with plastic applicator and patient instructions, or in twin pack with Mycelex 1% cream 7g tube.

Store Below 86°F (30°C).

U.S. Patent Numbers 3,660,577; 3,705,172; 3,839,573; 4,457,938.

Manufactured by
Bayer Corporation
Pharmaceutical Division
400 Morgan Lane
West Haven, CT 06516
PD500010 5/95 BAY 5097

 5213

Shown in Product Identification Guide, page 305

NIMOTOP® ℞
(nimodipine)
CAPSULES
For Oral Use

DESCRIPTION

Nimotop® (nimodipine) belongs to the class of pharmacological agents known as calcium channel blockers. Nimodipine is isopropyl (2 - methoxyethyl) 1, 4 - dihydro - 2, 6 - dimethyl - 4 - (3 - nitrophenyl) - 3, 5 - pyridine - dicarboxylate. It has a molecular weight of 418.5 and a molecular formula of $C_{21}H_{26}N_2O_7$. The structural formula is:

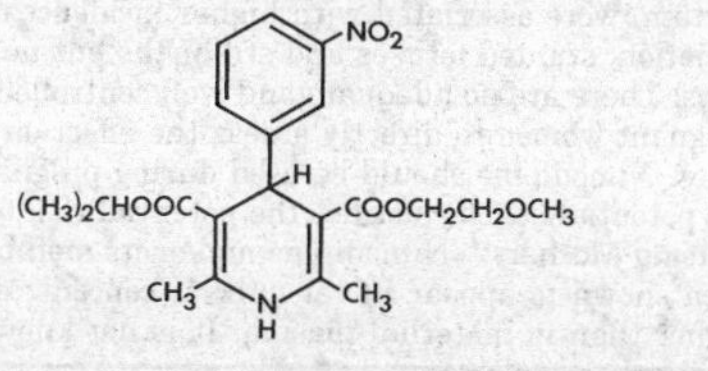

Nimodipine is a yellow crystalline substance, practically insoluble in water.

NIMOTOP® capsules are formulated as soft gelatin capsules for oral administration. Each liquid filled capsule contains 30 mg of nimodipine in a vehicle of glycerin, peppermint oil, purified water and polyethylene glycol 400. The soft gelatin capsule shell contains gelatin, glycerin, purified water and titanium dioxide.

CLINICAL PHARMACOLOGY

Mechanism of Action: Nimodipine is a calcium channel blocker. The contractile processes of smooth muscle cells are dependent upon calcium ions, which enter these cells during depolarization as slow ionic transmembrane currents. Nimodipine inhibits calcium ion transfer into these cells and thus inhibits contractions of vascular smooth muscle. In animal experiments, nimodipine had a greater effect on cerebral arteries than on arteries elsewhere in the body perhaps because it is highly lipophilic, allowing it to cross the blood-brain barrier; concentrations of nimodipine as high as 12.5 ng/mL have been detected in the cerebrospinal fluid of nimodipine treated subarachnoid hemorrhage (SAH) patients. Based on animal experiments, it was hoped that nimodipine would prevent cerebral arterial spasm in SAH patients. While the clinical studies described below demonstrate a favorable effect by nimodipine on the severity of neurological deficits caused by cerebral vasospasm following SAH, there is no arteriographic evidence that the drug either prevents or relieves the spasm of these arteries. The actual mechanism of action in humans is, therefore, unknown.

Pharmacokinetics and Metabolism: In man, nimodipine is rapidly absorbed after oral administration, and peak concentrations are generally attained within one hour. The terminal elimination half-life is approximately 8 to 9 hours but earlier elimination rates are much more rapid, equivalent to a half-life of 1–2 hours; a consequence is the need for frequent (every 4 hours) dosing. There were no signs of accumulation when nimodipine was given three times a day for seven days. Nimodipine is over 95% bound to plasma proteins. The binding was concentration independent over the range of 10 ng/mL to 10 µg/mL. Nimodipine is eliminated almost exclusively in the form of metabolites and less than 1% is recovered in the urine as unchanged drug. Numerous metabolites, all of which are either inactive or considerably less active than the parent compound, have been identified. Because of a high first-pass metabolism, the bioavailability of nimodipine averages 13% after oral administration. The bioavailability is significantly increased in patients with hepatic cirrhosis, with C_{max} approximately double that in normals which necessitates lowering the dose in this group of patients (see Dosage and Administration). In a study of 24 healthy male volunteers, administration of nimodipine capsules following a standard breakfast resulted in a 68% lower peak plasma concentration and 38% lower bioavailability relative to dosing under fasted conditions.

Clinical Trials: Nimodipine has been shown, in 4 randomized, placebo-controlled trials, to reduce the severity of neurological deficits resulting from vasospasm in patients who have had a recent subarachnoid hemorrhage (SAH). The trials used doses ranging from 20–30 mg to 90 mg every 4 hours, with drug given for 21 days in 3 studies, and for at least 18 days in the other. Three of the four trials followed patients for 3–6 months. Three of the trials studied relatively well patients, with all or most patients in Hunt and Hess Grades I–II (essentially free of focal deficits after the initial bleed); the fourth studied much sicker patients, Hunt and Hess Grades III–V. Two studies, one domestic, one French, were similar in design, with relatively unimpaired SAH patients randomized to nimodipine or placebo. In each, a judgment was made as to whether any late-developing deficit was due to spasm or other causes, and the deficits were graded. Both studies showed significantly fewer severe deficits due to spasm in the nimodipine group; the second (French) study showed fewer spasm-related deficits of all severities. No effect was seen on deficits not related to spasm.

[See table below]

A Canadian study entered much sicker patients, who had a high rate of death and disability, and used a dose of 90 mg every 4 hours, but was otherwise similar to the first two studies. Analysis of delayed ischemic deficits, many of which result from spasm, showed a significant reduction in spasm-related deficits. Among analyzed patients (72 nimodipine, 82 placebo), there were the following outcomes.

[See table at top of next page]

A fourth, large, study was performed in the United Kingdom in SAH patients with all grades of severity (but about 90% were in Grades I–III). Outcomes were not defined as spasm related or not but there was a significant reduction in the overall rate of infarction and severely disabling neurological outcome at 3 months:

	Nimodipine	Placebo
Total patients	278	276
Good recovery	199*	169

Continued on next page

			Patients		
Study	Dose	Grade*	Number Analyzed	Any Deficit Due to Spasm	Numbers With Severe Deficit
1.	20–30 mg	I–III	Nimodipine 56	13	1
			Placebo 60	16	8**
2.	60 mg	I–III	Nimodipine 31	4	2
			Placebo 39	11	10**

* Hunt and Hess Grade
** p = 0.03

Nimotop—Cont.

Moderate disability	24	16
Severe disability	12**	31
Death	43***	60

* p = 0.0444—good and moderate vs severe and dead
** p = 0.001—severe disability
*** p = 0.056—death

A dose-ranging study comparing 30, 60 and 90 mg doses found a generally low rate of spasm-related neurological deficits but no significant relation of response to dose.

The effect of nimodipine on mortality is not yet clear. The large United Kingdom study showed near-significantly improved survival. The two smaller studies (domestic, French) had too few deaths to contribute to this question. The Canadian study, despite showing markedly decreased spasm-related deficits, showed overall (all patients randomized) greater 90 day mortality, 49/91 (54%) on nimodipine vs 38/97 (39%) on placebo, a significant difference. Most of the deaths appeared, in this very severely ill group (Hunt and Hess Grades III–V), to be consequences of SAH, but a drug effect cannot be ruled out. In this study 90 mg every 4 hours was the dose used, perhaps too high for the very ill population studied. The 90 mg dose is not recommended nor is treatment of Hunt and Hess Grades IV–V patients.

INDICATIONS AND USAGE

Nimotop® (nimodipine) is indicated for the improvement of neurological outcome by reducing the incidence and severity of ischemic deficits in patients with subarachnoid hemorrhage from ruptured congenital aneurysms who are in good neurological condition post-ictus (e.g., Hunt and Hess Grades I–III).

CONTRAINDICATIONS

None known.

PRECAUTIONS

General: Blood Pressure: Nimodipine has the hemodynamic effects expected of a calcium channel blocker, although they are generally not marked. However, intravenous administration of the contents of Nimotop Capsules has resulted in serious adverse consequences including hypotension, cardiovascular collapse, and cardiac arrest. In patients with subarachnoid hemorrhage given Nimotop® in clinical studies, about 5% were reported to have had lowering of the blood pressure and about 1% left the study because of this (not all could be attributed to nimodipine). Nevertheless, blood pressure should be carefully monitored during treatment with Nimotop® based on its known pharmacology and the known effects of calcium channel blockers. Hepatic Disease: The metabolism of Nimotop® is decreased in patients with impaired hepatic function. Such patients should have their blood pressure and pulse rate monitored closely and should be given a lower dose (see Dosage and Administration).

Intestinal pseudo-obstruction and ileus have been reported rarely in patients treated with nimodipine. A causal relationship has not been established. The condition has responded to conservative management.

Laboratory Test Interactions: None known.

Drug Interaction: It is possible that the cardiovascular action of other calcium channel blockers could be enhanced by the addition of Nimotop®.

In Europe, Nimotop® was observed to occasionally intensify the effect of antihypertensive compounds taken concomi-

	Delayed Ischemic Deficits (DID)		Permanent Deficits	
	Nimodipine n (%)	Placebo n (%)	Nimodipine n (%)	Placebo n (%)
DID Spasm Alone	8 (11)*	25 (31)	5 (7)*	22 (27)
DID Spasm Contributing	18 (25)	21 (26)	16 (22)	17 (21)
DID Without Spasm	7 (10)	8 (10)	6 (8)	7 (9)
No DID	39 (54)	28 (34)	45 (63)	36 (44)

* P = 0.001, nimodipine vs placebo

tantly by patients suffering from hypertension; this phenomenon was not observed in North American clinical trials.

A study in eight healthy volunteers has shown a 50% increase in mean peak nimodipine plasma concentrations and a 90% increase in mean area under the curve, after a one-week course of cimetidine at 1,000 mg/day and nimodipine at 90 mg/day. This effect may be mediated by the known inhibition of hepatic cytochrome P-450 by cimetidine, which could decrease first-pass metabolism of nimodipine.

Carcinogenesis, Mutagenesis, Impairment of Fertility: In a two-year study, higher incidences of adenocarcinoma of the uterus and Leydig-cell adenoma of the testes were observed in rats given a diet containing 1800 ppm nimodipine (equivalent to 91 to 121 mg/kg/day nimodipine) than in placebo controls. The differences were not statistically significant, however, and the higher rates were well within historical control range for these tumors in the Wistar strain. Nimodipine was found not to be carcinogenic in a 91-week mouse study but the high dose of 1800 ppm nimodipine-in-feed (546 to 774 mg/kg/day) shortened the life expectancy of the animals. Mutagenicity studies, including the Ames, micronucleus and dominant lethal tests were negative.

Nimodipine did not impair the fertility and general reproductive performance of male and female Wistar rats following oral doses of up to 30 mg/kg/day when administered daily for more than 10 weeks in the males and 3 weeks in the females prior to mating and continued to day 7 of pregnancy. This dose in a rat is about 4 times the equivalent clinical dose of 60 mg q4h in a 50 kg patient.

Pregnancy: Pregnancy Category C. Nimodipine has been shown to have a teratogenic effect in Himalayan rabbits. Incidences of malformations and stunted fetuses were increased at oral doses of 1 and 10 mg/kg/day administered (by gavage) from day 6 through day 18 of pregnancy but not at 3.0 mg/kg/day in one of two identical rabbit studies. In the second study an increased incidence of stunted fetuses was seen at 1.0 mg/kg/day but not at higher doses. Nimodipine was embryotoxic, causing resorption and stunted growth of fetuses, in Long Evans rats at 100 mg/kg/day administered by gavage from day 6 through day 15 of pregnancy. In two other rat studies, doses of 30 mg/kg/day nimodipine administered by gavage from day 16 of gestation and continued until sacrifice (day 20 of pregnancy or day 21 post partum) were associated with higher incidences of skeletal variation, stunted fetuses and stillbirths but no malformations. There are no adequate and well controlled studies in pregnant women to directly assess the effect on human fetuses. Nimodipine should be used during pregnancy only if the potential benefit justifies the potential risk to the fetus.

Nursing Mothers: Nimodipine and/or its metabolites have been shown to appear in rat milk at concentrations much higher than in maternal plasma. It is not known whether

the drug is excreted in human milk. Because many drugs are excreted in human milk, nursing mothers are advised not to breast feed their babies when taking the drug.

Pediatric Use: Safety and effectiveness in children have not been established.

ADVERSE REACTIONS

Adverse experiences were reported by 92 of 823 patients with subarachnoid hemorrhage (11.2%) who were given nimodipine. The most frequently reported adverse experience was decreased blood pressure in 4.4% of these patients. Twenty-nine of 479 (6.1%) placebo treated patients also reported adverse experiences. The events reported with a frequency greater than 1% are displayed below by dose. [See table below]

There were no other adverse experiences reported by the patients who were given 0.35 mg/kg, 30 mg q4h or 120 mg q4h. Adverse experiences with an incidence rate of less than 1% in the 60 mg q4h dose group were: hepatitis; itching; gastrointestinal hemorrhage; thrombocytopenia; anemia; palpitations; vomiting; flushing; diaphoresis; wheezing; phenytoin toxicity; lightheadedness; dizziness; rebound vasospasm; jaundice; hypertension; hematoma.

Adverse experiences with an incidence rate less than 1% in the 90 mg q4h dose group were: itching, gastrointestinal hemorrhage; thrombocytopenia; neurological deterioration; vomiting; diaphoresis; congestive heart failure; hyponatremia; decreasing platelet count; disseminated intravascular coagulation; deep vein thrombosis.

As can be seen from the table, side effects that appear related to nimodipine use based on increased incidence with higher dose or a higher rate compared to placebo control, included decreased blood pressure, edema and headaches which are known pharmacologic actions of calcium channel blockers. It must be noted, however, that SAH is frequently accompanied by alterations in consciousness which lead to an under reporting of adverse experiences. Patients who received nimodipine in clinical trials for other indications reported flushing (2.1%), headache (4.1%) and fluid retention (0.3%), typical responses to calcium channel blockers. As a calcium channel blocker, nimodipine may have the potential to exacerbate heart failure in susceptible patients or to interfere with A-V conduction, but these events were not observed.

No clinically significant effects on hematologic factors, renal or hepatic function or carbohydrate metabolism have been causally associated with oral nimodipine. Isolated cases of non-fasting elevated serum glucose levels (0.8%), elevated LDH levels (0.4%), decreased platelet counts (0.3%), elevated alkaline phosphatase levels (0.2%) and elevated SGPT levels (0.2%) have been reported rarely.

DRUG ABUSE AND DEPENDENCE

There have been no reported instances of drug abuse or dependence with Nimotop®.

OVERDOSAGE

There have been no reports of overdosage from the oral administration of Nimotop®. Symptoms of overdosage would be expected to be related to cardiovascular effects such as excessive peripheral vasodilation with marked systemic hypotension. Clinically significant hypotension due to Nimotop® overdosage may require active cardiovascular support. Norepinephrine or dopamine may be helpful in restoring blood pressure. Since Nimotop® is highly protein-bound, dialysis is not likely to be of benefit.

DOSAGE AND ADMINISTRATION

Nimotop is given orally in the form of ivory colored, soft gelatin 30 mg capsules for subarachnoid hemorrhage.

The oral dose is 60 mg (two 30 mg capsules) every 4 hours for 21 consecutive days, preferably not less than one hour before or two hours after meals. Oral Nimotop® therapy should commence within 96 hours of the subarachnoid hemorrhage.

If the capsule cannot be swallowed, e.g., at the time of surgery, or if the patient is unconscious, a hole should be made in both ends of the capsule with an 18 gauge needle, and the contents of the capsule extracted into a syringe. The contents should then be emptied into the patient's in situ nasogastric tube and washed down the tube with 30 mL of normal saline (0.9%).

	DOSE q4h					
	Number of Patients (%)					
	Nimodipine					Placebo
Sign/Symptom	0.35 mg/kg (n = 82)	30 mg (n = 71)	60 mg (n = 494)	90 mg (n = 172)	120 mg (n = 4)	(n = 479)
Decreased Blood Pressure	1 (1.2)	0	19 (3.8)	14 (8.1)	2 (50.0)	6 (1.2)
Abnormal Liver Function Test	1 (1.2)	0	2 (0.4)	1 (0.6)	0	7 (1.5)
Edema	0	0	2 (0.4)	2 (1.2)	0	3 (0.6)
Diarrhea	0	3 (4.2)	0	3 (1.7)	0	3 (0.6)
Rash	2 (2.4)	0	3 (0.6)	2 (1.2)	0	3 (0.6)
Headache	0	1 (1.4)	6 (1.2)	0	0	1 (0.2)
Gastrointestinal Symptoms	2 (2.4)	0	0	2 (1.2)	0	0
Nausea	1 (1.2)	1 (1.4)	6 (1.2)	1 (0.6)	0	0
Dyspnea	1 (1.2)	0	0	0	0	0
EKG Abnormalities	0	1 (1.4)	0	1 (0.6)	0	0
Tachycardia	0	1 (1.4)	0	0	0	0
Bradycardia	0	0	5 (1.0)	1 (0.6)	0	0
Muscle Pain/Cramp	0	1 (1.4)	1 (0.2)	1 (0.6)	0	0
Acne	0	1 (1.4)	0	0	0	0
Depression	0	1 (1.4)	0	0	0	0

The contents of Nimotop Capsules must not be administered by intravenous injection or other parenteral routes. Patients with hepatic cirrhosis have substantially reduced clearance and approximately doubled C_{max}. Dosage should be reduced to 30 mg every 4 hours, with close monitoring of blood pressure and heart rate.

HOW SUPPLIED

Each ivory colored, soft gelatin NIMOTOP® capsule is imprinted with the word Nimotop and contains 30 mg of nimodipine. The 30 mg capsules are packaged in unit dose foil pouches and supplied in cartons containing 100 capsules. The product is also available in child resistant unit dose safety pak foil pouches containing 30 capsules per carton. The capsules should be stored in the manufacturer's original foil package at a controlled room temperature of 59°F to 86°F (15°C to 30°C).

Capsules should be protected from light and freezing.

	Strength	NDC Code	Capsule Identification
Unit Dose Package of 100:	30 mg	0026-2855-48	Nimotop
Unit Dose Package of 30:	30 mg	0026-2855-70	Nimotop

Manufactured by:
Bayer Corporation
Pharmaceutical Division
400 Morgan Lane
West Haven, CT 06516
Encapsulated by:
R.P. Scherer North America
Division of R.P. Scherer Corp.
Clearwater, FL 33518
Caution: Federal (USA) law prohibits dispensing without prescription.

PZ500057   12/96   BAY e 9736   5202-7-A-U.S.-6
© 1996 Bayer Corporation   7051
Shown in Product Identification Guide, page 305

Otic DOMEBORO®
Acetic Acid 2% in Aqueous Aluminum Acetate Otic Solution   ℞

DESCRIPTION

Otic Domeboro® solution contains 2% acetic acid as the active ingredient, in modified Burow's solution (water, aluminum acetate, and sodium acetate) with boric acid as a stabilizer. Otic Domeboro® solution is instilled in the external auditory canal. Acetic acid is an astringent and antimicrobial agent. The pH range is from 4.5 to 6.0.

Chemically, acetic acid is $C_2H_4O_2$ and has the following structural formula:

$$\begin{array}{c} \text{H} \\ | \\ \text{H---C---C---OH} \\ | \quad \| \\ \text{H} \quad \text{O} \end{array}$$

Molecular weight of acetic acid is 60.05.

CLINICAL PHARMACOLOGY

Acetic acid is antibacterial and antifungal; and is effective against microorganisms (bacteria and fungi) that infect the ears of patients with acute diffuse external otitis. In *in vitro* tests, minimum lethal-time was less than 0.25 minutes when bacteria and fungi isolated from patients with otitis externa were exposed to 2% acetic acid. Quantitative absorption of acetic acid 2% from external auditory canal is not known.

INDICATIONS AND USAGE

Otic Domeboro® solution is indicated for the treatment of superficial infections of the external auditory canal caused by organisms susceptible to the action of the antimicrobial.

CONTRAINDICATIONS

Hypersensitivity to acetic acid or any of the ingredients of this product. Perforated tympanic membrane is considered a contraindication to the use of any medication in the external ear canal.

WARNINGS

Avoid use or use with caution in patients with perforated tympanic membrane (see CONTRAINDICATIONS).
NOT FOR OPHTHALMIC USE.

PRECAUTIONS
General
Care should be taken to assure that the Otic Domeboro® solution gets into the ear canal and stays in contact with the affected area long enough for the drug to act.
Discontinue promptly if sensitization or irritation occurs.
Carcinogenesis, Mutagenesis, Impairment of Fertility: No long term studies in animals have been performed to evaluate the carcinogenic potential of Otic Domeboro® solution.

ADVERSE REACTIONS
Irritation may occur.

OVERDOSAGE
No toxic effect has been reported with overdosage of Otic Domeboro® solution.

DOSAGE AND ADMINISTRATION
Patient should lie on his side with affected ear uppermost. Instill 4 to 6 drops into the external auditory canal and maintain this position for five minutes. Repeat the procedure every 2 to 3 hours.

HOW SUPPLIED
Otic Domeboro® solution (Acetic Acid 2% in Aqueous Aluminum Acetate Otic solution) is supplied in 2 fl. oz. dropper bottle.
Store below (30°C), 86°F, avoid freezing.
Otic Domeboro® Solution is a clear colorless liquid.

	NDC
2 fl. oz.	0026-4312-02

Bayer Corporation
Pharmaceutical Division
400 Morgan Lane
West Haven, CT 06516 USA
CAUTION: Federal (USA) law prohibits dispensing without prescription.
PD500003 2/95   ©1995 Bayer Corporation   4787

PRECOSE®   ℞
(acarbose tablets)

DESCRIPTION

PRECOSE® (acarbose tablets) is an oral alpha-glucosidase inhibitor for use in the management of type 2 diabetes mellitus. Acarbose is an oligosaccharide which is obtained from fermentation processes of a microorganism, *Actinoplanes utahensis*, and is chemically known as O-4,6-dideoxy-4-[[(1S,4R,5S,6S)-4,5,6-trihydroxy-3-(hydroxymethyl)-2-cyclohexen-1-yl]amino]-α-D-glucopyranosyl-(1 → 4)-O-α-D-glucopyranosyl-(1 → 4)-D-glucose. It is a white to off-white powder with a molecular weight of 645.6. Acarbose is soluble in water and has a pK_a of 5.1. Its empirical formula is $C_{25}H_{43}NO_{18}$ and its chemical structure is as follows:

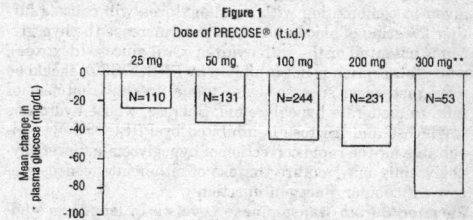

PRECOSE® is available as 25 mg, 50 mg and 100 mg tablets for oral use. The inactive ingredients are starch, microcrystalline cellulose, magnesium stearate, and colloidal silicon dioxide.

CLINICAL PHARMACOLOGY

Acarbose is a complex oligosaccharide that delays the digestion of ingested carbohydrates, thereby resulting in a smaller rise in blood glucose concentration following meals. As a consequence of plasma glucose reduction, PRECOSE® reduces levels of glycosylated hemoglobin in patients with Type 2 diabetes mellitus. Systemic non-enzymatic protein glycosylation, as reflected by levels of glycosylated hemoglobin, is a function of average blood glucose concentration over time.

Mechanism of Action: In contrast to sulfonylureas, PRECOSE® does not enhance insulin secretion. The antihyperglycemic action of acarbose results from a competitive, reversible inhibition of pancreatic alpha-amylase and membrane-bound intestinal alpha-glucoside hydrolase enzymes. Pancreatic alpha-amylase hydrolyzes complex starches to oligosaccharides in the lumen of the small intestine, while the membrane-bound intestinal alpha-glucosidases hydrolyze oligosaccharides, trisaccharides, and disaccharides to glucose and other monosaccharides in the brush border of the small intestine. In diabetic patients, this enzyme inhibition results in a delayed glucose absorption and a lowering of postprandial hyperglycemia.

Because its mechanism of action is different, the effect of PRECOSE® to enhance glycemic control is additive to that of sulfonylureas when used in combination. In addition, PRECOSE® diminishes the insulinotropic and weight-increasing effects of sulfonylureas.

Acarbose has no inhibitory activity against lactase and consequently would not be expected to induce lactose intolerance.

Pharmacokinetics:
Absorption: In a study of 6 healthy men, less than 2% of an oral dose of acarbose was absorbed as active drug, while

approximately 35% of total radioactivity from a ^{14}C-labeled oral dose was absorbed. An average of 51% of an oral dose was excreted in the feces as unabsorbed drug-related radioactivity within 96 hours of ingestion. Because acarbose acts locally within the gastrointestinal tract, this low systemic bioavailability of parent compound is therapeutically desired. Following oral dosing of healthy volunteers with ^{14}C-labeled acarbose, peak plasma concentrations of radioactivity were attained 14–24 hours after dosing, while peak plasma concentrations of active drug were attained at approximately 1 hour. The delayed absorption of acarbose-related radioactivity reflects the absorption of metabolites that may be formed by either intestinal bacteria or intestinal enzymatic hydrolysis.

Metabolism: Acarbose is metabolized exclusively within the gastrointestinal tract, principally by intestinal bacterial, but also by digestive enzymes. A fraction of these metabolites (approximately 34% of the dose) was absorbed and subsequently excreted in the urine. At least 13 metabolites have been separated chromatographically from urine specimens. The major metabolites have been identified as 4-methylpyrogallol derivatives (i.e., sulfate, methyl, and glucuronide conjugates). One metabolite (formed by cleavage of a glucose molecule from acarbose) also has alpha-glucosidase inhibitory activity. This metabolite, together with the parent compound, recovered from the urine, accounts for less than 2% of the total administered dose.

Excretion: The fraction of acarbose that is absorbed as intact drug is almost completely excreted by the kidneys. When acarbose was given *intravenously*, 89% of the dose was recovered in the urine as active drug within 48 hours. In contrast, less than 2% of an *oral* dose was recovered in the urine as active (i.e., parent compound and active metabolite) drug. This is consistent with the low bioavailability of the parent drug. The plasma elimination half-life of acarbose activity is approximately 2 hours in healthy volunteers. Consequently, drug accumulation does not occur with three times a day (t.i.d.) oral dosing.

Special Populations: The mean steady-state area under the curve (AUC) and maximum concentrations of acarbose were approximately 1.5 times higher in elderly compared to young volunteers; however, these differences were not statistically significant. Patients with severe renal impairment (Clcr<25 mL/min/1.73m²) attained about 5 times higher peak plasma concentrations of acarbose and 6 times larger AUCs than volunteers with normal renal function. No studies of acarbose pharmacokinetic parameters according to race have been performed. In U.S. controlled clinical studies of PRECOSE® in patients with type 2 diabetes mellitus, reductions in glycosylated hemoglobin levels were similar in Caucasians (n=478) and African-Americans (n=167), with a trend toward a better response in Latinos (n=132).

Drug-Drug Interactions: Studies in healthy volunteers have shown that PRECOSE® has no effect on either the pharmacokinetics or pharmacodynamics of digoxin, nifedipine, propranolol, or ranitidine. PRECOSE® did not interfere with the absorption or disposition of the sulfonylurea glyburide in diabetic patients.

CLINICAL TRIALS
Clinical Experience in Type 2 Diabetes Mellitus Patients on Dietary Treatment Only: Results from six controlled, fixed-dose, monotherapy studies of PRECOSE® in the treatment of type 2 diabetes mellitus, involving 769 PRECOSE®-treated patients, were combined and a weighted average of the difference from placebo in the mean change from baseline in glycosylated hemoglobin (HbA1c) was calculated for each dose level as presented below:
[See table 1 at top of next page]
Results from these six fixed-dose, monotherapy studies were also combined to derive a weighted average of the difference from placebo in mean change from baseline for one-hour postprandial plasma glucose levels as shown in the following figure:

Figure 1
Dose of PRECOSE® (t.i.d.)*

	25 mg	50 mg	100 mg	200 mg	300 mg**
	N=110	N=131	N=244	N=231	N=53

(y-axis: Mean change in plasma glucose (mg/dL), 0 to -100)

*PRECOSE® was statistically significantly different from placebo at all doses with respect to effect on one-hour postprandial plasma glucose.
**The 300 mg t.i.d. PRECOSE® regimen was superior to lower doses, but there were no statistically significant differences from 50 to 200 mg t.i.d.

Continued on next page

Precose—Cont.

Clinical Experience in Type 2 Diabetes Mellitus Patients Receiving Sulfonylureas: PRECOSE® was studied as adjunctive therapy to sulfonylurea treatment in two large, placebo-controlled, double-blind, randomized studies conducted in the United States in which 540 patients were included in the efficacy analysis. In addition, PRECOSE® was studied as adjunctive therapy to sulfonylurea treatment in a third study, conducted in Canada, in which patients were stratified according to background therapy. Study 1 (Table 2) involved patients under treatment at entry with diet alone who were subsequently randomized to four treatment groups. At the end of the study, patients in the PRECOSE® + tolbutamide group showed a mean treatment effect on glycosylated hemoglobin (HbA1c) of −1.78% and were receiving a significantly lower mean daily dose of tolbutamide than patients in the tolbutamide-alone group. Also, the efficacy in the PRECOSE® + tolbutamide group was significantly better than in the other three treatment groups. Study 2 (Table 2) involved patients taking background treatment with maximum daily doses of sulfonylureas. At the end of this study, the mean effect of the addition of PRECOSE® to maximum sulfonylurea therapy was a change in HbA1c of −0.54%. In addition, there was a significantly greater proportion of patients in the PRECOSE® + sulfonylurea group who reduced their sulfonylurea dose as compared to patients in the placebo + sulfonylurea group. In Study 3 (Table 2), the addition of PRECOSE® to a background treatment of sulfonylurea produced an additional change in mean HbA1c of −0.8%.
[See table 2 above]

INDICATIONS AND USAGE

PRECOSE®, as monotherapy, is indicated as an adjunct to diet to lower blood glucose in patients with type 2 diabetes mellitus whose hyperglycemia cannot be managed on diet alone. PRECOSE® may also be used in combination with a sulfonylurea when diet plus either PRECOSE® or a sulfonylurea do not result in adequate glycemic control. The effect of PRECOSE® to enhance glycemic control is additive to that of sulfonylureas when used in combination, presumably because its mechanism of action is different.

In initiating treatment for type 2 diabetes mellitus, diet should be emphasized as the primary form of treatment. Caloric restriction and weight loss are essential in the obese diabetic patient. Proper dietary management alone may be effective in controlling blood glucose and symptoms of hyperglycemia. The importance of regular physical activity when appropriate should also be stressed. If this treatment program fails to result in adequate glycemic control, the use of PRECOSE® should be considered. The use of PRECOSE® must be viewed by both the physician and patient as a treatment in addition to diet, and not as a substitute for diet or as a convenient mechanism for avoiding dietary restraint.

CONTRAINDICATIONS

PRECOSE® is contraindicated in patients with known hypersensitivity to the drug and in patients with diabetic ketoacidosis or cirrhosis. PRECOSE® is also contraindicated in patients with inflammatory bowel disease, colonic ulceration, partial intestinal obstruction or in patients predisposed to intestinal obstruction. In addition, PRECOSE® is contraindicated in patients who have chronic intestinal diseases associated with marked disorders of digestion or absorption and in patients who have conditions that may deteriorate as a result of increased gas formation in the intestine.

PRECAUTIONS

General

Hypoglycemia: Because of its mechanism of action, PRECOSE® when administered alone should not cause hypoglycemia in the fasted or postprandial state. Sulfonylurea agents may cause hypoglycemia. Because PRECOSE® given in combination with a sulfonylurea will cause a further lowering of blood glucose, it may increase the hypoglycemic potential or the sulfonylurea. Oral glucose (dextrose), whose absorption is not inhibited by PRECOSE®, should be used instead of sucrose (cane sugar) in the treatment of mild to moderate hypoglycemia. Sucrose, whose hydrolysis to glucose and fructose is inhibited by PRECOSE®, is unsuitable for the rapid correction of hypoglycemia. Severe hypoglycemia may require the use of either intravenous glucose infusion or glucagon injection.

Elevated Serum Transaminase Levels: In long-term studies (up to 12 months, and including PRECOSE® doses up to 300 mg t.i.d.) conducted in the United Stated, treatment-emergent elevations of serum transaminases (AST and/or ALT) above the upper limit of normal (ULN), greater than 1.8 times the ULN, and greater than 3 times the ULN occurred in 14%, 6%, and 3%, respectively, of PRECOSE®-treated patients as compared to 7%, 2%, and 1%, respectively, of placebo-treated patients. Although these differences between treatments were statistically significant, these elevations were asymptomatic, reversible, more com-

Table 1

Mean Change in HbA1c in Fixed-Dose Monotherapy Studies

Dose of PRECOSE®*	N	Change in HbA1c %	p-Value
25 mg t.i.d.	110	−0.44	0.0307
50 mg t.i.d.	131	−0.77	0.0001
100 mg t.i.d.	244	−0.74	0.0001
200 mg t.i.d.**	231	−0.86	0.0001
300 mg t.i.d.**	53	−1.00	0.0001

*PRECOSE® was statistically significantly different from placebo at all doses. Although there were no statistically significant differences among the mean results for doses ranging from 50 to 300 mg t.i.d., some patients may derive benefit by increasing the dosage from 50 to 100 mg t.i.d.
**Although studies utilized a maximum dose of 200 or 300 mg t.i.d., the maximum recommended dose for patients ≤ 60 kg is 50 mg t.i.d.; the maximum recommended dose for patients > 60 kg is 100 mg t.i.d.

Table 2

Study	Treatment	HbA1c(%)			p-Value
		Mean Baseline*	Mean Change from Baseline	Treatment Difference**	
1	Placebo	9.48	+0.05	—	—
	PRECOSE® 200† mg t.i.d.	9.19	−0.71	−0.76	0.0005
	Tolbutamide 250–1000 mg t.i.d. (mean dose 2.4 g/d)	9.28	−1.22	−1.27	0.0001
	PRECOSE® 200† mg t.i.d. + Tolbutamide 250–1000 mg t.i.d. (mean dose 1.9 g/d)	8.99	−1.73	−1.78	0.0001
2	Sulfonylurea + Placebo	9.56	+0.24	—	—
	Sulfonylurea + PRECOSE® 50–300† mg t.i.d.	9.64	−0.30	−0.54	0.0096
3	Sulfonylurea + Placebo Sulfonylurea + PRECOSE® 50–200† mg t.i.d.	8.00 8.10	+0.10 −0.80	— −0.90	0.0020

*Normal Range: 4–6%
**The result of subtracting the placebo group average.
†Although studies utilized a maximum dose of 200 or 300 mg t.i.d., the maximum recommended dose for patients ≤ 60 kg is 50 mg t.i.d.; the maximum recommended dose for patients > 60 kg is 100 mg t.i.d.

mon in females, and, in general, were not associated with other evidence of liver dysfunction. In addition, these serum transaminase elevations appeared to be dose related. In US studies including PRECOSE® doses up to the maximum approved dose of 100 mg t.i.d., treatment-emergent elevations of AST and/or ALT at any level of severity were similar between PRECOSE®-treated patients and placebo-treated patients (p >= 0.496).

In approximately 3 million patient-years of international post-marketing experience with PRECOSE®, 62 cases of serum transaminase elevations >500 IU/L (29 of which were associated with jaundice) have been reported. Forty-one of these 62 patients received treatment with 100 mg t.i.d. or greater and 33 of 45 patients for whom weight was reported weighed <60 kg. In the 59 cases where follow-up was recorded, hepatic abnormalities improved or resolved upon discontinuation of PRECOSE® in 55 and were unchanged in two. Two patients in Japan died of fulminant hepatitis; the relationship to acarbose is unclear.

Loss of Control of Blood Glucose: When diabetic patients are exposed to stress such as fever, trauma, infection, or surgery, a temporary loss of control of blood glucose may occur. At such times, temporary insulin therapy may be necessary.

Information for Patients: Patients should be told to take PRECOSE® orally three times a day at the start (with the first bite) of each main meal. It is important that patients continue to adhere to dietary instructions, a regular exercise program, and regular testing of urine and/or blood glucose.

PRECOSE® itself does not cause hypoglycemia even when administered to patients in the fasted state. Sulfonylurea drugs and insulin, however, can lower blood sugar levels enough to cause symptoms or sometimes life-threatening hypoglycemia. Because PRECOSE® given in combination with a sulfonylurea or insulin will cause a further lowering of blood sugar, it may increase the hypoglycemic potential of these agents. The risk of hypoglycemia, its symptoms and treatment, and conditions that predispose to its development should be well understood by patients and responsible family members. Because PRECOSE® prevents the break-

down of table sugar, patients should have a readily available source of glucose (dextrose, D-glucose) to treat symptoms of low blood sugar when taking PRECOSE® in combination with a sulfonylurea or insulin.

If side effects occur with PRECOSE®, they usually develop during the first few weeks of therapy. They are most commonly mild-to-moderate gastrointestinal effects, such as flatulence, diarrhea, or abdominal discomfort and generally diminish in frequency and intensity with time.

Laboratory Tests: Therapeutic response to PRECOSE® should be monitored by periodic blood glucose tests. Measurement of glycosylated hemoglobin levels is recommended for the monitoring of long-term glycemic control.

PRECOSE®, particularly at doses in excess of 50 mg t.i.d., may give rise to elevations of serum transaminases and, in rare instances, hyperbilirubinemia. It is recommended that serum transaminase levels be checked every 3 months during the first year of treatment with PRECOSE® and periodically thereafter. If elevated transaminases are observed, a reduction in dosage or withdrawal of therapy may be indicated, particularly if the elevations persist.

Renal Impairment: Plasma concentrations of PRECOSE® in renally impaired volunteers were proportionally increased relative to the degree of renal dysfunction. Long-term clinical trials in diabetic patients with significant renal dysfunction (serum creatinine >2.0 mg/dL) have not been conducted. Therefore, treatment of these patients with PRECOSE® is not recommended.

Drug Interactions: Certain drugs tend to produce hyperglycemia and may lead to loss of blood glucose control. These drugs include the thiazides and other diuretics, corticosteroids, phenothiazines, thyroid products, estrogens, oral contraceptives, phenytoin, nicotinic acid, sympathomimetics, calcium channel-blocking drugs, and isoniazid. When such drugs are administered to a patient receiving PRECOSE®, the patient should be closely observed for loss of blood glucose control. When such drugs are withdrawn from patients receiving PRECOSE® in combination with sulfonylureas or insulin, patients should be observed closely for any evidence of hypoglycemia.

Intestinal adsorbents (e.g., charcoal) and digestive enzyme preparations containing carbohydrate-splitting enzymes (e.g., amylase, pancreatin) may reduce the effect of PRECOSE® and should not be taken concomitantly.

Carcinogenesis, Mutagenesis, and Impairment of Fertility: Nine chronic toxicity/carcinogenicity studies were conducted in three animal species (rat, hamster, dog) including two rat strains (Sprague-Dawley and Wistar).

In the first rat study, Sprague-Dawley rats received acarbose in feed at high doses (up to approximately 500 mg/kg body weight) for 104 weeks. Acarbose treatment resulted in a significant increase in the incidence of renal tumors (adenomas and adenocarcinomas) and benign Leydig cell tumors. This study was repeated with a similar outcome. Further studies were performed to separate direct carcinogenic effects of acarbose from indirect effects resulting from the carbohydrate malnutrition induced by the large doses of acarbose employed in the studies. In one study using Sprague-Dawley rats, acarbose was mixed with feed but carbohydrate deprivation was prevented by the addition of glucose to the diet. In a 26-month study of Sprague-Dawley rats, acarbose was administered by daily postprandial gavage so as to avoid the pharmacologic effects of the drug. In both of these studies, the increased incidence of renal tumors found in the original studies did not occur.

Acarbose was also given in food and by postprandial gavage in two separate studies in Wistar rats. No increased incidence of renal tumors was found in either of these Wistar rat studies. In two feeding studies of hamsters, with and without glucose supplementation, there was also no evidence of carcinogenicity.

Acarbose showed no mutagenic activity when tested in six *in vitro* and three *in vivo* assays.

Fertility studies conducted in rats after oral administration produced no untoward effect on fertility or on the overall capability to reproduce.

Pregnancy:

Teratogenic Effects: Pregnancy Category B. The safety of PRECOSE® in pregnant women has not been established. Reproduction studies have been performed in rats at doses up to 480 mg/kg (corresponding to 9 times the exposure in humans, based on drug blood levels) and have revealed no evidence of impaired fertility or harm to the fetus due to acarbose. In rabbits, reduced maternal body weight gain, probably the result of the pharmacodynamic activity of high doses of acarbose in the intestines, may have been responsible for a slight increase in the number of embryonic losses. However, rabbits given 160 mg/kg acarbose (corresponding to 10 times the dose in man, based on body surface area) showed no evidence of embryotoxicity and there was no evidence of teratogenicity at a dose 32 times the dose in man (based on body surface area). There are, however, no adequate and well-controlled studies of PRECOSE® in pregnant women. Because animal reproduction studies are not always predictive of the human response, this drug should be used during pregnancy only if clearly needed. Because current information strongly suggests that abnormal blood glucose levels during pregnancy are associated with a higher incidence of congenital anomalies as well as increased neonatal morbidity and mortality, most experts recommend that insulin be used during pregnancy to maintain blood glucose levels as close to normal as possible.

Nursing Mothers: A small amount of radioactivity has been found in the milk of lactating rats after administration of radiolabeled acarbose. It is not known whether this drug is excreted in human milk. Because many drugs are excreted in human milk, PRECOSE® should not be administered to a nursing woman.

Pediatric Use: Safety and effectiveness of PRECOSE® in pediatric patients have not been established.

ADVERSE REACTIONS

Digestive Tract: Gastrointestinal symptoms are the most common reactions to PRECOSE®. In the U.S. placebo-controlled trials, the incidences of abdominal pain, diarrhea, and flatulence were 21%, 33%, and 77% respectively in 1075 patients treated with PRECOSE® 50–300 mg t.i.d., whereas the corresponding incidences were 9%, 12%, and 32% in 818 placebo-treated patients. Abdominal pain and diarrhea tended to return to pretreatment levels over time, and the frequency and intensity of flatulence tended to abate with time. The increased gastrointestinal tract symptoms in patients treated with PRECOSE® is a manifestation of the mechanism of action of PRECOSE® and is related to the presence of undigested carbohydrate in the lower GI tract. Rarely, these gastrointestinal events may be severe and might be confused with paralytic ileus.

Elevated Serum Transaminase Levels: See PRECAUTIONS.

Other Abnormal Laboratory Findings: Small reductions in hematocrit occurred more often in PRECOSE®-treated patients than in placebo-treated patients but were not associated with reductions in hemoglobin. Low serum calcium and low plasma vitamin B_6 levels were associated with PRECOSE® therapy but were thought to be either spurious or of no clinical significance.

	Strength	NDC	Tablet Identification
Bottles of 100:	25 mg	0026-2863-51	PRECOSE 25
	50 mg	0026-2861-51	PRECOSE 50
	100 mg	0026-2862-51	PRECOSE 100
Unit Dose Packages of 100:	50 mg	0026-2861-48	PRECOSE 50
	100 mg	0026-2862-48	PRECOSE 100

OVERDOSAGE

Unlike sulfonylureas or insulin, an overdose of PRECOSE® will not result in hypoglycemia. An overdose may result in transient increases in flatulence, diarrhea, and abdominal discomfort which shortly subside.

DOSAGE AND ADMINISTRATION

There is no fixed dosage regimen for the management of diabetes mellitus with PRECOSE® or any other pharmacologic agent. Dosage of PRECOSE® must be individualized on the basis of both effectiveness and tolerance while not exceeding the maximum recommended dose of 100 mg t.i.d. PRECOSE® should be taken three times daily at the start (with the first bite) of each main meal. PRECOSE® should be started at a low dose, with gradual dose escalation as described below, both to reduce gastrointestinal side effects and to permit identification of the minimum dose required for adequate glycemic control of the patient.

During treatment initiation and dose titration (see below), one-hour postprandial plasma glucose should be used to determine the therapeutic response to PRECOSE® and identify the minimum effective dose for the patient. Thereafter, glycosylated hemoglobin should be measured at intervals of approximately three months. The therapeutic goal should be to decrease both postprandial plasma glucose and glycosylated hemoglobin levels to normal or near normal by using the lowest effective dose of PRECOSE®, either as monotherapy or in combination with sulfonylureas.

Initial Dosage: The recommended starting dosage of PRECOSE® is 25 mg given orally three times daily at the start (with the first bite) of each main meal. However, some patients may benefit from more gradual dose titration to minimize gastrointestinal side effects. This may be achieved by initiating treatment at 25 mg once per day and subsequently increasing the frequency of administration to achieve 25 mg t.i.d.

Maintenance Dosage: Once a 25 mg t.i.d. dosage regimen is reached, dosage of PRECOSE® should be adjusted at 4–8 week intervals based on one-hour postprandial glucose levels and on tolerance. The dosage can be increased from 25 mg t.i.d. to 50 mg t.i.d. Some patients may benefit from further increasing the dosage to 100 mg t.i.d. The maintenance dose ranges from 50 mg t.i.d. to 100 mg t.i.d. However, since patients with low body weight may be at increased risk for elevated serum transaminases, only patients with body weight > 60 kg should be considered for dose titration above 50 mg t.i.d. (see PRECAUTIONS). If no further reduction in postprandial glucose or glycosylated hemoglobin levels is observed with titration to 100 mg t.i.d., consideration should be given to lowering the dose. Once an effective and tolerated dosage is established, it should be maintained.

Maximum Dosage: The maximum recommended dose for patients ≤ 60 kg is 50 mg t.i.d. The maximum recommended dose for patients > 60 kg is 100 mg t.i.d.

Patients Receiving Sulfonylureas: Sulfonylurea agents may cause hypoglycemia. PRECOSE® given in combination with a sulfonylurea will cause a further lowering of blood glucose and may increase the hypoglycemic potential of the sulfonylurea. If hypoglycemia occurs, appropriate adjustments in the dosage of these agents should be made.

HOW SUPPLIED

PRECOSE® is available as 25 mg, 50 mg or 100 mg round, unscored tablets. Each tablet strength is white to yellow-tinged in color. The 25 mg tablet is coded with the word "PRECOSE" on one side and "25" on the other side. The 50 mg tablet is coded with the word "PRECOSE" and "50" on the same side. The 100 mg tablet is coded with the word "PRECOSE" and "100" on the same side. PRECOSE® is available in bottles of 100 and unit dose packages of 100.

[See table above]

Do not store above 25°C (77°F). Protect from moisture. For bottles, keep container tightly closed.

Bayer Corporation
Pharmaceutical Division
400 Morgan Lane
West Haven, CT 06516 USA

Caution: Federal law prohibits dispensing without a prescription.

PZ500080 3/98 Bay g 5421 PRECOSE®/5202/0/8/USA-5
©1998 Bayer Corporation   8093

Shown in Product Identification Guide, page 305

TRASYLOL® ℞
(aprotinin injection)

DESCRIPTION

Trasylol® (aprotinin injection), $C_{284}H_{432}N_{84}O_{79}S_7$, is a natural proteinase inhibitor obtained from bovine lung. Aprotinin (molecular weight of 6512 daltons), consists of 58 amino acid residues that are arranged in a single polypeptide chain, cross-linked by three disulfide bridges. It is supplied as a clear, colorless, sterile isotonic solution for intravenous administration. Each milliliter contains 10,000 KIU (Kallikrein Inhibitor Units) (1.4 mg/ml) and 9 mg sodium chloride in water for injection. Hydrochloric acid and/or sodium hydroxide is used to adjust the pH to 4.5–6.5.

CLINICAL PHARMACOLOGY

Mechanism of Action: Aprotinin is a protease inhibitor with a variety of effects on the coagulation system. It inhibits plasmin and kallikrein, thus directly affecting fibrinolysis. It also inhibits the contact phase activation of coagulation which both initiates coagulation and promotes fibrinolysis. In addition to these effects on the clotting and lysis cascades in blood, aprotinin preserves the adhesive glycoproteins in the platelet membrane making them resistant to damage from the increased plasmin levels and mechanical injury that occur during cardiopulmonary bypass (CPB). The net effect is to inhibit both fibrinolysis and turnover of coagulation factors, and to decrease bleeding, although the precise mechanism of this effect is unclear.

Patients undergoing cardiac surgery with extracorporeal circulation by a heart-lung machine (cardiopulmonary bypass; CPB) develop adverse changes of their blood components, blood cells and specific coagulation proteins. These changes cause a transient hemostatic defect during the intraoperative and immediate postoperative period which may result in diffuse bleeding despite correct surgical technique. At times, this blood loss is severe enough to require multiple blood transfusions and even surgical re-exploration.

Pharmacokinetics: The studies comparing the pharmacokinetics of aprotinin in healthy volunteers, cardiac patients undergoing surgery with cardiopulmonary bypass, and women undergoing hysterectomy suggest linear pharmacokinetics over the dose range of 50,000 KIU to 2 million KIU. After intravenous (IV) injection, rapid distribution of aprotinin occurs into the total extracellular space, leading to a rapid initial decrease in plasma aprotinin concentration. Following this distribution phase, a plasma half-life of about 150 minutes is observed. At later time points, (i.e., beyond 5 hours after dosing) there is a terminal elimination phase with a half-life of about 10 hours.

Average steady state intraoperative plasma concentrations were 137 KIU/mL (n=10) after administration of the following dosage regimen: 1 million KIU IV loading dose, 1 million KIU into the pump prime volume, 250,000 KIU per hour of operation as continuous intravenous infusion (Regimen B). Average steady state intraoperative plasma concentrations were 250 KIU/mL in patients (n=20) treated with aprotinin during cardiac surgery by administration of Regimen A (exactly double Regimen B): 2 million KIU IV loading dose, 2 million KIU into the pump prime volume, 500,000 KIU per hour of operation as continuous intravenous infusion.

Following a single IV dose of radiolabelled aprotinin, approximately 25–40% of the radioactivity is excreted in the urine over 48 hours. After a 30 minute infusion of 1 million KIU, about 2% is excreted as unchanged drug. After a larger dose of 2 million KIU infused over 30 minutes, urinary excretion of unchanged aprotinin accounts for approximately 9% of the dose. Animal studies have shown that aprotinin is accumulated primarily in the kidney. Aprotinin, after being filtered by the glomeruli, is actively reabsorbed by the proximal tubules in which it is stored in phagolysosomes. Aprotinin is slowly degraded by lysosomal enzymes. The physiological renal handling of aprotinin is similar to that of other small proteins, e.g. insulin.

CLINICAL TRIALS

Three placebo-controlled, double-blind studies of Trasylol® were conducted in the United States involving 523 patients undergoing repeat coronary artery bypass graft (CABG) surgery, of whom 463 were valid for efficacy analysis. The following treatments were used in the studies: Trasylol® Regimen A (2 million KIU IV loading dose, 2 million KIU into the pump prime volume, 500,000 KIU per hour of surgery as a continuous intravenous infusion); Trasylol® Regimen B (1 million KIU IV loading dose, 1 million KIU into the pump prime volume, 250,000 KIU per hour of surgery as a continuous intravenous infusion); a pump prime regimen (2 million KIU into the pump prime volume only); and a placebo regimen (normal saline).

In the three studies, fewer patients receiving Trasylol® (either Regimen A or Regimen B) required any donor blood in comparison to the placebo regimen.

Continued on next page

Trasylol—Cont.

[See table below]

In these three studies there was no diminution of benefit with age. Male and female patients received benefits from Trasylol® in terms of a reduction in the average number of units of donor blood transfused. Male patients did better than female patients in terms of the percentage of patients who required any donor blood transfusions. However, the number of female patients studied was small.

A double-blind, randomized, Canadian study compared Trasylol® Regimen A (n=28) and placebo (n=23) in primary cardiac surgery patients (mainly CABG) requiring cardiopulmonary bypass who were treated with aspirin within 48 hours of surgery. The mean total blood loss (1209.7 mL vs. 2532.3 mL) and the mean number of units of packed red blood cells transfused (1.6 units vs. 4.3 units) were significantly less (p<0.008) in the Trasylol® group compared to the placebo group.

In a U.S. randomized study of Trasylol® Regimen A and Regimen B versus the placebo regimen in 212 patients undergoing primary aortic and/or mitral valve replacement or repair, no benefit was found for Trasylol® in terms of the need for transfusion or the number of units of blood required.

INDICATIONS AND USAGE

Trasylol® is indicated for prophylactic use to reduce perioperative blood loss and the need for blood transfusion in patients undergoing cardiopulmonary bypass in the course of repeat coronary artery bypass graft surgery. Trasylol® is also indicated in selected cases of primary coronary artery bypass graft surgery where the risk of bleeding is especially high (impaired hemostasis, e.g., presence of aspirin or coagulopathy of other origin) or where transfusion is unavailable or unacceptable. This selected use of Trasylol® in primary CABG patients is based on the risk of renal dysfunction and on the risk of anaphylaxis (should a second procedure be needed).

CONTRAINDICATIONS

Hypersensitivity to aprotinin.

WARNINGS

Anaphylactic or anaphylactoid reactions are possible when Trasylol® is administered. Hypersensitivity reactions are rare in patients with no prior exposure to aprotinin. Hypersensitivity reactions can range from skin eruptions, itching, dyspnea, nausea and tachycardia to fatal anaphylactic shock with circulatory failure. If a hypersensitivity reaction occurs during injection or infusion of Trasylol®, administration should be stopped immediately and emergency treatment should be initiated. It should be noted that severe (fatal) hypersensitivity/anaphylactic reactions can also occur in connection with application of the test dose. Even when a second exposure to aprotinin has been tolerated without symptoms, a subsequent administration may result in severe hypersensitivity/anaphylactic reactions.

Re-exposure to aprotinin: In a retrospective review of 387 European patient records with documented re-exposure to Trasylol®, the incidence of hypersensitivity/anaphylactic reactions per re-exposure was 2.7%. Two patients who experienced hypersensitivity/anaphylactic reactions subsequently died, 24 hours and five days after surgery, respectively. The relationship of these two deaths to Trasylol® is unclear. This retrospective review also showed that the incidence of a hypersensitivity or anaphylactic reaction following re-exposure is increased when the re-exposure occurs within six months of the initial administration (5.0% for re-exposures within six months and 0.9% for re-exposures greater than six months). Other smaller studies have confirmed that in case of re-exposure, the incidence of hypersensitivity/anaphylactic reactions may reach the five percent level. Before initiating treatment with Trasylol® in a patient with a history of prior exposure, the recommendations below should be followed to manage a potential hypersensitivity or anaphylactic reaction:

1) Have standard emergency treatments for hypersensitivity or anaphylactic reactions readily available in the operating room (e.g., epinephrine, corticosteroids).
2) Administration of the test dose and loading dose should be done only when the conditions for rapid cannulation (if necessary) are present.
3) Delay the addition of Trasylol® into the pump prime solution until after the loading dose has been safely administered.

Additionally, administration of H1 and H2 blockers 15 minutes before the test dose may be considered.

PRECAUTIONS

General: *Test Dose:* All patients treated with Trasylol® should first receive a test dose to assess the potential for allergic reactions. The test dose of 1 mL Trasylol® should be administered intravenously at least 10 minutes prior to the loading dose. However, even after the uneventful administration of the initial 1 mL-dose, the therapeutic dose may cause an anaphylactic reaction. If this happens the infusion of aprotinin should immediately be stopped, and standard emergency treatment for anaphylaxis should be applied. Patients who experience any allergic reaction to the test dose of aprotinin should not receive further administration of the drug. (see WARNINGS)

Allergic Reactions: Patients with a history of allergic reactions to drugs or other agents may be at greater risk of developing a hypersensitivity or anaphylactic reaction upon exposure to Trasylol® (see WARNINGS)

Loading Dose: The loading dose of Trasylol® should be given intravenously to patients in the supine position over a 20–30 minute period. Rapid intravenous administration of Trasylol® can cause a transient fall in blood pressure. (see DOSAGE AND ADMINISTRATION).

Use of Trasylol® in patients undergoing deep hypothermic circulatory arrest: An increase in both renal failure and mortality compared to age matched historical controls has been reported in patients receiving Trasylol® while undergoing deep hypothermic circulatory arrest in connection with surgery of the aortic arch. The strength of this association is uncertain because there are no data from randomized studies to confirm or refute these findings.

Drug Interactions: Trasylol® is known to have antifibrinolytic activity and, therefore, may inhibit the effects of fibrinolytic agents.

In a study of nine patients with untreated hypertension, Trasylol® infused intravenously in a dose of 2 million KIU over two hours blocked the acute hypotensive effect of 100 mg of captopril.

Trasylol®, in the presence of heparin, has been found to prolong the activated clotting time (ACT) as measured by a celite surface activation method. The kaolin activated clotting time appears to be much less affected. However, Trasylol® should not be viewed as a heparin sparing agent. (see Laboratory Monitoring of Anticoagulation During Cardiopulmonary Bypass).

Carcinogenesis, Mutagenesis, Impairment of Fertility: Long-term animal studies to evaluate the carcinogenic potential of Trasylol® or studies to determine the effect of Trasylol® on fertility have not been performed.

Results of microbial *in vitro* tests using *Salmonella typhimurium* and *Bacillus subtilis* indicate that Trasylol® is not a mutagen.

Pregnancy: Teratogenic Effects: Pregnancy Category B: Reproduction studies have been performed in rats at intravenous doses up to 200,000 KIU/kg/day for 11 days, and in rabbits at intravenous doses up to 100,000 KIU/kg/day for 13 days, 2.4 and 1.2 times the human dose on a mg/kg basis and 0.37 and 0.36 times the human mg/m² dose. They have revealed no evidence of impaired fertility or harm to the fetus due to Trasylol®. There are, however, no adequate and well-controlled studies in pregnant women. Because animal reproduction studies are not always predictive of human response, this drug should be used during pregnancy only if clearly needed.

Nursing Mother: Not applicable.

Pediatric Use: Safety and effectiveness in children have not been established.

Laboratory Monitoring of Anticoagulation during Cardiopulmonary Bypass: Trasylol® prolongs whole blood clotting times by a different mechanism than heparin. In the presence of aprotinin, prolongation is dependent on the type of whole blood clotting test employed. If an activated clotting time (ACT) is used to determine the effectiveness of heparin anticoagulation, the prolongation of the ACT by aprotinin may lead to an overestimation of the degree of anticoagula-

REPEAT CABG PATIENTS WHO REQUIRED DONOR BLOOD

	PLACEBO REGIMEN	TRASYLOL® PUMP PRIME REGIMEN	TRASYLOL® REGIMEN B	TRASYLOL® REGIMEN A
Study 1	40/52 (77%)	Not Studied	23/49 (47%)*	22/53 (42%)*
Study 2	23/32 (72%)	Not Studied	Not Studied	7/23 (30%)*
Study 3	49/65 (75%)	49/68 (72%)	28/60 (47%)*	33/61 (54%)*

* p≤0.007 compared to placebo

The number of units of donor blood required by patients was also reduced by Trasylol® Regimens A and B when compared to the placebo regimen:

UNITS OF DONOR BLOOD REQUIRED BY REPEAT CABG PATIENTS
Study 1

	PLACEBO REGIMEN	TRASYLOL® REGIMEN B	TRASYLOL® REGIMEN A
MEAN±SE	3.5±0.6	2.0±0.6**	1.8±0.6*
RANGE	0–34	0–18	0–24
MEDIAN	2	0	0

* p≤0.001 compared to placebo, ANOVA on ranks
** p=0.005 compared to placebo, ANOVA on ranks

Study 2

	PLACEBO REGIMEN	TRASYLOL® REGIMEN A
MEAN±SE	3.3±0.7	0.4±0.8*
RANGE	0–20	0–5
MEDIAN	4	0

* p=0.0001 compared to placebo, ANOVA on ranks

Study 3

	PLACEBO REGIMEN	TRASYLOL® PUMP PRIME REGIMEN	TRASYLOL® REGIMEN B	TRASYLOL® REGIMEN A
MEAN±SE	3.4±0.5	2.5±0.3	2.3±0.8*	1.6±0.2*
RANGE	0–17	0–13	0–46	0–6
MEDIAN	3.0	2.0	0.0	1.0

* p≤0.001 compared to placebo, ANOVA on ranks

Study 2 also included 151 patients undergoing primary CABG surgery; 74 of the patients receiving Trasylol® and 67 of the patients receiving placebo were valid for efficacy analysis. Fewer patients receiving Trasylol® required any donor blood:

PRIMARY CABG PATIENTS WHO REQUIRED DONOR BLOOD
Study 2

PLACEBO REGIMEN	TRASYLOL® REGIMEN A
35/67 (52%)	28/74 (38%)*

* p=0.052 compared to placebo

UNITS OF DONOR BLOOD REQUIRED BY PRIMARY CABG PATIENTS
Study 2

	PLACEBO REGIMEN	TRASYLOL® REGIMEN A
MEAN±SE	2.1±0.3	1.1±0.3*
RANGE	0–15	0–10
MEDIAN	1	0

* p=0.0246 compared to placebo, ANOVA on ranks

tion, thereby leading to inadequate anticoagulation. During extended extracorporeal circulation, patients may require additional heparin, even in the presence of ACT levels that appear adequate.

In patients undergoing CPB with Trasylol® therapy, one of the following methods may be employed to maintain adequate anticoagulation:

ACT—An ACT is not a standardized coagulation test, and different formulations of the assay are affected differently by the presence of aprotinin. The test is further influenced by variable dilution effects and the temperature experienced during cardiopulmonary bypass. It has been observed that kaolin-based ACTs are not increased to the same degree by aprotinin as are diatomaceous earth-based (celite) ACTs. While protocols vary, during bypass a minimal celite ACT of 750 seconds or kaolin-ACT of 480 seconds, independent of the effects of hemodilution and hypothermia, is recommended in the presence of aprotinin. Consult the manufacturer of the ACT test regarding the interpretation of the assay in the presence of Trasylol®.

Fixed Heparin Dosing—A standard loading dose of heparin, administered prior to cannulation of the heart, plus the quantity of heparin added to the prime volume of the CPB circuit, should total at least 350 IU/kg. Additional heparin should be administered in a fixed-dose regimen based on patient weight and duration of CPB.

Heparin Titration—Protamine titration, a method that is not affected by aprotinin, can be used to measure heparin levels. A heparin dose response, assessed by protamine titration, should be performed prior to administration of aprotinin to determine the heparin loading dose. Additional heparin should be administered on the basis of heparin levels measured by protamine titration. Heparin levels during bypass should not be allowed to drop below 2.7 U/mL (2.0 mg/kg) or below the level indicated by heparin dose-response testing performed prior to administration of aprotinin.

Protamine Administration—In patients treated with Trasylol®, the amount of protamine administered to reverse heparin activity should be based on the actual amount of heparin administered, and not on the ACT values.

ADVERSE REACTIONS

Studies analyzed to date indicate that Trasylol® is generally well tolerated. The adverse events reported are frequent sequelae of cardiac surgery and are not necessarily attributable to Trasylol® therapy. Adverse events reported, up to time of discharge from the hospital, from four double-blind, placebo-controlled studies conducted in the United States involving 2002 aprotinin patients are listed in the following tables. The tables list those events which occurred in patients treated with Trasylol® without regard to causal relationship.

[See table above]

In comparison to the placebo group, no increase in mortality in patients treated with Trasylol® was observed.

Additional events of particular interest from controlled US trials with an incidence of less than 2%, are listed below:

[See first table at top of next page]

Listed below are additional events, from controlled US trials with an incidence between 1 and 2%, and also from uncontrolled, compassionate use trials and spontaneous post-marketing reports. Estimates of frequency cannot be made for spontaneous post-marketing reports (italicized).

Body as a Whole: Sepsis, death, multi-system organ failure, immune system disorder, *hemoperitoneum*.

Cardiovascular: Ventricular fibrillation, heart arrest, bradycardia, congestive heart failure, hemorrhage, bundle branch block, myocardial ischemia, ventricular tachycardia, heart block, pericardial effusion, ventricular arrhythmia, shock, pulmonary hypertension.

Digestive: Dyspepsia, gastrointestinal hemorrhage, jaundice, hepatic failure.

Hematologic and Lymphatic: Although thrombosis was not reported more frequently in aprotinin versus placebo-treated patients in controlled trials, it has been reported in uncontrolled trials, compassionate use trials, and spontaneous post-marketing reporting. These reports of thrombosis encompass the following terms: thrombosis, occlusion, arterial thrombosis, *pulmonary thrombosis*, coronary occlusion, embolus, pulmonary embolus, thrombophlebitis, deep thrombophlebitis, cerebrovascular accident, cerebral embolism. Other hematologic events reported include leukocytosis, thrombocytopenia, coagulation disorder (which includes disseminated intravascular coagulation), decreased prothombin.

Metabolic and Nutritional: Hyperglycemia, hypokalemia, hypervolemia, acidosis.

Musculoskeletal: Arthralgia.

Nervous: Agitation, dizziness, anxiety, convulsion.

Respiratory: Pneumonia, apnea, increased cough, lung edema.

Skin: *Skin discoloration.*

Urogenital: Oliguria, kidney failure, acute kidney failure, kidney tubular necrosis.

INCIDENCE RATES OF ADVERSE EVENTS (> = 2%) BY BODY SYSTEM AND TREATMENT FOR ALL PATIENTS FROM US PLACEBO-CONTROLLED CLINICAL TRIALS

Adverse Event	Aprotinin (n = 2002) values in %	Placebo (n = 1084) values in %
Any Event	76	77
Body as a Whole		
Fever	15	14
Infection	6	7
Chest Pain	2	2
Asthenia	2	2
Cardiovascular		
Atrial Fibrillation	21	23
Hypotension	8	10
Myocardial Infarct	6	6
Atrial Flutter	6	5
Ventricular Extrasystoles	6	4
Tachycardia	6	7
Ventricular Tachycardia	5	4
Heart Failure	5	4
Pericarditis	5	5
Peripheral Edema	5	5
Hypertension	4	5
Arrhythmia	4	3
Supraventricular Tachycardia	4	3
Atrial Arrhythmia	3	3
Digestive		
Nausea	11	9
Constipation	4	5
Vomiting	3	4
Diarrhea	3	2
Liver Function Tests Abnormal	3	2
Hemic and Lymphatic		
Anemia	2	8
Metabolic & Nutritional		
Creatine Phosphokinase Increased	2	1
Musculoskeletal		
Any Event	2	3
Nervous		
Confusion	4	4
Insomnia	3	4
Respiratory		
Lung Disorder	8	8
Pleural Effusion	7	9
Atelectasis	5	6
Dyspnea	4	4
Pneumothorax	4	4
Asthma	2	3
Hypoxia	2	1
Skin and Appendages		
Rash	2	2
Urogenital		
Kidney Function Abnormal	3	2
Urinary Retention	3	3
Urinary Tract Infection	2	2

Myocardial Infarction: In a pooled analysis of all patients undergoing CABG surgery, there was no significant difference in the incidence of investigator-reported myocardial infarction (MI) in Trasylol® treated patients as compared to placebo treated patients. However, because no uniform criteria for the diagnosis of myocardial infarction were utilized by investigators, this issue was addressed prospectively in three later studies (two studies evaluated Regimen A, Regimen B, and pump prime regimen; one study evaluated only Regimen A) in which data were analyzed by a blinded consultant employing an algorithm for possible, probable or definite MI. Utilizing this method, the incidence of definite myocardial infarction was 5.9% in the aprotinin treated patients versus 4.7% in the placebo treated patients. This difference in the incidence rates was not statistically significant. Data from these three studies are summarized below.

[See second table at top of next page]

Graft Patency: In a recently completed multi-center, multi-national study to determine the effects of Trasylol® Regimen A vs. placebo on saphenous vein graft patency in patients undergoing primary CABG surgery, patients were subjected to routine postoperative angiography. Of the 13 study sites, 10 were in the United States and three were non-U.S. centers (Denmark (1), Israel (2)). The results of this study are summarized below.

Although there was a statistically significantly increased risk of graft closure for Trasylol® treated patients compared to patients who received placebo (p=0.035), further analysis showed a significant treatment by site interaction for one of the non-U.S. sites vs. the U.S. centers. When the analysis of graft closures was repeated for U.S. centers only, there was no statistically significant difference in graft closure rates in patients who received Trasylol® vs. placebo. These results are the same whether analyzed as the proportion of patients who experienced at least one graft closure postoperatively or as the proportion of grafts closed. There were no differences between treatment groups in the incidence of myocardial infarction as evaluated by the blinded consultant (2.9% Trasylol® vs. 3.8% placebo) or of death (1.4% Trasylol® vs. 1.6% placebo) in this study.

Hypersensitivity and Anaphylaxis: See WARNINGS.

Hypersensitivity and anaphylactic reactions during surgery were rarely reported in U.S. controlled clinical studies in patients with no prior exposure to Trasylol® (1/1424 patients or <0.1% on Trasylol® vs. 1/861 patients or 0.1% on placebo). In case of re-exposure the incidence of hypersensitivity/anaphylactic reactions has been reported to reach the 5% level.

[See third table at top of next page]

Laboratory Findings

Serum Creatinine: Pooled data from the four U.S. placebo-controlled studies showed a statistically significant increase in the incidence of post-operative renal dysfunction in patients treated with Trasylol®. The incidence of serum creatinine elevations ≥0.5 mg/dL above baseline was 21 percent in Regimen A, 18 percent in Regimen B compared to 14 percent in the placebo group (p=0.015 and p=0.495, respectively). In patients undergoing coronary artery bypass graft procedures only (Studies 1, 2, 3) the rates were 19 percent and 20 percent in the Trasylol® Regimen A and Regimen B groups and 15 percent in the placebo group (p≥0.345, versus placebo). Postoperative renal dysfunction was observed somewhat more frequently in association with primary cardiac valve procedures (30% for Trasylol® Regimen A, and 14% for Regimen B versus 8% for placebo). In the majority of instances the renal dysfunction was not severe and was reversible. A total of 4 percent of patients treated with Trasylol® Regimens A and B and 2 percent of the placebo group had a serum creatinine increase of ≥2 mg/dL above the pre-operative value.

Patients with baseline elevations in serum creatinine were not at increased risk of developing postoperative renal dysfunction following Trasylol® treatment although there were mean increases in creatinine of 0.11 mg/dL after the high dose regimen (A), and of 0.09 mg/dL after the low dose regimen (B), each of which was statistically significant compared to placebo.

Serum Glucose: In the hours after cardiopulmonary bypass surgery, the serum glucose levels increased; however,

Continued on next page

Trasylol—Cont.

the average increase in serum glucose in patients treated with the high dose regimen (61 mg/dL) was less than in the placebo treated group (78 mg/dL).

Serum Transaminases: In U.S. controlled studies, a significantly greater incidence of treatment emergent abnormal liver function tests was reported in all Trasylol® treated (Regimen A, Regimen B, and the pump prime regimen) patients (5%) compared to patients treated with the placebo regimen (2%). The percent of primary CABG patients developing an elevation of ALT (alanine amino transferase; formerly SGPT, serum glutamic pyruvic transaminase) greater than 1.8 times the upper limit of normal was higher in the Trasylol® treated group compared to the placebo group. Among the repeat CABG patients, the percent of subjects developing an elevation of ALT of this magnitude was significantly higher in the Trasylol® treated group. This suggests an indirect effect possibly related to the risk of repeated surgery and attendant myocardial dysfunction rather than a primary drug effect. There were no differences between the Trasylol® treated and placebo groups in the incidence of elevated ALT values greater than 3.0 times the upper limit of normal.

Serum Creatine Kinase (CK): There was a trend toward an increased incidence of elevated serum creatine kinase (CK) with increased MB fractions in Trasylol® treated patients.

Partial Thromboplastin Time (PTT) and Activated Clotting Time (ACT): Significant elevations in the partial thromboplastin time (PTT) and activated clotting time (ACT) in Trasylol® treated patients are expected in the hours after surgery due to circulating concentrations of Trasylol® which are known to inhibit activation of the intrinsic clotting system by contact with a foreign surface, a method used in these tests. (See Laboratory Monitoring of Anticoagulation During Cardiopulmonary Bypass.)

OVERDOSAGE

The maximum amount of Trasylol® that can be safely administered in single or multiple doses has not been determined. Doses up to 17.5 million KIU have been administered within a 24 hour period without any apparent toxicity. There is one poorly documented case, however, of a patient who received a large, but not well determined, amount of Trasylol® (in excess of 15 million KIU) in 24 hours. The patient, who had pre-existing liver dysfunction, developed hepatic and renal failure postoperatively and died. Autopsy showed hepatic necrosis and extensive renal tubular and glomerular necrosis. The relationship of these findings to Trasylol® therapy is unclear.

DOSAGE AND ADMINISTRATION

Trasylol® given prophylactically in both Regimen A and Regimen B (half Regimen A) to patients undergoing repeat CABG surgery significantly reduced the donor blood transfusion requirement relative to placebo treatment. In patients given aspirin preoperatively, while there was no difference in the number of patients requiring transfusion whether assigned to Regimen A or B, fewer units of blood and/or blood products were required by patients administered Regimen A. In high risk primary CABG surgery patients, only Regimen A was studied.

Trasylol® is supplied as a solution containing 10,000 KIU/mL, which is equal to 1.4 mg/mL. All intravenous doses of Trasylol® should be administered through a central line. **DO NOT ADMINISTER ANY OTHER DRUG USING THE SAME LINE.** Both regimens include a 1 mL test dose, a loading dose, a dose to be added to the priming fluid of the cardiopulmonary bypass circuit ("pump prime" dose), and a constant infusion dose. Regimens A and B (both incorporating a 1 mL test dose) are described in the table below:
[See fourth table from top of page]

The 1 mL test dose should be administered intravenously at least 10 minutes before the loading dose. With the patient in a supine position, the loading dose is given slowly over 20–30 minutes, after induction of anesthesia but prior to sternotomy. When the loading dose is complete, it is followed by the constant infusion dose, which is continued until surgery is complete and the patient leaves the operating room. The "pump prime" dose is added to the priming fluid of the cardiopulmonary bypass circuit, by replacement of an aliquot of the priming fluid, prior to the institution of cardiopulmonary bypass. Total doses of more than 7 million KIU have not been studied in controlled trials.

Parenteral drug products should be inspected visually for particulate matter and discoloration prior to administration whenever solution and container permit. Discard any unused portion.

Renal and Hepatic Impairment: No formal studies of the pharmacokinetics of aprotinin in patients with pre-existing renal insufficiency have been conducted. However, in the placebo-controlled clinical trials conducted in the United States, patients with mildly elevated pretreatment serum creatinine levels did not have a notably higher incidence of clinically significant post-treatment elevations in serum creatinine following either Trasylol® Regimen A or Regimen B compared to administration of the placebo regimen. Changes in aprotinin pharmacokinetics with age or impaired renal function are not great enough to require any dose adjustment. No pharmacokinetic data from patients with pre-existing hepatic disease treated with Trasylol® are available.

COMPATIBILITY

Trasylol® is incompatible *in vitro* with corticosteroids, heparin, tetracyclines, and nutrient solutions containing amino acids or fat emulsion. If Trasylol® is to be given concomitantly with another drug, each drug should be administered separately through different venous lines or catheters.

EVENT	Percentage of patients treated with Trasylol N = 2002	Percentage of patients treated with Placebo N = 1084
Thrombosis	1.0	0.6
Shock	0.7	0.4
Cerebrovascular Accident	0.7	2.1
Thrombophlebitis	0.2	0.5
Deep Thrombophlebitis	0.7	1.0
Lung Edema	1.3	1.5
Pulmonary Embolus	0.3	0.6
Kidney Failure	1.0	0.6
Acute Kidney Failure	0.5	0.6
Kidney Tubular Necrosis	0.8	0.4

Incidence of Myocardial Infarction by Treatment Group Population: All CABG Patients Valid for Safety Analysis

Treatment	Definite MI %	Definite or Probable MI %	Definite, Probable or Possible MI %
Pooled Data from Three Studies that Evaluated Regimen A			
Tryasylol® Regimen A n = 646	4.6	10.7	14.1
Placebo n = 661	4.7	11.3	13.4
Pooled Data from Two Studies that Evaluated Regimen B and Pump Prime Regimen			
Trasylol® Regimen B n = 241	8.7	15.9	18.7
Trasylol® Pump Prime Regimen n = 239	6.3	15.7	18.1
Placebo n = 240	6.3	15.1	15.8

Incidence of Graft Closure, Myocardial Infarction and Death by Treatment Group

	Overall Closure Rates*		Incidence of MI**	Incidence of Death***
	All Centers n = 703 %	U.S. Centers n = 381 %	All Centers n = 831 %	All Centers n = 870 %
Trasylol®	15.4	9.4	2.9	1.4
Placebo	10.9	9.5	3.8	1.6
Cl for the Difference (%) (Drug - Placebo)	(1.3, 9.6)†	(-3.8, 5.9)†	-3.3 to 1.5‡	-1.9 to 1.4‡

* Population: all patients with assessable saphenous vein grafts
** Population: all patients assessable by blinded consultant
*** All patients
† 90%; per protocol
‡ 95%; not specified in protocol

	TEST DOSE	LOADING DOSE	"PUMP PRIME" DOSE	CONSTANT INFUSION DOSE
TRASYLOL® REGIMEN A	1 mL (1.4 mg, or 10,000 KIU)	200 mL (280 mg, or 2.0 million KIU)	200 mL (280 mg, or 2.0 million KIU)	50 mL/hr (70 mg/hr, or 500,000 KIU/hr)
TRASYLOL® REGIMEN B	1 mL (1.4 mg, or 10,000 KIU)	100 mL (140 mg, or 1.0 million KIU)	100 mL (140 mg, or 1.0 million KIU)	25 mL/hr (35 mg/hr, or 250,000 KIU/hr)

HOW SUPPLIED

Size	Strength	NDC
100 mL vials	1,000,000 KIU	0026-8196-36
200 mL vials	2,000,000 KIU	0026-8197-63

STORAGE

Trasylol® should be stored between 2° and 25°C (36°–77°F). Protect from freezing.

Bayer Corporation
Pharmaceutical Division
400 Morgan Lane
West Haven, CT 06516

TRIDESILON® 0.05%
(desonide cream)   ℞

DESCRIPTION

Tridesilon® Cream contains microdispersed desonide (the active ingredient) in a compatible vehicle buffered to the pH range of normal skin. Each gram of Tridesilon® Cream contains 0.5 milligrams of desonide. Tridesilon® Cream is applied topically.

Tridesilon® (desonide) is a non-fluorinated corticosteroid. Chemically, desonide is Pregna-1,4-diene-3,20-dione,11,21-dihydroxy-16, 17-[(1-methylethylidene)bis(oxy)]-, (11β,16α)- with the following structural formula:

The vehicle for Tridesilon® Cream 0.05% contains glycerin, sodium lauryl sulfate, aluminum sulfate, calcium acetate, dextrin, purified water, cetyl stearyl alcohol, synthetic beeswax, (B-wax), white petrolatum, and light mineral oil. Preserved with methylparaben.

EMPIRICAL FORMULA	MOLECULAR WEIGHT	CAS REGISTRY NUMBER
$C_{24}H_{32}O_6$	416.51	638-94-8

CLINICAL PHARMACOLOGY

Topical corticosteroids share anti-inflammatory, anti-pruritic and vasoconstrictive actions.

The mechanism of anti-inflammatory activity of the topical corticosteroids is unclear. Various laboratory methods, including vasoconstrictor assays, are used to compare and predict potencies and/or clinical efficacies of the topical corticosteroids. There is some evidence to suggest that a recognizable correlation exists between vasoconstrictor potency and therapeutic efficacy in man.

Pharmacokinetics

The extent of percutaneous absorption of topical corticosteroids is determined by many factors including the vehicle, the integrity of the epidermal barrier, and the use of occlusive dressings.

Topical corticosteroids can be absorbed from normal intact skin. Inflammation and/or other disease processes in the skin increase percutaneous absorption. Occlusive dressings substantially increase the percutaneous absorption of topical corticosteroids.

Thus, occlusive dressings may be a valuable therapeutic adjunct for treatment of resistant dermatoses. (See DOSAGE AND ADMINISTRATION).

Once absorbed through the skin, topical corticosteroids are handled through pharmacokinetic pathways similar to systemically administered corticosteroids. Corticosteroids are bound to plasma proteins in varying degrees. Corticosteroids are metabolized primarily in the liver and are then excreted by the kidneys. Some of the topical corticosteroids and their metabolites are also excreted into the bile.

INDICATIONS AND USAGE

Topical corticosteroids are indicated for the relief of the inflammatory and pruritic manifestations of corticosteroid-responsive dermatoses.

CONTRAINDICATIONS

Topical corticosteroids are contraindicated in those patients with a history of hypersensitivity to any of the components of the preparation.

PRECAUTIONS
General

Systemic absorption of topical corticosteroids has produced reversible hypothalamic-pituitary-adrenal (HPA) axis suppression, manifestations of Cushing's syndrome, hyperglycemia, and glucosuria in some patients.

Conditions which augment systemic absorption include the application of the more potent steroids, use over large surface areas, prolonged use, and the addition of occlusive dressings.

Therefore, patients receiving a large dose of a potent topical steroid applied to a large surface area or under an occlusive dressing should be evaluated periodically for evidence of HPA axis suppression by using the urinary free cortisol and ACTH stimulation tests. If HPA axis suppression is noted, an attempt should be made to withdraw the drug, to reduce the frequency of application, or to substitute a less potent steroid.

Recovery of HPA axis function is generally prompt and complete upon discontinuation of the drug. Infrequently, signs and symptoms of steroid withdrawal may occur, requiring supplemental systemic corticosteroids.

Children may absorb proportionally larger amounts of topical corticosteroids and thus be more susceptible to systemic toxicity. (See PRECAUTIONS—Pediatric Use).

If irritation develops, topical corticosteroids should be discontinued and appropriate therapy instituted.

In the presence of dermatological infections, the use of an appropriate antifungal or antibacterial agent should be instituted. If a favorable response does not occur promptly, the corticosteroid should be discontinued until the infection has been adequately controlled.

Information for the Patient

Patients using topical corticosteroids should receive the following information and instructions:

1. This medication is to be used as directed by the physician. It is for external use only. Avoid contact with eyes.

2. Patients should be advised not to use this medication for any disorder other than for which it was prescribed.

3. The treated skin area should not be bandaged or otherwise covered or wrapped as to be occlusive unless directed by the physician.

4. Patients should report any signs of local adverse reactions especially under occlusive dressing.

5. Parents of pediatric patients should be advised not to use tight-fitting diapers or plastic pants on a child being treated in the diaper area, as these garments may constitute occlusive dressings.

Laboratory Tests

The following tests may be helpful in evaluating the HPA axis suppression:

Urinary free cortisol test
ACTH stimulation test

Carcinogenesis, Mutagenesis, and Impairment of Fertility

Long-term animal studies have not been performed to evaluate the carcinogenic potential or the effect on fertility of topical corticosteroids.

Studies to determine mutagenicity with prednisolone and hydrocortisone have revealed negative results.

Pregnancy Category C

Corticosteroids are generally teratogenic in laboratory animals when administered systemically at relatively low dosage levels. The more potent corticosteroids have been shown to be teratogenic after dermal application in laboratory animals. There are no adequate and well-controlled studies in pregnant women on teratogenic effects from topically applied corticosteroids. Therefore, topical corticosteroids should be used during pregnancy only if the potential benefit justifies the potential risk to the fetus. Drugs of this class should not be used extensively on pregnant patients, in large amounts, or for prolonged periods of time.

Nursing Mothers

It is not known whether topical administration of corticosteroids could result in sufficient systemic absorption to produce detectable quantities in breast milk. Systemically administered corticosteroids are secreted into breast milk in quantities *not* likely to have a deleterious effect on the infant. Nevertheless, caution should be exercised when topical corticosteroids are administered to a nursing woman.

Pediatric Use

Pediatric patients may demonstrate greater susceptibility to topical corticosteroid-induced HPA axis suppression and Cushing's syndrome than mature patients because of a larger skin surface area to body weight ratio.

Hypothalamic-pituitary-adrenal (HPA) axis suppression, Cushing's syndrome, and intracranial hypertension have been reported in children receiving topical corticosteroids. Manifestations of adrenal supression in children include linear growth retardation, delayed weight gain, low plasma cortisol levels, and absence of response to ACTH stimulation. Manifestations of intracranial hypertension include bulging fontanelles, headaches, and bilateral papilledema. Administration of topical corticosteroids to children should be limited to the least amount compatible with an effective therapeutic regimen. Chronic corticosteroid therapy may interfere with the growth and development of children.

ADVERSE REACTIONS

The following local adverse reactions are reported infrequently with topical corticosteroids, but may occur more frequently with the use of occlusive dressings. These reactions are listed in an approximate decreasing order of occurrence:

Burning
Itching
Irritation
Dryness
Folliculitis
Hypertrichosis
Acneiform eruptions
Hypopigmentation
Perioral dermatitis
Allergic contact dermatitis
Maceration of the skin
Secondary infection

Skin atrophy
Striae
Miliaria

OVERDOSAGE

Topically applied corticosteroids can be absorbed in sufficient amounts to produce systemic effects. (See PRECAUTIONS).

DOSAGE AND ADMINISTRATION

Topical corticosteroids are generally applied to the affected area as a thin film from two to four times daily depending on the severity of the condition.

Occlusive dressings may be used for management of psoriasis or recalcitrant conditions.

If an infection develops, the use of occlusive dressings should be discontinued and appropriate antimicrobial therapy instituted.

HOW SUPPLIED

Tridesilon® (desonide) Cream 0.05% is supplied in 15 and 60 gram tubes and in 5 pound jars. It is a white semi-solid.
Store below 86°F (30°C), avoid freezing.

	NDC Number
15g	0026-5561-61
60g	0026-5561-62
5lb	0026-5561-92

Bayer Corporation
Pharmaceutical Division
400 Morgan Lane
West Haven, CT 06516 USA

CAUTION

Federal (USA) law prohibits dispensing without a prescription.
PD500007   3/95   5064
© 1995 Bayer Corporation

TRIDESILON® 0.05%
(desonide ointment)   ℞

DESCRIPTION

Tridesilon® Ointment contains microdispersed desonide (the active ingredient) in white petrolatum. Each gram of Tridesilon® Ointment contains 0.5 milligrams of desonide. Tridesilon® Ointment is applied topically.

Tridesilon® (desonide) is a non-fluorinated corticosteroid. Chemically, desonide is Pregna-1,4-diene-3,20-dione, 11,21-dihydroxy-16,17- [(1-methylethylidene)bis(oxy)] -,11β, 16-α)- with the following structural formula:

EMPIRICAL FORMULA	MOLECULAR WEIGHT	CAS REGISTRY NUMBER
$C_{24}H_{32}O_6$	416.51	638-94-8

CLINICAL PHARMACOLOGY

Topical corticosteroids share anti-inflammatory, anti-pruritic and vasoconstrictive actions.

The mechanism of anti-inflammatory activity of the topical corticosteroids is unclear. Various laboratory methods, including vasoconstrictor assays, are used to compare and predict potencies and/or clinical efficacies of the topical corticosteroids. There is some evidence to suggest that a recognizable correlation exists between vasoconstrictor potency and therapeutic efficacy in man.

Pharmacokinetics

The extent of percutaneous absorption of topical corticosteroids is determined by many factors including the vehicle, the integrity of the epidermal barrier, and the use of occlusive dressings.

Topical corticosteroids can be absorbed from normal intact skin. Inflammation and/or other disease processes in the skin increase percutaneous absorption. Occlusive dressings substantially increase the percutaneous absorption of topical corticosteroids. Thus, occlusive dressings may be a valuable therapeutic adjunct for treatment of resistant dermatoses. (See DOSAGE AND ADMINISTRATION).

Once absorbed through the skin, topical corticosteroids are handled through pharmacokinetic pathways similar to systemically administered corticosteroids. Corticosteroids are bound to plasma proteins in varying degrees. Corticosteroids are metabolized primarily in the liver and are then excreted by the kidneys. Some of the topical corticosteroids and their metabolites are also excreted into the bile.

Continued on next page

Tridesilon Ointment—Cont.

INDICATIONS AND USAGE

Topical corticosteroids are indicated for the relief of the inflammatory and pruritic manifestations of corticosteroid-responsive dermatoses.

CONTRAINDICATIONS

Topical corticosteroids are contraindicated in those patients with a history of hypersensitivity to any of the components of the preparation.

PRECAUTIONS

General

Systemic absorption of topical corticosteroids has produced reversible hypothalamic-pituitary-adrenal (HPA) axis suppression, manifestations of Cushing's syndrome, hyperglycemia, and glucosuria in some patients.

Conditions which augment systemic absorption include the application of the more potent steroids, use over large surface areas, prolonged use, and the addition of occlusive dressings.

Therefore, patients receiving a large dose of a potent topical steroid applied to a large surface area or under an occlusive dressing should be evaluated periodically for evidence of HPA axis suppression by using the urinary free cortisol and ACTH stimulation tests. If HPA axis suppression is noted, an attempt should be made to withdraw the drug, to reduce the frequency of application, or to substitute a less potent steroid.

Recovery of HPA axis function is generally prompt and complete upon discontinuation of the drug. Infrequently, signs and symptoms of steroid withdrawal may occur, requiring supplemental systemic corticosteroids.

Children may absorb proportionally larger amounts of topical corticosteroids and thus be more susceptible to systemic toxicity. (See PRECAUTIONS—Pediatric Use.)

If irritation develops, topical corticosteroids should be discontinued and appropriate therapy instituted.

In the presence of dermatological infections, the use of an appropriate antifungal or antibacterial agent should be instituted. If a favorable response does not occur promptly, the corticosteroid should be discontinued until the infection has been adequately controlled.

Information for the Patient

Patients using topical corticosteroids should receive the following information and instructions:

1. This medication is to be used as directed by the physician. It is for external use only. Avoid contact with the eyes.
2. Patients should be advised not to use this medication for any disorder other than for which it was prescribed.
3. The treated skin area should not be bandaged or otherwise covered or wrapped as to be occlusive unless directed by the physician.
4. Patients should report any signs of local adverse reactions especially under occlusive dressing.
5. Parents of pediatric patients should be advised not to use tight-fitting diapers or plastic pants on a child being treated in the diaper area, as these garments may constitute occlusive dressings.

Laboratory Tests

The following tests may be helpful in evaluating the HPA axis suppression:

Urinary free cortisol test
ACTH stimulation test

Carcinogenesis, Mutagenesis, and Impairment of Fertility

Long-term animal studies have not been performed to evaluate the carcinogenic potential or the effect on fertility of topical corticosteroids.

Studies to determine mutagenicity with prednisolone and hydrocortisone have revealed negative results.

Pregnancy Category C

Corticosteroids are generally teratogenic in laboratory animals when administered systemically at relatively low dosage levels. The more potent corticosteroids have been shown to be teratogenic after dermal application in laboratory animals. There are no adequate and well-controlled studies in pregnant women on teratogenic effects from topically applied corticosteroids. Therefore, topical corticosteroids should be used during pregnancy only if the potential benefit justifies the potential risk to the fetus. Drugs of this class should not be used extensively on pregnant patients, in large amounts, or for prolonged periods of time.

Nursing Mothers

It is not known whether topical administration of corticosteroids could result in sufficient systemic absorption to produce detectable quantities in breast milk. Systemically administered corticosteroids are secreted into breast milk in quantities *not* likely to have a deleterious effect on the infant. Nevertheless, caution should be exercised when topical corticosteroids are administered to a nursing woman.

Pediatric Use

Pediatric patients may demonstrate greater susceptibility to topical corticosteroid-induced HPA axis suppression and Cushing's syndrome than mature patients because of a larger skin surface to body weight ratio.

Hypothalamic-pituitary-adrenal (HPA) axis suppression, Cushing's syndrome, and intracranial hypertension have

been reported in children receiving topical corticosteroids. Manifestations of adrenal suppression in children include linear growth retardation, delayed weight gain, low plasma cortisol levels, and absence of response to ACTH stimulation. Manifestations of intracranial hypertension include bulging fontanelles, headaches, and bilateral papilledema. Administration of topical corticosteroids to children should be limited to the least amount compatible with an effective therapeutic regimen. Chronic corticosteroid therapy may interfere with the growth and development of children.

ADVERSE REACTIONS

The following local adverse reactions are reported infrequently with topical corticosteroids, but may occur more frequently with the use of occlusive dressings. These reactions are listed in an approximate decreasing order of occurrence:

Burning
Itching
Irritation
Dryness
Folliculitis
Hypertrichosis
Acneiform eruptions
Hypopigmentation
Perioral dermatitis
Allergic contact dermatitis
Maceration of the skin
Secondary infection
Skin atrophy
Striae
Miliaria

OVERDOSAGE

Topically applied corticosteroids can be absorbed in sufficient amounts to produce systemic effects. (See PRECAUTIONS).

DOSAGE AND ADMINISTRATION

Topical corticosteroids are generally applied to the affected area as a thin film from two to four times daily depending on the severity of the condition.

Occlusive dressings may be used for the management of psoriasis or recalcitrant conditions.

If an infection develops, the use of occlusive dressings should be discontinued and appropriate antimicrobial therapy instituted.

HOW SUPPLIED

Tridesilon® (desonide) Ointment 0.05% is supplied in 15 and 60 gram tubes. It is white or faintly yellowish, transparent semisolid.

Store below 86°F (30°C). Avoid freezing.

	NDC Number
15g	0026-5591-61
60g	0026-5591-62

Bayer Corporation
Pharmaceutical Division
400 Morgan Lane
West Haven, CT 06516

CAUTION: Federal (USA) law prohibits dispensing without a prescription.

PD500008   3/95
© 1995 Bayer Corporation   5066

Bayer Corporation
Pharmaceutical Division
Allergy Products
**400 MORGAN LANE
WEST HAVEN, CT 06516**

For Medical Information Contact:
Director, Medical Services
(800) 468-0894
(203) 812-2000

ANA-KIT®   ℞
ANAPHYLAXIS EMERGENCY TREATMENT KIT

DESCRIPTION

Epinephrine Injection, USP, (1:1000), contained in a sterile, 1 mL syringe, designed to deliver 2 doses of 0.3 mL each. Product is intended for subcutaneous or intramuscular use. Each mL of Epinephrine Injection, USP, (1:1000) contains 1 mg *l*-epinephrine as the hydrochloride, 8.5 mg sodium chloride, not more than 5 mg chlorobutanol (chloral derivative) and 1.5 mg sodium bisulfite. Sealed under nitrogen.

Epinephrine is a sympathomimetic catecholamine. Its naturally occurring levo isomer, which is twenty times as active as the *d* isomer, is now obtained in pure form by separation from the synthetically produced racemate.

Chemically, epinephrine is 1-(3,4-dihydroxyphenyl)-2-(methylamino)ethanol with the following structure:

Chlo-Amine® Chlorpheniramine Maleate Tablets: 4 chewable tablets, each containing 2 mg chlorpheniramine maleate, USP, for oral administration. Contains FD&C Yellow No. 6 (Sunset Yellow) as a color additive. Chlorpheniramine maleate is an antihistamine having the chemical name *y*-(4-chlorophenyl)-N,N-dimethyl-2-pyridinepropanamine, (Z)-2-butenedioate(1:1) with the following structure:

DEVICES: 2 sterile pads containing isopropyl alcohol 70% by volume. One tourniquet.

CLINICAL PHARMACOLOGY

EPINEPHRINE: The most valuable drug for the emergency treatment of severe allergic reactions is epinephrine. The vasoconstrictor effect of epinephrine on the capillary directly antagonizes the generalized vasodilation produced by histamine. Epinephrine reverses the increased permeability of dilated capillaries to plasma. The shock of severe allergic reactions is due to the loss of circulating blood volume by pooling in the dilated capillary beds and loss of plasma into the tissues. Epinephrine quickly restores circulating blood volume and blood pressure by constricting the capillary bed. The itching during episodes of hives or angioedema is promptly relieved by epinephrine. Epinephrine is a powerful relaxer of the smooth muscle of the bronchioles, stomach, intestine, pregnant uterus and urinary bladder wall. The bronchospasm, wheezing and dyspnea of the acute allergic reactions are relieved. Where abdominal cramping, defecation or involuntary urination have occurred during severe allergic attacks, epinephrine rapidly produces relief. Subcutaneously or intramuscularly administered epinephrine has a rapid onset and short duration of action. Subcutaneous administration during asthmatic attacks may produce bronchodilation within 5 to 10 minutes, and maximal effects may occur within 20 minutes.

CHLO-AMINE®: Chlo-Amine® is an effective agent in nullifying the characteristic effects of histamine and is especially valuable in the prophylaxis and relief of many allergic symptoms. It is readily absorbed from the intestinal tract and released into the tissues from the bloodstream. This action is both prompt and sustained. Elimination of the drug is such that there is a low incidence of side effects.

INDICATIONS AND USAGE

Ana-Kit® Anaphylaxis Emergency Treatment Kit is indicated for use by adult and pediatric patients under the following situations:

1. Allergic reactions including anaphylactic shock due to stinging insects (primarily of the Hymenoptera order, which includes bees, wasps, hornets, yellow jackets, bumble bees, and fire ants).
2. Severe allergic or anaphylactoid reactions due to allergy injections, exposures to pollens, dusts, molds, foods, drugs, and exercise or unknown substances (so-called idiopathic anaphylaxis).
3. Severe, life-threatening asthma attacks characterized by wheezing, dyspnea and inability to breathe.

In the sensitive patient, severe allergic reactions and anaphylactic shock may occur within minutes of the insect sting or exposure to an allergenic substance.

Symptoms may include bronchoconstriction, wheezing, sneezing, hoarseness, urticaria, angioedema, erythema, pruritis, tachycardia, thready pulse, falling blood pressure, sense of oppression or impending doom, disorientation, cramping abdominal pain, incontinance, faintness, loss of consciousness.

The Ana-Kit® is compactly designed to be carried and used by patients when severe symptoms arise, and the patient is out of reach of immediate attention by a doctor or hospital.

CONTRAINDICATIONS

EPINEPHRINE: Epinephrine must not be given intra-arterially as marked vasoconstriction may result in gangrene. **This unit is not intended for intravenous use.** Further dilution would be necessary and is not practical with this emergency syringe.

Epinephrine Injection, USP, (1:1000) must not be used if there is hypersensitivity to any of the components.

Epinephrine is contraindicated in narrow-angle glaucoma; cardiogenic, traumatic, or hemorrhagic shock; cardiac dilation; cerebral arteriosclerosis; and organic brain damage.

Epinephrine should not be used to counteract circulatory collapse or hypotension due to phenothiazines, since such agents may reverse the pressor effect of epinephrine, leading to a further lowering of blood pressure.
Epinephrine should not be administered concomitantly with other sympathomimetic agents, since the effects are additive and may be detrimental to the patient.
CHLO-AMINE®: No known contraindications.

WARNINGS

EPINEPHRINE: Overdosage or accidental intravenous administration of conventional subcutaneous doses may induce severe or fatal hypertension, or cerebrovascular hemorrhage. Fatalities may also occur from pulmonary edema resulting from peripheral constriction and cardiac stimulation. The marked pressor effects may be counteracted by use of rapidly acting vasodilators, such as the nitrites and alpha-adrenergic blockers.
Deaths have been reported in asthmatics treated with epinephrine following the use of isoproterenol or orciprenaline.
Epinephrine is the preferred treatment for serious allergic or other emergency situations even though this product contains sodium bisulfite, a sulfite that may in other products cause allergic-type reactions including anaphylactic symptoms or life-threatening or less severe asthmatic episodes in certain susceptible persons. The alternatives to using epinephrine in a life-threatening situation may not be satisfactory. The presence of a sulfite(s) in this product should not deter administration of the drug for treatment of serious allergic or other emergency situations.
Epinephrine must be administered with great caution, if at all, in patients with cardiac arrhythmias, coronary artery or organic heart disease, and hypertension. In patients with coronary insufficiency or ischemic heart disease, epinephrine may precipitate or aggravate angina pectoris as well as produce potentially fatal ventricular arrhythmias. Epinephrine should be administered only with great caution to elderly patients, those with diabetes mellitus, hyperthyroidism or psychoneurotic disorders; also to those with longstanding bronchial asthma or emphysema if such individuals may also have degenerative heart disease, and to pregnant women (see "Pregnancy").
CHLO-AMINE®: Chlorpheniramine maleate should be used with extreme caution in patients with stenosing peptic ulcer, pyloroduodenal obstruction, prostatic hypertrophy, or bladder neck obstruction. These compounds have an atropine-like action and therefore should be used with caution in patients with a history of increased intraocular pressure, cardiovascular disease, or hypertension. The asthmatic patient should take the chlorpheniramine maleate tablets with caution.

PRECAUTIONS

GENERAL: Ana-Kit® is not intended to be a substitute for medical attention or hospital care. The kit is designed to be compact and easy to carry, and to provide emergency treatment when medical care is not immediately available.
Highly sensitive individuals should have the kit readily available at all times. Because of its small size it can be carried by outdoor sportsmen, golfers, gardeners, or any sensitive individual who may be exposed to stinging insects (wasps, hornets, yellow jackets, fire ants or bees) or other potentially life-threatening allergens. The drugs in the Ana-Kit®, when used as directed immediately following exposure to an allergen, may prove life-saving. Certain changes in the emergency instructions and in the kit itself may be made by the doctor according to the needs of the patient. IN ALL CASES THE PHYSICIAN SHOULD INSTRUCT THE PATIENT, AND/OR ANY OTHER PERSON WHO MIGHT BE IN A POSITION TO ADMINISTER THE EPINEPHRINE, IN THE PROPER USE OF THE SYRINGE AND THE OTHER COMPONENTS OF THIS KIT.
INFORMATION FOR PATIENTS: Complete patient information, including dosage, directions for proper administration, and precautions, can be found at the end of this package insert, as well as inside each Ana-Kit® kit.
Since epinephrine injection may produce disturbing or frightening reactions, it may be desirable to forewarn patients. Reactions commonly include an increase in pulse rate, a more forceful heartbeat, palpitations, a throbbing headache, pallor, feelings of overstimulation, anxiety, weakness, shakiness, dizziness, or nausea. Symptoms not involving an overdose generally do not indicate anything serious and usually subside rapidly with rest, quiet, and recumbency. Patients with hypertension or hyperthyroidism are prone to more severe or persistent effects, as are patients with coronary-artery disease, who may experience angina. Psychoneurotic patients may experience a worsening of symptoms. Diabetic patients may require an increased dose of insulin or other antidiabetic medication. Patients with Parkinson's disease may notice a temporary worsening of symptoms.
DRUG INTERACTIONS: Caution is indicated in patients receiving cardiac glycosides or mercurial diuretics, since these agents may sensitize the myocardium to beta-adrenergic stimulation and make cardiac arrhythmias more likely.
The effects of epinephrine may be potentiated by tricyclic antidepressants, sodium levothyroxine, and certain antihistamines, notably chlorpheniramine, tripelennamine, and diphenhydramine.
The cardiostimulating and bronchodilating effects of epinephrine are antagonized by beta-adrenergic blocking drugs, such as propranolol. The vasoconstricting and hypertensive effects are antagonized by alpha-adrenergic blocking drugs, such as phentolamine. Ergot alkaloids and phenothiazines may also reverse the pressor effects of epinephrine.
Diabetic patients receiving epinephrine may require an increased dose of insulin or oral hypoglycemic drugs.
Carcinogenesis, Mutagenesis, Impairment of Fertility: There are no data from either animal or human studies regarding the carcinogenicity or mutagenicity of epinephrine or Chlo-Amine®, and no studies have been conducted to determine their potential for the impairment of fertility.
Pregnancy: Teratogenic Effects. Pregnancy Category C—Epinephrine has been shown to be teratogenic in rats and hamsters at dose levels hundreds of times as high as the maximal human dose. Although there are no adequate or well-controlled studies in pregnant women, epinephrine crosses the placenta and its use during pregnancy may cause anoxia in the fetus. Epinephrine should be used in pregnancy only if the potential benefit justifies the potential risk to the fetus.
Pediatric Use: Administer Epinephrine or Chlo-Amine® with caution to infants and children (see "Dosage and Administration"). Syncope has occurred following the administration of epinephrine to asthmatic children.

ADVERSE REACTIONS

EPINEPHRINE: Adverse reactions include transient, moderate anxiety, apprehensiveness, restlessness, tremor, weakness, dizziness, sweating, palpitations, pallor, nausea and vomiting, headache, and respiratory difficulties. These symptoms occur in some persons receiving therapeutic doses of epinephrine, but are more likely to occur, or to occur in exaggerated form, in those with hypertension or hyperthyroidism. Excessive doses cause acute hypertension. Arrhythmias, including fatal ventricular fibrillation, have been reported, particularly in patients with underlying cardiac disease or those receiving certain drugs (see "Drug Interactions").
Rapid rises in blood pressure have produced cerebral hemorrhage, particularly in elderly patients with cerebrovascular disease. Angina may occur in patients with coronary-artery disease.
CHLO-AMINE®: Drowsiness, dizziness, blurred vision, dry mouth and gastrointestinal upsets may occur. Patients should not drive or operate machinery after taking the drug. Large doses produce central nervous system depression and occasionally tremors or convulsions. Reports of hematological disorders are rare.

OVERDOSAGE

EPINEPHRINE: Epinephrine is rapidly inactivated in the body, and treatment is primarily supportive. If necessary, pressor effects may be counteracted by rapidly acting vasodilators or alpha-adrenergic blocking drugs. If prolonged hypotension follows such measures, it may be necessary to administer another pressor drug, such as levarterenol.
Overdosage of epinephrine may produce extremely elevated arterial pressure, which may result in cerebrovascular hemorrhage, particularly in elderly patients.
If an epinephrine overdose induces pulmonary edema that interferes with respiration, treatment consists of a rapidly acting alpha-adrenergic blocking drug such as phentolamine and/or intermittent positive-pressure respiration.
Epinephrine overdosage can also cause transient bradycardia followed by tachycardia, and these may be accompanied by potentially fatal cardiac arrhythmias. Ventricular premature contractions may appear within one minute after injection and may be followed by multilocal ventricular tachycardia (prefibrillation rhythm). Subsidence of the ventricular effects may be followed by atrial tachycardia and occasionally by atrioventricular block. Treatment of arrhythmias consists of administration of beta-adrenergic blocking drug such as propranolol.
Overdosage sometimes also results in extreme pallor and coldness of the skin, metabolic acidosis, and kidney failure. Suitable corrective measures must be taken.
CHLO-AMINE®: Overdose symptoms may be sedation, apnea, cardiovascular collapse to stimulation, insomnia, hallucinations, tremors or convulsions. Also there may be dizziness, tinnitus, ataxia, blurred vision, hypotension, dry mouth, flushing, and abdominal symptoms.
Treatment—The patient should be induced to vomit, preferably with ipecac syrup—and large amounts of water. Prevent aspiration of vomitus. Gastric lavage may be necessary using activated charcoal and saline. Hyperosmotic cathartics such as Milk of Magnesia may hasten elimination of residual cling. Vasopressors can be used to correct hypotension. Diazepam may be used to control seizures. Hyperpyrexia can be treated with cool sponges or a hypothermic blanket.

DOSAGE AND ADMINISTRATION

Parenteral drug products should be inspected visually for particulate matter and discoloration prior to administration, whenever solution and container permit. Do not use Epinephrine Injection, USP, if it has a pinkish or darker than slightly yellow color or contains a precipitate.
The physician who prescribes the Ana-Kit® should review the package insert in detail with the patient. This review should include the proper use of the 2-dose epinephrine syringe to insure that subcutaneous or intramuscular injections are given into the deltoid region of the arm or the anteriolateral aspect of the thigh. See also the PATIENT DIRECTIONS FOR USE.
EPINEPHRINE: For subcutaneous or intramuscular injection only.
Adults and children over 12 years: 0.3 mL; 6–12 years: 0.2 mL; 2–6 years: 0.15 mL; Infants to 2 years: 0.05 to 0.1 mL.
When syringe is properly set up, as directed in the Patient Instruction Sheet, a 0.3 mL dose is administered when plunger is pushed until it stops. Syringe barrel has 0.1 mL graduations so that smaller doses can be measured. (Operation of syringe is explained in the Patient Directions For Use section at the end of this package insert.)
If after 10 minutes from the first injection symptoms are not noticeably improved, administer a second dose of epinephrine from the syringe.
CHLO-AMINE®: Tablets are chewable antihistamines. Adults and children over 12 years: 4 tablets; children 6–12 years: 2 tablets; children under 6 years: 1 tablet.

HOW SUPPLIED

ANA-KIT® ANAPHYLAXIS EMERGENCY TREATMENT KIT CONTAINS:
SYRINGE: One sterile syringe containing 1 mL Epinephrine Injection, USP, (1:1000). Syringe delivers two 0.3 mL doses.
TABLETS: Four 2 mg chewable Chlo-Amine® tablets, Chlorpheniramine Maleate Tablets.
DEVICES: Two sterile pads containing 70% isopropyl alcohol (by volume) and 1 tourniquet.
PROTECT FROM LIGHT. STORE AT ROOM TEMPERATURE, APPROX. 25°C (77°F). PROTECT FROM FREEZING.
CAUTION: U.S. Federal Law Prohibits Dispensing Without Prescription.

Epinephrine Mfg. by: Wyeth-Ayerst Laboratories,
Philadelphia, PA 19101
Pkgd. and Dist. by:
Bayer Corporation
Pharmaceutical Division
Spokane, WA 99207 USA

PATIENT DIRECTIONS FOR USE

ANA-KIT® Anaphylaxis Emergency Treatment Kit
(Please read entire direction sheet before an emergency arises.)

The Ana-Kit® **IS TO BE USED ONLY WHEN PRESCRIBED BY A PHYSICIAN,** for patients who are highly allergic to pollens, foods, dusts, insect stings, and drugs which may produce a life-threatening anaphylactic reaction, or have severe asthma attacks.
IN THE EVENT OF A LIFE-THREATENING SITUATION, FOLLOW THESE STEPS IMMEDIATELY TO ADMINISTER THE EPINEPHRINE.

1. **Remove (pull off) blue plastic needle cover. Hold syringe upright and push plunger to expel air and excess epinephrine (plunger will stop).**

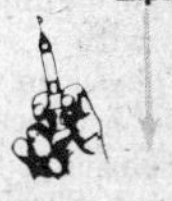

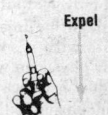

Expel

2. **Rotate rectangular plunger 1/4 turn to the right. Plunger will align with slot in barrel of syringe. Wipe injection site with alcohol swab.**

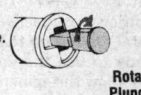

Rotate Plunger

3. **Insert needle straight into arm or thigh as illustrated.**

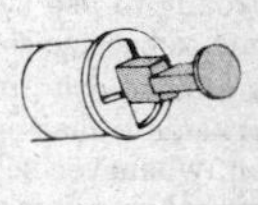

4. **Push plunger until it stops. Syringe will inject a 0.3 mL dose for adults and children over 12 years. Children: Syringe barrel has 0.1 mL graduations so that smaller doses can be measured. Administer to infants to 2 years: 0.05 to 0.1 mL; 2–6 years: 0.15 mL; and 6–12 years: 0.2 mL.**

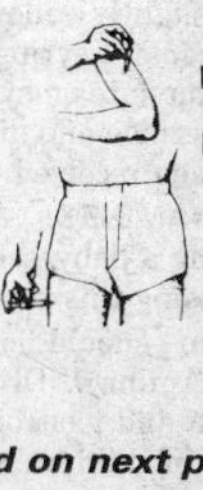

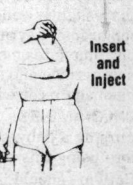

Insert and Inject

Continued on next page

Ana-Kit—Cont.

ONCE THE INITIAL EPINEPHRINE INJECTION HAS BEEN ADMINISTERED, FOLLOW THESE ADDITIONAL STEPS.

5. CONTACT PHYSICIAN, IF POSSIBLE.
6. REMOVE STINGER if stung by insect. (Use fingernails. DO NOT push, pinch or squeeze, or further imbed the stinger into the skin as this may cause further venom to be injected.)

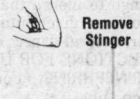
Remove Stinger

7. APPLY TOURNIQUET. If exposure to life-threatening agent was by injection (allergenic extract, drug) or insect sting on an arm or leg, place tourniquet between injection or sting site and body. Do not obstruct arterial blood flow with the tourniquet. (If exposure is elsewhere—neck, face, body—proceed immediately to Step 9.)

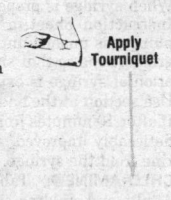
Apply Tourniquet

8. TIGHTEN TOURNIQUET. To tighten, pull on the end of ONE STRING. Then, at least every ten minutes, loosen the tourniquet by pulling on the small metal ring.
9. CHEW AND SWALLOW CHLO-AMINE® TABLETS. For adults and children over 12 years, take 4 tablets; children 6–12 years take 2 tablets; children under 6 years take 1 tablet. These tablets are chewable antihistamine which is generally tolerated.

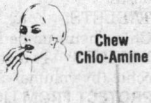
Chew Chlo-Amine

10. PREPARE SYRINGE FOR A POSSIBLE SECOND INJECTION. Turn the rectangular plunger $\frac{1}{4}$ turn to the right to line up with rectangular slot in the syringe. (A slight wiggling may aid the turning and alignment of the plunger.)

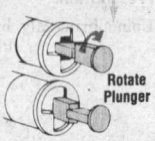
Rotate Plunger

11. THE SECOND INJECTION. If after 10 minutes from the first injection symptoms are not noticeably improved, a second injection is required. Cleanse skin area with alcohol swab and make second injection as in STEPS 3 and 4 for the first epinephrine injection. (A small amount of epinephrine will remain in syringe after the second dose and cannot be expelled.) **Note: Dispose of syringe and remaining contents if second injection is not required.**
12. APPLY ICE PACKS IF AVAILABLE, AT THE SITE OF THE DRUG OR ALLERGY INJECTION, OR INSECT STING (if applicable).
13. KEEP PATIENT WARM AND AVOID EXERTION.

PRECAUTIONS

EPINEPHRINE: For subcutaneous or intramuscular injection only. **Not intended for intravenous use.**

Epinephrine Injection, USP, contains sodium bisulfite. Patients with a suspected sulfite sensitivity should consult their physician well in advance before the need to use this product becomes critical.

Epinephrine is light sensitive and should be stored in box provided. STORE AT ROOM TEMPERATURE, approximately 25°C (77°F). Protect from freezing. Any epinephrine solution in contact with the needle may cause rusting of the metal. **Do not try to force air out of the syringe until you are ready to use the epinephrine.** This may rupture the seal and allow the epinephrine solution to contact the metal promoting deterioration. **Never remove cover from needle until ready to use syringe** as this may cause needle and contents to become contaminated.

Parenteral drug products should be inspected visually for particulate matter and discoloration prior to administration, whenever solution and container permit. Do not use Epinephrine Injection, USP, if it has a pinkish or darker than slightly yellow color or contains a precipitate. Obtain replacement syringe from physician. Periodically check expiration date on syringe. If expiration date is near, re-order new syringe and discard outdated syringe after new syringe has been received.

CHLO-AMINE®: As with any drug, if you are pregnant or nursing a baby, seek the advice of a health professional before using this product.

Patients should not drive or operate machinery after taking Chlo-Amine®. Drowsiness, dizziness, blurred vision, dry mouth and gastrointestinal upsets may occur. Keep out of reach of children.

The asthmatic patient should take the chlorpheniramine maleate tablets with caution.

LIMITED WARRANTY: A number of factors beyond our control could reduce the efficacy of this product or even result in an ill effect following its use. These include storage and handling of the product after it leaves our hands, diagnosis, dosage, method of administration and biological differences in individual patients. Because of these factors, it is important that this product be stored properly and that the directions be followed carefully during use.

No warranty, express or implied, including any warranty of merchantability or fitness, is made. Representatives or the Company are not authorized to vary the terms or the contents of any printed labeling, including the package insert, for this product except by printed notice from the Company's headquarters. The prescriber and user of this product must accept the terms hereof.

Epinephrine Mfg. by: Wyeth-Ayerst Laboratories, Philadelphia, PA 19101

Pkgd. and Dist. by:
Bayer Corporation
Pharmaceutical Division
Spokane, WA 99207 USA

Hollister-Stier®

From 471103 B07   12/95   Printed in U.S.A.
Shown in Product Identification Guide, page 305

Bayer Corporation Pharmaceutical Division Biological Products

400 MORGAN LANE
WEST HAVEN, CT 06516

For Medical Information Contact:
Director, Medical Services
(800) 468-0894
(203) 937-2000

BAYHEP B™   ℞
[*bāy-hep "*]
Hepatitis B Immune Globulin (Human)

DESCRIPTION

Hepatitis B Immune Globulin (Human)—BayHep B™ treated with solvent/detergent is a sterile solution of hepatitis B hyperimmune immune globulin for intramuscular administration; it contains no preservative. BayHep B is prepared by cold ethanol fractionation from the plasma of donors with high titers of antibody to the hepatitis B surface antigen (anti-HBs). The immune globulin is isolated from solubilized Cohn Fraction II. The Fraction II solution is adjusted to a final concentration of 0.3% tri-n-butyl phosphate (TNBP) and 0.2% sodium cholate. After the addition of solvent (TNBP) and detergent (sodium cholate), the solution is heated to 30°C and maintained at that temperature for not less than 6 hours. After the viral inactivation step, the reactants are removed by precipitation, filtration and finally ultrafiltration and diafiltration. BayHep B is formulated as a 15–18% protein solution at a pH of 6.4–7.2 in 0.21–0.32 M glycine. BayHep B is then incubated in the final container for 21–28 days at 20–27°C. Each vial contains anti-HBs antibody equivalent to or exceeding the potency of anti-HBs in a U.S. reference hepatitis B immune globulin (Center for Biologics Evaluation and Research, FDA). The U.S. reference has been tested against the World Health Organization standard Hepatitis B Immune Globulin and found to be equal to 217 international units (IU) per mL.

The removal and inactivation of spiked model enveloped and non-enveloped viruses during the manufacturing process for BayHep B has been validated in laboratory studies. Human Immunodeficiency Virus, Type 1 (HIV-1), was chosen as the relevant virus for blood products; Bovine Viral Diarrhea Virus (BVDV) was chosen to model Hepatitis C virus; Pseudorabies virus (PRV) was chosen to model Hepatitis B virus and the Herpes viruses; and Reo virus type 3 (Reo) was chosen to model non-enveloped viruses and for its resistance to physical and chemical inactivation. Significant removal of model enveloped and non-enveloped viruses is achieved at two steps in the Cohn fractionation process leading to the collection of Cohn Fraction II: the precipitation and removal of Fraction III in the processing of Fraction II + IIIW suspension to Effluent III and the filtration step in the processing of Effluent III to Filtrate III. Significant inactivation of enveloped viruses is achieved at the time of treatment of solubilized Cohn Fraction II with TNBP/sodium cholate.

CLINICAL PHARMACOLOGY

Hepatitis B Immune Globulin (Human) provides passive immunization for individuals exposed to the hepatitis B virus (HBV) as evidenced by a reduction in the attack rate of hepatitis B following its use.[1-6] The administration of the usual recommended dose of this immune globulin generally results in a detectable level of circulating anti-HBs which persists for approximately 2 months or longer. The highest antibody (IgG) serum levels were seen in the following distribution of subjects studied:[7]

DAY	% OF SUBJECTS
3	38%
7	41.7%
14	11.1%
21	8.3%

Mean values for half-life were between 17.5 and 25 days, with the shortest being 5.9 days and the longest 35 days.[7] Cases of type B hepatitis are rarely seen following exposure to HBV in persons with pre-existing anti-HBs. No confirmed instance of transmission of hepatitis B has been associated with this product.

In a clinical study in eight healthy human adults receiving another hyperimmune immune globulin product treated with solvent/detergent, Rabies Immune Globulin (Human), BayRab™, prepared by the same manufacturing process, detectable passive antibody titers were observed in the serum of all subjects by 24 hours post injection and persisted through the 21 day study period. These results suggest that passive immunization with immune globulin products is not affected by the solvent/detergent treatment.

INDICATIONS AND USAGE

Recommendations on post-exposure prophylaxis are based on available efficacy data and on the likelihood of future HBV exposure for the person requiring treatment. In all exposures, a regimen combining Hepatitis B Immune Globulin (Human) with hepatitis B vaccine will provide both short-and long-term protection, will be less costly than the two-dose Hepatitis B Immune Globulin (Human) treatment alone, and is the treatment of choice.[8]

BayHep B is indicated for post-exposure prophylaxis in the following situations:

Acute Exposure to Blood Containing HBsAg

After either parenteral exposure, e.g., by accidental "needlestick" or direct mucous membrane contact (accidental splash), or oral ingestion (pipetting accident) involving HBsAg-positive materials such as blood, plasma or serum. For inadvertent percutaneous exposure, a regimen of two doses of Hepatitis B Immune Globulin (Human), one given after exposure and one a month later, is about 75% effective in preventing hepatitis B in this setting.

Perinatal Exposure of Infants Born to HBsAg-positive Mothers

Infants born to HBsAg-positive mothers are at risk of being infected with hepatitis B virus and becoming chronic carriers.[5,8,9,10] This risk is especially great if the mother is HBeAg-positive.[11,12,13] For an infant with perinatal exposure to an HBsAg-positive and HBeAg-positive mother, a regimen combining one dose of Hepatitis B Immune Globulin (Human) at birth with the hepatitis B vaccine series started soon after birth is 85%–95% effective in preventing development of the HBV carrier state.[8,14] Regimens involving either multiple doses of Hepatitis B Immune Globulin (Human) alone or the vaccine series alone have 70%–90% efficacy, while a single dose of Hepatitis B Immune Globulin (Human) alone has only 50% efficacy.[8,15]

Sexual Exposure to an HBsAg-positive Person

Sex partners of HBsAg-positive persons are at increased risk of acquiring HBV infection. For sexual exposure to a person with acute hepatitis B, a single dose of Hepatitis B Immune Globulin (Human) is 75% effective if administered within 2 weeks of last sexual exposure.[8]

Household Exposure to Persons with Acute HBV Infection

Since infants have close contact with primary care-givers and they have a higher risk of becoming HBV carriers after acute HBV infection, prophylaxis of an infant less than 12 months of age with Hepatitis B Immune Globulin and hepatitis B vaccine is indicated if the mother or primary caregiver has acute HBV infection.[8] Administration of Hepatitis B Immune Globulin (Human) either preceding or concomitant with the commencement of active immunization with Hepatitis B Vaccine provides for more rapid achievement of protective levels of hepatitis B antibody, than when the vaccine alone is administered.[16] Rapid achievement of protective levels of antibody to hepatitis B virus may be desirable in certain clinical situations, as in cases of accidental inoculations with contaminated medical instruments.[16] Administration of Hepatitis B Immune Globulin (Human) either 1 month preceding or at the time of commencement of a program of active vaccination with Hepatitis B Vaccine has been shown not to interfere with the active immune response to the vaccine.[16]

CONTRAINDICATIONS

None known.

WARNINGS

BayHep B is made from human plasma. Products made from human plasma may contain infectious agents, such as viruses, that can cause disease. The risk that such products will transmit an infectious agent has been reduced by screening plasma donors for prior exposure to certain viruses, by testing for the presence of certain current virus infections, and by inactivating and/or removing certain viruses. Despite these measures, such products can still potentially transmit disease. There is also the possibility that unknown infectious agents may be present in such products. Individuals who receive infusions of blood or plasma products may develop signs and/or symptoms of some viral infections, particularly hepatitis C. ALL infections thought by a physician possibly to have been transmitted by this product should be reported by the physician or other healthcare provider to Bayer Corporation [1-888-765-3203].

The physician should discuss the risks and benefits of this product with the patient, before prescribing or administering it to the patient.

BayHep B should be given with caution to patients with a history of prior systemic allergic reactions following the administration of human immune globulin preparations. Epinephrine should be available.

In patients who have severe thrombocytopenia or any coagulation disorder that would contraindicate intramuscular injections, Hepatitis B Immune Globulin (Human) should be given only if the expected benefits outweigh the risks.

PRECAUTIONS

General

Hepatitis B Immune Globulin (Human)—BayHep B™ should **not** be administered intravenously because of the potential for serious reactions. Injections should be made intramuscularly, and care should be taken to draw back on the plunger of the syringe before injection in order to be certain that the needle is not in a blood vessel.

Intramuscular injections are preferably administered in the anterolateral aspects of the upper thigh and the deltoid muscle of the upper arm. The gluteal region should not be used routinely as an injection site because of the risk of injury to the sciatic nerve. An individual decision as to which muscle is injected must be made for each patient based on the volume of material to be administered. If the gluteal region is used when very large volumes are to be injected or multiple doses are necessary, the central region MUST be avoided; only the upper, outer quadrant should be used.[17]

Laboratory Tests

None required.

Drug Interactions

Although administration of Hepatitis B Immune Globulin (Human) did not interfere with measles vaccination,[18] it is not known whether Hepatitis B Immune Globulin (Human) may interfere with other live virus vaccines. Therefore, use of such vaccines should be deferred until approximately three months after Hepatitis B Immune Globulin (Human) administration. Hepatitis B Vaccine may be administered at the same time, but at a different injection site, without interfering with the immune response.[16] No interactions with other products are known.

Pregnancy Category C

Animal reproduction studies have not been conducted with BayHep B. It is also not known whether BayHep B can cause fetal harm when administered to a pregnant woman or can affect reproduction capacity. BayHep B should be given to a pregnant woman only if clearly needed.

Pediatric Use

Safety and effectiveness in the pediatric population have not been established.

ADVERSE REACTIONS

Local pain and tenderness at the injection site, urticaria and angioedema may occur; anaphylactic reactions, although rare, have been reported following the injection of human immune globulin preparations.[19]

OVERDOSAGE

Although no data are available, clinical experience with other immunoglobulin preparations suggests that the only manifestations would be pain and tenderness at the injection site.

DOSAGE AND ADMINISTRATION

Acute Exposure to Blood Containing HBsAg[15]

Table 1 summarizes prophylaxis for percutaneous (needle stick or bite), ocular, or mucous-membrane exposure to blood according to the source of exposure and vaccination status of the exposed person. For greatest effectiveness, passive prophylaxis with Hepatitis B Immune Globulin (Human) should be given as soon as possible after exposure (its value beyond 7 days of exposure is unclear). If Hepatitis B Immune Globulin (Human) is indicated (see Table 1 below), an injection of 0.06 mL/kg of body weight should be administered intramuscularly (see PRECAUTIONS) as soon as possible after exposure and within 24 hours, if possible. Consult Hepatitis B Vaccine package insert for dosage information regarding that product.
[See table 1 above]

Table 1. (adapted from[20])
Recommendations for Hepatitis B Prophylaxis Following Percutaneous or Permucosal Exposure

Source	Exposed Person	
	Unvaccinated	Vaccinated
HBsAg-Positive	1. Hepatitis B Immune Globulin (Human)×1 immediately* 2. Initiate HB Vaccine series†	1. Test exposed person for anti-HBs. 2. If inadequate antibody,‡ Hepatitis B Immune Globulin (Human) (×1) immediately plus HB Vaccine booster dose, or 2 doses of HBIG,* one as soon as possible after exposure and the second 1 month later.
Known Source (High Risk)	1. Initiate HB Vaccine series 2. Test source for HBsAg. If positive, Hepatitis B Immune Globulin (Human)×1	1. Test Source for HBsAg only if exposed is vaccine nonresponder; if source is HBsAg-positive, give Hepatitis B Immune Globulin (Human)×1 immediately plus HB Vaccine booster dose, or 2 doses of HBIG,* one as soon as possible after exposure and the second 1 month later.
Low Risk HBsAg-Positive	Initiate HB Vaccine series.	Nothing required.
Unknown Source	Initiate HB Vaccine series within 7 days of exposure.	Nothing required.

* Hepatitis B Immune Globulin (Human), dose 0.06 mL/kg IM.
† HB Vaccine dose 20 μg IM for adults; 10 μg IM for infants or children under 10 years of age. First dose within 1 week; second and third doses, 1 and 6 months later.
‡ Less than 10 sample ratio units (SRU) by radioimmunoassay (RIA), negative by enzyme immunoassay (EIA).

Table 2. (adapted from[21])
Recommendations for Postexposure Prophylaxis for Sexual Exposure to Hepatitis B

HBIG*		Vaccine	
Dose	Recommended timing	Dose	Recommended timing
0.06 mL/kg IM†	Single dose within 14 days of last sexual contact	1.0 mL IM†	First dose at time of HBIG* treatment¶

* HBIG = Hepatitis B Immune Globulin (Human)
† IM = intramuscularly
¶ The first dose can be administered the same time as the HBIG dose but at a different site; subsequent doses should be administered as recommended for specific vaccine.

For persons who refuse Hepatitis B Vaccine, a second dose of Hepatitis B Immune Globulin (Human)—BayHep B™ should be given 1 month after the first dose.

Prophylaxis of Infants Born to HBsAg and HBeAg Positive Mothers

Efficacy of prophylactic Hepatitis B Immune Globulin (Human) in infants at risk depends on administering Hepatitis B Immune Globulin (Human) on the day of birth. It is therefore vital that HBsAg-positive mothers be identified before delivery.

Hepatitis B Immune Globulin (Human) (0.5 mL) should be administered intramuscularly (IM) to the newborn infant after physiologic stabilization of the infant and preferably within 12 hours of birth. Hepatitis B Immune Globulin (Human) efficacy decreases markedly if treatment is delayed beyond 48 hours. Hepatitis B Vaccine should be administered IM in three doses of 0.5 mL of vaccine (10 μg) each. The first dose should be given within 7 days of birth and may be given concurrently with Hepatitis B Immune Globulin (Human) but at a separate site. The second and third doses of vaccine should be given 1 month and 6 months, respectively, after the first. If administration of the first dose of Hepatitis B Vaccine is delayed for as long as 3 months, then a 0.5 mL dose of Hepatitis B Immune Globulin (Human)—HyperHep® should be repeated at 3 months. If Hepatitis B Vaccine is refused, the 0.5 mL dose of Hepatitis B Immune Globulin (Human) should be repeated at 3 and 6 months. Hepatitis B Immune Globulin (Human) administered at birth should not interfere with oral polio and diphtheria-tetanus-pertussis vaccines administered at 2 months of age.[15]

Sexual Exposure to an HBsAg-positive Person

All susceptible persons whose sex partners have acute hepatitis B infection should receive a single dose of HBIG (0.06 mL/kg) and should begin the hepatitis B vaccine series if prophylaxis can be started within 14 days of the last sexual contact or if sexual contact with the infected person will continue (see Table 2 below). Administering the vaccine with HBIG may improve the efficacy of postexposure treatment. The vaccine has the added advantage of conferring long-lasting protection.[8]
[See table 2 above]

Household Exposure to Persons with Acute HBV Infection

Prophylactic treatment with a 0.5 mL dose of Hepatitis B Immune Globulin (Human) and hepatitis B vaccine is indicated for infants < 12 months of age who have been exposed to a primary care-giver who has acute hepatitis B. Prophylaxis for other household contacts of persons with acute HBV infection is not indicated unless they have had identifiable blood exposure to the index patient, such as by sharing toothbrushes or razors. Such exposures should be treated like sexual exposures. If the index patient becomes an HBV carrier, all household contacts should receive hepatitis B vaccine.[8]

Hepatitis B Immune Globulin (Human) may be administered at the same time (but at a different site), or up to 1 month preceding Hepatitis B Vaccination without impairing the active immune response from Hepatitis B Vaccination.[16] Parenteral drug products should be inspected visually for particulate matter and discoloration prior to administration, whenever solution and container permit.

Administer intramuscularly. Do not inject intravenously.

Directions for Syringe Usage

1. Remove the prefilled syringe from the package. Lift syringe by barrel, **not** by plunger.
2. Twist the plunger rod clockwise until the threads are seated.
3. With the rubber needle shield secured on the syringe tip, push the plunger rod forward a few millimeters to break any friction seal between the rubber stopper and the glass syringe barrel.
4. Remove the needle shield and expel air bubbles.
5. Proceed with hypodermic needle puncture.

Continued on next page

BayHep B—Cont.

6. Aspirate prior to injection to confirm that the needle is not in a vein or artery.
7. Inject the medication.
8. Withdraw the needle and dispose or destroy it.

HOW SUPPLIED

Hepatitis B Immune Globulin (Human)—BayHep B™ is supplied in a 0.5 mL neonatal single dose syringe with attached needle, a 1 mL and a 5 mL single dose vial.

NDC Number	Size
0026-0636-00	0.5 mL syringe
0026-0636-01	1 mL vial
0016-0636-05	5 mL vial

STORAGE

Store at 2°–8°C (36°–46°F). Do not freeze. Do not use after expiration date.

CAUTION

U.S. federal law prohibits dispensing without prescription.

LIMITED WARRANTY

A number of factors beyond our control could reduce the efficacy of this product or even result in an ill effect following its use. These include improper storage and handling of the product after it leaves our hands, diagnosis, dosage, method of administration and biological differences in individual patients. Because of these factors, it is important that this product be stored properly and that the directions be followed carefully during use.

No warranty, express or implied, including any warranty of merchantability or fitness is made. Representatives of the Company are not authorized to vary the terms or the contents of the printed labeling, including the package insert for this product, except by printed notice from the Company's headquarters. The prescriber and user of this product must accept the terms hereof.

REFERENCES

1. Grady GF, Lee VA: Hepatitis B immune globulin—prevention of hepatitis from accidental exposure among medical personnel. *N Engl J Med* 293(21): 1067-70, 1975.
2. Seeff LB, Zimmerman HJ, Wright EC, et al: Efficacy of hepatitis B immune serum globulin after accidental exposure. *Lancet* 2(7942):939-41, 1975.
3. Krugman S, Giles JP: Viral hepatitis, type B (MS-2-strain). Further observations on natural history and prevention. *N Engl J Med* 288(15):755-60, 1973.
4. Current trends: Health status of Indochinese refugees: malaria and hepatitis B. *MMWR* 28(39):463-4; 469-70, 1979.
5. Jhaveri R, Rosenfeld W, Salazar JD, et al: High titer multiple dose therapy with HBIG in newborn infants of HBsAg positive mothers. *J Pediatr* 97(2):305-8, 1980.
6. Hoofnagle JH, Seeff LB, Bales ZB, et al: Passive-active immunity from hepatitis B immune globulin. *Ann Intern Med* 91(6):813-8, 1979.
7. Scheiermann N, Kuwert EK: Uptake and elimination of hepatitis B immunoglobulins after intramuscular application in man. *Dev Biol Stand* 54:347-55, 1983.
8. Recommendations of the Immunization Practices Advisory Committee (ACIP): Hepatitis B Virus: A Comprehensive Strategy for Eliminating Transmission in the United States Through Universal Childhood Vaccination. Appendix A: Post-exposure Prophylaxis for Hepatitis B. *MMWR* 40(RR-13):21-25, 1991.
9. Stevens CE, Beasley RP, Tsui J, et al: Vertical transmission of hepatitis B antigen in Taiwan. *N Engl J Med* 292(15):771-4, 1975.
10. Shiraki K, Yoshihara N, Kawana T, et al: Hepatitis B surface antigen and chronic hepatitis in infants born to asymptomatic carrier mothers. *Am J Dis Child* 131(6): 644-7, 1977.
11. Recommendation of the Immunization Practices Advisory Committee (ACIP): Immune globulins for protection against viral hepatitis. *MMWR* 30(34):423-8; 433-5, 1981.
12. Okada K, Kamiyama I, Inomata M, et al: e antigen and anti-e in the serum of asymptomatic carrier mothers as indicators of positive and negative transmission of hepatitis B virus to their infants. *N Engl J Med* 294(14): 746-9, 1976.
13. Beasley RP, Trepo C, Stevens CE, et al: The e antigen and vertical transmission of hepatitis B surface antigen. *Am J Epidemiol* 105(2):94-8, 1977.
14. Beasley RP, Hwang LY, Lee GCY, et al: Prevention of perinatally transmitted hepatitis B virus infections with hepatitis B immune globulin and hepatitis B vaccine. *Lancet* 2(8359):1099-102, 1983.
15. Recommendation of the Immunization Practices Advisory Committee (ACIP): Recommendations for protection against viral hepatitis. *MMWR* 34(22):313-35, 1985.
16. Szmuness W, Stevens CE, Olesko WR, et al: Passive-active immunisation against hepatitis B: Immunogenicity studies in adult Americans. *Lancet* 1:575-77, 1981.
17. Recommendations of the Immunization Practices Advisory Committee (ACIP): General recommendations on immunization. *MMWR* 38(13):205-14; 219-27, 1989.
18. Beasley RP, Hwang LY: Measles vaccination not interfered with by hepatitis B immune globulin. *Lancet* 1:161, 1982.
19. Ellis EF, Henney CS: Adverse reactions following administration of human gamma globulin. *J Allerg* 43(1): 45-54, 1969.
20. Recommendations of the Immunization Practices Advisory Committee (ACIP): Update on Adult Immunization. Table 9. Recommendations for postexposure prophylaxis for percutaneous or permucosal exposure to hepatitis B, United States. *MMWR* 40(RR-12):70, 1991.
21. Recommendations of the Immunization Practices Advisory Committee (ACIP): Update on Adult Immunization. Table 10. Recommendations for postexposure prophylaxis for perinatal and sexual exposure to hepatitis B, United States. *MMWR* 40(RR-12):71, 1991.

BAYRAB™ ℞
[bāy - rab "]
Rabies Immune Globulin (Human)

DESCRIPTION

Rabies Immune Globulin (Human) — BayRab™ treated with solvent/detergent is a sterile solution of antirabies immune globulin for intramuscular administration; it contains no preservative. BayRab is prepared by cold ethanol fractionation from the plasma of donors hyperimmunized with rabies vaccine. The immune globulin is isolated from solubilized Cohn Fraction II. The Fraction II solution is adjusted to a final concentration of 0.3% tri-n-butyl phosphate (TNBP) and 0.2% sodium cholate. After the addition of solvent (TNBP) and detergent (sodium cholate), the solution is heated to 30°C and maintained at that temperature for not less than 6 hours. After the viral inactivation step, the reactants are removed by precipitation, filtration and finally ultrafiltration and diafiltration. BayRab is formulated as a 15–18% protein solution at a pH of 6.4–7.2 in 0.21–0.32 M glycine. BayRab is then incubated in the final container for 21–28 days at 20–27°C. The product is standardized against the U.S. Standard Rabies Immune Globulin to contain an average potency value of 150 IU/mL. The U.S. unit of potency is equivalent to the international unit (IU) for rabies antibody.

The removal and inactivation of spiked model enveloped and non-enveloped viruses during the manufacturing process for BayRab has been validated in laboratory studies. Human Immunodeficiency Virus, Type 1 (HIV-1), was chosen as the relevant virus for blood products; Bovine Viral Diarrhea Virus (BVDV) was chosen to model Hepatitis C virus; Pseudorabies virus (PRV) was chosen to model Hepatitis B virus and the Herpes viruses; and Reo virus type 3 (Reo) was chosen to model non-enveloped viruses and for its resistance to physical and chemical inactivation. Significant removal of model enveloped and non-enveloped viruses is achieved at two steps in the Cohn fractionation process leading to the collection of Cohn Fraction II: the precipitation and removal of Fraction III in the processing of Fraction II + IIIW suspension to Effluent III and the filtration step in the processing of Effluent III to Filtrate III. Significant inactivation of enveloped viruses is achieved at the time of treatment of solubilized Cohn Fraction II with TNBP/sodium cholate.

CLINICAL PHARMACOLOGY

The usefulness of prophylactic rabies antibody in preventing rabies in man when administered immediately after exposure was dramatically demonstrated in a group of persons bitten by a rabid wolf in Iran.[1,2] Similarly, beneficial results were later reported from the U.S.S.R.[3] Studies coordinated by WHO helped determine the optimal conditions under which antirabies serum of equine origin and rabies vaccine can be used in man.[4–7] These studies showed that serum can interfere to a variable extent with the active immunity induced by the vaccine, but could be minimized by booster doses of vaccine after the end of the usual dosage series.

Preparation of rabies immune globulin of human origin with adequate potency was reported by Cabasso et al.[8] In carefully controlled clinical studies, this globulin was used in conjunction with rabies vaccine of duck-embryo origin (DEV).[8,9] These studies determined that a human globulin dose of 20 IU/kg of rabies antibody, given simultaneously with the first DEV dose, resulted in amply detectable levels of passive rabies antibody 24 hours after injection in all recipients. The injections produced minimal, if any, interference with the subject's endogenous antibody response to DEV.

More recently, human diploid cell rabies vaccines (HDCV) prepared from tissue culture fluids containing rabies virus have received substantial clinical evaluation in Europe and the United States.[10–16] In a study in adult volunteers, the administration of Rabies Immune Globulin (Human) did not interfere with antibody formation induced by HDCV when given in a dose of 20 IU per kilogram body weight simultaneously with the first dose of vaccine.[15]

In a clinical study in eight healthy human adults receiving a 20 IU/kg intramuscular dose of Rabies Immune Globulin (Human) treated with solvent/detergent, BayRab™, detectable passive rabies antibody titers were observed in the serum of all subjects by 24 hours post injection and persisted through the 21 day study period. These results are consistent with prior studies[17,18] with non-solvent/detergent treated product.

INDICATIONS AND USAGE

Rabies vaccine and Rabies Immune Globulin (Human), BayRab™ should be given to all persons suspected of exposure to rabies with one exception: persons who have been previously immunized with rabies vaccine and have a confirmed adequate rabies antibody titer should receive only vaccine. BayRab should be administered as promptly as possible after exposure, but can be administered up to the eighth day after the first dose of vaccine is given.

Recommendations for use of passive and active immunization after exposure to an animal suspected of having rabies have been detailed by the U.S. Public Health Service Advisory Committee on Immunization Practices (ACIP).[19]

Every exposure to possible rabies infection must be individually evaluated. The following factors should be considered before specific antirabies treatment is initiated:

1. **Species of Biting Animal**
Carnivorous wild animals (especially skunks, foxes, coyotes, raccoons, and bobcats) and bats are the animals most commonly infected with rabies and have caused most of the indigenous cases of human rabies in the United States since 1960.[20] Unless the animal is tested and shown not to be rabid, postexposure prophylaxis should be initiated upon bite or nonbite exposure to these animals (see item 3 below). If treatment has been initiated and subsequent testing in a competent laboratory shows the exposing animal is not rabid, treatment can be discontinued.
In the United States, the likelihood that a domestic dog or cat is infected with rabies varies from region to region; hence, the need for postexposure prophylaxis also varies. However, in most of Asia and all of Africa and Latin America, the dog remains the major source of human exposure; exposures to dogs in such countries represent a special threat. Travelers to those countries should be aware that >50% of the rabies cases among humans in the United States result from exposure to dogs outside the United States.
Rodents (such as squirrels, hamsters, guinea pigs, gerbils, chipmunks, rats, and mice) and lagomorphs (including rabbits and hares) are rarely found to be infected with rabies and have not been known to cause human rabies in the United States. However, from 1971 through 1988, woodchucks accounted for 70% of the 179 cases of rabies among rodents reported to CDC.[21] In these cases, the state or local health department should be consulted before a decision is made to initiate postexposure antirabies prophylaxis.

2. **Circumstances of Biting Incident**
An unprovoked attack is more likely to mean that the animal is rabid. (Bites during attempts to feed or handle an apparently healthy animal may generally be regarded as provoked.)

3. **Type of Exposure**
Rabies is transmitted only when the virus is introduced into open cuts or wounds in skin or mucous membranes. If there has been no exposure (as described in this section), postexposure treatment is not necessary. Thus, the likelihood that rabies infection will result from exposure to a rabid animal varies with the nature and extent of the exposure. Two categories of exposure should be considered:
Bite: any penetration of the skin by teeth. Bites to the face and hands carry the highest risk, but the site of the bite should not influence the decision to begin treatment.[22]
Bat-associated strains of rabies can be transmitted to humans either directly through a bat's bite or indirectly through the bite of an animal previously infected by a bat. Because some bat bites may be less severe, and therefore more difficult to recognize, than bites inflicted by larger mammalian carnivores, rabies postexposure treatment should be considered for any physical contact with bats when bite or mucous membrane contact cannot be excluded.[23]
Nonbite: scratches, abrasions, open wounds or mucous membranes contaminated with saliva or any potentially infectious material, such as brain tissue, from a rabid animal constitute nonbite exposures. If the material containing the virus is dry, the virus can be considered noninfectious. Casual contact, such as petting a rabid animal and contact with the blood, urine, or feces (e.g., guano) of a rabid animal, does not constitute an exposure and is not an indication for prophylaxis. Instances of airborne rabies have been reported rarely. Adherence to respiratory

Rabies Postexposure Prophylaxis Guide[17]

Animal species	Condition of animal at time of attack	Treatment of exposed person [1]
Dog and cat	Healthy and available for 10 days of observation	None, unless animal develops rabies [2]
	Rabid or suspected rabid	RIGH [3] and HDCV
	Unknown (escaped)	Consult public health officials
Skunk, bat, fox, coyote, raccoon, bobcat, and other carnivores; woodchuck	Regard as rabid unless geographic area is known to be free of rabies or proven negative by laboratory tests [4]	RIGH [3] and HDCV
Livestock, rodents, and lagomorphs (rabbits and hares)	Consider individually. Local and state public health officials should be consulted on questions about the need for rabies prophylaxis. In most geographical areas bites of squirrels, hamsters, guinea pigs, gerbils, chipmunks, rats, mice, other rodents, rabbits, and hares almost never call for antirabies prophylaxis.	

[1] ALL BITES AND WOUNDS SHOULD IMMEDIATELY BE THOROUGHLY CLEANSED WITH SOAP AND WATER. If antirabies treatment is indicated, both Rabies Immune Globulin (Human) [RIGH] and human diploid cell rabies vaccine (HDCV) should be given as soon as possible, REGARDLESS of the interval from exposure.

[2] During the usual holding period of 10 days, begin treatment with RIGH and vaccine (HDCV) at first sign of rabies in a dog or cat that has bitten someone. The symptomatic animal should be killed immediately and tested.

[3] If RIGH is not available, use antirabies serum, equine (ARS). Do not use more than the recommended dosage.

[4] The animal should be killed and tested as soon as possible. Holding for observation is not recommended. Discontinue vaccine if immunofluorescence test results of the animal are negative.

precautions will minimize the risk of airborne exposure.[24] The only documented cases of rabies from human-to-human transmission have occurred in patients who received corneas transplanted from persons who died of rabies undiagnosed at the time of death. Stringent guidelines for acceptance of donor corneas have reduced this risk.

Bite and nonbite exposures from humans with rabies theoretically could transmit rabies, although no cases of rabies acquired this way have been documented.

4. Vaccination Status of Biting Animal
A properly immunized animal has only a minimal chance of developing rabies and transmitting the virus.

5. Presence of Rabies in Region
If adequate laboratory and field records indicate that there is no rabies infection in a domestic species within a given region, local health officials are justified in considering this in making recommendations on antirabies treatment following a bite by that particular species. Such officials should be consulted for current interpretations.

Rabies Postexposure Prophylaxis
The following recommendations are only a guide. In applying them, take into account the animal species involved, the circumstances of the bite or other exposure, the vaccination status of the animal, and presence of rabies in the region. Local or state public health officials should be consulted if questions arise about the need for rabies prophylaxis.

Local Treatment of Wounds: Immediate and thorough washing of all bite wounds and scratches with soap and water is perhaps the most effective measure for preventing rabies. In experimental animals, simple local wound cleansing has been shown to reduce markedly the likelihood of rabies. Tetanus prophylaxis and measures to control bacterial infection should be given as indicated.

Active Immunization: Active immunization should be initiated as soon as possible after exposure. Many dosage schedules have been evaluated for the currently available rabies vaccines and their respective manufacturers' literature should be consulted.

Passive Immunization: A combination of active and passive immunization (vaccine and immune globulin) is considered the acceptable postexposure prophylaxis except for those persons who have been previously immunized with rabies vaccine and who have documented adequate rabies antibody titer. These individuals should receive vaccine only. For passive immunization, Rabies Immune Globulin (Human) is preferred over antirabies serum, equine.[16,17] It is recommended both for treatment of all bites by animals suspected of having rabies and for nonbite exposure inflicted by animals suspected of being rabid. Rabies Immune Globulin (Human) should be used in conjunction with rabies vaccine and can be administered through the seventh day after the first dose of vaccine is given. Beyond the seventh day, Rabies Immune Globulin (Human) is not indicated since an antibody response to cell culture vaccine is presumed to have occurred.
[See table above]

CONTRAINDICATIONS
None known.

WARNINGS
Rabies Immune Globulin (Human)—BayRab™ is made from human plasma. Products made from human plasma may contain infectious agents, such as viruses, that can cause disease. The risk that such products will transmit an infectious agent has been reduced by screening plasma donors for prior exposure to certain viruses, by testing for the presence of certain current virus infections, and by inactivating and/or removing certain viruses. Despite these measures, such products can still potentially transmit disease. There is also the possibility that unknown infectious agents may be present in such products. Individuals who receive infusions of blood or plasma products may develop signs and/or symptoms of some viral infections, particularly hepatitis C. ALL infections thought by a physician possibly to have been transmitted by this product should be reported by the physician or other healthcare provider to Bayer Corporation [1-800-765-3203].

The physician should discuss the risks and benefits of this product with the patient, before prescribing or administering it to the patient.

Rabies Immune Globulin (Human) - BayRab™ should be given with caution to patients with a history of prior systemic allergic reactions following the administration of human immunoglobulin preparations.

The attending physician who wishes to administer BayRab to persons with isolated immunoglobulin A (IgA) deficiency must weigh the benefits of immunization against the potential risks of hypersensitivity reactions. Such persons have increased potential for developing antibodies to IgA and could have anaphylactic reactions to subsequent administration of blood products that contain IgA.[25]

As with all preparations administered by the intramuscular route, bleeding complications may be encountered in patients with thrombocytopenia or other bleeding disorders.

PRECAUTIONS
General
BayRab should **not** be administered intravenously because of the potential for serious reactions. Although systemic reactions to immunoglobulin preparations are rare, epinephrine should be available for treatment of acute anaphylactoid symptoms.

Drug Interactions
Repeated doses of Rabies Immune Globulin (Human) - BayRab™ should not be administered once vaccine treatment has been initiated as this could prevent the full expression of active immunity expected from the rabies vaccine.

Other antibodies in the BayRab preparation may interfere with the response to live vaccines such as measles, mumps, polio or rubella. Therefore, immunization with live vaccines should not be given within 3 months after BayRab administration.

Pregnancy Category C
Animal reproduction studies have not been conducted with BayRab. It is also not known whether BayRab can cause fetal harm when administered to a pregnant woman or can affect reproduction capacity. BayRab should be given to a pregnant woman only if clearly needed.

Pediatric Use
Safety and effectiveness in the pediatric population have not been established.

ADVERSE REACTIONS
Soreness at the site of injection and mild temperature elevations may be observed at times. Sensitization to repeated injections has occurred occasionally in immunoglobulin-deficient patients. Angioneurotic edema, skin rash, nephrotic syndrome, and anaphylactic shock have rarely been reported after intramuscular injection, so that a causal relationship between immunoglobulin and these reactions is not clear.

DOSAGE AND ADMINISTRATION
The recommended dose for BayRab is 20 IU/kg (0.133 mL/kg) of body weight given preferably at the time of the first vaccine dose.[8,9] It may also be given through the seventh day after the first dose of vaccine is given. If anatomically feasible, up to one-half the dose of BayRab should be thoroughly infiltrated in the area around the wound and the rest should be administered intramuscularly in the gluteal area. Because of risk of injury to the sciatic nerve, the central region of the gluteal area MUST be avoided; only the upper, outer quadrant should be used.[26] BayRab should never be administered in the same syringe or into the same anatomical site as vaccine.

Parenteral drug products should be inspected visually for particulate matter and discoloration prior to administration, whenever solution and container permit.

HOW SUPPLIED
BayRab is packaged in 2 mL and 10 mL vials with an average potency value of 150 International Units per mL (IU/mL). The 2 mL vial contains a total of 300 IU which is sufficient for a child weighing 15 kg. The 10 mL vial contains a total of 1500 IU which is sufficient for an adult weighing 75 kg.

NDC Number	Size
0026-0618-02	2 mL vial
0026-0618-10	10 mL vial

STORAGE
BayRab should be stored under refrigeration (2°–8°C, 36°–46°F). Solution that has been frozen should not be used.

CAUTION
U.S. federal law prohibits dispensing without prescription.

LIMITED WARRANTY
A number of factors beyond our control could reduce the efficacy of this product or even result in an ill effect following its use. These include improper storage and handling of the product after it leaves our hands, diagnosis, dosage, method of administration, and biological differences in individual patients. Because of these factors, it is important that this product be stored properly and that the directions be followed carefully during use.

No warranty, express or implied, including any warranty of merchantability or fitness is made. Representatives of the Company are not authorized to vary the terms or the contents of the printed labeling, including the package insert for this product, except by printed notice from the Company's headquarters. The prescriber and user of this product must accept the terms hereof.

REFERENCES
1. Baltazard M, Bahmanyar M, Ghodssi M, et al: Essai pratique du sérum antirabique chez les mordus par loups enragés. *Bull WHO* 13:747–72, 1955.
2. Habel K, Koprowski H: Laboratory data supporting the clinical trial of antirabies serum in persons bitten by a rabid wolf. *Bull WHO* 13:773–9, 1955.
3. Selimov M, Boltucij L, Semenova E, et al: [The use of antirabies gamma globulin in subjects severely bitten by rabid wolves or other animals.] *J Hyg Epidemiol Microbiol Immunol (Praha)* 3:168–80, 1959.
4. Atanasiu P, Bahmanyar M, Baltazard M, et al: Rabies neutralizing antibody response to different schedules of serum and vaccine inoculations in non-exposed persons. *Bull WHO* 14:593–611, 1956.
5. Atanasiu P, Bahmanyar M, Baltazard M, et al: Rabies neutralizing antibody response to different schedules of serum and vaccine inoculations in non-exposed persons: Part II. *Bull WHO* 17:911–32, 1957.
6. Atanasiu P, Cannon DA, Dean DJ, et al: Rabies neutralizing antibody response to different schedules of serum and vaccine inoculations in non-exposed persons: Part 3. *Bull WHO* 25:103–14, 1961.
7. Atanasiu P, Dean DJ, Habel K, et al: Rabies neutralizing antibody response to different schedules of serum and vaccine inoculations in non-exposed persons: Part 4. *Bull WHO* 36:361–5, 1967.

Continued on next page

BayRab—Cont.

8. Cabasso VJ, Loofbourow JC, Roby RE, et al: Rabies immune globulin of human origin: preparation and dosage determination in non-exposed volunteer subjects. *Bull WHO* 45:303–15, 1971.
9. Loofbourow JC, Cabasso VJ, Roby RE, et al: Rabies immune globulin (human): clinical trials and dose determination. *JAMA* 217(13): 1825–31, 1971.
10. Plotkin SA: New rabies vaccine halts disease — without severe reactions. *Mod Med* 45(20):45–8, 1977.
11. Plotkin SA, Wiktor TJ, Koprowski H, et al: Immunization schedules for the new human diploid cell vaccine against rabies. *Am J Epidemiol* 103(1):75–80, 1976.
12. Hafkin B, Hattwick MA, Smith JS, et al: A comparison of a WI-38 vaccine and duck embryo vaccine for preexposure rabies prophylaxis. *Am J Epidemiol* 107(5):439–43, 1978.
13. Kuwert EK, Marcus I, Höher PG; Neutralizing and complement-fixing antibody responses in pre- and post-exposure vaccinees to a rabies vaccine produced in human diploid cells. *J Biol Stand* 4(4):249–62, 1976.
14. Grandien M: Evaluation of tests for rabies antibody and analysis of serum responses after administration of three different types of rabies vaccines. *J Clin Microbiol* 5(3):263–7, 1977.
15. Kuwert EK, Marcus I, Werner J, et al: Postexpositionelle Schutzimpfung des Menschen gegen Tollwut mit einer neuentwickelten Gewebekulturvakzine (HDCS-Impfstoff). *Zentralbl Bakteriol [A]* 239(4):437–58, 1977.
16. Bahmanyar M, Fayaz A, Nour-Salehi S, et al: Successful protection of humans exposed to rabies infection: postexposure treatment with the new human diploid cell rabies vaccine and antirabies serum. *JAMA* 236(24): 2751–4, 1976.
17. American Society of Hospital Pharmacists: *Serums* 80: 04, 1983.
18. Rubin Rh, Sikes RK, Gregg MB: Human rabies immune globulin. Clinical trials and effects on serum anti-globulins. *JAMA*224:871–4, 1973.
19. Recommendations of the Immunization Practices Advisory Committee (ACIP): Rabies prevention—United States, 1991. *MMWR* 40(RR–3):1–19, 1991.
20. Reid-Sanden FL, Dobbins JG, Smith JS, et al: Rabies surveillance in the United States during 1989. *J Am Vet Med Assoc* 197(12):1571–83, 1990.
21. Fishbein DB, Belotto AJ, Pacer RE, et al: Rabies in rodents and lagomorphs in the United States, 1971–1984: increased cases in the woodchuck (*Marmota monax*) in mid-Atlantic states. *J Wildl Dis* 22(2):151–5, 1986.
22. Hattwick MAW: Human rabies. *Public Health Rev* 3(3): 229–74, 1974.
23. Epidemiologic Notes and Reports: Human Rabies—California, 1994. *MMWR* 43(25):455–457, 1994.
24. Garner JS, Simmons BP: Guideline for isolation precautions in hospitals. *Infect Control.*
25. Fudenberg HH: Sensitization to immunoglobulins and hazards of gamma globulin therapy. In: Merler E (ed.): Immunoglobulins: biologic aspects and clinical uses. Washington, DC, Nat Acad Sci, 1970, pp 211–20.
26. Recommendations of the Immunization Practices Advisory Committee (ACIP): General recommendations on immunization. *MMWR* 38(13):205–14; 219–27, 1989.

BAYRHO-D™ Mini-Dose ℞

[*bāy "rō-d*]

Rh_o(D) Immune Globulin (Human)

DESCRIPTION

Rh_o(D) Immune Globulin (Human) — BayRho-D™ Mini-Dose treated with solvent/detergent is a sterile solution of immune globulin containing antibodies to Rh_o(D) for intramuscular administration; it contains no preservative. BayRho-D Mini-Dose is prepared by cold ethanol fractionation from human plasma. The immune globulin is isolated from solubilized Cohn Fraction II. The Fraction II solution is adjusted to a final concentration of 0.3% tri-n-butyl phosphate (TNBP) and 0.2% sodium cholate. After the addition of solvent (TNBP) and detergent (sodium cholate), the solution is heated to 30°C and maintained at that temperature for not less than 6 hours. After the viral inactivation step, the reactants are removed by precipitation, filtration and finally ultrafiltration and diafiltration. BayRho-D Mini-Dose is then incubated in the final container for 21–28 days at 20–27°C. BayRho-D Mini-Dose is formulated as a 15–18% protein solution at a pH of 6.4–7.2 in 0.21–0.32 M glycine. One dose of BayRho-D Mini-Dose contains not less than one-sixth the quantity of Rh_o(D) antibody contained in one standard dose of Rh_o(D) Immune Globulin (Human), and it will suppress the immunizing potential of 2.5 mL of Rh_o(D) positive packed red blood cells or the equivalent of whole blood (5 mL). The quantity of Rh_o(D) antibody in BayRho-D Mini-Dose is not less than one-sixth of that contained in 1 mL of the U.S. Food and Drug Administration Reference Rh_o(D) Immune Globulin (Human).

The removal and inactivation of spiked model enveloped and non-enveloped viruses during the manufacturing process for BayRho-D Mini-Dose has been validated in laboratory studies. Human Immunodeficiency Virus, Type 1 (HIV-1), was chosen as the relevant virus for blood products; Bovine Viral Diarrhea Virus (BVDV) was chosen to model Hepatitis C virus; Pseudorabies virus (PRV) was chosen to model Hepatitis B virus and the Herpes viruses; and Reo virus type 3 (Reo) was chosen to model non-enveloped viruses and for its resistance to physical and chemical inactivation. Significant removal of model enveloped and non-enveloped viruses is achieved at two steps in the Cohn fractionation process leading to the collection of Cohn Fraction II: the precipitation and removal of Fraction III in the processing of Fraction II + IIIW suspension to Effluent III and the filtration step in the processing of Effluent III to Filtrate III. Significant inactivation of enveloped viruses is achieved at the time of treatment of solubilized Cohn Fraction II with TNBP/sodium cholate.

CLINICAL PHARMACOLOGY

Rh sensitization may occur in nonsensitized Rh_o(D) negative women following transplacental hemorrhage resulting from spontaneous or induced abortions.[1–2] The risk of sensitization is higher in women undergoing induced abortions than in those aborting spontaneously.[1–3]

BayRho-D Mini-Dose is used to prevent the formation of anti-Rh_o(D) antibody in Rh_o(D) negative women who are exposed to the Rh_o(D) antigen at the time of spontaneous or induced abortion (up to 12 weeks' gestation).[3–5] BayRho-D Mini-Dose suppresses the stimulation of active immunity by Rh_o(D) positive fetal erythrocytes that may enter the maternal circulation at the time of termination of the pregnancy.

The amount of anti-Rh_o(D) in BayRho-D Mini-Dose has been shown to effectively prevent maternal isosensitization to the Rh_o(D) antigens following spontaneous or induced abortion occurring up to the 12th week of gestation.[6–8] After the 12th week of gestation, a standard dose of BayRho-D™ Full Dose is indicated.

In a clinical study in eight healthy human adults receiving another hyperimmune immune globulin product treated with solvent/detergent, Rabies Immune Globulin (Human), BayRab™, prepared by the same manufacturing process, detectable passive antibody titers were observed in the serum of all subjects by 24 hours post injection and persisted through the 21 day study period. These results suggest that passive immunization with immune globulin products is not affected by the solvent/detergent treatment.

INDICATIONS AND USAGE

Rh_o(D) Immune Globulin (Human)—BayRho-D™ Mini-Dose is recommended to prevent the isoimmunization of Rh_o(D) negative women at the time of spontaneous or induced abortion of up to 12 weeks' gestation provided the following criteria are met:

1. The mother must be Rh_o(D) negative and must not already be sensitized to the Rh_o(D) antigen.
2. The father is not known to be Rh_o(D) negative.
3. Gestation is not more than 12 weeks at termination.

Note: Rh_o(D) Immune Globulin (Human) prophylaxis is not indicated if the fetus or father can be determined to be Rh negative. If the Rh status of the fetus is unknown, the fetus must be assumed to be Rh_o(D) positive, and BayRho-D Mini-Dose should be administered to the mother.

FOR ABORTIONS OR MISCARRIAGES OCCURRING AFTER 12 WEEKS' GESTATION, A STANDARD DOSE OF RH_O(D) IMMUNE GLOBULIN (HUMAN), IS INDICATED.

BayRho-D Mini-Dose should be administered within 3 hours or as soon as possible after spontaneous passage or surgical removal of the products of conception. However, if BayRho-D Mini-Dose is not given within this time period, consideration should still be given to its administration since clinical studies in male volunteers have demonstrated the effectiveness of Rh_o(D) Immune Globulin (Human), in preventing isoimmunization as long as 72 hours after infusion of Rh_o(D) positive red cells.[9]

CONTRAINDICATIONS

None known.

WARNINGS

BayRho-D Mini-Dose is made from human plasma. Products made from human plasma may contain infectious agents, such as viruses, that can cause disease. The risk that such products will transmit an infectious agent has been reduced by screening plasma donors for prior exposure to certain viruses, by testing for the presence of certain current virus infections, and by inactivating and/or removing certain viruses. Despite these measures, such products can still potentially transmit disease. There is also the possibility that unknown infectious agents may be present in such products. Individuals who receive infusions of blood or plasma products may develop signs and/or symptoms of some viral infections, particularly hepatitis C. ALL infections thought by a physician possibly to have been transmitted by this product should be reported by the physician or other healthcare provider to Bayer Corporation [1-888-765-3203].

The physician should discuss the risks and benefits of this product with the patient, before prescribing or administering it to the patient.

NEVER ADMINISTER BAYRHO-D MINI-DOSE INTRAVENOUSLY. INJECT ONLY INTRAMUSCULARLY. ADMINISTER ONLY TO WOMEN POST-ABORTION OR POST-MISCARRIAGE OF UP TO 12 WEEKS' GESTATION. NEVER ADMINISTER TO THE NEONATE.

BayRho-D Mini-Dose should be given with caution to patients with a history of prior systemic allergic reactions following the administration of human immune globulin preparations.

The attending physician who wishes to administer BayRho-D Mini-Dose to persons with isolated immunoglobulin A (IgA) deficiency must weigh the benefits of immunization against the potential risks of hypersensitivity reactions. Such persons have increased potential for developing antibodies to IgA and could have anaphylactic reactions to subsequent administration of blood products that contain IgA.

As with all preparations administered by the intramuscular route, bleeding complications may be encountered in patients with thrombocytopenia or other bleeding disorders.

PRECAUTIONS

General

Although systemic reactions to immunoglobulin preparations are rare, epinephrine should be available for treatment of acute anaphylactic symptoms.

Drug Interactions

Other antibodies in the Rh_o(D) Immune Globulin (Human)—BayRho-D™ Mini-Dose preparation may interfere with the response to live vaccines such as measles, mumps, polio or rubella. Therefore, immunization with live vaccines should not be given within 3 months after BayRho-D Mini-Dose administration.

Pregnancy Category C

Animal reproduction studies have not been conducted with BayRho-D Mini-Dose. It is also not known whether BayRho-D Mini-Dose can cause fetal harm when administered to a pregnant woman or can affect reproduction capacity.

It should be again noted, however, that BayRho-D Mini-Dose is **not** indicated for use during pregnancy and it should be administered only post-abortion or post-miscarriage.

Pediatric Use

Safety and effectiveness in the pediatric population have not been established.

ADVERSE REACTIONS

Reactions to $BayRh_o$-D Mini-Dose are infrequent in Rh_o (D) negative individuals and consist primarily of slight soreness at the site of injection and slight temperature elevation. While sensitization to repeated injections of human globulin is extremely rare, it has occurred.

DOSAGE AND ADMINISTRATION

One syringe of BayRho-D Mini-Dose provides sufficient antibody to prevent Rh sensitization to 2.5 mL Rh_o(D) positive packed red cells or the equivalent (5 mL) of whole blood. This dose is sufficient to provide protection against maternal Rh sensitization for women undergoing spontaneous or induced abortion of up to 12 weeks' gestation.

BayRho-D Mini-Dose should be administered within 3 hours or as soon as possible following spontaneous or induced abortion. If prompt administration is not possible, BayRho-D Mini-Dose should be given within 72 hours following termination of the pregnancy.

BayRho-D Mini-Dose is administered **intramuscularly**, preferably in the anterolateral aspects of the upper thigh and the deltoid muscle of the upper arm. The gluteal region should not be used routinely as an injection site because of the risk of injury to the sciatic nerve. If the gluteal region is used, the central region must be avoided; only the upper, outer quadrant should be used.[10]

Parenteral drug products should be inspected visually for particulate matter and discoloration prior to administration, whenever solution and container permit.

Directions for Syringe Usage

1. Remove the prefilled syringe from the package. Lift syringe by barrel, **not** by plunger.
2. Twist the plunger rod clockwise until the threads are seated.
3. With the rubber needle shield secured on the syringe tip, push the plunger rod forward a few millimeters to break any friction seal between the rubber stopper and the glass syringe barrel.
4. Remove the needle shield and expel air bubbles.
5. Proceed with hypodermic needle puncture.
6. Aspirate prior to injection to confirm that the needle is not in a vein or artery.
7. Inject the medication.
8. Withdraw the needle and dispose or destroy it.

HOW SUPPLIED

BayRho-D Mini-Dose package contains 10 single dose syringes

NDC Number	Size
0026-0631-05	Syringe (10 pack)

STORAGE

Store at 2°–8°C (36°–46°F). Do not freeze.

CAUTION

U.S. federal law prohibits dispensing without prescription.

LIMITED WARRANTY

A number of factors beyond our control could reduce the efficacy of this product or even result in an ill effect following its use. These include improper storage and handling of the product after it leaves our hands, diagnosis, dosage, method of administration, and biological differences in individual patients. Because of these factors, it is important that this product be stored properly and that the directions be followed carefully during use.

No warranty, express or implied, including any warranty of merchantability or fitness is made. Representatives of the Company are not authorized to vary the terms or the contents of the printed labeling, including the package insert for this product, except by printed notice from the Company's headquarters. The prescriber and user of this product must accept the terms hereof.

REFERENCES

1. Queenan JT, Shah S, Kubarych SF, *et al*: Role of induced abortion in rhesus immunisation. *Lancet* 1(7704): 815–7, 1971.
2. Goldman JA, Eckerling B: Prevention of Rh immunization after abortion with anti-Rh$_o$(D)-immunoglobulin. *Obstet Gynecol* 40(3):366–70, 1972.
3. The selective use of Rho(D) immune globulin (RhIG). *ACOG Tech Bull* 61, 1981.
4. Prevention of Rh sensitization. *WHO Tech Rep Ser* 468, 1971.
5. Recommendation of the Public Health Service Advisory Committee on Immunization Practices: Rh immune globulin. *MMWR* 21(15):126–7, 1972.
6. Stewart FH, Burnhill MS, Bozorgi N: Reduced dose of Rh immunoglobulin following first trimester pregnancy termination. *Obstet Gynecol* 51(3):318–22, 1978.
7. McMaster conference on prevention of Rh immunization, 28-30 September, 1977. *Vox Sang* 36(1):50–64, 1979.
8. Simonovits I: Efficiency of anti-D IgG prevention after induced abortion. *Vox Sang* 26(4):361–7, 1974.
9. Freda VJ, Gorman JG, Pollack W: Prevention of Rh-hemolytic disease with Rh-immune globulin. *Am J Obstet Gynecol* 128(4):456–60, 1977.
10. Recommendations of the Immunization Practices Advisory Committee (ACIP): General recommendations on immunization. *MMWR* 38(13):205–14; 219–27, 1989.

BAYRHO-D™ Full Dose

[bāy"rhō-d]

Rh$_o$(D) Immune Globulin (Human)

DESCRIPTION

Rh$_o$(D) Immune Globulin (Human) — BayRho-D™ Full Dose treated with solvent/detergent is a sterile solution of immune globulin containing antibodies to Rh$_o$(D) for intramuscular administration; it contains no preservative. BayRho-D Full Dose is prepared by cold ethanol fractionation from human plasma. The immune globulin is isolated from solubilized Cohn fraction II. The fraction II solution is adjusted to a final concentration of 0.3% tri-n-butyl phosphate (TNBP) and 0.2% sodium cholate. After the addition of solvent (TNBP) and detergent (sodium cholate), the solution is heated to 30°C and maintained at that temperature for not less than 6 hours. After the viral inactivation step, the reactants are removed by precipitation, filtration and finally ultrafiltration and diafiltration. BayRho-D Full Dose is formulated as a 15–18% protein solution at a pH of 6.4–7.2 in 0.21–0.32 M glycine. BayRho-D Full Dose is then incubated in the final container for 21–28 days at 20–27°C.

The potency is equal to or greater than that of the U.S. Food and Drug Administration Reference Rh$_o$(D) Immune Globulin. Each single dose vial or syringe contains sufficient anti-Rh$_o$(D) (approximately 300 µg*) to effectively suppress the immunizing potential of 15 mL of Rh$_o$(D) positive red blood cells.[2-4]

The removal and inactivation of spiked model enveloped and non-enveloped viruses during the manufacturing process for BayRho-D Full Dose has been validated in laboratory studies. Human Immunodeficiency Virus, Type 1 (HIV-1), was chosen as the relevant virus for blood products; Bovine Viral Diarrhea Virus (BVDV) was chosen to model Hepatitis C virus; Pseudorabies virus (PRV) was chosen to model Hepatitis B virus and the Herpes viruses; and Reo virus type 3 (Reo) was chosen to model non-enveloped viruses and for its resistance to physical and chemical inacti-

vation. Significant removal of model enveloped and non-enveloped viruses is achieved at two steps in the Cohn fractionation process leading to the collection of Cohn Fraction II: the precipitation and removal of Fraction III in the processing of Fraction II + IIIW suspension to Effluent III and the filtration step in the processing of Effluent III to Filtrate III. Significant inactivation of enveloped viruses is achieved at the time of treatment of solubilized Cohn Fraction II with TNBP/sodium cholate.

*A full dose of Rh$_o$(D) Immune Globulin (Human), has traditionally been referred to as a "300 µg" dose and this usage is employed here for convenience in terminology. **It should not be construed as the actual anti-D content.** Each full dose of Rh$_o$(D) Immune Globulin (Human), must contain at least as much anti-D as 1 mL of the U.S. Reference Rh$_o$(D) Immune Globulin. Studies performed at the FDA have shown that the U.S. Reference contains 820 international units (IU) of anti-D per mL. When the conversion factor determined for the International (WHO) Reference Preparation[1] is used, 820 IU per mL is equivalent to 164 µg per mL of anti-D.

CLINICAL PHARMACOLOGY

BayRho-D Full Dose is used to prevent isoimmunization in the Rh$_o$(D) negative individual exposed to Rh$_o$(D) positive blood as a result of a fetomaternal hemorrhage occurring during a delivery of an Rh$_o$(D) positive infant, abortion (either spontaneous or induced), or following amniocentesis or abdominal trauma. Similarly, immunization resulting in the production of anti-Rh$_o$(D) following transfusion of Rh positive red cells to an Rh$_o$(D) negative recipient may be prevented by administering Rh$_o$(D) Immune Globulin (Human).[5,6]

Rh hemolytic disease of the newborn is the result of the active immunization of an Rh$_o$(D) negative mother by Rh$_o$(D) positive red cells entering the maternal circulation during a previous delivery, abortion, amniocentesis, abdominal trauma, or as a result of red cell transfusion.[7,8] BayRho-D Full Dose acts by suppressing the immune response of Rh$_o$(D) negative individuals to Rh$_o$(D) positive red blood cells. The mechanism of action of BayRho-D Full Dose is not fully understood.

The administration of Rh$_o$(D) Immune Globulin (Human), within 72 hours of a full-term delivery of an Rh$_o$(D) positive infant by an Rh$_o$(D) negative mother reduces the incidence of Rh isoimmunization from 12%–13% to 1%–2%.[9]

The 1%–2% treatment failures are probably due to isoimmunization occurring during the latter part of pregnancy or following delivery.[10] Bowman and Pollock[11] have reported that the incidence of isoimmunization can be further reduced from approximately 1.6% to less than 0.1% by administering Rh$_o$(D) Immune Globulin (Human) in two doses, one antenatal at 28 weeks' gestation and another following delivery.

In a clinical study in eight healthy human adults receiving another hyperimmune immune globulin product treated with solvent/detergent, Rabies Immune Globulin (Human), BayRab™, prepared by the same manufacturing process, detectable passive antibody titers were observed in the serum of all subjects by 24 hours post injection and persisted through the 21 day study period. These results suggest that passive immunization with immune globulin products is not affected by the solvent/detergent treatment.

INDICATIONS AND USAGE

Pregnancy and Other Obstetric Conditions

Rh$_o$(D) Immune Globulin (Human), BayRho-D™ Full Dose is recommended for the prevention of Rh hemolytic disease of the newborn by its administration to the Rh$_o$(D) negative mother within 72 hours after birth of an Rh$_o$(D) positive infant,[12] providing the following criteria are met:

1. The mother must be Rh$_o$(D) negative, and must not already be sensitized to the Rh$_o$(D) factor.
2. Her child must be Rh$_o$(D) positive, and should have a negative direct antiglobulin test (see PRECAUTIONS).

If BayRho-D Full Dose is administered antepartum, it is essential that the mother receive another dose of BayRho-D Full Dose after delivery of an Rh$_o$(D) positive infant.

If the father can be determined to be Rh$_o$(D) negative, BayRho-D Full Dose need not be given.

BayRho-D Full Dose should be administered within 72 hours to all nonimmunized Rh$_o$(D) negative women who have undergone spontaneous or induced abortion, following ruptured tubal pregnancy, amniocentesis or abdominal trauma unless the blood group of the fetus or the father is known to be Rh$_o$(D) negative.[7,8] If the fetal blood group cannot be determined, one must assume that it is Rh$_o$(D) positive,[2] and BayRho-D Full Dose should be administered to the mother.

Transfusion

BayRho-D Full Dose may be used to prevent isoimmunization in Rh$_o$(D) negative individuals who have been transfused with Rh$_o$(D) positive red blood cells or blood components containing red blood cells.[5,13]

CONTRAINDICATIONS

None known.

WARNINGS

Rh$_o$(D) Immune Globulin (Human)—BayRho-D™ full dose is made from human plasma. Products made from human plasma may contain infectious agents, such as viruses, that can cause disease. The risk that such products will transmit an infectious agent has been reduced by screening plasma donors for prior exposure to certain viruses, by testing for the presence of certain current virus infections, and by inactivating and/or removing certain viruses. Despite these measures, such products can still potentially transmit disease. There is also the possibility that unknown infectious agents may be present in such products. Individuals who receive infusions of blood or plasma products may develop signs and/or symptoms of some viral infections, particularly hepatitis C. ALL infections thought by a physician possibly to have been transmitted by this product should be reported by the physician or other healthcare provider to Bayer Corporation [1-888-765-3203].

The physician should discuss the risks and benefits of this product with the patient, before prescribing or administering it to the patient.

NEVER ADMINISTER BAYRHO-D FULL DOSE INTRAVENOUSLY. INJECT ONLY INTRAMUSCULARLY. NEVER ADMINISTER TO THE NEONATE.

Rh$_o$(D) Immune Globulin (Human) should be given with caution to patients with a history of prior systemic allergic reactions following the administration of human immunoglobulin preparations.

The attending physician who wishes to administer Rh$_o$(D) Immune Globulin (Human) to persons with isolated immunoglobulin A (IgA) deficiency must weigh the benefits of immunization against the potential risks of hypersensitivity reactions. Such persons have increased potential for developing antibodies to IgA and could have anaphylactic reactions to subsequent administration of blood products that contain IgA.

As with all preparations administered by the intramuscular route, bleeding complications may be encountered in patients with thrombocytopenia or other bleeding disorders.

PRECAUTIONS

General

A large fetomaternal hemorrhage late in pregnancy or following delivery may cause a weak mixed field positive D^u test result. If there is any doubt about the mother's Rh type, she should be given Rh$_o$(D) Immune Globulin (Human). A screening test to detect fetal red blood cells may be helpful in such cases.

If more than 15 mL of D-positive fetal red blood cells are present in the mother's circulation, more than a single dose of Rh$_o$(D) Immune Globulin (Human), BayRho-D™ Full Dose is required. Failure to recognize this may result in the administration of an inadequate dose.

Although systemic reactions to human immunoglobulin preparations are rare, epinephrine should be available for treatment of acute anaphylactic reactions.

Drug Interactions

Other antibodies in the Rh$_o$(D) Immune Globulin (Human) preparation may interfere with the response to live vaccines such as measles, mumps, polio or rubella. Therefore, immunization with live vaccines should not be given within 3 months after Rh$_o$(D) Immune Globulin (Human) administration.

Drug/Laboratory Interactions

Babies born of women given Rh$_o$(D) Immune Globulin (Human) antepartum may have a weakly positive direct antiglobulin test at birth.

Passively acquired anti-Rh$_o$(D) may be detected in maternal serum if antibody screening tests are performed subsequent to antepartum or postpartum administration of Rh$_o$(D) Immune Globulin (Human).

Pregnancy Category C

Animal reproduction studies have not been conducted with BayRho-D Full Dose. It is also not known whether BayRho-D Full Dose can cause fetal harm when administered to a pregnant woman or can affect reproduction capacity. BayRho-D Full Dose should be given to a pregnant woman only if clearly needed.

Pediatric Use

Safety and effectiveness in the pediatric population have not been established.

ADVERSE REACTIONS

Reactions to Rh$_o$(D) Immune Globulin (Human) are infrequent in Rh$_o$(D) negative individuals and consist primarily of slight soreness at the site of injection and slight temperature elevation. While sensitization to repeated injections of human immune globulin is extremely rare, it has occurred. Elevated bilirubin levels have been reported in some individuals receiving multiple doses of Rh$_o$(D) Immune Globulin

Continued on next page

BayRho-D Full-Dose—Cont.

(Human) following mismatched tranfusions. This is believed to be due to a relatively rapid rate of foreign red cell destruction.

DOSAGE AND ADMINISTRATION

NEVER ADMINISTER BAYRHO-D FULL DOSE INTRAVENOUSLY. INJECT ONLY INTRAMUSCULARLY. NEVER ADMINISTER TO THE NEONATE.

Pregnancy and Other Obstetric Conditions

1. For postpartum prophylaxis, administer one vial or syringe of BayRho-D Full Dose (300 µg*), preferably within 72 hours of delivery. Although a lesser degree of protection is afforded if Rh antibody is administered beyond the 72-hour period, BayRho-D Full Dose may still be given.[7,14] Full-term deliveries can vary in their dosage requirements depending on the magnitude of the fetomaternal hemorrhage. One 300 µg* vial or syringe of BayRho-D Full Dose provides sufficient antibody to prevent Rh sensitization if the volume of red blood cells that has entered the circulation is 15 mL or less.[2-4] In instances where a large (greater than 30 mL of whole blood or 15 mL red blood cells) fetomaternal hemorrhage is suspected, a fetal red cell count by an approved laboratory technique (e.g., modified Kleihauer-Betke acid elution stain technique) should be performed to determine the dosage of immune globulin required.[8,15] The red blood cell volume of the calculated fetomaternal hemorrhage is divided by 15 mL to obtain the number of vials or syringes of Rh₀(D) Immune Globulin (Human), BayRho-D™ Full Dose for administration.[3,8,13] If more than 15 mL of red cells is suspected or if the dose calculation results in a fraction, administer the next higher whole number of vials or syringes (e.g., if 1.4, give 2 vials or syringes).

2. For antenatal prophylaxis, one 300 µg* vial or syringe of BayRho-D Full Dose is administered at approximately 28 weeks' gestation. This **must** be followed by another 300 µg* dose, preferably within 72 hours following delivery, if the infant is Rh positive.

3. Following threatened abortion at any stage of gestation with continuation of pregnancy, it is recommended that 300 µg* of BayRho-D Full Dose be given. If more than 15 mL of red cells is suspected due to fetomaternal hemorrhage, the same dose modification in No. 1 above applies.

4. Following miscarriage, abortion, or termination of ectopic pregnancy at or beyond 13 weeks' gestation, it is recommended that 300 µg* of BayRho-D Full Dose be given. If more than 15 mL of red blood cells is suspected due to fetomaternal hemorrhage, the same dose modification in No. 1 above applies. If pregnancy is terminated prior to 13 weeks' gestation, a single dose of BayRho-D Mini-Dose (approximately 50 µg*) may be used instead of BayRho-D Full Dose.

5. Following amniocentesis at either 15 to 18 weeks' gestation or during the third trimester, or following abdominal trauma in the second or third trimester, it is recommended that 300 µg* of BayRho-D Full Dose be administered. If there is a fetomaternal hemorrhage in excess of 15 mL of red cells, the same dose modification in No. 1 applies.

If abdominal trauma, amniocentesis, or other adverse event requires the administration of BayRho-D Full Dose at 13 to 18 weeks' gestation, another 300 µg* dose should be given at 26 to 28 weeks. To maintain protection throughout pregnancy, the level of passively acquired anti-Rh₀(D) should not be allowed to fall below the level required to prevent an immune response to Rh positive red cells. The half-life of IgG is 23 to 26 days. In any case, a dose of BayRho-D Full Dose should be given within 72 hours after delivery if the baby is Rh positive. If delivery occurs within 3 weeks after the last dose, the postpartum dose may be withheld unless there is a fetomaternal hemorrhage in excess of 15 mL of red blood cells.[16]

*See footnote under DESCRIPTION.

Transfusion

In the case of a transfusion of Rh₀(D) positive red cells to an Rh₀(D) negative recipient, the volume of Rh positive whole blood administered is multiplied by the hematocrit of the donor unit giving the volume of red blood cells transfused. The volume of red blood cells is divided by 15 mL which provides the number of vials or syringes of BayRho-D Full Dose to be administered.

If the dose calculated results in a fraction, the next higher whole number of vials or syringes should be administered (e.g., if 1.4, give 2 vials or 2 syringes). BayRho-D Full Dose should be administered within 72 hours after an incompatible transfusion, but preferably as soon as possible.

Injection Procedure

DO NOT INJECT INTRAVENOUSLY. DO NOT INJECT NEONATE. Rh₀(D) Immune Globulin (Human), BayRho-D™ Full Dose is administered **intramuscularly**, preferably in the anterolateral aspects of the upper thigh and the deltoid muscle of the upper arm. The gluteal region should not be used routinely as an injection site because of

the risk of injury to the sciatic nerve. If the gluteal region is used, the central region MUST be avoided; only the upper, outer quadrant should be used.[17]

A. Single Vial or Syringe Dose
   INJECT ENTIRE CONTENTS OF THE VIAL OR SYRINGE INTO THE INDIVIDUAL INTRAMUSCULARLY.

B. Multiple Vial or Syringe Dose
   1. Calculate the number of vials or syringes of BayRho-D Full Dose to be given (see Dosage section above).
   2. The total volume of BayRho-D Full Dose can be given in divided doses at different sites at one time or the total dose may be divided and injected at intervals, provided the total dosage is given within 72 hours of the fetomaternal hemorrhage or transfusion. USING STERILE TECHNIQUE, INJECT THE ENTIRE CONTENTS OF THE CALCULATED NUMBER OF VIALS OR SYRINGES INTRAMUSCULARLY INTO THE PATIENT.

Parenteral drug products should be inspected visually for particulate matter and discoloration prior to administration, whenever solution and container permit.

Directions for syringe Usage

1. Remove the prefilled syringe from the package. Lift syringe by barrel, **not** by plunger.
2. Twist the plunger rod clockwise until the threads are seated.
3. With the rubber needle shield secured on the syringe tip, push the plunger rod forward a few millimeters to break any friction seal between the rubber stopper and the glass syringe barrel.
4. Remove the needle shield and expel air bubbles.
5. Proceed with hypodermic needle puncture.
6. Aspirate prior to injection to confirm that the needle is not in a vein or artery.
7. Inject the medication.
8. Withdraw the needle and destroy it.

HOW SUPPLIED

BayRho-D Full Dose is available in individual and multiple-pack single dose syringes with attached needles and vials.

NDC Number	Size
0026-0631-01	Syringe
0026-0631-10	Vial (10 pack)
0026-0631-15	Vial
0026-0631-22	Syringe (10 pack)

STORAGE

Store at 2°–8°C (36°–46°F). Do not freeze.

CAUTION

U.S. federal law prohibits dispensing without prescription.

LIMITED WARRANTY

A number of factors beyond our control could reduce the efficacy of this product or even result in an ill effect following its use. These include improper storage and handling of the product after it leaves our hands, diagnosis, dosage, method of administration, and biological differences in individual patients. Because of these factors, it is important that this product be stored properly and that the directions be followed carefully during use.

No warranty, express or implied, including any warranty of merchantability or fitness is made. Representatives of the Company are not authorized to vary the terms or the contents of any printed labeling, including the package insert for this product, except by printed notice from the Company's headquarters. The prescriber and user of this product must accept the terms hereof.

REFERENCES

1. Gunson HH, Bowell PJ, Kirkwood TBL: Collaborative study to recalibrate the International Reference Preparation of Anti-D Immunoglobulin. *J Clin Pathol* 33:249–53, 1980.
2. Rh₀(D) immune globulin (human). *Med Lett Drugs Ther* 16(1):3–4, 1974.
3. Pollack W, Ascari WQ, Kochesky RJ, et al: Studies on Rh prophylaxis I. Relationship between doses of anti-Rh and size of antigenic stimulus. *Transfusion* 11(6):333–9, 1971.
4. Unpublished data in files of Bayer Corporation.
5. Pollack W, Asceri WQ, Crispen JF, et al: Studies on Rh prophylaxis. II. Rh immune prophylaxis after transfusion with Rh-positive blood. *Transfusion* 11 (6):340–4, 1971.
6. Keith LG, Houser GH: Anti-Rh immune globulin after a massive transfusion accident. *Transfusion* 11(3):176, 1971.
7. The selective use of Rh₀(D) Immune Globulin (RhIG). *ACOG Tech Bull* 61, 1981.
8. Current uses of Rh₀ immune globulin and detection of antibodies. *ACOG Tech Bull* 35, 1976.
9. Pollack W: Rh hemolytic disease of the newborn; its cause and prevention. *Prog Clin Biol Res* 70:185–203, 1981.
10. Bowman JM, Chown B, Lewis M, et al: Rh isoimmunization during pregnancy: antenatal prophylaxis. *Can Med Assoc J* 118(6):623–7, 1978.
11. Bowman JM, Pollock JM: Antenatal prophylaxis of Rh isommunization: 28-weeks'-gestation service program. *Can Med Assoc J* 118(6):627–30, 1978.
12. Ascari WQ, Allen AE, Baker WJ, et al: Rh₀(D) immune globulin (human): evaluation in women at risk of Rh immunization. *JAMA* 205(1): 1–4, 1968.
13. Prevention of Rh sensitization, *WHO Tech Rep Ser* 468: 25, 1971.
14. Samson D, Mollison PL: Effect on primary Rh immunization of delayed administration of anti-Rh. *Immunology* 28:349–57, 175.
15. Finn R, Harper DT, Stallings, SA, et al: Transplacental hemorrhage. *Transfusion* 3(2):114–24, 1963.
16. Garraty G (ed): Hemolytic disease of the newborn. Arlington, VA, American Association of Blood Banks, 1984, p 78.
17. Recommendations of the Immunization Practices Advisory Committee (ACIP): General recommendations on immunization. *MMWR* 38(13):205–14; 219–27, 1989.

BAYTET™   ℞

[*bāy 'tet* "]

Tetanus Immune Globulin (Human)
250 Units

DESCRIPTION

Tetanus Immune Globulin (Human) — BayTet™ treated with solvent/detergent is a sterile solution of tetanus hyperimmune immune globulin for intramuscular administration; it contains no preservative. BayTet is prepared by cold ethanol fractionation from the plasma of donors immunized with tetanus toxoid. The immune globulin is isolated from solubilized Cohn Fraction II. The Fraction II solution is adjusted to a final concentration of 0.3% tri-n-butyl phosphate (TNBP) and 0.2% sodium cholate. After the addition of solvent (TNBP) and detergent (sodium cholate), the solution is heated to 30°C and maintained at that temperature for not less than 6 hours. After the viral inactivation step, the reactants are removed by precipitation, filtration and finally ultrafiltration and diafiltration. BayTet is formulated as a 15–18% protein solution at a pH of 6.4–7.2 in 0.21–0.32 M glycine. BayTet is then incubated in the final container for 21–28 days at 20–27°C. The product is standardized against the U.S. Standard Antitoxin and the U.S. Control Tetanus Toxin and contains not less than 250 tetanus antitoxin units per container.

The removal and inactivation of spiked model enveloped and non-enveloped viruses during the manufacturing process for BayTet has been validated in laboratory studies. Human Immunodeficiency Virus, Type 1 (HIV-1), was chosen as the relevant virus for blood products; Bovine Viral Diarrhea Virus (BVDV) was chosen to model Hepatitis C virus; Pseudorabies virus (PRV) was chosen to model Hepatitis B and the Herpes viruses; and Reo virus type 3 (Reo) was chosen to model non-enveloped viruses and for its resistance to physical and chemical inactivation. Significant removal of model enveloped and non-enveloped viruses is achieved at two steps in the Cohn fractionation process leading to the collection of Cohn Fraction II: the precipitation and removal of Fraction III in the processing of Fraction II + IIIW suspension to Effluent III and the filtration step in the processing of Effluent III to Filtrate III. Significant inactivation of enveloped viruses is achieved at the time of treatment of solubilized Cohn Fraction II with TNBP/sodium cholate.

CLINICAL PHARMACOLOGY

The occurrence of tetanus in the United States has decreased dramatically from 560 reported cases in 1947, when national reporting began, to a record low of 48 reported cases in 1987.[1] The decline has resulted from widespread use of tetanus toxoid and improved wound management, including use of tetanus prophylaxis in emergency rooms.[2] BayTet supplies passive immunity to those individuals who have low or no immunity to the toxin produced by the tetanus organism, *Clostridium tetani*. The antibodies act to neutralize the free form of the powerful exotoxin produced by this bacterium. Historically, such passive protection was provided by antitoxin derived from equine or bovine serum; however, the foreign protein in these heterologous products often produced severe allergic manifestations, even in individuals who demonstrated negative skin and/or conjunctival tests prior to administration. Estimates of the frequency of these foreign protein reactions following antitoxin of equine origin varied from 5%–30%.[3–6] If passive immunization is needed, human tetanus immune globulin (TIG) is the product of choice. It provides protection longer than antitoxin of animal origin and causes few adverse reactions.[2] Several studies suggest the value of human tetanus antitoxin in the treatment of active tetanus.[7,8] In 1961 and 1962, Nation et al,[7] using Hyper-Tet® treated 20 patients with tetanus using single doses of 3,000 to 6,000 antitoxin units in combination with other accepted clinical and nursing procedures. Six patients, all over 45 years of age, died of causes other than tetanus. The authors felt that the morta-

Guide to Tetanus Prophylaxis in Wound Management[2]

History of Tetanus Immunization (Doses)	Clean, Minor Wounds		All Other Wounds*	
	Td†	TIG‡	Td	TIG
Uncertain or less than 3	Yes	No	Yes	Yes
3 or more§	No‖	No	No¶	No

* Such as, but not limited to, wounds contaminated with dirt, feces, soil, and saliva; puncture wounds; avulsions; and wounds resulting from missiles, crushing, burns and frostbite.
† Adult type tetanus and diphtheria toxoids. If the patient is less than 7 years old, DT or DTP is preferred to tetanus toxoid alone. For persons ≥ 7 years of age, Td is preferred to tetanus toxoid alone. (See Dosage and Administration)
‡ Tetanus Immune Globulin (Human).
§ If only three doses of fluid tetanus toxoid have been received, a fourth dose of toxoid, preferably an adsorbed toxoid, should be given.
‖ Yes if more than 10 years since the last dose.
¶ Yes if more than 5 years since the last dose. (More frequent boosters are not needed and can accentuate side effects).

lilty rate (30%) compared favorably with their previous experience using equine antitoxin in larger doses and that the results were much better than the 60% national death rate for tetanus reported from 1951 to 1954.[9] Blake et al,[10] however, found in a data analysis of 545 cases of tetanus reported to the Centers for Disease Control from 1965 to 1971 that survival was no better with 8,000 units of human tetanus immune globulin (TIG) than with 500 units; however, an optimal dose could not be determined.

Serologic tests indicate that naturally acquired immunity to tetanus toxin does not occur in the United States. Thus, universal primary vaccination, with subsequent maintenance of adequate antitoxin levels by means of appropriately timed boosters, is necessary to protect persons among all age groups. Tetanus toxoid is a highly effective antigen; a completed primary series generally induces protective levels of serum antitoxin that persist for ≥10 years.[2]

Passive immunization with BayTet may be undertaken concomitantly with active immunization using tetanus toxoid in those persons who must receive an immediate injection of tetanus antitoxin and in whom it is desirable to begin the process of active immunization. Based on the work of Rubbo,[11] McComb and Dwyer,[12] and Levine et al,[13] the physician may thus supply immediate passive protection against tetanus, and at the same time begin formation of active immunization in the injured individual which upon completion of a **full toxoid series** will preclude future need for antitoxin.

Peak blood levels of IgG are obtained approximately 2 days after intramuscular injection. The half-life of IgG in the circulation of individuals with normal IgG levels is approximately 23 days.[14]

In a clinical study in eight healthy human adults receiving another hyperimmune immune globulin product treated with solvent/detergent, Rabies Immune Globulin (Human), BayRab™, prepared by the same manufacturing process, detectable passive antibody titers were observed in the serum of all subjects by 24 hours post injection and persisted through the 21 day study period. These results suggest that passive immunization with immune globulin products is not affected by the solvent/detergent treatment.

INDICATIONS AND USAGE

BayTet is indicated for prophylaxis against tetanus following injury in patients whose immunization is incomplete or uncertain (see below). It is also indicated, although evidence of effectiveness is limited, in the regimen of treatment of active cases of tetanus.[7,8,15]

A thorough attempt must be made to determine whether a patient has completed primary vaccination. Patients with unknown or uncertain previous vaccination histories should be considered to have had no previous tetanus toxoid doses. Persons who had military service since 1941, can be considered to have received at least one dose, and although most of them may have completed a primary series of tetanus toxoid, this cannot be assumed for each individual. Patients who have not completed a primary series may require tetanus toxoid and passive immunization at the time of wound cleaning and debridement.[2]

The following table is a summary guide to tetanus prophylaxis in wound management:
[See table above]

CONTRAINDICATIONS

None known.

WARNINGS

BayTet is made from human plasma. Products made from human plasma may contain infectious agents, such as viruses, that can cause disease. The risk that such products will transmit an infectious agent has been reduced by screening plasma donors for prior exposure to certain viruses, by testing for the presence of certain current virus infections, and by inactivating and/or removing certain viruses. Despite these measures, such products can still potentially transmit disease. There is also the possibility that unknown infectious agents may be present in such products. Individuals who receive infusions of blood or plasma products may develop signs and/or symptoms of some viral infections, particularly hepatitis C. ALL infections thought by a physician possibly to have been transmitted by this product should be reported by the physician or other healthcare provider to Bayer Corporation [1-888-765-3203].

The physician should discuss the risks and benefits of this product with the patient, before prescribing or administering it to the patient.

BayTet should be given with caution to patients with a history of prior systemic allergic reactions following the administration of human immunoglobulin preparations.

In patients who have severe thrombocytopenia or any coagulation disorder that would contraindicate intramuscular injections, BayTet should be given only if the expected benefits outweigh the risks.

PRECAUTIONS

General

BayTet should not be given intravenously. Intravenous injection of immunoglobulin intended for intramuscular use can, on occasion, cause a precipitous fall in blood pressure, and a picture not unlike anaphylaxis. Injections should only be made **intramuscularly** and care should be taken to draw back on the plunger of the syringe before injection in order to be certain that the needle is not in a blood vessel. Intramuscular injections are preferably administered in the anterolateral aspects of the upper thigh and the deltoid muscle of the upper arm. The gluteal region should not be used routinely as an injection site because of the risk of injury to the sciatic nerve. If the gluteal region is used, the central region MUST be avoided; only the upper, outer quadrant should be used.[16]

Chemoprophylaxis against tetanus is neither practical nor useful in managing wounds. Wound cleaning, debridement when indicated, and proper immunization are important. The need for tetanus toxoid (active immunization), with or without TIG (passive immunization), depends on both the condition of the wound and the patient's vaccination history. Rarely has tetanus occurred among persons with documentation of having received a primary series of toxoid injections.[2] See table under INDICATIONS AND USAGE.

Skin tests should not be done. The intradermal injection of concentrated IgG solutions often causes a localized area of inflammation which can be misinterpreted as a positive allergic reaction. In actuality, this does not represent an allergy; rather, it is localized tissue irritation. Misinterpretation of the results of such tests can lead the physician to withhold needed human antitoxin from a patient who is not actually allergic to this material. True allergic responses to human IgG given in the prescribed intramuscular manner are rare.

Although systemic reactions to human immunoglobulin preparations are rare, epinephrine should be available for treatment of acute anaphylactic reactions.

Drug Interactions

Antibodies in immunoglobulin preparations may interfere with the response to live viral vaccines such as measles, mumps, polio, and rubella. Therefore, use of such vaccines should be deferred until approximately 3 months after Tetanus Immune Globulin (Human), BayTet™ administration. No interactions with other products are known.

Pregnancy Category C

Animal reproduction studies have not been conducted with BayTet. It is also not known whether BayTet can cause fetal harm when administered to a pregnant woman or can affect reproduction capacity. BayTet should be given to a pregnant woman only if clearly needed.

Pediatric Use

Safety and effectiveness in the pediatric population have not been established.

ADVERSE REACTIONS

Slight soreness at the site of injection and slight temperature elevation may be noted at times. Sensitization to repeated injections of human immunoglobulin is extremely rare.

In the course of routine injections of large numbers of persons with immunoglobulin there have been a few isolated occurrences of angioneurotic edema, nephrotic syndrome, and anaphylactic shock after injection.

OVERDOSAGE

Although no data are available, clinical experience with other immunoglobulin preparations suggests that the only manifestations would be pain and tenderness at the injection site.

DOSAGE AND ADMINISTRATION

Routine prophylactic dosage schedule:

Adults and children 7 years and older: BayTet, 250 units should be given by deep intramuscular injection (see PRECAUTIONS). At the same time, but in a different extremity and with a separate syringe, Tetanus and Diphtheria Toxoids Adsorbed (For Adult Use) (Td) should be administered according to the manufacturer's package insert. Adults with uncertain histories of a complete primary vaccination series should receive a primary series using the combined Td toxoid. To ensure continued protection, booster doses of Td should be given every 10 years.[2]

Children less than 7 years old: In small children the routine prophylactic dose of BayTet may be calculated by the body weight (4.0 units/kg). However, it may be advisable to administer the entire contents of the vial or syringe of BayTet (250 units) regardless of the child's size, since theoretically the same amount of toxin will be produced in the child's body by the infecting tetanus organism as it will in an adult's body. At the same time but in a different extremity and with a different syringe, Diphtheria and Tetanus Toxoids and Pertussis Vaccine Adsorbed (DTP) or Diphtheria and Tetanus Toxoids Adsorbed (For Pediatric Use) (DT), if pertussis vaccine is contraindicated, should be administered per the manufacturer's package insert.

Note: The single injection of tetanus toxoid only initiates the series for producing active immunity in the recipient. The physician must impress upon the patient the need for further toxoid injections in 1 month and 1 year. Without such, the active immunization series is incomplete. If a contraindication to using tetanus toxoid-containing preparations exists for a person who has not completed a primary series of tetanus toxoid immunization and that person has a wound that is neither clean nor minor, *only* passive immunization should be given using tetanus immune globulin.[2] See table under INDICATIONS AND USAGE.

Available evidence indicates that complete primary vaccination with tetanus toxoid provides long lasting protection ≥10 years for most recipients. Consequently, after complete primary tetanus vaccination, boosters–even for wound management–need be given only every 10 years when wounds are minor and uncontaminated. For other wounds, a booster is appropriate if the patient has not received tetanus toxoid within the preceding 5 years. Persons who have received at least two doses of tetanus toxoid rapidly develop antibodies.[2]

The prophylactic dosage schedule for these patients and for those with incomplete or uncertain immunity is shown on the table in INDICATIONS AND USAGE.

Since tetanus is actually a local infection, proper initial wound care is of paramount importance. The use of antitoxin is adjunctive to this procedure. However, in approximately 10% of recent tetanus cases, no wound or other breach in skin or mucous membrane could be implicated.[17]

Treatment of active cases of tetanus:

Standard therapy for the treatment of active tetanus including the use of BayTet must be implemented immediately. The dosage should be adjusted according to the severity of the infection.[7,8]

Parenteral drug products should be inspected visually for particulate matter and discoloration prior to administration, whenever solution and container permit. They should not be used if particulate matter and/or discoloration are present.

Directions for syrings Usage

1. Remove the prefilled syringe from the package. Lift syringe by barrel, **not** by plunger.
2. Twist the plunger rod clockwise until the threads are seated.
3. With the rubber needle shield secured on the syringe tip, push the plunger rod forward a few millimeters to break any friction seal between the rubber stopper and glass syringe barrel.
4. Remove the needle shield and expel air bubbles.
5. Proceed with hypodermic needle puncture.
6. Aspirate prior to injection to confirm that the needle is not in a vein or artery.
7. Inject the medication.
8. Withdraw the needle and dispose or destroy it.

Continued on next page

BayTet—Cont.

HOW SUPPLIED

BayTet is supplied in 250 unit prefilled disposable syringes with attached needles and 250 unit single dose vials.

NDC Number	Size
0026-0634-01	250 unit syringe
0026-0634-70	250 unit syringe (10 pack)
0026-0634-86	250 unit vial (10 pack)

Tetanus Immune Globulin (Human) —BayTet™ is supplied in 250 unit prefilled disposable syringes and 250 unit single dose vials.

STORAGE

Store at 2°–8°C (36°–46°F). Solution that has been frozen should not be used.

CAUTION

U.S. federal law prohibits dispensing without prescription.

LIMITED WARRANTY

A number of factors beyond our control could reduce the efficacy of this product or even result in an ill effect following its use. These include improper storage and handling of the product after it leaves our hands, diagnosis, dosage, method of administration, and biological differences in individual patients. Because of these factors it is important that this product be stored properly and that the directions be followed carefully during use.

No warranty, express or implied, including any warranty of merchantability or fitness is made. Representatives of the Company are not authorized to vary the terms or the contents of the printed labeling, including the package insert for this product, except by printed notice from the Company's headquarters. The prescriber and user of this product must accept the terms hereof.

REFERENCES

1. Tetanus — United States, 1987 and 1988, *MMWR* 39(3): 37–41, 1990.
2. Diphtheria, Tetanus, and Pertussis: Recommendations for Vaccine Use and Other Preventive Measures. Recommendations of the Immunization Practices Advisory Committee (ACIP). *MMWR* 40 (RR-10): 1–28, 1991.
3. Moynihan NH: Tetanus prophylaxis and serum sensitivity tests. *Br Med J* 1:260–4, 1956.
4. Scheibel I: The uses and results of active tetanus immunization. *Bull WHO* 13:381–94, 1955.
5. Edsall G: Specific prophylaxis of tetanus. *JAMA* 171(4): 417–27, 1959.
6. Bardenwerper HW: Serum neuritis from tetanus antitoxin. *JAMA* 179(10):763–6, 1962.
7. Nation NS, Pierce NF, Adler SJ, et al: Tetanus: the use of human hyperimmune globulin in treatment. *Calif Med* 98(6):305–6, 1963.
8. Ellis M: Human antitetanus serum in the treatment of tetanus. *Br Med J* 1(5338):1123–6, 1963.
9. Axnick NW, Alexander ER: Tetanus in the United States: A review of the problem. *Am J Public Health* 47(12):1493–1501, 1957.
10. Blake PA, Feldman RA, Buchanan TM, et al: Serologic therapy of tetanus in the United States, 1965–1971. *JAMA* 235(1):42–4, 1976.
11. Rubbo SD: New approaches to tetanus prophylaxis. *Lancet* 2(7461):449–53, 1966.
12. McComb JA, Dwyer RC: Passive-active immunization with tetanus immune globulin (human). *N Engl J Med* 268(16):857–62, 1963.
13. Levine L, McComb JA, Dwyer RC, et al: Active-passive tetanus immunization; choice of toxoid, dose of tetanus immune globulin and timing of injections. *N Engl J Med* 274(4);186–90, 1966.
14. Waldmann TA, Strober W, Blaese RM: Variations in the metabolism of immunoglobulins measured by turnover rates. In Merler E (ed.): Immunoglobulins: biologic aspects and clinical uses. Washington, DC, Nat Acad Sci, 1970, p 33–51.
15. McCracken GH Jr., Dowell DL, Marshall FN: Double-blind trial of equine antitoxin and human immune globulin in tetanus neonatorum. *Lancet* 1(7710):1146–9, 1971.
16. Recommendations of the Immunization Practices Advisory Committee (ACIP): General recommendations on immunization. *MMWR* 38(13): 205–14; 219–27, 1989.
17. Tetanus-Rates by year, United States, 1955–1984. Annual Summary 1984. *MMWR* 33 (54):61, 1986.

GAMIMUNE® N, 5% ℞

Immune Globulin Intravenous (Human), 5%
Solvent/Detergent Treated

DESCRIPTION

Immune Globulin Intravenous (Human), 5%—Gamimune® N, 5% treated with solvent/detergent is a sterile 4.5%–5.5% solution of human protein in 9%–11% maltose; it contains no preservative. Each milliliter (mL) contains approximately 50 mg of protein, not less than 98% of which has the electrophoretic mobility of gamma globulin. Not less than 90% of the IgG is monomer. Also present are traces of IgA and of IgM. The distribution of IgG subclasses is similar to that found in normal serum. Gamimune N, 5% has a buffer capacity of 16.5 mEq/L of solution (~0.33 mEq/g of protein). The calculated osmolality is 309 milliosmoles per kilogram of solvent (water) and the calculated osmolarity is 278 milliosmoles per liter of solution.

The product is made by cold ethanol fractionation of large pools of human plasm. Part of the fractionation may be performed by another licensed manufacturer. The immunoglobulin is isolated from Cohn Effluent III after limited diafiltration and ultrafiltration. The solution is adjusted to 0.3% tri-n-butyl phosphate (TNBP) and 0.2% sodium cholate. After addition of the solvent (TNBP) and the detergent (sodium cholate), the solution is heated to 30°C and maintained at that temperature for not less than 6 hours. After the viral inactivation step, the reactants are removed by precipitation, filtration, and finally diafiltration and ultrafiltration. The protein is stabilized during the process by adjusting the pH of the solution to 4.0–4.5.[1] Isotonicity is achieved by the addition of maltose. Gamimune N, 5% treated with solvent/detergent is then incubated in the final container (at the low pH of 4.25), for a minimum of 21 days at 20°C. The product is intended for intravenous administration.

The removal and inactivation of spiked model enveloped and non-enveloped viruses during the manufacturing process for Gamimune N, 5% has been validated in laboratory studies. Human Immunodeficiency Virus, Type 1 (HIV-1) was chosen as the relevant virus for blood products; Bovine Viral Diarrhea Virus (BVDV) was chosen to model for Hepatitis C virus; Pseudorabies virus (PRV) was chosen to model for Hepatitis B and the Herpes viruses; and Reo virus type 3 (Reo) was chosen to model non-enveloped viruses and for its resistance to physical and chemical inactivation. Significant removal of model enveloped and non-enveloped viruses is seen between the Fraction II + IIIW and Effluent III steps and between the Effluent III and Filtrate III steps. Significant inactivation of enveloped viruses is achieved at the time of treatment of Filtrate III with TNBP/sodium cholate and also at the time of low pH incubation in the final container.

CLINICAL PHARMACOLOGY

Primary Humoral Immunodeficiency

Gamimune N, 5% supplies a broad spectrum of opsonic and neutralizing IgG antibodies for the prevention or attenuation of a wide variety of infectious diseases. As Gamimune N, 5% is administered intravenously, essentially 100% of the infused IgG antibodies are immediately available in the recipient's circulation.[2] Studies using a modified intravenous immunoglobulin at pH 6.8 have shown that approximately 30% of the infused IgG disappeared from the circulation in the first 24 hours, due primarily to equilibration of the IgG between the plasma and the extravascular space.[2–5] A further decline to about 40% of the peak level found immediately post-infusion is to be expected during the first week.[2–5] The in vivo half-life of Gamimune N, 5% equals or exceeds the 3-week half-life reported for IgG in the literature, but individual patient variation in half-life has been observed.[2] Thus, this variable as well as the amount of immune globulin administered per dose is important in determining the frequency of administration of the drug for each individual patient. A comparative study of Gamimune N, 5% treated with solvent/detergent and Gamimune N, 5% in 16 subjects demonstrated bioequivalence.

Idiopathic Thrombocytopenic Purpura

While Gamimune N, 5% has been shown to be effective in some cases of idiopathic thrombocytopenic purpura (ITP) (see INDICATIONS AND USAGE), the mechanism of action has not been fully elucidated.

Bone Marrow Transplantation

Gamimune N, 5% has been shown to be effective in bone marrow transplant patients ≥20 years of age in the first 100 days posttransplant for the following: prevention of systemic and local infections, interstitial pneumonia of infectious and idiopathic etiologies and acute graft-versus-host disease (AGVHD)[6] (see INDICATIONS AND USAGE). Administration of Gamimune N, 5% to bone marrow transplant patients significantly increased IgG and IgG subclass levels while those seen in the control group fell below predicted levels. The mechanism of action of Gamimune N, 5% in reducing the incidence of AGVHD is presently unknown.

Pediatric HIV Infection

Children infected with human immunodeficiency virus (HIV) may display defects in both cellular and humoral immunity.[7–10] As a result, some children with HIV-1 infection experience serious, potentially life-threatening recurrent bacterial infections.[11–13] In one retrospective report, among 71 HIV-infected children observed over 3.5 years, 27 (37%) experienced serious documented bacterial infections.[12] The types of bacterial and viral infections observed in HIV-infected children are similar to those seen in children with primary hypogammaglobulinemia.[14] The replacement of opsonic and neutralizing IgG antibodies has been shown to reduce serious and minor bacterial infection in HIV-infected children.[15–16]

In a randomized, double-blind, placebo-controlled, multicenter study performed between March 7, 1988 and January 15, 1991, the efficacy of Gamimune N, 5% in pediatric HIV disease to decrease the frequency of serious and minor bacterial infections and the frequency of hospitalization, and to increase the time free of serious bacterial infection was documented in children with clinical or immunologic evidence of HIV disease (see INDICATIONS AND USAGE). The primary endpoint of this study was prospectively defined as a significant reduction in the proportion of subjects who develop at least one serious bacterial infection when compared to the control group of HIV-infected children who received placebo. Serious bacterial infections were defined as laboratory-proven and clinically diagnosed (i.e., radiologically proven acute pneumonia and sinusitis) infections. The Data Safety and Monitoring Board (DSMB) recommended early termination of the study based on data presented to them from an interim analysis in December 1990 which showed that treatment with Gamimune N, 5% increased the time free from serious infections in children with CD4+ counts ≥200/mm^3.

General

The intravenous administration of solutions of maltose has been studied by several investigators.[17–21] Healthy subjects tolerated the infusions well, and no adverse effects were observed at a rate of 0.25 g maltose/kg body weight per hour.[18] In safety studies conducted by Bayer Corporation, infusions of 10% maltose administered at 0.27–0.62 g maltose/kg per hour[21] to normal subjects produced either mild side effects (e.g., headache) or no adverse reaction.[2] Following intravenous administrations of maltose, maltose was detected in the peripheral blood; there was a dose-dependent excretion of maltose and glucose in the urine and a mild diuretic effect.[2] These alterations were well-tolerated without significant adverse effects.[2] The highest recommended infusion rate, 0.08 mL/kg body weight per minute (see DOSAGE AND ADMINISTRATION), is equivalent to 0.48 g maltose/kg body weight per hour.

The buffer capacity of Gamimune N, 5% is 16.5 mEq/L (~0.33 mEq/g protein); a dose of 1000 mg/kg body weight therefore represents an acid load of 0.33 mEq/kg body weight. The total buffering capacity of whole blood in a normal individual is 45–50 mEq/L of blood, or 3.6 mEq/kg body weight.[22] Thus, the acid load delivered with a dose of 1000 mg/kg of Gamimune N, 5% would be neutralized by the buffering capacity of whole blood alone, even if the dose were infused instantaneously. (An infusion usually lasts several hours.)

In Phase I human studies, no change in arterial blood pH measurements was detected following the intravenous administration of Gamimune N, 5% at a dose of 150 mg/kg body weight;[2] following a dose of 400 mg/kg body weight in 37 patients, there were no clinically important differences in mean venous pH or bicarbonate measurements in patients who received Gamimune N, 5% compared with those who received a chemically modified intravenous immunoglobulin preparation with a pH of 6.8.[2]

In patients with limited or compromised acid-base compensatory mechanisms, consideration should be given to the effect of the additional acid load Gamimune N, 5% might present.

INDICATIONS AND USAGE

Primary Humoral Immunodeficiency

Gamimune N, 5% is efficacious in the treatment of primary immunodeficiency states in which severe impairment of antibody forming capacity has been shown, such as: congenital agammaglobulinemias, common variable immunodeficiency. Wiskott-Aldrich syndrome, x-linked immunodeficiency with hyper IgM, and severe combined immunodeficiencies.[5,23–25] Gamimune N, 5% is especially useful when high levels or rapid elevation of circulating antibodies are desired or when intramuscular injections are contraindicated.

Idiopathic Thrombocytopenic Purpura (ITP)

In clinical situations in which a rapid rise in platelet count is needed to control bleeding or to allow a patient with ITP to undergo surgery, administration of Gamimune N, 5% should be considered; in patients in whom a response is achieved, the rise of platelets is generally rapid (within 1–5 days), transient (most often lasting from several days to several weeks) and should not be considered curative. It is presently not possible to predict which patients with ITP will respond to therapy, although the increase in platelet counts in children seems to be better than that of adults. Childhood ITP may, however, respond spontaneously without treatment.

Two different dosing regimens of Gamimune N, 5% have been studied in clinical investigations: a regimen consisting of 400 mg/kg body weight daily for 5 consecutive days, and a high dose treatment regimen consisting of 1,000 mg/kg body weight administered on either 1 day or 2 consecutive days.

In clinical studies of Gamimune N, 5% five of six (83.3%) children and 12 of 16 (75%) adults with acute or chronic ITP treated with 400 mg/kg body weight for 5 consecutive days demonstrated clinically significant platelet increments of ≥30,000/mm^3 over baseline. The mean platelet count in children with ITP rose from 27,800/mm^3 at baseline to 297,000/mm^3 (range 50,000–455,000/mm^3) and the mean platelet counts in adults with ITP rose from 27,900/mm^3 at baseline to 124,900/mm^3 (range 11,000–341,000/mm^3). Two of three children with acute ITP rapidly went into complete remission.

Thirteen of 14 children (92.9%) and 26 of 29 adults (89.7%) with acute or chronic ITP treated with Gamimune N, 5% 1,000 mg/kg body weight administered on either 1 day or 2 consecutive days responded to treatment with clinically significant platelet increments of ≥30,000/mm^3 over baseline. This included three of three patients with ITP that were human immunodeficiency virus (HIV) antibody positive and two of two patients with ITP that were pregnant. The mean platelet count in children with ITP treated with Gamimune N, 5% 1,000 mg/kg body weight on 1 day or 2 consecutive days rose from 44,400/mm^3 at baseline to 285,600/mm^3 (range 89,000–473,000/mm^3) and the mean platelet count in adults with ITP treated with the regimen rose from 23,400/mm^3 at baseline to 173,100/mm^3 (range 28,000–709,000/mm^3.

Two patients, one each with acute adult and chronic childhood ITP, entered complete remission with treatment.

Six of the 29 adult patients with ITP received Gamimune N, 5% 1,000 mg/kg on 1 day or 2 consecutive days to increase the platelet count prior to splenectomy. Mean platelet counts rose from 14,500/mm^3 at baseline to 129,300/mm^3 (range 51,000–242,000/mm^3) prior to surgery.

The duration of the platelet rise following treatment of ITP with either treatment regimen of Gamimune N, 5% was variable, ranging from several days to 12 months or more. Some ITP patients have demonstrated continuing responsiveness over many months to intermittent infusions of Gamimune N, 5% 400–1,000 mg/kg body weight, administered as a single maintenance dose, at intervals as indicated by the platelet count.

Bone Marrow Transplantation (BMT)

Gamimune N, 5% should be considered for use in bone marrow transplant patients ≥20 years of age to decrease the risk of septicemia and other infections, interstitial pneumonia of infectious or idiopathic etiologies and acute graft-versus-host disease (AGVHD) in the first 100 days post-transplant. Gamimune N, 5% is not indicated in bone marrow transplant patients below 20 years of age. In a controlled study of 369 evaluable BMT patients (184 treated and 185 controls) who either did or did not receive Gamimune N, 5% in doses of 500 mg/kg body weight on days –7 and –2 pretransplant, then weekly through day 90 post-transplant, posttransplant complications were evaluated in the entire study group and in patients under age 20 and age 20 or older. For patients ≥20 years of age (128 patients in the control group and 119 patients in the treated group), there was a statistically significant reduction in interstitial pneumonia from 21% in the control group to 9% in the treated group (p = 0.0032) during the first 100 days post-transplant. Also significantly reduced in this age group were: overall septicemia from 53 infections in the 128 patient control group to 26 infections in the 119 patient treated group (relative risk control:treated [RR] 2.36, p = 0.0025); gram-negative septicemia from 24 infections in the 128 patient control group to 9 infections in the 119 patient treated group (RR 2.53, p = 0.015); gram-positive septicemia from 16 infections in the 128 patient control group to 8 infections in the 119 patient treated group (RR 2.73, p = 0.046); and Grade II to IV AGVHD from an incidence of 58 of 110 in the control group to 38 of 108 in the treated group (p = 0.0051).

The given p-values do not take into account multiple end-points and subset analyses. Therefore, some of the p-values could occur by chance alone. There was no significant improvement in overall mortality in this study.

In patients below age 20, there appeared to be no benefit from treatment with Gamimune N, 5%, either in reducing the incidence of infections or the incidence of AGVHD.

Pediatric HIV Infection

Gamimune N, 5% 400 mg/kg every 28 days significantly decreased the frequency of serious and minor bacterial infections (laboratory-proven and clinically diagnosed) and the frequency of hospitalization, and increased the time free of serious bacterial infection. The effect of Gamimune N, 5% in preventing serious bacterial infections was especially apparent in preventing primary bacteremia (including *Streptococcus pneumoniae* bacteremia) and acute pneumonia.

In a randomized, double-blind, placebo-controlled, multicenter study, 394 HIV-infected, non-hemophilic, children less than 13 years of age were randomized. Of the children randomized, 369 were included in the efficacy analysis and 376 in the safety analysis. The study population had 1) a mean age of 40 months (range 2.4–136.8 months), 2) acquired HIV primarily through vertical transmission (91%), 3) a majority (87%) of CDC Class P-2 (symptomatic), and 4) had a median CD4+ count of 937 cells/mm^3 (range 0–6660 cells/mm^3). At the time of study entry, 14% (52 of 369) were receiving *Pneumocystis carinii* pneumonia (PCP) prophylaxis. During the course of the study, 51% (189 of 369) received PCP prophylaxis and 44% (164 of 369) received zidovudine (ZDV). Children with HIV-1 infection were initially stratified into two groups based upon CD4+ count (<200 cells/mm^3 versus ≥ 200 cells/mm^3) and CDC classification of pediatric HIV disease (history of opportunistic infections [P-2-D-1] and recurrent serious bacterial infections [P-2-D-2] versus others). Subjects received Gamimune N, 5% (400 mg/kg = 8mL/kg) (n=185) or an equivalent volume of placebo (0.1% Albumin [Human]) (n = 184) every 28 days. The mean follow-up for subjects receiving Gamimune N, 5% was 17.9 months and 17.8 months for patients on placebo. The number of subjects who had at least one serious bacterial infection was 86 of 184 (47%) in the placebo group and 55 of 185 (30%) in the Gamimune N, 5% group (p = 0.0009). All p-values reported are two-sided. Treatment with Gamimune N, 5% compared to placebo was also associated with a significant reduction in both the number of subjects with at least one laboratory-proven infection (36 of 184 vs. 18 of 185, p = 0.0081), and the number of subjects with at least one clinically diagnosed infection (71 of 184 vs. 45 of 185, p = 0.0036). Efficacy in patients with CDR+ counts < 200/mm^3 was not established, possibly because of the small number of subjects in this category.

The 2-year treatment period defined in the protocol was truncated for some patients by the DSMB based on data from the interim analysis. Rates of serious bacterial infections per 100 patient-years were computed and analyzed to take into account both the unequal duration of treatment and follow-up, as well as recurrent infections in individual subjects. Children treated with Gamimune N, 5% experienced a 50.5% lower frequency of laboratory-proven serious bacterial infection compared to the group treated with placebo (9.1 vs. 18.2 infections per 100 patient-years, p = 0.031), a 36.0% lower frequency of clinically diagnosed serious infections (24.0 vs. 37.5 infections per 100 patient-years, p = 0.013), a 40.6% reduction in total serious infections (laboratory-proven and clinically diagnosed) (33.1 vs. 55.7 infections per 100 patient-years, p = 0.003), a 60% lower frequency of primary bacteremias (5.8 vs. 14.5 infections per 100 patient-years, p = 0.009), a 75.6% lower frequency of *Streptococcus pneumoniae* bacteremia (1.1 vs. 4.5 bacteremias per 100 patient-years, p = 0.026), a 54.3% lower frequency of clinically diagnosed pneumonia (12.7 vs. 27.8 infections per 100 patient-years, p = 0.001), and a 22.5% lower frequency of minor bacterial infections (including otitis media, skin and soft tissue infections, and upper respiratory tract infections) (123.6 vs. 159.5 infections per 100 patient-years, p = 0.033).

In addition to a reduced frequency of infection, children treated with Gamimune N, 5% had a 36.8% lower number of hospitalizations per 100 patient-years (72 vs. 114 per 100 patient-years, p = 0.002) and a reduced number of hospital days (6.9 vs. 10.5 per patient-year, p = 0.030) than patients treated with placebo. Patients treated with Gamimune N, 5% had a higher probability of remaining free of laboratory-proven infections (p = 0.0093) and combined laboratory-proven and clinically diagnosed infections (p = 0.0015) for 24 months than the group of children treated with placebo. At 24 months, the estimated probabilities of remaining infection-free for the Gamimune N, 5% and placebo arms were 87.8% vs. 76.1%, respectively, for laboratory-proven infections and 63.5% vs. 44.5%, respectively, for combined laboratory-proven and clinically diagnosed infections.

There was no effect of Gamimune N, 5% therapy on mortality, which was low in both treatment groups (17%), or on the frequency of opportunistic or viral infections during the period of study.

Since antibacterial prophylaxis could also account for the observed reduction in the rate of serious bacterial infections, further analysis was performed to evaluate the role of *Pneumocystis carinii* pneumonia (PCP) prophylaxis on the efficacy of Gamimune N, 5%. PCP prophylaxis consisted primarily (96%) of trimethoprim/sulfamethoxazole given 3 successive days each week. This antibiotic combination could be active against the bacteria commonly encountered in this patient population. In the subgroup of patients receiving PCP prophylaxis at study entry, treatment with Gamimune N, 5% was associated with 44.0 infections per 100 patient-years, whereas placebo recipients had 64.7 infections per 100 patient-years (p = 0.047). In the subgroup of patients not receiving PCP prophylaxis at study entry, treatment with Gamimune N, 5% was associated with 22.1 infections per 100 patient-years, whereas placebo recipients had 44.9 infections per 100 patient-years on placebo (p = 0.024). Thus, Gamimune N, 5% benefited patients by reducing the rate of serious bacterial infections whether or not they were receiving PCP prophylactic treatment at study entry. However, it should be noted that the use of PCP prophylactic treatment in this study was not randomized and specific guidelines for its administration were not identified.

CONTRAINDICATION

Immune Globulin Intravenous (Human), 5%—Gamimune® N, 5% is contraindicated in individuals who are known to have had an anaphylactic or severe systemic response to Immune Globulin (Human). Individuals with selective IgA deficiencies who have known antibody against IgA (anti-IgA antibody) should not receive Gamimune N, 5% since these patients may experience severe reactions to the IgA which may be present.[23]

WARNINGS

Gamimune N, 5% is made from human plasma. Products made from human plasma may contain infectious agents, such as viruses, that can cause disease. The risk that such products will transmit an infectious agent has been reduced by screening plasma donors for prior exposure to certain viruses, by testing for the presence of certain current virus infections, and by inactivating and/or removing certain viruses. Despite these measures, such products can still potentially transmit disease. There is also the possibility that unknown infectious agents may be present in such products. Individuals who receive infusions of blood or plasma products may develop signs and/or symptoms of some viral infections, particularly hepatitis C. ALL infections thought by a physician possibly to have been transmitted by this product should be reported by the physician or other healthcare provider to Bayer Corporation [1-888-765-3203].

The physician should discuss the risks and benefits of this product with the patient, before prescribing or administering it to the patient.

Gamimune N, 5% should be administered only intravenously as the intramuscular and subcutaneous routes have not been evaluated.

Gamimune N, 5% may, on rare occasions, cause a precipitous fall in blood pressure and a clinical picture of anaphylaxis, even when the patient is not known to be sensitive to immune globulin preparations. These reactions may be related to the rate of infusion. Accordingly, the infusion rate given under DOSAGE AND ADMINISTRATION should be closely followed, at least until the physician has had sufficient experience with a given patient. The patient's vital signs should be monitored continuously and careful observation made for any symptoms throughout the entire infusion. Epinephrine should be available for the treatment of an acute anaphylactic reaction.

PRECAUTIONS

General

Any vial that has been entered should be used promptly. Partially used vials should be discarded. Do not use if turbid. Solution which has been frozen should not be used.

An aseptic meningitis syndrome (AMS) has been reported to occur infrequently in association with Immune Globulin Intravenous (Human) treatment. The syndrome usually begins within several hours to two days following Immune Globulin Intravenous (Human) treatment. It is characterized by symptoms and signs including severe headache, nuchal rigidity, drowsiness, fever, photophobia, painful eye movements, and nausea and vomiting. Cerebrospinal fluid studies are frequently positive with pleocytosis up to several thousand cells per mm^3, predominantly from the granulocytic series, and elevated protein levels up to several hundred mg/dL. Patients exhibiting such symptoms and signs should receive a thorough neurological examination, including CSF studies, to rule out other causes of meningitis. AMS may occur more frequently in association with high dose (2 g/kg) Immune Globulin Intravenous (Human) treatment. Discontinuation of Immune Globulin Intravenous (Human) treatment has resulted in remission of AMS within several days without sequelae.[26–29]

Isolated reports have appeared of transient and reversible renal insufficiency following administration of Immune Globulin Intravenous (Human) therapy.[30,31] The mechanics involved are uncertain.

Drug Interactions

Antibodies in Gamimune N, 5% may interfere with the response to live viral vaccines such as measles, mumps and rubella. Therefore, use of such vaccines should be deferred until approximately 6 months after Gamimune N, 5% administration.

Please see DOSAGE AND ADMINISTRATION for other drug interactions.

Pregnancy Category C

Animal reproduction studies have not been conducted with Gamimune N, 5%. It is not known whether Gamimune N, 5% can cause fetal harm when administered to a pregnant woman or can affect reproduction capacity. Gamimune N, 5% should be given to a pregnant woman only if clearly needed.

ADVERSE REACTIONS

Primary Humoral Immunodeficiency

In a study of 37 patients with immunodeficiency syndromes receiving Gamimune N, 5% at a monthly dose of 400 mg/kg body weight, reactions were seen in 5.2% of the infusions of Gamimune N, 5%. Symptoms reported with Gamimune N, 5% included malaise, a feeling of faintness, fever, chills, headache, nausea, vomiting, chest tightness, dyspnea and

Continued on next page

Gamimune N, 5%—Cont.

chest, back or hip pain. In addition, mild erythema following infiltration of Gamimune N, 5% at the infusion site was reported in some cases.

A safety study has been conducted in 16 adult and adolescent subjects with primary immunodeficiency syndrome, comparing side effects and bioequivalency of Gamimune N, 5% with those of Gamimune N, 5% treated with solvent/detergent. The incidence, nature and severity of reactions with Gamimune N, 5% treated with solvent/detergent were not different from those observed with Gamimune N, 5%.

Idiopathic Thrombocytopenic Purpura

In studies of Gamimune N, 5% administered at a dose of 400 mg/kg body weight in the treatment of adult and pediatric patients with ITP, systemic reactions were noted in only 4 of 154 (2.6%) infusions, and all but one occurred at rates of infusion greater than 0.04 mL/kg body weight per minute. The symptoms reported included chest tightness, a sense of tachycardia (pulse was 84 beats per minute), and a burning sensation in the head; these symptoms were all mild and transient.

In studies of Gamimune N, 5% administered at a dose of 1,000 mg/kg body weight either as a single dose or as two doses on consecutive days in the treatment of adult and pediatric patients with ITP, adverse reactions were noted in only 25 of 251 (10%) infusions. Symptoms reported included headache, nausea, fever, chills, back pain, chest tightness, and shortness of breath. In children, the high dose regimen has been well-tolerated at the highest rates of infusion. In adults, however, the frequency of adverse reactions tended to increase with infusion rates in excess of 0.06 mL/kg per minute. In general, reactions reported with infusion of Gamimune N, 5% in these studies were reported as mild or moderate, and responded to slowing of the infusion rate.

Bone Marrow Transplantation

In studies of Gamimune N, 5% administered to 185 bone marrow transplant recipients at doses of 500 mg/kg (10 mL/kg) body weight on day -7 and day -2 pretransplant, then weekly through day 90 posttransplant, adverse reactions were noted in 12 (6.5%) of the 185 patients that received Gamimune N, 5% and in 14 (0.6%) of 2,176 infusions. All reactions reported were rate-related and classified as mild. Chills were the most common symptom reported, occurring in nine patients. The other symptoms reported included headache, flushing, fever, pruritus and slight back discomfort. All reactions resolved satisfactorily, usually without treatment or decreasing the infusion rate.

Pediatric HIV Infection

Three hundred seventy-six (376) patients, 187 treated with Gamimune N, 5% and 189 treated with placebo (0.1% Albumin [Human]), were included in the safety analysis. Adverse reactions occurred during or within 24 hours of an infusion in 50 of 3,451 (1.4%) infusions of Gamimune N, 5% and 62 of 3,447 (1.8%) infusions of placebo. Fever was the most common adverse reaction and occurred in 30 of 105 (28.6%) patients receiving placebo and 19 of 78 (24.4%) patients treated with Gamimune N, 5%. Irritability was the second most common symptom reported, with 10 of 105 (9.5%) reports for the placebo group and 9 of 78 (11.5%) for the group treated with Gamimune N, 5%. A large number of diverse adverse reactions accounted for the remaining adverse reactions reported in both study groups. In general, the number of adverse events reported was comparable in both the placebo and Gamimune N, 5% treated groups. Three serious adverse reactions were reported. One patient experienced a hypersensitivity reaction and did not receive further Gamimune N, 5% treatment. A second patient developed tachycardia and was admitted to an intensive care unit, but later continued treatment with Gamimune N, 5%. A third patient had skin infiltration during infusion and developed a full thickness skin slough over the dorsum of the hand that required skin grafting.

General

In the studies undertaken to date, other types of reactions have not been reported with Gamimune N, 5%. It may be, however, that adverse effects will be similar to those previously reported with intravenous and intramuscular immunoglobulin administration. Potential reactions, therefore, may also include anxiety, flushing, wheezing, abdominal cramps, myalgias, arthralgia, and dizziness; rash has been reported only rarely. Reactions to intravenous immunoglobulin tend to be related to the rate of infusion.

True anaphylactic reactions to Gamimune N, 5% may occur in recipients with documented prior histories of severe allergic reactions to intramuscular immunoglobulin, but some patients may tolerate cautiously administered intravenous immunoglobulin without adverse effects.[2,32] Very rarely an anaphylactoid reaction may occur in patients with no prior history of severe allergic reactions to either intramuscular or intravenous immunoglobulin.[2]

DOSAGE AND ADMINISTRATION

General

Dosages for specific indications are indicated below, but in general, it is recommended that Gamimune N, 5% be ad-

ministered by itself at a rate of 0.01 to 0.02 mL/kg body weight per minute for 30 minutes; if well-tolerated, the rate may be **gradually** increased to a maximum of 0.08 mL/kg body weight per minute. Investigations indicate that Gamimune N, 5% is well-tolerated and less likely to produce side effects when infused at the indicated rate. If side effects occur, the rate may be reduced, or the infusion interrupted until symptoms subside. The infusion may then be resumed at the rate which is comfortable for the patient. Parenteral drug products should be inspected visually for particulate matter and discoloration prior to administration, whenever solution and container permit.

It is recommended that infusion of Gamimune N, 5% be given by a separate line, by itself, without mixing with other intravenous fluids or medications the patient might be receiving. Gamimune N, 5% should not be mixed with Immune Globulin Intravenous (Human) from another manufacturer. Gamimune N, 5% is not compatible with saline. If dilution is required, Gamimune N, 5% may be diluted with 5% dextrose in water (D5/W). No other drug interactions or compatibilities have been evaluated.

Primary Humoral Immunodeficiency

The usual dosage of Gamimune N, 5% for prophylaxis in primary immunodeficiency syndromes is 100–200 mg/kg (2–4 mL/kg) of body weight administered approximately once a month by intravenous infusion. The dosage may be given more frequently or increased as high as 400 mg/kg (8 mL/kg) body weight, if the clinical response is inadequate, or the level of IgG achieved in the circulation is felt to be insufficient. The minimum level of IgG required for protection has not been determined.

Idiopathic Thrombocytopenic Purpura (ITP)

Induction: An increase in platelet count has been observed in children and some adults with acute or chronic ITP receiving Gamimune N, 5% 400 mg/kg body weight daily for 5 days, or alternatively, 1,000 mg/kg body weight daily for 1 day or 2 consecutive days. In the latter treatment regimen, if an adequate increase in the platelet count is observed at 24 hours, the second dose of 1,000 mg/kg body weight may be withheld. The high dose regimen (1,000 mg/kg x 1–2 days) is not recommended for individuals with expanded fluid volumes or where fluid volume may be a concern. With both treatment regimens, a response usually occurs within several days and is maintained for a variable period of time. In general, a response is seen less often in adults than in children.

Maintenance: In adults and children with ITP, if after induction therapy the platelet count falls to less than 30,000/mm^3 and/or the patient manifests clinically significant bleeding, Gamimune N, 5% 400 mg/kg body weight may be given as a single infusion. If an adequate response does not result, the dose can be increased to 800–1,000 mg/kg of body weight given as a single infusion. Maintenance infusions may be administered intermittently as clinically indicated to maintain a platelet count greater than 30,000/mm^3

Bone Marrow Transplantation

Gamimune N, 5% should be administered in doses of 500 mg/kg (10 mL/kg) body weight beginning on days –7 and –2 pretransplant (or at the time conditioning therapy for transplantation is begun), then weekly through day 90 posttransplant. Gamimune N, 5% should be administered by itself through a Hickman line while it is in place, and thereafter through a peripheral vein. Please see DOSAGE AND ADMINISTRATION for other drug interactions.

Pediatric HIV Infection

A reduction in bacterial infections has been observed in children infected with HIV-1 receiving Gamimune N, 5% 400 mg/kg (8 mL/kg) body weight every 28 days.

HOW SUPPLIED

Gamimune N, 5% is supplied in the following sizes:

NDC Number	Size	Grams Protein
0026-0646-12	10 mL	0.5
0026-0646-20	50 mL	2.5
0026-0646-71	100 mL	5.0
0026-0646-24	200 mL	10.0
0026-0646-25	250 mL	12.5

STORAGE

Store at 2–8°C (36–46°F). Do not freeze. Do not use after expiration date.

CAUTION

U.S. federal law prohibits dispensing without prescription.

LIMITED WARRANTY

A number of factors beyond our control could reduce the efficacy of this product or even result in an ill effect following its use. These include improper storage and handling of the product after it leaves our hands, diagnosis, dosage, method of administration, and biological differences in individual patients. Because of these factors, it is important that this product be stored properly and that the directions be followed carefully during use.

No warranty, express or implied, including any warranty of merchantability or fitness is made. Representatives of the Company are not authorized to vary the terms or the contents of the printed labeling, including the package insert

for this product, except by printed notice from the Company's headquarters. The prescriber and user of this product must accept the terms hereof.

REFERENCES

1. Tenold RA, inventor; Cutter Laboratories, assignee. Intravenously injectable immune serum globulin. U.S. Patent 4,396,608, August 2, 1983

2. Data on file at Bayer Corporation

3. Pirofsky B, Campbell SM, Montanaro A: Individual patient variations in the kinetics of intravenous immune globulin administration. *J Clin Immunol* 2 (2): 7S-14S, 1982.

4. Pirofsky B: Intravenous immune globulin therapy in hypogammaglobulinemia. *Am J Med* 76 (3A): 53–60, 1984.

5. Pirofsky B, Anderson CJ, Bardana EJ Jr: Therapeutic and detrimental effects of intravenous immunoglobulin therapy. In: Alving BM (ed.): *Immunoglobulins: characteristics and uses of Intravenous preparations.* Washington, D.C., U.S. Government Printing Office, (1980), pp 15–22.

6. Sullivan KM, Kopecky KJ, Jocom J, et al: Immunomodulatory and antimicrobial efficacy of intravenous immunoglobulin in bone marrow transplantation, *N Engl J Med* 323(11):705–12, 1990.

7. Bernstein LJ, Ochs HD, Wedgwood RJ, et al; Defective humoral immunity in pediatric acquired immune deficiency syndrome. *J Pediatr* 107(3):352–7, 1985

8. Borkowsky W, Steele CJ, Grubman S. et al: Antibody responses to bacterial toxoids in children infected with human immunodeficiency virus. *J Pediatr* 110(4):563–6, 1987

9. Blanche S, Le Deist F, Fischer A, et al: Longitudinal study of 18 children with perinatal LAV/HTLV III infection: attempt at prognostic evaluation. *J Pediatr* 109(6): 965–70, 1986.

10. Pahwa S, Fikrig S, Menez R, et al: Pediatric acquired immunodeficiency syndrome demonstration of B-lymphocyte defects in vitro. *Diagn Immunol* 4(1):24–30, 1986.

11. Bernstein, LJ, Krieger BZ, Novick B, et al: Bacterial infections in the acquired immunodeficiency syndrome of children. *Pediatr Infect Dis* 4(5):472–5, 1985.

12. Krasinski K, Borkowsky W, Bonk S, et al: Bacterial infections in human immunodeficiency virus-infected children. *Pediatr Infect Dis J* 4(5):323–8, 1988.

13. Scott GB, Buck BE, Leterman JG, et al: Acquired immunodeficiency syndrome in infants. *N Engl J Med* 310(2): 76–81, 1984.

14. Mofenson LM, Willoughby A. Passive immunization. In: Pizzo PA, Wilfert CM, (eds.) *Pediatric AIDS: the challenge of HIV infection in infants, children and adolescents.* Baltimore: Williams & Wilkins (1991) pp 633–50.

15. National Institute of Child Health and Human Development Intravenous Immunoglobulin Study Group. Intravenous immune globulin for the prevention of bacterial infections in children with symptomatic human immunodeficiency virus infection. *N Engl J Med* 325(2):73–80, 1991.

16. Mofenson LM, Moye J Jr, Bethel J, et al: Prophylactic intravenous immunoglobulin in HIV-infected children with CD4+ counts of 0.20×10^9/L or more. Effect on viral, opportunistic, and bacterial infections. *JAMA* 268(4):483–88, 1992.

17. Berg G, Matzkies F: Wirkung von Maltose nach intravenöser Dauerinfusion auf den Stoffwechsel. *Z Ernährungswiss* 15:255–62, 1976.

18. Förster H, Hoos I, Boecker S: Versuche mit Probanden zur parenteralen Verwertung von Maltose. *Z Ernährungswiss* 15(3):284–93, 1976.

19. Finke C, Reinauer H: Utilization of maltose and oligosaccharides after intravenous infusion in man. *Nutr Metab* 21(Suppl 1):115–7, 1977.

20. Young EA, Drummond A, Cioletti L, et al: Metabolism of continuously infused intravenous maltose. [abstract] 25(3):543A, 1977.

21. Soroff HS, Hansen LM, Sasvary D, et al: Clinical pharmacology and metabolism of maltose in normal human volunteers, [abstract] *Clin Res* 26(3):286A, 1978.

22. Guyton AC: *Textbook of Medical Physiology.* 5th ed. Philadelphia, W.B. Saunders, 1976, pp 499–500.

23. Buckley RH: Immunoglobulin replacement therapy: Indications and contraindications for use and variable IgG levels achieved. In: Alving BM (ed): *immunoglobulins: characteristics and uses of intravenous preparations.* Washington, D.C., U.S. Government Printing Office, (1980), pp 3–8.

24. Nolte MT, Pirofsky B, Gerritz GA, et al: Intravenous immunoglobulin therapy for antibody deficiency. *Clin Exp Immunol* 36:237–43, 1979.

25. Ochs HD: Intravenous immunoglobulin therapy of patients with primary immunodeficiency syndromes: efficacy and safety of a new modified immune globulin preparation. In: Alving BM (ed.): *Immunoglobulins:*

characteristics and uses of intravenous preparations. Washington, D.C., U.S. Government Printing Office, (1980), pp 9–14.

26. Sekul E, Cupler E, Dalakas M: Aseptic meningitis associated with high-dose intravenous immunoglobulin therapy: Frequency and risk factors. *Ann Int Med* 121: 259–262, 1994.

27. Kato E, Shindo S, Eto Y, et al: Administration of Immune Globulin Associated with Aseptic Meningitis. *JAMA* 259(22):3269–3270, 1988.

28. Casteels-Van Daele M, Wijndaele L, Hunninck K, et al: Intravenous immune globulin and acute aseptic meningitis. *N Engl J Med* 323(9):614–615, 1990.

29. Scribner C, Kapit R, Phillips E, et al: Aseptic meningitis and intravenous immunoglobulin therapy. *Ann Intern Med* 121(4):305–306, 1994.

30. Schiavotto C, Ruggeri M, Rodeghiero F. Adverse reactions after high-dose intravenous immunoglobulin: Incidence in 83 patients treated for idiopathic thrombocytopenic purpura (ITP) and review of the literature. *Haematologica* 78(6:Suppl 2):35–40, 1993.

31. Pasatiempo AM, Kroser JA, Rudnick M, et al: Acute renal failure after intravenous immunoglobulin therapy. *J Rheumatol* 21(2):347–9, 1994.

32. Peerless AG, Stiehm ER: Intravenous gammaglobulin for reaction to intramuscular preparation. [letter] *Lancet* 2(8347):461, 1983.

Bayer Corporation
Pharmaceutical Division
Elkhart, IN 46515 USA
U.S. License No. 8

14-7646-002
(Rev. April 1998)
Shown in Product Identification Guide, page 305

GAMIMUNE® N, 10%   ℞
Immune Globulin Intravenous
(Human), 10%
Solvent/Detergent Treated

DESCRIPTION

Immune Globulin Intravenous (Human), 10%—Gamimune® N, 10% treated with solvent/detergent is a sterile solution of human protein containing no preservative. Gamimune N, 10% consists of 9%–11% protein in 0.16–0.24 M glycine. Not less than 98% of the protein has the electrophoretic mobility of gamma globulin. Not less than 90% of the IgG is monomer. Also present are traces of IgA and of IgM. The distribution of IgG subclasses is similar to that found in normal serum. The measured buffer capacity is 35 mEq/L and the osmolality is 274 mOsmol/kg solvent. The product is made by cold ethanol fractionation of large pools of human plasma. Part of the fractionation may be performed by another licensed manufacturer. The immunoglobulin is isolated from Cohn Effluent III after limited diafiltration and ultrafiltration. The solution is adjusted to 0.3% tri-n-butyl phosphate (TNBP) and 0.2% sodium cholate. After addition of the solvent (TNBP) and the detergent (sodium cholate), the solution is heated to 30°C and maintained at that temperature for not less than 6 hours. After the viral inactivation step, the reactants are removed by precipitation, filtration, and finally diafiltration and ultrafiltration. The protein is stabilized during the process by adjusting the pH of the solution to 4.0–4.5.[1] Isotonicity is achieved by the addition of glycine. Gamimune N, 10% treated with solvent/detergent is then incubated in the final container (at the low pH of 4.25), for a minimum of 21 days at 20°C. The product is intended for intravenous administration.

The removal and inactivation of spiked model enveloped and non-enveloped viruses during the manufacturing process for Gamimune N, 10% has been validated in laboratory studies. Human Immunodeficiency Virus, Type 1 (HIV-1) was chosen as the relevant virus for blood products; Bovine Viral Diarrhea Virus (BVDV) was chosen to model for Hepatitis C virus; Pseudorabies virus (PRV) was chosen to model for Hepatitis B and the Herpes viruses; and Reo virus type 3 (Reo) was chosen to model non-enveloped viruses and for its resistance to physical and chemical inactivation. Significant removal of model enveloped and non-enveloped viruses is seen between the Fraction II + IIIW and Effluent III steps and between the Effluent III and Filtrate III steps. Significant inactivation of enveloped viruses is achieved at the time of treatment of Filtrate III with TNBP/sodium cholate and also at the time of low pH incubation in the final container.

CLINICAL PHARMACOLOGY
Primary Humoral Immunodeficiency

Gamimune N, 10% supplies a broad spectrum of opsonic and neutralizing IgG antibodies for the prevention or attenuation of a wide variety of infectious diseases. Since Gamimune N, 10% is administered intravenously, essentially 100% of the infused IgG antibodies are immediately available in the recipient's circulation.[2] Studies using a modified intravenous immunoglobulin at pH 6.8 have shown that approximately 30% of the infused IgG disap-

peared from the circulation in the first 24 hours, due primarily to equilibration of the IgG between the plasma and the extravascular space.[2–5] A further decline to about 40% of the peak level found immediately post-infusion is to be expected during the first week.[2–5] The in vivo half-life of Immune Globulin Intravenous (Human), 5%—Gamimune® N, 5% equals or exceeds the 3-week half-life reported for IgG in the literature, but individual patient variation in half-life has been observed.[2] Thus, this variable as well as the amount of immune globulin administered per dose is important in determining the frequency of administration of the drug for each individual patient. A comparative study of Gamimune N, 10% with Gamimune N, 5% (in 10% maltose) in 18 subjects demonstrated equivalent post-infusion recovery for the two preparations. A comparative study of Gamimune N, 10% treated with solvent/detergent and Gamimune N, 10% in 17 subjects demonstrated bioequivalence.

Idiopathic Thrombocytopenic Purpura

While Gamimune N, 10% has been shown to be effective in some cases of idiopathic thrombocytopenic purpura (ITP) (see INDICATIONS AND USAGE), the mechanism of action has not been fully elucidated.

Bone Marrow Transplantation

Clinical studies with Gamimune N, 5% have shown that it is effective in bone marrow transplant patients ≥20 years of age in the first 100 days posttransplant for the following: prevention of systemic and local infections, interstitial pneumonia of infectious and idiopathic etiologies and acute graft-versus-host disease (AGVHD)[6] (see INDICATIONS AND USAGE). Administration of Gamimune N, 5% to bone marrow transplant patients significantly increased IgG and IgG subclass levels while those seen in the control group fell below predicted levels. The mechanism of action of Gamimune N, 5% in reducing the incidence of AGVHD is presently unknown.

Pediatric HIV Infection

Children infected with human immunodeficiency virus (HIV) may display defects in both cellular and humoral immunity.[7–10] As a result, some children with HIV-1 infection experience serious, potentially life-threatening recurrent bacterial infections.[11–13] In one retrospective report, among 71 HIV-infected children observed over 3.5 years, 27 (37%) experienced serious documented bacterial infections.[12] The types of bacterial and viral infections observed in HIV-infected children are similar to those seen in children with primary hypogammaglobulinemia.[14] The replacement of opsonic and neutralizing IgG antibodies has been shown to reduce serious and minor bacterial infection in HIV-infected children.[15,16]

In a randomized, double-blind, placebo-controlled, multicenter study performed between March 7, 1988 and January 15, 1991, the efficacy of Gamimune N, 5% in pediatric HIV disease to decrease the frequency of serious and minor bacterial infections and the frequency of hospitalization, and to increase the time free of serious bacterial infection was documented in children with clinical or immunologic evidence of HIV disease (see INDICATIONS AND USAGE). The primary endpoint of this study was prospectively defined as a significant reduction in the proportion of subjects who develop at least one serious bacterial infection when compared to the control group of HIV-infected children who received placebo. Serious bacterial infections were defined as laboratory-proven and clinically diagnosed (i.e., radiologically proven acute pneumonia and sinusitis) infections. The Data Safety and Monitoring Board (DSMB) recommended early termination of the study based on data presented to them from an interim analysis in December 1990 which showed that treatment with Gamimune N, 5% increased the time free from serious infections in children with CD4 + counts ≥ 200/mm³.

General

Glycine (aminoacetic acid) is a nonessential amino acid normally present in the body.[17] Glycine is a major ingredient in amino acid solutions employed in intravenous alimentation.[18] While toxic effects of glycine administration have been reported,[19] the doses and rates of administration were 3 – 4-fold greater than those for Gamimune N, 10%.

The buffer capacity of Gamimune N, 10% is 35.0 mEq/L (~0.35 mEq/g protein). A dose of 1000 mg/kg body weight therefore represents an acid load of 0.35 mEq/kg body weight. The total buffering capacity of whole blood in a normal individual is 45–50 mEq/L of blood, or 3.6 mEq/kg body weight.[20] Thus, the acid load delivered with a dose of 1000 mg/kg of Gamimune N, 10% would be neutralized by the buffering capacity of whole blood alone, even if the dose was infused instantaneously.

In Phase I human studies comparing Gamimune N, 10% with Gamimune N, 5% (in 10% maltose), venous blood measurements were taken following the intravenous administration of 400 mg/kg body weight in 18 patients. There were no clinically important changes in mean venous pH, bicarbonate, or base excess measurements in these patients receiving either preparation.[2]

In a similar, earlier Phase I study Gamimune N, 5% (in 10% maltose) was compared with a chemically modified 5% in-

travenous immunoglobulin preparation with a pH of 6.8. No clinically important changes in mean venous pH and bicarbonate measurements were detected following infusions of either preparation at doses of 400 mg/kg body weight in 37 patients.

In patients with limited or compromised acid-base compensatory mechanisms, consideration should be given to the effect of the additional acid load Gamimune N, 10% might present.

INDICATIONS AND USAGE
Primary Humoral Immunodeficiency

Gamimune N, 10% is efficacious in the treatment of primary immunodeficiency states in which severe impairment of antibody forming capacity has been shown, such as: congenital agammaglobulinemias, common variable immunodeficiency, Wiskott-Aldrich syndrome, x-linked immunodeficiency with hyper IgM, and severe combined immunodeficiencies.[5,21–23] Gamimune N, 10% is especially useful when high levels or rapid elevation of circulating antibodies are desired or when intramuscular injections are contraindicated.

Idiopathic Thrombocytopenic Purpura (ITP)

In clinical situations in which a rapid rise in platelet count is needed to control bleeding or to allow a patient with ITP to undergo surgery, administration of Gamimune N, 10% should be considered. Studies with Gamimune N, 5% demonstrate that in patients in whom a response was achieved, the rise of platelets was generally rapid (within 1–5 days), transient (most often lasting from several days to several weeks) and were not considered curative. It is presently not possible to predict which patients with ITP will respond to therapy, although the increase in platelet counts in children seems to be better than that in adults. Childhood ITP may, however, respond spontaneously without treatment.

Gamimune N, 10% has been studied in 31 adult and pediatric subjects with ITP using a dosage of 1,000 mg/kg body weight on either 1 day or 2 consecutive days. Fourteen of 16 children (87.5%) and 9 of 10 adults with platelet follow-up (90%) responded to treatment with clinically significant platelet increments of ≥ 30,000/mm³. In the 12 children with acute ITP, there was an average increase in platelet count above baseline of 274,000/mm³ (range 33,000–529,000/mm³).

Two different dosing regimens of Gamimune N, 5% have been studied in clinical investigations: a regimen consisting of 400 mg/kg body weight daily for 5 consecutive days, and a high dose treatment regimen consisting of 1,000 mg/kg body weight administered on either 1 day or 2 consecutive days (these studies are summarized below).

In clinical studies of Gamimune N, 5%, five of six (83.3%) children and 12 of 16 (75%) adults with acute or chronic ITP treated with 400 mg/kg body weight for 5 consecutive days demonstrated clinically significant platelet increments of ≥ 30,000/mm³ over baseline. The mean platelet count in children with ITP rose from 27,800/mm³ at baseline to 297,000/mm³ (range 50,000–455,000/mm³) and the mean platelet count in adults with ITP rose from 27,900/mm³ at baseline to 124,900/mm³ (range 11,000–341,000/mm³). Two of three children with acute ITP rapidly went into complete remission.

Thirteen of 14 children (92.9%) and 26 of 29 adults (89.7%) with acute or chronic ITP treated with Gamimune N, 5% 1,000 mg/kg body weight administered on either 1 day or 2 consecutive days responded to treatment with clinically significant platelet increments of ≥ 30,000/mm³ over baseline. This included three of three patients with ITP that were human immunodeficiency virus (HIV) antibody positive and two of two patients with ITP that were pregnant. The mean platelet count in children with ITP treated with Gamimune N, 5% 1,000 mg/kg body weight on 1 day or 2 consecutive days rose from 44,400/mm³ at baseline to 285,600/mm³ (range 89,000–473,000/mm³) and the mean platelet count in adults with ITP treated with the regimen rose from 23,400/mm³ at baseline to 173,100/mm³ (range 28,000–709,000/mm³). Two patients, one each with acute adult and chronic childhood ITP, entered complete remission with treatment.

Six of the 29 adult patients with ITP received Gamimune N, 5% 1,000 mg/kg on 1 day or 2 consecutive days to increase the platelet count prior to splenectomy. Mean platelet counts rose from 14,500/mm³ at baseline to 129,300/mm³ (range 51,000–242,000/mm³) prior to surgery.

The duration of the platelet rise following treatment of ITP with either treatment regimen of Gamimune N, 5% was variable, ranging from several days to 12 months or more. Some ITP patients have demonstrated continuing responsiveness over many months to intermittent infusions of Gamimune N, 5% 400–1,000 mg/kg body weight, administered as a single maintenance dose, at intervals as indicated by the platelet count.

Bone Marrow Transplantation (BMT)

In clinical studies in bone marrow transplant patients ≥ 20 years of age, Gamimune N, 5% decreased the risk of septicemia and other infections, interstitial pneumonia of infec-

Continued on next page

Gamimune N, 10%—Cont.

tious or idiopathic etiologies and acute graft-versus-host disease (AGVHD) in the first 100 days posttransplant. Gamimune N, 5% is not indicated in bone marrow transplant patients below 20 years of age. In a controlled study of 369 evaluable BMT patients (184 treated and 185 controls) who either did or did not receive Gamimune N, 5% in doses of 500 mg/kg body weight on days −7 and −2 pretransplant, then weekly through day 90 posttransplant, posttransplant complications were evaluated in the entire study group and in patients under age 20 and age 20 or older. For patients ≥ 20 years of age (128 patients in the control group and 119 patients in the treated group), there was a statistically significant reduction in interstitial pneumonia from 21% in the control group to 9% in the treated group (p = 0.0032) during the first 100 days posttransplant. Also significantly reduced in this age group were: overall septicemia from 53 infections in the 128 patient control group to 26 infections in the 119 patient treated group (relative risk control:treated [RR] 2.36, p = 0.0025); gram-negative septicemia from 24 infections in the 128 patient control group to 9 infections in the 119 patient treated group (RR 2.53, p = 0.015); gram-positive septicemia from 16 infections in the 128 patient control group to 8 infections in the 119 patient treated group (RR 2.73, p = 0.046); and Grade II to IV AGVHD from an incidence of 58 of 110 in the control group to 38 of 108 in the treated group (p = 0.0051).

The given p-values do not take into account multiple endpoints and subset analyses. Therefore, some of the p-values could occur by chance alone. There was no significant improvement in overall mortality in this study.

In patients below age 20, there appeared to be no benefit from treatment with Gamimune N, 5%, either in reducing the incidence of infections or the incidence of AGVHD.

Pediatric HIV Infection

Gamimune N, 5% 400 mg/kg every 28 days significantly decreased the frequency of serious and minor bacterial infections (laboratory-proven and clinically diagnosed) and the frequency of hospitalization, and increased the time free of serious bacterial infection. The effect of Gamimune N, 5% in preventing serious bacterial infections was especially apparent in preventing primary bacteremia (including *Streptococcus pneumoniae* bacteremia) and acute pneumonia.

In a randomized, double-blind, placebo-controlled, multicenter study, 394 HIV-infected, non-hemophilic, children less than 13 years of age were randomized. Of the children randomized, 369 were included in the efficacy analysis and 376 in the safety analysis. The study population had 1) a mean age of 40 months (range 2.4–136.8 months), 2) acquired HIV primarily through vertical transmission (91%), 3) a majority (87%) of CDC Class P-2 (symptomatic), and 4) had a median CD4 + count of 937 cells/mm^3 (range 0–6660 cells/mm^3). At the time of study entry, 14% (52 of 369) were receiving *Pneumocystis carinii* pneumonia (PCP) prophylaxis. During the course of the study, 51% (189 of 369) received PCP prophylaxis and 44% (164 of 369) received zidovudine (ZDV). Children with HIV-1 infection were initially stratified into two groups based upon CD4 + count (< 200 cells/mm^3 versus ≥ 200 cells/mm^3) and CDC classification of pediatric HIV disease (history of opportunistic infections [P-2-D-1] and recurrent serious bacterial infections [P-2-D-2] versus others). Subjects received Gamimune N, 5% (400 mg/kg = 8 mL/kg) (n = 185) or an equivalent volume of placebo (0.1% Albumin [Human]) (n = 184) every 28 days. The mean follow-up for subjects receiving Gamimune N, 5% was 17.9 months and 17.8 months for patients on placebo. The number of subjects who had at least one serious bacterial infection was 86 of 184 (47%) in the placebo group and 55 of 185 (30%) in the Gamimune N, 5% group (p = 0.0009). All p-values reported are two-sided. Treatment with Gamimune N, 5% compared to placebo was also associated with a significant reduction in both the number of subjects with at least one laboratory-proven infection (36 of 184 vs. 18 of 185, p = 0.0081), and the number of subjects with at least one clinically diagnosed infection (71 of 184 vs. 45 of 185, p = 0.0036). Efficacy in patients with CD4 + counts < 200/mm^3 was not established, possibly because of the small number of subjects in this category.

The 2-year treatment period defined in the protocol was truncated for some patients by the DSMB based on data from the interim analysis. Rates of serious bacterial infections per 100 patient-years were computed and analyzed to take into account both the unequal duration of treatment and follow-up, as well as recurrent infections in individual subjects. Children treated with Gamimune N, 5% experienced a 50.5% lower frequency of laboratory-proven serious bacterial infection compared to the group treated with placebo (9.1 vs. 18.2 infections per 100 patient-years, p = 0.031), a 36.0% lower frequency of clinically diagnosed serious infections (24.0 vs. 37.5 infections per 100 patient-years, p = 0.013), a 40.6% reduction in total serious infections (laboratory-proven and clinically diagnosed) (33.1 vs. 55.7 infections per 100 patient-years, p = 0.003), a 60% lower frequency of primary bacteremias (5.8 vs. 14.5 infections per

100 patient-years, p = 0.009), a 75.6% lower frequency of *Streptococcus pneumoniae* bacteremia (1.1 vs. 4.5 bacteremias per 100 patient-years, p = 0.026), a 54.3% lower frequency of clinically diagnosed pneumonia (12.7 vs. 27.8 infections per 100 patient-years, p = 0.001), and a 22.5% lower frequency of minor bacterial infections (including otitis media, skin and soft tissue infections, and upper respiratory tract infections) (123.6 vs. 159.5 infections per 100 patient-years, p = 0.033).

In addition to a reduced frequency of infection, children treated with Gamimune N, 5% had a 36.8% lower number of hospitalizations per 100 patient-years (72 vs. 114 per 100 patient-years, p = 0.002) and a reduced number of hospital days (6.9 vs. 10.5 per patient-year, p = 0.030) than patients treated with placebo. Patients treated with Gamimune N, 5% had a higher probability of remaining free of laboratory-proven infections (p = 0.0093) and combined laboratory-proven and clinically diagnosed infections (p = 0.0015) for 24 months than the group of children treated with placebo. At 24 months, the estimated probabilities of remaining infection-free for the Gamimune N, 5% and placebo arms were 87.8% vs. 76.1%, respectively, for laboratory-proven infections and 63.5% vs. 44.5%, respectively, for combined laboratory-proven and clinically diagnosed infections.

There was no effect of Gamimune N, 5% therapy on mortality, which was low in both treatment groups (17%), or on the frequency of opportunistic or viral infections during the period of study.

Since antibacterial prophylaxis could also account for the observed reduction in the rate of serious bacterial infections, further analysis was performed to evaluate the role of *Pneumocystis carinii* pneumonia (PCP) prophylaxis on the efficacy of Gamimune N, 5%. PCP prophylaxis consisted primarily (96%) of trimethoprim/sulfamethoxazole given 3 successive days each week. This antibiotic combination could be active against the bacteria commonly encountered in this patient population. In the subgroup of patients receiving PCP prophylaxis at study entry, treatment with Gamimune N, 5% was associated with 44.0 infections per 100 patient-years, whereas placebo recipients had 64.7 infections per 100 patient-years (p = 0.047). In the subgroup of patients not receiving PCP prophylaxis at study entry, treatment with Gamimune N, 5% was associated with 22.1 infections per 100 patient-years, whereas placebo recipients had 44.9 infections per 100 patient-years on placebo (p = 0.024). Thus, Gamimune N, 5% benefited patients by reducing the rate of serious bacterial infections whether or not they were receiving PCP prophylactic treatment at study entry. However, it should be noted that the use of PCP prophylactic treatment in this study was not randomized and specific guidelines for its administration were not identified.

CONTRAINDICATIONS

Gamimune N, 10% is contraindicated in individuals who are known to have had an anaphylactic or severe systemic response to Immune Globulin (Human). Individuals with selective IgA deficiencies who have known antibody against IgA (anti-IgA antibody) should not receive Gamimune N, 10% since these patients may experience severe reactions to the IgA which may be present.[22]

WARNINGS

Immune Globulin Intravenous (Human), 10%— Gamimune® N, 10% is made from human plasma. Products made from human plasma may contain infectious agents, such as viruses, that can cause disease. The risk that such products will transmit an infectious agent has been reduced by screening plasma donors for prior exposure to certain viruses, by testing for the presence of certain current virus infections, and by inactivating and/or removing certain viruses. Despite these measures, such products can still potentially transmit disease. There is also the possibility that unknown infectious agents may be present in such products. Individuals who receive infusions of blood or plasma products may develop signs and/or symptoms of some viral infections, particularly hepatitis C. ALL infections thought by a physician possibly to have been transmitted by this product should be reported by the physician or other healthcare provider to Bayer Corporation [1-888-765-3203].

The physician should discuss the risks and benefits of this product with the patient, before prescribing or administering it to the patient.

Gamimune N, 10% should be administered only intravenously as the intramuscular and subcutaneous routes have not been evaluated.

Immune Globulin Intravenous (Human), 5%—Gamimune® N, 5% has, on rare occasions, caused a precipitous fall in blood pressure and a clinical picture of anaphylaxis, even when the patient is not known to be sensitive to immune globulin preparations. These reactions may be related to the rate of infusion. Accordingly, the infusion rate given under DOSAGE AND ADMINISTRATION for Gamimune N, 10% should be closely followed, at least until the physician has had sufficient experience with a given patient. The patient's vital signs should be monitored continuously and careful ob-

servation made for any symptoms throughout the entire infusion. Epinephrine should be available for the treatment of an acute anaphylactic reaction.

PRECAUTIONS

General

Any vial that has been entered should be used promptly. Partially used vials should be discarded. Do not use if turbid. Solution which has been frozen should not be used.

An aseptic meningitis syndrome (AMS) has been reported to occur infrequently in association with Immune Globulin Intravenous (Human) treatment. The syndrome usually begins within several hours to two days following Immune Globulin Intravenous (Human) treatment. It is characterized by symptoms and signs including severe headache, nuchal rigidity, drowsiness, fever, photophobia, painful eye movements, and nausea and vomiting. Cerebrospinal fluid (CSF) studies are frequently positive with pleocytosis up to several thousand cells per mm^3, predominantly from the granulocytic series, and elevated protein levels up to several hundred mg/dL. Patients exhibiting such symptoms and signs should receive a thorough neurological examination, including CSF studies, to rule out other causes of meningitis. AMS may occur more frequently in association with high dose (2 g/kg) Immune Globulin Intravenous (Human) treatment. Discontinuation of Immune Globulin Intravenous (Human) treatment has resulted in remission of AMS within several days without sequelae.[24–27]

Isolated reports have appeared of transient and reversible renal insufficiency following administration of Immune Globulin Intravenous (Human) therapy. The mechanics involved are uncertain.[28,29]

Drug Interactions

Antibodies in Gamimune N, 10% may interfere with the response to live viral vaccines such as measles, mumps and rubella. Therefore, use of such vaccines should be deferred until approximately 6 months after Gamimune N, 10% administration.

Please see DOSAGE AND ADMINISTRATION for other drug interactions.

Pregnancy Category C

Animal reproduction studies have not been conducted with Gamimune N, 10%. It is not known whether Gamimune N, 10% can cause fetal harm when administered to a pregnant woman or can affect reproduction capacity. Gamimune N, 10% should be given to a pregnant woman only if clearly needed.

ADVERSE REACTIONS

Primary Humoral Immunodeficiency

A safety study has been conducted in 20 adult and pediatric subjects with primary immunodeficiency syndrome comparing side effects of Gamimune N, 5% with those of Gamimune N, 10%. The incidence, nature, or severity of reactions with Gamimune N, 10% were not different from those observed with Gamimune N, 5%, and were consistent with those observed in previous studies with Gamimune N, 5%. Symptoms related to the infusion of Gamimune N, 10% were observed in 9 (3.5%) of 255 infusions. These symptoms were all mild to moderate in severity and included chills, fever, headache and emesis.

In a study of 37 patients with immunodeficiency syndromes receiving Gamimune N, 5% in a monthly dose of 400 mg/kg body weight, reactions were seen in 5.2% of the infusions. Symptoms reported included malaise, a feeling of faintness, fever, chills, headache, nausea, vomiting, chest tightness, dyspnea and chest, back or hip pain. Mild erythema following infiltration of Gamimune N, 5% at the infusion site was reported in some cases.

A safety study has been conducted in 17 adult and adolescent subjects with primary immunodeficiency syndrome, comparing side effects and bioequivalency of Gamimune N, 10% with those of Gamimune N, 10% treated with solvent/detergent. The incidence, nature and severity of reactions with Gamimune N, 10% treated with solvent/detergent were not different from those observed with Gamimune N, 10%.

Idiopathic Thrombocytopenic Purpura

An investigation of Gamimune N, 10% in 31 adult and pediatric subjects with ITP encountered side effects in 17 of 119 (14.3%) infusions. The dosage in these studies was 1,000 mg/kg body weight for 1 day or 2 consecutive days. However, in the adult study, an induction dosage of 500 mg/kg body weight for 1 day or 2 consecutive days was associated with 17 of these infusions. Of those 17 infusions, three had adverse events. Overall, side effects included mild chest pain, mild and moderate emesis, moderate fever, mild or moderate headache (severe on one occasion) and a single incidence of hives, pruritus and rash. At least 17 of the 50 infusions in the pediatric study were given at rates of ≥ 0.1 mL/kg body weight per minute as part of a rate escalation investigation. Maximum infusion rates obtained were not limited by or interrupted due to adverse effects.

In studies of Gamimune N, 5% administered at a dose of 400 mg/kg body weight in the treatment of adult and pediatric patients with ITP, systemic reactions were noted in only 4 of 154 (2.6%) infusions, and all but one occurred at

rates of infusion greater than 0.04 mL/kg body weight per minute. The symptoms reported included chest tightness, a sense of tachycardia (pulse was 84 beats per minute), and a burning sensation in the head; these symptoms were all mild and transient.

In studies of Gamimune N, 5% administered at a dose of 1,000 mg/kg body weight either as a single dose or as two doses on consecutive days in the treatment of adult and pediatric patients with ITP, adverse reactions were noted in 25 of 251 (10%) infusions. Symptoms reported included headache, nausea, fever, chills, back pain, chest tightness, and shortness of breath. In children, the high dose regimen has been well-tolerated at the highest rates of infusion. In adults, however, the frequency of adverse reactions tended to increase with infusion rates in excess of 0.06 mL/kg body weight per minute. In general, reactions reported with infusion of Gamimune N, 5% in these studies were reported as mild or moderate, and responded to slowing of the infusion rate.

Bone Marrow Transplantation

In studies of Gamimune N, 5% administered to 185 bone marrow transplant recipients at doses of 500 mg/kg (10 mL/kg) body weight on day –7 and day –2 pretransplant, then weekly through day 90 posttransplant, adverse reactions were noted in 12 (6.5%) of the 185 patients that received Gamimune N, 5% and in 14 (0.6%) of 2,176 infusions. All reactions reported were rate-related and classified as mild. Chills were the most common symptom reported, occurring in nine patients. The other symptoms reported included headache, flushing, fever, pruritus and slight back discomfort. All reactions resolved satisfactorily, usually without treatment or decreasing the infusion rate.

Pediatric HIV Infection

Three hundred seventy-six (376) patients, 187 treated with Gamimune N, 5% and 189 treated with placebo (0.1% Albumin [Human]), were included in the safety analysis. Adverse reactions occurred during or within 24 hours of an infusion in 50 of 3,451 (1.4%) infusions of Gamimune N, 5% and 62 of 3,447 (1.8%) infusions of placebo. Fever was the most common adverse reaction and occurred 30 of 105 (28.6%) patients receiving placebo and 19 of 78 (24.4%) patients treated with Gamimune N, 5%. Irritability was the second most common symptom reported, with 10 of 105 (9.5%) reports for the placebo group and 9 of 78 (11.5%) for the group treated with Gamimune N, 5%. A large number of diverse adverse reactions accounted for the remaining adverse reactions reported in both study groups. In general, the number of adverse events reported was comparable in both the placebo and Gamimune N, 5% treated groups. Three serious adverse reactions were reported. One patient experienced a hypersensitivity reaction and did not receive further Gamimune N, 5% treatment. A second patient developed tachycardia and was admitted to an intensive care unit, but later continued treatment with Gamimune N, 5%. A third patient had skin infiltration during infusion and developed a full thickness skin slough over the dorsum of the hand that required skin grafting.

General

In the studies undertaken to date, other types of reactions have not been reported with Gamimune N, 5% or Gamimune N, 10%. It may be, however, that adverse effects will be similar to those previously reported with intravenous and intramuscular immunoglobulin administration. Potential reactions, therefore, may also include anxiety, flushing, wheezing, abdominal cramps, myalgias, arthralgia, and dizziness; rash has been reported only rarely. Reactions to intravenous immunoglobulin tend to be related to the rate of infusion.

True anaphylactic reactions to Gamimune N, 10% may occur in recipients with documented prior histories of severe allergic reactions to intramuscular immunoglobulin, but some patients may tolerate cautiously administered intravenous immunoglobulin without adverse effects.[2,30] Very rarely an anaphylactoid reaction may occur in patients with no prior history of severe allergic reactions to either intramuscular or intravenous immunoglobulin.[2]

DOSAGE AND ADMINISTRATION

General

Dosages for specific indications are indicated below, but in general, it is recommended that Gamimune N, 10% be infused by itself at a rate of 0.01 to 0.02 mL/kg body weight per minute for 30 minutes; if well-tolerated, the rate may be **gradually** increased to a maximum of 0.08 mL/kg body weight per minute. Investigations indicate that Gamimune N, 10% is well-tolerated and less likely to produce side effects when infused at the indicated rate. If side effects occur, the rate may be reduced, or the infusion interrupted until symptoms subside. The infusion may then be resumed at the rate which is comfortable for the patient. Parenteral drug products should be inspected visually for particulate matter and discoloration prior to administration, whenever solution and container permit.

It is recommended that infusion of Gamimune N, 10% be given by a separate line, by itself, without mixing with other intravenous fluids or medications the patient might be receiving. Gamimune N, 10% should not be mixed with Immune Globulin Intravenous (Human) from another manufacturer. Gamimune N, 10% is not compatible with saline. If dilution is required, Gamimune N, 10% may be diluted with 5% dextrose in water (D5/W). No other drug interactions or compatibilities have been evaluated.

Primary Humoral Immunodeficiency

The usual dosage of Gamimune N, 10% of prophylaxis in primary immunodeficiency syndromes is 100–200 mg/kg of body weight administered approximately once a month by intravenous infusion. The dosage may be given more frequently or increased as high as 400 mg/kg body weight, if the clinical response is inadequate, or the level of IgG achieved in the circulation is felt to be insufficient. The minimum level of IgG required for protection has not been determined.

Idiopathic Thrombocytopenic Purpura (ITP)

Induction: An increase in platelet count has been observed in children and some adults with acute or chronic ITP receiving Gamimune N, 5% 400 mg/kg body weight daily for 5 days. Alternatively, studies in adults and children with Gamimune N, 5% and Gamimune N, 10% using a dose of 1,000 mg/kg body weight daily for 1 day or 2 consecutive days have also shown increases in platelet count. In the latter treatment regimen, if an adequate increase in the platelet count is observed at 24 hours, the second dose of 1,000 mg/kg body weight may be withheld. The high dose regimen (1,000 mg/kg $\times$ 1–2 days) is not recommended for individuals with expanded fluid volumes or where fluid volume may be a concern. With both treatment regimens, a response usually occurs within several days and is maintained for a variable period of time. In general, a response is seen less often in adults than in children.

Maintenance: In adults and children with ITP, if after induction therapy the platelet count falls to less than 30,000/mm^3 and/or the patient manifests clinically significant bleeding, Gamimune N, 10% 400 mg/kg body weight may be given as a single infusion. If an adequate response does not result, the dose can be increased to 800–1,000 mg/kg of body weight given as a single infusion. Maintenance infusions may be administered intermittently as clinically indicated to maintain a platelet count greater than 30,000/mm^3.

Bone Marrow Transplantation

A reduction in posttransplant complications has been observed in bone marrow transplant patients $\geq$ 20 years of age receiving Gamimune N, 5%. An equivalent dosage of Gamimune N, 10% is recommended in doses of 500 mg/kg (5 mL/kg) body weight beginning on days –7 and –2 pretransplant (or at the time conditioning therapy for transplantation is begun), then weekly through day 90 posttransplant. Gamimune N, 10% should be administered by itself through a Hickman line while it is in place, and thereafter through a peripheral vein. Please see DOSAGE AND ADMINISTRATION for other drug interactions.

Pediatric HIV Infection

A reduction in bacterial infections has been observed in children infected with HIV-1 receiving Gamimune N, 5%. An equivalent dosage of Gamimune N, 10% is recommended in doses of 400 mg/kg (4 mL/kg) body weight every 28 days.

HOW SUPPLIED

Gamimune N, 10% is supplied in the following sizes:

NDC Number	Size	Grams Protein
0026-0648-12	10 mL	1.0
0026-0648-20	50 mL	5.0
0026-0648-71	100 mL	10.0
0026-0648-24	200 mL	20.0

STORAGE

Store at 2–8°C (36–46°F). Do not freeze. Do not use after expiration date.

CAUTION

U.S. federal law prohibits dispensing without prescription.

LIMITED WARRANTY

A number of factors beyond our control could reduce the efficacy of this product or even result in an ill effect following its use. These include improper storage and handling of the product after it leaves our hands, diagnosis, dosage, method of administration, and biological differences in individual patients. Because of these factors, it is important that this product be stored properly and that the directions be followed carefully during use.

No warranty, express or implied, including any warranty of merchantability or fitness is made. Representatives of the Company are not authorized to vary the terms or the contents of the printed labeling, including the package insert for this product, except by printed notice from the Company's headquarters. The prescriber and user of this product must accept the terms hereof.

REFERENCES

1. Tenold RA, Inventor: Cutter Laboratories, assignee, Intravenously injectable immune serum globulin. U.S. Patent 4,396,608, Aug. 2, 1983.
2. Data on file at Bayer Corporation.
3. Pirofsky B, Campbell SM, Montanaro A: Individual patient variations in the kinetics of intravenous immunoglobulin administration. *J Clin Immunol* 2(2): 7S-14S, 1982.
4. Pirofsky B: Intravenous immune globulin therapy in hypogammaglobulinemia. *Amer J Med* 76(3A):53–60, 1984.
5. Pirofsky B, Anderson CJ, Bardana EJ Jr.: Therapeutic and detrimental effects of intravenous immunoglobulin therapy. In: Alving BM (ed.): *Immunoglobulins: characteristics and uses of intravenous preparations.* Washington, D.C., U.S. Government Printing Office, (1980), pp 15–22.
6. Sullivan KM, Kopecky KJ, Jocom J, et al: Immunomodulatory and antimicrobial efficacy of intravenous immunoglobulin in bone marrow transplantation. *N Engl J Med* 323(11):705–12, 1990.
7. Bernstein LJ, Ochs HD, Wedgwood RJ, et al: Defective humoral immunity in pediatric acquired immune deficiency syndrome. *J Pediatr* 107(3):352–7, 1985.
8. Borlowsky W, Steele CJ, Grubman S, et al: Antibody responses to bacterial toxoids in children infected with human immunodeficiency virus. *J Pediatr* 110(4):563–6, 1987.
9. Blanche S, Le Deist F, Fischer A, et al: Longitudinal study of 18 children with perinatal LAV/HTLV III infection: attempt at prognostic evaluation. *J Pediatr* 109(6): 965–70, 1986.
10. Pahwa S, Fikrig S, Menez R, et al: Pediatric acquired immunodeficiency syndrome demonstration of B-lymphocyte defects in vitro. *Diagn Immunol* 4(1):24–30, 1986.
11. Bernstein LJ, Krieger BZ, Novick B, et al: Bacterial infections in the acquired immunodeficiency syndrome of children. *Pediatr Infect Dis* 4(5):472–5, 1985.
12. Krasinski K, Borkowsky W, Bonk S, et al: Bacterial infections in human immunodeficiency virus-infected children. *Pediatr Infect Dis J* 7(5):323–8, 1988.
13. Scott GB, Buck BE, Leterman JG, et al: Acquired immunodeficiency syndrome in infants. *N Engl J Med* 310(2): 76–81, 1984.
14. Mofenson LM, Willoughby A. Passive immunization. In: Pizzo PA, Wilfert CM, (eds.) *Pediatric AIDS: the challenge of HIV infection in infants, children and adolescents.* Baltimore: Williams & Wilkins (1991) pp 633–50.
15. National Institute of Child Health and Human Development Intravenous Immunoglobulin Study Group. Intravenous immune globulin for the prevention of bacterial infections in children with symptomatic human immunodeficiency virus infection. *N Engl J Med* 325(2):73–80, 1991.
16. Mofenson LM, Moye J Jr, Bethel J, et al: Prophylactic intravenous immunoglobulin in HIV-infected children with CD4 + counts of 0.20 $\times$ 10^9/L or more. Effect on viral, opportunistic, and bacterial infections. *JAMA* 268(4):483–88, 1992.
17. Glycine. In: Budavari S, O'Neil MJ, Smith A, et al, eds.: *Merck Index.* 11th ed. Rahway NJ, Merck & Co., 1989, p. 706.
18. Wretlind, A: Complete intravenous nutrition: theoretical and experimental background. *Nutr Metab* 14(Suppl):1–57, 1972.
19. Hahn RG, Stalberg HP, Gustafsson SA: Intravenous infusion of irrigating fluids containing glycine or mannitol with and without ethanol. *J Urol* 142(4):1102–1105, 1989.
20. Guyton AC: *Textbook of Medical Physiology.* 5th ed. Philadelphia, W.B. Saunders, 1976, pp 499–500.
21. Nolte MT, Pirofsky B, Gerritz GA, et al: Intravenous immunoglobulin therapy for antibody deficiency. *Clin Exp Immunol* 36: 237–43, 1979.
22. Buckley RH: Immunoglobulin replacement therapy: Indications and contraindications for use and variable IgG levels achieved. In: Alving BM (ed): *Immunoglobulins: characteristics and uses of intravenous preparations.* Washington, D.C., U.S. Government Printing Office, (1980), pp 3–8.
23. Ochs HD: Intravenous immunoglobulin therapy of patients with primary immunodeficiency syndromes: efficacy and safety of a new modified immune globulin preparation. In: Alving BM (ed.): *Immunoglobulins: characteristics and uses of intravenous preparations.* Washington, D.C., U.S. Government Printing Office, (1980), pp 9–14.
24. Sekul E, Cupler E, Dalakas M. Aseptic meningitis associated with high-dose intravenous immunoglobulin therapy: Frequency and risk factors. *Ann Int Med* 121: 259–262, 1994.
25. Kato E, Shindo S, Eto Y, et al: Administration of Immune Globulin Associated with Aseptic Meningitis. *JAMA* 259(22):3269–3270, 1988.

Continued on next page

Gamimune N, 10%—Cont.

26. Casteels-Van Daele M, Wijndaele L, Hunninck K, et al: Intravenous immune globulin and acute aseptic meningitis. *N Engl J Med* 323(9):614–615, 1990.
27. Scribner C, Kapit R, Phillips E, et al: Aseptic meningitis and intravenous immunoglobulin therapy. *Ann Intern Med* 121(4):305–306, 1994.
28. Schiavotto C, Ruggeri M, Rodeghiero F, Adverse reactions after high-dose intravenous immunoglobulin: incidence in 83 patients treated for idiopathic thrombocytopenic purpura (ITP) and review of the literature. *Haematologica* 78(6:Suppl 2):35–40, 1993.
29. Pasatiempo AM, Kroser JA, Rudnick M, et al: Acute renal failure after intravenous immunoglobulin therapy. *J Rheumatol* 21(2):347–9, 1994.
30. Peerless AG, Stiehm ER: Intravenous gammaglobulin for reaction to intramuscular preparation. [letter] *Lancet* 2(8347):461, 1983.

Bayer Corporation
Pharmaceutical Division
Elkhart, IN 46515 USA 14-7648-001
U.S. License No. 8 (Rev. April 1998)
Shown in Product Identification Guide, page 305

KOĀTE®-HP ℞
[*kō 'ate*]
Antihemophilic Factor (Human)
(Factor VIII, AHF, AHG)

DESCRIPTION

Antihemophilic Factor (Human), Koāte®-HP, is a sterile, stable, purified, dried concentrate of human Antihemophilic Factor (AHF, factor VIII, AHG) which has been treated with tri-n-butyl phosphate (TNBP) and polysorbate 80 and is intended for use in therapy of classical hemophilia (hemophilia A).

Koāte-HP is purified from the cold insoluble fraction of pooled fresh-frozen plasma by modification and refinements of the methods first described by Hershgold, Pool, and Pappenhagen.[1] Koāte-HP contains purified and concentrated factor VIII. The factor VIII is 300-1000 times purified over whole plasma. Part of the fractionation may be performed by another licensed manufacturer. When reconstituted as directed, Koāte-HP contains approximately 50-150 times as much factor VIII as an equal volume of fresh plasma. The specific activity, after addition of Albumin (Human), is in the range of 9-22 IU/mg protein. Koāte-HP must be administered by the intravenous route.

Each bottle of Koāte-HP contains the labeled amount of antihemophilic factor activity in International Units (IU). One IU, as defined by the World Health Organization Standard for Blood Coagulation factor VIII, human, is approximately equal to the level of AHF found in 1.0 mL of fresh pooled human plasma. The final product when reconstituted as directed contains not more than (NMT) 5 units heparin/mL, NMT 1500 ppm polyethylene glycol (PEG), NMT 0.05 M glycine, NMT 25 ppm polysorbate 80, NMT 5 ppm tri-n-butyl phosphate (TNBP), NMT 3 mM calcium chloride, NMT 1 ppm aluminum, NMT 0.06 M histidine, and NMT 10 mg/mL Albumin (Human).

CLINICAL PHARMACOLOGY

Hemophilia A is a hereditary bleeding disorder characterized by deficient coagulant activity of the specific plasma protein clotting factor, factor VIII. In afflicted individuals, hemorrhages may occur spontaneously or after only minor trauma. Surgery on such individuals is not feasible without first correcting the clotting abnormality. The administration of Koāte-HP provides an increase in plasma levels of factor VIII and can temporarily correct the coagulation defect in these patients.

After infusion of Koāte-HP, there is usually an instantaneous rise in the coagulant level followed by an initial rapid decrease in activity, and then a subsequent much slower rate of decrease in activity.[2–4] The early rapid phase may represent the time of equilibration with the extravascular compartment, and the second or slow phase of the survival curve presumably is the result of degradation and reflects the true biologic half-life of the infused Antihemophilic Factor (Human).[3] Studies with Koāte-HP in hemophilic patients have demonstrated a biologic half-life of approximately 9 to 14 hours.[2]

In 1984, Prince, et al[5] described the susceptibility of hepatitis B virus (HBV) and the Hutchinson strain of non-A, non-B hepatitis virus to inactivation by ether and polysorbate 80. This method is known to disrupt lipid-containing enveloped viruses. Subsequently, others[6,7] using tri-n-butyl phosphate as an alternative organic solvent to the hazardous ethyl ether in combination with a number of different detergents including polysorbate 80, sodium deoxycholate, sodium cholate, or Triton x-100, showed these forms of chemical treatment to be rapidly effective in inactivating certain lipid-enveloped viruses. These viruses included vesicular stomatitis virus (VSV), sindbis virus, and sendai virus[6] as well as, in a later study,[7] human immunodeficiency virus (HIV), HBV and non-A, non-B virus. Similar studies undertaken at Miles Inc. using TNBP and polysorbate 80 treatment of factor VIII concentrate immediately prior to a gel permeation chromatography purifying/concentrating procedure have confirmed the inactivation of VSV, visna, and sindbis viruses.

Antihemophilic Factor (Human), Koāte®-HP is purified by virtue of a gel permeation chromatography step serving the dual purpose of removing the TNBP and polysorbate 80 as well as increasing the purity of the Factor VIII. Recently, concerns have been expressed concerning alterations to immune function occurring in asymptomatic hemophiliacs,[8–15] with some of the abnormalities being independent of HIV exposure. It has been suggested that the underlying mechanisms might include repeated exposure to viral agents, repeated allostimulation and/or possible contaminants in factor VIII preparations (e.g., IgG aggregates). More highly purified preparations which have minimized risks of viral transmission may therefore be desirable.[6]

INDICATIONS AND USAGE

Koāte-HP is indicated for the treatment of classical hemophilia (hemophilia A) in which there is a demonstrated deficiency of activity of the plasma clotting factor, factor VIII. Koāte-HP provides a means of temporarily replacing the missing clotting factor in order to correct or prevent bleeding episodes, or in order to perform emergency and elective surgery on hemophiliacs.

Koāte-HP has not been investigated for efficacy in the treatment of von Willebrand's disease, and hence is not approved for such usage.

CONTRAINDICATIONS

None known.

WARNINGS

Koāte-HP is made from human plasma. Products made from human plasma may contain infectious agents, such as viruses, that can cause disease. The risk that such products will transmit an infectious agent has been reduced by screening plasma donors for prior exposure to certain viruses, by testing for the presence of certain current virus infections, and by inactivating and/or removing certain viruses. Despite these measures, such products can still potentially transmit disease. There is also the possibility that unknown infectious agents may be present in such products. ALL infections thought by a physician possibly to have been transmitted by this product should be reported by the physician or other healthcare provider to Bayer Corporation [1-888-765-3203]. The physician should discuss the risks and benefits of this product with the patient, before prescribing or administering it to the patient.

Individuals who receive infusions of blood or plasma products may develop signs and/or symptoms of some viral infections, particularly hepatitis C. It is emphasized that hepatitis B vaccination is essential for patients with hemophilia and it is recommended that this be done at birth or diagnosis.[16,17] Hepatitis A vaccination is also recommended for hemophilic patients who are hepatitis A seronegative.

No studies of CD4 cell count surveillance have been done in HIV seropositive patients treated exclusively with Koāte-HP; however, there have been several reports of increased rates of CD4 cell count decline in HIV seropositive hemophilia patients treated with conventionally purified FVIII concentrates compared to those treated with immunoaffinity purified products.[18–20] The clinical significance of these CD4 cell count findings remains uncertain.

PRECAUTIONS

General

1. Antihemophilic Factor (Human), Koāte-HP is intended for treatment of bleeding disorders arising from a deficiency in factor VIII. This deficiency should be proven prior to administering Koāte-HP.
2. Administer within 3 hours after reconstitution. Do not refrigerate after reconstitution.
3. Administer only by the intravenous route.
4. Filter needle should be used prior to administering.
5. Koāte-HP contains levels of blood group isoagglutinins which are not clinically significant when controlling relatively minor bleeding episodes. When large or frequently repeated doses are required, patients of blood groups A, B, or AB should be monitored by means of hematocrit for signs of progressive anemia, as well as by direct Coombs' tests.
6. Product administration and handling of the infusion set and needles must be done with caution. Percutaneous puncture with a needle contaminated with blood can transmit infectious viruses including HIV (AIDS) and hepatitis. Obtain immediate medical attention if injury occurs.

Place needles in sharps container after single use. Discard all equipment including any reconstituted Koāte-HP product in accordance with biohazard procedures.

Pregnancy Category C

Animal reproduction studies have not been conducted with Koāte-HP. It is also not known whether Koāte-HP can cause fetal harm when administered to a pregnant woman or can affect reproduction capacity. Koāte-HP should be given to a pregnant woman only if clearly needed.

Information for Patient

Some viruses, such as parvovirus B19 or hepatitis A, are particularly difficult to remove or inactivate at this time. Parvovirus B19 most seriously affects pregnant women, or immune-compromised individuals.

Symptoms of parvovirus B19 infection include fever, drowsiness, chills and runny nose followed about 2 weeks later by a rash and joint pain. Evidence of hepatitis A may include several days to weeks of poor appetite, tiredness, and low-grade fever followed by nausea, vomiting, and pain in the belly. Dark urine and a yellowed complexion are also common symptoms. Patients should be encouraged to consult their physician if such symptoms appear.

ADVERSE REACTIONS

Allergic-type reactions may result from the administration of Antihemophilic Factor (Human) preparations.[23,24]

DOSAGE AND ADMINISTRATION

Each bottle of Koāte-HP has the Antihemophilic Factor (Human) content in International Units per bottle stated on the label of the bottle. The reconstituted product must be administered intravenously by either direct syringe injection or drip infusion.

Shanbrom et al,[25] based upon studies in hemophiliacs, have suggested a linear dose-response relation with an approximate rise of 2.5% in Factor VIII activity for each unit of Antihemophilic Factor (Human) transfused per kg of body weight. Abildgaard et al,[26] in work with hemophilic children 8 months to 14 years of age, reported a response factor of 0.5 units/kg. Clinical experience with Koāte-HP has demonstrated a similar dose-response relationship.[2] The following formulas can provide a guide for dosage calculations:

$$\text{Expected factor VIII increase (\% of normal)} = \frac{\text{IU administered}}{\text{body weight (kg)} \times 0.4\ \text{IU/kg}}$$

$$\text{Example: } \frac{840\ \text{IU}}{70\ \text{kg} \times 0.4\ \text{IU/kg}} = 30\%$$

or

IU required = body weight (kg) × desired factor VIII increase (% normal) × 0.4 IU/kg
Example: 70 kg × 0.4 IU/kg × 30% = 840 IU

All efforts should be made to follow the course of therapy with factor VIII level assays. It may be dangerous to assume any certain level has been reached unless direct evidence is obtained.

Prophylaxis of Spontaneous Hemorrhage

The level of factor VIII required to prevent spontaneous hemorrhage is approximately 5% of normal, while a level of 30% of normal is the minimum required for hemostasis following trauma and surgery.[27–29] Mild superficial or early hemorrhages may respond to a single dose of 10 IU per kg,[4,30] leading to an in vivo rise of approximately 20% in the factor VIII level. In patients with early hemarthrosis (mild pain, minimal or no swelling, erythema, warmth, and minimal or no joint limitation), if treated promptly, even smaller doses may be adequate.[30–32]

Mild Hemorrhage

In cases of mild hemorrhage, therapy need not be repeated unless there is evidence of further bleeding.

Moderate Hemorrhage and Minor Surgery

For more serious hemorrhages and for minor surgical procedures, the patient's plasma factor VIII level should be raised to 30%–50% of normal for optimum hemostasis.[30,33] This usually requires an initial dose of 15–25 IU per kg; and if further therapy is required, a maintenance dose of 10–15 IU per kg every 8–12 hours.

Severe Hemorrhage

In patients with life-threatening bleeding, or hemorrhage involving vital structures (central nervous system, retropharyngeal and retroperitoneal spaces, iliopsoas sheath), it may be desirable to raise the factor VIII level to 80%–100% of normal in order to achieve hemostasis.[30,33–35] This may be achieved with an initial Koāte-HP dose of 40–50 IU per kg and a maintenance dose of 20–25 IU per kg every 8–12 hours.

Major Surgery

For major surgical procedures, Kasper[33] recommends that a dose of Antihemophilic Factor (Human) sufficient to achieve a level of 80%–100% of normal be given an hour before the procedure. It is recommended that the factor VIII level be checked prior to going to surgery to assure the expected level is achieved. A second dose, half the size of the priming dose, should be given about 5 hours after the first dose. The

factor VIII level should be maintained at a daily minimum of at least 30% for a healing period of 10–14 days, depending on the nature of the operative procedure.

The above discussion is presented as a reference and a guideline. It should be emphasized that the dosage of Antihemophilic Factor (Human), Koāte®-HP required for normalizing hemostasis must be individualized according to the needs of the patient. Factors to be considered include the weight of the patient, the severity of the deficiency, the severity of the hemorrhage, the presence of inhibitors, and the factor VIII level desired. All efforts should be made to follow the course of therapy with factor VIII level assays.

The clinical effect of Koāte-HP is the most important element in evaluating the effectiveness of treatment. It may be necessary to administer more Koāte-HP than would be estimated in order to attain satisfactory clinical results. If the calculated dose fails to attain the expected factor VIII levels, or if bleeding is not controlled after adequate calculated dosage, the presence of a factor VIII inhibitor should be suspected. Its presence should be substantiated and the inhibitor level quantitated by appropriate laboratory procedure. When an inhibitor is present, the dosage requirement for Koāte-HP is extremely variable and the dosage can be determined only by the clinical response.

Parenteral drug products should be inspected visually for particulate matter and discoloration prior to administration, whenever solution and container permit.

Reconstitution

Vacuum Transfer

1. Warm the unopened diluent and the concentrate to room temperature (NMT 37°C, 99°F).
2. After removing the plastic flip-top caps (Fig. A), aseptically cleanse the rubber stoppers of both bottles.
3. Remove the protective cover from the plastic transfer-needle cartridge with tamper-proof seal and penetrate the stopper of the diluent bottle (Fig. B).
4. Remove the remaining portion of the plastic cartridge, invert the diluent bottle and penetrate the rubber seal on the concentrate bottle (Fig. C) with the needle at an angle.
   Alternate method of transferring sterile water: With a sterile needle and syringe, withdraw the appropriate volume of diluent and transfer to the bottle of lyophilized concentrate.
5. The vacuum will draw the diluent into the concentrate bottle. Hold the diluent bottle at an angle to the concentrate bottle in order to direct the jet of diluent against the wall of the concentrate bottle (Fig. C). Avoid excessive foaming.
6. After removing the diluent bottle and transfer needle (Fig. D), swirl continuously until completely dissolved (Fig. E).
7. After the concentrate powder is completely dissolved, withdraw solution into the syringe through the filter needle which is supplied in the package (Fig. F). Replace the filter needle with the administration set provided and inject intravenously.
8. If the same patient is to receive more than one bottle, the contents of two bottles may be drawn into the same syringe through a separate unused filter needle before attaching the vein needle.

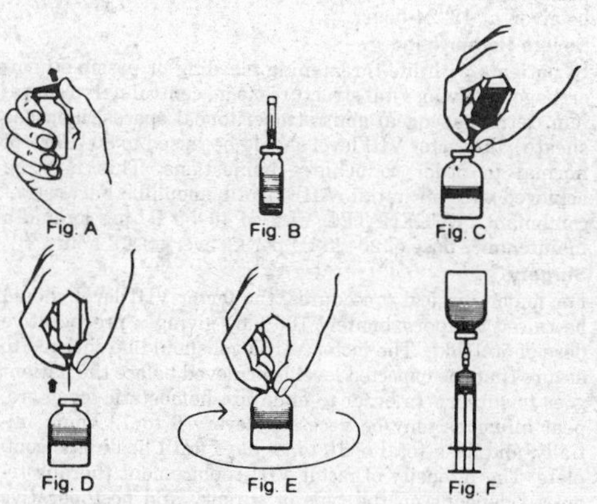

Fig. A Fig. B Fig. C Fig. D Fig. E Fig. F

Rate of Administration

The rate of administration should be adapted to the response of the individual patient, but administration of the entire dose in 5 to 10 minutes is generally well-tolerated.

HOW SUPPLIED

Antihemophilic Factor (Human), Koāte®-HP is supplied in the following single dose bottles with the total units of factor VIII activity stated on the label of each bottle. A suitable volume of Sterile Water for Injection, USP, a sterile double-ended transfer needle, a sterile filter needle, and a sterile administration set are provided.

NDC Number	Approximate Factor VIII Activity	Diluent
0026-0664-20	250 IU	5 mL
0026-0664-30	500 IU	5 mL
0026-0664-50	1000 IU	10 mL
0026-0664-60	1500 IU	10 mL

STORAGE

Koāte-HP should be stored under refrigeration (2–8°C; 36–46°F). Storage of lyophilized powder at room temperature (up to 25°C or 77°F) for 6 months, such as in home treatment situations, may be done without loss of factor VIII activity. Freezing should be avoided as breakage of the diluent bottle might occur.

CAUTION

U.S. federal law prohibits dispensing without prescription.

LIMITED WARRANTY

A number of factors beyond our control could reduce the efficacy of this product or even result in an ill effect following its use. These include improper storage and handling of the product after it leaves our hands, diagnosis, dosage, method of administration, and biological differences in individual patients. Because of these factors, it is important that this product be stored properly, that the directions be followed carefully during use, and that the risk of transmitting viruses be carefully weighed before the product is prescribed. No warranty, express or implied, including any warranty of merchantability or fitness is made. Representatives of the Company are not authorized to vary the terms or the contents of the printed labeling, including the package insert for this product, except by printed notice from the Company's headquarters. The prescriber and user of this product must accept the terms hereof.

REFERENCES

1. Hershgold EJ, Pool JG, Pappenhagen AR: The potent antihemophilic globulin concentrate derived from a cold insoluble fraction of human plasma: characterization and further data on preparation and clinical trial. *J Lab Clin Med* 67(1):23–32, 1966.
2. Unpublished data in files of Bayer Corporation.
3. Aronson DL: Factor VIII (antihemophilic globulin). *Semin Thromb Hemostas* 6(1):12–27, 1979.
4. Britton M, Harrison J, Abildgaard CF: Early treatment of hemophilic hemarthroses with minimal dose of new factor VIII concentrate. *J Pediatr* 85(2):245–7, 1974.
5. Prince AM, Horowitz B, Brotman B, et al: Inactivation of hepatitis B and Hutchinson strain non-A, non-B hepatitis viruses by exposure to Tween 80 and ether. *Vox Sang* 46:36–43, 1984.
6. Horowitz B, Wiebe ME, Lippin A, et al: Inactivation of viruses in labile blood derivatives. I. Disruption of lipid-enveloped viruses by tri(n-butyl) phosphate detergent combinations. *Transfusion* 25(6):516–22, 1985.
7. Piet MPJ, Chin S, Prince AM, et al: Inactivtion of viruses in plasma on treatment with tri(n-butyl) phosphate (TNBP) detergent mixtures. [abstract] *Thromb Haemost* 58(1):370, 1987.
8. Lederman MM, Ratnoff OD, Scillian JJ, et al: Impaired cell-mediated immunity in patients with classic hemophilia. *N Engl J Med* 308(2):79–83, 1983.
9. Weintrub PS, Koerper MA, Addiego JE Jr, et al: Immunologic abnormalities in patients with hemophilia A. *J Pediatr* 103(5):692–5, 1983.
10. Goldsmith JC, Moseley PL, Monick M, et al: T-lymphocyte subpopulation abnormalities in apparently healthy patients with hemophilia. *Ann Intern Med* 98:294–6, 1983.
11. Saidi P, Kim HC, Raska K Jr: T-cell subsets in hemophilia. [letter] *N Engl J Med* 308(21):1291–3, 1983.
12. Landay A, Poon MC, Abo T, et al: Immunologic studies in asymptomatic hemophilia patients: relationship to acquired immune deficiency syndrome (AIDS). *J Clin Invest* 71(5):1500–4, 1983.
13. Jones P, Proctor S, Dickinson A, et al: Altered immunology in haemophilia. [letter] *Lancet* 1:120–1, 1983.
14. Mannhalter JW, Zlabinger GJ, Ahmad R, et al: A functional defect in the early phase of the immune response observed in patients with hemophilia A. *Clin Immunol Immunopathol* 38:390–7, 1986.
15. Frydecka I, Kowalewska B, Lesiecki A, et al: Immunologic studies in asymptomatic hemophiliac patients. *Folia Haematol* 113(5):708–15, 1986.
16. National Hemophilia Foundation Medical and Scientific Advisory Council. Hemophilia Information Exchange—AIDS Update: Recommendations concerning HIV infection, AIDS and the treatment of hemophilia. Section I.G. (Rev. Jan., 1988).
17. Safety of therapeutic products used for hemophilia patients. *MMWR* 37(29):441–4, 449–50, 1988.
18. Fletcher ML, Trowell JM, Craske J, et al: Non-A, non-B hepatitis after transfusion of factor VIII in infrequently treated patients. *Br Med J* 287(6407):1754–7, 1983.
19. Kasper CK, Kipnis SA: Hepatitis and clotting-factor concentrates. *JAMA* 221(5):510, 1972.
20. Madhok R, Gracie A, Lowe GDO, et al: Impaired cell mediated immunity in haemophilia in the absence of infection with human immunodeficiency virus. *Br Med J* 239(6553):978–80, 1986.
21. Goldsmith JM, Deutsche J, Tang M, et al: CD4 cells in HIV-1 infected hemophiliacs: effect of factor VIII concentrates. *Thromb Haemost* 66(4):415–9, 1991.
22. Hilgartner MW, Buckley JD, Operskalski EA, et al: Purity of factor VIII concentrates and serial CD4 counts. *Lancet* 341(8857):1373–4, 1993.
23. Eyster ME, Bowman HS, Haverstick JN: Adverse reactions to factor VIII infusions. [letter] *Ann Intern Med* 87(2):248, 1977.
24. Prager D, Djerassi I, Eyster ME, et al: Pennsylvania state-wide hemophilia program: summary of immediate reactions with the use of factor VIII and factor IX concentrate. *Blood* 53(5):1012–3, 1979.
25. Shanbrom E, Thelin GM: Experimental prophylaxis of severe hemophilia with a factor VIII concentrate. *JAMA* 208(10):1853–6, 1969.
26. Abildgaard CF, Simone JV, Corrigan JJ, et al: Treatment of hemophilia with glycine-precipitated factor VIII. *N Engl J Med* 275(9):471–5, 1966.
27. Biggs R, MacFarlane RG: Haemophilia and related conditions: a survey of 187 cases. *Br J Haematol* 4(1):1–27, 1958.
28. Langdell RD, Wagner RH, Brinkhous KM: Antihemophilic factor (AHF) levels following transfusions of blood, plasma and plasma fractions. *Proc Soc Exp Biol Med* 88(2):212–5, 1955.
29. Shulman NR, Cowan DH, Libre EP, et al: The physiologic basis for therapy of classic hemophilia (factor VIII deficiency) and related disorders. *Ann Intern Med* 67(4): 856–82, 1967.
30. Abildgaard CF: Current concepts in the management of hemophilia. *Semin Hematol* 12(3):223–32, 1975.
31. Penner JA, Kelly PE: Low doses of factor VIII for hemophilia. [letter] *N Engl J Med* 297(7):401, 1977.
32. Ashenhurst JB, Langehennig PL, Seller RA: Early treatment of bleeding episodes with 10 U/kg of factor VIII. [letter] *Blood* 50(1):181–2, 1977.
33. Kasper CK: Hematologic care. In: Boone DC (ed.): Comprehensive management of hemophilia. Philadelphia, Davis, 1976, pp 3–17.
34. Edson JR: Hemophilia and related conditions. In: Conn HF (ed): Current therapy. Philadelphia, Saunders, 1980, pp 264–9.
35. Hilgartner MW; Management of hemophilia: the routine and the crises. *Drug Ther* 8(2):141–54, 1978.

KOGENATE® ℞

Antihemophilic Factor (Recombinant)

DESCRIPTION

Antihemophilic Factor (Recombinant), KOGENATE®, is a sterile, stable, purified, dried concentrate which has been manufactured by recombinant DNA technology. KOGENATE is intended for use in therapy of classical hemophilia (hemophilia A). KOGENATE is produced by Baby Hamster Kidney (BHK) cells into which the human factor VIII (FVIII) gene has been introduced.[1] KOGENATE is a highly purified glycoprotein consisting of multiple peptides including an 80 kD and various extensions of the 90 kD subunit. It has the same biological activity as FVIII derived from human plasma. In addition to the use of the classical purification methods of ion exchange chromatography and size exclusion chromatography, monoclonal antibody immunoaffinity chromatography is utilized along with other steps designed to purify recombinant factor VIII (rAHF) and remove contaminating substances. The final preparation is stabilized with Albumin (Human) and lyophilized. The concentration of KOGENATE is approximately 100 IU/mL. The product contains no preservatives.

Each vial of KOGENATE contains the labeled amount of rAHF in international units (IU). One IU, as defined by the World Health Organization standard for blood coagulation factor VIII, human, is approximately equal to the level of factor VIII activity found in 1.0 mL of fresh pooled human plasma. The final product when reconstituted as directed contains the following excipients: 10–30 mg glycine/mL, not more than (NMT) 500 µg imidazole/1000 IU, NMT 600 µg polysorbate 80/1000 IU, 2–5 mM calcium chloride, 100–130 mEq/L sodium, 100–130 mEq/L chloride and 4–10 mg Albumin (Human)/mL. KOGENATE must be administered by the intravenous route.

CLINICAL PHARMACOLOGY

The clinical trial of KOGENATE has included 168 patients, enrolled over a 55-month period. A total of 16,186 infusions have been utilized in this trial. The study was conducted in several stages.

Continued on next page

Kogenate—Cont.

Initial pharmacokinetic studies were conducted in 17 asymptomatic hemophilic patients, comparing pharmacokinetics of plasma-derived Antihemophilic Factor (Human) (pdAHF) and KOGENATE.[2] The mean biologic half-life of rAHF was 15.8 hours. The mean biologic half-life of pdAHF in the same individuals was 13.9 hours. A similar degree of shortening of the activated partial thromboplastin time was seen with both rAHF and pdAHF. The mean *in vivo* recovery of rAHF was similar to pdAHF, with a linear dose-response relationship. The recovery and half-life of rAHF was consistent with initial results following 13 weeks of exclusive treatment with KOGENATE. Subsequently, 826 recovery studies were conducted in 58 hemophilic patients participating in later clinical studies. Mean recovery from this group was 2.48% per IU/kg infused.

Fourteen (14) subjects from initial pharmacokinetic studies commenced home treatment with rAHF. Forty-four (44) additional subjects were then enrolled who treated themselves at home exclusively with rAHF. A total of 12,730 infusions have been administered under this portion of the study, of which 1,021 were given in clinic for recovery studies, 7,339 were given for treatment of bleeds, 4,361 were given as prophylaxis, 5 for minor surgery not requiring hospitalization, and 4 for unspecified reason.

Forty-eight (48) patients have received rAHF on 63 occasions for surgical procedures or in-hospital treatment of serious hemorrhage. Eleven (11) received rAHF for the first time in this study, while 37 were already on study or study participants under an investigation of previously untreated patients. Hemostatis has been satisfactory in all cases, with no adverse reactions.

In a study of previously untreated patients, a total of 3,254 infusions have been administered to 96 patients over a 48-month enrollment period. Hemostasis was successfully achieved in all cases.

During the analytical characterization of Antihemophilic Factor (Recombinant), KOGENATE®, analyses for carbohydrate structure revealed the presence of terminal galactose $\alpha1\rightarrow3$ galactose residues. Since naturally occurring antibody to this structure has been reported in humans, a trial in 18 patients was performed in which the half-life and recovery of rAHF with high levels on this carbohydrate residue was compared to that with KOGENATE, which contains low levels of this structure. As in the normal population, all patients had preexisting endogenous antibody to galactose $\alpha1\rightarrow3$ galactose in titers ranging from 1:320 to 1:5120 and no significant change in antibody level was noted during the study. While the mean recovery for KOGENATE in the study, 2.76%/IU/kg (N=43), was significantly different from that of rAHF with high levels of residues, 2.43%/IU/kg (N=155; p=0.0001), the recovery for rAHF with high levels of galactose $\alpha1\rightarrow3$ galactose is not significantly different from the 2.48%/IU/kg recovery obtained in the larger study from the 58 patients treated with KOGENATE mentioned above. Based on these results, the galactose $\alpha1\rightarrow3$ galactose residue appears to have no clinical significance.

INDICATIONS AND USAGE

KOGENATE is indicated for the treatment of classical hemophilia (hemophilia A) in which there is a demonstrated deficiency of activity of the plasma clotting factor, factor VIII. KOGENATE provides a means of temporarily replacing the missing clotting factor in order to correct or prevent bleeding episodes, or in order to perform emergency and elective surgery in hemophiliacs.

KOGENATE can also be used for treatment of hemophilia A in certain patients with inhibitors to factor VIII. In clinical studies of KOGENATE, patients who developed inhibitors on study continued to manifest a clinical response when inhibitor titers were less than 10 Bethesda Units (B.U.) per mL. When an inhibitor is present, the dosage requirement for factor VIII is variable. The dosage can be determined only by clinical response, and by monitoring of circulating factor VIII levels after treatment (see **DOSAGE AND ADMINISTRATION.)**

KOGENATE does not contain von Willebrand's factor and therefore is not indicated for the treatment of von Willebrand's disease.

CONTRAINDICATIONS

Due to the fact that Antihemophilic Factor (Recombinant) contains trace amounts of mouse protein (maximum 0.03 ng/IU rAHF) and hamster protein (maximum 0.04 ng/IU rAHF), KOGENATE should be administered with caution to individuals with previous hypersensitivity to pdAHF or known hypersensitivity to biologic preparations with trace amounts of murine or hamster proteins.

Assays to detect seroconversion to mouse and hamster protein were conducted on all patients on study. No patient has developed specific antibody titers against these proteins after commencing study, and no allergic reactions have been associated with rAHF infusions. Although no reactions were observed, patients should be warned of the theoretical possibility of a hypersensitivity reaction, and alerted to the early signs of such a reaction (e.g., hives, generalized urticaria, wheezing and hypotension). Patients should be advised to discontinue use of the product and contact their physician if such symptoms occur.

WARNINGS

None.

PRECAUTIONS

General

KOGENATE is intended for the treatment of bleeding disorders arising from a deficiency in factor VIII. This deficiency should be proven prior to administering KOGENATE.

The development of circulating neutralizing antibodies to factor VIII may occur during the treatment of patients with hemophilia A. In a study of previously untreated patients, inhibitor antibodies have developed in 17 of the 92 patients (18.5%) who have had at least one follow-up titer. The incidence of antibodies is 15/56 (26.7%) in patients with severe disease (<2% factor VIII), 2/18 (11%) in patients with moderate disease (2–5% factor VIII) and 0/18 in patients with mild disease (>5% factor VIII). Ten of the antibodies were high titer (>10 Bethesda Units), three were low titer, and four were low titer and transient. Studies most closely resembling the design of the study of inhibitor development with KOGENATE have reported incidences of inhibitor formation ranging between 18.4 and 52% for patients treated with pdAHF.[3–6] The incidence of inhibitor formation in previously untreated patients treated with Antihemophilic Factor (Recombinant), KOGENATE®, appears to be consistent with that reported in the literature, however the true immunogenicity of KOGENATE is not known at present. Patients treated with rAHF should be carefully monitored for the development of antibodies to rAHF by appropriate clinical observation and laboratory tests.

Product administration and handling of the infusion set and needles must be done with caution. Percutaneous puncture with a needle contaminated with blood can transmit infectious virus including HIV (AIDS) and hepatitis. Obtain immediate medical attention if injury occurs.

Place needles in sharps container after single use. Discard all equipment including any reconstituted KOGENATE product in accordance with biohazard procedures.

Carcinogenesis, Mutagenesis, Impairment of Fertility

In vitro evaluation of the mutagenic potential of KOGENATE failed to demonstrate reverse mutation or chromosomal aberrations at doses substantially greater than the maximum expected clinical dose. *In vivo* evaluation of rAHF using doses ranging between 10 and 40 times the expected clinical maximum also indicated that KOGENATE does not possess a mutagenic potential. Long-term investigations of carcinogenic potential in animals have not been performed.

Pediatric Use

KOGENATE has been proven to be safe and efficacious in newborns and the pediatric population while under investigation as previously treated (n=21) and previously untreated patients (n=96) (see **CLINICAL PHARMACOLOGY** and **PRECAUTIONS**).

Pregnancy Category C

Animal reproduction studies have not been conducted with KOGENATE. It is also not known whether KOGENATE can cause fetal harm when administered to a pregnant woman or can affect reproduction capacity. KOGENATE should be given to a pregnant woman only if clearly needed.

ADVERSE REACTIONS

During the clinical studies conducted in previously treated patients, 47 out of 12,932 infusions (0.36%) were associated with 58 reported minor adverse reactions. Of these, 19 reactions were local to the injection site (e.g., burning, pruritus, erythema); and 39 were systemic complaints (dizziness, nausea, chest discomfort, sore throat, cold feet, unusual taste in mouth, and slight decrease in blood pressure). In the study with previously untreated patients, 3,254 infusions have been associated with 11 minor adverse reactions (0.34%): two reports of erythema at the injection site, one of facial flushing related to the infusion, one report of diarrhea, two reports of nonspecific rash, two reports of fever, and three reports of emesis. No serious reactions have been reported, and all reactions have been self-limited.

DOSAGE AND ADMINISTRATION

Each bottle of KOGENATE has the rAHF content in international units per bottle stated on the label of the bottle. The reconstituted product must be administered intravenously by either direct syringe injection or drip infusion. The product must be administered within 3 hours after reconstitution.

General Approach to Treatment and Assessment of Treatment Efficacy

The dosages described below are presented as general guidance. It should be emphasized that the dosage of KOGENATE required for hemostasis must be individualized according to the needs of the patient, the severity of the deficiency, the severity of the hemorrhage, the presence of inhibitors, and the factor VIII level desired. It is often critical to follow the course of therapy with factor VIII level assays.

The clinical effect of KOGENATE is the most important element in evaluating the effectiveness of treatment. It may be necessary to administer more KOGENATE than would be estimated in order to attain satisfactory clinical results. If the calculated dose fails to attain the expected factor VIII levels, or if bleeding is not controlled after administration of the calculated dosage, the presence of a circulating inhibitor in the patient should be suspected. Its presence should be substantiated and the inhibitor level quantitated by appropriate laboratory tests. When an inhibitor is present, the dosage requirement for rAHF is extremely variable and the dosage can be determined only by the clinical response.

Some patients with low titer inhibitors (<10 B.U.) can be successfully treated with factor VIII without a resultant anamnestic rise in inhibitor titer.[7] Factor VIII levels and clinical response to treatment must be assessed to insure adequate response. Use of alternative treatment products, such as Factor IX Complex concentrates, Antihemophilic Factor (Porcine) or Anti-Inhibitor Coagulant Complex, may be necessary for patients with anamnestic responses to factor VIII treatment and/or high titer inhibitors.

Calculation of Dosage

The *in vivo* percent elevation in factor VIII level can be estimated by multiplying the dose of rAHF per kilogram of body weight (IU/kg) by 2%. This method of calculation is based on clinical findings by Abildgaard *et al.*,[8] and is illustrated in the following examples:

$$\text{Expected \% factor VIII increase} = \frac{\text{\# units administered} \times 2\%/\text{IU/kg}}{\text{body weight (kg)}}$$

Example for a 70 kg adult:

$$\frac{1400\ \text{IU} \times 2\%/\text{IU/kg}}{70\ \text{kg}} = 40\%$$

or

$$\text{Dosage required (IU)} = \frac{\text{body weight (kg)} \times \text{desired \% factor VIII increase}}{2\%/\text{IU/kg}}$$

Example for a 15 kg child:

$$\frac{15\ \text{kg} \times 100\%}{2\%/\text{IU/kg}} = 750\ \text{IU required}$$

The dosage necessary to achieve hemostasis depends upon the type and severity of the bleeding episode, according to the following general guidelines:

Mild Hemorrhage

Mild superficial or early hemorrhages may respond to a single dose of 10 IU per kg,[9] leading to an *in vivo* rise of approximately 20% in the factor VIII level. Therapy need not be repeated unless there is evidence of further bleeding.

Moderate Hemorrhage

For more serious bleeding episodes (e.g., definite hemarthroses, known trauma), the factor VIII level should be raised to 30–50% by administering approximately 15–25 IU per kg. If further therapy is required, a repeat infusion can be given at 12–24 hours.[10]

Severe Hemorrhage

In patients with life-threatening bleeding or possible hemorrhage involving vital structures (e.g., central nervous system, retropharyngeal and retroperitoneal spaces, iliopsoas sheath), the factor VIII level should be raised to 80–100% of normal in order to achieve hemostasis. This may be achieved with an initial rAHF (Antihemophilic Factor (Recombinant), KOGENATE®) dose of 40–50 IU per kg and a maintenance dose of 20–25 IU per kg every 8–12 hours.[11,12]

Surgery

For major surgical procedures, the factor VIII level should be raised to approximately 100% by giving a preoperative dose of 50 IU/kg. The factor VIII level should be checked to assure that the expected level is achieved before the patient goes to surgery. In order to maintain hemostatic levels, repeat infusions may be necessary every 6 to 12 hours initially, and for a total of 10 to 14 days until healing is complete. The intensity of factor VIII replacement therapy required depends on the type of surgery and postoperative regimen employed. For minor surgical procedures, less intensive treatment schedules may provide adequate hemostasis.[11,12]

Prophylaxis

Factor VIII concentrates may also be administered on a regular schedule for prophylaxis of bleeding, as reported by Nilsson, *et al.*[13]

Reconstitution

Vacuum Transfer

1. Warm the unopened diluent and the concentrate to room temperature (NMT 37°C, 99°F).
2. After removing the plastic flip-top caps (Fig. A), aseptically cleanse the rubber stoppers of both bottles.

3. Remove the protective cover from the plastic transfer-needle cartridge with tamper-proof seal and penetrate the stopper of the diluent bottle (Fig. B).

4. Remove the remaining portion of the plastic cartridge, invert the diluent bottle and penetrate the rubber seal on the concentrate bottle (Fig. C) with the needle at an angle.

   Alternate method of transferring sterile water: With a sterile needle and syringe, withdraw the appropriate volume of diluent and transfer to the bottle of lyophilized concentrate.

5. The vacuum will draw the diluent into the concentrate bottle. Hold the diluent bottle at an angle to the concentrate bottle in order to direct the jet of diluent against the wall of the concentrate bottle (Fig. C). Avoid excessive foaming.

6. After removing the diluent bottle and transfer needle (Fig. D), swirl continuously until completely dissolved (Fig. E).

7. After the concentrate powder is completely dissolved, withdraw solution into the syringe through the filter needle which is supplied in the package (Fig. F). Replace the filter needle with the administration set provided and inject intravenously. NOTE: Firmly grasp one or both wings to perform venipuncture; do not use the post-use needle shield for this purpose.

8. After infusion, lock post-use needle shield in place using one of the following methods:

   a. One-hand technique: Hold tubing in hand and advance needle shield with thumb and index finger until locked over needle tip (Fig. G).

   b. Two-hand technique: Hold wing stationary and slide needle shield forward with other hand until locked over needle tip (Fig. H).

9. If the same patient is to receive more than one bottle, the contents of two bottles may be drawn into the same syringe through a separate unused filter needle before attaching the vein needle.

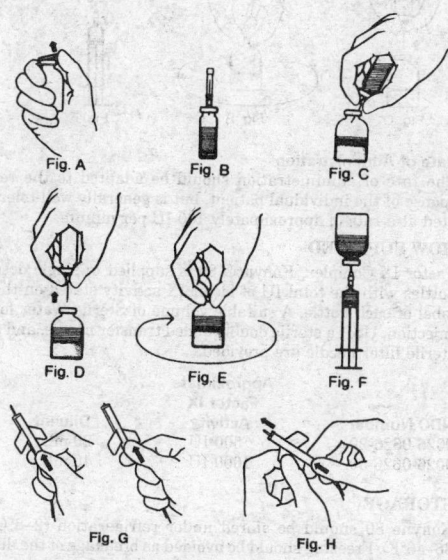

Fig. A   Fig. B   Fig. C

Fig. D   Fig. E   Fig. F

Fig. G   Fig. H

Rate of Administration

The rate of administration should be adapted to the response of the individual patient, but administration of the entire dose in 5 to 10 minutes or less is well-tolerated. Parenteral drug products should be inspected visually for particulate matter and discoloration prior to administration, whenever solution and container permit.

HOW SUPPLIED

Antihemophilic Factor (Recombinant), KOGENATE®, is supplied in the following single use bottles with the total units of factor VIII activity stated on the label of each bottle. A suitable volume of Sterile Water for Injection, USP, a sterile double-ended transfer needle, a sterile filter needle, and a sterile administration set are provided.

Product Code	Approximate Factor VIII Activity	Diluent
670-20	250 IU	2.5 mL
670-30	500 IU	5 mL
670-50	1000 IU	10 mL

STORAGE

KOGENATE should be stored under refrigeration (2–8°C; 36–46°F). Storage of lyophilized powder at room temperature (up to 25°C or 77°F) for 3 months, such as in home treatment situations, may be done without loss of factor

VIII activity. Freezing should be avoided, as breakage of the diluent bottle might occur. Do not use beyond the expiration date indicated on the bottle.

CAUTION

U.S. federal law prohibits dispensing without prescription.

REFERENCES

1. Lawn RM, Vehar GA: The molecular genetics of hemophilia. *Sci Am* 254(3):48–54, 1986.
2. Schwartz RS, Abildgaard CF, Aledort LM, et al: Human recombinant DNA-derived antihemophilic factor (factor VIII) in the treatment of hemophilia A. *N Engl J Med* 323(26):1800–5, 1990.
3. Lusher JM: Viral safaety and inhibitor development associated with monoclonal antibody-purified FVIIIc. *Ann Hematol* 63(3):138–41, 1991.
4. Addiego JE Jr, Gomperts E, Liu S-L, et al: Treatment of hemophilia A with a highly purified factor VIII concentrate prepared by anti-FVIIIc immunoaffinity chromatography. *Thromb Haemost* 67(1):19–27, 1992.
5. Schwarzinger I, Pabinger I, Korninger C, et al: Incidence of inhibitors in patients with severe and moderate hemophilia A treated with factor VIII concentrates. *Am J Hematol* 24(3):241–5, 1987.
6. Ehrenforth S, Kreuz W. Scharrer I, et al: Incidence of development of factor VIII and factor IX inhibitors in hemophiliacs. *Lancet* 339(8793):594–8, 1992.
7. Kasper CK: Complications of hemophilia A treatment: factor VIII inhibitors, *Ann NY Acad Sci* 614:97–105, 1991.
8. Abildgaard CF, Simone JV, Corrigan JJ, et al: Treatment of hemophilia with glycine-precipitated Factor VIII, *N Engl J Med* 275(9):471–5, 1966.
9. Britton M, Harrison J, Abildgaard CF: Early treatment of hemophilic hemarthroses with minimal dose of new factor VIII concentrate, *J Pediatr* 85(2):245–7, 1974.
10. Abildgaard CF: Current concepts in the management of hemophilia. *Semin Hematol* 12(3):223–32, 1975.
11. Hilgartner MW: Factor replacement therapy. In: Hilgartner MW, Pochedly C, eds.: Hemophilia in the child and adult. New York, Raven Press, 1989, pp 1–26.
12. Kasper CK, Dietrich SL: Comprehensive management of haemophilia. *Clin Haematol* 14(2):489–512, 1985.
13. Nilsson IM, Berntorp E, Lofqvist T, et al: Twenty-five years' experience of prophylactic treatment in severe haemophilia A and B. *J Intern Med* 232(1):25–32, 1992.

Factor IX Complex　　　　　　　　　　℞

KONYNE® 80

Heat-Treated at 80°C

DESCRIPTION

Factor IX Complex, Konyne® 80, heat-treated at 80°C for 72 hours, is a sterile, dried, plasma fraction comprising coagulation factors II, IX, X and low levels of factor VII.

	Nomenclature Synonyms:
Factor:	
II	prothrombin
VII	proconvertin
IX	plasma thromboplastin component, PTC, Christmas factor
X	Stuart-Prower factor

Konyne 80 is standardized in terms of factor IX content and each vial of Konyne 80 is labeled for factor IX. One international unit (IU) of factor IX as defined by the World Health Organization standard for blood coagulation factor IX is approximately equal to the level of factor IX found in 1.0 mL of fresh, normal plasma.

The factor IX content is approximately 50 times purified over whole plasma, and when reconstituted as directed, Konyne 80 contains 25 times as much factor IX as an equal volume of fresh plasma. Konyne 80, containing approximately 1000 IU of factor IX administered in 40 mL, contains the factor IX content of 1 liter of fresh plasma. Konyne 80 must be administered intravenously.

CLINICAL PHARMACOLOGY

Factor IX Complex raises the plasma level of factor IX and restores hemostasis in patients with factor IX deficiency. In general, a level of factor IX less than 5% of normal will give rise to spontaneous hemorrhage, while levels greater than 20% of normal will lead to satisfactory hemostasis even in the face of trauma or surgery. Approximately 30% to 50% of the factor IX activity can be detected in a hemophilia B (factor IX deficiency) recipient's plasma immediately after infusion.[1,2] The biological activity of the infused factor IX disappears from the plasma with a half-life of approximately 24 hours.[2] A pharmacokinetic study in six patients found similar recoveries and half-lives for Konÿ]ne 80 as for Konÿne®-HT. It must be noted that administration of Factor IX Complex causes an increase in blood levels of factors II, VII, IX and X.

Factors II, VII, IX and X are the vitamin K dependent coagulation factors and are synthesized in the liver. Congenital deficiencies of each of the four factors do occur and may result in a bleeding tendency. Naturally low levels of the vitamin K dependent factors may also be found in vitamin K deficiency and in severe liver disease.

This product has been heated at 80°C for 72 hours and there is no evidence of adverse effects upon the product. In a study[3] designed to assess the effectiveness of heat treatment at 68°C for 72 hours, hepatitis naive chimpanzees were inoculated with heated Antihemophilic Factor (Human) and Factor IX Complex preparations to which had been previously added non-A, non-B hepatitis Hutchinson Strain[4] to a total level of 2500 chimpanzee infectious doses (CID). The chimpanzees receiving heated preparations failed to exhibit any symptoms of non-A, non-B hepatitis. In contrast, one chimpanzee receiving Antihemophilic Factor (Human) concentrate which was not heated after the non-A, non-B inoculum was added, developed abnormally elevated alanine aminotransferase (ALT) levels beginning 10 weeks postinoculation and liver histopathology at 6 weeks. From these results, it was concluded that the heat treatment employed inactivated a known quantity of non-A, non-B hepatitis: at least 2500 CID.

Additional in vitro studies[5] on the effect of heating Factor IX Complex, Konyne® 80, in a dried state at 80°C for 72 hours, on virus inactivation were carried out with a number of viruses, including human immunodeficiency virus (HIV), added to Factor IX Complex prior to heating. The following table shows the amount of each model virus inactivated by the process:

Virus	Starting Amount Logs*	Logs Inactivated
Vesicular Stomatitis Virus	8.0	≥7.5
Vaccinia Virus	5.75	1.0
Sindbis Virus	7.25	≥6.75
Bovine Parvovirus	4.5	3.5
Human Immunodeficiency Virus (HIV), HIV-1	4.8	≥4.3

* $\log_{10}$ TCID$_{50}$/mL (for HIV-1, $\log_{10}$ TCID$_{50}$)

INDICATIONS AND USAGE

Factor IX Complex, Konÿne® 80 is indicated for the prevention and control of bleeding caused by Factor IX deficiency due to hemophilia B.

Konÿne 80 is not indicated for use in the treatment of factor VII deficiency.

Konÿne 80 is appropriate for use in:

1. Hemophilia B (Christmas disease); demonstrated factor IX deficiency in children or adults with real or impending bleeding episodes. Spontaneous bleeding can occur even in the absence of any trauma.

2. Reversal of coumarin anticoagulant induced hemorrhage; in situations where prompt reversal is required (e.g., preceding emergency surgery, trauma, etc.), administration of fresh-frozen plasma should be initially considered as treatment; however, Konÿne 80 may be considered as a secondary approach if the risk of transmitting hepatitis is considered justifiable in the face of a life-threatening situation.[6-8]

3. Treatment of bleeding episodes in patients with hemophilia A (factor VIII deficiency) who have inhibitors to factor VIII.[9]

   In addition to coumarin anticoagulant induced deficiencies, low levels of factors II, VII, IX and X may be found in vitamin K deficiency, in patients with gut sterilization due to oral antibiotics, in patients with liver disease, and in those with nephrotic syndrome. However, Factor IX Complex, Konÿne 80® is not indicated in these situations and treatment should be aimed at correcting the primary condition.

Note: For publications on the clinical use of Konÿne®, please refer to references 1,2, 6–17.

Continued on next page

Konȳne 80—Cont.

CONTRAINDICATIONS

None known.

WARNINGS

1. Hepatitis and Viral Diseases

Konȳne 80 is made from human plasma. Products made from human plasma may contain infectious agents, such as viruses, that can cause disease. The risk that such products will transmit an infectious agent has been reduced by screening plasma donors for prior exposure to certain viruses, by testing for the presence of certain current virus infections, and by inactivating certain viruses. Despite these measures, such products can still potentially transmit disease. There is also the possibility that unknown infectious agents may be present in such products. ALL infections thought by a physician possibly to have been transmitted by this product should be reported by the physician or other healthcare provider to Bayer Corporation [1-888-765-3203]. The physician should discuss the risks and benefits of this product with the patient, before prescribing or administering it to the patient.

Individuals who receive infusions of blood or plasma products may develop signs and/or symptoms of some viral infections, particularly hepatitis C. It is emphasized that hepatitis B vaccination is essential for patients with hemophilia and it is recommended that this be done at birth or diagnosis.[19,20] Hepatitis A vaccination is also recommended for hemophilic patients who are hepatitis A seronegative.

2. Thrombosis

Cases of patients developing postoperative thrombosis after treatment with Factor IX Complex have been described. Although thrombosis is a well-known risk of the postoperative period, it is found to be greater in these patients.[13-15] No other data are presently available. Until further surveys and more conclusive studies are available, Konȳne 80 is only advised for patients undergoing elective surgery where the expected beneficial effects of its use outweigh the increased risk of the possibility of thrombosis. This applies especially to those who may be predisposed to thrombosis. Do not use in cases of known liver disease where there is any suspicion of intravascular coagulation or fibrinolysis.

PRECAUTIONS

General

1. Reconstitute only with Sterile Water for Injection, USP.
2. Administer within 3 hours after reconstitution. Do not refrigerate after reconstitution.
3. Administer only by the intravenous route.
4. The administration equipment and any reconstituted Factor IX Complex, Konȳne® 80 not immediately used should be discarded.
5. E-aminocaproic acid should not be administered with Factor IX Complex as this may increase the risk of thrombosis.
6. Patients who receive Konȳne 80 either postoperatively or with known liver disease should be kept under close observation for signs and symptoms of intravascular coagulation or thrombosis. Any suspicious findings of this nature indicate the dosage should be markedly decreased if the patient's conditions are such that the treatment cannot be discontinued entirely. In the event of thrombohemorrhagic disorders occurring, reduction in dosage should be considered, and treatment with heparin may be warranted. Although this preparation does not contain heparin, it has been suggested that reconstitution with heparin in a concentration of 2–5 IU per mL may reduce the risk of development of thrombosis.[17] However, thrombosis can occur even in the presence of heparin.
7. Patients receiving Konȳne 80 for prolonged periods should be continually monitored at least for levels of factors II, IX and X. The same comments as in No. 6 above are indicated. Half-lives of factors II and X are considerably longer than the half-life of factor IX. Hence frequent repeated high-dose administration may result in build-up of factors II and X, with increasing risk of thrombotic side effects.
8. Product administration and handling of the needles must be done with caution. Percutaneous puncture with a needle contaminated with blood can transmit infectious viruses including HIV (AIDS) and hepatitis. Obtain immediate medical attention if injury occurs.

Place needles in sharps container after single use. Discard all equipment including any reconstituted Konȳne 80 product in accordance with biohazard procedures.

Pregnancy Category C

Animal reproduction studies have not been conducted with Konȳne 80. It is also not known whether Konȳne 80 can cause fetal harm when administered to a pregnant woman or can affect reproduction capacity. Konȳne 80 should be given to a pregnant woman only if clearly needed.

Information for Patient

Some viruses, such as parvovirus B19 or hepatitis A, are particularly difficult to remove or inactivate at this time. Parvovirus B19 most seriously affects pregnant women, or immune-compromised individuals.

Symptoms of parvovirus B19 infection include fever, drowsiness, chills and runny nose followed about 2 weeks later by a rash and joint pain. Evidence of hepatitis A may include several days to weeks of poor appetite, tiredness, and low-grade fever followed by nausea, vomiting, and pain in the belly. Dark urine and a yellowed complexion are also common symptoms. Patients should be encouraged to consult their physician if such symptoms appear.

ADVERSE REACTIONS

In some patients the rapid administration of Konȳne 80 can cause transient fever, chills, headache, flushing or tingling.

DOSAGE AND ADMINISTRATION

Each bottle of Konȳne 80 has the factor IX activity, in IU, stated on the bottle label. One IU is defined as the activity present in 1 mL of fresh, normal plasma. The potency is standardized in terms of factor IX content.

The amount of Konȳne 80 required for normalizing hemostasis will depend upon the patient and upon the circumstances. Sufficient Konȳne 80 should be administered to achieve and maintain a plasma level of at least 20% until hemostasis is achieved.

Levels of factor IX of 30 to 40 percent are considered effective in stopping hemorrhages.[1] Bleeds in life- or limb-threatening areas require factor IX levels of 50 to 80 percent which should be maintained at 30 to 40 percent for a few days.[1] The desired hemostatic plasma level in surgical patients for minor procedures or invasive dental surgery is between 30 and 40 percent of normal.[1] This can be achieved by a dosage not exceeding 30 to 40 units per kg body weight. In major hemorrhage, as during surgery or severe accidental trauma, plasma levels of 60 to 80 percent just prior to surgery, maintained above 30 percent for a further 5 to 7 days and then above 15 to 20 percent for 7 to 10 additional days, until healing occurs, are required.[1]

While the range of values in normal clinical practice is likely to vary depending upon differences between patients, their clinical condition and the type of assay employed, it is again stressed that high dosages, especially if frequently repeated (e.g., more than once per day) are hazardous. Such regimens can induce major thrombotic complications and hence must be avoided.

The following formulas may be used as guidelines to calculate an appropriate dose or to estimate the expected percentage increase obtained from a given dose.:

$$\text{Expected factor IX increase (in \% of normal)} = \frac{\text{IU administered} \times 1.0}{\text{body weight (in kg)}}$$

IU required = body weight (kg) × desired factor IX increase (% normal) × 1.0

Thus, in order to bring a 70 kg patient from 0% to 50% of normal, the patient would require 70 × 50 × 1.0 = 3500 IU or 50 IU/kg body weight.

Prophylaxis

The ideal treatment for proven congenital deficiency of procoagulants is prophylactic administration. For prophylaxis against hemorrhage during times of extensive physical activity, the plasma factor IX levels should be raised to 15 to 30 percent. Maintenance dosage should be adapted to the individual patient's needs. Additional Factor IX Complex, Konȳne® 80 should be administered when a patient on prophylaxis is exposed to trauma or surgery.

Maintenance Dose

Maintenance dosage should be administered according to the clinical response and the factor IX level achieved. Such dosage is usually about 10–20 IU per kg body weight per day.

Inhibitor Patients

For treatment of bleeding episodes in patients with hemophilia A (factor VIII deficiency) who have inhibitors to factor VIII, the recommended dose should be 75 IU/kg. A second dose may be administered after 12 hours if necessary.[9]

Reconstitution

Vacuum Transfer

1. Warm the unopened diluent and concentrate to room temperature (NMT 37°C, 99°F).
2. After removing the plastic flip-top caps (Fig. A) aseptically cleanse the rubber stoppers of both bottles.
3. Remove the protective cover from the plastic transfer-needle cartridge with tamper-proof seal and penetrate the stopper of the diluent bottle (Fig. B).
4. Remove the remaining portion of the plastic cartridge. Invert the diluent bottle and penetrate the rubber seal on the concentrate bottle (Fig. C) with the needle at an angle.

Alternate method of transferring sterile water: With a sterile needle and syringe, withdraw the appropriate volume of diluent and transfer to the bottle of lyophilized concentrate.

5. Hold the diluent bottle at an angle to the concentrate bottle in order to direct the jet of diluent against the wall of the concentrate bottle. The vacuum will draw the diluent into the concentrate bottle. Avoid excessive foaming. Do not shake the concentrate bottle.
6. After removing the diluent bottle and transfer-needle (Fig. D), optimal reconstitution time is achieved by swirling continuously until completely dissolved (Fig. E). Reconstitution can also be achieved by very gently agitating until dissolved.

Parenteral drug products should be inspected visually for particulate matter and discoloration prior to administration, whenever solution and container permit.

7. After the concentrate powder is completely dissolved, withdraw the Factor IX Complex, Konȳne® 80 solution into the syringe through the filter needle which is supplied in the package (Fig. F). Replace the filter needle with an appropriate sterile injection needle, e.g., 21 gauge × 1 inch, and inject intravenously.
8. If the same patient is to receive more than one bottle of Konȳne 80, the contents of two bottles may be drawn into the same syringe through filter needles before attaching the vein needle.

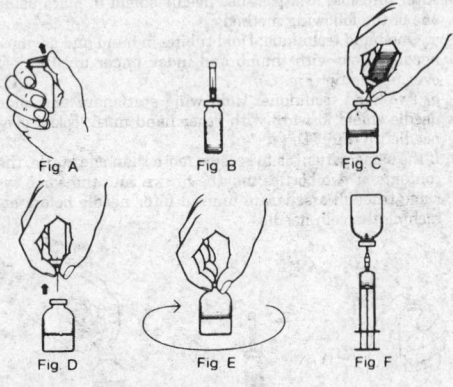

Fig A Fig B Fig C
Fig D Fig E Fig F

Rate of Administration

The rate of administration should be adapted to the response of the individual patient, but is generally well-tolerated at a rate of approximately 100 IU per minute.

HOW SUPPLIED

Factor IX Complex, Konȳne® 80 is supplied in single dose bottles with the total IU of factor IX activity stated on the label of each bottle. A suitable volume of Sterile Water for Injection, USP, a sterile double-ended transfer needle, and a sterile filter needle are provided.

NDC Number	Approximate Factor IX Activity	Diluent
0026-0626-20	500 IU	20 mL
0026-0626-50	1000 IU	40 mL

STORAGE

Konȳne 80 should be stored under refrigeration (2–8°C; 36–46°F). Freezing should be avoided as breakage of the diluent bottle might occur.

Konȳne 80 concentrate may be stored for a period of up to 1 month at temperatures not to exceed 25°C (77°F) during travel.

CAUTION

U.S. federal law prohibits dispensing without prescription.

LIMITED WARRANTY

A number of factors beyond our control could reduce the efficacy of this product or even result in an ill effect following its use. These include improper storage and handling of the product after it leaves our hands, diagnosis, dosage, method of administration, and biological differences in individual patients. Because of these factors it is important that this product be stored properly, that the directions be followed carefully during use, and that the risk of transmitting viruses be carefully weighed before the product is prescribed. No warranty, express or implied, including any warranty of merchantability or fitness is made. Representatives of the Company are not authorized to vary the terms or the contents of the printed labeling, including the package insert, for this product except by printed notice from the Company's headquarters. The prescriber and user of this product must accept the terms hereof.

REFERENCES

1. Johnson AJ, Aronson DL, Williams WJ: Preparation and clinical use of plasma and plasma fractions. In: Williams WJ (ed): *Hematology*, 4th ed, New York, McGraw-Hill, 1990, ch 170, pp 1659–1673.

2. Zauber NP, Levin J: Factor IX levels in patients with hemophilia B (Christmas disease) following transfusion with concentrates of factor IX or fresh frozen plasma (FFP). *Medicine* (Baltimore) 56(3): 213–24, 1977.
3. Mozen MM, Louie RE, Mitra G: Heat inactivation of viruses in antihemophilic factor concentrates. Abstracts, XVIth International Congress of the World Federation of Hemophilia, Rio de Janeiro, Aug. 24–28, 1984. Number 240.
4. Feinstone SM, Alter HJ, Dienes HP, et al: Non-A, non-B hepatitis in chimpanzees and marmosets. *J Infect Dis* 144(6):588–98, 1981.
5. Unpublished data in files of Bayer Corporation.
6. Taberner DA, Thompson JM, Poller L: Comparison of prothrombin complex concentrate and vitamin K_1 in oral anticoagulant reversal. *Br Med J* 2(6027):83–5, 1976.
7. Menache D, Roberts HR: Summary report and recommendations of the task force members and consultants. *Thromb Diath Haemorrh* 33:645–7, 1975.
8. Aronson DL: Factor IX Complex. *Semin Thromb Hemostas* 6(1):28–43, 1979.
9. Lusher JM, Shapiro SS, Palascak JE, et al: Efficacy of prothrombin-complex concentrates in hemophiliacs with antibodies to factor VIII: a multicenter therapeutic trial. *N Engl J Med* 303(8):421–5, 1980.
10. Hoag MS, Johnson FF, Robinson AJ, et al: Treatment of hemophilia B with a new clotting-factor concentrate. *N Engl J Med* 280(11):581–6, 1969.
11. Hoag MS, Johnson FF, Robinson AJ, et al: Use of plasma concentrate in congenital factor VII and IX deficiencies. *Clin Res* 17:152, 1969.
12. Breen FA Jr, Tullis JL: Prothrombin concentrates in treatment of Christmas disease and allied disorders. *JAMA* 208(10):1848–52, 1969.
13. Kasper CK: Postoperative thrombosis in hemophilia. *N Engl J Med* 289(3):160, 1973.
14. Kasper CK: Surgical operation in hemophilia B. Use of factor IX concentrate. *Calif Med* 113(1):4–8, 1970.
15. George JN, Breckenridge RT: The use of factor VIII and factor IX concentrates during surgery. *JAMA* 214(9): 1673–6, 1970.
16. Gunay U, Choi HS, Maurer HS, et al: Commercial preparations of prothrombin complex. A clinical comparison. *Am J Dis Child* 126(6):775–7, 1973.
17. White GC 2d, Lundblad RL, Kingdon HS: Prothrombin complex concentrates: preparation, properties, and clinical uses. *Curr Top Hematol* 2:203–44, 1979.
18. Colombo M, Mannucci PM, Carnelli V, et al: Transmission of non-A, non-B hepatitis by heat-treated factor VIII concentrate. *Lancet* 2(8445):1–4, 1985.
19. National Hemophilia Foundation Medical and Scientific Advisory Council. Hemophilia Information Exchange—AIDS Update: Recommendations concerning AIDS and the treatment of hemophilia. HIV infection, Section I.G. (Rev. Jan., 1988).

PROLASTIN® ℞
Alpha$_1$–Proteinase Inhibitor (HUMAN)
[*pro-las 'tin*]

DESCRIPTION

Alpha$_1$-Proteinase Inhibitor (Human), Prolastin®, is a sterile, stable, lyophilized preparation of purified human Alpha$_1$-Proteinase Inhibitor (alpha$_1$-PI), also known as alpha$_1$-antitrypsin. Alpha$_1$-Proteinase Inhibitor (Human) is intended for use in therapy of congenital alpha$_1$-antitrypsin deficiency.

Alpha$_1$-Proteinase Inhibitor (Human) is prepared from pooled human plasma of normal donors by modification and refinements of the cold ethanol method of Cohn.[1] Part of the fractionation may be performed by another licensed manufacturer. In order to reduce the potential risk of transmission of infectious agents, Alpha$_1$-Proteinase Inhibitor (Human) has been heat-treated in solution at 60±0.5°C for not less than 10 hours. However, no procedure has been found to be totally effective in removing viral infectivity from plasma fractionation products.

The specific activity of Alpha$_1$-Proteinase Inhibitor (Human) is ≥0.35 mg functional alpha$_1$-PI/mg protein and when reconstituted as directed, the concentration of alpha$_1$-PI is ≥20 mg/mL. When reconstituted, Alpha$_1$-Proteinase Inhibitor (Human) has a pH of 6.6–7.4, a sodium content of 100–210 mEq/L, a chloride content of 60–180 mEq/L, a sodium phosphate content of 0.015–0.025 M, a polyethylene glycol content of not more than (NMT) 5 ppm, NMT 0.1% sucrose. Alpha$_1$-Proteinase Inhibitor (Human) contains small amounts of other plasma proteins including alpha$_2$-plasmin inhibitor, alpha$_1$-antichymotrypsin, C_1-esterase inhibitor, haptoglobin, antithrombin III, alpha$_1$-lipoprotein, albumin, and IgA.[1]

Each vial of Prolastin contains the labeled amount of functionally active alpha$_1$-PI in milligrams per vial (mg/vial), as determined by capacity to neutralize porcine pancreatic elastase.[1] Alpha$_1$-Proteinase Inhibitor (Human) contains no preservative and must be administered by the intravenous route.

CLINICAL PHARMACOLOGY

Alpha$_1$-antitrypsin deficiency is a chronic, hereditary, usually fatal, autosomal recessive disorder in which a low concentration of alpha$_1$-PI (alpha$_1$-antitrypsin) is associated with slowly progressive, severe, panacinar emphysema that most often manifests itself in the third to fourth decades of life.[2–9][Although the terms "Alpha$_1$-Proteinase Inhibitor" and "alpha$_1$-antitrypsin" are used interchangeably in the scientific literature, the hereditary disorder associated with a reduction in the serum level of alpha$_1$-PI is conventionally referred to as "alpha$_1$-antitrypsin deficiency" while the deficient protein is referred to as "Alpha$_1$-Proteinase Inhibitor"[10]]. The emphysema is typically worse in the lower lung zones.[4,8,9] The pathogenesis of development of emphysema in alpha$_1$-antitrypsin deficiency is not well understood at this time. It is believed, however, to be due to a chronic biochemical imbalance between elastase (an enzyme capable of degrading elastin tissues, released by inflammatory cells, primarily neutrophils, in the lower respiratory tract) and alpha$_1$-PI (the principal inhibitor of neutrophil elastase) which is deficient in alpha$_1$-antitrypsin disease.[11–15] As a result, it is believed that alveolar structures are unprotected from chronic exposure to elastase released from a chronic, low level burden of neutrophils in the lower respiratory tract, resulting in progressive degradation of elastin tissues.[11–15] The eventual outcome is the development of emphysema. Neonatal hepatitis with cholestatic jaundice appears in approximately 10% of newborns with alpha$_1$-antitrypsin deficiency.[15] In some adults, alpha$_1$-antitrypsin deficiency is complicated by cirrhosis.[15]

A large number of phenotypic variants of alpha$_1$-antitrypsin deficiency exists.[15] The most severely affected individuals are those with the PiZZ variant, typically characterized by alpha$_1$-PI serum levels <35% normal.[15] Epidemiologic studies of individuals with various phenotypes of alpha$_1$-antitrypsin deficiency have demonstrated that individuals with endogenous serum levels of alpha$_1$-PI ≤50 mg/dL (based on commercial standards) have a risk of >80% of developing emphysema over a lifetime.[3–6,8,9,16] However, individuals with endogenous alpha$_1$-PI levels >80 mg/dL, in general, do not manifest an increased risk for development of emphysema above the general population background risk.[5,15] From these observations, it is believed that the "threshold" level of alpha$_1$-PI in the serum required to provide adequate anti-elastase activity in the lung of individuals with alpha$_1$-antitrypsin deficiency is about 80 mg/dL (based on commercial standards for immunologic assay of alpha$_1$-PI).[12,15,17]

In clinical studies of Alpha$_1$-Proteinase Inhibitor (Human), Prolastin®, 23 subjects with the PiZZ variant of congenital deficiency of alpha$_1$-antitrypsin deficiency and documented destructive lung disease participated in a study of acute and/or chronic replacement therapy with Alpha$_1$-Proteinase Inhibitor (Human).[18] The mean in vivo recovery of alpha$_1$-PI was 4.2 mg (immunologic)/dL per mg (functional)/kg body weight administered.[18,19] The half-life of alpha$_1$-PI in vivo was approximately 4.5 days.[18,19] Based on these observations, a program of chronic replacement therapy was developed. Nineteen of the subjects in these studies received Alpha$_1$-Proteinase Inhibitor (Human) replacement therapy, 60 mg/kg body weight, once weekly for up to 26 weeks (average 24 weeks of therapy). With this schedule of replacement therapy, blood levels of alpha$_1$-PI were maintained above 80 mg/dL (based on the commercial standards for alpha$_1$-PI immunologic assay).[18–20]. Within a few weeks of commencing this program, bronchoalveolar lavage studies demonstrated significantly increased levels of alpha$_1$-PI and functional antineutrophil elastase capacity in the epithelial lining fluid of the lower respiratory tract of the lung, as compared to levels prior to commencing the program of chronic replacement therapy with Alpha$_1$-Proteinase Inhibitor (Human).[18–20].

All 23 individuals who participated in the investigations were immunized with Hepatitis B Vaccine and received a single dose of Hepatitis B Immune Globulin (Human) on entry into the investigation. Although no other steps were taken to prevent hepatitis, neither hepatitis B nor non-A, non-B hepatitis occurred in any of the subjects.[18,19] All subjects remained seronegative for HIV antibody. None of the subjects developed any detectable antibody to alpha$_1$-PI or other serum protein.

Long-term controlled clinical trials to evaluate the effect of chronic replacement therapy with Alpha$_1$-Proteinase Inhibitor (Human), Prolastin®, on the development of or progression of emphysema in patients with congenital alpha$_1$-antitrypsin deficiency have not been performed. Estimates of the sample size required of this rare disorder and the slow, progressive nature of the clinical course have been considered impediments in the ability to conduct such a trial.[21] Studies to monitor the long-term effects will continue as part of the postapproval process.

INDICATIONS AND USAGE

Congenital Alpha$_1$-Antitrypsin Deficiency

Alpha$_1$-Proteinase Inhibitor (Human) is indicated for chronic replacement therapy of individuals having congenital deficiency of alpha$_1$-PI (alpha$_1$-antitrypsin deficiency) with clinically demonstrable panacinar emphysema. Clinical and biochemical studies have demonstrated that with such therapy, it is possible to increase plasma levels of alpha$_1$-PI, and that levels of functionally active alpha$_1$-PI in the lung epithelial lining fluid are increased proportionately.[18–20] As some individuals with alpha$_1$-antitrypsin deficiency will not go on to develop panacinar emphysema, only those with early evidence of such disease should be considered for chronic replacement therapy with Alpha$_1$-Proteinase Inhibitor (Human).[22] Subjects with the PiMZ or PiMS phenotypes of alpha$_1$-antitrypsin deficiency should not be considered for such treatment as they appear to be at small risk for panacinar emphysema.[22] Clinical data are not available as to the long-term effects derived from chronic replacement therapy of individuals with alpha$_1$-antitrypsin deficiency with Alpha$_1$-Proteinase Inhibitor (Human). Only adult subjects have received Alpha$_1$-Proteinase Inhibitor (Human) to date.

Alpha$_1$-Proteinase Inhibitor (Human) is not indicated for use in patients other than those with PiZZ, PiZ(null), or Pi(null)(null) phenotypes.

CONTRAINDICATIONS

Individuals with selective IgA deficiencies who have known antibody against IgA (anti-IgA antibody) should not receive Alpha$_1$-Proteinase Inhibitor (Human), since these patients may experience severe reactions, including anaphylaxis, to IgA which may be present.

WARNINGS

Alpha$_1$-Proteinase Inhibitor (Human), Prolastin® is made from human plasma. Products made from human plasma may contain infectious agents, such as viruses, that can cause disease. The risk that such products will transmit an infectious agent has been reduced by screening plasma donors for prior exposure to certain viruses, by testing for the presence of certain current virus infections, and by inactivating and/or removing certain viruses. Despite these measures, such products can still potentially transmit disease. There is also the possibility that unknown infectious agents may be present in such products. Individuals who receive infusions of blood or plasma products may develop signs and/or symptoms of some viral infections, particularly hepatitis C. ALL infections thought by a physician possibly to have been transmitted by this product should be reported by the physician or other healthcare provider to Bayer Corporation [1-888-765-3203].

The physician should discuss the risks and benefits of this product with the patient, before prescribing or administering it to a patient.

Prolastin has been heat-treated in solution at 60°C for 10 hours in order to reduce the potential for transmission of infectious agents.[1] No cases of hepatitis, either hepatitis B or hepatitis C, have been recorded to date in individuals receiving Prolastin.[18] However, as all individuals received prophylaxis against hepatitis B, no conclusion can be drawn at this time regarding potential transmission of hepatitis B virus.

PRECAUTIONS

General

1. Administer within 3 hours after reconstitution. Do not refrigerate after reconstitution.
2. Administer only by the intravenous route.
3. As with any colloid solution, there will be an increase in plasma volume following intravenous administration of Prolastin.[23] Caution should therefore be used in patients at risk for circulatory overload.
4. It is recommended that in preparation for receiving Prolastin, recipients be immunized against hepatitis B using a licensed Hepatitis B Vaccine according to the manufacturer's recommendations. Should it become necessary to treat an individual with Prolastin, and time is insufficient for adequate antibody response to vaccination, individuals should receive a single dose of Hepatitis B Immune Globulin (Human), 0.06 mL/kg body weight, intramuscularly, at the time of administration of the initial dose of Hepatitis B Vaccine.
5. Prolastin should be given alone, without mixing with other agents or diluting solutions.
6. Product administration and handling of the needles must be done with caution. Percutaneous puncture with a needle contaminated with blood can transmit infectious virus including HIV (AIDS) and hepatitis. Obtain immediate medical attention if injury occurs.
   Place needles in sharps container after single use. Discard all equipment including any reconstituted Prolastin product in accordance with biohazard procedures.

Carcinogenesis, Mutagenesis, Impairment of Fertility

Long-term studies in animals to evaluate carcinogenesis, mutagenesis or impairment of fertility have not been conducted.

Continued on next page

Prolastin—Cont.

Pregnancy Category C

Animal reproduction studies have not been conducted with Prolastin. It is also not known whether Prolastin can cause fetal harm when administered to a pregnant woman or can affect reproduction capacity. Prolastin should be given to a pregnant woman only if clearly needed.

Nursing Mothers

It is not known whether Prolastin is excreted in human milk. Because many drugs are excreted in human milk, caution should be exercised when Prolastin is administered to a nursing woman.

Pediatric Use

Safety and effectiveness in the pediatric population have not been established.

ADVERSE REACTIONS

Therapeutic administration of Alpha$_1$-Proteinase Inhibitor (Human), 60 mg/kg weekly, has been demonstrated to be well-tolerated. In clinical studies, six reactions were observed with 517 infusions of Alpha$_1$-Proteinase Inhibitor (Human), or 1.16%. None of the reactions was severe.[18] The adverse reactions reported included delayed fever (maximum temperature rise was 38.9°C, resolving spontaneously over 24 hours) occurring up to 12 hours following treatment (0.77%), light-headedness (0.19%), and dizziness (0.19%).[18] Mild transient leukocytosis and dilutional anemia several hours after infusion have also been noted.[18] Since market entry, occasional reports of other flu-like symptoms, allergic-like reactions, chills, dyspnea, rash, tachycardia, and, rarely, hypotension have also been received.

DOSAGE AND ADMINISTRATION

Each bottle of Alpha$_1$-Proteinase Inhibitor (Human) has the functional activity, as determined by inhibition of porcine pancreatic elastase,[1] stated on the label of the bottle.

The "threshold" level of alpha$_1$-PI in the serum believed to provide adequate anti-elastase activity in the lung of individuals with alpha$_1$-antitrypsin deficiency is 80 mg/dL (based on commercial standards for alpha$_1$-PI immunologic assay).[12,15,17] However, assays of alpha$_1$-PI based on commercial standards measure antigenic activity of alpha$_1$-PI, whereas the labeled potency value of alpha$_1$-PI is expressed as actual functional activity, i.e., actual capacity to neutralize porcine pancreatic elastase. As functional activity may be less than antigenic activity, serum levels of alpha$_1$-PI determined using commercial immunologic assays may not accurately reflect actual functional alpha$_1$-PI levels. Therefore, although it may be helpful to monitor serum levels of alpha$_1$-PI in individuals receiving Alpha$_1$-Proteinase Inhibitor (Human), Prolastin®, using currently available commercial assays of antigenic activity, results of these assays should not be used to determine the required therapeutic dosage.

The recommended dosage of Alpha$_1$-Proteinase Inhibitor (Human) is 60 mg/kg body weight administered once weekly. This dose is intended to increase and maintain a level of functional alpha$_1$-PI in the epithelial lining of the lower respiratory tract providing adequate anti-elastase activity in the lung of individuals with alpha$_1$-antitrypsin deficiency.

Alpha$_1$-Proteinase Inhibitor (Human) may be given at a rate of 0.08 mL/kg/min or greater and must be administered intravenously. The recommended dosage of 60 mg/kg takes approximately 30 minutes to infuse.

Parenteral drug products should be inspected visually for particulate matter and discoloration prior to administration, whenever solution and container permit.

Reconstitution

1. Warm the unopened diluent and concentrate to room temperature (NMT 37°C, 99°F).
2. After removing the plastic flip-top caps (Fig. A), aseptically cleanse rubber stoppers of both bottles.
3. Remove the protective cover from the plastic transfer needle cartridge with tamper-proof seal and penetrate the stopper of the diluent bottle (Fig. B).
4. Remove the remaining portion of the plastic cartridge. Invert the diluent bottle and penetrate the rubber seal on the concentrate bottle (Fig. C) with the needle at an angle.
   Alternate method of transferring sterile water: With a sterile needle and syringe, withdraw the appropriate volume of diluent and transfer to the bottle of lyophilized concentrate.
5. The vacuum will draw the diluent into the concentrate bottle. For best results, and to avoid foaming, hold the diluent bottle at an angle to the concentrate bottle in order to direct the jet of diluent against the wall of the concentrate bottle (Fig. C).
6. After removing the diluent bottle and transfer needle (Fig. D), gently swirl the concentrate bottle until the powder is completely dissolved (Fig. E).
7. Swab top of reconstituted bottle of Alpha$_1$-Proteinase Inhibitor (Human), Prolastin® again.
8. Attach the sterile filter needle provided to syringe. With

filter needle in place, insert syringe into reconstituted bottle of Prolastin and withdraw Prolastin solution into syringe (Fig. F).

9. To administer Prolastin, replace filter needle with appropriate injection needle and follow procedure for I.V. administration.
10. The contents of more than one bottle of Prolastin may be drawn into the same syringe before administration. If more than one bottle of Prolastin is used, withdraw contents from bottles using aseptic technique. Place contents into an administration container (plastic minibag or glass bottle) using a syringe.* Avoid pushing an I.V. administration set spike into the product container stopper as this has been known to force the stopper into the vial, with a resulting loss of sterility.

*For a patient of average weight (about 70 kg), the volume needed will exceed the limit of one syringe.

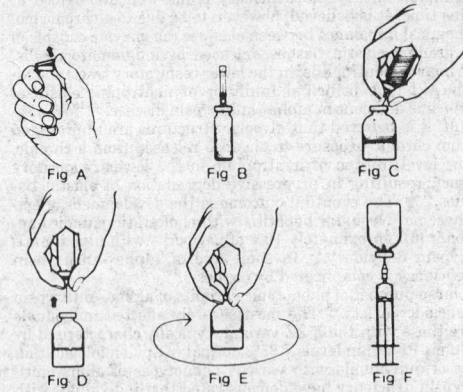

Fig A   Fig B   Fig C

Fig D   Fig E   Fig F

HOW SUPPLIED

Alpha$_1$-Proteinase Inhibitor (Human), Prolastin®, is supplied in the following single use vials with the total alpha$_1$-PI functional activity, in milligrams, stated on the label of each vial. A suitable volume of Sterile Water for Injection, USP, is provided.

NDC Number	Approximate Alpha$_1$-PI Functional Activity	Diluent
0026-0601-30	500 mg	20 mL
0026-0601-35	1000 mg	40 mL

STORAGE

Prolastin should be stored under refrigeration (2°–8°C; 36°–46°F) or at temperatures not to exceed 25°C (77°F). Freezing should be avoided as breakage of the diluent bottle might occur.

CAUTION

U.S. federal law prohibits dispensing without prescription.

LIMITED WARRANTY

A number of factors beyond our control could reduce the efficacy of this product or even result in an ill effect following its use. These include improper storage and handling of the product after it leaves our hands, diagnosis, dosage, method of administration, and biological differences in individual patients. Because of these factors, it is important that this product be stored properly, that the directions be followed carefully during use, and that the risk of transmitting viruses be carefully weighed before the product is prescribed. No warranty, express or implied, including any warranty of merchantability or fitness is made. Representatives of the Company are not authorized to vary the terms or the contents of the printed labeling, including the package insert for this product, except by printed notice from the Company's headquarters. The prescriber and user of this product must accept the terms hereof.

REFERENCES

1. Coan MH, Brockway WJ, Eguizabal H, et al: Preparation and properties of alpha$_1$-proteinase inhibitor concentrate from human plasma. Vox Sang 48(6):333–42, 1985.
2. Laurell CB, Eriksson S: The electrophoretic alpha$_1$-globulin pattern of serum in alpha$_1$-antitrypsin deficiency. Scand J Clin Lab Invest 15:132–40, 1963.
3. Eriksson S: Pulmonary emphysema and alpha$_1$-antitrypsin deficiency. Acta Med Scand 175(2):197–205, 1964.
4. Eriksson S: Studies in alpha$_1$-antitrypsin deficiency. Acta Med Scand Suppl 432:1–85, 1965.
5. Kueppers F, Black LF: Alpha$_1$-antitrypsin and its deficiency. Am Rev Respir Dis 110(2):176–94, 1974.
6. Morse JO: Alpha$_1$-antitrypsin deficiency. N Engl J Med 299:1045–8; 1099–105, 1978.
7. Black LF, Kueppers F: Alpha$_1$-antitrypsin deficiency in nonsmokers. Am Rev Respir Dis 117(3):421–8, 1978.
8. Tobin JM, Cook PJ, Hutchison DC: Alpha$_1$-antitrypsin deficiency: the clinical and physiological features of pulmonary emphysema in subjects homozygous for Pi type Z. A survey by the British Thoracic Association. Br J Dis Chest 77(1):14–27, 1983.
9. Larsson C. Natural history and life expectancy in severe alpha$_1$-antitrypsin deficiency, Pi Z. Acta Med Scand 204(5):345–51, 1978.
10. Pannell R, Johnson D, Travis J: Isolation and properties of human plasma alpha$_1$-proteinase inhibitor. Biochemistry 13(26):5439–45, 1974.
11. Lieberman J: Elastase, collagenase, emphysema, and alpha$_1$-antitrypsin deficiency. Chest 70(1):62–7, 1976.
12. Gadek JE, Fells GA, Zimmerman RL, et al: Antielastases of the human alveolar structures: implications for the protease-antiprotease theory of emphysema. J Clin Invest 68(4):889–98, 1981.
13. Beatty K, Bieth J, Travis J: Kinetics of association of serine proteinases with native and oxidized alpha-1-proteinase inhibitor and alpha-1-antichymotrypsin. J Biol Chem 255(9):3931–4, 1980.
14. Janoff A, White R, Carp H, et al: Lung injury induced by leukocytic proteases. Am J Pathol 97(1):111–36, 1979.
15. Gadek JE, Crystal RG: Alpha$_1$-antitrypsin deficiency. In: Stanbury JB, Wyngaarden JB, Frederickson DS, et al, eds.: The Metabolic Basis of Inherited Disease 5th ed. New York, McGraw-Hill, 1983, p. 1450–67.
16. Larsson C, Dirksen H, Sundstrom G, et al: Lung function studies in asymptomatic individuals with moderately (Pi SZ) and severely (Pi Z) reduced levels of alpha$_1$-antitrypsin. Scand J Respir Dis 57(6):267–80, 1976.
17. Gadek JE, Klein HG, Holland PV, et al: Replacement therapy of alpha$_1$-antitrypsin deficiency: reversal of protease-antiprotease imbalance within the alveolar structures of PiZ subjects. J Clin Invest 68(5):1158–65, 1981.
18. Data on file, Bayer Corporation.
19. Wewers MD, Casolaro MA, Sellers SE, et al: Replacement therapy for alpha$_1$-antitrypsin deficiency associated with emphysema. N Engl J Med 316(17):1055–62, 1987.
20. Wewers MD, Casolaro MA, Crystal RG: Comparison of alpha-1-antitrypsin levels and antineutrophil elastase capacity of blood and lung in a patient with the alpha-1-antitrypsin phenotype null-null before and during alpha-1-antitrypsin augmentation therapy. Am Rev Respir Dis 135(3):539–43, 1987.
21. Burrows B: A clinical trial of efficacy of antiproteolytic therapy: can it be done? Am Rev Respir Dis 127(2:2): S42–3, 1983.
22. Cohen AB: Unraveling the mysteries of alpha$_1$-antitrypsin deficiency. N Engl J Med 314(12):778–9, 1986.
23. Finlayson JS: Albumin products. Semin Thromb Hemost 6(2):85-120, 1980.

ANTITHROMBIN III (HUMAN)   ℞
THROMBATE III®

DESCRIPTION

Antithrombin III (Human), THROMBATE III®, is a sterile, stable, lyophilized preparation of purified human antithrombin III.

THROMBATE III is prepared from pooled units of human plasma from normal donors by modifications and refinements of the cold ethanol method of Cohn.[1] When reconstituted, THROMBATE III has a pH of 6.0–7.5, a sodium content of 110–210 mEq/L, a chloride content of 110–210 mEq/L, an alanine content of 0.075–0.125 M and a heparin content of not more than 0.004 unit/IU AT-III. THROMBATE III contains no preservative and must be administered by the intravenous route. In addition, THROMBATE III has been heat-treated in solution at 60°C ± 0.5°C for not less than 10 hours.

Each vial of THROMBATE III contains the labeled amount of antithrombin III in international units (IU) per vial. The potency assignment has been determined with a standard calibrated against a World Health Organization (WHO) antithrombin III reference preparation.

CLINICAL PHARMACOLOGY

Antithrombin III (AT-III), an alpha$_2$-glycoprotein of molecular weight 58,000, is normally present in human plasma at a concentration of approximately 12.5 mg/dL[2,3] and is the major plasma inhibitor of thrombin.[4] Inactivation of thrombin by AT-III occurs by formation of a covalent bond resulting in an inactive 1:1 stoichiometric complex between the two, involving an interaction of the active serine of thrombin and an arginine reactive site on AT-III.[4] AT-III is also capable of inactivating other components of the coagulation cascade including factors IXa, Xa, XIa, and XIIa, as well as plasmin.[4]

The neutralization rate of serine proteases by AT-III proceeds slowly in the absence of heparin, but is greatly accelerated in the presence of heparin.[4] As the therapeutic anti-

thrombotic effect in vivo of heparin is mediated by AT-III, heparin is ineffective in the absence or near absence of AT-III.[4–8]

The prevalence of the hereditary deficiency of AT-III is estimated to be one per 2000 to 5000 in the general population.[4,7] The pattern of inheritance is autosomal dominant. In affected individuals, spontaneous episodes of thrombosis and pulmonary embolism may be associated with AT-III levels of 40%–60% of normal.[7] These episodes usually appear after the age of 20, the risk increasing with age and in association with surgery, pregnancy and delivery. The frequency of thromboembolic events in hereditary antithrombin III (AT-III) deficiency during pregnancy has been reported to be 70%, and several studies of the beneficial use of Antithrombin III (Human) concentrates during pregnancy in women with hereditary deficiency have been reported.[9–11] In many cases, however, no precipitating factor can be identified for venous thrombosis or pulmonary embolism.[7] Greater than 85% of individuals with hereditary AT-III deficiency have had at least one thrombotic episode by the age of 50 years.[7] In about 60% of patients thrombosis is recurrent. Clinical signs of pulmonary embolism occur in 40% of affected individuals.[7] In some individuals, treatment with oral anticoagulants leads to an increase of the endogenous levels of AT-III, and treatment with oral anticoagulants may be effective in the prevention of thrombosis in such individuals.[6,7]

In clinical studies of Antithrombin III (Human), THROMBATE III® conducted in 10 asymptomatic subjects with hereditary deficiency of AT-III, the mean in vivo recovery of AT-III was 1.6% per unit per kg administered based on immunologic AT-III assays, and 1.4% per unit per kg administered based on functional AT-III assays.[12] The mean 50% disappearance time (the time to fall to 50% of the peak plasma level following an initial administration) was approximately 22 hours and the biologic half-life was 2.5 days based on immunologic assays and 3.8 days based on functional assays of AT-III.[12] These values are similar to the half-life for radiolabeled Antithrombin III (Human) reported in the literature of 2.8–4.8 days.[13–15]

In clinical studies of THROMBATE III, none of the 13 patients with hereditary AT-III deficiency and histories of thromboembolism treated prophylactically on 16 separate occasions with THROMBATE III for high thrombotic risk situations (11 surgical procedures, 5 deliveries) developed a thrombotic complication. Heparin was also administered in 3 of the 11 surgical procedures and all 5 deliveries. Eight patients with hereditary AT-III deficiency were treated therapeutically with THROMBATE III as well as heparin for major thrombotic or thromboembolic complications, with seven patients recovering. Treatment with THROMBATE III reversed heparin resistance in two patients with hereditary AT-III deficiency being treated for thrombosis or thromboembolism.

During clinical investigation of THROMBATE III, none of 12 subjects monitored for a median of 8 months (range 2–19 months) after receiving THROMBATE III, became antibody positive to human immunodeficiency virus (HIV-1). None of 14 subjects monitored for ≥ 3 months demonstrated any evidence of hepatitis, either non-A, non-B hepatitis or hepatitis B.

INDICATIONS AND USAGE

THROMBATE III is indicated for the treatment of patients with hereditary antithrombin III deficiency in connection with surgical or obstetrical procedures or when they suffer from thromboembolism.

Subjects with AT-III deficiency should be informed about the risk of thrombosis in connection with pregnancy and surgery and about the inheritance of the disease.

The diagnosis of hereditary antithrombin III (AT-III) deficiency should be based on a clear family history of venous thrombosis as well as decreased plasma AT-III levels, and the exclusion of acquired deficiency.

AT-III in plasma may be measured by amidolytic assays using synthetic chromogenic substrates, by clotting assays, or by immunoassays. The latter does not detect all hereditary AT-III deficiencies.[16]

The AT-III level in neonates of parents with hereditary AT-III deficiency should be measured immediately after birth. (Fatal neonatal thromboembolism, such as aortic thrombi in children of women with hereditary antithrombin III deficiency, has been reported.)[17]

Plasma levels of AT-III are lower in neonates than adults, averaging approximately 60% in normal term infants.[18,19] AT-III levels in premature infants may be much lower.[18,19] Low plasma AT-III levels, especially in a premature infant, therefore, do not necessarily indicate hereditary deficiency. It is recommended that testing and treatment with Antithrombin III (Human), THROMBATE III® of neonates be discussed with an expert on coagulation.[11]

CONTRAINDICATIONS

None known.

WARNINGS

THROMBATE III is made from human plasma. Products made from human plasma may contain infectious agents, such as viruses, that can cause disease. The risk that such products will trasmit an infectious agent has been reduced by screening plasma donors for prior exposure to certain viruses, by testing for the presence of certain current virus infections, and by inactivating and/or removing certain viruses. Despite these measures, such products can still potentially transmit disease. There is also the possibility that unknown infectious agents may be present in such products. Individuals who receive infusions of blood or plasma products may develop signs and/or symptoms of some viral infections, particularly hepatitis C. ALL infections thought by a physician possibly to have been transmitted by this product should be reported by the physician or other healthcare provider to Bayer Corporation [1-888-765-3203].

The physician should discuss the risks and benefits of this product with the patient, before prescribing or administering it to a patient.

The anticoagulant effect of heparin is enhanced by concurrent treatment with THROMBATE III in patients with hereditary AT-III deficiency. Thus, in order to avoid bleeding, reduced dosage of heparin is recommended during treatment with THROMBATE III.

PRECAUTIONS

General

1. Administer within 3 hours after reconstitution. Do not refrigerate after reconstitution.
2. Administer only by the intravenous route.
3. THROMBATE III, once reconstituted, should be given alone, without mixing with other agents or diluting solutions.
4. Product administration and handling of the needles must be done with caution. Percutaneous puncture with a needle contaminated with blood can transmit infectious virus including HIV (AIDS) and hepatitis. Obtain immediate medical attention if injury occurs.

   Place needles in sharps container after single use. Discard all equipment including any reconstituted THROMBATE III product in accordance with biohazard procedures.

The diagnosis of hereditary antithrombin III (AT-III) deficiency should be based on a clear family history of venous thrombosis as well as decreased plasma AT-III levels, and the exclusion of acquired deficiency.

Laboratory Tests

It is recommended that AT-III plasma levels be monitored during the treatment period. Functional levels of AT-III in plasma may be measured by amidolytic assays using chromogenic substrates or by clotting assays.

Drug Interactions

The anticoagulant effect of heparin is enhanced by concurrent treatment with THROMBATE III in patients with hereditary AT-III deficiency. Thus, in order to avoid bleeding, reduced dosage of heparin is recommended during treatment with THROMBATE III.

Pregnancy Category B

Reproduction studies have been performed in rats and rabbits at doses up to four times the human dose and have revealed no evidence of impaired fertility or harm to the fetus due to THROMBATE III. It is not known whether THROMBATE III can cause fetal harm when administered to a pregnant woman or can affect reproduction capacity. Because animal reproduction studies are not always predictive of human response, this drug should be used during pregnancy only if clearly needed.

Pediatric Use

Safety and effectiveness in the pediatric population have not been established. The AT-III level in neonates of parents with hereditary AT-III deficiency should be measured immediately after birth. (Fatal neonatal thromboembolism, such as aortic thrombi in children of women with hereditary antithrombin III deficiency, has been reported.)[17]

Plasma levels of AT-III are lower in neonates than adults, averaging approximately 60% in normal term infants.[18,19] AT-III levels in premature infants may be much lower.[18,19] Low plasma AT-III levels, especially in a premature infant, therefore, do not necessarily indicate hereditary deficiency. It is recommended that testing and treatment with Antithrombin III (Human), THROMBATE III® of neonates be discussed with an expert on coagulation.[11]

ADVERSE REACTIONS

In clinical studies involving THROMBATE III, adverse reactions were reported in association with 17 of the 340 infusions during the clinical studies. Included were dizziness (7), chest tightness (3), nausea (3), foul taste in mouth (3), chills (2), cramps (2), shortness of breath (1), chest pain (1), film over eye (1), light-headedness (1), bowel fullness (1), hives (1), fever (1), and oozing and hematoma formation (1). If adverse reactions are experienced, the infusion rate should be decreased, or if indicated, the infusion should be interrupted until symptoms abate.

DOSAGE AND ADMINISTRATION

Each bottle of THROMBATE III has the functional activity, in international units (IU), stated on the label of the bottle. The potency assignment has been determined with a standard calibrated against a World Health Organization antithrombin III reference preparation.

Dosage should be determined on an individual basis based on the pre-therapy plasma antithrombin III (AT-III) level, in order to increase plasma AT-III levels to the level found in normal human plasma (100%). Dosage of THROMBATE III can be calculated from the following formula:

$$\text{units required (IU)} = \frac{[\text{desired - baseline AT-III level}^*] \times \text{weight (kg)}}{1.4}$$

*expressed as % normal level based on functional AT-III assay

The above formula is based on an expected incremental in vivo recovery above baseline levels for THROMBATE III of 1.4% per IU per kg administered.[12] Thus, if a 70 kg individual has a baseline AT-III level of 57%, in order to increase plasma AT-III to 120%, the initial THROMBATE III dose would be [(120−57) × 70]/1.4 = 3150 IU total.

However, recovery may vary, and initially levels should be drawn at baseline and 20 minutes postinfusion. Subsequent doses can be calculated based on the recovery of the first dose. These recommendations are intended only as a guide for therapy. The exact loading dose and maintenance intervals should be individualized for each patient.

It is recommended that following an initial dose of THROMBATE III, plasma levels of AT-III be initially monitored at least every 12 hours and before the next infusion of THROMBATE III to maintain plasma AT-III levels greater than 80%. In some situations, e.g., following surgery,[20] hemorrhage or acute thrombosis, and during intravenous heparin administration,[13,21–23] the half-life of Antithrombin III (Human) has been reported to be shortened. In such conditions, plasma AT-III levels should be monitored more frequently, and Antithrombin III (Human), THROMBATE III® administered as necessary.

When an infusion of THROMBATE III is indicated for a patient with hereditary deficiency to control an acute thrombotic episode or prevent thrombosis following surgical or obstetrical procedures, it is desirable to raise the AT-III level to normal and maintain this level for 2 to 8 days, depending on the indication for treatment, type and extent of surgery, patient's medical condition, past history and physician's judgment. Concomitant administration of heparin in each of these situations should be based on the medical judgment of the physician.

As a general recommendation, the following therapeutic program may be utilized as a starting program for treatment, modifying the program based on the actual plasma AT-III levels achieved:

a) An initial loading dose of THROMBATE III calculated to elevate the plasma AT-III level to 120%, assuming an expected rise over the baseline plasma AT-III level of 1.4% (functional activity) per IU per kg of THROMBATE III administered. Thus, if an individual has a baseline AT-III level of 57%, the initial THROMBATE III dose would be (120−57)/1.4 = 45 IU/kg.
b) Measure preinfusion and 20 minutes postinfusion (peak) plasma antithrombin III levels following the initial dose, plasma antithrombin III level after 12 hours, then preceding the next infusion (trough level). Subsequently measure antithrombin III levels preceding and 20 minutes after each infusion until predictable peak and trough levels have been achieved, generally between 80%–120%. Plasma levels between 80%–120% may be maintained by administration of maintenance doses of 60% of the initial loading dose, administered every 24 hours. Adjustments in the maintenance dose and/or interval between doses should be made based on actual plasma AT-III levels achieved.

The above recommendations for dosing are provided as a general guideline for therapy only. The exact loading and maintenance dosages and dosing intervals should be individualized for each subject, based on the individual clinical conditions, response to therapy, and actual plasma AT-III levels achieved. In some situations, e.g., following surgery,[20] with hemorrhage or acute thrombosis and during intravenous heparin administration,[13,21–23] in vivo survival of infused THROMBATE III has been reported to be shortened, resulting in the need to administer THROMBATE III more frequently.

THROMBATE III should be reconstituted with Sterile Water for Injection, USP and brought to room temperature prior to administration. THROMBATE III should be filtered through a sterile filter needle as supplied in the package prior to use, and should be administered within 3 hours following reconstitution. THROMBATE III may be infused over 10–20 minutes. THROMBATE III must be administered intravenously.

Parenteral drug products should be inspected visually for particulate matter and discoloration prior to administration, whenever solution and container permit.

Continued on next page

Thrombate III—Cont.

Reconstitution
Vacuum Transfer
1. Warm the unopened diluent and the concentrate to room temperature (NMT 37°C, 99°F).
2. After removing the plastic flip-top caps (Fig. A), aseptically cleanse the rubber stoppers of both bottles.
3. Remove the protective cover from the plastic transfer needle cartridge with tamper-proof seal and penetrate the stopper of the diluent bottle (Fig. B).
4. Remove the remaining portion of the plastic cartridge, invert the diluent bottle and penetrate the rubber seal on the concentrate bottle (Fig. C) with the needle at an angle.
   Alternate method of transferring sterile water: With a sterile needle and syringe, withdraw the appropriate volume of diluent and transfer to the bottle of lyophilized concentrate.
5. The vacuum will draw the diluent into the concentrate bottle. Hold the diluent bottle at an angle to the concentrate bottle in order to direct the jet of diluent against the wall of the concentrate bottle (Fig. C). Avoid excessive foaming.
6. After removing the diluent bottle and transfer needle (Fig. D), swirl continuously until completely dissolved (Fig. E).
7. After the concentrate powder is completely dissolved, withdraw solution into the syringe through the filter needle which is supplied in the package (Fig. F). Replace the filter needle with an administration set (not provided) and inject intravenously.
8. If the same patient is to receive more than one bottle, the contents of two bottles may be drawn into the same syringe through a separate unused filter needle before attaching the vein needle.

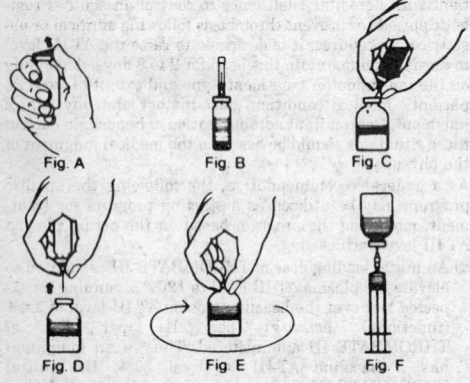

Fig. A   Fig. B   Fig. C
Fig. D   Fig. E   Fig. F

Rate of Administration
The rate of administration should be adapted to the response of the individual patient, but administration of the entire dose in 10 to 20 minutes is generally well-tolerated.

HOW SUPPLIED
Antithrombin III (Human), THROMBATE III® is supplied in the following single use vials with the potency in international units stated on the label of each vial. A suitable volume of Sterile Water for Injection, USP, a sterile double-ended transfer needle, and a sterile filter needle are provided.

NDC Number	Approximate Antithrombin III Potency	Diluent
0026-0603-20	500 IU	10 mL
0026-0603-30	1000 IU	20 mL

STORAGE
Antithrombin III (Human), THROMBATE III® should be stored under refrigeration (2–8°C; 36–46°F). Freezing should be avoided as breakage of the diluent bottle might occur.

CAUTION
U.S. federal law prohibits dispensing without prescription.

LIMITED WARRANTY
A number of factors beyond our control could reduce the efficacy of this product or even result in an ill effect following its use. These include improper storage and handling of the product after it leaves our hands, diagnosis, dosage, method of administration, and biological differences in individual patients. Because of these factors, it is important that this product be stored properly, that the directions be followed carefully during use, and that the risk of transmitting viruses be carefully weighed before the product is prescribed.

No warranty, express or implied, including any warranty of merchantability or fitness is made. Representatives of the Company are not authorized to vary the terms or the contents of the printed labeling, including the package insert for this product, except by printed notice from the Company's headquarters. The prescriber and user of this product must accept the terms hereof.

REFERENCES
1. Cohn EJ, Strong LE, Hughes WL Jr, et al: Preparation and properties of serum and plasma proteins. IV. A system for the separation into fractions of the protein and lipoprotein components of biological tissues and fluids. *J Am Chem Soc* 68(3):459–75, 1946.
2. Rosenberg RD, Bauer KA, Marcum JA: Antithrombin III "the heparin-antithrombin system." *Rev Hematol* 2:351–416, 1986.
3. Murano G, Williams L, Miller-Andersson M: Some properties of antithrombin-III and its concentration in human plasma. *Thromb Res* 18(1–2):259–62, 1980.
4. Rosenberg RD: Action and interactions of antithrombin and heparin. *N Engl J Med* 292(3):146–51, 1975.
5. Winter JH, Fenech A, Ridley W, et al: Familial antithrombin III deficiency. *Q J Med* 51(204):373–95, 1982.
6. Marciniak E, Farley CH, DeSimone PA: Familial thrombosis due to antithrombin III deficiency. *Blood* 43(2):219–31, 1974.
7. Thaler E, Lechner K: Antithrombin III deficiency and thromboembolism. *Clin Haematol* 10(2):369–90, 1981.
8. Blauhut B, Necek S, Kramar H, et al: Activity of antithrombin III and effect of heparin on coagulation in shock. *Thromb Res* 19(6):775–82, 1980.
9. Samson D, Stirling Y, Woolf L, et al: Management of planned pregnancy in a patient with congenital antithrombin III deficiency. *Br J Haematol* 56(2):243–9, 1984.
10. Brandt P: Observations during the treatment of antithrombin-III deficient women with heparin and antithrombin concentrate during pregnancy, parturition, and abortion. *Thromb Res* 22(1–2):15–24, 1981.
11. Hellgren M, Tengborn L, Abildgaard U: Pregnancy in women with congenital antithrombin III deficiency; experience of treatment with heparin and antithrombin. *Gynecol Obstet Invest* 14(2):127–41, 1982.
12. Schwartz RS, Bauer KA, Rosenberg RD, et al: Clinical experience with antithrombin III concentrate in treatment of congenital and acquired deficiency of antithrombin. *Am J Med* 87 (Suppl 3B): 53S–60S, 1989.
13. Collen D, Schetz J, de Cock F, et al: Metabolism of antithrombin III (heparin cofactor) in man; effects of venous thrombosis and of heparin administration. *Eur J Clin Invest* 7(1):27–35, 1977.
14. Knot EAR, de Jong E, ten Cate JW, et al: Purified radiolabeled antithrombin III metabolism in three families with hereditary AT III deficiency: application of a three-compartment model. *Blood* 67(1):93–8, 1986.
15. Tengborn L, Frohm B, Nilsson LE, et al: Antithrombin III concentrate; its catabolism in health and in antithrombin III deficiency. *Scand J Clin Lab Invest* 41(5):469–77, 1981.
16. Sas G, Blasko G, Banhegyi D, et al: Abnormal antithrombin III (antithrombin III "Budapest") as a cause of familial thrombophilia. *Thromb Diath Haemorrh* 32(1):105–15, 1974.
17. Bjarke B, Herin P, Blomback M: Neonatal aortic thrombosis. A possible clinical manifestation of congenital antithrombin III deficiency. *Acta Paediatr Scand* 63:297–301, 1974.
18. Hathaway WE, Bonnar J: Perinatal coagulation, New York, Grune & Stratton, 1978, p.68.
19. Peters M, Jansen E, ten Cate JW, et al: Neonatal antithrombin III. *Br J Haematol* 58(4):579–87, 1984.
20. Mannucci PM, Boyer C, Wolf M, et al: Treatment of congenital antithrombin III deficiency with concentrates. *Br J Haematol* 50(3):531–5, 1982.
21. Marciniak E, Gockerman JP: Heparin-induced decrease in circulating antithrombin-III. *Lancet* 2(8038):581–4, 1977.
22. O'Brien JR, Etherington MD: Effect of heparin and warfarin on antithrombin III. *Lancet* 2(8050):1232, 1977.
23. Kakkar VV, Bentley PG, Scully MF, et al: Antithrombin III and heparin. *Lancet* 1(8159):103–4, 1980.

For information on over-the-counter drugs, consult **PDR For Nonprescription Drugs.**

Beach Pharmaceuticals
Division of Beach Products, Inc.
5220 SOUTH MANHATTAN AVE.
TAMPA, FL 33611

Direct Inquiries to:
Richard Stephen Jenkins
(813) 839-6565
FAX (813) 837-2511

BEELITH Tablets   OTC
MAGNESIUM SUPPLEMENT
with PYRIDOXINE HCL
Each tablet supplies 362 mg (30 mEq) of magnesium and 25 mg of pyridoxine hydrochloride.

DESCRIPTION
Each tablet contains magnesium oxide 600 mg and pyridoxine hydrochloride (Vitamin B$_6$) 25 mg equivalent to Vitamin B$_6$ 20 mg. Each tablet yields 362 mg of magnesium and supplies 90% of the Adult U.S. Recommended Daily Allowance (RDA) for magnesium and 1000% of the Adult RDA for Vitamin B$_6$.

INDICATIONS
As a dietary supplement for patients with magnesium and/or Vitamin B$_6$ deficiencies resulting from malnutrition, alcoholism, magnesium depleting drugs, chemotherapy, and inadequate nutritional intake or absorption. Also, increases urinary magnesium levels.

DOSAGE
One tablet daily or as directed by a physician.

DRUG INTERACTION PRECAUTION
Do not take this product if you are presently taking a prescription drug without consulting your physician or other health professional.

WARNINGS
If you have kidney disease, take only under the supervision of a physician. Excessive dosage may cause laxation. **KEEP OUT OF THE REACH OF CHILDREN.** As with any drug, if you are pregnant or nursing a baby, seek the advice of a health professional before using this product.

HOW SUPPLIED
Golden yellow, film-coated tablet with the letters **BP** and the number **132** imprinted on each tablet. Packaged in bottles of 100 (NDC 0486-1132-01) tablets.
Shown in Product Identification Guide, page 306

CITROLITH TABLETS   ℞

DESCRIPTION
Each white, capsule-shaped tablet contains potassium citrate, anhydrous 50 mg, and sodium citrate, anhydrous 950 mg.

K-PHOS® M.F.   ℞
K-PHOS® No.2   ℞

DESCRIPTION
K-PHOS® M.F.: Each tablet contains potassium acid phosphate 155 mg and sodium acid phosphate, anhydrous 350 mg. Each tablet yields approximately 125.6 mg of phosphorus, 44.5 mg of potassium or 1.1 mEq and 67 mg of sodium or 2.9 mEq. **K-PHOS® No.2:** Each tablet contains potassium acid phosphate 305 mg and sodium acid phosphate, anhydrous 700 mg. Each tablet yields approximately 250 mg of phosphorus, 88 mg of potassium or 2.3 mEq and 134 mg of sodium or 5.8 mEq.
Shown in Product Identification Guide, page 306

K-PHOS® NEUTRAL   ℞
Supplies 250 mg of phosphorus per tablet.

DESCRIPTION
Each tablet contains 852 mg dibasic sodium phosphate anhydrous, 155 mg monobasic potassium phosphate, and 130 mg monobasic sodium phosphate monohydrate. Each tablet yields approximately 250 mg of phosphorus, 298 mg of sodium (13.0 mEq) and 45 mg of potassium (1.1 mEq).

CLINICAL PHARMACOLOGY
Phosphorus has a number of important functions in the biochemistry of the body. The bulk of the body's phosphorus is

located in the bones, where it plays a key role in osteoblastic and osteoclastic activities. Enzymatically catalyzed phosphate-transfer reactions are numerous and vital in the metabolism of carbohydrate, lipid and protein, and a proper concentration of the anion is of primary importance in assuring an orderly biochemical sequence. In addition, phosphorus plays an important role in modifying steady-state tissue concentrations of calcium. Phosphate ions are important buffers of the intracellular fluid, and also play a primary role in the renal excretion of hydrogen ion.

Oral administration of inorganic phosphates increases serum phosphate levels. Phosphates lower urinary calcium levels in idiopathic hypercalciuria.

In general, in adults, about two thirds of the ingested phosphate is absorbed from the bowel, most of which is rapidly excreted into the urine.

INDICATIONS AND USAGE

K-PHOS® NEUTRAL increases urinary phosphate and pyrophosphate. As a phosphorus supplement, each tablet supplies 25% of the U.S. Recommended Daily Allowance (U.S. RDA) of phosphorus for adults and children over 4 years of age.

CONTRAINDICATIONS

This product is contraindicated in patients with infected phosphate stones, in patients with severely impaired renal function (less than 30% of normal) and in the presence of hyperphosphatemia.

PRECAUTIONS

General: This product contains potassium and sodium and should be used with caution if regulation of these elements is desired. Occasionally, some individuals may experience a mild laxative effect during the first few days of phosphate therapy. If laxation persists to an unpleasant degree, reduce the daily dosage until this effect subsides or, if necessary, discontinue the use of this product.

Caution should be exercised when prescribing this product in the following conditions: Cardiac disease (particularly in digitalized patients); severe adrenal insufficiency (Addison's disease); acute dehydration; severe renal insufficiency; renal function impairment or chronic renal disease; extensive tissue breakdown (such as severe burns); myotonia congenita; cardiac failure; cirrhosis of the liver or severe hepatic disease; peripheral or pulmonary edema; hypernatremia; hypertension; toxemia of pregnancy; hypoparathyroidism; and acute pancreatitis. Rickets may benefit from phosphate therapy, but caution should be exercised. High serum phosphate levels may increase the incidence of extra-skeletal calcification.

Information for Patients: Patients with kidney stones may pass old stones when phosphate therapy is started and should be warned of this possibility. Patients should be advised to avoid the use of antacids containing aluminum, magnesium, or calcium which may prevent the absorption of phosphate.

Laboratory Tests: Careful monitoring of renal function and serum calcium, phosphorus, potassium, and sodium may be required at periodic intervals during phosphate therapy. Other tests may be warranted in some patients, depending on conditions.

Drug Interactions: The use of antacids containing magnesium, aluminum, or calcium in conjunction with phosphate preparations may bind the phosphate and prevent its absorption. Concurrent use of antihypertensives, especially diazoxide, guanethidine, hydralazine, methyldopa, or rauwolfia alkaloid; or corticosteroids, especially mineralocorticoids or corticotropin, with sodium phosphate may result in hypernatremia. Calcium-containing preparations and/or Vitamin D may antagonize the effects of phosphates in the treatment of hypercalcemia. Potassium-containing medications or potassium-sparing diuretics may cause hyperkalemia. Patients should have serum potassium level determinations at periodic intervals.

Carcinogenesis, Mutagenesis, Impairment of Fertility: No long term or reproduction studies in animals or humans have been performed with K-PHOS® NEUTRAL to evaluate its carcinogenic, mutagenic, or impairment of fertility potential.

Pregnancy: Teratogenic Effects: Pregnancy Category C. Animal reproduction studies have not been conducted with K-PHOS® NEUTRAL. It is also not known whether this product can cause fetal harm when administered to a pregnant woman or can affect reproductive capacity. This product should be given to a pregnant woman only if clearly needed.

Nursing Mothers: It is not known whether this drug is excreted in human milk. Because many drugs are excreted in human milk, caution should be exercised when this product is administered to a nursing woman.

Pediatric Use: See DOSAGE AND ADMINISTRATION.

ADVERSE REACTIONS

Gastrointestinal upset (diarrhea, nausea, stomach pain, and vomiting) may occur with phosphate therapy. Also, bone and joint pain (possible phosphate-induced osteomalacia)

could occur. The following adverse effects may be observed (primarily from sodium or potassium): headaches; dizziness; mental confusion; seizures; weakness or heaviness of legs; unusual tiredness or weakness; muscle cramps; numbness, tingling, pain, or weakness of hands or feet; numbness or tingling around lips; fast or irregular heartbeat; shortness of breath or troubled breathing; swelling of feet or lower legs; unusual weight gain; low urine output; unusual thirst.

DOSAGE AND ADMINISTRATION

K-PHOS® NEUTRAL tablets should be taken with a full glass of water, with meals and at bedtime. Adults: One or two tablets four times daily; Pediatric Patients over 4 years of age: One tablet four times daily. For Pediatric Patients under 4 years of age, use only as directed by a physician.

HOW SUPPLIED

White, film-coated, capsule-shaped tablet with the name BEACH and number 1125 imprinted on each tablet. Bottles of 100 (NDC 0486-1125-01) and 500 (NDC 0486-1125-05) tablets.

Rx ONLY

Shown in Product Identification Guide, page 306

K–PHOS® ORIGINAL (Sodium Free) ℞
(Potassium Acid Phosphate)
Urinary Acidifier
Supplies 114 mg of phosphorus per tablet.

DESCRIPTION

Each tablet contains potassium acid phosphate 500 mg. Each tablet yields approximately 114 mg of phosphorus and 144 mg of potassium or 3.7 mEq.

ACTIONS

K-PHOS® ORIGINAL (Sodium Free) is a highly effective urinary acidifier.

INDICATIONS AND USAGE

For use in patients with elevated urinary pH. Helps keep calcium soluble and reduces odor and rash caused by ammoniacal urine. Also, by acidifying the urine, it increases the antibacterial activity of methenamine mandelate and methenamine hippurate.

CONTRAINDICATIONS

This product is contraindicated in patients with infected phosphate stones; in patients with severely impaired renal function (less than 30% of normal) and in the presence of hyperphosphatemia and hyperkalemia.

PRECAUTIONS

General: This product contains potassium and should be used with caution if regulation of this element is desired. Occasionally, some individuals may experience a mild laxative effect during the first few days of phosphate therapy. If laxation persists to an unpleasant degree, reduce the daily dosage until this effect subsides or, if necessary, discontinue the use of this product.

Caution should be exercised when prescribing this product in the following conditions: Cardiac disease (particularly in digitalized patients); severe adrenal insufficiency (Addison's disease); acute dehydration; severe renal insufficiency or chronic renal disease; extensive tissue breakdown (such as severe burns); myotonia congenita; hypoparathyroidism; and acute pancreatitis. Rickets may benefit from phosphate therapy, but caution should be exercised. High serum phosphate levels may increase the incidence of extraskeletal calcification.

Information for Patients: Patients with kidney stones may pass old stones when phosphate therapy is started and should be warned of this possibility. Patients should be advised to avoid the use of antacids containing aluminum, calcium, or magnesium which may prevent the absorption of phosphate. To assure against gastrointestinal injury associated with oral ingestion of concentrated potassium salt preparations, patients should be instructed to dissolve tablets completely in an appropriate amount of water before taking.

Laboratory Tests: Careful monitoring of renal function and serum electrolytes (calcium, phosphorus, potassium) may be required at periodic intervals during potassium phosphate therapy. Other tests may be warranted in some patients, depending on conditions.

Drug Interactions: The use of antacids containing magnesium, calcium, or aluminum in conjunction with phosphate preparations may bind the phosphate and prevent its absorption. Potassium-containing medications or potassium-sparing diuretics may cause hyperkalemia when used concurrently with potassium salts. Patients should have serum potassium level determinations at periodic intervals. Concurrent use of salicylates may lead to increased serum salicylate levels since excretion of salicylates is reduced in acidified urine. Serum salicylate levels should be closely monitored to avoid toxicity.

Carcinogenesis, Mutagenesis, Impairment of Fertility: There have been no studies in animals or humans to evaluate the carcinogenesis, mutagenesis, or impairment of fertility for this product.

Pregnancy: Pregnancy Category C. Animal reproduction studies have not been conducted with this product. It is also not known whether this product can cause fetal harm when administered to a pregnant woman or can affect reproductive capacity. This product should be given to a pregnant woman only if clearly needed.

Nursing Mothers: It is not known whether this drug is excreted in human milk. Because many drugs are excreted in human milk, caution should be exercised when this product is administered to a nursing woman.

ADVERSE REACTIONS

Gastrointestinal upset (diarrhea, nausea, stomach pain, and vomiting) may occur with the use of potassium phosphate. Also, bone and joint pain (possible phosphate-induced osteomalacia) could occur. The following adverse effects may be observed with potassium administration: irregular heartbeat; dizziness; mental confusion; weakness or heaviness of legs; unusual tiredness; muscle cramps; numbness, tingling, pain, or weakness in hands or feet; numbness or tingling around lips; shortness of breath or troubled breathing.

DOSAGE AND ADMINISTRATION

Two tablets dissolved in 6–8 oz. of water 4 times daily with meals and at bedtime. For best results, let the tablets soak in water for 2 to 5 minutes, or more if necessary, and stir. If any tablet particles remain undissolved, they may be crushed and stirred vigorously to speed dissolution.

HOW SUPPLIED

White scored tablet with the name BEACH and the number 1111 imprinted on each tablet. Bottles of 100 (NDC 0486-1111-01) and bottles of 500 (NDC 0486-1111-05) tablets.

Rx ONLY

Shown in Product Identification Guide, page 306

UROQID-Acid® No.2 Tablets ℞

DESCRIPTION

Each UROQID-Acid® No.2 tablet contains methenamine mandelate 500 mg and sodium acid phosphate, monohydrate 500 mg.

CLINICAL PHARMACOLOGY

Methenamine mandelate is rapidly absorbed and excreted in the urine. Formaldehyde is released by acid hydrolysis from methenamine with bactericidal levels rapidly reached at pH 5.0–5.5. Proportionally less formaldehyde is released as urinary pH approaches 6.0 and insufficient quantities are released above this level for therapeutic response. In acid urine, mandelic acid exerts its antibacterial action and also contributes to the acidification of the urine. Mandelic acid is excreted by both glomerular filtration and tubular excretion. In acid urine, there is equally effective antibacterial activity against both gram-positive and gram-negative organisms, since the antibacterial action of mandelic acid and formaldehyde is nonspecific. With Proteus vulgaris and urea splitting strains of Pseudomonas and Aerobacter, results may be discouraging and particular attention is required in monitoring urinary pH and overall management.

INDICATIONS AND USAGE

For the suppression or elimination of bacteriuria associated with chronic and recurrent infections of the urinary tract, including pyelitis, pyelonephritis, cystitis, and infected residual urine accompanying neurogenic bladder. When used as recommended, UROQID-Acid® No.2 is particularly suitable for long-term therapy because of its relative safety and because resistance to the nonspecific bactericidal action of formaldehyde does not develop. Pathogens resistant to other antibacterial agents may respond because of the nonspecific effect of formaldehyde formed in an acid urine.

Prophylactic Use Rationale: Urine is a good culture medium for many urinary pathogens. Inoculation by a few organisms (relapse or reinfection) may lead to bacteriuria in susceptible individuals. Thus, the rationale of management in recurring urinary tract infection (bacteriuria) is to change the urine from a growth-supporting to a growth-inhibiting medium. There is a growing body of evidence that long-term administration of methenamine can prevent recurrence of bacteriuria in patients with chronic pyelonephritis.

Therapeutic Use Rationale: Helps to sterilize the urine and, in some situations in which underlying pathologic conditions prevent sterilization by any means, can help to suppress bacteriuria. As part of the overall management of the urinary tract infection, a thorough diagnostic evaluation should accompany the use of this product.

Continued on next page

Uroqid-Acid—Cont.

CONTRAINDICATIONS

UROQID-Acid® No.2 is contraindicated in patients with renal insufficiency, severe hepatic disease, severe dehydration, hyperphosphatemia, and in patients who have exhibited hypersensitivity to any components of this product.

PRECAUTIONS

General

This product should not be used as the sole therapeutic agent in acute parenchymal infections causing systemic symptoms such as chills and fever.

UROQID-Acid® No.2 contains approximately 83 mg of sodium per tablet and should be used with caution in patients on a sodium-restricted diet.

Sodium phosphates should be used with caution in the following conditions: cardiac failure; peripheral or pulmonary edema; hypernatremia; hypertension; toxemia of pregnancy; hypoparathyroidism; and acute pancreatitis. High serum phosphate levels increase the incidence of extraskeletal calcification.

Large doses of methenamine (8 grams daily for 3 to 4 weeks) have caused bladder irritation, painful and frequent micturition, albuminuria and gross hematuria. Dysuria may occur, although usually at higher than recommended doses, and can be controlled by reducing the dosage. This product contains a urinary acidifier and can cause metabolic acidosis.

Care should be taken to maintain an acidic urinary pH (below 5.5), especially when treating infections due to urea-splitting organisms such as Proteus and strains of Pseudomonas.

Drugs and/or foods which produce an alkaline urine should be restricted. Frequent urine pH tests are essential. If acidification of the urine is contraindicated or unattainable, use of this product should be discontinued.

Information For Patients: To assure an acidic pH, patients should be instructed to restrict or avoid most fruits, milk and milk products, and antacids containing sodium carbonate or bicarbonate.

Laboratory Tests: As with all urinary tract infections, the efficacy of therapy should be monitored by repeated urine cultures. During long-term therapy, careful monitoring of renal function, serum phosphorus and sodium may be required at periodic intervals.

Drug Interactions: Formaldehyde and sulfamethizole form an insoluble precipitate in acid urine and increase the risk of crystalluria; therefore, these products should not be used concurrently. Thiazide diuretics, carbonic anhydrase inhibitors, antacids, or urinary alkalinizing agents should not be used concurrently since they may cause the urine to become alkaline and reduce the effectiveness of methenamine by inhibiting its conversion to formaldehyde. Concurrent use of antihypertensives, especially diazoxide, guanethidine, hydralazine, methyldopa, or rauwolfia alkaloids; or corticosteroids, especially mineralocorticoids or corticotropin, with sodium phosphates may result in hypernatremia. Concurrent use of salicylates may lead to increased serum salicylate levels since excretion of salicylates is reduced in acidified urine. Serum salicylate levels should be closely monitored to avoid toxicity.

Laboratory Test Interactions: Formaldehyde interferes with fluorometric procedures for determination of urinary catecholamines and vanilmandelic acid (VMA) causing erroneously high results. Formaldehyde also causes falsely decreased urine estriol levels by reacting with estriol when acid hydrolysis techniques are used; estriol determinations which use enzymatic hydrolysis are unaffected by formaldehyde. Formaldehyde causes falsely elevated 17-hydroxycorticosteroid levels when the Porter-Silber method is used and falsely decreased 5-hydroxyindoleacetic acid (5HIAA) levels by inhibiting color development when nitrosonaphthol methods are used.

Carcinogenesis, Mutagenesis, Impairment Of Fertility: Long-term animal studies to evaluate the carcinogenic, mutagenic, or impairment of fertility potential of this product have not been performed.

Pregnancy: Teratogenic Effects. Pregnancy Category C. Animal reproduction studies have not been conducted with **UROQID-Acid® No.2**. It is also not known whether this product can cause fetal harm when administered to a pregnant woman or can affect reproductive capacity. Since methenamine is known to cross the placental barrier, this product should be given to a pregnant woman only if clearly needed.

Nursing Mothers: Methenamine is excreted in breast milk. Caution should be exercised when this product is administered to a nursing woman.

ADVERSE REACTIONS

Gastrointestinal disturbances (nausea, stomach upset), generalized skin rash, dysuria, painful or difficult urination may occur occasionally with the use of methenamine preparations. Microscopic and rarely, gross hematuria have also been reported.

Gastrointestinal upset (diarrhea, nausea, stomach pain, and vomiting) may occur with the use of sodium phosphates. Also, bone or joint pain (possible phosphate induced osteomalacia) could occur. The following adverse effects may be observed (primarily from sodium): headaches; dizziness; mental confusion; seizures; weakness or heaviness of legs; unusual tiredness or weakness; muscle cramps; numbness, tingling, pain, or weakness of hands or feet; numbness or tingling around lips; fast or irregular heartbeat; shortness of breath or troubled breathing; swelling of feet or lower legs; unusual weight gain; low urine output, unusual thirst.

DOSAGE AND ADMINISTRATION

UROQID-Acid® No.2: *Adults:* Initially, 2 tablets 4 times daily with a full glass of water. For maintenance, 2 to 4 tablets daily, in divided doses with a full glass of water.

HOW SUPPLIED

UROQID-Acid® No.2 is a yellow, film-coated, capsule-shaped tablet with the name **BEACH** and the number **1114** imprinted on each tablet. Packaged in bottles of 100 tablets (NDC 0486-1114-01).

Rx ONLY

Shown in Product Identification Guide, page 306

Bedford Laboratories

A Division of Ben Venue Laboratories, Inc.
300 NORTHFIELD ROAD
BEDFORD, OH 44146

Direct Inquiries to:
Customer Service: (800) 562-4797
FAX: (440) 232-6264
Professional Services: (800) 521-5169

CERUBIDINE® ℞

[sĭ-rew "bĭ 'dēan]
(daunorubicin HCl)
for Injection

> **WARNINGS**
>
> 1. Cerubidine must be given into a rapidly flowing intravenous infusion. It must *never* be given by the intramuscular or subcutaneous route. Severe local tissue necrosis will occur if there is extravasation during administration.
> 2. Myocardial toxicity manifested in its most severe form by potentially fatal congestive heart failure may occur either during therapy or months to years after termination of therapy. The incidence of myocardial toxicity increases after a total cumulative dose exceeding 400–550 mg/m^2 in adults, 300 mg/m^2 in children more than 2 years of age, or 10 mg/kg in children less than 2 years of age.
> 3. Severe myelosuppression occurs when used in therapeutic doses; this may lead to infection or hemorrhage.
> 4. It is recommended that Cerubidine be administered only by physicians who are experienced in leukemia chemotherapy and in facilities with laboratory and supportive resources adequate to monitor drug tolerance and protect and maintain a patient compromised by drug toxicity. The physician and institution must be capable of responding rapidly and completely to severe hemorrhagic conditions and/or overwhelming infection.
> 5. Dosage should be reduced in patients with impaired hepatic or renal function.

DESCRIPTION

Cerubidine (daunorubicin hydrochloride) is the hydrochloride salt of an anthracycline cytotoxic antibiotic produced by a strain of *Streptomyces coeruleorubidus*. It is provided as a sterile reddish lyophilized powder in vials for intravenous administration only. Each vial contains 21.4 mg daunorubicin hydrochloride, equivalent to 20 mg daunorubicin, and 100 mg of mannitol. It is soluble in water when adequately agitated and produces a reddish solution. It has the following structural formula which may be described with the chemical name of 7-(3-amino-2,3,6-trideoxy-L-lyxohexosyloxy)-9 -acetyl-7,8,9,10-tetrahydro-6,9,11-trihydroxy-4-methoxy-5, 12-naphthacenequinone hydrochloride. Its molecular formula is $C_{27}H_{29}NO_{10}HCl$ with a molecular weight of 563.99. It is a hygroscopic crystalline powder. The pH of a 5 mg/mL aqueous solution is 4.5 to 6.5.

[See chemical structure at top of next column]

ACTION

Cerubidine inhibits the synthesis of nucleic acids; its effect on deoxyribonucleic acid is particularly rapid and marked.

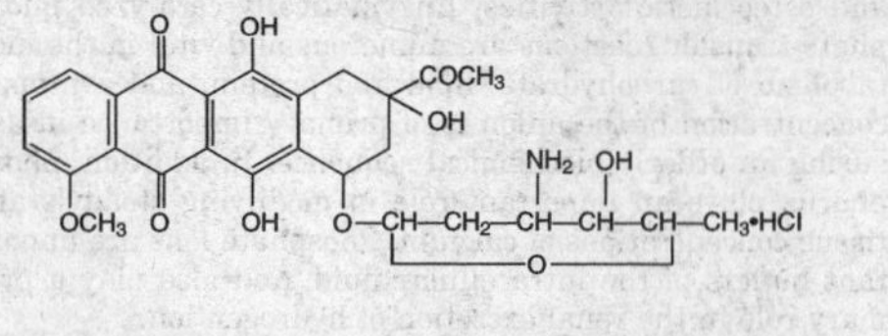

Cerubidine has antimitotic and cytotoxic activity although the precise mode of action is unknown. Cerubidine displays an immunosuppressive effect. It has been shown to inhibit the production of heterohemagglutinins in mice. *In vitro*, it inhibits blast-cell transformation of canine lymphocytes at 0.01 mcg/mL.

Cerubidine possesses a potent antitumor effect against a wide spectrum of animal tumors either grafted or spontaneous.

CLINICAL PHARMACOLOGY

Following intravenous injection of Cerubidine, plasma levels of daunorubicin decline rapidly, indicating rapid tissue uptake and concentration. Thereafter, plasma levels decline slowly with a half-life of 18.5 hours. By 1 hour after drug administration, the predominant plasma species is daunorubicinol, an active metabolite, which disappears with a half-life of 26.7 hours. Further metabolism via reduction cleavage of the glycosidic bond, 4-0 demethylation, and conjugation with both sulfate and glucuronide have been demonstrated. Simple glycosidic cleavage of daunorubicin or daunorubicinol is not a significant metabolic pathway in man. Twenty-five percent of an administered dose of Cerubidine is eliminated in an active form by urinary excretion and an estimated 40% by biliary excretion.

There is no evidence that Cerubidine crosses the blood-brain barrier.

In the treatment of adult acute nonlymphocytic leukemia, Cerubidine, used as a single agent, has produced complete remission rates of 40 to 50%, and in combination with cytarabine, has produced complete remission rates of 53 to 65%.

The addition of Cerubidine to the two-drug induction regimen of vincristine-prednisone in the treatment of childhood acute lymphocytic leukemia does not increase the rate of complete remission. In children receiving identical CNS prophylaxis and maintenance therapy (without consolidation), there is prolongation of complete remission duration (statistically significant, $p<0.02$) in those children induced with the three-drug (Cerubidine-vincristine-prednisone) regimen as compared to two drugs. There is no evidence of any impact of Cerubidine on the duration of complete remission when a consolidation (intensification) phase is employed as part of a total treatment program.

In adult acute lymphocytic leukemia, in contrast to childhood acute lymphocytic leukemia, Cerubidine during induction significantly increases the rate of complete remission, but not remission duration, compared to that obtained with vincristine, prednisone, and L-asparaginase alone. The use of Cerubidine in combination with vincristine, prednisone, and L-asparaginase has produced complete remission rates of 83% in contrast to a 47% remission in patients not receiving Cerubidine.

INDICATIONS AND USAGE

Cerubidine in combination with other approved anticancer drugs is indicated for remission induction in acute nonlymphocytic leukemia (myelogenous, monocytic, erythroid) of adults and for remission induction in acute lymphocytic leukemia of children and adults.

WARNINGS

Bone Marrow: Cerubidine is a potent bone marrow suppressant. Suppression will occur in all patients given a therapeutic dose of this drug. Therapy with Cerubidine should not be started in patients with pre-existing drug-induced bone marrow suppression unless the benefit from such treatment warrants the risk . Persistent, severe myelosuppression may result in superinfection or hemorrhage.

Cardiac Effects: Special attention must be given to the potential cardiac toxicity of Cerubidine, particularly in infants and children. Pre-existing heart disease and previous therapy with doxorubicin are co-factors of increased risk of Cerubidine-induced cardiac toxicity and the benefit-to-risk ratio of Cerubidine therapy in such patients should be weighed before starting Cerubidine. In adults, at total cumulative doses less than 550 mg/m^2, acute congestive heart failure is seldom encountered. However, rare instances of pericarditis-myocarditis, not dose-related, have been reported.

In adults, at cumulative doses exceeding 550 mg/m^2, there is an increased incidence of drug-induced congestive heart failure. Based on prior clinical experience with doxorubicin, this limit appears lower, namely 400 mg/m^2, in patients who received radiation therapy that encompassed the heart.[1]

In infants and children, there appears to be a greater susceptibility to anthracycline-induced cardiotoxicity compared

to that in adults, which is more clearly dose-related. Anthracycline therapy (including daunorubicin) in pediatric patients has been reported to produce impaired left ventricular systolic performance, reduced contractility, congestive heart failure or death. These conditions may occur months to years following cessation of chemotherapy. This appears to be dose-dependent and aggravated by thoracic irradiation. Long-term periodic evaluation of cardiac function in such patients should, thus, be performed.[2-7] In both children and adults, the total dose of Cerubidine administered should also take into account any previous or concomitant therapy with other potentially cardiotoxic agents or related compounds such as doxorubicin.

There is no absolutely reliable method of predicting the patients in whom acute congestive heart failure will develop as a result of the cardiac toxic effect of Cerubidine. However, certain changes in the electrocardiogram and a decrease in the systolic ejection fraction from pre-treatment baseline may help to recognize those patients at greatest risk to develop congestive heart failure. On the basis of the electrocardiogram, a decrease equal to or greater than 30% in limb lead QRS voltage has been associated with a significant risk of drug-induced cardiomyopathy. Therefore, an electrocardiogram and/or determination of systolic ejection fraction should be performed before each course of Cerubidine. In the event that one or the other of these predictive parameters should occur, the benefit of continued therapy must be weighed against the risk of producing cardiac damage. Early clinical diagnosis of drug-induced congestive heart failure appears to be essential for successful treatment with digitalis, diuretics, sodium restriction, and bed rest.

Evaluation of Hepatic and Renal Function: Significant hepatic or renal impairment can enhance the toxicity of the recommended doses of Cerubidine; therefore, prior to administration, evaluation of hepatic function and renal function using conventional clinical laboratory tests is recommended (See **"DOSAGE AND ADMINISTRATION"** Section).

Pregnancy: Cerubidine may cause fetal harm when administered to a pregnant woman because of its teratogenic potential. An increased incidence of fetal abnormalities (parieto-occipital cranioschisis, umbilical hernias, or rachischisis) and abortions was reported in rabbits. Decreases in fetal birth weight and post-delivery growth rate were observed in mice. There are no adequate and well-controlled studies in pregnant women. If this drug is used during pregnancy, or if the patient becomes pregnant while taking this drug, the patient should be apprised of the potential hazard to the fetus. Women of childbearing potential should be advised to avoid becoming pregnant.

Extravasation at Injection Site: Extravasation of Cerubidine at the site of intravenous administration can cause severe local tissue necrosis.

PRECAUTIONS

Therapy with Cerubidine requires close patient observation and frequent complete blood-count determinations. Cardiac, renal, and hepatic function should be evaluated prior to each course of treatment.

Cerubidine may induce hyperuricemia secondary to rapid lysis of leukemic cells. As a precaution, allopurinol administration is usually begun prior to initiating antileukemic therapy. Blood uric acid levels should be monitored and appropriate therapy initiated in the event that hyperuricemia develops.

Appropriate measures must be taken to control any systemic infection before beginning therapy with Cerubidine. Cerubidine may transiently impart a red coloration to the urine after administration, and patients should be advised to expect this.

Carcinogenesis, Mutagenesis, Impairment of Fertility: Cerubidine, when injected subcutaneously into mice, causes fibrosarcomas to develop at the injection site. When administered to mice orally or intraperitoneally, no carcinogenic effect was noted after 22 months of observation.

In male dogs at a daily dose of 0.25 mg/kg administered intravenously, testicular atrophy was noted at autopsy. Histologic examination revealed total aplasia of the spermatocyte series in the seminiferous tubules with complete aspermatogenesis.

Pregnancy Category D: See **"WARNINGS"** Section.

ADVERSE REACTIONS

Dose-limiting toxicity includes myelosuppression and cardiotoxicity (See **"WARNINGS"** Section). Other reactions include:

Cutaneous: Reversible alopecia occurs in most patients.
Gastrointestinal: Acute nausea and vomiting occur but are usually mild. Antiemetic therapy may be of some help. Mucositis may occur 3 to 7 days after administration. Diarrhea has occasionally been reported.
Local: If extravasation occurs during administration, tissue necrosis can result at the site.
Acute Reactions: Rarely, anaphylactoid reaction, fever, chills, and skin rash can occur.

DOSAGE AND ADMINISTRATION

Parenteral drug products should be inspected visually for particulate matter and discoloration prior to administration, whenever solution and container permit.

Principles: In order to eradicate the leukemic cells and induce a complete remission, a profound suppression of the bone marrow is usually required. Evaluation of both the peripheral blood and bone marrow is mandatory in the formulation of appropriate treatment plans.

It is recommended that the dosage of Cerubidine be reduced in instances of hepatic or renal impairment. For example, using serum bilirubin and serum creatinine as indicators of liver and kidney function, the following dose modifications are recommended:

Serum Bilirubin	Serum Creatinine	Recommended Dose
1.2 to 3.0 mg%		$3/4$ normal dose
>3 mg%	>3 mg%	$1/2$ normal dose

Representative Dose Schedules and Combination for the Approved Indication of Remission Induction in Adult Acute Nonlymphocytic Leukemia:

In Combination[8,9]: For patients under age 60, Cerubidine 45 mg/m²/day IV on days 1, 2, and 3 of the first course and on days 1, 2 of subsequent courses AND cytosine arabinoside 100 mg/m²/day IV infusion daily for 7 days for the first course and for 5 days for subsequent courses.

For patients 60 years of age and above, Cerubidine 30 mg/m²/day IV on days 1, 2, and 3 of the first course and on days 1, 2 of subsequent courses AND cytosine arabinoside 100 mg/m²/day IV infusion daily for 7 days for the first course and for 5 days for subsequent courses.[9] This Cerubidine dose-reduction is based on a single study and may not be appropriate if optimal supportive care is available.

The attainment of a normal-appearing bone marrow may require up to three courses of induction therapy. Evaluation of the bone marrow following recovery from the previous course of induction therapy determines whether a further course of induction treatment is required.

Representative Dose Schedule and Combination for the Approved Indication of Remission Induction in Pediatric Acute Lymphocytic Leukemia:

In Combination: Cerubidine 25 mg/m² IV on day 1 every week, vincristine 1.5 mg/m² IV on day 1 every week, prednisone 40 mg/m² PO daily. Generally, a complete remission will be obtained within four such courses of therapy; however, if after four courses the patient is in partial remission, an additional one or, if necessary, two courses may be given in an effort to obtain a complete remission.

In children less than 2 years of age or below 0.5 m² body surface area, it has been recommended that the Cerubidine dosage calculation should be based on weight (1 mg/kg) instead of body surface area.[17]

Representative Dose Schedules and Combination for the Approved Indication of Remission Induction in Adult Acute Lymphocytic Leukemia:

In Combination[10]: Cerubidine 45 mg/m²/day IV on days 1, 2, and 3 AND vincristine 2 mg IV on days 1, 8, and 15; prednisone 40 mg/m²/day PO on days 1 through 22, then tapered between days 22 to 29; L-asparaginase 500 IU/kg/day × 10 days IV on days 22 through 32.

The contents of a vial should be reconstituted with 4 mL of Sterile Water for Injection and agitated gently until the material has completely dissolved. The withdrawable vial contents provide 20 mg of daunorubicin activity, with 5 mg of daunorubicin activity per mL. The desired dose is withdrawn into a syringe containing 10 mL to 15 mL of normal saline and then injected into the tubing or sidearm in a rapidly flowing IV infusion of dextrose injection 5% or sodium chloride injection 0.9%. Cerubidine should not be administered mixed with other drugs or heparin. The reconstituted solution is stable for 24 hours at room temperature and 48 hours under refrigeration. It should be protected from exposure to sunlight.

Procedures for proper handling and disposal of anticancer drugs should be considered. Several guidelines on this subject have been published.[11-16] There is no general agreement that all of the procedures recommended in the guidelines are necessary or appropriate.

HOW SUPPLIED

Cerubidine® (daunorubicin hydrochloride) for Injection is available in butyl-rubber-stoppered vials, each containing 20 mg of base activity (21.4 mg as the hydrochloride salt) and 100 mg of mannitol, as a sterile reddish lyophilized powder. When reconstituted with 4 mL of Sterile Water for Injection, USP, each mL contains 5 mg of daunorubicin activity. Each package contains 10 vials.

NDC 55390-281-10   20 mg, single-use vials; carton of 10.

Store unreconstituted powder at controlled room temperature, 15° to 30°C (59° to 86°F).

REFERENCES

1. Gilladoga AC, Manuel C, Tan CTC, et al: The cardiotoxicity of Adriamycin and daunomycin in children. *Cancer* 37:1070-1078, 1976.
2. Bleyer WA: Delayed toxicities of chemotherapy on childhood tissues. *Front Radiat Ther Onc* 16:40-54, 1982.
3. Isner JM, Ferrans VJ, Cohen SR, et al: Clinical and morphological cardiac findings after anthracycline chemotherapy. *Am J Cardiol* 51:1167-1174, 1983.
4. Rhoden WE, Jenny M, Beton DC, et al: Long term effects on left ventricular function of treatment for childhood malignancy. *Br Heart J* 66:59, 1991.
5. Steinherz LJ, Steinherz PG, Tan CTC, et al: Cardiac toxicity 4 to 20 years after completing anthracycline therapy. *JAMA* 266:1672-1677, 1991.
6. Lipshultz SE, Colan SD, Gelber RD, et al: Late cardiac effects of doxorubicin therapy for acute lymphoblastic leukemia in childhood. *N Engl J Med* 324:808-815, 1991.
7. Steinherz L, Steinherz P: Delayed cardiac toxicity from anthracycline therapy. *Pediatrician* 18:49-52, 1991.
8. Rai KR, Holland JF, Glidewell O, et al: Treatment of acute myelocytic leukemia: a study by Cancer and Leukemia Group B. *Blood* 58:1203-1212, 1981.
9. Yates J, Glidewell O, Wiernik P, et al: Cytosine arabinoside with daunorubicin or adriamycin for therapy of acute myelocytic leukemia: a CALGB study. *Blood* 60:454-462, 1982.
10. Gottlieb AJ, Weinberg V, Ellison RR, et al: Efficacy of daunorubicin in the therapy of adult acute lymphocytic leukemia: a prospective randomized trial by Cancer and Leukemia Group B. *Blood* 64:267-274, 1984.
11. Recommendations for the Safe Handling of Parenteral Antineoplastic Drugs. NIH Publication No. 83-2621. For Sale by the Superintendent of Documents, U.S. Government Printing Office, Washington, D.C. 20402.
12. AMA Council Report. Guidelines for Handling Parenteral Antineoplastics. *JAMA*, March 15, 1985.
13. National Study Commission on Cytotoxic Exposure—Recommendations for Handling Cytotoxic Agents. Available from Louis P. Jeffrey, Sc.D., Chairman, National Study Commission on Cytotoxic Exposure, Massachusetts College of Pharmacy and Allied Health Sciences, 179 Longwood Avenue, Boston, Massachusetts 02115.
14. Clinical Oncological Society of Australia: Guidelines and recommendations for safe handling of antineoplastic agents. *Med J Australia* 1:426-428, 1983.
15. Jones RB, et al: Safe handling of chemotherapeutic agents: A report from the Mount Sinai Medical Center, *Ca—A Cancer Journal for Clinicians* Sept/Oct, 258-263, 1983.
16. American Society of Hospital Pharmacists technical assistance bulletin on handling cytotoxic and hazardous drugs. *Am J Hosp Pharm* 47:1033-1049, 1990.
17. Sallan SE: Personal communication, 1981.

MANUFACTURED BY:
Ben Venue Laboratories, Inc.
Bedford, OH 44146
MANUFACTURED FOR:
Bedford Laboratories™
Bedford, Ohio 44146
May, 1996   CRD-P00
A.H.F.S. CATEGORY 10:00

Beiersdorf Inc.
**P.O. BOX 5529
NORWALK, CT 06856-5529**

Direct Inquiries to:
Medical Division
(203) 563-5800

AQUAPHOR®—Original Ointment   OTC
NDC Numbers—10356-020-10

COMPOSITION

Petrolatum, Mineral Oil, Ceresin, Lanolin Alcohol.

ACTIONS AND USES

Aquaphor is a stable, neutral, odorless, anhydrous ointment base. It is miscible with water or aqueous solutions, forming smooth, creamy water-in-oil emulsions. In its pure form, Aquaphor is recommended for use as a topical preparation to help heal severely dry skin. Aquaphor contains no preservatives, fragrances or known irritants.

Continued on next page

Aquaphor-Original—Cont.

ADMINISTRATION AND DOSAGES

Use Aquaphor alone or in compounding virtually any ointment using aqueous solutions or in combination with other oil-based substances and all common topical medications. Apply Aquaphor liberally to affected area.

PRECAUTIONS

For external use only. Avoid contact with eyes. Not to be applied over deep or puncture wounds, infections or lacerations. If condition worsens or does not improve within 7 days, patient should consult a doctor.

HOW SUPPLIED

14 oz. jar—List No. 03147

AQUAPHOR® Healing Ointment   OTC
NDC Number—10356-021-01
             10356-021-05

COMPOSITION

Petrolatum, Mineral Oil, Ceresin, Lanolin Alcohol, Glycerin Panthenol, Bisabolol.

ACTIONS AND USES

Aquaphor Healing Ointment is specially formulated to help reduce healing time[1] on cracked, dry skin and minor burns. It is recommended for patients suffering from severe skin chapping and from skin disorders that result in severely cracked or dry skin. Because Aquaphor is free of fragrances and preservatives it is ideal for daily use.

ADMINISTRATION AND DOSAGE

Use Aquaphor Healing Ointment whenever a mild healing agent is needed. Apply liberally to affected dry skin areas two to three times a day. In the case of minor wounds, clean area prior to application.

PRECAUTIONS

For external use only. Avoid contact with the eyes. Not to be applied over deep or puncture wounds, infections or lacerations. If condition worsens or does not improve within seven days, patient should consult a physician.

HOW SUPPLIED

1.75 oz. tube—List No. 45231
1. Data on file, BDF Inc
3.5 oz. jar—List No. 03263

EUCERIN® Creme   OTC
[ū'sir-in]
Original Moisturizing Creme
NDC Numbers—10356-090-01
             10356-090-05
             10356-090-04
             10356-090-07

INDICATIONS

Use daily to help relieve dry and very dry skin conditions.

COMPOSITION

Water, Petrolatum, Mineral Oil, Ceresin, Lanolin Alcohol, Methylchloroisothiazolinone, Methylisothiazolinone.

ACTIONS AND USES

A gentle, non-comedogenic, fragrance-free unique, water-in-oil emulsion. Eucerin can be used for treating dry skin conditions associated with eczema, psoriasis, chapped or chafed skin, sunburn, windburn and itching associated with dryness.[1]

ADMINISTRATION AND DOSAGES

Apply freely to affected areas of the skin as often as necessary or as directed by a physician.

PRECAUTIONS

For external use only. Avoid contact with the eyes. Discontinue use if signs of irritation occur.

HOW SUPPLIED

16 oz. jar—List Number 00090
8 oz. jar—List Number 03774
4 oz. jar—List Number 03797
2 oz. tube—List Number 03868
1. Data on File.

EUCERIN®   OTC
FACIAL MOISTURIZING LOTION SPF 25
NDC Number—10356-972-01

INDICATIONS

Use daily to help relieve dry facial skin and provide broad spectrum sun protection.

COMPOSITION

Active Ingredients: Octyl Methoxcinnamate, Octyl Salicylate, Titanium Dioxide, Zinc Oxide.
Other Ingredients: Water, Octyldodecyl Neopentanoate, Dioctyl Malate, Glycerin, Petrolatum, Cetearyl Alcohol, DEA-Cetyl Phosphate, PEG-40 Castor Oil, Glyceryl Stearate SE, Sodium Hyaluronate, Lactic Acid, Lanolin Alcohol, Sodium Cetearyl Sulfate, Xanthan Gum, Methicone, Dimethicone, EDTA, Sodium Hydroxide, Methylchloroisothiazolinone, Methylisothiazolinone.

ACTIONS AND USES

Eucerin Facial Moisturizing Lotion SPF 25 is fragrance-free and non-comedogenic,[1] with a unique sun screen (titanium dioxide) to protect skin from UVA and UVB light.[1] It is specially formulated for dry, sensitive skin or for those undergoing therapies which irritate delicate facial skin. This light, oil-in-water formula is non-greasy and is easily absorbed into the skin.

ADMINISTRATION AND DOSAGE

Apply Eucerin Facial Moisturizing Lotion SPF 25 twice a day (especially in the morning), or as directed by a physician, to moisturize skin and protect it from harmful UVA and UVB rays.

PRECAUTIONS

For external use only. Avoid contact with eyes. Keep out of the reach of children. Discontinue use if signs of irritation or rash appear.

HOW SUPPLIED

4 fl. oz. bottle.—List No. 03972
1. Data on File

EUCERIN® LIGHT
MOISTURE-RESTORATIVE LOTION   OTC
[ū'sir-in]

INDICATIONS

For Daily Dry Skin Therapy

COMPOSITION

Active Ingredient: Dimethicone
Other Ingredients: Water, Sunflower Seed Oil (Helianthus Annuus), Petrolatum, Glycerin, Glyceryl Stearate SE, Octyldodecanol, Panthenol, Caprylic/Capric Triglyceride, Tocopheryl Acetate, Stearic Acid, Cholesterol, Triethanolamine, Carbomer, Disodium EDTA, BHT, Methylchloroisothiazolinone, Methylisothiazolinone.

ACTIONS AND USES

Lipid enhanced formula that is light and fast absorbing. Lotion proven to restore moisture and maintain the barrier function of the skin.[1]

ADMINISTRATION AND DOSAGE

Apply liberally as often as necessary or as directed by a physician.

PRECAUTIONS

For external use only. Avoid contact with eyes. If condition worsens or does not improve within 7 days, consult a doctor. Not to be applied over deep or puncture wounds, infections, or lacerations.

HOW SUPPLIED

8 fl. oz. — List Number 03276
NDC 10356-032-01
1. Data on File

EUCERIN® Lotion   OTC
[ū'sir-in]
Original Moisturizing Lotion
NDC Numbers—10356-793-01
             10356-793-04

INDICATIONS

Use daily to help relieve dry skin.

COMPOSITION

Water, Mineral Oil, Isopropyl Myristate, PEG-40 Sorbitan Peroleate, Glyceryl Lanolate, Sorbitol, Propylene Glycol, Cetyl Palmitate, Magnesium Sulfate, Aluminum Stearate, Lanolin Alcohol, BHT, Methylchloroisothiazolinone, Methylisothiazolinone.

ACTIONS AND USES

Eucerin Lotion is a non-comedogenic, fragrance-free, unique water-in-oil formulation that will help to alleviate and soothe dry skin, and provide long-lasting moisturization.

ADMINISTRATION AND DOSAGE

Use daily on dry skin or as directed by a physician.

PRECAUTIONS

For external use only. Avoid contact with the eyes. Discontinue use if signs of irritation occur.

HOW SUPPLIED

8 fl. oz. bottle—List Number 3793
16 fl. oz. bottle—List Number 3794

EUCERIN PLUS CREME   OTC
Alphahydroxy Moisturizing Creme
NDC 10356-036-01

INDICATIONS

Use daily to help relieve severely dry, flaky skin.

COMPOSITION

Water, Mineral Oil, Urea 10.0%, Magnesium Stearate, Ceresin, Polyglyceryl-3 Diisostearate, Sodium Lactate 2.5%, Isopropyl Palmitate, Benzyl Alcohol, Panthenol, Bisabolol, Lanolin Alcohol, Magnesium Sulfate.

ACTION AND USES

Eucerin Plus Creme is a unique alphahydroxy acid moisturizing creme (2.5% sodium lactate, 10% urea) that is clinically proven to help relieve severely dry, flaky skin conditions[1]. Unlike other alphahydroxy acid mositurizers, Eucerin Plus Creme has low irritation potential and is fragrance-free.

ADMINISTRATION AND DOSAGE

Use daily on severely dry, scaly skin or as directed by a physician.

PRECAUTIONS

Avoid contact with eyes or areas where skin is inflamed or cracked. Discontinue use if signs of irritation occur. For external use only. Keep out of reach of children.

HOW SUPPLIED

4 oz. jar—List No. 03611
1. Data on file.

EUCERIN PLUS FOR THE FACE
Alphahydroxy Moisturizing Lotion SPF 15   OTC
[ū'sir-in]

INDICATIONS

Moisturizes dry facial skin and helps improve texture and appearance of the skin. Helps protect from sun damage with SPF 15

COMPOSITION

Active Ingredient: Octyl Methoxcinnamate, Oxybenzone, Octyl Salicylate
Other Ingredients: Water, Sodium Lactate, Glycerin, Urea, Glyceryl Stearate PEG-5 Glyceryl Stearate, C12-15 Alkyl Benzoate, Octyldodecanol, Sodium PCA, Cyclomethicone, Cetyl Alcohol, Tocopheryl Acetate, Xanthan Gum, Lactic Acid, Methylchloroisothiazolinone, Methylisothiazolinone.

ACTIONS AND USES

Clinically proven to significantly increase skin hydration and improve skin texture, non-irritating, non-stinging.[1] Contains SPF 15 in a light cosmetically elegant formula. Non-comedogenic and fragrance free.[1]

ADMINISTRATION AND DOSAGE

Use daily to help moisturize dry facial skin or as directed by a physician.

PRECAUTIONS

For external use only. Avoid contact with eyes and areas where skin is inflamed or cracked. Keep out of the reach of children. Discontinue use if signs of irritation occur.

HOW SUPPLIED

4 fl. oz — List Number 03299
NDC 10356-299-01
1. Data on File

EUCERIN PLUS LOTION   OTC
Alphahydroxy Moisturizing Lotion
NDC 10356-967-01
        10356-967-03

INDICATIONS

Use daily to help relieve severely dry, flaky skin.

COMPOSITION

Water, Mineral Oil, PEG-7 Hydrogenated Castor Oil, Isohexadecane, Sodium Lactate 5%, Urea 5%, Glycerin, Isopro-

pyl Palmitate, Panthenol, Ozokerite, Magnesium Sulfate, Lanolin Alcohol, Bisabolol, Methylchloroisothiazolinone, Methylisothiazolinone.

ACTION AND USES

Eucerin Plus Lotion is a unique, patented alphahydroxy acid moisturizing lotion (5% Sodium Lactate, 5% Urea) that is clinically proven to help relieve severely dry, flaky skin conditions.[1] Unlike other alphahydroxy acid moisturizing lotions, Eucerin Plus has a very low irritation potential and is fragrance free.

ADMINISTRATION AND DOSAGE

Use daily on severely dry, flaky skin or as directed by a physician.

PRECAUTIONS

Avoid contact with eyes or areas where skin is inflamed or cracked. Discontinue use if signs of irritation occur. For external use only. Keep out of reach of children.

HOW SUPPLIED

6 fl. oz. bottle—List No. 03967
12 fl. oz. bottle—List No.–03321
1. Data on File.

Berlex Laboratories

300 FAIRFIELD ROAD
WAYNE, NJ 07470

Direct Inquiries to:
(973) 694-4100

For Medical Information and to report drug adverse events Contact:
Department of Epidemiology and Medical Affairs
300 Fairfield Road
Wayne, NJ 07470
(888) BERLEX-4

Betaseron for SC Injection Only: (Medical Information Only)
15049 San Pablo Avenue
Richmond, CA 94809-0099
(800) 888-4112

Fludara for Injection Only: (Medical Information Only)
15049 San Pablo Avenue
Richmond, CA 94809-0099
(800) 888-4112

BETAPACE®

[*bā '-tăh-pāce"*] ℞
(sotalol HCl)

DESCRIPTION

BETAPACE® (sotalol hydrochloride), is an antiarrhythmic drug with Class II (beta-adrenoreceptor blocking) and Class III (cardiac action potential duration prolongation) properties. It is supplied as a light-blue, capsule-shaped tablet for oral administration. Sotalol hydrochloride is a white, crystalline solid with a molecular weight of 308.8. It is hydrophilic, soluble in water, propylene glycol and ethanol, but is only slightly soluble in chloroform. Chemically, sotalol hydrochloride is d,l-N-[4-[l-hydroxy-2-[(l-methylethyl)amino] ethyl]phenyl]methane-sulfonamide monohydrochloride. The molecular formula is $C_{12}H_{20}N_2O_3S{\cdot}HCl$ and is represented by the following structural formula:

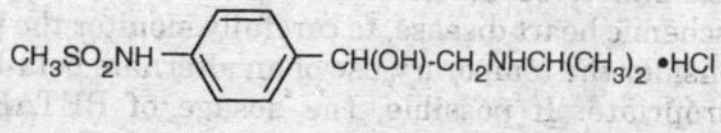
CH3SO2NH
CH(OH)-CH2NHCH(CH3)2 •HCl

BETAPACE® Tablets contain the following inactive ingredients: microcrystalline cellulose, lactose, starch, stearic acid, magnesium stearate, colloidal silicon dioxide, and FD&C blue color #2 (aluminum lake, conc.).

CLINICAL PHARMACOLOGY

Mechanism of Action: BETAPACE® (sotalol hydrochloride) has both beta-adrenoreceptor blocking (Vaughan Williams Class II) and cardiac action potential duration prolongation (Vaughan Williams Class III) antiarrhythmic properties. BETAPACE® (sotalol hydrochloride) is a racemic mixture of d- and l-sotalol. Both isomers have similar Class III antiarrhythmic effects, while the l-isomer is responsible for virtually all of the beta-blocking activity. The beta-blocking effect of sotalol is non-cardioselective, half maximal at about 80 mg/day and maximal at doses between 320 and 640 mg/day. Sotalol does not have partial agonist or membrane stabilizing activity. Although significant beta-blockade occurs at oral doses as low as 25 mg, Class III effects are seen only at daily doses of 160 mg and above.

Electrophysiology: Sotalol hydrochloride prolongs the plateau phase of the cardiac action potential in the isolated myocyte, as well as in isolated tissue preparations of ventricular or atrial muscle (Class III activity). In intact animals it slows heart rate, decreases AV nodal conduction and increases the refractory periods of atrial and ventricular muscle and conduction tissue.

In man, the Class II (beta-blockade) electrophysiological effects of BETAPACE® are manifested by increased sinus cycle length (slowed heart rate), decreased AV nodal conduction and increased AV nodal refractoriness. The Class III electrophysiological effects in man include prolongation of the atrial and ventricular monophasic action potentials, and effective refractory period prolongation of atrial muscle, ventricular muscle, and atrio-ventricular accessory pathways (where present) in both the anterograde and retrograde directions. With oral doses of 160 to 640 mg/day, the surface ECG shows dose–related mean increases of 40–100 msec in QT and 10–40 msec in QT_c. (See **WARNINGS** for description of relationship between QT_c and torsade de pointes type arrhythmias). No significant alteration in QRS interval is observed.

In a small study (n=25) of patients with implanted defibrillators treated concurrently with BETAPACE®, the average defibrillatory threshold was 6 joules (range 2–15 joules) compared to a mean of 16 joules for a non-randomized comparative group primarily receiving amiodarone.

Hemodynamics: In a study of systemic hemodynamic function measured invasively in 12 patients with a mean LV ejection fraction of 37% and ventricular tachycardia (9 sustained and 3 non-sustained), a median dose of 160 mg twice daily of BETAPACE® produced a 28% reduction in heart rate and a 24% decrease in cardiac index at 2 hours post dosing at steady-state. Concurrently, systemic vascular resistance and stroke volume showed non-significant increases of 25% and 8%, respectively. Pulmonary capillary wedge pressure increased significantly from 6.4 mmHg to 11.8 mmHg in the 11 patients who completed the study. One patient was discontinued because of worsening congestive heart failure. Mean arterial pressure, mean pulmonary artery pressure and stroke work index did not significantly change. Exercise and isoproterenol induced tachycardia are antagonized by BETAPACE®, and total peripheral resistance increases by a small amount.

In hypertensive patients, BETAPACE® (sotalol hydrochloride) produces significant reductions in both systolic and diastolic blood pressures. Although BETAPACE® (sotalol hydrochloride) is usually well-tolerated hemodynamically, caution should be exercised in patients with marginal cardiac compensation as deterioration in cardiac performance may occur. (See **WARNINGS: Congestive Heart Failure.**)

Clinical Actions: BETAPACE® (sotalol hydrochloride) has been studied in life-threatening and less severe arrhythmias. In patients with frequent premature ventricular complexes (VPC), BETAPACE® (sotalol hydrochloride) was significantly superior to placebo in reducing VPC's, paired VPCs and non-sustained ventricular tachycardia (NSVT); the response was dose-related through 640 mg/day with 80–85% of patients having at least a 75% reduction of VPCs. BETAPACE® (sotalol hydrochloride) was also superior, at the doses evaluated, to propranolol (40–80 mg TID) and similar to quinidine (200–400 mg QID) in reducing VPCs. In patients with life-threatening arrhythmias [sustained ventricular tachycardia/fibrillation (VT/VF)], BETAPACE® (sotalol hydrochloride) was studied acutely [by suppression of programmed electrical stimulation (PES) induced VT and by suppression of Holter monitor evidence of sustained VT] and, in acute responders, chronically.

In a double-blind, randomized comparison of BETAPACE® and procainamide given intravenously (total of 2 mg/kg BETAPACE® vs. 19 mg/kg of procainamide over 90 minutes), BETAPACE® suppressed PES induction in 30% of patients vs. 20% for procainamide (p=0.2).

In a randomized clinical trial [Electrophysiologic Study Versus Electrocardiographic Monitoring (ESVEM) Trial] comparing choice of antiarrhythmic therapy by PES suppression vs. Holter monitor selection (in each case followed by treadmill exercise testing) in patients with a history of sustained VT/VF who were also inducible by PES, the effectiveness acutely and chronically of BETAPACE® (sotalol hydrochloride) was compared with 6 other drugs (procainamide, quinidine, mexiletine, propafenone, imipramine and pirmenol). Overall response, limited to first randomized drug, was 39% for sotalol and 30% for the pooled other drugs. Acute response rate for first drug randomized using suppression of PES induction was 36% for BETAPACE® vs. a mean of 13% for the other drugs. Using the Holter monitoring endpoint (complete suppression of sustained VT, 90% suppression of NSVT, 80% suppression of VPC pairs, and at least 70% suppression of VPCs), BETAPACE® yielded 41% response vs. 45% for the other drugs combined. Among responders placed on long-term therapy identified acutely as effective (by either PES or Holter), BETAPACE®, when compared to the pool of other drugs, had the lowest two-year mortality (13% vs. 22%), the lowest two-year VT recurrence rate (30% vs. 60%), and the lowest withdrawal rate (38% vs. about 75–80%). The most commonly used doses of BETAPACE® (sotalol hydrochloride) in this trial were 320–480 mg/day (66% of patients), with 16% receiving 240 mg/day or less and 18% receiving 640 mg or more.

It cannot be determined, however, in the absence of a controlled comparison of BETAPACE® vs. no pharmacologic treatment (e.g., in patients with implanted defibrillators) whether BETAPACE® response causes improved survival or identifies a population with a good prognosis.

In a large double-blind, placebo controlled secondary prevention (post-infarction) trial (n=1,456), BETAPACE® (sotalol hydrochloride) was given as a non-titrated initial dose of 320 mg once daily. BETAPACE® did not produce a significant increase in survival (7.3% mortality on BETAPACE® vs 8.9% on placebo, p=0.3), but overall did not suggest an adverse effect on survival. There was, however, a suggestion of an early (i.e., first 10 days) excess mortality (3% on sotalol vs. 2% on placebo). In a second small trial (n=17 randomized to sotalol) where sotalol was administered at high doses (e.g., 320 mg twice daily) to high-risk post-infarction patients (ejection fraction <40% and either >10 VPC/hr or VT on Holter), there were 4 fatalities and 3 serious hemodynamic/electrical adverse events within two weeks of initiating sotalol.

Pharmacokinetics: In healthy subjects, the oral bioavailability of BETAPACE® (sotalol hydrochloride) is 90–100%. After oral administration, peak plasma concentrations are reached in 2.5 to 4 hours, and steady-state plasma concentrations are attained within 2–3 days (i.e., after 5–6 doses when administered twice daily). Over the dosage range 160–640 mg/day BETAPACE® (sotalol hydrochloride) displays dose proportionality with respect to plasma concentrations. Distribution occurs to a central (plasma) and to a peripheral compartment, with a mean elimination half-life of 12 hours. Dosing every 12 hours results in trough plasma concentrations which are approximately one-half of those at peak.

BETAPACE® (sotalol hydrochloride) does not bind to plasma proteins and is not metabolized. BETAPACE® (sotalol hydrochloride) shows very little intersubject variability in plasma levels. The pharmacokinetics of the d and l enantiomers of sotalol are essentially identical. BETAPACE® (sotalol hydrochloride) crosses the blood brain barrier poorly. Excretion is predominantly via the kidney in the unchanged form, and therefore lower doses are necessary in conditions of renal impairment (see **DOSAGE AND ADMINISTRATION**). Age per se does not significantly alter the pharmacokinetics of BETAPACE®, but impaired renal function in geriatric patients can increase the terminal elimination half-life, resulting in increased drug accumulation. The absorption of BETAPACE® (sotalol hydrochloride) was reduced by approximately 20% compared to fasting when it was administered with a standard meal. Since BETAPACE® (sotalol hydrochloride) is not subject to first-pass metabolism, patients with hepatic impairment show no alteration in clearance of BETAPACE®.

INDICATIONS AND USAGE

Oral BETAPACE® (sotalol hydrochloride) is indicated for the treatment of documented ventricular arrhythmias, such as sustained ventricular tachycardia, that in the judgment of the physician are life-threatening. Because of the proarrhythmic effects of BETAPACE® (See **WARNINGS**), including a 1.5 to 2% rate of torsade de pointes or new VT/VF in patients with either NSVT or supraventricular arrhythmias, its use in patients with less severe arrhythmias, even if the patients are symptomatic, is generally not recommended. Treatment of patients with asymptomatic ventricular premature contractions should be avoided.

Initiation of BETAPACE® treatment or increasing doses, as with other antiarrhythmic agents used to treat life-threatening arrhythmias, should be carried out in the hospital. The response to treatment should then be evaluated by a suitable method (e.g., PES or Holter monitoring) prior to continuing the patient on chronic therapy. Various approaches have been used to determine the response to antiarrhythmic therapy, including BETAPACE®.

In the ESVEM Trial, response by Holter monitoring was tentatively defined as 100% suppression of ventricular tachycardia, 90% suppression of non-sustained VT, 80% suppression of paired VPCs, and 75% suppression of total VPCs in patients who had at least 10 VPCs/hour at baseline; this tentative response was confirmed if VT lasting 5 or more beats was not observed during treadmill exercise testing us-

Continued on next page

Information on the Berlex products appearing here is based on the most current information available at the time of publication closing. Further information for these and other products may be obtained from the Medical Affairs Department, Berlex Laboratories, 300 Fairfield Road, Wayne, New Jersey 07470, 1-888-BERLEX-4. Information on Betaseron and Fludara may be obtained from Berlex Laboratories, 15049 San Pablo Avenue, Richmond, California 94804-0016, 1-800-888-4112.

Betapace—Cont.

ing a standard Bruce protocol. The PES protocol utilized a maximum of three extrastimuli at three pacing cycle lengths and two right ventricular pacing sites. Response by PES was defined as prevention of induction of the following: 1) monomorphic VT lasting over 15 seconds; 2) non-sustained polymorphic VT containing more than 15 beats of monomorphic VT in patients with a history of monomorphic VT; 3) polymorphic VT or VF greater than 15 beats in patients with VF or a history of aborted sudden death without monomorphic VT; and 4) two episodes of polymorphic VT or VF of greater than 15 beats in a patient presenting with monomorphic VT. Sustained VT or NSVT producing hypotension during the final treadmill test was considered a drug failure.

In a multicenter open-label long-term study of BETAPACE® in patients with life-threatening ventricular arrhythmias which had proven refractory to other antiarrhythmic medications, response by Holter monitoring was defined as in ESVEM. Response by PES was defined as non-inducibility of sustained VT by at least double extrastimuli delivered at a pacing cycle length of 400 msec. Overall survival and arrythmia recurrence rates in this study were similar to those seen in ESVEM, although there was no comparative group to allow a definitive assessment of outcome.

Antiarrhythmic drugs have not been shown to enhance survival in patients with ventricular arrhythmias.

CONTRAINDICATIONS

BETAPACE® (sotalol hydrochloride) is contraindicated in patients with bronchial asthma, sinus bradycardia, second and third degree AV block, unless a functioning pacemaker is present, congenital or acquired long QT syndromes, cardiogenic shock, uncontrolled congestive heart failure, and previous evidence of hypersensitivity to BETAPACE®.

WARNINGS

Mortality: The National Heart, Lung, and Blood Institute's Cardiac Arrhythmia Suppression Trial I (CAST I) was a long-term, multi-center, double-blind study in patients with asymptomatic, non-life-threatening ventricular arrhythmias, 1 to 103 weeks after acute myocardial infarction. Patients in CAST I were randomized to receive placebo or individually optimized doses of encainide, flecainide, or moricizine. The Cardiac Arrhythmia Suppression Trial II (CAST II) was similar, except that the recruited patients had had their index infarction 4 to 90 days before randomization, patients with left ventricular ejection fractions greater than 40% were not admitted, and the randomized regimens were limited to placebo and moricizine.

CAST I was discontinued after an average time-on-treatment of 10 months, and CAST II was discontinued after an average time-on-treatment of 18 months. As compared to placebo treatment, all three active therapies were associated with increases in short-term (14-day) mortality, and encainide and flecainide were associated with significant increases in longer-term mortality as well. The longer-term mortality rate associated with moricizine treatment could not be statistically distinguished from that associated with placebo.

The applicability of these results to other populations (e.g., those without recent myocardial infarction) and to other than Class I antiarrhythmic agents is uncertain. BETAPACE® (sotalol hydrochloride) is devoid of Class I effects, and in a large (n=1,456) controlled trial in patients with a recent myocardial infarction, who did not necessarily have ventricular arrhythmias, BETAPACE® did not produce increased mortality at doses up to 320 mg/day (see **Clinical Actions**). On the other hand, in the large post-infarction study using a non-titrated initial dose of 320 mg once daily and in a second small randomized trial in high-risk post-infarction patients treated with high doses (320 mg BID), there have been suggestions of an excess of early sudden deaths.

Proarrhythmia: Like other antiarrhythmic agents, BETAPACE® can provoke new or worsened ventricular arrhythmias in some patients, including sustained ventricular tachycardia or ventricular fibrillation, with potentially fatal consequences. Because of its effect on cardiac repolarization (QT_c interval prolongation), torsade de pointes, a polymorphic ventricular tachycardia with prolongation of the QT interval and a shifting electrical axis is the most common form of proarrhythmia associated with BETAPACE®, occurring in about 4% of high risk (history of sustained VT/VF) patients. The risk of torsade de pointes progressively increases with prolongation of the QT interval, and is worsened also by reduction in heart rate and reduction in serum potassium (See **Electrolyte Disturbances**.)

Because of the variable temporal recurrence of arrhythmias, it is not always possible to distinguish between a new or aggravated arrhythmic event and the patient's underlying rhythm disorder. (Note, however, that torsade de pointes is usually a drug-induced arrhythmia in people with an initially normal QT_c.) Thus, the incidence of drug-related events cannot be precisely determined, so that the occurrence rates provided must be considered approximations. Note also that drug-induced arrhythmias may often not be identified, particularly if they occur long after starting the drug, due to less frequent monitoring. It is clear from the NIH-sponsored CAST (see **WARNINGS: Mortality**) that some antiarrhythmic drugs can cause increased sudden death mortality, presumably due to new arrhythmias or asystole, that do not appear early in treatment but that represent a sustained increased risk.

Overall in clinical trials with sotalol, 4.3% of 3257 patients experienced a new or worsened ventricular arrhythmia. Of this 4.3%, there was new or worsened sustained ventricular tachycardia in approximately 1% of patients and torsade de pointes in 2.4%. Additionally, in approximately 1% of patients, deaths were considered possibly drug-related; such cases, although difficult to evaluate, may have been associated with proarrhythmic events. **In patients with a history of sustained ventricular tachycardia, the incidence of torsade de pointes was 4% and worsened VT in about 1%; in patients with other, less serious, ventricular arrhythmias and supraventricular arrhythmias, the incidence of torsade de pointes was 1% and 1.4%, respectively.**

Torsade de pointes arrhythmias were dose related, as is the prolongation of QT (QT_c) interval, as shown in the table below.

Percent incidence of Torsade de Pointes and Mean QT_c Interval by Dose For Patients With Sustained VT/VF

Daily Dose (mg)	Incidence of Torsade de pointes	Mean QT_c* (msec)
80	0 (69)	463 (17)
160	0.5 (832)	467 (181)
320	1.6 (835)	473 (344)
480	4.4 (459)	483 (234)
640	3.7 (324)	490 (185)
>640	5.8 (103)	512 (62)

( ) Number of patients assessed
*Highest on-therapy value

In addition to dose and presence of sustained VT, other risk factors for torsade de pointes were gender (females had a higher incidence), excessive prolongation of the QT_c interval (see table below) and history of cardiomegaly or congestive heart failure. Patients with sustained ventricular tachycardia and a history of congestive heart failure appear to have the highest risk for serious proarrhythmia (7%). Of the patients experiencing torsade de pointes, approximately two-thirds spontaneously reverted to their baseline rhythm. The others were either converted electrically (D/C cardioversion or overdrive pacing) or treated with other drugs (see **OVERDOSAGE**). It is not possible to determine whether some sudden deaths represented episodes of torsade de pointes, but in some instances sudden death did follow a documented episode of torsade de pointes. Although BETAPACE® therapy was discontinued in most patients experiencing torsade de pointes, 17% were continued on a lower dose. Nonetheless, BETAPACE® should be used with particular caution if the QT_c is greater than 500 msec on-therapy and serious consideration should be given to reducing the dose or discontinuing therapy when the QT_c exceeds 550 msec. Due to the multiple risk-factors associated with torsade de pointes, however, caution should be exercised regardless of the QT_c interval. The table below relates the incidence of torsade de pointes to on-therapy QT_c and change in QT_c from baseline. It should be noted, however, that the highest on-therapy QT_c was in many cases the one obtained at the time of the torsade de pointes event, so that the table overstates the predictive value of a high QT_c.

[See table below]

Proarrhythmic events must be anticipated not only on initiating therapy, but with every upward dose adjustment.

Proarrhythmic events most often occur within 7 days of initiating therapy or of an increase in dose; 75% of serious proarrhythmias (torsade de pointes and worsened VT) occurred within 7 days of initiating BETAPACE® therapy, while 60% of such events occurred within 3 days of initiation or a dosage change. Initiating therapy at 80 mg BID with gradual upward dose titration and appropriate evaluations for efficacy (e.g., PES or Holter) and safety (e.g., QT interval, heart rate and electrolytes) prior to dose escalation, should reduce the risk of proarrhythmia. Avoiding excessive accumulation of sotalol in patients with diminished renal function, by appropriate dose reduction, should also reduce the risk of proarrhythmia (see **DOSAGE AND ADMINISTRATION**).

Congestive Heart Failure: Sympathetic stimulation is necessary in supporting circulatory function in congestive heart failure, and beta-blockade carries the potential hazard of further depressing myocardial contractility and precipitating more severe failure. In patients who have congestive heart failure controlled by digitalis and/or diuretics, BETAPACE® should be administered cautiously. Both digitalis and sotalol slow AV conduction. As with all beta-blockers, caution is advised when initiating therapy in patients with any evidence of left ventricular dysfunction. In premarketing studies, new or worsened congestive heart failure (CHF) occurred in 3.3% (n=3257) of patients and led to discontinuation in approximately 1% of patients receiving BETAPACE®. The incidence was higher in patients presenting with sustained ventricular tachycardia/fibrillation (4.6%, n=1363), or a prior history of heart failure (7.3%, n=696). Based on a life-table analysis, the one-year incidence of new or worsened CHF was 3% in patients without a prior history and 10% in patients with a prior history of CHF. NYHA Classification was also closely associated to the incidence of new or worsened heart failure while receiving BETAPACE® (1.8% in 1395 Class I patients, 4.9% in 1254 Class II patients and 6.1% in 278 Class III or IV patients).

Electrolyte Disturbances: BETAPACE® should not be used in patients with hypokalemia or hypomagnesemia prior to correction of imbalance, as these conditions can exaggerate the degree of QT prolongation, and increase the potential for torsade de pointes. Special attention should be given to electrolyte and acid-base balance in patients experiencing severe or prolonged diarrhea or patients receiving concomitant diuretic drugs.

Conduction Disturbances: Excessive prolongation of the QT interval (>550 msec) can promote serious arrhythmias and should be avoided (see **Proarrhythmias** above). Sinus bradycardia (heart rate less than 50 bpm) occurred in 13% of patients receiving BETAPACE® in clinical trials, and led to discontinuation in about 3% of patients. Bradycardia itself increases the risk of torsade de pointes. Sinus pause, sinus arrest and sinus node dysfunction occur in less than 1% of patients. The incidence of 2nd- or 3rd-degree AV block is approximately 1%.

Recent Acute MI: BETAPACE® can be used safely and effectively in the long-term treatment of life-threatening ventricular arrhythmias following a myocardial infarction. However, experience in the use of BETAPACE® to treat cardiac arrhythmias in the early phase of recovery from acute MI is limited and at least at high initial doses is not reassuring. (See **WARNINGS: Mortality**.) In the first 2 weeks post-MI caution is advised and careful dose titration is especially important, particularly in patients with markedly impaired ventricular function.

The following warnings are related to the beta-blocking activity of BETAPACE®.

Abrupt Withdrawal: Hypersensitivity to catecholamines has been observed in patients withdrawn from beta-blocker therapy. Occasional cases of exacerbation of angina pectoris, arrhythmias and, in some cases, myocardial infarction have been reported after abrupt discontinuation of beta-blocker therapy. Therefore, it is prudent when discontinuing chronically administered BETAPACE®, particularly in patients with ischemic heart disease, to carefully monitor the patient and consider the temporary use of an alternate beta-blocker if appropriate. If possible, the dosage of BETAPACE® should be gradually reduced over a period of one to two

Relationship Between QT_c Interval Prolongation and Torsade de Pointes

On-Therapy QT_c Interval (msec)	Incidence of Torsade de pointes	Change in QT_c Interval From Baseline (msec)	Incidence of Torsade de pointes
less than 500	1.3% (1787)	less than 65	1.6% (1516)
500–525	3.4% (236)	65–80	3.2% (158)
525–550	5.6% (125)	80–100	4.1% (146)
>550	10.8% (157)	100–130	5.2% (115)
		>130	7.1% (99)

( ) Number of patients assessed

weeks. If angina or acute coronary insufficiency develops, appropriate therapy should be instituted promptly. Patients should be warned against interruption or discontinuation of therapy without the physician's advice. Because coronary artery disease is common and may be unrecognized in patients receiving BETAPACE®, abrupt discontinuation in patients with arrhythmias may unmask latent coronary insufficiency.

Non-Allergic Bronchospasm (e.g., chronic bronchitis and emphysema): **PATIENTS WITH BRONCHOSPASTIC DISEASES SHOULD IN GENERAL NOT RECEIVE BETA-BLOCKERS.** It is prudent, if BETAPACE® (sotalol hydrochloride) is to be administered, to use the smallest effective dose, so that inhibition of bronchodilation produced by endogenous or exogenous catecholamine stimulation of beta$_2$ receptors may be minimized.

Anaphylaxis: While taking beta-blockers, patients with a history of anaphylactic reaction to a variety of allergens may have a more severe reaction on repeated challenge, either accidental, diagnostic or therapeutic. Such patients may be unresponsive to the usual doses of epinephrine used to treat the allergic reaction.

Anesthesia: The management of patients undergoing major surgery who are being treated with beta-blockers is controversial. Protracted severe hypotension and difficulty in restoring and maintaining normal cardiac rhythm after anesthesia have been reported in patients receiving beta-blockers.

Diabetes: In patients with diabetes (especially labile diabetes) or with a history of episodes of spontaneous hypoglycemia, BETAPACE® should be given with caution since beta-blockade may mask some important premonitory signs of acute hypoglycemia; e.g., tachycardia.

Sick Sinus Syndrome: BETAPACE® should be used only with extreme caution in patients with sick sinus syndrome associated with symptomatic arrhythmias, because it may cause sinus bradycardia, sinus pauses or sinus arrest.

Thyrotoxicosis: Beta-blockade may mask certain clinical signs (e.g., tachycardia) of hyperthyroidism. Patients suspected of developing thyrotoxicosis should be managed carefully to avoid abrupt withdrawal of beta-blockade which might be followed by an exacerbation of symptoms of hyperthyroidism, including thyroid storm.

PRECAUTIONS

RENAL IMPAIRMENT: BETAPACE® (sotalol hydrochloride) is mainly eliminated via the kidneys through glomerular filtration and to a small degree by tubular secretion. There is a direct relationship between renal function, as measured by serum creatinine or creatinine clearance, and the elimination rate of BETAPACE®. Guidance for dosing in conditions of renal impairment can be found under "DOSAGE AND ADMINISTRATION."

DRUG INTERACTIONS

Antiarrhythmics: Class Ia antiarrhythmic drugs, such as disopyramide, quinidine and procainamide and other Class III drugs (e.g., amiodarone) are not recommended as concomitant therapy with BETAPACE®, because of their potential to prolong refractoriness (see **WARNINGS**). There is only limited experience with the concomitant use of Class Ib or Ic antiarrhythmics. Additive Class II effects would also be anticipated with the use of other beta-blocking agents concomitantly with BETAPACE®.

Digoxin: Single and multiple doses of BETAPACE® do not substantially affect serum digoxin levels. Proarrhythmic events were more common in BETAPACE® treated patients also receiving digoxin; it is not clear whether this represents an interaction or is related to the presence of CHF, a known risk factor for proarrhythmia, in the patients receiving digoxin.

Calcium blocking drugs: BETAPACE® should be administered with caution in conjunction with calcium blocking drugs because of possible additive effects on atrioventricular conduction or ventricular function. Additionally, concomitant use of these drugs may have additive effects on blood pressure, possibly leading to hypotension.

Catecholamine-depleting agents: Concomitant use of catecholamine-depleting drugs, such as reserpine and guanethidine, with a beta-blocker may produce an excessive reduction of resting sympathetic nervous tone. Patients treated with BETAPACE® plus a catecholamine depletor should therefore be closely monitored for evidence of hypotension and or marked bradycardia which may produce syncope.

Insulin and oral antidiabetics: Hyperglycemia may occur, and the dosage of insulin or antidiabetic drugs may require adjustment. Symptoms of hypoglycemia may be masked.

Beta-2-receptor stimulants: Beta-agonists such as salbutamol, terbutaline and isoprenaline may have to be administered in increased dosages when used concomitantly with BETAPACE®.

Clonidine: Beta-blocking drugs may potentiate the rebound hypertension sometimes observed after discontinuation of clonidine; therefore, caution is advised when discontinuing clonidine in patients receiving BETAPACE®.

Incidence (%) of Adverse Events and Discontinuations DAILY DOSE

Body System	160mg (n=832)	240mg (n=263)	320mg (n=835)	480mg (n=459)	640mg (n=324)	Any Dose* (n=1292)	% Patients Discontinued (n=1292)
Body as a whole							
infection	1	2	2	2	3	4	<1
fever	1	2	3	2	2	4	<1
localized pain	1	1	2	2	2	3	<1
Cardiovascular							
dyspnea	5	8	11	15	15	21	2
bradycardia	8	8	9	7	5	16	2
chest pain	4	3	10	10	14	16	<1
palpitation	3	3	8	9	12	14	<1
edema	2	2	5	3	5	8	1
ECG abnormal	4	2	4	2	2	7	1
hypotension	4	4	3	2	3	6	2
proarrhythmia	<1	<1	2	4	5	5	3
syncope	1	1	3	2	5	5	1
heart failure	2	3	2	2	2	5	1
presyncope	2	2	2	4	3	4	<1
peripheral vascular disorder	1	2	1	1	2	3	<1
cardiovascular disorder	1	<1	2	2	2	3	<1
vasodilation	1	<1	1	2	1	3	<1
AICD Discharge	<1	2	2	2	2	3	<1
hypertension	<1	1	1	1	2	2	<1
Nervous							
fatigue	5	8	12	12	13	20	2
dizziness	7	6	11	11	14	20	1
asthenia	4	5	7	8	10	13	1
light-headed	4	3	6	6	9	12	<1
headache	3	2	4	4	4	8	<1
sleep problem	1	1	5	4	6	8	<1
perspiration	1	2	3	4	5	6	<1
altered consciousness	2	3	1	2	3	4	<1
depression	1	2	2	2	3	4	<1
paresthesia	1	1	2	3	2	4	<1
anxiety	2	2	2	2	2	4	<1
mood change	<1	<1	1	3	2	3	<1
appetite disorder	1	2	2	1	3	3	<1
stroke	<1	<1	1	1	<1	1	<1
Digestive							
nausea/vomiting	5	4	4	6	6	10	1
diarrhea	2	3	3	3	5	7	<1
dyspepsia	2	3	3	3	3	6	<1
abdominal pain	<1	<1	2	2	2	3	<1
colon problem	2	1	1	<1	2	3	<1
flatulence	1	<1	1	1	2	2	<1
Respiratory							
pulmonary problem	3	3	5	3	4	8	<1
upper respiratory tract problem	1	1	3	4	3	5	<1
asthma	1	<1	1	1	1	2	<1
Urogenital							
genitourinary disorder	1	0	1	1	2	3	<1
sexual dysfunction	<1	1	1	1	3	2	<1
Metabolic							
abnormal lab value	1	2	3	2	1	4	<1
weight change	1	1	1	<1	2	2	<1
Musculoskeletal							
extremity pain	2	2	4	5	3	7	<1
back pain	1	<1	2	2	2	3	<1
Skin and Appendages							
rash	2	3	2	3	4	5	<1
Hematologic							
bleeding	1	<1	1	<1	2	2	<1
Special Senses							
visual problem	1	1	2	4	5	5	<1

* Because patients are counted at each dose level tested, the Any Dose column cannot be determined by adding across the doses.

Other: No pharmacokinetic interactions were observed with hydrochlorothiazide or warfarin.

Drugs prolonging the QT interval: BETAPACE® should be administered with caution in conjunction with other drugs known to prolong the QT interval such as Class I antiarrhythmic agents, phenothiazines, tricyclic antidepressants, terfenadine and astemizole (see **WARNINGS**).

DRUG/Laboratory Test Interactions

The presence of sotalol in the urine may result in falsely elevated levels of urinary metanephrine when measured by fluorimetric or photometric methods. In screening patients suspected of having a pheochromocytoma and being treated with sotalol, a specific method, using a high performance liquid chromatographic assay with solid phase extraction (e.g., J. Chromatogr. 385:241, 1987) should be employed in determining levels of catecholamines.

Carcinogenesis, Mutagenesis, Impairment of Fertility: No evidence of carcinogenic potential was observed in rats during a 24-month study at 137–275 mg/kg/day (approximately 30 times the maximum recommended human oral dose (MRHD) as mg/kg or 5 times the MRHD as mg/m^2) or in mice, during a 24-month study at 4141–7122 mg/kg/day (approximately 450–750 times the MRHD as mg/kg or 36–63 times the MRHD as mg/m^2).

Sotalol has not been evaluated in any specific assay of mutagenicity or clastogenicity.

Continued on next page

Information on the Berlex products appearing here is based on the most current information available at the time of publication closing. Further information for these and other products may be obtained from the Medical Affairs Department, Berlex Laboratories, 300 Fairfield Road, Wayne, New Jersey 07470, 1-888-BERLEX-4. Information on Betaseron and Fludara may be obtained from Berlex Laboratories, 15049 San Pablo Avenue, Richmond, California 94804-0016, 1-800-888-4112.

Betapace—Cont.

No significant reduction in fertility occurred in rats at oral doses of 1000 mg/kg/day (approximately 100 times the MRHD as mg/kg or 9 times the MRHD as mg/m^2) prior to mating, except for a small reduction in the number of offspring per litter.

Pregnancy Category B: Reproduction studies in rats and rabbits during organogenesis at 100 and 22 times the MRHD as mg/kg (9 and 7 times the MRHD as mg/m^2), respectively, did not reveal any teratogenic potential associated with sotalol HCl. In rabbits, a high dose of sotalol HCl (160 mg/kg/day) at 16 times the MRHD as mg/kg (6 times the MRHD as mg/m^2) produced a slight increase in fetal death likely due to maternal toxicity. Eight times the maximum dose (80 mg/kg/day or 3 times the MRHD as mg/m^2) did not result in an increased incidence of fetal deaths. In rats, 1000 mg/kg/day sotalol HCl, 100 times the MRHD (18 times the MRHD as mg/m^2), increased the number of early resorptions, while at 14 times the maximum dose (2.5 times the MRHD as mg/m^2), no increase in early resorptions was noted. However, animal reproduction studies are not always predictive of human response.

Although there are no adequate and well-controlled studies in pregnant women, sotalol HCl has been shown to cross the placenta, and is found in amniotic fluid. There has been a report of subnormal birth weight with BETAPACE®. Therefore, BETAPACE® should be used during pregnancy only if the potential benefit outweighs the potential risk.

Nursing Mothers: Sotalol is excreted in the milk of laboratory animals and has been reported to be present in human milk. Because of the potential for adverse reactions in nursing infants from BETAPACE®, a decision should be made whether to discontinue nursing or to discontinue the drug, taking into account the importance of the drug to the mother.

Pediatric Use: The safety and effectiveness of BETAPACE® in children have not been established.

ADVERSE REACTIONS

During premarketing trials, 3186 patients with cardiac arrhythmias (1363 with sustained ventricular tachycardia) received oral BETAPACE®, of whom 2451 received the drug for at least two weeks. The most important adverse effects are torsade de pointes and other serious new ventricular arrhythmias (see **WARNINGS**), occurring at rates of almost 4% and 1%, respectively, in the VT/VF population. Overall, discontinuation because of unacceptable side-effects was necessary in 17% of all patients in clinical trials, and in 13% of patients treated for at least two-weeks. The most common adverse reactions leading to discontinuation of BETAPACE® are as follows: fatigue 4%, bradycardia (less than 50 bpm) 3%, dyspnea 3%, proarrhythmia 3%, asthenia 2%, and dizziness 2%.

Occasional reports of elevated serum liver enzymes have occurred with BETAPACE® therapy but no cause and effect relationship has been established. One case of peripheral neuropathy which resolved on discontinuation of BETAPACE® and recurred when the patient was rechallenged with the drug was reported in an early dose tolerance study. Elevated blood glucose levels and increased insulin requirements can occur in diabetic patients.

The following table lists as a function of dosage the most common (incidence of 2% or greater) adverse events, regardless of relationship to therapy and the percent of patients discontinued due to the event, as collected from clinical trials involving 1292 patients with sustained VT/VF.

[See table at top of previous page]

Potential Adverse Effects: Foreign marketing experience with sotalol hydrochloride shows an adverse experience profile similar to that described above from clinical trials. Voluntary reports since introduction include rare reports (less than one report per 10,000 patients) of: emotional lability, slightly clouded sensorium, incoordination, vertigo, paralysis, thrombocytopenia, eosinophilia, leukopenia, photosensitivity reaction, fever, pulmonary edema, hyperlipidemia, myalgia, pruritis, alopecia.

The oculomucocutaneous syndrome associated with the beta-blocker practolol has not been associated with BETAPACE® during investigational use and foreign marketing experience.

OVERDOSAGE

Intentional or accidental overdosage with BETAPACE® (sotalol hydrochloride) has rarely resulted in death.

Symptoms and Treatment of Overdosage: The most common signs to be expected are bradycardia, congestive heart failure, hypotension, bronchospasm and hypoglycemia. In cases of massive intentional overdosage (2–16 grams) of BETAPACE® the following clinical findings were seen: hypotension, bradycardia, cardiac asystole, prolongation of QT interval, torsade de pointes, ventricular tachycardia, and premature ventricular complexes. If overdosage occurs, therapy with BETAPACE® should be discontinued and the patient observed closely. Because of the lack of protein binding, hemodialysis is useful for reducing sotalol plasma concentrations. Patients should be carefully observed until QT intervals are normalized and the heart rate returns to levels >50 bpm. In addition, if required, the following therapeutic measures are suggested:

Bradycardia or cardiac asystole: Atropine, another anticholinergic drug, a beta-adrenergic agonist or transvenous cardiac pacing.

Heart Block: (second and third degree) transvenous cardiac pacemaker.

Hypotension: (depending on associated factors) epinephrine rather than isoproterenol or norepinephrine may be useful.

Bronchospasm: Aminophylline or aerosol beta-2-receptor stimulant.

Torsade de pointes: DC cardioversion, transvenous cardiac pacing, epinephrine, magnesium sulfate.

DOSAGE AND ADMINISTRATION

As with other antiarrhythmic agents, BETAPACE® should be initiated and doses increased in a hospital with facilities for cardiac rhythm monitoring and assessment (see **INDICATIONS AND USAGE**). BETAPACE® should be administered only after appropriate clinical assessment (see **INDICATIONS AND USAGE**), and the dosage of BETAPACE® must be individualized for each patient on the basis of therapeutic response and tolerance. Proarrhythmic events can occur not only at initiation of therapy, but also with each upward dosage adjustment.

Dosage of BETAPACE® should be adjusted gradually, allowing 2–3 days between dosing increments in order to attain steady-state plasma concentrations, and to allow monitoring of QT intervals. Graded dose adjustment will help prevent the usage of doses which are higher than necessary to control the arrhythmia. The recommended initial dose is 80 mg twice daily. This dose may be increased, if necessary, after appropriate evaluation to 240 or 320 mg/day (120–160 mg twice daily). In most patients, a therapeutic response is obtained at a total daily dose of 160 to 320 mg/day, given in two or three divided doses. Some patients with life-threatening refractory ventricular arrhythmias may require doses as high as 480–640 mg/day; however, these doses should only be prescribed when the potential benefit outweighs the increased risk of adverse events, in particular proarrhythmia. Because of the long terminal elimination half-life of BETAPACE®, dosing on more than a BID regimen is usually not necessary.

DOSAGE IN RENAL IMPAIRMENT

Because sotalol is excreted predominantly in urine and its terminal elimination half-life is prolonged in conditions of renal impairment, the dosing interval (time between divided doses) of sotalol should be modified (when creatinine clearance is lower than 60 mL/min) according to the following table.

Creatinine Clearance mL/min	Dosing* Interval (hours)
>60	12
30–59	24
10–29	36–48
<10	Dose should be individualized

*The initial dose of 80 mg and subsequent doses should be administered at these intervals. See following paragraph for dosage escalations.

Since the terminal elimination half-life of BETAPACE® (sotalol hydrochloride) is increased in patients with renal impairment, a longer duration of dosing is required to reach steady-state. Dose escalations in renal impairment should be done after administration of at least 5–6 doses at appropriate intervals (see table above).

Extreme caution should be exercised in the use of sotalol in patients with renal failure undergoing hemodialysis. The half-life of sotalol is prolonged (up to 69 hours) in anuric patients. Sotalol, however, can be partly removed by dialysis with subsequent partial rebound in concentrations when dialysis is completed. Both safety (heart rate, QT interval) and efficacy (arrhythmia control) must be closely monitored.

Transfer to BETAPACE®

Before starting BETAPACE®, previous antiarrhythmic therapy should generally be withdrawn under careful monitoring for a minimum of 2–3 plasma half-lives if the patient's clinical condition permits (see **DRUG INTERACTIONS**). Treatment has been initiated in some patients receiving I.V. lidocaine without ill effect. After discontinuation of amiodarone, BETAPACE® should not be initiated until the QT interval is normalized (see **WARNINGS**).

HOW SUPPLIED

BETAPACE® (sotalol hydrochloride); capsule-shaped light-blue scored tablets imprinted with the strength and "BETAPACE", are available as follows:

NDC 50419–105–10 80 mg strength, bottle of 100
NDC 50419–105–11 80 mg strength, carton of 100 unit dose
NDC 50419–109–10 120 mg strength, bottle of 100
NDC 50419–109–11 120 mg strength, carton of 100 unit dose
NDC 50419–106–10 160 mg strength, bottle of 100
NDC 50419–106–11 160 mg strength, carton of 100 unit dose
NDC 50419–107–10 240 mg strength, bottle of 100
NDC 50419–107–11 240 mg strength, carton of 100 unit dose

Store at controlled room temperature, between 15° to 30°C (59° to 86°F).

Rx only

©1996, Berlex Laboratories. All rights reserved.

Manufactured by:

BERLEX Laboratories, Wayne, NJ 07470

6063801   Rev. 4/96

Shown in Product Identification Guide, page 306

CLIMARA® ℞
[clī-mär '-a]
(ESTRADIOL TRANSDERMAL SYSTEM)

PRESCRIBING INFORMATION

1. ESTROGENS HAVE BEEN REPORTED TO INCREASE THE RISK OF ENDOMETRIAL CARCINOMA IN POSTMENOPAUSAL WOMEN.
Close clinical surveillance of all women taking estrogens is important. Adequate diagnostic measures, including endometrial sampling when indicated, should be undertaken to rule out malignancy in all cases of undiagnosed persistent or recurring abnormal vaginal bleeding. There is currently no evidence that "natural" estrogens are more or less hazardous than "synthetic" estrogens at equiestrogenic doses.
2. ESTROGENS SHOULD NOT BE USED DURING PREGNANCY.
Estrogen therapy during pregnancy is associated with an increased risk of congenital defects in the reproductive organs of the fetus, and possibly upon other birth defects. Studies of women who received diethylstilbestrol (DES) during pregnancy have shown that female offspring have an increased risk of vaginal adenosis, squamous cell dysplasia of the uterine cervix, and clear cell vaginal cancer later in life; male offspring have an increased risk of urogenital abnormalities and possibly testicular cancer later in life. The 1985 DES Task Force concluded that use of DES during pregnancy is associated with a subsequent increased risk of breast cancer in the mothers, although a causal relationship remains unproven and the observed level of excess risk is similar to that for a number of other breast cancer risk factors.
There is no indication for estrogen therapy during pregnancy or during the immediate postpartum period. Estrogens are ineffective for the prevention or treatment of threatened or habitual abortion. Estrogens are not indicated for the prevention of postpartum breast engorgement.

DESCRIPTION

Climara®, estradiol transdermal system, is designed to release 17β-estradiol continuously upon application to intact skin. Three (12.5, 18.75 and 25.0 cm^2) systems are available to provide nominal *in vivo* delivery of 0.05, 0.075 or 0.1 mg respectively of estradiol per day. The period of use is 7 days. Each system has a contact surface area of either 12.5, 18.75 or 25.0 cm^2, and contains 3.9, 5.85 or 7.8 mg of estradiol USP respectively. The composition of the systems per unit area is identical.

Estradiol USP (17β-estradiol) is a white, crystalline powder, chemically described as estra-1,3,5(10)-triene-3,17β-diol. It has an empirical formula of $C_{18}H_{24}O_2$ and molecular weight of 272.37. The structural formula is:

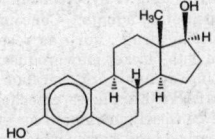

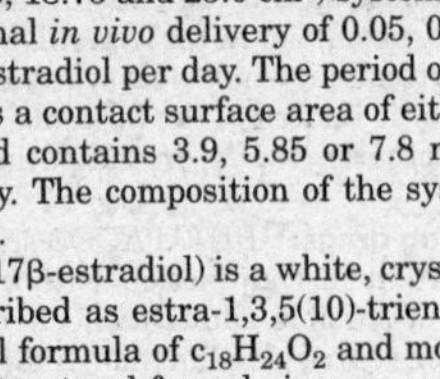

The Climara® system comprises two layers. Proceeding from the visible surface toward the surface attached to the skin, these layers are (1) a translucent polyethylene film, and (2) an acrylate adhesive matrix containing estradiol USP. A protective liner (3) of siliconized or fluoropolymer-coated polyester film is attached to the adhesive surface and must be removed before the system can be used.

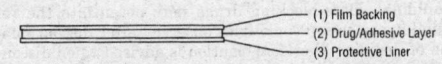

(1) Film Backing
(2) Drug/Adhesive Layer
(3) Protective Liner

The active component of the system is 17β-estradiol. The remaining components of the system (acrylate copolymer adhesive, fatty acid esters, and polyethylene backing) are pharmacologically inactive.

CLINICAL PHARMACOLOGY

The Climara® system provides systemic estrogen replacement therapy by releasing 17β-estradiol, the major estrogenic hormone secreted by the human ovary.

Estrogens are important in the development and maintenance of the female reproductive system and secondary sex characteristics. By a direct action, they cause growth and development of the uterus, fallopian tubes, and vagina. With other hormones, such as pituitary hormones and progesterone, they cause enlargement of the breasts through promotion of ductal growth, stromal development, and the accretion of fat. Estrogens are intricately involved with other hormones, especially progesterone, in the processes of the ovulatory menstrual cycle and pregnancy, and affect the release of pituitary gonadotropins. They also contribute to the shaping of the skeleton, maintenance of tone and elasticity of urogenital structures, changes in the epiphyses of the long bones that allow for the pubertal growth spurt and its termination, and pigmentation of the nipples and genitals.

Estrogens occur naturally in several forms. The primary source of estrogen in normally cycling adult women is the ovarian follicle, which secretes 70 to 500 micrograms of estradiol daily, depending on the phase of the menstrual cycle. This is converted primarily to estrone, which circulates in roughly equal proportion to estradiol, and to small amounts of estriol. After menopause, most endogenous estrogen is produced by conversion of androstenedione, secreted by the adrenal cortex, to estrone by peripheral tissues. Thus, estrone—especially in its sulfate ester form—is the most abundant circulating estrogen in postmenopausal women. Although circulating estrogens exist in a dynamic equilibrium of metabolic interconversions, estradiol is the principal intracellular human estrogen and is substantially more potent than estrone or estriol at the receptor.

Estrogen drug products act by regulating the transcription of a limited number of genes. Estrogens diffuse through cell membranes, distribute themselves throughout the cell, and bind to and activate the nuclear estrogen receptor, a DNA-binding protein which is found in estrogen-responsive tissues. The activated estrogen receptor binds to specific DNA sequences, or hormone-response elements, which enhance the transcription of adjacent genes and in turn lead to the observed effects. Estrogen receptors have been identified in tissues of the reproductive tract, breast, pituitary, hypothalamus, liver, and bone of women.

Estrogens used in therapy are well absorbed through the skin, mucous membranes, and gastrointestinal tract. Administered estrogens and their esters are handled within the body essentially the same as the endogenous hormones. Metabolic conversion of estrogens occurs primarily in the liver (first pass effect), but also at local target tissue sites. Complex metabolic processes result in a dynamic equilibrium of circulating conjugated and unconjugated estrogenic forms, which are continually interconverted, especially between estrone and estradiol and between esterified and unesterified forms. Although naturally-occurring estrogens circulate in the blood largely bound to sex hormone-binding globulin and albumin, only unbound estrogens enter target tissue cells. A significant proportion of the circulating estrogen exists as sulfate conjugates, especially estrone sulfate, which serves as a circulating reservior for the formation of more active estrogenic species. A certain proportion of the estrogen is excreted into the bile and then reabsorbed from the intestine. During this enterohepatic recirculation, estrogens are desulfated and resulfated and undergo degradation through conversion to less active estrogens (estriol and other estrogens), oxidation to nonestrogenic substances (catecholestrogens, which interact with catecholamine metabolism, especially in the central nervous system), and conjugation with glucuronic acids (which are then rapidly excreted in the urine).

When given orally, naturally-occurring estrogens and their esters are extensively metabolized (first pass effect) and circulate primarily as estrone sulfate, with smaller amounts of other conjugated and unconjugated estrogenic species. This results in limited oral potency. In contrast, the skin metabolizes estradiol only to a small extent. Therefore, transdermal administration produces therapeutic serum levels of estradiol with lower circulating levels of estrone and estrone conjugates, and requires smaller total doses than does oral therapy. Because estradiol has a short half-life, transdermal administration of estradiol allows a rapid decline in blood levels after the Climara® system is removed.

PHARMACOKINETICS

Transdermal administration of Climara® produces mean serum concentrations of estradiol comparable to those produced by premenopausal women in the early follicular phase of the ovulatory cycle. The pharmacokinetics of estradiol following application of the Climara® system were investigated in 173 healthy postmenopausal women in five studies. In four of the studies the Climara® system was applied to the abdomen and in a fifth study application to the buttocks and abdomen were compared.

Absorption: The Climara® transdermal delivery system continuously releases estradiol which is transported across intact skin leading to sustained circulating levels of estradiol during 7 day treatment period. The systemic availability of estradiol after transdermal administration is about 20 times higher than that after oral administration. This difference is due to the absence of first pass metabolism when estradiol is given by the transdermal route.

The bioavailability of Climara® was determined in two single dose studies after 1 week application of the Climara® system versus two consecutive 3 day and 4 day applications of the Estraderm® system. Mean estradiol serum concentrations observed during the treatment of the 25.0 and 12.5 cm^2 Climara® systems versus the 20 and 10 cm^2 Estraderm® systems are shown in Figures 1 and 2, respectively. Both sizes of Climara® maintained significantly lower peak and mean steady state estradiol levels than did the Estraderm® system; however, towards the end of each treatment period, the Climara® system maintained similar (day 6) or higher (day 7) serum estradiol levels than did the Estraderm® system. The fluctuation index was 3 to 4 times lower with the Climara® system.

Figure 1
Observed Mean (±S.E.)Estradiol Serum Concentrations for a One-Week Application of the Climara® System (25 cm²) and Consecutive Three-Day and Four-Day Application of the Estraderm® System (20 cm²) in 24 postmenopausal women.

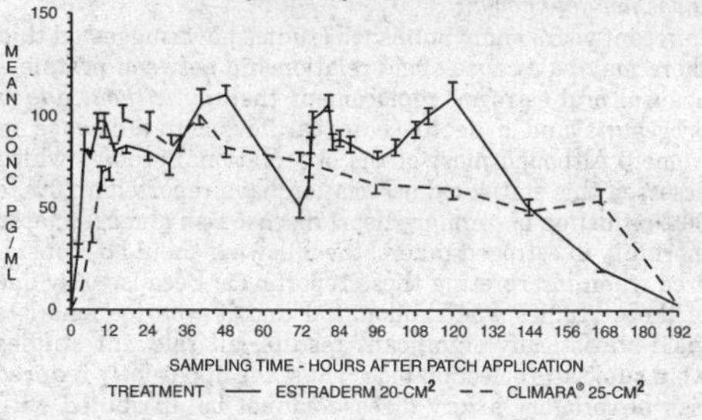

Figure 2
Observed Mean (±S.E.)Estradiol Serum Concentrations for a One-Week Application of the Climara® System (12.5 cm²) and Consecutive Three-Day and Four-Day Application of the Estraderm® System (10 cm²) in 26 postmenopausal women.

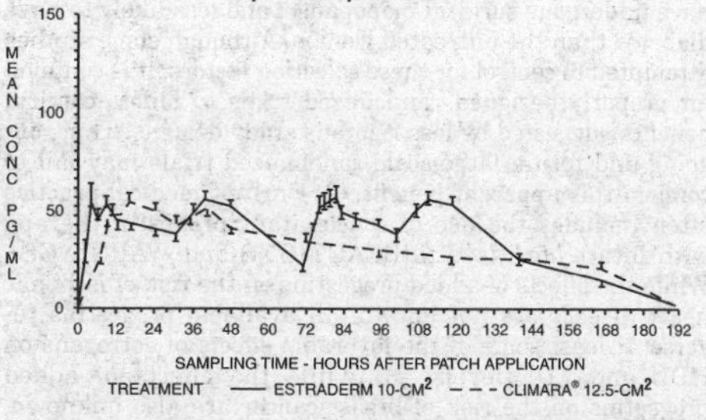

Dose proportionality was demonstrated for the Climara® system in a 1 week study conducted in 54 postmenopausal women. The mean steady state levels (Cavg) of the estradiol during the application of Climara 25 cm^2 and 12.5 cm^2 on the abdomen were about 80 and 40 pg/mL, respectively.

In a 3 week multiple application study in 24 postmenopausal women, the 25.0 cm^2 Climara® system produced average peak estradiol concentrations (Cmax) of approximately 100 pg/mL. Trough values at the end of each wear interval (Cmin) were approximately 35 pg/mL. Nearly identical serum curves were seen each week, indicating little or no accumulation of estradiol in the body. Serum estrone peak and trough levels were 60 and 40 pg/mL, respectively.

In a single dose randomized crossover study conducted to compare the effect of site of application, 38 postmenopausal women wore a single Climara® 25 cm^2 system for 1 week on the abdomen and buttocks. The estradiol serum concentration profiles are shown in Figure 3. Cmax and Cavg values were, respectively, 25% and 17% higher with the buttock application than with the abdomen application. Despite these pharmacokinetics differences, it is expected that Climara® applied to either of the two sites will have similar clinical effects.

Table 1
Pharmacokinetic Summary (Mean Estradiol Values)

Climara® Delivery Rate	Surface Area (cm^2)	Application Site	No. of Subjects	Dosing	Cmax (pg/mL)	Cmin (pg/mL)	Cavg (pg/mL)
0.05	12.5	Abdomen	78	Single	75	28	41
0.1	25	Abdomen	139	Single	147	60	87
0.1	25	Buttock	38	Single	174	71	106

Figure 3
Observed Mean (±S.E.)Estradiol Serum Concentrations for a One-Week Application of the Climara® System (25 cm²) to the abdomen and buttocks of 38 postmenopausal women.

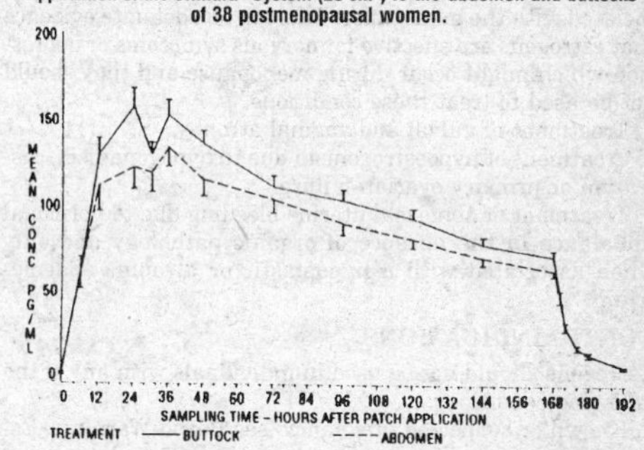

Table 1 provides a summary of estradiol pharmacokinetic parameters determined during evaluation of Climara.® [See table 1 above]

The relative standard deviation of each pharmacokinetic parameter after application to the abdomen averaged 50%, which is indicative of the considerable intersubject variability associated with transdermal drug delivery. The relative standard deviation of each pharmacokinetic parameter after application to the buttock was lower than that after application to the abdomen (e.g., for Cmax 39% vs 62%, and for Cavg 35% vs 48%).

Distribution: Estradiol circulates in blood bound to sex hormone binding globulin (SHBG) and albumin. Following transdermal administration of estradiol about 98% of estradiol and about 97% of estrone are reported to be bound to plasma proteins in postmenopausal women. The protein binding of estradiol and estrone as well as the concentration of SHBG were unchanged following three months of transdermal treatment. In postmenopausal women with end stage renal disease, the plasma protein binding of estradiol is reported to be decreased.

Metabolism: Circulating estrogens exist in a dynamic equilibrium of metabolic interconversions. These transformations take place mainly in the liver. Estradiol is converted reversibly to estrone, and both can be converted to estriol. Estrogens also undergo enterohepatic recirculation via sulfate and glucuronide conjugation in the liver, biliary excretion of conjugates into the intestine, and hydrolysis in the gut followed by reabsorption. In postmenopausal women a significant portion of the circulating estrogens exist as sulfate conjugates, especially estrone sulfate, which serves as a circulating reservoir for the formation of more active estrogens. The hepatic first pass effect is avoided with transdermal estrogens, but the clinical significance of this has not been fully established.

Excretion: Estradiol, estrone, and estriol are excreted in the urine mainly as glucuronide and sulfate conjugates and less than 1% as unconjugated steroids. After removal of the Climara® system, serum estradiol levels decline in about 12 hours to preapplication levels with an apparent half life of approximately 4 hours.

Continued on next page

Information on the Berlex products appearing here is based on the most current information available at the time of publication closing. Further information for these and other products may be obtained from the Medical Affairs Department, Berlex Laboratories, 300 Fairfield Road, Wayne, New Jersey 07470, 1-888-BERLEX-4. Information on Betaseron and Fludara may be obtained from Berlex Laboratories, 15049 San Pablo Avenue, Richmond, California 94804-0016, 1-800-888-4112.

Climara—Cont.

Special populations:

Race: There is no information to establish the relevance of race for the absorption and pharmacokinetics of estradiol following transdermal application.

Patients with Renal Impairment: Total estradiol serum levels are higher in postmenopausal women with end stage renal disease (ESRD) receiving maintenance hemodialysis than in normal subjects at baseline and following oral doses of estradiol. Therefore, conventional transdermal estradiol doses used in individuals with normal renal function may be excessive for postmenopausal women with ESRD receiving maintenance hemodialysis.

Patients with Hepatic Impairment: Estrogens may be poorly metabolized in patients with impaired liver function and should be administered with caution.

INDICATIONS AND USAGE

Climara® is indicated in the:

1. Treatment of moderate to severe vasomotor syptoms associated with the menopause. There is no adequate evidence that estrogens are effective for nervous symptoms or depression which might occur during menopause and they should not be used to treat these conditions.
2. Treatment of vulval and vaginal atrophy.
3. Treatment of hypoestrogenism due to hypogonadism, castration or primary ovarian failure.
4. Treatment of abnormal uterine bleeding due to hormonal imbalance in the absence of organic pathology and only when associated with a hypoplastic or atrophic endometrium.

CONTRAINDICATIONS

Estrogens should not be used in individuals with any of the following conditions:

1. Known or suspected pregnancy (see Boxed Warning). Estrogens may cause fetal harm when administered to a pregnant woman.
2. Undiagnosed abnormal genital bleeding.
3. Known or suspected cancer of the breast except in appropriately selected patients being treated for metastatic disease.
4. Known or suspected estrogen-dependent neoplasia.
5. Active thrombophlebitis or thromboembolic disorders.

WARNINGS

1. **Induction of malignant neoplasms.**

Endometrial cancer. The reported endometrial cancer risk among unopposed estrogen users is about 2 to 12 fold greater than in non-users, and appears dependent on duration of treatment and on estrogen dose. Most studies show no significant increased risk associated with use of estrogens for less than one year. The greatest risk appears associated with prolonged use—with increased risks of 15- to 24-fold for five to ten years or more. In three studies, persistence of risk was demonstrated for 8 to over 15 years after cessation of estrogen treatment. In one study a significant decrease in the incidence of endometrial cancer occurred six months after estrogen withdrawal. Concurrent progestin therapy may offset this risk but the overall health impact in postmenopausal women is not known (see Precautions).

Breast cancer. While the majority of studies have not shown an increased risk of breast cancer in women who have ever used estrogen replacement therapy, some have reported a moderately increased risk (relative risks of 1.3–2.0) in those taking higher doses or those taking lower doses for prolonged periods of time, especially in excess of 10 years. Other studies have not shown this relationship.

Congenital lesions with malignant potential. Estrogen therapy during pregnancy is associated with an increased risk of fetal congenital reproductive tract disorders, and possibly other birth defects. Studies of women who received DES during pregnancy have shown that female offspring have an increased risk of vaginal adenosis, squamous cell dysplasia of the uterine cervix, and clear cell vaginal cancer later in life; male offspring have an increased risk of urogenital abnormalities and possibly testicular cancer later in life. Although some of these changes are benign, others are precursors of malignancy.

2. **Gallbladder disease.** Two studies have reported a 2- to 4-fold increase in the risk of gallbladder disease requiring surgery in women receiving postmenopausal estrogens.

3. **Cardiovascular disease.** Large doses of estrogen (5 mg conjugated estrogens per day), comparable to those used to treat cancer of the prostate and breast, have been shown in a large prospective clinical trial in men to increase the risks of nonfatal myocardial infarction, pulmonary embolism, and thrombophlebitis. These risks cannot necessarily be extrapolated from men to women. However, to avoid the theoretical cardiovascular risk to women caused by high estrogen doses, the dose for estrogen replacement therapy should not exceed the lowest effective dose.

4. **Elevated blood pressure.** Occasional blood pressure increases during estrogen replacement therapy have been attributed to idiosyncratic reactions to estrogens. More often, blood pressure has remained the same or has dropped. One study showed that postmenopausal estrogen users have higher blood pressure than nonusers. Two other studies showed slightly lower blood pressure among estrogen users compared to nonusers. Postmenopausal estrogen use does not increase the risk of stroke. Nonetheless, blood pressure should be monitored at regular intervals with estrogen use. Ethinyl estradiol and conjugated estrogens have been shown to increase renin substrate. In contrast to these oral estrogens, transdermally administered estradiol has been reported not to affect renin substrate.

5. **Hypercalcemia.** Administration of estrogens may lead to severe hypercalcemia in patients with breast cancer and bone metastases. If this occurs, the drug should be stopped and appropriate measures taken to reduce the serum calcium level.

PRECAUTIONS

A. General

1. **Addition of a progestin.** Studies of the addition of a progestin for 10 or more days of a cycle of estrogen administration have reported a lowered incidence of endometrial hyperplasia than would be induced by estrogen treatment alone. Morphological and biochemical studies of endometria suggest that 10 to 14 days of progestin are needed to provide maximal maturation of the endometrium and to reduce the likelihood of hyperplastic changes.

There are, however, possible risks which may be associated with the use of progestins in estrogen replacement regimens. These include: (1) adverse effects on lipoprotein metabolism (lowering HDL and raising LDL) which could diminish the purported cardioprotective effect of estrogen therapy (see Precautions D.4., below); (2) impairment of glucose tolerance; and (3) possible enhancement of mitotic activity in breast epithelial tissue, although few epidemiological data are available to address this point (see Precautions below).

The choice of progestin, its dose, and its regimen may be important in minimizing these adverse effects, but these issues will require further study before they are clarified.

2. *Cardiovascular risk. A causal relationship between estrogen replacement therapy and reduction of cardiovascular disease in postmenopausal women has not been proven. Furthermore, the effect of added progestins on this putative benefit is not yet known.*

In recent years many published studies have suggested that there may be a cause-effect relationship between postmenopausal oral estrogen replacement therapy *without added progestins* and a decrease in cardiovascular disease in women. Although most of the observational studies which assessed this statistical association have reported a 20% to 50% reduction in coronary heart disease risk and associated mortality in estrogen takers, the following should be considered when interpreting these reports: (1) Because only one of these studies was randomized and it was too small to yield statistically significant results, all relevant studies were subject to selection bias. Thus, the apparently reduced risk of coronary artery disease cannot be attributed with certainty to estrogen replacement therapy. It may instead have been caused by life-style and medical characteristics of the women studied with the result that healthier women were selected for estrogen therapy. In general, treated women were of a higher socioeconomic and educational status, more slender, more physically active, more likely to have undergone surgical menopause, and less likely to have diabetes than the untreated women. Although some studies attempted to control for these selection factors, it is common for properly designed randomized trials to fail to confirm benefits suggested by less rigorous study designs. Thus, ongoing and future large-scale randomized trials may fail to confirm this apparent benefit. (2) Current medical practice often includes the use of concomitant progestin therapy with intact uteri (see PRECAUTIONS and WARNINGS). While the effects of added progestins on the risk of ischemic heart disease are not known, all available progestins reverse at least some of the favorable effects of estrogens on HDL and LDL levels. (3) While the effects of added progestins on the risk of breast cancer are also unknown, available epidemiological evidence suggests that progestins do not reduce, and may enhance, the moderately increased breast cancer incidence that has been reported with prolonged estrogen replacement therapy (see WARNINGS above).

Because relatively long-term use of estrogens by a woman with a uterus has been shown to induce endometrial cancer, physicians often recommend that women who are deemed candidates for hormone replacement should take progestins as well as estrogens. When considering prescribing concomitant estrogens and progestins for hormone replacement therapy, physicians and patients are advised to carefully weigh the potential benefits and risks of the added progestin. Large-scale randomized, placebo-controlled, prospective clinical trials are required to clarify these issues.

3. **Physical examination.** A complete medical and family history should be taken prior to the initiation of any estrogen therapy. The pretreatment and periodic physical examinations should include special reference to blood pressure, breasts, abdomen, and pelvic organs, and should include a Papanicolaou smear. As a general rule, estrogen should not be prescribed for longer than one year without reexamining the patient.

4. **Hypercoagulability.** Some studies have shown that women taking estrogen replacement therapy have hypercoagulability, primarily related to decreased antithrombin activity. This effect appears dose- and duration-dependent and is less pronounced than that associated with oral contraceptive use.

Also, postmenopausal women tend to have increased coagulation parameters at baseline compared to premenopausal women. There is some suggestion that low dose postmenopausal mestranol may increase the risk of thromboembolism, although the majority of studies (of primarily conjugated estrogens users) report no such increase. There is insufficient information on hypercoagulability in women who have had previous thromboembolic disease.

5. **Familial hyperlipoproteinemia.** Estrogen therapy may be associated with massive elevations of plasma triglycerides leading to pancreatitis and other complications in patients with familial defects of lipoprotein metabolism.

6. **Fluid retention.** Because estrogens may cause some degree of fluid retention, conditions which might be exacerbated by this factor, such as asthma, epilepsy, migraine, and cardiac or renal dysfunction, require careful observation.

7. **Uterine bleeding and mastodynia.** Certain patients may develop undesirable manifestations of estrogenic stimulation, such as abnormal uterine bleeding and mastodynia.

8. **Impaired liver function.** Estrogens may be poorly metabolized in patients with impaired liver function and should be administered with caution.

B. Information for the Patient. See text of Patient Package Insert after the How Supplied section.

C. Laboratory Tests. Estrogen administration should generally be guided by clinical response at the smallest dose, rather than laboratory monitoring, for relief of symptoms for those indications in which symptoms are observable.

D. Drug/Laboratory Test Interactions.

1. Accelerated prothrombin time, partial thromboplastin time, and platelet aggregation time; increased platelet count; increased factors II, VII antigen, VIII antigen, VIII coagulant activity, IX, X, XII, VII-X complex, II-VII-X complex, and betathromboglobulin; decreased levels of antifactor Xa and antithrombin III, decreased antithrombin III activity; increased levels of fibrinogen and fibrinogen activity; increased plasminogen antigen and activity.
2. Increased thyroid-binding globulin (TBG) leading to increased circulating total thyroid hormone, as measured by protein-bound iodine (PBI), T4 levels (by column or by radioimmunoassay) or T3 levels by radioimmunoassay. T3 resin uptake is decreased, reflecting the elevated TBG. Free T4 and free T3 concentrations are unaltered.
3. Other binding proteins may be elevated in serum, i.e., corticosteroid binding globulin (CBG), sex hormone-binding globulin (SHBG), leading to increased circulating corticosteroids and sex steroids respectively. Free or biologically active hormone concentrations are unchanged. Other plasma proteins may be increased (angiotensinogen/renin substrate, alpha-1-antitrypsin, ceruloplasmin).
4. Increased plasma HDL and HDL-2 subfraction concentrations, reduced LDL cholesterol concentration, increased triglycerides levels.
5. Impaired glucose tolerance.
6. Reduced response to metyrapone test.
7. Reduced serum folate concentration.

E. Carcinogenesis, Mutagenesis, and Impairment of Fertility. See CONTRAINDICATIONS and WARNINGS. Long term continuous administration of natural and synthetic estrogens in certain animal species increases the frequency of carcinomas of the breast, uterus, cervix, vagina, testis, and liver.

F. Pregnancy Category X. See CONTRAINDICATIONS and Boxed Warning. Estrogens should not be used during pregnancy.

G. Nursing Mothers. As a general principle, the administration of any drug to nursing mothers should be done only when clearly necessary since many drugs are excreted in human milk. In addition, estrogen administration to nursing mothers has been shown to decrease the quantity and quality of the milk.

ADVERSE REACTIONS

See WARNINGS and Boxed Warning regarding induction of neoplasia, adverse effects on the fetus, increased incidence of gallbladder disease, cardiovascular disease, elevated blood pressure, and hypercalcemia.

The most commonly reported adverse reaction to the Climara® system in clinical trials was skin irritation at the application site. In two well-controlled clinical studies, the overall rate of discontinuation due to skin irritation at the application site was 6.8%; 7.9% for the 12.5 cm² system and 5.3% for the 25.0 cm² system compared with 11.5% for the placebo system. In a 3-week comparative skin irritation study with the Estraderm® system, in 95 subjects, no statistically significant differences in irritation were observed.

Some degree of irritation at the end of week three was seen in 25% of Estraderm® and 31% of Climara® subjects. Clinically significant irritation (mild erythema associated with symptoms or moderate to severe erythema) was evident at the end of week three in 11% of Estraderm® and 9% of Climara® subjects.

The following additional adverse reactions have been reported with estrogen therapy:

1. **Genitourinary system.**
Changes in vaginal bleeding pattern and abnormal withdrawal bleeding or flow, breakthrough bleeding, spotting. Increase in size of uterine leiomyomata. Vaginal candidiasis. Change in amount of cervical secretion.

2. **Breasts.**
Tenderness, enlargement.

3. **Gastrointestinal.**
Nausea, vomiting. Abdominal cramps, bloating. Cholestatic jaundice. Increased incidence of gallbladder disease.

4. **Skin.**
Chloasma or melasma that may persist when drug is discontinued. Erythema multiforme. Erythema nodosum. Hemorrhagic eruption. Loss of scalp hair. Hirsutism.

5. **Eyes.**
Steepening of corneal curvature. Intolerance to contact lenses.

6. **Central nervous system.**
Headache, migraine, dizziness. Mental depression. Chorea.

7. **Miscellaneous.**
Increase or decrease in weight. Reduced carbohydrate tolerance. Aggravation of porphyria. Edema. Changes in libido.

OVERDOSAGE

Serious ill effects have not been reported following acute ingestion of large doses of estrogen-containing oral contraceptives by young children. Overdosage of estrogen may cause nausea and vomiting, and withdrawal bleeding may occur in females.

DOSAGE AND ADMINISTRATION

The adhesive side of the Climara® system should be placed on a clean, dry area of the lower abdomen or the upper quadrant of the buttock. *The Climara® system should not be applied to the breasts.* The sites of application must be rotated, with an interval of at least 1 week allowed between applications to a particular site. The area selected should not be oily, damaged, or irritated. The waistline should be avoided, since tight clothing may rub and remove the system. Applications to areas where sitting would dislodge the system should also be avoided.The system should be applied immediately after opening the pouch and removing the protective liner. The system should be pressed firmly in place with the fingers for about 10 seconds, making sure there is good contact, especially around the edges. If the system lifts, apply pressure to maintain adhesion. In the unlikely event that a system should fall off, a new system should be applied for the remainder of the 7-day dosing interval. Only one system should be worn at any one time during the 7-day dosing interval.

Initiation of Therapy

Three (12.5, 18.75 and 25.0 cm^2) Climara® systems are available. Treatment is usually initiated with the 12.5 cm^2 (0.05 mg/day) Climara® system applied to the skin once-weekly. The dose should be adjusted as necessary to control symptoms. Clinical responses (relief of symptoms) at the lowest effective dose should be the guide for establishing administration of the Climara® system, especially in women with an intact uterus. Attempts to taper or discontinue the medication should be made at 3- to 6-month intervals.

In women who are not currently taking oral estrogens, treatment with the Climara® system can be initiated at once. In women who are currently taking oral estrogen, treatment with the Climara® system can be initiated 1 week after withdrawal of oral therapy or sooner if symptoms reappear in less than 1 week.

Therapeutic Regimen

Therapy with the Climara® system is usually administered on a cyclic schedule (e.g., 3 weeks of therapy followed by 1 week without) especially in women with an intact uterus, who are not using concomitant progestin therapy.

HOW SUPPLIED

Climara® (estradiol transdermal system), 0.05 mg/day—each 12.5 cm^2 system contains 3.9 mg of estradiol

USP .... NDC 50419-451-04
Individual Carton of 4 systems
Shelf Pack Carton of 6 Individual Cartons of 4 systems

Climara® (estradiol transdermal system), 0.075 mg/day—each 18.75 cm^2 system contains 5.85 mg of estradiol

USP .... NDC 50419-453-04
Individual Carton of 4 systems
Shelf Pack Carton of 6 Individual Cartons of 4 systems

Climara® (estradiol transdermal system), 0.1 mg/day—each 25.0 cm^2 system contains 7.8 mg of estradiol

USP .... NDC 50419-452-04
Individual Carton of 4 systems
Shelf Pack Carton of 6 Individual Cartons of 4 systems

Do not store above 86°F (30°C). Do not store unpouched. Apply immediately upon removal from the protective pouch.
Rx only

INFORMATION FOR THE PATIENT

INTRODUCTION

The Climara® system that your doctor has prescribed for you releases small amounts of estradiol through the skin in a continuous way. Estradiol is the same hormone that your ovaries produce abundantly before menopause. The dose of estradiol you require will depend upon your individual response. The dose is adjusted by the size of the Climara® system used; the systems are available in three sizes.

This leaflet describes when and how to use estrogens, and the risks and benefits of estrogen treatment.

Estrogens have important benefits but also some risks. You must decide, with your doctor, whether the risks to you of estrogen use are acceptable because of their benefits. If you use estrogens, check with your doctor to be sure you are using the lowest possible dose that works, and that you don't use them longer than necessary. How long you need to use estrogens will depend on the reason for use.

INFORMATION ABOUT CLIMARA®

How The Climara® System Works

The Climara® system contains 17β-estradiol. When applied to the skin as directed below, the Climara® system releases 17β-estradiol, which flows through the skin into the bloodstream.

How and Where to Apply the Climara® System

Each Climara® system is individually sealed in a protective pouch. To open the pouch, hold it vertically with the Climara® name facing you. Tear left to right using the top tear notch. Tear from bottom to top using the side tear notch. Pull the pouch open. The Climara® patch is the translucent plastic film attached to the clear thicker plastic backing. There is a silver-foil sticker securely attached to the inside of the pouch. This contains a moisture protectant (desiccant). **Do not remove it. Carefully remove the Climara® patch.** You'll notice that the patch is attached to a thicker, hard-plastic backing and that the patch itself is oval and transparent.

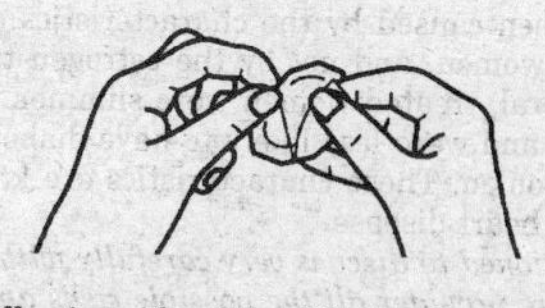

Apply the adhesive side of the Climara® system to a clean, dry area of the lower abdomen or the upper quadrant of the buttock. *Do not apply the Climara® system to your breasts.* The sites of application must be rotated, with an interval of at least 1 week allowed between applications to a particular site. The area selected should not be oily, damaged, or irritated. Avoid the waistline, since tight clothing may rub and remove the system. Application to areas where sitting would dislodge the system should also be avoided. Apply the system immediately after opening the pouch and removing the protective liner. Press the system firmly in place with the fingers for about 10 seconds, making sure there is good contact, especially around the edges.

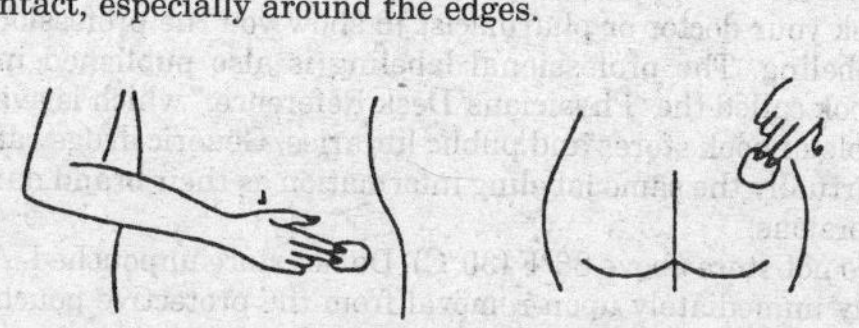

The Climara® system should be worn continuously for one week. You may wish to experiment with different locations when applying a new system, to find ones that are most comfortable for you and where clothing will not rub on the system.

When to Apply the Climara® System

The Climara® system should be changed once weekly.

When changing the system, remove the used Climara® system and discard it. Any adhesive that might remain on your skin can be easily rubbed off. Then place the new Climara® system on a different skin site. (The same skin site should not be used again for at least 1 week after removal of the system).

Contact with water when you are bathing, swimming, or showering will not affect the system. In the unlikely event that a system should fall off, a new system should be applied for the remainder of the 7-day dosing interval.

USES OF ESTROGEN

(Not every estrogen drug is approved for every use listed in this section. If you want to know which of these possible uses are approved for the medicine prescribed for you, ask your doctor or pharmacist to show you the professional labeling. You can also look up the specific estrogen product in a book called the "Physician's Desk Reference", which is available in many book stores and public libraries. Generic drugs carry virtually the same labeling information as their brand name versions.)

- **To reduce moderate or severe menopausal symptoms.** Estrogens are hormones made by the ovaries of normal women. Between ages 45 and 55, the ovaries normally stop making estrogens. This leads to a drop in body estrogen levels which causes the "change of life" or menopause (the end of monthly menstrual periods). If both ovaries are removed during an operation before natural menopause takes place, the sudden drop in estrogen levels causes "surgical menopause".
  When the estrogen levels begin dropping, some women develop very uncomfortable symptoms, such as feelings of warmth in the face, neck, and chest, or sudden intense episodes of heat and sweating ("hot flashes" or "hot flushes"). Using estrogen drugs can help the body adjust to lower estrogen levels and reduce these symptoms. Most women have only mild menopausal symptoms or none at all and do not need to use estrogen drugs for these symptoms. Others may need to take estrogens for a few months while their bodies adjust to lower estrogen levels. The majority of women do not need estrogen replacement for longer than six months for these symptoms.
- **To treat vulval and vaginal atrophy** (itching, burning, dryness in or around the vagina, difficulty or burning on urination) associated with menopause.
- **To treat certain conditions in which a young woman's ovaries do not produce enough estrogen naturally.**
- **To treat certain types of abnormal vaginal bleeding due to hormonal imbalance when your doctor has found no serious cause of the bleeding.**
- **To treat certain cancers in special situations, in men and women.**
- **To prevent thinning of bones.**
  Osteoporosis is a thinning of the bones that makes them weaker and allows them to break more easily. The bones of the spine, wrists and hips break most often in osteoporosis. Both men and women start to lose bone mass after about age 40, but women lose bone mass faster after the menopause. Using estrogens after the menopause slows down bone thinning and may prevent bones from breaking. Lifelong adequate calcium intake, either in the diet (such as dairy products) or by calcium supplements (to reach a total daily intake of 1000 milligrams per day before menopause or 1500 milligrams per day after menopause), may help to prevent osteoporosis. Regular weight-bearing exercise (like walking and running for an hour, two or three times a week) may also help to prevent osteoporosis. Before you change your calcium intake or exercise habits, it is important to discuss these lifestyle changes with your doctor to find out if they are safe for you.
  Since estrogen use has some risks, only women who are likely to develop osteoporosis should use estrogens for prevention. Women who are likely to develop osteoporosis often have the following characteristics: white or Asian race, slim, cigarette smokers, and a family history of osteoporosis in a mother, sister, or aunt. Women who have relatively early menopause, often because their ovaries were removed during an operation ("surgical menopause"), are more likely to develop osteoporosis than women whose menopause happens at the average age.

WHO SHOULD NOT USE ESTROGENS

Estrogens should not be used:

- **During pregnancy (see Boxed Warning).**
  If you think you may be pregnant, do not use any form of estrogen-containing drug. Using estrogens while you are pregnant may cause your unborn child to have birth defects. Estrogens do not prevent miscarriage.
- **If you have unusual vaginal bleeding which has not been evaluated by your doctor (see Boxed Warning).**
  Unusual vaginal bleeding can be a warning sign of cancer of the uterus, especially if it happens after menopause. Your doctor must find out the cause of the bleeding so that he or she can recommend the proper treatment. Taking estrogens without visiting your doctor can cause you serious harm if your vaginal bleeding is caused by cancer of the uterus.
- **If you have had cancer.**
  Since estrogens increase the risk of certain types of cancer, you should not use estrogens if you have ever had can-

Continued on next page

Information on the Berlex products appearing here is based on the most current information available at the time of publication closing. Further information for these and other products may be obtained from the Medical Affairs Department, Berlex Laboratories, 300 Fairfield Road, Wayne, New Jersey 07470, 1-888-BERLEX-4. Information on Betaseron and Fludara may be obtained from Berlex Laboratories, 15049 San Pablo Avenue, Richmond, California 94804-0016, 1-800-888-4112.

Climara—Cont.

cer of the breast or uterus, unless your doctor recommends that the drug may help in the cancer treatment. (For certain patients with breast or prostate cancer, estrogens may help).

• **If you have any circulation problems.**
Estrogen drugs should not be used except in unusually special situations in which your doctor judges that you need estrogen therapy so much that the risks are acceptable. Men and women with abnormal blood clotting conditions should avoid estrogen use (see Dangers of Estrogens, below).

• **When they do not work.**
During menopause, some women develop nervous symptoms or depression. Estrogens do not relieve these symptoms. You may have heard that taking estrogens for years after menopause will keep your skin soft and supple and keep you feeling young. There is no evidence for these claims and such long-term estrogen use may have serious risks.

• **After childbirth or when breastfeeding a baby.**
Estrogens should not be used to try to stop the breasts from filling with milk after a baby is born. Such treatment may increase the risk of developing blood clots (see Dangers of Estrogens, below).
If you are breastfeeding, you should avoid using any drugs because many drugs pass through to the baby in the milk. While nursing a baby, you should take drugs only on the advice of your health care provider.

DANGERS OF ESTROGENS

• **Cancer of the uterus.**
Your risk of developing cancer of the uterus gets higher the longer you use estrogens and the larger doses you use. One study showed that after women stop taking estrogens, this higher cancer risk quickly returns to the usual level of risk (as if you had never used estrogen therapy). Three other studies showed that the cancer risk stayed high for 8 to more than 15 years after stopping estrogen treatment. Because of this risk, **IT IS IMPORTANT TO TAKE THE LOWEST DOSE THAT WORKS AND TO TAKE IT ONLY AS LONG AS YOU NEED IT.**
Using progestin therapy together with estrogen therapy may reduce the higher risk of uterine cancer related to estrogen use (but see Other Information, below.)
If you have had your uterus removed (total hysterectomy), there is no danger of developing cancer of the uterus.

• **Cancer of the breast.**
Most studies have not shown a higher risk of breast cancer in women who have ever used estrogens. However, some studies have reported that breast cancer developed more often (up to twice the usual rate) in women who used estrogens for long periods of time (especially more than 10 years), or who used higher doses for shorter time periods.
Regular breast examinations by a health professional and monthly self-examination are recommended for all women.

• **Gallbladder disease.**
Women who use estrogens after menopause are more likely to develop gallbladder disease needing surgery than women who do not use estrogens.

• **Abnormal blood clotting.**
Taking estrogens may cause changes in your blood clotting system. These changes allow the blood to clot more easily, possibly allowing clots to form in your bloodstream. If blood clots do form in your bloodstream, they can cut off the blood supply to vital organs, causing serious problems. These problems may include a stroke (by cutting off blood to the brain), a heart attack (by cutting off blood to the heart), a pulmonary embolus (by cutting off blood to the lungs), or other problems. Any of these conditions may cause death or serious long-term disability. However, most studies of low dose estrogen usage by women do not show an increased risk of these complications.

SIDE EFFECTS

In addition to the risks listed above, the following side effects have been reported with estrogen use:
— Nausea and vomiting.
— Breast tenderness or enlargement.
— Enlargement of benign tumors ("fibroids") of the uterus.
— Retention of excess fluid. This may make some conditions worsen, such as asthma, epilepsy, migraine, heart disease, or kidney disease.
— A spotty darkening of the skin, particularly on the face.

REDUCING RISK OF ESTROGEN USE

If you use estrogens, you can reduce your risks by doing these things:

• **See your doctor regularly.**
While you are using estrogens, it is important to visit your doctor at least once a year for a check-up. If you develop vaginal bleeding while taking estrogens, you may need further evaluation. If members of your family have had breast cancer or if you have ever had breast lumps or an

abnormal mammogram (breast x-ray), you may need to have more frequent breast examinations.

• **Reassess your need for estrogens.**
You and your doctor should reevaluate whether or not you still need estrogens at least every six months.

• **Be alert for signs of trouble.**
If any of these warning signals (or any other unusual symptoms) happen while you are using estrogens, call your doctor immediately:
Abnormal bleeding from the vagina (possible uterine cancer)
Pains in the calves or chest, sudden shortness of breath, or coughing blood (possible clot in the legs, heart, or lungs)
Severe headache or vomiting, dizziness, faintness, changes in vision or speech, weakness or numbness of an arm or leg (possible clot in the brain or eye)
Breast lumps (possible breast cancer; ask your doctor or health professional to show you how to examine your breasts monthly)
Yellowing of the skin or eyes (possible liver problem)
Pain, swelling, or tenderness in the abdomen (possible gallbladder problem)

OTHER INFORMATION

1. Estrogens increase the risk of developing a condition (endometrial hyperplasia) that may lead to cancer of the lining of the uterus. Taking progestins, another hormone drug, with estrogens lowers the risk of developing this condition. Therefore, if your uterus has not been removed, your doctors may prescribe a progestin for you to take together with your estrogen.
You should know, however, that taking estrogens *with* progestins may have additional risks. These include:
— unhealthy effects on blood fats (especially a lowering of HDL blood cholesterol, the "good" blood fat which protects against heart disease);
— unhealthy effects on blood sugar (which might make a diabetic condition worse); and
— a possible further increase in breast cancer risk which may be associated with long-term estrogen use.
Some research has shown that estrogens taken *without* progestins may protect women against developing heart disease. However, this is not certain. The protection shown may have been caused by the characteristics of the estrogen-treated women, and not by the estrogen treatment itself. In general, treated women were slimmer, more physically active, and were less likely to have diabetes than the untreated women. These characteristics are known to protect against heart disease.
You are cautioned to discuss very carefully with your doctor or health care provider all the possible risks and benefits of long-term estrogen and progestin treatment as they affect you personally.
2. Your doctor has prescribed this drug for you and you alone. Do not give the drug to anyone else.
3. If you will be taking calcium supplements as part of the treatment to help prevent osteoporosis, check with your doctor about how much to take.
4. Keep this and all drugs out of the reach of children. In case of overdose, call your doctor, hospital or poison control center immediately.
5. This leaflet provides a summary of the most important information about estrogens. If you want more information, ask your doctor or pharmacist to show you the professional labeling. The professional labeling is also published in a book called the "Physicians' Desk Reference," which is available in book stores and public libraries. Generic drugs carry virtually the same labeling information as their brand name versions.
Do not store above 86°F (30°C). Do not store unpouched. Apply immediately upon removal from the protective pouch.

Rx only
Manufactured for Berlex Laboratories, Wayne, NJ 07470
Manufactured by 3M Pharmaceuticals, St. Paul, MN 55144
©1998, Berlex Laboratories.
All Rights Reserved.
6064303   April 1998
BERLEX LABORATORIES,
WAYNE, NJ 07470
Shown in Product Identification Guide, page 306

QUINAGLUTE   ℞
DURA-TABS® TABLETS
[kwĭn 'uh glōōt]
(BRAND OF QUINIDINE GLUCONATE EXTENDED-RELEASE TABLETS, USP)

DESCRIPTION

Quinidine is an antimalarial schizonticide and an antiarrhythmic agent with Class Ia activity; it is the d-isomer of quinine, and its molecular weight is 324.43. Quinidine gluconate is the gluconate salt of quinidine; its chemical name

is cinchonan-9-ol, 6'-methoxy-, (9S)-, mono-D-gluconate; its structural formula is:

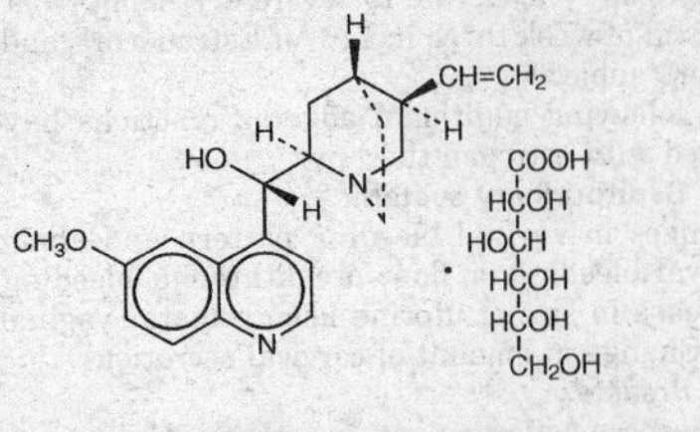

Its empirical formula is $C_{20}H_{24}N_2O_2 \cdot C_6H_{12}O_7$, and its molecular weight is 520.58, of which 62.3% is quinidine base. Each QUINAGLUTE DURA-TABS® tablet contains 324 mg of quinidine gluconate (202 mg of quinidine base) in a matrix to provide extended-release; the inactive ingredients include confectioner's sugar, magnesium stearate, corn starch and other ingredients. Meets USP Drug Release Test 4.

CLINICAL PHARMACOLOGY
Pharmacokinetics and Metabolism:
The absolute bioavailability of quinidine from QUINAGLUTE® is 70–80%. Relative to a solution of quinidine sulfate, the bioavailability of quinidine from QUINAGLUTE® is reported to be 1.03. The less-than-complete bioavailability is thought to be due to first-pass elimination by the liver. Peak serum levels generally appear 3–5 hours after dosing; when the drug is taken with food, absorption is increased in both rate (27%) and extent (17%). The rate and extent of absorption of quinidine from QUINAGLUTE® are not significantly affected by the coadministration of an aluminum-hydroxide antacid.

The **volume of distribution** of quinidine is 2–3 L/kg in healthy young adults, but this may be reduced to as little as 0.5 L/kg in patients with congestive heart failure, or increased to 3–5 L/kg in patients with cirrhosis of the liver. At concentrations of 2–5 mg/L (6.5–16.2 μmol/L), the fraction of quinidine bound to plasma proteins (mainly to α_1-acid glycoprotein and to albumin) is 80–88% in adults and older children, but it is lower in pregnant women, and in infants and neonates it may be as low as 50–70%. Because α_1-acid glycoprotein levels are increased in response to stress, serum levels of total quinidine may be greatly increased in settings such as acute myocardial infarction, even though the serum content of unbound (active) drug may remain normal. Protein binding is also increased in chronic renal failure, but binding abruptly descends toward or below normal when heparin is administered for hemodialysis.

Quinidine **clearance** typically proceeds at 3–5 ml/min/kg in adults, but clearance in children may be twice or three times as rapid. The elimination half-life is 6–8 hours in adults and 3–4 hours in children. Quinidine clearance is unaffected by hepatic cirrhosis, so the increased volume of distribution seen in cirrhosis leads to a proportionate increase in the elimination half-life.

Most quinidine is eliminated hepatically via the action of cytochrome P450IIIA4; there are several different hydroxylated metabolites, and some of these have antiarrhythmic activity.

The most important of quinidine's metabolites is 3-hydroxyquinidine (3HQ), serum levels of which can approach those of quinidine in patients receiving conventional doses of QUINAGLUTE®. The volume of distribution of 3HQ appears to be larger than that of quinidine, and the elimination half-life of 3HQ is about 12 hours.

As measured by antiarrhythmic effects on animals, by QT_c prolongation in human volunteers, or by various *in vitro* techniques, 3HQ has at least half the antiarrhythmic activity of the parent compound, so it may be responsible for a substantial fraction of the effect of QUINAGLUTE® in chronic use.

When the urine pH is less than 7, about 20% of administered quinidine appears unchanged in the urine, but this fraction drops to as little as 5% when the urine is more alkaline. Renal clearance involves both glomerular filtration and active tubular secretion, moderated by (pH-dependent) tubular reabsorption. The net renal clearance is about 1 ml/min/kg in healthy adults.

When renal function is taken into account, quinidine clearance is apparently independent of patient age.

Assays of serum quinidine levels are widely available, but the results of modern assays may not be consistent with results cited in the older medical literature. The serum levels of quinidine cited in this package insert are those derived from specific assays, using either benzene extraction or (preferably) reverse-phase high-pressure liquid chromatography. In matched samples, older assays might unpredictably have given results that were as much as two or three times higher. A typical "therapeutic" concentration range is 2–6 mg/L (6.2–18.5 μmol/L).

Mechanisms of action
In patients with malaria, quinidine acts primarily as an intraerythrocytic schizonticide, with little effect upon

sporozites or upon pre-erythrocytic parasites. Quinidine is gametocidal to *Plasmodium vivax* and *P. malariae*, but not to *P. falciparum*.

In cardiac muscle and in Purkinje fibers, quinidine depresses the rapid inward depolarizing sodium current, thereby slowing phase-0 depolarization and reducing the amplitude of the action potential without affecting the resting potential. In normal Purkinje fibers, it reduces the slope of phase-4 depolarization, shifting the threshold voltage upward toward zero. The result is slowed conduction and reduced automaticity in all parts of the heart, with increase of the effective refractory period relative to the duration of the action potential in the atria, ventricles, and Purkinje tissues. Quinidine also raises the fibrillation thresholds of the atria and ventricles, and it raises the ventricular *de*fibrillation threshold as well. Quinidine's actions fall into Class Ia in the Vaughan-Williams classification.

By slowing conduction and prolonging the effective refractory period, quinidine can interrupt or prevent reentrant arrhythmias and arrhythmias due to increased automaticity, including atrial flutter, atrial fibrillation, and paroxysmal supraventricular tachycardia.

In patients with sick sinus syndrome, quinidine can cause marked sinus node depression and bradycardia. In most patients, however, use of quinidine is associated with an increase in the sinus rate.

Like other antiarrhythmic drugs with Class Ia activity, quinidine prolongs the QT interval in a dose-related fashion. This may lead to increased ventricular automaticity and polymorphic ventricular tachycardias, including *torsades de pointes* (see **Warnings**).

In addition, quinidine has anticholinergic activity, it has negative inotropic activity, and it acts peripherally as an α-adrenergic antagonist (that is, as a vasodilator).

CLINICAL EFFECTS

Maintenance of sinus rhythm after conversion from atrial fibrillation: In six clinical trials (published between 1970 and 1984) with a total of 808 patients, quinidine (418 patients) was compared to nontreatment (258 patients) or placebo (132 patients) for the maintenance of sinus rhythm after cardioversion from chronic atrial fibrillation. Quinidine was consistently more efficacious in maintaining sinus rhythm, but a meta-analysis found that mortality in the quinidine-exposed patients (2.9%) was significantly greater than mortality in the patients who had not been treated with active drug (0.8%). Suppression of atrial fibrillation with quinidine has theoretical patient benefits (e.g., improved exercise tolerance; reduction in hospitalization for cardioversion; lack of arrhythmia-related palpitations, dyspnea and chest pain; reduced incidence of systemic embolism and/or stroke), but these benefits have never been demonstrated in clinical trials. Some of these benefits (e.g., reduction in stroke incidence) may be achievable by other means (anticoagulation).

By slowing the atrial rate in atrial flutter/fibrillation, quinidine can decrease the degree of atrioventricular block and cause an increase, sometimes marked, in the rate at which supraventricular impulses are successfully conducted by the atrioventricular node, with a resultant paradoxical increase in ventricular rate (see **Warnings**).

Non-life-threatening ventricular arrhythmias: In studies of patients with a variety of ventricular arrhythmias (mainly frequent ventricular premature beats and non-sustained ventricular tachycardia, quinidine (total n=502) has been compared with flecainide (n=141), mexiletine (n=246), propafenone (n=53), and tocainide (n=67). In each of these studies, the mortality in the quinidine group was numerically greater than the mortality in the comparator group. When the studies were combined in a meta-analysis quinidine was associated with a statistically significant threefold relative risk of death.

At therapeutic doses, quinidine's only consistent effect upon the surface electrocardiogram is an increase in the QT interval. This prolongation can be monitored as a guide to safety, and it may provide better guidance than serum drug levels (see **Warnings**).

INDICATIONS AND USAGE

Conversion of atrial fibrillation/flutter: In patients with symptomatic atrial fibrillation/flutter whose symptoms are not adequately controlled by measures that reduce the rate of ventricular response, QUINAGLUTE® is indicated as a means of restoring normal sinus rhythm. If this use of QUINAGLUTE® does not restore sinus rhythm within a reasonable time (see **Dosage and Administration**), then QUINAGLUTE® should be discontinued.

Reduction of frequency of relapse into atrial fibrillation/flutter: Chronic therapy with QUINAGLUTE® is indicated for some patients at high risk of symptomatic atrial fibrillation/flutter, generally patients who have had previous episodes of atrial fibrillation/flutter that were so frequent and poorly tolerated as to outweigh, in the judgment of the physician and the patient, the risks of prophylactic therapy with QUINAGLUTE®. The increased risk of death should specifically be considered. QUINAGLUTE® should

be used only after alternative measures (e.g., use of other drugs to control the ventricular rate) have been found to be inadequate.

In patients with histories of frequent symptomatic episodes of atrial fibrillation/flutter, the goal of therapy should be an increase in the average time between episodes. In most patients, the tachyarrhythmia *will recur* during therapy, and a single recurrence should not be interpreted as therapeutic failure.

Suppression of ventricular arrhythmias: QUINAGLUTE® is also indicated for the suppression of recurrent documented ventricular arrhythmias, such as sustained ventricular tachycardia, that in the judgment of the physician are life-threatening. Because of the proarrhythmic effects of quinidine, its use with ventricular arrhythmias of lesser severity is generally not reccommended and treatment of patients with asymptomatic ventricular premature contractions should be avoided. Where possible, therapy should be guided by the results of programmed electrical stimulation and/or Holter monitoring with exercise.

Antiarrhythmic drugs (including QUINAGLUTE®) have not been shown to enhance survival in patients with ventricular arrhythmias.

CONTRAINDICATIONS

Quinidine is contraindicated in patients who are known to be allergic to it, or who have developed thrombocytopenic purpura during prior therapy with quinidine or quinine.

In the absence of a functioning artificial pacemaker, quinidine is also contraindicated in any patient whose cardiac rhythm is dependent upon a junctional or idioventricular pacemaker, including patients in complete atrioventricular block.

Quinidine is also contraindicated in patients who, like those with myasthenia gravis, might be adversely affected by an anticholinergic agent.

WARNINGS
Mortality:

> In many trials of antiarrhythmic therapy for non-life-threatening arrhythmias, active antiarrhythmic therapy has resulted in increased mortality; the risk of active therapy is probably greatest in patients with structural heart disease.
>
> In the case of quinidine used to prevent or defer recurrence of atrial flutter/fibrillation, the best available data come from a meta-analysis described under *Clinical Pharmacology/Clinical Effects* above. In the patients studied in the trials there analyzed, the mortality associated with the use of quinidine was more than three times as great as the mortality associated with the use of placebo.
>
> Another meta-analysis, also described under *Clinical Pharmacology/Clinical Effects,* showed that in patients with various non-life-threatening ventricular arrhythmias, the mortality associated with the use of quinidine was consistently greater than that associated with the use of any of a variety of alternative antiarrhythmics.

Proarrhythmic effects: Like many other drugs (including all other Class Ia antiarrhythmics), quinidine prolongs the QT_c interval, and this can lead to *torsades de pointes*, a life-threatening ventricular arrhythmia (see **Overdosage**). The risk of *torsades* is increased by bradycardia, hypokalemia, hypomagnesemia or high serum levels of quinidine, but it may appear in the absence of any of these risk factors. The best predictor of this arrhythmia appears to be the length of QT_c interval, and quinidine should be used with extreme care in patients who have preexisting long-QT syndromes, who have histories of *torsades de pointes* of any cause, or who have previously responded to quinidine (or other drugs that prolong ventricular repolarization) with marked lengthening of the QT_c interval. Estimation of the incidence of *torsades* in patients with therapeutic levels of quinidine is not possible from the available data.

Other ventricular arrhythmias that have been reported with quinidine include frequent extrasystoles, ventricular tachycardia, ventricular flutter, and ventricular fibrillation.

Paradoxical increase in ventricular rate in atrial flutter/fibrillation: When quinidine is administered to patients with atrial flutter/fibrillation, the desired pharmacologic reversion to sinus rhythm may (rarely) be preceded by a slowing of the atrial rate with a consequent increase in the rate of beats conducted to the ventricles. The resulting ventricular rate may be very high (greater than 200 beats per minute) and poorly tolerated. This hazard may be decreased if partial atrioventricular block is achieved prior to initiation of quinidine therapy, using conduction-reducing drugs such as digitalis, verapamil, diltiazem, or a β-receptor blocking agent.

Exacerbated bradycardia in sick sinus syndrome: In patients with the sick sinus syndrome, quinidine has been associated with marked sinus node depression and bradycardia.

Pharmacokinetic considerations: Renal or hepatic dysfunction causes the elimination of quinidine to be slowed,

while congestive heart failure causes a reduction in quinidine's apparent volume of distribution. Any of these conditions can lead to quinidine toxicity if dosage is not appropriately reduced. In addition, interactions with coadministered drugs can alter the serum concentration and activity of quinidine, leading either to toxicity or to lack of efficacy if the dose of quinidine is not appropriately modified. (See **Precautions/Drug Interactions**.)

Vagolysis: Because quinidine opposes the atrial and A-V nodal effects of vagal stimulation, physical or pharmacological vagal maneuvers undertaken to terminate paroxysmal supraventricular tachycardia may be ineffective in patients receiving quinidine.

PRECAUTIONS
Heart block

In patients without implanted pacemakers who are at high risk of complete atrioventricular block (e.g., those with digitalis intoxication, second degree atrioventricular block, or severe intraventricular conduction defects), quinidine should be used only with caution.

Drug Interactions

Altered pharmacokinetics of quinidine: Diltiazem significantly decreases the clearance and increases the $t_{1/2}$ of quinidine, but quinidine does not alter the kinetics of diltiazem. Drugs that alkalinize the urine (**carbonic-anhydrase inhibitors, sodium bicarbonate, thiazide diuretics**) reduce renal elimination of quinidine.

By pharmacokinetic mechanisms that are not well understood, quinidine levels are increased by coadministration of **amiodarone** or **cimetidine**. Very rarely, and again by mechanisms not understood, quinidine levels are decreased by coadministration of **nifedipine**.

Hepatic elimination of quinidine may be accelerated by coadministration of drugs (**phenobarbital, phenytoin, rifampin**) that induce production of cytochrome P450IIIA4. Perhaps because of competition for the P450IIIA4 metabolic pathway, quinidine levels rise when **ketaconazole** is coadministered.

Coadministration of **propranolol** usually does not affect quinidine pharmacokinetics, but in some studies the β-blocker appeared to cause increases in the peak serum levels of quinidine, decreases in quinidine's volume of distribution, and decreases in total quinidine clearance. The effects (if any) of coadministration of **other β-blockers** on quinidine pharmacokinetics have not been adequately studied.

Hepatic clearance of quinidine is significantly reduced during coadministration of **verapamil**, with corresponding increases in serum levels and half-life.

Altered pharmacokinetics of other drugs: Quinidine slows the elimination of **digoxin** and simultaneously reduces digoxin's apparent volume of distribution. As a result, serum digoxin levels may be as much as doubled. When quinidine and digoxin are coadministered, digoxin doses usually need to be reduced. Serum levels of **digitoxin** are also raised when quinidine is coadministered, although the effect appears to be smaller.

By a mechanism that is not understood, quinidine potentiates the anticoagulatory action of **warfarin**, and the anticoagulant dosage may need to be reduced.

Cytochrome P450IID6 is an enzyme critical to the metabolism of many drugs, notably including **mexiletine**, some **phenothiazines**, and most **polycyclic antidepressants**. Constitutional deficiency of cytochrome P450IID6 is found in less than 1% of Orientals, in about 2% of American blacks, and in about 8% of American whites. Testing with debrisoquine is sometimes used to distinguish the P450IID6-deficient "poor metabolizers" from the majority-phenotype "extensive metabolizers."

When drugs whose metabolism is P450IID6-dependent are given to poor metabolizers, the serum levels achieved are higher, sometimes much higher, than the serum levels achieved when identical doses are given to extensive metabolizers. To obtain similar clinical benefit without toxicity, doses given to poor metabolizers may need to be greatly reduced. In the case of prodrugs whose actions are actually mediated by P450IID6-produced metabolites (for example, **codeine** and **hydrocodone**, whose analgesic and antitussive effects appear to be mediated by morphine and hydromorphone, respectively), it may be possible to achieve the desired clinical benefits in poor metabolizers.

Continued on next page

Information on the Berlex products appearing here is based on the most current information available at the time of publication closing. Further information for these and other products may be obtained from the Medical Affairs Department, Berlex Laboratories, 300 Fairfield Road, Wayne, New Jersey 07470, 1-888-BERLEX-4. Information on Betaseron and Fludara may be obtained from Berlex Laboratories, 15049 San Pablo Avenue, Richmond, California 94804-0016, 1-800-888-4112.

Quinaglute—Cont.

Quinidine is not metabolized by cytochrome P450IID6, but therapeutic serum levels of quinidine inhibit the action of cytochrome P450IID6, effectively converting extensive metabolizers into poor metabolizers. Caution must be exercised whenever quinidine is prescribed together with drugs metabolized by cytochrome P450IID6.

Perhaps by competing for pathways of renal clearance, coadministration of quinidine causes an increase in serum levels of **procainamide**.

Serum levels of **haloperidol** are increased when quinidine is coadministered.

Presumably because both drugs are metabolized by cytochrome P450IIIA4, coadministration of quinidine causes variable slowing of the metabolism of **nifedipine**. Interactions with other dihydropyridine calcium channel blockers have not been reported, but these agents (including **felodipine, nicardipine,** and **nimodipine**) are all dependent upon P450IIIA4 for metabolism, so similar interactions with quinidine should be anticipated.

Altered pharmacodynamics of other drugs: Quinidine's anticholinergic, vasodilating, and negative inotropic actions may be additive to those of other drugs with these effects, and antagonistic to those of drugs with cholinergic, vasoconstricting, and positive inotropic effects. For example, when quinidine and **verapamil** are coadministered in doses that are each well tolerated as monotherapy, hypotension attributable to additive peripheral α-blockade is sometimes reported.

Quinidine potentiates the actions of depolarizing (succinylcholine, decamethonium) and nondepolarizing (d-tubocurarine, pancuronium) **neuromuscular blocking agents.** These phenomena are not well understood, but they are observed in animal models as well as in humans. In addtion, *in vitro* addition of quinidine to the serum of pregnant women reduces the activity of pseudocholinesterase, an enzyme that is essential to the metabolism of succinylcholine.

Non-interactions of quinidine with other drugs: Quinidine has no clinically significant effect on the pharmacokinetics of **diltiazem, flecainide, mephenytoin, metoprolol, propafenone, propranolol, quinine, timolol,** or **tocainide.** Conversely, the pharmacokinetics of quinidine are not significantly affected by **caffeine, ciprofloxacin, digoxin, diltiazem, felodipine, omeprazole,** or **quinine.** Quinidine's pharmacokinetics are also unaffected by cigarette smoking.

INFORMATION FOR PATIENTS

Before prescibing QUINAGLUTE® as prophylaxis against recurrence of atrial fibrillation, the physician should inform the patient of the risks and benefits to be expected (see **Clinical Pharmacology**). Discussion should include the facts.

- that the goal of therapy will be a reduction (probably not to zero) in the frequency of episodes of atrial fibrillation; and
- that reduced frequency of fibrillatory episodes may be expected, if achieved, to bring symptomatic benefit; but
- that no data are available to show that reduced frequency of fibrillatory episodes will reduce the risks of irreversible harm through stroke or death; and in fact
- that such data as are available suggest that treatment with QUINAGLUTE® is likely to increase the patient's risk of death.

Carcinogenesis, mutagenesis, impairment of fertility

Animal studies to evaluate quinidine's carcinogenic or mutagenic potential have not been performed. Similarly, there are no animal data as to quinidine's potential to impair fertility.

Pregnancy

Pregnancy Category C. Animal reproductive studies have not been conducted with quinidine. There are no adequate and well-controlled studies in pregnant women. Quinidine should be given to a pregnant woman only if clearly needed. In one neonate whose mother had received quinidine throughout her pregnancy, the serum level of quinidine was equal to that of the mother, with no apparent ill effect. The level of quinidine in amniotic fluid was about three times higher than that found in serum.

Labor and Delivery

Quinine is said to be oxytocic in humans, but there are no adequate data as to quinidine's effects (if any) on human labor and delivery.

Nursing mothers

Quinidine is present in human milk at levels slightly lower than those in maternal serum; a human infant ingesting such milk should (scaling directly by weight) be expected to develop serum quinidine levels at least an order of magnitude lower than those of the mother. On the other hand, the pharmacokinetics and pharmacodynamics of quinidine in human infants have not been adequately studied, and neonates' reduced protein binding of quinidine may increase their risk of toxicity at low total serum levels. Administration of quinidine should (if possible) be avoided in lactating women who continue to nurse.

Geriatric use

Safety and efficacy of quinidine in elderly patients have not been systematically studied.

Pediatric use

In antimalarial trials, quinidine was as safe and effective in pediatric patients as in adults. Notwithstanding the known pharmacokinetic differences between children and adults (see **Parmacokinetics and Metabolism**), children in these trials received the same doses (on a mg/kg basis) as adults. Safety and effectiveness of antiarrhythmic use in children have not been established.

ADVERSE REACTIONS

Quinidine preparations have been used for many years, but there are only sparse data from which to estimate the incidence of various adverse reactions. The adverse reactions most frequently reported have consistently been gastrointestinal, including diarrhea, nausea, vomiting, and heartburn/esophagitis.

In the reported study that was closest in character to the predominant approved use of QUINAGLUTE®, 86 adult outpatients with atrial fibrillation were followed for six months while they received slow-release quinidine bisulfate tablets, 600 mg quinidine (approximately 400 mg of quinidine base) twice daily. The incidences of adverse experiences reported more than once were as shown in the table below. The most serious quinidine-associated adverse reactions are described above under **Warnings.**

ADVERSE EXPERIENCES REPORTED MORE THAN ONCE IN 86 PATIENTS WITH ATRIAL FIBRILLATION

	Incidence (%)
diarrhea	21 (24%)
fever	5 (6%)
rash	5 (6%)
arrhythmia	3 (3%)
abnormal electrocardiogram	3 (3%)
nausea/vomiting	3 (3%)
dizziness	3 (3%)
headache	3 (3%)
asthenia	2 (2%)
cerebral ischemia	2 (2%)

Vomiting and diarrhea can occur as isolated reactions to therapeutic levels of quinidine, but they may also be the first signs of **cinchonism,** a syndrome that may also include tinnitus, reversible high-frequency hearing loss, deafness, vertigo, blurred vision, diplopia, photophobia, headache, confusion, and delirium. Cinchonism is most often a sign of chronic quinidine toxicity, but it may appear in sensitive patients after a single moderate dose.

A few cases of **hepatotoxicity,** including granulomatous hepatitis, have been reported in patients receiving quinidine. All of these have appeared during the first few weeks of therapy, and most (not all) have remitted once quinidine was withdrawn.

Autoimmune and inflammatory syndromes associated with quinidine therapy have included fever, urticaria, flushing, exfoliative rash, bronchospasm, psoriasiform rash, pruritus and lymphadenopathy, hemolytic anemia, vasculitis, thrombocytopenic purpura, uveitis, angioedema, agranulocytosis, the sicca syndrome, arthralgia, myalgia, elevation in serum levels of skeletal-muscle enzymes, a disorder resembling systemic lupus erythematosus, and pneumonitis.

Convulsions, apprehension, and ataxia have been reported, but it is not clear that these were not simply the results of hypotension and consequent cerebral hypoperfusion. There are many reports of syncope. Acute psychotic reactions have been reported to follow the first dose of quinidine, but these reactions appear to be extremely rare.

Other adverse reactions occasionally reported include depression, mydriasis, disturbed color perception, night blindness, scotomata, optic neuritis, visual field loss, photosensitivity, and abnormalities of pigmentation.

OVERDOSAGE

Overdoses with various oral formulations of quinidine have been well described. Death has been described after a 5-gram ingestion by a toddler, while an adolescent was reported to survive after ingesting 8 grams of quinidine.

The most important ill effects of acute quinidine overdoses are ventricular arrhythmias and hypotension. Other signs and symptoms of overdose may include vomiting, diarrhea, tinnitus, high-frequency hearing loss, vertigo, blurred vision, diplopia, photophobia, headache, confusion and delirium.

Arrhythmias: Serum quinidine levels can be conveniently assayed and monitored, but the electrocardiographic QT_c interval is a better predictor of quinidine-induced ventricular arrhythmias.

The necessary treatment of hemodynamically unstable polymorphic ventricular tachycardia (including *torsades de pointes*) is withdrawal of treatment with quinidine and either immediate cardioversion or, if a cardiac pacemaker is in place or immediately available, immediate overdrive pacing. After pacing or cardioversion, further management must be guided by the length of the QT_c interval.

Quinidine-associated ventricular tachyarrhythmias with normal underlying QT_c intervals have not been adequately studied. Because of the theoretical possibility of QT-prolonging effects that might be additive to those of quinidine, other antiarrhythmics with Class I (disopyramide, procainamide) or Class III activities should (if possible) be avoided. Similarly, although the use of bretylium in quinidine overdose has not been reported, it is reasonable to expect that the α-blocking properties of bretylium might be additive to those of quinidine, resulting in problematic hypotension.

If the postcardioversion QT_c interval is prolonged, then the precardioversion polymorphic ventricular tachycardia was (by definition) *torsades de pointes.* In this case, lidocaine and bretylium are unlikely to be of value, and other Class I antiarrhythmics (disopyramide, procainamide) are likely to exacerbate the situation. Factors contributing to QT_c prolongation (especially hypokalemia and hypomagnesemia) should be sought out and (if possible) aggressively corrected. Prevention of recurrent *torsades* may require sustained overdrive pacing or the cautious administration of isoproterenol (30–150 ng/kg/min).

Hypotension: Quinidine-induced hypotension that is not due to an arrhythmia is likely to be a consequence of quinidine-related α-blockade and vasorelaxation. Simple repletion of central volume (Trendelenburg positioning, saline infusion) may be sufficient therapy; other interventions reported to have been beneficial in this setting are those that increase peripheral vascular resistance, including α-agonist catecholamines (norepinephrine, metaraminol) and the Military Anti-Shock Trousers.

Treatment:

To obtain up-to-date information about the treatment of overdose, a good resource is your certified Regional Poison-Control Center. Telephone numbers of certified poison-control centers are listed in the Physicians' Desk Reference (PDR). In managing overdose, consider the possibilities of multiple-drug overdoses, drug-drug interactions, and unusual drug kinetics in your patient.

Accelerated removal: Adequate studies of orally-administered activated charcoal in human overdoses of quinidine have not been reported, but there are animal data showing significant enhancement of systemic elimination following this intervention, and there is at least one human case report in which the elimination half-life of quinidine in the serum was apparently shortened by repeated gastric lavage. Activated charcoal should be avoided if an ileus is present; the conventional dose is 1 gram/kg administered every 2–6 hours as a slurry with 8 mL/kg of tap water.

Although renal elimination of quinidine might theoretically be accelerated by maneuvers to acidify the urine, such maneuvers are potentially hazardous and of no demonstrated benefit.

Quinidine is not usefully removed from the circulation by dialysis.

Following quinidine overdose, drugs that delay elimination of quinidine (cimetidine, carbonic-anhydrase inhibitors, thiazide diuretics) should be withdrawn unless absolutely required.

DOSAGE AND ADMINISTRATION

The dose of quinidine delivered by QUINAGLUTE DURA-TABS® tablets may be titrated by breaking a tablet in half. If tablets are crushed or chewed, their extended-release properties will be lost.

The dosage of quinidine varies considerably depending upon the general condition and the cardiovascular state of the patient.

Conversion of atrial fibrillation/flutter to sinus rhythm

Especially in patients with known structural heart disease or other risk factors for toxicity, initiation or dose-adjustment of treatment with QUINAGLUTE® should generally be performed in a setting where facilities and personnel for monitoring and resuscitation are continuously available. Patients with symptomatic atrial fibrillation/flutter should be treated with QUINAGLUTE® only after ventricular rate control (e.g., with digitalis or β-blockers) has failed to provide satisfactory control of symptoms.

Adequate trials have not identified an optimal regimen of QUINAGLUTE® for conversion of atrial fibrillation/flutter to sinus rhythm. In one reported regimen, the patient first receives two tablets (648 mg; 403 mg of quinidine base) of QUINAGLUTE® every eight hours. If this regimen has not resulted in conversion after 3 or 4 doses, then the dose is cautiously increased. If, at any point during administration, the QRS complex widens to 130% of its pre-treatment duration; the QT_c interval widens to 130% of its pre-treatment duration and is then longer than 500 ms; P waves disappear; or the patient develops significant tachycardia, symptomatic bradycardia, or hypotension, then QUINAGLUTE® is discontinued, and other means of conversion (e.g., direct-current cardioversion) are considered.

In another regimen sometimes used, the patient receives one tablet (324 mg; 202 mg of quinidine base) every eight hours for two days; then two tablets every twelve hours for two days; and finally two tablets every eight hours for up to four days. The four-day stretch may come at one of the lower doses if, in the judgment of the physician, the lower dose is the highest one that will be tolerated. The criteria for dis-

continuation of treatment with QUINAGLUTE® are the same as in the other regimen.

Reduction in the frequency of relapse into atrial fibrillation/flutter

In a patient with a history of frequent symptomatic episodes of atrial fibrillation/flutter, the goal of therapy with QUINAGLUTE® should be an increase in the average time between episodes. In most patients, the tachyarrhythmia *will recur* during therapy with QUINAGLUTE®, and a single recurrence should not be interpreted as therapeutic failure. Especially in patients with known structural heart disease or other risk factors for toxicity, initiation or dose adjustment of treatment with QUINAGLUTE® should generally be performed in a setting where facilities and personnel for monitoring and resuscitation are continuously available. Monitoring should be continued for two or three days after initiation of the regimen on which the patient will be discharged.

Therapy with QUINAGLUTE® should be begun with one tablet (324 mg; 202 mg of quinidine base) every eight or twelve hours. If this regimen is well tolerated, if the serum quinidine level is still well within the laboratory's therapeutic range, and if the average time between arrhythmic episodes has not been satisfactorily increased, then the dose may be cautiously raised. The total daily dosage should be reduced if the QRS complex widens to 130% of its pre-treatment duration; the QT_c interval widens to 130% of its pre-treatment duration and is then longer than 500 ms; P waves disappear; or the patient develops significant tachycardia, symptomatic bradycardia, or hypotension.

Suppression of life-threatening ventricular arrhythmias

Dosing regimens for the use of quinidine gluconate in suppressing life-threatening ventricular arrhythmias have not been adequately studied. Described regimens have generally been similar to the regimen described just above for the prophylaxis of symptomatic atrial fibrillation/flutter. Where possible, therapy should be guided by the results of programmed etetrical stimulation and/or Holter monitoring with exercise.

HOW SUPPLIED

QUINAGLUTE DURA-TABS® tablets are 324 mg white to off-white, round tablets embossed with **C** in a flask design on one side and with a clock-like design on the other.

  *

The tablets are available in bottles and unit-dose packages as follows:

bottle of 100 .... NDC 50419-101-10
bottle of 250 .... NDC 50419-101-25
bottle of 500 .... NDC 50419-101-50
unit-dose box of 100 .... NDC 50419-101-11

Store tablets at controlled room temperature (15–30°C; 59–86°F).

Rx only

*Tablet designs are registered trademarks of Berlex Laboratories

©1997, Berlex Laboratories. All rights reserved.

BERLEX® Laboratories, Wayne, NJ 07470

Rev. 11/97   6069503

Shown in Product Identification Guide, page 306

TRI-LEVLEN® 21   ℞
[trī-lĕvlĕn]
Tablets
(levonorgestrel and ethinyl estradiol tablets—triphasic regimen)

TRI-LEVLEN® 28   ℞
[trī-lĕvlĕn]
Tablets
(levonorgestrel and ethinyl estradiol tablets—triphasic regimen)

LEVLEN® 21   ℞
[lĕvlĕn]
Tablets
(levonorgestrel and ethinyl estradiol tablets)

LEVLEN® 28   ℞
[lĕvlĕn]
Tablets
(levonorgestrel and ethinyl estradiol tablets)

Patients should be counseled that this product does not protect against HIV infection (AIDS) and other sexually transmitted diseases.

DESCRIPTION

TRI-LEVLEN® 21 tablets

Each cycle of TRI-LEVLEN® 21 (Levonorgestrel and Ethinyl Estradiol Tablets—Triphasic Regimen) tablets consists of three different drug phases as follows: Phase 1 comprised of 6 brown film-coated tablets, each containing 0.050 mg of levonorgestrel (d(-)-13 beta-ethyl-17-alpha-ethinyl-17-beta-hydroxygon-4-en-3-one), a totally synthetic progestogen, and 0.030 mg of ethinyl estradiol (19-nor-17α-pregna-1,3,5(10)-trien-20-yne-3, 17-diol); phase 2 comprised of 5 white film-coated tablets, each containing 0.075 mg levonorgestrel and 0.040 mg ethinyl estradiol; and, phase 3 comprised of 10 light-yellow film-coated tablets, each containing 0.125 mg levonorgestrel and 0.030 mg ethinyl estradiol. The inactive ingredients present are cellulose, iron oxides, lactose, magnesium stearate, polacrilin potassium, polyethylene glycol, titanium dioxide, and hydroxypropyl methylcellulose.

TRI-LEVLEN® 28 tablets

Each cycle of TRI-LEVLEN® 28 (Levonorgestrel and Ethinyl Estradiol Tablets—Triphasic Regimen) tablets consists of three different drug phases as follows: Phase 1 comprised of 6 brown film-coated tablets, each containing 0.050 mg of levonorgestrel (d(-)-13 beta-ethyl-17-alpha-ethinyl-17-beta-hydroxygon-4-en-3-one), a totally synthetic progestogen, and 0.030 mg of ethinyl estradiol (19-nor-17 α-pregna-1,3,5(10)-trien-20-yne-3, 17-diol); phase 2 comprised of 5 white film-coated tablets, each containing 0.075 mg levonorgestrel and 0.040 mg ethinyl estradiol; and phase 3 comprised of 10 light-yellow film-coated tablets, each containing 0.125 mg levonorgestrel and 0.030 mg ethinyl estradiol; then followed by 7 light-green film-coated inert tablets. The inactive ingredients present are cellulose, F D & C Blue 1, iron oxides, lactose, magnesium stearate, polacrilin potassium, polyethylene glycol, titanium dioxide, and hydroxypropyl methylcellulose.

LEVLEN® 21 tablets:

Each LEVLEN® 21 tablet (Levonorgestrel and Ethinyl Estradiol Tablets) contains 0.15 mg of levonorgestrel (d(-)-13 beta-ethyl-17-alpha-ethinyl-17-beta-hydroxygon-4-en-3-one), a totally synthetic progestogen, and 0.03 mg of ethinyl estradiol (19-nor-17 α-pregna-1,3,5(10)-trien-20-yne-3, 17-diol). The inactive ingredients present are cellulose, FD&C Yellow 6, lactose, magnesium stearate, and polacrillin potassium.

LEVLEN® 28 tablets:

21 light-orange LEVLEN® tablets (Levonorgestrel and Ethinyl Estradiol Tablets), each containing 0.15 mg of levonorgestrel (d(-)-13 beta-ethyl-17-alpha-ethinyl-17-beta-hydroxygon-4-en-3-one), a totally synthetic progestogen, and 0.03 mg of ethinyl estradiol (19-nor-17 α-pregna-1,3,5(10)-trien-20-yne-3, 17-diol), and 7 pink inert tablets. The inactive ingredients present are cellulose, D&C Red 30, FD&C Yellow 6, lactose, magnesium stearate, and polacrillin potassium.

Levonorgestrel   Ethinyl Estradiol

CLINICAL PHARMACOLOGY

Combination oral contraceptives act by suppression of gonadotropins. Although the primary mechanism of this action is inhibition of ovulation, other alterations include changes in the cervical mucus (which increase the difficulty of sperm entry into the uterus) and the endometrium (which reduce the likelihood of implantation).

INDICATIONS AND USAGE

Oral contraceptives are indicated for the prevention of pregnancy in women who elect to use this product as a method of contraception.

Oral contraceptives are highly effective. Table I lists the typical accidental pregnancy rates for users of combination oral contraceptives and other methods of contraception. The efficacy of these contraceptive methods, except sterilization and the IUD, depends upon the reliability with which they are used. Correct and consistent use of methods can result in lower failure rates.

TABLE I: LOWEST EXPECTED AND TYPICAL FAILURE RATES DURING THE FIRST YEAR OF CONTINUOUS USE OF A METHOD

% of Women Experiencing an Accidental Pregnancy in the First Year of Continuous Use

Method	Lowest Expected*	Typical**
(No Contraception)	(85)	(85)
Oral contraceptives		
combined	0.1	N/A***
progestin only	0.5	N/A***
Diaphragm with spermicidal cream or jelly	6	18
Spermicides alone (foam, and vaginal suppositories)	3	21
Vaginal Sponge		
nulliparous	6	18
multiparous	9	28
Depo-Provera (injectable progestogen)	0.3	0.3
NORPLANT® SYSTEM (implants)	0.2#	0.2#
IUD		
progesterone	2	3
copper T 380A	0.8	N/A***
Condom without spermicides	2	12
Periodic abstinence (all methods)	1–9	20
Female sterilization	0.2	0.4
Male sterilization	0.1	0.15

Adapted from J. Trussell et al., Table I. Studies in Family Planning, *21(1):* Jan.–Feb. 1990.

* The authors' best guess of the percentage of women expected to experience an accidental pregnancy among couples who initiate a method (not necessarily for the first time) and who use it consistently and correctly during the first year if they do not stop use for any other reason.

** This term represents "typical" couples who initiate use of a method (not necessarily for the first time), who experience an accidental pregnancy during the first year if they do not stop use for any other reason.

*** N/A—Data not available.

This data is based on Norplant System clinical trials.

CONTRAINDICATIONS

Oral contraceptives should not be used in women with any of the following conditions:

Thrombophlebitis or thromboembolic disorders.

A past history of deep-vein thrombophlebitis or thromboembolic disorders.

Cerebral-vascular or coronary-artery disease.

Known or suspected carcinoma of the breast.

Carcinoma of the endometrium or other known or suspected estrogen-dependent neoplasia.

Undiagnosed abnormal genital bleeding.

Cholestatic jaundice of pregnancy or jaundice with prior pill use.

Hepatic adenomas or carcinomas.

Known or suspected pregnancy.

WARNINGS

Cigarette smoking increases the risk of serious cardiovascular side effects from oral-contraceptive use. This risk increases with age and with heavy smoking (15 or more cigarettes per day) and is quite marked in women over 35 years of age. Women who use oral contraceptives should be strongly advised not to smoke.

The use of oral contraceptives is associated with increased risks of several serious conditions including myocardial infarction, thromboembolism, stroke, hepatic neoplasia, gallbladder disease, and hypertension, although the risk of serious morbidity or mortality is very small in healthy women without underlying risk factors. The risk of morbidity and mortality increases significantly in the presence of other underlying risk factors such as hypertension, hyperlipidemias, obesity and diabetes.

Practitioners prescribing oral contraceptives should be familiar with the following information relating to these risks. The information contained in this package insert is based principally on studies carried out in patients who used oral contraceptives with higher formulations of estrogens and progestogens than those in common use today. The effect of

Continued on next page

Levlen/Tri-Levlen—Cont.

long-term use of the oral contraceptives with lower formulations of both estrogens and progestogens remains to be determined.

Throughout this labeling, epidemiological studies reported are of two types: retrospective or case control studies and prospective or cohort studies. Case control studies provide a measure of the relative risk of disease, namely, a ratio of the incidence of a disease among oral-contraceptive users to that among nonusers. The relative risk does not provide information on the actual clinical occurrence of a disease. Cohort studies provide a measure of attributable risk, which is the difference in the incidence of disease between oral-contraceptive users and nonusers. The attributable risk does provide information about the actual occurrence of a disease in the population. For further information, the reader is referred to a text on epidemiological methods.

1. THROMBOEMBOLIC DISORDERS AND OTHER VASCULAR PROBLEMS

a. *Myocardial Infarction*

An increased risk of myocardial infarction has been attributed to oral-contraceptive use. This risk is primarily in smokers or women with other underlying risk factors for coronary-artery disease such as hypertension, hypercholesterolemia, morbid obesity, and diabetes. The relative risk of heart attack for current oral-contraceptive users has been estimated to be two to six. The risk is very low under the age of 30.

Smoking in combination with oral-contraceptive use has been shown to contribute substantially to the incidence of myocardial infarctions in women in their mid-thirties or older with smoking accounting for the majority of excess cases. Mortality rates associated with circulatory disease have been shown to increase substantially in smokers over the age of 35 and nonsmokers over the age of 40 (Table II) among women who use oral contraceptives.

CIRCULATORY DISEASE MORTALITY RATES
PER 100,000 WOMEN YEARS BY AGE,
SMOKING STATUS AND ORAL-CONTRACEPTIVE USE

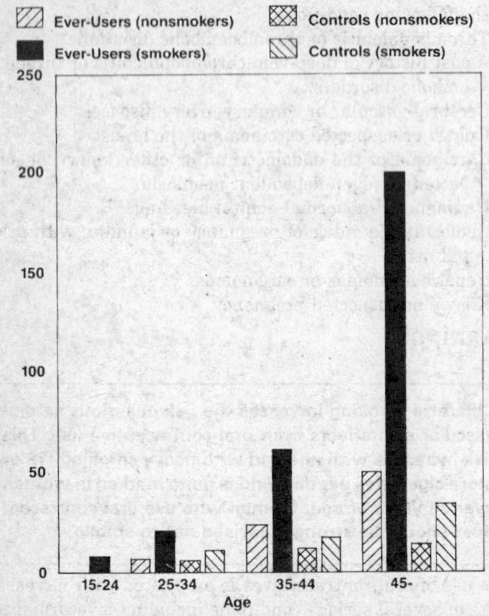

TABLE II. (Adapted from P.M. Layde and V. Beral, Lancet, *1*:541–546, 1981.)

Oral contraceptives may compound the effects of well-known risk factors, such as hypertension, diabetes, hyperlipidemias, age and obesity. In particular, some progestogens are known to decrease HDL cholesterol and cause glucose intolerance, while estrogens may create a state of hyperinsulinism. Oral contraceptives have been shown to increase blood pressure among users (see section 9 in "WARNINGS"). Similar effects on risk factors have been associated with an increased risk of heart disease. Oral contraceptives must be used with caution in women with cardiovascular disease risk factors.

b. *Thromboembolism*

An increased risk of thromboembolic and thrombotic disease associated with the use of oral contraceptives is well established. Case control studies have found the relative risk of users compared to nonusers to be 3 for the first episode of superficial venous thrombosis, 4 to 11 for deep vein thrombosis or pulmonary embolism, and 1.5 to 6 for women with predisposing conditions for venous thromboembolic disease. Cohort studies have shown the relative risk to be somewhat lower, about 3 for new cases and about 4.5 for new cases requiring hospitalization. The risk of thromboembolic disease due to oral contraceptives is not related to length of use and disappears after pill use is stopped.

TABLE III—ANNUAL NUMBER OF BIRTH-RELATED OR METHOD-RELATED DEATHS ASSOCIATED WITH CONTROL OF FERTILITY PER 100,000 NONSTERILE WOMEN, BY FERTILITY-CONTROL METHOD ACCORDING TO AGE

Method of control and outcome	15–19	20–24	25–29	30–34	35–39	40–44
No fertility—control methods*	7.0	7.4	9.1	14.8	25.7	28.2
Oral contraceptives nonsmoker**	0.3	0.5	0.9	1.9	13.8	31.6
Oral contraceptives smoker**	2.2	3.4	6.6	13.5	51.1	117.2
IUD**	0.8	0.8	1.0	1.0	1.4	1.4
Condom*	1.1	1.6	0.7	0.2	0.3	0.4
Diaphragm/spermicide*	1.9	1.2	1.2	1.3	2.2	2.8
Periodic abstinence*	2.5	1.6	1.6	1.7	2.9	3.6

* Deaths are birth related
** Deaths are method related

Adapted from H.W. Ory, Family Planning Perspectives *15*:57–63, 1983.

A two- to four-fold increase in relative risk of post-operative thromboembolic complications has been reported with the use of oral contraceptives. The relative risk of venous thrombosis in women who have predisposing conditions is twice that of women without such medical conditions. If feasible, oral contraceptives should be discontinued at least four weeks prior to and for two weeks after elective surgery of a type associated with an increase in risk of thromboembolism and during and following prolonged immobilization. Since the immediate postpartum period is also associated with an increased risk of thromboembolism, oral contraceptives should be started no earlier than four to six weeks after delivery in women who elect not to breast-feed, or a midtrimester pregnancy termination.

c. *Cerebrovascular diseases*

Oral contraceptives have been shown to increase both the relative and attributable risks of cerebrovascular events (thrombotic and hemorrhagic strokes), although, in general, the risk is greatest among older (>35 years), hypertensive women who also smoke. Hypertension was found to be a risk factor for both users and nonusers, for both types of strokes, while smoking interacted to increase the risk for hemorrhagic strokes.

In a large study, the relative risk of thrombotic strokes has been shown to range from 3 for normotensive users to 14 for users with severe hypertension. The relative risk of hemorrhagic stroke is reported to be 1.2 for nonsmokers who used oral contraceptives, 2.6 for smokers who did not use oral contraceptives, 7.6 for smokers who used oral contraceptives, 1.8 for normotensive users and 25.7 for users with severe hypertension. The attributable risk is also greater in older women.

d. *Dose-related risk of vascular disease from oral contraceptives*

A positive association has been observed between the amount of estrogen and progestogen in oral contraceptives and the risk of vascular disease. A decline in serum high-density lipoproteins (HDL) has been reported with many progestational agents. A decline in serum high-density lipoproteins has been associated with an increased incidence of ischemic heart disease. Because estrogens increase HDL cholesterol, the net effect of an oral contraceptive depends on a balance achieved between doses of estrogen and progestogen and the nature and absolute amount of progestogen used in the contraceptive. The amount of both hormones should be considered in the choice of an oral contraceptive.

Minimizing exposure to estrogen and progestogen is in keeping with good principles of therapeutics. For any particular estrogen/progestogen combination, the dosage regimen prescribed should be one which contains the least amount of estrogen and progestogen that is compatible with a low failure rate and the needs of the individual patient. New acceptors of oral-contraceptive agents should be started on preparations containing less than 50 mcg of estrogen.

e. *Persistence of risk of vascular disease*

There are two studies which have shown persistence of risk of vascular disease for ever-users of oral contraceptives. In a study in the United States, the risk of developing myocardial infarction after discontinuing oral contraceptives persists for at least 9 years for women 40–49 years who had used oral contraceptives for five or more years, but this increased risk was not demonstrated in other age groups. In another study in Great Britain, the risk of developing cerebrovascular disease persisted for at least 6 years after discontinuation of oral contraceptives, although excess risk was very small. However, both studies were performed with oral contraceptive formulations containing 50 micrograms or higher of estrogens.

2. ESTIMATES OF MORTALITY FROM CONTRACEPTIVE USE

One study gathered data from a variety of sources which have estimated the mortality rate associated with different methods of contraception at different ages (Table III). These estimates include the combined risk of death associated with contraceptive methods plus the risk attributable to pregnancy in the event of method failure. Each method of contraception has its specific benefits and risks. The study concluded that with the exception of oral-contraceptive users 35 and older who smoke and 40 and older who do not smoke, mortality associated with all methods of birth control is less than that associated with childbirth. The observation of a possible increase in risk of mortality with age for oral-contraceptive users is based on data gathered in the 1970's—but not reported until 1983. However, current clinical practice involves the use of lower estrogen dose formulations combined with careful restriction of oral-contraceptive use to women who do not have the various risk factors listed in this labeling.

Because of these changes in practice and, also, because of some limited new data which suggest that the risk of cardiovascular disease with the use of oral contraceptives may now be less than previously observed, the Fertility and Maternal Health Drugs Advisory Committee was asked to review the topic in 1989. The Committee concluded that although cardiovascular disease risks may be increased with oral-contraceptive use after age 40 in healthy nonsmoking women (even with the newer low-dose formulations), there are greater potential health risks associated with pregnancy in older women and with the alternative surgical and medical procedures which may be necessary if such women do not have access to effective and acceptable means of contraception.

Therefore, the Committee recommended that the benefits of oral-contraceptive use by healthy nonsmoking women over 40 may outweigh the possible risks. Of course, older women, as all women who take oral contraceptives, should take the lowest possible dose formulation that is effective.

[See table above]

3. CARCINOMA OF THE REPRODUCTIVE ORGANS

Numerous epidemiological studies have been performed on the incidence of breast, endometrial, ovarian and cervical cancer in women using oral contraceptives. The overwhelming evidence in the literature suggests that use of oral contraceptives is not associated with an increase in the risk of developing breast cancer, regardless of the age and parity of first use or with most of the marketed brands and doses. The Cancer and Steroid Hormone (CASH) study also showed no latent effect on the risk of breast cancer for at least a decade following long-term use. A few studies have shown a slightly increased relative risk of developing breast cancer, although the methodology of these studies, which included differences in examination of users and nonusers and differences in age at start of use, has been questioned. Some studies suggest that oral-contraceptive use has been associated with an increase in the risk of cervical intraepithelial neoplasia in some populations of women. However, there continues to be controversy about the extent to which such findings may be due to differences in sexual behavior and other factors.

In spite of many studies of the relationship between oral-contraceptive use and breast and cervical cancers, a cause-and-effect relationship has not been established.

4. HEPATIC NEOPLASIA

Benign hepatic adenomas are associated with oral-contraceptive use, although the incidence of benign tumors is rare in the United States. Indirect calculations have estimated the attributable risk to be in the range of 3.3 cases/100,000 for users, a risk that increases after four or more years of use. Rupture of rare, benign, hepatic adenomas may cause death through intra-abdominal hemorrhage.

Studies from Britain have shown an increased risk of developing hepatocellular carcinoma in long-term (>8 years) oral-contraceptive users. However, these cancers are extremely rare in the U.S. and the attributable risk (the excess incidence) of liver cancers in oral-contraceptive users approaches less than one per million users.

5. OCULAR LESIONS
There have been clincial case reports of retinal thrombosis associated with the use of oral contraceptives. Oral contraceptives should be discontinued if there is unexplained partial or complete loss of vision; onset of proptosis or diplopia; papilledema; or retinal vascular lesions. Appropriate diagnostic and therapeutic measures should be undertaken immediately.

6. ORAL-CONTRACEPTIVE USE BEFORE OR DURING EARLY PREGNANCY
Extensive epidemiological studies have revealed no increased risk of birth defects in women who have used oral contraceptives prior to pregnancy. Studies also do not suggest a teratogenic effect, particularly insofar as cardiac anomalies and limb-reduction defects are concerned, when taken inadvertently during early pregnancy.
The administration of oral contraceptives to induce withdrawal bleeding should not be used as a test for pregnancy. Oral contraceptives should not be used during pregnancy to treat threatened or habitual abortion.
It is recommended that for any patient who has missed two consecutive periods, pregnancy should be ruled out before continuing oral-contraceptive use. If the patient has not adhered to the prescribed schedule, the possibility of pregnancy should be considered at the time of the first missed period. Oral-contraceptive use should be discontinued if pregnancy is confirmed.

7. GALLBLADDER DISEASE
Earlier studies have reported an increased lifetime relative risk of gallbladder surgery in users of oral contraceptives and estrogens. More recent studies, however, have shown that the relative risk of developing gallbladder disease among oral-contraceptive users may be minimal. The recent findings of minimal risk may be related to the use of oral-contraceptive formulations containing lower hormonal doses of estrogens and progestogens.

8. CARBOHYDRATE AND LIPID METABOLIC EFFECTS
Oral contraceptives have been shown to cause glucose intolerance in a significant percentage of users. Oral contraceptives containing greater than 75 micrograms of estrogens cause hyperinsulinism, while lower doses of estrogen cause less glucose intolerance. Progestogens increase insulin secretion and create insulin resistance, this effect varying with different progestational agents. However, in the nondiabetic woman, oral contraceptives appear to have no effect on fasting blood glucose. Because of these demonstrated effects, prediabetic and diabetic women should be carefully observed while taking oral contraceptives.
A small proportion of women will have persistent hypertriglyceridemia while on the pill. As discussed earlier (see "WARNINGS" 1a. and 1d.), changes in serum triglycerides and lipoprotein levels have been reported in oral-contraceptive users.

9. ELEVATED BLOOD PRESSURE
An increase in blood pressure has been reported in women taking oral contraceptives and this increase is more likely in older oral-contraceptive users and with continued use. Data from the Royal College of General Practitioners and subsequent randomized trials have shown that the incidence of hypertension increases with increasing quantities of progestogens.
Women with a history of hypertension or hypertension-related diseases, or renal disease should be encouraged to use another method of contraception. If women with hypertension elect to use oral contraceptives, they should be monitored closely, and if significant elevation of blood pressure occurs, oral contraceptives should be discontinued. For most women, elevated blood pressure will return to normal after stopping oral contraceptives, and there is no difference in the occurrence of hypertension among ever- and never-users.

10. HEADACHE
The onset or exacerbation of migraine or development of headache with a new pattern that is recurrent, persistent, or severe requires discontinuation of oral contraceptives and evaluation of the case.

11. BLEEDING IRREGULARITIES
Breakthrough bleeding and spotting are sometimes encountered in patients on oral contraceptives, especially during the first three months of use. The type and dose of progestogen may be important. Nonhormonal causes should be considered and adequate diagnostic measures taken to rule out malignancy or pregnancy in the event of breakthrough bleeding, as in the case of any abnormal vaginal bleeding. If pathology has been excluded, time or a change to another formulation may solve the problem. In the event of amenorrhea, pregnancy should be ruled out.
Some women may encounter post-pill amenorrhea or oligomenorrhea, especially when such a condition was preexistent.

PRECAUTIONS

Patients should be counseled that this product does not protect against HIV infection (AIDS) and other sexually transmitted diseases.

1. PHYSICAL EXAMINATION AND FOLLOW UP
A complete medical history and physical examination should be taken prior to the initiation or reinstitution of oral contraceptives and at least annually during use of oral contraceptives. These physical examinations should include special reference to blood pressure, breasts, abdomen and pelvic organs, including cervical cytology, and relevant laboratory tests. In case of undiagnosed, persistent, or recurrent abnormal vaginal bleeding, appropriate diagnostic measures should be conducted to rule out malignancy. Women with a strong family history of breast cancer or who have breast nodules should be monitored with particular care.

2. LIPID DISORDERS
Women who are being treated for hyperlipidemias should be followed closely if they elect to use oral contraceptives. Some progestogens may elevate LDL levels and may render the control of hyperlipidemias more difficult. (See "WARNINGS" 1d.)

3. LIVER FUNCTION
If jaundice develops in any woman receiving such drugs, the medication should be discontinued. Steroid hormones may be poorly metabolized in patients with impaired liver function.

4. FLUID RETENTION
Oral contraceptives may cause some degree of fluid retention. They should be prescribed with caution, and only with careful monitoring, in patients with conditions which might be aggravated by fluid retention.

5. EMOTIONAL DISORDERS
Patients becoming significantly depressed while taking oral contraceptives should stop the medication and use an alternate method of contraception in an attempt to determine whether the symptom is drug related. Women with a history of depression should be carefully observed and the drug discontinued if depression recurs to a serious degree.

6. CONTACT LENSES
Contact-lens wearers who develop visual changes or changes in lens tolerance should be assessed by an ophthalmologist.

7. DRUG INTERACTIONS
Reduced efficacy and increased incidence of breakthrough bleeding and menstrual irregularities have been associated with concomitant use of rifampin. A similar association, though less marked, has been suggested with barbiturates, phenylbutazone, phenytoin sodium, and possibly with griseofulvin, ampicillin, and tetracyclines.

8. INTERACTIONS WITH LABORATORY TESTS
Certain endocrine- and liver-function tests and blood components may be affected by oral contraceptives:
a. Increased prothrombin and factors VII, VIII, IX, and X; decreased antithrombin 3; increased norepinephrine-induced platelet aggregability.
b. Increased thyroid-binding globulin (TBG) leading to increased circulating total thyroid hormone, as measured by protein-bound iodine (PBI), T4 by column or by radioimmunoassay. Free T3 resin uptake is decreased, reflecting the elevated TBG, free T4 concentration is unaltered.
c. Other binding proteins may be elevated in serum.
d. Sex-binding globulins are increased and result in elevated levels of total circulating sex steroids and corticoids; however, free or biologically active levels remain unchanged.
e. Triglycerides may be increased.
f. Glucose tolerance may be decreased.
g. Serum folate levels may be depressed by oral-contraceptive therapy. This may be of clinical significance if a woman becomes pregnant shortly after discontinuing oral contraceptives.

9. CARCINOGENESIS
See "WARNINGS" section.

10. PREGNANCY
Pregnancy Category X. See "CONTRAINDICATIONS" and "WARNINGS" sections.

11. NURSING MOTHERS
Small amounts of oral-contraceptive steroids have been identified in the milk of nursing mothers and a few adverse effects on the child have been reported, including jaundice and breast enlargement. In addition, oral contraceptives given in the postpartum period may interfere with lactation by decreasing the quantity and quality of breast milk. If possible, the nursing mother should be advised not to use oral contraceptives but to use other forms of contraception until she has completely weaned her child.

INFORMATION FOR THE PATIENT

See "Patient Labeling" printed below.

ADVERSE REACTIONS

An increased risk of the following serious adverse reactions has been associated with the use of oral contraceptives (see "WARNINGS" section).
- Thrombophlebitis
- Arterial thromboembolism
- Pulmonary embolism
- Myocardial infarction
- Cerebral hemorrhage
- Cerebral thrombosis
- Hypertension
- Gallbladder disease
- Hepatic adenomas or
- benign liver tumors

There is evidence of an association between the following conditions and the use of oral contraceptives, although additional confirmatory studies are needed:
- Mesenteric thrombosis
- Retinal thrombosis

The following adverse reactions have been reported in patients receiving oral contraceptives and are believed to be drug related:
- Nausea
- Vomiting
- Gastrointestinal symptoms (such as abdominal cramps and bloating)
- Breakthrough bleeding
- Spotting
- Change in menstrual flow
- Amenorrhea
- Temporary infertility after discontinuation of treatment
- Edema
- Melasma which may persist
- Breast changes: tenderness, enlargement, and secretion
- Change in weight (increase or decrease)
- Change in cervical erosion and cervical secretion
- Diminution in lactation when given immediately postpartum
- Cholestatic jaundice
- Migraine
- Rash (allergic)
- Mental depression
- Reduced tolerance to carbohydrates
- Vaginal candidiasis
- Change in corneal curvature (steepening)
- Intolerance to contact lenses

The following adverse reactions have been reported in users of oral contraceptives and the association has been neither confirmed nor refuted:
- Congenital anomalies
- Premenstrual syndrome
- Cataracts
- Optic neuritis
- Changes in appetite
- Cystitis-like syndrome
- Headache
- Nervousness
- Dizziness
- Hirsutism
- Loss of scalp hair
- Erythema multiforme
- Erythema nodosum
- Hemorrhagic eruption
- Vaginitis
- Porphyria
- Impaired renal function
- Hemolytic uremic syndrome
- Budd-Chiari syndrome
- Acne
- Changes in libido
- Colitis
- Sickle-Cell Disease
- Cerebral-vascular disease with mitral valve prolapse
- Lupus-like Syndromes

OVERDOSAGE

Serious ill effects have not been reported following acute ingestion of large doses of oral contraceptives by young children. Overdosage may cause nausea, and withdrawal bleeding may occur in females.

NONCONTRACEPTIVE HEALTH BENEFITS

The following noncontraceptive health benefits related to the use of oral contraceptives are supported by epidemiological studies which largely utilized oral-contraceptive formulations containing doses exceeding 0.035 mg of ethinyl estradiol or 0.05 mg of mestranol.
Effects on menses:
- increased menstrual cycle regularity
- decreased blood loss and decreased incidence of iron deficiency anemia
- decreased incidence of dysmenorrhea

Effects related to inhibition of ovulation:
- decreased incidence of functional ovarian cysts
- decreased incidence of ectopic pregnancies

Effects from long-term use:
- decreased incidence of fibroadenomas and fibrocystic disease of the breast
- decreased incidence of acute pelvic inflammatory disease
- decreased incidence of endometrial cancer
- decreased incidence of ovarian cancer

DOSAGE AND ADMINISTRATION

TRI-LEVLEN® 21 Tablets
To achieve maximum contraceptive effectiveness, TRI-LEVLEN® 21 Tablets (levonorgestrel and ethinyl es-

Continued on next page

Information on the Berlex products appearing here is based on the most current information available at the time of publication closing. Further information for these and other products may be obtained from the Medical Affairs Department, Berlex Laboratories, 300 Fairfield Road, Wayne, New Jersey 07470, 1-888-BERLEX-4. Information on Betaseron and Fludara may be obtained from Berlex Laboratories, 15049 San Pablo Avenue, Richmond, California 94804-0016, 1-800-888-4112.

Levlen/Tri-Levlen—Cont.

tradiol tablets—triphasic regimen) should be taken exactly as directed and at intervals not exceeding 24-hours.

TRI-LEVLEN® 21 Tablets are a three-phase preparation. The dosage of TRI-LEVLEN® 21 Tablets is **one tablet** daily for 21 consecutive days per menstrual cycle in the following order: 6 brown tablets (phase 1), followed by 5 white tablets (phase 2), and then followed by the last 10 light-yellow tablets (phase 3), according to the prescribed schedule. Tablets are then discontinued for 7 days (three weeks on, one week off).

It is recommended that TRI-LEVLEN® 21 Tablets be taken at the same time each day. During the first cycle of medication, the patient should be instructed to take one TRI-LEVLEN® 21 Tablet daily in the order of 6 brown, 5 white and, finally, 10 light-yellow tablets for twenty-one (21) consecutive days, beginning on day one (1) of her menstrual cycle. (The first day of menstruation is day one.) The tablets are then discontinued for one week (7 days). Withdrawal bleeding usually occurs within 3 days following discontinuation of TRI-LEVLEN® 21 Tablets. (If an alternate starting regimen is used [Sunday Start or postpartum], contraceptive reliance should not be placed on TRI-LEVLEN® 21 Tablets until after the first 7 consecutive days of administration. The possibility of ovulation and conception prior to initiation of medication should be considered.)

The patient begins her next and all subsequent 21-day courses of TRI-LEVLEN® 21 Tablets on the same day of the week that she began her first course, following the same schedule: 21 days on—7 days off. She begins taking her brown tablets on the 8th day after discontinuance, regardless of whether or not a menstrual period has occurred or is still in progress. Any time the next cycle of TRI-LEVLEN® 21 Tablets is started later than the 8th day, the patient should be protected by another means of contraception until she has taken a tablet daily for seven consecutive days.

If spotting or breakthrough bleeding occurs, the patient is instructed to continue on the same regimen. This type of bleeding is usually transient and without significance; however, if the bleeding is persistent or prolonged, the patient is advised to consult her physician. Although the occurrence of pregnancy is highly unlikely if TRI-LEVLEN® 21 Tablets are taken according to directions, if withdrawal bleeding does not occur, the possibility of pregnancy must be considered. If the patient has not adhered to the prescribed schedule (missed one or more tablets or started taking them on a day later than she should have), the probability of pregnancy should be considered at the time of the first missed period and appropriate diagnostic measures taken before the medication is resumed. If the patient has adhered to the prescribed regimen and misses two consecutive periods, pregnancy should be ruled out before continuing the contraceptive regimen.

The risk of pregnancy increases with each active (brown, white, or light-yellow) tablet missed. For additional patient instructions regarding missed pills, see the "WHAT TO DO IF YOU MISS PILLS" section in the DETAILED PATIENT LABELING below. If breakthrough bleeding occurs following missed active tablets, it will usually be transient and of no consequence. If the patient misses one or more light-green tablets, she is still protected against pregnancy **provided** she begins taking brown tablets again on the proper day.

In the nonlactating mother, TRI-LEVLEN® 21 Tablets may be initiated postpartum, for contraception. When the tablets are administered in the postpartum period, the increased risk of thromboembolic disease associated with the postpartum period must be considered. (See "CONTRAINDICATIONS", "WARNINGS", and "PRECAUTIONS" concerning thromboembolic disease.) It is to be noted that early resumption of ovulation may occur if Parlodel® (bromocriptine mesylate) has been used for the prevention of lactation.

TRI-LEVLEN® 28 Tablets
To achieve maximum contraceptive effectiveness, TRI-LEVLEN® 28 Tablets (levonorgestrel and ethinyl estradiol tablets—triphasic regimen) should be taken exactly as directed and at intervals not exceeding 24-hours.

TRI-LEVLEN® 28 Tablets are a three-phase preparation plus 7 inert tablets. The dosage of TRI-LEVLEN® 28 Tablets is one tablet daily for 28 consecutive days per menstrual cycle in the following order: 6 brown tablets (phase 1), followed by 5 white tablets (phase 2), followed by 10 light-yellow tablets (phase 3), plus 7 light-green inert tablets according to the prescribed schedule.

It is recommended that TRI-LEVLEN® 28 Tablets be taken at the same time each day. During the first cycle of medication, the patient should be instructed to take one TRI-LEVLEN® 28 Tablet daily in the order of 6 brown, 5 white, 10 light-yellow tablets and then 7 light-green inert tablets for twenty-eight (28) consecutive days, beginning on day one (1) of her menstrual cycle. (The first day of menstruation is day one.) Withdrawal bleeding usually occurs

within 3 days following the last light-yellow tablet. (If an alternate starting regimen is used [Sunday Start or postpartum], contraceptive reliance should not be placed on TRI-LEVLEN® 28 Tablets until after the first 7 consecutive days of administration. The possibility of ovulation and conception prior to initiation of medication should be considered.)

The patient begins her next and all subsequent 28-day courses of TRI-LEVLEN® 28 Tablets on the same day of the week that she began her first course, following the same schedule. She begins taking her brown tablets on the next day after ingestion of the last light-green tablet, regardless of whether or not a menstrual period has occurred or is still in progress. Any time a subsequent cycle of TRI-LEVLEN® 28 Tablets is started later than the next day, the patient should be protected by another means of contraception until she has taken a tablet daily for seven consecutive days.

If spotting or breakthrough bleeding occurs, the patient is instructed to continue on the same regimen. This type of bleeding is usually transient and without significance; however, if the bleeding is persistent or prolonged, the patient is advised to consult her physician. Although the occurrence of pregnancy is highly unlikely if TRI-LEVLEN® 28 Tablets are taken according to directions, if withdrawal bleeding does not occur, the possibility of pregnancy must be considered. If the patient has not adhered to the prescribed schedule (missed one or more active tablets or started taking them on a day later than she should have), the probability of pregnancy should be considered at the time of the first missed period and appropriate diagnostic measures taken before the medication is resumed. If the patient has adhered to the prescribed regimen and misses two consecutive periods, pregnancy should be ruled out before continuing the contraceptive regimen.

The risk of pregnancy increases with each active (brown, white, or light-yellow) tablet missed. For additional patient instructions regarding missed pills, see the "WHAT TO DO IF YOU MISS PILLS" section in the DETAILED PATIENT LABELING below. If breakthrough bleeding occurs following missed active tablets, it will usually be transient and of no consequence. If the patient misses one or more light-green tablets, she is still protected against pregnancy **provided** she begins taking brown tablets again on the proper day.

In the nonlactating mother, TRI-LEVLEN® 28 Tablets may be initiated postpartum, for contraception. When the tablets are administered in the postpartum period, the increased risk of thromboembolic disease associated with the postpartum period must be considered. (See "CONTRAINDICATIONS", "WARNINGS", and "PRECAUTIONS" concerning thromboembolic disease.) It is to be noted that early resumption of ovulation may occur if Parlodel® (bromocriptine mesylate) has been used for the prevention of lactation.

LEVLEN® 21 Tablets
To achieve maximum contraceptive effectiveness, LEVLEN® 21 Tablets (levonorgestrel and ethinyl estradiol tablets) should be taken exactly as directed and at intervals not exceeding 24-hours.

The dosage of LEVLEN® 21 Tablets is **one tablet** daily for 21 consecutive days per menstrual cycle according to the prescribed schedule. Tablets are then discontinued for 7 days (three weeks on, one week off).

It is recommended that LEVLEN® 21 Tablets be taken at the same time each day. During the first cycle of medication, the patient should be instructed to take one LEVLEN® 21 Tablet daily for twenty-one (21) consecutive days, beginning on day one (1) of her menstrual cycle. (The first day of menstruation is day one.) The tablets are then discontinued for one week (7 days). Withdrawal bleeding usually occurs within 3 days following discontinuation of LEVLEN® 21 Tablets. (If an alternate starting regimen is used [Sunday Start or postpartum], contraceptive reliance should not be placed on LEVLEN® 21 Tablets until after the first 7 consecutive days of administration. The possibility of ovulation and conception prior to initiation of medication should be considered.)

The patient begins her next and all subsequent 21-day courses of LEVLEN® 21 Tablets on the same day of the week that she began her first course, following the same schedule: 21 days on—7 days off. She begins taking her light-orange tablets on the 8th day after discontinuance, regardless of whether or not a menstrual period has occurred or is still in progress. Any time the next cycle of LEVLEN® 21 Tablets is started later than the 8th day, the patient should be protected by another means of contraception until she has taken a tablet daily for seven consecutive days.

If spotting or breakthrough bleeding occurs, the patient is instructed to continue on the same regimen. This type of bleeding is usually transient and without significance; however, if the bleeding is persistent or prolonged, the patient is advised to consult her physician. Although the occurrence of pregnancy is highly unlikely if LEVLEN® 21 Tablets are taken according to directions, if withdrawal bleeding does not occur, the possibility of pregnancy must be considered. If the patient has not adhered to the prescribed schedule (missed one or more tablets or started taking them on a day

later than she should have), the probability of pregnancy should be considered at the time of the first missed period and appropriate diagnostic measures taken before the medication is resumed. If the patient has adhered to the prescribed regimen and misses two consecutive periods, pregnancy should be ruled out before continuing the contraceptive regimen.

In the nonlactating mother, LEVLEN® 21 Tablets may be initiated postpartum, for contraception. When the tablets are administered in the postpartum period, the increased risk of thromboembolic disease associated with the postpartum period must be considered. (See "CONTRAINDICATIONS", "WARNINGS", and "PRECAUTIONS" concerning thromboembolic disease.)

LEVLEN® 28 Tablets
To achieve maximum contraceptive effectiveness, LEVLEN® 28 Tablets (levonorgestrel and ethinyl estradiol tablets) should be taken exactly as directed at intervals not exceeding 24-hours.

The dosage of LEVLEN® 28 Tablets is one light-orange tablet daily for 21 consecutive days per menstrual cycle, followed by 7 pink inert tablets according to the prescribed schedule.

It is recommended that LEVLEN® 28 Tablets be taken at the same time each day. During the first cycle of medication, the patient should be instructed to take one LEVLEN® 28 Tablet daily in the order of 21 light orange and then 7 pink inert tablets for twenty-eight (28) consecutive days, beginning on day one (1) of her menstrual cycle. (The first day of menstruation is day one.) Withdrawal bleeding usually occurs within 3 days following the last light-orange tablet. (If an alternate starting regimen is used [Sunday Start or postpartum], contraceptive reliance should not be placed on LEVLEN® 28 Tablets until after the first 7 consecutive days of administration. The possibility of ovulation and conception prior to initiation of medication should be considered.)

The patient begins her next and all subsequent 28-day courses of LEVLEN® 28 Tablets on the same day of the week that she began her first course, following the same schedule. She begins taking her light-orange tablets on the next day after ingestion of the last pink tablet, regardless of whether or not a menstrual period has occurred or is still in progress. Any time a subsequent cycle of LEVLEN® 28 Tablets is started later than the next day, the patient should be protected by another means of contraception until she has taken a tablet daily for seven consecutive days.

If spotting or breakthrough bleeding occurs, the patient is instructed to continue on the same regimen. This type of bleeding is usually transient and without significance; however, if the bleeding is persistent or prolonged, the patient is advised to consult her physician. Although the occurrence of pregnancy is highly unlikely if LEVLEN® 28 Tablets are taken according to directions, if withdrawal bleeding does not occur, the possibility of pregnancy must be considered. If the patient has not adhered to the prescribed schedule (missed one or more active tablets or started taking them on a day later than she should have), the probability of pregnancy should be considered at the time of the first missed period and appropriate diagnostic measures taken before the medication is resumed. If the patient has adhered to the prescribed regimen and misses two consecutive periods, pregnancy should be ruled out before continuing the contraceptive regimen.

Any time the patient misses two or more tablets, she should also use another method of contraception until she has taken a tablet daily for seven consecutive days. If breakthrough bleeding occurs following missed active tablets, it usually will be transient and of no consequence. If the patient misses one or more pink tablets, she is still protected against pregnancy provided she begins taking the light-orange tablets again on the proper day.

In the nonlactating mother, LEVLEN® 28 Tablets may be initiated postpartum, for contraception. When the tablets are administered in the postpartum period, the increased risk of thromboembolic disease associated with the postpartum period must be considered. (See "CONTRAINDICATIONS", "WARNINGS", and "PRECAUTIONS" concerning thromboembolic disease.)

HOW SUPPLIED

TRI-LEVLEN® 21 tablets (Levonorgestrel and Ethinyl Estradiol Tablets—Triphasic Regimen), are available in packages of 3 and 6 SLIDECASE® dispensers. Each cycle contains 21 round, film-coated tablets as follows:
NDC 50419-195, six brown tablets marked "B" on one side and "95" on the other side, each containing 0.050 mg levonorgestrel and 0.030 mg ethinyl estradiol;
NDC 50419-196, five white to off-white tablets marked "B" on one side and "96" on the other side, each containing 0.075 mg levonorgestrel and 0.040 mg ethinyl estradiol; and
NDC 50419-197, ten light-yellow tablets marked "B" on one side and "97" on the other side, each containing 0.125 mg levonorgestrel and 0.030 mg ethinyl estradiol.
In packages of:
3 SLIDECASE® dispensers .... NDC 50419-432-03
6 SLIDECASE® dispensers .... NDC 50419-432-06

TRI-LEVLEN® 28 tablets (Levonorgestrel and Ethinyl Estradiol Tablets—Triphasic Regimen), are available in packages of 3 and 6 SLIDECASE® dispensers. Each cycle contains 28 round, film-coated tablets as follows:
NDC 50419-195, six brown tablets marked "B" on one side and "95" on the other side, each containing 0.050 mg levonorgestrel and 0.030 mg ethinyl estradiol;
NDC 50419-196, five white to off-white tablets marked "B" on one side and "96" on the other side, each containing 0.075 mg levonorgestrel and 0.040 mg ethinyl estradiol;
NDC 50419-197, ten light-yellow tablets marked "B" on one side and "97" on the other side, each containing 0.125 mg levonorgestrel and 0.030 mg ethinyl estradiol; and
NDC 50419-111, seven light-green inert tablets marked "B" on one side and "11" on the other side.
In packages of:
3 SLIDECASE® dispensers .... NDC 50419-433-03
6 SLIDECASE® dispensers .... NDC 50419-433-06

LEVLEN® 21 tablets (Levonorgestrel and Ethinyl Estradiol Tablets), are available in packages of 3 SLIDECASE® dispensers. Each cycle contains 21 round, tablets as follows:
NDC 50419-021, 21 active, light-orange tablets marked "B" on one side and "21" on the other side, each containing 0.15 mg levonorgestrel and 0.03 mg ethinyl estradiol;
In packages of:
3 SLIDECASE® dispensers .... NDC 50419-410-21

LEVLEN® 28 tablets (Levonorgestrel and Ethinyl Estradiol Tablets), are available in packages of 3 SLIDECASE® dispensers. Each cycle contains 28 round tablets as follows:
NDC 50419-021, 21 active, light-orange tablets marked "B" on one side and "21" on the other side, each containing 0.15 mg levonorgestrel and 0.03 mg ethinyl estradiol;
NDC 50419-028, 7 inert pink tablets marked "B" on one side and "28" on the other side.
In packages of:
3 SLIDECASE® dispensers .... NDC 50419-411-28

REFERENCES

References furnished upon request.

BRIEF SUMMARY PATIENT PACKAGE INSERT

This product (like all oral contraceptives) is intended to prevent pregnancy. It does not protect against HIV infection (AIDS) and other sexually transmitted diseases.

Oral contraceptives, also known as "birth control pills" or "the pill," are taken to prevent pregnancy and when taken correctly, have a failure rate of less than 1% per year when used without missing any pills. The typical failure rate of large numbers of pill users is less than 3% per year when women who miss pills are included. For most women oral contraceptives are also free of serious or unpleasant side effects. However, forgetting to take pills considerably increases the chances of pregnancy.

For the majority of women, oral contraceptives can be taken safely. But there are some women who are at high risk of developing certain serious diseases that can be life-threatening or may cause temporary or permanent disability or death. The risks associated with taking oral contraceptives increase significantly if you:

- smoke
- have high blood pressure, diabetes, high cholesterol
- have or have had clotting disorders, heart attack, stroke, angina pectoris, cancer of the breast or sex organs, jaundice or malignant or benign liver tumors

You should not take the pill if you suspect you are pregnant or have unexplained vaginal bleeding.

Cigarette smoking increases the risk of serious adverse effects on the heart and blood vessels from oral-contraceptive use. This risk increases with age and with heavy smoking (15 or more cigarettes per day) and is quite marked in women over 35 years of age. Women who use oral contraceptives are strongly advised not to smoke.

Most side effects of the pill are not serious. The most common such effects are nausea, vomiting, bleeding between menstrual periods, weight gain, breast tenderness, and difficulty wearing contact lenses. These side effects, especially nausea, and vomiting, may subside within the first three months of use.

The serious side effects of the pill occur very infrequently, especially if you are in good health and do not smoke. However, you should know that the following medical conditions have been associated with or made worse by the pill:

1. Blood clots in the legs (thrombophlebitis), lungs (pulmonary embolism), stoppage or rupture of a blood vessel in the brain (stroke), blockage of blood vessels in the heart (heart attack or angina pectoris) or other organs of the body. As mentioned above, smoking increases the risk of heart attacks and strokes and subsequent serious medical consequences.
2. Liver tumors, which may rupture and cause severe bleeding. A possible but not definite association has been found with the pill and liver cancer. However, liver cancers are extremely rare. The chance of developing liver cancer from using the pill is thus even rarer.
3. High blood pressure, although blood pressure usually returns to normal when the pill is stopped.

The symptoms associated with these serious side effects are discussed in the detailed leaflet given to you with your supply of pills. Notify your doctor or health-care provider if you notice any unusual physical disturbances while taking the pill. In addition, drugs such as rifampin, as well as some anticonvulsants and some antibiotics may decrease oral contraceptive effectiveness.

Studies to date of women taking the pill have not shown an increase in the incidence of cancer of the breast or cervix. There is, however, insufficient evidence to rule out the possibility that pills may cause such cancers.

Taking the pill provides some important noncontraceptive benefits. These include less painful menstruation, less menstrual blood loss and anemia, fewer pelvic infections, and fewer cancers of the ovary and the lining of the uterus.

Be sure to discuss any medical condition you may have with your health-care provider. Your health-care provider will take a medical and family history before prescribing oral contraceptives and will examine you.

You should be reexamined at least once a year while taking oral contraceptives. The "Detailed Patient Labeling" gives you further information which you should read and discuss with your health-care provider.

DETAILED PATIENT LABELING

This product (like all oral contraceptives) is intended to prevent pregnancy. It does not protect against HIV infection (AIDS) and other sexually transmitted diseases.

INTRODUCTION

Any woman who considers using oral contraceptives (the "birth control pill" or the "pill") should understand the benefits and risks of using this form of birth control. This leaflet will give you much of the information you will need to make this decision and will also help you determine if you are at risk of developing any of the serious side effects of the pill. It will tell you how to use the pill properly so that it will be as effective as possible. However, this leaflet is not a replacement for a careful discussion between you and your health-care provider. You should discuss the information provided in this leaflet with him or her, both when you first start taking the pill and during your revisits. You should also follow your health-care provider's advice with regard to regular check-ups while you are on the pill.

EFFECTIVENESS OF ORAL CONTRACEPTIVES

Oral contraceptives or "birth control pills" or "the pill" are used to prevent pregnancy and are more effective than other nonsurgical methods of birth control. When they are taken correctly, the chance of becoming pregnant is less than 1% when used perfectly, without missing pills.

Typical failure rates are less than 3.0% per year. The chance of becoming pregnant increases with each missed pill during the menstrual cycle.

In comparison, typical failure rates for other nonsurgical methods of birth control during the first year of use are as follows:

Implant	<1%
Injection (Depo-Provera)	<1%
IUD	3%
Diaphragm with spermicides	18%
Spermicides alone	21%
Vaginal sponge	18%–28%
Condom alone	12%
Periodic abstinence	20%
No methods	85%

WHO SHOULD NOT TAKE ORAL CONTRACEPTIVES

Cigarette smoking increases the risk of serious adverse effects on the heart and blood vessels from oral-contraceptive use. This risk increases with age and with heavy smoking (15 or more cigarettes per day) and is quite marked in women over 35 years of age. Women who use oral contraceptives are strongly advised not to smoke.

Some women should not use the pill. For example, you should not take the pill if you are pregnant or think you may be pregnant. You should also not use the pill if you have had any of the following conditions:

- Heart attack or stroke
- Blood clots in the legs (thrombophlebitis), lungs (pulmonary embolism), or eyes
- Blood clots in the deep veins of your legs
- Known or suspected breast cancer or cancer of the lining of the uterus, cervix or vagina
- Liver tumor (benign or cancerous)

Or, if you have any of the following:

- Chest pain (angina pectoris)
- Unexplained vaginal bleeding (until a diagnosis is reached by your doctor)
- Yellowing of the whites of the eyes or of the skin (jaundice) during pregnancy or during previous use of the pill
- Known or suspected pregnancy

Tell your health-care provider if you have ever had any of these conditions. Your health-care provider can recommend another method of birth control.

OTHER CONSIDERATIONS BEFORE TAKING ORAL CONTRACEPTIVES

Tell your health-care provider if you or any family member has ever had:

- Breast nodules, fibrocystic disease of the breast, an abnormal breast x-ray or mammogram
- Diabetes
- Elevated cholesterol or triglycerides
- High blood pressure
- Migraine or other headaches or epilepsy
- Mental depression
- Gallbladder, heart or kidney disease
- History of scanty or irregular menstrual periods

Women with any of these conditions should be checked often by their health-care provider if they choose to use oral contraceptives. Also, be sure to inform your doctor or health-care provider if you smoke or are on any medications.

RISKS OF TAKING ORAL CONTRACEPTIVES

1. RISK OF DEVELOPING BLOOD CLOTS

Blood clots and blockage of blood vessels are the most serious side effects of taking oral contraceptives and can be fatal. In particular, a clot in the legs can cause thrombophlebitis and a clot that travels to the lungs can cause a sudden blocking of the vessel carrying blood to the lungs. Rarely, clots occur in the blood vessels of the eye and may cause blindness, double vision, or impaired vision.

If you take oral contraceptives and need elective surgery, need to stay in bed for a prolonged illness or have recently delivered a baby, you may be at risk of developing blood clots. You should consult your doctor about stopping oral contraceptives three to four weeks before surgery and not taking oral contraceptives for 2 weeks after surgery or during bed rest. You should also not take oral contraceptives soon after delivery of a baby or a midtrimester pregnancy termination. It is advisable to wait for at least 4 weeks after delivery if you are not breast-feeding. If you are breast-feeding, you should wait until you have weaned your child before using the pill. (See also the section on Breast-Feeding in "GENERAL PRECAUTIONS".)

2. HEART ATTACKS AND STROKES

Oral contraceptives may increase the tendency to develop strokes (stoppage or rupture of blood vessels in the brain) and angina pectoris and heart attacks (blockage of blood vessels in the heart). Any of these conditions can cause death or serious disability.

Smoking greatly increases the possibility of suffering heart attacks and strokes. Furthermore, smoking and the use of oral contraceptives greatly increase the chances of developing and dying of heart disease.

3. GALLBLADDER DISEASE

Oral-contraceptive users probably have a greater risk than nonusers of having gallbladder disease, although this risk may be related to pills containing high doses of estrogens.

4. LIVER TUMORS

In rare cases, oral contraceptives can cause benign but dangerous liver tumors. These benign liver tumors can rupture and cause fatal internal bleeding. In addition, a possible but not definite association has been found with the pill and liver cancers in two studies, in which a few women who developed these very rare cancers were found to have used oral contraceptives for long periods. However, liver cancers are extremely rare. The chance of developing liver cancer from using the pill is thus even rarer.

5. CANCER OF THE REPRODUCTIVE ORGANS

There is, at present, no confirmed evidence that oral contraceptives increase the risk of cancer of the reproductive organs in human studies. Several studies have found no overall increase in the risk of developing breast cancer. However, women who use oral contraceptives and have a strong family history of breast cancer or who have breast nodules or abnormal mammograms should be closely followed by their doctors.

Some studies have found an increase in the incidence of cancer of the cervix in women who use oral contraceptives. However, this finding may be related to factors other than the use of oral contraceptives.

Continued on next page

Information on the Berlex products appearing here is based on the most current information available at the time of publication closing. Further information for these and other products may be obtained from the Medical Affairs Department, Berlex Laboratories, 300 Fairfield Road, Wayne, New Jersey 07470, 1-888-BERLEX-4. Information on Betaseron and Fludara may be obtained from Berlex Laboratories, 15049 San Pablo Avenue, Richmond, California 94804-0016, 1-800-888-4112.

Levlen/Tri-Levlen—Cont.

ESTIMATED RISK OF DEATH FROM A BIRTH-CONTROL METHOD OR PREGNANCY

All methods of birth control and pregnancy are associated with a risk of developing certain diseases which may lead to disability or death. An estimate of the number of deaths associated with different methods of birth control and pregnancy has been calculated and is shown in the following table.

[See table below]

In the above table, the risk of death from any birth-control method is less than the risk of childbirth, except for oral contraceptive users over the age of 35 who smoke and pill users over the age of 40 even if they do not smoke. It can be seen in the table that for women aged 15 to 39, the risk of death is highest with pregnancy (7 to 26 deaths per 100,000 women, depending on age). Among pill users who do not smoke, the risk of death was always lower than that associated with pregnancy for any age group, except for those women over the age of 40 when the risk increases to 32 deaths per 100,000 women, compared to 28 associated with pregnancy at that age. However, for pill users who smoke and are over the age of 35, the estimated number of deaths exceeds those for other methods of birth control. If a woman is over the age of 40 and smokes, her estimated risk of death is four times higher (117/100,000 women) than the estimated risk associated with pregnancy (28/100,000 women) in that age group.

The suggestion that women over 40 who don't smoke should not take oral contraceptives is based on information from older high-dose pills and on less-selective use of pills than is practiced today. An Advisory Committee of the FDA discussed this issue in 1989 and recommended that the benefits of oral-contraceptive use by healthy, nonsmoking women over 40 years of age may outweigh the possible risks. However, all women, especially older women, are cautioned to use the lowest-dose pill that is effective.

WARNING SIGNALS

If any of these adverse effects occur while you are taking oral contraceptives, call your doctor immediately:

- Sharp chest pain, coughing of blood, or sudden shortness of breath (indicating a possible clot in the lung).
- Pain in the calf (indicating a possible clot in the leg).
- Crushing chest pain or heaviness in the chest (indicating a possible heart attack).
- Sudden severe headache or vomiting, dizziness or fainting, disturbances of vision or speech, weakness, or numbness in an arm or leg (indicating a possible stroke).
- Sudden partial or complete loss of vision (indicating a possible clot in the eye).
- Breast lumps (indicating possible breast cancer or fibrocystic disease of the breast; ask your doctor or health-care provider to show you how to examine your breasts).
- Severe pain or tenderness in the stomach area (indicating a possibly ruptured liver tumor).
- Difficulty in sleeping, weakness, lack of energy, fatigue, or change in mood (possibly indicating severe depression).
- Jaundice or a yellowing of the skin or eyeballs, accompanied frequently by fever, fatigue, loss of appetite, dark-colored urine, or light-colored bowel movements (indicating possible liver problems).

SIDE EFFECTS OF ORAL CONTRACEPTIVES

1. VAGINAL BLEEDING

Irregular vaginal bleeding or spotting may occur while you are taking the pills. Irregular bleeding may vary from slight staining between menstrual periods to breakthrough bleeding which is a flow much like a regular period. Irregular bleeding occurs most often during the first few months of oral contraceptive use, but may also occur after you have been taking the pill for some time. Such bleeding may be temporary and usually does not indicate any serious problems. It is important to continue taking your pills on schedule. If the bleeding occurs in more than one cycle or lasts for more than a few days, talk to your doctor or health-care provider.

2. CONTACT LENSES

If you wear contact lenses and notice a change in vision or an inability to wear your lenses, contact your doctor or health-care provider.

3. FLUID RETENTION

Oral contraceptives may cause edema (fluid retention) with swelling of the fingers or ankles and may raise your blood pressure. If you experience fluid retention, contact your doctor or health-care provider.

4. MELASMA

A spotty darkening of the skin is possible, particularly of the face.

5. OTHER SIDE EFFECTS

Other side effects may include change in appetite, headache, nervousness, depression, dizziness, loss of scalp hair, rash, and vaginal infections.

If any of these side effects bother you, call your doctor or health-care provider.

GENERAL PRECAUTIONS

1. Missed periods and use of oral contraceptives before or during early pregnancy.

There may be times when you may not menstruate regularly after you have completed taking a cycle of pills. If you have taken your pills regularly and miss one menstrual period, continue taking your pills for the next cycle but be sure to inform your health-care provider before doing so. If you have not taken the pills daily as instructed and missed a menstrual period, or if you missed two consecutive menstrual periods, you may be pregnant. Check with your health-care provider immediately to determine whether you are pregnant. Do not continue to take oral contraceptives until you are sure you are not pregnant, but continue to use another method of contraception.

There is no conclusive evidence that oral contraceptive use is associated with an increase in birth defects, when taken inadvertently during early pregnancy. Previously, a few studies had reported that oral contraceptives might be associated with birth defects, but these studies have not been confirmed. Nevertheless, oral contraceptives or any other drugs should not be used during pregnancy unless clearly necessary and prescribed by your doctor. You should check with your doctor about risks to your unborn child of any medication taken during pregnancy.

2. While breast-feeding

If you are breast-feeding, consult your doctor before starting oral contraceptives. Some of the drug will be passed on to the child in the milk. A few adverse effects on the child have been reported, including yellowing of the skin (jaundice) and breast enlargement. In addition, oral contraceptives may decrease the amount and quality of your milk. If possible, do not use oral contraceptives while breast-feeding. You should use another method of contraception since breast-feeding provides only partial protection from becoming pregnant and this partial protection decreases significantly as you breast-feed for longer periods of time. You should consider starting oral contraceptives only after you have weaned your child completely.

3. Laboratory tests

If you are scheduled for any laboratory tests, tell your doctor you are taking birth-control pills. Certain blood tests may be affected by birth-control pills.

4. Drug interactions

Certain drugs may interact with birth control pills to make them less effective in preventing pregnancy or cause an increase in breakthrough bleeding. Such drugs include rifampin, drugs used for epilepsy such as barbiturates (for example, phenobarbital) and phenytoin (Dilantin is one brand of this drug), phenylbutazone (Butazolidin is one brand) and possibly certain antibiotics. You may need to use an additional method of contraception during any cycle in which you take drugs that can make oral contraceptives less effective.

This product (like all oral contraceptives) is intended to prevent pregnancy. It does not protect against transmission of HIV (AIDS) and other sexually transmitted diseases such as Chlamydia, genital herpes, genital warts, gonorrhea, hepatitis B, and Syphilis.

HOW TO TAKE THE PILL

IMPORTANT POINTS TO REMEMBER

TRI-LEVLEN® and LEVLEN® Tablets
BEFORE YOU START TAKING YOUR PILLS:

1. BE SURE TO READ THESE DIRECTIONS:
   Before you start taking your pills.
   Anytime you are not sure what to do.
2. THE RIGHT WAY TO TAKE THE PILL IS TO TAKE ONE PILL EVERY DAY AT THE SAME TIME.
   If you miss pills you could get pregnant. This includes starting the pack late.
   The more pills you miss, the more likely you are to get pregnant.
3. MANY WOMEN HAVE SPOTTING OR LIGHT BLEEDING, OR MAY FEEL SICK TO THEIR STOMACH DURING THE FIRST 1-3 PACKS OF PILLS.
   If you do feel sick to your stomach, do not stop taking the pill. The problem will usually go away. If it doesn't go away, check with your doctor or clinic.
4. MISSING PILLS CAN ALSO CAUSE SPOTTING OR LIGHT BLEEDING, even when you make up these missed pills.
   On the days you take 2 pills, to make up for missed pills, you could also feel a little sick to your stomach.
5. IF YOU HAVE VOMITING OR DIARRHEA, for any reason, or IF YOU TAKE SOME MEDICINES, including some antibiotics, your pills may not work as well.
   Use a back-up method (such as condoms, foam, or sponge) until you check with your doctor or clinic.
6. IF YOU HAVE TROUBLE REMEMBERING TO TAKE THE PILL, talk to your doctor or clinic about how to make pill-taking easier or about using another method of birth control.
7. IF YOU HAVE ANY QUESTIONS OR ARE UNSURE ABOUT THE INFORMATION IN THIS LEAFLET, call your doctor or clinic.
8. THIS PRODUCT (LIKE ALL ORAL CONTRACEPTIVES) IS INTENDED TO PREVENT PREGNANCY. IT DOES NOT PROTECT AGAINST TRANSMISSION OF HIV (AIDS) AND OTHER SEXUALLY TRANSMITTED DISEASES SUCH AS CHLAMYDIA, GENITAL HERPES, GENITAL WARTS, GONORRHEA, HEPATITIS B, AND SYPHILIS.

BEFORE YOU START TAKING YOUR PILLS

TRI-LEVLEN® Tablets

1. DECIDE WHAT TIME OF DAY YOU WANT TO TAKE YOUR PILL.
   It is important to take it at about the same time every day.
2. LOOK AT YOUR PILL PACK TO SEE IF IT HAS 21 OR 28 PILLS:
   The 21-pill pack has 21 "active" (6 brown, 5 white and 10 light-yellow) pills (with hormones) to take for 3 weeks, followed by 1 week without pills.
   The 28-pill pack has 21 "active" (6 brown, 5 white and 10 light yellow) pills (with hormones) to take for 3 weeks, followed by 1 week of reminder (light-green) pills (without hormones).
3. ALSO FIND:
   1) where on the pack to start taking pills.
   2) in what order to take the pills (follow the arrows)

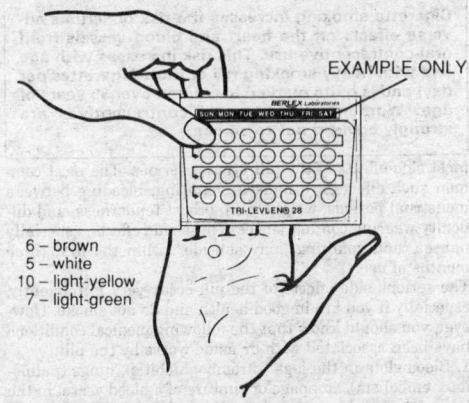

EXAMPLE ONLY

6 — brown
5 — white
10 — light-yellow
7 — light-green

4. BE SURE YOU HAVE READY AT ALL TIMES:
   ANOTHER KIND OF BIRTH CONTROL (such as condoms, foam or sponge) to use as a back-up in case you miss pills.
   AN EXTRA, FULL PILL PACK.

LEVLEN® Tablets
1. DECIDE WHAT TIME OF DAY YOU WANT TO TAKE YOUR PILL.

ANNUAL NUMBER OF BIRTH-RELATED OR METHOD-RELATED DEATHS ASSOCIATED WITH CONTROL OF FERTILITY PER 100,000 NONSTERILE WOMEN, BY FERTILITY-CONTROL METHOD ACCORDING TO AGE

Method of control and outcome	15–19	20–24	25–29	30–34	35–39	40–44
No fertility-control methods*	7.0	7.4	9.1	14.8	25.7	28.2
Oral contraceptives nonsmoker**	0.3	0.5	0.9	1.9	13.8	31.6
Oral contraceptives smoker**	2.2	3.4	6.6	13.5	51.1	117.2
IUD**	0.8	0.8	1.0	1.0	1.4	1.4
Condom*	1.1	1.6	0.7	0.2	0.3	0.4
Diaphragm/spermicide*	1.9	1.2	1.2	1.3	2.2	2.8
Periodic abstinence*	2.5	1.6	1.6	1.7	2.9	3.6

* Deaths are birth related
** Deaths are method related

It is important to take it at about the same time every day.

2. LOOK AT YOUR PILL PACK TO SEE IF IT HAS 21 OR 28 PILLS:

The 21-pill pack has 21 "active" (light-orange) pills (with hormones) to take for 3 weeks, followed by 1 week without pills.

The 28-pill pack has 21 "active" (light-orange) pills (with hormones) to take for 3 weeks, followed by 1 week of reminder (pink) pills (without hormones).

3. ALSO FIND:
   1) where on the pack to start taking pills.
   2) in what order to take the pills (follow the arrows).

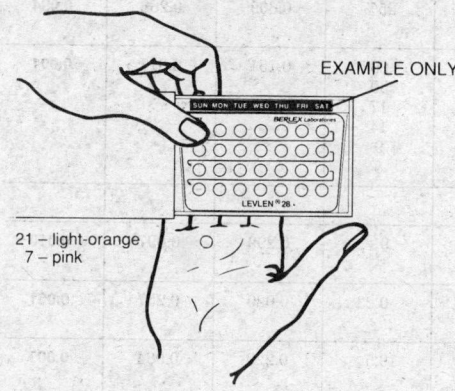

EXAMPLE ONLY

21 – light-orange
7 – pink

4. BE SURE YOU HAVE READY AT ALL TIMES:
ANOTHER KIND OF BIRTH CONTROL (such as condoms, foam or sponge) to use as a back-up in case you miss pills.
AN EXTRA, FULL PILL PACK.

WHEN TO START THE FIRST PACK OF PILLS

TRI-LEVLEN® Tablets
You have a choice for which day to start taking your first pack of pills. Decide with your doctor or clinic which is the best day for you. Pick a time of day which will be easy to remember.

DAY 1 START:
1. Take the first "active" (brown) pill of the first pack during the first 24 hours of your period.
2. You will not need to use a back-up method of birth control, since you are starting the pill at the beginning of your period.

SUNDAY START:
1. Take the first "active" (brown) pill of the first pack on the Sunday after your period starts, even if you are still bleeding. If your period begins on Sunday, start the pack that same day.
2. Use another method of birth control as a back-up method if you have sex anytime from the Sunday you start your first pack until the next Sunday (7 days). Condoms, foam, or the sponge are good back-up methods of birth control.

LEVLEN® Tablets
You have a choice for which day to start taking your first pack of pills. Decide with your doctor or clinic which is the best day for you. Pick a time of day which will be easy to remember.

DAY 1 START:
1. Take the first "active" (light-orange) pill of the first pack during the first 24 hours of your period.
2. You will not need to use a back-up method of birth control, since you are starting the pill at the beginning of your period.

SUNDAY START:
1. Take the first "active" (light-orange) pill of the first pack on the Sunday after your period starts, even if you are still bleeding. If your period begins on Sunday, start the pack that same day.
2. Use another method of birth control as a back-up method if you have sex anytime from the Sunday you start your first pack until the next Sunday (7 days). Condoms, foam, or the sponge are good back-up methods of birth control.

WHAT TO DO DURING THE MONTH

TRI-LEVLEN® and LEVLEN® Tablets
1. **TAKE ONE PILL AT THE SAME TIME EVERY DAY UNTIL THE PACK IS EMPTY.**
Do not skip pills even if you are spotting or bleeding between monthly periods or feel sick to your stomach (nausea).
Do not skip pills even if you do not have sex very often.
2. **WHEN YOU FINISH A PACK OR SWITCH YOUR BRAND OF PILLS:**
21 pills: Wait 7 days to start the next pack. You will prob-

ably have your period during that week. Be sure that no more than 7 days pass between 21-day packs.
28 pills: Start the next pack on the day after your last "reminder" pill.
Do not wait any days between packs.

WHAT TO DO IF YOU MISS PILLS

TRI-LEVLEN® Tablets
If you **MISS 1** (brown, white or light-yellow) "active" pill:
1. Take it as soon as you remember. Take the next pill at your regular time. This means you may take 2 pills in 1 day.
2. You do not need to use a back-up birth control method if you have sex.
If you **MISS 2** (brown or white) "active" pills in a row in **WEEK 1 OR WEEK 2** of your pack:
1. Take 2 pills on the day you remember and 2 pills the next day.
2. Then take 1 pill a day until you finish the pack.
3. YOU MAY BECOME PREGNANT if you have sex in the 7 days after you miss pills. You MUST use another birth control method (such as condoms, foam, or sponge) as a back-up for those 7 days.
If you **MISS 2** (light-yellow) "active" pills in a row in **THE 3rd WEEK:**
1. *If you are a Day 1 Starter:*
THROW OUT the rest of the pill pack and start a new pack that same day.
If you are a Sunday Starter:
Keep taking 1 pill every day until Sunday. On Sunday. THROW OUT the rest of the pack and start a new pack of pills that same day.
2. You may not have your period this month but this is expected. However, if you miss your period 2 months in a row, call your doctor or clinic because you might be pregnant.
3. You MAY BECOME PREGNANT if you have sex in the 7 days after you miss pills. You MUST use another birth control method (such as condoms, foam, or sponge) as a back-up for those 7 days.
If you **MISS 3 OR MORE** (brown, white or light-yellow) "active" pills in a row (during the first 3 weeks).
1. *If you are a Day 1 Starter:*
THROW OUT the rest of the pill pack and start a new pack that same day
If you are a Sunday Starter:
Keep taking 1 pill every day until Sunday. On Sunday. THROW OUT the rest of the pack and start a new pack of pills that same day.
2. You may not have your period this month but this is expected. However, if you miss your period 2 months in a row, call your doctor or clinic because you might be pregnant.
3. You MAY BECOME PREGNANT if you have sex in the 7 days after you miss pills. You MUST use another birth control method (such as condoms, foam, or sponge) as a back-up for those 7 days.

A REMINDER FOR THOSE ON 28-DAY PACKS:
If you forget any of the 7 (light-green) "reminder" pills in Week 4:
THROW AWAY the pills you missed.
Keep taking 1 pill each day until the pack is empty.
You do not need a back-up method if you start your next pack on time.

FINALLY, IF YOU ARE STILL NOT SURE WHAT TO DO ABOUT THE PILLS YOU HAVE MISSED:
Use a BACK-UP METHOD anytime you have sex.
KEEP TAKING ONE "ACTIVE" PILL EACH DAY until you can reach your doctor or clinic.

LEVLEN® Tablets
If you **MISS 1** (light-orange) "active" pill:
1. Take it as soon as you remember. Take the next pill at your regular time. This means you may take 2 pills in 1 day.
2. You do not need to use a back-up birth control method if you have sex.
If you **MISS 2** (light-orange) "active" pills in a row in **WEEK 1 OR WEEK 2** of your pack:
1. Take 2 pills on the day you remember and 2 pills the next day.
2. Then take 1 pill a day until you finish the pack.
3. You MAY BECOME PREGNANT if you have sex in the 7 days after you miss pills. You MUST use another birth control method (such as condoms, foam, or sponge) as a back-up for those 7 days.
If you **MISS 2** (light-orange) "active" pills in a row in **THE 3rd WEEK:**
1. *If you are a Day 1 Starter:*
THROW OUT the rest of the pill pack and start a new pack that same day.

If you are a Sunday Starter:
Keep taking 1 pill every day until Sunday. On Sunday. THROW OUT the rest of the pack and start a new pack of pills that same day.
2. You may not have your period this month but this is expected. However, if you miss your period 2 months in a row, call your doctor or clinic because you might be pregnant.
3. You MAY BECOME PREGNANT if you have sex in the 7 days after you miss pills. You MUST use another birth control method (such as condoms, foam, or sponge) as a back-up for those 7 days.
If you **MISS 3 OR MORE** (light-orange) "active" pills in a row (during the first 3 weeks).
1. *If you are a Day 1 Starter:*
THROW OUT the rest of the pill pack and start a new pack that same day
If you are a Sunday Starter:
Keep taking 1 pill every day until Sunday. On Sunday. THROW OUT the rest of the pack and start a new pack of pills that same day.
2. You may not have your period this month but this is expected. However, if you miss your period 2 months in a row, call your doctor or clinic because you might be pregnant.
3. You MAY BECOME PREGNANT if you have sex in the 7 days after you miss pills. You MUST use another birth control method (such as condoms, foam, or sponge) as a back-up for those 7 days.

A REMINDER FOR THOSE ON 28-DAY PACKS:
If you forget any of the 7 (pink) "reminder" pills in Week 4:
THROW AWAY the pills you missed.
Keep taking 1 pill each day until the pack is empty.
You do not need a back-up method if you start your next pack on time.

FINALLY, IF YOU ARE STILL NOT SURE WHAT TO DO ABOUT THE PILLS YOU HAVE MISSED:
Use a BACK-UP METHOD anytime you have sex.
KEEP TAKING ONE "ACTIVE" PILL EACH DAY until you can reach your doctor or clinic.

PREGNANCY DUE TO PILL FAILURE
The incidence of pill failure resulting in pregnancy is approximately less than 1.0% if taken every day as directed, but more typical failure rates are less than 3.0%. If failure does occur, the risk to the fetus is minimal.
RISKS TO THE FETUS
If you do become pregnant while using oral contraceptives, the risk to the fetus is small, on the order of no more than one per thousand. You should, however, discuss the risks to the developing child with your doctor.
PREGNANCY AFTER STOPPING THE PILL
There may be some delay in becoming pregnant after you stop using oral contraceptives, especially if you had irregular menstrual cycles before you used oral contraceptives. It may be advisable to postpone conception until you begin menstruating regularly once you have stopped taking the pill and desire pregnancy.
There does not appear to be any increase in birth defects in newborn babies when pregnancy occurs soon after stopping the pill.
OVERDOSAGE
Serious ill effects have not been reported following ingestion of large doses of oral contraceptives by young children. Overdosage may cause nausea and withdrawal bleeding in females. In case of overdosage, contact your health-care provider or pharmacist.
OTHER INFORMATION
Your health-care provider will take a medical and family history before prescribing oral contraceptives and will examine you. You should be reexamined at least once a year. Be sure to inform your health-care provider if there is a family history of any of the conditions listed previously in this leaflet. Be sure to keep all appointments with your health-care provider, because this is a time to determine if there are early signs of side effects of oral-contraceptive use. Do not use the drug for any condition other than the one for which it was prescribed. This drug has been prescribed specifically for you; do not give it to others who may want birth-control pills.

Continued on next page

Information on the Berlex products appearing here is based on the most current information available at the time of publication closing. Further information for these and other products may be obtained from the Medical Affairs Department, Berlex Laboratories, 300 Fairfield Road, Wayne, New Jersey 07470, 1-888-BERLEX-4. Information on Betaseron and Fludara may be obtained from Berlex Laboratories, 15049 San Pablo Avenue, Richmond, California 94804-0016, 1-800-888-4112.

Levlen/Tri-Levlen—Cont.

HEALTH BENEFITS FROM ORAL CONTRACEPTIVES

In addition to preventing pregnancy, use of oral contraceptives may provide certain benefits. They are:

- Menstrual cycles may become more regular.
- Blood flow during menstruation may be lighter and less iron may be lost. Therefore, anemia due to iron deficiency is less likely to occur.
- Pain or other symptoms during menstruation may be encountered less frequently.
- Ovarian cysts may occur less frequently.
- Ectopic (tubal) pregnancy may occur less frequently.
- Noncancerous cysts or lumps in the breast may occur less frequently.
- Acute pelvic inflammatory disease may occur less frequently.
- Oral-contraceptive use may provide some protection against developing two forms of cancer: cancer of the ovaries and cancer of the lining of the uterus.

If you want more information about birth-control pills, ask your doctor or pharmacist. They have a more technical leaflet called the "Professional Labeling", which you may wish to read.

© 1996, Berlex Laboratories, All Rights Reserved.

Manufactured for:

BERLEX Laboratories, Wayne, NJ 07470

Revised July 1996	6070001
Revised Sept. 1996	6065802

Shown in Product Identification Guide, page 306

Berlex Laboratories
15049 SAN PABLO AVENUE, P.O. BOX 4099 RICHMOND, CA 94804-0099

Direct Inquiries to:
(973) 694-4100

For Medical Information and to Report Drug Adverse Events Contact:
Department of Epidemiology and Medical Affairs
300 Fairfield Road
Wayne, NJ 07470
(800) 888-2407

Betaseron for SC Injection Only:
(Medical Information Only)
15049 San Pablo Avenue
P.O. Box 4099
Richmond, CA 94804-0099
(800) 888-4112

Fludara For Injection Only:
(Medical Information Only)
15049 San Pablo Avenue
P.O. Box 4099
Richmond, CA 94804-0099
(800) 888-4112

BETASERON®
(Interferon beta-1b)   ℞

DESCRIPTION

Betaseron® (Interferon beta-1b) is a purified, sterile, lyophilized protein product produced by recombinant DNA techniques and formulated for use by injection. Interferon beta-1b is manufactured by bacterial fermentation of a strain of *Escherichia coli* that bears a genetically engineered plasmid containing the gene for human interferon beta$_{ser17}$. The native gene was obtained from human fibroblasts and altered in a way that substitutes serine for the cysteine residue found at position 17. Interferon beta-1b is a highly purified protein that has 165 amino acids and an approximate molecular weight of 18,500 daltons. It does not include the carbohydrate side chains found in the natural material.

The specific activity of Betaseron is approximately 32 million international units (IU)/mg Interferon beta-1b. Each vial contains 0.3 mg of Interferon beta-1b. The unit measurement is derived by comparing the antiviral activity of the product to the World Health Organization (WHO) reference standard of recombinant human interferon beta. Dextrose and Albumin Human, USP (15 mg each/vial) are added as stabilizers. Prior to 1993, a different analytical standard was used to determine potency. It assigned 54 million IU to 0.3 mg Interferon beta-1b.

Lyophilized Betaseron is a sterile, white to off-white powder intended for subcutaneous injection after reconstitution with the diluent supplied (Sodium Chloride, 0.54% Solution).

TABLE 1
2 Year Study Results
Primary and Secondary Clinical Endpoints

Efficacy Parameters	Treatment Groups			Statistical Comparisons p-value		
Primary Endpoints	Placebo (N=123)	0.05 mg (N=125)	0.25 mg (N=124)	Placebo vs 0.05 mg	0.05 mg vs 0.25 mg	Placebo vs 0.25 mg
Annual exacerbation rate	1.31	1.14	0.90	0.005	0.113	**0.0001**
Proportion of exacerbation-free patients†	16%	18%	25%	0.609	0.288	**0.094**
Exacerbation frequency per patient 0†	20	22	29	0.151	0.077	**0.001**
1	32	31	39			
2	20	28	17			
3	15	15	14			
4	15	7	9			
≥5	21	16	8			
Secondary Endpoints††						
Median number of months to first on-study exacerbation	5	6	9	0.299	0.097	**0.010**
Rate of moderate or severe exacerbations per year	0.47	0.29	0.23	0.020	0.257	**0.001**
Mean number of moderate or severe exacerbation days per patient	44.1	33.2	19.5	0.229	0.064	**0.001**
Mean change in EDSS score‡ at endpoint	0.21	0.21	−0.07	0.995	0.108	**0.144**
Mean change in Scripps score‡‡ at endpoint	−0.53	−0.50	0.66	0.641	0.051	**0.126**
Median duration in days per exacerbation	36	33	35.5	ND	ND	**ND**
% change in mean MRI lesion area at endpoint	21.4%	9.8%	−0.9%	0.015	0.019	**0.0001**

ND -Not done
† 14 exacerbation-free patients (0 from placebo, 6 from 0.05 mg, and 8 from 0.25 mg) dropped out of the study before completing 6 months of therapy. These patients are excluded from this analysis.
†† Sequelae and Functional Neurologic Status, both required by protocol, were not analyzed individually but are included as a function of the EDSS.
‡ EDSS scores range from 0–10, with higher scores reflecting greater disability.
‡‡ Scripps neurologic rating scores range from 0–100, with smaller scores reflecting greater disability.

CLINICAL PHARMACOLOGY

General: Interferons are a family of naturally occurring proteins, which have molecular weights ranging from 15,000 to 21,000 daltons. Three major classes of interferons have been identified: alfa, beta, and gamma. Interferon beta-1b, interferon alfa, and interferon gamma have overlapping yet distinct biologic activities.[1-5] The activities of Interferon beta-1b are species-restricted and, therefore, the most pertinent pharmacologic information on Betaseron is derived from studies of human cells in culture and in humans.

Biologic Activities: Interferon beta-1b has been shown to possess both antiviral and immunoregulatory activities. The mechanisms by which Betaseron exerts its actions in multiple sclerosis (MS) are not clearly understood. However, it is known that the biologic response-modifying properties of Interferon beta-1b are mediated through its interactions with specific cell receptors found on the surface of human cells. The binding of Interferon beta-1b to these receptors induces the expression of a number of interferon-induced gene products (e.g., 2′, 5′-oligoadenylate synthetase, protein kinase, and indoleamine 2, 3-dioxygenase) that are believed to be the mediators of the biological actions of Interferon beta-1b.[1,3,6-10] A number of these interferon-induced products have been readily measured in the serum and cellular fractions of blood collected from patients treated with Interferon beta-1b.[11,12]

Pharmacokinetics: Because serum concentrations of Interferon beta-1b are low or not detectable following subcutaneous administration of 0.25 mg or less of Betaseron, pharmacokinetic information in patients with MS receiving the recommended dose of Betaseron is not available. Following single and multiple daily subcutaneous administrations of 0.5 mg Betaseron to healthy volunteers (N=12), serum Interferon beta-1b concentrations were generally below 100 IU/mL. Peak serum Interferon beta-1b concentrations occurred between 1 to 8 hours, with a mean peak serum interferon concentration of 40 IU/mL. Bioavailability, based on a total dose of 0.5 mg Betaseron given as two subcutaneous injections at different sites, was approximately 50%.

After intravenous administration of Betaseron (0.006 mg to 2.0 mg), similar pharmacokinetic profiles were obtained from healthy volunteers (N=12) and from patients with diseases other than MS (N=142). In patients receiving single intravenous doses up to 2.0 mg, increases in serum concentrations were dose proportional. Mean serum clearance values ranged from 9.4 mL/min·kg^{-1} to 28.9 mL/min·kg^{-1} and were independent of dose. Mean terminal elimination half-life values ranged from 8.0 minutes to 4.3 hours and mean steady-state volume of distribution values ranged from 0.25 L/kg to 2.88 L/kg. Three-times-a-week intravenous dosing for 2 weeks resulted in no accumulation of Interferon beta-1b in the serum of patients. Pharmacokinetic parameters after single and multiple intravenous doses of Betaseron were comparable.

Clinical Trials: The effectiveness of Betaseron in relapsing-remitting MS was evaluated in a double-blind, multiclinic (11 sites: 4 Canadian and 7 United States), randomized, parallel, placebo-controlled clinical investigation of 2 years duration. The study enrolled MS patients, aged 18 to 50, who were ambulatory (Kurtzke expanded disability status scale [EDSS] of ≤5.5), exhibited a relapsing-remitting clinical course, met Poser's criteria[13] for clinically definite and/or laboratory supported definite MS and had experienced at least two exacerbations over 2 years preceding the trial without exacerbation in the preceding month. Patients who had received prior immunosuppressant therapy were excluded.

An exacerbation was defined, per protocol, as the appearance of a new clinical sign/symptom or the clinical worsening of a previous sign/symptom (one that had been stable for at least 30 days) that persisted for a minimum of 24 hours. Patients selected for study were randomized to treatment with either placebo (N=123), 0.05 mg of Betaseron (N=125), or 0.25 mg of Betaseron (N=124) self-administered subcutaneously every other day. Outcome based on the 372 randomized patients was evaluated after 2 years.

Patients who required more than three 28-day courses of corticosteroids were removed from the study. Minor analgesics (acetaminophen, codeine), antidepressants, and oral baclofen were allowed ad libitum but chronic nonsteroidal anti-inflammatory drug (NSAID) use was not allowed.

The primary, protocol defined, outcome assessment measures were 1) frequency of exacerbations per patient and 2) proportion of exacerbation free patients. A number of secondary outcome measures were also employed as described in Table 1.

In addition to clinical measures, annual magnetic resonance imaging (MRI) was performed and quantitated for extent of disease as determined by changes in total area of lesions. In a substudy of patients (N=52) at one site, MRIs were performed every 6 weeks and quantitated for disease activity as determined by changes in size and number of lesions.

Results at the protocol designated endpoint of 2 years (see TABLE 1): In the 2-year analysis, there was a 31% reduction in annual exacerbation rate, from 1.31 in the placebo group to 0.9 in the 0.25 mg group. The p-value for this difference was 0.0001. The proportion of patients free of exacerbations was 16% in the placebo group, compared with 25% in the Betaseron® (Interferon beta-1b) 0.25 mg group.

Of the 372 patients randomized, 72 (19%) failed to complete 2 full years on their assigned treatments. The reasons given for withdrawal varied with treatment assignment. Excessive use of steroids accounted for 11 of the 26 placebo withdrawals, but only 2 of the 21 withdrawals from the 0.05 mg assigned group and 1 of the 25 withdrawals from the 0.25 mg assigned group. Withdrawals for adverse events attributed to study article, however, were more common among Betaseron-treated patients: 1, 5, and 10 withdrew from the placebo, 0.05 mg, and 0.25 mg groups, respectively.

Over the 2-year period, there were 25 MS-related hospitalizations in the 0.25 mg Betaseron-treated group compared to 48 hospitalizations in the placebo group. In comparison, non-MS hospitalizations were evenly distributed among the groups, with 16 in the 0.25 mg Betaseron group and 15 in the placebo group. The average number of days of MS-related steroid use was 41 days in the 0.25 mg Betaseron group and 55 days in the placebo group (p=0.004).

MRI data were also analyzed for patients in this study. A frequency distribution of the observed percent changes in MRI area at the end of 2 years was obtained by grouping the percentages in successive intervals of equal width. Figure 1 displays a histogram of the proportions of patients who fell into each of these intervals. The median percent change in MRI area for the 0.25 mg group was −1.1% which was significantly smaller than the 16.5% observed for the placebo group (p=0.0001).

[See table 1 at top of previous page]

Figure 1
Distribution of Change in MRI Area

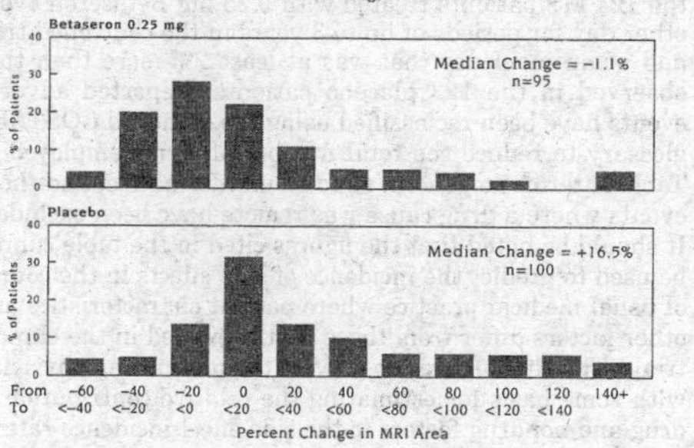

In an evaluation of frequent MRI scans (every 6 weeks) on 52 patients at one site, the percent of scans with new or expanding lesions was 29% in the placebo group and 6% in the 0.25 mg treatment group (p=0.006).

MRI scanning is viewed as a useful means to visualize changes in white matter that are believed to be a reflection of the pathologic changes that, appropriately located within the central nervous system (CNS), account for some of the signs and symptoms that typify relapsing-remitting MS. The exact relationship between MRI findings and the clinical status of patients is unknown. Changes in lesion area often do not correlate with clinical exacerbations probably because many of the lesions affect so-called "silent" regions of the CNS. Moreover, it is not clear what fraction of the lesions seen on MRI become foci of irreversible demyelinization (i.e., classic white matter plaques). The prognostic significance of the MRI findings in this study has not been evaluated.

At the end of 2 years on assigned treatment, patients in the study had the option of continuing on treatment under blinded conditions. Approximately 80% of patients under each treatment accepted. Although there was a trend toward patient benefit in the Betaseron groups during the third year, particularly in the 0.25 mg group, there was no statistically significant difference between the Betaseron-treated vs. placebo-treated patients in exacerbation rate, or in any of the secondary endpoints described in Table 1. As noted above, in the 2-year analysis, there was a 31% reduction in exacerbation rate in the 0.25 mg group, compared with placebo. The p-value for this difference was 0.0001. In the analysis of the third year alone, the difference between treatment groups was 28%. The p-value was 0.065. The lower number of patients may account for the loss of statistical significance, and lack of direct comparability among the patient groups in this extension study make the interpretation of these results difficult. The third year MRI data did not show a trend toward additional benefit in the Betaseron arm compared with the placebo arm.

Throughout the clinical trial, serum samples from patients were monitored for the development of antibodies to Interferon beta-1b. In patients receiving 0.25 mg of Betaseron (N=124) every other day in the clinical trial, 45% were found to have serum neutralizing activity at one or more of the time points tested. The relationship between antibody formation and clinical efficacy is not known.

INDICATIONS AND USAGE

Betaseron is indicated for use in ambulatory patients with relapsing-remitting multiple sclerosis to reduce the frequency of clinical exacerbations. (See **CLINICAL PHARMACOLOGY, Clinical Trials** section.) Relapsing-remitting MS is characterized by recurrent attacks of neurologic dysfunction followed by complete or incomplete recovery. The safety and efficacy of Betaseron in chronic-progressive MS has not been evaluated.

CONTRAINDICATIONS

Betaseron is contraindicated in patients with a history of hypersensitivity to natural or recombinant interferon beta, Albumin Human USP, or any other component of the formulation.

WARNINGS

One suicide and 4 attempted suicides were observed among 372 study patients during a 3-year period. All five patients received Betaseron (three in the 0.05 mg group and two in the 0.25 mg). There were no attempted suicides in patients on study who did not receive Betaseron. Depression and suicide have been reported to occur in patients receiving interferon alfa, a related compound. Patients to be treated with Betaseron should be informed that depression and suicidal ideation may be a side effect of the treatment and should report these symptoms immediately to the prescribing physician. Patients exhibiting depression should be monitored closely and cessation of therapy should be considered.

Injection site necrosis (ISN) has been reported in 5% of patients in controlled clinical trials (see **ADVERSE REACTIONS** section). Typically, injection site necrosis occurs within the first 4 months of therapy, although post-marketing reports have been received of ISN occurring over 1 year after initiation of therapy. Necrosis may occur at single or multiple injection sites. The necrotic lesions are typically 3 cm or less in diameter, but larger areas have been reported. While necrosis has commonly extended only to subcutaneous fat, there are also reports of necrosis extending to and including fascia overlaying muscle. In some lesions where biopsy results are available, vasculitis has been reported. For some lesions debridement and, infrequently, skin grafting has been required.

As with any open lesion, it is important to avoid infection and, if it occurs, to treat the infection. Time to healing has varied depending on the severity of the necrosis at the time treatment was begun. In most cases healing was associated with scarring.

Some patients have experienced healing of necrotic skin lesions while Betaseron therapy continued, others have not. Whether to discontinue therapy following a single site of necrosis is dependent on the extent of necrosis. For patients who continue therapy with Betaseron after injection site necrosis has occurred, Betaseron should not be administered into the afected area until it is fully healed. If multiple lesions occur, therapy should be discontinued until healing occurs.

Patient understanding and use of aseptic self-injection techniques and procedures should be periodically reevaluated, particularly if injection site necrosis has occured.

PRECAUTIONS

General: Patients should be instructed in injection techniques to assure the safe self-administration of Betaseron. (See **PRECAUTIONS: Information to patients,** and **Betaseron Patient Information** sheet.)

Information to patients:

Instruction on self-injection technique and procedures. Patients should be instructed in the use of aseptic technique when administering Betaseron. Appropriate instruction for reconstitution of Betaseron and self-injection should be given including careful review of the **Betaseron Patient Information** sheet. If possible, the first injection should be performed under the supervision of an appropriately qualified health care professional.

Patients should be cautioned against the re-use of needles or syringes and instructed in safe disposal procedures. A puncture resistant container for disposal of used needles and syringes should be supplied to the patient along with instructions for safe disposal of full containers.

Patients should be advised of the importance of rotating areas of injection with each dose, to minimize the likelihood of severe injection site reactions or necrosis (see **Rotating Injection Sites** section of **Patient Information** sheet).

Patients should be cautioned not to change the dosage or the schedule of administration without medical consultation.

Awareness of adverse reactions. Serious adverse reactions associated with the use of Betaseron have been reported including depression and injection site necrosis (see **WARNINGS** section).

Patients should immediately report symptoms of depression or suicidal ideation to their physician. The symptoms of depression should be closely monitored by a physician.

Injection site necrosis was reported in 5% of patients in a controlled MS trial. If the patient experiences any break in the skin, which may be associated with blue-black discoloration, swelling, or drainage of fluid from the injection site, the patient should be advised to promptly contact their physician prior to continuing their Betaseron therapy.

Other injection site reactions occurred in eighty-five percent of patients in the controlled MS trial, at one or more times during therapy. There was redness, pain, swelling and discoloration. In general, these were transient and did not require discontinuation of therapy, but the nature and severity of all reported reactions should be carefully assessed (see **ADVERSE REACTIONS** section).

Flu-like symptoms are common following initiation of therapy with Betaseron. In the controlled MS clinical trial, acetaminophen was permitted for relief of fever or myalgia (see **ADVERSE REACTIONS** section).

Patients should be cautioned about the abortifacient potential of Betaseron (see **PRECAUTIONS, Pregnancy - Teratogenic effects**).

Laboratory tests: The following laboratory tests are recommended prior to initiating Betaseron therapy and at periodic intervals thereafter: hemoglobin, complete and differential white blood cell counts, platelet counts and blood chemistries including liver function tests. In the controlled MS trial, patients were monitored every 3 months. The study protocol stipulated that Betaseron therapy be discontinued in the event the absolute neutrophil count fell below 750/mm^3. When the absolute neutrophil count had returned to a value greater than 750/mm^3, therapy could be restarted at a 50% reduced dose. No patients were withdrawn or dose reduced for neutropenia or lymphopenia.

Similarly, if hepatic transaminase (SGOT/SGPT) levels exceeded 10 times the upper limit of normal, or if the serum bilirubin exceeded 5 times the upper limit of normal, therapy was discontinued. In each instance during the controlled MS trial, hepatic enzyme abnormalities returned to normal following discontinuation of therapy. When measurements had decreased to below these levels, therapy could be restarted at a 50% dose reduction, if clinically appropriate. Two patients were dose reduced for increased liver enzymes; one continued on treatment and one was ultimately withdrawn.

Drug interactions: Interactions between Betaseron and other drugs have not been fully evaluated. Although studies designed to examine drug interactions have not been done, it was noted that corticosteroid or ACTH treatment of relapses for periods of up to 28 days has been administered to patients (N=180) receiving Betaseron.

Betaseron administration to three cancer patients over a dose range of 0.025 mg to 2.2 mg led to a dose-dependent inhibition of antipyrine elimination.[14] The effect of alternate-day administration of 0.25 mg of Betaseron on drug metabolism in MS patients is unknown.

Carcinogenesis: The carcinogenic potential of Betaseron was evaluated by studying its effect on the morphological transformation of the mammalian cell line BALBc-3T3. No significant increases in transformation frequency were noted. No carcinogenicity data are available in animals or humans.

Betaseron® (Interferon beta-1b) was not mutagenic when assayed for genotoxicity in the Ames bacterial test in the presence or absence of metabolic activation.

Impairment of fertility: Studies in rhesus monkeys at doses up to 0.33 mg/kg/day (32 times the recommended human dose based on body surface area comparison*) in normally cycling rhesus female monkeys had no apparent adverse effects on the menstrual cycle or on associated hor-

Continued on next page

Information on the Berlex products appearing here is based on the most current information available at the time of publication closing. Further information for these and other products may be obtained from the Medical Affairs Department, Berlex Laboratories, 300 Fairfield Road, Wayne, New Jersey 07470, 1-888-BERLEX-4. Information on Betaseron and Fludara may be obtained from Berlex Laboratories, 15049 San Pablo Avenue, Richmond, California 94804-0016, 1-800-888-4112.

Betaseron—Cont.

monal profiles (progesterone and estradiol) when administered over 3 consecutive menstrual cycles. The extrapolability of animal doses to human doses is not known. Effects of Betaseron on normal cycling human females are not known.

*body surface dose based on 70 kg female

Pregnancy - Teratogenic effects: Pregnancy Category C: Betaseron was not teratogenic at doses up to 0.42 mg/kg/day in rhesus monkeys, but demonstrated a dose-related abortifacient activity when administered at doses ranging from 0.028 mg/kg/day (2.8 times the recommended human dose based on body surface area comparison) to 0.42 mg/kg/day (40 times the recommended human dose based on body surface area comparison). The extrapolability of animal doses to human doses is not known. Lower doses were not studied in monkeys. Spontaneous abortions while on treatment were reported in patients (N=4) who participated in the Betaseron MS clinical trial. Betaseron given to rhesus monkeys on gestation days 20 to 70 did not cause teratogenic effects, however, it is not known if teratogenic effects exist in humans. There are no adequate and well-controlled studies in pregnant women. If the patient becomes pregnant or plans to become pregnant while taking Betaseron, the patient should be apprised of the potential hazard to the fetus and it should be recommended that the patient discontinue therapy.

Nursing mothers: It is not known whether Betaseron is excreted in human milk. Because many drugs are excreted in human milk and because of the potential for serious adverse reactions in nursing infants from Betaseron, a decision should be made as to whether either to discontinue nursing or discontinue the drug, taking into account the importance of drug to the mother.

Pediatric use: Safety and efficacy in children under 18 years of age have not been established.

ADVERSE REACTIONS

Experience with Betaseron in patients with MS is limited to a total of 147 patients at the recommended dose of 0.25 mg every other day or more (see **CLINICAL PHARMACOLOGY, Clinical Trials** section). Consequently, adverse events that are associated with the use of Betaseron in MS patients at a low incidence may not have been observed in pre-marketing studies. Clinical experience with Betaseron in other populations (patients with cancer, HIV positive patients, etc.) provides additional data regarding adverse reactions; however, experience in non-MS populations may not be fully applicable to the MS population.

Injection site reactions (85%) and injection site necrosis (5%) occurred after administration of Betaseron. Inflammation, pain, hypersensitivity, necrosis, and non-specific reactions were significantly associated (p<0.05) with the 0.25 mg Betaseron-treated group. Only inflammation, pain, and necrosis were reported as severe events (see **WARNINGS** and **PRECAUTIONS** sections). The incidence rate for injection site reactions was calculated over the course of 3 years. This incidence rate decreased over time, with 79% of patients experiencing the event during the first 3 months of treatment compared to 47% during the last 6 months. The median time to the first occurrence of an injection site reaction was 7 days. Patients with injection site reactions reported these events 183.7 days per year. Three patients withdrew from the 0.25 mg Betaseron-treated group for injection site pain.

Flu-like symptom complex was reported in 76% of the patients treated with 0.25 mg Betaseron. A patient was defined as having a flu-like symptom complex if flu-like symptoms or at least two of the following symptoms were concurrently reported: fever, chills, myalgia, malaise, or sweating. Only myalgia, fever, and chills were reported as severe in more than 5% of the patients. The incidence rate for flu-like symptom complex was also calculated over the course of 3 years. The incidence rate of these events decreased over time, with 60% of patients experiencing the event during the first 3 months of treatment compared to 10% during the last 6 months. The median time to the first occurrence of flu-like symptom complex was 3.5 days and the median duration per patient was 7.5 days per year.

Laboratory abnormalities included absolute neutrophil count less than 1500/mm³ (18%) (no patients had absolute neutrophil counts less than 500/mm³), WBC less than 3000/mm³ (16%), SGPT greater than 5 times baseline value (19%), and total bilirubin greater than 2.5 times baseline value (6%). Three patients were withdrawn from treatment with 0.25 mg Betaseron for abnormal liver enzymes including one following dose reduction (see **PRECAUTIONS, Laboratory Tests**).

Twenty-one (28%) of the 76 premenopausal females treated at 0.25 mg Betaseron and 10 (13%) of the 76 premenopausal females treated with placebo reported menstrual disorders. All of these reports were of mild to moderate severity and included: intermenstrual bleeding and spotting, early or delayed menses, decreased days of menstrual flow, and clotting and spotting during menstruation.

Mental disorders have been observed in patients in this study. Symptoms included depression, anxiety, emotional lability, depersonalization, suicide attempts, confusion, etc. In the treatment group, two patients withdrew for confusion. One suicide and four attempted suicides were also reported. It is not known whether these symptoms may be related to the underlying neurological basis of MS, to Betaseron treatment, or to a combination of both. Some similar symptoms have been noted in patients receiving interferon alfa and both interferons are thought to act through the same receptor. Patients who experience these symptoms should be closely monitored and cessation of therapy considered.

Additional common adverse clinical and laboratory events associated with the use of Betaseron are listed in the following paragraphs. These events occurred at an incidence of 5% or more in the 124 MS patients treated with 0.25 mg of Betaseron every other day for periods of up to 3 years in the controlled trial, and at an incidence that was at least twice that observed in the 123 placebo patients. Common adverse clinical and laboratory events associated with the use of Betaseron were: injection site reaction (85%), injection site necrosis (5%), palpitation (8%), hypertension (7%), tachycardia (6%), peripheral vascular disorders (5%), gastrointestinal disorders (6%), absolute neutrophil count <1500/mm³ (18%), WBC <3000/mm³ (16%), SGPT >5 times baseline value (19%), total bilirubin >2.5 times baseline value (6%), somnolence (6%), dyspnea (8%), laryngitis (6%), menstrual disorder (17%), cystitis (8%), breast pain (7%), pelvic pain (6%), and menorrhagia (6%).

TABLE 2
Adverse Reactions and Laboratory Abnormalities

Adverse Reaction	Placebo N=123	0.25 mg N=124
Body as a Whole		
Injection site reaction*	37%	85%
Headache	77%	84%
Fever*	41%	59%
Flu-like symptom complex*	56%	76%
Pain	48%	52%
Asthenia*	35%	49%
Chills*	19%	46%
Abdominal pain	24%	32%
Malaise*	3%	15%
Generalized edema	6%	8%
Pelvic pain	3%	6%
Injection site necrosis*	0%	5%
Cyst	2%	4%
Necrosis	0%	2%
Suicide attempt	0%	2%
Cardiovascular System		
Migraine	7%	12%
Palpitation*	2%	8%
Hypertension	2%	7%
Tachycardia	3%	6%
Peripheral vascular disorder	2%	5%
Hemorrhage	1%	3%
Digestive System		
Diarrhea	29%	35%
Constipation	18%	24%
Vomiting	19%	21%
Gastrointestinal disorder	3%	6%
Endocrine System		
Goiter	0%	2%
Hemic and Lymphatic System		
Lymphocytes less than 1500/mm³	67%	82%
ANC < 1500/mm³*	6%	18%
WBC < 3000/mm³*	5%	16%
Lymphadenopathy	11%	14%
Metabolic and Nutritional Disorders		
SGPT > 5 times baseline*	6%	19%
Glucose < 55 mg/dL	13%	15%
Total bilirubin > 2.5 times baseline	2%	6%
Urine protein > 1+	3%	5%
SGOT > 5 times baseline*	0%	4%
Weight gain	0%	4%
Weight loss	2%	4%
Musculoskeletal System		
Myalgia*	28%	44%
Myasthenia	10%	13%
Nervous System		
Dizziness	28%	35%
Hypertonia	24%	26%
Anxiety	13%	15%
Nervousness	5%	8%
Somnolence	3%	6%
Confusion	2%	4%
Speech disorder	1%	3%
Convulsion	0%	2%
Hyperkinesia	0%	2%
Amnesia	0%	2%
Respiratory System		
Sinusitis	26%	36%
Dyspnea*	2%	8%
Laryngitis	2%	6%
Skin and Appendages		
Sweating*	11%	23%
Alopecia	2%	4%
Special Senses		
Conjunctivitis	10%	12%
Abnormal vision	4%	7%
Urogenital System		
Dysmenorrhea	11%	18%
Menstrual disorder*	8%	17%
Metrorrhagia	8%	15%
Cystitis	4%	8%
Breast pain	3%	7%
Menorrhagia	3%	6%
Urinary urgency	2%	4%
Fibrocystic breast	1%	3%
Breast neoplasm	0%	2%

* Significantly associated with Betaseron treatment.

A total of 277 MS patients have been treated with Betaseron® (Interferon beta-1b) in doses ranging from 0.025 mg to 0.5 mg. During the first 3 years of treatment, withdrawals due to clinical adverse events or laboratory abnormalities not mentioned above included: fatigue (2%, 6 patients), cardiac arrhythmia (<1%, 1 patient), allergic urticarial skin reaction to injections (<1%, 1 patient), headache (<1%, 1 patient), unspecified adverse events (<1%, 1 patient), and "felt sick" (<1%, 1 patient).

Table 2 enumerates adverse events and laboratory abnormalities that occurred at an incidence of 2% or more among the 124 MS patients treated with 0.25 mg Betaseron every other day for periods of up to 3 years in the controlled trial and at an incidence that was at least 2% more than that observed in the 123 placebo patients. Reported adverse events have been reclassified using the standard COSTART glossary to reduce the total number of terms employed in Table 2, terms so general as to be uninformative, and those events where a drug cause was remote have been excluded. It should be noted that the figures cited in the table cannot be used to predict the incidence of side effects in the course of usual medical practice where patient characteristics and other factors differ from those that prevailed in the clinical trials. The cited figures do provide the prescribing physician with some basis for estimating the relative contribution of drug and nondrug factors to the side effect incidence rate in the population studied.

Other events observed during premarketing evaluation of various doses of Betaseron in 1440 patients are listed in the paragraph that follows. Because most of the events were observed in open and uncontrolled studies, the role of Betaseron in their causation cannot be reliably determined.

Body as a Whole: abscess, adenoma, anaphylactoid reaction, ascites, cellulitis, hernia, hydrocephalus, hypothermia, infection, peritonitis, photosensitivity, sarcoma, sepsis, and shock; **Cardiovascular System:** angina pectoris, arrhythmia, atrial fibrillation, cardiomegaly, cardiac arrest, cerebral hemorrhage, cerebral ischemia, endocarditis, heart failure, hypotension, myocardial infarct, pericardial effusion, postural hypotension, pulmonary embolus, spider angioma, subarachnoid hemorrhage, syncope, thrombophlebitis, thrombosis, varicose vein, vasospasm, venous pressure increased, ventricular extrasystoles, and ventricular fibrillation; **Digestive System:** aphthous stomatitis, cardiospasm, cheilitis, cholecystitis, cholelithiasis, duodenal ulcer, dry mouth, enteritis, esophagitis, fecal impaction, fecal incontinence, flatulence, gastritis, gastrointestinal hemorrhage, gingivitis, glossitis, hematemesis, hepatic neoplasia, hepatitis, hepatomegaly, ileus, increased salivation, intestinal obstruction, melena, nausea, oral leukoplakia, oral moniliasis, pancreatitis, periodontal abscess, proctitis, rectal hemorrhage, salivary gland enlargement, stomach ulcer, and tenesmus; **Endocrine System:** Cushing's Syndrome, diabetes insipidus, diabetes mellitus, hypothyroidism, and inappropriate ADH; **Hemic and Lymphatic System:** chronic lymphocytic leukemia, hemoglobin less than 9.4 g/100 mL, petechia, platelets less than 75,000/mm³, and splenomegaly; **Metabolic and Nutritional Disorders:** alcohol intolerance, alkaline phosphatase greater than 5 times baseline value,

BUN greater than 40 mg/dL, calcium greater than 11.5 mg/dL, cyanosis, edema, glucose greater than 160 mg/dL, glycosuria, hypoglycemic reaction, hypoxia, ketosis, and thirst; **Musculoskeletal System:** arthritis, arthrosis, bursitis, leg cramps, muscle atrophy, myopathy, myositis, ptosis, and tenosynovitis; **Nervous System:** abnormal gait, acute brain syndrome, agitation, apathy, aphasia, ataxia, brain edema, chronic brain syndrome, coma, delirium, delusions, dementia, depersonalization, diplopia, dystonia, encephalopathy, euphoria, facial paralysis, foot drop, hallucinations, hemiplegia, hypalgesia, hyperesthesia, incoordination, intracranial hypertension, libido decreased, manic reaction, meningitis, neuralgia, neuropathy, neurosis, nystagmus, oculogyric crisis, ophthalmoplegia, papilledema, paralysis, paranoid reaction, psychosis, reflexes decreased, stupor, subdural hematoma, torticollis, tremor, and urinary retention; **Respiratory System:** apnea, asthma, atelectasis, carcinoma of lung, hemoptysis, hiccup, hyperventilation, hypoventilation, interstitial pneumonia, lung edema, pleural effusion, pneumonia, and pneumothorax; **Skin and Appendages:** contact dermatitis, erythema nodosum, exfoliative dermatitis, furunculosis, hirsutism, leukoderma, lichenoid dermatitis, maculopapular rash, psoriasis, seborrhea, skin benign neoplasm, skin carcinoma, skin hypertrophy, skin necrosis, skin ulcer, urticaria, and vesiculobullous rash; **Special Senses:** blepharitis, blindness, deafness, dry eyes, ear pain, iritis, keratoconjunctivitis, mydriasis, otitis externa, otitis media, parosmia, photophobia, retinitis, taste loss, taste perversion, and visual field defect; **Urogenital System:** anuria, balanitis, breast engorgement, cervicitis, epididymitis, gynecomastia, hematuria, impotence, kidney calculus, kidney failure, kidney tubular disorder, leukorrhea, nephritis, nocturia, oliguria, polyuria, salpingitis, urethritis, urinary incontinence, uterine fibroids enlarged, uterine neoplasm, and vaginal hemorrhage.

DRUG ABUSE AND DEPENDENCE

No evidence or experience suggests that abuse or dependence occurs with Betaseron® (Interferon beta-1b) therapy; however, the risk of dependence has not been systematically evaluated.

DOSAGE AND ADMINISTRATION

The recommended dose of Betaseron for the treatment of ambulatory relapsing-remitting MS is 0.25 mg injected subcutaneously every other day. Limited data regarding the activity of a lower dose are presented above (see **CLINICAL PHARMACOLOGY, Clinical Trials**).

Evidence of efficacy beyond 2 years is not known since the primary evidence of efficacy derives from a 2-year, double-blind, placebo-controlled clinical trial (see **CLINICAL PHARMACOLOGY, Clinical Trials**). Safety data are not available beyond the third year. Patients were discontinued from this trial due to unremitting disease progression of 6 months or greater.

To reconstitute lyophilized Betaseron for injection, use a sterile syringe and needle to inject 1.2 mL of the diluent supplied, Sodium Chloride, 0.54% Solution, into the Betaseron vial. Gently swirl the vial of Betaseron to dissolve the drug completely; do not shake. Inspect the reconstituted product visually and discard the product before use if it contains particulate matter or is discolored. After reconstitution with accompanying diluent, Betaseron vials contain 0.25 mg Interferon beta-1b/mL of solution.

Withdraw 1 mL of reconstituted solution from the vial into a sterile syringe fitted with a 27-gauge needle and inject the solution subcutaneously. Sites for self-injection include arms, abdomen, hips, and thighs. A vial is suitable for single use only; unused portions should be discarded. (See **BETASERON PATIENT INFORMATION** sheet for **SELF-INJECTION PROCEDURE.**)

Stability:

The reconstituted product contains no preservative. Before reconstitution with diluent, store at 2° to 8°C (36° to 46°F). After reconstitution, if not used immediately, the product should be refrigerated and used within 3 hours. Avoid freezing.

If refrigeration is not possible, vials of Betaseron and diluent should be kept as cool as possible, below 30°C (86°F), away from heat and light, and used within 7 days.

HOW SUPPLIED

Betaseron is supplied as a lyophilized powder containing 0.3 mg of Interferon beta-1b, 15 mg Albumin Human USP, and 15 mg dextrose, USP. Drug is packaged in a clear glass, single-use vial (3 mL capacity); a separate vial containing 2 mL of diluent (Sodium Chloride, 0.54% solution) is included for each vial of drug. Store under refrigeration, between 2° to 8°C (36° to 46°F).

NDC 50419-521-03   0.3 mg/vial
NDC 50419-521-15   15 vials, 0.3 mg/vial

Caution: Federal law prohibits dispensing without prescription.

REFERENCES

1. Ruzicka FJ, et al. J Biol Chem, 1987; 262: 16142-16149. **2.** Uze G, et al. Cell, 1990; 60: 225-234. **3.** DeMaeyer E, et al. In: Interferons and other regulatory cytokines, NY, Wiley 1988. **4.** Colby CB, et al. J Immunol 1984; 133: 3091-3095. **5.** Pestka S, et al. Annu Rev Biochem 1987; 56: 727-777. **6.** Lengyel P, Annu Rev Biochem 1982; 51: 251-282. **7.** Witt PL, et al. J Interferon Res 1990; 10: 393-402. **8.** Schiller JH, et al. J Biol Resp Mod 1990; 9: 377-386. **9.** Rosenblum MG, et al. J Interferon Res 1990; 10: 141-151. **10.** Carlin JM, et al. J Immuno 1987; 130(7): 2414-2418. **11.** Witt PL, et al. J Immunotherapy 1993; 13: 191-200. **12.** Goldstein D, et al. J Natl Cancer Inst 1989; 81: 1061-1068. **13.** Poser CM, et al. Ann Neurol 1983; 13(3): 227-231. **14.** Blaschke TF, et al. Clinical Research 1985; 33(1): 19A.

Manufactured by:
CHIRON Corporation
Emeryville, CA 94608
U.S. License No. 1106
Distributed by:
BERLEX Laboratories
Richmond, CA 94804
U.S. Patent No. 4,588,585; 4,959,314; 4,737,462; 4,450,103
©1993 Berlex Laboratories All rights reserved.
Part Number L -1172.2   Revision date 10/96

BETASERON®
Interferon beta-1b

Read this patient information each time your prescription is filled because this information may have changed.

PATIENT INFORMATION

Betaseron® (Interferon beta-1b) is intended for use under the guidance and supervision of a physician. Your physician or his/her delegate should instruct you in the preparation of Betaseron for administration and in the technique of self injection. Do not attempt self-administration until you are sure that you understand the requirements for mixing the product and giving an injection to yourself.

Betaseron should be used as prescribed by your physician. However, if you miss a dose, take it as soon as you remember. Your next injection, however, should be scheduled about 48 hours later. While using Betaseron, please keep in mind the following facts:

• Betaseron must be kept cold. Be sure to store it in a refrigerator before and after reconstitution. Do not freeze.
• Keep syringes and needles away from children. Do not reuse needles or syringes. Discard used syringes and needles in a syringe disposal unit as instructed by your physician.
• Women: Betaseron should not be used during pregnancy or if you are trying to become pregnant. If you wish to become pregnant while using Betaseron, discuss the matter with your doctor. While using Betaseron, women of childbearing age should use birth control measures. If you do become pregnant you should discontinue treatment and contact your doctor immediately.
• Injection site reactions are common. They include redness, pain and swelling, and discoloration. Less frequently, injection site necrosis (skin breakdown and tissue destruction) has been observed. To minimize chances for a reaction you should rotate injection sites as described on pages 3 and 4 or as recommended by your physician. Do not make an injection into skin that is tender, red, or hard. If you experience a break in the skin or drainage of fluid from the injection site, you should promptly contact your physician before continuing injections with Betaseron.
• Flu-like symptoms are also common. They include fever, chills, sweating, fatigue, and muscle aches. Taking Betaseron at night may help lessen the impact of flu-like symptoms.
• Depression, including suicide attempts, has been reported by patients. If you experience such symptoms, contact your physician promptly.
• As with any prescription medication, side effects related to therapy can occur. Consult with your physician if you have any problems, whether or not you think they may be related to Betaseron® (Interferon beta-1b).

SELF-INJECTION PROCEDURE

To mix the contents of one vial

Only the vial of diluent (liquid) that comes inside your prescription package should be used to dissolve the white cake of drug in the Betaseron vial.

1. Wash your hands thoroughly with soap and water.
2. Collect all your equipment before you begin the process. You'll need:

• vial of Diluent for Betaseron (Sodium Chloride 0.54%)
• vial of Betaseron
• 3-mL syringe with 21-gauge needle (1)
• 1-mL syringe with 27-gauge needle (1)
• alcohol wipes
• disposal unit (an opaque, puncture-resistant, sealable container for used syringes/needles)

NOTE: Be sure needle guards are on the needles tightly.

3. Remove the protective caps from both vials.
4. Use alcohol wipes to clean the tops of the vials—move in one direction and use one wipe per vial.

NOTE: Leave an alcohol wipe on top of each vial until you are ready to use it.

5. Resting your hands on a stable surface, remove the needle cover on the 3-mL syringe by pulling the cover straight off the needle.

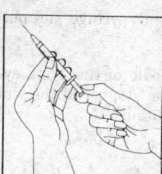

6. Pull back the plunger (on the 3-mL syringe) to the 1.2 mL mark.
NOTE: Read the labels on the vials—find the Diluent for Betaseron vial and throw away the alcohol wipe on top of it.
7. Holding the vial of Diluent for Betaseron on a stable surface, slowly insert the needle straight through the stopper, into the top of the vial.

NOTE: When inserting and removing needles from vials, be sure not to touch the needles or the rubber stoppers on the vials with your hands.
If you do touch a stopper, clean it with a fresh alcohol wipe. If you touch a needle, throw away the entire syringe into the disposal unit and start over with a new syringe.
If the needle touches any surface, throw away the entire syringe into the disposal unit and start over with a new syringe.

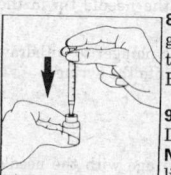

8. Push in the plunger all the way to gently inject air into the vial (leave the needle in the vial of Diluent for Betaseron).
9. Turn the vial of Diluent for Betaseron upside down.
NOTE: Keep the needle tip in the liquid.

10. Resting your hands on a stable surface, hold the vial and syringe in one hand and pull back the plunger on the syringe to the 1.2 mL mark (to draw up that amount of liquid) with your other hand.

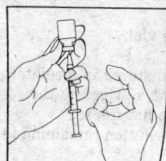

11. Keeping the vial upside down, gently tap the syringe until any air bubbles that formed rise to the top of the barrel of the syringe.

12. Carefully push in the plunger to eject ONLY THE AIR through the needle.

13. Remove the needle/syringe from the vial of Diluent for Betaseron.
NOTE: Find the Betaseron vial and throw away the alcohol wipe on top of it.
14. Holding the Betaseron vial on a stable surface, slowly insert the needle of the syringe (containing 1.2 mL of liquid) all the way through the stopper of the vial.

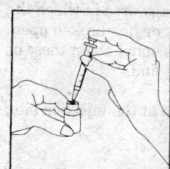

15. Push the plunger down slowly, directing the needle toward the side of the vial to allow the liquid to run down the inside wall (injecting Diluent for Betaseron directly onto the cake of drug will cause excess foaming).
16. Remove the needle/syringe from the Betaseron vial.

17. Throw away the 3 mL syringe into the disposal unit.
NOTE: Double-check that you are throwing away the correct syringe into the disposal unit.

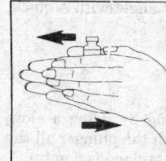

18. Roll the vial between your hands gently to completely dissolve the white cake of Betaseron (DO NOT SHAKE).
19. Look closely at the solution (it should be clear).
NOTE: If the mixture contains particles or is discolored, discard it and start again.

Continued on next page

Information on the Berlex products appearing here is based on the most current information available at the time of publication closing. Further information for these and other products may be obtained from the Medical Affairs Department, Berlex Laboratories, 300 Fairfield Road, Wayne, New Jersey 07470, 1-888-BERLEX-4. Information on Betaseron and Fludara may be obtained from Berlex Laboratories, 15049 San Pablo Avenue, Richmond, California 94804-0016, 1-800-888-4112.

Betaseron—Cont.

PREPARING THE INJECTION

1. Remove the needle guard of the 1 mL syringe and pull back the plunger to the 1 mL mark.

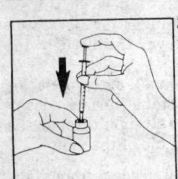

2. Insert the needle of the 1 mL syringe through the stopper of the vial of Betaseron solution.

3. Gently push the plunger all the way down to inject air into the vial (leave the needle in the vial).

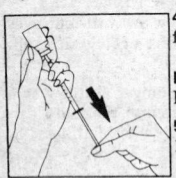

4. Turn the vial of Betaseron® (Interferon beta-1b) solution upside down.

NOTE: Keep the needle tip in the liquid.

5. Pull back the plunger to withdraw 1 mL of liquid into the syringe.

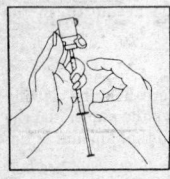

6. Hold the syringe with the needle pointing upward.

7. Tap the syringe gently until any air bubbles that formed rise to the top of the barrel of the syringe.

8. Carefully push in the plunger to eject ONLY THE AIR through the needle.

9. Remove the needle/syringe from the vial.
10. Recap the needle on the syringe.
NOTE: The injection should be administered immediately after mixing (if the injection is delayed, refrigerate the solution and inject it within 3 hours). Do not freeze.
11. Throw away unused portion of the solution remaining in the vial.

GIVING THE INJECTION

Subcutaneous (under the skin) self-administration
1. Choose an area for injection site (see diagrams for areas); use a different area each day.
- Abdomen—Areas 1 and 3
- Thighs— Areas 2 and 4
- Back of Arms—Areas 5 and 7
- Buttocks—Areas 6 and 8

NOTE: Do not use any areas in which you feel lumps, bumps, firm knots, or pain. Do not use any area in which the skin is discolored, depressed, scabbed, or has broken open. Talk to your doctor or healthcare professional about these or any other unusual conditions that you find.
Hold the syringe like a pencil or dart.
2. Use an alcohol wipe to clean the skin at the injection site; let it air dry.
3. Throw away the wipe.
4. Uncap the needle.

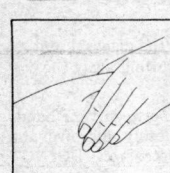

5. Gently pinch the skin together around the site (to lift it up a bit).

6. Resting your wrist on the skin near the site, stick the needle straight into the skin at a 90° angle with a quick, firm motion.

7. Inject the drug by using a slow, steady push (push the plunger all the way in until the syringe is empty).

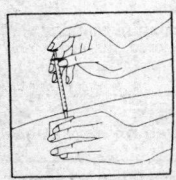

8. Hold a swab on the injection site. Remove the needle from the skin.

9. Gently massage the injection site with a dry cotton ball or gauze.
10. Throw away the 1 mL syringe in the disposal unit.

INJECTION SITE

Picking an injection site
Betaseron® (Interferon beta-1b) should be injected into subcutaneous tissue (into the fat layer between the skin and the muscles beneath). The best areas for injection are where the skin is loose and soft (flabby), away from joints, nerves, bones, and other important structures.
Each day of injection you can choose an injection site from the upper, middle, or lower section of an area shown in the accompanying diagrams. It is a good idea to know where your injection will be given before you prepare your syringe. If there are any sites that are difficult for you to reach, you can ask your support person (or someone who has been trained to give injections) to help you.

Rotating injection sites
Each day of injection you can choose an injection site from the upper, middle, or lower section of an area shown in the accompanying diagrams.
To help prevent injection site reactions, you need to select a site in an area different from the area where you last injected yourself. You should not choose the same area for two injections in a row. Keeping a record of your injections will help make sure you rotate areas.
On the accompanying diagrams of the body, the areas of injection are numbered 1 through 8. Each area may be divided into three sections—upper, middle, and lower. If self-administering Betaseron, areas 1 through 4 may be the most convenient. Use the 8 areas in the following sequence:
- Your first 8 injections should be in a site in the upper section of each area (Rotation 1);
- The next 8 injections should be in a site in the middle section of each area (Rotation 2);
- And the next 8 should be in a site in the lower section of each area (Rotation 3).

By following this schedule, you will come back to your first injection site after 24 injections (48 days). If there are any sites that are difficult for you to reach, you can ask your support person, or someone who has been trained to give injections, to help you.

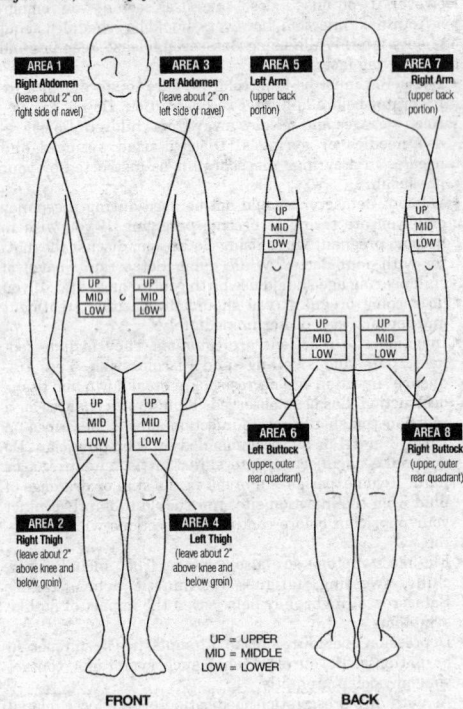

FRONT   BACK

UP = UPPER
MID = MIDDLE
LOW = LOWER

ROTATION 1	ROTATION 2	ROTATION 3
(Injections 1–8)	(Injections 9–16)	(Injections 17–24)
Upper Area 1	Middle Area 1	Lower Area 1
Upper Area 2	Middle Area 2	Lower Area 2
Upper Area 3	Middle Area 3	Lower Area 3
Upper Area 4	Middle Area 4	Lower Area 4
Upper Area 5	Middle Area 5	Lower Area 5
Upper Area 6	Middle Area 6	Lower Area 6
Upper Area 7	Middle Area 7	Lower Area 7
Upper Area 8	Middle Area 8	Lower Area 8

Manufactured by:
CHIRON Corporation
Emeryville, CA 94608
U.S. License No. 1106
Distributed by:
BERLEX Laboratories
Richmond, CA 94804
©1993 Berlex Laboratories   All rights reserved.

Part Number L-1171.2   Revision date 10/96
Shown in Product Identification Guide, page 306

FLUDARA®
(fludarabine phosphate)
FOR INJECTION
FOR INTRAVENOUS USE ONLY

℞

WARNING:
FLUDARA FOR INJECTION should be administered under the supervision of a qualified physician experienced in the use of antineoplastic therapy.
FLUDARA FOR INJECTION can severely suppress bone marrow function. When used at high doses in dose-ranging studies in patients with acute leukemia, FLUDARA FOR INJECTION was associated with severe neurologic effects, including blindness, coma, and death. This severe central nervous system toxicity occurred in 36% of patients treated with doses approximately four times greater (96 mg/m²/day for 5–7 days) than the recommended dose. Similar severe central nervous system toxicity has been rarely (≤0.2%) reported in patients treated at doses in the range of the dose recommended for chronic lymphocytic leukemia.
Instances of life-threatening and sometimes fatal autoimmune hemolytic anemia have been reported to occur after one or more cycles of treatment with FLUDARA FOR INJECTION. Patients undergoing treatment with FLUDARA FOR INJECTION should be evaluated and closely monitored for hemolysis.
In a clinical investigation using FLUDARA FOR INJECTION in combination with pentostatin (deoxycoformycin) for the treatment of refractory chronic lymphocytic leukemia (CLL), there was an unacceptably high incidence of fatal pulmonary toxicity. Therefore, the use of FLUDARA FOR INJECTION in combination with pentostatin is not recommended.

DESCRIPTION

FLUDARA FOR INJECTION contains fludarabine phosphate, a fluorinated nucleotide analog of the antiviral agent vidarabine, 9-β-D-arabinofuranosyladenine (ara-A) that is relatively resistant to deamination by adenosine deaminase. Each vial of sterile lyophilized solid cake contains 50 mg of the active ingredient fludarabine phosphate, 50 mg of mannitol, and sodium hydroxide to adjust pH to 7.7. The pH range for the final product is 7.2–8.2. Reconstitution with 2 mL of Sterile Water for Injection USP results in a solution containing 25 mg/mL of fludarabine phosphate intended for intravenous administration.
The chemical name for fludarabine phosphate is 9H-Purin-6-amine, 2-fluoro-9-(5-O-phosphono-β-D-arabinofuranosyl). The molecular formula of fludarabine phosphate is $C_{10}H_{13}FN_5O_7P$ (MW 365.2) and the structure is:

CLINICAL PHARMACOLOGY

Fludarabine phosphate is rapidly dephosphorylated to 2-fluoro-ara-A and then phosphorylated intracellularly by deoxycytidine kinase to the active triphosphate, 2-fluoro-ara-ATP. This metabolite appears to act by inhibiting DNA polymerase alpha, ribonucleotide reductase and DNA primase, thus inhibiting DNA synthesis. The mechanism of action of this antimetabolite is not completely characterized and may be multi-faceted.
Phase I studies in humans have demonstrated that fludarabine phosphate is rapidly converted to the active metabolite, 2-fluoro-ara-A, within minutes after intravenous infusion. Consequently, clinical pharmacology studies have focused on 2-fluoro-ara-A pharmacokinetics. In a study with 4 patients treated with 25 mg/m²/day for 5 days, the half-life of 2-fluoro-ara-A was approximately 10 hours. The mean total plasma clearance was 8.9 L/hr/m² and the mean volume of

distribution was 98 L/m². Approximately 23% of the dose was excreted in the urine as unchanged 2-fluoro-ara-A. The mean C_{max} after the Day 1 dose was 0.57 mcg/mL and after the Day 5 dose was 0.54 mcg/mL. No information is available on pharmacokinetic parameters, other than C_{max}, following the Day 5 dose of 25 mg/m². Total body clearance of 2-fluoro-ara-A has been shown to be inversely correlated with serum creatinine, suggesting renal elimination of the compound.

A correlation was noted between the degree of absolute granulocyte count nadir and increased area under the concentration × time curve (AUC).

Two single-arm open-label studies of FLUDARA FOR INJECTION have been conducted in patients with CLL refractory to at least one prior standard alkylating-agent containing regimen. In a study conducted by M.D. Anderson Cancer Center (MDAH), 48 patients were treated with a dose of 22–40 mg/m² daily for 5 days every 28 days. Another study conducted by the Southwest Oncology Group (SWOG) involved 31 patients treated with a dose of 15–25 mg/m² daily for 5 days every 28 days. The overall objective response rates were 48% and 32% in the MDAH and SWOG studies, respectively. The complete response rate in both studies was 13%; the partial response rate was 35% in the MDAH study and 19% in the SWOG study. These response rates were obtained using standardized response criteria developed by the National Cancer Institute CLL Working Group[1] and were achieved in heavily pre-treated patients. The ability of FLUDARA FOR INJECTION to induce a significant rate of response in refractory patients suggests minimal cross-resistance with commonly used anti-CLL agents.

The median time to response in the MDAH and SWOG studies was 7 weeks (range of 1 to 68 weeks) and 21 weeks (range of 1 to 53 weeks) respectively. The median duration of disease control was 91 weeks (MDAH) and 65 weeks (SWOG). The median survival of all refractory CLL patients treated with FLUDARA FOR INJECTION was 43 weeks and 52 weeks in the MDAH and SWOG studies, respectively.

Rai stage improved to Stage II or better in 7 of 12 MDAH responders (58%) and in 5 of 7 SWOG responders (71%) who were Stage III or IV at baseline. In the combined studies, mean hemoglobin concentration improved from 9.0 g/dL at baseline to 11.8 g/dL at the time of response, in a subgroup of anemic patients. Similarly, average platelet count improved from 63,500/mm³ to 103,300/mm³ at the time of response in a subgroup of patients who were thrombocytopenic at baseline.

INDICATIONS AND USAGE

FLUDARA FOR INJECTION is indicated for the treatment of patients with B-cell chronic lymphocytic leukemia (CLL) who have not responded to or whose disease has progressed during treatment with at least one standard alkylating-agent containing regimen. The safety and effectiveness of FLUDARA FOR INJECTION in previously untreated or non-refractory patients with CLL have not been established.

CONTRAINDICATIONS

FLUDARA FOR INJECTION is contraindicated in those patients who are hypersensitive to this drug or its components.

WARNINGS

(See boxed warning)

There are clear dose dependent toxic effects seen with FLUDARA FOR INJECTION. Dose levels approximately 4 times greater (96 mg/m²/day for 5 to 7 days) than that recommended for CLL (25 mg/m²/day for 5 days) were associated with a syndrome characterized by delayed blindness, coma and death. Symptoms appeared from 21 to 60 days following the last dose. Thirteen of 36 patients (36%) who received FLUDARA FOR INJECTION at high doses (96 mg/m²/day for 5 to 7 days) developed this severe neurotoxicity. This syndrome has been reported rarely in patients treated with doses in the range of the recommended CLL dose of 25 mg/m²/day for 5 days every 28 days. The effect of chronic administration of FLUDARA FOR INJECTION on the central nervous system is unknown, however, patients have received the recommended dose for up to 15 courses of therapy.

Severe bone marrow suppression, notably anemia, thrombocytopenia and neutropenia, has been reported in patients treated with FLUDARA FOR INJECTION. In a Phase I study in solid tumor patients, the median time to nadir counts was 13 days (range, 3–25 days) for granulocytes and 16 days (range, 2–32) for platelets. Most patients had hematologic impairment at baseline either as a result of disease or as a result of prior myelosuppressive therapy. Cumulative myelosuppression may be seen. While chemotherapy-induced myelosuppression is often reversible, administration of FLUDARA FOR INJECTION requires careful hematologic monitoring.

Instances of life-threatening and sometimes fatal autoimmune hemolytic anemia have been reported to occur after one or more cycles of treatment with FLUDARA FOR INJECTION in patients with or without a previous history of autoimmune hemolytic anemia or a positive Coombs' test and who may or may not be in remission for their disease. Steroids may or may not be effective in controlling these hemolytic episodes. The majority of patients rechallenged with FLUDARA FOR INJECTION developed a recurrence in the hemolytic process. The mechanism(s) which predispose patients to the development of this complication has not been identified. Patients undergoing treatment with FLUDARA FOR INJECTION should be evaluated and closely monitored for hemolysis.

In a clinical investigation using FLUDARA FOR INJECTION in combination with pentostatin (deoxycoformycin) for the treatment of refractory chronic lymphocytic leukemia (CLL), there was an unacceptably high incidence of fatal pulmonary toxicity. Therefore, the use of FLUDARA FOR INJECTION in combination with pentostatin is not recommended.

Of the 133 CLL patients in the two trials, there were 29 fatalities during study. Approximately 50% of the fatalities were due to infection and 25% due to progressive disease.

Pregnancy Category D: FLUDARA FOR INJECTION may cause fetal harm when administered to a pregnant woman. Fludarabine phosphate was teratogenic in rats and in rabbits. Fludarabine phosphate was administered intravenously at doses of 0, 1, 10 or 30 mg/kg/day to pregnant rats on days 6 to 15 of gestation. At 10 and 30 mg/kg/day in rats, there was an increased incidence of various skeletal malformations. Fludarabine phosphate was administered intravenously at doses of 0, 1, 5 or 8 mg/kg/day to pregnant rabbits on days 6 to 15 of gestation. Dose-related teratogenic effects manifested by external deformities and skeletal malformations were observed in the rabbits at 5 and 8 mg/kg/day. Drug-related deaths or toxic effects on maternal and fetal weights were not observed. There are no adequate and well-controlled studies in pregnant women.

If FLUDARA FOR INJECTION is used during pregnancy, or if the patient becomes pregnant while taking this drug, the patient should be apprised of the potential hazard to the fetus. Women of childbearing potential should be advised to avoid becoming pregnant.

PRECAUTIONS

General: FLUDARA FOR INJECTION is a potent antineoplastic agent with potentially significant toxic side effects. Patients undergoing therapy should be closely observed for signs of hematologic and nonhematologic toxicity. Periodic assessment of peripheral blood counts is recommended to detect the development of anemia, neutropenia and thrombocytopenia.

Tumor lysis syndrome associated with FLUDARA FOR INJECTION treatment has been reported in CLL patients with large tumor burdens. Since FLUDARA FOR INJECTION can induce a response as early as the first week of treatment, precautions should be taken in those patients at risk of developing this complication.

There are inadequate data on dosing of patients with renal insufficiency. FLUDARA FOR INJECTION must be administered cautiously in patients with renal insufficiency. The total body clearance of 2-fluoro-ara-A has been shown to be inversely correlated with serum creatinine, suggesting renal elimination of the compound.

Laboratory Tests: During treatment, the patient's hematologic profile (particularly neutrophils and platelets) should be monitored regularly to determine the degree of hematopoietic suppression.

Drug Interactions: The use of FLUDARA FOR INJECTION in combination with pentostatin is not recommended due to the risk of severe pulmonary toxicity (see WARNINGS section).

Carcinogenesis: No animal carcinogenicity studies with FLUDARA FOR INJECTION have been conducted.

Mutagenesis: Fludarabine phosphate has been shown to be non-mutagenic to several strains of Salmonella typhimurium, including TA-98, TA-100, TA-1535 and TA-1537. In addition, fludarabine phosphate was non-mutagenic to Chinese hamster ovary (CHO) cells at the hypoxanthine-guanine-phosphoribosyltransferase (HGPRT) locus under both activated and non-activated metabolic conditions. Fludarabine was determined to cause increased sister chromatid exchanges using an in vitro sister chromatid exchange (SCE) assay under both metabolically activated and non-activated conditions. In addition, fludarabine phosphate has also been shown to be mutagenic as indicated by an increase in the number of micronucleated erythrocytes in the in vivo mouse micronucleus test at doses up to 1000 mg/kg.

Impairment of Fertility: Studies in mice, rats and dogs have demonstrated dose-related adverse effects on the male reproductive system. Observations consisted of a decrease in mean testicular weights in mice and rats with a trend toward decreased testicular weights in dogs and degeneration and necrosis of spermatogenic epithelium of the testes in mice, rats and dogs. The possible adverse effects on fertility in humans have not been adequately evaluated.

Pregnancy: Pregnancy Category D: (See WARNINGS section).

Nursing Mothers: It is not known whether this drug is excreted in human milk. Because many drugs are excreted in human milk and because of the potential for serious adverse reactions in nursing infants from FLUDARA FOR INJECTION, a decision should be made to discontinue nursing or discontinue the drug, taking into account the importance of the drug for the mother.

Pediatric Use: The safety and effectiveness of FLUDARA FOR INJECTION in children have not been established.

ADVERSE REACTIONS:

The most common adverse events include myelosuppression (neutropenia, thrombocytopenia and anemia), fever and chills, infection, and nausea and vomiting. Other commonly reported events include malaise, fatigue, anorexia, and weakness. Serious opportunistic infections have occurred in CLL patients treated with FLUDARA FOR INJECTION. The most frequently reported adverse events and those reactions which are more clearly related to the drug are arranged below according to body system.

Hematopoietic Systems: Hematologic events (neutropenia, thrombocytopenia, and/or anemia) were reported in the majority of CLL patients treated with FLUDARA® FOR INJECTION. During FLUDARA FOR INJECTION treatment of 133 patients with CLL, the absolute neutrophil count decreased to less than 500/mm³ in 59% of patients, hemoglobin decreased from pretreatment values by at least 2 grams percent in 60%, and platelet count decreased from pretreatment values by at least 50% in 55%. Myelosuppression may be severe and cumulative. Bone marrow fibrosis occurred in one CLL patient treated with FLUDARA® FOR INJECTION.

Life-threatening and sometimes fatal autoimmune hemolytic anemia have been reported to occur in patients receiving FLUDARA FOR INJECTION (see WARNINGS section). The majority of patients rechallenged with FLUDARA FOR INJECTION developed a recurrence in the hemolytic process.

Metabolic: Tumor lysis syndrome has been reported in CLL patients treated with FLUDARA FOR INJECTION. This complication may include hyperuricemia, hyperphosphatemia, hypocalcemia, metabolic acidosis, hyperkalemia, hematuria, urate crystalluria, and renal failure. The onset of this syndrome may be heralded by flank pain and hematuria.

Nervous System: (See WARNINGS section) Objective weakness, agitation, confusion, visual disturbances, and coma have occurred in CLL patients treated with FLUDARA FOR INJECTION at the recommended dose. Peripheral neuropathy has been observed in patients treated with FLUDARA FOR INJECTION and one case of wrist-drop was reported.

Pulmonary System: Pneumonia, a frequent manifestation of infection in CLL patients, occurred in 16% and 22% of those treated with FLUDARA FOR INJECTION in the MDAH and SWOG studies, respectively. Pulmonary hypersensitivity reactions to FLUDARA FOR INJECTION characterized by dyspnea, cough and interstitial pulmonary infiltrate have been observed.

Gastrointestinal System: Gastrointestinal disturbances such as nausea and vomiting, anorexia, diarrhea, stomatitis and gastrointestinal bleeding have been reported in patients treated with FLUDARA FOR INJECTION.

Cardiovascular: Edema has been frequently reported. One patient developed a pericardial effusion possibly related to treatment with FLUDARA FOR INJECTION. No other severe cardiovascular events were considered to be drug related.

Genitourinary System: Rare cases of hemorrhagic cystitis have been reported in patients treated with FLUDARA FOR INJECTION.

Skin: Skin toxicity, consisting primarily of skin rashes, has been reported in patients treated with FLUDARA FOR INJECTION.

Data in the following table are derived from the 133 patients with CLL who received FLUDARA FOR INJECTION in the MDAH and SWOG studies.

PERCENT OF CLL PATIENTS REPORTING NON-HEMATOLOGIC ADVERSE EVENTS

ADVERSE EVENTS	MDAH (N=101)	SWOG (N=32)
ANY ADVERSE EVENT	88%	91%
BODY AS A WHOLE	72	84
FEVER	60	69

Continued on next page

Information on the Berlex products appearing here is based on the most current information available at the time of publication closing. Further information for these and other products may be obtained from the Medical Affairs Department, Berlex Laboratories, 300 Fairfield Road, Wayne, New Jersey 07470, 1-888-BERLEX-4. Information on Betaseron and Fludara may be obtained from Berlex Laboratories, 15049 San Pablo Avenue, Richmond, California 94804-0016, 1-800-888-4112.

Fludara—Cont.

CHILLS	11	19
FATIGUE	10	38
INFECTION	33	44
PAIN	20	22
MALAISE	8	6
DIAPHORESIS	1	13
ALOPECIA	0	3
ANAPHYLAXIS	1	0
HEMORRHAGE	1	0
HYPERGLYCEMIA	1	6
DEHYDRATION	1	0
NEUROLOGICAL	21	69
WEAKNESS	9	65
PARESTHESIA	4	12
HEADACHE	3	0
VISUAL DISTURBANCE	3	15
HEARING LOSS	2	6
SLEEP DISORDER	1	3
DEPRESSION	1	0
CEREBELLAR SYNDROME	1	0
IMPAIRED MENTATION	1	0
PULMONARY	35	69
COUGH	10	44
PNEUMONIA	16	22
DYSPNEA	9	22
SINUSITIS	5	0
PHARYNGITIS	0	9
UPPER RESPIRATORY INFECTION	2	16
ALLERGIC PNEUMONITIS	0	6
EPISTAXIS	1	0
HEMOPTYSIS	1	6
BRONCHITIS	1	0
HYPOXIA	1	0
GASTROINTESTINAL	46	63
NAUSEA/VOMITING	36	31
DIARRHEA	15	13
ANOREXIA	7	34
STOMATITIS	9	0
GI BLEEDING	3	13
ESOPHAGITIS	3	0
MUCOSITIS	2	0
LIVER FAILURE	1	0
ABNORMAL LIVER FUNCTION TEST	1	3
CHOLELITHIASIS	0	3
CONSTIPATION	1	3
DYSPHAGIA	1	0
CUTANEOUS	17	18
RASH	15	15
PRURITUS	1	3
SEBORRHEA	1	0
GENITOURINARY	12	22
DYSURIA	4	3
URINARY INFECTION	2	15
HEMATURIA	2	3
RENAL FAILURE	1	0
ABNORMAL RENAL FUNCTION TEST	1	0
PROTEINURIA	1	0
HESITANCY	0	3
CARDIOVASCULAR	12	38
EDEMA	8	19
ANGINA	0	6
CONGESTIVE HEART FAILURE	0	3
ARRHYTHMIA	0	3
SUPRAVENTRICULAR TACHYCARDIA	0	3
MYOCARDIAL INFARCTION	0	3
DEEP VENOUS THROMBOSIS	1	3
PHLEBITIS	1	3
TRANSIENT ISCHEMIC ATTACK	1	0
ANEURYSM	1	0
CEREBROVASCULAR ACCIDENT	0	3
MUSCULOSKELETAL	7	16
MYALGIA	4	16
OSTEOPOROSIS	1	0
ARTHRALGIA	1	0
TUMOR LYSIS SYNDROME	1	0

More than 3000 patients received FLUDARA FOR INJECTION in studies of other leukemias, lymphomas, and other solid tumors. The spectrum of adverse effects reported in these studies was consistent with the data presented above.

OVERDOSAGE

High doses of FLUDARA FOR INJECTION (see Warnings) have been associated with an irreversible central nervous system toxicity characterized by delayed blindness, coma and death. High doses are also associated with severe thrombocytopenia and neutropenia due to bone marrow suppression. There is no known specific antidote for FLUDARA FOR INJECTION overdosage. Treatment consists of drug discontinuation and supportive therapy.

DOSAGE AND ADMINISTRATION

Usual Dose:

The recommended dose of FLUDARA FOR INJECTION is 25 mg/m^2 administered intravenously over a period of approximately 30 minutes daily for five consecutive days. Each 5 day course of treatment should commence every 28 days. Dosage may be decreased or delayed based on evidence of hematologic or nonhematologic toxicity. Physicians should consider delaying or discontinuing the drug if neurotoxicity occurs.

A number of clinical settings may predispose to increased toxicity from FLUDARA FOR INJECTION. These include advanced age, renal insufficiency, and bone marrow impairment. Such patients should be monitored closely for excessive toxicity and the dose modified accordingly.

The optimal duration of treatment has not been clearly established. It is recommended that three additional cycles of FLUDARA FOR INJECTION be administered following the achievement of a maximal response and then the drug should be discontinued.

Preparation of Solutions:

FLUDARA FOR INJECTION should be prepared for parenteral use by aseptically adding Sterile Water for Injection USP. When reconstituted with 2 mL of Sterile Water for Injection, USP, the solid cake should fully dissolve in 15 seconds or less; each mL of the resulting solution will contain 25 mg of fludarabine phosphate, 25 mg of mannitol, and sodium hydroxide to adjust the pH to 7.7. The pH range for the final product is 7.2-8.2. In clinical studies, the product has been diluted in 100 cc or 125 cc of 5% Dextrose Injection USP or 0.9% Sodium Chloride USP.

Reconstituted FLUDARA FOR INJECTION contains no antimicrobial preservative and thus should be used within 8 hours of reconstitution. Care must be taken to assure the sterility of prepared solutions. Parenteral drug products should be inspected visually for particulate matter and discoloration prior to administration.

Handling and Disposal:

Procedures for proper handling and disposal should be considered. Consideration should be given to handling and disposal according to guidelines issued for cytotoxic drugs. Several guidelines on this subject have been published.[2-8] There is no general agreement that all of the procedures recommended in the guidelines are necessary or appropriate.

Caution should be exercised in the handling and preparation of FLUDARA FOR INJECTION solution. The use of latex gloves and safety glasses is recommended to avoid exposure in case of breakage of the vial or other accidental spillage. If the solution contacts the skin or mucous membranes, wash thoroughly with soap and water; rinse eyes thoroughly with plain water. Avoid exposure by inhalation or by direct contact of the skin or mucous membranes.

HOW SUPPLIED

FLUDARA FOR INJECTION is supplied as a white, lyophilized solid cake. Each vial contains 50 mg of fludarabine phosphate, 50 mg of mannitol and sodium hydroxide to adjust pH to 7.7. The pH range for the final product is 7.2-8.2. Store under refrigeration, between 2°-8°C (36°-46°F).

FLUDARA FOR INJECTION is supplied in a clear glass single dose vial (6 mL capacity) and packaged in a single dose vial carton in a shelf pack of five.

CAUTION: Federal law prohibits dispensing without prescription.

NDC 50419-511-06

Manufactured by: Ben Venue Laboratories, Bedford, OH 44146

Manufactured for: Berlex Laboratories, Richmond, CA 94804-0016

U.S. Patent Number: 4,357,324

RA 2/96

References: 1. Cheson B.D., Bennett J.M., Rai K.R. et al. Guidelines for clinical protocols for chronic lymphocytic leukemia: Recommendations of the National Cancer Institute-Sponsored Working Group. Amer J Hematol 29:152-163, 1988. **2.** Recommendations for the Safe Handling of Parenteral Antineoplastic Drugs. NIH Publication No. 83-2621. For sale by the Superintendent of Documents, U.S. Government Printing Office, Washington, D.C. 20402. **3.** AMA Council Report. Guidelines for Handling Parenteral Antineoplastics, JAMA, 1985; March 15. **4.** National Study Commission on Cytotoxic Exposure—Recommendations for Handling Cytotoxic Agents. Available from Louis P. Jeffrey, Sc.D., Chairman, National Study Commission on Cytotoxic Exposure, Massachusetts College of Pharmacy and Allied Health Sciences, 179 Longwood Avenue, Boston, Massachusetts 02115. **5.** Clinical Oncological Society of Australia: Guidelines and Recommendations for Safe Handling of Antineoplastic Agents, Med. J. Australia 1983;1:426-428. **6.** Jones, R.B. et al. Safe Handling of Chemotherapeutic Agents: A Report from the Mount Sinai Medical Center, Ca—A Cancer Journal for Clinicians 1983; Sept/Oct. 258-263. **7.** American Society of Hospital Pharmacists Technical Assistance Bulletin on Handling Cytotoxic Drugs in Hospitals, Am. J. Hosp. Pharm. 1985;42:131-137. **8.** OSHA Work-Practice Guidelines for Personnel Dealing with Cytotoxic (antineoplastic) Drugs. Am. J. Hosp. Pharm. 1986;43:1193-1204.

Shown in Product Identification Guide, page 306

Berna Products, Corp.

4216 PONCE DE LEON BLVD.
CORAL GABLES, FL 33146

Direct Inquiries to:
Michelle Moskowitz
(305) 443-2900
(800) 533-5899

For Medical Information Contact: Andres Murai, Jr
In Emergencies: Andres Murai, Jr.
(305) 443-2900
(800) 533-5899

TE ANATOXAL BERNA® ℞
Tetanus Toxoid Adsorbed

HOW SUPPLIED

Syringe 0.5 ml 10 ea UD (NDC: 58337-1301-02)
Vial 5 ml (NDC: 58337-1301-01)

Vivotif Berna® Vaccine
Typhoid Vaccine Live Oral Ty21a

DESCRIPTION

Vivotif Berna® (Typhoid Vaccine Live Oral Ty21a) is a live attenuated vaccine for oral administration only. The vaccine contains the attenuated strain *Salmonella typhi* Ty21a (1,2).

Vivotif Berna® Vaccine is manufactured by the Swiss Serum and Vaccine Institute. The vaccine strain is grown in fermentors under controlled conditions in medium containing a digest of yeast extract, an acid digest of casein, dextrose and galactose. The bacteria are collected by centrifugation, mixed with a stabilizer containing sucrose, ascorbic acid and amino acids, and lyophilized. The lyophilized bacteria are mixed with lactose and magnesium stearate and filled into gelatin capsules which are coated with an organic solution to render them resistant to dissolution in stomach acid. The enteric-coated, salmon/white capsules are then packaged in 4-capsule blisters for distribution. The contents of each enteric-coated capsule are shown in Table 1.

Table 1: Contents of one enteric-coated capsule of Vivotif Berna® Vaccine

Viable *S. typhi* Ty21a	2–6 ×10^9 colony-forming units*
Non-viable *S. typhi* Ty21a ..	5–50 ×10^9 bacterial cells
Sucrose	26–130 mg
Ascorbic acid	1–5 mg
Amino acid mixture	1.4–7 mg
Lactose	100–180 mg
Magnesium stearate	3.6–4.4 mg

* Vaccine potency (viable cell counts per capsule) is determined by inoculation of agar plates with appropriate dilutions of the vaccine suspended in physiological saline.

CLINICAL PHARMACOLOGY

Salmonella typhi is the etiological agent of typhoid fever, an acute, febrile enteric disease. Typhoid fever continues to be an important disease in many parts of the world. Travelers entering infected areas are at risk of contracting typhoid fever following the ingestion of contaminated food or water. Typhoid fever is considered to be endemic in most areas of Central and South America, the African continent, the Near East and the Middle East, Southeast Asia and the Indian subcontinent (3). There are approximately 500 cases of typhoid fever per year diagnosed in the United States (4). In 62% of these patients (data from 1975–1984) the disease was acquired outside of the United States while in 38% of the patients the disease was acquired within the United States (5). Of 340 cases acquired in the United States between 1977 and 1979, 23% of the cases were associated with typhoid carriers, 24% were due to food outbreaks, 23% were associated with the ingestion of contaminated food or water, 6% due to household contact with an infected person and 4% following exposure to *S. typhi* in a laboratory setting (6).

The majority of typhoid cases respond favorably to antibiotic therapy. However, the emergence of multi-drug resistant strains has greatly complicated therapy and cases of typhoid fever that are treated with ineffective drugs can be fatal (7). Approximately 2–4% of acute typhoid cases result in the development of a chronic carrier state (8). These non-symptomatic carriers are the natural reservoir for *S. typhi* and can serve to maintain the disease in its endemic state or to directly infect individuals (3).

Virulent strains of *S. typhi* upon ingestion are able to pass through the stomach acid barrier, colonize the intestinal tract, penetrate the lumen and enter the lymphatic system and blood stream, thereby causing disease. One possible mechanism by which disease may be prevented is by evoking a local immune response in the intestinal tract. Such local immunity may be induced by oral ingestion of a live attenuated strain of *S. typhi* undergoing an aborted infection. The ability of *S. typhi* to cause disease and to induce a protective immune response is dependent upon the bacteria possessing a complete lipopolysaccharide (1). The *S. typhi* Ty21a vaccine strain, by virtue of a reduction in enzymes essential for lipopolysaccharide biosynthesis, is restricted in its ability to produce complete lipopolysaccharide (1,2). However, a sufficient quantity of complete lipopolysaccharide is synthesized to evoke a protective immune response. Despite low levels of lipopolysaccharide synthesis, the cells lyse before regaining a virulent phenotype due to the intracellular build-up of intermediates during lipopolysaccharide synthesis (1,2).

Results from clinical studies indicate that adults and children greater than 6 years of age may be protected against typhoid fever following the oral ingestion of 4 doses of Vivotif Berna® Vaccine (Typhoid Vaccine Live Oral Ty21a). The efficacy of the *S. typhi* Ty21a strain has been evaluated in a series of randomized, double-blind, controlled field trials. Suspected typhoid cases, detected by passive surveillance, were confirmed bacteriologically either by blood or bone marrow culture. The first trial was performed in Alexandria, Egypt with a study population of 32,388 children aged 6 to 7 years. Three doses of vaccine, in the form of a freshly reconstituted suspension administered after ingestion of 1 g of bicarbonate, were given on alternate days. Immunization resulted in a 95% decrease (95% confidence interval (CI) = 77%–99%) in the incidence of typhoid fever over a 3-year period of surveillance (9). A series of field trials were subsequently performed in Santiago, Chile to evaluate efficacy when the vaccine strain was administered in the form of an acid-resistant enteric-coated capsule. The initial trial involved 82,543 school-aged children, and compared 1 or 2 doses of vaccine given one week apart. After 24 months of surveillance vaccine efficacy was 29% (95% CI = 4%–47%) for the single dose schedule and 59% (95% CI = 41%–71%) for the 2-dose schedule (10). A further field trial was performed in Santiago, Chile involving 109,594 school-aged children (11). Three doses of enteric-coated capsules were administered either on alternate days (short immunization schedule) or 21 days apart (long immunization schedule). Following 36 months of surveillance vaccination resulted in a 67% (95% CI = 47%–79%) decrease in the incidence of typhoid fever in the short immunization schedule group and a 49% reduction (95% CI = 24%–66%) in the long immunization schedule group. After 48 months of surveillance the short immunization schedule resulted in a 69% (95% CI = 55%–80%) decrease in typhoid fever (12). An undiminished level of protection was observed during the fifth year of surveillance. A field trial was next conducted in Santiago, Chile to determine the relative efficacy of 2, 3 and 4 doses of enteric-coated vaccine administered on alternate days to school-aged children. Relative vaccine efficacy as determined by comparison of disease incidence within the three vaccinated groups was highest for the four dose regimen (13). The incidence of typhoid fever per 10^5 study subjects was 160.5 (95% CI = 130–191) for the three dose regimen versus 95.8 (95% CI = 71–121) for the four dose regimen ($p<0.004$). An additional field trial to determine vaccine efficacy was conducted in Plaju, Indonesia involving 20,543 individuals approximately 3 to 44 years of age (14). Due to logistical considerations three doses of enteric-coated capsules were administered at weekly intervals, a schedule known to provide suboptimal protection (11). After 30 months of surveillance vaccine efficacy for all age groups was 42% (95% CI = 23%–57%). Vaccine organisms can be shed transiently in the stool of vaccine recipients (16). However, secondary transmission of vaccine organisms has not been documented. Ty21a has not been isolated from blood cultures following immunization. At present, the precise mechanism(s) by which Vivotif Berna® Vaccine confers protection against typhoid fever is unknown. However, it is known that immunization of adult subjects can elicit a humoral anti-*S. typhi* LPS antibody response. Taking advantage of this fact, the seroconversion rate (defined as a Ú0.15 increase in optical density units over baseline determined in an ELISA) was compared in an open study between adults living in an endemic area (Chile) and non-endemic areas (United States and Switzerland) after the ingestion of 3 doses of vaccine. Comparable seroconversion rates were seen between these groups (15). *S. typhi* Ty21a cultured in medium not containing BHI induced an anti-*S. typhi* LPS antibody response comparable to that obtained with vaccine organisms cultured in medium containing BHI (15). Challenge studies in North American volunteers have shown that the Ty21a strain is capable of providing significant protection to an experimental challenge of *S. typhi* (16). Because of the very low incidence of typhoid fever in United States citizens, efficacy studies are not currently feasible in this population. However, the above observations support the expectation that Vivotif Berna® Vaccine will provide protection to recipients from non-typhoid endemic areas such as the United States.

INDICATIONS AND USAGE

Vivotif Berna® Vaccine (Typhoid Vaccine Live Oral Ty21a) is indicated for immunization of adults and children greater than 6 years of age against disease caused by *Salmonella typhi*. Routine typhoid vaccination is not recommended in the United States of America. Selective immunization against typhoid fever is recommended for the following groups: 1) travelers to areas in which there is a recognized risk of exposure to *S. typhi*, 2) persons with intimate exposure (e.g. household contact) to a *S. typhi* carrier, and 3) microbiology laboratorians who work frequently with *S. typhi*(7). There is no evidence to support the use of typhoid vaccine to control common source outbreaks, disease following natural disasters or in persons attending rural summer camps.

Not all recipients of Vivotif Berna® Vaccine will be fully protected against typhoid fever. Vaccinated individuals should continue to take personal precautions against exposure to typhoid organisms. The vaccine will not afford protection against species of *Salmonella* other than *Salmonella typhi* or other bacteria that cause enteric disease. The vaccine is not suitable for treatment of acute infections with *S. typhi*.

CONTRAINDICATIONS

Hypersensitivity to any component of the vaccine or the enteric-coated capsule. The vaccine should not be administered to persons during an acute febrile illness. Safety of the vaccine has not been demonstrated in persons deficient in their ability to mount a humoral or cell-mediated immune response, due to either a congenital or acquired immunodeficient state including treatment with immunosuppressive or antimitotic drugs. The vaccine should not be administered to these persons regardless of benefits.

WARNINGS

Vivotif Berna® (Typhoid Vaccine Live Oral Ty21a) is not to be taken during an acute gastrointestinal illness. The vaccine should not be administered to individuals receiving sulfonamides and antibiotics since these agents may be active against the vaccine strain and prevent a sufficient degree of multiplication to occur in order to induce a protective immune response. Postpone taking the vaccine if persistent diarrhea or vomiting is occurring. Unless a complete immunization schedule is followed, an optimum immune response may not be achieved. Not all recipients of Vivotif Berna® Vaccine will be fully protected against typhoid fever. Vaccinated individuals should continue to take personal precautions against exposure to typhoid organisms, i.e. travelers should take all necessary precautions to avoid contact or ingestion of potentially contaminated food or water.

Drug-Interactions

Several anti-malaria drugs, such as mefloquine, chloroquine and proguanil (not approved for use in US) possess antibacterial activity which may interfere with the immunogenicity of Vivotif Berna® Vaccine (17, 18). To determine the effect of these anti-malaria drugs on the humoral IgG or IgA anti-*S. typhi* immune response, healthy adult subjects were given mefloquine (250mg at weekly intervals; N=30) chloroquine (150mg at weekly intervals; N=30) or proguanil (200mg daily; N=30) together with the *S. typhi* Ty21a vaccine strain (19). Concomitant treatment with mefloquine or chloroquine did not result in a significant reduction in the serum anti-*S. typhi* immune response compared to subjects receiving vaccine strain only (N=45). The simultaneous administration of proguanil did effect a significant decrease in the immune response rate. These findings indicate that mefloquine and chloroquine can be administered together with Vivotif Berna® Vaccine. Proguanil should be administered only if 10 days or more have elapsed since the final dose of Vivotif Berna® Vaccine was ingested. The concomitant administration of oral polio vaccine or yellow fever vaccine does not suppress the immune response elicited by the Ty21a vaccine strain (19). There are no data regarding simultaneous administration of other parenteral vaccines or immunoglobulins with Vivotif Berna® Vaccine.

PRECAUTIONS

General

The health care provider should take all necessary precautions to ensure the safe and effective use of the vaccine. Patients should be questioned about previous reactions to this or similar products. The previous immunization history of the patient and current antibiotic usage should be obtained by the health care provider.

Information for Patients

It is essential that all 4 doses of vaccine be taken at the prescribed alternate day interval to obtain a maximal protective immune response. Vaccine potency is dependent upon storage under refrigeration [between 2°C and 8°C (35.6°F–46.4°F)]. The vaccine should be stored under refrigeration at all times. It is essential to replace unused vaccine in the refrigerator between doses. The vaccine capsule should be swallowed approximately 1 hour before a meal with a cold or luke-warm (temperature not to exceed body temperature, e.g., 37°C (98.6°F) drink. Care should be taken not to chew the vaccine capsule. The vaccine capsule should be swallowed as soon after placing in the mouth as possible. Not all recipients of Vivotif Berna® Vaccine (Typhoid Vaccine Live Oral Ty21a) will be fully protected against typhoid fever. Travelers should take all necessary precautions to avoid contact or ingestion of potentially contaminated food or water.

Several anti-malaria drugs, such as mefloquine, chloroquine and proguanil (not approved for use in US) possess antibacterial activity which may interfere with the immunogenicity of Vivotif Berna® Vaccine. Clinical results (see Warnings - Drug-Interactions) indicate that mefloquine and chloroquine can be administered together with Vivotif Berna® Vaccine. Proguanil should be administered only if 10 days or more have elapsed since the final dose of Vivotif Berna® Vaccine was ingested. Any serious adverse reactions related to the administration of the vaccine should be reported to your health care provider. You may also report an adverse reaction directly to the Vaccine Adverse Event Reporting System (1-800-822-7967) (20). Your health care provider should inform you of the benefits and risks of the vaccine, the importance of taking all 4 capsules in the correct schedule, and the importance of proper storage temperature of the capsules.

Carcinogenesis, Mutagenesis, Impairment of Fertility

Long-term studies in animals with Vivotif Berna® Vaccine have not been performed to evaluate carcinogenic potential, mutagenic potential or impairment of fertility.

Pregnancy

Category C

Animal reproduction studies have not been conducted with Vivotif Berna® Vaccine. It is not known whether Vivotif Berna® Vaccine can cause fetal harm when administered to pregnant woman or can affect reproduction capacity. Vivotif Berna® Vaccine should be given to a pregnant woman only if clearly needed.

Nursing Mothers

There is no data to warrant the use of this product in nursing mothers. It is not known if Vivotif Berna® Vaccine is excreted in human milk.

Pediatric Use

The safety and efficacy of Vivotif Berna® Vaccine has not been established in children under 6 years of age. This product is not indicated for use in children under 6 years of age.

ADVERSE REACTIONS

More than 1.4 million doses of Ty21a have been administered in controlled clinical trials and more than 150 million doses of Vivotif Berna® Vaccine (Typhoid Vaccine Live Oral Ty21a) have been marketed world-wide. Active surveillance for adverse reactions of enteric-coated capsules was performed in a pilot study (21) and in a subgroup of a large field trial (14) involving a total of 483 individuals receiving three vaccine doses. The overall symptom rates from both studies when vaccinated with capsules were combined and shown to be: abdominal pain (6.4%), nausea (5.8%), headache (4.8%), fever (3.3%), diarrhea (2.9%), vomiting (1.5%) and skin rash (1.0%). Only the incidence of nausea occured at a statistically higher frequency in the vaccinated group as compared to the placebo group (14). Administration of vaccine doses more than 5-fold higher than the currently recommended dose caused only mild reactions in an open study involving 155 healthy adult males (16).

Post-marketing surveillance has revealed that adverse reactions are infrequent and mild (17). Adverse reactions reported to the manufacturer during 1991-1995, during which time over 60 million doses (capsules) were administered, included: diarrhea (N=45), abdominal pain (N=42), nausea (N=35), fever (N=34), headache (N=26), skin rash (N=26), vomiting (N=18), or urticaria in the trunk and/or extremities (N=13). One isolated, non-fatal anaphylactic shock considered to be an allergic reaction to the vaccine was reported.

DOSAGE AND ADMINISTRATION

One capsule is to be swallowed approximately 1 hour before a meal with a cold or luke-warm [temperature not to exceed body temperature, e.g., 37 °C (98.6 °F)] drink on alternate days, e.g., days 1, 3, 5 and 7. Immunization (ingestion of all 4 doses of Vivotif Berna® Vaccine - Typhoid Vaccine Live Oral Ty21a) should be completed at least 1 week prior to potential exposure to *S. typhi*.

Continued on next page

Vivotif Berna—Cont.

The blister containing the vaccine capsules should be inspected to ensure that the foil seal and capsules are intact. The vaccine capsule should not be chewed and should be swallowed as soon after placing in the mouth as possible. A complete immunization schedule is the ingestion of 4 vaccine capsules as described above.

Re-immunization

The optimum booster schedule for Vivotif Berna® Vaccine has not been determined. Efficacy has been shown to persist for at least 5 years. Further, there is no experience with Vivotif Berna® Vaccine as a booster in persons previously immunized with parenteral typhoid vaccine. It is recommended that a re-immunization dose consisting of four vaccine capsules taken on alternate days be given every 5 years under conditions of repeated or continued exposure to typhoid fever (7).

HOW SUPPLIED

A single foil blister contains 4 doses of vaccine in a single package. (NDC: 58337-0003-01)

STORAGE

Vivotif Berna® Vaccine (Typhoid Vaccine Live Oral Ty21a) is not stable when exposed to ambient temperatures. Vivotif Berna® Vaccine should therefore be shipped and stored between 2°C and 8°C (35.6–46.4°F). Each package of vaccine shows an expiration date. This expiration date is valid only if the product has been maintained at 2°C–8°C (35.6–46.4°F).

Vivotif Berna® Vaccine is manufactured by Swiss Serum and Vaccine Institute Berne, Switzerland, and distributed by Berna Products Corp., Coral Gables, FL 33146.

REFERENCES

1. Germanier R., E. Fürer. Isolation and characterisation of Gal E mutant Ty21a of *Salmonella typhi*: a candidate strain for a live, oral typhoid vaccine. J. Infect. Dis. 131: 553¤558, 1975.
2. Germanier R., E. Fürer. Characteristics of the attenuated oral vaccine strain *S. typhi* Ty21a. Develop. Biol. Standard 53: 3–7, 1983.
3. Miller S.I., E.L. Hohmann, D.A. Pegues. *Salmonella* (including *Salmonella typhi*). In: Principles and practice of infectious diseases. G.L. Mandell, J.E. Bennett, R. Dolin (ed.) fourth edition, Churchill Livingstone Inc. 2013-2033, 1995.
4. Centers for Disease Control. Summary of notifiable diseases, United States 1995. MMWR 44 (Supplement), 1996.
5. Ryan C.A., N.T. Hargrett-Bean, P.A. Blake. *Salmonella typhi* infections in the United States, 1975-1984: Increasing role of foreign travel. Rev. Infect. Dis. 11: 1 - 8, 1989.
6. Taylor D.N., R.A. Pollard, P.A. Blake. Typhoid in the United States and the Risk to the International Traveler. J. Infect. Dis. 148: 599–602, 1983.
7. Recommendations of the Advisory Committee on Immunization Practices (ACIP): Typhoid Immunization. MMWR 43 (RR-14), 1994
8. Ames, W.R., M. Robbins. Age and sex as factors in the development of the typhoid carrier state, and a model for estimating carrier prevalence. Am. J. Public Health 33: 221–230, 1943.
9. Wahdan M.H., C. Sérié, Y. Cerisier, S. Sallam, R. Germanier. A controlled field trial of live Salmonella typhi strain Ty21a oral vaccine against typhoid: three-year results. J. Infect. Dis. 145: 292–296, 1982.
10. Black R.E., M.M. Levine, C. Ferreccio, M.L. Clements, C. Lanata, J. Rooney, R. Germanier, Chilean Typhoid Committee. Efficacy of one or two doses of Ty21a *Salmonella typhi* vaccine in enteric-coated capsules in a controlled field trial. Vaccine 8: 81-84, 1990.
11. Levine M.M., C. Ferreccio, R.E. Black, R. Germanier, Chilean Typhoid Committee. Large-Scale Field Trial of Ty21a Live Oral Typhoid Vaccine in Enteric-Coated Capsule Formulation. Lancet 1: 1049–1052, 1987.
12. Levine M.M., C. Ferreccio, R.E. Black, C.O. Tacket, R. Germanier, Chilean Typhoid Committee. Progress in vaccines against typhoid fever. Rev. Inf. Dis. 11 (Supplement 3): S552-S567, 1989.
13. Ferreccio C., M.M. Levine, H. Rodriguez, R. Contreras, Chilean Typhoid Committee. Comparative efficacy of two, three, or four doses of Ty21a live oral typhoid vaccine in enteric-coated capsules: a field trial in endemic area. J. Inf. Dis. 159: 766-769, 1989.
14. Simanjuntak C.H., F.P. Paleologo, N.H. Punjabi, R. Darmowigoto, Soeprawoto, H. Totosudirjo, P. Haryanto, E. Suprijanto, N.D. Witham, S.L. Hoffman. Oral immunisation against typhoid fever in Indonesia with Ty21a vaccine. Lancet 38: 1055-1059, 1991.
15. Data on File, Swiss Serum and Vaccine Institute Berne, Switzerland.
16. Gilman R.H., R.B. Hornick, W.E. Woodward, H.L. DuPont, M.J. Snyder, M.M. Levine, J.P. Libonati. Evaluation of a UDP-glucose-4-epimeraseless mutant of *Salmonella typhi* as a live oral vaccine. J. Infect. Dis. 136: 717-723, 1977.
17. Cryz S.J. Jr., Post-marketing experience with live oral Ty21a Vaccine. Lancet; 341: 49-50, 1993. Data on File, Swiss Serum and Vaccine Institute Berne, Switzerland.
18. Horowitz H., CA. Carbonaro, Inhibition of the *Salmonella typhi* oral vaccine strain Ty21a, by mefloquine and chloroquine. J. Infect. Dis. 166: 1462-1464, 1992.
19. Kollaritsch H., J.U. Que, C. Kunz, G. Wiedermann, C. Herzog, S.J. Cryz Jr. Safety and immunogenicity of live oral cholera and typhoid vaccines administered alone or in combination with anti-malarial drugs, oral polio vaccine or yellow fever vaccine. J. Infect. Dis. (in press).
20. Vaccine Adverse Event Reporting System - United States. MMWR 39: 730–733, 1990.
21. Levine M.M., R.E. Black, C. Ferreccio, M.L. Clements, C. Lanata, J. Rooney, R. Gemanier. The efficacy of attenuated *Salmonella typhi* oral vaccine strain Ty21a evaluated in controlled field trials. In: Development of Vaccines and Drugs against Diarrhea. 11th Noble Conference, Stockholm, 1985, p. 90-101. J. Holmgren, A. Lindberg and R. Möllby (eds.). Studentlitteratur, Lund, Sweden, 1986.

Manufactured by:
Swiss Serum and Vaccine Institute Berne, Switzerland
US-Licence No. 21
Distributed by: Version:
Berna Products Corp., Coral Gables, FL 33146 April 1997
Shown in Product Identification Guide, page 306

Bertek Pharmaceuticals, Inc.
10410 CORORATE DRIVE
SUGAR LAND, TX 77478-2825

Direct Inquiries to:
(888) 823-7835
Fax: (304) 285-6453

Other Products Available:
NITREK® ℞

CLORPRES™ ℞
[klŏr prĕs]
(Clonidine Hydrochloride and Chlorthalidone)
TABLETS, USP
0.1 mg/15 mg, 0.2 mg/15 mg and 0.3 mg/15 mg

DESCRIPTION

CLORPRES™ is a combination of clonidine hydrochloride (a centrally acting antihypertensive agent) and chlorthalidone (a diuretic). CLORPRES™ is available as tablets for oral administration in three dosage strengths: 0.1 mg/15 mg, 0.2 mg/15 mg and 0.3 mg/15 mg of clonidine hydrochloride/chlorthalidone, respectively.

The inactive ingredients are ammonium chloride, colloidal silicon dioxide, croscarmellose sodium (Type A), magnesium stearate, microcrystalline cellulose, sodium lauryl sulfate, D&C yellow #10.

Clonidine Hydrochloride: Clonidine hydrochloride is an imidazoline derivative and exists as a mesomeric compound. The chemical name is 2-[(2,6-dichlorophenyl)imino]imidazoline monohydrochloride. The following are the structural formula, molecular formula and molecular weight:
[See structural formula at top of next column]
Clonidine hydrochloride is an odorless, bitter, white crystalline substance soluble in water and alcohol.

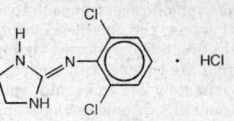

$C_9H_9Cl_2N_3$•HCl
M.W. 266.56

Chlorthalidone: Chlorthalidone is a monosulfamyl diuretic that differs chemically from thiazide diuretics in that a double ring system is incorporated in its structure. It is 2-chloro-5-(1-hydroxy-3-oxo-1-isoindolinyl) benzenesulfonamide with the following structural formula, molecular formula and molecular weight:

$C_{14}H_{11}Cl\,N_2O_4S$
M.W. 338.76

Chlorthalidone is practically insoluble in water, in ether and in chloroform; soluble in methanol; slightly soluble in alcohol.

CLINICAL PHARMACOLOGY

CLORPRES™: Clorpres produces a more pronounced antihypertensive response than occurs after either clonidine hydrochloride or chlorthalidone alone in equivalent doses.

Clonidine Hydrochloride: Clonidine hydrochloride acts relatively rapidly. The patient's blood pressure declines within 30 to 60 minutes after an oral dose, the maximum decrease occurring within 2 to 4 hours. The plasma level of clonidine hydrochloride peaks in approximately 3 to 5 hours and the plasma half-life ranges from 12 to 16 hours. The half-life increases up to 41 hours in patients with severe impairment of renal function. Following oral administration about 40 to 60% of the absorbed dose is recovered in the urine as unchanged drug in 24 hours. About 50% of the absorbed dose is metabolized in the liver.

Clonidine stimulates alpha-adrenoreceptors in the brain stem, resulting in reduced sympathetic outflow from the central nervous system and a decrease in peripheral resistance, renal vascular resistance, heart rate, and blood pressure. Renal blood flow and glomerular filtration rate remain essentially unchanged. Normal postural reflexes are intact and therefore orthostatic symptoms are mild and infrequent.

Acute studies with clonidine hydrochloride in humans have demonstrated a moderate reduction (15 to 20%) of cardiac output in the supine position with no change in the peripheral resistance; at a 45° tilt there is a smaller reduction in cardiac output and a decrease of peripheral resistance. During long-term therapy, cardiac output tends to return to control values, while peripheral resistance remains decreased. Slowing of the pulse rate has been observed in most patients given clonidine but the drug does not alter normal hemodynamic response to exercise.

Other studies in patients have provided evidence of a reduction in plasma renin activity and in the excretion of aldosterone and catecholamines, but the exact relationship of these pharmacologic actions to the antihypertensive effect has not been fully elucidated.

Clonidine acutely stimulates growth hormone release in both children and adults, but does not produce a chronic elevation of growth hormone with long-term use.

Tolerance may develop in some patients, necessitating a re-evaluation of therapy.

Chlorthalidone: Chlorthalidone is a long-acting oral diuretic with antihypertensive activity. Its diuretic action commences a mean of 2.6 hours after dosing and continues for up to 72 hours. The drug produces diuresis with increased excretion of sodium and chloride. The diuretic effects of chlorthalidone and the benzothiadiazine (thiazide) diuretics appear to arise from similar mechanisms and the maximal effect of chlorthalidone and the thiazides appears to be similar. The site of action appears to be the distal convoluted tubule of the nephron. The diuretic effects of chlorthalidone lead to decreased extracellular fluid volume, plasma volume, cardiac output, total exchangeable sodium, glomerular filtration rate, and renal plasma flow. Although the mechanism of action of chlorthalidone and related drugs is not wholly clear, sodium and water depletion appear to provide a basis for its antihypertensive effect. Like the thiazide diuretics, chlorthalidone produces dose-related reductions in serum potassium levels, elevations in serum uric acid and blood glucose, and it can lead to decreased sodium and chloride levels.

The mean plasma half-life of chlorthalidone is about 40 to 60 hours. It is eliminated primarily as unchanged drug in the urine. Non-renal routes of elimination have yet to be clarified. In the blood, approximately 75% of the drug is bound to plasma proteins.

INDICATIONS AND USAGE

CLORPRES™ (clonidine hydrochloride USP/chlorthalidone USP) is indicated in the treatment of hypertension. **This fixed combination drug is not indicated for initial therapy of hypertension. Hypertension requires therapy titrated to the individual patient. If the fixed combination represents the dosage so determined, its use may be more convenient in patient management. The treatment of hypertension is not static, but must be reevaluated as conditions in each patient warrant.**

CONTRAINDICATIONS

Anuria: CLORPRES™ is contraindicated in patients with known hypersensitivity to chlorthalidone or other sulfonamide-derived drugs.

WARNINGS

Chlorthalidone should be used with caution in severe renal disease. In patients with renal disease, chlorthalidone or related drugs may precipitate azotemia. Cumulative effects of the drug may develop in patients with impaired renal function. Chlorthalidone should be used with caution in patients with impaired hepatic function or progressive liver disease, because minor alterations of fluid and electrolyte balance may precipitate hepatic coma.

Sensitivity reactions may occur in patients with a history of allergy or bronchial asthma.

The possibility of exacerbation or activation of systemic lupus erythematosus has been reported with thiazide diuretics which are structurally related to chlorthalidone. However, systemic lupus erythematosus has not been reported following chlorthalidone administration.

PRECAUTIONS

Clonidine Hydrochloride: *General:* In patients who have developed localized contact sensitization to transdermal clonidine, substitution of oral clonidine hydrochloride therapy may be associated with the development of a generalized skin rash.

In patients who develop an allergic reaction from transdermal clonidine that extends beyond the local patch site (such as generalized skin rash, urticaria or angioedema), oral clonidine hydrochloride substitution may elicit a similar reaction.

As with all antihypertensive therapy, clonidine hydrochloride should be used with caution in patients with severe coronary insufficiency, recent myocardial infarction, cerebrovascular disease or chronic renal failure.

Withdrawal: Patients should be instructed not to discontinue therapy without consulting their physician. Sudden cessation of clonidine treatment has resulted in subjective symptoms such as nervousness, agitation and headache, accompanied or followed by a rapid rise in blood pressure and elevated catecholamine concentrations in the plasma, but such occurrences have usually been associated with previous administration of high oral doses (exceeding 1.2 mg/day) and/or with continuation of concomitant beta-blocker therapy. Rare instances of hypertensive encephalopathy and death have been reported. When discontinuing therapy with clonidine hydrochloride, the physician should reduce the dose gradually over 2 to 4 days to avoid withdrawl symptomatology.

An excessive rise in blood pressure following clonidine hydrochloride discontinuance can be reversed by administration of oral clonidine or by intravenous phentolamine. If therapy is to be discontinued in patients receiving beta-blockers and clonidine concurrently, beta-blockers should be discontinued several days before the gradual withdrawal of clonidine hydrochloride.

Perioperative Use: Administration of clonidine hydrochloride should be continued to within four hours of surgery and resumed as soon as possible thereafter. The blood pressure should be carefully monitored and appropriate measures instituted to control it as necessary.

Information for Patients: Patients who engage in potentially hazardous activities, such as operating machinery or driving, should be advised of a potential sedative effect of clonidine. Patients should be cautioned against interruption of clonidine hydrochloride therapy without a physician's advice.

Drug Interactions: If a patient receiving clonidine hydrochloride is also taking tricyclic antidepressants, the effect of clonidine may be reduced, thus necessitating an increase in dosage. Clonidine hydrochloride may enhance the CNS-depressive effects of alcohol, barbiturates or other sedatives. Amitriptyline in combination with clonidine enhances the manifestation of corneal lesions in rats (see Ocular Toxicity).

Ocular Toxicity: In several studies, oral clonidine hydrochloride produced a dose-dependent increase in the incidence and severity of spontaneously occurring retinal degeneration in albino rats treated for six months or longer. Tissue distribution studies in dogs and monkeys revealed that clonidine hydrochloride was concentrated in the choroid of the eye. In view of the retinal degeneration observed in rats, eye examinations were performed in 908 patients prior to the start of clonidine hydrochloride therapy, who were then examined periodically thereafter. In 353 of these 908 patients, examinations were performed for periods of 24 months or longer. Except for some dryness of the eyes, no drug-related abnormal ophthalmologic findings were recorded and clonidine hydrochloride did no alter retinal function as shown by specialized tests such as the electroretinogram and macular dazzle.

In rats, clonidine hydrochloride in combination with amitriptyline produced corneal lesions within 5 days.

Carcinogenesis, Mutagenesis, Impairment of Fertility: In a 132-week (fixed concentration) dietary administration study in rats, clonidine hydrochloride administered at 32 to 46 times the maximum recommended daily human oral dose was unassociated with evidence of carcinogenic potential.

Fertility of male or female rats was unaffected by clonidine hydrochloride doses as high as 150 mcg/kg or about 3 times the maximum recommended daily human oral dose (MRDHD). Fertility of female rats did, however, appear to be affected (in another experiment) at dose levels of 500 to 2000 mcg/kg or 10 to 40 times the MRDHD.

Usage in Pregnancy: *Teratogenic Effect. Pregnancy Category C:* Reproduction studies performed in rabbits at doses up to approximately 3 times the maximum recommended daily human dose (MRDHD) of clonidine hydrochloride have revealed no evidence of teratogenic or embryotoxic potential. In rats however, doses as low as 1/3 the MRDHD were associated with increased resorptions in a study in which dams were treated continuously from 2 months prior to mating. Increased resorptions were not associated with treatment at the same or at higher dose levels (up to 3 times the MRDHD) when dams were treated days 6 to 15 of gestation. Increased resorptions were observed at much higher levels (40 times the MRDHD) in rats and mice treated days 1 to 14 of gestation (lowest dose employed in that study was 500 mcg/kg). There are, however, no adequate and well-controlled studies in pregnant women. Because animal reproduction studies are not always predictive of human response, this drug should be used during pregnancy only if clearly needed.

Nursing Mothers: As clonidine hydrochloride is excreted in human milk, caution should be exercised when it is administered to a nursing woman.

Pediatric Use: Safety and effectiveness in the pediatric population have not been established.

Chlorthalidone: *General:* Hypokalemia and other electrolyte abnormalities, including hyponatremia and hypochloremic alkalosis, are common in patients receiving chlorthalidone. These abnormalities are dose-related but may occur even at the lowest marketed doses of chlorthalidone. Serum electrolytes should be determined before initiating therapy and at periodic intervals during therapy. Serum and urine electrolyte determinations are particularly important when the patient is vomiting excessively or receiving parenteral fluids. All patients taking chlorthalidone should be observed for clinical signs of electrolyte imbalance, including dryness of mouth, thirst, weakness, lethargy, drowsiness, muscle pains or cramps, muscular fatigue, hypotension, oliguria, tachycardia, palpitations and gastrointestinal disturbances, such as nausea and vomiting. Digitalis therapy may exaggerate metabolic effects of hypokalemia especially with reference to myocardial activity.

Any chloride deficit is generally mild and usually does not require specific treatment except under extraordinary circumstances (as in liver disease or renal disease). Dilutional hyponatremia may occur in edematous patients in hot weather: appropriate therapy is water restriction rather than administration of salt, except in rare instances when the hyponatremia is life-threatening. In cases of actual salt depletion, appropriate replacement is the therapy of choice.

Uric Acid: Hyperuricemia may occur or frank gout may be precipitated in certain patients receiving chlorthalidone.

Other: Increases in serum glucose may occur and latent diabetes mellitus may become manifest during chlorthalidone therapy (see PRECAUTIONS: Chlorthalidone: Drug Interactions). Chlorthalidone and related drugs may decrease serum PBI levels without signs of thyroid disturbance.

Information for Patients: Patients should inform their doctor if they have: 1) had an allergic reaction to chlorthalidone or other diuretics or have asthma 2) kidney disease 3) liver disease 4) gout 5) systemic lupus erythematosus, or 6) been taking other drugs such as cortisone, digitalis, lithium carbonate, or drugs for diabetes.

Patients should be cautioned to contact their physician if they experience any of the following symptoms of potassium loss: excess thirst, tiredness, drowsiness, restlessness, muscle pains or cramps, nausea, vomiting or increased heart rate or pulse.

Patients should also be cautioned that taking alcohol can increase the chance of dizziness occurring.

Laboratory Tests: Periodic determination of serum electrolytes to detect possible electrolyte imbalance should be performed at appropriate intervals.

All patients receiving chlorthalidone should be observed for clinical signs of fluid or electrolyte imbalance: namely, hyponatremia, hypochloremic alkalosis and hypokalemia. Serum and urine electrolyte determinations are particularly important when the patient is vomiting excessively or receiving parenteral fluids.

Drug Interactions: Chlorthalidone may add to or potentiate the action of other antihypertensive drugs. Insulin requirements in diabetic patients may be increased, decreased or unchanged. Higher dosage of oral hypoglycemic agents may be required. Chlorthalidone and related drugs may increase the responsiveness to tubocurarine. Clorthalidone and related drugs may decrease arterial responsiveness to norepinephrine. This diminution is not sufficient to preclude effectiveness of the pressor agent for therapeutic use. Lithium renal clearance is reduced by clorthalidone, increasing the risk of lithium toxicity.

Drug/Laboratory Test Interactions: Clorthalidone and related drugs may decrease serum PBI levels without signs of thyroid disturbance.

Carcinogenesis, Mutagenesis, Impairment of Fertility: No information is available.

Usage in Pregnancy: *Teratogenic Effects. Pregnancy Category B:* Reproduction studies have been performed in the rat and the rabbit at doses up to 420 times the human dose and have revealed no evidence of harm to the fetus due to clorthalidone. There are, however, no adequate and well-controlled studies in pregnant women. Because animal reproduction studies are not always predictive of human response, this drug should be used during pregnancy only if clearly needed.

Non-Teratogenic Effects: Thiazides cross the placental barrier and appear in cord blood. The use of clorthalidone and related drugs in pregnant women requires that the anticipated benefits of the drug be weighed against possible hazards to the fetus. These hazards include fetal or neonatal jaundice, thrombocytopenia, and possibly other adverse reactions that have occurred in the adult.

Nursing Mothers: Thiazides are excreted in human milk. Because of the potential for serious adverse reactions in nursing infants from clorthalidone, a decision should be made whether to discontinue nursing or to discontinue the drug, taking into account the importance of the drug to the mother.

Pediatric Use: Safety and effectiveness in the pediatric population have not been established.

ADVERSE REACTIONS

CLORPRES™ is generally well tolerated. Most adverse effects are mild and tend to diminish with continued therapy. The most frequent (which appears to be dose-related) are dry mouth, occurring in about 40 of 100 patients; drowsiness, about 33 in 100; dizziness, about 16 in 100; constipation and sedation, each about 10 in 100.

In addition to the reactions listed above, certain less frequent adverse experiences, which are shown below, have also been reported in patients receiving the component drugs of CLORPRES™ but in many cases patients were receiving concomitant medication and a causal relationship has not been established:

Clonidine Hydrochloride: *Gastrointestinal:* Nausea and vomiting, about 5 in 100 patients; anorexia and malaise, each about 1 in 100; mild transient abnormalities in liver function tests, about 1 in 100; rare reports of hepatitis; parotitis, rarely.

Metabolic: Weight gain, about 1 in 100 patients; gynecomastia, about 1 in 1000, transient elevation of blood glucose or serum creatinine phosphokinase, rarely.

Central Nervous System: Nervousness and agitation, about 3 in 100 patients; mental depression, about 1 in 100; headache, about 1 in 100; insomnia, about 5 in 1000. Vivid dreams or nightmares, other behavioral changes, restlessness, anxiety, visual and auditory hallucinations and delirium have been reported.

Cardiovascular: Orthostatic symptoms, about 3 in 100 patients; palpitations and tachycardia, and bradycardia, each about 5 in 1000. Raynaud's phenomenon, congestive heart failure, and electrocardiographic abnormalities, i.e., conduction disturbances and arrhythmias, have been reported rarely. Rare cases of sinus bradycardia and atrioventricular block have been reported, both with and without the use of concomitant digitalis.

Dermatological: Rash, about 1 in 100 patients; pruritus, about 7 in 1000; hives, angioneurotic edema and urticaria, about 5 in 1000, alopecia, about 2 in 1000.

Genitourinary: Decreased sexual activity, impotence and loss of libido, about 3 in 100 patients; nocturia, about 1 in 100; difficulty in micturition, about 2 in 1000; urinary retention, about 1 in 1000.

Other: Weakness, about 10 in 100 patients; fatigue, about 4 in 100; discontinuation syndrome, about 1 in 100; muscle or joint pain, about 6 in 1000 and cramps of the lower limbs, about 3 in 1000. Dryness, burning of the eyes, blurred vision, dryness of the nasal mucosa, pallor, weakly positive Coombs' test, increased sensitivity to alcohol and fever have been reported.

Continued on next page

Clorpres—Cont.

Chlorthalidone: ***Gastrointestinal:*** Anorexia, gastric irritation, nausea, vomiting, cramping, diarrhea, constipation, jaundice (intrahepatic cholestatic jaundice), pancreatitis.
Central Nervous System: Dizziness, vertigo, paresthesia, headache, xanthopsia.
Hematologic: Leukopenia, agranulocytosis, thrombocytopenia, aplastic anemia.
Dermatologic-Hypersensitivity: Purpura, photosensitivity, rash, urticaria, necrotizing angiitis (vasculitis) (cutaneous vasculitis), Lyell's syndrome (toxic epidermal necrolysis).
Cardiovascular: Orthostatic hypotension may occur and may be aggravated by alcohol, barbiturates or narcotics.
Other Adverse Reactions: Hyperglycemia, glycosuria, hyperuricemia, muscle spasm, weakness, restlessness, impotence.
Whenever adverse reactions are moderate or severe, chlorthalidone dosage should be reduced or therapy withdrawn.

OVERDOSAGE

Clonidine Hydrochloride: The signs and symptoms of clonidine hydrochloride ovedosage include hypotension, bradycardia, lethargy, irritability, weakness, somnolence, diminished or absent reflexes, miosis, vomiting and hypoventilation. With large overdoses, reversible cardiac conduction defects or arrhythmias, apnea, seizures and transient hypertension have been reported. The oral LD_{50} of clonidine in rats was 465 mg/kg, and in mice 206 mg/kg.
The general treatment of clonidine hydrochloride overdosage may include intravenous fluids as indicated. Bradycardia can be treated with intravenous atropine sulfate and hypotension with dopamine infusion in addition to intravenous fluids. Hypertension, associated with overdosage, has been treated with intravenous furosemide or diazoxide or alpha-blocking agents such as phentolamine. Tolazoline, an alpha-blocker, in intravenous doses of 10 mg at 30-minute intervals, may reverse clonidine's effects if other efforts fail. Routine hemodialysis is of limited benefit, since a maximum of 5% of circulating clonidine is removed.
In a patient who ingested 100 mg clonidine hydrochloride, plasma clonidine levels were 60 ng/mL (one hour), 190 ng/mL (1.5 hours), 370 ng/mL (two hours) and 120 ng/mL (5.5 and 6.5 hours). This patient developed hypertension followed by hypotension, bradycardia, apnea, hallucinations, semicoma, and premature ventricular contractions. The patient fully recovered after intensive treatment.
Chlorthalidone: Symptoms of acute overdosage include nausea, weakness, dizziness and disturbances of electrolyte balance. The oral LD_{50} of the drug in the mouse and the rat is more than 25,000 mg/kg body weight. The minimum lethal dose (MLD) in humans has not been established. There is no specific antidote but gastric lavage is recommended, followed by supportive treatment. Where necessary, this may include intravenous dextrose-saline with potassium, administered with caution.

DOSAGE AND ADMINISTRATION

The dosage must be determined by individual titration. (See INDICATIONS AND USAGE.)
Chlorthalidone is usually initiated at a dose of 25 mg once daily and may be increased to 50 mg if the response is insufficient after a suitable trial.
Clonidine hydrochloride is usually initiated at a dose of 0.1 mg twice daily. Elderly patients may benefit from a lower initial dose. Further increments of 0.1 mg/day may be made if necessary until the desired response is achieved. The therapeutic doses most commonly employed have ranged from 0.2 to 0.6 mg per day in divided doses.
One CLORPRES™ (clonidine hydrochloride/chlorthalidone) Tablet administered once or twice daily can be used to administer a minimum of 0.1 mg clonidine hydrochloride and 15 mg chlorthalidone to a maximum of 0.6 mg clonidine hydrochloride and 30 mg chlorthalidone.

HOW SUPPLIED

CLORPRES™ (clonidine hydrochloride and chlorthalidone) Tablets, USP are available containing:
0.1 mg clonidine hydrochloride, USP and 15 mg chlorthalidone, USP

or

0.2 mg clonidine hydrochloride, USP and 15 mg chlorthalidone, USP

or

0.3 mg clonidine hydrochloride, USP and 15 mg chlorthalidone, USP
The 0.1 mg/15 mg product is a yellow, round, scored tablet marked with M1. They are available as follows:

NDC 62794-001-01
bottles of 100 tablets

The 0.2 mg/15 mg product is a yellow, round, scored tablet marked with M27. They are available as follows:

NDC 62794-027-01
bottles of 100 tablets

The 0.3 mg/15 mg product is a yellow, round, scored tablet marked with M72. They are available as follows:

NDC 62794-072-01
bottles of 100 tablets

STORE AT CONTROLLED ROOM TEMPERATURE 15° to 30° C (59° to 86°F).
AVOID EXCESSIVE HUMIDITY.
Dispense in a tight, light-resistant container as defined in the USP using a child-resistant closure.
Rx only

BERTEK PHARMACEUTICALS INC.
Sugar Land, TX 77478
REVISED JUNE 1998
BKCLCH:R2

Shown in Product Identification Guide, page 306

GRANULEX ℞

COMPOSITION

Each 0.82 cc. of medication delivered to the wound site contains Trypsin crystallized 0.1 mg., Balsam Peru 72.5 mg., Castor Oil 650.0 mg., and an emulsifier.

ACTION

Trypsin is intended for debridement of eschar and other necrotic tissue. It appears that in many instances removal of wound debris strengthens humoral defense mechanisms sufficiently to retard proliferation of local pathogens. Balsam Peru is an effective capillary bed stimulant used to increase circulation in the wound site area. Also, Balsam Peru has a mildly bactericidal action. Castor Oil is used to improve epithelialization by reducing premature epithelial desiccation and cornification. Also, it can act as a protective covering and aids in the reduction of pain.

INDICATIONS

For the treatment of decubitus ulcers, varicose ulcers, debridement of eschar, dehiscent wounds and sunburn.

USES

Granulex is in aerosol form which can be important to healing. It must be remembered, healing starts with a thin sheath of epithelium no more than a cell or two thick. Any rough movement or trauma can quickly destroy the healing tissue. Aerosols have the advantage of eliminating all extraneous physical contact with the wound. Granulex is easy to apply and quickly reduces odor frequently accompanying a decubitus ulcer. The wound may be left open or a wet bandage may be applied. As a suggestion; keep in mind wounds heal poorly in the presence of hemoglobin or zinc deficiency.

WARNING

Do not spray on fresh arterial clots. Avoid spraying in eyes. Flammable, do not expose to fire or open flame. Contents under pressure. Do not puncture or incinerate. Do not store at temperature above 120°F. Keep out of reach of children. Use only as directed. Intentional misuse by deliberately concentrating and inhaling the contents can be harmful or fatal.

DOSAGE

Apply a minimum of twice daily or as often as necessary. Shake well, press the aerosol valve and coat the wound rapidly but not excessively.

HOW SUPPLIED

2 oz. Aerosol NDC 0514-0001-01
4 oz. Aerosol NDC 0514-0001-02

KRISTALOSE™ ℞

[krĭs' tă lōsē]
(LACTULOSE)
For Oral Solution

DESCRIPTION

KRISTALOSE™ (Lactulose) is a synethetic disaccharide in the form of crystals for reconstitution prior to use for oral administration. Each 10 g of lactulose contains less than 0.3 g galactose and lactose as a total sum. The pH range is 3.0 to 7.0
Lactulose is a colonic acidifier which promotes laxation.
The chemical name for lactulose is 4-O-β-D-Galactopyranosyl-D-fructofuranose. It has the following structural formula:

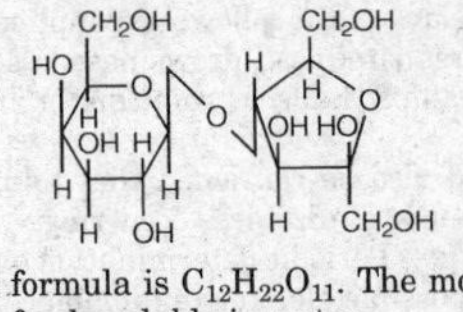

The molecular formula is $C_{12}H_{22}O_{11}$. The molecular weight is 342.30. It is freely soluble in water.

CLINICAL PHARMACOLOGY

KRISTALOSE™ (Lactulose) is poorly absorbed from the gastrointestinal tract and no enzyme capable of hydrolysis of this disaccharide is present in human gastrointestinal tissue. As a result, oral doses of lactulose reach the colon virtually unchanged. In the colon, lactulose is broken down primarily to lactic acid, and also to small amounts of formic and acetic acids, by the action of colonic bacteria, which results in an increase in osmotic pressure and slight acidification of the colonic contents. This in turn causes an increase in stool water content and softens the stool.
Since lactulose does not exert its effect until it reaches the colon, and since transit time through the colon may be slow, 24 to 48 hours may be required to produce desired bowel movement.
Lactulose given orally to man and experimental animals resulted in only small amounts reaching the blood. Urinary excretion has been determined to be 3% or less and is essentially complete within 24 hours.

INDICATIONS AND USAGE

KRISTALOSE™ (Lactulose) for Oral Solution is indicated for the treatment of constipation. In patients with a history of chronic constipation, lactulose therapy increases the number of bowel movements per day and the number of days on which bowel movements occur.

CONTRAINDICATIONS

Since KRISTALOSE™ (Lactulose) for Oral Solution contains galactose (less than 0.3 g/10 g as a total sum with lactose), it is contraindicated in patients who require a low galactose diet.

WARNINGS

A theoretical hazard may exist for patients being treated with lactulose who may be required to undergo electrocautery procedures during proctoscopy or colonoscopy. Accumulation of H_2 gas in significant concentration in the presence of an electrical spark may result in an explosive reaction. Although this complication has not been reported with lactulose, patients on lactulose therapy undergoing such procedures should have a thorough bowel cleansing with a non-fermentable solution. Insufflation of CO_2 as an additional safeguard may be pursued but is considered to be a redundant measure.

PRECAUTIONS

General
Since KRISTALOSE™ (Lactulose) for Oral Solution contains galactose and lactose (less than 0.3 g/10 g as a total sum), it should be used with caution in diabetics.
Information for patients
In the event that an unusual diarrheal condition occurs, contact your physician.
Laboratory Tests
Elderly, debilitated patients who receive lactulose for more than six months should have serum electrolytes (potassium, chloride, carbon dioxide) measured periodically.
Drug Interactions
Results of preliminary studies in humans and rats suggest that nonabsorbable antacids given concurrently with lactulose may inhibit the desired lactulose-induced drop in colonic pH. Therefore, a possible lack of desired effect of treatment should be taken into consideration before such drugs are given concomitantly with lactulose.
Carcinogenesis, Mutagenesis, Impairment of Fertility
There are no known human data on long-term potential for carcinogenicity, mutagenicity, or impairment of fertility.
There are no known animal data on long-term potential for mutagenicity.
Administration of lactulose syrup in the diet of mice for 18 months in concentrations of 3 and 10 percent (v/w) did not produce any evidence of carcinogenicity.
In studies in mice, rats, and rabbits, doses of lactulose syrup up to 6 or 12 mL/kg/day produced no deleterious effects in breeding, conception, or parturition.
Pregnancy
Teratogenic Effects
Pregnancy Category B
Reproduction studies have been performed in mice, rats, and rabbits at doses up to 3 or 6 times the usual human oral dose and have revealed no evidence of impaired fertility or harm to the fetus due to lactulose. There are, however, no adequate and well-controlled studies in pregnant women. Because animal reproduction studies are not always predictive of human response, this drug should be used during pregnancy only if clearly needed.
Nursing Mothers
It is not known whether this drug is excreted in human milk. Because many drugs are excreted in human milk, caution should be exercised when lactulose is administered to a nursing woman.
Pediatric Use
Safety and effectiveness in pediatric patients have not been established.

ADVERSE REACTIONS

Precise frequency data are not available.
Initial dosing may produce flatulence and intestinal

cramps, which are usually transient. Excessive dosage can lead to diarrhea with potential complications such as loss of fluids, hypokalemia, and hypernatremia.
Nausea and vomiting have been reported.

OVERDOSAGE

Signs and Symptoms
There have been no reports of accidental overdosage. In the event of overdosage, it is expected that diarrhea and abdominal cramps would be the major symptoms. Medication should be terminated.
Oral LD_{50}
The acute oral LD_{50} of the drug is 48.8 mL/kg in mice and greater than 30 mL/kg in rats.
Dialysis
Dialysis data are not available for lactulose. Its molecular similarity to sucrose, however, would suggest that it should be dialyzable.

DOSAGE AND ADMINISTRATION

The usual adult dosage is 10 g to 20 g of lactulose daily. The dose may be increased to 40 g daily if necessary. Twenty-four to forty-eight hours may be required to produce a normal bowel movement.

DIRECTIONS FOR PREPARATION
Dissolve contents of packet in half a glass (4 ounces) of water.
When Lactulose for Oral Solution is dissolved in water, the resulting solution may be colorless to a slightly pale yellow color.

HOW SUPPLIED

KRISTALOSE™ (Lactulose) for Oral Solution is available in 10 g and 20 g single dose packets in cartons of 30.
NDC 62794-501-17
Single dose packet of 10 g
NDC 62794-502-17
Single dose packet of 20 g

STORE AT ROOM TEMPERATURE, 15°–30°C (59°–86°F).
CAUTION: Federal law prohibits dispensing without prescription.
Distributed by
BERTEK PHARMACEUTICALS INC.
Sugar Land, TX 77478
Manufactured by
Inalco S.p.A.
Milan, Italy

BKKRST:R1
REVISED OCTOBER 1997

MAXZIDE® and MAXZIDE®-25 MG TABLETS ℞

[*măx 'zīde*]
BRAND OF (TRIAMTERENE AND HYDROCHLOROTHIAZIDE)

DESCRIPTION

MAXZIDE® (triamterene and hydrochlorothiazide) combines triamterene, a potassium-conserving diuretic, with the natriuretic agent, hydrochlorothiazide.
Each MAXZIDE® tablet contains:
Triamterene, USP .... 75 mg
Hydrochlorothiazide, USP .... 50 mg
Each MAXZIDE®-25 MG tablet contains:
Triamterene, USP .... 37.5 mg
Hydrochlorothiazide, USP .... 25 mg
MAXZIDE® and MAXZIDE®-25 MG tablets for oral administration contain the following inactive ingredients: Colloidal Silicon Dioxide, Croscarmellose Sodium, Magnesium Stearate, Microcrystalline Cellulose, Powdered Cellulose, Sodium Lauryl Sulfate and D&C Yellow #10. MAXZIDE®-25 MG tablets also contain FD&C Blue #1.
Triamterene is 2,4,7–triamino-6-phenylpteridine. Triamterene is practically insoluble in water, benzene, chloroform, ether and dilute alkali hydroxides. It is soluble in formic acid and sparingly soluble in methoxyethanol. Triamterene is very slightly soluble in acetic acid, alcohol and dilute mineral acids. Its molecular weight is 253.27. Its structural formula is:

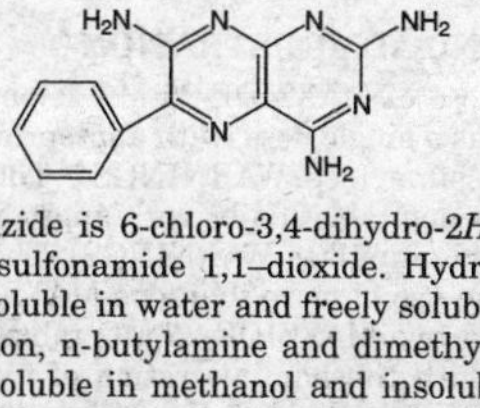

Hydrochlorothiazide is 6-chloro-3,4-dihydro-2*H*-1,2,4, benzothiadiazine-7-sulfonamide 1,1–dioxide. Hydrochlorothiazide is slightly soluble in water and freely soluble in sodium hydroxide solution, n-butylamine and dimethylformamide. It is sparingly soluble in methanol and insoluble in ether, chloroform and dilute mineral acids. Its molecular weight is 297.73. Its structural formula is:
[See chemical structure at top of next column]

CLINICAL PHARMACOLOGY

MAXZIDE (triamterene and hydrochlorothiazide) is a diuretic, antihypertensive drug product, principally due to its

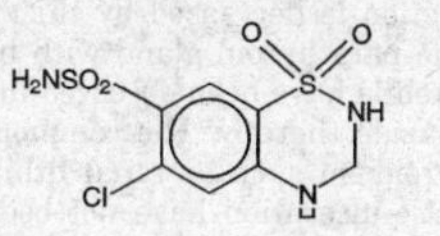

hydrochlorothiazide component; the triamterene component of MAXZIDE reduces the excessive potassium loss which may occur with hydrochlorothiazide use.

Hydrochlorothiazide
Hydrochlorothiazide is a diuretic and antihypertensive agent. It blocks the renal tubular absorption of sodium and chloride ions. This natriuresis and diuresis is accomplished by a secondary loss of potassium and bicarbonate. Onset of hydrochlorothiazide's diuretic effect occurs within two hours and the peak action takes place in four hours. Diuretic activity persists for approximately six to twelve hours.
The exact mechanism of hydrochlorothiazide's antihypertensive action is not known although it may relate to the excretion and redistribution of body sodium. Hydrochlorothiazide does not affect normal blood pressure.
Following oral administration, peak hydrochlorothiazide plasma levels are attained in approximately two hours. It is excreted rapidly and unchanged in the urine.
Well-controlled studies have demonstrated that doses of hydrochlorothiazide as low as 25 mg given once daily are effective in treating hypertension, but the dose response has not been clearly established.

Triamterene
Triamterene is a potassium-conserving (antikaliuretic) diuretic with relatively weak natriuretic properties. It exerts its diuretic effect on the distal renal tubule to inhibit the reabsorption of sodium in exchange for potassium and hydrogen. With this action, triamterene increases sodium excretion and reduces the excessive loss of potassium and hydrogen associated with hydrochlorothiazide. Triamterene is not a competitive antagonist of the mineralocorticoids and its potassium-conserving effect is observed in patients with Addison's disease, ie, without aldosterone. Triamterene's onset and duration of activity is similar to hydrochlorothiazide. No predictable antihypertensive effect has been demonstrated with triamterene.
Triamterene is rapidly absorbed following oral administration. Peak plasma levels are achieved within one hour after dosing. Triamterene is primarily metabolized to the sulfate conjugate of hydroxytriamterene. Both the plasma and urine levels of this metabolite greatly exceed triamterene levels.
The amount of triamterene added to 50 mg of hydrochlorothiazide in MAXZIDE tablets was determined from steady-state dose response evaluations in which various doses of liquid preparations of triamterene were administered to hypertensive persons who developed hypokalemia with hydrochlorothiazide (50 mg give once daily). Single daily doses of 75 mg triamterene resulted in greater increases in serum potassium than lower doses (25 mg and 50 mg), while doses greater than 75 mg of triamterene resulted in no additional levels in serum potassium levels. The amount of triamterene added to the 25 mg of hydrochlorothiazide in MAXZIDE-25 MG tablets was also determined from steady-state dose response evaluations in which various doses of liquid preparations of triamterene were administered to hypertensive persons who developed hypokalemia with hydrochlorothiazide (25 mg given once daily). Single daily doses of 37.5 mg triamterene resulted in greater increases in serum potassium than a lower dose (25 mg), while doses greater than 37.5 mg of triamterene, ie, 75 and 100 mg, resulted in no additional elevations in serum potassium levels. The dose response relationship of triamterene was also evaluated in patients rendered hypokalemic by hydrochlorothiazide given 25 mg twice daily. Triamterene given twice daily increased serum potassium levels in a dose-related fashion. However, the combination of triamterene and hydrochlorothiazide given twice daily also appeared to produce an increased frequency of elevation in serum BUN and creatinine levels. The largest increases in serum potassium, BUN and creatinine in this study were observed with 50 mg of triamterene given twice daily, the largest dose tested. Ordinarily, triamterene does not entirely compensate for the kaliuretic effect of hydrochlorothiazide and some patients may remain hypokalemic while receiving triamterene and hydrochlorothiazide. In some individuals, however, it may induce hyperkalemia (see WARNINGS).
The triamterene and hydrochlorothiazide components of MAXZIDE and MAXZIDE-25 MG are well absorbed and are bioequivalent to liquid preparations of the individual components administered orally. Food does not influence the absorption of triamterene or hydrochlorothiazide from MAXZIDE or MAXZIDE-25 MG tablets. The hydrochlorothiazide components of MAXZIDE is bioequivalent to single entity hydrochlorothiazide tablet formulations.

INDICATIONS AND USAGE

This fixed combination drug is not indicated for the initial therapy of edema or hypertension except in individuals in whom the development of hypokalemia cannot be risked.

1. MAXZIDE (triamterene and hydrochlorothiazide) is indicated for the treatment of hypertension or edema in patients who develop hypokalemia on hydrochlorothiazide alone.
2. MAXZIDE is also indicated for those patients who require a thiazide diuretic and in whom the development of hypokalemia cannot be risked (eg, patients on concomitant digitalis preparations, or with a history of cardiac arryhthmias, etc.).

MAXZIDE may be used alone or in combination with other antihypertensive drugs, such as beta-blockers. Since MAXZIDE (triamterene and hydrochlorothiazide) may enhance the actions of these drugs, dosage adjustments may be necessary.

Usage in Pregnancy
The routine use of diuretics in an otherwise healthy woman is inappropriate and exposes mother and fetus to unnecessary hazard. Diuretics do not prevent development of toxemia of pregnancy, and there is no satisfactory evidence that they are useful in the treatment of developed toxemia.
Edema during pregnancy may arise from pathological causes or from the physiologic and mechanical consequences of pregnancy. Thiazides are indicated in pregnancy when edema is due to pathologic causes, just as they are in absence of pregnancy. Dependent edema in pregnancy, resulting from restriction of venous return by the expanded uterus, is properly treated through elevation of the lower extremities and use of support hose; use of diuretics to lower intravascular volume in this case is illogical and unnecessary. There is hypervolemia during normal pregnancy which is harmful to neither the fetus nor the mother (in the absence of cardiovascular disease), but which is associated with edema, including generalized edema, in the majority of pregnant women. If this edema produces discomfort, increased recumbency will often provide relief. In rare instances, this edema may cause extreme discomfort which is not relieved by rest. In these cases, a short course of diuretics may provide relief and may be appropriate.

CONTRAINDICATIONS

Hyperkalemia
MAXZIDE (triamterene and hydrochlorothiazide) should not be used in the presence of elevated serum potassium levels (greater than or equal to 5.5 mEq/liter). If hyperkalemia develops, this drug should be discontinued and a thiazide alone should be substituted.

Antikaliuretic Therapy or Potassium Supplementation
MAXZIDE should not be given to patients receiving other potassium-conserving agents such as spironolactone, amiloride HCl or other formulations containing triamterene. Concomitant potassium supplementation in the form of medication, potassium-containing salt substitute or potassium-enriched diets should also not be used.

Impaired Renal Function
MAXZIDE is contraindicated in patients with anuria, acute and chronic renal insufficiency or significant renal impairment.

Hypersensitivity
MAXZIDE should not be used in patients who are hypersensitive to triamterene or hydrochlorothiazide or other sulfonamide-derived drugs.

WARNINGS

Hyperkalemia
Abnormal elevation of serum potassium levels (greater than or equal to 5.5 mEq/liter) can occur with all potassium-conserving diuretic combinations, including MAXZIDE. Hyperkalemia is more likely to occur in patients with renal impairment, diabetes (even without evidence of renal impairment), or elderly or severely ill patients. Since uncorrected hyperkalemia may be fatal, serum potassium levels must be monitored at frequent intervals especially in patients first receiving MAXZIDE, when dosages are changed or with any illness that may influence renal function.

If hyperkalemia is suspected, (warning signs include paresthesias, muscular weakness, fatigue, flaccid paralysis of the extremities, bradycardia and shock) an electrocardiogram (ECG) should be obtained. However, it is important to monitor serum potassium levels because mild hyperkalemia may not be associated with ECG changes.
If hyperkalemia is present, MAXZIDE (triamterene and hydrochlorothiazide) should be discontinued immediately and a thiazide alone should be substituted. If the serum potassium exceeds 6.5 mEq/liter, more vigorous therapy is required. The clinical situation dictates the procedures to be employed. These include the intravenous administration of calcium chloride solution, sodium bicarbonate solution and/or the oral or parenteral administration of glucose with a rapid-acting insulin preparation. Cationic exchange resins such as sodium polystyrene sulfonate may be orally or rectally administered. Persistent hyperkalemia may require dialysis.
The development of hyperkalemia associated with potassium-sparing diuretics is accentuated in the presence of renal

Continued on next page

Maxzide/Maxzide-25—Cont.

impairment (see CONTRAINDICATIONS). Patients with mild renal functional impairment should not receive this drug without frequent and continuing monitoring of serum electrolytes. Cumulative drug effects may be observed in patients with impaired renal function. The renal clearances of hydrochlorothiazide and the pharmacologically active metabolite of triamterene, the sulfate ester of hydroxytriamterene, have been shown to be reduced and the plasma levels increased following MAXZIDE (triamterene and hydrochlorothiazide) administration to elderly patients and patients with impaired renal function.

Hyperkalemia has been reported in diabetic patients with the use of potassium-conserving agents even in the absence of apparent renal impairment. Accordingly, MAXZIDE (triamterene and hydrochlorothiazide) should be avoided in diabetic patients. If it is employed, serum electrolytes must be frequently monitored.

Because of the potassium-sparing properties of angiotensin-converting enzyme (ACE) inhibitors, MAXZIDE should be used cautiously, if at all, with these agents (see PRECAUTIONS, Drug Interactions).

Metabolic or Respiratory Acidosis

Potassium-conserving therapy should also be avoided in severely ill patients in whom respiratory or metabolic acidosis may occur. Acidosis may be associated with rapid elevations in serum potassium levels. If MAXZIDE is employed, frequent evaluations of acid/base balance and serum electrolytes are necessary.

PRECAUTIONS

General

Electrolyte Imbalance and BUN Increases

Patients receiving MAXZIDE (triamterene and hydrochlorothiazide) should be carefully monitored for fluid or electrolyte imbalances, ie, hyponatremia, hypochloremic alkalosis, hypokalemia and hypomagnesemia. Determination of serum electrolytes to detect possible electrolyte imbalance should be performed at appropriate intervals. Serum and urine electrolyte determinations are especially important and should be frequently performed when the patient is vomiting or receiving parenteral fluids. Warning signs or symptoms of fluid and electrolyte imbalance include: dryness of mouth, thirst, weakness, lethargy, drowsiness, restlessness, muscle pains or cramps, muscular fatigue, hypotension, oliguria, tachycardia and gastrointestinal disturbances such as nausea and vomiting.

Any chloride deficit during thiazide therapy is generally mild and usually does not require any specific treatment except under extraordinary circumstances (as in liver disease or renal disease). Dilutional hyponatremia may occur in edematous patients in hot weather; appropriate therapy is water restriction, rather than administration of salt, except in rare instances when the hyponatremia is life threatening. In actual salt depletion, appropriate replacement is the therapy of choice.

Hypokalemia may develop with thiazide therapy, especially with brisk diuresis, when severe cirrhosis is present, or during concomitant use of corticosteroids, ACTH, amphotericin B or after prolonged thiazide therapy. However, hypokalemia of this type is usually prevented by the triamterene component of MAXZIDE (triamterene and hydrochlorothiazide).

Interference with adequate oral electrolyte intake will also contribute to hypokalemia. Hypokalemia can sensitize or exaggerate the response of the heart to the toxic effects of digitalis (eg, increased ventricular irritability).

MAXZIDE (triamterene and hydrochlorothiazide) may produce an elevated blood urea nitrogen level (BUN), creatinine level or both. This is probably not the result of renal toxicity but is secondary to a reversible reduction of the glomerular filtration rate or a depletion of the intravascular fluid volume. Elevations in BUN and creatinine levels may be more frequent in patients receiving divided dose diuretic therapy. Periodic BUN and creatinine determinations should be made especially in elderly patients, patients with suspected or confirmed hepatic disease or renal insufficiencies. If azotemia increases, MAXZIDE (triamterene and hydrochlorothiazide) should be discontinued.

Hepatic Coma

MAXZIDE should be used with caution in patients with impaired hepatic function or progressive liver disease, since minor alterations of fluid and electrolyte balance may precipitate hepatic coma.

Renal Stones

Triamterene has been reported in renal stones in association with other calculus components. MAXZIDE should be used with caution in patients with histories of renal lithiasis.

Folic Acid Deficiency

Triamterene is a weak folic acid antagonist and may contribute to the appearance of megaloblastosis in instances where folic acid stores are decreased. In such patients, periodic blood elevations are recommended.

Hyperuricemia

Hyperuricemia may occur or acute gout may be precipitated in certain patients receiving thiazide therapy.

Metabolic and Endocrine Effects

The thiazides may decrease serum PBI levels without signs of thyroid disturbance.

Calcium excretion is decreased by thiazides. Pathological changes in the parathyroid gland with hypercalcemia and hypophosphatemia have been observed in a few patients on prolonged thiazide therapy. The common complications of hyperparathyroidism such as renal lithiasis, bone resorption, and peptic ulceration have not been seen. Thiazides should be discontinued before carrying out tests for parathyroid function.

Insulin requirements in diabetic patients may be increased, decreased or unchanged. Diabetes mellitus which has been latent may become manifest during thiazide administration.

Hypersensitivity

Sensitivity reactions to thiazides may occur in patients with or without a history of allergy or bronchial asthma.

Possible exacerbation or activation of systemic lupus erythematosus by thiazides has been reported.

Drug Interactions

Thiazides may add to or potentiate the action of other antihypertensive drugs.

The thiazides may decrease arterial responsiveness to norepinephrine. This diminution is not sufficient to preclude effectiveness of the pressor agent for therapeutic use. Thiazides have also been shown to increase the responsiveness to tubocurarine.

Lithium generally should not be given with diuretics because they reduce its renal clearance and add a high risk of lithium toxicity. Refer to the package insert on lithium before use of such concomitant therapy.

Acute renal failure has been reported in a few patients receiving indomethacin and formulations containing triamterene and hydrochlorothiazide. Caution is therefore advised when administering nonsteroidal anti-inflammatory agents with MAXZIDE (triamterene and hydrochlorothiazide).

Potassium-sparing agents should be used very cautiously, if at all, in conjunction with angiotensin-converting enzyme (ACE) inhibitors due to a greatly increased risk of hyperkalemia. Serum potassium should be monitored frequently.

Drug/Laboratory Test Interactions

Triamterene and quinidine have similar fluorescence spectra; thus MAXZIDE (triamterene and hydrochlorothiazide) may interfere with the measurement of quinidine.

Carcinogenesis, Mutagenesis, Impairment of Fertility

Studies have not been performed to evaluate the mutagenic or carcinogenic potential of MAXZIDE.

Hydrochlorothiazide

Two-year feeding studies in mice and rats conducted under the auspices of the National Toxicology Program (NTP) uncovered no evidence of a carcinogenic potential of hydrochlorothiazide in female mice (at doses of up to approximately 600 mg/kg/day) or in male and female rats (at doses of up to approximately 100 mg/kg/day). The NTP, however, found equivocal evidence for hepatocarcinogenicity in male mice. Hydrochlorothiazide was not genotoxic in in vitro assays using strains TA 98, TA 100, TA 1535, TA 1537, and TA 1538 of Salmonella typhimurium (Ames assay) and in the Chinese Hamster Ovary (CHO) test for chromosomal aberrations, or in in vivo assays using mouse germinal cell chromosomes, Chinese hamster bone marrow chromosomes, and the Drosophila sex-linked recessive lethal trait gene. Positive test results were obtained only in the in vitro CHO Sister Chromatid Exchange (clastogenicity) and in the Mouse Lymphoma Cell (mutagenicity) assays, using concentrations of hydrochlorothiazide from 43 to 1300 µg/mL, and in the Aspergillus nidulans non-disjunction assay at an unspecified concentration.

Hydrochlorothiazide had no adverse effects on the fertility of mice and rats of either sex in studies wherein these species were exposed, via their diet, to doses of up to 100 and 4 mg/kg, respectively, prior to conception and throughout gestation.

Triamterene

Studies have not been performed to determine the carcinogenic or mutagenic potential of triamterene. Reproductive studies have been performed in rats at doses up to 30 times the human dose and have revealed no evidence of impaired fertility.

Pregnancy Category C

Teratogenic Effects—Animal reproduction studies have not been conducted with MAXZIDE. It is also not known if MAXZIDE can cause fetal harm when administered to a pregnant woman.

Hydrochlorothiazide

Studies in which hydrochlorothiazide was orally administered to pregnant mice and rats during their respective periods of major organogenesis at doses up to 3000 and 1000 mg hydrochlorothiazide/kg, respectively, provided no evidence of harm to the fetus. There are, however, no adequate and well-controlled studies in pregnant women.

Triamterene

Reproduction studies have been performed in rats at doses up to 30 times the human dose and have revealed no evidence of harm to the fetus due to triamterene. There are, however, no adequate and well-controlled studies in pregnant women.

Because animal reproduction studies are not always predictive of human response, MAXZIDE should be used during pregnancy only if clearly needed.

Nonteratogenic Effects

Thiazides and triamterene cross the placental barrier and appear in cord blood of animals. The use of MAXZIDE in pregnant women requires that the anticipated benefit be weighed against possible hazards to the fetus. These hazards include fetal or neonatal jaundice, thrombocytopenia following thiazides and possible other adverse reactions that have occurred in the adults.

Nursing Mothers

Thiazides appear and triamterene may appear in breast milk. If use of the drug product is deemed essential the patient should stop nursing.

Pediatric Use

The safety and effectiveness of MAXZIDE (triamterene and hydrochlorothiazide) in children has not been established.

ADVERSE REACTIONS

Side effects observed in association with the use of MAXZIDE, other combination products containing triamterene/hydrochlorothiazide, and products containing triamterene or hydrochlorothiazide include the following:

Gastrointestinal: jaundice (intrahepatic cholestatic jaundice), pancreatitis, nausea, appetite disturbance, taste alteration, vomiting, diarrhea, constipation, anorexia, gastric irritation, cramping.

Central Nervous System: drowsiness and fatigue, insomnia, headache, dizziness, dry mouth, depression, anxiety, vertigo, restlessness, paresthesias.

Cardiovascular: tachycardia, shortness of breath and chest pain, orthostatic hypotension (may be aggravated by alcohol, barbiturates or narcotics).

Renal: acute renal failure, acute interstitial nephritis, renal stones composed of triamterene in association with other calculus materials, urine discoloration.

Hematologic: leukopenia, agranulocytosis thrombocytopenia, aplastic anemia, hemolytic anemia and megaloblastosis.

Ophthalmic: xanthopsia, transient blurred vision.

Hypersensitivity: anaphylaxis, photosensitivity, rash, urticaria, purpura, necrotizing angiitis (vasculitis, cutaneous vasculitis), fever, respiratory distress including pneumonitis.

Other: muscle cramps and weakness, decreased sexual performance and sialadenitis.

Whenever adverse reactions are moderate to severe, therapy should be reduced or withdrawn.

Altered Laboratory Findings:

Serum Electrolytes: hyperkalemia, hypokalemia, hyponatremia, hypomagnesemia, hypochloremia (see WARNINGS, PRECAUTIONS).

Creatinine, Blood Urea Nitrogen: Reversible elevations in BUN and serum creatinine have been observed in hypertensive patients treated with MAXZIDE.

Glucose: hyperglycemia, glycosuria and diabetes mellitus (see PRECAUTIONS).

Serum Uric Acid, PBI and Calcium: (see PRECAUTIONS).

Other: Elevated liver enzymes have been reported in patients receiving MAXZIDE.

OVERDOSAGE

No specific data are available regarding MAXZIDE (triamterene and hydrochlorothiazide) overdosage in humans and no specific antidote is available.

Fluid and electrolyte imbalances are the most important concern. Excessive doses of the triamterene component may elicit hyperkalemia, dehydration, nausea, vomiting and weakness and possibly hypotension. Overdosing with hydrochlorothiazide has been associated with hypokalemia, hypochloremia, hyponatremia, dehydration, lethargy (may progress to coma) and gastrointestinal irritation. Treatment is symptomatic and supportive. Therapy with MAXZIDE (triamterene and hydrochlorothiazide) should be discontinued. Induce emesis or institute gastric lavage. Monitor serum electrolyte levels and fluid balance. Institute supportive measures as required to maintain hydration, electrolyte balance, respiratory, cardiovascular and renal function.

DOSAGE AND ADMINISTRATION

The usual dose of MAXZIDE-25 MG is one or two tablets daily, given as a single dose, with appropriate monitoring of serum potassium (see WARNINGS). The usual dose of MAXZIDE is one tablet daily, with appropriate monitoring of serum potassium (see WARNINGS). There is no experience with the use of more than one MAXZIDE tablet daily or more than two MAXZIDE-25 MG tablets daily. Clinical experience with the administration of two MAXZIDE-25 MG tablets daily in divided doses (rather than as a single dose) suggests an increased risk of electrolyte imbalance and renal dysfunction.

Patients receiving 50 mg of hydrochlorothiazide who become hypokalemic may be transferred to MAXZIDE (triamterene and hydrochlorothiazide) directly. Patients receiving 25 mg hydrochlorothiazide who become hypokalemic may be

transferred to MAXZIDE-25 MG (37.5 mg triamterene/25 mg hydrochlorothiazide) directly.
In patients requiring hydrochlorothiazide therapy and in whom hypokalemia cannot be risked therapy may be initiated with MAXZIDE-25 MG. If an optimal blood pressure response is not obtained with MAXZIDE-25 MG, the dose should be increased to two MAXZIDE-25 MG tablets daily as a single dose, or one MAXZIDE tablet daily. If blood pressure still is not controlled, another antihypertensive agent may be added (see PRECAUTIONS, Drug Interactions).
Clinical studies have shown that patients taking less bioavailable formulations of triamterene and hydrochlorothiazide in daily doses of 25–50 mg hydrochlorothiazide and 50–100 mg triamterene may be safely changed to one MAXZIDE-25 MG tablet daily. All patients changed from less bioavailable formulations to MAXZIDE should be monitored clinically for serum potassium after the transfer.

HOW SUPPLIED

MAXZIDE® (triamterene and hydrochlorothiazide) tablets are bowtie-shaped, flat-faced beveled, light yellow tablets, engraved with MAXZIDE on one side and scored on the other with B on the left and M8 on the right of the score. Each tablet contains 75 mg of triamterene, USP and 50 mg of hydrochlorothiazide, USP. They are supplied as follows:
NDC 62794-460-01—Bottle of 100 with CRC
NDC 62794-460-05—Bottle of 500
NDC 62794-460-88—Unit Dose 10 × 10s
MAXZIDE-25 MG (triamterene and hydrochlorothiazide) tablets are bowtie-shaped, flat-faced beveled, light green tablets, engraved with MAXZIDE on one side and scored on the other with B on the left and M9 on the right of the score. Each tablet contains 37.5 mg of triamterene, USP and 25 mg of hydrochlorothiazide, USP. They are supplied as follows:
NDC 62794-464-01—Bottle of 100 with CRC
NDC 62794-464-05—Bottle of 500
NDC 62794-464-88—Unit Dose 10 × 10s
Store at Controlled Room Temperature 15–30°C (59–86°F). Protect from Light.
Dispense in a tight, light-resistant, child-resistant container.
BERTEK PHARMACEUTICALS INC.
Sugar Land, TX 77478
REVISED SEPTEMBER 1996 BKMAX:R3

Shown in Product Identification Guide, page 306

SULFAMYLON® CREAM ℞

Brand of MAFENIDE ACETATE CREAM, USP
Topical Antibacterial Agent for Adjunctive Therapy in Second- and Third-Degree Burns

DESCRIPTION

SULFAMYLON Cream is a soft, white, nonstaining, water-miscible, anti-infective cream for topical administration to burn wounds.
SULFAMYLON Cream spreads easily, and can be washed off readily with water. It has a slight acetic odor. Each gram of SULFAMYLON Cream contains mafenide acetate equivalent to 85 mg of the base. The cream vehicle consists of cetyl alcohol, stearyl alcohol, cetyl esters wax, polyoxyl 40 stearate, polyoxyl 8 stearate, glycerin, and water, with methylparaben, propylparaben, sodium metabisulfite, and edetate disodium as preservatives.
Chemically, mafenide acetate is α-Amino-ρ-toluenesulfonamide monoacetate and has the following structural formula:

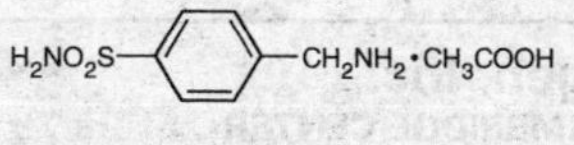
H2NO2S—
—CH2NH2•CH3COOH

CLINICAL PHARMACOLOGY

SULFAMYLON Cream, applied topically, produces a marked reduction in the bacterial population present in the avascular tissues of second- and third-degree burns. Reduction in bacterial growth after application of SULFAMYLON Cream has also been reported to permit spontaneous healing of deep partial-thickness burns, and thus prevent conversion of burn wounds from partial thickness to full thickness. It should be noted, however, that delayed eschar separation has occurred in some cases.
Absorption and Metabolism. Applied topically, SULFAMYLON Cream diffuses through devascularized areas, is absorbed, and rapidly converted to a metabolite (ρ-carboxybenzenesulfonamide) which is cleared through the kidneys. SULFAMYLON is active in the presence of pus and serum, and its activity is not altered by changes in the acidity of the environment.
Antibacterial Activity. SULFAMYLON exerts bacteriostatic action against many gram-negative and gram-positive organisms, including *Pseudomonas aeruginosa* and certain strains of anaerobes.

INDICATIONS AND USAGE

SULFAMYLON Cream is a topical agent indicated for adjunctive therapy of patients with second- and third-degree burns.

CONTRAINDICATIONS

SULFAMYLON is contraindicated in patients who are hypersensitive to it. It is not known whether there is cross sensitivity to other sulfonamides.

WARNINGS

Fatal hemolytic anemia with disseminated intravascular coagulation, presumably related to a glucose-6-phosphate dehydrogenase deficiency, has been reported following therapy with SULFAMYLON Cream.
Contains sodium metabisulfite, a sulfite that may cause allergic-type reactions including anaphylactic symptoms and life-threatening or less severe asthmatic episodes in certain susceptible people. The overall prevalence of sulfite sensitivity in the general population is unknown and probably low. Sulfite sensitivity is seen more frequently in asthmatic than in nonasthmatic people.

PRECAUTIONS

SULFAMYLON and its metabolite, ρ-carboxybenzenesulfonamide, inhibit carbonic anhydrase, which may result in metabolic acidosis, usually compensated by hyperventilation. In the presence of impaired renal function, high blood levels of SULFAMYLON and its metabolite may exaggerate the carbonic anhydrase inhibition. Therefore, close monitoring of acid-base balance is necessary, particularly in patients with extensive second-degree or partial thickness burns and in those with pulmonary or renal dysfunction. Some burn patients treated with SULFAMYLON Cream have also been reported to manifest an unexplained syndrome of marked hyperventilation with resulting respiratory alkalosis (slightly alkaline blood pH, low arterial pCO_2, and decreased total CO_2); change in arterial pO_2 is variable. The etiology and significance of these findings are unknown.
Mafenide acetate cream should be used with caution in burn patients with acute renal failure.
SULFAMYLON Cream should be administered with caution to patients with history of hypersensitivity to mafenide. It is not known whether there is cross sensitivity to other sulfonamides.
Fungal colonization in and below the eschar may occur concomitantly with reduction of bacterial growth in the burn wound. However, fungal dissemination through the infected burn wound is rare.
Carcinogenesis, Mutagenesis, Impairment of Fertility. No long-term animal studies have been performed to evaluate the drug's potential in these areas.
Pregnancy Category C. Animal reproduction studies have not been conducted with SULFAMYLON. It is also not known whether SULFAMYLON can cause fetal harm when administered to a pregnant woman or can affect reproduction capacity. Therefore, the preparation is not recommended for the treatment of women of childbearing potential, unless the burned area covers more than 20% of the total body surface, or the need for the therapeutic benefit of SULFAMYLON Cream is, in the physician's judgment, greater than the possible risk to the fetus.
Nursing Mothers. It is not known whether mafenide acetate is excreted in human milk. Because many drugs are excreted in human milk and because of the potential for serious adverse reaction in nursing infants from SULFAMYLON, a decision should be made whether to discontinue nursing or to discontinue the drug, taking into account the importance of the drug to the mother.
Pediatric Use. Same as for adults. (See DOSAGE AND ADMINISTRATION.)

ADVERSE REACTIONS

It is frequently difficult to distinguish between an adverse reaction to SULFAMYLON Cream and the effect of a severe burn. A single case of bone marrow depression and a single case of an acute attack of porphyria have been reported following therapy with SULFAMYLON Cream. Fatal hemolytic anemia with disseminated intravascular coagulation, presumably related to a glucose-6-phosphate dehydrogenase deficiency, has been reported following therapy with SULFAMYLON Cream.
Dermatologic: The most frequently reported reaction was pain on application or a burning sensation. Rare occurrences are excoriation of new skin, and bleeding of skin.
Allergic: Rash, itching, facial edema, swelling, hives, blisters, erythema, and eosinophilia.
Respiratory: Tachypnea or hyperventilation, decrease in arterial pCO_2.
Metabolic: Acidosis, increase in serum chloride.
Accidental ingestion of SULFAMYLON Cream has been reported to cause diarrhea.

DOSAGE AND ADMINISTRATION

Prompt institution of appropriate measures for controlling shock and pain is of prime importance. The burn wounds are then cleansed and debrided, and SULFAMYLON Cream is applied with a sterile gloved hand. Satisfactory results can be achieved with application of the cream once or twice daily, to a thickness of approximately 1/16 inch; thicker application is not recommended. The burned areas should be covered with SULFAMYLON Cream at all times. Therefore, whenever necessary, the cream should be reapplied to any areas from which it has been removed (eg, by patient activity). The routine of administration can be accomplished in minimal time, since dressings usually are not required. If individual patient demands make them necessary, however, only a thin layer of dressing should be used.
When feasible, the patient should be bathed daily, to aid in debridement. A whirlpool bath is particularly helpful, but the patient may be bathed in bed or in a shower.
The duration of therapy with SULFAMYLON Cream depends on each patient's requirements. Treatment is usually continued until healing is progressing well or until the burn site is ready for grafting. *SULFAMYLON Cream should not be withdrawn from the therapeutic regimen while there is the possibility of infection.* However, if allergic manifestations occur during treatment with SULFAMYLON Cream, discontinuation of treatment should be considered.
If acidosis occurs and becomes difficult to control, particularly in patients with pulmonary dysfunction, discontinuing therapy with SULFAMYLON Cream for 24 to 48 hours while continuing fluid therapy may aid in restoring acid-base balance.

HOW SUPPLIED

16 ounce plastic jar (453.6 g)—NDC 0514-0101-54
Collapsible tubes of 4 ounces (113.4 g)—NDC 0514-0101-51
Collapsible tubes of 2 ounces (56.7 g)—NDC 0514-0101-50
Avoid exposure to excessive heat (temperatures above 104°F or 40°C).
Caution: U.S. Federal law prohibits dispensing without prescription.
DISTRIBUTED BY:
BERTEK PHARMACEUTICALS INC.
SUGAR LAND, TX 77478
1-888-823-7835

Revised May 1995

SULFAMYLON® ℞

[*sulfă ' mylŏn*]
(Matenide Acetate, USP
FOR 5% TOPICAL SOLUTION

DESCRIPTION

Mafenide acetate, USP is a synthetic antimicrobial agent designated chemically as α-amino-*p*-toluenesulfonamide monoacetate. It has the following structural formula:

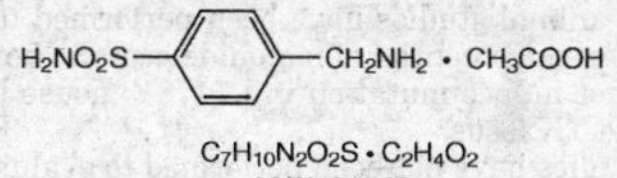
H2NO2S—
—CH2NH2 • CH3COOH

$C_7H_{10}N_2O_2S \cdot C_2H_4O_2$
M.W. 246.29

Mafenide acetate, USP is a white, crystalline powder which is freely soluble in water.
SULFAMYLON® For 5% Topical Solution is provided in packets containing 50 g of mafenide acetate to be reconstituted in 1000 mL of Sterile Water for Irrigation, USP or 0.9% Sodium Chloride Irrigation, USP. After mixing, the solution contains 5% w/v of mafenide acetate. The solution is an antimicrobial preparation suitable for topical administration. **The solution is not for injection.** The 5% topical solution is to be stored at room temperature, 25°–30°C (77°–86°F) and should be used within 48 hours after mixing.

CLINICAL PHARMACOLOGY

Mechanism of Action: The mechanism of action of mafenide is not known, but is different from that of the sulfonamides. Mafenide is not antagonized by pABA, serum, pus or tissue exudates, and there is no correlation between bacterial sensitivities to mafenide and to the sulfonamides. Its activity is not altered by changes in the acidity of the environment. The osmolality of the 5% topical solution is approximately 340 mOsm/kg.
Absorption and Metabolism: Applied topically, mafenide acetate diffuses through devascularized areas. Approximately 80% of a mafenide acetate dose is delivered to burned tissue over four hours following topical application of the 5% solution. Following application of mafenide acetate cream and solution, peak mafenide concentrations in human burned skin tissue occur at two and four hours, respectively. Peak tissue concentrations are similar following administration of the solution or cream. Once absorbed, mafenide is rapidly converted to an inactive metabolite (p-carboxybenzenesulfonamide) which is cleared through the kidneys. Clinical studies have shown that when applied topically to burns as an 11.2% mafenide acetate cream, blood levels of the parent drug peaked at 2-hours following appli-

Continued on next page

Sulfamylon—Cont.

cation, ranging from 26 to 197 µg/mL for single doses of 14 to 77 g of mafenide acetate. Metabolite levels peaked at 3 hours, ranging from 10 to 340 µg/mL. Twenty-four hours after application, combined parent and metabolite blood levels had fallen to pretreatment levels.

Antimicrobial Activity: Mafenide acetate exerts broad bacteriostatic action against many gram-negative and gram-positive organisms, including *Pseudomonas aeruginosa* and certain strains of anaerobes.

In Vitro **Cytotoxicity:** Data from *in vitro* studies on cell culture suggests that mafenide acetate may have a deleterious effect on human keratinocytes. The clinical significance of this information is unknown.

INDICATIONS AND USAGE

SULFAMYLON® For 5% Topical Solution is indicated for use as an adjunctive topical antimicrobial agent to control bacterial infection when used under moist dressings over meshed autografts on excised burn wounds.

CONTRAINDICATIONS

SULFAMYLON® For 5% Topical Solution is contraindicated in patients who are hypersensitive to mafenide acetate. It is not known whether there is cross sensitivity to other sulfonamides.

WARNINGS

Fatal hemolytic anemia with disseminated intravascular coagulation, presumably related to a glucose-6-phosphate dehydrogenase deficiency, has been reported following therapy with mafenide acetate.

PRECAUTIONS

General: Mafenide acetate and its metabolite, p-carboxy-benzenesulfonamide, inhibit carbonic anhydrase, which may result in metabolic acidosis, usually compensated by hyperventilation. In the presence of impaired renal function, high blood levels of mafenide acetate and its metabolite may exaggerate the carbonic anhydrase inhibition. Therefore, close monitoring of acid-base balance is necessary, particularly in patients with extensive second-degree or partial thickness burns and in those with pulmonary or renal dysfunction. Some burn patients treated with mafenide acetate have also been reported to manifest an unexplained syndrome of masked hyperventilation with resulting respiratory alkalosis (slightly alkaline blood pH, low arterial pCO_2, and decreased total CO_2); change in arterial pO_2 is variable. The etiology and significance of these findings are unknown.

Mafenide acetate should be used with caution in burn patients with acute renal failure.

Fungal colonization may occur concomitantly with reduction of bacterial growth in the burn wound. However, systemic fungal infection through the infected burn wound is rare.

Carcinogenesis, Mutagenesis, Impairment of Fertility: No long-term animal studies have been performed to evaluate the carcinogenic potential of mafenide acetate, however, the drug did not induce mutation in L5178Y mouse lymphoma cells at the TK locus.

Animal studies have not been performed to evaluate the potential effects of mafenide acetate on fertility.

Pregnancy: *Teratogenic Effects. Pregnancy Category C:* A teratology study performed in rats using oral doses of up to 600 mg/kg/day revealed no evidence of harm to the fetus due to mafenide acetate. There are no adequate data regarding the potential reproductive toxicity of mafenide acetate in a non-rodent species, nor are there adequate and well-controlled studies in pregnant women. Mafenide acetate should be used during pregnancy only if the potential benefit justifies the potential risk to the fetus.

Nursing Mothers: It is not known whether mafenide acetate is excreted in human milk. Because many drugs are excreted in human milk and because of the potential for serious adverse reactions in nursing infants from mafenide acetate, a decision should be made whether to discontinue nursing or to discontinue the drug, taking into account the importance of the drug to the mother.

Pediatric Use: The safety and effectiveness of SULFAMYLON® For 5% Topical Solution have been established in the age groups 3 months to 16 years.

Geriatric Use: No studies have been conducted to specifically examine the effects of mafenide acetate on burn wounds in geriatric patients.

ADVERSE REACTIONS

In the clinical setting of severe burns, it is often difficult to distinguish between an adverse reaction to mafenide acetate and burn sequelae. In a clinical study of pediatric patients with acute burns requiring autografts who received SULFAMYLON® 5% SOLUTION in addition to double antibiotic solution (DAB) wound therapy (neomycin sulfate 40 mg and polymyxin B 200,000 units/liter), the incidence of rash (4.6%) and itching (2.8%) in the group which received SULFAMYLON® 5% Solution was not different from that experienced with DAB dressings alone (5.7% and 1.3%, respectively).

From other clinical settings, a single case of bone marrow depression and a single case of an acute attack of porphyria

have been reported following therapy with mafenide acetate. Fatal hemolytic anemia with disseminated intravascular coagulation, presumably related to a glucose-6-phosphate dehydrogenase deficiency, has been reported following therapy with mafenide acetate. The following adverse reactions have been reported with topical mafenide acetate therapy:

Dermatologic and Allergic: Pain or burning sensation, rash and pruritus (often localized to the area covered by the wound dressing), erythema, skin maceration from prolonged wet dressings, facial edema, swelling, hives, blisters, eonsinophilia.

Respiratory or Metabolic: Tachypnea, hyperventilation, decrease in pCO_2, metabolic acidosis, increase in serum chloride.

OVERDOSAGE

Single oral doses of 2000 mg/kg of mafenide acetate as a 5% solution did not cause mortality or clinical symptoms of toxicity in rats.

DOSAGE AND ADMINISTRATION

SULFAMYLON® For 5% Topical Solution: *Directions for Preparation of the Solution:* SULFAMYLON® (Mafenide Acetate) For 5% Topical Solution is applied as a powder and is to be reconstituted with Sterile Water for Irrigation, USP or 0.9% Sodium Chloride Irrigation, USP. Aseptic techniques should be observed during preparation of the solution. Premeasured quantities of 50 g of mafenide acetate powder are provided in packets. The entire quantity of SULFAMYLON® should be emptied into a suitable container which contains 1000 mL of Sterile Water for Irrigation, USP or 0.9% Sodium Chloride Irrigation, USP and mixed until completely dissolved. **The resulting SULFAMYLON® (mafenide acetate, USP) 5% SOLUTION should be filtered through a 0.22 micron sterilizing grade filter prior to use.** The reconstituted/filtered solution should be stored at room temperature, 25°–30°C (77°–86°F), and should be used within 48 hours after preparation. **Not for Injection - For Topical Use Only.**

Directions for Use of the Solution: The grafted area should be covered with one layer of fine mesh gauze. An eight-ply burn dressing should be cut to the size of the graft and wetted with SULFAMYLON® 5% SOLUTION using an irrigation syringe and/or irrigation tubing until leaking is noticeable. If irrigation tubing is used, the tubing should be placed over the burn dressing in contact with the wound and covered with a second piece of eight-ply dressing. The irrigation dressing should be secured with a bolster dressing and wrapped as appropriate. The gauze dressing should be kept wet. In clinical studies, this has been accomplished by irrigating with a syringe or injecting the solution into the irrigation tubing every 4 hours or as necessary. If irrigation tubing is not used, the gauze dressing may be moistened every 6–8 hours or as necessary to keep wet.

Wound dressings may be left undisturbed, except for the irrigations, for up to five days. Additional soaks may be initiated until graft take is complete. Maceration of skin may result from wet dressings applied for intervals as short as 24 hours. Treatment is usually continued until autograft vascularization occurs and healing is progressing (typically occurring in about 5 days). Safety and effectiveness have not been established for longer than 5 days for an individual grafting procedure.

If allergic manifestations occur during treatment with SULFAMYLON® 5% SOLUTION, discontinuation of treatment should be considered. If acidosis occurs and becomes difficult to control, particularly in patients with pulmonary dysfunction, discontinuing the soaks with the mafenide acetate solution for 24 to 48 hours may aid in restoring acid-base balance (see PRECAUTIONS section). Dressing changes and monitoring the site for bacterial growth during this interruption should be adjusted accordingly.

HOW SUPPLIED

SULFAMYLON® (mafenide acetate, USP) For 5% Topical Solution is available in packets (NDC 62794-111-17) containing 50 g of mafenide acetate to be prepared using 1000 mL Sterile Water for Irrigation, USP or 0.9% Sodium Chloride Irrigation, USP. (See DOSAGE AND ADMINISTRATION: SULFAMYLON® For 5% Topical Solution: *Directions for Preparation of the Solution.*) The packets are supplied as follows:

Carton of five 50 g packets   NDC 62794-111-98

Recommended Storage:

Packets – STORE PACKETS IN A DRY PLACE AT ROOM TEMPERATURE, 25°–30°C (77°–86°F)

Prepared Solution – STORE AT ROOM TEMPERATURE, 25°–30°C (77°–86°F).

USE WITHIN 48 HOURS OF PREPARATION.

Distributed by: Bertek Pharmaceuticals Inc.

Sugar Land, TX 77478

1-888-823-7835

Rx only

BKSFMN:R3

REVISED MARCH 1998

Beutlich LP Pharmaceuticals
1541 SHIELDS DRIVE
WAUKEGAN, IL 60085-8304

Direct Inquiries to:
847-473-1100
800-238-8542
FAX 847–473-1122
E-mail fjb1541@worldnet.att.com
World Wide Web http://www.beutlich.com

CEO–TWO® EVACUANT SUPPOSITORY   OTC

NDC #0283-0763-09

COMPOSITION

Each adult rectal suppository contains sodium bicarbonate and potassium bitartrate in a water soluble polyethylene glycol base.

HOW SUPPLIED

In packages of 10, white opaque suppositories. Keep in cool, dry place.
DO NOT REFRIGERATE
(See PDR For Nonprescription Drugs)

HURRICAINE® TOPICAL ANESTHETIC   OTC

COMPOSITION

HURRICAINE contains 20% benzocaine in a flavored, water soluble polyethylene glycol base.

PACKAGING AVAILABLE

Gel
1 oz. Jar Wild Cherry NDC #0283-0871-31
1 oz. Jar Pina Colada NDC #0283-0886-31
1 oz. Jar Watermelon NDC #0283-0293-31
1/8 oz. Tube Wild Cherry NDC #0283-0871-12
1/8 oz. Tube Watermelon NDC #0283-0293-12
Liquid
1 fl. oz. Jar Wild Cherry NDC #0283-0569-31
1 fl. oz. Jar Pina Colada NDC #0283-1886-31
1/8 oz. Tube Wild Cherry NDC #0283-0569-12
.25 ml Dry Handle Swab Wild Cherry NDC #0283-0693-01
Spray
2 oz. Aerosol Wild Cherry NDC #0283-0679-02
Spray Kit
2 oz. Aerosol Wild Cherry NDC #0283-0183-02 with 200 Disposable Extension Tubes
(See PDR For Nonprescription Drugs)

PERIDIN-C®

Composition: Each orange colored tablet contains 2 popular antioxidants; Vitamin C and Bioflavonoids.

Ascorbic Acid 200 mg.
Hesperidin Complex 150 mg.
Hesperidin Methyl Chalcone 50 mg. F.D. & C. #6.

Dosage: 1 tablet daily or as directed.

How Supplied: In bottles of:
100 tablets NDC #0283-0597-01
500 tablets NDC #0283-0597-05

Biogen, Inc.
14 CAMBRIDGE CENTER
CAMBRIDGE, MA 02142

Direct Inquiries to:
Customer Service (800) 456-2255
Fax (617) 679-3100

AVONEX™   ℞
[ăv '-ə-nĕx]
INTERFERON BETA-1a

DESCRIPTION

AVONEX™ (Interferon beta-1a) is produced by recombinant DNA technology. Interferon beta-1a is a 166 amino acid glycoprotein with a predicted molecular weight of approximately 22,500 daltons. It is produced by mammalian cells (Chinese Hamster Ovary cells) into which the human interferon beta gene has been introduced. The amino acid sequence of AVONEX™ is identical to that of natural human interferon beta.

Using the World Health Organization (WHO) natural interferon beta standard, Second International Standard for Interferon, Human Fibroblast (Gb-23-902-531), AVONEX™ has a specific activity of approximately 200 million international units (IU) of antiviral activity per mg; 30 mcg of AVONEX™ contains 6 million IU of antiviral activity. The activity against other standards is not known.

AVONEX™ is formulated as a sterile, white to off-white lyophilized powder for intramuscular injection after reconstitution with supplied diluent or Sterile Water for Injection, USP, preservative-free.

Each 1.0 mL (1.0 cc) of reconstituted AVONEX™] contains 30 mcg of Interferon beta-1a, 15 mg Albumin Human, USP, 5.8 mg Sodium Chloride, USP, 5.7 mg Dibasic Sodium Phosphate, USP and 1.2 mg Monobasic Sodium Phosphate, USP at a pH of approximately 7.3.

CLINICAL PHARMACOLOGY
General
Interferons are a family of naturally occurring proteins and glycoproteins that are produced by eukaryotic cells in response to viral infection and other biological inducers. Interferon beta, one member of this family, is produced by various cell types including fibroblasts and macrophages. Natural interferon beta and Interferon beta-1a are glycosylated, with each containing a single N-linked complex carbohydrate moiety. Glycosylation of other proteins is known to affect their stability, activity, biodistribution and half-life in blood. However, the effects of glycosylation of interferon beta on these properties have not been fully defined.

Biologic Activities
Interferons are cytokines that mediate antiviral, antiproliferative and immunomodulatory activities in response to viral infection and other biological inducers. Three major interferons have been distinguished: alpha, beta and gamma. Interferons alpha and beta form the Type I class of interferons, and interferon gamma is a Type II interferon. These interferons have overlapping but clearly distinct biological activities.

Interferon beta exerts its biological effects by binding to specific receptors on the surface of human cells. This binding initiates a complex cascade of intracellular events that leads to the expression of numerous interferon-induced gene products and markers. These include 2′, 5′-oligoadenylate synthetase, β_2-microglobulin and neopterin. These products have been measured in the serum and cellular fractions of blood collected from patients treated with AVONEX™ (Interferon beta-1a).

The specific interferon-induced proteins and mechanisms by which AVONEX™ exerts its effects in multiple sclerosis have not been fully defined.

Pharmacokinetics
Pharmacokinetics of AVONEX™ in multiple sclerosis patients have not been evaluated. The pharmacokinetic and pharmacodynamic profiles of AVONEX™ in healthy subjects following doses of 30 mcg through 75 mcg have been investigated. Serum levels of Interferon beta-1a as measured by antiviral activity are slightly above detectable limits following a 30 mcg intramuscular (IM) dose, and increase with higher doses.

Table 1
Mean Single Dose Pharmacokinetic Parameters Following 60 mcg Administration

Route of Administration	AUC (IU·h/mL)	C_{max} (IU/mL)	T_{max} (Range) (h)	Elimination Half-life (h)
IM	1352	45	9.8 (3-15)	10.0
SC	478	30	7.8 (3-18)	8.6

Table 1 compares general pharmacokinetic parameters for AVONEX™ following administration of a 60 mcg dose by IM and subcutaneous (SC) routes to healthy volunteers. After an IM dose, serum levels of Interferon beta-1a typically peak between 3 and 15 hours and then decline at a rate consistent with a 10 hour elimination half-life. Serum levels of Interferon beta-1a may be sustained after IM administration due to prolonged absorption from the IM site. Systemic exposure, as determined by AUC and C_{max} values, is greater following IM than SC administration.

Biological response markers (e.g., neopterin and β_2-microglobulin) are induced by Interferon beta-1a following parenteral doses of 15 mcg through 75 mcg in healthy subjects and treated patients. Biological response marker levels increase within 12 hours of dosing and remain elevated for at least 4 days. Peak biological response marker levels are typically observed 48 hours after dosing. The relationship of serum Interferon beta-1a levels or levels of these induced biological response markers to the mechanisms by which AVONEX™] exerts its effects in multiple sclerosis is unknown.

Clinical Studies: Effects in Multiple Sclerosis
The clinical effects of AVONEX™ (Interferon beta-1a) in multiple sclerosis were studied in a randomized, multi-center, double-blind, placebo-controlled study in patients with relapsing (stable or progressive) multiple sclerosis[1]. In this study, 301 patients received either 6 million IU (30 mcg) of AVONEX™ (n=158) or placebo (n=143) by IM injection once weekly. Patients were entered into the trial over a $2\frac{1}{2}$ year period, received injections for up to 2 years, and continued to be followed until study completion. Two hundred eighty-two patients completed 1 year on study, and 172 patients completed 2 years on study. There were 144 patients treated with AVONEX™ for more than 1 year, 115 patients for more than 18 months and 82 patients for 2 years.

All patients had a definite diagnosis of multiple sclerosis of at least 1 year duration and had at least two exacerbations in the 3 years prior to study entry (or one per year if the duration of disease was less than 3 years). At entry, study participants were without exacerbation during the prior 2 months and had Kurtzke Expanded Disability Status Scale (EDSS[2]) scores ranging from 1.0 to 3.5. Patients with chronic progressive multiple sclerosis were excluded from this study.

The primary outcome assessment was time to progression in disability, measured as an increase in the EDSS of at least 1.0 point that was sustained for at least 6 months. An increase in EDSS score reflects accumulation of disability. This endpoint was used to assure that progression reflected permanent increase in disability rather than a transient effect due to an exacerbation.

Secondary outcomes included exacerbation frequency and results of magnetic resonance imaging (MRI) scans including gadolinium (Gd)-enhanced lesion number and volume and T2-weighted (proton density) lesion volume. Additional secondary endpoints included two upper limb (tested in both arms) and three lower limb function tests.

Twenty-three of the 301 patients (8%) discontinued treatment prematurely. Of these, one patient treated with placebo (1%) and six patients treated with AVONEX™ (4%) discontinued treatment due to adverse events. Thirteen of these 23 patients remained on study and were evaluated for clinical endpoints.

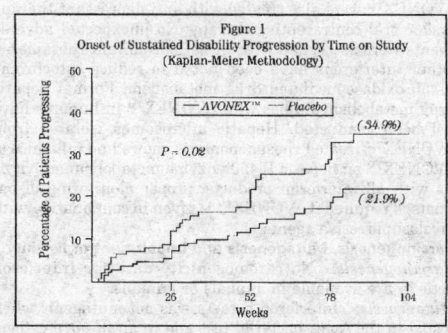

Figure 1
Onset of Sustained Disability Progression by Time on Study
(Kaplan-Meier Methodology)

— AVONEX™ — Placebo

P = 0.02

(34.9%)

(21.9%)

Note: Disability progression represents at least a 1.0 point increase in EDSS score sustained for at least 6 months.

Time to onset of sustained progression in disability was significantly longer in patients treated with AVONEX™ than in patients receiving placebo (p=0.02). The Kaplan-Meier plots of these data are presented in Figure 1. The Kaplan-Meier estimate of the percentage of patients progressing by the end of 2 years was 34.9% for placebo-treated patients and 21.9% for AVONEX™-treated patients, indicating a slowing of the disease process. This represents a 37% reduction in the risk of accumulating disability in the AVONEX™-treated group compared to the placebo-treated group.

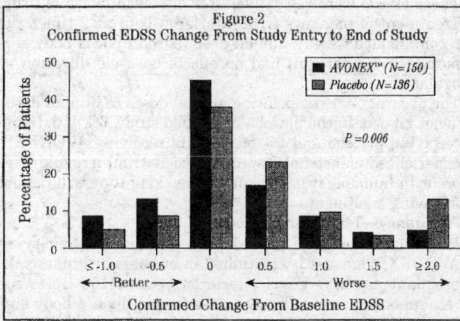

Figure 2
Confirmed EDSS Change From Study Entry to End of Study

■ AVONEX™ (N=150)
▨ Placebo (N=136)

P =0.006

← Better | Worse →
≤ -1.0 -0.5 0 0.5 1.0 1.5 ≥ 2.0

Confirmed Change From Baseline EDSS

The distribution of confirmed EDSS change from study entry to the end of the study is shown in Figure 2. There was a statistically significant difference between treatment groups in confirmed change for patients with at least two scheduled visits (136 placebo-treated and 150

AVONEX™-treated patients; p=0.006; see Table 2). Confirmed EDSS change was calculated as the difference between the EDSS score at study entry and one of the scores determined at the last two scheduled visits. If the EDSS score at either of the last two scheduled visits showed improvement (reduction in score) the higher score was used. Otherwise, the lower score was used. Nineteen patients had one score higher and one score lower than baseline; the higher score was used. The last two scheduled visits occurred at varying time points among patients.

Table 2
Major Clinical Endpoints

Endpoint	Placebo	AVONEX™	P-Value
PRIMARY ENDPOINT:			
Time to sustained progression in disability (N: 143, 158)[1]	—See Figure 1—		0.02[2]
Percentage of patients progressing in disability at 2 years (Kaplan-Meier estimate)[1]	34.9%	21.9%	
SECONDARY ENDPOINTS:DISABILITY			
Mean confirmed change in EDSS from study entry to end of study (N: 136, 150)[1]	0.50	0.20	0.006[3]
EXACERBATIONS			
Number of exacerbations in subset completing 2 years (N: 87, 85)			0.03[3]
0	26%	38%	
1	30%	31%	
2	11%	18%	
3	14%	7%	
≥4	18%	7%	
Percentage of patients exacerbation-free in subset completing 2 years (N: 87, 85)	26%	38%	0.10[4]
Annual exacerbation rate (N: 143, 158)[1]	0.82	0.67	0.04[5]
MRI			
Number of Gd-enhanced lesions:			
At study entry (N: 132, 141)			
Mean (Median)	2.3 (1.0)	3.2 (1.0)	
Range	0-23	0-56	
Year 1 (N: 123, 134)			
Mean (Median)	1.6 (0)	1.0 (0)	0.02[3]
Range	0-22	0-28	
Year 2 (N: 82, 83)			
Mean (Median)	1.6 (0)	0.8 (0)	0.05[3]
Range	0-34	0-13	
T2 lesion volume:			
Percentage change from study entry to year 1 (N: 116, 123)			
Median	−3.3%	−13.1%	0.02[3]
Percentage change from study entry to year 2 (N: 83, 81)			
Median	−6.5%	−13.2%	0.36[3]

Note: (N: ,) denotes the number of evaluable placebo and AVONEX™ (Interferon beta-1a) patients, respectively.
[1] *Patient data included in this analysis represent variable periods of time on study.*
[2] *Analyzed by Mantel-Cox (logrank) test.*
[3] *Analyzed by Mann-Whitney rank-sum test.*
[4] *Analyzed by Cochran-Mantel-Haenszel test.*
[5] *Analyzed by likelihood ratio test.*

The rate and frequency of exacerbations were determined as secondary outcomes. For all patients included in the study, irrespective of time on study, the annual exacerbation rate was 0.67 per year in the AVONEX™-treated group and 0.82 per year in the placebo-treated group (p=0.04).

AVONEX™ (Interferon beta-1a) treatment significantly decreased the frequency of exacerbations in the subset of patients who were enrolled in the study for at least 2 years (87 placebo-treated patients and 85 AVONEX™-treated patients; p=0.03; see Table 2).

Continued on next page

Avonex—Cont.

Gd-enhanced and T2-weighted (proton density) MRI scans of the brain were obtained in most patients at baseline and at the end of 1 and 2 years of treatment. Gd-enhancing lesions seen on brain MRI scans represent areas of breakdown of the blood brain barrier thought to be secondary to inflammation. Patients treated with AVONEX™ demonstrated significantly lower Gd-enhanced lesion number after 1 and 2 years of treatment ($p \leq 0.05$; see Table 2). The volume of Gd-enhanced lesions was also analyzed, and showed similar treatment effects ($p \leq 0.03$). Percentage change in T2-weighted lesion volume from study entry to year 1 was significantly lower in AVONEX™-treated than placebo-treated patients ($p=0.02$). A significant difference in T2-weighted lesion volume change was not seen between study entry and year 2.
The exact relationship between MRI findings and the clinical status of patients is unknown. Changes in lesion area often do not correlate with changes in disability progression. The prognostic significance of the MRI findings in this study has not been evaluated.
Of the limb function tests, only one demonstrated a statistically significant difference between treatment groups (favoring AVONEX™).
A summary of the effects of AVONEX™ on the primary and major secondary endpoints of this study is presented in Table 2.
Safety and efficacy of treatment with AVONEX™ beyond 2 years are not known.

INDICATIONS AND USAGE

AVONEX™ (Interferon beta-1a) is indicated for the treatment of relapsing forms of multiple sclerosis to slow the accumulation of physical disability and decrease the frequency of clinical exacerbations. Safety and efficacy in patients with chronic progressive multiple sclerosis have not been evaluated.

CONTRAINDICATIONS

AVONEX™ (Interferon beta-1a) is contraindicated in patients with a history of hypersensitivity to natural or recombinant interferon beta, human albumin, or any other component of the formulation.

WARNINGS

AVONEX™ (Interferon beta-1a) should be used with caution in patients with depression. Depression and suicide have been reported to occur in patients receiving other interferon compounds. Depression and suicidal ideation are known to occur at an increased frequency in the multiple sclerosis population. A relationship between occurrence of depression and/or suicidal ideation and the use of AVONEX™ has not been established. An equal incidence of depression was seen in the placebo-treated and AVONEX™-treated patients in the placebo-controlled multiple sclerosis study. Patients treated with AVONEX™ should be advised to report immediately any symptoms of depression and/or suicidal ideation to their prescribing physicians. If a patient develops depression, cessation of AVONEX™ therapy should be considered.

PRECAUTIONS

General

Caution should be exercised when administering AVONEX™ (Interferon beta-1a) to patients with pre-existing seizure disorder. In the placebo-controlled study, four patients receiving AVONEX™] experienced seizures, while no seizures occurred in the placebo group. Three of these four patients had no prior history of seizure. It is not known whether these events were related to the effects of multiple sclerosis alone, to AVONEX™, or to a combination of both. For patients with no prior history of seizure who develop seizures during therapy with AVONEX™], an etiologic basis should be established and appropriate anti-convulsant therapy instituted prior to considering resumption of AVONEX™ treatment. The effect of AVONEX™ administration on the medical management of patients with seizure disorder is unknown.

Patients with cardiac disease, such as angina, congestive heart failure or arrhythmia, should be closely monitored for worsening of their clinical condition during initiation of therapy with AVONEX™. AVONEX™ does not have any known direct-acting cardiac toxicity; however, symptoms of flu syndrome seen with AVONEX™ therapy may prove stressful to patients with severe cardiac conditions.

Information to Patients

Patients should be informed of the most common adverse events associated with AVONEX™ administration, including symptoms associated with flu syndrome (see Adverse Reactions section and precautions in Patient Information). Symptoms of flu syndrome are most prominent at the initiation of therapy and decrease in frequency with continued treatment. In the placebo-controlled study, patients were instructed to take 650 mg acetaminophen immediately prior to injection and for an additional 24 hours after each injection to modulate acute symptoms associated with AVONEX™ administration.
Patients should be cautioned to report depression or suicidal ideation (see Warnings).
Patients should be advised about the abortifacient potential of interferon beta (see Pregnancy—Teratogenic Effects).
When a physician determines that AVONEX™] can be used outside of the physician's office, persons who will be administering AVONEX™ should receive instruction in reconstitution and injection, including the review of the injection procedures (see Dosage and Administration). If a patient is to self-administer, the physical ability of that patient to self-inject intramuscularly should be assessed. The first injection should be performed under the supervision of a qualified health care professional. A puncture-resistant container for disposal of needles and syringes should be used. Patients should be instructed in the technique and importance of proper syringe and needle disposal and be cautioned against reuse of these items.

Laboratory Tests

In addition to those laboratory tests normally required for monitoring patients with multiple sclerosis, complete blood and differential white blood cell counts, platelet counts, and blood chemistries, including liver function tests, are recommended during AVONEX™ (Interferon beta-1a) therapy. During the placebo-controlled study, these tests were performed at least every 6 months. There were no significant differences between the placebo and AVONEX™ groups in the incidence of liver enzyme elevation, leukopenia or thrombocytopenia. However, these are known to be dose-related laboratory abnormalities associated with the use of interferons. Patients with myelosuppression may require more intensive monitoring of complete blood cell counts, with differential and platelet counts.

Drug Interactions

No formal drug interaction studies have been conducted with AVONEX™. In the placebo-controlled study, corticosteroids or ACTH were administered for treatment of exacerbations in some patients concurrently receiving AVONEX™. In addition, some patients receiving AVONEX™ were also treated with anti-depressant therapy and/or oral contraceptive therapy. No unexpected adverse events were associated with these concomitant therapies.
Other interferons have been noted to reduce cytochrome P-450 oxidase-mediated drug metabolism. Formal hepatic drug metabolism studies with AVONEX™ in humans have not been conducted. Hepatic microsomes isolated from AVONEX™-treated rhesus monkeys showed no influence of AVONEX™ on hepatic P-450 enzyme metabolism activity.
As with all interferon products, proper monitoring of patients is required if AVONEX™ is given in combination with myelosuppressive agents.

Carcinogenesis, Mutagenesis and Impairment of Fertility

Carcinogenesis: No carcinogenicity data for Interferon beta-1a are available in animals or humans.
Mutagenesis: Interferon beta-1a was not mutagenic when tested in the Ames bacterial test and in an *in vitro* cytogenetic assay in human lymphocytes in the presence and absence of metabolic activation. These assays are designed to detect agents that interact directly with and cause damage to cellular DNA. Interferon beta-1a is a glycosylated protein that does not directly bind to DNA.
Impairment of Fertility: No studies were conducted to evaluate the effects of interferon beta on fertility in normal women or women with multiple sclerosis. It is not known whether Interferon beta-1a can affect human reproductive capacity.
Menstrual irregularities were observed in monkeys administered interferon beta at a dose 100 times the recommended weekly human dose (based upon a body surface area comparison). Anovulation and decreased serum progesterone levels were also noted transiently in some animals. These effects were reversible after discontinuation of drug. Treatment of monkeys with interferon beta at 2 times the recommended weekly human dose (based upon a body surface area comparison) had no effects on cycle duration or ovulation.
The accuracy of extrapolating animal doses to human doses is not known. In the placebo-controlled study, 6% of patients receiving placebo and 5% of patients receiving AVONEX™ experienced menstrual disorder. If menstrual irregularities occur in humans, it is not known how long they will persist following treatment.

Pregnancy—Teratogenic Effects

Pregnancy Category C: The reproductive toxicity of AVONEX™ has not been studied in animals or humans. In pregnant monkeys given interferon beta at 100 times the recommended weekly human dose (based upon a body surface area comparison), no teratogenic or other adverse effects on fetal development were observed. Abortifacient activity was evident following 3 to 5 doses at this level. No abortifacient effects were observed in monkeys treated at 2 times the recommended weekly human dose (based upon a body surface area comparison). Although no teratogenic effects were seen in these studies, it is not known if teratogenic effects would be observed in humans. There are no adequate and well-controlled studies with interferons in pregnant women. If a woman becomes pregnant or plans to become pregnant while taking AVONEX™, she should be informed of the potential hazards to the fetus, and it should be recommended that the woman discontinue therapy.

Nursing Mothers

It is not known whether Interferon beta-1a is excreted in human milk. Because of the potential of serious adverse reactions in nursing infants, a decision should be made to either discontinue nursing or to discontinue AVONEX™.

Pediatric Use

Safety and effectiveness in pediatric patients below the age of 18 years have not been established.

ADVERSE REACTIONS

The safety data describing the use of AVONEX™ (Interferon beta-1a) in multiple sclerosis patients are based on the placebo-controlled trial in which 158 patients randomized to AVONEX™ were treated for up to 2 years (see Clinical Studies).
The five most common adverse events associated (at $p \leq 0.075$) with AVONEX™ treatment were flu-like symptoms (otherwise unspecified), muscle ache, fever, chills and asthenia. The incidence of all five adverse events diminished with continued treatment.
One patient in the placebo group attempted suicide; no AVONEX™-treated patient attempted suicide. The incidence of depression was equal in the two treatment groups. However, since depression and suicide have been reported with other interferon products, AVONEX™ should be used with caution in patients with depression (see Warnings).
In the placebo-controlled study, four patients receiving AVONEX™ experienced seizures, while no seizures occurred in the placebo group. Three of these four patients had no prior history of seizure. It is not known whether these events were related to the effects of multiple sclerosis alone, to AVONEX™, or to a combination of both (see Precautions).
Table 3 enumerates adverse events and selected laboratory abnormalities that occurred at an incidence of 2% or more among the 158 multiple sclerosis patients treated with 30 mcg of AVONEX™ once weekly by IM injection. Reported adverse events have been classified using standard COSTART terms. Terms so general as to be uninformative and those events that were equal in incidence or more common in the placebo-treated patients have been excluded.

Table 3
Adverse Events and Selected Laboratory Abnormalities in the Placebo-Controlled Study

Adverse Event	Placebo (N=143)	AVONEX™ (N=158)
Body as a Whole		
Headache	57%	67%
Flu-like symptoms (otherwise unspecified)*	40%	61%
Pain	20%	24%
Fever*	13%	23%
Asthenia	13%	21%
Chills*	7%	21%
Infection	6%	11%
Abdominal pain	6%	9%
Chest pain	4%	6%
Injection site reaction	1%	4%
Malaise	3%	4%
Injection site inflammation	0%	3%
Hypersensitivity reaction	0%	3%
Ovarian cyst	0%	3%
Cardiovascular System		
Syncope	2%	4%
Vasodilation	1%	4%
Digestive System		
Nausea	23%	33%
Diarrhea	10%	16%
Dyspepsia	7%	11%
Anorexia	6%	7%
Hemic and Lymphatic System		
Anemia*	3%	8%
Eosinophils ≥10%	4%	5%
HCT (%) ≤32 (females) or ≤37 (males)	1%	3%
Ecchymosis injection site	1%	2%
Metabolic andNutritional Disorders		
SGOT ≥3 × ULN	1%	3%
Musculoskeletal System		
Muscle ache*	15%	34%
Arthralgia	5%	9%
Nervous System		
Sleep difficult	16%	19%
Dizziness	13%	15%

Muscle spasm	6%	7%
Suicidal tendency	1%	4%
Seizure	0%	3%
Speech disorder	0%	3%
Ataxia	0%	2%
Respiratory System		
Upper respiratory tract infection	28%	31%
Sinusitis	17%	18%
Dyspnea	3%	6%
Skin and Appendages		
Urticaria	2%	5%
Alopecia	1%	4%
Nevus	0%	3%
Herpes zoster	2%	3%
Herpes simplex	1%	2%
Special Senses		
Otitis media	5%	6%
Hearing decreased	0%	3%
Urogenital		
Vaginitis	2%	4%

* *Significantly associated with AVONEX™ treatment (p ≤0.05).*

AVONEX™ (Interferon beta-1a) has also been evaluated in 290 patients with illnesses other than multiple sclerosis. The majority of these patients were enrolled in studies to evaluate AVONEX™ treatment of chronic viral hepatitis B and C, in which the doses studied ranged from 15 mcg to 75 mcg, given SC, 3 times a week, for up to 6 months. The incidence of common adverse events in these studies was generally seen at a frequency similar to that seen in the placebo-controlled multiple sclerosis study. In these non-multiple sclerosis studies, inflammation at the site of the SC injection was seen in 52% of treated patients. In contrast, injection site inflammation was seen in 3% of multiple sclerosis patients receiving AVONEX™, 30 mcg by IM injection. Subcutaneous injections were also associated with the following local reactions: injection site necrosis, injection site atrophy, injection site edema and injection site hemorrhage. None of the above was observed in the multiple sclerosis patients participating in the placebo-controlled study.

Other events observed during premarket evaluation of AVONEX™, administered either SC or IM in all patient populations studied, are listed in the paragraph that follows. Because most of the events were observed in open and uncontrolled studies, the role of AVONEX™ in their causation cannot be reliably determined. **Body as a Whole:** abscess, ascites, cellulitis, facial edema, hernia, injection site fibrosis, injection site hypersensitivity, lipoma, neoplasm, photosensitivity reaction, sepsis, sinus headache, toothache; **Cardiovascular System:** arrhythmia, arteritis, heart arrest, hemorrhage, hypotension, palpitation, pericarditis, peripheral ischemia, peripheral vascular disorder, postural hypotension, pulmonary embolus, spider angioma, telangiectasia, vascular disorder; **Digestive System:** blood in stool, colitis, constipation, diverticulitis, dry mouth, gallbladder disorder, gastritis, gastrointestinal hemorrhage, gingivitis, gum hemorrhage, hepatoma, hepatomegaly, increased appetite, intestinal perforation, intestinal obstruction, periodontal abscess, periodontitis, proctitis, thirst, tongue disorder; **Endocrine System:** hypothyroidism; **Hemic and Lymphatic System:** coagulation time increased, ecchymosis, lymphadenopathy, petechia; **Metabolic and Nutritional Disorders:** abnormal healing, dehydration, hypoglycemia, hypomagnesemia, hypokalemia; **Musculoskeletal System:** arthritis, bone pain, myasthenia, osteonecrosis, synovitis; **Nervous System:** abnormal gait, amnesia, Bell's Palsy, clumsiness, depersonalization, drug dependence, facial paralysis, hyperesthesia, increased libido, neurosis, psychosis; **Respiratory System:** emphysema, hemoptysis, hiccup, hyperventilation, laryngitis, pharyngeal edema, pneumonia; **Skin and Appendages:** basal cell carcinoma, blisters, cold clammy skin, contact dermatitis, erythema, furunculosis, genital pruritus, nevus, seborrhea, skin ulcer, skin discoloration; **Special Senses:** abnormal vision, conjunctivitis, earache, eye pain, labyrinthitis, vitreous floaters; **Urogenital:** breast fibroadenosis, breast mass, dysuria, epididymitis, fibrocystic change of the breast, fibroids, gynecomastia, hematuria, kidney calculus, kidney pain, leukorrhea, menopause, nocturia, pelvic inflammatory disease, penis disorder, Peyronies Disease, polyuria, postmenopausal hemorrhage, prostatic disorder, pyelonephritis, testis disorder, urethral pain, urinary urgency, urinary retention, urinary incontinence, vaginal hemorrhage.

Serum Neutralizing Activity

Throughout the placebo-controlled multiple sclerosis study, serum samples from patients were monitored for the development of Interferon beta-1a neutralizing activity. During the study, 24% of AVONEX™-treated patients were found to have serum neutralizing activity at one or more time points tested. Fifteen percent of AVONEX™-treated patients

tested positive for neutralizing activity at a level at which no placebo patient tested positive. The significance of the appearance of serum neutralizing activity is unknown.

DRUG ABUSE AND DEPENDENCE

There is no evidence that abuse or dependence occurs with AVONEX™ (Interferon beta-1a) therapy. However, the risk of dependence has not been systematically evaluated.

DOSAGE AND ADMINISTRATION

The recommended dosage of AVONEX™ (Interferon beta-1a) for the treatment of relapsing forms of multiple sclerosis is 30 mcg injected intramuscularly once a week (see Figure 3).

AVONEX™ is intended for use under the guidance and supervision of a physician. Patients may self-inject only if their physician determines that it is appropriate and with medical follow-up, as necessary, after proper training in intramuscular injection technique.

FIGURE 3
RECONSTITUTION AND INJECTION

Read through entire instructions prior to starting procedure.

Wash hands prior to preparing medication and after the medication has been administered. Allow the vial of AVONEX™ (Interferon beta-1a) and the vial of diluent to reach room temperature. Reconstitute AVONEX™ using sterile technique, as discussed below.

The following supplies will be needed:
• vial of AVONEX™
• vial of diluent, single-use (Sterile Water for Injection, USP, preservative-free)
• syringe
• blue MICRO PIN®
• sterile needle
• alcohol wipes
• syringe disposal container
• adhesive bandage

Reconstitution with diluent vial

1. Remove the cap from the vial of AVONEX™ and vial of diluent, and clean the rubber stopper of each vial with an alcohol wipe.

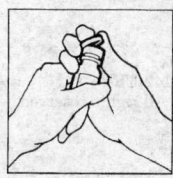

2. Remove the small protective cover from the syringe with a counterclockwise turn.

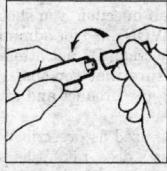

3. Attach the blue MICRO PIN® (vial access pin) to the syringe with a half turn clockwise.

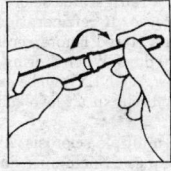

4. Remove the MICRO PIN® cover. Save for later use.

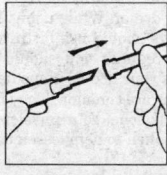

5. Pull back the syringe plunger to the 1.1 cc mark.

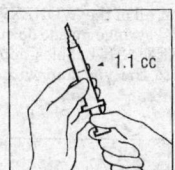

6. Push the MICRO PIN® down through the center of the rubber stopper of the diluent vial.

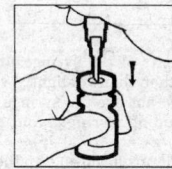

7. Inject air into the diluent vial by pushing down on the plunger until it cannot be pushed any further.
8. Turn the diluent vial and syringe upside down.
9. Keeping the MICRO PIN® in the fluid, withdraw 1.1 cc of diluent into the syringe by pulling back on the plunger.

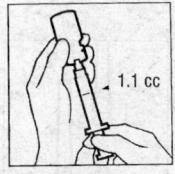

10. Tap the syringe gently to make any air bubbles rise to the top. If bubbles are present, press the plunger until the diluent is at the top of the syringe. Make sure there is still 1.1 cc of diluent in the syringe.

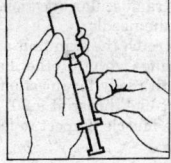

11. Pull the MICRO PIN® out of the diluent vial.
12. Insert the MICRO PIN® through the center of the rubber stopper of the vial of AVONEX™.
13. *Slowly* inject the diluent.
    CAUTION: Rapid addition of the diluent may cause foaming, making it difficult to withdraw AVONEX™.

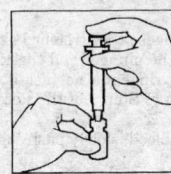

14. Without removing the syringe, *gently* swirl the vial until the white cake of AVONEX™ is dissolved.
    CAUTION: DO NOT SHAKE.

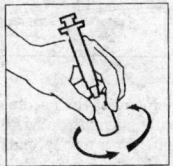

Continued on next page

Avonex—Cont.

15. Check to see that all of the AVONEX™ cake is dissolved.
16. Turn the vial and syringe upside down. Slowly withdraw 1.0 cc of AVONEX™. If bubbles appear, push solution *slowly* back into the vial and withdraw the solution again.

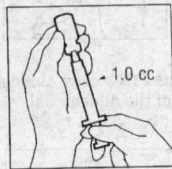

17. Check the contents of the syringe. If you see areas of discoloration (other than a slightly yellow solution) or solid particles do not use the syringe. Get a new set of materials, including syringe, and start again with Step 1.
18. With the vial still upside down, tap the syringe gently to make any air bubbles rise to the top. Then press the plunger until the AVONEX™ is at the top of the syringe. Check the volume (should be 1.0 cc) and withdraw more medication if necessary. Withdraw the MICRO PIN® and syringe from the vial.
19. Replace the cover on the MICRO PIN® and remove from the syringe with a counterclockwise turn.
20. Attach a needle to the syringe with a $^1/_2$ turn clockwise until the needle is secure.

Injection

1. Use a new alcohol wipe to clean the skin at one of the recommended intramuscular injection sites. Pull the protective cover off the needle.
2. With one hand stretch the skin taut around the injection site. Hold the syringe with the other hand, making sure it is horizontal, until ready for injection. Insert the needle with a quick dart-like thrust at a 90° angle, through the skin and into the muscle. Expect to feel some resistance.

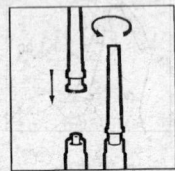

3. Once inserted, release the stretched skin and gently pull back slightly on the plunger and check for blood. If there is blood in the syringe, do not use it. Get a new set of materials, and go to Step 1 of the Reconstitution section and begin again.
4. If you do not see blood, slowly push the plunger until the syringe is empty.

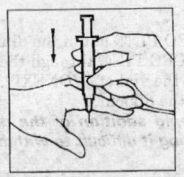

5. Hold an alcohol wipe near the needle at the injection site and pull the needle straight out. Use the wipe to apply pressure to the site for a few seconds or rub gently in a circular motion.
   [See figure at top of next column]
6. If there is bleeding at the site, wipe it off and, if necessary, apply an adhesive bandage.
7. Dispose of all supplies properly, including the diluent.

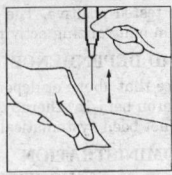

HOW SUPPLIED

AVONEX™ (Interferon beta-1a) is supplied as a lyophilized powder in a single-use vial containing 33 mcg (6.6 million IU) of Interferon beta-1a, 16.5 mg Albumin Human, USP, 6.4 mg Sodium Chloride, USP, 6.3 mg Dibasic Sodium Phosphate, USP, and 1.3 mg Monobasic Sodium Phosphate, USP, and is preservative-free. Diluent is supplied in a single-use vial (Sterile Water for Injection, USP, preservative-free). Reconstitute AVONEX™ with 1.1 mL (cc) of diluent and swirl gently to dissolve (approximate pH 7.3). Withdraw 1.0 mL (cc) for administration.
AVONEX™ is available in the following package configuration (NDC-59627-001-03): Package (Administration Pack) containing 4 Administration Dose Packs (each containing one vial of AVONEX™, one 10 mL (10 cc) diluent vial, two alcohol wipes, one 3 cc syringe, one Micro Pin® vial access pin, one needle and one adhesive bandage).

Stability and Storage
Vials of AVONEX™ (Interferon beta-1a) must be stored in a 2–8°C (36–46°F) refrigerator. Should refrigeration be unavailable, AVONEX™ can be stored at 25°C (77°F) for a period of up to 30 days. DO NOT EXPOSE TO HIGH TEMPERATURES. DO NOT FREEZE. Do not use beyond the expiration date stamped on the vial. Following reconstitution, it is recommended the product be used as soon as possible within 6 hours stored at 2–8°C (36–46°F). DO NOT FREEZE.

REFERENCES
1. Jacobs LD, *et al.* Ann Neurol 1996; 39: 285-294.
2. Kurtzke JF. Neurol 1983; 33: 1444-1452.

AVONEX™ (INTERFERON BETA-1a)

Manufactured by:

BIOGEN, INC.
14 Cambridge Center
Cambridge, MA 02142 USA
©1996 Biogen, Inc. All rights reserved.
1-800-456-2255
U.S. Patent Pending
I63000-1 (5/96)
Caution: Federal law prohibits dispensing without prescription.
Micro PIN® is the trademark of B. Braun Medical Inc.

Patient Information
AVONEX™ (Interferon beta-1a) is intended for use under the guidance and supervision of a physician. If your physician recommends self-injection, you should be instructed in the preparation of AVONEX™ for administration and in the technique of self-injection. Do not attempt self-administration until you are sure that you understand the requirements for preparing the product and giving an injection to yourself.
AVONEX™ must be used as prescribed by your physician. However, if you miss a dose, take it as soon as you remember. You may resume your regular schedule, but two injections should not be administered within 2 days of each other. While using AVONEX™, please keep in mind the following facts:

- AVONEX™ (Interferon beta-1a) must be kept cold. Be sure to store it in a refrigerator before and after reconstitution. Do not freeze. If refrigeration is not available, AVONEX™ can be stored before reconstitution at 25°C (77°F) for up to 30 days. When storing outside of a refrigerator, do not allow AVONEX™ to be exposed to high temperatures as may occur in a glove compartment or on a window sill.
- For treatment of multiple sclerosis, AVONEX™ must be injected into the muscle (intramuscular injection).
- Keep syringes and needles away from children. Do not reuse needles or syringes. Discard used syringes and needles in a syringe disposal unit as instructed by your health care professional.
- Women: AVONEX™] should not be used during pregnancy or if you are trying to become pregnant. If you wish to become pregnant while using AVONEX™, discuss the matter with your doctor. While using AVONEX™, women of childbearing age should use birth control measures. If you do become pregnant you should discontinue treatment and contact your doctor immediately.
- Flu-like symptoms are common. They include fever, chills, fatigue and muscle ache. Your physician may recommend taking acetaminophen to help lessen the impact of flu-like symptoms.

- Depression has been reported by patients treated with interferon drugs. If you experience such symptoms, contact your physician promptly.
- As with any prescription medication, side effects related to therapy can occur. Consult with your physician if you have any problems, whether or not you think they may be related to AVONEX™.

Shown in Product Identification Guide, page 306

Bioglan Pharma, Inc.
4902 EISENHOWER BOULEVARD
SUITE 150
TAMPA, FL 33634

Direct Inquiries to:
Bioglan Pharma, Inc.
(813) 243-8833
FAX: (813) 243-8832

MICANOL® ℞
(anthralin cream 1.0%, USP)
Topical treatment of psoriasis

DESCRIPTION
Micanol (anthralin cream 1.0%, USP) is a smooth, yellow cream containing 1% anthralin USP in an aqueous cream base of glyceryl monolaurate, glyceryl monomyristate, citric acid, sodium hydroxide and purified water.
The chemical name of anthralin is 1,8-dihydroxy-9-anthrone.

CLINICAL PHARMACOLOGY
Although the precise mechanism of anthralin's anti-psoriatic action is not fully understood, *in vitro* evidence suggests that its antimitotic effect results from inhibition of DNA synthesis. Additionally, the chemical reducing properties of anthralin may upset oxidative metabolic processes, providing a further slowing down of epidermal mitosis. Systemic absorption of anthralin after topical application of Micanol has not been determined in man.

INDICATIONS AND USAGE
For the topical treatment of psoriasis.

CONTRAINDICATIONS
Micanol is contraindicated for patients with acute or actively inflamed psoriatic eruptions, or a history of hypersensitivity to any of the ingredients.

WARNINGS
Avoid contact with the eyes or mucous membranes. Exercise care when applying Micanol cream to the face or intertriginous skin areas. Discontinue use if a sensitivity reaction occurs or if excessive irritation develops.

ADVERSE REACTIONS
Very few instances of contact allergic reactions to anthralin have been reported. However, transient primary irritation of the normal skin or uninvolved skin surrounding the treated lesions is more frequently seen. If the initial treatment produces excessive soreness or if the lesions spread, reduce frequency of application and, in extreme cases, discontinue use and consult a physician. Micanol cream may stain skin, hair or fabrics. Some temporary discoloration of hair and fingernails may arise during the period of treatment but should be minimized by careful application. Staining of fabrics may be permanent, so contact should be avoided.

DOSAGE AND ADMINISTRATION
Generally it is recommended that Micanol cream be applied once a day. Anthralin is known to be a potential skin irritant. The irritant potential of anthralin is directly related to the strength being used, the time of contact, and each patient's individual tolerance. Where the response to anthralin treatment has not previously been established, commence treatment using a short contact time for at least one week. When a short contact time is used initially, it can be increased stepwise to twenty to thirty minutes before removing the cream by washing or showering. The optimal period of contact will vary according to the patient's response to treatment. To open the tube, unscrew the cap and invert to puncture seal in tube.

FOR THE SKIN
Apply sparingly only to the psoriatic lesions and rub gently and carefully into the skin. Avoid applying an excessive quantity which may cause unnecessary soiling and staining of the clothing and/or bed linen.
At the end of each period of treatment, rinse the skin thoroughly with cool to lukewarm water before washing with soap.
The margins of the lesions may gradually become stained purple/brown as treatment progresses but this will disappear after cessation of treatment.

FOR THE SCALP

Wash hair with shampoo, rinse with water and apply Micanol cream while the hair is still damp. Rub the cream well into the psoriatic lesions. Keep Micanol cream away from the eyes. Care should be taken to avoid application of the cream to uninvolved scalp margins. Remove any unintended residue which may be deposited behind the ears. At the end of each period of contact, rinse hair and scalp thoroughly with cool to lukewarm water and then shampoo the hair and scalp to remove any surplus cream (which may have become red/brown in color). This treatment may be repeated on alternate days if necessary.

HOW SUPPLIED

Micanol (anthralin cream 1.0%, USP) is supplied in 50g tubes.
NDC 62436-401-01
Keep container tightly capped when not in use.
Avoid excessive heat.
For external use only.
Keep out of reach of children.
Store at controlled room temperature 59°F–86°F (15°C–30°C).
Caution: Federal (U.S.A.) law prohibits dispensing without prescription.
Manufactured for Bioglan Pharma, Inc., Tampa, FL 33634, by Bioglan AB, Sweden
June 1997   13212051

Blaine Company, Inc.
**1515 PRODUCTION DRIVE
BURLINGTON, KY 41005**

Inquiries or Medical Information Contact:
(606) 283-9437
(800) 633-9353
FAX: (606) 283-9460

MAG–OX 400   OTC

DESCRIPTION

Each tablet contains Magnesium Oxide 400 mg. U.S.P. (Heavy), or 241.3 mg. Elemental Magnesium (19.86 mEq.)

INDICATIONS AND USAGE

Hypomagnesemia, magnesium deficiencies and/or magnesium depletion resulting from malnutrition, restricted diet, alcoholism or magnesium depleting drugs. For increasing urinary magnesium excretion. Supplemental magnesium during pregnancy and/or as an antacid.

WARNINGS

Do not take more than 2 tablets in a 24 hour period, or use this maximum dosage for more than 2 weeks, except under the advice and supervision of a physician. Do not use this product except under the advice and supervision of a physician if you have a kidney disease. May have laxative effect. As with any drug, if you are pregnant or nursing a baby, seek professional advice before using this product. Keep this and all medicines out of children's reach.

DOSAGE

Adult dose 1 or 2 tablets daily or as directed by a physician.

HOW SUPPLIED

Bottles of 120 and 1000 and Hospital Unit Dose (UD).

URO–MAG   OTC

DESCRIPTION

Each capsule contains Magnesium Oxide 140 mg. U.S.P. (Heavy), or 84.5 mg. Elemental Magnesium (6.93 mEq.)

INDICATIONS AND USAGE

Hypomagnesemia, magnesium deficiencies and/or magnesium depletion resulting from malnutrition, restricted diet, alcoholism or magnesium depleting drugs. For increasing urinary magnesium excretion. Supplemental magnesium during pregnancy and/or as an antacid.

WARNINGS

Do not take more than 4 capsules in a 24 hour period, or use this maximum dosage for more than 2 weeks, except under the advice and supervision of a physician. Do not use this product except under the advice and supervision of a physician if you have a kidney disease. May have laxative effect. As with any drug, if you are pregnant or nursing a baby, seek professional advice before using this product. Keep this and all medicines out of children's reach.

DOSAGE

Adult dose 3–4 capsules daily or as directed by a physician.

HOW SUPPLIED

Bottles of 100 and 1000 and Hospital Unit Dose (UD).

EDUCATIONAL MATERIAL

Samples and anatomical charts available to physicians upon request.

Blansett Pharmacal
**P.O. BOX 638
N. LITTLE ROCK, AR 72115**

Direct Inquiries to:
Customer Service
(501) 758-8635
FAX: (501) 758-5369

ANOLOR® 300   ℞
(butalbital, acetaminophen & caffeine)

Each opaque white capsule imprinted light green ANOLOR 300 and 51674-0009 contains:
Butalbital* .... 50 mg
  *(WARNING: May be habit forming)
Acetaminophen .... 325 mg
Caffeine .... 40 mg

HOW SUPPLIED

Bottles of 100

CORTANE™-B OTIC   ℞
(chloroxylenol, hydrocortisone, pramoxine HCl)

Each 1 mL contains:
  Chloroxylenol .... 1 mg
  Pramoxine HCl .... 10 mg
  Hydrocortisone .... 10 mg

HOW SUPPLIED

Plastic dropper vials of 10 mL.

NALEX®-A TABLETS (Dye Free)   ℞
(Chlorpheniramine maleate, phenyltoloxamine citrate, phenylephrine HCl)

Each white timed release tablet embossed Blansett and 3 Bisect 08 contains:
  Phenylephrine HCl .... 20 mg
  Chlorpheniramine maleate .... 4 mg
  Phenyltoloxamine citrate .... 40 mg

HOW SUPPLIED

Bottles of 100

NALEX® CAPSULES   ℞
(pseudoephedrine HCl, guaifenesin)

Each opaque white-clear capsule imprinted Blansett and 30 contains:
  Pseudoephedrine HCl .... 120 mg
    In a special base providing prolonged action
  Guaifenesin .... 250 mg
    Designed for immediate release

NALEX® JR CAPSULES   ℞
(pseudoephedrine HCl, guaifenesin)

Each green-clear capsule imprinted Blansett and 33 contains:
Pseudoephedrine HCl .... 60 mg
  In a special base providing prolonged action
Guaifenesin .... 300 mg
  Designed for immediate release

HOW SUPPLIED

NALEX CAPSULES: Bottles of 100
NALEX JR: Bottles of 100

NALEX® DH LIQUID   Ⅽ
**Antitussive - Decongestant
(hydrocodone bitartrate, phenyphrine HCl)**

Each 5 mL cherry flavored alcohol-free, sugar-free red syrup contains:

Hydrocodone* Bitartrate .... 1.67 mg
  *(WARNING: May be habit forming)
Phenylephrine HCl .... 5 mg

HOW SUPPLIED

Bottles of 16 oz

Block Drug Company, Inc.
**257 CORNELISON AVENUE
JERSEY CITY, NJ 07302**

Direct Inquiries to:
Consumer Affairs
(201) 434-3000, Ext. 1308
FAX: (201) 434-5739
For Medical Information Contact:
Consumer Affairs
(800) 365-6500, Ext. 1308
FAX: (201) 434-5739

APHTHASOL®   ℞
[aph-thǎsōl]
**(amlexanox oral paste), 5%
For Oral Cavity Use Only
Not for Ophthalmic Use**

DESCRIPTION

Aphthasol contains 5% amlexanox in an adhesive oral paste. Chemically, amlexanox is 2-amino-7-isopropyl-5-oxo-5H-[1]benzopyrano[2,3-b] pyridine-3-carboxylic acid. It has a molecular formula of $C_{16}H_{14}N_2O_4$ and has a molecular weight of 298.30. Amlexanox is odorless, white to yellowish-white crystalline powder. The structural formula is:

Each gram of beige colored oral paste contains 50 mg of amlexanox in an adhesive oral paste base consisting of benzyl alcohol, gelatin, glyceryl monostearate, mineral oil, pectin, petrolatum, and sodium carboxymethylcellulose.

CLINICAL PHARMACOLOGY

The mechanism of action by which amlexanox accelerates healing of aphthous ulcers is unknown. *In vitro* studies have demonstrated amlexanox to be a potent inhibitor of the formation and/or release of inflammatory mediators (histamine and leukotrienes) from mast cells, neutrophils and mononuclear cells. Given orally to animals, amlexanox has demonstrated anti-allergic and anti-inflammatory activities and has been shown to suppress both immediate and delayed type hypersensitivity reactions. The relevance of these activities of amlexanox to its effects on aphthous ulcers has not been established.

Pharmacokinetics and Metabolism: After a single oral application of 100 mg of paste (5 mg amlexanox), maximal serum levels of approximately 120 ng/ml are observed at 2.4 hours. Most of the systemic absorption of amlexanox is via the gastrointestinal tract, and the amount absorbed directly through the active ulcer is not a significant portion of the applied dose. The half-life for elimination was 3.5 +/− 1.1 hours in healthy individuals. Approximately 17% of the dose is eliminated into the urine as unchanged amlexanox, a hydroxylated metabolite, and their conjugates. With multiple applications four times daily, steady state levels were reached within one week, and no accumulation was observed with up to four weeks of usage.

Clinical Studies: The safety of amlexanox oral paste, 5%, was established in a study in which 100 patients with aphthous ulcers applied the medication four times daily for 28 days with no significant topical or systemic adverse effects. The effectiveness was demonstrated in three controlled clinical studies of patients with mild to moderate aphthous ulcers which evaluated 464 patients receiving amlexanox oral paste, 5%, 465 patients receiving a placebo paste, and 195 patients receiving no treatment. Amlexanox oral paste, 5%, was shown to accelerate healing of aphthous ulcers in a statistically significant manner as compared to both vehicle and no treatment.

Amlexanox oral paste, 5%, versus no treatment: In the combined database of the two studies including a no treatment group, there was a significant difference in the rate of ulcer healing which translated to a reduction of 1.6 days in the median time to complete healing and a reduction of 1.3

Continued on next page

Aphthasol—Cont.

days in the median time to complete pain relief. After 3 days of treatment there was a significant difference in both percent of patients with complete healing of ulcers (21% vs. 8%) and percent of patients with complete resolution of pain (44% vs. 20%).

Amlexanox oral paste, 5%, versus vehicle: In the combined database of the three studies, there was a significant difference in the rate of ulcer healing which translated into a reduction of 0.7 days in the median time to complete healing, and a reduction of 0.7 days in the median time to complete pain relief. After 4 days of treatment there was a significant difference in both percent of patients with complete healing of ulcers (37% vs. 27%) and percent of patients with complete resolution of pain (60% vs. 49%).

Pain relief occurred in conjunction with healing of the ulcers. Amlexanox oral paste, 5%, by itself, was not shown to be an analgesic medication. The safety and effectiveness of the product in immunocompromised individuals has not been assessed.

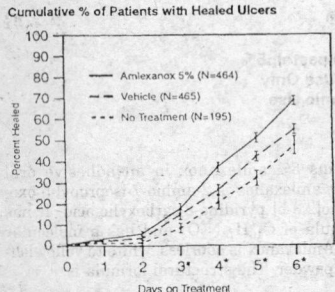

Cumulative % of Patients with Healed Ulcers

Results for amlexanox, 5%, vs. vehicle are based on three clinical trials. Results for amlexanox, 5%, vs. no treatment are based on two clinical trials.

* denotes statistically significant superiority of amlexanox, 5%, vs. vehicle and no treatment.

\# denotes statistically significant superiority of amlexanox, 5%, vs. no treatment.

Error bars represent Standard Error of the Mean.

INDICATIONS AND USAGE

Amlexanox oral paste, 5%, is indicated for the treatment of aphthous ulcers in people with normal immune systems.

CONTRAINDICATIONS

Amlexanox oral paste, 5%, is contraindicated in patients with known hypersensitivity to amlexanox or other ingredients in the formulation.

PRECAUTIONS

General: Wash hands immediately after applying amlexanox oral paste, 5%, directly to ulcers with the finger tips. In the event that a rash or contact mucositis occurs, discontinue use.

Information for Patients:
1. Apply the paste as soon as possible after noticing the symptoms of an aphthous ulcer. Continue to use the paste four times daily, preferably following oral hygiene after breakfast, lunch, dinner, and at bedtime.
2. Squeeze a dab of paste approximately 1/4 inch (0.5 cm) onto a finger tip. Dab the paste onto each ulcer in the mouth using gentle pressure.
3. Wash hands immediately after applying amlexanox oral paste, 5%.
4. Wash eyes promptly if they should come in contact with the paste.
5. Use the paste until the ulcer heals. If significant healing or pain reduction has not occurred in 10 days, consult your dentist or physician.
6. Keep out of reach of children.

Carcinogenesis, Mutagenesis, Impairment of Fertility: Amlexanox was not carcinogenic when administered orally to rats for two years and to mice for 18 months. *In vitro* (Ames) and *in vivo* (mouse micronucleus) mutagenicity tests of amlexanox were negative. Amlexanox at doses up to two hundred times the projected human daily dose, on a mg/m² basis, did not significantly affect fertility or general reproductive performance in rats.

Pregnancy Category B: Teratology studies were performed with rats and rabbits at doses up to two hundred and six hundred times, respectively, the projected human daily dose, on a mg/m² basis. No adverse fetal effects were observed. At doses up to two hundred times the projected human daily dose, on a mg/m² basis, amlexanox did not have significant effect on peri- and postnatal development of rat fetuses. There are no adequate and well-controlled studies in pregnant women. Because animal reproduction studies are not always predictive of human response, this drug should be used during pregnancy only if clearly needed.

Nursing Mothers: Amlexanox was found in the milk of lactating rats; therefore, caution should be exercised when administering amlexanox oral paste, 5%, to a nursing woman.

Pediatric Use: Safety and effectiveness of amlexanox oral paste, 5%, in pediatric patients have not been established.

ADVERSE REACTIONS

Adverse reactions considered related or possibly related to amlexanox oral paste, 5%, were not reported by more than

5% of patients. Adverse reactions reported by 1–2% of patients were transient pain, stinging and/or burning at the site of application. Infrequent (< 1%) adverse reactions in the clinical studies were contact mucositis, nausea, and diarrhea.

OVERDOSAGE

There are no reports of human ingestion overdosage. Ingestion of a full tube of 5 grams of paste would result in systemic exposure well below the maximum nontoxic dose of amlexanox in animals. Gastrointestinal upset such as diarrhea and vomiting could result from an overdose.

DOSAGE AND ADMINISTRATION

The paste should be applied as soon as possible after noticing the symptoms of an aphthous ulcer and should be used four times daily, preferably following oral hygiene after breakfast, lunch, dinner, and at bedtime. Squeeze a dab of paste approximately 1/4 inch (0.5 cm) onto a finger tip. With gentle pressure, dab the paste onto each ulcer in the mouth. Use of the medication should be continued until the ulcer heals. If significant healing or pain reduction has not occurred in 10 days, consult your dentist or physician.

HOW SUPPLIED

Amlexanox oral paste, 5%, is supplied in 5 gram tubes (NDC-10158-059-01). Amlexanox oral paste, 5%, should be stored at controlled room temperature, 15°–30°C (59°–86°F).

Caution: Federal law prohibits dispensing without prescription.

Manufactured for:

Oral Health Care Division
Block Drug Company, Inc.
Jersey City, NJ 07302

By Reedco, Inc.
Humacao, Puerto Rico 00791

Aphthasol® is a registered trademark of Block Drug Company, Inc.
© 1998 Block Drug Company, Inc.
December 1996

Bock Pharmacal Company
see Sanofi Pharmaceuticals, Inc.

Boehringer Ingelheim Pharmaceuticals, Inc.
A subsidiary of Boehringer Ingelheim Corporation
900 RIDGEBURY ROAD
POST OFFICE BOX 368
RIDGEFIELD, CT 06877-0368

For Medical Information Contact:
1-800-542-6257

ALUPENT®   ℞
[al 'u-pent]
(metaproterenol sulfate USP)
Bronchodilator

Tablets 10 mg		BI-CODE 74
Tablets 20 mg		BI-CODE 72
Inhalation Aerosol 10 ml		BI-CODE 70
Syrup 10 mg/5 ml		BI-CODE 73
Inhalation Solution 5%		BI-CODE 71
Inhalation Solution	0.6%	BI-CODE 69
Unit-dose Vials	0.4%	BI-CODE 78

DESCRIPTION

Alupent® (metaproterenol sulfate USP) Inhalation Aerosol is a bronchodilator administered by oral inhalation. The Alupent Inhalation Aerosol containing 150 mg of metaproterenol sulfate as micronized powder is sufficient medication for 200 inhalations. Each metered dose delivers through the mouthpiece 0.65 mg of metaproterenol sulfate (each ml contains 15 mg). The inert ingredients are dichlorodifluoromethane, dichlorotetrafluoroethane and trichloromonofluoromethane as propellants, and sorbitan trioleate.

Alupent Inhalation Solution is administered by oral inhalation with the aid of a nebulizer or an intermittent positive pressure breathing apparatus (IPPB). It contains Alupent 5% in a pH-adjusted aqueous solution containing benzalkonium chloride and edetate disodium as preservatives.

Alupent Inhalation Solution Unit-dose Vial is administered by oral inhalation with the aid of an IPPB. It contains Alupent 0.4% or 0.6% in a sterile pH-adjusted aqueous solution with edetate disodium and sodium chloride.

Alupent Syrup is an oral bronchodilator. Each teaspoonful (5 ml) of syrup contains 10 mg of metaproterenol sulfate. The inactive ingredients are edetate disodium, FD&C Red No. 40, hydroxyethylcellulose, imitation black cherry flavor, methylparaben, propylparaben, saccharin, sorbitol solution.

Alupent Tablets are administered orally. Each tablet contains metaproterenol sulfate 10 mg or 20 mg. The inactive ingredients are colloidal silicon dioxide, corn starch, dibasic calcium phosphate, lactose, magnesium stearate.

Chemically, Alupent is 1-(3,5 dihydroxyphenyl)-2-isopropylaminoethanol sulfate, a white crystalline, racemic mixture of two optically active isomers.

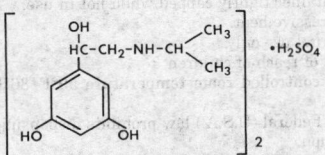

metaproterenol sulfate (Alupent)
$(C_{11}H_{17}NO_3)_2 \cdot H_2SO_4$
Mol. Wt. 520.59

CLINICAL PHARMACOLOGY

Alupent® (metaproterenol sulfate USP) is a potent beta-adrenergic stimulator. Alupent Inhalation Solutions have a rapid onset of action. It is postulated that beta-adrenergic stimulants produce many of their pharmacological effects by activation of adenyl cyclase, the enzyme which catalyzes the conversion of adenosine triphosphate to cyclic adenosine monophosphate.

In vitro studies and *in vivo* pharmacologic studies have demonstrated that Alupent® (metaproterenol sulfate USP) has a preferential effect on beta-2 adrenergic receptors compared with isoproterenol. While it is recognized that beta-2 adrenergic receptors are the predominant receptors in bronchial smooth muscle, recent data indicate that there is a population of beta-2 receptors in the human heart existing in a concentration between 10–50%. The precise function of these, however, is not yet established (see WARNINGS section).

The pharmacologic effects of beta adrenergic agonist drugs, including Alupent, are at least in part attributable to stimulation through beta adrenergic receptors of intracellular adenyl cyclase, the enzyme which catalyzes the conversion of adenosine triphosphate (ATP) to cyclic-3',5'-adenosine monophosphate (c-AMP). Increased c-AMP levels are associated with relaxation of bronchial smooth muscle and inhibition of release of mediators of immediate hypersensitivity from cells, especially from mast cells.

Pharmacokinetics: Absorption, biotransformation and excretion studies in humans following administration by inhalation have shown that approximately 3 percent of the actuated dose is absorbed intact through the lungs.

Absorption, biotransformation and excretion studies in humans following oral administration indicate that an average of less than 10% of the drug is absorbed intact; it is not metabolized by catechol-O-methyl-transferase nor converted to glucuronide conjugates but is excreted primarily as the sulfate conjugate formed in the gut.

When administered orally or by inhalation, Alupent decreases reversible bronchospasm. Pulmonary function tests performed concomitantly usually show improvement following aerosol Alupent administration, e.g., an increase in the one-second forced expiratory volume (FEV_1), an increase in maximum expiratory flow rate, an increase in peak expiratory flow rate, an increase in forced vital capacity, and/or a decrease in airway resistance. The resultant decrease in airway obstruction may relieve the dyspnea associated with bronchospasm.

Controlled single- and multiple-dose studies have been performed with pulmonary function monitoring. The duration of effect of a single dose of Alupent Tablets 20 mg or Alupent Syrup (that is, the period of time during which there is a 15% or greater increase in FEV_1) was up to 4 hours.

Controlled single- and multiple-dose studies have been performed with pulmonary function monitoring. The duration of effect of a single dose of two to three inhalations of Alupent Inhalation Aerosol (that is, the period of time during which there is a 20% or greater increase in FEV_1) has varied from 1 to 5 hours.

In repetitive-dosing studies (up to q.i.d.) the duration of effect for a similar dose of Alupent Inhalation Aerosol has ranged from about 1 to 2.5 hours. Present studies are inadequate to explain the divergence in duration of the FEV_1 effect between single- and repetitive-dosing studies, respectively.

Following controlled single dose studies with Alupent Inhalation Solution by an intermittent positive pressure breath-

ing apparatus (IPPB) and by hand-bulb nebulizers, significant improvement (15% or greater increase in FEV_1) occurred within 5 to 30 minutes and persisted for periods varying from 2 to 6 hours.

In these studies, the longer duration of effect occurred in the studies in which the drug was administered by IPPB, i.e., 6 hours, versus 2 to 3 hours when administered by hand-bulb nebulizer. In these studies, the doses used were 0.3 ml by IPPB and 10 inhalations by hand-bulb nebulizer.

In controlled repetitive-dosing studies with Alupent Inhalation Solution by IPPB and by hand-bulb nebulizer the onset of effect occurred within 5 to 30 minutes and duration ranged from 4 to 6 hours. In these studies, the doses used were 0.3 ml b.i.d. or t.i.d. when given by IPPB, and 10 inhalations q.i.d. (no more often than q4h) when given by hand-bulb nebulizer. As in the single dose studies, effectiveness was measured as a sustained increase in FEV_1 of 15% or greater. In these repetitive-dosing studies there was no apparent difference in duration between the two methods of delivery.

Clinical studies were conducted in which the effectiveness of Alupent® (metaproterenol sulfate USP) Inhalation Solution was evaluated by comparison with that of isoproterenol hydrochloride over periods of two to three months. Both drugs continued to produce significant improvement in pulmonary function throughout this period of treatment.

In two well-controlled studies in children 6 to 12 years of age with acute exacerbation of asthma, 70% of patients receiving Alupent Inhalation Solution (0.1 mL to 0.2 mL) showed improvement in pulmonary function as demonstrated by a 15% increase in FEV_1 above baseline.

Recent studies in laboratory animals (minipigs, rodents and dogs) recorded the occurrence of cardiac arrhythmias and sudden death (with histologic evidence of myocardial necrosis) when beta agonists and methylxanthines were administered concurrently. The significance of these findings when applied to humans is currently unknown.

INDICATIONS AND USAGE

Alupent® (metaproterenol sulfate USP) is indicated as a bronchodilator for bronchial asthma and for reversible bronchospasm which may occur in association with bronchitis and emphysema. Alupent Inhalation Solution 5% is additionally indicated for the treatment of acute asthmatic attacks in children age 6 years and older.

CONTRAINDICATIONS

Use in patients with cardiac arrhythmias associated with tachycardia is contraindicated.

Although rare, immediate hypersensitivity reactions and for Alupent Inhalation Solution 5% paradoxical bronchospasm can occur. Therefore, Alupent® (metaproterenol sulfate USP) is contraindicated in patients with a history of hypersensitivity to any of its components.

WARNINGS

Excessive use of adrenergic aerosols is potentially dangerous. Fatalities have been reported following excessive use of Alupent® (metaproterenol sulfate USP) as with other sympathomimetic inhalation preparations, and the exact cause is unknown. Cardiac arrest was noted in several cases.

Alupent, like other beta-adrenergic agonists, can produce a significant cardiovascular effect in some patients, as measured by pulse rate, blood pressure, symptoms and/or ECG changes. As with other beta-adrenergic aerosols, Alupent can produce paradoxical bronchospasm (which can be life threatening). If it occurs, the preparation should be discontinued immediately and alternative therapy instituted.

Alupent® (metaproterenol sulfate USP) should not be used more often than prescribed. Patients should be advised to contact their physician in the event that they do not respond to their usual dose of a sympathomimetic amine aerosol.

PRECAUTIONS

General: Extreme care must be exercised with respect to the administration of additional sympathomimetic agents. Since metaproterenol is a sympathomimetic amine it should be used with caution in patients with cardiovascular disorders, including ischemic heart disease, hypertension or cardiac arrhythmias, in patients with hyperthyroidism or diabetes mellitus, and in patients who are unusually responsive to sympathomimetic amines or who have convulsive disorders. Significant changes in systolic and diastolic blood pressure could be expected to occur in some patients after use of any beta-adrenergic bronchodilator.

Physicians should recognize that a single dose of nebulized Alupent® (metaproterenol sulfate USP) in the treatment of acute asthma may alleviate symptoms and improve pulmonary function temporarily but fail to completely abort an attack.

Information for Patients: Extreme care must be exercised with respect to the administration of additional sympathomimetic agents. A sufficient interval of time should elapse prior to administration of another sympathomimetic agent. Alupent Inhalation Solution 5% effects may last up to 6 hours or longer. It should not be used more often than recommended and the patient should not increase the number of inhalations or frequency of use without first consulting the physician. If symptoms of asthma get worse, adverse reactions occur, or the patient does not respond to the usual dose, the patient should be instructed to contact the physician immediately.

Alupent Tablets and Alupent Syrup should not be used more often than prescribed. If symptoms persist, patients should consult a physician promptly.

A single dose of nebulized Alupent in the treatment of an acute attack of asthma may not completely abort an attack.

Drug Interactions: Other beta-adrenergic aerosol bronchodilators should not be used concomitantly with Alupent® (metaproterenol sulfate USP) because they may have additive effects. Beta-adrenergic agonists should be administered with caution to patients being treated with monoamine oxidase inhibitors or tricyclic antidepressants, since the action of beta-adrenergic agonists on the vascular system may be potentiated.

Carcinogenesis/Mutagenesis/Impairment of Fertility: In an 18-month study in mice, Alupent produced a significant increase in benign hepatic adenomas in males and in benign ovarian tumors in females at doses corresponding to 31 and 62 times the maximum recommended dose (based on a 50 kg individual). In a 2-year study in rats, a nonsignificant incidence of benign leiomyomata of the mesovarium was noted at 62 times the maximum recommended dose. The relevance of these findings to man is not known. Mutagenic studies with Alupent have not been conducted. Reproduction studies in rats revealed no evidence of impaired fertility.

Pregnancy/Teratogenic Effects

PREGNANCY CATEGORY C: Alupent has been shown to be teratogenic and embryotoxic in rabbits when given orally in doses 620 times the human inhalation dose and 100 mg/kg or 62 times the maximum recommended human oral dose. These effects included skeletal abnormalities, hydrocephalus and skull bone separation.

Embryotoxicity has also been shown in mice when given orally at doses of 50 mg/kg or 31 times the maximum recommended human oral dose. Results of other oral reproduction studies in rats (40 mg/kg) and rabbits (50 mg/kg) have not revealed any teratogenic, embryotoxic or fetotoxic effects. There are no adequate and well-controlled studies in pregnant women. Alupent should be used during pregnancy only if the potential benefit justifies the potential risk to the fetus.

Nursing Mothers: It is not known whether Alupent is excreted in human milk; therefore, Alupent should be used during nursing only if the potential benefit justifies the possible risk to the newborn.

Pediatric Use: Safety and effectiveness in the pediatric population have not established under the age of 6 for Alupent Tablets, Syrup & Inhalation Solutions 5% and under the age of 12 for Inhalation Aerosol and Solution 0.4% & 0.6% UDV. See DOSAGE AND ADMINISTRATION.

ADVERSE REACTIONS

Adverse reactions are similar to those noted with other sympathomimetic agents. Adverse reactions such as tachycardia, hypertension, palpitations, nervousness, tremor, nausea and vomiting have been reported.

The most frequent adverse reaction to Alupent® (metaproterenol sulfate USP) administered by metered-dose inhaler among 251 patients in 90-day controlled clinical trials was nervousness. This was reported in 6.8% of patients. Less frequent adverse experiences, occurring in 1–4% of patients were headache, dizziness, palpitations, gastrointestinal distress, tremor, throat irritation, nausea, vomiting, cough and asthma exacerbation. Tachycardia occurred in less than 1% of patients.

Adverse experiences associated with Alupent Inhalation Solution 5% in at least 2% of 120 patients participating in multiple-dose clinical trial of 60 and 90-day (n=120) duration included nervousness (14.1%; n=17), cough (3.3%; n=4) headache (3.3%; n=4), tachycardia (2.5%; n=3) and tremor (2.5%; n=3).

Alupent Inhalation Solution 5% may be associated with a somewhat higher incidence of adverse reactions in children. In controlled clinical trials conducted in 160 pediatric patients the incidence of adverse reactions observed at the recommended doses was as follows: tachycardia, 16.6%; tremor, 33%; nausea, 14%; vomiting, 7.7%. The corresponding incidence in placebo-treated patients was: tachycardia, 7.6%; tremor, 20%; nausea, 7.7%; vomiting, 2.5%.

In two well-controlled studies in children 6 to 12 years of age with acute exacerbation of asthma, Alupent Inhalation Solution 5% was not efficacious in approximately 30% of patients, where efficacy was defined as a 15% increase in FEV_1 above baseline at two or more time points during the 1-hour testing period. In 8% of patients there was a decrease in FEV_1 of 10% or more from baseline at two or more time points during the testing period. Insufficient information exists to assess the relationship of drug administration to the decline in pulmonary function observed in these patients, but paradoxical bronchospasm is one possibility.

The most frequent adverse reactions to Alupent Inhalation Solution 0.4% and 0.6% are nervousness and tachycardia which occur in about 1 in 7 patients, tremor which occurs in about 1 in 20 patients and nausea which occurs in about 1 in 50 patients. Less frequent adverse reactions are hypertension, palpitations, vomiting and bad taste which occur in approximately 1 in 300 patients.

The following table of adverse experiences is derived from 26 controlled clinical trials with 496 patients treated with Alupent® (metaproterenol sulfate USP) Tablets:

ALUPENT® Tablets
Incidence of Adverse Events
Reported Among 496 Patients
Treated in 26 Controlled Clinical Trials

ADVERSE EXPERIENCE	Incidence Number of Patients	%
Cardiovascular		
Chest Pain	1	.2
Edema	1	.2
Hypertension	2	.4
Palpitations	19	3.8
Tachycardia	85	17.1
Central Nervous System		
Dizziness	12	2.4
Drowsiness	3	.6
Fatigue	7	1.4
Headache	35	7.0
Insomnia	9	1.8
Nervousness	100	20.2
Sensory disturbances	1	.2
Syncope	2	.4
Weakness	1	.2
Dermatological		
Diaphoresis	1	.2
Hives	1	.2
Pruritus	2	.4
Gastrointestinal		
Appetite changes	2	.4
Diarrhea	6	1.2
Gastrointestinal distress	15	3.0
Nausea	18	3.6
Vomiting	4	0.8
Musculoskeletal		
Pain	1	.2
Spasms	1	.2
Tremor	84	16.9
Ophthalmological		
Blurred vision	1	.2
Oro-Otolaryngeal		
Dry mouth/throat	2	.4
Laryngeal changes	1	.2
Bad taste	4	0.8
Respiratory		
Asthma exacerbation	10	2.0
Coughing	1	.2
Other		
Chatty	1	.2
Chills	1	.2
Clonus noted on flexing foot	1	.2
Feverish	2	.4
Flu symptoms	1	.2
Facial and finger puffiness	1	.2

The incidence of adverse events occurring in at least 1% of the 1,120 patients treated with Alupent Syrup in 44 clinical

Population	Method of Administration	Usual Single Dose	Range	Dilution
Adult	Hand-bulb nebulizer	10 inhalations	5–15 inhalations	No dilution
12 years and older	IPPB or nebulizer	0.3 ml	0.2–0.3 ml	Diluted in approx. 2.5 ml saline solution or other diluent
Pediatric 6–12 years	Nebulizer	0.1 ml	0.1–0.2 ml	Diluted in saline solution to a total volume of 3 ml

Continued on next page

Alupent—Cont.

trials are tachycardia (6.1%; n=68), nervousness (4.8%; n=54), tremor (1.6%; n=18), nausea (1.3%; n=15) and headache (1.1%; n=12).

It is important to recognize that adverse reactions from beta agonist bronchodilator solutions for nebulization may occur with the use of a new container of a product in patients who have previously tolerated that same product without adverse effect. There have been reports that indicate that such patients may subsequently tolerate replacement containers of the same product without adverse effect.

OVERDOSAGE

The expected symptoms with overdosage are those of excessive beta-adrenergic stimulation and/or any of the symptoms listed under adverse reactions, e.g. angina, hypertension or hypotension, arrhythmias, nervousness, headache, tremor, dry mouth, palpitation, nausea, dizziness, fatigue, malaise and insomnia.

Treatment consists of discontinuation of metaproterenol together with appropriate symptomatic therapy.

DOSAGE AND ADMINISTRATION

If Alupent® (metaproterenol sulfate USP) is administered before or after other sympathomimetic bronchodilators, caution should be exercised with respect to possible potentiation of adrenergic effects.

Inhalation Aerosol: The usual single dose is two to three inhalations. With repetitive dosing, inhalation should usually not be repeated more often than about every three to four hours. Total dosage per day should not exceed 12 inhalations. Alupent Inhalation Aerosol is not recommended for use in children under 12 years of age.

Usually, treatment need not be repeated more often than every four hours to relieve acute attacks of bronchospasm. As with all medications, the physician should begin therapy with the lowest effective dose and then titrate the dosage according to the individual patient's requirements.

Alupent Inhalation Solution 5% is administered by oral inhalation with the aid of a nebulizer or an intermittent positive pressure breathing apparatus (IPPB).

Alupent Inhalation Solution 5% may be administered three to four times a day for the treatment of reversible airways disease in adults. A single dose of nebulized Alupent in the treatment of an acute attack of asthma may not completely abort an attack.

The dosage and administration are summarized in the table below:

[See table at bottom of previous page]

Inhalation Solution 0.4% and 0.6% Unit-dose Vials: Alupent Inhalation Solution Unit-dose Vial is administered by oral inhalation using an IPPB device. The usual adult dose is one vial per nebulization treatment. Each vial of Alupent Inhalation Solution 0.4% is equivalent to 0.2 ml Alupent Inhalation Solution 5% diluted to 2.5 ml with normal saline; each vial of Alupent Inhalation Solution 0.6% is equivalent to 0.3 ml Alupent Inhalation Solution 5% diluted to 2.5 ml with normal saline.

Usually, treatment need not be repeated more often than every 4 hours to relieve acute attacks of bronchospasm. As part of a total treatment program in chronic bronchospastic pulmonary diseases, Alupent Inhalation Solution Unit-dose vials may be administered three to four times a day.

As with all medications, the physician should begin therapy with the lowest effective dose and then titrate the dosage according to the individual patient's requirements.

Alupent Inhalation Solution Unit-dose Vial is not recommended for use in children under 12 years of age.

Syrup: Children: Aged six to nine years or weight under 60 lbs—one teaspoonful three or four times a day. Children over nine years or weight over 60 lbs—two teaspoonfuls three or four times a day. Clinical trial experience in children under the age of 6 is limited. Of 40 children treated with Alupent® (metaproterenol sulfate USP) Syrup for at least 1 month, daily doses of approximately 1.3 to 2.6 mg/kg were well tolerated. Adults—two teaspoonfuls three or four times a day.

It is recommended that the physician titrate the dosage according to each individual patient's response to therapy.

Tablets: Adults: The usual dose is 20 mg three or four times a day. *Children:* Aged six to nine years or weight under 60 lbs—10 mg three or four times a day. Over nine years or weight over 60 lbs—20 mg three or four times a day. Alupent tablets are not recommended for use in children under six years at this time. (Please refer to the CLINICAL PHARMACOLOGY section for further information on clinical experience with this product.) It is recommended that the physician titrate the dosage according to each individual patient's response to therapy.

HOW SUPPLIED

Inhalation Aerosol: Each 200 inhalations of Alupent® (metaproterenol sulfate USP) Inhalation Aerosol contains 150 mg of metaproterenol sulfate as a micronized powder in inert propellants. Each metered dose delivers through the

mouthpiece 0.65 mg metaproterenol sulfate (each ml contains 15 mg). Alupent Inhalation Aerosol with Mouthpiece (NDC 0597-0070-17), net contents 14g (10 mL). The mouthpiece is white with a clear, colorless sleeve and a blue protective cap. Alupent Inhalation Aerosol Refill (NDC 0597-0070-18), net contents 14g (10 mL).

Note: The indented statement below is required by the Federal government's Clean Air Act for all products containing or manufactured with chlorofluorocarbons (CFCs).

> WARNING
> Contains trichloromonofluoromethane (CFC-11), dichlorodifluoromethane (CFC-12) and dichlorotetrafluoroethane (CFC-114), substances which harm public health and the environment by destroying ozone in the upper atmosphere.

A notice similar to the above WARNING has been placed in the "Instructions for Use" portion of the package insert pursuant to regulations of the United States Environmental Protection Agency.

Store between 59°F (15°C) and 77°F (25°C). Avoid excessive humidity.

Inhalation Solution: Alupent® (metaproterenol sulfate USP) Inhalation Solution is supplied as a 5% solution in bottles of 10 ml (NDC 0597-0071-75) or 30 ml (NDC 0597-0071-30) with accompanying calibrated dropper. Plastic cover on dropper should be discarded and not used to retain product. Store between 59°F (15°C) and 77°F (25°C). Protect from light. Do not use the solution if it is pinkish or darker than slightly yellow or contains a precipitate.

Alupent Inhalation Solution Unit-dose Vial is supplied as a 0.4% (NDC 0597-0078-62) or 0.6% (NDC 0597-0069-62) clear colorless or nearly colorless solution containing 2.5 ml with 25 vials per box. Each vial is made from a low-density polyethylene resin. Store below 77°F (25°C). Protect from light. Do not use the solution if it is pinkish or darker than slightly yellow or contains a precipitate.

Syrup: Alupent® (metaproterenol sulfate USP) is available as a cherry-flavored syrup, 10 mg per teaspoonful (5 ml) in 16 fl. oz. bottles (NDC 0597-0073-16). Store between 59°F (15°C) and 86°F (30°C). Protect from light.

Tablets: Alupent® (metaproterenol sulfate USP) is supplied in two dosage strengths as scored round white tablets in bottles of 100. Tablets of 10 mg coded BI/74 (NDC 0597-0074-01). Tablets of 20 mg coded BI/72 (NDC 0597-0072-01).

Storage for bottles: Store between 59°F (15°C) and 86°F (30°C). Protect from light. Blisters no longer distributed.

Rx Only.

AL-PI-7/95

Shown in Product Identification Guide, page 306

ATROVENT® ℞
[ă 'trō"vĕnt]
(ipratropium bromide)
Inhalation Aerosol
Bronchodilator .... BI-CODE 82

PRODUCT OVERVIEW

KEY FACTS

The active ingredient in Atrovent® (ipratropium bromide) Inhalation Aerosol is ipratropium bromide. It is an anticholinergic bronchodilator classified as a synthetic quaternary ammonium compound. The bronchodilating effect of Atrovent is primarily local and site specific. It is not well absorbed systemically, resulting in a low potential for toxicity.

MAJOR USES

Atrovent Inhalation Aerosol has proved to be clinically effective for maintenance treatment of bronchospasm associated with chronic obstructive pulmonary disease (COPD), including chronic bronchitis and emphysema.

SAFETY INFORMATION

Atrovent Inhalation Aerosol is contraindicated for patients with a hypersensitivity to atropine or its derivatives or to soya lecithin or related food products such as soybean or lecithin. It is not intended for the initial treatment of acute episodes of bronchospasm where rapid response is required. Before prescribing, please consult full Prescribing Information below.

PRESCRIBING INFORMATION

ATROVENT® ℞
[ă 'trō"vĕnt]
(ipratropium bromide)
Inhalation Aerosol
Bronchodilator

DESCRIPTION

The active ingredient in Atrovent® (ipratropium bromide) Inhalation Aerosol is ipratropium bromide. It is an anticholinergic bronchodilator chemically described as 8-azoniabicyclo (3.2.1)-octane, 3-(3-hydroxy -1- oxo-2-phenylpropoxy)-8-methyl-8(1-methylethyl)-, bromide, monohydrate

(endo, syn)-, (±)-: a synthetic quaternary ammonium compound, chemically related to atropine.

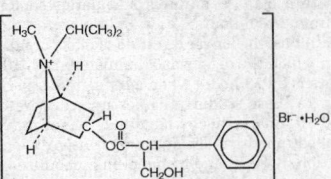

ipratropium bromide
(Atrovent)

$C_{20}H_{30}BrNO_3 \cdot H_2O$ Mol. Wt. 430.4

Ipratropium bromide is a white crystalline substance, freely soluble in water and lower alcohols but insoluble in lipophilic solvents such as ether, chloroform, and fluorocarbons. Atrovent Inhalation Aerosol is an inhalation aerosol for oral administration. The net weight is 14 grams; it yields 200 inhalations. Each actuation of the valve delivers 18 mcg of ipratropium bromide from the mouthpiece. The inert ingredients are dichlorodifluoromethane, dichlorotetrafluoroethane, and trichloromonofluoromethane as propellants and soya lecithin.

CLINICAL PHARMACOLOGY

Atrovent® (ipratropium bromide) is an anticholinergic (parasympatholytic) agent which, based on animal studies, appears to inhibit vagally mediated reflexes by antagonizing the action of acetylcholine, the transmitter agent released from the vagus nerve. Anticholinergics prevent the increases in intracellular concentration of cyclic guanosine monophosphate (cyclic GMP) which are caused by interaction of acetylcholine with the muscarinic receptor on bronchial smooth muscle.

The bronchodilation following inhalation of Atrovent is primarily a local, site-specific effect, not a systemic one. Much of an inhaled dose is swallowed as shown by fecal excretion studies. Atrovent is not readily absorbed into the systemic circulation either from the surface of the lung or from the gastrointestinal tract as confirmed by blood level and renal excretion studies.

The half-life of elimination is about 2 hours after inhalation or intravenous administration. Autoradiographic studies in rats have shown that Atrovent does not penetrate the blood-brain barrier.

In controlled 90-day studies in patients with bronchospasm associated with chronic obstructive pulmonary disease (chronic bronchitis and emphysema) significant improvements in pulmonary function (FEV_1 and $FEF_{25-75\%}$ increases of 15% or more) occurred within 15 minutes, reached a peak in 1–2 hours, and persisted for periods of 3 to 4 hours in the majority of patients and up to 6 hours in some patients. In addition, significant increases in Forced Vital Capacity (FVC) have been demonstrated.

Controlled clinical studies have demonstrated that Atrovent® (ipratropium bromide) does not alter either mucociliary clearance or the volume or viscosity of respiratory secretions. In studies without a positive control Atrovent did not alter pupil size, accommodation or visual acuity (See ADVERSE REACTIONS).

Ventilation/perfusion studies have shown no clinically significant effects on pulmonary gas exchange or arterial oxygen tension. Atrovent does not produce clinically significant changes in pulse rate or blood pressure.

INDICATIONS AND USAGE

Atrovent® (ipratropium bromide) Inhalation Aerosol is indicated as a bronchodilator for maintenance treatment of bronchospasm associated with chronic obstructive pulmonary disease, including chronic bronchitis and emphysema.

CONTRAINDICATIONS

Atrovent® (ipratropium bromide) Inhalation Aerosol is contraindicated in patients with a history of hypersensitivity to soya lecithin or related food products such as soybean and peanut. Atrovent should also not be taken by patients hypersensitive to any other components of the drug product or to atropine or its derivatives.

WARNINGS

Atrovent® (ipratropium bromide) is not indicated for the initial treatment of acute episodes of bronchospasm where rapid response is required. Immediate hypersensitivity reactions may occur after administration of ipratropium bromide, as demonstrated by rare cases of urticaria, angioedema, rash, bronchospasm and oropharyngeal edema.

PRECAUTIONS

General: Atrovent® (ipratropium bromide) should be used with caution in patients with narrow-angle glaucoma, prostatic hypertrophy or bladder-neck obstruction.

Information for Patients: Patients should be advised that temporary blurring of vision precipitation or worsening of narrow-angle glaucoma or eye pain may result if the aerosol is sprayed into the eyes.

If recommended dosage does not provide relief or symptoms become worse, patients should seek immediate medical attention. While taking Atrovent® Inhalation Aerosol, other inhaled drugs should not be used unless prescribed. (See illustrated Patient's Instructions for Use).

Drug Interactions: Atrovent has been used concomitantly with other drugs, including sympathomimetic bronchodilators, methylxanthines, steroids and cromolyn sodium, commonly used in the treatment of chronic obstructive pulmonary disease, without adverse drug reactions. There are no formal studies fully evaluating the interaction effects of Atrovent and these drugs with respect to effectiveness.

Carcinogenesis, Mutagenesis, Impairment of Fertility: Two-year oral carcinogenicity studies in rats and mice have revealed no carcinogenic potential at doses up to 1,250 times the maximum recommended human daily dose for Atrovent. Results of various mutagenicity studies were negative. Fertility of male or female rats at oral doses up to approximately 10,000 times the maximum recommended human daily dose was unaffected by Atrovent administration. At doses above 18,000 times the maximum recommended human daily dose, increased resorption and decreased conception rates were observed.

Pregnancy

TERATOGENIC EFFECTS Pregnancy Category B:

Oral reproduction studies performed in mice, rats and rabbits (at doses approximately 2,000, 200,000 and 26,000 times the maximum recommended human daily dose, respectively) and inhalation reproduction studies in rats and rabbits (at doses approximately 312 and 375 times the maximum recommended human daily dose, respectively) have demonstrated no evidence of teratogenic effects as a result of Atrovent® (ipratropium bromide). However, no adequate or well controlled studies have been conducted in pregnant women. Because animal reproduction studies are not always predictive of human response, Atrovent® (ipratropium bromide) should be used during pregnancy only if clearly needed.

Nursing Mothers: It is not known whether Atrovent is excreted in human milk. Although lipid-insoluble quaternary bases pass into breast milk, it is unlikely that Atrovent would reach the infant to an important extent, especially when taken by aerosol. However, because many drugs are excreted in human milk, caution should be exercised when Atrovent is administered to a nursing woman.

Pediatric Use: Safety and effectiveness in the pediatric population below the age of 12 have not been established.

ADVERSE REACTIONS

Adverse reaction information concerning Atrovent® (ipratropium bromide) is derived from 90 day controlled clinical trials (N = 254), other controlled clinical trials using recommended doses of Atrovent (N = 377) and an uncontrolled study (N = 1924). Additional information is derived from the foreign post-marketing experience and the published literature.

Adverse reactions occurring in greater than one percent of patients in the 90-day controlled clinical trials appear in the following table:

	Percent of Patients	
	Ipratropium bromide N = 254	**Metaproterenol sulfate N = 249**
Reaction		
Cardiovascular		
Palpitations	1.8	1.6
Central Nervous System		
Nervousness	3.1	6.8
Dizziness	2.4	2.8
Headache	2.4	2.0
Dermatological		
Rash	1.2	0.4
Gastrointestinal		
Nausea	2.8	1.2
Gastrointestinal distress	2.4	2.8
Vomiting	0	1.2
Musculoskeletal		
Tremor	0	2.4
Ophthalmological		
Blurred vision	1.2	0.8
Oro-Otolaryngeal		
Dry mouth	2.4	0.8
Irritation from aerosol	1.6	1.6
Respiratory		
Cough	5.9	1.2
Exacerbation of symptoms	2.4	3.6

Additional adverse reactions reported in less than one percent of the patients considered possibly due to Atrovent include urinary difficulty, fatigue, insomnia and hoarseness.

The large uncontrolled, open-label study included seriously ill patients. About 7% of patients treated discontinued the program because of adverse events.

Of the 2301 patients treated in the large uncontrolled study and in clinical trials other than the 90-day studies, the most common adverse reactions reported were: dryness of the oropharynx, about 5 in 100; cough, exacerbation of symptoms and irritation from aerosol, each about 3 in 100; headache, about 2 in 100; nausea, dizziness, blurred vision/difficulty in accommodation, and drying of secretions, each about 1 in 100. Less frequently reported adverse reactions that were possibly due to Atrovent® (ipratropium bromide) include tachycardia, paresthesias, drowsiness, coordination difficulty, itching, hives, flushing, alopecia, constipation, tremor, and mucosal ulcers.

Cases of precipitation or worsening of narrow-angle glaucoma, acute eye pain and hypotension have been reported. Allergic-type reactions such as skin rash, angioedema of tongue, lips and face, urticaria (including giant urticaria), laryngospasm and anaphylactic reaction have been reported, with positive rechallenge in some cases. Many of the patients had a history of allergies to other drugs and/or foods, including soybean. (See CONTRAINDICATIONS.)

OVERDOSAGE

Acute overdosage by inhalation is unlikely since Atrovent® (ipratropium bromide) is not well absorbed systemically after aerosol or oral administration. The oral LD_{50} of Atrovent ranged between 1001 and 2010 mg/kg in mice; between 1667 and more than 4000 mg/kg in rats; and between 400 and 1300 mg/kg in dogs.

DOSAGE AND ADMINISTRATION

The usual starting dose of Atrovent® (ipratropium bromide) is two inhalations (36 mcg) four times a day. Patients may take additional inhalations as required; however, the total number of inhalations should not exceed 12 in 24 hours.

HOW SUPPLIED

Atrovent® (ipratropium bromide) Inhalation Aerosol is supplied as a metered dose inhaler with a white mouthpiece which has a clear, colorless sleeve and a green protective cap.

Atrovent® Inhalation Aerosol with Mouthpiece (NDC 0597-0082-14), net contents 14 g. Atrovent® Inhalation Aerosol Refill (NDC 0597-0082-18), net contents 14 g.

Each 14 gram vial provides sufficient medication for 200 inhalations. Each actuation delivers 18 mcg of ipratropium bromide from the mouthpiece.

Note: The indented statement below is required by the Federal government's Clean Air Act for all products containing or manufactured with chlorofluorocarbons (CFCs):

> **WARNING**
> Contains trichloromonofluoromethane (CFC-11), dichlorodifluoromethane (CFC-12) and dichlorotetrafluoroethane (CFC-114), substances which harm public health and the environment by destroying ozone in the upper atmosphere.

A notice similar to the above WARNING has been placed in the information for the patient of this product under the Environmental Protection Agency's (EPA's) regulations. The patient's warning states that the patient should consult his or her physician if there are questions or alternatives.

Store between 59°F (15°C) and 86°F (30°C). Avoid excessive humidity.

Keep out of children's reach. Shake well before using. Patients should be reminded to read and follow the accompanying "Instructions for Use," which should be dispensed with the product. As with most inhaled medications in aerosol canisters, the therapeutic effect of this medication may decrease when the canister is cold.

Warning: Discard the canister after you have used the labeled number of inhalations. The correct amount of medication in each inhalation cannot be assured after this point.

Caution

Federal law prohibits dispensing without prescription.

AT-PI-11/96

Manufactured by Boehringer Ingelheim Pharmaceuticals, Inc., Ridgefield, CT 06877

Licensed from Boehringer Ingelheim International GmbH

Shown in Product Identification Guide, page 306

ATROVENT® ℞

[ă 'trō "vĕnt]

(ipratropium bromide)

Inhalation Solution .... BI-CODE 80

Prescribing Information

DESCRIPTION

The active ingredient in Atrovent® (ipratropium bromide) Inhalation Solution is ipratropium bromide monohydrate. It is an anticholinergic bronchodilator chemically described as 8-azoniabicyclo[3.2.1]-octane, 3-(3-hydroxy-1-oxo-2- phenylpropoxy)-8-methyl-8-(1-methylethyl)-, bromide, monohydrate *(endo, syn)*-, (±)-; a synthetic quaternary ammonium compound, chemically related to atropine.

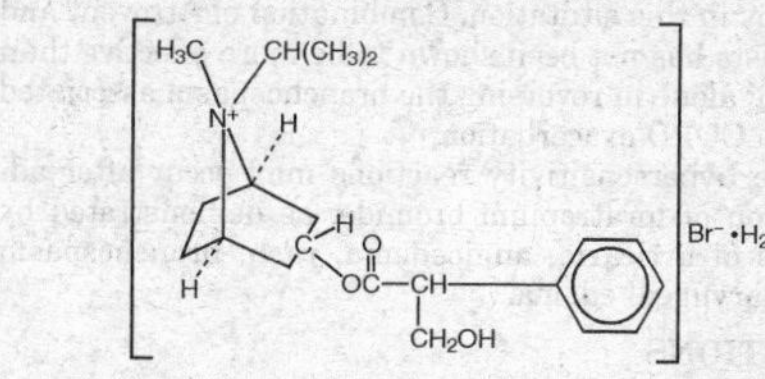

ipratropium bromide monohydrate (Atrovent)	$C_{20}H_{30}BrNO_3 \cdot H_2O$ Mol. Wt. 430.4

Ipratropium bromide is a white crystalline substance, freely soluble in water and lower alcohols. It is a quaternary ammonium compound and thus exists in an ionized state in aqueous solutions. It is relatively insoluble in non-polar media.

Atrovent Inhalation Solution is administered by oral inhalation with the aid of a nebulizer. It contains ipratropium bromide 0.02% (anhydrous basis) in a sterile, preservative-free, isotonic saline solution, pH-adjusted 3.4 (3 to 4) with hydrochloric acid.

CLINICAL PHARMACOLOGY

Atrovent® (ipratropium bromide) is an anticholinergic (parasympatholytic) agent that, based on animal studies, appears to inhibit vagally-mediated reflexes by antagonizing the action of acetylcholine, the transmitter agent released from the vagus nerve.

Anticholinergics prevent the increases in intracellular concentration of cyclic guanosine monophosphate (cyclic GMP) that are caused by interaction of acetylcholine with the muscarinic receptor on bronchial smooth muscle.

The bronchodilation following inhalation of Atrovent is primarily a local, site-specific effect, not a systemic one. Much of an administered dose is swallowed but not absorbed, as shown by fecal excretion studies. Following nebulization of a 2 mg dose, a mean 7% of the dose was absorbed into the systemic circulation either from the surface of the lung or from the gastrointestinal tract. The half-life of elimination is about 1.6 hours after intravenous administration. Ipratropium bromide is minimally (0 to 9% in vitro) bound to plasma albumin and α_1-acid glycoproteins. It is partially metabolized. Autoradiographic studies in rats have shown that Atrovent does not penetrate the blood-brain barrier. Atrovent has not been studied in patients with hepatic or renal insufficiency. It should be used with caution in those patient populations.

In controlled 12-week studies in patients with bronchospasm associated with chronic obstructive pulmonary disease (chronic bronchitis and emphysema) significant improvements in pulmonary function (FEV_1 increases of 15% or more) occurred within 15 to 30 minutes, reached a peak in 1–2 hours, and persisted for periods of 4–5 hours in the majority of patients, with about 25–38% of the patients demonstrating increases of 15% or more for at least 7–8 hours. Continued effectiveness of Atrovent Inhalation Solution was demonstrated throughout the 12-week period. In addition, significant increases in forced vital capacity (FVC) have been demonstrated. However, Atrovent did not consistently produce significant improvement in subjective symptom scores nor in quality of life scores over the 12-week duration of study.

Additional controlled 12-week studies were conducted to evaluate the safety and effectiveness of Atrovent Inhalation Solution administered concomitantly with the beta adrenergic bronchodilator solutions metaproterenol and albuterol compared with the administration of each of the beta agonists alone. Combined therapy produced significant additional improvement in FEV_1 and FVC. On combined therapy, the median duration of 15% improvement in FEV_1 was 5–7 hours, compared with 3–4 hours in patients receiving a beta agonist alone.

INDICATIONS AND USAGE

Atrovent® (ipratropium bromide) Inhalation Solution administered either alone or with other bronchodilators, especially beta adrenergics, is indicated as a bronchodilator for maintenance treatment of bronchospasm associated with chronic obstructive pulmonary disease, including chronic bronchitis and emphysema.

CONTRAINDICATIONS

Atrovent® (ipratropium bromide) is contraindicated in known or suspected cases of hypersensitivity to ipratropium bromide, or to atropine and its derivatives.

WARNINGS

The use of Atrovent® (ipratropium bromide) Inhalation Solution as a single agent for the relief of bronchospasm in acute COPD exacerbation has not been adequately studied. Drugs with faster onset of action may be preferable as ini-

Continued on next page

Atrovent Solution—Cont.

tial therapy in this situtation. Combination of Atrovent and beta agonists has not been shown to be more effective than either drug alone in reversing the bronchospasm associated with acute COPD exacerbation.

Immediate hypersensitivity reactions may occur after administration of ipratropium bromide, as demonstrated by rare cases of urticaria, angioedema, rash, bronchospasm and oropharyngeal edema.

PRECAUTIONS

General: Atrovent® (ipratropium bromide) should be used with caution in patients with narrow-angle glaucoma, prostatic hypertrophy or bladder-neck obstruction.

Information for Patients: Patients should be advised that temporary blurring of vision, precipitation or worsening of narrow-angle glaucoma or eye pain may result if the solution comes into direct contact with the eyes. Use of a nebulizer with mouthpiece rather than face mask may be preferable, to reduce the likelihood of the nebulizer solution reaching the eyes. Patients should be advised that Atrovent Inhalation Solution can be mixed in the nebulizer with albuterol or metaproterenol if used within one hour. Drug stability and safety of Atrovent® Inhalation Solution when mixed with other drugs in a nebulizer have not been established. Patients should be reminded that Atrovent Inhalation Solution should be used consistently as prescribed throughout the course of therapy.

Drug Interactions: Atrovent has been shown to be a safe and effective bronchodilator when used in conjuction with beta adrenergic bronchodilators. Atrovent has also been used with other pulmonary medications, including methylxanthines and corticosteroids, without adverse drug interactions.

Carcinogenesis, Mutagenesis, Impairment of Fertility: Two-year oral carcinogenicity studies in rats and mice have revealed no carcinogenic potential at doses up to 6 mg/kg/day of Atrovent.

Results of various mutagenicity studies (Ames test, mouse dominant lethal test, mouse micronucleus test and chromosome aberration of bone marrow in Chinese hamsters) were negative.

Fertility of male or female rats at oral doses up to 50 mg/kg/day was unaffected by Atrovent administration. At doses above 90 mg/kg, increased resorption and decreased conception rates were observed.

Pregnancy *TERATOGENIC EFFECTS*

Pregnancy Category B. Oral reproduction studies performed in mice, rats and rabbits at doses of 10, 100, and 125 mg/kg respectively, and inhalation reproduction studies in rats and rabbits at doses of 1.5 and 1.8 mg/kg (or approximately 38 and 45 times the recommended human daily dose) respectively, have demonstrated no evidence of teratogenic effects as a result of Atrovent. However, no adequate or well-controlled studies have been conducted in pregnant women. Because animal reproduction studies are not always predictive of human response, Atrovent should be used during pregnancy only if clearly needed.

Nursing Mothers: It is not known whether Atrovent is excreted in human milk. Although lipid-insoluble quaternary bases pass into breast milk, it is unlikely that Atrovent® (ipratropium bromide) would reach the infant to a significant extent, especially when taken by inhalation since Atrovent is not well absorbed systemically after inhalation or oral administration. However, because many drugs are excreted in human milk, caution should be exercised when Atrovent is administered to a nursing woman.

Pediatric Use: Safety and effectiveness in the pediatric population below the age of 12 have not been established.

ADVERSE REACTIONS

Adverse reaction information concerning Atrovent® (ipratropium bromide) Inhalation Solution is derived from 12-week active-controlled clinical trials. Additional information is derived from foreign post-marketing experience and the published literature.

All adverse events, regardless of drug relationship, reported by three percent or more patients in the 12-week controlled clinical trials appear in the table below:

[See table below]

Additional adverse reactions reported in less than three percent of the patients treated with Atrovent include tachycardia, palpitations, eye pain, urinary retention, urinary tract infection and urticaria. Cases of precipitation or worsening of narrow-angle glaucoma and acute eye pain have been reported.

Lower respiratory adverse reactions (bronchitis, dyspnea and bronchospasm) were the most common events leading to discontinuation of Atrovent therapy in the 12-week trials. Headache, mouth dryness and aggravation of COPD symptoms are more common when the total daily dose of Atrovent equals or exceeds 2,000 mcg.

Allergic-type reactions such a skin rash, angioedema of tongue, lips and face, urticaria, laryngospasm and anaphylactic reaction have been reported. Many of the patients had a history of allergies to other drugs and/or foods.

OVERDOSAGE

Acute systemic overdosage by inhalation is unlikely since Atrovent® (ipratropium bromide) is not well absorbed after inhalation at up to four-fold the recommended dose, or after oral administration at up to forty-fold the recommended dose. The oral LD_{50} of Atrovent ranged between 1001 and 2010 mg/kg in mice; between 1667 and more than 4000 mg/kg in rats; and between 400 and 1300 mg/kg in dogs.

DOSAGE AND ADMINISTRATION

The usual dosage of Atrovent® (ipratropium bromide) Inhalation Solution is 500 mcg (1 Unit-Dose Vial) administered three to four times a day by oral nebulization, with doses 6 to 8 hours apart. Atrovent Inhalation Solution Unit-Dose Vials contain 500 mcg ipratropium bromide anhydrous in 2.5 ml normal saline. Atrovent Inhalation Solution can be mixed in the nebulizer with albuterol or metaproterenol if used within one hour. Drug stability and safety of Atrovent Inhalation Solution when mixed with other drugs in a nebulizer have not been established.

HOW SUPPLIED

Atrovent® (ipratropium bromide) Inhalation Solution Unit Dose Vial is supplied as a 0.02% clear, colorless solution containing 2.5 ml with 25 vials per foil pouch (NDC 0597-0080-62).

Each vial is made from a low density polyethylene (LDPE) resin.

STORE BETWEEN 59°F (15°C) AND 86°F (30°C). PROTECT FROM LIGHT. STORE UNUSED VIALS IN THE FOIL POUCH. ATTENTION PHARMACIST: Detach "Patient's Instructions for Use" from Package Insert and dispense with solution.

Caution

Federal law prohibits dispensing without prescription.

AS-PI 6/96 Rev

Distributed by
Boehringer Ingelheim Pharmaceuticals, Inc. Ridgefield, CT 06877
Manufactured by Roxane Laboratories, Inc., Columbus, OH 43228
Licensed from Boehringer Ingelheim International GmbH

Shown in Product Identification Guide, page 306

ATROVENT®
(ipratropium bromide)
Nasal Spray 0.03%   ℞

Prescribing Information

DESCRIPTION

The active ingredient in ATROVENT® Nasal Spray is ipratropium bromide monohydrate. It is an anticholinergic agent chemically described as 8-azoniabicyclo (3.2.1) octane,3-(3-hydroxy-1-oxo-2-phenylpropoxy)-8-methyl-8-(1-methylethyl)-, bromide, monohydrate *(endo,syn)-*, (±)- :a synthetic quaternary ammonium compound, chemically related to atropine. Its structural formula is:

ipratropium bromide monohydrate $C_{20}H_{30}BrNO_3 \cdot H_2O$ Mol. Wt. 430.4

Ipratropium bromide is a white to off-white, crystalline substance. It is freely soluble in lower alcohols and water, existing in an ionized state in aqueous solutions, and relatively insoluble in non-polar media.

ATROVENT® (ipratropium bromide) Nasal Spray 0.03% is a metered-dose, manual pump spray unit which delivers 21 mcg (70μL) ipratropium bromide per spray on an anhydrous basis in an isotonic, aqueous solution with pH adjusted to 4.7. It also contains benzalkonium chloride, edetate disodium, sodium chloride, sodium hydroxide, hydrochloric acid, and purified water. Each bottle contains 345 sprays.

CLINICAL PHARMACOLOGY
Mechanism of Action
Ipratropium bromide is an anticholinergic agent that inhibits its vagally-mediated reflexes by antagonizing the action of

---

All Adverse Events, from a Double-blind, Parallel, 12-week Study of Patients with COPD*

PERCENT OF PATIENTS

	Atrovent® (500 mcg t.i.d) n=219	Alupent® 15 mg t.i.d) n=212	Atrovent®/Alupent® (500 mcg t.i.d/ 15 mg t.i.d) n=108	Albuterol (2.5 mg t.i.d) n=205	Atrovent®/ Albuterol (500 mcg t.i.d/ 2.5 mg t.i.d) n=100
Body as a Whole-General Disorders					
Headache	6.4	5.2	6.5	6.3	9.0
Pain	4.1	3.3	0.9	2.9	5.0
Influenza-like symptoms	3.7	4.7	6.5	0.5	1.0
Back pain	3.2	1.9	1.9	2.4	0.0
Chest pain	3.2	4.2	5.6	2.0	1.0
Cardiovascular Disorders					
Hypertension/Hypertension Aggravated	0.9	1.9	0.9	1.5	4.0
Central & Peripheral Nervous System					
Dizziness	2.3	3.3	1.9	3.9	4.0
Insomnia	0.9	0.5	4.6	1.0	1.0
Tremor	0.9	7.1	8.3	1.0	0.0
Nervousness	0.5	4.7	6.5	1.0	1.0
Gastrointestinal System Disorders					
Mouth Dryness	3.2	0.0	1.9	2.0	3.0
Nausea	4.1	3.8	1.9	2.9	2.0
Constipation	0.9	0.0	3.7	1.0	1.0
Musculo-Skeletal System Disorders					
Arthritis	0.9	1.4	0.9	0.5	3.0
Respiratory System Disorders (Lower)					
Coughing	4.6	8.0	6.5	5.4	6.0
Dyspnea	9.6	13.2	16.7	12.7	9.0
Bronchitis	14.6	24.5	15.7	16.6	20.0
Bronchospasm	2.3	2.8	4.6	5.4	5.0
Sputum Increased	1.4	1.4	4.6	3.4	0.0
Respiratory Disorder	0.0	6.1	6.5	2.0	4.0
Respiratory System Disorders (Upper)					
Upper Respiratory Tract Infection	13.2	11.3	9.3	12.2	16.0
Pharyngitis	3.7	4.2	5.6	2.9	4.0
Rhinitis	2.3	4.2	1.9	2.4	0.0
Sinusitis	2.3	2.8	0.9	5.4	4.0

* All adverse events, regardless of drug relationship, reported by three percent or more patients in the 12-week controlled clinical trials.

acetylcholine at the cholinergic receptor. In humans, ipratropium bromide has anti-secretory properties and, when applied locally, inhibits secretions from the serous and seromucous glands lining the nasal mucosa. Ipratropium bromide is a quaternary amine that minimally crosses the nasal and gastrointestinal membrane and the blood-brain barrier, resulting in a reduction of the systemic anticholinergic effects (e.g., neurologic, ophthalmic, cardiovascular, and gastrointestinal effects) that are seen with tertiary anticholinergic amines.

Pharmacokinetics

Absorption: Ipratropium bromide is poorly absorbed into the systemic circulation following oral administration (2–3%). Less than 20% of an 84 mcg per nostril dose was absorbed from the nasal mucosa of normal volunteers, induced-cold patients, or perennial rhinitis patients.

Distribution: Ipratropium bromide is minimally bound (0 to 9% *in vitro*) to plasma albumin and α1-acid glycoprotein. Its blood/plasma concentration ratio was estimated to be about 0.89. Studies in rats have shown that ipratropium bromide does not penetrate the blood-brain barrier.

Metabolism: Ipratropium bromide is partially metabolized to ester hydrolysis products, tropic acid and tropane. These metabolites appear to be inactive based on *in vitro* receptor affinity studies using rat brain tissue homogenates.

Elimination: After intravenous administration of 2 mg ipratropium bromide to 10 healthy volunteers, the terminal half-life of ipratropium was approximately 1.6 hours. The total body clearance and renal clearance were estimated to be 2,505 and 1,019 ml/min, respectively. The amount of the total dose excreted unchanged in the urine (Ae) within 24 hours was approximately one-half of the administered dose.

Pediatrics: Following administration of 42 mcg of ipratropium bromide per nostril two or three times a day in perennial rhinitis patients 6–18 years old, the mean amounts of the total dose excreted unchanged in the urine (8.6 to 11.1%) were higher than those reported in adult volunteers or adult perennial rhinitis patients (3.7 to 5.6%). Plasma ipratropium concentrations were relatively low (ranging from undetectable up to 0.49 ng/ml). No correlation of the amount of the total dose excreted unchanged in the urine (Ae) with age or gender was observed in the pediatric population.

Special Populations: Gender does not appear to influence the absorption or excretion of nasally administered ipratropium bromide. The pharmacokinetics of ipratropium bromide have not been studied in patients with hepatic or renal insufficiency or in the elderly.

Drug-Drug Interaction: No specific pharmacokinetic studies were conducted to evaluate potential drug-drug interactions.

Pharmacodynamics: In two single-dose trials (n=17), doses up to 336 mcg of ipratropium bromide did not significantly affect pupillary diameter, heart rate, or systolic/diastolic blood pressure. Similarly, in patients with induced-colds, ATROVENT (ipratropium bromide) Nasal Spray 0.06% (84 mcg/nostril four times a day), had no significant effects on pupillary diameter, heart rate or systolic/diastolic blood pressure.

Two nasal provocation trials in perennial rhinitis patients (n=44) using ipratropium bromide nasal spray showed a dose dependent increase in inhibition of methacholine induced nasal secretion with an onset of action within 15 minutes (time of first observation).

Controlled clinical trials demonstrated that intranasal fluorocarbon-propelled ipratropium bromide does not alter physiologic nasal functions (e.g., sense of smell, ciliary beat frequency, mucociliary clearance, or the air conditioning capacity of the nose).

Clinical Trials

The clinical trials for ATROVENT® (ipratropium bromide) Nasal Spray 0.03% were conducted in patients with nonallergic perennial rhinitis (NAPR) and in patients with allergic perennial rhinitis (APR). APR patients were those who experienced symptoms of nasal hypersecretion and nasal congestion or sneezing when exposed to specific perennial allergens (e.g., dust mites, molds) and were skin test positive to these allergens. NAPR patients were those who experienced symptoms of nasal hypersecretion and nasal congestion or sneezing throughout the year, but were skin test negative to common perennial allergens.

In four controlled, four- and eight-week comparisons of ATROVENT® (ipratropium bromide) Nasal Spray 0.03% (42 mcg per nostril, two or three times daily) with its vehicle, in patients with allergic or nonallergic perennial rhinitis, there was a statistically significant decrease in the severity and duration of rhinorrhea in the ATROVENT® group throughout the entire study period. An effect was seen as early as the first day of therapy. There was no effect of ATROVENT® (ipratropium bromide) Nasal Spray 0.03% on degree of nasal congestion, sneezing or postnasal drip. The response to ATROVENT® (ipratropium bromide) Nasal Spray 0.03% did not appear to be affected by the type of perennial rhinitis (NAPR or APR), age or gender. No controlled clinical trials directly compared the efficacy of BID versus TID treatment.

% of Patients Reporting Events+

	ATROVENT® Nasal Spray 0.03% (n=356)		Vehicle Control (n=347)	
	Incidence %	Discontinued %	Incidence %	Discontinued %
Headache	9.8	0.6	9.2	0
Upper respiratory tract infection	9.8	1.4	7.2	1.4
Epistaxis[1]	9.0	0.3	4.6	0.3
Rhinitis*				
Nasal dryness	5.1	0	0.9	0.3
Nasal irritation[2]	2.0	0	1.7	0.6
Other nasal symptoms[3]	3.1	1.1	1.7	0.3
Pharyngitis	8.1	0.3	4.6	0
Nausea	2.2	0.3	0.9	0

+ This table includes adverse events which occurred at an incidence rate of at least 2.0% in the ATROVENT® group and more frequently in the ATROVENT® group than in the vehicle group.

[1] Epistaxis reported by 7.0% of ATROVENT® patients and 2.3% of vehicle patients, blood-tinged mucus by 2.0% of ATROVENT® patients and 2.3% of vehicle patients.

[2] Nasal irritation includes reports of nasal itching, nasal burning, nasal irritation and ulcerative rhinitis.

[3] Other nasal symptoms include reports of nasal congestion, increased rhinorrhea, increased rhinitis, posterior nasal drip, sneezing, nasal polyps and nasal edema.

* All events are listed by their WHO term; rhinitis has been presented by descriptive terms for clarification.

INDICATIONS AND USAGE

ATROVENT® (ipratropium bromide) Nasal Spray 0.03% is indicated for the symptomatic relief of rhinorrhea associated with allergic and nonallergic perennial rhinitis in adults and children age 6 years and older. ATROVENT® (ipratropium bromide) Nasal Spray 0.03% does not relieve nasal congestion, sneezing or postnasal drip associated with allergic or nonallergic perennial rhinitis.

CONTRAINDICATIONS

ATROVENT® (ipratropium bromide) Nasal Spray 0.03% is contraindicated in patients with a history of hypersensitivity to atropine or its derivatives, or to any of the other ingredients.

WARNINGS

Immediate hypersensitivity reactions may occur after administration of ipratropium bromide, as demonstrated by rare cases of urticaria, angioedema, rash, bronchospasm and oropharyngeal edema.

PRECAUTIONS

General

ATROVENT® (ipratropium bromide) Nasal Spray 0.03% should be used with caution in patients with narrow-angle glaucoma, prostatic hypertrophy or bladder-neck obstruction, particularly if they are receiving an anticholinergic by another route. Cases of precipitation or worsening of narrow-angle glaucoma and acute eye pain have been reported with direct eye contact of ipratropium bromide administered by oral inhalation.

Information for Patients

Patients should be advised that temporary blurring of vision, precipitation or worsening of narrow-angle glaucoma, or eye pain may result if ATROVENT® (ipratropium bromide) Nasal Spray 0.03% comes into direct contact with the eyes. Patients should be instructed to avoid spraying ATROVENT® (ipratropium bromide) Nasal Spray 0.03% in or around their eyes. Patients who experience eye pain, blurred vision, excessive nasal dryness, or episodes of nasal bleeding should be instructed to contact their doctor. Patients should be reminded to carefully read and follow the accompanying Patient's Instructions for Use.

Drug Interactions

No controlled clinical trials were conducted to investigate drug-drug interactions. ATROVENT® (ipratropium bromide) Nasal Spray 0.03% is minimally absorbed into the systemic circulation; nonetheless, there is some potential for an additive interaction with other concomitantly administered anticholinergic medications, including ATROVENT® for oral inhalation.

Carcinogenesis, Mutagenesis, Impairment of Fertility

In two-year carcinogenicity studies in rats and mice, ipratropium bromide at oral doses up to 6 mg/kg (approximately 190 and 95 times the maximum recommended daily intranasal dose in adults, respectively, and approximately 110 and 60 times the maximum recommended daily intranasal dose in children, respectively, on a mg/m^2 basis) showed no carcinogenic activity. Results of various mutagenicity studies (Ames test, mouse dominant lethal test, mouse micronucleus test, and chromosome aberration of bone marrow in Chinese hamsters) were negative.

Fertility of male or female rats was unaffected by ipratropium bromide at oral doses up to 50 mg/kg (approximately 1,600 times the maximum recommended daily intranasal dose in adults on a mg/m^2 basis). At an oral dose of 500 mg/kg (approximately 16,000 times the maximum recommended daily intranasal dose in adults on a mg/m^2 basis), ipratropium bromide produced a decrease in the conception rate.

Pregnancy

TERATOGENIC EFFECTS Pregnancy Category B. Oral reproduction studies were performed at doses of 10 mg/kg in mice, 1000 mg/kg in rats and 125 mg/kg in rabbits. These doses correspond, in each species respectively, to approximately 160, 32,000 and 8,000 times the maximum recommended daily intranasal dose in adults on a mg/m^2 basis. Inhalation reproduction studies were conducted in rats and rabbits at doses of 1.5 and 1.8 mg/kg respectively, (approximately 50 and 120 times, respectively, the maximum recommended daily intranasal dose in adults on a mg/m^2 basis). These studies demonstrated no evidence of teratogenic effects as a result of ipratropium bromide. At oral doses above 90 mg/kg in rats (approximately 2,900 times the maximum recommended daily intranasal dose in adults on a mg/m^2 basis) embryotoxicity was observed as increased resorption. This effect is not considered relevant to human use due to the large doses at which it was observed and the difference in route of administration. However, no adequate or well controlled studies have been conducted in pregnant women. Because animal reproduction studies are not always predictive of human response, ATROVENT® (ipratropium bromide) Nasal Spray 0.03% should be used during pregnancy only if clearly needed.

Nursing Mothers

It is known that some ipratropium bromide is systemically absorbed following nasal adminstration; however the portion which may be excreted in human milk is unknown. Although lipid-insoluble quaternary bases pass into breast milk, the minimal systemic absorption makes it unlikely that ipratropium bromide would reach the infant in an amount sufficient to cause a clinical effect. However, because many drugs are excreted in human milk, caution should be exercised when ATROVENT® (ipratropium bromide) Nasal Spray 0.03% is administered to a nursing woman.

Pediatric Use

The safety of ATROVENT® (ipratropium bromide) Nasal Spray 0.03% at a dose of two sprays (42 mcg) per nostril two or three times daily (total dose 168 to 252 mcg/day) has been demonstrated in 77 pediatric patients 6–12 years of age in placebo-controlled, 4-week trials and in 55 pediatric patients in active-controlled, 6 month trials. The effectiveness of ATROVENT® (ipratropium bromide) Nasal Spray 0.03% for the treatment of rhinorrhea associated with allergic and nonallergic perennial rhinitis in this pediatric age group is based on an extrapolation of the demonstrated efficacy of ATROVENT® (ipratropium bromide) Nasal Spray 0.03% in adults with these conditions and the likelihood that the disease course, pathophysiology, and the drug's effects are substantially similar to that of the adults. The recommended dose for the pediatric population is based on within and cross-study comparisons of the efficacy of ATROVENT® (ipratropium bromide) Nasal Spray 0.03% in adults and pediatric patients and on its safety profile in both adults and pediatric patients. The safety and effectiveness of ATROVENT® (ipratropium bromide) Nasal Spray 0.03% in patients under 6 years of age have not been established.

ADVERSE REACTIONS

Adverse reaction information on ATROVENT® (ipratropium bromide) Nasal Spray 0.03% in patients with perennial rhinitis was derived from four multicenter, vehicle-controlled clinical trials involving 703 patients (356 patients on ATROVENT® and 347 patients on vehicle), and a one-year, open-label, follow-up trial. In three of the trials, patients received ATROVENT® (ipratropium bromide) Na-

Continued on next page

Atrovent Spray 0.03%—Cont.

sal Spray 0.03% three times daily, for eight weeks. In the other trial, ATROVENT® (ipratropium bromide) Nasal Spray 0.03% was given to patients two times daily for four weeks. Of the 285 patients who entered the open-label, follow-up trial, 232 were treated for 3 months, 200 for 6 months, and 159 up to one year. The majority (>86%) of patients treated for one year were maintained on 42 mcg per nostril, two or three times daily, of ATROVENT® (ipratropium bromide) Nasal Spray 0.03%.

The following table shows adverse events, and the frequency that these adverse events led to the discontinuation of treatment, reported for patients who received ATROVENT® (ipratropium bromide) Nasal Spray 0.03% at the recommended dose of 42 mcg per nostril, or vehicle two or three times daily for four or eight weeks. Only adverse events reported with an incidence of at least 2.0% in the ATROVENT® group and higher in the ATROVENT® group than in the vehicle group are shown.

[See table at top of previous page]

ATROVENT® (ipratropium bromide) Nasal Spray 0.03% was well tolerated by most patients. The most frequently reported nasal adverse events were transient episodes of nasal dryness or epistaxis. These adverse events were mild or moderate in nature, none was considered serious, none resulted in hospitalization and most resolved spontaneously or following a dose reduction. Treatment for nasal dryness and epistaxis was required infrequently (2% or less) and consisted of local application of pressure or a moisturizing agent (e.g., petroleum jelly or saline nasal spray). Patient discontinuation for epistaxis or nasal dryness was infrequent in both the controlled (0.3% or less) and one-year, open-label (2% or less) trials. There was no evidence of nasal rebound (i.e., a clinically significant increase in rhinorrhea, posterior nasal drip, sneezing or nasal congestion severity compared to baseline) upon discontinuation of double-blind therapy in these trials.

Adverse events reported by less than 2% of the patients receiving ATROVENT® (ipratropium bromide) Nasal Spray 0.03% during the controlled clinical trials or during the open-label follow-up trial, which are potentially related to systemic anticholinergic effects ATROVENT's® local effects or systemic anticholinergic effects include: dry mouth/throat, dizziness, ocular irritation, blurred vision, conjunctivitis, hoarseness, cough and taste perversion. Additional anticholinergic effects noted with other ATROVENT® dosage forms (ATROVENT® Inhalation Solution, ATROVENT® Inhalation Aerosol, and ATROVENT® Nasal Spray 0.06%) include: precipitation or worsening of narrow-angle glaucoma, urinary retention, prostatic disorders, tachycardia, constipation, and bowel obstruction.

There were infrequent reports of skin rash in both the controlled and uncontrolled clinical studies. Other allergic-type reactions such as angioedema of the throat, tongue, lips and face, urticaria, laryngospasm, and anaphylactic reactions have been reported with other ipratropium bromide products.

No controlled trial was conducted to address the relative incidence of adverse events of BID versus TID therapy.

OVERDOSAGE

Acute overdosage by intranasal administration is unlikely since ipratropium bromide is not well absorbed systemically after intranasal or oral administration. Following administration of a 20 mg oral dose (equivalent to ingesting more than four bottles of ATROVENT® Nasal Spray 0.03%) to 10 male volunteers, no change in heart rate or blood pressure was noted. Following a 2 mg intravenous infusion over 15 minutes to the same 10 male volunteers, plasma ipratropium concentrations of 22–45 ng/mL were observed (>100 times the concentrations observed following intranasal administration). Following intravenous infusion these 10 volunteers had a mean increase of heart rate of 50 bpm and less than 20 mmHg change in systolic or diastolic blood pressure at the time of peak ipratropium levels.

Oral median lethal doses of ipratropium bromide were greater than 1,000 mg/kg in mice (approximately 16,000 and 9,500 times the maximum recommended daily intranasal dose in adults and children, respectively, on a mg/m^2 basis), 1,700 mg/kg in rats (approximately 55,000 and 32,000 times the maximum recommended daily intranasal dose in adults and children, respectively, on a mg/m^2 basis), and 400 mg/kg in dogs (approximately 43,000 and 25,000 times the maximum recommended daily intranasal dose in adults and children, respectively, on a mg/m^2 basis).

DOSAGE AND ADMINISTRATION

The recommended dose of ATROVENT® (ipratropium bromide) Nasal Spray 0.03% is two sprays (42 mcg) per nostril two or three times daily (total dose 168 to 252 mcg/day) for the symptomatic relief of rhinorrhea associated with allergic and nonallergic perennial rhinitis in adults and children age 6 years and older. Optimum dosage varies with the response of the individual patient.

Initial pump priming requires seven sprays of the pump. If used regularly as recommended, no further priming is required. If not used for more than 24 hours, the pump will require two sprays, or if not used for more than seven days, the pump will require seven sprays to reprime.

HOW SUPPLIED

ATROVENT® (ipratropium bromide) Nasal Spray 0.03% is supplied in a white high density polyethylene (HDPE) bottle fitted with a white and clear metered nasal spray pump, a green safety clip to prevent accidental discharge of the spray, and a clear plastic dust cap. It contains 31.1 g of product formulation, 345 sprays, each delivering 21 mcg (70 µL) of ipratropium per spray, or 28 days of therapy at the maximum recommended dose (two sprays per nostril three times a day).

Store tightly closed between 59°F (15°C) and 86°F (30°C). Avoid freezing. Keep out of reach of children. Do not spray in the eyes.

Patients should be reminded to read and follow the accompanying Patient's Instructions for Use, which should be dispensed with the product.

Rx Only.

AN.03-PI-4/98

Manufactured by: Boehringer Ingelheim Pharmaceuticals, Inc.
Ridgefield, CT 06877
Licensed from: Boehringer Ingelheim International GmbH

Shown in Product Identification Guide, page 306

ATROVENT® ℞
(ipratropium bromide)
Nasal Spray 0.06%

Prescribing Information

DESCRIPTION

The active ingredient in ATROVENT® Nasal Spray is ipratropium bromide monohydrate. It is an anticholinergic agent chemically described as 8-azoniabicyclo (3.2.1) octane,3-(3-hydroxy-1-oxo-2-phenylpropoxy)-8-methyl-8-(1-methylethyl)-, bromide, monohydrate (*endo, syn*)-, (±)- : a synthetic quaternary ammonium compound, chemically related to atropine. Its structural formula is:

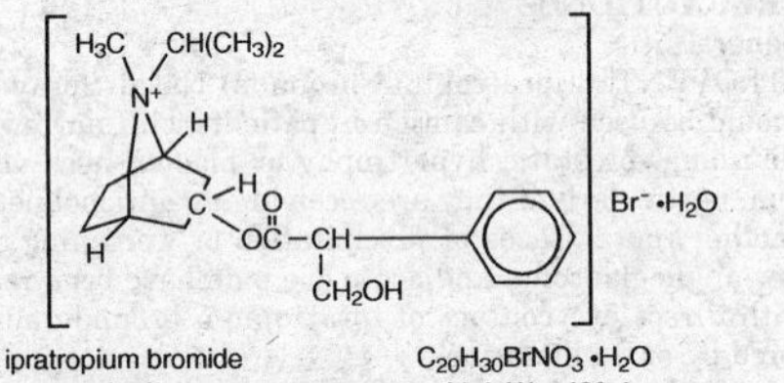

ipratropium bromide monohydrate
$C_{20}H_{30}BrNO_3 \cdot H_2O$
Mol. Wt. 430.4

Ipratropium bromide is a white to off-white, crystalline substance. It is freely soluble in lower alcohols and water, existing in an ionized state in aqueous solutions, and relatively insoluble in non-polar media.

ATROVENT® (ipratropium bromide) Nasal Spray 0.06% is intended for local administration to the nasal mucosa to control rhinorrhea in patients with the common cold. It contains 0.06% ipratropium bromide on an anhydrous basis (42 mcg/spray) in an isotonic, aqueous solution with pH adjusted to 4.7, which also contains benzalkonium chloride, edetate disodium, sodium chloride, sodium hydroxide, hydrochloric acid, and purified water.

CLINICAL PHARMACOLOGY

Mechanism of Action

Ipratropium bromide is an anticholinergic agent that inhibits vagally-mediated reflexes by antagonizing the action of acetylcholine at the cholinergic receptor. In humans, ipratropium bromide has anti-secretory properties and, when applied locally, inhibits secretions from the serous and seromucous glands lining the nasal mucosa. Ipratropium bromide is a quaternary amine that minimally crosses the nasal and gastrointestinal membrane and the blood-brain barrier, resulting in a reduction of the systemic anticholinergic effects (e.g., neurologic, ophthalmic, cardiovascular and gastrointestinal effects) that are seen with tertiary anticholinergic amines.

Pharmacokinetics

Ipratropium bromide is a quaternary amine that is poorly absorbed into the systemic circulation from the nasal mucosa. Less than 20% of an 84 mcg per nostril dose is absorbed from the nasal mucosa of normal volunteers, induced-cold patients or perennial rhinitis patients, but the amount of ipratropium bromide which is systemically absorbed from nasal administration exceeds the amount of ipratropium bromide absorbed from either ATROVENT® Inhalation Solution (2% of a 500 mcg dose) or ATROVENT® Inhalation Aerosol (20% of a 36 mcg mouthpiece dose).

The half-life of elimination of ipratropium is about 1.6 hours after intravenous administration. Ipratropium bromide is minimally bound (0 to 9% *in vitro*) to plasma albumin and α_1-acid glycoprotein. It is partially metabolized to inactive ester hydrolysis products. Following intravenous administration, approximately one-half of the dose is excreted unchanged in the urine. Studies in rats have shown that ipratropium bromide does not penetrate the blood-brain barrier. The pharmacokinetics of ipratropium bromide have not been studied in patients with hepatic or renal insufficiency or in the elderly. Gender does not seem to influence the absorption or excretion of nasally administered ipratropium bromide.

Pharmacodynamic data also indicate little systemic absorption. In two single-dose, pharmacokinetic trials (n = 17), solutions of up to 0.12% ipratropium bromide (336 mcg total nasal dose) did not significantly affect pupillary diameter, heart rate or systolic/diastolic blood pressure. Similarly, in an induced-cold, pharmacokinetic trial with ATROVENT® (ipratropium bromide) Nasal Spray 0.06% (84 mcg/nostril four times a day) no significant effects on pupillary diameter, heart rate or systolic/diastolic blood pressures were observed.

Controlled clinical trials demonstrated that intranasal fluorocarbon-propelled ipratropium bromide does not alter physiologic nasal functions (e.g., sense of smell, ciliary beat frequency, mucociliary clearance, or the air conditioning capacity of the nose).

Clinical Trials

The clinical trials for ATROVENT® (ipratropium bromide) Nasal Spray 0.06% were conducted in patients with rhinorrhea associated with naturally occurring common colds. In two controlled four-day comparisons of ATROVENT® (ipratropium bromide) Nasal Spray 0.06% (84 mcg per nostril, administered three or four times daily; n=352) with its vehicle (n=351), there was a statistically significant reduction of rhinorrhea, as measured by both nasal discharge weight and the patients' subjective assessment of severity of rhinorrhea using a visual analog scale. These significant differences were evident within one hour following dosing. There was no effect of ATROVENT® (ipratropium bromide) Nasal Spray 0.06% on degree of nasal congestion or sneezing. The response to ATROVENT® (ipratropium bromide) Nasal Spray 0.06% did not appear to be affected by age or gender. No controlled clinical trials directly compared the efficacy of TID versus QID treatment.

INDICATIONS AND USAGE

ATROVENT® (ipratropium bromide) Nasal Spray 0.06% is indicated for the symptomatic relief of rhinorrhea associated with the common cold for adults and children age 12 years and older. ATROVENT® (ipratropium bromide) Nasal Spray 0.06% does not relieve nasal congestion or sneezing associated with the common cold.

The safety and effectiveness of the use of ATROVENT® (ipratropium bromide) Nasal Spray 0.06% beyond four days in patients with the common cold has not been established.

CONTRAINDICATIONS

ATROVENT® (ipratropium bromide) Nasal Spray 0.06% is contraindicated in patients with a history of hypersensitivity to atropine or its derivatives, or to any of the other ingredients.

WARNINGS

Immediate hypersensitivity reactions may occur after administration of ipratropium bromide, as demonstrated by rare cases of urticaria, angioedema, rash, bronchospasm and oropharyngeal edema.

PRECAUTIONS

General

ATROVENT® (ipratropium bromide) Nasal Spray 0.06% should be used with caution in patients with narrow-angle glaucoma, prostatic hypertrophy or bladder-neck obstruction, particularly if they are receiving an anticholinergic by another route. Cases of precipitation or worsening of narrow-angle glaucoma and acute eye pain have been reported with direct eye contact of ipratropium bromide administered by oral inhalation.

Information for Patients

Patients should be advised that temporary blurring of vision, precipitation or worsening of narrow-angle glaucoma or eye pain may result if ATROVENT® (ipratropium bromide) Nasal Spray 0.06% comes into direct contact with the eyes. Patients should be instructed to avoid spraying ATROVENT® (ipratropium bromide) Nasal Spray 0.06% in or around the eyes. Patients who experience eye pain, blurred vision, excessive nasal dryness or episodes of nasal bleeding should be instructed to contact their doctor. Patients should be reminded to carefully read and follow the accompanying Patient's Instructions for Use.

Drug Interactions

No controlled clinical trials were conducted to investigate potential drug-drug interactions. ATROVENT® (ipratropium bromide) Nasal Spray 0.06% is minimally absorbed into the systemic circulation; nonetheless there is some po-

tential for an additive interaction with other concomitantly administered anticholinergic medications, including ATROVENT® for oral inhalation.

Carcinogenesis, Mutagenesis, Impairment of Fertility

Two-year oral carcinogenicity studies in rats and mice have revealed no carcinogenic activity at doses up to 6 mg/kg/day. This dose corresponds, in rats and mice respectively, to about 70 and 40 times the maximum recommended human daily dose (MRHD) on a mg/m^2 basis of ATROVENT® (ipratropium bromide) Nasal Spray 0.06%. Results of various mutagenicity studies (Ames test, mouse dominant lethal test, mouse micronucleus test and chromosome aberration of bone marrow in Chinese hamsters) were negative.

Fertility of male or female rats at oral doses up to 50 mg/kg/day (about 600 times the MRHD on a mg/m^2 basis) was unaffected by ipratropium bromide administration. At doses above 90 mg/kg/day (about 1,000 times the MRHD on a mg/m^2 basis) a decreased conception rate was observed.

Pregnancy

TERATOGENIC EFFECTS Pregnancy Category B. Oral reproduction studies were performed at doses of 10 mg/kg/day in mice, 100 mg/kg/day in rats and 125 mg/kg/day in rabbits. These doses correspond, in each species respectively, to about 60, 1,200 and 3,000 times the MRHD of ATROVENT® (ipratropium bromide) Nasal Spray 0.06% in the common cold (672 mcg/day) on a mg/m^2 basis. Inhalation reproduction studies in rats and rabbits at doses of 1.5 and 1.8 mg/kg/day (about 20 and 40 times the MRHD dose on a mg/m^2 basis for each species, respectively) have demonstrated no evidence of teratogenic effects as a result of ipratropium bromide. At oral doses above 90 mg/kg/day in rats (about 1,000 times the MRHD on a mg/m^2 basis) embryotoxicity was observed as increased resorption. This effect is not considered relevant to human use due to the large doses at which it was observed and the difference in route of administration. However, no adequate or well controlled studies have been conducted in pregnant women. Because animal reproduction studies are not always predictive of human response, ATROVENT® (ipratropium bromide) Nasal Spray 0.06% should be used during pregnancy only if clearly needed.

Nursing Mothers

It is known that some ipratropium bromide is systemically absorbed following nasal administration; however the portion which may be excreted in human milk is unknown. Although lipid-insoluble quaternary bases pass into breast milk, the minimal systemic absorption makes it unlikely that ipratropium bromide would reach the infant in an amount sufficient to cause a clinical effect. However, because many drugs are excreted in human milk, caution should be exercised when ATROVENT® (ipratropium bromide) Nasal Spray 0.06% is administered to a nursing woman.

Pediatric Use

Safety and effectiveness of ATROVENT® (ipratropium bromide) Nasal Spray 0.06% in patients below the age of 12 years have not been established.

ADVERSE REACTIONS

Adverse reaction information on ATROVENT® (ipratropium bromide) Nasal Spray 0.06% in patients with the common cold was derived from two multicenter, vehicle-controlled clinical trials involving 1276 patients (195 patients on ATROVENT® Nasal Spray 0.03%, 352 patients on ATROVENT® Nasal Spray 0.06%, 189 patients on ATROVENT® Nasal Spray 0.12%, 351 patients on vehicle and 189 patients receiving no treatment).

The following table shows adverse events reported for patients who received ATROVENT® (ipratropium bromide) Nasal Spray 0.06% at the recommended dose of 84 mcg per nostril, or vehicle, administered three or four times daily, where the incidence is 1% or greater in the ATROVENT® group, and higher in the ATROVENT® group than in the vehicle group.

% of Patients Reporting Events[1]

	ATROVENT® Nasal Spray 0.06% (n = 352)	Vehicle Control (n = 351)
Epistaxis[2]	8.2%	2.3%
Dry Mouth/Throat	1.4%	0.3%
Nasal Congestion	1.1%	0.0%
Nasal Dryness	4.8%	2.8%

1 This table includes adverse events for which the incidence was 1% or greater in the ATROVENT® group and higher in the ATROVENT® group than in the vehicle group.

2 Epistaxis reported by 5.4% of ATROVENT® patients and 1.4% of vehicle patients, blood-tinged nasal mucus by 2.8% of ATROVENT® patients and 0.9% of vehicle patients.

ATROVENT® (ipratropium bromide) Nasal Spray 0.06% was well tolerated by most patients. The most frequently reported adverse events were transient episodes of nasal dryness or epistaxis. The majority of these adverse events (96%) were mild or moderate in nature, none was considered serious and none resulted in hospitalization. No patient required treatment for nasal dryness and only three patients (<1%) required treatment for epistaxis, which consisted of local application of pressure or a moisturizing agent (e.g., petroleum jelly). No patient receiving ATROVENT® (ipratropium bromide) Nasal Spray 0.06% was discontinued from the trial due to other nasal dryness or bleeding.

Adverse events reported by less than 1% of the patients receiving ATROVENT® (ipratropium bromide) Nasal Spray 0.06% during the controlled clinical trials which are potentially related to ATROVENT's® local effects or systemic anticholinergic effects include: taste perversion, nasal burning, conjunctivitis, coughing, dizziness, hoarseness, palpitation, pharyngitis, tachycardia, thirst, tinnitus and blurred vision. Additional anticholinergic effects noted with other ATROVENT® dosage forms (ATROVENT® Inhalation Solution, ATROVENT® Inhalation Aerosol and ATROVENT® Nasal Spray 0.03%) include: precipitation or worsening of narrow-angle glaucoma, urinary retention, prostate disorders, constipation and bowel obstruction.

There were no reports of allergic-type reactions in the controlled clinical trials. Allergic-type reactions such as skin rash, angioedema of the tongue, lips and face, urticaria, laryngospasm and anaphylactic reactions have been reported with other ipratropium bromide products.

No controlled trial was conducted to address the relative incidence of adverse events for TID versus QID therapy.

OVERDOSAGE

Acute overdosage by intranasal administration is unlikely since ipratropium bromide is not well absorbed systemically after intranasal or oral administration. Following administration of a 20 mg oral dose (equivalent to ingesting more than two bottles of ATROVENT® Nasal Spray 0.06%) to 10 male volunteers, no change in heart rate or blood pressure was noted. Following a 2 mg intravenous infusion over 15 minutes to the same 10 male volunteers, plasma ipratropium concentrations of 22–45 ng/mL were observed (>100 times the concentrations observed following intranasal administration). Following intravenous infusion these 10 volunteers had a mean increase of heart rate of 50 bpm and less than 20 mm Hg change in systolic or diastolic blood pressure at the time of peak ipratropium levels.

The oral LD_{50} of ipratropium bromide ranged between 1000 and 2000 mg/kg in mice (about 2,000 and 4,000 times the MRHD on a mg/m^2 basis, respectively); between 1,700 and 4,000 mg/kg in rats (about 3,300 and 8,000 times the MRHD on a mg/m^2 basis, respectively); and between 400 and 1300 mg/kg in dogs (about 800 and 2,600 times the MRHD on a mg/m^2 basis, respectively). Target organs of toxicity at repeated doses were liver, GI tract, adrenals (rat), male reproductive organs and eyes (dog).

DOSAGE AND ADMINISTRATION

The recommended dose of ATROVENT® (ipratropium bromide) Nasal Spray 0.06% is two sprays (84 mcg) per nostril three or four times daily (total dose 504 to 672 mcg/day) for the symptomatic relief of rhinorrhea associated with the common cold in adults and children age 12 years and older. Optimum dosage varies with the response of the individual patient.

The safety and effectiveness of the use of ATROVENT® (ipratropium bromide) Nasal Spray 0.06% beyond four days in patients with the common cold have not been established.

Initial pump priming requires seven actuations of the pump. If used regularly as recommended, no further priming is required. If not used for more than 24 hours, the pump will require two actuations, or if not used for more than seven days, the pump will require seven actuations to reprime.

HOW SUPPLIED

ATROVENT® (ipratropium bromide) Nasal Spray 0.06% is supplied as 15 ml of solution in a high density polyethylene (HDPE) bottle fitted with a metered nasal spray pump, a safety clip to prevent accidental discharge of the spray, and a clear plastic dust cap. The 15 ml bottle of ATROVENT® Nasal Spray 0.06% is designed to deliver 165 sprays of 0.07 ml each (42 mcg ipratropium bromide).

Store tightly closed between 59°F (15°C) and 86°F (30°C). Avoid freezing. Keep out of reach of children. Avoid spraying in or around the eyes.

Patients should be reminded to read and follow the accompanying Patient's Instructions for Use, which should be dispensed with the product.

CAUTION Federal law prohibits dispensing without prescription.

AN.06-PI-9/95

Manufactured by
Boehringer Ingelheim Pharmaceuticals, Inc.
Ridgefield, CT 06877

Licensed from
Boehringer Ingelheim
International GmbH

Shown in Product Identification Guide, page 306

CATAPRES® ℞

[*kah 'tah-pres*]

(clonidine hydrochloride USP)

Oral Antihypertensive

Tablets of 0.1, 0.2 and 0.3 mg

Prescribing Information

DESCRIPTION

CATAPRES® (clonidine hydrochloride USP) is a centrally acting alpha-agonist hypotensive agent available as tablets for oral administration in three dosage strengths: 0.1 mg, 0.2 mg and 0.3 mg. The 0.1 mg tablet is equivalent to 0.087 mg of the free base.

The inactive ingredients are colloidal silicon dioxide, cornstarch, dibasic calcium phosphate, FD&C Yellow No. 6, gelatin, glycerin, lactose, magnesium stearate, methylparaben, propylparaben. The CATAPRES 0.1 mg tablet also contains FD&C Blue No. 1 and FD&C Red No. 3.

Clonidine hydrochloride is an imidazoline derivative and exists as a mesomeric compound. The chemical name is 2-(2,6-dichlorophenylamino)-2-imidazoline hydrochloride. The following is the structural formula:

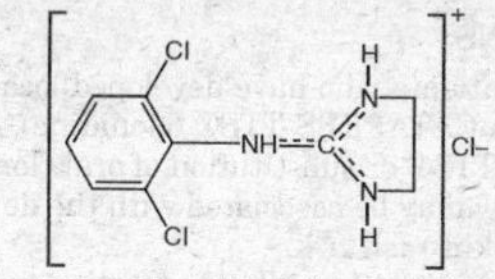

clonidine hydrochloride
(CATAPRES)

$C_9H_9Cl_2N_3{\cdot}HCl$ Mol. Wt. 266.56

Clonidine hydrochloride is an odorless, bitter, white, crystalline substance soluble in water and alcohol.

CLINICAL PHARMACOLOGY

Clonidine stimulates alpha-adrenoreceptors in the brain stem. This action results in reduced sympathetic outflow from the central nervous system and in decreases in peripheral resistance, renal vascular resistance, heart rate, and blood pressure. CATAPRES (clonidine hydrochloride USP) acts relatively rapidly. The patient's blood pressure declines within 30 to 60 minutes after an oral dose, the maximum decrease occurring within 2 to 4 hours. Renal blood flow and glomerular filtration rate remain essentially unchanged. Normal postural reflexes are intact; therefore, orthostatic symptoms are mild and infrequent.

Acute studies with clonidine hydrochloride in humans have demonstrated a moderate reduction (15% to 20%) of cardiac output in the supine position with no change in the peripheral resistance: at a 45° tilt there is a smaller reduction in cardiac output and a decrease of peripheral resistance. During long-term therapy, cardiac output tends to return to control values, while peripheral resistance remains decreased. Slowing of the pulse rate has been observed in most patients given clonidine, but the drug does not alter normal hemodynamic response to exercise.

Tolerance to the antihypertensive effect may develop in some patients, necessitating a reevaluation of therapy.

Other studies in patients have provided evidence of a reduction in plasma renin activity and in the excretion of aldosterone and catecholamines. The exact relationship of these pharmacologic actions to the antihypertensive effect of clonidine has not been fully elucidated.

Clonidine acutely stimulates growth hormone release in both children and adults, but does not produce a chronic elevation of growth hormone with long-term use.

Pharmacokinetics: The plasma level of clonidine peaks in approximately 3 to 5 hours and the plasma half-life ranges from 12 to 16 hours. The half-life increases up to 41 hours in patients with severe impairment of renal function. Following oral administration, about 40–60% of the absorbed dose is recovered in the urine as unchanged drug in 24 hours. About 50% of the absorbed dose is metabolized in the liver.

INDICATIONS AND USAGE

CATAPRES® (clonidine hydrochloride USP) is indicated in the treatment of hypertension. CATAPRES may be employed alone or concomitantly with other antihypertensive agents.

CONTRAINDICATIONS

CATAPRES® (clonidine hydrochloride USP) Tablets should not be used in patients with known hypersensitivity to clonidine (see PRECAUTIONS).

Continued on next page

Catapres—Cont.

WARNINGS

Withdrawal: Patients should be instructed not to discontinue therapy without consulting their physician. Sudden cessation of clonidine treatment has, in some cases, resulted in symptoms such as nervousness, agitation, headache, and tremor accompanied or followed by a rapid rise in blood pressure and elevated catecholamine concentrations in the plasma. The likelihood of such reactions to discontinuation of clonidine therapy appears to be greater after administration of higher doses or continuation of concomitant beta-blocker treatment and special caution is therefore advised in these situations. Rare instances of hypertensive encephalopathy, cerebrovascular accidents and death have been reported after clonidine withdrawal. When discontinuing therapy with CATAPRES®, the physician should reduce the dose gradually over 2 to 4 days to avoid withdrawal symptomatology.

An excessive rise in blood pressure following discontinuation of CATAPRES therapy can be reversed by administration of oral clonidine hydrochloride or by intravenous phentolamine. If therapy is to be discontinued in patients receiving a beta-blocker and clonidine concurrently, the beta-blocker should be withdrawn several days before the gradual discontinuation of CATAPRES.

Because children commonly have gastrointestinal illnesses that lead to vomiting, they may be particularly susceptible to hypertensive episodes resulting from abrupt inability to take medication.

PRECAUTIONS

General: In patients who have developed localized contact sensitization to CATAPRES-TTS® (clonidine), continuation of CATAPRES-TTS® or substitution of oral clonidine hydrochloride therapy may be associated with the development of a generalized skin rash.

In patients who develop an allergic reaction to CATAPRES-TTS, substitution of oral clonidine hydrochloride may also elicit an allergic reaction (including generalized rash, urticaria, or angioedema).

CATAPRES® (clonidine hydrochloride) should be used with caution in patients with severe coronary insufficiency, conduction disturbances, recent myocardial infarction, cerebrovascular disease or chronic renal failure.

Perioperative Use: Administration of CATAPRES should be continued to within four hours of surgery and resumed as soon as possible thereafter. Blood pressure should be carefully monitored during surgery and additional measures to control blood pressure should be available if required.

Information for Patients: Patients should be cautioned against interruption of CATAPRES therapy without their physician's advice.

Patients who engage in potentially hazardous activities, such as operating machinery or driving, should be advised of a possible sedative effect of clonidine. They should also be informed that this sedative effect may be increased by concomitant use of alcohol, barbiturates, or other sedating drugs.

Drug Interactions: Clonidine may potentiate the CNS-depressive effects of alcohol, barbiturates or other sedating drugs. If a patient receiving clonidine hydrochloride is also taking tricyclic antidepressants, the hypotensive effect of clonidine may be reduced, necessitating an increase in the clonidine dose.

Due to a potential for additive effects such as bradycardia and AV block, caution is warranted in patients receiving clonidine concomitantly with agents known to affect sinus node function or AV nodal conduction, e.g. digitalis, calcium channel blockers and beta-blockers.

Amitriptyline in combination with clonidine enhances the manifestation of corneal lesions in rats (See TOXICOLOGY).

Toxicology: In several studies with oral clonidine hydrochloride, a dose-dependent increase in the incidence and severity of spontaneous retinal degeneration was seen in albino rats treated for six months or longer. Tissue distribution studies in dogs and monkeys showed a concentration of clonidine in the choroid.

In view of the retinal degeneration seen in rats, eye examinations were performed during clinical trials in 908 patients before, and periodically after, the start of clonidine therapy. In 353 of these 908 patients, the eye examinations were carried out over periods of 24 months or longer. Except for some dryness of the eyes, no drug-related abnormal ophthalmological findings were recorded and, according to specialized tests such as electroretinography and macular dazzle, retinal function was unchanged.

In combination with amitriptyline, clonidine hydrochloride administration led to the development of corneal lesions in rats within five days.

Carcinogenesis, Mutagenesis, Impairment of Fertility: Chronic dietary administration of clonidine was not carcinogenic to rats (132 weeks) or mice (78 weeks) dosed, respectively, at up to 46 or 70 times the maximum recommended daily human dose (MRDHD) as mg/kg (9 or 6 times the MRDHD on a mg/m^2 basis). There was no evidence of genotoxicity in the Ames test for mutagenicity or mouse micronucleus test for clastogenicity.

Fertility of male or female rats was unaffected by clonidine doses as high as 150 mcg/kg (approximately 3 times the MRDHD). In a separate experiment, fertility of female rats appeared to be affected at dose levels of 500 to 2000 mcg/kg (10 to 40 times the oral MRDHD on a mg/kg basis; 2 to 8 times the MRDHD on a mg/m^2 basis).

Usage in Pregnancy: *TERATOGENIC EFFECTS Pregnancy Category C.* Reproduction studies performed in rabbits at doses up to approximately three times the oral maximum recommended daily human dose (MRDHD) of CATAPRES (clonidine hydrochloride) produced no evidence of a teratogenic or embryotoxic potential in rabbits. In rats, however, doses as low as $^1/_3$ the oral MRDHD ($^1/_{15}$ the MRDHD on a mg/m^2 basis) of clonidine were associated with increased resorptions in a study in which dams were treated continuously from two months prior to mating. Increased resorptions were not associated with treatment at the same time or at higher dose levels (up to three times the oral MRDHD) when the dams were treated on gestation days 6–15. Increases in resorption were observed at much higher dose levels (40 times the oral MRDHD on a mg/kg basis; 4 to 8 times the MRDHD on a mg/m^2 basis) in mice and rats treated on gestation days 1–14 (lowest dose employed in the study was 500 mcg/kg).

No adequate, well-controlled studies have been conducted in pregnant women. Because animal reproduction studies are not always predictive of human response, this drug should be used during pregnancy only if clearly needed.

Nursing Mothers: As clonidine hydrochloride is excreted in human milk, caution should be exercised when CATAPRES® (clonidine hydrochloride USP) is administered to a nursing woman.

Pediatric Use: Safety and effectiveness in pediatric patients below the age of 12 have not been established (See WARNINGS on Withdrawal).

ADVERSE REACTIONS

Most adverse effects are mild and tend to diminish with continued therapy. The most frequent (which appear to be dose-related) are dry mouth, occurring in about 40 of 100 patients; drowsiness, about 33 in 100; dizziness, about 16 in 100; constipation and sedation, each about 10 in 100.

The following less frequent adverse experiences have also been reported in patients receiving CATAPRES® (clonidine hydrochloride USP), but in many cases patients were receiving concomitant medication and a causal relationship has not been established.

Body as a Whole: Weakness, about 10 in 100 patients; fatigue, about 4 in 100; headache and withdrawal syndrome each about 1 in 100. Also reported were pallor; a weakly positive Coombs' test; increased sensitivity to alcohol; and fever.

Cardiovascular: Orthostatic symptoms, about 3 in 100 patients; palpitations and tachycardia, and bradycardia, each about 5 in 1000. Syncope, Raynaud's phenomenon, congestive heart failure, and electrocardiographic abnormalities (i.e., sinus node arrest, functional bradycardia, high degree AV block and arrhythmias) have been reported rarely. Rare cases of sinus bradycardia and atrioventricular block have been reported, both with and without the use of concomitant digitalis.

Central Nervous System: Nervousness and agitation, about 3 in 100 patients; mental depression, about 1 in 100 and insomnia, about 5 in 1000. Other behavioral changes, vivid dreams or nightmares, restlessness, anxiety, visual and auditory hallucinations and delirium have rarely been reported.

Dermatological: Rash, about 1 in 100 patients; pruritus, about 7 in 1000; hives, angioneurotic edema and urticaria, about 5 in 1000; alopecia, about 2 in 1000.

Gastrointestinal: Nausea and vomiting, about 5 in 100 patients; anorexia and malaise, each about 1 in 100; mild transient abnormalities in liver function tests, about 1 in 100; hepatitis, parotitis, constipation, pseudo-obstruction, and abdominal pain, rarely.

Genitourinary: Decreased sexual activity, impotence and loss of libido, about 3 in 100 patients; nocturia, about 1 in 100; difficulty in micturition, about 2 in 1000; urinary retention, about 1 in 1000.

Hematologic: Thrombocytopenia, rarely.

Metabolic: Weight gain, about 1 in 100 patients; gynecomastia, about 1 in 1000; transient elevation of blood glucose or serum creatine phosphokinase, rarely.

Musculoskeletal: Muscle or joint pain, about 6 in 1000 and leg cramps, about 3 in 1000.

Oro-otolaryngeal: Dryness of the nasal mucosa was rarely reported.

Ophthalmological: Dryness of the eyes, burning of the eyes and blurred vision were reported.

OVERDOSAGE

Hypertension may develop early and may be followed by hypotension, bradycardia, respiratory depression, hypothermia, drowsiness, decreased or absent reflexes, weakness, irritability and miosis. The frequency of CNS depression may be higher in children than adults. Large overdoses may result in reversible cardiac conduction defects or dysrhythmias, apnea, coma and seizures. Signs and symptoms of overdose generally occur within 30 minutes to two hours after exposure. As little as 0.1 mg of clonidine has produced signs of toxicity in children.

There is no specific antidote for clonidine overdose. Clonidine overdosage may result in the rapid development of CNS depression; therefore, induction of vomiting with ipecac syrup is not recommended. Gastric lavage may be indicated following recent and/or large ingestions. Administration of activated charcoal and/or a cathartic may be beneficial. Supportive care may include atropine sulfate for bradycardia, intravenous fluids and/or vasopressor agents for hypotension and vasodilators for hypertension. Naloxone may be a useful adjunct for the management of clonidine-induced respiratory depression, hypotension and/or coma; blood pressure should be monitored since the administration of naloxone has occasionally resulted in paradoxical hypertension. Tolazoline administration has yielded inconsistent results and is not recommended as first-line therapy. Dialysis is not likely to significantly enhance the elimination of clonidine.

The largest overdose reported to date involved a 28-year-old male who ingested 100 mg of clonidine hydrochloride powder. This patient developed hypertension followed by hypotension, bradycardia, apnea, hallucinations, semicoma, and premature ventricular contractions. The patient fully recovered after intensive treatment. Plasma clonidine levels were 60 ng/ml after 1 hour, 190 ng/ml after 1.5 hours, 370 ng/ml after 2 hours, and 120 ng/ml after 5.5 and 6.5 hours. In mice and rats, the oral LD_{50} of clonidine is 206 and 465 mg/kg, respectively.

DOSAGE AND ADMINISTRATION

Adults: The dose of CATAPRES® (clonidine hydrochloride USP) must be adjusted according to the patient's individual blood pressure response. The following is a general guide to its administration.

Initial Dose: 0.1 mg tablet twice daily (morning and bedtime). Elderly patients may benefit from a lower initial dose.

Maintenance Dose: Further increments of 0.1 mg per day may be made at weekly intervals if necessary until the desired response is achieved. Taking the larger portion of the oral daily dose at bedtime may minimize transient adjustment effects of dry mouth and drowsiness. The therapeutic doses most commonly employed have ranged from 0.2 mg to 0.6 mg per day given in divided doses. Studies have indicated that 2.4 mg is the maximum effective daily dose, but doses as high as this have rarely been employed.

Renal Impairment: Dosage must be adjusted according to the degree of impairment, and patients should be carefully monitored. Since only a minimal amount of clonidine is removed during routine hemodialysis, there is no need to give supplemental clonidine following dialysis.

HOW SUPPLIED

CATAPRES® (clonidine hydrochloride USP) is supplied in scored oval tablets containing 0.1 mg, 0.2 mg or 0.3 mg of clonidine hydrochloride.

[See table below]

Store below 86°F (30°C).

Dispense in tight, light-resistant container.

Caution: Federal law prohibits dispensing without prescription.

CA-PI-8/96

Boehringer Ingelheim Pharmacueticals, Inc.
Ridgefield, CT 06877
Licensed from Boehringer Ingelheim International GmbH
Shown in Product Identification Guide, page 306

Dose (mg)	Color	Marking	Bottle of 100	Bottle of 1000	Unit Dose of 100
0.1	Tan	BI 6	NDC0597-0006-01	NDC0597-0006-10	NDC0597-0006-61
0.2	Orange	BI 7	NDC0597-0007-01	NDC0597-0007-10	NDC0597-0007-61
0.3	Peach	BI 11	NDC0597-0011-01		

CATAPRES-TTS® ℞

[*căt-a 'prĕss*]
(clonidine)
Transdermal Therapeutic System
Catapres-TTS® -1
Catapres-TTS® -2
Catapres-TTS® -3

Programmed delivery *in vivo* of 0.1, 0.2 or 0.3 mg clonidine per day, for one week.

Prescribing Information

DESCRIPTION

Catapres-TTS® (clonidine) is a transdermal system providing continuous systemic delivery of clonidine for 7 days at an approximately constant rate. Clonidine is a centrally acting alpha-agonist hypotensive agent. It is an imidazoline derivative with the chemical name 2, 6-dichloro-N-2-imidazolidinylidenebenzenamine and has the following chemical structure:

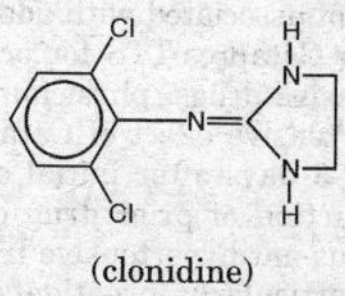

(clonidine)

System Structure and Components Catapres-TTS is a multilayered film, 0.2 mm thick, containing clonidine as the active agent. The system areas are 3.5 cm^2 (CATAPRES-TTS-1), 7.0 cm^2 (CATAPRES-TTS-2) and 10.5 cm^2 (CATAPRES-TTS-3) and the amount of drug released is directly proportional to the area (See Release Rate Concept). The composition per unit area is the same for all three doses.

Proceeding from the visible surface towards the surface attached to the skin, there are four consecutive layers: 1) a backing layer of pigmented polyester film; 2) a drug reservoir of clonidine, mineral oil, polyisobutylene, and colloidal silicon dioxide; 3) a microporous polypropylene membrane that controls the rate of delivery of clonidine from the system to the skin surface; 4) an adhesive formulation of clonidine, mineral oil, polyisobutylene, and colloidal silicon dioxide. Prior to use, a protective slit release liner of polyester that covers the adhesive layer is removed.

Cross section of the system:

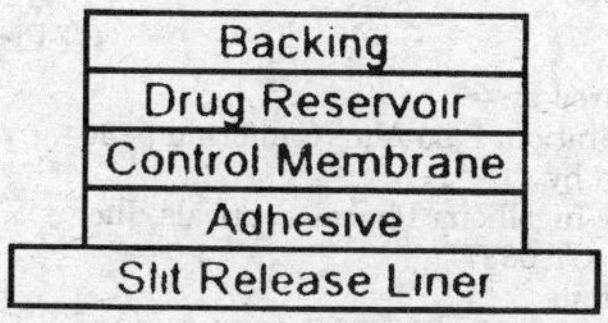

Release Rate Concept Catapres-TTS is programmed to release clonidine at an approximately constant rate for 7 days. The energy for drug release is derived from the concentration gradient existing between a saturated solution of drug in the system and the much lower concentration prevailing in the skin. Clonidine flows in the direction of the lower concentration at a constant rate, limited by the rate-controlling membrane, so long as a saturated solution is maintained in the drug reservoir.

Following system application to intact skin, clonidine in the adhesive layer saturates the skin site below the system. Clonidine from the drug reservoir then begins to flow through the rate-controlling membrane and the adhesive layer of the system into the systemic circulation via the capillaries beneath the skin. Therapeutic plasma clonidine levels are achieved 2 to 3 days after initial application of Catapres-TTS.

The 3.5, 7.0, and 10.5 cm^2 systems deliver 0.1, 0.2, and 0.3 mg of clonidine per day, respectively. To ensure constant release of drug for 7 days, the total drug content of the system is higher than the total amount of drug delivered. Application of a new system to a fresh skin site at weekly intervals continuously maintains therapeutic plasma concentrations of clonidine. If the Catapres-TTS is removed and not replaced with a new system, therapeutic plasma clonidine levels will persist for about 8 hours and then decline slowly over several days. Over this time period, blood pressure returns gradually to pretreatment levels.

CLINICAL PHARMACOLOGY

Clonidine stimulates alpha-adrenoreceptors in the brain stem. This action results in reduced sympathetic outflow from the central nervous system and in decreases in peripheral resistance, renal vascular resistance, heart rate, and blood pressure. Renal blood flow and glomerular filtration rate remain essentially unchanged. Normal postural reflexes are intact; therefore, orthostatic symptoms are mild and infrequent.

Acute studies with clonidine hydrochloride in humans have demonstrated a moderate reduction (15–20%) of cardiac output in the supine position with no change in peripheral resistance; at a 45° tilt there is a smaller reduction in cardiac output and a decrease of peripheral resistance.

During long-term therapy, cardiac output tends to return to control values, while peripheral resistance remains decreased. Slowing of the pulse rate has been observed in most patients given clonidine, but the drug does not alter normal hemodynamic responses to exercise.

Tolerance to the antihypertensive effect may develop in some patients, necessitating a reevaluation of therapy.

Other studies in patients have provided evidence of a reduction in plasma renin activity and in the excretion of aldosterone and catecholamines. The exact relationship of these pharmacologic actions to the antihypertensive effect of clonidine has not been fully elucidated.

Clonidine acutely stimulates the release of growth hormone in children as well as adults but does not produce a chronic elevation of growth hormone with long-term use.

Pharmacokinetics The plasma half-life of clonidine is 12.7 ± 7 hours. Following oral administration, about 40–60% of the absorbed dose is recovered in the urine as unchanged drug within 24 hours. The remainder of the absorbed dose is metabolized in the liver.

INDICATIONS AND USAGE

Catapres-TTS® (clonidine) is indicated in the treatment of hypertension. It may be employed alone or concomitantly with other antihypertensive agents.

CONTRAINDICATIONS

Catapres-TTS® (clonidine) should not be used in patients with known hypersensitivity to clonidine or to any other component of the therapeutic system.

WARNINGS

Withdrawal Patients should be instructed not to discontinue therapy without consulting their physician. Sudden cessation of clonidine treatment has, in some cases, resulted in symptoms such as nervousness, agitation, headache, and confusion accompanied or followed by a rapid rise in blood pressure and elevated catecholamine concentrations in the plasma. The likelihood of such reactions to discontinuation of clonidine therapy appears to be greater after administration of higher doses or continuation of concomitant beta-blocker treatment and special caution is therefore advised in these situations. Rare instances of hypertensive encephalopathy, cerebrovascular accidents and death have been reported after clonidine withdrawal. When discontinuing therapy with Catapres, the physician should reduce the dose gradually over 2 to 4 days to avoid withdrawal symptomatology.

An excessive rise in blood pressure following discontinuation of Catapres-TTS® therapy can be reversed by administration of oral clonidine hydrochloride or by intravenous phentolamine. If therapy is to be discontinued in patients receiving a beta-blocker and clonidine concurrently, the beta-blocker should be withdrawn several days before the gradual discontinuation of Catapres-TTS®.

PRECAUTIONS

General In patients who have developed localized contact sensitization to Catapres-TTS® (clonidine) continuation of Catapres-TTS or substitution of oral clonidine hydrochloride therapy may be associated with development of a generalized skin rash.

In patients who develop an allergic reaction to Catapres-TTS, substitution of oral clonidine hydrochloride may also elicit an allergic reaction (including generalized rash, urticaria, or angioedema).

Catapres-TTS should be used with caution in patients with severe coronary insufficiency, conduction disturbances, recent myocardial infarction, cerebrovascular disease, or chronic renal failure.

In rare instances, loss of blood pressure control has been reported in patients using Catapres-TTS according to the instructions for use.

Perioperative Use Catapres-TTS therapy should not be interrupted during the surgical period. Blood pressure should be carefully monitored during surgery and additional measures to control blood pressure should be available if required. Physicians considering starting Catapres-TTS therapy during the perioperative period must be aware that therapeutic plasma clonidine levels are not achieved until 2 to 3 days after initial application of Catapres-TTS (see DOSAGE AND ADMINISTRATION).

Defibrillation or Cardioversion The transdermal clonidine systems should be removed before attempting defibrillation or cardioversion because of the potential for altered electrical conductivity which may increase the risk of arcing, a phenomenon associated with the use of defibrillators.

Information for Patients Patients should be cautioned against interruption of Catapres-TTS therapy without their physician's advice.

Patients who engage in potentially hazardous activities, such as operating machinery or driving, should be advised of a possible sedative effect of clonidine. They should also be informed that this sedative effect may be increased by concomitant use of alcohol, barbiturates, or other sedating drugs.

Patients should be instructed to consult their physicians promptly about the possible need to remove the patch if they observe moderate to severe localized erythema and/or vesicle formation at the site of application or generalized skin rash.

If a patient experiences isolated, mild localized skin irritation before completing 7 days of use, the system may be removed and replaced with a new system applied to a fresh skin site.

If the system should begin to loosen from the skin after application, the patient should be instructed to place the adhesive overlay directly over the system to ensure adhesion during its 7-day use.

Used Catapres-TTS patches contain a substantial amount of their initial drug content which may be harmful to infants and children if accidentally applied or ingested. THEREFORE, PATIENTS SHOULD BE CAUTIONED TO KEEP BOTH USED AND UNUSED CATAPRES-TTS PATCHES OUT OF THE REACH OF CHILDREN. After use, Catapres-TTS should be folded in half with the adhesive sides together and discarded away from children's reach.

Instructions for use, storage and disposal of the system are provided at the end of this monograph. These instructions also are included in each box of Catapres-TTS.

Drug Interactions Clonidine may potentiate the CNS-depressive effects of alcohol, barbiturates or other sedating drugs. If a patient receiving clonidine is also taking tricyclic antidepressants, the hypotensive effect of clonidine may be reduced, necessitating an increase in the clonidine dose.

Due to potential for additive effects such as bradycardia and AV block, caution is warranted in patients receiving clonidine concomitantly with agents known to affect sinus node function or AV nodal conduction e.g., digitalis, calcium channel blockers and beta-blockers.

Amitriptyline in combination with clonidine enhances the manifestation of corneal lesions in rats (see TOXICOLOGY).

Toxicology In several studies with oral clonidine hydrochloride, a dose-dependent increase in the incidence and severity of spontaneous retinal degeneration was seen in albino rats treated for six months or longer. Tissue distribution studies in dogs and monkeys showed a concentration of clonidine in the choroid.

In view of the retinal degeneration seen in rats, eye examinations were performed during clinical trials in 908 patients before, and periodically after, the start of clonidine therapy. In 353 of these 908 patients, the eye examinations were carried out over periods of 24 months or longer. Except for some dryness of the eyes, no drug-related abnormal ophthalmological findings were recorded and, according to specialized tests such as electroretinography and macular dazzle, retinal function was unchanged.

In combination with amitriptyline, clonidine hydrochloride administration led to the development of corneal lesions in rats within 5 days.

Carcinogenesis, Mutagenesis, Impairment of Fertility Chronic dietary administration of clonidine was not carcinogenic to rats (132 weeks) or mice (78 weeks) dosed, respectively, at up to 46 to 70 times the maximum recommended daily human dose (MRDHD) as mg/kg (9 or 6 times the MRDHD on a mg/m^2 basis). There was no evidence of genotoxicity in the Ames test for mutagenicity or mouse micronucleus test for clastogenicity.

Fertility of male and female rats was unaffected by clonidine doses as high as 150 mcg/kg (approximately 3 times the MRDHD). In a separate experiment, fertility of female rats appeared to be affected at dose levels of 500 to 2000 mcg/kg (10 to 40 times the oral MRDHD on a mg/kg basis; 2 to 8 times the MRDHD on a mg/m^2 basis).

Pregnancy *TERATOGENIC EFFECTS Pregnancy Category C.* Reproduction studies performed in rabbits at doses up to approximately 3 times the oral maximum recommended daily human dose (MRDHD) of Catapres (clonidine hydrochloride) produced no evidence of a teratogenic or embryotoxic potential in rabbits. In rats, however, doses as low as $^1/_3$ the oral MRDHD ($^1/_{15}$ the MRDHD on a mg/m^2 basis) of clonidine were associated with increased resorptions in a study in which dams were treated continuously from 2 months prior to mating. Increased resorptions were not associated with treatment at the same time or at higher dose levels (up to 3 times the oral MRDHD) when the dams were treated on gestation days 6–15. Increases in resorption were observed at much higher dose levels (40 times the oral MRDHD on a mg/kg basis; 4 to 8 times the MRDHD on a mg/m^2 basis) in mice and rats treated on gestation days 1–14 (lowest dose employed in the study was 500 mcg/kg). No adequate, well-controlled studies have been conducted in pregnant women. Because animal reproduction studies are not always predictive of human response, this drug should be used during pregnancy only if clearly needed.

Nursing Mothers As clonidine is excreted in human milk, caution should be exercised when Catapres-TTS is administered to a nursing woman.

Pediatric Use Safety and effectiveness in pediatric patients below the age of 12 have not been established (See Warnings on Withdrawal).

ADVERSE REACTIONS

Clinical trial experience with Catapres-TTS® Most systemic adverse effects during Catapres-TTS therapy have been mild and have tended to diminish with continued therapy. In a 3-month multiclinic trial of Catapres-TTS in 101

Continued on next page

Catapres-TTS—Cont.

hypertensive patients, the systemic adverse reactions were, dry mouth (25 patients) and drowsiness (12) fatigue (6), headache (5), lethargy and sedation (3 each), insomnia, dizziness, impotence/sexual dysfunction, dry throat (2 each) and constipation, nausea, change in taste and nervousness (1 each).

In the above mentioned 3-month controlled clinical trial, as well as other uncontrolled clinical trials, the most frequent adverse reactions were dermatological and are described below.

In the 3-month trial, 51 of the 101 patients had localized skin reactions such as erythema (26 patients) and/or pruritus, particularly after using an adhesive overlay throughout the 7-day dosage interval. Allergic contact sensitization to Catapres-TTS was observed in 5 patients. Other skin reactions were localized vesiculation (7 patients), hyperpigmentation (5), edema (3), excoriation (3), burning (3), papules (1), throbbing (1), blanching (1), and a generalized macular rash (1).

In additional clinical experience, contact dermatitis resulting in treatment discontinuation was observed in 128 of 673 patients (about 19 in 100) after a mean duration of treatment of 37 weeks. The incidence of contact dermatitis was about 34 in 100 among white women, about 18 in 100 in white men, about 14 in 100 in black women, and approximately 8 in 100 in black men. Analysis of skin reaction data showed that the risk of having to discontinue Catapres-TTS treatment because of contact dermatitis was greatest between treatment weeks 6 and 26, although sensitivity may develop either earlier or later in treatment.

In a large-scale clinical acceptability and safety study by 451 physicians in a total of 3539 patients, other allergic reactions were recorded for which a causal relationship to Catapres-TTS was not established: maculopapular rash (10 cases); urticaria (2 cases); and angioedema of the face (2 cases), which also affected the tongue in one of the patients.

Marketing Experience with Catapres-TTS Other adverse effects reported since the drug has been marketed are listed below by body system. In this setting, an incidence or causal relationship cannot always be accurately determined. However, none of the events listed below occurred in a frequency greater than 0.5%.

Body as a Whole Fever, malaise, weakness and pallor, and withdrawal syndrome.

Cardiovascular Congestive heart failure; cerebrovascular accident; electrocardiographic abnormalities (i.e., bradycardia, sick sinus syndrome disturbances and arrhythmias); chest pain; orthostatic symptoms; syncope, increases in blood pressure; sinus bradycardia and atrioventricular block with and without the use of concomitant digitalis; Raynaud's phenomenon; tachycardia; bradycardia; and palpitations.

Central and Peripheral Nervous System/Psychiatric Delirium, mental depression, visual and auditory hallucinations, localized numbness, vivid dreams or nightmares, restlessness, anxiety, agitation, irritability, other behavioral changes, and drowsiness.

Dermatological Angioneurotic edema, localized or generalized rash, hives, urticaria, contact dermatitis, pruritus, alopecia, and localized hypo or hyperpigmentation.

Gastrointestinal Anorexia and vomiting.

Genitourinary Difficult micturition, loss of libido, and decreased sexual activity.

Metabolic Gynecomastia or breast enlargement and weight gain.

Musculoskeletal Muscle or joint pain, and leg cramps.

Ophthalmological Blurred vision, burning of the eyes and dryness of the eyes.

Adverse Events Associated with Oral Catapres Therapy Most adverse effects are mild and tend to diminish with continued therapy. The most frequent (which appear to be dose-related) are dry mouth, occurring in about 40 of 100 patients; drowsiness, about 33 in 100; dizziness, about 16 in 100; constipation and sedation, each about 10 in 100. The following less frequent adverse experiences have also been reported in patients receiving Catapres® (clonidine hydrochloride USP), but in many cases patients were receiving concomitant medication and a causal relationship has not been established.

Body as A Whole Weakness, about 10 in 100 patients; fatigue, about 4 in 100; headache and withdrawal syndrome, each about 1 in 100. Also reported were pallor, a weakly positive Coombs' test, increased sensitivity to alcohol, and fever.

Cardiovascular Orthostatic symptoms, about 3 in 100 patients; palpitations and tachycardia, and bradycardia, each about 5 in 1000. Syncope, Raynaud's phenomenon, congestive heart failure, and electrocardiographic abnormalities (i.e., sinus node arrest, functional bradycardia, high degree AV block and arrhythmias) have been reported rarely. Rare cases of sinus bradycardia and AV block have been reported, both with and without the use of concomitant digitalis.

Central Nervous System Nervousness and agitation, about 3 in 100 patients; mental depression, about 1 in 100; and insomnia, about 5 in 1000. Other behavioral changes, vivid dreams or nightmares, restlessness, anxiety, visual and auditory hallucinations and delirium have rarely been reported.

Dermatological Rash, about 1 in 100 patients; puritus, about 7 in 1000; hives, angioneurotic edema and urticaria, about 5 in 1000; alopecia, about 2 in 1000.

Gastrointestinal Nausea and vomiting, about 5 in 100 patients; anorexia and malaise, each about 1 in 100; mild transient abnormalities in liver function tests, about 1 in 100; hepatitis, parotitis, constipation, pseudo-obstruction, and abdominal pain, rarely.

Genitourinary Decreased sexual activity, impotence and loss of libido, about 3 in 100 patients; nocturia, about 1 in 100; difficulty in micturition, about 2 in 1000; urinary retention, about 1 in 1000.

Hematologic Thrombocytopenia, rarely.

Metabolic Weight gain, about 1 in 100 patients; gynecomastia, about 1 in 1000; transient elevation of blood glucose or serum creatine phosphokinase, rarely.

Musculoskeletal Muscle or joint pain, about 6 in 1000 and leg cramps, about 3 in 1000.

Oro-otolaryngeal Dryness of the nasal mucosa was rarely reported.

Ophthalmological Dryness of the eyes, burning of the eyes and blurred vision were reported.

OVERDOSAGE

Hypertension may develop early and may be followed by hypotension, bradycardia, respiratory depression, hypothermia, drowsines, decreased or absent reflexes, weakness, irritability and miosis. The frequency of CNS depression may be higher in children than adults. Large overdoses may result in reversible cardiac conduction defects or dysrhythmias, apnea, coma and seizures. Signs and symptoms of overdose generally occur within 30 minutes to two hours after exposure. As little as 0.1 mg of clonidine has produced signs of toxicity in children.

If symptoms of poisoning occur following dermal exposure, remove all Catapres-TTS systems. After their removal, the plasma clonidine levels will persist for about 8 hours, then decline slowly over a period of several days. Rare cases of Catapres-TTS poisoning due to accidental or deliberate mouthing or ingestion of the patch have been reported, many of them involving children.

There is no specific antidote for clonidine overdosage. Ipecac syrup-induced vomiting and gastric lavage would not be expected to remove significant amounts of clonidine following dermal exposure. If the patch is ingested, whole bowel irrigation may be considered and the administration of activated charcoal and/or cathartic may be beneficial. Supportive care may include atropine sulfate for bradycardia, intravenous fluids and/or vasopressor agents for hypotension and vasodilators for hypertension. Naloxone may be a useful adjunct for the management of clonidine-induced respiratory depression, hypotension and/or coma; blood pressure should be monitored since the administration of naloxone has occasionally resulted in paradoxical hypertension. Tolazoline administration has yielded inconsistent results and is not recommended as first-line therapy. Dialysis is not likely to significantly enhance the elimination of clonidine.

The largest overdose reported to date, involved a 28-year-old male who ingested 100 mg of clonidine hydrochloride powder. This patient developed hypertension followed by hypotension, bradycardia, apnea, hallucinations, semicoma, and premature ventricular contractions. The patient fully recovered after intensive treatment. Plasma clonidine levels were 60 ng/mL after 1 hour, 190 ng/mL after 1.5 hours, 370 ng/mL after 2 hours, and 120 ng/mL after 5.5 and 6.5 hours. In mice and rats, the oral LD_{50} of clonidine is 206 and 465 mg/kg, respectively.

DOSAGE AND ADMINISTRATION

Apply Catapres-TTS® (clonidine) once every 7 days to a hairless area of intact skin on the upper outer arm or chest. Each new application of Catapres-TTS should be on a different skin site from the previous location. If the system loosens during 7-day wearing, the adhesive overlay should be applied directly over the system to ensure good adhesion. There have been rare reports of the need for patch changes prior to 7 days to maintain blood pressure control.

To initiate therapy, Catapres-TTS dosage should be titrated according to individual therapeutic requirements, starting with Catapres-TTS-1. If after one or two weeks the desired reduction in blood pressure is not achieved, increase the dosage by adding another Catapres-TTS-1 or changing to a larger system. An increase in dosage above two Catapres-TTS-3 is usually not associated with additional efficacy.

When substituting Catapres-TTS for oral clonidine or for other antihypertensive drugs, physicians should be aware that the antihypertensive effect of Catapres-TTS may not commence until 2–3 days after initial application. Therefore, gradual reduction of prior drug dosage is advised. Some or all previous antihypertensive treatment may have to be continued, particularly in patients with more severe forms of hypertension.

Renal Impairment Dosage must be adjusted according to the degree of impairment, and patients should be carefully monitored. Since only a minimal amount of clonidine is removed during routine hemodialysis, there is no need to give supplemental clonidine following dialysis.

HOW SUPPLIED

Catapres-TTS-1® (clonidine) and Catapres-TTS-2 are supplied as 4 pouched systems and 4 adhesive overlays per carton, 3 cartons per shipper (NDC 0597-0031-12 and 0597-0032-12, respectively). Catapres-TTS-3 is supplied as 4 pouched systems and 4 adhesive overlays per carton (NDC 0597-0033-34). See chart below.

[See table below]

	Programmed Delivery Clonidine *in vivo* Per Day Over 1 Week	Clonidine Content	Size	Code
Catapres-TTS®-1 (clonidine)	0.1 mg	2.5 mg	3.5 cm^2	BI-31
Catapres-TTS®-2 (clonidine)	0.2 mg	5.0 mg	7.0 cm^2	BI-32
Catapres-TTS®-3 (clonidine)	0.3 mg	7.5 mg	10.5 cm^2	BI-33

STORAGE AND HANDLING

Store below 86° F (30° C).

CAUTION Federal law prohibits dispensing without prescription.

CT-PI-10/96 Rev

Manufactured by
Alza Corporation, Palo Alto, California 94304
Distributed by
Boehringer Ingelheim Pharmaceuticals, Inc.
Ridgefield, CT 06877
Licensed from
Boehringer Ingelheim International GmbH

Shown in Product Identification Guide, page 306

COMBIPRES® ℞

[kom 'be-pres]

Each tablet contains: 0.1/15 mg, 0.2/15 mg, 0.3/15 mg of clonidine hydrochloride/chlorthalidone, respectively

Oral Antihypertensive

Tablets 0.1 .... BI-CODE 08
Tablets 0.2 .... BI-CODE 09
Tablets 0.3 .... BI-CODE 10

Prescribing Information

DESCRIPTION

Combipres® is a combination of clonidine hydrochloride (a centrally acting antihypertensive agent) and chlorthalidone (a diuretic). Combipres® is available as tablets for oral administration in three dosage strengths: 0.1/15 mg, 0.2/15 mg and 0.3/15 mg of clonidine hydrochloride/chlorthalidone, respectively.

The inactive ingredients are colloidal silicon dioxide, corn starch, dibasic calcium phosphate, gelatin, glycerin, lactose, magnesium stearate, methylparaben and propylparaben. The Combipres 0.1/15 mg tablet also contains FD&C Red No. 3. The Combipres 0.2/15 mg tablet also contains FD&C Blue No. 1.

Clonidine hydrochloride:

Clonidine hydrochloride is an imidazoline derivative and exists as a mesomeric compound. The chemical name is 2-(2,6-dichlorophenylamino)-2-imidazoline hydrochloride. The following is the structural formula:

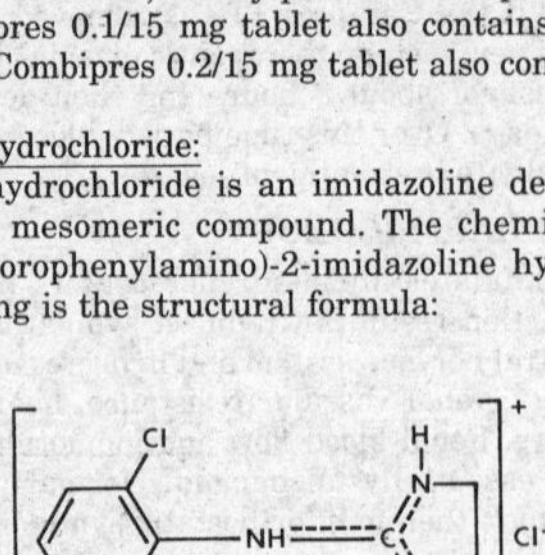

$C_9H_9Cl_2N_3 \cdot HCl$
Mol. Wt. 266.56

Clonidine hydrochloride is an odorless, bitter, white crystalline substance soluble in water and alcohol.

Chlorthalidone

Chlorthalidone is a monosulfamyl diuretic that differs chemically from thiazide diuretics in that a double ring system is incorporated in its structure. It is a racemic mixture

of 2-chloro-5-(1- hydroxy-3-oxo-1-isoindolinyl) benzenesulfonamide with the following structural formula:

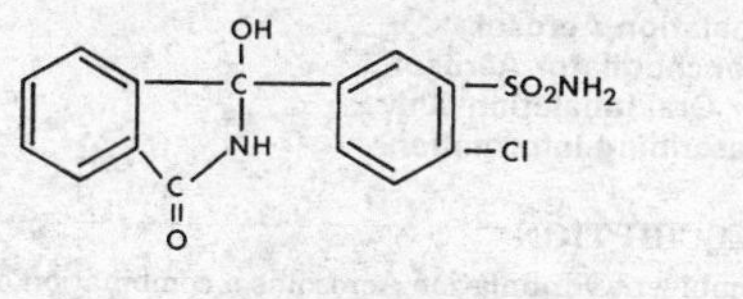

$C_{14}H_{11}Cl\,N_2O_4S$
Mol. Wt. 338.76

Chlorthalidone is practically insoluble in water, in ether and in chloroform; soluble in methanol; slightly soluble in alcohol.

CLINICAL PHARMACOLOGY

Combipres®:

Combipres produces a more pronounced antihypertensive response than occurs after either clonidine hydrochloride or chlorthalidone alone in equivalent doses.

Clonidine hydrochloride:

Clonidine hydrochloride acts relatively rapidly. The patient's blood pressure declines within 30 to 60 minutes after an oral dose, the maximum decrease occurring within 2 to 4 hours. The plasma level of clonidine hydrochloride peaks in approximately 3 to 5 hours and the plasma half-life ranges from 12 to 16 hours. The half-life increases up to 41 hours in patients with severe impairment of renal function. Following oral administration about 40–60% of the absorbed dose is recovered in the urine as unchanged drug in 24 hours. About 50% of the absorbed dose is metabolized in the liver.

Clonidine stimulates alpha-adrenoreceptors in the brain stem, resulting in reduced sympathetic outflow from the central nervous system and a decrease in peripheral resistance, renal vascular resistance, heart rate, and blood pressure. Renal blood flow and glomerular filtration rate remain essentially unchanged. Normal postural reflexes are intact and therefore orthostatic symptoms are mild and infrequent.

Acute studies with clonidine hydrochloride in humans have demonstrated a moderate reduction (15 to 20%) of cardiac output in the supine position with no change in the peripheral resistance; at a 45° tilt there is a smaller reduction in cardiac output and a decrease of peripheral resistance. During long-term therapy, cardiac output tends to return to control values, while peripheral resistance remains decreased. Slowing of the pulse rate has been observed in most patients given clonidine but the drug does not alter normal hemodynamic response to exercise.

Other studies in patients have provided evidence of a reduction in plasma renin activity and in the excretion of aldosterone and catecholamines, but the exact relationship of these pharmacologic actions to the antihypertensive effect has not been fully elucidated.

Clonidine acutely stimulates growth hormone release in both children and adults, but does not produce a chronic elevation of growth hormone with long-term use.

Tolerance may develop in some patients, necessitating a reevaluation of therapy.

Chlorthalidone:

Chlorthalidone is a long-acting oral diuretic with antihypertensive activity. Its diuretic action commences a mean of 2.6 hours after dosing and continues for up to 72 hours. The drug produces diuresis with increased excretion of sodium and chloride. The diuretic effects of chlorthalidone and the benzothiadiazine (thiazide) diuretics appear to arise from similar mechanisms and the maximal effect of chlorthalidone and the thiazides appears to be similar. The site of action appears to be the distal convoluted tubule of the nephron. The diuretic effects of chlorthalidone lead to decreased extracellular fluid volume, plasma volume, cardiac output, total exchangeable sodium, glomerular filtration rate, and renal plasma flow. Although the mechanism of action of chlorthalidone and related drugs is not wholly clear, sodium and water depletion appear to provide a basis for its antihypertensive effect. Like the thiazide diuretics, chlorthalidone produces dose-related reductions in serum potassium levels, elevations in serum uric acid and blood glucose, and it can lead to decreased sodium and chloride levels.

The mean plasma half-life of chlorthalidone is about 40 to 60 hours. It is eliminated primarily as unchanged drug in the urine. Non-renal routes of elimination have yet to be clarified. In the blood, approximately 75% of the drug is bound to plasma proteins.

INDICATIONS AND USAGE

Combipres® (clonidine hydrochloride USP/chlorthalidone USP) is indicated in the treatment of hypertension. **This fixed combination drug is not indicated for initial therapy of hypertension. Hypertension requires therapy titrated to the individual patient. If the fixed combination represents the dosage so determined, its use may be more convenient in patient management. The treatment of hypertension is not static, but must be reevaluated as conditions in each patient warrant.**

CONTRAINDICATIONS

Anuria. Combipres® is contraindicated in patients with known hypersensitivity to chlorthalidone or other sulfonamide-derived drugs.

WARNINGS

Chlorthalidone should be used with caution in severe renal disease. In patients with renal disease, chlorthalidone or related drugs may precipitate azotemia. Cumulative effects of the drug may develop in patients with impaired renal function. Chlorthalidone should be used with caution in patients with impaired hepatic function or progressive liver disease, because minor alterations of fluid and electrolyte balance may precipitate hepatic coma.

Sensitivity reactions may occur in patients with a history of allergy or bronchial asthma. The possibility of exacerbation or activation of systemic lupus erythematosus has been reported with thiazide diuretics which are structurally related to chlorthalidone. However, systemic lupus erythematosus has not been reported following chlorthalidone administration.

PRECAUTIONS

Clonidine hydrochloride:

General: In patients who have developed localized contact sensitization to Catapres-TTS® (clonidine), substitution of oral clonidine hydrochloride therapy may be associated with the development of a generalized skin rash.

In patients who develop an allergic reaction from Catapres-TTS® (clonidine) that extends beyond the local patch site (such as generalized skin rash, urticaria, or angioedema), oral clonidine hydrochloride substitution may elicit a similar reaction.

As with all antihypertensive therapy, clonidine hydrochloride should be used with caution in patients with severe coronary insufficiency, recent myocardial infarction, cerebrovascular disease or chronic renal failure.

Withdrawal Patients should be instructed not to discontinue therapy without consulting their physician. Sudden cessation of clonidine treatment has resulted in subjective symptoms such as nervousness, agitation and headache, accompanied or followed by a rapid rise in blood pressure and elevated catecholamine concentrations in the plasma, but such occurrences have usually been associated with previous administration of high oral doses (exceeding 1.2 mg/day) and/or with continuation of concomitant beta-blocker therapy. Rare instances of hypertensive encephalopathy and death have been reported. When discontinuing therapy with clonidine hydrochloride, the physician should reduce the dose gradually over 2 to 4 days to avoid withdrawal symptomatology.

An excessive rise in blood pressure following clonidine hydrochloride discontinuance can be reversed by administration of oral clonidine or by intravenous phentolamine. If therapy is to be discontinued in patients receiving beta-blockers and clonidine concurrently, beta-blockers should be discontinued several days before the gradual withdrawal of clonidine hydrochloride.

Perioperative Use Administration of clonidine hydrochloride should be continued to within four hours of surgery and resumed as soon as possible thereafter. The blood pressure should be carefully monitored and appropriate measures instituted to control it as necessary.

Information for Patients Patients who engage in potentially hazardous activities, such as operating machinery or driving, should be advised of a potential sedative effect of clonidine. Patients should be cautioned against interruption of clonidine hydrochloride therapy without a physician's advice.

Drug Interactions If a patient receiving clonidine hydrochloride is also taking tricyclic antidepressants, the effect of clonidine may be reduced, thus necessitating an increase in dosage. Clonidine hydrochloride may enhance the CNS-depressive effects of alcohol, barbiturates or other sedatives. Amitriptyline in combination with clonidine enhances the manifestation of corneal lesions in rats (see OCULAR TOXICITY).

OCULAR TOXICITY

In several studies, oral clonidine hydrochloride produced a dose-dependent increase in the incidence and severity of spontaneously occurring retinal degeneration in albino rats treated for six months or longer. Tissue distribution studies in dogs and monkeys revealed that clonidine hydrochloride was concentrated in the choroid of the eye. In view of the retinal degeneration observed in rats, eye examinations were performed in 908 patients prior to the start of clonidine hydrochloride therapy, who were then examined periodically thereafter. In 353 of these 908 patients, examinations were performed for periods of 24 months or longer. Except for some dryness of the eyes, no drug-related abnormal ophthalmologic findings were recorded and clonidine hydrochloride did not alter retinal function as shown by specialized tests such as the electroretinogram and macular dazzle.

In rats, clonidine hydrochloride in combination with amitriptyline produced corneal lesions within 5 days.

Carcinogenesis, Mutagenesis, Impairment of Fertility In a 132-week (fixed concentration) dietary administration study in rats, clonidine hydrochloride administered at 32 to 46 times the maximum recommended daily human oral dose was unassociated with evidence of carcinogenic potential. Fertility of male or female rats was unaffected by clonidine hydrochloride doses as high as 150 mcg/kg or about 3 times the maximum recommended daily human oral dose (MRDHD). Fertility of female rats did, however, appear to be affected (in another experiment) at dose levels of 500 to 2000 mcg/kg or 10 to 40 times the MRDHD.

Usage in Pregnancy

TERATOGENIC EFFECTS Pregnancy Category C. Reproduction studies performed in rabbits at doses up to approximately 3 times the maximum recommended daily human dose (MRDHD) of clonidine hydrochloride have revealed no evidence of teratogenic or embryotoxic potential. In rats however, doses as low as 1/3 the MRDHD were associated with increased resorptions in a study in which dams were treated continuously from 2 months prior to mating. Increased resorptions were not associated with treatment at the same or at higher dose levels (up to 3 times the MRDHD) when dams were treated days 6–15 of gestation. Increased resorptions were observed at much higher levels (40 times the MRDHD) in rats and mice treated days 1–14 of gestation (lowest dose employed in that study was 500 mcg/kg). There are, however, no adequate and well-controlled studies in pregnant women. Because animal reproduction studies are not always predictive of human response, this drug should be used during pregnancy only if clearly needed.

Nursing Mothers As clonidine hydrochloride is excreted in human milk, caution should be exercised when it is administered to a nursing woman.

Pediatric Use Safety and effectiveness in the pediatric population have not been established.

Chlorthalidone: **General**

Hypokalemia and other electrolyte abnormalities, including hyponatremia and hypochloremic alkalosis, are common in patients receiving chlorthalidone. These abnormalities are dose-related but may occur even at the lowest marketed doses of chlorthalidone. Serum electrolytes should be determined before initiating therapy and at periodic intervals during therapy. Serum and urine electrolyte determinations are particularly important when the patient is vomiting excessively or receiving parenteral fluids. All patients taking chlorthalidone should be observed for clinical signs of electrolyte imbalance, including dryness of mouth, thirst, weakness, lethargy, drowsiness, restlessness, muscle pains or cramps, muscular fatigue, hypotension, oliguria, tachycardia, palpitations and gastrointestinal disturbances, such as nausea and vomiting. Digitalis therapy may exaggerate metabolic effects of hypokalemia especially with reference to myocardial activity.

Any chloride deficit is generally mild and usually does not require specific treatment except under extraordinary circumstances (as in liver disease or renal disease). Dilutional hyponatremia may occur in edematous patients in hot weather: appropriate therapy is water restriction, rather than administration of salt, except in rare instances when the hyponatremia is life-threatening. In cases of actual salt depletion, appropriate replacement is the therapy of choice.

Uric Acid Hyperuricemia may occur or frank gout may be precipitated in certain patients receiving chlorthalidone.

Other Increases in serum glucose may occur and latent diabetes mellitus may become manifest during chlorthalidone therapy (see PRECAUTIONS Drug Interactions). Chlorthalidone and related drugs may decrease serum PBI levels without signs of thyroid disturbance.

Information for Patients Patients should inform their doctor if they have: 1) had an allergic reaction to chlorthalidone or other diuretics or have asthma 2) kidney disease 3) liver disease 4) gout 5) systemic lupus erythematosus, or 6) been taking other drugs such as cortisone, digitalis, lithium carbonate, or drugs for diabetes.

Patients should be cautioned to contact their physician if they experience any of the following symptoms of potassium loss: excess thirst, tiredness, drowsiness, restlessness, muscle pains or cramps, nausea, vomiting or increased heart rate or pulse.

Patients should also be cautioned that taking alcohol can increase the chance of dizziness occurring.

Laboratory Tests Periodic determination of serum electrolytes to detect possible electrolyte imbalance should be performed at appropriate intervals.

All patients receiving chlorthalidone should be observed for clinical signs of fluid or electrolyte imbalance: namely, hyponatremia, hypochloremic alkalosis and hypokalemia. Serum and urine electrolyte determinations are particularly important when the patient is vomiting excessively or receiving parenteral fluids.

Drug Interactions Chlorthalidone may add to or potentiate the action of other antihypertensive drugs. Insulin requirements in diabetic patients may be increased, decreased or

Continued on next page

Combipres—Cont.

unchanged. Higher dosage of oral hypoglycemic agents may be required. Chlorthalidone and related drugs may increase the responsiveness to tubocurarine. Chlorthalidone and related drugs may decrease arterial responsiveness to norepinephrine. This diminution is not sufficient to preclude effectiveness of the pressor agent for therapeutic use. Lithium renal clearance is reduced by chlorthalidone, increasing the risk of lithium toxicity.

Drug/Laboratory Test Interactions Chlorthalidone and related drugs may decrease serum PBI levels without signs of thyroid disturbance.

Carcinogenesis, Mutagenesis, Impairment of Fertility No information is available.

Usage in Pregnancy

TERATOGENIC EFFECTS Pregnancy Category B. Reproduction studies have been performed in the rat and the rabbit at doses up to 420 times the human dose and have revealed no evidence of harm to the fetus due to chlorthalidone. There are, however, no adequate and well-controlled studies in pregnant women. Because animal reproduction studies are not always predictive of human response, this drug should be used during pregnancy only if clearly needed.

NON-TERATOGENIC EFFECTS Thiazides cross the placental barrier and appear in cord blood. The use of chlorthalidone and related drugs in pregnant women requires that the anticipated benefits of the drug be weighed against possible hazards to the fetus. These hazards include fetal or neonatal jaundice, thrombocytopenia, and possibly other adverse reactions that have occurred in the adult.

Nursing Mothers Thiazides are excreted in human milk. Because of the potential for serious adverse reactions in nursing infants from chlorthalidone, a decision should be made whether to discontinue nursing or to discontinue the drug, taking into account the importance of the drug to the mother.

Pediatric Use Safety and effectiveness in the pediatric population have not been established.

ADVERSE REACTIONS

Combipres® is generally well tolerated. Most adverse effects are mild and tend to diminish with continued therapy. The most frequent (which appear to be dose-related) are dry mouth, occurring in about 40 to 100 patients; drowsiness, about 33 in 100; dizziness, about 16 in 100; constipation and sedation, each about 10 in 100.

In addition to the reactions listed above, certain less frequent adverse experiences, which are shown below, have also been reported in patients receiving the component drugs of Combipres® but in many cases patients were receiving concomitant medication and a causal relationship has not been established:

Clonidine hydrochloride:

Gastrointestinal Nausea and vomiting, about 5 in 100 patients; anorexia and malaise, each about 1 in 100; mild transient abnormalities in liver function tests, about 1 in 100; rare reports of hepatitis; parotitis, rarely.

Metabolic Weight gain, about 1 in 100 patients; gynecomastia, about 1 in 1000, transient elevation of blood glucose or serum creatine phosphokinase, rarely.

Central Nervous System Nervousness and agitation, about 3 in 100 patients; mental depression, about 1 in 100; headache, about 1 in 100; insomnia, about 5 in 1000. Vivid dreams or nightmares, other behavioral changes, restlessness, anxiety, visual and auditory hallucinations and delirium have been reported.

Cardiovascular Orthostatic symptoms, about 3 in 100 patients; palpitations and tachycardia, and bradycardia, each about 5 in 1000. Raynaud's phenomenon, congestive heart failure, and electrocardiographic abnormalities i.e. conduction disturbances and arrhythmias have been reported rarely. Rare cases of sinus bradycardia and atrioventricular block have been reported, both with and without the use of concomitant digitalis.

Dermatological Rash, about 1 in 100 patients; pruritus, about 7 in 1000; hives, angioneurotic edema and urticaria, about 5 in 1000, alopecia, about 2 in 1000.

Genitourinary Decreased sexual activity, impotence and loss of libido, about 3 in 100 patients; nocturia, about 1 in 100; difficulty in micturition, about 2 in 1000; urinary retention, about 1 in 1000.

Other Weakness, about 10 in 100 patients; fatigue, about 4 in 100; discontinuation syndrome, about 1 in 100; muscle or joint pain, about 6 in 1000 and cramps of the lower limbs, about 3 in 1000. Dryness, burning of the eyes, blurred vision, dryness of the nasal mucosa, pallor, weakly positive Coombs' test, increased sensitivity to alcohol and fever have been reported.

Chlorthalidone:

Gastrointestinal: Anorexia, gastric irritation, nausea, vomiting, cramping, diarrhea, constipation, jaundice (intrahepatic cholestatic jaundice), pancreatitis.

Central Nervous System: Dizziness, vertigo, paresthesias, headache, xanthopsia.

Hematologic: Leukopenia, agranulocytosis, thrombocytopenia, aplastic anemia.

Dermatologic-Hypersensitivity: Purpura, photosensitivity, rash, urticaria, necrotizing angiitis (vasculitis) (cutaneous vasculitis), Lyell's syndrome (toxic epidermal necrolysis).

Cardiovascular: Orthostatic hypotension may occur and may be aggravated by alcohol, barbiturates or narcotics.

Other adverse reactions: Hyperglycemia, glycosuria, hyperuricemia, muscle spasm, weakness, restlessness, impotence. Whenever adverse reactions are moderate or severe, chlorthalidone dosage should be reduced or therapy withdrawn.

OVERDOSAGE

Clonidine hydrochloride:

The signs and symptoms of clonidine hydrochloride overdosage include hypotension, bradycardia, lethargy, irritability, weakness, somnolence, diminished or absent reflexes, miosis, vomiting and hypoventilation. With large overdoses, reversible cardiac conduction defects or arrhythmias, apnea, seizures and transient hypertension have been reported. The oral LD_{50} of clonidine in rats was 465 mg/kg, and in mice 206 mg/kg.

The general treatment of clonidine hydrochloride overdosage may include intravenous fluids as indicated. Bradycardia can be treated with intravenous atropine sulfate and hypotension with dopamine infusion in addition to intravenous fluids. Hypertension, associated with overdosage, has been treated with intravenous furosemide or diazoxide or alpha-blocking agents such as phentolamine. Tolazoline, an alpha-blocker, in intravenous doses of 10 mg at 30-minute intervals, may reverse clonidine's effects if other efforts fail. Routine hemodialysis is of limited benefit, since a maximum of 5% of circulating clonidine is removed.

In a patient who ingested 100 mg clonidine hydrochloride, plasma clonidine levels were 60 ng/ml (one hour), 190 ng/ml (1.5 hours), 370 ng/ml (two hours) and 120 ng/ml (5.5 and 6.5 hours). This patient developed hypertension followed by hypotension, bradycardia, apnea, hallucinations, semicoma, and premature ventricular contractions. The patient fully recovered after intensive treatment.

Chlorthalidone:

Symptoms of acute overdosage include nausea, weakness, dizziness and disturbances of electrolyte balance. The oral LD_{50} of the drug in the mouse and the rat is more than 25,000 mg/kg body weight. The minimum lethal dose (MLD) in humans has not been established. There is no specific antidote but gastric lavage is recommended, followed by supportive treatment. Where necessary, this may include intravenous dextrose-saline with potassium, administered with caution.

DOSAGE AND ADMINISTRATION

The dosage must be determined by individual titration. (See INDICATIONS AND USAGE.)

Chlorthalidone is usually initiated at a dose of 25 mg once daily and may be increased to 50 mg if the response is insufficient after a suitable trial.

Clonidine hydrochloride is usually initiated at a dose of 0.1 mg twice daily. Elderly patients may benefit from a lower initial dose. Further increments of 0.1 mg/day may be made if necessary until the desired response is achieved. The therapeutic doses most commonly employed have ranged from 0.2 to 0.6 mg per day in divided doses.

One Combipres® (clonidine hydrochloride/chlorthalidone) Tablet administered once or twice daily can be used to administer a minimum of 0.1 mg clonidine hydrochloride and 15 mg chlorthalidone to a maximum of 0.6 mg clonidine hydrochloride and 30 mg chlorthalidone.

HOW SUPPLIED

Combipres® 0.1/15 mg (each tablet contains clonidine hydrochloride USP, 0.1 mg + chlorthalidone USP, 15 mg) tablets are pink, oval shaped and single scored with the marking Bl 8. Available in bottles of 100 (NDC 0597-0008-01) and 1000 (NDC 0597-0008-10).

Combipres® 0.2/15 mg (each tablet contains clonidine hydrochloride USP 0.2 mg +chlorthalidone USP, 15 mg) tablets are blue, oval shaped and single scored with the marking Bl 9. Available in bottles of 100 (NDC 0597-0009-01) and 1000 (NDC 0597-0009-10).

Combipres® 0.3/15 mg (each tablet contains clonidine hydrochloride USP, 0.3 mg + chlorthalidone USP, 15 mg) tablets are white, oval shaped and single scored with the marking Bl 10. Available in bottles of 100 (NDC 0597-0010-01).

Store below 86°F (30°C). Avoid excessive humidity.

Dispense in tight, light-resistant container.

Caution: Federal law prohibits dispensing without prescription.

CM-PI-2/95 Rev.

Boehringer Ingelheim Pharmaceuticals, Inc.
Ridgefield, CT 06877
Licensed from Boehringer Ingelheim International GbmH

Shown in Product Identification Guide, page 306

COMBIVENT® ℞

[*cŏmbēvant*]
(ipratropium bromide and albuterol sulfate)
Inhalation Aerosol
Bronchodilator Aerosol
For Oral Inhalation Only
Prescribing Information

DESCRIPTION

Combivent® Inhalation Aerosol is a combination of ipratropium bromide and albuterol sulfate. Ipratropium bromide is an anticholinergic bronchodilator chemically described as 8-azoniabicyclo[3.2.1]octane, 3-(3-hydroxy-1-oxo-2-phenylpropoxy)-8-methyl-8-(1-methylethyl)-, bromide, monohydrate *(endo,syn)*-,(±): a synthetic quaternary ammonium compound chemically related to atropine. Ipratropium bromide is a white to off-white crystalline substance, freely soluble in water and lower alcohols but insoluble in lipophilic solvents such as ether, chloroform and fluorocarbons. The structural formula is:

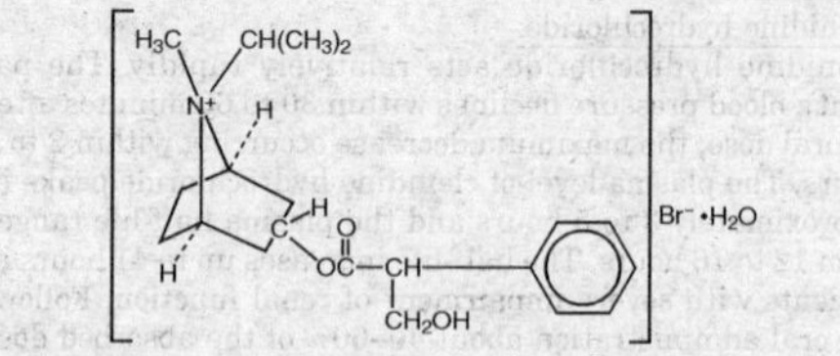

$C_{20}H_{30}BrNO_3 \cdot H_2O$ ipratropium bromide Mol. Wt. 430.4

Albuterol sulfate, chemically known as (1,3-benzenedimethanol, α'-[[(1,1-dimethylethyl) amino] methyl]-4-hydroxy, sulfate (2:1)(salt), (±)- is a relatively selective beta$_2$-adrenergic bronchodilator. Albuterol is the official generic name in the United States. The World Health Organization recommended name for the drug is salbutamol. Albuterol sulfate is a white to off-white crystalline powder, soluble in water and slightly soluble in ethanol. The structural formula is:

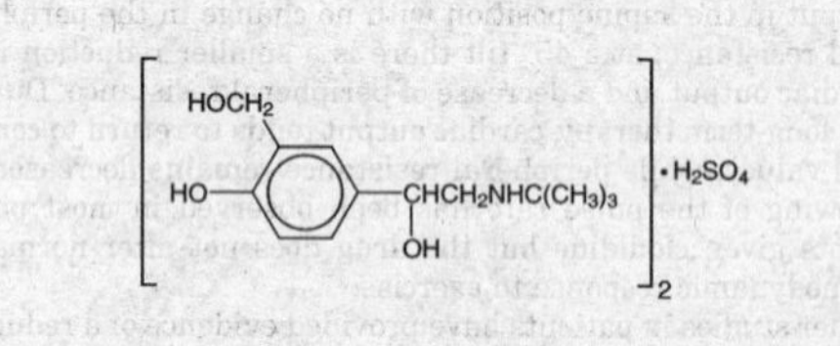

$(C_{13}H_{21}NO_3)_2 \cdot H_2SO_4$ albuterol sulfate Mol. Wt. 576.7

Combivent® Inhalation Aerosol contains a microcrystalline suspension of ipratropium bromide and albuterol sulfate in a pressurized metered-dose aerosol unit for oral inhalation administration. The 200 inhalation unit has a net weight of 14.7 grams. Each actuation meters 21 mcg of ipratropium bromide and 120 mcg of albuterol sulfate from the valve and delivers 18 mcg of ipratropium bromide and 103 mcg of albuterol sulfate (equivalent to 90 mcg albuterol base) from the mouthpiece. The excipients are dichlorodifluoromethane, dichlorotetrafluoroethane, and trichloromonofluoromethane as propellants and soya lecithin.

CLINICAL PHARMACOLOGY

Combivent® Inhalation Aerosol is a combination of the anticholinergic bronchodilator, ipratropium bromide, and the beta$_2$-adrenergic bronchodilator, albuterol sulfate.

Ipratropium Bromide:

Mechanism of Action

Ipratropium bromide is an anticholinergic (parasympatholytic) agent which, based on animal studies, appears to inhibit vagally mediated reflexes by antagonizing the action of acetylcholine, the transmitter agent released from the vagus nerve. Anticholinergics prevent the increases in intracellular concentration of cyclic guanosine monophosphate (cyclic GMP) which are caused by interaction of acetylcholine with the muscarinic receptor on bronchial smooth muscle.

Pharmacokinetics

The bronchodilation following inhalation of ipratropium bromide is primarily a local, site-specific effect, not a systemic one. Much of an administered dose is swallowed as shown by fecal excretion studies. Ipratropium bromide is a quaternary amine. It is not readily absorbed into the systemic circulation either from the surface of the lung or from the gastrointestinal tract as confirmed by blood level and renal excretion studies. Plasma levels of ipratropium bromide were below the assay sensitivity limit of 100 pg/mL. The half-life of elimination is about 2 hours after inhalation or intravenous administration. Ipratropium bromide is minimally bound (0 to 9% *in vitro*) to plasma albumin and α_1-acid glycoprotein. It is partially metabolized to inactive ester hydrolysis products. Following intravenous administra-

tion, approximately one-half of the dose is excreted unchanged in the urine. Studies in rats have shown that ipratropium bromide does not penetrate the blood-brain barrier. The pharmacokinetics of Combivent® Inhalation Aerosol or ipratropium bromide have not been studied in patients with hepatic or renal insufficiency or in the elderly (See PRECAUTIONS).

Controlled clinical studies have demonstrated that ipratropium bromide does not alter either mucociliary clearance or the volume or viscosity of respiratory secretions. In studies without a positive control, ipratropium bromide did not alter pupil size, accommodation or visual acuity (See ADVERSE REACTIONS).

Ventilation/perfusion studies have shown no clinically significant effects on pulmonary gas exchange or arterial oxygen tension. At recommended doses, ipratropium bromide does not produce clinically significant changes in pulse rate or blood pressure.

Albuterol Sulfate:
Mechanism of Action
In-vitro studies and *in-vivo* pharmacologic studies have demonstrated that albuterol has a preferential effect on beta$_2$-adrenergic receptors compared with isoproterenol. While it is recognized that beta$_2$-adrenergic receptors are the predominant receptors on bronchial smooth muscle, recent data indicate that there is a population of beta$_2$-receptors in the human heart which comprise between 10% and 50% of cardiac beta-adrenergic receptors. The precise function of these receptors, however, is not yet established (See WARNINGS).

Activation of beta$_2$-adrenergic receptors on airway smooth muscle leads to the activation of adenylyl cyclase and to an increase in the intracellular concentration of cyclic-3',5'-adenosine monophosphate (cyclic AMP). This increase of cyclic AMP leads to the activation of protein kinase A, which inhibits the phosphorylation of myosin and lowers intracellular ionic calcium concentrations, resulting in relaxation. Albuterol relaxes the smooth muscles of all airways, from the trachea to the terminal bronchioles. Albuterol acts as a functional antagonist to relax the airway irrespective of the spasmogen involved, thus protecting against all bronchoconstrictor challenges. Increased cyclic AMP concentrations are also associated with the inhibition of release of mediators from mast cells in the airway.

Albuterol has been shown in most clinical trials to have more bronchial smooth muscle relaxation effect than isoproterenol at comparable doses while producing fewer cardiovascular effects. However, all beta-adrenergic drugs, including albuterol sulfate, can produce a significant cardiovascular effect in some patients (See PRECAUTIONS).

Pharmacokinetics
Albuterol is longer acting than isoproterenol in most patients because it is not a substrate for the cellular uptake processes for catecholamines nor for metabolism by catechol-O-methyl transferase. Instead, the drug is conjugatively metabolized to albuterol 4'-O-sulfate.

In a pharmacokinetic study in 12 healthy male volunteers of two inhalations of albuterol sulfate, 103 mcg dose/inhalation through the mouthpiece, peak plasma albuterol concentrations ranging from 419 to 802 pg/mL (mean 599 ± 122 pg/mL) were obtained within three hours post-administration. Following this single-dose administration, 30.8 ± 10.2% of the estimated mouthpiece dose was excreted unchanged in the 24-hour urine. Since albuterol sulfate is rapidly and completely absorbed, this study could not distinguish between pulmonary and gastrointestinal absorption. Intravenous pharmacokinetics of albuterol were studied in a comparable group of 16 healthy male volunteers; the mean terminal half-life following a 30-minute infusion of 1.5 mg was 3.9 hours with a mean clearance of 439 mL/min/1.73 m^2.

Intravenous albuterol studies in rats demonstrated that albuterol crossed the blood-brain barrier and reached brain concentrations amounting to about 5% of the plasma concentrations. In structures outside the blood-brain barrier (pineal and pituitary glands), the drug achieved concentrations more than 100 times those in whole brain.

Studies in pregnant rats with tritiated albuterol demonstrated that approximately 10% of the circulating maternal drug was transferred to the fetus. Disposition in fetal lungs was comparable to maternal lungs, but fetal liver disposition was 1% of maternal liver levels.

Studies in laboratory animals (minipigs, rodents, and dogs) have demonstrated the occurrence of cardiac arrhythmias and sudden death (with histologic evidence of myocardial necrosis) when beta-agonists and methylxanthines were administered concurrently. The significance of these findings when applied to humans is unknown.

Combivent® Inhalation Aerosol:
Mechanism of Action
Combivent® Inhalation Aerosol is expected to maximize the response to treatment in patients with chronic obstructive pulmonary disease (COPD) by reducing bronchospasm through two distinctly different mechanisms, anticholinergic (parasympatholytic) and sympathomimetic. Simultaneous administration of both an anticholinergic (ipratro-

pium bromide) and a beta$_2$-sympathomimetic (albuterol sulfate) is designed to benefit the patient by producing a greater bronchodilator effect than when either drug is utilized alone at its recommended dosage.

Pharmacokinetics
In a crossover pharmacokinetic study in 12 healthy male volunteers comparing the pattern of absorption and excretion of two inhalations of Combivent® Inhalation Aerosol to the two active components individually, the co-administration of ipratropium bromide and albuterol sulfate from a single canister did not significantly alter the systemic absorption of either component. Ipratropium bromide levels remained below detectable limits (<100 pg/mL). Peak albuterol level obtained within 3 hours post-administration was 492 ± 132 pg/mL. Following this single administration, 27.1 ± 5.7% of the estimated mouthpiece dose was excreted unchanged in the 24 hour urine. From a pharmacokinetic perspective, the synergistic efficacy of Combivent® Inhalation Aerosol is likely to be due to a local effect on the muscarinic and beta$_2$-adrenergic receptors in the lung.

Clinical Trials
In two 12-week randomized, double-blind, active-controlled clinical trials, 1067 patients with chronic obstructive pulmonary disease (COPD) were evaluated for the bronchodilator efficacy of Combivent® Inhalation Aerosol (358 patients) in comparison to its components, ipratropium bromide (362 patients) and albuterol sulfate (347 patients).

Serial FEV$_1$ measurements (shown below as a percent change from test-day baseline) demonstrated that Combivent® Inhalation Aerosol produced significantly greater improvement in pulmonary function than either ipratropium bromide or albuterol sulfate when given separately. The median time to onset of a 15% increase in FEV$_1$ was 15 minutes and the median time to peak FEV$_1$ was one hour for Combivent® Inhalation Aerosol and its components. The median duration of effect as measured by FEV$_1$ was 4–5 hours for Combivent® Inhalation Aerosol compared to 4 hours for ipratropium bromide and 3 hours for albuterol sulfate.

Percent Change in Adjusted Mean[a] FEV$_1$ From Test-Day Baseline–Endpoint Analysis of the Evaluable Data Set

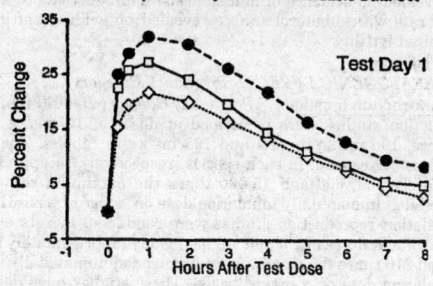

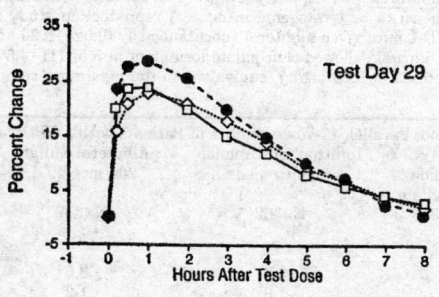

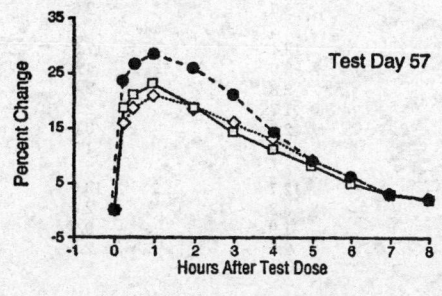

[See figure at top of next column]

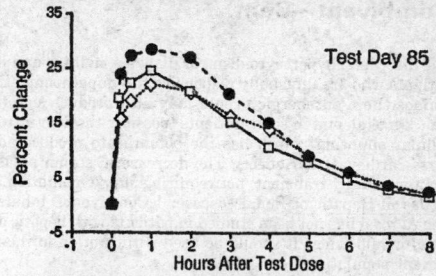

● Combivent (n=347) ◇ Ipratropium (n=355) □ Albuterol (n=331)
[a] Adjusted for test-day baseline FEV$_1$, center and treatment-by-center interaction

These studies demonstrated that each component of Combivent® Inhalation Aerosol contributed to the improvement in pulmonary function produced by the combination, especially during the first 4–5 hours after dosing, and that Combivent® Inhalation Aerosol was significantly more effective than ipratropium bromide or albuterol sulfate administered alone.

In the two controlled twelve-week studies, Combivent® Inhalation Aerosol did not produce any change in the secondary efficacy parameters including symptom scores, physician global assessments and morning PEFR, all of which were monitored throughout the study period.

INDICATIONS AND USAGE
Combivent® Inhalation Aerosol is indicated for use in patients with chronic obstructive pulmonary disease (COPD) on a regular aerosol bronchodilator who continue to have evidence of bronchospasm and who require a second bronchodilator.

CONTRAINDICATIONS
Combivent® Inhalation Aerosol is contraindicated in patients with a history of hypersensitivity to soya lecithin or related food products such as soybean and peanut. Combivent® Inhalation Aerosol is also contraindicated in patients hypersensitive to any other components of the drug product or to atropine or its derivatives.

WARNINGS
1. Paradoxical Bronchospasm: Combivent® Inhalation Aerosol can produce paradoxical bronchospasm that can be life threatening. If it occurs, the preparation should be discontinued immediately and alternative therapy instituted. It should be recognized that paradoxical bronchospasm, when associated with inhaled formulations, frequently occurs with the first use of a new canister.

2. Cardiovascular Effect: The albuterol sulfate contained in Combivent® Inhalation Aerosol, like other beta-adrenergic agonists, can produce a clinically significant cardiovascular effect in some patients, as measured by pulse rate, blood pressure and/or symptoms. Although such effects are uncommon after administration of Combivent® Inhalation Aerosol at recommended doses, if they occur, discontinuation of the drug may be indicated. In addition, beta-adrenergic agents have been reported to produce ECG changes, such as flattening of the T wave, prolongation of the QTc interval, and ST segment depression. Therefore, Combivent® Inhalation Aerosol should be used with caution in patients with cardiovascular disorders, especially coronary insufficiency, cardiac arrhythmias and hypertension.

3. Do Not Exceed Recommended Dose: Fatalities have been reported in association with excessive use of inhaled sympathomimetic drugs, in patients with asthma. The exact cause of death is unknown, but cardiac arrest following an unexpected development of a severe acute asthmatic crisis and subsequent hypoxia is suspected.

4. Immediate Hypersensitivity Reactions: Immediate hypersensitivity reactions may occur after administration of ipratropium bromide or albuterol sulfate, as demonstrated by rare cases of urticaria, angioedema, rash, bronchospasm, anaphylaxis and oropharyngeal edema.

5. Storage Conditions: The contents of Combivent® Inhalation Aerosol are under pressure. Do not puncture. Do not use or store near heat or open flame. Exposure to temperatures above 120°F may cause bursting. Never throw the container into a fire or incinerator. Keep out of reach of children.

PRECAUTIONS
General
1. Effects Seen with Anticholinergic Drugs: Combivent® Inhalation Aerosol contains ipratropium bromide and, therefore, should be used with caution in patients with narrow-angle glaucoma, prostatic hypertrophy or bladder-neck obstruction.

2. Effects Seen with Sympathomimetic Drugs: Preparations containing sympathomimetic amines such as albuterol sulfate should be used with caution in patients with convul-

Continued on next page

Combivent—Cont.

sive disorders, hyperthyroidism, or diabetes mellitus and in patients who are unusually responsive to sympathomimetic amines. Beta-adrenergic agents may also produce significant hypokalemia in some patients (possibly through intracellular shunting) which has the potential to produce adverse cardiovascular effects. The decrease in serum potassium is usually transient, not requiring supplementation.

3. Use in Hepatic or Renal Disease: Combivent® Inhalation Aerosol has not been studied in patients with hepatic or renal insufficiency. It should be used with caution in those patient populations.

Information for Patients

Patients should be cautioned to avoid spraying the aerosol into their eyes and be advised that this may result in precipitation or worsening of narrow-angle glaucoma, eye pain or discomfort, temporary blurring of vision, visual halos or colored images in association with red eyes from conjunctival and corneal congestion. Should any combination of these symptoms develop, consult your physician immediately.

The action of Combivent® Inhalation Aerosol should last 4–5 hours or longer. Combivent® Inhalation Aerosol should not be used more frequently than recommended. Do not increase the dose or frequency of Combivent® Inhalation Aerosol without consulting your physician. If you find that treatment with Combivent® Inhalation Aerosol becomes less effective for symptomatic relief, your symptoms become worse, and/or you need to use the product more frequently than usual, medical attention should be sought immediately. While you are taking Combivent® Inhalation Aerosol, other inhaled drugs should be taken only as directed by your physician. If you are pregnant or nursing, contact your physician about use of Combivent® Inhalation Aerosol. Appropriate use of Combivent® Inhalation Aerosol includes an understanding of the way it should be administered (See Patient's Instructions for Use).

Drug Interactions

Combivent® Inhalation Aerosol has been used concomitantly with other drugs, including sympathomimetic bronchodilators, methylxanthines and steroids, commonly used in the treatment of COPD, without adverse drug reactions. No formal drug interaction studies have been performed with Combivent® Inhalation Aerosol and these or other medications commonly used in the treatment of COPD.

Anticholinergic agents: Although ipratropium bromide is minimally absorbed into the systemic circulation, there is some potential for an additive interaction with concomitantly used anticholinergic medications. Caution is therefore advised in the co-administration of Combivent® Inhalation Aerosol with other anticholinergic-containing drugs.

Beta-adrenergic agents: Caution is advised in the co-administration of Combivent® Inhalation Aerosol and other sympathomimetic agents due to the increased risk of adverse cardiovascular effects.

Beta-receptor blocking agents and albuterol inhibit the effect of each other. Beta-receptor blocking agents should be used with caution in patients with hyperreactive airways.

Diuretics: The ECG changes and/or hypokalemia which may result from the administration of non-potassium sparing diuretics (such as loop or thiazide diuretics) can be acutely worsened by beta-agonists, especially when the recommended dose of the beta-agonist is exceeded. Although the clinical significance of these effects is not known, caution is advised in the co-administration of beta-agonist-containing drugs, such as Combivent® Inhalation Aerosol, with non-potassium sparing diuretics.

Monoamine oxidase inhibitors or tricyclic antidepressants: Combivent® Inhalation Aerosol should be administered with extreme caution to patients being treated with monoamine oxidase inhibitors or tricyclic antidepressants or within two weeks of discontinuation of such agents because the action of albuterol on the cardiovascular system may be potentiated.

Carcinogenesis, Mutagenesis, Impairment of Fertility

Ipratropium bromide: Two-year oral carcinogenicity studies in rats and mice have revealed no carcinogenic potential at doses up to 6 mg/kg/day. This dose corresponds to approximately 360 and 180 times the maximum recommended human daily inhalation dose in rats and mice respectively, on a mg/m^2 basis. Results of various mutagenicity studies (Ames test, mouse dominant lethal test, mouse micronucleus test and chromosome aberration of bone marrow in Chinese hamsters) were negative. Fertility of male or female rats at oral doses up to 50 mg/kg/day (approximately 3000 times the maximum recommended human daily inhalation dose on a mg/m^2 basis) was unaffected by ipratropium bromide administration. At doses above 90 mg/kg/day (approximately 5400 times the maximum recommended human daily inhalation dose on a mg/m^2 basis), increased resorption and decreased conception rates were observed.

Albuterol: Like other agents in its class, albuterol caused a significant dose-related increase in the incidence of benign leiomyomas of the mesovarium in a two-year study in the rat at dietary doses of 2, 10 and 50 mg/kg/day (approximately 20, 100 and 500 times the maximum recommended human daily inhalation dose on a mg/m^2 basis). In another study this effect was blocked by the co-administration of propranolol. The relevance of these findings to humans is not known. An 18-month study in mice at dietary doses up to 500 mg/kg/day (approximately 2500 times the maximum recommended human daily inhalation dose on a mg/m^2 basis) and a 99-week study in hamsters at oral doses up to 50 mg/kg/day (approximately 375 times the maximum recommended human daily inhalation dose on a mg/m^2 basis) revealed no evidence of tumorigenicity. Studies with albuterol revealed no evidence of mutagenesis. Reproduction studies in rats with albuterol sulfate revealed no evidence of impaired fertility.

Pregnancy

TERATOGENIC EFFECTS Pregnancy Category C.

Ipratropium bromide: *Pregnancy Category B.* Oral reproduction studies were performed at doses of 10 mg/kg in mice, 100 mg/kg in rats and 125 mg/kg in rabbits. These doses correspond, in each species, respectively, to approximately 300, 600 and 15,000 times the maximum recommended human daily inhalation dose on a mg/m^2 basis. Inhalation reproduction studies were conducted in rats and rabbits at doses of 1.5 and 1.8 mg/kg/day (approximately 90 and 210 times the maximum recommended human daily inhalation dose on a mg/m^2 basis). These studies have demonstrated no evidence of teratogenic effects as a result of ipratropium bromide.

Albuterol: *Pregnancy Category C.* Albuterol has been shown to be teratogenic in mice. A reproduction study in CD-1 mice given albuterol subcutaneously (0.025, 0.25 and 2.5 mg/kg) showed cleft palate formation in 5 of 111 (4.5%) fetuses at 0.25 mg/kg (equivalent to the maximum recommended human daily inhalation dose on a mg/m^2 basis) and in 10 of 108 (9.3%) fetuses at 2.5 mg/kg (approximately 10 times the maximum recommended human daily inhalation dose on a mg/m^2 basis). None was observed at 0.025 mg/kg (approximately one-tenth the maximum recommended human daily inhalation dose). Cleft palate also occurred in 22 of 72 (30.5%) fetuses treated with 2.5 mg/kg isoproterenol (positive control). A reproduction study with oral albuterol in Stride Dutch rabbits revealed cranioschisis in 7 of 19 (37%) fetuses at 50 mg/kg (approximately 1000 times the maximum recommended human daily inhalation dose on a mg/m^2 basis).

There are, however, no adequate and well-controlled studies of Combivent® Inhalation Aerosol, ipratropium bromide or albuterol sulfate, in pregnant women. Because animal reproduction studies are not always predictive of human response, Combivent® Inhalation Aerosol should be used during pregnancy only if the potential benefit justifies the potential risk to the fetus.

Labor and Delivery

Because of the potential for beta-agonist interference with uterine contractility, use of Combivent® Inhalation Aerosol for the treatment of COPD during labor should be restricted to those patients in whom the benefits clearly outweigh the risk.

Nursing Mothers

It is not known whether the components of Combivent® Inhalation Aerosol are excreted in human milk.

Ipratropium bromide: Although lipid-insoluble quaternary bases pass into breast milk, it is unlikely that the active component ipratropium bromide, would reach the infant to an important extent, especially when taken by aerosol. However, because many drugs are excreted in human milk, caution should be exercised when Combivent® Inhalation Aerosol is administered to a nursing mother.

Albuterol: Because of the potential for tumorigenicity shown for albuterol in animal studies, a decision should be made whether to discontinue nursing or to discontinue the drug, taking into account the importance of the drug to the mother.

Pediatric Use

Safety and effectiveness of Combivent® Inhalation Aerosol in pediatric patients have not been established.

ADVERSE REACTIONS

Adverse reaction information concerning Combivent® Inhalation Aerosol is derived from two 12-week controlled clinical trials (N=358 for Combivent® Inhalation Aerosol). [See table below]

All Adverse Events (in percentages), from Two Large Double-Blind, Parallel, 12-Week Studies of Patients with COPD*

	Combivent® Ipratropium Bromide 36 mcg/Albuterol Sulfate 206 mcg q.i.d. N=358	Ipratropium Bromide 36 mcg q.i.d. N=362	Albuterol Sulfate 206 mcg q.i.d. N=347
Body as A Whole— General Disorders			
Headache	5.6	3.9	6.6
Pain	2.5	1.9	1.2
Influenza	1.4	2.2	2.9
Chest Pain	0.3	1.4	2.9
Gastrointestinal System Disorders			
Nausea	2.0	2.5	2.6
Respiratory System Disorders (Lower)			
Bronchitis	12.3	12.4	17.9
Dyspnea	4.5	3.9	4.0
Coughing	4.2	2.8	2.6
Respiratory Disorders	2.5	1.7	2.3
Pneumonia	1.4	2.5	0.6
Bronchospasm	0.3	3.9	1.7
Respiratory System Disorders (Upper)			
Upper Resp. Tract Infection	10.9	12.7	13.0
Pharyngitis	2.2	3.3	2.3
Sinusitis	2.3	1.9	0.9
Rhinitis	1.1	2.5	2.3

* All adverse events, regardless of drug relationship, reported by two percent or more patients in one or more treatment group in the 12-week controlled clinical trials.

Additional adverse reactions, reported in less than two percent of the patients in the Combivent® Inhalation Aerosol treatment group include edema, fatigue, hypertension, dizziness, nervousness, paresthesia, tremor, dysphonia, insomnia, diarrhea, dry mouth, dyspepsia, vomiting, arrhythmia, palpitation, tachycardia, arthralgia, angina, increased sputum, taste perversion, and urinary tract infection/dysuria. Allergic-type reactions such as skin rash, angioedema of tongue, lips and face, urticaria (including giant urticaria), laryngospasm and anaphylactic reaction have been reported, with positive rechallenge in some cases. Many of these patients had a history of allergies to other drugs and/or foods including soybean (See CONTRAINDICATIONS).

Additional information derived from the published literature and post-marketing surveillance on the use of ipratropium or albuterol inhalation aerosol singly or in combination that is not included in the lists above includes: cases of precipitation or worsening of narrow-angle glaucoma, acute eye pain, blurred vision, nasal congestion, drying of secretions, mucosal ulcers, irritation from aerosol, paradoxical bronchospasm, wheezing, exacerbation of COPD symptoms, heartburn, drowsiness, CNS stimulation, coordination difficulty, weakness, itching, flushing, alopecia, hypotension, gastrointestinal distress, constipation, and urinary difficulties.

OVERDOSAGE

The effects of overdosage are expected to be related primarily to albuterol sulfate. Acute overdosage with ipratropium bromide is unlikely since ipratropium bromide is not well absorbed systemically after aerosol or oral administration. The oral median lethal dose of ipratropium bromide ranged between 1001 and 2010 mg/kg in mice (approximately 30,000 and 60,000 times the maximum recommended human daily inhalation dose on a mg/m^2 basis, respectively); between 1667 and 4000 mg/kg in rats (approximately 100,000 and 240,000 times the maximum recommended human daily inhalation dose, respectively, on a mg/m^2 basis); and between 400 and 1300 mg/kg (approximately 80,000 and 260,000 times the maximum recommended human daily inhalation dose, respectively, on a mg/m^2 basis) in dogs. Whereas the oral median lethal dose of albuterol sulfate in mice and rats was greater than 2,000 mg/kg (approximately 10,000 and 20,000 times the maximum recommended human daily inhalation dose, respectively, on a mg/m^2 basis), the inhalational median lethal dose could not be determined. Manifestations of overdosage with albuterol

may include anginal pain, hypertension, hypokalemia, tachycardia with rates up to 200 beats per minute and exaggeration of the pharmacologic effects listed in ADVERSE REACTIONS. As with all sympathomimetic aerosol medications, cardiac arrest and even death may be associated with abuse. Dialysis is not appropriate treatment for overdosage of albuterol as an inhalation aerosol; the judicious use of a cardiovascular beta-receptor blocker, such as metoprolol tartrate may be indicated.

DOSAGE AND ADMINISTRATION

The dose of Combivent® Inhalation Aerosol is two inhalations four times a day. Patients may take additional inhalations as required; however, the total number of inhalations should not exceed 12 in 24 hours. Safety and efficacy of additional doses of Combivent® Inhalation Aerosol beyond 12 puffs/24 hours have not been studied. Also, safety and efficacy of extra doses of ipratropium or albuterol in addition to the recommended doses of Combivent® Inhalation Aerosol have not been studied. It is recommended to "test-spray" three times before using for the first time and in cases where the aerosol has not been used for more than 24 hours.

HOW SUPPLIED

Combivent® Inhalation Aerosol is supplied as a metered-dose inhaler with a white mouthpiece which has a clear, colorless sleeve and an orange protective cap. The Combivent® Inhalation Aerosol canister should be used with the Combivent® Inhalation Aerosol actuator only. The actuator should not be used with other aerosol medications. Each actuation meters 21 mcg of ipratropium bromide and 120 mcg of albuterol sulfate from the valve and delivers 18 mcg of ipratropium bromide and 103 mcg of albuterol sulfate (equivalent to 90 mcg albuterol base) from the mouthpiece. Each 14.7 gram canister provides sufficient medication for 200 inhalations (NDC 0597-0013-14).

The canister should be discarded after the labeled number of actuations have been used. The amount of medication in each actuation cannot be assured after this point.

Store between 59° F (15° C) and 86° F (30° C). Avoid excessive humidity. For optimal results, the canister should be at room temperature before use. Shake well before using.

Note: The indented statement below is required by the Federal government's Clean Air Act for all products containing or manufactured with chlorofluorocarbons (CFCs):

> **Warning:** Contains trichloromonofluoromethane (CFC-11), dichlorodifluoromethane (CFC-12) and dichlorotetrafluoroethane (CFC-114), substances which harm public health and the environment by destroying ozone in the upper atmosphere.

A notice similar to the above **Warning** has been placed in the information for the patient of this product under the Environmental Protection Agency's (EPA's) regulations. The patient's warning states that the patient should consult his or her physician if there are any questions about alternatives.

CAUTION

Federal law prohibits dispensing without prescription.

CB-5/97-PI

Manufactured by: 3M Pharmaceuticals, St. Paul, MN 55144
Ipratropium bromide licensed from: Boehringer Ingelheim International GmbH

Shown in Product Identification Guide, page 306

FLOMAX® ℞

[*flŏ-max*]
(tamsulosin hydrochloride)
Capsules

Prescribing Information

DESCRIPTION

Tamsulosin hydrochloride is an antagonist of $alpha_{1A}$adrenoceptors in the prostate. Tamsulosin HCl is (-)-(*R*)-5-[2-[[2-(0-ethoxyphenoxy) ethyl]amino]propyl]-2-methoxybenzenesulfonamide, monohydrochloride. Tamsulosin HCl occurs as white crystals that melt with decomposition at approximately 230°C. It is sparingly soluble in water and in methanol, slightly soluble in glacial acetic acid and in ethanol, and practically insoluble in ether.

The empirical formula of tamsulosin HCl is $C_{20}H_{28}N_2O_5S \cdot HCl$.

The molecular weight of tamsulosin HCl is 444.98. Its structural formula is:

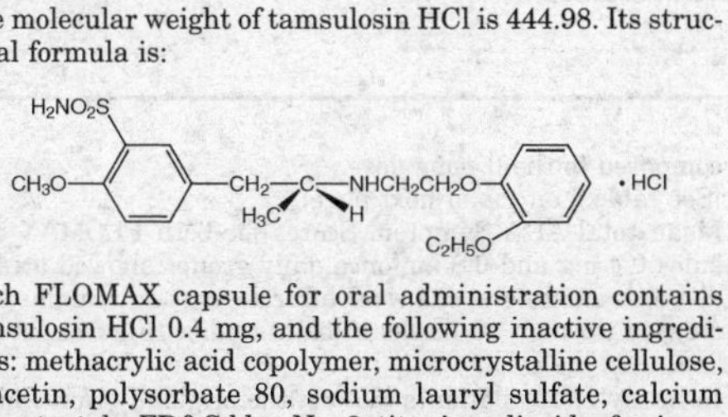

Each FLOMAX capsule for oral administration contains tamsulosin HCl 0.4 mg, and the following inactive ingredients: methacrylic acid copolymer, microcrystalline cellulose, triacetin, polysorbate 80, sodium lauryl sulfate, calcium stearate, talc, FD&C blue No. 2, titanium dioxide, ferric oxide, gelatin, and trace amounts of shellac, industrial methylated spirit 74OP, soya lecithin, 1-ethoxyethanol, dimethylpolysiloxane, and black iron oxide E172.

TABLE 1 Mean (± S.D.) Pharmacokinetic Parameters Following FLOMAX capsules 0.4 mg Once Daily or 0.8 mg Once Daily with a Light Breakfast, High-Fat Breakfast or Fasted

Pharmacokinetic Parameter	0.4 mg q.d. to healthy volunteers; n=23 (age range 18-32 years)		0.8 mg q.d. to healthy volunteers; n=22 (age range 55-75 years)		
	Light Breakfast	Fasted	Light Breakfast	High-Fat Breakfast	Fasted
Cmin (ng/mL)	4.0 ± 2.6	3.8 ± 2.5	12.3 ± 6.7	13.5 ± 7.6	13.3 ± 13.3
Cmax (ng/mL)	10.1 ± 4.8	17.1 ± 17.1	29.8 ± 10.3	29.1 ± 11.0	41.6 ± 15.6
Cmax/Cmin Ratio	3.1 ± 1.0	5.3 ± 2.2	2.7 ± 0.7	2.5 ± 0.8	3.6 ± 1.1
Tmax (hours)	6.0	4.0	7.0	6.6	5.0
T1/2 (hours)	–	–	–	–	14.9 ± 3.9
AUCτ (ng·hr/mL)	151 ± 81.5	199 ± 94.1	440 ± 195	449 ± 217	557 ± 257

Cmin = observed minimum concentration
Cmax = observed maximum tamsulosin HCl plasma concentration
Tmax = median time-to-maximum concentration
T1/2 = observed half-life
AUCτ = Area under the tamsulosin HCl plasma time curve over the dosing interval

CLINICAL PHARMACOLOGY

The symptoms associated with benign prostatic hyperplasia (BPH) are related to bladder outlet obstruction, which is comprised of two underlying components: static and dynamic. The static component is related to an increase in prostate size caused, in part, by a proliferation of smooth muscle cells in the prostatic stroma. However, the severity of BPH symptoms and the degree of urethral obstruction do not correlate well with the size of the prostate. The dynamic component is a function of an increase in smooth muscle tone in the prostate and bladder neck leading to constriction of the bladder outlet. Smooth muscle tone is mediated by the sympathetic nervous stimulation of $alpha_1$ adrenoceptors, which are abundant in the prostate, prostatic capsule, prostatic urethra, and bladder neck. Blockade of these adrenoceptors can cause smooth muscles in the bladder neck and prostate to relax, resulting in an improvement in urine flow rate and a reduction in symptoms of BPH.

Tamsulosin, an $alpha_1$ adrenoceptor blocking agent, exhibits selectivity for $alpha_1$ receptors in the human prostate. At least three discrete $alpha_1$ adrenoceptor subtypes have been identified: $alpha_{1A}$, $alpha_{1B}$ and $alpha_{1D}$; their distribution differs between human organs and tissue. Approximately 70% of the $alpha_1$- receptors in human prostate are of the $alpha_{1A}$ subtype.

FLOMAX capsules are not intended for use as an antihypertensive drug.

Pharmacokinetics The pharmacokinetics of tamsulosin HCl have been evaluated in adult healthy volunteers and patients with BPH after single and/or multiple administration with doses ranging from 0.1 mg to 1 mg.

Absorption: Absorption of tamsulosin HCl from FLOMAX capsules 0.4 mg is essentially complete (>90%) following oral administration under fasting conditions. Tamsulosin HCl exhibits linear kinetics following single and multiple dosing, with achievement of steady-state concentrations by the fifth day of once-a-day dosing.

Effect of Food: The time to maximum concentration (T_{max}) is reached by four to five hours under fasting conditions and by six to seven hours when FLOMAX capsules are administered with food. Taking FLOMAX capsules under fasted conditions results in a 30% increase in bioavailability (AUC) and 40% to 70% increase in peak concentrations (C_{max}) compared to fed conditions (Figure 1).

Figure 1: Mean Plasma Tamsulosin HCl Concentrations Following Single-Dose Administration of FLOMAX capsules 0.4 mg Under Fasted and Fed Conditions (n=8).

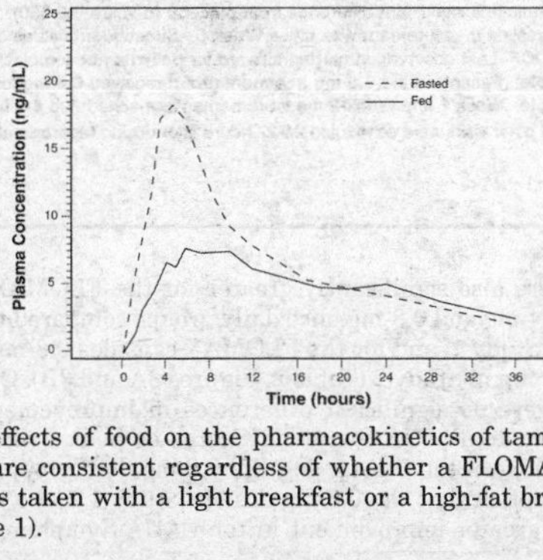

The effects of food on the pharmacokinetics of tamsulosin HCl are consistent regardless of whether a FLOMAX capsule is taken with a light breakfast or a high-fat breakfast (Table 1).

[See table above]

Distribution: The mean steady-state apparent volume of distribution of tamsulosin HCl after intravenous administration to ten healthy male adults was 16L, which is suggestive of distribution into extracellular fluids in the body. Additionally, whole body autoradiographic studies in mice and rats and tissue distribution in rats and dogs indicate that tamsulosin HCl is widely distributed to most tissues including kidney, prostate, liver, gall bladder, heart, aorta, and brown fat, and minimally distributed to the brain, spinal cord, and testes.

Tamsulosin HCl is extensively bound to human plasma proteins (94% to 99%), primarily alpha-1 acid glycoprotein (AAG), with linear binding over a wide concentration range (20 to 600 ng/mL). The results of two-way *in vitro* studies indicate that the binding of tamsulosin HCl to human plasma proteins is not affected by amitriptyline, diclofenac, glyburide, simvastatin plus simvastatin-hydroxy acid metabolite, warfarin, diazepam, propranolol, trichlormethiazide, or chlormadinone. Likewise, tamsulosin HCl had no effect on the extent of binding of these drugs.

Metabolism: There is no enantiometric bioconversion from tamsulosin HCl [R(-) isomer] to the S(+) isomer in humans. Tamsulosin HCl is extensively metabolized by cytochrome P450 enzymes in the liver and less than 10% of the dose is excreted in urine unchanged. However, the pharmacokinetic profile of the metabolites in humans has not been established. Additionally, the cytochrome P450 enzymes that primarily catalyze the Phase I metabolism of tamsulosin HCl have not been conclusively identified. Therefore, possible interactions with other cytochrome P450 metabolized compounds cannot be discerned with current information. The metabolites of tamsulosin HCl undergo extensive conjugation to glucuronide or sulfate prior to renal excretion.

Incubations with human liver microsomes showed no evidence of clinically significant metabolic interactions between tamsulosin HCl and amitriptyline, albuterol (beta agonist), glyburide (glibenclamide) and finasteride (5alpha-reductase inhibitor for treatment of BPH). However, results of the *in vitro* testing of the tamsulosin HCl interaction with diclofenac and warfarin were equivocal.

Excretion: On administration of the radiolabeled dose of tamsulosin HCl to four healthy volunteers, 97% of the administered radioactivity was recovered, with urine (76%) representing the primary route of excretion compared to feces (21%) over 168 hours.

Following intravenous or oral administration of an immediate-release formulation, the elimination half-life of tamsulosin HCl in plasma range from five to seven hours. Because of absorption rate-controlled pharmacokinetics with FLOMAX capsules, the apparent half-life of tamsulosin HCl is approximately 9 to 13 hours in healthy volunteers and 14 to 15 hours in the target population. Tamsulosin HCl undergoes restrictive clearance in humans, with a relatively low systemic clearance (2.88 L/h).

Special Populations: Geriatrics (Age): Cross-study comparison of FLOMAX capsules overall exposure (AUC) and half-life indicate that the pharmacokinetic disposition of tamsulosin HCl may be slightly prolonged in geriatric males compared to young, healthy male volunteers. Intrinsic clearance is independent of tamsulosin HCl binding to AAG, but diminishes with age, resulting in a 40% overall higher exposure (AUC) in subjects of age 55 to 75 years compared to subjects of age 20 to 32 years.

Renal Dysfunction: The pharmacokinetics of tamsulosin HCl have been compared in 6 subjects with mild - moderate (30≤CLcr < 70 mL/min/1.73m²) or moderate - severe (10

Continued on next page

Flomax—Cont.

≤CLcr < 30 mL/min/1.73m²) renal impairment and 6 normal subjects (CLcr < 90 mL/min/1.73m²). While a change in the overall plasma concentration of tamsulosin HCl was observed as the result of altered binding to AAG, the unbound (active) concentration of tamsulosin HCl, as well as the intrinsic clearance, remained relatively constant. Therefore, patients with renal impairment do not require an adjustment in FLOMAX capsules dosing. However, patients with endstage renal disease (CLcr < 10 mL/min/1.73m²) have not been studied.

Hepatic Dysfunction: The pharmacokinetics of tamsulosin HCl have been compared in 8 subjects with moderate hepatic dysfunction (Child-Pugh's classification: Grades A and B) and 8 normal subjects. While a change in the overall plasma concentration of tamsulosin HCl was observed as the result of altered binding to AAG, the unbound (active) concentration of tamsulosin HCl does not change significantly with only a modest (32%) change in intrinsic clearance of unbound tamsulosin HCl. Therefore, patients with moderate hepatic dysfunction do not require an adjustment in FLOMAX capsules dosage.

Drug-Drug Interactions: Nifedipine, Atenolol, Enalapril: In three studies in hypertensive subjects (age range 47–79 years) whose blood pressure was controlled with stable doses of Procardia XL®, atenolol, or enalapril for at least three months, FLOMAX capsules 0.4 mg for seven days followed by FLOMAX capsules 0.8 mg for another seven days (n=8 per study) resulted in no clinically significant effects on blood pressure and pulse rate compared to placebo (n=4 per study). Therefore, dosage adjustments are not necessary when FLOMAX capsules are administered concomitantly with Procardia XL®, atenolol, or enalapril.

Warfarin: A definitive drug-drug interaction study between tamsulosin HCl and warfarin was not conducted. Results from limited *in vitro* and *in vivo* studies are inconclusive. Therefore, caution should be exercised with concomitant administration of warfarin and FLOMAX capsules.

Digoxin and Theophylline: In two studies in healthy volunteers (n=10 per study; age range 19–39 years) receiving FLOMAX capsules 0.4 mg/day for two days, followed by FLOMAX capsules 0.8 mg/day for five to eight days, single intravenous doses of digoxin 0.5 mg or theophylline 5 mg/kg resulted in no change in the pharmacokinetics of digoxin or theophylline. Therefore, dosage adjustments are not necessary when a FLOMAX capsule is administered concomitantly with digoxin or theophylline.

Furosemide: The pharmacokinetic and pharmacodynamic interaction between FLOMAX capsules 0.8 mg/day (steady-state) and furosemide 20 mg intravenously (single dose) was evaluated in ten healthy volunteers (age range 21–40 years). FLOMAX capsules had no effect on the pharmacodynamics (excretion of electrolytes) of furosemide. While furosemide produced an 11% to 12% reduction in tamsulosin HCl Cmax and AUC, these changes are expected to be clinically insignificant and do not require adjustment of the FLOMAX capsules dosage.

Cimetidine: The effects of cimetidine at the highest recommended dose (400 mg every six hours for six days) on the pharmacokinetics of a single FLOMAX capsule 0.4 mg dose was investigated in ten healthy volunteers (age range 21–38 years). Treatment with cimetidine resulted in a significant decrease (26%) in the clearance of tamsulosin HCl which resulted in a moderate increase in tamsulosin HCl AUC (44%). Therefore, FLOMAX capsules should be used with caution in combination with cimetidine, particularly at doses higher than 0.4 mg.

Clinical Studies Four placebo-controlled clinical studies and one active-controlled clinical study enrolled a total of 2296 patients (1003 received FLOMAX capsules 0.4 mg once daily, 491 received FLOMAX capsules 0.8 mg once daily, and 802 were control patients) in the U.S. and Europe.

In the two U.S. placebo-controlled, double-blind, 13-week, multicenter studies [Study 1 (US92-03A) and Study 2 (US93-01)], 1486 men with the signs and symptoms of BPH were enrolled. In both studies, patients were randomized to either placebo, FLOMAX capsules 0.4 mg once daily, or FLOMAX capsules 0.8 mg once daily. Patients in FLOMAX capsules 0.8-mg once daily treatment groups received a dose of 0.4 mg once daily for one week before increasing to the 0.8-mg once daily dose. The primary efficacy assessments included 1) total American Urological Association (AUA) Symptom Score questionnaire, which evaluated irritative (frequency, urgency, and nocturia), and obstructive (hesitancy, incomplete emptying, intermittency, and weak stream) symptoms, where a decrease in score is consistent with improvement in symptoms; and 2) peak urine flow rate, where an increased peak urine flow rate value over baseline is consistent with decreased urinary obstruction.

Mean changes from baseline to week 13 in total AUA Symptom Score were significantly greater for groups treated with FLOMAX capsules 0.4 mg and 0.8 mg once daily compared to placebo in both U.S. studies (Table 2, Figures 2A and 2B). The changes from baseline to week 13 in peak urine flow

rate were also significantly greater for the FLOMAX capsules 0.4-mg and 0.8-mg once daily groups compared to placebo in Study 1, and for the FLOMAX capsules 0.8-mg once daily group in Study 2 (Table 2, Figures 3A and 3B). Overall there were no significant differences in improvement observed in total AUA Symptom Scores or peak urine flow rates between the 0.4-mg and the 0.8-mg dose groups with the exception that the 0.8-mg dose in Study 1 had a significantly greater improvement in total AUA Symptom Score

compared to the 0.4-mg dose.
[See table 2 on top of next page]
Mean total AUA Symptom Scores for both FLOMAX capsules 0.4-mg and 0.8-mg once daily groups showed a rapid decrease starting at one week after dosing and remained decreased through 13 weeks in both studies (Figures 2A and 2B).

In Study 1, 400 patients (53% of the originally randomized group) elected to continue in their originally assigned treat-

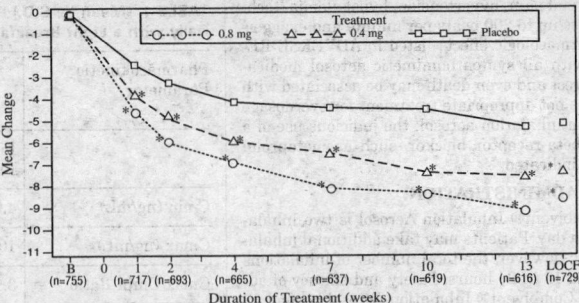

FIGURE 2A:
Mean Change from Baseline in Total AUA Symptom Score (0-35) Study 1

* indicates significant difference from placebo (p-value ≤0.050).
B=Baseline determined approximately one week prior to the initial dose of double-blind medication at Week 0. Subsequent values are observed cases.
LOCF= Last observation carried forward for patients not completing the 13-week study.
Note: Patients in the 0.8 mg treatment group received 0.4 mg for the first week.
Note: Total AUA Symptom Scores range from 0 to 35.

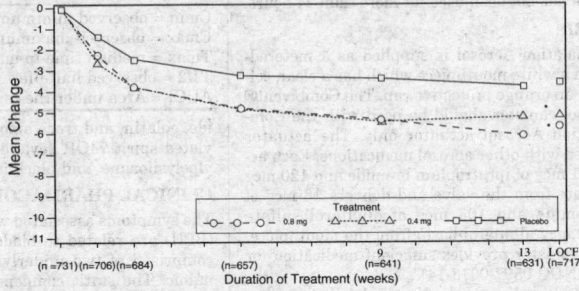

FIGURE 2B:
Mean Change from Baseline in Total AUA Symptom Score (0-35) Study 2

* indicates significant difference from placebo (p-value ≤0.050).
Baseline measurement was taken Week 0. Subsequent values are observed cases.
LOCF= Last observation carried forward for patients not completing the 13-week study.
Note: Patients in the 0.8 mg treatment group received 0.4 mg for the first week.
Note: Total AUA Symptom Scores range from 0 to 35.

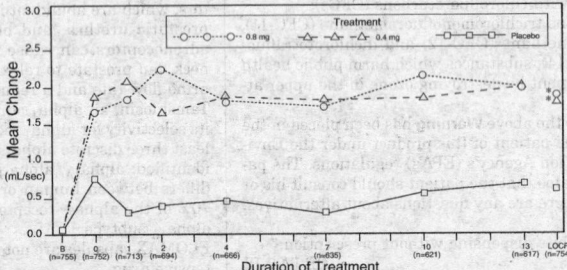

FIGURE 3A:
Mean Increase in Peak Urine Flow Rate (mL/Sec) Study 1

* indicates significant difference from placebo (p-value ≤0.050).
B=Baseline determined approximately one week prior to the initial dose of double-blind medication at Week 0. Subsequent values are observed cases.
LOCF= Last observation carried forward for patients not completing the 13-week study.
Note: The uroflowmetry assessments at week 0 were recorded 4-8 hours after patients received the first dose of double-blind medication.
Measurements at each visit were scheduled 4-8 hours after dosing (approximately peak plasma tamsulosin HCl concentration).
Note: Patients in the 0.8 mg treatment groups received 0.4 for the first week.

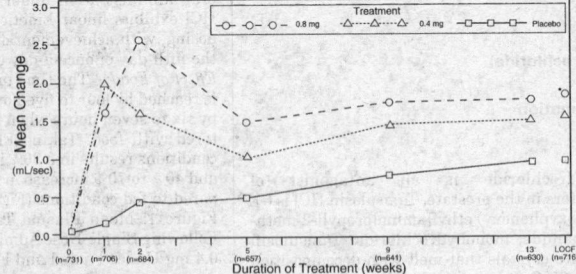

FIGURE 3B:
Mean Increase in Peak Urine Flow Rate (mL/Sec) Study 2

* indicates significant difference from placebo (p-value ≤0.050).
Baseline measurement was taken Week 0. Subsequent values are observed cases.
LOCF=Last observation carried forward for patients not completing the 13-week study.
Note: Patients in the 0.8 mg treatment group received 0.4 mg for the first week.
Note: Week 1 and Week 2 measurements were scheduled 4-8 hours after dosing (approximate peak plasma tamsulosin HCl concentration).
All other visits were scheduled 24-27 hours after dosing (approximate trough tamsulosin HCl concentration).

TABLE 2 MEAN (±S.D.) CHANGES FROM BASELINE TO WEEK 13 IN TOTAL AUA SYMPTOM SCORE ** AND PEAK URINE FLOW RATE (ML/SEC)

	Total AUA Symptom Score		Peak Urine Flow Rate	
	Mean Baseline Value	Mean Change	Mean Baseline Value	Mean Change
Study 1 †				
FLOMAX capsules 0.8 mg once daily	19.9±4.9 n=247	-9.6*±6.7 n=237	9.57±2.51 n=247	1.78*±3.35 n=247
FLOMAX capsules 0.4 mg once daily	19.8±5.0 n=254	-8.3*±6.5 n=246	9.46±2.49 n=254	1.75*±3.57 n=254
Placebo	19.6±4.9 n=254	-5.5±6.6 n=246	9.75±2.54 n=254	0.52±3.39 n=253
Study 2 ‡				
FLOMAX capsules 0.8 mg once daily	18.2±5.6 n=244	-5.8*±6.4 n=238	9.96±3.16 n=244	1.79*±3.36 n=237
FLOMAX capsules 0.4 mg once daily	17.9±5.8 n=248	-5.1*±6.4 n=244	9.94±3.14 n=248	1.52±3.64 n=244
Placebo	19.2±6.0 n=239	-3.6±5.7 n=235	9.95±3.12 n=239	0.93±3.28 n=235

* Statistically significant difference from placebo (p-value ≤0.050; Bonferroni-Holm multiple test procedure);
**Total AUA Symptom Scores ranged from 0 to 35
† Peak urine flow rate measured 4 to 8 hours post dose at week 13
‡ Peak urine flow rate measured 24 to 27 hours post dose at week 13
Week 13: For patients not completing the 13 week study the last observation was carried forward.

TABLE 3. TREATMENT EMERGENT[1] ADVERSE EVENTS OCCURRING IN ≥2% OF FLOMAX CAPSULES OR PLACEBO PATIENTS IN TWO U.S. SHORT-TERM, PLACEBO-CONTROLLED CLINICAL STUDIES

BODY SYSTEM/ ADVERSE EVENT	FLOMAX CAPSULES GROUPS		PLACEBO
	0.4 mg n=502	0.8 mg n=492	n=493
BODY AS A WHOLE			
Headache	97 (19.3%)	104 (21.1%)	99 (20.1%)
Infection	45 (9.0%)	53 (10.8%)	37 (7.5%)
Asthenia	39 (7.8%)	42 (8.5%)	27 (5.5%)
Back Pain	35 (7.0%)	41 (8.3%)	27 (5.5%)
Chest Pain	20 (4.0%)	20 (4.1%)	18 (3.7%)
NERVOUS SYSTEM			
Dizziness	75 (14.9%)	84 (17.1%)	50 (10.1%)
Somnolence	15 (3.0%)	21 (4.3%)	8 (1.6%)
Insomnia	12 (2.4%)	7 (1.4%)	3 (0.6%)
Libido Decreased	5 (1.0%)	10 (2.0%)	6 (1.6%)
RESPIRATORY SYSTEM			
Rhinitis	66 (13.1%)	88 (17.9%)	41 (8.3%)
Pharyngitis	29 (5.8%)	25 (5.1%)	23 (4.7%)
Cough Increased	17 (3.4%)	22 (4.5%)	12 (2.4%)
Sinusitis	11 (2.2%)	18 (3.7%)	8 (1.6%)
DIGESTIVE SYSTEM			
Diarrhea	31 (6.2%)	21 (4.3%)	22 (4.5%)
Nausea	13 (2.6%)	19 (3.9%)	16 (3.2%)
Tooth Disorder	6 (1.2%)	10 (2.0%)	7 (1.4%)
UROGENITAL SYSTEM			
Abnormal Ejaculation	42 (8.4%)	89 (18.1%)	1 (0.2%)
SPECIAL SENSES			
Amblyopia	1 (0.2%)	10 (2.0%)	2 (0.4%)

[1] A treatment-emergent adverse event was defined as any event satisfying one of the following criteria:
• The adverse event occurred for the first time after initial dosing with double-blind study medication.
• The adverse event was present prior to or at the time of initial dosing with double-blind study medication and subsequently increased in severity during double-blind treatment;
or
• The adverse event was present prior to or at the time of initial dosing with double-blind study medication, disappeared completely, and then reappeared during double-blind treatment.

ment groups in a double-blind, placebo controlled, 40 week extension trial (138 patients on 0.4 mg, 135 patients on 0.8 mg and 127 patients on placebo). Three hundred and twenty-three patients (43% of the originally randomized group) completed one year. Of these, 81% (97 patients) on 0.4 mg, 74% (75 patients) on 0.8 mg and 56% (57 patients) on placebo had a response ≥25% above baseline in total AUA Symptom Score at one year.
[See figures 2A, 2B, 3A & 3B on previous page]

INDICATIONS AND USAGE

FLOMAX® (tamsulosin HCl) capsules are indicated for the treatment of the signs and symptoms of benign prostatic hyperplasia (BPH). FLOMAX capsules are not indicated for the treatment of hypertension.

CONTRAINDICATIONS

FLOMAX capsules are contraindicated in patients known to be hypersensitive to tamsulosin HCl or any component of FLOMAX capsules.

WARNINGS

The signs and symptoms of orthostasis (postural hypotension, dizziness and vertigo) were detected more frequently in FLOMAX capsule treated patients than in placebo recipients. As with other alpha-adrenergic blocking agents there is a potential risk of syncope (see ADVERSE REACTIONS). Patients beginning treatment with FLOMAX capsules should be cautioned to avoid situations where injury could result should syncope occur.

PRECAUTIONS

General

1) Carcinoma of the prostate: Carcinoma of the prostate and BPH cause many of the same symptoms. These two diseases frequently co-exist. Patients should be evaluated prior to the start of FLOMAX capsules therapy to rule out the presence of carcinoma of the prostate.
2) Drug-Drug Interactions: The pharmacokinetic and pharmacodynamic interactions between FLOMAX capsules and other alpha-adrenergic blocking agents have not been determined. However, interactions may be expected and FLOMAX capsules should NOT be used in combination with other alpha-adrenergic blocking agents.

The pharmacokinetic interaction between cimetidine and FLOMAX capsules was investigated. The results indicate significant changes in tamsulosin HCl clearance (26% decrease) and AUC (44% increase). Therefore, FLOMAX capsules should be used with caution in combination with cimetidine, particularly at doses higher than 0.4 mg.

Results from limited *in vitro* and *in vivo* drug-drug interaction studies between tamsulosin HCl and warfarin are inconclusive. Therefore, caution should be exercised with concomitant administration of warfarin and FLOMAX capsules.

(See also drug-drug interaction studies in CLINICAL PHARMACOLOGY, Pharmacokinetics subsection.)

Information for Patients (see Patient Package Insert)

Patients should be told about the possible occurrence of symptoms related to postural hypotension such as dizziness when taking FLOMAX capsules, and they should be cautioned about driving, operating machinery or performing hazardous tasks.

Patients should be advised not to crush, chew or open the FLOMAX capsules.

Laboratory Tests

No laboratory test interactions with FLOMAX capsules are known. Treatment with FLOMAX capsules for up to 12 months had no significant effect on prostate-specific antigen (PSA).

Pregnancy Teratogenic Effects, Pregnancy Category B. Administration of tamsulosin HCl to pregnant female rats at dose levels up to 300 mg/kg/day (approximately 50 times the human therapeutic AUC exposure) revealed no evidence of harm to the fetus. Administration of tamsulosin HCl to pregnant rabbits at dose levels up to 50 mg/kg/day produced no evidence of fetal harm. FLOMAX capsules are not indicated for use in women.

Nursing Mothers FLOMAX capsules are not indicated for use in women.

Pediatric Use FLOMAX capsules are not indicated for use in pediatric populations.

Carcinogenesis, Mutagenesis, and Impairment of Fertility
Rats administered doses up to 43 mg/kg/day in males and 52 mg/kg/day in females had no increases in tumor incidence with the exception of a modest increase in the frequency of mammary gland fibroadenomas in female rats receiving doses ≥ 5.4 mg/kg (P < 0.015). The highest doses of tamsulosin HCl evaluated in the rat carcinogenicity study produced systemic exposures (AUC) in rats 3 times the exposures in men receiving the maximum therapeutic dose of 0.8 mg/day.

Mice were administered doses up to 127 mg/kg/day in males and 158 mg/kg/day in females. There were no significant tumor findings in male mice. Female mice treated for 2 years with the two highest doses of 45 and 158 mg/kg/day had statistically significant increases in the incidence of mammary gland fibroadenomas (P< 0.0001) and adenocarcinomas (P< 0.0075). The highest dose levels of tamsulosin HCl evaluated in the mice carcinogenicity study produced systemic exposures (AUC) in mice 8 times the exposures in men receiving the maximum therapeutic dose of 0.8 mg/day.

The increased incidences of mammary gland neoplasms in female rats and mice were considered secondary to tamsulosin HCl-induced hyperprolactinemia. It is not known if FLOMAX capsules elevate prolactin in humans. The relevance for human risk of the findings of prolactin-mediated endocrine tumors in rodents is not known.

Tamsulosin HCl produced no evidence of mutagenic potential *in vitro* in the Ames reverse mutation test, mouse lymphoma thymidine kinase assay, unscheduled DNA repair synthesis assay, and chromosomal aberration assays in Chinese hamster ovary cells or human lymphocytes. There were no mutagenic effects in the *in vivo* sister chromatid exchange and mouse micronucleus assay.

Studies in rats revealed significantly reduced fertility in males dosed with single or multiple daily doses of 300 mg/kg/day of tamsulosin HCl (AUC exposure in rats about 50 times the human exposure with the maximum therapeutic dose). The mechanism of decreased fertility in male rats is considered to be an effect of the compound on the vaginal plug formation possibly due to changes of semen content or impairment of ejaculation. The effects on fertility were reversible showing improvement by 3 days after a single dose and 4 weeks after multiple dosing. Effects on fertility in males were completely reversed within nine weeks of discontinuation of multiple dosing. Multiple doses of 10 and 100 mg/kg/day tamsulosin HCl (1/5 and 16 times the anticipated human AUC exposure) did not significantly alter fertility in male rats. Effects of tamsulosin HCl on sperm counts or sperm function have not been evaluated.

Continued on next page

Flomax—Cont.

Studies in females rats revealed significant reductions in fertility after single or multiple dosing with 300 mg/kg/day of the R-isomer or racemic mixture of tamsulosin HCl, respectively. In female rats, the reductions in fertility after single doses were considered to be associated with impairments in fertilization. Multiple dosing with 10 or 100 mg/kg/day of the racemic mixture did not significantly alter fertility in female rats.

ADVERSE REACTIONS

The incidence of treatment-emergent adverse events has been ascertained from six short-term U.S. and European placebo-controlled clinical trials in which daily doses of 0.1 to 0.8 mg FLOMAX capsules were used. These studies evaluated safety in 1783 patients treated with FLOMAX capsules and 798 patients administered placebo. Table 3 summarizes the treatment-emergent adverse events that occurred in ≥ 2% of patients receiving either FLOMAX capsules 0.4 mg or 0.8 mg and at an incidence numerically higher than that in the placebo group during two 13-week U.S. trials (US92-03A and US93-01) conducted in 1487 men. [See table 3 on previous page]

Signs and Symptoms of Orthostasis In the two U.S. studies, symptomatic postural hypotension was reported by 0.2% of patients (1 of 502) in the 0.4-mg group, 0.4% of patients (2 of 492) in the 0.8-mg group, and by no patients in the placebo group. Syncope was reported by 0.2% of patients (1 of 502) in the 0.4-mg group, 0.4% of patients (2 of 492) in the 0.8-mg group and 0.6% of patients (3 of 493) in the placebo group. Dizziness was reported by 15% of patients (75 of 502) in the 0.4-mg group, 17% of patients (84 of 492) in the 0.8-mg group, and 10% of patients (50 of 493) in the placebo group. Vertigo was reported by 0.6% of patients (3 of 502) in the 0.4-mg group, 1% of patients (5 of 492) in the 0.8 mg group and by 0.6% of patients (3 of 493) in the placebo group.

Multiple testing for orthostatic hypotension was conducted in a number of studies. Such a test was considered positive if it met one or more of the following criteria: (1) a decrease in systolic blood pressure of ≥20 mmHg upon standing from the supine position during the orthostatic tests; (2) a decrease in diastolic blood pressure ≥10 mmHg upon standing, with the standing diastolic blood pressure <65 mmHg during the orthostatic test; (3) an increase in pulse rate of ≥20 bpm upon standing with a standing pulse rate ≥100 bpm during the orthostatic test; and (4) the presence of clinical symptoms (faintness, lightheadedness/lightheaded, dizziness, spinning sensation, vertigo, or postural hypotension) upon standing during the orthostatic test.

Following the first dose of double-blind medication in Study 1, a positive orthostatic test result at 4 hours post-dose was observed in 7% of patients (37 of 498) who received FLOMAX capsules 0.4 mg once daily and in 3% of the patients (8 of 253) who received placebo. At 8 hours post-dose, a positive orthostatic test result was observed for 6% of the patients (31 of 498) who received FLOMAX capsules 0.4 mg once daily and 4% (9 of 250) who received placebo. (Note: patients in the 0.8-mg group received 0.4 mg once daily for the first week of Study 1.)

In Studies 1 and 2, at least one positive orthostatic test result was observed during the course of these studies for 81 of the 502 patients (16%) in the FLOMAX 0.4-mg once daily group, 92 of the 491 patients (19%) in the FLOMAX 0.8-mg once daily group and 54 of the 493 patients (11%) in the placebo group.

Because orthostasis was detected more frequently in FLOMAX capsule-treated patients than in placebo recipients, there is a potential risk of syncope (see WARNINGS).

Abnormal Ejaculation Abnormal ejaculation includes ejaculation failure, ejaculation disorder, retrograde ejaculation and ejaculation decrease. As shown in Table 3, abnormal ejaculation was associated with FLOMAX capsules administration and was dose-related in the U.S. studies. Withdrawal from these clinical studies of FLOMAX capsules because of abnormal ejaculation was also dose-dependent with 8 of 492 patients (1.6%) in the 0.8-mg group, and no patients in the 0.4-mg or placebo groups discontinuing treatment due to abnormal ejaculation.

Post-Marketing Experience Allergic-type reactions such as skin rash, pruritus angioedema of tongue, lips and face and urticaria have been reported with positive rechallenge in some cases.

OVERDOSAGE

Should overdosage of FLOMAX capsules lead to hypotension (See WARNINGS and ADVERSE REACTIONS), support of the cardiovascular system is of first importance. Restoration of blood pressure and normalization of heart rate may be accomplished by keeping the patient in the supine position. If this measure is inadequate, then administration of intravenous fluids should be considered. If necessary, vasopressors should then be used and renal function should be monitored and supported as needed. Laboratory data indicate that tamsulosin HCl is 94% to 99% protein bound; therefore, dialysis is unlikely to be of benefit.

One patient reported an overdose of thirty 0.4-mg FLOMAX capsules. Following the ingestion of the capsules, the patient reported a severe headache.

DOSAGE AND ADMINISTRATION FLOMAX capsules 0.4 mg once daily is recommended as the dose for the treatment of the signs and symptoms of BPH. It should be administered approximately one-half hour following the same meal each day.

For those patients who fail to respond to the 0.4-mg dose after two to four weeks of dosing, the dose of FLOMAX capsules can be increased to 0.8 mg once daily. If FLOMAX capsules administration is discontinued or interrupted for several days at either the 0.4-mg or 0.8-mg dose, therapy should be started again with the 0.4-mg once daily dose.

HOW SUPPLIED: FLOMAX capsules 0.4 mg are supplied in high density polyethylene bottles containing 100 or 1000 hard gelatin capsules with olive green opaque cap and orange opaque body. The capsules are imprinted on one side with "Flomax 0.4 mg" and on the other side with "BI 58."

NDC 0597-0058-01
FLOMAX Capsules
0.4 mg, 100 Capsules
NDC 0597-0058-10
FLOMAX Capsules
0.4 mg, 1000 Capsules

Rx Only

Store at controlled room temperature 20°–25°C (68°–77°F).
Keep FLOMAX capsules and all medicines out of reach of children. FL-PI-4/98

Distributed by: Boehringer Ingelheim Pharmaceuticals, Inc.
Ridgefield, CT 06877, U.S.A.

Licensed from and Manufactured by:
Yamanouchi Pharmaceutical Co., Ltd.
3-11 Nihonbashi-Honcho 2-Chome
Chuo-ku, Tokyo 103, Japan

Shown in Product Identification Guide, page 307

MEXITIL® ℞

[mex' ĭ-til]
(mexiletine hydrochloride, USP)
Oral Antiarrhythmic
Capsules of

150 mg	**BI-CODE 66**
200 mg	**BI-CODE 67**
250 mg	**BI-CODE 68**

Prescribing Information

DESCRIPTION

Mexitil® (mexiletine hydrochloride, USP) is an orally active antiarrhythmic agent available as 150 mg, 200 mg and 250 mg capsules. 100 mg of mexiletine hydrochloride is equivalent to 83.31 mg of mexiletine base. It is a white to off-white crystalline powder with slightly bitter taste, freely soluble in water and in alcohol. Mexitil® has a pKa of 9.2.

Chemically, Mexitil® is 1-methyl-2-(2,6-xylyloxy)ethylamine hydrochloride and has the following structural formula:

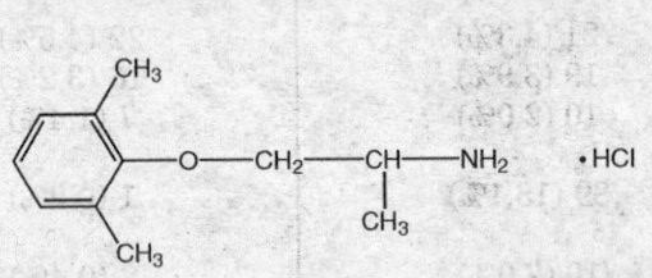

$C_{11}H_{17}NO{\cdot}HCl$ mexiletine hydrochloride, USP
Mol. Wt. 215.73 (Mexitil)

Mexitil® Capsules contain the following inactive ingredients: colloidal silicon dioxide, corn starch, magnesium stearate, titanium dioxide, gelatin, FD&C Red No. 40, D&C Red No. 28, and FD&C Blue No. 1; the Mexitil® 150 mg and 250 mg capsules also contain FD&C Yellow No. 10. Mexitil® capsules may contain one or more of the following components: sodium lauryl sulfate, sodium proprionate, edetate calcium disodium, benzyl alcohol, carboxymethylcellulose sodium, glycerin, butylparaben, propylparaben, methylparaben, pharmaceutical glaze, ethylene glycol monoethylether, soya lecithin, dimethylpolysiloxane, refined shellac (food grade) and other inactive ingredients.

CLINICAL PHARMACOLOGY

Mechanism of Action

Mexitil® (mexiletine hydrochloride, USP) is a local anesthetic, antiarrhythmic agent, structurally similar to lidocaine, but orally active. In animal studies, Mexitil® has been shown to be effective in the suppression of induced ventricular arrhythmias, including those induced by glycoside toxicity and coronary artery ligation. Mexitil®, like lidocaine, inhibits the inward sodium current, thus reducing the rate of rise of the action potential, Phase 0. Mexitil® decreased the effective refractory period (ERP) in Purkinje fibers. The decrease in ERP was of lesser magnitude than the decrease in action potential duration (APD), with a resulting increase in the ERP/APD ratio.

Electrophysiology in Man Mexiletine is a Class 1B antiarrhythmic compound with electrophysiologic properties in man similar to lidocaine, but dissimilar from quinidine, procainamide, and disopyramide.

In patients with normal conduction systems, Mexitil® has a minimal effect on cardiac impulse generation and propagation. In clinical trials, no development of second-degree or third-degree AV block was observed. Mexitil® did not prolong ventricular depolarization (QRS duration) or repolarization (QT intervals) as measured by electrocardiography. Theoretically, therefore, Mexitil® may be useful in the treatment of ventricular arrhythmias associated with a prolonged QT interval.

In patients with pre-existing conduction defects, depression of the sinus rate, prolongation of sinus node recovery time, decreased conduction velocity and increased effective refractory period of the intraventricular conduction system have occasionally been observed.

The antiarrhythmic effect of Mexitil® has been established in controlled comparative trials against placebo, quinidine, procainamide and disopyramide. Mexitil®, at doses of 200–400 mg q8h, produced a significant reduction of ventricular premature beats, paired beats, and episodes of non-sustained ventricular tachycardia compared to placebo and was similar in effectiveness to the active agents. Among all patients entered into the studies, about 30% in each treatment group had a 70% or greater reduction in PVC count and about 40% failed to complete the 3 month studies because of adverse effects. Follow-up of patients from the controlled trials has demonstrated continued effectiveness of mexitil® in long-term use.

Hemodynamics Hemodynamic studies in a limited number of patients, with normal or abnormal myocardial function, following oral administration of Mexitil® have shown small, usually not statistically significant, decreases in cardiac output and increases in systemic vascular resistance, but no significant negative inotropic effect. Blood pressure and pulse rate remain essentially unchanged. Mild depression of myocardial function, similar to that produced by lidocaine, has occasionally been observed following intravenous Mexitil® therapy in patients with cardiac disease.

Pharmacokinetics Mexitil® is well absorbed (~90%) from the gastrointestinal tract. Unlike lidocaine, its first-pass metabolism is low. Peak blood levels are reached in two to three hours. In normal subjects, the plasma elimination half-life of Mexitil® is approximately 10–12 hours. It is 50–60% bound to plasma protein, with a volume of distribution of 5–7 liters/kg. Mexitil® is metabolized in the liver. Approximately 10% is excreted unchanged by the kidney. While urinary pH does not normally have much influence on elimination, marked changes in urinary pH influence the rate of excretion: acidification accelerates excretion, while alkalinization retards it.

Several metabolites of mexiletine have shown minimal antiarrhythmic activity in animal models. The most active is the minor metabolite N-methylmexiletine, which is less than 20% as potent as mexiletine. The urinary excretion of N-methylmexiletine in man is less than 0.5%. Thus the therapeutic activity of Mexitil® is due to the parent compound.

Hepatic impairment prolongs the elimination half-life of Mexitil®. In eight patients with moderate to severe liver disease, the mean half-life was approximately 25 hours.

Consistent with the limited renal elimination of Mexitil®, little change in the half-life has been detected in patients with reduced renal function. In eight patients with creatinine clearance less than 10 ml/min, the mean plasma elimination half-life was 15.7 hours; in seven patients with creatinine clearance between 11–40 ml/min, the mean half-life was 13.4 hours.

The absorption rate of Mexitil® is reduced in clinical situations such as acute myocardial infarction in which gastric emptying time is increased. Narcotics, atropine and magnesium-aluminum hydroxide have also been reported to slow the absorption of Mexitil®. Metoclopramide has been reported to accelerate absorption.

Mexiletine plasma levels of at least 0.5 mcg/ml are generally required for therapeutic response. An increase in the frequency of central nervous system adverse effects has been observed when plasma levels exceed 2.0 mcg/ml. Thus the therapeutic range is approximately 0.5 to 2.0 mcg/ml. Plasma levels within the therapeutic range can be attained with either three times daily or twice daily dosing but peak to trough differences are greater with the latter regimen, creating the possibility of adverse effects at peak and arrhythmic escape at trough. Nevertheless, some patients may be transferred successfully to the twice daily regimen (See DOSAGE AND ADMINISTRATION).

INDICATIONS AND USAGE

Mexitil® is indicated for the treatment of documented ventricular arrhythmias, such as sustained ventricular tachycardia, that, in the judgement of the physician, are life-threatening. Because of the proarrhythmic effects of Mexitil®, its use with lesser arrhythmias is generally not recommended. Treatment of patients with asymptomatic ventricular premature contractions should be avoided.

Initiation of Mexitil® treatment, as with other antiarrhythmic agents used to treat life-threatening arrhythmias, should be carried out in the hospital.

Antiarrhythmic drugs have not been shown to enhance survival in patients with ventricular arrhythmias.

CONTRAINDICATIONS

Mexitil® (mexiletine hydrochloride, USP) is contraindicated in the presence of cardiogenic shock or pre-existing second- or third-degree AV block (if no pacemaker is present).

WARNINGS: Mortality: In the National Heart, Lung and Blood Institute's Cardiac Arrhythmia Suppression Trial (CAST), a long-term, multicentered, randomized, double-blind study in patients with asymptomatic non-life-threatening ventricular arrhythmias who had a myocardial infarction more than six days but less than two years previously, an excessive mortality or non-fatal cardiac arrest rate (7.7%) was seen in patients treated with encainide or flecainide compared with that seen in patients assigned to carefully matched placebo-treated groups (3.0%). The average duration of treatment with encainide or flecainide in this study was ten months.

The applicability of the CAST results to other populations (e.g., those without recent myocardial infarction) is uncertain. Considering the known proarrhythmic properties of Mexitil® and the lack of evidence of improved survival for any antiarrhythmic drug in patients without life-threatening arrhythmias, the use of Mexitil® as well as other antiarrhythmic agents should be reserved for patients with life-threatening ventricular antiarrhythmia.

Acute Liver Injury In postmarketing experience abnormal liver function tests have been reported, some in the first few weeks of therapy with Mexitil® (mexiletine hydrochloride, USP). Most of these have been observed in the setting of congestive heart failure or ischemia and their relationship to Mexitil® has not been established.

PRECAUTIONS

General If a ventricular pacemaker is operative, patients with second or third degree heart block may be treated with Mexitil® (mexiletine hydrochloride, USP) if continuously monitored. A limited number of patients (45 of 475 in controlled clinical trials) with pre-existing first degree AV block were treated with Mexitil®; none of these patients developed second or third degree AV block. Caution should be exercised when it is used in such patients or in patients with pre-existing sinus node dysfunction or intraventricular conduction abnormalities.

Like other antiarrhythmics Mexitil® (mexiletine hydrochloride, USP) can cause worsening of arrhythmias. This has been uncommon in patients with less serious arrhythmias (frequent premature beats or non-sustained ventricular tachycardia: see ADVERSE REACTIONS), but is of greater concern in patients with life-threatening arrhythmias such as sustained ventricular tachycardia. In patients with such arrhythmias subjected to programmed electrical stimulation or to exercise provocation, 10–15% of patients had exacerbation of the arrhythmia, a rate not greater than that of other agents.

Mexitil® should be used with caution in patients with hypotension and severe congestive heart failure because of the potential for aggravating these conditions.

Since Mexitil® is metabolized in the liver, and hepatic impairment has been reported to prolong the elimination half-life of Mexitil®, patients with liver disease should be followed carefully while receiving Mexitil®. The same caution should be observed in patients with hepatic dysfunction secondary to congestive heart failure.

Concurrent drug therapy or dietary regimens which may markedly alter urinary pH should be avoided during Mexitil® therapy. The minor fluctuations in urinary pH associated with normal diet do not affect the excretion of Mexitil®.

SGOT Elevation and Liver Injury: In three-month controlled trials, elevations of SGOT greater than three times the upper limit of normal occurred in about 1% of both mexiletine-treated and control patients. Approximately 2% of patients in the mexiletine compassionate use program had elevations of SGOT greater than or equal to three times the upper limit of normal. These elevations frequently occurred in association with identifiable clinical events and therapeutic measures such as congestive heart failure, acute myocardial infarction, blood transfusions and other medications. These elevations were often asymptomatic and transient, usually not associated with elevated bilirubin levels and usually did not require discontinuation of therapy. Marked elevations of SGOT (>1000 U/L) were seen before death in four patients with end-stage cardiac disease (severe congestive heart failure, cardiogenic shock).

Rare instances of severe liver injury, including hepatic necrosis, have been reported in association with Mexitil® treatment. It is recommended that patients in whom an abnormal liver test has occurred, or who have signs or symptoms suggesting liver dysfunction, be carefully evaluated. If persistent or worsening elevation of hepatic enzymes is detected, consideration should be given to discontinuing therapy.

Blood Dyscrasias: Among 10,867 patients treated with mexiletine in the compassionate use program, marked leukopenia (neutrophils less than 1000/mm^3) or agranulocytosis were seen in 0.06% and milder depressions of leukocytes were seen in 0.08%, and thrombocytopenia was observed in 0.16%. Many of these patients were seriously ill and receiving concomitant medications with known hematologic adverse effects. Rechallenge with mexiletine in several cases was negative. Marked leukopenia or agranulocytosis did not occur in any patient receiving Mexitil® alone; five of the six cases of agranulocytosis were associated with procainamide (sustained release preparations in four) and one with vinblastine. If significant hematologic changes are observed, the patient should be carefully evaluated, and, if warranted, Mexitil® should be discontinued. Blood counts usually return to normal within one month of discontinuation. (See ADVERSE REACTIONS.)

Convulsions (seizures) did not occur in Mexitil® controlled clinical trials. In the compassionate use program, convulsions were reported in about 2 of 1000 patients. Twenty-eight percent of these patients discontinued therapy. Convulsions were reported in patients with and without a prior history of seizures. Mexiletine should be used with caution in patients with known seizure disorder.

Drug Interactions In a large compassionate use program Mexitil® has been used concurrently with commonly employed antianginal, antihypertensive, and anticoagulant drugs without observed interactions. A variety of antiarrhythmics such as quinidine or propranolol were also added, sometimes with improved control of ventricular ectopy. When phenytoin or other hepatic enzyme inducers such as rifampin and phenobarbital have been taken concurrently with Mexitil®, lowered Mexitil® plasma levels have been reported. Monitoring of Mexitil® plasma levels is recommended during such concurrent use to avoid ineffective therapy.

In a formal study, benzodiazepines were shown not to affect Mexitil® plasma concentrations. ECG intervals (PR, QRS and QT) were not affected by concurrent Mexitil® and digoxin, diuretics, or propranolol.

Concurrent administration of cimetidine and Mexitil® has been reported to increase, decrease, or leave unchanged Mexitil® plasma levels; therefore patients should be followed carefully during concurrent therapy.

Mexitil® does not alter serum digoxin levels but magnesium-aluminum hydroxide, when used to treat gastrointestinal symptoms due to Mexitil®, has been reported to lower serum digoxin levels.

Concurrent use of Mexitil® and theophylline may lead to increased plasma theophylline levels. One controlled study in eight normal subjects showed a 72% mean increase (range 35–136%) in plasma theophylline levels. This increase was observed at the first test point which was the second day after starting Mexitil®. Theophylline plasma levels returned to pre-Mexitil® values within 48 hours after discontinuing Mexitil®. If Mexitil® and theophylline are to be used concurrently, theophylline blood levels should be monitored, particularly when the Mexitil® dose is changed. An appropriate adjustment in theophylline dose should be considered.

Additionally, in one controlled study in five normal subjects and seven patients, the clearance of caffeine was decreased 50% following the administration of Mexitil®.

Carcinogenesis, Mutagenesis and Impairment of Fertility Studies of carcinogenesis in rats (24 months) and mice (18 months) did not demonstrate any tumorigenic potential. Mexitil® was found to be non-mutagenic in the Ames test. Mexitil® did not impair fertility in the rat.

Pregnancy/Teratogenic Effects *PREGNANCY CATEGORY C:* Reproduction studies performed with Mexitil® (mexiletine hydrochloride, USP) in rats, mice and rabbits at doses up to four times the maximum human oral dose (24 mg/kg in a 50 kg patient) revealed no evidence of teratogenicity or impaired fertility but did show an increase in fetal resorption. There are no adequate and well-controlled studies in pregnant women; this drug should be used in pregnancy only if the potential benefit justifies the potential risk to the fetus.

Nursing Mothers Mexitil® appears in human milk in concentrations similar to those observed in plasma. Therefore, if the use of Mexitil® is deemed essential, an alternative method of infant feeding should be considered.

Pediatric Use Safety and effectiveness in the pediatric population have not been established.

ADVERSE REACTIONS

Mexitil® (mexiletine hydrochloride, USP) commonly produces reversible gastrointestinal and nervous system adverse reactions but is otherwise well tolerated. Mexitil® has been evaluated in 483 patients in one-month and three-

COMPARATIVE INCIDENCE (%) OF ADVERSE EVENTS AMONG PATIENTS TREATED WITH MEXILETINE OR CONTROL DRUGS IN THE 12-WEEK, DOUBLE-BLIND TRIALS

	Mexiletine N = 430	Quinidine N = 262	Procainamide N = 78	Disopyramide N = 69
Cardiovascular				
Palpitations	4.3	4.6	1.3	5.8
Chest Pain	2.6	3.4	1.3	2.9
Angina/Angina-like Pain	1.7	1.9	2.6	2.9
Increased Ventricular Arrhythmias/PVC's	1.0	2.7	2.6	—
Digestive				
Nausea/Vomiting/Heartburn	39.3	21.4	33.3	14.5
Diarrhea	5.2	33.2	2.6	8.7
Constipation	4.0	—	6.4	11.6
Changes in Appetite	2.6	1.9	—	—
Abdominal Pain/Cramps/Discomfort	1.2	1.5	—	1.4
Central Nervous System				
Dizziness/Lightheadedness	18.9	14.1	14.1	2.9
Tremor	13.2	2.3	3.8	1.4
Coordination Difficulties	9.7	1.1	1.3	—
Changes in Sleep Habits	7.1	2.7	11.5	8.7
Weakness	5.0	5.3	7.7	2.9
Nervousness	5.0	1.9	6.4	5.8
Fatigue	3.8	5.7	5.1	1.4
Speech Difficulties	2.6	0.4	—	—
Confusion/Clouded Sensorium	2.6	—	3.8	—
Paresthesias/Numbness	2.4	2.3	2.6	—
Tinnitus	2.4	1.5	—	—
Depression	2.4	1.1	1.3	1.4
Other				
Blurred Vision/Visual Disturbances	5.7	3.1	5.1	7.2
Headache	5.7	6.9	7.7	4.3
Rash	4.2	3.8	10.3	1.4
Dyspnea/Respiratory	3.3	3.1	5.1	2.9
Dry Mouth	2.8	1.9	5.1	14.5
Arthralgia	1.7	2.3	5.1	1.4
Fever	1.2	3.1	2.6	—

Continued on next page

Mexitil—Cont.

month controlled studies and in over 10,000 patients in a large compassionate use program. Dosages in the controlled studies ranged from 600–1200 mg/day; some patients (8%) in the compassionate use program were treated with higher daily doses (1600–3200 mg/day). In the three-month controlled trials comparing Mexitil® to quinidine, procainamide and disopyramide, the most frequent adverse reactions were upper gastrointestinal distress (41%), lightheadedness (10.5%), tremor (12.6%) and coordination difficulties (10.2%). Similar frequency and incidence were observed in the one-month placebo-controlled trial. Although these reactions were generally not serious, and were dose-related and reversible with a reduction in dosage, by taking the drug with food or antacid or by therapy discontinuation, they led to therapy discontinuation in 40% of patients in the controlled trials. A tabulation of the adverse events reported in the one-month placebo-controlled trial follows:

COMPARATIVE INCIDENCE (%) OF ADVERSE EVENTS AMONG PATIENTS TREATED WITH MEXILETINE AND PLACEBO IN THE 4-WEEK, DOUBLE-BLIND CROSSOVER TRIAL

	Mexiletine N = 53	Placebo N = 49
Cardiovascular		
Palpitations	7.5	10.2
Chest Pain	7.5	4.1
Increased Ventricular Arrhythmias/PVC's	1.9	—
Digestive		
Nausea/Vomiting/Heartburn	39.6	6.1
Central Nervous System		
Dizziness/ Lightheadedness	26.4	14.3
Tremor	13.2	—
Nervousness	11.3	6.1
Coordination Difficulties	9.4	—
Changes in Sleep Habits	7.5	16.3
Paresthesias/Numbness	3.8	2.0
Weakness	1.9	4.1
Fatigue	1.9	2.0
Tinnitus	1.9	4.1
Confusion/ Clouded Sensorium	1.9	2.0
Other		
Headache	7.5	6.1
Blurred Vision/Visual Disturbances	7.5	2.0
Dyspnea/Respiratory	5.7	10.2
Rash	3.8	2.0
Non-specific Edema	3.8	—

A tabulation of adverse reactions occurring in one percent or more of patients in the three-month controlled studies follows:

[See table at top of previous page]

Less than 1%: Syncope, edema, hot flashes, hypertension, short-term memory loss, loss of consciousness, other psychological changes, diaphoresis, urinary hesitancy/retention, malaise, impotence/decreased libido, pharyngitis, congestive heart failure.

An additional group of over 10,000 patients has been treated in a program allowing administration of Mexitil® (mexiletine hydrochloride, USP) under compassionate use circumstances. These patients were seriously ill with the large majority on multiple drug therapy. Twenty-four percent of the patients continued in the program for one year or longer. Adverse reactions leading to therapy discontinuation occurred in 15 percent of patients (usually upper gastrointestinal system or nervous system effects). In general, the more common adverse reactions were similar to those in the controlled trials. Less common adverse events possibly related to Mexitil® use include:

Cardiovascular System: Syncope and hypotension, each about 6 in 1000; bradycardia, about 4 in 1000; angina/angina-like pain, about 3 in 1000; edema, atrioventricular block/conduction disturbances and hot flashes, each about 2 in 1000; atrial arrhythmias, hypertension and cardiogenic shock, each about 1 in 1000.

Central Nervous System: Short-term memory loss, about 9 in 1000 patients; hallucinations and other psychological changes, each about 3 in 1000; psychosis and convulsions/seizures, each about 2 in 1000; loss of consciousness, about 6 in 10,000.

Digestive: Dysphagia, about 2 in 1000; peptic ulcer, about 8 in 10,000; upper gastrointestinal bleeding, about 7 in 10,000; esophageal ulceration, about 1 in 10,000. Rare cases of severe hepatitis/acute hepatic necrosis.

Skin: Rare cases of exfoliative dermatitis and Stevens-Johnson Syndrome with Mexitil® (mexiletine hydrochloride, USP) treatment have been reported.

Laboratory: Abnormal liver function tests, about 5 in 1000 patients; positive ANA and thrombocytopenia, each about 2 in 1000; leukopenia (including neutropenia and agranulocytosis), about 1 in 1000; myelofibrosis, about 2 in 10,000 patients.

Other: Diaphoresis, about 6 in 1000; altered taste, about 5 in 1000; salivary changes, hair loss and impotence/decreased libido, each about 4 in 1000; malaise, about 3 in 1000; urinary hesitancy/retention, each about 2 in 1000; hiccups, dry skin, laryngeal and pharyngeal changes and changes in oral mucous membranes, each about 1 in 1000; SLE syndrome, about 4 in 10,000.

Hematology: Blood dyscrasias were not seen in the controlled trials but did occur among the 10,867 patients treated with mexiletine in the compassionate use program (see PRECAUTIONS).

Myelofibrosis was reported in two patients in the compassionate use program: one was receiving long-term thiotepa therapy and the other had pretreatment myeloid abnormalities.

In postmarketing experience, there have been isolated, spontaneous reports of pulmonary changes including pulmonary fibrosis during Mexitil® therapy with or without other drugs or diseases that are known to produce pulmonary toxicity. A causal relationship to Mexitil® therapy has not been established. In addition, there have been isolated reports of exacerbation of congestive heart failure in patients with pre-existing compromised ventricular function. There have been rare reports of pancreatitis associated with Mexitil® treatment.

OVERDOSAGE

Clinical findings associated with Mexitil® overdosage have included nausea, hypotension, sinus bradycardia, paresthesia, seizures, bundle branch block, AV heart block, asystole, ventricular tachyarrhythmia, including ventricular fibrillation, cardiovascular collapse and coma. The lowest known dose in a fatality case was 4.4g with postmortem serum mexiletine level of 34–37 mcg/ml (Jequier P. et al. Lancet 1976: 1 (7956): 429). Patients have recovered from ingestion of 4g to 18g of mexiletine (Frank S.E. et al. *Am J Emerg Med* 1991: 9:43–48).

There is no specific antidote for Mexitil®. Management of Mexitil® overdosage includes general supportive measures, close observation and monitoring of vital signs. In addition, the use of pharmacologic interventions (e.g., pressor agents, atropine or anticonvulsants) or transvenous cardiac pacing is suggested, depending on the patient's clinical condition.

DOSAGE AND ADMINISTRATION

The dosage of Mexitil® (mexiletine hydrochloride, USP) must be individualized on the basis of response and tolerance, both of which are dose-related. Administration with food or antacid is recommended. Initiate Mexitil® therapy with 200 mg every eight hours when rapid control of arrhythmia is not essential. A minimum of two to three days between dose adjustments is recommended. Dose may be adjusted in 50 or 100 mg increments up or down.

As with any antiarrhythmic drug, clinical and electrocardiographic evaluation (including Holter monitoring if necessary for evaluation) are needed to determine whether the desired antiarrhythmic effect has been obtained and to guide titration and dose adjustment.

Satisfactory control can be achieved in most patients by 200 to 300 mg given every eight hours with food or antacid. If satisfactory response has not been achieved at 300 mg q8h, and the patient tolerates Mexitil® well, a dose of 400 mg q8h may be tried. As the severity of CNS side effects increases with total daily dose, the dose should not exceed 1200 mg/day.

In general, patients with renal failure will require the usual doses of Mexitil®. Patients with severe liver disease, however, may require lower doses and must be monitored closely. Similarly, marked right-sided congestive heart failure can reduce hepatic metabolism and reduce the needed dose. Plasma level may also be affected by certain concomitant drugs (see PRECAUTIONS: Drug Interactions).

Loading Dose: When rapid control of ventricular arrhythmia is essential, an initial loading dose of 400 mg of Mexitil® may be administered, followed by a 200 mg dose in eight hours. Onset of therapeutic effect is usually observed within 30 minutes to two hours.

Q12H Dosage Schedule: Some patients responding to Mexitil® may be transferred to a 12-hour dosage schedule to improve convenience and compliance. If adequate suppression is achieved on a Mexitil® dose of 300 mg or less every eight hours, the same total daily dose may be given in divided doses every 12 hours while carefully monitoring the degree of suppression of ventricular ectopy. This dose may be adjusted up to a maximum of 450 mg every 12 hours to achieve the desired response.

Transferring to Mexitil: The following dosage schedule, based on theoretical considerations rather than experimental data, is suggested for transferring patients from other Class I oral antiarrhythmic agents to Mexitil®: Mexitil® treatment may be initiated with a 200 mg dose, and titrated to response as described above, 6–12 hours after the last dose of quinidine sulfate, 3–6 hours after the last dose of procainamide, 6–12 hours after the last dose of disopyramide or 8–12 hours after the last dose of tocainide.

In patients in whom withdrawal of the previous antiarrhythmic agent is likely to produce life-threatening arrhythmias, hospitalization of the patient is recommended.

When transferring from lidocaine to Mexitil®, the lidocaine infusion should be stopped when the first oral dose of Mexitil® is administered. The infusion line should be left open until suppression of the arrhythmia appears to be satisfactorily maintained. Consideration should be given to the similarity of the adverse effects of lidocaine and Mexitil® and the possibility that they may be additive.

HOW SUPPLIED

Mexitil® (mexiletine hydrochloride, USP) is supplied in hard gelatin capsules containing 150 mg, 200 mg or 250 mg of mexiletine hydrochloride:

Mexitil® 150 mg capsules are red and caramel with the marking BI 66. Available in bottles of 100 (NDC 0597-0066-01) and individually blister-sealed unit-dose cartons of 100 (NDC 0597-0066-61).

Mexitil® 200 mg capsules are red with the marking BI 67. Available in bottles of 100 (NDC 0597-0067-01) and individually blister-sealed unit-dose cartons of 100 (NDC 0597-0067-61).

Mexitil® 250 mg capsules are red and aqua green with the marking BI 68. Available in bottles of 100 (NDC 0597-0068-01) and individually blister-sealed unit-dose cartons of 100 (NDC 0597-0068-61).

Store at room temperature 20–25°C (68–77°F).

Caution: Federal law prohibits dispensing without prescription.

ME-PI-7/96 Rev.

Boehringer Ingelheim
Pharmaceuticals, Inc.
Ridgefield, Connecticut 06877
Licensed from
Boehringer Ingelheim
International GmbH

Shown in Product Identification Guide, page 307

PERSANTINE® ℞

[per-san 'tēn]
(dipyridamole USP)

Tablets of 25 mg .... BI-CODE 17
Tablets of 50 mg .... BI-CODE 18
Tablets of 75 mg .... BI-CODE 19

Prescribing Information

DESCRIPTION

Persantine® (dipyridamole USP) is a platelet inhibitor chemically described as 2,6-bis-(diethanolamino)-4,8-dipiperidino-pyrimido-(5,4-d) pyrimidine. It has the following structural formula:

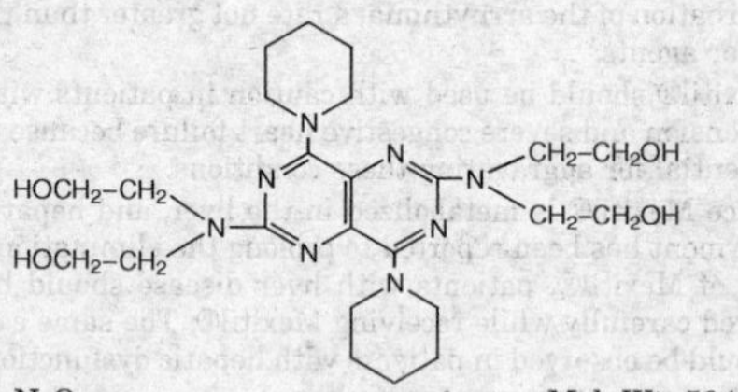

$C_{24}H_{40}N_8O_4$ Mol. Wt. 504.63

Dipyridamole is an odorless yellow crystalline powder, having a bitter taste. It is soluble in dilute acids, methanol and chloroform, and practically insoluble in water.

Persantine tablets for oral administration contain:

Active Ingredient: *TABLETS 25, 50 and 75 mg:* dipyridamole USP 25, 50 and 75 mg respectively.

Inactive Ingredients: *TABLETS 25, 50 and 75 mg:* acacia, carnauba wax, cornstarch, FD&C blue No. 1 aluminum lake, D&C yellow No. 10 aluminum lake, D&C red No. 30 aluminum lake, lactose, magnesium stearate, polyethylene glycol, povidone, shellac, sodium benzoate, sucrose, talc, titanium dioxide, white wax.

CLINICAL PHARMACOLOGY

It is believed that platelet reactivity and interaction with prosthetic cardiac valve surfaces, resulting in abnormally shortened platelet survival time, is a significant factor in thromboembolic complications occurring in connection with prosthetic heart valve replacement.

Persantine® (dipyridamole USP) has been found to lengthen abnormally shortened platelet survival time in a dose-dependent manner.

In three randomized controlled clinical trials involving 854 patients who had undergone surgical placement of a prosthetic heart valve, Persantine, in combination with warfa-

rin, decreased the incidence of postoperative thromboembolic events by 62% to 91% compared to warfarin treatment alone. The incidence of thromboembolic events in patients receiving the combination of Persantine and warfarin ranged from 1.2% to 1.8%. In three additional studies involving 392 patients taking Persantine and coumarin-like anticoagulants, the incidence of thromboembolic events ranged from 2.3% to 6.9%.

In these trials, the coumarin anticoagulant was begun between 24 hours and 4 days postoperatively, and the Persantine® (dipyridamole USP) was begun between 24 hours and 10 days postoperatively. The length of follow-up in these trials varied from 1 to 2 years.

Persantine does not influence prothrombin time or activity measurements when administered with warfarin.

Mechanism of Action: Persantine is a platelet adhesion inhibitor, although the mechanism of action has not been fully elucidated. The mechanism may relate to inhibition of red blood cell uptake of adenosine, itself an inhibitor of platelet reactivity, phosphodiesterase inhibition leading to increased cyclic-3', 5'-adenosine monophosphate within platelets, and inhibition of thromboxane A_2 formation, which is a potent stimulator of platelet activation.

Hemodynamics: In dogs intraduodenal doses of Persantine of 0.5 to 4.0 mg/kg produced dose-related decreases in systemic and coronary vascular resistance leading to decreases in systemic blood pressure and increases in coronary blood flow. Onset of action was in about 24 minutes and effects persisted for about 3 hours.

Similar effects were observed following IV Persantine in doses ranging from 0.025 to 2.0 mg/kg.

In man the same qualitative hemodynamic effects have been observed. However, acute intravenous administration of Persantine may worsen regional myocardial perfusion distal to partial occlusion of coronary arteries.

Pharmacokinetics and Metabolism: Following an oral dose of Persantine, the average time to peak concentration is about 75 minutes. The decline in plasma concentration following a dose of Persantine fits a two-compartment model. The alpha half-life (the initial decline following peak concentration) is approximately 40 minutes. The beta half-life (the terminal decline in plasma concentration) is approximately 10 hours. Persantine is highly bound to plasma proteins. It is metabolized in the liver where it is conjugated as a glucuronide and excreted with the bile.

INDICATIONS AND USAGE

Persantine® (dipyridamole USP) is indicated as an adjunct to coumarin anticoagulants in the prevention of postoperative thromboembolic complications of cardiac valve replacement.

CONTRAINDICATIONS

None known.

PRECAUTIONS

General: Persantine® (dipyridamole USP) should be used with caution in patients with hypotension since it can produce peripheral vasodilation.

Carcinogenesis, Mutagenesis, Impairment of Fertility: In a 111 week oral study in mice and in a 128-142 week oral study in rats, Persantine® (dipyridamole USP) produced no significant carcinogenic effects at doses of 8, 25 and 75 mg/kg (1, 3.1 and 9.4 times the maximum recommended daily human dose). Mutagenicity testing with Persantine was negative. Reproduction studies with Persantine revealed no evidence of impaired fertility in rats at dosages up to 60 times the maximum recommended human dose. A significant reduction in number of corpora lutea with consequent reduction in implantations and live fetuses was, however, observed at 155 times the maximum recommended human dose.

Teratogenic Effects: *PREGNANCY CATEGORY B.* Reproduction studies have been performed in mice at doses up to 125 mg/kg (15.6 times the maximum recommended daily human dose), rats at doses up to 1000 mg/kg (125 times the maximum recommended daily human dose) and rabbits at doses up to 40 mg/kg (5 times the maximum recommended daily human dose) and have revealed no evidence of harm to the fetus due to Persantine. There are, however, no adequate and well-controlled studies in pregnant women. Because animal reproduction studies are not always predictive of human response, this drug should be used during pregnancy only if clearly needed.

Nursing Mothers: As dipyridamole is excreted in human milk, caution should be exercised when Persantine is administered to a nursing woman.

Pediatric Use: Safety and effectiveness in the pediatric population below the age of 12 years has not been established.

ADVERSE REACTIONS

Adverse reactions at therapeutic doses are usually minimal and transient. On long-term use of Persantine® (dipyridamole USP) initial side effects usually disappear. The following reactions were reported in two heart valve replacement trials comparing Persantine and warfarin therapy to either warfarin alone or warfarin and placebo:

	Persantine/ Warfarin (N=147)	Placebo/ Warfarin (N=170)
Dizziness	13.6%	8.2%
Abdominal distress	6.1%	3.5%
Headache	2.3%	0.0
Rash	2.3%	1.1%

Other reactions from uncontrolled studies include diarrhea, vomiting, flushing and pruritus. In addition, angina pectoris has been reported rarely and there have been rare reports of liver dysfunction. On those uncommon occasions when adverse reactions have been persistent or intolerable, they have ceased on withdrawal of the medication.

When Persantine® (dipyridamole USP) was administered concomitantly with warfarin, bleeding was no greater in frequency or severity than that observed when warfarin was administered alone.

OVERDOSAGE

Hypotension, if it occurs, is likely to be of short duration, but a vasopressor drug may be used if necessary. The oral LD_{50} in mice is 2,150 mg/kg. Single oral doses of 6,000 mg/kg in rats and 350 mg/kg in dogs were lethal. Symptoms of acute toxicity included ataxia, decreased locomotion and diarrhea in rodents and emesis, ataxia and depression in dogs. Since Persantine® (dipyridamole USP) is highly protein bound, dialysis is not likely to be of benefit.

DOSAGE AND ADMINISTRATION

Adjunctive Use in Prophylaxis of Thromboembolism after Cardiac Valve Replacement. The recommended dose is 75-100 mg four times daily as an adjunct to the usual warfarin therapy. Please note that aspirin is not to be administered concomitantly with coumarin anticoagulants.

HOW SUPPLIED

Persantine® (dipyridamole USP) is available as round, orange, sugar-coated tablets of 25 mg, 50 mg and 75 mg coded BI/17, BI/18 and BI/19 respectively.

They are available in the following package sizes:

25 mg Tablets	
Bottles of 100	(NDC 0597-0017-01)
Bottles of 1000	(NDC 0597-0017-10)
Unit Dose Packages of 100	(NDC 0597-0017-61)
50 mg Tablets	
Bottles of 100	(NDC 0597-0018-01)
Bottles of 1000	(NDC 0597-0018-10)
Unit Dose Packages of 100	(NDC 0597-0018-61)
75 mg Tablets	
Bottles of 100	(NDC 0597-0019-01)
Bottles of 500	(NDC 0597-0019-05)
Unit Dose Packages of 100	(NDC 0597-0019-61)

Store below 86°F (30°C).

Caution: Federal law prohibits dispensing without prescription.

PE-PI-4/95 Rev

Boehringer Ingelheim
Pharmaceuticals, Inc.
Ridgefield, CT 06877

Licensed from
Boehringer Ingelheim
International GmbH

Shown in Product Identification Guide, page 307

PRELU-2® Ⓒ℞

[pra´lu (2)]
(phendimetrazine tartrate)
Timed Release Capsules .... BI-CODE 64
105 mg

DESCRIPTION

Chemical name: phendimetrazine tartrate (+) 3, 4 dimethyl-2-phenylmorpholine tartrate. Phendimetrazine tartrate is a white, odorless powder with a bitter taste. It is soluble in water, methanol and ethanol. It has a molecular weight of 341, and has the following molecular structure:

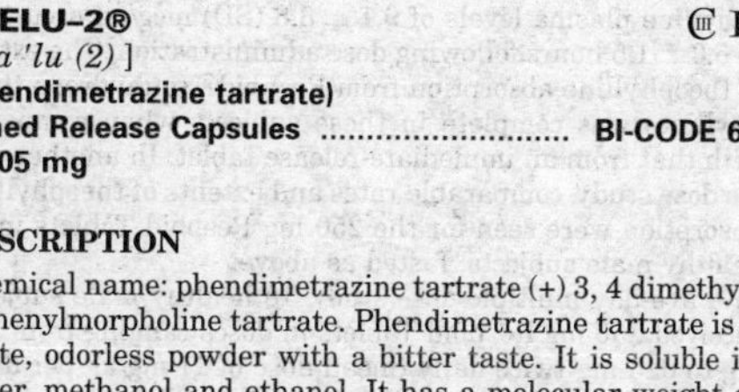

d-3, 4-dimethyl-2-phenylmorpholine tartrate

The capsule is manufactured in a special base which is designed for prolonged release.

Active Ingredient: Each timed-release capsule contains phendimetrazine tartrate 105 mg.

Inactive Ingredients: D&C Red No. 33, D&C Yellow No. 10, FD&C Blue No. 1, FD&C Yellow No. 6, gelatin, povidone, shellac, silica gel, starch, sucrose, talc, titanium dioxide.

CLINICAL PHARMACOLOGY

Phendimetrazine tartrate is a sympathomimetic amine with pharmacologic activity similar to the prototype of drugs of this class used in obesity, the amphetamines. Actions include central nervous system stimulation and elevation of blood pressure. Tachyphylaxis and tolerance have been demonstrated with all drugs of this class in which these phenomena have been looked for.

Drugs of this class used in obesity are commonly known as 'anorectics' or 'anorexigenics.' It has not been established, however, that the action of such drugs in treating obesity is primarily one of appetite suppression. Other central nervous system actions, or metabolic effects, may be involved, for example.

Adult obese subjects instructed in dietary management and treated with 'anorectic' drugs lose more weight on the average than those treated with placebo and diet, as determined in relatively short-term clinical trials.

The magnitude of increased weight loss of drug-treated patients over placebo-treated patients is only a fraction of a pound a week. The rate of weight loss is greatest in the first weeks of therapy for both drug and placebo subjects and tends to decrease in succeeding weeks. The possible origins of the increased weight loss due to the various drug effects are not established. The amount of weight loss associated with the use of an 'anorectic' drug varies from trial to trial, and the increased weight loss appears to be related in part to variables other than the drug prescribed, such as the physician-investigator, the population treated, and the diet prescribed. Studies do not permit conclusions as to the relative importance of the drug and non-drug factors on weight loss.

The natural history of obesity is measured in years, whereas the studies cited are restricted to a few weeks duration; thus, the total impact of drug-induced weight loss over that of diet alone must be considered clinically limited.

The active drug, 105 mg of phendimetrazine tartrate in each capsule of this special timed release dosage form approximates the action of three 35 mg non-timed doses taken at four-hour intervals.

The major route of elimination is via the kidneys where most of the drug and metabolites are excreted. Some of the drug is metabolized to phenmetrazine and also phendimetrazine-N-oxide.

The average half-life of elimination when studied under controlled conditions is about 3.7 hours for both the timed and non-timed forms. The absorption half-life of the drug from conventional non-timed 35 mg phendimetrazine tablets is appreciably more rapid than the absorption rate of the drug from the timed release formulation.

INDICATIONS AND USAGE

Phendimetrazine tartrate is indicated in the management of exogenous obesity as a short term adjunct (a few weeks) in a regimen of weight reduction based on caloric restriction. The limited usefulness of agents of this class (see Clinical Pharmacology) should be measured against possible risk factors inherent in their use such as those described below.

CONTRAINDICATIONS

Advanced arteriosclerosis, symptomatic cardiovascular disease, moderate to severe hypertension, hyperthyroidism, known hypersensitivity, or idiosyncrasy to the sympathomimetic amines, glaucoma.

Agitated states.

Patients with a history of drug abuse.

During or within 14 days following the administration of monoamine oxidase inhibitors (hypertensive crises may result).

WARNINGS

Tolerance to the anorectic effect usually develops within a few weeks. When this occurs, the recommended dose should not be exceeded in an attempt to increase the effect; rather, the drug should be discontinued.

Phendimetrazine tartrate may impair the ability of the patient to engage in potentially hazardous activities such as operating machinery or driving a motor vehicle; the patient should therefore be cautioned accordingly.

DRUG DEPENDENCE

Phendimetrazine tartrate is related chemically and pharmacologically to the amphetamines. Amphetamines and related stimulant drugs have been extensively abused, and the possibility of abuse of phendimetrazine tartrate should be kept in mind when evaluating the desirability of including a drug as part of a weight reduction program. Abuse of amphetamines and related drugs may be associated with intense psychological dependence and severe social dysfunc-

Continued on next page

Prelu-2—Cont.

tion. There are reports of patients who have increased the dosage to many times that recommended. Abrupt cessation following prolonged high dosage administration results in extreme fatigue and mental depression; changes are also noted on the sleep EEG. Manifestations of chronic intoxication with anorectic drugs include severe dermatosis, marked insomnia, irritability, hyperactivity, and personality changes. The most severe manifestation of chronic intoxications is psychosis, often clinically indistinguishable from schizophrenia.

Usage in Pregnancy: The safety of phendimetrazine tartrate in pregnancy and lactation has not been established. Therefore phendimetrazine tartrate should not be taken by women who are or may become pregnant.

Pediatric Use: Phendimetrazine tartrate is not recommended for use in the pediatric population under 12 years of age.

PRECAUTIONS

Caution is to be exercised in prescribing phendimetrazine tartrate for patients with even mild hypertension.

Insulin requirements in diabetes mellitus may be altered in association with the use of phendimetrazine tartrate and the concomitant dietary regimen.

Phendimetrazine tartrate may decrease the hypotensive effect of guanethidine.

The least amount feasible should be prescribed or dispensed at one time in order to minimize the possibility of overdosage.

ADVERSE REACTIONS

Cardiovascular: Palpitation, tachycardia, elevation of blood pressure.

Central Nervous System: Overstimulation, restlessness, dizziness, insomnia, euphoria, dysphoria, tremor, headache; rarely psychotic episodes at recommended doses.

Gastrointestinal: Dryness of the mouth, unpleasant taste, diarrhea, constipation, other gastrointestinal disturbances.

Allergic: Urticaria.

Endocrine: Impotence, changes in libido.

OVERDOSAGE

Manifestations of acute overdosage with phendimetrazine tartrate include restlessness, tremor, hyperreflexia, rapid respiration, confusion, assaultiveness, hallucinations, panic states.

Fatigue and depression usually follow the central stimulation.

Cardiovascular effects include arrhythmias, hypertension or hypotension and circulatory collapse. Gastrointestinal symptoms include nausea, vomiting, diarrhea, and abdominal cramps. Fatal poisoning usually terminates in convulsions and coma. Management of acute phendimetrazine tartrate intoxication is largely symptomatic and includes lavage and sedation with a barbiturate. Experience with hemodialysis or peritoneal dialysis is inadequate to permit recommendation in this regard. Acidification of the urine increases phendimetrazine tartrate excretion. Intravenous phentolamine (Regitine) has been suggested for possible acute, severe hypertension, if this complicates phendimetrazine tartrate overdosage.

DOSAGE AND ADMINISTRATION

Since this product is a timed release dosage form, limit to one timed release capsule (105 mg phendimetrazine tartrate) in the morning.

Phendimetrazine tartrate is not recommended for use in children under 12 years of age.

HOW SUPPLIED

105 mg capsules (celery and green) in bottles of 100.

Store at controlled room temperature 15°–30°C (59°–86°F).

Federal law prohibits dispensing without prescription.

P2-PI-10/93 Rev.

Distributed by
Boehringer Ingelheim
Pharmaceuticals, Inc.
Ridgefield, CT 06877
Manufactured by
Eon Labs Manufacturing, Inc.
Laurelton, NY 11413

Shown in Product Identification Guide, page 307

RESPBID® ℞

[*resp 'bid*]

(anhydrous theophylline, sustained release)

TABLETS

250 mg .... **BI-CODE 48**

500 mg .... **BI-CODE 49**

Oral Bronchodilator

Prescribing Information

DESCRIPTION

Theophylline is a bronchodilator structurally classified as a xanthine derivative. It occurs as a white, odorless, crystalline powder having a bitter taste. Theophylline anhydrous has the chemical name, 1*H*-Purine-2, 6-dione, 3,7-dihydro-1,3-dimethyl-, and is represented by the following structural formula:

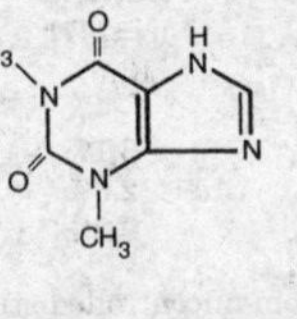

$C_7H_8N_4O_2$ Molecular Weight 180.17

Respbid® (anhydrous theophylline) Tablets contain 250 or 500 mg theophylline anhydrous, in a sustained-release formulation for oral administration. Respbid Tablets also contain: cellulose acetate phthalate, lactose, and magnesium stearate.

CLINICAL PHARMACOLOGY

Theophylline directly relaxes the smooth muscle of the bronchial airways and pulmonary blood vessels, thus acting mainly as a bronchodilator and smooth muscle relaxant. It has also been demonstrated that aminophylline has a potent effect on diaphragmatic contractility in normal persons and may then be capable of reducing fatigability and thereby improve contractility in patients with chronic obstructive airways disease. The exact mode of action remains unsettled. Although theophylline does cause inhibition of phosphodiesterase with a resultant increase in intracellular cyclic AMP, other agents similarly inhibit the enzyme producing a rise of cyclic AMP but are unassociated with any demonstrable bronchodilation. Other mechanisms proposed include an effect on translocation of intracellular calcium; prostaglandin antagonism; stimulation of catecholamines endogenously; inhibition of cyclic guanosine monophosphate metabolism and adenosine receptor antagonism. None of these mechanisms has been proved, however.

In vitro, theophylline has been shown to act synergistically with beta agonists and there are now available data which do demonstrate an additive effect *in vivo* with combined use.

Pharmacokinetics: The half-life of theophylline is influenced by a number of known variables. It may be prolonged in chronic alcoholics, particularly those with liver disease (cirrhosis or alcoholic liver disease), in patients with congestive heart failure, and in those patients taking certain other drugs (see PRECAUTIONS, Drug Interactions). Newborns and neonates have extremely slow clearance rates compared to older infants and children, i.e., those over 1 year. Older children have rapid clearance rates while most nonsmoking adults have clearance rates between these two extremes. In premature neonates clearance is related to oxidative pathways that have yet to be established.

Theophylline Elimination Characteristics

	Half-Life (in Hours) Range	Mean
Children	1–9	3.7
Adults	3–15	7.7

In cigarette smokers (1–2 packs/day) the mean half-life is 4–5 hours, much shorter than in nonsmokers. The increase in clearance associated with smoking is presumably due to stimulation of the hepatic metabolic pathway by components of cigarette smoke. The duration of this effect after cessation of smoking is unknown but may require 6 months to 2 years before the rate approaches that of the nonsmoker.

A single 500 mg dose of Respbid® (anhydrous theophylline) in 8 healthy male subjects fasted for 10 hours predose (overnight) through 4 hours postdose resulted in mean peak theophylline plasma levels of 9.1 ± 3.8 (SD) mcg/ml occurring at 5.0 ± 1.5 hours following dose administration. The extent of theophylline absorption from Respbid® (anhydrous theophylline) was complete in these subjects when compared with that from an immediate-release tablet. In another single dose study, comparable rates and extents of theophylline absorption were seen for the 250 mg Respbid Tablets in 18 healthy male subjects, fasted as above.

In a five-day multiple-dose study, 18 healthy male subjects received 250 mg Respbid Tablets in doses ranging from 375 mg to 625 mg twice daily (mean dose of 11 mg/kg per day). Subjects were allowed to take drug with milk and were permitted their normal daily meals except for fasting from 10 hours before through 4 hours after the morning dose on day 5. Following that dose, mean minimum and maximum plasma theophylline levels were 7.3 ± 2.3 mcg/ml and 10.8 ± 3.1 mcg/ml, respectively. The average percent fluctuation $[(C_{max} - C_{min}/C_{min}) \times 100]$ was 48%. The extent of theophylline absorption from Respbid averaged 94 ± 19% of that from an immediate-release liquid given four times daily.

In other studies: A single 500 mg dose of Respbid was administered to 35 healthy volunteers in both a fasting state and with a high-fat content breakfast. The resultant pharmacokinetic values recorded a delay in the rate of absorption (but not the extent) for the fed group.

In a multiple-dose study involving 12 adolescent patients, the rate and extent of absorption was similar whether the drug was taken immediately after, or two hours after, a low-fat content breakfast (see PRECAUTIONS, Drug/Food Interactions).

INDICATIONS AND USAGE

For relief and/or prevention of symptoms from asthma and reversible bronchospasm associated with chronic bronchitis and emphysema.

CONTRAINDICATIONS

Respbid® (anhydrous theophylline) Tablets are contraindicated in individuals who are hypersensitive to theophylline or any of the tablet components. It is also contraindicated in patients with active peptic ulcer disease, and in individuals with underlying seizure disorders (unless receiving appropriate anticonvulsant therapy).

WARNINGS

Serum levels above 20 mcg/ml are rarely found after appropriate administration of the recommended doses. However, in individuals in whom theophylline plasma clearance is reduced for any reason, even conventional doses may result in increased serum levels and potential toxicity. Reduced theophylline clearance has been documented in the following readily identifiable groups: 1) patients with impaired liver function; 2) patients over 55 years of age, particularly males and those with chronic lung disease; 3) those with cardiac failure from any cause; 4) patients with sustained high fever; 5) neonates and infants under 1 year of age; and 6) those patients taking certain drugs (see PRECAUTIONS, Drug Interactions). Frequently, such patients have markedly prolonged theophylline serum levels following discontinuation of the drug.

Reduction of dosage and laboratory monitoring is especially appropriate in the above individuals.

Serious side effects such as ventricular arrhythmias, convulsions or even death may appear as the first sign of toxicity without any previous warning. Less serious signs of theophylline toxicity (i.e., nausea and restlessness) may occur frequently when initiating therapy, but are usually transient; when such signs are persistent during maintenance therapy; they are often associated with serum concentrations above 20 mcg/ml. Stated differently: serious toxicity is not reliably preceded by less severe side effects. A serum concentration measurement is the only reliable method of predicting potentially life-threatening toxicity.

Many patients who require theophylline exhibit tachycardia due to their underlying disease process so that the cause/effect relationship to elevated serum theophylline concentrations may not be appreciated.

Theophylline products may cause or worsen arrhythmias and any significant change in rate and/or rhythm warrants monitoring and further investigation.

Studies in laboratory animals (minipigs, rodents, and dogs) recorded the occurrence of cardiac arrhythmias and sudden death (with histologic evidence of myocardial necrosis) when beta-agonists and methylxanthines were administered concurrently. The significance of these findings when applied to humans is currently unknown.

PRECAUTIONS

General: On the average, theophylline half-life is shorter in cigarette and marijuana smokers than in nonsmokers, but smokers can have half-lives as long as nonsmokers. Theophylline should not be administered concurrently with other xanthines. Use with caution in patients with hypoxemia, hypertension, or those with history of peptic ulcer. Theophylline may occasionally act as a local irritant to G.I. tract although gastrointestinal symptoms are more commonly centrally mediated and associated with serum drug concentrations over 20 mcg/ml.

Information for Patients: If nausea, vomiting, restlessness, irregular heartbeat, or convulsions occur, contact a physician immediately.

Take only the amount of drug that has been prescribed. Do not take a larger dose, or take the drug more often, or for a longer time than recommended.

Take this drug consistently with respect to food: either with meals, or fasted (at least two hours pre- or 2 hours post-meals).

Do not take other medicines, especially those for pulmonary disorders, except on the advice of a physician.

Contact your physician if pulmonary symptoms occur repeatedly, especially at the end of a dosing interval.

Avoid drinking large amounts of caffeine-containing beverages, such as coffee, tea, cocoa, or cola, or eating large quantities of chocolate while taking this medicine, since these foods increase the side effects of theophylline.

Respbid® (anhydrous theophylline) Tablets should not be chewed or crushed.

Laboratory Tests: Serum levels should be monitored periodically to determine the theophylline level associated with observed clinical response and as the method of predicting toxicity. For such measurements, the serum sample should be obtained four to six hours after administration of Resp-

bid Tablets. It is important that the patient will not have missed or taken additional doses during the previous 48 hours and that dosing intervals will have been reasonably equally spaced. DOSAGE ADJUSTMENT BASED ON SERUM THEOPHYLLINE MEASUREMENTS WHEN THESE INSTRUCTIONS HAVE NOT BEEN FOLLOWED MAY RESULT IN RECOMMENDATIONS THAT PRESENT RISK OF TOXICITY TO THE PATIENT.

Drug Interactions: *Drug/Drug*—Toxic synergism with ephedrine has been documented and may occur with other sympathomimetic bronchodilators. In addition, the following drug interactions have been demonstrated:

Theophylline with:	
Allopurinol (high dose)	Increased serum theophylline levels
Cimetidine	Increased serum theophylline levels
Ciprofloxacin	Increased serum theophylline levels
Erythromycin, Troleandomycin	Increased serum theophylline levels
Lithium carbonate	Increased renal excretion of lithium
Oral Contraceptives	Increased serum theophylline levels
Phenytoin	Decreased theophylline and phenytoin serum levels
Propranolol	Increased serum theophylline levels
Rifampin	Decreased serum theophylline levels

Drug/Food—Administration of a single dose of Respbid immediately after a high-fat content breakfast (8 ounces of whole milk, 2 fried eggs, 2 bacon strips, 2 ounces of hash browns and 2 slices of buttered toast, which equates to approximately 71 grams of fat and 985 calories) to 35 healthy volunteers resulted in plasma concentration levels (for the first 8 hours) of 40–60% of those noted during the fasted state and a delay in the time to peak plasma level (T-max) of 17.1 hours in contrast to the 5.1 hours observed during the fasted state.
However, when Respbid was administered on an every 12 hour schedule for 5 days, no consequential effect on absorption was noted following similar high-fat content breakfast, and the time to peak concentration averaged 5.4 hours. The rate and extent of absorption seen was similar when the drug was taken immediately after, and two hours after, a low-fat content breakfast.
The effect of other types and amounts of food, and the pharmacokinetic profile following an evening meal is not presently known.

Drug-Laboratory Test Interactions: Currently available analytical methods, including high pressure liquid chromatography and immunoassay techniques, for measuring serum theophylline levels are specific. Metabolites and other drugs generally do not affect the results. Other new analytic methods are also now in use. The physician should be aware of the laboratory method used and whether other drugs will interfere with the assay for theophylline.

Carcinogenesis, Mutagenesis, and Impairment of Fertility: Long-term carcinogenicity studies have not been performed with theophylline.
Chromosome-breaking activity was detected in human cell cultures at concentrations of theophylline up to 50 times the therapeutic serum concentration in humans. Theophylline was not mutagenic in the dominant lethal assay in male mice given theophylline intraperitoneally in doses up to 30 times the maximum daily human oral dose.
Studies to determine the effect on fertility have not been performed with theophylline.

Pregnancy: *Category C*—Animal reproduction studies have not been conducted with theophylline. It is also not known whether theophylline can cause fetal harm when administered to a pregnant woman or can affect reproduction capacity. Xanthines should be given to a pregnant woman only if clearly needed.

Nursing Mothers: Theophylline is distributed into breast milk and may cause irritability or other signs of toxicity in nursing infants. Because of the potential for serious adverse reactions in nursing infants from theophylline, a decision should be made whether to discontinue nursing or to discontinue the drug, taking into account the importance of the drug to the mother.

Pediatric Use: Respbid® (anhydrous theophylline) Tablets are not recommended for administration to the pediatric population less than six years of age.

ADVERSE REACTIONS

The following adverse reactions have been observed, but there has not been enough systematic collection of data to support an estimate of their frequency. The most consistent adverse reactions are usually due to overdosage.

1. Gastrointestinal: nausea, vomiting, epigastric pain, hematemesis, diarrhea.

If serum theophylline is:		Directions:
Within desired range		Maintain dosage if tolerated. Recheck serum theophylline concentration at 6- to 12-month intervals.*
Too high	20 to 25 mcg/ml	Decrease doses by about 10% and recheck serum level after 3 days.
	25 to 30 mcg/ml	Skip the next dose and decrease subsequent doses by about 25%. Recheck serum level after 3 days.
	Over 30 mcg/ml	Skip next two doses and decrease subsequent doses by 50%. Recheck serum level after 3 days.
Too low		Increase dosage by 25% at 3 day intervals until either the desired serum concentration and/or clinical response is achieved.* The total daily dose may need to be administered at more frequent intervals if symptoms occur repeatedly at the end of the dosing interval.

The serum concentration may be rechecked at appropriate intervals, but at least at the end of any adjustment period. When the patient's condition is otherwise clinically stable, and none of the recognized factors which alter elimination are present, measurement of serum levels need be repeated only every 6 to 12 months.

* Finer adjustments in dosage may be needed for some patients.

2. Central nervous system: headaches, irritability, restlessness, insomnia, reflex hyperexcitability, muscle twitching, clonic and tonic generalized convulsions.
3. Cardiovascular: palpitation, tachycardia, extrasystoles, flushing, hypotension, circulatory failure, ventricular arrhythmias.
4. Respiratory: tachypnea.
5. Renal: potentiation of diuresis.
6. Others: alopecia, hyperglycemia, inappropriate ADH syndrome, rash.

OVERDOSAGE

Management: It is suggested that the management principles (consistent with the clinical status of the patient when first seen) outlined below be instituted and that simultaneous contact with a Regional Poison Control Center be established. In this way both updated information and individualization regarding required therapy may be provided.

1. When potential oral overdose is established and seizure has not occurred:

a) If patient is alert and seen within the early hours after ingestion, induction of emesis may be of value. Gastric lavage has been demonstrated to be of no value in influencing outcome in patients who present more than 1 hour after ingestion.
b) Administer a cathartic. Sorbitol solution is reported to be of value.
c) Administer repeated doses of activated charcoal and monitor theophylline serum levels.
d) Prophylactic administration of phenobarbital has been shown to increase the seizure threshold in laboratory animals, and administration of this drug can be considered.

2. If patient presents with a seizure:

a) Establish an airway.
b) Administer oxygen.
c) Treat the seizure with intravenous diazepam, 0.1 to 0.3 mg/kg up to 10 mg. If seizures cannot be controlled, the use of general anesthesia should be considered.
d) Monitor vital signs, maintain blood pressure and provide adequate hydration.

3. If post-seizure coma is present:

a) Maintain airway and oxygenation.
b) If a result of oral medication, follow above recommendations to prevent absorption of the drug, but intubation and lavage will have to be performed instead of inducing emesis, and the cathartic and charcoal will need to be introduced via a large bore gastric lavage tube.
c) Continue to provide full supportive care and adequate hydration until the drug is metabolized. In general, drug metabolism is sufficiently rapid so as not to warrant dialysis. If repeated oral activated charcoal is ineffective (as noted by stable or rising serum levels) charcoal hemoperfusion may be indicated.

DOSAGE AND ADMINISTRATION

Effective use of theophylline (i.e., the concentration of drug in the serum associated with optimal benefit and minimal risk of toxicity) is considered to occur when the theophylline concentration is maintained from 10 to 20 mcg/ml. The early studies from which these levels were derived were carried out in patients immediately or shortly after recovery from acute exacerbations of their disease (some hospitalized with status asthmaticus).
Although the 20 mcg/ml level remains appropriate as a critical value (above which toxicity is more likely to occur) for safety purposes, additional data are now available which indicate that the serum theophylline concentrations required to produce maximum physiologic benefit may, in fact, fluctuate with the degree of bronchospasm present and are variable. Therefore, the physician should individualize the range appropriate to the patient's requirements, based on both symptomatic response and improvement in pulmonary function. It should be stressed that serum theophylline concentrations maintained at the upper level of the 10 to 20 mcg/ml range may be associated with potential toxicity when factors known to reduce theophylline clearance are operative (see WARNINGS).
If it is not possible to obtain serum level determinations, restriction of the daily dose (in otherwise healthy adults) to not greater than 13 mg/kg/day, to a maximum of 900 mg, in divided doses, will result in relatively few patients exceeding serum levels of 20 mcg/ml and the resultant greater risk of toxicity.
Caution should be exercised for younger children who cannot complain of minor side effects. Older adults, those with cor pulmonale, congestive heart failure, and/or liver diseases may have unusually low dosage requirements and thus may experience toxicity at the maximal dosage recommended below.
Theophylline does not distribute into fatty tissue. Dosage should be calculated on the basis of lean (ideal) body weight where mg/kg doses are presented.
Dosage guidelines are approximations only and the wide range of theophylline clearance between individuals (particularly those with concomitant disease) makes indiscriminate usage hazardous.
Respbid® (anhydrous theophylline) Tablets Should Not Be Chewed or Crushed.

Dosage Guidelines: There is information which shows that taking Respbid consistently after both high-fat and low-fat content breakfasts does not result in a decrease in peak concentration or delay in time to peak concentration that are seen when a single dose of Respbid is taken immediately after a high-fat content breakfast. Therefore, Respbid® (anhydrous theophylline) should be administered consistently with respect to food: either with meals, or fasted (at least 2 hours pre- or 2 hours post-meals). (See PRECAUTIONS, Drug/Food Interactions.)
Status asthmaticus should be considered a medical emergency and is defined as that degree of bronchospasm which is not rapidly responsive to usual doses of conventional bronchodilators. Optimal therapy for such patients frequently requires both additional medication, parenterally administered, and close monitoring, preferably in an intensive care setting.
Acute Symptoms—Respbid Tablets are not intended for patients experiencing an acute episode of bronchospasm (associated with asthma, chronic bronchitis, or emphysema). Such patients require rapid relief of symptoms and should be treated with an immediate-release theophylline preparation, an intravenous theophylline preparation or other bronchodilators, and not with controlled-release products.
Chronic Symptoms—Theophylline administration is a treatment for the management of reversible bronchospasm (asthma, chronic bronchitis and emphysema) to prevent symptoms and maintain patent airways. The appropriate dosage of theophylline can be established using an immediate-release preparation. Slow clinical titration is preferred to help assure acceptance and safety of the medication. When appropriate theophylline serum levels have been attained and clinical improvement has been maintained, the patient can usually be switched to Respbid Tablets by dividing the total daily dose of immediate-release theophylline by two and administering the appropriate Respbid Tablet every 12 hours. (see conversion chart below). However, certain patients, such as the young, smokers, or some non-smoking adults are likely to metabolize theophylline rapidly and require the total daily dose administered as three equal doses at eight-hour intervals. Such patients can generally be identified as having trough serum levels lower than desired or repeatedly exhibiting symptoms near the end of a dosing interval.

If the established daily dose is:	The q 12 hr regimen is: no. tablets:	strength:
500 mg	1	Respbid 250 mg
1000 mg	1	Respbid 500 mg

Alternatively, therapy can be initiated with Respbid since it is available in dosage strengths which permit titration and adjustment of dosage as noted above. A liquid preparation should be considered for children to permit both greater ease of and more accurate dosage adjustment.

Recommended Doses for Initiating Therapy with Respbid: *Initial Dose*—As an initial dose, 16 mg/kg per 24 hours or

Continued on next page

Respbid—Cont.

400 mg per 24 hours (whichever is less) of Respbid® (anhydrous theophylline) Tablets in divided doses at 8– or 12–hour intervals, as appropriate (see DOSAGE AND ADMINISTRATION).

Increasing Dose—The above dosage may be increased in approximately 25% increments at three-day intervals so long as the drug is tolerated, until clinical response is satisfactory or the maximum dose as indicated in the following section is reached. The serum concentration may be checked at these intervals, but at a minimum, should be determined at the end of this adjustment period.

IT IS IMPORTANT THAT NO PATIENT BE MAINTAINED ON ANY DOSAGE THAT IS NOT TOLERATED. In instructing patients to increase dosage, they should be instructed not to take a subsequent dose if side effects occur and to resume therapy at a lower dose once adverse effects have disappeared.

Maximum Dose Where the Serum Concentration Is Not Measured:

WARNING: DO NOT ATTEMPT TO MAINTAIN ANY DOSE THAT IS NOT TOLERATED.

Do not exceed the following (or 900 mg, whichever is less):

Age 6 to under 9 years	24 mg/kg/day
Age 9 to under 12 years	20 mg/kg/day
Age 12 to under 16 years	18 mg/kg/day
Age 16 years and older	13 mg/kg/day

Measurement of Serum Theophylline Concentrations During Chronic Therapy: If the above maximum doses are to be maintained or exceeded, serum theophylline measurement is essential (see PRECAUTIONS, Laboratory Tests, for guidance).

Dosage Adjustment After Serum Theophylline Measurement:

[See table at top of previous page]

HOW SUPPLIED

Respbid® brand theophylline is supplied as 250 mg white, round, scored sustained release tablets imprinted with "BI 48" (NDC 0597-0048-01) and 500 mg white, capsule-shaped, scored sustained-release tablets imprinted with "BI 49" (NDC 0597-0049-01) in bottles of 100.

STORE AT CONTROLLED ROOM TEMPERATURE 15°–30°C (59°–86°F).

Caution: Federal law prohibits dispensing without prescription.

RE-PI-Rev 10/95

Distributed by
Boehringer Ingelheim
Pharmaceuticals, Inc.
Ridgefield, CT 06877
Manufactured by
3M Pharmaceuticals
St. Paul, MN 55144-1000

Shown in Product Identification Guide, page 307

SERENTIL® ℞

[seh-ren 'til]

(mesoridazine besylate) USP

Tablets, 10 mg	**BI-CODE 20**
Tablets, 25 mg	**BI-CODE 21**
Tablets, 50 mg	**BI-CODE 22**
Tablets, 100 mg	**BI-CODE 23**
Concentrate of 25 mg/ml	**BI-CODE 25**
Ampuls of 1 ml (25 mg)	**BI-CODE 27**

Prescribing Information

Caution:

Federal law prohibits dispensing without prescription.

DESCRIPTION

Serentil® (mesoridazine besylate), the besylate salt of a metabolite of thioridazine, is a phenothiazine tranquilizer which is effective in the treatment of schizophrenia, organic brain disorders, alcoholism and psychoneuroses. Serentil® (mesoridazine besylate) is 10-[2(1-methyl-2-piperidyl) ethyl]-2- (methyl-sulfinyl)-phenothiazine [as the besylate].

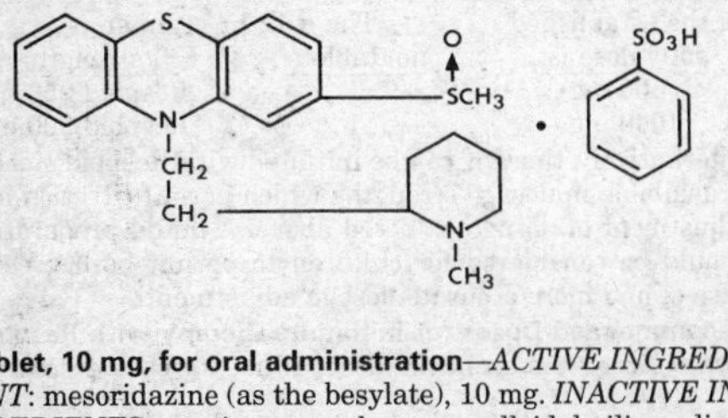

Tablet, 10 mg, for oral administration—*ACTIVE INGREDIENT*: mesoridazine (as the besylate), 10 mg. *INACTIVE INGREDIENTS*: acacia, carnauba wax, colloidal silicon dioxide, FD&C Red No. 40 aluminum lake, lactose, microcrystalline cellulose, povidone, sodium benzoate, starch, stearic acid, sucrose, synthetic black iron oxide, talc, titanium dioxide and other ingredients.

Tablet, 25 mg, for oral administration—*ACTIVE INGREDIENT*: mesoridazine (as the besylate), 25 mg. *INACTIVE INGREDIENTS*: acacia, carnauba wax, colloidal silicon dioxide, FD&C Red No. 40 aluminum lake, lactose, microcrystalline cellulose, povidone, sodium benzoate, stearic acid, sucrose, synthetic black iron oxide, talc, titanium dioxide and other ingredients.

Tablet, 50 mg, for oral administration—*ACTIVE INGREDIENT*: mesoridazine (as the besylate), 50 mg. *INACTIVE INGREDIENTS*: acacia, carnauba wax, colloidal silicon dioxide, FD&C Red No. 40 aluminum lake, gelatin, lactose, microcrystalline cellulose, povidone, sodium benzoate, starch, stearic acid, sucrose, synthetic black iron oxide, talc, titanium dioxide and other ingredients.

Tablet, 100 mg, for oral administration—*ACTIVE INGREDIENT*: mesoridazine (as the besylate), 100 mg. *INACTIVE INGREDIENTS*: acacia, carnauba wax, colloidal silicon dioxide, FD&C Red No. 40 aluminum lake, gelatin, lactose, microcrystalline cellulose, povidone, sodium benzoate, starch, stearic acid, sucrose, synthetic black iron oxide, talc, titanium dioxide, and other ingredients.

Ampuls, 1 ml, for intramuscular administration—*ACTIVE INGREDIENT*: mesoridazine (as the besylate), 25 mg. *INACTIVE INGREDIENTS*: edetate disodium USP, 0.5 mg; sodium chloride USP, 7.2 mg; carbon dioxide gas (bone dry) q.s., water for injection USP, q.s. to 1 ml.

Concentrate, for oral administration—*ACTIVE INGREDIENT*: mesoridazine (as the besylate), 25 mg per ml. *INACTIVE INGREDIENTS*: alcohol, 0.61% by volume; citric acid; FD&C Red No. 40; flavors; methylparaben; propylparaben; purified water; sodium citrate, sorbitol.

ACTIONS

Based upon animal studies, Serentil® (mesoridazine besylate), as with other phenothiazines, acts indirectly on reticular formation, whereby neuronal activity into reticular formation is reduced without affecting its intrinsic ability to activate the cerebral cortex. In addition, the phenothiazines exhibit at least part of their activities through depression of hypothalamic centers. Neurochemically, the phenothiazines are thought to exert their effects by a central adrenergic blocking action.

INDICATIONS

In clinical studies Serentil® (mesoridazine besylate) has been found useful in the following disease states:

Schizophrenia: Serentil® (mesoridazine besylate) is effective in the treatment of schizophrenia. It substantially reduces the severity of emotional withdrawal, conceptual disorganization, anxiety, tension, hallucinatory behavior, suspiciousness and blunted affect in schizophrenic patients. As with other phenothiazines, patients refractory to previous medication may respond to Serentil® (mesoridazine besylate).

Behavioral Problems in Mental Deficiency and Chronic Brain Syndrome: The effect of Serentil® (mesoridazine besylate) was found to be excellent or good in the management of hyperactivity and uncooperativeness associated with mental deficiency and chronic brain syndrome.

Alcoholism—Acute and Chronic: Serentil® (mesoridazine besylate) ameliorates anxiety, tension, depression, nausea and vomiting in both acute and chronic alcoholics without producing hepatic dysfunction or hindering the functional recovery of the impaired liver.

Psychoneurotic Manifestations: Serentil® (mesoridazine besylate) reduces the symptoms of anxiety and tension, prevalent symptoms often associated with neurotic components of many disorders, and benefits personality disorders in general.

CONTRAINDICATIONS

As with other phenothiazines, Serentil® (mesoridazine besylate) is contraindicated in severe central nervous system depression or comatose states from any cause including drug induced central nervous system depression (see WARNINGS).

Serentil® (mesoridazine besylate) is contraindicated in individuals who have previously shown hypersensitivity to the drug.

WARNINGS

Tardive Dyskinesia: Tardive dyskinesia, a syndrome consisting of potentially irreversible, involuntary, dyskinetic movements may develop in patients treated with neuroleptic (antipsychotic) drugs. Although the prevalence of the syndrome appears to be highest among the elderly, especially elderly women, it is impossible to rely upon prevalence estimates to predict, at the inception of neuroleptic treatment, which patients are likely to develop the syndrome. Whether neuroleptic drug products differ in their potential to cause tardive dyskinesia is unknown.

Both the risk of developing the syndrome and the likelihood that it will become irreversible are believed to increase as the duration of treatment and the total cumulative dose of neuroleptic drugs administered to the patient increase. However, the syndrome can develop, although much less commonly, after relatively brief treatment periods at low doses.

There is no known treatment for established cases of tardive dyskinesia, although the syndrome may remit, partially or completely, if neuroleptic treatment is withdrawn. Neuroleptic treatment itself, however, may suppress (or partially suppress) the signs and symptoms of the syndrome and thereby may possibly mask the underlying disease process. The effect that symptomatic suppression has upon the long-term course of the syndrome is unknown.

Given these considerations, neuroleptics should be prescribed in a manner that is most likely to minimize the occurrence of tardive dyskinesia. Chronic neuroleptic treatment should generally be reserved for patients who suffer from a chronic illness 1) that is known to respond to neuroleptic drugs, and 2) for which alternative, equally effective but potentially less harmful treatments are *not* available or appropriate. In patients who do require chronic treatment, the smallest dose and the shortest duration of treatment producing a satisfactory clinical response should be sought. The need for continued treatment should be reassessed periodically.

If signs and symptoms of tardive dyskinesia appear in a patient on neuroleptics, drug discontinuation should be considered. However, some patients may require treatment despite the presence of the syndrome.

(For further information about the description of tardive dyskinesia and its clinical detection, please refer to the sections on Information for Patients and Adverse Reactions).

Neuroleptic Malignant Syndrome (NMS): A potentially fatal symptom complex sometimes referred to as Neuroleptic Malignant Syndrome (NMS) has been reported in association with antipsychotic drugs. Clinical manifestations of NMS are hyperpyrexia, muscle rigidity, altered mental status and evidence of autonomic instability (irregular pulse or blood pressure, tachycardia, diaphoresis, and cardiac dysrhythmias).

The diagnostic evaluation of patients with this syndrome is complicated. In arriving at a diagnosis, it is important to identify cases where the clinical presentation includes both serious medical illness (e.g., pneumonia, systemic infection, etc.) and untreated or inadequately treated extrapyramidal signs and symptoms (EPS). Other important considerations in the differential diagnosis include central anticholinergic toxicity, heat stroke, drug fever and primary central nervous system (CNS) pathology.

The management of NMS should include 1) immediate discontinuation of antipsychotic drugs and other drugs not essential to concurrent therapy, 2) intensive symptomatic treatment and medical monitoring, and 3) treatment of any concomitant serious medical problems for which specific treatments are available. There is no general agreement about specific pharmacological treatment regimens for uncomplicated NMS.

If a patient requires antipsychotic drug treatment after recovery from NMS, the potential reintroduction of drug therapy should be carefully considered. The patient should be carefully monitored, since recurrences of NMS have been reported.

Where patients are participating in activities requiring complete mental alertness (e.g., driving), it is advisable to administer the phenothiazines cautiously and to increase the dosage gradually.

Central Nervous System Depressants: As in the case of other phenothiazines, Serentil® (mesoridazine besylate) is capable of potentiating central nervous system depressants (e.g., alcohol, anesthetics, barbiturates, narcotics, opiates, other psychoactive drugs, etc.) as well as atropine and phosphorus insecticides. Severe respiratory depression and respiratory arrest have been reported when a patient was given Serentil® (mesoridazine besylate) and a concomitant high dose of a barbiturate.

Usage in Pregnancy: The safety of this drug in pregnancy has not been established; hence, it should be given only when the anticipated benefits to be derived from treatment exceed the possible risks to mother and fetus.

Pediatric Use: Safety and effectiveness in pediatric patients have not been established.

PRECAUTIONS

While ocular changes have not to date been related to Serentil® (mesoridazine besylate), one should be aware that such changes have been seen with other drugs of this class. Because of possible hypotensive effects, reserve parenteral administration for bedfast patients or for acute ambulatory cases, and keep patient lying down for at least one-half hour after injection.

Leukopenia and/or agranulocytosis have been attributed to phenothiazine therapy. A single case of transient granulocytopenia has been associated with Serentil® (mesoridazine besylate). Since convulsive seizures have been reported, patients receiving anticonvulsant medication should be maintained on that regimen while receiving Serentil® (mesoridazine besylate).

Neuroleptic drugs elevate prolactin levels; the elevation persists during chronic administration. Tissue culture experiments indicate that approximately one-third of human breast cancers are prolactin dependent in vitro, a factor of potential importance if the prescription of these drugs is contemplated in a patient with a previously detected breast cancer. Although disturbances such as galactorrhea, amenorrhea, gynecomastia, and impotence have been reported, the clinical significance of elevated serum prolactin levels is unknown for most patients. An increase in mammary neoplasms has been found in rodents after chronic administration of neuroleptic drugs. Neither clinical studies nor epidemiologic studies conducted to date, however, have shown an association between chronic administration of these drugs and mammary tumorigenesis; the available evidence is considered too limited to be conclusive at this time.

INFORMATION FOR PATIENTS: Given the likelihood that some patients exposed chronically to neuroleptics will develop tardive dyskinesia, it is advised that all patients in whom chronic use is contemplated be given, if possible, full information about this risk.

ADVERSE REACTIONS

Drowsiness and hypotension were the most prevalent side effects encountered. Side effects tended to reach their maximum level of severity early with the exception of a few (rigidity and motoric effects) which occurred later in therapy. With the exceptions of tremor and rigidity, adverse reactions were generally found among those patients who received relatively high doses early in treatment. Clinical data showed no tendency for the investigators to terminate treatment because of side effects.

Serentil® (mesoridazine besylate) has demonstrated a remarkably low incidence of adverse reactions when compared with other phenothiazine compounds.

Central Nervous System: Drowsiness, Parkinson's syndrome, dizziness, weakness, tremor, restlessness, ataxia, dystonia, rigidity, slurring, akathisia, and motoric reactions (opisthotonos) have been reported.

Autonomic Nervous System: Dry mouth, nausea and vomiting, fainting, stuffy nose, photophobia, constipation and blurred vision have occurred in some instances.

Genitourinary System: Inhibition of ejaculation, impotence, enuresis, incontinence, and priapism have been reported.

Skin: Itching, rash, hypertrophic papillae of the tongue and angioneurotic edema have been reported.

Cardiovascular System: Hypotension and tachycardia have been reported. EKG changes have occurred in some instances (see PHENOTHIAZINE DERIVATIVES: Cardiovascular Effects).

PHENOTHIAZINE DERIVATIVES: It should be noted that efficacy, indications and untoward effects have varied with the different phenothiazines. The physician should be aware that the following have occurred with one or more phenothiazines and should be considered whenever one of these drugs is used.

Autonomic Reactions: Miosis, obstipation, anorexia, paralytic ileus.

Cutaneous Reactions: Erythema, exfoliative dermatitis, contact dermatitis.

Blood Dyscrasias: Agranulocytosis, leukopenia, eosinophilia, thrombocytopenia, anemia, aplastic anemia, pancytopenia.

Allergic Reactions: Fever, laryngeal edema, angioneurotic edema, asthma.

Hepatotoxicity: Jaundice, biliary stasis.

Cardiovascular Effects: Changes in the terminal portion of the electrocardiogram, including prolongation of the Q-T interval, lowering and inversion of the T wave and appearance of a wave tentatively identified as a bifid T or a U wave have been observed in some patients receiving the phenothiazine tranquilizers, including Serentil® (mesoridazine besylate). To date, these appear to be due to altered repolarization and not related to myocardial damage. They appear to be reversible. While there is no evidence at present that these changes are in any way precursors of any significant disturbance of cardiac rhythm, it should be noted that sudden and unexpected deaths apparently due to cardiac arrest have occurred in patients previously showing characteristic electrocardiographic changes while taking the drug. The use of periodic electrocardiograms has been proposed but would appear to be of questionable value as a predictive device. Hypotension, rarely resulting in cardiac arrest, has been noted.

Extrapyramidal Symptoms: Akathisia, agitation, motor restlessness, dystonic reactions, trismus, torticollis, opisthotonos, oculogyric crises, tremor, muscular rigidity, akinesia.

Tardive Dyskinesia: Chronic use of neuroleptics may be associated with the development of tardive dyskinesia. The salient features of this syndrome are described in the WARNINGS section and below.

The syndrome is characterized by involuntary choreoathetoid movements which variously involve the tongue, face, mouth, lips, or jaw (e.g., protrusion of the tongue, puffing of cheeks, puckering of the mouth, chewing movements), trunk and extremities. The severity of the syndrome and the degree of impairment produced vary widely.

The syndrome may become clinically recognizable either during treatment, upon dosage reduction, or upon withdrawal of treatment. Movements may decrease in intensity and may disappear altogether if further treatment with neuroleptics is withheld. It is generally believed that reversibility is more likely after short rather than long-term neuroleptic exposure. Consequently, early detection of tardive dyskinesia is important. To increase the likelihood of detecting the syndrome at the earliest possible time, the dosage of neuroleptic drug should be reduced periodically (if clinically possible) and the patient observed for signs of the disorder. This maneuver is critical, for neuroleptic drugs may mask the signs of the syndrome.

Endocrine Disturbances: Menstrual irregularities, altered libido, gynecomastia, lactation, weight gain, edema. False positive pregnancy tests have been reported.

Urinary Disturbances: Retention, incontinence.

Others: Hyperpyrexia. Behavioral effects suggestive of a paradoxical reaction have been reported. These include excitement, bizarre dreams, aggravation of psychoses and toxic confusional states. More recently, a peculiar skin-eye syndrome has been recognized as a side effect following long-term treatment with phenothiazines. This reaction is marked by progressive pigmentation of areas of the skin or conjunctiva and/or accompanied by discoloration of the exposed sclera and cornea. Opacities of the anterior lens and cornea described as irregular or stellate in shape have also been reported. Systemic lupus erythematosus-like syndrome.

OVERDOSAGE

Symptoms of Acute Overdosage

— Drowsiness, confusion, disorientation, agitation, coma, death.

— Dryness of mouth, edema of glottis, laryngeal spasms, nasal congestion, blurred vision, vomiting.

— Hyperpyrexia, dilated pupils, muscle rigidity, hyperactive reflexes, areflexia.

— Stupor, and CNS depression or stimulation with convulsions followed by respiratory depression.

— Cardiac abnormalities, including Q.R.S. changes, tachycardia, hypotension, bilateral bundle branch block, ventricular fibrillation, shock, cardiac arrest and congestive heart failure. (See case descriptions below).

Treatment of Acute Overdosage: No specific antidote is known. The drug is not dialyzable. Treatment should include:

— *General supportive* measures with *emesis* and *gastric lavage*.

— *Respiratory assistance* is apparently the most effective measure when indicated.

— The *administration of barbiturates* for control of convulsions alleviates an increase in the cardiac work load, but should be undertaken with caution to avoid potentiation of respiratory depression.

— *Intramuscular paraldehyde* or *diazepam* provides anticonvulsant activity with less respiratory depression than do the barbiturates; diazepam seems to be preferred.

— The use of *digitalis and/or physostigmine* may be considered in case of serious cardiovascular abnormalities or cardiac failure.

— Due to several cases of severe cardiotoxicity following Serentil® (mesoridazine besylate) overdose, *continuous ECG monitoring* of these patients is recommended. Two cases are described below:

Marrs-Simon P.A. et al ("Cardiotoxic Manifestations of Mesoridazine Overdose" *Ann Emerg Med.* 1988;17:1074-1078) describes the management of a 20-year-old female who experienced severe cardiotoxicity following an overdose of mesoridazine. The paper also describes similar cases from the published literature.

The serum mesoridazine level in a 115 lb. patient following ingestion of 4.5 to 6.0 grams of Serentil® (mesoridazine besylate) was 2.5 mcg/mL. She was comatose, hypotensive, convulsing, and had ECG changes. Twenty-four hours later, after hemoperfusion with activated charcoal, the mesoridazine blood levels fell to 1.3 mcg/mL and the patient was normotensive and responsive.

DOSAGE AND ADMINISTRATION

The dosage of Serentil® (mesoridazine besylate) as in most medications, should be adjusted to the needs of the individual. The lowest effective dosage should always be used. When maximum response is achieved, dosage may be reduced gradually to a maintenance level.

Schizophrenia: For most patients, regardless of severity, a starting dose of 50 mg t.i.d. is recommended. The usual optimum total daily dose range is 100-400 mg per day.

Behavioral Problems in Mental Deficiency and Chronic Brain Syndrome: For most patients a starting dose of 25 mg t.i.d. is recommended. The usual optimum total daily dose range is 75-300 mg per day.

Alcoholism: For most patients the usual starting dose is 25 mg b.i.d. The usual optimum total daily dose range is 50-200 mg per day.

Psychoneurotic Manifestations: For most patients the usual starting dose is 10 mg t.i.d. The usual optimum total daily dose range is 30-150 mg per day.

Injectable Form: In those situations in which an intramuscular form of medication is indicated, Serentil® (mesoridazine besylate) injectable is available. For most patients a starting dose of 25 mg is recommended. The dose may be repeated in 30 to 60 minutes, if necessary. The usual optimum total daily dose range is 25-200 mg per day.

HOW SUPPLIED

Tablets 10 mg (NDC 0597-0020-01), 25 mg (NDC 0597-0021-01), 50 mg (NDC 0597-0022-01), and 100 mg (NDC 0597-0023-01) mesoridazine (as the besylate). Bottles of 100.

Ampuls 1 mL [25 mg mesoridazine (as the besylate)]. Boxes of 20 (NDC 0597-0027-02).

Concentrate Contains 25 mg mesoridazine (as the besylate) per mL, alcohol, USP, 0.61% by volume. Immediate containers: Amber glass bottles of 4 fl oz (118 mL) packaged in cartons of 12 bottles, with an accompanying dropper graduated to deliver 10 mg, 25 mg, and 50 mg of mesoridazine (as the besylate) (NDC 0597-0025-04).

STORAGE

Tablets: Below 86°F (30°C). Injection: Below 86°F (30°C); protect from light. Oral Solution: Below 77°F (25°C); protect from light; dispense in amber glass bottles only.

The concentrate may be diluted with distilled water, acidified tap water, orange juice or grape juice.

Each dose should be diluted just prior to administration. Preparation and storage of bulk dilutions is not recommended.

Additional information available to physicians.

PHARMACOLOGY

Pharmacological studies in laboratory animals have established that Serentil® (mesoridazine besylate) has a spectrum of pharmacodynamic actions typical of a major tranquilizer. In common with other tranquilizers it inhibits spontaneous motor activity in mice, prolongs thiopental and hexobarbital sleeping time in mice and produces spindles and block of arousal reaction in the EEG of rabbits. It is effective in blocking spinal reflexes in the cat and antagonizes d-amphetamine excitation and toxicity in grouped mice. It shows a moderate adrenergic blocking activity in vitro and in vivo and antagonizes 5-hydroxytryptamine in vivo. Intravenously administered, it lowers the blood pressure of anesthetized dogs. It has a weak antiacetylcholine effect in vitro.

The most outstanding activity of Serentil® (mesoridazine besylate) is seen in tests developed to investigate antiemotive activity of drugs. Such tests are those in which the rat reacts to acute or chronic stress by increased defecation (emotogenic defecation) or tests in which "emotional mydriasis" is elicited in the mouse by an electric shock. In both of these tests Serentil® (mesoridazine besylate) is effective in reducing emotive reactions. Its ED_{50} in inhibiting emotogenic defecation in the rat is 0.053 mg/kg (subcutaneous administration). Serentil® (mesoridazine besylate) has a potent antiemetic action. The intravenous ED_{50} against apomorphine-induced emesis in the dog is 0.64 mg/kg. Serentil® (mesoridazine besylate), in common with other phenothiazines, demonstrates antiarrhythmic activity in anesthetized dogs.

Metabolic studies in the dog and rabbit with tritium labeled mesoridazine demonstrate that the compound is well absorbed from the gastrointestinal tract. The biological half-life of Serentil® (mesoridazine besylate) in these studies appears to be somewhere between 24 and 48 hours. Although significant urinary excretion was observed following the administration of Serentil® (mesoridazine besylate), these studies also suggest that biliary excretion is an important excretion route for mesoridazine and/or its metabolites.

Toxicity Studies
Acute LD_{50} (mg/kg):

Route	Mouse	Rat	Rabbit	Dog
Oral	560±62.5	644±48	MLD=800	MLD=800
I.M.	—	509M 584 F	405	
I.V.	26±0.08	—	—	—

Chronic toxicity studies were conducted in rats and dogs. Rats were administered Serentil® (mesoridazine besylate) orally seven days per week for a period of seventeen months in doses up to 160 mg/kg per day. Dogs were administered

Continued on next page

Serentil—Cont.

Serentil® (mesoridazine besylate) orally seven days per week for a period of thirteen months. The daily dosage of the drug was increased during the period of this test such that the "top-dose" group received a daily dose of 120 mg/kg of mesoridazine for the last month of the study.

Untoward effects that occurred upon chronic administration of high dose levels included:

Rats: Reduction of food intake, slowed weight gain, morphological changes in pituitary-supported endocrine organs, and melanin-like pigment deposition in renal tissues.

Dogs: Emesis, muscle tremors, decreased food intake and death associated with aspiration of oral-gastric contents into the respiratory system.

Increased intrauterine resorptions were seen with Serentil® (mesoridazine besylate) in rats at 70 mg/kg and in rabbits at 125 mg/kg but not at 60 and 100 mg/kg, respectively. No drug related teratology was suggested by these reproductive studies.

Local irritation from the intramuscular injection of Serentil® (mesoridazine besylate) was of the same order of magnitude as with other phenothiazines.

SE-PI-7/96 Rev

Manufactured by
Sandoz Pharmaceuticals Corporation
East Hanover, NJ 07936
Distributed by
Boehringer Ingelheim Pharmaceuticals, Inc.
Ridgefield, CT 06877
Shown in Product Identification Guide, page 307

Boehringer Mannheim Corporation Therapeutics

(See Roche Laboratories Inc. for Demadex Tablets and Injection)

Braintree Laboratories, Inc.

P.O. BOX 850929
BRAINTREE, MA 02185-0929

Direct Inquiries to:
Harry P. Keegan, President
(781) 843-2202

For Medical Information Contact:
In Emergencies:
Jack DiPalma, M.D.
(800) 874-6756

GoLYTELY®   ℞
[go-līt 'lē]
PEG–3350 and Electrolytes For Oral Solution

DESCRIPTION

A white powder in a 4 liter jug for reconstitution, containing 236 g polyethylene glycol 3350, 22.74 g sodium sulfate (anhydrous), 6.74 g sodium bicarbonate, 5.86 g sodium chloride and 2.97 g potassium chloride. When dissolved in water to a volume of 4 liters, GoLYTELY is an isosmotic solution having a mildly salty taste. GoLYTELY is administered orally or via nasogastric tube.

CLINICAL PHARMACOLOGY

GoLYTELY induces a diarrhea which rapidly cleanses the bowel, usually within four hours. The osmotic activity of polyethylene glycol 3350 and the electrolyte concentration result in virtually no net absorption or excretion of ions or water. Accordingly, large volumes may be administered without significant changes in fluid or electrolyte balance.

INDICATIONS AND USAGE

GoLYTELY is indicated for bowel cleansing prior to colonoscopy and barium enema X-ray examination.

CONTRAINDICATIONS

GoLYTELY is contraindicated in patients with gastrointestinal obstruction, gastric retention, bowel perforation, toxic colitis, toxic megacolon or ileus.

WARNINGS

No additional ingredients, e.g. flavorings, should be added to the solution. GoLYTELY should be used with caution in patients with severe ulcerative colitis.

PRECAUTIONS

General: Patients with impaired gag reflex, unconscious, or semiconscious patients, and patients prone to regurgita-

tion or aspiration, should be observed during the administration of GoLYTELY, especially if it is administered via nasogastric tube. If a patient experiences severe bloating, distention or abdominal pain, administration should be slowed or temporarily discontinued until the symptoms abate. If gastrointestinal obstruction or perforation is suspected, appropriate studies should be performed to rule out these conditions before administration of GoLYTELY.

Information for patients: GoLYTELY produces a watery stool which cleanses the bowel before examination. Prepare the solution according to the instructions on the bottle. It is more palatable if chilled. For best results, no solid food should be consumed during the 3 to 4 hour period before drinking the solution, but in no case should solid foods be eaten within 2 hours of taking GoLYTELY.

Drink 240 mL (8 oz.) every 10 minutes. Rapid drinking of each portion is better than drinking small amounts continuously. The first bowel movement should occur approximately one hour after the start of GoLYTELY administration. You may experience some abdominal bloating and distention before the bowels start to move. If severe discomfort or distention occur, stop drinking temporarily or drink each portion at longer intervals until these symptoms disappear. Continue drinking until the watery stool is clear and free of solid matter. This usually requires at least 3 liters and it is best to drink all of the solution. Any unused portion should be discarded.

Drug Interactions: Oral medication administered within one hour of the start of administration of GoLYTELY may be flushed from the gastrointestinal tract and not absorbed.

Carcinogenesis, Mutagenesis, Impairment of Fertility: Carcinogenic and reproductive studies with animals have not been performed.

Pregnancy: Category C. Animal reproduction studies have not been conducted with GoLYTELY. It is also not known whether GoLYTELY can cause fetal harm when administered to a pregnant woman or can affect reproductive capacity. GoLYTELY should be given to a pregnant woman only if clearly needed.

Pediatric Use: Safety and effectiveness in children have not been established.

ADVERSE REACTIONS

Nausea, abdominal fullness and bloating are the most common adverse reactions (occurring in up to 50% of patients) to administration of GoLYTELY. Abdominal cramps, vomiting and anal irritation occur less frequently. These adverse reactions are transient and subside rapidly. Isolated cases of urticaria, rhinorrhea, dermatitis and (rarely) anaphylactic reaction have been reported which may represent allergic reactions.

DOSAGE AND ADMINISTRATION

The recommended dose for adults is 4 liters of GoLYTELY solution prior to gastrointestinal examination, as ingestion of this dose produces a satisfactory preparation in over 95% of patients. Ideally, the patient should fast for approximately three or four hours prior to GoLYTELY administration, but in no case should solid food be given for at least two hours before the solution is given.

GoLYTELY is usually administered orally, but may be given via nasogastric tube to patients who are unwilling or unable to drink the solution. **Oral administration** is at a rate of 240 mL (8 oz.) every 10 minutes, until 4 liters are consumed or the rectal effluent is clear. Rapid drinking of each portion is preferred to drinking small amounts continuously. **Nasogastric tube administration** is at the rate of 20–30 mL per minute (1.2–1.8 liters per hour). The first bowel movement should occur approximately one hour after the start of GoLYTELY administration.

Various regimens have been used. One method is to schedule patients for examination in midmorning or later, allowing the patients three hours for drinking and an additional one hour period for complete bowel evacuation. Another method is to administer GoLYTELY on the evening before the examination, particularly if the patient is to have a barium enema.

Preparation of the solution: GoLYTELY solution is prepared by filling the container to the 4 liter mark with water and shaking vigorously several times to insure that the ingredients are dissolved. Dissolution is facilitated by using lukewarm water. The solution is more palatable if chilled before administration. The reconstituted solution should be refrigerated and used within 48 hours. Discard any unused portion.

HOW SUPPLIED

In powdered form, for oral administration as a solution following reconstitution. GoLYTELY® is available in a disposable jug and a packet in powdered form containing:

Disposable Jug: polyethylene glycol 3350 236 g, sodium sulfate (anhydrous) 22.74 g, sodium bicarbonate 6.74 g, sodium chloride 5.86 g, potassium chloride 2.97 g. When made up to 4 liters volume with water, the solution contains PEG 3350 17.6 mmol/L, sodium 125 mmol/L, sulfate 40 mmol/L, chloride 35 mmol/L, bicarbonate 20 mmol/L and potassium 10 mmol/L.

Packet: polyethylene glycol 3350 227.1 g, anhydrous sodium sulfate 21.5 g, sodium bicarbonate 6.36 g, sodium chloride 5.53 g, potassium chloride 2.82 g. When made up to 1 gallon volume with water, the solution contains PEG 3350 60 g/L, sodium sulfate 5.68 g/L, sodium bicarbonate 1.68 g/L, sodium chloride 1.46 g/L and potassium chloride 0.745 g/L.

Rx only

STORAGE

Store in sealed container at 59°–86°F. When reconstituted, keep solution refrigerated. Use within 48 hours. Discard unused portion.

NDC 52268-100-01

Revised 8/96

Distributed by Braintree Laboratories, Inc.,
Braintree, MA 02185-0929
Shown in Product Identification Guide, page 307

NuLYTELY®   ℞
[new-līt ' lē]
PEG 3350, Sodium Chloride, Sodium Bicarbonate and Potassium Chloride for Oral Solution

CHERRY FLAVOR
NuLYTELY®   ℞
PEG 3350, Sodium Chloride, Sodium Bicarbonate and Potassium Chloride for Oral Solution

DESCRIPTION

A white powder for reconstitution containing 420 g polyethylene glycol 3350, 5.72 g sodium bicarbonate, 11.2 g sodium chloride, 1.48 g potassium chloride and 2 g flavoring ingredients (Cherry Flavor NuLYTELY). When dissolved in water to a volume of 4 liters, NuLYTELY is an isosmotic solution. NuLYTELY has a pleasant mineral water taste and Cherry Flavor NuLYTELY has a pleasant cherry flavored taste. NuLYTELY is administered orally or via nasogastric tube.

CLINICAL PHARMACOLOGY

NuLYTELY induces a diarrhea which rapidly cleanses the bowel, usually within four hours. The osmotic activity of polyethylene glycol 3350 and the electrolyte concentration result in virtually no net absorption or excretion of ions or water. Accordingly, large volumes may be administered without significant changes in fluid or electrolyte balance.

INDICATIONS AND USAGE

NuLYTELY is indicated for bowel cleansing prior to colonoscopy.

CONTRAINDICATIONS

NuLYTELY is contraindicated in patients with gastrointestinal obstruction, gastric retention, bowel perforation, toxic colitis or toxic megacolon.

WARNINGS

No additional ingredients, e.g. flavorings, should be added to the solution. NuLYTELY should be used with caution in patients with severe ulcerative colitis. Use of NuLYTELY in children younger than 2 years of age should be carefully monitored for occurrence of possible hypoglycemia, as this solution has no caloric substrate. Dehydration has been reported in 1 child and hypokalemia has been reported in 3 children.

PRECAUTIONS

General: Patients with impaired gag reflex, unconscious, or semiconscious patients, and patients prone to regurgitation or aspiration should be observed during the administration of NuLYTELY, especially if it is administered via nasogastric tube. If a patient experiences severe bloating, distention or abdominal pain, administration should be slowed or temporarily discontinued until the symptoms abate. If gastrointestinal obstruction or perforation is suspected, appropriate studies should be performed to rule out these conditions before administration of NuLYTELY.

Information for patients: NuLYTELY produces a watery stool which cleanses the bowel before examination. Prepare the solution according to the instructions on the bottle. It is more palatable if chilled. For best results, no solid food should be consumed during the 3 to 4 hour period before drinking the solution, but in no case should solid foods be eaten within 2 hours of taking NuLYTELY.

Adults drink 240 mL (8 oz.) every 10 minutes. Pediatric patients (aged 6 months or greater) drink 25 mL/kg/hour. Rapid drinking of each portion is better than drinking small amounts continuously. The first bowel movement should occur approximately one hour after the start of NuLYTELY administration. You may experience some abdominal bloating and distention before the bowels start to move. If severe discomfort or distention occur, stop drinking temporarily or drink each portion at longer intervals until these symptoms disappear. Continue drinking until the watery stool is clear and free of solid matter. This usually requires at least 3 liters. Any unused portion should be discarded.

Use of NuLYTELY in children younger than 2 years of age should be carefully monitored for occurrence of possible hypoglycemia, as this solution has no caloric substrate. Dehydration has been reported in 1 child and hypokalemia has been reported in 3 children.

Drug Interactions: Oral medication administered within one hour of the start of administration of NuLYTELY may be flushed from the gastrointestinal tract and not absorbed.

Carcinogenesis, Mutagenesis, Impairment of Fertility: Carcinogenic and reproductive studies with animals have not been performed.

Pregnancy: Category C. Animal reproduction studies have not been conducted with NuLYTELY. It is also not known whether NuLYTELY can cause fetal harm when administered to a pregnant woman or can affect reproductive capacity. NuLYTELY should be given to a pregnant woman only if clearly needed.

Pediatric Use: Safety and effectiveness of NuLYTELY in pediatric patients aged 6 months and older is supported by evidence from adequate and well controlled clinical trials of NuLYTELY in adults with additional safety and efficacy data from published studies of similar formulations.

ADVERSE REACTIONS

Nausea, abdominal fullness and bloating are the most common adverse reactions (occurring in up to 50% of patients) to administration of NuLYTELY. Abdominal cramps, vomiting and anal irritation occur less frequently. These adverse reactions are transient and subside rapidly. Isolated cases of urticaria, rhinorrhea, dermatitis and (rarely) anaphylactic reaction have been reported which may represent allergic reactions.

DOSAGE AND ADMINISTRATION

NuLYTELY is usually administered orally, but may be given via nasogastric tube to patients who are unwilling or unable to drink the solution. Ideally, the patient should fast for approximately three or four hours prior to NuLYTELY administration, but in no case should solid food be given for at least two hours before the solution is given.

Oral administration: Adults: At a rate of 240 mL (8 oz.) every 10 minutes, until the rectal effluent is clear or 4 liters are consumed. **Pediatric patients (aged 6 months or greater):** At a rate of 25 mL/kg/hour, until the rectal effluent is clear or 4 liters are consumed. Rapid drinking of each portion is preferred to drinking small amounts continuously.

Nasogastric tube administration: Adults: At a rate of 20–30 mL per minute (1.2–1.8 liters per hour). **Pediatric patients (aged 6 months or greater):** At a rate of 25 mL/kg/hour, until the rectal effluent is clear or 4 liters are consumed. The first bowel movement should occur approximately one hour after the start of NuLYTELY administration. Ingestion of 4 liters of NuLYTELY solution prior to gastrointestinal examination produces satisfactory preparation in over 95% of patients.

Various regimens have been used. One method is to schedule patients for examination in midmorning or later, allowing the patients three hours for drinking and an additional one hour period for complete bowel evacuation. Another method is to administer NuLYTELY on the evening before the examination.

Preparation of the solution: NuLYTELY solution is prepared by filling the container to the 4 liter mark with water and shaking vigorously several times to insure that the ingredients are dissolved. Dissolution is facilitated by using lukewarm water. The solution is more palatable if chilled before administation. However, chilled solution is not recommended for infants. The reconstituted solution should be refrigerated and used within 48 hours. Discard any unused portion.

HOW SUPPLIED

NuLYTELY and Cherry NuLYTELY are available in a disposable jug, in powdered form, for oral administration as a solution following reconstitution. Each jug contains:

NuLYTELY: polyethylene glycol 3350 420 g, sodium bicarbonate 5.72 g, sodium chloride 11.2 g, potassium chloride 1.48 g. When made up to 4 liters volume with water, the solution contains PEG 3350 31.3 mmol/L, sodium 65 mmol/L, chloride 53 mmol/L, bicarbonate 17 mmol/L, and potassium 5 mmol/L.

Cherry NuLYTELY: polyethylene glycol 3350 420 g, sodium bicarbonate 5.72 g, sodium chloride 11.2 g, potassium chloride 1.48 g, and flavoring ingredients 2g. When made up to 4 liters volume with water, the solution contains PEG 3350 31.3 mmol/L, sodium 65 mmol/L, chloride 53 mmol/L, bicarbonate 17 mmol/L, and potassium 5 mmol/L.

Rx only

STORAGE: Store in sealed container at 25°C. When reconstituted, keep solution refrigerated. Use within 48 hours. Discard unused portion.

NDC NuLYTELY 52268-300-01
NDC Cherry NuLYTELY 52268-301-01
Distributed by Braintree Laboratories, Inc.,
Braintree, MA 02185-0929 Revised 1/98

Shown in Product Identification Guide, page 307

PhosLo® ℞

[*phos "lō '*]

Calcium Acetate Tablets

DESCRIPTION

Each white round tablet (stamped "BRA 200") contains 667 mg of calcium acetate, USP (anhydrous; $Ca(CH_3COO)_2$; MW=158.17 grams) equal to 169 mg (8.45 mEq) calcium, and 10 mg of the inert binder, polyethylene glycol 8000 NF.

CLINICAL PHARMACOLOGY

Patients with advanced renal insufficiency (creatinine clearance less than 30 ml/min) exhibit phosphate retention and some degree of hyperphosphatemia. The retention of phosphate plays a pivotal role in causing secondary hyperparathyroidism associated with osteodystrophy, and soft tissue calcification. The mechanism by which phosphate retention leads to hyperparathyroidism is not clearly delineated. Therapeutic efforts directed toward the control of hyperphosphatemia include reduction in the dietary intake of phosphate, inhibition of absorption of phosphate in the intestine with phosphate binders, and removal of phosphate from the body by more efficient methods of dialysis. The rate of removal of phosphate by dietary manipulation or by dialysis is insufficient. Dialysis patients absorb 40% to 80% of dietary phosphorus. Therefore, the fraction of dietary phosphate absorbed from the diet needs to be reduced by using phopsphate binders in most renal failure patients on maintenance dialysis. Calcium acetate (PhosLo) when taken with meals, combines with dietary phosphate to form insoluble calcium phosphate which is excreted in the feces. Maintenance of serum phosphorus below 6.0 mg/dl is generally considered as a clinically acceptable outcome of treatment with phosphate binders. PhosLo is highly soluble at neutral pH, making the calcium readily available for binding to phosphate in the proximal small intestine.

Orally administered calcium acetate from pharmaceutical dosage forms has been demonstrated to be systemically absorbed up to approximately 40% under fasting conditions and up to approximately 30% under nonfasting conditions. This range represents data from both healthy subjects and renal dialysis patients under various conditions.

INDICATIONS AND USAGE

PhosLo is indicated for the control of hyperphosphatemia in end stage renal failure and does not promote aluminum absorption.

CONTRAINDICATIONS

Patients with hypercalcemia.

WARNINGS

Patients with end stage renal failure may develop hypercalcemia when given calcium with meals. No other calcium supplements should be given concurrently with PhosLo. Progressive hypercalcemia due to overdose of PhosLo may be severe as to require emergency measures. Chronic hypercalcemia may lead to vascular calcification, and other soft-tissue calcification. The serum calcium level should be monitored twice weekly during the early dose adjustment period. **The serum calcium times phosphate (CaXP) product should not be allowed to exceed 66.** Radiographic evaluation of suspect anatomical region may be helpful in early detection of soft-tissue calcification.

PRECAUTIONS

General: Excessive dosage of PhosLo induces hypercalcemia; therefore, early in the treatment during dosage adjustment serum calcium should be determined twice weekly. Should hypercalcemia develop, the dosage should be reduced or the treatment discontinued immediately depending on the severity of hypercalcemia. PhosLo should not be given to patients on digitalis, because hypercalcemia may precipitate cardiac arrhythmias. PhosLo therapy should always be started at low dose and should not be increased without careful monitoring of serum calcium. An estimate of daily dietary calcium intake should be made initially and the intake adjusted as needed. Serum phosphorus should also be determined periodically.

Information for the patient: The patient should be informed about compliance with dosage instructions, adherence to instructions about diet and avoidance of the use of nonprescription anatacids. Patients should be informed about the symptoms of hypercalcemia (see ADVERSE REACTIONS section).

Drug interactions: PhosLo may decrease the bioavailability of tetracyclines.

Carcinogenesis, mutagenesis, impairment of fertility: Long term animal studies have not been performed to evaluate the carcinogenic potential or effect on fertility of PhosLo.

Pregnancy: teratogenic effects: Category C. Animal reproduction studies have not been conducted with PhosLo. It is also not known whether PhosLo can cause fetal harm when administered to a pregnant woman or can affect reproduction capacity. PhosLo should be given to a pregnant woman only if clearly needed.

Pediatric use: Safety and efficacy of PhosLo have not been established.

ADVERSE REACTIONS

In clinical studies, patients have occasionally experienced nausea during PhosLo therapy. Hypercalcemia may occur during treatment with PhosLo. Mild hypercalcemia (Ca>10.5 mg/dl) may be asymptomatic or manifest itself as constipation, anorexia, nausea and vomiting. More severe hypercalcemia (Ca>12 mg/dl) is associated with confusion, delerium, stupor and coma. Mild hypercalcemia is easily controlled by reducing the PhosLo dose or temporarily discontinuing therapy. Severe hypercalcemia can be treated by acute hemodialysis and discontinuing PhosLo therapy.

Decreasing dialysate calcium concentration could reduce the incidence and severity of PhosLo induced hypercalcemia. The long-term effect of PhosLo on the progression of vascular or soft-tissue calcification has not been determined. Isolated cases of pruritus have been reported which may represent allergic reactions.

OVERDOSAGE

Administration of PhosLo in excess of the appropriate daily dosage can cause severe hypercalcemia (See Adverse Reactions).

DOSAGE AND ADMINISTRATION

The recommended initial dose of PhosLo for the adult dialysis patient is 2 tablets with each meal. The dosage may be increased gradually to bring serum phosphate value below 6 mg/dl, as long as hypercalcemia does not develop. Most patients require 3–4 tablets with each meal.

Store at controlled room temperature, 15°–30°C.

HOW SUPPLIED

In tablet form for oral administration. Each white round tablet contains 667 mg of calcium acetate (anhydrous; $Ca(CH_3COO)_2$; MW=158.17 grams equal to 169 mg (8.45 mEq) calcium, and 10 mg of the inert binder, polyethylene glycol 8000.

NDC 52268-200-01 R 7/96

Rx only

Manufactured for Braintree Laboratories, Inc.,
Braintree, MA 02185-0929

Shown in Product Identification Guide, page 307

Breckenridge Pharmaceutical, Inc.

P.O. BOX 206
BOCA RATON, FL 33429

Direct Inquiries to:
Customer Service Dept.
(561) 367-8512

DOUBLECAP™ OTC

[*dōublekăp*]

Topical Analgesic Cream
ODOR FREE

DESCRIPTION

DoubleCap™ contains 0.05% capsaicin cream.

INDICATIONS AND USAGE

DoubleCap™ Cream contains purified capsaicin, a natural ingredient, derived from the pepper plant, which provides odor-free penetrating, temporary pain relief of muscles and joints associated with arthritis, simple backache, sprains and strains. Capsaicin is so effective it is the #1 doctor recommended topical analgesic.

In order for DoubleCap™ Cream to work best, it must be used as outlined in the DIRECTIONS section below. When applying DoubleCap™ Cream on hands, allow 30 minutes for it to penetrate and then wash hands thoroughly. When applying to other areas of the body, immediately afterwards, wash your hands thoroughly. Do not use warm compresses over the area where DoubleCap™ Cream has been applied.

WARNINGS:

- FOR EXTERNAL USE ONLY.
- Avoid contact with the eyes and any mucous membranes.
- If condition worsens, or if symptoms persist for more than 7 days or clear up and occur again within a few days, discontinue use of this product and consult a doctor.
- Do not apply to wounds, damaged or broken (open), irritated skin or if excessive irritation develops.
- Do not bandage tightly.
- Do not use with a heating pad.
- Temporary burning may occur upon application, but generally disappears in several days.

Continued on next page

DoubleCap—Cont.

- If pregnant or breast feeding, ask a health professional before use.

Keep out of reach of children. In case of ingestion, get medical help right away.

DIRECTIONS:

Adults and children 2 years of age and older: Apply a thin film of DoubleCap Cream™ to affected area 3 to 4 times daily. For maximum relief, continue to apply every day, 3 to 4 times daily. Children under 2 years of age: Ask a doctor. **WASH HANDS WITH SOAP AND WATER IMMEDIATELY AFTER APPLYING. Read package insert before using.**
Store at controlled room temperature 15°–30°C (59°–86°F). Close cap tightly after use.

HOW SUPPLIED

Doublecap Cream™ is supplied in a 2 oz. tube (NDC 51991-340-22)

Information on the Origin and Action of Capsaicin

Capsicum is the fruit of a number of naturally occurring plant species (paprika, chili peppers) and has been recognized for many years as an effective topical treatment of pain associated with, amongst others, arthritis. The key components of capsicum are capsaicinoids.

Mechanism of Action: The mechanism of action of capsaicinoids in the relief of pain is presumed to be their inhibition of neurotransmitter release from afferent pain-receptors. The available evidence indicates that capsaicinoids directly open non-selective action channels in the peripheral nerve terminals to slow down conduction and block release of substance P and other neuropeptides. Release of these neuropeptides from unmyelinated primary afferent nerve fibers mediates pain and neurogenic inflammation. The antinociceptive effects of capsaicinoids are subsequent to initial nerve stimulation which may evoke the sensation of warmth and stinging. This agonism is seen during the first part of therapy and may cause initial discomfort. Because capsaicinoids prevent neuropeptide re-accumulation, any initial pain and stinging progressively decrease.

©Breckenridge Pharmaceutical, Inc., 1998

PRODIUM™   OTC
[prō 'dē um]
(Phenazopyridine HCl 95 mg)
FOR URINARY TRACT DISCOMFORT

DESCRIPTION

Each analgesic tablet contains 95 mg Phenazopyridine HCl.

INDICATIONS AND USAGE

Phenazopyridine HCl is indicated for the temporary relief of minor pain, urgency, frequency, and burning on urination. Treatment of a urinary tract infection with Phenazopyridine HCl should not exceed 2 days because there is a lack of evidence that the combined administration of Phenazopyridine HCl and an antibacterial provides greater benefit than administration of the antibacterial alone after 2 days.

CONTRAINDICATIONS

Phenazopyridine HCl should not be used in patients who have previously exhibited hypersensitivity to it. Its use is also contraindicated in patients with hepatitis or renal insufficiency.

PRECAUTIONS

Do not administer to children under 12 years of age unless directed by physician. Individuals with any hepatic or renal trouble should not use this product unless directed by a physician. If symptoms persist for more than 2 days, consult a physician. The decline in renal function associated with advanced age should be kept in mind. A yellowish tinge of the skin or sclera may indicate accumulation due to impaired renal excretion and the need to discontinue therapy.

NOTE:

Phenazopyridine HCl produces an orange to red color in the urine and may stain fabric. Staining of contact lenses has been reported.

Phenazopyridine HCl is known to cause gastrointestinal upset in some individuals; discontinue use if symptoms occur. Taking with or following meals will reduce gastric upset.

Carcinogenesis: Long-term administration of phenazopyridine hydrochloride has induced neoplasia in rats (large intestine) and mice (liver). Although no association between phenazopyridine hydrochloride and human neoplasia has been reported, adequate epidemiological studies along these lines have not been conducted.

WARNING

As with any drug, if you are pregnant or nursing a baby, seek the advice of a health professional before using this product. If symptoms persist for more than 2 days, consult a physician. Keep this and all medicines out of the reach of children.

DOSAGE AND ADMINISTRATION

95 mg tablets — adult dosage is two tablets 3 times a day after meals and administration should not exceed 2 days. Store at room temperature.

HOW SUPPLIED

Prodium™ is supplied in cartons of 30 tablets (ND 51991-240-30) and cartons of 12 tablets (NDC 51991-240-12).
©Breckenridge Pharmaceutical, Inc., 1998

Bristol-Myers Squibb Oncology/ Immunology Division

A Bristol-Myers Squibb Company
P.O. BOX 4500
PRINCETON, NJ 08543-4500

For Medical Information Contact:
Generally:
Bristol-Myers Squibb Drug Information Department
P.O. Box 4500
Princeton, NJ 08543-4500
(800) 426-7644
Adverse Drug Experiences
and Product Defects Reporting call
during business hours only:
(609) 818-3737

Sales and Ordering:
Orders may be placed by:
1. Calling the following toll-free number between 8:30 AM– 6:00 PM EST:
 Continental U.S.: (800) 631-5244
 Alaska-Hawaii: (800) 631-5244
2. Mail orders and all inquiries should be sent to:
 Bristol-Myers Squibb Oncology Division
 Attn: Customer Service
 P.O. Box 5250
 Princeton, NJ 08543-5250
3. Faxing your purchase orders to:
 (800) 523-2965
4. Transmitting computer-to-computer on the NWDA and UCS formats through Ordernet Services use: DEA #PE0048579

BiCNU®   ℞
(sterile carmustine [BCNU])

CAUTION: FEDERAL LAW PROHIBITS DISPENSING WITHOUT PRESCRIPTION.

> **WARNINGS**
> BiCNU® (sterile carmustine [BCNU]) should be administered under the supervision of a qualified physician experienced in the use of cancer chemotherapeutic agents.
> Bone marrow suppression, notably thrombocytopenia and leukopenia, which may contribute to bleeding and overwhelming infections in an already compromised patient, is the most common and severe of the toxic effects of BiCNU (see **"WARNINGS"** and **"ADVERSE REACTIONS"**).
> Since the major toxicity is delayed bone marrow suppression, blood counts should be monitored weekly for at least 6 weeks after a dose (see **"ADVERSE REACTIONS"**). At the recommended dosage, courses of BiCNU should not be given more frequently than every 6 weeks.
> The bone marrow toxicity of BiCNU is cumulative and therefore dosage adjustment must be considered on the basis of nadir blood counts from prior dose (see "Dosage Adjustment Table" under **"DOSAGE AND ADMINISTRATION"**).
> Pulmonary toxicity from BiCNU appears to be dose related. Patients receiving greater than 1400 mg/m² cumulative dose are at significantly higher risk than those receiving less.
> Delayed pulmonary toxicity can occur years after treatment, and can result in death, particularly in patients treated in childhood (see **"ADVERSE REACTIONS"**, and **"PRECAUTIONS: Pediatric Use"**).

DESCRIPTION

BiCNU® (sterile carmustine [BCNU]) is one of the nitrosoureas used in the treatment of certain neoplastic diseases. It is 1,3-bis (2-chloroethyl)-1-nitrosourea. It is lyophilized pale yellow flakes or congealed mass with a molecular weight of 214.06. It is highly soluble in alcohol and lipids, and poorly soluble in water. BiCNU is administered by intravenous infusion after reconstitution as recommended. The structural formula is:

$$Cl\text{-}CH_2\text{-}CH_2\text{-}\overset{\displaystyle O}{\overset{\|}{C}}\text{-}NH\text{-}CH_2\text{-}CH_2\text{-}Cl$$
$$\underset{NO}{|}$$

Sterile BiCNU is available in 100 mg single dose vials of lyophilized material.

CLINICAL PHARMACOLOGY

Although it is generally agreed that carmustine alkylates DNA and RNA, it is not cross resistant with other alkylators. As with other nitrosoureas, it may also inhibit several key enzymatic processes by carbamoylation of amino acids in proteins.

Intravenously administered carmustine is rapidly degraded, with no intact drug detectable after 15 minutes. However, in studies with C^{14}- labeled drug, prolonged levels of the isotope were detected in the plasma and tissue, probably representing radioactive fragments of the parent compound.

It is thought that the antineoplastic and toxic activities of carmustine may be due to metabolites. Approximately 60% to 70% of a total dose is excreted in the urine in 96 hours and about 10% as respiratory CO_2. The fate of the remainder is undetermined.

Because of the high lipid solubility and the relative lack of ionization at physiological pH, carmustine crosses the blood-brain barrier quite effectively. Levels of radioactivity in the CSF are $\geq$ 50% of those measured concurrently in plasma.

INDICATIONS AND USAGE

BiCNU is indicated as palliative therapy as a single agent or in established combination therapy with other approved chemotherapeutic agents in the following:
1. Brain tumors-glioblastoma, brainstem glioma, medulloblastoma, astrocytoma, ependymoma, and metastatic brain tumors.
2. Multiple myeloma-in combination with prednisone.
3. Hodgkin's Disease-as secondary therapy in combination with other approved drugs in patients who relapse while being treated with primary therapy, or who fail to respond to primary therapy.
4. Non-Hodgkin's lymphomas-as secondary therapy in combination with other approved drugs for patients who relapse while being treated with primary therapy, or who fail to respond to primary therapy.

CONTRAINDICATIONS

BiCNU should not be given to individuals who have demonstrated a previous hypersensitivity to it.

WARNINGS

Since the major toxicity is delayed bone marrow suppression, blood counts should be monitored weekly for at least 6 weeks after a dose (see **"ADVERSE REACTIONS"**). At the recommended dosage, courses of BiCNU should not be given more frequently than every 6 weeks.

The bone marrow toxicity of BiCNU is cumulative and therefore dosage adjustment must be considered on the basis of nadir blood counts from prior dose (see "Dosage Adjustment Table" under **"DOSAGE AND ADMINISTRATION"**).

Pulmonary toxicity from BiCNU appears to be dose related. Patients receiving greater than 1400 mg/m² cumulative dose are at significantly higher risk than those receiving less. Additionally delayed onset pulmonary fibrosis occurring up to 17 years after treatment has been reported in patients who receive BiCNU in childhood and early adolescence (see **"ADVERSE REACTIONS"**).

Long term use of nitrosoureas has been reported to be associated with the development of secondary malignancies.

Liver and renal function tests should be monitored periodically (see **"ADVERSE REACTIONS"**).

BiCNU may cause fetal harm when administered to a pregnant woman. BiCNU has been shown to be embryotoxic in rats and rabbits and teratogenic in rats when given in doses equivalent to the human dose. There are no adequate and well-controlled studies in pregnant women. If this drug is used during pregnancy, or if the patient becomes pregnant while taking (receiving) this drug, the patient should be apprised of the potential hazard to the fetus. Women of childbearing potential should be advised to avoid becoming pregnant.

BiCNU (sterile carmustine [BCNU]) has been administered through an intraarterial intracarotid route; this procedure is investigational and has been associated with ocular toxicity.

PRECAUTIONS

General: In all instances where the use of BiCNU is considered for chemotherapy, the physician must evaluate the need and usefulness of the drug against the risks of toxic effects or adverse reactions. Most such adverse reactions are reversible if detected early. When such effects or reactions

do occur, the drug should be reduced in dosage or discontinued and appropriate corrective measures should be taken according to the clinical judgment of the physician. Reinstitution of BiCNU therapy should be carried out with caution, and with adequate consideration of the further need for the drug and alertness as to possible recurrence of toxicity.

Laboratory Tests: Due to delayed bone marrow suppression, blood counts should be monitored weekly for at least 6 weeks after a dose.

Baseline pulmonary function studies should be conducted along with frequent pulmonary function tests during treatment. Patients with a baseline below 70% of the predicted Forced Vital Capacity (FVC) or Carbon Monoxide Diffusing Capacity (DL_{co}) are particularly at risk.

Since BiCNU may cause liver dysfunction, it is recommended that liver function tests be monitored.

Renal function tests should also be monitored periodically.

Carcinogenesis, Mutagenesis, Impairment of Fertility: BiCNU is carcinogenic in rats and mice, producing a marked increase in tumor incidence in doses approximating those employed clinically. Nitrosourea therapy does have carcinogenic potential in humans (see **"ADVERSE REACTIONS"**). BiCNU also affects fertility in male rats at doses somewhat higher than the human dose.

Pregnancy: Pregnancy "Category D" (see **"WARNINGS"**).

Nursing Mothers: It is not known whether this drug is excreted in human milk. Because of the potential for serious adverse events in nursing infants, nursing should be discontinued while taking BiCNU.

Pediatric Use: Safety and effectiveness in children have not been established. Delayed onset pulmonary fibrosis occurring up to 17 years after treatment, has been reported in a long term study of patients who received BiCNU in childhood and early adolescence (1–16 years). Eight out of the 17 patients (47%) who survived childhood brain tumors, including all the five patients initially treated at less than five years of age, died of pulmonary fibrosis. Therefore, the risks and benefits of BiCNU therapy must be carefully considered, due to the extremely high risk of pulmonary toxicity. (See **"ADVERSE REACTIONS: Pulmonary Toxicity"**).

ADVERSE REACTIONS

Pulmonary Toxicity: Pulmonary toxicity characterized by pulmonary infiltrates and/or fibrosis has been reported to occur from 9 days to 43 months after treatment with BiCNU and related nitrosoureas. Most of these patients were receiving prolonged therapy with total doses of BiCNU greater than 1400 mg/m². However, there have been reports of pulmonary fibrosis in patients receiving lower total doses. Other risk factors include past history of lung disease and duration of treatment. Cases of fatal pulmonary toxicity with BiCNU have been reported.

Additionally, delayed onset pulmonary fibrosis occurring up to 17 years after treatment has been reported in a long-term study with 17 patients who received BiCNU in childhood and early adolescence (1–16 years) in cumulative doses ranging from 770 to 1800 mg/m² combined with cranial radiotherapy for intracranial tumors. Chest x-rays demonstrated pulmonary hypoplasia with upper zone contraction. Gallium scans were normal in all cases. Thoracic CT scans have demonstrated an unusual pattern of upper zone fibrosis. There was some late reduction of pulmonary function in all long-term survivors. This form of lung fibrosis may be slowly progressive and has resulted in death in some cases. In this long-term study, 8 of 17 died of delayed pulmonary lung fibrosis, including all those initially treated (5 of 17) at less than 5 years of age.

Hematologic Toxicity: A frequent and serious toxicity of BiCNU is delayed myelosuppression. It usually occurs 4 to 6 weeks after drug administration and is dose related. Thrombocytopenia occurs at about 4 weeks postadministration and persists for 1 to 2 weeks. Leukopenia occurs at 5 to 6 weeks after a dose of BiCNU and persists for 1 to 2 weeks. Thrombocytopenia is generally more severe than leukopenia. However, both may be dose-limiting toxicities.

BiCNU may produce cumulative myelosuppression, manifested by more depressed indices or longer duration of suppression after repeated doses.

The occurrence of acute leukemia and bone marrow dysplasias have been reported in patients following long term nitrosourea therapy.

Anemia also occurs, but is less frequent and less severe than thrombocytopenia or leukopenia.

Gastrointestinal Toxicity: Nausea and vomiting after IV administration of BiCNU are noted frequently. This toxicity appears within 2 hours of dosing, usually lasting 4 to 6 hours, and is dose related. Prior administration of antiemetics is effective in diminishing and sometimes preventing this side effect.

Hepatotoxicity: A reversible type of hepatic toxicity, manifested by increased transaminase, alkaline phosphatase, and bilirubin levels, has been reported in a small percentage of patients receiving BiCNU.

Nephrotoxicity: Renal abnormalities consisting of progressive azotemia, decrease in kidney size and renal failure have been reported in patients who received large cumula-

tive doses after prolonged therapy with BiCNU and related nitrosoureas. Kidney damage has also been reported occasionally in patients receiving lower total doses.

Other Toxicities: Accidental contact of reconstituted BiCNU with skin has caused burning and hyperpigmentation of the affected areas.

Rapid IV infusion of BiCNU may produce intensive flushing of the skin and suffusion of the conjunctiva within 2 hours, lasting about 4 hours. It is also associated with burning at the site of injection although true thrombosis is rare.

Neuroretinitis, chest pain, headache, allergic reaction, hypotension and tachycardia have been reported as part of ongoing surveillance.

OVERDOSAGE

No proven antidotes have been established for BiCNU overdosage.

DOSAGE AND ADMINISTRATION

The recommended dose of BiCNU as a single agent in previously untreated patients is 150 to 200 mg/m² intravenously every 6 weeks. This may be given as a single dose or divided into daily injections such as 75 to 100 mg/m² on 2 successive days. When BiCNU is used in combination with other myelosuppressive drugs or in patients in whom bone marrow reserve is depleted, the doses should be adjusted accordingly.

Doses subsequent to the initial dose should be adjusted according to the hematologic response of the patient to the preceding dose. The following schedule is suggested as a guide to dosage adjustment:

Nadir After Prior Dose		Percentage of Prior Dose to be Given
Leukocytes/mm³	Platelets/mm³	
>4000	>100,000	100%
3000–3999	75,000–99,999	100%
2000–2999	25,000–74,999	70%
<2000	<25,000	50%

A repeat course of BiCNU (sterile carmustine [BCNU]) should not be given until circulating blood elements have returned to acceptable levels (platelets above 100,000/mm³, leukocytes above 4,000/mm³), and this is usually in 6 weeks. Adequate number of neutrophils should be present on a peripheral blood smear. Blood counts should be monitored weekly and repeat courses should not be given before 6 weeks because the hematologic toxicity is delayed and cumulative.

Administration Precautions: As with other potentially toxic compounds, caution should be exercised in handling BiCNU and preparing the solution of BiCNU. Accidental contact of reconstituted BiCNU with the skin has caused transient hyperpigmentation of the affected areas. The use of gloves is recommended. If BiCNU lyophilized material or solution contacts the skin or mucosa, immediately wash the skin or mucosa thoroughly with soap and water.

The reconstituted solution should be used intravenously only and should be administered by IV drip. Injection of BiCNU over shorter periods of time than 1 to 2 hours may produce intense pain and burning at the site of injection.

Preparation of Intravenous Solutions: First, dissolve BiCNU with 3 mL of the supplied sterile diluent (Dehydrated Alcohol Injection, USP). Second, aseptically add 27 mL Sterile Water for Injection, USP. Each mL of resulting solution contains 3.3 mg of BiCNU in 10% ethanol, pH 5.6 to 6.0. Such solutions should be protected from light.

Reconstitution as recommended results in a clear, colorless to yellowish solution which may be further diluted with 5% Dextrose Injection, USP. Parenteral drug products should be inspected visually for particulate matter and discoloration prior to administration, whenever solution and container permit.

Important Note: The lyophilized dosage formulation contains no preservatives and is not intended for use as a multiple dose vial.

Stability: Unopened vials of the dry drug must be stored in a refrigerator (2°C to 8°C, 36°F to 46°F). The recommended storage of unopened vials provides a stable product for 2 years. After reconstitution as recommended, BiCNU is stable for 8 hours at room temperature (25°C, 77°F), protected from light.

Vials reconstituted as directed and further diluted to a concentration of 0.2 mg/mL in 5% Dextrose Injection, USP, should be stored at room temperature, protected from light and utilized within 8 hours.

Glass containers were used for the stability data provided in this section. Only use glass containers for BiCNU administration.

Important Note: BiCNU has a low melting point (30.5° to 32.0°C or 86.9° to 89.6°F). Exposure of the drug to this temperature or above will cause the drug to liquefy and appear as an oil film on the vials. This is a sign of decomposition and vials should be discarded. If there is a question of adequate refrigeration upon receipt of this product, immedi-

ately inspect the larger vial in each individual carton. Hold the vial to the bright light for inspection. The BiCNU will appear as a very small amount of dry flakes or dry congealed mass. If this is evident, the BiCNU is suitable for use and should be refrigerated immediately.

Procedures for proper handling and disposal of anticancer drugs should be considered. Several guidelines on this subject have been published.[1-7] There is no general agreement that all of the procedures recommended in the guidelines are necessary or appropriate.

HOW SUPPLIED

BiCNU® (sterile carmustine [BCNU]). Each package includes a vial containing 100 mg carmustine and a vial containing 3 mL sterile diluent.

NDC 0015-3012-38

Store dry powder in refrigerator (2° to 8°C, 36° to 46°F). For information on package sizes available refer to the current price schedule.

REFERENCES

1. Recommendations for the Safe Handling of Parenteral Antineoplastic Drugs. NIH Publication No. 83-2621. For sale by the Superintendent of Documents, U.S. Government Printing Office, Washington, DC 20402.
2. AMA Council Report. Guidelines for Handling Parenteral Antineoplastics. JAMA 1985; 253(11): 1590-1592.
3. National Study Commission on Cytotoxic Exposure–Recommendations for Handling Cytotoxic Agents. Available from Louis P. Jeffrey, ScD Chairman, National Study Commission on Cytotoxic Exposure, Massachusetts College of Pharmacy and Allied Health Sciences, 179 Longwood Avenue, Boston, Massachusetts 02115.
4. Clinical Oncological Society of Australia. Guidelines and Recommendations for Safe Handling of Antineoplastic Agents. Med J Australia 1983; 1:426–428.
5. Jones, RB, et al: Safe Handling of Chemotherapeutic Agents. A Report from the Mount Sinai Medical Center. CA–A Cancer Journal for Clinicians 1983; (Sept/Oct)258-263.
6. American Society of Hospital Pharmacists Technical Assistance Bulletin on Handling Cytotoxic and Hazardous Drugs. Am J Hosp Pharm 1990; 47:1033–1049.
7. Controlling occupational exposure to hazardous drugs. (OSHA WORK PRACTICE GUIDELINES). Am J Health-Syst Pharm 1996; 53:1669–1685.

Manufactured by:
Ben Venue Laboratories, Inc., Bedford, Ohio 44146
Distributed by:
BRISTOL LABORATORIES®
ONCOLOGY PRODUCTS
A Bristol-Myers Squibb Company
Princeton, NJ 08543
U.S.A.
H1-B001-3-97   P7980-05
                        Latest Revised: December 1996

BLENOXANE®   ℞
(sterile bleomycin sulfate, USP)

CAUTION: FEDERAL LAW PROHIBITS DISPENSING WITHOUT PRESCRIPTION.

> **WARNING**
> It is recommended that BLENOXANE® (sterile bleomycin sulfate, USP) be administered under the supervision of a qualified physician experienced in the use of cancer chemotherapeutic agents. Appropriate management of therapy and complications is possible only when adequate diagnostic and treatment facilities are readily available.
> Pulmonary fibrosis is the most severe toxicity associated with BLENOXANE. The most frequent presentation is pneumonitis occasionally progressing to pulmonary fibrosis. Its occurrence is higher in elderly patients and in those receiving greater than 400 units total dose, but pulmonary toxicity has been observed in young patients and those treated with low doses.
> A severe idiosyncratic reaction consisting of hypotension, mental confusion, fever, chills, and wheezing has been reported in approximately 1% of lymphoma patients treated with BLENOXANE.

DESCRIPTION

BLENOXANE® (sterile bleomycin sulfate, USP) is a mixture of cytotoxic glycopeptide antibiotics isolated from a strain of *Streptomyces verticillus*. It is freely soluble in water.

Note: A unit of bleomycin is equal to the formerly used milligram activity. The term milligram activity is a misnomer and was changed to units to be more precise.

Continued on next page

Blenoxane—Cont.

CLINICAL PHARMACOLOGY

Although the exact mechanism of action of BLENOXANE is unknown, available evidence would seem to indicate that the main mode of action is the inhibition of DNA synthesis with some evidence of lesser inhibition of RNA and protein synthesis.

In mice, high concentrations of BLENOXANE are found in the skin, lungs, kidneys, peritoneum, and lymphatics. Tumor cells of the skin and lungs have been found to have high concentrations of BLENOXANE in contrast to the low concentrations found in hematopoietic tissue. The low concentrations of BLENOXANE found in bone marrow may be related to high levels of BLENOXANE degradative enzymes found in that tissue.

In patients with normal renal function, 60 to 70% of an administered dose is recovered in the urine as active bleomycin. In patients with a creatinine clearance of > 35 mL per minute, the serum or plasma terminal elimination half-life of bleomycin is approximately 115 minutes. In patients with a creatinine clearance of < 35 mL per minute, the plasma or serum terminal elimination half-life increases exponentially as the creatinine clearance decreases. It was reported that patients with moderately severe renal failure excreted less than 20% of the dose in the urine. This result would suggest that severe renal impairment could lead to accumulation of the drug in blood.

Information on the dose proportionally of bleomycin is not available.

When administered intrapleurally for the treatment of malignant pleural effusion, BLENOXANE acts as a sclerosing agent.

Following intrapleural administration to a limited number of patients (n=4), the resultant bleomycin plasma concentrations suggest a systemic absorption of approximately 45%.

The safety and efficacy of BLENOXANE 60 units and tetracycline (1 gm) as treatment for malignant pleural effusion were evaluated in a multicenter, randomized trial. Patients were required to have cytologically positive pleural effusion, good performance status (0,1,2), lung re-expansion following tube thoracostomy with drainage rates of 100 mL/24 hr or less, no prior intrapleural therapy, no prior systemic BLENOXANE therapy, no chest irradiation and no recent change in systemic therapy. Overall survival did not differ between the BLENOXANE 60 units (n=44) and tetracycline (n=41) groups. Of patients evaluated within 30 days of instillation, the recurrence rate was 36% (10/28) with BLENOXANE and 67% (18/27) with tetracycline (p=0.023). Toxicity was similar between groups.

INDICATIONS & USAGE

BLENOXANE should be considered a palliative treatment. It has been shown to be useful in the management of the following neoplasms either as a single agent or in proven combinations with other approved chemotherapeutic agents:

Squamous Cell Carcinoma—Head and neck (including mouth, tongue, tonsil, nasopharynx, oropharynx, sinus, palate, lip, buccal mucosa, gingivae, epiglottis, skin, larynx), penis, cervix, and vulva. The response to BLENOXANE is poorer in patients with previously irradiated head and neck cancer.

Lymphomas—Hodgkin's Disease, non-Hodgkin's lymphoma.

Testicular Carcinoma—Embryonal cell, choriocarcinoma, and teratocarcinoma.

BLENOXANE has also been shown to be useful in the management of:

Malignant Pleural Effusion—BLENOXANE is effective as a sclerosing agent for the treatment of malignant pleural effusion and prevention of recurrent pleural effusions.

CONTRAINDICATIONS

BLENOXANE is contraindicated in patients who have demonstrated a hypersensitive or an idiosyncratic reaction to it.

WARNINGS

Patients receiving BLENOXANE must be observed carefully and frequently during and after therapy. It should be used with extreme caution in patients with significant impairment of renal function or compromised pulmonary function.

Pulmonary toxicities occur in 10% of treated patients. In approximately 1%, the nonspecific pneumonitis induced by BLENOXANE progresses to pulmonary fibrosis, and death. Although this is age and dose related, the toxicity is unpredictable. Frequent roentgenograms are recommended.

A severe idiosyncratic reaction (similar to anaphylaxis) consisting of hypotension, mental confusion, fever, chills, and wheezing has been reported in approximately 1% of lymphoma patients treated with BLENOXANE. Since these reactions usually occur after the first or second dose, careful monitoring is essential after these doses.

Renal or hepatic toxicity, beginning as a deterioration in renal or liver function tests, have been reported, infrequently. These toxicities may occur, however, at any time after initiation of therapy.

Usage in Pregnancy

Pregnancy "Category D"—BLENOXANE (sterile bleomycin sulfate, USP) can cause fetal harm when administered to a pregnant woman. It has been shown to be teratogenic in rats. Administration of intraperitoneal doses of 1.5 mg/kg/day to rats (about 1.6 times the recommended human dose on a unit/m² basis) on days 6-15 of gestation caused skeletal malformations, shortened innominate artery and hydroureter. BLENOXANE is abortifacient but not teratogenic in rabbits, at intravenous doses of 1.2 mg/kg/day (about 2.4 times the recommended human dose on a unit/m² basis) given on gestation days 6-18.

There have been no studies in pregnant women. If BLENOXANE is used during pregnancy, or if the patient becomes pregnant while receiving this drug, the patient should be apprised of the potential hazard to the fetus. Women of childbearing potential should be advised to avoid becoming pregnant during therapy with BLENOXANE.

PRECAUTIONS

General—Bleomycin clearance may be reduced in patients with impaired renal function. No guidelines have been established for dose adjustments, but bleomycin should be used with extreme caution in patients with significant renal impairment.

Carcinogenesis, Mutagenesis, and Impairment of Fertility—The carcinogenic potential of BLENOXANE in humans is unknown. A study in F344-type male rats demonstrated an increased incidence of nodular hyperplasia after induced lung carcinogenesis by nitrosamines, followed by treatment with bleomycin. In another study where the drug was administered to rats by subcutaneous injection at 0.35mg/kg weekly (3.82 units/m² weekly or about 30% at the recommended human dose), necropsy findings included dose related injection site fibrosarcomas as well as various renal tumors. Bleomycin has been shown to be mutagenic both *in vitro* and *in vivo*. The effects of bleomycin on fertility have not been studied.

Pregnancy—Pregnancy "Category D". (See **"WARNINGS"** section.)

Nursing Mothers—It is not known whether the drug is excreted in human milk. Because many drugs are excreted in human milk and because of the potential for serious adverse reactions in nursing infants, it is recommended that nursing be discontinued by women receiving BLENOXANE therapy.

Pediatric Use—Safety and effectiveness of BLENOXANE in pediatric patients have not been established.

ADVERSE REACTIONS

Pulmonary—This is potentially the most serious side effect, occurring in approximately 10% of treated patients. The most frequent presentation is pneumonitis occasionally progressing to pulmonary fibrosis. Approximately 1% of patients treated have died of pulmonary fibrosis. Pulmonary toxicity is both dose and age related, being more common in patients over 70 years of age and in those receiving over 400 units total dose. This toxicity, however, is unpredictable and has been seen occasionally in young patients receiving low doses. Some published reports have suggested that the risk of pulmonary toxicity may be increased when bleomycin is used in combination with G-CSF (filgrastim) or other cytokines. However, randomized clinical studies completed to date have not demonstrated an increased risk of pulmonary complications in patients treated with bleomycin and G-CSF.

Because of lack of specificity of the clinical syndrome, the identification of patients with pulmonary toxicity due to BLENOXANE has been extremely difficult. The earliest symptom associated with BLENOXANE pulmonary toxicity is dyspnea. The earliest sign is fine rales.

Radiographically, BLENOXANE-induced pneumonitis produces nonspecific patchy opacities, usually of the lower lung fields. The most common changes in pulmonary function tests are a decrease in total lung volume and a decrease in vital capacity. However, these changes are not predictive of the development of pulmonary fibrosis.

The microscopic tissue changes due to BLENOXANE toxicity include bronchiolar squamous metaplasia, reactive macrophages, atypical alveolar epithelial cells, fibrinous edema, and interstitial fibrosis. The acute stage may involve capillary changes and subsequent fibrinous exudation into alveoli producing a change similar to hyaline membrane formation and progressing to a diffuse interstitial fibrosis resembling the Hamman-Rich syndrome. These microscopic findings are nonspecific; e.g., similar changes are seen in radiation pneumonitis and pneumocystic pneumonitis.

To monitor the onset of pulmonary toxicity, roentgenograms of the chest should be taken every 1 to 2 weeks. If pulmonary changes are noted, treatment should be discontinued until it can be determined if they are drug related. Recent studies have suggested that sequential measurement of the pulmonary diffusion capacity for carbon monoxide (DL_{co})

during treatment with BLENOXANE may be an indicator of subclinical pulmonary toxicity. It is recommended that the DL_{co} be monitored monthly if it is to be employed to detect pulmonary toxicities, and thus the drug should be discontinued when the DL_{co} falls below 30 to 35% of the pretreatment value.

Because of bleomycin's sensitization of lung tissue, patients who have received bleomycin are at greater risk of developing pulmonary toxicity when oxygen is administered in surgery. While long exposure to very high oxygen concentrations is a known cause of lung damage, after bleomycin administration, lung damage can occur at lower concentrations that are usually considered safe. Suggested preventive measures are:

1. Maintain Fl O_2 at concentrations approximating that of room air (25%) during surgery and the postoperative period.
2. Monitor carefully fluid replacement, focusing more on colloid administration rather than crystalloid.

Sudden onset of an acute chest pain syndrome suggestive of pleuropericarditis has been rarely reported during BLENOXANE infusions. Although each patient must be individually evaluated, further courses of BLENOXANE do not appear to be contraindicated.

Pulmonary adverse events which may be related to the intrapleural administration of BLENOXANE have been reported only rarely.

Idiosyncratic Reactions—In approximately 1% of the lymphoma patients treated with BLENOXANE, an idiosyncratic reaction, similar to anaphylaxis clinically, has been reported. The reaction may be immediate or delayed for several hours, and usually occurs after the first or second dose. It consists of hypotension, mental confusion, fever, chills, and wheezing. Treatment is symptomatic including volume expansion, pressor agents, antihistamines, and corticosteroids.

Integument and Mucous Membranes—These are the most frequent side effects, being reported in approximately 50% of treated patients. These consist of erythema, rash, striae, vesiculation, hyperpigmentation, and tenderness of the skin. Hyperkeratosis, nail changes, alopecia, pruritus, and stomatitis have also been reported. It was necessary to discontinue BLENOXANE (sterile bleomycin sulfate, USP) therapy in 2% of treated patients because of these toxicities. Skin toxicity is a relatively late manifestation usually developing in the 2nd and 3rd week of treatment after 150 to 200 units of BLENOXANE have been administered and appears to be related to the cumulative dose.

Intrapleural administration of BLENOXANE has occasionally been associated with local pain. Hypotension possibly requiring symptomatic treatment has been reported infrequently. Death has been very rarely reported in association with BLENOXANE pleurodesis in these very seriously ill patients.

Other—Vascular toxicities coincident with the use of BLENOXANE in combination with other antineoplastic agents have been reported rarely. The events are clinically heterogeneous and may include myocardial infarction, cerebrovascular accident, thrombotic microangiopathy (HUS) or cerebral arteritis. Various mechanisms have been proposed for these vascular complications. There are also reports of Raynaud's phenomenon occurring in patients treated with BLENOXANE in combination with vinblastine with or without cisplatin or, in a few cases, with BLENOXANE as a single agent. It is currently unknown if the cause of Raynaud's phenomenon in these cases is the disease, underlying vascular compromise, BLENOXANE, vinblastine, hypomagnesemia, or a combination of any of these factors.

Fever, chills, and vomiting were frequently reported side effects. Anorexia and weight loss are common and may persist long after termination of this medication. Pain at tumor site, phlebitis, and other local reactions were reported infrequently.

DOSAGE & ADMINISTRATION

Because of the possibility of an anaphylactoid reaction, lymphoma patients should be treated with 2 units or less for the first two doses. If no acute reaction occurs, then the regular dosage schedule may be followed.

The following dose schedule is recommended: **Squamous cell carcinoma, non-Hodgkin's lymphoma, testicular carcinoma**—0.25 to 0.50 units/kg (10 to 20 units/m²) given intravenously, intramuscularly, or subcutaneously weekly or twice weekly.

Hodgkin's Disease—0.25 to 0.50 units/kg (10 to 20 units/m²) given intravenously, intramuscularly, or subcutaneously weekly or twice weekly. After a 50% response, a maintenance dose of 1 unit daily or 5 units weekly intravenously or intramuscularly should be given.

Pulmonary toxicity of BLENOXANE appears to be dose related with a striking increase when the total dose is over 400 units. Total doses over 400 units should be given with great caution.

Note: When BLENOXANE is used in combination with other antineoplastic agents, pulmonary toxicities may occur at lower doses.

Improvement of Hodgkin's Disease and testicular tumors is prompt and noted within 2 weeks. If no improvement is seen by this time, improvement is unlikely. Squamous cell cancers respond more slowly, sometimes requiring as long as 3 weeks before any improvement is noted.

Malignant Pleural Effusion—60 units administered as a single dose bolus intrapleural injection.

ADMINISTRATION

BLENOXANE may be given by the intramuscular, intravenous, subcutaneous or intrapleural routes.

Intramuscular or Subcutaneous—The BLENOXANE 15 units vial should be reconstituted with 1 to 5 mL of Sterile Water for Injection, USP, Sodium Chloride for Injection, 0.9%, USP, or Bacteriostatic Water for Injection, USP. The BLENOXANE 30 units vial should be reconstituted with 2 to 10 mL of the above diluents.

Intravenous—The contents of the 15 units or 30 units vial should be dissolved in 5 mL or 10 mL, respectively of Sodium Chloride for Injection, 0.9%, USP and administered slowly over a period of 10 minutes.

Intrapleural—60 units of BLENOXANE is dissolved in 50-100 mL sodium chloride injection 0.9%, and administered through a thoracostomy tube following drainage of excess pleural fluid and confirmation of complete lung expansion. The literature suggests that successful pleurodesis is, in part, dependent upon complete drainage of the pleural fluid and reestablishment of negative intrapleural pressure prior to instillation of a sclerosing agent. Therefore, the amount of drainage from the chest tube should be as minimal as possible prior to instillation of BLENOXANE. Although there is no conclusive evidence to support this contention, it is generally accepted that chest tube drainage should be less than 100 mL in a 24 hour period prior to sclerosis. However, BLENOXANE instillation may be appropriate when drainage is between 100-300 mL under clinical conditions that necessitate sclerosis therapy. The thoracostomy tube is clamped after BLENOXANE instillation. The patient is moved from the supine to the left and right lateral positions several times during the next four hours. The clamp is then removed and suction reestablished. The amount of time the chest tube remains in place following sclerosis is dictated by the clinical situation.

The intrapleural injection of topical anesthetics or systemic narcotic analgesia is generally not required.

Parenteral drug products should be inspected visually for particulate matter and discoloration prior to administration, whenever solution and container permit.

HOW SUPPLIED

BLENOXANE® is available as follows:

NDC 0015-3010-20, 15 units per vial as sterile bleomycin sulfate, USP.

NDC 0015-3063-01, 30 units per vial as sterile bleomycin sulfate, USP.

Stability—The sterile powder is stable under refrigeration 2°C (36°F) to 8°C (46°F) and should not be used after the expiration date is reached.

BLENOXANE should not be reconstituted or diluted with D_5W or other dextrose containing diluents. When reconstituted in D_5W and analyzed by HPLC, BLENOXANE demonstrates a loss of A_2 and B_2 potency that does not occur when BLENOXANE is reconstituted in 0.9% sodium chloride.

BLENOXANE is stable for 24 hours at room temperature in Sodium Chloride.

Procedures for proper handling and disposal of anticancer drugs should be considered. Several guidelines on this subject have been published.[1-7] There is no general agreement that all of the procedures recommended in the guidelines are necessary or appropriate.

REFERENCES

1. Recommendations for the Safe Handling of Parenteral Antineoplastic Drugs. NIH Publication No. 83-2621. For sale by the Superintendent of Documents, US Government Printing Office, Washington, DC 20402.
2. AMA Council Report. Guidelines for Handling Parenteral Antineoplastics. JAMA 1985; 253(11):1590-1592.
3. National Study Commission on Cytotoxic Exposure–Recommendations for Handling Cytotoxic Agents. Available from Louis P. Jeffrey, ScD, Chairman, National Study Commission on Cytotoxic Exposure, Massachusetts College of Pharmacy and Allied Health Sciences, 179 Longwood Avenue, Boston, Massachusetts 02115.
4. Clinical Oncological Society of Australia: Guidelines and Recommendations for Safe Handling of Antineoplastic Agents. Med J Australia 1983; 1:426–428.
5. Jones RB, et al: Safe Handling of Chemotherapeutic Agents: A Report from the Mount Sinai Medical Center. CA–A Cancer Journal for Clinicians 1983; (Sept/Oct) 258–263.
6. American Society of Hospital Pharmacists Technical Assistance Bulletin on Handling Cytotoxic and Hazardous Drugs. Am J Hosp Pharm 1990; 47:1033–1049.
7. OSHA Work-Practice Guidelines for Personnel Dealing with Cytotoxic (Antineoplastic) Drugs. Am J Hosp Pharm 1986; 43:1193–1204.

Manufactured by:
Nippon Kayaku Co., Ltd.
Tokyo, Japan
Distributed by:
MeadJohnson
ONCOLOGY PRODUCTS
A Bristol-Myers Squibb Company
Princeton, NJ 08543
U.S.A.
H2-B001-3-96   P7514-01
                                  Revised: March 1996
Shown in Product Identification Guide, page 308

CeeNU®   ℞
[cē ′nū]
(lomustine [CCNU]) Capsules

CAUTION: FEDERAL LAW PROHIBITS DISPENSING WITHOUT A PRESCRIPTION.

> ## WARNINGS
> CeeNU® (lomustine [CCNU]) Capsules should be administered under the supervision of a qualified physician experienced in the use of cancer chemotherapeutic agents.
>
> Bone marrow suppression, notably thrombocytopenia and leukopenia, which may contribute to bleeding and overwhelming infections in an already compromised patient, is the most common and severe of the toxic effects of CeeNU (see "**WARNINGS**" and "**ADVERSE REACTIONS**" section).
>
> Since the major toxicity is delayed bone marrow suppression, blood counts should be monitored weekly for at least 6 weeks after a dose (see "**ADVERSE REACTIONS**" section). At the recommended dosage, courses of CeeNU should not be given more frequently than every 6 weeks.
>
> The bone marrow toxicity of CeeNU is cumulative and therefore dosage adjustment must be considered on the basis of nadir blood counts from prior dose (see dosage-adjustment table under "**DOSAGE AND ADMINISTRATION**" section).

DESCRIPTION

CeeNU® (lomustine [CCNU]) Capsules is one of the nitrosoureas used in the treatment of certain neoplastic diseases. It is 1-(2-chloroethyl)-3-cyclohexyl-1-nitrosourea. It is a yellow powder with the empirical formula of $C_9H_{16}ClN_3O_2$ and a molecular weight of 233.71. CeeNU is soluble in 10% ethanol (0.05 mg per mL) and in absolute alcohol (70 mg per mL). CeeNU is relatively insoluble in water (< 0.05 mg per mL).

It is relatively unionized at a physiological pH.

Inactive ingredients in CeeNU capsules are: magnesium stearate and mannitol.

The structural formula is:

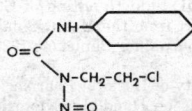

CeeNU is available in 10 mg, 40 mg, and 100 mg capsules for oral administration.

CLINICAL PHARMACOLOGY

Although it is generally agreed that CeeNU alkylates DNA and RNA, it is not cross resistant with other alkylators. As with other nitrosoureas, it may also inhibit several key enzymatic processes by carbamoylation of amino acids in proteins.

CeeNU may be given orally. Following oral administration of radioactive CeeNU at doses ranging from 30 mg/m^2 to 100 mg/m^2, about half of the radioactivity given was excreted in the form of degradation products within 24 hours.

The serum half-life of the metabolites ranges from 16 hours to 2 days. Tissue levels are comparable to plasma levels at 15 minutes after intravenous administration.

Because of the high lipid solubility and the relative lack of ionization at physiological pH, CeeNU crosses the blood-brain barrier quite effectively. Levels of radioactivity in the CSF are 50% or greater than those measured concurrently in plasma.

INDICATIONS AND USAGE

CeeNU has been shown to be useful as a single agent in addition to other treatment modalities, or in established combination therapy with other approved chemotherapeutic agents in the following:

Brain tumors - both primary and metastatic, in patients who have already received appropriate surgical and/or radiotherapeutic procedures.

Hodgkin's Disease - secondary therapy in combination with other approved drugs in patients who relapse while being treated with primary therapy, or who fail to respond to primary therapy.

CONTRAINDICATIONS

CeeNU should not be given to individuals who have demonstrated a previous hypersensitivity to it.

WARNINGS

Since the major toxicity is delayed bone marrow suppression, blood counts should be monitored weekly for at least 6 weeks after a dose (see "**ADVERSE REACTIONS**" section). At the recommended dosage, courses of CeeNU should not be given more frequently than every 6 weeks.

The bone marrow toxicity of CeeNU is cumulative and therefore dosage adjustment must be considered on the basis of nadir blood counts from prior dose (see dosage adjustment table under "**DOSAGE AND ADMINISTRATION**" section).

Pulmonary toxicity from CeeNU appears to be dose related (see "**ADVERSE REACTIONS**" section).

Long term use of nitrosoureas has been reported to be possibly associated with the development of secondary malignancies.

Liver and renal function tests should be monitored periodically (see "**ADVERSE REACTIONS**" section).

Pregnancy: Pregnancy "Category D". CeeNU can cause fetal harm when administered to a pregnant woman. CeeNU is embryotoxic and teratogenic in rats and embryotoxic in rabbits at dose levels equivalent to the human dose. There are no adequate and well controlled studies in pregnant women. If this drug is used during pregnancy, or if the patient becomes pregnant while taking (receiving) this drug, the patient should be apprised of the potential hazard to the fetus. Women of childbearing potential should be advised to avoid becoming pregnant.

PRECAUTIONS

General: In all instances where the use of CeeNU is considered for chemotherapy, the physician must evaluate the need and usefulness of the drug against the risks of toxic effects or adverse reactions. Most such adverse reactions are reversible if detected early. When such effects or reactions do occur, the drug should be reduced in dosage or discontinued and appropriate corrective measures should be taken according to the clinical judgment of the physician. Reinstitution of CeeNU therapy should be carried out with caution and with adequate consideration of the further need for the drug and alertness as to possible recurrence of toxicity.

Laboratory Tests: Due to delayed bone marrow suppression, blood counts should be monitored weekly for at least 6 weeks after a dose.

Baseline pulmonary function studies should be conducted along with frequent pulmonary function tests during treatment. Patients with a baseline below 70% of the predicted Forced Vital Capacity (FVC) or Carbon Monoxide Diffusing Capacity (DL_{co}) are particularly at risk.

Since CeeNU (lomustine [CCNU]) Capsules may cause liver dysfunction, it is recommended that liver function tests be monitored periodically.

Renal function tests should also be monitored periodically.

Carcinogenesis, Mutagenesis, Impairment of Fertility: CeeNU is carcinogenic in rats and mice, producing a marked increase in tumor incidence in doses approximating those employed clinically. Nitrosourea therapy does have carcinogenic potential in humans (see "**ADVERSE REACTIONS**" section). CeeNU also affects fertility in male rats at doses somewhat higher than the human dose.

Pregnancy: Pregnancy "Category D". (See "**WARNINGS**" section.)

Nursing Mothers: It is not known whether this drug is excreted in human milk. Because many drugs are excreted in human milk and because of the potential for serious adverse reactions in nursing infants from CeeNU, a decision should be made whether to discontinue nursing or to discontinue the drug, taking into account the importance of the drug to the mother.

Pediatric Use: See "**ADVERSE REACTIONS, Pulmonary Toxicity**" subsection, and "**DOSAGE AND ADMINISTRATION**" section.

Information for the Patient: Patients receiving CeeNU should be given the following information and instructions by the physician:

1. Patients should be told that CeeNU is an anticancer drug and belongs to the group of medicines known as alkylating agents.

2. In order to provide the proper dose of CeeNU, patients should be aware that there may be two or more different types and colors of capsules in the container dispensed by the pharmacist.

Continued on next page

CeeNU—Cont.

3. Patients should be told that CeeNU is given as a single oral dose and will not be repeated for at least 6 weeks.
4. Patients should be told that nausea and vomiting usually last less than 24 hours, although loss of appetite may last for several days.
5. If any of the following reactions occur, notify the physician: fever, chills, sore throat, unusual bleeding or bruising, shortness of breath, dry cough, swelling of feet or lower legs, mental confusion, or yellowing of eyes and skin.

ADVERSE REACTIONS

Hematologic Toxicity - The most frequent and most serious toxicity of CeeNU is delayed myelosuppression. It usually occurs 4 to 6 weeks after drug administration and is dose related. Thrombocytopenia occurs at about 4 weeks postadministration and persists for 1 to 2 weeks. Leukopenia occurs at 5 to 6 weeks after a dose of CeeNU and persists for 1 to 2 weeks. Approximately 65% of patients receiving 130 mg/m^2 develop white blood counts below 5000 wbc/mm^3. Thirty-six percent develop white blood counts below 3000 wbc/mm^3. Thrombocytopenia is generally more severe than leukopenia. However, both may be dose-limiting toxicities.
CeeNU may produce cumulative myelosuppression, manifested by more depressed indices or longer duration of suppression after repeated doses.
The occurrence of acute leukemia and bone marrow dysplasias have been reported in patients following long term nitrosourea therapy.
Anemia also occurs, but is less frequent and less severe than thrombocytopenia or leukopenia.

Pulmonary Toxicity: Pulmonary toxicity characterized by pulmonary infiltrates and/or fibrosis has been reported rarely with CeeNU. Onset of toxicity has occurred after an interval of 6 months or longer from the start of therapy with cumulative doses of CeeNU usually greater than 1100 mg/m^2. There is one report of pulmonary toxicity at a cumulative dose of only 600 mg.
Delayed onset pulmonary fibrosis occurring up to 17 years after treatment has been reported in patients who received related nitrosoureas in childhood and early adolescence (1–16) years combined with cranial radiotherapy for intracranial tumors. There appeared to be some late reduction of pulmonary function of all long-term survivors. This form of lung fibrosis may be slowly progressive and has resulted in death in some cases. In this long-term study of carmustine, all those initially treated at less than five years of age died of delayed pulmonary fibrosis.

Gastrointestinal Toxicity: Nausea and vomiting may occur 3 to 6 hours after an oral dose and usually lasts less than 24 hours. Prior administration of antiemetics is effective in diminishing and sometimes preventing this side effect. Nausea and vomiting can also be reduced if CeeNU is administered to fasting patients.

Hepatotoxicity: A reversible type of hepatic toxicity, manifested by increased transaminase, alkaline phosphatase and bilirubin levels, has been reported in a small percentage of patients receiving CeeNU.

Nephrotoxicity: Renal abnormalities consisting of progressive azotemia, decrease in kidney size and renal failure have been reported in patients who received large cumulative doses after prolonged therapy with CeeNU. Kidney damage has also been reported occasionally in patients receiving lower total doses.

Other Toxicities: Stomatitis, alopecia, optic atrophy, and visual disturbances such as blindness have been reported infrequently.
Neurological reactions such as disorientation, lethargy, ataxia, and dysarthria have been noted in some patients receiving CeeNU. However, the relationship to medication in these patients is unclear.

OVERDOSAGE

No proven antidotes have been established for CeeNU overdosage.

DOSAGE AND ADMINISTRATION

The recommended dose of CeeNU in adult and pediatric patients as a single agent in previously untreated patients is 130 mg/m^2 as a single oral dose every 6 weeks. In individuals with compromised bone marrow function, the dose should be reduced to 100 mg/m^2 every 6 weeks. When CeeNU is used in combination with other myelosuppressive drugs, the doses should be adjusted accordingly.
Doses subsequent to the initial dose should be adjusted according to the hematologic response of the patient to the preceding dose. The following schedule is suggested as a guide to dosage adjustment:

Nadir After Prior Dose		Percentage of Prior Dose to be Given
Leukocytes	Platelets	
> 4000	> 100,000	100%
3000–3999	75,000–99,999	100%
2000–2999	25,000–74,999	70%
< 2000	< 25,000	50%

A repeat course of CeeNU (lomustine [CCNU]) should not be given until circulating blood elements have returned to acceptable levels (platelets above 100,000/ mm^3; leukocytes above 4000/mm^3) and this is usually in 6 weeks. Adequate number of neutrophils should be present on a peripheral blood smear. Blood counts should be monitored weekly and repeat courses should not be given before 6 weeks because the hematologic toxicity is delayed and cumulative.

HOW SUPPLIED

The dose pack of CeeNU® (lomustine [CCNU]) Capsules **NDC** 0015-3034-10 Capsules contains:
2–100 mg capsules (Green/Green)
2–40 mg capsules (White/Green)
2–10 mg capsules (White/White)

Stability: CeeNU Capsules are stable for the lot life indicated on package labeling when stored at room temperature in well closed containers. Avoid excessive heat (over 40°C, 104°F).

Directions to the Pharmacist: The dose pack contains a total of 300 mg and will provide enough medication for titration of a single dose. The total dose prescribed by the physician can be obtained (to within 10 mg) by determining the appropriate combination of the enclosed capsule strengths.
The appropriate number of capsules of each size should be placed in a single vial to which the patient information label (gummed label provided) explaining the differences in the appearance of the capsules is affixed. Each color-coded capsule is imprinted with the dose in milligrams.
A patient information sticker, to be placed on dispensing container, is enclosed.

Also available: Individual bottles of 20 capsules each.
NDC 0015-3032-20—100 mg capsules (Green/Green)
NDC 0015-3031-20—40 mg capsules (White/Green)
NDC 0015-3030-20—10 mg capsules (White/White)

Procedures for proper handling and disposal of anticancer drugs should be considered. Several guidelines on this subject have been published.[1-7] There is no general agreement that all of the procedures recommended in the guidelines are necessary or appropriate.

REFERENCES

1. Recommendations for the Safe Handling of Parenteral Antineoplastic Drugs. NIH Publication No. 83–2621. For sale by the Superintendent of Documents, US Government Printing Office, Washington, DC 20402.
2. AMA Council Report. Guidelines for Handling Parenteral Antineoplastics. JAMA, 1985; 253 (11):1590–1592.
3. National Study Commission on Cytotoxic Exposure-Recommendations for Handling Cytotoxic Agents. Available from Louis P. Jeffrey, ScD, Chairman, National Study Commission on Cytotoxic Exposure, Massachusetts College of Pharmacy and Allied Health Sciences, 179 Longwood Avenue, Boston, Massachusetts 02115.
4. Clinical Oncological Society of Australia. Guidelines and Recommendations for Safe Handling of Antineoplastic Agents. Med J Australia 1983; 1:426–428.
5. Jones RB, et al: Safe Handling of Chemotherapeutic Agents: A Report from the Mount Sinai Medical Center. CA-A Cancer Journal for Clinicians 1983; (Sept/Oct)258–263.
6. American Society of Hospital Pharmacists Technical Assistance Bulletin on Handling Cytotoxic and Hazardous Drugs. Am J Hosp Pharm 1990; 47:1033–1049.
7. Controlling occupational exposure to hazardous drugs. (OSHA WORK PRACTICE GUIDELINES). Am J Health-Syst Pharm 1996; 53:1669–1685.

BRISTOL LABORATORIES®
ONCOLOGY PRODUCTS
A Britol-Myers Squibb Company
Princeton, NJ 08543
U.S.A.
H3-B001-12-96 P6047-03
Revised December 1996

Lyophilized CYTOXAN® for Injection ℞

[sī-taks 'an]
(cyclophosphamide for injection, USP)
CYTOXAN® Tablets
(cyclophosphamide tablets, USP)

CAUTION: FEDERAL LAW PROHIBITS DISPENSING WITHOUT PRESCRIPTION.

DESCRIPTION

Lyophilized CYTOXAN® for Injection (cyclophosphamide for injection, USP) is a sterile white lyophilized cake or partially broken cake, containing 75 mg mannitol per 100 mg cyclophosphamide (anhydrous). CYTOXAN® Tablets (cyclophosphamide tablets, USP) are for oral use and contain 25 mg or 50 mg cyclophosphamide (anhydrous). Inactive ingredients in CYTOXAN tablets are: acacia, FD&C Blue No. 1, D&C Yellow No. 10 Aluminum Lake, lactose, magnesium stearate, starch, stearic acid, and talc. Cyclophosphamide is a synthetic antineoplastic drug chemically related to the nitrogen mustards. Cyclophosphamide is a white crystalline powder with the molecular formula of $C_7H_{15}C_{12}N_2O_2P{\bullet}H_2O$ and a molecular weight of 279.1. The chemical name for cyclophosphamide is 2-[bis(2-chloroethyl)amino]tetrahydro-2H-1,3,2-oxazaphosphorine 2-oxide monohydrate. Cyclophosphamide is soluble in water, saline, or ethanol and has the following structural formula:

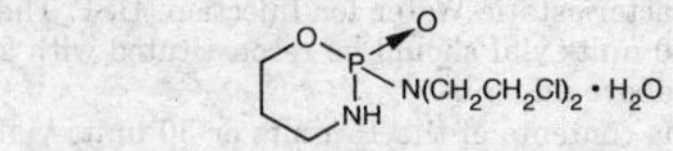
O
P
O
N(CH2CH2Cl)2 • H2O
NH

CLINICAL PHARMACOLOGY

CYTOXAN (cyclophosphamide, USP) is biotransformed principally in the liver to active alkylating metabolites by a mixed function microsomal oxidase system. These metabolites interfere with the growth of susceptible rapidly proliferating malignant cells. The mechanism of action is thought to involve cross-linking of tumor cell DNA.
CYTOXAN is well absorbed after oral administration with a bioavailability greater than 75%. The unchanged drug has an elimination half-life of 3 to 12 hours. It is eliminated primarily in the form of metabolites, but from 5 to 25% of the dose is excreted in urine as unchanged drug. Several cytotoxic and noncytotoxic metabolites have been identified in urine and in plasma. Concentrations of metabolites reach a maximum in plasma 2 to 3 hours after an intravenous dose. Plasma protein binding of unchanged drug is low but some metabolites are bound to an extent greater than 60%. It has not been demonstrated that any single metabolite is responsible for either the therapeutic or toxic effects of cyclophosphamide. Although elevated levels of metabolites of cyclophosphamide have been observed in patients with renal failure, increased clinical toxicity in such patients has not been demonstrated.

INDICATIONS AND USAGE

Malignant Diseases-CYTOXAN, although effective alone in susceptible malignancies, is more frequently used concurrently or sequentially with other antineoplastic drugs. The following malignancies are often susceptible to CYTOXAN treatment:
1. Malignant lymphomas (Stages III and IV of the Ann Arbor staging system), Hodgkin's disease, lymphocytic lymphoma (nodular or diffuse), mixed-cell type lymphoma, histiocytic lymphoma, Burkitt's lymphoma. **2.** Multiple myeloma. **3.** Leukemias: Chronic lymphocytic leukemia, chronic granulocytic leukemia (it is usually ineffective in acute blastic crisis), acute myelogenous and monocytic leukemia, acute lymphoblastic (stem-cell) leukemia in children (CYTOXAN given during remission is effective in prolonging its duration). **4.** Mycosis fungoides (advanced disease). **5.** Neuroblastoma (disseminated disease). **6.** Adenocarcinoma of the ovary. **7.** Retinoblastoma. **8.** Carcinoma of the breast.
Nonmalignant Disease: Biopsy Proven "Minimal Change" Nephrotic Syndrome in Children-CYTOXAN is useful in carefully selected cases of biopsy proven "minimal change" nephrotic syndrome in children but should not be used as primary therapy. In children whose disease fails to respond adequately to appropriate adrenocorticosteroid therapy or in whom the adrenocorticosteroid therapy produces or threatens to produce intolerable side effects, CYTOXAN may induce a remission. CYTOXAN is not indicated for the nephrotic syndrome in adults or for any other renal disease.

CONTRAINDICATIONS

Continued use of cyclophosphamide is contraindicated in patients with severely depressed bone marrow function. Cyclophosphamide is contraindicated in patients who have demonstrated a previous hypersensitivity to it. (See **"WARNINGS"** and **"PRECAUTIONS"** sections.)

WARNINGS

Carcinogenesis, Mutagenesis, Impairment of Fertility–Second malignancies have developed in some patients treated with cyclophosphamide used alone or in association with other antineoplastic drugs and/or modalities. Most frequently, they have been urinary bladder, myeloproliferative, or lymphoproliferative malignancies. Second malignancies most frequently were detected in patients treated for primary myeloproliferative or lymphoproliferative malignancies or nonmalignant disease in which immune processes are believed to be involved pathologically. In some cases, the second malignancy developed several years after cyclophosphamide treat ment had been discontinued. In a single breast cancer trial utilizing two to four times the standard dose of cyclophosphamide, in conjunction with doxorubicin, a small number of cases of secondary acute myeloid leukemia occurred within two years of treatment initiation. Urinary bladder malignancies generally have occurred in pa-

tients who previously had hemorrhagic cystitis. In patients treated with cyclophosphamide-containing regimens for a variety of solid tumors, isolated case reports of secondary malignancies have been published. One case of carcinoma of the renal pelvis was reported in a patient receiving long-term cyclophosphamide therapy for cerebral vasculitis. The possibility of cyclophosphamide-induced malignancy should be considered in any benefit-to-risk assessment for use of the drug.

Cyclophosphamide can cause fetal harm when administered to a pregnant woman and such abnormalities have been reported following cyclophosphamide therapy in pregnant women. Abnormalities were found in two infants and a 6-month-old fetus born to women treated with cyclophosphamide. Ectrodactylia was found in two of the three cases. Normal infants have also been born to women treated with cyclophos phamide during pregnancy, including the first trimester. If this drug is used during pregnancy, or if the patient becomes pregnant while taking (receiving) this drug, the patient should be apprised of the potential hazard to the fetus. Women of childbearing potential should be advised to avoid becoming pregnant.

Cyclophosphamide interferes with oogenesis and spermatogenesis. It may cause sterility in both sexes. Development of sterility appears to depend on the dose of cyclophosphamide, duration of therapy, and the state of gonadal function at the time of treatment. Cyclophosphamide-induced sterility may be irreversible in some patients.

Amenorrhea associated with decreased estrogen and increased gonadotropin secretion develops in a significant proportion of women treated with cyclophosphamide. Affected patients generally resume regular menses within a few months after cessation of therapy. Girls treated with cyclophosphamide during prepubescence generally develop secondary sexual characteristics normally and have regular menses. Ovarian fibrosis with apparently complete loss of germ cells after prolonged cyclophosphamide treatment in late prepubescence has been reported. Girls treated with cyclophosphamide during prepubescence subsequently have conceived.

Men treated with cyclophosphamide may develop oligospermia or azoospermia associated with increased gonadotropin but normal testosterone secretion. Sexual potency and libido are unimpaired in these patients. Boys treated with cyclophosphamide during prepubescence develop secondary sexual characteristics normally, but may have oligospermia or azoospermia and increased gonadotropin secretion. Some degree of testicular atrophy may occur. Cyclophosphamide-induced azoospermia is reversible in some patients, though the reversibility may not occur for several years after cessation of therapy. Men temporarily rendered sterile by cyclophosphamide have subsequently fathered normal children.

Urinary System–Hemorrhagic cystitis may develop in patients treated with cyclophosphamide. Rarely, this condition can be severe and even fatal. Fibrosis of the urinary bladder, sometimes extensive, also may develop with or without accompanying cystitis. Atypical urinary bladder epithelial cells may appear in the urine. These adverse effects appear to depend on the dose of cyclophosphamide and the duration of therapy. Such bladder injury is thought to be due to cyclophosphamide metabolites excreted in the urine. Forced fluid intake helps to assure an ample output of urine, necessitates frequent voiding, and reduces the time the drug remains in the bladder. This helps to prevent cystitis. Hematuria usually resolves in a few days after cyclophosphamide treatment is stopped, but it may persist. Medical and/or surgical supportive treatment may be required, rarely, to treat protracted cases of severe hemorrhagic cystitis. It is usually necessary to discontinue cyclophosphamide therapy in instances of severe hemorrhagic cystitis.

Cardiac Toxicity–Although a few instances of cardiac dysfunction have been reported following use of recommended doses of cyclophosphamide, no causal relationship has been established. Acute cardiac toxicity has been reported with doses as low as 2.4 g/m^2 to as high as 26 g/m^2, usually as a portion of an intensive antineoplastic multidrug regimen or in conjunction with transplantation procedures. In a few instances with high doses of cyclophosphamide, severe, and sometimes fatal, congestive heart failure has occurred after the first cyclophosphamide dose. Histopathologic examination has primarily shown hemorrhagic myocarditis. Hemopericardium has occurred secondary to hemorrhagic myocarditis and myocardial necrosis. Pericarditis has been reported independent of any hemopericardium.

No residual cardiac abnormalities, as evidenced by electrocardiogram or echocardiogram appear to be present in patients surviving episodes of apparent cardiac toxicity associated with high doses of cyclophosphamide.

Cyclophosphamide has been reported to potentiate doxorubicin-induced cardiotoxicity.

Infections–Treatment with cyclophosphamide may cause significant suppression of immune responses. Serious, sometimes fatal, infections may develop in severely immunosuppressed patients. Cyclophosphamide treatment may not be indicated or should be interrupted or the dose reduced in patients who have or who develop viral, bacterial, fungal, protozoan, or helminthic infections.

Other–Rare instances of anaphylactic reaction including one death have been reported. One instance of possible cross-sensitivity with other alkylating agents has been reported.

PRECAUTIONS

General–Special attention to the possible development of toxicity should be exercised in patients being treated with cyclophosphamide if any of the following conditions are present.

1. Leukopenia **2.** Thrombocytopenia **3.** Tumor cell infiltration of bone marrow **4.** Previous X-ray therapy **5.** Previous therapy with other cytotoxic agents **6.** Impaired hepatic function **7.** Impaired renal function

Laboratory Tests–During treatment, the patient's hematologic profile (particularly neutrophils and platelets) should be monitored regularly to determine the degree of hematopoietic suppression. Urine should also be examined regularly for red cells which may precede hemorrhagic cystitis.

Drug Interactions–The rate of metabolism and the leukopenic activity of cyclophosphamide reportedly are increased by chronic administration of high doses of phenobarbital.

The physician should be alert for possible combined drug actions, desirable or undesirable, involving cyclophosphamide even though cyclophosphamide has been used successfully concurrently with other drugs, including other cytotoxic drugs.

Cyclophosphamide treatment, which causes a marked and persistent inhibition of cholinesterase activity, potentiates the effect of succinylcholine chloride.

If a patient has been treated with cyclophosphamide within 10 days of general anesthesia, the anesthesiologist should be alerted.

Adrenalectomy–Since cyclophosphamide has been reported to be more toxic in adrenalectomized dogs, adjustment of the doses of both replacement steroids and cyclophosphamide may be necessary for the adrenalectomized patient.

Wound Healing–Cyclophosphamide may interfere with normal wound healing.

Carcinogenesis, Mutagenesis, Impairment of Fertility–See "**WARNINGS**" section for information on carcinogenesis, mutagenesis, and impairment of fertility.

Pregnancy– Pregnancy "Category D". (See "**WARNINGS**" section.)

Nursing Mothers–Cyclophosphamide is excreted in breast milk. Because of the potential for serious adverse reactions and the potential for tumorigenicity shown for cyclophosphamide in humans, a decision should be made whether to discontinue nursing or to discontinue the drug, taking into account the importance of the drug to the mother.

ADVERSE REACTIONS

Information on adverse reactions associated with the use of CYTOXAN (cyclophosphamide, USP) is arranged according to body system affected or type of reaction. The adverse reactions are listed in order of decreasing incidence. The most serious adverse reactions are described in the "**WARNINGS**" section.

Reproductive System–See "**WARNINGS**" section for information on impairment of fertility.

Digestive System–Nausea and vomiting commonly occur with cyclophosphamide therapy. Anorexia and, less frequently, abdominal discomfort or pain and diarrhea may occur. There are isolated reports of hemorrhagic colitis, oral mucosal ulceration and jaundice occurring during therapy. These adverse drug effects generally remit when cyclophosphamide treatment is stopped.

Skin and Its Structures–Alopecia occurs commonly in patients treated with cyclophosphamide. The hair can be expected to grow back after treatment with the drug or even during continued drug treatment, though it may be different in texture or color. Skin rash occurs occasionally in patients receiving the drug. Pigmentation of the skin and changes in nails can occur.

Hematopoietic System–Leukopenia occurs in patients treated with cyclophosphamide, is related to the dose of drug, and can be used as a dosage guide. Leukopenia of less than 2000 cells/mm^3 develops commonly in patients treated with an initial loading dose of the drug, and less frequently in patients maintained on smaller doses. The degree of neutropenia is particularly important because it correlates with a reduction in resistance to infections. Fever without documented infection has been reported in neutropenic patients. Thrombocytopenia or anemia develop occasionally in patients treated with CYTOXAN. These hematologic effects usually can be reversed by reducing the drug dose or by interrupting treatment. Recovery from leukopenia usually begins in 7 to 10 days after cessation of therapy.

Urinary System–See "**WARNINGS**" section for information on cystitis and urinary bladder fibrosis.

Hemorrhagic ureteritis and renal tubular necrosis have been reported to occur in patients treated with cyclophosphamide. Such lesions usually resolve following cessation of therapy.

Infections–See "**WARNINGS**" section for information on reduced host resistance to infections.

Carcinogenesis–See "**WARNINGS**" section for information on carcinogenesis.

Respiratory System–Interstitial pulmonary fibrosis has been reported in patients receiving high doses of cyclophosphamide over a prolonged period.

Other–Rare instances of anaphylactic reaction including one death have been reported. One instance of possible cross-sensitivity with other alkylating agents has been reported. SIADH (syndrome of inappropriate ADH secretion) has been reported with the use of cyclophosphamide.

OVERDOSAGE

No specific antidote for cyclophosphamide is known. Overdosage should be managed with supportive measures, including appropriate treatment for any concurrent infection, myelosuppression, or cardiac toxicity should it occur.

DOSAGE AND ADMINISTRATION

Treatment of Malignant Diseases: Adults and Children–When used as the only oncolytic drug therapy, the initial course of CYTOXAN (cyclophosphamide, USP) for patients with no hematologic deficiency usually consists of 40 to 50 mg/kg given intravenously in divided doses over a period of 2 to 5 days. Other intravenous regimens include 10 to 15 mg/kg given every 7 to 10 days or 3 to 5 mg/kg twice weekly. Oral CYTOXAN dosing is usually in the range of 1 to 5 mg/kg/day for both initial and maintenance dosing.

Many other regimens of intravenous and oral CYTOXAN have been reported. Dosages must be adjusted in accord with evidence of antitumor activity and/or leukopenia. The total leukocyte count is a good, objective guide for regulating dosage. Transient decreases in the total white blood cell count to 2000 cells/mm^3 (following short courses) or more persistent reduction to 3000 cells/mm^3 (with continuing therapy) are tolerated without serious risk of infection if there is no marked granulocytopenia.

When CYTOXAN is included in combined cytotoxic regimens, it may be necessary to reduce the dose of CYTOXAN as well as that of the other drugs.

CYTOXAN and its metabolites are dialyzable although there are probably quantitative differences depending upon the dialysis system being used. Patients with compromised renal function may show some measurable changes in pharmacokinetic parameters of CYTOXAN metabolism, but there is no consistent evidence indicating a need for CYTOXAN dosage modification in patients with renal function impairment.

Treatment of Nonmalignant Diseases: Biopsy Proven "Minimal Change" Nephrotic Syndrome In Children–An oral dose of 2.5 to 3 mg/kg daily for a period of 60 to 90 days is recommended. In males, the incidence of oligospermia and azoospermia increases if the duration of CYTOXAN treatment exceeds 60 days. Treatment beyond 90 days increases the probability of sterility. Adrenocorticosteroid therapy may be tapered and discontinued during the course of CYTOXAN therapy. See "**PRECAUTIONS**" section concerning hematologic monitoring.

Preparation and Handling of Solutions–Parenteral drug products should be inspected visually for particulate matter and discoloration prior to administration, whenever solution and container permit.

Lyophilized CYTOXAN for Injection should be prepared for parenteral use by adding Sterile Water for Injection, USP to the vial and shaking to dissolve. Use the quantity of diluent shown below to reconstitute the product.

Double Strength	**Lyophilized CYTOXAN for Injection** Quantity of Diluent
100 mg	5 mL
200 mg	10 mL
500 mg	20-25 mL
1 g	50 mL
2 g	80-100 mL

Solutions of Lyophilized CYTOXAN for Injection may be injected intravenously, intramuscularly, intraperitoneally, or intrapleurally or it may be infused intravenously in the following:

Dextrose Injection, USP (5% dextrose)
Dextrose and Sodium Chloride Injection, USP (5% dextrose and 0.9% sodium chloride)
5% Dextrose and Ringer's Injection
Lactated Ringer's Injection, USP
Sodium Chloride Injection, USP (0.45% sodium chloride)
Sodium Lactate Injection, USP (1/6 molar sodium lactate)

Reconstituted Lyophilized CYTOXAN for Injection is chemically and physically stable for 24 hours at room temperature or for 6 days in the refrigerator; it does not contain any antimicrobial preservative and thus care must be taken to assure the sterility of prepared solutions.

The osmolarities of solutions of Lyophilized CYTOXAN for Injection, and normal saline are found in the following table:

Continued on next page

Cytoxan—Cont.

	m0sm/L
Lyophilized CYTOXAN for Injection	
4 mL diluent per 100 mg cyclophosphamide	219
5 mL diluent per 100 mg cyclophosphamide	172

Lyophilized CYTOXAN for Injection is slightly hypotonic. Extemporaneous liquid preparations of CYTOXAN for oral administration may be prepared by dissolving Lyophilized CYTOXAN for Injection in Aromatic Elixir, N.F. Such preparations should be stored under refrigeration in glass containers and used within 14 days.

HOW SUPPLIED

Lyophilized CYTOXAN for Injection contains 75 mg of mannitol per 100 mg of cyclophosphamide (anhydrous) and is supplied in vials for single-dose use.

Lyophilized CYTOXAN® for Injection (cyclophosphamide for injection, USP). U.S. Patent No. 4,537,883

NDC 0015-0539-41 100 mg vials, carton of 12, case of 1 carton

NDC 0015-0546-41 200 mg vials, carton of 12, case of 1 carton

NDC 0015-0547-41 500 mg vials, carton of 12, case of 1 carton

NDC 0015-0548-41 1 g vials, carton of 6

NDC 0015-0549-41 2 g vials, carton of 6

CYTOXAN Tablets (cyclophosphamide tablets, USP), 25 mg, and CYTOXAN Tablets, 50 mg, are white tablets with blue flecks containing 25 mg and 50 mg cyclophosphamide (anhydrous), respectively.

CYTOXAN® Tablets (cyclophosphamide tablets, USP).

NDC 0015-0503-01 50 mg, bottles of 100

NDC 0015-0503-02 50 mg, bottles of 1000

NDC 0015-0504-01 25 mg, bottles of 100

Storage at or below 77°F (25°C) is recommended; this product will withstand brief exposure to temperatures up to 86°F (30°C) but should be protected from temperatures above 86°F (30°C).

Procedures for proper handling and disposal of anticancer drugs should be considered. Several guidelines on this subject have been published.[1-7] There is no general agreement that all of the procedures recommended in the guidelines are necessary or appropriate.

REFERENCES

1. Recommendations for the Safe Handling of Parenteral Antineoplastic Drugs. NIH Publication No. 83-2621. For sale by the Superintendent of Documents, US Government Printing Office, Washington, DC 20402.
2. AMA Council Report. Guidelines for Handling Parenteral Antineoplastics. JAMA 1985; 253 (11):1590-1592.
3. National Study Commission on Cytotoxic Exposure-Recommendations for Handling Cytotoxic Agents. Available from Louis P. Jeffrey, ScD, Chairman, National Study Commission on Cytotoxic Exposure, Massachusetts College of Pharmacy and Allied Health Sciences, 179 Longwood Avenue, Boston, Massachusetts 02115.
4. Clinical Oncological Society of Australia. Guidelines and Recommendations for Safe Handling of Antineoplastic Agents. Med J Australia 1983; 1:426-428.
5. Jones RB, et al: Safe Handling of Chemotherapeutic Agents: A Report from the Mount Sinai Medical Center. CA-A Cancer Journal for Clinicians 1983; (Sept/Oct)258-263.
6. American Society of Hospital Pharmacists Technical Assistance Bulletin on Handling Cytotoxic and Hazardous Drugs. Am J Hosp Pharm 1990; 47:1033-1049.
7. OSHA Work-Practice Guidelines for Personnel Dealing with Cytotoxic (Antineoplastic) Drugs. Am J Hosp Pharm 1986; 43:1193-1204.

MeadJohnson
ONCOLOGY PRODUCTS
A Bristol-Myers Squibb company
Princeton, NJ 08543
U.S.A.
H4-B001-8-96   0539DIM-06
51-001103-03   Revised July 1996
Shown in Product Identification Guide, page 308

DROXIA™   ℞ ONLY
(hydroxyurea capsules, USP)

CAUTION: FEDERAL LAW PROHIBITS DISPENSING WITHOUT A PRESCRIPTION.

WARNING

Treatment of patients with DROXIA™ (hydroxyurea capsules, USP) may be complicated by severe, sometimes life-threatening, adverse effects. DROXIA should be administered under the supervision of a physician experienced in the use of this medication for the treatment of sickle cell anemia.

Hydroxyurea is mutagenic and clastogenic, and causes cellular transformation to a tumorigenic phenotype. Hydroxyurea is thus unequivocally genotoxic and a presumed transspecies carcinogen which implies a carcinogenic risk to humans. In patients receiving long term hydroxyurea for myeloproliferative disorders, such as polcythemia vera and thrombocythemia, secondary leukemias have been reported. It is unknown whether this leukemogenic effect is secondary to hydroxyurea or is associated with the patients' underlying disease. The physician and patient must very carefully consider the potential benefits of DROXIA relative to the undefined risk of developing secondary malignancies.

DESCRIPTION

DROXIA™ (hydroxyurea capsules, USP) is available for oral use as capsules providing 200 mg, 300 mg and 400 mg hydroxyurea. Inactive ingredients: citric acid, gelatin, lactose, magnesium stearate, sodium phosphate, titanium dioxide and capsule colorants: FD&C Blue #1 and FD&C Green #3 (200 mg capsules): D&C Red #28, D&C Red #33 and FD&C Blue #1 (300 mg capsules); D&C Red #28, D&C Red #33 and D&C Yellow #10 (400 mg capsules).

Hydroxyurea is an essentially tasteless, white crystalline powder. Its structural formula is:

$$H_2N-\overset{\overset{\displaystyle O}{\|}}{C}-NH-OH$$

CLINICAL PHARMACOLOGY

Mechanism of Action: The precise mechanism by which hydroxyurea produces its cytotoxic and cytoreductive effects is not known. However, various studies support the hypothesis that hydroxyurea causes an immediate inhibition of DNA synthesis by acting as a ribonucleotide reductase inhibitor, without interfering with the synthesis of ribonucleic acid or of protein.

The mechanisms by which DROXIA produces its beneficial effects in patients with sickle cell anemia (SCA) are uncertain. Known pharmacologic effects of DROXIA that may contribute to its beneficial effects include increasing hemoglobin F levels in RBCs, decreasing neutrophils, increasing the water content of RBCs, increasing deformability of sickled cells, and altering the adhesion of RBCs to endothelium.

Pharmacokinetics:

Absorption—Hydroxyurea is readily absorbed after oral administration. Peak plasma levels are reached in 1 to 4 hours after an oral dose. With increasing doses, disproportionately greater mean peak plasma concentrations and AUCs are observed.

There are no data on the effect of food on the absorption of hydroxyurea.

Distribution—Hydroxyurea distributes rapidly and widely in the body with an estimated volume of distribution approximating total body water.

Plasma to ascites fluid ratios range from 2:1 to 7.5:1. Hydroxyurea concentrates in leukocytes and erythrocytes.

Metabolism—Up to 50% of an oral dose undergoes conversion through metabolic pathways that are not fully characterized. In one minor pathway, hydroxyurea may be degraded by urease found in intestinal bacteria. Acetohydroxamic acid was found in the serum of three leukemic patients receiving hydroxyurea and may be formed from hydroxylamine resulting from action of urease on hydroxyurea.

Excretion—Excretion of hydroxyurea in humans is a nonlinear process occurring through two pathways. One is saturable, probably hepatic metabolism; the other is first-order re-

nal excretion. In adults with SCA, mean cumulative urinary hydroxyurea excretion was 62% of the administered dose at 8-hours.

Special Populations:

Geriatric, Gender, Race—No information is available regarding pharmacokinetic differences due to age, gender or race.

Pediatric—No pharmacokinetic data are available in pediatric patients treated with hydroxyurea for SCA.

Renal Insufficiency—There are no data that support specific guidance for dosage adjustment in patients with renal impairment. As renal excretion is a pathway of elimination, consideration should be given to decreasing the dosage of hydroxyurea in patients with renal impairment. Close monitoring of hematologic parameters is advised in these patients.

Hepatic Insufficiency—There are no data that support specific guidance for dosage adjustment in patients with hepatic impairment. Close monitoring of hematologic parameters is advised in these patients.

Drug Interactions—There are no data on concomitant use of hydroxyurea with other drugs in humans.

CLINICAL STUDIES

The efficacy of hydroxyurea in sickle cell anemia was assessed in a large clinical study (Multicenter Study of Hydroxyurea in Sickle Cell Anemia)[1].

The study was a randomized, double-blind, placebo-controlled trial that evaluated 299 adult patients (≥ 18 years) with moderate to severe disease (≥ 3 painful crises yearly). The trial was stopped by the Data Safety Monitoring Committee, after accrual was completed but before the scheduled 24 months of follow-up was completed in all patients, based on observations of fewer painful crises among patients receiving hydroxyurea.

Compared to placebo treatment, treatment with hydroxyurea resulted in a significant decrease in the yearly rate of painful crises, the yearly rate of painful crises requiring hospitalization, the incidence of chest syndrome, the number of patients transfused, and units of blood transfused. Hydroxyurea treatment significantly increased the median time to both first and second painful crises.

Although patients with 3 or more painful crises during the preceding 12 months were eligible for the study, most of the benefit in crisis reduction was seen in the patients with 6 or more painful crises during the preceding 12 months.

[See table below]

No deaths were attributed to treatment with hydroxyurea, and none of the patients developed neoplastic disorders during the study. Treatment was permanently stopped for medical reasons in 14 hydroxyurea-treated (2 patients with myelotoxicity) and 6 placebo-treated patients. (See **"ADVERSE REACTIONS"** section.)

Fetal Hemoglobin—In patients with SCA treated with hydroxyurea, fetal hemoglobin (HbF) increases 4 to 12 weeks after initiation of treatment. In general, average HbF levels correlate with dose and plasma level with possible plateauing at higher dosages.

A clear relation between reduction in crisis frequency and increased HbF or F-cell levels has not been demonstrated. The dose-related cytoreductive effects of hydroxyurea, particularly on neutrophils, was the factor most strongly correlated with reduced crisis frequency.

INDICATIONS AND USAGE

DROXIA (hydroxyurea capsules, USP) is indicated to reduce the frequency of painful crises and to reduce the need for

Event	Hydroxyurea (N=152)	Placebo (N=147)	Percent Change vs Placebo	P Value
Median yearly rate of painful crises*	2.5	4.6	−46	=0.001
Median yearly rate of painful crises requiring hospitalization	1.0	2.5	−60	=0.0027
Median time to first painful crisis (months)	2.76	1.35	+104	=0.014
Median time to second painful crisis (months)	6.58	4.13	+59	=0.0024
Incidence of chest syndrome (# episodes)	56	101	−45	=0.003
Number of patients transfused	55	79	−30	=0.002
Number of units of blood transfused	423	670	−37	=0.003

* A painful crisis was defined in the study as acute sickling-related pain that resulted in a visit to a medical facility, that lasted more than 4 hours, and that required treatment with a parenteral narcotic or NSAID. Chest syndrome, priapism, and hepatic sequestration were included in this definition.

blood transfusions in adult patients with sickle cell anemia with recurrent moderate to severe painful crises (generally at least 3 during the preceding 12 months).

CONTRAINDICATIONS

DROXIA is contraindicated in patients who have demonstrated a previous hypersensitivity to hydroxyurea or any other component of its formulation.

WARNINGS

DROXIA is a cytotoxic and myelosuppresive agent. DROXIA should not be given if bone marrow function is markedly depressed, as indicated by neutrophils below 2000 cells/mm^3; a platelet count below 80,000/mm^3; a hemoglobin level below 4.5 g/dL; or reticulocytes below 80,000/mm^3 when the hemoglobin concentration is below 9 g/dL. Neutropenia is generally the first and most common manifestation of hematologic suppression. (See **"DOSAGE AND ADMINISTRATION"** section.) Thrombocytopenia and anemia occur less often, and are seldom seen without a preceding leukopenia. Recovery from myelosuppression is usually rapid when therapy is interrupted. DROXIA causes macrocytosis, which may mask the incidental development of folic acid deficiency. Prophylactic administration of folic acid is recommended.

Hydroxyurea should be used with caution in patients with renal dysfunction. (See **"DOSAGE AND ADMINISTRATION"** section.)

Carcinogenesis and Mutagenesis: (See **"Boxed WARNING"** section.) Hydroxyurea is genotoxic in a wide range of test systems and is thus presumed to be a human carcinogen. In patients receiving long-term hydroxyurea for myeloproliferative disorders, such as polycythemia vera and thrombocythemia, secondary leukemia has been reported. It is unknown whether this leukemogenic effect is secondary to hydroxyurea or is associated with the patients' underlying disease. Skin cancer has also been reported in patients receiving long-term hydroxyurea.

Conventional long-term studies to evaluate the carcinogenic potential of DROXIA have not been performed. However, intraperitoneal administration of 125–250 mg/kg hydroxyurea (about 0.6–1.2 times the maximum recommended human oral daily dose on a mg/m^2 basis) thrice weekly for 6 months to female rats increased the incidence of mammary tumors in rats surviving to 18 months compared to control. Hydroxyurea is mutagenic *in vitro* to bacteria, fungi, protozoa, and mammalian cells. Hydroxyurea is clastogenic *in vitro* (hamster cells, human lymphoblasts) and *in vivo* (SCE assay in rodents, mouse micronucleus assay). Hydroxyurea causes the transformation of rodent embryo cells to a tumorigenic phenotype.

Pregnancy: DROXIA can cause fetal harm when administered to a pregnant woman. Hydroxyurea is embryotoxic and causes fetal malformations (partially ossified cranial bones, absence of eye sockets, hydrocephaly, bipartite sternebrae, missing lumbar vertebrae) at 180 mg/kg/day (about 0.8 times the maximum recommended human daily dose on a mg/m^2 basis) in rats and at 30 mg/kg/day (about 0.3 times the maximum recommended human daily dose on a mg/m^2 basis) in rabbits. Embryotoxicity was characterized by decreased fetal viability, reduced live litter sizes, and developmental delays. Hydroxyurea crosses the placenta. Single doses of ≥ 375 mg/kg (about 1.7 times the maximum recommended human daily dose on a mg/m^2 basis) to rats caused growth retardation and impaired learning ability. There are no adequate and well-controlled studies in pregnant women. If this drug is used during pregnancy or if the patient becomes pregnant while taking this drug, the patient should be apprised of the potential harm to the fetus. Women of childbearing potential should be advised to avoid becoming pregnant.

PRECAUTIONS

Therapy with DROXIA requires close supervision. Some patients treated at the recommended initial dose of 15 mg/kg/day have experienced severe or life-threatening myelosuppression, requiring interruption of treatment and dose reduction. The hematologic status of the patient, as well as kidney and liver function should be determined prior to, and repeatedly during treatment. Treatment should be interrupted if neutrophil levels fall to < 2000/mm^3; platelets fall to < 80,000/mm^3; hemoglobin declines to less than 4.5 g/dL; or if reticulocytes fall below 80,000/mm^3 when the hemoglobin concentration is below 9 g/dL. Following recovery, treatment may be resumed at lower doses (see **"DOSAGE AND ADMINISTRATION"** section).

Patients must be able to follow directions regarding drug administration and their monitoring and care.

Carcinogenesis, Mutagenesis, and Impairment of Fertility: See **"WARNINGS"** and **"Boxed WARNING"** sections for Carcinogenesis and Mutagenesis information.

Impairment of Fertility—Hydroxyurea administered to male rats at 60 mg/kg/day (about 0.3 times the maximum recommended human daily dose on a mg/m^2 basis) produced testicular atrophy, decreased spermatogenesis, and significantly reduced their ability to impregnate females.

Pregnancy: Pregnancy "Category D". (See **"WARNINGS"** section.)

Nursing Mothers: Hydroxyurea is excreted in human milk. Because of the potential for serious adverse reactions with hydroxyurea, a decision should be made either to discontinue nursing or to discontinue the drug, taking into account the importance of the drug to the mother.

Pediatric Use: Safety and effectiveness in pediatric patients have not been established.

Drug Interactions: Prospective studies on the potential for hydroxyurea to interact with other drugs have not been performed.

Information for Patients: (See **"MEDICATION GUIDE"** at end of labeling). Patients should be reminded that this medication must be handled with care. People who are not taking DROXIA (hydroxyurea capsules, USP) should not be exposed to it. If the powder from the capsule is spilled, it should be wiped up immediately with a damp disposable towel and discarded in a closed container, such as a plastic bag. The medication should be kept away from children and pets.

The necessity of monitoring blood counts every two weeks, throughout the duration of therapy, should be emphasized. For additional information, see the accompanying **"MEDICATION GUIDE"**.

ADVERSE REACTIONS

Sickle Cell Anemia: In patients treated for sickle cell anemia in the Multicenter Study of Hydroxyurea in Sickle Cell Anemia[1], the most common adverse reactions were hematologic, with neutropenia, and low reticulocyte and platelet levels necessitating temporary cessation in almost all patients. Hematologic recovery usually occurred in two weeks. Non-hematologic events that possibly were associated with treatment include hair loss, skin rash, fever, gastrointestinal disturbances, weight gain, bleeding and parvovirus B-19 infection; however, these non-hematologic events occurred with similar frequencies in the hydroxyurea and placebo treatment groups. Melanonychia has also been reported in patients receiving DROXIA for SCA.

Other: Adverse events associated with the use of hydroxyurea in the treatment of neoplastic diseases, in addition to hematologic effects include: gastrointestinal symptoms (stomatitis, anorexia, nausea, vomiting, diarrhea, and constipation), and dermatological reactions such as maculopapular rash, skin ulceration, dermatomyositis-like skin changes, peripheral erythema and facial erythema. Hyperpigmentation, atrophy of skin and nails, scaling and violet papules have been observed in some patients after several years of long-term daily maintenance therapy with hydroxyurea. Skin cancer has been reported. Dysuria and alopecia occur very rarely. Large doses may produce moderate drowsiness. Neurological disturbances have occurred extremely rarely and were limited to headache, dizziness, disorientation, hallucinations, and convulsions. Hydroxyurea occasionally may cause temporary impairment of renal tubular function accompanied by elevations in serum uric acid, BUN, and creatinine levels. Abnormal BSP retention has been reported. Fever, chills, malaise, edema, asthenia, and elevation of hepatic enzymes have also been reported.

The association of hydroxyurea with the development of acute pulmonary reactions consisting of diffuse pulmonary infiltrates, fever and dyspnea has been rarely reported. Pulmonary fibrosis also has been reported rarely.

OVERDOSAGE

Acute mucocutaneous toxicity has been reported in patients receiving hydroxyurea at dosages several times the therapeutic dose. Soreness, violet erythema, edema on palms and soles followed by scaling of hands and feet, severe generalized hyperpigmentation of the skin, and stomatitis have been observed.

DOSAGE AND ADMINISTRATION

Dosage should be based on the patient's actual or ideal weight, whichever is less. The initial dose of DROXIA is 15 mg/kg/day as a single dose. The patient's blood count must be monitored every two weeks. (See **"WARNINGS"** section.)

If blood counts are in an **acceptable range***, the dose may be increased by 5 mg/kg/day every 12 weeks until a maximum tolerated dose (the highest dose that does not produce **toxic**** blood counts over 24 consecutive weeks), or 35 mg/kg/day, is reached.

If blood counts are between the **acceptable range** and **toxic**, the dose is not increased.

If blood counts are considered **toxic****, DROXIA should be discontinued until hematologic recovery. Treatment may then be resumed after reducing the dose by 2.5 mg/kg/day from the dose associated with hematologic toxicity. DROXIA may then be titrated up or down, every 12 weeks in 2.5 mg/kg/day increments, until the patient is at a stable dose that does not result in hematologic toxicity for 24 weeks. Any dosage on which a patient develops hematologic toxicity twice should not be tried again.

***acceptable range =**
neutrophils ≥ 2500 cells/mm^3,
platelets ≥ 95,000/mm^3,
hemoglobin > 5.3 g/dL and
reticulocytes ≥ 95,000/mm^3 if the hemoglobin concentration < 9 g/dL.

****toxic =**
neutrophils < 2000 cells/mm^3,
platelets < 80,000/mm^3,
hemoglobin < 4.5 g/dL and
reticulocytes < 80,000/mm^3 if the hemoglobin concentration < 9 g/dL.

Renal Insufficiency

There are no data that support specific guidance for dosage adjustment in patients with renal impairment. As renal excretion is a pathway of elimination, consideration should be given to decreasing the dosage of DROXIA in patients with renal impairment. Close monitoring of hematologic parameters is advised in these patients.

Hepatic Insufficiency

There are no data that support specific guidelines for dosage adjustment in patients with hepatic impairment. Close monitoring of hematologic parameters is advised in these patients.

Procedures for proper handling and disposal of cytotoxic drugs should be considered. Several guidelines on this subject have been published.[2–8] There is no general agreement that all of the procedures recommended in the guidelines are necessary or appropriate.

HOW SUPPLIED

DROXIA™ (hydroxyurea capsules, USP).

200 mg capsules packaged in HDPE bottles of 60 with a plastic safety screw cap. (NDC 0003-6335-17). The cap and body are opaque blue-green. The capsule is marked in black ink on both the cap and body with **DROXIA** and **6335**.

300 mg capsules packaged in HDPE bottles of 60 with a plastic safety screw cap. (NDC 0003-6336-17). The cap and body are opaque purple. The capsule is marked in black ink on both the cap and body with **DROXIA** and **6336**.

400 mg capsules packaged in HDPE bottles of 60 with a plastic safety screw cap. (NDC 0003-6337-17). The cap and body are opaque reddish-orange. The capsule is marked in black ink on both the cap and body with **DROXIA** and **6337**.

Storage: Store at 25°C (77°F); excursions permitted to 15–30°C (59–86°F). Keep tightly closed.

REFERENCES

1. Charache, S, et al: Hydroxyurea and Sickle Cell Anemia: Clinical Utility of a Myelosuppressive "Switching" Agent. Medicine 1996; 75:300–326.
2. Recommendations for the Safe Handling of Parenteral Antineoplastic Drugs. NIH Publications. No. 83–2621. For sale by the Superintendent of Documents, US Government Printing Office, Washington, DC 20402.
3. AMA Council Report: Guidelines for Handling Parenteral Antineoplastics. JAMA 1985; 253(11):1590–1592.
4. National Study Commission on Cytotoxic Exposure-Recommendations for Handling Cytotoxic Agents. Available from Louis P. Jeffrey, ScD, Chairman, National Study Commission on Cytotoxic Exposure, Massachusetts College of Pharmacy and Allied Health Sciences, 179 Longwood Avenue, Boston, MA 02115
5. Clinical Oncological Society of Australia: Guidelines and Recommendations for Safe Handling of Antineoplastic Agents. Med J Australia 1983; 1:426–428.
6. Jones RB, et al: Safe Handling of Chemotherapeutic Agents: A Report from the Mount Sinai Medical Center, CA-A Cancer Journal for Clinicians 1983; (Sept./Oct.) 258–263.
7. American Society of Hospital Pharmacists Technical Assistance Bulletin on Handling Cytotoxic and Hazardous Drugs. Am J Hosp Pharm 1990; 47:1033–1049.
8. Controlling Occupational Exposure to Hazardous Drugs. (OSHA Work-Practice Guidelines) Am J Health-Syst Pharm 1996; 53:1669–1685.

MEDICATION GUIDE

***DROXIA*™ Capsules**
(generic name = hydroxyurea)

WHAT IS THE MOST IMPORTANT INFORMATION I SHOULD KNOW ABOUT DROXIA?

DROXIA (pronounced drock-SEE-yuh) capsules are used to treat sickle cell anemia in adults. DROXIA reduces the frequency of painful crises and reduces the need for blood transfusions.

It is VERY IMPORTANT that you have regular blood counts so that your doctor can decrease or increase the DROXIA dose as needed to avoid serious complications. The most serious side effects of DROXIA involve the blood and may include severely low white blood cell counts (leukopenia, neutropenia), which can decrease your resistance to infections; severely low red blood cell counts (anemia); or severely low platelet counts (thrombocytopenia), which can cause bleeding. Almost all patients who received DROXIA in clinical studies needed

Continued on next page

Droxia—Cont.

to have their medication stopped for a time to allow their low blood counts to return to acceptable levels.
If you get pregnant, DROXIA may harm or cause death to your unborn child. You should not become pregnant while taking DROXIA. Make sure you use a contraceptive method. *Tell your doctor if you become pregnant or plan to become pregnant while taking DROXIA.*
DROXIA may decrease the ability of men to father children and women to have children.
Laboratory tests and reports in humans suggest DROXIA may increase your risk of developing cancer, especially if it is taken for a long time. However, it is still uncertain whether DROXIA causes cancer.

WHAT IS DROXIA?
DROXIA is a prescription medicine that is used to reduce the frequency of painful crises and reduce the need for blood transfusions in adults with sickle cell anemia. How DROXIA works is not certain but it may work by reducing the number of white blood cells and/or increasing red blood cells that carry fetal hemoglobin (HbF). Fetal hemoglobin may prevent sickling.

WHAT IS SICKLE CELL ANEMIA?
Sickle cell anemia is an inherited disorder of the red blood cells. Red blood cells carry oxygen to all parts of the body by using a protein called hemoglobin. Normal red blood cells contain only normal hemoglobin and are shaped like indented disks. These cells are very flexible and move easily through small blood vessels.
In sickle cell anemia, the red blood cells contain sickle hemoglobin, which causes them to change to a rigid, spiked shape (sickle shape) after oxygen is released. Sickled cells get stuck and form plugs in small blood vessels. These plugs restrict blood flow. causing damage to surrounding tissues resulting in a painful crisis.
Because there are blood vessels in all parts of the body, painful crises can occur anywhere in your body. In addition, sickle cells are trapped and destroyed in the liver and spleen. This results in a shortage of red blood cells (anemia).

WILL DROXIA CURE MY SICKLE CELL ANEMIA?
No. However, DROXIA may help you better control your sickle cell anemia, but it is important to follow your doctor's instructions carefully.
In a study of adults taking recommended doses, daily treatment with DROXIA resulted in fewer painful crises, fewer patients with "acute chest syndromes" (a pneumonia-like condition that leads to difficulty in breathing) and less need for blood transfusions.

WHO SHOULD NOT TAKE DROXIA CAPSULES?
Do not take DROXIA capsules if you are allergic to any of the ingredients. Besides the active ingredient hydroxyurea. DROXIA capules contain the following inactive ingredients: citric acid, gelatin, lactose, magnesium stearate, sodium phosphate, titanium dioxide and capsule colorants. Tell your doctor if you think you have ever had an allergic reaction.
If you get pregnant, DROXIA may harm or cause death to your unborn child. You should not become pregnant while taking DROXIA. Make sure you use a contraceptive method. *Tell your doctor if you become pregnant or plan to become pregnant while taking DROXIA.*

HOW DO I TAKE DROXIA CAPSULES?
Always follow your doctor's instructions carefully when taking DROXIA capsules or any prescription medication. The usual dose of DROXIA may range from as few as one to several capsules per day. DROXIA is usually taken once a day. You should try to take it at the same time each day. Your doctor will determine the proper starting dose of DROXIA for you based on your weight and blood count. The dose will then be increased slowly to your maximum tolerated dose (maximum dose that does NOT produce severely low blood counts). **Your doctor should measure your blood counts every two weeks after you begin treatment with DROXIA.** Depending on the results, your dosage may be adjusted or the drug may be stopped for a while.
DROXIA is a medication that must be handled with care. People who are not taking DROXIA should not be exposed to it. If the powder from the capsule is spilled, it should be wiped up immediately with a damp disposable towel and discarded in a closed container, such as a plastic bag.
If you accidentally take an overdose of DROXIA capsules, seek medical attention immediately. Contact your doctor, local poison control center, or emergency room.

WHAT IF I MISS A DOSE OF DROXIA CAPSULES?
Try not to miss your dose of DROXIA, but if you do, take it as soon as possible. If it is almost time for your next dose, skip the missed dose and resume your regular dosing schedule. *Do not take two doses during the same day.* If you miss more than one dose, call your doctor for instructions.

WHAT SHOULD I AVOID WHILE TAKING DROXIA CAPSULES?
Some other medicines can increase your risk of experiencing serious side effects from DROXIA. While you are taking DROXIA capsules, you should inform your doctor of all prescription and over-the-counter medicines that you are taking.
In nursing mothers, DROXIA is present in breast milk. Because of the potential for side effects in the newborn, you should discontinue nursing your baby while taking DROXIA.

WHAT ARE THE POSSIBLE SIDE EFFECTS OF DROXIA CAPSULES?
As with other medicines, DROXIA may cause unwanted effects, although it is not always possible to tell whether such effects are caused by DROXIA, another medication you may be taking, or your sickle cell anemia. Any side effects or unusual symptoms that you experience should be reported to your doctor, particularly if they persist or are troublesome.
The most serious side effects of DROXIA involve the blood, and may include severely low white blood cell counts (leukopenia, neutropenia), which can decrease your resistance to infections; severely low red blood cell counts (anemia); or severely low platelet counts (thrombocytopenia), which can cause bleeding. Almost all patients who received DROXIA in clinical studies needed to have their medication stopped for a time to allow their low blood counts to return to acceptable levels.
The side effects reported most often by adults with sickle cell anemia participating in studies of DROXIA included hair loss, skin rash, fever, stomach and/or bowel disturbances, weight gain, bleeding, virus infection, and discolored nails (melanonychia), but these were equally common in people getting a placebo (sugar pill).
Skin cancer and leukemia, which can be fatal, have been reported in patients, receiving long-term hydroxyurea for conditions other than sickle cell anemia. In laboratory tests DROXIA causes changes in chromosomes and DNA (genetic material) that strongly suggest it can cause cancer in people, especially if it is taken for a long time.

ARE REGULAR BLOOD COUNTS NECESSARY WHILE TAKING DROXIA CAPSULES?
Yes. Your doctor should measure your blood counts every two weeks while you are taking DROXIA. Your DROXIA dose will require adjustment based on these regular blood counts. Serious problems can occur if the DROXIA dose is not adjusted on time.

WHAT ELSE SHOULD I KNOW ABOUT DROXIA CAPSULES?
If you have kidney or liver disease, close monitoring of your blood count, kidney and liver function will be required.
Because it may not be possible to detect a deficiency of folic acid in patients taking DROXIA, your doctor may prescribe a folic acid supplement for you.

WHAT ELSE SHOULD I DO TO CONTROL MY SICKLE CELL CRISES?
Because painful crises can be brought on by factors such as infection, dehydration, worsening anemia, emotional stress, extreme temperature exposure, or ingestion of substances such as alcohol or other recreational drugs, you should be aware of the following general guidelines that will help keep you pain-free:

- Seek immediate medical attention when a fever develops or signs of infection appear.
- Avoid smoking and drinking more than 1–2 alcoholic beverages a day.
- Drink 8 to 10 glasses of water or other fluid each day.
- Avoid any types of physical exertion that seem to bring on painful crises or other discomfort.
- Avoid extreme temperature changes and dress appropriately in hot and cold weather.

This medicine was prescribed for your particular condition. Do not use DROXIA Capsules for another condition or give it to others. Keep DROXIA Capsules and all medicines out of the reach of children. Discard DROXIA Capsules when they are outdated or no longer needed by flushing the contents of your bottle down the toilet.
This Medication Guide has been approved by the U.S. Food and Drug Administration.

BRISTOL LABORATORIES®
ONCOLOGY PRODUCTS
A Bristol-Myers Squibb Company
Princeton, NJ 08543
U.S.A.
U3-B001-3-98 N1219-00
Issued: March 1998

Shown in Product Identification Guide, page 308

ETOPOPHOS® ℞
[ē-top-ō-phos]
(etoposide phosphate) for Injection

PHARMACY BULK PACKAGE IS NOT FOR DIRECT INFUSION

WARNINGS
ETOPOPHOS® (etoposide phosphate) for Injection should be administered under the supervision of a qualified physician experienced in the use of cancer chemotherapeutic agents. Severe myelosuppression with resulting infection or bleeding may occur.

DESCRIPTION
ETOPOPHOS® (etoposide phosphate) for Injection is an antineoplastic agent which is available for intravenous infusion as a sterile lyophile in single-dose vials containing etoposide phosphate equivalent to 100 mg etoposide, 32.7 mg sodium citrate, USP and 300 mg dextran 40; and in pharmacy-bulk vials containing etoposide phosphate equivalent to 500 mg or 1000 mg etoposide, sodium citrate, USP (163.5 mg, or 327 mg, respectively), and dextran 40 (1500 mg or 3000 mg, respectively).
Etoposide phosphate is a water soluble ester of etoposide (commonly known as VP-16), a semi-synthetic derivative of podophyllotoxin. The water solubility of etoposide phosphate lessens the potential for precipitation following dilution and during intravenous administration.
The chemical name for etoposide phosphate is: 4'-Demethylepipodophyllotoxin 9-[4,6-O-(R)-ethylidene-β-D-glucopyranoside], 4'-(dihydrogen phosphate).
Etoposide phosphate has the following structure:

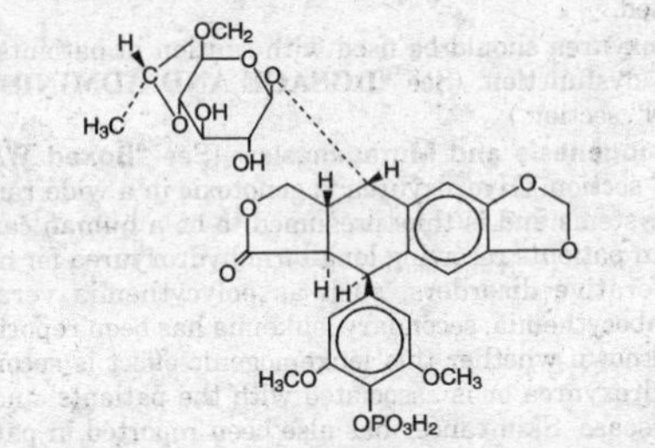

CLINICAL PHARMACOLOGY
The *in vitro* cytotoxicity observed for etoposide phosphate is significantly less than that seen with etoposide which is believed due to the necessity for conversion *in vivo* to the active moiety, etoposide, by dephosphorylation. The mechanism of action is believed to be the same as that of etoposide. Etoposide has been shown to cause metaphase arrest in chick fibroblasts. Its main effect, however, appears to be at the G_2 portion of the cell cycle in mammalian cells. Two different dose-dependent responses are seen. At high concentrations (10 µg/mL or more), lysis of cells entering mitosis is observed. At low concentrations (0.3 to 10 µg/mL), cells are inhibited from entering prophase. It does not interfere with microtubular assembly. The predominant macromolecular effect of etoposide appears to be the induction of DNA strand breaks by an interaction with DNA-topoisomerase II or the formation of free radicals.

ETOPOPHOS Bioequivalence: Following intravenous administration of ETOPOPHOS, etoposide phosphate is rapidly and completely converted to etoposide in plasma. A direct comparison of the pharmacokinetic parameters [area under the concentration time curve (AUC) and the maximum plasma concentration (C_{max})] of etoposide following intravenous administration of molar equivalent doses of ETOPOPHOS and VePesid® (etoposide) was made in two randomized cross-over studies in patients with a variety of malignancies. In the first study of 41 evaluable patients, the etoposide mean ± S.D. AUC values were 168.3 ± 48.2 µg•hr/mL and 156.7 ± 43.4 µg•hr/mL following administration of molar equivalent doses of 150 mg/m^2 ETOPOPHOS or VePesid with a 3.5 hour infusion time; the corresponding mean ± S.D. C_{max} values were 20.0 ± 3.7 µg/mL and 19.6 ± 4.2 µg/mL, respectively. The point estimate (90% confidence interval) for the bioavailability of etoposide from ETOPOPHOS, relative to VePesid, was 107% (105%, 110%) for AUC and 103% (99%, 106%) for C_{max}. In the second study of 29 evaluable patients following intravenous administration of 90, 100 and 110 mg/m^2 molar equivalents of ETOPOPHOS or VePesid with a 60 minute infusion time, the etoposide mean ± S.D. AUC values (normalized to the 100 mg/m^2 dose) were 96.1 ± 22.6 µg•hr/mL and 86.5 ± 25.8 µg•hr/mL, respectively; the corresponding mean ± S.D. C_{max} values (normalized to the 100 mg/m^2 dose) were 20.1 ± 4.1 µg/mL and 19.0 ± 5.1 µg/mL, respectively. The point estimate (90% confidence interval) for the bioavailability of etoposide from ETOPOPHOS, relative to VePesid, was 113% (107%, 119%) for AUC and 107% (101%, 113%) for C_{max} indicating bioequivalence. Results from both studies demonstrated no statistically significant differences in the AUC and C_{max} parameters for etoposide when administered as ETOPOPHOS or VePesid. In addition, in the latter study, there were no statistically significant differences in the pharmacodynamic parameters (hematologic toxicity) after administration of ETOPOPHOS or VePesid. Following VePesid administration, the mean nadir values (expressed as percent decrease from baseline) for leukocytes, granulocytes, hemoglobin and thrombocytes were 67.2 ± 17.0%, 84.1 ± 14.6%, 22.6 ± 9.8% and 46.4 ± 21.9%, respectively; the corresponding values after administration of ETOPO-

PHOS were 67.3 ± 14.2%, 81.0 ± 16.5%, 21.4 ± 9.9% and 44.1 ± 20.7%, respectively.

Because of the similarity of pharmacokinetics and pharmacodynamics of etoposide after administration of either ETOPOPHOS or VePesid, the following information on VePesid should be considered:

VePesid Pharmacokinetics: On intravenous administration, the disposition of etoposide is best described as a biphasic process with a distribution half-life of about 1.5 hours and terminal elimination half-life ranging from 4 to 11 hours. Total body clearance values range from 33 to 48 mL/min or 16 to 36 mL/min/m^2 and, like the terminal elimination half-life, are independent of dose over a range 100-600 mg/m^2. Over the same dose range, the AUC and the C_{max} values increase linearly with dose. Etoposide does not accumulate in the plasma following daily administration of 100 mg/m^2 for 4 to 5 days. After intravenous infusion the C_{max} and AUC values exhibit marked intra- and inter-subject variability.

The mean volumes of distribution at steady state fall in the range of 18 to 29 liters or 7 to 17 L/m^2. Etoposide enters the CSF poorly. Although it is detectable in CSF and intracerebral tumors, the concentrations are lower than in extracerebral tumors and in plasma. Etoposide concentrations are higher in normal lung than in lung metastases and are similar in primary tumors and normal tissues of the myometrium. In vitro, etoposide is highly protein bound (97%) to human plasma proteins. An inverse relationship between plasma albumin levels and etoposide renal clearance is found in children. In a study determining the effect of other therapeutic agents on the in vitro binding of carbon-14 labeled etoposide to human serum proteins, only phenylbutazone, sodium salicylate, and aspirin displaced protein-bound etoposide at concentrations achieved in vivo.

Etoposide binding ratio correlates directly with serum albumin in patients with cancer and in normal volunteers. The unbound fraction of etoposide significantly correlated with bilirubin in a population of cancer patients. Data have suggested a significant inverse correlation between serum albumin concentration and free fraction of etoposide (see "**PRECAUTIONS**" section).

After intravenous administration of ^{3}H-etoposide (70-290 mg/m^2), mean recoveries of radioactivity in the urine range from 42 to 67%, and fecal recoveries range from 0 to 16% of the dose. Less than 50% of an intravenous dose is excreted in the urine as etoposide with mean recoveries of 8 to 35% within 24 hours.

In children, approximately 55% of the dose of VePesid (etoposide) is excreted in the urine as etoposide in 24 hours. The mean renal clearance of etoposide is 7 to 10 mL/min/m^2 or 35% of the total body clearance over a dose of 80 to 600 mg/m^2. Etoposide, therefore, is cleared by both renal and nonrenal processes, i.e., metabolism and biliary excretion. The effect of renal disease on plasma etoposide clearance is not known in children.

Biliary excretion appears to be a minor route of etoposide elimination. Only 6% or less of an intravenous dose is recovered in the bile as etoposide. Metabolism accounts for most of the nonrenal clearance of etoposide. The major urinary metabolite of etoposide in adults and children is the hydroxy acid [4'-demethylepipodophyllic acid-9-(4,6-0-(R)-ethylidene-β-D-glucopyranoside)], formed by opening of the lactone ring. It is also present in human plasma, presumably as the **trans** isomer. Glucuronide and/or sulfate conjugates of etoposide are excreted in human urine and represent 5 to 22% of the dose. In addition, O-demethylation of the dimethoxyphenol ring occurs through the CYP450 3A4 isoenzyme pathway to produce the corresponding catechol.

In adults, the total body clearance of etoposide is correlated with creatinine clearance, serum albumin concentration, and nonrenal clearance. Patients with impaired renal function receiving etoposide have exhibited reduced total body clearance, increased AUC and a lower volume of distribution at steady state (see "**PRECAUTIONS**" section). Use of cisplatin therapy is associated with reduced total body clearance. In children, elevated serum SGPT levels are associated with reduced drug total body clearance. Prior use of cisplatin may also result in a decrease of etoposide total body clearance in children.

Although some minor differences in pharmacokinetic parameters between age and gender have been observed, these differences were not considered clinically significant.

Clinical Studies: A total of 7 clinical trials with 365 patients treated (368 entered) provide the data base for the human experience summarized in this insert. Five phase I trials evaluated etoposide phosphate given on a days 1, 3 and 5 or days 1 through 5 schedule. In two trials the drug was given over 5 minutes and in three over 30 minutes. The following table summarizes the doses, schedules, infusion times and numbers of patients entered in the phase I experience.

Response to Treatment for All Patients

	Etoposide Phosphate plus Cisplatin	Etoposide plus Cisplatin	P-value
Complete Responses:	15%	15%	1.000*
Partial Response:	46%	43%	0.855*
Overall Response Rate:	61%	58%	0.854*
Median Time to Response:	48 days	46 days	0.596**
Median Response Duration:	273 days	241 days	0.141***
Median Time to Progression:	211 days	213 days	0.500***
Median Time to Worsening Performance Status:	210 days	149 days	0.472***
Median Survival:	348 days	318 days	0.780***

* Fisher's Exact test
** Wilcoxon Rank Sum test
*** Logrank test

Dose Escalation (Phase I) Trials of Etoposide Phosphate

Study	Schedule Q 21 days	Infusion Time	Dose Range (mg/m^2)	Number of Patients Entered
002	Days 1-5	30 minutes	25 - 110	68
005	Days 1, 3, 5	30 minutes	50 - 175	39
006	Days 1-5	30 minutes	50 - 125	28
008	Days 1, 3, 5	5 minutes	50 - 200	36
009	Days 1-5	5 minutes	50 - 125	27

Two trials evaluated the pharmacokinetic equivalence of etoposide and etoposide phosphate. A phase I study (002) was expanded at the higher doses to compare the pharmacokinetic profile of etoposide following administration of etoposide or etoposide phosphate. Another, multi-institutional trial (012), was conducted at a dose of 150 mg/m^2 using a day 1, 3 and 5 schedule and a crossover design.

The seventh trial (011) was a randomized study in which patients with limited or extensive small cell lung cancer and no prior therapy were treated with either cisplatin plus etoposide or cisplatin plus etoposide phosphate. Patients received 20 mg/m^2/day of cisplatin for 5 days and 80 mg/m^2/day of etoposide or etoposide phosphate. A total of 121 patients were randomized and 120 treated (60 per group). Response rates, time to response, duration of response, time to progression, time to worsening performance status and survival were similar in the two groups whether the analysis was done for patients with limited or extensive disease or for the entire population. The following table summarizes the results regardless of disease extent.

[See table at top of page]

The most prominent side effects were myelosuppression and GI toxicity. Sixty-eight percent of patients treated with etoposide phosphate plus cisplatin had neutrophils less than 500/mm^3 at some time during treatment as did 88% of those getting etoposide and cisplatin. Over 85% in each group had nausea and/or vomiting. No differences in the pattern or severity of side effects were observed.

INDICATION AND USAGE

ETOPOPHOS (etoposide phosphate) for Injection is indicated in the management of the following neoplasms:

Refractory Testicular Tumors: ETOPOPHOS for Injection in combination therapy with other approved chemotherapeutic agents in patients with refractory testicular tumors who have already received appropriate surgical, chemotherapeutic, and radiotherapeutic therapy.

Small Cell Lung Cancer: ETOPOPHOS for Injection in combination with other approved chemotherapeutic agents as first line treatment in patients with small cell lung cancer.

CONTRAINDICATIONS

ETOPOPHOS (etoposide phosphate) for Injection is contraindicated in patients who have demonstrated a previous hypersensitivity to etoposide, etoposide phosphate, or any other component of the formulations.

WARNINGS

Patients being treated with ETOPOPHOS must be frequently observed for myelosuppression both during and after therapy. Myelosuppression resulting in death has been reported following etoposide administration. Dose-limiting bone marrow suppression is the most significant toxicity associated with ETOPOPHOS therapy. Therefore, the following studies should be obtained at the start of therapy and prior to each subsequent cycle of ETOPOPHOS: platelet count, hemoglobin, white blood cell count, and differential.

The occurrence of a platelet count below 50,000/mm^3 or an absolute neutrophil count below 500/mm^3 is an indication to withhold further therapy until the blood counts have sufficiently recovered. The toxicity of rapidly infused ETOPOPHOS in patients with impaired renal or hepatic function has not been adequately evaluated. The toxicity profile of ETOPOPHOS when infused at doses >175 mg/m^2 has not been delineated.

Physicians should be aware of the possible occurrence of an anaphylactic reaction manifested by chills, fever, tachycardia, bronchospasm, dyspnea and hypotension. Higher rates of anaphylactic-like reactions have been reported in children who received infusions of etoposide at concentrations higher than those recommended. The role that concentration of infusion (or rate of infusion) plays in the development of anaphylactic-like reactions is uncertain. (See "**ADVERSE REACTIONS**" section.) Treatment is symptomatic. The infusion should be terminated immediately, followed by the administration of pressor agents, corticosteroids, antihistamines, or volume expanders at the discretion of the physician.

ETOPOPHOS can cause fetal harm when administered to a pregnant woman. Etoposide has been shown to be teratogenic in mice and rats, and it is therefore likely that ETOPOPHOS is also teratogenic.

In rats, an intravenous etoposide dose of 0.4 mg/kg/day (about 1/20th of the human dose on a mg/m^2 basis) during organogenesis caused maternal toxicity, embryotoxicity, and teratogenicity (skeletal abnormalities, exencephaly, encephalocele, and anophthalmia); higher doses of 1.2 and 3.6 mg/kg/day (about 1/7th and 1/2 of the human dose on a mg/m^2 basis) resulted in 90 and 100% embryonic resorptions. In mice, a single 1.0 mg/kg (1/16th of the human dose on a mg/m^2 basis) dose of etoposide administered intraperitoneally on days 6, 7, or 8 of gestation caused embryotoxicity, cranial abnormalities, and major skeletal malformations. An i.p. dose of 1.5 mg/kg (about 1/10th of the human dose on a mg/m^2 basis) on day 7 of gestation caused an increase in the incidence of intrauterine death and fetal malformations and a significant decrease in the average fetal body weight. If this drug is used during pregnancy, or if the patient becomes pregnant while receiving this drug, the patient should be warned of the potential hazard to the fetus. Women of childbearing potential should be advised to avoid becoming pregnant.

ETOPOPHOS should be considered a potential carcinogen in humans. The occurrence of acute leukemia with or without a preleukemic phase has been reported in rare instances in patients treated with etoposide alone or in association with other neoplastic agents. The risk of development of a preleukemic or leukemic syndrome is unclear. Carcinogenicity tests with ETOPOPHOS have not been conducted in laboratory animals.

PRECAUTIONS

General: In all instances where the use of ETOPOPHOS is considered for chemotherapy, the physician must evaluate the need and usefulness of the drug against the risk of adverse reactions. Most such adverse reactions are reversible if detected early. If severe reactions occur, the drug should be reduced in dosage or discontinued and appropriate corrective measures should be taken according to the clinical judgement of the physician. Reinstitution of ETOPOPHOS therapy should be carried out with caution, and with adequate consideration of the further need for the drug and alertness as to possible recurrence of toxicity.

Patients with low serum albumin may be at an increased risk for etoposide associated toxicities.

Laboratory Tests: Periodic complete blood counts should be done during the course of ETOPOPHOS treatment. They should be performed prior to each cycle of therapy and at appropriate intervals during and after therapy.

Continued on next page

Etopophos—Cont.

Carcinogenesis (see "WARNINGS" section), Mutagenesis, Impairment of Fertility: ETOPOPHOS was non-mutagenic in *in vitro* Ames microbial mutagenicity assay and the *E. coli* WP2 uvrA reverse mutation assay. Since ETOPOPHOS is rapidly and completely converted to etoposide *in vivo* and etoposide has been shown to be mutagenic in Ames assay, ETOPOPHOS should be considered as a potential mutagen *in vivo*.

In rats, an oral dose of ETOPOPHOS at 86.0 mg/kg/day (about 10 times the human dose on a mg/m^2 basis) or above administered for 5 consecutive days resulted in irreversible testicular atrophy. Irreversible testicular atrophy was also present in rats treated with ETOPOPHOS intravenously for 30 days at 5.11 mg/kg/day (about 1/2 of the human dose on a mg/m^2 basis).

Pregnancy: Pregnancy "Category D." (See "**WARNINGS**" section.)

Nursing Mothers: It is not known whether this drug is excreted in human milk. Because many drugs are excreted in human milk and because of the potential for serious adverse reactions in nursing infants from ETOPOPHOS, a decision should be made whether to discontinue nursing or to discontinue the drug, taking into account the importance of the drug to the mother.

Pediatric Use: Safety and effectiveness in pediatric patients have not been established. Anaphylactic reactions have been reported in pediatric patients who received etoposide (see "**WARNINGS**" section).

Drug Interactions: Caution should be exercised when administering ETOPOPHOS with drugs that are known to inhibit phosphatase activities (e.g., levamisole hydrochloride). High-dose cyclosporin A resulting in concentrations above 2000 ng/mL administered with oral etoposide has led to an 80% increase in etoposide exposure with a 38% decrease in total body clearance of etoposide compared to etoposide alone.

Renal Impairment: In patients with impaired renal function, the following initial dose modification should be considered based on measured creatinine clearance:

Measured Creatinine Clearance	>50 mL/min	15–50 mL/min
etoposide	100% of dose	75% of dose

Subsequent etoposide dosing should be based on patient tolerance and clinical effect. Equivalent dose adjustments of ETOPOPHOS should be used.

Data are not available in patients with creatinine clearances <15 mL/min and further dose reduction should be considered in these patients.

ADVERSE REACTIONS

ETOPOPHOS has been found to be well tolerated as a single agent in clinical studies involving 206 patients with a wide variety of malignancies, and in combination with cisplatin in 60 patients with small cell lung cancer. The most frequent clinically significant adverse experiences were leukopenia and neutropenia.

The incidences of adverse experiences in the table that follows are derived from studies in which ETOPOPHOS (etoposide phosphate) for Injection was administered as a single agent. A total of 98 patients received total doses at or above 450 mg/m^2 on a 5 consecutive day or day 1, 3 and 5 schedule during the first course of therapy.

Summary of Adverse Events Reported with Single Agent ETOPOPHOS Following Course 1 at Total Five Day Doses of ≥ 450 mg/m^2

		Percent of Patients
Hematologic toxicity		
Leukopenia	<4000 /mm^3	91
	<1000 /mm^3	17
Neutropenia	<2000 /mm^3	88
	<500 /mm^3	37
Thrombocytopenia	<100,000 /mm^3	23
	<50,000 /mm^3	9
Anemia	<11 g/dL	72
	<8 g/dL	19
Gastrointestinal toxicity		
Nausea and/or Vomiting		37
Anorexia		16
Mucositis		11
Constipation		8
Abdominal Pain		7
Diarrhea		6
Taste Alteration		6
Asthenia/Malaise		39
Alopecia		33
Chills and/or Fever		24
Dizziness		5
Extravasation/Phlebitis		5

Since etoposide phosphate is converted to etoposide, those adverse experiences that are associated with VePesid (etoposide) can be expected to occur with ETOPOPHOS.

Hematologic Toxicity: Myelosuppression after ETOPOPHOS administration is dose related and dose limiting with the leukocyte nadir counts occurring from day 15 to day 22 after initiation of drug therapy, granulocyte nadir counts occurring day 12–19 after initiation of drug therapy, and platelet nadirs occurring from day 10–15. Bone marrow recovery usually occurs by day 21 but may be delayed, and no cumulative toxicity has been reported. Fever and infection have also been reported in patients with neutropenia. Death associated with myelosuppression has been reported following etoposide administration.

Gastrointestinal Toxicity: Nausea and vomiting are the major gastrointestinal toxicities. The severity of such nausea and vomiting is generally mild to moderate with treatment discontinuation required in 1% of patients. Nausea and vomiting can usually be controlled with standard antiemetic therapy.

Blood Pressure Changes: In clinical studies, one hundred fifty-one patients were treated with ETOPOPHOS with infusion times ranging from thirty minutes to three and one-half hours. Sixty-three patients received ETOPOPHOS as a five minute bolus infusion. Four patients experienced one or more episodes of hypertension and eight patients experienced one or more episodes of hypotension, which may or may not be drug related. One episode of hypotension was reported among those patients who received a five minute bolus infusion. If clinically significant hypotension or hypertension occurs with ETOPOPHOS, appropriate supportive therapy should be initiated.

Allergic Reactions: Anaphylactic type reactions characterized by chills, rigors, tachycardia, bronchospasm, dyspnea, diaphoresis, fever, pruritus, hypertension or hypotension, loss of consciousness, nausea, and vomiting have been reported to occur in 3% (7/245) of all patients treated with ETOPOPHOS. Facial flushing was reported in 2% and skin rashes in 3% of patients receiving ETOPOPHOS. These reactions have usually responded promptly to the cessation of the infusion and administration of pressor agents, corticosteroids, antihistamines, or volume expanders as appropriate; however, the reactions can be fatal. Hypertension and/or flushing have also been reported. Blood pressure usually normalizes within a few hours after cessation of the initial infusion.

Anaphylactic-like reactions have occurred during the initial infusion of ETOPOPHOS (see "**WARNINGS**" section). Facial/tongue swelling, coughing, diaphoresis, cyanosis, tightness in throat, laryngospasm, back pain, and/or loss of consciousness have sometimes occurred in association with the above reactions. In addition, an apparent hypersensitivity-associated apnea has been reported rarely.

Rash, urticaria, and/or pruritus have infrequently been reported at recommended doses. At investigational doses, a generalized pruritic erythematous maculopapular rash, consistent with perivasculitis, has been reported.

Alopecia: Reversible alopecia, sometimes progressing to total baldness, was observed in up to 44% of patients.

Other Toxicities: The following adverse reactions have been infrequently reported: abdominal pain, aftertaste, constipation, dysphagia, fever, transient cortical blindness, interstitial pneumonitis/pulmonary fibrosis, optic neuritis, pigmentation, seizure (occasionally associated with allergic reactions), Stevens-Johnson Syndrome, toxic epidermal necrolysis, and a single report of radiation recall dermatitis. Rarely, hepatic toxicity may be seen.

The incidences of adverse reactions in the table that follows are derived from multiple data bases from studies in 2,081 patients when VePesid (etoposide) was used either orally or by injection as a single agent.

Adverse Drug Effects Observed with Single Agent VePesid		Percent Range of Reported Incidence
Hematologic toxicity		
Leukopenia	< 1,000 /mm^3	3–17
	< 4,000 /mm^3	60–91
Thrombocytopenia	< 50,000 /mm^3	1–20
	< 100,000 /mm^3	22–41
Anemia		0–33
Gastrointestinal toxicity		
Nausea and Vomiting		31–43
Abdominal Pain		0–2
Anorexia		10–13
Diarrhea		1–13
Stomatitis		1–6
Hepatic		0–3
Alopecia		8–66
Peripheral Neurotoxicity		1–2
Hypotension		1–2
Allergic Reaction		1–2

OVERDOSAGE

No proven antidotes have been established for ETOPOPHOS (etoposide phosphate) for Injection overdosage in humans. In mice, a single intravenous dose of rapidly administered ETOPOPHOS was lethal at or above 120 mg/kg (about 7 times human dose on a mg/m^2 basis) and was associated with clinical signs of neurotoxicity.

DOSAGE AND ADMINISTRATION

The usual dose of VePesid for Injection in testicular cancer in combination with other approved chemotherapeutic agents ranges from 50 to 100 mg/m^2/day on days 1 through 5 to 100 mg/m^2/day on days 1, 3, and 5. Equivalent doses of ETOPOPHOS should be used.

In small cell lung cancer, the VePesid for Injection dose in combination with other approved chemotherapeutic drugs ranges from 35 mg/m^2/day for 4 days to 50 mg/m^2/day for 5 days. Equivalent doses of ETOPOPHOS should be used.

For recommended dosing adjustments in patients with renal impairment, see "**PRECAUTIONS**" section.

ETOPOPHOS solutions may be administered at infusion rates from 5 to 210 minutes. Chemotherapy courses are repeated at 3- to 4-week intervals after adequate recovery from any toxicity.

The dosage should be modified to take into account the myelosuppressive effect of other drugs in the combination or the effects of prior x-ray therapy or chemotherapy which may have compromised bone marrow reserve.

Administration Precautions: As with other potentially toxic compounds, caution should be exercised in handling and preparing the solution of ETOPOPHOS. Skin reactions associated with accidental exposure to ETOPOPHOS may occur. The use of gloves is recommended. If ETOPOPHOS solution contacts the skin or mucosa, immediately and thoroughly wash the skin with soap and water and flush the mucosa with water.

Preparation for Intravenous Administration: Prior to use, the content of each vial must be reconstituted with Sterile Water for Injection, USP; 5% Dextrose Injection, USP; 0.9% Sodium Chloride Injection, USP; Sterile Bacteriostatic Water for Injection with Benzyl Alcohol; or Bacteriostatic Sodium Chloride for Injection with Benzyl Alcohol to a concentration equivalent to 20 mg/mL or 10 mg/mL etoposide (22.7 mg/mL or 11.4 mg/mL etoposide phosphate, respectively). Use the quantity of diluent shown below to reconstitute the products.

Vial Strength	Volume of Diluent	Final Concentration
100 mg	5 mL	20 mg/mL
	10 mL	10 mg/mL
500 mg	25 mL	20 mg/mL
	50 mL	10 mg/mL
1000 mg	50 mL	20 mg/mL
	100 mL	10 mg/mL

Following reconstitution, ETOPOPHOS can be further diluted to concentrations as low as 0.1 mg/mL etoposide with either 5% Dextrose Injection, USP or 0.9% Sodium Chloride Injection, USP.

Directions for Dispensing: Pharmacy Bulk Vial - Not for Direct Infusion: CONTENTS SHOULD BE USED AS SOON AS POSSIBLE FOLLOWING INITIAL PUNCTURE OF THE CLOSURE. DISCARD ANY UNUSED PORTION WITHIN 24 HOURS OF FIRST ENTRY (i.e., RECONSTITUTION). The 500 mg and 1000 mg pharmacy bulk vials are for use in a pharmacy admixture service only under a laminar flow hood. The closure should be penetrated only once with a sterile transfer set or other sterile dispensing device, which allows measured distribution of the contents, and the contents dispensed in aliquots using aseptic technique. Following the first penetration of the closure, container should be maintained at controlled room temperature 20°-25° C (68° to 77° F) under a laminar flow hood until contents are dispensed.

Stability: Unopened vials of ETOPOPHOS (etoposide phosphate) for Injection are stable until the date indicated on the package when stored under refrigeration 2°–8° C (36°–46° F) in the original package. When reconstituted as directed, ETOPOPHOS solutions can be stored in glass or plastic containers under refrigeration 2°–8° C (36° to 46° F) for 7 days; at controlled room temperature 20°–25° C (68° to 77° F) for 24 hours following reconstitution with Sterile Water for Injection, USP, 5% Dextrose Injection, USP, or 0.9% Sodium Chloride Injection, USP; or at controlled room temperature 20°–25° C (68° to 77° F) for 48 hours following reconstitution with Sterile Bacteriostatic Water for Injection with Benzyl Alcohol or Bacteriostatic Sodium Chloride for Injection with Benzyl Alcohol. ETOPOPHOS solutions further diluted as directed can be stored under refrigeration 2°–8° C (36° to 46° F) or at controlled room temperature 20°–25° C (68° to 77° F) for 24 hours.

HOW SUPPLIED

ETOPOPHOS® (etoposide phosphate) for Injection is supplied as individual cartoned vials with flip-off seals containing etoposide phosphate equivalent to 100 mg, 500 mg, or 1000 mg etoposide as follows:

NDC 0015-3404-20	100 mg single-dose vial	(White flip-off seal)
NDC 0015-3405-12	500 mg pharmacy bulk vial	(Slate flip-off seal)
NDC 0015-3406-13	1000 mg pharmacy bulk vial	(Dark grey flip-off seal)

STORAGE

Store the unopened vials under refrigeration 2°–8° C (36°–46° F). Retain in original package to protect from light.

HANDLING AND DISPOSAL

Procedures for proper handling and disposal of anticancer drugs should be considered. Several guidelines on this subject have been published.[1-7] There is no general agreement that all of the procedures recommended in the guidelines are necessary or appropriate.

REFERENCES

1. Recommendations for the Safe Handling of Parenteral Antineoplastic Drugs. NIH Publication No. 83-2621. For sale by the Superintendent of Documents, US Government Printing Office, Washington, DC 20402.
2. AMA Council Report. Guidelines for Handling Parenteral Antineoplastics. JAMA 1985; 253(11):1590-1592.
3. National Study Commission on Cytotoxic Exposure – Recommendations for Handling Cytotoxic Agents. Available from Louis P. Jeffrey, ScD, Chairman, National Study Commission on Cytotoxic Exposure, Massachusetts College of Pharmacy and Allied Health Sciences, 179 Longwood Avenue, Boston, Massachusetts 02115.
4. Clinical Oncological Society of Australia. Guidelines and Recommendations for Safe Handling of Antineoplastic Agents. Med J Australia 1983; 1:426-428.
5. Jones RB, et al: Safe Handling of Chemotherapeutic Agents: A Report from the Mount Sinai Medical Center. CA-A Cancer Journal for Clinicians 1983; (Sept/Oct)258-263.
6. American Society of Hospital Pharmacists Technical Assistance Bulletin on Handling Cytotoxic and Hazardous Drugs. Am J Hosp Pharm 1990; 47:1033–1049.
7. Controlling Occupational Exposure to Hazardous Drugs. (OSHA Work–Practice Guidelines). Am J Health-Syst Pharm 1996; 53:1669-1685.

BRISTOL LABORATORIES®
ONCOLOGY PRODUCTS
A Bristol-Myers Squibb Company
Princeton, NJ 08543
U.S.A.
U2-B001-6-98
51-004164-04
3404DIM-05
Revised: April 1998
Shown in Product Identification Guide, page 308

FUNGIZONE® ORAL SUSPENSION ℞
Amphotericin B Oral Suspension

CAUTION: Federal law prohibits dispensing without prescription.

DESCRIPTION

Fungizone Oral Suspension (Amphotericin B Oral Suspension) contains amphotericin B, an antifungal polyene antibiotic obtained from a strain of *Streptomyces nodosus*. Amphotericin B is designated chemically as [1R (1R*,3S*,5R*,6R*,9R*,11R*, 15S*,16R*,17R*,18S*,19E, 21E,23E,25E,27E,29E,31E,33R*,35S*,36R*,37S*)]-33-[(3-Amino-3,6-dideoxy-β-(D -mannopyranosyl)oxy]-1,3,5,6,9,11,17,37-octahydroxy-15,16,18-trimethyl -13- oxo-14,39-dioxabicyclo [33.3.1] nonatriaconta-19,21,23,25,27,29,31-heptaene-36-carboxylic acid.
Structural formula:

Fungizone [amphotericin B]

$C_{47}H_{73}NO_{17}$ MW=924.10

Fungizone Oral Suspension is a flavored aqueous suspension providing 100 mg amphotericin B per mL. Inactive ingredients: not more than 0.55 percent alcohol, carboxymethylcellulose sodium, citric acid, flavors, glycerin, methyl- and propylparaben, mono- and dibasic sodium phosphate, potassium chloride, sodium benzoate, sodium metabisulfite, and purified water.

MICROBIOLOGY
Mechanism of Action

Amphotericin B exhibits antifungal activity by binding to sterols in the cell membrane of susceptible fungi with a resultant change of membrane permeability allowing leakage of intracellular components.

Anti-Candida activity *in vitro*

Candida species are inhibited by concentrations of amphotericin B ranging from 0.03 to 2.0 µg/mL *in vitro*. While *Candida albicans* is generally quite susceptible to amphotericin B, non-*albicans* species may be less susceptible. The activity of amphotericin B is fungistatic or fungicidal depending on the concentration at the site of infection and the susceptibility of the fungal organism. However, standardized techniques for susceptibility testing of antifungal agents have not been established and results of susceptibility studies have not been correlated with clinical outcomes. The antibiotic is without effect against bacteria, rickettsiae and viruses.

Drug Resistance

Mutants with decreased susceptibility to amphotericin B have been isolated from several fungal species after serial passage *in vitro* in the presence of the drug, and from some patients receiving prolonged therapy. However, the clinical relevance of drug resistance to clinical outcome has not been established.

Drug Interaction

Antagonism between amphotericin B and imidazole derivatives, such as miconazole, and ketoconazole, which inhibit ergosterol synthesis, has been reported. However, the clinical significance of this phenomena has not been demonstrated.

CLINICAL PHARMACOLOGY
Pharmacokinetics

Amphotericin B administered as Fungizone Oral Suspension is poorly absorbed from the gastrointestinal tract. In limited studies conducted in both pediatric and adult patients administered Fungizone Oral Suspension (dose 100 mg four to six times a day), the average amphotericin B serum concentration measured by microbiological assay following at least 14 days of therapy was 0.05 µg/mL (range <0.01–0.15). Serum concentrations did not show evidence of significant antibiotic accumulation over a period of two weeks. Metabolic pathways have not been elucidated.

INDICATIONS AND USAGE

Fungizone Oral Suspension (Amphotericin B Oral Suspension) is indicated for the treatment of oral candidiasis caused by susceptible strains of *Candida albicans*.
When appropriate, it is recommended that identification of the causative pathogen be obtained by means of suitable mycologic techniques before the initiation of treatment.

CONTRAINDICATIONS

Fungizone Oral Suspension is contraindicated in patients with a history of hypersensitivity to any of its components.

PRECAUTIONS
General

Fungizone Oral Suspension is not to be used for the treatment of systemic mycoses. If a systemic mycosis is suspected or documented, appropriate therapy should be instituted. Superficial candidal lesions present in addition to the oral infection should be treated concomitantly with an appropriate topical anti-candidal preparation.
If irritation or hypersensitivity develops with Fungizone Oral Suspension, treatment should be discontinued and appropriate therapy instituted.

Information for Patients

Patients taking this medication should be provided the following information:
1. Use as directed by your physician. This medication is only for the treatment of oral candidiasis and should not be used for any other diseases or symptoms.
2. The medication works by direct contact with the oral *Candida* lesions; you should try to swish the medication around in your mouth as long as reasonably possible before swallowing.
3. If symptoms of local irritation develop, preexisting symptoms worsen, or new symptoms develop, your physician should be notified promptly.
4. Notify your physician if symptoms recur after discontinuation of medication.

Carcinogenesis, Mutagenesis, Impairment of Fertility

No long-term studies have been performed to evaluate carcinogenic or mutagenic potential of Fungizone Oral Suspension. Animal studies of Fungizone Oral Suspension have shown effects on reproduction.

Pregnancy: Category C

Fungizone Oral Suspension has been shown to cause a significantly higher incidence of stillborn fetuses when administered to pregnant rats at a dose of 200 mg/kg/day (4x the human dose, based on body surface area considerations). No signs of fetal abnormalities were observed. An increased number of deaths occurred in pregnant rabbits administered 50 mg/kg/day (2x the human dose) and 100 mg/kg/day (4x the human dose). The number of births were also reduced at those doses and one stillbirth occurred at the lower dose. No fetal abnormalities were observed. There are no adequate and well-controlled studies in pregnant women. Fungizone Oral Suspension should be used during pregnancy only if the potential benefit justifies the potential risk to the fetus.

Nursing Mothers

Though systemic absorption is poor, it is not known whether amphotericin B is excreted in human milk. Because many drugs are excreted in human milk and because of the potential for serious adverse reactions in nursing infants from Fungizone Oral Suspension, a decision should be made whether to discontinue nursing or to discontinue the drug taking into account the importance of the drug to the mother.

Pediatric Use

There has been limited study of Fungizone Oral Suspension in pediatric patients, although studies have included premature infants. Doses used have been 100 mg four times per day regardless of age. Mycological eradication of oral *Candida* in these studies has been in the range of 10 to 20%, although clinical responses are more frequent.

ADVERSE REACTIONS

Rash, gastrointestinal symptoms, including nausea, vomiting, steatorrhea, and diarrhea have been reported following administration of Fungizone Oral Suspension. Rare occurrences of urticaria, angioedema, Stevens-Johnson Syndrome and toxic epidermal necrolysis have also been reported.

DOSAGE AND ADMINISTRATION

The recommended dosage for Fungizone Oral Suspension in adults and pediatric patients is 1 mL (100 mg), four times daily. If possible, the suspension should be administered between meals to permit prolonged contact with the oral lesions.
Shake well before using. The suspension should be dropped directly on the tongue with the calibrated dropper. Patients should be directed to swish the medication in the mouth for as long as is reasonably possible before swallowing. If application by swabbing is desired, a non-absorbent swab should be used in applying medication.
The recommended duration of therapy is 2 weeks, although longer treatment may be necessary based on clinical response. Recurrence of oral candidiasis may be common depending on patient risk factors.

HOW SUPPLIED

Fungizone Oral Suspension (Amphotericin B Oral Suspension)
100 mg per mL is available in bottles of 24 mL
NDC 0087-1162-10
A dropper calibrated for 1 mL is supplied with each 24 mL bottle.
Storage
Store at controlled room temperature 15° C (59° F) to 30° C (86° F); avoid freezing. Protect from direct sunlight. Keep tightly closed.
BRISTOL-MYERS SQUIBB
Immunology
A Bristol-Myers Squibb Company
Princeton, New Jersey 08543
U.S.A.
Made in UK
Revised January 1996
51-004179-00

HYDREA® ℞
[hī-drea]
(hydroxyurea capsules, USP)

CAUTION: FEDERAL LAW PROHIBITS DISPENSING WITHOUT PRESCRIPTION.

DESCRIPTION

HYDREA® (hydroxyurea capsules, USP) is an antineoplastic agent, available for oral use as capsules providing 500 mg hydroxyurea. Inactive ingredients: citric acid, colorants (D&C Yellow No. 10, FD&C Blue No. 1, FD&C Red 40 and D&C Red 28), gelatin, lactose, magnesium stearate, sodium phosphate, and titanium dioxide.

Continued on next page

Hydrea—Cont.

Hydroxyurea occurs as an essentially tasteless, white crystalline powder. Its structural formula is:

$$H_2N-\overset{\displaystyle O}{\overset{\displaystyle \|}{C}}-NH-OH$$

ACTIONS

Mechanism of Action—The precise mechanism by which hydroxyurea produces its cytotoxic effects cannot, at present, be described. However, the reports of various studies in tissue culture in rats and man lend support to the hypothesis that hydroxyurea causes an immediate inhibition of DNA synthesis without interfering with the synthesis of ribonucleic acid or of protein. This hypothesis explains why, under certain conditions, hydroxyurea may induce teratogenic effects.

Three mechanisms of action have been postulated for the increased effectiveness of concomitant use of hydroxyurea therapy with irradiation on squamous cell (epidermoid) carcinomas of the head and neck. *In vitro* studies utilizing Chinese hamster cells suggest that hydroxyurea (1) is lethal to normally radioresistant S-stage cells, and (2) holds other cells of the cell cycle in the G1 or pre-DNA synthesis stage where they are most susceptible to the effects of irradiation. The third mechanism of action has been theorized on the basis of *in vitro* studies of HeLa cells: it appears that hydroxyurea, by inhibition of DNA synthesis, hinders the normal repair process of cells damaged but not killed by irradiation, thereby decreasing their survival rate; RNA and protein syntheses have shown no alteration.

Absorption, Metabolism, Fate and Excretion—After oral administration in man, hydroxyurea is readily absorbed from the gastrointestinal tract. The drug reaches peak serum concentrations within 2 hours; by 24 hours the concentration in the serum is essentially zero. Approximately 80 percent of an oral or intravenous dose of 7 to 30 mg/kg may be recovered in the urine within 12 hours.

Animal Pharmacology and Toxicology—The oral LD_{50} of hydroxyurea is 7330 mg/kg in mice and 5780 mg/kg in rats, given as a single dose.

In subacute and chronic toxicity studies in the rat, the most consistent pathological findings were an apparent dose-related mild to moderate bone marrow hypoplasia as well as pulmonary congestion and mottling of the lungs. At the highest dosage levels (1260 mg/kg/day for 37 days then 2520 mg/kg/day for 40 days), testicular atrophy with absence of spermatogenesis occurred; in several animals, hepatic cell damage with fatty metamorphosis was noted. In the dog, mild to marked bone marrow depression was a consistent finding except at the lower dosage levels. Additionally, at the higher dose levels (140 to 420 mg or 140 to 1260 mg/kg/week given 3 or 7 days weekly for 12 weeks), growth retardation, slightly increased blood glucose values, and hemosiderosis of the liver or spleen were found; reversible spermatogenic arrest was noted. In the monkey, bone marrow depression, lymphoid atrophy of the spleen, and degenerative changes in the epithelium of the small and large intestines were found. At the higher, often lethal, doses (400 to 800 mg/kg/day for 7 to 15 days), hemorrhage and congestion were found in the lungs, brain, and urinary tract. Cardiovascular effects (changes in heart rate, blood pressure, orthostatic hypotension, EKG changes) and hematological changes (slight hemolysis, slight methemoglobinemia) were observed in some species of laboratory animals at doses exceeding clinical levels.

INDICATIONS AND USAGE

Significant tumor response to HYDREA has been demonstrated in melanoma, resistant chronic myelocytic leukemia, and recurrent, metastatic, or inoperable carcinoma of the ovary.

Hydroxyurea used concomitantly with irradiation therapy is intended for use in the local control of primary squamous cell (epidermoid) carcinomas of the head and neck, excluding the lip.

CONTRAINDICATIONS

Hydroxyurea is contraindicated in patients with marked bone marrow depression, i.e., leukopenia (<2500 WBC) or thrombocytopenia (<100,000), or severe anemia.

WARNINGS

Treatment with hydroxyurea should not be initiated if bone marrow function is markedly depressed (see "CONTRAINDICATIONS" section). Bone marrow suppression may occur, and leukopenia is generally its first and most common manifestation. Thrombocytopenia and anemia occur less often, and are seldom seen without a preceding leukopenia. However, the recovery from myelosuppression is rapid when therapy is interrupted. It should be borne in mind that bone marrow depression is more likely in patients who have previously received radiotherapy of cytotoxic cancer chemotherapeutic agents; hydroxyurea should be used cautiously in such patients.

Patients who have received irradiation therapy in the past may have an exacerbation of postirradiation erythema.

Severe anemia must be corrected with whole blood replacement before initiating therapy with hydroxyurea.

Erythrocytic abnormalities: megaloblastic erythropoiesis, which is self-limiting, is often seen early in the course of hydroxyurea therapy. The morphologic change resembles pernicious anemia, but is not related to vitamin B12 or folic acid deficiency. Hydroxyurea may also delay plasma iron clearance and reduce the rate of iron utilization by erythrocytes, but it does not appear to alter the red blood cell survival time.

Hydroxyurea should be used with caution in patients with marked renal dysfunction.

Elderly patients may be more sensitive to the effects of hydroxyurea, and may require a lower dose regimen.

Usage in Pregnancy—Drugs which affect DNA synthesis, such as hydroxyurea, may be potential mutagenic agents. The physician should carefully consider this possibility before administering this drug to male or female patients who may contemplate conception.

Hydroxyurea is a known teratogenic agent in animals. Therefore, hydroxyurea should not be used in women who are or may become pregnant unless in the judgment of the physician the potential benefits outweigh the possible hazards.

PRECAUTIONS

Therapy with hydroxyurea requires close supervision. The complete status of the blood, including bone marrow examination, if indicated, as well as kidney function and liver function should be determined prior to, and repeatedly during, treatment. The determination of the hemoglobin level, total leukocyte counts, and platelet counts should be performed at least once a week throughout the course of hydroxyurea therapy. If the white blood cell count decreases to less than 2500/mm³, or the platelet count to less than 100,000/mm³, therapy should be interrupted until the values rise significantly toward normal levels. Anemia, if it occurs, should be managed with whole blood replacement, without interrupting hydroxyurea therapy.

Information for Patients—Patients who take the drug by emptying the contents of the capsule into water (see "DOSAGE AND ADMINISTRATION" section) should be reminded that this is a potent medication that must be handled with care. Patients must be cautioned not to allow the powder to come in contact with the skin or mucous membranes, and must be told not to inhale the powder when opening the capsules. If the powder is spilled, it should be immediately wiped up with a damp towel and disposed of, as should the empty capsules. The medication, particularly open capsules, should be kept away from children and pets.

ADVERSE REACTIONS

Adverse reactions have been primarily bone marrow depression (leukopenia, anemia, and occasionally thrombocytopenia), and less frequently gastrointestinal symptoms (stomatitis, anorexia, nausea, vomiting, diarrhea, and constipation), and dermatological reactions such as maculopapular rash, skin ulceration and facial erythema. Dysuria and alopecia occur very rarely. Large doses may produce moderate drowsiness. Neurological disturbances have occurred extremely rarely and were limited to headache, dizziness, disorientation, hallucinations, and convulsions. HYDREA (hydroxyurea capsules, USP) occasionally may cause temporary impairment of renal tubular function accompanied by elevations in serum uric acid, BUN, and creatinine levels. Abnormal BSP retention has been reported. Fever, chills, malaise, and elevation of hepatic enzymes have also been reported.

Adverse reactions observed with combined hydroxyurea and irradiation therapy are similar to those reported with the use of hydroxyurea alone. These effects primarily include bone marrow depression (anemia and leukopenia), and gastric irritation. Almost all patients receiving an adequate course of combined hydroxyurea and irradiation therapy will demonstrate concurrent leukopenia. Platelet depression (<100,000 cells/mm³) has occurred rarely and only in the presence of marked leukopenia. Gastric distress has also been reported with irradiation alone and in combination with hydroxyurea therapy.

It should be borne in mind that therapeutic doses of irradiation alone produce the same adverse reactions as hydroxyurea; combined therapy may cause an increase in the incidence and severity of these side effects.

Although inflammation of the mucous membranes at the irradiated site (mucositis) is attributed to irradiation alone, some investigators believe that the more severe cases are due to combination therapy.

The association of hydroxyurea with the development of acute pulmonary reactions consisting of diffuse pulmonary infiltrates, fever and dyspnea has been rarely reported.

DOSAGE AND ADMINISTRATION

Procedures for proper handling and disposal of antineoplastic drugs should be considered. Several guidelines on this subject have been published.[1-7] There is no general agreement that all of the procedures recommended in the guidelines are necessary or appropriate.

Because of the rarity of melanoma, resistant chronic myelocytic leukemia, carcinoma of the ovary, and carcinomas of the head and neck in children, dosage regimens have not been established.

All dosage should be based on the patient's actual or ideal weight, whichever is less.

NOTE: If the patient prefers, or is unable to swallow capsules, the contents of the capsules may be emptied into a glass of water and taken immediately. (See "PRECAUTIONS: Information for Patients" section.) Some inert material used as a vehicle in the capsule may not dissolve, and may float on the surface.

SOLID TUMORS

Intermittent Therapy—80 mg/kg administered orally as a *single* dose every *third* day.

Continuous Therapy—20 to 30 mg/kg administered orally as a *single* dose *daily*. The intermittent dosage schedule offers the advantage of reduced toxicity since patients on this dosage regimen have rarely required complete discontinuance of therapy because of toxicity.

Concomitant Therapy with Irradiation *Carcinoma of the head and neck*—80 mg/kg administered orally as a *single* dose every *third* day.

Administration of hydroxyurea should be begun at least seven days before initiation of irradiation and continued during radiotherapy as well as indefinitely afterwards provided that the patient may be kept under adequate observation and evidences no unusual or severe reactions.

Irradiation should be given at the maximum dose considered appropriate for the particular therapeutic situation; adjustment of irradiation dosage is not usually necessary when hydroxyurea is used concomitantly.

RESISTANT CHRONIC MYELOCYTIC LEUKEMIA

Until the intermittent therapy regimen has been evaluated, CONTINUOUS therapy (20 to 30 mg/kg administered orally as a *single dose daily*) is recommended.

An adequate trial period for determining the antineoplastic effectiveness of hydroxyurea is six weeks of therapy. When there is regression in tumor size or arrest in tumor growth, therapy should be continued indefinitely. Therapy should be interrupted if the white blood cell count drops below 2500/mm³ or the platelet count below 100,000/mm³. In these cases, the counts should be rechecked after three days, and therapy resumed when the counts rise significantly toward normal values. Since the hematopoietic rebound is prompt, it is usually necessary to omit only a few doses. If prompt rebound has not occurred during combined HYDREA and irradiation therapy, irradiation may also be interrupted. However, the need for postponement of irradiation has been rare; radiotherapy has usually been continued using the recommended dosage and technique. Anemia, if it occurs, should be corrected with whole blood replacement, without interrupting hydroxyurea therapy. Because hematopoiesis may be compromised by extensive irradiation or by other antineoplastic agents, it is recommended that hydroxyurea be administered cautiously to patients who have recently received extensive radiation therapy or chemotherapy with other cytotoxic drugs.

Pain or discomfort from inflammation of the mucous membranes at the irradiated site (mucositis) is usually controlled by measures such as topical anesthetics and orally administered analgesics. If the reaction is severe, hydroxyurea therapy may be temporarily interrupted; if it is extremely severe, irradiation dosage may, in addition, be temporarily postponed. However, it has rarely been necessary to terminate these therapies.

Severe gastric distress, such as nausea, vomiting, and anorexia, resulting from combined therapy may usually be controlled by temporary interruption of hydroxyurea administration; rarely has the additional interruption of irradiation been necessary.

HOW SUPPLIED

HYDREA® (hydroxyurea capsules, USP)

500 mg capsules in bottles of 100 (**NDC** 0003-0830-50).

Capsule identification number: 830.

Storage: Store at room temperature; avoid excessive heat. Keep tightly closed.

REFERENCES:

1. Recommendations for the Safe Handling of Parenteral Antineoplastic Drugs. NIH Publication No. 83-2621. For sale by the Superintendent of Documents, US Government Printing Office, Washington, DC 20402.
2. AMA Council Report. Guidelines for Handling Parenteral Antineoplastics. JAMA 1985; 253(11):1590-1592.
3. National Study Commission on Cytotoxic Exposure — Recommendations for Handling Cytotoxic Agents. Available from Louis P. Jeffrey, ScD, Chairman, National Study Commission on Cytotoxic Exposure, Massachusetts College of Pharmacy and Allied Health Sciences, 179 Longwood Avenue, Boston, MA 02115.

4. Clinical Oncological Society of Australia. Guidelines and Recommendations for Safe Handling of Antineoplastic Agents. Med J Australia 1983; 1:426-428.
5. Jones RB, et al. Safe Handling of Chemotherapeutic Agents: A Report from the Mount Sinai Medical Center, CA-A Cancer Journal for Clinicians 1983; (Sept/Oct) 258-263.
6. American Society of Hospital Pharmacists Technical Assistance Bulletin on Handling Cytotoxic and Hazardous Drugs. Am J Hosp Pharm 1990; 47:1033-1049.
7. OSHA Work-Practice Guidelines for Personnel Dealing with Cytotoxic (Antineoplastic) Drugs. Am J Hosp Pharm 1986; 43:1193-1204.

BRISTOL LABORATORIES®
ONCOLOGY PRODUCTS
A Bristol-Myers Squibb Company
Princeton, NJ 08543
U.S.A.
K8-B001-5-96 P9281-02
Revised: March 1996

IFEX® ℞

[*i-fĕx*]
(ifosfamide for injection)

CAUTION: FEDERAL LAW PROHIBITS DISPENSING WITHOUT PRESCRIPTION.

WARNING
IFEX® (ifosfamide for injection) should be administered under the supervision of a qualified physician experienced in the use of cancer chemotherapeutic agents. Urotoxic side effects, especially hemorrhagic cystitis, as well as CNS toxicities such as confusion and coma have been associated with the use of IFEX. When they occur, they may require cessation of IFEX therapy. Severe myelosuppression has been reported. (See **"ADVERSE REACTIONS"** section.)

DESCRIPTION

IFEX® (ifosfamide for injection) single-dose vials for constitution and administration by intravenous infusion each contain 1 gram or 3 grams of sterile ifosfamide. Ifosfamide is a chemotherapeutic agent chemically related to the nitrogen mustards and a synthetic analog of cyclophosphamide. Ifosfamide is 3-(2-chloroethyl)-2-[(2-chloroethyl)amino]tetrahydro-2H-1,3,2-oxazaphosphorine 2-oxide. The molecular formula is $C_7H_{15}Cl_2N_2O_2P$ and its molecular weight is 261.1. Its structural formula is:

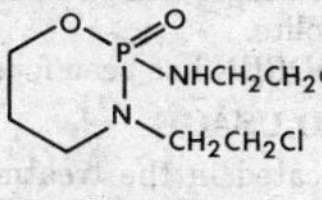

Ifosfamide is a white crystalline powder that is soluble in water.

CLINICAL PHARMACOLOGY

Ifosfamide has been shown to require metabolic activation by microsomal liver enzymes to produce biologically active metabolites. Activation occurs by hydroxylation at the ring carbon atom 4 to form the unstable intermediate 4-hydroxyifosfamide. This metabolite rapidly degrades to the stable urinary metabolite 4-ketoifosfamide. Opening of the ring results in formation of the stable urinary metabolite, 4-carboxyifosfamide. These urinary metabolites have not been found to be cytotoxic. N, N-*bis*(2-chloroethyl)-phosphoric acid diamide (ifosphoramide) and acrolein are also found. Enzymatic oxidation of the chloroethyl side chains and subsequent dealkylation produces the major urinary metabolites, dechloroethyl ifosfamide and dechloroethyl cyclophosphamide. The alkylated metabolites of ifosfamide have been shown to interact with DNA.
In vitro incubation of DNA with activated ifosfamide has produced phosphotriesters. The treatment of intact cell nuclei may also result in the formation of DNA-DNA cross-links. DNA repair most likely occurs in G-1 and G-2 stage cells.

Pharmacokinetics: Ifosfamide exhibits dose-dependent pharmacokinetics in humans. At single doses of 3.8–5.0 g/m^2, the plasma concentrations decay biphasically and the mean terminal elimination half-life is about 15 hours. At doses of 1.6–2.4 g/m^2/day, the plasma decay is monoexponential and the terminal elimination half-life is about 7 hours. Ifosfamide is extensively metabolized in humans and the metabolic pathways appear to be saturated at high doses.
After administration of doses of 5 g/m^2 of ^{14}C-labeled ifosfamide, from 70 to 86% of the dosed radioactivity was recovered in the urine, with about 61% of the dose excreted as parent compound. At doses of 1.6–2.4 g/m^2 only 12 to 18% of the dose was excreted in the urine as unchanged drug within 72 hours.

Adverse Reaction	*Incidence (%)	Adverse Reaction	*Incidence (%)
Alopecia	83	Coagulopathy	< 1
Nausea-Vomiting	58	Constipation	< 1
Hematuria	46	Dermatitis	< 1
Gross Hematuria	12	Diarrhea	< 1
CNS Toxicity	12	Fatigue	< 1
Infection	8	Hypertension	< 1
Renal Impairment	6	Hypotension	< 1
Liver Dysfunction	3	Malaise	< 1
Plebitis	2	Polyneuropathy	< 1
Fever	1	Pulmonary Symptoms	< 1
Allergic Reaction	< 1	Salivation	< 1
Anorexia	< 1	Stomatitis	< 1
Cardiotoxicity	< 1		

*Based upon 2,070 patients from the published literature in 30 single agent studies.

Two different dechloroethylated derivatives of ifosfamide, 4-carboxyifosfamide, thiodiacetic acid and cysteine conjugates of chloroacetic acid have been identified as the major urinary metabolites of ifosfamide in humans and only small amounts of 4-hydroxy ifosfamide and acrolein are present. Small quantities (nmole/mL) of ifosfamide mustard and 4-hydroxyifosfamide are detectable in human plasma. Metabolism of ifosfamide is required for the generation of the biologically active species and while metabolism is extensive, it is also quite variable among patients.
In a study at Indiana University, 50 fully evaluable patients with germ cell testicular cancer were treated with IFEX in combination with cisplatin and either vinblastine or etoposide after failing (47 of 50 patients) at least two prior chemotherapy regimens consisting of cisplatin/vinblastine/bleomycin, (PVB), cisplatin/vinblastine/actinomycin D/bleomycin/cyclophosphamide, (VAB6), or the combination of cisplatin and etoposide. Patients were selected for remaining cisplatin sensitivity because they had previously responded to a cisplatin containing regimen and had not progressed while on the cisplatin containing regimen or within 3 weeks of stopping it. Patients served as their own control based on the premise that long term complete responses could not be achieved by retreatment with a regimen to which they had previously responded and subsequently relapsed.
Ten of 50 fully evaluable patients were still alive 2 to 5 years after treatment. Four of the 10 long term survivors were rendered free of cancer by surgical resection after treatment with the ifosfamide regimen; median survival for the entire group of 50 fully evaluable patients was 53 weeks.

INDICATION AND USAGE

IFEX, used in combination with certain other approved antineoplastic agents, is indicated for third line chemotherapy of germ cell testicular cancer. It should ordinarily be used in combination with a prophylactic agent for hemorrhagic cystitis, such as mesna.

CONTRAINDICATIONS

Continued use of IFEX is contraindicated in patients with severely depressed bone marrow function (See **"WARNINGS"** and **"PRECAUTIONS"** sections.) IFEX is also contraindicated in patients who have demonstrated a previous hypersensitivity to it.

WARNINGS

Urinary System: Urotoxic side effects, especially hemorrhagic cystitis, have been frequently associated with the use of IFEX. It is recommended that a urinalysis should be obtained prior to each dose of IFEX. If microscopic hematuria (greater than 10 RBCs per high power field), is present, then subsequent administration should be withheld until complete resolution.
Further administration of IFEX should be given with vigorous oral or parenteral hydration.

Hematopoietic System: When IFEX is given in combination with other chemotherapeutic agents, severe myelosuppression is frequently observed. Close hematologic monitoring is recommended. White blood cell (WBC) count, platelet count and hemoglobin should be obtained prior to each administration and at appropriate intervals. Unless clinically essential, IFEX should not be given to patients with a WBC count below 2000/µL and/or a platelet count below 50,000/µL.

Central Nervous System: Neurologic manifestations consisting of somnolence, confusion, hallucinations and in some instances, coma, have been reported following IFEX (ifosfamide for injection) therapy. The occurrence of these symptoms requires discontinuing IFEX therapy. The symptoms have usually been reversible and supportive therapy should be maintained until their complete resolution.

Pregnancy: Animal studies indicate that the drug is capable of causing gene mutations and chromosomal damage *in vivo*. Embryotoxic and teratogenic effects have been observed in mice, rats and rabbits at doses 0.05 to 0.075 times the human dose. Ifosfamide can cause fetal damage when administered to a pregnant woman. If IFEX is used during pregnancy, or if the patient becomes pregnant while taking this drug, the patient should be apprised of the potential hazard to the fetus.

PRECAUTIONS

General: IFEX should be given cautiously to patients with impaired renal function as well as to those with compromised bone marrow reserve, as indicated by: leukopenia, granulocytopenia, extensive bone marrow metastases, prior radiation therapy, or prior therapy with other cytotoxic agents.

Laboratory Tests: During treatment, the patient's hematologic profile (particularly neutrophils and platelets) should be monitored regularly to determine the degree of hematopoietic suppression. Urine should also be examined regularly for red cells which may precede hemorrhagic cystitis.

Drug Interactions: The physician should be alert for possible combined drug actions, desirable or undesirable, involving ifosfamide even though ifosfamide has been used successfully concurrently with other drugs, including other cytotoxic drugs.

Wound Healing: Ifosfamide may interfere with normal wound healing.

Pregnancy: Pregnancy "Category D". (See **"WARNINGS"** section.)

Nursing Mothers: Ifosfamide is excreted in breast milk. Because of the potential for serious adverse events and the tumorigenicity shown for ifosfamide in animal studies, a decision should be made whether to discontinue nursing or to discontinue the drug, taking into account the importance of the drug to the mother.

Carcinogenesis, Mutagenesis, Impairment of Fertility: Ifosfamide has been shown to be carcinogenic in rats, with female rats showing a significant incidence of leiomyosarcomas and mammary fibroadenomas.
The mutagenic potential of ifosfamide has been documented in bacterial systems *in vitro* and mammalian cells *in vivo*. *In vivo*, ifosfamide has induced mutagenic effects in mice and *Drosophila melanogaster* germ cells, and has induced a significant increase in dominant lethal mutations in male mice as well as recessive sex-linked lethal mutations in *Drosophila*.
In pregnant mice, resorptions increased and anomalies were present at day 19 after a 30 mg/m^2 dose of ifosfamide was administered on day 11 of gestation. Embryolethal effects were observed in rats following the administration of 54 mg/m^2 doses of ifosfamide from the 6th through the 15th day of gestation and embryotoxic effects were apparent after dams received 18 mg/m^2 doses over the same dosing period. Ifosfamide is embryotoxic to rabbits receiving 88 mg/m^2/day doses from the 6th through the 18th day after mating. The number of anomalies was also significantly increased over the control group.

Pediatric Use: Safety and effectiveness in pediatric patients have not been established.

ADVERSE REACTIONS

In patients receiving IFEX as a single agent, the dose-limiting toxicities are myelosuppression and urotoxicity. Dose fractionation, vigorous hydration, and a protector such as mesna can significantly reduce the incidence of hematuria, especially gross hematuria, associated with hemorrhagic cystitis. At a dose of 1.2 g/m^2 daily for 5 consecutive days, leukopenia, when it occurs, is usually mild to moderate. Other significant side effects include alopecia, nausea, vomiting, and central nervous system toxicities.
[See table above]

Hematologic Toxicity: Myelosuppression was dose related and dose limiting. It consisted mainly of leukopenia and, to a lesser extent, thrombocytopenia. A WBC count < 3000/µL is expected in 50% of the patients treated with IFEX single agent at doses of 1.2 g/m^2 per day for 5 consecutive days. At this dose level, thrombocytopenia (platelets < 100,000/µL) occurred in about 20% of the patients. At higher dosages, leukopenia was almost universal, and at total dosages of 10–12 g/m^2/cycle, one half of the patients had a WBC count below 1000/µL and 8% of patients had platelet counts less

Continued on next page

Ifex—Cont.

than 50,000/μL. Myelosuppression was usually reversible and treatment can be given every 3 to 4 weeks. When IFEX is used in combination with other myelosuppressive agents, adjustments in dosing may be necessary. Patients who experience severe myelosuppression are potentially at increased risk for infection.

Digestive System: Nausea and vomiting occurred in 58% of the patients who received IFEX. They were usually controlled by standard antiemetic therapy. Other gastrointestinal side effects include anorexia, diarrhea, and in some cases, constipation.

Urinary System: Urotoxicity consisted of hemorrhagic cystitis, dysuria, urinary frequency and other symptoms of bladder irritation. Hematuria occurred in 6% to 92% of patients treated with IFEX. The incidence and severity of hematuria can be significantly reduced by using vigorous hydration, a fractionated dose schedule and a protector such as mesna. At daily doses of 1.2 g/m^2 for 5 consecutive days without a protector, microscopic hematuria is expected in about one half of the patients and gross hematuria in about 8% of patients.

Renal toxicity occurred in 6% of the patients treated with ifosfamide as a single agent. Clinical signs, such as elevation in BUN or serum creatinine or decrease in creatinine clearance, were usually transient. They were most likely to be related to tubular damage. One episode of renal tubular acidosis which progressed into chronic renal failure was reported. Proteinuria and acidosis also occurred in rare instances. Metabolic acidosis was reported in 31% of patients in one study when IFEX was administered at doses of 2.0 to 2.5 g/m^2/day for 4 days. Renal tubular acidosis, Fanconi syndrome and renal rickets have been reported. Close clinical monitoring of serum and urine chemistries including phosphorus, potassium, alkaline phosphatase and other appropriate laboratory studies is recommended. Appropriate replacement therapy should be administered as indicated.

Central Nervous System: CNS side effects were observed in 12% of patients treated with IFEX. Those most commonly seen were somnolence, confusion, depressive psychosis, and hallucinations. Other less frequent symptoms include dizziness, disorientation, and cranial nerve dysfunction. Seizures and coma with death were occasionally reported. The incidence of CNS toxicity may be higher in patients with altered renal function.

Other: Alopecia occurred in approximately 83% of the patients treated with IFEX (ifosfamide for injection) as a single agent. In combination, this incidence may be as high as 100%, depending on the other agents included in the chemotherapy regimen. Increases in liver enzymes and/or bilirubin were noted in 3% of the patients. Other less frequent side effects included phlebitis, pulmonary symptoms, fever of unknown origin, allergic reactions, stomatitis, cardiotoxicity, and polyneuropathy.

OVERDOSAGE

No specific antidote for IFEX is known. Management of overdosage would include general supportive measures to sustain the patient through any period of toxicity that might occur.

DOSAGE AND ADMINISTRATION

IFEX should be administered intravenously at a dose of 1.2 g/m^2 per day for 5 consecutive days. Treatment is repeated every 3 weeks or after recovery from hematologic toxicity (Platelets ≥ 100,000/μL, WBC ≥ 4,000/μL). In order to prevent bladder toxicity, IFEX should be given with extensive hydration consisting of at least 2 liters of oral or intravenous fluid per day. A protector, such as mesna, should also be used to prevent hemorrhagic cystitis. IFEX should be administered as a slow intravenous infusion lasting a minimum of 30 minutes. Although IFEX has been administered to a small number of patients with compromised hepatic and/or renal function, studies to establish optimal dose schedules of IFEX in such patients have not been conducted.

Preparation for Intravenous Administration/Stability: Injections are prepared for parenteral use by adding *Sterile Water for Injection, USP*, or *Bacteriostatic Water for Injection, USP* (benzyl alcohol or parabens preserved), to the vial and shaking to dissolve. Use the quantity of diluent shown below to constitute the product:

Dosage Strength	Quantity of Diluent	Final Concentration
1 gram	20 mL	50 mg/mL
3 grams	60 mL	50 mg/mL

Solutions of ifosfamide may be diluted further to achieve concentrations of 0.6 to 20 mg/mL in the following fluids:

5% Dextrose Injection, USP
0.9% Sodium Chloride Injection, USP
Lactated Ringer's Injection, USP
Sterile Water for Injection, USP

Because essentially identical stability results were obtained for Sterile Water admixtures as for the other admixtures (5% Dextrose Injection, 0.9% Sodium Chloride Injection, and Lactated Ringer's Injection), the use of large volume parenteral glass bottles, Viaflex bags or PAB™ bags that contain intermediate concentrations or mixtures of excipients (eg, 2.5% Dextrose Injection, 0.45% Sodium Chloride Injection, or 5% Dextrose and 0.9% Sodium Chloride Injection) is also acceptable.

Constituted or constituted and further diluted solutions of IFEX should be refrigerated and used within 24 hours.

Parenteral drug products should be inspected visually for particulate matter and discoloration prior to administration.

HOW SUPPLIED

IFEX® (ifosfamide for injection) is only available in combination packages with the uroprotective agent Mesnex® (mesna) Injection.

IFEX (ifosamide for injection)/MESNEX® (mesna) Injection.

NDC 0015-3556-26 – 5 × 1-gram Single Dose Vial of IFEX – 3 × 1-gram Multidose Vial of MESNEX

NDC 0015-3554-27 – 10 × 1-gram Single Dose Vial of IFEX – 10 × 1-gram Multidose Vial of MESNEX

NDC 0015-3564-15 – 2 × 3-gram Single Dose Vial of IFEX – 6 × 1-gram Multidose Vial of MESNEX

Store at controlled room temperature 20°C to 25°C (68°F to 77°F). Protect from temperatures above 30°C (86°F).

Procedures for proper handling and disposal of anticancer drugs should be considered. Skin reactions associated with accidental exposure to IFEX may occur. The use of gloves is recommended. If IFEX solution contacts the skin or mucosa, immediately wash the skin thoroughly with soap and water or rinse the mucosa with copious amounts of water. Several guidelines on this subject have been published.[1–7] There is no general agreement that all of the procedures recommended in the guidelines are necessary or appropriate.

REFERENCES

1. Recommendations for the Safe Handling of Parenteral Antineoplastic Drugs. NIH Publication No. 83-2621. For sale by the Superintendent of Documents, US Government Printing Office, Washington, DC 20402.
2. AMA Council Report. Guidelines for Handling Parenteral Antineoplastics. JAMA 1985; 253 (11):1590-1592.
3. National Study Commission on Cytotoxic Exposure-Recommendations for Handling Cytotoxic Agents. Available from Louis P. Jeffrey, ScD, Chairman, National Study Commission on Cytotoxic Exposure, Massachusetts College of Pharmacy and Allied Health Sciences, 179 Longwood Avenue, Boston, Massachusetts 02115.
4. Clinical Oncological Society of Australia. Guidelines and Recommendations for Safe Handling of Antineoplastic Agents. Med J Australia 1983; 1:426-428.
5. Jones, RB, et al: Safe Handling of Chemotherapeutic Agents: A Report from the Mount Sinai Medical Center. CA-A Cancer Journal for Clinicians 1983; (Sept/Oct)258-263.
6. American Society of Hospital Pharmacists Technical Assistance Bulletin on Handling Cytotoxic and Hazardous Drugs. Am J Hosp Pharm 1990; 47:1033-1049.
7. Controlling occupational exposure to hazardous drugs. (OSHA WORK PRACTICE GUIDELINES). Am J Health Syst-Pharm 1996; 53:1669-1685.

Distributed by:
MeadJohnson
ONCOLOGY PRODUCTS
A Bristol-Myers Squibb Company
Princeton, NJ 08543
U.S.A.

Manufactured by:
ASTA MEDICA
A Degussa Company
Frankfurt am Mein
Germany

H5-B001-3-97 N0054-00
51-006149-00 Revised: February 1997

Shown in Product Identification Guide, page 308

LYSODREN® ℞ ONLY

[*lī-so'dren*]
(mitotane tablets, USP)

WARNINGS

LYSODREN® (mitotane tablets, USP) should be administered under the supervision of a qualified physician experienced in the uses of cancer chemotherapeutic agents. LYSODREN should be temporarily discontinued immediately following shock or severe trauma since adrenal suppression is its prime action. Exogenous steroids should be administered in such circumstances, since the depressed adrenal may not immediately start to secrete steroids.

DESCRIPTION

LYSODREN® (mitotane tablets, USP) is an oral chemotherapeutic agent. It is best known by its trivial name, o,p'-DDD, and is chemically, 1,1-dichloro-2-(o-chlorophenyl)-2-(p-chlorophenyl) ethane. The chemical structure is shown below.

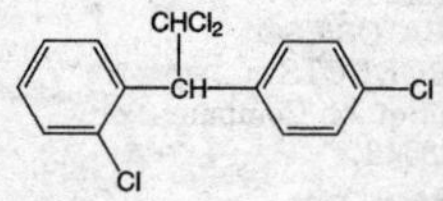

LYSODREN is a white granular solid composed of clear colorless crystals. It is tasteless and has a slight pleasant aromatic odor. It is soluble in ethanol, isoctane and carbon tetrachloride. It has a molecular weight of 320.05.

Inactive ingredients in LYSODREN tablets are: avicel, Polyethylene Glycol 3350, silicon dioxide, and starch.

LYSODREN is available as 500 mg scored tablets for oral administration.

CLINICAL PHARMACOLOGY

LYSODREN can best be described as an adrenal cytotoxic agent, although it can cause adrenal inhibition, apparently without cellular destruction. Its biochemical mechanism of action is unknown. Data are available to suggest that the drug modifies the peripheral metabolism of steroids as well as directly suppressing the adrenal cortex. The administration of LYSODREN alters the extra-adrenal metabolism of cortisol in man; leading to a reduction in measurable 17-hydroxy corticosteroids, even though plasma levels of corticosteroids do not fall. The drug apparently causes increased formation of 6-B-hydroxyl cortisol.

Data in adrenal carcinoma patients indicate that about 40% of oral LYSODREN is absorbed and approximately 10% of administered dose is recovered in the urine as a water-soluble metabolite. A variable amount of metabolite (1 to 17%) is excreted in the bile and the balance is apparently stored in the tissues.

Following discontinuation of LYSODREN, the plasma terminal half-life has ranged from 18 to 159 days. In most patients blood levels become undetectable after 6 to 9 weeks. Autopsy data have provided evidence that LYSODREN is found in most tissues of the body; however, fat tissues are the primary site of storage. LYSODREN is converted to a water-soluble metabolite.

No unchanged LYSODREN has been found in urine or bile.

INDICATIONS AND USAGE

LYSODREN is indicated in the treatment of inoperable adrenal cortical carcinoma of both functional and nonfunctional types.

CONTRAINDICATIONS

LYSODREN should not be given to individuals who have demonstrated a previous hypersensitivity to it.

WARNINGS

LYSODREN should be temporarily discontinued immediately following shock or severe trauma, since adrenal suppression is its prime action. Exogenous steroids should be administered in such circumstances, since the depressed adrenal may not immediately start to secrete steroids.

LYSODREN should be administered with care to patients with liver disease other than metastatic lesions from the adrenal cortex, since the metabolism of LYSODREN may be interfered with and the drug may accumulate.

All possible tumor tissues should be surgically removed from large metastatic masses before LYSODREN administration is instituted. This is necessary to minimize the possibility of infarction and hemorrhage in the tumor due to a rapid cytotoxic effect of the drug.

Long-term continuous administration of high doses of LYSODREN may lead to brain damage and impairment of function. Behavioral and neurological assessments should be made at regular intervals when continuous LYSODREN treatment exceeds 2 years.

A substantial percentage of the patients treated show signs of adrenal insufficiency. It therefore appears necessary to watch for and institute steroid replacement in those patients. However, some investigators have recommended that steroid replacement therapy be administered concomitantly with LYSODREN. It has been shown that the metabolism of exogenous steroids is modified and consequently somewhat higher doses than normal replacement therapy may be required.

PRECAUTIONS

General: Adrenal insufficiency may develop in patients treated with LYSODREN (mitotane tablets, USP), and

adrenal steroid replacement should be considered for these patients.

Since sedation, lethargy, vertigo, and other CNS side effects can occur, ambulatory patients should be cautioned about driving, operating machinery, and other hazardous pursuits requiring mental and physical alertness.

Drug Interactions: LYSODREN has been reported to accelerate the metabolism of warfarin by the mechanism of hepatic microsomal enzyme induction, leading to an increase in dosage requirements for warfarin. Therefore, physicians should closely monitor patients for a change in anticoagulant dosage requirements when administering LYSODREN to patients on coumarin-type anticoagulants. In addition, LYSODREN should be given with caution to patients receiving other drugs susceptible to the influence of hepatic enzyme induction.

Carcinogenesis, Mutagenesis, Impairment of Fertility: The carcinogenic and mutagenic potentials of LYSODREN are unknown. However, the mechanism of action of this compound suggests that it probably has less carcinogenic potential than other cytotoxic chemotherapeutic drugs.

Pregnancy: Pregnancy "Category C". Animal reproduction studies have not been conducted with LYSODREN. It is also not known whether LYSODREN can cause fetal harm when administered to a pregnant woman or can affect reproduction capacity. LYSODREN should be given to a pregnant woman only if clearly needed.

Nursing Mothers: It is not known whether this drug is excreted in human milk. Because many drugs are excreted in human milk and because of the potential for adverse reactions in nursing infants from mitotane, a decision should be made whether to discontinue nursing or to discontinue the drug, taking into account the importance of the drug to the mother.

Pediatric Use: Safety and effectiveness in pediatric patients have not been established.

ADVERSE REACTIONS

A very high percentage of patients treated with LYSODREN have shown at least one type of side effect. The main types of adverse reactions consist of the following:

1. Gastrointestinal disturbances, which consist of anorexia, nausea or vomiting, and in some cases diarrhea, occur in about 80% of the patients.
2. Central nervous system side effects occur in 40% of the patients. These consist primarily of depression as manifested by lethargy and somnolence (25%), and dizziness or vertigo (15%).
3. Skin toxicity has been observed in about 15% of the cases. These skin changes consist primarily of transient skin rashes which do not seem to be dose related. In some instances, this side effect subsided while the patients were maintained on the drug without a change of dose.

Infrequently occurring side effects involve the eye (visual blurring, diplopia, lens opacity, toxic retinopathy); the genitourinary system (hematuria, hemorrhagic cystitis, and albuminuria); cardiovascular system (hypertension, orthostatic hypotension, and flushing); and some miscellaneous effects including generalized aching, hyperpyrexia, and lowered protein bound iodine (PBI).

OVERDOSAGE

No proven antidotes have been established for LYSODREN overdosage.

DOSAGE AND ADMINISTRATION

The recommended treatment schedule is to start the patient at 2 to 6 g of LYSODREN per day in divided doses, either three or four times a day. Doses are usually increased incrementally to 9 to 10 g per day. If severe side effects appear, the dose should be reduced until the maximum tolerated dose is achieved. If the patient can tolerate higher doses and improved clinical response appears possible, the dose should be increased until adverse reactions interfere. Experience has shown that the maximum tolerated dose (MTD) will vary from 2 to 16 g per day, but has usually been 9 to 10 g per day. The highest doses used in the studies to date were 18 to 19 g per day.

Treatment should be instituted in the hospital until a stable dosage regimen is achieved.

Treatment should be continued as long as clinical benefits are observed. Maintenance of clinical status or slowing of growth of metastatic lesions can be considered clinical benefits if they can clearly be shown to have occurred.

If no clinical benefits are observed after 3 months at the maximum tolerated dose, the case would generally be considered a clinical failure. However, 10% of the patients who showed a measurable response required more than 3 months at the MTD. Early diagnosis and prompt institution of treatment improve the probability of a positive clinical response. Clinical effectiveness can be shown by reduction in tumor mass; reduction in pain, weakness or anorexia; and reduction of symptoms and signs due to excessive steroid production.

A number of patients have been treated intermittently with treatment being restarted when severe symptoms have reappeared. Patients often do not respond after the third or fourth such course. Experience accumulated to date suggests that continuous treatment with the maximum possible dosage of LYSODREN is the best approach.

Procedures for proper handling and disposal of anticancer drugs should be considered. Several guidelines on this subject have been published.[1-7] There is no general agreement that all of the procedures recommended in the guidelines are necessary or appropriate.

HOW SUPPLIED

LYSODREN® (mitotane tablets, USP)

NDC 0015-3080-60–500 mg Tablets, bottle of 100

STORAGE

Tablets may be stored at room temperature.

REFERENCES

1. Recommendations for the Safe Handling of Parenteral Antineoplastic Drugs. NIH Publication No. 83-2621. For sale by the Superintendent of Documents, US Government Printing Office, Washington, DC 20402.
2. AMA Council Report. Guidelines for Handling Parenteral Antineoplastics. JAMA 1985; 253(11) 1590–1592.
3. National Study Commission on Cytotoxic Exposure—Recommendations for Handling Cytotoxic Agents. Available from Louis P. Jeffrey, ScD, Chairman, National Study Commission on Cytotoxic Exposure, Massachusetts College of Pharmacy and Allied Health Sciences, 179 Longwood Avenue, Boston, Massachusetts 02115.
4. Clinical Oncological Society of Australia. Guidelines and Recommendations for Safe Handling of Antineoplastic Agents. Med J Australia 1983; 1:426–428.
5. Jones, RB, et al: Safe Handling of Chemotherapeutic Agents: A Report from the Mount Sinai Medical Center. CA-A Cancer Journal for Clinicians 1983; (Sept/Oct) 258–263.
6. American Society of Hospital Pharmacists Technical Assistance Bulletin on Handling Cytotoxic Drugs in Hospitals. Am J Hosp Pharm 1990; 47:1033–1049.
7. OSHA Work-Practice Guidelines for Personnel Dealing with Cytotoxic (Antineoplastic) Drugs. Am J Hosp Pharm 1986; 43:1193–1204.

Manufactured by: Anabolic, Inc.
Irvine, California 92614

Distributed by:
BRISTOL LABORATORIES
ONCOLOGY PRODUCTS
A Bristol-Myers Squibb Company
Princeton, NJ 08543
U.S.A.

H6-B001-5-98 P5260-08
51-004805-02 Revised January 1998

MEGACE® ORAL SUSPENSION ℞ ONLY

[mĕg ′ace]
(megestrol acetate)

> **WARNING**
> **THE USE OF MEGACE® (megestrol acetate) Oral Suspension IS CONTRAINDICATED IN PREGNANCY.**
> Progestational agents have been used beginning with the first trimester of pregnancy in an attempt to prevent habitual abortion. There is no evidence that the use of a high dose progestational agent such as MEGACE Oral Suspension during any phase of pregnancy is effective for this purpose. Furthermore, in the vast majority of women, the cause of abortion is a defective ovum, which progestational agents could not be expected to influence. In addition, the use of progestational agents, with their uterine-relaxant properties, in patients with fertilized defective ova may cause a delay in spontaneous abortion.
> Several reports suggest an association between intrauterine exposure to progestational drugs in the first trimester of pregnancy and genital abnormalities in male and female fetuses. The risk of hypospadias, 5 to 8 per 1,000 male births in the general population, may be approximately doubled with exposure to these drugs. There are insufficient data to quantify the risk to exposed female fetuses. Because of increased genital abnormalities in male and female fetuses induced by some progestational drugs, it is prudent to avoid the use of MEGACE Oral Suspension during pregnancy.
> If the patient is exposed to MEGACE Oral Suspension during pregnancy or if she becomes pregnant while taking this drug, she should be apprised of the potential risks to the fetus.

DESCRIPTION

MEGACE® (megestrol acetate) Oral Suspension contains megestrol acetate, a synthetic derivative of the naturally occurring steroid hormone, progesterone. Megestrol acetate is a white, crystalline solid chemically designated as 17α-(acetyloxy)-6-methylpregna-4,6-diene-3,20-dione. Solubility at 37°C in water is 2 μg per mL, solubility in plasma is 24 μg per mL. Its molecular weight is 384.51.

The empirical formula is $C_{24}H_{32}O_4$ and the structural formula is represented as follows:

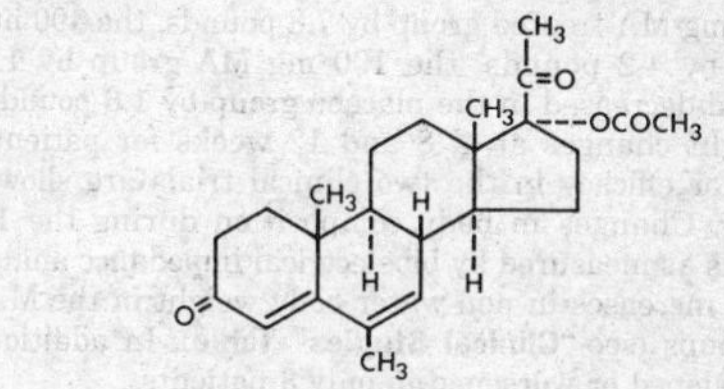

MEGACE Oral Suspension is supplied as an oral suspension containing 40 mg of micronized megestrol acetate per mL.

MEGACE Oral Suspension contains the following inactive ingredients: alcohol (max. 0.06% v/v from flavor), citric acid, lemon-lime flavor, polyethylene glycol, polysorbate 80, purified water, sodium benzoate, sodium citrate, sucrose and xanthan gum.

CLINICAL PHARMACOLOGY

Several investigators have reported on the appetite enhancing property of megestrol acetate and its possible use in cachexia. The precise mechanism by which megestrol acetate produces effects in anorexia and cachexia is unknown at the present time.

There are several analytical methods used to estimate megestrol acetate plasma concentrations, including gas chromatography-mass fragmentography (GC-MF), high pressure liquid chromatography (HPLC) and radioimmunoassay (RIA). The GC-MF and HPLC methods are specific for megestrol acetate and yield equivalent concentrations. The RIA method reacts to megestrol acetate metabolites and is, therefore, non-specific and indicates higher concentrations than the GC-MF and HPLC methods. Plasma concentrations are dependent, not only on the method used, but also on intestinal and hepatic inactivation of the drug, which may be affected by factors such as intestinal tract motility, intestinal bacteria, antibiotics administered, body weight, diet and liver function.

The major route of drug elimination in humans is urine. When radiolabeled megestrol acetate was administered to humans in doses of 4 to 90 mg, the urinary excretion within 10 days ranged from 56.5 to 78.4% (mean 66.4%) and fecal excretion ranged from 7.7 to 30.3% (mean 19.8%). The total recovered radioactivity varied between 83.1 and 94.7% (mean 86.2%). Megestrol acetate metabolites which were identified in urine constituted 5 to 8% of the dose administered. Respiratory excretion as labeled carbon dioxide and fat storage may have accounted for at least part of the radioactivity not found in urine and feces.

Plasma steady state pharmacokinetics of megestrol acetate were evaluated in 10 adult, cachectic male patients with acquired immunodeficiency syndrome (AIDS) and an involuntary weight loss greater than 10% of baseline. Patients received single oral doses of 800 mg/day of MEGACE Oral Suspension for 21 days. Plasma concentration data obtained on day 21 were evaluated for up to 48 hours past the last dose.

Mean (±1SD) peak plasma concentration (C_{max}) of megestrol acetate was 753 (±539) ng/mL. Mean area under the concentration time-curve (AUC) was 10476 (±7788) ng x hr/mL. Median T_{max} value was five hours. Seven of 10 patients gained weight in three weeks.

Additionally, 24 adult, asymptomatic HIV seropositive male subjects were dosed once daily with 750 mg of MEGACE Oral Suspension. The treatment was administered for 14 days. Mean C_{max} and AUC values 490 (±238) ng/mL and 6779 (±3048) hr × ng/mL, respectively. The median T_{max} value was three hours. The mean C_{min} value was 202 (±101) ng/mL. The mean % of fluctuation value was 107 (±40).

The relative bioavailability of MEGACE 40 mg tablets and MEGACE Oral Suspension has not been evaluated. The effect of food on the bioavailability of MEGACE Oral Suspension has not been evaluated.

DESCRIPTION OF CLINICAL STUDIES

The clinical efficacy of MEGACE Oral Suspension was assessed in two clinical trials. One was a multicenter, randomized, double-blind, placebo-controlled study comparing megestrol acetate (MA) at doses of 100 mg, 400 mg, and 800 mg per day versus placebo in AIDS patients with anorexia/cachexia and significant weight loss. Of the 270 patients entered on study, 195 met all inclusion/exclusion criteria, had at least two additional post baseline weight measurements over a 12 week period or had one post baseline weight measurement but dropped out for therapeutic failure. The percent of patients gaining five or more pounds at maximum

Continued on next page

Megace O.S.—Cont.

weight gain in 12 study weeks was statistically significantly greater for the 800 mg (64%) and 400 mg (57%) MA-treated groups than for the placebo group (24%). Mean weight increased from baseline to last evaluation in 12 study weeks in the 800 mg MA-treated group by 7.8 pounds, the 400 mg MA group by 4.2 pounds, the 100 mg MA group by 1.9 pounds, and decreased in the placebo group by 1.6 pounds. Mean weight changes at 4, 8 and 12 weeks for patients evaluable for efficacy in the two clinical trials are shown graphically. Changes in body composition during the 12 study weeks as measured by bioelectrical impedance analysis showed increases in non-water body weight in the MA-treated groups (see "**Clinical Studies**" Table). In addition, edema developed or worsened in only 3 patients.

Greater percentages of MA-treated patients in the 800 mg group (89%), the 400 mg group (68%) and the 100 mg group (72%), than in the placebo group (50%), showed an improvement in appetite at last evaluation during the 12 study weeks. A statistically significant difference was observed between the 800 mg MA-treated group and the placebo group in the change in caloric intake from baseline to time of maximum weight change. Patients were asked to assess weight change, appetite, appearance, and overall perception of well-being in a 9 question survey. At maximum weight change only the 800 mg MA-treated group gave responses that were statistically significantly more favorable to all questions when compared to the placebo-treated group. A dose response was noted in the survey with positive responses correlating with higher dose for all questions.

The second trial was a multicenter, randomized, double-blind, placebo-controlled study comparing megestrol acetate 800 mg/day versus placebo in AIDS patients with anorexia/cachexia and significant weight loss. Of the 100 patients entered on study, 65 met all inclusion/exclusion criteria, had at least two additional post baseline weight measurements over a 12 week period or had one post baseline weight measurement but dropped out for therapeutic failure. Patients in the 800 mg MA-treated group had a statistically significantly larger increase in mean maximum weight change than patients in the placebo group. From baseline to study week 12, mean weight increased by 11.2 pounds in the MA-treated group and decreased 2.1 pounds in the placebo group. Changes in body composition as measured by bioelectrical impedance analysis showed increases in non-water weight in the MA-treated group (see "**Clinical Studies**" Table). No edema was reported in the MA-treated group. A greater percentage of MA-treated patients (67%) than placebo-treated patients (38%) showed an improvement in appetite at last evaluation during the 12 study weeks; this difference was statistically significant. There were no statistically significant differences between treatment groups in mean caloric change or in daily caloric intake at time to maximum weight change. In the same 9 question survey referenced in the first trial, patients' assessments of weight change, appetite, appearance, and overall perception of well-being showed increases in mean scores in MA-treated patients as compared to the placebo group.

In both trials, patients tolerated the drug well and no statistically significant differences were seen between the treatment groups with regard to laboratory abnormalities, new opportunistic infections, lymphocyte counts, T_4 counts, T_8 counts, or skin reactivity tests (see "**ADVERSE REACTIONS**" section).
[See table below]
The following figures are the results of mean weight changes for patients evaluable for efficacy in trials 1 and 2.
[See figures at top of next column]

INDICATIONS AND USAGE

MEGACE (megestrol acetate) Oral Suspension is indicated for the treatment of anorexia, cachexia, or an unexplained, significant weight loss in patients with a diagnosis of acquired immunodeficiency syndrome (AIDS).

CONTRAINDICATIONS

History of hypersensitivity to megestrol acetate or any component of the formulation. As a diagnostic test for pregnancy. Known or suspected pregnancy.

WARNINGS

Megestrol acetate may cause fetal harm when administered to a pregnant woman. For animal data on fetal effects (see **PRECAUTIONS: "Impairment of Fertility"** section). There are no adequate and well-controlled studies in pregnant women. If this drug is used during pregnancy, or if the patient becomes pregnant while taking (receiving) this drug, the patient should be apprised of the potential hazard to the fetus. Women of childbearing potential should be advised to avoid becoming pregnant.

Megestrol acetate is not intended for prophylactic use to avoid weight loss.

(See also **PRECAUTIONS: "Carcinogenesis, Mutagenesis, and Impairment of Fertility"** sections.)

Although the glucocorticoid activity of MEGACE Oral Suspension has not been fully evaluated, laboratory evidence of adrenal suppression has been observed. Clinical cases of new onset diabetes, exacerbation of pre-existing diabetes, and Cushing's syndrome have been reported in association with the use of MEGACE. Rare cases of clinically apparent adrenal insufficiency have also been reported in association with MEGACE. The possibility of adrenal suppression should be considered in any patient taking or withdrawing from chronic MEGACE therapy who presents with symptoms of adrenal insufficiency such as hypotension, nausea, vomiting, dizziness, or weakness. Laboratory evaluation for adrenal insufficiency and replacement stress doses of a rapidly acting glucocorticoid may be indicated for such patients.

PRECAUTIONS

General: Therapy with MEGACE Oral Suspension for weight loss should only be instituted after treatable causes of weight loss are sought and addressed. These treatable causes include possible malignancies, systemic infections, gastrointestinal disorders affecting absorption, endocrine disease and renal or psychiatric diseases.

Effects on HIV viral replication have not been determined. Use with caution in patients with a history of thromboembolic disease.

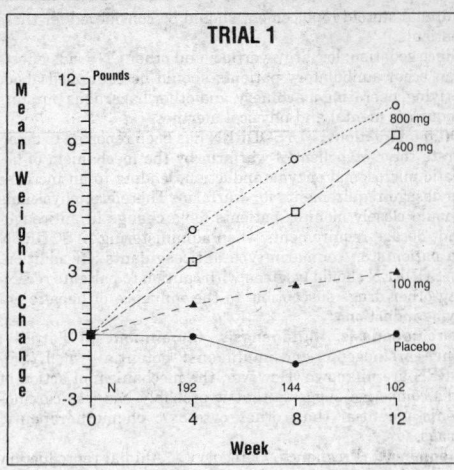

TRIAL 1

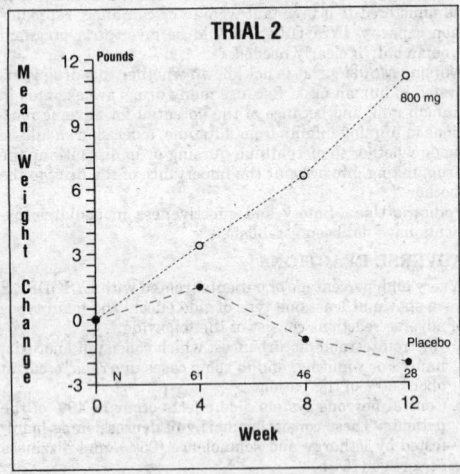

TRIAL 2

Use in Diabetics: Exacerbation of pre-existing diabetes with increased insulin requirements have been reported in association with the use of MEGACE.

Information for the Patients: Patients using megestrol acetate should receive the following instructions:
1. This medication is to be used as directed by the physician.
2. Report any adverse reaction experiences while taking this medication.
3. Use contraception while taking this medication if you are a woman capable of becoming pregnant.
4. Notify your physician if you become pregnant while taking this medication.

Drug Interactions: Pharmacokinetic studies show that there are no significant alterations in pharmacokinetic parameters of zidovudine or with rifabutin to warrant dosage adjustment when megestrol acetate is administered with these drugs. The effects of zidovudine or rifabutin on the pharmacokinetics of megestrol acetate were not studied.

Animal Toxicology: Long-term treatment with MEGACE may increase the risk of respiratory infections. A trend toward increased frequency of respiratory infections, decreased lymphocyte counts and increased neutrophil counts was observed in a two-year chronic toxicity/carcinogenicity study of megestrol acetate conducted in rats.

Carcinogenesis, Mutagenesis, and Impairment of Fertility:
Carcinogenesis-Data on carcinogenesis were obtained from studies conducted in dogs, monkeys and rats treated with megestrol acetate at doses 53.2, 26.6 and 1.3 times *lower* than the proposed dose (13.3 mg/kg/day) for humans. No males were used in the dog and monkey studies. In female beagles, megestrol acetate (0.01, 0.1 or 0.25 mg/kg/day) administered for up to 7 years induced both benign and malignant tumors of the breast. In female monkeys, no tumors were found following 10 years of treatment with 0.01, 0.1 or 0.5 mg/kg/day megestrol acetate. Pituitary tumors were observed in female rats treated with 3.9 or 10 mg/kg/day of megestrol acetate for 2 years. The relationship of these tumors in rats and dogs to humans is unknown but should be considered in assessing the risk-to-benefit ratio when prescribing MEGACE Oral Suspension and in surveillance of patients on therapy. (See "**WARNINGS**" section.)

Mutagenesis-No mutagenesis data are currently available.

Impairment of Fertility-Perinatal/postnatal (segment III) toxicity studies were performed in rats at doses (0.05–12.5 mg/kg) less than that indicated for humans (13.3 mg/kg); in

MEGACE (megestrol acetate) Oral Suspension Clinical Efficacy Trials

	Trial 1 Study Accrual Dates 11/88 to 12/90				Trial 2 Study Accrual Dates 5/89 to 4/91	
Megestrol Acetate, mg/day	0	100	400	800	0	800
Entered Patients	38	82	75	75	48	52
Evaluable Patients	28	61	53	53	29	36
Mean Change in Weight (lb.) Baseline to 12 Weeks	0.0	2.9	9.3	10.7	-2.1	11.2
% Patients ≥5 Pound Gain at Last Evaluation in 12 Weeks	21	44	57	64	28	47
Mean Changes in Body Composition*: Fat Body Mass (lb.)	0.0	2.2	2.9	5.5	1.5	5.7
Lean Body Mass (lb.)	-1.7	-0.3	1.5	2.5	-1.6	-0.6
Water (liters)	-1.3	-0.3	0.0	0.0	-0.1	-0.1
% Patients With Improved Appetite: At time of Max. Wt. Change	50	72	72	93	48	69
At Last Evaluation in 12 Wk.	50	72	68	89	38	67
Mean Change in Daily Caloric Intake: Baseline to Time of Maximum Weight Change	-107	326	308	646	30	464

*Based on bioelectrical impedence analysis determinations at last evaluation in 12 weeks.

Adverse Events
% of Patients Reporting

Megestrol Acetate mg/day No. of Patients	Trial 1 (N=236)				Trial 1 (N=87)		Open Label Trial
	Placebo 0 N=34	100 N=68	400 N=69	800 N=65	Placebo 0 N=38	800 N=49	1200 N=176
Diarrhea	15	13	8	15	8	6	10
Impotence	3	4	6	14	0	4	7
Rash	9	9	4	12	3	2	6
Flatulence	9	0	1	9	3	10	6
Hypertension	0	0	0	8	0	0	4
Asthenia	3	2	3	6	8	4	5
Insomnia	0	3	4	6	0	0	1
Nausea	9	4	0	5	3	4	5
Anemia	6	3	3	5	0	0	0
Fever	3	6	4	5	3	2	1
Libido Decreased	3	4	0	5	0	2	1
Dyspepsia	0	0	3	3	5	4	2
Hyperglycemia	3	0	6	3	0	0	3
Headache	6	10	1	3	0	0	3
Pain	6	0	0	2	5	6	4
Vomiting	9	3	0	2	3	6	4
Pneumonia	6	2	0	2	3	0	1
Urinary Freq.	0	0	1	2	5	2	1

these low dose studies, the reproductive capability of male offspring of megestrol acetate-treated females was impaired. Similar results were obtained in dogs. Pregnant rats treated with megestrol acetate showed a reduction in fetal weight and number of live births, and feminization of male fetuses. No toxicity data are currently available on male reproduction (spermatogenesis).

Pregnancy: Pregnancy "Category X". (See **WARNINGS** and **"PRECAUTIONS": Impairment of Fertility** sections.) No adequate animal teratology information is available at clinically relevant doses.

Nursing Mothers: Because of the potential for adverse effects on the newborn, nursing should be discontinued if MEGACE (megestrol acetate) Oral Suspension is required.

Use in HIV-Infected Women: Although megestrol acetate has been used extensively in women for the treatment of endometrial and breast cancers, its use in HIV-infected women has been limited.

All 10 women in the clinical trials reported breakthrough bleeding.

Pediatric Use: Safety and effectiveness in pediatric patients have not been established.

ADVERSE REACTIONS

Clinical Adverse Events: Adverse events which occurred in at least 5% of patients in any arm of the two clinical efficacy trials and the open trial are listed below by treatment group. All patients listed had at least one post baseline visit during the 12 study weeks. These adverse events should be considered by the physician when prescribing MEGACE Oral Suspension.

[See table above]

Adverse events which occurred in 1 to 3% of all patients enrolled in the two clinical efficacy trials with at least one follow-up visit during the first 12 weeks of the study are listed below by body system. Adverse events occurring less than 1% are not included. There were no significant differences between incidence of these events in patients treated with megestrol acetate and patients treated with placebo.

Body as a Whole-abdominal pain, chest pain, infection, moniliasis and sarcoma

Cardiovascular System-cardiomyopathy and palpitation

Digestive System-constipation, dry mouth, hepatomegaly, increased salivation and oral moniliasis

Hemic and Lymphatic System-leukopenia

Metabolic and Nutritional-LDH increased, edema and peripheral edema

Nervous System-paresthesia, confusion, convulsion, depression, neuropathy, hypesthesia and abnormal thinking

Respiratory System-dyspnea, cough, pharyngitis and lung disorder

Skin and Appendages-alopecia, herpes, pruritus, vesiculobullous rash, sweating and skin disorder

Special Senses-amblyopia

Urogenital System-albuminuria, urinary incontinence, urinary tract infection and gynecomastia

Postmarketing-Postmarketing reports associated with MEGACE Oral Suspension included thromboembolic phenomena including thrombophlebitis, pulmonary embolism and glucose intolerance (see **WARNINGS** and **PRECAUTIONS** sections).

OVERDOSAGE

No serious unexpected side effects have resulted from studies involving MEGACE Oral Suspension administered in dosages as high as 1200 mg/day. Megestrol acetate has not been tested for dialyzability; however, due to its low solubility it is postulated that dialysis would not be an effective means of treating overdose.

DOSAGE AND ADMINISTRATION

The recommended adult initial dosage of MEGACE Oral Suspension, is 800 mg/day (20 mL/day). Shake container well before using.

In clinical trials evaluating different dose schedules, daily doses of 400 and 800 mg/day were found to be clinically effective.

A plastic dosage cup with 10 mL and 20 mL markings is provided for convenience.

HOW SUPPLIED

MEGACE® Oral Suspension is available as a lemon-lime flavored oral suspension containing 40 mg of micronized megestrol acetate per mL.
NDC 0015-0508-42   Bottles of 240 mL (8 fl. oz.)

STORAGE
Store MEGACE Oral Suspension between 15°–25°C (59°–77°F) and dispense in a tight container. Protect from heat.

SPECIAL HANDLING
Health Hazard Data: There is no threshold limit value established by OSHA, NIOSH, or ACGIH.

Exposure or "overdose" at levels approaching recommended dosing levels could result in side effects described above (see **"WARNINGS"** and **"ADVERSE REACTIONS"** sections). Women at risk of pregnancy should avoid such exposure.

MeadJohnson
ONCOLOGY PRODUCTS
A Bristol-Myers Squibb Company
Princeton, NJ 08543
U.S.A.
H7-B001A-3-98   P5745-02
52-004083-00   Revised: January 1998
Shown in Product Identification Guide, page 308

MEGACE®   ℞
[mĕg 'ace]
(megestrol acetate tablets, USP)

CAUTION: FEDERAL LAW PROHIBITS DISPENSING WITHOUT PRESCRIPTION.

> **WARNING**
> **THE USE OF MEGACE® (megestrol acetate tablets, USP) DURING THE FIRST 4 MONTHS OF PREGNANCY IS NOT RECOMMENDED.**
> Progestational agents have been used beginning with the first trimester of pregnancy in an attempt to prevent habitual abortion. There is no adequate evidence that such use is effective when such drugs are given during the first 4 months of pregnancy. Furthermore, in the vast majority of women, the cause of abortion is a defective ovum, which progestational agents could not be expected to influence. In addition, the use of progestational agents, with their uterine-relaxant properties, in patients with fertilized defective ova may cause a delay in spontaneous abortion. Therefore, the use of such drugs during the first 4 months of pregnancy is not recommended.
> Several reports suggest an association between intrauterine exposure to progestational drugs in the first trimester of pregnancy and genital abnormalities in male and female fetuses. The risk of hypospadias, 5 to 8 per 1,000 male births in the general population, may be approximately doubled with exposure to these drugs. There are insufficient data to quantify the risk to exposed female fetuses, but insofar as some of these drugs

induce mild virilization of the external genitalia of the female fetus, and because of the increased association of hypospadias in the male fetus, it is prudent to avoid the use of these drugs during the first trimester of pregnancy.

If the patient is exposed to MEGACE during the first 4 months of pregnancy or if she becomes pregnant while taking this drug, she should be apprised of the potential risks to the fetus.

DESCRIPTION

MEGACE® (megestrol acetate tablets, USP) is a synthetic, antineoplastic and progestational drug. Megestrol acetate is a white, crystalline solid chemically designated as 17α-acetyloxy-6-methylpregna-4,6-diene-3, 20-dione. Solubility at 37°C in water is 2 mcg per mL, solubility in plasma is 24 mcg per mL. Its molecular weight is 384.51. The empirical formula is $C_{24}H_{32}O_4$ and the structural formula is represented as follows:

MEGACE is supplied as tablets for oral administration containing 20 mg and 40 mg megestrol acetate.

MEGACE Tablets contain the following inactive ingredients: acacia, calcium phosphate, FD&C Blue No. 1 Aluminum Lake, lactose, magnesium stearate, silicon dioxide colloidal, and starch.

CLINICAL PHARMACOLOGY

While the precise mechanism by which MEGACE produces its antineoplastic effects against endometrial carcinoma is unknown at the present time, inhibition of pituitary gonadotropin production and resultant decrease in estrogen secretion may be factors. There is evidence to suggest a local effect as a result of the marked changes brought about by the direct instillation of progestational agents into the endometrial cavity. The antineoplastic action of megestrol acetate on carcinoma of the breast is effected by modifying the action of other steroid hormones and by exerting a direct cytotoxic effect on tumor cells.[1] In metastatic cancer, hormone receptors may be present in some tissues but not others. The receptor mechanism is a cyclic process whereby estrogen produced by the ovaries enters the target cell, forms a complex with cytoplasmic receptor and is transported into the cell nucleus. There it induces gene transcription and leads to the alteration of normal cell functions. Pharmacologic doses of megestrol acetate not only decrease the number of hormone-dependent human breast cancer cells but also is capable of modifying and abolishing the stimulatory effects of estrogen on these cells. It has been suggested[2] that progestins may inhibit in one of two ways: by interfering with either the stability, availability, or turnover of the estrogen receptor complex in its interaction with genes or in conjunction with the progestin receptor complex, by interacting directly with the genome to turn off specific estrogen-responsive genes.

There are several analytical methods used to estimate MEGACE plasma levels, including mass fragmentography, gas chromatography (GC), high pressure liquid chromatography (HPLC), and radioimmunoassay. The plasma levels by HPLC assay or radioimmunoassay methods are about one-sixth those obtained by the GC method. The plasma levels are dependent not only on the method used, but also on intestinal and hepatic inactivation of the drug, which may be affected by factors such as intestinal tract motility, intestinal bacteria, antibiotics administered, body weight, diet, and liver function.[3,4]

Metabolites account for only 5 to 8% of the administered dose and are considered negligible.[5] The major route of drug elimination in humans is the urine.

When radiolabeled megestrol acetate was administered to humans in doses of 4 to 90 mg, the urinary excretion within 10 days ranged from 56.5 to 78.4% (mean 66.4%) and fecal excretion ranged from 7.7 to 30.3% (mean 19.8%). The total recovered radioactivity varied between 83.1 and 94.7% (mean 86.2%). Respiratory excretion as labeled carbon dioxide and fat storage may have accounted for at least part of the radioactivity not found in the urine and feces.

In normal male volunteers (n=23) who received 160 mg of megestrol acetate given as a 40 mg qid regimen, the oral absorption of MEGACE (megestrol acetate tablets, USP) appeared to be variable. Plasma levels were assayed by a high

Continued on next page

Megace Tablets—Cont.

pressure liquid chromatographic (HPLC) procedure. Peak drug levels for the first 40 mg dose ranged from 10 to 56 ng/mL (mean 27.6 ng/mL) and the times to peak concentrations ranged from 1.0 to 3.0 hours (mean 2.2 hours). Plasma elimination half-life ranged from 13.0 to 104.9 hours (mean 34.2 hours). The steady state plasma concentrations for a 40 mg qid regimen have not been established.

INDICATION AND USAGE

MEGACE is indicated for the palliative treatment of advanced carcinoma of the breast or endometrium (i.e., recurrent, inoperable, or metastatic disease). It should not be used in lieu of currently accepted procedures such as surgery, radiation, or chemotherapy.

CONTRAINDICATIONS

History of hypersensitivity to megestrol acetate or any component of the formulation. As a diagnostic test for pregnancy.

WARNINGS

Megestrol acetate may cause fetal harm when administered to a pregnant woman. Fertility and reproduction studies with high doses of megestrol acetate have shown a reversible feminizing effect on some male rat fetuses.[6] There are no adequate and well-controlled studies in pregnant women. If this drug is used during pregnancy, or if the patient becomes pregnant while taking (receiving) this drug, the patient should be apprised of the potential hazard to the fetus. Women of childbearing potential should be advised to avoid becoming pregnant.

The use of MEGACE in other types of neoplastic disease is not recommended. (See also **"PRECAUTIONS: Carcinogenesis, Mutagenesis, and Impairment of Fertility"** subsection.)

Although the glucocorticoid activity of MEGACE tablets has not been fully evaluated, laboratory evidence of adrenal suppression has been observed. Clinical cases of new onset diabetes, exacerbation of pre-existing diabetes, and Cushing's syndrome have been reported in association with the use of MEGACE. Rare cases of clinically apparent adrenal insufficiency have also been reported in association with MEGACE. The possibility of adrenal suppression should be considered in any patient taking or withdrawing from chronic MEGACE therapy who presents with symptoms of adrenal insufficiency such as hypotension, nausea, vomiting, dizziness, or weakness. Laboratory evaluation for adrenal insufficiency and replacement stress doses of a rapidly acting glucocorticoid may be indicated for such patients.

PRECAUTIONS

General: Close surveillance is indicated for any patient treated for recurrent or metastatic cancer. Use with caution in patients with a history of thromboembolic disease.

Use in Diabetics: Exacerbation of pre-existing diabetes with increased insulin requirements has been reported in association with the use of MEGACE.

Information for the Patients: Patients using megestrol acetate should receive the following instructions:

1. This medication is to be used as directed by the physician.
2. Report any adverse reaction experiences while taking this medication.

Laboratory Tests: Breast malignancies in which estrogen and/or progesterone receptors are positive are more likely to respond to MEGACE.[7, 8, 9]

Carcinogenesis, Mutagenesis, and Impairment of Fertility: Administration of megestrol acetate to female dogs for up to 7 years is associated with an increased incidence of both benign and malignant tumors of the breast.[10] Comparable studies in rats and studies in monkeys are not associated with an increased incidence of tumors. The relationship of the dog tumors to humans is unknown but should be considered in assessing the benefit-to-risk ratio when prescribing MEGACE and in surveillance of patients on therapy.[10,11] (See **"WARNINGS"** section.)

Pregnancy: Pregnancy "Category D". (See **"WARNINGS"** section.)

Nursing Mothers: Because of the potential for adverse effects on the newborn, nursing should be discontinued if MEGACE is required for treatment of cancer.

Pediatric Use: Safety and effectiveness in pediatric patients have not been established.

ADVERSE REACTIONS

Weight Gain: Weight gain is a frequent side effect of MEGACE.[12,13] This gain has been associated with increased appetite and is not necessarily associated with fluid retention.

Thromboembolic Phenomena: Thromboembolic phenomena including thrombophlebitis and pulmonary embolism (in some cases fatal) have been reported.

Glucocorticoid Effects: (See **"WARNINGS"** and **"PRECAUTIONS"**sections.)

Other Adverse Reactions: Heart failure, nausea and vomiting, edema, breakthrough menstrual bleeding, dyspnea, tumor flare (with or without hypercalcemia), hyperglycemia, glucose intolerance, alopecia, hypertension, carpal tunnel syndrome, mood changes, hot flashes, sweating and rash.

OVERDOSAGE

No serious unexpected side effects have resulted from studies involving MEGACE administered in dosages as high as 1600 mg/day. Oral administration of large, single doses of megestrol acetate (5 g/kg) did not produce toxic effects in mice.[6] Megestrol acetate has not been tested for dialyzability; however, due to its low solubility it is postulated that this would not be an effective means of treating overdose.

DOSAGE AND ADMINISTRATION

Breast Cancer: 160 mg/day (40 mg qid).
Endometrial Carcinoma: 40 to 320 mg/day in divided doses.
At least 2 months of continuous treatment is considered an adequate period for determining the efficacy of MEGACE (megestrol acetate tablets, USP).

HOW SUPPLIED

MEGACE® (megestrol acetate tablets, USP) is available as light blue, scored tablets containing 20 mg or 40 mg megestrol acetate.

NDC 0015-0595-01 20 mg tablet, bottles of 100
NDC 0015-0596-41 40 mg tablet, bottles of 100
NDC 0015-0596-45 40 mg tablet, bottles of 500
NDC 0015-0596-46 40 mg tablet, bottles of 250

STORAGE

Store MEGACE (megestrol acetate tablets, USP) at room temperature; protect from temperatures above 40°C (104°F).

SPECIAL HANDLING

Health Hazard Data: There is no threshold limit value established by OSHA, NIOSH, or ACGIH.

Exposure or "overdose" at levels approaching recommended dosing levels could result in side effects described above (see **"WARNINGS"**and **"ADVERSE REACTIONS"** sections). Women at risk of pregnancy should avoid such exposure.

REFERENCES

1. Allegra JC, Kiefer SM: Mechanisms of Action of Progestational Agents. Semin Oncol 1985; 12(Suppl 1):3.
2. DeSombre ER, Kuivanen PC: Progestin Modulation of Estrogen-Dependent Marker Protein Synthesis in the Endometrium. Semin Oncol 1985; 12(Suppl 1):6.
3. Alexieva-Figusch J, et al: Treatment of Metastatic Breast Cancer Patients with Different Dosages of Megestrol Acetate: Dose Relations, Metabolic and Endocrine Effects. Eur J Cancer Clin Oncol 1984; 20:33-40.
4. Gaver RC, et al: Liquid Chromatographic Procedure for the Quantitative Analysis of Megestrol Acetate in Human Plasma. J Pharm Sci 1985; 74:664.
5. Cooper JM, Kellie AE: The Metabolism of Megestrol Acetate (17-alpha-acetoxy-6-methylpregna-4,6-diene-3, 20-dione) in Women. Steroids 1968;11:133.
6. David A, et al: Anti-Ovulatory and Other Biological Properties of Megestrol Acetate. J Reprod Fertil 1963; 5:331.
7. McGuire WL, Clark GM: The Prognostic Role of Progesterone Receptors in Human Breast Cancer. Semin Oncol 1983; 10(suppl 4):2.
8. Horwitz KB: The Central Role of Progesterone Receptors and Progestational Agents in the Management and Treatment of Breast Cancer. Semin Oncol 1988; 15(Suppl 1):14.
9. Bonomi P, et al: Primary Hormonal Therapy of Advanced Breast Cancer with Megestrol Acetate: Predictive Value of Estrogen Receptor and Progesterone Receptor Levels. Semin Oncol 1985; 12(Suppl 1):48-54.
10. Nelson LW, et al: Mammary Nodules in Dogs During Four Years' Treatment with Megestrol Acetate or Chlormadinone Acetate. J Natl Cancer Inst 1973; 51:1303.
11. Owen LN, Briggs MH: Contraceptive Steroid Toxicology in the Beagle Dog and its Relevance to Human Carcinogenicity. Curr Med Res Opin 1976; 4:309.
12. Ansfield FJ, et al: Clinical Results with Megestrol Acetate in Patients with Advanced Carcinoma of the Breast. Surg Gynecol Obstet 1982; 155:888.
13. Alexieva-Figusch J, et al: Progestin Therapy in Advanced Breast Cancer: Megestrol Acetate—An Evaluation of 160 Treated Cases. Cancer 1980; 46:2369.

Mead Johnson
ONCOLOGY PRODUCTS
A Bristol-Myers Squibb Company
Princeton, NJ 08543
U.S.A.
H7-B001-7-96 P6842-00
Latest Revision: July 1996

Shown in Product Identification Guide, page 308

MESNEX® Rx ONLY

[mĕs-nĕx]
(Mesna) Injection

DESCRIPTION

MESNEX® (mesna) Injection is a detoxifying agent to inhibit the hemorrhagic cystitis induced by ifosfamide (IFEX®). The active ingredient mesna is a synthetic sulfhydryl compound designated as sodium 2-mercaptoethane sulfonate with a molecular formula of $C_2H_5NaO_3S_2$ and a molecular weight of 164.18. Its structural formula is as follows:

$$HS\text{-}CH_2\text{-}CH_2SO_3\text{-}Na^+$$

MESNEX Injection is a sterile, nonpyrogenic, aqueous solution of clear and colorless appearance in clear glass single dose ampules or multidose vials for intravenous administration. MESNEX Injection contains 100 mg/mL mesna, 0.25 mg/mL edetate disodium and sodium hydroxide for pH adjustment. MESNEX Injection multidose vials also contain 10.4 mg of benzyl alcohol as a preservative. The solution has a pH range of 6.5–8.5.

CLINICAL PHARMACOLOGY

MESNEX was developed as a prophylactic agent to prevent the hemorrhagic cystitis induced by ifosfamide.

Analogous to the physiological cysteine-cystine system, following intravenous administration, mesna is rapidly oxidized to its only metabolite, mesna disulfide (dimesna). Mesna disulfide remains in the intravascular compartment and is rapidly eliminated by the kidneys.

In the kidney, the mesna disulfide is reduced to the free thiol compound, mesna, which reacts chemically with the urotoxic ifosfamide metabolites (acrolein and 4-hydroxy-ifosfamide) resulting in their detoxification. The first step in the detoxification process is the binding of mesna to 4-hydroxy-ifosfamide forming a nonurotoxic 4-sulfoethylthioifosfamide. Mesna also binds to the double bonds of acrolein and other urotoxic metabolites.

After administration of an 800 mg dose the half-lives of mesna and dimesna in the blood are 0.36 hours and 1.17 hours respectively. Approximately 32% and 33% of the administered dose was eliminated in the urine in 24 hours as mesna and dimesna respectively. The majority of the dose recovered was eliminated within 4 hours. Mesna has a volume of distribution of 0.652 L/kg and a plasma clearance of 1.23 L/kg/hour.

Ifosfamide has been shown to have dose dependent pharmacokinetics in humans. At doses of 2–4 g, its terminal elimination half-life is about 7 hours. As a result, in order to maintain adequate levels of mesna in the urinary bladder during the course of elimination of the urotoxic ifosfamide metabolites, repeated doses of MESNEX are required.

Based on the pharmacokinetic profiles of mesna and ifosfamide as discussed above, MESNEX was given as bolus doses prior to ifosfamide and at 4 and 8 hours after ifosfamide administration. The hemorrhagic cystitis produced by ifosfamide is dose dependent. At a dose of 1.2 g/m^2 ifosfamide administered daily for 5 days, 16–26% of the patients who received conventional uroprophylaxis (high fluid intake, alkalinization of the urine and the administration of diuretics) developed hematuria > 50 rbc/hpf or macrohematuria). In contrast, none of the patients who received MESNEX together with this dose of ifosfamide developed hematuria. Higher doses of ifosfamide from 2 to 4 g/m^2 administered for three to five days, produced hematuria in 31 to 100% of the patients. When MESNEX was administered together with these doses of ifosfamide the incidence of hematuria was less than 7%.

INDICATIONS AND USAGE

MESNEX has been shown to be effective as a prophylactic agent in reducing the incidence of ifosfamide-induced hemorrhagic cystitis.

CONTRAINDICATIONS

MESNEX is contraindicated in patients known to be hypersensitive to mesna or other thiol compounds.

WARNINGS

Allergic reactions to mesna were reported in patients with autoimmune disorders. The majority of the patients received high doses of mesna orally. The symptoms ranged from mild hypersensitivity to systemic anaphylactic reactions.

MESNEX has been developed as an agent to prevent ifosfamide-induced hemorrhagic cystitis. It will not prevent or alleviate any of the other adverse reactions or toxicities associated with ifosfamide therapy.

MESNEX does not prevent hemorrhagic cystitis in all patients. Up to 6% of patients treated with mesna have developed hematuria (> 50 rbc/hpf or WHO grade 2 and above). As a result, a morning specimen of urine should be examined for the presence of hematuria (red blood cells) each day prior to ifosfamide therapy. If hematuria develops when MESNEX is given with ifosfamide according to the recommended dosage schedule, depending on the severity of the hematuria, dosage reductions or discontinuation of ifosfamide therapy may be initiated.

In order to obtain adequate protection, MESNEX must be administered with each dose of ifosfamide as outlined in the **"DOSAGE AND ADMINISTRATION"** section. MESNEX is not effective in preventing hematuria due to other pathological conditions such as thrombocytopenia.

Because of the benzyl alcohol content, the multidose vial should not be used in neonates or infants and should be used with caution in older pediatric patients.

PRECAUTIONS

Laboratory Tests: A false positive test for urinary ketones may arise in patients treated with MESNEX (mesna) Injection. In this test, a red-violet color develops which, with the addition of glacial acetic acid, will return to violet.

Pediatrics: Because of the benzyl alcohol content, the multidose vial should not be used in neonates or infants and should be used with caution in older pediatric patients.

Drug Interactions: *In vitro* and *in vivo* animal tumor models have shown that mesna does not have any effect on the antitumor efficacy of concomitantly administered cytotoxic agents.

Carcinogenesis, Mutagenesis and Impairment of Fertility: No long term animal studies have been performed to evaluate the carcinogenic potential of mesna. The Ames Salmonella typhimurium test, mouse micronucleus assay and frequency of sister chromatid exchange and chromosomal aberrations in PHA-stimulated lymphocytes *in vitro* assays revealed no mutagenic activity.

Pregnancy: Pregnancy "Category B". Reproduction studies in rats and rabbits with oral doses up to 1000 mg/kg have revealed no harm to the fetus due to mesna. It is not known whether MESNEX can cause fetal harm when administered to a pregnant woman or can affect reproductive capacity. MESNEX should be given to a pregnant woman only if the benefits clearly outweigh any possible risks.

Teratology studies in rats and rabbits have shown no effects.

Nursing Mothers: It is not known whether mesna or dimesna is excreted in human milk. Because many drugs are excreted in human milk and because of the potential for adverse reactions in nursing infants from mesna, a decision should be made whether to discontinue nursing or discontinue the drug, taking into account the importance of the drug to the mother.

ADVERSE REACTIONS

Because mesna is used in combination with ifosfamide and other chemotherapeutic agents with documented toxicities, it is difficult to distinguish the adverse reactions which may be due to MESNEX from those caused by the concomitantly administered cytostatic agents. As a result, the adverse reaction profile of MESNEX was determined in three Phase I studies (16 subjects) utilizing intravenous and oral administration and two controlled studies in which ifosfamide and mesna were compared to ifosfamide and standard prophylaxis.

In Phase I studies in which I.V. bolus doses of 0.8 to 1.6 g/m^2 MESNEX were administered as single or three repeated doses to a total of 10 patients, a bad taste in the mouth (100%) and soft stools (70%) were reported. At intravenous and oral bolus doses of 2.4 g/m^2 which are approximately 10 times the recommended clinical doses (0.24 g/m^2) headache (50%), fatigue (33%), nausea (33%), diarrhea (83%), limb pain (50%), hypotension (17%) and allergy (17%) have also been reported in the 6 patients who participated in this study.

In controlled clinical studies, adverse reactions which can be reasonably associated with mesna were vomiting, diarrhea and nausea.

OVERDOSAGE

There is no known antidote for MESNEX.

DOSAGE AND ADMINISTRATION

For the prophylaxis of ifosfamide-induced hemorrhagic cystitis, MESNEX may be given on a fractionated dosing schedule of bolus intravenous injections as outlined below.

MESNEX is given as intravenous bolus injections in a dosage equal to 20% of the ifosfamide dosage (w/w) at the time of ifosfamide administration and 4 and 8 hours after each dose of ifosfamide. The total daily dose of mesna is 60% of the ifosfamide dose.

The recommended dosing schedule is outlined below:

	0 hours	4 hours	8 hours
Ifosfamide	1.2 g/m^2	–	–
MESNEX	240 mg/m^2	240 mg/m^2	240 mg/m^2

In order to maintain adequate protection, this dosing schedule should be repeated on each day that ifosfamide is administered. When the dosage of ifosfamide is adjusted (either increased or decreased), the dose of MESNEX should be modified accordingly. When exposed to oxygen, mesna is oxidized to the disulfide, dimesna. As a result, if the ampules are used, any unused mesna remaining in the ampules after dosing should be discarded and new ampules used for each administration.

The MESNEX multidose vials may be stored and used for up to 8 days.

PREPARATION OF INTRAVENOUS SOLUTIONS/STABILITY

For I.V. administration the drug can be diluted by adding the MESNEX Injection solution to any of the following fluids obtaining final concentrations of 20 mg mesna/mL fluid:

5% Dextrose Injection, USP
5% Dextrose and 0.2% Sodium Chloride Injection, USP
5% Dextrose and 0.33% Sodium Chloride Injection, USP
5% Dextrose and 0.45% Sodium Chloride Injection, USP
0.92% Sodium Chloride Injection, USP
Lactated Ringer's Injection, USP

For example:
One mL of MESNEX (mesna) Injection multidose vial 100 mg/mL may be added to 4 mL, or one ampule of MESNEX Injection 200 mg/2 mL may be added to 8 mL of any of the solutions listed above to create a final concentration of 20 mg mesna/mL fluid.

Diluted solutions are chemically and physically stable for 24 hours at 25°C (77°F).

Mesna is not compatible with cisplatin.

Parenteral drug products should be inspected visually for particulate matter and discoloration prior to administration.

HOW SUPPLIED

MESNEX® (mesna) Injection 100 mg/mL
NDC 0015-3560-41
200 mg Single Dose Ampule, Box of 15 Ampules of 2-mL (color-ring coding: turquoise/yellow)
NDC 0015-3563-02
1 g Multidose Vial,
Box of 1 vial of 10 mL
NDC 0015-3563-03
1 g Multidose Vial,
Box of 10 vials of 10 mL

Store at controlled room temperature 15–30°C (59°–86°F).
U.S. Patent No.: 4,220,660

Distributed by:
Mead Johnson
ONCOLOGY PRODUCTS
A Bristol-Myers Squibb Company
Princeton, NJ 08543
U.S.A.

Manufactured by:
ASTA MEDICA
A Degussa Company
Frankfurt am Mein
Germany
H8-B001-5-98 N1217-00

Revised: March 1998

Shown in Product Identification Guide, page 308

MUTAMYCIN® ℞

[*mū"-tĕ-mī'-sĭn*]
(mitomycin for injection, USP)

CAUTION: FEDERAL LAW PROHIBITS DISPENSING WITHOUT PRESCRIPTION.

WARNING

MUTAMYCIN® (mitomycin for injection, USP) should be administered under the supervision of a qualified physician experienced in the use of cancer chemotherapeutic agents. Appropriate management of therapy and complications is possible only when adequate diagnostic and treatment facilities are readily available.

Bone marrow suppression, notably thrombocytopenia and leukopenia, which may contribute to overwhelming infections in an already compromised patient, is the most common and severe of the toxic effects of MUTAMYCIN (see "**WARNINGS**" and "**ADVERSE REACTIONS**" sections).

Hemolytic Uremic Syndrome (HUS), a serious complication of chemotherapy, consisting primarily of microangiopathic hemolytic anemia, thrombocytopenia, and irreversible renal failure has been reported in patients receiving systemic MUTAMYCIN. The syndrome may occur at any time during systemic therapy with MUTAMYCIN as a single agent or in combination with other cytotoxic drugs, however, most cases occur at doses ≥ 60 mg of MUTAMYCIN. Blood product transfusion may exacerbate the symptoms associated with this syndrome.

The incidence of the syndrome has not been defined.

DESCRIPTION

MUTAMYCIN® (mitomycin for injection, USP) (also known as mitomycin and/or mitomycin-C) is an antibiotic isolated from the broth of *Streptomyces caespitosus* which has been shown to have antitumor activity. The compound is heat stable, has a high melting point, and is freely soluble in organic solvents.

ACTION

MUTAMYCIN selectively inhibits the synthesis of deoxyribonucleic acid (DNA). The guanine and cytosine content correlates with the degree of MUTAMYCIN-induced cross-linking. At high concentrations of the drug, cellular RNA and protein synthesis are also suppressed.

In humans, MUTAMYCIN is rapidly cleared from the serum after intravenous administration. Time required to reduce the serum concentration by 50% after a 30 mg bolus injection is 17 minutes. After injection of 30 mg, 20 mg, or 10 mg I.V., the maximal serum concentrations were 2.4 µg/mL, 1.7 µg/mL, and 0.52 µg/mL, respectively. Clearance is effected primarily by metabolism in the liver, but metabolism occurs in other tissues as well. The rate of clearance is inversely proportional to the maximal serum concentration because, it is thought, of saturation of the degradative pathways.

Approximately 10% of a dose of MUTAMYCIN is excreted unchanged in the urine. Since metabolic pathways are saturated at relatively low doses, the percent of a dose excreted in urine increases with increasing dose. In children, excretion of intravenously administered MUTAMYCIN is similar.

Animal Toxicology—MUTAMYCIN has been found to be carcinogenic in rats and mice. At doses approximating the recommended clinical dose in man, it produces a greater than 100% increase in tumor incidence in male Sprague-Dawley rats, and a greater than 50% increase in tumor incidence in female Swiss mice.

INDICATIONS

MUTAMYCIN is not recommended as single-agent, primary therapy. It has been shown to be useful in the therapy of disseminated adenocarcinoma of the stomach or pancreas in proven combinations with other approved chemotherapeutic agents and as palliative treatment when other modalities have failed. MUTAMYCIN is not recommended to replace appropriate surgery and/or radiotherapy.

CONTRAINDICATIONS

MUTAMYCIN is contraindicated in patients who have demonstrated a hypersensitive or idiosyncratic reaction to it in the past.

MUTAMYCIN is contraindicated in patients with thrombocytopenia, coagulation disorder, or an increase in bleeding tendency due to other causes.

WARNINGS

Patients being treated with MUTAMYCIN must be observed carefully and frequently during and after therapy.

The use of MUTAMYCIN results in a high incidence of bone marrow suppression, particularly thrombocytopenia and leukopenia. Therefore, the following studies should be obtained repeatedly during therapy and for at least eight weeks following therapy: platelet count, white blood cell count, differential, and hemoglobin. The occurrence of a platelet count below 100,000/mm^3 or a WBC below 4,000/mm^3 or a progressive decline in either is an indication to withhold further therapy until blood counts have recovered above these levels.

Patients should be advised of the potential toxicity of this drug, particularly bone marrow suppression. Deaths have been reported due to septicemia as a result of leukopenia due to the drug.

Patients receiving MUTAMYCIN should be observed for evidence of renal toxicity. MUTAMYCIN should not be given to patients with a serum creatinine greater than 1.7 mg %.

Usage in Pregnancy—Safe use of MUTAMYCIN in pregnant women has not been established. Teratological changes have been noted in animal studies. The effect of MUTAMYCIN on fertility is unknown.

Pediatric Use—Safety and effectiveness in pediatric patients have not been established.

PRECAUTIONS

Acute shortness of breath and severe bronchospasm have been reported following the administration of vinca alkaloids in patients who had previously or simultaneously received MUTAMYCIN. The onset of this acute respiratory distress occurred within minutes to hours after the vinca alkaloid injection. The total number of doses for each drug has varied considerably. Bronchodilators, steroids and/or oxygen have produced symptomatic relief.

A few cases of adult respiratory distress syndrome have been reported in patients receiving MUTAMYCIN in combination with other chemotherapy and maintained at FIO_2 concentrations greater than 50% perioperatively. Therefore, caution should be exercised using only enough oxygen to provide adequate arterial saturation since oxygen itself is toxic to the lungs. Careful attention should be paid to fluid balance and overhydration should be avoided.

ADVERSE REACTIONS

Bone Marrow Toxicity—This was the most common and most serious toxicity, occurring in 605 of 937 patients (64.4%). Thrombocytopenia and/or leukopenia may occur anytime within 8 weeks after onset of therapy with an average time of 4 weeks. Recovery after cessation of therapy was within 10 weeks. About 25% of the leukopenic or thrombocytopenic episodes did not recover. MUTAMYCIN produces cumulative myelosuppression.

Integument and Mucous Membrane Toxicity—This has occurred in approximately 4% of patients treated with

Continued on next page

Mutamycin—Cont.

MUTAMYCIN (mitomycin for injection, USP). Cellulitis at the injection site has been reported and is occasionally severe. Stomatitis and alopecia also occur frequently. Rashes are rarely reported. The most important dermatological problem with this drug, however, is the necrosis and consequent sloughing of tissue which results if the drug is extravasated during injection. Extravasation may occur with or without an accompanying stinging or burning sensation and even if there is adequate blood return when the injection needle is aspirated. There have been reports of delayed erythema and/or ulceration occurring either at or distant from the injection site, weeks to months after MUTAMYCIN, even when no obvious evidence of extravasation was observed during administration. Skin grafting has been required in some of the cases.

Renal Toxicity–2% of 1,281 patients demonstrated a statistically significant rise in creatinine. There appeared to be no correlation between total dose administered or duration of therapy and the degree of renal impairment.

Pulmonary Toxicity—This has occurred infrequently but can be severe and may be life threatening. Dyspnea with a nonproductive cough and radiographic evidence of pulmonary infiltrates may be indicative of MUTAMYCIN-induced pulmonary toxicity. If other etiologies are eliminated, MUTAMYCIN therapy should be discontinued. Steriods have been employed as treatment of this toxicity, but the therapeutic value has not been determined. A few cases of adult respiratory distress syndrome have been reported in patients receiving MUTAMYCIN in combination with other chemotherapy and maintained at FIO_2 concentrations greater than 50% perioperatively.

Hemolytic Uremic Syndrome (HUS)—This serious complication of chemotherapy, consisting primarily of microangiopathic hemolytic anemia (hematocrit $\leq$ 25%), thrombocytopenia ($\leq$ 100,000/mm^3), and irreversible renal failure (serum creatinine $\geq$ 1.6 mg/dL) has been reported in patients receiving systemic MUTAMYCIN. Microangiopathic hemolysis with fragmented red blood cells on peripheral blood smears has occurred in 98% of patients with the syndrome. Other less frequent complications of the syndrome may include pulmonary edema (65%), neurologic abnormalities (16%), and hypertension. Exacerbation of the symptoms associated with HUS has been reported in some patients receiving blood product transfusions. A high mortality rate (52%) has been associated with this syndrome.

The syndrome may occur at any time during systemic therapy with MUTAMYCIN as a single agent or in combination with other cytotoxic drugs. Less frequently, HUS has also been reported in patients receiving combinations of cytotoxic drugs not including MUTAMYCIN. Of 83 patients studied, 72 developed the syndrome at total doses exceeding 60 mg of MUTAMYCIN. Consequently, patients receiving $\geq$ 60 mg of MUTAMYCIN should be monitored closely for unexplained anemia with fragmented cells on peripheral blood smear, thrombocytopenia, and decreased renal function.

The incidence of the syndrome has not been defined.

Therapy for the syndrome is investigational.

Cardiac Toxicity—Congestive heart failure, often treated effectively with diuretics and cardiac glycosides, has rarely been reported. Almost all patients who experienced this side effect had received prior doxorubicin therapy.

Acute Side Effects Due to MUTAMYCIN were fever, anorexia, nausea, and vomiting. They occurred in about 14% of 1,281 patients.

Other Undesirable Side Effects that have been reported during MUTAMYCIN therapy have been headache, blurring of vision, confusion, drowsiness, syncope, fatigue, edema, thrombophlebitis, hematemesis, diarrhea, and pain. These did not appear to be dose related and were not unequivocally drug related. They may have been due to the primary or metastatic disease processes.

DOSAGE AND ADMINISTRATION

MUTAMYCIN should be given intravenously only, using care to avoid extravasation of the compound. If extravasation occurs, cellulitis, ulceration, and slough may result.

Each vial contains either mitomycin 5 mg and mannitol 10 mg, mitomycin 20 mg and mannitol 40 mg, or mitomycin 40 mg and mannitol 80 mg. To administer, add Sterile Water for Injection, 10 mL, 40 mL, or 80 mL respectively. Shake to dissolve. If product does not dissolve immediately, allow to stand at room temperature until solution is obtained.

After full hematological recovery (see guide to dosage adjustment) from any previous chemotherapy, the following dosage schedule may be used at 6 to 8 week intervals:

20 mg/m^2 intravenously as a single dose via a functioning intravenous catheter.

Because of cumulative myelosuppression, patients should be fully reevaluated after each course of MUTAMYCIN, and the dose reduced if the patient has experienced any toxicities. Doses greater than 20 mg/m^2 have not been shown to be more effective, and are more toxic than lower doses.

The following schedule is suggested as a guide to dosage adjustment:

Nadir After Prior Dose		
Leukocytes/ mm^3	**Platelets/ mm^3**	**Percentage of Prior Dose to be Given**
>4000	>1,000,000	100%
3000–3999	75,000–99,999	100%
2000–2999	25,000–74,999	70%
<2000	<25,000	50%

No repeat dosage should be given until leukocyte count has returned to 4000/mm^3 and platelet count to 100,000/mm^3. When MUTAMYCIN is used in combination with other myelosuppressive agents, the doses should be adjusted accordingly. If the disease continues to progress after two courses of MUTAMYCIN, the drug should be stopped since chances of response are minimal.

STABILITY

1. **Unreconstituted** MUTAMYCIN stored at room temperature is stable for the lot life indicated on the package. Avoid excessive heat (over 40°C).
2. **Reconstituted** with Sterile Water for Injection to a concentration of 0.5 mg per mL, MUTAMYCIN is stable for 14 days refrigerated or 7 days at room temperature.
3. **Diluted** in various I.V. fluids at room temperature, to a concentration of 20 to 40 micrograms per mL:

I.V. Fluid	Stability
5% Dextrose Injection	3 hours
0.9% Sodium Chloride Injection	12 hours
Sodium Lactate Injection	24 hours

4. The combination of MUTAMYCIN (5 mg to 15 mg) and heparin (1,000 units to 10,000 units) in 30 mL of 0.9% Sodium Chloride Injection is stable for 48 hours at room temperature.

Procedures for proper handling and disposal of anticancer drugs should be considered. Several guidelines on this subject have been published.[1–7] There is no general agreement that all of the procedures recommended in the guidelines are necessary or appropriate.

HOW SUPPLIED

MUTAMYCIN® (mitomycin for injection, USP)

NDC 0015-3001-20—Each vial contains 5 mg mitomycin.
NDC 0015-3002-20—Each vial contains 20 mg mitomycin.
NDC 0015-3059-20—Each vial contains 40 mg mitomycin.

For information on package sizes available, refer to the current price schedule.

REFERENCES:

1. Recommendations for the Safe Handling of Parenteral Antineoplastic Drugs. NIH Publication No. 83–2621. For sale by the Superintendent of Documents, US Government Printing Office, Washington, DC 20402.
2. AMA Council Report. Guidelines for Handling Parenteral Antineoplastics. JAMA 1985; 253 (11):1590–1592.
3. National Study Commission on Cytotoxic Exposure—Recommendations for Handling Cytotoxic Agents. Available from Louis P. Jeffrey, ScD, Chairman, National Study Commission on Cytotoxic Exposure, Massachusetts College of Pharmacy and Allied Health Sciences, 179 Longwood Avenue, Boston, Massachusetts 02115.
4. Clinical Oncological Society of Australia. Guidelines and Recommendations for Safe Handling of Antineoplastic Agents. Med J Australia 1983; 1:426–428.
5. Jones RB, et al: Safe Handling of Chemotherapeutic Agents: A Report from the Mount Sinai Medical Center. CA-A Cancer Journal for Clinicians 1983; (Sept/Oct) 258–263.
6. American Society of Hospital Pharmacists Technical Assistance Bulletin on Handling Cytotoxic and Hazardous Drugs. Am J Hosp Pharm 1990; 47:1033–1049.
7. OSHA Work-Practice Guidelines for Personnel Dealing with Cytotoxic (Antineoplastic) Drugs. Am J Hosp Pharm 1986; 43: 1193–1204.

BRISTOL LABORATORIES®
ONCOLOGY PRODUCTS
A Bristol-Myers Squibb Company
Princeton, NJ 08543
U.S.A.
H9-B001-10-96	3001DIM-29
51-001114-01	Revised September 1996

Shown in Product Identification Guide, page 308

MYCOSTATIN® PASTILLES ℞

[mīk 'ō-stat "in]
Nystatin

DESCRIPTION

Nystatin is a polyene antifungal antibiotic obtained from *Streptomyces noursei.* Structural formula:

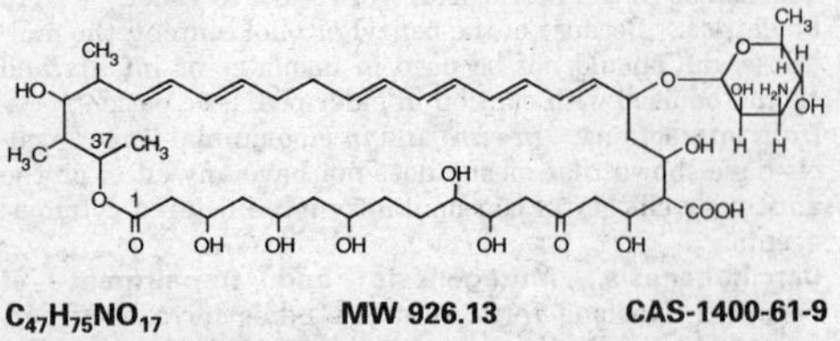

$C_{47}H_{75}NO_{17}$	**MW 926.13**	**CAS-1400-61-9**

MYCOSTATIN (nystatin) Pastilles are round, light to dark gold-colored troches designed to dissolve slowly in the mouth. Each pastille provides 200,000 units nystatin. Inactive ingredients: anise oil, cinnamon oil, gelatin, sucrose, and other ingredients.

CLINICAL PHARMACOLOGY

Nystatin is both fungistatic and fungicidal *in vitro* against a wide variety of yeasts and yeast-like fungi. *Candida albicans* demonstrates no significant resistance to nystatin *in vitro* on repeated subculture in increasing levels of nystatin; other *Candida* species become quite resistant. Generally, resistance does not develop *in vivo.* Nystatin acts by binding to sterols in the cell membrane of susceptible fungi with a resultant change in membrane permeability allowing leakage of intracellular components. Nystatin exhibits no activity against bacteria, protozoa, trichomonads, or viruses.

Pharmacokinetics

Gastrointestinal absorption of nystatin is insignificant. Most orally administered nystatin is passed unchanged in the stool. Significant concentrations of nystatin may appear occasionally in the plasma of patients with renal insufficiency during oral therapy with conventional dosage forms. Mean nystatin concentrations in excess of those required *in vitro* to inhibit growth of clinically significant *Candida* persisted in saliva for approximately two hours after the start of oral dissolution of two nystatin pastilles (400,000 units nystatin) administered simultaneously to 12 healthy volunteers.

INDICATIONS AND USAGE

Mycostatin (nystatin) Pastilles are indicated for the treatment of candidiasis in the oral cavity.

CONTRAINDICATIONS

The pastille is contraindicated in those patients with a history of hypersensitivity to any of its components.

PRECAUTIONS

General

This medication is not to be used for the treatment of systemic mycoses.

In order to achieve maximum effect from the medication, pastilles must be allowed to dissolve slowly in the mouth; therefore, patients for whom the pastille is prescribed, including children and the elderly, must be competent to utilize the dosage form as intended.

If irritation or hypersensitivity develops with nystatin pastilles, treatment should be discontinued and appropriate therapy instituted.

Information for the Patient

Patients taking this medication should receive the following information and instructions:

1. Use as directed; the medication is not for any disorder other than for which it was prescribed.
2. Allow pastille to dissolve slowly in the mouth; **do not chew or swallow the pastille.**
3. The patient should be advised regarding replacement of any missed doses.
4. There should be no interruption or discontinuation of medication until the prescribed course of treatment is completed even though symptomatic relief may occur within a few days.
5. If symptoms of local irritation develop, the physician should be notified promptly.
6. Good oral hygiene, including proper care of dentures, is particularly important for denture wearers.

Laboratory Tests

If there is a lack of therapeutic response, appropriate microbiological studies (eg, KOH smears and/or cultures) should be repeated to confirm the diagnosis of candidiasis and rule out other pathogens before instituting another course of therapy.

Carcinogenesis, Mutagenesis, Impairment of Fertility

Studies have not been performed to evaluate carcinogenic or mutagenic potential, or possible impairment of fertility in males or females.

Pregnancy: Teratogenic Effects

Category C. Animal reproduction studies have not been conducted with nystatin pastilles. It is also not known whether

nystatin pastilles can cause fetal harm when administered to a pregnant woman or can affect reproduction capacity. Nystatin pastilles should be dispensed to a pregnant woman only if clearly needed.

Pediatric Use
See PRECAUTIONS, General.

ADVERSE REACTIONS
Nystatin is generally well-tolerated by all age groups, even during prolonged use. Rarely, oral irritation or sensitization may occur. Nausea has been reported occasionally during therapy.
Large oral doses of nystatin have occasionally produced diarrhea, gastrointestinal distress, nausea and vomiting. Rash, including urticaria, has been reported rarely. Stevens-Johnson syndrome has been reported very rarely.

OVERDOSAGE
Oral doses of nystatin in excess of five million units daily have caused nausea and gastrointestinal upset. There have been no reports of serious toxic effects or superinfections (see CLINICAL PHARMACOLOGY, Pharmacokinetics).

DOSAGE AND ADMINISTRATION
Children and Adults: The recommended dose is one or two pastilles (200,000 or 400,000 units nystatin) four or five times daily for as long as 14 days if necessary. The dosage regimen should be continued for at least 48 hours after disappearance of oral symptoms.
Dosage should be discontinued if symptoms persist after the initial 14 day period of treatment (see PRECAUTIONS, Laboratory Tests).
Administration: Pastilles must be allowed to dissolve slowly in the mouth, and should not be chewed or swallowed whole.

HOW SUPPLIED
Mycostatin (nystatin) Pastilles, 200,000 units nystatin each, in packages containing 30 pleasant-tasting pastilles (NDC 0003-0543-20).

ALSO AVAILABLE
Mycostatin (Nystatin, USP) is also available as a ready-to-use oral suspension, oral tablets, vaginal tablets, and topical powder, cream, and ointment (see package inserts accompanying those products for complete information).
Storage
Refrigerate between 2° and 8°C (36° and 46°F).
Manufactured by Ernest Jackson & Co., Ltd.
Crediton, Devon, England
(P9297-01)
April 1992

PARAPLATIN®   ℞
[păr-a-plătin]
(carboplatin for injection)

CAUTION: FEDERAL LAW PROHIBITS DISPENSING WITHOUT A PRESCRIPTION.

> **WARNING**
> PARAPLATIN® (carboplatin for injection) should be administered under the supervision of a qualified physician experienced in the use of cancer chemotherapeutic agents. Appropriate management of therapy and complications is possible only when adequate treatment facilities are readily available.
> Bone marrow suppression is dose related and may be severe, resulting in infection and/or bleeding. Anemia may be cumulative and may require transfusion support. Vomiting is another frequent drug-related side effect.
> Anaphylactic-like reactions to PARAPLATIN have been reported and may occur within minutes of PARAPLATIN administration. Epinephrine, corticosteroids, and antihistamines have been employed to alleviate symptoms.

DESCRIPTION
PARAPLATIN® (carboplatin for injection) is supplied as a sterile, lyophilized white powder available in single-dose vials containing 50 mg, 150 mg, and 450 mg of carboplatin for administration by intravenous infusion. Each vial contains equal parts by weight of carboplatin and mannitol.
Carboplatin is a platinum coordination compound that is used as a cancer chemotherapeutic agent. The chemical name for carboplatin is platinum, diammine [1,1-cyclobutane-dicarboxylato(2-)-0,0']-, (SP-4-2), and has the following structural formula:

Carboplatin is a crystalline powder with the molecular formula of $C_6H_{12}N_2O_4Pt$ and a molecular weight of 371.25. It is soluble in water at a rate of approximately 14 mg/mL, and the pH of a 1% solution is 5-7. It is virtually insoluble in ethanol, acetone, and dimethylacetamide.

CLINICAL PHARMACOLOGY
Carboplatin, like cisplatin, produces predominantly interstrand DNA cross-links rather than DNA-protein cross-links. This effect is apparently cell-cycle nonspecific. The aquation of carboplatin, which is thought to produce the active species, occurs at a slower rate than in the case of cisplatin. Despite this difference, it appears that both carboplatin and cisplatin induce equal numbers of drug-DNA cross-links, causing equivalent lesions and biological effects. The differences in potencies for carboplatin and cisplatin appear to be directly related to the difference in aquation rates.
In patients with creatinine clearances of about 60 mL/min or greater, plasma levels of intact carboplatin decay in a biphasic manner after a 30-minute intravenous infusion of 300 to 500 mg/m² of PARAPLATIN. The initial plasma half-life (alpha) was found to be 1.1 to 2 hours (N = 6), and the postdistribution plasma half-life (beta) was found to be 2.6 to 5.9 hours (N = 6). The total body clearance, apparent volume of distribution and mean residence time for carboplatin are 4.4 L/hour, 16 L and 3.5 hours, respectively. The C_{max} values and areas under the plasma concentration vs time curves from 0 to infinity (AUC inf) increase linearly with dose, although the increase was slightly more than dose proportional. Carboplatin, therefore, exhibits linear pharmacokinetics over the dosing range studied (300-500 mg/m²).
Carboplatin is not bound to plasma proteins. No significant quantities of protein-free, ultrafilterable platinum-containing species other than carboplatin are present in plasma. However, platinum from carboplatin becomes irreversibly bound to plasma proteins and is slowly eliminated with a minimum half-life of 5 days.
The major route of elimination of carboplatin is renal excretion. Patients with creatinine clearances of approximately 60 mL/min or greater excrete 65% of the dose in the urine within 12 hours and 71% of the dose within 24 hours. All of the platinum in the 24-hour urine is present as carboplatin. Only 3 to 5% of the administered platinum is excreted in the urine between 24 and 96 hours. There are insufficient data to determine whether biliary excretion occurs.
In patients with creatinine clearances below 60 mL/min the total body and renal clearances of carboplatin decrease as the creatinine clearance decreases. PARAPLATIN dosages should therefore be reduced in these patients (See "DOSAGE AND ADMINISTRATION" section).

CLINICAL STUDIES
Use with cyclophosphamide for initial treatment of ovarian cancer: In two prospectively randomized, controlled studies conducted by the National Cancer Institute of Canada, Clinical Trials Group (NCIC) and the Southwest Oncology Group (SWOG), 789 chemotherapy naive patients with advanced ovarian cancer were treated with PARAPLATIN or cisplatin, both in combination with cyclophosphamide, every 28 days for six courses before surgical reevaluation. The following results were obtained from both studies:

COMPARATIVE EFFICACY

Overview of Pivotal Trials

	NCIC	SWOG
Number of patients randomized	447	342
Median age (years)	60	62
Dose of cisplatin	75 mg/m²	100 mg/m²
Dose of carboplatin	300 mg/m²	300 mg/m²
Dose of Cytoxan	600 mg/m²	600 mg/m²
Residual tumor < 2 cm (number of patients)	39% (174/447)	14% (49/342)

Clinical Response in Measurable Disease Patients

	NCIC	SWOG
Carboplatin (number of patients)	60% (48/80)	58% (49/83)
Cisplatin (number of patients)	58% (49/85)	43% (33/76)
95% C.I. of difference (Carboplatin - Cisplatin)	(−13.9%, 18.6%)	(−2.3%, 31.1%)

Pathologic Complete Response*

	NCIC	SWOG
Carboplatin (number of patients)	11% (24/224)	10% (17/171)
Cisplatin (number of patients)	15% (33/223)	10% (17/171)
95% C.I. of difference (Carboplatin - Cisplatin)	(−10.7%, 2.5%)	(−6.9%, 6.9%)

---

* 114 PARAPLATIN and 109 Cisplatin patients did not undergo second look surgery in NCIC study, 90 PARAPLATIN and 106 Cisplatin patients did not undergo second look surgery in SWOG study

Progression-Free Survival (PFS)

	NCIC	SWOG
Median		
Carboplatin	59 weeks	49 weeks
Cisplatin	61 weeks	47 weeks
2-year PFS*		
Carboplatin	31%	21%
Cisplatin	31%	21%
95% C.I. of difference (Carboplatin - Cisplatin)	(−9.3, 8.7)	(−9.0, 9.4)
3-year PFS*		
Carboplatin	19%	8%
Cisplatin	23%	14%
95% C.I. of difference (Carboplatin - Cisplatin)	(−11.5, 4.5)	(−14.1, 0.3)
Hazard Ratio**	1.10	1.02
95% C.I. (Carboplatin - Cisplatin)	(0.89, 1.35)	(0.81, 1.29)

---

*Kaplan-Meier Estimates
Unrelated deaths occurring in the absence of progression were counted as events (progression) in this analysis.
**Analysis adjusted for factors found to be of prognostic significance were consistent with unadjusted analysis.

Survival

	NCIC	SWOG
Median		
Carboplatin	110 weeks	86 weeks
Cisplatin	99 weeks	79 weeks
2-year Survival*		
Carboplatin	51.9%	40.2%
Cisplatin	48.4%	39.0%
95% C.I. of difference (Carboplatin - Cisplatin)	(−6.2, 13.2)	(−9.8, 12.2)
3-year Survival*		
Carboplatin	34.6%	18.3%
Cisplatin	33.1%	24.9%
95% C.I. of difference (Carboplatin - Cisplatin)	(−7.7, 10.7)	(−15.9, 2.7)
Hazard Ratio**	0.98	1.01
95% C.I. (Carboplatin - Cisplatin)	(0.78, 1.23)	(0.78, 1.30)

---

*Kaplan-Meier Estimates
**Analysis adjusted for factors found to be of prognostic significance were consistent with unadjusted analysis.

COMPARATIVE TOXICITY
The pattern of toxicity exerted by the PARAPLATIN (carboplatin for injection)-containing regimen was significantly different from that of the cisplatin-containing combinations. Differences between the two studies may be explained by different cisplatin dosages and by different supportive care. The PARAPLATIN-containing regimen induced significantly more thrombocytopenia and, in one study, significantly more leukopenia and more need for transfusional support. The cisplatin-containing regimen produced significantly more anemia in one study. However, no significant differences occurred in incidences of infections and hemorrhagic episodes.
Non-hematologic toxicities (emesis, neurotoxicity, ototoxicity, renal toxicity, hypomagnesemia, and alopecia) were significantly more frequent in the cisplatin-containing arms. [See table at top of next page]
[See table at bottom of page 791]
Use as a single agent for secondary treatment of advanced ovarian cancer:
In two prospective, randomized controlled studies in patients with advanced ovarian cancer previously treated with chemotherapy, PARAPLATIN (carboplatin for injection) achieved six clinical complete responses in 47 patients. The duration of these responses ranged from 45 to 71+ weeks.

INDICATIONS
Initial treatment of advanced ovarian carcinoma: PARAPLATIN is indicated for the initial treatment of advanced ovarian carcinoma in established combination with other approved chemotherapeutic agents. One established combination regimen consists of PARAPLATIN and cyclophosphamide (CYTOXAN®). Two randomized controlled studies conducted by the NCIC and SWOG with PARAPLATIN vs. cisplatin, both in combination with cyclophosphamide, have demonstrated equivalent overall survival between the two groups (see "CLINICAL STUDIES" section).
There is limited statistical power to demonstrate equivalence in overall pathologic complete response rates and long term survival (≥ 3 years) because of the small number of

Continued on next page

Paraplatin—Cont.

patients with these outcomes: the small number of patients with residual tumor < 2 cm after initial surgery also limits the statistical power to demonstrate equivalence in this subgroup.

Secondary treatment of advanced ovarian carcinoma: PARAPLATIN is indicated for the palliative treatment of patients with ovarian carcinoma recurrent after prior chemotherapy, including patients who have been previously treated with cisplatin.

Within the group of patients previously treated with cisplatin, those who have developed progressive disease while receiving cisplatin therapy may have a decreased response rate.

CONTRAINDICATIONS

PARAPLATIN is contraindicated in patients with a history of severe allergic reactions to cisplatin or other platinum-containing compounds, or mannitol.

PARAPLATIN should not be employed in patients with severe bone marrow depression or significant bleeding.

WARNINGS

Bone marrow suppression (leukopenia, neutropenia, and thrombocytopenia) is dose-dependent and is also the dose-limiting toxicity. Peripheral blood counts should be frequently monitored during PARAPLATIN treatment and, when appropriate, until recovery is achieved. Median nadir occurs at day 21 in patients receiving single-agent PARAPLATIN. In general, single intermittent courses of PARAPLATIN should not be repeated until leukocyte, neutrophil, and platelet counts have recovered.

Since anemia is cumulative, transfusions may be needed during treatment with PARAPLATIN, particularly in patients receiving prolonged therapy.

Bone marrow suppression is increased in patients who have received prior therapy, especially regimens including cisplatin. Marrow suppression is also increased in patients with impaired kidney function. Initial PARAPLATIN dosages in these patients should be appropriately reduced (See "DOSAGE AND ADMINISTRATION" section) and blood counts should be carefully monitored between courses. The use of PARAPLATIN in combination with other bone marrow suppressing therapies must be carefully managed with respect to dosage and timing in order to minimize additive effects. PARAPLATIN has limited nephrotoxic potential, but concomitant treatment with aminoglycosides has resulted in increased renal and/or audiologic toxicity, and caution must be exercised when a patient receives both drugs.

PARAPLATIN can induce emesis, which can be more severe in patients previously receiving emetogenic therapy. The incidence and intensity of emesis have been reduced by using premedication with antiemetics. Although no conclusive efficacy data exist with the following schedules of PARAPLATIN, lengthening the duration of single intravenous administration to 24 hours or dividing the total dose over five consecutive daily pulse doses has resulted in reduced emesis.

Although peripheral neurotoxicity is infrequent, its incidence is increased in patients older than 65 years and in patients previously treated with cisplatin. Pre-existing cisplatin-induced neurotoxicity does not worsen in about 70% of the patients receiving PARAPLATIN as secondary treatment.

Loss of vision, which can be complete for light and colors, has been reported after the use of PARAPLATIN (carboplatin for injection) with doses higher than those recommended in the package insert. Vision appears to recover totally or to a significant extent within weeks of stopping these high doses.

As in the case of other platinum coordination compounds, allergic reactions to PARAPLATIN have been reported. These may occur within minutes of administration and should be managed with appropriate supportive therapy.

High dosages of PARAPLATIN (more than four times the recommended dose) have resulted in severe abnormalities of liver function tests.

PARAPLATIN may cause fetal harm when administered to a pregnant woman. PARAPLATIN has been shown to be embryotoxic and teratogenic in rats. There are no adequate and well-controlled studies in pregnant women. If this drug is used during pregnancy, or if the patient becomes pregnant while receiving this drug, the patient should be apprised of the potential hazard to the fetus. Women of childbearing potential should be advised to avoid becoming pregnant.

PRECAUTIONS

General: Needles or intravenous administration sets containing aluminum parts that may come in contact with PARAPLATIN should not be used for the preparation or administration of the drug. Aluminum can react with carboplatin causing precipitate formation and loss of potency.

Drug interactions: The renal effects of nephrotoxic compounds may be potentiated by PARAPLATIN.

ADVERSE EXPERIENCES IN PATIENTS WITH OVARIAN CANCER NCIC STUDY

		PARAPLATIN Arm Percent*	Cisplatin Arm Percent*	P-Values**
Bone Marrow				
Thrombocytopenia,	<100,000/mm³	70	29	<0.001
	<50,000/mm³	41	6	<0.001
Neutropenia,	<2,000 cells/mm³	97	96	n.s.
	<1,000 cells/mm³	81	79	n.s.
Leukopenia,	<4,000 cells/mm³	98	97	n.s.
	<2,000 cells/mm³	68	52	0.001
Anemia,	<11 g/dL	91	91	n.s.
	<8 g/dL	18	12	n.s.
Infections		14	12	n.s.
Bleeding		10	4	n.s.
Transfusions		42	31	0.018
Gastrointestinal				
Nausea and vomiting		93	98	0.010
Vomiting		84	97	<0.001
Other GI side effects		50	62	0.013
Neurologic				
Peripheral neuropathies		16	42	<0.001
Ototoxicity		13	33	<0.001
Other sensory side effects		6	10	n.s.
Central neurotoxicity		28	40	0.009
Renal				
Serum creatinine elevations		5	13	0.006
Blood urea elevations		17	31	<0.001
Hepatic				
Bilirubin elevations		5	3	n.s.
SGOT elevations		17	13	n.s.
Alkaline phosphatase elevations		–	–	–
Electrolytes loss				
Sodium		10	20	0.005
Potassium		16	22	n.s.
Calcium		16	19	n.s.
Magnesium		63	88	<0.001
Other side effects				
Pain		36	37	n.s.
Asthenia		40	33	n.s.
Cardiovascular		15	19	n.s.
Respiratory		8	9	n.s.
Allergic		12	9	n.s.
Genitourinary		10	10	n.s.
Alopecia+		50	62	0.017
Mucositis		10	9	n.s.

* Values are in percent of evaluable patients
**n.s. = not significant, p > 0.05
+ May have been affected by cyclophosphamide dosage delivered

Carcinogenesis, mutagenesis, impairment of fertility: The carcinogenic potential of carboplatin has not been studied, but compounds with similar mechanisms of action and mutagenicity profiles have been reported to be carcinogenic. Carboplatin has been shown to be mutagenic both *in vitro* and *in vivo*. It has also been shown to be embryotoxic and teratogenic in rats receiving the drug during organogenesis.

Pregnancy: Pregnancy "Category D". (See "**WARNINGS**" section.)

Nursing mothers: It is not known whether carboplatin is excreted in human milk. Because there is a possibility of toxicity in nursing infants secondary to PARAPLATIN treatment of the mother, it is recommended that breast-feeding be discontinued if the mother is treated with PARAPLATIN.

Pediatric Use: Safety and effectiveness in pediatric patients have not been established.

ADVERSE REACTIONS

For a comparison of toxicities when carboplatin or cisplatin was given in combination with cyclophosphamide, see the "**COMPARATIVE TOXICITY**" subsection of the "**CLINICAL STUDIES**" section.

[See table at top of page 792]

In the narrative section that follows, the incidences of adverse events are based on data from 1,893 patients with various types of tumors who received PARAPLATIN as single-agent therapy.

Hematologic toxicity: Bone marrow suppression is the dose-limiting toxicity of PARAPLATIN. Thrombocytopenia with platelet counts below 50,000/mm³ occurs in 25% of the patients (35% of pretreated ovarian cancer patients); neutropenia with granulocyte counts below 1,000/mm³ occurs in 16% of the patients (21% of pretreated ovarian cancer patients); leukopenia with WBC counts below 2,000/mm³ occurs in 15% of the patients (26% of pretreated ovarian cancer patients). The nadir usually occurs about day 21 in patients receiving single-agent therapy. By day 28, 90% of patients have platelet counts above 100,000/mm³; 74% have neutrophil counts above 2,000/mm³; 67% have leukocyte counts above 4,000/mm³.

Marrow suppression is usually more severe in patients with impaired kidney function. Patients with poor performance status have also experienced a higher incidence of severe leukopenia and thrombocytopenia.

The hematologic effects, although usually reversible, have resulted in infectious or hemorrhagic complications in 5% of the patients treated with PARAPLATIN (carboplatin for injection), with drug related death occurring in less than 1% of the patients. Fever has also been reported in patients with neutropenia.

Anemia with hemoglobin less than 11 g/dL has been observed in 71% of the patients who started therapy with a baseline above that value. The incidence of anemia increases with increasing exposure to PARAPLATIN. Transfusions have been administered to 26% of the patients treated with PARAPLATIN (44% of previously treated ovarian cancer patients).

Bone marrow depression may be more severe when PARAPLATIN is combined with other bone marrow suppressing drugs or with radiotherapy.

Gastrointestinal toxicity: Vomiting occurs in 65% of the patients (81% of previously treated ovarian cancer patients) and in about one-third of these patients it is severe. Carboplatin, as a single agent or in combination, is significantly less emetogenic than cisplatin; however, patients previously treated with emetogenic agents, especially cisplatin, appear to be more prone to vomiting. Nausea alone occurs in an additional 10 to 15% of patients. Both nausea and vomiting usually cease within 24 hours of treatment and are often responsive to antiemetic measures. Although no conclusive efficacy data exist with the following schedules, prolonged administration of PARAPLATIN, either by continuous 24-hour infusion or by daily pulse doses given for five consecutive days, was associated with less severe vomiting than the single dose intermittent schedule. Emesis was increased when PARAPLATIN was used in combination with other emetogenic compounds. Other gastrointestinal effects observed frequently were pain, in 17% of the patients; diarrhea, in 6%; and constipation, also in 6%.

Neurologic toxicity: Peripheral neuropathies have been observed in 4% of the patients receiving PARAPLATIN (6% of pretreated ovarian cancer patients) with mild paresthe-

sias occurring most frequently. Carboplatin therapy produces significantly fewer and less severe neurologic side effects than does therapy with cisplatin. However, patients older than 65 years and/or previously treated with cisplatin appear to have an increased risk (10%) for peripheral neuropathies. In 70% of the patients with pre-existing cisplatin-induced peripheral neurotoxicity, there was no worsening of symptoms during therapy with PARAPLATIN. Clinical ototoxicity and other sensory abnormalities such as visual disturbances and change in taste have been reported in only 1% of the patients. Central nervous system symptoms have been reported in 5% of the patients and appear to be most often related to the use of antiemetics.

Although the overall incidence of peripheral neurologic side effects induced by PARAPLATIN is low, prolonged treatment, particularly in cisplatin pretreated patients, may result in cumulative neurotoxicity.

Nephrotoxicity: Development of abnormal renal function test results is uncommon, despite the fact that carboplatin, unlike cisplatin, has usually been administered without high-volume fluid hydration and/or forced diuresis. The incidences of abnormal renal function tests reported are 6% for serum creatinine and 14% for blood urea nitrogen (10% and 22%, respectively, in pretreated ovarian cancer patients). Most of these reported abnormalities have been mild and about one-half of them were reversible.

Creatinine clearance has proven to be the most sensitive measure of kidney function in patients receiving PARAPLATIN, and it appears to be the most useful test for correlating drug clearance and bone marrow suppression. Twenty-seven percent of the patients who had a baseline value of 60 mL/min or more demonstrated a reduction below this value during PARAPLATIN therapy.

Hepatic toxicity: The incidences of abnormal liver function tests in patients with normal baseline values were reported as follows: total bilirubin, 5%; SGOT, 15%; and alkaline phosphatase, 24%; (5%, 19%, and 37%, respectively, in pretreated ovarian cancer patients). These abnormalities have generally been mild and reversible in about one-half of the cases, although the role of metastatic tumor in the liver may complicate the assessment in many patients. In a limited series of patients receiving very high dosages of PARAPLATIN and autologous bone marrow transplantation, severe abnormalities of liver function tests were reported.

Electrolyte changes: The incidences of abnormally decreased serum electrolyte values reported were as follows: sodium, 29%; potassium, 20%; calcium, 22%; and magnesium, 29%; (47%, 28%, 31%, and 43%, respectively, in pretreated ovarian cancer patients). Electrolyte supplementation was not routinely administered concomitantly with PARAPLATIN, and these electrolyte abnormalities were rarely associated with symptoms.

Allergic reactions: Hypersensitivity to PARAPLATIN has been reported in 2% of the patients. These allergic reactions have been similar in nature and severity to those reported with other platinum-containing compounds, i.e., rash, urticaria, erythema, pruritus, and rarely bronchospasm and hypotension. These reactions have been successfully managed with standard epinephrine, corticosteroid, and antihistamine therapy.

Other events: Pain and asthenia were the most frequently reported miscellaneous adverse effects; their relationship to the tumor and to anemia was likely. Alopecia was reported (3%). Cardiovascular, respiratory, genitourinary, and mucosal side effects have occurred in 6% or less of the patients. Cardiovascular events (cardiac failure, embolism, cerebrovascular accidents) were fatal in less than 1% of the patients and did not appear to be related to chemotherapy. Cancer-associated hemolytic uremic syndrome has been reported rarely.

OVERDOSAGE

There is no known antidote for PARAPLATIN overdosage. The anticipated complications of overdosage would be secondary to bone marrow suppression and/or hepatic toxicity.

DOSAGE AND ADMINISTRATION

NOTE: **Aluminum reacts with carboplatin causing precipitate formation and loss of potency, therefore, needles or intravenous sets containing aluminum parts that may come in contact with the drug must not be used for the preparation or administration of PARAPLATIN.**

Single agent therapy: PARAPLATIN, as a single agent, has been shown to be effective in patients with recurrent ovarian carcinoma at a dosage of 360 mg/m² I.V. on day 1 every 4 weeks (Alternatively see **Formula Dosing**). In general, however, single intermittent courses of PARAPLATIN should not be repeated until the neutrophil count is at least 2,000 and the platelet count is at least 100,000.

Combination therapy with cyclophosphamide: In the chemotherapy of advanced ovarian cancer, an effective combination for previously untreated patients consists of:
PARAPLATIN-300 mg/m² I.V. on day 1 every 4 weeks for six cycles (Alternatively see **Formula Dosing**).
Cyclophosphamide (CYTOXAN®)-600 mg/m² I.V. on day 1 every 4 weeks for six cycles. For directions regarding the use and administration of cyclophosphamide (CYTOXAN®), please refer to its package insert. (See "**CLINICAL STUDIES**" section).
Intermittent courses of PARAPLATIN in combination with cyclophosphamide should not be repeated until the neutrophil count is at least 2,000 and the platelet count is at least 100,000.

Dose Adjustment Recommendations: Pretreatment platelet count and performance status are important prognostic factors for severity of myelosuppression in previously treated patients.
The suggested dose adjustments for single agent or combination therapy shown in the table below are modified from controlled trials in previously treated and untreated patients with ovarian carcinoma. Blood counts were done weekly, and the recommendations are based on the lowest post-treatment platelet or neutrophil value.

Platelets	Neutrophils	Adjusted Dose* (From Prior Course)
>100,000	>2,000	125%
50-100,000	500-2,000	No Adjustment
<50,000	<500	75%

* Percentages apply to PARAPLATIN (carboplatin for injection) as a single agent or to both PARAPLATIN and cyclophosphamide in combination. In the controlled studies, dosages were also adjusted at a lower level (50 to 60%) for severe myelosuppression. Escalations above 125% were not recommended for these studies.

PARAPLATIN is usually administered by an infusion lasting 15 minutes or longer. No pre- or post-treatment hydration or forced diuresis is required.

Patients with impaired kidney function: Patients with creatinine clearance values below 60 mL/min are at increased risk of severe bone marrow suppression. In renally-impaired patients who received single agent PARAPLATIN therapy, the incidence of severe leukopenia, neutropenia, or thrombocytopenia has been about 25% when the dosage modifications in the table below have been used.

Baseline Creatinine Clearance	Recommended Dose on Day 1
41-59 mL/min	250 mg/m²
16-40 mL/min	200 mg/m²

The data available for patients with severely impaired kidney function (creatinine clearance below 15 mL/min) are too limited to permit a recommendation for treatment.[1,2]
These dosing recommendations apply to the initial course of treatment. Subsequent dosages should be adjusted according to the patient's tolerance based on the degree of bone marrow suppression.

Formula Dosing: Another approach for determining the initial dose of PARAPLATIN is the use of mathematical formulae, which are based on a patient's pre-existing renal function[3-5] or renal function and desired platelet nadir.[6] Renal excretion is the major route of elimination for carboplatin. (see "**CLINICAL PHARMACOLOGY**" section). The use of dosing formulae, as compared to empirical dose calculation based on body surface area, allows compensation for patient variations in pretreatment renal function that might otherwise result in either underdosing (in patients with above average renal function) or overdosing (in patients with impaired renal function).
A simple formula for calculating dosage, based upon a patient's glomerular filtration rate (GFR in mL/min) and PARAPLATIN target area under the concentration versus time curve (AUC in mg/mL•min), has been proposed by Calvert[3-5]. In these studies, GFR was measured by ^{51}Cr-EDTA, which has a good correlation with creatinine clearance[7].

CALVERT FORMULA FOR CARBOPLATIN DOSING

Total Dose (mg)=(target AUC) × (GFR + 25)

Note: With the Calvert formula, the total dose of PARAPLATIN is calculated in mg, **not** mg/m².

ADVERSE EXPERIENCES IN PATIENTS WITH OVARIAN CANCER SWOG STUDY

		PARAPLATIN Arm Percent*	Cisplatin Arm Percent*	P-Values**
Bone Marrow				
Thrombocytopenia,	<100,000/mm³	59	35	<0.001
	<50,000/mm³	22	11	0.006
Neutropenia,	<2,000 cells/mm³	95	97	n.s.
	<1,000 cells/mm³	84	78	n.s.
Leukopenia,	<4,000 cells/mm³	97	97	n.s.
	<2,000 cells/mm³	76	67	n.s.
Anemia,	<11 g/dL	88	87	n.s.
	<8 g/dL	8	24	<0.001
Infections		18	21	n.s.
Bleeding		6	4	n.s.
Transfusions		25	33	n.s.
Gastrointestinal				
Nausea and vomiting		94	96	n.s.
Vomiting		82	91	0.007
Other GI side effects		40	48	n.s.
Neurologic				
Peripheral neuropathies		13	28	0.001
Ototoxicity		12	30	<0.001
Other sensory side effects		4	6	n.s.
Central neurotoxicity		23	29	n.s.
Renal				
Serum creatinine elevations		7	38	<0.001
Blood urea elevations		–	–	–
Hepatic				
Bilirubin elevations		5	3	n.s.
SGOT elevations		23	16	n.s.
Alkaline phosphatase elevations		29	20	n.s.
Electrolytes loss				
Sodium		–	–	–
Potassium		–	–	–
Calcium		–	–	–
Magnesium		58	77	<0.001
Other side effects				
Pain		54	52	n.s.
Asthenia		43	46	n.s.
Cardiovascular		23	30	n.s.
Respiratory		12	11	n.s.
Allergic		10	11	n.s.
Genitourinary		11	13	n.s.
Alopecia+		43	57	0.009
Mucositis		6	11	n.s.

* Values are in percent of evaluable patients
**n.s. = not significant, p>0.05
+ May have been affected by cyclophosphamide dosage delivered

Continued on next page

Paraplatin—Cont.

The target AUC of 4-6 mg/mL•min using single agent PARAPLATIN appears to provide the most appropriate dose range in previously treated patients[4]. This study also showed a trend between the AUC of single agent PARAPLATIN administered to previously treated patients and the likelihood of developing toxicity[1].

% Actual Toxicity in Previously Treated Patients

AUC (mg/mL•min)	Gr 3 or Gr 4 Thrombocytopenia	Gr 3 or Gr 4 Leukopenia
4 to 5	16%	13%
6 to 7	33%	34%

PREPARATION OF INTRAVENOUS SOLUTIONS

Immediately before use, the content of each vial must be reconstituted with either Sterile Water for Injection, USP, 5% Dextrose in Water (D_5W), or 0.9% Sodium Chloride Injection, USP, according to the following schedule:

Vital Strength	Diluent Volume
50 mg	5 mL
150 mg	15 mL
450 mg	45 mL

These dilutions all produce a carboplatin concentration of 10 mg/mL.

PARAPLATIN can be further diluted to concentrations as low as 0.5 mg/mL with 5% Dextrose in Water (D_5W) or 0.9% Sodium Chloride Injection, USP.

STABILITY

Unopened vials of PARAPLATIN for Injection are stable for the life indicated on the package when stored at controlled room temperature 15°–30°C (59°–86°F), and protected from light.

When prepared as directed, PARAPLATIN solutions are stable for 8 hours at room temperature (25°C). Since no antibacterial preservative is contained in the formulation, it is recommended that PARAPLATIN solutions be discarded 8 hours after dilution.

Parenteral drug products should be inspected visually for particulate matter and discoloration prior to administration.

HOW SUPPLIED

NDC	
0015-3213-30	50 mg vials, individually cartoned, shelf packs of 10 cartons, 10 shelf packs per case. (Yellow flip-off seals)
NDC 0015-3214-30	150 mg vials, individually cartoned, shelf packs of 10 cartons, 10 shelf packs per case. (Violet flip-off seals)
NDC 0015-3215-30	450 mg vials, individually cartoned, shelf packs of 6 cartons, 10 shelf packs per case. (Blue flip-off seals)

STORAGE

Store the unopened vials at controlled room temperature 15°–30°C (59°–86°F). Protect unopened vials from light. Solutions for infusion should be discarded 8 hours after preparation.

HANDLING AND DISPOSAL

Procedures for proper handling and disposal of anti-cancer drugs should be considered. Several guidelines on this subject have been published.[8–14] There is no general agreement that all of the procedures recommended in the guidelines are necessary or appropriate.

REFERENCES

1. Egorin MJ, et al: Pharmacokinetics and Dosage Reduction of cis-diamine(1,1-cyclobutanedicarboxylato) Platinum in Patients with Impaired Renal Function. Cancer Res 1984; 44:5432-5438.
2. Carboplatin, Etoposide, and Bleomycin for Treatment of Stage IIC Seminoma Complicated by Acute Renal Failure. Cancer Treatment Reports, Vol. 71, No. 11, pp. 1123-1124, November 1987.
3. Calvert AH, et al: Carboplatin dosage: Prospective evaluation of a simple formula based on renal function. J Clin Oncol. 1989; 7:1748-1756.
4. Jodrell DI, et al: Relationships between carboplatin exposure and tumor response and toxicity in patients with ovarian cancer. J Clin Oncol. 1992; 10:520-528.
5. Sorensen BT, et al: Dose-toxicity relationship of carboplatin in combination with cyclophosphamide in ovarian cancer patients. Cancer Chemother Pharmacol. 1991; 28:397-401.
6. Egorin MJ, et al: Prospective validation of a pharmacologically based dosing scheme for the cis-diam-minedichloroplatinum (II) analogue diamminecyclobutanedicarboxylatoplatinum. Cancer Res. 1985; 45:6502-6506.
7. Daugaard G, et al: Effects of cisplatin on different measures of glomerular function in the human kidney with special emphasis on high-dose. Cancer Chemother Pharmacol. 1988; 21:163-167.
8. Recommendations for the Safe Handling of Parenteral Antineoplastic Drugs. NIH Publication No. 83-2621. For sale by the Superintendent of Documents, US Government Printing Office, Washington, DC 20402.
9. AMA Council Report. Guidelines for Handling Parenteral Antineoplastics. JAMA 1985; 253(11):1590-1592.
10. National Study Commission on Cytotoxic Exposure—Recommendations for Handling Cytotoxic Agents. Available from Louis P. Jeffrey, ScD, Chairman, National Study Commission on Cytotoxic Exposure, Massachusetts College of Pharmacy and Allied Health Sciences, 179 Longwood Avenue, Boston, Massachusetts 02115.
11. Clinical Oncological Society of Australia: Guidelines and Recommendations for Safe Handling of Antineoplastic Agents. Med J Australia 1983; 1:426-428.
12. Jones RB, et al: Safe Handling of Chemotherapeutic Agents: A Report from the Mount Sinai Medical Center. CA-A Cancer Journal for Clinicians 1983; (Sept/Oct) 258-263.
13. American Society of Hospital Pharmacists Technical Assistance Bulletin on Handling Cytotoxic and Hazardous Drugs. Am J Hosp Pharm 1990; 47:1033-1049.
14. Controlling occupational exposure to hazardous drugs. (OSHA WORK PRACTICE GUIDELINES). Am J Health-Syst Pharm 1996; 53:1669-1685.

U.S. Patent Nos. 4,140,707
4,657,927

ADVERSE EXPERIENCES IN PATIENTS WITH OVARIAN CANCER

		First Line Combination Therapy* Percent	Second Line Single Agent Therapy** Percent
Bone Marrow			
Thrombocytopenia,	<100,000/mm^3	66	62
	<50,000/mm^3	33	35
Neutropenia,	<2,000 cells/mm^3	96	67
	<1,000 cells/mm^3	82	21
Leukopenia,	<4,000 cells/mm^3	97	85
	<2,000 cells/mm^3	71	26
Anemia,	<11 /dL	90	90
	<8 g/dL	14	21
Infections		16	5
Bleeding		8	5
Transfusions		35	44
Gastrointestinal			
Nausea and vomiting		93	92
Vomiting		83	81
Other GI side effects		46	21
Neurologic			
Peripheral neuropathies		15	6
Ototoxicity		12	1
Other sensory side effects		5	1
Central neurotoxicity		26	5
Renal			
Serum creatinine elevations		6	10
Blood urea elevations		17	22
Hepatic			
Bilirubin elevations		5	5
SGOT elevations		20	19
Alkaline phosphatase elevations		29	37
Electrolytes loss			
Sodium		10	47
Potassium		16	28
Calcium		16	31
Magnesium		61	43
Other side effects			
Pain		44	23
Asthenia		41	11
Cardiovascular		19	6
Respiratory		10	6
Allergic		11	2
Genitourinary		10	2
Alopecia		49	2
Mucositis		8	1

* **Use with cyclophosphamide for initial treatment of ovarian cancer:** Data are based on the experience of 393 patients with ovarian cancer (regardless of baseline status) who received initial combination therapy with PARAPLATIN and cyclophosphamide in two randomized controlled studies conducted by SWOG and NCIC (see **"CLINICAL STUDIES"** section). Combination with cyclophosphamide as well as duration of treatment may be responsible for the differences that can be noted in the adverse experience table.

****Single agent use for the secondary treatment of ovarian cancer:** Data are based on the experience of 553 patients with previously treated ovarian carcinoma (regardless of baseline status) who received single-agent PARAPLATIN.

BRISTOL LABORATORIES®
ONCOLOGY PRODUCTS
A Bristol-Myers Squibb Company
Princeton, NJ 08543
U.S.A.
K2-B001-12-96   3213DIM-O9
51-002473-01   Revised December 1996
Shown in Product Identification Guide, page 308

PLATINOL®   ℞

[plă 'tĭ-nŏl]
(cisplatin for injection, USP)

CAUTION: FEDERAL LAW PROHIBITS DISPENSING WITHOUT PRESCRIPTION.

> **WARNING**
> PLATINOL® (cisplatin for injection, USP) should be administered under the supervision of a qualified physician experienced in the use of cancer chemotherapeutic agents. Appropriate management of therapy and complications is possible only when adequate diagnostic and treatment facilities are readily available.
> Cumulative renal toxicity associated with PLATINOL is severe. Other major dose-related toxicities are myelosuppression, nausea, and vomiting.
> Ototoxicity, which may be more pronounced in children, and is manifested by tinnitus, and/or loss of high frequency hearing and occasionally deafness, is significant.
> *Anaphylactic-like* reactions to PLATINOL have been reported. Facial edema, bronchoconstriction, tachycardia, and hypotension may occur within minutes of PLATINOL administration. Epinephrine, corticoster-

oids, and antihistamines have been effectively employed to alleviate symptoms (see **"Warnings"** and **"Adverse Reactions"** sections).

Exercise caution to prevent inadvertent PLATINOL overdose. Doses greater than 100 mg/m²/cycle once every 3 to 4 weeks are rarely used. Care must be taken to avoid inadvertent PLATINOL overdose due to confusion with PARAPLATIN® (carboplatin for injection) or prescribing practices that fail to differentiate daily doses from total dose per cycle.

DESCRIPTION

PLATINOL® (cisplatin for injection, USP) (cis-diamminedichloroplatinum) is a heavy metal complex containing a central atom of platinum surrounded by two chloride atoms and two ammonia molecules in the cis position. It is a white to light yellow lyophilized powder with the molecular formula Pt $Cl_2H_6N_2$, and a molecular weight of 300.1. It is soluble in water or saline at 1 mg/mL and in dimethylformamide at 24 mg/mL. It has a melting point of 207°C. Each vial of PLATINOL contains either 10 mg cisplatin, 90 mg Sodium Chloride, USP, and 100 mg Mannitol, USP or 50 mg cisplatin, 450 mg Sodium Chloride, USP, and 500 mg Mannitol, USP.

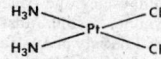

CLINICAL PHARMACOLOGY

Plasma concentrations of the parent compound, cisplatin, decay monoexponentially with a half-life of about 20 to 30 minutes following bolus administrations of 50 or 100 mg/m² doses. Monoexponential decay and plasma half-lives of about 0.5 hour are also seen following two hour or seven hour infusions of 100 mg/m². After the latter, the total-body clearances and volumes of distribution at steady-state for cisplatin are about 15 to 16 L/h/m² and 11 to 12 L/m².

Due to its unique chemical structure, the chlorine atoms of cisplatin are more subject to chemical displacement reactions by nucleophiles, such as water or sulfhydryl groups, than to enzyme-catalyzed metabolism. At physiological pH in the presence of 0.1M NaCl, the predominant molecular species are cisplatin and monohydroxymonochloro cis-diammine platinum (II) in nearly equal concentrations. The latter, combined with the possible direct displacement of the chlorine atoms by sulfhydryl groups of amino acids or proteins, accounts for the instability of cisplatin in biological matrices. The ratios of cisplatin to total free (ultrafilterable) platinum in the plasma vary considerably between patients and range from 0.5 to 1.1 after a dose of 100 mg/m².

Cisplatin does not undergo the instantaneous and reversible binding to plasma proteins that is characteristic of normal drug-protein binding. However, the platinum from cisplatin, but not cisplatin itself, becomes bound to several plasma proteins including albumin, transferrin, and gamma globulin. Three hours after a bolus injection and two hours after the end of a three-hour infusion, 90% of the plasma platinum is protein bound. The complexes between albumin and the platinum from cisplatin do not dissociate to a significant extent and are slowly eliminated with a minimum half-life of five days or more.

Following cisplatin doses of 20 to 120 mg/m², the concentrations of platinum are highest in liver, prostate, and kidney, somewhat lower in bladder, muscle, testicle, pancreas, and spleen and lowest in bowel, adrenal, heart, lung, cerebrum, and cerebellum. Platinum is present in tissues for as long as 180 days after the last administration. With the exception of intracerebral tumors, platinum concentrations in tumors are generally somewhat lower than the concentrations in the organ where the tumor is located. Different metastatic sites in the same patient may have different platinum concentrations. Hepatic metastases have the highest platinum concentrations, but these are similar to the platinum concentrations in normal liver. Maximum red blood cell concentrations of platinum are reached within 90 to 150 minutes after a 100 mg/m² dose of cisplatin and decline in a biphasic manner with a terminal half-life of 36 to 47 days.

Over a dose range of 40 to 140 mg/m² cisplatin given as a bolus injection or as infusions varying in length from 1 hour to 24 hours, from 10% to about 40% of the administered platinum is excreted in the urine in 24 hours. Over five days following administration of 40 to 100 mg/m² doses given as rapid, 2 to 3 hour, or 6 to 8 hour infusions, a mean of 35 to 51% of the dosed platinum is excreted in the urine. Similar mean urinary recoveries of platinum of about 14 to 30% of the dose are found following five daily administrations of 20, 30, or 40 mg/m²/day. Only a small percentage of the administered platinum is excreted beyond 24 hours post-infusion and most of the platinum excreted in the urine in 24 hours is excreted within the first few hours. Platinum-containing species excreted in the urine are the same as those found following the incubation of cisplatin with urine from healthy subjects, except that the proportions are different.

The parent compound, cisplatin, is excreted in the urine and accounts for 13 to 17% of the dose excreted within one hour after administration of 50 mg/m². The mean renal clearance of cisplatin exceeds creatinine clearance and is 62 and 50 mL/min/m² following administration of 100 mg/m² as 2 hour or 6 to 7 hour infusions, respectively.

The renal clearance of free (ultrafilterable) platinum also exceeds the glomerular filtration rate indicating that cisplatin or other platinum-containing molecules are actively secreted by the kidneys. The renal clearance of free platinum is nonlinear and variable and is dependent on dose, urine flow rate, and individual variability in the extent of active secretion and possible tubular reabsorption.

There is a potential for accumulation of ultrafilterable platinum plasma concentrations whenever cisplatin is administered on a daily basis but not when dosed on an intermittent basis.

No significant relationships exist between the renal clearance of either free platinum or cisplatin and creatinine clearance.

Although small amounts of platinum are present in the bile and large intestine after administration of cisplatin, the fecal excretion of platinum appears to be insignificant.

INDICATIONS

PLATINOL (cisplatin for injection, USP) is indicated as therapy to be employed as follows:

Metastatic Testicular Tumors – In established combination therapy with other approved chemotherapeutic agents in patients with metastatic testicular tumors who have already received appropriate surgical and/or radiotherapeutic procedures.

Metastatic Ovarian Tumors – In established combination therapy with other approved chemotherapeutic agents in patients with metastatic ovarian tumors who have already received appropriate surgical and/or radiotherapeutic procedures. An established combination consists of PLATINOL and CYTOXAN (cyclophosphamide). PLATINOL, as a single agent, is indicated as secondary therapy in patients with metastatic ovarian tumors refractory to standard chemotherapy who have not previously received PLATINOL therapy.

Advanced Bladder Cancer – PLATINOL is indicated as a single agent for patients with transitional cell bladder cancer which is no longer amenable to local treatments such as surgery and/or radiotherapy.

CONTRAINDICATIONS

PLATINOL is contraindicated in patients with preexisting renal impairment.

PLATINOL should not be employed in myelosuppressed patients, or patients with hearing impairment.

PLATINOL is contraindicated in patients with a history of allergic reactions to PLATINOL or other platinum-containing compounds.

WARNINGS

PLATINOL produces cumulative nephrotoxicity which is potentiated by aminoglycoside antibiotics. The serum creatinine, BUN, creatinine clearance, and magnesium, sodium, potassium, and calcium levels should be measured prior to initiating therapy, and prior to each subsequent course. At the recommended dosage, PLATINOL should not be given more frequently than once every 3 to 4 weeks (See **"ADVERSE REACTIONS"** section).

There are reports of severe neuropathies in patients in whom regimens are employed using higher doses of PLATINOL or greater dose frequencies than those recommended. These neuropathies may be irreversible and are seen as paresthesias in a stocking-glove distribution, areflexia, and loss of proprioception and vibratory sensation.

Loss of motor function has also been reported.

Anaphylactic-like reactions to PLATINOL have been reported. These reactions have occurred within minutes of administration to patients with prior exposure to PLATINOL, and have been alleviated by administration of epinephrine, corticosteroids, and antihistamines.

Since ototoxicity of PLATINOL is cumulative, audiometric testing should be performed prior to initiating therapy and prior to each subsequent dose of drug (See **"ADVERSE REACTIONS"** section).

PLATINOL can cause fetal harm when administered to a pregnant woman. PLATINOL is mutagenic in bacteria and produces chromosome aberrations in animal cells in tissue culture. In mice PLATINOL is teratogenic and embryotoxic. If this drug is used during pregnancy or if the patient becomes pregnant while taking this drug, the patient should be apprised of the potential hazard to the fetus. Patients should be advised to avoid becoming pregnant.

The carcinogenic effect of PLATINOL was studied in BD IX rats. PLATINOL was administered i.p. to 50 BD IX rats for 3 weeks, 3 × 1 mg/kg body weight per week. Four hundred and fifty-five days after the first application, 33 animals died, 13 of them related to malignancies: 12 leukemias and 1 renal fibrosarcoma.

The development of acute leukemia coincident with the use of PLATINOL has rarely been reported in humans. In these reports, PLATINOL was generally given in combination with other leukemogenic agents.

PRECAUTIONS

Peripheral blood counts should be monitored weekly. Liver function should be monitored periodically. Neurologic examination should also be performed regularly (See **"ADVERSE REACTIONS"** section).

Drug Interactions – Plasma levels of anticonvulsant agents may become subtherapeutic during cisplatin therapy.

In a randomized trial in advanced ovarian cancer, response duration was adversely affected when pyridoxine was used in combination with altretamine (hexamethylmelamine) and PLATINOL.[1]

Carcinogenesis, Mutagenesis, Impairment of Fertility – See "WARNINGS" section.

Pregnancy—"Category D". (See **"WARNINGS"** section.)

Pediatric Use—Safety and effectiveness in pediatric patients have not been established.

ADVERSE REACTIONS

Nephrotoxicity – Dose-related and cumulative renal insufficiency is the major dose-limiting toxicity of PLATINOL. Renal toxicity has been noted in 28 to 36% of patients treated with a single dose of 50 mg/m². It is first noted during the second week after a dose and is manifested by elevations in BUN and creatinine, serum uric acid and/or a decrease in creatinine clearance. **Renal toxicity becomes more prolonged and severe with repeated courses of the drug. Renal function must return to normal before another dose of PLATINOL can be given.**

Impairment of renal function has been associated with renal tubular damage. The administration of PLATINOL using a 6- to 8-hour infusion with intravenous hydration, and mannitol has been used to reduce nephrotoxicity. However, renal toxicity still can occur after utilization of these procedures.

Ototoxicity – Ototoxicity has been observed in up to 31% of patients treated with a single dose of PLATINOL 50 mg/m², and is manifested by tinnitus and/or hearing loss in the high frequency range (4,000 to 8,000 Hz). Decreased ability to hear normal conversational tones may occur occasionally. Deafness after the initial dose of PLATINOL has been reported rarely. Ototoxic effects may be more severe in children receiving PLATINOL. Hearing loss can be unilateral or bilateral and tends to become more frequent and severe with repeated doses. Ototoxicity may be enhanced with prior or simultaneous cranial irradiation. It is unclear whether PLATINOL induced ototoxicity is reversible. Ototoxic effects may be related to the peak plasma concentration of PLATINOL. Careful monitoring of audiometry should be performed prior to initiation of therapy and prior to subsequent doses of PLATINOL.

Vestibular toxicity has also been reported.

Ototoxicity may become more severe in patients being treated with other drugs with nephrotoxic potential.

Hematologic – Myelosuppression occurs in 25 to 30% of patients treated with PLATINOL. The nadirs in circulating platelets and leukocytes occur between days 18 to 23 (range 7.5 to 45) with most patients recovering by day 39 (range 13 to 62). Leukopenia and thrombocytopenia are more pronounced at higher doses (>50 mg/m²). Anemia (decrease of 2 g hemoglobin/100 mL) occurs at approximately the same frequency and with the same timing as leukopenia and thrombocytopenia. Fever and infection have been reported in patients with neutropenia.

In addition to anemia secondary to myelosuppression, a Coombs' positive hemolytic anemia has been reported. In the presence of cisplatin hemolytic anemia, a further course of treatment may be accompanied by increased hemolysis and this risk should be weighed by the treating physician. The development of acute leukemia coincident with the use of PLATINOL has rarely been reported in humans. In these reports, PLATINOL was generally given in combination with other leukemogenic agents.

Gastrointestinal – Marked nausea and vomiting occur in almost all patients treated with PLATINOL, and are occasionally so severe that the drug must be discontinued. Nausea and vomiting usually begin within 1 to 4 hours after treatment and last up to 24 hours. Various degrees of vomiting, nausea and/or anorexia may persist for up to 1 week after treatment.

Delayed nausea and vomiting (begins or persists 24 hours or more after chemotherapy) has occurred in patients attaining complete emetic control on the day of PLATINOL (cisplatin for injection, USP) therapy.

Diarrhea has also been reported.

OTHER TOXICITIES

Vascular toxicities coincident with the use of PLATINOL in combination with other antineoplastic agents have been reported rarely. The events are clinically heterogeneous and may include myocardial infarction, cerebrovascular accident, thrombotic microangiopathy (HUS), or cerebral arteritis. Various mechanisms have been proposed for these vascular complications. There are also reports of Raynaud's phenomenon occurring in patients treated with the combi-

Continued on next page

Platinol—Cont.

nation of bleomycin, vinblastine with or without PLATINOL. It has been suggested that hypomagnesemia developing coincident with the use of PLATINOL may be an added, although not essential, factor associated with this event. However, it is currently unknown if the cause of Raynaud's phenomenon in these cases is the disease, underlying vascular compromise, bleomycin, vinblastine, hypomagnesemia, or a combination of any of these factors.

Serum Electrolyte Disturbances – Hypomagnesemia, hypocalcemia, hyponatremia, hypokalemia, and hypophosphatemia have been reported to occur in patients treated with PLATINOL and are probably related to renal tubular damage. Tetany has occasionally been reported in those patients with hypocalcemia and hypomagnesemia. Generally, normal serum electrolyte levels are restored by administering supplemental electrolytes and discontinuing PLATINOL. Inappropriate antidiuretic hormone syndrome has also been reported.

Hyperuricemia – Hyperuricemia has been reported to occur at approximately the same frequency as the increases in BUN and serum creatinine.

It is more pronounced after doses greater than 50 mg/m^2, and peak levels of uric acid generally occur between 3 to 5 days after the dose. Allopurinol therapy for hyperuricemia effectively reduces uric acid levels.

Neurotoxicity (See "WARNINGS" section)– Neurotoxicity, usually characterized by peripheral neuropathies, has been reported. The neuropathies usually occur after prolonged therapy (4 to 7 months); however, neurologic symptoms have been reported to occur after a single dose. Although symptoms and signs of PLATINOL neuropathy usually develop during treatment, symptoms of neuropathy may begin 3 to 8 weeks after the last dose of PLATINOL, although this is rare. PLATINOL therapy should be discontinued when the symptoms are first observed. The neuropathy, however, may progress further even after stopping treatment. Preliminary evidence suggests peripheral neuropathy may be irreversible in some patients.

Lhermitte's sign, dorsal column myelopathy, and autonomic neuropathy have also been reported.

Loss of taste and seizures have also been reported.

Muscle cramps, defined as localized, painful, involuntary skeletal muscle contractions of sudden onset and short duration, have been reported and were usually associated in patients receiving a relatively high cumulative dose of PLATINOL and with a relatively advanced symptomatic stage of peripheral neuropathy.

Ocular Toxicity – Optic neuritis, papilledema, and cerebral blindness have been reported infrequently in patients receiving standard recommended doses of PLATINOL. Improvement and/or total recovery usually occurs after discontinuing PLATINOL. Steroids with or without mannitol have been used; however, efficacy has not been established.

Blurred vision and altered color perception have been reported after the use of regimens with higher doses of PLATINOL or greater dose frequencies than those recommended in the package insert. The altered color perception manifests as a loss of color discrimination, particularly in the blue-yellow axis. The only finding on funduscopic exam is irregular retinal pigmentation of the macular area.

Anaphylactic-like Reactions – Anaphylactic-like reactions have been occasionally reported in patients previously exposed to PLATINOL. The reactions consist of facial edema, wheezing, tachycardia, and hypotension within a few minutes of drug administration. Reactions may be controlled by intravenous epinephrine with corticosteroids and/or antihistamines as indicated. Patients receiving PLATINOL should be observed carefully for possible anaphylactic-like reactions and supportive equipment and medication should be available to treat such a complication.

Hepatotoxicity – Transient elevations of liver enzymes, especially SGOT, as well as bilirubin, have been reported to be associated with PLATINOL administration at the recommended doses.

Other Events – Other toxicities reported to occur infrequently are cardiac abnormalities, hiccups, elevated serum amylase, and rash. Alopecia has also been reported.

Local soft tissue toxicity has rarely been reported following extravasation of PLATINOL. Severity of the local tissue toxicity appears to be related to the concentration of the PLATINOL solution. Infusion of solutions with a PLATINOL concentration greater than 0.5 mg/mL may result in tissue cellulitis, fibrosis, and necrosis.

OVERDOSAGE

Caution should be exercised to prevent inadvertent overdosage with PLATINOL. Acute overdosage with this drug may result in kidney failure, liver failure, deafness, ocular toxicity (including detachment of the retina), significant myelosuppression, intractable nausea and vomiting and/or neuritis. In addition, death can occur following overdosage. No proven antidotes have been established for PLATINOL overdosage. Hemodialysis, even when initiated four hours after the overdosage, appears to have little effect on remov-

ing platinum from the body because of PLATINOL's rapid and high degree of protein binding. Management of overdosage should include general supportive measures to sustain the patient through any period of toxicity that may occur.

DOSAGE AND ADMINISTRATION

Note: Needles or intravenous sets containing aluminum parts that may come in contact with PLATINOL should not be used for preparation or administration. Aluminum reacts with PLATINOL, causing precipitate formation and a loss of potency.

Metastatic Testicular Tumors – The usual PLATINOL dose for the treatment of testicular cancer in combination with other approved chemotherapeutic agents is 20 mg/m^2 I.V. daily for 5 days per cycle.

Metastatic Ovarian Tumors – The usual PLATINOL dose for the treatment of metastatic ovarian tumors in combination with CYTOXAN (cyclophosphamide) is 75–100 mg/m^2 I.V. per cycle once every 4 weeks, (Day 1).[2,3]

The dose of CYTOXAN when used in combination with PLATINOL is 600 mg/m^2 I.V. once every 4 weeks, (Day 1).[2,3] For directions for the administration of CYTOXAN, refer to the CYTOXAN package insert.

In combination therapy, PLATINOL and CYTOXAN are administered sequentially.

As a single agent, PLATINOL should be administered at a dose of 100 mg/m^2 I.V. per cycle once every 4 weeks.

Advanced Bladder Cancer – PLATINOL should be administered as a single agent at a dose of 50–70 mg/m^2 I.V. per cycle once every 3 to 4 weeks depending on the extent of prior exposure to radiation therapy and/or prior chemotherapy. For heavily pre-treated patients an initial dose of 50 mg/m^2 per cycle repeated every 4 weeks is recommended.

Pretreatment hydration with 1 to 2 liters of fluid infused for 8 to 12 hours prior to a PLATINOL (cisplatin for injection, USP) dose is recommended. The drug is then diluted in 2 liters of 5% Dextrose in 1/2 or 1/3 normal saline containing 37.5 g of mannitol, and infused over a 6- to 8-hour period. If diluted solution is not to be used within 6 hours, protect solution from light. Adequate hydration and urinary output must be maintained during the following 24 hours.

A repeat course of PLATINOL should not be given until the serum creatinine is below 1.5 mg/100 mL, and/or the BUN is below 25 mg/100 mL. A repeat course should not be given until circulating blood elements are at an acceptable level (platelets ≥ 100,000/mm^3, WBC ≥ 4,000/mm^3). Subsequent doses of PLATINOL should not be given until an audiometric analysis indicates that auditory acuity is within normal limits.

As with other potentially toxic compounds, caution should be exercised in handling the powder and preparing the solution of cisplatin. Skin reactions associated with accidental exposure to cisplatin may occur. The use of gloves is recommended. If cisplatin powder or solution contacts the skin or mucosae, immediately wash the skin or mucosae thoroughly with soap and water.

PREPARATION OF INTRAVENOUS SOLUTIONS

The 10 and 50 mg vials should be reconstituted with 10 mL or 50 mL of Sterile Water for Injection, USP, respectively. Each mL of the resulting solution will contain 1 mg of PLATINOL.

Reconstitution as recommended results in a clear, colorless to slight yellow solution.

The reconstituted solution should be used intravenously only and should be administered by I.V. infusion over a 6- to 8-hour period. (See "DOSAGE AND ADMINISTRATION.")

NOTE TO PHARMACIST: Exercise caution to prevent inadvertent PLATINOL overdosage. Please call prescriber if dose greater than 100 mg/m^2 per cycle. Aluminum and flip-off seal of vial have been imprinted with the following statement: **CALL DR. IF DOSE>100 MG/M^2/CYCLE.**

STABILITY

Unopened vials of dry powder are stable for the lot life indicated on the package when stored at room temperature (27°C).

The reconstituted solution is stable for 20 hours at room temperature (27°C). Solution removed from the amber vial should be protected from light if it is not to be used within six hours.

Important Note: Once reconstituted, the solution should be kept at room temperature (27°C). If the reconstituted solution is refrigerated, a precipitate will form.

Procedures for proper handling and disposal of anticancer drugs should be considered. Several guidelines on this subject have been published.[4–10] There is no general agreement that all of the procedures recommended in the guidelines are necessary or appropriate.

HOW SUPPLIED

PLATINOL® (cisplatin for injection, USP)

NDC 0015-3070-20—Each amber vial contains 10 mg of cisplatin

NDC 0015-3070-20—Each amber vial contains 50 mg of cisplatin

REFERENCES

1. Wiernik PH: Hexamethylmelamine and Low or Moderate Dose Cisplatin With or Without Pyridoxine for Treatment of Advanced Ovarian Carcinoma: A Study of the Eastern Oncology Group. Cancer Invest, 1992; 10: 1-9.
2. Alberts DS, et al: Improved Therapeutic Index of Carboplatin Plus Cyclophosphamide verses Cisplatin Plus Cyclophosphamide: Final Report by the Southwest Oncology Group of a Phase III Randomized Trial in Stages III and IV Ovarian Cancer. J Clin Oncol. 1992; 10:706-717.
3. Swenerton K, et al: Cisplatin-Cyclophosphamide verses Carboplatin-Cyclophosphamide in Advanced Ovarian Cancer: A Randomized Phase III Study of the National Cancer Institute of Canada Clinical Trials Group. J Clin Oncol. 1992; 10:718-726.
4. Recommendations for the Safe Handling of Parenteral Antineoplastic Drugs. NIH Publication No. 83-2621. For sale by the Superintendent of Documents, US Government Printing Office, Washington, DC 20402.
5. AMA Council Report. Guidelines for Handling Parenteral Antineo plastics. JAMA 1985; 253(11):1590-1592.
6. National Study Commission on Cytotoxic Exposure — Recommendations for Handling Cytotoxic Agents. Available from Louis P. Jeffrey, ScD, Chairman, National Study Commission on Cytotoxic Exposure. Massachusetts College of Pharmacy and Allied Health Sciences, 179 Longwood Avenue, Boston, Massachusetts 02115.
7. Clinical Oncological Society of Australia. Guidelines and Recommendations for Safe Handling of Antineoplastic Agents. Med J Australia 1983; 1:426-428.
8. Jones RB, et al: Safe Handling of Chemotherapeutic Agents: A Report from the Mount Sinai Medical Center. CA–A Cancer Journal for Clinicians 1983; (Sept/Oct) 258–263.
9. American Society of Hospital Pharmacists Technical Assistance Bulletin on Handling Cytotoxic and Hazardous Drugs. Am J Hosp Pharm 1990; 47:1033–1049.
10. Controlling occupations exposure to hazardous drugs. (OSHA WORK PRACTICE GUIDELINES). Am J Health-Syst Pharm 1996; 53:1669-1685.

BRISTOL LABORATORIES
ONCOLOGY PRODUCTS
A Bristol-Myers Squibb Company
Princeton, NJ 08543
U.S.A.

K3-B001-12-96   3070DIM-37
51-001105-02   Revised December 1996

PLATINOL®-AQ   ℞
[pla-ti-nol-AQ]
(cisplatin injection)

CAUTION: FEDERAL LAW PROHIBITS DISPENSING WITHOUT PRESCRIPTION.

WARNING

PLATINOL®-AQ (cisplatin injection) should be administered under the supervision of a qualified physician experienced in the use of cancer chemotherapeutic agents. Appropriate management of therapy and complications is possible only when adequate diagnostic and treatment facilities are readily available.

Cumulative renal toxicity associated with PLATINOL-AQ is severe. Other major dose-related toxicities are myelosuppression, nausea, and vomiting. Ototoxicity, which may be more pronounced in children, and is manifested by tinnitus, and/or loss of high frequency hearing and occasionally deafness, is significant. *Anaphylactic-like* reactions to PLATINOL-AQ have been reported. Facial edema, bronchoconstriction, tachycardia, and hypotension may occur within minutes of PLATINOL-AQ administration. Epinephrine, corticosteroids, and antihistamines have been effectively employed to alleviate symptoms (see "WARNINGS" and "ADVERSE REACTIONS" sections).

Exercise caution to prevent inadvertent PLATINOL-AQ overdose. Doses greater than 100 mg/m^2/cycle once every 3 to 4 weeks are rarely used. Care must be taken to avoid inadvertent PLATINOL-AQ overdose due to confusion with PARAPLATIN® (carboplatin for injection) or prescribing practices that fail to differentiate daily doses from total dose per cycle.

DESCRIPTION

Cisplatin (cis-diamminedichloroplatinum) is a heavy metal complex containing a central atom of platinum surrounded by two chloride atoms and two ammonia molecules in the cis position. It is a white powder with the molecular formula PtCl$_2$H$_6$N$_2$, and molecular weight of 300.1. It is soluble in water or saline at 1 mg/mL and in dimethylformamide at 24 mg/mL. It has a melting point of 207°C. PLATINOL-AQ (cisplatin injection) is a sterile aqueous solution, each mL con-

taining 1 mg cisplatin and 9 mg sodium chloride. HCl and/or sodium hydroxide added to adjust pH.

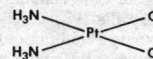

CLINICAL PHARMACOLOGY

Plasma concentrations of the parent compound, cisplatin, decay monoexponentially with a half-life of about 20 to 30 minutes following bolus administrations of 50 or 100 mg/m^2 doses. Monoexponential decay and plasma half-lives of about 0.5 hour are also seen following two hour or seven hour infusions of 100 mg/m^2. After the latter, the total-body clearances and volumes of distribution at steady-state for cisplatin are about 15 to 16 L/h/m^2 and 11 to 12 L/m^2.

Due to its unique chemical structure, the chlorine atoms of cisplatin are more subject to chemical displacement reactions by nucleophiles, such as water or sulfhydryl groups, than to enzyme-catalyzed metabolism. At physiological pH in the presence of 0.1M NaCl, the predominant molecular species are cisplatin and monohydroxymonochloro cis-diammine platinum (II) in nearly equal concentrations. The latter, combined with the possible direct displacement of the chlorine atoms by sulfhydryl groups of amino acids or proteins, accounts for the instability of cisplatin in biological matrices. The ratios of cisplatin to total free (ultrafilterable) platinum in the plasma vary considerably between patients and range from 0.5 to 1.1 after a dose of 100 mg/m^2.

Cisplatin does not undergo the instantaneous and reversible binding to plasma proteins that is characteristic of normal drug-protein binding. However, the platinum from cisplatin, but not cisplatin itself, becomes bound to several plasma proteins including albumin, transferrin, and gamma globulin. Three hours after a bolus injection and two hours after the end of a three-hour infusion, 90% of the plasma platinum is protein bound. The complexes between albumin and the platinum from cisplatin do not dissociate to a significant extent and are slowly eliminated with a minimum half-life of five days or more.

Following cisplatin doses of 20 to 120 mg/m^2, the concentrations of platinum are highest in liver, prostate, and kidney, somewhat lower in bladder, muscle, testicle, pancreas, and spleen and lowest in bowel, adrenal, heart, lung, cerebrum, and cerebellum. Platinum is present in tissues for as long as 180 days after the last administration. With the exception of intracerebral tumors, platinum concentrations in tumors are generally somewhat lower than the concentrations in the organ where the tumor is located. Different metastatic sites in the same patient may have different platinum concentrations. Hepatic metastases have the highest platinum concentrations, but these are similar to the platinum concentrations in normal liver. Maximum red blood cell concentrations of platinum are reached within 90 to 150 minutes after a 100 mg/m^2 dose of cisplatin and decline in a biphasic manner with a terminal half-life of 36 to 47 days.

Over a dose range of 40 to 140 mg cisplatin/m^2 given as a bolus injection or as infusions varying in length from 1 hour to 24 hours, from 10% to about 40% of the administered platinum is excreted in the urine in 24 hours. Over five days following administration of 40 to 100 mg/m^2 doses given as rapid, 2 to 3 hour, or 6 to 8 hour infusions, a mean of 35 to 51% of the dosed platinum is excreted in the urine. Similar mean urinary recoveries of platinum of about 14 to 30% of the dose are found following five daily administrations of 20, 30, or 40 mg/m^2/day. Only a small percentage of the administered platinum is excreted beyond 24 hours post-infusion and most of the platinum excreted in the urine in 24 hours is excreted within the first few hours. Platinum-containing species excreted in the urine are the same as those found following the incubation of cisplatin with urine from healthy subjects, except that the proportions are different. The parent compound, cisplatin, is excreted in the urine and accounts for 13 to 17% of the dose excreted within one hour after administration of 50 mg/m^2. The mean renal clearance of cisplatin exceeds creatinine clearance and is 62 and 50 mL/min/m^2 following administration of 100 mg/m^2 as 2 hour or 6 to 7 hour infusions, respectively.

The renal clearance of free (ultrafilterable) platinum also exceeds the glomerular filtration rate indicating that cisplatin or other platinum-containing molecules are actively secreted by the kidneys. The renal clearance of free platinum is nonlinear and variable and is dependent on dose, urine flow rate, and individual variability in the extent of active secretion and possible tubular reabsorption.

There is a potential for accumulation of ultrafilterable platinum plasma concentrations whenever cisplatin is administered on a daily basis but not when dosed on an intermittent basis.

No significant relationships exist between the renal clearance of either free platinum or cisplatin and creatinine clearance.

Although small amounts of platinum are present in the bile and large intestine after administration of cisplatin, the fecal excretion of platinum appears to be insignificant.

INDICATIONS

PLATINOL-AQ is indicated as therapy to be employed as follows:

Metastatic Testicular Tumors – In established combination therapy with other approved chemotherapeutic agents in patients with metastatic testicular tumors who have already received appropriate surgical and/or radiotherapeutic procedures.

Metastatic Ovarian Tumors – In established combination therapy with other approved chemotherapeutic agents in patients with metastatic ovarian tumors who have already received appropriate surgical and/or radiotherapeutic procedures. An established combination consists of PLATINOL-AQ (cisplatin injection) and CYTOXAN® (cyclophosphamide). PLATINOL-AQ, as a single agent, is indicated as secondary therapy in patients with metastatic ovarian tumors refractory to standard chemotherapy who have not previously received PLATINOL-AQ therapy.

Advanced Bladder Cancer – PLATINOL-AQ is indicated as a single agent for patients with transitional cell bladder cancer which is no longer amenable to local treatments such as surgery and/or radiotherapy.

CONTRAINDICATIONS

PLATINOL-AQ is contraindicated in patients with preexisting renal impairment. PLATINOL-AQ should not be employed in myelosuppressed patients, or patients with hearing impairment.

PLATINOL-AQ is contraindicated in patients with a history of allergic reactions to PLATINOL-AQ or other platinum-containing compounds.

WARNINGS

PLATINOL-AQ produces cumulative nephrotoxicity which is potentiated by aminoglycoside antibiotics. The serum creatinine, BUN, creatinine clearance, and magnesium, sodium, potassium, and calcium levels should be measured prior to initiating therapy, and prior to each subsequent course. At the recommended dosage, PLATINOL-AQ should not be given more frequently than once every 3 to 4 weeks (See **"ADVERSE REACTIONS"**).

There are reports of severe neuropathies in patients in whom regimens are employed using higher doses of PLATINOL-AQ or greater dose frequencies than those recommended. These neuropathies may be irreversible and are seen as paresthesias in a stocking-glove distribution, areflexia, and loss of proprioception and vibratory sensation. Loss of motor function has also been reported.

Anaphylactic-like reactions to PLATINOL-AQ have been reported. These reactions have occurred within minutes of administration to patients with prior exposure to PLATINOL-AQ, and have been alleviated by administration of epinephrine, corticosteroids, and antihistamines.

Since ototoxicity of PLATINOL-AQ is cumulative, audiometric testing should be performed prior to initiating therapy and prior to each subsequent dose of drug (See **"ADVERSE REACTIONS"**).

PLATINOL-AQ can cause fetal harm when administered to a pregnant woman. PLATINOL-AQ is mutagenic in bacteria and produces chromosome aberrations in animal cells in tissue culture. In mice PLATINOL-AQ is teratogenic and embryotoxic. If this drug is used during pregnancy or if the patient becomes pregnant while taking this drug, the patient should be apprised of the potential hazard to the fetus. Patients should be advised to avoid becoming pregnant.

The carcinogenic effect of PLATINOL-AQ was studied in BD IX rats. PLATINOL-AQ was administered i.p. to 50 BD IX rats for 3 weeks, 3 x 1 mg/kg body weight per week. Four hundred and fifty-five days after the first application, 33 animals died, 13 of them related to malignancies: 12 leukemias and 1 renal fibrosarcoma.

The development of acute leukemia coincident with the use of PLATINOL-AQ has rarely been reported in humans. In these reports, PLATINOL-AQ was generally given in combination with other leukemogenic agents.

PRECAUTIONS

Peripheral blood counts should be monitored weekly. Liver function should be monitored periodically. Neurologic examination should also be performed regularly (See **"ADVERSE REACTIONS"**).

Drug Interactions – Plasma levels of anticonvulsant agents may become subtherapeutic during cisplatin therapy.

In a randomized trial in advanced ovarian cancer, response duration was adversely affected when pyridoxine was used in combination with altretamine (hexamethylmelamine) and PLATINOL-AQ.[1]

Carcinogenesis, Mutagenesis, Impairment of Fertility —See **"WARNINGS"** section.

Pregnancy—Pregnancy "Category D". (See **"WARNINGS"** section.)

Pediatric Use—Safety and effectiveness in pediatric patients have not been established.

ADVERSE REACTIONS

Nephrotoxicity – Dose-related and cumulative renal insufficiency is the major dose-limiting toxicity of PLATINOL-AQ. Renal toxicity has been noted in 28 to 36% of patients treated with a single dose of 50 mg/m^2. It is first noted during the second week after a dose and is manifested by elevations in BUN and creatinine, serum uric acid and/or a decrease in creatinine clearance. **Renal toxicity becomes more prolonged and severe with repeated courses of the drug. Renal function must return to normal before another dose of PLATINOL-AQ can be given.**

Impairment of renal function has been associated with renal tubular damage. The administration of PLATINOL-AQ using a 6- to 8-hour infusion with intravenous hydration, and mannitol has been used to reduce nephrotoxicity. However, renal toxicity still can occur after utilization of these procedures.

Ototoxicity – Ototoxicity has been observed in up to 31% of patients treated with a single dose of PLATINOL-AQ 50 mg/m^2, and is manifested by tinnitus and/or hearing loss in the high frequency range (4,000 to 8,000 Hz). Decreased ability to hear normal conversational tones may occur occasionally. Deafness after the initial dose of PLATINOL-AQ has been reported rarely. Ototoxic effects may be more severe in children receiving PLATINOL-AQ. Hearing loss can be unilateral or bilateral and tends to become more frequent and severe with repeated doses. Ototoxicity may be enhanced with prior or simultaneous cranial irradiation. It is unclear whether PLATINOL-AQ induced ototoxicity is reversible. Ototoxic effects may be related to the peak plasma concentration of PLATINOL-AQ. Careful monitoring of audiometry should be performed prior to initiation of therapy and prior to subsequent doses of PLATINOL-AQ.

Vestibular toxicity has also been reported.

Ototoxicity may become more severe in patients being treated with other drugs with nephrotoxic potential.

Hematologic – Myelosuppression occurs in 25 to 30% of patients treated with PLATINOL-AQ. The nadirs in circulating platelets and leukocytes occur between days 18 to 23 (range 7.5 to 45) with most patients recovering by day 39 (range 13 to 62). Leukopenia and thrombocytopenia are more pronounced at higher doses (>50 mg/m^2). Anemia (decrease of 2 g hemoglobin/100 mL) occurs at approximately the same frequency and with the same timing as leukopenia and thrombocytopenia. Fever and infection have also been reported in patients with neutropenia.

In addition to anemia secondary to myelosuppression, a Coombs' positive hemolytic anemia has been reported. In the presence of cisplatin hemolytic anemia, a further course of treatment may be accompanied by increased hemolysis and this risk should be weighed by the treating physician. The development of acute leukemia coincident with the use of PLATINOL-AQ has rarely been reported in humans. In these reports, PLATINOL-AQ was generally given in combination with other leukemogenic agents.

Gastrointestinal – Marked nausea and vomiting occur in almost all patients treated with PLATINOL-AQ, and are occasionally so severe that the drug must be discontinued. Nausea and vomiting usually begin within 1 to 4 hours after treatment and last up to 24 hours. Various degrees of vomiting, nausea and/or anorexia may persist for up to 1 week after treatment.

Delayed nausea and vomiting (begins or persists 24 hours or more after chemotherapy) has occurred in patients attaining complete emetic control on the day of PLATINOL-AQ (cisplatin injection) therapy.

Diarrhea has also been reported.

OTHER TOXICITIES

Vascular toxicities coincident with the use of PLATINOL-AQ in combination with other antineoplastic agents have been reported rarely. The events are clinically heterogeneous and may include myocardial infarction, cerebrovascular accident, thrombotic microangiopathy (HUS), or cerebral arteritis. Various mechanisms have been proposed for these vascular complications. There are also reports of Raynaud's phenomenon occurring in patients treated with the combination of bleomycin, vinblastine with or without PLATINOL-AQ. It has been suggested that hypomagnesemia developing coincident with the use of PLATINOL-AQ may be an added, although not essential, factor associated with this event. However, it is currently unknown if the cause of Raynaud's phenomenon in these cases is the disease, underlying vascular compromise, bleomycin, vinblastine, hypomagnesemia, or a combination of any of these factors.

Serum Electrolyte Disturbances – Hypomagnesemia, hypocalcemia, hyponatremia, hypokalemia, and hypophosphatemia have been reported to occur in patients treated with PLATINOL-AQ and are probably related to renal tubular damage. Tetany has occasionally been reported in those patients with hypocalcemia and hypomagnesemia. Generally, normal serum electrolyte levels are restored by administering supplemental electrolytes and discontinuing PLATINOL-AQ.

Inappropriate antidiuretic hormone syndrome has also been reported.

Continued on next page

Platinol-AQ—Cont.

Hyperuricemia – Hyperuricemia has been reported to occur at approximately the same frequency as the increases in BUN and serum creatinine.

It is more pronounced after doses greater than 50 mg/m^2, and peak levels of uric acid generally occur between 3 to 5 days after the dose. Allopurinol therapy for hyperuricemia effectively reduces uric acid levels.

Neurotoxicity (See **"WARNINGS"** section) – Neurotoxicity, usually characterized by peripheral neuropathies, has been reported. The neuropathies usually occur after prolonged therapy (4 to 7 months); however, neurologic symptoms have been reported to occur after a single dose. Although symptoms and signs of PLATINOL-AQ neuropathy usually develop during treatment, symptoms of neuropathy may begin 3 to 8 weeks after the last dose of PLATINOL-AQ, although this is rare. PLATINOL-AQ therapy should be discontinued when the symptoms are first observed. The neuropathy, however, may progress further even after stopping treatment. Preliminary evidence suggests peripheral neuropathy may be irreversible in some patients.

Lhermitte's sign, dorsal column myelopathy, and autonomic neuropathy have also been reported.

Loss of taste and seizures have also been reported.

Muscle cramps, defined as localized, painful, involuntary skeletal muscle contractions of sudden onset and short duration, have been reported and were usually associated in patients receiving a relatively high cumulative dose of PLATINOL-AQ and with a relatively advanced symptomatic stage of peripheral neuropathy.

Ocular Toxicity – Optic neuritis, papilledema, and cerebral blindness have been reported infrequently in patients receiving standard recommended doses of PLATINOL-AQ. Improvement and/or total recovery usually occurs after discontinuing PLATINOL-AQ. Steroids with or without mannitol have been used; however, efficacy has not been established.

Blurred vision and altered color perception have been reported after the use of regimens with higher doses of PLATINOL-AQ or greater dose frequencies than those recommended in the package insert. The altered color perception manifests as a loss of color discrimination, particularly in the blue-yellow axis. The only finding on funduscopic exam is irregular retinal pigmentation of the macular area.

Anaphylactic-like Reactions – Anaphylactic-like reactions have been occasionally reported in patients previously exposed to PLATINOL-AQ. The reactions consist of facial edema, wheezing, tachycardia, and hypotension within a few minutes of drug administration. Reactions may be controlled by intravenous epinephrine with corticosteroids and/or antihistamines as indicated. Patients receiving PLATINOL-AQ should be observed carefully for possible anaphylactic-like reactions and supportive equipment and medication should be available to treat such a complication.

Hepatotoxicity – Transient elevations of liver enzymes, especially SGOT, as well as bilirubin, have been reported to be associated with PLATINOL-AQ administration at the recommended doses.

Other Events – Other toxicities reported to occur infrequently are cardiac abnormalities, hiccups, elevated serum amylase, and rash. Alopecia has also been reported.

Local soft tissue toxicity has rarely been reported following extravasation of PLATINOL-AQ. Severity of the local tissue toxicity appears to be related to the concentration of the PLATINOL-AQ solution. Infusion of solutions with a PLATINOL-AQ concentration greater than 0.5 mg/mL may result in tissue cellulitis, fibrosis, and necrosis.

OVERDOSAGE

Caution should be exercised to prevent inadvertent overdosage with PLATINOL-AQ. Acute overdosage with this drug may result in kidney failure, liver failure, deafness, ocular toxicity (including detachment of the retina), significant myelosuppression, intractable nausea and vomiting and/or neuritis. In addition, death can occur following overdosage.

No proven antidotes have been established for PLATINOL-AQ overdosage. Hemodialysis, even when initiated four hours after the overdosage, appears to have little effect on removing platinum from the body because of PLATINOL-AQ's rapid and high degree of protein binding. Management of overdosage should include general supportive measures to sustain the patient through any period of toxicity that may occur.

DOSAGE AND ADMINISTRATION

Note: Needles or intravenous sets containing aluminum parts that may come in contact with PLATINOL-AQ should not be used for preparation or administration. Aluminum reacts with PLATINOL-AQ, causing precipitate formation and a loss of potency.

Metastatic Testicular Tumors – The usual PLATINOL-AQ dose for the treatment of testicular cancer in combination with other approved chemotherapeutic agents is 20 mg/m^2 I.V. daily for 5 days per cycle.

Metastatic Ovarian Tumors – The usual PLATINOL-AQ dose for the treatment of metastatic ovarian tumors in combination with CYTOXAN (cyclophosphamide) is 75-100 mg/m^2 I.V. per cycle once every 4 weeks, (Day 1).[2,3]

The dose of CYTOXAN when used in combination with PLATINOL-AQ is 600 mg/m^2 I.V. once every 4 weeks, (Day 1).[2,3]

For directions for the administration of CYTOXAN, refer to the CYTOXAN package insert.

In combination therapy, PLATINOL-AQ and CYTOXAN are administered sequentially.

As a single agent, PLATINOL-AQ should be administered at a dose of 100 mg/m^2 I.V. per cycle once every 4 weeks.

Advanced Bladder Cancer – PLATINOL-AQ should be administered as a single agent at a dose of 50-70 mg/m^2 I.V. per cycle once every 3 to 4 weeks depending on the extent of prior exposure to radiation therapy and/or prior chemotherapy. For heavily pre-treated patients an initial dose of 50 mg/m^2 per cycle repeated every 4 weeks is recommended.

Pretreatment hydration with 1 to 2 liters of fluid infused for 8 to 12 hours prior to a PLATINOL-AQ dose is recommended. The drug is then diluted in 2 liters of 5% Dextrose in 1/2 or 1/3 normal saline containing 37.5 g of mannitol, and infused over a 6- to 8-hour period. If diluted solution is not to be used within 6 hours, protect solution from light. Do not dilute PLATINOL-AQ in just 5% Dextrose Injection. Adequate hydration and urinary output must be maintained during the following 24 hours.

A repeat course of PLATINOL-AQ (cisplatin injection) should not be given until the serum creatinine is below 1.5 mg/100 mL, and/or the BUN is below 25 mg/100 mL. A repeat course should not be given until circulating blood elements are at an acceptable level (platelets $\geq$ 100,000/mm^3, WBC $\geq$ 4,000/mm^3). Subsequent doses of PLATINOL-AQ should not be given until an audiometric analysis indicates that auditory acuity is within normal limits.

As with other potentially toxic compounds, caution should be exercised in handling the aqueous solution. Skin reactions associated with accidental exposure to cisplatin may occur. The use of gloves is recommended. If cisplatin solution contacts the skin or mucosae, immediately wash the skin or mucosae thoroughly with soap and water.

The aqueous solution should be used intravenously only and should be administered by I.V. infusion over a 6- to 8-hour period.

NOTE TO PHARMACIST: Exercise caution to prevent inadvertent PLATINOL-AQ overdosage. Please call prescriber if dose greater than 100 mg/m^2 per cycle. Aluminum and flip-off seal of vial have been imprinted with the following statement: **CALL DR. IF DOSE>100 MG/M^2/CYCLE.**

STABILITY

PLATINOL-AQ (cisplatin injection) is a sterile, multidose vial without preservatives.

Store at 15°C–25°C. Do not refrigerate. Protect unopened container from light.

The cisplatin remaining in the amber vial following initial entry is stable for 28 days protected from light or for 7 days under fluorescent room light.

Procedures for proper handling and disposal of anticancer drugs should be considered. Several guidelines on this subject have been published.[4–10] There is no general agreement that all of the procedures recommended in the guidelines are necessary or appropriate.

HOW SUPPLIED

PLATINOL®-AQ (cisplatin injection)

NDC 0015-3220-22 – Each multidose vial contains 50 mg of cisplatin

NDC 0015-3221-22 – Each multidose vial contains 100 mg of cisplatin

REFERENCES

1. Wiernik PH: Hexamethylmelamine and Low or Moderate Dose Cisplatin With or Without Pyridoxine for Treatment of Advanced Ovarian Carcinoma: A Study of the Eastern Oncology Group. Cancer Invest, 1992; 10: 1-9.
2. Alberts DS, et al: Improved Therapeutic Index of Carboplatin Plus Cyclophosphamide verses Cisplatin Plus Cyclophosphamide: Final Report by the Southwest Oncology Group of a Phase III Randomized Trial in Stages III and IV Ovarian Cancer. J Clin Oncol. 1992; 10:706-717.
3. Swenerton K, et al: Cisplatin-Cyclophosphamide verses Carboplatin-Cyclophosphamide in Advanced Ovarian Cancer: A Randomized Phase III Study of the National Cancer Institute of Canada Clinical Trials Group. J Clin Oncol. 1992; 10:718-726.
4. Recommendations for the Safe Handling of Parenteral Antineoplastic Drugs. NIH Publication No. 83-2621. For sale by the Superintendent of Documents, US Government Printing Office, Washington, DC 20402.
5. AMA Council Report. Guidelines for Handling Parenteral Antineoplastics. JAMA1985; 253(11):1590-1592.
6. National Study Commission on Cytotoxic Exposure – Recommendations for Handling Cytotoxic Agents. Available from Louis P. Jeffrey, ScD, Chairman, National Study Commission on Cytotoxic Exposure. Massachusetts College of Pharmacy and Allied Health Sciences, 179 Longwood Avenue, Boston, Massachusetts 02115.
7. Clinical Oncological Society of Australia. Guidelines and Recommendations for Safe Handling of Antineoplastic Agents. Med J Australia 1983; 1:426-428.
8. Jones RB, et al: Safe Handling of Chemotherapeutic Agents: A Report from the Mount Sinai Medical Center. CA-A Cancer Journal for Clinicians 1983; (Sept/Oct) 258-263.
9. American Society of Hospital Pharmacists Technical Assistance Bulletin on Handling Cytotoxic and Hazardous Drugs. Am J Hosp Pharm 1990; 47:1033-1049.
10. OSHA Work-Practice Guidelines for Personnel Dealing with Cytotoxic (Antineoplastic) Drugs. Am J Hosp Pharm 1986; 43:1193-1204.

BRISTOL LABORATORIES®
ONCOLOGY PRODUCTS
A Bristol-Myers Squibb Company
Princeton, NJ 08543
U.S.A.
K3-B002-9-96 3220DIM-16
51-001108-03 Revised September 1996

Shown in Product Identification Guide, page 308

RUBEX® ℞

[*rū-bex*]
(doxorubicin hydrochloride for injection, USP)

FOR INTRAVENOUS USE ONLY

CAUTION: FEDERAL LAW PROHIBITS DISPENSING WITHOUT PRESCRIPTION.

WARNINGS

1. Severe local tissue necrosis will occur if there is extravasation during administration (see **"DOSAGE AND ADMINISTRATION"** section). Doxorubicin must not be given by the intramuscular or subcutaneous route.
2. Myocardial toxicity manifested in its most severe form by potentially fatal congestive heart failure may occur either during therapy or months to years after termination of therapy. The probability of developing impaired myocardial function based on a combined index of signs, symptoms and decline in left ventricular ejection fraction (LVEF) is estimated to be 1 to 2% at a total cumulative dose of 300 mg/m^2 of doxorubicin, 3 to 5% at a dose of 400 mg/m^2, 5 to 8% at 450 mg/m^2 and 6 to 20% at 500 mg/m^2. The risk of developing CHF increases rapidly with increasing total cumulative doses of doxorubicin in excess of 450 mg/m^2. This toxicity may occur at lower cumulative doses in patients with prior mediastinal irradiation or on concurrent cyclophosphamide therapy or with pre-existing heart disease.
3. Dosage should be reduced in patients with impaired hepatic function.
4. Severe myelosuppression may occur.
5. Doxorubicin should be administered only under the supervision of a physician who is experienced in the use of cancer chemotherapeutic agents.

DESCRIPTION

Doxorubicin is a cytotoxic anthracycline antibiotic isolated from cultures of **Streptomyces peucetius** var. **caesius**. Doxorubicin consists of a naphthacenequinone nucleus linked through a glycosidic bond at ring atom 7 to an amino sugar, daunosamine. Chemically, doxorubicin hydrochloride is: (8S, 10S)-10-[(3-Amino-2,3,6-trideoxy-α-L-*lyxo*-hexopyranosyl)-oxy]-8-glycoloyl-7,8,9,10-tetrahydro-6,8,11-trihydroxy-1-methoxy-5, 12-naphthacenedione hydrochloride [*25316-40-9*].

The structural formula is as follows:

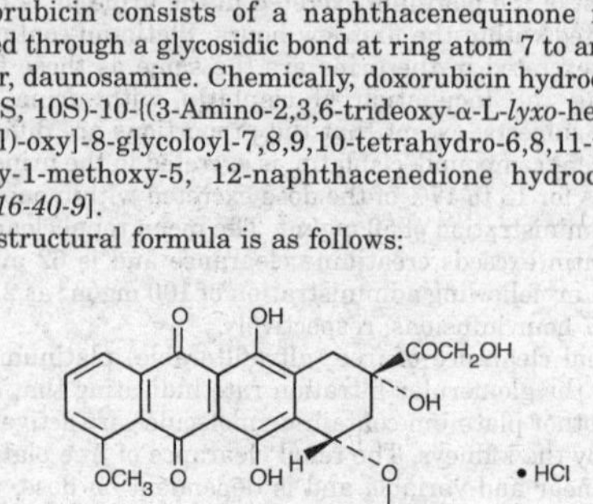

$C_{27}H_{29}NO_{11}$ ·HCl Molecular Weight 579.99

Doxorubicin binds to nucleic acids, presumably by specific intercalation of the planar anthracycline nucleus with the DNA double helix. The anthracycline ring is lipophilic but

the saturated end of the ring system contains abundant hydroxyl groups adjacent to the amino sugar, producing a hydrophilic center. The molecule is amphoteric, containing acidic functions in the ring phenolic groups and a basic function in the sugar amino group. It binds to cell membranes as well as plasma proteins. RUBEX® (doxorubicin hydrochloride for injection, USP) is for intravenous use only. It is available in 50 mg and 100 mg single dose vials as a lyophilized, sterile powder with added lactose (anhydrous), 250 mg and 500 mg, respectively.

CLINICAL PHARMACOLOGY

The cytotoxic effect of doxorubicin on malignant cells and its toxic effects on various organs are thought to be related to nucleotide base intercalation and cell membrane lipid binding activities of doxorubicin. Intercalation inhibits nucleotide replication and action of DNA and RNA polymerases. The interaction of doxorubicin with topoisomerase II to form DNA-cleavable complexes appears to be an important mechanism of doxorubicin cytocidal activity. Doxorubicin cellular membrane binding may effect a variety of cellular functions. Enzymatic electron reduction of doxorubicin by a variety of oxidases, reductases and dehydrogenases generate highly reactive species including the hydroxyl free radical OH^-. Free radical formation has been implicated in doxorubicin cardiotoxicity by means of Cu (II) and Fe (III) reduction at the cellular level.

Animal studies have shown activity in a spectrum of experimental tumors, immunosuppression, carcinogenic properties in rodents, induction of a variety of toxic effects, including delayed and progressive cardiac toxicity, myelosuppression in all species and atrophy to testes in rats and dogs.

Pharmacokinetic studies, determined in patients with various types of tumors undergoing either single or multi-agent therapy, have shown that doxorubicin follows a multiphasic disposition after intravenous injection. The initial distributive half-life of approximately 5.0 minutes suggests rapid tissue uptake of doxorubicin, while its slow elimination from tissues is reflected by a terminal half-life of 20 to 48 hours. Steady-state distribution volumes exceed 20 to 30 L/kg and are indicative of extensive drug uptake into tissues. Plasma clearance is in the range of 8 to 20 mL/min/kg and is predominately by metabolism and biliary excretion. Approximately 40% of the dose appears in the bile in 5 days while only 5 to 12% of the drug and its metabolites appear in the urine during the same time period. Binding of doxorubicin and its major metabolite, doxorubicinol to plasma proteins is about 74 to 76% and is independent of plasma concentration of doxorubicin up to 2 µM. Enzymatic reduction at the 7 position and cleavage of the daunosamine sugar yields aglycones which are accompanied by free radical formation, the local production of which may contribute to the cardiotoxic activity of doxorubicin. Disposition of doxorubicinol (DOX-OL) in patients is formation rate limited. The terminal half-life of DOX-OL is similar to doxorubicin. The relative exposure of DOX-OL, compared to doxorubicin ranges between 0.4 to 0.6. In urine, <3% of the dose was recovered as DOX-OL over 7 days. The literature contains no information regarding gender related differences in the pharmacokinetics of doxorubicin and doxorubicinol.

In four patients dose-independent pharmacokinetics have been shown for doxorubicin in the dose range of 30 to 70 mg/m^2. Systemic clearance of doxorubicin is significantly reduced in obese women with ideal body weight greater than 130%. There was a significant reduction in clearance without any change in volume of distribution in obese patients when compared with normal patients with less than 115% ideal body weight. The clearance of doxorubicin and doxorubicinol was also reduced in patients with impaired hepatic function. Doxorubicin was excreted in the milk of one lactating patient, with peak milk concentration at 24 hours after treatment being approximately 4.4-fold greater than the corresponding plasma concentration. Doxorubicin was detectable in the milk up to 72 hours after therapy with 70 mg/m^2 of doxorubicin given as a 15 minute intravenous infusion and 100 mg/m^2 of cisplatin as a 26 hour intravenous infusion. The peak concentration of doxorubicinol in milk at 24 hours was 0.2 µM and AUC up to 24 hours was 16.5 µM.hr while the AUC for doxorubicin was 9.9 µM.hr. Doxorubicin does not cross the blood brain barrier.

INDICATIONS AND USAGE

RUBEX (doxorubicin hydrochloride for injection, USP) has been used successfully to produce regression in disseminated neoplastic conditions such as acute lymphoblastic leukemia, acute myeloblastic leukemia, Wilms' tumor, neuroblastoma, soft tissue and bone sarcomas, breast carcinoma, ovarian carcinoma, transitional cell bladder carcinoma, thyroid carcinoma, gastric carcinoma, Hodgkin's disease, malignant lymphoma and bronchogenic carcinoma in which the small cell histologic type is the most responsive compared to other cell types.

CONTRAINDICATIONS

Doxorubicin therapy should not be started in patients who have marked myelosuppression induced by previous treatment with other antitumor agents or by radiotherapy. Doxorubicin treatment is contraindicated in patients who received previous treatment with complete cumulative doses of doxorubicin, daunorubicin, idarubicin and/or other anthracyclines and anthracenes.

WARNINGS

Special attention must be given to the cardiotoxicity induced by doxorubicin. Irreversible myocardial toxicity, manifested in its most severe form by life-threatening and potentially fatal congestive heart failure, may occur either during therapy or months to years after termination of therapy. The probability of developing impaired myocardial function, based on a combined index of signs, symptoms and decline in left ventricular ejection fraction (LVEF) is estimated to be 1 to 2% at a total cumulative dose of 300 mg/m^2 of doxorubicin, 3 to 5% at a dose of 400 mg/m^2, 5 to 8% at a dose of 450 mg/m^2 and 6 to 20% at a dose of 500 mg/m^2 given in a schedule of a bolus injection once every 3 weeks. In a retrospective review by Von Hoff *et al*, the probability of developing congestive heart failure was reported to be 5/168 (3%) at a cumulative dose of 430 mg/m^2 of doxorubicin, 8/110 (7%) at 575 mg/m^2 and 3/14 (21%) at 728 mg/m^2. The cumulative incidence of CHF was 2.2%. In a prospective study of doxorubicin in combination with cyclophosphamide, fluorouracil and/or vincristine in patients with breast cancer or small cell lung cancer, the cumulative incidence of congestive heart failure was 5 to 6%. The probability of CHF at various cumulative doses of doxorubicin was 1.5% at 300 mg/m^2, 4.9% at 400 mg/m^2, 7.7% at 450 mg/m^2 and 20.5% at 500 mg/m^2.

Cardiotoxicity may occur at lower doses in patients with prior mediastinal irradiation, concurrent cyclophosphamide therapy and advanced age. Data also suggest that pre-existing heart disease is a co-factor for increased risk of doxorubicin cardiotoxicity. In such cases, cardiac toxicity may occur at doses lower than the respective recommended cumulative dose of doxorubicin. Studies have suggested that concomitant administration of doxorubicin and calcium channel entry blockers may increase the risk of doxorubicin cardiotoxicity. The total dose of doxorubicin administered to the individual patient should also take into account previous or concomitant therapy with related compounds such as daunorubicin, idarubicin and mitoxantrone. Cardiomyopathy and/or congestive heart failure may be encountered several months or years after discontinuation of doxorubicin therapy.

The risk of congestive heart failure and other acute manifestations of doxorubicin cardiotoxicity in children may be as much or lower than in adults. Children appear to be at particular risk for developing delayed cardiac toxicity in that doxorubicin induced cardiomyopathy impairs myocardial growth as children mature, subsequently leading to possible development of congestive heart failure during early adulthood. As many as 40% of children may have subclinical cardiac dysfunction and 5 to 10% of children may develop congestive heart failure on long term follow-up. This late cardiac toxicity may be related to the dose of doxorubicin. The longer the length of follow-up the greater the increase in the detection rate.

Treatment of doxorubicin induced congestive heart failure includes the use of digitalis, diuretics, after load reducers such as angiotensin I converting enzyme (ACE) inhibitors, low salt diet, and bed rest. Such intervention may relieve symptoms and improve the functional status of the patient.

Monitoring Cardiac Function

In adult patients severe cardiac toxicity may occur precipitously without antecedent ECG changes. Cardiomyopathy induced by anthracyclines is usually associated with very characteristic histopathologic changes on an endomyocardial biopsy (EM biopsy), and a decrease of left ventricular ejection fraction (LVEF), as measured by multi-gated radionuclide angiography (MUGA scans) and/or echocardiogram (ECHO), from pretreatment baseline values. However, it has not been demonstrated that monitoring of the ejection fraction will predict when individual patients are approaching their maximally tolerated cumulative dose of doxorubicin. Cardiac function should be carefully monitored during treatment to minimize the risk of cardiac toxicity. A baseline cardiac evaluation with an ECG, LVEF, and /or an echocardiogram (ECHO) is recommended especially in patients with risk factors for increased cardiac toxicity (pre-existing heart disease, mediastinal irradiation, or concurrent cyclophosphamide therapy). Subsequent evaluations should be obtained at a cumulative dose of doxorubicin of at least 400 mg/m^2 and periodically thereafter during the course of therapy. Children are at increased risk for developing delayed cardiotoxicity following doxorubicin administration and therefore a follow-up cardiac evaluation is recommended periodically to monitor for this delayed cardiotoxicity.

In adults, a 10% decline in LVEF to below the lower limit of normal or an absolute LVEF of 45%, or a 20% decline in LVEF at any level is indicative of deterioration in cardiac function. In children, deterioration in cardiac function during or after the completion of therapy with doxorubicin is indicated by a drop in fractional shortening (FS) by an absolute value of ≥ 10 percentile units or below 29%, and a decline in LVEF of 10 percentile units or an LVEF below 55%. In general, if test results indicate deterioration in cardiac function associated with doxorubicin, the benefit of continued therapy should be carefully evaluated against the risk of producing irreversible cardiac damage.

Acute life-threatening arrhythmias have been reported to occur during or within a few hours after doxorubicin administration.

There is a high incidence of bone marrow depression, primarily of leukocytes, requiring careful hematologic monitoring. With the recommended dose schedule, leukopenia is usually transient, reaching its nadir 10 to 14 days after treatment with recovery usually occurring by the 21st day. White blood counts as low as 1000/mm^3 are to be expected during treatment with appropriate doses of doxorubicin. Red blood cell and platelet levels should also be monitored since they may also be depressed. Hematologic toxicity may require dose reduction or suspension or delay of doxorubicin therapy. Persistent severe myelosuppression may result in superinfection or hemorrhage.

Doxorubicin may potentiate the toxicity of other anticancer therapies. Exacerbation of cyclophosphamide induced hemorrhagic cystitis and enhancement of the hepatotoxicity of 6-mercaptopurine have been reported. Radiation induced toxicity to the myocardium, mucosae, skin and liver have been reported to be increased by the administration of doxorubicin.

Since metabolism and excretion of doxorubicin occurs predominantly by the hepatobiliary route, toxicity to recommended doses of doxorubicin can be enhanced by hepatic impairment, therefore, prior to the individual dosing, evaluation of hepatic function is recommended using conventional laboratory tests such as SGOT, SGPT, alkaline phosphatase and bilirubin (see "**DOSAGE AND ADMINISTRATION**" section).

Necrotizing colitis manifested by typhlitis (cecal inflammation), bloody stools and severe and sometimes fatal infections have been associated with a combination of doxorubicin given by I.V. push daily for 3 days and cytarabine given by continuous infusion daily for 7 or more days.

On intravenous administration of doxorubicin, extravasation may occur with or without an accompanying stinging or burning sensation, even if blood returns well on aspiration of the infusion needle (see "**DOSAGE AND ADMINISTRATION**" section). If any signs or symptoms of extravasation have occurred, the injection or infusion should be immediately terminated and restarted in another vein.

Pregnancy "Category D" – Safe use of doxorubicin in pregnancy has not been established. Doxorubicin is embryotoxic and teratogenic in rats and embryotoxic and abortifacient in rabbits. There are no adequate and well-controlled studies in pregnant women. If doxorubicin is to be used during pregnancy, or if the patient becomes pregnant during therapy, the patient should be apprised of the potential hazard to the fetus. Women of childbearing age should be advised to avoid becoming pregnant.

PRECAUTIONS

General – Doxorubicin is not an anti-microbial agent.

Information for Patients – RUBEX (doxorubicin hydrochloride for injection, USP) imparts a red coloration to the urine for 1 to 2 days after administration, and patients should be advised to expect this during active therapy.

Drug Interactions – Literature contain the following drug interactions with doxorubicin in humans: cyclosporine (Sandimmune) may induce coma and/or seizures, phenobarbital increases the elimination of doxorubicin, phenytoin levels may be decreased by doxorubicin, streptozocin (Zanosar) may inhibit the hepatic metabolism, and administration of live vaccines to immunosuppressed patients, including those undergoing cytotoxic chemotherapy, may be hazardous. Information on other potential drug interactions may be found in the literature.

Laboratory Tests – Initial treatment with doxorubicin requires observation of the patient and periodic monitoring of complete blood counts, hepatic function tests, and radionuclide left ventricular ejection fraction (See "**WARNINGS**" section).

Like other cytotoxic drugs, doxorubicin may induce "tumor lysis syndrome" and hyperuricemia in patients with rapidly growing tumors. Appropriate supportive and pharmacologic measures may prevent or alleviate this complication.

Carcinogenesis, Mutagenesis, Impairment of Fertility – Formal long-term carcinogenicity studies have not been conducted with doxorubicin. Doxorubicin and related compounds have been shown to have mutagenic and carcinogenic properties when tested in experimental models (including bacterial systems, mammalian cells in culture, and female Sprague-Dawley rats).

The possible adverse effect on fertility in males and females in humans or experimental animals have not been adequately evaluated. Testicular atrophy was observed in rats and dogs.

Continued on next page

Rubex—Cont.

A variant of chemotherapy-related acute non-lymphocytic leukemia has been reported to occur infrequently a few years after multiple drug treatment of some neoplasms, which sometimes included doxorubicin. The exact role of doxorubicin has not been elucidated.

Pregnancy "Category D". (See "**WARNINGS**" section.)

Nursing Mothers: Because of the potential for serious adverse reactions in nursing infants from doxorubicin, mothers should be advised to discontinue nursing during doxorubicin therapy.

ADVERSE REACTIONS

Dose-limiting toxicities of therapy are myelosuppression and cardiotoxicity. Other reactions reported are:

Cardiotoxicity – (See "**WARNINGS**" section.)

Cutaneous – Reversible complete alopecia occurs in most cases. Hyperpigmentation of nailbeds and dermal creases, primarily in children, and onycholysis have been reported in a few cases. Recall of skin reaction due to prior radiotherapy has occurred with doxorubicin administration.

Gastrointestinal – Acute nausea and vomiting occurs frequently and may be severe. This may be alleviated by antiemetic therapy. Mucositis (stomatitis and esophagitis) may occur 5 to 10 days after administration. The effect may be severe leading to ulceration and represents a site of origin for severe infections. The dosage regimen consisting of administration of doxorubicin on three successive days results in greater incidence and severity of mucositis. Ulceration and necrosis of the colon, especially the cecum, may occur leading to bleeding or severe infections which can be fatal. This reaction has been reported in patients with acute nonlymphocytic leukemia treated with a 3-day course of doxorubicin combined with cytarabine. Anorexia and diarrhea have been occasionally reported.

Vascular – Phlebosclerosis has been reported especially when small veins are used or a single vein is used for repeated administration. Facial flushing may occur if the injection is given too rapidly.

Local – Severe cellulitis, vesication and tissue necrosis will occur if extravasation of doxorubicin occurs during administration. Erythematous streaking along the vein proximal to the site of the injection has been reported (see "**DOSAGE AND ADMINISTRATION**" section).

Hematologic – The occurrence of secondary acute myeloid leukemia with or without a preleukemic phase has been reported rarely in patients concurrently treated with doxorubicin in association with DNA-damaging antineoplastic agents. Such cases could have a short (1–3 years) latency period.

Hypersensitivity – Fever, chills and urticaria have been reported occasionally. Anaphylaxis may occur. A case of apparent cross sensitivity to lincomycin has been reported.

Other – Conjunctivitis and lacrimation occur rarely.

OVERDOSAGE

Acute overdosage with doxorubicin enhances the toxic effects of mucositis, leukopenia and thrombocytopenia. Treatment of acute overdosage consists of treatment of the severely myelosuppressed patient with hospitalization, antimicrobials, platelet transfusions and symptomatic treatment of mucositis. Use of hemopoietic growth factor (G-CSF, GM-CSF) may be considered.

Cumulative dosage with doxorubicin increases the risk of cardiomyopathy and resultant congestive heart failure (See "**WARNINGS**" section). Treatment consists of vigorous management of congestive heart failure with digitalis preparations, diuretics, and after load reducers such as ACE inhibitors.

DOSAGE AND ADMINISTRATION

Care in the administration of doxorubicin hydrochloride will reduce the chance of perivenous infiltration (See "**WARNINGS**" section). It may also decrease the chance of local reactions such as urticaria and erythematous streaking. On intravenous administration of doxorubicin, extravasation may occur with or without an accompanying burning or stinging sensation, even if blood returns well on aspiration of the infusion needle. If any signs or symptoms of extravasation have occurred, the injection or infusion should be immediately terminated and restarted in another vein. If extravasation is suspected, intermittent application of ice to the site for 15 min., q.i.d. × 3 days may be useful. The benefit of local administration of drugs has not been clearly established. Because of the progressive nature of extravasation reactions, close observation and plastic surgery consultation is recommended. Blistering, ulceration and/or persistent pain are indications for wide excision surgery, followed by split-thickness skin grafting.[1]

The most commonly used dose schedule when used as a single agent is 60 to 75 mg/m^2 as a single intravenous injection administered at 21-day intervals. The lower dosage should be given to patients with inadequate marrow reserves due to old age, or prior therapy, or neoplastic marrow infiltration. RUBEX has been used concurrently with other approved chemotherapeutic agents. Evidence is available that in some types of neoplastic disease combination chemotherapy is superior to single agents. The benefits and risks of such therapy continue to be elucidated. When used in combination with other chemotherapy drugs, the most commonly used dosage of doxorubicin is 40 to 50 mg/m^2 given as a single intravenous injection every 21 to 28 days. Doxorubicin dosage must be reduced in case of hyperbilirubinemia as follows:

Plasma bilirubin concentrate (mg/dL)	Dosage reduction (%)
1.2-3.0	50
3.1-5.0	75

Reconstitution Directions – RUBEX (doxorubicin hydrochloride for injection, USP) 50 mg and 100 mg vials should be reconstituted with 25 mL and 50 mL, respectively, of Sodium Chloride Injection, USP (0.9%) to give a final concentration of 2 mg/mL of doxorubicin hydrochloride. An appropriate volume of air should be withdrawn from the vial during reconstitution to avoid excessive pressure buildup. Bacteriostatic diluents are not recommended.

After adding the diluent, the vial should be shaken and the contents allowed to dissolve. The reconstituted solution is stable for 7 days at room temperature and 15 days under refrigeration 2°–8°C (36°–46°F). It should be protected from exposure to sunlight and any unused solution should be discarded.

It is recommended that doxorubicin be slowly administered into the tubing of a freely running intravenous infusion of Sodium Chloride Injection, USP or 5% Dextrose Injection, USP. The tubing should be attached to a Butterfly® needle inserted preferably into a large vein. If possible, avoid veins over joints or in extremities with compromised venous or lymphatic drainage. The rate of administration is dependent on the size of the vein and the dosage. However, the dose should be administered in not less than 3 to 5 minutes. Local erythematous streaking along the vein as well as facial flushing may be indicative of too rapid an administration. A burning or stinging sensation may be indicative of perivenous infiltration and the infusion should be immediately terminated and restarted in another vein. Perivenous infiltration may occur painlessly.

Doxorubicin should not be mixed with heparin or fluorouracil since it has been reported that these drugs are incompatible to the extent that a precipitate may form. Until specific compatibility data are available, it is not recommended that doxorubicin be mixed with other drugs.

Parenteral drug products should be inspected visually for particulate matter and discoloration prior to administration, whenever solution and container permit.

Handling and Disposal – Skin reactions associated with doxorubicin have been reported. Skin accidently exposed to doxorubicin should be rinsed copiously with soap and warm water, and if the eyes are involved, standard irrigation techniques should be used immediately. The use of goggles, gloves, and protective gowns is recommended during preparation and administration of the drug.

Procedures for proper handling and disposal of anticancer drugs should be considered. Several guidelines on this subject have been published.[2–8] There is no general agreement that all of the procedures recommended in the guidelines are necessary or appropriate.

HOW SUPPLIED

RUBEX® (doxorubicin hydrochloride for injection, USP) is available as follows:

50 mg – Each single-dose vial contains 50 mg of doxorubicin HCl, USP as a sterile red-orange lyophilized powder, **NDC** 0015-3352-22. Available as one individually cartoned vial.

100 mg – Each single-dose vial contains 100 mg of doxorubicin HCl, USP as a sterile red-orange lyophilized powder, **NDC** 0015-3353-22. Available as one individually cartoned vial.

Store dry powder at controlled room temperature 15°–30°C (59°–86°F).

The reconstituted solution is stable for 7 days at room temperature or 15 days under refrigeration 2°–8°C (36°–46°F). Protect from exposure to sunlight. Retain in carton until time of use.

REFERENCES

1. Rudolph R, Larson DL: Etiology and Treatment of Chemotherapeutic Agent Extravasation Injuries: A Review. J Clin Oncol 1987; 5:1116-1126.
2. Recommendations for the Safe Handling of Parenteral Antineoplastic Drugs. NIH Publication No. 83-2621. For sale by the Superintendent of Documents, US Government Printing Office, Washington, DC 20402.
3. AMA Council Report. Guidelines for Handling Parenteral Antineoplastics. JAMA 1985; 253 (11):1590-1592.
4. National Study Commission on Cytotoxic Exposure – Recommendations for Handling Cytotoxic Agents. Available from Louis P. Jeffrey, ScD, Chairman, National Study Commission on Cytotoxic Exposure, Massachusetts College of Pharmacy and Allied Health Sciences, 179 Longwood Avenue, Boston, Massachusetts 02115.
5. Clinical Oncological Society of Australia. Guidelines and Recommendations for Safe Handling of Antineoplastic Agents. Med J Australia 1983; 1:426-428.
6. Jones RB, et al: Safe Handling of Chemotherapeutic Agents: A Report from the Mount Sinai Medical Center. CA-A Cancer Journal for Clinicians 1983; (Sept/Oct) 258-263.
7. American Society of Hospital Pharmacists Technical Assistance Bulletin on Handling Cytotoxic and Hazardous Drugs. Am J Hosp Pharm 1990; 47:1033-1049.
8. Controlling Occupational Exposure to Hazardous Drugs. (OSHA Work-Practice Guidelines). Am J Health-Syst Pharm 1996;53:1169-1685.

MeadJohnson
ONCOLOGY PRODUCTS
A Bristol-Myers Squibb Company
Princeton, NJ 08543
U.S.A.
K9-B001-5-97 3351DIM-05
51-004726-01 Revised: March 1997

TAXOL® ℞ ONLY

[*tăx-all*]
(paclitaxel) Injection

> **WARNING**
>
> TAXOL® (paclitaxel) Injection should be administered under the supervision of a physician experienced in the use of cancer chemotherapeutic agents. Appropriate management of complications is possible only when adequate diagnostic and treatment facilities are readily available.
>
> Anaphylaxis and severe hypersensitivity reactions characterized by dyspnea and hypotension requiring treatment, angioedema, and generalized urticaria have occurred in 2% of patients receiving TAXOL in clinical trials. Fatal reactions have occurred in patients despite premedication. All patients should be pretreated with corticosteroids, diphenhydramine, and H_2 antagonists. (See "**DOSAGE AND ADMINISTRATION**" section.)
>
> Patients who experience severe hypersensitivity reactions to TAXOL should not be rechallenged with the drug.
>
> TAXOL therapy should not be given to patients with solid tumors who have baseline neutrophil counts of less than 1,500 cells/mm^3 and should not be given to patients with AIDS-related Kaposi's sarcoma if the baseline neutrophil count is less than 1000 cells/mm^3. In order to monitor the occurrence of bone marrow suppression, primarily neutropenia, which may be severe and result in infection, it is recommended that frequent peripheral blood cell counts be performed on all patients receiving TAXOL.

DESCRIPTION

TAXOL® (paclitaxel) Injection is a clear colorless to slightly yellow viscous solution. It is supplied as a nonaqueous solution intended for dilution with a suitable parenteral fluid prior to intravenous infusion. TAXOL is available in 30 mg (5 mL), 100 mg (16.7 mL), and 300 mg (50 mL) multidose vials. Each mL of sterile nonpyrogenic solution contains 6 mg paclitaxel, 527 mg of purified Cremophor® EL* (polyoxyethylated castor oil) and 49.7% (v/v) dehydrated alcohol, USP.

Paclitaxel is a natural product with antitumor activity. TAXOL is obtained via a semi-synthetic process from *Taxus baccata*. The chemical name for paclitaxel is 5β,20-Epoxy-1,2α,4,7β,10β,13α-hexahydroxytax-11-en-9-one 4,10-diacetate 2-benzoate 13-ester with (2*R*,3*S*)-*N*-benzoyl-3-phenylisoserine.

Paclitaxel has the following structural formula:

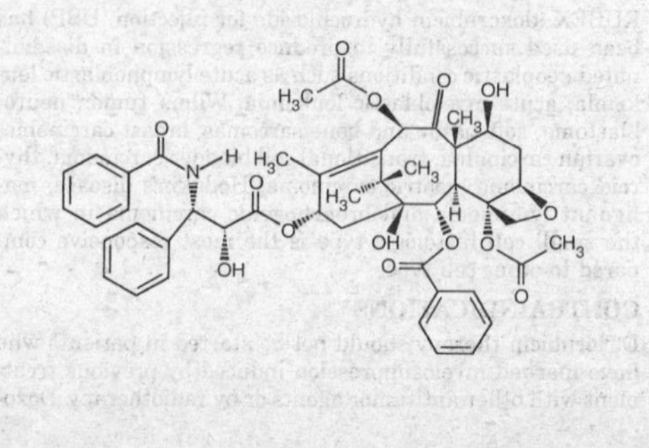

Paclitaxel is a white to off-white crystalline powder with the empirical formula $C_{47}H_{51}NO_{14}$ and a molecular weight of 853.9. It is highly lipophilic, insoluble in water, and melts at around 216–217°C.

CLINICAL PHARMACOLOGY

Paclitaxel is a novel antimicrotubule agent that promotes the assembly of microtubules from tubulin dimers and stabilizes microtubules by preventing depolymerization. This stability results in the inhibition of the normal dynamic reorganization of the microtubule network that is essential for vital interphase and mitotic cellular functions. In addition, paclitaxel induces abnormal arrays or "bundles" of microtubules throughout the cell cycle and multiple asters of microtubules during mitosis.

Following intravenous administration of TAXOL, paclitaxel plasma concentrations declined in a biphasic manner. The initial rapid decline represents distribution to the peripheral compartment and elimination of the drug. The later phase is due, in part, to a relatively slow efflux of paclitaxel from the peripheral compartment.

Pharmacokinetic parameters of paclitaxel following 3- and 24-hour infusions of TAXOL at dose levels of 135 and 175 mg/m^2 were determined in a Phase 3 randomized study in ovarian cancer patients and are summarized in the following table:

[See table above]

Summary of Pharmacokinetic Parameters - Mean Values

Dose (mg/m^2)	Infusion Duration (h)	N (patients)	C_{max} (mg/mL)	AUC (0-∞) (ng•h/mL)	T-HALF (h)	CL_T (L/h/m^2)
135	24	2	195	6300	52.7	21.7
175	24	4	365	7993	15.7	23.8
135	3	7	2170	7952	13.1	17.7
175	3	5	3650	15007	20.2	12.2

C_{max} = Maximum plasma concentration
AUC (0-∞) = Area under the plasma concentration-time curve from time 0 to infinity
CL_T = Total body clearance

It appeared that with the 24-hour infusion of TAXOL, a 30% increase in dose (135 mg/m^2 versus 175 mg/m^2) increased the C_{max} by 87%, whereas the AUC (0-∞) remained proportional. However, with a 3-hour infusion, for a 30% increase in dose, the C_{max} and AUC (0-∞) were increased by 68% and 89%, respectively. The mean apparent volume of distribution at steady state, with the 24-hour infusion of TAXOL, ranged from 227 to 688 L/m^2, indicating extensive extravascular distribution and/or tissue binding of paclitaxel.

The pharmacokinetics of paclitaxel were also evaluated in adult cancer patients who received single doses of 15–135 mg/m^2 given by 1-hour infusions (n=15), 30-275 mg/m^2 given by 6-hour infusions (n=36), and 200–275 mg/m^2 given by 24-hour infusions (n=54) in Phase 1 & 2 studies. Values for CL_T and volume of distribution were consistent with the findings in the Phase 3 study. The pharmacokinetics of TAXOL in patients with AIDS-related Kaposi's sarcoma have not been studied.

In vitro studies of binding to human serum proteins, using paclitaxel concentrations ranging from 0.1 to 50 µg/mL, indicate that between 89–98% of drug is bound; the presence of cimetidine, ranitidine, dexamethasone, or diphenhydramine did not affect protein binding of paclitaxel.

After intravenous administration of 15–275 mg/m^2 doses of TAXOL as 1-, 6-, or 24-hour infusions, mean values for cumulative urinary recovery of unchanged drug ranged from 1.3 to 12.6% of the dose, indicating extensive non-renal clearance. In five patients administered a 225 or 250 mg/m^2 dose of radiolabeled TAXOL as a 3-hour infusion, a mean of 71% of the radioactivity was excreted in the feces in 120 hours, and 14% was recovered in the urine. Total recovery of radioactivity ranged from 56 to 101% of the dose. Paclitaxel represented a mean of 5% of the administered radioactivity recovered in the feces, while metabolites, primarily 6α-hydroxypaclitaxel, accounted for the balance. *In vitro* studies with human liver microsomes and tissue slices showed that paclitaxel was metabolized primarily to 6α-hydroxypaclitaxel by the cytochrome P450 isozyme CYP2C8; and to two minor metabolites, 3'-*p*-hydroxypaclitaxel and 6α, 3'-*p*-dihydroxypaclitaxel, by CYP3A4. *In vitro*, the metabolism of paclitaxel to 6α-hydroxypaclitaxel was inhibited by a number of agents (ketoconazole, verapamil, diazepam, quinidine, dexamethasone, cyclosporin, teniposide, etoposide, and vincristine), but the concentrations used exceeded those found *in vivo* following normal therapeutic doses. Testosterone, 17α-ethinyl estradiol, retinoic acid, and quercetin, a specific inhibitor of CYP2C8, also inhibited the formation of 6α-hydroxypaclitaxel *in vitro*. The pharmacokinetics of paclitaxel may also be altered *in vivo* as a result of interactions with compounds that are substrates, inducers, or inhibitors of CYP2C8 and/or CYP3A4. (See **"PRECAUTIONS: Drug Interactions"** section.) The effect of renal or hepatic dysfunction on the disposition of paclitaxel has not been investigated.

Possible interactions of paclitaxel with concomitantly administered medications have not been formally investigated.

* Cremophor® EL is the registered trademark of BASF Aktiengesellschaft.
Cremophor® EL is further purified by a Bristol-Myers Squibb Company proprietary process before use.

CLINICAL STUDIES

Ovarian Carcinoma: Data from five Phase 1 and 2 clinical studies (189 patients), a multicenter, randomized Phase 3 study (407 patients), as well as an interim analysis of data from more than 300 patients enrolled in a treatment referral center program were used in support of the use of TAXOL (paclitaxel) Injection in patients who have failed initial or subsequent chemotherapy for metastatic carcinoma of the ovary. Two of the Phase 2 studies (92 patients) utilized an initial dose of 135 to 170 mg/m^2 in most patients (> 90%) administered over 24 hours by continuous infusion. Response rates in these two studies were 22% (95% CI = 11–37%) and 30% (95% CI = 18–46%) with a total of six complete and 18 partial responses in 92 patients. The median duration of overall response in these two studies measured from the first day of treatment was 7.2 months (range: 3.5–15.8 months) and 7.5 months (range: 5.3–17.4 months), respectively. The median survival was 8.1 months (range: 0.2–36.7 months) and 15.9 months (range: 1.8–34.5+ months).

The Phase 3 study had a bifactorial design and compared the efficacy and safety of TAXOL, administered at two different doses (135 or 175 mg/m^2) and schedules (3- or 24-hour infusion). The overall response rate for the 407 patients was 16.2% (95% CI = 12.8–20.2%), with 6 complete and 60 partial responses. Duration of response, measured from the first day of treatment was 8.3 months (range: 3.2–21.6 months). Median time to progression was 3.7 months (range: 0.1+ –25.1+ months). Median survival was 11.5 months (range: 0.2–26.3+ months).

Response rates, median survival and median time to progression for the 4 arms are given in the following table.

[See first table at top of next page]

Analyses were performed as planned by the study protocol, by comparing the two doses (135 or 175 mg/m^2) irrespective of the schedule (3 or 24 hours) and the two schedules irrespective of dose. Patients receiving the 175 mg/m^2 dose achieved a higher response rate than those receiving the 135 mg/m^2 dose: 18 vs. 14% (p=0.28). No difference in response rate was detected when comparing the 3-hour with the 24-hour infusion: 15 vs. 17% (p=0.50). Patients receiving the 175 mg/m^2 dose of TAXOL had a longer time to progression than those receiving the 135 mg/m^2 dose: median 4.2 vs. 3.1 months (p=0.03). Time to progression was longer for patients receiving the 3-hour vs. the 24-hour infusion: 4.0 months vs. 3.7 months (p=0.08). No difference in survival according to dose or schedule was observed. These statistical analyses should be viewed with caution because of the multiple comparisons made.

TAXOL remained active in patients who had developed resistance to platinum-containing therapy (defined as tumor progression while on, or tumor relapse within 6 months from completion of, a platinum-containing regimen) with response rates of 14% in the Phase 3 study and 31% in the Phase 1 & 2 clinical studies.

The adverse event profile in the Phase 3 study was consistent with that seen for a pooled analysis performed on 812 patients treated in ten clinical studies (see **"ADVERSE REACTIONS"** section). For the 403 patients who received TAXOL in the Phase 3 study, the following table shows the incidence of several important adverse events.

[See second table at top of next page]

Myelosuppression was dose and schedule related, with the schedule effect being more prominent. The development of severe hypersensitivity reactions (HSRs) was rare; 1% of the patients and 0.2% of the courses overall. There was no apparent dose or schedule effect seen for the HSRs. Peripheral neuropathy was clearly dose-related, but schedule did not appear to affect the incidence.

The results of the randomized study support the use of TAXOL at doses of 135 or 175 mg/m^2, administered by a 3-hour intravenous infusion. The same doses administered by 24-hour infusion were more toxic.

Breast Carcinoma: Data from 83 patients accrued in three phase 2 open label studies and from 471 patients enrolled in a phase 3 randomized study were available to support the use of TAXOL in patients with metastatic breast carcinoma.

Phase 2 open label studies- Two studies were conducted in 53 patients previously treated with a maximum of one prior chemotherapeutic regimen. TAXOL was administered in these 2 trials as a 24-hour infusion at initial doses of 250 mg/m^2 (with G-CSF support) or 200 mg/m^2. The response rates were 57% (95% CI: 37–75%) and 52% (95% CI: 32–72%), respectively. The third phase 2 study was conducted in extensively pretreated patients who had failed anthracycline therapy and who had received a minimum of 2 chemotherapy regimens for the treatment of metastatic disease. The dose of TAXOL was 200 mg/m^2 as a 24-hour infusion with G-CSF support. Nine of the 30 patients achieved a partial response, for a response rate of 30% (95% CI: 15–50%).

Phase 3 randomized study- This multicenter trial was conducted in patients previously treated with one or two regimens of chemotherapy. Patients were randomized to receive TAXOL at a dose of either 175 mg/m^2 or 135 mg/m^2 given as a 3-hour infusion. In the 471 patients enrolled, 60% had symptomatic disease with impaired performance status at study entry, and 73% had visceral metastases. These patients had failed prior chemotherapy either in the adjuvant setting (30%), the metastatic setting (39%), or both (31%). Sixty-seven percent of the patients had been previously exposed to anthracyclines and 23% of them had disease considered resistant to this class of agents.

The overall response rate for the 454 evaluable patients was 26% (95% CI: 22–30%), with 17 complete and 99 partial responses. The median duration of response, measured from the first day of treatment, was 8.1 months (range: 3.4–18.1+ months). Overall for the 471 patients, the median time to progression was 3.5 months (range: 0.03–17.1 months). Median survival was 11.7 months (range: 0–18.9 months).

Response rates, median survival and median time to progression for the 2 arms are given in the following table.

Efficacy in the Phase 3 Breast Carcinoma Study

	175/3 (n=235)	135/3 (n=236)
• **Response**		
- rate (percent)	28	22
- 95% Confidence Interval	(22–34)	(17–27)
• **Time to Progression**		
- median (months)	4.2	3.0
- 95% Confidence Interval	(3.2–4.6)	(2.5–3.8)
• **Survival**		
- median (months)	11.7	10.5
- 95% Confidence Interval	(10.0–13.8)	(9.0–12.8)

For the 458 patients who received TAXOL (paclitaxel) Injection in the Phase 3 study, the following table shows the incidence of several important adverse events by treatment arm (each arm was administered by a 3-hour infusion).

[See third table at top of next page]

Myelosuppression and peripheral neuropathy were dose related. There was one severe hypersensitivity reaction (HSR) observed at the dose of 135 mg/m^2.

AIDS-Related Kaposi's Sarcoma: Data from two Phase 2 open label studies support the use of TAXOL as second-line therapy in patients with AIDS-related Kaposi's sarcoma. Fifty-nine of the 85 patients enrolled in these studies had previously received systemic therapy, including interferon alpha (32%), DaunoXome® (31%), DOXIL® (2%) and doxorubicin containing chemotherapy (42%), with 64% having received prior anthracyclines. Eighty-five percent of the pretreated patients had progressed on, or could not tolerate, prior systemic therapy.

In Study CA139-174 patients received TAXOL at 135 mg/m^2 as a 3-hour infusion every 3 weeks (intended dose intensity 45 mg/m^2/week). If no dose-limiting toxicity was observed, patients were to receive 155 mg/m^2 and 175 mg/m^2 in subsequent courses. Hematopoietic growth factors were not to be used initially. In Study CA139-281 patients received TAXOL at 100 mg/m^2 as a 3-hour infusion every 2 weeks (intended dose intensity 50 mg/m^2/week). In this study patients could be receiving hematopoietic growth factors before the start of TAXOL therapy, or this support was to be initiated as indicated; the dose of TAXOL was not increased. The dose intensity of TAXOL used in this patient population was lower than the dose intensity recommended for other solid tumors.

All patients had widespread and poor risk disease. Applying the ACTG staging criteria to patients with prior systemic therapy, 93% were poor risk for extent of disease (T_1), 88% had a CD4 count <200 cells/mm^3 (I_1), and 97% had poor risk considering their systemic illness (S_1).

DaunoXome® is a registered trademark of NeXstar Pharmaceuticals, Inc.
DOXIL® is a registered trademark of Sequus Pharmaceuticals, Inc.

Continued on next page

Taxol—Cont.

All patients in Study CA139-174 had a Karnofsky performance status of 80 or 90 at baseline; in Study CA139-281, there were 26 (46%) patients with a Karnofsky performance status of 70 or worse at baseline.
[See fourth table below]
Although the planned dose intensity in the two studies was slightly different (45 mg/m²/week in Study CA139-174 and 50 mg/m²/week in Study CA139-281), delivered dose intensity was 38–39 mg/m²/week in both studies, with a similar range (20–24 to 51–61).
Efficacy- The efficacy of TAXOL was evaluated by assessing cutaneous tumor response according to the amended ACTG criteria and by seeking evidence of clinical benefit in patients in six domains of symptoms and/or conditions that are commonly related to AIDS-related Kaposi's sarcoma.
Cutaneous Tumor Response (Amended ACTG Criteria)- The objective response rate was 59% (95% CI: 46 to 72%)(35 of 59 patients) in patients with prior systemic therapy. Cutaneous responses were primarily defined as flattening of more than 50% of previously raised lesions.

Overall Best Response (Amended ACTG Criteria)

	Percent of Patients Prior Systemic Therapy (n=59)
Complete response	3
Partial response	56
Stable disease	29
Progression	8
Early death/toxicity	3

The median time to response was 8.1 weeks and the median duration of response measured from the first day of treatment was 10.4 months (95% CI: 7.0 to 11.0 months) for the patients who had previously received systemic therapy. The median time to progression was 6.2 months (95% CI: 4.6 to 8.7 months).
Additional Clinical Benefit- Most data on patient benefit were assessed retrospectively (plans for such analyses were not included in the study protocols). Nonetheless, clinical descriptions and photographs indicated clear benefit in some patients, including instances of improved pulmonary function in patients with pulmonary involvement, improved ambulation, resolution of ulcers, and decreased analgesic requirements in patients with KS involving the feet and resolution of facial lesions and edema in patients with KS involving the face, extremities and genitalia.
Safety- The adverse event profile of TAXOL (paclitaxel) Injection administered to patients with advanced HIV disease and poor-risk AIDS-related Kaposi's sarcoma was generally similar to that seen in a pooled analysis of 812 patients with solid tumors (see "ADVERSE REACTIONS" section). In this immunosuppressed patient population, however, a lower dose intensity of TAXOL and supportive therapy including hematopoietic growth factors in patients with severe neutropenia are recommended. Patients with AIDS-related Kaposi's sarcoma may have more severe hematologic toxicities than patients with solid tumors.

INDICATIONS

TAXOL is indicated, after failure of first-line or subsequent chemotherapy for the treatment of metastatic carcinoma of the ovary.
TAXOL is indicated for the treatment of breast cancer after failure of combination chemotherapy for metastatic disease or relapse within 6 months of adjuvant chemotherapy. Prior therapy should have included an anthracycline unless clinically contraindicated.
TAXOL is indicated for the second-line treatment of AIDS-related Kaposi's sarcoma.

CONTRAINDICATIONS

TAXOL is contraindicated in patients who have a history of hypersensitivity reactions to TAXOL or other drugs formulated in Cremophor® EL (polyoxyethylated castor oil).
TAXOL should not be used in patients with solid tumors who have baseline neutrophil counts of <1500 cells/mm³ or in patients with AIDS-related Kaposi's sarcoma with baseline neutrophil counts of <1000 cells/mm³.

WARNINGS

Anaphylaxis and severe hypersensitivity reactions characterized by dyspnea and hypotension requiring treatment, angioedema, and generalized urticaria have occurred in 2% of patients receiving TAXOL in clinical trials. Fatal reactions have occurred in patients despite premedication. All patients should be pretreated with corticosteroids, diphenhydramine, and H_2 antagonists. (See "DOSAGE AND ADMINISTRATION" section.) Patients who experience severe hypersensitivity reactions to TAXOL should not be rechallenged with the drug.
Bone marrow suppression (primarily neutropenia) is dose-dependent and is the dose-limiting toxicity. Neutrophil na-

Efficacy in the Phase 3 Ovarian Carcinoma Study

	175/3 (n=96)	175/24 (n=106)	135/3 (n=99)	135/24 (n=106)
• Response				
- rate (percent)	14.6	21.7	15.2	13.2
- 95% Confidence Interval	(8.5–23.6)	(14.5–31.0)	(9.0–24.1)	(7.7–21.5)
• Time to Progression				
- median (months)	4.4	4.2	3.4	2.8
- 95% Confidence Interval	(3.0–5.6)	(3.5–5.1)	(2.8–4.2)	(1.9–4.0)
• Survival				
- median (months)	11.5	11.8	13.1	10.7
- 95% Confidence Interval	(8.4–14.4)	(8.9–14.6)	(9.1–14.6)	(8.1–13.6)

Frequency* of Important Adverse Events in the Phase 3 Ovarian Carcinoma Study

		Percent of Patients			
		175/3 (n=95)	175/24 (n=105)	135/3 (n=98)	135/24 (n=105)
• Bone Marrow					
- Neutropenia	< 2,000/mm³	78	98	78	98
	< 500/mm³	27	75	14	67
- Thrombocytopenia	< 100,000/mm³	4	18	8	6
	< 50,000/mm³	1	7	2	1
- Anemia	< 11 g/dL	84	90	68	88
	< 8 g/dL	11	12	6	10
- Infections		26	29	20	18
• Hypersensitivity Reaction**					
- All		41	45	38	45
- Severe		2	0	2	1
• Peripheral Neuropathy					
- Any symptoms		63	60	55	42
- Severe symptoms		1	2	0	0
• Mucositis					
- Any symptoms		17	35	21	25
- Severe symptoms		0	3	0	2

* Based on worst course analysis
** All patients received premedication

Frequency* of Important Adverse Events in the Phase 3 Breast Carcinoma Study

		Percent of Patients	
		175 mg/m² (n=229)	135 mg/m² (n=229)
• Bone Marrow			
- Neutropenia	< 2,000/mm³	90	81
	< 500/mm³	28	19
- Thrombocytopenia	< 100,000/mm³	11	7
	< 50,000/mm³	3	2
- Anemia	< 11 g/dL	55	47
	< 8 g/dL	4	2
- Infections		23	15
- Febrile Neutropenia		2	2
• Hypersensitivity Reaction**			
- All		36	31
- Severe		0	<1
• Peripheral Neuropathy			
- Any symptoms		70	46
- Severe symptoms		7	3
• Mucositis			
- Any symptoms		23	17
- Severe symptoms		3	<1

* Based on worst course analysis
** All patients received premedication

Extent of Disease at Study Entry

	Percent of Patients Prior Systemic Therapy (n=59)
Visceral ± edema ± oral ± cutaneous	42
Edema or lymph nodes oral ± cutaneous	41
Oral ± cutaneous	10
Cutaneous only	7

dirs occurred at a median of 11 days. TAXOL should not be administered to patients with baseline neutrophil counts of less than 1500 cells/mm³ (<1000 cells/mm³ for patients with KS). Frequent monitoring of blood counts should be instituted during TAXOL treatment. Patients should not be re-treated with subsequent cycles of TAXOL until neutrophils recover to a level >1500 cells/mm³ (>1000 cells/mm³ for patients with KS) and platelets recover to a level >100,000 cells/mm³.
Severe conduction abnormalities have been documented in <1% of patients during TAXOL therapy and in some cases requiring pacemaker placement. If patients develop significant conduction abnormalities during TAXOL infusion, appropriate therapy should be administered and continuous cardiac monitoring should be performed during subsequent therapy with TAXOL.
Pregnancy: TAXOL can cause fetal harm when administered to a pregnant woman. Administration of paclitaxel during the period of organogenesis to rabbits at doses of 3.0 mg/kg/day (about 0.2 the daily maximum recommended human dose on a mg/m² basis) caused embryo-and fetotoxicity, as indicated by intrauterine mortality, increased resorptions and increased fetal deaths. Maternal toxicity was also observed at this dose. No teratogenic effects were observed at 1.0 mg/kg/day (about 1/15 the daily maximum recommended human dose on a mg/m² basis); teratogenic potential could not be assessed at higher doses due to extensive fetal mortality.

There are no adequate and well-controlled studies in pregnant women. If TAXOL is used during pregnancy, or if the patient becomes pregnant while receiving this drug, the patient should be apprised of the potential hazard to the fetus. Women of childbearing potential should be advised to avoid becoming pregnant.

PRECAUTIONS

Contact of the undiluted concentrate with plasticized polyvinyl chloride (PVC) equipment or devices used to prepare solutions for infusion is not recommended. In order to minimize patient exposure to the plasticizer DEHP [di-(2-ethylhexyl)phthalate], which may be leached from PVC infusion bags or sets, diluted TAXOL solutions should preferably be stored in bottles (glass, polypropylene) or plastic bags (polypropylene, polyolefin) and administered through polyethylene-lined administration sets.

TAXOL should be administered through an in-line filter with a microporous membrane not greater than 0.22 microns. Use of filter devices such as IVEX-2® filters which incorporate short inlet and outlet PVC-coated tubing has not resulted in significant leaching of DEHP.

Drug Interaction: In a Phase I trial using escalating doses of TAXOL (110-200 mg/m^2) and cisplatin (50 or 75 mg/m^2) given as sequential infusions, myelosuppression was more profound when TAXOL was given after cisplatin than with the alternate sequence (i.e., TAXOL before cisplatin). Pharmacokinetic data from these patients demonstrated a decrease in paclitaxel clearance of approximately 33% when TAXOL was administered following cisplatin.

The metabolism of TAXOL is catalyzed by cytochrome P450 isoenzymes CYP2C8 and CYP3A4. In the absence of formal clinical drug interaction studies, caution should be exercised when administering TAXOL concomitantly with known substrates or inhibitors of the cytochrome P450 isoenzymes CYP2C8 and CYP3A4. (See **"CLINICAL PHARMACOLOGY"** section.)

Potential interactions between paclitaxel, a substrate of CYP3A4 and protease inhibitors (ritonavir, saquinavir, indinavir, and nelfinavir), which are substrates and/or inhibitors of CYP3A4 have not been evaluated in clinical trials.

Reports in the literature suggest that plasma levels of doxorubicin (and its active metabolite doxorubicinol) may be increased when paclitaxel and doxorubicin are used in combination.

Hematology: TAXOL therapy should not be administered to patients with baseline neutrophil counts of less than 1,500 cells/mm^3. In order to monitor the occurrence of myelotoxicity, it is recommended that frequent peripheral blood cell counts be performed on all patients receiving TAXOL. Patients should not be re-treated with subsequent cycles of TAXOL until neutrophils recover to a level >1500 cells/mm^3 and platelets recover to a level >100,000 cells/mm^3. In the case of severe neutropenia (<500 cells/mm^3 for seven days or more) during a course of TAXOL therapy, a 20% reduction in dose for subsequent courses of therapy is recommended.

For patients with advanced HIV disease and poor-risk AIDS-related Kaposi's sarcoma, TAXOL, at the recommended dose for this disease, can be initiated and repeated if the neutrophil count is at least 1000 cells/mm^3.

Hypersensitivity Reactions: Patients with a history of severe hypersensitivity reactions to products containing Cremophor® EL (e.g., cyclosporin for injection concentrate and teniposide for injection concentrate) should not be treated with TAXOL. In order to avoid the occurrence of severe hypersensitivity reactions, all patients treated with TAXOL should be premedicated with corticosteroids (such as dexamethasone), diphenhydramine and H_2 antagonists (such as cimetidine or ranitidine). Minor symptoms such as flushing, skin reactions, dyspnea, hypotension or tachycardia do not require interruption of therapy. However, severe reactions, such as hypotension requiring treatment, dyspnea requiring bronchodilators, angioedema or generalized urticaria require immediate discontinuation of TAXOL (paclitaxel) Injection and aggressive symptomatic therapy. Patients who have developed severe hypersensitivity reactions should not be rechallenged with TAXOL.

Cardiovascular: Hypotension, bradycardia, and hypertension have been observed during administration of TAXOL, but generally do not require treatment. Occasionally TAXOL infusions must be interrupted or discontinued because of initial or recurrent hypertension. Frequent vital sign monitoring, particularly during the first hour of TAXOL infusion, is recommended. Continuous cardiac monitoring is not required except for patients with serious conduction abnormalities. (See **"WARNINGS"** section.)

Nervous System: Although, the occurrence of peripheral neuropathy is frequent, the development of severe symptomatology is unusual and requires a dose reduction of 20% for all subsequent courses of TAXOL.

TAXOL contains dehydrated alcohol USP, 396 mg/mL; consideration should be given to possible CNS and other effects of alcohol. (See **"PRECAUTIONS: Pediatric Use"** section.)

Hepatic: There is evidence that the toxicity of TAXOL is enhanced in patients with elevated liver enzymes. Caution should be exercised when administering TAXOL to patients with moderate to severe hepatic impairment and dose adjustments should be considered.

Injection Site Reaction: Injection site reactions, including reactions secondary to extravasation, were usually mild and consisted of erythema, tenderness, skin discoloration, or swelling at the injection site. These reactions have been observed more frequently with the 24-hour infusion than with the 3-hour infusion. Recurrence of skin reactions at a site of previous extravasation following administration of TAXOL at a different site, i.e., "recall", has been reported rarely. Rare reports of more severe events such as phlebitis, cellulitis, induration, skin exfoliation, necrosis and fibrosis have been received as part of the continuing surveillance of TAXOL safety. In some cases the onset of the injection site reaction either occurred during a prolonged infusion or was delayed by a week to ten days.

A specific treatment for extravasation reactions is unknown at this time. Given the possibility of extravasation, it is advisable to closely monitor the infusion site for possible infiltration during drug administration.

Carcinogenesis, Mutagenesis, Impairment of Fertility: The carcinogenic potential of TAXOL has not been studied.

Paclitaxel has been shown to be clastogenic *in vitro* (chromosome aberrations in human lymphocytes) and *in vivo* (micronucleus test in mice). Paclitaxel was not mutagenic in the Ames test or the CHO/HGPRT gene mutation assay.

Administration of paclitaxel prior to and during mating produced impairment of fertility in male and female rats at doses equal to or greater than 1 mg/kg/day (about 0.04 the daily maximum recommended human dose on a mg/m^2 basis). At this dose, paclitaxel caused reduced fertility and reproductive indices, and increased embryo- and fetotoxicity. (See **"WARNINGS"** section.)

Pregnancy: Pregnancy "Category D". (See **"WARNINGS"** section.)

Nursing Mothers: It is not known whether the drug is excreted in human milk. Following intravenous administration of carbon-14 labeled TAXOL to rats on days 9 to 10 postpartum, milk concentrations of radioactivity exceeded and declined in parallel with the plasma concentrations. Because many drugs are excreted in human milk and because of the potential for serious adverse reactions in nursing infants, it is recommended that nursing be discontinued when receiving TAXOL therapy.

Pediatric Use: The safety and effectiveness of TAXOL in pediatric patients have not been established.

There have been reports of central nervous system (CNS) toxicity in an ongoing investigational clinical trial in pediatric patients in which TAXOL was infused intravenously over 3 hours at doses ranging from 350 mg/m^2 to 420 mg/m^2. The toxicity is most likely attributable to the high dose of the ethanol component of the TAXOL vehicle given over a short infusion time. The use of concomitant antihistamines may intensify this effect. Although a direct effect of the paclitaxel itself cannot be discounted, the high doses used in this study (over twice the recommended adult dosage) must be considered in assessing the safety of TAXOL for use in this population.

ADVERSE REACTIONS

Data in the following table are based on the experience of 812 patients (493 with ovarian carcinoma and 319 with breast carcinoma) enrolled in 10 studies. Two hundred and seventy-five patients were treated in 8 Phase 2 studies with TAXOL doses ranging from 135 to 300 mg/m^2 administered over 24 hours (in 4 of these studies, G-CSF was administered as hematopoietic support). Three hundred and one patients were treated in the randomized Phase 3 ovarian carcinoma study which compared two doses (135 or 175 mg/m^2) and two schedules (3 or 24 hours) of TAXOL. Two hundred and thirty-six patients with breast carcinoma received TAXOL (135 or 175 mg/m^2) administered over 3 hours in a controlled study.

Summary of Adverse Events in 812 Patients With Solid Tumors Receiving Single-Agent TAXOL

		% Incidence
• Bone Marrow		
- Neutropenia	< 2,000/mm^3	90
	< 500/mm^3	52
- Leukopenia	< 4,000/mm^3	90
	< 1,000/mm^3	17
- Thrombocytopenia	< 100,000/mm^3	20
	< 50,000/mm^3	7
- Anemia	< 11 g/dL	78
	< 8 g/dL	16
- Infections		30
- Bleeding		14
- Red Cell Transfusions		25
- Platelet Transfusions		2
• Hypersensitivity Reaction[1]		
- All		41
- Severe		2
• Cardiovascular		
- Vital Sign Changes[2]		
- Bradycardia (N=537)		3
- Hypotension (N=532)		12
- Significant Cardiovascular Events		1
• Abnormal ECG		
- All Pts		23
- Pts with normal baseline (N=559)		14
• Peripheral Neuropathy		
- Any symptoms		60
- Severe symptoms		3
• Myalgia/Arthralgia		
- Any symptoms		60
- Severe symptoms		8
• Gastrointestinal		
- Nausea and vomiting		52
- Diarrhea		38
- Mucositis		31
• Alopecia		87
• Hepatic (Pts with normal baseline and on study data)		
- Bilirubin elevations (N=765)		7
- Alkaline Phosphatase elevations (N=575)		22
- AST (SGOT) elevations (N=591)		19
• Injection Site Reaction		13

[1] *All patients received premedication*
[2] *During the first 3-hours of infusion*

None of the observed toxicities were clearly influenced by age.

The following table shows the frequency of important adverse events in the 85 patients with KS treated with two different TAXOL (paclitaxel) Injection regimens.

[See table at top of next page]

As demonstrated in this table, toxicity was more pronounced in the study utilizing TAXOL at a dose of 135 mg/m^2 every 3 weeks than in the study utilizing TAXOL at a dose of 100 mg/m^2 every 2 weeks. Notably, severe neutropenia (76% versus 35%), febrile neutropenia (55% versus 9%), and opportunistic infections (76% versus 54%) were more common with the former dose and schedule. The differences between the two studies with respect to dose escalation and use of hematopoietic growth factors, as described above, should be taken into account. (See **"CLINICAL STUDIES: AIDS-Related Kaposi's Sarcoma"** section.) Note also that only 26% of the 85 patients in these studies received concomitant treatment with protease inhibitors, whose effect on paclitaxel metabolism has not yet been studied.

The following discussion refers to the overall safety database of 812 patients with solid tumors treated in clinical studies. The frequency and severity of adverse events have been generally similar for patients receiving TAXOL for the treatment of ovarian or breast carcinoma or for Kaposi's sarcoma, but patients with AIDS-related Kaposi's sarcoma may have more frequent and severe hematologic toxicity, infections, and febrile neutropenia. These patients require a lower dose intensity and supportive care. (See **"CLINICAL STUDIES: AIDS-Related Kaposi's Sarcoma"** section.) In addition, rare events have been reported from the postmarketing experience or from other clinical studies; toxicities that were observed only in the population with Kaposi's sarcoma or that occurred with greater severity in this population are also described. The frequency and severity of important adverse events for the Phase 3 ovarian and breast carcinoma studies are presented in tabular form by treatment arm in the **CLINICAL STUDIES** section.

Hematologic: Bone marrow suppression was the major dose-limiting toxicity of TAXOL. Neutropenia, the most important hematologic toxicity, was dose and schedule dependent and was generally rapidly reversible. Among patients treated in the Phase 3 ovarian study with a 3-hour infusion, neutrophil counts declined below 500 cells/mm^3 in 13% of the patients treated with a dose of 135 mg/m^2 compared to 27% at a dose of 175 mg/m^2 (p=0.05). In the same study, severe neutropenia (<500 cells/mm^3) was more frequent with the 24-hour than with the 3-hour infusion; infusion duration had a greater impact on myelosuppression than dose. Neutropenia did not appear to increase with cumulative exposure and did not appear to be more frequent nor more severe for patients previously treated with radiation therapy. Fever was frequent (12% of all treatment courses). Infectious episodes occurred in 30% of all patients and 9% of all courses; these episodes were fatal in 1% of all patients, and included sepsis, pneumonia and peritonitis. In the Phase 3 ovarian study, infectious episodes were reported in 19% of the patients given either 135 or 175 mg/m^2 dose by a 3-hour infusion. Urinary tract infections and upper respiratory tract infections were the most frequently reported infectious complications. In the immunosuppressed patient population

Continued on next page

Taxol—Cont.

with advanced HIV disease and poor-risk AIDS-related Kaposi's sarcoma, 61% of the patients reported at least one opportunistic infection. (See **"CLINICAL STUDIES: AIDS-Related Kaposi's Sarcoma"** section.) The use of supportive therapy, including G-CSF, is recommended for patients who have experienced severe neutropenia. (See **"DOSAGE AND ADMINISTRATION"** section.)

Thrombocytopenia was uncommon, and almost never severe ($<$50,000 cells/mm^3). Twenty percent of the patients experienced a drop in their platelet count below 100,000 cells/mm^3 at least once while on treatment; 7% had a platelet count $<$50,000 cells/mm^3 at the time of their worst nadir. Among the 812 patients, bleeding episodes were reported in 4% of all courses and by 14% of all patients but most of the hemorrhagic episodes were localized and the frequency of these events was unrelated to the TAXOL dose and schedule. In the Phase 3 ovarian study, bleeding episodes were reported in 10% of the patients receiving either the 135 or 175 mg/m^2 dose given by a 3-hour infusion; no patients treated with the 3-hour infusion received platelet transfusions.

Anemia (Hb $<$11 g/dL) was observed in 78% of all patients and was severe (Hb $<$8 g/dL) in 16% of the cases. No consistent relationship between dose or schedule and the frequency of anemia was observed. Among all patients with normal baseline hemoglobin, 69% became anemic on study but only 7% had severe anemia. Red cell transfusions were required in 25% of all patients and in 12% of those with normal baseline hemoglobin levels.

Hypersensitivity Reactions (HSRs): All patients received premedication prior to TAXOL (see **"WARNINGS"** and **"PRECAUTIONS: Hypersensitivity Reactions"** sections). The frequency and severity of HSRs were not affected by the dose or schedule of TAXOL (paclitaxel) Injection administration. In the Phase 3 ovarian study the 3-hour infusion was not associated with a greater increase in HSRs when compared to the 24-hour infusion. Hypersensitivity reactions were observed in 20% of all courses and in 41% of all patients. These reactions were severe in less than 2% of the patients and 1% of the courses. No severe reactions were observed after course 3 and severe symptoms occurred generally within the first hour of TAXOL infusion. The most frequent symptoms observed during these severe reactions were dyspnea, flushing, chest pain and tachycardia.

The minor hypersensitivity reactions consisted mostly of flushing (28%), rash (12%), hypotension (4%), dyspnea (2%), tachycardia (2%) and hypertension (1%). The frequency of hypersensitivity reactions remained relatively stable during the entire treatment period.

Rare reports of chills and reports of back pain in association with hypersensitivity reactions have been received as part of the continuing surveillance of TAXOL safety.

Cardiovascular: Hypotension, during the first 3 hours of infusion, occurred in 12% of all patients and 3% of all courses administered. Bradycardia, during the first 3 hours of infusion, occurred in 3% of all patients and 1% of all courses. In the Phase 3 ovarian study, neither dose nor schedule had an effect on the frequency of hypotension and bradycardia. These vital sign changes most often caused no symptoms and required neither specific therapy nor treatment discontinuation. The frequency of hypotension and bradycardia were not influenced by prior anthracycline therapy.

Significant cardiovascular events possibly related to TAXOL occurred in approximately 1% of all patients. These events included syncope, rhythm abnormalities, hypertension and venous thrombosis. One of the patients with syncope treated with TAXOL at 175 mg/m^2 over 24 hours had progressive hypotension and died. The arrhythmias included asymptomatic ventricular tachycardia, bigeminy and complete AV block requiring pacemaker placement.

Electrocardiogram (ECG) abnormalities were common among patients at baseline. ECG abnormalities on study did not usually result in symptoms, were not dose-limiting, and required no intervention. ECG abnormalities were noted in 23% of all patients. Among patients with a normal ECG prior to study entry, 14% of all patients developed an abnormal tracing while on study. The most frequently reported ECG modifications were non-specific repolarization abnormalities, sinus bradycardia, sinus tachycardia and premature beats. Among patients with normal ECGs at baseline, prior therapy with anthracyclines did not influence the frequency of ECG abnormalities.

Cases of myocardial infarction have been reported rarely. Congestive heart failure has been reported typically in patients who have received other chemotherapy, notably anthracyclines. (See **"PRECAUTIONS: Drug Interactions"** section.)

Rare reports of atrial fibrillation and supraventricular tachycardia have been received as part of the continuing surveillance of TAXOL safety.

Respiratory: Rare reports of interstitial pneumonia, lung fibrosis and pulmonary embolism have been received as part of the continuing surveillance of TAXOL safety. Rare

Frequency* of Important Adverse Events in the AIDS-Related Kaposi's Sarcoma Studies

		Percent of Patients	
		Study CA139–174 135 mg/m^{2}q 3 wk (n=29)	**Study CA139–281** 100 mg/m^{2}q 2 wk (n=56)
• **Bone Marrow**			
- Neutropenia	$<$ 2,000/mm^3	100	95
	$<$ 500/mm^3	76	35
- Thrombocytopenia	$<$ 100,000/mm^3	52	27
	$<$ 50,000/mm^3	17	5
- Anemia	$<$ 11 g/dL	86	73
	$<$ 8 g/dL	34	25
- Febrile Neutropenia		55	9
• **Opportunistic Infection**			
- Any		76	54
- Cytomegalovirus		45	27
- Herpes Simplex		38	11
- *Pneumocystis carinii*		14	21
- M. avium intracellulare		24	4
- Candidiasis, esophageal		7	9
- Cryptosporidiosis		7	7
- Cryptococcal meningitis		3	2
- Leukoencephalopathy		–	2
• **Hypersensitivity Reaction****			
- All		14	9
• **Cardiovascular**			
- Hypotension		17	9
- Bradycardia		3	–
• **Peripheral Neuropathy**			
- Any		79	46
- Severe		10	2
• **Myalgia/Arthralgia**			
- Any		93	48
- Severe		14	16
• **Gastrointestinal**			
- Nausea and Vomiting		69	70
- Diarrhea		90	73
- Mucositis		45	20
• **Renal (creatinine elevation)**			
- Any		34	18
- Severe (grade III/IV)		7	5
• **Discontinuation for drug toxicity**		7	16

* Based on worst course analysis
** All patients received premedication

reports of radiation pneumonitis have been received in patients receiving concurrent radiotherapy.

Neurologic: The frequency and severity of neurologic manifestations were dose-dependent, but were not influenced by infusion duration. Peripheral neuropathy was observed in 60% of all patients (3% severe) and in 52% (2% severe) of the patients without pre-existing neuropathy.

The frequency of peripheral neuropathy increased with cumulative dose. Neurologic symptoms were observed in 27% of the patients after the first course of treatment and in 34–51% from course 2 to 10.

Peripheral neuropathy was the cause of TAXOL discontinuation in 1% of all patients. Sensory symptoms have usually improved or resolved within several months of TAXOL discontinuation. The incidence of neurologic symptoms did not increase in the subset of patients previously treated with cisplatin. Pre-existing neuropathies resulting from prior therapies are not a contraindication for TAXOL therapy.

Other than peripheral neuropathy, serious neurologic events following TAXOL administration have been rare ($<$1%) and have included grand mal seizures, syncope, ataxia and neuroencephalopathy.

Rare reports of autonomic neuropathy resulting in paralytic ileus have been received as part of the continuing surveillance of TAXOL safety. Optic nerve and/or visual disturbances (scintillating scotomata) have also been reported, particularly in patients who have received higher doses than those recommended. These effects generally have been reversible. However, rare reports in the literature of abnormal visual evoked potentials in patients have suggested persistent optic nerve damage.

Arthralgia/Myalgia: There was no consistent relationship between dose or schedule of TAXOL and the frequency or severity of arthralgia/myalgia. Sixty percent of all patients treated experienced arthralgia/myalgia; 8% experienced severe symptoms. The symptoms were usually transient, occurred two or three days after TAXOL administration, and resolved within a few days. The frequency and severity of musculoskeletal symptoms remained unchanged throughout the treatment period.

Hepatic: No relationship was observed between liver function abnormalities and either dose or schedule of TAXOL administration. Among patients with normal baseline liver function 7%, 22% and 19% had elevations in bilirubin, alkaline phosphatase and AST (SGOT), respectively. Prolonged exposure to TAXOL was not associated with cumulative hepatic toxicity.

Rare reports of hepatic necrosis and hepatic encephalopathy leading to death have been received as part of the continuing surveillance of TAXOL safety.

Renal: Among the patients treated for Kaposi's sarcoma with TAXOL, five patients had renal toxicity of grade III or IV severity. One patient with suspected HIV nephropathy of grade IV severity had to discontinue therapy. The other four patients had renal insufficiency with reversible elevations of serum creatinine.

Gastrointestinal (GI): Nausea/vomiting, diarrhea and mucositis were reported by 52%, 38% and 31% of all patients, respectively. These manifestations were usually mild to moderate. Mucositis was schedule dependent and occurred more frequently with the 24-hour than with the 3-hour infusion.

In patients with poor-risk AIDS-related Kaposi's sarcoma, nausea/vomiting, diarrhea, and mucositis were reported by 69%, 79%, and 28% of patients, respectively. One third of patients with Kaposi's sarcoma complained of diarrhea prior to study start. (See **"CLINICAL STUDIES: AIDS-Related Kaposi's Sarcoma"** section.)

Rare reports of intestinal obstruction, intestinal perforation, pancreatitis, ischemic colitis, and dehydration have been received as part of the continuing surveillance of TAXOL safety. Rare reports of neutropenic enterocolitis (typhlitis), despite the coadministration of G-CSF, were observed in patients treated with TAXOL alone and in combination with other chemotherapeutic agents.

Injection Site Reaction: Injection site reactions, including reactions secondary to extravasation, were usually mild and consisted of erythema, tenderness, skin discoloration, or swelling at the injection site. These reactions have been observed more frequently with the 24-hour infusion than with the 3-hour infusion. Recurrence of skin reactions at a site of previous extravasation following administration of TAXOL at a different site, i.e., "recall", has been reported rarely. Rare reports of more severe events such as phlebitis, cellulitis, induration, skin exfoliation, necrosis and fibrosis have been received as part of the continuing surveillance of TAXOL safety. In some cases the onset of the injection site reaction either occurred during a prolonged infusion or was delayed by a week to ten days.

A specific treatment for extravasation reactions is unknown at this time. Given the possibility of extravasation, it is advisable to closely monitor the infusion site for possible infiltration during drug administration.

Other Clinical Events: Alopecia was observed in almost all (87%) of the patients. Transient skin changes due to

TAXOL-related hypersensitivity reactions have been observed, but no other skin toxicities were significantly associated with TAXOL (paclitaxel) Injection administration. Nail changes (changes in pigmentation or discoloration of nail bed) were uncommon (2%). Edema was reported in 21% of all patients (17% of those without baseline edema); only 1% had severe edema and none of these patients required treatment discontinuation. Edema was most commonly focal and disease-related. Edema was observed in 5% of all courses for patients with normal baseline and did not increase with time on study.

Rare reports of skin abnormalities related to radiation recall as well as reports of maculopapular rash and pruritus have been received as part of the continuing surveillance of TAXOL safety.

Reports of asthenia and malaise have been received as part of the continuing surveillance of TAXOL safety.

Accidental Exposure: Upon inhalation, dyspnea, chest pain, burning eyes, sore throat and nausea have been reported. Following topical exposure, events have included tingling, burning and redness.

OVERDOSAGE

There is no known antidote for TAXOL overdosage. The primary anticipated complications of overdosage would consist of bone marrow suppression, peripheral neurotoxicity and mucositis.

DOSAGE AND ADMINISTRATION

Note: Contact of the undiluted concentrate with plasticized PVC equipment or devices used to prepare solutions for infusion is not recommended. In order to minimize patient exposure to the plasticizer DEHP [di-(2-ethylhexyl)phthalate], which may be leached from PVC infusion bags or sets, diluted TAXOL solutions should be stored in bottles (glass, polypropylene) or plastic bags (polypropylene, polyolefin) and administered through polyethylene-lined administration sets.

All patients should be premedicated prior to TAXOL administration in order to prevent severe hypersensitivity reactions. Such premedication may consist of dexamethasone 20 mg PO administered approximately 12 and 6 hours before TAXOL, diphenhydramine (or its equivalent) 50 mg I.V. 30 to 60 minutes prior to TAXOL, and cimetidine (300 mg) or ranitidine (50 mg) I.V. 30 to 60 minutes before TAXOL.

In patients with carcinoma of the ovary, TAXOL has been used at several doses and schedules; however, the optimal regimen is not yet clear. (See **"CLINICAL STUDIES: Ovarian Carcinoma"** section.) In patients previously treated with chemotherapy for ovarian cancer, the recommended regimen is TAXOL 135 mg/m^2 or 175 mg/m^2 administered intravenously over 3 hours every 3 weeks.

For patients with carcinoma of the breast, TAXOL at a dose of 175 mg/m^2 administered intravenously over 3 hours every 3 weeks has been shown to be effective after failure of chemotherapy for metastatic disease or relapse within 6 months of adjuvant chemotherapy.

For patients with AIDS-related Kaposi's sarcoma, TAXOL administered at a dose of 135 mg/m^2 given intravenously over 3 hours every 3 weeks or at a dose of 100 mg/m^2 given intravenously over 3 hours every 2 weeks is recommended (dose intensity 45–50 mg/m^2/week). In the two clinical trials evaluating these schedules (see **"CLINICAL STUDIES: AIDS-Related Kaposi's Sarcoma"** section), the former schedule (135 mg/m^2 every 3 weeks) was more toxic than the latter. In addition, all patients with low performance status were treated with the latter schedule (100 mg/m^2 every 2 weeks).

Based upon the immunosuppression in patients with advanced HIV disease, the following modifications are recommended in these patients:

1) Reduce the dose of dexamethasone as one of the three premedication drugs to 10 mg PO (instead of 20 mg PO);
2) Initiate or repeat treatment with TAXOL only if the neutrophil count is at least 1000 cells/mm^3;
3) Reduce the dose of subsequent courses of TAXOL by 20% for patients who experience severe neutropenia (neutrophil <500 cells/mm^3 for a week or longer); and
4) Initiate concomitant hematopoietic growth factor (G-CSF) as clinically indicated.

For the therapy of patients with solid tumors (ovary and breast), courses of TAXOL should not be repeated until the neutrophil count is at least 1,500 cells/mm^3 and the platelet count is at least 100,000 cells/mm^3 and TAXOL should not be given to patients with AIDS-related Kaposi's sarcoma if the baseline or subsequent neutrophil count is less than 1000 cells/mm^3. Patients who experience severe neutropenia (neutrophil <500 cells/mm^3 for a week or longer) or severe peripheral neuropathy during TAXOL therapy should have dosage reduced by 20% for subsequent courses of TAXOL. The incidence of neurotoxicity and the severity of neutropenia increase with dose.

Preparation and Administration Precautions: TAXOL is a cytotoxic anticancer drug and, as with other potentially toxic compounds, caution should be exercised in handling TAXOL. The use of gloves is recommended. If TAXOL solution contacts the skin, wash the skin immediately and thoroughly with soap and water. Following topical exposure, events have included tingling, burning and redness. If TAXOL contacts mucous membranes, the membranes should be flushed thoroughly with water. Upon inhalation, dyspnea, chest pain, burning eyes, sore throat, and nausea have been reported.

Given the possibility of extravasation, it is advisable to closely monitor the infusion site for possible infiltration during drug administration. (See **"PRECAUTIONS: Injection Site Reaction"** section.)

Preparation for Intravenous Administration: TAXOL must be diluted prior to infusion. TAXOL should be diluted in 0.9% Sodium Chloride Injection, USP; 5% Dextrose Injection, USP; 5% Dextrose and 0.9% Sodium Chloride Injection, USP or 5% Dextrose in Ringer's Injection to a final concentration of 0.3 to 1.2 mg/mL. The solutions are physically and chemically stable for up to 27 hours at ambient temperature (approximately 25°C) and room lighting conditions. Parenteral drug products should be inspected visually for particulate matter and discoloration prior to administration whenever solution and container permit.

Upon preparation, solutions may show haziness, which is attributed to the formulation vehicle. No significant losses in potency have been noted following simulated delivery of the solution through I.V. tubing containing an in-line (0.22 micron) filter.

Data collected for the presence of the extractable plasticizer DEHP [di-(2-ethylhexyl)phthalate] show that levels increase with time and concentration when dilutions are prepared in PVC containers. Consequently, the use of plasticized PVC containers and administration sets is not recommended. TAXOL solutions should be prepared and stored in glass, polypropylene, or polyolefin containers. Non-PVC containing administration sets, such as those which are polyethylene-lined, should be used.

TAXOL should be administered through an in-line filter with a microporous membrane not greater than 0.22 microns. Use of filter devices such as IVEX-2® filters which incorporate short inlet and outlet PVC-coated tubing has not resulted in significant leaching of DEHP.

The Chemo Dispensing Pin™ device or similar devices with spikes should not be used with vials of TAXOL since they can cause the stopper to collapse resulting in the loss of sterile integrity of the TAXOL solution.

Stability: Unopened vials of TAXOL Injection are stable until the date indicated on the package when stored between 20°–25°C (68°–77°F), in the original package. Neither freezing nor refrigeration adversely affects the stability of the product. Upon refrigeration components in the TAXOL vial may precipitate, but will redissolve upon reaching room temperature with little or no agitation. There is no impact on product quality under these circumstances. If the solution remains cloudy or if an insoluble precipitate is noted, the vial should be discarded. Solutions for infusion prepared as recommended are stable at ambient temperature (approximately 25°C) and lighting conditions for up to 27 hours.

IVEX-2® is the registered trademark of the Millipore Corporation.

Chemo Dispensing Pin™ is a trademark of B. Braun Medical Incorporated.

HOW SUPPLIED

NDC 0015-3475-30	30 mg/5 mL multidose vial individually packaged in a carton.
NDC 0015-3476-30	100 mg/16.7 mL multidose vial individually packaged in a carton.
NDC 0015-3479-11	300 mg/50 mL multidose vial individually packaged in a carton.

U.S. Patent Nos.: 5,496,804 and 5,641,803.

Storage: Store the vials in original cartons between 20°–25°C (68°–77°F). Retain in the original package to protect from light.

Handling and Disposal: Procedures for proper handling and disposal of anticancer drugs should be considered. Several guidelines on this subject have been published.[1–7] There is no general agreement that all of the procedures recommended in the guidelines are necessary or appropriate.

REFERENCES

1. Recommendations for the Safe Handling of Parenteral Antineoplastic Drugs. NIH Publication No. 83-2621. For sale by the Superintendent of Documents, US Government Printing Office, Washington, DC 20402.
2. AMA Council Report. Guidelines for Handling Parenteral Antineoplastics. JAMA 1985; 253 (11):1590-1592.
3. National Study Commission on Cytotoxic Exposure - Recommendations for Handling Cytotoxic Agents. Available from Louis P. Jeffrey, ScD, Chairman, National Study Commission on Cytotoxic Exposure. Massachusetts College of Pharmacy and Allied Health Sciences, 179 Longwood Avenue, Boston, Massachusetts, 02115.
4. Clinical Oncological Society of Australia. Guidelines and Recommendations for Safe Handling of Antineoplastic Agents. Med J Australia 1983; 1:426-428.
5. Jones RB, et al: Safe Handling of Chemotherapeutic Agents: A Report from the Mount Sinai Medical Center. CA-A Cancer Journal for Clinicians 1983; (Sept/Oct) 258-263.
6. American Society of Hospital Pharmacists Technical Assistance Bulletin on Handling Cytotoxic and Hazardous Drugs. Am J Hosp Pharm 1990; 47:1033-1049.
7. OSHA Work-Practice Guidelines for Personnel Dealing with Cytotoxic (Antineoplastic) Drugs. Am J Hosp Pharm 1986; 43:1193-1204.

MeadJohnson
ONCOLOGY PRODUCTS
A Bristol-Myers Squibb Company
Princeton, NJ 08543
U.S.A.
K4-B001-5-98 347630DIM-04
51-006186-03 Revised April 1998

Shown in Product Identification Guide, page 308

TESLAC® Ⓒ℞

(testolactone tablets, USP)

CAUTION: FEDERAL LAW PROHIBITS DISPENSING WITHOUT PRESCRIPTION.

DESCRIPTION

Teslac® (testolactone tablets, USP) is available for oral administration as tablets providing 50 mg testolactone per tablet. Testolactone is a synthetic antineoplastic agent that is structurally distinct from the androgen steroid nucleus in possessing a six-membered lactone ring in place of the usual five-membered carbocyclic D-ring. Testolactone is chemically designated as 13-hydroxy-3-oxo-13,17-secoandrosta-1,4-dien-17-oic acid δ-lactone. Graphic formula:

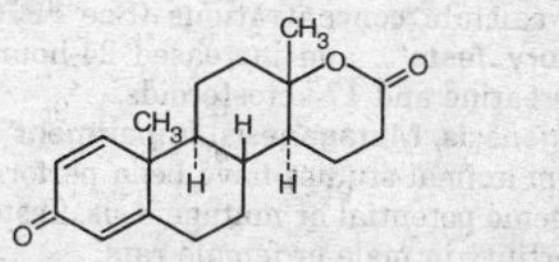

$C_{19}H_{24}O_3$ MW 300.40 CAS-968-93-4

Inactive ingredients: calcium stearate, cornstarch, gelatin, and lactose. Testolactone is a white, odorless, crystalline solid, soluble in ethanol and slightly soluble in water.

CLINICAL PHARMACOLOGY

Although the precise mechanism by which testolactone produces its clinical antineoplastic effects has not been established, its principal action is reported to be inhibition of steroid aromatase activity and consequent reduction in estrone synthesis from adrenal androstenedione, the major source of estrogen in postmenopausal women. Based on *in vitro* studies, the aromatase inhibition may be noncompetitive and irreversible. This phenomenon may account for the persistence of testolactone's effect on estrogen synthesis after drug withdrawal.

Despite some similarity to testosterone, testolactone has no *in vivo* androgenic effect. No other hormonal effects have been reported in clinical studies in patients receiving testolactone. In one study, testolactone administered orally (1000 mg/day) was reported to increase renal tubular reabsorption of calcium but to have no effect on serum calcium concentration. The mechanism of the hypocalciuric effect is unknown. No clinical effects in humans of testolactone on adrenal function have been reported; however, one study noted an increase in urinary excretion of 17-ketosteroids in most of the patients treated with 150 mg/day orally.

Testolactone is well absorbed from the gastrointestinal tract. It is metabolized to several derivatives in the liver, all of which preserve the lactone D-ring. These metabolites, as well as some unmetabolized drug, are excreted in the urine. Additional pharmacokinetic data in humans are unavailable.

For information concerning carcinogenesis, mutagenesis, pregnancy, and lactation, see the corresponding **"PRECAUTIONS"** sections.

In animals, parenteral but not oral testolactone reduced cortisone acetate induced hepatic glycogen deposits. In animal tests conducted to detect any hormonal activity for testolactone, some evidence of antiandrogenic and antiglucocorticoid activity was seen; increased growth rate in the newborn was suggested. However there was no clear manifestation of androgenic, estrogenic or antiestrogenic, progestational or antiprogestational, gonadotropin-like or antigonadotropic effects. Testolactone did not demonstrate anti-inflammatory, mineralocorticoid-like, or glucocorticoid-like properties.

INDICATIONS AND USAGE

TESLAC (testolactone tablets, USP) is recommended as adjunctive therapy in the palliative treatment of advanced or

Continued on next page

Teslac—Cont.

disseminated breast cancer in postmenopausal women when hormonal therapy is indicated. It may also be used in women who were diagnosed as having had disseminated breast carcinoma when premenopausal, in whom ovarian function has been subsequently terminated.
TESLAC was found to be effective in approximately 15 percent of patients with advanced or disseminated mammary cancer evaluated according to the following criteria: 1) those with a measurable decrease in size of all demonstrable tumor masses; 2) those in whom more than 50 percent of nonosseous lesions decreased in size although all bone lesions remained static; and 3) those in whom more than 50 percent of total lesions improved while the remainder were static.

CONTRAINDICATIONS

Testolactone is contraindicated in the treatment of breast cancer in men and in patients with a history of hypersensitivity to the drug.

PRECAUTIONS

Information for Patients–The physician should be consulted regarding missed doses. Notify the physician if adverse reactions occur or become more pronounced.
Laboratory Tests – Plasma calcium levels should be routinely determined in any patient receiving therapy for mammary cancer, particularly during periods of active remission of bony metastases. If hypercalcemia occurs, appropriate measures should be instituted.
Drug Interactions– When administered concurrently, testolactone may increase the effects of oral anticoagulants; monitor and adjust anticoagulant dosage accordingly.
Drug/Laboratory Test Interactions – Physiologic effects of testolactone may result in decreased estradiol concentrations with radioimmunoassays for estradiol, increased plasma calcium concentrations (See **"PRECAUTIONS, Laboratory Tests"**), and increased 24-hour urinary excretion of creatine and 17-ketosteroids.
Carcinogenesis, Mutagenesis, Impairment of Fertility – No long-term animal studies have been performed to evaluate carcinogenic potential or mutagenesis. Testolactone did not affect fertility in male or female rats.
Pregnancy: Teratogenic Effects, "Category C" – In rats, testolactone has been shown to produce increased fetal mortality, increased abnormal fetal development, and increased mortality in growing pups when given at doses 5 to 15 times the recommended human dose. In rabbits, no teratologic effects were observed at doses 2.5 to 7.5 times the recommended human dose. There are no adequate and well controlled studies in pregnant women. Testolactone is intended for use only in postmenopausal women and should not be used during pregnancy.
Nursing Mothers – It is not known whether this drug is excreted in human milk. Because many drugs are excreted in human milk, a decision should be made whether or not to discontinue nursing.
Pediatric Use–Safety and effectiveness in children have not been established.

ADVERSE REACTIONS

Certain signs and symptoms have been reported in association with the use of this drug but, in these instances, it is often impossible to determine the relationship of the underlying disease and drug administration to the reported reaction. Such reactions include maculopapular erythema, increase in blood pressure, paresthesia, aches and edema of the extremities, glossitis, anorexia and nausea and vomiting. Alopecia alone and with associated nail growth disturbance have been reported rarely; these side effects subsided without interruption of treatment.

DRUG ABUSE AND DEPENDENCE

TESLAC is classified as a controlled substance under the Anabolic Steroids Control Act of 1990 and has been assigned to Schedule III.

OVERDOSAGE

There have been no reports of acute overdosage with testolactone tablets.

DOSAGE AND ADMINISTRATION

The recommended oral dose is 250 mg qid.
In order to evaluate the response, therapy with testolactone should be continued for a minimum of three months unless there is active progression of the disease.

HOW SUPPLIED

TESLAC® (testolactone tablets, USP) **50 mg/tablet**: bottles of 100 (**NDC** 0003-0690-50). Each round, white, biconvex tablet is imprinted with the identification number 690.
Storage
Store at room temperature 25°C (77°F).

MeadJohnson
ONCOLOGY PRODUCTS
A Bristol-Myers Squibb Company
Princeton, NJ 08543
U.S.A.

K5-B001-5-96 P1-1944-00
Issued November 1994

VePesid® ℞

[*vě-pesid*]
(etoposide)
For Injection and Capsules

CAUTION: FEDERAL LAW PROHIBITS DISPENSING WITHOUT PRESCRIPTION.

> **WARNINGS**
> VePesid® (etoposide) should be administered under the supervision of a qualified physician experienced in the use of cancer chemotherapeutic agents. Severe myelosuppression with resulting infection or bleeding may occur.

DESCRIPTION

VePesid® (etoposide) (also commonly known as VP-16) is a semisynthetic derivative of podophyllotoxin used in the treatment of certain neoplastic diseases. It is 4′-demethylepipodophyllotoxin 9-[4,6-0-(R)-ethylidene-β-D-glucopyranoside]. It is very soluble in methanol and chloroform, slightly soluble in ethanol, and sparingly soluble in water and ether. It is made more miscible with water by means of organic solvents. It has a molecular weight of 588.58 and a molecular formula of $C_{29}H_{32}O_{13}$.
VePesid may be administered either intravenously or orally.
VePesid for Injection is available in 100 mg (5 mL), 150 mg (7.5 mL), 500 mg (25 mL), or 1 gram (50 mL), sterile, multiple dose vials. The pH of the clear, nearly colorless to yellow liquid is 3 to 4. Each mL contains 20 mg etoposide, 2 mg citric acid, 30 mg benzyl alcohol, 80 mg modified polysorbate 80/Tween 80, 650 mg polyethylene glycol 300, and 30.5 percent (v/v) alcohol. Vial headspace contains nitrogen.
VePesid is also available as 50 mg pink capsules. Each liquid filled, soft gelatin capsule contains 50 mg of etoposide in a vehicle consisting of citric acid, glycerin, purified water, and polyethylene glycol 400. The soft gelatin capsules contain gelatin, glycerin, sorbitol, purified water, and parabens (ethyl and propyl) with the following dye system: iron oxide (red) and titanium dioxide; the capsules are printed with edible ink.
The structural formula is:

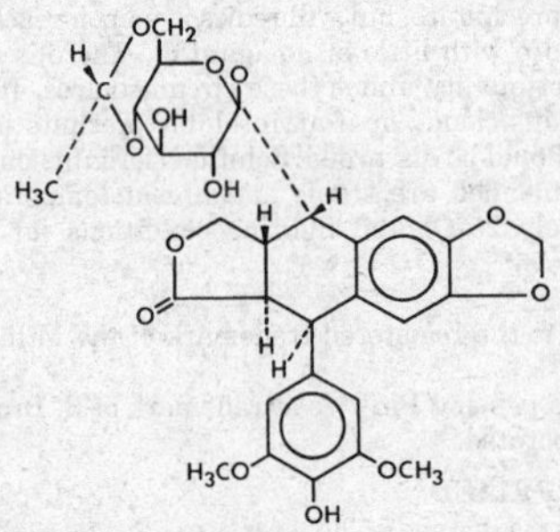

CLINICAL PHARMACOLOGY

VePesid has been shown to cause metaphase arrest in chick fibro blasts. Its main effect, however, appears to be at the G_2 portion of the cell cycle in mammalian cells. Two different dose-dependent responses are seen. At high concentrations (10 µg/mL or more), lysis of cells entering mitosis is observed. At low concentrations (0.3 to 10 µg/mL), cells are inhibited from entering prophase. It does not interfere with microtubular assembly. The predominant macromolecular effect of etoposide appears to be the induction of DNA strand breaks by an interaction with DNA topoisomerase II or the formation of free radicals.

Pharmacokinetics: On intravenous administration, the disposition of etoposide is best described as a biphasic process with a distribution half-life of about 1.5 hours and terminal elimination half-life ranging from 4 to 11 hours. Total body clearance values range from 33 to 48 mL/min or 16 to 36 mL/min/m^2 and, like the terminal elimination half-life, are independent of dose over a range 100–600 mg/m^2. Over the same dose range, the areas under the plasma concentration vs time curves (AUC) and the maximum plasma concentration (C_{max}) values increase linearly with dose. Etoposide does not accumulate in the plasma following daily administration of 100 mg/m^2 for 4 to 5 days.
The mean volumes of distribution at steady state fall in the range of 18 to 29 liters or 7 to 17 L/m^2. Etoposide enters the CSF poorly. Although it is detectable in CSF and intracerebral tumors, the concentrations are lower than in extracerebral tumors and in plasma. Etoposide concentrations are higher in normal lung than in lung metastases and are similar in primary tumors and normal tissues of the myometrium. *In vitro*, etoposide is highly protein bound (97%) to human plasma proteins. An inverse relationship between plasma albumin levels and etoposide renal clearance is found in children. In a study determining the effect of other therapeutic agents on the *in vitro* binding of carbon-14 labeled etoposide to human serum proteins, only phenylbutazone, sodium salicylate, and aspirin displaced protein-bound etoposide at concentrations achieved *in vivo*.[1]
Etoposide binding ratio correlates directly with serum albumin in patients with cancer and in normal volunteers. The unbound fraction of etoposide significantly correlated with bilirubin in a population of cancer patients.[2,3] Data have suggested a significant inverse correlation between serum albumin concentration and free fraction of etoposide (see **"PRECAUTIONS"** section).
After intravenous administration of ^{3}H-etoposide (70–290 mg/m^2), mean recoveries of radioactivity in the urine range from 42 to 67%, and fecal recoveries range from 0 to 16% of the dose. Less than 50% of an intravenous dose is excreted in the urine as etoposide with mean recoveries of 8 to 35% within 24 hours.
In children, approximately 55% of the dose is excreted in the urine as etoposide in 24 hours. The mean renal clearance of etoposide is 7 to 10 mL/min/m^2 or about 35% of the total body clearance over a dose range of 80 to 600 mg/m^2. Etoposide, therefore, is cleared by both renal and nonrenal processes, i.e., metabolism and biliary excretion. The effect of renal disease on plasma etoposide clearance is not known.
Biliary excretion appears to be a minor route of etoposide elimination. Only 6% or less of an intravenous dose is recovered in the bile as etoposide. Metabolism accounts for most of the nonrenal clearance of etoposide. The major urinary metabolite of etoposide in adults and children is the hydroxy acid [4′-demethylepipodophyllic acid-9-(4,6-0-(R)-ethylidene-β-D-glucopyranoside)], formed by opening of the lactone ring. It is also present in human plasma, presumably as the trans isomer. Gluc uronide and/or sulfate conjugates of etoposide are excreted in human urine and represent 5 to 22% of the dose. In addition, O-demethylation of the dimethoxyphenol ring occurs through the CYP450 3A4 isoenzyme pathway to produce the corresponding catechol.
After either intravenous infusion or oral capsule administration, the C_{max} and AUC values exhibit marked intra- and inter-subject variability. This results in variability in the estimates of the absolute oral bioavailability of etoposide oral capsules.
C_{max} and AUC values for orally administered etoposide capsules consistently fall in the same range as the C_{max} and AUC values for an intravenous dose of one-half the size of the oral dose. The overall mean value of oral capsule bioavailability is approximately 50% (range 25–75%). The bioavailability of etoposide capsules appears to be linear up to a dose of at least 250 mg/m^2.
There is no evidence of a first-pass effect for etoposide. For example, no correlation exists between the absolute oral bioavailability of etoposide capsules and nonrenal clearance. No evidence exists for any other differences in etoposide metabolism and excretion after administration of oral capsules as compared to intravenous infusion.
In adults, the total body clearance of etoposide is correlated with creatinine clearance, serum albumin concentration, and nonrenal clearance. Patients with impaired renal function receiving etoposide have exhibited reduced total body clearance, increased AUC and a lower volume of distribution at steady state (see **"PRECAUTIONS"** section). Use of cisplatin therapy is associated with reduced total body clearance. In children, elevated serum SGPT levels are associated with reduced drug total body clearance. Prior use of cisplatin may also result in a decrease of etoposide total body clearance in children.
Although some minor differences in pharmacokinetic parameters between age and gender have been observed, these differences were not considered clinically significant.

INDICATIONS AND USAGE

VePesid (etoposide) is indicated in the management of the following neoplasms:
Refractory Testicular Tumors — VePesid for Injection in combination therapy with other approved chemotherapeutic agents in patients with refractory testicular tumors who have already received appropriate surgical, chemotherapeutic, and radiotherapeutic therapy.
Adequate data on the use of VePesid Capsules in the treatment of testicular cancer are not available.
Small Cell Lung Cancer — VePesid for Injection and/or Capsules in combination with other approved chemotherapeutic agents as first line treatment in patients with small cell lung cancer.

CONTRAINDICATIONS

VePesid is contraindicated in patients who have demonstrated a previous hypersensitivity to etoposide or any component of the formulation.

WARNINGS

Patients being treated with VePesid must be frequently observed for myelosuppression both during and after therapy.

Myelosuppression resulting in death has been reported. Dose-limiting bone marrow suppression is the most significant toxicity associated with VePesid therapy. Therefore, the following studies should be obtained at the start of therapy and prior to each subsequent cycle of VePesid: platelet count, hemoglobin, white blood cell count, and differential. The occurrence of a platelet count below 50,000/mm^3 or an absolute neutrophil count below 500/mm^3 is an indication to withhold further therapy until the blood counts have sufficiently recovered.

Physicians should be aware of the possible occurrence of an anaphylactic reaction manifested by chills, fever, tachycardia, bronchospasm, dyspnea, and hypotension. Higher rates of anaphylactic-like reactions have been reported in children who received infusions at concentrations higher than those recommended. The role that concentration of infusion (or rate of infusion) plays in the development of anaphylactic-like reactions is uncertain. (See "ADVERSE REACTIONS" section.) Treatment is symptomatic. The infusion should be terminated immediately, followed by the administration of pressor agents, corticosteroids, antihistamines, or volume expanders at the discretion of the physician.

For parenteral administration, VePesid should be given only by slow intravenous infusion (usually over a 30 to 60 minute period) since hypotension has been reported as a possible side effect of rapid intravenous injection.

Pregnancy: VePesid can cause fetal harm when administered to a pregnant woman. Etoposide has been shown to be teratogenic in mice and rats.

In rats, an intravenous etoposide dose of 0.4 mg/kg/day (about 1/20th of the human dose on a mg/m^2 basis) during organogenesis caused maternal toxicity, embryotoxicity, and teratogenicity (skeletal abnormalities, exencephaly, encephalocele, and anophthalmia); higher doses of 1.2 and 3.6 mg/kg/day (about 1/7th and 1/2 of human dose on a mg/m^2 basis) resulted in 90 and 100% embryonic resorptions. In mice, a single 1.0 mg/kg (1/16th of human dose on a mg/m^2 basis) dose of etoposide administered intraperitoneally on days 6, 7, 8 of gestation caused embryotoxicity, cranial abnormalities, and major skeletal malformations. An i.p. dose of 1.5 mg/kg (about 1/10th of human dose on a mg/m^2 basis) on day 7 of gestation caused an increase in the incidence of intrauterine death and fetal malformations and a significant decrease in the average fetal body weight.

Women of childbearing potential should be advised to avoid becoming pregnant. If this drug is used during pregnancy, or if the patient becomes pregnant while receiving this drug, the patient should be warned of the potential hazard to the fetus.

VePesid should be considered a potential carcinogen in humans. The occurrence of acute leukemia with or without a preleukemic phase has been reported in rare instances in patients treated with etoposide alone or in association with other neo-plastic agents. The risk of development of a preleukemic or leukemic syndrome is unclear. Carcinogenicity tests with VePesid have not been conducted in laboratory animals.

PRECAUTIONS

General: In all instances where the use of VePesid is considered for chemotherapy, the physician must evaluate the need and usefulness of the drug against the risk of adverse reactions. Most such adverse reactions are reversible if detected early. If severe reactions occur, the drug should be reduced in dosage or discontinued and appropriate corrective measures should be taken according to the clinical judgment of the physician. Reinstitution of VePesid therapy should be carried out with caution, and with adequate consideration of the further need for the drug and alertness as to possible recurrence of toxicity.

Patients with low serum albumin may be at an increased risk for etoposide-associated toxicities.

Laboratory Tests: Periodic complete blood counts should be done during the course of VePesid treatment. They should be performed prior to each cycle of therapy and at appropriate intervals during and after therapy. At least one determination should be done prior to each dose of VePesid.

Renal Impairment: In patients with impaired renal function, the following initial dose modification should be considered based on measured creatinine clearance:

Measured Creatinine Clearance	> 50 mL/min	15–50 mL/min
etoposide	100% of dose	75% of dose

Subsequent VePesid dosing should be based on patient tolerance and clinical effect.

Data are not available in patients with creatinine clearances <15 mL/min and further dose reduction should be considered in these patients.

Carcinogenesis, (see "WARNINGS" section) **Mutagenesis, Impairment of Fertility:** Etoposide has been shown to be mutagenic in Ames assay.

Treatment of Swiss-Albino mice with 1.5 mg/kg IP of VePesid on day 7 of gestation increased the incidence of intra-

uterine death and fetal malformations as well as significantly decreased the average fetal body weight. Maternal weight gain was not affected.

Irreversible testicular atrophy was present in rats treated with etoposide intravenously for 30 days at 0.5 mg/kg/day (about 1/16th of the human dose on a mg/m^2 basis).

Pregnancy Pregnancy "Category D". (See "WARNINGS" section.)

Nursing Mothers: It is not known whether this drug is excreted in human milk. Because many drugs are excreted in human milk and because of the potential for serious adverse reactions in nursing infants from VePesid (etoposide), a decision should be made whether to discontinue nursing or to discontinue the drug, taking into account the importance of the drug to the mother.

Pediatric Use: Safety and effectiveness in pediatric patients have not been established.

VePesid for Injection contains polysorbate 80. In premature infants, a life-threatening syndrome consisting of liver and renal failure, pulmonary deterioration, thrombocytopenia, and ascites has been associated with an injectable vitamin E product containing polysorbate 80. Anaphylactic reactions have been reported in pediatric patients. (See "WARNINGS" section.)

ADVERSE REACTIONS

The following data on adverse reactions are based on both oral and intravenous administration of VePesid as a single agent, using several different dose schedules for treatment of a wide variety of malignancies.

Hematologic Toxicity: Myelosuppression is dose related and dose limiting, with granulocyte nadirs occurring 7 to 14 days after drug administration and platelet nadirs occurring 9 to 16 days after drug administration. Bone marrow recovery is usually complete by day 20, and no cumulative toxicity has been reported. Fever and infection have also been reported in patients with neutropenia. Death associated with myelosuppression has been reported.

The occurrence of acute leukemia with or without a preleukemic phase has been reported rarely in patients treated with VePesid in association with other antineoplastic agents. (See "WARNINGS" section.)

Gastrointestinal Toxicity: Nausea and vomiting are the major gastrointestinal toxicities. The severity of such nausea and vomiting is generally mild to moderate with treatment discontinuation required in 1% of patients. Nausea and vomiting can usually be controlled with standard antiemetic therapy. Gastrointestinal toxicities are slightly more frequent after oral administration than after intravenous infusion.

Hypotension: Transient hypotension following rapid intravenous administration has been reported in 1 to 2% of patients. It has not been associated with cardiac toxicity or electrocardiographic changes. No delayed hypotension has been noted. To prevent this rare occurrence, it is recommended that VePesid be administered by slow intravenous infusion over a 30- to 60-minute period. If hypotension occurs, it usually responds to cessation of the infusion and administration of fluids or other supportive therapy as appropriate. When restarting the infusion, a slower administration rate should be used.

Allergic Reactions: Anaphylactic-like reactions characterized by chills, fever, tachycardia, bronchospasm, dyspnea, and/or hypotension have been reported to occur in 0.7 to 2% of patients receiving intravenous VePesid and in less than 1% of the patients treated with the oral capsules. These reactions have usually responded promptly to the cessation of the infusion and administration of pressor agents, corticosteroids, antihistamines, or volume expanders as appropriate; however, the reactions can be fatal. Hypertension and/or flushing have also been reported. Blood pressure usually normalizes within a few hours after cessation of the infusion. Anaphylactic-like reactions have occurred during the initial infusion of VePesid.

Facial/tongue swelling, coughing, diaphoresis, cyanosis, tightness in throat, laryngospasm, back pain, and/or loss of consciousness have sometimes occurred in association with the above reactions. In addition, an apparent hypersensitivity-associated apnea has been reported rarely.

Rash, urticaria, and/or pruritus have infrequently been reported at recommended doses. At investigational doses, a generalized pruritic erythematous maculopapular rash, consistent with perivasculitis, has been reported.

Alopecia: Reversible alopecia, sometimes progressing to total baldness, was observed in up to 66% of patients.

Other Toxicities: The following adverse reactions have been infrequently reported: abdominal pain, aftertaste, constipation, dysphagia, fever, transient cortical blindness, interstitial pneumonitis/pulmonary fibrosis, optic neuritis, pigmentation, seizure (occasionally associated with allergic reactions), and a single report of radiation recall dermatitis.

Hepatic toxicity, generally in patients receiving higher doses of the drug than those recommended, has been reported with VePesid. Metabolic acidosis has also been reported in patients receiving higher doses.

The incidences of adverse reactions in the table that follows are derived from multiple data bases from studies in 2,081 patients when VePesid was used either orally or by injection as a single agent.

ADVERSE DRUG EFFECT	PERCENT RANGE OF REPORTED INCIDENCE
Hematologic toxicity	
Leukopenia (less than 1,000 WBC/mm^3)	3–17
Leukopenia (less than 4,000 WBC/mm^3)	60–91
Thrombocytopenia (less than 50,000 platelets/mm^3)	1–20
Thrombocytopenia (less than 100,000 platelets/mm^3)	22–41
Anemia	0–33
Gastrointestinal toxicity	
Nausea and vomiting	31–43
Abdominal pain	0–2
Anorexia	10–13
Diarrhea	1–13
Stomatitis	1–6
Hepatic	0–3
Alopecia	8–66
Peripheral neurotoxicity	1–2
Hypotension	1–2
Allergic reaction	1–2

OVERDOSAGE

No proven antidotes have been established for VePesid overdosage.

DOSAGE AND ADMINISTRATION

Note: Plastic devices made of acrylic or ABS (a polymer composed of acrylonitrile, butadiene, and styrene) have been reported to crack and leak when used with *undiluted* VePesid for Injection.

VePesid for Injection: The usual dose of VePesid for Injection in testicular cancer in combination with other approved chemotherapeutic agents ranges from 50 to 100 mg/m^2/day on days 1 through 5 to 100 mg/m^2/day on days 1, 3, and 5. In small cell lung cancer, the VePesid for Injection dose in combination with other approved chemotherapeutic drugs ranges from 35 mg/m^2/day for 4 days to 50 mg/m^2/day for 5 days.

For recommended dosing adjustments in patients with renal impairment, (see "PRECAUTIONS" section).

Chemotherapy courses are repeated at 3- to 4-week intervals after adequate recovery from any toxicity.

VePesid Capsules: In small cell lung cancer, the recommended dose of VePesid Capsules is two times the I.V. dose rounded to the nearest 50 mg.

The dosage, by either route, should be modified to take into account the myelosuppressive effects of other drugs in the combination or the effects of prior x-ray therapy or chemotherapy which may have compromised bone marrow reserve.

Administration Precautions: As with other potentially toxic compounds, caution should be exercised in handling and preparing the solution of VePesid (etoposide). Skin reactions associated with accidental exposure to VePesid may occur. The use of gloves is recommended. If VePesid solution contacts the skin or mucosa, immediately and thoroughly wash the skin with soap and water and flush the mucosa with water.

Preparation for Intravenous Administration: VePesid for Injection must be diluted prior to use with either 5% Dextrose Injection, USP, or 0.9% Sodium Chloride Injection, USP, to give a final concentration of 0.2 to 0.4 mg/mL. If solutions are prepared at concentrations above 0.4 mg/mL, precipitation may occur. Hypotension following rapid intravenous administration has been reported, hence, it is recommended that the VePesid solution be administered over a 30- to 60-minute period. A longer duration of administration may be used if the volume of fluid to be infused is a concern. **VePesid should not be given by rapid intravenous injection.** Parenteral drug products should be inspected visually for particulate matter and discoloration (see "DESCRIPTION" section) prior to administration whenever solution and container permit.

Stability: Unopened vials of VePesid for Injection are stable for 24 months at room temperature (25°C). Vials diluted as recommended to a concentration of 0.2 or 0.4 mg/mL are stable for 96 and 24 hours, respectively, at room temperature (25°C) under normal room fluorescent light in both glass and plastic containers.

Continued on next page

VePesid—Cont.

VePesid (etoposide) Capsules must be stored under refrigeration 2°–8°C (36°–46°F). The capsules are stable for 24 months under such refrigeration conditions.

Procedures for proper handling and disposal of anticancer drugs should be considered. Several guidelines on this subject have been published.[4-10] There is no general agreement that all of the procedures recommended in the guidelines are necessary or appropriate.

HOW SUPPLIED

VePesid® (etoposide) For Injection

NDC 0015-3095-20 — 100 mg/5 mL Sterile, Multiple Dose Vial, 10's

NDC 0015-3084-20 — 150 mg/7.5 mL Sterile, Multiple Dose Vial

NDC 0015-3061-20 — 500 mg/25 mL Sterile, Multiple Dose Vial

NDC 0015-3062-20 — 1 gram/50 mL Sterile, Multiple Dose Vial

VePesid® (etoposide) Capsules

NDC 0015-3091-45 — 50 mg pink capsules with "BRISTOL 3091" printed in black in blisterpacks of 20 individually labeled blisters, each containing one capsule.

Capsules are to be stored under refrigeration 2°–8°C (36°–46°F).

DO NOT FREEZE.

Dispense in child-resistant containers.

For information on package size s available, refer to the current price schedule.

REFERENCES

1. Gaver RC, Deeb G: The Effect of Other Drugs on the *in vitro* Binding of 14C-Etoposide to Human Serum Proteins. Proc Am Assoc Cancer Res 1989; 30:A2132.
2. Stewart CF, et al: Altered Protein Binding of Etoposide in Patients with Cancer. Clin Pharmacol Ther 1989; 45: 49-55.
3. Stewart CF, et al: Prospective Evaluation of a Model for Predicting Etoposide Plasma Protein Binding in Cancer Patients. Proc Am Assoc Cancer Res 1989; 30:A958.
4. Recommendations for the Safe Handling of Parenteral Antineoplastic Drugs. NIH Publication No. 83-2621. For sale by the Superintendent of Documents, US Government Printing Office, Washington, DC 20402.
5. AMA Council Report. Guidelines for Handling Parenteral Antineo plastics. JAMA 1985; 253 (11):1590-1592.
6. National Study Commission on Cytotoxic Exposure – Recommendations for Handling Cytotoxic Agents. Available from Louis P. Jeffrey, ScD, Chairman, National Study Commission on Cytotoxic Exposure, Massachusetts College of Pharmacy and Allied Health Sciences, 179 Longwood Avenue, Boston, Massachusetts 02115.
7. Clinical Oncological Society of Australia. Guidelines and Recommendations for Safe Handling of Antineoplastic Agents. Med J Australia 1983; 1:426-428.
8. Jones RB, et al: Handling of Chemotherapeutic Agents: A Report from the Mount Sinai Medical Center. CA-A Cancer Journal for Clinicians 1983; (Sept/Oct) 258–263.
9. American Society of Hospital Pharmacists Technical Assistance Bulletin on Handling Cytotoxic and Hazardous Drugs. Am J Hosp Pharm 1990; 47:1033-1049.
10. Controlling occupational exposure to hazardous drugs. (OSHA WORK PRACTICE GUIDELINES). Am J Health-Syst Pharm 1996; 53:1669-1685.

Capsules:
Manufactured by:
R.P. Scherer GmbH
Eberback/Baden, Germany

Injection:
BRISTOL LABORATORIES
Oncology Products
A Bristol-Myers Squibb Co.
Princeton, New Jersey 08543 U.S.A.

Distributed by:
BRISTOL LABORATORIES®
ONCOLOGY PRODUCTS
A Bristol-Myers Squibb Company
Princeton, NJ 08543
U.S.A.

K6-B001-3-97   P0566-01
52-005874-00   Revised March 1997
Shown in Product Identification Guide, page 308

VIDEX®   ℞ ONLY
[*vī-dex*]
(didanosine)

VIDEX® (didanosine) Chewable/Dispersible Buffered Tablets
VIDEX® (didanosine) Buffered Powder for Oral Solution
VIDEX® (didanosine) Pediatric Powder for Oral Solution

> **WARNING**
> **PANCREATITIS, WHICH HAS BEEN FATAL IN SOME CASES, HAS OCCURRED DURING THERAPY WITH VIDEX. VIDEX USE SHOULD BE SUSPENDED IN PATIENTS WITH SIGNS OR SYMPTOMS OF PANCREATITIS AND DISCONTINUED IN PATIENTS WITH CONFIRMED PANCREATITIS (SEE "WARNINGS" SECTION).**
> **LACTIS ACIDOSIS AND SEVERE HEPATOMEGALY WITH STEATOSIS INCLUDING FATAL CASES HAVE BEEN REPORTED WITH THE USE OF ANTIRETROVIRAL NUCLEOSIDE ANALOGUES ALONE OR IN COMBINATION, INCLUDING DIDANOSINE (SEE "WARNINGS" SECTION).**

DESCRIPTION

VIDEX® (didanosine) is the brand name for didanosine [formerly called dideoxyinosine (ddI)], a synthetic purine nucleoside analogue active against the Human Immunodeficiency Virus (HIV). VIDEX Chewable/Dispersible Buffered Tablets are available for oral administration in strengths of 25, 50, 100, or 150 mg of didanosine. Each tablet is buffered with calcium carbonate and magnesium hydroxide. VIDEX tablets also contain aspartame, sorbitol, microcrystalline cellulose, polyplasdone, mandarin-orange flavor, and magnesium stearate.

VIDEX Buffered Powder for Oral Solution is supplied for oral administration in single-dose packets containing 100, 167, or 250 mg of didanosine. Packets of each product strength also contain a citrate-phosphate buffer (composed of dibasic sodium phosphate, sodium citrate, and citric acid) and sucrose.

VIDEX Pediatric Powder for Oral Solution is supplied for oral administration in 4- or 8-ounce glass bottles containing 2 or 4 grams of didanosine, respectively.

The chemical name for didanosine is 2',3'-dideoxyinosine. The structural formula is:

Didanosine is a white crystalline powder with the molecular formula $C_{10}H_{12}N_4O_3$ and a molecular weight of 236.2. The aqueous solubility of didanosine at 25°C and pH of approximately 6 is 27.3 mg/mL. Didanosine is unstable in acidic solutions. For example, at pH <3 and 37°C, 10 percent of didanosine decomposes to hypoxanthine in less than 2 minutes.

MICROBIOLOGY

Mechanism of Action: Didanosine is a synthetic nucleoside analogue of the naturally occurring nucleoside deoxyadenosine in which the 3'-hydroxyl (OH) group is replaced by hydrogen. Intracellularly, didanosine is converted by cellular enzymes to the active metabolite, dideoxyadenosine 5'-triphosphate (ddATP). Dideoxyadenosine 5'-triphosphate inhibits the activity of HIV-1 reverse transcriptase both by competing with the natural substrate, deoxyadenosine 5'-triphosphate (dATP), and by its incorporation into viral DNA. The lack of a 3'-OH group in the incorporated nucleoside analogue prevents the formation of the 5' to 3' phosphodiester linkage essential for DNA chain elongation and, therefore, the viral DNA growth is terminated.

***In Vitro* HIV Susceptibility:** The *in vitro* anti-HIV-1 activity of didanosine was evaluated in a variety of HIV-1 infected lymphoblastic cell lines and monocyte/macrophage cell cultures. Didanosine has shown antiviral activity against laboratory and clinical isolates of HIV-1. The concentration of drug necessary to inhibit viral replication by 50 percent (IC_{50}) ranged from 2.5 to 10 μM (1 μM = 0.24 μg/mL) in lymphoblastic cell lines and 0.01 to 0.1 μM in monocyte/macrophage cell cultures. The relationship between *in vitro* susceptibility of HIV to didanosine and the inhibition of HIV replication in humans has not been established.

Drug Resistance: HIV-1 isolates with reduced sensitivity to didanosine have been selected *in vitro* and were also obtained from patients treated with didanosine. Genetic analysis of these isolates showed a predominant mutation at Leu 74 (Leu 74 Val) and another mutation at Met 184 (Met 184 Val) in the Pol gene that encodes for the reverse transcriptase.

Cross-resistance: The potential for cross-resistance between reverse transcriptase inhibitors and protease inhibitors is low because of the different enzyme targets involved. Mutations in the reverse transcriptase gene at both codons 74 and 184 are associated with cross-resistance to zalcitabine. Lamivudine-resistant isolates containing only the Met 184 Val mutation have been recovered and these isolates showed a 4- to 8-fold decrease in didanosine sensitivity. HIV-1 isolates with multidrug resistance mutations to zidovudine, didanosine, zalcitabine, stavudine and lamivudine have been reported (2/39 isolates) following combination therapy with zidovudine and didanosine for 2 years. Multidrug resistance was dependent on five mutations (Ala 62 Val, Val 75 Ile, Phe 77 Leu, Phe 116 Tyr and Gln 151 Met) in the reverse transcriptase gene. Of these, the mutation at codon position 151 (Q151M) played a significant role in the development of viable virus with a multidrug resistance phenotype.

CLINICAL PHARMACOLOGY

Animal Toxicology: Evidence of a dose-limiting skeletal muscle toxicity has been observed in mice and rats (but not in dogs) following long-term (greater than 90 days) dosing with didanosine at doses that were approximately 1.2 to 12 times the estimated human exposure. The relationship of this finding to the potential of VIDEX to cause myopathy in humans is unclear. However, human myopathy has been associated with administration of other nucleoside analogues.

Pharmacokinetics: The pharmacokinetic parameters of didanosine are summarized in Table 1. Didanosine is rapidly absorbed, with peak plasma concentrations generally observed from 0.25 to 1.50 hours following oral dosing. In-

---

Table 1

Mean ± SD Pharmacokinetic Parameters for Didanosine in Adult and Pediatric Patients

Parameter	Adult Patients	n	Pediatric Patients	n
Oral bioavailability	42±12%	6	25±20%	46
Apparent volume of distribution[a]	1.08±0.22 L/kg	6	28±15 L/m²	49
CSF-plasma ratio[b]	21±0.03%[c]	5	46% (range 12 –85%)	7
Systemic clearance[a]	13.0±1.6 mL/min/kg	6	516±184 mL/min/m²	49
Renal clearance[d]	5.5±2.1 mL/min/kg	6	240±90 mL/min/m²	15
Elimination half-life[d]	1.5±0.4 hr	6	0.8±0.3 hr	60
Urine recovery of didanosine[d]	18±8%	6	18±10%	15

CSF = cerebrospinal fluid
[a] following I.V. administration
[b] following I.V. administration in adults and I.V. or oral administration in pediatric patients
[c] mean ± SE
[d] following oral administration

creases in plasma didanosine concentrations were dose proportional over the range of oral doses administered in clinical practice. Steady-state pharmacokinetic parameters did not differ significantly from values obtained after a single dose. Binding of didanosine to plasma proteins *in vitro* was low (<5%). Based on data from *in vitro* and animal studies, it is presumed that the metabolism of didanosine in man occurs by the same pathways responsible for the elimination of endogenous purines.
[See table 1 at bottom of previous page]

Effect of Food on Absorption of Didanosine- Didanosine peak plasma concentrations (C_{max}) and area under the plasma concentration time curve (AUC) were decreased by approximately 55% when VIDEX (didanosine) tablets were administered up to 2 hours after a meal. Administration of VIDEX tablets up to 30 minutes before a meal did not result in any significant changes in bioavailability. VIDEX should be taken on an empty stomach, at least 30 minutes before or 2 hours after eating. (See "**DOSAGE AND ADMINISTRATION**" section.)

Special Populations:
Renal Insufficiency- It is recommended that the VIDEX dose be modified in patients with reduced creatinine clearance and in patients receiving maintenance hemodialysis (see "**DOSAGE AND ADMINISTRATION**" section). Data from two studies indicated that the apparent oral clearance of didanosine decreased and the terminal elimination half-life increased as creatinine clearance decreased (see Table 2). Following oral administration, didanosine was not detectable in peritoneal dialysate fluid (n=6); recovery in hemodialysate (n=5) ranged from 0.6% to 7.4% of the dose over a 3–4 hour dialysis period. The absolute bioavailability of didanosine was not affected in patients requiring dialysis.
[See table 2 above]

Pediatric Patients- The pharmacokinetics of didanosine have been evaluated in HIV-infected pediatric patients from 0.7 to 18.9 years of age (see Table 1). Overall, the pharmacokinetics of didanosine in pediatric patients greater than 0.7 years of age are similar to those of didanosine in adults. Didanosine plasma concentrations increased in proportion to oral doses ranging from 80 to 180 mg/m². For information on controlled clinical trials in pediatric patients, see "**PRECAUTIONS, Pediatric Use**" section.

Geriatric Patients- Didanosine pharmacokinetics have not been studied in patients over 65 years of age.

Gender- The effects of gender on didanosine pharmacokinetics have not been studied.

Drug Interactions- Drug interaction studies have demonstrated that there are no clinically significant pharmacokinetic interactions between VIDEX and the following: dapsone, loperamide, metoclopramide, ranitidine, rifabutin, stavudine, sulfamethoxazole, trimethoprim, and zidovudine. Studies with loperamide, metoclopramide, ranitidine, sulfamethoxazole, trimethoprim were single-dose studies, and effects on pharmacokinetics at steady-state are not known.

INDICATIONS AND USAGE

VIDEX is indicated for the treatment of HIV infection when antiretroviral therapy is warranted.

Description of Clinical Data

Controlled Clinical Trial ACTG 175
ACTG 175 was a randomized, double-blind, controlled trial that compared zidovudine 200 mg TID; VIDEX 200 mg BID; zidovudine + VIDEX; and zidovudine + zalcitabine 0.75 mg TID. A total of 2467 HIV-infected adults with baseline CD4 counts of 200–500 cells/mm³ (mean=352) and no prior AIDS-defining event enrolled with the following demographics: male (82%), Caucasian (70%), mean age of 35 years, asymptomatic HIV infection (81%) and prior antiretroviral use (57%, mean duration = 89.5 weeks). The overall mean duration of study treatment was 99 weeks.
Results: The incidence of AIDS-defining events or death is shown in the following table:
[See table 3 above]

Controlled Clinical Trial ACTG 116A
ACTG 116A was a randomized, double-blind, controlled trial that compared high and recommended doses of VIDEX (didanosine) to zidovudine in patients who had received up to 16 weeks of zidovudine therapy. 617 HIV-infected adults enrolled with the following demographics: male (92%), Caucasian (73%), mean age of 36 years, median CD4 cell count of 130 cells/mm³, symptomatic HIV infection (67%) or AIDS (26%) and median duration of prior antiretroviral use of 8 weeks. The median duration of study treatment was 60 weeks.
Results: In the three treatment groups, the time until development of a first new AIDS-defining event or death was similar. Patients randomized to zidovudine had longer survival times than patients randomized to VIDEX recommended dose with mortality rates of 26% and 21% for VIDEX recommended dose and zidovudine, respectively.

Controlled Clinical Trial ACTG 116B/117
ACTG 116B/117 was a randomized, double-blind, controlled clinical trial that compared high and recommended doses of VIDEX to zidovudine in patients who had tolerated four

Table 2

Mean ± SD Pharmacokinetic Parameters for Didanosine Following a Single Oral Dose

| Parameter | Creatinine Clearance (mL/min) | | | | |
	≥ 90 (n=12)	60–90 (n=6)	30–59 (n=6)	10–29 (n=3)	Dialysis Patients (n=11)
CL_{cr} (mL/min)	112±22	68±8	46±8	13±5	ND[a]
CL/F (mL/min)	2164±638	1566±833	1023±378	628±104	543±174
CL_R (mL/min)	485±164	247±153	100±44	20±8	<10
$T_{1/2}$ (hr)	1.42±0.33	1.59±0.13	1.75±0.43	2.0±0.3	4.1±1.2

[a]ND = not determined due to anuria
CL_{cr} = creatinine clearance
CL/F = apparent oral clearance
CL_R = renal clearance

Table 3

First AIDS-defining Event or Death and Death Only by Study Arm and Antiretroviral Experience

| Antiretroviral Experience | Event | Treatment [n (%)] | | | |
		zidovudine	VIDEX	zidovudine + VIDEX	zidovudine + zalcitabine
Overall	n	619	620	613	615
	AIDS/Death	96 (16)	71 (11)	65 (11)	76 (12)
	Death Only	54 (9)	29 (5)	31 (5)	40 (7)
Naive	n	269	268	263	267
	AIDS/Death	32 (12)	23 (9)	20 (8)	16 (6)
	Death Only	18 (7)	11 (4)	11 (4)	9 (3)
Experienced	n	350	352	350	348
	AIDS/Death	64 (18)	48 (14)	45 (13)	60 (17)
	Death Only	36 (10)	18 (5)	20 (6)	31 (9)

months or greater of prior zidovudine therapy. 913 HIV-infected adults enrolled with the following demographics: male (96%), Caucasian (82%), mean age of 37 years, median CD4 cell count of 95 cells/mm³, symptomatic HIV infection (60%) or AIDS (30%) and median duration of prior antiretroviral use of 59.4 weeks. The median duration of study treatment was 49.7 weeks.
Results: Subjects randomized to the currently recommended dose of VIDEX had a lower rate of progression to a new AIDS-defining event or death compared to those randomized to zidovudine (32% vs. 41%, respectively). Survival rates were similar for the two treatment groups.

CONTRAINDICATION

VIDEX is contraindicated in patients with previously demonstrated clinically significant hypersensitivity to any of the components of the formulations.

WARNINGS

1. Pancreatitis
PANCREATITIS, WHICH HAS BEEN FATAL IN SOME CASES, HAS OCCURRED DURING THERAPY WITH VIDEX. VIDEX USE SHOULD BE SUSPENDED IN PATIENTS WITH SIGNS OR SYMPTOMS OF PANCREATITIS AND DISCONTINUED IN PATIENTS WITH CONFIRMED PANCREATITIS. When treatment with other drugs known to cause pancreatic toxicity is required, suspension of VIDEX therapy is recommended. In patients with risk factors for pancreatitis, VIDEX should be used with extreme caution and only if clearly indicated. Patients with advanced HIV infection are at increased risk of pancreatitis and should be followed closely. Patients with renal impairment may be at greater risk for pancreatitis if treated without dose adjustment. The frequency of pancreatitis is dose-related. In phase 3 studies, incidence ranged from 1 to 10% with high dose and 1 to 7% with recommended dose.
In pediatric studies, pancreatitis occurred in 3% (2/60) of patients treated at entry doses below 300 mg/m²/day and in 13% (5/38) of patients treated at higher doses. VIDEX use should be suspended in pediatric patients with signs or symptoms of pancreatitis and discontinued in pediatric patients with confirmed pancreatitis.

2. Lactic Acidosis/Severe Hepatomegaly with Steatosis
Lactic acidosis and severe hepatomegaly with steatosis, including fatal cases, have been reported with the use of antiretroviral nucleoside analogues alone or in combination, including didanosine. A majority of these cases have been in women. Caution should be exercised when administering VIDEX to any patient, and particularly to those with known risk factors for liver disease. Treatment with VIDEX should be suspended in any patient who develops clinical or laboratory findings suggestive of lactic acidosis or hepatotoxicity.

3. Retinal and Visual Changes
Retinal changes and optic neuritis have been reported in adult and pediatric patients. Periodic retinal examinations should be considered for patients receiving VIDEX. (See "**ADVERSE REACTIONS**" section.)

PRECAUTIONS

General: The duration of clinical benefit from antiretroviral therapy may be limited. Patients receiving VIDEX or any other antiretroviral therapy may continue to develop opportunistic infections and other complications of HIV infection, and therefore should remain under close clinical observation by physicians experienced in the treatment of patients with associated HIV diseases.
VIDEX should be taken on an empty stomach, at least 30 minutes before or 2 hours after eating.

Patients with Phenylketonuria: VIDEX Chewable/Dispersible Buffered Tablets contain the following quantities of phenylalanine:

Table 4

	All Strengths
Phenylalanine per 2-tablet dose	73 mg
Phenylalanine per tablet	36.5 mg

Patients on Sodium-Restricted Diets: VIDEX Buffered Powder for Oral Solution: Each single-dose packet of VIDEX Buffered Powder for Oral Solution contains 1380 mg sodium.

Patients with Renal Impairment: Patients with renal impairment (creatinine clearance < 60 mL/min) may be at greater risk of toxicity from VIDEX due to decreased drug clearance (see "**CLINICAL PHARMACOLOGY**" section). A dose reduction is recommended in these patients (see "**DOSAGE AND ADMINISTRATION**" section). The magnesium content of each buffered tablet of VIDEX is 8.6 mEq. This may present an excessive load of magnesium to patients with significant renal impairment, particularly after prolonged dosing.

Patients with Hepatic Impairment: It is unknown if hepatic impairment significantly affects didanosine pharmacokinetics. Therefore, these patients should be monitored closely for evidence of didanosine toxicity.

Hyperuricemia: VIDEX has been associated with asymptomatic hyperuricemia; treatment suspension may be nec-

Continued on next page

Videx—Cont.

essary if clinical measures aimed at reducing uric acid levels fail.

Diarrhea: VIDEX Buffered Powder for Oral Solution was associated with diarrhea in 34% of patients in phase 1 adult studies (see "**ADVERSE REACTIONS**" section).

Pediatric Use
Results from Controlled Clinical Trial ACTG 152
ACTG 152 was a randomized, double-blind, controlled trial that compared zidovudine 180 mg/m² q6h; VIDEX 120 mg/m² q12h; and zidovudine (120 mg/m² q6h) + VIDEX (90 mg/m² q12h). A total of 831 HIV-infected pediatric patients were enrolled with the following demographics: male (50%), racial minority groups (86%), mean age of 3.8 years (54% were <30 months of age), perinatally acquired infection (90%), naive to antiretroviral treatment (89%). The overall median duration of study treatment was 20 months.
Results: The incidence of clinical progression or death is shown in the following table:
[See table 5 above]

Information for Patients
VIDEX is not a cure for HIV infection, and patients may continue to develop HIV-associated illnesses, including opportunistic infection. Therefore, patients should remain under the care of a physician when using VIDEX. Patients should be advised that VIDEX therapy has not been shown to reduce the risk of transmission of HIV to others through sexual contact or blood contamination.
Patients should be informed that the major toxicity of VIDEX is pancreatitis, which has been fatal in some patients. Patients should also be aware that peripheral neuropathy may develop. Patients should be counseled that these toxicities occur with greatest frequency in patients with a history of these events, and that dose modification and/or discontinuation of VIDEX may be required if toxicity develops. They should be cautioned about the use of other medications that may exacerbate the VIDEX toxicity, including alcohol.

Drug Interactions
(see also "CLINICAL PHARMACOLOGY, Drug Interactions" section)
Coadministration of VIDEX with drugs that are known to cause pancreatitis may increase the risk of this toxicity (see "WARNINGS" section) and should be done with extreme caution and only if clearly indicated. Neuropathy has occurred more frequently in patients with a history of neuropathy or neurotoxic drug therapy and these patients may be at increased risk of neuropathy during VIDEX therapy (see "**ADVERSE REACTIONS**" section).
Allopurinol- The AUC of didanosine was increased about 4-fold when allopurinol at 300 mg/day was coadministered with a single 200-mg dose of VIDEX to two patients with renal impairment (Cl$_{cr}$=15 and 18 mL/min). The effects of allopurinol on didanosine pharmacokinetics in subjects with normal renal function are not known.
Antacids- Concomitant administration of antacids containing magnesium or aluminum with VIDEX Chewable/Dispersible Buffered Tablets or Pediatric Powder for Oral Solution may potentiate adverse events associated with the antacid components.
Drugs Whose Absorption Can Be Affected by the Level of Acidity in the Stomach- Drugs such as ketoconazole and itraconazole should be administered at least 2 hours prior to dosing with VIDEX.
Ganciclovir- Administration of VIDEX 2 hours prior to or concurrent with oral ganciclovir was associated with a 111 (±114)% increase in the steady-state AUC of didanosine (n=12). A 21 (±17)% decrease in the steady-state AUC of ganciclovir was observed when VIDEX was administered 2 hours prior to ganciclovir, but not when the two drugs were administered simultaneously (n=12).
Quinolone Antibiotics- VIDEX should be administered at least 2 hours after or 6 hours before dosing with ciprofloxacin because plasma concentrations of ciprofloxacin are decreased when administered with antacids containing magnesium, calcium, or aluminum. In eight HIV-infected patients, the steady-state AUC of ciprofloxacin was decreased an average of 26% (95% Cl = 14%, 37%) when ciprofloxacin was administered 2 hours prior to a marketed chewable/dispersible tablet formulation of VIDEX. The AUC of ciprofloxacin was decreased an average of 15-fold in 12 healthy subjects given ciprofloxacin and didanosine-placebo tablets concurrently. In a single subject given one dose of ciprofloxacin 2 hours after a dose of didanosine-placebo tablets, a greater than 50% reduction in the AUC of ciprofloxacin was observed.
Plasma concentrations of quinolone antibiotics are decreased when administered with antacids containing magnesium, calcium, or aluminum. The optimal dosing interval for coadministration with VIDEX should be determined by consulting the appropriate quinolone package insert.

Carcinogenesis and Mutagenesis
Lifetime carcinogenicity studies were conducted in mice and rats for 22 and 24 months, respectively. In the mouse study,

Table 5
Clinical Progression or Death and Death Only by Study Arm

	Treatment [n (%)]		
Event	zidovudine n=276	VIDEX n=281	VIDEX (didanosine) + zidovudine n=274
Disease Progression† or Death	74 (27)	54 (19)	48 (18)
Death Only	31 (11)	20 (7)	23 (8)

† Disease Progression was defined as any of the following: weight growth failure, brain growth failure, ≥2 opportunistic infections or malignancy.

Table 6
Clinical Adverse Events: Cumulative Incidence ≥5%

	Percent of Patients			
	VIDEX		zidovudine	
Adverse Events	116A n=197	116B/117 n=298	116A n=212	116B/117 n=304
Diarrhea	19	28	15	21
Neuropathy (all grades)	17	20	14	12
Chills/Fever	9	12	12	11
Rash/Pruritus	7	9	8	5
Abdominal Pain	13	7	8	8
Asthenia	4	7	8	9
Headache	6	7	12	7
Pain	6	7	6	3
Nausea & Vomiting	7	7	14	6
Pancreatitis	7	6	3	2

initial doses of 120, 800 and 1200 mg/kg/day for each sex, were lowered after 8 months to 120, 210 and 210 mg/kg/day for females and 120, 300 and 600 mg/kg/day for males. The two higher doses exceeded the maximally tolerated dose in females and the high dose exceeded the maximally tolerated dose in males. The low dose in females represented the 0.68-fold maximum human exposure and the intermediate dose in males represented 1.7-fold maximum human exposure. In the rat study, initial doses were 100, 250, and 1000 mg/kg/day, and the high dose was lowered to 500 mg/kg/day after 18 months. The upper dose in male and female rats represented 3-fold maximum human exposure.
Didanosine induced no significant increase in neoplastic lesions in mice or rats at maximally tolerated doses.
No evidence of mutagenicity (with or without metabolic activation) was observed in Ames *Salmonella* mutagenicity assays or in a mutagenicity assay conducted with *Escherichia coli* tester strain WP2 uvrA where only a slight increase in revertants was observed with didanosine. In a mammalian cell gene mutation assay conducted in L5178Y/TK+/−mouse lymphoma cells, didanosine was weakly positive both in the absence and presence of metabolic activation at concentrations of approximately 2000 μg/mL and above. In an *in vitro* cytogenic study performed in cultured human peripheral lymphocytes, high concentrations of didanosine (≥500 μg/mL) elevated the frequency of cells bearing chromosome aberrations. Another *in vitro* mammalian cell chromosome aberration study using Chinese Hamster Lung cells revealed that didanosine produces chromosome aberrations at ≥500 μg/mL after 48 hours of exposure. However, no significant elevations in the frequency of cells with chromosome aberrations were seen at didanosine concentrations up to 250 μg/mL. In a BALB/c 3T3 *in vitro* transformation assay, didanosine was considered positive only at concentrations of 3000 μg/mL and above. No evidence of genotoxicity was observed in rat and mouse micronucleus assays.
The results from the genotoxicity studies suggest that didanosine is not mutagenic at biologically and pharmacologically relevant doses. At significantly elevated doses *in vitro*, the genotoxic effects of didanosine are similar in magnitude to those seen with natural DNA nucleosides.

Pregnancy, Reproduction and Fertility
Pregnancy "Category B". Reproduction studies have been performed in rats and rabbits at doses up to 12 and 14.2 times the estimated human exposure (based upon plasma levels), respectively, and have revealed no evidence of impaired fertility or harm to the fetus due to didanosine. At approximately 12 times the estimated human exposure, didanosine was slightly toxic to female rats and their pups during mid and late lactation. These rats showed reduced food intake and body weight gains but the physical and functional development of the offspring was not impaired and there were no major changes in the F2 generation. A study in rats showed that didanosine and/or its metabolites are transferred to the fetus through the placenta. There are no adequate and well-controlled studies in pregnant

women. Because animal reproduction studies are not always predictive of human response, this drug should be used during pregnancy only if clearly needed.

Antiretroviral Pregnancy Registry
To monitor maternal-fetal outcomes of pregnant women exposed to didanosine and other antiretroviral agents, an Antiretroviral Pregnancy Registry has been established. Physicians are encouraged to register patients by calling (800) 258-4263.

Nursing Mothers
A study in rats showed that following oral administration, didanosine and/or its metabolites were excreted into the milk of lactating rats. Although it is not known if didanosine is excreted in human milk, there is the potential for adverse effects from didanosine in nursing infants. Mothers should be instructed to discontinue nursing if they are receiving didanosine. This instruction is consistent with the Centers for Disease Control recommendation that HIV-infected mothers not breast feed their infants to avoid risking postnatal transmission of HIV infection.

ADVERSE REACTIONS
THE MAJOR TOXICITY OF VIDEX (DIDANOSINE) IS PANCREATITIS. OTHER IMPORTANT TOXICITIES INCLUDE LACTIC ACIDOSIS/SEVERE HEPATOMEGALY WITH STEATOSIS AND RETINAL/VISUAL CHANGES (see "**WARNINGS**" section).
Adults: Clinical adverse events that occurred in at least 5% of adult patients in clinical trials with VIDEX monotherapy are provided in Table 6. The types of adverse events reported to occur in the ACTG 175 trial in VIDEX-treated patients were generally similar to those events reported in other controlled clinical trials, although the incidence of adverse events was generally lower in all treatment groups in this population with less advanced HIV disease. Adverse events reported to occur in patients treated with VIDEX + zidovudine combination therapy in the ACTG 175 clinical trial were generally similar to those reported in patients treated with either individual drug.
[See table 6 above]
The frequency of peripheral neuropathy is related to dose and stage of disease. Patients should be monitored for the development of a neuropathy that is usually characterized by numbness, tingling or pain in the feet or hands. Neuropathy has occurred more frequently in patients with a history of neuropathy or neurotoxic drug therapy and these patients may be at increased risk of neuropathy during VIDEX therapy.
The cumulative incidences of serious laboratory abnormalities in clinical trials with VIDEX monotherapy are listed in Table 7. The types of serious laboratory abnormalities reported in the ACTG 175 trial in VIDEX-treated patients were generally similar to those reported in other controlled clinical trials. Serious laboratory abnormalities reported in patients treated with VIDEX + zidovudine combination

Table 7
Cumulative Incidences of Serious Laboratory Abnormalities

Lab Tests (Seriously Abnormal Level)	Percent of Patients			
	VIDEX		zidovudine	
	116A n=197	116B/117 n=298	116A n=212	116B/117 n=304
Hemoglobin (<8.0 g/dL)	6	3	8	5
Leukopenia (<2000/mL)	13	16	26	22
Granulocytopenia (<750/mL)	6	8	19	15
Thrombocytopenia (<50,000/mL)	2	2	4	3
SGOT (AST) (>5 × ULN)	9	7	4	6
SGPT (ALT) (>5 × ULN)	9	6	6	6
Alkaline phosphatase (>5 × ULN)	4	1	1	1
Bilirubin (>2.6 × ULN)	1	1	1	1
Amylase (≥1.4 × ULN)	17	15	12	5
Uric Acid (>12 mg/dL)	3	2	1	1

Table 8
Pediatric Patient Serious Laboratory Abnormalities in ACTG 152 (Cumulative Incidences)

Laboratory Test (Seriously Abnormal Level)	Percent of Patients		
	VIDEX n=281	VIDEX + zidovudine n=274	zidovudine n=276
Hemoglobin (<7.5 g/dL)	5	7	10
Leukopenia (<2000/mL)	<1	<1	1
Granulocytopenia (<500/mL)	11	16	27
Thombocytopenia (<50,000/mL)	6	7	7
SGOT (AST) (≥5 × ULN)	14	10	16
SGPT (ALT) (≥10 × ULN)	5	2	7
Alkaline Phosphatase (≥2 × ULN)	7	9	10
Bilirubin (≥2.6 × ULN)	6	3	4
Amylase (≥3.1 × ULN)	5	6	7
Creatine Kinase (≥5.1 × ULN)	6	8	8
Uric Acid (≥3.5 × ULN)	<1	<1	<1

Table 11

NDC No.	Packaging Information	Product Strength
VIDEX® Chewable/Dispersible Buffered Tablets		
0087-6650-01	60 tablets/bottle	25 mg/tablet
0087-6651-01	60 tablets/bottle	50 mg/tablet
0087-6652-01	60 tablets/bottle	100 mg/tablet
0087-6653-01	60 tablets/bottle	150 mg/tablet
VIDEX® Buffered Powder for Oral Solution		
0087-6614-43	One single-dose foil packet*	100 mg/packet
0087-6615-43	One single-dose foil packet*	167 mg/packet
0087-6616-43	One single-dose foil packet*	250 mg/packet
VIDEX® Pediatric Powder for Oral Solution		
0087-6632-41	One bottle per carton	2 g/bottle
0087-6633-41	One bottle per carton	4 g/bottle

*Packaged as 30 packets per carton.

therapy in the ACTG 175 clinical trial were generally similar to those reported in patients treated with either individual drug.
[See table 7 above]

Observed during Clinical Practice: The following events have been identified during postapproval use of VIDEX. Because they are reported voluntarily from a population of unknown size, estimates of frequency cannot be made. These events have been chosen for inclusion due to their seriousness, frequency of reporting, causal connection to VIDEX, or a combination of these factors.

Body as a Whole- alopecia and anaphylactoid reaction.
Digestive Disorders- anorexia, dyspepsia, and flatulence.
Exocrine Gland Disorders- sialoadenitis, parotid gland enlargement, dry mouth and dry eyes.
Liver- lactic acidosis and hepatic steatosis (see "WARNINGS" section); hepatitis and liver failure.
Metabolic Disorders- diabetes mellitus, hypoglycemia, and hyperglycemia.
Musculoskeletal Disorders- myalgia (with or without increases in creatinine phosphokinase), rhabdomyolysis including acute renal failure and hemodialysis, arthralgia, and myopathy.

Optical Disorders- Retinal depigmentation and optic neuritis (see "WARNINGS" section).
Pediatric Patients: Adverse events reported to occur in the pediatric patients in the ACTG 152 trial were generally similar to those reported in adults.
In pediatric phase I studies, pancreatitis occurred in 2 of 60 (3 percent) patients treated at entry doses below 300 mg/m²/day and in 5 of 38 (13 percent) patients treated at higher doses.
Retinal changes and optic neuritis have been reported in pediatric patients.
Serious laboratory abnormalities experienced by the pediatric patients in the ACTG 152 clinical trial are listed in Table 8.
[See table 8 above]

OVERDOSAGE
There is no known antidote for VIDEX (didanosine) overdosage. In phase 1 studies, in which VIDEX was initially administered at doses ten times the currently recommended dose, toxicities included: pancreatitis, peripheral neuropathy, diarrhea, hyperuricemia and hepatic dysfunction.

Didanosine is not dialyzable by peritoneal dialysis, although there is some clearance by hemodialysis (see "CLINICAL PHARMACOLOGY, Pharmacokinetics" section).

DOSAGE AND ADMINISTRATION
Dosage:
Adults- The dosing interval should be 12 hours. **All VIDEX formulations should be administered on an empty stomach, at least 30 minutes before or 2 hours after eating. Adult patients should take 2 tablets at each dose so that adequate buffering is provided to prevent gastric acid degradation of didanosine.** The recommended starting dose in adults is dependent on weight as outlined in the table below:

Table 9
Adult Dosing

Patient Weight	VIDEX Tablets	VIDEX Buffered Powder
≥60 kg	200 mg BID	250 mg BID
<60 kg	125 mg BID	167 mg BID

Pediatric Patients- The recommended dosing interval is 12 hours. **All VIDEX formulations should be administered on an empty stomach, at least 30 minutes before or 2 hours after eating.** The recommended dose of VIDEX monotherapy in pediatric patients is 120 mg/m² BID.
Dose Adjustment: Clinical signs suggestive of pancreatitis should prompt dose suspension and careful evaluation of the possibility of pancreatitis. VIDEX use should be discontinued in patients with confirmed pancreatitis.
Patients who have presented with symptoms of neuropathy may tolerate a reduced dose of VIDEX after resolution of these symptoms upon drug discontinuation.
In adult patients with impaired renal function, the dose of VIDEX should be adjusted to compensate for the slower rate of elimination. The recommended doses and dosing intervals of VIDEX in adult patients with renal insufficiency are presented in Table 10.

Table 10
Recommended Dose (mg) of VIDEX by Body Weight

Creatinine Clearance (mL/min)	≥60 kg		<60 kg		Interval (hr)
	Tablet[a]	Solution[b]	Tablet[a]	Solution[b]	
≥60	200	250	125	167	12
30–59	100	100	75	100	12
10–29	150	167	100	100	24
<10	100	100	75	100	24

[a] VIDEX Chewable/Dispersible Buffered Tablet. Two VIDEX tablets must be taken with each dose; different strengths of tablets may be combined to yield the recommended dose.
[b] VIDEX Buffered Powder for Oral Solution

Urinary excretion is also a major route of elimination of didanosine in pediatric patients; therefore, the clearance of didanosine may be altered in children with renal impairment. Although there are insufficient data to recommend a specific dose adjustment of VIDEX in this patient population, a reduction in the dose and/or an increase in the interval between doses should be considered.
Patients Requiring Continuous Ambulatory Peritoneal Dialysis (CAPD) or Hemodialysis- It is recommended that one fourth of the total daily dose of VIDEX be administered once a day (see Table 10, recommended dosage for patients with CL_CR <10 mL/min). It is not necessary to administer a supplemental dose of VIDEX following hemodialysis.
Hepatic Impairment- See "PRECAUTIONS" section.
Method of Preparation:
VIDEX Chewable/Dispersible Buffered Tablets
Adult Dosing- Two tablets should be thoroughly chewed, manually crushed, or dispersed in at least 1 ounce of water prior to consumption. To disperse tablets, add 2 tablets to at least 1 ounce of drinking water. Stir until a uniform dispersion forms, and drink the entire dispersion immediately. If additional flavoring is desired, the dispersion may be diluted with one ounce of clear apple juice. Stir the further diluted dispersion just prior to consumption. The dispersion with clear apple juice is stable at room temperature, 62–73°F (17–23°C), for up to one hour.
VIDEX Buffered Powder for Oral Solution
1. Open packet carefully and pour contents into a container with approximately 4 ounces of drinking water. Do not mix with fruit juice or other acid-containing liquid.

Continued on next page

Videx—Cont.

2. Stir until the powder completely dissolves (approximately 2 to 3 minutes).
3. Drink the entire solution immediately.

VIDEX Pediatric Powder for Oral Solution

Prior to dispensing, the pharmacist must constitute dry powder with Purified Water, USP, to an initial concentration of 20 mg/mL and immediately mix the resulting solution with antacid to a final concentration of 10 mg/mL as follows:

20 mg/mL Initial Solution- Constitute the product to 20 mg/mL by adding 100 mL or 200 mL of Purified Water, USP, to the 2 g or 4 g of VIDEX powder, respectively, in the product bottle.

10 mg/mL Final Admixture- 1. Immediately mix one part of the 20 mg/mL initial solution with one part of either Mylanta® Double Strength Liquid (Mylanta® is a registered trademark of Stuart Pharmaceuticals, a business unit of Zeneca, Inc. Mylanta® Double Strength, formerly Mylanta® II, is distributed by Johnson & Johnson/Merck, Consumer Pharmaceuticals Company, Fort Washington, PA 19034 [USA]), Extra Strength Maalox® Plus Suspension, or Maalox® TC Suspension (Maalox® is a registered trademark of William H. Rorer Inc., Unit of Rhone-Poulenc) for a final dispensing concentration of 10 mg VIDEX (didanosine) per mL. For patient home use, the admixture should be dispensed in appropriately sized, flint-glass or plastic (HDPE, PET, or PETG) bottles with child-resistant closures. This admixture is stable for 30 days under refrigeration, 36° to 46°F (2° to 8°C).

2. Instruct the patient to shake the admixture thoroughly prior to use and to store the tightly closed container in the refrigerator, 36° to 46°F (2° to 8°C), up to 30 days.

HOW SUPPLIED

VIDEX® (didanosine) Chewable/Dispersible Buffered Tablets are round, off white to light orange/yellow with a mottled appearance, orange-flavored, tablets embossed with "VIDEX" on one side and the product strength on the other. The tablets are available in the following strengths of VIDEX: 25, 50, 100, or 150 mg. Sixty tablets are packaged in bottles with child-resistant closures.

The tablets should be stored in tightly closed bottles at 59° to 86°F (15° to 30°C). If dispersed in water, the dose may be held for up to 1 hour at ambient temperature.

VIDEX® (didanosine) Buffered Powder for Oral Solution is supplied in single-dose, child-resistant foil packets in the following strengths of VIDEX : 100, 167, or 250 mg. Each product strength provides a sweetened, buffered solution of VIDEX.

The packets should be stored at 59° to 86°F (15° to 30°C). After dissolving in water, the solution may be stored at ambient room temperature for up to 4 hours.

VIDEX® (didanosine) Pediatric Powder for Oral Solution is supplied in 4- and 8-ounce glass bottles containing 2 g or 4 g of VIDEX, respectively.

The bottles of powder should be stored at 59° to 86°F (15° to 30°C). The VIDEX admixture may be stored up to 30 days in a refrigerator, 36° to 46°F (2° to 8°C). Discard any unused portion after 30 days.

The NDC numbers for the previously described VIDEX products are:

[See table 11 on previous page]

US Patent Nos.: 4,861,759 and 5,616,566.

HANDLING AND DISPOSAL

Spill, Leak and Disposal Procedure

Avoid generating dust during clean-up of powdered products; use wet mop or damp sponge. Clean surface with soap and water as necessary. Containerize larger spills.

There is no single preferred method of disposal of containerized waste. Disposal options include incineration, landfill, or sewer as dictated by specific circumstances and relevant national, state, and local regulations.

BRISTOL-MYERS SQUIBB
Immunology
Bristol-Myers Squibb Company
Princeton, NJ 08543
U.S.A.

F8-B001-6-98 P9691-02

Revised May 1998

Shown in Product Identification Guide, page 308

VUMON® ℞

[*vū 'mŏn*]

(teniposide) for Injection Concentrate

WARNING

Vumon (teniposide) for Injection Concentrate is a cytotoxic drug, which should be administered under the supervision of a qualified physician experienced in the use of cancer chemotherapeutic agents. Appropriate management of therapy and complications is possible only when adequate treatment facilities are readily available.

Severe myelosuppression with resulting infection or bleeding may occur. Hypersensitivity reactions, including anaphylaxis-like symptoms, may occur with initial dosing or at repeated exposure to Vumon. Epinephrine, with or without corticosteroids and antihistamines has been employed to alleviate hypersensitivity reaction symptoms.

DESCRIPTION

Vumon (teniposide) for Injection Concentrate (also commonly known as VM-26), is supplied as a sterile nonpyrogenic solution in a nonaqueous medium intended for dilution with a suitable parenteral vehicle prior to intravenous infusion. Vumon is available in 50 mg (5 mL) ampules. Each mL contains 10 mg teniposide, 30 mg benzyl alcohol, 60 mg N,N-dimethylacetamide, 500 mg Cremophor® EL (polyoxyethylated castor oil)* and 42.7 percent (V/V) dehydrated alcohol. The pH of the clear solution is adjusted to approximately 5 with maleic acid.

Teniposide is a semisynthetic derivative of podophyllotoxin. The chemical name for teniposide is 4′-demethylepipodophyllotoxin 9-[4,6-0-(R)-2-thenylidene-β-D-glucopyranoside]. Teniposide differs from etoposide, another podophyllotoxin derivative, by the substitution of a thenylidene group on the glucopyranoside ring.

Teniposide has the following structural formula:

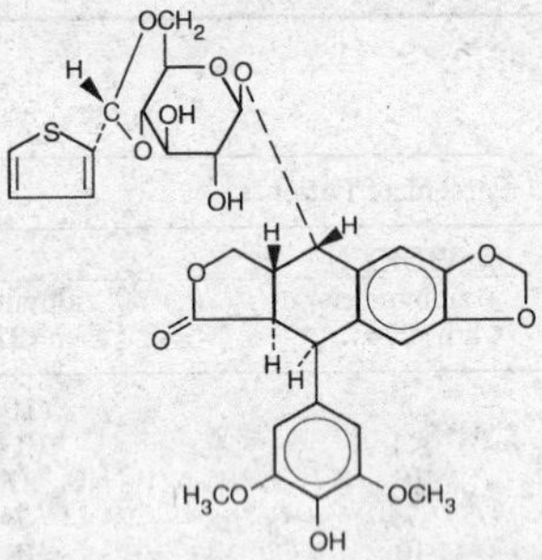

Teniposide is a white to off-white crystalline powder with the empirical formula $C_{32}H_{32}O_{13}S$ and a molecular weight of 656.66. It is a lipophilic compound with a partition coefficient value (octanol/water) of approximately 100. Teniposide is insoluble in water and ether. It is slightly soluble in methanol and very soluble in acetone and dimethylformamide.

CLINICAL PHARMACOLOGY

Teniposide is a phase-specific cytotoxic drug, acting in the late S or early G_2 phase of the cell cycle, thus preventing cells from entering mitosis.

Teniposide causes dose-dependent single- and double-stranded breaks in DNA and DNA: protein cross-links. The mechanism of action appears to be related to the inhibition of type II topoisomerase activity since teniposide does not intercalate into DNA or bind strongly to DNA. The cytotoxic effects of teniposide are related to the relative number of double-stranded DNA breaks produced in cells, which are a reflection of the stabilization of a topoisomerase II-DNA intermediate.

Teniposide has a broad spectrum of *in vivo* antitumor activity against murine tumors, including hematologic malignancies and various solid tumors. Notably, teniposide is active against sublines of certain murine leukemias with acquired resistance to cisplatin, doxorubicin, amsacrine, daunorubicin, mitoxantrone or vincristine.

Plasma drug levels declined biexponentially following intravenous infusion (155 mg/m^2 over 1 to 2.5 hours) of Vumon given to eight children (4–11 years old) with newly diagnosed acute lymphoblastic leukemia (ALL). The observed average pharmacokinetic parameters and associated coefficients of variation (CV^6/$_9$) based on a two-compartmental model analysis of the data are as follows:

[See table at top of next page]

There appears to be some association between an increase in serum alkaline phosphatase or gamma glutamyl-transpeptidase and a decrease in plasma clearance of teniposide. Therefore, caution should be exercised if Vumon is to be administered to patients with hepatic dysfunction.

In adults, at doses of 100 to 333 mg/m^2/day, plasma levels increased linearly with dose. Drug accumulation in adult patients did not occur after daily administration of Vumon for 3 days. In pediatric patients, maximum plasma concentrations (Cmax) after infusions of 137 to 203 mg/m^2 over a period of one to two hours exceeded 40 μg/mL; by 20 to 24 hours after infusion plasma levels were generally $<$2μg/mL. Renal clearance of parent teniposide accounts for about 10 percent of total body clearance. In adults, after intravenous administration of 10 mg/kg or 67 mg/m^2 of tritium-labeled teniposide, 44 percent of the radiolabel was recovered in urine (parent drug and metabolites) within 120 hours after dosing. From 4 to 12 percent of a dose is excreted in urine as parent drug. Fecal excretion of radioactivity within 72 hours after dosing accounted for 0 to 10 percent of the dose. Mean steady-state volumes of distribution range from 8 to 44 L/m^2 for adults and 3 to 11 L/m^2 for children. The blood-brain barrier appears to limit diffusion of teniposide into the brain, although in a study in patients with brain tumors, CSF levels of teniposide were higher than CSF levels reported in other studies of patients who did not have brain tumors.

Teniposide is highly protein bound. *In vitro* plasma protein binding of teniposide is > 99 percent. The high affinity of teniposide for plasma proteins may be an important factor in limiting distribution of drug within the body. Steady state volume of distribution of the drug increases with a decrease in plasma albumin levels. Therefore, careful monitoring of children with hypoalbuminemia is indicated during therapy. Levels of teniposide in saliva, CSF and malignant ascites fluid are low relative to simultaneously measured plasma levels.

The pharmacokinetic characteristics of teniposide differ from those of etoposide, another podophyllotoxin. Teniposide is more extensively bound to plasma proteins, and its cellular uptake is greater. Teniposide also has a lower systemic clearance, a longer elimination half-life, and is excreted in the urine as parent drug to a lesser extent than etoposide.

In a study at St. Jude Children's Research Hospital (SJCRH), 9 children with acute lymphocytic leukemia (ALL) failing induction therapy with a cytarabine-containing regimen, were treated with Vumon plus cytarabine. Three of these patients were induced into complete remission with durations of remission of 30 weeks, 59 weeks, and 13 years. In another study at SJCRH, 16 children with ALL refractory to vincristine/prednisone-containing regimens were treated with Vumon plus vincristine and prednisone. Three of these patients were induced into complete remission with durations of remission of 5, 5, 37, and 73 weeks. In these two studies patients served as their own control based on the premise that long term complete remissions could not be achieved by re-treatment with drugs to which they had previously failed to respond.

INDICATIONS AND USAGE

Vumon, in combination with other approved anticancer agents, is indicated for induction therapy in patients with refractory childhood acute lymphoblastic leukemia.

CONTRAINDICATIONS

Vumon is generally contraindicated in patients who have demonstrated a previous hypersensitivity to teniposide and/or Cremophor® EL (polyoxyethylated castor oil).

WARNINGS

Vumon is a potent drug and should be used only by physicians experienced in the administration of cancer chemotherapeutic drugs. Blood counts as well as renal and hepatic function tests should be carefully monitored prior to and during therapy.

Patients being treated with Vumon (teniposide) should be observed frequently for myelosuppression both during and after therapy. Dose-limiting bone marrow suppression is the most significant toxicity associated with Vumon therapy. Therefore, the following studies should be obtained at the start of therapy and prior to each subsequent dose of Vumon: hemoglobin, white blood cell count and differential and platelet count. If necessary, repeat bone marrow examination should be performed prior to the decision to continue therapy in the setting of severe myelosuppression.

Physicians should be aware of the possible occurrence of a hypersensitivity reaction variably manifested by chills, fever, urticaria, tachycardia, bronchospasm, dyspnea, hypertension or hypotension and facial flushing. This reaction may occur with the first dose of Vumon and may be life threatening if not treated promptly with antihistamines, corticosteroids, epinephrine, intravenous fluids and other supportive measures as clinically indicated. The exact cause of these reactions is unknown. They may be due to the Cremophor® EL (polyoxyethylated castor oil) component of the vehicle or to teniposide itself[1]. Patients who have experienced prior hypersensitivity reactions to Vumon are at risk for recurrence of symptoms and should only be re-treated with Vumon if the antileukemic benefit already demonstrated clearly outweighs the risk of a probable hypersensitivity reaction for that patient. When a decision is made to re-treat a patient with Vumon in spite of an earlier hypersensitivity reaction, the patient should be pretreated with corticosteroids and antihistamines and receive careful clinical observation during and after Vumon infusion. In the clinical experience with Vumon at SJCRH and the National Cancer Institute (NCI), re-treatment of patients with prior hypersensitivity reactions has been accomplished using measures described above. To date, there is no evidence to suggest cross-sensitization between Vumon and VePesid.

One episode of sudden death, attributed to probable arrhythmia and intractable hypotension has been reported in

Parameter	Mean	CV%
Total body clearance (mL/min/m^2)	10.3	25
Volume at steady-state (L/m^2)	3.1	30
Terminal half-life (hours)	5.0	44
Volume of central compartment (L/m^2)	1.5	36
Rate constant, central to peripheral (1/hours)	0.47	62
Rate constant, peripheral to central (1/hours)	0.42	37

an elderly patient receiving Vumon combination therapy for a nonleukemic malignancy. (See "ADVERSE REACTIONS" section.) Patients receiving Vumon treatment should be under continuous observation for at least the first 60 minutes following the start of the infusion and at frequent intervals thereafter. If symptoms or signs of anaphylaxis occur, the infusion should be stopped immediately, followed by the administration of epinephrine, corticosteroids, antihistamines, pressor agents, or volume expanders at the discretion of the physician. An aqueous solution of epinephrine 1:1000 and a source of oxygen should be available at the bedside.

For parenteral administration, Vumon should be given only by slow intravenous infusion (lasting at least 30- to 60-minutes) since hypotension has been reported as a possible side effect of rapid intravenous injection, perhaps due to a direct effect of Cremophor® EL[2,3]. If clinically significant hypotension develops, the Vumon infusion should be discontinued. The blood pressure usually normalizes within hours in response to cessation of the infusion and administration of fluids or other supportive therapy as appropriate. If the infusion is restarted, a slower administration rate should be used and the patient should be carefully monitored.

Acute central nervous system depression and hypotension have been observed in patients receiving investigational infusions of high-dose Vumon who were pretreated with antiemetic drugs. The depressant effects of the antiemetic agents and the alcohol content of the Vumon formulation may place patients receiving higher than recommended doses of Vumon at risk for central nervous system depression.

Pregnancy: Pregnancy "Category D."

Vumon may cause fetal harm when administered to a pregnant woman. Vumon has been shown to be teratogenic and embryotoxic in laboratory animals. In pregnant rats intravenous administration of Vumon, 0. 1–3 mg/kg (0.6–18 mg/m^2), every second day from day 6 to day 16 post coitum caused dose-related embryotoxicity and teratogenicity. Major anomalies included spinal and rib defects, deformed extremities, anophthalmia and celosomia.

There are no adequate and well-controlled studies in pregnant women. If Vumon is used during pregnancy, or if the patient becomes pregnant while receiving this drug, the patient should be apprised of the potential hazard to the fetus. Women of childbearing potential should be advised to avoid becoming pregnant during therapy with Vumon.

*Cremophor®EL is the registered trademark of BASF Aktiengesellschaft

PRECAUTIONS

General: In all instances where the use of Vumon is considered for chemotherapy, the physician must evaluate the need and usefulness of the drug against the risk of adverse reactions. Most such adverse reactions are reversible if detected early. If severe reactions occur, the drug should be reduced in dosage or discontinued and appropriate corrective measures should be taken according to the clinical judgment of the physician. Reinstitution of Vumon therapy should be carried out with caution, and with adequate consideration of the further need for the drug and alertness as to possible recurrence of toxicity.

Vumon must be administered as an intravenous infusion. Care should be taken to ensure that the intravenous catheter or needle is in the proper position and functional prior to infusion. Improper administration of Vumon may result in extravasation causing local tissue necrosis and/or thrombophlebitis. In some instances, occlusion of central venous access devices has occurred during 24-hour infusion of Vumon at a concentration of 0.1 to 0.2 mg/mL. Frequent observation during these infusions is necessary to minimize this risk[4,5].

Laboratory Tests: Periodic complete blood counts and assessments of renal and hepatic function should be done during the course of Vumon treatment. They should be performed prior to therapy and at clinically appropriate intervals during and after therapy. There should be at least one determination of hematologic status prior to therapy with Vumon.

Drug Interactions: In a study in which 34 different drugs were tested, therapeutically relevant concentrations of tolbutamide, sodium salicylate and sulfamethizole displaced protein-bound teniposide in fresh human serum to a small but significant extent. Because of the extremely high binding of teniposide to plasma proteins, these small decreases in binding could cause substantial increases in free drug levels in plasma which could result in potentiation of drug toxicity. Therefore, caution should be used in administering Vumon to patients receiving these other agents. There was no change in the plasma kinetics of teniposide when coadministered with methotrexate. However, the plasma clearance of methotrexate was slightly increased. An increase in intracellular levels of methotrexate was observed *in vitro* in the presence of teniposide.

Carcinogenesis, Mutagenesis, Impairment of Fertility: Children at SJCRH with ALL in remission who received maintenance therapy with Vumon at weekly or twice weekly doses (plus other chemotherapeutic agents), had a relative risk of developing secondary acute nonlymphocytic leukemia (ANLL) approximately 12 times that of patients treated according to other less intensive schedules[6].

A short course of Vumon for remission-induction and/or consolidation therapy was not associated with an increased risk of secondary ANLL, but the number of patients assessed was small. The potential benefit from Vumon must be weighed on a case by case basis against the potential risk of the induction of a secondary leukemia. The carcinogenicity of teniposide has not been studied in laboratory animals. Compounds with similar mechanisms of action and mutagenicity profiles have been reported to be carcinogenic and teniposide should be considered a potential carcinogen in humans. Teniposide has been shown to be mutagenic in various bacterial and mammalian genetic toxicity tests. These include positive mutagenic effects in the Ames/Salmonella and *B. subtilis* bacterial mutagenicity assays. Teniposide caused gene mutations in both Chinese hamster ovary cells and mouse lymphoma cells and DNA damage as measured by alkaline elution in human lung carcinoma derived cell lines. In addition, teniposide induced aberrations in chromosome structure in primary cultures of human lymphocytes *in vitro* and in L5178y/TK + /-mouse lymphoma cells *in vitro*. Chromosome aberrations were observed *in vivo* in the embryonic tissue of pregnant Swiss albino mice treated with teniposide. Teniposide also caused a dose-related increase in sister chromatid exchanges in Chinese hamster ovary cells and it has been shown to be embryotoxic and teratogenic in rats receiving teniposide during organogenesis. Treatment of pregnant rats IV with doses between 1.0 and 3.0 mg/kg/day on alternate days from day 6 to 16 post coitum caused retardation of embryonic development, prenatal mortality and fetal abnormalities.

Pregnancy: Pregnancy "Category D." (See "WARNINGS" section.)

Nursing Mothers: It is not known whether this drug is excreted in human milk. Because many drugs are excreted in human milk and because of the potential for serious adverse reactions in nursing infants, a decision should be made whether to discontinue nursing or to discontinue the drug, taking into account the importance of Vumon therapy to the mother.

Patients with Down's Syndrome: Patients with both Down's Syndrome and leukemia may be especially sensitive to myelosuppressive chemotherapy. therefore, initial dosing with Vumon should be reduced in these patients. It is suggested that the first course of Vumon should be given at half the usual dose. Subsequent courses may be administered at higher dosages depending on the degree of myelosuppression and mucositis encountered in earlier courses in an individual patient.

ADVERSE REACTIONS

The table below presents the incidences of adverse reactions derived from an anlysis of data contained within literature reports of 7 studies involving 303 pediatric patients in which Vumon was administered by injection as a single agent in a variety of doses and schedules for a variety of hematologic malignancies and solid tumors. The total number of patients evaluable for a given event was not 303 since the individual studies did not address the occurrence of each event listed. Five of these 7 studies assessed Vumon activity in hematologic malignancies, such as leukemia. Thus, many of these patients had abnormal hematologic status at start of therapy with Vumon and were expected to develop significant myelosuppression as an endpoint of treatment.

Single-Agent Vumon (teniposide)
Summary of Toxicity for All Evaluable Pediatric Patients

Toxicity	Incidence in Evaluable Patients (%)
Hematologic toxicity	
Myelosuppression, nonspecified	75
Leukopenia (<3,000 WBC/µL)	89
Neutropenia (<2,000 ANC/µL)	95
Thrombocytopenia (<100,000 plt/µL)	85
Anemia	88
Non-Hematologic Toxicity	
Mucositis	76
Diarrhea	33
Nausea/vomiting	29
Infection	12
Alopecia	9
Bleeding	5
Hypersensitivity reactions	5
Rash	3
Fever	3
Hypotension/Cardiovascular	2
Neurotoxicity	<1
Hepatic dysfunction	<1
Renal dysfunction	<1
Metabolic abnormalities	<1

Hematologic Toxicity: Vumon, when used with other chemotherapeutic agents for the treatment of ALL, results in severe myelosuppression. Early onset of profound myelosuppression with delayed recovery can be expected when using the doses and schedules of Vumon necessary for treatment of refractory ALL, since bone marrow hypoplasia is a desired endpoint of therapy. The occurrence of acute nonlymphocytic leukemia (ANLL), with or without a preleukemic phase, has been reported in patients treated with Vumon in combination with other antineoplastic agents. See "PRECAUTIONS" subsection "Carcinogenesis, Mutagenesis, Impairment of fertility".

Gastrointestinal Toxicity: Nausea and vomiting are the most common gastrointestinal toxicities, having occurred in 29 percent of evaluable pediatric patients. The severity of this nausea and vomiting is generally mild to moderate.

Hypotension: Transient hypotension following rapid intravenous administration has been reported in 2 percent of evaluable pediatric patients. One episode of sudden death, attributed to probable arrhythmia and intractable hypotension, has been reported in an elderly patient receiving Vumon combination therapy for a non-leukemic malignancy. No other cardiac toxicity or electrocardiographic changes have been documented. No delayed hypotension has been noted.

Allergic Reactions: Hypersensitivity reactions characterized by chills, fever, tachycardia, flushing, bronchospasm, dyspnea, and blood pressure changes (hypertension or hypotension) have been reported to occur in approximately 5 percent of evaluable pediatric patients receiving intravenous Vumon. The incidence of hypersensitivity reactions to Vumon appears to be increased in patients with brain tumors, and in patients with neuroblastoma[1].

Central Nervous System: Acute central nervous system depression and hypotension have been observed in patients receiving investigational infusions of high-dose Vumon who were pretreated with antiemetic drugs. The depressant effects of the antiemetic agents and the alcohol content of the Vumon formulation may place patients receiving higher than recommended doses of Vumon at risk for central nervous system depression.

Alopecia: Alopecia, sometimes progressing to total baldness, was observed in 9 percent of evaluable pediatric patients who received Vumon as single agent therapy. It was usually reversible.

OVERDOSAGE

There is no known antidote for Vumon overdosage. The anticipated complications of overdosage are secondary to bone marrow suppression. Treatment should consist of supportive care including blood products and antibiotics as indicated.

DOSAGE AND ADMINISTRATION

NOTE: Contact of undiluted Vumon (teniposide) for injection Concentrate with plastic equipment or devices used to prepare solutions for infusion may result in softening or cracking and possible drug product leakage. This effect has *not* been reported with *diluted solutions* of Vumon.

In order to prevent extraction of the plasticizer DEHP [di(2-ethylhexyl)phtalate], solutions of Vumon for injection Concentrate should be prepared in non-DEHP containing LVP containers such as glass or polyolefin plastic bags or containers.

Vumon solutions should be administered with non-DEHP containing IV administration sets.

Continued on next page

Vumon—Cont.

In one study, childhood ALL patients failing induction therapy with a cytarabine-containing regimen were treated with the combination of Vumon 165 mg/m^2 and cytarabine 300 mg/m^2 intravenously, twice weekly for 8–9 doses. In another study, patients with childhood ALL refractory to vincristine/prednisone-containing regimens were treated with the combination of Vumon 250 mg/m^2 and vincristine 1.5 mg/m^2 intravenously, weekly for 4–8 weeks and prednisone 40 mg/m^2 orally × 28 days.

Adequate data in patients with hepatic insufficiency and/or renal insufficiency are lacking, but dose adjustments may be necessary for patients with significant renal or hepatic impairment.

Preparation and Administration Precautions: Vumon is a cytotoxic anticancer drug and as with other potentially toxic compounds, caution should be exercised in handling and preparing the solution of Vumon. Skin reactions associated with accidental exposure to Vumon may occur. The use of gloves is recommended. If Vumon solution contacts the skin, immediately wash the skin thoroughly with soap and water. If Vumon contacts mucous membranes, the membranes should be flushed thoroughly with water.

Preparation for Intravenous Administration: Vumon must be diluted with either 5 percent Dextrose Injection, USP or 0.9 percent Sodium Chloride Injection, USP, to give final teniposide concentrations of 0.1 mg/mL, 0.2 mg/mL, 0.4 mg/mL or 1.0 mg/mL. Solutions prepared in 5 percent Dextrose Injection, USP or 0.9 percent Sodium Chloride Injection, USP at teniposide concentrations of 0.1 mg/mL, 0.2 mg/mL or 0.4 mg/mL are stable at room temperature for up to 24 hours after preparation. Vumon solutions prepared at a final teniposide concentration of 1.0 mg/mL should be administered within 4 hours of preparation to reduce the potential for precipitation. **Refrigeration of Vumon solutions is not recommended.** Stability and use times are identical in glass and plastic parenteral solution containers.

Although solutions are chemically stable under the conditions indicated, precipitation of teniposide may occur at the recommended concentrations, especially if the diluted solution is subjected to more agitation than is recommended to prepare the drug solution for parenteral administration[7]. In addition, storage time prior to administration should be minimized and care should be taken to avoid contact of the diluted solution with other drugs or fluids. Parenteral drug products should be inspected visually for particulate matter and discoloration prior to administration whenever solution and container permit. **Precipitation has been reported during 24-hour infusions of Vumon diluted to teniposide concentrations of 0.1 to 0.2 mg/mL, resulting in occlusion of central venous access catheters in several patients[4,5]. Heparin solution can cause precipitation of teniposide, therefore, the administration apparatus should be flushed thoroughly with 5 percent Dextrose Injection or 0.9 percent Sodium Chloride Injection, USP before and after administration of Vumon[5].**

Hypotension has been reported following rapid intravenous administration; it is recommended that the Vumon solution be administered over at least a 30 to 60-minute period. **Vumon should not be given by rapid intravenous injection.**

In a 24-hour study under simulated conditions of actual use of the product relative to dilution strength, diluent and administration rates, dilutions at 0.1 to 1.0 mg/mL were chemically stable for at least 24 hours. Data collected for the presence of the extractable DEHP [di(2-ethylhexyl)phtalate] from PVC containers show that levels increased with time and concentration of the solutions. The data appeared similar for 0.9 percent Sodium Chloride Injection, USP, and 5 percent Dextrose Injection, USP. Consequently, the use of PVC containers is not recommended.

Similarly, the use of non-DEHP IV administration sets is recommended. Lipid administration sets or low DEHP containing nitroglycerin sets will keep patients' exposure to DEHP at low levels and are suitable for use. The diluted solutions are chemically and physically compatible with the recommended IV administration sets and LVP containers for up to 24 hours at ambient room temperature and lighting conditions. **Because of the potential for precipitation, compatibility with other drugs, infusion materials or IV pumps cannot be assured.**

Stability: Unopened ampules of Vumon (teniposide) for Injection Concentrate are stable until the date indicated on the package when stored under refrigeration (2°–8°C) in the original package. Freezing does not adversely affect the product.

HOW SUPPLIED

NDC 0015-3075-19 50 mg/5 mL sterile clear, colorless glass ampules individually packaged in a carton.

NDC 0015-3075-97 50 mg/5 mL sterile clear, colorless glass ampules individually nested in a carton tray of 10 ampules per tray.

Storage: Store the unopened ampules under refrigeration (2°–8°C). Retain in original package to protect from light.

Handling and Disposal: Procedures for proper handling and disposal of anticancer drugs should be considered. Several guidelines on this subject have been published[6–14]. There is no general agreement that all of the procedures recommended in the guidelines are necessary or appropriate.

REFERENCES

1. O'Dwyer PJ, King SA, Fortner CL and Leyland-Jones B: Hypersensitivity reactions to teniposide (VM-26): an analysis. *J Clin Oncol.* 1986; 4(8):1262–1269.
2. Lorenz W, Perlmann H-J, Schmall A, et al: Histamine release in dogs by Cremophor® EL and its derivatives. *Agents and Actions.* 1977; 7(1):63–67.
3. Lassus M, Scott D, and Leyland-Jones B: Allergic reactions associated with cremophor containing antineoplastics. *Proc Am Soc Clin Oncol* 1985; 4:268 (Abstract C-1042).
4. Strong D, Morris L: Precipitation of teniposide during infusion. *Am J Hosp Pharm* Mar 1990: Letter, 47:512,518.
5. Bogardus J, Kaplan M, Carpenter J: Precipitation of Teniposide During Infusion. *Am J Hosp Pharm;* Mar 1990: Letter, 47:518–519.
6. Pul C-H, et al: Acute Myeloid Leukemia in Children Treated with Epipodophyllotoxins for Acute Lymphoblastic Leukemia. *N Engl J Med.* 1991; 325:1682–1687.
7. Deardoff D, Schmidt C: Mixing additives in plastic LVPs. *Am J Hosp Phar.* Dec 1980: Letter, 37:1610, 1613.
8. Recommendations for the Safe Handling of Parenteral Antineoplastic Drugs. NIH Publication No. 83–2621. For sale by the Superintendent of Documents, US Government Printing office, Washington, DC 20402.
9. AMA Council Report. Guidelines for handling parenteral antineoplastics. *JAMA* 1985; 253 (11): 1590–1592.
10. National Study Commission on Cytotoxic Exposure—Recommendations for Handling Cytotoxic Agents. Available from Louis P. Jeffrey, Chairman, ScD, National Study Commission on Cytotoxic Exposure. Massachusetts College of Pharmacy and Allied Health Sciences, 179 Longwood Avenue, Boston, Massachusetts, 02115.
11. Clinical Oncological Society of Australia. Guidelines and Recommendations for Safe Handling of Antineoplastic Agents. *Med J Australia* 1983; 1:426–428.
12. Jones RB, et al: Safe handling of chemotherapeutic agents: a report from the Mount Sinai Medical Center. *CA-A Cancer Journal for Clinicians* 1983; Sept./Oct. 258–263.
13. American Society of Hospital Pharmacists Technical Assistance Bulletin on Handling Cytotoxic Drugs in Hospitals. *Am J Hosp Pharm* 1990; 47:1033–1049.
14. OSHA Work-Practice Guidelines for Personnel Dealing With Cytotoxic (Antineoplastic) drugs. *Am J Hosp Pharm* 1986; 43:1193–1204.

February 1994 P9819-02

ZERIT® (stavudine)

℞ ONLY

[zə' rit]

ZERIT® (stavudine) Capsules

ZERIT® (stavudine) for Oral Solution

WARNING

LACTIC ACIDOSIS AND SEVERE HEPATOMEGALY WITH STEATOSIS, INCLUDING FATAL CASES, HAVE BEEN REPORTED WITH THE USE OF ANTIRETROVIRAL NUCLEOSIDE ANALOGUES ALONE OR IN COMBINATION, INCLUDING STAVUDINE (SEE "WARNINGS" SECTION).

DESCRIPTION

ZERIT is the brand name for stavudine (formerly called d4T), a synthetic thymidine nucleoside analogue, active against the Human Immunodeficiency Virus (HIV).

ZERIT® (stavudine) Capsules are supplied for oral administration in strengths of 15, 20, 30, and 40 mg of stavudine. Each capsule also contains inactive ingredients microcrystalline cellulose, sodium starch glycolate, lactose, and magnesium stearate. The hard gelatin shell consists of gelatin, methylparaben, propylparaben, titanium dioxide, and iron oxides.

ZERIT (stavudine) for Oral Solution is supplied as a dye-free, fruit-flavored powder in bottles with child-resistant closures providing 200 mL of a 1 mg/mL stavudine solution upon constitution with water per label instructions. The powder for oral solution contains the following inactive ingredients: methylparaben, propylparaben, sodium carboxymethylcellulose, sucrose, and antifoaming and flavoring agents.

The chemical name for stavudine is 2',3'-didehydro-3'-deoxythymidine. Stavudine has the following structural formula:

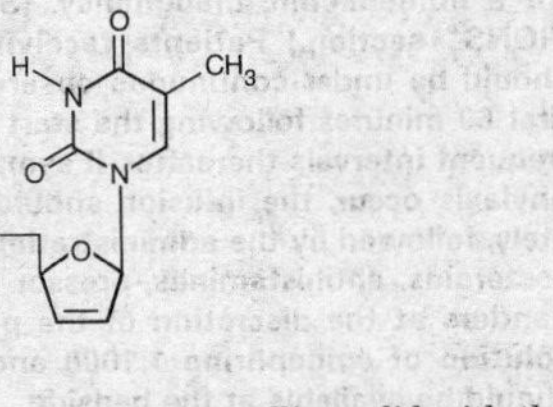

Stavudine is a white to off-white crystalline solid with the molecular formula $C_{10}H_{12}N_2O_4$ and a molecular weight of 224.2. The solubility of stavudine at 23°C is approximately 83 mg/mL in water and 30 mg/mL in propylene glycol. The n-octanol/water partition coefficient of stavudine at 23°C is 0.144.

MICROBIOLOGY

Mechanism of Action: Stavudine, a nucleoside analogue of thymidine, inhibits the replication of HIV in human cells *in vitro*. Stavudine is phosphorylated by cellular kinases to stavudine triphosphate which exerts antiviral activity. Stavudine triphosphate inhibits HIV replication by two known mechanisms: 1) it inhibits HIV reverse transcriptase by competing with the natural substrate deoxythymidine triphosphate (K_i=0.0083 to 0.032 µM); and 2) it inhibits viral DNA synthesis by causing DNA chain termination because stavudine lacks the 3'-hydroxyl group necessary for DNA elongation. In addition to the inhibitory effect on HIV reverse transcriptase, stavudine triphosphate inhibits cellular DNA polymerase beta and gamma, and markedly reduces the synthesis of mitochondrial DNA.

***In vitro* HIV Susceptibility:** The relationship between *in vitro* susceptibility of HIV to stavudine and the inhibition of HIV replication in humans has not been established. The *in vitro* antiviral activity of stavudine was measured in peripheral blood mononuclear cells, monocytic cells, and lymphoblastoid cell lines. ED_{50} values (50% inhibitory concentration) ranged from 0.009 - 4 mM against laboratory and clinical isolates of HIV-1. In CEM cells, stavudine demonstrated additive and synergistic activity against HIV in drug combination regimens with didanosine and zalcitabine, respectively. Stavudine combined with zidovudine demonstrated additive or antagonistic activity depending upon the molar ratios of the agents tested.

Drug Resistance:

Preclinical studies- The potential for development of resistance to stavudine has been investigated *in vitro*. Selection studies performed with HIV-1 strains HXB2 and IIIb have produced viral isolates with reduced (7- to 30-fold) sensitivity to stavudine.

Clinical studies-Limited phenotypic and genotypic resistance studies (20 paired HIV isolates) have shown that 4- to 12-fold decreases (3/20 isolates) in stavudine susceptibility are possible; however, the genetic basis for the observed susceptibility changes has not been identified. The clinical relevance of changes in stavudine susceptibility has not been established.

Cross-Resistance: Five of 11 stavudine post-treatment isolates developed moderate resistance to zidovudine (9- to 176-fold) and 3 of those 11 isolates developed moderate resistance to didanosine (7- to 29-fold). The clinical relevance of these findings is unknown.

CLINICAL PHARMACOLOGY

Pharmacokinetics in Adults: The pharmacokinetics of stavudine have been evaluated in HIV-infected adult and pediatric patients (Table 1). Peak plama concentrations (C_{max}) and area under the plasma concentration-time curve (AUC) increased in proportion to dose after both single and multiple doses ranging from 0.03 to 4 mg/kg. There was no significant accumulation of stavudine with repeated administration every 6, 8, or 12 hours.

Absorption: Following oral administration, stavudine is rapidly absorbed, with peak plasma concentrations occurring within 1 hour after dosing. The systemic exposure to stavudine is the same following administration as capsules or solution.

Distribution: Binding of stavudine to serum proteins was negligible over the concentration range of 0.01 to 11.4 µg/mL. Stavudine distributes equally between red blood cells and plasma.

Metabolism: The metabolic fate of stavudine has not been elucidated in humans.

Excretion: Renal elimination accounted for about 40% of the overall clearance regardless of the route of administration. The mean renal clearance was about twice the average

Table 1
Mean ± SD Pharmacokinetic Parameters of Stavudine In Adult and Pediatric HIV-Infected Patients

Parameter	Adult Patients	n	Pediatric Patients	n
Oral bioavailability (F)	86.4 ± 18.2%	25	76.9 ± 31.7%	20
Volume of distribution[a] (VD)	58 ± 21 L	44	18.5 ± 9.2 L/m²	21
Apparent oral volume of distribution[b] (VD/F)	66 ± 22 L	71	not determined	-
Ratio of CSF: plasma concentrations (as %)[c]	not determined	-	59 ± 35%	8
Total body clearance[a] (CL)	8.3 ± 2.3 mL/min/kg	44	247 ± 94 mL/min/m²	21
Apparent oral clearance[b] (CL/F)	8.0 ± 2.6 mL/min/kg	113	333 ± 87 mL/min/m²	20
Elimination half-life ($T_{1/2}$), I.V. dose[a]	1.15 ± 0.35 hr	44	1.11 ± 0.28 hr	21
Elimination half-life ($T_{1/2}$), oral dose[b]	1.44 ± 0.30 hr	115	0.96 ± 0.26 hr	20
Urinary recovery of stavudine (% of dose)	39 ± 23%	88	34 ± 16%	19

[a] following 1 hour I.V. infusion
[b] following single oral dose
[c] following multiple oral doses

Table 2
**Mean ± SD Pharmacokinetic Parameter Values
Single 40-mg Oral Dose of ZERIT**

	Creatinine Clearance			
	>50 mL/min (n=10)	26–50 mL/min (n=5)	9–25 mL/min (n=5)	Hemodialysis Patients* (n=11)
CL_{cr} (mL/min)	104 ± 28	41 ± 5	17 ± 3	NA
CL/F (mL/min)	335 ± 57	191 ± 39	116 ± 25	105 ± 17
CL_R (mL/min)	167 ± 65	73 ± 18	17 ± 3	NA
$T_{1/2}$ (h)	1.7 ± 0.4	3.5 ± 2.5	4.6 ± 0.9	5.4 ± 1.4

CL_{cr}=creatinine clearance
CL/F=apparent oral clearance
CL_R=renal clearance
$T_{1/2}$=terminal elimination half-life
NA=not applicable

*Determined while patients were off dialysis.

endogenous creatinine clearance, indicating active tubular secretion in addition to glomerular filtration.
[See table 1 above]
Special Populations:
Pediatric- For pharmacokinetic properties of stavudine in pediatric patients, see Table 1.
Renal Insufficiency: Data from two studies indicated that the apparent oral clearance of stavudine decreased and the terminal elimination half-life increased as creatinine clearance decreased (see Table 2). C_{max} and T_{max} were not significantly altered by renal insufficiency. The mean ± SD hemodialysis clearance value of stavudine was 120 ± 18 mL/min (n=12); the mean ± SD percentage of the stavudine dose recovered in the dialysate, timed to occur between 2-6 hours post-dose, was 31 ± 5%. Based on these observations, it is recommended that ZERIT (stavudine) dosage be modified in patients with reduced creatinine clearance and in patients receiving maintenance hemodialysis (see **"DOSAGE AND ADMINISTRATION"** section).
[See table 2 above]
Hepatic Insufficiency: Stavudine pharmacokinetics were not altered in 5 non-HIV-infected patients with hepatic impairment secondary to cirrhosis (Child-Pugh classification B or C) following the administration of a single 40 mg dose.
Geriatric: Stavudine pharmacokinetics have not been studied in patients >65 years of age.
Gender: The effects of gender on stavudine pharmacokinetics are not known.
Race: The effects of race on stavudine pharmacokinetics are not known.

INDICATIONS AND USAGE
ZERIT is indicated for the treatment of HIV-infected patients who have received prolonged prior zidovudine therapy.

CLINICAL STUDIES
Study AI455-019 was a multi-center, randomized, double-blind trial of ZERIT Capsules vs zidovudine for the treatment of HIV-infected adults with CD4 counts of 50 to 500 cells/mm³ who had received at least six months prior zidovudine treatment. ZERIT was administered in dosages of 40 mg BID for patients weighing ≥60 kg, and 30 mg BID for those weighing <60 kg. The zidovudine dosage was 200 mg TID.
The study enrolled 822 patients with a median baseline CD4 count of 235 cells/mm³ (range: 10 to 735 cells/mm³), and a median duration of prior zidovudine treatment of 88 weeks (range 11 to 356 weeks). Fourteen percent of subjects had AIDS at baseline, 50% had HIV-related symptoms and 36% were asymptomatic.
Table 3 gives the Kaplan-Meier estimates for the time to disease progression.

Table 3
Incidence of Disease Progression

	First AIDS-Defining Event or Death[a]	
	ZERIT	zidovudine
6 months	4.4%	5.7%
12 months	10.4%	14.1%
18 months	18.5%	23.3%
24 months	26.6%	31.8%

[a] Kaplan-Meier estimates; the overall difference between stavudine and zidovudine was not significant.

CONTRAINDICATIONS
ZERIT is contraindicated in patients with clinically significant hypersensitivity to stavudine or to any of the components contained in the formulation.

WARNINGS
Lactic Acidosis/Severe Hepatomegaly with Steatosis: Lactic acidosis and severe hepatomegaly with steatosis, including fatal cases, have been reported with the use of antiretroviral nucleoside analogues alone or in combination, including stavudine. A majority of these cases have been in women. Caution should be exercised when administering ZERIT to any patient, and particularly to those with known risk factors for liver disease. Treatment with ZERIT should be discontinued in any patient who develops clinical or laboratory findings suggestive of lactic acidosis or hepatotoxicity.
Peripheral Neuropathy: ZERIT (stavudine) therapy can be associated with severe peripheral neuropathy, which is dose-related and occurs more frequently in patients with advanced HIV infection or who have previously experienced peripheral neuropathy (see Table 4).

PRECAUTIONS
Information for Patients: Patients should be informed that the most common toxicity of ZERIT is peripheral neuropathy. Symptoms of peripheral neuropathy usually include tingling, burning, pain, or numbness in the hands or feet. Patients should be counseled that this toxicity occurs with greater frequency in patients with a history of peripheral neuropathy. They should be advised that these symptoms should be reported to their physicians and that dose changes may be necessary. They should also be cautioned about the use of other medications that may exacerbate peripheral neuropathy.
Caregivers of young children receiving ZERIT therapy should be instructed regarding detection and reporting of peripheral neuropathy.
The duration of clinical benefit from antiretroviral therapy may be limited. Patients should be informed that ZERIT is not a cure for HIV infection, and that they may continue to acquire illnesses associated with HIV infection, including opportunistic infections. Patients should be advised to remain under the care of a physician when using ZERIT. They should be advised that ZERIT therapy has not been shown to reduce the risk of transmission of HIV to others through sexual contact or blood contamination. Patients should be informed that long-term effects of ZERIT are unknown at this time.
Patients should be informed that the Centers for Disease Control and Prevention (CDC) recommend that HIV-infected mothers not nurse newborn infants to reduce the risk of postnatal transmissions of HIV infection.
Carcinogenesis, Mutagenesis, Impairment of Fertility: In 2-year carcinogenicity studies in mice and rats, stavudine was noncarcinogenic at doses which produced exposures (AUC) 39 and 168 times, respectively, human exposure at the recommended clinical dose. Benign and malignant liver tumors in mice and rats and malignant urinary bladder tumors in male rats occurred at levels of exposure, 250 (mice) and 732 (rats) times human exposure at the recommended clinical dose.
Stavudine was not mutagenic in the Ames, *E. coli* reverse mutation, or the CHO/HGPRT mammalian cell forward mutation assays, with and without metabolic activation. Stavudine produced positive results in the *in vitro* human lymphocyte clastogenesis and mouse fibroblast assays, and in the *in vivo* mouse micronucleus test. In the *in vitro* assays, stavudine elevated the frequency of chromosome aberrations in human lymphocytes (concentrations of 25 to 250 μg/mL, without metabolic activation) and increased the frequency of transformed foci in mouse fibroblast cells (concentrations of 25 to 2500 μg/mL, with and without metabolic activation). In the *in vivo* micronucleus assay, stavudine was clastogenic in bone marrow cells following oral stavudine administration to mice at dosages of 600 to 2000 mg/kg/day for 3 days.
No evidence of impaired fertility was seen in rats with exposures (based on C_{max}) up to 216 times that observed following a clinical dosage of 1 mg/kg/day.
Pregnancy: Pregnancy "Category C". Reproduction studies have been performed in rats and rabbits with exposures (based on C_{max}) up to 399 and 183 times, respectively, of that seen at a clinical dosage of 1 mg/kg/day and have revealed no evidence of teratogenicity. The incidence in fetuses of a common skeletal variation, unossified or incomplete ossification of sternebra, was increased in rats at 399 times human exposure, while no effect was observed at 216 times human exposure. A slight post-implantation loss was noted at 216 times the human exposure with no effect noted at approximately 135 times the human exposure. An increase in early rat neonatal mortality (birth to 4 days of age)

Continued on next page

Zerit—Cont.

occurred at 399 times the human exposure, while survival of neonates was unaffected at approximately 135 times the human exposure. A study in rats showed that stavudine is transferred to the fetus through the placenta. The concentration in fetal tissue was approximately one-half the concentration in maternal plasma. There are no adequate and well-controlled studies in pregnant women. Because animal reproduction studies are not always predictive of human response, stavudine should be used during pregnancy only if clearly needed.

Antiretroviral Pregnancy Registry: To monitor maternal-fetal outcomes of pregnant women exposed to stavudine and other antiretroviral agents, an Antiretroviral Pregnancy Registry has been established. Physicians are encouraged to register patients by calling (800) 258-4263.

Nursing Mothers: Studies in lactating rats demonstrated that stavudine is excreted in milk. Although it is not known whether stavudine is excreted in human milk, there exists the potential for adverse effects from stavudine in nursing infants. Mothers should be instructed to discontinue nursing if they are receiving stavudine. This is consistent with the recommendation by the U.S. Public Health Service Centers for Disease Control and Prevention that HIV-infected mothers not breast-feed their infants to avoid risking postnatal transmission of HIV.

Pediatric Use: Use of stavudine in pediatric patients is supported by evidence from adequate and well-controlled studies of stavudine in adults with additional safety data in 115 pediatric patients.

Stavudine pharmacokinetics have been evaluated in 25 HIV-infected pediatric patients ranging in age from 5 weeks to 15 years and in weight from 2 to 43 kg after I.V. or oral administration of single doses and BID regimen (see "CLINICAL PHARMACOLOGY" section, Table 1).

ADVERSE REACTIONS

Adults: ZERIT therapy can be associated with severe peripheral neuropathy, which is dose related and occurs more frequently in patients with advanced HIV infection or who have previously experienced peripheral neuropathy (see Table 4).

Table 4
Peripheral Neuropathy Leading to Dose Modification

	Percent (%)			
	Study AI455-019		Parallel Track Program	
	ZERIT (40 mg BID) (n=412)	zidovudine (200 mg TID) (n=402)	ZERIT (40 mg BID) (n=5905)	ZERIT (20 mg BID) (n=5879)
Peripheral Neuropathy				
Grade 1–2	11	3	20	17
Grade 3–4	2	1	4	2
Total	13	4	24	19

Patients should be monitored for the development of neuropathy that is usually characterized by numbness, tingling, or pain in the feet or hands. Stavudine-related peripheral neuropathy may resolve if therapy is withdrawn promptly. In some cases, symptoms may worsen temporarily following discontinuation of therapy. If symptoms resolve completely, resumption of treatment may be considered at a reduced dose (see "DOSAGE AND ADMINISTRATION" section).

Selected adverse events that occurred in adult patients receiving ZERIT (stavudine) in the Phase 3 controlled comparative trial (Study AI455-019) are provided in Table 5.

Table 5
Selected Clinical Adverse Events in the Phase 3 Controlled Clinical Trial[a]

	Percent (%)	
	Study AI455-019[b]	
Adverse Events	ZERIT (40 mg BID) (n=412)	zidovudine (200 mg TID) (n=402)
Headache	54	49
Chills/Fever	50	51
Diarrhea	50	43
Rash	40	35
Nausea and Vomiting	38	44
Abdominal Pain	34	27
Myalgia	32	35
Insomnia	29	31
Anorexia	19	22

Allergic Reaction	9	8
Pancreatitis	*	*

* This event was reported in fewer than 1% of patients.
[a] Includes all clinical complaints.
[b] Median duration of stavudine therapy =79 weeks; median duration of zidovudine therapy = 53 weeks.

Laboratory abnormalities reported in the Phase 3 controlled comparative trial (Study AI455-019) are shown in Table 6.

Table 6
Controlled Clinical Trial: Incidence of Adult Laboratory Abnormalities*

	Percent (%)	
	Study AI455-019[b]	
Lab Tests (units)	ZERIT (40 mg BID) (n=412)	zidovudine (200 mg TID) (n=402)
AST (SGOT) (>5.0 × ULN[c])	11	10
ALT (SGPT) (>5.0 × ULN)	13	11
Bilirubin (>5.0 × ULN)	2	2
Anemia (<8.0 × g/dL)	*	3
Neutropenia (neutrophils <750/mm³)	5	9
Thrombocytopenia (platelets <50,000/mm³)	3	3
Amylase (>1.4 × ULN)	14	13

* This abnormality was reported in fewer than 1% of patients.
[a] Data presented for patients for whom laboratory evaluations were performed.
[b] Median duration of stavudine therapy =79 weeks; mediation duration of zidovudine therapy =53 weeks.
[c] ULN =upper limit of normal.

Observed During Clinical Practice: The following events have been identified during post-approval use of ZERIT. Because they are reported voluntarily from a population of unknown size, estimates of frequency cannot be made. These events have been chosen for inclusion due to their seriousness, frequency of reporting, causal connection to ZERIT, or a combination of these factors.

Lactic acidosis and hepatic steatosis (see "WARNINGS" section), hepatitis and liver failure.

Pediatric Patients: Adverse reactions and serious laboratory abnormalities in pediatric patients were similar in type and frequency to those seen in adult patients.

OVERDOSAGE

Experience with adults treated with 12 to 24 times the recommended daily dosage revealed no acute toxicity. Complications of chronic overdosage include peripheral neuropathy and hepatic toxicity. Stavudine can be removed by hemodialysis; the mean ± SD hemodialysis clearance of stavudine is 120 ± 18 mL/min. Whether stavudine is eliminated by peritoneal dialysis has not been studied.

DOSAGE AND ADMINISTRATION

The interval between doses of ZERIT should be 12 hours. ZERIT may be taken without regard to meals.

Adults: The recommended starting dose based on body weight is as follows:

    40 mg twice daily for patients ≥60 kg.
    30 mg twice daily for patients <60 kg.

Pediatrics: The recommended starting dose for pediatric patients weighing less than 30 kg is 1mg/kg/dose, given every 12 hours. Pediatric patients weighing 30 kg or greater should receive the recommended adult dosage.

Dosage Adjustment: Patients should be monitored for the development of peripheral neuropathy, which is usually characterized by numbness, tingling, or pain in the feet or hands. These symptoms may be difficult to detect in young children (see "WARNINGS" section). If these symptoms develop on treatment, stavudine therapy should be interrupted. Symptoms may resolve if therapy is withdrawn promptly. In some cases, symptoms may worsen temporarily following discontinuation of therapy. If symptoms resolve completely, resumption of treatment may be considered using the following dosage schedule for adults:

    20 mg twice daily for patients ≥ 60 kg.
    15 mg twice daily for patients < 60 kg.

For pediatric patients, resumption of treatment may be considered at one-half the recommended dose.

Renal Impairment: Zerit (stavudine) may be administered to adult patients with impaired renal function with adjustment in dose as shown in Table 7:

Table 7
Recommended Dosage Adjustment for Renal Impairment

Creatinine Clearance	Recommended ZERIT Dose by Patient Weight	
(mL/min)	≥60 kg	<60 kg
>50	40 mg every 12 hours	30 mg every 12 hours
26–50	20 mg every 12 hours	15 mg every 12 hours
10–25	20 mg every 24 hours	15 mg every 24 hours

Since urinary excretion is also a major route of elimination of stavudine in pediatric patients, the clearance of stavudine may be altered in children with renal impairment. Although there are insufficient data to recommend a specific dose adjustment of ZERIT in this patient population, a reduction in the dose and/or an increase in the interval between doses should be considered.

Hemodialysis Patients: The recommended dose is 20 mg every 24 hours (≥60 kg) or 15 mg every 24 hours (<60 kg), administered after the completion of hemodialysis and at the same time of day on non-dialysis days.

Method of Preparation:
ZERIT (stavudine) for Oral Solution
Prior to dispensing, the pharmacist must constitute the dry powder with purified water to a concentration of 1 mg stavudine per mL of solution, as follows:
1. Add 202 mL of purified water to the container.
2. Shake container vigorously until the powder dissolves completely. Constitution in this way produces 200 mL (deliverable volume) of 1 mg/mL stavudine solution. The solution may appear slightly hazy.
3. Dispense solution in original container with measuring cup provided. Instruct patient to shake the container vigorously prior to measuring each dose and to store the tightly closed container in a refrigerator, 36° to 46°F (2° to 8°C). Discard any unused portion after 30 days.

HOW SUPPLIED

ZERIT® (stavudine) Capsules are available in the following strengths and configurations of plastic bottles with child-resistant closures:
[See table 8 below]
ZERIT® (stavudine) for Oral Solution is a dye-free, fruit-flavored powder that provides 1 mg of stavudine per mL of solution upon constitution with water. Directions for solution preparation are included on the product label and in the **DOSAGE AND ADMINISTRATION** section of this insert. ZERIT for Oral Solution (NDC No. 0003-1968-01) is available in child-resistant containers that provide 200 mL of solution after constitution with water.
US Patent No.: 4,978,655

Table 8

Product Strength	Capsule Shell Color	Markings on Capsule (in Black Ink)		Capsules per bottle	NDC No.
15 mg	Light yellow & dark red	BMS 1964	15	60	0003-1964-01
20 mg	Light brown	BMS 1965	20	60	0003-1965-01
30 mg	Light orange & dark orange	BMS 1966	30	60	0003-1966-01
40 mg	Dark orange	BMS 1967	40	60	0003-1967-01

Storage: ZERIT Capsules should be stored in tightly closed containers at controlled room temperature, 59° to 86°F (15° to 30°C).

ZERIT for Oral Solution should be protected from excessive moisture and stored in tightly closed containers at controlled room temperature, 59° to 86°F (15° to 30°C). After constitution, store tightly closed containers of ZERIT for Oral Solution in a refrigerator, 36° to 46°F (2° to 8°C). Discard any unused portion after 30 days.

BRISTOL-MYERS SQUIBB
Immunology
Bristol-Myers Squibb Company
Princeton, NJ 08543
U.S.A.
F9-B001-6-98 P4577-06
Revised May 1998

Shown in Product Identification Guide, page 308

Bristol-Myers Products
(A Bristol-Myers Squibb Company)
345 PARK AVENUE
NEW YORK, NY 10154

Direct Inquiries to:
Products Division
Consumer Affairs Department
1350 Liberty Avenue
Hillside, NJ 07207
(800) 468-7746

Aspirin Free EXCEDRIN® OTC

COMPOSITION

Each caplet and geltab contains Acetaminophen 500 mg. and Caffeine 65 mg. Other Ingredients (caplet): Benzoic Acid, Carnauba Wax, Corn starch, D&C Red No. 27 Lake, D&C Yellow No. 10 Lake, FD&C Blue No. 1 Lake, Hydroxypropyl methylcellulose, Magnesium stearate, Methylparaben, Microcrystalline Cellulose, Mineral Oil, Polysorbate 20, Povidone, Propylene Glycol, Propylparaben, Simethicone Emulsion, Sorbitan Monolaurate, Stearci Acid, Titanium Dioxide.

May also contain: Croscarmellose sodium, FD&C Red No. 40, Saccharin sodium, Sodium starch glycolate

Other Ingredients: (geltab) Benzoic Acid, Corn Starch, FD&C Blue No. 1., FD&C Red No. 40, FD&C Yellow No. 6, Gelatin, Glycerin, Hydroxypropyl methylcellulose, Magnesium stearate, Methylparaben, Microcrystalline cellulose, Mineral oil, Polysorbate 20, Povidone, Propylene glycol, Propylparaben, Simethicone emulsion, Sorbitan monolaurate, Stearic acid, Titanium dioxide.

May also contain: Croscarmellose sodium, Sodium starch glycolate

INDICATIONS

For temporary relief of the minor pain of headache, sinusitis, colds, muscular aches, menstrual discomfort, toothaches and arthritis pain.

DIRECTIONS

Adults: 2 caplets or geltabs every 6 hours while symptoms persist, not to exceed 8 caplets or geltabs in 24 hours, or as directed by a doctor. Children under 12 years of age: Consult a doctor.

WARNINGS

Keep this and all drugs out of the reach of children. In case of accidental overdose, seek professional assistance or contact a poison control center immediately. Prompt medical attention is critical for adults as well as for children even if you do not notice any signs or symptoms. As with any drug, if you are pregnant or nursing a baby, seek the advice of a health professional before using this product. Do not take this product for pain for more than 10 days or for fever for more than 3 days unless directed by a doctor. If pain or fever persists or gets worse, if new symptoms occur, of if redness or swelling is present, consult a doctor because these could be signs of a serious condition. Consult a dentist promptly for toothache. If you generally consume 3 or more alcohol-containing drinks per day, you should consult your physician for advice on when and how you should take Aspirin Free Excedrin and other pain relievers.

OVERDOSE

(Acetylcysteine As An Antidote For Acetaminophen Overdose)

Acetaminophen is rapidly absorbed from the upper gastrointestinal tract with peak plasma levels occurring between 30 and 60 minutes after therapeutic doses and usually within 4 hours following an overdose. The parent compound, which is nontoxic, is extensively metabolized in the liver to form principally the sulfate and glucuronide conjugates which are also nontoxic and are rapidly excreted in the urine. A small fraction of an ingested dose is metabolized in the liver by the cytochrome P-450 mixed function oxidase enzyme system to form a reactive, potentially toxic, intermediate metabolite which preferentially conjugates with hepatic glutathione to form the nontoxic cysteine and mercapturic acid derivatives which are then excreted by the kidney. Therapeutic doses of acetaminophen do not saturate the glucuronide and sulfate conjugation pathways and do not result in the formation of sufficient reactive metabolite to deplete glutathione stores. However, following ingestion of a large overdose (150 mg/kg or greater) the glucuronide and sulfate conjugation pathways are saturated resulting in a larger fraction of the drug being metabolized via the P-450 pathway. The increased formation of reactive metabolite may deplete the hepatic stores of glutathione with subsequent binding of the metabolite to protein molecules within the hepatocyte resulting in cellular necrosis. Acetylcysteine has been shown to reduce the extent of liver injury following acetaminophen overdose. Early symptoms following a potentially hepatotoxic overdose may include: nausea, vomiting, diaphoresis and general malaise. Clinical and laboratory evidence of hepatic toxicity may not be apparent until 48 to 72 hours postingestion. In most adults and adolescents, regardless of the quantity of acetaminophen reported to have been ingested, administer acetylcysteine immediately. Acetylcysteine therapy should be initiated and continued for a full course of therapy. Its effectiveness depends on early administration, with benefit seen principally in patients treated within 16 hours of the overdose.

If acetaminophen plasma assay capability is not available, and the estimated acetaminophen ingestion exceeds 150 mg/kg, acetylcysteine therapy should be initiated and continued for a full course of therapy.

For full prescribing information, refer to the acetylcysteine package insert. Do not await the results of assays for acetaminophen level before initiating treatment with acetylcysteine. The following additional procedures are recommended: The stomach should be emptied promptly by lavage or by induction of emesis with syrup of ipecac. A serum acetaminophen assay should be obtained as early as possible, but no sooner than four hours following ingestion. Liver function studies should be obtained initially and repeated at 24-hour intervals.

For additional emergency information call your regional poison center or toll-free (1-800-525-6115) to the Rocky Mountain Poison and Drug Center for assistance in diagnosis and for directions in the use of acetylcysteine as an antidote.

HOW SUPPLIED

Aspirin Free EXCEDRIN® is supplied as: Coated red caplets with AFE debossed on one side

Supplied in bottles of 24's, 50's, 100's

All sizes packaged in child resistant closures except 100's size for caplets which is recommended for households without young children.

Easy to swallow red geltabs with "AF Excedrin" printed in white on one side

Supplied in bottles of 20's, 40's, 80's

All sizes packaged in child resistant closures except 40's which is recommended for households without young children.

Store at room temperature.

Shown in Product Identification Guide, page 307

EXCEDRIN® Extra-Strength OTC
Analgesic
[ĕx″cĕd′rĭn]

COMPOSITION

Each tablet, caplet, or geltab contains Acetaminophen 250 mg.; Aspirin 250 mg.; and Caffeine 65 mg.

Other ingredients (tablet, caplet): Benzoic Acid, Hydroxypropylcellulose, Hydroxypropyl methylcellulose, Microcrystalline Cellulose, Mineral Oil, Polysorbate 20, Povidone, Propylene Glycol, Simethicone Emulsion, Sorbitan Monolaurate, Stearic Acid.

Tablets and caplets may also contain: Carnauba wax, FD&C Blue No. 1, Saccharin Sodium, Titanium Dioxide.

Other ingredients (geltab): Benzoic Acid, D&C Yellow # 10 Lake, Disodium EDTA, FD&C Blue # 1 Lake, FD&C Red # 40 Lake, Ferric Oxide, Gelatin, Glycerin, Hydroxypropylcellulose, Hydroxypropyl Methylcellulose, Maltitol Solution, Microcrystalline Cellulose, Mineral Oil, Pepsin, Polysorbate 20, Povidone, Propylene Glycol, Propyl Gallate, Simethicone Emulsion, Sorbitan Monolaurate, Stearic Acid, Titanium Dioxide

INDICATIONS

For temporary relief of the pain of headache, sinusitis, colds, muscular aches, menstrual discomfort, toothache and minor arthritis pain.

WARNINGS

Children and teenagers should not use this medicine for chicken pox or flu symptoms before a doctor is consulted about Reye syndrome, a rare but serious illness reported to be associated with aspirin. Keep this and all drugs out of the reach of children. In case of accidental overdose, seek professional assistance or contact a poison control center immediately. Prompt medical attention is critical for adults as well as for children even if you do not notice any signs or symptoms. As with any drug, if you are pregnant or nursing a baby, seek the advice of a health professional before using this product. IT IS ESPECIALLY IMPORTANT NOT TO USE ASPIRIN DURING THE LAST 3 MONTHS OF PREGNANCY UNLESS SPECIFICALLY DIRECTED TO DO SO BY A DOCTOR BECAUSE IT MAY CAUSE PROBLEMS IN THE UNBORN CHILD OR COMPLICATIONS DURING DELIVERY. Do not take this product for pain for more than 10 days or for fever for more than 3 days unless directed by a doctor. If pain or fever persists or gets worse if new symptoms occur, or if redness or swelling is present, consult a doctor because these could be signs of a serious condition. Consult a dentist promptly for toothache. Do not take this product if you are allergic to aspirin, have asthma, have stomach problems (such as heartburn, upset stomach or stomach pain) that persist or recur, or if you have ulcers or bleeding problems, unless directed by a doctor. If ringing in the ears or loss of hearing occurs, consult a doctor before taking any more of this product. If you generally consume 3 or more alcohol-containing drinks per day, you should consult your physician for advice on when and how you should take Excedrin and other pain relievers.

DRUG INTERACTION PRECAUTION

Do not take this product if you are taking a prescription drug for anticoagulation (thinning of blood), diabetes, gout or arthritis unless directed by a doctor.

DIRECTIONS

Adults: 2 tablets, caplets or geltabs with water every 6 hours while symptoms persist, not to exceed 8 tablets, caplets or geltabs in 24 hours, or as directed by a doctor. Children under 12 years of age: Consult a doctor.

OVERDOSE

(Acetylcysteine As An Antidote For Acetaminophen Overdose)

Acetaminophen is rapidly absorbed from the upper gastrointestinal tract with peak plasma levels occurring between 30 and 60 minutes after therapeutic doses and usually within 4 hours following an overdose. The parent compound, which is nontoxic, is extensively metabolized in the liver to form principally the sulfate and glucuronide conjugates which are also nontoxic and are rapidly excreted in the urine. A small fraction of an ingested dose is metabolized in the liver by the cytochrome P-450 mixed function oxidase enzyme system to form a reactive, potentially toxic, intermediate metabolite which preferentially conjugates with hepatic glutathione to form the nontoxic cysteine and mercapturic acid derivatives which are then excreted by the kidney. Therapeutic doses of acetaminophen do not saturate the glucuronide and sulfate conjugation pathways and do not result in the formation of sufficient reactive metabolite to deplete glutathione stores. However, following ingestion of a large overdose (150 mg/kg or greater) the glucuronide and sulfate conjugation pathways are saturated resulting in a larger fraction of the drug being metabolized via the P-450 pathway. The increased formation of reactive metabolite may deplete the hepatic stores of glutathione with subsequent binding of the metabolite to protein molecules within the hepatocyte resulting in cellular necrosis. Acetylcysteine has been shown to reduce the extent of liver injury following acetaminophen overdose. Early symptoms following a potentially hepatotoxic overdose may include: nausea, vomiting, diaphoresis and general malaise. Clinical and laboratory evidence of hepatic toxicity may not be apparent until 48 to 72 hours postingestion. In adults and adolescents, regardless of the quantity of acetaminophen reported to have been ingested, administer acetylcysteine immediately. Acetylcysteine therapy should be initiated and continued for a full course of therapy. Its effectiveness depends on early administration, with benefit seen principally in patients treated within 16 hours of the overdose.

If acetaminophen plasma assay capability is not available, and the estimated acetaminophen ingestion exceeds 150 mg/kg, acetylcysteine therapy should be initiated and continued for a full course of therapy.

For full prescribing information, refer to the acetylcysteine package insert. Do not await the results of assays for acetaminophen level before initiating treatment with acetylcysteine. The following additional procedures are recommended: The stomach should be emptied promptly by la-

Continued on next page

Excedrin E-S—Cont.

vage or by induction of emesis with syrup of ipecac. A serum acetaminophen assay should be obtained as early as possible, but no sooner than four hours following ingestion. Liver function studies should be obtained initially and repeated at 24-hour intervals.

For additional emergency information call your regional poison center or toll-free (1-800-525-6115) to the Rocky Mountain Poison and Drug Center for assistance in diagnosis and for directions in the use of acetylcysteine as an antidote.

HOW SUPPLIED

Extra Strength EXCEDRIN® is supplied as:
White circular tablet with letter "E" debossed on one side. Supplied in bottles of 12's, 24's, 50's, 100's, 175's, 275's and metal tins of 12's.
Coated white caplets with "E" debossed on one side.
Supplied in bottles of 24's, 50's, 100's and 175's, and 275's.
Coated round geltabs–green on one side, white on the other Tablets printed with black "E" on one side.
Supplied in bottles of 20's, 40's, 80's.
All sizes packaged in child resistant closures except 100's for tablets, 50's for caplets which are sizes recommended for households without young children.
Shown in Product Identification Guide, page 307

EXCEDRIN® MIGRAINE   OTC
Pain Reliever/Pain Reliever Aid

ACTIVE INGREDIENTS

Each tablet or caplet contains Acetaminophen 250mg, Aspirin 250mg and Caffeine 65mg.

INACTIVE INGREDIENTS

Benzoic acid, carnauba wax, hydroxypropylcellulose, hydroxypropyl methylcellulose, microcrystalline cellulose, mineral oil, polysorbate 20, povidone, propylene glycol, stearate acid, simethicone emulsion, sorbitan monolaurate. May also contain: FD&C blue no. 1, titanium dioxide.

USE

For the temporary relief of mild to moderate pain associated with migraine headache.

WARNINGS

Children and teenagers should not use this medication for chicken pox, or flu symptoms, before a doctor is consulted about Reye syndrome, a rare but serious illness reported to be associated with aspirin.
Allergy Alert: If after taking a pain reliever or fever reducer, you have ever had hives, facial swelling, asthma or shock, do not take Excedrin Migraine. You may have a serious reaction.
Alcohol Warning: If you drink 3 or more alcoholic beverages daily, ask your doctor whether you should take Excedrin Migraine or other pain relievers. Excedrin Migraine may increase your risk of liver damage and stomach bleeding.
The recommended dose of this product contains about as much caffeine as a cup of coffee. Limit the use of caffeine-containing medications, foods, or beverages while taking this product because too much caffeine may cause nervousness, irritability, sleeplessness, and, occasionally, rapid heart beat.
Ask a Doctor Before Use If You Have: The worst headache of your life; fever and stiff neck; bleeding problems; ulcers; asthma; liver disease; renal disease; stomach problems such as heartburn, upset stomach, or stomach pain that do not go away or recur, daily headaches; headaches beginning after or are caused by head injury, exertion, coughing or bending; experienced your first headache after the age of 50; migraine headaches so severe as to require bed rest; vomiting with your migraine headache
Ask a Doctor Before Use If You Are: Taking a prescription drug for anticoagulation (thinning of the blood), diabetes, gout or arthritis
Stop Using This Product and See a Doctor If: Migraine headache pain worsens or continues for more than 48 hours; new or unexpected symptoms occur; ringing of the ears or loss of hearing occurs.
As with any drug, if you are pregnant or nursing a baby, seek the advice of a health professional before using this product. **IT IS ESPECIALLY IMPORTANT NOT TO USE ASPIRIN DURING THE LAST 3 MONTHS OF PREGNANCY UNLESS SPECIFICALLY DIRECTED TO DO SO BY A DOCTOR BECAUSE IT MAY CAUSE PROBLEMS IN THE UNBORN CHILD OR COMPLICATIONS DURING DELIVERY. Keep this and all drugs out of the reach of children.** In case of accidental overdose, seek professional assistance or contact a Poison Control Center immediately. Prompt medical attention is critical for adults as well as for children even if you do not notice any signs or symptoms.

DIRECTIONS

Adults and children over 12 years: 2 tablets or caplets with a full glass of water every 6 hours while symptoms persist, not to exceed 8 tablets or caplets in 24 hours, or as directed by a doctor. Do not take for more than 48 hours for the pain of migraine. Children: Do not give to children under 12 unless directed by a doctor.

OVERDOSE
Acetylcysteine As An Antidote For Acetaminophen Overdose
Acetaminophen is rapidly absorbed from the upper gastrointestinal tract with peak plasma levels occurring between 30 and 60 minutes after therapeutic doses and usually within 4 hours following an overdose. The parents compound, which is nontoxic, is extensively metabolized in the liver to form principally the sulfate and glucuronide conjugates which are also nontoxic and are rapidly excreted in the urine. A small fraction of an ingested dose is metabolized in the liver by the cytochrome P-450 mixed function oxidase enzyme system to form a reactive, potentially toxic, intermediate metabolite which preferentially conjugates with hepatic glutathione to form the nontoxic cysteine and mercapturic acid derivatives which are then excreted by the kidney. Therapeutic doses of acetaminophen do not saturate the glucuronide and sulfate conjunction pathways and do not result in the formation of sufficient reactive metabolite to deplete glutathione stores. However, following ingestion of a large overdose (150 mg/kg or greater) the glucuronide and sulfate conjugation pathways are saturated resulting in a larger fraction of the drug being metabolized via te P-450 pathway. The increased formation of reactive metabolite may deplete the hepatic stores of glutathione with subsequent binding of the metabolite to protein molecules within the hepatocyte resulting in cellular necrosis. Acetylcysteine has been shown to reduce the extent of liver injury following acetaminophen overdose. Early symptoms following a potentially hepatotoxic overdose may include: nausea, vomiting, diaphoresis and general malaise. Clinical and laboratory evidence of hepatic toxicity may not be apparent until 48 to 72 hours postingestion. In most adults and adolescents, regardless of the quantity of acetaminophen reported to have been ingested, administer acetylcysteine immediately. Acetylcysteine therapy should be initiated and continued for a full course of therapy. Its effectiveness depends on early administration, with benefit seen principally in patients treated within 16 hours of the overdose. If acetaminophen plasma assay capability is not available, and the estimated acetaminophen ingestion exceeds 150 mg/kg, acetylcysteine therapy should be initiated and continued for a full course of therapy.
For full prescription information, refer to the acetylcysteine package insert. Do not await the results of assays for acetaminophen level before initiating treatment with acetylcysteine. The following additional procedures are recomended: The stomach should be emptied promptly by lavage or by induction of emesis with syrup of ipecac. A serum acetaminophen assay should be obtained as early as possible, but no sooner than four hours following ingestion. Liver function studies should be obtained initially and repeated at 24-hour intervals. For additional emergency information call your regional poison center or toll-free (1-800-525-6115) to the Rocky Mountain Poison and Drug Center for assistance in diagnosis and for directions in the use of acetylcysteine as an antidote.

HOW SUPPLIED

EXCEDRIN® MIGRAINE is supplied as:
Coated white circular tablets or coated white caplets with letter "E" debossed on one side. Supplied in bottles of 24's, 50's, and 100's. All sizes packaged in child resistance closures except 100's tablets, 50's caplets which are sizes recommended for households without young children.
Shown in Product Identification Guide, page 307

EXCEDRIN P.M.®   OTC
[ex "cĕd 'rĭn]
Analgesic Sleeping Aid

COMPOSITION

Each tablet, caplet, or geltab contains:

	EXCEDRIN®PM Per Tablet or Caplet
Acetaminophen	500 mg.
Diphenhydramine Citrate:	38 mg.

Other Ingredients:
Tablet or Caplet
  benzoic acid
  carnauba wax
  corn starch
  D&C yellow no. 10

D&C yellow no. 10 aluminum lake
FD&C blue no. 1
FD&C blue no. 1 aluminum lake
hydroxypropyl methylcellulose
magnesium stearate
methylparaben
pregelatinized starch
propylene glycol
propylparaben
simethicone emulsion
stearic acid
titanium dioxide
May also contain:
  mineral oil
  polysorbate 20
  povidone
  sodium citrate
  sorbitan monolaurate

	EXCEDRIN®PM Per Geltab
Acetaminophen	500 mg.
Diphenhydramine Citrate	38 mg.

Other Ingredients:
Geltab
  Benzoic Acid
  Corn Starch
  D&C Red No. 33 Lake
  D&C Yellow No. 10
  D&C Yellow No. 10 Lake
  Edetate Disodium
  Fd&C Blue No. 1
  Fd&C Blue No. 1 Lake
  Gelatin
  Glycerin
  Hydroxypropyl Methylcellulose
  Magnesium Stearate
  Methylparaben
  Mineral Oil
  Polysorbate 20
  Povidone
  Pregelatinized Starch
  Propylene Glycol
  Propylparaben
  Simethicone Emulsion
  Sorbitan Monolaurate
  Stearic Acid
  Titanium Dioxide

INDICATIONS

For temporary relief of occasional headaches and minor aches and pains with accompanying sleeplessness.

WARNINGS

Keep this and all drugs out of the reach of children. In case of accidental overdose, seek professional assistance or contact a poison control center immediately. Prompt medical attention is critical for adults as well as for children even if you do not notice any signs or symptoms. As with any drug, if you are pregnant or nursing a baby, seek the advice of a health professional before using this product. Do not give to children under 12 years of age or use for more than 10 days unless directed by a doctor. If symptoms persist or get worse, if new ones occur, or if sleeplessness persists continuously for more than 2 weeks, consult your doctor. Insomnia may be a symptom of a serious underlying medical illness. Do not take this product, unless directed by a doctor, if you have a breathing problem such as emphysema or chronic bronchitis, or if you have gluacoma or difficulty in urination due to enlargement of the prostate gland. Avoid alcoholic beverages while taking this product. Do not take this product if you are taking sedatives or tranquilizers, without first consulting your doctor. If you generally consume 3 or more alcohol-containing drinks per day, you should consult your physician for advice on when and how you should take Excedrin PM and other pain relievers.

DIRECTIONS

Adults and children 12 years of age and over: 2 tablets, caplets, or geltabs at bedtime if needed or as directed by a doctor.

OVERDOSE
(Acetylcysteine As An Antidote For Acetaminophen Overdose)
Acetaminophen is rapidly absorbed from the upper gastrointestinal tract with peak plasma levels occurring between 30 and 60 minutes after therapeutic doses and usually within 4 hours following an overdose. The parent compound, which is nontoxic, is extensively metabolized in the liver to form principally the sulfate and glucuronide conjugates which are also nontoxic and are rapidly excreted in the urine. A small fraction of an ingested dose is metabo-

lized in the liver by the cytochrome P-450 mixed function oxidase enzyme system to form a reactive, potentially toxic, intermediate metabolite which preferentially conjugates with hepatic glutathione to form the nontoxic cysteine and mercapturic acid derivatives which are then excreted by the kidney. Therapeutic doses of acetaminophen do not saturate the glucuronide and sulfate conjugation pathways and do not result in the formation of sufficient reactive metabolite to deplete glutathione stores. However, following ingestion of a large overdose (150 mg/kg or greater) the glucuronide and sulfate conjugation pathways are saturated resulting in a larger fraction of the drug being metabolized via the P-450 pathway. The increased formation of reactive metabolite may deplete the hepatic stores of glutathione with subsequent binding of the metabolite to protein molecules within the hepatocyte resulting in cellular necrosis. Acetylcysteine has been shown to reduce the extent of liver injury following acetaminophen overdose. Early symptoms following a potentially hepatotoxic overdose may include: nausea, vomiting, diaphoresis and general malaise. Clinical and laboratory evidence of hepatic toxicity may not be apparent until 48 to 72 hours postingestion. In adults and adolescents, regardless of the quantity of acetaminophen reported to have been ingested, administer acetylcysteine immediately. Acetylcysteine therapy should be initiated and continued for a full course of therapy. Its effectiveness depends on early administration, with benefit seen principally in patients treated within 16 hours of the overdose.

If acetaminophen plasma assay capability is not available, and the estimated acetaminophen ingestion exceeds 150 mg/kg, acetylcysteine therapy should be initiated and continued for a full course of therapy.

For full prescribing information, refer to the acetylcysteine package insert. Do not await the results of assays for acetaminophen level before initiating treatment with acetylcysteine. The following additional procedures are recommended: The stomach should be emptied promptly by lavage or by induction of emesis with syrup of ipecac. A serum acetaminophen assay should be obtained as early as possible, but no sooner than four hours following ingestion. Liver function studies should be obtained initially and repeated at 24-hour intervals.

For additional emergency information call your regional poison center or toll-free (1-800-525-6115) to the Rocky Mountain Poison and Drug Center for assistance in diagnosis and for directions in the use of acetylcysteine as an antidote.

For overdose treatment information, consult a regional poison control center.

HOW SUPPLIED

EXCEDRIN P.M.® is supplied as:
Light blue circular coated tablets with "PM" debossed on one side.
Supplied in bottles of 10's, 24's, 50's, 100's, 150's
Light blue coated caplet with "PM" debossed on one side.
Supplied in bottles of 24's, 50's, and 100's.
Light blue and white geltabs with "PM" printed in black on one side.
Supplied in bottles of 24's, 50's, and 100's.
All sizes packaged in child resistant closures except 50's, which are recommended for households without young children.
Store at room temperature.

VAGISTAT®-1   OTC
vaginal ointment
(tioconazole 6.5%)

DESCRIPTION

Tioconazole, 1-[2-2(2,4-dichlorophenyl)ethyl]-1H-imidazole, is a topical antifungal agent which is now available over-the-counter. Its chemical formula is $C_{16}H_{13}Cl_3N_2OS$ with a molecular weight of 387.7. The structural formula is given below:

VAGISTAT-1 (tioconazole 6.5%) is formulated in a base of white petrolatum and magnesium aluminum silicate with butylated hydroxyanisole (BHA) added as a preservative. Each applicatorful of VAGISTAT-1 provides approximately 4.6 grams of ointment containing 300 mg of tioconazole.

CLINICAL PHARMACOLOGY

Tioconazole is a broad-spectrum antifungal agent that inhibits the growth of human pathogenic yeasts. Tioconazole

exhibits fungicidal activity *in vitro* against *Candida albicans,* other species of the genus *Candida,* and against *Torulopsis glabrata.*

Pharmacokinetics

Systemic absorption of tioconazole after a single intravaginal application of VAGISTAT-1 in non-pregnant patients is negligible.

INDICATIONS

VAGISTAT-1 is indicated for the treatment of recurrent vaginal yeast infections (candidiasis) previously diagnosed by a physician. If this is the first time vaginal itch and discomfort have been present, a doctor should be consulted. If you have had a doctor diagnose a vaginal yeast infection before and have the same symptoms now, use this ointment as directed.

Studies have shown that women taking oral contraceptives have cure rates similar to those not taking such agents when treated with VAGISTAT-1.

Safety and effectiveness in pregnant and diabetic patients have not been established.

CONTRAINDICATIONS

VAGISTAT-1 is contraindicated in individuals who have been shown to be sensitive to imidazole antifungal agents or to other components of the ointment.

PRECAUTIONS

General

VAGISTAT-1 is intended for intravaginal administration only. Applicators should be opened just prior to administration to prevent contamination.

If clinical symptoms persist, appropriate microbiological tests should be repeated to rule out other pathogens and to confirm the diagnosis.

Pregnancy

There are no adequate and well-controlled studies in pregnant women. VAGISTAT-1 (tioconazole 6.5%) should be used during pregnancy only if the physician believes the potential benefit justifies the potential risk to the fetus.

Nursing Mothers:

It is not known whether this drug is excreted in human milk. Because many drugs are excreted in human milk, nursing should be temporarily discontinued while VAGISTAT-1 is administered.

Pediatric Use:

Safety and effectiveness in children have not been established.

WARNINGS

- Do not use if you have abdominal pain, fever (higher than 100 °F orally), chills, nausea, vomiting, diarrhea, or foul-smelling discharge. Contact your doctor immediately.
- If your symptoms do not improve in 3 days or if you still have symptoms after 7 days, consult your doctor. Your doctor may recommend other treatment, or you may have a condition other than a yeast infection.
- If your symptoms return within 2 months or if you think you have been exposed to the human immunodeficiency virus (HIV) that causes AIDS, consult your doctor immediately. Recurring yeast infections may be a sign of pregnancy or a serious condition, such as AIDS or diabetes.
- Do not use if you are pregnant or think you may be pregnant, have diabetes, a positive HIV test, or AIDS. Consult your doctor.
- Do not use tampons while using this medicine. Use sanitary napkins instead.
- Do not rely on condoms or diaphragms to prevent sexually transmitted diseases or pregnancy while using VAGISTAT-1. This product may damage condoms and diaphragms and may cause them to fail. You should wait 3 days after treatment to resume using condoms or your diaphragm.
- Do not use in girls under 12 years of age.
- Keep this and all drugs out of the reach of children.
- VAGISTAT-1 is for vaginal use only. Do not use in eyes or take by mouth. In case of accidental ingestion, seek professional assistance or contact a Poison Control Center immediately.

ADVERSE REACTIONS

The incidence of adverse reactions to VAGISTAT-1 is based on clinical trials involving 1000 patients. Burning and itching were the most frequent side effects occurring in approximately 6% and 5% of patients, respectively. In most instances these did not interfere with the course of therapy. There were occasional reports (less than 1%) of other side effects including irritation, discharge, vulvar swelling, vaginal pain, dysuria, nocturia, dyspareunia, dryness of vaginal secretions, desquamation, and burning sensation.

In two clinical trials involving 1060 patients which supported the Rx to OTC switch, the most frequently reported side effects were vaginitis (5%), headache (5%), infection (3%), and abdominal pain (2%). There were also occasional reports (less than 2%) of pharyngitis, rhinitis, vulvovaginal disorder, rash and dysuria.

DOSAGE AND ADMINISTRATION

Using the prefilled applicator, insert one applicatorful intravaginally.

Remove prefilled applicator and plunger from foil packet. Hold blue capped end of applicator and push tip of plunger into base of applicator. Remove the blue cap with a pull twist action. Insert applicatorful intravaginally while lying on your back with knees bent. Push plunger into applicator until it will go no further. Withdraw applicator and plunger and dispose of in wastebasket. Administration of VAGISTAT-1 just prior to bedtime is recommended.

HOW SUPPLIED

VAGISTAT-1 is supplied in a ready-to-use, prefilled, single-dose vaginal applicator. Each applicatorful will deliver approximately 4.6 grams of VAGISTAT-1 containing 65 mg of tioconazole per gram of ointment.
Store at controlled room temperature 15°–30°C (59°–86°F).
Shown in Product Identification Guide, page 307

Bristol-Myers Squibb Company
**P.O. BOX 4500
PRINCETON, NJ 08543-4500**

For Medical Information Contact:
Generally:
Bristol-Myers Squibb Drug Information Department
P.O. Box 4500
Princeton, NJ 08543-4500
(800) 321–1335

Adverse Drug Experiences
and Product Defects Reporting call
between 8:30 AM–6:00 PM EST:
(609) 818-3737

Sales and Ordering:
Orders may be placed by:
1. Calling your purchase orders toll-free between 8:30 AM–6:00 PM EST:
(800) 631-5244
2. Mailing your purchase orders to:
Bristol-Myers Squibb U.S. Pharmaceuticals
Attn: Customer Service
P.O. Box 5250
Princeton, NJ 08543-5250
3. Faxing your purchase orders to:
(800) 523-2965
4. Transmitting computer-to-computer on the NWDA and UCS formats through Ordernet Services use: DEA# PE0048579

AVAPRO®   Rx
(irbesartan) Tablets

USE IN PREGNANCY
When used in pregnancy during the second and third trimesters, drugs that act directly on the renin-angiotensin system can cause injury and even death to the developing fetus. When pregnancy is detected, AVAPRO should be discontinued as soon as possible. See **WARNINGS: Fetal/Neonatal Morbidity and Mortality.**

DESCRIPTION

AVAPRO* (irbesartan) is an angiotensin II receptor (AT_1 subtype) antagonist.

Irbesartan is a non-peptide compound, chemically described as a 2-butyl-3-[[2'-(1H-tetrazol-5-yl) [1, 1'-biphenyl]-4-yl]methyl]-1,3-diazaspiro [4,4] non-1-en-4-one.

Its empirical formula is $C_{25}H_{28}N_6O$, and the structural formula:

Continued on next page

Avapro—Cont.

Irbesartan is a white to off-white crystalline powder with a molecular weight of 428.5. It is a nonpolar compound with a partition coefficient (octanol/water) of 10.1 at pH of 7.4. Irbesartan is slightly soluble in alcohol and methylene chloride and practically insoluble in water.
AVAPRO is available for oral administration in unscored tablets containing 75 mg, 150 mg, or 300 mg of irbesartan. Inactive ingredients include: lactose, microcrystalline cellulose, pregelatinized starch, croscarmellose sodium, poloxamer 188, silicon dioxide and magnesium stearate.

CLINICAL PHARMACOLOGY

Mechanism of Action

Angiotensin II is a potent vasoconstrictor formed from angiotensin I in a reaction catalyzed by angiotensin-converting enzyme (ACE, kininase II). Angiotensin II is the principal pressor agent of the renin-angiotensin system (RAS) and also stimulates aldosterone synthesis and secretion by adrenal cortex, cardiac contraction, renal resorption of sodium, activity of the sympathetic nervous system, and smooth muscle cell growth. Irbesartan blocks the vasoconstrictor and aldosterone-secreting effects of angiotensin II by selectively binding to the AT_1 angiotensin II receptor. There is also an AT_2 receptor in many tissues, but it is not involved in cardiovascular homeostasis.
Irbesartan is a specific competitive antagonist of AT_1 receptors with a much greater affinity (more than 8500-fold) for the AT_1 receptor than for the AT_2 receptor and no agonist activity.
Blockade of the AT_1 receptor removes the negative feedback of angiotensin II on renin secretion, but the resulting increased plasma renin activity and circulating angiotensin II do not overcome the effects of irbesartan on blood pressure.
Irbesartan does not inhibit ACE or renin or affect other hormone receptors or ion channels known to be involved in the cardiovascular regulation of blood pressure and sodium homeostasis. Because irbesartan does not inhibit ACE, it does not affect the response to bradykinin; whether this has clinical relevance is not known.

*Registered trademark of Sanofi

Pharmacokinetics

Irbesartan is an orally active agent that does not require biotransformation into an active form. The oral absorption of irbesartan is rapid and complete with an average absolute bioavailability of 60–80%. Following oral administration of AVAPRO (irbesartan), peak plasma concentrations of irbesartan are attained at 1.5–2 hours after dosing. Food does not affect the bioavailability of AVAPRO.
Irbesartan exhibits linear pharmacokinetics over the therapeutic dose range.
The terminal elimination half-life of irbesartan averaged 11–15 hours. Steady-state concentrations are achieved within 3 days. Limited accumulation of irbesartan (<20%) is observed in plasma upon repeated once-daily dosing.

Metabolism and Elimination

Irbesartan is metabolized via glucuronide conjugation and oxidation. Following oral or intravenous administration of ^{14}C-labeled irbesartan, more than 80% of the circulating plasma radioactivity is attributable to unchanged irbesartan. The primary circulating metabolite is the inactive irbesartan glucuronide conjugate (approximately 6%). The remaining oxidative metabolites do not add appreciably to irbesartan's pharmacologic activity.
Irbesartan and its metabolites are excreted by both biliary and renal routes. Following either oral or intravenous administration of ^{14}C-labeled irbesartan, about 20% of radioactivity is recovered in the urine and the remainder in the feces, as irbesartan or irbesartan glucuronide.
In vitro studies of irbesartan oxidation by cytochrome P450 isoenzymes indicated irbesartan was oxidized primarily by 2C9; metabolism by 3A4 was negligible. Irbesartan was neither metabolized by, nor did it substantially induce or inhibit, isoenzymes commonly associated with drug metabolism (1A1, 1A2, 2A6, 2B6, 2D6, 2E1). There was no induction or inhibition of 3A4.

Distribution

Irbesartan is 90% bound to serum proteins (primarily albumin and α_1-acid glycoprotein) with negligible binding to cellular components of blood. The average volume of distribution is 53–93 liters. Total plasma and renal clearances are in the range of 157–176 and 3.0–3.5 mL/min, respectively. With repetitive dosing, irbesartan accumulates to no clinically relevant extent.
Studies in animals indicate that radiolabeled irbesartan weakly crosses the blood brain barrier and placenta. Irbesartan is excreted in the milk of lactating rats.

Special Populations

Pediatric: Irbesartan pharmacokinetics have not been investigated in patients <18 years of age.
Gender: No gender related differences in pharmacokinetics were observed in healthy elderly (age 65–80 years) or in healthy young (age 18–40 years) subjects. In studies of hypertensive patients, there was no gender difference in half-life or accumulation, but somewhat higher plasma concentrations of irbesartan were observed in females (11–44%). No gender-related dosage adjustment is necessary.
Geriatric: In elderly subjects (age 65–80 years), irbesartan elimination half-life was not significantly altered, but AUC and C_{max} values were about 20–50% greater than those of young subjects (age 18–40 years). No dosage adjustment is necessary in the elderly.
Race: In healthy black subjects, irbesartan AUC values were approximately 25% greater than whites; there were no differences in C_{max} values.
Renal Insufficiency: The pharmacokinetics of irbesartan were not altered in patients with renal impairment or in patients on hemodialysis. Irbesartan is not removed by hemodialysis. No dosage adjustment is necessary in patients with mild to severe renal impairment unless a patient with renal impairment is also volume depleted. (See **WARNINGS: Hypotension in Volume- or Salt-depleted Patients** and **DOSAGE AND ADMINISTRATION**.)
Hepatic Insufficiency: The pharmacokinetics of irbesartan following repeated oral administration were not significantly affected in patients with mild to moderate cirrhosis of the liver. No dosage adjustment is necessary in patients with hepatic insufficiency.
Drug Interactions: (See **PRECAUTIONS: Information for Patients, Drug Interactions.**)

Pharmacodynamics

In healthy subjects, single oral irbesartan doses of up to 300 mg produced dose-dependent inhibition of the pressor effect of angiotensin II infusions. Inhibition was complete (100%) 4 hours following oral doses of 150 mg or 300 mg and partial inhibition was sustained for 24 hours (60% and 40% at 300 mg and 150 mg, respectively).
In hypertensive patients, angiotensin II receptor inhibition following chronic administration of irbesartan causes a 1.5–2 fold rise in angiotensin II plasma concentration and a 2–3 fold increase in plasma renin levels. Aldosterone plasma concentrations generally decline following irbesartan administration, but serum potassium levels are not significantly affected at recommended doses.
In hypertensive patients, chronic oral doses of irbesartan (up to 300 mg) had no effect on glomerular filtration rate, renal plasma flow or filtration fraction. In multiple dose studies in hypertensive patients, there were no clinically important effects on fasting triglycerides, total cholesterol, HDL-cholesterol, or fasting glucose concentrations. There was no effect on serum uric acid during chronic oral administration, and no uricosuric effect.

Clinical Studies

The antihypertensive effects of AVAPRO (irbesartan) were examined in seven (7) major placebo-controlled 8–12 week trials in patients with baseline diastolic blood pressures of 95–110 mmHg. Doses of 1–900 mg were included in these trials in order to fully explore the dose-range of irbesartan. These studies allowed comparison of once- or twice-daily regimens at 150 mg/day, comparisons of peak and trough effects, and comparisons of response by gender, age, and race. Two of the seven placebo-controlled trials identified above examined the antihypertensive effects of irbesartan and hydrochlorothiazide in combination.
The seven (7) studies of irbesartan monotherapy included a total of 1915 patients randomized to irbesartan (1–900 mg) and 611 patients randomized to placebo. Once-daily doses of 150 and 300 mg provided statistically and clinically significant decreases in systolic and diastolic blood pressure with trough (24 hours post-dose) effects after 6-12 weeks of treatment compared to placebo, of about 8–10/5–6 and 8–12/5–8 mmHg, respectively. No further increase in effect was seen at dosages greater than 300 mg. The dose-response relationships for effects on systolic and diastolic pressure are shown in Figures 1 and 2.

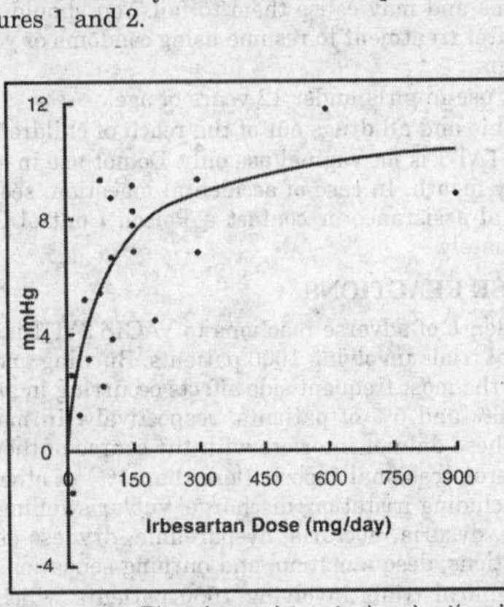

Figure 1. Placebo-subtracted reduction in trough SeSBP; integrated analysis

[See figure at top of next column]

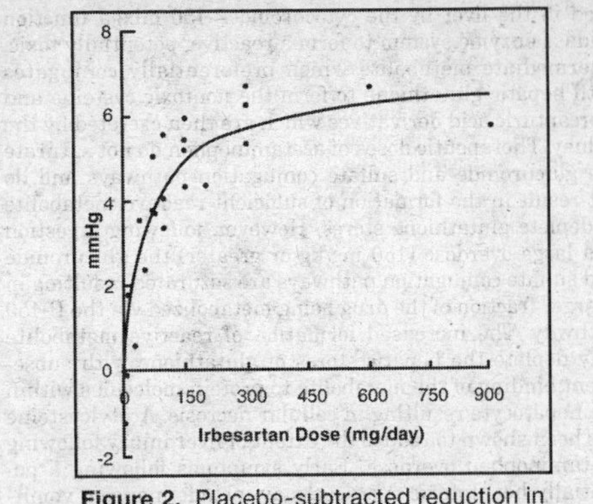

Figure 2. Placebo-subtracted reduction in trough SeDBP; integrated analysis

Once-daily administration of therapeutic doses of irbesartan gave peak effects at around 3–6 hours and, in one ambulatory blood pressure monitoring study, again around 14 hours. This was seen with both once-daily and twice-daily dosing. Trough-to-peak ratios for systolic and diastolic response were generally between 60–70%. In a continuous ambulatory blood pressure monitoring study, once-daily dosing with 150 mg gave trough and mean 24-hour responses similar to those observed in patients receiving twice-daily dosing at the same total daily dose.
In controlled trials, the addition of irbesartan to hydrochlorothiazide doses of 6.25, 12.5, or 25 mg produced further dose-related reductions in blood pressure similar to those achieved with the same monotherapy dose of irbesartan. HCTZ also had an approximately additive effect.
Analysis of age, gender, and race subgroups of patients showed that men and women, and patients over and under 65 years of age, had generally similar responses. Irbesartan was effective in reducing blood pressure regardless of race, although the effect was somewhat less in blacks (usually a low-renin population).
The effect of irbesartan is apparent after the first dose and it is close to its full observed effect at 2 weeks. At the end of an 8-week exposure, about 2/3 of the antihypertensive effect was still present one week after the last dose. Rebound hypertension was not observed. There was essentially no change in average heart rate in irbesartan-treated patients in controlled trials.

INDICATIONS AND USAGE

AVAPRO (irbesartan) is indicated for the treatment of hypertension. It may be used alone or in combination with other antihypertensive agents.

CONTRAINDICATIONS

AVAPRO is contraindicated in patients who are hypersensitive to any component of this product.

WARNINGS

Fetal/Neonatal Morbidity and Mortality

Drugs that act directly on the renin-angiotensin system can cause fetal and neonatal morbidity and death when administered to pregnant women. Several dozen cases have been reported in the world literature in patients who were taking angiotensin-converting-enzyme inhibitors. When pregnancy is detected, AVAPRO should be discontinued as soon as possible.
The use of drugs that act directly on the renin-angiotensin system during the second and third trimesters of pregnancy has been associated with fetal and neonatal injury, including hypotension, neonatal skull hypoplasia, anuria, reversible or irreversible renal failure, and death. Oligohydramnios has also been reported, presumably resulting from decreased fetal renal function; oligohydramnios in this setting has been associated with fetal limb contractures, craniofacial deformation, and hypoplastic lung development. Prematurity, intrauterine growth retardation, and patent ductus arteriosus have also been reported, although it is not clear whether these occurrences were due to exposure to the drug.
These adverse effects do not appear to have resulted from intrauterine drug exposure that has been limited to the first trimester.
Mothers whose embryos and fetuses are exposed to an angiotensin II receptor antagonist only during the first trimester should be so informed. Nonetheless, when patients become pregnant, physicians should have the patient discontinue the use of AVAPRO as soon as possible.
Rarely (probably less often than once in every thousand pregnancies), no alternative to a drug acting on the renin-angiotensin system will be found. In these rare cases, the mothers should be apprised of the potential hazards to their fetuses, and serial ultrasound examinations should be performed to assess the intraamniotic environment.
If oligohydramnios is observed, AVAPRO should be discontinued unless it is considered life-saving for the mother.

Contraction stress testing (CST), a non-stress test (NST), or biophysical profiling (BPP) may be appropriate depending upon the week of pregnancy. Patients and physicians should be aware, however, that oligohydramnios may not appear until after the fetus has sustained irreversible injury.

Infants with histories of in utero exposure to an angiotensin II receptor antagonist should be closely observed for hypotension, oliguria, and hyperkalemia. If oliguria occurs, attention should be directed toward support of blood pressure and renal perfusion. Exchange transfusion or dialysis may be required as means of reversing hypotension and/or substituting for disordered renal function.

When pregnant rats were treated with irbesartan from day 0 to day 20 of gestation (oral doses of 50, 180, and 650 mg/kg/day), increased incidences of renal pelvic cavitation, hydroureter and/or absence of renal papilla were observed in fetuses at doses ≥50 mg/kg/day [approximately equivalent to the maximum recommended human dose (MRHD), 300 mg/day, on a body surface area basis]. Subcutaneous edema was observed in fetuses at doses ≥180 mg/kg/day (about 4 times the MRHD on a body surface area basis). As these anomalies were not observed in rats in which irbesartan exposure (oral doses of 50, 150 and 450 mg/kg/day) was limited to gestation days 6–15, they appear to reflect late gestational effects of the drug. In pregnant rabbits, oral doses of 30 mg irbesartan/kg/day were associated with maternal mortality and abortion. Surviving females receiving this dose (about 1.5 times the MRHD on a body surface area basis) had a slight increase in early resorptions and a corresponding decrease in live fetuses. Irbesartan was found to cross the placental barrier in rats and rabbits.

Radioactivity was present in the rat and rabbit fetus during late gestation and in rat milk following oral doses of radiolabeled irbesartan.

Hypotension in Volume- or Salt-depleted Patients

Excessive reduction of blood pressure was rarely seen (<0.1%) in patients with uncomplicated hypertension. Initiation of antihypertensive therapy may cause symptomatic hypotension in patients with intravascular volume- or sodium-depletion, e.g., in patients treated vigorously with diuretics or in patients on dialysis. Such volume depletion should be corrected prior to administration of AVAPRO (irbesartan), or a low starting dose should be used (see **DOSAGE AND ADMINISTRATION**).

If hypotension occurs, the patient should be placed in the supine position and, if necessary, given an intravenous infusion of normal saline. A transient hypotensive response is not a contraindication to further treatment, which usually can be continued without difficulty once the blood pressure has stabilized.

PRECAUTIONS

Impaired Renal Function

As a consequence of inhibiting the renin-angiotensin-aldosterone system, changes in renal function may be anticipated in susceptible individuals. In patients whose renal function may depend on the activity of the renin-angiotensin-aldosterone system (e.g., patients with severe congestive heart failure), treatment with angiotensin-converting-enzyme inhibitors has been associated with oliguria and/or progressive azotemia and (rarely) with acute renal failure and/or death. AVAPRO would be expected to behave similarly. In studies of ACE inhibitors in patients with unilateral or bilateral renal artery stenosis, increases in serum creatinine or BUN have been reported. There has been no known use of AVAPRO in patients with unilateral or bilateral renal artery stenosis, but a similar effect should be anticipated.

Information for Patients

Pregnancy: Female patients of childbearing age should be told about the consequences of second- and third-trimester exposure to drugs that act on the renin-angiotensin system, and they should also be told that these consequences do not appear to have resulted from intrauterine drug exposure that has been limited to the first trimester. These patients should be asked to report pregnancies to their physicians as soon as possible.

Drug Interactions

No significant drug-drug pharmacokinetic (or pharmacodynamic) interactions have been found in interaction studies with hydrochlorothiazide, digoxin, warfarin, and nifedipine.

In vitro studies show significant inhibition of the formation of oxidized irbesartan metabolites with the known cytochrome CYP 2C9 substrates/inhibitors sulphenazole, tolbutamide and nifedipine. However, in clinical studies the consequences of concomitant irbesartan on the pharmacodynamics of warfarin were negligible. Based on *in vitro* data, no interaction would be expected with drugs whose metabolism is dependent upon cytochrome P450 isozymes 1A1, 1A2, 2A6, 2B6, 2D6, 2E1, or 3A4.

In separate studies of patients receiving maintenance doses of warfarin, hydrochlorothiazide, or digoxin, irbesartan administration for 7 days had no effect on the pharmacodynamics of warfarin (prothrombin time) or pharmacokinetics of digoxin. The pharmacokinetics of irbesartan were not affected by coadministration of nifedipine or hydrochlorothiazide.

Carcinogenesis, Mutagenesis, Impairment of Fertility

No evidence of carcinogenicity was observed when irbesartan was administered at doses of up to 500/1000 mg/kg/day (males/females, respectively) in rats and 1000 mg/kg/day in mice for up to two years. For male and female rats, 500 mg/kg/day provided an average systemic exposure to irbesartan (AUC_{0-24h}, bound plus unbound) about 3 and 11 times, respectively, the average systemic exposure in humans receiving the maximum recommended dose (MRD) of 300 mg irbesartan/day, whereas 1000 mg/kg/day (administered to females only) provided an average systemic exposure about 21 times that reported for humans at the MRD. For male and female mice, 1000 mg/kg/day provided an exposure to irbesartan about 3 and 5 times, respectively, the human exposure at 300 mg/day.

Irbesartan was not mutagenic in a battery of *in vitro* tests (Ames microbial test, rat hepatocyte DNA repair test, V79 mammalian-cell forward gene-mutation assay). Irbesartan was negative in several tests for induction of chromosomal aberrations (*in vitro*-human lymphocyte assay; *in vivo*-mouse micronucleus study).

Irbesartan had no adverse effects on fertility or mating of male or female rats at oral doses ≤650 mg/kg/day, the highest dose providing a systemic exposure to irbesartan (AUC_{0-24h}, bound plus unbound) about 5 times that found in humans receiving the maximum recommended dose of 300 mg/day.

Pregnancy

Pregnancy Categories C (first trimester) and D (second and third trimester). See **WARNINGS: Fetal/Neonatal Morbidity and Mortality**.

Nursing Mothers

It is not known whether irbesartan is excreted in human milk, but irbesartan or some metabolite of irbesartan is secreted at low concentration in the milk of lactating rats. Because of the potential for adverse effects on the nursing infant, a decision should be made whether to discontinue nursing or discontinue the drug, taking into account the importance of the drug to the mother.

Pediatric Use

Safety and effectiveness in pediatric patients have not been established.

Geriatric Use

Of the total number of patients receiving AVAPRO (irbesartan) in controlled clinical studies, 911 patients (18.5%) were 65 years and over, while 150 patients (3.0%) were 75 years and over. No overall differences in effectiveness or safety were observed between these patients and younger patients, but greater sensitivity of some older individuals cannot be ruled out.

ADVERSE REACTIONS

AVAPRO has been evaluated for safety in more than 4300 patients with hypertension and about 5000 subjects overall. This experience includes 1303 patients treated for over 6 months and 407 patients for 1 year or more. Treatment with AVAPRO was well-tolerated, with an incidence of adverse events similar to placebo. These events generally were mild and transient with no relationship to the dose of AVAPRO. In placebo-controlled clinical trials, discontinuation of therapy due to a clinical adverse event was required in 3.3 percent of patients treated with AVAPRO, versus 4.5 percent of patients given placebo.

In placebo-controlled clinical trials, the adverse event experiences that occurred in at least 1% of patients treated with AVAPRO (n=1965) and at a higher incidence versus placebo (n=641) included diarrhea (3% vs. 2%), dyspepsia/heartburn (2% vs. 1%), musculoskeletal trauma (2% vs. 1%), fatigue (4% vs. 3%), and upper respiratory infection (9% vs. 6%). None of these differences were significant.

The following adverse events occurred at an incidence of 1% or greater in patients treated with irbesartan, but were at least as frequent or more frequent in patients receiving placebo: abdominal pain, anxiety/nervousness, chest pain, dizziness, edema, headache, influenza, musculoskeletal pain, pharyngitis, nausea/vomiting, rash, rhinitis, sinus abnormality, tachycardia and urinary tract infection.

Irbesartan use was not associated with an increased incidence of dry cough, as is typically associated with ACE inhibitor use. In placebo controlled studies, the incidence of cough in irbesartan treated patients was 2.8% versus 2.7% in patients receiving placebo.

The incidence of hypotension or orthostatic hypotension was low in irbesartan treated patients (0.4%), unrelated to dos-

age, and similar to the incidence among placebo treated patients (0.2%). Dizziness, syncope, and vertigo were reported with equal or less frequency in patients receiving irbesartan compared with placebo.

In addition, the following potentially important events occurred in less than 1% of the 1965 patients and at least 5 patients (0.3%) receiving irbesartan in clinical studies, and those less frequent, clinically significant events (listed by body system). It cannot be determined whether these events were causally related to irbesartan:

Body as a Whole: fever, chills, facial edema, upper extremity edema;

Cardiovascular: flushing, hypertension, cardiac murmur, myocardial infarction, angina pectoris, arrhythmic/conduction disorder, cardio-respiratory arrest, heart failure, hypertensive crisis;

Dermatologic: pruritus, dermatitis, ecchymosis, erythema face, urticaria;

Endocrine/Metabolic/Electrolyte Imbalances: sexual dysfunction, libido change, gout;

Gastrointestinal: constipation, oral lesion, gastroenteritis, flatulence, abdominal distention;

Musculoskeletal/Connective Tissue: extremity swelling, muscle cramp, arthritis, muscle ache, musculoskeletal chest pain, joint stiffness, bursitis, muscle weakness;

Nervous System: sleep disturbance, numbness, somnolence, emotional disturbance, depression, paresthesia, tremor, transient ischemic attack, cerebrovascular accident;

Renal/Genitourinary: abnormal urination, prostate disorder;

Respiratory: epistaxis, tracheobronchitis, congestion, pulmonary congestion, dyspnea, wheezing;

Special Senses: vision disturbance, hearing abnormality, ear infection, ear pain, conjunctivitis, other eye disturbance, eyelid abnormality, ear abnormality.

Laboratory Test Findings

In controlled clinical trials, clinically important differences in laboratory tests were rarely associated with administration of AVAPRO (irbesartan).

Creatinine, Blood Urea Nitrogen: Minor increases in blood urea nitrogen (BUN) or serum creatinine were observed in less than 0.7% of patients with essential hypertension treated with AVAPRO alone versus 0.9% on placebo. (See **PRECAUTIONS: Impaired Renal Function.**)

Hematologic: Mean decreases in hemoglobin of 0.2 g/dL were observed in 0.2% of patients receiving AVAPRO compared to 0.3% of placebo treated patients. Neutropenia (<1000 cells/mm³) occurred at similar frequencies among patients receiving AVAPRO (0.3%) and placebo treated patients (0.5%).

OVERDOSAGE

No data are available in regard to overdosage in humans. However, daily doses of 900 mg for 8 weeks were well-tolerated. The most likely manifestations of overdosage are expected to be hypotension and tachycardia; bradycardia might also occur from overdose. Irbesartan is not removed by hemodialysis.

To obtain up-to-date information about the treatment of overdosage, a good resource is a certified Regional Poison-Control Center. Telephone numbers of certified poison-control centers are listed in the *Physicians' Desk Reference* (PDR). In managing overdose, consider the possibilities of multiple-drug interactions, drug-drug interactions, and unusual drug kinetics in the patient.

Laboratory determinations of serum levels of irbesartan are not widely available, and such determinations have, in any event, no known established role in the management of irbesartan overdose.

Acute oral toxicity studies with irbesartan in mice and rats indicated acute lethal doses were in excess of 2000 mg/kg, about 25- and 50-fold the maximum recommended human dose (300 mg) on a mg/m² basis, respectively.

DOSAGE AND ADMINISTRATION

The recommended initial dose of AVAPRO is 150 mg once daily. Patients requiring further reduction in blood pressure should be titrated to 300 mg once daily.

A low dose of a diuretic may be added, if blood pressure is not controlled by AVAPRO alone. Hydrochlorothiazide has

Continued on next page

	75 mg	150 mg	300 mg
Debossing	2771	2772	2773
Bottle of 30	0087-2771-31	0087-2772-31	0087-2773-31
Bottle of 90	0087-2771-32	0087-2772-32	0087-2773-32
Bottle of 500	0087-2771-15	0087-2772-15	0087-2773-15
Blister of 100	0087-2771-35	0087-2772-35	0087-2773-35

Consult 1999 PDR® supplements and future editions for revisions

Avapro—Cont.

been shown to have an additive effect (see **CLINICAL PHARMACOLOGY: Clinical Studies**). Patients not adequately treated by the maximum dose of 300 mg once daily are unlikely to derive additional benefit from a higher dose or twice-daily dosing.
No dosage adjustment is necessary in elderly patients, or in patients with hepatic impairment or mild to severe renal impairment.
AVAPRO may be administered with other antihypertensive agents.
AVAPRO may be administered with or without food.

Volume- and Salt-depleted Patients
A lower initial dose of AVAPRO (75 mg) is recommended in patients with depletion of intravascular volume or salt (e.g., patients treated vigorously with diuretics or on hemodialysis) (see **WARNINGS: Hypotension in Volume- or Salt-depleted Patients**).

HOW SUPPLIED

AVAPRO® (irbesartan) is available as white to off-white biconvex oval tablets, debossed with a heart shape on one side and a portion of the NDC code on the other. Unit-of-use bottles contain 30, 90, or 500 tablets and blister packs contain 100 tablets, as follows:
[See table at bottom of previous page]

Storage
Store at a temperature between 15° C and 30° C (59° F and 86° F) [USP].

Manufactured and Distributed by:
Bristol-Myers Squibb Company
Princeton, NJ 08543-4500
Comarketed by:
sanofi
New York, NY 10016

Issued October 1997 P0617-00
Shown in Product Identification Guide, page 307

AZACTAM® ℞

[a-zak 'tam]
(aztreonam for injection, USP)

CAUTION: Federal law prohibits dispensing without prescription.

DESCRIPTION

AZACTAM (aztreonam for injection, USP) contains the active ingredient, aztreonam, a monobactam. It was originally isolated from *Chromobacterium violaceum*. It is a synthetic bactericidal antibiotic.
The monobactams, having a unique monocyclic beta-lactam nucleus, are structurally different from other beta-lactam antibiotics (e.g., penicillins, cephalosporins, cephamycins). The sulfonic acid substituent in the 1-position of the ring activates the beta-lactam moiety; an aminothiazolyl oxime side chain in the 3-position and a methyl group in the 4-position confer the specific antibacterial spectrum and beta-lactamase stability.
Aztreonam is designated chemically as (Z)-2-[[[(2-amino-4-thiazolyl)[[(2S,-3S)-2-methyl-4-oxo-1-sulfo-3-azetidinyl]carbamoyl]methylene]amino]oxy]-2-methylpropionic acid.
AZACTAM is a sterile, nonpyrogenic, sodium-free, white to yellowish-white lyophilized cake containing approximately 780 mg arginine per gram of aztreonam. Following constitution, the product is for intramuscular or intravenous use. Aqueous solutions of the product have a pH in the range of 4.5 to 7.5.

CLINICAL PHARMACOLOGY

Single 30-minute intravenous infusions of 500 mg, 1 g and 2 g doses of AZACTAM (aztreonam for injection, USP) in healthy subjects produced peak serum levels of 54, 90 and 204 µg/mL, respectively, immediately after administration; at eight hours, serum levels were 1, 3 and 6 µg/mL, respectively (Figure 1). Single 3-minute intravenous injections of the same doses resulted in serum levels of 58, 125 and 242 µg/mL at five minutes following completion of injection.
Serum concentrations of aztreonam in healthy subjects following completion of single intramuscular injections of 500 mg and 1 g doses are depicted in Figure 1; maximum serum concentrations occur at about one hour. After identical single intravenous or intramuscular doses of AZACTAM, the serum concentrations of aztreonam are comparable at one hour (1.5 hours from start of intravenous infusion) with similar slopes of serum concentrations thereafter.
[See figure at top of next column]
The serum levels of aztreonam following single 500 mg or 1 g (intramuscular or intravenous) or 2 g (intravenous) doses of AZACTAM exceed the MIC_{90} for *Neisseria* sp., *H. influenzae* and most genera of the *Enterobacteriaceae* for eight hours (for *Enterobacter* sp., the eight hour serum levels exceed the MIC for 80 percent of strains). For *Ps. aeruginosa*, a single 2 g intravenous dose produces serum levels that exceed the MIC_{90} for approximately four to six hours. All of

FIGURE 1

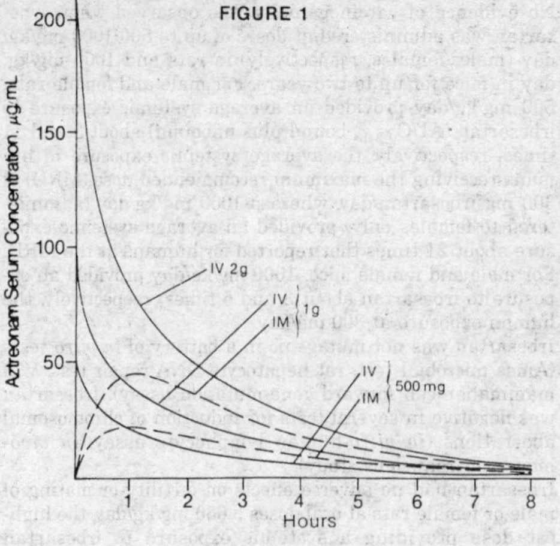

the above doses of AZACTAM (aztreonam for injection, USP) result in average urine levels of aztreonam that exceed the MIC_{90} for the same pathogens for up to 12 hours.
When aztreonam pharmacokinetics were assessed for adult and pediatric patients, they were found to be comparable (down to 9 months old). The serum half-life of aztreonam averaged 1.7 hours (1.5 to 2.0) in subjects with normal renal function, independent of the dose and route of administration. In healthy subjects, based on a 70 kg person, the serum clearance was 91 mL/min and renal clearance was 56 mL/min; the apparent mean volume of distribution at steady-state averaged 12.6 liters, approximately equivalent to extracellular fluid volume.
In a study of healthy elderly male subjects (65 to 75 years of age), the average elimination half-life of aztreonam was slightly longer than in young healthy males.
In patients with impaired renal function, the serum half-life of aztreonam is prolonged (see **DOSAGE AND ADMINISTRATION, Renal Impairment**). The serum half-life of aztreonam is only slightly prolonged in patients with hepatic impairment since the liver is a minor pathway of excretion.
Average urine concentrations of aztreonam were approximately 1100, 3500 and 6600 µg/mL within the first two hours following single 500 mg, 1 g and 2 g intravenous doses of AZACTAM (30-minute infusions), respectively. The range of average concentrations for aztreonam in the 8 to 12 hour urine specimens in these studies was 25 to 120 µg/mL. After intramuscular injection of single 500 mg and 1 g doses of AZACTAM (aztreonam for injection, USP), urinary levels were approximately 500 and 1200 µg/mL, respectively, within the first two hours, declining to 180 and 470 µg/mL in the six to eight hour specimens. In healthy subjects, aztreonam is excreted in the urine about equally by active tubular secretion and glomerular filtration. Approximately 60 to 70 percent of an intravenous or intramuscular dose was recovered in the urine by eight hours. Urinary excretion of a single parenteral dose was essentially complete by 12 hours after injection. About 12 percent of a single intravenous radiolabeled dose was recovered in the feces. Unchanged aztreonam and the inactive beta-lactam ring hydrolysis product of aztreonam were present in feces and urine.
Intravenous or intramuscular administration of a single 500 mg or 1 g dose of AZACTAM every eight hours for seven days to healthy subjects produced no apparent accumulation of aztreonam or modification of its disposition characteristics; serum protein binding averaged 56 percent and was independent of dose. An average of about 6 percent of a 1 g intramuscular dose was excreted as a microbiologically inactive open beta-lactam ring hydrolysis product (serum half-life approximately 26 hours) of aztreonam in the zero to eight hour urine collection on the last day of multiple dosing.
Renal function was monitored in healthy subjects given aztreonam; standard tests (serum creatinine, creatinine clearance, BUN, urinalysis and total urinary protein excretion) as well as special tests (excretion of N-acetyl-β-glucosaminidase, alanine aminopeptidase and β_2-microglobulin) were used. No abnormal results were obtained.
Aztreonam achieves measurable concentrations in the following body fluids and tissues:
[See table at bottom of next page]
The concentration of aztreonam in saliva at 30 minutes after a single 1 g intravenous dose (9 patients) was 0.2 µg/mL; in breast milk at two hours after a single 1 g intravenous dose (6 patients), 0.2 µg/mL, and at six hours after a single 1 g intramuscular dose (6 patients), 0.3 µg/mL; in amniotic fluid at six to eight hours after a single 1 g intravenous dose (5 patients), 2 µg/mL. The concentration of aztreonam in peritoneal fluid obtained one to six hours after multiple 2 g intravenous doses ranged between 12 and 90 µg/mL in 7 of 8 patients studied.
Aztreonam given intravenously rapidly reaches therapeutic concentrations in peritoneal dialysis fluid; conversely, aztreonam given intraperitoneally in dialysis fluid rapidly produces therapeutic serum levels.
Concomitant administration of probenecid or furosemide and AZACTAM (aztreonam for injection, USP) causes clinically insignificant increases in the serum levels of aztreonam. Single-dose intravenous pharmacokinetic studies have not shown any significant interaction between aztreonam and concomitantly administered gentamicin, nafcillin sodium, cephradine, clindamycin or metronidazole. No reports of disulfiram-like reactions with alcohol ingestion have been noted; this is not unexpected since aztreonam does not contain a methyl-tetrazole side chain.

Microbiology
Aztreonam exhibits potent and specific activity *in vitro* against a wide spectrum of gram-negative aerobic pathogens including *Pseudomonas aeruginosa*. The bactericidal action of aztreonam results from the inhibition of bacterial cell wall synthesis due to a high affinity of aztreonam for penicillin binding protein 3 (PBP3). Aztreonam, unlike the majority of beta-lactam antibiotics, does not induce beta-lactamase activity and its molecular structure confers a high degree of resistance to hydrolysis by beta-lactamases (i.e., penicillinases and cephalosporinases) produced by most gram-negative and gram-positive pathogens; it is therefore usually active against gram-negative aerobic organisms that are resistant to antibiotics hydrolyzed by beta-lactamases. Aztreonam maintains its antimicrobial activity over a pH range of 6 to 8 *in vitro*, as well as in the presence of human serum and under anaerobic conditions. Aztreonam is active *in vitro* and is effective in laboratory animal models and clinical infections against most strains of the following organisms, including many that are multiply-resistant to other antibiotics (i.e., certain cephalosporins, penicillins, and aminoglycosides):

Escherichia coli
Enterobacter species
Klebsiella pneumoniae and *K. oxytoca*
Proteus mirabilis
Pseudomonas aeruginosa
Serratia marcescens
Haemophilus influenzae (including ampicillin-resistant and other penicillinase-producing strains)
Citrobacter species

While *in vitro* studies have demonstrated the susceptibility to aztreonam of most strains of the following organisms, clinical efficacy for infections other than those included in the **INDICATIONS AND USAGE** section has not been documented:

Neisseria gonorrhoeae (including penicillinase-producing strains)
Proteus vulgaris
Morganella morganii (formerly *Proteus morganii*)
Providencia species, including *P. stuartii and P. rettgeri* (formerly *Proteus rettgeri*)
Pseudomonas species
Shigella species
Pasteurella multocida
Yersinia enterocolitica
Aeromonas hydrophila
Neisseria meningitidis

Aztreonam and aminoglycosides have been shown to be synergistic *in vitro* against most strains of *Ps. aeruginosa*, many strains of *Enterobacteriaceae*, and other gram-negative aerobic bacilli.
Alterations of the anaerobic intestinal flora by broad spectrum antibiotics may decrease colonization resistance, thus permitting overgrowth of potential pathogens, e.g., *Candida* and Clostridia species. Aztreonam has little effect on the anaerobic intestinal microflora in *in vitro* studies. *Clostridium difficile* and its cytotoxin were not found in animal models following administration of aztreonam. (See **ADVERSE REACTIONS**, Gastrointestinal.)

Susceptibility Testing
Diffusion Technique: Quantitative procedures that require measurement of zone diameters give precise estimates of microbial susceptibility to antibiotics. One such method, recommended for use with the aztreonam 30 µg disk, is the National Committee of Clinical Laboratory Standards (NCCLS) approved procedure. Only a 30 µg aztreonam disk should be used; there are no suitable surrogate disks.
Results of laboratory tests using 30 µg aztreonam disks should be interpreted using the following criteria:

Zone Diameter (mm)	Interpretation
≥22	(S) Susceptible
16–21	(I) Intermediate (Moderate Susceptibility)
≤15	(R) Resistant

Dilution Technique: Broth or agar dilution methods may be used to determine the minimal inhibitory concentration (MIC) of aztreonam.
MIC test results should be interpreted according to the concentrations of aztreonam that can be attained in serum, tissues and body fluids.

MIC (µg/mL)	Interpretation
≤8	(S) Susceptible
16	(I) Intermediate
	(Moderate Susceptibility)
≥32	(R) Resistant

For any susceptibility test, a report of "susceptible" indicates that the pathogen is likely to respond to AZACTAM (aztreonam for injection, USP) therapy; a report of "resistant" indicates that the pathogen is not likely to respond. A report of "intermediate" (moderate susceptibility) indicates that the pathogen is expected to be susceptible to AZACTAM if high dosages are used, or if the infection is confined to tissues and fluids (e.g., urine, bile) in which high aztreonam levels are attained.

The quality control cultures should have the following assigned daily ranges for aztreonam:

		Disks	Mode MIC (µg/mL)
E. coli	(ATCC 25922)	28–36 mm	0.06–0.25
Ps. aeruginosa	(ATCC 27853)	23–29 mm	2.0–8.0

INDICATIONS AND USAGE

Before initiating treatment with AZACTAM, appropriate specimens should be obtained for isolation of the causative organism(s) and for determination of susceptibility to aztreonam. Treatment with AZACTAM may be started empirically before results of the susceptibility testing are available; subsequently, appropriate antibiotic therapy should be continued.

AZACTAM is indicated for the treatment of the following infections caused by susceptible gram-negative microorganisms:

Urinary Tract Infections (complicated and uncomplicated), including pyelonephritis and cystitis (initial and recurrent) caused by Escherichia coli, Klebsiella pneumoniae, Proteus mirabilis, Pseudomonas aeruginosa, Enterobacter cloacae, Klebsiella oxytoca*, Citrobacter species*and Serratia marcescens*.

Lower Respiratory Tract Infections, including pneumonia and bronchitis caused by Escherichia coli, Klebsiella pneumoniae, Pseudomonas aeruginosa, Haemophilus influenzae, Proteus mirabilis, Enterobacter species and Serratia marcescens*.

Septicemia caused by Escherichia coli, Klebsiella pneumoniae, Pseudomonas aeruginosa, Proteus mirabilis*, Serratia marcescens* and Enterobacter species.

Skin and Skin-Structure Infections, including those associated with postoperative wounds, ulcers and burns caused by Escherichia coli, Proteus mirabilis, Serratia marcescens, Enterobacter species, Pseudomonas aeruginosa, Klebsiella pneumoniae and Citrobacter species*.

Intra-abdominal Infections, including peritonitis caused by Escherichia coli, Klebsiella species including K. pneumoniae, Enterobacter species including E. cloacae*, Pseudomonas aeruginosa, Citrobacter species* including C. freundii* and Serratia species* including S. marcescens*.

Gynecologic Infections, including endometritis and pelvic cellulitis caused by Escherichia coli, Klebsiella pneumoni-ae*, Enterobacter species* including E. cloacae* and Proteus mirabilis*.

*Efficacy for this organism in this organ system was studied in fewer than ten infections.

AZACTAM (aztreonam) is indicated for adjunctive therapy to surgery in the management of infections caused by susceptible organisms, including abscesses, infections complicating hollow viscus perforations, cutaneous infections and infections of serous surfaces. AZACTAM is effective against most of the commonly encountered gram-negative aerobic pathogens seen in general surgery.

Concurrent Therapy

Concurrent initial therapy with other antimicrobial agents and AZACTAM (aztreonam for injection, USP) is recommended before the causative organism(s) is known in seriously ill patients who are also at risk of having an infection due to gram-positive aerobic pathogens. If anaerobic organisms are also suspected as etiologic agents, therapy should be initiated using an anti-anaerobic agent concurrently with AZACTAM (see **DOSAGE AND ADMINISTRATION**). Certain antibiotics (e.g., cefoxitin, imipenem) may induce high levels of beta-lactamase in vitro in some gram-negative aerobes such as Enterobacter and Pseudomonas species, resulting in antagonism to many beta-lactam antibiotics including aztreonam. These in vitro findings suggest that such beta-lactamase inducing antibiotics not be used concurrently with aztreonam. Following identification and susceptibility testing of the causative organism(s), appropriate antibiotic therapy should be continued.

CONTRAINDICATIONS

This preparation is contraindicated in patients with known hypersensitivity to aztreonam or any other component in the formulation.

WARNINGS

Both animal and human data suggest that AZACTAM (aztreonam for injection, USP) is rarely cross-reactive with other beta-lactam antibiotics and weakly immunogenic. Treatment with aztreonam can result in hypersensitivity reactions in patients with or without prior exposure. (See **CONTRAINDICATIONS**.)

Careful inquiry should be made to determine whether the patient has any history of hypersensitivity reactions to any allergens.

While cross-reactivity of aztreonam with other beta-lactam antibiotics is rare, this drug should be administered with caution to any patient with a history of hypersensitivity to beta-lactams (e.g., penicillins, cephalosporins, and/or carbapenems). Treatment with aztreonam can result in hypersensitivity reactions in patients with or without prior exposure to aztreonam. If an allergic reaction to aztreonam occurs, discontinue the drug and institute supportive treatment as appropriate (e.g., maintenance of ventilation, pressor amines, antihistamines, corticosteroids). Serious hypersensitivity reactions may require epinephrine and other emergency measures. (See **ADVERSE REACTIONS**.)

Pseudomembranous colitis has been reported with nearly all antibacterial agents, including aztreonam, and may range in severity from mild to life-threatening. Therefore, it is important to consider this diagnosis in patients who present with diarrhea subsequent to the administration of antibacterial agents.

Treatment with antibacterial agents alters the normal flora of the colon and may permit overgrowth of Clostridia. Studies indicate that a toxin produced by Clostridium difficile is one primary cause of "antibiotic-associated colitis."

After the diagnosis of pseudomembranous colitis has been established, therapeutic measures should be initiated. Mild cases of pseudomembranous colitis usually respond to drug discontinuation alone. In moderate to severe cases, consideration should be given to management with fluids and electrolytes, protein supplementation, and treatment with an antibacterial drug clinically effective against C. difficile colitis.

Rare cases of toxic epidermal necrolysis have been reported in association with aztreonam in patients undergoing bone marrow transplant with multiple risk factors including sepsis, radiation therapy and other concomitantly administered drugs associated with toxic epidermal necrolysis.

PRECAUTIONS

General

In patients with impaired hepatic or renal function, appropriate monitoring is recommended during therapy.

If an aminoglycoside is used concurrently with aztreonam, especially if high dosages of the former are used or if therapy is prolonged, renal function should be monitored because of the potential nephrotoxicity and ototoxicity of aminoglycoside antibiotics.

The use of antibiotics may promote the overgrowth of nonsusceptible organisms, including gram-positive organisms (Staphylococcus aureus and Streptococcus faecalis) and fungi. Should superinfection occur during therapy, appropriate measures should be taken.

Carcinogenesis, Mutagenesis, Impairment of Fertility

Carcinogenicity studies in animals have not been performed.

Genetic toxicology studies performed in vivo and in vitro with aztreonam in several standard laboratory models revealed no evidence of mutagenic potential at the chromosomal or gene level.

Two-generation reproduction studies in rats at daily doses up to 20 times the maximum recommended human dose, prior to and during gestation and lactation, revealed no evidence of impaired fertility. There was a slightly reduced survival rate during the lactation period in the offspring of rats that received the highest dosage, but not in offspring of rats that received five times the maximum recommended human dose.

Pregnancy

Pregnancy Category B

Aztreonam crosses the placenta and enters the fetal circulation.

Studies in pregnant rats and rabbits, with daily doses up to 15 and 5 times, respectively, the maximum recommended human dose, revealed no evidence of embryo- or fetotoxicity or teratogenicity. No drug induced changes were seen in any of the maternal, fetal, or neonatal parameters that were monitored in rats receiving 15 times the maximum recommended human dose of aztreonam during late gestation and lactation.

There are no adequate and well-controlled studies in pregnant women. Because animal reproduction studies are not always predictive of human response, aztreonam should be used during pregnancy only if clearly needed.

Nursing Mothers

Aztreonam is excreted in breast milk in concentrations that are less than 1 percent of concentrations determined in simultaneously obtained maternal serum; consideration should be given to temporary discontinuation of nursing and use of formula feedings.

Pediatric Use

The safety and effectiveness of intravenous AZACTAM (aztreonam for injection, USP) have been established in the age groups 9 months to 16 years. Use of AZACTAM in these age groups is supported by evidence from adequate and well-controlled studies of AZACTAM in adults with additional efficacy, safety, and pharmacokinetic data from noncomparative clinical studies in pediatric patients. Sufficient data are not available for pediatric patients under 9 months of age or for the following treatment indications/pathogens: septicemia and skin and skin-structure infections (where the skin infection is believed or known to be due to H. influenzae type b). In pediatric patients with cystic fibrosis, higher doses of AZACTAM may be warranted. (See **CLINICAL PHARMACOLOGY, DOSAGE AND ADMINISTRATION**, and **CLINICAL STUDIES**.)

ADVERSE REACTIONS

Local reactions such as phlebitis/thrombophlebitis following IV administration, and discomfort/swelling at the injection site following IM administration occurred at rates of approximately 1.9 percent and 2.4 percent, respectively.

EXTRAVASCULAR CONCENTRATIONS OF AZTREONAM AFTER A SINGLE PARENTERAL DOSE[1]

Fluid or Tissue	Dose (g)	Route	Hours Postinjection	Number of Patients	Mean Concentration (µg/mL or µg/g)
Fluids					
bile	1	IV	2	10	39
blister fluid	1	IV	1	6	20
bronchial secretion	2	IV	4	7	5
cerebrospinal fluid (inflamed meninges)	2	IV	0.9–4.3	16	3
pericardial fluid	2	IV	1	6	33
pleural fluid	2	IV	1.1–3.0	3	51
synovial fluid	2	IV	0.8–1.9	11	83
Tissues					
atrial appendage	2	IV	0.9–1.6	12	22
endometrium	2	IV	0.7–1.9	4	9
fallopian tube	2	IV	0.7–1.9	8	12
fat	2	IV	1.3–2.0	10	5
femur	2	IV	1.0–2.1	15	16
gallbladder	2	IV	0.8–1.3	4	23
kidney	2	IV	2.4–5.6	5	67
large intestine	2	IV	0.8–1.9	9	12
liver	2	IV	0.9–2.0	6	47
lung	2	IV	1.2–2.1	6	22
myometrium	2	IV	0.7–1.9	9	11
ovary	2	IV	0.7–1.9	7	13
prostate	1	IM	0.8–3.0	8	8
skeletal muscle	2	IV	0.3–0.7	6	16
skin	2	IV	0.0–1.0	8	25
sternum	2	IV	1	6	6

[1]Tissue penetration is regarded as essential to therapeutic efficacy, but specific tissue levels have not been correlated with specific therapeutic effects.

Continued on next page

Azactam—Cont.

Systemic reactions (considered to be related to therapy or of uncertain etiology) occurring at an incidence of 1 to 1.3 percent include diarrhea, nausea and/or vomiting, and rash. Reactions occurring at an incidence of less than 1 percent are listed within each body system in order of decreasing severity:

Hypersensitivity—anaphylaxis, angioedema, bronchospasm.

Hematologic—pancytopenia, neutropenia, thrombocytopenia, anemia, eosinophilia, leukocytosis, thrombocytosis.

Gastrointestinal—abdominal cramps; rare cases of *C. difficile*-associated diarrhea, including pseudomembraneous colitis, or gastrointestinal bleeding have been reported. Onset of pseudomembranous colitis symptoms may occur during or after antibiotic treatment. (See **WARNINGS**.)

Dermatologic—toxic epidermal necrolysis (see **WARNINGS**), purpura, erythema multiforme, exfoliative dermatitis, urticaria, petechiae, pruritus, diaphoresis.

Cardiovascular—hypotension, transient ECG changes (ventricular bigeminy and PVC), flushing.

Respiratory—wheezing, dyspnea, chest pain.

Hepatobiliary—hepatitis, jaundice.

Nervous System—seizure, confusion, vertigo, paresthesia, insomnia, dizziness.

Musculoskeletal—muscular aches.

Special Senses—tinnitus, diplopia, mouth ulcer, altered taste, numb tongue, sneezing, nasal congestion, halitosis.

Other—vaginal candidiasis, vaginitis, breast tenderness.

Body as a Whole—weakness, headache, fever, malaise.

Pediatric Adverse Reactions

Of the 612 pediatric patients who were treated with AZACTAM (aztreonam for injection, USP) in clinical trials, less than 1% required discontinuation of therapy due to adverse events. The following systemic adverse events, regardless of drug relationship, occurred in at least 1% of treated patients in domestic clinical trials: rash (4.3%), diarrhea (1.4%), and fever (1.0%). These adverse events were comparable to those observed in adult clinical trials.

In 343 pediatric patients receiving intravenous therapy, the following local reactions were noted: pain (12%), erythema (2.9%), induration (0.9%), and phlebitis (2.1%). In the US patient population, pain occurred in 1.5% of patients, while each of the remaining three local reactions had an incidence of 0.5%.

The following laboratory adverse events, regardless of drug relationship, occurred in at least 1% of treated patients: increased eosinophils (6.3%), increased platelets (3.6%), neutropenia (3.2%), increased AST (3.8%), increased ALT (6.5%), and increased serum creatinine (5.8%).

In US pediatric clinical trials, neutropenia (absolute neutrophil count less than 1000/mm³) occurred in 11.3% of patients (8/71) younger than 2 years receiving 30 mg/kg q6h. AST and ALT elevations to greater than 3 times the upper limit of normal were noted in 15–20% of patients aged 2 years or above receiving 50 mg/kg q6h. The increased frequency of these reported laboratory adverse events may be due to either increased severity of illness treated or higher doses of AZACTAM (aztreonam for injection, USP) administered.

Adverse Laboratory Changes

Adverse laboratory changes without regard to drug relationship that were reported during clinical trials were:

Hepatic—elevations of AST (SGOT), ALT (SGPT), and alkaline phosphatase; signs or symptoms of hepatobiliary dysfunction occurred in less than 1 percent of recipients (see above).

Hematologic—increases in prothrombin and partial thromboplastin times, positive Coombs test.

Renal—increases in serum creatinine.

OVERDOSAGE

If necessary, aztreonam may be cleared from the serum by hemodialysis and/or peritoneal dialysis.

DOSAGE AND ADMINISTRATION

Dosage in Adult Patients

AZACTAM may be administered intravenously or by intramuscular injection. Dosage and route of administration should be determined by susceptibility of the causative organisms, severity and site of infection, and the condition of the patient.

The intravenous route is recommended for patients requiring single doses greater than 1 g or those with bacterial septicemia, localized parenchymal abscess (e.g., intra-abdominal abscess), peritonitis or other severe systemic or life-threatening infections.

The duration of therapy depends on the severity of infection. Generally, AZACTAM should be continued for at least 48 hours after the patient becomes asymptomatic or evidence of bacterial eradication has been obtained. Persistent infections may require treatment for several weeks. Doses smaller than those indicated should not be used.

Renal Impairment in Adult Patients

Prolonged serum levels of aztreonam may occur in patients with transient or persistent renal insufficiency. Therefore, the dosage of AZACTAM should be halved in patients with estimated creatinine clearances between 10 and 30 mL/min/1.73 m² after an initial loading dose of 1 g or 2 g.

When only the serum creatinine concentration is available, the following formula (based on sex, weight, and age of the patient) may be used to approximate the creatinine clearance (Clcr). The serum creatinine should represent a steady state of renal function.

$$\text{Males: Clcr} = \frac{\text{weight (kg)} \times (140\text{-age})}{72 \times \text{serum creatinine (mg/dL)}}$$

Females: 0.85 × above value

In patients with severe renal failure (creatinine clearance less than 10 mL/min/1.73 m²), such as those supported by hemodialysis, the usual dose of 500 mg, 1 g or 2 g should be given initially. The maintenance dose should be one-fourth of the usual initial dose given at the usual fixed interval of 6, 8 or 12 hours. For serious or life-threatening infections, in addition to the maintenance doses, one-eighth of the initial dose should be given after each hemodialysis session.

Dosage in The Elderly

Renal status is a major determinant of dosage in the elderly; these patients in particular may have diminished renal function. Serum creatinine may not be an accurate determinant of renal status. Therefore, as with all antibiotics eliminated by the kidneys, estimates of creatinine clearance should be obtained, and appropriate dosage modifications made if necessary.

Dosage in Pediatric Patients

AZACTAM (aztreonam for injection, USP) should be administered intravenously to pediatric patients with normal renal function. There are insufficient data regarding intramuscular administration to pediatric patients or dosing in pediatric patients with renal impairment. (See **PRECAUTIONS: Pediatric Use**.)

[See table below]

Because of the serious nature of infections due to *Pseudomonas aeruginosa*, dosage of 2 g every six or eight hours is recommended, at least upon initiation of therapy, in systemic infections caused by this organism in adults.

CLINICAL STUDIES

A total of 612 pediatric patients aged 1 month to 12 years were enrolled in uncontrolled clinical trials of aztreonam in the treatment of serious gram-negative infections, including urinary tract, lower respiratory tract, skin and skin-structure, and intra-abdominal infections.

Preparation Of Parenteral Solutions

General

Upon the addition of the diluent to the container, contents should be shaken **immediately** and **vigorously**. Constituted solutions are not for multiple-dose use; should the entire volume in the container not be used for a single-dose, the unused solution must be discarded.

Depending upon the concentration of aztreonam and diluent used, constituted AZACTAM For Injection yields a colorless to light straw yellow solution which may develop a slight pink tint on standing (potency is not affected). Parenteral drug products should be inspected visually for particulate matter and discoloration whenever solution and container permit.

Admixtures With Other Antibiotics

Intravenous infusion solutions of AZACTAM not exceeding 2% w/v prepared with Sodium Chloride Injection USP 0.9% or Dextrose Injection USP 5%, to which clindamycin phosphate, gentamicin sulfate, tobramycin sulfate, or cefazolin sodium have been added at concentrations usually used clinically, are stable for up to 48 hours at room temperature or seven days under refrigeration. Ampicillin sodium admixtures with aztreonam in Sodium Chloride Injection USP 0.9% are stable for 24 hours at room temperature and 48 hours under refrigeration; stability in Dextrose Injection USP 5% is two hours at room temperature and eight hours under refrigeration.

Aztreonam-cloxacillin sodium and aztreonam-vancomycin hydrochloride admixtures are stable in Dianeal® 137 (Peritoneal Dialysis Solution) with 4.25% Dextrose for up to 24 hours at room temperature.

Aztreonam is incompatible with nafcillin sodium, cephradine, and metronidazole.

Other admixtures are not recommended since compatibility data are not available.

Intravenous (IV) Solutions

For Bolus Injection: The contents of an AZACTAM (aztreonam for injection, USP) 15 mL or 30 mL capacity vial should be constituted with 6 to 10 mL Sterile Water for Injection USP. *For Infusion*: Contents of the 100 mL capacity bottle should be constituted to a final concentration not exceeding 2% w/v (at least 50 mL of any appropriate infusion solution listed below per gram aztreonam). These solutions may be frozen immediately after constitution in the original container. (See **Stability** below.)

If the contents of a 15 mL or 30 mL capacity vial are to be transferred to an appropriate infusion solution, each gram of aztreonam should be initially constituted with at least 3 mL Sterile Water for Injection USP. Further dilution may be obtained with one of the following intravenous infusion solutions:

Sodium Chloride Injection USP, 0.9%
Ringer's Injection USP
Lactated Ringer's Injection USP
Dextrose Injection USP, 5% or 10%
Dextrose and Sodium Chloride Injection USP, 5%:0.9%, 5%:0.45% or 5%:0.2%
Sodium Lactate Injection USP (M/6 Sodium Lactate)
Ionosol® B and 5% Dextrose
Isolyte® E
Isolyte® E with 5% Dextrose
Isolyte® M with 5% Dextrose
Normosol®-R
Normosol®-R and 5% Dextrose
Normosol®-M and 5% Dextrose
Mannitol Injection USP, 5% or 10%
Lactated Ringer's and 5% Dextrose Injection
Plasma-Lyte® M and 5% Dextrose
10% Travert® Injection
10% Travert® and Electrolyte No. 1 Injection
10% Travert® and Electrolyte No. 2 Injection
10% Travert® and Electrolyte No. 3 Injection

Intramuscular (IM) Solutions

The contents of an AZACTAM (aztreonam for injection, USP) 15 mL or 30 mL capacity vial should be constituted with at least 3 mL of an appropriate diluent per gram aztreonam. The following diluents may be used:

Sterile Water for Injection USP
Sterile Bacteriostatic Water for Injection, USP (with benzyl alcohol or with methyl- and propylparabens)
Sodium Chloride Injection USP, 0.9%
Bacteriostatic Sodium Chloride Injection USP (with benzyl alcohol)

Stability Of IV And IM Solutions

AZACTAM solutions for IV infusion at concentrations not exceeding 2% w/v must be used within 48 hours following constitution if kept at controlled room temperature (59°–86° F/15°–30° C) or within seven days if refrigerated (36°–46° F/ 2°–8° C).

Frozen aztreonam infusion solutions may be stored for up to three months at −4° F/−20° C; frozen solutions may be thawed at controlled room temperature or by overnight refrigeration. Solutions that have been thawed and maintained at controlled room temperature or under refrigeration should be used within 24 or 72 hours after removal from the freezer, respectively. Solutions should not be refrozen.

AZACTAM solutions at concentrations exceeding 2% w/v, except those prepared with Sterile Water for Injection USP or Sodium Chloride Injection USP, should be used promptly after preparation; the two excepted solutions must be used within 48 hours if stored at controlled room temperature or within seven days if refrigerated.

AZACTAM DOSAGE GUIDELINES

Type of Infection	Dose	Frequency (hours)
ADULTS*		
Urinary tract infections	500 mg or 1 g	8 or 12
Moderately severe systemic infections	1 g or 2 g	8 or 12
Severe systemic or life-threatening infections	2 g	6 or 8
*Maximum recommended dose is 8 per day		
PEDIATRIC PATIENTS**		
Mild to moderate infections	30 mg/kg	8
Moderate to severe infections	30 mg/kg	6 or 8
**Maximum recommended dose is 120 mg/kg/day.		

Intravenous Administration

Bolus Injection: A bolus injection may be used to initiate therapy. The dose should be **slowly** injected directly into a vein, or the tubing of a suitable administration set, over a period of three to five minutes (see next paragraph regarding flushing of tubing).

Infusion: With any intermittent infusion of aztreonam and another drug with which it is not pharmaceutically compatible, the common delivery tube should be flushed before and after delivery of aztreonam with any appropriate infusion solution compatible with both drug solutions; the drugs should not be delivered simultaneously. Any AZACTAM infusion should be completed within a 20 to 60 minute period. With use of a *Y-type administration set*, careful attention should be given to the calculated volume of aztreonam solution required so that the entire dose will be infused. A volume control administration set may be used to deliver an initial dilution of AZACTAM (see **Preparation Of Parenteral Solutions, For Infusion**) into a compatible infusion solution during administration; in this case, the final dilution of aztreonam should provide a concentration not exceeding 2% w/v.

Intramuscular Administration

The dose should be given by deep injection into a large muscle mass (such as the upper outer quadrant of the gluteus maximus or lateral part of the thigh). Aztreonam is well tolerated and should not be admixed with any local anesthetic agent.

HOW SUPPLIED

AZACTAM® (aztreonam for injection, USP)-Lyophilized

Single-dose 15 mL capacity vials:

500 mg/vial: Packages of 10 (NDC 0003-2550-10)

1 g/vial: Packages of 10 (NDC 0003-2560-10)

Single-dose 30 mL capacity vial:

2 g/vial: Packages of 10 (NDC 0003-2570-10)

Single-dose 100 mL capacity intravenous infusion bottles with bail bands:

1 g/bottle: Packages of 10 (NDC 0003-2560-20)

2 g/bottle: Packages of 10 (NDC 0003-2570-20)

Storage

Store original packages at room temperature; avoid excessive heat.

ALSO SUPPLIED AS:

AZACTAM® (aztreonam injection) in Galaxy® plastic container (PL 2040) as a frozen, 50 mL single-dose intravenous solution as follows:

1 g aztreonam/50 mL container:	Packages of 24 (NDC 0003-2231-01)
2 g aztreonam/50 mL container:	Packages of 24 (NDC 0003-2241-01)

Bristol-Myers Squibb Company
Princeton, NJ 08543, U.S.A.
1-246-797 Revised July 1997
E1-B001

BUSPAR® ℞

[*bus-pär*]
(buspirone HCl, USP)

Rx only

DESCRIPTION

BuSpar® (buspirone hydrochloride tablets, USP) is an antianxiety agent that is not chemically or pharmacologically related to the benzodiazepines, barbiturates, or other sedative/anxiolytic drugs.

Buspirone hydrochloride is a white crystalline, water soluble compound with a molecular weight of 422.0. Chemically, buspirone hydrochloride is 8-[4-[4-(2-pyrimidinyl)-1-piperazinyl]butyl]-8-azaspiro[4.5]decane-7,9-dione monohydrochloride. The empirical formula $C_{21}H_{31}N_5O_2 \bullet HCl$ is represented by the following structural formula:

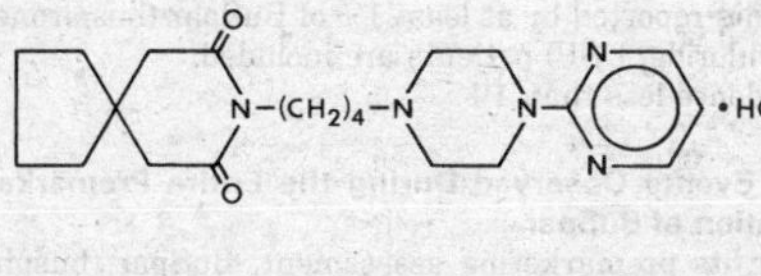

BuSpar is supplied as tablets for oral administration containing 5 mg, 10 mg, or 15 mg of buspirone hydrochloride, USP (equivalent to 4.6 mg, 9.1 mg, and 13.7 mg of buspirone free base respectively). The 15 mg tablet is provided in DIVIDOSE® tablet design. This tablet is scored so it can be either bisected or trisected. Thus, a single tablet can provide the following doses: 15 mg (entire tablet), 10 mg (two-thirds of a tablet), 7.5 mg (one-half of a tablet), or 5 mg (one-third of a tablet). BuSpar Tablets contain the following inactive ingredients: colloidal silicon dioxide, lactose, magnesium stearate, microcrystalline cellulose, and sodium starch glycolate.

CLINICAL PHARMACOLOGY

The mechanism of action of buspirone is unknown. Buspirone differs from typical benzodiazepine anxiolytics in that it does not exert anticonvulsant or muscle relaxant effects. It also lacks the prominent sedative effect that is associated with more typical anxiolytics. *In vitro* preclinical studies have shown that buspirone has a high affinity for serotonin ($5\text{-}HT_{1A}$) receptors. Buspirone has no significant affinity for benzodiazepine receptors and does not affect GABA binding *in vitro* or *in vivo* when tested in preclinical models.

Buspirone has moderate affinity for brain D_2-dopamine receptors. Some studies do suggest that buspirone may have indirect effects on other neurotransmitter systems.

BuSpar is rapidly absorbed in man and undergoes extensive first-pass metabolism. In a radiolabeled study, unchanged buspirone in the plasma accounted for only about 1% of the radioactivity in the plasma. Following oral administration, plasma concentrations of unchanged buspirone are very low and variable between subjects. Peak plasma levels of 1 to 6 ng/mL have been observed 40 to 90 minutes after single oral doses of 20 mg. The single-dose bioavailability of unchanged buspirone when taken as a tablet is on the average about 90% of an equivalent dose of solution, but there is large variability.

The effects of food upon the bioavailability of BuSpar have been studied in eight subjects. They were given a 20-mg dose with and without food; the area under the plasma concentration-time curve (AUC) and peak plasma concentration (C_{max}) of unchanged buspirone increased by 84% and 116% respectively, but the total amount of buspirone immunoreactive material did not change. This suggests that food may decrease the extent of presystemic clearance of buspirone, but the clinical significance of these findings is unknown.

A multiple-dose study conducted in 15 subjects suggests that buspirone has nonlinear pharmacokinetics. Thus, dose increases and repeated dosing may lead to somewhat higher blood levels of unchanged buspirone than would be predicted from results of single-dose studies.

An *in vitro* protein binding study indicated that approximately 86% of buspirone is bound to plasma proteins. It was also observed that aspirin increased the plasma levels of free buspirone by 23%, while flurazepam decreased the plasma levels of free buspirone by 20%. However, it is not known whether these drugs cause similar effects on plasma levels of free buspirone *in vivo*, or whether such changes, if they do occur, cause clinically significant differences in treatment outcome. An *in vitro* study indicated that buspirone did not displace highly protein-bound drugs such as phenytoin, warfarin, and propranolol from plasma protein, and that buspirone may displace digoxin.

Buspirone is metabolized primarily by oxidation, which *in vitro* has been shown to be mediated by cytochrome P450 3A4 (CYP3A4). (See **PRECAUTIONS, Drug Interactions** section.) Several hydroxylated derivatives and a pharmacologically active metabolite, 1-pyrimidinylpiperazine (1-PP), are produced. In animal models predictive of anxiolytic potential, 1-PP has about one quarter of the activity of buspirone, but is present in up to 20-fold greater amounts. However, this is probably not important in humans: blood samples from humans chronically exposed to BuSpar do not exhibit high levels of 1-PP; mean values are approximately 3ng/mL and the highest human blood level recorded among 108 chronically dosed patients was 17ng/mL, less than 1/200th of 1-PP levels found in animals given large doses of buspirone without signs of toxicity.

In a single-dose study using ^{14}C-labeled buspirone, 29% to 63% of the dose was excreted in the urine within 24 hours, primarily as metabolites; fecal excretion accounted for 18% to 38% of the dose. The average elimination half-life of unchanged buspirone after single doses of 10 to 40 mg is about 2 to 3 hours.

Special Populations

Age and Gender Effects

After single or multiple doses in adults, no significant differences in buspirone pharmacokinetics (AUC and C_{max}) were observed between elderly and younger subjects or between men and women.

Hepatic Impairment

After multiple-dose administration of buspirone to patients with hepatic impairment, steady-state AUC of buspirone increased 13-fold compared with healthy subjects (see **PRECAUTIONS** section).

Renal Impairment

After multiple-dose administration of buspirone to renally impaired (Cl_{cr} = 10–70 mL/min/1.73 m^2) patients, steady-state AUC of buspirone increased 4-fold compared with healthy ($Cl_{cr} \geq 80$ mL/min/1.73 m^2) subjects (see **PRECAUTIONS** section).

Race Effects

The effects of race on the pharmacokinetics of buspirone have not been studied.

INDICATIONS AND USAGE

BuSpar (buspirone hydrochloride, USP) is indicated for the management of anxiety disorders or the short-term relief of the symptoms of anxiety. Anxiety or tension associated with the stress of everyday life usually does not require treatment with an anxiolytic.

The efficacy of BuSpar has been demonstrated in controlled clinical trials of outpatients whose diagnosis roughly corresponds to Generalized Anxiety Disorder (GAD). Many of the patients enrolled in these studies also had coexisting depressive symptoms and BuSpar relieved anxiety in the presence of these coexisting depressive symptoms. The patients evaluated in these studies had experienced symptoms for periods of 1 month to over 1 year prior to the study, with an average symptom duration of 6 months. Generalized Anxiety Disorder (300.02) is described in the American Psychiatric Association's Diagnostic and Statistical Manual, III[1] as follows:

Generalized, persistent anxiety (of at least 1 month continual duration), manifested by symptoms from three of the four following categories:

1. Motor tension: shakiness, jitteriness, jumpiness, trembling, tension, muscle aches, fatigability, inability to relax, eyelid twitch, furrowed brow, strained face, fidgeting, restlessness, easy startle.
2. Autonomic hyperactivity: sweating, heart pounding or racing, cold, clammy hands, dry mouth, dizziness, lightheadedness, paresthesias (tingling in hands or feet), upset stomach, hot or cold spells, frequent urination, diarrhea, discomfort in the pit of the stomach, lump in the throat, flushing, pallor, high resting pulse, and respiration rate.
3. Apprehensive expectation: anxiety, worry, fear, rumination, and anticipation of misfortune to self or others.
4. Vigilance and scanning: hyperattentiveness resulting in distractibility, difficulty in concentrating, insomnia, feeling "on edge," irritability, impatience.

The above symptoms would not be due to another mental disorder, such as a depressive disorder or schizophrenia. However, mild depressive symptoms are common in GAD.

The effectiveness of BuSpar (buspirone hydrochloride, USP) in long-term use, that is, for more than 3 to 4 weeks, has not been demonstrated in controlled trials. There is no body of evidence available that systematically addresses the appropriate duration of treatment for GAD. However, in a study of long-term use, 264 patients were treated with BuSpar for 1 year without ill effect. Therefore, the physician who elects to use BuSpar for extended periods should periodically reassess the usefulness of the drug for the individual patient.

CONTRAINDICATIONS

BuSpar is contraindicated in patients hypersensitive to buspirone hydrochloride.

WARNINGS

The administration of BuSpar to a patient taking a monoamine oxidase inhibitor (MAOI) may pose a hazard. There have been reports of the occurrence of elevated blood pressure when BuSpar has been added to a regimen including an MAOI. Therefore, it is recommended that BuSpar not be used concomitantly with an MAOI.

Because BuSpar has no established antipsychotic activity, it should not be employed in lieu of appropriate antipsychotic treatment.

PRECAUTIONS

General

Interference with Cognitive and Motor Performance

Studies indicate that BuSpar is less sedating than other anxiolytics and that it does not produce significant functional impairment. However, its CNS effects in any individual patient may not be predictable. Therefore, patients should be cautioned about operating an automobile or using complex machinery until they are reasonably certain that buspirone treatment does not affect them adversely.

While formal studies of the interaction of BuSpar with alcohol indicate that buspirone does not increase alcohol-induced impairment in motor and mental performance, it is prudent to avoid concomitant use of alcohol and buspirone.

Potential for Withdrawal Reactions in Sedative/Hypnotic/Anxiolytic Drug-Dependent Patients

Because BuSpar does not exhibit cross-tolerance with benzodiazepines and other common sedative/hypnotic drugs, it will not block the withdrawal syndrome often seen with cessation of therapy with these drugs. Therefore, before starting therapy with BuSpar, it is advisable to withdraw patients gradually, especially patients who have been using a CNS-depressant drug chronically, from their prior treatment. Rebound or withdrawal symptoms may occur over varying time periods, depending in part on the type of drug, and its effective half-life of elimination.

The syndrome of withdrawal from sedative/hypnotic/anxiolytic drugs can appear as any combination of irritability, anxiety, agitation, insomnia, tremor, abdominal cramps, muscle cramps, vomiting, sweating, flu-like symptoms without fever, and occasionally, even as seizures.

Possible Concerns Related to Buspirone's Binding to Dopamine Receptors

Because buspirone can bind to central dopamine receptors, a question has been raised about its potential to cause acute

Continued on next page

BuSpar—Cont.

and chronic changes in dopamine-mediated neurological function (e.g., dystonia, pseudo-parkinsonism, akathisia, and tardive dyskinesia). Clinical experience in controlled trials has failed to identify any significant neuroleptic-like activity; however, a syndrome of restlessness, appearing shortly after initiation of treatment, has been reported in some small fraction of buspirone-treated patients. The syndrome may be explained in several ways. For example, buspirone may increase central noradrenergic activity; alternatively, the effect may be attributable to dopaminergic effects (i.e., represent akathisia). Obviously, the question cannot be totally resolved at this point in time. Generally, long-term sequelae of any drug's use can be identified only after several years of marketing.

Information for Patients

To assure safe and effective use of BuSpar (buspirone hydrochloride, USP), the following information and instructions should be given to patients:

1. Inform your physician about any medications, prescription or nonprescription, alcohol, or drugs that you are now taking or plan to take during your treatment with BuSpar.
2. Inform your physician if you are pregnant, or if you are planning to become pregnant, or if you become pregnant while you are taking BuSpar.
3. Inform your physician if you are breast-feeding an infant.
4. Until you experience how this medication affects you, do not drive a car or operate potentially dangerous machinery.

Laboratory Tests

There are no specific laboratory tests recommended.

Drug Interactions

MAO Inhibitors: It is recommended that BuSpar (buspirone hydrochloride, USP) *not* be used concomitantly with MAO inhibitors (see **WARNINGS** section).

Trazadone: There is one report suggesting that the concomitant use of Desyrel® (trazodone hydrochloride) and BuSpar may have caused 3- to 6-fold elevations on SGPT (ALT) in a few patients. In a similar study attempting to replicate this finding, no interactive effect on hepatic transaminases was identified.

Haloperidol: In a study in normal volunteers, concomitant administration of BuSpar and haloperidol resulted in increased serum haloperidol concentrations. The clinical significance of this finding is not clear.

Amitriptyline: After addition of buspirone to the amitriptyline dose regimen, no statistically significant differences in the steady-state pharmacokinetic parameters (C_{max}, AUC, and C_{min}) of amitriptyline or its metabolite nortriptyline were observed.

Diazepam: After addition of buspirone to the diazepam dose regimen, no statistically significant differences in the steady-state pharmacokinetic parameters (C_{max}, AUC, and C_{min}) were observed for diazepam, but increases of about 15% were seen for nordiazepam, and minor adverse clinical effects (dizziness, headache, and nausea) were observed.

Triazolam/Flurazepam: Coadministration of buspirone with either triazolam or flurazepam did not appear to prolong or intensify the sedative effects of either benzodiazepine.

Nefazodone: In a study of steady-state pharmacokinetics in healthy volunteers, coadministration of buspirone (2.5 or 5 mg b.i.d.) with nefazodone (250 mg b.i.d.) resulted in marked increases in plasma buspirone concentrations (increases up to 20-fold in C_{max} and up to 50-fold in AUC) and statistically significant decreases (~50%) in plasma concentrations of the buspirone metabolite 1-PP. With 5-mg b.i.d. doses of buspirone, slight increases in AUC were observed for nefazodone (23%) and its metabolites hydroxynefazodone (17%) and meta-chlorophenylpiperazine (9%). The side effect profile for subjects receiving buspirone 2.5 mg b.i.d. and nefazodone 250 mg b.i.d. was similar to that for subjects receiving either drug alone. Subjects receiving buspirone 5 mg b.i.d. and nefazodone 250 mg b.i.d. experienced side effects such as lightheadedness, asthenia, dizziness, and somnolence. If the two drugs are to be used in combination, a low dose of buspirone (eg, 2.5 mg b.i.d.) is recommended. Subsequent dose adjustment of either drug should be based on clinical assessment.

Other Psychotropics: Because the effects of concomitant administration of BuSpar (buspirone hydrochloride, USP) with most other psychotropic drugs have not been studied, the concomitant use of BuSpar with other CNS-active drugs should be approached with caution.

Cimetidine: Coadministration of buspirone with cimetidine was found to increase C_{max} (40%) and T_{max} (2-fold), but had minimal effects on the AUC of buspirone.

Erythromycin: In a study in healthy volunteers, coadministration of BuSpar (10 mg/day) with erythromycin (1.5 g/day) increased plasma buspirone concentrations (fivefold increase in C_{max} and sixfold increase in AUC). These pharmacokinetic interactions were accompanied by an increased incidence of side effects attributable to buspirone. If the two drugs are to be used in combination, a low dose of buspirone (eg, 2.5 mg b.i.d.) is recommended. Subsequent dose adjustment of either drug should be based on clinical assessment.

Itraconazole: In a study in healthy volunteers, coadministration of BuSpar (10 mg/day) with itraconazole (200 mg/day) increased plasma buspirone concentrations (13-fold increase in C_{max} and 19-fold increase in AUC). These pharmacokinetic interactions were accompanied by an increased incidence of side effects attributable to buspirone. If the two drugs are to be used in combination, a low dose of buspirone (eg, 2.5 mg b.i.d.) is recommended. Subsequent dose adjustment of either drug should be based on clinical assessment.

Potential Interaction with Drugs That Inhibit Cytochrome P450 3A4 (CYP3A4): Buspirone has been shown *in vitro* to be metabolized by CYP3A4. This is consistent with the interaction observed between buspirone and erythromycin, itraconazole, and nefazodone, drugs that inhibit this isozyme. Consequently, if BuSpar is to be used in combination with a potent inhibitor of CYP3A4, a low dose of buspirone (eg, 2.5 mg b.i.d.) is recommended. Subsequent dose adjustment of either drug should be based on clinical assessment.

Protein Binding: In vitro, buspirone does not displace tightly bound drugs like phenytoin, propranolol, and warfarin from serum proteins. However, there has been one report of prolonged prothrombin time when buspirone was added to the regimen of a patient with warfarin. The patient was also chronically receiving phenytoin, phenobarbital, digoxin, and Synthroid®. *In vitro*, buspirone may displace less firmly bound drugs like digoxin. The clinical significance of this property is unknown.

Therapeutic levels of aspirin, desipramine, diazepam, flurazepam, ibuprofen, propranolol, thioridazine, and tolbutamide had only a limited effect on the extent of binding buspirone to plasma proteins (see **CLINICAL PHARMACOLOGY** section).

Drug/Laboratory Test Interactions

Buspirone is not known to interfere with commonly employed clinical laboratory tests.

Carcinogenesis, Mutagenesis, Impairment of Fertility

No evidence of carcinogenic potential was observed in rats during a 24-month study at approximately 133 times the maximum recommended human oral dose; or in mice, during an 18-month study at approximately 167 times the maximum recommended human oral dose.

With or without metabolic activation, buspirone did not induce point mutations in five strains of *Salmonella typhimurium* (Ames Test) or mouse lymphoma L5178YTK+ cell cultures, nor was DNA damage observed with buspirone in Wi-38 human cells. Chromosomal aberrations or abnormalities did not occur in bone marrow cells of mice given one or five daily doses of buspirone.

Pregnancy: Teratogenic Effects

Pregnancy Category B: No fertility impairment or fetal damage was observed in reproduction studies performed in rats and rabbits at buspirone doses of approximately 30 times the maximum recommended human dose. In humans, however, adequate and well-controlled studies during pregnancy have *not* been performed. Because animal reproduction studies are not always predictive of human response, this drug should be used during pregnancy only if clearly needed.

Labor and Delivery

The effect of BuSpar on labor and delivery in women is unknown. No adverse effects were noted in reproduction studies in rats.

Nursing Mothers

The extent of the excretion in human milk of buspirone or its metabolites is not known. In rats, however, buspirone and its metabolites are excreted in milk. BuSpar (buspirone hydrochloride, USP) administration to nursing women should be avoided if clinically possible.

Pediatric Use

The safety and effectiveness of BuSpar have not been determined in individuals below 18 years of age.

Use in the Elderly

The safety and efficacy profiles of buspirone in 605 anxious, elderly patients (mean age = 70.8 years) were similar to those in a younger population (mean age = 43.3 years). There were no effects of age on the pharmacokinetics of buspirone.

Use in Patients With Impaired Hepatic or Renal Function

Buspirone is metabolized by the liver and excreted by the kidneys. A pharmacokinetic study in patients with impaired hepatic or renal function demonstrated increased plasma levels and a lengthened half-life of buspirone. Therefore, the administration of BuSpar to patients with severe hepatic or renal impairment cannot be recommended (see **CLINICAL PHARMACOLOGY** section).

ADVERSE REACTIONS (See also PRECAUTIONS)

Commonly Observed

The more commonly observed untoward events associated with the use of BuSpar not seen at an equivalent incidence among placebo-treated patients include dizziness, nausea, headache, nervousness, lightheadedness, and excitement.

Associated With Discontinuation of Treatment

One guide to the relative clinical importance of adverse events associated with BuSpar is provided by the frequency with which they caused drug discontinuation during clinical testing. Approximately 10% of the 2200 anxious patients who participated in the BuSpar premarketing clinical efficacy trials in anxiety disorders lasting 3 to 4 weeks discontinued treatment due to an adverse event. The more common events causing discontinuation included: central nervous system disturbances (3.4 %), primarily dizziness, insomnia, nervousness, drowsiness, and lightheaded feeling; gastrointestinal disturbances (1.2%), primarily nausea; and miscellaneous disturbances (1.1%), primarily headache and fatigue. In addition, 3.4% of patients had multiple complaints, none of which could be characterized as primary.

Incidence in Controlled Clinical Trials

The table that follows enumerates adverse events that occurred at a frequency of 1% or more among BuSpar patients who participated in 4-week, controlled trials comparing BuSpar with placebo. The frequencies were obtained from pooled data for 17 trials. The prescriber should be aware that these figures cannot be used to predict the incidence of side effects in the course of usual medical practice where patient characteristics and other factors differ from those which prevailed in the clinical trials. Similarly, the cited frequencies cannot be compared with figures obtained from other clinical investigations involving different treatments, uses, and investigators. Comparison of the cited figures, however, does provide the prescribing physician with some basis for estimating the relative contribution of drug and nondrug factors to the side-effect incidence rate in the population studied.

TREATMENT-EMERGENT ADVERSE EXPERIENCE INCIDENCE IN PLACEBO-CONTROLLED CLINICAL TRIALS*
(Percent of Patients Reporting)

Adverse Experience	BuSpar (n= 477)	Placebo (n= 464)
Cardiovascular		
Tachycardia/Palpitations	1	1
CNS		
Dizziness	12	3
Drowsiness	10	9
Nervousness	5	1
Insomnia	3	3
Lightheadedness	3	—
Decreased Concentration	2	2
Excitement	2	—
Anger/Hostility	2	—
Confusion	2	—
Depression	2	2
EENT		
Blurred Vision	2	—
Gastrointestinal		
Nausea	8	5
Dry Mouth	3	4
Abdominal/Gastric Distress	2	2
Diarrhea	2	—
Constipation	1	2
Vomiting	1	2
Musculoskeletal		
Musculoskeletal Aches/Pains	1	—
Neurological		
Numbness	2	—
Paresthesia	1	—
Incoordination	1	—
Tremor	1	—
Skin		
Skin Rash	1	—
Miscellaneous		
Headache	6	3
Fatigue	4	4
Weakness	2	—
Sweating/Clamminess	1	—

* Events reported by at least 1% of BuSpar (buspirone hydrochloride, USP) patients are included.
—Incidence less than 1%.

Other Events Observed During the Entire Premarketing Evaluation of BuSpar

During its premarketing assessment, BuSpar (buspirone hydrochloride, USP) was evaluated in over 3500 subjects. This section reports event frequencies for adverse events occurring in approximately 3000 subjects from this group who took multiple doses of BuSpar in the dose range for which BuSpar is being recommended (i.e., the modal daily dose of BuSpar fell between 10 and 30 mg for 70% of the patients studied) and for whom safety data were systematically collected. The conditions and duration of exposure to BuSpar varied greatly, involving well-controlled studies as well as experience in open and uncontrolled clinical settings. As part of the total experience gained in clinical studies, various adverse events were reported. In the absence of appro-

priate controls in some of the studies, a causal relationship to BuSpar treatment cannot be determined. The list includes all undesirable events reasonably associated with the use of the drug.

The following enumeration by organ system describes events in terms of their relative frequency of reporting in this data base. Events of major clinical importance are also described in the **PRECAUTIONS** section.

The following definitions of frequency are used: Frequent adverse events are defined as those occurring in at least 1/100 patients. Infrequent adverse events are those occurring in 1/100 to 1/1000 patients, while rare events are those occurring in less than 1/1000 patients.

Cardiovascular

Frequent was nonspecific chest pain; infrequent were syncope, hypotension, and hypertension; rare were cerebrovascular accident, congestive heart failure, myocardial infarction, cardiomyopathy, and bradycardia.

Central Nervous System

Frequent were dream disturbances; infrequent were depersonalization, dysphoria, noise intolerance, euphoria, akathisia, fearfulness, loss of interest, dissociative reaction, hallucinations, involuntary movements, slowed reaction time, suicidal ideation, and seizures; rare were feelings of claustrophobia, cold intolerance, stupor, and slurred speech and psychosis.

EENT

Frequent were tinnitus, sore throat, and nasal congestion; infrequent were redness and itching of the eyes, altered taste, altered smell, and conjunctivitis; rare were inner ear abnormality, eye pain, photophobia, and pressure on eyes.

Endocrine

Rare were galactorrhea and thyroid abnormality.

Gastrointestinal

Infrequent were flatulence, anorexia, increased appetite, salivation, irritable colon, and rectal bleeding; rare was burning of the tongue.

Genitourinary

Infrequent were urinary frequency, urinary hesitancy, menstrual irregularity and spotting, and dysuria; rare were amenorrhea, pelvic inflammatory disease, enuresis, and nocturia.

Musculoskeletal

Infrequent were muscle cramps, muscle spasms, rigid/stiff muscles, and arthralgias; rare was muscle weakness.

Respiratory

Infrequent were hyperventilation, shortness of breath, and chest congestion; rare was epistaxis.

Sexual Function

Infrequent were decreased or increased libido; rare were delayed ejaculation and impotence.

Skin

Infrequent were edema, pruritus, flushing, easy bruising, hair loss, dry skin, facial edema, and blisters; rare were acne and thinning of nails.

Clinical Laboratory

Infrequent were increases in hepatic aminotransferases (SGOT, SGPT); rare were eosinophilia, leukopenia, and thrombocytopenia.

Miscellaneous

Infrequent were weight gain, fever, roaring sensation in the head, weight loss, and malaise; rare were alcohol abuse, bleeding disturbance, loss of voice, and hiccoughs.

POSTINTRODUCTION CLINICAL EXPERIENCE

Postmarketing experience has shown an adverse experience profile similar to that given above. Voluntary reports since introduction have included rare occurrences of allergic reactions (including urticaria), angioedema, cogwheel rigidity, dizziness (rarely reported as vertigo), dystonic reactions, ataxias, extrapyramidal symptoms, dyskinesias (acute and tardive), ecchymosis, emotional lability, serotonin syndrome, transient difficulty with recall, urinary retention, and visual changes (including tunnel vision). Because of the uncontrolled nature of these spontaneous reports, a causal relationship to BuSpar (buspirone hydrochloride, USP) treatment has not been determined.

DRUG ABUSE AND DEPENDENCE

Controlled Substance Class

BuSpar is not a controlled substance.

Physical and Psychological Dependence

In human and animal studies, buspirone has shown no potential for abuse or diversion and there is no evidence that it causes tolerance, or either physical or psychological dependence. Human volunteers with a history of recreational drug or alcohol usage were studied in two double-blind clinical investigations. None of the subjects were able to distinguish between BuSpar (buspirone hydrochloride, USP) and placebo. By contrast, subjects showed a statistically significant preference for methaqualone and diazepam. Studies in monkeys, mice, and rats have indicated that buspirone lacks potential for abuse.

Following chronic administration in the rat, abrupt withdrawal of buspirone did not result in the loss of body weight commonly observed with substances that cause physical dependency.

Although there is no direct evidence that BuSpar causes physical dependence or drug-seeking behavior, it is difficult to predict from experiments the extent to which a CNS-active drug will be misused, diverted, and/or abused once marketed. Consequently, physicians should carefully evaluate patients for a history of drug abuse and follow such patients closely, observing them for signs of BuSpar misuse or abuse (e.g., development of tolerance, incrementation of dose, drug-seeking behavior).

OVERDOSAGE

Signs and Symptoms

In clinical pharmacology trials, doses as high as 375 mg/day were administered to healthy male volunteers. As this dose was approached, the following symptoms were observed: nausea, vomiting, dizziness, drowsiness, miosis, and gastric distress. A few cases of overdosage have been reported, with complete recovery as the usual outcome. No deaths have been reported following overdosage with BuSpar alone. Rare cases of intentional overdosage with a fatal outcome were invariably associated with ingestion of multiple drugs and/or alcohol, and a causal relationship to buspirone could not be determined. Toxicology studies of buspirone yielded the following LD_{50} values: mice, 655 mg/kg; rats, 196 mg/kg; dogs, 586 mg/kg; and monkeys, 356 mg/kg. These dosages are 160 to 550 times the recommended human daily dose.

Recommended Overdose Treatment

General symptomatic and supportive measures should be used along with immediate gastric lavage. Respiration, pulse, and blood pressure should be monitored as in all cases of drug overdosage. No specific antidote is known to buspirone, and dialyzability of buspirone has not been determined.

DOSAGE AND ADMINISTRATION

The recommended initial dose is 15 mg daily (7.5 mg b.i.d.) To achieve an optimal therapeutic response, at intervals of 2 to 3 days the dosage may be increased 5 mg per day, as needed. The maximum daily dosage should not exceed 60 mg per day. In clinical trials allowing dose titration, divided doses of 20 to 30 mg per day were commonly employed.

HOW SUPPLIED

BuSpar® (buspirone hydrochloride tablets, USP)

Tablets, 5 mg and 10 mg (white, ovoid-rectangular with score, MJ logo, strength and the name BuSpar embossed) are available in bottles of 100 and 500, and in cartons containing 100 individually packaged tablets.

5 mg tablets

NDC 0087-0818-41	Bottles of 100
NDC 0087-0818-44	Bottles of 500
NDC 0087-0818-43	Cartons of 100 unit dose

10 mg tablets

NDC 0087-0819-41	Bottles of 100
NDC 0087-0819-44	Bottles of 500
NDC 0087-0819-43	Cartons of 100 unit dose

Tablets, 15 mg white, in the DIVIDOSE® tablet design imprinted with the MJ logo, are available in bottles of 60 and 180. The 15 mg tablet is scored so that it can be either bisected or trisected. It has ID number 822 on one side and on the reverse side, the number 5 on each trisect segment.

15 mg tablets

NDC 0087-0822-32	Bottles of 60
NDC 0087-0822-33	Bottles of 180
NDC 0087-0822-34	First Month Pack (one bottle of 7 and one bottle of 42)

U.S. Patent Nos. 4,182,763 and 5,015,646; (DIVIDOSE®) 4,215,104 and 4,258,027

Store at Room Temperature—Protect from temperatures greater than 86°F (30°C). Dispense in a tight, light-resistant container (USP).

REFERENCE

1. American Psychiatric Association, Ed.: Diagnostic and Statistical Manual of Mental Disorders—III, American Psychiatric Association, May 1980.

Synthroid® is the registered trademark of Knoll Pharmaceutical Company

Bristol-Myers Squibb Company
Princeton, NJ 08543
U.S.A.

N0184-02 Revised May 1998
51-000649-04 D1-B001A

Shown in Product Identification Guide, page 307

CEFZIL® ℞
[sĕf-zil]
(CEFPROZIL) Tablets
250 mg and 500 mg
CEFZIL® ℞
(CEFPROZIL)
for Oral Suspension
125 mg/5 mL and 250 mg/5 mL

Rx only

DESCRIPTION

CEFZIL® (cefprozil) is a semi-synthetic broad-spectrum cephalosporin antibiotic.

Cefprozil is a cis and trans isomeric mixture (≥ 90% cis). The chemical name for the monohydrate is (6R, 7R)-7-[(R)-2-amino-2-(p-hydroxyphenyl)acetamido]-8-oxo-3-propenyl-5-thia-1-azabicyclo[4.2.0]oct-2-ene-2-carboxylic acid monohydrate, and the structural formula is:

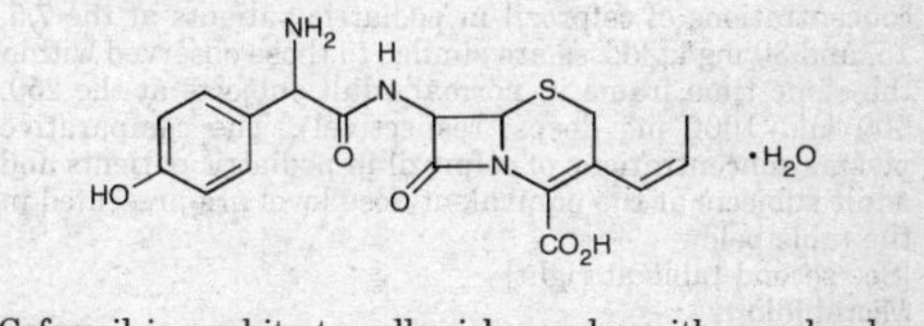

Cefprozil is a white to yellowish powder with a molecular formula for the monohydrate of $C_{18}H_{19}N_3O_5S \cdot H_2O$ and a molecular weight of 407.45.

CEFZIL (cefprozil) tablets and CEFZIL for oral suspension are intended for oral administration.

CEFZIL tablets contain cefprozil equivalent to 250 mg or 500 mg of anhydrous cefprozil. In addition, each tablet contains the following inactive ingredients: cellulose, hydroxypropylmethylcellulose, magnesium stearate, methylcellulose, simethicone, sodium starch glycolate, polyethylene glycol, polysorbate 80, sorbic acid and titanium dioxide. The 250 mg tablets also contain FD&C Yellow No. 6.

CEFZIL for oral suspension contains cefprozil equivalent to 125 mg or 250 mg anhydrous cefprozil per 5 mL constituted suspension. In addition, the oral suspension contains the following inactive ingredients: aspartame, cellulose, citric acid, colloidal silicone dioxide, FD&C Red No. 3, flavors (natural and artificial), glycine, polysorbate 80, simethicone, sodium benzoate, sodium carboxymethylcellulose, sodium chloride, and sucrose.

CLINICAL PHARMACOLOGY

The pharmacokinetic data were derived from the capsule formulation; however, bioequivalence has been demonstrated for the oral solution, capsule, tablet and suspension formulations under fasting conditions.

Following oral administration of cefprozil to fasting subjects, approximately 95% of the dose was absorbed. The average plasma half-life in normal subjects was 1.3 hours, while the steady state volume of distribution was estimated to be 0.23 L/kg. The total body clearance and renal clearance rates were approximately 3 mL/min/kg and 2.3 mL/min/kg, respectively.

Average peak plasma concentrations after administration of 250 mg, 500 mg, or 1 g doses of cefprozil to fasting subjects were approximately 6.1, 10.5, and 18.3 µg/mL, respectively, and were obtained within 1.5 hours after dosing. Urinary recovery accounted for approximately 60% of the administered dose. (See Table.)

[See table at top of next page]

During the first four-hour period after drug administration, the average urine concentrations following 250 mg, 500 mg, and 1 g doses were approximately 700 µg/mL, 1000 µg/mL, and 2900 µg/mL, respectively.

Administration of CEFZIL® (cefprozil) tablet or suspension formulation with food did not affect the extent of absorption (AUC) or the peak plasma concentration (C_{max}) of cefprozil. However, there was an increase of 0.25 to 0.75 hours in the time to maximum plasma concentration of cefprozil (T_{max}). The bioavailability of the capsule formulation of cefprozil was not affected when administered 5 minutes following an antacid.

Plasma protein binding is approximately 36% and is independent of concentration in the range of 2 µg/mL to 20 µg/mL.

There was no evidence of accumulation of cefprozil in the plasma in individuals with normal renal function following multiple oral doses of up to 1000 mg every 8 hours for 10 days.

In patients with reduced renal function, the plasma half-life may be prolonged up to 5.2 hours depending on the degree of the renal dysfunction. In patients with complete absence of renal function, the plasma half-life of cefprozil has been shown to be as long as 5.9 hours. The half-life is shortened during hemodialysis. Excretion pathways in patients with markedly impaired renal function have not been determined. (See **PRECAUTIONS** and **DOSAGE AND ADMINISTRATION**.)

In patients with impaired hepatic function, the half-life increases to approximately 2 hours. The magnitude of the changes does not warrant a dosage adjustment for patients with impaired hepatic function.

The average AUC observed in elderly subjects (≥ 65 years of age) is approximately 35–60% higher relative to young adults, and the average AUC in females is approximately 15–20% higher than in males. The magnitude of these age- and gender-related changes in the pharmacokinetics of cefprozil is not sufficient to necessitate dosage adjustments.

Continued on next page

Cefzil—Cont.

Adequate data on CSF levels of cefprozil are not available. Comparable pharmacokinetic parameters of cefprozil are observed between pediatric patients (6 months–12 years) and adults following oral administration of selected matched doses. The maximum concentrations are achieved at 1–2 hours after dosing. The plasma elimination half-life is approximately 1.5 hours. In general, the observed plasma concentrations of cefprozil in pediatric patients at the 7.5, 15, and 30 mg/kg doses are similar to those observed within the same time frame in normal adult subjects at the 250, 500 and 1000 mg doses, respectively. The comparative plasma concentrations of cefprozil in pediatric patients and adult subjects at the equivalent dose level are presented in the table below.
[See second table at right]

Microbiology

Cefprozil has in vitro activity against a broad range of gram-positive and gram-negative bacteria. The bactericidal action of cefprozil results from inhibition of cell-wall synthesis. Cefprozil has been shown to be active against most strains of the following microorganisms both in vitro and in clinical infections as described in the INDICATIONS AND USAGE section.

Aerobic gram-positive microorganisms:

Staphylococcus aureus (including β-lactamase-producing strains)
NOTE: Cefprozil is inactive against methicillin-resistant staphylococci.
Streptococcus pneumoniae
Streptococcus pyogenes

Aerobic gram-negative microorganisms:

Haemophilus influenzae (including β-lactamase-producing strains)
Moraxella (Branhamella) catarrhalis (including β-lactamase-producing strains)
The following in vitro data are available; however, their clinical significance is unknown. Cefprozil exhibits in vitro minimum inhibitory concentrations (MIC's) of 8 µg/mL or less against most (≥90%) strains of the following microorganisms; however, the safety and effectiveness of cefprozil in treating clinical infections due to these microorganisms have not been established in adequate and well-controlled clinical trials.

Aerobic gram-positive microorganisms:

Enterococcus durans
Enterococcus faecalis
Listeria monocytogenes
Staphylococcus epidermidis
Staphylococcus saprophyticus
Staphylococcus warneri
Streptococcus agalactiae
Streptococci (Groups C, D, F, and G)
viridans group Streptococci
NOTE: Cefprozil is inactive against *Enterococcus faecium*.

Aerobic gram-negative microorganisms:

Citrobacter diversus
Escherichia coli
Klebsiella pneumoniae
Neisseria gonorrhoeae (including β-lactamase-producing strains)
Proteus mirabilis
Salmonella spp.
Shigella spp.
Vibrio spp.
NOTE: Cefprozil is inactive against most strains of *Acinetobacter, Enterobacter, Morganella morganii, Proteus vulgaris, Providencia, Pseudomonas,* and *Serratia*.

Anaerobic microorganisms:

Prevotella (Bacteroides) melaninogenicus
Clostridium difficile
Clostridium perfringens
Fusobacterium spp.
Peptostreptococcus spp.
Propionibacterium acnes
NOTE: Most strains of the *Bacteroides fragilis* group are resistant to cefprozil.

Susceptibility Tests

Dilution Techniques: Quantitative methods are used to determine antimicrobial minimal inhibitory concentrations (MIC's). These MIC's provide estimates of the susceptibility of bacteria to antimicrobial compounds. The MIC's should be determined using a standardized procedure. Standardized procedures are based on a dilution method[1,2] (broth or agar) or equivalent with standardized inoculum concentrations and standardized concentrations of cefprozil powder. The MIC values should be interpreted according to the following criteria:

MIC (µg/mL)	Interpretation
≤ 8	Susceptible (S)
16	Intermediate (I)
≥ 32	Resistant (R)

Dosage (mg)	Peak appx. 1.5 hr	Mean Plasma Cefprozil* Concentration (µg/mL) 4 hr	8 hr	8-hour Urinary Excretion (%)
250 mg	6.1	1.7	0.2	60%
500 mg	10.5	3.2	0.4	62%
1000 mg	18.3	8.4	1.0	54%

* Data represent mean values of 12 healthy volunteers.

Population	Dose	Mean (SD) Plasma Cefprozil Concentrations (µg/mL) 1 hr	2 hr	4 hr	6 hr	$T_{1/2}$ (hr)
children (n = 18)	7.5 mg/kg	4.70 (1.57)	3.99 (1.24)	0.91 (0.30)	0.23[a] (0.13)	0.94 (0.32)
adults (n =12)	250 mg	4.82 (2.13)	4.92 (1.13)	1.70[b] (0.53)	0.53 (0.17)	1.28 (0.34)
children (n = 19)	15 mg/kg	10.86 (2.55)	8.47 (2.03)	2.75 (1.07)	0.61[c] (0.27)	1.24 (0.43)
adults (n = 12)	500 mg	8.39 (1.95)	9.42 (0.98)	3.18[d] (0.76)	1.00[d] (0.24)	1.29 (0.14)
children (n = 10)	30 mg/kg	6.69 (4.26)	17.61 (6.39)	8.66 (2.70)	–	2.06 (0.21)
adults (n = 12)	1000 mg	11.99 (4.67)	16.95 (4.07)	8.36 (4.13)	2.79 (1.77)	1.27 (0.12)

[a] n = 11; [b] n = 5; [c] n = 9; [d] n = 11.

A report of "Susceptible" indicates that the pathogen is likely to be inhibited if the antimicrobial compound in the blood reaches the concentrations usually achievable. A report of "Intermediate" indicates that the result should be considered equivocal, and, if the microorganism is not fully susceptible to alternative, clinically feasible drugs, the test should be repeated. This category implies possible clinical applicability in body sites where the drug is physiologically concentrated or in situations where high dosage of drug can be used. This category also provides a buffer zone which prevents small uncontrolled technical factors from causing major discrepancies in interpretation. A report of "Resistant" indicates that the pathogen is not likely to be inhibited if the antimicrobial compound in the blood reaches the concentrations usually achievable; other therapy should be selected.

Standardized susceptibility test procedures require the use of laboratory control microorganisms to control the technical aspects of the laboratory procedures. Standard cefprozil powder should provide the following MIC values:

Microorganism	MIC (µg/mL)
Enterococcus faecalis ATCC 29212	4–16
Escherichia coli ATCC 25922	1–4
Haemophilus influenzae ATCC 49766	1–4
Staphylococcus aureus ATCC 29213	0.25–1
Streptococcus pneumoniae ATCC 49619	0.25–1

Diffusion Techniques: Quantitative methods that require measurement of zone diameters also provide reproducible estimates of the susceptibility of bacteria to antimicrobial compounds. One such standardized procedure[3] requires the use of standardized inoculum concentrations. This procedure uses paper disks impregnated with 30 µg cefprozil to test the susceptibility of microorganisms to cefprozil.
Reports from the laboratory providing results of the standard single-disk susceptibility test with a 30 µg cefprozil disk should be interpreted according to the following criteria:

Zone diameter (mm)	Interpretation
≥ 18	Susceptible (S)
15–17	Intermediate (I)
≤ 14	Resistant (R)

Interpretation should be as stated above for results using dilution techniques. Interpretation involves correlation of the diameter obtained in the disk test with the MIC for cefprozil.
As with standardized dilution techniques, diffusion methods require the use of laboratory control microorganisms that are used to control the technical aspects of the laboratory procedures. For the diffusion technique, the 30 µg cefprozil disk should provide the following zone diameters in these laboratory test quality control strains.

Microorganism	Zone diameter (mm)
Escherichia coli ATCC 25922	21–27
Haemophilus influenzae ATCC 49766	20–27
Staphylococcus aureus ATCC 25923	27–33
Streptococcus pneumoniae ATCC 49619	25–32

INDICATIONS AND USAGE

CEFZIL (cefprozil) is indicated for the treatment of patients with mild to moderate infections caused by susceptible strains of the designated microorganisms in the conditions listed below:

UPPER RESPIRATORY TRACT

Pharyngitis/tonsillitis caused by *Streptococcus pyogenes*.
NOTE: The usual drug of choice in the treatment and prevention of streptococcal infections, including the prophylaxis of rheumatic fever, is penicillin given by the intramuscular route. Cefprozil is generally effective in the eradication of *Streptococcus pyogenes* from the nasopharynx; however, substantial data establishing the efficacy of cefprozil in the subsequent prevention of rheumatic fever are not available at present.

Otitis Media caused by *Streptococcus pneumoniae, Haemophilus influenzae* (including β-lactamase-producing strains) and *Moraxella (Branhamella) catarrhalis* (including β-lactamase-producing strains). (See CLINICAL STUDIES section.)
NOTE: In the treatment of otitis media due to β-lactamase producing organisms, cefprozil had bacteriologic eradication rates somewhat lower than those observed with a product containing a specific β-lactamase inhibitor. In considering the use of cefprozil, lower overall eradication rates should be balanced against the susceptibility patterns of the common microbes in a given geographic area and the increased potential for toxicity with products containing β-lactamase inhibitors.

Acute Sinusitis caused by *Streptococcus pneumoniae, Haemophilus influenzae* (including β-lactamase-producing strains) and *Moraxella (Branhamella) catarrhalis* (including β-lactamase-producing strains).

LOWER RESPIRATORY TRACT

Secondary Bacterial Infection of Acute Bronchitis and Acute Bacterial Exacerbation of Chronic Bronchitis caused by *Streptococcus pneumoniae, Haemophilus influenzae* (including β-lactamase-producing strains), and *Moraxella (Branhamella) catarrhalis* (including β-lactamase-producing strains).

SKIN AND SKIN STRUCTURE

Uncomplicated Skin and Skin-Structure Infections caused by *Staphylococcus aureus* (including penicillinase-producing strains), and *Streptococcus pyogenes*. Abscesses usually require surgical drainage.
Culture and susceptiblity testing should be performed when appropriate to determine susceptibility of the causative organism to cefprozil.

CONTRAINDICATIONS

CEFZIL (cefprozil) is contraindicated in patients with known allergy to the cephalosporin class of antibiotics.

WARNINGS

BEFORE THERAPY WITH CEFZIL IS INSTITUTED, CAREFUL INQUIRY SHOULD BE MADE TO DETERMINE WHETHER THE PATIENT HAS HAD PREVIOUS HYPERSENSITIVITY REACTIONS TO CEFZIL, CEPHALOSPORINS, PENICILLINS, OR OTHER DRUGS. IF THIS PRODUCT IS TO BE GIVEN TO PENICILLIN-SENSITIVE PATIENTS, CAUTION SHOULD BE EXERCISED BECAUSE CROSS-SENSITIVITY AMONG β-LACTAM ANTIBIOTICS HAS BEEN CLEARLY DOCUMENTED AND MAY OCCUR IN UP TO 10% OF PATIENTS WITH A HISTORY OF PENICILLIN ALLERGY. IF AN ALLERGIC REACTION TO CEFZIL OCCURS, DISCONTINUE THE DRUG. SERIOUS ACUTE HYPERSENSITIVITY REACTIONS MAY REQUIRE TREATMENT WITH EPINEPHRINE AND OTHER EMERGENCY MEASURES, INCLUDING OXYGEN,

INTRAVENOUS FLUIDS, INTRAVENOUS ANTIHISTAMINES, CORTICOSTEROIDS, PRESSOR AMINES, AND AIRWAY MANAGEMENT, AS CLINICALLY INDICATED.

Pseudomembranous colitis has been reported with nearly all antibacterial agents, including cefprozil, and may range in severity from mild to life threatening. Therefore, it is important to consider this diagnosis in patients who present with diarrhea subsequent to the administration of antibacterial agents.

Treatment with antibacterial agents alters the normal flora of the colon and may permit overgrowth of clostridia. Studies indicate that a toxin produced by *Clostridium difficile* is one primary cause of "antibiotic-associated" colitis.

After the diagnosis of pseudomembranous colitis has been established, appropriate therapeutic measures should be initiated. Mild cases of pseudomembranous colitis usually respond to drug discontinuation alone. In moderate to severe cases, consideration should be given to management with fluids and electrolytes, protein supplementation, and treatment with an antibacterial drug clinically effective against *Clostridium difficile* colitis.

PRECAUTIONS

General

In patients with known or suspected renal impairment (see **DOSAGE AND ADMINISTRATION**), careful clinical observation and appropriate laboratory studies should be done prior to and during therapy. The total daily dose of CEFZIL (cefprozil) should be reduced in these patients because high and/or prolonged plasma antibiotic concentrations can occur in such individuals from usual doses. Cephalosporins, including CEFZIL, should be given with caution to patients receiving concurrent treatment with potent diuretics since these agents are suspected of adversely affecting renal function.

Prolonged use of CEFZIL may result in the overgrowth of nonsusceptible organisms. Careful observation of the patient is essential.

If superinfection occurs during therapy, appropriate measures should be taken.

Cefprozil should be prescribed with caution in individuals with a history of gastrointestinal disease particularly colitis.

Positive direct Coombs' tests have been reported during treatment with cephalosporin antibiotics.

Information for Patients

Phenylketonurics: CEFZIL (cefprozil) for oral suspension contains phenylalanine 28 mg per 5 mL (1 teaspoonful) constituted suspension for both the 125 mg/5 mL and 250 mg/5 mL dosage forms.

Drug Interactions

Nephrotoxicity has been reported following concomitant administration of aminoglycoside antibiotics and cephalosporin antibiotics. Concomitant administration of probenecid doubled the AUC for cefprozil.

The bioavailability of the capsule formulation of cefprozil was not affected when administered 5 minutes following an antacid.

Drug/Laboratory Test Interactions

Cephalosporin antibiotics may produce a false positive reaction for glucose in the urine with copper reduction tests (Benedict's or Fehling's solution or with Clinitest®[4] tablets), but not with enzyme-based tests for glycosuria (e.g., TesTape®[5]). A false negative reaction may occur in the ferricyanide test for blood glucose. The presence of cefprozil in the blood does not interfere with the assay of plasma or urine creatinine by the alkaline picrate method.

Carcinogenesis, Mutagenesis, and Impairment of Fertility

Long term *in vivo* studies have not been performed to evaluate the carcinogenic potential of cefprozil.

Cefprozil was not found to be mutagenic in either the Ames *Salmonella* or *E. coli* WP2 urvA reversion assays or the Chinese hamster ovary cell HGPRT forward gene mutation assay and it did not induce chromosomal abnormalities in Chinese hamster ovary cells or unscheduled DNA synthesis in rat hepatocytes *in vitro*. Chromosomal aberrations were not observed in bone marrow cells from rats dosed orally with over 30 times the highest recommended human dose based upon mg/m². Impairment of fertility was not observed in male or female rats given oral doses of cefprozil up to 18.5 times the highest recommended human dose based upon mg/m².

Pregnancy: Teratogenic Effects. Pregnancy Category B

Reproduction studies have been performed in rabbits, mice and rats using oral doses of cefprozil of 0.8, 8.5 and 18.5 times the maximum daily human dose (1000 mg) based upon mg/m², and have revealed no harm to the fetus. There are, however, no adequate and well-controlled studies in pregnant women. Because animal reproduction studies are

Population/Infection	Dosage (mg)	Duration (days)
ADULTS (13 years and older)		
UPPER RESPIRATORY TRACT		
Pharyngitis/Tonsillitis	500 q 24h	10*
Acute Sinusitis	250 q 12h or	10
(For moderate to severe infections, the higher dose should be used)	500 q 12h	
LOWER RESPIRATORY TRACT		
Secondary Bacterial Infection of Acute Bronchitis and Acute Bacterial Exacerbation of Chronic Bronchitis	500 q 12h	10
SKIN AND SKIN STRUCTURE		
Uncomplicated Skin and Skin Structure Infections	250 q 12h or 500 q 24h or 500 q 12h	10
CHILDREN (2 years – 12 years)		
UPPER RESPIRATORY TRACT†		
Pharyngitis/Tonsillitis	7.5 mg/kg q 12h	10*
SKIN AND SKIN STRUCTURE†		
Uncomplicated Skin and Skin Structure Infections	20 mg/kg q 24h	10
INFANTS & CHILDREN (6 months – 12 years)		
UPPER RESPIRATORY TRACT†		
Otitis Media (See **INDICATIONS AND USAGE** and **CLINICAL STUDIES** sections)	15 mg/kg q 12h	10
Acute Sinusitis (For moderate to severe infections, the higher dose should be used	7.5 mg/kg q 12h 15 mg/kg	10

* In the treatment of infections due to *Streptococcus pyogenes*, CEFZIL should be administered for at least 10 days.
† Not to exceed recommended adult doses.

U.S. Acute Otitis Media Study
Cefprozil vs β-lactamase inhibitor-containing control drug

EFFICACY:

Pathogen	% of Cases with Pathogen (n = 155)	Outcome
S. pneumoniae	48.4%	cefprozil success rate 5% better than control
H. influenzae	35.5%	cefprozil success rate 17% less than control
M. catarrhalis	13.5%	cefprozil success rate 12% less than control
S. pyogenes	2.6%	cefprozil equivalent to control
Overall	100.0%	cefprozil success rate 5% less than control

SAFETY:
The incidence of adverse events, primarily diarrhea and rash*, were clinically and statistically significantly higher in the control arm versus the cefprozil arm.

not always predictive of human response, this drug should be used during pregnancy only if clearly needed.

Labor and Delivery

Cefprozil has not been studied for use during labor and delivery. Treatment should only be given if clearly needed.

Nursing Mothers

Small amounts of cefprozil (< 0.3% of dose) have been detected in human milk following administration of a single 1 gram dose to lactating women. The average levels over 24 hours ranged from 0.25 to 3.3 μg/mL. Caution should be exercised when CEFZIL is administered to a nursing woman, since the effect of cefprozil on nursing infants is unknown.

Pediatric Use: (See **INDICATIONS AND USAGE** and **DOSAGE AND ADMINISTRATION**.)

The safety and effectiveness of cefprozil in the treatment of otitis media have been established in the age groups 6 months to 12 years. Use of CEFZIL for the treatment of otitis media is supported by evidence from adequate and well-controlled studies of cefprozil in pediatric patients. (See **CLINICAL STUDIES** section.)

The safety and effectiveness of cefprozil in the treatment of pharyngitis/ tonsillitis or uncomplicated skin and skin structure infections have been established in the age groups 2 to 12 years. Use of CEFZIL for the treatment of these infections is supported by evidence from adequate and well-controlled studies of cefprozil in pediatric patients.

The safety and effectiveness of cefprozil in the treatment of acute sinusitis have been established in the age groups 6 months to 12 years. Use of CEFZIL in these age groups is supported by evidence from adequate and well-controlled studies of cefprozil in adults.

Safety and effectiveness in pediatric patients below the age of 6 months have not been established for the treatment of otitis media or acute sinusitis or below the age of 2 years for the treatment of pharyngitis/tonsillitis or uncomplicated skin and skin structure infections. However, accumulation

of other cephalosporin antibiotics in newborn infants (resulting from prolonged drug half-life in this age group) has been reported.

Geriatric Use

Healthy geriatric volunteers (≥ 65 years old) who received a single 1 g dose of cefprozil had 35%–60% higher AUC and 40% lower renal clearance values when compared to healthy adult volunteers 20–40 years of age. In clinical studies, when geriatric patients received the usual recommended adult doses, clinical efficacy and safety were acceptable and comparable to results in non-geriatric adult patients.

ADVERSE REACTIONS

The adverse reactions to cefprozil are similar to those observed with other orally administered cephalosporins. Cefprozil was usually well tolerated in controlled clinical trials. Approximately 2% of patients discontinued cefprozil therapy due to adverse events.

The most common adverse effects observed in patients treated with cefprozil are:

Gastrointestinal: Diarrhea (2.9%), nausea (3.5%), vomiting (1%) and abdominal pain (1%).

Hepatobiliary: Elevations of AST (SGOT) (2%), ALT (SGPT) (2%), alkaline phosphatase (0.2%), and bilirubin values (<0.1%). As with some penicillins and some other cephalosporin antibiotics, cholestatic jaundice has been reported rarely.

Hypersensitivity: Rash (0.9%), urticaria (0.1%). Such reactions have been reported more frequently in children than in adults. Signs and symptoms usually occur a few days after initiation of therapy and subside within a few days after cessation of therapy.

CNS: Dizziness (1%). Hyperactivity, headache, nervousness, insomnia, confusion, and somnolence have been reported rarely (<1%). All were reversible.

Continued on next page

Cefzil—Cont.

Hematopoietic: Decreased leukocyte count (0.2%), eosinophilia (2.3%).
Renal: Elevated BUN (0.1%), serum creatinine (0.1%).
Other: Diaper rash and superinfection (1.5%), genital pruritus and vaginitis (1.6%).
The following adverse events, regardless of established causal relationship to CEFZIL, have been rarely reported during post-marketing surveillance: anaphylaxis, angioedema, colitis (including pseudomembranous colitis), erythema multiforme, fever, serum-sickness like reactions, Stevens-Johnson Syndrome and thrombocytopenia.

Cephalosporin class paragraph

In addition to the adverse reactions listed above which have been observed in patients treated with cefprozil, the following adverse reactions and altered laboratory tests have been reported for cephalosporin-class antibiotics: Aplastic anemia, hemolytic anemia, hemorrhage, renal dysfunction, toxic epidermal necrolysis, toxic nephropathy, prolonged prothrombin time, positive Coombs' test, elevated LDH, pancytopenia, neutropenia, agranulocytosis. Several cephalosporins have been implicated in triggering seizures, particularly in patients with renal impairment, when the dosage was not reduced. (See **DOSAGE AND ADMINISTRATION** and **OVERDOSAGE**.) If seizures associated with drug therapy occur, the drug should be discontinued. Anticonvulsant therapy can be given if clinically indicated.

OVERDOSAGE

Single 5000 mg/kg oral doses of cefprozil caused no mortality or signs of toxicity in adult, weanling, or neonatal rats, or adult mice. A single oral dose of 3000 mg/kg caused diarrhea and loss of appetite in cynomolgus monkeys, but no mortality.
Cefprozil is eliminated primarily by the kidneys. In case of severe overdosage, especially in patients with compromised renal function, hemodialysis will aid in the removal of cefprozil from the body.

DOSAGE AND ADMINISTRATION

CEFZIL (cefprozil) is administered orally.
[See first table at top of previous page]

Renal Impairment

Cefprozil may be administered to patients with impaired renal function. The following dosage schedule should be used.

Creatinine Clearance (mL/min)	Dosage (mg)	Dosing Interval
30–120	standard	standard
0–29*	50% of standard	standard

* Cefprozil is in part removed by hemodialysis; therefore, cefprozil should be administered after the completion of hemodialysis.

Hepatic Impairment

No dosage adjustment is necessary for patients with impaired hepatic function.

HOW SUPPLIED

CEFZIL® (Cefprozil) Tablets
Each light orange film-coated tablet, imprinted with "7720" on one side and "250" on the other, contains the equivalent of 250 mg anhydrous cefprozil.

Bottles of 100 Tablets	NDC 0087-7720-60
Cartons of 100 Tablets	NDC 0087-7720-66

(10 strips containing 10 tablets on each strip)
Each white film-coated tablet, imprinted with "7721" on one side and "500" on the other, contains the equivalent of 500 mg anhydrous cefprozil.

Bottles of 50 Tablets	NDC 0087-7721-50
Bottles of 100 Tablets	NDC 0087-7721-60
Cartons of 100 Tablets	NDC 0087-7721-66

(10 strips containing 10 tablets on each strip)
Store at controlled room temperature, 59° to 86° F (15° to 30° C).
CEFZIL® (Cefprozil) For Oral Suspension
Each 5 mL of constituted suspension contains the equivalent of 125 mg anhydrous cefprozil.

50 mL Bottle	NDC 0087-7718-40
75 mL Bottle	NDC 0087-7718-62
100 mL Bottle	NDC 0087-7718-64

Each 5 mL of constituted suspension contains the equivalent of 250 mg anhydrous cefprozil.

50 mL Bottle	NDC 0087-7719-40
75 mL Bottle	NDC 0087-7719-62
100 mL Bottle	NDC 0087-7719-64

All powder formulations for oral suspension contain cefprozil in a bubble-gum flavored mixture.
Reconstitution Directions for Oral Suspension
Prepare the suspension at the time of dispensing; for ease in preparation, add water in two portions and shake well after each aliquot.

Total Amount of Water Required for Reconstitution

Bottle Size	Final Concentration 125 mg/ 5 mL	Final Concentration 250 mg/5 mL
50 mL	36 mL	36 mL
75 mL	54 mL	54 mL
100 mL	72 mL	72 mL

After mixing, store in a refrigerator and discard unused portion after 14 days.
Store at 59° to 77° F (15° to 25° C) prior to constitution.
U.S. Patent No. 4,520,022

CLINICAL STUDIES

Study One:
In a controlled clinical study of **acute otitis media** performed in the United States where significant rates of β-lactamase producing organisms were found, cefprozil was compared to an oral antimicrobial agent that contained a specific β-lactamase inhibitor. In this study, using very strict evaluability criteria and microbiologic and clinical response criteria at the 10-16 days post-therapy follow-up, the following presumptive bacterial eradication/clinical cure outcomes (i.e. clinical success) and safety results were obtained:
[See second table at top of previous page]

Age Group	Cefprozil	Control
6 months-2 years	21%	41%
3–12 years	10%	19%

*The majority of these involved the diaper area in young children.

Study Two:
In a controlled clinical study of **acute otitis media** performed in Europe, cefprozil was compared to an oral antimicrobial agent that contained a specific β-lactamase inhibitor. As expected in a European population, this study population had a lower incidence of β-lactamase-producing organisms than usually seen in U.S. trials. In this study, using very strict evaluability criteria and microbiologic and clinical response criteria at the 10–16 days post-therapy follow-up, the following presumptive bacterial eradication/clinical cure outcomes (i.e. clinical success) were obtained:
[See table below]

REFERENCES

1. National Committee for Clinical Laboratory Standards. *Methods for Dilution Antimicrobial Susceptibility Tests for Bacteria that Grow Aerobically*—Third Edition. Approved Standard NCCLS Document M7-A3, Vol. 13, No. 25, NCCLS, Villanova, PA, December, 1993.
2. National Committee for Clinical Laboratory Standards. *Methods for Antimicrobial Susceptibility Testing of Anaerobic Bacteria*—Third Edition. Approved Standard NCCLS Document M11-A3, Vol. 13, No. 26, NCCLS, Villanova, PA, December, 1993.
3. National Committee for Clinical Laboratory Standards. *Performance Standards for Antimicrobial Disk Susceptibility Tests*—Fifth Edition. Approved Standard NCCLS Document M2-A5, Vol. 13, No. 24, NCCLS, Villanova, PA, December, 1993.
4. Clinitest® is a registered trademark of the Bayer Corporation.
5. Tes-Tape® is a registered trademark of Eli Lilly and Company.

7718DIM-12
51-004077-03
Revised March 1998
Bristol-Myers Squibb Company
Princeton, New Jersey 08543
USA
Shown in Product Identification Guide, page 307

DURICEF® ℞

[dur 'ĭ-sef]
(cefadroxil monohydrate, USP)
500-mg capsules, 1-g tablets, oral suspensions
Rx only

DESCRIPTION

DURICEF® (cefadroxil monohydrate, USP) is a semisynthetic cephalosporin antibiotic intended for oral administration. It is a white to yellowish-white crystalline powder. It is soluble in water and it is acid-stable. It is chemically designated as 5-Thia-1-azabicyclo[4.2.0]oct-2-ene-2-carboxylic acid, 7-[[amino(4-hydroxyphenyl)acetyl] amino]-3-methyl-8-oxo-, monohydrate, [6R-[6α,7β(R*)]]-. It has the formula $C_{16}H_{17}N_3O_5S•H_2O$ and the molecular weight of 381.40. It has the following structural formula:

DURICEF film-coated tablets, 1 g, contain the following inactive ingredients: microcrystalline cellulose, hydroxypropyl methylcellulose, magnesium stearate, polyethylene glycol, polysorbate 80, simethicone emulsion, and titanium dioxide.
DURICEF for Oral Suspension contains the following inactive ingredients: FD&C Yellow No. 6, flavors (natural and artificial), polysorbate 80, sodium benzoate, sucrose, and xanthan gum.
DURICEF capsules contain the following inactive ingredients: D&C Red No. 28, FD&C Blue No. 1, FD&C Red No. 40, gelatin, magnesium stearate, and titanium dioxide.

CLINICAL PHARMACOLOGY

DURICEF is rapidly absorbed after oral administration. Following single doses of 500 and 1000 mg, average peak serum concentrations were approximately 16 and 28 μg/mL, respectively. Measurable levels were present 12 hours after administration. Over 90% of the drug is excreted unchanged in the urine within 24 hours. Peak urine concentrations are approximately 1800 μg/mL during the period following a single 500-mg oral dose. Increases in dosage generally produce a proportionate increase in DURICEF urinary concentration. The urine antibiotic concentration, following a 1-g dose, was maintained well above the MIC of susceptible urinary pathogens for 20 to 22 hours.

Microbiology

In vitro tests demonstrate that the cephalosporins are bactericidal because of their inhibition of cell-wall synthesis. Cefadroxil has been shown to be active against the following organisms both *in vitro* and in clinical infections (see INDICATIONS AND USAGE):
Beta-hemolytic streptococci
Staphylococci, including penicillinase-producing strains
Streptococcus (Diplococcus) pneumoniae
Escherichia coli
Proteus mirabilis
Klebsiella species
Moraxella (Branhamella) catarrhalis
Note: Most strains of *Enterococcus faecalis* (formerly *Streptococcus faecalis*) and *Enterococcus faecium* (formerly *Streptococcus faecium*) are resistant to DURICEF (cefadroxil monohydrate, USP). It is not active against most strains of *Enterobacter* species, *Morganella morganii* (formerly *Proteus morganii*), and *P. vulgaris*. It has no activity against *Pseudomonas* species and *Acinetobacter calcoaceticus* (formerly *Mima* and *Herellea* species).
Susceptibility tests: Diffusion techniques
The use of antibiotic disk susceptibility test methods which measure zone diameter give an accurate estimation of antibiotic susceptibility. One standard procedure[1] which has been recommended for use with disks to test susceptibility of organisms to cefadroxil uses the cephalosporin class (cephalothin) disk. Interpretation involves the correlation of the diameters obtained in the disk test with the minimum inhibitory concentration (MIC) for cefadroxil.
Reports from the laboratory giving results of the standard single-disk susceptibility test with a 30 μg cephalothin disk should be interpreted according to the following criteria:

European Acute Otitis Media Study
Cefprozil vs β-lactamase inhibitor-containing control drug

EFFICACY:

Pathogen	% of Cases with Pathogen (n = 47)	Outcome
S. pneumoniae	51.0%	cefprozil equivalent to control
H. influenzae	29.8%	cefprozil equivalent to control
M. catarrhalis	6.4%	cefprozil equivalent to control
S. pyogenes	12.8%	cefprozil equivalent to control
Overall	100.0%	cefprozil equivalent to control

SAFETY:
The incidence of adverse events in the cefprozil arm was comparable to the incidence of adverse events in the control arm (agent that contained a specific β-lactamase inhibitor).

Zone Diameter (mm)	Interpretation
≥ 18	(S) Susceptible
15-17	(I) Intermediate
≤ 14	(R) Resistant

A report of "Susceptible" indicates that the pathogen is likely to be inhibited by generally achievable blood levels. A report of "Intermediate susceptibility" suggests that the organism would be susceptible if high dosage is used or if the infection is confined to tissue and fluids (eg, urine) in which high antibiotic levels are attained. A report of "Resistant" indicates that achievable concentrations of the antibiotic are unlikely to be inhibitory and other therapy should be selected.
Standardized procedures require the use of laboratory control organisms. The 30 µg cephalothin disk should give the following zone diameters:

Organism	Zone Diameter (mm)
Staphylococcus aureus ATCC 25923	29-37
Escherichia coli ATCC 25922	17-22

Dilution Techniques
When using the NCCLS agar dilution or broth dilution (including microdilution) method[2] or equivalent, a bacterial isolate may be considered susceptible if the MIC (minimum inhibitory concentration) value for cephalothin is 8 µg/mL or less. Organisms are considered resistant if the MIC is 32 µg/mL or greater. Organisms with an MIC value of less than 32 µg/mL but greater than 8 µg/mL are intermediate.
As with standard diffusion methods, dilution procedures require the use of laboratory control organisms. Standard cephalothin powder should give MIC values in the range of 0.12 µg/mL and 0.5 µg/mL for *Staphylococcus aureus* ATCC 29213. For *Escherichia coli* ATCC 25922, the MIC range should be between 4.0 µg/mL and 16.0 µg/mL. For *Streptococcus faecalis* ATCC 29212, the MIC range should be between 8.0 and 32.0 µg/mL.

INDICATIONS AND USAGE

DURICEF (cefadroxil monohydrate, USP) is indicated for the treatment of patients with infection caused by susceptible strains of the designated organisms in the following diseases:
Urinary tract infections caused by *E. coli, P. mirabilis,* and *Klebsiella* species.
Skin and skin structure infections caused by staphylococci and/or streptococci.
Pharyngitis and/or tonsillitis caused by *Streptococcus pyogenes* (Group A beta-hemolytic streptococci).
Note: Only penicillin by the intramuscular route of administration has been shown to be effective in the prophylaxis of rheumatic fever. DURICEF is generally effective in the eradication of streptococci from the oropharynx. However, data establishing the efficacy of DURICEF for the prophylaxis of subsequent rheumatic fever are not available.
Note: Culture and susceptibility tests should be initiated prior to and during therapy. Renal function studies should be performed when indicated.

CONTRAINDICATIONS

DURICEF (cefadroxil monohydrate, USP) is contraindicated in patients with known allergy to the cephalosporin group of antibiotics.

WARNINGS

BEFORE THERAPY WITH DURICEF IS INSTITUTED, CAREFUL INQUIRY SHOULD BE MADE TO DETERMINE WHETHER THE PATIENT HAS HAD PREVIOUS HYPERSENSITIVITY REACTIONS TO CEFADROXIL, CEPHALOSPORINS, PENICILLINS, OR OTHER DRUGS. IF THIS PRODUCT IS TO BE GIVEN TO PENICILLIN-SENSITIVE PATIENTS, CAUTION SHOULD BE EXERCISED BECAUSE CROSS-SENSITIVITY AMONG BETA-LACTAM ANTIBIOTICS HAS BEEN CLEARLY DOCUMENTED AND MAY OCCUR IN UP TO 10% OF PATIENTS WITH A HISTORY OF PENICILLIN ALLERGY.
IF AN ALLERGIC REACTION TO DURICEF OCCURS, DISCONTINUE THE DRUG. SERIOUS ACUTE HYPERSENSITIVITY REACTIONS MAY REQUIRE TREATMENT WITH EPINEPHRINE AND OTHER EMERGENCY MEASURES, INCLUDING OXYGEN, INTRAVENOUS FLUIDS, INTRAVENOUS ANTIHISTAMINES, CORTICOSTEROIDS, PRESSOR AMINES, AND AIRWAY MANAGEMENT, AS CLINICALLY INDICATED.
Pseudomembranous colitis has been reported with nearly all antibacterial agents, including cefadroxil, and may range from mild to life-threatening. Therefore, it is important to consider this diagnosis in patients who present with diarrhea subsequent to the administration of antibacterial agents.
Treatment with antibacterial agents alters the normal flora of the colon and may permit overgrowth of clostridia. Studies indicate that a toxin produced by *Clostridium difficile* is a primary cause of "antibiotic-associated colitis."
After the diagnosis of pseudomembranous colitis has been established, therapeutic measures should be initiated. Mild cases of pseudomembranous colitis usually respond to discontinuation of the drug alone. In moderate to severe cases, consideration should be given to management with fluids and electrolytes, protein supplementation and treatment with an antibacterial drug effective against *Clostridium difficile.*

PRECAUTIONS

General
DURICEF should be used with caution in the presence of markedly impaired renal function (creatinine clearance rate of less than 50 mL/min/1.73 M^2). (See DOSAGE AND ADMINISTRATION.) In patients with known or suspected renal impairment, careful clinical observation and appropriate laboratory studies should be made prior to and during therapy.
Prolonged use of DURICEF may result in the overgrowth of nonsusceptible organisms. Careful observation of the patient is essential. If superinfection occurs during therapy, appropriate measures should be taken.
DURICEF® (cefadroxil monohydrate, USP) should be prescribed with caution in individuals with history of gastrointestinal disease, particularly colitis.
Drug/Laboratory Test Interactions
Positive direct Coombs' tests have been reported during treatment with the cephalosporin antibiotics. In hematologic studies or in transfusion cross-matching procedures when anti globulin tests are performed on the minor side or in Coombs' testing of newborns whose mothers have received cephalosporin antibiotics before parturition, it should be recognized that a positive Coombs' test may be due to the drug.
Carcinogenesis, Mutagenesis, and Impairment of Fertility: No long-term studies have been performed to determine carcinogenic potential. No genetic toxicity tests have been performed.
Pregnancy: Pregnancy Category B: Reproduction studies have been performed in mice and rats at doses up to 11 times the human dose and have revealed no evidence of impaired fertility or harm to the fetus due to cefadroxil monohydrate. There are, however, no adequate and well controlled studies in pregnant women. Because animal reproduction studies are not always predictive of human response, this drug should be used during pregnancy only if clearly needed.
Labor and Delivery: DURICEF (cefadroxil monohydrate, USP) has not been studied for use during labor and delivery. Treatment should only be given if clearly needed.
Nursing Mothers: Caution should be exercised when cefadroxil monohydrate is administered to a nursing mother.
Pediatric Use: (See DOSAGE AND ADMINISTRATION.)

ADVERSE REACTIONS

Gastrointestinal
Onset of pseudomembranous colitis symptoms may occur during or after antibiotic treatment (see WARNINGS). Dyspepsia, nausea and vomiting have been reported rarely. Diarrhea has also occurred.
Hypersensitivity
Allergies (in the form of rash, urticaria, angioedema, and pruritis) have been observed. These reactions usually subsided upon discontinuation of the drug. Anaphylaxis has also been reported.
Other
Other reactions have included hepatic dysfunction including cholestasis and elevations in serum transaminase, genital pruritus, genital moniliasis, vaginitis, moderate transient neutropenia, fever. Agranulocytosis, thrombocytopenia, idiosyncratic hepatic failure, erythema multiforme, Stevens-Johnson syndrome, serum sickness, and arthralgia have been rarely reported.
In addition to the adverse reactions listed above which have been observed in patients treated with cefadroxil, the following adverse reactions and altered laboratory tests have been reported for cephalosporin-class antibiotics:
Toxic epidermal necrolysis, abdominal pain, superinfection, renal dysfunction, toxic nephropathy, aplastic anemia, hemolytic anemia, hemorrhage, prolonged prothrombin time, positive Coombs test, increased BUN, increased creatinine, elevated alkaline phosphatase, elevated aspartate aminotransferase (AST), elevated alanine aminotransferase (ALT), elevated bilirubin, elevated LDH, eosinophilia, pancytopenia, neutropenia.
Several cephalosporins have been implicated in triggering seizures, particularly in patients with renal impairment, when the dosage was not reduced (see DOSAGE AND ADMINISTRATION and OVERDOSAGE). If seizures associated with drug therapy occur, the drug should be discontinued. Anticonvulsant therapy can be given if clinically indicated.

OVERDOSAGE

A study of children under six years of age suggested that ingestion of less than 250 mg/kg of cephalosporins is not associated with significant outcomes. No action is required other than general support and obser vation. For amounts greater than 250 mg/kg, induce gastric emptying.
In five anuric patients, it was demonstrated that an average of 63% of a 1 g oral dose is extracted from the body during a 6-8 hour hemodialysis session.

DOSAGE AND ADMINISTRATION

DURICEF is acid-stable and may be administered orally without regard to meals. Administration with food may be helpful in diminishing potential gastrointestinal complaints occasionally associated with oral cephalosporin therapy.
Adults
Urinary Tract Infections: For uncomplicated lower urinary tract infections (i.e., cystitis) the usual dosage is 1 or 2 g per day in single (q.d.) or divided doses (b.i.d.).
For all other urinary tract infections the usual dosage is 2 g per day in divided doses (b.i.d.).
Skin and Skin Structure Infections: For skin and skin structure infections the usual dosage is 1 g per day in single (q.d.) or divided doses (b.i.d.).
Pharyngitis and Tonsillitis: Treatment of group A beta-hemolytic streptococcal pharyngitis and tonsillitis—1 g per day in single (q.d.) or divided doses (b.i.d.) for 10 days.
Children
For urinary tract infections, the recommended daily dosage for children is 30 mg/kg/day in divided doses every 12 hours. For pharyngitis, tonsillitis, and impetigo, the recommended daily dosage for children is 30 mg/kg/day in a single dose or in equally divided doses every 12 hours. For other skin and skin structure infections, the recommended daily dosage is 30 mg/kg/day in equally divided doses every 12 hours. In the treatment of beta-hemolytic streptococcal infections, a therapeutic dosage of DURICEF should be administered for at least 10 days.
See chart for total daily dosage for children.

DAILY DOSAGE OF DURICEF® SUSPENSION

Child's Weight				
lbs	kg	125 mg/ 5 mL	250 mg/ 5 mL	500 mg/ 5 mL
10	4.5	1 tsp	—	
20	9.1	2 tsp	1 tsp	
30	13.6	3 tsp	1½ tsp	
40	18.2	4 tsp	2 tsp	1 tsp
50	22.7	5 tsp	2½ tsp	1¼ tsp
60	27.3	6 tsp	3 tsp	1½ tsp
70 & above	31.8+	—	—	2 tsp

In patients with renal impairment, the dosage of cefadroxil monohydrate should be adjusted according to creatinine clearance rates to prevent drug accumulation. The following schedule is suggested. In adults, the initial dose is 1000 mg of DURICEF (cefadroxil monohydrate, USP) and the maintenance dose (based on the creatinine clearance rate [mL/min/1.73 M^2]) is 500 mg at the time intervals listed below.

Creatinine Clearances	Dosage Interval
0-10 mL/min	36 hours
10-25 mL/min	24 hours
25-50 mL/min	12 hours

Patients with creatinine clearance rates over 50 mL/min may be treated as if they were patients having normal renal function.

Reconstitution Directions for Oral Suspension

Bottle Size	Reconstitution Directions
100 mL	Suspend in a total of 67 mL water. Method: Tap bottle lightly to loosen powder. Add 67 mL of water in two portions. Shake well after each addition.
75 mL	Suspend in a total of 51 mL water. Method: Tap bottle lightly to loosen powder. Add 51 mL of water in two portions. Shake well after each addition.
50 mL	Suspend in a total of 34 mL water. Method: Tap bottle lightly to loosen powder. Add 34 mL of water in two portions. Shake well after each addition.

After reconstitution, store in refrigerator. Shake well before using. Keep container tightly closed. Discard unused portion after 14 days.

Continued on next page

Duricef—Cont.

HOW SUPPLIED

DURICEF® (cefadroxil monohydrate, USP) 500 mg Capsules: opaque, maroon and white hard gelatin capsules, imprinted with "PPP" and "784" on one end and with "DURICEF" and "500 mg" on the other end. Capsules are supplied as follows:

NDC 0087-0784-07	Bottle of 20
NDC 0087-0784-46	Bottle of 50
NDC 0087-0784-42	Bottle of 100
NDC 0087-0784-44	10 strips of 10 individually labeled blisters with 1 capsule per blister

Store at controlled room temperature (15°-30° C).
DURICEF® 1 gram Tablets: white to off white, top bisected, oval shaped, imprinted with "PPP" on one side of the bisect and "785" on the other side of the bisect. Tablets are supplied as follows:

NDC 0087-0785-43	Bottle of 50
NDC 0087-0785-42	Bottle of 100
NDC 0087-0785-45	4 packs of 10 individually labeled blisters with 1 tablet per blister

Store at controlled room temperature (15°-30° C).
DURICEF® for Oral Suspension is orange-pineapple flavored, and is supplied as follows:

125 mg/5 mL	**NDC** 0087-0786-42	50 mL Bottle
	NDC 0087-0786-41	100 mL Bottle
250 mg/5 mL	**NDC** 0087-0782-42	50 mL Bottle
	NDC 0087-0782-41	100 mL Bottle
500 mg/5 mL	**NDC** 0087-0783-42	50 mL Bottle
	NDC 0087-0783-05	75 mL Bottle
	NDC 0087-0783-41	100 mL Bottle

Prior to reconstitution: Store at controlled room temperature (15°-30° C).

REFERENCES

1. National Committee for Clinical Laboratory Standards, Approved Standard, *Performance Standards for Antimicrobial Disk Susceptibility Test*, 4th Edition, Vol. 10 (7): M2-A4, Villanova, PA, April, 1990. **2.** National Committee for Clinical Laboratory Standards, Approved Standard: *Methods for Dilution Antimicrobial Susceptibility Tests for Bacteria that Grow Aerobically*, 2nd Edition, Vol. 10 (8): M7-A2, Villanova, PA, April, 1990.

0782DIM-05 Revised March 1998
E3-B001-3-98

Bristol-Myers Squibb Company
Princeton, NJ 08543
USA

Shown in Product Identification Guide, page 307

ESTRACE® ℞
(ESTRADIOL VAGINAL CREAM, USP, 0.01%)
[es'trāce]

ESTRACE® ℞
(ESTRADIOL TABLETS, USP)

Rx only

WARNINGS

1. ESTROGENS HAVE BEEN REPORTED TO INCREASE THE RISK OF ENDOMETRIAL CARCINOMA IN POSTMENOPAUSAL WOMEN.
Close clinical surveillance of all women taking estrogens is important. Adequate diagnostic measures, including endometrial sampling when indicated, should be undertaken to rule out malignancy in all cases of undiagnosed persistent or recurring abnormal vaginal bleeding. There is no evidence that "natural" estrogens are more or less hazardous than "synthetic" estrogens at equiestrogenic doses.

2. ESTROGENS SHOULD NOT BE USED DURING PREGNANCY.
There is no indication for estrogen therapy during pregnancy or during the immediate postpartum period. Estrogens are ineffective for the prevention or treatment of threatened or habitual abortion. Estrogens are not indicated for the prevention of postpartum breast engorgement.
Estrogen therapy during pregnancy is associated with an increased risk of congenital defects in the reproductive organs of the fetus, and possibly other birth defects. Studies of women who received diethylstilbestrol (DES) during pregnancy have shown that female offspring have an increased risk of vaginal adenosis, squamous cell dysplasia of the uterine cervix, and clear cell vaginal cancer later in life; male offspring have an increased risk of urogenital abnormalities and possibly testicular cancer later in life. The 1985 DES Task Force concluded that use of DES during pregnancy is associated with a subsequent increased risk of breast cancer in the mothers, although a causal relationship remains unproven and the observed level of excess risk is similar to that for a number of other breast cancer risk factors.

DESCRIPTION

Estradiol (17β-estradiol) is a white, crystalline solid, chemically described as estra-1,3,5(10)-triene-3,17β-diol. It has an empirical formula of $C_{18}H_{24}O_2$ and molecular weight of 272.37. The structural formula is:

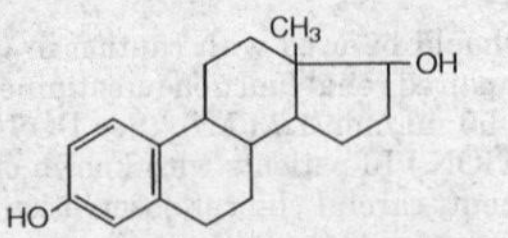

ESTRACE® (Estradiol Vaginal Cream, USP) contains 0.1 mg estradiol per gram in a nonliquefying base containing purified water, propylene glycol, stearyl alcohol, white ceresin wax, glyceryl monostearate, hydroxypropyl methylcellulose, 2208 4000 cps, sodium lauryl sulfate, methylparaben, edetate disodium and *tertiary*-butylhydroquinone.
ESTRACE® (Estradiol Tablets, USP) for oral administration contains 0.5, 1 or 2 mg of micronized estradiol per tablet.
ESTRACE Tablets, 0.5 mg, contain the following inactive ingredients: acacia, dibasic calcium phosphate, lactose, magnesium stearate, colloidal silicon dioxide, starch (corn), and talc.
ESTRACE Tablets, 1 mg, contain the following inactive ingredients: acacia, D&C Red No. 27 (aluminum lake), dibasic calcium phosphate, FD&C Blue No. 1 (aluminum lake), lactose, magnesium stearate, colloidal silicon dioxide, starch (corn), and talc.
ESTRACE Tablets, 2 mg, contain the following inactive ingredients: acacia, dibasic calcium phosphate, FD&C Blue No. 1 (aluminum lake), FD&C Yellow No. 5 (tartrazine) (aluminum lake), lactose, magnesium stearate, colloidal silicon dioxide, starch (corn), and talc.

CLINICAL PHARMACOLOGY

Estrogen drug products act by regulating the transcription of a limited number of genes. Estrogens diffuse through cell membranes, distribute themselves throughout the cell, and bind to and activate the nuclear estrogen receptor, a DNA-binding protein which is found in estrogen-responsive tissues. The activated estrogen receptor binds to specific DNA sequences, or hormone-response elements, which enhance the transcription of adjacent genes and in turn lead to the observed effects. Estrogen receptors have been identified in tissues of the reproductive tract, breast, pituitary, hypothalamus, liver, and bone of women.
Estrogens are important in the development and maintenance of the female reproductive system and secondary sex characteristics. By a direct action, they cause growth and development of the uterus, fallopian tubes, and vagina. With other hormones, such as pituitary hormones and progesterone, they cause enlargement of the breasts through promotion of ductal growth, stromal development, and the accretion of fat. Estrogens are intricately involved with other hormones, especially progesterone, in the processes of the ovulatory menstrual cycle and pregnancy, and affect the release of pituitary gonadotropins. They also contribute to the shaping of the skeleton, maintenance of tone and elasticity of urogenital structures, changes in the epiphyses of the long bones that allow for the pubertal growth spurt and its termination, and pigmentation of the nipples and genitals.
Estrogens occur naturally in several forms. The primary source of estrogen in normally cycling adult women is the ovarian follicle, which secretes 70 to 500 micrograms of estradiol daily, depending on the phase of the menstrual cycle. This is converted primarily to estrone, which circulates in roughly equal proportion to estradiol, and to small amounts of estriol. After menopause, most endogenous estrogen is produced by conversion of androstenedione, secreted by the adrenal cortex, to estrone by peripheral tissues. Thus, estrone—especially in its sulfate ester form—is the most abundant circulating estrogen in postmenopausal women. Although circulating estrogens exist in a dynamic equilibrium of metabolic interconversions, estradiol is the principal intracellular human estrogen and is substantially more potent than estrone or estriol at the receptor.
Estrogens used in therapy are well absorbed through the skin, mucous membranes, and gastrointestinal tract. When applied for a local action, absorption is usually sufficient to cause systemic effects. When conjugated with aryl and alkyl groups for parenteral administration, the rate of absorption of oily preparations is slowed with a prolonged duration of action, such that a single intramuscular injection of estradiol valerate or estradiol cypionate is absorbed over several weeks.
Administered estrogens and their esters are handled within the body essentially the same as the endogenous hormones. Metabolic conversion of estrogens occurs primarily in the liver (first pass effect), but also at local target tissue sites. Complex metabolic processes result in a dynamic equilibrium of circulating conjugated and unconjugated estrogenic forms which are continually interconverted, especially between estrone and estradiol and between esterified and non-esterified forms. Although naturally-occurring estrogens circulate in the blood largely bound to sex hormone-binding globulin and albumin, only unbound estrogens enter target tissue cells. A significant proportion of the circulating estrogen exists as sulfate conjugates, especially estrone sulfate, which serves as a circulating reservoir for the formation of more active estrogenic species. A certain proportion of the estrogen is excreted into the bile and then reabsorbed from the intestine. During this enterohepatic recirculation, estrogens are desulfated and resulfated and undergo degradation through conversion to less active estrogens (estriol and other estrogens), oxidation to nonestrogenic substances (catecholestrogens, which interact with catecholamine metabolism, especially in the central nervous system), and conjugation with glucuronic acids (which are then rapidly excreted in the urine).
When given orally, naturally-occurring estrogens and their esters are extensively metabolized (first pass effect) and circulate primarily as estrone sulfate, with smaller amounts of other conjugated and unconjugated estrogenic species. This results in limited oral potency. By contrast, synthetic estrogens, such as ethinyl estradiol and the nonsteroidal estrogens, are degraded very slowly in the liver and other tissues, which results in their high intrinsic potency. Estrogen drug products administered by non-oral routes are not subject to first-pass metabolism, but also undergo significant hepatic uptake, metabolism, and enterohepatic recycling.

INDICATIONS AND USAGE

ESTRACE® (Estradiol Vaginal Cream, USP, 0.01%) is indicated in the treatment of vulval and vaginal atrophy.
ESTRACE® (Estradiol Tablets, USP) is indicated in the:
1. Treatment of moderate to severe vasomotor symptoms associated with the menopause. There is no adequate evidence that estrogens are effective for nervous symptoms or depression which might occur during menopause and they should not be used to treat these conditions.
2. Treatment of vulval and vaginal atrophy.
3. Treatment of hypoestrogenism due to hypogonadism, castration or primary ovarian failure.
4. Treatment of breast cancer (for palliation only) in appropriately selected women and men with metastatic disease.
5. Treatment of advanced androgen-dependent carcinoma of the prostate (for palliation only).
6. Prevention of osteoporosis.
Since estrogen administration is associated with risk, selection of patients should ideally be based on prospective identification of risk factors for developing osteoporosis. Unfortunately, there is no certain way to identify those women who will develop osteoporotic fractures. Most prospective studies of efficacy for this indication have been carried out in white menopausal women, without stratification by other risk factors, and tend to show a universally salutary effect on bone. Thus, patient selection must be individualized based on the balance of risks and benefits. A more favorable risk/benefit ratio exists in a hysterectomized woman because she has no risk of endometrial cancer (see BOXED WARNINGS).
Estrogen replacement therapy reduces bone resorption and retards or halts postmenopausal bone loss. Case-control studies have shown an approximately 60 percent reduction in hip and wrist fractures in women whose estrogen replacement was begun within a few years of menopause. Studies also suggest that estrogen reduces the rate of vertebral fractures. Even when started as late as 6 years after menopause, estrogen prevents further loss of bone mass for as long as the treatment is continued. The results of a two-year, randomized, placebo-controlled, double-blind, dose-ranging study have shown that treatment with 0.5 mg estradiol daily for 23 days (of a 28 day cycle) prevents vertebral bone mass loss in postmenopausal women. When estrogen therapy is discontinued, bone mass declines at a rate comparable to the immediate postmenopausal period. There is no evidence that estrogen replacement therapy restores bone mass to premenopausal levels.
At skeletal maturity there are sex and race differences in both the total amount of bone present and its density, in favor of men and blacks. Thus, women are at higher risk than men because they start with less bone mass and, for several years following natural or induced menopause, the rate of bone mass decline is accelerated. White and Asian women are at higher risk than black women. Early menopause is one of the strongest predictors for the development of osteoporosis. In addition, other factors affecting the skeleton which are associated with osteoporosis include genetic factors (small build, family history), and endocrine factors (nulliparity, thyrotoxicosis, hyperparathyroidism, Cushing's syndrome, hyperprolactinemia, Type I diabetes), lifestyle (cigarette smoking, alcohol abuse, sedentary exercise habits) and nutrition (below average body weight, dietary calcium intake).
The mainstays of prevention and management of osteoporosis are estrogen, adequate lifetime calcium intake, and ex-

ercise. Postmenopausal women absorb dietary calcium less efficiently than premenopausal women and require an average of 1500 mg/day of elemental calcium to remain in neutral calcium balance. By comparison, premenopausal women require about 1000 mg/day and the average calcium intake in the USA is 400–600 mg/day. Therefore, when not contraindicated, calcium supplementation may be helpful. Weight-bearing exercise and nutrition may be important adjuncts to the prevention and management of osteoporosis. Immobilization and prolonged bed rest produce rapid bone loss, while weight-bearing exercise has been shown both to reduce bone loss and to increase bone mass. The optimal type and amount of physical activity that would prevent osteoporosis have not been established, however in two studies, an hour of walking and running exercise twice or three times weekly significantly increased lumbar spine bone mass.

CONTRAINDICATIONS

Estrogens should not be used in individuals with any of the following conditions:

1. Known or suspected pregnancy (see BOXED WARNINGS). Estrogens may cause fetal harm when administered to a pregnant woman.
2. Undiagnosed abnormal genital bleeding.
3. Known or suspected cancer of the breast except in appropriately selected patients being treated for metastatic disease.
4. Known or suspected estrogen-dependent neoplasia.
5. Active thrombophlebitis or thromboembolic disorders.

WARNINGS

1. Induction of malignant neoplasms.

Endometrial cancer. The reported endometrial cancer risk among unopposed estrogen users is about 2- to 12-fold greater than in non-users, and appears dependent on duration of treatment and on estrogen dose. Most studies show no significant increased risk associated with use of estrogens for less than one year. The greatest risk appears associated with prolonged use—with increased risks of 15- to 24-fold for five to ten years or more. In three studies, persistence of risk was demonstrated for 8 to over 15 years after cessation of estrogen treatment. In one study a significant decrease in the incidence of endometrial cancer occurred six months after estrogen withdrawal. Concurrent progestin therapy may offset this risk but the overall health impact in postmenopausal women is not known (see PRECAUTIONS).

Breast Cancer. While the majority of studies have not shown an increased risk of breast cancer in women who have ever used estrogen replacement therapy, some have reported a moderately increased risk (relative risks of 1.3-2.0) in those taking higher doses or those taking lower doses for prolonged periods of time, especially in excess of 10 years. Other studies have not shown this relationship.

While the effects of added progestins on the risk of breast cancer are also unknown, available epidemiological evidence suggests that progestins do not reduce, and may enhance, the moderately increased breast cancer incidence that has been reported with prolonged estrogen replacement therapy (see PRECAUTIONS).

Congenital lesions with malignant potential. Estrogen therapy during pregnancy is associated with an increased risk of fetal congenital reproductive tract disorders, and possibly other birth defects. Studies of women who received DES during pregnancy have shown that female offspring have an increased risk of vaginal adenosis, squamous cell dysplasia of the uterine cervix, and clear cell vaginal cancer later in life; male offspring have an increased risk of urogenital abnormalities and possibly testicular cancer later in life. Although some of these changes are benign, others are precursors of malignancy.

2. Gallbladder disease. Two studies have reported a 2- to 4-fold increase in the risk of gallbladder disease requiring surgery in women receiving postmenopausal estrogens.

3. Cardiovascular disease. Large doses of estrogen (5 mg conjugated estrogens per day), comparable to those used to treat cancer of the prostate and breast, have been shown in a large prospective clinical trial in men to increase the risks of nonfatal myocardial infarction, pulmonary embolism, and thrombophlebitis. These risks cannot necessarily be extrapolated from men to women. However, to avoid the theoretical cardiovascular risk to women caused by high estrogen doses, the dose for estrogen replacement therapy should not exceed the lowest effective dose.

4. Elevated blood pressure. Occasional blood pressure increases during estrogen replacement therapy have been attributed to idiosyncratic reactions to estrogens. More often, blood pressure has remained the same or has dropped. One study showed that postmenopausal estrogen users have higher blood pressure than nonusers. Two other studies showed slightly lower blood pressure among estrogen users compared to nonusers. Postmenopausal estrogen use does not increase the risk of stroke. Nonetheless, blood pressure should be monitored at regular intervals with estrogen use.

5. Hypercalcemia. Administration of estrogens may lead to severe hypercalcemia in patients with breast cancer and bone metastases. If this occurs, the drug should be stopped and appropriate measures taken to reduce the serum calcium level.

PRECAUTIONS

A. General

1. Addition of a progestin. Studies of the addition of a progestin for 10 or more days of a cycle of estrogen administration have reported a lowered incidence of endometrial hyperplasia than would be induced by estrogen treatment alone. Morphological and biochemical studies of endometria suggest that 10 to 14 days of progestin are needed to provide maximal maturation of the endometrium and to reduce the likelihood of hyperplastic changes.

There are, however, possible risks which may be associated with the use of progestins in estrogen replacement regimens. These include: (1) adverse effects on lipoprotein metabolism (lowering HDL and raising LDL) which could diminish the purported cardioprotective effect of estrogen therapy (see PRECAUTIONS below); (2) impairment of glucose tolerance; and (3) possible enhancement of mitotic activity in breast epithelial tissue, although few epidemiological data are available to address this point (see WARNINGS).

The choice of progestin, its dose, and its regimen may be important in minimizing these adverse effects, but these issues will require further study before they are clarified.

2. Cardiovascular risk. *A causal relationship between estrogen replacement therapy and reduction of cardiovascular disease in postmenopausal women has not been proven. Furthermore, the effect of added progestins on this putative benefit is not yet known.*

In recent years many published studies have suggested that there may be a cause-effect relationship between postmenopausal oral estrogen replacement therapy *without added progestins* and a decrease in cardiovascular disease in women. Although most of the observational studies which assessed this statistical association have reported a 20% to 50% reduction in coronary artery disease risk and associated mortality in estrogen takers, the following should be considered when interpreting these reports:

(1) Because only one of these studies was randomized and it was too small to yield statistically significant results, all relevant studies were subject to selection bias. Thus, the apparently reduced risk of coronary artery disease cannot be attributed with certainty to estrogen replacement therapy. It may instead have been caused by life-style and medical characteristics of the women studied with the result that healthier women were selected for estrogen therapy. In general, treated women were of higher socioeconomic and educational status, more slender, more physically active, more likely to have undergone surgical menopause, and less likely to have diabetes than the untreated women. Although some studies attempted to control for these selection factors, it is common for properly designed randomized trials to fail to confirm benefits suggested by less rigorous study designs. Thus, ongoing and future large-scale randomized trials may fail to confirm this apparent benefit.

(2) Current medical practice often includes the use of concomitant progestin therapy in women with intact uteri (see PRECAUTIONS and WARNINGS). While the effects of added progestins on the risk of ischemic heart disease are not known, all available progestins reverse at least some of the favorable effects of estrogens on HDL and LDL levels.

3. Physical examination. A complete medical and family history should be taken prior to the initiation of any estrogen therapy. The pretreatment and periodic physical examinations should include special reference to blood pressure, breasts, abdomen, and pelvic organs, and should include a Papanicolaou smear. As a general rule, estrogen should not be prescribed for longer than one year without reexamining the patient.

4. Hypercoagulability. Some studies have shown that women taking estrogen replacement therapy have hypercoagulability, primarily related to decreased antithrombin activity. This effect appears dose- and duration-dependent and is less pronounced than that associated with oral contraceptive use. Also, postmenopausal women tend to have increased coagulation parameters at baseline compared to pre-menopausal women. There is some suggestion that low dose postmenopausal mestranol may increase the risk of thromboembolism, although the majority of studies (of primarily conjugated estrogens users) report no such increase. There is insufficient information on hypercoagulability in women who have had previous thromboembolic disease.

5. Familial hyperlipoproteinemia. Estrogen therapy may be associated with massive elevations of plasma triglycerides leading to pancreatitis and other complications in patients with familial defects of lipoprotein metabolism.

6. Fluid retention. Because estrogens may cause some degree of fluid retention, conditions which might be exacerbated by this factor, such as asthma, epilepsy, migraine, and cardiac or renal dysfunction, require careful observation.

7. Uterine bleeding and mastodynia. Certain patients may develop undesirable manifestations of estrogenic stimulation, such as abnormal uterine bleeding and mastodynia.

8. Impaired liver function. Estrogens may be poorly metabolized in patients with impaired liver function and should be administered with caution.

ESTRACE® (Estradiol Tablets, USP), 2 mg, contain FD&C Yellow No. 5 (tartrazine) which may cause allergic-type reactions (including bronchial asthma) in certain susceptible individuals. Although the overall incidence of FD&C Yellow No. 5 (tartrazine) sensitivity in the general population is low, it is frequently seen in patients who also have aspirin hypersensitivity.

B. Information for the Patient. See text of Patient Package Insert below.

Advise patients that the number of doses per tube of ESTRACE® (Estradiol Vaginal Cream, USP, 0.01%) will vary with dosage requirements and patient handling.

C. Laboratory Tests. Estrogen administration should generally be guided by clinical response at the smallest dose, rather than laboratory monitoring, for relief of symptoms for those indications in which symptoms are observable. For prevention of osteoporosis, however, see DOSAGE AND ADMINISTRATION section under ESTRACE® (Estradiol Tablets, USP) item 5.

D. Drug/Laboratory Test Interactions.

1. Accelerated prothrombin time, partial thromboplastin time, and platelet aggregation time; increased platelet count; increased factors II, VII antigen, VIII antigen, VIII coagulant activity, IX, X, XII, VII-X complex, II-VII-X complex, and beta-thromboglobulin; decreased levels of antifactor Xa and antithrombin III, decreased antithrombin III activity; increased levels of fibrinogen and fibrinogen activity; increased plasminogen antigen and activity.

2. Increased thyroid-binding globulin (TBG) leading to increased circulating total thyroid hormone, as measured by protein-bound iodine (PBI), T4 levels (by column or by radioimmunoassay) or T3 levels by radioimmunoassay. T3 resin uptake is decreased, reflecting the elevated TBG. Free T4 and free T3 concentrations are unaltered.

3. Other binding proteins may be elevated in serum, i.e., corticosteroid binding globulin (CBG), sex hormone-binding globulin (SHBG), leading to increased circulating corticosteroids and sex steroids, respectively. Free or biologically active hormone concentrations are unchanged. Other plasma proteins may be increased (angiotensinogen/renin substrate, alpha-1-antitrypsin, ceruloplasmin).

4. Increased plasma HDL and HDL-2 subfraction concentrations, reduced LDL cholesterol concentration, increased triglycerides levels.

5. Impaired glucose tolerance.

6. Reduced response to metyrapone test.

7. Reduced serum folate concentration.

E. Carcinogenesis, Mutagenesis, and Impairment of Fertility. Long term continuous administration of natural and synthetic estrogens in certain animal species increases the frequency of carcinomas of the breast, uterus, cervix, vagina, testis, and liver. See CONTRAINDICATIONS and WARNINGS.

F. Pregnancy Category X. Estrogens should not be used during pregnancy. See CONTRAINDICATIONS and BOXED WARNINGS.

G. Nursing Mothers. As a general principle, the administration of any drug to nursing mothers should be done only when clearly necessary since many drugs are excreted in human milk. In addition, estrogen administration to nursing mothers has been shown to decrease the quantity and quality of the milk.

F. Pediatric Use. Safety and effectiveness in pediatric patients have not been established. Large and repeated doses of estrogen over an extended period of time have been shown to accelerate epiphyseal closure, resulting in short adult stature if treatment is initiated before the completion of physiologic puberty in normally developing children. In patients in whom bone growth is not complete, periodic monitoring of bone maturation and effects on epiphyseal centers is recommended.

Estrogen treatment of prepubertal children also induces premature breast development and vaginal cornification, and may potentially induce vaginal bleeding in girls. In boys, estrogen treatment may modify the normal pubertal process. All other physiological and adverse reactions shown to be associated with estrogen treatment of adults could potentially occur in the pediatric population, including thromboembolic disorders and growth stimulation of certain tumors. Therefore, estrogens should only be administered to pediatric patients when clearly indicated and the lowest effective dose should always be utilized.

ADVERSE REACTIONS

The following additional adverse reactions have been reported with estrogen therapy (see WARNINGS regarding induction of neoplasia, adverse effects on the fetus, increased incidence of gallbladder disease, cardiovascular disease, elevated blood pressure, and hypercalcemia).

1. **Genitourinary system.**

Changes in vaginal bleeding pattern and abnormal withdrawal bleeding or flow; breakthrough bleeding, spotting.

Increase in size of uterine leiomyomata.

Vaginal candidiasis.

Change in amount of cervical secretion.

Continued on next page

Estrace—Cont.

2. **Breasts.**
Tenderness, enlargement.
3. **Gastrointestinal.**
Nausea, vomiting.
Abdominal cramps, bloating.
Cholestatic jaundice.
Increased incidence of gallbladder disease.
4. **Skin.**
Chloasma or melasma that may persist when drug is discontinued.
Erythema multiforme.
Erythema nodosum.
Hemorrhagic eruption.
Loss of scalp hair.
Hirsutism.
5. **Eyes.**
Steepening of corneal curvature.
Intolerance to contact lenses.
6. **Central Nervous System.**
Headache, migraine, dizziness.
Mental depression.
Chorea.
7. **Miscellaneous.**
Increase or decrease in weight.
Reduced carbohydrate tolerance.
Aggravation of porphyria.
Edema.
Changes in libido.

OVERDOSAGE

Serious ill effects have not been reported following acute ingestion of large doses of estrogen-containing oral contraceptives by young children. Overdosage of estrogen may cause nausea and vomiting, and withdrawal bleeding may occur in females.

DOSAGE AND ADMINISTRATION

ESTRACE® (Estradiol Vaginal Cream, USP, 0.01%) .
For treatment of vulval and vaginal atrophy associated with the menopause, the lowest dose and regimen that will control symptoms should be chosen and medication should be discontinued as promptly as possible.
Attempts to discontinue or taper medication should be made at 3-month to 6-month intervals.
Usual Dosage: The usual dosage range is 2 to 4 g (marked on the applicator) daily for one or two weeks, then gradually reduced to one half initial dosage for a similar period. A maintenance dosage of 1 g, one to three times a week, may be used after restoration of the vaginal mucosa has been achieved.
NOTE: The number of doses per tube will vary with dosage requirements and patient handling.
Patients with intact uteri should be monitored closely for signs of endometrial cancer and appropriate diagnostic measures should be taken to rule out malignancy in the event of persistent or recurring abnormal vaginal bleeding.

ESTRACE® (Estradiol Tablets, USP)
1. For treatment of moderate to severe vasomotor symptoms, vulval and vaginal atrophy associated with the menopause, the lowest dose and regimen that will control symptoms should be chosen and medication should be discontinued as promptly as possible.
Attempts to discontinue or taper medication should be made at 3-month to 6-month intervals.
The usual initial dosage range is 1 to 2 mg daily of estradiol adjusted as necessary to control presenting symptoms. The minimal effective dose for maintenance therapy should be determined by titration. Administration should be cyclic (e.g., 3 weeks on and 1 week off).
2. For treatment of female hypoestrogenism due to hypogonadism, castration, or primary ovarian failure.
Treatment is usually initiated with a dose of 1 to 2 mg daily of estradiol, adjusted as necessary to control presenting symptoms; the minimal effective dose for maintenance therapy should be determined by titration.
3. For treatment of breast cancer, for palliation only, in appropriately selected women and men with metastatic disease.
Suggested dosage is 10 mg three times daily for a period of at least three months.
4. For treatment of advanced androgen-dependent carcinoma of the prostate, for palliation only.
Suggested dosage is 1 to 2 mg three times daily. The effectiveness of therapy can be judged by phosphatase determinations as well as by symptomatic improvement of the patient.
5. For prevention of osteoporosis.
Therapy with ESTRACE® (Estradiol Tablets, USP) to prevent postmenopausal bone loss should be initiated as soon as possible after menopause. A daily dosage of 0.5 mg should be administered cyclically (i.e., 23 days on and 5 days off). The dosage may be adjusted if necessary to control concur-

rent menopausal symptoms. Discontinuation of estrogen replacement therapy may re-establish the natural rate of bone loss.

HOW SUPPLIED

ESTRACE® (Estradiol Vaginal Cream, USP, 0.01%)
NDC 0087-0754-42: Tube containing 1½ oz (42.5 g) with a calibrated plastic applicator for delivery of 1,2,3, or 4 g. Store at room temperature. Protect from temperatures in excess of 40°C (104°F).
ESTRACE® (Estradiol Tablets, USP) 0.5 mg: round, white scored tablets imprinted with **021** and **MJ** on one side.
NDC 0087-0021-41   Bottles of 100
ESTRACE® (Estradiol Tablets, USP) 1 mg: round, lavender scored tablets imprinted with **755** and **MJ** on one side.
NDC 0087-0755-01   Bottles of 100
NDC 0087-0755-48   Bottles of 500
ESTRACE® (Estradiol Tablets, USP) 2 mg: round, turquoise scored tablets imprinted with **756** and **MJ** on one side.
NDC 0087-0756-01   Bottles of 100
NDC 0087-0756-48   Bottles of 500
Store at controlled room temperature 15°–30°C (59°–86°F). Dispense in a tight, light-resistant container as defined in the USP.

INFORMATION FOR THE PATIENT
INTRODUCTION

NOTE: The number of doses per tube of ESTRACE® (Estradiol Vaginal Cream, USP, 0.01%) will vary with dosage requirements and patient handling.
This leaflet describes when and how to use estrogens, and the risks and benefits of estrogen treatment.
Estrogens have important benefits but also some risks. You must decide, with your doctor, whether the risks to you of estrogen use are acceptable because of their benefits. If you use estrogens, check with your doctor to be sure you are using the lowest possible dose that works, and that you don't use them longer than necessary. How long you need to use estrogens will depend on the reason for use.

WARNINGS
1. ESTROGENS INCREASE THE RISK OF CANCER OF THE UTERUS IN WOMEN WHO HAVE HAD THEIR MENOPAUSE ("CHANGE OF LIFE").
If you use any estrogen-containing drug, it is important to visit your doctor regularly and report any unusual vaginal bleeding right away. Vaginal bleeding after menopause may be a warning sign of uterine cancer. Your doctor should evaluate any unusual vaginal bleeding to find out the cause.
2. ESTROGENS SHOULD NOT BE USED DURING PREGNANCY.
Estrogens do not prevent miscarriage (spontaneous abortion) and are not needed in the days following childbirth. If you take estrogens during pregnancy, your unborn child has a greater than usual chance of having birth defects. The risk of developing these defects is small, but clearly larger than the risk in children whose mothers did not take estrogens during pregnancy. These birth defects may affect the baby's urinary system and sex organs. Daughters born to mothers who took DES (an estrogen drug) have a higher than usual chance of developing cancer of the vagina or cervix when they become teenagers or young adults. Sons may have a higher than usual chance of developing cancer of the testicles when they become teenagers or young adults.

USES OF ESTROGEN
(Not every estrogen drug is approved for every use listed in this section. If you want to know which of these possible uses are approved for the medicine prescribed for you, ask your doctor or pharmacist to show you the professional labeling. You can also look up the specific estrogen product in a book called the "Physicians' Desk Reference", which is available in many book stores and public libraries. Generic drugs carry virtually the same labeling information as their brand name versions.)
• **To reduce moderate or severe menopausal symptoms.** Estrogens are hormones made by the ovaries of normal women. Between ages 45 and 55, the ovaries normally stop making estrogens. This leads to a drop in body estrogen levels which causes the "change of life" or menopause (the end of monthly menstrual periods). If both ovaries are removed during an operation before natural menopause takes place, the sudden drop in estrogen levels causes "surgical menopause."
When the estrogen levels begin dropping, some women develop very uncomfortable symptoms, such as feelings of warmth in the face, neck, and chest, or sudden intense episodes of heat and sweating ("hot flashes" or "hot flushes"). Using estrogen drugs can help the body adjust to lower estrogen levels and reduce these symptoms. Most women have only mild menopausal symptoms or none at all and do not need to use estrogen drugs for these symptoms. Others may need to take estrogens for a few months while their bodies adjust to lower estrogen levels. The ma-

jority of women do not need estrogen replacement for longer than six months for these symptoms.
• **To treat vulval and vaginal atrophy** (itching, burning, dryness in or around the vagina, difficulty or burning on urination) associated with menopause.
• **To treat certain conditions in which a young woman's ovaries do not produce enough estrogen naturally.**
• **To treat certain types of abnormal vaginal bleeding due to hormonal imbalance when your doctor has found no serious cause of the bleeding.**
• **To treat certain cancers in special situations, in men and women.**
• **To prevent thinning of bones.**
Osteoporosis is a thinning of the bones that makes them weaker and allows them to break more easily. The bones of the spine, wrists and hips break most often in osteoporosis. Both men and women start to lose bone mass after about age 40, but women lose bone mass faster after the menopause. Using estrogens after the menopause slows down bone thinning and may prevent bones from breaking. Lifelong adequate calcium intake, either in the diet (such as dairy products) or by calcium supplements (to reach a total daily intake of 1000 milligrams per day before menopause or 1500 milligrams per day after menopause), may help to prevent osteoporosis. Regular weight-bearing exercise (like walking and running for an hour, two or three times a week) may also help to prevent osteoporosis. Before you change your calcium intake or exercise habits, it is important to discuss these lifestyle changes with your doctor to find out if they are safe for you.
Since estrogen use has some risks, only women who are likely to develop osteoporosis should use estrogens for prevention. Women who are likely to develop osteoporosis often have the following characteristics: white or Asian race, slim, cigarette smokers, and a family history of osteoporosis in a mother, sister, or aunt. Women who have relatively early menopause, often because their ovaries were removed during an operation ("surgical menopause"), are more likely to develop osteoporosis than women whose menopause happens at the average age.

WHO SHOULD NOT USE ESTROGENS
Estrogens should not be used:
• **During pregnancy (see Boxed Warnings).** If you think you may be pregnant, do not use any form of estrogen-containing drug. Using estrogens while you are pregnant may cause your unborn child to have birth defects. Estrogens do not prevent miscarriage.
• **If you have unusual vaginal bleeding which has not been evaluated by your doctor (see Boxed Warnings).** Unusual vaginal bleeding can be a warning sign of cancer of the uterus, especially if it happens after menopause. Your doctor must find out the cause of the bleeding so that he or she can recommend the proper treatment. Taking estrogens without visiting your doctor can cause you serious harm if your vaginal bleeding is caused by cancer of the uterus.
• **If you have had cancer.** Since estrogens increase the risk of certain types of cancer, you should not use estrogens if you have ever had cancer of the breast or uterus, unless your doctor recommends that the drug may help in the cancer treatment. (For certain patients with breast or prostate cancer, estrogens may help.)
• **If you have any circulation problems.** Estrogen drugs should not be used except in unusually special situations in which your doctor judges that you need estrogen therapy so much that the risks are acceptable. Men and women with abnormal blood clotting conditions should avoid estrogen use (see Dangers of Estrogens, below).
• **When they do not work.** During menopause, some women develop nervous symptoms or depression. Estrogens do not relieve these symptoms. You may have heard that taking estrogens for years after menopause will keep your skin soft and supple and keep you feeling young. There is no evidence for these claims and such long-term estrogen use may have serious risks.
• **After childbirth or when breastfeeding a baby.** Estrogens should not be used to try to stop the breasts from filling with milk after a baby is born. Such treatment may increase the risk of developing blood clots (see Dangers of Estrogens, below).
If you are breastfeeding, you should avoid using any drugs because many drugs pass through to the baby in the milk. While nursing a baby, you should take drugs only on the advice of your health care provider.

DANGERS OF ESTROGENS
• **Cancer of the uterus.** Your risk of developing cancer of the uterus gets higher the longer you use estrogens and the larger doses you use. One study showed that after women stop taking estrogens, this higher cancer risk quickly returns to the usual level of risk (as if you had never used estrogen therapy). Three other studies showed that the cancer risk stayed high for 8 to more than 15 years after stopping estrogen treatment. Because of this risk, **IT IS IMPORTANT TO TAKE THE LOWEST DOSE THAT WORKS AND TO TAKE IT ONLY AS LONG AS YOU NEED IT.**
Using progestin therapy together with estrogen therapy

may reduce the higher risk of uterine cancer related to estrogen use (but see Other Information, below).
If you have had your uterus removed (total hysterectomy), there is no danger of developing cancer of the uterus.

- **Cancer of the breast.** Most studies have not shown a higher risk of breast cancer in women who have ever used estrogens. However, some studies have reported that breast cancer developed more often (up to twice the usual rate) in women who used estrogens for long periods of time (especially more than 10 years), or who used higher doses for shorter time periods.
Regular breast examinations by a health professional and monthly self-examination are recommended for all women.
- **Gallbladder disease.** Women who use estrogens after menopause are more likely to develop gallbladder disease needing surgery than women who do not use estrogens.
- **Abnormal blood clotting.** Taking estrogens may cause changes in your blood clotting system. These changes allow the blood to clot more easily, possibly allowing clots to form in your bloodstream. If blood clots do form in your bloodstream, they can cut off the blood supply to vital organs, causing serious problems. These problems may include a stroke (by cutting off blood to the brain), a heart attack (by cutting off blood to the heart), a pulmonary embolus (by cutting off blood to the lungs), or other problems. Any of these conditions may cause death or serious long term disability. However, most studies of low dose estrogen usage by women do not show an increased risk of these complications.

SIDE EFFECTS
In addition to the risks listed above, the following side effects have been reported with estrogen use:
— Nausea and vomiting.
— Breast tenderness or enlargement.
— Enlargement of benign tumors ("fibroids") of the uterus.
— Retention of excess fluid. This may make some conditions worsen, such as asthma, epilepsy, migraine, heart disease, or kidney disease.
— A spotty darkening of the skin, particularly of the face.

REDUCING RISK OF ESTROGEN USE
If you use estrogens, you can reduce your risks by doing these things:

- **See your doctor regularly.** While you are using estrogens, it is important to visit your doctor at least once a year for a check-up. If you develop vaginal bleeding while taking estrogens, you may need further evaluation. If members of your family have had breast cancer or if you have ever had breast lumps or an abnormal mammogram (breast x-ray), you may need to have more frequent breast examinations.
- **Reassess your need for estrogens.** You and your doctor should reevaluate whether or not you still need estrogens at least every six months.
- **Be alert for signs of trouble.** If any of these warning signals (or any other unusual symptoms) happen while you are using estrogens, call your doctor immediately:
— Abnormal bleeding from the vagina (possible uterine cancer)
— Pains in the calves or chest, sudden shortness of breath, or coughing blood (possible clot in the legs, heart, or lungs)
— Severe headache or vomiting, dizziness, faintness, changes in vision or speech, weakness or numbness of an arm or leg (possible clot in the brain or eye)
— Breast lumps (possible breast cancer; ask your doctor or health professional to show you how to examine your breasts monthly)
— Yellowing of the skin or eyes (possible liver problem)
— Pain, swelling, or tenderness in the abdomen (possible gallbladder problem)

OTHER INFORMATION
1. Estrogens increase the risk of developing a condition (endometrial hyperplasia) that may lead to cancer of the lining of the uterus. Taking progestins, another hormone drug, with estrogens lowers the risk of developing this condition. Therefore, if your uterus has not been removed, your doctor may prescribe a progestin for you to take together with the estrogen.
You should know, however, that taking estrogens **with** progestins may have additional risks. These include: (a) unhealthy effects on blood fats (especially the lowering of HDL blood cholesterol, the "good" blood fat which protects against heart disease); (b) unhealthy effects on blood sugar (which might make a diabetic condition worse); and (c) a possible further increase in breast cancer risk which may be associated with long-term estrogen use.
Some research has shown that estrogens taken **without** progestins may protect women against developing heart disease. However, this is not certain. The protection shown may have been caused by the characteristics of the estrogen-treated women, and not by the estrogen treatment itself. In general, treated women were slimmer, more physically active, and were less likely to have diabetes than the untreated women. These characteristics are known to be associated with a reduced risk for heart disease.
You are cautioned to discuss very carefully with your doctor or health care provider all the possible risks and benefits of long-term estrogen and progestin treatment as they affect you personally.
2. Your doctor has prescribed this drug for you and you alone. Do not give the drug to anyone else.
3. If you will be taking calcium supplements as part of the treatment to help prevent osteoporosis, check with your doctor about how much to take.
4. Keep this and all drugs out of the reach of children. In case of overdose, call your doctor, hospital or poison control center immediately.
5. This leaflet provides a summary of the most important information about estrogens. If you want more information, ask your doctor or pharmacist to show you the professional labeling. The professional labeling is also published in a book called the "Physicians' Desk Reference", which is available in book stores and public libraries. Generic drugs carry virtually the same labeling information as their brand name versions.

Bristol-Myers Squibb Company
Princeton, New Jersey 08543
U.S.A.
A1-B001C-05-98 0755DIM-05-06-98
J4503E

GLUCOPHAGE® ℞
[glü-kō-faj]
(metformin hydrochloride tablets)
500 mg and 850 mg

DESCRIPTION
GLUCOPHAGE (metformin hydrochloride tablets) is an oral antihyperglycemic drug used in the management of non-insulin-dependent diabetes mellitus (NIDDM). Metformin hydrochloride (N,N-dimethylimidodicarbonimidic diamide hydrochloride) is not chemically or pharmacologically related to the oral sulfonylureas. The structural formula is as shown:

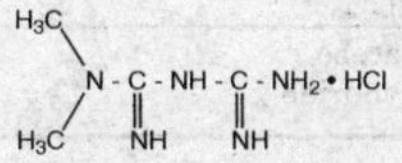

Metformin hydrochloride is a white to off-white crystalline compound with a molecular formula of $C_4H_{11}N_5$•HCl and a molecular weight of 165.63. Metformin hydrochloride is freely soluble in water and is practically insoluble in acetone, ether and chloroform. The pK_a of metformin is 12.4. The pH of a 1% aqueous solution of metformin hydrochloride is 6.68.
GLUCOPHAGE tablets contain 500 mg and 850 mg of metformin hydrochloride. In addition, each tablet contains the following inactive ingredients: povidone, magnesium stearate and hydroxypropyl methylcellulose (hypromellose) coating.

CLINICAL PHARMACOLOGY:
Antidiabetic Activity
GLUCOPHAGE is an antihyperglycemic agent which improves glucose tolerance in NIDDM subjects, lowering both basal and postprandial plasma glucose. Its pharmacologic mechanisms of action are different from those of sulfonylureas. GLUCOPHAGE decreases hepatic glucose production, decreases intestinal absorption of glucose and improves insulin sensitivity (increases peripheral glucose uptake and utilization). Unlike sulfonylureas, GLUCOPHAGE does not produce hypoglycemia in either diabetic or nondiabetic subjects (except in special circumstances, see PRECAUTIONS) and does not cause hyperinsulinemia. With metformin therapy, insulin secretion remains unchanged while fasting insulin levels and day-long plasma insulin response may actually decrease.
In a double-blind, placebo-controlled, multicenter U.S. clinical trial involving obese NIDDM patients whose hyperglycemia was not adequately controlled with dietary management alone (baseline fasting plasma glucose [FPG] of approximately 240 mg/dL), treatment with GLUCOPHAGE (up to 2.55 g/day) for 29 weeks resulted in significant mean net reductions in fasting and postprandial plasma glucose (PPG) and HbA_{1c} of 59 mg/dL, 83 mg/dL, and 1.8%, respectively, compared to placebo group (see Table 1).
[See table 1 below]
Monotherapy with GLUCOPHAGE may be effective in patients who have not responded to sulfonylureas or who have only a partial response to sulfonylureas or who have ceased to respond to sulfonylureas. In such patients, if adequate glycemic control is not attained with GLUCOPHAGE monotherapy, the combination of GLUCOPHAGE and a sulfonylurea may have a synergistic effect, since both agents act to improve glucose tolerance by different but complementary mechanisms.
A 29-week, double-blind, placebo-controlled study of GLUCOPHAGE and glyburide, alone and in combination, was conducted in obese NIDDM patients who had failed to achieve adequate glycemic control while on maximum doses of glyburide (baseline FPG of approximately 250 mg/dL) (see Table 2). Patients randomized to continue on glyburide experienced worsening of glycemic control, with mean increases in FPG, PPG and HbA_{1c} of 14 mg/dL, 3 mg/dL and 0.2%, respectively. In contrast, those randomized to GLUCOPHAGE (metformin hydrochloride tablets) (up to 2.5 g/day) did not experience a deterioration in glycemic control, but rather a slight improvement, with mean reductions in FPG, PPG and HbA_{1c} of 1 mg/dL, 6 mg/dL and 0.4%, respectively. The combination of GLUCOPHAGE and glyburide was synergistic in reducing FPG, PPG and HbA_{1c} levels by 63 mg/dL, 65 mg/dL, and 1.7%, respectively. Compared to results of glyburide treatment alone, the net differences with combination treatment were -77 mg/dL, -68 mg/dL and -1.9%, respectively (see Table 2).
[See table 2 at top of next page]
The magnitude of the decline in fasting blood glucose concentration following the institution of GLUCOPHAGE (metformin hydrochloride tablets) therapy is proportional to the level of fasting hyperglycemia. Non-insulin-dependent diabetics with higher fasting glucose concentrations will experience greater declines in plasma glucose and glycosylated hemoglobin.
GLUCOPHAGE has a modest favorable effect on serum lipids, which are often abnormal in NIDDM patients. In clinical studies, particularly when baseline levels were abnormally elevated, GLUCOPHAGE, alone or in combination with a sulfonylurea, lowered mean fasting serum triglycerides, total cholesterol and LDL cholesterol levels and had no adverse effects on other lipid levels (see Table 3).
[See table 3 on next page]
In contrast to sulfonylureas, body weight of individuals on GLUCOPHAGE tends to remain stable or may even decrease somewhat (see Tables 1 and 2).
In summary, metformin-treated patients showed significant improvement in all parameters of glycemic control (FPG, PPG and HbA_{1c}), stabilization or decrease in body weight, and a tendency to improvement in the lipid profile, particularly when baseline values are abnormally elevated.
Pharmacokinetics
Absorption and Bioavailability:
The absolute bioavailability of a 500 mg metformin hydrochloride tablet given under fasting conditions is approximately 50–60%. Studies using single oral doses of met-

Continued on next page

Table 1. GLUCOPHAGE vs Placebo
Summary of Mean Changes from Baseline* in Plasma Glucose
HbA_{1C} and Body Weight, at Final Visit (29-week study)

	GLUCOPHAGE (n = 141)	Placebo (n = 145)	P-Value
FPG (mg/dL)			
Baseline	241.5	237.7	NS
Change at FINAL VISIT	−53.0	6.3	0.001**
Hemoglobin A_{1C} (%)			
Baseline	8.4	8.2	NS
Change at FINAL VISIT	−1.4	0.4	0.001**
Body Weight (lbs)			
Baseline	201.0	206.0	NS
Change at FINAL VISIT	−1.4	−2.4	NS

*All patients on diet therapy at Baseline
**Statistically significant

Glucophage—Cont.

formin tablets of 500 mg and 1500 mg, and 850 mg to 2550 mg, indicate that there is a lack of dose proportionality with increasing doses, which is due to decreased absorption rather than an alteration in elimination. Food decreases the extent and slightly delays the absorption of metformin, as shown by approximately a 40% lower peak concentration and 25% lower AUC in plasma and a 35 minute prolongation of time to peak plasma concentration following administration of a single 850 mg tablet of metformin with food, compared to the same tablet strength administered fasting. The clinical relevance of these decreases is unknown.

Distribution:
The apparent volume of distribution (V/F) of metformin following single oral doses of 850 mg averaged 654 ± 358 L. Metformin is negligibly bound to plasma proteins in contrast to sulfonylureas which are more than 90% protein bound. Metformin partitions into erythrocytes, most likely as a function of time. At usual clinical doses and dosing schedules of GLUCOPHAGE (metformin hydrochloride tablets), steady state plasma concentrations of metformin are reached within 24–48 hours and are generally < 1 µg/mL. During controlled clinical trials, maximum metformin plasma levels did not exceed 5 µg/mL, even at maximum doses.

Metabolism and Elimination:
Intravenous single-dose studies in normal subjects demonstrate that metformin is excreted unchanged in the urine and does not undergo hepatic metabolism (no metabolites have been identified in humans) nor biliary excretion. Renal clearance (see Table 4) is approximately 3.5 times greater than creatinine clearance which indicates that tubular secretion is the major route of metformin elimination. Following oral administration, approximately 90% of the absorbed drug is eliminated via the renal route within the first 24 hours, with a plasma elimination half-life of approximately 6.2 hours. In blood, the elimination half-life is approximately 17.6 hours, suggesting that the erythrocyte mass may be a compartment of distribution.

Special Populations:
NIDDM Subjects:
In the presence of normal renal function, there are no differences between single or multiple dose pharmacokinetics of metformin between diabetics and nondiabetics (see Table 4), nor is there any accumulation of metformin in either group at usual clinical doses.

Renal Insufficiency:
In subjects with decreased renal function (based on measured creatinine clearance), the plasma and blood half-life of metformin is prolonged and the renal clearance is decreased in proportion to the decrease in creatinine clearance (see Table 4).

Hepatic Insufficiency:
No pharmacokinetic studies have been conducted in subjects with hepatic insufficiency.

Geriatrics:
Limited data from controlled pharmacokinetic studies of metformin in healthy elderly subjects suggest that total plasma clearance is decreased, the half-life is prolonged and C_{max} is increased, compared to healthy young subjects. From these data, it appears that the change in metformin pharmacokinetics with aging is primarily accounted for by a change in renal function (see Table 4).
[See table 4 at right]

Pediatrics:
No pharmacokinetic studies have been conducted in pediatric subjects.

Gender:
Metformin pharmacokinetic parameters did not differ significantly in diabetic and nondiabetic subjects when analyzed according to gender (males = 19, females = 16). Similarly, in controlled clinical studies in patients with NIDDM, the antihyperglycemic effect of GLUCOPHAGE (metformin hydrochloride tablets) was comparable in males and females.

Race:
No studies of metformin pharmacokinetic parameters according to race have been performed. In controlled clinical studies of GLUCOPHAGE in patients with NIDDM, the antihyperglycemic effect was comparable in whites (n = 249), blacks (n = 51) and hispanics (n = 24).

INDICATIONS AND USE

GLUCOPHAGE (metformin hydrochloride tablets), as monotherapy, is indicated as an adjunct to diet to lower blood glucose in patients with NIDDM whose hyperglycemia cannot be satisfactorily managed on diet alone.
GLUCOPHAGE may be used concomitantly with a sulfonylurea when diet and GLUCOPHAGE or a sulfonylurea alone do not result in adequate glycemic control.
In initiating treatment for NIDDM, diet should be emphasized as the primary form of treatment. Caloric restriction and weight loss are essential in the obese diabetic patient. Proper dietary management alone may be effective in controlling the blood glucose and symptoms of hyperglycemia.

Loss of blood glucose control in diet-managed patients may be transient, thus requiring only short-term pharmacologic therapy. The importance of regular physical activity should also be stressed, and cardiovascular risk factors should be identified and corrective measures taken where possible. If this treatment program fails to reduce symptoms and/or blood glucose, the use of GLUCOPHAGE alone or GLUCOPHAGE plus a sulfonylurea should be considered. If, after a suitable trial of such treatments, glucose control still has not been achieved, consideration should be given to the use of insulin. Judgments should be based on regular clinical and laboratory evaluations.

CONTRAINDICATIONS:

GLUCOPHAGE is contraindicated in patients with:
1. Renal disease or renal dysfunction (e.g., as suggested by serum creatinine levels ≥ 1.5 mg/dL [males], ≥ 1.4 mg/dL [females] or abnormal creatinine clearance) which may also result from conditions such as cardiovascular collapse (shock), acute myocardial infarction, and septicemia (see WARNINGS and PRECAUTIONS).
2. Congestive heart failure requiring pharmacologic treatment.

Table 2. Combined GLUCOPHAGE/Glyburide (Comb) vs Glyburide (Glyb) or Glucophage (GLU) Monotherapy: Summary of Mean Changes from Baseline* in Plasma Glucose, HbA$_{1C}$ and Body Weight, at Final Visit (29-week study)

	Comb (n = 213)	Glyb (n = 209)	GLU (n = 210)	Glyb vs Comb	P-values GLU vs Comb	GLU vs Glyb
Fasting Plasma Glucose (mg/dL)						
Baseline	250.5	247.5	253.9	NS	NS	NS
Change at FINAL VISIT	−63.5	13.7	−0.9	0.001**	0.001**	0.025**
Hemoglobin A$_{1C}$ (%)						
Baseline	8.8	8.5	8.9	NS	NS	0.007**
Change at FINAL VISIT	−1.7	0.2	−0.4	0.001**	0.001**	0.001**
Body Weight (lbs)						
Baseline	202.2	203.0	204.0	NS	NS	NS
Change at FINAL VISIT	0.9	−0.7	−8.4	0.011**	0.001**	0.001**

*All patients on glyburide, 20 mg/day, at Baseline
**Statistically significant

Table 3. Summary of Mean Percent Reduction of Major Serum Lipid Variables at Final Visit (29-week study)

	Glucophage vs. Placebo (% Change from Baseline)		Combined Glucophage/Glyburide vs. Monotherapy (% Change from Baseline)		
	Glucophage (n = 141)	Placebo (n = 145)	Glucophage (n = 210)	Glucophage/ Glyburide (n = 213)	Glyburide (n = 209)
Total Cholesterol	−5%*	1%	−2%	−4%**	1%
Total Triglycerides	−16%	1%	−3%**	−8%**	4%
LDL- Cholesterol	−8%*	1%	−4%**	−6%**	3%
HDL- Cholesterol	2%	−1%	5%	3%	1%

*P < 0.05 vs. Placebo
**P < 0.05 vs. Glyburide

Table 4. Select Mean (± S.D.) Metformin Pharmacokinetic Parameters Following Single or Multiple Oral Doses of GLUCOPHAGE

Subject Groups: GLUCOPHAGE dose[a] (number of subjects)	C_{max}[b] (µg/mL)	t_{max}[c] (hrs)	Renal Clearance (mL/min)
Healthy, nondiabetic adults:			
500 mg SD[d] (24)	1.03 (± 0.33)	2.75 (± 0.81)	600 (± 132)
850 mg SD (74)[e]	1.60 (± 0.38)	2.64 (± 0.82)	552 (± 139)
850 mg t.i.d. for 19 doses[f] (9)	2.01 (± 0.42)	1.79 (± 0.94)	642 (± 173)
Adults with NIDDM:			
850 mg SD (23)	1.48 (± 0.5)	3.32 (± 1.08)	491 (± 138)
850 mg t.i.d. for 19 doses[f] (9)	1.90 (± 0.62)	2.01 (± 1.22)	550 (± 160)
Elderly[g], healthy nondiabetic adults:			
850 mg SD (12)	2.45 (± 0.70)	2.71 (± 1.05)	412 (± 98)
Renal-impaired adults: 850 mg SD			
Mild (CL$_{cr}$[h] 61–90 mL/min) (5)	1.86 (± 0.52)	3.20 (± 0.45)	384 (± 122)
Moderate (CL$_{cr}$ 31–60 mL/min) (4)	4.12 (± 1.83)	3.75 (± 0.50)	108 (± 57)
Severe (CL$_{cr}$ 10–30 mL/min) (6)	3.93 (± 0.92)	4.01 (± 1.10)	130 (± 90)

[a]–All doses given fasting except the first 18 doses of the multiple dose studies;
[b]–Peak plasma concentration;
[c]–Time to peak plasma concentration;
[d]–SD = single dose;
[e]–Combined results (average means) of five studies: mean age 32 years (range 23–59 yrs).
[f]–Kinetic study done following dose 19, given fasting.
[g]–Elderly subjects, mean age 71 years (range 65–81 years).
[h]–CL$_{cr}$ = creatinine clearance normalized to body surface area of 1.73 m^2.

3. GLUCOPHAGE should be temporarily discontinued in patients undergoing radiologic studies involving intravascular administration of iodinated contrast materials, because use of such products may result in acute alteration of renal function. (See also PRECAUTIONS).

4. Known hypersensitivity to metformin hydrochloride.

5. Acute or chronic metabolic acidosis, including diabetic ketoacidosis, with or without coma. Diabetic ketoacidosis should be treated with insulin.

WARNINGS

Lactic Acidosis:

Lactic acidosis is a rare, but serious, metabolic complication that can occur due to metformin accumulation during treatment with GLUCOPHAGE; when it occurs, it is fatal in approximately 50% of cases. Lactic acidosis may also occur in association with a number of pathophysiologic conditions, including diabetes mellitus, and whenever there is significant tissue hypoperfusion and hypoxemia. Lactic acidosis is characterized by elevated blood lactate levels (>5 mmol/L), decreased blood pH, electrolyte disturbances with an increased anion gap, and an increased lactate/pyruvate ratio. When metformin is implicated as the cause of lactic acidosis, metformin plasma levels >5 µg/mL are generally found.

The reported incidence of lactic acidosis in patients receiving metformin hydrochloride is very low (approximately 0.03 cases/1,000 patient-years, with approximately 0.015 fatal cases/1,000 patient-years). Reported cases have occurred primarily in diabetic patients with significant renal insufficiency, including both intrinsic renal disease and renal hypoperfusion, often in the setting of multiple concomitant medical/surgical problems and multiple concomitant medications. Patients with congestive heart failure requiring pharmacologic management, in particular those with unstable or acute congestive heart failure who are at risk of hypoperfusion and hypoxemia are at increased risk of lactic acidosis. The risk of lactic acidosis increases with the degree of renal dysfunction and the patient's age. The risk of lactic acidosis may, therefore, be significantly decreased by regular monitoring of renal function in patients taking GLUCOPHAGE and by use of the minimum effective dose of GLUCOPHAGE. In particular, treatment of the elderly should be accompanied by careful monitoring of renal function. GLUCOPHAGE treatment should not be initiated in patients ≥ 80 years of age unless measurement of creatinine clearance demonstrates that renal function is not reduced, as these patients are more susceptible to developing lactic acidosis. In addition, GLUCOPHAGE should be promptly withheld in the presence of any condition associated with hypoxemia, dehydration or sepsis. Because impaired hepatic function may significantly limit the ability to clear lactate, GLUCOPHAGE should generally be avoided in patients with clinical or laboratory evidence of hepatic disease. Patients should be cautioned against excessive alcohol intake, either acute or chronic, when taking GLUCOPHAGE (metformin hydrochloride tablets), since alcohol potentiates the effects of metformin hydrochloride on lactate metabolism. In addition, GLUCOPHAGE should be temporarily discontinued prior to any intravascular radiocontrast study and for any surgical procedure (see also PRECAUTIONS).

The onset of lactic acidosis often is subtle, and accompanied only by nonspecific symptoms such as malaise, myalgias, respiratory distress, increasing somnolence and nonspecific abdominal distress. There may be associated hypothermia, hypotension and resistant bradyarrhythmias with more marked acidosis. The patient and the patient's physician must be aware of the possible importance of such symptoms and the patient should be instructed to notify the physician immediately if they occur (see also PRECAUTIONS). GLUCOPHAGE (metformin hydrochloride tablets) should be withdrawn until the situation is clarified. Serum electrolytes, ketones, blood glucose and, if indicated, blood pH, lactate levels and even blood metformin levels may be useful. Once a patient is stabilized on any dose level of GLUCOPHAGE, gastrointestinal symptoms, which are common during initiation of therapy, are unlikely to be drug related. Later occurrence of gastrointestinal symptoms could be due to lactic acidosis or other serious disease.

Levels of fasting venous plasma lactate above the upper limit of normal but less than 5 mmol/L in patients taking GLUCOPHAGE do not necessarily indicate impending lactic acidosis and may be explainable by other mechanisms, such as poorly controlled diabetes or obesity, vigorous physical activity or technical problems in sample handling. (See also PRECAUTIONS.)

Lactic acidosis should be suspected in any diabetic patient with metabolic acidosis lacking evidence of ketoacidosis (ketonuria and ketonemia).

Lactic acidosis is a medical emergency that must be treated in a hospital setting. In a patient with lactic acidosis who is taking GLUCOPHAGE, the drug should be discontinued immediately and general supportive measures promptly instituted. Because metformin hydrochloride is dialyzable (with a clearance of up to 170 mL/min under good hemodynamic conditions), prompt hemodialysis is recommended to correct the acidosis and remove the accumulated metformin. Such management often results in prompt reversal of symptoms and recovery. (See also CONTRAINDICATIONS and PRECAUTIONS).

SPECIAL WARNING ON INCREASED RISK OF CARDIOVASCULAR MORTALITY:

The administration of oral antidiabetic drugs has been reported to be associated with increased cardiovascular mortality as compared to treatment with diet alone or diet plus insulin. This warning is based on the study conducted by the University Group Diabetes Program (UGDP), a long-term prospective clinical trial designed to evaluate the effectiveness of glucose-lowering drugs in preventing or delaying vascular complications in patients with non-insulin-dependent diabetes. The study involved 1027 patients who were randomly assigned to one of five treatment groups (*Diabetes*, 19 (Suppl.2):747–830, 1970; *Diabetes*, 24 (Suppl.1):65–184, 1975).

The UGDP reported that patients treated for 5 to 8 years with diet plus a fixed dose of tolbutamide (1.5 g per day) or diet plus a fixed dose of phenformin (100 mg per day), had a rate of cardiovascular mortality approximately 2.5 times that of patients treated with diet alone, resulting in discontinuation of both these treatments in the UGDP study. Total mortality was increased in both the tolbutamide- and phenformin-treated groups and this increase was statistically significant in the phenformin-treated group. Despite controversy regarding the interpretation of these results, the findings of the UGDP study provide an adequate basis for this warning. The patient should be informed of the potential risks and benefits of GLUCOPHAGE and alternative modes of therapy.

Although only one drug in the sulfonylurea category (tolbutamide) and one in the biguanide category (phenformin) were included in this study, it is prudent from a safety standpoint to consider that this warning may also apply to other related oral antidiabetic drugs, in view of the similarities in mode of action and chemical structure among the drugs in each category.

PRECAUTIONS

General:

Monitoring of renal function – GLUCOPHAGE is known to be substantially excreted by the kidney, and the risk of metformin accumulation and lactic acidosis increases with the degree of impairment of renal function. Thus, patients with serum creatinine levels above the upper limit of normal for their age should not receive GLUCOPHAGE. In patients with advanced age, GLUCOPHAGE should be carefully titrated to establish the minimum dose for adequate glycemic effect, because aging is associated with reduced renal function. In elderly patients, renal function should be monitored regularly and, generally, GLUCOPHAGE should not be titrated to the maximum dose (see DOSAGE AND ADMINISTRATION). For patients ≥ 80 years of age, see WARNINGS. Before initiation of GLUCOPHAGE therapy and at least annually thereafter, renal function should be assessed and verified as normal. In patients in whom development of renal dysfunction is anticipated, renal function should be assessed more frequently and GLUCOPHAGE discontinued if evidence of renal impairment is present.

Use of concomitant medications that may affect renal function or metformin disposition — Concomitant medication(s) that may affect renal function or result in significant hemodynamic change or may interfere with the disposition of GLUCOPHAGE, such as cationic drugs that are eliminated by renal tubular secretion (See Drug Interactions), should be used with caution.

Radiologic studies involving the use of intravascular iodinated contrast materials (for example, intravenous urogram, intravenous cholangiography, angiography, and computed tomography (CT) scans with intravascular contrast materials) — Intravascular contrast studies with iodinated materials can lead to acute alteration of renal function and have been associated with lactic acidosis in patients receiving GLUCOPHAGE (see CONTRAINDICATIONS). Therefore, in patients in whom any such study is planned, GLUCOPHAGE should be discontinued at the time of or prior to the procedure, and withheld for 48 hours subsequent to the procedure and reinstituted only after renal function has been re-evaluated and found to be normal.

Hypoxic states — Cardiovascular collapse (shock) from whatever cause, acute congestive heart failure, acute myocardial infarction and other conditions characterized by hypoxemia have been associated with lactic acidosis and may also cause prerenal azotemia. When such events occur in patients on GLUCOPHAGE therapy, the drug should be promptly discontinued.

Surgical procedures — GLUCOPHAGE therapy should be temporarily suspended for any surgical procedure (except minor procedures not associated with restricted intake of food and fluids) and should not be restarted until the patient's oral intake has resumed and renal function has been evaluated as normal.

Alcohol intake — Alcohol is known to potentiate the effect of metformin on lactate metabolism. Patients, therefore, should be warned against excessive alcohol intake, acute or chronic, while receiving GLUCOPHAGE.

Impaired hepatic function — Since impaired hepatic function has been associated with some cases of lactic acidosis, GLUCOPHAGE should generally be avoided in patients with clinical or laboratory evidence of hepatic disease.

Vitamin B₁₂ levels — A decrease to subnormal levels of previously normal serum vitamin B_{12} levels, without clinical manifestations, is observed in approximately 7% of patients receiving GLUCOPHAGE in controlled clinical trials of 29 weeks duration. Such decrease, possibly due to interference with B_{12} absorption from the B_{12}-intrinsic factor complex, is, however, very rarely associated with anemia and appears to be rapidly reversible with discontinuation of GLUCOPHAGE (metformin hydrochloride tablets) or vitamin B_{12} supplementation. Measurement of hematologic parameters on an annual basis is advised in patients on GLUCOPHAGE and any apparent abnormalities should be appropriately investigated and managed (see Laboratory Tests).

Certain individuals (those with inadequate vitamin B_{12} or calcium intake or absorption) appear to be predisposed to developing subnormal vitamin B_{12} levels. In these patients, routine serum vitamin B_{12} measurements at two- to three-year intervals may be useful.

Change in clinical status of previously controlled diabetic — A diabetic patient previously well controlled on GLUCOPHAGE (metformin hydrochloride tablets) who develops laboratory abnormalities or clinical illness (especially vague and poorly defined illness) should be evaluated promptly for evidence of ketoacidosis or lactic acidosis. Evaluation should include serum electrolytes and ketones, blood glucose and, if indicated, blood pH, lactate, pyruvate and metformin levels. If acidosis of either form occurs, GLUCOPHAGE must be stopped immediately and other appropriate corrective measures initiated (see also WARNINGS).

Hypoglycemia — Hypoglycemia does not occur in patients receiving GLUCOPHAGE alone under usual circumstances of use, but could occur when caloric intake is deficient, when strenuous exercise is not compensated by caloric supplementation, or during concomitant use with other glucose-lowering agents (such as sulfonylureas) or ethanol.

Elderly, debilitated or malnourished patients, and those with adrenal or pituitary insufficiency or alcohol intoxication are particularly susceptible to hypoglycemic effects. Hypoglycemia may be difficult to recognize in the elderly, and in people who are taking beta-adrenergic blocking drugs.

Loss of control of blood glucose — When a patient stabilized on any diabetic regimen is exposed to stress such as fever, trauma, infection, or surgery, a temporary loss of glycemic control may occur. At such times, it may be necessary to withhold GLUCOPHAGE and temporarily administer insulin. GLUCOPHAGE may be reinstituted after the acute episode is resolved.

The effectiveness of oral antidiabetic drugs in lowering blood glucose to a targeted level decreases in many patients over a period of time. This phenomenon, which may be due to progression of the underlying disease or to diminished responsiveness to the drug, is known as secondary failure, to distinguish it from primary failure in which the drug is ineffective during initial therapy. Should secondary failure occur with GLUCOPHAGE or sulfonylurea monotherapy, combined therapy with GLUCOPHAGE and sulfonylurea may result in a response. Should secondary failure occur with combined GLUCOPHAGE/sulfonylurea therapy, it may be necessary to initiate insulin therapy.

Information for Patients:

Patients should be informed of the potential risks and advantages of GLUCOPHAGE and of alternative modes of therapy. They should also be informed about the importance of adherence to dietary instructions, of a regular exercise program, and of regular testing of blood glucose, glycosylated hemoglobin, renal function and hematologic parameters.

The risks of lactic acidosis, its symptoms, and conditions that predispose to its development, as noted in the WARNINGS and PRECAUTIONS sections should be explained to patients. Patients should be advised to discontinue GLUCOPHAGE immediately and to promptly notify their health practitioner if unexplained hyperventilation, myalgia, malaise, unusual somnolence or other nonspecific symptoms occur. Once a patient is stabilized on any dose level of GLUCOPHAGE, gastrointestinal symptoms, which

Continued on next page

Glucophage—Cont.

are common during initiation of therapy, are unlikely to be drug related. Later occurrence of gastrointestinal symptoms could be due to lactic acidosis or other serious disease. Patients should be counselled against excessive alcohol intake, either acute or chronic, while receiving GLUCOPHAGE.

GLUCOPHAGE alone does not usually cause hypoglycemia, although it may occur when GLUCOPHAGE is used in conjunction with oral sulfonylureas. When initiating combination therapy, the risks of hypoglycemia, its symptoms and treatment, and conditions that predispose to its development should be explained to patients.
(See Patient Labeling Printed Below)

Laboratory Tests:
Response to all diabetic therapies should be monitored by periodic measurements of fasting blood glucose and glycosylated hemoglobin levels, with a goal of decreasing these levels toward the normal range. During initial dose titration, fasting glucose can be used to determine the therapeutic response. Thereafter, both glucose and glycosylated hemoglobin should be monitored. Measurements of glycosylated hemoglobin may be especially useful for evaluating long-term control (see also DOSAGE AND ADMINISTRATION).

Initial and periodic monitoring of hematologic parameters (e.g., hemoglobin/hematocrit and red blood cell indices) and renal function (serum creatinine) should be performed, at least on an annual basis. While megaloblastic anemia has rarely been seen with GLUCOPHAGE therapy, if this is suspected, vitamin B_{12} deficiency should be excluded.

Drug Interactions:
Glyburide: In a single-dose interaction study in NIDDM subjects, co-administration of metformin and glyburide did not result in any changes in either metformin pharmacokinetics or pharmacodynamics. Decreases in glyburide AUC and C_{max} were observed, but were highly variable. The single-dose nature of this study and the lack of correlation between glyburide blood levels and pharmacodynamic effects, makes the clinical significance of this interaction uncertain (see DOSAGE AND ADMINISTRATION, Concomitant Glucophage and Oral Sulfonylurea Therapy).

Furosemide: A single-dose, metformin-furosemide drug interaction study in healthy subjects demonstrated that pharmacokinetic parameters of both compounds were affected by co-administration. Furosemide increased the metformin plasma and blood C_{max} by 22% and blood AUC by 15%, without any significant change in metformin renal clearance. When administered with metformin, the C_{max} and AUC of furosemide were 31% and 12% smaller, respectively, than when administered alone, and the terminal half-life was decreased by 32%, without any significant change in furosemide renal clearance. No information is available about the interaction of metformin and furosemide when co-administered chronically.

Nifedipine: A single-dose, metformin-nifedipine drug interaction study in normal healthy volunteers demonstrated that co-administration of nifedipine increased plasma metformin C_{max} and AUC by 20% and 9%, respectively, and increased the amount excreted in the urine. T_{max} and half-life were unaffected. Nifedipine appears to enhance the absorption of metformin. Metformin had minimal effects on nifedipine.

Cationic Drugs: Cationic drugs (e.g., amiloride, digoxin, morphine, procainamide, quinidine, quinine, ranitidine, triamterene, trimethoprim, and vancomycin) that are eliminated by renal tubular secretion theoretically have the potential for interaction with metformin by competing for common renal tubular transport systems. Such interaction between metformin and oral cimetidine has been observed in normal healthy volunteers in both single- and multiple-dose, metformin-cimetidine drug interaction studies, with a 60% increase in peak metformin plasma and whole blood concentrations and a 40% increase in plasma and whole blood metformin AUC. There was no change in elimination half-life in the single-dose study. Metformin had no effect on cimetidine pharmacokinetics. Although such interactions remain theoretical (except for cimetidine), careful patient monitoring and dose adjustment of GLUCOPHAGE and/or the interfering drug is recommended in patients who are taking cationic medications that are excreted via the proximal renal tubular secretory system.

Other: Certain drugs tend to produce hyperglycemia and may lead to loss of glycemic control. These drugs include thiazide and other diuretics, corticosteroids, phenothiazines, thyroid products, estrogens, oral contraceptives, phenytoin, nicotinic acid, sympathomimetics, calcium channel blocking drugs, and isoniazid. When such drugs are administered to a patient receiving GLUCOPHAGE, the patient should be closely observed to maintain adequate glycemic control.

In healthy volunteers, the pharmacokinetics of metformin and propranolol and metformin and Ibuprofen were not affected when co-administered in single-dose interaction studies.

Metformin is negligibly bound to plasma proteins and is, therefore, less likely to interact with highly protein-bound drugs such as salicylates, sulfonamides, chloramphenicol, and probenecid, as compared to the sulfonylureas, which are extensively bound to serum proteins.

Carcinogenesis, Mutagenesis, Impairment of Fertility:
Long-term carcinogenicity studies have been performed in rats (dosing duration of 104 weeks) and mice (dosing duration of 91 weeks) at doses up to and including 900 mg/kg/day and 1500 mg/kg/day, respectively. These doses are both approximately three times the maximum recommended human daily dose on a body surface area basis. No evidence of carcinogenicity with metformin was found in either male or female mice. Similarly, there was no tumorigenic potential observed with metformin in male rats. However, an increased incidence of benign stromal uterine polyps was seen in female rats treated with 900 mg/kg/day.

No evidence of a mutagenic potential of metformin was found in the Ames test (*S. typhimurium*), gene mutation test (mouse lymphoma cells), chromosomal aberrations test (human lymphocytes), or *in-vivo* micronuclei formation test (mouse bone marrow).

Fertility of male or female rats was unaffected by metformin administration at doses as high as 600 mg/kg/day, or approximately two times the maximum recommended human daily dose on a body surface area basis.

Pregnancy:
Teratogenic effects:
Pregnancy Category B. Safety in pregnant women has not been established. Metformin was not teratogenic in rats and rabbits at doses up to 600 mg/kg/day, or about two times the maximum recommended human daily dose on a body surface area basis. Determination of fetal concentrations demonstrated a partial placental barrier to metformin. Because animal reproduction studies are not always predictive of human response, any decision to use this drug should be balanced against the benefits and risks.

Because recent information suggests that abnormal blood glucose levels during pregnancy are associated with a higher incidence of congenital abnormalities, there is a consensus among experts that insulin be used during pregnancy to maintain blood glucose levels as close to normal as possible.

Nursing Mothers:
Studies in lactating rats show that metformin is excreted into milk and reaches levels comparable to those in plasma. Similar studies have not been conducted in nursing mothers, but caution should be exercised in such patients, and a decision should be made whether to discontinue nursing or to discontinue the drug, taking into account the importance of the drug to the mother.

Pediatric Use:
Safety and effectiveness in pediatric patients have not been established. Studies in maturity-onset diabetes of the young (MODY) have not been conducted.

Geriatric Use:
Controlled clinical studies of GLUCOPHAGE (metformin hydrochloride tablets) did not include sufficient numbers of elderly patients to determine whether they respond differently from younger patients, although other reported clinical experience has not identified differences in responses between the elderly and younger patients. GLUCOPHAGE is known to be substantially excreted by the kidney and because the risk of serious adverse reactions to the drug is greater in patients with impaired renal function, it should only be used in patients with normal renal function (see CONTRAINDICATIONS, CLINICAL PHARMACOLOGY, Pharmacokinetics). Because aging is associated with reduced renal function, GLUCOPHAGE should be used with caution as age increases. Care should be taken in dose selection and should be based on careful and regular monitoring of renal function. Generally, elderly patients should not be titrated to the maximum dose of GLUCOPHAGE (see also WARNINGS and DOSAGE AND ADMINISTRATION).

ADVERSE REACTIONS

Lactic Acidosis: See WARNINGS, PRECAUTIONS and OVERDOSAGE Sections.

Gastrointestinal Reactions: Gastrointestinal symptoms (diarrhea, nausea, vomiting, abdominal bloating, flatulence, and anorexia) are the most common reactions to GLUCOPHAGE and are approximately 30% more frequent in patients on GLUCOPHAGE monotherapy than in placebo-treated patients, particularly during initiation of GLUCOPHAGE therapy. These symptoms are generally transient and resolve spontaneously during continued treatment. Occasionally, temporary dose reduction may be useful. In controlled trials, GLUCOPHAGE was discontinued due to gastrointestinal reactions in approximately 4% of patients.

Because gastrointestinal symptoms during therapy initiation appear to be dose-related, they may be decreased by gradual dose escalation and by having patients take GLUCOPHAGE with meals (see DOSAGE AND ADMINISTRATION).

Because significant diarrhea and/or vomiting may cause dehydration and prerenal azotemia, under such circumstances, GLUCOPHAGE should be temporarily discontinued.

For patients who have been stabilized on GLUCOPHAGE, nonspecific gastrointestinal symptoms should not be attributed to therapy unless intercurrent illness or lactic acidosis have been excluded.

Special Senses: During initiation of GLUCOPHAGE therapy, approximately 3% of patients may complain of an unpleasant or metallic taste, which usually resolves spontaneously.

Dermatologic Reactions: The incidence of rash/dermatitis in controlled clinical trials was comparable to placebo for GLUCOPHAGE monotherapy and to sulfonylurea for GLUCOPHAGE/sulfonylurea therapy.

Hematologic: (See also PRECAUTIONS). During controlled clinical trials of 29 weeks duration, approximately 9% of patients on GLUCOPHAGE monotherapy and 6% of patients on GLUCOPHAGE/sulfonylurea therapy developed asymptomatic subnormal serum vitamin B_{12} levels; serum folic acid levels did not decrease significantly. However, only five cases of megaloblastic anemia have been reported with metformin administration (none during U.S. clinical studies) and no increased incidence of neuropathy has been observed. Therefore, serum B_{12} levels should be appropriately monitored or periodic parenteral B_{12} supplementation considered.

DRUG ABUSE AND DEPENDENCE:

GLUCOPHAGE possesses no pharmacodynamic properties, either primary or secondary, which could be expected to result in abuse as a recreational drug or addiction.

OVERDOSAGE:

Hypoglycemia has not been seen even with ingestion of up to 85 grams of GLUCOPHAGE, although lactic acidosis has occurred in such circumstances (see WARNINGS). Metformin is dialyzable with a clearance of up to 170 mL/min under good hemodynamic conditions. Therefore, hemodialysis may be useful for removal of accumulated drug from patients in whom metformin overdosage is suspected.

DOSAGE AND ADMINISTRATION:

There is no fixed dosage regimen for the management of hyperglycemia in diabetes mellitus with GLUCOPHAGE or any other pharmacologic agent. Dosage of GLUCOPHAGE must be individualized on the basis of both effectiveness and tolerance, while not exceeding the maximum recommended daily dose of 2550 mg. GLUCOPHAGE should be given in divided doses with meals and should be started at a low dose, with gradual dose escalation, as described below, both to reduce gastrointestinal side effects and to permit identification of the minimum dose required for adequate glycemic control of the patient.

During treatment initiation and dose titration (see below, USUAL STARTING DOSE), fasting plasma glucose should be used to determine the therapeutic response to GLUCOPHAGE and identify the minimum effective dose for the patient. Thereafter, glycosylated hemoglobin should be measured at intervals of approximately three months. **The therapeutic goal should be to decrease both fasting plasma glucose and glycosylated hemoglobin levels to normal or near normal by using the lowest effective dose of GLUCOPHAGE (metformin hydrochloride tablets), either when used as monotherapy or in combination with sulfonylurea.**

Monitoring of blood glucose and glycosylated hemoglobin will also permit detection of primary failure, i.e., inadequate lowering of blood glucose at the maximum recommended dose of medication, and secondary failure, i.e., loss of an adequate blood glucose lowering response after an initial period of effectiveness.

Short-term administration of GLUCOPHAGE may be sufficient during periods of transient loss of control in patients usually well-controlled on diet alone.

Usual Starting Dose:
In general, clinically significant responses are not seen at doses below 1500 mg per day. However, a lower recommended starting dose and gradually increased dosage is advised to minimize gastrointestinal symptoms.

GLUCOPHAGE 500 mg Tablets:
The usual starting dose of GLUCOPHAGE 500 mg tablets is one tablet b.i.d., given with the morning and evening meals. Dosage increases should be made in increments of one tablet every week, given in divided doses, up to a maximum of 2500 mg per day. GLUCOPHAGE can be administered twice a day up to 2000 mg per day (e.g., 1000 mg b.i.d. with morning and evening meals). If a 2500 mg daily dose is required, it may be better tolerated given t.i.d. with meals.

GLUCOPHAGE 850 mg Tablets:
The usual starting dose of GLUCOPHAGE 850 mg tablets is one tablet daily, given with the morning meal. Dosage increases should be made in increments of one tablet every OTHER week, given in divided doses, up to a maximum of 2550 mg per day. The usual maintenance dose is 850 mg b.i.d. with the morning and evening meals. When necessary, patients may be given 850 mg t.i.d. with meals.

Transfer from Other Antidiabetic Therapy:
When transferring patients from standard oral hypoglycemic agents other than chlorpropamide to GLUCOPHAGE, no transition period generally is necessary. When transferring patients from chlorpropamide, care should be exercised during the first two weeks because of the prolonged retention of chlorpropamide in the body, leading to overlapping drug effects and possible hypoglycemia.

Concomitant GLUCOPHAGE and Oral Sulfonylurea Therapy:
If patients have not responded to four weeks of the maximum dose of GLUCOPHAGE monotherapy, consideration should be given to gradual addition of an oral sulfonylurea while continuing GLUCOPHAGE at the maximum dose, even if prior primary or secondary failure to a sulfonylurea has occurred. Clinical and pharmacokinetic drug-drug interaction data are currently available only for metformin plus glyburide (glibenclamide). Published clinical information exists for the use of metformin with either chlorpropamide, tolbutamide or glipizide. No published clinical information exists regarding concomitant use of metformin with acetohexamide or tolazamide.
With concomitant GLUCOPHAGE and sulfonylurea therapy, the desired control of blood glucose may be obtained by adjusting the dose of each drug. However, attempts should be made to identify the minimum effective dose of each drug to achieve this goal. With concomitant GLUCOPHAGE and sulfonylurea therapy, the risk of hypoglycemia associated with sulfonylurea therapy continues and may be increased. Appropriate precautions should be taken. (See Package Insert of the respective sulfonylurea).
If patients have not satisfactorily responded to one to three months of concomitant therapy with the maximum dose of GLUCOPHAGE and the maximum dose of an oral sulfonylurea, institution of insulin therapy and discontinuation of these oral agents should be considered.

Specific Patient Populations:
GLUCOPHAGE is not recommended for use in pregnancy or for use in pediatric patients.
The initial and maintenance dosing of GLUCOPHAGE should be conservative in patients with advanced age, due to the potential for decreased renal function in this population. Any dosage adjustment should be based on a careful assessment of renal function. Generally, elderly patients should not be titrated to the maximum dose of GLUCOPHAGE.
Monitoring of renal function is necessary to aid in prevention of lactic acidosis, particularly in the elderly. (see WARNINGS.)
In debilitated or malnourished patients, the dosing should also be conservative and based on a careful assessment of renal function.

HOW SUPPLIED

GLUCOPHAGE® (brand of metformin hydrochloride tablets) is supplied as round, white to off-white, film-coated tablets, available in the following strengths:

500 mg	Bottles of 100	NDC 0087-6060-05
500 mg	Bottles of 500	NDC 0087-6060-10
850 mg	Bottles of 100	NDC 0087-6070-05
850 mg	Bottles of 300	NDC 0087-6070-10

GLUCOPHAGE 500 mg tablets are debossed with BMS 6060 around the periphery of the tablet on one side and 500 across the face of the other side. GLUCOPHAGE 850 mg tablets are debossed with BMS 6070 around the periphery of the tablet on one side and 850 across the face of the other side.

Storage
Store between 15°–30° C (59°–86° F).

PATIENT INFORMATION ABOUT GLUCOPHAGE®

(metformin hydrochloride tablets)
500 mg and 850 mg

> **WARNING: A small number of people who have taken Glucophage have developed a serious condition called lactic acidosis. Properly functioning kidneys are needed to help prevent lactic acidosis. Most people with kidney problems should not take Glucophage. (See Question Nos. 7–11)**

Q1. Why do I need to take GLUCOPHAGE?
Your doctor has prescribed GLUCOPHAGE (GLUE-coe-fahj) to treat your type II diabetes. This is also known as non-insulin-dependent diabetes mellitus (NIDDM).

Q2. What is type II diabetes?
People with diabetes are not able to make enough insulin and/or respond normally to the insulin their body does make. When this happens, sugar (glucose) builds up in the blood. This can lead to serious medical problems including kidney damage, amputations and blindness. Diabetes is also closely linked to heart disease. The main goal of treating diabetes is to lower your blood sugar to a normal level.

Q3. How is type II diabetes usually controlled?
High blood sugar can be lowered by diet and exercise, by a number of oral medications and by insulin injections. Before taking GLUCOPHAGE you should first try to control your diabetes by exercise and weight loss. Even if you are taking GLUCOPHAGE, you should still exercise and follow the diet recommended for your diabetes.

Q4. Does GLUCOPHAGE work differently from other glucose-control medications?
Yes it does. Until GLUCOPHAGE (metformin hydrochloride tablets) was introduced, all the available oral glucose-control medications were from the same chemical group called sulfonylureas. These drugs lower blood sugar primarily by causing more of the body's own insulin to be released. GLUCOPHAGE lowers the amount of sugar in your blood by helping your body respond better to its own insulin. GLUCOPHAGE (metformin hydrochloride tablets) does not cause your body to produce more insulin. Therefore, GLUCOPHAGE rarely causes hypoglycemia (low blood sugar) and it doesn't usually cause weight gain.

Q5. What happens if my blood sugar is still too high?
When blood sugar cannot be lowered enough by either GLUCOPHAGE or a sulfonylurea, the two medications may be effective taken together. However, if you are unable to maintain your blood sugar with diet, exercise and glucose-control medication taken orally, then your doctor may prescribe injectable insulin to control your diabetes.

Q6. Can GLUCOPHAGE cause side effects?
GLUCOPHAGE, like all blood-sugar lowering medications, can cause side effects in some patients. Most of these side effects are minor and will go away after you've taken GLUCOPHAGE for a while. However, there are also serious, but rare side effects related to GLUCOPHAGE (see below).

Q7. What kind of side effects can GLUCOPHAGE cause?
If side effects occur, they usually occur during the first few weeks of therapy. They are normally minor ones such as diarrhea, nausea and upset stomach. Taking your GLUCOPHAGE with meals can help reduce these side effects.
Although these side effects are likely to go away, call your doctor if you have severe discomfort or if these effects last for more than a few weeks. Some patients may need to have their dose lowered or stop taking GLUCOPHAGE, either temporarily or permanently. Although these problems occur in up to one-third of patients when they first start taking GLUCOPHAGE, you should tell your doctor if the problems come back or start later on during the therapy.
About three out of one hundred people report having a temporary unpleasant or metallic taste when they start taking GLUCOPHAGE.

Q8. Are there any serious side effects that GLUCOPHAGE can cause?
GLUCOPHAGE rarely causes serious side effects. The most serious side effect that GLUCOPHAGE can cause is called lactic acidosis.

Q9. What is lactic acidosis and can it happen to me?
Lactic acidosis is caused by a buildup of lactic acid in the blood. Lactic acidosis associated with GLUCOPHAGE is rare and has occurred mostly in people whose kidneys were not working normally. Lactic acidosis has been reported in about one in 33,000 patients taking GLUCOPHAGE over the course of a year. Although rare, if lactic acidosis does occur, it can be fatal in up to half the cases.
It's also important for your liver to be working normally when you take GLUCOPHAGE. Your liver helps remove lactic acid from your bloodstream.
Your doctor will monitor your diabetes and may perform blood tests on you from time to time to make sure your kidneys and your liver are functioning normally.
There is no evidence that GLUCOPHAGE causes harm to the kidneys or liver.

Q10. Are there other risk factors for lactic acidosis?
Your risk of developing lactic acidosis from taking GLUCOPHAGE is very low as long as your kidneys and liver are healthy. However, some factors can increase your risk because they can affect kidney and liver function. You should discuss your risk with your physician. You should not take GLUCOPHAGE if:

- You have chronic kidney or liver problems
- You have congestive heart failure which is treated with medications, e.g., digoxin (Lanoxin®) or furosemide (Lasix®)
- You drink alcohol excessively (all the time or short-term "binge" drinking)
- You are seriously dehydrated (have lost a large amount of body fluids)
- You are going to have certain x-ray procedures with injectable contrast agents
- You are going to have surgery
- You develop a serious condition such as a heart attack, severe infection, or a stroke
- You are ≥ 80 years of age and have NOT had your kidney function tested.

Q11. What are the symptoms of lactic acidosis?
Some of the symptoms include: feeling very weak, tired or uncomfortable; unusual muscle pain, trouble breathing, unusual or unexpected stomach discomfort, feeling cold, feeling dizzy or lightheaded, or suddenly developing a slow or irregular heartbeat.
If you notice these symptoms, or if your medical condition has suddenly changed, stop taking GLUCOPHAGE and call your doctor right away. Lactic acidosis is a medical emergency that must be treated in a hospital.

Q12. What does my doctor need to know to decrease my risk of lactic acidosis?
Tell your doctor if you have an illness that results in severe vomiting, diarrhea and/or fever, or if your intake of fluids is significantly reduced. These situations can lead to severe dehydration, and it may be necessary to stop taking GLUCOPHAGE temporarily.
You should let your doctor know if you are going to have any surgery or specialized x-ray procedures that require injection of contrast agents. GLUCOPHAGE therapy will need to be stopped temporarily in such instances.

Q13. Can I take GLUCOPHAGE with other medications?
Remind your doctor that you are taking GLUCOPHAGE when any new drug is prescribed or a change is made in how you take a drug already prescribed. GLUCOPHAGE may interfere with the way some drugs work and some drugs may interfere with the action of GLUCOPHAGE.

Q14. What if I become pregnant while taking GLUCOPHAGE?
Tell your doctor if you plan to become pregnant or have become pregnant. As with other oral glucose-control medications, you should not take GLUCOPHAGE during pregnancy.
Usually your doctor will prescribe insulin while you are pregnant. As with all medications, you and your doctor should discuss the use of GLUCOPHAGE if you are nursing a child.

Q15. Are there other risks associated with GLUCOPHAGE?
There is some evidence that any oral diabetes drug may increase the risk of heart problems. Experts are not sure what the real risk is for heart problems, if any, from taking oral diabetes medicine.

Q16. How do I take GLUCOPHAGE?
Your doctor will tell you how many GLUCOPHAGE tablets to take and how often. This should also be printed on the label of your prescription. You will probably be started on a low dose of GLUCOPHAGE and your dosage will be increased gradually until your blood sugar is controlled.

Q17. Where can I get more information about GLUCOPHAGE?
This leaflet is a summary of the most important information about GLUCOPHAGE. If you have any questions or problems, you should talk to your doctor or other healthcare provider about type II diabetes as well as GLUCOPHAGE and its side effects. There is also a leaflet (package insert) written for health professionals that your pharmacist can let you read.

Glucophage is a registered trademark of LIPHA s.a. Licensed to Bristol-Myers Squibb Company.

Revised March 1998 6060DIM-04
F5-B001R-03-98

Distributed by
Bristol-Myers Squibb Company
Princeton, NJ 08543 USA

Shown in Product Identification Guide, page 307

MAXIPIME® ℞

[max-ə-pīme]
(Cefepime Hydrochloride) for Injection
For Intravenous or Intramuscular Use

Rx only

DESCRIPTION

Cefepime hydrochloride is a semi-synthetic, broad spectrum, cephalosporin antibiotic for parenteral administration. The chemical name is 1-[[(6R,7R)-7-[2-(2-amino-4-thiazolyl)-glyoxylamido]-2-carboxy-8-oxo-5-thia-1-azabicyclo-[4.2.0]oct-2-en-3-yl]methyl]-1-methylpyrrolidinium chloride, 7^2-(Z)- (O-methyloxime), monohydrochloride, monohydrate.
Cefepime hydrochloride is a white to pale yellow powder with a molecular formula of $C_{19}H_{25}ClN_6O_5S_2 \bullet HCl \bullet H_20$ and a molecular weight of 571.5. It is highly soluble in water.
MAXIPIME® (cefepime hydrochloride) for Injection, is supplied for intramuscular or intravenous administration in strengths equivalent to 500 mg, 1 g and 2 g of cefepime. (See **DOSAGE AND ADMINISTRATION**.) MAXIPIME is a sterile, dry mixture of cefepime hydrochloride and L-arginine. The L-arginine, at an approximate concentration of 725 mg/g of cefepime, is added to control the pH of the constituted solution at 4.0–6.0. Freshly constituted solutions of MAXIPIME will range in color from colorless to amber.

Continued on next page

Maxipime—Cont.

CLINICAL PHARMACOLOGY

Pharmacokinetics: The average plasma concentrations of cefepime observed in healthy adult male volunteers (n=9) at various times following single 30-minute infusions (IV) of cefepime 500 mg, 1 g, and 2 g are summarized in Table 1. Elimination of cefepime is principally via renal excretion with an average ($\pm$ SD) half-life of 2.0 ($\pm$0.3) hours and total body clearance of 120.0 ($\pm$ 8.0) mL/min in healthy volunteers. Cefepime pharmacokinetics are linear over the range 250 mg to 2 g. There is no evidence of accumulation in healthy adult male volunteers (n=7) receiving clinically relevant doses for a period of 9 days.

Absorption: The average plasma concentrations of cefepime and its derived pharmacokinetic parameters after intravenous administration are portrayed in Table 1.

TABLE 1
Average Plasma Concentrations in μg/mL of Cefepime and Derived Pharmacokinetic Parameters (±SD), Intravenous Administration

Parameter	MAXIPIME		
	500 mg IV	1 g IV	2 g IV
0.5 hr	38.2	78.7	163.1
1.0 hr	21.6	44.5	85.8
2.0 hr	11.6	24.3	44.8
4.0 hr	5.0	10.5	19.2
8.0 hr	1.4	2.4	3.9
12.0 hr	0.2	0.6	1.1
C_{max}, μg/mL	39.1 (3.5)	81.7 (5.1)	163.9 (25.3)
AUC, hr•μg/mL	70.8 (6.7)	148.5 (15.1)	284.8 (30.6)
Number of subjects (male)	9	9	9

Following intramuscular (IM) administration, cefepime is completely absorbed. The average plasma concentrations of cefepime at various times following a single IM injection are summarized in Table 2. The pharmacokinetics of cefepime are linear over the range of 500 mg to 2 g IM and do not vary with respect to treatment duration.

Table 2
Average Plasma Concentrations in μg/mL of Cefepime and Derived Pharmacokinetic Parameters (±SD), Intramuscular Administration

Parameter	MAXIPIME (cefepime hydrochloride)		
	500 mg IM	1 g IM	2 g IM
0.5 hr	8.2	14.8	36.1
1.0 hr	12.5	25.9	49.9
2.0 hr	12.0	26.3	51.3
4.0 hr	6.9	16.0	31.5
8.0 hr	1.9	4.5	8.7
12.0 hr	0.7	1.4	2.3
C_{max}, μg/mL	13.9 (3.4)	29.6 (4.4)	57.5 (9.5)
T_{max}, hr	1.4 (0.9)	1.6 (0.4)	1.5 (0.4)
AUC, hr•μg/mL	60.0 (8.0)	137.0 (11.0)	262.0 (23.0)
Number of subjects (male)	6	6	12

Distribution: The average steady state volume of distribution of cefepime is 18.0 ($\pm$ 2.0)L. The serum protein binding of cefepime is approximately 20% and is independent of its concentration in serum.

Cefepime is excreted in human milk. A nursing infant consuming approximately 1000 mL of human milk per day would receive approximately 0.5 mg of cefepime per day. (See **PRECAUTIONS, Nursing Mothers.**)

Table 3
Average Concentrations of Cefepime in Specific Body Fluids (μg/mL) or Tissues (μg/g)

Tissue or Fluid	Dose/Route	# of Patients	Average Time of Sample Post-Dose (hr)	Average Concentration
Blister Fluid	2 g IV	6	1.5	81.4 μg/mL
Bronchial Mucosa	2 g IV	20	4.8	24.1 μg/g
Sputum	2 g IV	5	4.0	7.4 μg/mL
Urine	500 mg IV	8	0-4	292 μg/mL
	1 g IV	12	0-4	926 μg/mL
	2 g IV	12	0-4	3120 μg/mL
Bile	2 g IV	26	9.4	17.8 μg/mL
Peritoneal Fluid	2 g IV	19	4.4	18.3 μg/mL
Appendix	2 g IV	31	5.7	5.2 μg/g
Gallbladder	2 g IV	38	8.9	11.9 μg/g
Prostate	2 g IV	5	1.0	31.5 μg/g

TABLE 4

Microorganism	MIC (μg/mL)		
	Susceptible (S)	Intermediate (I)	Resistant (R)
Microorganisms other than Haemophilus spp.* and S. pneumoniae*	≤8	16	≥32
Haemophilus spp.*	≤2	—*	—*
Streptococcus pneumoniae*	≤0.5	1	≥2

* NOTE: Isolates from these species should be tested for susceptibility using specialized dilution testing methods.[1] Also, strains of Haemophilus spp. with MIC's greater than 2 μg/mL should be considered equivocal and should be further evaluated.

Concentrations of cefepime achieved in specific tissues and body fluids are listed in Table 3.
[See table 3 above]
Data suggest that cefepime does cross the inflamed blood-brain barrier. **The clinical relevance of these data are uncertain at this time.**

Metabolism and Excretion: Cefepime is metabolized to N-methylpyrrolidine (NMP) which is rapidly converted to the N-oxide (NMP-N-oxide). Urinary recovery of unchanged cefepime accounts for approximately 85% of the administered dose. Less than 1% of the administered dose is recovered from urine as NMP, 6.8% as NMP-N-oxide, and 2.5% as an epimer of cefepime. Because renal excretion is a significant pathway of elimination, patients with renal dysfunction and patients undergoing hemodialysis require dosage adjustment. (See **DOSAGE AND ADMINISTRATION.**)

Special Populations: *Geriatric patients:* Cefepime pharmacokinetics have been investigated in elderly (65 years of age and older) men (n=12) and women (n=12) whose creatinine clearance was 74.0 ($\pm$ 15.0) mL/min. There appeared to be a decrease in cefepime total body clearance as a function of creatinine clearance. Therefore, dosage administration of cefepime in the elderly should be adjusted as appropriate if the patient's creatinine clearance is 60 mL/min or less. (See **DOSAGE AND ADMINISTRATION.**)

Renal Insufficiency: Cefepime pharmacokinetics have been investigated in patients with various degrees of renal insufficiency (n=30). The average half-life in patients requiring hemodialysis was 13.5 ($\pm$ 2.7) hours and in patients requiring continuous peritoneal dialysis was 19.0 ($\pm$ 2.0) hours. Cefepime total body clearance decreased proportionally with creatinine clearance in patients with abnormal renal function, which serves as the basis for dosage adjustment recommendations in this group of patients. (See **DOSAGE AND ADMINISTRATION.**)

Hepatic Insufficiency: The pharmacokinetics of cefepime were unaltered in patients with impaired hepatic function who received a single 1 g dose (n=11).

Microbiology: Cefepime is a bactericidal agent that acts by inhibition of bacterial cell wall synthesis. Cefepime has a broad spectrum of *in vitro* activity that encompasses a wide range of gram-positive and gram-negative bacteria. Cefepime has a low affinity for chromosomally-encoded beta-lactamases. Cefepime is highly resistant to hydrolysis by most beta-lactamases and exhibits rapid penetration into gram-negative bacterial cells. Within bacterial cells, the molecular targets of cefepime are the penicillin binding proteins (PBP).

Cefepime has been shown to be active against most strains of the following micro organisms, both *in vitro* and in clinical infections as described in the **INDICATIONS AND USAGE** section.

Aerobic Gram-Negative Microorganisms:
Enterobacter
Escherichia coli
Klebsiella pneumoniae
Proteus mirabilis
Pseudomonas aeruginosa

Aerobic Gram-Positive Microorganisms:
Staphylococcus aureus (methicillin-susceptible strains only)
Streptococcus pneumoniae
Streptococcus pyogenes (Lancefield's Group A streptococci)

The following *in vitro* data are available, **but their clinical significance is unknown.** Cefepime has been shown to have *in vitro* activity against most strains of the following microorganisms; however, the safety and effectiveness of cefepime in treating clinical infections due to these microorganisms have not been established in adequate and well-controlled trials.

Aerobic Gram-Positive Microorganisms:
Staphylococcus epidermidis (methicillin-susceptible strains only)
Staphylococcus saprophyticus
Streptococcus agalactiae (Lancefield's Group B streptococci)
Viridans group streptococci

NOTE: Most strains of enterococci, e.g. *Enterococcus faecalis*, and methicillin-resistant staphylococci are resistant to cefepime.

Aerobic Gram-Negative Microorganisms:
Acinetobacter calcoaceticus subsp. *lwoffi*
Citrobacter diversus
Citrobacter freundii
Enterobacter agglomerans
Haemophilus influenzae (including beta-lactamase producing strains)
Hafnia alvei
Klebsiella oxytoca
Moraxella catarrhalis (including beta-lactamase producing strains)
Morganella morganii
Proteus vulgaris
Providencia rettgeri
Providencia stuartii
Serratia marcescens

NOTE: Cefepime is inactive against many strains of *Stenotrophomonas* (formerly *Xanthomonas maltophilia* and *Pseudomonas maltophilia*).

Anaerobic Microorganisms:

NOTE: Cefepime is inactive against most strains of *Clostridium difficile*.

Susceptibility Tests

Dilution Techniques: Quantitative methods are used to determine antimicrobial minimum inhibitory concentrations (MIC's). These MIC's provide estimates of the susceptibility of bacteria to antimicrobial compounds. The MIC's should be determined using a standardized procedure. Standardized procedures are based on a dilution method[1] (broth or agar) or equivalent with standardized inoculum concentrations and standardized concentrations of cefepime powder. The MIC values should be interpreted according to the following criteria:

[See table 4 on previous page]

A report of "Susceptible" indicates that the pathogen is likely to be inhibited if the antimicrobial compound in the blood reaches the concentrations usually achievable. A report of "Intermediate" indicates that the result should be considered equivocal, and, if the microorganism is not fully susceptible to alternative, clinically feasible drugs, the test should be repeated. This category implies possible clinical applicability in body sites where the drug is physiologically concentrated or in situations where high dosage of drug can be used. This category also provides a buffer zone which prevents small uncontrolled technical factors from causing major discrepancies in interpretation. A report of "Resistant" indicates that the pathogen is not likely to be inhibited if the antimicrobial compound in the blood reaches the concentrations usually achievable; other therapy should be selected.

Standardized susceptibility test procedures require the use of laboratory control microorganisms to control the technical aspects of the laboratory procedures. Laboratory control microorganisms are specific strains of microbiological assay organisms with intrinsic biological properties relating to resistance mechanisms and their genetic expression within bacteria; the specific strains are not clinically significant in their current microbiological status. Standard cefepime powder should provide the following MIC values (Table 5) when tested against the designated quality control strains:

TABLE 5

Microorganism	ATCC	MIC (µg/mL)
Escherichia coli	25922	0.015-0.06
Staphylococcus aureus	29213	1-4
Pseudomonas aeruginosa	27853	1-4
Haemophilus influenzae	49247	0.5-2
Streptococcus pneumoniae	49619	0.06-0.25

Diffusion Techniques: Quantitative methods that require measurement of zone diameters also provide reproducible estimates of the susceptibility of bacteria to antimicrobial compounds. One such standardized procedure[2] requires the use of standardized inoculum concentrations. This procedure uses paper disks impregnated with 30 µg of cefepime to test the susceptibility of microorganisms to cefepime. Interpretation is identical to that stated above for results using dilution techniques.

Reports from the laboratory providing results of the standard single-disk susceptibility test with a 30-µg cefepime disk should be interpreted according to the following criteria:

[See table 6 below]

As with standardized dilution techniques, diffusion methods require the use of laboratory control microorganisms to control the technical aspects of the laboratory procedures. Laboratory control microorganisms are specific strains of microbiological assay organisms with intrinsic biological properties relating to resistance mechanisms and their genetic expression within bacteria; the specific strains are not clinically significant in their current microbiological status. For the diffusion technique, the 30-µg cefepime disk should provide the following zone diameters in these laboratory test quality control strains (Table 7):

TABLE 7

Microorganism	ATCC	Zone Size Range (mm)
Escherichia coli	25922	29 - 35
Staphylococcus aureus	25923	23 - 29
Pseudomonas aeruginosa	27853	24 - 30
Haemophilus influenza	49247	25 - 31

TABLE 6

Microorganism	Zone Diameter (mm)		
	Susceptible (S)	Intermediate (I)	Resistant (R)
Microorganisms other than *Haemophilus* spp.* and *S. pneumoniae**	≥ 18	15-17	≤ 14
Haemophilus spp.*	≥ 26	—*	—*

* NOTE: Isolates from these species should be tested for susceptibility using specialized diffusion testing methods[2]. Isolates of *Haemophilus* spp. with zones smaller than 26 mm should be considered equivocal and should be further evaluated. Isolates of *S. pneumoniae* should be tested against a 1 µg oxacillin disk; isolates with oxacillin zone sizes larger than or equal to 20 mm may be considered susceptible to cefepime.

INDICATIONS AND USAGE

MAXIPIME (cefepime hydrochloride) is indicated in the treatment of the following infections caused by susceptible strains of the designated microorganisms:

Pneumonia (moderate to severe) caused by *Streptococcus pneumoniae*, including cases associated with concurrent bacteremia, *Pseudomonas aeruginosa*, *Klebsiella pneumoniae*, or *Enterobacter* species.

Empiric Therapy for Febrile Neutropenic Patients. Cefepime as monotherapy is indicated for empiric treatment of febrile neutropenic patients. In patients at high risk for severe infection (including patients with a history of recent bone marrow transplantation, with hypotension at presentation, with an underlying hematologic malignancy, or with severe or prolonged neutropenia), antimicrobial monotherapy may not be appropriate. Insufficient data exist to support the efficacy of cefepime monotherapy in such patients. (See **CLINICAL STUDIES**.)

Uncomplicated and Complicated Urinary Tract Infections (including pyelonephritis) caused by *Escherichia coli* or *Klebsiella pneumoniae*, when the infection is severe, or caused by *Escherichia coli*, *Klebsiella pneumoniae*, or *Proteus mirabilis*, when the infection is mild to moderate, including cases associated with concurrent bacteremia with these microorganisms.

Uncomplicated Skin and Skin Structure Infections caused by *Staphylococcus aureus* (methicillin-susceptible strains only) or *Streptococcus pyogenes*.

Complicated Intra-abdominal Infections (used in combination with metronidazole) caused by *Escherichia coli*, viridans group streptococci, Pseudomonas aeruginosa, Klebsiella pneumoniae, Enterobacter species, or *Bacteroides fragilis*. (See **CLINICAL STUDIES**.)

Culture and susceptibility testing should be performed where appropriate to determine the susceptibility of the causative microorganism(s) to cefepime.

Therapy with MAXIPIME may be instituted before results of susceptibility studies are known; however, once these results become available, the antibiotic treatment should be adjusted accordingly.

CLINICAL STUDIES

Febrile Neutropenic Patients

The safety and efficacy of empiric cefepime monotherapy of febrile neutropenic patients have been assessed in two multicenter, randomized trials, comparing cefepime monotherapy (at a dose of 2 g IV q8h) to ceftazidime monotherapy (at a dose of 2 g IV q8h). These studies comprised 317 evaluable patients. Table 8 describes the characteristics of the evaluable patient population.

[See table 8 at top of next page]

Table 9 describes the clinical response rates observed. For all outcome measures, cefepime was therapeutically equivalent to ceftazidime.

[See table 9 on next page]

Insufficient data exist to support the efficacy of cefepime monotherapy in patients at high risk for severe infection (including patients with a history of recent bone marrow transplantation, with hypotension at presentation, with an underlying hematologic malignancy, or with severe or prolonged neutropenia). No data are available in patients with septic shock.

Complicated Intra-abdominal Infections

Patients hospitalized with complicated intra-abdominal infections participated in a randomized, double-blind, multicenter trial comparing the combination of cefepime (2 g q12h) plus intravenous metronidazole (500 mg q6h) versus imipenem/cilastatin (500 mg q6h) for a maximum duration of 14 days of therapy. The study was designed to demonstrate equivalence of the two therapies. The primary analyses were conducted on the protocol-valid population, which consisted of those with a surgically confirmed complicated infection, at least one pathogen isolated pretreatment, at least 5 days of treatment, and a 4–6 week follow-up assessment for cured patients. Subjects in the imipenem/cilastatin arm had higher APACHE II scores at baseline. The treatment groups were otherwise generally comparable with regard to their pretreatment characteristics. The overall clinical cure rate among the protocol-valid patients was 81% (51 cured/63 evaluable patients) in the cefepime plus metronidazole group and 66% (62/94) in the imipenem/cilastatin group. The observed differences in efficacy may have been due to a greater proportion of patients with high APACHE II scores in the imipenem/cilastatin group.

CONTRAINDICATIONS

MAXIPIME (cefepime hydrochloride) is contraindicated in patients who have shown immediate hypersensitivity reactions to cefepime or the cephalosporin class of antibiotics, penicillins or other beta-lactam antibiotics.

WARNINGS

BEFORE THERAPY WITH MAXIPIME (CEFEPIME HYDROCHLORIDE) FOR INJECTION IS INSTITUTED, CAREFUL INQUIRY SHOULD BE MADE TO DETERMINE WHETHER THE PATIENT HAS HAD PREVIOUS IMMEDIATE HYPERSENSITIVITY REACTIONS TO CEFEPIME, CEPHALOSPORINS, PENICILLINS, OR OTHER DRUGS. IF THIS PRODUCT IS TO BE GIVEN TO PENICILLIN-SENSITIVE PATIENTS, CAUTION SHOULD BE EXERCISED BECAUSE CROSS-HYPERSENSITIVITY AMONG BETA-LACTAM ANTIBIOTICS HAS BEEN CLEARLY DOCUMENTED AND MAY OCCUR IN UP TO 10% OF PATIENTS WITH A HISTORY OF PENICILLIN ALLERGY. IF AN ALLERGIC REACTION TO MAXIPIME OCCURS, DISCONTINUE THE DRUG. SERIOUS ACUTE HYPERSENSITIVITY REACTIONS MAY REQUIRE TREATMENT WITH EPINEPHRINE AND OTHER EMERGENCY MEASURES INCLUDING OXYGEN, CORTICOSTEROIDS, INTRAVENOUS FLUIDS, INTRAVENOUS ANTIHISTAMINES, PRESSOR AMINES, AND AIRWAY MANAGEMENT, AS CLINICALLY INDICATED.

Pseudomembranous colitis has been reported with nearly all antibacterial agents, including MAXIPIME, and may range in severity from mild to life-threatening. Therefore, it is important to consider this diagnosis in patients who present with diarrhea subsequent to the administration of antibacterial agents.

Treatment with antibacterial agents alters the normal flora of the colon and may permit overgrowth of clostridia. Studies indicate that a toxin produced by *Clostridium difficile* is a primary cause of "antibiotic-associated colitis".

After the diagnosis of pseudomembranous colitis has been established, therapeutic measures should be initiated. Mild cases of pseudomembranous colitis usually respond to drug discontinuation alone. In moderate-to-severe cases, consideration should be given to management with fluids and electrolytes, protein supplementation, and treatment with an antibacterial drug clinically effective against *Clostridium difficile* colitis.

PRECAUTIONS

General: As with other antimicrobials, prolonged use of MAXIPIME may result in overgrowth of nonsusceptible microorganisms. Repeated evaluation of the patient's condition is essential. Should superinfection occur during therapy, appropriate measures should be taken.

Many cephalosporins, including cefepime, have been associated with a fall in prothrombin activity. Those at risk include patients with renal or hepatic impairment, or poor nutritional state, as well as patients receiving a protracted course of antimicrobial therapy. Prothrombin time should be monitored in patients at risk, and exogenous vitamin K administered as indicated.

Positive direct Coombs' tests have been reported during treatment with MAXIPIME. In hematologic studies or in transfusion cross-matching procedures when antiglobulin tests are performed on the minor side or in Coombs' testing of newborns whose mothers have received cephalosporin antibiotics before parturition, it should be recognized that a positive Coombs' test may be due to the drug.

Continued on next page

Maxipime—Cont.

MAXIPIME should be prescribed with caution in individuals with a history of gastrointestinal disease, particularly colitis.

Arginine has been shown to alter glucose metabolism and elevate serum potassium transiently when administered at 33 times the amount provided by the maximum recommended human dose of MAXIPIME. The effect of lower doses is not presently known.

In patients with impaired renal function (creatinine clearance ≤60 mL/min), the dose of MAXIPIME should be adjusted to compensate for the slower rate of renal elimination. Because high and prolonged serum antibiotic concentrations can occur from usual dosages in patients with renal insufficiency or other conditions that may compromise renal function, the maintenance dosage should be reduced when cefepime is administered to such patients. Serious adverse events including encephalopathy, myoclonus, seizures, and/or renal failure have been reported postmarketing in patients with renal impairment treated with unadjusted doses of cefepime (see **ADVERSE REACTIONS**: In Postmarketing Experience and OVERDOSAGE). Continued dosage should be determined by degree of renal impairment, severity of infection, and susceptibility of the causative organisms. (See specific recommendations for dosing adjustment in **DOSAGE AND ADMINISTRATION.**)

Drug Interactions

Renal function should be monitored carefully if high doses of aminoglycosides are to be administered with MAXIPIME because of the increased potential of nephrotoxicity and ototoxicity of aminoglycoside antibiotics. Nephrotoxicity has been reported following concomitant administration of other cephalosporins with potent diuretics such as furosemide.

Drug/Laboratory Test Interactions

The administration of cefepime may result in a false-positive reaction for glucose in the urine when using Clinitest® tablets. It is recommended that glucose tests based on enzymatic glucose oxidase reactions (such as Clinistix® or Tes-Tape®) be used.

Carcinogenesis, Mutagenesis, and Impairment of Fertility

No long-term animal carcinogenicity studies have been conducted with cefepime. A battery of *in vivo* and *in vitro* genetic toxicity tests, including the Ames Salmonella reverse mutation assay, CHO/HGPRT mammalian cell forward gene mutation assay, chromosomal aberration and sister chromatid exchange assays in human lymphocytes, CHO fibroblast clastogenesis assay, and cytogenetic and micronucleus assays in mice were conducted. The overall conclusion of these tests indicated no definitive evidence of genotoxic potential. No untoward effects on fertility or reproduction have been observed in rats, mice, and rabbits when cefepime is administered subcutaneously at 1 to 4 times the recommended maximum human dose calculated on a mg/m^2 basis.

Usage in Pregnancy—Teratogenic effects—Pregnancy Category B

Cefepime was not teratogenic or embryocidal when administered during the period of organogenesis to rats at doses up to 1000 mg/kg/day (4 times the recommended maximum human dose calculated on a mg/m^2 basis) or to mice at doses up to 1200 mg/kg (2 times the recommended maximum human dose calculated on a mg/m^2 basis) or to rabbits at a dose level of 100 mg/kg (approximately equal to the recommended maximum human dose calculated on a mg/m^2 basis).

There are, however, no adequate and well-controlled studies of cefepime use in pregnant women. Because animal reproduction studies are not always predictive of human response, this drug should be used during pregnancy only if clearly needed.

Nursing Mothers

Cefepime is excreted in human breast milk in very low concentrations [0.5 μg/mL]. Caution should be exercised when cefepime is administered to a nursing woman.

Labor and Delivery

Cefepime has not been studied for use during labor and delivery. Treatment should only be given if clearly indicated.

Pediatric Use

The safety and efficacy of MAXIPIME (cefepime hydrochloride) in pediatric patients below the age of 12 years have not been established. This product is intended for use in patients 12 years of age and older.

Geriatric Use

In clinical studies, when geriatric patients received the usual recommended adult dose, clinical efficacy and safety were comparable to clinical efficacy and safety in non-geriatric adult patients.

In elderly patients, dosage and administration of cefepime should be adjusted in the presence of renal insufficiency. (See **DOSAGE and ADMINISTRATION.**)

ADVERSE REACTIONS

Clinical Trials: In clinical trials using multiple doses of cefepime, 4137 patients were treated with the recommended dosages of cefepime (500 mg to 2 g IV q12h). There

TABLE 8
Demographics of Evaluable Patients (First Episodes Only)

	Cefepime	Ceftazidime
Total	164	153
Median age (yr)	56.0 (range, 18-82)	55.0 (range, 16-84)
Male	86 (52%)	85 (56%)
Female	78 (48%)	68 (44%)
Leukemia	65 (40%)	52 (34%)
Other hematologic malignancies	43 (26%)	36 (24%)
Solid tumor	54 (33%)	56 (37%)
Median ANC nadir (cells/μL)	20.0 (range, 0-500)	20.0 (range, 0-500)
Median duration of neutropenia (days)	6.0 (range, 0–39)	6.0 (range, 0-32)
Indwelling venous catheter	97 (59%)	86 (56%)
Prophylactic antibiotics	62 (38%)	64 (42%)
Bone marrow graft	9 (5%)	7 (5%)
SBP < 90 mm Hg at entry	7 (4%)	2 (1%)

ANC = absolute neutropil count; SBP = systolic blood pressure.

TABLE 9
Pooled Response Rates For Empiric Therapy of Febrile Neutropenic Patients

	% Response	
	Cefepime	Ceftazidime
Outcome Measures	**(N=164)**	**(N=153)**
Primary episode resolved with no treatment modification, no new febrile episodes or infection, and oral antibiotics allowed for completion of treatment	51	55
Primary episode resolved with no treatment modification, no new febrile episodes or infection, and no post-treatment oral antibiotics	34	39
Survival, any treatment modification allowed	93	97
Primary episode resolved with no treatment modification and oral antibiotics allowed for completion of treatment	62	67
Primary episode resoled with no treatment modification and no post-treatment oral antibiotics	46	51

TABLE 10
Adverse Clinical Reactions
Cefepime Multiple-Dose
Dosing Regimens Clinical Trials—North America

INCIDENCE EQUAL TO OR GREATER THAN 1%	Local reactions (3.0%), including phlebitis (1.3%), pain and/or inflammation (0.6%)*; rash (1.1%)
INCIDENCE LESS THAN 1% BUT GREATER THAN 0.1%	Colitis (including pseudomembranous colitis), diarrhea, fever, headache, nausea, oral moniliasis, pruritus, urticarial, vaginitis, vomiting

* local reactions, irrespective of relationship to cefepime in those patients who received intravenous infusion (n = 3048).

TABLE 11
Adverse Laboratory Changes
Cefepime Multiple-Dose Dosing Regimens
Clinical Trials—North America

INCIDENCE EQUAL TO OR GREATER THAN 1%	Positive Coombs' test (without hemolysis) (16.2%); decreased phosphorous (2.8%); increased ALT/SGPT (2.8%), AST/SGOT (2.4%), eosinophils (1.7%); abnormal PTT (1.6%), PT (1.4%)
INCIDENCE LESS THAN 1% BUT GREATER THAN 0.1%	Increased alkaline phosphatase, BUN, calcium, creatinine, phosphorous, potassium, total bilirubin; decreased calcium*, hematocrit, neutrophils, platelets, WBC

* Hypocalcemia was more common among elderly patients. Clinical consequences from changes in either calcium or phosphorus were not reported.

were no deaths or permanent disabilities thought related to drug toxicity. Sixty-four (1.5%) patients discontinued medication due to adverse events thought by the investigators to be possibly, probably, or almost certainly related to drug toxicity. Thirty-three (51%) of these 64 patients who discontinued therapy did so because of rash. The percentage of cefepime-treated patients who discontinued study drug because of drug-related adverse events was very similar at daily doses of 500 mg, 1 g and 2 g q12h (0.8%, 1.1%, and 2.0%, respectively). However, the incidence of discontinuation due to rash increased with the higher recommended doses.

The following adverse events were thought to be probably related to cefepime during evaluation of the drug in clinical trials conducted in North America (n=3125 cefepime-treated patients).
[See table 10 above]

At the higher dose of 2 g q8h, the incidence of probably-related adverse events was higher among the 795 patients who received this dose of cefepime. They consisted of rash (4%), diarrhea (3%), nausea (2%), vomiting (1%), pruritus (1%), fever (1%), and headache (1%).

The following adverse laboratory changes, irrespective of relationship to therapy with cefepime, were seen during clinical trials conducted in North America.
[See table 11 above]

In Postmarketing Experience: In addition to the events reported during North American clinical trials with cefepime, the following adverse experiences have been reported during worldwide postmarketing experience. Because of the uncontrolled nature of spontaneous reports, a causal relationship to MAXIPIME (cefepime hydrochloride) treatment has not been determined.

Encephalopathy, myoclonus, and seizures have been reported in renally impaired patients treated with unadjusted dosing regimens of cefepime. Several cephalosporins have been implicated in triggering seizures, particularly in patients with renal impairment when the dosage

was not reduced. (See **DOSAGE AND ADMINISTRATION** and **OVERDOSAGE**.) If seizures associated with drug therapy occur, the drug should be discontinued. Anticonvulsant therapy can be given if clinically indicated. Precautions should be taken to adjust daily dosage in patients with renal insufficiency or other conditions that may compromise renal function to reduce antibiotic concentrations that can lead or contribute to these and other serious adverse events, including renal failure.

As with other cephalosporins, transient leukopenia, neutropenia, agranulocytosis and thrombocytopenia have been reported.

Cephalosporin-class adverse reactions: In addition to the adverse reactions listed above that have been observed in patients treated with cefepime, the following adverse reactions and altered laboratory tests have been reported for cephalosporin-class antibiotics:

Stevens-Johnson syndrome, erythema multiforme, toxic epidermal necrolysis, renal dysfunction, toxic nephropathy, aplastic anemia, hemolytic anemia, hemorrhage, hepatic dysfunction including cholestasis, and pancytopenia.

OVERDOSAGE

Patients who receive an overdose should be carefully observed and given supportive treatment. In the presence of renal insufficiency, hemodialysis, not peritoneal dialysis, is recommended to aid in the removal of cefepime from the body.

Accidental overdosing might occur if large doses are given to patients with reduced renal function. In clinical trials, MAXIPIME overdosage occurred in a patient with renal failure (creatinine clearance <11 mL/min) who received 2 g q24h for 7 days. The patient exhibited seizures, encephalopathy, and neuromuscular excitability. (See **PRECAUTIONS**, **ADVERSE REACTIONS**, and **DOSAGE AND ADMINISTRATION**.)

DOSAGE AND ADMINISTRATION

The recommended adult dosages and routes of administration are outlined in the following table. MAXIPIME should be administered intravenously over approximately 30 minutes.

[See table 12 above]

Impaired Hepatic Function—No adjustment is necessary for patients with impaired hepatic function.

Impaired Renal Function—In patients with impaired renal function (creatinine clearance ≤60 mL/min), the dose of MAXIPIME (cefepime hydrochloride) should be adjusted to compensate for the slower rate of renal elimination. The recommended initial dose of MAXIPIME should be the same as in patients with normal renal function. The recommended maintenance doses of MAXIPIME in patients with renal insufficiency are presented in Table 13.

[See table 13 above]

When only serum creatinine is available, the following formula (Cockcroft and Gault equation)[3] may be used to estimate creatinine clearance. The serum creatinine should represent a steady state of renal function:

[See third table from top of page]

In patients undergoing hemodialysis, approximately 68% of the total amount of cefepime present in the body at the start of dialysis will be removed during a 3-hour dialysis period. A repeat dose, equivalent to the initial dose, should be given at the completion of each dialysis session.

In patients undergoing continuous ambulatory peritoneal dialysis, MAXIPIME may be administered at normally recommended doses at a dosage interval of every 48 hours.

Administration:

For Intravenous Infusion, constitute the 1 g or 2 g piggyback (100 mL) bottle with 50 or 100 mL of a compatible IV fluid listed in the **Compatibility and Stability** subsection. Alternatively, constitute the 500 mg, 1 g, or 2 g vial, and add an appropriate quantity of the resulting solution to an IV container with one of the compatible IV fluids. **THE RESULTING SOLUTION SHOULD BE ADMINISTERED OVER APPROXIMATELY 30 MINUTES.**

Intermittent IV infusion with a Y-type administration set can be accomplished with compatible solutions. However, during infusion of a solution containing cefepime, it is desirable to discontinue the other solution.

ADD-Vantage® vials are to be constituted only with 50 or 100 mL of 5% Dextrose Injection or 0.9% Sodium Chloride Injection in Abbott ADD-Vantage® flexible diluent containers. (See ADD-Vantage® Vial Instructions for Use.)

Intramuscular Administration: For IM administration, MAXIPIME (cefepime hydrochloride) should be constituted with one of the following diluents: Sterile Water for Injection, 0.9% Sodium Chloride, 5% Dextrose Injection, 0.5% or 1.0% Lidocaine Hydrochloride, or Sterile Bacteriostatic Water for Injection with Parabens or Benzyl Alcohol (refer to Table 14). Preparation of MAXIPIME solutions is summarized in Table 14.

[See table 14 above]

Compatibility and Stability:

Intravenous: MAXIPIME is compatible at concentrations between 1 and 40 mg/mL with the following IV infusion fluids: 0.9% Sodium Chloride Injection, 5% and 10% Dextrose Injection, M/6 Sodium Lactate Injection, 5% Dextrose and 0.9% Sodium Chloride Injection, Lactated Ringers and 5% Dextrose Injection, Normosol-R®, and Normosol-M® in 5% Dextrose Injection. These solutions may be stored up to 24 hours at controlled room temperature 20°–25° C (68°–77° F) or 7 days in a refrigerator 2°–8° C (36°–46° F). MAXIPIME in ADD-Vantage® vials is stable at concentrations of 10–40 mg/mL in 5% Dextrose Injection or 0.9% Sodium Chloride Injection for 24 hours at controlled room temperature 20°–25° C or 7 days in a refrigerator 2°–8° C.

MAXIPIME admixture compatibility information is summarized in Table 15.

[See table 15 on next page]

Table 12
Recommended Dosage Schedule for MAXIPIME

Site and Type of Infection	Dose	Frequency	Duration (days)
Moderate to Severe Pneumonia due to *S. pneumoniae**, *P. aeruginosa, K. pneumoniae,* or *Enterobacter* species	1–2 g IV	q12h	10
Empiric therapy for febrile neutropenic patients (See **INDICATIONS AND USAGE** and **CLINICAL STUDIES**.)	2 g IV	q8h	7**
Mild to Moderate Uncomplicated or Complicated Urinary Tract Infections, including pyelonephritis, due to *E. coli, K. pneumoniae,* or *P. mirabilis**	0.5–1 g IV/IM***	q12h	7–10
Severe Uncomplicated or Complicated Urinary Tract Infections, including pyelonephritis, due to *E. coli* or *K. pneumoniae**	2 g IV	q12h	10
Moderate to Severe Uncomplicated Skin and Skin Structure Infections due to *S. aureus* or *S. pyogenes*	2 g IV	q12h	10
Complicated Intra-abdominal Infections (used in combination with metronidazole) caused by *E. coli,* viridans group streptococci, *P. aeruginosa, K. pneumoniae, Enterobacter* species, or *B. fragilis.* (See **CLINICAL STUDIES**.)	2 g IV	q12h	7–10

* including cases associated with concurrent bacteremia
** or until resolution of neutropenia. In patients whose fever resolves but who remain neutropenic for more than 7 days, the need for continued antimicrobial therapy should be re-evaluated frequently.
***IM route of administration is indicated only for mild to moderate, uncomplicated or complicated UTI's due to *E. coli* when the IM route is considered to be a more appropriate route of drug administration.

TABLE 13
Recommended Maintenance Schedule in Adult Patients with Renal Impairment Relative to Normal Recommended Dosing Schedule

Creatinine Clearance (mL/min)	Recommended Maintenance Schedule			
> 60 Normal recommended dosing schedule	500 mg q12h	1 g q12h	2 g q12h	2 g q8h
30 – 60	500 mg q24h	1 g q24h	2 g q24h	2 g q12h
11 – 29	500 mg q24h	500 mg q24h	1 g q24h	2 g q24h
< 11	250 mg q24h	250 mg q24h	500 mg q24h	1 g q24h

Males: Creatinine Clearance (mL/min) $= \dfrac{\text{Weight (kg)} \times (140 - \text{age})}{72 \times \text{serum creatinine (mg/dL)}}$

Females: 0.85 × above value

TABLE 14
Preparation of Solutions of Maxipime

Single Dose Vials for Intravenous/Intramuscular Administration	Amount of Diluent to be added (mL)	Approximate Available Volume (mL)	Approximate Cefepime Concentration (mg/mL)
cefepime vial content			
500 mg (IV)	5.0	5.6	100
500 mg (IM)	1.3	1.8	280
1 g (IV)	10.0	11.3	100
1 g (IM)	2.4	3.6	280
2 g (IV)	10.0	12.5	160
Piggyback (100 mL)			
1 g bottle	50	50	20
1 g bottle	100	100	10
2 g bottle	50	50	40
2 g bottle	100	100	20
ADD-Vantage®			
1 g vial	50	50	20
1 g vial	100	100	10
2 g vial	50	50	40
2 g vial	100	100	20

Continued on next page

Maxipime—Cont.

Solutions of MAXIPIME, like those of most beta-lactam antibiotics, should not be added to solutions of ampicillin at a concentration greater than 40 mg/mL, and should not be added to metronidazole, vancomycin, gentamicin, tobramycin, netilmicin sulfate or aminophylline because of potential interaction. However, if concurrent therapy with MAXIPIME is indicated, each of these antibiotics can be administered separately.

Intramuscular: MAXIPIME (cefepime hydrochloride) constituted as directed is stable for 24 hours at controlled room temperature 20°–25° C (68°–77° F) or for 7 days in a refrigerator 2°–8° C (36°–46° F) with the following diluents: Sterile Water for Injection, 0.9% Sodium Chloride Injection, 5% Dextrose Injection, Sterile Bacteriostatic Water for Injection with Parabens or Benzyl Alcohol, or 0.5% or 1% Lidocaine Hydrochloride.

NOTE: PARENTERAL DRUGS SHOULD BE INSPECTED VISUALLY FOR PARTICULATE MATTER BEFORE ADMINISTRATION.

As with other cephalosporins, the color of MAXIPIME powder, as well as its solutions, tend to darken depending on storage conditions; however, when stored as recommended, the product potency is not adversely affected.

HOW SUPPLIED

MAXIPIME® (cefepime hydrochloride) for Injection is supplied as follows:
[See table at bottom of page]

Storage
MAXIPIME IN THE DRY STATE SHOULD BE STORED BETWEEN 2°–25° C (36°–77° F) AND PROTECTED FROM LIGHT.
U.S. Patent No. 4,406,899; 4,910,301; 4,994,451 and 5,244,891

REFERENCES

(1) National Committee for Clinical Laboratory *Standards. Methods for Dilution Antimicrobial Susceptibility Tests for Bacteria that Grow Aerobically*—Third Edition. Approved Standard NCCLS Document M7-A3, Vol. 13, No. 25, NCCLS, Villanova, PA, December, 1993.
(2) National Committee for Clinical Laboratory Standards. *Performance Standards for Antimicrobial Disk Susceptibility Tests*—Fifth Edition. Approved Standard NCCLS Document M2-A5, Vol. 13, No. 24, NCCLS, Villanova, PA, December, 1993.
(3) Cockcroft DW, Gault MH. Prediction of creatinine clearance from serum creatinine. *Nephron.* 1976; 16:31–41.

ADD-Vantage® is a registered trademark of Abbott Laboratories.
Normosol-R® is a registered trademark of Abbott Laboratories.
Normosol-M® is a registered trademark of Abbott Laboratories.
Aminosyn® is a registered trademark of Abbott Laboratories.
Inpersol® is a registered trademark of Abbott Laboratories.
Clinitest® and Clinistix® are registered trademarks of the Bayer Corporation.
Tes-Tape® is a registered trademark of Eli Lilly and Company.

Bristol-Myers Squibb Company
Princeton, NJ 08543
U.S.A.
Revised: January 1998
7733DIM-06
51-004476-04
E4-B001-1-98

Shown in Product Identification Guide, page 307

MONOPRIL® ℞
Fosinopril Sodium Tablets

CAUTION: Federal law prohibits dispensing without prescription.

> **USE IN PREGNANCY**
> When used in pregnancy during the second and third trimesters, ACE inhibitors can cause injury and even death to the developing fetus. When pregnancy is detected, MONOPRIL should be discontinued as soon as possible. **See WARNINGS: Fetal/Neonatal Morbidity and Mortality**

DESCRIPTION
MONOPRIL (fosinopril sodium tablets) is the sodium salt of fosinopril, the ester prodrug of an angiotensin converting enzyme (ACE) inhibitor, fosinoprilat. It contains a phosphinate group capable of specific binding to the active site of angiotensin converting enzyme. Fosinopril sodium is designated chemically as: L-proline, 4-cyclohexyl-1-[[[2-methyl-1-(1-oxopropoxy) propoxy] (4-phenylbutyl) phosphinyl]acetyl]-, sodium salt, *trans*-.
Fosinopril sodium is a white to off-white crystalline powder. It is soluble in water (100 mg/mL), methanol, and ethanol and slightly soluble in hexane.
Its empiric formula is $C_{30}H_{45}NNaO_7P$, and its molecular weight is 585.65.
MONOPRIL is available for oral administration as 10 mg, 20 mg, and 40 mg tablets. Inactive ingredients include: lactose, microcrystalline cellulose, crospovidone, povidone, and sodium stearyl fumarate.

CLINICAL PHARMACOLOGY
Mechanism of Action
In animals and humans, fosinopril sodium is hydrolyzed by esterases to the pharmacologically active form, fosinoprilat, a specific competitive inhibitor of angiotensin converting enzyme (ACE).
ACE is a peptidyl dipeptidase that catalyzes the conversion of angiotensin I to the vasoconstrictor substance, angiotensin II. Angiotensin II also stimulates aldosterone secretion by the adrenal cortex. Inhibition of ACE results in decreased plasma angiotensin II, which leads to decreased vasopressor activity and to decreased aldosterone secretion. The latter decrease may result in a small increase of serum potassium.
In 647 hypertensive patients treated with fosinopril alone for an average of 29 weeks, mean increases in serum potassium of 0.1 mEq/L were observed. Similar increases were observed among all patients treated with fosinopril, including those receiving concomitant diuretic therapy. Removal of angiotensin II negative feedback on renin secretion leads to increased plasma renin activity.
ACE is identical to kininase, an enzyme that degrades bradykinin. Whether increased levels of bradykinin, a potent vasodepressor peptide, play a role in the therapeutic effects of MONOPRIL remains to be elucidated.
While the mechanism through which MONOPRIL lowers blood pressure is believed to be primarily suppression of the renin-angiotensin-aldosterone system, MONOPRIL has an antihypertensive effect even in patients with low-renin hypertension. Although MONOPRIL was antihypertensive in all races studied, black hypertensive patients (usually a low-renin hypertensive population) had a smaller average response to ACE inhibitor monotherapy than non-black patients.
In patients with heart failure, the beneficial effects of MONOPRIL are thought to result primarily from suppression of the renin-angiotensin-aldosterone system; inhibition of the angiotensin-converting enzyme produces decreases in both preload and afterload.

Pharmacokinetics and Metabolism
Following oral administration, fosinopril (the prodrug) is absorbed slowly. The absolute absorption of fosinopril averaged 36% of an oral dose. The primary site of absorption is the proximal small intestine (duodenum/jejunum). While the rate of absorption may be slowed by the presence of food in the gastrointestinal tract, the extent of absorption of fosinopril is essentially unaffected.
Fosinoprilat is highly protein-bound (approximately 99.4%), has a relatively small volume of distribution, and has negligible binding to cellular components in blood. After single and multiple oral doses, plasma levels, areas under plasma concentration-time curves (AUCs) and peak concentrations (Cmaxs) are directly proportional to the dose of fosinopril. Times to peak concentrations are independent of dose and are achieved in approximately 3 hours.
After an oral dose of radiolabeled fosinopril, 75% of radioactivity in plasma was present as active fosinoprilat, 20–30%

Table 15
Cefepime Admixture Stability

Maxipime Concentration	Admixture and Concentration	IV Infusion Solutions	Stability Time for	
			RT/L (20°–25° C)	Refrigeration (2°–8° C)
40 mg/mL	Amikacin 6 mg/mL	NS or D5W	24 hours	7 days
40 mg/mL	Ampicillin 1 mg/mL	D5W	8 hours	8 hours
40 mg/mL	Ampicillin 10 mg/mL	D5W	2 hours	8 hours
40 mg/mL	Ampicillin 1 mg/mL	NS	24 hours	48 hours
40 mg/mL	Ampicillin 10 mg/mL	NS	8 hours	48 hours
4 mg/mL	Ampicillin 40 mg/mL	NS	8 hours	8 hours
4–40 mg/mL	Clindamycin Phosphate 0.25–6 mg/mL	NS or D5W	24 hours	7 days
4 mg/mL	Heparin 10–50 units/mL	NS or D5W	24 hours	7 days
4 mg/mL	Potassium Chloride 10–40 mEq/L	NS or D5W	24 hours	7 days
4 mg/mL	Theophylline 0.8 mg/mL	D5W	24 hours	7 days
1–4 mg/mL	na	Aminosyn® II 4.25% with electrolytes and calcium	8 hours	3 days
0.125–0.25 mg/mL	na	Inpersol® with 4.25% dextrose	24 hours	7 days

NS = 0.9% Sodium Chloride Injection
D5W = 5% Dextrose Injection
na = not applicable
RT/L = Ambient room temperature and light

NDC 0003-7731-99	500 mg*	15 mL vial (tray of 10)
NDC 0003-7732-95	1 g*	Piggyback bottle 100 mL (tray of 10)
NDC 0003-7732-89	1 g*	ADD-Vantage® vial (tray of 10)
NDC 0003-7732-99	1 g*	15 mL vial (tray of 10)
NDC 0003-7733-95	2 g*	Piggyback bottle 100 mL (tray of 10)
NDC 0003-7733-31	2 g*	ADD-Vantage® vial (tray of 10)
NDC 0003-7733-99	2 g*	20 mL vial (tray of 10)

*Based on cefepime activity

as a glucuronide conjugate of fosinoprilat, and 1–5% as a *p*-hydroxy metabolite of fosinoprilat. Since fosinoprilat is not biotransformed after intravenous administration, fosinopril, not fosinoprilat, appears to be the precursor for the glucuronide and *p*-hydroxy metabolites. In rats, the *p*-hydroxy metabolite of fosinoprilat is as potent an inhibitor of ACE as fosinoprilat; the glucuronide conjugate is devoid of ACE inhibitory activity.

After intravenous administration, fosinoprilat was eliminated approximately equally by the liver and kidney. After oral administration of radiolabeled fosinopril, approximately half of the absorbed dose is excreted in the urine and the remainder is excreted in the feces. In two studies involving healthy subjects, the mean body clearance of intravenous fosinoprilat was between 26 and 39 mL/min.

In healthy subjects, the terminal elimination half-life ($t^1/_2$) of an intravenous dose of radiolabeled fosinoprilat is approximately 12 hours. In hypertensive patients with normal renal and hepatic function, who received repeated doses of fosinopril, the effective $t^1/_2$ for accumulation of fosinoprilat averaged 11.5 hours. In patients with heart failure, the effective $t^1/_2$ was 14 hours.

In patients with mild to severe renal insufficiency (creatinine clearance 10–80 mL/min/1.73m²), the clearance of fosinoprilat does not differ appreciably from normal, because of the large contribution of hepatobiliary elimination. In patients with end-stage renal disease (creatinine clearance <10 mL/min/1.73m²), the total body clearance of fosinoprilat is approximately one-half of that in patients with normal renal function. (See DOSAGE AND ADMINISTRATION.)

Fosinopril is not well dialyzed. Clearance of fosinoprilat by hemodialysis and peritoneal dialysis averages 2% and 7%, respectively, of urea clearances.

In patients with hepatic insufficiency (alcoholic or biliary cirrhosis), the extent of hydrolysis of fosinopril is not appreciably reduced, although the rate of hydrolysis may be slowed; the apparent total body clearance of fosinoprilat is approximately one-half of that in patients with normal hepatic function.

In elderly (male) subjects (65–74 years old) with clinically normal renal and hepatic function, there appear to be no significant differences in pharmacokinetic parameters for fosinoprilat compared to those of younger subjects (20–35 years old).

Fosinoprilat was found to cross the placenta of pregnant animals.

Studies in animals indicate that fosinopril and fosinoprilat do not cross the blood-brain barrier.

Pharmacodynamics and Clinical Effects

Serum ACE activity was inhibited by ≥90% at 2 to 12 hours after single doses of 10 to 40 mg of fosinopril. At 24 hours, serum ACE activity remained suppressed by 85%, 93%, and 93% in the 10, 20, and 40 mg dose groups, respectively.

Hypertension

Administration of MONOPRIL (fosinopril sodium tablets) to patients with mild to moderate hypertension results in a reduction of both supine and standing blood pressure to about the same extent with no compensatory tachycardia. Symptomatic postural hypotension is infrequent, although it can occur in patients who are salt- and/or volume-depleted (see WARNINGS.) Use of MONOPRIL in combination with thiazide diuretics gives a blood pressure-lowering effect greater than that seen with either agent alone.

Following oral administration of single doses of 10–40 mg, MONOPRIL lowered blood pressure within one hour, with peak reductions achieved 2–6 hours after dosing. The antihypertensive effect of a single dose persisted for 24 hours. Following four weeks of monotherapy in placebo-controlled trials in patients with mild to moderate hypertension, once daily doses of 20–80 mg lowered supine or seated systolic and diastolic blood pressures 24 hours after dosing by an average of 8–9/6–7 mmHg more than placebo. The trough effect was about 50–60% of the peak diastolic response and about 80% of the peak systolic response.

In most trials, the antihypertensive effect of MONOPRIL increased during the first several weeks of repeated measurements. The antihypertensive effect of MONOPRIL has been shown to continue during long-term therapy for at least 2 years. Abrupt withdrawal of MONOPRIL has not resulted in a rapid increase in blood pressure.

Limited experience in controlled and uncontrolled trials combining fosinopril with a calcium channel blocker or a loop diuretic has indicated no unusual drug-drug interactions. Other ACE inhibitors have had less than additive effects with beta-adrenergic blockers, presumably because both drugs lower blood pressure by inhibiting parts of the renin-angiotensin system.

ACE inhibitors are generally less effective in blacks than in non-blacks. The effectiveness of MONOPRIL was not influenced by age, sex, or weight.

In hemodynamic studies in hypertensive patients, after three months of therapy, responses (changes in BP, heart rate, cardiac index, and PVR) to various stimuli (e.g.: isometric exercise, 45° head-up tilt, and mental challenge) were unchanged compared to baseline, suggesting that MONOPRIL does not affect the activity of the sympathetic nervous system. Reduction in systemic blood pressure appears to have been mediated by a decrease in peripheral vascular resistance without reflex cardiac effects. Similarly, renal, splanchnic, cerebral, and skeletal muscle blood flow were unchanged compared to baseline, as was glomerular filtration rate.

Heart Failure

In a randomized, double-blind, placebo-controlled trial, 179 patients with heart failure, all receiving diuretics and some receiving digoxin, were administered single doses of 1, 20 or 40 mg of MONOPRIL or placebo. Doses of 20 and 40 mg of MONOPRIL resulted in acute decreases in pulmonary capillary wedge pressure (preload) and mean arterial blood pressure and systemic vascular resistance (afterload). One hundred fifty-five of these patients were re-randomized to once daily therapy with MONOPRIL (1, 20, or 40 mg) for an additional 10 weeks. Hemodynamic measurements made 24 hours after dosing showed (relative to baseline) continued reduction in pulmonary capillary wedge pressure, mean arterial blood pressure, right atrial pressure and an increase in cardiac index and stroke volume for the 20 and 40 mg dose groups. No tachyphylaxis was seen.

MONOPRIL was studied in 3 double-blind, placebo-controlled, 12–24 week trials including a total of 734 patients with heart failure, with MONOPRIL doses from 10 to 40 mg daily. Concomitant therapy in 2 of these 3 trials included diuretics and digitalis; in the third trial patients were receiving only diuretics. All 3 trials showed statistically significant benefits of MONOPRIL therapy, compared to placebo, in one or more of the following: exercise tolerance (one study), symptoms of dyspnea, orthopnea and paroxysmal nocturnal dyspnea (2 studies), NYHA classification (2 studies), hospitalization for heart failure (2 studies), study withdrawals for worsening heart failure (2 studies), and/or need for supplemental diuretics (2 studies). Favorable effects were maintained for up to two years. Effects of MONOPRIL on long-term mortality in heart failure have not been evaluated. The once daily dosage for the treatment of congestive heart failure was the only dosage regimen used during clinical trial development and was determined by the measurement of hemodynamic responses.

INDICATIONS AND USAGE

MONOPRIL is indicated for the treatment of hypertension. It may be used alone or in combination with thiazide diuretics.

MONOPRIL is indicated in the management of heart failure as adjunctive therapy when added to conventional therapy including diuretics with or without digitalis (see DOSAGE AND ADMINISTRATION).

In using MONOPRIL (fosinopril sodium tablets), consideration should be given to the fact that another angiotensin converting enzyme inhibitor, captopril, has caused agranulocytosis, particularly in patients with renal impairment or collagen-vascular disease. Available data are insufficient to show that MONOPRIL does not have a similar risk (see WARNINGS).

In considering use of MONOPRIL, it should be noted that in controlled trials ACE inhibitors have an effect on blood pressure that is less in black patients than in non-blacks. In addition, ACE inhibitors (for which adequate data are available) cause a higher rate of angioedema in black than in non-black patients (see **WARNINGS: Angioedema**).

CONTRAINDICATIONS

MONOPRIL is contraindicated in patients who are hypersensitive to this product or to any other angiotensin converting enzyme inhibitor (e.g., a patient who has experienced angioedema with any other ACE inhibitor therapy).

WARNINGS

Anaphylactoid and Possibly Related Reactions

Presumably because angiotensin-converting enzyme inhibitors affect the metabolism of eicosanoids and polypeptides, including endogenous bradykinin, patients receiving ACE inhibitors (including MONOPRIL) may be subject to a variety of adverse reactions, some of them serious.

Angioedema: Angioedema involving the extremities, face, lips, mucous membranes, tongue, glottis or larynx has been reported in patients treated with ACE inhibitors. If angioedema involves the tongue, glottis or larynx, airway obstruction may occur and be fatal. If laryngeal stridor or angioedema of the face, lips, mucous membranes, tongue, glottis or extremities occurs, treatment with MONOPRIL should be discontinued and appropriate therapy instituted immediately. **Where there is involvement of the tongue, glottis, or larynx, likely to cause airway obstruction, appropriate therapy, e.g., subcutaneous epinephrine solution 1:1000 (0.3 mL to 0.5 mL) should be promptly administered** (See PRECAUTIONS: Information for Patients and ADVERSE REACTIONS).

Anaphylactoid reactions during desensitization: Two patients undergoing desensitizing treatment with hymenoptera venom while receiving ACE inhibitors sustained life-threatening anaphylactoid reactions. In the same patients, these reactions were avoided when ACE inhibitors were temporarily withheld, but they reappeared upon inadvertent rechallenge.

Anaphylactoid reactions during membrane exposure: Anaphylactoid reactions have been reported in patients dialyzed with high-flux membranes and treated concomitantly with an ACE inhibitor. Anaphylactoid reactions have also been reported in patients undergoing low-density lipoprotein apheresis with dextran sulfate absorption.

Hypotension

MONOPRIL can cause symptomatic hypotension. Like other ACE inhibitors, fosinopril has been only rarely associated with hypotension in uncomplicated hypertensive patients. Symptomatic hypotension is most likely to occur in patients who have been volume- and/or salt-depleted as a result of prolonged diuretic therapy, dietary salt restriction, dialysis, diarrhea, or vomiting. Volume and/or salt depletion should be corrected before initiating therapy with MONOPRIL.

In patients with heart failure, with or without associated renal insufficiency, ACE inhibitor therapy may cause excessive hypotension, which may be associated with oliguria or azotemia and, rarely, with acute renal failure and death. In such patients, MONOPRIL therapy should be started under close medical supervision; they should be followed closely for the first 2 weeks of treatment and whenever the dose of fosinopril or diuretic is increased. Consideration should be given to reducing the diuretic dose in patients with normal or low blood pressure who have been treated vigorously with diuretics or who are hyponatremic.

If hypotension occurs, the patient should be placed in a supine position, and, if necessary, treated with intravenous infusion of physiological saline. MONOPRIL treatment usually can be continued following restoration of blood pressure and volume.

Neutropenia/Agranulocytosis

Another angiotensin converting enzyme inhibitor, captopril, has been shown to cause agranulocytosis and bone marrow depression, rarely in uncomplicated patients, but more frequently in patients with renal impairment, especially if they also have a collagen-vascular disease such as systemic lupus erythematosus or scleroderma. Available data from clinical trials of fosinopril are insufficient to show that fosinopril does not cause agranulocytosis at similar rates. Monitoring of white blood cell counts should be considered in patients with collagen-vascular disease, especially if the disease is associated with impaired renal function.

Fetal/Neonatal Morbidity and Mortality

ACE inhibitors can cause fetal and neonatal morbidity and death when administered to pregnant women. Several dozen cases have been reported in the world literature. When pregnancy is detected, ACE inhibitors should be discontinued as soon as possible.

The use of ACE inhibitors during the second and third trimesters of pregnancy has been associated with fetal and neonatal injury, including hypotension, neonatal skull hypoplasia, anuria, reversible or irreversible renal failure, and death. Oligohydramnios has also been reported, presumably resulting from decreased fetal renal function; oligohydramnios in this setting has been associated with fetal limb contractures, craniofacial deformation, and hypoplastic lung development. Prematurity, intrauterine growth retardation, and patent ductus arteriosus have also been reported, although it is not clear whether these occurrences were due to the ACE-inhibitor exposure.

These adverse effects do not appear to have resulted from intrauterine ACE-inhibitor exposure that has been limited to the first trimester. Mothers whose embryos and fetuses are exposed to ACE inhibitors only during the first trimester should be so informed. Nonetheless, when patients become pregnant, physicians should make every effort to discontinue the use of fosinopril as soon as possible.

Rarely (probably less often than once in every thousand pregnancies), no alternative to ACE inhibitors will be found. In these rare cases, the mothers should be apprised of the potential hazards to their fetuses, and serial ultrasound examinations should be performed to assess the intraamniotic environment.

If oligohydramnios is observed, fosinopril should be discontinued unless it is considered life-saving for the mother. Contraction stress testing (CST), a non-stress test (NST), or biophysical profiling (BPP) may be appropriate, depending upon the week of pregnancy. Patients and physicians should be aware, however, that oligohydramnios may not appear until after the fetus has sustained irreversible injury.

Infants with histories of *in utero* exposure to ACE inhibitors should be closely observed for hypotension, oliguria, and hyperkalemia. If oliguria occurs, attention should be directed toward support of blood pressure and renal perfusion. Exchange transfusion or dialysis may be required as a means of reversing hypotension and/or substituting for disordered renal function. Fosinopril is poorly dialyzed from the circulation of adults by hemodialysis and peritoneal dialysis. There is no experience with any procedure for removing fosinopril from the neonatal circulation.

When fosinopril was given to pregnant rats at doses about 80 to 250 times (on a mg/kg basis) the maximum recommended human dose, three similar orofacial malformations and one fetus with *situs inversus* were observed among the offspring. No teratogenic effects of fosinopril were seen in studies in pregnant rabbits at doses up to 25 times (on a mg/kg basis) the maximum recommended human dose.

Hepatic Failure

Rarely, ACE Inhibitors have been associated with a syndrome that starts with cholestatic jaundice and progresses

Continued on next page

Monopril—Cont.

to fulminant hepatic necrosis and (sometimes) death. The mechanism of this syndrome is not understood. Patients receiving ACE inhibitors who develop jaundice or marked elevations of hepatic enzymes should discontinue the ACE inhibitor and receive appropriate medical follow-up.

PRECAUTIONS

General

Impaired Renal Function: As a consequence of inhibiting the renin-angiotensin-aldosterone system, changes in renal function may be anticipated in susceptible individuals. In patients with severe congestive heart failure whose renal function may depend on the activity of the renin-angiotensin-aldosterone system, treatment with angiotensin converting enzyme inhibitors, including MONOPRIL (fosinopril sodium tablets), may be associated with oliguria and/or progressive azotemia and (rarely) with acute renal failure and/or death.

In hypertensive patients with renal artery stenosis in a solitary kidney or bilateral renal artery stenosis, increases in blood urea nitrogen and serum creatinine may occur. Experience with another angiotensin converting enzyme inhibitor suggests that these increases are usually reversible upon discontinuation of ACE inhibitor and/or diuretic therapy. In such patients, renal function should be monitored during the first few weeks of therapy. Some hypertensive patients with no apparent pre-existing renal vascular disease have developed increases in blood urea nitrogen and serum creatinine, usually minor and transient, especially when MONOPRIL has been given concomitantly with a diuretic. This is more likely to occur in patients with preexisting renal impairment. Dosage reduction of MONOPRIL and/or discontinuation of the diuretic may be required.

Evaluation of patients with hypertension or heart failure should always include assessment of renal function (see DOSAGE AND ADMINISTRATION).

Impaired renal function decreases total clearance of fosinoprilat and approximately doubles AUC. In general, no adjustment of dosing is needed. However, patients with heart failure and severely reduced renal function may be more sensitive to the hemodynamic effects (e.g., hypotension) of ACE inhibition (see CLINICAL PHARMACOLOGY).

Hyperkalemia: In clinical trials, hyperkalemia (serum potassium greater than 10% above the upper limit of normal) has occurred in approximately 2.6% of hypertensive patients receiving MONOPRIL. In most cases, these were isolated values which resolved despite continued therapy. In clinical trials, 0.1% of patients (two patients) were discontinued from therapy due to an elevated serum potassium. Risk factors for the development of hyperkalemia include renal insufficiency, diabetes mellitus, and the concomitant use of potassium-sparing diuretics, potassium supplements, and/or potassium-containing salt substitutes, which should be used cautiously, if at all, with MONOPRIL (see PRECAUTIONS: Drug Interactions).

Cough: Presumably due to the inhibition of the degradation of endogenous bradykinin, persistent nonproductive cough has been reported with all ACE inhibitors, always resolving after discontinuation of therapy. ACE inhibitor-induced cough should be considered in the differential diagnosis of cough.

Impaired Liver Function: Since fosinopril is primarily metabolized by hepatic and gut wall esterases to its active moiety, fosinoprilat, patients with impaired liver function could develop elevated plasma levels of unchanged fosinopril. In a study in patients with alcoholic or biliary cirrhosis, the extent of hydrolysis was unaffected, although the rate was slowed. In these patients, the apparent total body clearance of fosinoprilat was decreased and the plasma AUC approximately doubled.

Surgery/Anesthesia: In patients undergoing surgery or during anesthesia with agents that produce hypotension, fosinopril will block the angiotensin II formation that could otherwise occur secondary to compensatory renin release. Hypotension that occurs as a result of this mechanism can be corrected by volume expansion.

Hemodialysis

Recent clinical observations have shown an association of hypersensitivity-like (anaphylactoid) reactions during hemodialysis with high-flux dialysis membranes (e.g., AN69) in patients receiving ACE inhibitors as medication. In these patients, consideration should be given to using a different type of dialysis membrane or a different class of medication. (See WARNINGS: Anaphylactoid reactions during membrane exposure.)

Information for Patients

Angioedema: Angioedema, including laryngeal edema, can occur with treatment with ACE inhibitors, especially following the first dose. Patients should be advised to immediately report to their physician any signs or symptoms suggesting angioedema (e.g., swelling of face, eyes, lips, tongue, larynx, mucous membranes, and extremities; difficulty in swallowing or breathing; hoarseness) and to discontinue therapy. (See WARNINGS: Angioedema and ADVERSE REACTIONS.)

Symptomatic Hypotension: Patients should be cautioned that light-headedness can occur, especially during the first days of therapy, and it should be reported to a physician. Patients should be told that if syncope occurs, MONOPRIL (fosinopril sodium tablets) should be discontinued until the physician has been consulted.

All patients should be cautioned that inadequate fluid intake or excessive perspiration, diarrhea, or vomiting can lead to an excessive fall in blood pressure, with the same consequences of lightheadedness and possible syncope.

Hyperkalemia: Patients should be told not to use potassium supplements or salt substitutes containing potassium without consulting the physician.

Neutropenia: Patients should be told to promptly report any indication of infection (e.g., sore throat, fever), which could be a sign of neutropenia.

Pregnancy: Female patients of childbearing age should be told about the consequences of second- and third-trimester exposure to ACE inhibitors, and they should also be told that these consequences do not appear to have resulted from intrauterine ACE-inhibitor exposure that has been limited to the first trimester. These patients should be asked to report pregnancies to their physicians as soon as possible.

Drug Interactions

With diuretics: Patients on diuretics, especially those with intravascular volume depletion, may occasionally experience an excessive reduction of blood pressure after initiation of therapy with MONOPRIL. The possibility of hypotensive effects with MONOPRIL can be minimized by either discontinuing the diuretic or increasing salt intake prior to initiation of treatment with MONOPRIL. If this is not possible, the starting dose should be reduced and the patient should be observed closely for several hours following an initial dose and until blood pressure has stabilized (see DOSAGE AND ADMINISTRATION).

With potassium supplements and potassium-sparing diuretics: MONOPRIL can attenuate potassium loss caused by thiazide diuretics. Potassium-sparing diuretics (spironolactone, amiloride, triamterene, and others) or potassium supplements can increase the risk of hyperkalemia. Therefore, if concomitant use of such agents is indicated, they should be given with caution, and the patient's serum potassium should be monitored frequently.

With lithium: Increased serum lithium levels and symptoms of lithium toxicity have been reported in patients receiving ACE inhibitors during therapy with lithium. These drugs should be coadministered with caution, and frequent monitoring of serum lithium levels is recommended. If a diuretic is also used, the risk of lithium toxicity may be increased.

With antacids: In a clinical pharmacology study, coadministration of an antacid (aluminum, hydroxide, magnesium hydroxide, and simethicone) with fosinopril reduced serum levels and urinary excretion of fosinoprilat as compared with fosinopril administrated alone, suggesting that antacids may impair absorption of fosinopril.Therefore, if concomitant administration of these agents is indicated, dosing should be separated by 2 hours.

Other: Neither MONOPRIL nor its metabolites have been found to interact with food. In separate single or multiple dose pharmacokinetic interaction studies with chlorthalidone, nifedipine, propranolol, hydrochlorothiazide, cimetidine, metoclopramide, propantheline, digoxin, and warfarin, the bioavailability of fosinoprilat was not altered by coadministration of fosinopril with any one of these drugs. In a study with concomitant administration of aspirin and MONOPRIL the bioavailability of unbound fosinoprilat was not altered.

In a pharmacokinetic interaction study with warfarin, bioavailability parameters, the degree of protein binding, and the anticoagulant effect (measured by prothrombin time) of warfarin were not significantly changed.

Drug/Laboratory Test Interaction

Fosinopril may cause a false low measurement of serum digoxin levels with the Digi-Tab® RIA Kit for Digoxin. Other kits, such as the Coat-A-Count® RIA Kit, may be used.

Carcinogenesis, Mutagenesis, and Impairment of Fertility

No evidence of a carcinogenic effect was found when fosinopril was given in the diet to mice and rats for up to 24 months at doses up to 400 mg/kg/day. On a body weight basis, the highest dose in mice and rats is about 250 times the maximum human dose of 80 mg, assuming a 50 kg subject. On a body surface area basis, in mice, this dose is 20 times the maximum human dose; in rats, this dose is 40 times the maximum human dose. Male rats given the highest dose level had a slightly higher incidence of mesentery/omentum lipomas.

Neither fosinopril nor the active fosinoprilat was mutagenic in the Ames microbial mutagen test, the mouse lymphoma forward mutation assay, or a mitotic gene conversion assay. Fosinopril was also not genotoxic in a mouse micronucleus test *in vivo* and a mouse bone marrow cytogenetic assay *in vivo*.

In the Chinese hamster ovary cell cytogenetic assay, fosinopril increased the frequency of chromosomal aberrations when tested without metabolic activation at a concentration that was toxic to the cells. However, there was no increase in chromosomal aberrations at lower drug concentrations without metabolic activation or at any concentration with metabolic activation.

There were no adverse reproductive effects in male and female rats treated with 15 or 60 mg/kg daily. On a body weight basis, the high dose of 60 mg/kg is about 38 times the maximum recommended human dose. On a body surface area basis, this dose is 6 times the maximum recommended human dose. There was no effect on pairing time prior to mating in rats until a daily dose of 240 mg/kg, a toxic dose, was given; at this dose, a slight increase in pairing time was observed. On a body weight basis, this dose is 150 times the maximum recommended human dose. On a body surface area basis, this dose is 24 times the maximum recommended human dose.

Pregnancy Categories C (first trimester) and D (second and third trimesters)

See WARNINGS: Fetal/Neonatal Morbidity and Mortality.

Nursing Mothers

Ingestion of 20 mg daily for three days resulted in detectable levels of fosinoprilat in breast milk. MONOPRIL (fosinopril sodium tablets) should not be administered to nursing mothers.

Geriatric Use

Of the total number of patients who received fosinopril in US clinical studies of MONOPRIL, 13% were 65 and older while 1.3% were 75 and older. No overall differences in effectiveness or safety were observed between these patients and younger patients, and other reported clinical experience has not identified differences in response between the elderly and younger patients, but greater sensitivity of some older individuals cannot be ruled out.

In a pharmacokinetic study comparing elderly (65–74 years old) and non-elderly (20–35 years old) healthy volunteers, there were no differences between the groups in peak fosinoprilat levels or area under the plasma concentration time curve (AUC).

Pediatric Use

Safety and effectiveness in pediatric patients have not been established.

ADVERSE REACTIONS

MONOPRIL has been evaluated for safety in more than 2100 individuals in hypertension and heart failure trials, including approximately 530 patients treated for a year or more. Generally adverse events were mild and transient, and their frequency was not prominently related to dose within the recommended daily dosage range.

Hypertension

In placebo-controlled clinical trials (688 MONOPRIL-treated patients), the usual duration of therapy was two to three months. Discontinuations due to any clinical or laboratory adverse event were 4.1 and 1.1 percent in MONOPRIL-treated and placebo-treated patients, respectively. The most frequent reasons (0.4 to 0.9%) were headache, elevated transaminases, fatigue, cough (see PRECAUTIONS: General, Cough), diarrhea, and nausea and vomiting.

During clinical trials with any MONOPRIL regimen, the incidence of adverse events in the elderly (≥65 years old) was similar to that seen in younger patients.

Clinical adverse events probably or possibly related or of uncertain relationship to therapy, occurring in at least 1% of patients treated with MONOPRIL alone and at least as frequent on MONOPRIL as on placebo in placebo-controlled clinical trials are shown in the table below.

Clinical Adverse Events in Placebo-Controlled Trials (Hypertension)

	MONOPRIL (N = 688) Incidence (Discontinuation)		Placebo (N = 184) Incidence (Discontinuation)
Cough	2.2	(0.4)	0.0 (0.0)
Dizziness	1.6	(0.0)	0.0 (0.0)
Nausea/ Vomiting	1.2	(0.4)	0.5 (0.0)

The following events were also seen at >1% on MONOPRIL but occurred in the placebo group at a greater rate: headache, diarrhea, fatigue, and sexual dysfunction. Other clinical events probably or possibly related, or of uncertain relationship to therapy occurring in 0.2 to 1.0% of patients (except as noted) treated with MONOPRIL in controlled or uncontrolled clinical trials (N=1479) and less frequent, clinically significant events include (listed by body system):

General: Chest pain, edema, weakness, excessive sweating.

Cardiovascular: Angina/myocardial infarction, cerebrovascular accident, hypertensive crisis, rhythm disturbances, palpitations, hypotension, syncope, flushing, claudication.

Orthostatic hypotension occurred in 1.4% of patients treated with fosinopril monotherapy. Hypotension or orthostatic hypotension was a cause for discontinuation of therapy in 0.1% of patients.
Dermatologic: Urticaria, rash, photosensitivity, pruritis.
Endocrine/Metabolic: Gout, decreased libido.
Gastrointestinal: Pancreatitis, hepatitis, dysphagia, abdominal distention, abdominal pain, flatulence, constipation, heartburn, appetite/weight change, dry mouth.
Hematologic: Lymphadenopathy.
Immunologic: Angioedema. (See WARNINGS: Angioedema).
Musculoskeletal: Arthralgia, musculoskeletal pain, myalgia/muscle cramp.
Nervous/Psychiatric: Memory disturbance, tremor, confusion, mood change, paresthesia, sleep disturbance, drowsiness, vertigo.
Respiratory: Bronchospasm, pharyngitis, sinusitis/rhinitis, laryngitis/hoarseness, epistaxis. A symptom-complex of cough, bronchospasm, and eosinophilia has been observed in two patients treated with fosinopril.
Special Senses: Tinnitus, vision disturbance, taste disturbance, eye irritation.
Urogenital: Renal insufficiency, urinary frequency.

Heart Failure

In placebo-controlled clinical trials (361 MONOPRIL-treated patients), the usual duration of therapy was 3–6 months. Discontinuations due to any clinical or laboratory adverse event, except for heart failure, were 8.0% and 7.5% in MONOPRIL-treated and placebo-treated patients, respectively. The most frequent reason for discontinuation of MONOPRIL was angina pectoris (1.1%). Significant hypotension after the first dose of MONOPRIL occurred in 14/590 (2.4%) of patients; 5/590 (0.8%) patients discontinued due to first dose hypotension.

Clinical adverse events probably or possibly related or of uncertain relationship to therapy, occurring in at least 1% of patients treated with MONOPRIL and at least as common as the placebo group, in placebo-controlled trials are shown in the table below.

Clinical Adverse Events in Placebo-Controlled Trials (Heart Failure)

	MONOPRIL (N =361) Incidence (Discontinuation)	Placebo (N =373) Incidence (Discontinuation)
Dizziness	11.9 (0.6)	5.4 (0.3)
Cough	9.7 (0.8)	5.1 (0.0)
Hypotension	4.4 (0.8)	0.8 (0.0)
Musculoskeletal Pain	3.3 (0.0)	2.7 (0.0)
Nausea/Vomiting	2.2 (0.6)	1.6 (0.3)
Diarrhea	2.2 (0.0)	1.3 (0.0)
Chest Pain (non-cardiac)	2.2 (0.0)	1.6 (0.0)
Upper Respiratory Infection	2.2 (0.0)	1.3 (0.0)
Orthostatic Hypotension	1.9 (0.0)	0.8 (0.0)
Subjective Cardiac Rhythm Disturbance	1.4 (0.6)	0.8 (0.3)
Weakness	1.4 (0.3)	0.5 (0.0)

The following events also occurred at a rate of 1% or more on MONOPRIL (fosinopril sodium tablets) but occurred on placebo more often: fatigue, dyspnea, headache, rash, abdominal pain, muscle cramp, angina pectoris, edema, and insomnia.

The incidence of adverse events in the elderly (≥65 years old) was similar to that seen in younger patients.

Other clinical events probably or possibly related, or of uncertain relationship to therapy occurring in 0.4 to 1.0% of patients (except as noted) treated with MONOPRIL in controlled clinical trials (N=516) and less frequent, clinically significant events include (listed by body system):
General: Fever, influenza, weight gain, hyperhidrosis, sensation of cold, fall, pain.
Cardiovascular: Sudden death, cardiorespiratory arrest, shock (0.2%), atrial rhythm disturbance, cardiac rhythm disturbances, non anginal chest pain, edema lower extremity, hypertension, syncope, conduction disorder, bradycardia, tachycardia.
Dermatologic: Pruritus.
Endocrine/Metabolic: Gout, sexual dysfunction.
Gastrointestinal: Hepatomegaly, abdominal distension, decreased appetite, dry mouth, constipation, flatulence.
Immunologic: Angioedema. (0.2%).
Musculoskeletal: Muscle ache, swelling of an extremity, weakness of an extremity.
Nervous/Psychiatric: Cerebral infarction, TIA, depression, numbness, paresthesia, vertigo, behavior change, tremor.
Respiratory: Abnormal vocalization, rhinitis, sinus abnormality, tracheobronchitis, abnormal breathing, pleuritic chest pain.
Special Senses: Visual disturbance, taste disturbance.
Urogenital: Abnormal urination, kidney pain.

Fetal/Neonatal Morbidity and Mortality

See WARNINGS: Fetal/Neonatal Morbidity and Mortality.

Potential Adverse Effects Reported with ACE Inhibitors

Body as a whole: Anaphylactoid reactions (see WARNINGS: Anaphylactoid and possible related reactions and PRECAUTIONS: Hemodialysis).

Other medically important adverse effects reported with ACE inhibitors include: Cardiac arrest; eosinophilic pneumonitis; neutropenia/agranulocytosis, pancytopenia, anemia (including hemolytic and aplastic), thrombocytopenia; acute renal failure; hepatic failure, jaundice (hepatocellular or cholestatic); symptomatic hyponatremia; bullous pemphigus, exfoliative dermatitis; a syndrome which may include: arthralgia/arthritis, vasculitis, serositis, myalgia, fever, rash or other dermatologic manifestations, a positive ANA, leukocytosis, eosinophilia, or an elevated ESR.

Laboratory Test Abnormalities

Serum Electrolytes: Hyperkalemia, (see PRECAUTIONS); hyponatremia, (see PRECAUTIONS: Drug Interactions, With diuretics).
BUN/Serum Creatinine: Elevations, usually transient and minor, of BUN or serum creatinine have been observed. In placebo-controlled clinical trials, there were no significant differences in the number of patients experiencing increases in serum creatinine (outside the normal range or 1.33 times the pre-treatment value) between the fosinopril and placebo treatment groups. Rapid reduction of long-standing or markedly elevated blood pressure by any antihypertensive therapy can result in decreases in the glomerular filtration rate and, in turn, lead to increases in BUN or serum creatinine. (See PRECAUTIONS: General.)
Hematology: In controlled trials, a mean *hemoglobin* decrease of 0.1 g/dL was observed in fosinopril-treated patients. In individual patients decreases in hemoglobin or hematocrit were usually transient, small, and not associated with symptoms. No patient was discontinued from therapy due to the development of anemia. *Other:* Neutropenia (see WARNINGS), leukopenia and eosinophilia.
Liver Function Tests: Elevations of transaminases, LDH, alkaline phosphatase and serum bilirubin have been reported. Fosinopril therapy was discontinued because of serum transaminase elevations in 0.7% of patients. In the majority of cases, the abnormalities were either present at baseline or were associated with other etiologic factors. In those cases which were possibly related to fosinopril therapy, the elevations were generally mild and transient and resolved after discontinuation of therapy.

OVERDOSAGE

Oral doses of fosinopril at 2600 mg/kg in rats were associated with significant lethality. Human overdoses of fosinopril have not been reported, but the most common manifestations of human fosinopril overdosage is likely to be hypotension.

Laboratory determinations of serum levels of fosinoprilat and its metabolites are not widely available, and such determinations have, in any event, no established role in the management of fosinopril overdose. No data are available to suggest physiological maneuvers (e.g., maneuvers to change the pH of the urine) that might accelerate elimination of fosinopril and its metabolites. Fosinoprilat is poorly removed from the body by both hemodialysis and peritoneal dialysis.

Angiotensin II could presumably serve as a specific antagonist-antidote in the setting of fosinopril overdose, but angiotensin II is essentially unavailable outside of scattered research facilities. Because the hypotensive effect of fosinopril is achieved through vasodilation and effective hypovolemia, it is reasonable to treat fosinopril overdose by infusion of normal saline solution.

DOSAGE AND ADMINISTRATION

Hypertension

The recommended initial dose of MONOPRIL (fosinopril sodium tablets) is 10 mg once a day, both as monotherapy and when the drug is added to a diuretic. Dosage should then be adjusted according to blood pressure response at peak (2–6 hours) and trough (about 24 hours after dosing) blood levels. The usual dosage range needed to maintain a response at trough is 20–40 mg but some patients appear to have a further response to 80 mg. In some patients treated with once daily dosing, the antihypertensive effect may diminish toward the end of the dosing interval. If trough response is inadequate, dividing the daily dose should be considered. If blood pressure is not adequately controlled with MONOPRIL alone, a diuretic may be added.

Concomitant administration of MONOPRIL with potassium supplements, potassium salt substitutes, or potassium-sparing diuretics can lead to increases of serum potassium (see PRECAUTIONS).

In patients who are currently being treated with a diuretic, symptomatic hypotension occasionally can occur following the initial dose of MONOPRIL. To reduce the likelihood of hypotension, the diuretic should, if possible, be discontinued two to three days prior to beginning therapy with MONOPRIL (see WARNINGS). Then, if blood pressure is not controlled with MONOPRIL alone, diuretic therapy should be resumed. If diuretic therapy cannot be discontinued, an initial dose of 10 mg of MONOPRIL should be used with careful medical supervision for several hours and until blood pressure has stabilized. (See WARNINGS; PRECAUTIONS: Information for Patients and Drug Interactions.)

Since concomitant administration of MONOPRIL with potassium supplements, or potassium-containing salt substitutes or potassium-sparing diuretics may lead to increases in serum potassium, they should be used with caution (see PRECAUTIONS).

Heart Failure

Digitalis is not required for MONOPRIL to manifest improvements in exercise tolerance and symptoms. Most placebo-controlled clinical trial experience has been with both digitalis and diuretics present as background therapy.

The usual starting dose of MONOPRIL should be 10 mg once daily. Following the initial dose of MONOPRIL, the patient should be observed under medical supervision for at least two hours for the presence of hypotension or orthostasis and, if present, until blood pressure stabilizes. An initial dose of 5 mg is preferred in heart failure patients with moderate to severe renal failure or those who have been vigorously diuresed.

Dosage should be increased, over a several week period, to a dose that is maximal and tolerated but not exceeding 40 mg once daily. The usual effective dosage range is 20 to 40 mg once daily.

The appearance of hypotension, orthostasis, or azotemia early in dose titration should not preclude further careful dose titration. Consideration should be given to reducing the dose of concomitant diuretic.

For Hypertensive or Heart Failure Patients With Renal Impairment: In patients with impaired renal function, the total body clearance of fosinoprilat is approximately 50% slower than in patients with normal renal function. Since hepatobiliary elimination partially compensates for diminished renal elimination, the total body clearance of fosinoprilat does not differ appreciably with any degree of renal insufficiency (creatinine clearances <80 mL/min/1.73m^2), including end-stage renal failure (creatinine clearance <10 mL/min/1.73m^2). This relative constancy of body clearance of active fosinoprilat, resulting from the dual route of elimination, permits use of the usual dose in patients with any degree of renal impairment. (See WARNINGS: Anaphylactoid reactions during membrane exposure and PRECAUTIONS: Hemodialysis).

HOW SUPPLIED

10 mg tablets: White to off-white, biconvex flat-end diamond shaped, compressed partially scored tablets with **BMS** on one side and **Monopril 10** on the other. They are supplied in bottles of 30 (NDC 0087-0158-22), bottles of 90 (NDC 0087-0158-46) and 1000 (NDC 0087-0158-85). Bottles contain a desiccant canister.

20 mg tablets: White to off-white, oval shaped, compressed tablets with **BMS** on one side and **Monopril 20** on the other. They are supplied in bottles of 30 (NDC 0087-0609-41), bottles of 90 (NDC 0087-0609-42) and 1000 (NDC 0087-0609-85). Bottles contain a desiccant canister.

40 mg tablets: White to off-white, biconvex hexagonal shaped, compressed tablets with **BMS** on one side and **Monopril 40** on the other. They are supplied in bottles of 30 (NDC 0087-1202-12), bottles of 90 (NDC 0087-1202-13) and 1000 (NDC 0087-1202-51). Bottles contain a desiccant canister.

UNIMATIC® unit-dose packs containing 100 tablets are also available for each potency: **10 mg** (NDC 0087-0158-45), **20 mg** (NDC 0087-0609-45) and **40 mg** (NDC 0087-1202-45).

STORAGE

Store between 15°C (59°F) and 30°C (86°F). Avoid prolonged exposure to temperatures above 30°C (86°F). Keep bottles tightly closed (protect from moisture).

J4-502H

F4-B001-11-96 Revised: November 1996

Bristol-Myers Squibb Company

Shown in Product Identification Guide, page 307

OVCON® 35 ℞

[*ov-cŏn*]

OVCON® 50

(NORETHINDRONE AND ETHINYL ESTRADIOL TABLETS, USP)

21- and 28-DAY REGIMENS

Rx only

Patients should be counseled that this product does not protect against HIV infection (AIDS) and other sexually transmitted diseases.

Continued on next page

Ovcon 35—Cont.

DESCRIPTION

21-Day OVCON 35 provides a regimen for oral contraception derived from 21 tablets composed of norethindrone and ethinyl estradiol. The chemical name for norethindrone is 17-hydroxy-19-nor-17α-pregn-4-en-20-yn-3-one and for ethinyl estradiol the chemical name is 19-nor-17α-pregna-1,3,5 (10)-trien-20-yne-3,17-diol.

28-Day OVCON® 35 and OVCON® 50 (norethindrone and ethinyl estradiol tablets, USP) provide a continuous regimen for oral contraception derived from 21 tablets composed of norethindrone and ethinyl estradiol to be followed by 7 green tablets of inert ingredients. The structural formulas are:

NORETHINDRONE

ETHINYL ESTRADIOL

The active OVCON 35 tablets contain 0.4 mg norethindrone and 0.035 mg ethinyl estradiol. The active OVCON 50 tablets contain 1 mg norethindrone and 0.05 mg ethinyl estradiol.

The green tablets contain inert ingredients.

OVCON 35, 21-Day contains the following inactive ingredients: dibasic calcium phosphate, FD&C Yellow No. 6 (aluminum lake), lactose, magnesium stearate, povidone, and sodium starch glycolate.

OVCON 35, 28-Day contains the following inactive ingredients: acacia, dibasic calcium phosphate, D&C Yellow No. 10 (aluminum lake), FD&C Blue No. 1 (aluminum lake), FD&C Yellow No. 6 (aluminum lake), lactose, magnesium stearate, povidone, sodium starch glycolate, starch (corn), and talc.

OVCON 50, 28-Day contains the following inactive ingredients: acacia, dibasic calcium phosphate, D&C Yellow No. 10 (aluminum lake), FD&C Blue No.1 (aluminum lake), FD&C Yellow No. 6 (aluminum lake), lactose, magnesium stearate, povidone, sodium starch glycolate, starch (corn), and talc.

CLINICAL PHARMACOLOGY

Combination oral contraceptives act by suppression of gonadotropins. Although the primary mechanism of this action is inhibition of ovulation, other alterations include changes in the cervical mucus (which increase the difficulty of sperm entry into the uterus) and the endometrium (which reduce the likelihood of implantation).

INDICATIONS AND USAGE

Oral contraceptives are indicated for the prevention of pregnancy in women who elect to use this product as a method of contraception. Oral contraceptive products such as Ovcon 50, 28-day, which contain 50 mcg of estrogen, should not be used unless medically indicated.

Oral contraceptives are highly effective. Table 1 lists the typical accidental pregnancy rates for users of combination oral contraceptives and other methods of contraception. The efficacy of these contraceptive methods, except sterilization, depends upon the reliability with which they are used. Correct and consistent use of methods can result in lower failure rates.

TABLE 1
LOWEST EXPECTED AND TYPICAL FAILURE RATES DURING THE FIRST YEAR OF CONTINUOUS USE OF A METHOD

% of Women Experiencing an Accidental Pregnancy in the First Year of Continuous Use

Method	Lowest Expected*	Typical**
(No contraception)	(85)	(85)
Oral contraceptives combined	0.1	3***
progestin only	0.5	3***
Diaphragm with spermicidal cream or jelly	6	18
Spermicides alone (foam, creams, jellies and vaginal suppositories)	3	21

Vaginal sponge		
nulliparous	6	18
multiparous	9	28
IUD	0.8-2.0	3#
Condom without spermicides	2	12
Periodic abstinence (all methods)	1-9	20
Injectable progestogen	0.3-0.4	0.3-0.4
Implants		
6 capsules	0.04	0.04
2 rods	0.03	0.03
Female sterilization	0.2	0.4
Male sterilization	0.1	0.15

Reproduced with permission of the Population Council from J. Trussell, et al: Contraceptive failure in the United States: An update. Studies in Family Planning, 21 (1), January-February 1990.

* The authors' best guess of the percentage of women expected to experience an accidental pregnancy among couples who initiate a method (not necessarily for the first time) and who use it consistently and correctly during the first year if they do not stop for any reason other than pregnancy.

** This term represents "typical" couples who initiate use of a method (not necessarily for the first time), who experience an accidental pregnancy during the first year if they do not stop use for any reason other than pregnancy.

*** Combined typical rate for both combined and progestin only.

\# Combined typical rate for both medicated and nonmedicated IUD.

CONTRAINDICATIONS

Oral contraceptives should not be used in women who currently have the following conditions:

• Thrombophlebitis or thromboembolic disorders
• A past history of deep vein thrombophlebitis or thromboembolic disorders
• Cerebrovascular or coronary artery disease
• Known or suspected carcinoma of the breast
• Carcinoma of the endometrium or other known or suspected estrogen-dependent neoplasia
• Undiagnosed abnormal genital bleeding
• Cholestatic jaundice of pregnancy or jaundice with prior pill use
• Hepatic adenomas or carcinomas
• Known or suspected pregnancy

WARNINGS

> Cigarette smoking increases the risk of serious cardiovascular side effects from oral contraceptive use. This risk increases with age and with heavy smoking (15 or more cigarettes per day) and is quite marked in women over 35 years of age. Women who use oral contraceptives should be strongly advised not to smoke.

The use of oral contraceptives is associated with increased risk of several serious conditions including myocardial infarction, thromboembolism, stroke, hepatic neoplasia, and gallbladder disease, although the risk of serious morbidity or mortality is very small in healthy women without underlying risk factors. The risk of morbidity and mortality increases significantly in the presence of other underlying risk factors such as hypertension, hyperlipidemias, obesity and diabetes.

Practitioners prescribing oral contraceptives should be familiar with the following information relating to these risks. The information contained in this package insert is principally based on studies carried out in patients who used oral contraceptives with higher formulations of estrogens and progestogens than those in common use today. The effect of long-term use of the oral contraceptives with lower formulations of both estrogens and progestogens remains to be determined.

Throughout this labeling, epidemiological studies reported are of two types: retrospective or case control studies and prospective or cohort studies. Case control studies provide a measure of the relative risk of a disease, namely, a *ratio* of the incidence of a disease among oral contraceptive users to that among nonusers. The relative risk does not provide information on the actual clinical occurrence of a disease. Cohort studies provide a measure of attributable risk, which is the *difference* in the incidence of disease between oral contraceptive users and nonusers. The attributable risk does provide information about the actual occurrence of a disease in the population. *For further information, the reader is referred to a text on epidemiological methods.

*Adapted from Stadel BB: Oral contraceptives and cardiovascular disease. *N Engl J Med*, 1981;305:612–618, 672–677; with author's permission.

1. THROMBOEMBOLIC DISORDERS AND OTHER VASCULAR PROBLEMS

The physician should be alert to the earliest manifestations of thromboembolic thrombotic disorders as discussed below. Should any of these occur or be suspected the drug should be discontinued immediately.

a. Myocardial Infarction

An increased risk of myocardial infarction has been attributed to oral contraceptive use. This risk is primarily in smokers or women with other underlying risk factors for coronary artery disease such as hypertension, hypercholesterolemia, morbid obesity, and diabetes. The relative risk of heart attack for current oral contraceptive users has been estimated to be two to six. The risk is very low under the age of 30.

Smoking in combination with oral contraceptive use has been shown to contribute substantially to the incidence of myocardial infarctions in women in their mid-thirties or older, with smoking accounting for the majority of excess cases. Mortality rates associated with circulatory disease have been shown to increase substantially in smokers over the age of 35 and nonsmokers over the age of 40 (Figure 1) among women who use oral contraceptives.

FIGURE 1
CIRCULATORY DISEASE MORTALITY RATES PER 100,000 WOMAN-YEARS BY AGE, SMOKING STATUS AND ORAL CONTRACEPTIVE USE

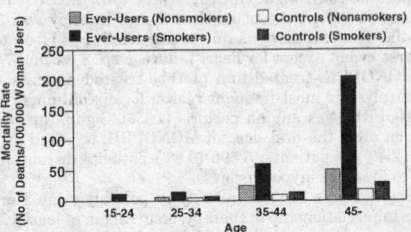

Layde PM, Beral V: Further analyses of mortality in oral contraceptive users: Royal College of General Practitioners' oral contraception study. (Table 5) *Lancet* 1981;1:541–546.

Oral contraceptives may compound the effects of well-known risk factors, such as hypertension, diabetes, hyperlipidemias, age, and obesity. In particular, some progestogens are known to decrease HDL cholesterol and cause glucose intolerance, while estrogens may create a state of hyperinsulinism. Oral contraceptives have been shown to increase blood pressure among users (see section 9 in Warnings). Such increases in risk factors have been associated with an increased risk of heart disease and the risk increases with the number of risk factors present. Oral contraceptives must be used with caution in women with cardiovascular disease risk factors.

b. Thromboembolism

An increased risk of thromboembolic and thrombotic disease associated with the use of oral contraceptives is well established. Case control studies have found the relative risk of users compared to nonusers to be 3 for the first episode of superficial venous thrombosis, 4 to 11 for deep vein thrombosis or pulmonary embolism, and 1.5 to 6 for women with predisposing conditions for venous thromboembolic disease. Cohort studies have shown the relative risk to be somewhat lower, about 3 for new cases and about 4.5 for new cases requiring hospitalization. The risk of thromboembolic disease due to oral contraceptives is not related to length of use and disappears after pill use is stopped.

A two- to four-fold increase in relative risk of postoperative thromboembolic complications has been reported with the use of oral contraceptives. The relative risk of venous thrombosis in women who have predisposing conditions is twice that of women without such medical conditions. If feasible, oral contraceptives should be discontinued at least four weeks prior to and for two weeks after elective surgery of a type associated with an increase in risk of thromboembolism and during and following prolonged immobilization. Since the immediate postpartum period is also associated with an increased risk of thromboembolism, oral contraceptives should be started no earlier than four to six weeks after delivery in women who elect not to breastfeed.

c. Cerebrovascular diseases

Oral contraceptives have been shown to increase both the relative and attributable risk of cerebrovascular events (thrombotic and hemorrhagic strokes); although, in general, the risk is greatest among older (>35 years) hypertensive women who also smoke. Hypertension was found to be a risk factor for both users and nonusers, for both types of strokes, while smoking interacted to increase the risk for hemorrhagic strokes.

In a large study, the relative risk of thrombotic strokes has been shown to range from 3 for normotensive users to 14 for users with severe hypertension. The relative risk of hemorrhagic stroke is reported to be 1.2 for nonsmokers who used oral contraceptives, 2.6 for smokers who did not use oral contraceptives, 7.6 for smokers who used oral contraceptives, 1.8 for normotensive users and 25.7 for users with severe hypertension. The attributable risk is also greater in older women.

d. **Dose-related risk of vascular disease from oral contraceptives**

A positive association has been observed between the amount of estrogen and progestogen in oral contraceptives and the risk of vascular disease. A decline in serum high density lipoproteins (HDL) has been reported with many progestational agents. A decline in serum high density lipoproteins has been associated with an increased incidence of ischemic heart disease. Because estrogens increase HDL cholesterol, the net effect of an oral contraceptive depends on a balance achieved between doses of estrogen and progestogen and the nature and absolute amount of progestogens used in the contraceptive. The amount of both hormones should be considered in the choice of an oral contraceptive.

Minimizing exposure to estrogen and progestogen is in keeping with good principles of therapeutics. For any particular estrogen/progestogen combination, the dosage regimen prescribed should be one which contains the least amount of estrogen and progestogen that is compatible with a low failure rate and the needs of the individual patient. New acceptors of oral contraceptive agents should be started on preparations containing 0.05 mg or less of estrogen. Products containing 50 mcg estrogen should be used only when medically indicated.

e. **Persistence of risk**

There are two studies which have shown persistence of risk of vascular disease for ever-users of oral contraceptives. In a study in the United States, the risk of developing myocardial infarction after discontinuing oral contraceptives persists for at least 9 years for women 40–49 years old who had used oral contraceptives for 5 or more years, but this increased risk was not demonstrated in other age groups. In another study in Great Britain, the risk of developing cerebrovascular disease persisted for at least 6 years after discontinuation of oral contraceptives, although excess risk was very small. However, both studies were performed with oral contraceptive formulations containing 50 micrograms or higher of estrogens.

2. ESTIMATES OF MORTALITY FROM CONTRACEPTIVE USE

One study gathered data from a variety of sources which have estimated the mortality rate associated with different methods of contraception at different ages (Table 2).

[See table above]

TABLE 2

ANNUAL NUMBER OF BIRTH-RELATED OR METHOD-RELATED DEATHS ASSOCIATED WITH CONTROL OF FERTILITY PER 100,000 NONSTERILE WOMEN, BY FERTILITY CONTROL METHOD ACCORDING TO AGE

Method of control and outcome	AGE 15–19	20–24	25–29	30–34	35–39	40–44
No fertility control methods*	7.0	7.4	9.1	14.8	25.7	28.2
Oral contraceptives nonsmoker**	0.3	0.5	0.9	1.9	13.8	31.6
Oral contraceptives smoker**	2.2	3.4	6.6	13.5	51.1	117.2
IUD**	0.8	0.8	1.0	1.0	1.4	1.4
Condom*	1.1	1.6	0.7	0.2	0.3	0.4
Diaphragm/ spermicide*	1.9	1.2	1.2	1.3	2.2	2.8
Periodic abstinence*	2.5	1.6	1.6	1.7	2.9	3.6

*Deaths are birth related

**Deaths are method related

Ory HW: Mortality associated with fertility and fertility control: 1983. *Fam Plann Perspect* 1983;15:50–56.

These estimates include the combined risk of death associated with contraceptive methods plus the risk attributable to pregnancy in the event of method failure. Each method of contraception has its specific benefits and risk. The study concluded that with the exception of oral contraceptive users 35 and older who smoke and 40 and older who do not smoke, mortality associated with all methods of birth control is low and below that associated with childbirth.

The observation of a possible increase in risk of mortality with age for oral contraceptive users is based on data gathered in the 1970s—but not reported until 1983. However, current clinical practice involves the use of lower estrogen dose formulations combined with careful restriction of oral contraceptive use to women who do not have the various risk factors listed in this labeling.

Because of these changes in practice and, also, because of some limited new data which suggest that the risk of cardiovascular disease with the use of oral contraceptives may now be less than previously observed (Porter JB, Hunter J, Jick H, et al. Oral contraceptives and nonfatal vascular disease. *Obstet Gynecol* 1985;66:1-4 and Porter JB, Jick H, Walker AM. Mortality among oral contraceptive users. *Obstet Gynecol* 1987;70:29-32), the Fertility and Maternal Health Drugs Advisory Committee was asked to review the topic in 1989. The Committee concluded that although cardiovascular disease risk may be increased with oral contraceptive use after age 40 in healthy nonsmoking women (even with the newer low-dose formulations), there are greater potential health risks associated with pregnancy in older women and with the alternative surgical and medical procedures which may be necessary if such women do not have access to effective and acceptable means of contraception.

Therefore, the Committee recommended that the benefits of oral contraceptive use by healthy nonsmoking women over 40 may outweigh the possible risks. Of course, older women, as all women who take oral contraceptives, should take the lowest possible dose formulation that is effective.

3. CARCINOMA OF THE REPRODUCTIVE ORGANS

Numerous epidemiological studies have been performed on the incidence of breast, endometrial, ovarian, and cervical cancer in women using oral contraceptives. The overwhelming evidence in the literature suggests that use of oral contraceptives is not associated with an increase in the risk of developing breast cancer, regardless of the age and parity of first use or with most of the marketed brands and doses. The Cancer and Steroid Hormone (CASH) study also showed no latent effect on the risk of breast cancer for at least a decade following long-term use. A few studies have shown a slightly increased relative risk of developing breast cancer, although the methodology of these studies, which included differences in examination of users and nonusers and differences in age at start of use, has been questioned. Some studies suggest that oral contraceptive use has been associated with an increase in the risk of cervical intraepithelial neoplasia in some populations of women. However, there continues to be controversy about the extent to which such findings may be due to differences in sexual behavior and other factors.

In spite of many studies of the relationship between oral contraceptive use and breast cancer and cervical cancers, a cause-and-effect relationship has not been established.

4. HEPATIC NEOPLASIA

Benign hepatic adenomas are associated with oral contraceptive use, although their occurrence is rare in the United States. Indirect calculations have estimated the attributable risk to be in the range of 3.3 cases/100,000 for users, a risk that increases after four or more years of use. Rupture of hepatic adenomas may cause death through intra-abdominal hemorrhage.

Studies from Britain have shown an increased risk of developing hepatocellular carcinoma in long-term (>8 years) oral contraceptive users. However, these cancers are extremely rare in the U.S. and the attributable risk (the excess incidence) of liver cancers in oral contraceptive users approaches less than one per million users.

5. OCULAR LESIONS

There have been clinical case reports of retinal thrombosis associated with the use of oral contraceptives. Oral contraceptives should be discontinued if there is unexplained partial or complete loss of vision; onset of proptosis or diplopia; papilledema; or retinal vascular lesions. Appropriate diagnostic and therapeutic measures should be undertaken immediately.

6. ORAL CONTRACEPTIVE USE BEFORE OR DURING EARLY PREGNANCY

Extensive epidemiological studies have revealed no increased risk of birth defects in women who have used oral contraceptives prior to pregnancy. Studies also do not suggest a teratogenic effect, particularly in so far as cardiac anomalies and limb reduction defects are concerned, when taken inadvertently during early pregnancy.

The administration of oral contraceptives to induce withdrawal bleeding should not be used as a test for pregnancy. Oral contraceptives should not be used during pregnancy to treat threatened or habitual abortion.

It is recommended that for any patient who has missed two consecutive periods, pregnancy should be ruled out before continuing oral contraceptive use. If the patient has not adhered to the prescribed schedule, the possibility of pregnancy should be considered at the time of the first missed period. Oral contraceptive use should be discontinued if pregnancy is confirmed.

7. GALLBLADDER DISEASE

Earlier studies have reported an increased lifetime relative risk of gallbladder surgery in users of oral contraceptives and estrogens. More recent studies, however, have shown that the relative risk of developing gallbladder disease among oral contraceptive users may be minimal.

The recent findings of minimal risk may be related to the use of oral contraceptive formulations containing lower hormonal doses of estrogens and progestogens.

8. CARBOHYDRATE AND LIPID METABOLIC EFFECTS

Oral contraceptives have been shown to cause glucose intolerance in a significant percentage of users. Oral contraceptives containing greater than 75 micrograms of estrogens cause hyperinsulinism, while lower doses of estrogen cause less glucose intolerance. Progestogens increase insulin secretion and create insulin resistance, this effect varying with different progestational agents.

However, in the nondiabetic woman, oral contraceptives appear to have no effect on fasting blood glucose. Because of these demonstrated effects, prediabetic and diabetic women should be carefully observed while taking oral contraceptives.

A small proportion of women will have persistent hypertriglyceridemia while on the pill. As discussed earlier (see Warnings 1.a. and 1.d.), changes in serum trigylcerides and lipoprotein levels have been reported in oral contraceptive users.

9. ELEVATED BLOOD PRESSURE

An increase in blood pressure has been reported in women taking oral contraceptives and this increase is more likely in older oral contraceptive users and with continued use. Data from the Royal College of General Practitioners and subsequent randomized trials have shown that the incidence of hypertension increases with increasing concentrations of progestogens.

Women with a history of hypertension or hypertension-related diseases, or renal disease should be encouraged to use another method of contraception. If women elect to use oral contraceptives, they should be monitored closely and if significant elevation of blood pressure occurs, oral contraceptives should be discontinued. For most women, elevated blood pressure will return to normal after stopping oral contraceptives, and there is no difference in the occurrence of hypertension among ever- and never-users.

10. HEADACHE

The onset or exacerbation of migraine or development of headache with a new pattern which is recurrent, persistent, or severe requires discontinuation of oral contraceptives and evaluation of the cause.

11. BLEEDING IRREGULARITIES

Breakthrough bleeding and spotting are sometimes encountered in patients on oral contraceptives, especially during the first three months of use. Nonhormonal causes should be considered and adequate diagnostic measures taken to rule out malignancy or pregnancy in the event of breakthrough bleeding, as in the case of any abnormal vaginal bleeding. If pathology has been excluded, time or a change to another formulation may solve the problem. In the event of amenorrhea, pregnancy should be ruled out.

Women with a history of oligomenorrhea or secondary amenorrhea or young women without regular cycles prior to taking oral contraceptives may again have irregular bleeding or amenorrhea after discontinuation of oral contraceptives.

PRECAUTIONS

1. SEXUALLY-TRANSMITTED DISEASES

Patients should be counseled that this product does not protect against HIV infection (AIDS) and other sexually transmitted diseases.

2. PHYSICAL EXAMINATION AND FOLLOW-UP

It is good medical practice for all women to have annual history and physical examinations, including women using oral contraceptives. The physical examination, however, may be deferred until after initiation of oral contraceptives if requested by the woman and judged appropriate by the clinician. The physical examination should include special reference to blood pressure, breasts, abdomen, and pelvic organs, including cervical cytology, and relevant laboratory tests. In case of undiagnosed, persistent, or recurrent abnormal vaginal bleeding, appropriate measures should be conducted to rule out malignancy. Women with a strong family history of breast cancer or who have breast nodules should be monitored with particular care.

3. LIPID DISORDERS

Women who are being treated for hyperlipidemias should be followed closely if they elect to use oral contraceptives. Some progestogens may elevate LDL levels and may render the control of hyperlipidemias more difficult.

Continued on next page

Ovcon 35—Cont.

4. LIVER FUNCTION
If jaundice develops in any woman receiving such drugs, the medication should be discontinued. Steroid hormones may be poorly metabolized in patients with impaired liver function.

5. FLUID RETENTION
Oral contraceptives may cause some degree of fluid retention. They should be prescribed with caution, and only with careful monitoring, in patients with conditions which might be aggravated by fluid retention.

6. EMOTIONAL DISORDERS
Women with a history of depression should be carefully observed and the drug discontinued if depression recurs to a serious degree.

Patients becoming significantly depressed while taking oral contraceptives should stop the medication and use an alternate method of contraception in an attempt to determine whether the symptom is drug related.

7. CONTACT LENSES
Contact lens wearers who develop visual changes or changes in lens tolerance should be assessed by an ophthalmologist.

8. DRUG INTERACTIONS
Reduced efficacy and increased incidence of breakthrough bleeding and menstrual irregularities have been associated with concomitant use of rifampin. A similar association, though less marked, has been suggested with barbiturates, phenylbutazone, phenytoin sodium, and possibly with griseofulvin, ampicillin, and tetracyclines.

9. INTERACTIONS WITH LABORATORY TESTS
Certain endocrine and liver function tests and blood components may be affected by oral contraceptives:

a. Increased prothrombin and factors VII, VIII, IX, and X; decreased antithrombin 3; increased norepinephrine-induced platelet aggregability.

b. Increased thyroid-binding globulin (TBG) leading to increased circulating total thyroid hormone, as measured by protein-bound iodine (PBI), T4 by column or by radioimmunoassay. Free T3 resin uptake is decreased, reflecting the elevated TBG, free T4 concentration is unaltered.

c. Other binding proteins may be elevated in serum.

d. Sex-binding globulins are increased and result in elevated levels of total circulating sex steroids and corticoids; however, free or biologically active levels remain unchanged.

e. Triglycerides may be increased.

f. Glucose tolerance may be decreased.

g. Serum folate levels may be depressed by oral contraceptive therapy. This may be of clinical significance if a woman becomes pregnant shortly after discontinuing oral contraceptives.

10. CARCINOGENESIS
See WARNINGS section.

11. PREGNANCY
Pregnancy Category X. See CONTRAINDICATIONS and WARNINGS sections.

12. NURSING MOTHERS
Small amounts of oral contraceptive steroids have been identified in the milk of nursing mothers and a few adverse effects on the child have been reported, including jaundice and breast enlargement. In addition, oral contraceptives given in the postpartum period may interfere with lactation by decreasing the quantity and quality of breast milk. If possible, the nursing mother should be advised not to use oral contraceptives but to use other forms of contraception until she has completely weaned her child.

13. VOMITING AND/OR DIARRHEA
Although a cause-and-effect relationship has not been clearly established, several cases of oral contraceptive failure have been reported in association with vomiting and/or diarrhea. If significant gastrointestinal disturbance occurs in any woman receiving contraceptive steroids, the use of a back-up method of contraception for the remainder of that cycle is recommended.

14. PEDIATRIC CARE
Safety and efficacy of OVCON 35 and OVCON 50 have been established in women of reproductive age. Safety and efficacy are expected to be the same in postpubertal adolescents under the age of 16 years and in users 16 years and older. Use of this product before menarche is not indicated.

INFORMATION FOR THE PATIENT
See Patient Labeling Printed Below

ADVERSE REACTIONS
An increased risk of the following serious adverse reactions has been associated with the use of oral contraceptives (see WARNINGS section):
- Thrombophlebitis
- Arterial thromboembolism
- Pulmonary embolism
- Myocardial infarction
- Cerebral hemorrhage
- Cerebral thrombosis
- Hypertension

- Gallbladder disease
- Hepatic adenomas or benign liver tumors

There is evidence of an association between the following conditions and the use of oral contraceptives, although additional confirmatory studies are needed:
- Mesenteric thrombosis
- Retinal thrombosis

The following adverse reactions have been reported in patients receiving oral contraceptives and are believed to be drug related:
- Nausea
- Vomiting
- Gastrointestinal symptoms (such as abdominal cramps and bloating)
- Breakthrough bleeding
- Spotting
- Change in menstrual flow
- Amenorrhea
- Temporary infertility after discontinuation of treatment
- Edema
- Melasma which may persist
- Breast changes: tenderness, enlargement, and secretion
- Change in weight (increase or decrease)
- Change in cervical ectropion and secretion
- Possible diminution in lactation when given immediately postpartum
- Cholestatic jaundice
- Migraine
- Rash (allergic)
- Mental depression
- Reduced tolerance to carbohydrates
- Vaginal candidiasis
- Change in corneal curvature (steepening)
- Intolerance to contact lenses

The following adverse reactions have been reported in users of oral contraceptives, and the association has been neither confirmed nor refuted:
- Premenstrual syndrome
- Cataracts
- Changes in appetite
- Cystitis-like syndrome
- Headache
- Nervousness
- Dizziness
- Hirsutism
- Loss of scalp hair
- Erythema multiforme
- Erythema nodosum
- Hemorrhagic eruption
- Vaginitis
- Porphyria
- Impaired renal function
- Hemolytic uremic syndrome
- Budd-Chiari syndrome
- Acne
- Changes in libido
- Colitis

OVERDOSAGE
Serious ill effects have not been reported following acute ingestion of large doses of oral contraceptives by young children. Overdosage may cause nausea, and withdrawal bleeding may occur in females.

NONCONTRACEPTIVE HEALTH EFFECTS
The following noncontraceptive health benefits related to the use of oral contraceptives are supported by epidemiological studies which largely utilized oral contraceptive formulations containing estrogen doses exceeding 0.035 mg of ethinyl estradiol or 0.05 mg of mestranol.

Effects on menses:
- Increased menstrual cycle regularity
- Decreased blood loss and decreased incidence of iron deficiency anemia
- Decreased incidence of dysmenorrhea

Effects related to inhibition of ovulation:
- Decreased incidence of functional ovarian cysts
- Decreased incidence of ectopic pregnancies

Effects from long-term use:
- Decreased incidence of fibroadenomas and fibrocystic disease of the breast
- Decreased incidence of acute pelvic inflammatory disease
- Decreased incidence of endometrial cancer
- Decreased incidence of ovarian cancer

DOSAGE AND ADMINISTRATION
The following is a summary of the instructions given to the patient in the "HOW TO TAKE THE PILL" section of the DETAILED PATIENT PACKAGE INSERT.

The patient is given instructions in five (5) categories.

1. IMPORTANT POINTS TO REMEMBER: The patient is told (a) that she should take one pill every day at the same time, (b) many women have spotting or light bleeding or gastric distress during the first one to three cycles, (c) missing pills can also cause spotting or light bleeding, (d) she should use a back-up method for contraception if she has vomiting or diarrhea or takes some concomitant medica-

tions, and/or if she has trouble remembering the pill, (e) if she has any other questions, she should consult her physician.

2. BEFORE SHE STARTS TAKING HER PILLS: She should decide what time of day she wishes to take the pill, check whether her pill pack has 21 or 28 pills, and note the order in which she should take the pills (diagrammatic drawings of the pill pack are included in the patient insert).

3. WHEN SHE SHOULD START THE FIRST PACK: The Day-One start is listed as the first choice and the Sunday start (the Sunday after her period starts) is given as the second choice. If she uses the Sunday start she should use a back-up method in the first cycle if she has intercourse before she has taken seven pills.

4. WHAT TO DO DURING THE CYCLE: The patient is advised to take one pill at the same time every day until the pack is empty. If she is on a 21 day regimen, she should wait seven days to start the next pack. If she is on the 28 day regimen, she should start the next pack the day after the last inactive tablet and not wait any days between packs.

5. WHAT TO DO IF SHE MISSED A PILL OR PILLS: The patient is given instructions about what she should do if she misses one, two or more than two pills at varying times in her cycle for both the Day-One and the Sunday start. The patient is warned that she may become pregnant if she has unprotected intercourse in the seven days after missing pills. To avoid this, she must use another birth control method such as condom, foam, or sponge in these seven days.

HOW SUPPLIED
OVCON®35 (norethindrone and ethinyl estradiol tablets, USP) is available in 21- and 28-day regimens. Each package contains 21 round, peach tablets of 0.4 mg norethindrone and 0.035 mg ethinyl estradiol, imprinted with MJ on one side and 583 on the other. Each round, green tablet in the 28-day regimen contains inert ingredients and is imprinted with MJ on one side and 850 on the other.

OVCON 35, 21-Day
NDC 0087-0583-42 Carton of 6 compacts
OVCON 35, 28-Day
NDC 0087-0578-41 Carton of 6 compacts
OVCON® 50 (norethindrone and ethinyl estradiol tablets, USP) is available in 28-day regimens. Each package contains 21 round, yellow tablets of 1.0 mg norethindrone and 0.05 mg ethinyl estradiol, imprinted with MJ on one side and 584 on the other. Each round, green tablet in the 28-day regimen contains inert ingredients and is imprinted with MJ on one side and 850 on the other.

OVCON 50, 28-Day
NDC 0087-0579-41 Carton of 6 compacts
Store below 30°C (86°F)
References are available upon request.

PATIENT PACKAGE INSERT BRIEF SUMMARY
This product (like all oral contraceptives) is intended to prevent pregnancy. It does not protect against HIV infection (AIDS) and other sexually transmitted diseases.

Oral contraceptives, also known as "birth control pills" or "the pill," are taken to prevent pregnancy and when taken correctly, have a failure rate of about 1% per year when used without missing any pills. The typical failure rate of large numbers of pill users is less than 3% per year when women who miss pills are included.

Oral contraceptive use is associated with certain serious diseases that can be life-threatening or may cause temporary or permanent disability. The risks associated with taking oral contraceptives increase significantly if you:
- Smoke
- Have high blood pressure, diabetes, high cholesterol
- Have or have had clotting disorders, heart attack, stroke, angina pectoris, cancer of the breast or sex organs, jaundice or malignant or benign liver tumors.

You should not take the pill if you suspect you are pregnant or have unexplained vaginal bleeding.

> Cigarette smoking increases the risk of serious cardiovascular side effects from oral contraceptive use. This risk increases with age and with heavy smoking (15 or more cigarettes per day) and is quite marked in women over 35 years of age. Women who use oral contraceptives should not smoke.

Most side effects of the pill are not serious. The most common such effects are nausea, vomiting, bleeding between menstrual periods, weight gain, breast tenderness, and difficulty wearing contact lenses. These side effects, especially nausea and vomiting, may subside within the first three months of use.

The serious side effects of the pill occur very infrequently, especially if you are in good health and are young. However, you should know that the following medical conditions have been associated with or made worse by the pill:

1. Blood clots in the legs (thrombophlebitis), lungs (pulmonary embolism), stoppage or rupture of a blood vessel in the brain (stroke), blockage of blood vessels in the heart (heart attack or angina pectoris), or other organs of the body. As

ANNUAL NUMBER OF BIRTH-RELATED OR METHOD-RELATED DEATHS ASSOCIATED WITH CONTROL OF FERTILITY PER 100,000 NONSTERILE WOMEN, BY FERTILITY CONTROL METHOD ACCORDING TO AGE

Method of control and outcome	AGE 15–19	20–24	25–29	30–34	35–39	40–44
No fertility control methods*	7.0	7.4	9.1	14.8	25.7	28.2
Oral contraceptives nonsmoker**	0.3	0.5	0.9	1.9	13.8	31.6
Oral contraceptives smoker**	2.2	3.4	6.6	13.5	51.1	117.2
IUD**	0.8	0.8	1.0	1.0	1.4	1.4
Condom*	1.1	1.6	0.7	0.2	0.3	0.4
Diaphragm/spermicide*	1.9	1.2	1.2	1.3	2.2	2.8
Periodic abstinence*	2.5	1.6	1.6	1.7	2.9	3.6

*Deaths are birth related
**Deaths are method related

mentioned above, smoking increases the risk of heart attacks and strokes and subsequent serious medical consequences.

2. Liver tumors, which may rupture and cause severe bleeding. A possible but not definite association has been found with the pill and liver cancer. However, liver cancers are extremely rare. The chance of developing liver cancer from using the pill is thus even rarer.

3. High blood pressure, although blood pressure usually returns to normal when the pill is stopped.

The symptoms associated with these serious side effects are discussed in the detailed leaflet given to you with your supply of pills. Notify your doctor or health care provider if you notice any unusual physical disturbances while taking the pill. In addition, drugs such as rifampin, as well as some anticonvulsants and some antibiotics may decrease oral contraceptive effectiveness.

Studies to date of women taking the pill have not shown an increase in the incidence of cancer of the breast or cervix. There is, however, insufficient evidence to rule out the possibility that the pill may cause such cancers.

Taking the pill provides some important noncontraceptive effects. These include less painful menstruation, less menstrual blood loss and anemia, fewer pelvic infections, and fewer cancers of the ovary and the lining of the uterus.

Be sure to discuss any medical condition you may have with your health care provider. Your health care provider will take a medical and family history before prescribing oral contraceptives and will examine you. The physical examination may be delayed to another time if you request it and the health care provider believes that it is a good medical practice to postpone it. You should be reexamined at least once a year while taking oral contraceptives. The detailed patient information booklet gives you further information which you should read and discuss with your health care professional.

DOSAGE AND ADMINISTRATION

HOW TO TAKE THE PILL

The instructions given in the DETAILED PATIENT PACKAGE INSERT are also given in the **BRIEF SUMMARY** included inside each compact. In the event the patient may read only the brief summary, these instructions include the directions on starting the first pack on Day-One (first choice) of her period and the Sunday start (Sunday after period starts). The patient is advised that, if she used the Sunday start, she should use a back-up method in the first cycle if she has intercourse before she has taken seven pills. The patient is also instructed as to what she should do if she misses a pill or pills. The patient is warned that she may become pregnant if she misses a pill or pills and that she should use a back-up method of birth control in the event she has intercourse any time during the seven day period following the missed pill or pills.

A diagrammatic drawing of the specific pill pack is included in the **BRIEF SUMMARY**.

PATIENT PACKAGE INSERT

This product (like all oral contraceptives) is intended to prevent pregnancy. It does not protect against HIV infection (AIDS) and other sexually transmitted diseases.

INTRODUCTION

You should not use Ovcon 50, 28-day, which contains higher doses of estrogen than other oral contraceptives, unless specifically recommended by your health care provider.

Any woman who considers using oral contraceptives (the birth control pill or the pill) should understand the benefits and risks of using this form of birth control.

Although the oral contraceptives have important advantages over other methods of contraception, they have certain risks that no other method has and some of these risks may continue after you have stopped using the oral contraceptive. This booklet will give you much of the information you will need to make this decision and will also help you determine if you are at risk of developing any of the serious side effects of the pill. It will tell you how to use the pill properly so that it will be as effective as possible. However, this booklet is not a replacement for a careful discussion between you and your health care professional. You should discuss the information provided in this booklet with him or her, both when you first start taking the pill and during your revisits. You should also follow your health care professional's advice with regard to regular check-ups while you are on the pill.

EFFECTIVENESS OF ORAL CONTRACEPTIVES

Oral contraceptives or "birth control pills" or "the pill" are used to prevent pregnancy and are more effective than other nonsurgical methods of birth control. The chance of becoming pregnant is less than 1% (1 pregnancy per 100 women per year of use) when the pills are used correctly and no pills are missed. Typical failure rates are actually 3% per year. The chance of becoming pregnant increases with each missed pill during a menstrual cycle.

In comparison, typical accidental pregnancy rates for other nonsurgical methods of birth control during the first year of use are as follows:

IUD: 3%
Diaphragm with spermicides: 18%
Spermicides alone: 21%
Vaginal sponge: 18% to 28%
Condom alone: 12%
Periodic abstinence: 20%
Injectible progestogen: 0.3% to 0.4%
Implants: 0.03% to 0.04%
No methods: 85%

WHO SHOULD NOT TAKE ORAL CONTRACEPTIVES

Cigarette smoking increases the risk of serious cardiovascular side effects from oral contraceptive use. This risk increases with age and with heavy smoking (15 or more cigarettes per day) and is quite marked in women over 35 years of age. Women who use oral contraceptives should not smoke.

Some women should not use the pill. For example, you should not take the pill if you are pregnant or think you may be pregnant. You should also not use the pill if you have or have ever had any of the following conditions:

- A history of heart attack or stroke
- Blood clots in the legs (thrombophlebitis), lungs (pulmonary embolism), or eyes
- A history of blood clots in the deep veins of your legs
- Chest pain (angina pectoris)
- Known or suspected breast cancer or cancer of the lining of the uterus
- Unexplained vaginal bleeding (until a diagnosis is reached by your doctor)
- Yellowing of the whites of the eyes or of the skin (jaundice) during pregnancy or during previous use of the pill
- Liver tumor (benign or cancerous)

Tell you health care professional if you have ever had any of these conditions. Your health care professional can recommend a safer method of birth control.

OTHER CONSIDERATIONS BEFORE TAKING ORAL CONTRACEPTIVES

Tell your health care professional if you have:

- Breast nodules, fibrocystic disease of the breast or an abnormal breast x-ray or mammogram
- Diabetes
- Elevated cholesterol or triglycerides
- High blood pressure
- Migraine or other headaches or epilepsy
- Mental depression
- Gallbladder, heart, or kidney disease
- History of scanty or irregular menstrual periods

Women with any of these conditions should be checked often by their health care professional if they choose to use oral contraceptives.

Also, be sure to inform your doctor or health care professional if you smoke or are on any medications.

RISKS OF TAKING ORAL CONTRACEPTIVES

1. Risk of developing blood clots.

Blood clots and blockage of blood vessels are the most serious side effects of taking oral contraceptives. In particular, a clot in the legs can cause thrombophlebitis and a clot that travels to the lungs can cause a sudden blockage of the vessel carrying blood to the lungs. Either of these can cause death or disability. Rarely, clots occur in the blood vessels of the eye and may cause blindness, double vision, or impaired vision.

If you take oral contraceptives and need elective surgery, need to stay in bed for a prolonged illness, or have recently delivered a baby, you may be at risk of developing blood clots. You should consult your doctor about stopping oral contraceptives three to four weeks before surgery and not taking oral contraceptives for two weeks after surgery or during bed rest. You should also not take oral contraceptives soon after delivery of a baby. It is advisable to wait for at least four weeks after delivery if you are not breastfeeding. If you are breastfeeding see the section on Breastfeeding in **GENERAL PRECAUTIONS**.

2. Heart attacks and strokes

Oral contraceptives may increase the tendency of developing strokes (stoppage or rupture of blood vessels in the brain) and angina pectoris and heart attacks (blockage of blood vessels in the heart). Any of these conditions can cause death or disability.

Smoking greatly increases the possibility of suffering heart attacks and strokes. Furthermore, smoking and the use of oral contraceptives greatly increase the chances of developing and dying of heart disease.

3. Gallbladder disease

Oral contraceptive users probably have a greater risk than nonusers of having gallbladder disease, although this risk may be related to pills containing high doses of estrogens.

4. Liver tumors

In rare cases, oral contraceptives can cause benign but dangerous liver tumors. These benign liver tumors can rupture and cause fatal internal bleeding. In addition, a possible, but not definite, association has been found with the pill and liver cancers in two studies, in which a few women who developed these very rare cancers were found to have used oral contraceptives for long periods. However, liver cancers in general are extremely rare and the chance of developing liver cancer from using the pill is thus even rarer.

5. Cancer of the reproductive organs

There is, at present, no confirmed evidence that oral contraceptives increase the risk of cancer of the reproductive organs and breasts in human studies. Several studies have found no overall increase in the risk of developing breast cancer. However, women who use oral contraceptives and have a strong family history of breast cancer, or who have breast nodules or abnormal mammograms, should be closely followed by their doctors.

Some studies have found an increase in the incidence of cancer of the cervix in women who use oral contraceptives. However, this finding may be related to factors other than the use of oral contraceptives.

ESTIMATED RISK OF DEATH FROM A BIRTH CONTROL METHOD OR PREGNANCY

All methods of birth control and pregnancy are associated with a risk of developing certain diseases which may lead to disability or death. An estimate of the number of deaths associated with different methods of birth control and pregnancy has been calculated and is shown in the following table.

[See table above]

It can be seen in the table that for women aged 15 to 39, the risk of death was highest with pregnancy (7–26 deaths per 100,000 women, depending on age). Among pill users who do not smoke, the risk of death was always lower than that associated with pregnancy for any age group, although over the age of 40, the risk increases to 32 deaths per 100,000 women, compared to 28 associated with pregnancy at that age. However, for pill users who smoke and are over the age of 35, the estimated number of deaths exceeds those for other methods of birth control. If a woman is over the age of 40 and smokes, her estimated risk of death is four times higher (117/100,000 women) than the estimated risk associated with pregnancy (28/100,000 women) in that age group.

The suggestion that women over 40 who don't smoke should not take oral contraceptives is based on information from older high-dose pills and on less selective use of pills than is practiced today.

An Advisory Committee of the FDA discussed this issue in 1989 and recommended that the benefits of oral contraceptive use by healthy, nonsmoking women over 40 years of age may outweigh the possible risks. However, all women, especially older women, are cautioned to use the lowest dose pill that is effective.

Continued on next page

Ovcon 35—Cont.

In the above table, the risk of death from any birth control method is less than the risk of childbirth, except for oral contraceptive users over the age of 35 who smoke and pill users over the age of 40 even if they do not smoke.

You should discuss this information with your health care professional.

WARNING SIGNALS

If any of these adverse conditions occur while you are taking oral contraceptives, call your doctor immediately.

- Sharp chest pain, coughing of blood, or sudden shortness of breath (indicating a possible clot in the lung)
- Pain in the calf (indicating a possible clot in the leg)
- Crushing chest pain or heaviness in the chest (indicating a possible heart attack)
- Sudden severe headache or vomiting, dizziness or fainting, disturbances of vision or speech, weakness, or numbness in an arm or leg (indicating a possible stroke)
- Sudden partial or complete loss of vision (indicating a possible clot in the eye)
- Breast lumps (indicating possible breast cancer or fibrocystic disease of the breast; ask your doctor or health care professional to show you how to examine your breasts)
- Severe pain or tenderness in the stomach area (indicating a possibly ruptured liver tumor)
- Difficulty in sleeping, weakness, lack of energy, fatigue, or change in mood (possibly indicating severe depression)
- Jaundice or a yellowing of the skin or eyeballs, accompanied frequently by fever, fatigue, loss of appetite, dark-colored urine, or light-colored bowel movements (indicating possible liver problems).
- Abnormal vaginal bleeding (See SIDE EFFECTS OF ORAL CONTRACEPTIVES, 1. Vaginal bleeding, below).

SIDE EFFECTS OF ORAL CONTRACEPTIVES

In addition to the risks and more serious side effects discussed above (See RISKS OF TAKING ORAL CONTRACEPTIVES, ESTIMATED RISK OF DEATH FROM A BIRTH CONTROL METHOD OR PREGNANCY and WARNING SIGNALS sections, above), the following may also occur:

1. Vaginal bleeding

Irregular vaginal bleeding or spotting may occur while you are taking the pills. Irregular bleeding may vary from slight staining between menstrual periods to breakthrough bleeding which is a flow much like a regular period. Irregular bleeding occurs most often during the first few months of oral contraceptive use, but may also occur after you have been taking the pill for some time. Such bleeding may be temporary and usually does not indicate any serious problems. It is important to continue taking your pills on schedule. If the bleeding occurs in more than one cycle or lasts for more than a few days, talk to your doctor or health care professional.

2. Gastrointestinal effects

The most frequent, unpleasant side effects are nausea and vomiting, stomach cramps, bloating, and a change in appetite.

3. Contact lenses

If you wear contact lenses and notice a change in vision or an inability to wear your lenses, contact your doctor or health care professional.

4. Fluid retention

Oral contraceptives may cause edema (fluid retention) with swelling of the fingers or ankles and may raise your blood pressure. If you experience fluid retention, contact your doctor or health care professional.

5. Melasma

A spotty darkening of the skin is possible, particularly of the face.

6. Other side effects

Other side effects may include change in appetite, headache, nervousness, depression, dizziness, loss of scalp hair, rash, and vaginal infections.

If any of these side effects bother you, call your doctor or health care professional.

GENERAL PRECAUTIONS

1. Missed periods and use of oral contraceptives before or during early pregnancy

There may be times when you may not menstruate regularly after you have completed taking a cycle of pills. If you have taken your pills regularly and miss one menstrual period, continue taking your pills for the next cycle but be sure to inform your health care professional before doing so. If you have not taken the pills daily as instructed and missed a menstrual period, or if you missed two consecutive menstrual periods, you may be pregnant. Check with your health care professional immediately to determine whether you are pregnant. Do not continue to take oral contraceptives until you are sure you are not pregnant, but continue to use another method of contraception.

There is no conclusive evidence that oral contraceptive use is associated with an increase in birth defects, when taken inadvertently during early pregnancy. Previously, a few studies had reported that oral contraceptives might be associated with birth defects, but these studies have not been

confirmed. Nevertheless, oral contraceptives or any other drugs should not be used during pregnancy unless clearly necessary and prescribed by your doctor. You should check with your doctor about risks to your unborn child of any medication taken during pregnancy.

2. While breastfeeding

If you are breastfeeding, consult your doctor before starting oral contraceptives. Some of the drug will be passed on to the child in the milk. A few adverse effects on the child have been reported, including yellowing of the skin (jaundice) and breast enlargement. In addition, oral contraceptives may decrease the amount and quality of your milk. If possible, do not use oral contraceptives while breastfeeding. You should use another method of contraception since breastfeeding provides only partial protection from becoming pregnant and this partial protection decreases significantly as you breastfeed for longer periods of time. You should consider starting oral contraceptives only after you have weaned your child completely.

3. Laboratory tests

If you are scheduled for any laboratory tests, tell your doctor you are taking birth control pills. Certain blood tests may be affected by birth control pills.

4. Drug interactions

Certain drugs may interact with birth control pills to make them less effective in preventing pregnancy or cause an increase in breakthrough bleeding. Such drugs include rifampin, drugs used for epilepsy such as barbiturates (for example, phenobarbital) and phenytoin (Dilantin is one brand of this drug), phenylbutazone (Butazolidin is one brand) and possibly ampicillin and tetracyclines (several brand names). You may need to use an additional method of contraception when you take drugs which can make oral contraceptives less effective.

HOW TO TAKE THE PILL

IMPORTANT POINTS TO REMEMBER

SEXUALLY-TRANSMITTED DISEASES

This product (like all oral contraceptives) is intended to prevent pregnancy. It does not protect against transmission of HIV (AIDS) and other sexually transmitted diseases such as chlamydia, genital herpes, genital warts, gonorrhea, hepatitis B, and syphilis.

BEFORE YOU START TAKING YOUR PILLS

1. BE SURE TO READ THESE DIRECTIONS:
Before you start taking your pills.
Anytime you are not sure what to do.

2. THE RIGHT WAY TO TAKE THE PILL IS TO TAKE ONE PILL EVERY DAY AT THE SAME TIME.
If you miss pills you could get pregnant. This includes starting the pack late. The more pills you miss, the more likely you are to get pregnant.

3. MANY WOMEN HAVE SPOTTING OR LIGHT BLEEDING, OR MAY FEEL SICK TO THEIR STOMACH DURING THE FIRST 1–3 PACKS OF PILLS.
If you do feel sick to your stomach, do not stop taking the pill. The problem will usually go away. If it doesn't go away, check with your doctor or clinic.

4. MISSING PILLS CAN ALSO CAUSE SPOTTING OR LIGHT BLEEDING, even when you make up these missed pills.
On the days you take 2 pills to make up for missed pills, you could also feel a little sick to you stomach.

5. IF YOU HAVE VOMITING OR DIARRHEA, for any reason, or IF YOU TAKE SOME MEDICINES, including some antibiotics, your pills may not work as well.
Use a back-up method (such as condoms, foam, or sponge) until you check with your doctor or clinic.

6. IF YOU HAVE TROUBLE REMEMBERING TO TAKE THE PILL, talk to your doctor or clinic about how to make pill-taking easier or about using another method of birth control.

7. IF YOU HAVE ANY QUESTIONS OR ARE UNSURE ABOUT THE INFORMATION IN THIS LEAFLET, call your doctor or clinic.

BEFORE YOU START TAKING YOUR PILLS

---

1. DECIDE WHAT TIME OF DAY YOU WANT TO TAKE YOUR PILL.
It is important to take it at about the same time every day.

2. LOOK AT YOUR PILL PACK TO SEE IF IT HAS 21 or 28 PILLS:
The 21-pill pack has 21 "active" peach pills (with hormones) to take for 3 weeks, followed by 1 week without pills.
The 28-pill pack has 21 "active" peach or yellow pills (with hormones) to take for 3 weeks, followed by 1 week of reminder green pills (without hormones).
[See figure at top of next column]

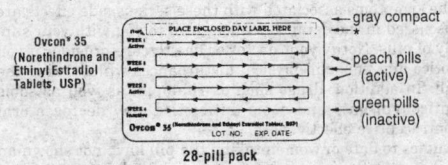

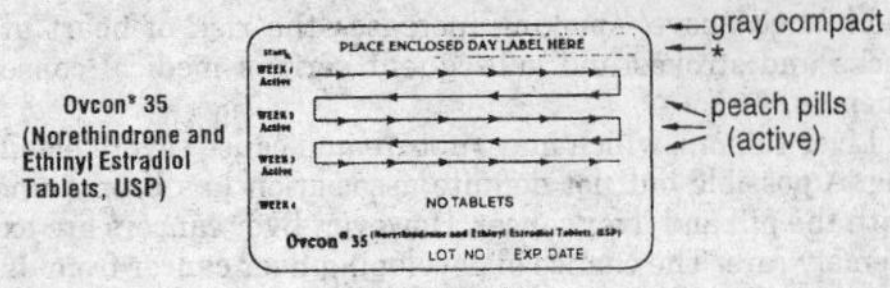

Ovcon® 35 (Norethindrone and Ethinyl Estradiol Tablets, USP)

21-pill pack

Each of the 21 peach pills contains norethindrone (0.4 mg) and ethinyl estradiol (0.035 mg).

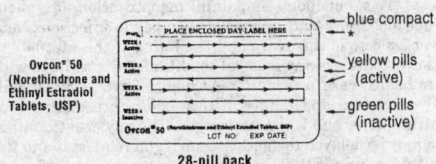

Ovcon® 35 (Norethindrone and Ethinyl Estradiol Tablets, USP)

28-pill pack

Each of the 21 peach pills contains norethindrone (0.4 mg) and ethinyl estradiol (0.035 mg). Each green pill in the 28-day regimen contains inert ingredients.

Ovcon® 50 (Norethindrone and Ethinyl Estradiol Tablets, USP)

28-pill pack

Each of the 21 yellow pills contains norethindrone (1 mg) and ethinyl estradiol (0.05 mg). Each green pill in the 28-day regimen contains inert ingredients.

* For use of day labels, see WHEN TO START THE FIRST PACK OF PILLS below.

3. BE SURE YOU HAVE READY AT ALL TIMES: ANOTHER KIND OF BIRTH CONTROL (such as condoms, foam, or sponge) to use as a back-up in case you miss pills. AN EXTRA, FULL PILL PACK.

WHEN TO START THE FIRST PACK OF PILLS

You have a choice of which day to start taking your first pack of pills. Decide with your doctor or clinic which is the best day for you. Once you have decided which day you will begin taking your pills, immediately do the following: remove the Brief Summary from inside the compact and look for the day label sheet attached; peel the day label from the sheet which has the start day printed on the left hand side; affix the label to the blister card in the designated location. Take your pill daily in the order indicated by the arrows on the blister card. Pick a time of day which will be easy to remember.

DAY 1 START:
1. Take the first "active" peach or yellow pill of the first pack during the first 24 hours of your period.
2. You will not need to use a back-up method of birth control, since you are starting the pill at the beginning of your period.

SUNDAY START:
1. Take the first "active" peach or yellow pill of the first pack on the Sunday after your period starts, even if you are still bleeding. If your period begins on Sunday, start the pack that same day.
2. Use another method of birth control as a back-up method if you have sex anytime from the Sunday you start your first pack until the next Sunday (7 days). Condoms, foam, or the sponge are good back-up methods of birth control.

WHAT TO DO DURING THE MONTH

---

1. TAKE ONE PILL AT THE SAME TIME EVERY DAY UNTIL THE PACK IS EMPTY.
Do not skip pills even if you are spotting or bleeding between monthly periods or feel sick to your stomach (nausea).
Do not skip pills even if you do not have sex very often.

2. WHEN YOU FINISH A PACK OR SWITCH YOUR BRAND OF PILLS:
21 pills: Wait 7 days to start the next pack. You will probably have your period during that week. Be sure that no more than 7 days pass between the 21-day packs.
28 pills: Start the next pack on the day after your last "reminder" pill. Do not wait any days between packs.

WHAT TO DO IF YOU MISS PILLS

If you MISS 1 peach or yellow "active" pill:
1. Take it as soon as you remember. Take the next pill at your regular time. This means you may take 2 pills in 1 day.
2. You do not need to use a back-up birth control method if you have sex.

If you MISS 2 peach or yellow "active" pills in a row in WEEK 1 or WEEK 2 of your pack:

1. Take 2 pills on the day you remember and 2 pills the next day.
2. Then take 1 pill a day until you finish the pack.
3. You MAY BECOME PREGNANT if you have sex in the *7 days* after you miss pills. You MUST use another birth control method (such as condoms, foam, or sponge) as a back-up for those 7 days.

If you MISS 2 peach or yellow "active" pills in a row in the 3rd WEEK:

1. If you are a DAY 1 Starter:
THROW OUT the rest of the pill pack and start a new pack that same day.
If you are a Sunday Starter:
Keep taking 1 pill every day until Sunday.
On Sunday, THROW OUT the rest of the pack and start a new pack of pills that same day.
2. You may not have your period this month but this is expected. However, if you miss your period 2 months in a row, call your doctor or clinic because you might be pregnant.
3. You MAY BECOME PREGNANT if you have sex in the *7 days* after you miss pills. You MUST use another birth control method (such as condoms, foam, or sponge) as a back-up for those 7 days.

If you MISS 3 OR MORE peach or yellow "active" pills in a row (during the first 3 weeks):

1. If you are a DAY 1 Starter:
THROW OUT the rest of the pill pack and start a new pack that same day.

If you are a Sunday Starter:
Keep taking 1 pill every day until Sunday.
On Sunday, THROW OUT the rest of the pack and start a new pack of pills that same day.

2. You may not have your period this month but this is expected. However, if you miss your period 2 months in a row, call your doctor or clinic because you might be pregnant.
3. You MAY BECOME PREGNANT if you have sex in the *7 days* after you miss pills. You MUST use another birth control method (such as condoms, foam, or sponge) as a back-up for those 7 days.

A REMINDER FOR THOSE ON 28-DAY PACKS: If you forget any of the 7 green "reminder" pills in Week 4:
THROW AWAY the pills you missed.
Keep taking 1 pill each day until the pack is empty.
You do not need a back-up method.

FINALLY, IF YOU ARE STILL NOT SURE WHAT TO DO ABOUT THE PILLS YOU HAVE MISSED:
Use a BACK-UP METHOD anytime you have sex.
KEEP TAKING ONE "ACTIVE" PILL EACH DAY until you can reach your doctor or clinic.

GENERAL

1. Pregnancy due to pill failure

The incidence of pill failure resulting in pregnancy is approximately 1% (i.e., one pregnancy per 100 women per year) if taken every day as directed, but more typical failure rates are about 3%. If failure does occur, the risk to the fetus is minimal.

2. Pregnancy after stopping the pill

There may be some delay in becoming pregnant after you stop using oral contraceptives, especially if you had irregular menstrual cycles before you used oral contraceptives. It may be advisable to postpone conception until you begin menstruating regularly once you have stopped taking the pill and desire pregnancy.

There does not appear to be any increase in birth defects in newborn babies when pregnancy occurs soon after stopping the pill.

3. Other

a. Overdosage

Serious ill effects have not been reported following ingestion of large doses of oral contraceptives by young children. Overdosage may cause nausea and withdrawal bleeding in females. In case of overdosage, contact your poison control center, health care professional, or nearest emergency room.
KEEP THIS DRUG AND ALL DRUGS OUT OF THE REACH OF CHILDREN.

b. General medical information

Your health care professional will take a medical and family history before prescribing oral contraceptives and will examine you. The physical examination may be delayed to another time if you request it and the health care provider believes that it is a good medical practice to postpone it. You should be reexamined at least once a year. Be sure to inform your health care professional if there is a family history of any of the conditions listed previously in this leaflet. Be sure to keep all appointments with your health care professional, because this is a time to determine if there are early signs of side effects of oral contraceptive use.

Do not use the drug for any condition other than the one for which it was prescribed. This drug has been prescribed specifically for you; do not give it to others who may want birth control pills.

NONCONTRACEPTIVE EFFECTS OF ORAL CONTRACEPTIVES

In addition to preventing pregnancy, use of oral contraceptives may provide certain benefits. They are:

- Menstrual cycles may become more regular
- Blood flow during menstruation may be lighter and less iron may be lost. Therefore, anemia due to iron deficiency is less likely to occur
- Pain or other symptoms during menstruation may be encountered less frequently
- Ectopic (tubal) pregnancy may occur less frequently
- Noncancerous cysts or lumps in the breast may occur less frequently
- Acute pelvic inflammatory disease may occur less frequently
- Oral contraceptive use may provide some protection against developing two forms of cancer: cancer of the ovaries and cancer of the lining of the uterus.

If you want more information about birth control pills, ask your doctor or pharmacist. They have a more technical leaflet called the Professional Labeling, which you may wish to read.

Bristol-Myers Squibb Company
Princeton, NJ 08543
U.S.A.
Revised June 1998
57841DIM-8
A3-B001-6-98

Shown in Product Identification Guide, page 307

PLAVIX® ℞
[*plă vĭks*]
clopidogrel bisulfate tablets

DESCRIPTION

PLAVIX (clopidogrel bisulfate) is an inhibitor of ADP-induced platelet aggregation acting by direct inhibition of adenosine diphosphate (ADP) binding to its receptor and of the subsequent ADP-mediated activation of the glycoprotein GPIIb/IIIa complex. Chemically it is methyl (+)-(*S*)-α-(2-chlorophenyl)-6,7-dihydrothieno[3,2-c]pyridine-5(4*H*)-acetate sulfate (1:1). The empirical formula of clopidogrel bisulfate is $C_{16}H_{16}Cl\ NO_2S \bullet H_2SO_4$ and its molecular weight is 419.9.

The structural formula is as follows:

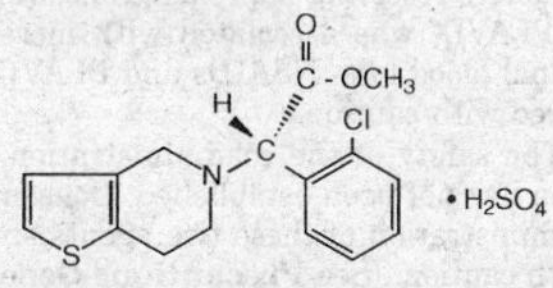

Clopidogrel bisulfate is a white to off-white powder. It is practically insoluble in water at neutral pH but freely soluble at pH 1. It also dissolves freely in methanol, dissolves sparingly in methylene chloride, and is practically insoluble in ethyl ether. It has a specific optical rotation of about +56°.

PLAVIX for oral administration is provided as pink, round, biconvex, engraved film-coated tablets containing 97.875 mg of clopidogrel bisulfate which is the molar equivalent of 75 mg of clopidogrel base.

Each tablet contains anhydrous lactose, hydrogenated castor oil, microcrystalline cellulose, polyethylene glycol 6000 and pregelatinized starch as inactive ingredients. The pink film coating contains ferric oxide (red), hydroxypropyl methylcellulose 2910, polyethylene glycol 6000 and titanium dioxide. The tablets are polished with Carnauba wax.

CLINICAL PHARMACOLOGY

Mechanism of Action

Clopidogrel is an inhibitor of platelet aggregation. A variety of drugs that inhibit platelet function have been shown to decrease morbid events in people with established atherosclerotic cardiovascular disease as evidenced by stroke or transient ischemic attacks, myocardial infarction, or need for bypass or angioplasty. This indicates that platelets participate in the initiation and/or evolution of these events and that inhibiting them can reduce the event rate.

Pharmacodynamic Properties

Clopidogrel selectively inhibits the binding of adenosine diphosphate (ADP) to its platelet receptor and the subsequent ADP-mediated activation of the glycoprotein GPIIb/IIIa complex, thereby inhibiting platelet aggregation. Biotransformation of clopidogrel is necessary to produce inhibition of platelet aggregation, but an active metabolite responsible for the activity of the drug has not been isolated. Clopidogrel also inhibits platelet aggregation induced by agonists other than ADP by blocking the amplification of platelet activation by released ADP. Clopidogrel does not inhibit phosphodiesterase activity.

Clopidogrel acts by irreversibly modifying the platelet ADP receptor. Consequently, platelets exposed to clopidogrel are affected for the remainder of their lifespan.

Dose dependent inhibition of platelet aggregation can be seen 2 hours after single oral doses of PLAVIX. Repeated doses of 75 mg PLAVIX per day inhibit ADP-induced platelet aggregation on the first day, and inhibition reaches steady state between Day 3 and Day 7. At steady state, the average inhibition level observed with a dose of 75 mg PLAVIX per day was between 40% and 60%. Platelet aggregation and bleeding time gradually return to baseline values after treatment is discontinued, generally in about 5 days.

Pharmacokinetics and Metabolism

After repeated 75-mg oral doses of clopidogrel (base), plasma concentrations of the parent compound, which has no platelet inhibiting effect, are very low and are generally below the quantification limit (0.00025 mg/L) beyond 2 hours after dosing. Clopidogrel is extensively metabolized by the liver. The main circulating metabolite is the carboxylic acid derivative, and it too has no effect on platelet aggregation. It represents about 85% of the circulating drug-related compounds in plasma.

Following an oral dose of ^{14}C-labeled clopidogrel in humans, approximately 50% was excreted in the urine and approximately 46% in the feces in the 5 days after dosing. The elimination half-life of the main circulating metabolite was 8 hours after single and repeated administration. Covalent binding to platelets accounted for 2% of radiolabel with a half-life of 11 days.

Effect of Food: Administration of PLAVIX (clopidogrel bisulfate) with meals did not significantly modify the bioavailability of clopidogrel as assessed by the pharmacokinetics of the main circulating metabolite.

Absorption and Distribution: Clopidogrel is rapidly absorbed after oral administration of repeated doses of 75 mg clopidogrel (base), with peak plasma levels (≅3 mg/L) of the main circulating metabolite occurring approximately 1 hour after dosing. The pharmacokinetics of the main circulating metabolite are linear (plasma concentrations increased in proportion to dose) in the dose range of 50 to 150 mg of clopidogrel. Absorption is at least 50% based on urinary excretion of clopidogrel-related metabolites.

Clopidogrel and the main circulating metabolite bind reversibly *in vitro* to human plasma proteins (98% and 94%, respectively). The binding is nonsaturable *in vitro* up to a concentration of 100 µg/mL.

Metabolism and Elimination: *In vitro* and *in vivo*, clopidogrel undergoes rapid hydrolysis into its carboxylic acid derivative. In plasma and urine, the glucuronide of the carboxylic acid derivative is also observed.

Special Populations

Geriatric Patients: Plasma concentrations of the main circulating metabolite are significantly higher in elderly (≥75 years) compared to young healthy volunteers but these higher plasma levels were not associated with differences in platelet aggregation and bleeding time. No dosage adjustment is needed for the elderly.

Renally Impaired Patients: After repeated doses of 75 mg PLAVIX per day, plasma levels of the main circulating metabolite were lower in patients with severe renal impairment (creatinine clearance from 5 to 15 mL/min) compared to subjects with moderate renal impairment (creatinine clearance 30 to 60 mL/min) or healthy subjects. Although inhibition of ADP-induced platelet aggregation was lower (25%) than that observed in healthy volunteers, the prolongation of bleeding time was similar to healthy volunteers receiving 75 mg of PLAVIX per day. No dosage adjustment is needed in renally impaired patients.

Gender: No significant difference was observed in the plasma levels of the main circulating metabolite between males and females. In a small study comparing men and women, less inhibition of ADP-induced platelet aggregation was observed in women, but there was no difference in prolongation of bleeding time. In the large, controlled clinical study (Clopidogrel vs. Aspirin in Patients at Risk of Ischemic Events; CAPRIE), the incidence of clinical outcome events, other adverse clinical events, and abnormal clinical laboratory parameters was similar in men and women.

Race: Pharmacokinetic differences due to race have not been studied.

CLINICAL STUDIES

The clinical evidence for the efficacy of PLAVIX is derived from the CAPRIE (Clopidogrel vs. Aspirin in Patients at Risk of Ischemic Events) trial. This was a 19,185-patient, 304-center, international, randomized, double-blind, parallel-group study comparing PLAVIX (75 mg daily) to aspirin (325 mg daily). The patients randomized had: 1) recent histories of myocardial infarction (within 35 days); 2) recent histories of ischemic stroke (within 6 months) with at least a week of residual neurological signs; or 3) objectively established peripheral arterial disease. Patients received randomized treatment for an average of 1.6 years (maximum of 3 years).

The trial's primary outcome was the time to first occurrence of new ischemic stroke (fatal or not), new myocardial infarction (fatal or not), or other vascular death. Deaths not easily attributable to nonvascular causes were all classified as vascular.

Continued on next page

Plavix—Cont.

Outcome Events of the Primary Analysis

Patients	PLAVIX 9599	aspirin 9586
IS (fatal or not)	438 (4.56%)	461 (4.81%)
MI (fatal or not)	275 (2.86%)	333 (3.47%)
Other vascular death	226 (2.35%)	226 (2.36%)
Total	939 (9.78%)	1020 (10.64%)

As shown in the table, PLAVIX (clopidogrel bisulfate) was associated with a lower incidence of outcome events of every kind. The overall risk reduction (9.78% vs. 10.64%) was 8.7%, P=0.045. Similar results were obtained when all-cause mortality and all-cause strokes were counted instead of vascular mortality and ischemic strokes (risk reduction 6.9%). In patients who survived an on-study stroke or myocardial infarction, the incidence of subsequent events was again lower in the PLAVIX group.

The curves showing the overall event rate are shown in the figure. The event curves separated early and continued to diverge over the 3-year follow-up period.

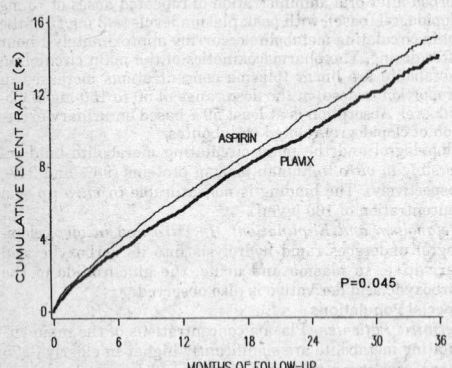

FATAL OR NON-FATAL VASCULAR EVENTS

Although the statistical significance favoring PLAVIX over aspirin was marginal (P=0.045), and represents the result of a single trial that has not been replicated, the comparator drug, aspirin, is itself effective (vs. placebo) in reducing cardiovascular events in patients with recent myocardial infarction or stroke. Thus, the difference between PLAVIX and placebo, although not measured directly, is substantial. The CAPRIE trial included a population that was randomized on the basis of 3 entry criteria. The efficacy of PLAVIX relative to aspirin was heterogeneous across these randomized subgroups (P=0.043). It is not clear whether this difference is real or a chance occurrence. Although the CAPRIE trial was not designed to evaluate the relative benefit of PLAVIX over aspirin in the individual patient subgroups, the benefit appeared to be strongest in patients who were enrolled because of peripheral vascular disease (especially those who also had a history of myocardial infarction) and weaker in stroke patients. In patients who were enrolled in the trial on the sole basis of a recent myocardial infarction, PLAVIX was not numerically superior to aspirin.

In the meta-analyses of studies of aspirin vs. placebo in patients similar to those in CAPRIE, aspirin was associated with a reduced incidence of atherothrombotic events. There was a suggestion of heterogeneity in these studies too, with the effect strongest in patients with a history of myocardial infarction, weaker in patients with a history of stroke, and not discernible in patients with a history of peripheral vascular disease. With respect to the inferred comparison of PLAVIX to placebo, there is no indication of heterogeneity.

INDICATIONS AND USAGE

PLAVIX (clopidogrel bisulfate) is indicated for the reduction of atherosclerotic events (myocardial infarction, stroke, and vascular death) in patients with atherosclerosis documented by recent stroke, recent myocardial infarction, or established peripheral arterial disease.

CONTRAINDICATIONS

The use of PLAVIX is contraindicated in the following conditions:
- Hypersensitivity to the drug substance or any component of the product.
- Active pathological bleeding such as peptic ulcer or intracranial hemorrhage.

WARNINGS

None.

PRECAUTIONS

General

As with other anti-platelet agents, PLAVIX should be used with caution in patients who may be at risk of increased bleeding from trauma, surgery, or other pathological conditions. If a patient is to undergo elective surgery and an antiplatelet effect is not desired, PLAVIX should be discontinued 7 days prior to surgery.

GI Bleeding: PLAVIX prolongs the bleeding time. In CAPRIE, PLAVIX was associated with a rate of gastrointestinal bleeding of 2.0%, vs. 2.7% on aspirin. PLAVIX should be used with caution in patients who have lesions with a propensity to bleed (such as ulcers). Drugs that might induce such lesions (such as aspirin and other nonsteroidal anti-inflammatory drugs [NSAIDs]) should be used with caution in patients taking PLAVIX.

Use in Hepatically Impaired Patients: Experience is limited in patients with severe hepatic disease, who may have bleeding diatheses. PLAVIX should be used with caution in this population.

Information for Patients

Patients should be told that it may take them longer than usual to stop bleeding when they take PLAVIX, and that they should report any unusual bleeding to their physician. Patients should inform physicians and dentists that they are taking PLAVIX before any surgery is scheduled and before any new drug is taken.

Drug Interactions

Study of specific drug interactions yielded the following results:

Aspirin: Aspirin did not modify the clopidogrel-mediated inhibition of ADP-induced platelet aggregation. Concomitant administration of 500 mg of aspirin twice a day for 1 day did not significantly increase the prolongation of bleeding time induced by PLAVIX. PLAVIX potentiated the effect of aspirin on collagen-induced platelet aggregation. The safety of chronic concomitant administration of aspirin and PLAVIX has not been established.

Heparin: In a study in healthy volunteers, PLAVIX did not necessitate modification of the heparin dose or alter the effect of heparin on coagulation. Coadministration of heparin had no effect on inhibition of platelet aggregation induced by PLAVIX. The safety of this combination has not been established, however, and concomitant use should be undertaken with caution.

Nonsteroidal Anti-Inflammatory Drugs (NSAIDs): In healthy volunteers receiving naproxen, concomitant administration of PLAVIX was associated with increased occult gastrointestinal blood loss. NSAIDs and PLAVIX should be coadministered with caution.

Warfarin: The safety of the coadministration of PLAVIX with warfarin has not been established. Consequently, concomitant administration of these two agents should be undertaken with caution. (See **Precautions-General**).

Other Concomitant Therapy: No clinically significant pharmacodynamic interactions were observed when PLAVIX was coadministered with **atenolol, nifedipine,** or both atenolol and nifedipine. The pharmacodynamic activity of PLAVIX was also not significantly influenced by the coadministration of **phenobarbital, cimetidine** or **estrogen.**

The pharmacokinetics of **digoxin** or **theophylline** were not modified by the coadministration of PLAVIX (clopidogrel bisulfate).

At high concentrations *in vitro,* clopidogrel inhibits P_{450} (2C9). Accordingly, PLAVIX may interfere with the metabolism of **phenytoin, tamoxifen, tolbutamide, warfarin, torsemide, fluvastatin,** and many **non-steroidal anti-inflammatory agents,** but there are no data with which to predict the magnitude of these interactions. Caution should be used when any of these drugs is coadministered with PLAVIX.

In addition to the above specific interaction studies, patients entered into CAPRIE received a variety of concomitant medications **including diuretics, beta-blocking agents, angiotensin converting enzyme inhibitors, calcium antagonists, cholesterol lowering agents, coronary vasodilators, antidiabetic agents, antiepileptic agents** and **hormone replacement therapy** without evidence of clinically significant adverse interactions.

Drug/Laboratory Test Interactions

None known.

Carcinogenesis, Mutagenesis, Impairment of Fertility

There was no evidence of tumorigenicity when clopidogrel was administered for 78 weeks to mice and 104 weeks to rats at dosages up to 77 mg/kg per day, which afforded plasma exposures >25 times that in humans at the recommended daily dose of 75 mg.

Clopidogrel was not genotoxic in four *in vitro* tests (Ames test, DNA-repair test in rat hepatocytes, gene mutation assay in Chinese hamster fibroblasts, and metaphase chromosome analysis of human lymphocytes) and in one *in vivo* test (micronucleus test by oral route in mice).

Clopidogrel was found to have no effect on fertility of male and female rats at oral doses up to 400 mg/kg per day (52 times the recommended human dose on a mg/m² basis).

Pregnancy

Pregnancy Category B. Reproduction studies performed in rats and rabbits at doses up to 500 and 300 mg/kg/day (respectively, 65 and 78 times the recommended daily human dose on a mg/m² basis), revealed no evidence of impaired fertility or fetotoxicity due to clopidogrel. There are, however, no adequate and well-controlled studies in pregnant women. Because animal reproduction studies are not always predictive of a human response, PLAVIX should be used during pregnancy only if clearly needed.

Nursing Mothers

Studies in rats have shown that clopidogrel and/or its metabolites are excreted in the milk. It is not known whether this drug is excreted in human milk. Because many drugs are excreted in human milk and because of the potential for serious adverse reactions in nursing infants, a decision should be made whether to discontinue nursing or to discontinue the drug, taking into account the importance of the drug to the nursing woman.

Pediatric Use

Safety and effectiveness in the pediatric population have not been established.

ADVERSE REACTIONS

PLAVIX has been evaluated for safety in more than 11,300 patients, including over 7,000 patients treated for 1 year or more. The overall tolerability of PLAVIX was similar to that of aspirin regardless of age, gender and race, with an approximately equal incidence (13%) of patients withdrawing from treatment because of adverse reactions. The clinically important adverse events observed in CAPRIE are discussed below.

Hemorrhagic: In patients receiving PLAVIX in CAPRIE, gastrointestinal hemorrhage occurred at a rate of 2.0%, and required hospitalization in 0.7%. In patients receiving aspirin, the corresponding rates were 2.7% and 1.1%, respectively. The incidence of intracranial hemorrhage was 0.4% for PLAVIX compared to 0.5% for aspirin.

Neutropenia/agranulocytosis: Ticlopidine, a drug chemically similar to PLAVIX, is associated with a 0.8% rate of severe neutropenia (less than 450 neutrophils/µL). Patients in CAPRIE (see Clinical Trials) were intensively monitored for neutropenia. Severe neutropenia was observed in six patients, four on PLAVIX and two on aspirin. Two of the 9599 patients who received PLAVIX and none of the 9586 patients who received aspirin had neutrophil counts of zero. One of the four PLAVIX patients was receiving cytotoxic chemotherapy, and another recovered and returned to the trial after only temporarily interrupting treatment with PLAVIX.

Although the risk of myelotoxicity with PLAVIX thus appears to be quite low, this possibility should be considered when a patient receiving PLAVIX demonstrates fever or other sign of infection.

Gastrointestinal: Overall, the incidence of gastrointestinal events (e.g. abdominal pain, dyspepsia, gastritis and constipation) in patients receiving PLAVIX (clopidogrel bisulfate) was 27.1%, compared to 29.8% in those receiving aspirin. The incidence of peptic, gastric or duodenal ulcers was 0.7% for PLAVIX and 1.2% for aspirin.

Cases of diarrhea were reported in 4.5% of patients in the PLAVIX group compared to 3.4% in the aspirin group. However, these were rarely severe (PLAVIX=0.2% and aspirin=0.1%).

The incidence of patients withdrawing from treatment because of gastrointestinal adverse reactions was 3.2% for PLAVIX and 4.0% for aspirin.

Rash and Other Skin Disorders: The incidence of skin and appendage disorders in patients receiving PLAVIX was 15.8% (0.7% serious); the corresponding rate in aspirin patients was 13.1% (0.5% serious).

The overall incidence of patients withdrawing from treatment because of skin and appendage disorders adverse reactions was 1.5% for PLAVIX and 0.8% for aspirin.

Adverse events occurring in ≥2.5% of patients on PLAVIX in the CAPRIE controlled clinical trial are shown below regardless of relationship to PLAVIX. The median duration of therapy was 20 months, with a maximum of 3 years.

[See table at bottom of next page]

Other adverse experiences of potential importance occurring in 1% to 2.5% of patients receiving PLAVIX (clopidogrel bisulfate) in the CAPRIE controlled clinical trial are listed below regardless of relationship to PLAVIX. In general, the incidence of these events was similar in the aspirin-treated group.

Autonomic Nervous System Disorders: Syncope, Palpitation. *Body as a Whole - general disorders:* Asthenia, Hernia. *Cardiovascular disorders:* Cardiac failure. *Central and peripheral nervous system disorders:* Cramps legs, Hypoaesthesia, Neuralgia, Paraesthesia, Vertigo. *Gastrointestinal system disorders:* Constipation, Vomiting. *Heart rate and rhythm disorders:* Fibrillation atrial. *Liver and biliary system disorders:* Hepatic enzymes increased. *Metabolic and nutritional disorders:* Gout, hyperuricemia, non-protein nitrogen (NPN) increased. *Musculo-skeletal system disorders:* Arthritis, Arthrosis. *Platelet, bleeding & clotting disorders:* GI hemorrhage, hematoma, platelets decreased. *Psychiatric disorders:* Anxiety, Insomnia. *Red blood cell disorders:* Anemia. *Respiratory system disorders:* Pneumonia, Sinusitis.

Skin and appendage disorders: Eczema, Skin ulceration. *Urinary system disorders:* Cystitis. *Vision disorders:* Cataract, Conjunctivitis.

Other potentially serious adverse events which may be of clinical interest but were rarely reported (<1%) in patients who received PLAVIX are listed below regardless of relationship to PLAVIX. In general, the incidence of these events was similar in the aspirin group.

Body as a whole: Allergic reaction, necrosis ischemic. *Cardiovascular disorders:* Edema generalized. *Gastrointestinal system disorders:* Gastric ulcer perforated, gastritis hemorrhagic, upper GI ulcer hemorrhagic. *Liver and Biliary system disorders:* Bilirubinemia, hepatitis infectious, liver fatty. *Platelet, bleeding and clotting disorders:* hemarthrosis, hematuria, hemoptysis, hemorrhage intracranial, hemorrhage retroperitoneal, hemorrhage of operative wound, ocular hemorrhage, pulmonary hemorrhage, purpura allergic, thrombocytopenia. *Red blood cell disorders:* Anemia aplastic, anemia hypochromic. *Reproductive disorders, female:* Menorrhagia. *Respiratory system disorders:* Hemothorax. *Skin and appendage disorders:* Bullous eruption, rash erythematous, rash maculopapular, urticaria. *White cell and reticuloendothelial system disorders:* Agranulocytosis, granulocytopenia, leukemia, leukopenia, neutrophils decreased.

OVERDOSAGE

One case of deliberate overdosage with PLAVIX was reported in the large, controlled clinical study. A 34-year-old woman took a single 1,050-mg dose of PLAVIX (equivalent to 14 standard 75-mg tablets). There were no associated adverse events. No special therapy was instituted, and she recovered without sequelae.

No adverse events were reported after single oral administration of 600 mg (equivalent to 8 standard 75-mg tablets) of PLAVIX in healthy volunteers. The bleeding time was prolonged by a factor of 1.7, which is similar to that typically observed with the therapeutic dose of 75 mg of PLAVIX per day.

A single oral dose of clopidogrel at 1500 or 2000 mg/kg was lethal to mice and to rats and at 3000 mg/kg to baboons. Symptoms of acute toxicity were vomiting (in baboons), prostration, difficult breathing, and gastrointestinal hemorrhage in all species.

Recommendations About Specific Treatment:
Based on biological plausibility, platelet transfusion may be appropriate to reverse the pharmacological effects of PLAVIX if quick reversal is required.

DOSAGE AND ADMINISTRATION

The recommended dose of PLAVIX is 75 mg once daily with or without food.

No dosage adjustment is necessary for elderly patients or patients with renal disease. (See **Clinical Pharmacology: Special Populations.**)

HOW SUPPLIED

PLAVIX (clopidogrel bisulfate) is available as a pink, round, biconvex, film-coated tablet engraved with "75" on one side. Tablets are provided as follows:
   NDC 63653-1171-4 bottles of 100
   NDC 63653-1171-5 bottles of 500
   NDC 63653-1171-3 blisters of 100

Storage
Store at 25° C (77° F); excursions permitted to 15°–30° C (59°–86° F) [See USP Controlled Room Temperature]
Caution: Federal law prohibits dispensing without a prescription.
Manufactured by:
   Sanofi Pharmaceuticals, Inc.
   New York, NY 10016
Distributed by:
   Bristol-Myers Squibb/Sanofi Pharmaceuticals Partnership
   New York, NY 10016
69-257757   B1-B001
   PLAVIX® is a registered trademark of Sanofi
Issued November 1997   J4-643   51-006857-00
   Shown in Product Identification Guide, page 307

Adverse Events Occurring in ≥2.5% of PLAVIX Patients

Body System Event	% Incidence (% Discontinuation)	
	PLAVIX [n=9599]	Aspirin [n=9586]
Body as a Whole – general disorders		
Chest Pain	8.3 (0.2)	8.3 (0.3)
Accidental Injury	7.9 (0.1)	7.3 (0.1)
Influenza-like symptoms	7.5 (<0.1)	7.0 (<0.1)
Pain	6.4 (0.1)	6.3 (0.1)
Fatigue	3.3 (0.1)	3.4 (0.1)
Cardiovascular disorders, general		
Edema	4.1 (<0.1)	4.5 (<0.1)
Hypertension	4.3 (<0.1)	5.1 (<0.1)
Central & peripheral nervous system disorders		
Headache	7.6 (0.3)	7.2 (0.2)
Dizziness	6.2 (0.2)	6.7 (0.3)
Gastrointestinal system disorders		
Abdominal pain	5.6 (0.7)	7.1 (1.0)
Dyspepsia	5.2 (0.6)	6.1 (0.7)
Diarrhea	4.5 (0.4)	3.4 (0.3)
Nausea	3.4 (0.5)	3.8 (0.4)
Metabolic & nutritional disorders		
Hypercholesterolemia	4.0 (0)	4.4 (<0.1)
Musculo-skeletal system disorders		
Arthralgia	6.3 (0.1)	6.2 (0.1)
Back Pain	5.8 (0.1)	5.3 (<0.1)
Platelet, bleeding, & clotting disorders		
Purpura	5.3 (0.3)	3.7 (0.1)
Epistaxis	2.9 (0.2)	2.5 (0.1)
Psychiatric disorders		
Depression	3.6 (0.1)	3.9 (0.2)
Respiratory system disorders		
Upper resp tract infection	8.7 (<0.1)	8.3 (<0.1)
Dyspnea	4.5 (0.1)	4.7 (0.1)
Rhinitis	4.2 (0.1)	4.2 (<0.1)
Bronchitis	3.7 (0.1)	3.7 (0)
Coughing	3.1 (<0.1)	2.7 (<0.1)
Skin & appendage disorders		
Rash	4.2 (0.5)	3.5 (0.2)
Pruritus	3.3 (0.3)	1.6 (0.1)
Urinary system disorders		
Urinary tract infection	3.1 (0)	3.5 (0.1)

Incidence of discontinuation, regardless of relationship to therapy, is shown in parentheses.

PRAVACHOL®   ℞
[pră-vă-chol]
(pravastatin sodium) tablets

Rx only

DESCRIPTION

PRAVACHOL® (pravastatin sodium) is one of a new class of lipid-lowering compounds, the HMG-CoA reductase inhibitors, which reduce cholesterol biosynthesis. These agents are competitive inhibitors of 3-hydroxy-3-methylglutaryl-coenzyme A (HMG-CoA) reductase, the enzyme catalyzing the early rate-limiting step in cholesterol biosynthesis, conversion of HMG-CoA to mevalonate.

Pravastatin sodium is designated chemically as 1-Naphthalene-heptanoic acid, 1,2,6,7,8,8a-hexahydro-β,δ,6-trihydroxy-2-methyl-8-(2-methyl-1-oxobutoxy)-, monosodium salt, [1S-[1α(βS*,δS*),2α,6α,8β(R*),8aα]]-.

Pravastatin sodium is an odorless, white to off-white, fine or crystalline powder. It is a relatively polar hydrophilic compound with a partition coefficient (octanol/water) of 0.59 at a pH of 7.0. It is soluble in methanol and water (>300 mg/mL), slightly soluble in isopropanol, and practically insoluble in acetone, acetonitrile, chloroform, and ether.

PRAVACHOL is available for oral administration as 10 mg, 20 mg and 40 mg tablets. Inactive ingredients include: croscarmellose sodium, lactose, magnesium oxide, magnesium stearate, microcrystalline cellulose, and povidone. The 10 mg tablet also contains Red Ferric Oxide, the 20 mg tablet also contains Yellow Ferric Oxide, and the 40 mg tablet also contains Green Lake Blend (mixture of D&C Yellow No. 10-Aluminum Lake and FD&C Blue No. 1-Aluminum Lake).

CLINICAL PHARMACOLOGY

Cholesterol and triglycerides in the bloodstream circulate as part of lipoprotein complexes. These complexes can be separated by density ultracentrifugation into high (HDL), intermediate (IDL), low (LDL), and very low (VLDL) density lipoprotein fractions. Triglycerides (TG) and cholesterol synthesized in the liver are incorporated into very low density lipoproteins (VLDLs) and released into the plasma for delivery to peripheral tissues. In a series of subsequent steps, VLDLs are transformed into intermediate density lipoproteins (IDLs), and cholesterol-rich low density lipoproteins (LDLs). High density lipoproteins (HDLs), containing apolipoprotein A, are hypothesized to participate in the reverse transport of cholesterol from tissues back to the liver.

PRAVACHOL produces its lipid-lowering effect in two ways. First, as a consequence of its reversible inhibition of HMG-CoA reductase activity, it effects modest reductions in intracellular pools of cholesterol. This results in an increase in the number of LDL-receptors on cell surfaces and enhanced receptor-mediated catabolism and clearance of circulating LDL. Second, pravastatin inhibits LDL production by inhibiting hepatic synthesis of VLDL, the LDL precursor.

Clinical and pathologic studies have shown that elevated levels of total cholesterol (Total-C), low density lipoprotein cholesterol (LDL-C), and apolipoprotein B (a membrane transport complex for LDL) promote human atherosclerosis. Similarly, decreased levels of HDL-cholesterol (HDL-C) and its transport complex, apolipoprotein A, are associated with the development of atherosclerosis. Epidemiologic investigations have established that cardiovascular morbidity and mortality vary directly with the level of Total-C and LDL-C and inversely with the level of HDL-C. Though frequently found in association with low HDL, elevated plasma triglyceride (TG) has not been established as an independent risk factor for coronary heart disease. The independent effect of raising HDL or lowering TG on the risk of coronary and cardiovascular morbidity and mortality has not been determined. In both normal volunteers and patients with hyper cholesterolemia, treatment with PRAVACHOL reduced Total-C, LDL-C, and apolipoprotein B. PRAVACHOL also reduced VLDL-C and TG and produced variable increases in HDL-C and apolipoprotein A. The effects of pravastatin on Lp (a), fibrinogen, and certain other independent biochemical risk markers for coronary heart disease are unknown. Although pravastatin is relatively more hydrophilic than other HMG-CoA reductase inhibitors, the effect of relative hydrophilicity, if any, on either efficacy or safety has not been established.

In the Pravastatin Primary Prevention Study (West of Scotland Coronary Prevention Study – WOS), the effect of improving lipoprotein levels with PRAVACHOL on fatal and nonfatal coronary heart disease (CHD) was assessed in 6595 men, without a previous myocardial infarction, and with LDL-C levels between 156–254 mg/dL (4–6.7 mmol/L). The patients were followed for a median of 4.8 years. In this randomized, double-blind, placebo-controlled study, PRAVACHOL reduced the risk of a first coronary event [either CHD death or nonfatal myocardial infarction (MI)] by

Continued on next page

Pravachol—Cont.

31% [7.9% vs 5.5%, placebo vs PRAVACHOL, p=0.0001: 248 events in the placebo group (CHD death=44, nonfatal MI=204) vs 174 events in the PRAVACHOL group (CHD death=31, nonfatal MI=143)]. PRAVACHOL also decreased the risk for undergoing myocardial revascularization procedures (coronary artery bypass graft surgery or coronary angioplasty) by 37% (2.5% vs 1.7%, p=0.009) and coronary angiography by 31% (4.2% vs 2.8%, p=0.007). Cardiovascular deaths were decreased by 32% (2.3% vs 1.6%, p=0.03) and there was no increase in death from non-cardiovascular causes.

Pharmacokinetics/Metabolism

PRAVACHOL (pravastatin sodium) is administered orally in the active form. In clinical pharmacology studies in man, pravastatin is rapidly absorbed, with peak plasma levels of parent compound attained 1 to 1.5 hours following ingestion. Based on urinary recovery of radiolabeled drug, the average oral absorption of pravastatin is 34% and absolute bioavailability is 17%. While the presence of food in the gastrointestinal tract reduces systemic bioavailability, the lipid-lowering effects of the drug are similar whether taken with, or 1 hour prior, to meals.

Pravastatin undergoes extensive first-pass extraction in the liver (extraction ratio 0.66), which is its primary site of action, and the primary site of cholesterol synthesis and of LDL-C clearance. *In vitro* studies demonstrated that pravastatin is transported into hepatocytes with substantially less uptake into other cells. In view of pravastatin's apparently extensive first-pass hepatic metabolism, plasma levels may not necessarily correlate perfectly with lipid-lowering efficacy. Pravastatin plasma concentrations [including: area under the concentration-time curve (AUC), peak (C_{max}), and steady-state minimum (C_{min})] are directly proportional to administered dose. Systemic bioavailability of pravastatin administered following a bedtime dose was decreased 60% compared to that following an AM dose. Despite this decrease in systemic bioavailability, the efficacy of pravastatin administered once daily in the evening, although not statistically significant, was marginally more effective than that after a morning dose. This finding of lower systemic bioavailability suggests greater hepatic extraction of the drug following the evening dose. Steady-state AUCs, C_{max} and C_{min} plasma concentrations showed no evidence of pravastatin accumulation following once or twice daily administration of PRAVACHOL (pravastatin sodium) tablets. Approximately 50% of the circulating drug is bound to plasma proteins. Following single dose administration of ^{14}C-pravastatin, the elimination half-life (t½) for total radioactivity (pravastatin plus metabolites) in humans is 77 hours. Pravastatin, like other HMG-CoA reductase inhibitors, has variable bioavailability. The coefficient of variation, based on between-subject variability, was 50% to 60% for AUC.

Approximately 20% of a radiolabeled oral dose is excreted in urine and 70% in the feces. After intravenous administration of radiolabeled pravastatin to normal volunteers, approximately 47% of total body clearance was via renal excretion and 53% by non-renal routes (i.e., biliary excretion and biotransformation). Since there are dual routes of elimination, the potential exists both for compensatory excretion by the alternate route as well as for accumulation of drug and/or metabolites in patients with renal or hepatic insufficiency.

In a study comparing the kinetics of pravastatin in patients with biopsy confirmed cirrhosis (N=7) and normal subjects (N=7), the mean AUC varied 18-fold in cirrhotic patients and 5-fold in healthy subjects. Similarly, the peak pravastatin values varied 47-fold for cirrhotic patients compared to 6-fold for healthy subjects.

Biotransformation pathways elucidated for pravastatin include: (a) isomerization to 6-epi pravastatin and the 3α-hydroxyisomer of pravastatin (SQ 31,906), (b) enzymatic ring hydroxylation to SQ 31,945, (c) ω-1 oxidation of the ester side chain, (d) β-oxidation of the carboxy side chain, (e) ring oxidation followed by aromatization, (f) oxidation of a hydroxyl group to a keto group, and (g) conjugation. The major degradation product is the 3α-hydroxy isomeric metabolite, which has one-tenth to one-fortieth the HMG-CoA reductase inhibitory activity of the parent compound.

Clinical Studies

PRAVACHOL (pravastatin sodium) is highly effective in reducing Total-C, LDL-C and Triglycerides (TG) in patients with heterozygous familial, presumed familial combined and non-familial (non-FH) forms of primary hypercholesterolemia, and mixed dyslipidemia. A therapeutic response is seen within 1 week, and the maximum response usually is achieved within 4 weeks. This response is maintained during extended periods of therapy. In addition, PRAVACHOL is effective in reducing the risk of acute coronary events in hypercholesterolemic patients with and without previous myocardial infarction.

A single daily dose administered in the evening (the recommended dosing) is as effective as the same total daily dose given twice a day. Once daily administration in the evening appears to be marginally more effective than once daily administration in the morning, perhaps because hepatic cholesterol is synthesized mainly at night. In multicenter, double-blind, placebo-controlled studies of patients with primary hypercholesterolemia, trea tment with pravastatin in daily doses ranging from 10 mg to 40 mg consistently and significantly decreased Total-C, LDL-C, TG, and Total-C/HDL-C and LDL-C/HDL-C ratios; modestly decreased VLDL-C and produced variable increases in HDL-C.

Primary Hypercholesterolemia Study
Dose Response of PRAVACHOL*
Once Daily Administration At Bedtime

Dose	Total-C	LDL-C	HDL-C	TG
10 mg	−16%	−22%	+ 7%	−15%
20 mg	−24%	−32%	+ 2%	−11%
40 mg	−25%	−34%	+12%	−24%

*Mean percent change from baseline after 8 weeks

In another clinical trial, patients treated with pravastatin in combination with cholestyramine (70% of patients were taking cholestyramine 20 or 24 g per day) had reductions equal to or greater than 50% in LDL-C. Furthermore, pravastatin attenuated cholestyramine-induced increases in TG levels (which are themselves of uncertain clinical significance).

Prevention of Coronary Heart Disease

In the Pravastatin Primary Prevention Study (West of Scotland Coronary Prevention Study — WOS)[1], the effect of PRAVACHOL on fatal and nonfatal coronary heart disease (CHD) was assessed in 6595 men 45–64 years of age, without a previous MI, and with LDL-C levels between 156–254 mg/dL (4–6.7 mmol/L). In this randomized, double-blind, placebo-controlled study, patients were treated with standard care, including dietary advice, and either PRAVACHOL 40 mg daily (N=3302) or placebo (N=3293) and followed for a median duration of 4.8 years.

PRAVACHOL significantly reduced the rate of first coronary events (either CHD death or nonfatal MI) by 31% [248 events in the placebo group (CHD death=44, nonfatal MI=204) vs 174 events in the PRAVACHOL group (CHD death=31, nonfatal MI=143), p=0.0001 (see figure below)]. The risk reduction with PRAVACHOL was similar and significant throughout the entire range of baseline LDL cholesterol levels. This reduction was also similar and significant across the age range studied with a 40% risk reduction for patients younger than 55 years and a 27% risk reduction for patients 55 years and older. The Pravastatin Primary Prevention Study included only men and therefore it is not clear to what extent these data can be extrapolated to a similar population of female patients.

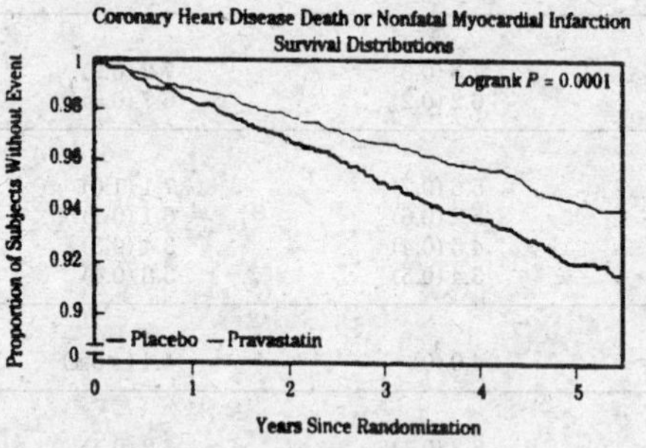
Coronary Heart Disease Death or Nonfatal Myocardial Infarction
Survival Distributions
Logrank P = 0.0001
Proportion of Subjects Without Event
1
0.98
0.96
0.94
0.92
0.9
0
— Placebo — Pravastatin
0
1
2
3
4
5
Years Since Randomization

PRAVACHOL (pravastatin sodium) also significantly decreased the risk for undergoing myocardial revascularization procedures (coronary artery bypass graft surgery or coronary angioplasty) by 37% (80 vs 51 patients, p=0.009) and coronary angiography by 31% (128 vs 90, p=0.007). Cardiovascular deaths were decreased by 32% (73 vs 50, p=0.03) and there was no increase in death from non-cardiovascular causes.

Atherosclerosis and Myocardial Infarction

In the Pravastatin Limitation of Atherosclerosis in the Coronary Arteries (PLAC I)[2] study, the effect of pravastatin therapy on coronary atherosclerosis was assessed by coronary angiography in patients with coronary disease and moderate hypercholesterolemia (baseline LDL-C range = 130-190 mg/dL). In this double-blind, multicenter, controlled clinical trial angiograms were evaluated at baseline and at three years in 264 patients. Although the difference between pravastatin and placebo for the primary endpoint (per-patient change in mean coronary artery diameter) and one of two secondary endpoints (change in percent lumen diameter stenosis) did not reach statistical significance, for the secondary endpoint of change in minimum lumen diameter, statistically significant slowing of disease was seen in the pravastatin treatment group (p=0.02).

In the Regression Growth Evaluation Statin Study (REGRESS)[3], the effect of pravastatin on coronary atherosclerosis was assessed by coronary angiography in 885 patients with angina pectoris, angiographically documented coronary artery disease and hypercholesterolemia (baseline total cholesterol range = 160-310 mg/dL). In this double-blind, multicenter, controlled clinical trial, angiograms were evaluated at baseline and at two years in 653 patients (323 treated with pravastatin). Progression of coronary atherosclerosis was significantly slowed in the pravastatin group as assessed by changes in mean segment diameter (p=0.037) and minimum obstruction diameter (p=0.001).

Analysis of pooled events from PLAC I, the Pravastatin, Lipids and Atherosclerosis in the Carotids Study (PLAC II)[4], REGRESS, and the Kuopio Atherosclerosis Prevention Study (KAPS)[5] (combined N=1891) showed that treatment with pravastatin was associated with a statistically significant reduction in the composite event rate of fatal and nonfatal myocardial infarction (46 events or 6.4% for placebo versus 21 events or 2.4% for pravastatin, p=0.001). The predominant effect of prava statin was to reduce the rate of nonfatal myocardial infarction.

In the Cholesterol and Recurrent Events (CARE)[6] study the effect of PRAVACHOL, 40 mg daily, on coronary heart disease death and nonfatal MI was assessed in 4159 patients (3583 men and 576 women) who had experienced a myocardial infarction in the preceding 3–20 months and who had normal (below the 75th percentile of the general population) plasma total cholesterol levels. Patients in this double-blind, placebo controlled study participated for an average of 4.9 years and had a mean baseline total cholesterol of 209 mg/dL. LDL cholesterol levels in this patient population ranged from 101 mg/dL–180 mg/dL (mean = 139 mg/dL). At baseline, 84% of patients were receiving aspirin and 82% were taking antihypertensive medications. Treatment with PRAVACHOL significantly reduced the rate of first recurrent coronary events (either CHD death or nonfatal MI) by 24% [274 patients with events (13.3%) in the placebo group vs 212 patients with events (10.4%) in the PRAVACHOL group, p=0.003]. The reduction in risk was consistent in both sexes. The risk of undergoing revascularization procedures (coronary artery bypass grafting or percutaneous transluminal coronary angioplasty) was significantly reduced by 27% (p<0.001) in the PRAVACHOL treated patients [391 (19.6%) vs 294 (14.2%) patients]. PRAVACHOL also significantly reduced the risk for stroke or transient ischemic attack (TIA) by 26% [124 (6.3%) vs 93 (4.7%) patients, p=0.029].

INDICATIONS AND USAGE

Therapy with lipid-altering agents should be considered in those individuals at increased risk for atherosclerosis-related clinical events as a function of cholesterol level, the presence or absence of coronary heart disease, and other risk factors. Lipid-altering agents should be used in addition to a diet restricted in saturated fat and cholesterol when the response to diet and other nonpharmacological measures alone has been inadequate (see NCEP Guidelines below).

Primary Prevention of Coronary Events

In hypercholesterolemic patients without clinically evident coronary heart disease, PRAVACHOL is indicated to:

— Reduce the risk of myocardial infarction
— Reduce the risk of undergoing myocardial revascularization procedures
— Reduce the risk of cardiovascular mortality with no increase in death from non-cardiovascular causes

Secondary Prevention of Cardiovascular Events

Atherosclerosis

In hypercholesterolemic patients *with* clinically evident coronary artery disease, including prior MI, PRAVACHOL is indicated to:

— Slow the progression of coronary atherosclerosis
— Reduce the risk of acute coronary events

Myocardial Infarction

In patients with previous myocardial infarction, and normal (below the 75th percentile of the general population) cholesterol levels, PRAVACHOL is indicated to:

— Reduce the risk of recurrent myocardial infarction
— Reduce the risk of undergoing myocardial revascularization procedures
— Reduce the risk of stroke or transient ischemic attack (TIA)

Hypercholesterolemia and Mixed Dyslipidemia

PRAVACHOL is indicated as an adjunct to diet to reduce elevated Total-C, LDL-C, and TG levels in patients with primary hypercholesterolemia and mixed dyslipidemia (Frederickson Type IIa and IIb)[7].

Prior to initiating therapy with pravastatin, secondary causes for hypercholesterolemia (e.g., poorly controlled diabetes mellitus, hypothyroidism, nephrotic syndrome, dysproteinemias, obstructive liver disease, other drug therapy, alcoholism) should be excluded, and a lipid profile performed to measure Total-C, HDL-C, and TG. For patients with triglycerides (TG) <400 mg/dL (<4.5 mmol/L), LDL-C can be estimated using the following equation:

$$LDL\text{-}C = Total\ \text{-}C - HDL\text{-}C - 1/5\ TG$$

For TG levels >400 mg/dL (>4.5 mmol/L), this equation is less accurate and LDL-C concentrations should be determined by ultracentrifugation. In many hypertriglyceridemic patients, LDL-C may be low or normal despite elevated Total-C. In such cases, HMG-CoA reductase inhibitors are not indicated.

Lipid determinations should be performed at intervals of no less than four weeks and dosage adjusted according to the patient's response to therapy.

The National Cholesterol Education Program's Treatment Guidelines are summarized below:

		LDL Cholesterol mg/dL (mmol/L)	
Definite Atherosclerotic Disease*	Two or more Other Risk Factors**	Initiation Level	Goal
NO	NO	≥190 (>4.9)	<160 (<4.1)
NO	YES	≥160 (≥4.1)	<130 (<3.4)
YES	YES or NO	≥130 (≥3.4)	≤100 (≤2.6)

* Coronary heart disease or peripheral vascular disease (including symptomatic carotid artery disease).

**Other risk factors for coronary heart disease (CHD) include: age (males: ≥45 years; females: ≥55 years or premature menopause without estrogen replacement therapy); family history of premature CHD; current cigarette smoking; hypertension; confirmed HDL-C <35 mg/dL (<0.91 mmol/L); and diabetes mellitus. Subtract one risk factor if HDL-C is ≥60 mg/dL (≥1.6 mmol/L).

Since the goal of treatment is to lower LDL-C, the NCEP recommends that LDL-C levels be used to initiate and assess treatment response. Only if LDL-C levels are not available, should the Total-C be used to monitor therapy.

As with other lipid-lowering therapy, PRAVACHOL (pravastatin sodium) is not indicated when hypercholesterolemia is due to hyperalphalipoproteinemia (elevated HDL-C). The efficacy of pravastatin has not been evaluated in patients with combined elevated Total-C and hypertriglyceridemia [>500 mg/dL (>5.7 mmol/L)] or in patients with elevated intermediate density lipoproteins as their primary lipid abnormality.

CONTRAINDICATIONS

Hypersensitivity to any component of this medication.

Active liver disease or unexplained, persistent elevations in liver function tests (see **WARNINGS**).

Pregnancy and lactation. Atherosclerosis is a chronic process and discontinuation of lipid-lowering drugs during pregnancy should have little impact on the outcome of long-term therapy of primary hypercholesterolemia. Cholesterol and other products of cholesterol biosynthesis are essential components for fetal development (including synthesis of steroids and cell membranes). Since HMG-CoA reductase inhibitors decrease cholesterol synthesis and possibly the synthesis of other biologically active substances derived from cholesterol, they may cause fetal harm when administered to pregnant women. Therefore, HMG-CoA reductase inhibitors are contraindicated during pregnancy and in nursing mothers. **Pravastatin should be administered to women of childbearing age only when such patients are highly unlikely to conceive and have been informed of the potential hazards.** If the patient becomes pregnant while taking this class of drug, therapy should be discontinued and the patient apprised of the potential hazard to the fetus.

WARNINGS

Liver Enzymes

HMG-CoA reductase inhibitors, like some other lipid-lowering therapies, have been associated with biochemical abnormalities of liver function. Increases of serum transaminase (ALT, AST) values to more than 3 times the upper limit of normal occurring on 2 or more (not necessarily sequential) occasions have been reported in 1.3% of patients treated with pravastatin in the US over an average period of 18 months. These abnormalities were not associated with cholestasis and did not appear to be related to treatment duration. In those patients in whom these abnormalities were believed to be related to pravastatin and who were discontinued from therapy, the transaminase levels usually fell slowly to pretreatment levels. These biochemical findings are usually asymptomatic although worldwide experience indicates that anorexia, weakness, and/or abdominal pain may also be present in rare patients.

In the largest long-term placebo-controlled clinical trial with pravastatin (Pravastatin Primary Prevention Study; see **Clinical Pharmacology**), the overall incidence of AST and/or ALT elevations to greater than three times the upper limit of normal was 1.05% in the pravastatin group as compared to 0.75% in the placebo group. One (0.03%) pravasta-

tin-treated patient and 2 (0.06%) placebo-treated patients were discontinued because of transaminase elevations. Of the patients with normal liver function at week 12, three of 2875 treated with pravastatin (0.10%) and one of the 2919 placebo patients (0.03%) had elevations of AST greater than three times the upper limit of normal on two consecutive measurements and/or discontinued due to elevations in transaminase levels during the 4.8 years (median treatment) of the study.

It is recommended that liver function tests be performed prior to and at 12 weeks following initiation of therapy or the elevation of dose. Patients who develop increased transaminase levels or signs and symptoms of liver disease should be monitored with a second liver function evaluation to confirm the finding and be followed thereafter with frequent liver function tests until the abnormality(ies) return to normal. Should an increase in AST or ALT of three times the upper limit of normal or greater persist, withdrawal of pravastatin therapy is recommended.

Active liver disease or unexplained transaminase elevations are contraindications to the use of pravastatin (see **CONTRAINDICATIONS**). Caution should be exercised when pravastatin is administered to patients with a history of liver disease or heavy alcohol ingestion (see **CLINICAL PHARMACOLOGY: Pharmacokinetics/Metabolism**). Such patients should be closely monitored, started at the lower end of the recommended dosing range, and titrated to the desired therapeutic effect.

Skeletal Muscle

Rare cases of rhabdomyolysis with acute renal failure secondary to myoglobinuria have been reported with pravastatin and other drugs in this class. Uncomplicated myalgia has also been reported in pravastatin-treated patients (see **ADVERSE REACTIONS**). Myopathy, defined as muscle aching or muscle weakness in conjunction with increases in creatine phosphokinase (CPK) values to greater than 10 times the upper normal limit, was rare (<0.1%) in pravastatin clinical trials. Myopathy should be considered in any patient with diffuse myalgias, muscle tenderness or weakness, and/or marked elevation of CPK. Patients should be advised to report promptly unexplained muscle pain, tenderness or weakness, particularly if accompanied by malaise or fever. **Pravastatin therapy should be discontinued if markedly elevated CPK levels occur or myopathy is diagnosed or suspected. Pravastatin therapy should also be temporarily withheld in any patient experiencing an acute or serious condition predisposing to the development of renal failure secondary to rhabdomyolysis, e.g., sepsis; hypotension; major surgery; trauma; severe metabolic, endocrine, or electrolyte disorders; or uncontrolled epilepsy.**

The risk of myopathy during treatment with another HMG-CoA reductase inhibitor is increased with concurrent therapy with either erythromycin, cyclosporine, niacin, or fibrates. However, neither myopathy nor significant increases in CPK levels have been observed in three reports involving a total of 100 post-transplant patients (24 renal and 76 cardiac) treated for up to two years concurrently with pravastatin 10–40 mg and cyclosporine. Some of these patients also received other concomitant immunosuppressive therapies. Further, in clinical trials involving small numbers of patients who were treated concurrently with pravastatin and niacin, there were no reports of myopathy. Also, myopathy was not reported in a trial of combination pravastatin (40 mg/day) and gemfibrozil (1200 mg/day), although 4 of 75 patients on the combination showed marked CPK elevations versus one of 73 patients receiving placebo. There was a trend toward more frequent CPK elevations and patient withdrawals due to musculoskeletal symptoms in the group receiving combined treatment as compared with the groups receiving placebo, gemfibrozil, or pravastatin monotherapy (see **PRECAUTIONS: Drug Interactions**). The use of fibrates alone may occasionally be associated with myopathy. The combined use of pravastatin and fibrates should be avoided unless the benefit of further alterations in lipid levels is likely to outweigh the increased risk of this drug combination.

PRECAUTIONS

General

Pravastatin (pravastatin sodium) may elevate creatine phosphokinase and transaminase levels (see **ADVERSE REACTIONS**). This should be considered in the differential diagnosis of chest pain in a patient on therapy with pravastatin.

Homozygous Familial Hypercholesterolemia. Pravastatin has not been evaluated in patients with rare homozygous familial hypercholesterolemia. In this group of patients, it has been reported that HMG-CoA reductase inhibitors are less effective because the patients lack functional LDL receptors.

Renal Insufficiency. A single 20 mg oral dose of pravastatin was administered to 24 patients with varying degrees of renal impairment (as determined by creatinine clearance). No effect was observed on the pharmacokinetics of pravastatin or its 3α-hydroxy isomeric metabolite (SQ 31,906). A small increase was seen in mean AUC values and half-life (t½) for

the inactive enzymatic ring hydroxylation metabolite (SQ 31,945). Given this small sample size, the dosage administered, and the degree of individual variability, patients with renal impairment who are receiving pravastatin should be closely monitored.

Information for Patients

Patients should be advised to report promptly unexplained muscle pain, tenderness or weakness, particularly if accompanied by malaise or fever.

Drug Interactions

Immunosuppressive Drugs, Gemfibrozil, Niacin (Nicotinic Acid), Erythromycin: See **WARNINGS: Skeletal Muscle.**

Cytochrome P450 3A4 Inhibitors: In vitro and in vivo data indicate that pravastatin is not metabolized by cytochrome P450 3A4 to a clinically significant extent. This has been shown in studies with known cytochrome P450 3A4 inhibitors (see diltiazem and itraconazole below). Other examples of cytochrome P450 3A4 inhibitors include ketoconazole, mibefradil, and erythromycin. Diltiazem—Steady-state levels of diltiazem (a known, weak inhibitor of P450 3A4) had no effect on the pharmacokinetics of pravastatin. In this study, the AUC and C_{max} of another HMG-CoA reductase inhibitor which is known to be metabolized by cytochrome P450 3A4 increased by factors of 3.6 and 4.3, respectively. Itraconazole—The mean AUC and C_{max} for pravastatin were increased by factors of 1.7 and 2.5, respectively, when given with itraconazole (a potent P450 3A4 inhibitor which also inhibits p-glycoprotein transport) as compared to placebo. The mean t½ was not affected by itraconazole, suggesting that the relatively small increases in C_{max} and AUC were due solely to increased bioavailability rather than a decrease in clearance, consistent with inhibition of p-glycoprotein transport by itraconazole. This drug transport system is thought to affect bioavailability and excretion of HMG-CoA reductase inhibitors, including pravastatin. The AUC and C_{max} of another HMG-CoA reductase inhibitor which is known to be metabolized by cytochrome P450 3A4 increased by factors of 19 and 17, respectively, when given with itraconazole.

Antipyrine: Since concomitant administration of pravastatin had no effect on the clearance of antipyrine, interactions with other drugs metabolized via the same hepatic cytochrome isozymes are not expected.

Cholestyramine/Colestipol: Concomitant administration resulted in an approximately 40 to 50% decrease in the mean AUC of pravastatin. However, when pravastatin was administered 1 hour before or 4 hours after cholestyramine or 1 hour before colestipol and a standard meal, there was no clinically significant decrease in bioavailability or therapeutic effect. (See **DOSAGE AND ADMINISTRATION: Concomitant Therapy.**)

Warfarin: Pravastatin had no clinically significant effect on prothrombin time when administered in a study to normal elderly subjects who were stabilized on warfarin.

Cimetidine: The $AUC_{0-12\ hr}$ for pravastatin when given with cimetidine was not significantly different from the AUC for pravastatin when given alone. A significant difference was observed between the AUC's for pravastatin when given with cimetidine compared to when administered with antacid.

Digoxin: In a crossover trial involving 18 healthy male subjects given pravastatin and digoxin concurrently for 9 days, the bioavailability parameters of digoxin were not affected. The AUC of pravastatin tended to increase, but the overall bioavailability of pravastatin plus its metabolites SQ 31,906 and SQ 31,945 was not altered.

Cyclosporine: Some investigators have measured cyclosporine levels in patients on pravastatin, and to date, these results indicate no clinically meaningful elevations in cyclosporine levels. In one single-dose study, pravastatin levels were found to be increased in cardiac transplant patients receiving cyclosporine.

Gemfibrozil: In a crossover study in 20 healthy male volunteers given concomitant single doses of pravastatin and gemfibrozil, there was a significant decrease in urinary excretion and protein binding of pravastatin. In addition, there was a significant increase in AUC, C_{max}, and T_{max} for the pravastatin metabolite SQ 31,906. Combination therapy with pravastatin and gemfibrozil is generally not recommended.

In interaction studies with *aspirin, antacids* (1 hour prior to PRAVACHOL), *cimetidine, nicotinic acid,* or *probucol,* no statistically significant differences in bioavailability were seen when PRAVACHOL (pravastatin sodium) was administered.

Endocrine Function

HMG-CoA reductase inhibitors interfere with cholesterol synthesis and lower circulating cholesterol levels and, as such, might theoretically blunt adrenal or gonadal steroid hormone production. Results of clinical trials with pravastatin in males and post-menopausal females were inconsistent with regard to possible effects of the drug on basal steroid hormone levels. In a study of 21 males, the mean tes-

Continued on next page

Pravachol—Cont.

tosterone response to human chorionic gonadotropin was significantly reduced ($p<0.004$) after 16 weeks of treatment with 40 mg of pravastatin. However, the percentage of patients showing a ≥50% rise in plasma testosterone after human chorionic gonadotropin stimulation did not change significantly after therapy in these patients. The effects of HMG-CoA reductase inhibitors on spermatogenesis and fertility have not been studied in adequate numbers of patients. The effects, if any, of pravastatin on the pituitary-gonadal axis in pre-menopausal females are unknown. Patients treated with pravastatin who display clinical evidence of endocrine dysfunction should be evaluated appropriately. Caution should also be exercised if an HMG-CoA reductase inhibitor or other agent used to lower cholesterol levels is administered to patients also receiving other drugs (e.g., ketoconazole, spironolactone, cimetidine) that may diminish the levels or activity of steroid hormones.

CNS Toxicity

CNS vascular lesions, characterized by perivascular hemorrhage and edema and mononuclear cell infiltration of perivascular spaces, were seen in dogs treated with pravastatin at a dose of 25 mg/kg/day, a dose that produced a plasma drug level about 50 times higher than the mean drug level in humans taking 40 mg/day. Similar CNS vascular lesions have been observed with several other drugs in this class.

A chemically similar drug in this class produced optic nerve degeneration (Wallerian degeneration of retinogeniculate fibers) in clinically normal dogs in a dose-dependent fashion starting at 60 mg/kg/day, a dose that produced mean plasma drug levels about 30 times higher than the mean drug level in humans taking the highest recommended dose (as measured by total enzyme inhibitory activity). This same drug also produced vestibulocochlear Wallerian-like degeneration and retinal ganglion cell chromatolysis in dogs treated for 14 weeks at 180 mg/kg/day, a dose which resulted in a mean plasma drug level similar to that seen with the 60 mg/kg/day dose.

Carcinogenesis, Mutagenesis, Impairment of Fertility

In a 2-year study in rats fed pravastatin at doses of 10, 30, or 100 mg/kg body weight, there was an increased incidence of hepatocellular carcinomas in males at the highest dose ($p<0.01$). Although rats were given up to 125 times the human dose (HD) on a mg/kg body weight basis, serum drug levels were only 6 to 10 times higher than those measured in humans given 40 mg pravastatin as measured by AUC.

The oral administration of 10, 30, or 100 mg/kg (producing plasma drug levels approximately 0.5 to 5.0 times the human drug levels at 40 mg) of pravastatin to mice for 22 months resulted in a statistically significant increase in the incidence of malignant lymphomas in treated females when all treatment groups were pooled and compared to controls ($p<0.05$). The incidence was not dose-related and male mice were not affected.

A chemically similar drug in this class was administered to mice for 72 weeks at 25, 100, and 400 mg/kg body weight, which resulted in mean serum drug levels approximately 3, 15, and 33 times higher than the mean human serum drug concentration (as total inhibitory activity) after a 40 mg oral dose. Liver carcinomas were significantly increased in high-dose females and mid- and high-dose males, with a maximum incidence of 90 percent in males. The incidence of adenomas of the liver was significantly increased in mid- and high-dose females. Drug treatment also significantly increased the incidence of lung adenomas in mid- and high-dose males and females. Adenomas of the eye Harderian gland (a gland of the eye of rodents) were significantly higher in high-dose mice than in controls.

No evidence of mutagenicity was observed *in vitro*, with or without rat-liver metabolic activation, in the following studies: microbial mutagen tests, using mutant strains of *Salmonella typhimurium* or *Escherichia coli*; a forward mutation assay in L5178Y TK +/- mouse lymphoma cells; a chromosomal aberration test in hamster cells; and a gene conversion assay using *Saccharomyces cerevisiae*. In addition, there was no evidence of mutagenicity in either a dominant lethal test in mice or a micronucleus test in mice.

In a study in rats, with daily doses up to 500 mg/kg, pravastatin did not produce any adverse effects on fertility or general reproductive performance. However, in a study with another HMG-CoA reductase inhibitor, there was decreased fertility in male rats treated for 34 weeks at 25 mg/kg body weight, although this effect was not observed in a subsequent fertility study when this same dose was administered for 11 weeks (the entire cycle of spermatogenesis, including epididymal maturation). In rats treated with this same reductase inhibitor at 180 mg/kg/day, seminiferous tubule degeneration (necrosis and loss of spermatogenic epithelium) was observed. Although not seen with pravastatin, two similar drugs in this class caused drug-related testicular atrophy, decreased spermatogenesis, spermatocytic degeneration, and giant cell formation in dogs. The clinical significance of these findings is unclear.

Pregnancy

Pregnancy Category X.

See **CONTRAINDICATIONS.**

Safety in pregnant women has not been established. Pravastatin was not teratogenic in rats at doses up to 1000 mg/kg daily or in rabbits at doses of up to 50 mg/kg daily. These doses resulted in 20x (rabbit) or 240x (rat) the human exposure based on surface area (mg/meter^2). However, in studies with another HMG-CoA reductase inhibitor, skeletal malformations were observed in rats and mice. There has been one report of severe congenital bony deformity, tracheo-esophageal fistula, and anal atresia (Vater association) in a baby born to a woman who took another HMG-CoA reductase inhibitor with dextroamphetamine sulfate during the first trimester of pregnancy. PRAVACHOL (pravastatin sodium) should be administered to women of child-bearing potential only when such patients are highly unlikely to conceive and have been informed of the potential hazards. If the woman becomes pregnant while taking PRAVACHOL (pravastatin sodium), it should be discontinued and the patient advised again as to the potential hazards to the fetus.

Nursing Mothers

A small amount of pravastatin is excreted in human breast milk. Because of the potential for serious adverse reactions in nursing infants, women taking PRAVACHOL should not nurse (see **CONTRAINDICATIONS**).

Pediatric Use

Safety and effectiveness in individuals less than 18 years old have not been established. Hence, treatment in patients less than 18 years old is not recommended at this time.

ADVERSE REACTIONS

Pravastatin is generally well tolerated; adverse reactions have usually been mild and transient. In 4-month long placebo-controlled trials, 1.7% of pravastatin-treated patients and 1.2% of placebo-treated patients were discontinued from treatment because of adverse experiences attributed to study drug therapy; this difference was not statistically significant. In long-term studies, the most common reasons for discontinuation were asymptomatic serum transaminase increases and mild, non-specific gastrointestinal complaints. During clinical trials the overall incidence of adverse events in the elderly was not different from the incidence observed in younger patients.

Adverse Clinical Events

All adverse clinical events (regardless of attribution) reported in more than 2% of pravastatin-treated patients in the placebo-controlled trials are identified in the table below; also shown are the percentages of patients in whom these medical events were believed to be related or possibly related to the drug:

[See table below]

Body System/Event	All Events: Pravastatin (N = 900) %	All Events: Placebo (N = 411) %	Events Attributed to Study Drug: Pravastatin (N = 900) %	Events Attributed to Study Drug: Placebo (N = 411) %
Cardiovascular				
Cardiac Chest Pain	4.0	3.4	0.1	0.0
Dermatologic Rash	4.0*	1.1	1.3	0.9
Gastrointestinal				
Nausea/Vomiting	7.3	7.1	2.9	3.4
Diarrhea	6.2	5.6	2.0	1.9
Abdominal Pain	5.4	6.9	2.0	3.9
Constipation	4.0	7.1	2.4	5.1
Flatulence	3.3	3.6	2.7	3.4
Heartburn	2.9	1.9	2.0	0.7
General				
Fatigue	3.8	3.4	1.9	1.0
Chest Pain	3.7	1.9	0.3	0.2
Influenza	2.4*	0.7	0.0	0.0
Musculoskeletal				
Localized Pain	10.0	9.0	1.4	1.5
Myalgia	2.7	1.0	0.6	0.0
Nervous System				
Headache	6.2	3.9	1.7*	0.2
Dizziness	3.3	3.2	1.0	0.5
Renal/Genitourinary				
Urinary Abnormality	2.4	2.9	0.7	1.2
Respiratory				
Common Cold	7.0	6.3	0.0	0.0
Rhinitis	4.0	4.1	0.1	0.0
Cough	2.6	1.7	0.1	0.0

*Statistically significantly different from placebo.

In the Pravastatin Primary Prevention Study (West of Scotland Coronary Prevention Study) involving 6595 patients treated with PRAVACHOL (N=3302) or placebo (N=3293) for a median of 4.8 years and in the Cholesterol and Recurrent Events (CARE) study, involving 4159 men and women treated with PRAVACHOL (N=2081) or placebo (N=2078) for an average of 4.9 years the adverse event profile in the PRAVACHOL (pravastatin sodium) group was comparable to that of placebo for the duration of the studies.

The following effects have been reported with drugs in this class; not all the effects listed below have necessarily been associated with pravastatin therapy:

Skeletal: myopathy, rhabdomyolysis, arthralgia.

Neurological: dysfunction of certain cranial nerves (including alteration of taste, impairment of extra-ocular movement, facial paresis), tremor, vertigo, memory loss, paresthesia, peripheral neuropathy, peripheral nerve palsy, anxiety, insomnia, depression.

Hypersensitivity Reactions: An apparent hypersensitivity syndrome has been reported rarely which has included one or more of the following features: anaphylaxis, angioedema, lupus erythematous-like syndrome, polymyalgia rheumatica, dermatomyositis, vasculitis, purpura, thrombocytopenia, leukopenia, hemolytic anemia, positive ANA, ESR increase, eosinophilia, arthritis, arthralgia, urticaria, asthenia, photosensitivity, fever, chills, flushing, malaise, dyspnea, toxic epidermal necrolysis, erythema multiforme, including Stevens-Johnson syndrome.

Gastrointestinal: pancreatitis, hepatitis, including chronic active hepatitis, cholestatic jaundice, fatty change in liver, and rarely, cirrhosis, fulminant hepatic necrosis, and hepatoma; anorexia, vomiting.

Skin: alopecia, pruritus. A variety of skin changes (e.g., nodules, discoloration, dryness of skin/mucous membranes, changes to hair/nails) have been reported.

Reproductive: gynecomastia, loss of libido, erectile dysfunction.

Eye: progression of cataracts (lens opacities), ophthalmoplegia.

Laboratory Abnormalities: elevated transaminases, alkaline phosphatase, and bilirubin; thyroid function abnormalities.

Laboratory Test Abnormalities

Increases in serum transaminase (ALT, AST) values and CPK have been observed (see **WARNINGS**).

Transient, asymptomatic eosinophilia has been reported. Eosinophil counts usually returned to normal despite continued therapy. Anemia, thrombocytopenia, and leukopenia have been reported with HMG-CoA reductase inhibitors.

Concomitant Therapy

Pravastatin has been administered concurrently with cholestyramine, colestipol, nicotinic acid, probucol and gemfibrozil. Preliminary data suggest that the addition of either probucol or gemfibrozil to therapy with lovastatin or pravastatin is **not** associated with greater reduction in LDL-cholesterol than that achieved with lovastatin or pravastatin alone. No adverse reactions unique to the combination or in addition to those previously reported for each drug alone have been reported. Myopathy and rhabdomyolysis (with or without acute renal failure) have been reported when another HMG-CoA reductase inhibitor was used in combination with immunosuppressive drugs, gemfibrozil, erythromycin, or lipid-lowering doses of nicotinic acid. Concomitant therapy with HMG-CoA reductase inhibitors and these agents is generally not recommended. (See **WARNINGS: Skeletal Muscle** and **PRECAUTIONS: Drug Interactions.**)

OVERDOSAGE

To date, there are two reported cases of overdosage with pravastatin, both of which were asymptomatic and not associated with clinical laboratory abnormalities. If an overdose occurs, it should be treated symptomatically and supportive measures should be instituted as required.

DOSAGE AND ADMINISTRATION

The patient should be placed on a standard cholesterol-lowering diet before receiving PRAVACHOL (pravastatin sodium) and should continue on this diet during treatment with PRAVACHOL (see NCEP Treatment Guidelines for details on dietary therapy).

The recommended starting dose is 10 or 20 mg once daily at bedtime. In primary hypercholesterolemic patients with a history of significant renal or hepatic dysfunction, and in the elderly, a starting dose of 10 mg daily at bedtime is recommended. PRAVACHOL (pravastatin sodium) may be taken without regard to meals.

Since the maximal effect of a given dose is seen within 4 weeks, periodic lipid determinations should be performed at this time and dosage adjusted according to the patient's response to therapy and established treatment guidelines. The recommended dosage range is generally 10 to 40 mg administered once a day at bedtime. In the elderly, maximum reductions in LDL-cholesterol may be achieved with daily doses of 20 mg or less.

In patients taking immunosuppressive drugs such as cyclosporine (see **WARNINGS**: **Skeletal Muscle**) concomitantly with pravastatin, therapy should begin with 10 mg of pravastatin once-a-day at bedtime and titration to higher doses should be done with caution. Most patients treated with this combination received a maximum pravastatin dose of 20 mg/day.

Concomitant Therapy

The lipid-lowering effects of PRAVACHOL on total and LDL cholesterol are enhanced when combined with a bile-acid-binding resin. When administering a bile-acid-binding resin (e.g., cholestyramine, colestipol) and pravastatin, PRAVACHOL should be given either 1 hour or more before or at least 4 hours following the resin. See also **ADVERSE REACTIONS**: **Concomitant Therapy**.

HOW SUPPLIED

PRAVACHOL® (pravastatin sodium) Tablets are supplied as:

10 mg tablets: Pink to peach, rounded, rectangular-shaped, biconvex with a P embossed on one side and PRAVACHOL 10 engraved on the opposite side. They are supplied in bottles of 90 (NDC 0003-5154-05). Bottles contain a desiccant canister.

20 mg tablets: Yellow, rounded, rectangular-shaped, biconvex with a P embossed on one side and PRAVACHOL 20 engraved on the opposite side. They are supplied in bottles of 90 (NDC 0003-5178-05) and bottles of 1000 (NDC 0003-5178-75). Bottles contain a desiccant canister.

40 mg tablets: Green, rounded, rectangular-shaped, biconvex with a P embossed on one side and PRAVACHOL 40 engraved on the opposite side. They are supplied in bottles of 90 (NDC 0003-5194-10). Bottles contain a desiccant canister.

Unimatic® unit-dose packs containing 100 tablets are also available for each potency: **10 mg** (NDC 0003-5154-06), **20 mg** (NDC 0003-5178-06) and **40 mg** (NDC 0003-5194-11).

Storage

Do not store above 86° F (30°C). Keep tightly closed (protect from moisture). Protect from light.

REFERENCES

1. Shepherd J, et al. Prevention of coronary heart disease with pravastatin in men with hypercholesterolemia. *N Engl J Med* 1995;333:1301–7.
2. Pitt, B, et al. Pravastatin Limitation of Atherosclerosis in the Coronary Arteries (PLAC I): Reduction in Atherosclerosis Progression and Clinical Events. *J Am Coll Cardiol* 1995;26:1133–9.
3. Jukema JW, et al. Effects of Lipid Lowering by Pravastatin on Progression and Regression of Coronary Artery Disease in Symptomatic Man With Normal to Moderately Elevated Serum Cholesterol Levels. The Regression Growth Evaluation Statin Study (REGRESS). *Circulation* 1995;91:2528–2540.
4. Crouse JR, et al. Pravastatin, lipids, and atherosclerosis in the carotid arteries: design features of a clinical trial with carotid atherosclerosis outcome, *Controlled Clinical Trials* 13:495, 1992.
5. Salonen R, et al. Kuopio Atherosclerosis Prevention Study (KAPS). A population-based primary preventive trial of the effect of LDL lowering on atherosclerotic progression in carotid and femoral arteries. Research Institute of Public Health, University of Kuopio, Finland. *Circulation* 92:1758, 1995.
6. Sacks FM, et al. The effect of pravastatin on coronary events after myocardial infarction in patients with average cholesterol levels. *N Engl J Med.* 1996;335:1001-9.
7. Frederickson classification: Type IIa-elevation of LDL; Type IIb-elevation of LDL and VLDL. Type III (familial dysbetalipoproteinemia)-elevation of IDL. Frederickson, DS, Fat transport in lipoproteins-an integrated approach to mechanism and disorders, *N Engl J Med* 276:34, 1967.

5154DIM-09

51-000876-07 Revised May 1998

D3-B001-5-98

Bristol-Myers Squibb Company
Princeton, NJ 08543 U.S.A.

Shown in Product Identification Guide, page 307

QUESTRAN® POWDER ℞

[*quĕs'trăn*]

QUESTRAN® LIGHT

(Cholestyramine for Oral Suspension, USP)

CAUTION: FEDERAL LAW PROHIBITS DISPENSING WITHOUT PRESCRIPTION.

DESCRIPTION

QUESTRAN® (Cholestyramine for Oral Suspension, USP), the chloride salt of a basic anion exchange resin, a cholesterol lowering agent, is intended for oral administration. Cholestyramine resin is quite hydrophilic, but insoluble in water. The cholestyramine resin in QUESTRAN is not absorbed from the digestive tract. Nine grams of QUESTRAN POWDER contain 4 grams of anhydrous cholestyramine resin. Five grams of QUESTRAN LIGHT contain 4 grams of anhydrous cholestyramine resin. It is represented by the following structural formula:

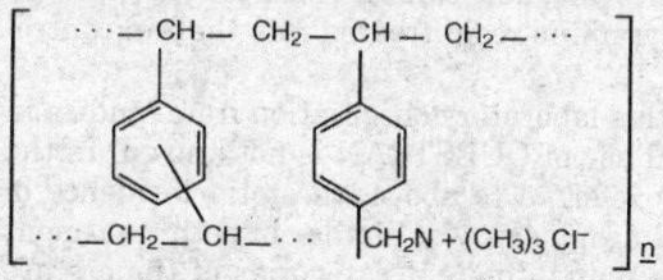

Representation of structure of main polymeric groups

QUESTRAN POWDER contains the following inactive ingredients: acacia, citric acid, D&C Yellow No. 10, FD&C Yellow No. 6, flavor (natural and artificial), polysorbate 80, propylene glycol alginate, and sucrose (421 mg/g powder). QUESTRAN LIGHT contains the following inactive ingredients: aspartame, citric acid, D&C Yellow No. 10, FD&C Red No. 40, flavor (natural and artificial), propylene glycol alginate, colloidal silicon dioxide and sucrose (144 mg/g powder), and xanthan gum.

ACTIONS/CLINICAL PHARMACOLOGY

Cholesterol is probably the sole precursor of bile acids. During normal digestion, bile acids are secreted into the intestines. A major portion of the bile acids is absorbed from the intestinal tract and returned to the liver via the enterohepatic circulation. Only very small amounts of bile acids are found in normal serum.

QUESTRAN resin adsorbs and combines with the bile acids in the intestine to form an insoluble complex which is excreted in the feces. This results in a partial removal of bile acids from the enterohepatic circulation by preventing their absorption.

The increased fecal loss of bile acids due to QUESTRAN administration leads to an increased oxidation of cholesterol to bile acids, a decrease in beta lipoprotein or low density lipoprotein plasma levels and a decrease in serum cholesterol levels. Although in man, QUESTRAN produces an increase in hepatic synthesis of cholesterol, plasma cholesterol levels fall.

In patients with partial biliary obstruction, the reduction of serum bile acid levels by QUESTRAN reduces excess bile acids deposited in the dermal tissue with resultant decrease in pruritus.

Clinical Studies

In a large, placebo-controlled, multi-clinic study, LRC-CPPT[1], hypercholesterolemic subjects treated with QUESTRAN had mean reductions in total and low-density lipoprotein cholesterol (LDL-C) which exceeded those for diet and placebo treatment by 7.2% and 10.4%, respectively. Over the seven-year study period the QUESTRAN group experienced a 19% reduction (relative to the incidence in the placebo group) in the combined rate of coronary heart disease death plus non-fatal myocardial infarction (cumulative incidences of 7% QUESTRAN and 8.6% placebo). The subjects included in the study were men aged 35–59 with serum cholesterol levels above 265 mg/dL and no previous history of heart disease. It is not clear to what extent these findings can be extrapolated to females and other segments of the hypercholesterolemic population. (See also **PRECAUTIONS**: **Carcinogenesis, Mutagenesis, and Impairment of Fertility**.)

Two controlled clinical trials have examined the effects of QUESTRAN monotherapy upon coronary atherosclerotic lesions using coronary arteriography. In the NHLBI Type II Coronary Intervention Trial[2], 116 patients (80% male) with coronary artery disease (CAD) documented by arteriography were randomized to QUESTRAN or placebo for five years of treatment. Final study arteriography revealed progression of coronary artery disease in 49% of placebo patients compared to 32% of the QUESTRAN group ($p<0.05$). In the St. Thomas Atherosclerosis Regression Study (STARS)[3], 90 hypercholesterolemic men with CAD were randomized to three blinded treatments: usual care, lipid-lowering diet, and lipid-lowering diet plus QUESTRAN. After 36 months, follow-up coronary arteriography revealed progression of disease in 46% of usual care patients, 15% of patients on lipid-lowering diet and 12% of those receiving diet plus QUESTRAN ($p<0.02$). The mean absolute width of coronary segments decreased in the usual care group, increased slightly (0.003mm) in the diet group and increased by 0.103mm in the diet plus QUESTRAN group ($p<0.05$). Thus in these randomized controlled clinical trials using coronary arteriography, QUESTRAN monotherapy has been demonstrated to slow progression [2,3] and promote regression[3] of atherosclerotic lesions in the coronary arteries of patients with coronary artery disease.

The effect of intensive lipid-lowering therapy on coronary atherosclerosis has been assessed by arteriography in hyperlipidemic patients. In these randomized, controlled clinical trials, patients were treated for two to four years by either conventional measures (diet, placebo, or in some cases low dose resin), or intensive combination therapy using diet plus colestipol (an anion exchange resin with a mechanism of action and an effect on serum lipids similar to that of QUESTRAN and QUESTRAN LIGHT) plus either nicotinic acid or lovastatin. When compared to conventional measures, intensive lipid-lowering combination therapy significantly reduced the frequency of progression and increased the frequency of regression of coronary atherosclerotic lesions in patients with or at risk for coronary artery disease.

INDICATIONS AND USAGE

1) QUESTRAN is indicated as adjunctive therapy to diet for the reduction of elevated serum cholesterol in patients with primary hypercholesterolemia (elevated low density lipoprotein [LDL] cholesterol) who do not respond adequately to diet. QUESTRAN may be useful to lower LDL cholesterol in patients who also have hypertriglyceridemia, but it is not indicated where hypertriglyceridemia is the abnormality of most concern.

Therapy with lipid-altering agents should be a component of multiple risk factor intervention in those individuals at significantly increased risk for atherosclerotic vascular disease due to hypercholesterolemia. Treatment should begin and continue with dietary therapy specific for the type of hyperlipoproteinemia determined prior to initiation of drug therapy. Excess body weight may be an important factor and caloric restriction for weight normalization should be addressed prior to drug therapy in the overweight.

Prior to initiating therapy with QUESTRAN (Cholestyramine for Oral Suspension, USP), secondary causes of hypercholesterolemia (e.g., poorly controlled diabetes mellitus, hypothyroidism, nephrotic syndrome, dysproteinemias, obstructive liver disease, other drug therapy, alcoholism), should be excluded, and a lipid profile performed to assess Total cholesterol, HDL-C, and triglycerides (TG). For individuals with TG less than 400 mg/dL (<4.5 mmol/L), LDL-C can be estimated using the following equation:-

$$\text{LDL-C} = \text{Total cholesterol} - [(\text{TG}/5) + \text{HDL-C}]$$

For TG levels >400 mg/dL, this equation is less accurate and LDL-C concentrations should be determined by ultracentrifugation. In hypertriglyceridemic patients, LDL-C may be low or normal despite elevated Total-C. In such cases QUESTRAN may not be indicated.

Serum cholesterol and triglyceride levels should be determined periodically based on NCEP guidelines to confirm initial and adequate long-term response. A favorable trend in cholesterol reduction should occur during the first month of QUESTRAN therapy. The therapy should be continued to sustain cholesterol reduction. If adequate cholesterol reduction is not attained, increasing the dosage of QUESTRAN or adding other lipid-lowering agents in combination with QUESTRAN should be considered.

Since the goal of treatment is to lower LDL-C, the NCEP[4] recommends that LDL-C levels be used to initiate and assess treatment response. If LDL-C levels are not available then Total-C alone may be used to monitor long-term therapy. A lipoprotein analysis (including LDL-C determination) should be carried out once a year. The NCEP treatment guidelines are summarized below.

Definite Atherosclerotic Disease*	Two or More Other Risk Factors**	LDL-Cholesterol mg/dl (mmol/L) Initiation Level	Goal
NO	NO	≥190 (≥4.9)	<160 (<4.1)
NO	YES	≥160 (≥4.1)	<130 (<3.4)
YES	YES or NO	≥130 (≥3.4)	≤100 (≤2.6)

*Coronary heart disease or peripheral vascular disease (including symptomatic carotid artery disease).

Continued on next page

Questran—Cont.

**Other risk factors for coronary heart disease (CHD) include: age (males: ≥45 years; females: ≥55 years or premature menopause without estrogen replacement therapy); family history of premature CHD; current cigarette smoking; hypertension; confirmed HDL-C <35 mg/dL (<0.91 mmol/L); and diabetes mellitus. Subtract one risk factor if HDL-C is ≥60 mg/dL (≥1.6 mmol/L).

QUESTRAN monotherapy has been demonstrated to retard the rate of progression[2,3] and increase the rate of regression[3] of coronary atherosclerosis.
2) QUESTRAN is indicated for the relief of pruritus associated with partial biliary obstruction. QUESTRAN has been shown to have a variable effect on serum cholesterol in these patients. Patients with primary biliary cirrhosis may exhibit an elevated cholesterol as part of their disease.

CONTRAINDICATIONS

QUESTRAN is contraindicated in patients with complete biliary obstruction where bile is not secreted into the intestine and in those individuals who have shown hypersensitivity to any of its components.

WARNING

PHENYLKETONURICS: QUESTRAN LIGHT CONTAINS 16.8 mg PHENYLALANINE PER 5-GRAM DOSE.

PRECAUTIONS

General

Chronic use of QUESTRAN may be associated with increased bleeding tendency due to hypoprothrombinemia associated with Vitamin K deficiency. This will usually respond promptly to parenteral Vitamin K_1 and recurrences can be prevented by oral administration of Vitamin K_1. Reduction of serum or red cell folate has been reported over long term administration of QUESTRAN. Supplementation with folic acid should be considered in these cases.
There is a possibility that prolonged use of QUESTRAN, since it is a chloride form of anion exchange resin, may produce hyperchloremic acidosis. This would especially be true in younger and smaller patients where the relative dosage may be higher. Caution should also be exercised in patients with renal insufficiency or volume depletion, and in patients receiving concomitant spironolactone.
QUESTRAN may produce or worsen pre-existing constipation. The dosage should be increased gradually in patients to minimize the risk of developing fecal impaction. In patients with pre-existing constipation, the starting dose should be 1 packet or 1 scoop once daily for 5–7 days, increasing to twice daily with monitoring of constipation and of serum lipoproteins, at least twice, 4–6 weeks apart. Increased fluid intake and fiber intake should be encouraged to alleviate constipation and a stool softener may occasionally be indicated. If the initial dose is well tolerated, the dose may be increased as needed by one dose/day (at monthly intervals) with periodic monitoring of serum lipoproteins. If constipation worsens or the desired therapeutic response is not achieved at one to six doses/day, combination therapy or alternate therapy should be considered. Particular effort should be made to avoid constipation in patients with symptomatic coronary artery disease. Constipation associated with QUESTRAN may aggravate hemorrhoids.

Information for Patients

Inform your physician if you are pregnant or plan to become pregnant or are breastfeeding. Drink plenty of fluids and mix each 9-gram dose of QUESTRAN POWDER in at least 2 to 6 ounces of fluid or 5-gram dose of QUESTRAN LIGHT in at least 2 to 3 ounces of fluid before taking. Sipping or holding the resin suspension in the mouth for prolonged periods may lead to changes in the surface of the teeth resulting in discoloration, erosion of enamel or decay; good oral hygiene should be maintained.

Laboratory Tests

Serum cholesterol levels should be determined frequently during the first few months of therapy and periodically thereafter. Serum triglyceride levels should be measured periodically to detect whether significant changes have occurred.
The LRC-CPPT showed a dose-related increase in serum triglycerides of 10.7%–17.1% in the cholestyramine-treated group, compared with an increase of 7.9%–11.7% in the placebo group. Based on the mean values and adjusting for the placebo group, the cholestyramine-treated group showed an increase of 5% over pre-entry levels the first year of the study and an increase of 4.3% the seventh year.

Drug Interactions

QUESTRAN (Cholestyramine for Oral Suspension, USP) may delay or reduce the absorption of concomitant oral medication such as phenylbutazone, warfarin, thiazide diuretics (acidic), or propranolol (basic), as well as tetracycline, penicillin G, phenobarbital, thyroid and thyroxine preparations, estrogens and progestins, and digitalis. Interference with the absorption of oral phosphate supplements has been observed with another positively-charged bile acid sequestrant. QUESTRAN may interfere with the pharmacokinetics of drugs that undergo enterohepatic circulation. The discontinuance of QUESTRAN could pose a hazard to health if a potentially toxic drug such as digitalis has been titrated to a maintenance level while the patient was taking QUESTRAN.
Because cholestyramine binds bile acids, QUESTRAN may interfere with normal fat digestion and absorption and thus may prevent absorption of fat-soluble vitamins such as A, D, E and K. When QUESTRAN is given for long periods of time, concomitant supplementation with water-miscible (or parenteral) forms of fat-soluble vitamins should be considered.
SINCE QUESTRAN MAY BIND OTHER DRUGS GIVEN CONCURRENTLY, IT IS RECOMMENDED THAT PATIENTS TAKE OTHER DRUGS AT LEAST ONE HOUR BEFORE OR 4 TO 6 HOURS AFTER QUESTRAN (OR AT AS GREAT AN INTERVAL AS POSSIBLE) TO AVOID IMPEDING THEIR ABSORPTION.

Carcinogenesis, Mutagenesis, and Impairment of Fertility

In studies conducted in rats in which cholestyramine resin was used as a tool to investigate the role of various intestinal factors, such as fat, bile salts and microbial flora, in the development of intestinal tumors induced by potent carcinogens, the incidence of such tumors was observed to be greater in cholestyramine resin-treated rats than in control rats.
The relevance of this laboratory observation from studies in rats to the clinical use of QUESTRAN is not known. In the LRC-CPPT study referred to above, the total incidence of fatal and nonfatal neoplasms was similar in both treatment groups. When the many different categories of tumors are examined, various alimentary system cancers were somewhat more prevalent in the cholestyramine group. The small numbers and the multiple categories prevent conclusions from being drawn. However, in view of the fact that cholestyramine resin is confined to the GI tract and not absorbed, and in light of the animal experiments referred to above, a six-year post-trial follow-up of the LRC-CPPT[5] patient population has been completed (a total of 13.4 years of in-trial plus post-trial follow-up) and revealed no significant difference in the incidence of cause-specific mortality or cancer morbidity between cholestyramine and placebo treated patients.

Pregnancy

Pregnancy Category C

There are no adequate and well controlled studies in pregnant women. The use of QUESTRAN in pregnancy or lactation or by women of childbearing age requires that the potential benefits of drug therapy be weighed against the possible hazards to the mother and child. QUESTRAN is not absorbed systemically, however, it is known to interfere with absorption of fat-soluble vitamins; accordingly, regular prenatal supplementation may not be adequate (see **PRECAUTIONS: Drug Interactions**).

Nursing Mothers

Caution should be exercised when QUESTRAN is administered to a nursing mother. The possible lack of proper vitamin absorption described in the "**Pregnancy**" section may have an effect on nursing infants.

Pediatric Use

Although an optimal dosage schedule has not been established, standard texts[6,7] list a usual pediatric dose of 240 mg/kg/day of anhydrous cholestyramine resin in two to three divided doses, normally not to exceed 8 gm/day with dose titration based on response and tolerance.
In calculating pediatric dosages, 44.4 mg of anhydrous cholestyramine resin are contained in 100 mg of QUESTRAN POWDER and 80 mg of anhydrous cholestyramine are contained in 100 mg of QUESTRAN LIGHT.
The effects of long-term administration, as well as its effect in maintaining lowered cholesterol levels in pediatric patients, are unknown. (Also see **ADVERSE REACTIONS**.)

ADVERSE REACTIONS

The most common adverse reaction is constipation. When used as a cholesterol-lowering agent predisposing factors for most complaints of constipation are high dose and increased age (more than 60 years old). Most instances of constipation are mild, transient, and controlled with conventional therapy. Some patients require a temporary decrease in dosage or discontinuation of therapy.
Less Frequent Adverse Reactions: Abdominal discomfort and/or pain, flatulence, nausea, vomiting, diarrhea, eructation, anorexia, and steatorrhea, bleeding tendencies due to hypoprothrombinemia (Vitamin K deficiency) as well as Vitamin A (one case of night blindness reported) and D deficiencies, hyperchloremic acidosis in children, osteoporosis, rash and irritation of the skin, tongue and perianal area. Rare reports of intestinal obstruction, including two deaths, have been reported in pediatric patients.
Occasional calcified material has been observed in the biliary tree, including calcification of the gallbladder, in patients to whom QUESTRAN has been given. However, this may be a manifestation of the liver disease and not drug related.
One patient experienced biliary colic on each of three occasions on which he took QUESTRAN. One patient diagnosed as acute abdominal symptom complex was found to have a "pasty mass" in the transverse colon on x-ray.
Other events (not necessarily drug related) reported in patients taking QUESTRAN include:
Gastrointestinal—GI-rectal bleeding, black stools, hemorrhoidal bleeding, bleeding from known duodenal ulcer, dysphagia, hiccups, ulcer attack, sour taste, pancreatitis, rectal pain, diverticulitis.
Laboratory test changes—Liver function abnormalities.
Hematologic—Prolonged prothrombin time, ecchymosis, anemia.
Hypersensitivity—Urticaria, asthma, wheezing, shortness of breath.
Musculoskeletal—Backache, muscle and joint pains, arthritis.
Neurologic—Headache, anxiety, vertigo, dizziness, fatigue, tinnitus, syncope, drowsiness, femoral nerve pain, paresthesia.
Eye—Uveitis.
Renal—Hematuria, dysuria, burnt odor to urine, diuresis.
Miscellaneous—Weight loss, weight gain, increased libido, swollen glands, edema, dental bleeding, dental caries, erosion of tooth enamel, tooth discoloration.

OVERDOSAGE

Overdosage with QUESTRAN has been reported in a patient taking 150% of the maximum recommended daily dosage for a period of several weeks. No ill effects were reported. Should an overdosage occur, the chief potential harm would be obstruction of the gastrointestinal tract. The location of such potential obstruction, the degree of obstruction, and the presence or absence of normal gut motility would determine treatment.

DOSAGE AND ADMINISTRATION

The recommended starting adult dose for QUESTRAN POWDER is one packet or one level scoopful (9 grams of QUESTRAN contains 4 grams of anhydrous cholestyramine resin) once or twice a day. The recommended starting adult dose for QUESTRAN LIGHT is one packet or one level scoopful (5 grams of QUESTRAN LIGHT contains 4 grams of anhydrous cholestyramine resin) once or twice a day. The recommended maintenance dose for QUESTRAN POWDER and QUESTRAN LIGHT is 2 to 4 packets or scoopfuls daily (8–16 grams anhydrous cholestyramine resin) divided into two doses. It is recommended that increases in dose be gradual with periodic assessment of lipid/lipoprotein levels at intervals of not less than 4 weeks. The maximum recommended daily dose is six packets or scoopfuls of QUESTRAN (24 grams of anhydrous cholestyramine resin). The suggested time of administration is at mealtime but may be modified to avoid interference with absorption of other medications. Although the recommended dosing schedule is twice daily, QUESTRAN may be administered in 1–6 doses per day.

QUESTRAN should not be taken in its dry form. Always mix QUESTRAN with water or other fluids before ingesting. See Preparation Instructions.

Concomitant Therapy

Preliminary evidence suggests that the lipid-lowering effects of QUESTRAN on total and LDL-cholesterol are enhanced when combined with a HMG-CoA reductase inhibitor, e.g., pravastatin, lovastatin, simvastatin, and fluvastatin. Additive effects on LDL-cholesterol are also seen with combined nicotinic acid/QUESTRAN therapy. See the **Drug Interactions** subsection of the **PRECAUTIONS** section for recommendations on administering concomitant therapy.

PREPARATION

The color of QUESTRAN may vary somewhat from batch to batch but this variation does not affect the performance of the product. Place the contents of one single-dose packet or one level scoopful of QUESTRAN in a glass or cup. Add at least 2 to 6 ounces of water or the beverage of your choice. Stir to a uniform consistency.
QUESTRAN may also be mixed with highly fluid soups or pulpy fruits with a high moisture content such as applesauce or crushed pineapple.

HOW SUPPLIED

QUESTRAN® POWDER (Cholestyramine for Oral Suspension, USP) is available in cartons of sixty 9-gram packets and in cans containing 378 grams. Nine grams of QUESTRAN POWDER contain 4 grams of anhydrous cholestyramine resin.

NDC 0087-0580-05	Can, 378 g
NDC 0087-0580-11	Carton of 60, 9 g packets

QUESTRAN LIGHT (Cholestyramine for Oral Suspension, USP) is available in cartons of sixty 5-gram packets and in cans containing 210 grams. Five grams of QUESTRAN LIGHT contain 4 grams of anhydrous cholestyramine resin.

NDC 0087-0589-01	Can, 210 g
NDC 0087-0589-03	Carton of 60, 5 g packets

Storage

Store at room temperature.

REFERENCES

1. The Lipid Research Clinics Coronary Primary Prevention Trial Results: (I) Reduction in Incidence of Coronary Heart

Disease; (II) The Relationship of Reduction in Incidence of Coronary Heart Disease to Cholesterol Lowering. *JAMA* 1984; 251:351–374.
2. Brensike JF, Levy RI, Kelsey SF, et al. Effects of therapy with cholestyramine on progression of coronary arteriosclerosis: results of the NHLBI type II coronary intervention study. *Circulation*1984;69:313-24.
3. Watts, GF, Lewis B, Brunt JNH, Lewis ES, et al. Effects on coronary artery disease of lipid-lowering diet, or diet plus cholestyramine, in the St Thomas Atherosclerosis Regression Study (STARS). *Lancet* 1992;339:563-69.
4. National Cholesterol Education Program. Second Report of the Expert Panel on Detection, Evaluation, and Treatment of High Blood Cholesterol in Adults (Adult Treatment Panel II). *Circulation* 1994 Mar; 89(3):1333-445.
5. The Lipid Research Clinics Investigators. The Lipid Research Clinics Coronary Primary Prevention Trial: Results of 6 Years of Post-Trial Follow-up. *Arch Intern Med* 1992; 152:1399-1410.
6. Behrman RE et al (eds): *Nelson, Textbook of Pediatrics,* ed 15. Philadelphia, PA, WB Saunders Company, 1996.
7. Takemoto CK et al (eds): *Pediatric Dosage Handbook,* ed 3. Cleveland/Akron, OH, Lexi-Comp, Inc., 1996-1997.
BRISTOL LABORATORIES®
A Bristol-Myers Squibb Co.
Princeton, New Jersey 08543
USA

Revised: November 1997
58901DIM-11 51-000638-04
Shown in Product Identification Guide, page 307

SERZONE® ℞
[*sĕr-zonē*]
(nefazodone hydrochloride) Tablets

Rx only

DESCRIPTION

SERZONE (nefazodone hydrochloride) is an antidepressant for oral administration with a chemical structure unrelated to selective serotonin reuptake inhibitors, tricyclics, tetracyclics, or monoamine oxidase inhibitors (MAOI).
Nefazodone hydrochloride is a synthetically derived phenylpiperazine antidepressant. The chemical name for nefazodone hydrochloride is 2-[3-[4-(3-chlorophenyl)-1-piperazinyl]propyl]-5-ethyl-2,4-dihydro-4-(2-phenoxyethyl)-3H-1,2,4-triazol-3-one monohydrochloride. The molecular formula is $C_{25}H_{32}ClN_5O_2 \bullet HCl$, which corresponds to a molecular weight of 506.5.
Nefazodone hydrochloride is a nonhygroscopic, white crystalline solid. It is freely soluble in chloroform, soluble in propylene glycol, and slightly soluble in polyethylene glycol and water.
SERZONE is supplied as hexagonal tablets containing 50 mg, 100 mg, 150 mg, 200 mg, or 250 mg of nefazodone hydrochloride and the following inactive ingredients: microcrystalline cellulose, povidone, sodium starch glycolate, colloidal silicon dioxide, magnesium stearate, and iron oxides (red and/or yellow) as colorants.

CLINICAL PHARMACOLOGY

Pharmacodynamics

The mechanism of action of nefazodone, as with other antidepressants, is unknown.
Preclinical studies have shown that nefazodone inhibits neuronal uptake of serotonin and norepinephrine.
Nefazodone occupies central 5-HT_2 receptors at nanomolar concentrations, and acts as an antagonist at this receptor. Nefazodone was shown to antagonize alpha$_1$-adrenergic receptors, a property which may be associated with postural hypotension. *In vitro* binding studies showed that nefazodone had no significant affinity for the following receptors: alpha$_2$ and beta adrenergic, 5-HT_{1A}, cholinergic, dopaminergic, or benzodiazepine.

Pharmacokinetics

Nefazodone hydrochloride is rapidly and completely absorbed but is subject to extensive metabolism, so that its absolute bioavailability is low, about 20%, and variable. Peak plasma concentrations occur at about one hour and the half-life of nefazodone is 2-4 hours.
Both nefazodone and its pharmacologically similar metabolite, hydroxynefazodone, exhibit nonlinear kinetics for both dose and time, with AUC and C_{max} increasing more than proportionally with dose increases and more than expected upon multiple dosing over time, compared to single dosing. For example, in a multiple-dose study involving BID dosing with 50, 100, and 200 mg, the AUC for nefazodone and hydroxynefazodone increased by about 4-fold with an increase in dose from 200 to 400 mg per day; C_{max} increased by about 3-fold with the same dose increase. In a multiple-dose study involving BID dosing with 25, 50, 100, and 150 mg, the accumulation ratios for nefazodone and hydroxynefazodone AUC, after 5 days of BID dosing relative to the first dose, ranged from approximately 3 to 4 at the lower doses (50-100 mg/day) and from 5 to 7 at the higher doses (200-300 mg/day); there were also approximately 2- to 4-fold increases in C_{max} after 5 days of BID dosing relative to the first dose, suggesting extensive and greater than predicted accumulation of nefazodone and its hydroxy metabolite with multiple dosing. Steady-state plasma nefazodone and metabolite concentrations are attained within 4 to 5 days of initiation of BID dosing or upon dose increase or decrease.
Nefazodone is extensively metabolized after oral administration by n-dealkylation and aliphatic and aromatic hydroxylation, and less than 1% of administered nefazodone is excreted unchanged in urine. Attempts to characterize three metabolites identified in plasma, hydroxynefazodone (HO-NEF), meta-chlorophenylpiperazine (mCPP), and a triazoledione metabolite, have been carried out. The AUC (expressed as a multiple of the AUC for nefazodone dosed at 100 mg BID) and elimination half-lives for these three metabolites were as follows:

AUC Multiples and T1/2 for
Three Metabolites of Nefazodone (100 mg BID)

Metabolite	AUC Multiple	T1/2
HO-NEF	0.4	1.5-4 hrs
mCPP	0.07	4-8 hrs
Triazole-dione	4.0	18 hrs

HO-NEF possesses a pharmacological profile qualitatively and quantitatively similar to that of nefazodone. mCPP has some similarities to nefazodone, but also has agonist activity at some serotonergic receptor subtypes. The pharmacological profile of the triazole-dione metabolite has not yet been well characterized. In addition to the above compounds, several other metabolites were present in plasma but have not been tested for pharmacological activity.
After oral administration of radiolabelled nefazodone, the mean half-life of total label ranged between 11 and 24 hours. Approximately 55% of the administered radioactivity was detected in urine and about 20-30% in feces.
Distribution—Nefazodone is widely distributed in body tissues, including the central nervous system (CNS). In humans the volume of distribution of nefazodone ranges from 0.22 to 0.87 L/kg.
Protein Binding—At concentrations of 25-2500 ng/mL nefazodone is extensively (> 99%) bound to human plasma proteins *in vitro.* While nefazodone did not alter the *in vitro* protein binding of chlorpromazine, desipramine, diazepam, diphenylhydantoin, lidocaine, prazosin, propranolol, verapamil, or warfarin, it is unknown whether or not displacement of either nefazodone or other drugs occurs *in vivo.* There was a 5% decrease in the protein binding of haloperidol; this is probably of no clinical significance.
Effect of Food—Food delays the absorption of nefazodone and decreases the bioavailability of nefazodone by approximately 20%.
Renal Disease—In studies involving 29 renally-impaired patients, renal impairment (creatinine clearances ranging from 7 to 60 mL/min/1.73m^2) had no effect on steady-state nefazodone plasma concentrations.
Liver Disease—In a multiple-dose study of patients with liver cirrhosis, the AUC values for nefazodone and HO-NEF at steady state were approximately 25% greater than those observed in normal volunteers.
Age/Gender Effects—After single doses of 300 mg to younger and older patients, C_{max} and AUC for nefazodone and hydroxynefazodone were up to twice as high in the older patients. With multiple doses, however, differences were much smaller, 10-20%. A similar result was seen for gender, with a higher C_{max} and AUC in women after single doses but no difference after multiple doses.
Treatment with SERZONE (nefazodone hydrochloride) should be initiated at half the usual dose in elderly patients, especially women (see **DOSAGE AND ADMINISTRATION** Section), but the therapeutic dose range is similar in younger and older patients.

Clinical Efficacy Trial Results

Studies in Outpatients with Depression
During its premarketing development, the efficacy of SERZONE (nefazodone hydrochloride) was evaluated at doses within the therapeutic range in five well-controlled, short-term (6-8 weeks) clinical investigations. These trials enrolled outpatients meeting DSM-III or DSM-IIIR criteria for major depression. Among these trials, two demonstrated the effectiveness of SERZONE, and two provided additional support for that conclusion.
One trial was a 6-week dose-titration study comparing SERZONE in two dose ranges (up to 300 mg/day and up to 600 mg/day [mean modal dose for this group was about 400 mg/day], on a BID schedule) and placebo. The second trial was an 8-week dose-titration study comparing SERZONE (up to 600 mg/day; mean modal dose was 375 mg/day), imipramine (up to 300 mg/day), and placebo, all on a BID schedule. Both studies demonstrated SERZONE, at doses titrated between 300 mg to 600 mg/day (therapeutic dose range), to be superior to placebo on at least three of the following four measures: 17-Item Hamilton Depression Rating Scale or HDRS (total score), Hamilton Depressed Mood item, Clinical Global Impressions (CGI) Severity score, and CGI Improvement score. Significant differences were also found for certain factors of the HDRS (e.g., anxiety factor, sleep disturbance factor, and retardation factor). In the two supportive studies, SERZONE was titrated up to 500 or 600 mg/day (mean modal doses of 462 mg/day and 363 mg/day). In the fifth study, the differentiation in response rates between SERZONE and placebo was not statistically significant. Three additional trials were conducted using subtherapeutic doses of SERZONE.
There were no efficacy studies focusing specifically on the elderly or on men and women separately. Overall, approximately two-thirds of patients in these trials were women, and an analysis of the effects of gender on outcome did not suggest any differential responsiveness on the basis of sex. There were too few elderly patients in these trials to reveal possible age-related differences in response.
Since its initial marketing as an antidepressant drug product, additional clinical investigations of SERZONE have been conducted. These studies explored SERZONE's use under conditions not evaluated fully at the time initial marketing approval was granted.
Studies in "Inpatients"
Two studies were conducted to evaluate SERZONE's effectiveness in hospitalized depressed patients. These were 6-week, dose-titration trials comparing SERZONE (up to 600 mg/day) and placebo, on a BID schedule. In one study, SERZONE was superior to placebo. In this study, the mean modal dose of SERZONE was 503 mg/day, and 85% of these inpatients were melancholic; at baseline, patients were distributed at the higher end of the 7-point CGI Severity scale, as follows: 4=moderately ill (17%); 5=markedly ill (48%); 6=severely ill (32%). In the other study, the differentiation in response rates between SERZONE and placebo was not statistically significant. This result may be explained by the "high" rate of spontaneous improvement among the patients randomized to placebo.
Studies in "Relapse Prevention in Patients Recently Recovered (Clinically) from Depression"
Two studies were conducted to assess SERZONE's capacity to maintain a clinical remission in acutely depressed patients who were judged to have responded adequately (HDRS total score ≤10) after a 16-week period of open treatment with SERZONE (titration up to 600 mg/day). In one study, SERZONE was superior to placebo. In this study, patients (n=131) were randomized to continuation on SERZONE or placebo for an additional 36 weeks (1 year total). This study demonstrated a significantly lower relapse rate (HDRS total score ≥18) for patients taking SERZONE compared to those on placebo. The second study was of appropriate design and power, but the sample of patients admitted for evaluation did not suffer relapses at a high enough incidence to provide a meaningful test of SERZONE's efficacy for this use.
Comparisons of Clinical Trial Results
Highly variable results have been seen in the clinical development of all antidepressant drugs. Further more, in those circumstances when the drugs have not been studied in the same controlled clinical trial(s), comparisons among the findings of studies evaluating the effectiveness of different antidepressant drug products are inherently unreliable. Because conditions of testing (e.g., patient samples, investigators, doses of the treatments administered and compared, outcome measures, etc.) vary among trials, it is virtually impossible to distinguish a difference in drug effect from a difference due to one or more of the confounding factors just enumerated.

INDICATIONS AND USAGE

SERZONE is indicated for the treatment of depression.
The efficacy of SERZONE in the treatment of depression was established in 6–8 week controlled trials of outpatients and in a 6-week controlled trial of depressed inpatients whose diagnoses corresponded most closely to the DSM-III or DSM-IIIR category of major depressive disorder (see **CLINICAL PHARMACOLOGY** Section).
A major depressive episode implies a prominent and relatively persistent depressed or dysphoric mood that usually interferes with daily functioning (nearly every day for at least 2 weeks). It must include either depressed mood or loss of interest or pleasure and at least 5 of the following nine symptoms: depressed mood, loss of interest in usual activities, significant change in weight and/or appetite, insomnia or hypersomnia, psychomotor agitation or retardation, increased fatigue, feelings of guilt or worthlessness, slowed thinking or impaired concentration, a suicide attempt or suicidal ideation.
The efficacy of SERZONE in reducing relapse in patients with major depression who were judged to have had a satisfactory clinical response to 16 weeks of open-label

Continued on next page

Serzone—Cont.

SERZONE treatment for an acute depressive episode has been demonstrated in a randomized placebo-controlled trial (see **CLINICAL PHARMACOLOGY** Section). Although remitted patients were followed for as long as 36 weeks in the study cited (i.e., 52 weeks total), the physician who elects to use SERZONE for extended periods should periodically reevaluate the long-term usefulness of the drug for the individual patient.

CONTRAINDICATIONS

Coadministration of terfenadine, astemizole or cisapride with SERZONE (nefazodone hydrochloride) is contraindicated (see **WARNINGS** and **PRECAUTIONS** Sections).

SERZONE is contraindicated in patients with known hypersensitivity to nefazodone or other phenylpiperazine antidepressants.

The coadministration of triazolam and nefazodone causes a significant increase in the plasma level of triazolam (see **WARNINGS** and **PRECAUTIONS** Sections), and a 75% reduction in the initial triazolam dosage is recommended if the two drugs are to be given together. Because not all commercially available dosage forms of triazolam permit a sufficient dosage reduction, the coadministration of triazolam and SERZONE should be avoided for most patients, including the elderly.

WARNINGS

Potential for Interaction with Monoamine Oxidase Inhibitors

In patients receiving antidepressants with pharmacological properties similar to nefazodone in combination with a monoamine oxidase inhibitor (MAOI), there have been reports of serious, sometimes fatal, reactions. For a selective serotonin reuptake inhibitor, these reactions have included hyperthermia, rigidity, myoclonus, autonomic instability with possible rapid fluctuations of vital signs, and mental status changes that include extreme agitation progressing to delirium and coma. These reactions have also been reported in patients who have recently discontinued that drug and have been started on a MAOI. Some cases presented with features resembling neuroleptic malignant syndrome. Severe hyperthermia and seizures, sometimes fatal, have been reported in association with the combined use of tricyclic antidepressants and MAOIs. These reactions have also been reported in patients who have recently discontinued these drugs and have been started on an MAOI.

Although the effects of combined use of nefazodone and MAOI have not been evaluated in humans or animals, because nefazodone is an inhibitor of both serotonin and norepinephrine reuptake, it is recommended that nefazodone not be used in combination with an MAOI, or within 14 days of discontinuing treatment with an MAOI. At least 1 week should be allowed after stopping nefazodone before starting a MAOI.

Interaction with Triazolobenzodiazepines

Interaction studies of nefazodone with two triazolobenzodiazepines, i.e., triazolam and alprazolam, metabolized by cytochrome $P_{450}IIIA_4$, have revealed substantial and clinically important increases in plasma concentrations of these compounds when administered concomitantly with nefazodone.

Triazolam

When a single oral 0.25-mg dose of triazolam was coadministered with nefazodone (200 mg BID) at steady state, triazolam half-life and AUC increased 4-fold and peak concentrations increased 1.7-fold. Nefazodone plasma concentrations were unaffected by triazolam. *Coadministration of nefazodone potentiated the effects of triazolam on psychomotor performance tests.* If triazolam is coadministered with SERZONE (nefazodone hydrochloride), a 75% reduction in the initial triazolam dosage is recommended. Because not all commercially available dosage forms of triazolam permit sufficient dosage reduction, coadministration of triazolam with SERZONE should be avoided for most patients, including the elderly. In the exceptional case where coadministration of triazolam with SERZONE (nefazodone hydrochloride) may be considered appropriate, only the lowest possible dose of triazolam should be used (see **CONTRAINDICATIONS** and **PRECAUTIONS** Sections).

Alprazolam

When alprazolam (1 mg BID) and nefazodone (200 mg BID) were coadministered, steady-state peak concentrations, AUC and half-life values for alprazolam increased by approximately 2-fold. Nefazodone plasma concentrations were unaffected by alprazolam. If alprazolam is coadministered with SERZONE, a 50% reduction in the initial alprazolam dosage is recommended. No dosage adjustment is required for SERZONE.

Potential Terfenadine, Astemizole, and Cisapride Interactions

Terfenadine, astemizole, and cisapride are all metabolized by the cytochrome $P_{450}IIIA_4$ isozyme, and it has been demonstrated that ketoconazole, erythromycin, and other inhibitors of $IIIA_4$ can block the metabolism of these drugs,

resulting in increased plasma concentrations of parent drug. Increased plasma concentrations of terfenadine, astemizole, and cisapride are associated with QT prolongation and with rare cases of serious cardiovascular adverse events, including death, due principally to ventricular tachycardia of the torsades de pointes type. Nefazodone has been shown *in vitro* to be an inhibitor of $IIIA_4$. Consequently, it is recommended that nefazodone not be used in combination with either terfenadine, astemizole, or cisapride (see **CONTRAINDICATIONS** and **PRECAUTIONS** Sections).

PRECAUTIONS
General
Postural Hypotension

A pooled analysis of the vital signs monitored during placebo-controlled premarketing studies revealed that 5.1% of nefazodone patients compared to 2.5% of placebo patients ($p \leq 0.01$) met criteria for a potentially important decrease in blood pressure at some time during treatment (systolic blood pressure ≤ 90 mmHg *and* a change from baseline of ≥ 20 mmHg). While there was no difference in the proportion of nefazodone and placebo patients having adverse events characterized as 'syncope' (nefazodone, 0.2%; placebo, 0.3%), the rates for adverse events characterized as 'postural hypotension' were as follows: nefazodone (2.8%), tricyclic antidepressants (10.9%), SSRI (1.1%), and placebo (0.8%). Thus, the prescriber should be aware that there is some risk of postural hypotension in association with nefazodone use. SERZONE should be used with caution in patients with known cardiovascular or cerebrovascular disease that could be exacerbated by hypotension (history of myocardial infarction, angina, or ischemic stroke) and conditions that would predispose patients to hypotension (dehydration, hypovolemia, and treatment with antihypertensive medication).

Activation of Mania/Hypomania

During premarketing testing, hypomania or mania occurred in 0.3% of nefazodone-treated unipolar patients, compared to 0.3% of tricyclic- and 0.4% of placebo-treated patients. In patients classified as bipolar the rate of manic episodes was 1.6% for nefazodone, 5.1% for the combined tricyclic-treated groups, and 0% for placebo-treated patients. Activation of mania/hypomania is a known risk in a small proportion of patients with major affective disorder treated with other marketed antidepressants. As with all antidepressants, SERZONE should be used cautiously in patients with a history of mania.

Suicide

The possibility of a suicide attempt is inherent in depression and may persist until significant remission occurs. Close supervision of high risk patients should accompany initial drug therapy. Prescriptions for SERZONE should be written for the smallest quantity of tablets consistent with good patient management in order to reduce the risk of overdose.

Seizures

During premarketing testing, a recurrence of a petit mal seizure was observed in a patient receiving nefazodone who had a history of such seizures. In addition, one nonstudy participant reportedly experienced a convulsion (type not documented) following a multiple-drug overdose (see **OVERDOSAGE** Section). Rare occurrences of convulsions (including grand mal seizures) following nefazodone administration have been reported since market introduction. A causal relationship to nefazodone has not been established (see **ADVERSE REACTIONS** Section).

Priapism

While priapism did not occur during premarketing experience with nefazodone, rare reports of priapism have been received since market introduction. A causal relationship to nefazodone has not been established (see **ADVERSE REACTIONS** Section). If patients present with prolonged or inappropriate erections, they should discontinue therapy immediately and consult their physicians. If the condition persists for more than 24 hours, a urologist should be consulted to determine appropriate management.

Use in Patients with Concomitant Illness

SERZONE has not been evaluated or used to any appreciable extent in patients with a recent history of myocardial infarction or unstable heart disease. Patients with these diagnoses were systematically excluded from clinical studies during the product's premarketing testing. Evaluation of electrocardiograms of 1153 patients who received nefazodone in 6- to 8-week, double-blind, placebo-controlled trials did not indicate that nefazodone is associated with the development of clinically important ECG abnormalities. However, sinus bradycardia, defined as heart rate ≤ 50 bpm and a decrease of at least 15 bpm from baseline, was observed in 1.5% of nefazodone-treated patients compared to 0.4% of placebo-treated patients ($p \leq 0.05$). Because patients with a recent history of myocardial infarction or unstable heart disease were excluded from clinical trials, such patients should be treated with caution.

In patients with cirrhosis of the liver, the AUC values of nefazodone and HO-NEF were increased by approximately 25%.

Information for Patients

Physicians are advised to discuss the following issues with patients for whom they prescribe SERZONE:

Time to Response/Continuation

As with all antidepressants, several weeks on treatment may be required to obtain the full antidepressant effect. Once improvement is noted, it is important for patients to continue drug treatment as directed by their physician.

Interference With Cognitive and Motor Performance

Since any psychoactive drug may impair judgment, thinking, or motor skills, patients should be cautioned about operating hazardous machinery, including automobiles, until they are reasonably certain that SERZONE (nefazodone hydrochloride) therapy does not adversely affect their ability to engage in such activities.

Pregnancy

Patients should be advised to notify their physician if they become pregnant or intend to become pregnant during therapy.

Nursing

Patients should be advised to notify their physician if they are breast-feeding an infant (see **PRECAUTIONS** Section, **Nursing Mothers** Subsection).

Concomitant Medication

Patients should be advised to inform their physicians if they are taking, or plan to take, any prescription or over-the-counter drugs, since there is a potential for interactions. Significant caution is indicated if SERZONE is to be used in combination with XANAX®[1], concomitant use with HALCION®[1] should be avoided for most patients including the elderly, and concomitant use with SELDANE®[2], HISMANAL®[3], or PROPULSID®[3] is contraindicated (see **CONTRAINDICATIONS** and **WARNINGS** Sections).

Alcohol

Patients should be advised to avoid alcohol while taking SERZONE.

Allergic Reactions

Patients should be advised to notify their physician if they develop a rash, hives, or a related allergic phenomenon.

Laboratory Tests

There are no specific laboratory tests recommended.

Drug Interactions

Drugs Highly Bound to Plasma Protein

Because nefazodone is highly bound to plasma protein (see **CLINICAL PHARMACOLOGY** Section, **Pharmacokinetics** Subsection), administration of SERZONE to a patient taking another drug that is highly protein bound may cause increased free concentrations of the other drug, potentially resulting in adverse events. Conversely, adverse effects could result from displacement of nefazodone by other highly bound drugs.

CNS Active Drugs

Monoamine Oxidase Inhibitors—See **WARNINGS** Section Haloperidol—When a single oral 5-mg dose of haloperidol was coadministered with nefazodone (200 mg BID) at steady state, haloperidol apparent clearance decreased by 35% with no significant increase in peak haloperidol plasma concentrations or time of peak. This change is of unknown clinical significance. Pharmacodynamic effects of haloperidol were generally not altered significantly. There were no changes in the pharmacokinetic parameters for nefazodone. Dosage adjustment of haloperidol may be necessary when coadministered with nefazodone.

Lorazepam—When lorazepam (2 mg BID) and nefazodone (200 mg BID) were coadministered to steady state, there was no change in any pharmacokinetic parameter for either drug compared to each drug administered alone. Therefore, dosage adjustment is not necessary for either drug when coadministered.

Triazolam/Alprazolam—See **CONTRAINDICATIONS** and **WARNINGS** Sections

Alcohol—Although nefazodone did not potentiate the cognitive and psychomotor effects of alcohol in experiments with normal subjects, the concomitant use of SERZONE and alcohol in depressed patients is not advised.

General Anesthetics—Little is known about the potential for interaction between nefazodone and general anesthetics; therefore, prior to elective surgery, SERZONE should be discontinued for as long as clinically feasible.

Other CNS Active Drugs—The use of nefazodone in combination with other CNS-active drugs has not been systematically evaluated. Consequently, caution is advised if concomitant administration of SERZONE and such drugs is required.

Cimetidine

When nefazodone (200 mg BID) and cimetidine (300 mg QID) were coadministered for one week, no change in the steady-state pharmacokinetics of either nefazodone or cimetidine was observed compared to each dosed alone. Therefore, dosage adjustment is not necessary for either drug when coadministered.

Cardiovascular Active Drugs

Digoxin—When nefazodone (200 mg BID) and digoxin (0.2 mg QD) were coadministered for 9 days to healthy male volunteers (n = 18) who were phenotyped as $P_{450}IID_6$ extensive metabolizers, C_{max}, C_{min}, and AUC of digoxin were increased by 29%, 27%, and 15%, respectively. Digoxin had no

effects on the pharmacokinetics of nefazodone and its active metabolites. Because of the narrow therapeutic index of digoxin, caution should be exercised when nefazodone and digoxin are coadministered; plasma level monitoring for digoxin is recommended.

Propranolol—The coadministration of nefazodone (200 mg BID) and propranolol (40 mg BID) for 5.5 days to healthy male volunteers (n = 18), including 3 poor and 15 extensive $P_{450}IID_6$ metabolizers, resulted in 30% and 14% reductions in C_{max} and AUC of propranolol, respectively, and a 14% reduction in C_{max} for the metabolite, 4-hydroxypropranolol. The kinetics of nefazodone, hydroxynefazodone, and triazole-dione were not affected by coadministration of propranolol. However, C_{max}, C_{min}, and AUC of m-chlorophenylpiperazine were increased by 23%, 54%, and 28%, respectively. No change in initial dose of either drug is necessary and dose adjustments should be made on the basis of clinical response.

HMG-CoA Reductase Inhibitors—There have been rare reports of rhabdomyolysis involving patients receiving the combination of SERZONE and either of the HMG-CoA reductase inhibitors lovastatin or simvastatin, known substrates of cytochrome $P_{450}IIIA_4$ (see ADVERSE REACTIONS: Postintroduction Clinical Experience Section). Rhabdomyolysis has been observed in patients receiving HMG-CoA reductase inhibitors administered alone (at recommended dosages) and in particular, for certain drugs in this class, when given in combination with inhibitors of the $IIIA_4$ isozyme. Since nefazodone is known to inhibit this isozyme, caution should be used if SERZONE is administered in combination with simvastatin, lovastatin, or atorvastatin. Metabolic interactions are unlikely between nefazodone and HMG-CoA reductase inhibitors that undergo little or no metabolism by the $IIIA_4$ isozyme, such as pravastatin or fluvastatin.

Pharmacokinetics of Nefazodone in 'Poor Metabolizers' and Potential Interaction with Drugs That Inhibit and/or are Metabolized by Cytochrome P_{450} Isozymes

$IIIA_4$ Isozyme—Nefazodone has been shown in vitro to be an inhibitor of cytochrome $P_{450}IIIA_4$. This is consistent with the interaction observed between nefazodone and the benzodiazepines triazolam and alprazolam, drugs metabolized by this isozyme. Consequently, caution is indicated in the combined use of nefazodone with any drugs known to be metabolized by the $IIIA_4$ isozyme. In particular, the combined use of nefazodone with triazolam should be avoided for most patients, including the elderly. The combined use of nefazodone with terfenadine, astemizole, or cisapride is contraindicated (see CONTRAINDICATIONS and WARNINGS Sections).

IID_6 Isozyme—A subset (3% to 10%) of the population has reduced activity of the drug-metabolizing enzyme cytochrome $P_{450}IID_6$. Such individuals are referred to commonly as "poor metabolizers" of drugs such as debrisoquin, dextromethorphan, and the tricyclic antidepressants. The pharmacokinetics of nefazodone and its major metabolites are not altered in these "poor metabolizers." Plasma concentrations of one minor metabolite (mCPP) are increased in this population; the adjustment of SERZONE (nefazodone hydrochloride) dosage is not required when administered to "poor metabolizers." Nefazodone and its metabolites have been shown in vitro to be extremely weak inhibitors of $P_{450}IID_6$. Thus, it is not likely that nefazodone will decrease the metabolic clearance of drugs metabolized by this isozyme.

IA_2 Isozyme—Nefazodone and its metabolites have been shown in vitro not to inhibit cytochrome $P_{450}IA_2$. Thus, metabolic interactions between nefazodone and drugs metabolized by this isozyme are unlikely.

Electro-Convulsive Therapy (ECT)

There are no clinical studies of the combined use of ECT and nefazodone.

Carcinogenesis, Mutagenesis, Impairment of Fertility

Carcinogenesis

There is no evidence of carcinogenicity with nefazodone. The dietary administration of nefazodone to rats and mice for 2 years at daily doses of up to 200 mg/kg and 800 mg/kg, respectively, which are approximately 3 and 6 times, respectively, the maximum human daily dose on a mg/m² basis, produced no increase in tumors.

Mutagenesis

Nefazodone has been shown to have no genotoxic effects based on the following assays: bacterial mutation assays, a DNA repair assay in cultured rat hepatocytes, a mammalian mutation assay in Chinese hamster ovary cells, an in vivo cytogenetics assay in rat bone marrow cells, and a rat dominant lethal study.

Impairment of Fertility

A fertility study in rats showed a slight decrease in fertility at 200 mg/kg/day (approximately three times the maximum human daily dose on a mg/m² basis) but not at 100 mg/kg/day (approximately 1.5 times the maximum human daily dose on a mg/m² basis).

Pregnancy

Teratogenic Effects - Pregnancy Category C

Reproduction studies have been performed in pregnant rabbits and rats at daily doses up to 200 and 300 mg/kg, respec-

tively (approximately 6 and 5 times, respectively, the maximum human daily dose on a mg/m² basis). No malformations were observed in the offspring as a result of nefazodone treatment. However, increased early pup mortality was seen in rats at a dose approximately five times the maximum human dose, and decreased pup weights were seen at this and lower doses, when dosing began during pregnancy and continued until weaning. The cause of these deaths is not known. The no-effect dose for rat pup mortality was 1.3 times the human dose on a mg/m² basis. There are no adequate and well-controlled studies in pregnant women. Nefazodone should be used during pregnancy only if the potential benefit justifies the potential risk to the fetus.

Labor and Delivery

The effect of SERZONE on labor and delivery in humans is unknown.

Nursing Mothers

It is not known whether SERZONE or its metabolites are excreted in human milk. Because many drugs are excreted in human milk, caution should be exercised when SERZONE is administered to a nursing woman.

Pediatric Use

Safety and effectiveness in individuals below 18 years of age have not been established.

Geriatric Use

Over 500 elderly (≥ 65 years) individuals participated in clinical studies with nefazodone. No unusual adverse age-related phenomena were identified in this cohort of elderly patients treated with nefazodone. Due to the increased systemic exposure to nefazodone seen in single dose studies in elderly patients (see CLINICAL PHARMACOLOGY Section, Pharmacokinetics Subsection), treatment should be initiated at half the usual dose, but titration upward should take place over the same range as in younger patients (see DOSAGE AND ADMINISTRATION Section). The usual precautions should be observed in elderly patients who have concomitant medical illnesses or who are receiving concomitant drugs.

ADVERSE REACTIONS

Associated with Discontinuation of Treatment

Approximately 16% of the 3496 patients who received SERZONE in worldwide premarketing clinical trials discontinued treatment due to an adverse experience. The more common (≥ 1%) events in clinical trials associated with discontinuation and considered to be drug related (i.e., those events associated with dropout at a rate approximately twice or greater for SERZONE compared to placebo) included: nausea (3.5%), dizziness (1.9%), insomnia (1.5%), asthenia (1.3%), and agitation (1.2%).

Incidence in Controlled Trials

Commonly Observed Adverse Events in Controlled Clinical Trials:

The most commonly observed adverse events associated with the use of SERZONE (incidence of 5% or greater) and not seen at an equivalent incidence among placebo-treated patients (i.e., significantly higher incidence for SERZONE compared to placebo, p ≤ 0.05), derived from the table below, were: somnolence, dry mouth, nausea, dizziness, constipation, asthenia, lightheadedness, blurred vision, confusion, and abnormal vision.

Adverse Events Occurring at an Incidence of 1% or More Among SERZONE-Treated Patients:

The table that follows enumerates adverse events that occurred at an incidence of 1% or more, and were more frequent than in the placebo group, among SERZONE-treated patients who participated in short-term (6- to 8-week) placebo-controlled trials in which patients were dosed with SERZONE to ranges of 300 to 600 mg/day. This table shows the percentage of patients in each group who had at least one episode of an event at some time during their treatment. Reported adverse events were classified using a standard COSTART-based Dictionary terminology.

The prescriber should be aware that these figures cannot be used to predict the incidence of side effects in the course of usual medical practice where patient characteristics and other factors differ from those which prevailed in the clinical trials. Similarly, the cited frequencies cannot be compared with figures obtained from other clinical investigations involving different treatments, uses, and investigators. The cited figures, however, do provide the prescribing physician with some basis for estimating the relative contribution of drug and nondrug factors to the side-effect incidence rate in the population studied.

[See table at top of next page]

Dose Dependency of Adverse Events

The table that follows enumerates adverse events that were more frequent in the SERZONE dose range of 300 to 600 mg/day than in the SERZONE dose range of up to 300 mg/day. This table shows only those adverse events for which there was a statistically significant difference (p ≤ 0.05) in incidence between the SERZONE dose ranges as well as a difference between the high dose range and placebo.

[See second table at top of next page]

Vital Sign Changes

(See PRECAUTIONS Section, Postural Hypotension Subsection)

Weight Changes

In a pooled analysis of placebo-controlled premarketing studies, there were no differences between nefazodone and placebo groups in the proportions of patients meeting criteria for potentially important increases or decreases in body weight (a change of ≥ 7%).

Laboratory Changes

Of the serum chemistry, serum hematology, and urinalysis parameters monitored during placebo-controlled premarketing studies with nefazodone, a pooled analysis revealed a statistical trend between nefazodone and placebo for hematocrit, i.e., 2.8% of nefazodone patients met criteria for a potentially important decrease in hematocrit (≤ 37% male or ≤ 32% female) compared to 1.5% of placebo patients (0.05 < p ≤ 0.10). Decreases in hematocrit, presumably dilutional, have been reported with many other drugs that block alpha₁-adrenergic receptors. There was no apparent clinical significance of the observed changes in the few patients meeting these criteria.

ECG Changes

Of the ECG parameters monitored during placebo-controlled premarketing studies with nefazodone, a pooled analysis revealed a statistically significant difference between nefazodone and placebo for sinus bradycardia, i.e., 1.5% of nefazodone patients met criteria for a potentially important decrease in heart rate (≤ 50 bpm and a decrease of ≥ 15 bpm) compared to 0.4% of placebo patients (p < 0.05). There was no obvious clinical significance of the observed changes in the few patients meeting these criteria.

Other Events Observed During the Premarketing Evaluation of SERZONE

During its premarketing assessment, multiple doses of SERZONE (nefazodone hydrochloride) were administered to 3496 patients in clinical studies, including more than 250 patients treated for at least one year. The conditions and duration of exposure to SERZONE varied greatly, and included (in overlapping categories) open and double-blind studies, uncontrolled and controlled studies, inpatient and outpatient studies, fixed-dose and titration studies. Untoward events associated with this exposure were recorded by clinical investigators using terminology of their own choosing. Consequently, it is not possible to provide a meaningful estimate of the proportion of individuals experiencing adverse events without first grouping similar types of untoward events into a smaller number of standardized event categories.

In the tabulations that follow, reported adverse events were classified using a standard COSTART-based Dictionary terminology. The frequencies presented, therefore, represent the proportion of the 3496 patients exposed to multiple doses of SERZONE who experienced an event of the type cited on at least one occasion while receiving SERZONE. All reported events are included except those already listed in the Treatment-Emergent Adverse Experience Incidence table, those events listed in other safety-related sections of this insert, those adverse experiences subsumed under COSTART terms that are either overly general or excessively specific so as to be uninformative, those events for which a drug cause was very remote, and those events which were not serious and occurred in fewer than two patients.

It is important to emphasize that, although the events reported occurred during treatment with SERZONE, they were not necessarily caused by it.

Events are further categorized by body system and listed in order of decreasing frequency according to the following definitions: frequent adverse events are those occurring on one or more occasions in at least 1/100 patients (only those not already listed in the tabulated results from placebo-controlled trials appear in this listing); infrequent adverse events are those occurring in 1/100 to 1/1000 patients; rare events are those occurring in fewer than 1/1000 patients.

Body as a whole — Infrequent: allergic reaction, malaise, photosensitivity reaction, face edema, hangover effect, abdomen enlarged, hernia, pelvic pain, and halitosis. *Rare:* cellulitis.

Cardiovascular system — Infrequent: tachycardia, hypertension, syncope, ventricular extrasystoles, and angina pectoris. *Rare:* AV block, congestive heart failure, hemorrhage, pallor, and varicose vein.

Dermatological system — Infrequent: dry skin, acne, alopecia, urticaria, maculopapular rash, vesiculobullous rash, and eczema.

Gastrointestinal system — Frequent: gastroenteritis. *Infrequent:* eructation, periodontal abscess, abnormal liver function tests, gingivitis, colitis, gastritis, mouth ulceration, stomatitis, esophagitis, peptic ulcer, and rectal hemorrhage. *Rare:* glossitis, hepatitis, dysphagia, gastrointestinal hemorrhage, oral moniliasis, and ulcerative colitis.

Continued on next page

Serzone—Cont.

Hemic and lymphatic system — *Infrequent:* ecchymosis, anemia, leukopenia, and lymphadenopathy.

Metabolic and nutritional system — *Infrequent:* weight loss, gout, dehydration, lactic dehydrogenase increased, SGOT increased, and SGPT increased. *Rare:* hypercholesteremia and hypoglycemia.

Musculoskeletal system — *Infrequent:* arthritis, tenosynovitis, muscle stiffness, and bursitis. *Rare:* tendinous contracture.

Nervous system — *Infrequent:* vertigo, twitching, depersonalization, hallucinations, suicide attempt, apathy, euphoria, hostility, suicidal thoughts, abnormal gait, thinking abnormal, attention decreased, derealization, neuralgia, paranoid reaction, dysarthria, increased libido, suicide, and myoclonus. *Rare:* hyperkinesia, increased salivation, cerebrovascular accident, hyperesthesia, hypotonia, ptosis, and neuroleptic malignant syndrome.

Respiratory system — *Frequent:* dyspnea and bronchitis. Infrequent: asthma, pneumonia, laryngitis, voice alteration, epistaxis, hiccup. *Rare:* hyperventilation and yawn.

Special senses — *Frequent:* eye pain. Infrequent: dry eye, ear pain, abnormality of accommodation, diplopia, conjunctivitis, mydriasis, keratoconjunctivitis, hyperacusis, and photophobia. *Rare:* deafness, glaucoma, night blindness, and taste loss.

Urogenital system — *Frequent:* impotence.[a] Infrequent: cystitis, urinary urgency, metrorrhagia[a], amenorrhea[a], polyuria, vaginal hemorrhage[a], breast enlargement[a], menorrhagia[a], urinary incontinence, abnormal ejaculation[a], hematuria, nocturia, and kidney calculus. *Rare:* uterine fibroids enlarged[a], uterine hemorrhage[a], anorgasmia, and oliguria.

---
[a]Adjusted for gender.

Postintroduction Clinical Experience

Postmarketing experience with SERZONE has shown an adverse experience profile similar to that seen during the premarketing evaluation of nefazodone. Voluntary reports of adverse events temporally associated with SERZONE have been received since market introduction that are not listed above and for which a causal relationship has not been established. These include:

Rare occurrences of convulsions (including grand mal seizures) and priapism (see **PRECAUTIONS** Section);

Rare reports of rhabdomyolysis involving patients receiving the combination of SERZONE and lovastatin or simvastatin (see **PRECAUTIONS** Section).

DRUG ABUSE AND DEPENDENCE

Controlled Substance Class

SERZONE (nefazodone hydrochloride) is not a controlled substance.

Physical and Psychological Dependence

In animal studies, nefazodone did not act as a reinforcer for intravenous self-administration in monkeys trained to self-administer cocaine, suggesting no abuse liability. In a controlled study of abuse liability in human subjects, nefazodone showed no potential for abuse.

Nefazodone has not been systematically studied in humans for its potential for tolerance, physical dependence, or withdrawal. While the premarketing clinical experience with nefazodone did not reveal any tendency for a withdrawal syndrome or any drug-seeking behavior, it is not possible to predict on the basis of this limited experience the extent to which a CNS-active drug will be misused, diverted, and/or abused once marketed. Consequently, physicians should carefully evaluate patients for a history of drug abuse and follow such patients closely, observing them for signs of misuse or abuse of SERZONE (e.g., development of tolerance, dose escalation, drug-seeking behavior).

OVERDOSAGE

Human Experience

There is very limited experience with nefazodone overdose. In premarketing clinical studies, there were seven reports of nefazodone overdose alone or in combination with other pharmacological agents. The amount of nefazodone ingested ranged from 1000 mg to 11,200 mg. Commonly reported symptoms from overdose of nefazodone included nausea, vomiting, and somnolence. One nonstudy participant took 2000-3000 mg of nefazodone with methocarbamol and alcohol; this person reportedly experienced a convulsion (type not documented). None of the patients died.

Overdose Management

Overdosage may cause an increase in incidence or severity of any of the reported adverse reactions (see **ADVERSE REACTIONS** Section).

There is no specific antidote for SERZONE (nefazodone hydrochloride). Treatment should be symptomatic and supportive in the case of hypotension or excessive sedation. Any patient suspected of having taken an overdose should have the stomach emptied by gastric lavage.

In managing overdosage, consider the possibility of multiple drug involvement. The physician should consider contacting a poison control center on the treatment of any overdose.

DOSAGE AND ADMINISTRATION

Initial Treatment

The recommended starting dose for SERZONE is 200 mg/day, administered in two divided doses (BID). In the controlled clinical trials establishing the antidepressant efficacy of SERZONE, the effective dose range was generally 300 to 600 mg/day. Consequently, most patients, depending on tolerability and the need for further clinical effect, should have their dose increased. Dose increases should occur in increments of 100 mg/day to 200 mg/day, again on a BID schedule, at intervals of no less than 1 week. As with all antidepressants, several weeks on treatment may be required to obtain a full antidepressant response.

Dosage for Elderly or Debilitated Patients

The recommended initial dose for elderly or debilitated patients is 100 mg/day on a BID schedule. These patients often have reduced nefazodone clearance and/or increased sensitivity to the side effects of CNS-active drugs. It may also be appropriate to modify the rate of subsequent dose titration. As steady-state plasma levels do not change with age, the final target dose based on a careful assessment of the patient's clinical response may be similar in healthy younger and older patients.

Treatment-Emergent Adverse Experience Incidence in
6- to 8-Week Placebo-Controlled Clinical Trials[1]
SERZONE 300 to 600 mg/day Dose Range

Body System	Preferred Term	SERZONE (n = 393)	Placebo (n = 394)
Body as a Whole	Headache	36%	33%
	Asthenia	11%	5%
	Infection	8%	6%
	Flu syndrome	3%	2%
	Chills	2%	1%
	Fever	2%	1%
	Neck Rigidity	1%	0
Cardiovascular	Postural hypotension	4%	1%
	Hypotension	2%	1%
Dermatological	Pruritus	2%	1%
	Rash	2%	1%
Gastrointestinal	Dry mouth	25%	13%
	Nausea	22%	12%
	Constipation	14%	8%
	Dyspepsia	9%	7%
	Diarrhea	8%	7%
	Increased appetite	5%	3%
	Nausea & Vomiting	2%	1%
Metabolic	Peripheral edema	3%	2%
	Thirst	1%	<1%
Musculoskeletal	Arthralgia	1%	<1%
Nervous	Somnolence	25%	14%
	Dizziness	17%	5%
	Insomnia	11%	9%
	Lightheadedness	10%	3%
	Confusion	7%	2%
	Memory Impairment	4%	2%
	Paresthesia	4%	2%
	Vasodilatation[2]	4%	2%
	Abnormal dreams	3%	2%
	Concentration decreased	3%	1%
	Ataxia	2%	0
	Incoordination	2%	1%
	Psychomotor retardation	2%	1%
	Tremor	2%	1%
	Hypertonia	1%	0
	Libido decreased	1%	<1%
Respiratory	Pharyngitis	6%	5%
	Cough increased	3%	1%
Special Senses	Blurred vision	9%	3%
	Abnormal vision[3]	7%	1%
	Tinnitus	2%	1%
	Taste perversion	2%	1%
	Visual field defect	2%	0
Urogenital	Urinary frequency	2%	1%
	Urinary tract infection	2%	1%
	Urinary retention	2%	1%
	Vaginitis[4]	2%	1%
	Breast pain[4]	1%	<1%

[1] Events reported by at least 1% of patients treated with SERZONE (nefazodone hydrochloride) and more frequent than the placebo group are included; incidence is rounded to the nearest 1% (<1% indicates an incidence less than 0.5%). Events for which the SERZONE incidence was equal to or less than placebo are not listed in the table, but included the following: abdominal pain, pain, back pain, accidental injury, chest pain, neck pain, palpitation, migraine, sweating, flatulence, vomiting, anorexia, tooth disorder, weight gain, edema, myalgia, cramp, agitation, anxiety, depression, hypesthesia, CNS stimulation, dysphoria, emotional lability, sinusitis, rhinitis, dysmenorrhea[4], dysuria.
[2] Vasodilatation—flushing, feeling warm.
[3] Abnormal vision—scotoma, visual trails.
[4] Incidence adjusted for gender.

Dose Dependency of Adverse Events in Placebo-Controlled Trials[1]

Body System	Preferred Term	SERZONE 300–600 mg/day (n = 209)	SERZONE ≤ 300 mg/day (n = 211)	Placebo (n = 212)
Gastrointestinal	Nausea	23%	14%	12%
	Constipation	17%	10%	9%
Nervous	Somnolence	28%	16%	13%
	Dizziness	22%	11%	4%
	Confusion	8%	2%	1%
Special Senses	Abnormal vision	10%	0	2%
	Blurred vision	9%	3%	2%
	Tinnitus	3%	0	1%

[1] Events for which there was a statistically significant difference (p ≤ 0.05) between the nefazodone dose groups.

Maintenance/Continuation/Extended Treatment

There is no body of evidence available from controlled trials to indicate how long the depressed patient should be treated with SERZONE. It is generally agreed, however, that pharmacological treatment for acute episodes of depression should continue for up to 6 months or longer. Whether the dose of antidepressant needed to induce remission is identical to the dose needed to maintain euthymia is unknown. Systematic evaluation of the efficacy of SERZONE has shown that efficacy is maintained for periods of up to 36 weeks following 16 weeks of open-label acute treatment (treated for 52 weeks total) at dosages that averaged 438 mg/day. For most patients, their maintenance dose was that associated with response during acute treatment. (See **CLINICAL PHARMACOLOGY** Section.) The safety of SERZONE in long-term use is supported by data from both double-blind and open-label trials involving more than 250 patients treated for at least one year.

Switching Patients to or from a Monoamine Oxidase Inhibitor

At least 14 days should elapse between discontinuation of an MAOI and initiation of therapy with SERZONE. In addition, at least 7 days should be allowed after stopping SERZONE before starting an MAOI.

HOW SUPPLIED

SERZONE® (nefazodone hydrochloride) tablets are hexagonal tablets imprinted with BMS and the strength (i.e., 100 mg) on one side and the identification code number on the other. The100 mg and 150 mg tablets are bisect scored on both tablet faces. The 50 mg, 200 mg and 250 mg tablets are unscored.

NDC CODE	DESCRIPTION
NDC 0087-0031-47	50 mg light pink tablet, bottle of 60
NDC 0087-0032-31	100 mg white tablet, bottle of 60
NDC 0087-0032-44	100 mg white tablet, blister pack of 100
NDC 0087-0039-31	150 mg peach tablet, bottle of 60
NDC 0087-0039-01	150 mg peach tablet, blister pack of 100
NDC 0087-0033-31	200 mg light yellow tablet, bottle of 60
NDC 0087-0033-44	200 mg light yellow tablet, blister pack of 100
NDC 0087-0041-31	250 mg white tablet, bottle of 60

U.S. Patent No. 4,338,317
Store at room temperature, below 40° C (104° F) and dispense in a tight container.
Revised May 1998
P4460-07

REFERENCES

1. HALCION® and XANAX® are registered trademarks of the Upjohn Company.
2. SELDANE® is a registered trademark of Merrell Pharmaceuticals, Incorporated, a subsidiary of Hoechst Marion Roussel.
3. HISMANAL® and PROPULSID® are registered trademarks of Janssen Pharmaceutica, Incorporated.

Bristol Myers Squibb Co
Princeton, NJ 08543
U.S.A.

Shown in Product Identification Guide, page 308

STADOL NS® Ⓒ Ⓡ
[stā '-dŏl]
(butorphanol tartrate)
Nasal Spray

DESCRIPTION

Butorphanol tartrate is a synthetically derived opioid agonist-antagonist analgesic of the phenanthrene series. The chemical name is (-)-17-(cyclobutylmethyl) morphinan-3, 14-diol [S-(R*,R*)] - 2,3 - dihydroxybutanedioate (1:1) (salt). The molecular formula is $C_{21}H_{29}NO_2,C_4H_6O_6$, which corresponds to a molecular weight of 477.55. Butorphanol tartrate is a white crystalline substance. The dose is expressed as the tartrate salt. One milligram of the salt is equivalent to 0.68 mg of the free base. The n-octanol/aqueous buffer partition coefficient of butorphanol is 180:1 at pH 7.5. STADOL NS (butorphanol tartrate) is an aqueous solution of butorphanol tartrate for administration as a metered spray to the nasal mucosa. Each bottle of STADOL NS contains 2.5 mL of a 10 mg/mL solution of butorphanol tartrate with sodium chloride, citric acid, and benzethonium chloride in purified water with sodium hydroxide and/or hydrochloric acid added to adjust the pH to 5.0. The pump reservoir must be fully primed (see **PATIENT INSTRUCTIONS**) prior to initial use. After initial priming each metered spray delivers an average of 1.0 mg of butorphanol tartrate and the 2.5 mL bottle will deliver an average of 14–15 doses of STADOL NS. If not used for 48 hours or longer, the unit must be reprimed (see **PATIENT IN-**

Table 1—
Mean Pharmacokinetic Parameters of Butorphanol in Young and Elderly Subjects[a]

Parameters	Intravenous		Nasal	
	Young	Elderly	Young	Elderly
T_{max}[b] (hr)			0.62 (0.32)[e] (0.15–1.50)[g]	1.03 (0.74) (0.25–3.00)
C_{max}[c] (ng/mL)			1.04 (0.40) (0.35–1.97)	0.90 (0.57) (0.10–2.68)
AUC (inf)[d] (hr•ng/mL)	7.24 (1.57) (4.40–9.77)	8.71 (2.02) (4.76–13.03)	4.93 (1.24) (2.16–7.27)	5.24 (2.27) (0.30–10.34)
Half-life (hr)	4.56 (1.67) (2.06–8.70)	5.61 (1.36) (3.25–8.79)	4.74 (1.57) (2.89–8.79)	6.56 (1.51) (3.75–9.17)
Absolute Bioavailability (%)			69 (16) (44–113)	61 (25) (3–121)
Volume of Distribution[f] (L)	487 (155) (305–901)	552 (124) (305–737)		
Total Body Clearance (L/hr)	99 (23) (70–154)	82 (21) (52–143)		

(a) Young subjects (n = 24) are from 20 to 40 years old and elderly (n = 24) are greater than 65 years of age.
(b) Time to peak plasma concentration.
(c) Peak plasma concentration normalized to 1 mg dose.
(d) Area under the plasma concentration-time curve after a 1 mg dose.
(e) Mean (1 S.D.)
(f) Derived from IV data.
(g) (range of observed values).

STRUCTIONS). With intermittent use requiring repriming before each dose, the 2.5 mL bottle will deliver an average of 8–10 doses of STADOL NS depending on how much repriming is necessary.

CLINICAL PHARMACOLOGY

General Pharmacology and Mechanism of Action: Butorphanol and its major metabolites are agonists at κ-opioid receptors and mixed agonist-antagonists at μ-opioid receptors. Its interactions with these receptors in the central nervous system apparently mediate most of its pharmacologic effects, including analgesia. In addition to analgesia, CNS effects include depression of spontaneous respiratory activity and cough, stimulation of the emetic center, miosis and sedation. Effects possibly mediated by non-CNS mechanisms include alteration in cardiovascular resistance and capacitance, bronchomotor tone, gastrointestinal secretory and motor activity and bladder sphincter activity. In an animal model, the dose of butorphanol tartrate required to antagonize morphine analgesia by 50% was similar to that for nalorphine, less than that for pentazocine and more than that for naloxone. The pharmacological activity of butorphanol metabolites has not been studied in humans; in animal studies, butorphanol metabolites have demonstrated some analgesic activity. In human studies of butorphanol (see **Clinical Trials**), sedation is commonly noted at doses of 0.5 mg or more. Narcosis is produced in 10–12 mg doses of butorphanol administered over 10–15 minutes intravenously. Butorphanol, like other mixed agonist-antagonists with a high affinity for the κ-receptor, may produce unpleasant psychotomimetic effects in some individuals. Nausea and/or vomiting may be produced by doses of 1 mg or more administered by any route. In human studies involving individuals without significant respiratory dysfunction, 2 mg of butorphanol IV and 10 mg of morphine sulfate IV depressed respiration to a comparable degree. At higher doses, the magnitude of respiratory depression with butorphanol is not appreciably increased; however, the duration of respiratory depression is longer. Respiratory depression noted after administration of butorphanol to humans by any route is reversed by treatment with naloxone, a specific opioid antagonist (see **Treatment** in **OVERDOSAGE** section). Butorphanol tartrate demonstrates antitussive effects in animals at doses less than those required for analgesia. Hemodynamic changes noted during cardiac catheterization in patients receiving single 0.025 mg/kg intravenous doses of butorphanol have included increases in pulmonary artery pressure, wedge pressure and vascular resistance, increases in left ventricular end diastolic pressure and in systemic arterial pressure.

Pharmacodynamics: The analgesic effect of butorphanol is influenced by the route of administration. Onset of analgesia is within a few minutes for intravenous administration, within 10–15 minutes for intramuscular injection, and within 15 minutes for the nasal spray doses. Peak analgesic activity occurs within 30–60 minutes following intravenous and intramuscular administration and within 1–2 hours following the nasal spray administration. The duration of analgesia varies depending on the pain model as well as the route of administration, but is generally 3–4 hours with IM and IV doses as defined by the time 50% of patients required remedication. In postoperative studies, the duration of analgesia with IV or IM butorphanol was similar to morphine,

meperidine and pentazocine when administered in the same fashion at equipotent doses (see **Clinical Trials**). Compared to the injectable form and other drugs in this class, STADOL NS (butorphanol tartrate) has a longer duration of action (4–5 hours) (see **Clinical Trials**).

Pharmacokinetics: STADOL Injection is rapidly absorbed after IM injection and peak plasma levels are reached in 20–40 minutes. After nasal administration, mean peak blood levels of 0.9–1.04 ng/mL occur at 30–60 minutes after a 1 mg dose (see Table 1). The absolute bioavailability of STADOL NS is 60–70% and is unchanged in patients with allergic rhinitis. In patients using a nasal vasoconstrictor (oxymetazoline) the fraction of the dose absorbed was unchanged, but the rate of absorption was slowed. The peak plasma concentrations were approximately half those achieved in the absence of the vasoconstrictor. Following its initial absorption/distribution phase, the single dose pharmacokinetics of butorphanol by the intravenous, intramuscular, and nasal routes of administration are similar (see Figure 1).

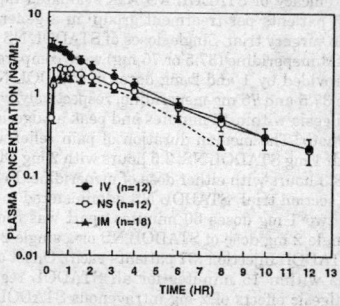

Figure 1—Butorphanol Plasma Levels After IV, IM and Nasal Spray Administration of 2 mg Dose

Serum protein binding is independent of concentration over the range achieved in clinical practice (up to 7 ng/mL) with a bound fraction of approximately 80%.
The volume of distribution of butorphanol varies from 305–901 liters and total body clearance from 52–154 liters/hr (see Table 1).
[See table above]
Dose proportionality for STADOL NS has been determined at steady state in doses up to 4 mg at 6 hour intervals. Steady state is achieved within 2 days. The mean peak plasma concentration at steady state was 1.8-fold (maximal 3-fold) following a single dose. The drug is transported across the blood-brain and placental barriers and into human milk (see **Labor and Delivery** and **Nursing Mothers** in the **PRECAUTIONS** section). Butorphanol is extensively metabolized in the liver. Metabolism is qualitatively and quantitatively similar following intravenous, intramuscular, or nasal administration. Oral bioavailability is only 5–17% because of extensive first-pass metabolism of butorphanol. The major metabolite of butorphanol is hydroxybutorphanol, while norbutorphanol is produced in small

Continued on next page

Stadol/Stadol NS—Cont.

amounts. Both have been detected in plasma following administration of butorphanol. Preliminary evidence suggests the elimination half-life of hydroxybutorphanol may be greater than that of its parent. Elimination occurs by urine and fecal excretion. When ^{3}H labelled butorphanol is administered to normal subjects, most (70–80%) of the dose is recovered in the urine, while approximately 15% is recovered in the feces. About 5% of the dose is recovered in the urine as butorphanol. Forty-nine percent is eliminated in the urine as hydroxybutorphanol. Less than 5% is excreted in the urine as norbutorphanol. Butorphanol pharmacokinetics in the elderly differ from younger patients (see Table 1). The mean absolute bioavailability of STADOL NS (butorphanol tartrate) in elderly women (48%) was less than that in elderly men (75%), young men (68%) or young women (70%). Elimination half-life is increased in the elderly (6.6 hours as opposed to 4.7 hours in younger subjects). In renally impaired patients with creatinine clearances < 30 mL/min the elimination half-life is approximately doubled and the total body clearance is approximately one half (10.5 hours [clearance 150 L/h] as compared to 5.8 hours [clearance 260 L/h] in normals). No effect was observed on C_{max} or T_{max} after a single dose. For further recommendations refer to statements on use in Geriatric Patients, Renal Disease, Hepatic Disease, and statement on Drug Interactions in the **Individualization of Dosage** and **PRECAUTIONS** sections below.

Clinical Trials: The effectiveness of opioid analgesics varies in different pain syndromes. Studies with STADOL Injection have been performed in postoperative (primarily abdominal and orthopedic) pain and pain during labor and delivery, as preoperative and preanesthetic medication, and as a supplement to balanced anesthesia (see below). Studies with STADOL NS have been performed in postoperative (general, orthopedic, oral, cesarean section) pain, in postepisiotomy pain, in pain of musculoskeletal origin, and in migraine headache pain (see below).

Use in the Management of Pain: *Postoperative Pain:* The analgesic efficacy of STADOL Injection (butorphanol tartrate) in postoperative pain was investigated in several double-blind active-controlled studies involving 958 butorphanol-treated patients. The following doses were found to have approximately equivalent analgesic effect: 2 mg butorphanol, 10 mg morphine, 40 mg pentazocine and 80 mg meperidine. After intravenous administration of STADOL Injection, onset and peak analgesic effect occurred by the time of first observation (30 minutes). After intramuscular administration, pain relief onset occurred at 30 minutes or less, and peak effect occurred between 30 minutes and 1 hour. The duration of action of STADOL Injection was 3–4 hours when defined as the time necessary for pain intensity to return to pretreatment level or the time to retreatment. The analgesic efficacy of STADOL NS was evaluated (approximately 35 patients per treatment group) in a general and orthopedic surgery trial. Single doses of STADOL NS (1 or 2 mg) and IM meperidine (37.5 or 75 mg) were compared. Analgesia provided by 1 and 2 mg doses of STADOL NS was similar to 37.5 and 75 mg meperidine, respectively, with onset of analgesia within 15 minutes and peak analgesic effect within 1 hour. The median duration of pain relief was 2.5 hours with 1 mg STADOL NS, 3.5 hours with 2 mg STADOL NS, and 3.3 hours with either dose of meperidine. In a postcesarean section trial, STADOL NS administered to 35 patients as two 1 mg doses 60 minutes apart was compared with a single 2 mg dose of STADOL NS or a single 2 mg IV dose of STADOL Injection (37 patients each). Onset of analgesia was within 15 minutes for all STADOL regimens. Peak analgesic effects of 2 mg intravenous STADOL Injection and STADOL NS were similar in magnitude. The duration of pain relief provided by both 2 mg STADOL NS regimens was approximately 4.5 hours and was greater than intravenous STADOL Injection (2.6 hours). *Migraine Headache Pain:* The analgesic efficacy of two 1 mg doses 1 hour apart of STADOL NS in migraine headache pain was compared with a single dose of 10 mg IM methadone (31 and 32 patients, respectively). Significant onset of analgesia occurred within 15 minutes for both STADOL NS and IM methadone. Peak analgesic effect occurred at 2 hours for STADOL NS and 1.5 hours for methadone. The median duration of pain relief was 6 hours with STADOL NS and 4 hours with methadone as judged by the time when approximately half of the patients remedicated. In two other trials in patients with migraine headache pain, a 2 mg initial dose of STADOL NS followed by an additional 1 mg dose 1 hour later (76 patients) was compared with either 75 mg IM meperidine (24 patients) or placebo (72 patients). Onset, peak activity and duration were similar with both active treatments; however, the incidence of adverse experiences (nausea, vomiting, dizziness) was higher in these two trials with the 2 mg initial dose of STADOL NS than in the trial with the 1 mg initial dose.

Preanesthetic Medication: STADOL Injection (2 mg and 4 mg) and meperidine (80 mg) were studied for use as preanesthetic medication in hospitalized surgical patients. Pa-

tients received a single intramuscular dose of either STADOL Injection or meperidine approximately 90 minutes prior to anesthesia. The anesthesia regimen included barbiturate induction, followed by nitrous oxide and oxygen with halothane or enflurane, with or without a muscle relaxant. Anesthetic preparation was rated as satisfactory in all 42 STADOL Injection patients regardless of the type of surgery.

Balanced Anesthesia: STADOL Injection administered intravenously (mean dose 2 mg) was compared to intravenous morphine sulfate (mean dose 10 mg) as premedication shortly before thiopental induction, followed by balanced anesthesia in 50 ASA Class 1 and 2 patients. Anesthesia was then maintained by repeated intravenous doses, averaging 4.6 mg STADOL Injection and 22.8 mg morphine per patient. Anesthetic induction and maintenance were generally rated as satisfactory with both STADOL Injection (25 patients) and morphine (25 patients) regardless of the type of surgery performed. Emergence from anesthesia was comparable with both agents.

Labor (see **PRECAUTIONS**): The analgesic efficacy of intravenous STADOL Injection was studied in pain during labor. In a total of 145 patients STADOL Injection (1 mg and 2 mg) was as effective as 40 mg and 80 mg of meperidine (144 patients) in the relief of pain in labor with no effect on the duration or progress of labor. Both drugs readily crossed the placenta and entered fetal circulation. The condition of the infants in these studies, determined by Apgar scores at 1 and 5 minutes (8 or above) and time to sustained respiration, showed that STADOL Injection had the same effects on the infants as meperidine. In these studies neurobehavioral testing in infants exposed to STADOL Injection at a mean of 18.6 hours after delivery, showed no significant differences between treatment groups.

Individualization of Dosage: The usual starting dose of butorphanol is 1 mg followed by 1 mg in 60–90 minutes nasally repeated every 3–4 hours (see **DOSAGE AND ADMINISTRATION**). Use of butorphanol in geriatric patients, patients with renal impairment, patients with hepatic impairment, and during labor requires extra caution (see below and the appropriate sections in **PRECAUTIONS**). Since STADOL NS does not require an injection, it allows the physician to initiate therapy with a low dose and repeat the dose if needed. The usual recommended dose for initial nasal administration is 1 mg (1 spray in **one** nostril). If adequate pain relief is not achieved within 60–90 minutes, an additional 1 mg dose may be given. The initial dose sequence outlined above may be repeated in 3–4 hours as required. For the management of severe pain, an initial dose of 2 mg (1 spray in **each** nostril) may be used in patients who will be able to remain recumbent in the event drowsiness or dizziness occur. In such patients additional doses should not be given for 3–4 hours. The incidence of adverse events is higher with an initial 2 mg dose (see **Clinical Trials**). The initial dose sequence in elderly patients and patients with renal or hepatic impairment should be limited to 1 mg followed by 1 mg in 90–120 minutes. The repeat dose sequence in these patients should be determined by the patient's response rather than at fixed times but will generally be no less than at 6 hour intervals (see **PRECAUTIONS**).

INDICATIONS AND USAGE

STADOL NS (butorphanol tartrate) is indicated for the management of pain when the use of an opioid analgesic is appropriate.

CONTRAINDICATIONS

STADOL NS is contraindicated in patients hypersensitive to butorphanol tartrate or the preservative benzethonium chloride in STADOL NS or STADOL Injection in the multidose vial.

WARNINGS

Patients Dependent on Narcotics: Because of its opioid antagonist properties, butorphanol is not recommended for use in patients dependent on narcotics. Such patients should have an adequate period of withdrawal from opioid drugs prior to beginning butorphanol therapy. In patients taking opioid analgesics chronically, butorphanol has precipitated withdrawal symptoms such as anxiety, agitation, mood changes, hallucinations, dysphoria, weakness and diarrhea. Because of the difficulty in assessing opioid tolerance in patients who have recently received repeated doses of narcotic analgesic medication, caution should be used in the administration of butorphanol to such patients.

Drug Abuse and Dependence: Butorphanol tartrate has been associated with episodes of abuse and dependence with most reports involving outpatient treatment of chronic painful conditions. Of the cases received, there were more reports of abuse with the nasal spray formulation than with the injectable formulation. In general, patients receiving opioid treatment for an extended period of time are at a higher risk for abuse and dependence. Proper patient selection, dose and prescribing limitations, appropriate directions for use, and frequent monitoring are important to min-

imize the risk of abuse and dependence. (See **DRUG ABUSE AND DEPENDENCE** section below.)

PRECAUTIONS

General: Hypotension associated with syncope during the first hour of dosing with STADOL NS has been reported rarely, particularly in patients with past history of similar reactions to opioid analgesics. Therefore, patients should be advised to avoid activities with potential risks. **Head Injury and Increased Intracranial Pressure:** As with other opioids, the use of butorphanol in patients with head injury may be associated with carbon dioxide retention and secondary elevation of cerebrospinal fluid pressure, drug-induced miosis, and alterations in mental state that would obscure the interpretation of the clinical course of patients with head injuries. In such patients, butorphanol should be used only if the benefits of use outweigh the potential risks. **Disorders of Respiratory Function or Control:** Butorphanol may produce respiratory depression, especially in patients receiving other CNS active agents, or patients suffering from CNS diseases or respiratory impairment. **Hepatic and Renal Disease:** In patients with severe hepatic or renal disease the initial dosage interval for STADOL NS (butorphanol tartrate) should be increased to 6–8 hours until the response has been well characterized. Subsequent doses should be determined by patient response rather than being scheduled at fixed intervals (see **Individualization of Dosage** in **CLINICAL PHARMACOLOGY** section). **Cardiovascular Effects:** Because butorphanol may increase the work of the heart, especially the pulmonary circuit (see **CLINICAL PHARMACOLOGY**), the use of butorphanol in patients with acute myocardial infarction, ventricular dysfunction, or coronary insufficiency should be limited to those situations where the benefits clearly outweigh the risk. Severe hypertension has been reported rarely during butorphanol therapy. In such cases, butorphanol should be discontinued and the hypertension treated with antihypertensive drugs. In patients who are not opioid dependent, naloxone has also been reported to be effective.

Information for Patients: 1. Opioid analgesics impair the mental or physical abilities required for the performance of potentially dangerous tasks such as driving a car or operating machinery. Effects such as drowsiness or dizziness can appear, usually within the first hour after dosing, and may last up to several hours. Patients who have taken butorphanol should not drive or operate dangerous machinery for at least 1 hour and until the effects of the drug are no longer present. 2. Alcohol should not be consumed while using butorphanol. Concurrent use of butorphanol with drugs that affect the central nervous system (e.g., alcohol, barbiturates, tranquilizers, and antihistamines) may result in increased central nervous system depressant effects such as drowsiness, dizziness and impaired mental function. 3. Patients should be instructed on the proper use of STADOL NS (see **PATIENT INSTRUCTIONS**). 4. While addiction to STADOL NS in the treatment of pain is uncommon, this is one of a class of drugs known to be abused and thus should be handled accordingly.

Drug Interactions: Concurrent use of butorphanol with central nervous system depressants (e.g., alcohol, barbiturates, tranquilizers, and antihistamines) may result in increased central nervous system depressant effects. When used concurrently with such drugs, the dose of butorphanol should be the smallest effective dose and the frequency of dosing reduced as much as possible when administered concomitantly with drugs that potentiate the action of opioids. It is not known if the effects of butorphanol are altered by concomitant medications that affect hepatic metabolism of drugs (cimetidine, erythromycin, theophylline, etc.), but physicians should be alert to the possibility that a smaller initial dose and longer intervals between doses may be needed. The fraction of STADOL NS absorbed is unaffected by the concomitant administration of a nasal vasoconstrictor (oxymetazoline), but the rate of absorption is decreased. Therefore, a slower onset can be anticipated if STADOL NS is administered concomitantly with, or immediately following, a nasal vasoconstrictor. No information is available about the use of butorphanol concurrently with MAO inhibitors.

Use in Ambulatory Patients: Opioid analgesics impair the mental or physical abilities required for the performance of potentially dangerous tasks such as driving a car or operating machinery. Effects such as drowsiness or dizziness can appear, usually within the first hour after dosing, and may last up to several hours. Patients who have taken butorphanol should not drive or operate dangerous machinery for at least 1 hour and until the effects of the drug are no longer present. Alcohol should not be consumed while using butorphanol. Concurrent use of butorphanol with central nervous system depressants (e.g., alcohol, barbiturates, tranquilizers, and antihistamines) may result in increased central nervous system depressant effects. While addiction to STADOL NS in the treatment of pain is uncommon, this is one of a class of drugs known to be abused and thus should be handled accordingly. Patients should be instructed on the proper use of STADOL NS (see **PATIENT INSTRUCTIONS**). **Carcinogenesis, Mutagenesis, Impairment of Fertility:** The carcinogenic potential of butorphanol has not been

adequately evaluated. Butorphanol was not genotoxic in *S. typhimurium* or *E. coli* assays or in unscheduled DNA synthesis and repair assays conducted in cultured human fibroblast cells. Rats treated orally with 160 mg/kg/day (944 mg/m²) had a reduced pregnancy rate. However, a similar effect was not observed with a 2.5 mg/kg/day (14.75 mg/m²) subcutaneous dose.

Pregnancy: Pregnancy Category C: Reproduction studies in mice, rats and rabbits during organogenesis did not reveal any teratogenic potential to butorphanol. However, pregnant rats treated subcutaneously with butorphanol at 1 mg/kg (5.9 mg/m²) had a higher frequency of stillbirths than controls. Butorphanol at 30 mg/kg/oral (5.1 mg/m²) and 60 mg/kg/oral (10.2 mg/m²) also showed higher incidences of post-implantation loss in rabbits. There are no adequate and well-controlled studies of STADOL in pregnant women before 37 weeks' gestation. STADOL should be used during pregnancy only if the potential benefit justifies the potential risk to the infant.

Labor and Delivery: Although there have been rare reports of infant respiratory distress/apnea following the administration of STADOL (butorphanol tartrate) Injection during labor, this adverse effect was not attributed to STADOL Injection as used during controlled clinical trials. The reports of respiratory distress/apnea have been associated with administration of a dose within 2 hours of delivery, use of multiple doses, use with additional analgesic or sedative drugs, or use in preterm pregnancies. In a study of 119 patients, the administration of 1 mg of IV STADOL Injection during labor was associated with transient (10–90 minutes) sinusoidal fetal heart rate patterns, but was not associated with adverse neonatal outcomes. In the presence of an abnormal fetal heart rate pattern, STADOL Injection should be used with caution. STADOL NS is not recommended during labor or delivery because there is no clinical experience with its use in this setting.

Nursing Mothers: Butorphanol has been detected in milk following administration of STADOL Injection to nursing mothers. The amount an infant would receive is probably clinically insignificant (estimated 4 µg/L of milk in a mother receiving 2 mg IM four times a day). Although there is no clinical experience with the use of STADOL NS in nursing mothers, it should be assumed that butorphanol will appear in the milk in similar amounts following the nasal route of administration.

Pediatric Use: Butorphanol is not recommended for use in patients below 18 years of age because safety and efficacy have not been established in this population.

Geriatric Use: The initial dose of STADOL Injection recommended for elderly patients is half the usual dose at twice the usual interval. Subsequent doses and intervals should be based on the patient response (see **Individualization of Dosage** in **CLINICAL PHARMACOLOGY** section). Initially a 1 mg dose of STADOL NS should generally be used in geriatric patients and 90–120 minutes should elapse before deciding whether a second 1 mg dose is needed (see **Individualization of Dosage** in **CLINICAL PHARMACOLOGY** section). Due to changes in clearance, the mean half-life of butorphanol is increased by 25% (to over 6 hours) in patients over the age of 65 years. Elderly patients may be more sensitive to its side effects. Results from a long-term clinical safety trial suggest that elderly patients may be less tolerant of dizziness due to STADOL NS than younger patients.

ADVERSE REACTIONS

A total of 2446 patients were studied in butorphanol clinical trials. Approximately half received STADOL Injection with the remainder receiving STADOL NS. In nearly all cases the type and incidence of side effects with butorphanol by any route were those commonly observed with opioid analgesics. The adverse experiences described below are based on data from short- and long-term clinical trials as well as postmarketing experience in patients receiving butorphanol by any route. There has been no attempt to correct for placebo effect or to subtract the frequencies reported by placebo treated patients in controlled trials. The most frequently reported adverse experiences across all clinical trials with STADOL Injection and STADOL NS were somnolence (43%), dizziness (19%), nausea and/or vomiting (13%). In long-term trials with STADOL NS only, nasal congestion (13%) and insomnia (11%) were frequently reported. The following adverse experiences were reported at a frequency of 1% or greater in clinical trials, and were considered to be probably related to the use of butorphanol: **Body as a Whole:** asthenia/lethargy*, headache*, sensation of heat **Cardiovascular:** VASODILATION*, PALPITATIONS **Digestive:** ANOREXIA*, CONSTIPATION*, dry mouth*, nausea and/or vomiting (13%), stomach pain **Nervous:** anxiety, confusion*, dizziness (19%), euphoria, floating feeling, INSOMNIA (11%), nervousness, paresthesia, somnolence (43%), TREMOR **Respiratory:** BRONCHITIS, COUGH, DYSPNEA*, EPISTAXIS*, NASAL CONGESTION (13%), NASAL IRRITATION*, PHARYNGITIS*, RHINITIS*, SINUS CONGESTION*, SINUSITIS, UPPER RESPIRATORY INFECTION* **Skin and Appendages:** sweating/clammy*, pruritus **Special Senses:** blurred vision, EAR PAIN, TINNITUS*, UNPLEASANT TASTE* (also seen in short-term trials with STADOL NS). (Reactions occurring with a frequency of 3–9% are marked with an asterisk.* Reactions reported predominantly from long-term trials with STADOL NS are CAPITALIZED). The following adverse experiences were reported from postmarketing experience or with a frequency of less than 1% in clinical trials, and were considered to be probably related to the use of butorphanol. **Body as a Whole:** *excessive drug effect associated with transient difficulty speaking and/or executing purposeful movements* **Cardiovascular:** hypotension, syncope **Nervous:** abnormal dreams, agitation, *drug dependence*, dysphoria, hallucinations, hostility, *vertigo*, withdrawal symptoms **Skin and Appendages:** rash/hives **Urogenital:** impaired urination (Reactions reported only from postmarketing experience are *italicized*.) The following infrequent additional adverse experiences were reported in a frequency of less than 1% of the patients studied in short-term STADOL NS trials and from postmarketing experiences under circumstances where the association between these events and butorphanol administration is unknown. They are being listed as alerting information for the physician. **Body as a Whole:** edema **Cardiovascular:** chest pain, hypertension, tachycardia **Nervous:** *convulsion, delusion,* depression **Respiratory:** *apnea,* shallow breathing (Reactions reported only from postmarketing experience are *italicized*.)

DRUG ABUSE AND DEPENDENCE

STADOL NS (butorphanol tartrate) is classified by the Drug Enforcement Administration as Schedule IV. Although the mixed agonist-antagonist opioid analgesics, as a class, have lower abuse potential than morphine, all such drugs can be and have been reported to be abused.

Clinical Trial Experience: Probable withdrawal symptoms were reported in <1% of patients using STADOL NS in controlled clinical trials. However, in one study where patients with chronic pain were treated with STADOL NS for up to 6 months, overuse and probable withdrawal symptoms were each reported in approximately 3% of patients. Patients abruptly discontinuing STADOL NS after extended use or high doses were at greatest risk for symptoms.

Postmarketing Experience: Butorphanol tartrate has been associated with episodes of abuse and dependence. Of the cases received, there were more reports of abuse with the nasal spray formulation than with the injectable formulation. Proper patient selection, dose and prescribing limitations, appropriate directions for use, and frequent monitoring are important to minimize the risk of abuse and dependence with butorphanol tartrate. Special care should be exercised in administering butorphanol to patients with a history of drug abuse or to patients receiving the drug on a repeated basis for an extended period of time.

OVERDOSAGE

Clinical Manifestations: The clinical manifestations of overdose are those of opioid drugs, the most serious of which are hypoventilation, cardiovascular insufficiency and/or coma. Rare cases of overdosage with a fatal outcome were usually associated with ingestion of multiple drugs, and a causal relationship to butorphanol could not be determined. Overdose can occur due to accidental or intentional misuse of butorphanol, especially in young children who may gain access to the drug in the home.

Treatment: The management of suspected butorphanol overdosage includes maintenance of adequate ventilation, peripheral perfusion, normal body temperature, and protection of the airway. Patients should be under continuous observation with adequate serial measures of mental state, responsiveness and vital signs. Oxygen and ventilatory assistance should be available with continual monitoring by pulse oximetry if indicated. In the presence of coma, placement of an artificial airway may be required. An adequate intravenous portal should be maintained to facilitate treatment of hypotension associated with vasodilation. The use of a specific opioid antagonist such as naloxone should be considered. As the duration of butorphanol action usually exceeds the duration of action of naloxone, repeated dosing with naloxone may be required.

DOSAGE AND ADMINISTRATION

Factors to be considered in determining the dose are age, body weight, physical status, underlying pathological condition, use of other drugs, type of anesthesia to be used, and surgical procedure involved. Use in the elderly, patients with hepatic or renal disease or in labor requires extra caution (see **PRECAUTIONS** section and **Individualization of Dosage** in **CLINICAL PHARMACOLOGY** section). The following doses are for patients who do not have impaired hepatic or renal function and who are not on CNS active agents.

Use for Pain: The usual recommended dose for initial nasal administration is 1 mg (1 spray in **one** nostril). Adherence to this dose reduces the incidence of drowsiness and dizziness. If adequate pain relief is not achieved within 60–90 minutes, an additional 1 mg dose may be given. The initial two dose sequence outlined above may be repeated in 3–4 hours as needed. Depending on the severity of the pain, an initial dose of 2 mg (1 spray in **each** nostril) may be used in patients who will be able to remain recumbent in the event drowsiness or dizziness occurs. In such patients single additional 2 mg doses should not be given for 3–4 hours.

Use in Balanced Anesthesia: The use of STADOL NS is not recommended because it has not been studied in induction or maintenance of anesthesia. **Labor:** The use of STADOL NS (butorphanol tartrate) is not recommended as it has not been studied in labor.

Safety and Handling: STADOL NS is an open delivery system with increased risk of exposure to health care workers. In the priming process, a certain amount of butorphanol may be aerosolized; therefore, the pump sprayer should be aimed away from the patient or other people or animals. The disposal of Schedule IV controlled substances must be consistent with State and Federal Regulations.

HOW SUPPLIED

STADOL NS® (butorphanol tartrate) Nasal Spray is supplied in a child-resistant prescription vial containing a metered-dose spray pump with protective clip and dust cover, a bottle of nasal spray solution, and a patient instruction leaflet. On average, one bottle will deliver 14–15 doses if no repriming is necessary. NDC 0087-5650-41 - 10 mg per mL, 2.5 mL bottle

PHARMACIST ASSEMBLY INSTRUCTIONS FOR STADOL NS NASAL SPRAY: The pharmacist will assemble STADOL NS prior to dispensing to the patient, according to the following instructions: 1. Open the child-resistant prescription vial and remove the spray pump and solution bottle. 2. Assemble STADOL NS by first unscrewing the white cap from the solution bottle and screwing the pump unit tightly onto the bottle. Make sure the clear cover is on the pump unit. 3. Return the STADOL NS bottle to the child-resistant prescription vial for dispensing to the patient. **Storage Conditions:** Store below 86°F (30°C). Parenteral drug products should be inspected visually for particulate matter and discoloration prior to administration, whenever solution and container permit.

CAUTION: FEDERAL LAW PROHIBITS DISPENSING WITHOUT PRESCRIPTION

Revised August 1997   5644DIM-06
53-006093-01
STADOL NS also promoted by:
Cephalon, Inc.
Bristol-Myers Squibb Company
Princeton, New Jersey 08543-4500
USA

Shown in Product Identification Guide, page 308

BTG Pharmaceuticals
70 WOOD AVENUE SOUTH
ISELIN, NJ 08830

For Medical Information or Emergencies Contact:
(800) 741-2698

For Customer Service and Ordering:
(800) 741-2698
FAX: (800) 741-2696

DELATESTRYL®   Ⓒ Ⅲ ℞
Testosterone Enanthate Injection USP

DESCRIPTION

DELATESTRYL (Testosterone Enanthate Injection) provides testosterone enanthate, a derivative of the primary endogenous androgen testosterone, for intramuscular administration. In their active form, androgens have a 17-beta-hydroxy group. Esterification of the 17-beta-hydroxy group increases the duration of action of testosterone; hydrolysis to free testosterone occurs *in vivo*. Each mL of sterile, colorless to pale yellow solution provides 200 mg testosterone enanthate in sesame oil with 5 mg chlorobutanol (chloral derivative) as a preservative.

HOW SUPPLIED

DELATESTRYL (Testosterone Enanthate Injection USP) is available in 1 mL (200 mg/mL) Unimatic single dose syringes (NDC 54396-328-16). Each syringe is supplied with a sterile disposable 20-gauge. 1½-inch needle. DELATESTRYL is also available in 5 mL (200 mg/mL) multiple dose vials (NDC 54396-328-40).

Storage

DELATESTRYL (Testosterone Enanthate Injection USP) should be stored at room temperature. Warming and rotating the syringe unit or vial between the palms of the hands

Continued on next page

Delatestryl—Cont.

will redissolve any crystals that may have formed during storage at low temperatures.

Manufactured for
BTG Pharmaceuticals
Iselin, NJ 08830
by: Bristol-Myers Squibb
Princeton, NJ 08543

J4-484D   Revised October 1995

OXANDRIN®   Ⓒ Ⅲ ℞
(oxandrolone tablets, USP)

DESCRIPTION

Oxandrin® oral tablets contain 2.5 mg of the anabolic steroid oxandrolone. Oxandrolone is 17β-hydroxy-17α-methyl-2-oxa-5α-androstan-3-one with the following structural formula:

Inactive ingredients include cornstarch, lactose, magnesium stearate, and hydroxypropyl methylcellulose.

CLINICAL PHARMACOLOGY

Anabolic steroids are synthetic derivatives of testosterone. Certain clinical effects and adverse reactions demonstrate the androgenic properties of this class of drugs. Complete dissociation of anabolic and androgenic effects has not been achieved. The actions of anabolic steroids are therefore similar to those of male sex hormones with the possibility of causing serious disturbances of growth and sexual development if given to young children. Anabolic steroids suppress the gonadotropic functions of the pituitary and may exert a direct effect upon the testes.

During exogenous administration of anabolic androgens, endogenous testosterone release is inhibited through inhibition of pituitary luteinizing hormone (LH). At large doses, spermatogenesis may be suppressed through feedback inhibition of pituitary follicle-stimulating hormone (FSH).

Anabolic steroids have been reported to increase low-density lipoproteins and decrease high-density lipoproteins. These levels revert to normal on discontinuation of treatment.

INDICATIONS AND USAGE

Oxandrin is indicated as adjunctive therapy to promote weight gain after weight loss following extensive surgery, chronic infections, or severe trauma, and in some patients who without definite pathophysiologic reasons fail to gain or to maintain normal weight, to offset the protein catabolism associated with prolonged administration of corticosteroids, and for the relief of the bone pain frequently accompanying osteoporosis (See **DOSAGE AND ADMINISTRATION**).

DRUG ABUSE AND DEPENDENCE

Oxandrolone is classified as a controlled substance under the Anabolic Steroids Control Act of 1990 and has been assigned to Schedule III (non-narcotic).

CONTRAINDICATIONS

1. Known or suspected carcinoma of the prostate or the male breast.
2. Carcinoma of the breast in females with hypercalcemia (androgenic anabolic steroids may stimulate osteolytic bone resorption).
3. Pregnancy, because of possible masculinization of the fetus. Oxandrin has been shown to cause embryotoxicity, fetotoxicity, infertility, and masculinization of female animal offspring when given in doses 9 times the human dose.
4. Nephrosis, the nephrotic phase of nephritis.
5. Hypercalcemia.

WARNINGS

PELIOSIS HEPATIS, A CONDITION IN WHICH LIVER AND SOMETIMES SPLENIC TISSUE IS REPLACED WITH BLOOD-FILLED CYSTS, HAS BEEN REPORTED IN PATIENTS RECEIVING ANDROGENIC ANABOLIC STEROID THERAPY. THESE CYSTS ARE SOMETIMES PRESENT WITH MINIMAL HEPATIC DYSFUNCTION, BUT AT OTHER TIMES THEY HAVE BEEN ASSOCIATED WITH

LIVER FAILURE. THEY ARE OFTEN NOT RECOGNIZED UNTIL LIFE-THREATENING LIVER FAILURE OR INTRA-ABDOMINAL HEMORRHAGE DEVELOPS. WITHDRAWAL OF DRUG USUALLY RESULTS IN COMPLETE DISAPPEARANCE OF LESIONS.

LIVER CELL TUMORS ARE ALSO REPORTED. MOST OFTEN THESE TUMORS ARE BENIGN AND ANDROGEN-DEPENDENT, BUT FATAL MALIGNANT TUMORS HAVE BEEN REPORTED. WITHDRAWAL OF DRUG OFTEN RESULTS IN REGRESSION OR CESSATION OF PROGRESSION OF THE TUMOR. HOWEVER, HEPATIC TUMORS ASSOCIATED WITH ANDROGENS OR ANABOLIC STEROIDS ARE MUCH MORE VASCULAR THAN OTHER HEPATIC TUMORS AND MAY BE SILENT UNTIL LIFE-THREATENING INTRA-ABDOMINAL HEMORRHAGE DEVELOPS. BLOOD LIPID CHANGES THAT ARE KNOWN TO BE ASSOCIATED WITH INCREASED RISK OF ATHEROSCLEROSIS ARE SEEN IN PATIENTS TREATED WITH ANDROGENS OR ANABOLIC STEROIDS. THESE CHANGES INCLUDE DECREASED HIGH-DENSITY LIPOPROTEINS AND SOMETIMES INCREASED LOW-DENSITY LIPOPROTEINS. THE CHANGES MAY BE VERY MARKED AND COULD HAVE A SERIOUS IMPACT ON THE RISK OF ATHEROSCLEROSIS AND CORONARY ARTERY DISEASE.

Cholestatic hepatitis and jaundice may occur with 17-alpha-alkylated androgens at a relatively low dose. If cholestatic hepatitis with jaundice appears or if liver function tests become abnormal, oxandrolone should be discontinued and the etiology should be determined. Drug-induced jaundice is reversible when the medication is discontinued.

In patients with breast cancer, anabolic steroid therapy may cause hypercalcemia by stimulating osteolysis. Oxandrolone therapy should be discontinued if hypercalcemia occurs.

Edema with or without congestive heart failure may be a serious complication in patients with pre-existing cardiac, renal, or hepatic disease. Concomitant administration of adrenal cortical steroid or ACTH may increase the edema.

In children, androgen therapy may accelerate bone maturation without producing compensatory gain in linear growth. This adverse effect results in compromised adult height. The younger the child, the greater the risk of compromising final mature height. The effect on bone maturation should be monitored by assessing bone age of the left wrist and hand every 6 months (See **PRECAUTIONS: Laboratory tests**).

Geriatric patients treated with androgenic anabolic steroids may be at an increased risk for the development of prostatic hypertrophy and prostatic carcinoma.

ANABOLIC STEROIDS HAVE NOT BEEN SHOWN TO ENHANCE ATHLETIC ABILITY.

PRECAUTIONS

General:

Women should be observed for signs of virilization (deepening of the voice, hirsutism, acne, clitoromegaly). Discontinuation of drug therapy at the time of evidence of mild virilism is necessary to prevent irreversible virilization. Some virilizing changes in women are irreversible even after prompt discontinuance of therapy and are not prevented by concomitant use of estrogens. Menstrual irregularities may also occur.

Anabolic steroids may cause suppression of clotting factors II, V, VII, and X, and an increase in prothrombin time.

Information for patients:

The physician should instruct patients to report any of the following side effects of androgens:

Males: Too frequent or persistent erections of the penis, appearance or aggravation of acne.

Females: Hoarseness, acne, changes in menstrual periods, or more facial hair.

All patients: Nausea, vomiting, changes in skin color, or ankle swelling.

Laboratory tests:

Women with disseminated breast carcinoma should have frequent determination of urine and serum calcium levels during the course of therapy (See **WARNINGS**).

Because of the hepatotoxicity associated with the use of 17-alpha-alkylated androgens, liver function tests should be obtained periodically.

Periodic (every 6 months) x-ray examinations of bone age should be made during treatment of children to determine the rate of bone maturation and the effects of androgen therapy on the epiphyseal centers.

Serum lipids and high-density lipoprotein cholesterol determinations should be done periodically as androgenic anabolic steroids have been reported to increase low-density lipoproteins. Serum cholesterol levels may increase during therapy. Therefore, caution is required when administering these agents to patients with a history of myocardial infarc-

tion or coronary artery disease. Serial determinations of serum cholesterol should be made and therapy adjusted accordingly.

Hemoglobin and hematocrit should be checked periodically for polycythemia in patients who are receiving high doses of anabolic steroids.

Drug interactions
Anticoagulants:

Anabolic steroids may increase sensitivity to oral anticoagulants. Dosage of the anticoagulant may have to be decreased in order to maintain desired prothrombin time. Patients receiving oral anticoagulant therapy require close monitoring, especially when anabolic steroids are started or stopped.

Oral hypoglycemic agents:

Oxandrolone may inhibit the metabolism of oral hypoglycemic agents.

Adrenal steroids or ACTH:

In patients with edema, concomitant administration with adrenal cortical steroids or ACTH may increase the edema.

Drug/Laboratory test interactions:

Anabolic steroids may decrease levels of thyroxine-binding globulin, resulting in decreased total T_4 serum levels and increased resin uptake of T_3 and T_4. Free thyroid hormone levels remain unchanged. In addition, a decrease in PBI and radioactive iodine uptake may occur.

Carcinogenesis, mutagenesis, impairment of fertility
Animal data:

Oxandrolone has not been tested in laboratory animals for carcinogenic or mutagenic effects. In 2-year chronic oral rat studies, a dose-related reduction of spermatogenesis and decreased organ weights (testes, prostate, seminal vesicles, ovaries, uterus, adrenals, and pituitary) were shown.

Human data:

Liver cell tumors have been reported in patients receiving long-term therapy with androgenic anabolic steroids in high doses (See **WARNINGS**). Withdrawal of the drugs did not lead to regression of the tumors in all cases.

Geriatric patients treated with androgenic anabolic steroids may be at an increased risk for the development of prostatic hypertrophy and prostatic carcinoma.

Pregnancy:

Teratogenic effects—Pregnancy Category X (See **CONTRAINDICATIONS**).

Nursing mothers:

It is not known whether anabolic steroids are excreted in human milk. Because of the potential for serious adverse reactions in nursing infants from oxandrolone, a decision should be made whether to discontinue nursing or to discontinue the drug, taking into account the importance of the drug to the mother.

Pediatric use:

Anabolic agents may accelerate epiphyseal maturation more rapidly than linear growth in children and the effect may continue for 6 months after the drug has been stopped. Therefore, therapy should be monitored by x-ray studies at 6-month intervals in order to avoid the risk of compromising adult height. Androgenic anabolic steroid therapy should be used very cautiously in children and only by specialists who are aware of the effects on bone maturation (See **WARNINGS**).

ADVERSE REACTIONS

The following adverse reactions have been associated with use of anabolic steroids:

Hepatic: Cholestatic jaundice with, rarely, hepatic necrosis and death. Hepatocellular neoplasms and peliosis hepatis with long-term therapy (See **WARNINGS**). Reversible changes in liver function tests also occur including increased bromsulphthalein (BSP) retention, and increases in serum bilirubin, aspartate aminotransferase (AST, SGOT) and alkaline phosphatase.

In *males:*
  Prepubertal: Phallic enlargement and increased frequency or persistence of erections.
  Postpubertal: Inhibition of testicular function, testicular atrophy and oligospermia, impotence, chronic priapism, epididymitis, and bladder irritability.

In *females:*
Clitoral enlargement, menstrual irregularities.

CNS: Habituation, excitation, insomnia, depression, and changes in libido.

Hematologic: Bleeding in patients on concomitant anticoagulant therapy.

Breast: Gynecomastia.

Larynx: Deepening of the voice in females.

Hair: Hirsutism and male pattern baldness in females.

Skin: Acne (especially in females and prepubertal males).

Skeletal: Premature closure of epiphyses in children (See **PRECAUTIONS: Pediatric use**).

Fluid and electrolytes: Edema, retention of serum electrolytes (sodium chloride, potassium, phosphate, calcium).

Metabolic/Endocrine: Decreased glucose tolerance (See **PRECAUTIONS: Laboratory tests**), increased creatinine excretion, increased serum levels of creatinine phosphokinase (CPK). Masculinization of the fetus. Inhibition of gonadotropin secretion.

OVERDOSAGE

No symptoms or signs associated with overdosage have been reported. It is possible that sodium and water retention may occur.

The oral LD_{50} of oxandrolone in mice and dogs is greater than 5,000 mg/kg. No specific antidote is known, but gastric lavage may be used.

DOSAGE AND ADMINISTRATION

Therapy with anabolic steroids is adjunctive to and not a replacement for conventional therapy. The duration of therapy with Oxandrin (oxandrolone) will depend on the response of the patient and the possible appearance of adverse reactions. Therapy should be intermittent.

Adults: The *usual adult* dosage of Oxandrin is one 2.5-mg tablet 2 to 4 times daily. However, the response of individuals to anabolic steroids varies, and a daily dosage of as little as 2.5 mg or as much as 20 mg may be required to achieve the desired response. A course of therapy of 2 to 4 weeks is usually adequate. This may be repeated intermittently as indicated.

Children: For children the total daily dosage of Oxandrin is ≤ 0.1 mg per kilogram body weight or ≤ 0.045 mg per pound of body weight. This may be repeated intermittently as indicated.

HOW SUPPLIED

Oxandrin 2.5-mg tablets are oval, white, and scored with BTG on one side and "11" on each side of the scoreline on the other side; bottles of 100 (NDC 54396-111-11).

Rx only

Revised: Apr. 17, 1998

Manufactured for
BTG Pharmaceuticals by:
G.D. Searle & Co.
Chicago, IL 60680
Address medical inquires to:
BTG Pharmaceuticals
Medical Affairs
70 Wood Avenue South
Iselin, NJ 08830
BTG PHARMACEUTICALS
©1996, BTG Pharmaceuticals
BTG PHARMACEUTICALS
OXANDRIN®
(oxandrolone tablets, USP)

A05268-1

J.R. Carlson Laboratories, Inc.
15 COLLEGE DR.
ARLINGTON HEIGHTS, IL 60004-1985

Direct Inquiries to:
Customer Service
(847) 255-1600
FAX: (847) 255-1605

For Medical Information Contact:
In Emergencies:
Customer Service
(847) 255-1600
FAX: (847) 255-1605

ACES®   OTC

DESCRIPTION

ACES provides four natural antioxidant nutrients.

Two Soft Gels Contain:		% U.S. RDA
Beta-Carotene (Pro-Vitamin A)	10,000 IU	200%
Vitamin C (Calcium Ascorbate)	1000 mg	1667%
Vitamin E (d-Alpha Tocopherol)	400 IU	1333%
Selenium (L-selenomethionine)	100 mcg	*

RDA: Recommended Daily Allowance—Adults
*U.S. RDA not determined

The nutrients in ACES are: Beta Carotene—(Pro-vitamin A) derived from tiny sea plants or algae (*D. salina*) grown in the fresh ocean waters off southern Australia; Vitamin C provided as the gentle, buffered calcium ascorbate; Vitamin E 100% natural-source from soy, the most biologically active form; And Selenium—organically bound with the essential nutrient methionine to promote assimilation.

Suggested Use: For dietary supplementation, take two soft gels daily, preferably at mealtime.
Corn-free. Wheat-free. Milk-free. Sugar-free. Yeast-free. Preservative-free. Soft Gel Contents: Nutrients listed above, soybean oil, vegetable stearin, lecithin, beeswax. Soft Gel Shell: Beef gelatin, glycerin, water, carob.

HOW SUPPLIED

In bottles of 50, 90, 200, and 360.
Also available as *ACES® plus ZINC.*

CO-Q10   OTC

As a key component of the electron transport chain, Co-Enzyme Q-10 plays an important role in the production of ATP energy. Carlson Co-Q10 is in opaque soft-gels, which protect against degradation by heat, light, and air. Natural Vitamin E is added to protect freshness and potency. Available in 10 mg, 30 mg, 50 mg, 100 mg strengths.

HOW SUPPLIED

Bottles of 30, 50, 60, 90, 100, 120, 240, 300, 360.

E-GEMS®   OTC

DESCRIPTION

100% natural-source vitamin E (d-alpha tocopheryl acetate) soft gels. Available in 8 strengths: 30 IU, 100 IU, 200 IU, 400 IU, 600 IU, 800 IU, 1000 IU, 1200 IU.

HOW SUPPLIED

Supplied in a variety of bottle sizes.

Carnrick Laboratories, Inc.
65 HORSE HILL ROAD
CEDAR KNOLLS, NJ 07927

Direct Inquiries to:
(973) 267-2670
FAX: (973) 267-2289

For Medical Information Contact:
Technical Service Dept.
(973) 267-2670
FAX: (973) 267-2289

AMEN®   ℞
[ā 'men ']
(medroxyprogesterone acetate
tablets USP 10 mg)

CAUTION

Federal Law Prohibits Dispensing Without Prescription

WARNING
THE USE OF AMEN® (MEDROXYPROGESTERONE ACETATE) DURING THE FIRST FOUR MONTHS OF PREGNANCY IS NOT RECOMMENDED.
Progestational agents have been used beginning with the first trimester of pregnancy in an attempt to prevent habitual abortion. There is no adequate evidence that such use is effective when such drugs are given during the first four months of pregnancy. Furthermore, in the vast majority of women, the cause of abortion is a defective ovum, which progestational agents could not be expected to influence. In addition, the use of progestational agents, with their uterine-relaxant properties, in patients with fertilized defective ova may cause a delay in spontaneous abortion. Therefore, the use of such drugs during the first four months of pregnancy is not recommended.
Several reports suggest an association between intrauterine exposure to progestational drugs in the first trimester of pregnancy and genital abnormalities in male and female fetuses. The risk of hypospadias, 5 to 8 per 1,000 male births in the general population, may be approximately doubled with exposure to these drugs. There are insufficient data to quantify the risk to exposed female fetuses, but insofar as some of these drugs induce mild virilization of the external genitalia of the female fetus, and because of the increased association of hypospadias in the male fetus, it is prudent to avoid the use of these drugs during the first trimester of pregnancy.
If the patient is exposed to AMEN® Tablets (medroxyprogesterone acetate) during the first four months of pregnancy or if she becomes pregnant while taking this drug, she should be apprised of the potential risks to the fetus.

DESCRIPTION

AMEN® tablets contain medroxyprogesterone acetate, which is a derivative of progesterone. It is a white to off-white, odorless crystalline powder, stable in air, melting between 200° and 210°C. It is freely soluble in chloroform, soluble in acetone and in dioxane, sparingly soluble in alcohol and in methanol, slightly soluble in ether, and insoluble in water.

The chemical name for medroxyprogesterone acetate is pregn-4-ene-3,20-dione, 17-(acetyloxy)-6-methyl-, (6α)- with molecular formula $C_{24}H_{34}O_4$ and a molecular weight of 386.53. The structural formula is:

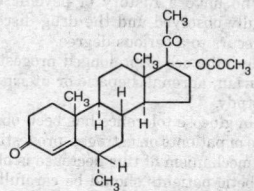

Each AMEN® tablet for oral administration contains 10 mg of medroxyprogesterone acetate.

AMEN® tablets contain Anhydrous Lactose, Colloidal Silicon Dioxide, Magnesium Stearate, Microcrystalline Cellulose, D&C Yellow #10, FD&C Blue #1, FD&C Red #40, and FD&C Yellow #6 as color additives.

CLINICAL PHARMACOLOGY

Medroxyprogesterone acetate administered orally or parenterally in the recommended doses to women with adequate endogenous estrogen, transforms proliferative into secretory endometrium. Androgenic and anabolic effects have been noted, but the drug is apparently devoid of significant estrogenic activity. While parenterally administered medroxyprogesterone acetate inhibits gonadotropin production, which in turn prevents follicular maturation and ovulation, available data indicate that this does not occur when the usually recommended oral dosage is given as single daily doses.

INDICATIONS AND USAGE

Secondary amenorrhea; abnormal uterine bleeding due to hormonal imbalance in the absence of organic pathology, such as fibroids or uterine cancer.

CONTRAINDICATIONS

1. Thrombophlebitis, thromboembolic disorders, cerebral apoplexy or patients with a past history of these conditions. **2.** Liver dysfunction or disease. **3.** Known or suspected malignancy of breast or genital organs. **4.** Undiagnosed vaginal bleeding. **5.** Missed abortion. **6.** As a diagnostic test for pregnancy. **7.** Known sensitivity to AMEN® (medroxyprogesterone acetate tablets).

WARNINGS

1. The physician should be alert to the earliest manifestations of thrombotic disorders (thrombophlebitis, cerebrovascular disorders, pulmonary embolism, and retinal thrombosis). Should any of these occur or be suspected, the drug should be discontinued immediately.
2. Beagle dogs treated with medroxyprogesterone acetate developed mammary nodules, some of which were malignant. Although nodules occasionally appeared in control animals, they were intermittent in nature, whereas the nodules in the drug treated animals were larger, more numerous, persistent, and there were some breast malignancies with metastases. Their significance with respect to humans has not been established.
3. Discontinue medication pending examination if there is sudden partial or complete loss of vision, or if there is a sudden onset of proptosis, diplopia or migraine. If examination reveals papilledema, or retinal vascular lesions, medication should be withdrawn.
4. Detectable amounts of progestin have been identified in the milk of mothers receiving the drug. The effect of this on the nursing infant has not been determined.
5. Usage in pregnancy is not recommended (See WARNING Box).
6. Retrospective studies of morbidity and mortality in Great Britain and studies of morbidity in the United States have shown a statistically significant association between thrombophlebitis, pulmonary embolism, and cerebral thrombosis and embolism and the use of oral contraceptives.[1-4] The estimate of the relative risk of thromboembolism in the study by Vessey and Doll[3] was about sevenfold, while Sartwell and associates[4] in the United States found a relative risk of 4.4, meaning that the users are several times as likely to undergo thromboembolic disease without evident cause as nonusers. The American study also indicated that the risk did not persist after discontinuation of administration, and that it was not enhanced by long continued administration. The American study was not designed to evaluate a difference between products.

PRECAUTIONS

1. The pretreatment physical examination should include special reference to breast and pelvic organs, as well as Papanicolaou smear.

Continued on next page

Amen—Cont.

2. Because progestogens may cause some degree of fluid retention, conditions which might be influenced by this factor, such as epilepsy, migraine, asthma, cardiac or renal dysfunction require careful observation.
3. In cases of breakthrough bleeding, as in all cases of irregular bleeding per vaginum, nonfunctional causes should be borne in mind. In cases of undiagnosed vaginal bleeding adequate diagnostic measures are indicated.
4. Patients who have a history of psychic depression should be carefully observed and the drug discontinued if the depression recurs to a serious degree.
5. Any possible influence of prolonged progestin therapy on pituitary, ovarian, adrenal, hepatic or uterine functions awaits further study.
6. A decrease in glucose tolerance has been observed in a small percentage of patients on estrogen-progestin combination drugs. The mechanism of this decrease is obscure. For this reason, diabetic patients should be carefully observed while receiving progestin therapy.
7. The age of the patient constitutes no absolute limiting factor although treatment with progestins may mask the onset of the climacteric.
8. The pathologist should be advised of progestin therapy when relevant specimens are submitted.
9. Because of the occasional occurrence of thrombotic disorders, (thrombophlebitis, pulmonary embolism, retinal thrombosis, and cerebrovascular disorders) in patients taking estrogen-progestin combinations and since the mechanism is obscure, the physician should be alert to the earliest manifestation of these disorders.
10. Studies of the addition of a progestin product to an estrogen replacement regimen for seven or more days of a cycle of estrogen administration have reported a lowered incidence of endomentrial hyperplasia. Morphological and biochemical studies of endometrium suggest that 10–13 days of a progestin are needed to provide maximal maturation of the endometrium and to eliminate any hyperplastic changes. Whether this will provide protection from endometrial carcinoma has not been clearly established. There are possible additional risks which may be associated with the inclusion of progestin in estrogen replacement regimens. The potential risks include adverse effects on carbohydrate and lipid metabolism. The dosage used may be important in minimizing these adverse effects.
11. Aminoglutethimide administered concomitantly with AMEN® may significantly depress the bioavailability of AMEN®.

Carcinogenesis, Mutagenesis, Impairment of Fertility.
Long-term intramuscular administration of medroxyprogesterone acetate has been shown to produce mammary tumors in beagle dogs (see WARNINGS). There was no evidence of a carcinogenic effect associated with the oral administration of medroxyprogesterone acetate to rats and mice. Medroxyprogesterone acetate was not mutagenic in a battery of *in vitro* or *in vivo* genetic toxicity assays.
Medroxyprogesterone acetate at high doses is an antifertility drug and high doses would be expected to impair fertility until the cessation of treatment.

Information for the Patient
See Patient Information at end of insert.

ADVERSE REACTIONS

Pregnancy—(See WARNING Box for possible adverse effects on the fetus).
Breast—Breast tenderness or galactorrhea has been reported rarely.
Skin—Sensitivity reactions consisting of urticaria, pruritus, edema and generalized rash have occured in an occasional patient. Acne, alopecia and hirsutism have been reported in a few cases.
Thromboembolic Phenomena—Thromboembolic phenomena including thrombophlebitis and pulmonary embolism have been reported.
The following adverse reactions have been observed in women taking progestins including medroxyprogesterone acetate tablets: breakthrough bleeding; spotting; change in menstrual flow; amenorrhea; edema; change in weight (increase or decrease); changes in cervical erosion and cervical secretions; cholestatic jaundice; anaphylactoid reactions and anaphylaxis; rash (allergic) with and without pruritus; mental depression; pyrexia; insomnia; nausea; somnolence.
A statistically significant association has been demonstrated between use of estrogen-progestin combination drugs and the following serious adverse reactions: thrombophlebitis, pulmonary embolism and cerebral thrombosis and embolism. For this reason patients on progestin therapy should be carefully observed.
Although available evidence is suggestive of an association, such a relationship has been neither confirmed nor refuted for the following serious adverse reactions: neuro-ocular lesions, eg. retinal thrombosis and optic neuritis.
The following adverse reactions have been observed in patients receiving estrogen-progestin combination drugs: rise in blood pressure in susceptible individuals; premenstrual-like syndrome; changes in libido; changes in appetite; cystitis-like syndrome; headache; nervousness; fatigue; backache; hirsutism; loss of scalp hair; erythema multiforme; erythema nodosum; hemorrhagic eruption; itching; dizziness. In view of these observations, patients on progestin therapy should be carefully observed.
The following laboratory results may be altered by the use of estrogen-progestin combination drugs:
Increased sulfobromophthalein retention and other hepatic function tests.
Coagulation tests: increase in prothrombin factors VII, VIII, IX and X.
Metyrapone test.
Pregnanediol determination.
Thyroid function: increase in PBI, and butanol extractable protein bound iodine and decrease in T^3 uptake values.

DOSAGE AND ADMINISTRATION

Secondary Amenorrhea—AMEN® (medroxyprogesterone acetate tablets) may be given in dosages of 5 to 10 mg daily for from 5 to 10 days. A dose for inducing an optimum secretory transformation of an endometrium that has been adequately primed with either endogenous or exogenous estrogen is 10 mg of AMEN® daily for 10 days. In cases of seconary amenorrhea, therapy may be started at any time. Progestin withdrawal bleeding usually occurs within three to seven days after discontinuing AMEN® therapy.
Abnormal Uterine Bleeding Due to Hormonal Imbalance in the Absence of Organic Pathology—Beginning on the calculated 16th or 21st day of the menstrual cycle, 5 to 10 mg of medroxyprogesterone acetate may be given daily for from 5 to 10 days. To produce an optimum secretory transformation of an endometrium that has been adequately primed with either endogenous or exogenous estrogen, 10 mg of medroxyprogesterone acetate daily for 10 days beginning on the 16th day of the cycle is suggested. Progestin withdrawal bleeding usually occurs within three to seven days after discontinuing therapy with AMEN®. Patients with a past history of recurrent episodes of abnormal uterine bleeding may benefit from planned menstrual cycling with AMEN®.

HOW SUPPLIED

Two-layered peach and white scored tablet with "C" on one side and "AMEN" on the other. AMEN® tablets containing 10 mg of medroxyprogesterone acetate USP are available in bottles of 50 (NDC 0086-0049-05), 100 (NDC 0086-0049-10) and 1000 (NDC 0086-0049-90).
Store at controlled room temperature 15°–30°C (59°–86°F).

REFERENCES

1. Royal College of General Practitioners: Oral contraception and thromboembolic disease. J Coll Gen Prac *13*:267–279, 1967.
2. Inman WHW, Vessey MP: Investigation of deaths from pulmonary, coronary, and cerebral thrombosis and embolism in women of child-bearing age. Br Med J *2*:193–199, 1968.
3. Vessey MP, Doll R: Investigation of relation between use of oral contraceptives and thromboembolic disease. A further report. Br Med J *2*:651–657, 1969.
4. Sartwell PE, Masi AT, Arthes FG, et al: Thromboembolism and oral contraceptives: An epidemiological case-control study. Am J Epidemiol *90*:365–380, 1969.

The text of the patient insert for progesterone and progesterone-like drugs is set forth below.

PATIENT INFORMATION: AMEN® Tablets contain medroxyprogesterone acetate, a progesterone. The information below is that which the U.S. Food and Drug Administration requires be provided for all patients taking progesterones. The information below relates only to the risk to the unborn child associated with use of progesterone during pregnancy. For further information on the use, side effects and other risks associated with this product, ask your doctor.

WARNING FOR WOMEN
Progesterone or progesterone-like drugs have been used to prevent miscarriage in the first few months of pregnancy. No adequate evidence is available to show that they are effective for this purpose. Furthermore, most cases of early miscarriage are due to causes which could not be helped by these drugs.
There is an increased risk of minor birth defects in children whose mothers take this drug during the first 4 months of pregnancy. Several reports suggest an association between mothers who take these drugs in the first trimester of pregnancy and genital abnormalities in male and female babies. The risk to the male baby is the possibility of being born with a condition in which the opening of the penis is on the underside rather than the tip of the penis (hypospadias). Hypospadias occurs in about 5 to 8 per 1,000 male births and is about doubled with exposure to these drugs. There is not enough information to quantify the risk to exposed female fetuses, but enlargement of the clitoris and fusion of the labia may occur, although rarely.
Therefore, since drugs of this type may induce mild masculinization of the external genitalia of the female fetus, as well as hypospadias in the male fetus, it is wise to avoid using the drug during the first trimester of pregnancy.
These drugs have been used as a test for pregnancy but such use is no longer considered safe because of possible damage to a developing baby. Also, more rapid methods for testing for pregnancy are now available.
If you take AMEN® (medroxyprogesterone acetate tablets) and later find you were pregnant when you took it, be sure to discuss this with your doctor as soon as possible.
Manufactured for Carnrick Laboratories, Inc.
Revised September 1994
Shown in Product Identification Guide, page 308

BONTRIL® PDM Ⓒ III

[*bŏn 'tril*]
(phendimetrazine tartrate tablets, USP 35 mg)

HOW SUPPLIED

Three-layered green, white and yellow tablet with 8648 on the scored side and the letter "C" on the other. Bontril® PDM tablets containing 35 mg of phendimetrazine tartrate are available in bottles of 100 (NDC 0086-0048-10) and 1,000 (NDC 0086-0048-90).

CAUTION

Federal law prohibits dispensing without prescription.
See product insert for complete information.
Manufactured for Carnrick Laboratories, Inc.
Shown in Product Identification Guide, page 308

BONTRIL® SLOW-RELEASE Ⓒ III

[*bŏn 'tril*]
(brand of phendimetrazine tartrate slow-release capsules 105 mg)

DESCRIPTION

Phendimetrazine tartrate, as the dextro isomer, has the chemical name of (+)-3,4-Dimethyl-2-phenylmorpholine Tartrate.
The structural formula is as follows:

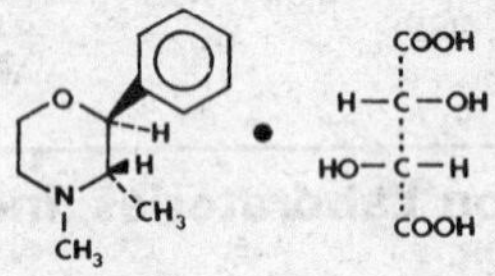

M.W. 341

Phendimetrazine tartrate is a white, odorless powder with a bitter taste. It is soluble in water, methanol and ethanol. Bontril Slow-Release capsules contain FD&C Yellow No. 6 as a color additive.

ACTIONS

Phendimetrazine tartrate is a sympathomimetic amine with pharmacological activity similar to the prototype drugs of this class used in obesity, the amphetamines. Actions include central nervous system stimulation and elevation of blood pressure. Tachyphylaxis and tolerance have been demonstrated with all drugs of this class in which these phenomena have been looked for.
Drugs of this class used in obesity are commonly known as "anorectics" or "anorexigenics". It has not been established, however, that the action of such drugs in treating obesity is primarily one of appetite suppression. Other central nervous system actions or metabolic effects may be involved.
Adult obese subjects instructed in dietary management and treated with anorectic drugs lose more weight on the average than those treated with placebo and diet, as determined in relatively short term clinical trials.
The magnitude of increased weight loss of drug-treated patients over placebo-treated patients is only a fraction of a pound a week. The rate of weight loss is greatest in the first weeks of therapy for both drug and placebo subjects and tends to decrease in succeeding weeks. The possible origin of the increased weight loss due to the various drug effects is not established. The amount of weight loss associated with the use of an anorectic drug varies from trial to trial, and the increased weight loss appears to be related in part to variables other than the drug prescribed, such as the physician investigator, the population treated, and the diet prescribed. Studies do not permit conclusions as to the relative importance of the drug and non-drug factors on weight loss.
The natural history of obesity is measured in years, whereas the studies cited are restricted to a few weeks duration; thus, the total impact of drug-induced weight loss over that of diet alone must be considered clinically limited.
The active drug 105 mg of phendimetrazine tartrate in each capsule of this special slow-release dosage form approximates the action of three 35 mg non-time release doses taken at 4 hours intervals.

The major route of elimination is via the kidneys where most of the drug and metabolites are excreted. Some of the drug is metabolized to phenmetrazine and also phendimetrazine-N-oxide.

The average half-life of elimination when studied under controlled conditions is about 1.9 hours for the non-time and 9.8 hours for the slow-release dosage form. The absorption half-life of the drug from conventional non-time 35 mg phendimetrazine tartrate tablets is approximately the same. These data indicate that the slow-release product has a similar onset of action to the conventional non-time-release product and, in addition, has a prolonged therapeutic effect.

INDICATIONS

Phendimetrazine tartrate is indicated in the management of exogenous obesity as a short term adjunct (a few weeks) in a regimen of weight reduction based on caloric restriction. The limited usefulness of agents of this class (see ACTIONS) should be measured against possible risk factors inherent in their use such as those described below.

CONTRAINDICATIONS

Advanced arteriosclerosis, symptomatic cardiovascular disease, moderate and severe hypertension, hyperthyroidism, known hypersensitivity, or idiosyncrasy to the sympathomimetic amines, glaucoma. Agitated states. Patients with a history of drug abuse. Use in patients taking other CNS stimulants including monoamine oxidase inhibitors.

WARNINGS

Tolerance to the anorectic effect usually develops within a few weeks. When this occurs, the recommended dose should not be exceeded in an attempt to increase the effect; rather, the drug should be discontinued.

Use of phendimetrazine tartrate within 14 days following the administration of monoamine oxidase inhibitors may result in a hypertensive crisis.

Abrupt cessation of administration following prolonged high dosage results in extreme fatigue and depression. Because of the effect on the central nervous system phendimetrazine tartrate may impair the ability of the patient to engage in potentially hazardous activities such as operating machinery or driving a motor vehicle; the patient should therefore be cautioned accordingly.

PRECAUTIONS

Caution is to be exercised in prescribing phendimetrazine tartrate for patients with even mild hypertension.

Insulin requirements in diabetes mellitus may be altered in association with the use of phendimetrazine tartrate and the concomitant dietary regimen.

Phendimetrazine tartrate may decrease the hypotensive effect of guanethidine.

The least amount feasible should be prescribed or dispensed at one time in order to minimize the possibility of overdosage.

Usage in Pregnancy: Safe use in pregnancy has not been established. Until more information is available, phendimetrazine tartrate should not be taken by women who are or may become pregnant unless, in the opinion of the physician, the potential benefits outweigh the possible hazards.

Usage in Children: Phendimetrazine tartrate is not recommended for use in children under 12 years of age.

ADVERSE REACTIONS

Cardiovascular: Palpitation, tachycardia, elevation of blood pressure.

Central Nervous System: Overstimulation, restlessness, dizziness, insomnia, tremor, headache; rarely psychotic episodes at recommended doses, agitation, flushing, sweating, blurring of vision.

Gastrointestinal: Dryness of the mouth, diarrhea, constipation, nausea, stomach pain.

Genitourinary: Changes in libido, urinary frequency, dysuria.

DRUG ABUSE AND DEPENDENCE

Controlled Substance: Phendimetrazine tartrate is a Schedule III controlled substance.

Dependence: Phendimetrazine Tartrate is related chemically and pharmacologically to the amphetamines. Amphetamines and related stimulant drugs have been extensively abused, and the possibility of abuse of phendimetrazine should be kept in mind when evaluating the desirability of including a drug as part of a weight reduction program. Abuse of amphetamines and related drugs may be associated with intense psychological dependence and severe social dysfunction. There are reports of patients who have increased the dosage to many times that recommended. Abrupt cessation following prolonged high dosage administration results in extreme fatigue and mental depression; changes are also noted on the sleep EEG. Manifestations of chronic intoxication with anorectic drugs include severe dermatoses, marked insomnia, irritability, hyperactivity and personality changes. The most severe manifestation of chronic intoxications is psychosis, often clinically indistinguishable from schizophrenia.

OVERDOSAGE

Manifestations of acute overdosage may include restlessness, tremor, hyperreflexia, rapid respiration, confusion, assaultiveness, hallucinations, panic states.

Fatigue and depression usually follow the central stimulation.

Cardiovascular effects include arrhythmias, hypertension, or hypotension and circulatory collapse. Gastrointestinal symptoms include nausea, vomiting, diarrhea, and abdominal cramps. Poisoning may result in convulsions, coma, and death.

Management of acute intoxication is largely symptomatic and includes lavage and sedation with a barbiturate. Experience with hemodialysis or peritoneal dialysis is inadequate to permit recommendation in this regard.

Acidification of the urine increases phendimetrazine tartrate excretion.

Intravenous phentolamine (Regitine) has been suggested for possible acute, severe hypertension, if this complicates overdosage.

DOSAGE AND ADMINISTRATION

One Slow-Release Capsule (105 mg) in the morning, taken 30-60 minutes before the morning meal.

Phendimetrazine Tartrate is not recommended for use in children under twelve years of age.

HOW SUPPLIED

Phendimetrazine Tartrate Slow-Release Capsules, 105 mg is supplied in bottles of 100 opaque green and clear yellow capsules, imprinted with the letter "C" and 8647. NDC # 0086-0047-10.

Store at controlled room temperature, 15°–30°C(59°–86°F). The most recent revision of this labeling is Nov. 1990.

CAUTION

Federal law prohibits dispensing without prescription.
Manufactured for Carnrick Laboratories, Inc.
Shown in Product Identification Guide, page 308

CAPITAL® AND CODEINE ORAL
SUSPENSION
(acetaminophen and codeine phosphate oral suspension USP)

HOW SUPPLIED

CAPITAL® AND CODEINE ORAL SUSPENSION contains 120 mg of acetaminophen and 12 mg of codeine phosphate/5 mL and is given orally. CAPITAL® AND CODEINE ORAL SUSPENSION is a fruit punch-flavored pink suspension available in 16 fluid oz. (473 mL) bottles, NDC 0086-0046-16.

SHAKE WELL BEFORE USING

Store at controlled room temperature 15°–30°C (59°–86°F). Dispense in tight, light-resistant glass container and label "Shake Well Before Using."

CAUTION

Federal law prohibits dispensing without prescription.
See product insert for complete information.
Manufactured for Carnrick Laboratories, Inc.
Shown in Product Identification Guide, page 308

EXGEST® LA ℞
(phenylpropanolamine hydrochloride/guaifenesin)

DESCRIPTION

Each EXGEST® LA white, lightly blue-speckled, oval, scored, long-acting tablet for oral administration contains:
phenylpropanolamine hydrochloride .... 75 mg
guaifenesin .... 400 mg
in a special base to provide a prolonged therapeutic effect. This product contains ingredients of the following therapeutic classes: decongestant and expectorant.

Phenylpropanolamine hydrochloride is a decongestant having the chemical name, benzenemethanol, α-(l-aminoethyl)-, hydrochloride (R*, S*), (±), with the following structure:

CH–CH–CH₃ · HCl
OH NH₂

Guaifenesin is an expectorant having the chemical name, 1,2-propanediol, 3-(2-methoxyphenoxy)-, with the following structure:
[See chemical structure at top of next column]

CLINICAL PHARMACOLOGY

Phenylpropanolamine hydrochloride is an α-adrenergic receptor agonist (sympathomimetic) which produces vasoconstriction by stimulating α-receptors within the mucosa of

OH
OCH₂CHCH₂OH
OCH₃

the respiratory tract. Clinically, phenylpropanolamine shrinks swollen mucous membranes, reduces tissue hyperemia, edema, and nasal congestion, and increases nasal airway patency. Guaifenesin promotes lower respiratory tract drainage by thinning bronchial secretions, lubricates irritated respiratory tract membranes through increased mucous flow, and facilitates removal of viscous, inspissated mucus. As a result, sinus and bronchial drainage is improved, and dry, nonproductive coughs become more productive and less frequent.

INDICATIONS AND USAGE

EXGEST® LA is indicated for the symptomatic relief of sinusitis, bronchitis, pharyngitis, and coryza when these conditions are associated with nasal congestion and viscous mucus in the lower respiratory tract.

CONTRAINDICATIONS

EXGEST® LA is contraindicated in individuals with known hypersensitivity to sympathomimetics, severe hypertension, or in patients receiving monoamine oxidase inhibitors.

WARNINGS

Sympathomimetic amines should be used with caution in patients with hypertension, diabetes mellitus, heart disease, peripheral vascular disease, increased intraocular pressure, hyperthyroidism, or prostatic hypertrophy.

PRECAUTIONS

Information for Patients: Do not crush or chew EXGEST® LA tablets prior to swallowing.

Drug Interactions: EXGEST® LA should not be used in patients taking monoamine oxidase inhibitors or other sympathomimetics.

Drug/Laboratory Test Interactions: Guaifenesin has been reported to interfere with clinical laboratory determinations of urinary 5-hydroxyindoleacetic acid (5-HIAA) and urinary vanillylmandelic acid (VMA).

Pregnancy: Pregnancy Category C. Animal reproduction studies have not been conducted with EXGEST® LA. It is also not known whether EXGEST® LA can cause fetal harm when administered to a pregnant woman or can affect reproduction capacity. EXGEST® LA should not be given to a pregnant woman, unless clearly needed.

Nursing Mothers: It is not known whether the drugs in EXGEST® LA are excreted in human milk. Because many drugs are excreted in human milk and because of the potential for serious adverse reactions in nursing infants, a decision should be made whether to discontinue nursing or to discontinue the product, taking into account the importance of the drug to the mother.

Pediatric Use: Safety and effectivness of EXGEST® LA tablets in children below the age of 6 have not been established.

ADVERSE REACTIONS

Possible adverse reactions include nervousness, insomnia, restlessness, headache, nausea, or gastric irritation. These reactions seldom, if ever, require discontinuation of therapy. Urinary retention may occur in patients with prostatic hypertrophy.

OVERDOSAGE

The treatment of overdosage should provide symptomatic and supportive care. If the amount ingested is considered dangerous or excessive, induce vomiting with ipecac syrup unless the patient is convulsing, comatose, or has lost the gag reflex, in which case perform gastric lavage using a large-bore tube. If indicated, follow with activated charcoal and a saline cathartic. Since the effects of EXGEST® LA may last up to 12 hours, treatment should be continued for at least that length of time.

DOSAGE AND ADMINISTRATION

Adults and children 12 years of age and older—one tablet twice daily (every 12 hours); **children 6 to under 12 years**—one-half (¹/₂) tablet twice daily (every 12 hours). EXGEST® LA is not recommended for children under 6 years of age. Tablets may be broken in half for ease of administration without affecting release of medication but should not be crushed or chewed prior to swallowing.

HOW SUPPLIED

EXGEST® LA is available as a white, lightly blue-speckled, oval, scored, long-acting tablet for oral administration. It is inscribed with "8673" on the scored side and "C" on the other. Each long-acting tablet contains phenylpropanol-

Continued on next page

Exgest LA—Cont.

amine hydrochloride 75 mg and guaifenesin 400 mg. Supplied in bottles of 100 tablets (NDC 0086-0063-10) and in bottles of 500 tablets (NDC 0086-0063-50).
Store at controlled room temperature, 15°–30°C (59°–86°F.)

CAUTION

Federal law prohibits dispensing without prescription.
Manufactured for Carnrick Laboratories, Inc.
7/95

Shown in Product Identification Guide, page 308

HYDROCET® CAPSULES (HYDROCODONE BITARTRATE AND ACETAMINOPHEN CAPSULES) Ⓒ III

CAUTION Federal law prohibits dispensing without prescription.

DESCRIPTION

Hydrocodone bitartrate and acetaminophen is supplied in capsule form for oral administration.
Hydrocodone bitartrate is an opioid analgesic and antitussive and occurs as fine, white crystals or as a crystalline powder. It is affected by light. The chemical name is 4,5α-epoxy-3 methoxy-17-methylmorphinan-6-one tartrate (1:1) hydrate (2:5). It has the following structural formula:

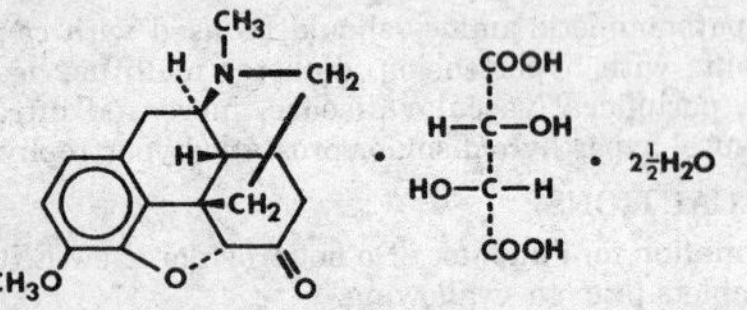

$C_{18}H_{21}NO_3 \cdot C_4H_6O_6 \cdot 2^1/_2\ H_2O$ MW = 494.50

Acetaminophen, 4'-hydroxyacetanilide, a slightly bitter, white, odorless, crystalline powder, is a non-opiate, non-salicylate analgesic and antipyretic. It has the following structural formula:

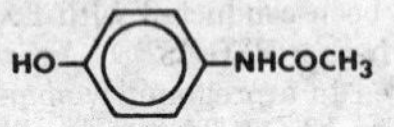

$C_8H_9NO_2$ MW = 151.16

Each Hydrocet® Capsule contains:
Hydrocodone Bitartrate*, USP .... 5 mg
*(WARNING: MAY BE HABIT FORMING)
Acetaminophen, USP .... 500 mg
In addition, each imprinted capsule contains the following inactive ingredients: Deionized Water, Ethylene Glycol Monoethyl Ether, FD&C Blue #1, Lecithin, Pharmaceutical Glaze (Modified), Simethicone, Sodium Propionate, and Titanium Dioxide.

CLINICAL PHARMACOLOGY

Hydrocodone is a semisynthetic narcotic analgesic and antitussive with multiple actions qualitatively similar to those of codeine. Most of these involve the central nervous system and smooth muscle. The precise mechanism of action of hydrocodone and other opiates is not known, although it is believed to relate to the existence of opiate receptors in the central nervous system. In addition to analgesia, narcotics may produce drowsiness, changes in mood and mental clouding.
The analgesic action of acetaminophen involves peripheral influences, but the specific mechanism is as yet undetermined. Antipyretic activity is mediated through hypothalamic heat regulating centers. Acetaminophen inhibits prostaglandin synthetase. Therapeutic doses of acetaminophen have negligible effects on the cardiovascular or respiratory systems; however, toxic doses may cause circulatory failure and rapid, shallow breathing.
Pharmacokinetics: The behavior of the individual components is described below.
Hydrocodone: Following a 10 mg oral dose of hydrocodone administered to five adult male subjects, the mean peak concentration was 23.6 ± 5.2 ng/mL. Maximum serum levels were achieved at 1.3 ± 0.3 hours and the half-life was determined to be 3.8 ± 0.3 hours. Hydrocodone exhibits a complex pattern of metabolism including O-demethylation, N-demethylation and 6-keto reduction to the corresponding 6-α-and 6-β-hydroxymetabolites.
See OVERDOSAGE for toxicity information.
Acetaminophen: Acetaminophen is rapidly absorbed from the gastrointestinal tract and is distributed throughout most body tissues. The plasma half-life is 1.25 to 3 hours, but may be increased by liver damage and following overdosage. Elimination of acetaminophen is principally by liver metabolism (conjugation) and subsequent renal excretion of metabolites. Approximately 85% of an oral dose appears in the urine within 24 hours of administration, most as the glucuronide conjugate, with small amounts of other conjugates and unchanged drug.
See OVERDOSAGE for toxicity information.

INDICATIONS AND USAGE

Hydrocet® Capsules (Hydrocodone bitartrate and acetaminophen) are indicated for the relief of moderate to moderately severe pain.

CONTRAINDICATIONS

This product should not be administered to patients who have previously exhibited hypersensitivity to hydrocodone or acetaminophen.

WARNINGS

Respiratory Depression: At high doses or in sensitive patients, hydrocodone may produce dose-related respiratory depression by acting directly on the brain stem respiratory center. Hydrocodone also affects the center that controls respiratory rhythm, and may produce irregular and periodic breathing.
Head Injury and Increased Intracranial Pressure: The respiratory depressant effects of narcotics and their capacity to elevate cerebrospinal fluid pressure may be markedly exaggerated in the presence of head injury, other intracranial lesions or a preexisting increase in intracranial pressure. Furthermore, narcotics produce adverse reactions which may obscure the clinical course of patients with head injuries.
Acute Abdominal Conditions: The administration of narcotics may obscure the diagnosis or clinical course of patients with acute abdominal conditions.

PRECAUTIONS

General: Special Risk Patients: As with any narcotic analgesic agent, Hydrocet® Capsules (hydrocodone bitartrate and acetaminophen) should be used with caution in elderly or debilitated patients, and those with severe impairment of hepatic or renal function, hypothyroidism, Addison's disease, prostatic hypertrophy or urethral stricture. The usual precautions should be observed and the possibility of respiratory depression should be kept in mind.
Cough reflex: Hydrocodone suppresses the cough reflex; as with all narcotics, caution should be exercised when Hydrocet® Capsules (hydrocodone bitartrate and acetaminophen) are used postoperatively and in patients with pulmonary disease.
Information for Patients: Hydrocodone, like all narcotics, may impair mental and/or physical abilities required for the performance of potentially hazardous tasks such as driving a car or operating machinery; patients should be cautioned accordingly.
Alcohol and other CNS depressants may produce an additive CNS depression, when taken with this combination product, and should be avoided.
Hydrocodone may be habit-forming. Patients should take the drug only for as long as it is prescribed, in the amounts prescribed, and no more frequently than prescribed.
Laboratory Tests: In patients with severe hepatic or renal disease, effects of therapy should be monitored with serial liver and/or renal function tests.
Drug Interactions: Patients receiving narcotics, antihistamines, antipsychotics, antianxiety agents, or other CNS depressants (including alcohol) concomitantly with Hydrocet® Capsules (hydrocodone bitartrate and acetaminophen) may exhibit an additive CNS depression. When combined therapy is contemplated, the dose of one or both agents should be reduced.
The use of MAO inhibitors or tricyclic antidepressants with hydrocodone preparations may increase the effect of either the antidepressant or hydrocodone.
Drug/Laboratory Test Interactions: Acetaminophen may produce false-positive test results for urinary 5-hydroxyindoleacetic acid.
Carcinogenesis, Mutagenesis, Impairment of Fertility: No adequate studies have been conducted in animals to determine whether hydrocodone or acetaminophen have a potential for carcinogenesis, mutagenesis, or impairment of fertility.
Pregnancy:
Teratogenic Effects: Pregnancy Category C: There are no adequate and well-controlled studies in pregnant women. Hydrocet® Capsules (hydrocodone bitartrate and acetaminophen) should be used during pregnancy only if the potential benefit justifies the potential risk to the fetus.
Nonteratogenic Effects: Babies born to mothers who have been taking opioids regularly prior to delivery will be physically dependent. The withdrawal signs include irritability and excessive crying, tremors, hyperactive reflexes, increased respiratory rate, increased stools, sneezing, yawning, vomiting and fever. The intensity of the syndrome does not always correlate with the duration of maternal opioid use or dose. There is no consensus on the best method of managing withdrawal.
Labor and Delivery: As with all narcotics, administration of this product to the mother shortly before delivery may result in some degree of respiratory depression in the newborn, especially if higher doses are used.
Nursing Mothers: Acetaminophen is excreted in breast milk in small amounts, but the significance of its effects on nursing infants is not known. It is not known whether hydrocodone is excreted in human milk. Because many drugs are excreted in human milk and because of the potential for serious adverse reactions in nursing infants from hydrocodone and acetaminophen, a decision should be made whether to discontinue nursing or to discontinue the drug, taking into account the importance of the drug to the mother.
Pediatric Use: Safety and effectiveness in pediatric patients have not been established.

ADVERSE REACTIONS

The most frequently reported adverse reactions are lightheadedness, dizziness, sedation, nausea and vomiting. These effects seem to be more prominent in ambulatory than in non-ambulatory patients, and some of these adverse reactions may be alleviated if the patient lies down.
Other adverse reactions include:
Central Nervous System: Drowsiness, mental clouding, lethargy, impairment of mental and physical performance, anxiety, fear, dysphoria, psychic dependence, mood changes.
Gastrointestinal System: Prolonged administration of Hydrocet® Capsules (hydrocodone bitartrate and acetaminophen) may produce constipation.
Genitourinary System: Ureteral spasm, spasm of vesical sphincters and urinary retention have been reported with opiates.
Respiratory Depression: Hydrocodone bitartrate may produce dose-related respiratory depression by acting directly on brain stem respiratory centers (see OVERDOSAGE).
Dermatological: Skin rash, pruritis.
The following adverse drug events may be borne in mind as potential effects of acetaminophen: allergic reactions, rash, thrombocytopenia, agranulocytosis.
Potential effects of high dosage are listed in the OVERDOSAGE section.

DRUG ABUSE AND DEPENDENCE

Controlled Substance: Hydrocet® Capsules (hydrocodone bitartrate and acetaminophen) are classified as a Schedule III controlled substance.
Abuse and Dependence: Psychic dependence, physical dependence, and tolerance may develop upon repeated administration of narcotics; therefore, this product should be prescribed and administered with caution. However, psychic dependence is unlikely to develop when Hydrocet® Capsules (hydrocodone bitartrate and acetaminophen) are used for a short time for the treatment of pain.
Physical dependence, the condition in which continued administration of the drug is required to prevent the appearance of a withdrawal syndrome, assumes clinically significant proportions only after several weeks of continued narcotic use, although some mild degree of physical dependence may develop after a few days of narcotic therapy. Tolerance, in which increasingly large doses are required in order to produce the same degree of analgesia, is manifested initially by a shortened duration of analgesic effect, and subsequently by decreases in the intensity of analgesia. The rate of development of tolerance varies among patients.

OVERDOSAGE

Following an acute overdosage, toxicity may result from hydrocodone or acetaminophen.
Signs and Symptoms:
Hydrocodone: Serious ovedose with hydrocodone is characterized by respiratory depression (a decrease in respiratory rate and/or tidal volume, Cheyne-Stokes respiration, cyanosis) extreme somnolence progressing to stupor or coma, skeletal muscle flaccidity, cold and clammy skin, and sometimes bradycardia and hypotension. In severe overdosage, apnea, circulatory collapse, cardiac arrest and death may occur.
Acetaminophen: In acetaminophen overdosage; dose-dependent, potentially fatal hepatic necrosis is the most serious adverse effect. Renal tubular necrosis, hypoglycemic coma and thrombocytopenia may also occur.
Early symptoms following a potentially hepatotoxic overdose may include: nausea, vomiting, diaphoresis and general malaise. Clinical and laboratory evidence of hepatic toxicity may not be apparent until 48 to 72 hours post-ingestion.
In adults, hepatic toxicity has rarely been reported with acute overdoses of less than 10 grams or fatalities with less than 15 grams.
Treatment: A single or multiple overdose with hydrocodone and acetaminophen is a potentially lethal polydrug overdose, and consultation with a regional poison control center is recommended.
Immediate treatment includes support of cardiorespiratory function and measures to reduce drug absorption. Vomiting should be induced mechanically, or with syrup of ipecac, if

the patient is alert (adequate pharyngeal and laryngeal reflexes). Oral activated charcoal (1g/kg) should follow gastric emptying. The first dose should be accompanied by an appropriate cathartic. If repeated doses are used, the cathartic might be included with alternate doses as required. Hypotension is usually hypovolemic and should respond to fluids. Vasopressors and other supportive measures should be employed as indicated. A cuffed endo-tracheal tube should be inserted before gastric lavage of the unconscious patient and, when necessary, to provide assisted respiration.

Meticulous attention should be given to maintaining adequate pulmonary ventilation. In severe cases of intoxication, peritoneal dialysis, or preferably hemodialysis may be considered. If hypoprothrombinemia occurs due to acetaminophen overdose, vitamin K should be administered intravenously.

Naloxone, a narcotic antagonist, can reverse respiratory depression and coma associated with opioid overdose. Naloxone hydrochloride 0.4 mg to 2 mg is given parenterally. Since the duration of action of hydrocodone may exceed that of the naloxone, the patient should be kept under continuous surveillance and repeated doses of the antagonist should be administered as needed to maintain adequate respiration. A narcotic antagonist should not be administered in the absence of clinically significant respiratory or cardiovascular depression.

If the dose of acetaminophen may have exceeded 140 mg/kg, acetylcysteine should be administered as early as possible. Serum acetaminophen levels should be obtained, since levels four or more hours following ingestion help predict acetaminophen toxicity. Do not await acetaminophen assay results before initiating treatment. Hepatic enzymes should be obtained initially, and repeated at 24-hour intervals. Methemoglobinemia over 30% should be treated with methylene blue by slow intravenous administration.

The toxic dose for adults for acetaminophen is 10 g.

DOSAGE AND ADMINISTRATION

Dosage should be adjusted according to severity of pain and response of the patient. However, it should be kept in mind that tolerance to hydrocodone can develop with continued use and that the incidence of untoward effects is dose related.

The usual adult dosage is one or two capsules every four to six hours as needed for pain. The total daily dosage should not exceed 8 capsules.

HOW SUPPLIED

Blue and white, opaque capsules imprinted with the letter "C" and 8657.

Each capsule contains Hydrocodone Bitartrate*, USP 5 mg *(WARNING: MAY BE HABIT FORMING.) and Acetaminophen, USP 500 mg. Keep in tight, light resistant containers. Supplied in bottles of 100 capsules NDC 0086-0057-10. Store at controlled room temperature, 15°–30°C (59°–86°F). The most recent revision of this labeling is August 1997.
Manufactured for:

Carnrick Laboratories, Inc.
Shown in Product Identification Guide, page 308

MIDRIN®
[mid 'rin]   ℞

CAUTION

Federal law prohibits dispensing without prescription.

DESCRIPTION

Each red capsule with pink band contains Isometheptene Mucate 65 mg., Dichloralphenazone 100 mg., and Acetaminophen 325 mg.

Isometheptene Mucate is a white crystalline powder having a characteristic aromatic odor and bitter taste. It is an unsaturated aliphatic amine with sympathomimetic properties.

Dichloralphenazone is a white, microcrystalline powder, with slight odor and tastes saline at first, becoming acrid. It is a mild sedative.

Acetaminophen, a non-salicylate, occurs as a white, odorless, crystalline powder possessing a slightly bitter taste. Midrin® capsules contain FD&C Yellow No. 6 as a color additive.

ACTIONS

Isometheptene Mucate, a sympathomimetic amine, acts by constricting dilated cranial and cerebral arterioles, thus reducing the stimuli that lead to vascular headaches. Dichloralphenazone, a mild sedative, reduces the patient's emotional reaction to the pain of both vascular and tension headaches. Acetaminophen raises the threshold to painful stimuli, thus exerting an analgesic effect against all types of headaches.

INDICATIONS

For relief of tension and vascular headaches.*

* Based on a review of this drug (isometheptene mucate) by the National Academy of Sciences-National Research Council and/or other information, FDA has classified the other indication as "possibly" effective in the treatment of migraine headache.
Final classification of the less-than-effective indication requires further investigation.

CONTRAINDICATIONS

Midrin® is contraindicated in glaucoma and/or severe cases of renal disease, hypertension, organic heart disease, hepatic disease and in those patients who are on monoamineoxidase (MAO) inhibitor therapy.

PRECAUTIONS

Caution should be observed in hypertension, peripheral vascular disease and after recent cardiovascular attacks.

ADVERSE REACTIONS

Transient dizziness and skin rash may appear in hypersensitive patients. This can usually be eliminated by reducing the dose.

DOSAGE AND ADMINISTRATION

FOR RELIEF OF MIGRAINE HEADACHE: The usual adult dosage is two capsules at once, followed by one capsule every hour until relieved, up to 5 capsules within a twelve hour period.

FOR RELIEF OF TENSION HEADACHE: The usual adult dosage is one or two capsules every four hours up to 8 capsules a day.

HOW SUPPLIED

Red capsules imprinted with pink band, the letter "C" and 86120. Bottles of 50 capsules, NDC 0086-0120-05. Bottles of 100 capsules, NDC 0086-0120-10. Bottles of 250 capsules, NDC 0086-0120-25. Store at controlled room temperature 15°–30°C (59°–86°F) in a dry place.

The most recent revision of this labeling is July 1997.
Manufactured for Carnrick Laboratories, Inc.
Shown in Product Identification Guide, page 308

MOTOFEN®   Ⓒ
Tablets
(difenoxin hydrochloride with atropine sulfate)
antidiarrheal

DESCRIPTION

Each five-sided dye free MOTOFEN® tablet contains:
Difenoxin (as the hydrochloride) .... 1.0 mg
Warning —May be habit forming.
Atropine sulfate .... 0.025 mg
Difenoxin hydrochloride, 1-(3-cyano-3,3-diphenylpropyl)-4-phenyl-4-piperidinecarboxylic acid monohydrochloride, is an orally administered antidiarrheal agent which is chemically related to the narcotic meperidine.

The structural formula is:

Difenoxin Hydrochloride

Atropine sulfate is present to discourage deliberate overdosage.

Atropine sulfate, an anticholinergic, is endo ($\pm$)-α-(hydroxymethyl) benzeneacetic acid 8-methyl-8-azabicyclo[3.2.1] oct-3-yl ester sulfate (2:1) (salt) monohydrate and has the following structural formula:

Atropine Sulfate

Inactive ingredients: calcium stearate, cellulose, lactose, corn starch.

CLINICAL PHARMACOLOGY

Animal studies have shown that difenoxin hydrochloride manifests its antidiarrheal effect by slowing intestinal motility. The mechanism of action is by a local effect on the gastrointestinal wall.

Difenoxin is the principal active metabolite of diphenoxylate.

Following oral administration of MOTOFEN®, difenoxin is rapidly and extensively absorbed. Mean peak plasma levels of approximately 160 ng/mL occurred within 40 to 60 minutes in most patients following an oral dose of 2mg. Plasma levels decline to less than 10% of their peak values within 24 hours and to less than 1% of their peak values within 72 hours. This decline parallels the appearance of difenoxin and its metabolites in the urine. Difenoxin is metabolized to an inactive hydroxylated metabolite. Both the drug and its metabolites are excreted, mainly as conjugates, in urine and feces.

INDICATIONS AND USAGE

MOTOFEN® (difenoxin hydrochloride with atropine sulfate) is indicated as adjunctive therapy in the management of acute nonspecific diarrhea and acute exacerbations of chronic functional diarrhea.

CONTRAINDICATIONS

MOTOFEN® is contraindicated in patients with diarrhea associated with organisms that penetrate the intestinal mucosa (toxigenic *E. coli, Salmonella* species, *Shigella*) and pseudomembranous colitis associated with broad spectrum antibiotics. Antiperistaltic agents should not be used in these conditions because they may prolong and/or worsen diarrhea.

MOTOFEN® is *contraindicated in children under 2 years of age* because of the decreased margin of safety of drugs in this class in younger age groups.

MOTOFEN® is contraindicated in patients with a known hypersensitivity to difenoxin, atropine, or any of the inactive ingredients, and in patients who are jaundiced.

WARNINGS

MOTOFEN® IS *NOT* AN INNOCUOUS DRUG AND DOSAGE RECOMMENDATIONS SHOULD BE STRICTLY ADHERED TO. MOTOFEN IS NOT RECOMMENDED FOR CHILDREN UNDER 2 YEARS OF AGE. OVERDOSAGE MAY RESULT IN SEVERE RESPIRATORY DEPRESSION AND COMA, POSSIBLY LEADING TO PERMANENT BRAIN DAMAGE OR DEATH (SEE *OVERDOSAGE*). THEREFORE, KEEP THIS MEDICATION OUT OF THE REACH OF CHILDREN.

FLUID AND ELECTROLYTE BALANCE—THE USE OF MOTOFEN® DOES NOT PRECLUDE THE ADMINISTRATION OF APPROPRIATE FLUID AND ELECTROLYTE THERAPY. DEHYDRATION, PARTICULARLY IN CHILDREN, MAY FURTHER INFLUENCE THE VARIABILITY OF RESPONSE TO MOTOFEN AND MAY PREDISPOSE TO DELAYED DIFENOXIN INTOXICATION. DRUG-INDUCED INHIBITION OF PERISTALSIS MAY RESULT IN FLUID RETENTION IN THE COLON, AND THIS MAY FURTHER AGGRAVATE DEHYDRATION AND ELECTROLYTE IMBALANCE.

IF SEVERE DEHYDRATION OR ELECTROLYTE IMBALANCE IS MANIFESTED, MOTOFEN® SHOULD BE WITHHELD UNTIL APPROPRIATE CORRECTIVE THERAPY HAS BEEN INITIATED.

Ulcerative Colitis —In some patients with acute ulcerative colitis, agents which inhibit intestinal motility or delay intestinal transit time have been reported to induce toxic megacolon. Consequently, patients with acute ulcerative colitis should be carefully observed and MOTOFEN® therapy should be discontinued promptly if abdominal distention occurs or if other untoward symptoms develop.

Liver and Kidney Disease —MOTOFEN® (difenoxin hydrochloride with atropine sulfate) should be used with extreme caution in patients with advanced hepatorenal disease and in all patients with abnormal liver function tests since hepatic coma may be precipitated.

Atropine —A subtherapeutic dose of atropine has been added to difenoxin hydrochloride to discourage deliberate overdosage. Usage of MOTOFEN® in recommended doses is not likely to cause prominent anticholinergic side effects, but MOTOFEN® should be avoided in patients in whom anticholinergic drugs are contraindicated. The warnings and precautions for use of anticholinergic agents should be observed. In children, signs of atropinism may occur even with recommended doses of MOTOFEN®, particularly in patients with Down's Syndrome.

PRECAUTIONS

Information for Patients
CAUTION PATIENTS TO ADHERE STRICTLY TO RECOMMENDED DOSAGE SCHEDULES. THE MEDICATION SHOULD BE KEPT OUT OF REACH OF CHILDREN SINCE ACCIDENTAL OVERDOSAGE MAY RESULT IN SEVERE, EVEN FATAL, RESPIRATORY DEPRESSION.

MOTOFEN® may produce drowsiness or dizziness. The patient should be cautioned regarding activities requiring mental alertness, such as driving or operating dangerous machinery.

Continued on next page

Motofen—Cont.

Drug Interactions
Since the chemical structure of difenoxin hydrochloride is similar to meperidine hydrochloride, the concurrent use of MOTOFEN® with monoamine oxidase inhibitors may, in theory, precipitate a hypertensive crisis.
MOTOFEN® may potentiate the action of barbiturates, tranquilizers, narcotics, and alcohol. When these medications are used concomitantly with MOTOFEN®, the patient should be closely monitored.
Diphenoxylate hydrochloride, from which the principal active metabolite difenoxin is derived, was found to inhibit the hepatic microsomal enzyme system at a dose of 2 mg/kg/day in studies conducted with male rats. Therefore, difenoxin has the potential to prolong the biological half-lives of drugs for which the rate of elimination is dependent on the microsomal drug metabolizing enzyme system.

Carcinogenesis, Mutagenesis, Impairment of Fertility
No evidence of carcinogenesis was found in a long-term study of difenoxin hydrochloride/atropine in the rat. In this 104 week study, rats received dietary doses of 0, 1.25, 2.5, or 5 mg/kg/day difenoxin/atropine (20:1 ratio).
No experiments have been conducted to determine the mutagenic potential of MOTOFEN®. MOTOFEN® did not significantly impair fertility in rats.

Pregnancy/Teratogenic Effects
Pregnancy Category C. Reproduction studies in rats and rabbits with doses at 31 and 61 times the human therapeutic dose respectively, on a mg/kg basis, demonstrated no evidence of teratogenesis due to MOTOFEN® (difenoxin hydrochloride with atropine sulfate).
Pregnant rats receiving oral doses of difenoxin hydrochloride/atropine 20 times the maximum human dose had an increase in delivery time as well as a significant increase in the percent of stillbirths.
Neonatal survival in rats was also reduced with most deaths occurring within four days of delivery.
There are no well controlled studies in pregnant women. MOTOFEN® should be used during pregnancy only if the potential benefit justifies the potential risk to the fetus.

Nursing Mothers
Because of the potential for serious adverse reactions in nursing infants from MOTOFEN®, a decision should be made whether to discontinue nursing or to discontinue the drug, taking into account the importance of the drug to the mother.

Pediatric Use
SAFETY AND EFFECTIVENESS IN CHILDREN BELOW THE AGE OF 12 HAVE NOT BEEN ESTABLISHED. MOTOFEN® IS CONTRAINDICATED IN CHILDREN UNDER 2 YEARS OF AGE. See OVERDOSAGE section for information on hazards from accidental poisoning in children.

ADVERSE REACTIONS
In view of the small amount of atropine present (0.025 mg/tablet), effects such as dryness of the skin and mucous membranes, flushing, hyperthermia, tachycardia and urinary retention are very unlikely to occur, except perhaps in children.
Many of the adverse effects reported during clinical investigation of MOTOFEN® are difficult to distinguish from symptoms associated with the diarrheal syndrome. However, the following events were reported at the stated frequencies:
Gastrointestinal: Nausea, 1 in 15 patients; vomiting, 1 in 30 patients; dry mouth, 1 in 30 patients; epigastric distress, 1 in 100 patients; and constipation, 1 in 300 patients.
Central Nervous System: Dizziness and light-headedness, 1 in 20 patients; drowsiness, 1 in 25 patients; and headache, 1 in 40 patients; tiredness, nervousness, insomnia and confusion ranged from 1 in 200 to 1 in 600 patients.
Other less frequent reactions: Burning eyes and blurred vision occurred in a few cases.
The following adverse reactions have been reported in patients receiving chemically-related drugs: numbness of extremities, euphoria, depression, sedation, anaphylaxis, angioneurotic edema, urticaria, swelling of the gums, pruritus, toxic megacolon, paralytic ileus, pancreatitis, and anorexia.
THIS MEDICATION SHOULD BE KEPT IN A CHILD-RESISTANT CONTAINER AND OUT OF THE REACH OF CHILDREN SINCE AN OVERDOSAGE MAY RESULT IN SEVERE RESPIRATORY DEPRESSION AND COMA, POSSIBLY LEADING TO PERMANENT BRAIN DAMAGE OR DEATH.

DRUG ABUSE AND DEPENDENCE
MOTOFEN® (difenoxin hydrochloride with atropine sulfate) tablets are a Schedule IV controlled substance.
Addiction to (dependence on) difenoxin hydrochloride is theoretically possible at high dosage. Therefore, the recommended dosage should not be exceeded. Because of the structural and pharmacological similarities of difenoxin hydrochloride to drugs with a definite addiction potential, MOTOFEN® should be administered with considerable caution to patients who are receiving addicting drugs, to individuals known to be addiction prone, or to those in whom histories suggest may increase the dosage on their own initiative.

OVERDOSAGE
Diagnosis and Treatment
In the event of overdosage (initial signs may include dryness of the skin and mucous membranes, flushing, hyperthermia and tachycardia followed by lethargy or coma, hypotonic reflexes, nystagmus, pinpoint pupils and respiratory depression) gastric lavage, establishment of a patent airway and possibly mechanically assisted respiration are advised. The narcotic antagonist naloxone may be used in the treatment of respiratory depression caused by narcotic analgesics or pharmacologically related compounds such as MOTOFEN® tablets. When naloxone is administered intravenously, the onset of action is generally apparent within two minutes. Naloxone may also be administered subcutaneously or intramuscularly providing a slightly less rapid onset of action but a more prolonged effect.
To counteract respiratory depression caused by MOTOFEN® overdosage, the following dosage schedule for naloxone should be followed:
Adult Dosage: The usual initial adult dose of naloxone is 0.4 mg (one mL) administered intravenously. If respiratory function does not adequately improve after the initial dose, the same IV dose may be repeated at two-to-three minute intervals.
Children: The usual adult dose of naloxone for children is 0.01 mg/kg of body weight administered intravenously and repeated at two-to-three minute intervals if necessary.
Since the duration of action of difenoxin hydrochloride is longer than that of naloxone, improvement of respiration following administration may be followed by recurrent respiratory depression. Consequently, continuous observation is necessary until the effect of difenoxin hydrochloride on respiration (which effect may persist for many hours) has passed. Supplemental intramuscular doses of naloxone may be utilized to produce a longer lasting effect. TREAT ALL POSSIBLE MOTOFEN® OVERDOSAGES AS SERIOUS AND MAINTAIN MEDICAL OBSERVATION FOR AT LEAST 48 HOURS, PREFERABLY UNDER CONTINUOUS HOSPITAL CARE.
Although signs of overdosage and respiratory depression may not be evident soon after ingestion of difenoxin hydrochloride, respiratory depression may occur from 12 to 30 hours later.

DOSAGE AND ADMINISTRATION
The recommended starting dose of MOTOFEN® tablets in adults is 2 tablets (2 mg), then 1 tablet (1 mg) after each loose stool or 1 tablet (1 mg) every 3 to 4 hours as needed, but the total dosage during any 24-hour treatment period should not exceed 8 tablets (8 mg). In the treatment of diarrhea, if clinical improvement is not observed in 48 hours, continued administration of this type medication is not recommended. For acute diarrheas and acute exacerbations of functional diarrhea, treatment beyond 48 hours is usually not necessary.
Studies in children below the age of 12 have been inadequate to evaluate the safety and effectiveness of MOTOFEN® in this age group. MOTOFEN® is contraindicated in children under 2 years of age.

HOW SUPPLIED
MOTOFEN® is available as a white, dye-free, five-sided, scored tablet with "8674" on the scored side and "C" on the other. Each tablet contains 1.0 mg difenoxin (as the hydrochloride salt) and 0.025 mg atropine sulfate. Supplied in bottles of 100 tablets (NDC 0086-0074-10) and in bottles of 50 tablets (NDC 0086-0074-05).
Store at controlled room temperature, 15°–30°C (59°–86°F).
CAUTION: FEDERAL LAW PROHIBITS DISPENSING WITHOUT PRESCRIPTION
Manufactured for: Carnrick Laboratories, Inc.
6/95

Shown in Product Identification Guide, page 308

NOLAHIST® OTC
[*nō 'lă-hist*]
(phenindamine tartrate)
ANTIHISTAMINE
Alcohol-free
Allergy Tablets

DESCRIPTION
Each dye-free, alcohol-free NOLAHIST® tablet contains:
Phenindamine Tartrate .... 25 mg

INDICATIONS
Temporarily relieves runny nose, sneezing, itching of the nose or throat, and itchy, watery eyes due to hay fever or other upper respiratory allergies or allergic rhinitis.

WARNINGS
May cause excitability especially in children. Do not take this product if you have a breathing problem such as emphysema or chronic bronchitis, or if you have glaucoma or difficulty in urination due to enlargement of the prostate gland, unless directed by a doctor. May cause drowsiness; alcohol, sedatives, and tranquilizers may increase the drowsiness effect. Avoid alcoholic beverages while taking this product. Do not take this product if you are taking sedatives or tranquilizers without first consulting your doctor. Use caution when driving a motor vehicle or operating machinery. May cause nervousness and insomnia in some individuals. As with any drug, if you are pregnant or nursing a baby, seek the advice of a health professional before using this product. Keep this and all medication out of the reach of children. In case of accidental overdose, seek professional assistance or contact a Poison Control Center immediately.

DIRECTIONS
Adults and children 12 years of age and over: oral dosage is one tablet every 4 to 6 hours, not to exceed six tablets in 24 hours, or as directed by a doctor. Children 6 to under 12 years of age: oral dosage is one-half tablet every 4 to 6 hours, not to exceed 3 tablets in 24 hours, or as directed by a doctor. Children under 6 years of age: consult a doctor.
TAMPER-RESISTANT PACKAGE FEATURE
Bottle of 100—If printed outer wrap on carton is broken or removed, do not purchase. Blisters—Tablets are individually sealed with Nolahist® identifying copy on the back. If seal is broken, do not use.

HOW SUPPLIED
White, capsule-shaped, scored tablet inscribed with 8652 on one side and C logo on the other side in bottles of 100 (NDC 0086-0052-10) and 7 boxes of 24 blisters (NDC 0086-0052-24). Each tablet contains phenindamine tartrate 25 mg. Store at 15°–30°C (59°–86°F) and keep tightly closed away from light.
Manufactured for Carnrick Laboratories, Inc. 6/96

Shown in Product Identification Guide, page 308

NOLAMINE® ℞
[*nō 'lă-mēn '*]

DESCRIPTION
Each timed-release tablet contains:

Phenindamine tartrate	24 mg
Chlorpheniramine maleate	4 mg
Phenylpropanolamine hydrochloride	50 mg

Formulated to provide 8 to 12 hours of continuous relief.

CAUTION
Federal law prohibits dispensing without prescription.

INDICATIONS
As a nasal decongestant associated with the common cold, sinusitis, hay fever and other allergies.

CONTRAINDICATIONS
Hypersensitivity to any of the components. Contraindicated in concurrent MAO inhibitor therapy.

SIDE EFFECTS
Nervousness, insomnia, tremors, dizziness and drowsiness may occur occasionally.

PRECAUTIONS
Antihistamines may cause drowsiness and should be used with caution in patients who operate motor vehicles or dangerous machinery. Use with caution in patients with hypertension, cardiovascular disease, diabetes or hyperthyroidism. This product should be used with caution in patients with prostatic hypertrophy or glaucoma.

DOSAGE
Usual adult dose: Orally, one tablet every 8 hours. In mild cases, one tablet every 10 to 12 hours.
WARNING: Keep this and all medication out of the reach of children.

HOW SUPPLIED
Pink, timed release tablets coded C 86204 in bottles of 100 (NDC 0086-0204-10) and 250 (NDC 0086-0204-25). Store at controlled room temperature, 15°–30°C (59°–86°F) and keep away from light.
Manufactured for Carnrick Laboratories, Inc. 6/90

Shown in Product Identification Guide, page 308

PHRENILIN® ℞
[fren 'ĭ-lin]
(Butalbital* 50 mg and Acetaminophen 325 mg Tablet) and
PHRENILIN® FORTE ℞
(Butalbital* 50 mg and Acetaminophen 650 mg Capsule)
***(WARNING—May be habit forming)**

DESCRIPTION

PHRENILIN®: Each PHRENILIN® tablet, for oral administration, contains Butalbital*, USP 50 mg *(WARNING—May be habit forming), Acetaminophen, USP 325 mg.
In addition each PHRENILIN® Tablet contains the following inactive ingredients: alginic acid, cornstarch, D&C Red No. 27—Aluminum Lake, FD&C Blue No. 1—Aluminum Lake, gelatin, magnesium stearate, microcrystalline cellulose and pregelatinized starch.
PHRENILIN® FORTE: Each PHRENILIN® FORTE capsule, for oral administration, contains Butalbital*, USP 50 mg *(WARNING—May be habit forming), Acetaminophen, USP 650 mg.
In addition each PHRENILIN® FORTE capsule may also contain the following inactive ingredients: benzyl alcohol, butylparaben, D&C Red No. 28, D&C Red No. 33, edetate calcium disodium, FD&C Blue No. 1, FD&C Red No. 40, gelatin, methylparaben, propylparaben, silicon dioxide, sodium lauryl sulfate, sodium propionate and titanium dioxide.
Butalbital (5-allyl-5-isobutylbarbituric acid), a slightly bitter, white, odorless, crystalline powder, is a short to intermediate-acting barbiturate. It has the following structural formula:

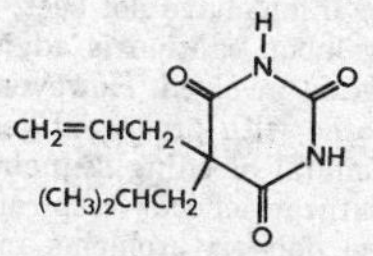

$C_{11}H_{16}N_2O_3$ MW = 224.26

Acetaminophen, (4'-hydroxyacetanilide), a slightly bitter, white, odorless, crystalline powder, is a non-opiate, nonsalicylate analgesic and antipyretic. It has the following structural formula:

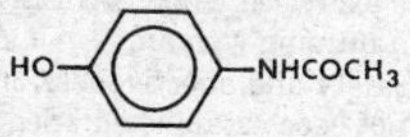

$C_8H_9NO_2$ MW = 151.16

CLINICAL PHARMACOLOGY

This combination drug product is intended as a treatment for tension headache.
It consists of a fixed combination of butalbital and acetaminophen. The role each component plays in the relief of the complex of symptoms known as tension headache is incompletely understood.
Pharmacokinetics: The behavior of the individual components is described below.
Butalbital: Butalbital is well absorbed from the gastrointestinal tract and is expected to distribute to most tissues in the body. Barbiturates in general may appear in breast milk and readily cross the placental barrier. They are bound to plasma and tissue proteins to a varying degree and binding increases directly as a function of lipid solubility.
Elimination of butalbital is primarily via the kidney (59% to 88% of the dose) as unchanged drug or metabolites. The plasma half-life is about 35 hours. Urinary excretion products include parent drug (about 3.6% of the dose), 5-isobutyl-5-(2,3-dihydroxypropyl) barbituric acid (about 24% of the dose), 5-allyl-5(3-hydroxy-2- methyl-1-propyl) barbituric acid (about 4.8% of the dose), products with the barbituric acid ring hydrolyzed with excretion of urea (about 14% of the dose), as well as unidentified materials. Of the material excreted in the urine, 32% is conjugated.
See OVERDOSAGE for toxicity information.
Acetaminophen: Acetaminophen is rapidly absorbed from the gastrointestinal tract and is distributed throughout most body tissues. The plasma half-life is 1.25 to 3 hours, but may be increased by liver damage and following overdosage. Elimination of acetaminophen is principally by liver metabolism (conjugation) and subsequent renal excretion of metabolites. Approximately 85% of an oral dose appears in the urine within 24 hours of administration, most as the glucuronide conjugate, with small amounts of other conjugates and unchanged drug.
See OVERDOSAGE for toxicity information.

INDICATIONS AND USAGE

PHRENILIN® tablets & PHRENILIN® FORTE capsules are indicated for the relief of the symptom complex of tension (or muscle contraction) headache.
Evidence supporting the efficacy and safety of this combination product in the treatment of multiple recurrent headaches is unavailable. Caution in this regard is required because butalbital is habit-forming and potentially abusable.

CONTRAINDICATIONS

This product is contraindicated under the following conditions:

- Hypersensitivity or intolerance to any component of this product.
- Patients with porphyria.

WARNINGS

Butalbital is habit-forming and potentially abusable. Consequently, the extended use of this product is not recommended.

PRECAUTIONS

General: PHRENILIN® tablets & PHRENILIN® FORTE capsules (Butalbital and Acetaminophen) should be prescribed with caution in certain special-risk patients, such as the elderly or debilitated, and those with severe impairment of renal or hepatic function, or acute abdominal conditions.
Information for Patients: This product may impair mental and/or physical abilities required for the performance of potentially hazardous tasks such as driving a car or operating machinery. Such tasks should be avoided while taking this product.
Alcohol and other CNS depressants may produce an additive CNS depression, when taken with this combination product, and should be avoided.
Butalbital may be habit-forming. Patients should take the drug only for as long as it is prescribed, in the amounts prescribed, and no more frequently than prescribed.
Laboratory Tests: In patients with severe hepatic or renal disease, effects of therapy should be monitored with serial liver and/or renal function tests.
Drug Interactions: The CNS effects of butalbital may be enhanced by monoamine oxidase (MAO) inhibitors.
Butalbital and acetaminophen may enhance the effects of: other narcotic analgesics, alcohol, general anesthetics, tranquilizers such as chlordiazepoxide, sedative-hypnotics, or other CNS depressants, causing increased CNS depression.
Drug/Laboratory Test Interactions: Acetaminophen may produce false-positive test results for urinary 5-hydroxyindoleacetic acid.
Carcinogenesis, Mutagenesis, Impairment of Fertility: No adequate studies have been conducted in animals to determine whether acetaminophen or butalbital have a potential for carcinogenesis, mutagenesis or impairment of fertility.
Pregnancy: ***Teratogenic Effects:*** Pregnancy Category C: Animal reproduction studies have not been conducted with this combination product. It is also not known whether butalbital and acetaminophen can cause fetal harm when administered to a pregnant woman or can affect reproduction capacity. These products should be given to a pregnant woman only when clearly needed.
Nonteratogenic Effects: Withdrawal seizures were reported in a two-day-old male infant whose mother had taken a butalbital-containing drug during the last two months of pregnancy. Butalbital was found in the infant's serum. The infant was given phenobarbital 5 mg/kg, which was tapered without further seizure or other withdrawal symptoms.
Nursing Mothers: Barbiturates and acetaminophen are excreted in breast milk in small amounts, but the significance of their effects on nursing infants is not known. Because of potential for serious adverse reactions in nursing infants from butalbital and acetaminophen, a decision should be made whether to discontinue nursing or to discontinue the drug, taking into account the importance of the drug to the mother.
Pediatric Use: Safety and effectiveness in children below the age of 12 have not been established.

ADVERSE REACTIONS

Frequently Observed: The most frequently reported adverse reactions are drowsiness, lightheadedness, dizziness, sedation, shortness of breath, nausea, vomiting, abdominal pain, and intoxicated feeling.
Infrequently Observed: All adverse events tabulated below are classified as infrequent.
Central Nervous: headache, shaky feeling, tingling, agitation, fainting, fatigue, heavy eyelids, high energy, hot spells, numbness, sluggishness, seizure. Mental confusion, excitement or depression can also occur due to intolerance, particularly in elderly or debilitated patients, or due to overdosage of butalbital.
Autonomic Nervous: dry mouth, hyperhidrosis.
Gastrointestinal: difficulty swallowing, heartburn, flatulence, constipation.
Cardiovascular: tachycardia.
Musculoskeletal: leg pain, muscle fatigue.
Genitourinary: diuresis.
Miscellaneous: pruritus, fever, earache, nasal congestion, tinnitus, euphoria, allergic reactions.
Several cases of dermatological reactions, including toxic epidermal necrolysis and erythema multiforme, have been reported.
The following adverse drug events may be borne in mind as potential effects of the components of this product. Potential effects of high dosage are listed in the OVERDOSAGE section.
Acetaminophen: allergic reactions, rash, thrombocytopenia, agranulocytosis.

DRUG ABUSE AND DEPENDENCE

Abuse and Dependence:
Butalbital: *Barbiturates may be habit-forming:* Tolerance, psychological dependence, and physical dependence may occur especially following prolonged use of high doses of barbiturates. The average daily dose for the barbiturate addict is usually about 1500 mg. As tolerance to barbiturates develops, the amount needed to maintain the same level of intoxication increases; tolerance to a fatal dosage, however, does not increase more than two-fold. As this occurs, the margin between an intoxication dosage and fatal dosage becomes smaller. The lethal dose of a barbiturate is far less if alcohol is also ingested. Major withdrawal symptoms (convulsions and delirium) may occur within 16 hours and last up to 5 days after abrupt cessation of these drugs. Intensity of withdrawal symptoms gradually declines over a period of approximately 15 days. Treatment of barbiturate dependence consists of cautious and gradual withdrawal of the drug. Barbiturate-dependent patients can be withdrawn by using a number of different withdrawal regimens. One method involves initiating treatment at the patient's regular dosage level and gradually decreasing the daily dosage as tolerated by the patient.

OVERDOSAGE

Following an acute overdosage of butalbital and acetaminophen, toxicity may result from the barbiturate or acetaminophen.
Signs and Symptoms: Toxicity from barbiturate poisoning include drowsiness, confusion, and coma; respiratory depression; hypotension; and hypovolemic shock.
In acetaminophen overdosage: dose-dependent, potentially fatal hepatic necrosis is the most serious adverse effect. Renal tubular necroses, hypoglycemic coma and thrombocytopenia may also occur. Early symptoms following a potentially hepatotoxic overdose may include: nausea, vomiting, diaphoresis and general malaise. Clinical and laboratory evidence of hepatic toxicity may not be apparent until 48 to 72 hours post-ingestion. In adults hepatic toxicity has rarely been reported with acute overdoses of less than 10 grams, or fatalities with less than 15 grams.
Treatment: A single or multiple overdose with these combination products is a potentially lethal polydrug overdose, and consultation with a regional poison control center is recommended.
Immediate treatment includes support of cardiorespiratory function and measures to reduce drug absorption. Vomiting should be induced mechanically, or with syrup of ipecac, if the patient is alert (adequate pharyngeal and laryngeal reflexes). Oral activated charcoal (1 g/kg) should follow gastric emptying. The first dose should be accompanied by an appropriate cathartic. If repeated doses are used, the cathartic might be included with alternate doses as required. Hypotension is usually hypovolemic and should respond to fluids. Pressors should be avoided. A cuffed endotracheal tube should be inserted before gastric lavage of the unconscious patient and, when necessary, to provide assisted respiration. If renal function is normal, forced diuresis may aid in the elimination of the barbiturate. Alkalinization of the urine increases renal excretion of some barbiturates, especially phenobarbital.
Meticulous attention should be given to maintaining adequate pulmonary ventilation. In severe cases of intoxication, peritoneal dialysis, or preferably hemodialysis may be considered. If hypoprothrombinemia occurs due to acetaminophen overdose, vitamin K should be administered intravenously.
If the dose of acetaminophen may have exceeded 140 mg/kg, acetylcysteine should be administered as early as possible. Serum acetaminophen levels should be obtained, since levels four or more hours following ingestion help predict acetaminophen toxicity. Do not await acetaminophen assay results before initiating treatment. Hepatic enzymes should be obtained initially, and repeated at 24-hour intervals.
Methemoglobinemia over 30% should be treated with methylene blue by slow intravenous administration.
Toxic Doses (for adults):
PHRENILIN® tablets (Butalbital 50 mg and Acetaminophen 325 mg tablets)
Butalbital: toxic dose 1 g (20 tablets)
Acetaminophen: toxic dose 10 g (30 tablets)
PHRENILIN® FORTE capsules (Butalbital 50 mg and Acetaminophen 650 mg capsules)
Butalbital: toxic dose 1 g (20 capsules)
Acetaminophen: toxic dose 10 g (15 capsules)

Continued on next page

Phrenilin/Phrenilin Forte—Cont.

DOSAGE AND ADMINISTRATION

PHRENILIN®: One or two tablets every four hours. Total daily dosage should not exceed 6 tablets.
PHRENILIN® FORTE: One capsule every four hours. Total daily dosage should not exceed 6 capsules.
Extended and repeated use of these products is not recommended because of the potential for physical dependence.

HOW SUPPLIED

PHRENILIN®: Pale violet scored tablets with the letter C on one side and 8650 on the other, in bottles of 100 (NDC 0086-0050-10) in bottles of 500 (NDC 0086-0050-50). Each tablet contains butalbital, USP 50 mg (WARNING: May be habit forming) and acetaminophen, USP 325 mg.
PHRENILIN® FORTE: Amethyst, opaque capsules imprinted with the letter C and 8656, in bottles of 100 (NDC 0086-0056-10) in bottles of 500 (NDC 0086-0056-50). Each capsule contains butalbital, USP 50 mg (WARNING: May be habit forming) and acetaminophen USP 650 mg.
Store PHRENILIN® and PHRENILIN® FORTE (Butalbital and Acetaminophen) at controlled room temperature, 15°–30°C (59°–86°F). Dispense in a tight container as defined in the USP.
Caution: Federal Law Prohibits Dispensing Without Prescription
The most recent revision of this labeling is June 1997.
Manufactured for Carnrick Laboratories, Inc.
Shown in Product Identification Guide, page 308

PROPAGEST® OTC
(Phenylpropanolamine HCl)
Alcohol-free
NASAL DECONGESTANT TABLETS

DESCRIPTION

Each alcohol-free tablet contains:
Phenylpropanolamine HCl .... 25 mg

INDICATIONS

For the temporary relief of nasal congestion associated with the common cold, sinusitis, hay fever or other upper respiratory allergies.

DOSAGE

Adult oral dosage is one tablet every 4 hours not to exceed 6 tablets in 24 hours. Children 6 to under 12 years oral dosage is one-half tablet every 4 hours not to exceed 3 tablets in 24 hours. For children under 6 years, there is no recommended dosage except under the advice and supervision of a doctor.

WARNINGS

Do not exceed recommended dosage because at higher doses nervousness, dizziness, sleeplessness, rapid pulse or high blood pressure may occur.
Do not take this product for more than 7 days. If symptoms do not improve or are accompanied by fever, consult a doctor.
Do not take this product if you have heart disease, high blood pressure, thyroid disease, glaucoma, diabetes, or difficulty in urination due to enlargement of the prostate gland unless directed by a doctor.
As with any drug, if you are pregnant or nursing a baby, seek the advice of a health professional before using this product.
Keep this and all medication out of the reach of children.
In case of accidental overdose, seek professional assistance or contact a Poison Control Center immediately.
Drug Interaction Precaution: Do not take this product if you are presently taking a prescription drug for high blood pressure or depression, without first consulting your doctor.
Do not take this product concurrently with other medication except on the advice of a doctor.
TAMPER-RESISTANT PACKAGE FEATURE:
Bottle of 100—If printed outer wrap on carton is broken or removed, do not purchase.

HOW SUPPLIED

White, oval, scored tablets inscribed with 8651 on one side and "C" logo on the other, containing 25 mg phenylpropanolamine HCl in bottles of 100. (NDC 0086-0051-10). Keep tightly closed, away from light and store at room temperature. 1/96
Manufactured for Carnrick Laboratories, Inc.
Shown in Product Identification Guide, page 308

SALFLEX® ℞
(salsalate tablets USP)

DESCRIPTION

SALFLEX® (salsalate) is a nonsteroidal anti-inflammatory agent for oral administration. Chemically, salsalate (salicylic acid or 2-hydroxy-benzoic acid, 2-carboxyphenyl ester) is a dimer of salicylic acid; its structural formula is shown below.
Chemical Structure:

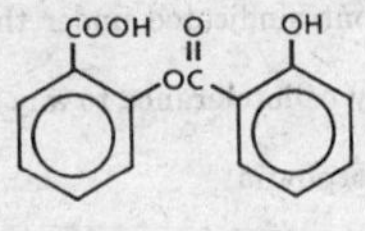

Each round, white, dye-free, film-coated SALFLEX® tablet contains 500 mg salsalate.
Each oval, white, dye-free, film-coated SALFLEX® tablet contains 750 mg salsalate. (See HOW SUPPLIED.)

CLINICAL PHARMACOLOGY

Salsalate is insoluble in acid gastric fluids (<0.1 mg/ml at pH 1.0), but readily soluble in the small intestine where it is partially hydrolyzed to two molecules of salicylic acid. A significant portion of the parent compound is absorbed unchanged and undergoes rapid esterase hydrolysis in the body; its half-life is about one hour. About 13% is excreted through the kidneys as a glucuronide conjugate of the parent compound, the remainder as salicylic acid and its metabolites. Thus, the amount of salicylic acid available from SALFLEX® (salsalate) is about 15% less than from aspirin, when the two drugs are administered on a salicylic acid molar equivalent basis (3.6 g salsalate/5 g aspirin). Salicylic acid biotransformation is saturated at anti-inflammatory doses of salsalate. Such capacity-limited biotransformation results in an increase in the half-life of salicylic acid from 3.5 to 16 or more hours. Thus, dosing with SALFLEX® twice a day will satisfactorily maintain blood levels within the desired therapeutic range (10 to 30 mg/100 ml) throughout the 12-hour intervals. Therapeutic blood levels continue for up to 16 hours after the last dose. The parent compound does not show capacity-limited biotransformation, nor does it accumulate in the plasma on multiple dosing. Food slows the absorption of all salicylates including salsalate.
The mode of anti-inflammatory action of salsalate and other nonsteroidal anti-inflammatory drugs is not fully defined. Although salicylic acid (the primary metabolite of salsalate) is a weak inhibitor of prostaglandin synthesis **in vitro**, salsalate appears to selectively inhibit prostaglandin synthesis **in vivo**,[1] providing anti-inflammatory activity equivalent to aspirin[2] and indomethacin.[3] Unlike aspirin, salsalate does not inhibit platelet aggregation.[4]
The usefulness of salicylic acid, the active **in vivo** product of salsalate, in the treatment of arthritic disorders has been established.[5,6] In contrast to aspirin, salsalate causes no greater fecal gastrointestinal blood loss than placebo.[7]

INDICATIONS AND USAGE

SALFLEX® (salsalate) is indicated for relief of the signs and symptoms of rheumatoid arthritis, osteoarthritis and related rheumatic disorders.

CONTRAINDICATIONS

SALFLEX® is contraindicated in patients hypersensitive to salsalate.

WARNINGS

Reye Syndrome may develop in individuals who have chicken pox, influenza, or flu symptoms. Some studies suggest possible association between the development of Reye Syndrome and the use of medicines containing salicylate or aspirin. SALFLEX® contains a salicylate and therefore is not recommended for use in patients with chicken pox, influenza or flu symptoms. See PRECAUTIONS.

PRECAUTIONS

General Precautions: Patients on treatment with SALFLEX® should be warned not to take other salicylates so as to avoid potentially toxic concentrations. Great care should be exercised when SALFLEX® is prescribed in the presence of chronic renal insufficiency or peptic ulcer disease. Protein binding of salicylic acid can be influenced by nutritional status, competitive binding of other drugs, and fluctuations in serum proteins caused by disease (rheumatoid arthritis, etc.). Although cross reactivity, including bronchospasm, has been reported occasionally with non-acetylated salicylates including salsalate, in aspirin-sensitive patients,[8,9] salsalate is less likely than aspirin to induce asthma in such patients.[10]
Laboratory Tests: Plasma salicylic acid concentrations should be periodically monitored during long-term treatment with SALFLEX® to aid maintenance of therapeutically effective levels: 10 to 30 mg/100 ml. Toxic manifestations are not usually seen until plasma concentrations exceed 30 mg/100 ml (see OVERDOSAGE). Urinary pH should also be regularly monitored: sudden acidification, as from pH 6.5 to 5.5, can double the plasma level, resulting in toxicity.
Drug Interactions: Salicylates antagonize the uricosuric action of drugs used to treat gout. ASPIRIN AND OTHER SALICYLATE DRUGS WILL BE ADDITIVE TO SALFLEX® (salsalate) AND MAY INCREASE PLASMA CONCENTRATIONS OF SALICYLIC ACID TO TOXIC LEVELS. Drugs and foods that raise urine pH will increase renal clearance and urinary excretion of salicylic acid, thus lowering plasma levels; acidifying drugs or foods will decrease urinary excretion and increase plasma levels. Salicylates given concomitantly with anticoagulant drugs may predispose to systemic bleeding. Salicylates may enhance the hypoglycemic effect of oral antidiabetic drugs of the sulfonylurea class. Salicylate competes with a number of drugs for protein binding sites, notably penicillin, thiopental, thyroxine, triiodothyronine, phenytoin, sulfinpyrazone, naproxen, warfarin, methotrexate, and possibly corticosteroids.
Drug/Laboratory Test Interactions: Salicylate competes with thyroid hormone for binding to plasma proteins, which may be reflected in a depressed plasma T_4 value in some patients; thyroid function and basal metabolism are unaffected.
Carcinogenesis: No long-term animal studies have been performed with salsalate to evaluate its carcinogenic potential.
Use in Pregnancy: Pregnancy Category C: Salsalate and salicylic acid have been shown to be teratogenic and embryocidal in rats when given in doses 4 to 5 times the usual human dose. These effects were not observed at doses twice as great as the usual human dose. There are no adequate and well-controlled studies in pregnant women. SALFLEX® should be used during pregnancy only if the potential benefit justifies the potential risk to the fetus.
Labor and Delivery: There exist no adequate and well-controlled studies in pregnant women. Although adverse effects on mother or infant have not been reported with salsalate use during labor, caution is advised when anti-inflammatory dosage is involved. However, other salicylates have been associated with prolonged gestation and labor, maternal and neonatal bleeding sequelae, potentiation of narcotic and barbiturate effects (respiratory or cardiac arrest in the mother), delivery problems and stillbirth.
Nursing Mothers: It is not known whether salsalate per se is excreted in human milk; salicylic acid, the primary metabolite of salsalate, has been shown to appear in human milk in concentrations approximating the maternal blood level. Thus the infant of a mother on SALFLEX® therapy might ingest in mother's milk 30 to 80% as much salicylate per kg body weight as the mother is taking. Accordingly, caution should be exercised when SALFLEX® (salsalate) is administered to a nursing woman.
Pediatric Use: Safety and effectiveness of SALFLEX® use in children have not been established. (See WARNINGS section.)

ADVERSE REACTIONS

In two well-controlled clinical trials, the following reversible adverse experiences characteristic of salicylates were most commonly reported with salsalate (n=280 pts; listed in descending order of frequency): tinnitus, nausea, hearing impairment, rash, and vertigo. These common symptoms of salicylates, i.e., tinnitus or reversible hearing impairment, are often used as a guide to therapy.
Although cause-and-effect relationships have not been established, spontaneous reports over a ten-year period have included the following additional medically significant adverse experiences: abdominal pain, abnormal hepatic function, anaphylactic shock, angioedema, bronchospasm, decreased creatinine clearance, diarrhea, G.I. bleeding, hepatatis, hypotension, nephritis and urticaria.

DRUG ABUSE AND DEPENDENCE

Drug abuse and dependence have not been reported with salsalate.

OVERDOSAGE

Death has followed ingestion of 10 to 30 g of salicylates in adults, but much larger amounts have been ingested without fatal outcome.
Symptoms: The usual symptoms of salicylism—tinnitus, vertigo, headache, confusion, drowsiness, sweating, hyperventilation, vomiting and diarrhea—will occur. More severe intoxication will lead to disruption of electrolyte balance and blood pH, and hyperthermia and dehydration.
Treatment: Further absorption of salsalate from the G.I. tract should be prevented by emesis (syrup of ipecac) and, if necessary, by gastric lavage.
Fluid and electrolyte imbalance should be corrected by the administration of appropriate I.V. therapy. Adequate renal function should be maintained. Hemodialysis or peritoneal dialysis may be required in extreme cases.

DOSAGE AND ADMINISTRATION

Adults: The usual dosage is 3000 mg daily, given in divided doses as follows:
1) two doses of two 750 mg tablets;
2) two doses of three 500 mg tablets; or
3) three doses of two 500 mg tablets.

Some patients, e.g., the elderly, may require a lower dosage to achieve therapeutic blood concentrations and to avoid the more common side effects such as auditory.

Alleviation of symptoms is gradual, and full benefit may not be evident for 3 to 4 days, when plasma salicylate levels have achieved steady state. There is no evidence for development of tissue tolerance (tachyphylaxis), but salicylate therapy may induce increased activity of metabolizing liver enzymes, causing a greater rate of salicyluric acid production and excretion, with a resultant increase in dosage requirement for maintenance of therapeutic serum salicylate levels.

Children: Dosage recommendations and indications for SALFLEX® use in children have not been established.

HOW SUPPLIED

SALFLEX® 500 mg tablets:
Each round, white, dye-free, film-coated SALFLEX® tablet is inscribed with 8671 on one side and "C" on the other. Each tablet contains 500 mg salsalate and is available in bottles of 100 tablets (NDC 0086-0071-10).

SALFLEX® 750 mg tablets:
Each oval, white, dye-free, film-coated SALFLEX® tablet is inscribed with 8672 on the scored side and "C" on the other. Each tablet contains 750 mg salsalate and is available in bottles of 100 tablets (NDC 0086-0072-10) and 500 tablets (NDC 0086-0072-50).

Store at controlled room temperature, 15°–30°C (59°–86°F). Dispense in a tight container as defined in the USP.

CAUTION: Federal law prohibits dispensing without prescription.

REFERENCES

1. Morris HG, Sherman NA, McQuain C., et al: Effects of Salsalate (Nonacetylated) Salicylate and Aspirin on Serum Prostaglandins in Humans. Ther. Drug Monit. 7:435-438, 1985.
2. April PA, Curran NJ, Ekholm BP, et al: Multicenter Comparative Study of Salsalate (SSA) vs Aspirin (ASA) in Rheumatoid Arthritis (RA), Arthritis Rheumatism 30(4 supplement):S93, 1987.
3. Deodhar SD, McLeod MM, Dick WC, et al: A Short-Term Comparative Trial of Salsalate and Indomethacin in Rheumatoid Arthritis. Curr. Med. Res. Opin. 5:185–188, 1977.
4. Estes D, Kaplan K: Lack of Platelet Effect With the Aspirin Analog, Salsalate, Arthritis and Rheumatism, 23:1303–1307, 1980.
5. Dick C, Dick PH, Nuki G, et al: Effect of Anti-inflammatory Drug Therapy on Clearance of ^{133}Xe from Knee Joints of Patients with Rheumatoid Arthritis. British Med. J. 3:278–280, 1969.
6. Dick WC, Grayson MF, Woodburn A, et al: Indices of Inflammatory Activity. Ann. of the Rheum. Dis. 29:643–648, 1970.
7. Cohen, A: Fecal Blood Loss and Plasma Salicylate Study of Salicylsalicylic Acid and Aspirin. J. Clin. Pharmacol. 19:242–247, 1979.
8. Chudwin DS, Strub M, Golden HE, et al: Sensitivity to Non-Acetylated Salicylates in a Patient with Asthma, Nasal Polyps, and Rheumatoid Arthritis. Annals of Allergy 57:133–134, 1986.
9. Spector SL, Wangaard CH, Farr RS: Aspirin and Concomitant Idiosyncrasies in Adult Asthmatic Patients. J. Allergy Clin. Immunol. 64:500–506, 1979.
10. Stevenson DD, Schrank PJ, Hougham AJ, et al: Salsalate Cross Sensitivity in Aspirin-Sensitive Asthmatics. J. Allergy Clin. Immunol. 81:181, 1988.

June 1993

Shown in Product Identification Guide, page 309

SINULIN®   OTC
Alcohol-free
Analgesic • Antihistamine • Decongestant

DESCRIPTION
SINULIN® contains acetaminophen, an analgesic and antipyretic that relieves pain, sinus headache and reduces fever; phenylpropanolamine HCl, a decongestant that promotes nasal drainage and relieves sinus pressure; and chlorpheniramine maleate, an antihistamine that helps control allergic symptoms.

ACTIVE INGREDIENTS
Each alcohol-free tablet contains: acetaminophen 650 mg. (650 mg. is a nonstandard strength of acetaminophen per tablet compared to the established standard of 325 mg. acetaminophen per tablet), chlorpheniramine maleate 4 mg., phenylpropanolamine HCl 25 mg.

INDICATIONS
For the temporary relief of nasal and sinus congestion, runny nose, sneezing, itching of the nose or throat, itchy watery eyes, headache and fever associated with the common cold, sinusitis, hay fever or other upper respiratory allergies.

WARNINGS

Sinulin® tablets contain FD&C Yellow No. 6 as a color additive. Do not exceed recommended dosage because severe liver damage may occur and at higher doses, nervousness, dizziness, sleeplessness, rapid pulse or high blood pressure may occur. Adults should not take this product for more than 7 days. Children 6 to under 12 years of age should not take this product for more than 5 days. If fever persists for more than 3 days, or recurs, consult a doctor. If symptoms persist, do not improve, or new ones occur, consult a doctor. Do not take this product if you have high blood pressure; heart disease; diabetes; thyroid disease; glaucoma; a breathing problem such as emphysema or chronic bronchitis, asthma, chronic pulmonary disease, shortness of breath or difficulty in breathing; or difficulty in urination due to enlargement of the prostate gland, or if you are presently taking a prescription drug for high blood pressure or depression, unless directed by a doctor. May cause drowsiness; alcohol, sedatives and tranquilizers may increase the drowsiness effect. Avoid alcoholic beverages while taking this product. Do not take this product if you are taking sedatives or tranquilizers, without first consulting your doctor. Use caution when driving a motor vehicle or operating machinery. May cause excitability especially in children. If a rare sensitivity reaction occurs, discontinue use and consult a doctor. As with any drug, if you are pregnant or nursing a baby, seek the advice of a health professional before using this product. Keep this and all medication out of the reach of children. In case of accidental overdose, seek professional assistance or contact a Poison Control Center immediately.

DRUG INTERACTION PRECAUTION

Do not take this product if you are presently taking a prescription drug for high blood pressure or depression, or if you are taking a sedative or tranquilizer, without first consulting your doctor. Do not take this product concurrently with other medication except on the advise of a doctor.

DIRECTIONS

Adults: oral dosage is one tablet every 4 to 6 hours, or as directed by a doctor. Do not exceed 6 tablets in 24 hours. Children 6 to under 12 years of age: oral dosage is one-half tablet every 4 to 6 hours, or as directed by a doctor. Do not exceed 3 tablets in 24 hours.
Children under 6 years of age: do not use unless directed by a doctor.

TAMPER-RESISTANT PACKAGE FEATURE

Bottles of 20's & 100's—If printed outer wrap on carton is broken or removed, do not purchase. Blisters—Tablets are individually sealed with Sinulin® identifying copy on the back. If seal is broken, do not use.

HOW SUPPLIED

Peach color, scored tablets inscribed with 8666 on one side and C logo on the other. Bottles of 20 (NDC 0086-0066-02),7 boxes of 24 blisters (NDC 0086-0066-24), and Bottles of 100 (NDC 0086-0066-10). Store at controlled room temperature (59°–86°F).   9/95
Manufactured for Carnrick Laboratories, Inc.
Shown in Product Identification Guide, page 309

SKELAXIN®   ℞
brand of metaxalone

CAUTION
Federal law prohibits dispensing without prescription.

DESCRIPTION
Each pale rose, scored tablet contains: metaxalone, 400 mg. Skelaxin® (metaxalone) has the following chemical structure and name:
5-[(3,4-dimethylphenoxy)methyl]-2 oxazolidinone

ACTIONS
The mechanism of action of metaxalone in humans has not been established, but may be due to general central nervous system depression. It has no direct action on the contractile mechanism of striated muscle, the motor end plate or the nerve fiber.

INDICATIONS
Skelaxin® (metaxalone) is indicated as an adjunct to rest, physical therapy, and other measures for the relief of discomforts associated with acute, painful musculoskeletal

conditions. The mode of action of this drug has not been clearly identified, but may be related to its sedative properties. Metaxalone does not directly relax tense skeletal muscles in man.

CONTRAINDICATIONS

Metaxalone is contraindicated in individuals who have shown hypersensitivity to the drug. Metaxalone should not be administered to patients with a known tendency to drug-induced, hemolytic, or other anemias. It is contraindicated in patients with significantly impaired renal or hepatic function.

PRECAUTIONS

Elevation in cephalin flocculation tests without concurrent changes in other liver function parameters have been noted. Hence, it is recommended that metaxalone be administered with great care to patients with pre-existing liver damage and that serial liver function studies be performed as required.

False-positive Benedict's tests, due to an unknown reducing substance, have been noted. A glucose-specific test will differentiate findings.

Pregnancy: Reproduction studies have been performed in rats and have revealed no evidence of impaired fertility or harm to the fetus due to metaxalone. Reactions reports from marketing experience have not revealed evidence of fetal injury, but such experience cannot exclude the possibility of infrequent or subtle damage to the human fetus. Safe use of metaxalone has not been established with regard to possible adverse effects upon fetal development. Therefore, metaxalone tablets should not be used in women who are or may become pregnant and particularly during early pregnancy unless in the judgment of the physician the potential benefits outweigh the possbile hazards.

Nursing Mothers: It is not known whether this drug is secreted in human milk. As a general rule, nursing should not be undertaken while a patient is on a drug since many drugs are excreted in human milk.

Pediatric Use: Safety and effectiveness in children 12 years of age and below have not been established.

ADVERSE REACTIONS

The most frequent reactions to metaxalone include nausea, vomiting, gastrointestinal upset, drowsiness, dizziness, headache, and nervousness or "irritability." Other adverse reactions are: hypersensitivity reaction, characterized by a light rash with or without pruritus; leukopenia; hemolytic anemia; jaundice.

DOSAGE

The recommended dose for adults and children over 12 years of age is two tablets (800 mg) three to four times a day.

MANAGEMENT OF OVERDOSAGE

Gastric lavage and supportive therapy as indicated. (When determining the LD_{50} in rats and mice, progressive sedation, hypnosis and finally respiratory failure were noted as the dosage increased. In dogs, no LD_{50} could be determined as the higher doses produced an emetic action in 15 to 30 minutes. No documented case of major toxicity has been reported.

HOW SUPPLIED

Skelaxin® (metaxalone) is available as a 400 mg. pale rose tablet, inscribed with 8662 on the scored side and "C" on the other. Available in bottles of 100 (NDC 0086-0062-10) and in bottles of 500 (NDC 0086-0062-50).

Store at Controlled Room Temperature, between 15°C and 30°C (59°F and 86°F).

1/98

Manufactured for Carnrick Laboratories, Inc.
Shown in Product Identification Guide, page 309

THEO-X®   ℞
(Theophylline Extended-Release Tablets)

DESCRIPTION

Theophylline is a bronchodilator structurally classified as a xanthine derivative. It occurs as a white, odorless, crystalline powder having a bitter taste. Theophylline anhydrous has the chemical name 1H-Purine-2, 6-dione, 3,7-dihydro-1, 3-dimethyl-, and is represented by the following structural formula:

$C_7H_8N_4O_2$ 180.17

Continued on next page

Theo-X—Cont.

This product allows a 12-hour dosing interval for a majority of patients and a 24-hour dosing interval for selected patients (see DOSAGE AND ADMINISTRATION section for description of appropriate patient populations).

This product is available as extended-release tablets intended for oral administration, containing 100 mg, 200 mg, or 300 mg of theophylline anhydrous. Also contains Povidone, USP, Hydroxypropyl Methylcellulose, USP, Lactose Anhydrous, NF, and Magnesium Stearate, NF.

CLINICAL PHARMACOLOGY

Theophylline directly relaxes the smooth muscle of the bronchial airways and pulmonary blood vessels, thus acting mainly as a bronchodilator and smooth muscle relaxant. It has also been demonstrated that aminophylline has a potent effect on diaphragmatic contractility in normal persons and may then be capable of reducing fatigability and thereby improve contractility in patients with chronic obstructive airways disease. The exact mode of action remains unsettled. Although theophylline does cause inhibition of phosphodiesterase with a resultant increase in intracellular cyclic AMP, other agents similarly inhibit the enzyme, producing a rise of cyclic AMP, but are unassociated with any demonstrable bronchodilation. Other mechanisms proposed include an effect on translocation of intracellular calcium, prostaglandin antagonism, stimulation of catecholamines endogenously; inhibition of cyclic guanosine monophosphate metabolism, and adenosine receptor antagonism. None of these mechanisms has been proved, however.

In vitro, theophylline has been shown to act synergistically with beta agonists, and there are now available data which demonstrate an additive effect *in vivo* with combined use.

Pharmacokinetics: The half-life of theophylline is influenced by a number of known variables. It may be prolonged in chronic alcoholics, particularly those with liver disease (cirrhosis or alcoholic liver disease), in patients with congestive heart failure, and in those patients taking certain other drugs (see **PRECAUTIONS, Drug interactions**).

Newborns and neonates have extremely slow clearance rates compared to older infants and children, ie, those over 1 year. Older children have rapid clearance rates while most non-smoking adults have clearance rates between these two extremes. In premature neonates the decreased clearance is related to oxidative pathways that have yet to be established.

Theophylline Elimination Characteristics
Theophylline

	Half-Life (in hours) Range	Mean
Children	1–9	3.7
Adults	3–15	7.7

In cigarette smokers (1–2 packs/day) the mean half-life is 4–5 hours, much shorter than in nonsmokers. The increase in clearance associated with smoking is presumably due to stimulation of the hepatic metabolic pathway by components of cigarette smoke. The duration of this effect after cessation of smoking is unknown but may require 6 months to 2 years before the rate approaches that of the nonsmoker.

Single-Dose Study:

A single-dose crossover study was conducted in twelve healthy male volunteers to compare pharmacokinetic parameters when theophylline extended-release tablets were administered with and without food. Subjects were fasted overnight and received a single 300 mg tablet early the following morning.

When dosing was done under fed conditions, the subjects received a standard breakfast consisting of 2 fried eggs, 2 strips of bacon, 4 oz. hash brown potatoes, 1 slice of toast with a pat of butter, and 8 oz. whole milk 15 minutes predosing. No food was allowed for five hours post-dosing then a standard lunch was served; at ten hours post-dosing a standard supper was served. Mean peak theophylline serum levels for the two treatments were 3.7 mcg/mL (fasting) and 4.4 mcg/mL (with food). The time of peak serum level varied from subject to subject, occurring from 4 to 14 hours after dosing. However, 92% of the subjects had serum levels at least 75% of the maximum value at 4 to 8 hours after dosing, during each phase.

Thus, blood samples taken 4 to 8 hours post-dosing should reference the peak serum level for most patients. The mean T_{max} was 6.2 hours (fasting) and 8.7 hours (with food). The respective AUC (0- inf.) for these treatments were 73.3 mcg × hr/mL and 82.2 mcg × hr/mL, respectively.

Multiple-Dose Study:

(300 mg)

A multiple-dose, steady-state study was conducted under fed conditions. Three high fat content meals were served at 6:30 a.m., 12 noon and 6:30 p.m. Nineteen normal subjects were dosed as 300 mg every 12 hours (7 p.m. and 7 a.m.) for eight doses. Dosing began one-half hour after the evening

meal with the test dose occurring one-half hour after breakfast. At steady-state, the mean peak concentration was 8.8 mcg/mL and the mean trough concentration was 5.9 mcg/mL.

The time of peak concentration (T_{max}) was 6.2 hours. The average percent fraction of fluctuation [(C_{max}- C_{min}/C_{min}) × 100] was 49% for this formulation and dosing regimen.

The subjects used for this study exhibited a mean half-life of 8.3 hours (range 5.2–12.2) and a mean clearance of 3.5 L/hour (range 2.3–5.6) as determined in a separate single-dose clearance study using 500 mg of immediate release theophylline, prior to this multiple-dose study.

(200 mg)

A multiple-dose steady-state study was conducted in sixteen normal subjects, with one 200 mg tablet given every 12 hours for eight doses. Three high fat content meals were served at 6:30 a.m., 12 noon and 6:30 p.m. Dosing began one-half hour after the evening meal with the test dose occurring one-half hour after breakfast. At steady-state following the eighth dose, the mean C_{max} was 5.1 mcg/mL and the mean C_{min} was 3.7 mcg/mL. The mean time to peak concentration was 6.2 hours. The average percent fraction of fluctuation was 39%.

The subjects used for this study exhibited a mean half-life of 8.7 hours (range 5.0–14.6) and a mean clearance of 3.6 L/hour (range 2.2–6.1).

(100 mg)

A multiple-dose steady-state study was conducted in sixteen normal subjects, with three 100 mg tablets given every 12 hours for eight doses. Three high fat content meals were served at 6:30 a.m., 12 noon and 6:30 p.m. Dosing began one-half hour after the evening meal with the test dose occurring one-half hour after breakfast. At steady-state following the eighth dose, the mean C_{max} was 8.1 mcg/mL and the mean C_{min} was 5.6 mcg/mL. The mean time to peak concentration was 6.2 hours. The average percent fraction of fluctuation was 45%.

The subjects used for this study were the same as those used in the previously cited 200 mg study.

Once-a-Day Dosing:

A multiple-dose, steady-state study was conducted under fed conditions with once-a-day dosing. Fed conditions were the same as those previously cited. Sixteen subjects were dosed as 2 × 300 mg tablets every morning at 8 a.m. for five doses. At steady-state, the mean C_{max} was 11.7 mcg/mL, and the mean C_{min} was 3.4 mcg/mL. The average percent fraction of fluctuation was 244%. The mean t_{max} was 8.7 hours. The subjects used in the above study exhibited a mean half-life of 7.9 hours (range 5.3–13.4) and a mean clearance of 3.8 L/hour (range 2.3–5.7).

INDICATIONS AND USAGE

For relief and/or prevention of symptoms from asthma and reversible bronchospasm associated with chronic bronchitis and emphysema.

CONTRAINDICATIONS

This product is contraindicated in individuals who have shown hypersensitivity to its components. It is also contraindicated in patients with active peptic ulcer disease, and in individuals with underlying seizure disorders (unless receiving appropriate anticonvulsant medication).

WARNINGS

Serum levels above 20 mcg/mL are rarely found after appropriate administration of the recommended doses. However, in individuals in whom theophylline plasma clearance is reduced *for any reason*, even conventional doses may result in increased serum levels and potential toxicity. Reduced theophylline clearance has been documented in the following readily identifiable groups: 1) patients with impaired renal or liver function; 2) patients over 55 years of age, particularly males and those with chronic lung disease; 3) those with cardiac failure from any cause; 4) patients with sustained high fever; 5) neonates and infants under 1 year of age; and 6) those patients taking certain drugs (see **PRECAUTIONS, Drug Interactions**). Frequently, such patients have markedly prolonged theophylline serum levels following discontinuation of the drug.

Reduction of dosage and laboratory monitoring are especially appropriate in the above individuals.

Serious side effects such as ventricular arrhythmias, convulsions, or even death may appear as the first sign of theophylline toxicity without any previous warning. Less serious signs of theophylline toxicity (ie, nausea and restlessness) may occur frequently when initiating therapy, but are usually transient; when such signs are persistent during maintenance therapy, they are often associated with serum concentrations above 20 mcg/mL.

Stated differently, *serious toxicity is not reliably preceded by less severe side-effects.* A serum concentration measurement is the only reliable method of predicting potentially life-threatening toxicity.

Many patients who require theophylline may exhibit tachycardia due to their underlying disease process so that the cause/effect relationship to elevated serum theophylline concentrations may not be appreciated.

Theophylline products may cause or worsen arrhythmias and any significant change in rate and/or rhythm warrants monitoring and further investigation.

Studies in laboratory animals (minipigs, rodents, and dogs) recorded the occurrence of cardiac arrhythmias and sudden death (with histologic evidence of myocardial necrosis) when beta-agonists and methylxanthines were administered concurrently. The significance of these findings when applied to humans is currently unknown.

PRECAUTIONS

THEO-X TABLETS SHOULD NOT BE CHEWED OR CRUSHED.

General: On the average, theophylline half-life is shorter in cigarette and marijuana smokers than in non-smokers, but smokers can have half-lives as long as non-smokers. Theophylline should not be administered concurrently with other xanthines. Use with caution in patients with hypoxemia, hypertension, or those with history of peptic ulcer. Theophylline may occasionally act as a local irritant to the G.I. tract although gastrointestinal symptoms are more commonly centrally mediated and associated with serum drug concentrations over 20 mcg/mL.

Information for Patients: The importance of taking only the prescribed dose and time interval between doses should be reinforced. THEO-X Extended-Release Tablets should not be chewed or crushed. When dosing THEO-X on a once daily (q24h) basis, tablets should be taken whole and not split. The patient should alert the physician if symptoms occur repeatedly, especially near the end of a dosing interval.

Laboratory Tests: Serum levels should be monitored periodically to determine the theophylline level associated with observed clinical response and as the method of predicting toxicity. For such measurements, the serum sample should be obtained at the time of peak concentration, under steady-state conditions at approximately 6 hours after administration for this sustained-release product. It is important that the patient will not have missed or taken additional doses during the previous 48 hours and that dosing intervals will have been reasonably equally spaced. DOSAGE ADJUSTMENT BASED ON SERUM THEOPHYLLINE MEASUREMENTS WHEN THESE INSTRUCTIONS HAVE NOT BEEN FOLLOWED MAY RESULT IN RECOMMENDATIONS THAT PRESENT RISK OF TOXICITY TO THE PATIENT.

Drug Interactions:

Drug-Drug: Toxic synergism with ephedrine has been documented and may occur with some other sympathomimetic bronchodilators. In addition, the following drug interactions have been demonstrated:

Theophylline with:	
Allopurinol (high-dose)	Increased serum theophylline levels
Cimetidine	Increased serum theophylline levels
Ciprofloxacin	Increased serum theophylline levels
Erythromycin, Troleandomycin	Increased serum theophylline levels
Lithium carbonate	Increased renal excretion of lithium
Oral contraceptives	Increased serum theophylline levels
Phenytoin	Decreased theophylline and pheyntoin serum levels
Propranolol	Increased serum theophylline levels
Rifampin	Decreased serum theophylline levels

Drug-Food: Taking THEO-X Extended-Release Tablets immediately after ingesting a high fat content meal (45 g fat, 55 g carbohydrates, 28 g protein, 789 calories) may result in a somewhat higher C_{max} and delayed T_{max}, and a somewhat greater extent of absorption when compared to taking in the fasting state. The influence of the type and amount of other foods, as well as the time interval between drug and food, has not been studied.

Drug-Laboratory Tests Interactions: Currently available analytical methods, including high pressure liquid chromatography and immunoassay techniques, for measuring serum theophylline levels are specific. Metabolites and other drugs generally do not affect the results. Other new

analytic methods are also now in use. The physician should be aware of the laboratory method used and whether other drugs will interfere with the assay for theophylline.

Carcinogenesis, Mutagenesis, and Impairment of Fertility: Long-term carcinogenicity studies have not been performed with theophylline.

Chromosome-breaking activity was detected in human cell cultures at concentrations of theophylline up to 50 times the therapeutic serum concentrations in humans. Theophylline was not mutagenic in the dominant lethal assay in male mice given theophylline intraperitoneally in doses up to 30 times the maximum daily human oral dose.

Studies to determine the effect on fertility have not been performed with theophylline.

Pregnancy: Category C—Animal reproduction studies have not been conducted with theophylline. It is also not known whether theophylline can cause fetal harm when administered to a pregnant woman or can affect reproduction capacity. Xanthines should be given to a pregnant woman only if clearly needed.

Nursing Mothers: Theophylline is distributed into breast milk and may cause irritability or other signs of toxicity in nursing infants. Because of the potential for serious adverse reactions in nursing infants from theophylline, a decision should be made whether to discontinue nursing or to discontinue the drug, taking into account the importance of the drug to the mother.

Pediatric Use: Safety and effectiveness of THEO-X Extended-Release Tablets administered:
1. Every 24 hours in children under 12 years of age, have not been established.
2. Every 12 hours in children under 6 years of age, have not been established.

ADVERSE REACTIONS

The following adverse reactions have been observed, but there has not been enough systematic collection of data to support an estimate of their frequency. The most consistent adverse reactions are usually due to overdosage.
1. *Gastrointestinal:* nausea, vomiting, epigastric pain, hematemesis, diarrhea.
2. *Central nervous system:* headaches, irritability, restlessness, insomnia, reflex hyperexcitability, muscle twitching, clonic and tonic generalized convulsions.
3. *Cardiovascular:* palpitation, tachycardia, extrasystoles, flushing, hypotension, circulatory failure, ventricular arrhythmias.
4. *Respiratory:* tachypnea.
5. *Renal:* potentiation of diuresis.
6. *Others:* alopecia, hyperglycemia, inappropriate ADH syndrome, rash.

OVERDOSAGE

Management: It is suggested that the management principles (consistent with the clinical status of the patient when first seen) outlined below be instituted and that simultaneous contact with a Regional Poison Control Center be established. In this way both updated information and individualization regarding required therapy may be provided.
1. When potential oral overdose is established and seizure has not occurred:
   a. If patient is alert and seen within the early hours after ingestion, induction of emesis may be of value. Gastric lavage has been demonstrated to be of no value in influencing outcome in patients who present more than 1 hour after ingestion.
   b. Administer a cathartic. Sorbitol solution is reported to be of value.
   c. Administer repeated doses of activated charcoal and monitor theophylline serum levels.
   d. Prophylactic administration of phenobarbital has been shown to increase the seizure threshold in laboratory animals and administration of this drug can be considered.
2. If patient presents with a seizure:
   a. Establish an airway.
   b. Administer oxygen.
   c. Treat the seizure with intravenous diazepam, 0.1 to 0.3 mg/kg up to 10 mg. If seizures cannot be controlled, the use of general anesthesia should be considered.
   d. Monitor vital signs, maintain blood pressure, and provide adequate hydration.
3. If postseizure coma is present:
   a. Maintain airway and oxygenation.
   b. If a result of oral medication, follow above recommendations to prevent absorption of the drug, but intubation and lavage will have to be performed instead of inducing emesis, and the cathartic and charcoal will need to be introduced via a large bore gastric lavage tube.
   c. Continue to provide full supportive care and adequate hydration until the drug is metabolized. In general, drug metabolism is sufficiently rapid so as not to warrant dialysis. If repeated oral activated charcoal is ineffective (as noted by stable or rising serum levels) charcoal hemoperfusion may be indicated.

DOSAGE AND ADMINISTRATION

Taking THEO-X Extended-Release Tablets immediately after a high-fat content meal may result in a somewhat higher C_{max} and delayed T_{max}, and somewhat greater extent of absorption. However, the differences are usually not great and this product may normally be administered without regard to meals.

Effective use of theophylline (ie, the concentration of drug in the serum associated with optimal benefit and minimal risk of toxicity) is considered to occur when the theophylline concentration is maintained from 10 to 20 mcg/mL. The early studies from which these levels were derived were carried out in patients immediately or shortly after recovery from acute exacerbations of their disease (some hospitalized with status asthmaticus).

Although the 20 mcg/mL level remains appropriate as a critical value (above which toxicity is more likely to occur) for safety purposes, additional data are now available which indicate that the serum theophylline concentrations required to produce maximum physiologic benefit may, in fact, fluctuate with the degree of bronchospasm present and are variable. Therefore, the physician should individualize the range appropriate to the patient's requirements, based on both symptomatic response and improvement in pulmonary function. It should be stressed that serum theophylline concentrations maintained at the upper level of the 10 to 20 mcg/mL range may be associated with potential toxicity when factors known to reduce theophylline clearance are operative. (See **WARNINGS**).

If it is not possible to obtain serum level determinations, restriction of the daily dose (in otherwise healthy adults) to not greater than 13 mg/kg/day, to a maximum of 900 mg in divided doses will result in relatively few patients exceeding serum levels of 20 mcg/mL and the resultant greater risk of toxicity.

Caution should be exercised for younger children who cannot complain of minor side-effects. Older adults, those with cor pulmonale, congestive heart failure, and/or liver disease may have unusually low dosage requirements, and thus, may experience toxicity at the maximal dosage recommended below.

Theophylline does not distribute into fatty tissue. Dosage should be calculated on the basis of lean (ideal) body weight were mg/kg doses are presented.

THEO-X (Theophylline Extended-Release Tablets) are recommended for chronic or long-term management and prevention of symptoms, and not for use in treating acute symptoms of asthma and reversible bronchospasm.

Dosage Guidelines:
WARNING: DO NOT ATTEMPT TO MAINTAIN ANY DOSE THAT IS NOT TOLERATED.

Dosage guidelines are approximations only and the wide range of theophylline clearance between individuals (particularly those with concomitant disease) makes indiscriminate usage hazardous.

I. Acute Symptoms:
NOTE: Status asthmaticus should be considered a medical emergency and is defined as that degree of bronchospasm that is not rapidly responsive to usual doses of conventional bronchodilators. Optimal therapy for such patients frequently requires both **additional medication** parenterally administered, and **close** **monitoring**, preferably in an intensive care setting.

THEO-X (Theophylline Extended-Release Tablets) are not intended for patients experiencing an acute episode of bronchospasm (associated with asthma, chronic bronchitis, or emphysema). Such patients require rapid relief of symptoms and should be treated with an immediate-release or intravenous theophylline preparation (or other bronchodilators) and not with extended-release products.

II. Chronic Therapy:
A. Initiating Therapy with an Immediate-Release Product: It is recommended that the appropriate dosage be established using an immediate-release preparation. A dosage form which allows small incremental doses is desirable for initiating therapy. A liquid preparation should be considered for children to permit easier and more accurate dosage adjustment. Slow clinical titration is generally preferred to help assure acceptance and safety of the medication and to allow the patient to develop tolerance to transient caffeine-like side-effects. Then, if the total 24-hour dose can be given by use of the available strengths of this product, the patient can usually be switched to THEO-X Extended-Release Tablets giving one-half of the daily dose at 12 hour intervals or one-third daily dose at 8-hour intervals. Patients who metabolize theophylline rapidly, such as the young, smokers and some non-smoking adults, are the most likely candidates for dosing at 8-hour intervals. Such patients can generally be identified as having trough serum concentrations lower than desired or repeatedly exhibiting symptoms near the end of a dosing interval.

B. Initiating Therapy with THEO-X (Theophylline Extended-Release Tablets):
Alternatively, therapy can be initiated with THEO-X (Theophylline Extended-Release Tablets) since it is available in

dosage forms/strengths which permit titration and adjustment of dosage as outlined in the following dosing guidelines. It is recommended that for children under 25 kg proper dosage be established with a liquid preparation to permit titration in small increments.

Initial Dose:
16 mg/kg/24 hours or 400 mg/24 hours (whichever is less) of theophylline in divided doses at 12 hours intervals.

Increasing Dose:
The above dosage may be increased in approximately 25 percent increments at 3 day intervals so long as the drug is tolerated. Following each adjustment, if the clinical response is satisfactory and serum levels can be measured, then such measurements should be obtained, then that dosage level should be maintained. Dosage increases may be made in this manner until the maximum dose indicated in section III below is reached.

It is important that no patient be maintained on any dosage that is not tolerated. When instructing patients to increase dosage according to the schedule above, they should be told not to take a subsequent dose if apparent side effects occur and to resume therapy at a lower dose once adverse effects have disappeared.

Titration and Adjustment and Chronic Maintenance:
If the desired response is not achieved with the above AVERAGE INITIAL DOSE recommendations, there are no adverse reactions and the serum theophylline level cannot be measured, dosage adjustment should proceed by increasing the dose in approximately 25% increments at three-day intervals. Following each adjustment, if the clinical response is satisfactory, then the dosage level should be maintained. DOSAGE increases may be made in this manner up to the following.

III. Maximum Dose of Theophylline Where the Serum Concentration is not Measured:
WARNING: DO NOT ATTEMPT TO MAINTAIN ANY DOSE THAT IS NOT TOLERATED.

Not to exceed the following: (or 900 mg, whichever is less)

Age 6 to under 9 years	24 mg/kg/day
Age 9 to under 12 years	20 mg/kg/day
Age 12 to under 16 Years	18 mg/kg/day
Age 16 years and older	13 mg/kg/day

IV. Measurement of Serum Theophylline Concentrations During Chronic Therapy:
If the above maximum doses are to be maintained or exceeded, serum theophylline measurement is essential (see **PRECAUTIONS, Laboratory Tests,** for guidance).

V. Final Adjustment of Dosage:
Dosage adjustment after serum theophylline measurement:

If serum theophylline is:		Directions:
Within desired range		Maintain dosage if tolerated.
Too high	20 to 25 mcg/mL	Decrease doses by about 10% and recheck serum level after 3 days.
	25 to 30 mcg/mL	Skip the next dose and decrease subsequent doses by about 25%. Recheck serum level after 3 days.
	Over 30 mcg/mL	Skip the next 2 doses and decrease subsequent doses by 50%. Recheck serum level after 3 days.
Too low		Increase dosage by 25% at 3-day intervals until either the desired serum concentration and/or clinical response is achieved. The total daily dose may need to be administered at more frequent intervals if symptoms occur repeatedly at the end of a dosing interval.

The serum concentration may be rechecked at appropriate intervals, but at least at the end of any adjustment period. When the patient's condition is otherwise clinically stable and none of the recognized factors which alter elimination are present, measurement of serum levels need be repeated only every 6 to 12 months.
DOSAGE ADJUSTMENT BASED ON SERUM THEOPHYLLINE CONCENTRATION MEASUREMENTS WHEN THESE INSTRUCTIONS HAVE NOT BEEN FOLLOWED MAY RESULT IN RECOMMENDATIONS THAT PRESENT RISK OF TOXICITY TO THE PATIENT.

Once-Daily Dosing: The slow absorption rate of this preparation may allow once-daily administration in adult non-smokers with appropriate total body clearance and other

Continued on next page

Theo-X—Cont.

patients with low dosage requirements. Once-daily dosing should be considered only after the patient has been gradually and satisfactorily titrated to therapeutic levels with q12h dosing. Once-daily dosing should be based on twice the q12h dose and should be initiated at the end of the last q12h dosing interval. The trough concentration (C_{min}) obtained following conversion to once-daily dosing may be lower (especially in high clearance patients) and the peak concentration (C_{max}) may be higher (especially in low clearance patients) than that obtained with q12h dosing. If symptoms recur, or signs of toxicity appear during the once-daily dosing interval, dosing on the q12h basis should be reinstituted.

It is essential that serum theophylline concentrations be monitored before and after transfer to once-daily dosing.

Food and posture, along with changes associated with circadian rhythm, may influence the rate of absorpiton and/or clearance rates of theophylline from extended-release dosage forms administered at night. The exact relationship of these and other factors to nighttime serum concentrations and the clinical significance of such findings require additional study. Therefore, it is not recommended that THEO-X, when used as a once-a-day product, be administered at night.

HOW SUPPLIED

THEO-X (Theophylline Extended-Release Tablets) for oral administration is available as:

100 mg—White, dye-free, round, bisected, extended-release tablets inscribed with "C" on one side and "8631" on the scored side. Supplied in bottles of 100 (NDC 0086-0031-10) and 500 (NDC 0086-0031-50).

200 mg—White, dye-free, oval-shaped, bisected, extended-release tablets inscribed with "C" on one side and "8632" on the scored side. Supplied in bottles of 100 (NDC 0086-0032-10), 500 (NDC 0086-0032-50) and 1,000 (NDC 0086-0032-90).

300 mg—White, dye-free, capsule-shaped, bisected, extended-release tablets inscribed with "C" on one side and "8633" on the scored side. Supplied in bottles of 100 (NDC 0086-0033-10), 500 (NDC 0086-0033-50) and 1,000 (NDC 0086-0033-90).

Dispense in a well-closed container as defined in the USP.
Store at controlled room temperature 15°–30°C (59°–86°F).

CAUTION: Federal law prohibits dispensing without prescription.

Issued 6/93

Shown in Product Identification Guide, page 309

Centeon L.L.C.

1020 FIRST AVENUE
KING OF PRUSSIA, PA 19406-1310

Direct Inquiries to:
(610) 878-4000

For Medical Information Contact:
(800) 504-5434

Sales and Ordering:
Customer Support Center
(800) 683-1288
Fax: (610) 878-4888

ALBUMIN (HUMAN) U.S.P., 5% ALBUMINAR®-5 ℞

DESCRIPTION

Albumin (Human) 5%, ALBUMINAR®-5 is a sterile solution of albumin obtained from large pools of adult human venous plasma by low temperature controlled fractionation according to the Cohn process. It is heated at 60°C for 10 hours and stabilized with 0.004 M sodium acetyltryptophanate and 0.004 M sodium caprylate.

Each 50 mL bottle of 5% solution contains 2.5 grams of albumin in normal saline. Each 250 mL bottle of 5% solution contains 12.5 grams of albumin in normal saline. Each 500 mL bottle of 5% solution contains 25 grams of albumin in normal saline. Each 1000 mL bottle of 5% solution contains 50 grams of albumin in normal saline. The 5% solution is osmotically equivalent with citrated plasma. The pH of the solution is adjusted to 6.9 ± 0.5 with sodium bicarbonate, sodium hydroxide, or acetic acid. Approximate concentrations of significant electrolytes per liter are: Sodium 130–160 mEq; and Potassium-n.m.t. 1mEq. The solution contains no preservative. This product has been prepared in accordance with the requirements established by the Food and Drug Administration and is in compliance with the standards of the United States Pharmacopeia.

Albumin (Human) 5%, ALBUMINAR®-5, is to be administered by the intravenous route.

CLINICAL PHARMACOLOGY

Albumin (Human) 5%, ALBUMINAR®-5, being active osmotically, is useful in regulating the volume of circulating blood. It is a valuable therapeutic aid for the treatment of conditions that will be benefited by its marked osmotic effect. When the circulating blood volume has been depleted, the hemodilution following albumin administration persists for many hours. In individuals with normal blood volume, it usually lasts only a few hours.

Albumin (Human), unlike whole blood or plasma, is considered free of the danger of viral hepatitis because it is heated at 60°C for 10 hours. It is convenient to use since no crossmatching is required and the absence of cellular elements removes the danger of sensitization with repeated infusions.

INDICATIONS AND USAGE

Shock—Albumin (Human) 5% is indicated in the emergency treatment of shock due to burns, trauma, operations and infections, in the treatment of severe injuries, and in other similar conditions where the restoration of blood volume is urgent. The primary function is maintenance of colloid osmotic pressure. If there has been considerable loss of red blood cells, transfusion with whole blood is indicated.

Burns—Albumin (Human) 5% is indicated in conjunction with adequate infusions of crystalloid to counteract hemoconcentration and the loss of protein, electrolytes and water that usually follow severe burns. Because of changes in permeability, little administered albumin is likely to be retained intravenously in the first 12 hours after a major burn. However, an optimum regimen for the use of colloid, electrolytes and water in the treatment of burns has not been established.

Hypoproteinemia—Albumin (Human) 5%, ALBUMINAR®-5 may be used in acutely hypoproteinemic patients, provided sodium restriction is not a problem.

CONTRAINDICATIONS

Albumin (Human) 5%, ALBUMINAR®-5 is contraindicated in patients with severe anemia or cardiac failure and in patients with a history of allergic reactions to human albumin.

WARNINGS

Do not use if the solution is turbid or if there is a sediment in the bottle. Since the product contains no antimicrobial preservative, do not begin administration more than 4 hours after the container has been entered. Destroy unused portions to prevent the possibility of subsequent use of a solution that may have become contaminated.

PRECAUTIONS

General—Administration of large quantities of albumin should be supplemented with red blood cells or replaced by whole blood to combat the relative anemia which would follow such use. The quick response of blood pressure, which may follow the rapid administration of albumin, necessitates careful observation of the injured patient to detect bleeding points which failed to bleed at lower blood pressure. Albumin (Human) 5%, ALBUMINAR®-5 should be administered with caution to patients with low cardiac reserve or with no albumin deficiency because a rapid increase in plasma volume may cause circulatory embarrassment or pulmonary edema.

PREGNANCY CATEGORY C—Animal reproduction studies have not been conducted with Albumin (Human) 5%, ALBUMINAR®-5. It is also not known whether ALBUMINAR®-5 can cause fetal harm when administered to a pregnant woman or can affect reproduction capacity. ALBUMINAR®-5 should be given to a pregnant woman only if clearly needed.

ADVERSE REACTIONS

The incidence of untoward reactions to Albumin (Human) 5% is low although nausea, vomiting, increased salivation, chills and febrile reactions occasionally may occur. Urticaria and skin rash have been reported following administration of albumin.

DOSAGE AND ADMINISTRATION

Albumin (Human) 5%, ALBUMINAR®-5 may be given intravenously without further dilution. This concentration is approximately isotonic and iso-osmotic with citrated plasma. Albumin (Human) in this concentration provides additional fluid for plasma volume expansion. Therefore, when it is administered to patients with normal blood volume, the rate of infusion should be slow enough to prevent too rapid expansion of plasma volume.

In the treatment of shock in an adult patient an initial dose of 500 mL of the 5% albumin solution is given as rapidly as tolerated. If response within 30 minutes is inadequate, an additional 500 mL of 5% albumin solution may be given. The 50 mL dosage form would be appropriate for pediatric use, with a dose of 10–20 mL per Kg of body weight infused intravenously at a rate of up to 5–10 mL per minute. Therapy should be guided by the clinical response, blood pressure and an assessment of relative anemia. If more than 1000 mL are given, or if hemorrhage has occurred, the administration of Whole Blood or Red Blood Cells may be desirable.

In severe burns, immediate therapy should include large volumes of crystalloid with lesser amounts of 5% albumin solution to maintain an adequate plasma volume. After the first 24 hours, the ratio of albumin to crystalloid may be increased to establish and maintain a plasma albumin level of about 2.5g/100 mL or a total serum protein level of about 5.2g/100 mL. However, an optimal regimen for the use of colloids, electrolytes and water after severe burns has not been established.

The infusion of Albumin (Human) as a nutrient in the treatment of chronic hypoproteinemia is not recommended. In acute hypoproteinemia, 5% albumin may be used in replacing the protein lost in hypoproteinemic conditions. However, if edema is present or if large amounts of albumin are lost, Albumin (Human) 25% is preferred because of a greater amount of protein in the concentrated solution.

Parenteral drug products should be inspected visually for particulate matter and discoloration prior to administration, whenever solution and container permit.

HOW SUPPLIED

Albumin (Human) 5%, ALBUMINAR®-5 is supplied as a 5% solution in:

NDC0053-7670-06
50 mL bottles containing 2.5 grams of albumin
NDC0053-7670-01
250 mL bottles containing 12.5 grams of albumin
NDC0053-7670-02
500 mL bottles containing 25.0 grams of solution
NDC0053-7670-03
1000 mL bottles containing 50.0 grams of albumin

Store at controlled room temperature—between 15°–30 °C (59°–86 °F).

CAUTION: FEDERAL (U.S.A.) LAW PROHIBITS DISPENSING WITHOUT PRESCRIPTION.

REFERENCES

1. Finlayson, J.S.: Albumin Products. Seminars in Thrombosis and Hemostasis 6:85-120, 1980.
2. Tullis, J.L.: Albumin. JAMA 237:355-360 and 460-463, 1977.
3. Rudolph, A.M.: Pediatrics. 18th ED., p. 1839, Appleton and Lange, 1987.

Revised: June, 1996 IBM 12602

CENTEON L.L.C.
Kankakee, Illinois 60901 U.S.A.
U.S. Government License No. 149

ALBUMIN (HUMAN) U.S.P., 25% ALBUMINAR®-25 ℞

DESCRIPTION

Albumin (Human) 25%, ALBUMINAR®-25 is a sterile aqueous solution of albumin obtained from large pools of adult human plasma by low temperature controlled fractionation according to the Cohn process. It is stabilized with 0.02 M sodium acetyltryptophanate and 0.02 M sodium caprylate and pasteurized at 60 °C for 10 hours.

Albumin (Human) 25%, ALBUMINAR®-25 is a solution containing in each 100 mL, 25 grams of serum albumin, osmotically equivalent to 500 mL of normal human plasma. The pH of the solution is adjusted with sodium bicarbonate, sodium hydroxide, or acetic acid. Approximate concentrations of significant electrolytes per liter are: sodium – 130-160 mEq; and potassium – n.m.t. 1 mEq. The solution contains no preservative. This product has been prepared in accordance with the requirements established by the Food and Drug Administration and is in compliance with the standards of the United States Pharmacopeia.

Albumin (Human) 25%, ALBUMINAR®-25, is to be administered by the intravenous route.

CLINICAL PHARMACOLOGY

ALBUMINAR®-25 is active osmotically and is therefore important in regulating the volume of circulating blood. When injected intravenously, 50 mL of 25% albumin draws approximately 175 mL of additional fluid into the circulation within 15 minutes, except in the presence of marked dehydration. This extra fluid reduces hemoconcentration and blood viscosity. The degree of volume expansion is dependent on the initial blood volume. When the circulating blood volume has been depleted, the hemodilution following albumin administration persists for many hours. In individuals with normal blood volume, it usually lasts only a few hours. Albumin, unlike whole blood or plasma, is considered free of the danger of homologous serum hepatitis. Albumin (Human) 25%, ALBUMINAR®-25 may be given in conjunction with other parenteral fluids – such as saline, glucose or sodium lactate. It is convenient to use since no crossmatching is required and the absence of cellular elements removes the danger of sensitization with repeated infusions.

INDICATIONS AND USAGE

SHOCK – Albumin is indicated in the emergency treatment of shock and in other similar conditions where the restoration of blood volume is urgent. If there has been considerable loss of red blood cells, transfusion with whole blood is indicated.

BURNS – Albumin or Albumin in either normal saline or glucose is indicated to prevent marked hemoconcentration and to maintain appropriate electrolyte balance.

HYPOPROTEINEMIA with or without edema – Albumin is indicated in those clinical situations usually associated with a low concentration of plasma protein and a resulting decreased circulating blood volume. Although diuresis may occur soon after albumin administration has been instituted, best results are obtained if albumin is continued until the normal serum protein level is regained.

CONTRAINDICATIONS

Albumin (Human) 25%, ALBUMINAR®-25 may be contraindicated in patients with severe anemia or cardiac failure.

WARNING

Do not use if the solution is turbid. Since this product contains no antimicrobial preservative, do not begin administration more than 4 hours after the container has been entered.

PRECAUTIONS
GENERAL

If dehydration is present additional fluids must accompany or follow the administration of albumin. Administration of large quantities of albumin should be supplemented with or replaced by whole blood to combat the relative anemia which would follow such use. The quick response of blood pressure which may follow the rapid administration of concentrated albumin necessitates careful observation of the injured patient to detect bleeding points which failed to bleed at lower blood pressure. Albumin (Human) 25% should be administered with caution to patients with low cardiac reserve or with no albumin deficiency because a rapid increase in plasma volume may cause circulatory embarrassment or pulmonary edema. In cases of hypertension, a slower rate of administration is desired – 200 mL of albumin solution may be mixed with 300 mL of 10% glucose solution and administered at a rate of 10 grams of albumin (100 mL) per hour.

PREGNANCY CATEGORY C

Animal reproduction studies have not been conducted with Albumin (Human) 25%, ALBUMINAR®-25. It is also not known whether ALBUMINAR®-25 can cause fetal harm when administered to a pregnant woman or can affect reproduction capacity. ALBUMINAR®-25 should be given to a pregnant woman only if clearly needed.

ADVERSE REACTIONS

The incidence of untoward reactions to Albumin (Human) 25% is low although nausea, vomiting, increased salivation and febrile reactions occasionally may occur.

DOSAGE AND ADMINISTRATION

Albumin (Human) 25%, ALBUMINAR®-25 may be given intravenously without dilution or it may be diluted with normal saline or 5% glucose before administration. Two hundred mL per liter gives a solution which is approximately isotonic and iso-osmotic with citrated plasma.

When undiluted albumin solution is administered in patients with normal blood volume, the rate of infusion should be slow enough (1 mL per minute) to prevent too rapid expansion of plasma volume.

In the treatment of shock the amount of albumin and duration of therapy must be based on the responsiveness of the patient as indicated by blood pressure, degree of pulmonary congestion, and hematocrit. The initial dose may be followed by additional albumin within 15–30 minutes if the response is deemed inadequate. If there is continued loss of protein, it also may be desirable to give whole blood and/or other blood fractions.

In the treatment of burns an optimal regimen involving use of albumin, crystalloids, electrolytes and water has not been established. Suggested therapy during the first 24 hours includes administration of large volumes of crystalloid solution to maintain an adequate plasma volume. Continuation of therapy beyond 24 hours usually requires more albumin and less crystalloid solution to prevent marked hemoconcentration and maintain electrolyte balance. Duration of treatment varies depending upon the extent of protein loss through renal excretion, denuded areas of skin and decreased albumin synthesis. Attempts to raise the albumin level above 4.0 g/100 mL may only result in an increased rate of catabolism.

In the treatment of hypoproteinemia, 200 to 300 mL of 25% albumin may be required to reduce edema and to bring serum protein values to normal. Since such patients usually have approximately normal blood volume, doses of more than 100 mL of 25% albumin should not be given faster than 100 mL in 30 to 45 minutes to avoid circulatory embarrassment. If slower administration is desired, 200 mL of 25% albumin may be mixed with 300 mL of 10% glucose solution and administered by continuous drip at a rate of 100 mL of this glucose solution an hour.

Parenteral drug products should be inspected visually for particulate matter and discoloration prior to administration, whenever solution and container permit.

HOW SUPPLIED

Albumin (Human), ALBUMINAR®-25 is supplied as a 25% solution in:

NDC0053-7680-01
20 mL vials containing 5.0 grams of albumin.
NDC0053-7680-02
50 mL vials containing 12.5 grams of albumin.
NDC0053-7680-03
100 mL vials containing 25.0 grams of albumin.

Store at controlled room temperature–between 15°–30 °C (59°–86 °F).

CAUTION: FEDERAL (U.S.A.) LAW PROHIBITS DISPENSING WITHOUT PRESCRIPTION.

Revised: June, 1996   IBM 12522
CENTEON L.L.C.
Kankakee, Illinois 60901 U.S.A.
U.S. Government License No. 149

Immune Globulin
(Human) U.S.P.
GAMMAR®-P I.M.   ℞

DESCRIPTION

Immune Globulin (Human), Gammar®-P I.M., is a sterile solution of immunoglobulin, primarily immunoglobulin G (IgG), containing $16.5 \pm 1.5\%$ protein. It is prepared by cold alcohol fractionation of pooled plasma. Immune Globulin (Human), Gammar®-P I.M., also contains approximately 0.45% sodium chloride, the mercurial preservative, thimerosal, at a concentration of 0.01% (0.1 mg per milliliter) and is stabilized with 0.3 M glycine. The pH of the solution is 6.8 ± 0.4 and may have been adjusted with sodium carbonate, and/or acetic acid. The product is intended for the intramuscular route of administration.

The heat treatment step employed in the manufacture of Immune Globulin (Human), Gammar®-P I.M., pasteurization at 60°C for 10 hours of a stabilized, aqueous solution, has been validated in a series of in vitro experiments for its capacity to inactivate Human Immunodeficiency Virus (HIV) and the following model viruses: Sindbis Virus, Vesicular Stomatitis Virus (VSV), Bovine Viral Diarrhea Virus (BVDV), Vaccinia Virus, Pseudorabies Virus (PrV) and Murine Encephalomyocarditis Virus (EMC), a non-enveloped model virus. HIV was reduced from 6.0 and 5.4 $\log_{10}$ to an undetectable level after 0.5 hours of heating in two independent experiments. For each of the model viruses studied, two independent experiments were also conducted with the following results: Sindbis Virus was reduced from 7.5 and 7.9 $\log_{10}$ to an undetectable level after two hours of heating, VSV was reduced from 6.8 and 7.2 $\log_{10}$ to an undetectable level after 0.5 hours of heating, BVDV, a model for hepatitis C virus, was reduced from 6.4 and 6.5 $\log_{10}$ to an undetectable level after four hours of heating, Vaccinia Virus was reduced from 5.6 and 5.6 $\log_{10}$ to an undetectable level after two hours of heating, PrV was reduced from 4.9 and 3.6 $\log_{10}$ to an undetectable level after six hours of heating and EMC, a non-enveloped model virus, was reduced by 4.5 and 4.8 $\log_{10}$ after ten hours of heating.[1]

The viral reduction capacity of the purification procedures used in the manufacture of Immune Globulin (Human), Gammar®-P I.M., exclusive of heat treatment, was also studied in a series of in vitro experiments using HIV and three model viruses: Murine Encephalomyocarditis Virus (EMC), a non-enveloped virus, Bovine Viral Diarrhea Virus (BVDV), a model for hepatitis C virus, and Pseudorabies (PrV), a large DNA virus. HIV was reduced by at least 6.7 $\log_{10}$ by the cold, alcohol fractionation process used to isolate Cohn Fraction II from pooled plasma during the initial purification of Gammar®-P I.M. Additionally, an alcohol purification step performed subsequent to heat treatment was found to have the following viral reduction capacities when challenged with HIV and the three model viruses in three replicate experiments each: HIV (reductions of 3.4, 4.0, >4.6 $\log_{10}$), EMC (reductions of 3.4, 1.0, 1.5 $\log_{10}$) BVDV (reductions of 3.5, 3.6, 3.5 $\log_{10}$) and PrV (reductions of >5.3, >5.5, >5.4 $\log_{10}$).[1]

The results of these validation studies document an HIV viral reduction capacity of > 15.5 $\log_{10}$ and a viral reduction capacity of >7.5 $\log_{10}$ for Sindbis Virus, >6.8 $\log_{10}$ for VSV, >9.9 $\log_{10}$ for BVDV, >5.6 $\log_{10}$ for Vaccinia Virus, >8.9 $\log_{10}$ for PrV, and 5.5 $\log_{10}$ for EMC. These viral reduction data are summarized in Table 1 below.
[See table below]

CLINICAL PHARMACOLOGY

Peak blood levels of immunoglobulin G are obtained approximately 2 days after intramuscular injection of Immune Globulin (Human).[2] The half-life of IgG in the circulation of individuals with normal IgG levels is 23 days.[3]

Gammar®-P I.M. is prepared from a plasma pool composed of donations from at least 1000 donors and, consequently, represents the expected diversity of antibodies in that population. Each lot must conform to standards for antibody potencies including Hepatitis A and measles antibodies.

Passive immunization with Immune Globulin (Human) prevents or modifies hepatitis A, prevents or modifies measles, and provides replacement therapy in persons with hypo- or agammaglobulinemia. Gammar®-P I.M. is not standardized with respect to antibody titers against hepatitis B surface antigen (HBsAg) and should not be used for prophylaxis of viral hepatitis B. Prophylactic treatment to prevent hepatitis B can best be accomplished with the use of Hepatitis B Immune Globulin, often in combination with Hepatitis B Vaccine.[4,5]

Gammar®-P I.M. is not indicated for routine prophylaxis or treatment of rubella, poliomyelitis, mumps or varicella. It is not indicated for allergy or asthma in patients who have normal levels of immunoglobulin.[6]

Gammar®-P I.M., Immune Globulin (Human), was evaluated for safety and tolerance in a Phase I, open label, single dose study using 12 healthy volunteers composed equally of male and female subjects. Each subject received a dose of 0.25 mL/Kg (with a maximum of 15 mL total) divided across the following three injection sites, i.e., the right and left dorsal gluteal areas and the right vastus lateralis region. This dose was selected to allow for an effective examination of the safety and tolerability of the product. While it corresponds to the recommended dose for prevention or modification of measles, it is approximately 4–12 times the dose range prescribed for the product's most common indication, prophylaxis in cases of hepatitis A exposure. Each patient was followed for 30 days. There were no clinically significant changes from baseline noted in physical examinations, ECG or laboratory testing. There were no serious or unexpected adverse experiences reported. Assessment of the sites of injection found the expected occurrence of local pain and tenderness, erythema, pruritus and induration associated with products of this type. (See **ADVERSE REACTIONS**).

INDICATIONS AND USAGE

HEPATITIS A—The prophylactic value of Immune Globulin (Human) Gammar®-P I.M. is greatest when given before or soon after exposure to hepatitis A. Gammar®-P I.M. is not indicated in persons with clinical manifestations of hepatitis A or in those exposed more than 2 weeks previously.

MEASLES (RUBEOLA)—Gammar®-P I.M. should be given to prevent or modify measles in a susceptible person exposed less than 6 days previously.[7,8] (A susceptible person is one who has not been vaccinated or has not had an appropriate immune response to vaccination and has not had measles previously). Gammar®-P I.M. may be especially indicated for susceptible household contacts of measles patients, particularly contacts under one year of age, for whom the risk of complications is highest.[7] Gammar®-P I.M. and measles vaccine should not be given at the same time.[7,8] If a child is older than 12 months and has received Immune Globulin (Human), the child should be given measles vaccine at least 3 months later, when the neutralizing measles antibody titer will have decreased, based on the original dosage of Immune Globulin administered.[9,10] (See **PRECAUTIONS—DRUG INTERACTIONS**).

If a susceptible child exposed to measles is immunocompromised, Immune Globulin (Human), Gammar®-P I.M. should be given immediately.[11,12] Children who are immunocompromised should not receive measles vaccine or any other live viral vaccine.

IMMUNOGLOBULIN DEFICIENCY—In patients with immunoglobulin deficiencies, replacement therapy can best be accomplished by use of Immune Globulin Intravenous (Human) (IGIV). If IGIV is unavailable, Gammar®-P I.M. may prevent serious infection. However, Immune Globulin (Human), Gammar®-P I.M. may not prevent chronic infections

Continued on next page

Table 1[1]

	HIV	Sindbis	VSV	BVDV	Vacc	PrV	EMC
Cohn Plasma Fractionation	>6.7	*	*	*	*	*	*
Heat Treatment	>5.4	>7.5	>6.8	>6.4	>5.6	>3.6	4.5
Post-Heat Treatment Purification	3.4	*	*	3.5	*	>5.3	1.0
Total $\log_{10}$ Reduction	>15.5	>7.5	>6.8	>9.9	>5.6	>8.9	5.5

*Step not studied with this virus

Gammar-P I.M.—Cont.

of the external secretory tissues such as the respiratory and gastrointestinal tract.

Prophylactic therapy, especially against infections due to encapsulated bacteria, is effective in Bruton-type, sex-linked congenital agammaglobulinemia, agammaglobulinemia and severe combined immunodeficiency.

CONTRAINDICATIONS

Immune Globulin (Human), Gammar®-P I.M., should not be given to persons with isolated immunoglobulin A (IgA) deficiency. Such persons have the potential for developing antibodies to IgA and could have anaphylactic reactions to subsequent administration of blood products that contain IgA.[13, 14]

Gammar®-P I.M. should not be administered to patients who have severe thrombocytopenia or any coagulation disorder that would contraindicate intramuscular injections.

WARNINGS

Immune Globulin (Human), Gammar®-P I.M. is made from human plasma. Products made from human plasma may contain infectious agents, such as viruses, that can cause disease. The risk that such products will transmit an infectious agent has been reduced by screening plasma donors for prior exposure to certain viruses, by testing for the presence of certain current virus infections, and by inactivating and/or removing certain viruses during manufacture. (See DESCRIPTION section for viral reduction measures.) The manufacturing procedure for Immune Globulin (Human), Gammar®-P I.M., includes processing steps designed to reduce further risk of viral transmission. Stringent procedures utilized at plasma collection centers, plasma testing laboratories, and fractionation facilities are designed to reduce the risk of viral transmission. The primary viral reduction step of the Gammar®-P I.M. manufacturing process is the heat treatment of the purified, stabilized aqueous solution at $60.0 \pm 0.05°C$ for 10–11 hours. In addition, the purification procedures used in the manufacture of Immune Globulin (Human), Gammar®-P I.M., also provide viral reduction capacity. Despite these measures, such products may still potentially contain human pathogenic agents, including those not yet known or identified. Thus the risk of transmission of infectious agents cannot be totally eliminated. Any infections thought by a physician possibly to have been transmitted by this product should be reported by the physician or other healthcare provider to Centeon at (800) 504-5434 in the U.S. and Canada. The physician should discuss the risks and benefits of this product with the patient.

Gammar®-P I.M. should be given with caution to patients with a history of prior systemic allergic reactions following the administration of human immunoglobulin preparations.[13]

Gammar®-P I.M. is for intramuscular injection only.

PRECAUTIONS

GENERAL—Gammar®-P I.M. should not be administered intravenously because of the potential for serious adverse reactions. Injections must be made intramuscularly, and care should be taken to draw back on the plunger of the syringe before injection in order to be certain that the needle is not in a blood vessel.

Although systemic reactions to intramuscularly administered immunoglobulin preparations are rare, epinephrine should be available for treatment of acute allergic symptoms.

LABORATORY TESTS—None are required.

DRUG INTERACTIONS—Antibodies in the globulin preparation may interfere with the response to live viral vaccines such as measles, mumps, rubella, and varicella. Therefore, use of such vaccines should be deferred until at least three months after Gammar®-P I.M. administration, based on the original dosage of immune globulin administered.[9, 10] The reduced immunogenicity of hepatitis A vaccine that occurs with concurrent administration of Immune Globulin (Human) is not expected to be clinically significant. If Immune Globulin (Human) is recommended for a person being given hepatitis A vaccine, it may be administered simultaneously with the hepatitis A vaccine at a separate anatomic injection site.[9, 14]

No interactions with other products are known.

PREGNANCY CATEGORY C—Animal reproduction studies have not been performed with Immune Globulin (Human) U.S.P., Gammar®-P I.M. It is also not known whether Gammar®-P I.M. can cause fetal harm when administered to a pregnant woman or can affect reproduction capacity. Gammar®-P I.M. should be given to a pregnant woman only if clearly needed.

PEDIATRIC USE—No clinical studies using Gammar®-P I.M. have been conducted in pediatric patients. Safety and effectiveness in pediatric patients have not been established.

ADVERSE REACTIONS

Local pain and tenderness at the injection site, urticaria, and angioedema may occur. Anaphylactic reactions, although rare, have been reported following the injection of human immune globulin preparations.[13] Anaphylaxis is more likely to occur if Gammar®-P I.M. is given intravenously; therefore Gammar®-P I.M. must be administered only intramuscularly.

Potential reactions to Immune Globulin (Human) may include: local pain, erythema, induration and pruritus at the site of injection, headache, nausea, dizziness, flushing, emesis, diaphoresis, hypotension, and body aches and pains such as back pain.

An open label, single dose study in 12 healthy volunteers was conducted with evaluations of adverse experiences inclusive of an assessment of the site of injection for erythema, pruritus, induration and local pain. Each subject received a dose of 0.25 mL/Kg (with a maximum of 15 mL total) divided across three injection sites, i.e., the right and left dorsal gluteal areas and the right vastus lateralis region. The dose employed (0.25 mL/Kg) is 4 to 12 times the dose recommended for prophylaxis of hepatitis A exposure. The results of this clinical study are described below.

The injection site assessment in this clinical study included observations at the following times post-infusion: 10, 20, and 30 minutes and 1, 4, 8, 12 and 24 hours and on Day 30. The predominant injection site reactions were moderate local pain and mild erythema with mild induration and pruritus being observed less frequently. Local pain was reported for 11/12 subjects. Most of these subjects (7/11) reported pain of moderate intensity. Two had mild pain and two others reported constant pain at the injection site which was associated with a restriction of activities. The median time for resolution of the injection site pain was 47 hours. Erythema was reported for 9/12 subjects. Most (8/9) were mild in intensity and one consisted of an area raised by more than a millimeter, extending beyond the injection site. The median time for resolution of the erythema was 1 hour. Induration was reported by 5/12 subjects, all mild, with a median time for resolution of 1 hour. Finally, mild pruritus was reported by 2/12 subjects with a median time for resolution of 22 hours.

In this clinical study, adverse reactions reported and related to study product, other than those noted at the site of injection, included headache, nausea, dizziness, vasodilation, vomiting, sweating, hypotension, myalgia and pain. The patient incidence of the most frequent of these reactions, were headache (3/12), nausea (2/12), vasodilation (2/12) and pain (2/12); all other related adverse events occurred in 1/12 subjects. A total of 18 adverse reactions were reported by 5 of 12 patients in the study, which were related to the study product, other than those noted at the site of injection. These adverse experiences were predominantly mild in severity, 14/18 (78%), with the remainder being moderate.

DOSAGE AND ADMINISTRATION

Dosage

HEPATITIS A—Gammar®-P I.M. in a dose of 0.01 mL/Lb (0.02 mL/Kg) is recommended for household and institutional hepatitis A contacts.

The following doses of Gammar®-P I.M. are recommended for persons who plan to travel in areas where hepatitis A is common.[14, 15]

Length of Stay	Dose Volume
Less than 3 months	0.02 mL/Kg
3 months or longer	0.06 mL/Kg
	(repeat every 4–6 months)

MEASLES (Rubeola)—Gammar®-P I.M. should be given in a dose of 0.11 mL/Lb (0.25 mL/Kg) to prevent or modify measles in a susceptible person exposed less than 6 days previously.[7, 8]

If a susceptible child who is also immunocompromised is exposed, Immune Globulin (Human) in a dose of 0.5 mL/Kg (maximum 15 mL) should be given immediately.[11, 12]

IMMUNOGLOBULIN DEFICIENCY—In patients with immunoglobulin deficiencies, replacement therapy can best be accomplished by use of Immune Globulin Intravenous (Human) (IGIV). If IGIV is unavailable, Gammar®-P I.M. may prevent serious infection in patients with immunoglobulin deficiencies if circulating IgG levels of approximately 200 mg/100mL plasma are maintained. The recommended dosage is 0.66 mL/Kg (at least 100 mg/Kg) given every 3 to 4 weeks.[6] A double dose is given at onset of therapy: some patients may require more frequent injections.

Administration

Gammar®-P I.M. is administered intramuscularly (see PRECAUTIONS), preferably in the gluteal region. Doses over 10 mL should be divided, so that no more than 5 mL is injected into any one site, and injected into several muscle sites to reduce local pain and discomfort.[16]

Parenteral drug products should be inspected visually for particulate matter and discoloration prior to administration whenever solution and container permit.

HOW SUPPLIED

Immune Globulin (Human), Gammar®-P I.M. is available as:

NDC0053-7576-01   2mL vial
NDC0053-7576-02   10mL vial

STORAGE

Vials should be stored at 2–8°C (36–46°F). Do not freeze. Do not use after expiration date.

CAUTION: FEDERAL LAW PROHIBITS DISPENSING WITHOUT PRESCRIPTION.

REFERENCES

1. Data on File: **Centeon L.L.C.**
2. Smith, GN, Mollison, D, Griffiths, B, and Mollison, PL; Uptake of IgG after intramuscular and subcutaneous injection. Lancet i; 1208–1212, 1972.
3. Waldmann, TA, Strober, W, and Blaese, RM: Variations in the metabolism of immunoglobulins measured by turnover rates, in Immunoglobulins. Biologic Aspects and Clinical Uses. Edited by Ezio Merler, National Academy of Sciences, Washington, D.C., 1970, pp. 33–51.
4. CDC. Post-Exposure Prophylaxis of Hepatitis B: Recommendations of the Immunization Practices Advisory Committee (ACIP). MMWR 1984;33, (No.21).
5. CDC. Protection Against Viral Hepatitis: Recommendations of the Immunization Practices Advisory Committee (ACIP). MMWR 1990;39 (No. RR-2).
6. Report of the Committee on Infectious Diseases, American Academy of Pediatrics, 1994, Red Book pp. 40–43.
7. CDC. Measles Prevention: Recommendations of the Immunization Practices Advisory Committee (ACIP). MMWR 1982;31 (No.17).
8. CDC. Measles Prevention: Recommendations of the Immunization Practices Advisory Committee (AICP). MMWR 1989;38 (NO. S-9).
9. Immune Globulin Monograph in AHFS Drug Information® 97. American Society of Health System Pharmacists, 1997©, pp. 2536-2545.
10. CDC. Update: Vaccine Side Effects, Adverse Reactions, Contraindications and Precautions—Recommendations of the Advisory Committee on Immunization Practices (ACIP). MMWR 1996;45 (No. RR-12).
11. Report of the Committee on Infectious Diseases, American Academy of Pediatrics, 1982, Red Bood pp. 134–135.
12. CDC. Recommendations of the Advisory Committee on Immunization Practices (ACIP): Use of Vaccines and Immune Globulins in Persons with Altered Immunocompetence. MMWR 1993;42 (No. RR-4).
13. Fudenberg, HH: Sensitization to immunoglobulins and hazards of gamma globulin therapy, in Immunoglobulins. Biologic Aspects and Clinical Uses. Edited by Ezio Merler. National Academy of Sciences, Washington, D.C., 1970, pp. 211–220.
14. CDC. Prevention of Hepatitis A Through Active or Passive Immunization: Recommendations of the Advisory Committee on Immunization Practices (ACIP). MMWR 1996;45 (No. RR-15).
15. CDC. Immune Globulins for Protection against Viral Hepatitis: Recommendations of the Advisory Committee on Immunization Practices (ACIP). MMWR 1981 (Vol. 30, No. 34).
16. CDC. General Recommendations on Immunization: Recommendations of the Advisory Committee on Immunization Practices (ACIP). MMWR 1994;43 (No. RR-1).

Revised: December, 1997   IBM 12250
Centeon L.L.C.
Kankakee, Illinois 60901 U.S.A.
U.S. License No. 149

Immune Globulin
Intravenous
(Human)
GAMMAR®-P I.V.   ℞

DESCRIPTION

Immune Globulin Intravenous (Human), Gammar®-P I.V., is a sterile, lyophilized preparation of intact, unmodified, immunoglobulin, primarily IgG, stabilized with Albumin (Human) and sucrose. The distribution of IgG subclasses is similar to that present in normal human plasma. It is prepared by cold alcohol fractionation of pooled plasma and is not chemically altered or enzymatically degraded. When reconstituted with the appropriate volume of Sterile Water for Injection, USP, Gammar®-P I.V. contains 5% IgG, 3% Albumin (Human), 5% sucrose, and 0.5% sodium chloride. The pH of the solution has been adjusted to 6.8 ± 0.4 with citric acid and/or sodium carbonate. Gammar®-P I.V. contains no preservative. This product is intended for intravenous administration.

The heat treatment step employed in the manufacture of Immune Globulin Intravenous (Human), Gammar®-P I.V., pasteurization at 60°C for 10 hours in aqueous solution form with stabilizers, has been validated in a series of *in vitro* experiments for its capacity to inactivate Human Immunodeficiency Virus (HIV) and the following model viruses: Sindbis, Vesicular Stomatitis (VSV), Bovine Viral Diarrhea Virus (BVD), Vaccinia, Pseudorabies and Murine Encephalomyocarditis (EMC), a non-lipid enveloped model

virus. HIV was reduced by 6.0 and 5.4 $\log_{10}$ to an undetectable level after 0.5 hours of heating in two independent experiments. For each of the model viruses studied, two independent experiments were also conducted with the following results: Sindbis was reduced by 7.5 and 7.9 $\log_{10}$ to an undetectable level after two hours of heating, VSV was reduced by 6.8 and 7.2 $\log_{10}$ to an undetectable level after 0.5 hours of heating, BVD, a model for hepatitis C virus, was reduced by 6.4 and 6.5 $\log_{10}$ to an undetectable level after four hours of heating, Vaccinia was reduced by 5.6 and 5.6 $\log_{10}$ to an undetectable level after two hours of heating, Pseudorabies was reduced by 4.9 and 3.6 $\log_{10}$ to an undetectable level after six hours of heating and EMC, a non-lipid enveloped model virus, was reduced by 4.5 and 4.8 $\log_{10}$ after ten hours of heating.[1]

The viral reduction capacity of the purification procedures used in the manufacture of Immune Globulin Intravenous (Human), Gammar®-P I.V., exclusive of heat treatment, was also studied in a series of *in vitro* experiments using HIV and the model virus EMC, a non-lipid enveloped virus. EMC was reduced by 4.9 $\log_{10}$ and 3.4 $\log_{10}$ by two, independent purification steps which are conducted before and after heat treatment, respectively. HIV was reduced by at least 6.7 $\log_{10}$ by the processing steps employed to isolate Cohn Fraction II from pooled plasma during the initial purification of Gammar®-P I.V. The total viral reduction capacity for HIV and EMC attributable to the Gammar®-P I.V. manufacturing procedure, inclusive of both the heat treatment protocol and the fractionation steps studied, is, therefore, ≥ 12.1 $\log_{10}$ for HIV and ≥ 12.8 $\log_{10}$ for EMC.[1]

CLINICAL PHARMACOLOGY

The half-life of Immune Globulin Intravenous (Human), Gammar®-P I.V., was evaluated in a double blind clinical study in which it was compared to Gammar® I.V.. The mean half-life of Gammar®-P I.V. in nine patients was determined to be approximately 40 days and was not statistically different from the mean half-life of 34 days found for Gammar® I.V. in seven patients; however, the half-life of IgG can vary considerably from patient to patient.[1]

Immune Globulin Intravenous (Human), Gammar®-P I.V., is a native, non-chemically modified IgG fractionated from pooled human donor plasma. The distribution of IgG subclasses (IgG_1, IgG_2, IgG_3, IgG_4) is similar to that present in Cohn Fraction II. Since the IgG concentrate is prepared from a large pool of at least 1000 donors, it represents the expected diversity of antibodies in that population. In a study of an unheated version of this product, Gammar® I.V., it was found that Gammar® I.V. provided a broad range of antibodies, capable of opsonization and neutralization of microbes and toxins, against bacterial and viral antigens for prevention or attenuation of infectious diseases.[2] In *in vitro* testing, Gammar®-P I.V. has been shown to provide equivalent levels of a broad range of antibodies when compared to Gammar® I.V.[1]

Albumin (Human) and sucrose are added to the formulation in order to provide adequate stabilization of the IgG molecules and the reconstituted product. Because sucrose, when given intravenously, is excreted unchanged in the urine, Immune Globulin Intravenous (Human), Gammar®-P I.V., may be given to diabetics without compensatory changes in insulin dosage regimen.[3]

INDICATIONS AND USAGE

Gammar®-P I.V. is indicated for patients with primary defective antibody synthesis such as agammaglobulinemia or hypogammaglobulinemia, who are at increased risk of infection. When high levels or rapid elevation of circulating gamma globulins are desired, intravenous administration is more desirable than intramuscular therapy.

CONTRAINDICATIONS

Gammar®-P I.V. is contraindicated in individuals with a history of anaphylactic or severe systemic response to immune globulin intramuscular or intravenous preparations or in individuals with a history of allergic reactions to human albumin.

Immune Globulin Intravenous (Human), Gammar®-P I.V., should not be given to persons with isolated immunoglobulin A (IgA) deficiency. These persons have the potential for developing antibodies to IgA and could have anaphylactic reactions to subsequent administration of blood products that contain IgA.[4]

WARNINGS

If anaphylactic or severe anaphylactoid reactions occur, discontinue infusion immediately. Epinephrine should be available for the treatment of any acute anaphylactoid reactions.

Patients with agammaglobulinemia or extreme hypogammaglobulinemia who have never received immunoglobulin substitution therapy before or who have not received immunoglobulin therapy within the preceding 8 weeks may be at risk of developing inflammatory reactions upon the infusion of human immunoglobulins. These reactions are manifested by a rise in temperature, chills, nausea and vomiting, and appear to be related to the rate of infusion.

NDC	Product	Diluent
NDC0053-7486-01	1 g immune globulin/vial	20 mL
NDC0053-7486-02	2.5 g immune globulin/vial	50 mL
NDC0053-7486-05	5 g immune globulin/vial	100 mL
NDC0053-7486-10	10 g immune globulin/vial	200 mL

Infusion rates and the patient's clinical state should be monitored closely during infusion. (See **Administration** section under **DOSAGE AND ADMINISTRATION**)

PRECAUTIONS

GENERAL – Epinephrine should be available for treatment of acute allergic reactions.

See **DOSAGE AND ADMINISTRATION** section for product compatibility information.

DRUG INTERACTIONS – It is reported that antibodies in immune globulin preparations may interfere with the response by pediatric patients to live viral vaccines such as measles, mumps and rubella. Immunizing physicians should be informed of recent therapy with Immune Globulin Intravenous (Human) so that appropriate precautions may be taken.

PREGNANCY CATEGORY C – Animal reproduction studies have not been performed with Immune Globulin Intravenous (Human), Gammar®-P I.V. It is also not known whether Immune Globulin Intravenous (Human), Gammar®-P I.V., can cause fetal harm when administered to a pregnant woman or can affect reproduction capacity. Gammar®-P I.V. should be given to a pregnant woman only if clearly needed.

ASEPTIC MENINGITIS SYNDROME – An aseptic meningitis syndrome (AMS) has been reported to occur infrequently in association with Immune Globulin Intravenous (Human) (IGIV) treatment. The syndrome usually begins within several hours to two days following IGIV treatment. It is characterized by symptoms and signs including severe headache, nuchal rigidity, drowsiness, fever, photophobia, painful eye movements, and nausea and vomiting. Cerebrospinal fluid (CSF) studies are frequently positive with pleocytosis up to several thousand cells per cubic millimeter, predominantly from the granulocytic series, and elevated protein levels up to several hundred mg/dl. Patients exhibiting such symptoms and signs should receive a thorough neurological examination, including CSF studies, to rule out other causes of meningitis. AMS may occur more frequently in association with high dose (2 g/kg) IGIV treatment. Discontinuation of IGIV treatment has resulted in remission of AMS within several days without sequelae.[5-8]

ACUTE RENAL FAILURE – Recently, there have been several reports in the literature of patients who experienced acute renal failure after receiving Immune Globulin Intravenous (Human), particularly in patients with compromised renal function.[9]

ADVERSE REACTIONS

Potential reactions for all Immune Globulin Intravenous (Human) products are often related to infusion rate and may include: nausea, vomiting, abdominal cramps, chills, pyrexia, chest tightness, palpitations, tachycardia, blood pressure changes, edema, flushing, diaphoresis, acute renal failure, rash, erythemia, pruritus, cyanosis, dizziness, headache, backache or other body aches, anxiety, wheezing (and other respiratory events), myalgia, shaking, fatigue, malaise and arthralgia, usually beginning within one hour of the start of the infusion.

A double blind study comparing Gammar® I.V. and Gammar® P I.V. as replacement therapy was conducted in 19 patients (108 infusions) with primary defective antibody synthesis, such as common variable or X-linked hypogammaglobulinemia. The types of infusion related adverse reactions noted were similar in frequency and nature. For the ten patients receiving only Gammar® P I.V. (56 infusions), all of the infusion related adverse reactions were characterized as mild and of short duration. These included the following most frequent reactions: Chills 8.9% (5/56), Headache 5.4% (3/56), and Pain: Back/Neck 3.6% (2/56). The overall incidence of infusions associated with an adverse reaction was 16% (9/56 infusions) for Gammar®-P I.V. which compared favorably with the overall incidence of infusions associated with an adverse reaction for Gammar® I.V. (25%; 13/52 infusions).[1]

True anaphylactic reactions may occur in patients with a history of prior systemic allergic reactions or seizure following administration of human immunoglobulin preparations. Very rarely an anaphylactoid reaction may occur in patients with no prior history of severe allergic reactions to human immunoglobulin preparations. Patients previously sensitized to certain antigens, most commonly IgA, may be at risk of immediate anaphylactoid and hypersensitivity reactions.[4] Epinephrine should be available for the treatment of any acute anaphylactoid reaction. (See **WARNINGS** and **CONTRAINDICATIONS**)

Infusion rates and clinical state should be monitored closely during infusion. If an adverse reaction occurs, the infusion rate should be reduced or the infusion stopped until the symptoms have subsided. (See **DOSAGE AND ADMINISTRATION**)

DOSAGE AND ADMINISTRATION

The usual dose of Immune Globulin Intravenous (Human), Gammar®-P I.V., is directed toward restoration of the immune deficient patient's circulating IgG level to near-normal levels. Use of 200–400 mg/kg body weight every three to four weeks is recommended although some patients may require 600 mg/Kg every three to four weeks. An initial loading dose of at least 200 mg/kg at more frequent intervals, proceeding to 200–600 mg/kg at three week intervals once a therapeutic plasma level has been established can be used. However, treatment must be individualized for each patient due to variation among patients in catabolic rate of IgG.

PRODUCT COMPATIBILITY – It is recommended that Immune Globulin Intravenous (Human), Gammar®-P I.V., be administered by a separate infusion line without admixture with other drugs or medications which the patient may be receiving. However, based upon compatibility studies, Gammar®-P I.V. may be infused sequentially into a primary i.v. line containing either 0.9% sodium chloride injection or 5% dextrose injection or flushed with 0.9% sodium chloride injection or 5% dextrose injection. **Do not mix Immune Globulin Intravenous (Human) products of differing formulations.** If several doses of Immune Globulin Intravenous (Human), Gammar®-P I.V. are to be administered, several reconstituted vials of identical formulation and diluent may be pooled, using proper aseptic technique. As described under **Reconstitution,** below, do not shake or cause excessive foaming. Swirl gently to mix. Filtration is acceptable but not required; pore sizes of greater than or equal to 15 microns will be less likely to slow infusion.

Reconstitution

CAUTION: **Reconstitution instructions must be followed exactly.** Please read the following instructions in their entirety before attempting to reconstitute product.

1) Bring both product vial and diluent vial to room temperature prior to reconstitution.
2) Examine product vial to ensure no product powder or cake is wedged in the neck of the vial. If so, gently tap the vial to dislodge the product.
3) Remove plastic flip-off caps from both vials.
4) Treat rubber stoppers with antiseptic solution and allow to dry.

CAUTION: The double ended vented transfer spike (see diagram below), provided in the package is comprised of a **white** (diluent) end, which has a double orifice, and a **green** (product) end, which has a single orifice. Incorrect use of the transfer spike will result in loss of vacuum, and prevent transfer of diluent thereby preventing reconstitution of the product.

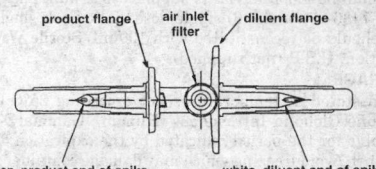

product flange — air inlet filter — diluent flange

green, product end of spike — white, diluent end of spike

The transfer spike is sterile. Do not touch the exposed ends of the spike after removing the guards.

5) Remove the guard from the **white** (diluent) end of the transfer spike. Insert the **white** end of the transfer spike into the center of the stopper of the upright **diluent** vial first.
6) Remove the guard from the **green** (product) end of the transfer spike. Invert the diluent vial with the attached transfer spike and, using minimum force, insert the **green** end into the center of the stopper of the upright **product** vial. The flange of the transfer spike should rest on the surface of the stopper and the diluent will begin to transfer into the **product** vial.
7) Allow the vacuum in the product vial to pull the diluent into the product vial.
8) During diluent transfer, wet the lyophilized cake completely by gently tilting the product vial. Do not allow the air inlet filter to face downward. Care should be taken not to lose the vacuum, as this will prolong reconstitution of the product.
9) After diluent transfer is complete, the transfer spike will allow filtered air into the product vial through the air filter. Additional venting of the product vial after diluent transfer is complete, is not required. When diluent transfer is complete, withdraw and properly discard transfer spike and diluent bottle.

Continued on next page

Gammar-P I.V.—Cont.

10) Allow the product vial to remain undisturbed for 5 minutes after diluent addition. Do not touch or mix during this time.
11) After 5 minutes, mix the product vial by gently swirling the vial without creating excessive foam. Never shake the product vial.

Note: A syrup-like layer may remain on the bottom of the vial following reconstitution. Swirl gently to disperse this layer until a homogenous solution is obtained.

12) Examine solution. All unreconstituted product should dissolve with gentle swirling and the solution should be clear and ready to administer in 20 minutes or less.
13) Product contains no preservative. Infusion must be initiated within 3 hours of reconstitution. If not used within this time frame, it should be properly disposed of and not administered.
14) Reconstituted product does not need to be filtered. If a filter is used, it should be a 15 micron filter or larger.
15) If several doses of Immune Globulin Intravenous (Human), Gammar®-P I.V., are to be pooled aseptically for administration, avoid excessive formation of foam in the pooling container and gently swirl the pooling container to mix. **DO NOT SHAKE THE POOLING CONTAINER.**

Administration

CAUTION: When entering the product stopper with an IV set spike for administration, care should be taken to follow the path made by the transfer spike (see Reconstitution).

Immune Globulin Intravenous (Human), Gammar®-P I.V., is to be administered by intravenous infusion. The infusion should begin at a rate of 0.01 mL/Kg/minute, increasing to 0.02 mL/Kg/minute after 15 to 30 minutes. Most patients tolerate a gradual increase to 0.03 – 0.06 mL/Kg/minute. For the average 70 kg person this is equivalent to 2 to 4 mL/minute. If adverse reactions develop, slowing the infusion rate will usually eliminate the reaction. Discard any unused solution.

Parenteral drug products should be inspected visually for particulate matter and discoloration prior to administration whenever solution and container permit.

HOW SUPPLIED

Individual Vial Packages

Immune Globulin Intravenous (Human), Gammar®-P I.V., is supplied in single dose vials, with diluent and sterile, vented transfer spike for reconstitution. The 10 g dosage form package also contains an administration set. The following dosage forms are available:

[See table at top of previous page]

Bulk Package

Immune Globulin Intravenous (Human), Gammar®-P I.V., 5 g immune globulin/vial is supplied in a bulk pack (NDC 0053-7486-06) of six (6) single dose vials. Each single dose vial should be reconstituted with 100 mL Sterile Water for Injection, U.S.P. (not supplied).

STORAGE

When stored at temperatures not exceeding 25°C (77°F), Immune Globulin Intravenous (Human), Gammar®-P I.V., is stable for the period indicated by the expiration date on its label. Avoid freezing which may damage container for the diluent.

CAUTION: FEDERAL LAW PROHIBITS DISPENSING WITHOUT PRESCRIPTION.

REFERENCES

1. Data on File: Armour Pharmaceutical Company.
2. Steele RW, Augustine RA, Tannenbaum AS, Marmer DJ. Intravenous Immune Globulin for Hypogammaglobulinemia: A Comparison of Opsonizing Capacity in Recipient Sera. *Clin. Immunol. Immunopathol.* 1985; 34:275–283.
3. Martindale. *The Extra Pharmacopoeia* 27th ed. Edited by Wade A. London: The Pharmaceutical Press. 1979; 65.
4. Fudenberg HH. Sensitization to Immunoglobulins and Hazards of Gamma Globulin Therapy. *Immunoglobulins, Biologic Aspects and Clinical Uses.* 1970; 211–220. Edited by Merler E. National Academy of Sciences, Washington, D.C.
5. Sekul EA, Cupler EJ, Dalakas, MC. Aseptic Meningitis Associated with High Dose Intravenous Immunoglobulin Therapy: Frequency and Risk Factors. *Ann Int Med* 1994; 121:4, 259–262.
6. Kato E, Shindo S, Eto Y, et al. Administration of Immune Globulin Associated with Aseptic Meningitis. *JAMA* 1988; 259:3269–3271.
7. Casteels-Van Daele M, Wijndaele L, Hunninck K, Gillis P, Ziekenhuis V. Intravenous Immune Globulin and Acute Aseptic Meningitis. *N Engl J Med* 1990; 323:614–615.
8. Scribner C, Kapit R, Phillips E, Rickels N. Aseptic Meningitis and Intravenous Immunoglobulin Therapy. *Ann Int Med* 1994; 121:305–306.
9. Tan E, et al. Acute Renal Failure Resulting from Intravenous Immunoglobulin Therapy. *Arch Neurol.* 1993; 50(2): 137–139.

BIBLIOGRAPHY

Polley MJ, Fischetti VA, Landaburu PH. Native Intravenous IgG Exhibits Greater Biological Activity than Modified IgG. From the *XX Cong. Int. Soc. of Hematology;* 1984.

Revised: June, 1997 IBM 12173

CENTEON L.L.C.
Kankakee, Illinois 60901 U.S.A.
U.S. License No. 149

Antihemophilic Factor (Recombinant)
HELIXATE® ℞

DESCRIPTION

Antihemophilic Factor (Recombinant), HELIXATE® is a sterile, stable, purified, non-pyrogenic, dried concentrate which has been manufactured by recombinant DNA technology. HELIXATE is intended for use in therapy of classical hemophilia (hemophilia A). HELIXATE is produced by Baby Hamster Kidney (BHK) cells into which the human factor VIII (FVIII) gene has been introduced.[1] HELIXATE is a highly purified glycoprotein consisting of multiple peptides including an 80 kD and various extensions of the 90 kD subunit. It has the same biological activity as FVIII derived from human plasma. In addition to the use of the classical purification methods of ion exchange chromatography and size exclusion chromatography, monoclonal antibody immunoaffinity chromatography is utilized along with other steps designed to purify recombinant factor VIII (rAHF) and remove contaminating substances. The final preparation is stabilized with Albumin (Human) and lyophilized. The concentration of HELIXATE is approximately 100 IU/mL. The product contains no preservatives.

Each vial of HELIXATE contains the labeled amount of rAHF in international units (IU). One IU, as defined by the World Health Organization standard for blood coagulation factor VIII, human, is approximately equal to the level of factor VIII activity found in 1.0 mL of fresh pooled human plasma. The final product when reconstituted as directed contains the following excipients: 10–30 mg glycine/mL, not more than (NMT) 500 µg imidazole/1000 IU, NMT 600 µg polysorbate 80/1000 IU, 2–5 mM calcium chloride, 100–130 mEq/L sodium, 100–130 mEq/L chloride, and 4–10 mg Albumin (Human)/mL. HELIXATE must be administered by the intravenous route.

CLINICAL PHARMACOLOGY

The clinical trial of HELIXATE has included 168 patients, enrolled over a 55-month period. A total of 16,186 infusions have been utilized in this trial. The study was conducted in several stages.

Initial pharmacokinetic studies were conducted in 17 asymptomatic hemophilic patients, comparing pharmacokinetics of plasma-derived Antihemophilic Factor (Human) (pdAHF) and HELIXATE.[2] The mean biologic half-life of rAHF was 15.8 hours. The mean biologic half-life of pdAHF in the same individuals was 13.9 hours. A similar degree of shortening of the activated partial thromboplastin time was seen with both rAHF and pdAHF. The mean in vivo recovery of rAHF was similar to pdAHF, with a linear dose-response relationship. The recovery and half-life of rAHF was consistent with initial results following 13 weeks of exclusive treatment with HELIXATE. Subsequently, 826 recovery studies were conducted in 58 hemophilic patients participating in later clinical studies. Mean recovery from this group was 2.48% per IU/kg infused.

Fourteen (14) subjects from initial pharmacokinetic studies commenced home treatment with rAHF. Forty-four (44) additional subjects were then enrolled who treated themselves at home exclusively with rAHF. A total of 12,730 infusions have been administered under this portion of the study, of which 1,021 were given in clinic for recovery studies, 7,339 were given for treatment of bleeds, 4,361 were given as prophylaxis, 5 for minor surgery not requiring hospitalization, and 4 for unspecified reason.

Forty-eight (48) patients have received rAHF on 63 occasions for surgical procedures or in-hospital treatment of serious hemorrhage. Eleven (11) received rAHF for the first time in this study, while 37 were already on study or study participants under an investigation of previously untreated patients. Hemostasis has been satisfactory in all cases, with no adverse reactions.

In a study of previously untreated patients, a total of 3,254 infusions have been administered to 96 patients over a 48-month enrollment period. Hemostasis was successfully achieved in all cases.

During the analytical characterization of Antihemophilic Factor (Recombinant), HELIXATE®, analyses for carbohydrate structure revealed the presence of terminal galactose $\alpha 1 \rightarrow 3$ galactose residues. Since naturally occurring antibody to this structure has been reported in humans, a trial in 18 patients was performed in which the half-life and recovery of rAHF with high levels of this carbohydrate residue was compared to that with HELIXATE, which contains low levels of this structure. As in the normal population, all patients had preexisting endogenous antibody to galactose $\alpha 1 \rightarrow 3$ galactose in titers ranging from 1:320 to 1:5120 and no significant change in antibody level was noted during the study. While the mean recovery for HELIXATE in the study, 2.76%/IU/kg (N = 43), was significantly different from that of rAHF with high levels of residues, 2.43%/IU/kg (N = 155; p = 0.0001), the recovery for rAHF with high levels of galactose $\alpha 1 \rightarrow 3$ galactose is not significantly different from the 2.48%/IU/kg recovery obtained in the larger study from the 58 patients treated with HELIXATE mentioned above. Based on these results, the galactose $\alpha 1 \rightarrow 3$ galactose residue appears to have no clinical significance.

INDICATIONS AND USAGE

HELIXATE is indicated for the treatment of classical hemophilia (hemophilia A) in which there is a demonstrated deficiency of activity of the plasma clotting factor, factor VIII. HELIXATE provides a means of temporarily replacing the missing clotting factor in order to correct or prevent bleeding episodes, or in order to perform emergency and elective surgery in hemophiliacs.

HELIXATE can also be used for treatment of hemophilia A in certain patients with inhibitors to factor VIII. In clinical studies of HELIXATE, patients who developed inhibitors on study continued to manifest a clinical response when inhibitor titers were less than 10 Bethesda Units (B.U.) per mL. When an inhibitor is present, the dosage requirement for factor VIII is variable. The dosage can be determined only by clinical response, and by monitoring of circulating factor VIII levels after treatment (see **DOSAGE AND ADMINISTRATION**).

HELIXATE does not contain von Willebrand's factor and therefore is not indicated for the treatment of von Willebrand's disease.

CONTRAINDICATIONS

Due to the fact that Antihemophilic Factor (Recombinant) contains trace amounts of mouse protein (maximum 0.03 ng/IU rAHF) and hamster protein (maximum 0.04 ng/IU rAHF), HELIXATE should be administered with caution to individuals with previous hypersensitivity to pdAHF or known hypersensitivity to biologic preparations with trace amounts of murine or hamster proteins.

Assays to detect seroconversion to mouse and hamster protein were conducted on all patients on study. No patient has developed specific antibody titers against these proteins after commencing study, and no allergic reactions have been associated with rAHF infusions. Although no reactions were observed, patients should be warned of the theoretical possibility of a hypersensitivity reaction, and alerted to the early signs of such a reaction (e.g., hives, generalized urticaria, wheezing and hypotension). Patients should be advised to discontinue use of the product and contact their physician if such symptoms occur.

WARNINGS

None.

PRECAUTIONS

General

HELIXATE is intended for the treatment of bleeding disorders arising from a deficiency in factor VIII. This deficiency should be proven prior to administering HELIXATE.

The development of circulating neutralizing antibodies to factor VIII may occur during the treatment of patients with hemophilia A. In a study of previously untreated patients, inhibitor antibodies have developed in 17 of the 92 patients (18.5%) who have had at least one follow-up titer. The incidence of antibodies is 15/56 (26.7%) in patients with severe disease (<2% factor VIII), 2/18 (11%) in patients with moderate disease (2–5% factor VIII) and 0/18 in patients with mild disease (>5% factor VIII). Ten of the antibodies were high titer (>10 Bethesda Units), three were low titer, and four were low titer and transient. Studies most closely resembling the design of the study of inhibitor development with Antihemophilic Factor (Recombinant), HELIXATE® have reported incidences of inhibitor formation ranging between 18.4 and 52% for patients treated with pdAHF.[3-6] The incidence of inhibitor formation in previously untreated patients treated with HELIXATE appears to be consistent with that reported in the literature, however the true immunogenicity of HELIXATE is not known at present. Patients treated with rAHF should be carefully monitored for the development of antibodies to rAHF by appropriate clinical observation and laboratory tests.

Product administration and handling of the infusion set and needles must be done with caution. Percutaneous puncture with a needle contaminated with blood can transmit infectious virus including HIV (AIDS) and hepatitis. Obtain immediate medical attention if injury occurs.

Place needles in sharps container after single use. Discard all equipment including any reconstituted HELIXATE product in accordance with biohazard procedures.

Carcinogenesis, Mutagenesis, Impairment of Fertility

In vitro evaluation of the mutagenic potential of HELIXATE failed to demonstrate reverse mutation or chromosomal aberrations at doses substantially greater than the maximum expected clinical dose. In vivo evaluation of rAHF using doses ranging between 10 and 40 times the expected clinical maximum also indicated that HELIXATE does not possess a mutagenic potential. Long-term investigations of carcinogenic potential in animals have not been performed.

Pediatric Use

HELIXATE has been proven to be safe and efficacious in newborns and children while under investigation as previously treated (n=21) and previously untreated patients (n=96) (see **CLINICAL PHARMACOLOGY** and **PRECAUTIONS**).

Pregnancy Category C

Animal reproduction studies have not been conducted with HELIXATE. It is also not known whether HELIXATE can cause fetal harm when administered to a pregnant woman or can affect reproduction capacity. HELIXATE should be given to a pregnant woman only if clearly needed.

ADVERSE REACTIONS

During the clinical studies conducted in previously treated patients, 47 out of 12,932 infusions (0.36%) were associated with 58 reported minor adverse reactions. Of these, 19 reactions were local to the injection site (e.g., burning, pruritus, erythema); and 39 were systemic complaints (dizziness, nausea, chest discomfort, sore throat, cold feet, unusual taste in mouth, and slight decrease in blood pressure). In the study with previously untreated patients, 3,254 infusions have been associated with 11 minor adverse reactions (0.34%): two reports of erythema at the injection site, one of facial flushing related to the infusion, one report of diarrhea, two reports of nonspecific rash, two reports of fever, and three reports of emesis. No serious reactions have been reported, and all reactions have been self-limited.

DOSAGE AND ADMINISTRATION

Each bottle of HELIXATE has the rAHF content in international units per bottle stated on the label of the bottle. The reconstituted product must be administered intravenously by either direct syringe or drip infusion. The product must be administered within 3 hours after reconstitution.

General Approach to Treatment and Assessment of Treatment Efficacy

The dosages described below are presented as general guidance. It should be emphasized that the dosage of HELIXATE required for hemostasis must be individualized according to the needs of the patient, the severity of the deficiency, the severity of the hemorrhage, the presence of inhibitors, and the factor VIII level desired. It is often critical to follow the course of therapy with factor VIII level assays. The clinical effect of HELIXATE is the most important element in evaluating the effectiveness of treatment. It may be necessary to administer more HELIXATE than would be estimated in order to attain satisfactory clinical results. If the calculated dose fails to attain the expected factor VIII levels, or if bleeding is not controlled after administration of the calculated dosage, the presence of a circulating inhibitor in the patient should be suspected. Its presence should be substantiated and the inhibitor level quantitated by appropriate laboratory tests. When an inhibitor is present, the dosage requirement for rAHF is extremely variable and the dosage can be determined only by the clinical response.

Some patients with low titer inhibitors (<10 B.U.) can be successfully treated with factor VIII without a resultant amnestic rise in inhibitor titer.[7] Factor VIII levels and clinical response to treatment must be assessed to insure adequate response. Use of alternative treatment products, such as Factor IX Complex concentrates, Antihemophilic Factor (Porcine) or Anti-Inhibitor Coagulant Complex, may be necessary for patients with anamnestic responses to factor VIII treatment and/or high titer inhibitors.

Calculation of Dosage

The in vivo percent elevation in factor VIII level can be estimated by multiplying the dose of rAHF per kilogram of body weight (IU/kg) by 2%. This method of calculation is based on clinical findings by Abildgaard et al,[8] and is illustrated in the following examples:

[See first table above]
[See second table above]
or
[See third table above]
[See fourth table above]

The dosage necessary to achieve hemostasis depends upon the type and severity of the bleeding episode, according to the following general guidelines:

Mild Hemorrhage

Mild superficial or early hemorrhages may respond to a single dose of 10 IU per kg,[9] leading to an in vivo rise of approximately 20% in the factor VIII level. Therapy need not be repeated unless there is evidence of further bleeding.

Moderate Hemorrhage

For more serious bleeding episodes (e.g., definite hemarthroses, known trauma), the factor VIII level should be

---

$$\text{Expected \% factor VIII increase} = \frac{\text{\# units administered} \times 2\%/\text{IU/kg}}{\text{body weight (kg)}}$$

$$\text{Example for a 70 kg adult:} = \frac{1400 \text{ IU} \times 2\%/\text{IU/kg}}{70 \text{ kg}} = 40\%$$

$$\text{Dosage required (IU)} = \frac{\text{body weight (kg)} \times \text{desired \% factor VIII increase}}{2\%/\text{IU/kg}}$$

$$\text{Example for a 15 kg child:} = \frac{15 \text{ kg} \times 100\%}{2\%/\text{IU/kg}} = 750 \text{ IU required}$$

Product Code	Approximate Factor VIII Activity	Diluent
NDC 0053-8120-01	250 IU	2.5 mL
NDC 0053-8120-02	500 IU	5 mL
NDC 0053-8120-04	1000 IU	10 mL

---

raised to 30–50% by administering approximately 15–25 IU per kg. If further therapy is required, a repeat infusion can be given at 12–24 hours.[10]

Severe Hemorrhage

In patients with life-threatening bleeding or possible hemorrhage involving vital structures (e.g., central nervous system, retropharyngeal and retroperitoneal spaces, iliopsoas sheath), the factor VIII level should be raised to 80–100% of normal in order to achieve hemostasis. This may be achieved with an initial rAHF (Antihemophilic Factor (Recombinant), HELIXATE®) dose of 40–50 IU per kg and a maintenance dose of 20–25 IU per kg every 8–12 hours.[11, 12]

Surgery

For major surgical procedures, the factor VIII level should be raised to approximately 100% by giving a preoperative dose of 50 IU/kg. The factor VIII level should be checked to assure that the expected level is achieved before the patient goes to surgery. In order to maintain hemostatic levels, repeat infusions may be necessary every 6 to 12 hours initially, and for a total of 10 to 14 days until healing is complete. The intensity of factor VIII replacement therapy required depends on the type of surgery and postoperative regimen employed. For minor surgical procedures, less intensive treatment schedules may provide adequate hemostasis.[11, 12]

Prophylaxis

Factor VIII concentrates may also be administered on a regular schedule for prophylaxis of bleeding, as reported by Nilsson et al.[13]

Reconstitution

Vacuum Transfer

1. Warm the unopened diluent and the concentrate to room temperature (NMT 37°C, 99°F).
2. After removing the plastic flip-top caps (Fig. A), aseptically cleanse the rubber stoppers of both bottles.
3. Remove the protective cover from the plastic transfer needle cartridge with tamper-proof seal and penetrate the stopper of the diluent bottle (Fig. B).
4. Remove the remaining portion of the plastic cartridge, invert the diluent bottle and penetrate the rubber seal on the concentrate bottle (Fig. C) with the needle at an angle.

   Alternate method of transferring sterile water: With a sterile needle and syringe, withdraw the appropriate volume of diluent and transfer to the bottle of lyophilized concentrate.
5. The vacuum will draw the diluent into the concentrate bottle. Hold the diluent bottle at an angle to the concentrate bottle in order to direct the jet of diluent against the wall of the concentrate bottle (Fig. C). Avoid excessive foaming.
6. After removing the diluent bottle and transfer needle (Fig. D), swirl continuously until completely dissolved (Fig. E).
7. After the concentrate powder is completely dissolved, withdraw solution into the syringe through the filter needle which is supplied in the package (Fig. F). Replace the filter needle with the administration set provided and inject intravenously.
8. If the same patient is to receive more than one bottle, the contents of two bottles may be drawn into the same syringe through a separate unused filter needle before attaching the vein set.

   [See figures A-F in next column]

Rate of Administration

The rate of administration should be adapted to the response of the individual patient. Administration of the entire dose in 5 to 10 minutes or less is well tolerated. Parenteral drug products should be inspected visually for particulate matter and discoloration prior to administration, whenever solution and container permit.

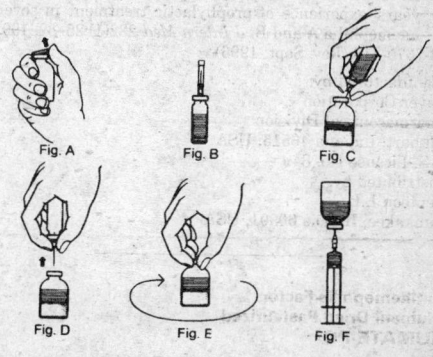

Fig. A   Fig. B   Fig. C

Fig. D   Fig. E   Fig. F

HOW SUPPLIED

Antihemophilic Factor (Recombinant), HELIXATE® is supplied in the following single use bottles with the total units of factor VIII activity stated on the label of each bottle. A suitable volume of Sterile Water for Injection, USP, a sterile double-ended transfer needle, a sterile filter needle, and a sterile administration set are provided.

[See fifth table above]

STORAGE

HELIXATE should be stored under refrigeration (2°–8°C; 36°–46°F). Storage of lyophilized powder at room temperature (up to 25°C or 77°F) for 3 months, such as in home treatment situations, may be done without loss of factor VIII activity. Freezing should be avoided, as breakage of the diluent bottle might occur. Do not use beyond the expiration date indicated on the bottle.

CAUTION

U.S. federal law prohibits dispensing without prescription.

LIMITED WARRANTY

A number of factors beyond our control could reduce the efficacy of this product or even result in an ill effect following its use. These include improper storage and handling of the product after it leaves our hands, diagnosis, dosage, method of administration, and biological differences in individual patients. Because of these factors, it is important that this product be stored properly, and that the directions be followed carefully during use.

No warranty, express or implied, including any warranty of merchantability or fitness is made. Representatives of the Company are not authorized to vary the terms or the contents of the printed labeling, including the package insert for this product, except by printed notice from the Company's headquarters. The prescriber and use of this product must accept the terms hereof.

REFERENCES

1. Lawn RM, Vehar GA: The molecular genetics of hemophilia. *Sci Am* 254(3):48–54, 1986.
2. Schwartz RS, Abildgaard CF, Aledort LM, et al: Human recombinant DNA-derived antihemophilic factor (factor VIII) in the treatment of hemophilia A. *N Engl J Med* 323(26):1800–5, 1990.
3. Lusher JM: Viral safety and inhibitor development associated with monoclonal antibody-purified FVIIIc. *Ann Hematol* 63(3):138–41, 1991.
4. Addiego JE Jr, Gomperts E, Liu S-L, et al: Treatment of hemophilia A with a highly purified factor VIII concentrate prepared by anti-FVIIIc immunoaffinity chromatography. *Thromb Haemost* 67(1):19–27, 1992.

Continued on next page

Helixate—Cont.

5. Schwarzinger I, Pabinger I, Korninger C, et al: Incidence of inhibitors in patients with severe and moderate hemophilia A treated with factor VIII concentrates. *Am J Hematol* 24(3):241–5, 1987.
6. Ehrenforth S, Kreuz W, Scharrer I, et al: Incidence of development of factor VIII and factor IX inhibitors in hemophiliacs. *Lancet* 339(8793):594–8, 1992.
7. Kasper CK: Complications of hemophilia A treatment: factor VIII inhibitors. *Ann NY Acad Sci* 614:97–105, 1991.
8. Abildgaard CF, Simone JV, Corrigan JJ, et al: Treatment of hemophilia with glycine-precipitated Factor VIII. *N Engl J Med* 275(9):471–5, 1966.
9. Britton M, Harrison J, Abildgaard CF: Early treatment of hemophilic hemarthroses with minimal dose of new factor VIII concentrate. *J Pediatr* 85(2):245–7, 1974.
10. Abildgaard CF: Current concepts in the management of hemophilia. *Semin Hematol* 12(3):223–32, 1975.
11. Hilgartner MW: Factor replacement therapy. In: Hilgartner MW, Pochedly C, eds.: Hemophilia in the child and adult. New York, Raven Press, 1989, pp 1–26.
12. Kasper CK, Dietrich SL: Comprehensive management of haemophilia. *Clin Haematol* 14(2):489–512, 1985.
13. Nilsson IM, Berntorp E, Löfqvist T, et al: Twenty-five years' experience of prophylactic treatment in severe haemophilia A and B. *J Intern Med* 232(1):25–32, 1992.

14-7670-213 (Rev. Sept. 1996)

Manufactured by:
Bayer Corporation
Pharmaceutical Division
Elkhart, Indiana 46515, USA
U.S. License No. 8
Distributed by:
Centeon L.L.C.
Kankakee, Illinois 60901, USA

Antihemophilic Factor (Human) Dried Pasteurized
HUMATE-P® ℞

DESCRIPTION

Antihemophilic Factor (Human), Pasteurized, Humate-P® is a stable, purified, sterile, lyophilized concentrate of Antihemophilic Factor (Human) (Factor VIII, AHF) to be administered by the intravenous route in the treatment of patients with classical hemophilia (hemophilia A).
Humate-P® is purified from the cold insoluble fraction of pooled human fresh-frozen plasma and contains highly purified and concentrated Antihemophilic Factor (Human). Humate-P® has a high degree of purity with a low amount of non-factor VIII proteins and contains no fibrinogen (as detected by the Clauss method). Humate-P® has a higher AHF potency than cryoprecipitate preparations. Each bottle of Humate-P® contains the labeled amount of antihemophilic activity in international units. The Unit (IU) is defined by an international standard established by the World Health Organization: one AHF international unit is approximately equal to the level of AHF found in 1.0 mL of fresh-pooled human plasma.
Each 100 IU of Antihemophilic Factor (Human) contains 60 to 100 mg of glycine, 14 to 28 mg of sodium citrate, 8 to 16 mg of sodium chloride, 16 to 24 mg of albumin (human), 4 to 20 mg of other proteins and 20 to 44 mg of total proteins.
This product is prepared from pooled human plasma collected in the United States. Humate-P® may also be prepared from source material supplied by other U.S. licensed manufacturers.
Antihemophilic Factor (Human), Pasteurized, Humate-P® is pasteurized by a new procedure: heating to 60°C for 10 hours in aqueous solution form.[1] This procedure has been shown to inactivate several DNA viruses (cytomegalovirus, herpes, and hepatitis B) and RNA viruses (rubella, mumps, measles, and poliomyelitis). However, no procedure has been shown to be totally effective in removing hepatitis infectivity from Antihemophilic Factor (Human) (See Clinical Pharmacology and Warnings).
Humate-P® contains anti-A and anti-B blood group isoagglutinins (see PRECAUTIONS).

CLINICAL PHARMACOLOGY

After I.V. injection in humans, there is a rapid increase in plasma Antihemophilic Factor followed by a rapid decrease in activity (time of equilibration with the extravascular compartment) and a subsequent slower rate of decrease in activity (biological half-life). Studies with Humate-P® in hemophilic patients have demonstrated a mean initial half-disappearance time of 8 hours and a mean half-life of 12 hours.
Tests of infectivity on chimpanzees have confirmed the reliability of this pasteurization method in eliminating the risk of transmission of hepatitis B virus. Two chimpanzee studies were used to evaluate the efficacy of the pasteurization process in inactivating hepatitis B virus. In studies of six and nine months duration, cryoprecipitate was infected with hepatitis B virus to give a concentration of 3000 infectious units/mL. All chimpanzees injected with either cryoprecipitate or non-pasteurized Antihemophilic Factor (Human) developed hepatitis B markers (HbsAg, Anti-Hbs, Anti-Hbc). All chimpanzees injected with the pasteurized Antihemophilic Factor (Human) product consistently remained serologically negative.
The pasteurization process used in the manufacture of this product has demonstrated *in vitro* inactivation of a number of infectious agents, including HIV, Epstein-Barr virus, cytomegalovirus, herpes simplex virus, rubella virus, measles virus, mumps virus, and poliomyelitis virus. *In vivo* experiments have demonstrated inactivation of hepatitis B virus and at least one type of nonA, nonB-hepatitis virus. Furthermore, clinical studies using this product have indicated an absence of transmission of HIV, hepatitis B virus, and nonA, nonB-hepatitis.
Clinical evidence confirms the hepatitis B safety of the pasteurization procedure. Of the 34 patients who had serological follow-up for hepatitis B markers, none had developed sero-conversion of the antibodies. Anti-Hbs or Anti-Hbc caused by the administration of Antihemophilic Factor (Human), Pasteurized, Humate-P®.[2]
A total of 24 lots of Humate-P® were administered to a cohort of 16 patients who had not previously received any blood products. The study showed no elevation in ALT levels over observation periods ranging from 2 months to 12 months.
In a retrospective study of 56 patients all have remained negative for the presence of HIV-1 antibody for time periods ranging from 2 months to 5 years from initial administration of product.

INDICATIONS AND USAGE

The usage of Humate-P® is indicated in hemophilia A (classical hemophilia) for the prevention and control of hemorrhagic episodes. Antihemophilic Factor (Human) is not indicated in von Willebrands disease.

CONTRAINDICATIONS

None known.

WARNINGS

This product is prepared from pooled human plasma which may contain the causative agents of hepatitis and other viral diseases. Prescribed manufacturing procedures utilized at the plasma collection centers, plasma testing laboratories, and the fractionation facilities are designed to reduce the risk of transmitting viral infection. However, the risk of viral infectivity from this product cannot be totally eliminated. Accordingly, the benefits and risks of treatment with this concentrate should be carefully assessed prior to use. Individuals who receive infusions of blood or plasma products may develop signs and/or symptoms of some viral infections, particularly nonA, and nonB hepatitis.

PRECAUTIONS

It is important to determine that the coagulation disorder is caused by factor VIII deficiency, since no benefit in treating other deficiencies can be expected.
This Antihemophilic Factor (Human), Pasteurized, Humate-P® preparation contains blood group isoagglutinins (anti-A and anti-B). When large or frequently repeated doses are needed, as when inhibitors are present or when pre- and post-surgical care is involved, patients of blood groups A, B and AB should be monitored for signs of intravascular hemolysis and decreasing hematocrit values. In the event of severe hemolysis, type-specific cryoprecipitate can be given instead. Hemolytic anemia, when present, may be corrected by the administration of compatible Group O Red Blood Cells (Human).
Other precautions are as follows:

- The filter needle should only be used to transfer solution from the preparation vial to a syringe or infusion bottle or bag. The filter needle must not be used for injection.
- The administration equipment and any unused Antihemophilic Factor (Human), Pasteurized, Humate-P® should be discarded.

Pregnancy Category C.
Animal reproduction studies have not been conducted with Antihemophilic Factor (Human). It is also not known whether Antihemophilic Factor (Human) can cause fetal harm when administered to a pregnant woman or can affect reproduction capacity. Antihemophilic Factor (Human) should be given to a pregnant woman only if clearly needed.

ADVERSE REACTIONS

Antihemophilic Factor (Human), Pasteurized, Humate-P®, is usually tolerated without reaction. Rare cases of allergic reaction and rise in temperature have been observed.

DOSAGE AND ADMINISTRATION

Humate-P® is for intravenous administration only. Although dosage must be individualized according to the needs of the patient (weight, severity of hemorrhage, presence of inhibitors), the following general dosages are suggested:

1. OVERT BLEEDING — Initially 15 units per kg of body weight followed by 8 units per kg every 8 hours for the first 24 hours and the same dose every 12 hours for 3 or 4 days.
2. MUSCLE HEMORRHAGES —
   a. Minor hemorrhages in extremities or non-vital areas: 8 units per kg once a day for 2 or 3 days.
   b. Massive hemorrhages in non-vital area: 8 units per kg by infusion at 12 hours intervals for 2 days and then one a day for 2 more days.
   c. Hemorrhages near vital organs (neck, throat, subperitoneal), 15 units per kg initially, then 8 units per kg every 8 hours.
   After 2 days the dose may be reduced by one-half.
3. JOINT HEMORRHAGES — The usual dose is 8 units per kg every 8 hours for 1 day; then every 12 hours for 1 or 2 days. However, recent experience suggests that a substantially lower dose, 5–8 units per kg given once, may be sufficient for most hemorrhages. If aspiration is carried out, 8 units per kg are given just prior to aspiration; 8 hours later and again on the following day.
4. SURGERY — Dosages of 26 to 30 units per kg body weight prior to surgery are recommended. After surgery, 15 units per kg every 8 hours should be administered. Close laboratory control to maintain the blood AHF at the level deemed appropriate for the surgical procedure is recommended for at least 10 days postoperatively. As a general rule, 1 unit of AHF activity per kg will increase the circulating AHF level by 2%. Adequacy of treatment must be judged by the clinical effects — thus the dosage may vary with individual cases.

Reconstitution

1. Warm both diluent and Antihemophilic Factor (Human), Pasteurized, Humate-P® in unopened vials to room temperature [not above 37°C (98°F)].
2. Remove caps from both vials to expose central portions of the rubber stoppers.
3. Treat surface of rubber stoppers with antiseptic solution and allow to dry.
4. Using aseptic technique, pierce the double needle of the blue transfer set into the diluent vial. Remove the protective cap and insert the exposed (longer) needle into the upright Antihemophilic Factor (Human), Pasteurized, Humate-P® vial. The diluent will be transferred into the Humate-P® by vacuum.
5. Remove the diluent vial, then the transfer set, from the Humate-P® vial.
6. Gently rotate the vial. DO NOT SHAKE VIAL. Vigorous shaking will prolong the reconstitution time. Continue swirling until the powder is dissolved and the solution is ready for administration. To assure product sterility, Humate-P® should be administered within three hours after reconstitution.
7. Parenteral drug products should be inspected visually for particulate matter and discoloration prior to administration, whenever solution and container permit.

Administration

INTRAVENOUS INJECTION

Plastic disposable syringes are recommended with Antihemophilic Factor (Human), Pasteurized, Humate-P® solution. The ground glass surface of all-glass syringes tend to stick with solutions of this type.

1. Open the package containing the disposable filter. Attach the filter to a sterile disposable syringe and take the filter out of the package.
2. Remove the protective cap and — without touching the tip of the filter — insert the disposable filter into the stopper of the Humate-P® vial; inject air.
3. Draw up the solution slowly (when using several syringes leave the filter in the vial). Discard the filter.
4. Slowly inject the solution (maximally 4 mL/minute) intravenously with an infusion kit or with a suitable injection needle. Aspiration of blood into the filled syringe must be avoided.

HOW SUPPLIED

Antihemophilic Factor (Human), Pasteurized, Humate-P®, is supplied in a single dose vial with a vial of diluent and sterile needles for reconstitution and withdrawal. I.U. activity is stated on the carton and label of each vial.

STORAGE

When stored at refrigerator temperature, 2°–8°C (36°–46°F), Antihemophilic Factor (Human), Pasteurized, Humate-P® is stable for the period indicated by the expiration date on its label. Within this period, Humate-P® may be stored at room temperature not to exceed 30°C (86°F), for up to 6 months. Avoid freezing, which may damage container for the diluent.

CAUTION: FEDERAL LAW PROHIBITS DISPENSING WITHOUT PRESCRIPTION.

REFERENCES

1. Heimburger N, Schwinn H, Gratz P, et al: Factor VIII Concentrate — highly purified and heated in solution. Arzneim Forsch 31(1): 619–22, 1981.
2. Experimental and clinical studies of a new pasteurized antihemophilic factor concentrate. In press.
3. Abildgaard CF, Simone JV, Corrigan JJ, et al: Treatment of hemophilia with glycine-precipitated factor VIII, New Engl J Med 275: 471–475, 1966.
4. Hilgartner MW: Current Therapy, in Hilgartner MW (ed): Hemophilia in children. Littleton, MA, Publishing Sciences Group Inc., 1976, p 158.
5. Schimpf K, Rothman P, Zimmermann K: Factor VIII dosis in prophylaxis of hemophilia A; A further controlled study, Proc XIth Cong W.F.H. Tokyo, Academia Press, 1976, p 363.

Revised: August, 1996   8700 A 2

Manufactured by:
Centeon Pharma GmbH
D-35002 Marburg, Germany
U.S. Government License N. 1202

Distributed by:
Centeon L.L.C.
Kankakee, Illinois 60901, U.S.A.

ANTIHEMOPHILIC FACTOR (HUMAN)
MONOCLATE-P®   ℞
FACTOR VIII:C PASTEURIZED
MONOCLONAL ANTIBODY PURIFIED

DESCRIPTION

Antihemophilic Factor (Human), MONOCLATE-P,® Factor VIII:C Pasteurized, Monoclonal Antibody Purified is a sterile, stable, lyophilized concentrate of Factor VIII:C with reduced amounts of vWf:Ag and purified of extraneous plasma-derived protein by use of affinity chromatography. A murine monoclonal antibody to vWf:Ag is used as an affinity ligand to first isolate the Factor VIII Complex. Factor VIII:C is then dissociated from vWf:Ag, recovered, formulated and provided as a sterile lyophilized powder.[1,2,3] The concentrate as formulated contains Albumin (Human) as a stabilizer, resulting in a concentrate with a specific activity between 5 and 10 units/mg of total protein. In the absence of this added Albumin (Human) stabilizer, specific activity has been determined to exceed 3000 units/mg of protein.[4] MONOCLATE-P® has been prepared from pooled human plasma and is intended for use in therapy of classical hemophilia (Hemophilia A).

This concentrate has been pasteurized by heating at 60°C for 10 hours in aqueous solution form during its manufacture in order to further reduce the risk of viral transmission.[5] However, no procedure has been shown to be totally effective in removing viral infectivity from coagulant factor concentrates. (See CLINICAL PHARMACOLOGY and WARNINGS)

MONOCLATE-P® is a highly purified preparation of Factor VIII:C.

When stored as directed, it will maintain its labeled potency for the period indicated on the container and package labels.[8,9]

Upon reconstitution, a clear, colorless solution is obtained, containing 50 to 150 times as much Factor VIII:C as does an equal volume of plasma.

Each vial contains the labeled amount of antihemophilic factor (AHF) activity as expressed in terms of International Units of antihemophilic activity. One unit of antihemophilic activity is equivalent to that quantity of AHF present in one mL of normal human plasma. When reconstituted as recommended, the resulting solution contains approximately 300 to 450 millimoles of sodium ions per liter and has 2 to 3 times the tonicity of saline. It contains approximately 2–5 millimoles of calcium ions per liter, contributed as calcium chloride, approximately 1 to 2% Albumin (Human), 0.8% mannitol, and 1.2 mM histidine. The pH is adjusted with hydrochloric acid and/or sodium hydroxide. MONOCLATE-P® also contains trace amounts (≤ 50 ng per 100 I.U. of AHF) of the murine monoclonal antibody used in its purification (see CLINICAL PHARMACOLOGY).

MONOCLATE-P® is to be administered only intravenously.

CLINICAL PHARMACOLOGY

Factor VIII:C is the coagulant portion of the Factor VIII complex circulating in plasma. It is noncovalently associated with the von Willebrand protein responsible for von Willebrand factor activity. These two proteins have distinct biochemical and immunological properties and are under separate genetic control. Factor VIII:C act as a cofactor for Factor IX to activate Factor X in the intrinsic pathway of blood coagulation.[6] Hemophilia A, an hereditary disorder of blood coagulation due to decreased levels of Factor VIII:C, results in profuse bleeding into joints, muscles or internal organs as a result of a trauma. Antihemophilic Factor (Human), MONOCLATE-P,® Factor VIII:C Pasteurized, Mono-

clonal Antibody Purified provides an increase in plasma levels of AHF, thereby enabling temporary correction of Hemophilia A bleeding.

Clinical evaluation of MONOCLATE-P,® Factor VIII:C Pasteurized, Monoclonal Antibody Purified concentrate for its half-life characteristics in hemophilic patients showed it to be comparable to other commercially available Antihemophilic Factor (Human) concentrates. The mean half-life obtained from six patients was 17.5 hours with a mean recovery of 1.9 Units/dl rise/U/kg.

The pasteurization process used in the manufacture of this concentrate has demonstrated *in vitro* inactivation of human immunodeficiency virus (HIV) and several model viruses. In two separate studies, HIV was reduced by ≥7.0 $\log_{10}$ to an undetectable level and by 10.5 $\log_{10}$, respectively. In addition to HIV, studies were also performed using three lipid containing model viruses and one non-lipid, encapsulated model virus. Vesicular stomatitis (VSV) was reduced by ≥6.79 $\log_{10}$ to undetectable, Sindbis was reduced by ≥6.48 $\log_{10}$ to undetectable and Vaccinia was reduced by ≥5.36 $\log_{10}$ to undetectable. Murine encephalomyocarditis (EMC), a non-lipid, encapsulated model virus, was reduced by ≥7.1 $\log_{10}$ to undetectable.

Evidence of the capability of the purification and preparative steps used in the production of Antihemophilic Factor (Human), MONOCLATE-P,® Factor VIII:C Pasteurized, Monoclonal Antibody Purified to reduce viral bioburden was obtained in studies involving the addition of known quantities of virus to cryoprecipitate. These studies were conducted using an earlier form of the concentrate which had not undergone liquid pasteurization (Antihemophilic Factor (Human), MONOCLATE,® Monoclonal Antibody Purified, Factor VIII:C, Heat-Treated). These studies provide evidence of the viral removal potential of the purification and preparative steps of the manufacturing process (exclusive of heat treatment) which are common to both concentrates. In one study, the viruses used were human immunodeficiency virus (HIV), sindbis virus, vesicular stomatitis virus (VSV) and pseudorabies virus (PsRV). A comparison of the cumulative mean reductions for all viruses tested with the individual values obtained in each experiment indicates that the combined effects of the manufacturing steps, which purify the Factor VIII:C and prepare the concentrate in a final sterile container as a lyophilized powder, contribute viral reduction capabilities of approximately 5 to 6 logs. In a separate study, aluminum hydroxide treatment followed by antibody affinity chromatography reduced vaccinia virus infectivity by 4.81 logs. These studies indicate that the purification and preparative steps of the manufacturing process are capable of providing a non-specific, viral reduction of approximately 5 to 6 logs, independent of the pasteurization process.

MONOCLATE-P® contains trace amounts of mouse protein[7] (≤50 ng per 100 I.U. of AHF). In a study using an earlier form of the concentrate which had not undergone pasteurization (MONOCLATE®), a number of patients seronegative for Anti-HIV-1 were monitored to determine whether they would develop antibody or experience adverse reactions as a result of repeated exposure. These patients were treated on multiple occasions. Pre-study serum measurements of 27 patients for human anti-mouse IgG showed that, prior to treatment, 6 of them had either detectable antibody to mouse proteins or cross-reactive proteins. These patients continued to demonstrate similar or lower antibody levels during the study. Of the remaining 21 patients, 6 were shown to have low antibody levels on one or more occasions. In no case was observance of low antibody level associated with an anamnestic response or with any clinical adverse reaction. Patients were observed for time periods ranging from 2 to 30 months.

INDICATIONS AND USAGE

Antihemophilic Factor (Human), MONOCLATE-P,® Factor VIII:C Pasteurized, Monoclonal Antibody Purified is indicated for treatment of classical hemophilia (Hemophilia A). Affected individuals frequently require therapy following minor accidents. Surgery, when required in such individuals, must be preceded by temporary corrections of the clotting abnormality. Presurgical correction of severe AHF deficiency can be accomplished with a small volume of MONOCLATE-P®.

MONOCLATE-P® is not effective in controlling the bleeding of patients with von Willebrand's disease.

CONTRAINDICATIONS

Known hypersensitivity to mouse protein is a contraindication to Antihemophilic Factor (Human), MONOCLATE-P,® Factor VIII:C Pasteurized, Monoclonal Antibody Purified.

WARNINGS

This product is prepared from pooled human plasma which may contain the causative agents of hepatitis and other viral diseases. Prescribed manufacturing procedures utilized at the plasma collection centers, plasma testing laborato-

ries, and the fractionation facilities are designed to reduce the risk of transmitting viral infection. However, the risk of viral infectivity from this product cannot be totally eliminated. Accordingly, the benefits and risks of treatment with this concentrate should be carefully assessed prior to use. Individuals who receive infusions of blood or plasma products may develop signs and/or symptoms of some viral infections, particularly nonA, nonB hepatitis.

PRECAUTIONS

General—Most Antihemophilic Factor (Human) concentrates contain naturally occurring blood group specific antibodies. However, the processing of MONOCLATE-P® significantly reduces the presence of blood group specific antibodies in the final product. Nevertheless, when large or frequently repeated doses of product are needed, patients should be monitored by means of hematocrit and direct Coombs tests for signs of progressive anemia.

Formation of Antibodies to Mouse Protein—Although no hypersensitivity reactions have been observed, because MONOCLATE-P® contains trace amounts of mouse protein (≤ 50 ng per 100 I.U. of AHF), the possibility exists that patients treated with MONOCLATE-P® may develop hypersensitivity to the mouse proteins.

Information For Patients—Patients should be informed of the early signs of hypersensitivity reactions including hives, generalized urticaria, tightness of the chest, wheezing, hypotension, and anaphylaxis, and should be advised to discontinue use of the concentrate and contact their physician if these symptoms occur.

Pregnancy Category C—Animal reproduction studies have not been conducted with Antihemophilic Factor (Human), MONOCLATE-P,® Factor VIII:C Pasteurized, Monoclonal Antibody Purified. It is also not known whether MONOCLATE-P® can cause fetal harm when administered to a pregnant woman or can affect reproduction capacity. MONOCLATE-P® should be given to a pregnant woman only if clearly needed.

ADVERSE REACTIONS

Products of this type are known to cause allergic reactions, mild chills, nausea or stinging at the infusion site.

DOSAGE AND ADMINISTRATION

Antihemophilic Factor (Human), MONOCLATE-P,® Factor VIII:C Pasteurized, Monoclonal Antibody Purified is for intravenous administration only. As a general rule 1 unit of AHF activity per kg will increase the circulating AHF level by 2%.[10] The following formula provides a guide of dosage calculations:

$$\text{Number of AHF I.U. Required} = \text{Body weight (in kg)} \times \text{desired Factor VIII increase (\% normal)} \times 0.5^{10}$$

Although dosage must be individualized according to the needs of the patient (weight, severity of hemorrhage, presence of inhibitors), the following general dosages are suggested.[11]

1. MILD HEMORRHAGES—Minor hemorrhagic episodes will generally subside with a single infusion if a level of 30% or more is attained.
2. MODERATE HEMORRHAGE AND MINOR SURGERY—For more serious hemorrhages and minor surgical procedures, the patient's Factor VIII level should be raised to 30–50% of normal, which usually requires an initial dose of 15–25 I.U. per kg. If further therapy is required a maintenance dose is 10–15 I.U. per kg every 8–12 hours.
3. SEVERE HEMORRHAGE—In hemorrhages near vital organs (neck, throat, subperitoneal) it may be desirable to raise the Factor VIII level to 80–100% of normal which can be achieved with an initial dose of 40–50 I.U. per kg and a maintenance dose of 20–25 I.U. per kg every 8–12 hours.
4. MAJOR SURGERY—For surgical procedures a dose of AHF sufficient to achieve a level 80–100% of normal should be given an hour prior to surgery. A second dose, half the size of the priming dose, should be given five hours after the first dose. Factor VIII levels should be maintained at a daily minimum of at least 30% for a period of 10–14 days postoperatively. Close laboratory control to maintain AHF plasma levels deemed appropriate to maintain hemostasis is recommended.

Reconstitution

1. Warm both the diluent and Antihemophilic Factor (Human), MONOCLATE-P,® Factor VIII:C Pasteurized, Monoclonal Antibody Purified in unopened vials to room temperature [not above 37°C (98°F)].
2. Remove the caps from both vials to expose the central portions of the rubber stoppers.
3. Treat the surface of the rubber stoppers with antiseptic solution and allow them to dry.
4. Using aseptic technique, insert one end of the double-end needle into the rubber stopper of the diluent vial. Invert the diluent vial and insert the other end of the double-

Continued on next page

Monoclate-P—Cont.

end needle into the rubber stopper of the MONOCLATE-P® vial. Direct the diluent, which will be drawn in by vacuum, over the entire surface of the MONOCLATE-P® cake. (In order to assure transfer of all the diluent, adjust the position of the tip of the needle in the diluent vial to the inside edge of the diluent stopper.) Rotate the vial to ensure complete wetting of the cake during the transfer process.

5. Remove the diluent vial to release the vacuum, then remove the double-end needle, from the MONOCLATE-P® vial.
6. Gently swirl the vial until the powder is dissolved and the solution is ready for administration. The concentrate routinely and easily reconstitutes within one minute. To assure sterility, MONOCLATE-P® should be administered within three hours after reconstitution.
7. Parenteral drug preparations should be inspected visually for particulate matter and discoloration prior to administration, whenever solution and container permit.

Administration

CAUTION: This kit contains two devices, a stainless steel 5 micron filter needle, individually labeled as a 5 micron filter needle and contained in a separate blister pack, and an all plastic 5 micron vented filter spike which is supplied with the four-item administration components blister pack, either of which may be used to withdraw the reconstituted product for administration. The withdrawal directions specific for each of these alternate devices must be followed exactly for whichever device is chosen for use as described below. Product loss or inability to withdraw product will result if the improper instructions are followed.

A. Administration using the Stainless Steel Filter Needle for Withdrawal (This item is individually packaged in a separate, labeled blister pack.)

Intravenous Injection

Plastic disposable syringes are recommended with Antihemophilic Factor (Human), MONOCLATE-P,® Factor VIII:C Pasteurized, Monoclonal Antibody Purified solution. The ground glass surface of all-glass syringes tend to stick with solutions of this type.

1. Using aseptic technique, attach the filter needle to a sterile disposable syringe.
2. Draw air into the syringe equal to or greater than the contents of the vial.
3. Insert the filter needle into the stopper of the MONOCLATE-P® vial, invert the vial, position the filter needle above the level of the liquid and inject all of the air into the vial.
4. Pull the filter needle back down below the level of the liquid until the tip is at the inside edge of the stopper.
5. Withdraw the reconstituted solution into the syringe being careful to always keep the tip of the needle below the level of the liquid.
   CAUTION: Failure to inject air into the vial, or allowing air to pass through the filter needle while filling the syringe with reconstituted solution, may cause the needle to clog.
6. Discard the filter needle. Perform venipuncture using the enclosed winged needle with microbore tubing. Attach the syringe to the luer end of the tubing.
   CAUTION: Use of other winged needles without microbore tubing, although compatible with the concentrate, will result in a larger retention of solution within the winged infusion set.
7. **Administer solution intravenously at a rate (approximately 2 mL/minute) comfortable to the patient.**

B. Administration using the all plastic Vented Filter Spike for Withdrawal (This spike is supplied in the four-item Administration Components pack.)

Intravenous Injection

Plastic disposable syringes are recommended with Antihemophilic Factor (Human), MONOCLATE-P,® Factor VIII:C Pasteurized, Monoclonal Antibody Purified solution. The ground glass surface of all-glass syringes tend to stick with solutions of this type.

1. Using aseptic technique, attach the vented filter spike to a sterile disposable syringe.
   CAUTION: DO NOT INJECT AIR INTO THE MONOCLATE-P® VIAL. The self-venting feature of the vented filter spike precludes the need to inject air in order to facilitate withdrawal of the reconstituted solution. The injection of air could cause partial product loss through the vent filter.
   CAUTION: The use of other, non-vented filter needles or spikes without the proper procedure may result in an air lock and prevent the complete transfer of the concentrate.
2. Insert the vented filter spike into the stopper of the MONOCLATE-P® vial, invert the vial, and position the filter spike so that the orifice is at the inside edge of the stopper.
3. Withdraw the reconstituted solution into the syringe.
4. Discard the filter spike. Perform venipuncture using the enclosed winged needle with microbore tubing. Attach the syringe to the luer end of the tubing.
   CAUTION: Use of other winged needles without microbore tubing, although compatible with the concentrate, will result in a larger retention of solution within the winged infusion set.
5. **Administer solution intravenously at a rate (approximately 2 mL/minute) comfortable to the patient.**

STORAGE

When stored at refrigerator temperature, 2°–8°C (36°–46°F), Antihemophilic Factor (Human), MONOCLATE-P,® Factor VIII:C Pasteurized, Monoclonal Antibody Purified is stable for the period indicated by the expiration date on its label. Within this period, MONOCLATE-P® may be stored at room temperature not to exceed 30°C (86°F), for up to 6 months.

Avoid freezing which may damage container for the diluent.

HOW SUPPLIED

MONOCLATE-P® is supplied in a single dose vial with diluent, double-ended needle for reconstitution, vented filter spike for withdrawal, filter needle for withdrawal, winged infusion set and alcohol swabs. I.U. activity is stated on the label of each vial.

CAUTION: FEDERAL (U.S.A.) LAW PROHIBITS DISPENSING WITHOUT PRESCRIPTION.

REFERENCES

1. W. Terry, A. Schreiber, C. Tarr, M. Hrinda, W. Curry, and F. Feldman, "Human Factor VIII:C Produced Using Monoclonal Antibodies," in *Research in Clinic and Laboratory*, Vol. XVI, (#1), 202 (1986) from the XVIIth International Congress of the World Federation of Hemophilia.
2. A.B. Schreiber, "The Preclinical Characterization of Monoclate Factor VIII C Antihemophilic Factor Human," *Semin Hematol* 25 (2 Suppl. 1), 1988, pp. 27–32.
3. E. Berntorp and I.M. Nilsson, "Biochemical Properties of Human Factor VIII C Monoclate Purified Using Monoclonal Antibody to VWF," *Thromb Res* O (Suppl. 7), 1987, p. 60, from the Satellite Symposia of the XIth International Congress on Thrombosis and Haemostasis, Brussels, Belgium, July 11, 1987.
4. S. Chandra, C.C. Huang, R.L. Weeks, K. Beatty and F. Feldman, " Purity of a Factor VIII:C Preparation (Monoclate) Manufactured by Monoclonal Immunoaffinity Chromatography Technique," from the XVIII International Congress of the World Federation of Hemophilia, May 1988.
5. B. Spire, D. Dormont, F. Barre-Sinousii, L. Montagnier, and J.C. Chermann, "Inactivation of Lymphadenopathy Associated Virus by Heat, Gamma Rays, and Ultraviolet Light," *Lancet*, Jan. 26, 1985, p. 188.
6. L.W. Hoyer, "The Factor VIII Complex: Structure and Function," *Blood* 58 (1981), p. 1.
7. F.Feldman, S. Chandra, R. Kleszynski, C.C. Huang and R.L. Weeks, "Measurement of Murine Protein Levels in Monoclonal Antibody Purified Coagulation Factor," from the XVIII International Congress of the World Federation of Hemophilia, May 1988.
8. F. Feldman, R. Kleszynski, L. Ho, R. Kling, S. Chandra and C.C. Huang, "Validation of Coagulation Test Methods for Evaluation of Monoclate (Factor VIII:C) Potencies," from the XVIII International Congress of the World Federation of Hemophilia, May 1988.
9. S. Chandra, C.C. Huang, L. Ho, R. Kling, R.L. Weeks and F. Feldman, "Studies on the Stability of Factor VIII:C (Monoclate) in Lyophilized and Solution Form," from the XVIII International Congress of the World Federation of Hemophilia, May 1988.
10. C.F. Abilgaard, J.V. Simone, J.J. Corrigan, et al., "Treatment of Hemophilia with Glycine—Precipitated Factor VIII," *New Eng J Med*, 275 (1966), p. 471.
11. C.K. Kasper, "Hematologic Care," *Comprehensive Management of Hemophilia*, ed. Boone, D.C., Philadelphia, F.A. Davis Co., (1976) pp. 2–20.

BIBLIOGRAPHY

Hershman, R.J., Naconti, S.B., and Shulman, N.R. "Prophylactic Treatment of Factor VIII Deficiency." *Blood* 35 (1970), p. 189.

Kasper, C.K., Dietrich, S.I. and Rapaport, S.K. "Hemophilia Prophylaxis in Factor VIII Concentrate." *Arch. Int. Med.* 125 (1970), p. 1004.

Biggs, R., ed. "The Treatment of Hemophilia A and B and von Willebrands Disease." Oxford: Blackwell, 1978.

Fulcher, C.A., Zimmerman, T.S., "Characterization of the Human Factor VII Procoagulant Protein With a Heterologous Precipitating Antibody." *Proc. Natl. Acad. Sci.* 79 (1982), pp. 1648–1652.

Levine, P.H., "Factor VIII C Purified from Plasma Via Monoclonal Antibodies Human Studies." *Semin Hematol* 25 (2 Suppl. 1), 1988, pp. 38–41.

Revised: June, 1996 IBM 12810

CENTEON L.L.C.
Kankakee, Illinois 60901 U.S.A.

U.S. Patent No. Re. 32,011
U.S. Government License No. 149
U.S. Patent No. 4,876,241

COAGULATION FACTOR IX (HUMAN) MONONINE® MONOCLONAL ANTIBODY PURIFIED

℞

DESCRIPTION

Coagulation Factor IX (Human), Mononine®, is a sterile, stable, lyophilized concentrate of Factor IX prepared from pooled human plasma and is intended for use in therapy of Factor IX deficiency, known as Hemophilia B or Christmas disease. Coagulation Factor IX (Human), Mononine®, is purified of extraneous plasma-derived proteins, including Factors II, VII and X, by use of immunoaffinity chromatography. A murine monoclonal antibody to Factor IX is used as an affinity ligand to isolate Factor IX from the source material. Factor IX is then dissociated from the monoclonal antibody, recovered, purified further, formulated and provided as a sterile, lyophilized powder. The immunoaffinity protocol utilized results in a highly pure Factor IX preparation. It shows predominantly a single component by SDS polyacrylamide electrophoretic evaluation and has a specific activity of not less than 190 Factor IX units per mg total protein.

This concentrate has been processed by monoclonal antibody immunoaffinity chromatography during its manufacture which has been shown to be capable of reducing the risk of viral transmission. Additionally, a chemical treatment protocol and two sequential ultrafiltration steps used in its manufacture have also been shown to be capable of significant viral reductions. However, no procedure has been shown to be totally effective in removing the risk of viral infectivity from coagulation factor concentrates (See **CLINICAL PHARMACOLOGY** and **WARNINGS**).

Mononine® is a highly purified preparation of Factor IX. When stored as directed, it will maintain its labeled potency for the period indicated on the container label.

Each vial contains the labeled amount of Factor IX activity expressed in International Units (IU). One IU represents the activity of Factor IX present in 1 mL of normal, pooled plasma. When reconstituted as recommended, the resulting solution is a clear, colorless, isotonic preparation of neutral pH, containing approximately 100 times the Factor IX potency found in an equal volume of plasma. Each mL of the reconstituted concentrate contains approximately, 100 IU of Factor IX and non-detectable levels of Factors II, VII and X (<0.0025 IU per Factor IX unit using standard coagulation assays). It also contains histidine (approx. 10mM), sodium chloride (approx. 0.066M) and mannitol (approx. 3%). Hydrochloric acid and/or sodium hydroxide may have been used to adjust pH. Mononine® also contains trace amounts (≤50 ng mouse protein/100 Factor IX activity units) of the murine monoclonal antibody used in its purification (See **CLINICAL PHARMACOLOGY).**

Mononine® is to be administered only intravenously.

CLINICAL PHARMACOLOGY

Hemophilia B, or Christmas disease, is an X-linked recessively inherited disorder of blood coagulation characterized by insufficient or abnormal synthesis of the clotting protein Factor IX. Factor IX is a vitamin K-dependent coagulation factor which is synthesized in the liver. Factor IX is activated by Factor XIa in the intrinsic coagulation pathway. Activated Factor IX (IXa), in combination with Factor VIII:C, activates Factor X to Xa, resulting ultimately in the conversion of prothrombin to thrombin and the formation of a fibrin clot. The infusion of exogenous Factor IX to replace the deficiency present in Hemophilia B temporarily restores hemostasis. Depending upon the patient's level of biologically active Factor IX, clinical symptoms range from moderate skin bruising or excessive hemorrhage after trauma or surgery to spontaneous hemorrhage into joints, muscles or internal organs including the brain. Severe or recurring hemorrhages can produce death, organ dysfunction or orthopedic deformity.

Infusion of Factor IX Complex concentrates that contain varying but significant amounts of the other liver-dependent blood coagulation proteins, Factors II, VII and X, into patients with Hemophilia B results in Factor IX recoveries ranging from approximately 0.57–1.1 IU/dL rise per IU/Kg body weight infused with plasma half-lives for Factor IX ranging from approximately 23 hours to 31 hours.[1,2] Infusion of Coagulation Factor IX (Human), Mononine®, into ten patients with severe or moderate Hemophilia B has shown a mean recovery of 0.67 IU/dL rise per IU/Kg body weight infused and a mean half-life of 22.6 hours.[3] After six months of experience with repeated infusions performed on the nine patients who remained in the study, it was shown that the half-life and recovery was maintained at a level comparable to that found with the initial infusion. The six-month data showed a mean recovery of 0.68 IU/dL rise per

IU/Kg body weight infused and a mean half-life of 25.3 hours.[3] The data show no statistically significant differences between the initial and six-month values.

Two studies were conducted to provide Mononine® for compassionate treatment of hemophilia B patients who required extensive Factor IX replacement for surgery, trauma, or spontaneous bleeding (73 unique patients and eight patients enrolled twice for a total of 81 patients), as well as to evaluate the safety and efficacy of Mononine®. The overall mean recovery during treatment was determined to be 1.23 ± 0.42 IU/dL rise/IU/Kg (K) (range = 0.59 to 2.92 K) among the 55 patients included in recovery analyses in the one study and to be 1.12 ± 0.52 K (range = 0.61 to 2.08 K) among 10 patients included in these analyses in the second study. Five (5/81, 6%) patients reported adverse events attributed to Mononine® across the two studies. In these studies, 100 doses of Mononine® were administered at what are considered high doses for a Factor IX concentrate, a range of 71 to 161 IU/Kg to a total of 36 patients. Sixty-seven (67) of these infusions were the subject of recovery analyses. Mean recovery tended to decrease as the dose of Mononine® increased: 1.09 ± 0.52 K at doses > 75-95 IU/Kg (n=38), 0.98 ± 0.45 K at doses >95–115 IU/Kg (n=21), 0.70 ± 0.38 K at doses >115–135 IU/Kg (n=2), 0.67 K at doses >135–155 IU/Kg (n=1), and 0.73 ± 0.34 K at doses >155 IU/Kg (n=5). Among the 36 patients who received these high doses, only one (2.8%) reported an adverse experience with a possible relationship to Mononine® ("difficulty in concentrating", patient recovered). In no patients were thrombogenic complications observed or reported.[4]

The manufacturing procedure for Coagulation Factor IX (Human), Mononine®, includes multiple processing steps that have been designed to reduce the risk of viral transmission. Validation studies of the monoclonal antibody (MAb) immunoaffinity chromatography/chemical treatment steps and two sequential ultrafiltration steps used in the production of Mononine® document the viral reduction capacity of the processes employed. These studies were conducted using the Human Immunodeficiency Virus (HIV) and four model viruses representing a broad range of viral characteristics, i.e., Sindbis, Vaccinia, Vesicular Stomatitis (VSV) and Murine Encephalomyocarditis (EMC), a non-lipid encapsulated model virus.

The results of these validation studies (see Table 1 below) document cumulative viral reduction capacities of ≥11.56 log_{10} for HIV, 10.24 log_{10} for Sindbis, 11.64 log_{10} for EMC, ≥14.23 log_{10} for VSV, and ≥ 10.90 log_{10} for Vaccinia.
[See table 1 above]

Similar viral reduction studies were conducted using porcine parvovirus (used as a model for human parvovirus B19). The results for these validation studies (see Table 2 below) document cumulative viral reduction capacity of ≥11.64 log_{10} for porcine parvovirus.

Viral Reduction Studies Table 1
(Log_{10} Reduction)

Processing Step	HIV	Sindbis	EMC	VSV	Vaccinia
MAb Chromatography	*	2.76	3.89	≥7.18**	≥3.60
Sodium thiocyanate Chemical Treatment	≥4.16	0	0	**	0
Ultrafiltration ***	≥7.4	7.48	7.75	7.05	≥7.30
Total Log_{10} Reduction	≥11.56	10.24	11.64	≥14.23	≥10.90

* MAb Chromatography not studied.
** Results are for combined MAb chromatography/sodium thiocyanate step.
*** For VSV and Vaccinia these data are results for a single ultrafiltration; the data for HIV, Sindbis, and EMC are results for double ultrafiltration.

Viral Reduction Studies Table 2
(Log_{10} Reduction)

Processing Step	Porcine Parvovirus
Combined MAb Chromatography and Sodium Thiocyanate Chemical Treatment	>4.28
AH Sepharose Chromatography	2.26
Ultrafiltration	5.10
Total Log_{10} Reduction	≥11.64

CLINICAL STUDIES

The viral safety of Coagulation Factor IX (Human), Mononine®, has been studied in clinical trials of two cohorts of hemophilia B patients previously unexposed to blood or blood products.[5] One cohort of patients included those with moderate to severe factor IX deficiency requiring chronic replacement therapy (36 patients dosed thus far); the second cohort included patients with a mild deficiency requiring factor IX replacement for surgical procedures (nine patients dosed thus far).

These patients were followed for serum ALT elevations, as well as for a range of viral serologies. Thirty-two (32) patients (25 with a moderate to severe deficiency and seven with a mild deficiency) were evaluable for assessment of viral hepatitis safety by ISTH-SSC criteria. None of these patients showed evidence of transmission of hepatitis B, hepatitis C, or HIV. In two of the evaluable patients, ALT elevations were attributed to causes other than Mononine®. In addition, one patient considered unevaluable for assessment of viral safety was found to have persistent and significant ALT elevations after infusion. This patient received hepatitis B hyperimmune immunoglobulin and his first injection of hepatitis B vaccine approximately three days after his first infusion. As a result, definitive conclusions regarding the occurrence of hepatitis B in this patient cannot be made.

Coagulation Factor IX (Human), Mononine®, contains trace amounts of the murine monoclonal antibody (MAb) used in its purification (≤50 ng mouse protein/100 IU). While the levels of mouse protein are extremely low, infusion of such proteins might theoretically induce human anti-mouse antibody (HAMA) responses. To test this possibility, human IgG, IgM, and IgE antibodies to mouse IgG were assessed by immunoradiometric assay (IRMA) in 11 hemophilia B patients who received Mononine® and were previously untreated with other blood products. HAMAs were evaluated prior to the first infusion and at 2 to 42 months after initial treatment. Human IgE antibodies to mouse IgG were below the level of detectability at all time points for all patients, and there were no statistically significant increases in either human IgG antibodies or human IgM antibodies to mouse protein. In addition, an analysis of clinical data shows that no replacement factor-related adverse events occurred that might have been considered as allergic or anaphylactoid reactions.[6]

In clinical studies of Coagulation Factor IX (Human), Mononine®, patients were monitored for evidence of disseminated intravascular coagulation. In six patients evaluated after infusion, fibrinogen levels and platelet counts were unchanged, and fibrin degradation products did not appear.[3]

In further clinical evaluations of Coagulation Factor IX (Human), Mononine®, in a crossover study with a Factor IX Complex concentrate, Mononine® was not associated with the formation of prothrombin activation fragment (F_{1+2}) whereas the Factor IX Complex was associated with the formation of prothrombin activation fragment (F_{1+2}).[3,7] Prothrombin activation fragment (F_{1+2}) is indicative of activation of prothrombin.

INDICATIONS AND USAGE

Coagulation Factor IX (Human), Mononine®, is indicated for the prevention and control of bleeding in Factor IX deficiency, also known as Hemophilia B or Christmas disease. Mononine® is not indicated in the treatment or prophylaxis of Hemophilia A patients with inhibitors to Factor VIII.

Coagulation Factor IX (Human), Mononine®, contains non-detectable levels of Factors II, VII and X (<0.0025 IU per Factor IX unit using standard coagulation assays) and is, therefore, not indicated for replacement therapy of these clotting factors.

Mononine® is also not indicated in the treatment or reversal of coumarin-induced anticoagulation or in a hemorrhagic state caused by hepatitis-induced lack of production of liver dependent coagulation factors.

CONTRAINDICATIONS

Known hypersensitivity to mouse protein is a contraindication to Coagulation Factor IX (Human), Mononine®.

WARNINGS

Coagulation Factor IX (Human), Mononine®, is derived from human plasma that may contain human pathogenic agents, including those not yet known or identified. Thus, the risk of transmission of infectious agents can not be totally eliminated. Stringent procedures, designed to reduce the risk of adventitious agent transmission, have been employed in the manufacture of this product from the collection and testing of plasma, through to the application of viral elimination/reduction steps. As with any pharmaceutical, the physician should weigh the risks and benefits of administration.

Individuals who receive infusions of blood or plasma products may develop signs and/or symptoms of some viral infections, particularly nonA, nonB hepatitis.

Since the use of Factor IX Complex concentrates has historically been associated with the development of thromboembolic complications, the use of Factor IX-containing products may be potentially hazardous in patients with signs of fibrinolysis and in patients with disseminated intravascular coagulation (DIC).

PRECAUTIONS

Extensive clinical experience suggests that there is a lower risk of thromboembolic complications with the use of Mononine® than with prothrombin complex concentrates. However, as with all products containing Factor IX, caution should be exercised when administering Mononine® to patients with liver disease, to patients post-operatively, to neonates, or to patients at risk of thromboembolic phenomena or DIC.[8,9] In each of these situations, the potential benefit of treatment with Mononine® should be weighed against the potential risk of these complications.

Coagulation Factor IX (Human), Mononine®, should be administered intravenously at a rate that will permit observation of the patient for any immediate reaction. Rates of infusion of up to 225 IU per minute have been regularly tolerated with no adverse reactions. If any reaction takes place that is thought to be related to the administration of Mononine®, the rate of infusion should be decreased or the infusion stopped, as dictated by the response of the patient. During the course of treatment, determination of daily Factor IX levels is advised to guide the dose to be administered and the frequency of repeated infusions. Individual patients may vary in their response to Mononine®, achieving different levels of in vivo recovery and demonstrating different half-lives.

The use of high doses of Factor IX Complex concentrates has been reported to be associated with instances of myocardial infarction, disseminated intravascular coagulation, venous thrombosis and pulmonary embolism. Generally a Factor IX level of 25% to 50% is considered adequate for hemostasis, including major hemorrhages and surgery. Attempting to maintain Factor IX levels of >75% to 100% during treatment is not routinely recommended nor required. To achieve Factor IX levels that will remain about 25% between once a day administrations, each daily dose should attempt to raise the level to 50% – 60%. (See **DOSAGE AND ADMINISTRATION**)

No controlled studies have been available regarding the use of ε-amino caproic acid or other antifibrinolytic agents following an initial infusion of Mononine® for the prevention or treatment of oral bleeding following trauma or dental procedures such as extractions.

Information For Patients

Patients should be informed of the early signs of hypersensitivity reactions including hives, generalized urticaria, tightness of the chest, wheezing, hypotension, and anaphylaxis, and should be advised to discontinue use of the concentrate and contact their physician if these symptoms occur.

Pregnancy Category C

Animal reproduction studies have not been conducted with Coagulation Factor IX (Human), Mononine®. It is also not known whether Mononine® can cause fetal harm when administered to a pregnant woman or can affect reproduction capacity. Mononine® should be given to a pregnant woman only if clearly needed.

Pediatric Use

Evaluation of the safety and effectiveness of Mononine® treatment in 51 pediatric patients between the ages of 1 day and 20 years, as a part of viral safety trials and trials for surgery, trauma or spontaneous bleeding, showed that excellent hemostasis was achieved with no thrombotic complications.[10] Included in the experience with patients aged birth to 20 years are two long-term viral safety studies demonstrating lack of viral transmission. Dosing in children is based on body weight and is generally based on the same guidelines as for adults (see below).

ADVERSE REACTIONS

As with the administration of any product intravenously, the following reactions may be observed following administration: headache, fever, chills, flushing, nausea, vomiting, tingling, lethargy, hives, stinging or burning at the infusion site or other manifestations of allergic reactions including anaphylaxis.

There is a potential risk of thromboembolic episodes following the administration of Mononine® (See **WARNINGS** and **PRECAUTIONS**).

Continued on next page

Mononine—Cont.

The patient should be monitored closely during the infusion of Mononine® to observe for the development of any reaction. If any reaction takes place that is thought to be related to the administration of Mononine®, the rate of infusion should be decreased or the infusion stopped, as dictated by the response of the patient.

DOSAGE AND ADMINISTRATION

Coagulation Factor IX (Human), Mononine®, is intended for intravenous administration only. It should be reconstituted with the volume of Sterile Water for Injection, USP supplied with the lot, and administered within three hours of reconstitution. Do not refrigerate after reconstitution. After administration, any unused solution and the administration equipment should be discarded.

As a general rule, 1 IU of Factor IX activity per Kg can be expected to increase the circulating level of Factor IX by 1% of normal. The following formula provides a guide to dosage calculations:

$$\begin{array}{l}\text{Number of Factor IX} \\ = \text{IU required}\end{array} = \begin{array}{l}\text{Body Weight (in Kg)}\end{array} \times \begin{array}{l}\text{desired Factor IX increase (\% normal)}\end{array} \times 1.0\ \text{IU/Kg}$$

The amount of Coagulation Factor IX (Human), Mononine®, to be infused, as well as the frequency of infusions, will vary with each patient and with the clinical situation.[11,12]

As a general rule, the level of Factor IX required for treatment of different conditions is as follows:

[See table below]

Recovery of the loading dose varies from patient to patient. Doses administered should be titrated to the patient's response. Mononine® administered in doses of ≥ 75 IU/Kg were well tolerated (See CLINICAL PHARMACOLOGY). In the presence of an inhibitor to Factor IX, higher doses of Mononine® might be necessary to overcome the inhibitor (See PRECAUTIONS). No data on the treatment of patients with inhibitors to Factor IX with Mononine® are available.

For information on rate of administration, see Rate of Administration, below.

Reconstitution

1. Warm both the diluent and Coagulation Factor IX (Human), Mononine®, in unopened vials to room temperature [not above 37°C (98°F)].
2. Remove the caps from both vials to expose the central portions of the rubber stoppers.
3. Treat the surface of the rubber stoppers with antiseptic solution and allow them to dry.
4. Using aseptic technique, insert one end of the double-end needle into the rubber stopper of the diluent vial. Invert the diluent vial and insert the other end of the double-end needle into the rubber stopper of the Mononine® vial. Direct the diluent, which will be drawn in by vacuum, over the entire surface of the Mononine® cake. (In order to assure transfer of all the diluent, adjust the position of the tip of the needle in the diluent vial to the inside edge of the diluent stopper.) Rotate the vial to ensure complete wetting of the cake during the transfer process.
5. Remove the diluent vial to release the vacuum, then remove the double-end needle from the Mononine® vial.
6. Gently swirl the vial until the powder is dissolved and the solution is ready for administration. The concentrate routinely and easily reconstitutes within one minute. To assure sterility, Mononine® should be administered within three hours after reconstitution.
7. Product should be filtered prior to use as described under Administration. Parenteral drug preparations

should be inspected visually for particulate matter and discoloration prior to administration, whenever solution and container permit.

Administration
Intravenous Injection

Parenteral drug products should be inspected visually for particulate matter and discoloration prior to administration, whenever solution and container permit.

Plastic disposable syringes are recommended with Coagulation Factor IX (Human), Mononine®, solution. The ground glass surface of all-glass syringes tend to stick with solutions of this type. Please note, this concentrate is supplied with a SELF-VENTING filter spike.

1. Using aseptic technique, attach the vented filter spike to a sterile disposable syringe.

    CAUTION: The use of other, non-vented filter needles or spikes without the proper procedure may result in an air lock and prevent the complete transfer of the concentrate.

    CAUTION: DO NOT INJECT AIR INTO THE MONONINE® VIAL. The self-venting feature of the vented filter spike precludes the need to inject air in order to facilitate withdrawal of the reconstituted solution. The injection of air could cause partial product loss through the vent filter.

2. Insert the vented filter spike into the stopper of the Mononine® vial, invert the vial, and position the filter spike so that the orifice is at the inside edge of the stopper.
3. Withdraw the reconstituted solution into the syringe.
4. Discard the filter spike. Perform venipuncture using the enclosed winged needle with microbore tubing. Attach the syringe to the luer end of the tubing.

    CAUTION: Use of other winged needles without microbore tubing, although compatible with the concentrate, will result in a larger retention of solution within the winged infusion set.

Rate of Administration

The rate of administration should be determined by the response and comfort of the patient; intravenous dosage administration rates of up to 225 IU/minute have been regularly tolerated without incident. When reconstituted as directed, i.e., to approximately 100 IU/mL, Mononine® should be administered at a rate of approximately 2.0 mL per minute.

STORAGE

When stored at refrigerator temperature, 2°–8°C (36°–46°F), Coagulation Factor IX (Human), Mononine®, is stable for the period indicated by the expiration date on its label. Within this period, Mononine® may be stored at room temperature not to exceed 30°C (86°F), for up to one month. Avoid freezing, which may damage container of the diluent.

HOW SUPPLIED

Mononine® is supplied in a single dose vial with diluent, double-ended needle for reconstitution, vented filter spike for withdrawal, winged infusion set and alcohol swabs. Factor IX activity in IU is stated on the label of each vial.

The following dosage forms are available:

NDC 0053-7668-01 in 10 mL vials containing approximately 250 IU

NDC 0053-7668-02 in 10 mL vials containing approximately 500 IU

NDC 0053-7668-04 in 20 mL vials containing approximately 1,000 IU

CAUTION: FEDERAL LAW PROHIBITS DISPENSING WITHOUT PRESCRIPTION.

REFERENCES

1. Zauber NP, Levin J. Factor IX levels in patients with hemophilia B (Christmas disease) following transfusion with concentrates of Factor IX or fresh frozen plasma (FFP), Medicine (Baltimore) 56(3): 213-24, 1977.
2. Smith KJ, Thompson AR. Labeled Factor IX Kinetics in Patients with Hemophilia-B. Blood 58(3): 625-629, 1981.
3. Kim HC, McMillan CW, White GC, Horton MW, Saidi P. Purified Factor IX Using Monoclonal Immunoaffinity Technique: Clinical Trials in Hemophilia B and Comparison to Prothrombin Complex Concentrates. Blood 79(3): 568-575, 1992.
4. Warrier I, Kasper CK, White II GC, Shapiro AD, Bergman GE, the Mononine® Study Group. Safety of high doses of a monoclonal antibody-purified factor IX concentrate, Am J Hematol 49:92-94, 1995.
5. Shapiro AD, Ragni MV, Lusher JM, Culbert S, Koerper MA, Bergman GE, Hannan MM. Safety and Efficacy of Monoclonal Antibody Purified Factor IX Concentrate in Previously Untreated Patients with Hemophilia B. Thrombosis and Haemostasis, 75:30-35, 1996.
6. Davis HM, Nash DW, Clymer MD, Frigo ML, Bergman GE. Lack of immune response to mouse IgG in previously untreated haemophilia A and haemophilia B patients treated with monoclonal antibody purified factor VIII and factor IX preparations. Haemophilia. 3(2): 102-107, April 1997.
7. Kim HC, Matts L, Eisele J, Czachur M, Saidi P. Monoclonal Antibody Purified Factor IX-Comparative Thrombogenicity to Prothrombin Complex Concentrate. Seminars in Hematology, 28 (Suppl. 6 to no.3) : 15–20, July 1991.
8. Aledort LM. Factor IX and Thrombosis. Scand J. Haematology Suppl. 30:40, 1977.
9. Cederbaum Al, Blatt PM, Roberts HR. Intravascular coagulation with use of human prothrombin complex concentrates. Ann. Intern. Med. 84: 683-687, 1976.
10. Kurczynski E, Lusher JM, Pitel P, Shapiro AD, Bergman GE, the Mononine® Study Group. Safety and efficacy of monoclonal antibody-purified factor IX concentrate for management of bleeding and surgical prophylaxis in previously treated children with hemophilia B. Int J Ped Hemat/Oncol. 2:211-216, 1995.
11. Kasper CK, Dietrich SL. Comprehensive Management of Hemophilia. Clin. Haematol. 14(2): 489-512, 1985.
12. Johnson AJ, Aronson DL, Williams WJ. Preparation and clinical use of plasma and plasma fractions. Chap 167 in Hematology 3rd Edition, Williams WJ, Beutler E, Erslev AJ, Lichtman MA (Eds), McGraw Hill Book Co., New York: 1563-1583.

Revised: April, 1997   IBM 12835

CENTEON L.L.C.
Kankakee, Illinois 60901 U.S.A.
U.S. Government License No. 149 U.S. Patent No. 5,055,557

STIMATE™   ℞
(desmopressin acetate)
Nasal Spray, 1.5 mg/mL

DESCRIPTION

Stimate™ (desmopressin acetate) is a synthetic analogue of the natural pituitary hormone 8-arginine vasopressin (ADH), an antidiuretic hormone affecting renal water conservation. Stimate™ Nasal Spray contains 1.5 mg/mL desmopressin acetate in a pH-adjusted aqueous solution with chlorobutanol and sodium chloride as inactive ingredients. Stimate™ Nasal Spray's compression pump delivers 0.1 mL (150 µg) of solution per spray. It is chemically defined as follows:

Mol. Wt. 1183.34   Empirical formula: $C_{46}H_{64}N_{14}O_{12}S_2 \cdot C_2H_4O_2 \cdot 3H_2O$

SCH₂CH₂C - Tyr - Phe - Gln - Asn - Cys - Pro - D - Arg - Gly - NH₂ · CH₃COOH · 3H₂O
   1   2   3   4   5   6   7   8   9

1-(3-mercaptopropionic acid)-8-D-arginine vasopressin monoacetate (salt) trihydrate. Stimate™ Nasal Spray is provided as an aqueous solution for intranasal use.

Each mL contains:

Desmopressin acetate	1.5 mg
Chlorobutanol	5.0 mg
Sodium Chloride	9.0 mg
Hydrochloric acid to adjust pH to approximately 4	

CLINICAL PHARMACOLOGY

Stimate™ Nasal Spray contains as active substance, desmopressin acetate, which is a synthetic analogue of the natural hormone arginine vasopressin. One spray or 0.1 mL (150 µg) of Stimate™ Nasal Spray solution has an antidiuretic activity of about 600 IU.

Desmopressin acetate has been shown to be more potent than arginine vasopressin in increasing plasma levels of Factor VIII activity in patients with hemophilia and von Willebrand's disease Type I.

Dose-response studies were performed in healthy persons using doses of 150 to 450 µg, administered as one to three

	Minor Spontaneous Hemorrhage, Prophylaxis	Major Trauma or Surgery
Desired levels of Factor IX for Hemostasis	15%–25%	25%–50%
Initial loading dose to achieve desired level	up to 20–30 IU/Kg	up to 75 IU/Kg
Frequency of dosing	once; repeated in 24 hours if necessary	every 18–30 hours, depending on T½ and measured Factor IX levels
Duration of treatment	once; repeated if necessary	up to ten days, depending upon nature of insult

sprays. The response to **Stimate™ Nasal Spray** is dose-related, with maximal plasma levels of 150 to 250 percent of initial concentrations achieved for both Factor VIII and von Willebrand factor [1]. The increase is rapid and evident within 30 minutes, reaching a maximum at about 1.5 hours [1].

The percentage increase of Factor VIII and von Willebrand factor levels in patients with mild hemophilia A and von Willebrand's disease was not notably different from that observed in normal healthy individuals when treated with 300 µg of **Stimate™ Nasal Spray** [1–4]. In patients with von Willebrand's disease, levels of Factor VIII coagulant activity and von Willebrand factor antigen remained greater than 30 U/dL for 8 hours after a 300 µg dose of **Stimate™ Nasal Spray** [7]. After 300 µg of **Stimate™ Nasal Spray**, the percentage increase of Factor VIII and von Willebrand factor levels in patients with mild hemophilia A and von Willebrand's disease was less than observed after 0.3 µg/kg of intravenous desmopressin acetate [2–4].

Plasminogen activator activity increases rapidly after intravenous desmopressin acetate infusion, but there has been no clinically significant fibrinolysis in patients treated with desmopressin acetate.

The effect of repeated intravenous desmopressin acetate administration when doses were given every 12 to 24 hours has generally shown a diminution of the Factor VIII activity increase noted after a single dose. It is possible to reproduce the initial response in some patients after an interval of one week, but other patients may require as long as 6 weeks [2, 4,6].

The half-life of **Stimate™ Nasal Spray** was between 3.3 and 3.5 hours, over the range of intranasal doses, 150 to 450 µg [1]. Plasma concentrations of **Stimate™ Nasal Spray** were maximal approximately 40 to 45 minutes after dosing [1].

The bioavailability of **Stimate™ Nasal Spray** when administered by the intranasal route as a 1.5 mg/mL solution is between 3.3 and 4.1 percent [1].

The change in structure of arginine vasopressin to desmopressin acetate has resulted in a decreased vasopressor action and decreased actions on visceral smooth muscle relative to the enhanced antidiuretic activity, so that clinically effective antidiuretic doses are usually below threshold levels for effects on vascular or visceral smooth muscle.

INDICATIONS AND USAGE

Before the initial therapeutic administration of **Stimate™ Nasal Spray,** the physician should establish that the patient shows an appropriate change in the coagulation profile following a test dose of intranasal administration of **Stimate™ Nasal Spray** [2–4].

Desmopressin acetate is also available as a solution for injection (DDAVP® Injection) when the intranasal route may be compromised. These situations include nasal congestion and blockage, nasal discharge, atrophy of nasal mucosa, and severe atrophic rhinitis. Intranasal delivery may also be inapproriate where there is an impaired level of consciousness.

Hemophilia A

Stimate™ Nasal Spray is indicated for patients with hemophilia A with Factor VIII coagulant activity levels greater than 5%.

Desmopressin acetate will also stop bleeding in patients with hemophilia A with episodes of spontaneous or trauma-induced injuries such as hemarthroses, intramuscular hematomas or mucosal bleeding [2,3].

In the outpatient setting during two clinical trials where patients recorded bleeding episodes, **Stimate™ Nasal Spray** provided effective hemostasis 100% of the time in 2 of the 5 patients. For those patients not responding in 100% of bleeding occasions, 45% (14 of 31) of bleeding episodes were effectively controlled with **Stimate™ Nasal Spray.**

Desmopressin acetate is not indicated for the treatment of hemophilia A with Factor VIII coagulant activity levels equal to or less than 5%, or for the treatment of hemophilia B, or in patients who have Factor VIII antibodies.

von Willebrand's Disease (Type I)

Stimate™ Nasal Spray is indicated for patients with mild to moderate classic von Willebrand's disease (Type 1) with Factor VIII levels greater than 5%.

Desmopressin acetate will also stop bleeding in mild to moderate von Willebrand's disease patients with episodes of spontaneous or trauma-induced injuries such as hemarthroses, intramuscular hematomas, mucosal bleeding or menorrhagia [2,3].

In the outpatient setting during two clinical trials where patients recorded bleeding episodes, **Stimate™ Nasal Spray** provided effective hemostasis 100% of the time in 75% of the patients (n=16). For those patients not responding in 100% of bleeding occasions, 78% (64 of 82) of bleeding episodes were effectively controlled with **Stimate™ Nasal Spray.**

Patients may respond in a variable fashion depending on the type of molecular defect they have. Bleeding time and Factor VIII coagulant activity, ristocetin cofactor activity, and von Willebrand factor antigen should be checked after initial administration of **Stimate™ Nasal Spray** to ensure that adequate levels have been achieved.

Stimate™ Nasal Spray is not indicated for the treatment of severe classic von Willebrand's disease (Type I) and when there is evidence of an abnormal molecular form of Factor VIII antigen. See WARNING.

CONTRAINDICATIONS

Stimate™ Nasal Spray is contraindicated in individuals with known hypersensitivity to desmopressin acetate or to any of the components of **Stimate™ Nasal Spray.**

WARNINGS

For intranasal use only.

Patients who do not have need of antidiuretic hormone for its antidiuretic effect, in particular those who are young or elderly, should be cautioned to ingest only enough fluid to satisfy thirst, in order to decrease the potential occurrence of water intoxication and hyponatremia.

Fluid intake should be adjusted downward, particularly in very young and elderly patients, in order to decrease the potential occurrence of water intoxication and hyponatremia [1]. Particular attention should be paid to the possibility of the rare occurrence of an extreme decrease in plasma osmolality that may result in seizures which could lead to coma.

Stimate™ Nasal Spray should not be used to treat patients with Type IIB von Willebrand's disease since platelet aggregation may be induced.

PRECAUTIONS

General

Desmopressin acetate has infrequently produced changes in blood pressure causing either a slight elevation in blood pressure or a transient fall in blood pressure and a compensatory increase in heart rate. The drug should be used with caution in patients with coronary artery insufficiency and/or hypertensive cardiovascular disease.

Stimate™ Nasal Spray should be used with caution in patients with conditions associated with fluid and electrolyte imbalance, such as cystic fibrosis, because these patients are prone to hyponatremia.

There have been rare reports of thrombotic events (thrombosis [9], acute cerebrovascular thrombosis, acute myocardial infarction) following desmopressin acetate injection in patients predisposed to thrombus formation. No causality has been determined; however, the drug should be used with caution in these patients.

Severe allergic reactions have been reported rarely [2, 11–13]. Fatal anaphylaxis has been reported in one patient who received intravenous DDAVP® (desmopressin acetate). It is not known whether antibodies to desmopressin acetate are produced after repeated administration.

Since **Stimate™ Nasal Spray** is used intranasally, changes in the nasal mucosa such as scarring, edema, or other disease may cause erratic, unreliable absorption in which case **Stimate™ Nasal Spray** should be discontinued until the nasal problems resolve. For such situations, DDAVP® Injection should be considered.

Information for Patients: Patients should be informed that the bottle accurately delivers 25 doses of 150 µg each. Any solution remaining after 25 doses should be discarded since the amount delivered thereafter may be substantially less than 150 µg of drug. No attempt should be made to transfer remaining solution to another bottle. Patients should be instructed to read accompanying directions on use of the spray pump carefully before use.

Patients should also be advised that if bleeding is not controlled, the physician should be contacted [2,3].

Hemophilia A

Laboratory tests for assessing patient status levels of Factor VIII coagulant, Factor VIII antigen and Factor VIII ristocetin cofactor (von Willebrand factor) as well as activated partial thromboplastin time. Factor VIII coagulant activity should be determined before giving **Stimate™ Nasal Spray** for hemostasis. If Factor VIII coagulant activity is present at less than 5% of normal, **Stimate™ Nasal Spray** should not be relied on.

von Willebrand's Disease

Laboratory tests for assessing patient status include levels of Factor VIII coagulant activity, Factor VIII ristocetin cofactor activity, and Factor VIII von Willebrand factor antigen. The skin bleeding time may be helpful in following these patients.

Drug Interactions

Although the pressor activity of desmopressin acetate is very low, its use with other pressor agents should be done only with careful patient monitoring.

DDAVP® Injection has been used with epsilon aminocaproic acid without adverse effects.

Carcinogenicity, Mutagenicity, Impairment of Fertility: There have been no long-term studies in animals to assess the carcinogenic, mutagenic or impairment of fertility potential of **Stimate™ Nasal Spray.**

Pregnancy Category B: Reproduction studies performed in rats and rabbits by the subcutaneous route at doses up to 10 µg/kg/day have revealed no evidence of harm to the fetus due to desmopressin acetate. This dose is equivalent to 10 times (for Factor VIII stimulation) or 38 times (for diabetes insipidus) the systemic human dose based on a mg/M^2 surface area.

There are no adequate and well-controlled studies in pregnant women. Several publications of desmopressin acetate's use in the management of diabetes insipidus during pregnancy are available; these include a few anecdotal reports of congenital anomalies and low birth weight babies. However, no causal connection between these events and desmopressin acetate has been established. A 15-year, Swedish epidemiologic study of the use of desmopressin acetate in pregnant women with diabetes insipidus found the rate of birth defects to be no greater than that in the general population. As opposed to preparations containing natural hormones, desmopressin acetate in antidiuretic doses has no uterotonic action and the physician will have to weigh the therapeutic advantages against the possible risks in each case.

Nursing Mothers: There have been no controlled studies in nursing mothers. A single study in postpartum women demonstrated a marked change in plasma, but little if any change in assayable DDAVP in breast milk following an intranasal dose of 10 µg. It is not known whether this drug is excreted in human milk. Because many drugs are excreted in human milk, caution should be exercised when **Stimate™ Nasal Spray** is administered to a nursing woman.

Pediatric Use: Use in infants and children will require careful fluid intake restriction to prevent possible hyponatremia and water intoxication. **Stimate™ Nasal Spray** should not be used in infants younger than 11 months in the treatment of hemophilia A or von Willebrand's disease; safety and effectiveness in children between 11 months and 12 years of age has been demonstrated [2–4].

ADVERSE REACTIONS

Infrequently, DDAVP® Injection has produced transient headache, nausea, mild abdominal cramps and vulval pain. These symptoms disappeared with reduction in dosage. Occasional facial flushing has been reported with the administration of DDAVP® Injection. Infrequently, high doses of intranasal DDAVP® have produced transient headache and nausea. Nasal congestion, rhinitis and flushing have also been reported occasionally along with mild abdominal cramps. These symptoms disappeared with reduction in dosage. Nosebleed, sore throat, cough and upper respiratory infections have also been reported.

In addition to those listed above, the following have also been reported in clinical trials with **Stimate™ Nasal Spray:** Somnolence, dizziness, itchy or light-sensitive eyes, insomnia, chills, warm feeling, pain, chest pain, palpitations, tachycardia, dyspepsia, edema, vomiting, agitation and balanitis [1–4].

DDAVP® Injection (desmopressin acetate) has infrequently produced changes in blood pressure causing either a slight elevation or a transient fall and a compensatory increase in heart rate. Severe allergic reactions including anaphylaxis have been reported rarely with DDAVP® Injection.

See WARNING for the possibility of water intoxication, hyponatremia and coma [10].

OVERDOSAGE

See ADVERSE REACTIONS above. In cases of overdosage, the dosage should be reduced, frequency of administration decreased, or the drug withdrawn according to the severity of the condition.

There is no known specific antidote for desmopressin acetate or **Stimate™ Nasal Spray.**

An oral LD_{50} has not been established. An intravenous dose of 2 mg/kg in mice demonstrated no effect.

DOSAGE AND ADMINISTRATION

Hemophilia A and von Willebrand's Disease (Type I)

Stimate™ Nasal Spray is administered by nasal insufflation, one spray per nostril, to provide a total dose of 300 µg. In patients weighing less than 50 kg, 150 µg administered as a single spray provided the expected effect on Factor VIII coagulant activity, Factor VIII ristocetin cofactor activity and skin bleeding time [3,4]. If **Stimate™ Nasal Spray** is used preoperatively, it should be administered 2 hours prior to the scheduled procedure [5,8].

The necessity for repeat administration of **Stimate™ Nasal Spray** or use of any blood products for hemostasis should be determined by laboratory response as well as the clinical condition of the patient. The tendency toward tachyphylaxis (lessening of response) with repeated administration given more frequently than every 48 hours should be considered in treating each patient.

The nasal spray pump can only delivery doses of 0.1 mL (150 µg) or multiples of 0.1 mL. If doses other than these are required, DDAVP® Injection may be used.

The spray pump must be primed prior to the first use. To prime pump, press down 4 times. The bottle should be discarded after 25 doses since the amount delivered thereafter per spray may be substantially less than 150 µg of drug.

Continued on next page

Stimate—Cont.

HOW SUPPLIED

A 2.5 mL bottle with spray pump capable of delivering 25 doses of 150 μg (NDC 0053-2453-00).
KEEP REFRIGERATED AT 2°–8°C (36°–46°F). When traveling, product will maintain stability for up to 3 weeks when stored at room temperature, 22°C (72°F).
Caution: Federal (U.S.A.) law prohibits dispensing without prescription.

REFERENCES

1. RHÔNE-POULENC RORER STUDY RG-83884-141: An Open-Label Pharmacokinetic Comparison of Desmopressin Acetate Administration by Intranasal (1.5 mg/mL) and Intravenous Routes: A Dose-Proportionality Trial.
2. RHÔNE-POULENC RORER STUDY RG-83884-142: Nasal Spray Desmopressin (DDAVP). A simple Technique for Treatment of Mild Hemophilia A and von Willebrand's disease.
3. RHÔNE-POULENC RORER STUDY RG-83884-143: Intranasal Desmopression (DDAVP) by spray in Mild Hemophilia A and von Willebrand's disease Type I.
4. RHÔNE-POULENC RORER STUDY RG-83884-144: Evaluation of Intranasal Spray DDAVP in Patients with Mild or Moderate Hemophilia A or von Willebrand's disease: Inpatient Trial.
5. Chistolini A, Dragoni F, Ferrari A, La Verde G, Arcieri R, Mohamud AE and Mazzucconi MG: Intranasal DDAVP: Biological and clinical evaluation in mild Factor VIII deficiency. Haemostasis, 21: 273-277, 1991.
6. Lethagen S, Harris AS, Sjörin E and Nilsson IM: Intranasal and intravenous administration of desmopressin: Effect on FVIII/vWF, pharmacokinetics and reproducibility. Thromb. Haemost., 58:1033-1036, 1987.
7. Lethagen S, Harris AS and Nilsson IM: Intranasal desmopressin (DDAVP) by spray in mild hemophilia A and von Willebrand's disease type I. Blut, 60: 187-191, 1990.
8. Rose EH and Aledort LM: Nasal spray desmopressin (DDAVP) for mild hemophilia A and von Willebrand's disease. Ann. Int. Med., 114: 563-568, 1991.
9. Viron B, Michel C, Serrato T and Verdy E: Risque thrombogene du D.D.A.V.P. dans l'insuffisance rénale chronique (Thrombogenic risk of DDAVP in chronic renal failure). Néphrologie, 8: 225, 1987.
10. RHÔNE-POULENC RORER PHARMACEUTICALS INC. ADVERSE REACTION REPORT No. 01-003827; Coma, grand mal seizure, etc.
11. RHÔNE-POULENC RORER PHARMACEUTICALS INC. ADVERSE REACTION REPORT No. 01-000657; Anaphylaxis, etc.
12. RHÔNE-POULENC RORER PHARMACEUTICALS INC. ADVERSE REACTION REPORT No. 01-001182; Anaphylactoid reaction.
13. RHÔNE-POULENC RORER PHARMACEUTICALS INC. ADVERSE REACTION REPORT No. US-870671; Erythema, rash.

Rev. 3/95   IN-8155B

Manufactured for
CENTEON L.L.C.
1020 FIRST AVENUE
KING OF PRUSSIA, PA 19406-1310
By Ferring Pharmaceuticals, Malmö, Sweden

Celgene Corporation
7 POWDER HORN DRIVE
WARREN, NJ 07059

Direct Inquiries to:
Ph: (732) 271–1001

THALOMID™   ℞
(thalidomide) Capsules

For full prescribing information, please look under Celgene Corporation at the end of the Product Information section

For information on over-the-counter drugs, consult **PDR For Nonprescription Drugs.**

Centocor, Inc.
200 GREAT VALLEY PARKWAY
MALVERN, PA 19355

Direct General Inquiries to:
Ph: (610) 651-6000
    (888) 874-3083
Fax: (610) 651-6100

Medical Emergency Contact:
Ph: 1-800-457-6399
For Medical Information/Adverse Experience Reporting Contact:
Medical Information & Product Surveillance
Ph: (800) 457-6399
Fax: (610) 651-6197

REOPRO®   ℞
Abciximab
For intravenous administration

DESCRIPTION

Abciximab, ReoPro®, is the Fab fragment of the chimeric human-murine monoclonal antibody 7E3. Abciximab binds to the glycoprotein (GP) IIb/IIIa ($\alpha_{IIb}\beta_3$) receptor of human platelets and inhibits platelet aggregation. Abciximab also binds to the vitronectin ($\alpha_v\beta_3$) receptor found on platelets and vessel wall endothelial and smooth muscle cells.
The chimeric 7E3 antibody is produced by continuous perfusion in mammalian cell culture. The 47,615 dalton Fab fragment is purified from cell culture supernatant by a series of steps involving specific viral inactivation and removal procedures, digestion with papain, and column chromatography.
ReoPro® is a clear, colorless, sterile, non-pyrogenic solution for intravenous (IV) use. Each single-use vial contains 2 mg/mL of Abciximab in a buffered solution (pH 7.2) of 0.01 M sodium phosphate, 0.15 M sodium chloride and 0.001% polysorbate 80 in Water for Injection. No preservatives are added.

CLINICAL PHARMACOLOGY

General: Abciximab binds to the intact platelet GPIIb/IIIa receptor, which is a member of the integrin family of adhesion receptors and the major platelet surface receptor involved in platelet aggregation. Abciximab inhibits platelet aggregation by preventing the binding of fibrinogen, von Willebrand factor, and other adhesive molecules to GPIIb/IIIa receptor sites on activated platelets. The mechanism of action is thought to involve steric hindrance and/or conformational effects to block access of large molecules to the receptor rather than direct interaction with the RGD (arginine-glycine-aspartic acid) binding site of GPIIb/IIIa. Abciximab binds with similar affinity to the vitronectin receptor, also known as the $\alpha_v\beta_3$ integrin. The vitronectin receptor mediates the procoagulant properties of platelets and the proliferative properties of vascular endothelial and smooth muscle cells. In *in vitro* studies using a model cell line derived from melanoma cells, Abciximab blocked $\alpha_v\beta_3$-mediated effects including cell adhesion (IC$_{50}$=0.34 μg/mL). At concentrations which, *in vitro*, provide >80% GPIIb/IIIa receptor blockade, but above the *in vivo* therapeutic range, Abciximab more effectively blocked the burst of thrombin generation that followed platelet activation than select comparator antibodies which inhibit GPIIb/IIIa alone(1). The relationship of these *in vitro* data to clinical efficacy is uncertain.
Pre-clinical experience: Maximal inhibition of platelet aggregation was observed when ≥ 80% of GPIIb/IIIa receptors were blocked by Abciximab. In non-human primates, Abciximab bolus doses of 0.25 mg/kg generally achieved a blockade of at least 80% of platelet receptors and fully inhibited platelet aggregation. Inhibition of platelet function was temporary following a bolus dose, but receptor blockade could be sustained at ≥ 80% by continuous intravenous infusion. The inhibitory effects of Abciximab were substantially reversed by the transfusion of platelets in monkeys. The antithrombotic efficacy of prototype antibodies [murine 7E3 Fab and F(ab')$_2$] and Abciximab was evaluated in dog, monkey and baboon models of coronary, carotid, and femoral artery thrombosis. Doses of the murine version of 7E3 or Abciximab sufficient to produce high-grade (≥ 80%) GPIIb/IIIa receptor blockade prevented acute thrombosis and yielded lower rates of thrombosis compared with aspirin and/or heparin.
Pharmacokinetics: Following intravenous bolus administration, free plasma concentrations of Abciximab decrease rapidly with an initial half-life of less than 10 minutes and a second phase half-life of about 30 minutes, probably related to rapid binding to the platelet GPIIb/IIIa receptors. Platelet function generally recovers over the course of 48 hours (2,3), although Abciximab remains in the circulation for 15 days or more in a platelet-bound state. Intravenous

administration of a 0.25 mg/kg bolus dose of Abciximab followed by continuous infusion of 10 μg/min (or a weight-adjusted infusion of 0.125 μg/kg/min to a maximum of 10 μg/min) produces approximately constant free plasma concentrations throughout the infusion. At the termination of the infusion period, free plasma concentrations fall rapidly for approximately six hours then decline at a slower rate.
Pharmacodynamics: Intravenous administration in humans of single bolus doses of Abciximab from 0.15 mg/kg to 0.30 mg/kg produced rapid dose-dependent inhibition of platelet function as measured by *ex vivo* platelet aggregation in response to adenosine diphosphate (ADP) or by prolongation of bleeding time. At the two highest doses (0.25 and 0.30 mg/kg) at two hours post injection, over 80% of the GPIIb/IIIa receptors were blocked and platelet aggregation in response to 20 μM ADP was almost abolished. The median bleeding time increased to over 30 minutes at both doses compared with a baseline value of approximately five minutes.
Intravenous administration in humans of a single bolus dose of 0.25 mg/kg followed by a continuous infusion of 10 μg/min for periods of 12 to 96 hours produced sustained high-grade GPIIb/IIIa receptor blockade (≥ 80%) and inhibition of platelet function (*ex vivo* platelet aggregation in response to 5 μM or 20 μM ADP less than 20% of baseline and bleeding time greater than 30 minutes) for the duration of the infusion in most patients. Similar results were obtained when a weight-adjusted infusion dose (0.125 μg/kg/min to a maximum of 10 μg/min) was used in patients weighing up to 80 kg. Results in patients who received the 0.25 mg/kg bolus followed by a 5 μg/min infusion for 24 hours showed a similar initial receptor blockade and inhibition of platelet aggregation, but the response was not maintained throughout the infusion period.
Low levels of GPIIb/IIIa receptor blockade are present for more than 10 days following cessation of the infusion. After discontinuation of Abciximab infusion, platelet function returns gradually to normal. Bleeding time returned to ≤ 12 minutes within 12 hours following the end of infusion in 15 of 20 patients (75%), and within 24 hours in 18 of 20 patients (90%). *Ex vivo* platelet aggregation in response to 5 μM ADP returned to ≥ 50% of baseline within 24 hours following the end of infusion in 11 of 32 patients (34%) and within 48 hours in 23 of 32 patients (72%). In response to 20 μM ADP, *ex vivo* platelet aggregation returned to ≥ 50% of baseline within 24 hours in 20 of 32 patients (62%) and within 48 hours in 28 of 32 patients (88%).

CLINICAL STUDIES

Abciximab has been studied in three Phase 3 clinical trials, all of which evaluated the effect of Abciximab in patients undergoing percutaneous coronary intervention: in patients at high risk for abrupt closure of the treated coronary vessel (EPIC), in a broader group of patients (EPILOG), and in unstable angina patients not responding to conventional medical therapy (CAPTURE). Percutaneous intervention included balloon angioplasty, atherectomy, or stent placement. All trials involved the use of various, concomitant heparin dose regimens and, unless contraindicated, aspirin (325 mg) was administered orally two hours prior to the planned procedure and then once daily.
EPIC was a multicenter, double-blind, placebo-controlled trial of Abciximab in patients undergoing percutaneous transluminal coronary angioplasty or atherectomy (4). In the EPIC trial, 2099 patients between 26 and 83 years of age who were at high risk for abrupt closure of the treated coronary vessel were randomly allocated to one of three treatments: 1) an Abciximab bolus (0.25 mg/kg) followed by an Abciximab infusion (10 μg/min) for 12 hours (bolus plus infusion group); 2) an Abciximab bolus (0.25 mg/kg) followed by a placebo infusion (bolus group); or, 3) a placebo bolus followed by a placebo infusion (placebo group). Patients at high risk during or following percutaneous coronary intervention were defined as those with unstable angina or non-Q wave myocardial infarction (n=489), those with an acute Q-wave myocardial infarction within 12 hours of symptom onset (n=66), and those who were at high risk because of coronary morphology and/or clinical characteristics (n=1544). Treatment with study agent in each of the three arms was initiated 10–60 minutes before the onset of percutaneous coronary intervention. All patients initially received an intravenous heparin bolus (10,000 to 12,000 units) and boluses of up to 3,000 units thereafter to a maximum of 20,000 units during percutaneous coronary intervention. Heparin infusion was continued for 12 hours to maintain a therapeutic elevation of activated partial thromboplastin time (APTT, 1.5–2.5 times normal).
The primary endpoint was the occurrence of any of the following events within 30 days of percutaneous coronary intervention: death, myocardial infarction (MI), or the need for urgent intervention for recurrent ischemia [i.e., urgent percutaneous transluminal coronary angioplasty, urgent coronary artery bypass graft (CABG) surgery, a coronary stent, or an intra-aortic balloon pump]. The 30-day (Kaplan-Meier) primary endpoint event rates for each treatment group by intention-to-treat analysis of all randomized pa-

tients are shown in Table 1. The 4.5% lower incidence of the primary endpoint rates in the bolus plus infusion treatment group, compared with the placebo group, was statistically significant, whereas the 1.3% lower incidence in the bolus treatment group was not. A lower incidence of the primary endpoint was observed in the bolus plus infusion treatment arm for all three high-risk subgroups: patients with unstable angina, patients presenting within 12 hours of the onset of symptoms of an acute myocardial infarction, and patients with other high-risk clinical and/or morphologic characteristics (4). The treatment effect was largest in the first two subgroups and smallest in the third subgroup.

[See table 1 above]

Table 1
PRIMARY ENDPOINT EVENT RATE AT 30 DAYS - EPIC TRIAL

	Placebo (n=696)	Abciximab Bolus (n=695)	Abciximab Bolus + Infusion (n=708)
	Number of Patients (%)		
Death, MI, or urgent intervention[a]	89 (12.8)	79 (11.5)	59 (8.3)
p-value vs. placebo		0.428	0.008
Components of Primary Endpoint[b]			
Death	12 (1.7)	9 (1.3)	12 (1.7)
Acute myocardial infarctions in surviving patients	55 (7.9)	40 (5.8)	31 (4.4)
Urgent intervention in surviving patients without acute MI	22 (3.2)	30 (4.4)	16 (2.2)

[a]Patients who experienced more than one event in the first 30 days are counted only once.
[b]Patients are counted only once under the most serious component (death > acute MI > urgent intervention).

The primary endpoint event rates in the bolus plus infusion treatment group were reduced mostly in the first 48 hours and this benefit was sustained through blinded evaluations at 30 days(4), six months(5) and three years(6). At the six-month follow-up visit this event rate remained lower in the bolus plus infusion arm (12.3%) than in the placebo arm (17.6%) (p=0.006 vs. placebo). Median long-term follow up was 3.1 years (99% of patients had follow up between 2.5 and 3.5 years). Using Kaplan-Meier estimates, at 3 years the absolute reduction in events was maintained with an event rate of 19.6% in the bolus plus infusion arm and 24.4% in the placebo arm (p=0.027 vs. placebo).

EPILOG was a randomized, double-blind, multicenter, placebo-controlled trial which evaluated Abciximab in a broad population of patients undergoing percutaneous coronary intervention (excluding patients with myocardial infarction and unstable angina meeting the EPIC high-risk criteria)(7). EPILOG tested the hypothesis that use of a low-dose, weight-adjusted heparin regimen, early femoral arterial sheath removal, improved access site management and weight-adjustment of the Abciximab infusion dose could significantly lower the bleeding rate yet maintain the efficacy seen in the EPIC trial. EPILOG was a three-treatment-arm trial: Abciximab plus standard-dose, weight-adjusted heparin[1]; Abciximab plus low-dose, weight-adjusted heparin[2]; and placebo plus standard-dose, weight-adjusted heparin. The Abciximab bolus dose was the same as that used in the EPIC trial (0.25 mg/kg), but the continuous infusion dose was weight adjusted in patients up to 80 kg[3] (0.125 μg/kg/min). Specific patient and access site management procedures as well as a strong recommendation for early sheath removal were also incorporated into the trial as described in PRECAUTIONS. The EPILOG trial achieved the objective of lowering the bleeding rate while maintaining efficacy: in the Abciximab treatment arms major bleeding was not significantly different from that in the placebo arm (see ADVERSE REACTIONS: Bleeding).

[1] Bolus administration of 100 U/kg weight-adjusted heparin to achieve an activated clotting time (ACT) of 300 seconds (maximum initial bolus 10,000 units).
[2] Bolus administration of 70 U/kg weight-adjusted heparin to achieve an activated clotting time (ACT) of 200 seconds (maximum initial bolus 7,000 units).
[3] Bolus administration of 0.25 mg/kg Abciximab 10 to 60 minutes before percutaneous coronary intervention immediately followed by a 0.125 μg/kg/min infusion (maximum 10 μg/min) for 12 hours.

The primary endpoint of the EPILOG trial was the composite of death or MI occurring within 30 days of percutaneous coronary intervention. The composite of death, MI, or urgent intervention was an important secondary endpoint. As seen in the EPIC trial, the endpoint events in the Abciximab treatment group were reduced mostly in the first 48 hours and this benefit was sustained through blinded evaluations at 30 days and six months. The (Kaplan-Meier) endpoint event rates at 30 days are shown in Table 2 for each treatment group by intention-to-treat analysis of all 2792 randomized patients. At the six-month follow-up visit, the event rate for death, MI, or repeat (urgent or non-urgent) intervention remained lower in the Abciximab treatment arms (22.3% and 22.8%, respectively, for the standard- and low-dose heparin arms) than in the placebo arm (25.8%) and the event rate for death, MI, or urgent intervention was substantially lower in the Abciximab treatment arms (8.3% and 8.4%, respectively, for the standard- and low-dose heparin arms) than in the placebo arm (14.7%). The proportionate reductions in endpoint event rates were similar irrespective of the type of coronary intervention used (balloon angioplasty, atherectomy, or stent placement). Risk assessment using the American College of Cardiology/American Heart Association clinical/morphological criteria had large inter-observer variability. Consequently, a low risk subgroup could not be reproducibly identified in which to evaluate efficacy.

[See table 2 at top of next page]

CAPTURE was a randomized, double-blind, multicenter, placebo-controlled trial of the use of Abciximab in unstable angina patients not responding to conventional medical therapy for whom percutaneous coronary intervention was planned, but not immediately performed(8) In contrast to the EPIC and EPILOG trials, the CAPTURE trial involved the administration of placebo or Abciximab starting 18 to 24 hours prior to percutaneous coronary intervention and continuing until one hour after completion of the intervention. Patients were assessed as having unstable angina not responding to conventional medical therapy if they had at least one episode of myocardial ischemia despite bed rest and at least two hours of therapy with intravenous heparin and oral or intravenous nitrates. These patients were enrolled into the CAPTURE trial if, during a screening angiogram, they were determined to have a coronary lesion amenable to percutaneous coronary intervention. Patients received a bolus dose and intravenous infusion of placebo or Abciximab for 18 to 24 hours. At the end of the infusion period, the intervention was performed. The Abciximab or placebo infusion was discontinued one hour following the intervention. Patients were treated with intravenous heparin and oral or intravenous nitrates throughout the 18 to 24-hour Abciximab infusion period prior to the percutaneous coronary intervention.

The Abciximab dose was a 0.25 mg/kg bolus followed by a continuous infusion at a rate of 10 μg/min. The CAPTURE trial incorporated weight adjustment of the standard heparin dose only during the performance of the intervention, but did not investigate the effect of a lower heparin dose, and arterial sheaths were left in place for approximately 40 hours. The primary endpoint of the CAPTURE trial was the occurrence of any of the following events within 30 days of percutaneous coronary intervention: death, MI, or urgent intervention. The 30-day (Kaplan-Meier) primary endpoint event rates for each treatment group by intention-to-treat analysis of all 1265 randomized patients are shown in Table 3.

[See table 3 on next page]

The 30-day results are consistent with EPIC results, with the greatest effects on the myocardial infarction and urgent intervention components of the composite endpoint. As secondary endpoints, the components of the composite endpoint were analyzed separately for the period prior to the percutaneous coronary intervention and the period from the beginning of the intervention through Day 30. The greatest difference in MI occurred in the post-intervention period: the rates of MI were lower in the Abciximab group compared with placebo (Abciximab 3.6%, placebo 6.1%). There was also a reduction in MI occurring prior to the percutaneous coronary intervention (Abciximab 0.6%, placebo 2.0%). An Abciximab-associated reduction in the incidence of urgent intervention occurred in the post-intervention period. No effect on mortality was observed in either period. At six months of follow up, the composite endpoint of death, MI, or repeat intervention (urgent or non-urgent) was not different between the Abciximab and placebo groups (Abciximab 31.0%, placebo 30.8%, p=0.77).

Mortality was uncommon in all three trials, EPIC, EPILOG and CAPTURE. Similar mortality rates were observed in all arms within each trial. In all three trials, the rates of acute MI were significantly lower in the groups treated with Abciximab. Urgent intervention rates were also lower in Abciximab-treated groups in these trials.

Anticoagulation: Due to the incidence of bleeding seen in the EPIC trial, the dosing regimens of concomitant heparin and the target levels for anticoagulation were successively varied in the CAPTURE and EPILOG trials. These modified dosing regimens combined with other measures for patient management were associated with reduced bleeding rates (see ADVERSE REACTIONS: Bleeding)

EPILOG trial: Heparin was weight adjusted in all treatment arms. A baseline ACT was determined prior to percutaneous coronary intervention. In the low-dose heparin arm of the trial, heparin was administered as follows:

The initial heparin bolus was based upon the results of the baseline ACT, according to the following regimen:

ACT < 150 seconds: administer 70 U/kg heparin
ACT 150 - 199 seconds: administer 50 U/kg heparin
ACT ≥ 200 seconds: administer no heparin

Additional 20 U/kg heparin boluses were given to achieve and maintain an ACT of 200 seconds during the procedure.

Discontinuation of heparin immediately after the procedure and removal of the arterial sheath within six hours were strongly recommended in the trial. If prolonged heparin therapy or delayed sheath removal was clinically indicated, heparin was adjusted to keep the APTT at a target of 60 to 85 seconds.

CAPTURE trial: Anticoagulation was initiated prior to the administration of Abciximab. Anticoagulation was initiated with an intravenous heparin infusion to achieve a target APTT of 60 to 85 seconds. The heparin infusion was not uniformly weight adjusted in this trial. The heparin infusion was maintained during the Abciximab infusion and was adjusted to achieve an ACT of 300 seconds or an APTT of 70 seconds during the percutaneous coronary intervention. Following the intervention, heparin management was as outlined above for the EPILOG trial.

INDICATIONS AND USAGE

Abciximab is indicated as an adjunct to percutaneous coronary intervention for the prevention of cardiac ischemic complications.

- in patients undergoing percutaneous coronary intervention
- in patients with unstable angina not responding to conventional medical therapy when percutaneous coronary intervention is planned within 24 hours

Abciximab use in patients not undergoing percutaneous coronary intervention has not been studied.

Abciximab is intended for use with aspirin and heparin and has been studied only in that setting, as described in CLINICAL STUDIES.

CONTRAINDICATIONS

Because Abciximab may increase the risk of bleeding, Abciximab is contraindicated in the following clinical situations:

- Active internal bleeding
- Recent (within six weeks) gastrointestinal (GI) or genitourinary (GU) bleeding of clinical significance
- History of cerebrovascular accident (CVA) within two years, or CVA with a significant residual neurological deficit
- Bleeding diathesis
- Administration of oral anticoagulants within seven days unless prothrombin time is ≤ 1.2 times control
- Thrombocytopenia (< 100,000 cells/μL)
- Recent (within six weeks) major surgery or trauma
- Intracranial neoplasm, arteriovenous malformation, or aneurysm
- Severe uncontrolled hypertension
- Presumed or documented history of vasculitis
- Use of intravenous dextran before percutaneous coronary intervention, or intent to use it during an intervention

Abciximab is also contraindicated in patients with known hypersensitivity to any component of this product or to murine proteins.

WARNINGS

Abciximab has the potential to increase the risk of bleeding, particularly in the presence of anticoagulation, e.g., from heparin, other anticoagulants, or thrombolytics (see ADVERSE REACTIONS: Bleeding).

The risk of major bleeds due to Abciximab therapy may be increased in patients receiving thrombolytics and should be weighed against the anticipated benefits.

Should serious bleeding occur that is not controllable with pressure, the infusion of Abciximab and any concomitant heparin should be stopped.

Continued on next page

ReoPro—Cont.

PRECAUTIONS

Bleeding Precautions: Results of the EPILOG trial show that bleeding can be reduced by the use of low-dose, weight-adjusted heparin regimens, adherence to stricter anticoagulation guidelines, early femoral arterial sheath removal, careful patient and access site management and weight-adjustment of the Abciximab infusion dose.

Therapy with Abciximab requires careful attention to all potential bleeding sites (including catheter insertion sites, arterial and venous puncture sites, cutdown sites, needle puncture sites, and gastrointestinal, genitourinary, and retroperitoneal sites).

Arterial and venous punctures, intramuscular injections, and use of urinary catheters, nasotracheal intubation, nasogastric tubes and automatic blood pressure cuffs should be minimized. When obtaining intravenous access, noncompressible sites (e.g., subclavian or jugular veins) should be avoided. Saline or heparin locks should be considered for blood drawing. Vascular puncture sites should be documented and monitored. Gentle care should be provided when removing dressings.

Femoral artery access site:
Arterial access site care is important to prevent bleeding. Care should be taken when attempting vascular access that only the anterior wall of the femoral artery is punctured, avoiding a Seldinger (through and through) technique for obtaining sheath access. Femoral vein sheath placement should be avoided unless needed. While the vascular sheath is in place, patients should be maintained on complete bed rest with the head of the bed ≤30° and the affected limb restrained in a straight position. Patients may be medicated for back/groin pain as necessary.

Discontinuation of heparin immediately upon completion of the procedure and removal of the arterial sheath within six hours is strongly recommended if APTT ≤ 50 sec or ACT ≤ 175 sec (See PRECAUTIONS: Laboratory Tests). In all circumstances, heparin should be discontinued at least two hours prior to arterial sheath removal.

Following sheath removal, pressure should be applied to the femoral artery for at least 30 minutes using either manual compression or a mechanical device for hemostasis. A pressure dressing should be applied following hemostasis. The patient should be maintained on bed rest for six to eight hours following sheath removal or discontinuation of Abciximab, or four hours following discontinuation of heparin, whichever is later. The pressure dressing should be removed prior to ambulation. The sheath insertion site and distal pulses of affected leg(s) should be frequently checked while the femoral artery sheath is in place and for six hours after femoral artery sheath removal. Any hematoma should be measured and monitored for enlargement.

The following conditions have been associated with an increased risk of bleeding and may be additive with the effect of Abciximab in the angioplasty setting: percutaneous coronary intervention within 12 hours of the onset of symptoms for acute myocardial infarction, prolonged percutaneous coronary intervention (lasting more than 70 minutes) and failed percutaneous coronary intervention.

Use of Thrombolytics, Anticoagulants and Other Antiplatelet Agents: In the EPIC, EPILOG and CAPTURE trials, Abciximab was used concomitantly with heparin and aspirin. For details of the anticoagulation algorithms used in these clinical trials, see CLINICAL STUDIES: Anticoagulation. Because Abciximab inhibits platelet aggregation, caution should be employed when it is used with other drugs that affect hemostasis, including thrombolytics, oral anticoagulants, non-steroidal anti-inflammatory drugs, dipyridamole, and ticlopidine.

In the EPIC trial, there was limited experience with the administration of Abciximab with low molecular weight dextran. Low molecular weight dextran was usually given for the deployment of a coronary stent, for which oral anticoagulants were also given. In the 11 patients who received low molecular weight dextran with Abciximab, five had major bleeding events and four had minor bleeding events. None of the five placebo patients treated with low molecular weight dextran had a major or minor bleeding event (see CONTRAINDICATIONS).

There are limited data on the use of Abciximab in patients receiving thrombolytic agents. Because of concern about synergistic effects on bleeding, systemic thrombolytic therapy should be used judiciously.

Thrombocytopenia: Platelet counts should be monitored prior to treatment, two to four hours following the bolus dose of Abciximab and at 24 hours or prior to discharge, whichever is first. If a patient experiences an acute platelet decrease (e.g., a platelet decrease to less than 100,000 cells/µL and a decrease of at least 25% from pre-treatment value), additional platelet counts should be determined. These platelet counts should be drawn in three separate tubes containing ethylenediaminetetraacetic acid (EDTA), citrate and heparin, respectively, to exclude pseudothrombocytopenia due to *in vitro* anticoagulant interaction. If true

Table 2
ENDPOINT EVENT RATES AT 30 DAYS - EPILOG TRIAL

	Placebo + Standard Dose Heparin (n=939)	Abciximab + Standard Dose Heparin (n=918)	Abciximab + Low Dose Heparin (n=935)
	Number of Patients (%)		
Death or MI[a]	85 (9.1)	38 (4.2)	35 (3.8)
p-value vs. placebo		<0.001	<0.001
Death, MI, or urgent intervention[a]	109 (11.7)	49 (5.4)	48 (5.2)
p-value vs. placebo		<0.001	<0.001
Components of Composite Endpoints[b]			
Death	7 (0.8)	4 (0.4)	3 (0.3)
Acute myocardial infarctions in surviving patients	78 (8.4)	34 (3.7)	32 (3.4)
Urgent intervention in surviving patients without acute MI	24 (2.6)	11 (1.2)	13 (1.4)

[a]Patients who experienced more than one event in the first 30 days are counted only once.
[b]Patients are counted only once under the most serious component (death > acute MI > urgent intervention).

Table 3
PRIMARY ENDPOINT EVENT RATE AT 30 DAYS - CAPTURE TRIAL

	Placebo (n=635)	Abciximab (n=630)
	Number of Patients (%)	
Death, MI, or urgent intervention[a]	101 (15.9)	71 (11.3)
p-value vs. placebo		0.012
Components of Primary Endpoint[b]		
Death	8 (1.3)	6 (1.0)
MI in surviving patients	49 (7.7)	24 (3.8)
Urgent intervention in surviving patients without acute MI	44 (6.9)	41 (6.6)

[a] Patients who experienced more than one event in the first 30 days are counted only once. Urgent interventions included any unplanned percutaneous coronary intervention after the planned intervention, as well as any stent placement for immediate patency and any unplanned CABG or use of an intra-aortic balloon pump.
[b] Patients are counted only once under the most serious component (death>acute MI>urgent intervention).

Table 4
NON-CABG BLEEDING IN THE EPIC, EPILOG AND CAPTURE TRIALS
Number of Patients with Bleeds (%)
EPIC:

	Placebo (n = 696)	Abciximab (Bolus + Infusion) (n = 708)
Major[a]	23 (3.3)	75 (10.6)
Minor	64 (9.2)	119 (16.8)
Requiring Transfusion[b]	14 (2.0)	55 (7.8)

CAPTURE:

	Placebo (n = 635)	Abciximab (n = 630)
Major[a]	12 (1.9)	24 (3.8)
Minor	13 (2.0)	30 (4.8)
Requiring Transfusion[b]	9 (1.4)	15 (2.4)

EPILOG:

	Placebo (n = 939)	Abciximab + Standard-dose Heparin (n = 918)	Abciximab + Low-dose Heparin (n = 935)
Major[a]	10 (1.1)	17 (1.9)	10 (1.1)
Minor	32 (3.4)	70 (7.6)	37 (4.0)
Requiring Transfusion[b]	10 (1.1)	7 (0.8)	6 (0.6)

[a] Patients who had bleeding in more than one classification are counted only once according to the most severe classification. Patients with multiple bleeding events of the same classification are also counted once within that classification.
[b] Packed red blood cells or whole blood

thrombocytopenia is verified, Abciximab should be immediately discontinued and the condition appropriately monitored and treated. For patients with thrombocytopenia in the clinical trials, a daily platelet count was obtained until it returned to normal. If a patient's platelet count dropped to 60,000 cells/µL, heparin and aspirin were discontinued. If a patient's platelet count dropped below 50,000 cells/µL, platelets were transfused. Most cases of severe thrombocytopenia (<50,000 cells/µL) occurred within the first 24 hours of Abciximab administration.

Restoration of Platelet Function: In the event of serious uncontrolled bleeding or the need for emergency surgery, Abciximab should be discontinued. If platelet function does not return to normal, it may be restored, at least in part, with platelet transfusions.

Laboratory Tests: Before infusion of Abciximab, platelet count, prothrombin time, ACT and APTT should be measured to identify pre-existing hemostatic abnormalities.

Based on an integrated analysis of data from all studies, the following guidelines may be utilized to minimize the risk for bleeding:

When Abciximab is initiated 18 to 24 hours before percutaneous coronary intervention, the APTT should be maintained between 60 and 85 seconds during the Abciximab and heparin infusion period.

During percutaneous coronary intervention, the ACT should be maintained between 200 and 300 seconds.

If anticoagulation is continued in these patients following percutaneous coronary intervention, the APTT should be maintained between 60 and 85 seconds.

The APTT or ACT should be checked prior to arterial sheath removal. The sheath should not be removed unless APTT ≤ 50 seconds or ACT ≤ 175 seconds.

Readmistration: Administration of Abciximab may result in human anti-chimeric antibody (HACA) formation that could potentially cause allergic or hypersensitivity re-

actions (including anaphylaxis), thrombocytopenia or diminished benefit upon readministration of Abciximab. In the EPIC, EPILOG, and CAPTURE trials, positive HACA responses occurred in approximately 5.8% of the Abciximab-treated patients. There was no excess of hypersensitivity or allergic reactions related to Abciximab treatment.

Readministration of Abciximab to 29 healthy volunteers who had not developed a HACA response after first administration has not led to any change in Abciximab pharmacokinetics or to any reduction in antiplatelet potency. However, results in this small group of patients suggest that the incidence of HACA response may be increased after readministration. Readministration to patients who have developed a positive HACA response after initial administration has not been evaluated in clinical trials.

Allergic Reactions: Anaphylaxis has not been reported for Abciximab-treated patients in any of the Phase 3 clinical trials. However, anaphylaxis may occur. If it does, administration of Abciximab should be immediately stopped and standard appropriate resuscitative measures should be initiated.

Drug Interactions: Although drug interactions with Abciximab have not been studied systematically, Abciximab has been administered to patients with ischemic heart disease treated concomitantly with a broad range of medications used in the treatment of angina, myocardial infarction and hypertension. These medications have included heparin, warfarin, beta-adrenergic receptor blockers, calcium channel antagonists, angiotensin converting enzyme inhibitors, intravenous and oral nitrates, and aspirin. Heparin, other anticoagulants, thrombolytics, and antiplatelet agents may be associated with an increase in bleeding. Patients with HACA titers may have allergic or hypersensitivity reactions when treated with other diagnostic or therapeutic monoclonal antibodies.

Carcinogenesis, Mutagenesis and Impairment of Fertility: In vitro and in vivo mutagenicity studies have not been demonstrated any mutagenic effect. Long-term studies in animals have not been performed to evaluate the carcinogenic potential or effects on fertility in male or female animals.

Pregnancy Category C: Animal reproduction studies have not been conducted with Abciximab. It is also not known whether Abciximab can cause fetal harm when administered to a pregnant woman or can affect reproduction capacity. Abciximab should be given to a pregnant woman only if clearly needed.

Nursing Mothers: It is not known whether this drug is excreted in human milk or absorbed systemically after ingestion. Because many drugs are excreted in human milk, caution should be exercised when Abciximab is administered to a nursing woman.

Pediatric Use: Safety and effectiveness in pediatric patients have not been studied.

ADVERSE REACTIONS

Bleeding: Abciximab has the potential to increase the risk of bleeding, particularly in the presence of anticoagulation, e.g. from heparin, other anticoagulants or thrombolytics. Bleeding in the Phase 3 trials was classified as major, minor or insignificant by the criteria of the Thrombolysis in Myocardial Infarction study group(9). Major bleeding events were defined as either an intracranial hemorrhage or a decrease in hemoglobin greater than 5 g/dL. Minor bleeding events included spontaneous gross hematuria, spontaneous hematemesis, observed blood loss with a hemoglobin decrease of more than 3 g/dL, or a decrease in hemoglobin of at least 4 g/dL without an identified bleeding site. Insignificant bleeding events were defined as a decrease in hemoglobin of less than 3 g/dL or a decrease in hemoglobin between 3–4 g/dL without observed bleeding. In patients who received transfusions, the number of units of blood lost was estimated through an adaptation of the method of Landefeld, et al.(10).

In the EPIC trial, in which a non-weight-adjusted, standard heparin dose regimen was used, the most common complication during Abciximab therapy was bleeding during the first 36 hours. The incidences of major bleeding, minor bleeding and transfusion of blood products were significantly increased. Approximately 70% of Abciximab-treated patients with major bleeding had bleeding at the arterial access site in the groin. Abciximab-treated patients also had a higher incidence of major bleeding events from gastrointestinal, genitourinary, retroperitoneal, and other sites.

Bleeding rates were reduced in the CAPTURE trial, and further reduced in the EPILOG trial by use of modified dosing regimens and specific patient management techniques. In EPILOG, using the heparin and Abciximab dosing, sheath removal and arterial access site guidelines described under PRECAUTIONS, the incidence of major bleeding in patients treated with Abciximab and low-dose, weight-adjusted heparin was not significantly different from that in patients receiving placebo.

Subgroup analyses in the EPIC and CAPTURE trials showed that non-CABG major bleeding was more common in Abciximab patients weighing ≤ 75 kg. In the EPILOG

trial which used weight-adjusted heparin dosing, the non-CABG major bleeding rates for Abciximab-treated patients did not differ substantially by weight subgroup.

Although data are limited, Abciximab treatment was not associated with excess major bleeding in patients who underwent CABG surgery. (The range among all treatment arms was 3–5% in EPIC and 1–2% in the CAPTURE and EPILOG trials.) Some patients with prolonged bleeding times received platelet transfusions to correct the bleeding time prior to surgery. (See PRECAUTIONS: Restoration of Platelet Function.)

The rates of major bleeding, minor bleeding and bleeding events requiring transfusions in the EPIC, CAPTURE and EPILOG trials are shown in Table 4. The rates of insignificant bleeding events are not included in Table 4.

[See table 4 on previous page]

Intracranial Hemorrhage and Stroke: The total incidence of intracranial hemorrhage and non-hemorrhagic stroke across all three trials was not significantly different, 7/2225 for placebo patients and 10/3112 for Abciximab-treated patients. The incidence of intracranial hemorrhage was 3/2225 for placebo patients and 6/3112 for Abciximab patients.

Thrombocytopenia: In the clinical trials, patients treated with Abciximab were more likely than patients treated with placebo to experience decreases in platelet counts. The rates of thrombocytopenia and transfusions were lower in the subsequent CAPTURE and EPILOG trials (Table 5).

[See table 5 above]

Other Adverse Reactions: Table 6 shows adverse events other than bleeding and thrombocytopenia from the combined EPIC, EPILOG and CAPTURE trials which occurred in patients in the bolus plus infusion arm at an incidence of more than 0.5% higher than in those treated with placebo.

[See table 6 above]

The following additional adverse events from the EPIC, EPILOG and CAPTURE trials were reported by investigators in the patients treated with a bolus plus infusion of Abciximab at incidences which were less than 0.5% higher than for patients in the placebo arm.

Cardiovascular System—ventricular tachycardia (1.4%), pseudoaneurysm (0.8%), palpitation (0.5%), arteriovenous fistula (0.4%), incomplete AV block (0.3%), nodal arrhythmia (0.2%), complete AV block (0.1%), embolism (limb)(0.1%); thrombophlebitis (0.1%);

Gastrointestinal System—dyspepsia (2.1%), diarrhea (1.1%), ileus (0.1%), gastroesophageal reflux (0.1%);

Hemic and Lymphatic System—anemia (1.3%), leukocytosis (0.5%), petechiae (0.2%);

Nervous System—dizziness (2.9%), anxiety (1.7%), abnormal thinking (1.3%), agitation (0.7%), hypesthesia (0.6%), confusion (0.5%), muscle contractions (0.4%), coma (0.2%), hypertonia (0.2%), diplopia (0.1%);

Respiratory System—pneumonia (0.4%), rales (0.4%), pleural effusion (0.3%), bronchitis (0.3%) bronchospasm (0.3%), pleurisy (0.2%), pulmonary embolism (0.2%), rhonchi (0.1%);

Musculoskeletal System—myalgia (0.2%);

Urogenital System—urinary retention (0.7%), dysuria (0.4%), abnormal renal function (0.4%), frequent micturition (0.1%), cystalgia (0.1%), urinary incontinence (0.1%), prostatitis (0.1%);

Miscellaneous—pain (5.4%), sweating increased (1.0%), asthenia (0.7%), incisional pain (0.6%), pruritus (0.5%), abnormal vision (0.3%), edema (0.3%), wound (0.2%), abscess (0.2%), cellulitis (0.2%), peripheral coldness (0.2%), injection site pain (0.1%), dry mouth (0.1%), pallor (0.1%), diabetes mellitus (0.1%), hyperkalemia (0.1%), enlarged abdomen (0.1%), bullous eruption (0.1%), inflammation (0.1%), drug toxicity (0.1%).

OVERDOSAGE

There has been no experience of overdosage in human clinical trials.

DOSAGE AND ADMINISTRATION

The safety and efficacy of Abciximab have only been investigated with concomitant administration of heparin and aspirin as described in CLINICAL STUDIES.

In patients with failed percutaneous coronary interventions, the continuous infusion of Abciximab should be stopped because there is no evidence for Abciximab efficacy in that setting.

Table 5
THROMBOCYTOPENIA AND PLATELET TRANSFUSIONS[a]

	Placebo + Standard-dose Heparin	Abciximab + Standard-dose Heparin	Abciximab + Low-dose Heparin
	Total number of patients enrolled		
EPIC	n = 696	n = 708	—
CAPTURE	n = 635	n = 630	—
EPILOG	n = 939	n = 918	n = 935
Patients with decrease of platelets to <50,000 cells/µL[a]	% of patients with events		
EPIC	0.7	1.6	—
CAPTURE	0.3	1.7	—
EPILOG	0.4	0.9	0.4
Patients with decrease of platelets to <100,000 cells/µL[a]			
EPIC	3.4	5.2	—
CAPTURE	1.3	5.6	—
EPILOG	1.5	2.6	2.5
Patients who received platelet transfusions[b]			
EPIC	2.6	5.5	—
CAPTURE	0.3	2.1	—
EPILOG	1.1	1.6	0.9

[a] Patients with a platelet count of <50,000 cells/µL are also included in the category of patients with a platelet count of <100,000 cells/µL.

[b] Includes patients receiving platelet transfusions for thrombocytopenia or any other reason.

Table 6
ADVERSE EVENTS AMONG TREATED PATIENTS IN THE EPIC, EPILOG AND CAPTURE TRIALS

Event	Placebo (n = 2226)	Bolus + Infusion (n = 3111)
	Number of Patients (%)	
Cardiovascular System		
Hypotension	230 (10.3)	447 ((14.4)
Bradycardia	79 (3.5)	140 (4.5)
Gastrointestinal System		
Nausea	255 (11.5)	423 (13.6)
Vomiting	152 (6.8)	226 (7.3)
Abdominal Pain	49 (2.2)	97 (3.1)
Miscellaneous		
Back Pain	304 (13.7)	546 (17.6)
Chest Pain	208 (9.3)	356 (11.4)
Headache	122 (5.5)	200 (6.4)
Puncture Site Pain	58 (2.6)	113 (3.6)
Peripheral Edema	25 (1.1)	49 (1.6)

Continued on next page

ReoPro—Cont.

In the event of serious bleeding that cannot be controlled by compression, Abciximab and heparin should be discontinued immediately.

The recommended dosage of Abciximab in adults is a 0.25 mg/kg intravenous bolus administered 10–60 minutes before the start of percutaneous coronary intervention, followed by a continuous intravenous infusion of 0.125 µg/kg/min (to a maximum of 10 µg/min) for 12 hours.

Patients with unstable angina not responding to conventional medical therapy and who are planned to undergo percutaneous coronary intervention within 24 hours may be treated with an Abciximab 0.25 mg/kg intravenous bolus followed by an 18 to 24-hour intravenous infusion of 10 µg/min, concluding one hour after the percutaneous coronary intervention.

Instructions for Administration

1. Parenteral drug products should be inspected visually for particulate matter prior to administration. Preparations of Abciximab containing visibly opaque particles should NOT be used.
2. Hypersensitivity reactions should be anticipated whenever protein solutions such as Abciximab are administered. Epinephrine, dopamine, theophylline, antihistamines and corticosteroids should be available for immediate use. If symptoms of an allergic reaction or anaphylaxis appear, the infusion should be stopped and appropriate treatment given.
3. As with all parenteral drug products, aseptic procedures should be used during the administration of Abciximab.
4. Withdraw the necessary amount of Abciximab for bolus injection into a syringe. Filter the bolus injection using a sterile, non-pyrogenic, low-protein-binding 0.2 or 0.22 µm filter (Millipore SLGV025LS or equivalent).
5. Withdraw the necessary amount of Abciximab for the continuous infusion into a syringe. Inject into an appropriate container of sterile 0.9% saline or 5% dextrose and infuse at the calculated rate via a continuous infusion pump. The continuous infusion should be filtered either upon admixture using a sterile, non-pyrogenic, low-protein-binding 0.2 or 0.22 µm syringe filter (Millipore SLGV025LS or equivalent) or upon administration using an in-line, sterile, non-pyrogenic, low-protein-binding 0.2 or 0.22 µm filter (Abbott #4524 or equivalent). Discard the unused portion at the end of the infusion.
6. No incompatibilities have been shown with intravenous infusion fluids or commonly used cardiovascular drugs. Nevertheless, Abciximab should be administered in a separate intravenous line whenever possible and not mixed with other medications.
7. No incompatibilities have been observed with glass bottles or polyvinyl chloride bags and administration sets.

HOW SUPPLIED

Abciximab (ReoPro®) 2 mg/mL is supplied in 5 mL vials containing 10 mg (NDC 0002-7140-01).

Vials should be stored at 2 to 8°C (36 to 46°F). Do not freeze. Do not shake. Do not use beyond the expiration date. Discard any unused portion left in the vial.

REFERENCES

1. Reverter JC, Beguin S, Kessels H, Kumar R, Hemmer HC, Coller BS. Inhibition of platelet-mediated, tissue-factor-induced thrombin generation by the mouse/human chimeric 7E3 antibody; potential implications for the effect of c7E3 Fab treatment on acute thrombosis and "clinical restenosis". *J Clin Invest;*1996;**98**:863–874.
2. Tcheng J, Ellis SG, George BS. Pharmacodynamics of chimeric glycoprotein IIb/IIIa integrin antiplatelet antibody Fab 7E3 in high risk coronary angioplasty. *Circulation;*1994;**90**:1757–1764.
3. Simoons ML, de Boer MJ, van der Brand MJBM, et al. Randomized trial of a GPIIb/IIIa platelet receptor blocker in refractory unstable angina. *Circulation;*1994;**89**:596–603.
4. EPIC Investigators. Use of a monoclonal antibody directed against the platelet glycoprotein IIb/IIIa receptor in high-risk coronary angioplasty. *N Engl J Med* 1994;**330**:956–961.
5. Topol EJ, Califf RM, Weisman HF, et al. Randomised trial of coronary intervention with antibody against platelet IIb/IIIa integrin for reduction of clinical restenosis: results at six months. *Lancet* 1994;**343**:881–886.
6. Topol EJ, Ferguson JJ, Weisman HF, et al. for the EPIC Investigators. Long term protection from myocardial ischemic events in a randomized trial of brief integrin blockade with percutaneous coronary intervention. *JAMA.*1997;**278**:479–484.
7. EPILOG Investigators. Platelet glycoprotein IIb/IIIa receptor blockade and low dose heparin during percutaneous coronary revascularization. *N Eng J Med.* 1997;**336**:1689–1696.
8. CAPTURE Investigators. Randomised placebo-controlled trial of abciximab before, during and after coronary intervention in refractory unstable angina: the CAPTURE study. *Lancet* 1997;**349**;1429–1435.
9. Rao, AK, Pratt C, Berke A, et al. Thrombolysis in Myocardial Infarction (TIMI) Trial – Phase I: Hemorrhagic manifestations and changes in plasma fibrinogen and the fibrinolytic system in patients treated with recombinant tissue plasminogen activator and streptokinase. *J Am Coll Cardiol* 1988;**11**:1–11.
10. Landefeld, CS, Cook EF, Flatley M, et al. Identification and preliminary validation of predictors of major bleeding in hospitalized patients starting anticoagulant therapy. *Am J Med.* 1987;**82**:703–713.

Manufactured by:

Centocor B.V.
Leiden, The Netherlands
U.S. License Number: 1178

Distributed by:

Eli Lilly and Company
Indianapolis, IN 46285

Shown in Product Identification Guide, page 309

Central Pharmaceuticals, Inc.

**1101 "C" AVENUE WEST
FREEMAN FIELD
PO BOX 328
SEYMOUR, IN 47274**

For product information, please see Schwarz Pharma, Inc.

Cetylite Industries, Inc.

**9051 RIVER ROAD
P.O. BOX 90006
PENNSAUKEN, NJ 08110-0700**

Direct Inquiries to:

Mr. Stanley L. Wachman, President
(609) 665-6111
(800) 257-7740
FAX: (609) 665-5408

CETACAINE®   ℞
[set 'a-cane "]
TOPICAL ANESTHETIC

ACTIVE INGREDIENTS

Benzocaine	14.0%
Butyl Aminobenzoate	2.0%
Tetracaine Hydrochloride	2.0%

CONTAINS

Benzalkonium Chloride	0.5%
Cetyl Dimethyl Ethyl Ammonium Bromide	0.005%

In a bland water soluble base.

ACTION

Cetacaine produces anesthesia rapidly in approximately 30 seconds.

INDICATIONS

Cetacaine is a topical anesthetic indicated for the production of anesthesia of accessible mucous membrane.

Cetacaine Spray is indicated for use to control pain or gagging. Cetacaine in all forms is indicated for use to control pain.

DOSAGE AND ADMINISTRATION

Cetacaine Spray should be applied for approximately one second or less for normal anesthesia. Only limited quantity of Cetacaine is required for anesthesia. Spray in excess of two seconds is contraindicated. Average expulsion rate of residue from spray, at normal temperatures, is 200 mg. per second.

Tissue need not be dried prior to application of Cetacaine. Cetacaine should be applied directly to the site where pain control is required.

Cetacaine Liquid or Cetacaine Ointment may be applied with a cotton pledget or directly to tissue. Cotton pledget should not be held in position for extended periods of time, since local reactions to benzoate topical anesthetics are related to the length of time of application.

ADVERSE REACTION

Systemic reactions to Cetacaine have not been reported. Localized allergic reactions may occur after prolonged or repeated use. Dehydration of the epithelium or an escharotic effect may result from prolonged contact. Allergic reactions are known to occur in some patients with preparations containing benzocaine.

Usage in Pregnancy: Safe use of Cetacaine has not been established with respect to possible adverse effects upon fetal development. Therefore Cetacaine should not be used during early pregnancy, unless in the judgment of a physician the potential benefits outweigh the unknown hazards.

Routine precaution for the use of any topical anesthetic should be observed when Cetacaine is used.

CONTRAINDICATIONS

Cetacaine is not for injection.

Do not use on the eyes.

To avoid excessive systemic absorption, Cetacaine should not be applied to large areas of denuded or inflamed tissue. Cetacaine should not be administered to patients who are hypersensitive to any of its ingredients.

Individual dosage of tetracaine hydrochloride in excess of 20 mg. is contraindicated. Cetacaine should not be used under dentures or cotton rolls, as retention of the active ingredients under a denture or cotton roll could possibly cause an escharotic effect.

Jetco-Spray® Cannula

The autoclavable, stainless steel Jetco cannula for Cetacaine Spray is specially designed for accessibility and application of Cetacaine, at the required site of pain control. The Jetco cannula is supplied in various lengths and shapes.

The Jetco cannula is inserted firmly onto the protruding plastic tubing on each bottle of Cetacaine Spray.

The Jetco cannula may be removed and re-inserted as many times as required for cleansing or sterilization.

PACKAGING AVAILABLE

Cetacaine Spray 56 g. including propellant.
Cetacaine Liquid 56 g.
Cetacaine Hospital Gel 29 g Tube.
Cetacaine Ointment 37 g Jar.

CAUTION

Federal law prohibits dispensing Cetacaine without prescription.

Made in U.S.A.   (Rev. 7/93)

Shown in Product Identification Guide, page 309

Chiron Corporation

**4560 HORTON STREET
EMERYVILLE, CA 94608-2997**

For Medical Information Contact:

Generally:
Professional Services (6:00 AM to 5:00 PM PST):
(800) CHIRON-8 selection #2
(800) 244-7668 selection #2
FAX: (510) 923-3435
e-mail: drug__info@cc.chiron.com

In Emergencies:
(6:00 AM to 5:00 PM PST):
(800) CHIRON-8 selection #3
(800) 244-7668 selection #3

After Hours and Weekend Emergencies:
(415) 885-8777

Sales and Ordering:
(800) CHIRON-8 selection #1
(800) 244-7668 selection #1
FAX: (510) 923-3434

PROLEUKIN®   ℞
[prō-lū '-kin]
Aldesleukin For Injection

WARNINGS

Therapy with PROLEUKIN® (aldesleukin) for injection should be restricted to patients with normal cardiac and pulmonary functions as defined by thallium stress testing and formal pulmonary function testing. Extreme caution should be used in patients with a normal thallium stress test and a normal pulmonary function test who have a history of cardiac or pulmonary disease.

PROLEUKIN should be administered in a hospital setting under the supervision of a qualified physician experienced in the use of anti cancer agents. An intensive care facility and specialists skilled in cardiopulmonary or intensive care medicine must be available.

PROLEUKIN administration has been associated with capillary leak syndrome (CLS) which is characterized by a loss of vascular tone and extravasation of plasma proteins and fluid into the extravascular space. CLS results in hypotension and reduced organ perfusion which may be severe and can result in death. CLS may be associated with cardiac arrhythmias (supraventricular and ventricular), angina, myocardial infarction, respiratory insufficiency requiring intubation, gastrointestinal bleeding or infarction, renal insufficiency, edema, and mental status changes.

PROLEUKIN treatment is associated with impaired neutrophil function (reduced chemotaxis) and with an increased risk of disseminated infection, including sepsis and bacterial endocarditis. Consequently, preexisting bacterial infections should be adequately treated prior to initiation of PROLEUKIN therapy. Patients with indwelling central lines are particularly at risk for infection with gram positive microorganisms. Antibiotic prophylaxis with oxacillin, nafcillin, ciprofloxacin, or vancomycin has been associated with a reduced incidence of staphylococcal infections.

PROLEUKIN administration should be withheld in patients developing moderate to severe lethargy or somnolence; continued administration may result in coma.

DESCRIPTION

PROLEUKIN® (aldesleukin) for injection, a human recombinant interleukin-2 product, is a highly purified protein with a molecular weight of approximately 15,300 daltons. The chemical name is des-alanyl-1, serine-125 human interleukin-2. PROLEUKIN, a lymphokine, is produced by recombinant DNA technology using a genetically engineered *E. coli* strain containing an analog of the human interleukin-2 gene. Genetic engineering techniques were used to modify the human IL-2 gene, and the resulting expression clone encodes a modified human interleukin-2. This recombinant form differs from native interleukin-2 in the following ways: a) PROLEUKIN is not glycosylated because it is derived from *E. coli*; b) the molecule has no N-terminal alanine; the codon for this amino acid was deleted during the genetic engineering procedure; c) the molecule has serine substituted for cysteine at amino acid position 125; this was accomplished by site specific manipulation during the genetic engineering procedure; and d) the aggregation state of PROLEUKIN is likely to be different from that of native interleukin-2.

The *in vitro* biological activities of the native nonrecombinant molecule have been reproduced with PROLEUKIN.[1,2]

PROLEUKIN is supplied as a sterile, white to off-white, lyophilized cake in single-use vials intended for intravenous (IV) administration. When reconstituted with 1.2 mL Sterile Water for Injection, USP, each mL contains 18 million IU (1.1 mg) PROLEUKIN, 50 mg mannitol, and 0.18 mg sodium dodecyl sulfate, buffered with approximately 0.17 mg monobasic and 0.89 mg dibasic sodium phosphate to a pH of 7.5 (range 7.2 to 7.8). The manufacturing process for PROLEUKIN involves fermentation in a defined medium containing tetracycline hydrochloride. The presence of the antibiotic is not detectable in the final product. PROLEUKIN contains no preservatives in the final product.

PROLEUKIN biological potency is determined by a lymphocyte proliferation bioassay and is expressed in International Units (IU) as established by the World Health Organization 1st International Standard for Interleukin-2 (human). The relationship between potency and protein mass is as follows:

18 million (18 X 10^6) IU PROLEUKIN = 1.1 mg protein

CLINICAL PHARMACOLOGY

PROLEUKIN® (aldesleukin) has been shown to possess the biological activities of human native interleukin-2.[1,2]

In vitro studies performed on human cell lines demonstrate the immunoregulatory properties of PROLEUKIN, including: a) enhancement of lymphocyte mitogenesis and stimulation of long-term growth of human interleukin-2 dependent cell lines; b) enhancement of lymphocyte cytotoxicity; c) induction of killer cell (lymphokine-activated (LAK) and natural (NK)) activity; and d) induction of interferon-gamma production.

The *in vivo* administration of PROLEUKIN in animals and humans produces multiple immunological effects in a dose dependent manner. These effects include activation of cellular immunity with profound lymphocytosis, eosinophilia, and thrombocytopenia, and the production of cytokines including tumor necrosis factor, IL-1 and gamma interferon.[3]

In vivo experiments in murine tumor models have shown inhibition of tumor growth.[4] The exact mechanism by which PROLEUKIN mediates its antitumor activity in animals and humans is unknown.

Pharmacokinetics: PROLEUKIN exists as biologically active, non-covalently bound microaggregates with an average size of 27 recombinant interleukin-2 molecules. The solubilizing agent, sodium dodecyl sulfate, may have an effect on the kinetic properties of this product.

TABLE I

PROLEUKIN CLINICAL RESPONSE DATA

	METASTATIC RCC		METASTATIC MELANOMA	
	Number of Responding Patients (response rate)	**Median Response Duration in Months (range)**	**Number of Responding Patients (response rate)**	**Median Response Duration in Months (range)**
CR's	17 (7%)	54+* (7 to 107+)	17 (6%)	40+* (3 to 106+)
PR's	20 (8%)	20 (3 to 97+)	26 (10%)	6 (2 to 92+)
PR's + CR's	37 (15%)	54 (3 to 107+)	43 (16%)	9 (2 to 106+)

(+) sign means ongoing

* Median duration not yet observed; a conservative value is presented which represents the minimum median duration of response.

The pharmacokinetic profile of PROLEUKIN is characterized by high plasma concentrations following a short IV infusion, rapid distribution into the extravascular space and elimination from the body by metabolism in the kidneys with little or no bioactive protein excreted in the urine. Studies of IV PROLEUKIN in sheep and humans indicate that upon completion of infusion, approximately 30% of the administered dose is detectable in plasma. This finding is consistent with studies in rats using radiolabeled PROLEUKIN, which demonstrate a rapid (<1 min) uptake of the majority of the label into the lungs, liver, kidney, and spleen.

The serum half-life (T 1/2) curves of PROLEUKIN remaining in the plasma are derived from studies done in 52 cancer patients following a 5-minute IV infusion. These patients were shown to have a distribution and elimination T 1/2 of 13 and 85 minutes, respectively.

Following the initial rapid organ distribution, the primary route of clearance of circulating PROLEUKIN is the kidney. In humans and animals, PROLEUKIN is cleared from the circulation by both glomerular filtration and peritubular extraction in the kidney.[5–8] This dual mechanism for delivery of PROLEUKIN to the proximal tubule may account for the preservation of clearance in patients with rising serum creatinine values. Greater than 80% of the amount of PROLEUKIN distributed to plasma, cleared from the circulation and presented to the kidney is metabolized to amino acids in the cells lining the proximal convoluted tubules. In humans, the mean clearance rate in cancer patients is 268 mL/min.

The relatively rapid clearance of PROLEUKIN has led to dosage schedules characterized by frequent, short infusions. Observed serum levels are proportional to the dose of PROLEUKIN.

Immunogenicity: Fifty-seven of 77 (74%) metastatic renal cell carcinoma patients treated with an every 8-hour PROLEUKIN regimen and 33 of 50 (66%) metastatic melanoma patients treated with a variety of IV regimens developed low titers of non-neutralizing anti-PROLEUKIN antibodies. Neutralizing antibodies were not detected in this group of patients, but have been detected in 1/106 (<1%) patients treated with IV PROLEUKIN using a wide variety of schedules and doses. The clinical significance of anti-PROLEUKIN antibodies is unknown.

Clinical Experience: Two hundred fifty-five patients with metastatic renal cell cancer (metastatic RCC) were treated with single agent PROLEUKIN in 7 clinical studies conducted at 21 institutions. Two hundred seventy patients with metastatic melanoma were treated with single agent PROLEUKIN in 8 clinical studies conducted at 22 institutions. Patients enrolled in trials of single agent PROLEUKIN were required to have an Eastern Cooperative Oncology Group (ECOG) Performance Status (PS) of 0 or 1 and normal organ function as determined by cardiac stress test, pulmonary function tests, and creatinine ≤1.5 mg/dL. Patients with brain metastases, active infections, organ allografts and diseases requiring steroid treatment were excluded.

PROLEUKIN was given by 15 min IV infusion every 8 hours for up to 5 days (maximum of 14 doses). No treatment was given on days 6 to 14 and then dosing was repeated for up to 5 days on days 15 to 19 (maximum of 14 doses). These 2 cycles constituted 1 course of therapy. Patients could receive a maximum of 28 doses during a course of therapy. In practice >90% of patients had doses withheld. Metastatic RCC patients received a median of 20 of 28 scheduled doses of PROLEUKIN. Metastatic melanoma patients received a median of 18 of 28 scheduled doses of PROLEUKIN during the first course of therapy. Doses were withheld for specific toxicities (See "**DOSAGE AND ADMINISTRATION**" section, "**Dose Modifications**" subsection and "**ADVERSE REACTIONS**" section).

In the renal cell cancer studies (n=255), objective response was seen in 37 (15%) patients, with 17 (7%) complete and 20 (8%) partial responders. The 95% confidence interval for objective response was 11% to 20%. Onset of tumor regression was observed as early as 4 weeks after completion of the first course of treatment, and in some cases, tumor regression continued for up to 12 months after the start of treatment. The median duration of objective complete responses has not been observed and for partial response was 20 months. Thirteen patients who achieved a complete response and seven patients who achieved a partial response had responses ongoing at the time of last contact. The median progression-free survival for all responding patients was 55 months. Responses were observed in both lung and non-lung sites (e.g., liver, lymph node, renal bed occurrences, soft tissue). Some patients with individual bulky lesions and high tumor burden achieved responses.

In the metastatic melanoma studies (n=270), objective response was seen in 43 (16%) patients, with 17 (6%) complete and 26 (10%) partial responders. The 95% confidence interval for objective response was 12% to 21%. The median duration of objective (partial or complete) response was 9 months (2 to 106+ months); the median duration of objective complete responses has not been observed and the median duration for partial response was 6 months. Ten patients who achieved a complete response and two patients who achieved a partial response had responses ongoing at the time of last contact. The median progression-free survival for the 43 responding patients was 13 months. Responses in metastatic melanoma patients were observed in both visceral and non-visceral sites (e.g., lung, liver, lymph node, soft tissue, adrenal, subcutaneous). Some patients with individual bulky lesions and large cumulative tumor burden achieved responses.

[See table I above]

An analysis of prognostic factors showed that a better ECOG performance status (see Table II) was significantly associated with response.

[See table II at top of next page]

INDICATIONS AND USAGE

PROLEUKIN® (aldesleukin) is indicated for the treatment of adults with metastatic renal cell carcinoma (metastatic RCC).

PROLEUKIN is indicated for the treatment of adults with metastatic melanoma.

Careful patient selection is mandatory prior to the administration of PROLEUKIN. See "**CONTRAINDICATIONS**", "**WARNINGS**" and "**PRECAUTIONS**" sections regarding patient screening, including recommended cardiac and pulmonary function tests and laboratory tests.

Evaluation of clinical studies to date reveals that patients with more favorable ECOG performance status (ECOG PS O) at treatment initiation respond better to PROLEUKIN, with a higher response rate and lower toxicity (See "**CLINICAL PHARMACOLOGY**" section, "**Clinical Experience**" subsection and "**ADVERSE REACTIONS**" section). Therefore, selection of patients for treatment should include assessment of performance status.

Experience in patients with ECOG PS >1 is extremely limited.

CONTRAINDICATIONS

PROLEUKIN® (aldesleukin) is contraindicated in patients with a known history of hypersensitivity to interleukin-2 or any component of the PROLEUKIN formulation.

PROLEUKIN is contraindicated in patients with an abnormal thallium stress test or abnormal pulmonary function tests and those with organ allografts. Retreatment with PROLEUKIN is contraindicated in patients who have experienced the following drug-related toxicities while receiving an earlier course of therapy:

- Sustained ventricular tachycardia (≥5 beats)
- Cardiac arrhythmias not controlled or unresponsive to management
- Chest pain with ECG changes, consistent with angina or myocardial infarction
- Cardiac tamponade
- Intubation for >72 hours
- Renal failure requiring dialysis >72 hours
- Coma or toxic psychosis lasting >48 hours
- Repetitive or difficult to control seizures
- Bowel ischemia/perforation
- GI bleeding requiring surgery

Continued on next page

Proleukin—Cont.

WARNINGS

See boxed "WARNINGS"

Because of the severe adverse events which generally accompany PROLEUKIN® (aldesleukin) therapy at the recommended dosages, thorough clinical evaluation should be performed to identify patients with significant cardiac, pulmonary, renal, hepatic, or CNS impairment in whom PROLEUKIN is contraindicated. Patients with normal cardiovascular, pulmonary, hepatic, and CNS function may experience serious, life threatening or fatal adverse events. Adverse events are frequent, often serious, and sometimes fatal.

Should adverse events, which require dose modification occur, dosage should be withheld rather than reduced (See "DOSAGE AND ADMINISTRATION" section, "Dose Modifications" subsection).

PROLEUKIN has been associated with exacerbation of pre-existing or initial presentation of autoimmune disease and inflammatory disorders. Exacerbation of Crohn's disease, scleroderma, thyroiditis, inflammatory arthritis, diabetes mellitus, oculo-bulbar myasthenia gravis, crescentic IgA glomerulonephritis, cholecystitis, cerebral vasculitis, Stevens-Johnson syndrome and bullous pemphigoid, has been reported following treatment with IL-2.

All patients should have thorough evaluation and treatment of CNS metastases and have a negative scan prior to receiving PROLEUKIN therapy. New neurologic signs, symptoms, and anatomic lesions following PROLEUKIN therapy have been reported in patients without evidence of CNS metastases. Clinical manifestations included changes in mental status, speech difficulties, cortical blindness, limb or gait ataxia, hallucinations, agitation, obtundation, and coma. Radiological findings included multiple and, less commonly, single cortical lesions on MRI and evidence of demyelination. Neurologic signs and symptoms associated with PROLEUKIN therapy usually improve after discontinuation of PROLEUKIN therapy; however, there are reports of permanent neurologic defects. One case of possible cerebral vasculitis, responsive to dexamethasone, has been reported. In patients with known seizure disorders, extreme caution should be exercised as PROLEUKIN may cause seizures.

PRECAUTIONS

General: Patients should have normal cardiac, pulmonary, hepatic, and CNS function at the start of therapy. (See "PRECAUTIONS" section, "Laboratory Tests" subsection).

Capillary leak syndrome (CLS) begins immediately after PROLEUKIN® (aldesleukin) treatment starts and is marked by increased capillary permeability to protein and fluids and reduced vascular tone. In most patients, this results in a concomitant drop in mean arterial blood pressure within 2 to 12 hours after the start of treatment. With continued therapy, clinically significant hypotension (defined as systolic blood pressure below 90 mm Hg or a 20 mm Hg drop from baseline systolic pressure) and hypoperfusion will occur. In addition, extravasation of protein and fluids into the extravascular space will lead to the formation of edema and creation of new effusions.

Medical management of CLS begins with careful monitoring of the patient's fluid and organ perfusion status. This is achieved by frequent determination of blood pressure and pulse, and by monitoring organ function, which includes assessment of mental status and urine output. Hypovolemia is assessed by catheterization and central pressure monitoring.

Flexibility in fluid and pressor management is essential for maintaining organ perfusion and blood pressure. Consequently, extreme caution should be used in treating patients with fixed requirements for large volumes of fluid (e.g., patients with hypercalcemia). Administration of IV fluids, either colloids or crystalloids is recommended for treatment of hypovolemia. Correction of hypovolemia may require large volumes of IV fluids but caution is required because unrestrained fluid administration may exacerbate problems associated with edema formation or effusions. With extravascular fluid accumulation, edema is common and ascites, pleural or pericardial effusions may develop. Management of these events depends on a careful balancing of the effects of fluid shifts so that neither the consequences of hypovolemia (e.g., impaired organ perfusion) nor the consequences of fluid accumulations (e.g., pulmonary edema) exceed the patient's tolerance.

Clinical experience has shown that early administration of dopamine (1 to 5 µg/kg/min) to patients manifesting capillary leak syndrome, before the onset of hypotension, can help to maintain organ perfusion particularly to the kidney and thus preserve urine output. Weight and urine output should be carefully monitored. If organ perfusion and blood pressure are not sustained by dopamine therapy, clinical investigators have increased the dose of dopamine to 6 to 10 µg/kg/min or have added phenylephrine hydrochloride (1 to 5 µg/kg/min) to low dose dopamine (See "ADVERSE REACTIONS" section). Prolonged use of pressors, either in combination or as individual agents, at relatively high doses, may be associated with cardiac rhythm disturbances. If there has been excessive weight gain or edema formation, particularly if associated with shortness of breath from pulmonary congestion, use of diuretics, once blood pressure has normalized, has been shown to hasten recovery. **NOTE: Prior to the use of any product mentioned, the physician should refer to the package insert for the respective product.**

PROLEUKIN® (aldesleukin) treatment should be withheld for failure to maintain organ perfusion as demonstrated by altered mental status, reduced urine output, a fall in the systolic blood pressure below 90 mm Hg or onset of cardiac arrhythmias (See "DOSAGE AND ADMINISTRATION" section, "Dose Modifications" subsection). Recovery from CLS begins soon after cessation of PROLEUKIN therapy. Usually, within a few hours, the blood pressure rises, organ perfusion is restored and reabsorption of extravasated fluid and protein begins.

Kidney and liver function are impaired during PROLEUKIN treatment. Use of concomitant nephrotoxic or hepatotoxic medications may further increase toxicity to the kidney or liver.

Mental status changes including irritability, confusion, or depression which occur while receiving PROLEUKIN may be indicators of bacteremia or early bacterial sepsis, hypoperfusion, occult CNS malignancy, or direct PROLEUKIN-induced CNS toxicity. Alterations in mental status due solely to PROLEUKIN therapy may progress for several days before recovery begins. Rarely, patients have sustained permanent neurologic deficits (See "PRECAUTIONS" section "Drug Interactions" subsection).

Exacerbation of preexisting autoimmune disease or initial presentation of autoimmune and inflammatory disorders has been reported following PROLEUKIN alone or in combination with interferon (See "PRECAUTIONS" section "Drug Interactions" subsection and "ADVERSE REACTIONS" section). Impairment of thyroid function, sometimes preceded by hyperthyroidism, has been reported following PROLEUKIN treatment. Some of these patients required thyroid replacement therapy. Changes in thyroid function may be a manifestation of autoimmunity. Onset of symptomatic hyperglycemia and/or diabetes mellitus has been reported during PROLEUKIN therapy.

PROLEUKIN enhancement of cellular immune function may increase the risk of allograft rejection in transplant patients.

Laboratory Tests: The following clinical evaluations are recommended for all patients, prior to beginning treatment and then daily during drug administration.

- Standard hematologic tests-including CBC, differential and platelet counts
- Blood chemistries-including electrolytes, renal and hepatic function tests
- Chest x-rays

Serum creatinine should be ≤1.5 mg/dL prior to initiation of PROLEUKIN treatment.

All patients should have baseline pulmonary function tests with arterial blood gases. Adequate pulmonary function should be documented (FEV$_1$ >2 liters or ≥75% of predicted for height and age) prior to initiation therapy.

All patients should be screened with a stress thallium study. Normal ejection fraction and unimpaired wall motion should be documented. If a thallium stress test suggests minor wall motion abnormalities further testing is suggested to exclude significant coronary artery disease.

Daily monitoring during therapy with PROLEUKIN should include vital signs (temperature, pulse, blood pressure, and respiration rate), weight, and fluid intake and output. In a patient with a decreased systolic blood pressure, especially less than 90 mm Hg, constant cardiac monitoring should be conducted. If an abnormal complex or rhythm is seen, an ECG should be performed. Vital signs in these hypotensive patients should be taken hourly.

During treatment, pulmonary function should be monitored on a regular basis by clinical examination, assessment of vital signs and pulse oximetry. Patients with dyspnea or clinical signs of respiratory impairment (tachypnea or rales) should be further assessed with arterial blood gas determination. These tests are to be repeated as often as clinically indicated.

Cardiac function should be assessed daily by clinical examination and assessment of vital signs. Patients with signs or symptoms of chest pain, murmurs, gallops, irregular rhythm or palpitations should be further assessed with an ECG examination and cardiac enzyme evaluation. Evidence of myocardial injury, including findings compatible with myocardial infarction or myocarditis, has been reported. Ventricular hypokinesia due to myocarditis may be persistent for several months. If there is evidence of cardiac ischemia or congestive heart failure, PROLEUKIN therapy should be held, and a repeat thallium study should be done.

Drug Interactions: PROLEUKIN may affect central nervous function. Therefore, interactions could occur following

TABLE II
PROLEUKIN CLINICAL RESPONSE BY ECOG PERFORMANCE STATUS (PS)

Pre Treatment ECOG PS	METASTATIC RCC		METASTATIC MELANOMA	
	CR	PR	CR	PR
0	14/166 (8%)	16/166 (10%)	14/191 (7%)	22/191 (12%)
≥1	3/89 (3%)	4/89 (4%)	3/79 (4%)	4/79 (5%)

TABLE III
ADVERSE EVENTS OCCURRING IN ≥10% OF PATIENTS
(n=525)

Body System	% Patients	Body System	% Patients
Body as a Whole		Metabolic and Nutritional Disorders	
Chills	52	Bilirubinemia	40
Fever	29	Creatinine increase	33
Malaise	27	Peripheral edema	28
Asthenia	23	SGOT increase	23
Infection	13	Weight gain	16
Pain	12	Edema	15
Abdominal pain	11	Acidosis	12
Abdomen enlarged	10	Hypomagnesium	12
Cardiovascular		Hypocalcemia	11
Hypotension	71	Alkaline phosphatase increase	10
Tachycardia	23	Nervous	
Vasodilation	13	Confusion	34
Supraventricular tachycardia	12	Somnolence	22
Cardiovascular disorder[a]	11	Anxiety	12
Arrhythmia	10	Dizziness	11
Digestive		Respiratory	
Diarrhea	67	Dyspnea	43
Vomiting	50	Lung disorder[b]	24
Nausea	35	Respiratory disorder[c]	11
Stomatitis	22	Cough increase	11
Anorexia	20	Rhinitis	10
Nausea and vomiting	19	Skin and Appendages	
Hemic and Lymphatic		Rash	42
Thrombocytopenia	37	Pruritus	24
Anemia	29	Exfoliative dermatitis	18
Leukopenia	16	Urogenital	
		Oliguria	63

[a] Cardiovascular disorder: fluctuations in blood pressure, asymptomatic ECG changes, CHF.
[b] Lung disorder: physical findings associated with pulmonary congestion, rales, rhonchi.
[c] Respiratory disorder: ARDS, CXR infiltrates, unspecified pulmonary changes.

concomitant administration of psychotropic drugs (e.g., narcotics, analgesics, antiemetics, sedatives, tranquilizers).

Concurrent administration of drugs possessing nephrotoxic (e.g., aminoglycosides, indomethacin), myelotoxic (e.g., cytotoxic chemotherapy), cardiotoxic (e.g., doxorubicin) or hepatotoxic (e.g., methotrexate, asparaginase) effects with PROLEUKIN may increase toxicity in these organ systems. The safety and efficacy of PROLEUKIN in combination with any antineoplastic agents have not been established.

In addition, reduced kidney and liver function secondary to PROLEUKIN treatment may delay elimination of concomitant medications and increase the risk of adverse events from those drugs.

Hypersensitivity reactions have been reported in patients receiving combination regimens containing sequential high dose PROLEUKIN and antineoplastic agents, specifically, dacarbazine, cis-platinum, tamoxifen and interferon-alfa. These reactions consisted of erythema, pruritus, and hypotension and occurred within hours of administration of chemotherapy. These events required medical intervention in some patients.

Myocardial injury, including myocardial infarction, myocarditis, ventricular hypokinesia, and severe rhabdomyolysis appear to be increased in patients receiving PROLEUKIN and interferon-alfa concurrently.

Exacerbation or the initial presentation of a number of autoimmune and inflammatory disorders has been observed following concurrent use of interferon-alfa and PROLEUKIN, including crescentic IgA glomerulonephritis, oculobulbar myasthenia gravis, inflammatory arthritis, thyroiditis, bullous pemphigoid, and Stevens-Johnson syndrome.

Although glucocorticoids have been shown to reduce PROLEUKIN-induced side effects including fever, renal insufficiency, hyperbilirubinemia, confusion, and dyspnea, concomitant administration of these agents with PROLEUKIN may reduce the antitumor effectiveness of PROLEUKIN and thus should be avoided.[12]

Beta-blockers and other antihypertensives may potentiate the hypotension seen with PROLEUKIN.

Delayed Adverse Reactions to Iodinated Contrast Media: A review of the literature revealed that 12.6% (range 11–28%) of 501 patients treated with various interleukin-2 containing regimens who were subsequently administered radiographic iodinated contrast media experienced acute, atypical adverse reactions. The onset of symptoms usually occurred within hours (most commonly 1 to 4 hours) following administration of contrast media. These reactions include fever, chills, nausea, vomiting, pruritus, rash, diarrhea, hypotension, edema, and oliguria. Some clinicians have noted that these reactions resemble the immediate side effects caused by interleukin-2 administration, however the cause of contrast reactions after interleukin-2 therapy is unknown. Most events were reported to occur when contrast media was given within 4 weeks after the last dose of interleukin-2. These events were also reported to occur when contrast media was given several months after interleukin-2 treatment.[13]

Carcinogenesis, Mutagenesis, Impairment of Fertility: There have been no studies conducted assessing the carcinogenic or mutagenic potential of PROLEUKIN.

There have been no studies conducted assessing the effect of PROLEUKIN on fertility. It is recommended that this drug not be administered to fertile persons of either gender not practicing effective contraception.

Pregnancy: *Pregnancy Category C.* PROLEUKIN has been shown to have embryolethal effects in rats when given in doses at 27 to 36 times the human dose (scaled by body weight). Significant maternal toxicities were observed in pregnant rats administered PROLEUKIN by IV injection at doses 2.1 to 36 times higher than the human dose during critical period of organogenesis. No evidence of teratogenicity was observed other than that attributed to maternal toxicity. There are no adequate well-controlled studies of PROLEUKIN in pregnant women. PROLEUKIN should be used during pregnancy only if the potential benefit justifies the potential risk to the fetus.

Nursing Mothers: It is not known whether this drug is excreted in human milk. Because many drugs are excreted in human milk and because of the potential for serious adverse reactions in nursing infants from PROLEUKIN, a decision should be made whether to discontinue nursing or to discontinue the drug, taking into account the importance of the drug to the mother.

Pediatric Use: Safety and effectiveness in children under 18 years of age have not been established.

ADVERSE REACTIONS

The rate of drug-related deaths in the 255 metastatic RCC patients who received single-agent PROLEUKIN® (aldesleukin) was 4% (11/255); the rate of drug-related deaths in the 270 metastatic melanoma patients who received single-agent PROLEUKIN was 2% (6/270).

The following data on common adverse events (reported in greater than 10% of patients, any grade), presented by body system, decreasing frequency and by preferred term (COSTART) are based on 525 patients (255 with renal cell cancer and 270 with metastatic melanoma) treated with the recommended infusion dosing regimen.

[See table III on previous page]

The following data on life-threatening adverse events (reported in greater than 1% of patients, grade 4), presented by body system, and by preferred term (COSTART) are based on 525 patients (255 with renal cell cancer and 270 with metastatic melanoma) treated with the recommended infusion dosing regimen.

[See table IV above]

TABLE IV
LIFE-THREATENING (GRADE 4) ADVERSE EVENTS
(n=525)

Body System	# (%) Patients	Body System	# (%) Patients
Body as a Whole		Metabolic and Nutritional Disorders	
Fever	5 (1%)	Bilirubinemia	13 (2%)
Infection	7 (1%)	Creatinine increase	5 (1%)
Sepsis	6 (1%)	SGOT increase	3 (1%)
Cardiovascular		Acidosis	4 (1%)
Hypotension	15 (3%)	Nervous	
Supraventricular tachycardia	3 (1%)	Confusion	5 (1%)
Cardiovascular disorder[a]	7 (1%)	Stupor	3 (1%)
Myocardial Infarction	7 (1%)	Coma	8 (2%)
Ventricular tachycardia	5 (1%)	Psychosis	7 (1%)
Heart arrest	4 (1%)	Respiratory	
Digestive		Dyspnea	5 (1%)
Diarrhea	10 (2%)	Respiratory disorder[c]	14 (3%)
Vomiting	7 (1%)	Apnea	5 (1%)
Hemic and Lymphatic		Urogenital	
Thrombocytopenia	5 (1%)	Oliguria	33 (6%)
Coagulation disorder[b]	4 (1%)	Anuria	25 (5%)
		Acute kidney failure	3 (1%)

[a] Cardiovascular disorder: fluctuations in blood pressure.
[b] Coagulation disorder: intravascular coagulopathy.
[c] Respiratory disorder: ARDS, respiratory failure, intubation.

Retreatment with PROLEUKIN is contraindicated in patients who have experienced the following toxicities:

Body System	
Cardiovascular	Sustained ventricular tachycardia (≥5 beats)
	Cardiac rhythm disturbances not controlled or unresponsive to management
	Chest pain with ECG changes, consistent with angina or myocardial infarction
	Cardiac tamponade
Respiratory	Intubation for >72 hours
Urogenital	Renal failure requiring dialysis >72 hours
Nervous	Coma or toxic psychosis lasting >48 hours
	Repetitive or difficult to control seizures
Digestive	Bowel ischemia/perforation
	GI bleeding requiring surgery

The following life-threatening (grade 4) events were reported by <1% of the 525 patients: reaction unevaluable; hypothermia; shock; bradycardia; ventricular extrasystoles; myocardial ischemia; syncope; hemorrhage; atrial arrhythmia; phlebitis; AV block second degree; endocarditis; pericardial effusion; peripheral gangrene; thrombosis; coronary artery disorder; stomatitis; nausea and vomiting; liver function test abnormalities; gastrointestinal hemorrhage; hematemesis; bloody diarrhea; gastrointestinal disorder; intestinal perforation; pancreatitis; anemia; leukopenia; leukocytosis; hypocalcemia; alkaline phosphatase increase; BUN increase; hyperuricemia; NPN increase; respiratory acidosis; somnolence; agitation; neuropathy; paranoid reaction; convulsion; grand mal convulsion; delirium; lung edema; hyperventilation; hypoxia; hemoptysis; hypoventilation; pneumothorax; mydriasis; pupillary disorder; kidney function abnormalities; kidney failure; acute tubular necrosis.

In an additional population of greater than 1,800 patients treated with PROLEUKIN-based regimens using a variety of doses and schedules (e.g., subcutaneous, continuous infusion, administration with LAK cells) the following serious adverse events were reported: duodenal ulceration; bowel necrosis; myocarditis; tachycardia; permanent or transient blindness secondary to optic neuritis; transient ischemic attacks; meningitis; cerebral edema; pericarditis; allergic interstitial nephritis; tracheo-esophageal fistula.

In the same clinical population, the following adverse events which were fatal or resulted in death occurred with a frequency of <1%: liver or renal failure; intestinal perforation; cardiac arrest; myocardial infarction; malignant hyperthermia; pulmonary edema; respiratory arrest; respiratory failure; stroke; pulmonary emboli; severe depression leading to suicide.

In patients with both metastatic RCC and metastatic melanoma, those with ECOG PS of 1 or higher had a higher treatment-related mortality, and serious adverse events.

Most adverse reactions are self-limiting and, usually, but not invariably, reverse or improve within 2 or 3 days of discontinuation of therapy. Examples of adverse reactions with permanent sequelae include: myocardial infarction, bowel perforation/infarction, and gangrene.

In post marketing experience, the following serious adverse events have been reported in a variety of treatment regimens that include interleukin-2: hypertension; pneumonia (bacterial, fungal, viral); neutropenia; cholecystitis; colitis; gastritis; hepatitis; hepatosplenomegaly; intestinal obstruction; retroperitoneal hemorrhage; cerebral lesions; cerebral hemorrhage; encephalopathy; extrapyramidal syndrome; neuralgia; neuritis; neuropathy (demyelination); rhabdomyolysis; myopathy; myositis; hyperthyroidism; anaphylaxis; cellulitis; injection site necrosis; insomnia.

Exacerbation or initial presentation of a number of autoimmune disorders have been reported (See **"WARNINGS"** section, **"PRECAUTIONS"** section, **"Drug Interactions"** subsection). Persistent but nonprogressive vitiligo has been observed in malignant melanoma patients treated with interleukin-2. Synergistic, additive and novel toxicities have been reported with PROLEUKIN used in combination with other drugs. Novel toxicities include delayed adverse reactions to iodinated contrast media and hypersensitivity reactions to antineoplastic agents (See **"PRECAUTIONS"** section, **"Drug Interactions"** subsection).

Experience has shown the following concomitant medications to be useful in the management of patients on PROLEUKIN therapy: a) standard antipyretic therapy, including nonsteroidal anti-inflammatories (NSAIDs), started immediately prior to PROLEUKIN to reduce fever. Renal function should be monitored as some NSAIDs may case synergistic nephrotoxicity; b) meperidine used to control the rigors associated with fever; c) H_2 antagonists given for prophylaxis of gastrointestinal irritation and bleeding; d) antiemetics and antidiarrheals used as needed to treat other gastrointestinal side effects. Generally these medications were discontinued 12 hours after the last dose of PROLEUKIN.

Patients with indwelling central lines have a higher risk of infection with gram positive organisms.[9–11] A reduced incidence of staphylococcal infections in PROLEUKIN studies has been associated with the use of antibiotic prophylaxis which includes the use of oxacillin, nafcillin, ciprofloxacin, or vancomycin. Hydroxyzine or diphenhydramine has been used to control symptoms from pruritic rashes and continued until resolution of pruritus. Topical creams and ointments should be applied as needed for skin manifestations. Preparations containing a steroid (e.g., hydrocortisone) should be avoided. **NOTE: Prior to the use of any product mentioned, the physician should refer to the package insert for the respective product.**

OVERDOSAGE

Side effects following the use of PROLEUKIN® (aldesleukin) appear to be dose-related. Exceeding the recommended

Continued on next page

Proleukin—Cont.

dose has been associated with a more rapid onset of expected dose-limiting toxicities. Symptoms which persist after cessation of PROLEUKIN should be monitored and treated supportively. Life-threatening toxicities may be ameliorated by the intravenous administration of dexamethasone, which may also result in loss of the therapeutic effects of PROLEUKIN.[12] NOTE: Prior to the use of dexamethasone, the physician should refer to the package insert for this product.

DOSAGE AND ADMINISTRATION

The recommended PROLEUKIN® (aldesleukin) for injection treatment regimen is administered by a 15-minute IV infusion every 8 hours. Before initiating treatment, carefully review the "INDICATIONS AND USAGE", "CONTRAINDICATIONS", "WARNINGS", "PRECAUTIONS", and "ADVERSE REACTIONS" sections, particularly regarding patient selection, possible serious adverse events, patient monitoring and withholding dosage. The following schedule has been used to treat adult patients with metastatic renal cell carcinoma (metastatic RCC) or metastatic melanoma. Each course of treatment consists of two 5-day treatment cycles separated by a rest period.

600,000 IU/kg (0.037 mg/kg) dose administered every 8 hours by a 15-minute IV infusion for a maximum of 14 doses. Following 9 days of rest, the schedule is repeated for another 14 doses, for a maximum of 28 doses per course, as tolerated. During clinical trials, doses were frequently withheld for toxicity (See "Clinical Experience" and "Dose Modifications" subsections). Metastatic RCC patients treated with this schedule received a median of 20 of the 28 doses during the first course of therapy.

Retreatment: Patients should be evaluated for response approximately 4 weeks after completion of a course of therapy and again immediately prior to the scheduled start of the next treatment course. Additional courses of treatment should be given to patients only if there is some tumor shrinkage following the last course and retreatment is not contraindicated (See "CONTRAINDICATIONS" section). Each treatment course should be separated by a rest period of at least 7 weeks from the date of hospital discharge.

Dose Modifications: Dose modification for toxicity should be accomplished by withholding or interrupting a dose rather than reducing the dose to be given. Decisions to stop, hold, or restart PROLEUKIN therapy must be made after a global assessment of the patient. With this in mind, the following guidelines should be used:
[See second table on previous page]
[See table below]

Reconstitution and Dilution Directions: Reconstitution and dilution procedures other than those recommended may alter the delivery and/or pharmacology of PROLEUKIN and thus should be avoided.

1. PROLEUKIN® (aldesleukin) is a sterile, white to off-white, preservative-free, lyophilized powder suitable for IV infusion upon reconstitution and dilution. EACH VIAL CONTAINS 22 MILLION IU (1.3 MG) OF PROLEUKIN AND SHOULD BE RECONSTITUTED ASEPTICALLY WITH 1.2 ML OF STERILE WATER FOR INJECTION, USP. WHEN RECONSTITUTED AS DIRECTED, EACH ML CONTAINS 18 MILLION IU (1.1 MG) PROLEUKIN. The resulting solution should be a clear, colorless to slightly yellow liquid. The vial is used for single-use only and any unused portion should be discarded.

2. During reconstitution, the Sterile Water for Injection, USP should be directed at the side of the vial and the contents gently swirled to avoid excess foaming. DO NOT SHAKE.

3. The dose of PROLEUKIN, reconstituted with Sterile Water for Injection, USP (without preservative) should be diluted aseptically in 50 mL of 5% Dextrose Injection, USP (D5W) and infused over a 15-minute period.
In cases where the total dose of PROLEUKIN is 1.5 mg or less (e.g., a patient with a body weight of less than 40 kilograms), the dose of PROLEUKIN should be diluted in a smaller volume of D5W. Concentrations of PROLEUKIN below 30 μg/mL and above 70 μg/mL have shown increased variability in drug delivery. Dilution and delivery of PROLEUKIN outside of this concentration range should be avoided.

4. Glass bottles and plastic (polyvinyl chloride) bags have been used in clinical trials with comparable results. It is recommended that plastic bags be used as the dilution container since experimental studies suggest that use of plastic containers results in more consistent drug delivery. In-line filters should not be used when administering PROLEUKIN.

5. Before and after reconstitution and dilution, store in a refrigerator at 2° to 8°C (36° to 46°F). Do not freeze. Administer PROLEUKIN within 48 hours of reconstitution. The solution should be brought to room temperature prior to infusion in the patient.

6. Reconstitution or dilution with Bacteriostatic Water for Injection, USP, or 0.9% Sodium Chloride Injection, USP should be avoided because of increased aggregation. PROLEUKIN should not be coadministered with other drugs in the same container.

7. Parenteral drug products should be inspected visually for particulate matter and discoloration prior to administration, whenever solution and container permit.

HOW SUPPLIED

PROLEUKIN® (aldesleukin) for injection is supplied in individually boxed single-use vials. Each vial contains 22 × 10⁶ IU of PROLEUKIN. Discard unused portion.
NDC 63905-991-01   Individually boxed single-use vial
Store vials of lyophilized PROLEUKIN in a refrigerator at 2° to 8°C (36° to 46°F).
Reconstituted or diluted PROLEUKIN is stable for up to 48 hours at refrigerated and room temperatures, 2° to 25°C (36° to 77°F). However, since this product contains no preservative, the reconstituted and diluted solutions should be stored in the refrigerator.
Do not use beyond the expiration date printed on the vial.
NOTE: This product contains no preservative.
CAUTION: Federal law (USA) prohibits dispensing without a prescription.

REFERENCES

1. Doyle MV, Lee MT, Fong S. Comparison of the biological activities of human recombinant interleukin-2¹²⁵ and native interleukin-2. *J Biol Response Mod* 1985; 4:96-109.
2. Ralph P, Nakoinz I, Doyle M, et al. Human B and T lymphocyte stimulating properties of interleukin-2 (IL-2) muteins. In: *Immune Regulation by Characterized Polypeptides.* Alan R. Liss, Inc. 1987; 453-62.
3. Winkelhake JL and Gauny SS. Human recombinant interleukin-2 as an experimental therapeutic. *Pharmacol Rev* 1990; 42:1-28.
4. Rosenburg SA, Mule JJ, Spiess PJ, et al. Regression of established pulmonary metastases and subcutaneous tumor mediated by the systemic administration of high-dose recombinant interleukin-2. *J Exp Med* 1985; 161:1169-88.
5. Konrad MW, Hemstreet G, Hersh EM, et al. Pharmacokinetics of recombinant interleukin-2 in humans. *Cancer Res* 1990; 50:2009-17.
6. Donohue JH and Rosenburg SA. The fate of interleukin-2 after *in vivo* administration. *J Immunol* 1983; 130:2203-8.
7. Koths K, Halenback R. Pharmacokinetic studies on ³⁵S-labeled recombinant interleukin-2 in mice. In: Sorg C and Schimpl A, eds. *Cellular And Molecular Biology Of Lymphokines.* Academic Press: Orlando, FL, 1985;779.
8. Gibbons JA, Luo ZP, Hansen ER et al. Quantitation of the renal clearance of interleukin-2 using nephrectomized and ureter ligated rats. *J Pharmacol Exp Ther* 1995; 272: 119-125.
9. Bock SN, Lee RE, Fisher B, et al. A prospective randomized trial evaluating prophylactic antibiotics to prevent triple-lumen catheter-related spesis in patients treated with immunotherapy. *J Clin Oncol* 1990; 8:161-69.
10. Hartman LC, Urba WJ, Steis RG, et al. Use of prophylactic antibiotics for prevention of intravascular catheter-related infections in interleukin-2-treated patients. *J Natl Cancer Inst* 81:1190-93.
11. Snydman DR, Sullivan B, Gill M, et al. Nosocomial sepsis associated with interleukin-2. *Ann Intern Med* 1990; 112:102-07.
12. Mier JW, Vachino G, Klempner MS, et al. Inhibition of interleukin-2-induced tumor necrosis factor release by dexamethasone: Prevention of an acquired neutrophil chemotaxis defect and differential suppression of interleukin-2 associated side effects. *Blood* 1990; 76:1933-40.
13. Choyke PL, Miller DL, Lotze MT, et al. Delayed reactions to contrast media after interleukin-2-immunotherapy. *Radiology* 1992; 183:111-114.

Manufactured by:
Chiron Corporation
Emeryville, CA 94608
U.S. License No. 1106
Distributed by:
Chiron Therapeutics
Emeryville, CA 94608
For additional information, contact Chiron Therapeutics Professional Services 1-800-244-7668, selection 2.
U.S. Patent Nos. RE 33653; 4,530,787; 4,569,790; 4,604,377; 4,748,234; 4,572,798; 4,959,314; 6,464,939
© 1998 Chiron Corporation
L-7271   Revised February 1998

Doses should be held and restarted according to the following:

Body System	Hold dose for	Subsequent doses may be given if
Cardiovascular	Atrial fibrillation, supraventricular tachycardia, or bradycardia that requires treatment or is recurrent or persistent	Patient is asymptomatic with full recovery to normal sinus rhythm
	Systolic bp <90 mm Hg with increasing requirements for pressors	Systolic bp ≥90 mmHg and stable or improving requirements for pressors
	Any ECG change consistent with MI, ischemia or myocarditis with or without chest pain; suspicion of cardiac ischemia	Patient is asymptomatic, MI and myocarditis have been ruled out, clinical suspicion of angina is low; there is no evidence of ventricular hypokinesia
Respiratory	O₂ saturation <94% on room air or <90% with 2 liters O₂ by nasal prongs	O₂ saturation >94% on room air or >90% with 2 liters O₂ by nasal prongs
Nervous	Mental status changes, including moderate confusion or agitation	Mental status changes completely resolved
Body as a Whole	Sepsis syndrome, patient is clinically unstable	Sepsis syndrome has resolved, patient is clinically stable, infection is under treatment
Urogenital	Serum creatinine > 4.5 mg/dL or a serum creatinine of ≥4 mg/dL in the presence of severe volume overload, acidosis, or hyperkalemia Persistent oliguria, urine output of <10 mL/hour for 16 to 24 hours with rising serum creatinine	Serum creatinine <4 mg/dL and fluid and electrolyte status is stable Urine output >10 mL/hour with a decrease of serum creatinine >1.5 mg/dL or normalization of serum creatinine
Digestive	Signs of hepatic failure including encephalopathy, increasing ascites, liver pain, hypoglycemia Stool guaiac repeatedly >3-4+	All signs of hepatic failure have resolved* Stool guaiac negative
Skin	Bullous dermatitis or marked worsening of preexisting skin condition, avoid topical steroid therapy	Resolution of all signs of bullous dermatitis

* Discontinue all further treatment for that course. A new course of treatment, if warranted, should be initiated no sooner than 7 weeks after cessation of adverse event and hospital discharge.

Rabies Vaccine
RABAVERT™
Rabies Vaccine for Human Use   ℞

DESCRIPTION

RabAvert, rabies vaccine, produced by Chiron Behring GmbH & Co is a sterile freeze-dried vaccine obtained by

growing the fixed-virus strain Flury LEP in primary cultures of chicken fibroblasts. The strain Flury LEP was obtained from American Type Culture Collection as the 59th egg passage. The growth medium for propagation of the virus is a synthetic cell culture medium with the addition of human albumin, polygeline (processed bovine gelatin) and antibiotics. The virus is inactivated with β-propiolactone, and further processed by zonal centrifugation in a sucrose density-gradient. The vaccine is lyophilized after addition of a stabilizer solution which consists of buffered polygeline and potassium glutamate. One dose of reconstituted vaccine contains less than 12 mg polygeline (processed bovine gelatin), 1 mg potassium glutamate and 0.3 mg sodium EDTA. Small quantities of bovine serum are used in the cell culture process. Testing of the product components and excipients using currently available methods has not detected any adventitious agents. Further, bovine components originate only from source countries known to be free of bovine spongioform encephalopathy. Minimal amounts of chicken protein may be present in the final product; ovalbumin content is less than 3 ng/dose (1 mL), based on ELISA. Antibiotics (neomycin, chlortetracycline, amphotericin B) added during cell and virus propagation are largely removed during subsequent steps in the manufacturing process. In the final vaccine, neomycin is present at <1 µg, chlortetracycline at < 20 ng, and amphotericin B at < 2 ng per dose. RabAvert is intended for intramuscular (IM) injection. The vaccine contains no preservative and should be used immediately after reconstitution with the supplied diluent (Water For Injection, USP). The potency of the final product is determined by the NIH mouse potency test using the US reference standard. The potency of one dose (1.0 mL) RabAvert is at least 2.5 IU of rabies antigen. RabAvert is a white, freeze-dried vaccine for reconstitution with the diluent prior to use; the reconstituted vaccine is a clear to slightly opaque, colorless suspension.

Table 1: Criteria for Pre-exposure immunization

Risk Category and Nature of Risk	Typical Populations	Pre-exposure regimen
Continuous. Virus present continuously, often in high concentrations. Aerosol, mucous membrane, bite, or nonbite exposures may go unrecognized.	Rabies research lab workers,* rabies biologics production workers.	Primary course. Serologic testing every 6 months; booster vaccination when antibody level falls below acceptable level.*
Frequent. Exposure usually episodic, with source recognized, but exposure may also be unrecognized. Aerosol, mucous membrane, bite or nonbite exposure.	Rabies, diagnostic lab workers,* spelunkers, veterinarians and staff, and animal-control and wildlife workers in rabies enzootic areas. Travelers visiting foreign areas of enzootic rabies for more than 30 days.	Primary course. Booster vaccination or serologic testing every 2 years.**
Infrequent (greater than population-at large). Exposure nearly always episodic with source recognized. Mucous membrane, bite, or nonbite exposure.	Veterinarians and animal-control and wildlife workers in areas of low rabies enzooticity. Veterinary students.	Primary course. No routine booster vaccination or serologic testing.**
Rare (population-at-large). Exposures always episodic. Mucous membrane, or bite with source unrecognized.	US population-at-large, including individuals in rabies epizootic areas.	No vaccination necessary.

Adapted from the recommendations of the Immunization Practices Advisory Committee (ACIP) on rabies prevention. MMWR, 1991; 40 (Suppl. RR-3): 1–19.

* Judgment of relative risk and extra monitoring of vaccination status of laboratory workers is the responsibility of the laboratory supervisor (see US Department of Health and Human Service's Biosafety in Microbiological and Biomedical Laboratories, 1984).

** Minimal acceptable antibody level is complete virus neutralization at a 1:5 serum dilution by RFFIT. Booster dose should be administered if the titer falls below this level.

CLINICAL PHARMACOLOGY

Rabies in the United States

Over the last 100 years, the epidemiology of rabies in animals in the United States has changed dramatically. More than 90% of all animal rabies cases reported annually to the Centers for Disease Control and Prevention (CDC) now occur in wildlife, whereas before 1960 the majority were in domestic animals. The principal rabies hosts today are wild carnivores and bats. Annual human deaths have fallen from more than a hundred at the turn of the century to one to two per year despite major outbreaks of animal rabies in several geographic areas. Within the United States, only Hawaii has remained rabies free. Although rabies among humans is rare in the United States, every year tens of thousands of people receive rabies vaccine for post-exposure prophylaxis. Rabies is almost invariably fatal due to encephalomyelitis. Modern day prophylaxis has proven nearly 100% successful; most human fatalities now occur in people who fail to seek medical treatment, usually because they do not recognize a risk in the animal contact leading to the infection. Inappropriate post-exposure prophylaxis may also result in clinical rabies. Survival after clinical rabies is extremely rare, and is associated with severe brain damage and permanent disability.

RabAvert (in combination with passive immunization with Human Rabies Immune Globulin (HRIG) and local wound treatment) in post-exposure immunization against rabies has been shown to protect patients of all age groups from rabies, when the vaccine was administered according to the World Health Organization (WHO) guidelines and as soon as possible after rabid animal contact. Anti-rabies antibody titers after immunization have been shown to reach levels well above the minimal protective level of 0.5 IU/mL within 14 days after initiating the immunization series. The minimal antibody titer accepted as seroconversion is 0.5 IU, measured by the rapid fluorescent inhibition test (RFFIT) as specified by the WHO (1, 2) or a 1:5 titer (complete inhibition of RFFIT at 1:5 dilution) as specified by the CDC. Vaccine failure has only been reported when key elements of rabies post-exposure regimens were omitted or when the vaccine has been incorrectly administered.

Pre-exposure Immunization

The immunogenicity of RabAvert has been demonstrated in clinical trials conducted in different countries such as the USA (3, 4), UK (5), Croatia (6), and Thailand (7, 8, 9). When administered according to the recommended immunization schedule (days 0, 7, 21), 100% of subjects attained a protective titer. Two studies carried out in the USA in 101 subjects antibody titers > 0.5 IU/mL were obtained by day 28 in all subjects. In studies carried out in Thailand in 22 subjects, and in Croatia in 25 subjects, antibody titers of > 0.5 IU/mL were obtained by day 14 (injections on days 0, 7, 21) in all subjects.

The ability of RabAvert to boost previously immunized subjects was evaluated in three clinical trials. In the Thailand study, pre-exposure booster doses were administered to 10 individuals. Antibody titers of > 0.5 IU/mL were present at baseline on day 0 in all subjects (8). Titers after a booster dose were enhanced from geometric mean titers (GMT) of 1.91 IU/mL to 23.66 IU/mL on day 30. In an additional booster study, individuals known to have been immunized with Human Diploid Cell Vaccine (HDCV) were boosted with RabAvert. In this study, a booster response was observed on day 14 for all (22/22) individuals (10). In a trial carried out in the USA (3), a RabAvert IM booster dose resulted in a significant increase in titers in all (35/35) subjects, regardless of whether they had received RabAvert or HDCV as the primary vaccine.

Persistence of antibody after immunization with RabAvert has been evaluated. In a trial performed in the UK, neutralizing antibody titers > 0.5 IU/mL were present 2 years after immunization in all sera (6/6) tested.

Post-exposure Immunization

RabAvert, when used in the recommended post-exposure WHO program of 5 to 6 IM injections of 1 mL (days 0, 3, 7, 14, 30, and one optionally on day 90) provided protective titers of neutralizing antibody (> 0.5 IU/mL) in 158/160 patients (7, 8, 11–14) within 14 days and in 215/216 patients by day 28–38.

Of these, 203 were followed for at least 10 months. No case of rabies was observed (7, 8, 11–18). Some patients received HRIG, 20–30 IU per kg body weight, or Equine Rabies Immune Globulin (ERIG), 40 IU per kg body weight, at the time of the first dose. In most studies (7, 8, 11, 15), the addition of either HRIG or ERIG caused a slight decrease in GMTs which was neither clinically relevant nor statistically significant. In one study (14), patients receiving HRIG had significantly lower ($p < 0.05$) GMTs on day 14; however, again this was not clinically relevant. After day 14 there was no statistical significance.

The results of several studies of normal volunteers who have been given the WHO regimen of vaccine for post-exposure use (10, 19–22) i.e., "simulated" post-exposure use, show that with sampling by day 28–30, 205/208 vaccinees had protective titers > 0.5 IU/mL.

Over a 10 year (7/85 – 6/95) period, 46 reports of suspected post-exposures vaccine failure have been evaluated (11.8 million doses, distributed). In each use, post-exposure treatment had not been in compliance with WHO recommendations.

INDICATIONS AND USAGE

RabAvert is indicated for pre-exposure immunization, in both primary series and booster dose, and for post-exposure prophylaxis against rabies.

There are no data on the interchangeable use of different rabies vaccines in a single pre- or post-exposure series. Therefore the vaccine from a single manufactured should be used for the complete series whenever possible. If vaccines from other manufacturers are administered during the immunization series, an adequate antibody response should be confirmed by appropriate serologic tests. However, for booster immunization, RabAvert was shown to elicit satisfactory antibody level responses in 41 persons who received a primary series with HDCV (3, 10).

A. Pre-exposure Immunization—See Table 1

Pre-exposure Immunization Schedule

Pre-exposure Immunization consists of three doses of RabAvert 1.0 mL, intramuscularly (deltoid region), one each on days 0, 7, and 21 or 28 ([23] see also Table 1 for criteria for pre-exposure immunization).

Pre-exposure immunization should be offered to persons in high-risk groups, such as veterinarians, animal handlers, wildlife officers, certain laboratory workers, and persons spending time in foreign countries where rabies is endemic. Persons whose activities bring them into contact with potentially rabid dogs, cats, foxes, skunks, bats, or other species at risk of having rabies should also be considered for pre-exposure prophylaxis.

Pre-exposure immunization is given for several reasons. First, it may provide protection to persons with inapparent exposure to rabies. Second, it may protect persons whose post-exposure therapy might be expected to be delayed. Finally, although it does not eliminate the need for prompt therapy after a rabies exposure, it simplifies therapy by eliminating the need for globulin and decreasing the number of doses of vaccine needed. This is of particular importance for persons at high risk of being exposed in countries where the available rabies immunizing products may carry a higher risk of adverse reactions.

In some instances, pre-exposure immunization should be boosted periodically in an effort to provide continuous protection (see Table 1); each booster immunization consists of a single dose. See **Clinical Pharmacology**. Serum antibody determinations before and after booster immunization may be helpful in determining both the need for a booster dose and the timing of such a dose.

[See table 1 above]

B. Post-exposure Immunization—See Table 2

The following recommendations are only a guide. In applying them, take into account the animal species involved, the circumstances of the bit or other exposure, the immunization status of the animal, and presence of rabies in the region (as outlined below). Local or state public health officials should be consulted if questions arise about the need for rabies prophylaxis (23).

[See table 2 at top of next page]

In the United States, the following factors should be considered before antirabies treatment is initiated.

Species of Biting Animal

Carnivorous wild animals (especially skunks, raccoons, foxes and coyotes) and bats are the animals most commonly infected with rabies and have caused most of the indigenous cases of human rabies in the United States since 1960. Unless an animal is tested and shown not to be rabid, post-exposure prophylaxis should be initiated upon bite or nonbite exposure to the animals. (See definition in "Type of Exposure" below). If treatment has been initiated and subsequent testing in a qualified laboratory shows the exposing animal is not rabid, treatment can be discontinued (23).

The likelihood that a domestic dog or cat is infected with rabies varies from region to region; hence the need for post-exposure prophylaxis also varies (23).

Rodents (such as squirrels, hamsters, guinea pigs, gerbils, chipmunks, rats, and mice) and lagomorphs (including rabbits and hares) are rarely found to be infected with rabies and have not been known to cause human rabies in the United States. In these cases, the state or local health department should be consulted before a decision is made to initiate post-exposure antirabies prophylaxis (23).

Continued on next page

RabAvert—Cont.

Circumstances of Biting Incident
An UNPROVOKED attack is more likely than a provoked attack to indicate the animal is rabid. Bites inflicted on a person attempting to feed or handle an apparently healthy animal should generally be regarded as PROVOKED.
Type of Exposure
Rabies is transmitted by introducing the virus into open cuts or wounds in skin or via mucous membranes. The likelihood of rabies infection varies with the nature and extent of exposure. Two categories of exposure should be considered:
Bite: Any penetration of the skin by teeth. Bites to the face and hands carry the highest risk, but the site of the bite should not influence the decision to begin treatment (23).
Nonbite: Scratches, abrasions, open wounds, or mucous membranes contaminated with saliva or other potentially infectious material, such as brain tissue, from a rabid animal. Casual contact, such as petting a rabid animal (without a bite or nonbite exposure as described above), does not constitute an exposure and is not an indication for prophylaxis. There have been two instances of airborne rabies acquire in laboratories and two probably airborne rabies cases acquired in a bat-infested cave in Texas (23).
The only documented cases for rabies from human-to-human transmission occurred in four patients in the United States and overseas who received corneas transplanted from persons who died of rabies undiagnosed at the time of death (2). Stringent guidelines for acceptance of donor corneas should reduce this risk.
Bite and nonbite exposure from humans with rabies theoretically could transmit rabies, although no cases of rabies acquired this way have been documented. Each potential exposure to human rabies should be carefully evaluated to minimize unnecessary rabies prophylaxis (23).
Post-exposure Immunization Schedule
The essential components of rabies post-exposure prophylaxis are prompt local treatment of wounds and immunization, including administration, in most instances of both globulin and vaccine (Table 2).
A complete course of post-exposure immunization for previously unvaccinated adults and children consists of a total of 5 doses, each 1.0 mL; one IM injection on each of days 0, 3, 7, 14 and 28.
1. Local Treatment of Wounds
Immediate and thorough washing of all bite wounds and scratches with soap and water is an important measure for preventing rabies. In animal studies, simple local wound cleansing has been shown to reduce markedly the likelihood of rabies. Whenever possible, bite injuries should not be sutured to avoid further and/or deeper contamination. Tetanus prophylaxis and measures to control bacterial infection should be given as indicated (23).
2. Specific Treatment of Rabies
The injection schedule for post-exposure prophylaxis depends on whether the patient has had or has not had previous immunization against rabies. For persons who have not previously been immunized against rabies, the schedule consists of an initial injection IM of HRIG exactly 20 IU per kilogram body weight in total. If anatomically feasible, up to half of the dose of HRIG should be thoroughly infiltrated in and around the wound(s) and the remainder should be administered IM in the gluteal region. HRIG is administered only once (for specific instructions for HRIG use, see the product package insert). The HRIG injection is followed by a series of 5 individual injections of RabAvert (1.0 mL each) given IM on days 0, 3,7, 14 and 28. Administration of HRIG and RabAvert should be given at separate sites using separate syringes. Post-exposure rabies prophylaxis should begin the same day exposure occurred or as soon after exposure as possible. The combined use of HRIG and RabAvert is recommended for both bite and non-bite exposures, regardless of the interval between exposure and initiation of treatment.
In the event that HRIG is not readily available for the initiation of treatment, it can be given through the seventh day after administration of the first dose of vaccine. HRIG is not indicated beyond the seventh day because an antibody response to RabAvert is presumed to have begun by that time (23).
The sooner treatment is begun after exposure, the better. However, there have been instances in which the decision to begin treatment was made as late as 6 months or longer after exposure due to delay in recognition that passive antibody and immunization with the exception of persons who have previously received complete immunization regimens (pre-exposure or post-exposure) with a cell culture vaccine, or persons, who have been immunized with other types of vaccines and have had documented rabies antibody titers. Persons who have previously received rabies immunization should receive 2 IM doses of RabAvert: 1 on day 0 and another on day 3. They should not be given HRIG.
3. Treatment Outside the United States
If post-exposure immunization is begun outside the United States with regimens or products that are not used in the United States, it may be desirable to provide additional treatment when the patient reaches the USA. State or local health departments should be contacted for specific advice in such cases (23).

Table 2: Rabies Post-exposure Prophylaxis Guide (Advisory Committee on Immunization Practices [ACIP]) (23)

Animal type	Evaluation and disposition of animal	Post-exposure prophylaxis recommendations
Dogs and cats	Healthy and available for 10 days observation Rabid or suspected rabid Unknown (escaped)	Should not begin prophylaxis unless animal develops symptoms of rabies* Immediate immunization Consult public health officials
Skunks, raccoons, bats, foxes, and most other carnivores; woodchucks	Regarded as rabid unless geographic area is known to be free of rabies or until animal proven negative by laboratory tests**	Immediate immunization
Livestock, rodents, and lagomorphs (rabbits and hares)	Consider individually	Consult public health officials. Bites of squirrels, hamsters, guinea pigs, gerbils, chipmunks, rats, mice, other rodents, rabbits, and hares almost never require antirabies treatment

* During the 10-day holding period, begin treatment with HRIG and RabAvert rabies vaccine at first sign of rabies in a dog or cat that has bitten someone. The symptomatic animal should be killed immediately and tested.
**The animal should be killed and tested as soon as possible. Holding for observation is not recommended. Discontinue vaccine if immunofluorescence test results of the animal are negative.

CONTRAINDICATIONS
In view of the almost invariably fatal outcome of rabies, there is no contraindication to post-exposure immunization. However, if an alternative product (e.g., HDCV or Rabies Vaccine Adsorbed [RVA]) is not available, care should be taken if the vaccine is to be administered to persons known to be sensitive to processed bovine gelatin, chicken protein, neomycin, chlortetracycline and amphotericin B in trace amounts, which may be present in the vaccine and may cause an allergic reaction in such individuals.

WARNINGS
Serious systemic anaphylactic reactions have been reported and neuroparalytic events have been reported in temporal association with RabAvert, rabies vaccine, administration. Against the background of 11.8 million doses distributed worldwide as of June 30, 1995, 10 cases of encephalitis (1 death) or meningitis, 7 cases of transient paralysis (including 2 cases of Guillain-Barré Syndrome), 1 case of myelitis, 1 case of retrobulbar neuritis, and 2 cases of suspected multiple sclerosis have been temporally associated with the use of RabAvert. Also 2 cases of anaphylactic shock have been reported. Such events pose a dilemma for the attending physician. A patient's risk of developing rabies must be carefully considered, however, before deciding to discontinue immunization.
RABAVERT MUST NOT BE USED SUBCUTANEOUSLY OR INTRADERMALLY!
RabAvert must be injected intramuscularly. For adults, the deltoid area is the preferred site of immunization; for small children, administration into the anterolateral zone of the thigh is preferred. The use of the gluteal region should be avoided, since administration in this area may result in lower neutralizing antibody titers (2).
DO NOT INJECT INTRAVASCULARLY!
Unintentional intravascular injection may result in systemic reactions, including shock. Immediate measures include catecholamines, volume replacement, high doses of corticosteroids, and oxygen.
Development of active immunity after vaccination may be impaired in immune-compromised individuals. Please refer to *Drug Interactions*, under **Precautions.**

PRECAUTIONS
General
Care is to be taken by the heath care provider for the safe and effective use of the product. The health care provider should also question the patient, parent or guardian about 1) the current health status of the vaccinee; and 2) reactions to a previous dose of RabAvert, or a similar product. Pre-exposure vaccination should be postponed in the case of sick and convalescent persons, and those considered to be in the incubation stage of an infectious disease. A separate, sterile syringe and needle or a sterile disposable unit should be used for each patient to prevent transmission of hepatitis and other infectious agents from person to person. Needles should not be recapped and should be properly disposed of. As with any vaccine, vaccination with RabAvert may not protect 100% of susceptible individuals.
Hypersensitivity
RabAvert is produced in chick embryo cell culture. Persons with a history of anaphylactic, anaphylactoid, or other immediate reactions (e.g., hives, swelling of the mouth and throat, difficulty breathing, hypotension, or shock) subsequent to egg ingestion should not be immunized with this vaccine. At present there is no evidence that persons are at increased risk if they have egg hypersensitivities that are not anaphylactic or anaphylactoid in nature; however, in this case, HDCV rabies vaccines or RVA should be administered. There is no evidence to indicate that persons with allergies to chickens or feathers are at increased risk of reaction to vaccines produced in chick embryo cell culture.
Since reconstituted RabAvert contains traces of processed bovine gelatin, chicken protein, neomycin, chlortetracycline and amphotericin B, the possibility of allergic reactions in individuals sensitive to these substances should be considered when administering the vaccine.
Epinephrine injection (1:1000) must be immediately available should anaphylactic or other allergic reactions occur.
When a person with a history of hypersensitivity must be given RabAvert, antihistamines may be given; epinephrine (1:1000), volume replacement, corticosteroids and oxygen should be readily available to counteract anaphylactic reactions.
Drug Interactions
Corticosteroids, other immunosuppressive agents, antimalarials and immunosuppressive illnesses can interfere with the development of active immunity after vaccination, and may diminish the protective efficacy of the vaccine. Pre-exposure prophylaxis should be administered to such persons with the awareness that the immune response may be inadequate. Immunosuppressive agents should not be administered during post-exposure therapy unless essential for the treatment of other conditions. When rabies post-exposure prophylaxis is administered to persons receiving corticosteroids or other immunosuppressive therapy, or who are immunosuppressed, it is important that a serum sample be tested for rabies antibody to ensure that an acceptable antibody response has been induced (23).
Rabies Immune Globulin must not be administered at more than the recommended dose, since response to active immunization may be impaired.
Use in Pregnancy
Category C. Animal reproduction studies have not been conducted with RabAvert. It is also not known whether RabAvert can cause fetal harm when administered to a pregnant woman or can affect reproduction capacity. RabAvert should be given to a pregnant woman only if clearly needed. However, because of the potential consequences of inadequately treated rabies exposure, and limited data which indicate that fetal abnormalities have not been associated with rabies vaccination, pregnancy is not considered a contraindication to post-exposure prophylaxis. If there is substantial risk of exposure to rabies, pre-exposure prophylaxis may also be indicated during pregnancy. However, in such instances, consideration should be given to removing the pregnant woman from the high risk environment.
Carcinogenesis, Mutagenesis, Impairment of Fertility
Long-term studies with RabAvert have not been conducted to assess the potential for carcinogenesis, mutagenesis, or impairment of fertility.

ADVERSE REACTIONS
SEE ALSO **WARNINGS** AND **CONTRAINDICATIONS** SECTIONS FOR ADDITIONAL STATEMENTS
Local reactions such as induration, swelling and reddening have been reported more often than systemic reactions. In a comparative trial in normal volunteers, Dreesen *et al.* (3, 24) described their experience with RabAvert compared to a HDCV rabies vaccine. Nineteen subjects received RabAvert and 20 received HDCV. The most commonly reported adverse reaction was pain at the injection site, reported in 45% of the HDCV group, and 34% of the RabAvert group. Localized lymphadenopathy was reported in about 15% of each group. The most common systemic reactions were malaise (15% RabAvert group vs. 25% HDCV group), headache (10% RabAvert group vs. 20% HDCV group), and dizziness

(15% RabAvert group vs. 10% HDCV group). In a recent study in the USA (4), 83 subjects received RabAvert and 82 received HDCV. Again the most common adverse reaction was pain at the injection site in 80% in the HDCV group and 84% in the RabAvert group. the most common systemic reactions were headache (52% RabAvert group vs. 45% HDCV group), myalgia (53% RabAvert group vs. 38% HDCV group) and malaise (20% RabAvert group vs. 17% HDCV group). None of the adverse events was serious, almost all adverse events were of mild or moderate intensity. Statistically significant differences between vaccination groups were not found. Both vaccines were generally well tolerated.

Uncommonly observed adverse events include temperatures above 38°C (100°F), swollen lymph nodes, and gastrointestinal complaints. In rare cases, patients have experienced severe headache, fatigue, circulatory reactions, sweating, chills, monoarthritis and allergic reactions; transient paresthesias and one case of suspected urticaria pigmentosa have also been reported.

Type III hypersensitivity reactions in pre-exposure booster immunizations have been reported with one HDCV rabies vaccine (25–27). These reactions are thought to be due to small amounts of human serum albumin (HSA) rendered allergenic by β-propiolactone (23, 28, 29). Human serum albumin (HSA) is present in RabAvert at concentrations less than 0.3µg/dose. No type III hypersensitivity reactions have been observed with RabAvert (30).

Serious systemic anaphylactic reactions or neuroparalytic events have been reported in association with RabAvert administration. Against a background of 11.8 million doses distributed world-wide 10 cases of encephalitis (1 death) or meningitis, 7 cases of transient paralysis including 2 cases of Guillaine-Barré Syndrome, 1 case of myelitis, 1 case of retrobulbar neuritis, and 2 cases of suspected multiple sclerosis have been temporally associated with the use of RabAvert. Also, 2 cases of anaphylactic shock have been reported. A patient's risk of developing rabies must be carefully considered, however, before deciding to discontinue immunization (see **Warnings**).

The use of corticosteroids to treat life-threatening neuroparalytic reactions may inhibit the development of immunity to rabies (see **Precautions,** Drug Interactions).

Once initiated, rabies prophylaxis should not be interrupted or discontinued because of local or mild systemic adverse reactions to rabies vaccine. Usually such reactions can be successfully managed with anti-inflammatory and antipyretic agents.

Reporting of Adverse Events
Adverse events should be reported by the health care provider or patient to the US Department of Health and Human Services (DHHS) Vaccine Adverse Event Reporting System (VAERS). Report forms and information about reporting requirements or completion of the form can be obtained from VAERS by calling the toll-free number 1-800-822-7967 (26). In the USA, such events can be reported to the Professional Services Department, Chiron Corporation: phone: 1-800-CHIRON8.

DOSAGE AND ADMINISTRATION

The individual dose is 1 mL, given intramuscularly.
Administer in adults by IM injection into the deltoid muscle or, in the case of small children, into the anterolateral zone of the thigh. The gluteal area should be avoided for vaccine injections, since administration in this area may result in lower neutralizing antibody titers. Care should be taken to avoid injection into or near blood vessels and nerves. After aspiration, if blood or any suspicious discoloration appears in the syringe, do not inject but discard contents and repeat procedure using a new dose of vaccine, at a different site.

Instructions for Reconstituting RabAvert
Using the longer of the 2 needles supplied, transfer the entire contents of the diluent vial into the vaccine vial. Mix gently to avoid foaming. The white, freeze-dried vaccine dissolves to give a clear or slightly opaque suspension. Withdraw the total amount of dissolved vaccine into the syringe and replace the long needle with the small needle for IM injection. The reconstituted vaccine should be used immediately.

Parenteral drug products should be inspected visually for particulate matter and discoloration prior to administration. If either of these conditions exists, the vaccine should not be administered. A separate, sterile syringe and needle or a sterile disposable unit should be used for each patient to prevent transmission of hepatitis and other infectious agents from person to person. Needles should not be recapped and should be properly disposed of. No data are available regarding the concurrent administration of RabAvert rabies vaccine with other vaccines.

Pediatric Use
Children and adults receive the same dose of 1 mL, given IM.
Only limited data on the safety and efficacy of RabAvert in the pediatric age group are available. However, in four studies some pre-exposure and post-exposure experience has been gained (17, 31, 32, 33).

Pre-exposure:
Pre-exposure administration of RabAvert in 11 Thai children from the age of 2 years and older resulted in antibody levels higher than 0.5 IU/mL on day 14 in all children (32). In another study in Mexico, 15/21 children aged 7–18 years had antibody titers of ≥ 0.5 IU/mL on day 14 and all 21 children had antibody titers of ≥ 0.5 IU/mL on day 30. Only mild local pain was noted in approximately one quarter of the children (33).

Post-exposure:
In a 10-year serosurveillance study, RabAvert has been administered to 91 children aged 1 to 5 years and 436 children and adolescents aged 6 to 20 years (17). The vaccine was effective in both age groups. None of these patients developed rabies.

One newborn has received RabAvert on an immunization schedule of day 0, 3, 7, 14 and 30; the antibody concentration on day 37 was 2.34 IU/mL. There were no clinically significant adverse events (31).

A. Pre-exposure Dosage
1. Primary Immunization
In the United States, the Advisory Committee on Immunization Practices (ACIP) recommends three injections of 1.0 mL each: one injection on day 0 and one on day 7, and one either on day 21 or 28 (for criteria for pre-exposure immunization, see Table 1).
2. Booster Immunization
The individual booster dose is 1 mL, given intramuscularly. Booster immunization is given to persons who have received previous rabies immunization and remain at increased risk of rabies exposure by reasons of occupation.

Persons who work with live rabies virus in research laboratories or vaccine production facilities (continuous-risk category: see Table 1) should have a serum sample tested for rabies antibodies every 6 months. Booster doses of vaccine should be given to maintain a serum titer > 1:5 serum dilution by the RFFIT.

The frequent-risk category includes other laboratory workers such as those doing rabies diagnostic testing, spelunkers, veterinarians and staff, animal-control and wildlife officers in areas where rabies is epizootic, and international travelers living or visiting (for > 30 days) in areas where canine rabies is endemic. Persons among this group should have a serum sample tested for rabies antibodies every 2 years and, if the titer is less than complete neutralization at a 1:5 serum dilution by RFFIT, should have a booster dose of vaccine. Alternatively, a booster can be administered in the absence of a titer determination.

Veterinarians and animal-control and wildlife officers working in areas of low rabies enzooticity (infrequent-exposure group) do not require routine pre-exposure booster doses of RabAvert after completion of a full primary pre-exposure immunization scheme (Table 1).

B. Post-exposure Dosage
Immunization should begin as soon as possible after exposure. A complete course of immunization consists of a total of 5 injections of 1 mL each: one injection on each of days 0, 3, 7, 14 and 28 in conjunction with the administration of HRIG on day 0. For children, see *Pediatric Use* section, above.

Begin with the administration of HRIG. Give 20 IU/kg body weight.

This formula is applicable to all age groups, including children. The recommended dosage of HRIG should not exceed 20 IU/kg body weight because it may otherwise interfere with active antibody production. Since vaccine-induced antibody appears within 1 week, HRIG is not indicated more than 7 days after initiating post-exposure immunization with RabAvert. If possible, up to one-half the dose of HRIG should be thoroughly infiltrated in the area around the wound and the rest should be administered IM, in a different site from the rabies vaccine, preferably in the gluteal area.

Because the antibody response following the recommended immunization regimen with RabAvert has been satisfactory, routine post-immunization serologic testing is not recommended. Serologic testing is indicated in unusual circumstances, as when the patient is known to be immunosuppressed. Contact state health department or CDC for recommendations.

C. Post-exposure Therapy of Previously Immunized Persons
When rabies exposure occurs in an immunized person who was vaccinated according to the recommended regimen with RabAvert or other tissue culture vaccines or who had previously demonstrated rabies antibody, that person should receive two IM doses (1.0 mL each) of RabAvert: one immediately and one 3 days later. HRIG should not be given in these cases. Persons should be considered to have been immunized previously if they received pre- or post-exposure prophylaxis with RabAvert or other tissue culture vaccines or have been documented to have had an adequate antibody response to duck embryo rabies vaccine. If the immune status of a previously vaccinated person is not known, full primary post-exposure antirabies treatment (HRIG plus 5 doses of vaccine) may be necessary. In such cases, if anti-

bodies can be demonstrated in a serum sample collected before vaccine is given, treatment can be discontinued after at least two doses of vaccine.

HOW SUPPLIED

Package with:
1 vial of freeze-dried vaccine containing a single dose
1 disposable syringe
1 longer needle for reconstitution, 21 gauge × 1.5"
1 vial of sterile Water For Injection, USP (1 mL)
1 smaller needle for injection, 25 gauge × 1"
N.D.C.# 53905-501-01 CAUTION: Federal law prohibits dispensing without a prescription
Storage
RabAvert should be stored protected from light at 2°C to 8°C (36°F to 46°F). After reconstitution the vaccine is to be used immediately. The vaccine may not be used after the expiration date given on package and container.

REFERENCES

1. Smith JS, Yager, PA & Baer, GM. A rapid reproducible test for determining rabies neutralisation antibody. Bull WHO. 1973; 48: 535–541.
2. Eighth Report of the WHO Expert Committee on Rabies. WHO Technical Report Series, no. 824; 1992.
3. Dreesen DW, et al. Two-year comparative trial on the immunogenicity and adverse effects of purified chick embryo cell rabies vaccine for pre-exposure immunization. Vaccine. 1989; 7: 397–400.
4. Dreesen DW. Investigation of antibody response to purified chick embryo cell tissue culture vaccine (PCECV) or human diploid cell culture vaccine (HDCV) in health volunteers. Study synopsis 7USA401RA, September 1996–December 1996 (unpublished)
5. Nicholson KG, et al. Pre-exposure studies with purified chick embryo cell culture rabies vaccine and human diploid cell vaccine: serological and clinical responses in man. Vaccine. 1987; 5: 208–210.
6. Vodopija I, et al. An evaluation of second generation tissue culture rabies vaccine for use in man: a four-vaccine comparative immunogenicity study using a pre-exposure vaccination schedule and an abbreviated 2-1-1 post-exposure schedule. Vaccine. 1986; 4: 245–248
7. Wasi C, et al. Purified chick embryo cell rabies vaccine (letter). Lancet. 1986; 1: 40.
8. Wasi C. Rabies prophylaxis with purified chick embryo (PCEC) rabies vaccine. Protocol 8T–201RA, 1983–1984 (unpublished).
9. Wasi C. Personal communication to Behringwerke AG, 1990.
10. Bijok U, et al. Clinical trials in healthy volunteers with the new purified chick embryo cell rabies vaccine for man: J Commun Dis. 1984; 16: 61–69.
11. Vodopija I. Post-exposure rabies prophylaxis with purified chick embryo cell (PCEC) rabies vaccine. Protocol 7YU-201RA, 1983–1985 (unpublished).
12. John J. Evaluation of purified chick embryo cell culture (PCEC) rabies vaccine, 1987 (unpublished).
13. Tanphaichitra D, Siristonpun Y. Study of the efficacy of a purified chick embryo cell vaccine in patients bitten by rabid animals. Intern Med. 1987; 3: 158–160.
14. Thongcharoen P, et al. Effectiveness of new economical schedule of rabies postexposure prophylaxis using purified chick embryo cell tissue culture rabies vaccine. Protocol 7T–301IP, 1993 (unpublished).
15. Ljubicic M, et al. Efficacy of PCEC vaccines in post-exposure rabies prophylaxis. In: Vodopija, Nicholson, Smerdel & Bijok (eds.): Improvements in rabies post-exposure treatment (Proceedings of a meeting in Dubrovnik, Yugoslavia). Zagreb Institute of Public Health 1985.
16. Madhusudana SN, Tripathi KK. Post exposure studies with human diploid cell rabies vaccine and purified chick embryo cell vaccine: Comparative Serological Responses in Man. Int. Med Microbiol. 1989; 271: 345–350.
17. Sehgal S, et al. Ten year longitudinal study of efficacy and safety of purified chick embryo cell vaccine for pre- and post-exposure prophylaxis of rabies in Indian population. J Commun Dis. 1995; 27: 36–43.
18. Sehgal S, et al. Cinical evaluation of purified chick embryo cell antirabies vaccine for post-exposure treatment. J Commun Dis. 1988; 20: 293–300.
19. Suntharasamai P, et al: Purified chick embryo cell rabies vaccine: economical multisite intradermal regimen for post-exposure prophylaxis. Epidemiol Infect. 1987; 99; (3): 755–765.
20. Meesomboon V, et al. Antibody response to PCEC-rabies vaccine. J. Commun.Dis. 1987; 13: 130–136.
21. Sehgal S. Report of the trials of PCEC (Purified Chick Embryo Cell) rabies vaccine in India. In: Vodopija, Nicholson, Smerdel & Bijok (eds.): Improvements in rabies post-exposure treatment (Proceedings of a meeting in Dubrovnik, Yugoslavia). Zagreb Institute of Public Heath 1985 pp. 71–75.

Continued on next page

RabAvert—Cont.

22. Lesic L, Petrovic M. Study Report: Findings of Clinical Trials on Rabipur PCEC, Rabies Vaccine, National Reference Laboratory for Rabies, Novi Sad, Yugoslavia, 1988 (unpublished).
23. Centers for Disease Control. Rabies Prevention – United States, 1991. Recommendations of the Immunization Practices Advisory Committee (ACIP). MMWR, 1991; 40 (RR-3): 1–19.
24. Dreesen D, et al.: A comparative study of cell culture rabies vaccine: Immunogenicity and safety. Protocol 8USA301RA, 1985–1986 (unpublished).
25. Centers for Disease Control. Systemic allergic reactions following immunization with HDC rabies vaccine. MMWR. 1984; 33: 185–187.
26. Centers for Disease Control. Rabies Prevention - United States, MMWR. 1984; 33: 393–402.
27. Dreesen DW, et al. Immune complex-like disease in 23 persons following a booster dose of rabies HDC vaccine. Vaccine. 1986; 4: 45–49.
28. Anderson, MC, et al: The role of specific IgE and beta-propiolactone in reactions resulting from booster dose of human diploid rabies cell vaccine. J Allergy Clin. Immunol. 1987; 80: 861–868.
29. Swanson MC, et al. IgE and IgG antibodies to beta-propiolactone and human serum albumin associated with urticarial reactions to rabies vaccine. J Infect Dis. 1987; 155: 909–913.
30. Marwick C. Changes recommended in use of human diploid cell rabies vaccine (news). JAMA. 1985; 245: 14–15.
31. Lumbiganon P, Wasi C. Survival after rabies immunisation in newborn infant of affected mother. Lancet. 1990; 336: 319–332.
32. Lumbiganon P, et al. Pre-exposure vaccination with purified chick embryo cell rabies vaccines in children. Asian Pacific J Allergy Immunol, 1989; 7: 99–101.
33. Gonzales de Ciso. Comparative evaluation of PCEC and Fluenzalida vaccines. Protocol 8Mex201RA, 1983–1984 (unpublished).

Manufactured by:
Chiron Behring GmbH & Co.
D-35006 Marburg, Germany
Distributed by:
Chiron Corporation
Emeryville, CA 94608, USA

Rev. 10/97

Shown in Product Identification Guide, page 309

CibaGeneva Pharmaceuticals

Ciba-Geigy Corporation

Geneva Pharmaceuticals, Inc.

PLEASE NOTE:
Due to the merger of CibaGeneva Pharmaceuticals and Sandoz Pharmaceuticals Corporation, please refer to **Novartis Pharmaceuticals Corporation** for branded product information and **Geneva Pharmaceuticals, Inc.** for branded generic product information.

Colgate Oral Pharmaceuticals, Inc.

a subsidiary of Colgate-Palmolive Company
ONE COLGATE WAY
CANTON, MA 02021 U.S.A.

Direct Inquiries to:
Professional Services Department
(800) 226-5428

For Medical Information Contact:
In Emergencies:
Pittsburgh Poison Control
(412) 692-5596

LURIDE® DROPS ℞
brand of sodium fluoride
oral solution

1.69 fl oz (50 mL) bottles, calibrated dropper

LURIDE® LOZI-TABS® ℞
brand of sodium fluoride

120 tablet bottles 0.25 mg F vanilla
120 tablet bottles 0.5 mg F grape
120 tablet bottles 1 mg F cherry

PERIOGARD® ℞
(chlorhexidine gluconate oral rinse, 0.12%)

16 fl oz bottles

PREVIDENT® 5000 PLUS™ ℞
brand of 1.1% Sodium Fluoride prescription dental cream

DESCRIPTION
Self-topical neutral fluoride dentifrice containing 1.1% (w/w) sodium fluoride for use as a dental caries preventive in adults and pediatric patients.
Active Ingredient: Sodium Fluoride, 1.1% (w/w).
Inactive Ingredients: Purified Water, Sorbitol, Hydrated Silica, PEG-12, Tetrapotassium Pyrophosphate, Xanthan Gum, Flavor, Sodium Benzoate, Sodium Lauryl Sulfate, Sodium Saccharin, Titanium Dioxide, Sodium Hydrochloride, FD&C Blue #1.

CLINICAL PHARMACOLOGY
Frequent topical applications to the teeth with preparations having a relatively high fluoride content increase tooth resistance to acid dissolution and enhance penetration of the fluoride ion into tooth enamel.

INDICATIONS AND USAGE
A dental caries preventive, for once daily self-applied topical use. It is well established that 1.1% sodium fluoride is safe and extraordinarily effective as a caries preventive when applied frequently with mouthpiece applicators.[1-4] PreviDent 5000 Plus brand of 1.1% sodium fluoride in a squeeze-tube is easily applied onto a toothbrush. This prescription dental cream should be used once daily in place of your regular toothpaste unless otherwise instructed by your dental professional. May be used whether or not drinking water is fluoridated, since topical fluoride cannot produce fluorosis. (See WARNINGS for exception.)

CONTRAINDICATIONS
Do not use in pediatric patients under 6 years unless recommended by a dentist or physician.

WARNINGS
Prolonged daily ingestion may result in various degrees of dental fluorosis in pediatric patients under age 6 years, especially if the water fluoridation exceeds 0.6 ppm, since younger pediatric patients frequently cannot perform the brushing process without significant swallowing. Use in pediatric patients under age 6 years requires special supervision to prevent repeated swallowing of dental cream which could cause dental fluorosis. Read directions carefully before using. Keep out of reach of infants and children.

PRECAUTIONS
Not for systemic treatment. DO NOT SWALLOW
Carcinogenesis, Mutagenesis, Impairment of Fertility: In a study conducted in rodents, no carcinogenesis was found in male and female mice and female rats treated with fluoride at dose levels ranging from 4.1 to 9.1 mg/kg of body weight. Equivocal evidence of carcinogenesis was reported in male rats treated with 2.5 and 4.1 mg/kg of body weight. In a second study, no carcinogenesis was observed in rats, males or females, treated with fluoride up to 11.3 mg/kg of body weight. Epidemiological data provide no credible evidence for an association between fluoride either naturally occurring or added to drinking water, and risk of human cancer. Fluoride ion is not mutagenic in standard bacterial systems. It has been shown that fluoride ion has potential to induce chromosome aberrations in cultured human and rodent cells at doses much higher than those to which humans are exposed. *In vivo* data are conflicting. Some studies report chromosome damage in rodents while other studies using similar protocols report negative results.
Potential adverse reproductive effects of fluoride exposure in humans has not been adequately evaluated. Adverse effects on reproduction were reported for rats, mice, fox, and cattle exposed to 100 ppm or greater concentrations of fluoride in their diet or drinking water. Other studies conducted in rats demonstrated that lower concentrations of fluoride (5 mg/kg body weight) did not result in impaired fertility and reproductive capabilities.
Pregnancy: Pregnancy Category B. It has been shown that fluoride crosses the placenta of rats, but only 0.01% of the amount administered is incorporated in fetal tissue. Animal studies (rats, mice, rabbits) have shown that fluoride is not a teratogen. Maternal exposure to 12.2 mg fluoride/kg of body weight (rats) or 13.1 mg/kg of body weight (rabbits) did not affect the litter size or fetal weight and did not increase the frequency of skeletal or visceral malformations. Epidemiological studies conducted in areas with high levels of naturally fluoridated water showed no increase in birth defects. Heavy exposure to fluoride during *in utero* development may result in skeletal fluorosis which becomes evident in childhood.
Nursing Mothers: It is not known if fluoride is excreted in human milk. However, many drugs are excreted in milk and caution should be exercised when products containing fluoride are administered to a nursing woman. Reduced milk production was reported in farm-raised fox when the animals were fed a diet containing a high concentration of fluoride (98–137 mg/kg of body weight). No adverse effects on parturition, lactation, or offspring were seen in rats administered fluoride up to 5 mg/kg of body weight.
Pediatric Use: The use of PreviDent 5000 Plus in pediatric age groups 6 to 16 years as a caries preventive is supported by pioneering clinical studies with 1.1% sodium fluoride gels in mouthtrays in students age 11–14 years conducted by Englander, et al,[2,3,4]. Safety and effectiveness in pediatric patients below the age of 6 years have not been established. Please refer to the CONTRAINDICATIONS and WARNINGS sections.

ADVERSE REACTIONS
Allergic reactions and other idiosyncrasies have been rarely reported.

OVERDOSAGE
Accidental ingestion of large amounts of fluoride may result in acute burning in the mouth and sore tongue. Nausea, vomiting, and diarrhea may occur soon after ingestion (within 30 minutes) and are accompanied by salivation, hematemesis, and epigastric cramping abdominal pain. These symptoms may persist for 24 hours. If less than 5 mg fluoride/kg body weight (i.e., less than 2.3 mg fluoride/lb body weight) have been ingested, give calcium (e.g., milk) orally to relieve gastrointestinal symptoms and observe for a few hours. If more than 5 mg fluoride/kg body weight (i.e., more than 2.3 mg fluoride/lb body weight) have been ingested, induce emesis, give orally soluble calcium (e.g., milk, 5% calcium gluconate or calcium lactate solution) and immediately seek medical assistance. For accidental ingestion of more than 15 mg fluoride/kg of body weight (i.e., more than 6.9 mg fluoride/lb body weight), induce vomiting and admit immediately to a hospital facility.
A treatment dose (a thin ribbon) of PreviDent 5000 Plus contains 2.5 mg fluoride. A 1.8 oz. tube contains 255 mg fluoride.

DOSAGE AND ADMINISTRATION
Follow these instructions unless otherwise instructed by your dental professional: 1. Adults and pediatric patients 6 years of age or older, apply a thin ribbon of PreviDent 5000 Plus to a toothbrush. Brush thoroughly once daily for two minutes, preferably at bedtime. 2. After use, adults expectorate. For best results, do not eat, drink, or rinse for 30 minutes. Pediatric patients, age 6–16, expectorate after use and rinse mouth thoroughly.

HOW SUPPLIED
1.8 oz. (51g) net wt. tubes.
NDC# 0126-0287-66
Twin Pack (two 1.8 oz.(51g) net wt. tubes.)
NDC# 0126-0287-33
STORAGE: Store at Controlled Room Temperature, 20–25°C (68–77°F).
CAUTION: Rx only

REFERENCES
1. Accepted Dental Therapeutics, Ed. 40, ADA, Chicago. P. 405-407, 1984. 2. Englander HR, Keyes et al: JADA 75:638-644, 1967. 3. Englander HR, et al: JADA 78:783-787, 1969. 4. Englander HR, et al: JADA 83:354-358, 1971.
Part # P005202
Rev 8/97

For information on over-the-counter drugs, consult **PDR For Nonprescription Drugs**.

Connetics Corporation
3400 WEST BAYSHORE ROAD
PALO ALTO, CA 94303

Direct Inquiries to:
(650) 843–2800

RIDAURA® ℞
[*rĭ-dăură*]
auranofin
Capsules

PRESCRIBING INFORMATION

> Ridaura (auranofin) contains gold and, like other gold-containing drugs, can cause gold toxicity, signs of which include: fall in hemoglobin, leukopenia below 4,000 WBC/cu mm, granulocytes below 1,500/cu mm, decrease in platelets below 150,000/cu mm, proteinuria, hematuria, pruritus, rash, stomatitis or persistent diarrhea. Therefore, the results of recommended laboratory work (See PRECAUTIONS) should be reviewed before writing each *Ridaura* prescription. Like other gold preparations, *Ridaura* is only indicated for use in selected patients with active rheumatoid arthritis. Physicians planning to use *Ridaura* should be experienced with chrysotherapy and should thoroughly familiarize themselves with the toxicity and benefits of *Ridaura*.
> In addition, the following precautions should be routinely employed:
> 1. The possibility of adverse reactions should be explained to patients before starting therapy.
> 2. Patients should be advised to report promptly any symptoms suggesting toxicity. (See PRECAUTIONS—Information for Patients.)

DESCRIPTION
Radaura (auranofin) is available in oral form as capsules containing 3 mg auranofin.
Auranofin is (2,3,4,6–tetra-O-acetyl-1-thio-β-D-glucopyranosato-S-) (triethylphosphine) gold.
Auranofin contains 29% gold and has the following chemical structure:

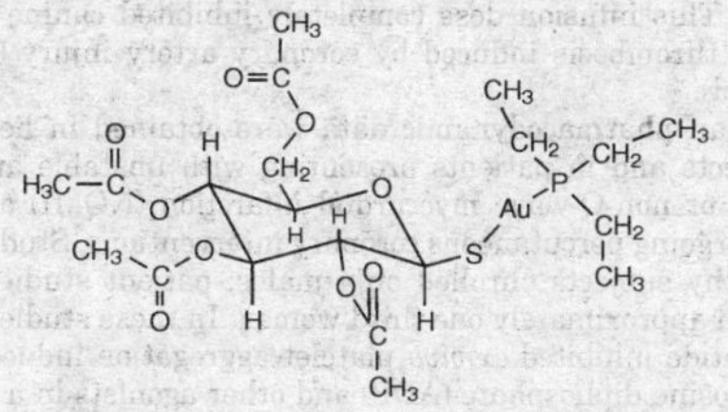

Each *Ridaura* capsule, with opaque brown cap and opaque tan body, contains auranofin, 3 mg, and is imprinted with the product name RIDAURA. Inactive ingredients consist of benzyl alcohol, cellulose, cetylpyridinium chloride, D&C Red No. 33, FD&C Blue No. 1, FD&C Red No. 40, FD&C Yellow No. 6, gelatin, lactose, magnesium stearate, povidone, sodium lauryl sulfate, sodium starch glycolate, starch, titanium dioxide and trace amounts of other inactive ingredients.

CLINICAL PHARMACOLOGY
The mechanism of action of Ridaura (auranofin) is not understood. In patients with adult rheumatoid arthritis, *Ridaura* may modify disease activity as manifested by synovitis and associated symptoms, and reflected by laboratory parameters such as ESR. There is no substantial evidence, however, that gold-containing compounds induce remission of rheumatoid arthritis.
Pharmacokinetics: Pharmacokinetic studies were performed in rheumatoid arthritis patients, not in normal volunteers. Auranofin is rapidly metabolized and intact auranofin has never been detected in the blood. Thus, studies of the pharmacokinetics of auranofin have involved measurement of gold concentrations. Approximately 25% of the gold in auranofin is absorbed.
The mean terminal plasma half-life of auranofin gold at steady state was 26 days (range 21 to 31 days; n=5). The mean terminal body half-life was 80 days (range 42 to 128; n=5). Approximately 60% of the absorbed gold (15% of the administered dose) from a single dose of auranofin is excreted in urine, the remainder is excreted in the feces.
In clinical studies, steady state blood-gold concentrations are achieved in about three months. In patients on 6 mg auranofin/day, mean steady state blood-gold concentrations were 0.68 ±0.45 mcg/mL (n=63 patients). In blood, approximately 40% of auranofin gold is associated with red cells, and 60% associated with serum proteins. In contrast, 99% of injectable gold is associated with serum proteins.
Mean blood-gold concentrations are proportional to dose; however, no correlation between blood-gold concentrations and safety or efficacy has been established.

INDICATIONS AND USAGE
Ridaura (auranofin) is indicated in the management of adults with active classical or definite rheumatoid arthritis (ARA criteria) who have had an insufficient therapeutic response to, or are intolerant of, an adequate trial of full doses of one or more nonsteroidal anti-inflammatory drugs. *Ridaura* should be added to a comprehensive baseline program, including non-drug therapies.
Unlike anti-inflammatory drugs, *Ridaura* does not produce an immediate response. Therapeutic effects may be seen after three to four months of treatment, although improvement has not been seen in some patients before six months. When cartilage and bone damage has already occurred, gold cannot reverse structural damage to joints caused by previous disease. The greatest potential benefit occurs in patients with active synovitis, particularly in its early stage. In controlled clinical trials comparing *Ridaura* with injectable gold, *Ridaura* was associated with fewer dropouts due to adverse reactions, while injectable gold was associated with fewer dropouts for inadequate or poor therapeutic effect. Physicians should consider these findings when deciding on the use of *Ridaura* in patients who are candidates for chrysotherapy.

CONTRAINDICATIONS
Ridaura (auranofin) is contraindicated in patients with a history of any of the following gold-induced disorders: anaphylactic reactions, necrotizing enterocolitis, pulmonary fibrosis, exfoliative dermatitis, bone marrow aplasia or other severe hematologic disorders.

WARNINGS
Danger signs of possible gold toxicity include fall in hemoglobin, leukopenia below 4,000 WBC/cu mm, granulocytes below 1,500/cu mm, decrease in platelets below 150,000/cu mm, proteinuria, hematuria, pruritus, rash, stomatitis or persistent diarrhea.
Thrombocytopenia has occurred in 1–3% of patients (See ADVERSE REACTIONS) treated with Ridaura (auranofin), some of whom developed bleeding. The thrombocytopenia usually appears to be peripheral in origin and is usually reversible upon withdrawal of *Ridaura*. Its onset bears no relationship to the duration of *Ridaura* therapy and its course may be rapid. While patients' platelet counts should normally be monitored at least monthly (See PRECAUTIONS—Laboratory Tests), the occurrence of a precipitous decline in platelets or a platelet count less than 100,000/cu mm or signs and symptoms (e.g., purpura, ecchymoses or petechiae) suggestive of thrombocytopenia indicates a need to immediately withdraw *Ridaura* and other therapies with the potential to cause thrombocytopenia, and to obtain additional platelet counts. No additional *Ridaura* should be given unless the thrombocytopenia resolves and further studies show it was not due to gold therapy.
Proteinuria has developed in 3–9% of patients (See ADVERSE REACTIONS) treated with *Ridaura*. If clinically significant proteinuria or microscopic hematuria is found (See PRECAUTIONS—Laboratory Tests), *Ridaura* and other therapies with the potential to cause proteinuria or microscopic hematuria should be stopped immediately.

PRECAUTIONS
General: The safety of concomitant use of Ridaura (auranofin) with injectable gold, hydroxychloroquine, penicillamine, immunosuppressive agents (e.g., cyclophosphamide, azathioprine, or methotrexate) or high doses of corticosteroids has not been established.
Medical problems that might affect the signs or symptoms used to detect *Ridaura* toxicity should be under control before starting Ridaura (auranofin).
The potential benefits of using *Ridaura* in patients with progressive renal disease, significant hepatocellular disease, inflammatory bowel disease, skin rash or history of bone marrow depression should be weighed against 1) the potential risks of gold toxicity on organ systems previously compromised or with decreased reserve, and 2) the difficulty in quickly detecting and correctly attributing the toxic effect.
The following adverse reactions have been reported with the use of gold preparations and require modification of *Ridaura* treatment or additional monitoring. See ADVERSE REACTIONS for the approximate incidence of those reactions specifically reported with *Ridaura*.
Gastrointestinal Reactions: Gastrointestinal reactions reported with gold therapy include diarrhea/loose stools, nausea, vomiting, anorexia and abdominal cramps. The most common reaction to *Ridaura* is diarrhea/loose stools reported in approximately 50% of the patients. This is generally manageable by reducing the dosage (e.g., from 6 mg to 3 mg) and in only 6% of the patients is it necessary to discontinue Ridaura (auranofin) permanently.
Ulcerative enterocolitis is a rare serious gold reaction. Therefore, patients with gastrointestinal symptoms should be monitored for the appearance of gastrointestinal bleeding.
Cutaneous Reactions: Dermatitis is the most common reaction to injectable gold therapy and the second most common reaction to *Ridaura*. *Any eruption, especially if pruritic, that develops during treatment should be considered a gold reaction until proven otherwise.* Pruritus often exists before dermatitis becomes apparent, and therefore should be considered to be a warning signal of a cutaneous reaction. Gold dermatitis may be aggravated by exposure to sunlight or an actinic rash may develop. The most serious form of cutaneous reaction reported with injectable gold is generalized exfoliative dermatitis.
Mucous Membrane Reactions: Stomatitis, another common gold reaction, may be manifested by shallow ulcers on the buccal membranes, on the borders of the tongue, and on the palate or in the pharynx. Stomatitis may occur as the only adverse reaction or with a dermatitis. Sometimes diffuse glossitis or gingivitis develops. A metallic taste may precede these oral mucous membrane reactions and should be considered a warning signal.
Renal Reactions: Gold can produce a nephrotic syndrome or glomerulitis with proteinuria and hematuria. These renal reactions are usually relatively mild and subside completely if recognized early and treatment is discontinued. They may become severe and chronic if treatment is continued after the onset of the reaction. *Therefore it is important to perform urinalyses regularly* and to discontinue treatment promptly if proteinuria or hematuria develops.
Hematologic Reactions: Blood dyscrasias including leukopenia, granulocytopenia, thrombocytopenia and aplastic anemia have all been reported as reactions to injectable gold and *Ridaura*. These reactions may occur separately or in combination at anytime during treatment. Because they have potentially serious consequences, *blood dyscrasias should be constantly watched for through regular monitoring (at least monthly) of the formed elements of the blood throughout treatment.*
Miscellaneous Reactions: Rare reactions attributed to gold include cholestatic jaundice; gold bronchitis and interstitial pneumonitis and fibrosis; peripheral neuropathy; partial or complete hair loss; fever.
Information for Patients: Patients should be advised of the possibility of toxicity from *Ridaura* and of the signs and symptoms that they should report promptly. (Patient information sheets are available.)
Women of childbearing potential should be warned of the potential risks of *Ridaura* therapy during pregnancy (See PRECAUTIONS—Pregnancy).
Laboratory Tests: CBC with differential, platelet count, urinalysis, and renal and liver function tests should be performed prior to Ridaura (auranofin) therapy to establish a baseline and to identify any preexisting conditions.
CBC with differential, platelet count and urinalysis should then be monitored at least monthly; other parameters should be monitored as appropriate.
Drug Interactions: In a single patient-report, there is the suggestion that concurrent administration of *Ridaura* and phenytoin may have increased phenytoin blood levels.
Carcinogenesis/Mutagenesis: In a 24-month study in rats, animals treated with auranofin at 0.4, 1.0 or 2.5 mg/kg/day orally (3, 8 or 21 times the human dose) or gold sodium thiomalate at 2 or 6 mg/kg injected twice weekly (4 or 12 times the human dose) were compared to untreated control animals.
There was a significant increase in the frequency of renal tubular cell karyomegaly and cytomegaly and renal adenoma in the animals treated with 1.0 or 2.5 mg/kg/day of auranofin and 2 or 6 mg/kg twice weekly of gold sodium thiomalate. Malignant renal epithelial tumors were seen in the 1.0 mg/kg/day and the 2.5 mg/kg/day auranofin and in the 6 mg/kg twice weekly gold sodium thiomalate-treated animals.
In a 12-month study, rats treated with auranofin at 23 mg/kg/day (192 times the human dose) developed tumors of the renal tubular epithelium, whereas those treated with 3.6 mg/kg/day (30 times the human dose) did not.
In an 18-month study in mice given oral auranofin at doses of 1, 3 and 9 mg/kg/day (8, 24 and 72 times the human dose), there was no statistically significant increase above controls in the instances of tumors.
In the mouse lymphoma forward mutation assay, auranofin at high concentrations (313 to 700 ng/mL) induced increases in the mutation frequencies in the presence of a rat liver microsomal preparation. Auranofin produced no mutation effects in the Ames test (Salmonella), in the *in vitro* assay (Forward and Reverse Mutation Inducement Assay with Saccharomyces), in the *in vitro* transformation of BALB/T3 cell mouse assay or in the Dominant Lethal Assay.
Pregnancy: Teratogenic Effects—Pregnancy Category C. Use of Ridaura (auranofin) by pregnant women is not recommended. Furthermore, women of childbearing potential

Continued on next page

Ridaura—Cont.

should be warned of the potential risks of *Ridaura* therapy during pregnancy (See below.)

Pregnant rabbits given auranofin at doses of 0.5, 3 or 6 mg/kg/day (4.2 to 50 times the human dose) had impaired food intake, decreased maternal weights, decreased fetal weights and an increase above controls in the incidence of resorptions, abortions and congenital abnormalities, mainly abdominal defects such as gastroschisis and umbilical hernia.

Pregnant rats given auranofin at a dose of 5 mg/kg/day (42 times the human dose) had an increase above controls in the incidence of resorptions and a decrease in litter size and weight linked to maternal toxicity. No such effects were found in rats given 2.5 mg/kg/day (21 times the human dose).

Pregnant mice given auranofin at a dose of 5 mg/kg/day (42 times the human dose) had no teratogenic effects.

There are no adequate and well-controlled *Ridaura* studies in pregnant women.

Nursing Mothers: Nursing during *Ridaura* therapy is not recommended. Following auranofin administration to rats and mice, gold is excreted in milk. Following the administration of injectable gold, gold appears in the milk of nursing women; human data on auranofin are not available.

Pediatric Use: Riduara (auranofin) is not recommended for use in pediatric patients because its safety and effectiveness have not been established.

ADVERSE REACTIONS

The adverse reactions incidences listed below are based on observations of 1) 4,784 *Ridaura*-treated patients in clinical trials (2,474 U.S., 2,310 foreign), of whom 2,729 were treated more than one year and 573 for more than three years; and 2) postmarketing experience. The highest incidence is during the first six months of treatment; however, reactions can occur after many months of therapy. With rare exceptions, all patients were on concomitant nonsteroidal anti-inflammatory therapy; some of them were also taking low dosages of corticosteroids

Reactions occurring in more than 1% of *Ridaura*-treated patients

Gastrointestinal: loose stools or diarrhea (47%); abdominal pain (14%); nausea with or without vomiting (10%); constipation; anorexia*; flatulence*; dyspepsia*; dysgeusia.

Dermatological: rash (24%); pruritus (17%); hair loss; urticaria.

Mucous Membrane: stomatitis (13%); conjunctivitis*; glossitis.

Hematological: anemia; leukopenia; thrombocytopenia; eosinophilia.

Renal: proteinuria*; hematuria.

Hepatic: elevated liver enzymes.

---

* Reactions marked with an asterisk occurred in 3–9% of the patients. The other reactions listed occurred in 1–3%.

Reactions occurring in less than 1% of *Ridaura*-treated patients

Gastrointestinal: dysphagia; gastointestinal bleeding†; melena†; positive stool for occult blood†; ulcerative enterocolitis.

Dermatological: angioedema.

Mucous Membrane: gingivitis†.

Hematological: aplastic anemia; neutropenia†; agranulocytosis; pure red call aplasia; pancytopenia.

Hepatic: jaundice.

Respiratory: interstitial pneumonitis.

Neurological: peripheral neuropathy.

Ocular: gold deposits in the lens or cornea unassociated clinically with eye disorders or visual impairment.

---

† Reactions marked with a dagger occurred in 0.1–1% of the patients. The other reactions listed occurred in less than 0.1%.

Reactions reported with injectable gold preparations, but not with Ridaura (auranofin) (based on clinical trials and on postmarketing experience)

Cutaneous Reactions: generalized exfoliative dermatitis.

Incidence of Adverse Reactions for Specific Categories— 18 Comparative Trials

	Ridaura (445 patients)	Injectable Gold (445 patients)
Proteinuria	0.9%	5.4%
Rash	26%	39%
Diarrhea	42.5%	13%
Stomatitis	13%	18%
Anemia	3.1%	2.7%
Leukopenia	1.3%	2.2%
Thrombocytopenia	0.9%	2.2%

Elevated liver function tests	1.9%	1.7%
Pulmonary	0.2%	0.2%

OVERDOSAGE

The acute oral LD_{50} for auranofin is 310 mg/kg in adult mice and 265 mg/kg in adult rats. The minimum lethal dose in rats is 30 mg/kg.

In case of acute overdosage, immediate induction of emesis or gastric lavage and appropriate supportive therapy are recommended.

Ridaura overdosage experience is limited. A 50-year-old female, previously on 6 mg *Ridaura* daily, took 27 mg (9 capsules) daily for 10 days and developed an encephalopathy and peripheral neuropathy. *Ridaura* was discontinued and she eventually recovered.

There has been no experience with treating *Ridaura* overdosage with modalities such as chelating agents. However, they have been used with injectable gold and may be considered for *Ridaura* overdosage.

DOSAGE AND ADMINISTRATION

Usual Adult Dosage: The usual adult dosage of Ridaura (auranofin) is 6 mg daily, given either as 3 mg twice daily or 6 mg once daily. Initiation of therapy at dosages exceeding 6 mg daily is not recommended because it is associated with an increased incidence of diarrhea. If response is inadequate after six months, an increase to 9 mg (3 mg three times daily) may be tolerated. If response remains inadequate after a three-month trial of 9 mg daily, *Ridaura* therapy should be discontinued. Safety at dosages exceeding 9 mg daily has not been studied.

Transferring from Injectable Gold: In controlled clinical studies, patients on injectable gold have been transferred to Ridaura (auranofin) by discontinuing the injectable agent and starting oral therapy with *Ridaura*, 6 mg daily. When patients are transferred to *Ridaura*, they should be informed of its adverse reaction profile, in particular the gastrointestinal reactions. (See PRECAUTIONS—Information for Patients.) At six months, control of disease activity of patients transferred to *Ridaura* and those maintained on the injectable agent was not different. Data beyond six months are not available.

HOW SUPPLIED

Capsules, containing 3 mg auranofin, in bottles of 60.

NDC 63032-011-60

STORAGE AND HANDLING

Store between 15° and 30°C (59° and 86°F). Dispense in a tight, light-resistant container.

REVISED JANUARY, 1998

© Connetics, 1998

Manufactured for
Connetics Corporation
Palo Alto, CA 94303

by SmithKline Beecham
Pharmaceuticals
Philadelphia, PA 19101
RI:L33
685700
LB0101

Shown in Product Identification Guide, page 309

COR Therapeutics, Inc.
**256 EAST GRAND AVENUE
SOUTH SAN FRANCISCO, CA 94080**

Direct Inquiries to:
Ph: 1-888-267-4-MED

INTEGRILIN™   ℞
[*in-tĕg-rĭl-in*]
**(eptifibatide)
Injection**

For Intravenous Administration

DESCRIPTION

Eptifibatide is a cyclic heptapeptide containing six amino acids and one mercaptopropionyl (des-amino cysteinyl) residue. An interchain disulfide bridge is formed between the cysteine amide and the mercaptopropionyl moieties. Chemically it is N^6-(aminoiminomethyl)-N^2-(3-mercapto-1-oxopropyl-L-lysylglycyl-L-α-aspartyl-L-tryptophyl-L-prolyl-L-cysteinamide, cyclic (1→6)-disulfide. Eptifibatide binds to the platelet receptor glycoprotein (GP) IIb/IIIa of human platelets and inhibits platelet aggregation.

The eptifibatide peptide is produced by solution-phase peptide synthesis, and is purified by preparative reverse-phase liquid chromatography and lyophilized. The structural formula is:

$C_{35}H_{49}N_{11}O_9S_2$ Mol Wt. 831.96

INTEGRILIN (eptifibatide) Injection is a clear, colorless, sterile, non-pyrogenic solution for intravenous (IV) use. Each 10-mL vial contains 2 mg/mL of eptifibatide and each 100-mL vial contains 0.75 mg/mL of eptifibatide. Each vial of either size also contains 5.25 mg/mL citric acid and sodium hydroxide to adjust the pH to 5.25.

CLINICAL PHARMACOLOGY

Mechanism of Action. Eptifibatide reversibly inhibits platelet aggregation by preventing the binding of fibrinogen, von Willebrand factor, and other adhesive ligands to GP IIb/IIIa. When administered intravenously, eptifibatide inhibits *ex vivo* platelet aggregation in a dose- and concentration-dependent manner. Platelet aggregation inhibition is reversible following cessation of the eptifibatide infusion; this is thought to result from dissociation of eptifibatide from the platelet.

Pharmacodynamics. Infusion of eptifibatide into baboons caused a dose-dependent inhibition of *ex vivo* platelet aggregation, with complete inhibition of aggregation achieved at infusion rates greater than 5 µg/kg/min. In a baboon model that is refractory to aspirin and heparin, doses of eptifibatide that inhibit aggregation prevented acute thrombosis with only a modest prolongation (2- to 3-fold) of the bleeding time. Platelet aggregation in dogs was also inhibited by infusions of eptifibatide, with complete inhibition at 2 µg/kg/min. This infusion dose completely inhibited canine coronary thrombosis induced by coronary artery injury (Folts model).

Human pharmacodynamic data were obtained in healthy subjects and in patients presenting with unstable angina (UA) or non-Q-wave myocardial infarction (NQMI) and/or undergoing percutaneous coronary interventions. Studies in healthy subjects enrolled only males; patient studies enrolled approximately one third women. In these studies, eptifibatide inhibited *ex vivo* platelet aggregation induced by adenosine diphosphate (ADP) and other agonists in a dose- and concentration-dependent manner. The effect of eptifibatide was observed immediately after administration of a 180 µg/kg intravenous bolus. Table 1 shows the effects on platelet function and bleeding time of the doses of eptifibatide used in the two principal clinical studies.

Table 1
Platelet Inhibition and Bleeding Time

	IMPACT II 135/0.5	PURSUIT 180/2.0
Inhibition of platelet aggregation 15 min. after bolus	69%	84%
Inhibition of platelet aggregation at steady state	40–50%	>90%
Bleeding-time prolongation at steady state	<5×	<5×
Inhibition of platelet aggregation 4h after infusion discontinuation	<30%	<50%
Bleeding-time prolongation 6h after infusion discontinuation	1×	1.4×

When administered alone, eptifibatide has no measurable effect on prothrombin time (PT) or activated partial thromboplastin time (aPTT). (See also PRECAUTIONS: Drug Interactions.)

There were no important differences between men and women or between age groups in the pharmacodynamics properties of eptifibatide. Differences among ethnic groups have not been assessed.

Pharmacokinetics. The pharmacokinetics of eptifibatide are linear and dose-proportional for bolus doses ranging from 90 to 250 µg/kg and infusion rates from 0.5 to 3 µg/kg/min. Plasma elimination half-life is approximately 2.5

hours. The recommended regimens of a bolus followed by an infusion produce an early peak level, followed by a small decline with attainment of steady state within 4–6 hours. The extent of eptifibatide binding to human plasma protein is about 25%.

Excretion and Metabolism. Clearance in patients with coronary artery disease is 55–58 mL/kg/h. In healthy subjects, renal clearance accounts for approximately 50% of total body clearance, with the majority of the drug excreted in the urine as eptifibatide, deamidated eptifibatide, and other, more polar metabolites. No major metabolites have been detected in human plasma. Clinical studies have included 2418 patients with serum creatinine between 1 and 2 mg/dL (for the 180 µg/kg bolus and the 2 µg/kg/min infusion) and 7 patients with serum creatinine between 2 and 4 mg/dL (for the 135 µg/kg bolus and the 0.5 µg/kg/min infusion), without dose adjustment. No data are available in patients with more severe degrees of renal impairment, but plasma eptifibatide levels are expected to be higher in such patients (see CONTRAINDICATIONS).

Special Populations. Patients in clinical studies were older than the subjects in clinical pharmacology studies, and they had lower total body eptifibatide clearance and higher eptifibatide plasma levels. Clinical studies were conducted in patients aged 20 to 94 years with coronary artery disease without dose adjustment for age. Because patients over 75 years of age were enrolled into the PURSUIT clinical study only if their body weight exceeded 50 kg, minimal data are available on lighter-weight patients over 75 years of age. Men and women showed no important differences in the pharmacokinetics of eptifibatide.

CLINICAL STUDIES

Eptifibatide was studied in two placebo-controlled, randomized studies, one (PURSUIT) in patients with acute coronary syndrome (unstable angina (UA) or non-Q-wave myocardial infarction (NQMI)), the other (IMPACT II) in patients about to undergo a percutaneous cardiovascular intervention (PCI; balloon angioplasty in most cases, but sometimes directional atherectomy, transluminal extraction catheter atherectomy, rotational ablation atherectomy, or excimer-laser angioplasty).

Acute coronary syndrome is defined as prolonged (≥10 minutes) symptoms of cardiac ischemia within the previous 24 hours associated with either ST-segment changes (elevation between 0.6 mm and 1 mm or depression >0.5 mm), T-wave inversion (>1 mm), or positive CK-MB. This definition includes "unstable angina" and "non-Q-wave myocardial infarction" but excludes myocardial infarction that is associated with Q waves or greater degrees of ST-segment elevation.

PURSUIT was a 726-center, 27-country, double-blind, randomized, placebo-controlled study in 10,948 patients presenting with UA or NQMI. Patients could be enrolled only if they had experienced cardiac ischemia at rest (≥10 minutes) within the previous 24 hours and had either ST-segment changes (elevations between 0.6 mm and 1 mm or depression >0.5 mm), T-wave inversion (>1 mm), or increased CK-MB. Important exclusion criteria included a history of bleeding diathesis, evidence of abnormal bleeding within the previous 30 days, uncontrolled hypertension, major surgery within the previous 6 weeks, stroke within the previous 30 days, any history of hemorrhagic stroke, serum creatinine >2 mg/dL, dependency on renal dialysis, or platelet count <100,000/mm³.

Patients were randomized to either placebo, eptifibatide 180 µg/kg bolus followed by a 2 µg/kg/min infusion (180/2.0), or eptifibatide 180 µg/kg bolus followed by a 1.3 µg/kg/min infusion (180/1.3). The infusion was continued for 72 hours, until hospital discharge, or until the time of coronary artery bypass grafting (CABG), whichever occurred first, except that if PCI was performed, the eptifibatide infusion was continued for 24 hours after the procedure, allowing for a duration of infusion up to 96 hours.

The lower-infusion-rate arm was stopped after the first interim analysis when the two active-treatment arms appeared to have the same incidence of bleeding.

Patient age ranged from 20 to 94 (mean 63) years, and 65% were male. The patients were 89% Caucasian, 6% Hispanic, and 5% Black, recruited in the United States and Canada (40%), Western Europe (39%), Eastern Europe (16%), and Latin America (5%).

This was a "real world" study; each patient was managed according to the usual standards of the investigational site; frequencies of angiography, PCI, and CABG therefore differed widely from site to site and from country to country. Of the patients in PURSUIT, 13% were managed with PCI during drug infusion, of whom 50% received intracoronary stents; 87% were managed medically (without PCI during drug infusion).

The majority of patients received aspirin (75–325 mg once daily). Heparin was administered intravenously or subcutaneously, at the physician's discretion, most commonly as an intravenous bolus of 5000 U followed by a continuous infusion of 1000 U/h. For patients weighing less than 70 kg, the recommended heparin bolus dose was 60 U/kg followed by a

continuous infusion of 12 U/kg/h. A target aPTT of 50–70 seconds was recommended. A total of 1250 patients underwent PCI within 72 hours after randomization, in which case they received intravenous heparin to maintain an activated clotting time (ACT) of 300–350 seconds.

The primary endpoint of the study was the occurrence of death from any cause or new myocardial infarction (MI) (evaluated by a blinded Clinical Endpoints Committee) within 30 days of randomization.

Compared to placebo, eptifibatide administered as a 180 µg/kg bolus followed by a 2 µg/kg/min infusion significantly (p=0.042) reduced the incidence of endpoint events (see Table 2). The reduction in the incidence of endpoint events in patients receiving eptifibatide was evident early during treatment, and this reduction was maintained through at least 30 days (see Figure 1). Table 2 also shows the incidence of the components of the primary endpoint, death (whether or not preceded by an MI) and new MI in surviving patients at 30 days.

[See table 2 above]

Figure 1
Kaplan-Meier Plot of Time to Death or Myocardial Infarction Within 30 Days of Randomization

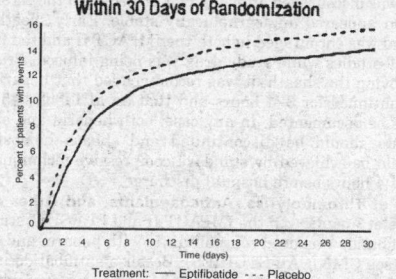

Treatment: —— Eptifibatide - - - Placebo

The effect of eptifibatide in PURSUIT did not appear to vary with patients' age. There were too few non-Caucasian patients to reach any conclusion as to possible differences related to race. Analysis of the PURSUIT results reveals a complex interaction of treatment, gender, and region. Throughout the world, eptifibatide was significantly less beneficial in women than in men, and in the overall study eptifibatide in women was nonsignificantly worse than placebo. These results were, however, strikingly heterogeneous across the several regions; eptifibatide appeared much worse than placebo in women in Latin America, while effects in men and women were scarcely distinguishable (rel-

ative risk reductions of 23% and 18%, respectively) in the U.S. and Canada. These results may reflect (a) genuine biological interactions between eptifibatide and gender, (b) interactions between eptifibatide and unknown international differences in concomitant therapy delivered to men and women, and (c) the play of chance, but the relative contributions of these possible factors are unknown. Treatment with eptifibatide reduced clinical events in patients undergoing PCI during drug administration and in those receiving medical management alone. Table 3 shows the incidence of death or MI within 72 hours of randomization.

Table 3
Clinical Events (Death or MI) in the PURSUIT Study Within 72 Hours of Randomization

	Placebo	Eptifibatide 180/2.0
Overall Patient Population	n=4739	n=4722
–At 72 hours	7.6%	5.9%
Patients undergoing early PCI	n=631	n=619
–Pre-procedure (nonfatal MI only)	5.5%	1.8%
–At 72 hours	14.4%	9.0%
Patients not undergoing early PCI	n=4108	n=4103
–At 72 hours	6.5%	5.4%

All of the effect of eptifibatide was established within 72 hours (during the period of drug infusion), regardless of management strategy. Moreover, for patients undergoing early PCI, a reduction in events was evident prior to the procedure.

IMPACT II was a multi-center, double-blind, randomized, placebo-controlled study conducted in the United States in 4010 patients undergoing PCI. Major exclusion criteria included a history of bleeding diathesis, major surgery within 6 weeks of treatment, gastrointestinal bleeding within 30 days, any stroke or structural CNS abnormality, uncontrolled hypertension, PT >1.2 times control, hematocrit <30%, platelet count <100,000/mm³, and pregnancy. Patient age ranged from 24 to 89 (mean 60) years, and 75% were male. The patients were 92% Caucasian, 5% Black, and 3% Hispanic. Patients were randomly assigned to one of three treatment regimens, each incorporating a bolus dose initiated immediately prior to PCI followed by a continuous infusion lasting 20–24 hours: 1) 135 µg/kg bolus followed by

Table 2
Clinical Events in The PURSUIT Study

Death or MI	Placebo (n = 4739) n (%)	Eptifibatide (180/2.0) (n = 4722) n (%)	p-value
3 days	359 (7.6%)	279 (5.9%)	0.001
7 days	552 (11.6%)	477 (10.1%)	0.016
30 days			
Death or MI (Primary Endpoint)	745 (15.7%)	672 (14.2%)	0.042
Death	177 (3.7%)	165 (3.5%)	
Nonfatal MI	568 (12.0%)	507 (10.7%)	

Table 4
Clinical Events in the IMPACT II Study

	Placebo n (%)	Eptifibatide (135/0.5) n (%)	Eptifibatide (135/0.75) n (%)
Patients	1285	1300	1286
Abrupt Closure	65 (5.1%)	36 (2.8%)	43 (3.3%)
p-value vs. placebo		0.003	0.030
Death, MI, or Urgent Intervention			
24 hours	123 (9.6%)	86 (6.6%)	89 (6.9%)
p-value vs. placebo		0.006	0.014
48 hours	131 (10.2%)	99 (7.6%)	102 (7.9%)
p-value vs. placebo		0.021	0.045
30 days (primary endpoint)	149 (11.6%)	118 (9.1%)	128 (10.0%)
p-value vs. placebo		0.035	0.179
Death or MI			
30 days	110 (8.6%)	89 (6.8%)	95 (7.4%)
p-value vs. placebo		0.102	0.272
6 months	151 (11.9%)*	136 (10.6%)*	130 (10.3%)*
p-value vs. placebo		0.297	0.182

*Kaplan-Meier estimate of event rate

Continued on next page

Consult 1999 PDR® supplements and future editions for revisions

Integrilin—Cont.

a continuous infusion of 0.5 µg/kg/min of eptifibatide (135/0.5); 2) 135 µg/kg bolus followed by a continuous infusion of 0.75 µg/kg/min of eptifibatide (135/0.75); or 3) a matching placebo bolus followed by a matching placebo continuous infusion. Each patient received aspirin and an intravenous heparin bolus of 100 U/kg, with additional bolus infusions of up to 2000 additional units of heparin every 15 minutes to maintain an activated clotting time (ACT) of 300–350 seconds.

The primary endpoint was the composite of death, MI, or urgent revascularization, analyzed at 30 days after randomization in all patients who received at least one dose of study drug.

As shown in Table 4, each eptifibatide regimen reduced the rate of death, MI, or urgent intervention, although at 30 days, this finding was statistically significant only in the lower-dose eptifibatide group. As in the PURSUIT study, the effects of eptifibatide were seen early and persisted throughout the 30-day period.

[See table 4 on previous page]

At the time of randomization, approximately 25% of the IMPACT II patients suffered from only chronic stable angina, or had had no angina at all since a remote (more than 14 days prior) myocardial infarction. At the other extreme, approximately 40% of the IMPACT II patients had ongoing acute coronary syndromes, including patients with rest angina, others with refractory recurrent angina, others with early post-infarction angina, and others about to receive percutaneous interventions during or immediately following acute myocardial infarction. The remaining patients had various histories of recent and remote acute coronary syndromes; data are not available to describe what fraction of these underwent PCI within only a day or two of an acute episode. The IMPACT II study was not powered to obtain stable estimates of efficacy in subpopulations defined by degree of acuity, but (as shown in Table 5) the data suggest that the benefit of eptifibatide was not limited to patients with ongoing acute coronary syndromes.

[See table 5 above]

INDICATIONS AND USAGE

INTEGRILIN is indicated:
- For the treatment of patients with acute coronary syndrome (UA/NQMI), including patients who are to be managed medically and those undergoing percutaneous coronary intervention (PCI). In this setting, INTEGRILIN has been shown to decrease the rate of a combined endpoint of death or new myocardial infarction.
- For the treatment of patients undergoing PCI. In this setting, INTEGRILIN has been shown to decrease the rate of a combined endpoint of death, new myocardial infarction, or need for urgent intervention.

In the clinical studies of eptifibatide, most patients received heparin and aspirin, as described in CLINICAL TRIALS.

CONTRAINDICATIONS

Treatment with eptifibatide is contraindicated in patients with:
- A history of bleeding diathesis, or evidence of active abnormal bleeding within the previous 30 days.
- Severe hypertension (systolic blood pressure >200 mm Hg or diastolic blood pressure >110 mm Hg) not adequately controlled on antihypertensive therapy.
- Major surgery within the preceding 6 weeks.
- History of stroke within 30 days or any history of hemorrhagic stroke.
- Current or planned administration of another parenteral GP IIb/IIIa inhibitor.
- Platelet count <100,000/mm^3.
- Serum creatinine ≥2.0 mg/dL (for the 180 µg/kg bolus and the 2 µg/kg/min infusion) or ≥4.0 mg/dL (for the 135 µg/kg bolus and the 0.5 µg/kg/min infusion).
- Dependency on renal dialysis.
- Known hypersensitivity to any component of the product.

WARNINGS

Bleeding. Bleeding is the most common complication encountered during eptifibatide therapy. Administration of eptifibatide is associated with an increase in major and minor bleeding, as classified by the criteria of the Thrombolysis in Myocardial Infarction Study group (TIMI), (see ADVERSE REACTIONS). Most major bleeding associated with eptifibatide has been at the arterial access site for cardiac catheterization or from the gastrointestinal or genitourinary tract.

In patients undergoing percutaneous coronary interventions, patients receiving eptifibatide experience an increased incidence of major bleeding compared to those receiving placebo. Special care should be employed to minimize the risk of bleeding among these patients (see PRECAUTIONS).

If bleeding cannot be controlled with pressure, infusion of eptifibatide and concomitant heparin should be stopped immediately.

PRECAUTIONS

Bleeding Precautions
Care of the Femoral Artery Access Site in Patients Undergoing Percutaneous Coronary Intervention (PCI). In patients undergoing PCI, treatment with eptifibatide is

Table 5
Clinical Events at 30 Days in the IMPACT II Study, Stratified by Acuity at Time of Randomization

Classification of Patients (%)	Placebo n (%)	Eptifibatide 135/0.5 n (%)	Eptifibatide 135/0.75 n (%)
Ongoing ACS, MI ongoing or within past 24h(41.3%)	538 (11.5%)	532 (10.0%)	527 (10.6%)
Others (58.7%)	747 (11.6%)	768 (8.5%)	759 (9.5%)

Table 6
Major Bleeding by Maximal aPTT Within 72 Hours in the PURSUIT Study

	Placebo n (%)	Eptifibatide 180/1.3* n (%)	Eptifibatide 180/2.0 n (%)
Maximum aPTT (seconds)			
<50	44/721(6.1%)	21/244(8.6%)	44/743(5.9%)
50–70 (recommended)	92/908(10.1%)	28/259(10.8%)	99/883(11.2%)
>70	281/2786(10.1%)	99/891(11.1%)	345/2811(12.3%)

*Administered only until the first interim analysis

Table 7
Bleeding Events and Transfusions in the PURSUIT and IMPACT II Studies

PURSUIT

	Placebo n (%)	Eptifibatide 180/1.3* n (%)	Eptifibatide 180/2.0 n (%)
Patients	4696	1472	4679
Major bleeding[a]	425 (9.3%)	152 (10.5%)	498 (10.8%)
Minor bleeding[a]	347 (7.6%)	152 (10.5%)	604 (13.1%)
Requiring Transfusions[b]	490 (10.4%)	188 (12.8%)	601 (12.8%)

IMPACT II

	Placebo n (%)	Eptifibatide 135/0.5 n (%)	Eptifibatide 135/0.75 n (%)
Patients	1285	1300	1286
Major bleeding[a]	55 (4.5%)	55 (4.4%)	58 (4.7%)
Minor bleeding[a]	115 (9.3%)	146 (11.7%)	177 (14.2%)
Requiring Transfusions[b]	66 (5.1%)	71 (5.5%)	74 (5.8%)

Note: denominator is based on patients for whom data are available
* Administered only until the first interim analysis
[a] For major and minor bleeding, patients are counted only once according to the most severe classification.
[b] Includes transfusions of whole blood, packed red blood cells, fresh frozen plasma, cryoprecipitate, platelets, and autotransfusion during the initial hospitalization.

associated with an increase in major and minor bleeding at the site of arterial sheath placement. After PCI, eptifibatide infusion should be continued for 20–24 hours. The femoral artery sheath may be removed during treatment with eptifibatide, but only after heparin has been discontinued and its effects largely reversed. In the IMPACT II study, heparin use was discouraged after the PCI procedure if the coronary lesion appeared angiographically stable. Early sheath removal was encouraged in both the IMPACT II and the PURSUIT studies while study drug was being infused. Prior to removing the sheath, it was recommended that heparin be discontinued for 3–4 hours and that an aPTT of <45 seconds be documented. In any case, both heparin and eptifibatide should be discontinued and sheath hemostasis should be achieved by standard compressive techniques at least 4 hours before hospital discharge.

Use of Thrombolytics, Anticoagulants, and Other Antiplatelet Agents. In the IMPACT II and PURSUIT studies, eptifibatide was used concomitantly with heparin and aspirin (see CLINICAL STUDIES). Because eptifibatide inhibits platelet aggregation, caution should be employed when it is used with other drugs that affect hemostasis, including **thrombolytics, oral anticoagulants, non-steroidal anti-inflammatory drugs, dipyridamole, ticlopidine,** and **clopidogrel.** To avoid potentially additive pharmacologic effects, concomitant treatment with **other inhibitors of platelet receptor GP IIb/IIIa** should be avoided.

There is only a small experience with concomitant use of eptifibatide and **thrombolytics.** In a study of 180 patients with acute myocardial infarction (AMI), eptifibatide (in regimens up to a bolus of 180 µg/kg followed by a continuous infusion of 0.75 µg/kg/min for 24 hours) was administered concomitantly with the approved "accelerated" regimen of alteplase, a thrombolytic agent. The studied regimens of ep-

tifibatide did not increase the incidence of major bleeding or transfusion compared to the incidence seen when alteplase was given alone.

In the IMPACT II study, 15 patients received a thrombolytic agent in conjunction with the 135/0.5 dosing regimen, 2 of whom experienced a major bleed. In the PURSUIT study, 40 patients who received eptifibatide at the 180/2.0 dosing regimen received a thrombolytic agent, 10 of whom experienced a major bleed.

In another AMI study involving 181 patients, eptifibatide (in regimens up to a bolus of 180 µg/kg followed by a continuous infusion of up to 2.0 µg/kg/min for up to 72 hours) was administered concomitantly with streptokinase (1.5 million units over 60 minutes), another thrombolytic agent. At the highest studied infusion rates (1.3 µg/kg/min and 2.0 µg/kg/min), eptifibatide was associated with an increase in the incidence of bleeding and transfusions compared to the incidence seen when streptokinase was given alone.

These limited data on the use of eptifibatide in patients receiving thrombolytic agents do not allow an estimate of the bleeding risk associated with concomitant use of thrombolytics. Systemic thrombolytic therapy should be used with caution in patients who have received eptifibatide.

Minimization of Vascular and Other Trauma. Arterial and venous punctures, intramuscular injections, and the use of urinary catheters, nasotracheal intubation, and nasogastric tubes should be minimized. When obtaining intravenous access, noncompressible sites (e.g., subclavian or jugular veins) should be avoided.

Laboratory Tests. Before infusion of eptifibatide, the following laboratory tests should be performed to identify preexisting hemostatic abnormalities: hematocrit or hemoglobin, platelet count, serum creatinine, and PT/aPTT. In patients undergoing PCI, the activated clotting time (ACT) should also be measured.

Maintaining Target aPTT and ACT. The aPTT should be maintained between 50 and 70 seconds unless PCI is to be performed. During PCI, the ACT should be maintained between 300 and 350 seconds.

The aPTT should be checked prior to arterial sheath removal. The sheath should not be removed unless the aPTT is <45 seconds. In patients treated with heparin, bleeding can be minimized by close monitoring of the aPTT. Table 6 displays the risk of major bleeding according to the maximum aPTT attained within 72 hours in the PURSUIT study.

[See table 6 on previous page]

Thrombocytopenia. If the patient experiences a confirmed platelet decrease to <100,000/mm^3, INTEGRILIN and heparin should be discontinued and the condition appropriately monitored and treated.

Renal Insufficiency. Based on results of clinical studies with eptifibatide (which did not adjust dose for renal function) and the fact that the drug is cleared equally by renal and nonrenal mechanisms, dose adjustment is unnecessary for patients with mild to moderate renal impairment (serum creatinine <2 mg/dL for the 180 μg/kg bolus and the 2.0 μg/kg/min infusion and <4 mg/dL for the 135 μg/kg bolus and the 0.5 μg/kg/min infusion). Plasma eptifibatide levels are expected to be higher in patients with more severe renal impairment, but no data are available for such patients or for patients on renal dialysis. *In vitro* studies have indicated that eptifibatide may be cleared from plasma by dialysis.

Geriatric Use. The PURSUIT and IMPACT II clinical studies enrolled patients up to the age of 94 years (45% were age 65 and over; 12% were age 75 and older). There was no apparent difference in efficacy between older and younger patients treated with eptifibatide. The incidence of bleeding complications was higher in the elderly in both placebo and eptifibatide groups, and the incremental risk of eptifibatide-associated bleeding was greater in the older patients. No dose adjustment was made for elderly patients, but patients over 75 years of age had to weigh at least 50 kg to be enrolled in the PURSUIT study because of concern about an increased risk of bleeding in this subgroup (see also ADVERSE REACTIONS).

Carcinogenesis, Mutagenesis, Impairment of Fertility. No long-term studies in animals have been performed to evaluate the carcinogenic potential of eptifibatide. Eptifibatide was not genotoxic in the Ames test, the mouse lymphoma cell (L5178Y, TK$^{+/-}$) forward mutation test, the human lymphocyte chromosome aberration test, or the mouse micronucleus test. Administered by continuous intravenous infusion at total daily doses up to 72 mg/kg/day (about 4 times the recommended maximum daily human dose on a body surface area basis), eptifibatide had no effect on fertility and reproductive performance of male and female rats.

Pregnancy. Pregnancy Category B. Teratology studies have been performed by continuous intravenous infusion of eptifibatide in pregnant rats at total daily doses of up to 72 mg/kg/day (about 4 times the recommended maximum daily human dose on a body surface area basis) and in pregnant rabbits at total daily doses of up to 36 mg/kg/day (also about 4 times the recommended maximum daily human dose on a body surface area basis). These studies revealed no evidence of harm to the fetus due to eptifibatide. There are, however, no adequate and well-controlled studies in pregnant women with eptifibatide. Because animal reproduction studies are not always predictive of human response, eptifibatide should be used during pregnancy only if clearly needed.

Pediatric Use. Safety and effectiveness of eptifibatide in pediatric patients have not been studied.

Nursing Mothers. It is not known whether eptifibatide is excreted in human milk. Because many drugs are excreted in human milk, caution should be exercised when eptifibatide is administered to a nursing mother.

ADVERSE REACTIONS

A total of 14,718 patients were treated in the two Phase III clinical trials (PURSUIT and IMPACT II). Of these, 8737 received eptifibatide: 1300 at 135/0.5 for up to 24 hours, 1286 at 135/0.75 for up to 24 hours, 1472 at 180/1.3 for up to 72 hours, and 4679 at 180/2.0 for up to 72 hours. The other 5981 patients received placebo. These 14,718 patients had a mean age of 62 years (range 20 to 94 years). Eighty-nine percent of the patients were Caucasian, with the remainder being predominantly Black (5%) and Hispanic (5%). Sixty-seven percent were men.

Because of the different regimens used in PURSUIT and IMPACT II, data from the two studies were not pooled.

Bleeding. The incidences of bleeding events and transfusions in the PURSUIT and IMPACT II studies are shown in Table 7. Bleeding was classified as major or minor by the criteria of the TIMI study group. Major bleeding events consisted of intracranial hemorrhage and other bleeding that led to decreases in hemoglobin greater than 5 g/dL. Minor bleeding events included spontaneous gross hematuria, spontaneous hematemesis, other observed blood loss with a hemoglobin decrease of more than 3 g/dL, and other hemoglobin decreases that were greater than 4 g/dL but less than 5 g/dL. In patients who received transfusions, the corre-

sponding loss in hemoglobin was estimated through an adaptation period of the method of Landefeld *et al.*

[See table 7 on previous page]

As shown in Tables 8 and 9, the overall incidence of major bleeding in these studies was strongly related to the incidence of coronary artery bypass graft (CABG) surgery; the excess bleeding seen with eptifibatide, however, was seen only among the patients who did not undergo CABG.

In the PURSUIT study, the greatest increase in major bleeding in eptifibatide-treated patients compared to placebo was associated with bleeding at the femoral artery access site (2.8% versus 1.3%). Oropharyngeal (primarily gingival), genitourinary, gastrointestinal, and retroperitoneal bleeding were also seen more commonly in eptifibatide-treated patients compared to placebo. Among patients experiencing a major bleed in the IMPACT II study, an increase in bleeding on eptifibatide versus placebo was observed only for the femoral artery access site (3.2% versus 2.8%).

Tables 8 and 9 display the incidence of TIMI major bleeding according to the cardiac procedures carried out in the PURSUIT and IMPACT II studies, respectively. The most common bleeding complications were related to cardiac revascularization (CABG-related or femoral artery access site bleeding).

[See table 8 above]

[See table 9 above]

In the PURSUIT study, the risk of major bleeding with eptifibatide increased inversely with patient weight. This relationship was most apparent for patients weighing less than 70 kg. These trends were not apparent in the IMPACT II study.

Bleeding adverse events resulting in discontinuation of study drug were more frequent among patients receiving eptifibatide than placebo (8% versus 1% in PURSUIT, 3.5% versus 1.9% in IMPACT II).

Intracranial Hemorrhage and Stroke. Intracranial hemorrhage was rare in the PURSUIT clinical study, with only 3 patients in the placebo group, 1 patient in the group treated with eptifibatide 180/1.3 and 5 patients in the group treated with eptifibatide 180/2.0 experiencing a hemorrhagic stroke. The overall incidence of stroke was 0.5% in patients receiving eptifibatide 180/1.3, 0.7% in patients receiving eptifibatide 180/2.0, and 0.8% in placebo patients.

In the IMPACT II study, intracranial hemorrhage was experienced by 1 patient treated with eptifibatide 135/0.5, 2 patients treated with eptifibatide 135/0.75 and 2 patients in the placebo group. The overall incidence of stroke was 0.5% in patients receiving 135/0.5 eptifibatide, 0.7% in patients receiving eptifibatide 135/0.75 and 0.7% in the placebo group.

Thrombocytopenia. In the PURSUIT and IMPACT II studies, the incidence of thrombocytopenia (<100,000/mm^3 or ≥50% reduction from baseline) and the incidence of platelet transfusions were similar between patients treated with eptifibatide and placebo.

Allergic Reactions. In the IMPACT II study, anaphylaxis was reported in 1 patient (0.08%) on placebo and in no patients on eptifibatide. In the PURSUIT study, anaphylaxis was reported in 7 patients receiving placebo (0.15%) and 7 patients receiving eptifibatide 180/2.0 (0.16%). In the IM-

Table 8
Major Bleeding by Procedures in the PURSUIT Study

	Placebo n (%)	Eptifibatide 180/1.3* n (%)	Eptifibatide 180/2.0 n (%)
Patients	4577	1451	4604
Overall Incidence of Major Bleeding	425 (9.3%)	152 (10.5%)	498 (10.8%)
Breakdown by Procedure:			
CABG	375 (8.2%)	123 (8.5%)	377 (8.2%)
Angioplasty without CABG	27 (0.6%)	16 (1.1%)	64 (1.4%)
Angiography without angioplasty or CABG	11 (0.2%)	7 (0.5%)	29 (0.6%)
Medical Therapy Only	12 (0.3%)	6 (0.4%)	28 (0.6%)

Denominators are based on the total number of patients whose TIMI classification was resolved.
*Administered only until the first interim analysis

Table 9
Major Bleeding by Procedures in the IMPACT II Study

	Placebo n (%)	Eptifibatide 135/0.5 n (%)	Eptifibatide 135/0.75 n (%)
Patients	1230	1249	1245
Overall Incidence of Major Bleeding	55 (4.5%)	55 (4.4%)	58 (4.7%)
Breakdown of Bleeding by Procedure:			
CABG	35 (2.8%)	23 (1.8%)	26 (2.1%)
Angioplasty without CABG	20 (1.6%)	32 (2.6%)	32 (2.7%)

Denominators are based on the total number of patients whose TIMI classification was resolved.

1. INTEGRILIN Dosing Chart by Weight for Patients With Acute Coronary Syndrome (180 μg/kg Bolus and 2μg/kg/min Infusion)

Patient Weight (kg)	Bolus Volume (2 mg/mL)	Infusion Rate (0.75 mg/mL)
37–41	3.4 mL	6 mL/h
42–46	4	7
47–53	4.5	8
54–59	5	9
60–65	5.6	10
66–71	6.2	11
72–78	6.8	12
79–84	7.3	13
85–90	7.9	14
91–96	8.5	15
97–103	9	16
104–109	9.5	17
110–115	10.2	18
116–121	10.7	19
>121	11.3	20

Continued on next page

Integrilin—Cont.

PACT II study, 2 patients (1 patient (0.04%) receiving eptifibatide and 1 patient (0.08%) receiving placebo) discontinued study drug because of allergic reactions. In the PURSUIT study, anaphylaxis was given as a reason for drug discontinuation in 3 patients (0.05%) who received eptifibatide and in none of the patients who received placebo.

Other Adverse Reactions. Serious non-bleeding events occurred in 19% of the eptifibatide and 19% of the placebo patients in the PURSUIT study. The only serious non-bleeding adverse event that occurred at a rate of at least 1% and was more common with eptifibatide than placebo (7% versus 6%) was hypotension. Most of the serious non-bleeding events consisted of cardiovascular events typical of an unstable angina population. In the IMPACT II study, serious non-bleeding events that occurred in greater than 1% of patients were uncommon and similar in incidence between placebo- and eptifibatide-treated patients.

Discontinuation of study drug due to adverse events other than bleeding was uncommon in both the PURSUIT and IMPACT II studies, with no single event occurring in >0.5% of the study population. In the PURSUIT study, non-bleeding adverse events leading to discontinuation occurred in the eptifibatide and placebo groups in the following body systems with an incidence of ≥0.1%: cardiovascular system (0.3% and 0.3%), digestive system (0.1% and 0.1%), hemic/lymphatic system (0.1% and 0.1%), nervous system (0.3% and 0.4%), urogenital system (0.1% and 0.1%), and whole body system (0.2% and 0.2%). In the IMPACT II study, non-bleeding adverse events leading to discontinuation occurred in the 135/0.5 eptifibatide and placebo groups in the following body systems with an incidence of ≥0.1%: whole body (0.3% and 0.1%), cardiovascular system (1.4% and 1.4%), digestive system (0.2% and 0%), hemic/lymphatic system (0.2% and 0%), nervous system (0.3% and 0.2%), and respiratory system (0.1% and 0.1%).

OVERDOSAGE

There has been only limited experience with overdosage of eptifibatide. There were 8 patients in the IMPACT II study and 9 patients in the PURSUIT study who received bolus doses and/or infusion doses more than double those called for in the protocols, or who were identified by the investigator as having received an overdose. None of these patients experienced an intracranial bleed or other major bleeding. Eptifibatide was not lethal to rats, rabbits, or monkeys when administered by continuous intravenous infusion for 90 minutes at a total dose of 45 mg/kg (about 2 to 5 times the recommended maximum daily human dose on a body surface area basis). Symptoms of acute toxicity were loss of righting reflex, dyspnea, ptosis, and decreased muscle tone in rabbits and petechial hemorrhages in the femoral and abdominal areas of monkeys.

DOSAGE AND ADMINISTRATION

The safety and efficacy of eptifibatide has been established in clinical studies that employed concomitant use of heparin and aspirin. Different dose regimens of eptifibatide were used in the major clinical studies. (See CLINICAL STUDIES.)

Acute Coronary Syndrome. The recommended adult dosage of eptifibatide in patients with acute coronary syndrome is an intravenous bolus of 180 µg/kg as soon as possible following diagnosis, followed by a continuous infusion of 2 µg/kg/min until hospital discharge or initiation of CABG surgery, up to 72 hours. If a patient is to undergo a percutaneous coronary intervention (PCI) while receiving eptifibatide, consideration can be given to decreasing the infusion rate to 0.5 µg/kg/min (the infusion rate in IMPACT II) at the time of the procedure. Infusion should be continued for an additional 20–24 hours after the procedure, allowing for up to 96 hours of therapy. In the PURSUIT study, patients weighing more than 121 kg received a maximum bolus of 22.6 mg (11.3 mL of the 2 mg/mL injection) followed by a maximum infusion of 15 mg (20 mL of the 0.75 mg/mL injection) per hour.

Percutaneous Coronary Intervention (PCI) in patients not presenting with an acute coronary syndrome. The recommended adult dosage of eptifibatide in patients undergoing PCI and not presenting with an acute coronary syndrome is an intravenous bolus of 135 µg/kg administered immediately before the initiation of PCI followed by a continuous infusion of 0.5 µg/kg/min for 20–24 hours. In the IMPACT II study, there was little experience in patients weighing more than 143 kg.

In patients who undergo coronary artery bypass graft surgery, eptifibatide infusion should be discontinued prior to surgery.

In the clinical trials that showed eptifibatide to be effective, most patients received concomitant aspirin and heparin. The aspirin doses used in the clinical studies were as follows:

Acute Coronary Syndrome (PURSUIT Study)	Angioplasty (IMPACT II Study)
160 mg initially, then 75–325 mg daily	75–325 mg 1–24 hours prior to intervention

The initial target aPTT in the PURSUIT study was 50–70 seconds, and the recommended heparin dosing was:
- if weight ≥70 kg, 5000 U bolus followed by infusion of 1000 U/h
- if weight <70 kg, 60 U/kg bolus followed by infusion of 12 U/kg/h

When these patients were to undergo PCI, the target ACT was 300–350 seconds, and the recommended heparin doses were:

	Initial Heparin Bolus
ACT (seconds)	**Heparin Bolus**
<150	100 U/kg (10,000 U maximum)
151–225	75 U/kg
226–299	50 U/kg
≥300	none

	Repeat Heparin Bolus*
ACT (seconds)	**Heparin Bolus**
<275	50 U/kg
275–299	25 U/kg
≥300	none

*based on hourly ACT determinations

In the IMPACT II study, the target ACT was 300–350 seconds before the procedure and ≤ 350 seconds thereafter. The recommended heparin doses were:
- prior to intervention: 100 U/kg bolus
- during intervention: up to 2000 U bolus q15min
- after intervention: infusion at physician's discretion

Patients requiring thrombolytic therapy had eptifibatide infusions stopped and were discontinued from the studies.

Instructions for Administration

1. Like other parenteral drug products, INTEGRILIN solutions should be inspected visually for particulate matter and discoloration prior to administration, whenever solution and container permit.
2. INTEGRILIN may be administered in the same intravenous line as alteplase, atropine, dobutamine, heparin, lidocaine, meperidine, metoprolol, midazolam, morphine, nitroglycerin, or verapamil. INTEGRILIN should not be administered through the same intravenous line as furosemide.
3. INTEGRILIN may be administered in the same IV line with 0.9% NaCl or 0.9% NaCl/5% dextrose. With either vehicle, the infusion may also contain up to 60 mEq/L of potassium chloride. No incompatibilities have been observed with intravenous administration sets. No compatibility studies have been performed with PVC bags.
4. The bolus dose of INTEGRILIN should be withdrawn from the 10-mL vial into a syringe. The bolus dose should be administered by IV push over 1–2 minutes.
5. Immediately following the bolus dose administration, a continuous infusion of INTEGRILIN should be initiated. When using an intravenous infusion pump, INTEGRILIN should be administered undiluted directly from the 100-mL vial. The 100-mL vial should be spiked with a vented infusion set. Care should be taken to center the spike within the circle on the stopper top.

INTEGRILIN is to be administered by volume according to patient weight. Patients should receive study drug according to the following table:

2. INTEGRILIN Dosing Chart by Weight for Patients Without Acute Coronary Syndromes Undergoing PCI (135 µg/kg Bolus and 0.5 µg/kg/min Infusion)

Patient Weight (kg)	Bolus Volume (2 mg/mL)	Infusion Rate (0.75 mg/mL)
40–55	3.4 mL	2 mL/h
56–68	4.2	2.5
69–80	5.1	3
81–93	5.9	3.5
94–105	6.8	4
106–118	7.6	4.5
119–131	8.4	5
132–143	9.2	5.5

[See third table on previous page]
[See table below]

HOW SUPPLIED

INTEGRILIN (eptifibatide) Injection is supplied as a sterile solution in 10-mL vials containing 20 mg of eptifibatide (NDC 0085-1177-01) and 100-mL vials containing 75 mg of eptifibatide (NDC 0085-1136-01).

Vials should be stored refrigerated at 2–8°C (36–46°F). Protect from light until administration. Do not use beyond the expiration date. Discard any unused portion left in the vial.

Rx only

Marketed By:
COR Therapeutics, Inc.
South San Francisco, CA 94080
and
Key Pharmaceuticals, Inc.
Kenilworth, NJ 07033

Distributed By:
Key Pharmaceuticals, Inc.
Kenilworth, NJ 07033

Issued May 1998
Rev 0

Shown in Product Identification Guide, page 309

Cypros Pharmaceutical Corporation
2714 LOKER AVENUE WEST
CARLSBAD, CA 92008

Direct Inquiries to:
(800) 411-3065
(760) 929-9500
FAX: (760) 929-8038

ETHAMOLIN®   ℞
[ē-tham-ō-lin]
(ethanolamine oleate)
Injection, 5%
For Local Intravenous Use Only

DESCRIPTION

ETHAMOLIN® (ethanolamine oleate) Injection is a mild sclerosing agent.
Chemically it is $C_{17}H_{33}COOH \cdot NH_2CH_2CH_2OH$. It has the following structure:

The empirical formula is $C_{20}H_{41}NO_3$, representing a molecular weight of 343.55.

ETHAMOLIN Injection consists of ethanolamine, a basic substance, which when combined with oleic acids forms a clear, straw to pale yellow colored, deliquescent oleate. The pH ranges from 8.0 to 9.0.

ETHAMOLIN Injection is a sterile, apyrogenic, aqueous solution containing in each mL approximately 50 mg of ethanolamine oleate with benzyl alcohol 2% by volume as preservative.

HOW SUPPLIED

ETHAMOLIN® (ethanolamine oleate) Injection, 5% is available in 2 mL ampules in boxes of 10 (NDC 63004-4790-6).

Store at Controlled Room Temperature, 15°–30°C (59°–86°F). Protect from light.

GLOFIL-125   ℞
[glōw-fill]
Sodium Iothalamate I-125
Injection, USP

INULIN AND SODIUM CHLORIDE   ℞
INJECTION USP
[in-ū-lynn]
For Intravenous Injection

Daiichi Pharmaceutical Corp.
11 PHILLIPS PARKWAY
MONTVALE, NJ 07645

Direct Inquiries to:
Medical Services Department
Ph: (877) 324-4244 (877-DAIICHI)
Fax: (888) 727-5666
For Medical Emergencies and Product Information Contact:
Medical Services Department
Ph: (888) 727-2500
Fax: (888) 272-7979

FLOXIN® Otic ℞
[*flox-in*]
(ofloxacin otic solution) 0.3%

DESCRIPTION

FLOXIN® Otic (ofloxacin otic solution) 0.3% is a sterile aqueous anti-infective (anti-bacterial) solution for otic use. Chemically, ofloxacin has three condensed 6-membered rings made up of a fluorinated Carboxyquinolone with a benzoxazine ring. The chemical name of ofloxacin is: (±)-9-fluoro-2,3-dihydro-3-methyl-10-(4-methyl-1-piperazinyl)-7-oxo-7*H*-pyrido [1,2,3-*de*]-1,4-benzoxazine- 6-carboxylic acid. The empirical formula of ofloxacin is $C_{18}H_{20}FN_3O_4$ and its molecular weight is 361.38. The structural formula is:

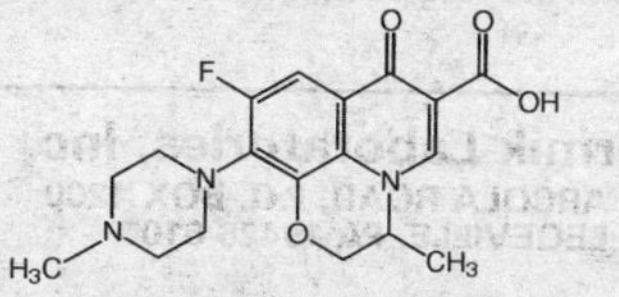

FLOXIN® Otic contains 0.3% (3mg/mL) ofloxacin with benzalkonium chloride (0.0025%), sodium chloride (0.9%), and water for injection. Hydrochloric acid and sodium hydroxide are added to adjust the pH to 6.5 ± 0.5.

CLINICAL PHARMACOLOGY

Pharmacokinetics: Drug concentrations in serum (in subjects with tympanostomy tubes and perforated tympanic membranes), in otorrhea, and in mucosa of the middle ear (in subjects with perforated tympanic membranes) were determined following otic administration of ofloxacin solution. In two single-dose studies, mean ofloxacin serum concentrations were low in adult patients with tympanostomy tubes, with and without otorrhea, after otic administration of a 0.3% solution (4.1 ng/mL (n=3) and 5.4 ng/mL (n=5), respectively). In adults with perforated tympanic membranes, the maximum serum drug level of ofloxacin detected was 10 ng/mL after administration of a 0.3% solution. Ofloxacin was detectable in the middle ear mucosa of some adult subjects with perforated tympanic membranes (11 of 16 subjects). The variability of ofloxacin concentration in middle ear mucosa was high. The concentrations ranged from 1.2 to 602 µg/g after otic administration of a 0.3% solution. Ofloxacin was present in high concentrations in otorrhea (389–2850 µg/g, n=13) 30 minutes after otic administration of a 0.3% solution in subjects with chronic suppurative otitis media and perforated tympanic membranes. However, the measurement of ofloxacin in the otorrhea does not necessarily reflect the exposure of the middle ear to ofloxacin.

Microbiology: Ofloxacin has *in vitro* activity against a wide range of gram-negative and gram-positive microorganisms. Ofloxacin exerts its antibacterial activity by inhibiting DNA gyrase, a bacterial topoisomerase. DNA gyrase is an essential enzyme which controls DNA topology and assists in DNA replication, repair, deactivation, and transcription. Cross-resistance has been observed between ofloxacin and other fluoroquinolones. There is generally no cross-resistance between ofloxacin and other classes of antibacterial agents such as beta-lactams or aminoglycosides.

Ofloxacin has been shown to be active against most strains of the following microorganisms, both *in vitro* and clinically in otic infections as described in the **INDICATIONS AND USAGE** section.

AEROBES, GRAM-POSITIVE:
Staphylococcus aureus
Streptococcus pneumoniae

AEROBES, GRAM-NEGATIVE:
Haemophilus influenzae
Moraxella catarrhalis
Proteus mirabilis
Pseudomonas aeruginosa

INDICATIONS AND USAGE

FLOXIN® Otic (ofloxacin otic solution) 0.3% is indicated for the treatment of infections caused by susceptible strains of the designated microorganisms in the specific conditions listed below:

Otitis Externa in adults and pediatric patients, one year and older, due to *Staphylococcus aureus* and *Pseudomonas aeruginosa.*

Chronic Suppurative Otitis Media in patients 12 years and older with perforated tympanic membranes due to *Staphylococcus aureus, Proteus mirabilis, and Pseudomonas aeruginosa.*

Acute Otitis Media in pediatric patients one year and older with tympanostomy tubes due to *Staphylococcus aureus, Streptococcus pneumoniae, Haemophilus influenzae, Moraxella catarrhalis,* and *Pseudomonas aeruginosa.*

CONTRAINDICATIONS

FLOXIN® Otic (ofloxacin otic solution) 0.3% is contraindicated in patients with a history of hypersensitivity to ofloxacin, to other quinolones, or to any of the components in this medication.

WARNINGS

NOT FOR OPHTHALMIC USE.
NOT FOR INJECTION.

Serious and occasionally fatal hypersensitivity (anaphylactic) reactions, some following the first dose, have been reported in patients receiving systemic quinolones, including ofloxacin. Some reactions were accompanied by cardiovascular collapse, loss of consciousness, angioedema (including laryngeal, pharyngeal or facial edema), airway obstruction, dyspnea, urticaria, and itching. If an allergic reaction to ofloxacin is suspected, stop the drug. Serious acute hypersensitivity reactions may require immediate emergency treatment. Oxygen and airway management, including intubation, should be administered as clinically indicated.

PRECAUTIONS

General: As with other anti-infective preparations, prolonged use may result in over-growth of nonsusceptible organisms, including fungi. If the infection is not improved after one week, cultures should be obtained to guide further treatment. If otorrhea persists after a full course of therapy, or if two or more episodes of otorrhea occur within six months, further evaluation is recommended to exclude an underlying condition such as cholesteatoma, foreign body, or a tumor.

The systemic administration of quinolones, including ofloxacin at doses much higher than given or absorbed by the otic route, has led to lesions or erosions of the cartilage in weight-bearing joints and other signs of arthropathy in immature animals of various species.

Young growing guinea pigs dosed in the middle ear with 0.3% ofloxacin otic solution showed no systemic effects, lesions or erosions of the cartilage in weight-bearing joints, or other signs of arthropathy. No drug-related structural or functional changes of the cochlea and no lesions in the ossicles were noted in the guinea pig following otic administration of 0.3% ofloxacin for one month.

No signs of local irritation were found when 0.3% ofloxacin was applied topically in the rabbit eye. Ofloxacin was also shown to lack dermal sensitizing potential in the guinea pig maximization study.

Information for Patients: Avoid contaminating the applicator tip with material from the fingers or other sources. This precaution is necessary if the sterility of the drops is to be preserved. Systemic quinolones, including ofloxacin, have been associated with hypersensitivity reactions, even following a single dose. Discontinue use immediately and contact your physician at the first sign of a rash or allergic reaction.

Otitis Externa

Prior to administration of FLOXIN® Otic in patients with otitis externa, the solution should be warmed by holding the bottle in the hand for one or two minutes to avoid dizziness which may result from the instillation of a cold solution. The patient should lie with the affected ear upward, and then the drops should be instilled. This position should be maintained for five minutes to facilitate penetration of the drops into the ear canal. Repeat, if necessary, for the opposite ear (see **DOSAGE AND ADMINISTRATION**).

Acute Otitis Media and Chronic Suppurative Otitis Media

In pediatric patients (from 1 to 12 years old) with acute otitis media with tympanostomy tubes and in patients with chronic suppurative otitis media with perforated tympanic membranes, prior to administration, the solution should be warmed by holding the bottle in the hand for one or two minutes to avoid dizziness which may result from the instillation of a cold solution. The patient should lie with the affected ear upward, and then the drops should be instilled. The tragus should then be pumped 4 times by pushing inward to facilitate penetration of the drops into the middle ear. This position should be maintained for five minutes. Repeat, if necessary, for the opposite ear (see **DOSAGE AND ADMINISTRATION**).

Drug Interactions: Specific drug interactions studies have not been conducted with FLOXIN® Otic.

Carcinogenesis, Mutagenesis, Impairment of Fertility

Long-term studies to determine the carcinogenic potential of ofloxacin have not been conducted. Ofloxacin was not mutagenic in the Ames test, the sister chromatid exchange assay (Chinese hamster and human cell lines), the unscheduled DNA synthesis (UDS) assay using human fibroblasts, the dominant lethal assay, or the mouse micronucleus assay. Ofloxacin was positive in the rat hepatocyte UDS assay, and in the mouse lymphoma assay. In rats, ofloxacin did not affect male or female reproductive performance at oral doses up to 360 mg/kg/day. This would be over 1000 times the maximum recommended clinical dose, based upon body surface area, assuming total absorption of ofloxacin from the ear of a patient treated with FLOXIN® Otic twice per day.

Pregnancy

Teratogenic Effects: Pregnancy Category C. Ofloxacin has been shown to have an embryocidal effect in rats at a dose of 810 mg/kg/day and in rabbits at 160 mg/kg/day. These dosages resulted in decreased fetal body weights and increased fetal mortality in rats and rabbits, respectively. Minor fetal skeletal variations were reported in rats receiving doses of 810 mg/kg/day. Ofloxacin has not been shown to be teratogenic at doses as high as 810 mg/kg/day and 160 mg/kg/day when administered to pregnant rats and rabbits, respectively.

Ofloxacin has not been shown to have any adverse effects on the developing embryo or fetus at doses relevant to the amount of ofloxacin that will be delivered ototopically at the recommended clinical doses.

Nonteratogenic Effects: Additional studies in the rat demonstrated that doses up to 360 mg/kg/day during late gestation had no adverse effects on late fetal development, labor, delivery, lactation, neonatal viability, or growth of the newborn. There are, however, no adequate and well-controlled studies in pregnant women. FLOXIN® Otic should be used during pregnancy only if the potential benefit justifies the potential risk to the fetus.

Nursing Mothers: In nursing women, a single 200 mg oral dose resulted in concentrations of ofloxacin in milk which were similar to those found in plasma. It is not known whether ofloxacin is excreted in human milk following topical otic administration. Because of the potential for serious adverse reactions from ofloxacin in nursing infants, a decision should be made whether to discontinue nursing or to discontinue the drug, taking into account the importance of the drug to the mother.

Pediatric Use: No changes in hearing function occurred in 30 pediatric subjects treated with ofloxacin otic and tested for audiometric parameters. Although safety and efficacy have been demonstrated in pediatric patients one year and older, safety and effectiveness in infants below the age of one year have not been established. Although quinolones, including ofloxacin, have been shown to cause arthropathy in immature animals after systemic administration, young growing guinea pigs dosed in the middle ear with 0.3% ofloxacin otic solution for one month showed no systemic effects, quinolone-induced lesions, erosions of the cartilage in weight-bearing joints, or other signs of arthropathy.

ADVERSE REACTIONS

In the Phase III registration trials, a total of 885 subjects were treated with ofloxacin otic solution. This included 229 subjects with otitis externa (with intact tympanic membranes) and 656 subjects with acute otitis media with tympanostomy tubes or chronic suppurative otitis media with perforated tympanic membranes. The reported treatment-related adverse events are listed below:

<u>Subjects with Otitis Externa</u>

The following treatment-related adverse events occurred in 1% or more of the subjects with intact tympanic membranes.

Adverse Event	Frequency (n=229)
Pruritus	4%
Application Site Reaction	3%
Dizziness	1%
Earache	1%
Vertigo	1%

The following treament-related adverse events were each reported in a single subject: dermatitis, eczema, erythematous rash, follicular rash, rash, hypoaesthesia, tinnitus, dyspepsia, hot flushes, flushing, and otorrhagia.

<u>Subjects with Acute Otitis Media with Tympanostomy Tubes and Subjects with Chronic Suppurative Otitis Media with Perforated Tympanic Membranes</u>

The following treatment-related adverse events occurred in 1% or more of the subjects with non-intact tympanic membranes.

Adverse Event	Frequency (n=656)
Taste Perversion	7%
Earache	1%
Pruritus	1%
Paraesthesia	1%

Continued on next page

Floxin Otic—Cont.

Rash   1%
Dizziness   1%

Other treatment-related adverse reactions reported in subjects with non-intact tympanic membranes included: diarrhea (0.6%), nausea (0.3%), vomiting (0.3%), dry mouth (0.5%), headache (0.3%), vertigo (0.5%), otorrhagia (0.6%), tinnitus (0.3%), fever (0.3%). The following treatment-related adverse events were each reported in a single subject: application site reaction, otitis externa, urticaria, abdominal pain, dysaesthesia, hyperkinesia, halitosis, inflammation, pain, insomnia, coughing, pharyngitis, rhinitis, sinusitis, and tachycardia.

DOSAGE AND ADMINISTRATION

Otitis Externa: The recommended dosage regimen for the treatment of otitis externa is:

For pediatric patients (from 1 to 12 years old): Five drops (0.25 mL, 0.75 mg ofloxacin) instilled into the affected ear twice daily for ten days. For patients 12 years and older: Ten drops (0.5 mL, 1.5 mg ofloxacin) instilled into the affected ear twice daily for ten days. The solution should be warmed by holding the bottle in the hand for one or two minutes to avoid dizziness which may result from the instillation of a cold solution. The patient should lie with the affected ear upward, and then the drops should be instilled. This position should be maintained for five minutes to facilitate penetration of the drops into the ear canal. Repeat, if necessary, for the opposite ear.

Acute Otitis Media in Pediatric Patients with Tympanostomy Tubes: The recommended dosage regimen for the treatment of acute otitis media in pediatric patients (from one to 12 years old) with tympanostomy tubes is:

Five drops (0.25 mL, 0.75 mg ofloxacin) instilled into the affected ear twice daily for ten days. The solution should be warmed by holding the bottle in the hand for one or two minutes to avoid dizziness which may result from the instillation of a cold solution. The patient should lie with the affected ear upward, and then the drops should be instilled. The tragus should then be pumped 4 times by pushing inward to facilitate penetration of the drops into the middle ear. This position should be maintained for five minutes. Repeat, if necessary, for the opposite ear.

Chronic Suppurative Otitis Media with perforated tympanic membranes: The recommended dosage regimen for the treatment of chronic suppurative otitis media with perforated tympanic membranes in patients 12 years and older is:

Ten drops (0.5 mL, 1.5 mg ofloxacin) instilled into the affected ear twice daily for fourteen days. The solution should be warmed by holding the bottle in the hand for one or two minutes to avoid dizziness which may result from the instillation of a cold solution. The patient should lie with the affected ear upward, before instilling the drops. The tragus should then be pumped 4 times by pushing inward to facilitate penetration into the middle ear. This position should be maintained for five minutes. Repeat, if necessary, for the opposite ear.

HOW SUPPLIED

FLOXIN® Otic (ofloxacin otic solution) 0.3% is supplied in plastic dropper bottles containing 5 mL. The NDC code is: 63395-101-05 FLOXIN® OTIC
Note: Store at 15–25°C (59–77°F).
Caution: Federal (U.S.A.) law prohibits dispensing without prescription.

DAIICHI PHARMACEUTICAL CORPORATION
Fort Lee, NJ 07024
January 29, 1998

Medication Guide

FLOXIN® (FLOX-IN) Otic
(ofloxacin otic solution) 0.3%

IMPORTANT PATIENT INFORMATION AND INSTRUCTIONS. READ BEFORE USE.

What is FLOXIN Otic?
FLOXIN Otic is an antibiotic in a sterile solution used to treat ear infections caused by certain bacteria found in:
- Patients (12 years and older) who have a middle ear infection and have a hole in the eardrum.
- Pediatric patients (between 1 and 12) who have a middle ear infection and have a tube in the eardrum.
- Patients (1 year and older) who have an infection in the ear canal.

Middle Ear Infection: A middle ear infection is a bacterial infection behind the eardrum. People with a hole or a tube in the eardrum may notice a discharge (fluid draining) in the ear canal.

Ear Canal Infection: An ear canal infection (also known as "Swimmer's Ear") is a bacterial infection of the ear canal. The ear canal and the outer part of the ear may swell, turn red, and be painful. Also, a fluid discharge may appear in the ear canal.

Who should NOT use FLOXIN Otic?
- Do not use this product if allergic to ofloxacin or to other quinolone antibiotics.
- Do not give this product to pediatric patients who are less than one year old.

How should FLOXIN Otic be given?

1. Wash hands
The person giving FLOXIN Otic should wash his/her hands with soap and water.

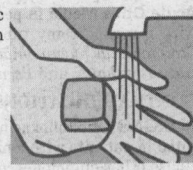

2. Clean ear
Gently clean any discharge that can be removed easily from the outer ear. DO NOT INSERT ANY OBJECT OR SWAB INTO THE EAR CANAL.

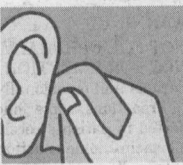

3. Add drops
The person receiving FLOXIN Otic should lie on his/her side with the infected ear up. Patients (12 and older) should have **10 drops** of FLOXIN Otic put into the infected ear. Pediatric patients under 12 should have **5 drops** put into the infected ear. The tip of the bottle should not touch the fingers or the ear or any other surfaces.

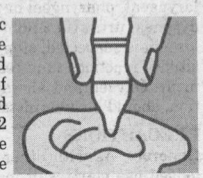

BE SURE TO FOLLOW INSTRUCTIONS BELOW FOR THE PATIENT'S SPECIFIC EAR INFECTION.

4. Press ear or pull ear
For a **Middle Ear Infection:** While the person receiving FLOXIN Otic lies on his/her side, the person giving the drops should gently press the

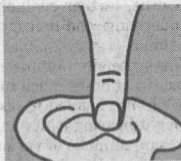

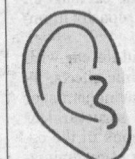

TRAGUS (see diagram) 4 times in a pumping motion. This will allow the drops to pass through the hole or tube in the eardrum and into the middle ear.

For an **Ear Canal Infection ("Swimmer's Ear"):** While the person receiving the drops lies on his/her side, the person giving the drops should gently pull the outer ear upward and backward. This will allow the ear drops to flow down into the ear canal.

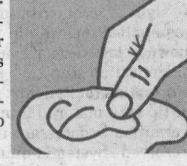

5. Stay on side
The person who received the ear drops should remain on his/her side for at least 5 minutes.
Repeat Steps 2–5 for the other ear if both ears are infected.

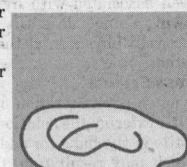

How often should FLOXIN® Otic be given?
FLOXIN Otic ear drops should be given 2 times each day (about 12 hours apart, for example, 8 AM and 8 PM) in each infected ear unless the doctor has instructed otherwise. The best times to use the ear drops are in the morning and at night. It is very important to use the ear drops for as long as the doctor has instructed, **even if the symptoms improve.** If FLOXIN Otic ear drops are not used for as long as the doctor has instructed, the infection may return.

What if a dose is missed?
If a dose of FLOXIN Otic is missed, it should be given as soon as possible. If it is almost time for the next dose, skip the missed dose and go back to the regular dosing schedule. Do not use a double dose unless the doctor has instructed you to do so. If the infection is not improved after one week, you should consult your doctor. If you have two or more episodes of drainage within six months, it is recommended you see your doctor for further evaluation.

What activities should be avoided while using FLOXIN Otic?
It is important that the infected ear(s) remain clean and dry. When bathing, avoid getting the infected ear(s) wet. Avoid swimming unless the doctor has instructed otherwise.

What are the possible side effects of FLOXIN Otic?
During the testing of FLOXIN Otic, the most common side effect was a bitter taste which happened in 7% of patients

with a middle ear infection. This may occur when some of the drops pass from the middle ear to the back of the mouth. This side effect is not serious and there is no need to stop the medicine if this should happen. Other side effects were:
For Middle Ear Infections: Earache (1%), itching (1%), abnormal sensation (1%), rash (1%) and dizziness (1%).
For Ear Canal Infections: Itching (4%), discomfort upon application (3%), dizziness (1%), earache (1%) and light headedness (1%).
If any of these side effects occur, call the doctor.
If an allergic reaction to FLOXIN Otic occurs, stop using the product and contact your doctor.
DO NOT TAKE FLOXIN Otic BY MOUTH.
If FLOXIN Otic is accidentally swallowed or overdose occurs, call the doctor immediately. This medicine is available only with a doctor's prescription. Use only as directed. Do not use this medicine if outdated. If you wish to learn more about FLOXIN Otic ask the doctor or pharmacist.
Store at 15° to 25° C (59°–77° F)

FLOXIN Otic is manufactured for:
Daiichi Pharmaceutical Corp.
Fort Lee, NJ
07024

By:
Warner-Lambert
Morris Plains, NJ
07950

This Medication Guide has been approved by the U.S. Food and Drug Administration.
Revised: (12/15/97)
Shown in Product Identification Guide, page 309

Dermik Laboratories, Inc.
500 ARCOLA ROAD, P.O. BOX 1200
COLLEGEVILLE, PA 19426-0107

Direct Inquiries to:
QUALITY ASSURANCE QUESTIONS:
John Chiles, Manager, Quality Control
(610) 454-3130
REGULATORY AFFAIRS QUESTIONS:
Ron Panner, Director, Regulatory Affairs
(610) 454-3026

For Medical Information Contact:
PRODUCT INFORMATION/ADVERSE DRUG EXPERIENCES/EMERGENCIES
Medical Information and Education
(800) 340-7502
(610) 454-8110

5 BENZAGEL®   ℞
[ben-za-jel]
(5% benzoyl peroxide) and
10 BENZAGEL®   ℞
(10% benzoyl peroxide)
MICROGEL™ FORMULA
Acne Gels

DESCRIPTION

Each gram of **5 Benzagel®** and **10 Benzagel®** contains 50 mg and 100 mg respectively, of benzoyl peroxide in a gel vehicle of purified water, carbomer 940, 14% alcohol, sodium hydroxide, dioctyl sodium sulfosuccinate and fragrances. Benzoyl peroxide is an antibacterial and keratolytic agent.

HOW SUPPLIED

5 & 10 Benzagel® are available in 1.5 oz (42.5 g) and 3 oz (85 g) plastic tubes; 5 Benzagel® contains 50 mg benzoyl peroxide per gram and 10 Benzagel® contains 100 mg benzoyl peroxide per gram.
Store at room temperature.
5-Benzagel 1.5 oz NDC 0066-0430-15
5-Benzagel 3.0 oz NDC 0066-0430-30
10-Benzagel 1.5 oz NDC 0066-0431-15
10 Benzagel 3.0 oz NDC 0066-0431-30
CR-5733N   Rev. 12/96

BENZAMYCIN®   ℞
[ben 'za-mi "sin]
(erythromycin-benzoyl peroxide topical gel)
Topical gel: erythromycin (3%), benzoyl peroxide (5%)
For Dermatological Use Only - Not for Ophthalmic Use
Reconstitute Before Dispensing

DESCRIPTION

BENZAMYCIN® Topical Gel contains erythromycin [(3R*, 4S*, 5S*, 6R*, 7R*, 9R*, 11R*, 12R*, 13S*, 14R*)-4-[(2,6-

Dideoxy-3-*C*-methyl-3-*O*-methyl-α-L-*ribo*-hexopyranosyl)oxy]-14-ethyl-7,12,13-trihydroxy-3,5,7,9,11,13-hexamethyl-6-[[3,4,6-trideoxy-3-(dimethylamino)-β-D-*xylo*-hexopyranosyl]oxy]oxacyclotetradecane-2,10-dione]. Erythromycin is a macrolide antibiotic produced from a strain of *Saccharopolyspora erythraea* (formerly *Streptomyces erythreus*). It is a base and readily forms salts with acids.

Chemically, erythromycin is ($C_{37}H_{67}NO_{13}$). It has the following structural formula:

Erythromycin has the molecular weight of 733.94. It is a white crystalline powder and has a solubility of approximately 1 mg/mL in water and is soluble in alcohol at 25°C. BENZAMYCIN Topical Gel also contains benzoyl peroxide for topical use. Benzoyl peroxide is an antibacterial and keratolytic agent.

Chemically, benzoyl peroxide is ($C_{14}H_{10}O_4$). It has the following structural formula:

Benzoyl peroxide has the molecular weight of 242.23. It is a white granular powder and is sparingly soluble in water and alcohol and soluble in acetone, chloroform and ether. Each gram of BENZAMYCIN Topical Gel contains, as dispensed, 30 mg (3%) of erythromycin and 50 mg (5%) of benzoyl peroxide in a base of purified water USP, carbomer 940 NF, alcohol 20%, sodium hydroxide NF, docusate sodium and fragrance.

CLINICAL PHARMACOLOGY

The exact mechanism by which erythromycin reduces lesions of acne vulgaris is not fully known; however, the effect appears to be due in part to the antibacterial activity of the drug.

Benzoyl peroxide has a keratolytic and desquamative effect which may also contribute to its efficacy. Benzoyl peroxide has been shown to be absorbed by the skin where it is converted to benzoic acid.

MICROBIOLOGY

Erythromycin acts by inhibition of protein synthesis in susceptible organisms by reversibly binding to 50 **S** ribosomal subunits, thereby inhibiting translocation of aminoacyl transfer-RNA and inhibiting polypeptide synthesis. Antagonism has been demonstrated *in vitro* between erythromycin, lincomycin, chloramphenicol and clindamycin.

Benzoyl peroxide is an antibacterial agent which has been shown to be effective against *Propionibacterium acnes*, an anaerobe found in sebaceous follicles and comedones. The antibacterial action of benzoyl peroxide is believed to be due to the release of active oxygen.

INDICATIONS AND USAGE

BENZAMYCIN Topical Gel is indicated for the topical treatment of acne vulgaris.

CONTRAINDICATIONS

BENZAMYCIN Topical Gel is contraindicated in those individuals who have shown hypersensitivity to any of its components.

WARNINGS

Pseudomembranous colitis has been reported with nearly all antibacterial agents, including erythromycin, and may range in severity from mild to life-threatening. Therefore, it is important to consider this diagnosis in patients who present with diarrhea subsequent to the administration of antibacterial agents.

Treatment with antibacterial agents alters the normal flora of the colon and may permit overgrowth of clostridia. Studies indicate that a toxin produced by *Clostridium difficile* is one primary cause of "antibiotic-associated colitis."

After the diagnosis of pseudomembranous colitis has been established, therapeutic measures should be initiated. Mild cases of pseudomembranous colitis usually respond to drug discontinuation alone. In moderate to severe cases, consideration should be given to management with fluids and electrolytes, protein supplementation and treatment with an antibacterial drug clinically effective against *C. difficile* colitis.

Size (Net Weight)	NDC 0066-	Benzoyl Peroxide Gel	Active Erythromycin Powder (In Plastic Vial)	Ethyl Alcohol (70%) To Be Added
11.65 grams (as dispensed) SAMPLE	0510-05	10 grams	0.4 grams	1.5 mL
23.3 grams (as dispensed)	0510-23	20 grams	0.8 grams	3 mL
46.6 grams (as dispensed)	0510-46	40 grams	1.6 grams	6 mL

PRECAUTIONS

General: For topical use only; not for ophthalmic use. Concomitant topical acne therapy should be used with caution because a possible cumulative irritancy effect may occur, especially with the use of peeling, desquamating or abrasive agents. If severe irritation develops, discontinue use and institute appropriate therapy.

The use of antibiotic agents may be associated with the overgrowth of nonsusceptible organisms including fungi. If this occurs, discontinue use and take appropriate measures. Avoid contact with eyes and all mucous membranes.

Information for Patients: Patients using BENZAMYCIN Topical Gel should receive the following information and instructions:

1. This medication is to be used as directed by the physician. It is for external use only. Avoid contact with the eyes, nose, mouth, and all mucous membranes.
2. This medication should not be used for any disorder other than that for which it was prescribed.
3. Patients should not use any other topical acne preparation unless otherwise directed by physician.
4. Patients should report to their physician any signs of local adverse reactions.
5. BENZAMYCIN® Topical Gel may bleach hair or colored fabric.
6. Keep product refrigerated and discard after 3 months.

CARCINOGENESIS, MUTAGENESIS AND IMPAIRMENT OF FERTILITY

Data from a study using mice known to be highly susceptible to cancer suggests that benzoyl peroxide acts as a tumor promoter. The clinical significance of this is unknown.

No animal studies have been performed to evaluate the carcinogenic and mutagenic potential or effects on fertility of topical erythromycin. However, long-term (2-year) oral studies in rats with erythromycin ethylsuccinate and erythromycin base did not provide evidence of tumorigenicity. There was no apparent effect on male or female fertility in rats fed erythromycin (base) at levels up to 0.25% of diet.

Pregnancy: Teratogenic Effects: Pregnancy CATEGORY C: Animal reproduction studies have not been conducted with BENZAMYCIN Topical Gel or benzoyl peroxide.

There was no evidence of teratogenicity or any other adverse effect on reproduction in female rats fed erythromycin base (up to 0.25% diet) prior to and during mating, during gestation and through weaning of two successive litters.

There are no well-controlled trials in pregnant women with BENZAMYCIN Topical Gel. It also is not known whether BENZAMYCIN Topical Gel can cause fetal harm when administered to a pregnant woman or can affect reproductive capacity. BENZAMYCIN Topical Gel should be given to a pregnant woman only if clearly needed.

Nursing Women: It is not known whether BENZAMYCIN Topical Gel is excreted in human milk after topical application. However, erythromycin is excreted in human milk following oral and parenteral erythromycin administration. Therefore, caution should be exercised when erythromycin is administered to a nursing woman.

Pediatric Use: Safety and effectiveness of this product in pediatric patients below the age of 12 have not been established.

ADVERSE REACTIONS

In controlled clinical trials, the total incidence of adverse reactions associated with the use of BENZAMYCIN Topical Gel was approximately 3%. These were dryness and urticarial reaction.

The following additional local adverse reactions have been reported occasionally: irritation of the skin including peeling, itching, burning sensation, erythema, inflammation of the face, eyes and nose, and irritation of the eyes. Skin discoloration, oiliness and tenderness of the skin have also been reported.

DOSAGE AND ADMINISTRATION

BENZAMYCIN Topical Gel should be applied twice daily, morning and evening, or as directed by a physician, to affected areas after the skin is thoroughly washed, rinsed with warm water and gently patted dry.

How Supplied and Compounding Directions:
[See table above]
Prior to dispensing, tap vial until powder flows freely. Add indicated amount of ethyl alcohol (70%) to vial (to the

mark) and immediately shake to completely dissolve erythromycin. Add this solution to gel and stir until homogeneous in appearance (1 to 1 1/2 minutes). BENZAMYCIN Topical Gel should then be stored under refrigeration. Do not freeze. Place a 3-month expiration date on the label.

NOTE: *Prior to reconstitution*, store at room temperature between 15° and 30°C (59°–86°F).

After reconstitution, store under refrigeration between 2° and 8°C (36°–46°F).

Do not freeze. Keep tightly closed. Keep out of the reach of children.

Caution: Federal (U.S.A.) law prohibits dispensing without prescription.

U.S. Patent Nos. 4,387,107 and 4,497,794.
Manufactured by Rhône-Poulenc Rorer Puerto Rico Inc.
Manati, Puerto Rico
For Dermik Laboratories, Inc.
A Rhône-Poulenc Rorer Company
Collegeville, PA 19426
Rev. 2/96   IN-7121P
BENZAMYCIN®
(erythromycin-benzoyl
peroxide topical gel)

PLEASE READ COMPLETE COMPOUNDING DIRECTIONS

NOTE: TAP VIAL UNTIL ALL POWDER FLOWS FREELY. ADD ETHYL ALCOHOL (70%) TO VIAL (TO THE MARK) AND **IMMEDIATELY** SHAKE/DISSOLVE **COMPLETELY**.

DRITHOCREME®   ℞
[*drĭth'ocrēm*]
(anthralin) 0.1%, 0.25%, 0.5%, 1.0% (HP)

DESCRIPTION

Drithocreme® is a pale yellow topical cream containing 0.1%, 0.25%, 0.5% or 1.0% (HP) anthralin USP in a base of white petrolatum, sodium lauryl sulfate, cetostearyl alcohol, ascorbic acid, salicylic acid, chlorocresol and purified water. The chemical name of anthralin is 1,8-dihydroxy-9-anthrone.

HOW SUPPLIED

50g tubes
Drithocreme 0.1% NDC 0066-7200-50
Drithocreme 0.25% NDC 0066-7201-50
Drithocreme 0.5% NDC 0066-7202-50
Drithocreme HP 1% NDC 0066-7203-50

Caution: Federal law prohibits dispensing without prescription.
Distributed by
DERMIK LABORATORIES, INC.
A RHÔNE-POULENC RORER COMPANY
COLLEGEVILLE, PA 19426
Made in UK.   Rev. 1/97   IN-1660B (LTF 089)

DRITHO-SCALP®   ℞
(anthralin) 0.25%, 0.5%

DESCRIPTION

Dritho-Scalp® is a pale yellow topical cream containing 0.25% or 0.5% anthralin USP in a base of white petrolatum, mineral oil, sodium lauryl sulfate, cetostearyl alcohol, ascorbic acid, salicylic acid, chlorocresol and purified water. The chemical name of anthralin is 1,8-dihydroxy-9-anthrone.

HOW SUPPLIED

50g tube with special applicator
Dritho-Scalp 0.25% NDC 0066-7204-50
Dritho-Scalp 0.5% NDC 0066-7205-50

Caution: Federal law prohibits dispensing without prescription.

Continued on next page

Dritho-Scalp—Cont.

Distributed by
DERMIK LABORATORIES, INC.
A RHÔNE-POULENC RORER COMPANY
COLLEGEVILLE, PA 19426
Made in UK.   Rev. 1/97   IN-1663B (LTF 090)

HYTONE®   ℞
[hĭ-tōne]
(hydrocortisone)
Cream, Lotion

DESCRIPTION

Each gram of Hytone® (hydrocortisone) Cream 2 1/2% contains 25 mg of hydrocortisone in a water-washable base of purified water, propylene glycol, glyceryl monostearate SE, cholesterol and related sterols, isopropyl myristate, polysorbate 60, cetyl alcohol, sorbitan monostearate, polyoxyl 40 stearate and sorbic acid.
Each mL of Hytone (hydrocortisone) Lotion 2 1/2% contains 25 mg of hydrocortisone in a vehicle consisting of carbomer 940, propylene glycol, polysorbate 40, propylene glycol stearate, cholesterol and related sterols, isopropyl myristate, sorbitan palmitate, cetyl alcohol, triethanolamine, sorbic acid, simethicone, and purified water.

HOW SUPPLIED

Cream-2 1/2% Tube 1 OZ NDC 0066-0095-01;
          2 1/2% Tube 2 OZ NDC 0066-0095-02
Lotion-2 1/2% bottle 2 FL OZ NDC 0066-0098-02
Caution: Federal law prohibits dispensing without prescription.
Keep out of the reach of children.
Marketed by
Dermik Laboratories, Inc.
A Rhône-Poulenc Rorer Company
Collegeville, PA 19426
Rev. 12/96   IN-7245D

HYTONE®   ℞
[hĭ-tōne]
(hydrocortisone)
Ointment

DESCRIPTION

The topical corticosteroids constitute a class of primarily synthetic steroids used as anti-inflammatory and antipruritic agents. Hytone® 2 1/2% (hydrocortisone ointment, USP) contains Hydrocortisone [Pregn-4-ene-3,20-dione,11,17,21-trihydroxy-,(11β)-], with the molecular formula $C_{21}H_{30}O_5$ and a molecular weight of 362.47. CAS 50-23-7. Each gram of the ointment contains 25 mg of hydrocortisone in a base of white petrolatum and mineral oil.

HOW SUPPLIED

Hytone® 2 1/2% (hydrocortisone ointment, USP) in 1 oz (28.35 g) tubes, NDC 0066-9997-01.
Store at controlled room temperature 15°-30°C (59°-86°F).
Caution: Federal law prohibits dispensing without prescription.
Marketed by
Dermik Laboratories, Inc.
A Rhône-Poulenc Rorer Company
Collegeville, PA 19426
Rev. 3/96   IN-5609

KLARON®   ℞
[klă - rŏn]
(sodium sulfacetamide lotion)
Lotion, 10%

DESCRIPTION

Each mL of **Klaron®** (sodium sulfacetamide lotion) **Lotion, 10%** contains 100 mg of sodium sulfacetamide in a vehicle consisting of purified water; propylene glycol; lauramide DEA (and) diethanolamine; polyethylene glycol 400, monolaurate; hydroxyethyl cellulose; sodium chloride; sodium metabisulfite; methylparaben; xanthan gum; EDTA and simethicone.
Sodium sulfacetamide is a sulfonamide with antibacterial activity. Chemically, sodium sulfacetamide is N' -[(4-aminophenyl) sulfonyl] - acetamide, monosodium salt, monohydrate. The structural formula is:

CLINICAL PHARMACOLOGY

The most widely accepted mechanism of action of sulfonamides is the Woods-Fildes theory, based on sulfonamides acting as a competitive inhibitor of para-aminobenzoic acid (PABA) utilization, an essential component for bacterial growth. While absorption through intact skin in humans has not been determined, in vitro studies with human cadaver skin indicated a percutaneous absorption of about 4%. Sodium sulfacetamide is readily absorbed from the gastrointestinal tract when taken orally and excreted in the urine largely unchanged. The biological half-life has been reported to be between 7 to 13 hours.

INDICATIONS

Klaron Lotion is indicated in the topical treatment of acne vulgaris.

CONTRAINDICATIONS

Klaron Lotion is contraindicated for use by patients having known hypersensitivity to sulfonamides or any other component of this preparation (see **WARNINGS** section).

WARNINGS

Fatalities have occurred, although rarely, due to severe reactions to sulfonamides including Stevens-Johnson syndrome, toxic epidermal necrolysis, fulminant hepatic necrosis, agranulocytosis, aplastic anemia, and other blood dyscrasias. Hypersensitivity reactions may occur when a sulfonamide is readministered, irrespective of the route of administration. Sensitivity reactions have been reported in individuals with no prior history of sulfonamide hypersensitivity. At the first sign of hypersensitivity, skin rash or other reactions, discontinue use of this preparation (see **ADVERSE REACTIONS** section).
Klaron Lotion contains sodium metabisulfite, a sulfite that may cause allergic-type reactions including anaphylactic symptoms and life-threatening or less severe asthmatic episodes in certain susceptible people. The overall prevalence of sulfite sensitivity in the general population is unknown and probably low. Sulfite sensitivity is seen more frequently in asthmatic than in non-asthmatic people (see **CONTRAINDICATIONS** section).

PRECAUTIONS

General: For external use only. Keep away from eyes. If irritation develops, use of the product should be discontinued and appropriate therapy instituted. Patients should be carefully observed for possible local irritation or sensitization during long-term therapy. Hypersensitivity reactions may occur when a sulfonamide is readministered irrespective of the route of administration, and cross-sensitivity between different sulfonamides may occur. Sodium sulfacetamide can cause reddening and scaling of the skin. Particular caution should be employed if areas of involved skin to be treated are denuded or abraded.
Keep out of reach of children.
Carcinogenesis, Mutagenesis and Impairment of Fertility: Long-term studies in animals have not been performed to evaluate carcinogenic potential.
Pregnancy - Category C: Animal reproduction studies have not been conducted with **Klaron® Lotion**. It is also not known whether **Klaron Lotion** can cause fetal harm when administered to a pregnant woman or can affect reproductive capacity. **Klaron Lotion** should be given to a pregnant woman only if clearly needed.
Kernicterus may occur in the newborn as a result of treatment of a pregnant woman at term with orally administered sulfonamide. There are no adequate and well controlled studies of **Klaron Lotion** in pregnant women, and it is not known whether topically applied sulfonamides can cause fetal harm when administered to a pregnant woman.
Nursing Mothers: It is not known whether sodium sulfacetamide is excreted in the human milk following topical use of **Klaron Lotion**. Systemically administered sulfonamides are capable of producing kernicterus in the infants of lactating women. Small amounts of orally administered sulfonamides have been reported to be eliminated in human milk. Because many drugs are excreted in human milk, caution should be exercised in prescribing for nursing women.
Pediatric Use: Safety and effectiveness in pediatric patients under the age of 12 have not been established.

ADVERSE REACTIONS

In controlled clinical trials for the management of acne vulgaris, the occurrence of adverse reactions associated with the use of **Klaron Lotion** was infrequent and restricted to local events. The total incidence of adverse reactions reported in these studies was less than 2%. Only one of 105 patients treated with **Klaron Lotion** had adverse reactions of erythema, itching and edema. It has been reported that sodium sulfacetamide may cause local irritation, stinging and burning. While the irritation may be transient, occasionally, the use of medication has to be discontinued.

DOSAGE AND ADMINISTRATION

Apply a thin film to affected areas twice daily.

HOW SUPPLIED

2 FL OZ (59 mL) bottles (**NDC** 0066-7500-02).
Store at room temperature.
Caution: Federal law prohibits dispensing without prescription.
Marketed by
Dermik Laboratories, Inc.
A Rhône-Poulenc Rorer Company
Collegeville, PA, USA 19426
Rev. 12/96   IN-5178C

NORITATE™   ℞
(metronidazole cream)
Cream, 1%
FOR TOPICAL USE ONLY
(NOT FOR OPHTHALMIC USE)

DESCRIPTION

NORITATE™ (metronidazole cream) **Cream, 1%**, contains metronidazole, USP. Chemically, metronidazole is 2-methyl-5-nitro-1H-imidazole-1-ethanol. The molecular formula for metronidazole is $C_6H_9N_3O_3$. It has the following structural formula:

Metronidazole has a molecular weight of 171.16. It is a white to pale yellow crystalline powder. It is slightly soluble in alcohol and has a solubility in water of 10 mg/mL at 20°C. Metronidazole is a member of the imidazole class of antibacterial agents and is classified as an antiprotozoal and anti-bacterial agent.
NORITATE is an emollient cream; each gram contains 10 mg micronized metronidazole USP, in a base of purified water USP, stearic acid NF, glyceryl monostearate NF, glycerin USP, methylparaben NF, triethanolamine NF and propylparaben NF.

CLINICAL PHARMACOLOGY

Pharmacokinetics: When one gram dose of NORITATE cream, 1%, was applied in a single application to the face of 16 healthy volunteers, low concentrations of metronidazole were detected in the plasma of 7 of the volunteers. The mean ± SD C_{max} of metronidazole was 27.6 ± 7.3 ng/mL, which is about 1% of the value reported for a single 250 mg oral dose of metronidazole. The time to maximum plasma concentration (T_{max}) in the volunteers with detectable metronidazole was 8–12 hours after topical application.
Pharmacodynamics: The mechanisms by which metronidazole acts in reducing inflammatory lesions of rosacea are unknown.
Clinical Studies: Safety and efficacy of NORITATE were evaluated in two randomized vehicle-controlled clinical studies for the treatment of rosacea, which excluded patients who had nodules, moderate or severe rhinophyma, dense telangiectases, plaque-like facial edema or ocular involvement and those who had a history of not responding to metronidazole therapy for rosacea. Of the patients included in the efficacy database (n=416), there were 142 men and 274 women. Endpoint efficacy data comparisons for patients treated with daily NORITATE or vehicle applications are listed below.
[See table at top of next page]
Safety Studies: Studies of contact sensitization (n=258), phototoxicity (n=21), and photocontact sensitization (n=29) of NORITATE were conducted. No evidence of sensitization or phototoxicity was seen in these studies.

INDICATIONS AND USAGE

NORITATE is indicated for the topical treatment of inflammatory lesions and erythema of rosacea.

CONTRAINDICATIONS

NORITATE is contraindicated in those patients with a history of hypersensitivity to metronidazole or to any other ingredient in this formulation.

PRECAUTIONS

General: If a reaction suggesting local skin irritation occurs, patients should be directed to discontinue use of the medication. Conjunctivitis associated with topical use of

Inflammatory Lesion Counts and Erythema Severity Scores in Two Clinical Trials for Rosacea

	Noritate				Vehicle			
	Study 1		Study 2		Study 1		Study 2	
	N	Result	N	Result	N	Result	N	Result
Papules + Pustules Count								
Baseline	89	15	92	19	50	18	49	17
Week-10	80	7*	82	8	45	15	41	12
Reduction		49%*		58%*		17%		30%
Papules Count								
Baseline	89	13	92	17	50	15	49	15
Week-10	80	7*	82	7	45	12	41	11
Reduction		41%*		55%*		14%		28%
Erythema Score								
Baseline	89	2.2	92	2.3	50	2.2	49	2.2
Week-10	80	1.3*	82	1.4*	45	1.7	40	1.8
Reduction		42%*		40%*		25%		19%

* Statistically significant differences between NORITATE and vehicle groups with $p \leq 0.05$. Erythema scores: 0=none, 1=mild, 2=moderate and 3=severe.

metronidazole on the face has been reported. Contact with the eyes should be avoided. Metronidazole is a nitroimidazole and should be used with care in patients with evidence of, or history of, blood dyscrasia.

Information for Patients: Patients using NORITATE™ should receive the following information and instructions:

1. This medication is to be used as directed.
2. It is for external use only.
3. Avoid contact with the eyes.
4. Cleanse affected area(s) before applying NORITATE.
5. This medication should not be used for any disorder other than that for which it is prescribed.
6. Patients should report any adverse reaction to their physician.

Drug Interactions: Oral metronidazole has been reported to potentiate the anticoagulant effect of coumarin and warfarin resulting in a prolongation of prothrombin time. Drug interactions should be kept in mind when NORITATE is prescribed for patients who are receiving anticoagulant treatment, although they are less likely to occur with topical metronidazole administration because of low absorption. (See **CLINICAL PHARMACOLOGY**, **Pharmacokinetics** section)

Carcinogenesis, Mutagenesis and Impairment of Fertility: Metronidazole has shown evidence of carcinogenic activity in a number of studies involving chronic, oral administration in mice and rats but not in studies involving hamsters. In several long term studies in mice, oral doses of approximately 225 mg/m^2/day or greater (approximately 37 times the human topical dose on a mg/m^2 basis) were associated with an increase in pulmonary tumors and lymphomas. Several long term oral studies in the rat have shown statistically significant increases in mammary and hepatic tumors at doses >885 mg/m^2/day (144 times the topical human dose).

Metronidazole has shown evidence of mutagenic activity in several *in vitro* bacterial assay systems. In addition, a dose-related increase in the frequency of micronuclei was observed in mice after intraperitoneal injections. An increase in chromosomal aberrations in peripheral blood lymphocytes was reported in patients with Crohn's disease who were treated with 200 to 1200 mg/day of metronidazole for 1 to 24 months. However, in another study, no increase in chromosomal aberrations in circulating lymphocytes was observed in patients with Crohn's disease treated with the drug for 8 months.

In one published study, using albino hairless mice, intraperitoneal administration of metronidazole at a dose of 45 mg/m^2/day (approximately 7 times the human topical dose on a mg/m^2 basis) was associated with an increase in ultraviolet radiation-induced skin carcinogenesis. Neither dermal carcinogenicity nor photocarcinogenicity studies have been performed with NORITATE or any marketed metronidazole formulations.

Pregnancy: *Teratogenic Effects*: Pregnancy Category B. There are no adequate and well controlled studies with the use of NORITATE in pregnant women.

Metronidazole crosses the placental barrier and enters the fetal circulation rapidly. No fetotoxicity was observed after oral administration of metronidazole to rats or mice at 200 and 20 times, respectively, the expected clinical dose. However, oral metronidazole has shown carcinogenic activity in rodents. Because animal reproduction studies are not always predictive of human response, NORITATE should be used during pregnancy only if clearly needed.

Nursing Mothers: After oral administration, metronidazole is secreted in breast milk in concentrations similar to those found in the plasma. Even though blood levels taken after topical metronidazole application are significantly lower than those achieved after oral metronidazole, a decision should be made whether to discontinue nursing or to discontinue the drug, taking into account the importance of the drug to the mother and the risk to the infant.

Pediatric Use: Safety and effectiveness in pediatric patients have not been established.

ADVERSE REACTIONS

Safety data from 302 patients who used NORITATE (n=200) or vehicle control (n=102) once daily in clinical trials and experienced an adverse event considered to be treatment-related include: application site reaction (NORITATE 1, vehicle 1), condition aggravated (NORITATE 1, vehicle 0), paresthesia (NORITATE 0, vehicle 1), acne (NORITATE 1, vehicle 0), dry skin (NORITATE 0, vehicle 2). The majority of adverse reactions were mild to moderate in severity.

Two patients treated with NORITATE once daily discontinued treatment because of adverse events: one for a severe flare of comedonal acne and one for rosacea aggravated.

DOSAGE AND ADMINISTRATION

Areas to be treated should be cleansed before application of NORITATE. Apply and rub in a thin film of NORITATE once daily to entire affected area(s). Patients may use cosmetics after application of NORITATE.

HOW SUPPLIED

Cream—30 gram aluminum tube NDC 0066-9850-30.

Caution: Federal law prohibits dispensing without a prescription. Keep out of the reach of children.

Storage Conditions: Store at controlled room temperature: 20 to 25°C (68 to 77°F).

Marketed by:
Dermik Laboratories, Inc.
A Rhône-Poulenc Rorer Company
Collegeville, PA 19426 Rev. 09/97
Made in Canada IN-0040
688097-20-0

PSORCON® CREAM ℞

[*sŏr-kon*]
(diflorasone diacetate cream) 0.05%

Caution: Federal law prohibits dispensing without prescription.

For Dermatological Use Only—Not for Ophthalmic Use.

DESCRIPTION

psorcon (diflorasone diacetate cream) contains the active compound diflorasone diacetate, a synthetic corticosteroid for topical dermatological use.

Chemically, diflorasone diacetate is 6α, 9α-difluoro-11β,17,21-trihydroxy-16-methylpregna-1,4-diene-3,20-dione 17,21 diacetate, with the empirical formula $C_{26}H_{32}F_2O_7$, a molecular weight of 494.5, and the following structural formula:

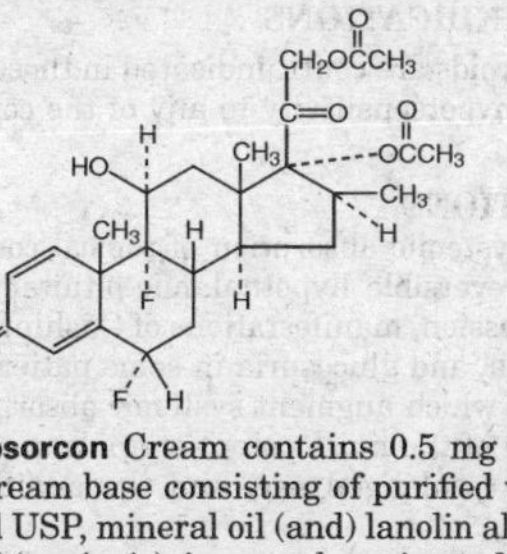

Each gram of **psorcon** Cream contains 0.5 mg diflorasone diacetate in a cream base consisting of purified water USP, propylene glycol USP, mineral oil (and) lanolin alcohol, glyceryl stearate SE (nonionic), isopropyl myristate NF, polysorbate 60 NF, sorbitan monostearate NF, polyoxyl 40 stearate NF, cetyl alcohol NF, monobasic sodium phosphate USP, vegetable oil, monoglyceride citrate, BHT and citric acid.

CLINICAL PHARMACOLOGY

Like other topical corticosteroids, diflorasone diacetate has anti-inflammatory, anti-pruritic, and vasoconstrictive actions. The mechanism of the anti-inflammatory activity of the topical corticosteroids, in general, is unclear. However, corticosteroids are thought to act by the induction of phospholipase A_2 inhibitory proteins collectively called lipocortins. It is postulated that these proteins control the biosynthesis of potent mediators of inflammation such as prostaglandins and leukotrienes by inhibiting the release of their common precursor, arachidonic acid. Arachidonic acid is released from membrane phospholipids by phospholipase A_2.

Pharmacokinetics: The extent of percutaneous absorption of topical corticosteroids is determined by many factors including the vehicle and the integrity of the epidermal barrier. Occlusive dressings with hydrocortisone for up to 24 hours have not been demonstrated to increase penetration; however, occlusion of hydrocortisone for 96 hours markedly enhances penetration. Topical corticosteroids can be absorbed from normal intact skin. Inflammation and/or other disease processes in the skin may increase percutaneous absorption. Studies performed with **psorcon** Cream indicate that it is in the high range of potency as compared with other topical corticosteroids.

INDICATION AND USAGE

psorcon (diflorasone diacetate cream), 0.05% is a high potency corticosteroid indicated for the relief of the inflammatory and pruritic manifestations of corticosteroid-responsive dermatoses.

CONTRAINDICATIONS

psorcon (diflorasone diacetate cream) is contraindicated in those patients with a history of hypersensitivity to any of the components of the preparation.

PRECAUTIONS

General: Systemic absorption of topical corticosteroids can produce reversible hypothalamic-pituitary-adrenal (HPA) axis suppression with the potential for glucocorticosteroid insufficiency after withdrawal of treatment. Manifestations of Cushing's syndrome, hyperglycemia, and glucosuria can also be produced in some patients by systemic absorption of topical corticosteroids while on treatment. Patients receiving a large dose of a higher potency topical steroid applied to a large surface area or under an occlusive dressing should be evaluated periodically for evidence of HPA axis suppression. This may be done by using the ACTH-stimulation, A.M. plasma cortisol, and urinary free-cortisol tests.

This product has a greater ability to produce adrenal suppression than does **psorcon** (diflorasone diacetate) Ointment, 0.05%. At 30 g per day (applied as 15 g twice daily) **psorcon** Cream, 0.05% was shown to cause inhibition of the HPA axis in one of two patients following application for one week to psoriatic skin. At 15 g per day (applied as 7.5 g twice daily) **psorcon** Cream was shown to cause mild inhibition of the HPA axis in one of five patients following application for one week to diseased skin (psoriasis or atopic dermatitis). These effects were reversible upon discontinuation of treatment. By comparison, **psorcon** (diflorasone diacetate) Ointment, 0.05% did not produce significant HPA axis suppression when used in divided doses at 30 g per day for one week in patients with psoriasis or atopic dermatitis.

If HPA axis suppression is noted, an attempt should be made to withdraw the drug, to reduce the frequency of application, or to substitute a less potent corticosteroid. Recovery of HPA axis function is generally prompt and complete upon discontinuation of topical corticosteroids. Infrequently, signs and symptoms of glucocorticosteroid insufficiency may occur, requiring supplemental systemic corticosteroids. For information on systemic supplementation, see prescribing information for those products.

Pediatric patients may be more susceptible to systemic toxicity from equivalent doses due to their larger skin surface to body mass ratios (see PRECAUTIONS: Pediatric Use).

If irritation develops, **psorcon** (diflorasone diacetate cream) should be discontinued and appropriate therapy instituted. Allergic contact dermatitis with corticosteroids is usually diagnosed by observing failure to heal rather than noting a clinical exacerbation as with most topical products not containing corticosteroids. Such an observation should be corroborated with appropriate diagnostic patch testing.

If concomitant skin infections are present or develop, an appropriate antifungal or antibacterial agent should be used. If a favorable response does not occur promptly, use of **psorcon** (diflorasone diacetate cream) should be discontinued until the infection has been adequately controlled.

psorcon (diflorasone diacetate cream) should not be used in the treatment of rosacea or perioral dermatitis, and it should not be used on the face, groin, or axillae.

Information for Patients: Patients using topical corticosteroids should receive the following information and instructions:

Continued on next page

Psorcon Cream—Cont.

1. The medication is to be used as directed by the physician. It is for external use only. Avoid contact with the eyes.
2. The medication should not be used for any disorder other than that for which it was prescribed.
3. The treated skin area should not be bandaged or otherwise covered or wrapped so as to be occlusive unless directed by the physician.
4. Patients should report to their physician any signs of local adverse reactions.

Laboratory Tests: The following tests may be helpful in evaluating patients for HPA axis suppression: ACTH-stimulation test; A.M. plasma-cortisol test; Urinary free-cortisol test.

Carcinogenesis, Mutagenesis and Impairment of Fertility: Long-term animal studies have not been performed to evaluate the carcinogenic potential of diflorasone diacetate.
Diflorasone diacetate was not found to be mutagenic in a micronucleus test in rats at dosages of 2400 mg/kg.
Studies in the rat following topical administration at doses up to 0.5 mg/kg revealed no effects on fertility.

Pregnancy: Teratogenic effects. Pregnancy Category C. Corticosteroids have been shown to be teratogenic in laboratory animals when administered systemically at relatively low dosage levels. Some corticosteroids have been shown to be teratogenic after dermal application to laboratory animals.
Diflorasone diacetate has been shown to be teratogenic (cleft palate) in rats when applied topically at a dose of approximately 0.001 mg/kg/day to the shaven thorax of pregnant animals. This is approximately 0.3 times the human topical dose of **psorcon** (diflorasone diacetate cream). When pregnant rats were treated topically with approximately 0.5 mg/kg/day, uterine deaths were higher in the treated animals than in control animals.
In rabbits, cleft palate was seen when diflorasone diacetate was applied in topical doses as low as 20 mg/kg/day. In addition, fetal weight was depressed and litter sizes were smaller.
There are no adequate and well-controlled studies of the teratogenic potential of diflorasone diacetate in pregnant women. **psorcon** Cream should be used during pregnancy only if the potential benefit justifies the potential risk to the fetus.

Nursing Mothers: Systemically administered corticosteroids appear in human milk and could suppress growth, interfere with endogenous corticosteroid production, or cause other untoward effects. It is not known whether topical administration of corticosteroids could result in sufficient systemic absorption to produce detectable quantities in human milk. Because many drugs are excreted in human milk, caution should be exercised when **psorcon** (diflorasone diacetate cream) is administered to a nursing woman.

Pediatric Use: Safety and effectiveness of **psorcon** (diflorasone diacetate cream) in pediatric patients have not been established. Because of a higher ratio of skin surface area to body mass, pediatric patients are at a greater risk than adults of HPA-axis suppression when they are treated with topical corticosteroids. They are, therefore, also at greater risk of glucocorticosteroid insufficiency after withdrawal of treatment and of Cushing's syndrome while on treatment. Adverse effects including striae have been reported with inappropriate use of topical corticosteroids in pediatric patients.
HPA axis suppression, Cushing's syndrome, and intracranial hypertension have been reported in pediatric patients receiving topical corticosteroids. Manifestations of adrenal suppression in pediatric patients include linear growth retardation, delayed weight gain, low plasma cortisol levels, and absence of response to ACTH stimulation. Manifestations of intracranial hypertension include bulging fontanelles, headaches, and bilateral papilledema.

ADVERSE REACTIONS

The following local adverse reactions have been reported infrequently with other topical corticosteroids, and they may occur more frequently with the use of occlusive dressings, especially with higher potency corticosteroids. These reactions are listed in an approximate decreasing order of occurrence: burning, itching, irritation, dryness, folliculitis, acneiform eruptions, hypopigmentation, perioral dermatitis, allergic contact dermatitis, secondary infections, skin atrophy, striae, and miliaria.

OVERDOSAGE

Topically applied **psorcon** (diflorasone diacetate cream) can be absorbed in sufficient amounts to produce systemic effects (see PRECAUTIONS).

DOSAGE AND ADMINISTRATION

psorcon (diflorasone diacetate cream) should be applied to the affected area twice daily.

HOW SUPPLIED

psorcon Cream 0.05% is available in the following size tubes:
15 gram NDC 0066-0069-17
30 gram NDC 0066-0069-31
60 gram NDC 0066-0069-60
Store at or below 25°C (77°F).
Manufactured by
Pharmacia & Upjohn Company
Kalamazoo, MI, USA 49001
For **Dermik Laboratories, Inc.**
A Rhône-Poulenc Rorer Company
Collegeville, PA 19426
US Patent No. 3,980,778
Revised January 1997 815 437 103α
691694
IN-1193D

PSORCON® OINTMENT ℞

[*sŏr-kon*]
(diflorasone diacetate ointment) 0.05%
Not for Ophthalmic Use

DESCRIPTION

Each gram of **psorcon** Ointment contains 0.5 mg diflorasone diacetate in an ointment base.
Chemically, diflorasone diacetate is 6α, 9-difluoro-11β,17,21-trihydroxy-16β-methylpregna-1,4-diene-3,20-dione 17,21-diacetate. The structural formula is represented below:

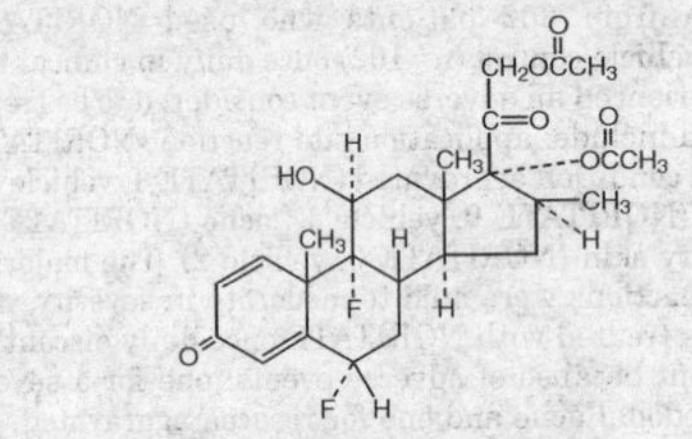

Each gram of **psorcon** Ointment contains 0.5 mg diflorasone diacetate in an ointment base of propylene glycol, glyceryl monostearate and white petrolatum.

CLINICAL PHARMACOLOGY

Topical corticosteroids share anti-inflammatory, antipruritic and vasoconstrictive actions.
The mechanism of anti-inflammatory activity of the topical corticosteroids is unclear. Various laboratory methods, including vasoconstrictor assays, are used to compare and predict potencies and/or clinical efficacies of the topical corticosteroids. There is some evidence to suggest that a recognizable correlation exists between vasoconstrictor potency and therapeutic efficacy in man.

Pharmacokinetics: The extent of percutaneous absorption of topical corticosteroids is determined by many factors including the vehicle, the integrity of the epidermal barrier, and the use of occlusive dressings.
Topical corticosteroids can be absorbed from normal intact skin. Inflammation and/or other disease processes in the skin increase percutaneous absorption. Occlusive dressings substantially increase the percutaneous absorption of topical corticosteroids. Thus, occlusive dressings may be a valuable therapeutic adjunct for treatment of resistant dermatoses. (See DOSAGE AND ADMINISTRATION.)
Once absorbed through the skin, topical corticosteroids are handled through pharmacokinetic pathways similar to systemically administered corticosteroids. Corticosteroids are bound to plasma proteins in varying degrees. They are metabolized primarily in the liver and are then excreted by the kidneys. Some of the topical corticosteroids and their metabolites are also excreted into the bile.

INDICATIONS AND USAGE

Topical corticosteroids are indicated for relief of the inflammatory and pruritic manifestations of corticosteroid-responsive dermatoses.

CONTRAINDICATIONS

Topical steroids are contraindicated in those patients with a history of hypersensitivity to any of the components of the preparation.

PRECAUTIONS

General: Systemic absorption of topical corticosteroids has produced reversible hypothalamic-pituitary-adrenal (HPA) axis suppression, manifestations of Cushing's syndrome, hyperglycemia, and glucosuria in some patients.
Conditions which augment systemic absorption include the application of the more potent steroids, use over large surface areas, prolonged use, and the addition of occlusive dressings.
Therefore, patients receiving a large dose of a potent topical steroid applied to a large surface area or under an occlusive dressing should be evaluated periodically for evidence of HPA axis suppression by using the urinary free cortisol and ACTH stimulation tests. If HPA axis suppression is noted, an attempt should be made to withdraw the drug, to reduce the frequency of application, or to substitute a less potent steroid.
Recovery of HPA axis function is generally prompt and complete upon discontinuation of the drug. Infrequently, signs and symptoms of steroid withdrawal may occur, requiring supplemental systemic corticosteroids.
Pediatric patients may absorb proportionally larger amounts of topical corticosteroids and thus be more susceptible to systemic toxicity. (See PRECAUTIONS—Pediatric Use.)
If irritation develops, topical corticosteroids should be discontinued and appropriate therapy instituted.
In the presence of dermatological infections, the use of an appropriate antifungal or antibacterial agent should be instituted. If a favorable response does not occur promptly, the corticosteroid should be discontinued until the infection has been adequately controlled.

Information for the Patient: Patients using topical corticosteroids should receive the following information and instructions:

1. This medication is to be used as directed by the physician. It is for external use only. Avoid contact with the eyes.
2. Patients should be advised not to use this medication for any disorder other than for which it was prescribed.
3. The treated skin area should not be bandaged or otherwise covered or wrapped as to be occlusive unless directed by the physician.
4. Patients should report any signs of local adverse reactions especially under occlusive dressing.
5. Parents of pediatric patients should be advised not to use tight-fitting diapers or plastic pants on an infant or child being treated in the diaper area, as these garments may constitute occlusive dressings.

Laboratory Tests: The following tests may be helpful in evaluating the HPA axis suppression:
Urinary free cortisol test
ACTH stimulation test

Carcinogenesis, Mutagenesis, and Impairment of Fertility: Long-term animal studies have not been performed to evaluate the carcinogenic potential or the effect on fertility of topical corticosteroids.
Studies to determine mutagenicity with prednisolone and hydrocortisone have revealed negative results.

Pregnancy Category C: Corticosteroids are generally teratogenic in laboratory animals when administered systemically at relatively low dosage levels. The more potent corticosteroids have been shown to be teratogenic after dermal application in laboratory animals. There are no adequate and well-controlled studies in pregnant women on teratogenic effects from topically applied corticosteroids. Therefore, topical corticosteroids should be used during pregnancy only if the potential benefit justifies the potential risk to the fetus. Drugs of this class should not be used extensively on pregnant patients, in large amounts, or for prolonged periods of time.

Nursing Mothers: It is not known whether topical administration of corticosteroids could result in sufficient systemic absorption to produce detectable quantities in breast milk. Systemically administered corticosteroids are secreted into breast milk in quantities **not** likely to have a deleterious effect on the infant. Nevertheless, caution should be exercised when topical corticosteroids are administered to a nursing woman.

Pediatric Use: *Pediatric patients may demonstrate greater susceptibility to topical corticosteroid-induced HPA axis suppression and Cushing's syndrome than mature patients because of a larger skin surface area to body weight ratio.*
Hypothalamic-pituitary-adrenal (HPA) axis suppression, Cushing's syndrome, and intracranial hypertension have been reported in pediatric patients receiving topical corticosteroids. Manifestations of adrenal suppression in pediatric patients include linear growth retardation, delayed weight gain, low plasma cortisol levels, and absence of response to ACTH stimulation. Manifestations of intracranial hypertension include bulging fontanelles, headaches, and bilateral papilledema.
Administration of topical corticosteroids to pediatric patients should be limited to the least amount compatible with an effective therapeutic regimen. Chronic corticosteroid therapy may interfere with the growth and development of pediatric patients.

ADVERSE REACTIONS

The following local adverse reactions have been reported with topical corticosteroids, but may occur more frequently with the use of occlusive dressings. These reactions are listed in approximate decreasing order of occurrence:

1. Burning
2. Itching
3. Irritation
4. Dryness
5. Folliculitis
6. Hypertrichosis

7. Acneiform eruptions
8. Hypopigmentation
9. Perioral dermatitis
10. Allergic contact dermatitis
11. Maceration of the skin
12. Secondary infection
13. Skin atrophy
14. Striae
15. Miliaria

OVERDOSAGE

Topically applied corticosteroids can be absorbed in sufficient amounts to produce systemic effects. (See PRECAUTIONS.)

DOSAGE AND ADMINISTRATION

psorcon Ointment should be applied to the affected area as a thin film from one to three times daily depending on the severity or resistant nature of the condition.
Occlusive dressings may be used for the management of psoriasis or recalcitrant conditions.
If an infection develops, the use of occlusive dressings should be discontinued and appropriate antimicrobial therapy initiated.

HOW SUPPLIED

psorcon Ointment 0.05% is available in the following size tubes:

15 gram	NDC 0066-0071-17
30 gram	NDC 0066-0071-31
60 gram	NDC 0066-0071-60

Store at controlled room temperature 20° to 25°C (68° to 77°F) [see USP].
Caution: Federal law prohibits dispensing without prescription.
Manufactured by
Pharmacia & Upjohn Company
Kalamazoo, MI, USA 49001
For
Dermik Laboratories, Inc.
A Rhône-Poulenc Rorer Company
Collegeville, PA, USA 19426
Revised October 1996
IN-7191J

813 377 208α
691694

SULFACET-R® Lotion ℞
[sul-fa-set]
(Sodium Sulfacetamide 10% and Sulfur 5%)

DESCRIPTION

Each mL of **Sulfacet-R® Lotion** (sodium sulfacetamide 10% and sulfur 5%) as dispensed contains 100 mg of sodium sulfacetamide and 50 mg of sulfur in a tinted lotion of 2-bromo-2-nitropropane-1, 3 diol, attapulgite, butylparaben, hydroxyethyl cellulose, iron oxides, lauramide DEA (and) diethanolamine, methylparaben, polyethylene glycol 400 monolaurate, propylene glycol, purified water, silicone emulsion, sodium chloride, sodium metabisulfite, sodium polynaphthalenesulfonate, talc, titanium dioxide, xanthan gum, and zinc oxide. Color Blender contains an additional inactive ingredient, polyethylene glycol 400, NF.
Sodium sulfacetamide is a sulfonamide with antibacterial activity while sulfur acts as a keratolytic agent. Chemically sodium sulfacetamide is N'-[(4-aminophenyl) sulfonyl]-acetamide, monosodium salt, monohydrate.
The structural formula is:
Sulfacetamide Sodium

$$NH_2 - - SO_2NCOCH_3 \cdot H_2O$$

CLINICAL PHARMACOLOGY

The most widely accepted mechanism of action of sulfonamides is the Woods-Fildes theory which is based on the fact that sulfonamides act as competitive antagonists to para-aminobenzoic acid (PABA), an essential component for bacterial growth. While absorption through intact skin has not been determined, sodium sulfacetamide is readily absorbed from the gastrointestinal tract when taken orally and excreted in the urine, largely unchanged. The biological half-life has variously been reported as 7 to 12.8 hours.
The exact mode of action of sulfur in the treatment of acne is unknown, but it has been reported that it inhibits the growth of *p. acnes* and the formation of free fatty acids.

INDICATIONS

Sulfacet-R® Lotion is indicated in the topical control of acne vulgaris, acne rosacea and seborrheic dermatitis.

CONTRAINDICATIONS

Sulfacet-R Lotion is contraindicated for use by patients having known hypersensitivity to sulfonamides, sulfur, or any other component of this preparation. **Sulfacet-R Lotion** is not to be used by patients with kidney disease.

WARNINGS

Although rare, sensitivity to sodium sulfacetamide may occur. Therefore, caution and careful supervision should be observed when prescribing this drug for patients who may be prone to hypersensitivity to topical sulfonamides. Systemic toxic reactions such as agranulocytosis, acute hemolytic anemia, purpura hemorrhagica, drug fever, jaundice, and contact dermatitis indicate hypersensitivity to sulfonamides. Particular caution should be employed if areas of denuded or abraded skin are involved.
Contains sodium metabisulfite, a sulfite that may cause allergic-type reactions including anaphylactic symptoms and life-threatening or less severe asthmatic episodes in certain susceptible people. The overall prevalence of sulfite sensitivity in the general population is unknown and probably low. Sulfite sensitivity is seen more frequently in asthmatic than in nonasthmatic people.

PRECAUTIONS

General: If irritation develops, use of the product should be discontinued and appropriate therapy instituted. For external use only. Keep away from eyes. Patients should be carefully observed for possible local irritation or sensitization during long-term therapy. The object of this therapy is to achieve desquamation without irritation, but sodium sulfacetamide and sulfur can cause reddening and scaling of epidermis. These side effects are not unusual in the treatment of acne vulgaris, but patients should be cautioned about the possibility. Keep out of the reach of children.
Carcinogenesis, Mutagenesis and Impairment of Fertility: Long-term studies in animals have not been performed to evaluate carcinogenic potential.
Pregnancy: Category C. Animal reproduction studies have not been conducted with Sulfacet-R Lotion. It is also not known whether Sulfacet-R Lotion can cause fetal harm when administered to a pregnant woman or can affect reproduction capacity. Sulfacet-R Lotion should be given to a pregnant woman only if clearly needed.
Nursing Mothers: It is not known whether sodium sulfacetamide is excreted in the human milk following topical use of Sulfacet-R Lotion. However, small amounts of orally administered sulfonamides have been reported to be eliminated in human milk. In view of this and because many drugs are excreted in human milk, caution should be exercised when Sulfacet-R Lotion is administered to a nursing woman.
Pediatric Use: Safety and effectiveness in pediatric patients under the age of 12 have not been established.

ADVERSE REACTIONS

Although rare, sodium sulfacetamide may cause local irritation.

DOSAGE AND ADMINISTRATION

Shake well before using. Apply a thin film to affected areas with light massaging to blend in each application 1 to 3 times daily. Each package contains a Dermik Color Blender-trademark which enables the patient to alter the basic shade of the lotion so that it matches the skin color exactly.
(Important to the Pharmacist: At the time of dispensing, add contents of Sulfa-Pak™ vial* to the bottle. Shake well and/or stir with a glass rod to insure uniform dispersion. Place expiration date of four (4) months on bottle label.)
*Sulfa-Pak™ vial contains 2.1 g of sodium sulfacetamide.

HOW SUPPLIED

25 g bottles (NDC 0066-0028-25).
CAUTION: Federal law prohibits dispensing without prescription.
Dermik Laboratories, Inc.
A Rhône-Poulenc Rorer Company
Collegeville, PA, USA 19426

Rev. 11/96
CR-5055R

SULFACET-R® TINT FREE LOTION ℞
[sul-fā-set]
(Sodium Sulfacetamide 10% and Sulfur 5%)

DESCRIPTION

Each mL of **Sulfacet-R® Tint Free Lotion**e (sodium sulfacetamide 10% and sulfur 5%) as dispensed contains 100 mg of sodium sulfacetamide and 50 mg of sulfur in a lotion of 2-bromo-2-nitropropane-1, 3 diol, attapulgite, butylparaben, hydroxyethyl cellulose, iron oxides, lauramide DEA (and) diethanolamine, methylparaben, polyethylene glycol 400 monolaurate, propylene glycol, purified water, silicone emulsion, sodium chloride, sodium metabisulfite, sodium polynaphthalenesulfonate, talc, xanthan gum, and zinc oxide.
Sodium sulfacetamide is a sulfonamide with antibacterial activity while sulfur acts as a keratolytic agent. Chemically sodium sulfacetamide is N'-[(4-aminophenyl) sulfonyl]-acetamide, monosodium salt, monohydrate.

HOW SUPPLIED

25 g bottles (NDC 0066-9028-25).
Store at room temperature. Keep tightly closed.

Caution: Federal law prohibits dispensing without prescription.
Dermik Laboratories, Inc.
A Rhône-Poulenc Rorer Company
Collegeville, PA 19426

Rev. 11/96
CR-5380A

VANOXIDE®-HC LOTION ℞
[vă-noxĭde]
(benzoyl peroxide 50 mg, hydrocortisone 5 mg)

DESCRIPTION

Each mL of **Vanoxide®-HC Lotion** contains, as dispensed, 50 mg benzoyl peroxide and 5 mg hydrocortisone in a water washable vanishing lotion of BHA/BHT, caprylic/capric triglyceride, cetyl alcohol, decyl oleate, dibasic sodium phosphate, edetic acid, hydroxyethyl cellulose, methylparaben, mineral oil (and) lanolin oil, monobasic sodium phosphate, monoglyceride citrate, polysorbate 20, polysorbate 80 (and) cetyl acetate (and) acetylated lanolin alcohol, propyl gallate, propylene glycol, propylene glycol monostearate, propylparaben, purified water, simethicone, sodium hydroxide, stearyl heptanoate, tetrasodium EDTA, and vegetable oil.
The structural formula for benzoyl peroxide is:

$$O=C-O-O-C=O$$

The structural formula for hydrocortisone, chemically 11β, 17, 21-trihydroxypregn-4-ene-3, 20-dione, is:

CLINICAL PHARMACOLOGY

Benzoyl peroxide is an antibacterial agent which has been shown to be effective against *Propionibacterium acnes*. This action is believed to be largely responsible for its usefulness. In addition, benzoyl peroxide exerts a desquamative and keratolytic action. One study in the rhesus monkey demonstrated a percutaneous absorption of about 1.8 µg per cm^2 of benzoyl peroxide or 45% of the applied dose in a 24-hour period. The absorbed benzoyl peroxide was completely converted in the skin to benzoic acid.
Topical steroids are primarily effective because of their anti-inflammatory, antipruritic and vasoconstrictive actions.

INDICATION AND USAGE

Treatment of acne vulgaris and oily skin.

CONTRAINDICATIONS

Vanoxide-HC Lotion is contraindicated in individuals having known sensitivity to benzoyl peroxide, hydrocortisone or any of the components of the product. Topical steroids are contraindicated in viral diseases of the skin, such as varicella or vaccinia.

WARNINGS

If itching, redness, swelling or undue dryness occurs, discontinue use.

PRECAUTIONS

For external use only. Keep away from the eyes and mucosae. Very fair individuals should begin with a single application at bedtime allowing overnight medication. May bleach colored fabrics.
Carcinogenesis, Mutagenesis, Impairment of Fertility: Long-term studies in animals have not been performed to evaluate carcinogenic potential.
Pregnancy, Category C: Animal reproduction studies have not been conducted with Vanoxide-HC Lotion. It is not known whether Vanoxide-HC Lotion can cause fetal harm when administered to a pregnant woman or can affect reproduction capacity. Vanoxide-HC Lotion should be given to a pregnant woman only if clearly needed.
Nursing Mothers: It is not known whether this drug is excreted in human milk. Because many drugs are excreted in human milk, caution should be exercised when Vanoxide-HC Lotion is administered to a nursing woman.
Pediatric Use: Safety and effectiveness in pediatric patients under the age of 12 have not been established.

ADVERSE REACTIONS

Irritation and contact dermatitis are the most frequent side reactions to benzoyl peroxide. Although 0.5% hydrocortisone

Continued on next page

Vanoxide-HC—Cont.

is considered safe, the following adverse reactions have been reported with topical corticosteriods, especially under occlusive dressings: burning, itching, irritation, dryness, folliculitis, hypertrichosis, acneform eruptions, hypopigmentation, perioral dermatitis, allergic contact dermatitis, maceration of the skin, secondary infection, skin atrophy, striae, miliaria.

DOSAGE AND ADMINISTRATION

Shake well before using. Apply a thin film 1 to 3 times daily with gentle massaging to blend with skin, or as directed by physician.

HOW SUPPLIED

Bottles, 25 grams net weight as dispensed. Package contains a bottle of lotion base and a **Benzie-Pak™** vial containing a mixture of 35% benzoyl peroxide, 64% calcium phosphate and 1% silica. Net weight of vial is 3.8 grams.
To the Pharmacist: At the time of dispensing, add contents of **Benzie-Pak™** to the lotion in the bottle. Shake well and/or stir with glass rod to ensure uniform dispersion. Place expiration date of three (3) months on bottle label.
Caution: Federal law prohibits dispensing without prescription.
KEEP THIS AND ALL MEDICATIONS OUT OF THE REACH OF CHILDREN.
Marketed by
Dermik Laboratories, Inc.
A Rhône-Poulenc Rorer Company   Rev. 8/96
Collegeville, PA 19426   CR-5043L

VYTONE® CREAM 1%   ℞
[*vī-tōne*]
(hydrocortisone-iodoquinol)

DESCRIPTION

Each gram of Vytone® Cream 1% contains 10 mg of hydrocortisone and 10 mg of iodoquinol in a greaseless base of purified water, propylene glycol, glyceryl monostearate SE, cholesterol and related sterols, isopropyl myristate, polysorbate 60, cetyl alcohol, sorbitan monostearate, polyoxyl 40 stearate, sorbic acid, and polysorbate 20.

HOW SUPPLIED

1%—Tube 1 oz NDC 0066-0051-01
CAUTION: Federal law prohibits dispensing without prescription.
Dermik Laboratories, Inc.   IN-5357K
A Rhône-Poulenc Rorer Company   Rev. 12/96
Collegeville, PA 19426

ZETAR® EMULSION (Coal Tar)   ℞
[*zē-tar*]

DESCRIPTION

Zetar® Emulsion, coal tar, is a liquid for topical application, following dilution in aqueous media. Each ml contains 300 mg whole coal tar in polysorbates. It is a topical anti-eczematic. The complete chemical composition of coal tar has not been ascertained; components are grouped into six categories: aromatic hydrocarbons, acidic phenolic compounds, cyclic nitrogen compounds, organic sulfur compounds, nonacidic phenolics and nonbasic nitrogen compounds.

HOW SUPPLIED

Zetar® Emulsion (coal tar) is available in 6 fl oz (177 ml) plastic bottles. The strength of the preparation is 300 mg coal tar/mL.

IDENTIFICATION PROBLEM?
Turn to the **Product Identification Guide,**
where you'll find more than
1600 products pictured in actual
size and full color.

Dey
2751 NAPA VALLEY CORPORATE DRIVE
NAPA, CA 94558

Direct Inquiries to:
Russ Johnston
(800) 755-5560
FAX: (707) 224-8918
For Medical Information Contact:
In Emergencies:
Cal McGoogan
(707) 224-3200
FAX: (707) 224-3235

Brand Name or Generic Name	Concentration Or Size	NDC or Product #
Acetylcysteine Solution USP (Mucosil™)	Acetylcysteine Solution 10%	
	Twelve 4 mL Vials	49502-181-04
	Three 10 mL Vials	49502-181-10
	Three 30 mL Vials	49502-181-30
Acetylcysteine Solution USP (Mucosil™)	Acetylcysteine Solution 20%	
	Twelve 4 mL Vials	49502-182-04
	Three 10 mL Vials	49502-182-10
	Three 30 mL Vials	49502-182-30
	One 100 mL Vial	49502-182-00
Albuterol Inhalation Aerosol (℞)	One 17 g Inhaler 200 Metered Inhalations	49502-303-17
	One 17g Refill	49502-303-27

Shown in Product Identification Guide, page 309

Albuterol Sulfate Inhalation Solution (℞)	Twenty-Five 3 mL Vials 0.083% (expressed as Albuterol)	49502-697-03
	Thirty 3 mL Vials 0.083% (expressed as Albuterol)	49502-697-33
	Sixty 3 mL Vials 0.083% (expressed as Albuterol)	49502-697-60

Shown in Product Identification Guide, page 309

Albuterol Sulfate Inhalation Solution 0.5% (℞)	One 20 mL Concentrate	49502-196-20

Shown in Product Identification Guide, page 309

Cromolyn Sodium Inhalation Solution USP (℞)	Sixty 2 mL Vials 20 mg/2mL	49502-689-02
	One Hundred Twenty 2 mL Vials 20 mg/2mL	49502-689-12

Shown in Product Identification Guide, page 309

Ipratropium Bromide Inhalation Solution (℞)	Twenty-five 2.5 mL Vials (0.5 mg/2.5 mL)	49502-685-03
	Thirty 2.5 ml vials (0.5/2.5 mL)	49502-685-33
	Sixty 2.5 mL Vials (0.5/2.5 mL)	49502-685-60

Shown in Product Identification Guide, page 309

Metaproterenol Sulfate Inhalation Solution USP (℞)	Twenty-five 2.5 mL Vials 0.4%	49502-678-03
	Twenty-five 2.5 mL Vials 0.6%	49502-676-03

Shown in Product Identification Guide, page 309

Sodium Chloride Inhalation Solution USP (OTC)	One Hundred 3 mL Vials 0.45%	49502-820-03
	One Hundred 5 mL Vials 0.45%	49502-820-05
	One Hundred 3 mL Vials 0.9%	49502-830-03
	One Hundred 5 mL Vials 0.9%	49502-830-05
	Twenty Four 15 mL Vials 0.9%	49502-830-15
Sodium Chloride Solution (℞)	Fifty 15 mL Vials 3%	49502-640-15
	Fifty 15 mL Vials 10%	49502-641-15
Sterile Water For Inhalation USP (OTC)	One Hundred 3 mL Vials	49502-810-03
	One Hundred 5 mL Vials	49502-810-05

EPIPEN® 0.3-mg   ℞
EPINEPHRINE AUTO-INJECTOR
Auto-Injector for Intramuscular Injection of EPINEPHRINE
For the Emergency Treatment of Allergic Reactions (Anaphylaxis)
Delivers 0.3 mg intramuscular dose of epinephrine from epinephrine injection, USP, 1:1000 (0.3 mL).

EPIPEN® JR. 0.15 mg   ℞
EPINEPHRINE AUTO-INJECTOR
Auto-Injector for Intramuscular Injection of EPINEPHRINE
For the Emergency Treatment of Allergic Reactions (Anaphylaxis)
Delivers 0.15 mg intramuscular dose of epinephrine from epinephrine injection, USP, 1:2000 (0.3 mL).

IMPORTANT INFORMATION
- **DO NOT REMOVE SAFETY CAP UNTIL READY FOR USE.**
- **ONLY 0.3 ML OF SOLUTION IS DISPENSED. THE MAJORITY OF THE DRUG PRODUCT, 1.7 ML, REMAINS IN THE AUTO-INJECTOR AFTER ACTIVATION.**
- **THE UNIT CONTAINS NO LATEX.**

DESCRIPTION

The EpiPen and EpiPen Jr. Auto-Injectors contain 2 mL epinephrine injection for emergency intramuscular use. Each EpiPen auto-injector delivers a single dose of 0.3 mg epinephrine from epinephrine injection, USP, 1:1000 (0.3 mL) in a sterile solution.
Each EpiPen Jr. auto-injector delivers a single dose of 0.15 mg epinephrine from epinephrine injection, USP, 1:2000 (0.3 mL) in a sterile solution.
For stability purposes, approximately 1.7 mL remains in the auto-injector after activation.
Each 0.3 mL in the EpiPen contains 0.3 mg epinephrine, 1.8 mg sodium chloride, 0.5 mg sodium metabisulfite, hydrochloric acid to adjust pH, and Water for Injection. The pH range is 2.2–5.0.
Each 0.3 mL in the EpiPen Jr. contains 0.15 mg epinephrine, 1.8 mg sodium chloride, 0.5 mg sodium metabisulfite, hydrochloric acid to adjust pH, and Water for Injection. The pH range is 2.2–5.0.
Epinephrine is a sympathomimetic catecholamine. Chemically, epinephrine is B-(3, 4-dihydroxyphenyl)-a-methylaminoethanol, with the following structure:

$$HO-C_6H_3(OH)-\overset{OH}{\underset{H}{C}}-CH_2NHCH_3$$

It deteriorates rapidly on exposure to air or light, turning pink from oxidation to adrenochrome and brown from the formation of melanin. Epinephrine solutions which show evidence of discoloration should be replaced.

CLINICAL PHARMACOLOGY

Epinephrine is a sympathomimetic drug, acting on both alpha and beta receptors. It is the drug of choice for the emergency treatment of severe allergic reactions (Type I) to insect stings or bites, foods, drugs, and other allergens. It can also be used in the treatment of idiopathic or exercise-induced anaphylaxis. Epinephrine when given subcutaneously or intramuscularly has a rapid onset and short duration of action. The strong vasoconstrictor action of epinephrine through its effect on alpha adrenergic receptors acts quickly to counter vasodilation and increased vascular permeability which can lead to loss of intravascular fluid volume and hypotension during anaphylactic reactions. Epinephrine through its action on beta receptors on bronchial smooth muscle causes bronchial smooth muscle relaxation which alleviates wheezing and dyspnea. Epinephrine also alleviates pruritis, urticaria, and angioedema and may be effective in relieving gastrointestinal and genitourinary symptoms associated with anaphylaxis.

INDICATIONS AND USAGE

Epinephrine is indicated in the emergency treatment of allergic reactions (anaphylaxis) to insect stings or bites, foods, drugs and other allergens as well as idiopathic or exercise-induced anaphylaxis. The EpiPen and EpiPen Jr. auto-injectors are intended for immediate self-administration by a person with a history of an anaphylactic reaction. Such reactions may occur within minutes after exposure and consist of flushing, apprehension, syncope, tachycardia, thready or unobtainable pulse associated with a fall in blood pressure, convulsions, vomiting, diarrhea and abdominal cramps, involuntary voiding, wheezing, dyspnea due to laryngeal spasm, pruritis, rashes, uticaria or angioedema. The EpiPen and EpiPen Jr. are designed as emergency supportive therapy only and are not a replacement or substitute for immediate medical or hospital care.

CONTRAINDICATIONS

There are no absolute contraindications to the use of epinephrine in a life-threatening situation.

WARNINGS

Epinephrine is light sensitive and should be stored in the tube provided. Store at room temperature (15°–30°C/59°–86°F). Do not refrigerate. Before using, check to make sure solution in auto-injector is not discolored. Replace the auto-injector if the solution is discolored or contains a precipitate. Avoid possible inadvertent intravascular administration. EpiPen and EpiPen Jr. should **only** be injected into the anterolateral aspect of the thigh. DO NOT INJECT INTO THE BUTTOCK.

Large doses or accidental intravenous injection of epinephrine may result in cerebral hemorrhage due to sharp rise in blood pressure. DO NOT INJECT INTRAVENOUSLY. Rapidly acting vasodilators can counteract the marked pressor effects of epinephrine.

Epinephrine is the preferred treatment for serious allergic or other emergency situations even through this product contains sodium metabisulfite, a sulfite that may in other products cause allergic-type reactions including anaphylactic symptoms or life-threatening or less severe asthmatic episodes in certain susceptible persons. The alternatives to using epinephrine in a life-threatening situation may not be satisfactory. The presence of a sulfite in this product should not deter administration of the drug for treatment of serious allergic or other emergency situations.

Accidental injection into the hands or feet may result in loss of blood flow to the affected area and should be avoided. If there is an accidental injection into these areas, advise the patient to go immediately to the nearest emergency room for treatment. EpiPen and EpiPen Jr. should **only** be injected into the anterolateral aspect of the thigh.

PRECAUTIONS

Epinephrine is essential for the treatment of anaphylaxis. Patients with a history of severe allergic reactions (anaphylaxis) to insect stings or bites, foods, drugs, and other allergens as well as idiopathic and exercise-induced anaphylaxis should be carefully instructed about the circumstances under which this life-saving medication should be used. It must be clearly determined that the patient is at risk of future anaphylaxis, since the following risks may be associated with epinephrine administration (see Dosage and Administration).

Epinephrine is ordinarily administered with extreme caution to patients who have heart disease. Use of epinephrine with drugs that may sensitize the heart to arrhythmias, e.g., digitalis, mercurial diuretics, or quinidine, ordinarily is not recommended. Anginal pain may be induced by epinephrine in patients with coronary insufficiency.

The effects of epinephrine may be potentiated by tricyclic antidepressants and monoamine oxidase inhibitors.

Some patients may be theoretically at greater risk of developing adverse reactions after epinephrine administration. These include: hyperthyroid individuals, individuals with cardiovascular disease, hypertension, or diabetes, elderly individuals, pregnant women, pediatric patients under 30 kg (66 lbs.) body weight using EpiPen and pediatric patients under 15 kg (33 lbs.) body weight using EpiPen Jr.

Despite these concerns, epinephrine is essential for the treatment of anaphylaxis. Therefore, patients with these conditions, and/or any other person who might be in a position to administer EpiPen or EpiPen Jr. to a patient experiencing anaphylaxis should be carefully instructed in regard to the circumstances under which this life-saving medication should be used.

CARCINOGENESIS, MUTAGENESIS, IMPAIRMENT OF FERTILITY

Studies of epinephrine in animals to evaluate the carcinogenic and mutagenic potential or the effect on fertility have not been conducted. This should not prevent the use of this life-saving medication under the conditions noted in INDICATIONS AND USAGE and as indicated under PRECAUTIONS above.

USAGE IN PREGNANCY

Pregnancy Category C: Epinephrine has been shown to be teratogenic in rats when given in doses about 25 times the human dose. There are no adequate and well-controlled studies in pregnant women. Epinephrine should be used during pregnancy only if the potential benefit justifies the potential risk to the fetus.

PEDIATRIC USE

Epinephrine may be given safely to pediatric patients at a dosage appropriate to body weight (see Dosage and Administration).

ADVERSE REACTIONS

Side effects of epinephrine may include palpitations, tachycardia, sweating, nausea and vomiting, respiratory difficulty, pallor, dizziness, weakness, tremor, headache, apprehension, nervousness and anxiety.

Cardiac arrhythmias may follow administration of epinephrine.

OVERDOSAGE

Overdosage or inadvertent intravascular injection of epinephrine may cause cerebral hemorrhage resulting from a sharp rise in blood pressure. Fatalities may also result from pulmonary edema because of peripheral vascular constriction together with cardiac stimulation.

DOSAGE AND ADMINISTRATION

A physician who prescribes EpiPen or EpiPen Jr. should take appropriate steps to insure that the patient understands the indications and use of this device thoroughly. The physician should review with the patient or any other person who might be in a position to administer EpiPen or EpiPen Jr. to a patient experiencing anaphylaxis, in detail, the patient instructions and operation of the EpiPen or EpiPen Jr. auto-injector. Inject the delivered dose of the EpiPen auto-injector (0.3 mL epinephrine injection, USP, 1:1000) or the EpiPen Jr. auto-injector (0.3 mL epinephrine injection, USP, 1:2000) intramuscularly into the anterolateral aspect of the thigh, through clothing if necessary. See detailed Directions for Use on the accompanying Patient Instructions.

Usual epinephrine adult dose for allergic emergencies is 0.3 mg. For pediatric use, the appropriate dosage may be 0.15 or 0.30 mg depending upon the body weight of the patient. A dosage of 0.01 mg/kg body weight is recommended. EpiPen Jr., which provides a dosage of 0.15 mg, may be more appropriate for patients weighing less than 30 kg. However the prescribing physician has the option of prescribing more or less than these amounts, based on careful assessment of each individual patient and recognizing the life-threatening nature of the reactions for which this drug is being prescribed. The physician should consider using other forms of injectable epinephrine if doses lower than 0.15 mg are felt to be necessary.

With severe persistent anaphylaxis, repeat injections with an additional EpiPen may be necessary.

Parenteral drug products should be periodically inspected visually by the patient for particulate matter or discoloration and should be replaced if these are present.

HOW SUPPLIED

EpiPen auto-injectors (epinephrine injection, USP, 1:1000, 0.3 mL) are available singly or in packages of twelve (pharmacy pack), NDC 49502-500-01.

EpiPen Jr. auto-injectors (epinephrine injection, USP, 1:2000, 0.3 mL) are available singly or in packages of twelve (pharmacy Pack), NDC 49502-501-01.

Store in a dark place at room temperature (15°–30°C/59°–86°F). Do not refrigerate. Contains no latex.

Rx only.

DEY

Manufactured for Dey, Napa, California, 94558, U.S.A by Meridian Medical Technologies, Inc., Columbia, MD 21046, U.S.A.

Shown in Product Identification Guide, page 309

Dista Products Company
Division of Eli Lilly and Company
General Offices
LILLY CORPORATE CENTER
INDIANAPOLIS, INDIANA 46285

Direct Inquiries to:
Dista Products and Eli Lilly and Company
Lilly Corporate Center
Indianapolis, IN 46285
(317) 276-2000

For Medical Information Contact:
Lilly Research Laboratories
Lilly Corporate Center
Indianapolis, IN 46285
(800) 545-5979

LEGEND

Identi-Code®—*Formula Identification Code, Dista*
Identi-Dose®—*Unit Dose Medication, Dista*
Pulvules®—*Filled Gelatin Capsules, Dista*
R̥Pak—*Prescription Package, Dista*

IDENTI-CODE® Index
(formula identification code, Dista)
Provides Positive Product Identification

A letter-number symbol, a 4-digit number, the name of the product, the strength of the product, or a combination of these appears on each Dista capsule and tablet and on each label of pediatric liquids and powders for oral suspension. The letter/number or 4-digit number identifies the product.

Identi-Code® Product Name		
Coated		**Tablets**

Pulvules®

3104 Prozac®
Composition (Each Pulvule®): fluoxetine hydrochloride, 10 mg (equiv. to fluoxetine)

3105 Prozac®
Composition (Each Pulvule®): fluoxetine hydrochloride, 20 mg (equiv. to fluoxetine)

H09 Ilosone®
Composition (Each Pulvule®): Erythromycin Estolate, USP, 250 mg (equiv. to erythromycin)

H69 Keflex®
Composition (Each Pulvule®): Cephalexin, USP, 250 mg

H71 Keflex®
Composition (Each Pulvule®): Cephalexin, USP, 500 mg

Compressed Tablets

U26 Ilosone®
Composition (Each Compressed Tablet): Erythromycin Estolate, USP, 500 mg (equiv. to erythromycin)

Miscellaneous

W15 Ilosone® Liquid, Oral Suspension
Composition: Each 5 mL contain erythromycin estolate equivalent to 125 mg erythromycin (USP).

W17 Ilosone® Liquid, Oral Suspension
Composition: Each 5 mL contain erythromycin estolate equivalent to 250 mg erythromycin (USP).

W21 Keflex®, for Oral Suspension
Composition (When Mixed as Directed): Each 5 mL contain 125 mg cephalexin (USP).

W68 Keflex®, for Oral Suspension
Composition (When Mixed as Directed): Each 5 mL contain 250 mg cephalexin (USP).

UNIT-DOSE PACKAGING

Identi-Dose® (unit dose medication, Dista) Closed-circuit control of medication from pharmacy to nurse to patient and return. Simplifies counting and dispensing whether in single-unit or prescription-size quantities. Fits into any dispensing system for ready identification and legibility, better inventory control, protection from contamination, easier handling and recording under Medicare, prevention of drug loss through pilferage or spilling, better control of Federal Controlled Substances, and less chance of medication errors.

The following products are available through normal channels of supply:
Identi-Dose®
Pulvules®
No.
3105 Prozac®, 20 mg

ILOSONE®   R̥
[ī′lō-sōn]
ERYTHROMYCIN ESTOLATE, USP

WARNING

Hepatic dysfunction with or without jaundice has occurred, chiefly in adults, in association with erythromycin estolate administration. It may be accompanied by malaise, nausea, vomiting, abdominal colic, and fever. In some instances, severe abdominal pain may simulate an abdominal surgical emergency.

If the above findings occur, discontinue Ilosone® (Erythromycin Estolate, USP) promptly.

Ilosone is contraindicated for patients with a known history of sensitivity to this drug and for those with preexisting liver disease.

Continued on next page

This product information was prepared in June 1998. Current information on these and other products of Dista Products Company may be obtained by direct inquiry to Lilly Research Laboratories, Lilly Corporate Center, Indianapolis, Indiana 46285, (800) 545-5979.

Ilosone—Cont.

DESCRIPTION

Erythromycin is produced by a strain of *Saccharopolyspora erythraea* (formerly *Streptomyces erythraeus*) and belongs to the macrolide group of antibiotics. It is basic and readily forms salts with acids. The base, the stearate salt, and the esters are poorly soluble in water and are suitable for oral administration.

Chemically, erythromycin estolate is erythromycin 2′-propionate, dodecyl sulfate (salt). The structural formula is as follows:

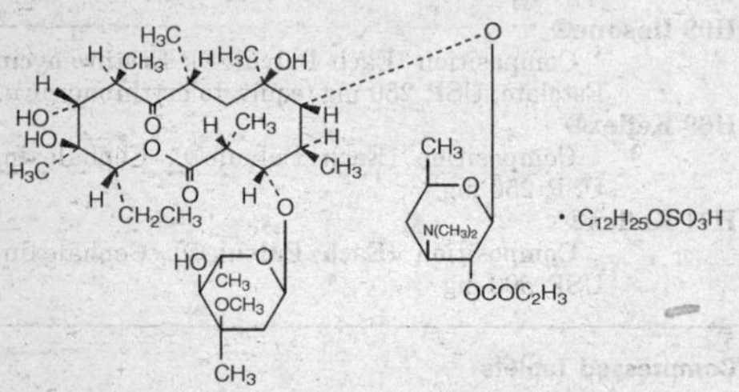

Erythromycin estolate has the empirical formula of $C_{40}H_{71}NO_{14} \bullet C_{12}H_{26}O_4S$ representing a molecular weight of 1056.39.

Erythromycin estolate, the lauryl sulfate salt of the propionyl ester of erythromycin, occurs as a white, nearly odorless, crystalline powder. The drug is essentially tasteless.

Erythromycin estolate has a pH between 4.5 and 7.0, in an aqueous suspension containing 10 mg/mL.

The Pulvules® contain erythromycin estolate equivalent to 250 mg of erythromycin. They also contain F D & C Red No. 3, F D & C Yellow No. 6, gelatin, iron oxides, magnesium stearate, mineral oil, silica gel, talc, titanium dioxide, and other inactive ingredients.

The tablets contain erythromycin estolate equivalent to 500 mg of erythromycin. They also contain starch, magnesium stearate, povidone, titanium dioxide, methylcellulose, benzyl alcohol, polyethylene glycol, and white colo̲r mixture.

The suspensions contain erythromycin estolate equivalent to 125 mg or 250 mg of erythromycin per 5 mL. The suspensions also contain butylparaben, carboxymethylcellulose, cellulose, citric acid, edetate calcium disodium, flavors, methylparaben, propylparaben, silicone, sodium chloride, sodium citrate, sodium lauryl sulfate, sucrose, and water. The 125-mg suspension also contains F D & C Yellow No. 6. The 250-mg suspension also contains F D & C Red No. 40, and saccharin sodium.

CLINICAL PHARMACOLOGY

Orally administered erythromycin estolate is readily and reliably absorbed. Because of acid stability, plasma concentrations are comparable whether the estolate is taken in the fasting state or after food. After a single 250-mg dose, blood concentrations averaged 0.29, 1.2, and 1.2 µg/mL at 2, 4, and 6 hours, respectively. Following administration of a single 500-mg dose to 12 healthy adults in the fasting state, the mean peak concentration of erythromycin estolate in plasma was 3.1 µg/mL, time to peak concentration in plasma averaged 2.7 h, and half-life measured 3 h. The volume of distribution was 2.1 L/kg, with an apparent total clearance of 572 mL/min, which was primarily non-renal.

When administered in multiple doses (500 mg q8h for 3 days) to 12 healthy adults, the mean peak concentration of erythromycin estolate in plasma measured 5.9 µg/mL, time to peak concentration in plasma averaged 2.0 h, and half-life measured 5.5 h. The volume of distribution at steady state was 1.8 L/kg with an apparent total clearance of 314 mL/min, which was also primarily non-renal.

After oral administration, plasma antibiotic concentrations consist of erythromycin base and propionyl erythromycin ester. The propionyl ester continuously hydrolyzes to the base form of erythromycin to maintain an equilibrium ratio of approximately 30% to 47% base and 53% to 57% ester in plasma.

After administration of erythromycin base, erythromycin is largely bound to plasma proteins, with freely dissociating bound fraction representing 90% of the total erythromycin absorbed.

After absorption, erythromycin diffuses readily into most body fluids. In the absence of meningeal inflammation, low concentrations are normally achieved in the spinal fluid, but passage of the drug across the blood-brain barrier increases when the meninges are inflamed. In the presence of normal hepatic function, erythromycin is concentrated in the liver and excreted in the bile; the effect of hepatic dysfunction on excretion of erythromycin by the liver is not known. After oral administration, less than 5% of the administered dose can be recovered as the active form in the urine.

Erythromycin crosses the placental barrier, but fetal plasma levels are low.

The drug is excreted in human milk.

Microbiology—Erythromycin acts by inhibition of protein synthesis by binding 50 *S* ribosomal subunits of susceptible organisms. It does not affect nucleic acid synthesis. Antagonism has been demonstrated *in vitro* between erythromycin and clindamycin, lincomycin, and chloramphenicol.

Many strains of *Haemophilus influenzae* are resistant to erythromycin alone but are susceptible to erythromycin and sulfonamides used concomitantly.

Staphylococci resistant to erythromycin may emerge during a course of therapy.

Erythromycin has been shown to be active against most strains of the following microorganisms, both *in vitro* and in clinical infections as described in the **INDICATIONS AND USAGE** section.

Gram-positive Organisms:
Corynebacterium diphtheriae
Corynebacterium minutissimum
Listeria monocytogenes
Staphylococcus aureus (resistant organisms may emerge during treatment)
Streptococcus pneumoniae
Streptococcus pyogenes

Gram-negative Organisms:
Bordetella pertussis
Legionella pneumophila
Neisseria gonorrhoeae

Other Microorganisms:
Chlamydia trachomatis
Entamoeba histolytica
Mycoplasma pneumoniae
Treponema pallidum
Ureaplasma urealyticum

Susceptibility Tests

Dilution techniques: Quantitative methods are used to determine antimicrobial minimal inhibitory concentrations (MIC's). These MIC's provide estimates of the susceptibility of bacteria to antimicrobial compounds. The MIC's should be determined using a standardized procedure. Standardized procedures are based on a dilution method[1] (broth or agar) or equivalent with standardized inoculum concentrations and standardized concentrations of erythromycin powder. The MIC values obtained should be interpreted according to the following criteria:

MIC (µg/mL)	Interpretation
≤0.5	Susceptible (S)
1-4	Intermediate (I)
≥8	Resistant (R)

A report of "Susceptible" indicates that the pathogen is likely to be inhibited if the antimicrobial compound in the blood reaches the concentrations usually achievable. A report of "Intermediate" indicates that the result should be considered equivocal, and, if the microorganism is not fully susceptible to alternative, clinically feasible drugs, the test should be repeated. This category implies possible clinical applicability in body sites where the drug is physiologically concentrated or in situations where high dosage of drug can be used. This category also provides a buffer zone which prevents small uncontrolled technical factors from causing major discrepancies in interpretation. A report of "Resistant" indicates that the pathogen is not likely to be inhibited if the antimicrobial compound in the blood reaches the concentrations usually achievable; other therapy should be selected.

Standardized susceptibility test procedures require the use of laboratory control microorganisms to control the technical aspects of the laboratory procedures. Standard erythromycin powder should provide the following MIC values:

Microorganism	MIC (µg/mL)
E. faecalis ATCC 29212	1-4
S. aureus ATCC 29213	0.12-0.5

Diffusion techniques: Quantitative methods that require measurement of zone diameters also provide reproducible estimates of the susceptibility of bacteria to antimicrobial compounds. One such standardized procedure[2] requires the use of standardized inoculum concentrations. This procedure uses paper disks impregnated with 15-µg erythromycin to test the susceptibility of microorganisms to erythromycin.

Reports from the laboratory providing results of the standard single-disk susceptibility test with a 15-µg erythromycin disk should be interpreted according to the following criteria:

Zone Diameter (mm)	Interpretation
≤13	Resistant (R)
14-17	Intermediate (I)
≥18	Susceptible (S)

Interpretation should be as stated above for results using dilution techniques. Interpretation involves correlation of the diameter obtained in the disk test with the MIC for erythromycin.

As with standardized dilution techniques, diffusion methods require the use of laboratory control microorganisms that are used to control the technical aspects of the laboratory procedures. For the diffusion technique, the 15-µg erythromycin disk should provide the following zone diameters in these laboratory test quality control strains:

Microorganism	Zone Diameter (mm)
S. aureus ATCC 25923	22-30

INDICATIONS AND USAGE

Ilosone is indicated in the treatment of infections caused by susceptible strains of the designated organisms in the diseases listed below:

Upper respiratory tract infections of mild to moderate severity caused by *Streptococcus pyogenes, Streptococcus pneumoniae*, or *Haemophilus influenzae* (when used concomitantly with adequate doses of sulfonamides, since many strains of *H. influenzae* are not susceptible to the erythromycin concentrations ordinarily achieved). (See appropriate sulfonamide labeling for prescribing information.)

Lower respiratory tract infections of mild to moderate severity caused by *Streptococcus pneumoniae* or *Streptococcus pyogenes*.

Listeriosis caused by *Listeria monocytogenes*.

Pertussis (whooping cough) caused by *Bordetella pertussis*. Erythromycin is effective in eliminating the organism from the nasopharynx of infected individuals rendering them noninfectious. Some clinical studies suggest that erythromycin may be helpful in the prophylaxis of pertussis in exposed susceptible individuals.

Respiratory tract infections due to *Mycoplasma pneumoniae*.

Skin and skin structure infections of mild to moderate severity caused by *Streptococcus pyogenes* or *Staphylococcus aureus* (resistant staphylococci may emerge during treatment).

Diphtheria: Infections due to *Corynebacterium diphtheriae*, as an adjunct to antitoxin to prevent establishment of carriers and to eradicate the organism in carriers.

Erythrasma: In the treatment of infections due to *Corynebacterium minutissimum*.

Syphilis caused by *Treponema pallidum:* Erythromycin is an alternate choice of treatment for primary syphilis in penicillin-allergic patients. In primary syphilis, spinal-fluid examinations should be done before treatment and as part of follow-up after therapy.

Intestinal amebiasis caused by *Entamoeba histolytica* (oral erythromycins only). Extraenteric amebiasis requires treatment with other agents.

Acute pelvic inflammatory disease caused by *Neisseria gonorrhoeae*: As an alternative drug in the treatment of acute pelvic inflammatory disease caused by *N. gonorrhoeae* in female patients with a history of sensitivity to penicillin. Patients should have a serologic test for syphilis before receiving erythromycin as treatment of gonorrhea and a follow-up serologic test for syphilis after 3 months.

Erythromycins are indicated for the treatment of the following infections caused by *Chlamydia trachomatis:* conjunctivitis of the newborn, pneumonia of infancy, and urogenital infections during pregnancy. When tetracyclines are contraindicated or not tolerated, erythromycin is indicated for the treatment of uncomplicated urethral, endocervical, or rectal infections due to *C. trachomatis*.

When tetracyclines are contraindicated or not tolerated, erythromycin is indicated for the treatment of nongonococcal urethritis caused by *Ureaplasma urealyticum*.

Legionnaires' Disease caused by *Legionella pneumophila*. Although no controlled clinical efficacy studies have been conducted, *in vitro* and limited preliminary clinical data suggest that erythromycin may be effective in treating Legionnaires' disease.

Prophylaxis

Prevention of Initial Attacks of Rheumatic Fever: Penicillin is considered by the American Heart Association to be the drug of choice in the prevention of initial attacks of rheumatic fever (treatment of *Streptococcus pyogenes* infections of the upper respiratory tract, e.g., tonsillitis or pharyngitis). Erythromycin is indicated for the prevention of rheumatic fever in penicillin-allergic patients. A therapeutic dose should be administered for 10 days.

Prevention of Recurrent Attacks of Rheumatic Fever: Penicillin or sulfonamides are considered by the American Heart Association to be the drugs of choice in the prevention of recurrent attacks of rheumatic fever. In patients who are allergic to penicillin and sulfonamides, oral erythromycin is recommended by the American Heart Association in the long-term prophylaxis of streptococcal pharyngitis (for the prevention of recurrent attacks of rheumatic fever).[3]

Prevention of Bacterial Endocarditis: Although no controlled clinical efficacy trials have been conducted, oral erythromycin has been recommended by the American Heart Association for prevention of bacterial endocarditis in penicillin-allergic patients with prosthetic cardiac valves, most congenital cardiac malformations, surgically constructed systemic pulmonary shunts, rheumatic or other acquired valvular dysfunction, idiopathic hypertrophic subaortic stenosis (IHSS), previous history of bacte-

rial endocarditis or mitral valve prolapse with insufficiency when they undergo dental procedures or surgical procedures of the upper respiratory tract.[4]

CONTRAINDICATIONS

Erythromycin is contraindicated in patients with known hypersensitivity to this antibiotic.

Erythromycin is contraindicated in patients taking terfenadine or astemizole. (See **PRECAUTIONS** - *Drug Interactions*.)

WARNINGS

(*See* boxed **WARNING**.) The administration of erythromycin estolate has been associated with the infrequent occurrence of cholestatic hepatitis. Laboratory findings have been characterized by abnormal hepatic function test values, peripheral eosinophilia, and leukocytosis. Symptoms may include malaise, nausea, vomiting, abdominal cramps, and fever. Jaundice may or may not be present. In some instances, severe abdominal pain may simulate the pain of biliary colic, pancreatitis, perforated ulcer, or an acute abdominal surgical problem. In other instances, clinical symptoms and results of liver function tests have resembled findings in extrahepatic obstructive jaundice.

Initial symptoms have developed in some cases after a few days of treatment but generally have followed 1 or 2 weeks of continuous therapy. Symptoms reappear promptly, usually within 48 hours after the drug is readministered to sensitive patients. The syndrome seems to result from a form of sensitization, occurs chiefly in adults, and has been reversible when medication is discontinued.

There have been reports suggesting that erythromycin does not reach the fetus in adequate concentration to prevent congenital syphilis. Infants born to women treated for early syphilis during pregnancy with oral erythromycin should be treated with an appropriate penicillin regimen.

Rhabdomyolysis with or without renal impairment has been reported in seriously ill patients receiving erythromycin concomitantly with lovastatin. Therefore, patients receiving concomitant lovastatin and erythromycin should be carefully monitored for creatine kinase (CK) and serum transaminase levels. (See package insert for lovastatin.)

Pseudomembranous colitis has been reported with nearly all antibacterial agents, including erythromycin estolate, and may range in severity from mild to life-threatening. Therefore, it is important to consider this diagnosis in patients who present with diarrhea subsequent to the administration of antibacterial agents.

Treatment with antibacterial agents alters the normal flora of the colon and may permit overgrowth of clostridia. Studies indicate that a toxin produced by *Clostridium difficile* is a primary cause of "antibiotic-associated colitis".

After the diagnosis of pseudomembranous colitis has been established, therapeutic measures should be initiated. Mild cases of pseudomembranous colitis usually respond to drug discontinuation alone. In moderate to severe cases, consideration should be given to management with fluids and electrolytes, protein supplementation, and treatment with an antibacterial drug clinically effective against *C. difficile* colitis.

PRECAUTIONS

General—Since erythromycin is principally excreted by the liver, caution should be exercised when erythromycin is administered to patients with impaired hepatic function. (*See* **CLINICAL PHARMACOLOGY** and **WARNINGS** sections.)

When indicated, incision and drainage or other surgical procedures should be performed in conjunction with antibiotic therapy.

There have been reports that erythromycin may aggravate the weakness of patients with myasthenia gravis.

Prolonged or repeated use of erythromycin may result in overgrowth of nonsusceptible bacteria or fungi. If superinfection occurs, erythromycin should be discontinued and appropriate therapy instituted.

Drug Interactions—Erythromycin has been reported to significantly alter the metabolism of the nonsedating antihistamines, terfenadine and astemizole when taken concomitantly. Rare cases of serious cardiovascular adverse events, including electrocardiographic QT/QT$_c$ interval prolongation, cardiac arrest, torsades de pointes, and other ventricular arrhythmias, have been observed. (See **CONTRAINDICATIONS**.) In addition, deaths have been reported rarely with concomitant administration of terfenadine and erythromycin.

Erythromycin and lincomycin or clindamycin may under some conditions be antagonistic.

Erythromycin use in patients who are receiving high doses of theophylline may be associated with an increase in serum theophylline levels and potential theophylline toxicity. In case of theophylline toxicity and/or elevated serum theophylline levels, the dose of theophylline should be reduced while the patient is receiving concomitant erythromycin therapy.

Concomitant administration of erythromycin and digoxin has been reported to result in elevated digoxin serum levels.

There have been reports of increased anticoagulant effects when erythromycin and oral anticoagulants were used concomitantly. Increased anticoagulation effects due to this drug interaction may be more pronounced in the elderly.

Concurrent use of erythromycin and ergotamine or dihydroergotamine has been associated in some patients with acute ergot toxicity characterized by severe peripheral vasospasm and dysesthesia.

Erythromycin has been reported to decrease the clearance of triazolam and midazolam and, thus, may increase the pharmacologic effect of these benzodiazepines.

The use of erythromycin in patients concurrently taking drugs metabolized by the cytochrome P-450 system may be associated with elevations in serum levels of these other drugs. There have been reports of interactions of erythromycin with carbamazepine, cyclosporine, hexobarbital, phenytoin, alfentanil, disopyramide, lovastatin, bromocriptine, valproate, terfenadine, cisapride, pimozide, and astemizole. Serum concentrations of drugs metabolized by the cytochrome P-450 system should be monitored closely in patients concurrently receiving erythromycin.

Drug / Laboratory Test Interactions—Erythromycin may interfere with AST (SGOT) determinations if azone-fast violet B or diphenylhydrazine colorimetric determinations are used.

Erythromycin interferes with the fluorometric determination of urinary catecholamines.

Carcinogenesis, Mutagenesis, and Impairment of Fertility—Two-year oral studies conducted in rats with erythromycin did not provide evidence of tumorigenicity or mutagenicity. Reproduction studies have been performed in rats, mice, and rabbits using erythromycin and its various salts and esters at doses several times the usual human dose. No evidence of impaired fertility or harm to the fetus that appeared to be related to erythromycin was reported in these studies.

Pregnancy: Teratogenic Effects: Pregnancy Category B—Teratogenic studies performed in animals have not revealed evidence of harm to the fetus. There are, however, no adequate and well-controlled studies in pregnant women. Because animal reproductive studies are not always predictive of human response, this drug should be used during pregnancy only if clearly needed.

Erythromycin has been reported to cross the placental barrier in humans, but fetal plasma levels are generally low.

Labor and Delivery—The effect of erythromycin estolate on labor and delivery is unknown.

Nursing Mothers—Erythromycin is excreted in human milk. Caution should be exercised when erythromycin is administered to a nursing woman.

Pediatric Use—See **INDICATIONS AND USAGE** and **DOSAGE AND ADMINISTRATION** sections.

ADVERSE REACTIONS

The most frequent side effects of erythromycin preparations are gastrointestinal (eg, abdominal cramping and discomfort) and are dose related. Nausea, vomiting, and diarrhea occur infrequently with usual oral doses. Onset of pseudomembranous colitis symptoms may occur during or after antibacterial treatment. (*See* **WARNINGS**.)

During prolonged or repeated therapy, there is a possibility of overgrowth of nonsusceptible bacteria or fungi. If such infections arise, the drug should be discontinued and appropriate therapy instituted.

Allergic reactions ranging from urticaria to anaphylaxis have occurred. Skin reactions ranging from mild eruptions to erythema multiforme, Stevens-Johnson syndrome, and toxic epidermal necrolysis have been reported rarely.

There have been isolated reports of hearing loss and/or tinnitus in patients receiving erythromycin. The ototoxic effect of the drug is usually reversible with drug discontinuance; however, in rare instances involving intravenous administration, the ototoxic effect has been irreversible. Ototoxic effects occur chiefly in patients with renal or hepatic insufficiency and in patients receiving high doses of erythromycin.

Rarely, erythromycin has been associated with the production of ventricular arrhythmias, including ventricular tachycardia and torsades de pointes, in individuals with prolonged QT$_c$ intervals.

OVERDOSAGE

In the case of overdosage, erythromycin should be discontinued. Overdosage should be handled with the prompt elimination of unabsorbed drug, and all other appropriate measures should be instituted. Erythromycin is not removed by peritoneal dialysis or hemodialysis.

DOSAGE AND ADMINISTRATION

Adults—The usual dosage is 250 mg every 6 hours. This may be increased up to 4 g/day or more according to the severity of the infection.

Pediatric Patients—Age, weight, and severity of the infection are important factors in determining the proper dosage. The usual regimen is 30 to 50 mg/kg/day in divided doses. For more severe infections, this dosage may be doubled.

If administration is desired on a twice-a-day schedule in either adults or pediatric patients, ½ of the total daily dose may be given every 12 hours.

Twice-a-day dosing is not recommended when doses larger than 1 g daily are administered.

Streptococcal Infections—For the treatment of streptococcal pharyngitis and tonsillitis, the usual dosage range is 20 to 50 mg/kg/day in divided doses.

Body Weight	Total Daily Dose
10 kg or less (less than 25 lb)	250 mg
11–18 kg (25–40 lb)	375 mg
18–25 kg (40–55 lb)	500 mg
25–36 kg (55–80 lb)	750 mg
36 kg or more (more than 80 lb)	1,000 mg (adult dose)

In the treatment of *S. pyogenes* infections, a therapeutic dosage of erythromycin should be administered for 10 days. In continuous prophylaxis of streptococcal infections in persons with a history of rheumatic heart disease, the dosage is 250 mg twice a day.

For prophylaxis against bacterial endocarditis[5] in penicillin-allergic patients with congenital heart disease or rheumatic or other acquired valvular heart disease when undergoing dental procedures or surgical procedures of the upper respiratory tract, the dosage schedule for adults is 1 g (20 mg/kg for pediatric patients) orally 1 hour before the procedure and then 500 mg (10 mg/kg for pediatric patients) orally 6 hours later.

Primary Syphilis—A regimen of 20 g of erythromycin estolate in divided doses over a period of 10 days has been shown to be effective in the treatment of primary syphilis.

Dysenteric Amebiasis—Dosage for adults is 250 mg 4 times daily for 10 to 14 days; for pediatric patients, 30 to 50 mg/kg/day in divided doses for 10 to 14 days.

Pertussis—Although optimum dosage and duration have not been established, the dosage of erythromycin utilized in reported clinical studies was 40 to 50 mg/kg/day, given in divided doses for 5 to 14 days.

Legionnaires' Disease—Although optimum doses have not been established, doses utilized in reported clinical data were those recommended above (1 to 4 g erythromycin estolate daily in divided doses).

Conjunctivitis of the Newborn Caused by C. trachomatis—Oral erythromycin suspension, 50 mg/kg/day in 4 divided doses for at least 2 weeks.

Pneumonia of Infancy Caused by C. trachomatis—Although the optimum duration of therapy has not been established, the recommended therapy is oral erythromycin suspension, 50 mg/kg/day in 4 divided doses for at least 3 weeks.

Urogenital Infections During Pregnancy Due to C. trachomatis—Although the optimum dose and duration of therapy have not been established, the suggested treatment is erythromycin, 500 mg orally 4 times a day for at least 7 days. For women who cannot tolerate this regimen, a decreased dose of 250 mg orally 4 times a day should be used for at least 14 days.

For adults with uncomplicated urethral, endocervical, or rectal infections caused by *C. trachomatis* in whom tetracyclines are contraindicated or not tolerated: 500 mg orally 4 times a day for at least 7 days.

HOW SUPPLIED

Pulvules, ivory and red
  250 mg* (No. 375)—(100s) NDC 0777-0809-02
Tablets, specially coated, white (capsule-shaped, scored)
  500 mg* (No. 1863)—(50s) NDC 0777-2126-50
Store at controlled room temperature, 59° to 86°F (15° to 30°C).
Liquid, Oral Suspension
  125 mg*/5 mL, orange-flavored vehicle (M-148)†—(16 fl oz) NDC 0777-2315-05
  250 mg*/5 mL, cherry-flavored vehicle (M-153)†—(100 mL) NDC 0777-2317-48; (16 fl oz) NDC 0777-2317-05

* Equivalent to erythromycin.
† Shake well before using. Refrigerate to maintain optimum taste.

Continued on next page

This product information was prepared in June 1998. Current information on these and other products of Dista Products Company may be obtained by direct inquiry to Lilly Research Laboratories, Lilly Corporate Center, Indianapolis, Indiana 46285, (800) 545-5979.

Consult 1999 PDR® supplements and future editions for revisions

Ilosone—Cont.

REFERENCES

1. National Committee for Clinical Laboratory Standards. Methods for Dilution Antimicrobial Susceptibility Tests for Bacteria that Grow Aerobically--Third Edition. Approved Standard NCCLS Document M7-A3, Vol. 13, No. 25, NCCLS, Villanova, PA, December 1993.
2. National Committee for Clinical Laboratory Standards. Performance Standards for Antimicrobial Disk Susceptibility Tests—Fifth Edition. Approved Standard NCCLS Document M2-A5, Vol. 13, No. 24, NCCLS, Villanova, PA, December 1993.
3. Committee on Rheumatic Fever, Endocarditis, and Kawasaki Disease of the Council on Cardiovascular Disease in the Young, the American Heart Association: Prevention of rheumatic fever. **Special Report**, *Circulation* 78(4): 1082-1086, October 1988.
4. Dajani, Adnan S., M.D., et al: Prevention of Bacterial Endocarditis. Recommendations by the American Heart Association. *JAMA* 264 (22):2919-2922, December 12, 1990.
5. American Heart Association: Prevention of Bacterial Endocarditis. *Circulation* 1984;70:1123A.

CAUTION—Federal (USA) law prohibits dispensing without prescription.
Literature revised July 28, 1997
PV 2105 DPP   [072897]

ILOTYCIN®   ℞
[ī-lō-tī '-sīn]
(erythromycin)
Ophthalmic Ointment, USP, 0.5%
(Sterile)

DESCRIPTION

Ilotycin® (Erythromycin Ophthalmic Ointment, USP) belongs to the macrolide group of antibiotics. It is basic and readily forms a salt when combined with an acid. The base, as crystals or powder, is slightly soluble in water, moderately soluble in ether, and readily soluble in alcohol or chloroform. Erythromycin is an antibiotic produced from a strain of *Streptomyces erythraeus*. The special sterile ophthalmic ointment base flows freely over the conjunctiva. It has the following structural formula:

erythromycin

$C_{37}H_{67}NO_{13}$ Mol. Wt. 733.94

Chemical Name: (3R*, 4S*, 5S*, 6R*, 7R*, 9R*, 11R*, 12R*, 13S*, 14R*)-4-[(2,6-Dideoxy-3-C-methyl-3-O-methyl-α-L-*ribo*-hexopyranosyl)oxy]-14-ethyl-7,12,13-trihydroxy-3,5,7, 9,11,13-hexamethyl-6-[[3,4,6-trideoxy-3-(dimethylamino)-β-D-*xylo*-hexopyranosyl]oxy]oxacyclotetradecane-2,10-dione. Each Gram Contains: ACTIVE: Erythromycin, USP, 5 mg (0.5%); INACTIVES: White Petrolatum, Mineral Oil.

CLINICAL PHARMACOLOGY

Microbiology—Erythromycin inhibits protein synthesis without affecting nucleic acid synthesis. Erythromycin is usually active against the following organisms *in vitro* and in clinical infections:

  Streptococcus pyogenes (group A β-hemolytic)
  Alpha-hemolytic streptococci (viridans group)
  Staphylococcus aureus, including penicillinase-producing strains (methicillin-resistant staphylococci are uniformly resistant to erythromycin)
  Streptococcus pneumoniae
  Mycoplasma pneumoniae (Eaton Agent, PPLO)
  Haemophilus influenzae (not all strains of this organism are susceptible at the erythromycin concentrations ordinarily achieved)
  Treponema pallidum
  Corynebacterium diphtheriae
  Neisseria gonorrhoeae
  Chlamydia trachomatis

INDICATIONS AND USAGE

For the treatment of superficial ocular infections involving the conjunctiva and/or cornea caused by organisms susceptible to Ilotycin®.
For prophylaxis of ophthalmia neonatorum due to *N. gonorrhoeae* or *C. trachomatis*.

The effectiveness of erythromycin in the prevention of ophthalmia caused by penicillinase-producing *N. gonorrhoeae* is not established.
For infants born to mothers with clinically apparent gonorrhea, intravenous or intramuscular injections of aqueous crystalline penicillin G should be given; a single dose of 50,000 units for term infants or 20,000 units for infants of low birth weight. Topical prophylaxis alone is inadequate for these infants.

CONTRAINDICATION

This drug is contraindicated in patients with a history of hypersensitivity to erythromycin.

PRECAUTIONS

General—The use of antimicrobial agents may be associated with the overgrowth of nonsusceptible organisms including fungi; in such a case, antibiotic administration should be stopped and appropriate measures taken.
Information for Patients—Avoid contaminating the tip of container with material from the eye, fingers, or other source.
Carcinogenesis, Mutagenesis, Impairment of Fertility —Two year oral studies conducted in rats with erythromycin did not provide evidence of tumorigenicity. Mutagenicity studies have not been conducted. No evidence of impaired fertility or harm to the fetus that appeared related to erythromycin was reported in these studies.
Pregnancy—Pregnancy Category B—Reproduction studies have been performed in rats, mice, and rabbits using erythromycin and its various salts and esters, at doses that were several multiples of the usual human dose. There are, however, no adequate and well-controlled studies in pregnant women. Because animal reproductive studies are not always predictive of human response, the erythromycins should be used during pregnancy only if clearly needed.
Nursing Mothers—Caution should be exercised when erythromycin is administered to a nursing woman.
Pediatric Use—See INDICATIONS AND USAGE and DOSAGE AND ADMINISTRATION.

ADVERSE REACTIONS

The most frequently reported adverse reactions are minor ocular irritations, redness, and hypersensitivity reactions.

DOSAGE AND ADMINISTRATION

In the treatment of superficial ocular infections, Ophthalmic Ointment ILOTYCIN® approximately 1 cm in length should be applied directly to the infected eye(s) up to six times daily, depending on the severity of the infection.
For prophylaxis of neonatal gonococcal or chlamydial ophthalmia, a ribbon of ointment approximately 1 cm in length should be instilled into each lower conjunctival sac. The ointment should not be flushed from the eye following instillation. A new tube should be used for each infant.
Directions For Use for 1 Gram Plastic Tube: DO NOT PULL CAP OFF. Twist cap to verify that a click is heard and/or resistance is felt. Either indicates that the plastic tip under cap was intact. The twisting motion breaks the seal and the tip remains in the cap. Dispense product and discard after use.

HOW SUPPLIED

ILOTYCIN® (Erythromycin Ophthalmic Ointment, USP, 0.5%) No. 52 is available in the following sizes:
$^1/_8$ oz. (3.5 g) tamper-resistant tube—(NDC 0777-1863-17—Prod. No. FL09234

DO NOT USE IF BOTTOM RIDGE OF TUBE CAP IS EXPOSED.

---

1 g plastic container (in cartons of 50)—(NDC 0777-1863-52)—Prod. No. FL09232

DO NOT USE IF CLICK IS NOT HEARD AND/OR RESISTANCE IS NOT FELT.

Storage: Store between 15°–30°C (59°–86°F).
KEEP OUT OF REACH OF CHILDREN.

Caution: Federal law prohibits dispensing without prescription.
                                                              [050095]

KEFLEX®   ℞
[kĕf 'lĕks]
(cephalexin)
USP

DESCRIPTION

Keflex® (Cephalexin, USP) is a semisynthetic cephalosporin antibiotic intended for oral administration. It is 7-(D-α-Amino-α-phenylacetamido)-3-methyl-3-cephem-4-carboxylic acid monohydrate. Cephalexin has the molecular formula $C_{16}H_{17}N_3O_4S \cdot H_2O$ and the molecular weight is 365.41.

Cephalexin has the following structural formula:

The nucleus of cephalexin is related to that of other cephalosporin antibiotics. The compound is a zwitterion; ie, the molecule contains both a basic and an acidic group. The isoelectric point of cephalexin in water is approximately 4.5 to 5.
The crystalline form of cephalexin which is available is a monohydrate. It is a white crystalline solid having a bitter taste. Solubility in water is low at room temperature; 1 or 2 mg/mL may be dissolved readily, but higher concentrations are obtained with increasing difficulty.
The cephalosporins differ from penicillins in the structure of the bicyclic ring system. Cephalexin has a D-phenylglycyl group as substituent at the 7-amino position and an unsubstituted methyl group at the 3-position.
Each Pulvule® contains cephalexin monohydrate equivalent to 250 mg (720 µmol) or 500 mg (1,439 µmol) of cephalexin. The Pulvules also contain cellulose, D & C Yellow No. 10, F D & C Blue No. 1, F D & C Yellow No. 6, gelatin, magnesium stearate, silicone, titanium dioxide, and other inactive ingredients.
After mixing, each 5 mL of Keflex, for Oral Suspension, will contain cephalexin monohydrate equivalent to 125 mg (360 µmol) or 250 mg (720 µmol) of cephalexin. The suspensions also contain flavors, methylcellulose, silicone, sodium lauryl sulfate, and sucrose. The 125-mg suspension contains F D & C Red No. 40, and the 250-mg suspension contains F D & C Yellow No. 6.

CLINICAL PHARMACOLOGY

Human Pharmacology—Keflex is acid stable and may be given without regard to meals. It is rapidly absorbed after oral administration. Following doses of 250 mg, 500 mg, and 1 g, average peak serum levels of approximately 9, 18, and 32 µg/mL respectively were obtained at 1 hour. Measurable levels were present 6 hours after administration. Cephalexin is excreted in the urine by glomerular filtration and tubular secretion. Studies showed that over 90% of the drug was excreted unchanged in the urine within 8 hours. During this period, peak urine concentrations following the 250-mg, 500-mg, and 1-g doses were approximately 1,000, 2,200, and 5,000 µg/mL respectively.
Microbiology—In vitro tests demonstrate that the cephalosporins are bactericidal because of their inhibition of cell-wall synthesis. Cephalexin has been shown to be active against most strains of the following microorganisms both *in vitro* and in clinical infections as described in the INDICATIONS AND USAGE section.
Aerobes, Gram-positive:
Staphylococcus aureus (including penicillinase-producing strains)
Staphylococcus epidermidis (penicillin-susceptible strains)
Streptococcus pneumoniae
Streptococcus pyogenes
Aerobes, Gram-negative:
Escherichia coli
Haemophilus influenzae
Klebsiella pneumoniae
Moraxella (Branhamella) catarrhalis
Proteus mirabilis
Note—Methicillin-resistant staphylococci and most strains of enterococci (*Enterococcus faecalis* [formerly *Streptococcus faecalis*]) are resistant to cephalosporins, including cephalexin. It is not active against most strains of *Enterobacter* spp, *Morganella morganii* and *Proteus vulgaris*. It has no activity against *Pseudomonas* spp or *Acinetobacter calcoaceticus*.
Susceptibility Tests —**Diffusion techniques:** Quantitative methods that require measurement of zone diameters provide reproducible estimates of the susceptibility of bacteria to antimicrobial compounds. One such standardized procedure[1] that has been recommended for use with disks to test the susceptibility of microorganisms to cephalexin uses the 30-µg cephalothin disk. Interpretation involves correlation of the diameter obtained in the disk test with the minimal inhibitory concentration (MIC) for cephalexin.
Reports from the laboratory providing results of the standard single-disk susceptibility test with a 30-µg cephalothin disk should be interpreted according to the following criteria:

Zone Diameter (mm)	Interpretation
≥18	(S) Susceptible
15–17	(I) Intermediate
≤14	(R) Resistant

A report of "Susceptible" indicates that the pathogen is likely to be inhibited by usually achievable concentrations of the antimicrobial compound in blood. A report of "Inter-

mediate" indicates that the result should be considered equivocal, and, if the microorganism is not fully susceptible to alternative, clinically feasible drugs, the test should be repeated. This category implies possible clinical applicability in body sites where the drug is physiologically concentrated or in situations where high dosage of drug can be used. This category also provides a buffer zone that prevents small uncontrolled technical factors from causing major discrepancies in interpretation. A report of "Resistant" indicates that usually achievable concentrations of the antimicrobial compound in the blood are unlikely to be inhibitory and that other therapy should be selected.

Measurement of MIC or MBC and achieved antimicrobial compound concentrations may be appropriate to guide therapy in some infections. (See CLINICAL PHARMACOLOGY section for information on drug concentrations achieved in infected body sites and other pharmacokinetic properties of this antimicrobial drug product.)

Standardized susceptibility test procedures require the use of laboratory control microorganisms. The 30-µg cephalothin disk should provide the following zone diameters in these laboratory test quality control strains:

Microorganism	Zone Diameter (mm)
E. coli ATCC 25922	15–21
S. aureus ATCC 25923	29–37

Dilution techniques:

Quantitative methods that are used to determine MICs provide reproducible estimates of the susceptibility of bacteria to antimicrobial compounds. One such standardized procedure uses a standardized dilution method[2] (broth, agar, microdilution) or equivalent with cephalothin powder. The MIC values obtained should be interpreted according to the following criteria:

MIC (µg/mL)	Interpretation
≤8	(S) Susceptible
16	(I) Intermediate
≥32	(R) Resistant

Interpretation should be as stated above for results using diffusion techniques.

As with standard diffusion techniques, dilution methods require the use of laboratory control organisms. Standard cephalothin powder should provide the following MIC values:

Microorganism	MIC (µg/mL)
E. coli ATCC 25922	4–16
S. aureus ATCC 29213	0.12–0.5

INDICATIONS AND USAGE

Keflex is indicated for the treatment of the following infections when caused by susceptible strains of the designated microorganisms:

Respiratory tract infections caused by S. pneumoniae and S. pyogenes (Penicillin is the usual drug of choice in the treatment and prevention of streptococcal infections, including the prophylaxis of rheumatic fever. Keflex is generally effective in the eradication of streptococci from the nasopharynx; however, substantial data establishing the efficacy of Keflex in the subsequent prevention of rheumatic fever are not available at present.)

Otitis media due to S. pneumoniae, H. influenzae, staphylococci, streptococci, and M. catarrhalis

Skin and skin structure infections caused by staphylococci and/or streptococci

Bone infections caused by staphylococci and/or P. mirabilis

Genitourinary tract infections, including acute prostatitis, caused by E. coli, P. mirabilis, and K. pneumoniae

Note —Culture and susceptibility tests should be initiated prior to and during therapy. Renal function studies should be performed when indicated.

CONTRAINDICATIONS

Keflex is contraindicated in patients with known allergy to the cephalosporin group of antibiotics.

WARNINGS

BEFORE CEPHALEXIN THERAPY IS INSTITUTED, CAREFUL INQUIRY SHOULD BE MADE CONCERNING PREVIOUS HYPERSENSITIVITY REACTIONS TO CEPHALOSPORINS AND PENICILLIN. CEPHALOSPORIN C DERIVATIVES SHOULD BE GIVEN CAUTIOUSLY TO PENICILLIN-SENSITIVE PATIENTS.

SERIOUS ACUTE HYPERSENSITIVITY REACTIONS MAY REQUIRE EPINEPHRINE AND OTHER EMERGENCY MEASURES.

There is some clinical and laboratory evidence of partial cross-allergenicity of the penicillins and the cephalosporins. Patients have been reported to have had severe reactions (including anaphylaxis) to both drugs.

Any patient who has demonstrated some form of allergy, particularly to drugs, should receive antibiotics cautiously. No exception should be made with regard to Keflex.

Pseudomembranous colitis has been reported with nearly all antibacterial agents, including cephalexin, and may range from mild to life threatening. Therefore, it is important to consider this diagnosis in patients with diarrhea subsequent to the administration of antibacterial agents.

Treatment with antibacterial agents alters the normal flora of the colon and may permit overgrowth of clostridia. Studies indicate that a toxin produced by Clostridium difficile is one primary cause of antibiotic-associated colitis.

After the diagnosis of pseudomembranous colitis has been established, appropriate therapeutic measures should be initiated. Mild cases of pseudomembranous colitis usually respond to drug discontinuation alone. In moderate to severe cases, consideration should be given to management with fluids and electrolytes, protein supplementation, and treatment with an antibacterial drug clinically effective against Clostridium difficile colitis.

Usage in Pregnancy —Safety of this product for use during pregnancy has not been established.

PRECAUTIONS

General —Patients should be followed carefully so that any side effects or unusual manifestations of drug idiosyncrasy may be detected. If an allergic reaction to Keflex occurs, the drug should be discontinued and the patient treated with the usual agents (eg, epinephrine or other pressor amines, antihistamines, or corticosteroids).

Prolonged use of Keflex may result in the overgrowth of nonsusceptible organisms. Careful observation of the patient is essential. If superinfection occurs during therapy, appropriate measures should be taken.

Positive direct Coombs' tests have been reported during treatment with the cephalosporin antibiotics. In hematologic studies or in transfusion cross-matching procedures when antiglobulin tests are performed on the minor side or in Coombs' testing of newborns whose mothers have received cephalosporin antibiotics before parturition, it should be recognized that a positive Coombs' test may be due to the drug.

Keflex should be administered with caution in the presence of markedly impaired renal function. Under such conditions, careful clinical observation and laboratory studies should be made because safe dosage may be lower than that usually recommended.

Indicated surgical procedures should be performed in conjunction with antibiotic therapy.

As a result of administration of Keflex, a false-positive reaction for glucose in the urine may occur. This has been observed with Benedict's and Fehling's solutions and also with Clinitest® tablets.

As with other β-lactams, the renal excretion of cephalexin is inhibited by probenecid.

Broad-spectrum antibiotics should be prescribed with caution in individuals with a history of gastrointestinal disease, particularly colitis.

Usage in Pregnancy —Pregnancy Category B —The daily oral administration of cephalexin to rats in doses of 250 or 500 mg/kg prior to and during pregnancy, or to rats and mice during the period of organogenesis only, had no adverse effect on fertility, fetal viability, fetal weight, or litter size. Note that the safety of cephalexin during pregnancy in humans has not been established.

Cephalexin showed no enhanced toxicity in weanling and newborn rats as compared with adult animals. Nevertheless, because the studies in humans cannot rule out the possibility of harm, Keflex should be used during pregnancy only if clearly needed.

Nursing Mothers —The excretion of cephalexin in the milk increased up to 4 hours after a 500-mg dose; the drug reached a maximum level of 4 µg/mL, then decreased gradually, and had disappeared 8 hours after administration. Caution should be exercised when Keflex is administered to a nursing woman.

ADVERSE REACTIONS

Gastrointestinal —Symptoms of pseudomembranous colitis may appear either during or after antibiotic treatment. Nausea and vomiting have been reported rarely. The most frequent side effect has been diarrhea. It was very rarely severe enough to warrant cessation of therapy. Dyspepsia, gastritis, and abdominal pain have also occurred. As with some penicillins and some other cephalosporins, transient hepatitis and cholestatic jaundice have been reported rarely.

Hypersensitivity —Allergic reactions in the form of rash, urticaria, angioedema and, rarely, erythema multiforme, Stevens-Johnson syndrome, or toxic epidermal necrolysis have been observed. These reactions usually subsided upon discontinuation of the drug. In some of these reactions, supportive therapy may be necessary. Anaphylaxis has also been reported.

Other reactions have included genital and anal pruritus, genital moniliasis, vaginitis and vaginal discharge, dizziness, fatigue, headache, agitation, confusion, hallucinations, arthralgia, arthritis, and joint disorder. Reversible interstitial nephritis has been reported rarely. Eosinophilia, neutropenia, thrombocytopenia, and slight elevations in AST and ALT have been reported.

OVERDOSAGE

Signs and Symptoms —Symptoms of oral overdose may include nausea, vomiting, epigastric distress, diarrhea, and

hematuria. If other symptoms are present, it is probably secondary to an underlying disease state, an allergic reaction, or toxicity due to ingestion of a second medication.

Treatment —To obtain up-to-date information about the treatment of overdose, a good resource is your certified Regional Poison Control Center. Telephone numbers of certified poison control centers are listed in the Physicians' Desk Reference (PDR). In managing overdosage, consider the possibility of multiple drug overdoses, interaction among drugs, and unusual drug kinetics in your patient.

Unless 5 to 10 times the normal dose of cephalexin has been ingested, gastrointestinal decontamination should not be necessary.

Protect the patient's airway and support ventilation and perfusion. Meticulously monitor and maintain, within acceptable limits, the patient's vital signs, blood gases, serum electrolytes, etc. Absorption of drugs from the gastrointestinal tract may be decreased by giving activated charcoal, which, in many cases, is more effective than emesis or lavage; consider charcoal instead of or in addition to gastric emptying. Repeated doses of charcoal over time may hasten elimination of some drugs that have been absorbed. Safeguard the patient's airway when employing gastric emptying or charcoal.

Forced diuresis, peritoneal dialysis, hemodialysis, or charcoal hemoperfusion have not been established as beneficial for an overdose of cephalexin; however, it would be extremely unlikely that one of these procedures would be indicated.

The oral median lethal dose of cephalexin in rats is >5,000 mg/kg.

DOSAGE AND ADMINISTRATION

Keflex is administered orally.

Adults —The adult dosage ranges from 1 to 4 g daily in divided doses. The usual adult dose is 250 mg every 6 hours. For the following infections, a dosage of 500 mg may be administered every 12 hours: streptococcal pharyngitis, skin and skin structure infections, and uncomplicated cystitis in patients over 15 years of age. Cystitis therapy should be continued for 7 to 14 days. For more severe infections or those caused by less susceptible organisms, larger doses may be needed. If daily doses of Keflex greater than 4 g are required, parenteral cephalosporins, in appropriate doses, should be considered.

Pediatric Patients —The usual recommended daily dosage for pediatric patients is 25 to 50 mg/kg in divided doses. For streptococcal pharyngitis in patients over 1 year of age and for skin and skin structure infections, the total daily dose may be divided and administered every 12 hours.

Keflex Suspension

Weight	125 mg/5 mL
10 kg (22 lb)	1/2 to 1 tsp q.i.d.
20 kg (44 lb)	1 to 2 tsp q.i.d.
40 kg (88 lb)	2 to 4 tsp q.i.d
Weight	250 mg/5 mL
10 kg (22 lb)	1/4 to 1/2 tsp q.i.d.
20 kg (44 lb)	1/2 to 1 tsp q.i.d.
40 kg (88 lb)	1 to 2 tsp q.i.d.

or

Weight	125 mg/5 mL
10 kg (22 lb)	1 to 2 tsp b.i.d.
20 kg (44 lb)	2 to 4 tsp b.i.d.
40 kg (88 lb)	4 to 8 tsp b.i.d.
Weight	250 mg/5 mL
10 kg (22 lb)	1/2 to 1 tsp b.i.d.
20 kg (44 lb)	1 to 2 tsp b.i.d.
40 kg (88 lb)	2 to 4 tsp b.i.d.

In severe infections, the dosage may be doubled.

In the therapy of otitis media, clinical studies have shown that a dosage of 75 to 100 mg/kg/day in 4 divided doses is required.

In the treatment of β-hemolytic streptococcal infections, a therapeutic dosage of Keflex should be administered for at least 10 days.

HOW SUPPLIED

Keflex® For Oral Suspension, (or cephalexin, USP), is available in:

The 125 mg per 5 mL oral suspension* is available as follows:

100-mL Bottles	NDC 0777-2321-48 (M-201)
200-mL Bottles	NDC 0777-2321-89 (M-201)

The 250 mg per 5 mL oral suspension* is available as follows:

100-mL Bottles	NDC 0777-2368-48 (M-202)

Continued on next page

This product information was prepared in June 1998. Current information on these and other products of Dista Products Company may be obtained by direct inquiry to Lilly Research Laboratories, Lilly Corporate Center, Indianapolis, Indiana 46285, (800) 545-5979.

Keflex—Cont.

200-mL Bottles	NDC 0777-2368-89	(M-202)
ID†100	NDC 0777-2368-33	(M-202)

Keflex® Pulvules®, (or cephalexin, USP), are available in: The 250 mg Pulvules are a white powder filled into size 2 Para-Posilok® Caps (opaque white and opaque light green) that are imprinted with "Dista" and identity code "H69" on the green cap, and Keflex 250 on the white body in edible black ink. They are available as follows:

Bottles of 20	NDC 0777-0869-20	(PU402)
Bottles of 100	NDC 0777-0869-02	(PU402)
ID†100	NDC 0777-0869-33	(PU402)

The 500 mg Pulvules are a white powder filled into an elongated, size 0 Para-Posilok Caps (opaque light green and opaque dark green) that are imprinted with "Dista" and identity code "H71" on the light green cap, and Keflex 500 on the dark green body in edible black ink. They are available as follows:

Bottles of 20	NDC 0777-0871-20	(PU403)
Bottles of 100	NDC 0777-0871-02	(PU403)
ID†100	NDC 0777-0871-33	(PU403)

* After mixing, store in a refrigerator. May be kept for 14 days without significant loss of potency. Shake well before using. Keep tightly closed.

† Identi-Dose® (unit dose medication, Dista).

Store at controlled room temperature, 15° to 30°C (59° to 86°F).

REFERENCES

1. National Committee for Clinical Laboratory Standards: Performance standards for antimicrobial disk susceptibility tests—5th ed. Approved Standard NCCLS Document M2-A5, Vol 13, No 24, NCCLS, Villanova, PA, 1993.
2. National Committee for Clinical Laboratory Standards: Methods for dilution antimicrobial susceptibility tests for bacteria that grow aerobically—3rd ed. Approved Standard NCCLS Document M7-A3, Vol 13, No 25, NCCLS, Villanova, PA, 1993.

CAUTION—Federal (USA) law prohibits dispensing without prescription.

Literature revised September 3, 1996.

PV 0368 DPP [090396]

NALFON® ℞

[*năl 'fŏn*]

(fenoprofen calcium)

USP

DESCRIPTION

Nalfon® (Fenoprofen Calcium, USP) is a nonsteroidal, anti-inflammatory, antiarthritic drug. Pulvules® Nalfon contain fenoprofen calcium as the dihydrate in an amount equivalent to 200 mg (0.826 mmol) or 300 mg (1.24 mmol) of fenoprofen. The Pulvules also contain cellulose, gelatin, iron oxides, silicone, titanium dioxide, and other inactive ingredients. The 300-mg Pulvules also contain D & C Yellow No. 10 and F D & C Yellow No. 6.

Tablets Nalfon contain fenoprofen calcium as the dihydrate in an amount equivalent to 600 mg (2.48 mmol) of fenoprofen. The tablets also contain amberlite, benzyl alcohol, calcium phosphate, corn starch, D & C Yellow No. 10, F D & C Yellow No. 6, hydroxypropyl methylcellulose, magnesium stearate, polyethylene glycol, stearic acid, titanium dioxide, and other inactive ingredients.

Chemically, Nalfon is an arylacetic acid derivative.

The structural formula is as follows:

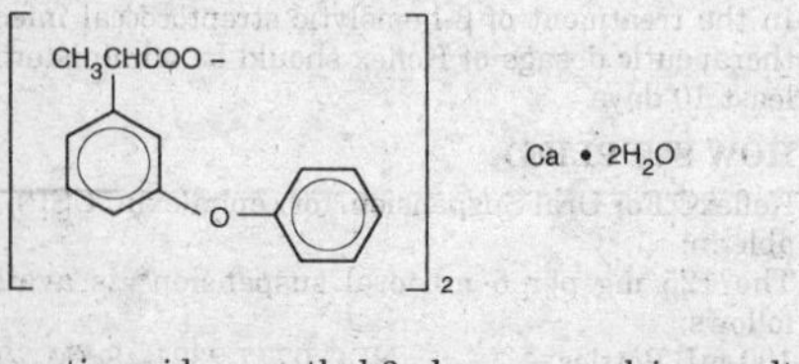

CH3CHCOO –
Ca • 2H2O
O
2

Benzeneacetic acid, α-methyl-3-phenoxy-, calcium salt dihydrate, (±)-

Nalfon is a white crystalline powder that has the empirical formula $C_{30}H_{26}CaO_6 \bullet 2H_2O$ representing a molecular weight of 558.65. At 25°C, it dissolves to a 15 mg/mL solution in alcohol (95%). It is slightly soluble in water and insoluble in benzene.

The *p*Ka of Nalfon is 4.5 at 25°C.

CLINICAL PHARMACOLOGY

Nalfon is a nonsteroidal, anti-inflammatory, antiarthritic drug that also possesses analgesic and antipyretic activities. Its exact mode of action is unknown, but it is thought that prostaglandin synthetase inhibition is involved. Nalfon has been shown to inhibit prostaglandin synthetase isolated from bovine seminal vesicles. Reproduction studies in rats have shown Nalfon to be associated with prolonged labor and difficult parturition when given during late pregnancy. Evidence suggests that this may be due to decreased uterine contractility resulting from the inhibition of prostaglandin synthesis. Its action is not mediated through the adrenal gland.

Fenoprofen shows anti-inflammatory effects in rodents by inhibiting the development of redness and edema in acute inflammatory conditions and by reducing soft-tissue swelling and bone damage associated with chronic inflammation. It exhibits analgesic activity in rodents by inhibiting the writhing response caused by the introduction of an irritant into the peritoneal cavities of mice and by elevating pain thresholds that are related to pressure in edematous hindpaws of rats. In rats made febrile by the subcutaneous administration of brewer's yeast, fenoprofen produces antipyretic action. These effects are characteristic of nonsteroidal, anti-inflammatory, antipyretic, analgesic drugs.

The results in humans confirmed the anti-inflammatory and analgesic actions found in animals. The emergence and degree of erythemic response were measured in adult male volunteers exposed to ultraviolet irradiation. The effects of Nalfon, aspirin, and indomethacin were each compared with those of a placebo. All 3 drugs demonstrated antierythemic activity.

In patients with rheumatoid arthritis, the anti-inflammatory action of Nalfon has been evidenced by relief of pain, increase in grip strength, and reductions in joint swelling, duration of morning stiffness, and disease activity (as assessed by both the investigator and the patient). The anti-inflammatory action of Nalfon has also been evidenced by increased mobility (ie, a decrease in the number of joints having limited motion).

The use of Nalfon in combination with gold salts or corticosteroids has been studied in patients with rheumatoid arthritis. The studies, however, were inadequate in demonstrating whether further improvement is obtained by adding Nalfon to maintenance therapy with gold salts or steroids. Whether or not Nalfon used in conjunction with partially effective doses of a corticosteroid has a "steroid-sparing" effect is unknown.

In patients with osteoarthritis, the anti-inflammatory and analgesic effects of Nalfon have been demonstrated by reduction in tenderness as a response to pressure and reductions in night pain, stiffness, swelling, and overall disease activity (as assessed by both the patient and the investigator). These effects have also been demonstrated by relief of pain with motion and at rest and increased range of motion in involved joints.

In patients with rheumatoid arthritis and osteoarthritis, clinical studies have shown Nalfon to be comparable to aspirin in controlling the aforementioned measures of disease activity, but mild gastrointestinal reactions (nausea, dyspepsia) and tinnitus occurred less frequently in patients treated with Nalfon than in aspirin-treated patients. It is not known whether Nalfon causes less peptic ulceration than does aspirin.

In patients with pain, the analgesic action of Nalfon has produced a reduction in pain intensity, an increase in pain relief, improvement in total analgesia scores, and a sustained analgesic effect.

Under fasting conditions, Nalfon is rapidly absorbed, and peak plasma levels of 50 µg/mL are achieved within 2 hours after oral administration of 600-mg doses. Good dose proportionality was observed between 200-mg and 600-mg doses in fasting male volunteers. The plasma half-life is approximately 3 hours. About 90% of a single oral dose is eliminated within 24 hours as fenoprofen glucuronide and 4′-hydroxyfenoprofen glucuronide, the major urinary metabolites of fenoprofen. Fenoprofen is highly bound (99%) to albumin.

The concomitant administration of antacid (containing both aluminum and magnesium hydroxide) does not interfere with absorption of Nalfon.

There is less suppression of collagen-induced platelet aggregation with single doses of Nalfon than there is with aspirin.

INDICATIONS AND USAGE

Nalfon is indicated for relief of the signs and symptoms of rheumatoid arthritis and osteoarthritis. It is recommended for the treatment of acute flare-ups and exacerbations and for the long-term management of these diseases.

Nalfon is also indicated for the relief of mild to moderate pain.

CONTRAINDICATIONS

Nalfon is contraindicated in patients who have shown hypersensitivity to it.

The drug should not be administered to patients with a history of significantly impaired renal function.

Nalfon should not be given to patients in whom aspirin and other nonsteroidal anti-inflammatory drugs induce the symptoms of asthma, rhinitis, or urticaria, because cross-sensitivity to these drugs occurs in a high proportion of such patients.

WARNINGS

Risk of GI Ulceration, Bleeding, and Perforation with NSAID Therapy —Serious gastrointestinal toxicity, such as bleeding, ulceration, and perforation, can occur at any time, with or without warning symptoms, in patients treated chronically with NSAID therapy. Although minor upper gastrointestinal problems, such as dyspepsia, are common, usually developing early in therapy, physicians should remain alert for ulceration and bleeding in patients treated chronically with NSAIDs, even in the absence of previous GI tract symptoms. In patients observed in clinical trials of several months to 2 years duration, symptomatic upper GI ulcers, gross bleeding, or perforation appear to occur in approximately 1% of patients treated for 3 to 6 months, and in about 2% to 4% of patients treated for 1 year. Physicians should inform patients about the signs and/or symptoms of serious GI toxicity and what steps to take if they occur.

Studies to date have not identified any subset of patients not at risk of developing peptic ulceration and bleeding. Except for a prior history of serious GI events and other risk factors known to be associated with peptic ulcer disease, such as alcoholism, smoking, etc, no risk factors (eg, age, sex) have been associated with increased risk. Elderly or debilitated patients seem to tolerate ulceration or bleeding less well than other individuals and most spontaneous reports of fatal GI events are in this population. Studies to date are inconclusive concerning the relative risk of various NSAIDs in causing such reactions. High doses of any NSAID probably carry a greater risk of these reactions, although controlled clinical trials showing this do not exist in most cases. In considering the use of relatively large doses (within the recommended dosage range), sufficient benefit should be anticipated to offset the potential increased risk of GI toxicity.

Since Nalfon has been marketed, there have been reports of genitourinary tract problems in patients taking it. The most frequently reported problems have been episodes of dysuria, cystitis, hematuria, interstitial nephritis, and nephrotic syndrome. This syndrome may be preceded by the appearance of fever, rash, arthralgia, oliguria, and azotemia and may progress to anuria. There may also be substantial proteinuria, and, on renal biopsy, electron microscopy has shown foot process fusion and T-lymphocyte infiltration in the renal interstitium. Early recognition of the syndrome and withdrawal of the drug have been followed by rapid recovery. Administration of steroids and the use of dialysis have also been included in the treatment. Because a syndrome with some of these characteristics has also been reported with other nonsteroidal anti-inflammatory drugs, it is recommended that patients who have had these reactions with other such drugs not be treated with Nalfon. In patients with possibly compromised renal function, periodic renal function examinations should be done.

PRECAUTIONS

General —Renal Effects —There have been reports of acute interstitial nephritis and nephrotic syndrome (*see* Contraindications *and* Warnings).

A second form of renal toxicity has been seen in patients with prerenal conditions leading to a reduction in renal blood flow or blood volume, in which renal prostaglandins play a supportive role in the maintenance of renal perfusion. In these patients, administration of an NSAID may cause a dose-dependent reduction in prostaglandin formation and may precipitate overt renal decompensation at any time. Patients at greatest risk for this reaction are those with impaired renal function, heart failure, liver dysfunction, those taking diuretics, and the elderly. Discontinuation of NSAID therapy is typically followed by recovery to the pretreatment state.

Since Nalfon is primarily eliminated by the kidneys, patients with possibly compromised renal function (such as the elderly) should be monitored periodically, especially during long-term therapy. For such patients, it may be anticipated that a lower daily dosage will avoid excessive drug accumulation.

Miscellaneous —Peripheral edema has been observed in some patients taking Nalfon; therefore, Nalfon should be used with caution in patients with compromised cardiac function or hypertension. The possibility of renal involvement should be considered.

Studies to date have not shown changes in the eyes attributable to the administration of Nalfon. However, adverse ocular effects have been observed with other anti-inflammatory drugs. Eye examinations, therefore, should be performed if visual disturbances occur in patients taking Nalfon.

Caution should be exercised by patients whose activities require alertness if they experience CNS side effects while taking Nalfon.

Since the safety of Nalfon has not been established in patients with impaired hearing, these patients should have periodic tests of auditory function during prolonged therapy with Nalfon.

Information for Patients —Nalfon, like other drugs of its class, is not free of side effects. The side effects of these drugs can cause discomfort and, rarely, there are more serious side effects, such as gastrointestinal bleeding, which may result in hospitalization and even fatal outcomes.
NSAIDs (Nonsteroidal Anti-Inflammatory Drugs) are often essential agents in the management of arthritis and have a major role in the treatment of pain, but they also may be commonly employed for conditions which are less serious. Physicians may wish to discuss with their patients the potential risks (*see* Warnings, Precautions, *and* Adverse Reactions sections) and likely benefits of NSAID treatment, particularly when the drugs are used for less serious conditions where treatment without NSAIDs may represent an acceptable alternative to both the patient and physician.
Laboratory Tests —In chronic studies in rats, high doses of Nalfon caused elevation of serum transaminase and hepatocellular hypertrophy. In clinical trials, some patients developed elevation of serum transaminase, LDH, and alkaline phosphatase that persisted for some months and usually, but not always, declined despite continuation of the drug. The significance of this is unknown. It is recommended, therefore, that Nalfon be discontinued if any significant liver abnormality occurs.
As with other nonsteroidal anti-inflammatory drugs, borderline elevations in 1 or more liver tests may occur in up to 15% of patients. These abnormalities may progress, may remain essentially unchanged, or may be transient with continued therapy. The SGPT (ALT) test is probably the most sensitive indicator of liver dysfunction. Meaningful (ie, 3 times the upper limit of normal) elevations of SGPT or SGOT (AST) occurred in controlled clinical trials in less than 1% of patients. A patient with symptoms and/or signs suggesting liver dysfunction, or in whom an abnormal liver test has occurred, should be evaluated for evidence of the development of more severe hepatic reactions while using Nalfon.
Severe hepatic reactions, including jaundice and cases of fatal hepatitis, have been reported with Nalfon, as with other nonsteroidal anti-inflammatory drugs. As a result, during long-term therapy, liver function tests should be monitored periodically. Although such reactions are rare, if liver tests continue to be abnormal or worsen, if clinical signs and symptoms consistent with liver disease develop, or if systemic manifestations occur (eg, eosinophilia and rash), Nalfon should be discontinued. If this drug is to be used in the presence of impaired liver function, it must be done under strict observation.
Patients with initial low hemoglobin values who are receiving long-term therapy with Nalfon should have a hemoglobin determination made at reasonable intervals.
Nalfon decreases platelet aggregation and may prolong bleeding time. Patients who may be adversely affected by prolongation of the bleeding time should be carefully observed when Nalfon is administered.
Because serious GI tract ulceration and bleeding can occur without warning symptoms, physicians should follow chronically treated patients for the signs and symptoms of ulceration and bleeding and should inform them of the importance of this follow-up (*see* Risk of GI Ulcerations, Bleeding and Perforation with NSAID Therapy *under* Warnings).
Laboratory Test Interactions —Amerlex-M kit assay values of total and free triiodothyronine in patients receiving Nalfon have been reported as falsely elevated on the basis of a chemical cross-reaction that directly interferes with the assay. Thyroid-stimulating hormone, total thyroxine, and thyrotropin-releasing hormone response are not affected.
Drug Interactions —The coadministration of aspirin decreases the biologic half-life of fenoprofen because of an increase in metabolic clearance that results in a greater amount of hydroxylated fenoprofen in the urine. Although the mechanism of interaction between fenoprofen and aspirin is not totally known, enzyme induction and displacement of fenoprofen from plasma albumin binding sites are possibilities. Because Nalfon has not been shown to produce any additional effect beyond that obtained with aspirin alone and because aspirin increases the rate of excretion of Nalfon, the concomitant use of Nalfon and salicylates is not recommended.
Chronic administration of phenobarbital, a known enzyme inducer, may be associated with a decrease in the plasma half-life of fenoprofen. When phenobarbital is added to or withdrawn from treatment, dosage adjustment of Nalfon may be required.
In vitro studies have shown that fenoprofen, because of its affinity for albumin, may displace from their binding sites other drugs that are also albumin bound, and this may lead to drug interaction. Theoretically, fenoprofen could likewise be displaced. Patients receiving hydantoin, sulfonamides, or sulfonylureas should be observed for increased activity of these drugs and, therefore, signs of toxicity from these drugs. In patients receiving coumarin-type anticoagulants, the addition of Nalfon to therapy could prolong the prothrombin time. Patients receiving both drugs should be under careful observation. Patients treated with Nalfon may be resistant to the effects of loop diuretics.

In patients receiving Nalfon and a steroid concomitantly, any reduction in steroid dosage should be gradual in order to avoid the possible complications of sudden steroid withdrawal.
Usage in Pregnancy —Safe use of Nalfon during pregnancy and lactation has not been established; therefore, administration to pregnant patients and nursing mothers is not recommended. Reproduction studies have been performed in rats and rabbits. When fenoprofen was given to rats during pregnancy and continued until the time of labor, parturition was prolonged. Similar results have been found with other nonsteroidal anti-inflammatory drugs that inhibit prostaglandin synthetase.
Usage in Pediatric Patients —Safety and effectiveness in pediatric patients have not been established.

ADVERSE REACTIONS

During clinical studies for rheumatoid arthritis, osteoarthritis, or mild to moderate pain and studies of pharmacokinetics, complaints were compiled from a checklist of potential adverse reactions, and the following data emerged. These encompass observations in 6,786 patients, including 188 observed for at least 52 weeks. For comparison, data are also presented from complaints received from the 266 patients who received placebo in these same trials. During short-term studies for analgesia, the incidence of adverse reactions was markedly lower than that seen in longer-term studies.
INCIDENCE GREATER THAN 1%
Probable Causal Relationship
Digestive System —During clinical trials with Nalfon, the most common adverse reactions were gastrointestinal in nature and occurred in 20.8% of patients receiving Nalfon as compared to 16.9% of patients receiving placebo. In descending order of frequency, these reactions included dyspepsia (10.3%, Nalfon, vs 2.3%, placebo), nausea (7.7% vs 7.1%), constipation (7% vs 1.5%), vomiting (2.6% vs 1.9%), abdominal pain (2% vs 1.1%), and diarrhea (1.8% vs 4.1%). The drug was discontinued because of adverse gastrointestinal reactions in less than 2% of patients during premarketing studies.
Nervous System —The most frequent adverse neurologic reactions were headache (8.7% treated vs 7.5% placebo) and somnolence (8.5% vs 6.4%). Dizziness (6.5% vs 5.6%), tremor (2.2% vs 0.4%), and confusion (1.4% vs none) were noted less frequently.
Nalfon was discontinued in less than 0.5% of patients because of these side effects during premarketing studies.
Skin and Appendages —Increased sweating (4.6% vs 0.4%), pruritus (4.2% vs 0.8%), and rash (3.7% vs 0.4%) were reported.
Nalfon was discontinued in about 1% of patients because of an adverse effect related to the skin during premarketing studies.
Special Senses —Tinnitus (4.5% vs 0.4%), blurred vision (2.2% vs none), and decreased hearing (1.6% vs none) were reported.
Nalfon was discontinued in less than 0.5% of patients because of adverse effects related to the special senses during premarketing studies.
Cardiovascular —Palpitations (2.5% vs 0.4%).
Nalfon was discontinued in about 0.5% of patients because of adverse cardiovascular reactions during premarketing studies.
Miscellaneous —Nervousness (5.7% vs 1.5%), asthenia (5.4% vs 0.4%), peripheral edema (5.0% vs 0.4%), dyspnea (2.8% vs none), fatigue (1.7% vs 1.5%), upper respiratory infection (1.5% vs 5.6%), and nasopharyngitis (1.2% vs none).
INCIDENCE LESS THAN 1%
Probable Causal Relationship
The following adverse reactions, occurring in less than 1% of patients, were reported in controlled clinical trials and voluntary reports made since Nalfon was initially marketed. The probability of a causal relationship exists between Nalfon and these adverse reactions:
Digestive System —Gastritis, peptic ulcer with/without perforation, gastrointestinal hemorrhage, anorexia, flatulence, dry mouth, and blood in the stool. Increases in alkaline phosphatase, LDH, and SGOT, jaundice, and cholestatic hepatitis were observed (*see* Precautions).
Genitourinary Tract —Renal failure, dysuria, cystitis, hematuria, oliguria, azotemia, anuria, interstitial nephritis, nephrosis, and papillary necrosis (*see* Warnings).
Hypersensitivity —Angioedema (angioneurotic edema).
Hematologic —Purpura, bruising, hemorrhage, thrombocytopenia, hemolytic anemia, aplastic anemia, agranulocytosis, and pancytopenia.
Miscellaneous —Anaphylaxis, urticaria, malaise, insomnia, and tachycardia.
INCIDENCE LESS THAN 1%
Causal Relationship Unknown
Other reactions reported either in clinical trials or spontaneously, occurred in circumstances in which a causal relationship could not be established. However, with these

rarely reported reactions, the possibility of such a relationship cannot be excluded. Therefore, these observations are listed to alert the physician.
Skin and Appendages —Exfoliative dermatitis, toxic epidermal necrolysis, Stevens-Johnson syndrome, and alopecia.
Digestive System —Aphthous ulcerations of the buccal mucosa, metallic taste, and pancreatitis.
Cardiovascular —Atrial fibrillation, pulmonary edema, electrocardiographic changes, and supraventricular tachycardia.
Nervous System —Depression, disorientation, seizures, and trigeminal neuralgia.
Special Senses —Burning tongue, diplopia, and optic neuritis.
Miscellaneous —Personality change, lymphadenopathy, mastodynia, and fever.

OVERDOSAGE

Signs and Symptoms —Symptoms of overdose appear within several hours and generally involve the gastrointestinal and central nervous systems. They include dyspepsia, nausea, vomiting, abdominal pain, dizziness, headache, ataxia, tinnitus, tremor, drowsiness, and confusion. Hyperpyrexia, tachycardia, hypotension, and acute renal failure may occur rarely following overdose. Respiratory depression and metabolic acidosis have also been reported following overdose with certain NSAIDs.
Treatment —To obtain up-to-date information about the treatment of overdose, a good resource is your certified Regional Poison Control Center. Telephone numbers of certified poison control centers are listed in the *Physicians' Desk Reference (PDR)*. In managing overdosage, consider the possibility of multiple drug overdoses, interaction among drugs, and unusual drug kinetics in your patient.
Protect the patient's airway and support ventilation and perfusion. Meticulously monitor and maintain, within acceptable limits, the patient's vital signs, blood gases, serum electrolytes, etc. Absorption of drugs from the gastrointestinal tract may be decreased by giving activated charcoal, which, in many cases, is more effective than emesis or lavage; consider charcoal instead of or in addition to gastric emptying. Repeated doses of charcoal over time may hasten elimination of some drugs that have been absorbed. Safeguard the patient's airway when employing gastric emptying or charcoal.
Alkalinization of the urine, forced diuresis, peritoneal dialysis, hemodialysis, and charcoal hemoperfusion do not enhance systemic drug elimination.

DOSAGE AND ADMINISTRATION

Analgesia —For the treatment of mild to moderate pain, the recommended dosage is 200 mg every 4 to 6 hours, as needed.
Rheumatoid Arthritis and Osteoarthritis —The suggested dosage is 300 to 600 mg, 3 or 4 times a day. The dose should be tailored to the needs of the patient and may be increased or decreased depending on the severity of the symptoms. Dosage adjustments may be made after initiation of drug therapy or during exacerbations of the disease. Total daily dosage should not exceed 3,200 mg.
If gastrointestinal complaints occur, Nalfon may be administered with meals or with milk. Although the total amount absorbed is not affected, peak blood levels are delayed and diminished.
Patients with rheumatoid arthritis generally seem to require larger doses of Nalfon than do those with osteoarthritis. The smallest dose that yields acceptable control should be employed.
Although improvement may be seen in a few days in many patients, an additional 2 to 3 weeks may be required to gauge the full benefits of therapy.

HOW SUPPLIED

Pulvules:
200 mg* (white and ocher) (No. 415)—(Identi-Code† H76) (RxPak‡ of 100) NDC 0777-0876-02
300 mg* (yellow and ocher) (No. 416)—(Identi-Code H77) (RxPak of 100) NDC 0777-0877-02; (500s) NDC 0777-0877-03
Tablets (DISTA imprinted on one side, NALFON on other side):
600 mg* (yellow, paracapsule-shaped, scored) (No. 1900)—(RxPak of 100) NDC 0777-2159-02; (500s) NDC 0777-2159-03

* Equivalent to fenoprofen.
† Identi-Code® (formula identification code, Dista).

Continued on next page

This product information was prepared in June 1998. Current information on these and other products of Dista Products Company may be obtained by direct inquiry to Lilly Research Laboratories, Lilly Corporate Center, Indianapolis, Indiana 46285, (800) 545-5979.

Nalfon—Cont.

‡ All RxPaks (prescription packages, Dista) have safety closures.

Store at controlled room temperature, 59° to 86°F (15° to 30°C).

CAUTION—Federal (USA) law prohibits dispensing without prescription.

Literature revised August 30, 1996

PV 1025 DPP [083096]

PROZAC® ℞

[*prō 'zăk*]

(fluoxetine hydrochloride)

DESCRIPTION

Prozac® (Fluoxetine Hydrochloride) is an antidepressant for oral administration; it is chemically unrelated to tricyclic, tetracyclic, or other available antidepressant agents. It is designated (±)-N-methyl-3-phenyl-3-[(α,α,α-trifluoro-*p*-tolyl)oxy]propylamine hydrochloride and has the empirical formula of $C_{17}H_{18}F_3NO \cdot HCl$. Its molecular weight is 345.79. The structural formula is:

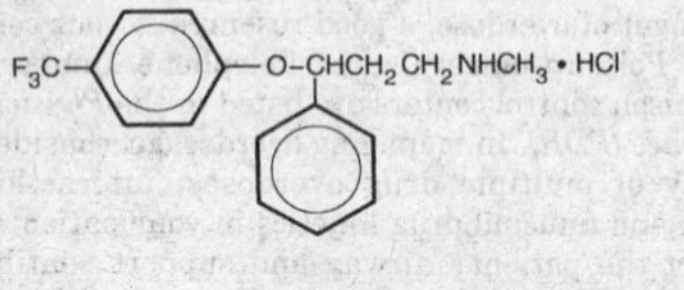

Fluoxetine hydrochloride is a white to off-white crystalline solid with a solubility of 14 mg/mL in water.

Each Pulvule® contains fluoxetine hydrochloride equivalent to 10 mg (32.3 µmol) or 20 mg (64.7 µmol) of fluoxetine. The Pulvules also contain F D & C Blue No. 1, gelatin, iron oxide, silicone, starch, titanium dioxide, and other inactive ingredients.

The oral solution contains fluoxetine hydrochloride equivalent to 20 mg/5 mL (64.7 µmol) of fluoxetine. It also contains alcohol 0.23%, benzoic acid, flavoring agent, glycerin, purified water, and sucrose.

CLINICAL PHARMACOLOGY

Pharmacodynamics:

The antidepressant, antiobsessive-compulsive, and antibulimic actions of fluoxetine are presumed to be linked to its inhibition of CNS neuronal uptake of serotonin. Studies at clinically relevant doses in man have demonstrated that fluoxetine blocks the uptake of serotonin into human platelets. Studies in animals also suggest that fluoxetine is a much more potent uptake inhibitor of serotonin than of norepinephrine.

Antagonism of muscarinic, histaminergic, and α_1-adrenergic receptors has been hypothesized to be associated with various anticholinergic, sedative, and cardiovascular effects of classical tricyclic antidepressant drugs. Fluoxetine binds to these and other membrane receptors from brain tissue much less potently in vitro than do the tricyclic drugs.

Absorption, Distribution, Metabolism, and Excretion:

Systemic Bioavailability—In man, following a single oral 40-mg dose, peak plasma concentrations of fluoxetine from 15 to 55 ng/mL are observed after 6 to 8 hours.

The Pulvule and oral solution dosage forms of fluoxetine are bioequivalent. Food does not appear to affect the systemic bioavailability of fluoxetine, although it may delay its absorption inconsequentially. Thus, fluoxetine may be administered with or without food.

Protein Binding—Over the concentration range from 200 to 1,000 ng/mL, approximately 94.5% of fluoxetine is bound in vitro to human serum proteins, including albumin and α_1-glycoprotein. The interaction between fluoxetine and other highly protein-bound drugs has not been fully evaluated, but may be important (*see* Precautions).

Enantiomers—Fluoxetine is a racemic mixture (50/50) of *R*-fluoxetine and *S*-fluoxetine enantiomers. In animal models, both enantiomers are specific and potent serotonin uptake inhibitors with essentially equivalent pharmacologic activity. The *S*-fluoxetine enantiomer is eliminated more slowly and is the predominant enantiomer present in plasma at steady state.

Metabolism—Fluoxetine is extensively metabolized in the liver to norfluoxetine and a number of other, unidentified metabolites. The only identified active metabolite, norfluoxetine, is formed by demethylation of fluoxetine. In animal models, *S*-norfluoxetine is a potent and selective inhibitor of serotonin uptake and has activity essentially equivalent to *R*- or *S*-fluoxetine. *R*-norfluoxetine is significantly less potent than the parent drug in the inhibition of serotonin uptake. The primary route of elimination appears to be hepatic metabolism to inactive metabolites excreted by the kidney.

Clinical Issues Related to Metabolism/Elimination—The complexity of the metabolism of fluoxetine has several consequences that may potentially affect fluoxetine's clinical use.

Variability in Metabolism—A subset (about 7%) of the population has reduced activity of the drug metabolizing enzyme cytochrome P450IID6. Such individuals are referred to as "poor metabolizers" of drugs such as debrisoquin, dextromethorphan, and the tricyclic antidepressants. In a study involving labeled and unlabeled enantiomers administered as a racemate, these individuals metabolized *S*-fluoxetine at a slower rate and thus achieved higher concentrations of *S*-fluoxetine. Consequently, concentrations of *S*-norfluoxetine at steady state were lower. The metabolism of *R*-fluoxetine in these poor metabolizers appears normal. When compared with normal metabolizers, the total sum at steady state of the plasma concentrations of the 4 active enantiomers was not significantly greater among poor metabolizers. Thus, the net pharmacodynamic activities were essentially the same. Alternative, nonsaturable pathways (non-IID6) also contribute to the metabolism of fluoxetine. This explains how fluoxetine achieves a steady-state concentration rather than increasing without limit.

Because fluoxetine's metabolism, like that of a number of other compounds including tricyclic and other selective serotonin antidepressants, involves the P450IID6 system, concomitant therapy with drugs also metabolized by this enzyme system (such as the tricyclic antidepressants) may lead to drug interactions (*see* Drug Interactions *under* Precautions).

Accumulation and Slow Elimination—The relatively slow elimination of fluoxetine (elimination half-life of 1 to 3 days after acute administration and 4 to 6 days after chronic administration) and its active metabolite, norfluoxetine (elimination half-life of 4 to 16 days after acute and chronic administration), leads to significant accumulation of these active species in chronic use and delayed attainment of steady state, even when a fixed dose is used. After 30 days of dosing at 40 mg/day, plasma concentrations of fluoxetine in the range of 91 to 302 ng/mL and norfluoxetine in the range of 72 to 258 ng/mL have been observed. Plasma concentrations of fluoxetine were higher than those predicted by single-dose studies, because fluoxetine's metabolism is not proportional to dose. Norfluoxetine, however, appears to have linear pharmacokinetics. Its mean terminal half-life after a single dose was 8.6 days and after multiple dosing was 9.3 days. Steady state levels after prolonged dosing are similar to levels seen at 4–5 weeks.

The long elimination half-lives of fluoxetine and norfluoxetine assure that, even when dosing is stopped, active drug substance will persist in the body for weeks (primarily depending on individual patient characteristics, previous dosing regimen, and length of previous therapy at discontinuation). This is of potential consequence when drug discontinuation is required or when drugs are prescribed that might interact with fluoxetine and norfluoxetine following the discontinuation of Prozac.

Liver Disease—As might be predicted from its primary site of metabolism, liver impairment can affect the elimination of fluoxetine. The elimination half-life of fluoxetine was prolonged in a study of cirrhotic patients, with a mean of 7.6 days compared to the range of 2 to 3 days seen in subjects without liver disease; norfluoxetine elimination was also delayed, with a mean duration of 12 days for cirrhotic patients compared to the range of 7 to 9 days in normal subjects. This suggests that the use of fluoxetine in patients with liver disease must be approached with caution. If fluoxetine is administered to patients with liver disease, a lower or less frequent dose should be used (*see* Precautions *and* Dosage and Administration).

Renal Disease—In depressed patients on dialysis (N=12), fluoxetine administered as 20 mg once daily for two months produced steady-state fluoxetine and norfluoxetine plasma concentrations comparable to those seen in patients with normal renal function. While the possibility exists that renally excreted metabolites of fluoxetine may accumulate to higher levels in patients with severe renal dysfunction, use of a lower or less frequent dose is not routinely necessary in renally impaired patients (*see* Use in Patients With Concomitant Illness *under* Precautions *and* Dosage and Administration).

Age—The disposition of single doses of fluoxetine in healthy elderly subjects (greater than 65 years of age) did not differ significantly from that in younger normal subjects. However, given the long half-life and nonlinear disposition of the drug, a single-dose study is not adequate to rule out the possibility of altered pharmacokinetics in the elderly, particularly if they have systemic illness or are receiving multiple drugs for concomitant diseases. The effects of age upon the metabolism of fluoxetine have been investigated in 260 elderly but otherwise healthy depressed patients (≥60 years of age) who received 20 mg fluoxetine for 6 weeks. Combined fluoxetine plus norfluoxetine plasma concentrations were 209.3 ± 85.7 ng/mL at the end of 6 weeks. No unusual age-associated pattern of adverse events was observed in those elderly patients.

Clinical Trials:

Depression—The efficacy of Prozac for the treatment of patients with depression (≥18 years of age) has been studied in 5- and 6-week placebo-controlled trials. Prozac was shown to be significantly more effective than placebo as measured by the Hamilton Depression Rating Scale (HAM-D). Prozac was also significantly more effective than placebo on the HAM-D subscores for depressed mood, sleep disturbance, and the anxiety subfactor.

Two 6-week controlled studies comparing Prozac, 20mg, and placebo have shown Prozac, 20 mg daily, to be effective in the treatment of elderly patients (≥60 years of age) with depression. In these studies, Prozac produced a significantly higher rate of response and remission as defined respectively by a 50% decrease in the HAM-D score and a total endpoint HAM-D score of ≤7. Prozac was well tolerated and the rate of treatment discontinuations due to adverse events did not differ between Prozac (12%) and placebo (9%).

A study was conducted involving depressed outpatients who had responded (modified HAMD-17 score of ≤ 7 during each of the last 3 weeks of open-label treatment and absence of major depression by DSM-III-R criteria) by the end of an initial 12–week open treatment phase on Prozac 20 mg/day. These patients (N=298) were randomized to continuation on double-blind Prozac 20 mg/day or placebo. At 38 weeks (50 weeks total), a statistically significantly lower relapse rate (defined as symptoms sufficient to meet a diagnosis of major depression for 2 weeks or a modified HAMD-17 score of ≥ 14 for 3 weeks) was observed for patients taking Prozac compared to those on placebo.

Obsessive-Compulsive Disorder—The effectiveness of Prozac for the treatment for obsessive-compulsive disorder (OCD) was demonstrated in two 13-week, multicenter, parallel group studies (Studies 1 and 2) of adult outpatients who received fixed Prozac doses of 20, 40, or 60 mg/day (on a once a day schedule, in the morning) or placebo. Patients in both studies had moderate to severe OCD (DSM-III-R), with mean baseline ratings on the Yale-Brown Obsessive Compulsive Scale (YBOCS, total score) ranging from 22 to 26. In Study 1, patients receiving Prozac experienced mean reductions of approximately 4 to 6 units on the YBOCS total score, compared to a 1-unit reduction for placebo patients. In Study 2, patients receiving Prozac experienced mean reductions of approximately 4 to 9 units on the YBOCS total score, compared to a 1-unit reduction for placebo patients. While there was no indication of a dose response relationship for effectiveness in Study 1, a dose response relationship was observed in Study 2, with numerically better responses in the 2 higher dose groups. The following table provides the outcome classification by treatment group on the Clinical Global Impression (CGI) improvement scale for studies 1 and 2 combined:

Outcome Classification (%) on CGI Improvement Scale for Completers in Pool of Two OCD Studies

Outcome Classification	Placebo	Prozac 20 mg	40 mg	60 mg
Worse	8%	0%	0%	0%
No Change	64%	41%	33%	29%
Minimally Improved	17%	23%	28%	24%
Much Improved	8%	28%	27%	28%
Very Much Improved	3%	8%	12%	19%

Exploratory analyses for age and gender effects on outcome did not suggest any differential responsiveness on the basis of age or sex.

Bulimia Nervosa—The effectiveness of Prozac for the treatment of bulimia was demonstrated in two 8-week and one 16-week, multicenter, parallel group studies of adult outpatients meeting DSM-III-R criteria for bulimia. Patients in the 8-week studies received either 20 mg/day or 60 mg/day of Prozac or placebo in the morning. Patients in the 16-week study received a fixed Prozac dose of 60 mg/day (once a day) or placebo. Patients in these 3 studies had moderate to severe bulimia with median binge-eating and vomiting frequencies ranging from 7 to 10 per week and 5 to 9 per week, respectively. In these 3 studies, Prozac, 60 mg, but not 20 mg, was statistically significantly superior to placebo in reducing the number of binge-eating and vomiting episodes per week. The statistically significantly superior effect of 60 mg vs placebo was present as early as week 1 and persisted throughout each study. The Prozac related reduction in bulimic episodes appeared to be independent of baseline depression as assessed by the Hamilton Depression Rating Scale. In each of these 3 studies, the treatment effect, as measured by differences between Prozac, 60 mg, and placebo on median reduction from baseline in frequency of bulimic behaviors at endpoint, ranged from 1 to 2 episodes per week for binge-eating and 2 to 4 episodes per week for vomiting. The size of the effect was related to baseline fre-

quency, with greater reductions seen in patients with higher baseline frequencies. Although some patients achieved freedom from binge-eating and purging as a result of treatment, for the majority, the benefit was a partial reduction in the frequency of binge-eating and purging.

INDICATIONS AND USAGE

Depression—Prozac is indicated for the treatment of depression. The efficacy of Prozac was established in 5- and 6-week trials with depressed outpatients (≥18 years of age) whose diagnoses corresponded most closely to the DSM-III category of major depressive disorder (*see* Clinical Trials *under* Clinical Pharmacology).

A major depressive episode implies a prominent and relatively persistent depressed or dysphoric mood that usually interferes with daily functioning (nearly every day for at least 2 weeks); it should include at least 4 of the following 8 symptoms: change in appetite, change in sleep, psychomotor agitation or retardation, loss of interest in usual activities or decrease in sexual drive, increased fatigue, feelings of guilt or worthlessness, slowed thinking or impaired concentration, and a suicide attempt or suicidal ideation.

The antidepressant action of Prozac in hospitalized depressed patients has not been adequately studied.

The efficacy of Prozac in maintaining an antidepressant response for up to 38 weeks following 12 weeks of open-label acute treatment (50 weeks total) was demonstrated in a placebo-controlled trial. The usefulness of the drug in patients receiving Prozac for extended periods should be reevaluated periodically (*see* Clinical Trials *under* Clinical Pharmacology).

Obsessive-Compulsive Disorder—Prozac is indicated for the treatment of obsessions and compulsions in patients with obsessive-compulsive disorder (OCD), as defined in the DSM-III-R; ie, the obsessions or compulsions cause marked distress, are time-consuming, or significantly interfere with social or occupational functioning.

The efficacy of Prozac was established in 13-week trials with obsessive-compulsive outpatients whose diagnoses corresponded most closely to the DSM-III-R category of obsessive-compulsive disorder (*see* Clinical Trials *under* Clinical Pharmacology).

Obsessive-compulsive disorder is characterized by recurrent and persistent ideas, thoughts, impulses, or images (obsessions) that are ego-dystonic and/or repetitive, purposeful, and intentional behaviors (compulsions) that are recognized by the person as excessive or unreasonable.

The effectiveness of Prozac in long-term use, ie, for more than 13 weeks, has not been systematically evaluated in placebo-controlled trials. Therefore, the physician who elects to use Prozac for extended periods should periodically reevaluate the long-term usefulness of the drug for the individual patient (*see* Dosage and Administration).

Bulimia Nervosa—Prozac is indicated for the treatment of binge-eating and vomiting behaviors in patients with moderate to severe bulimia nervosa.

The efficacy of Prozac was established in 8 to 16 week trials for adult outpatients with moderate to severe bulimia nervosa, ie, at least 3 bulimic episodes per week for 6 months (*see* Clinical Trials *under* Clinical Pharmacology).

The effectiveness of Prozac in long-term use, ie, for more than 16 weeks, has not been systematically evaluated in placebo-controlled trials. Therefore, the physician who elects to use Prozac for extended periods should periodically reevaluate the long-term usefulness of the drug for the individual patient (*see* Dosage and Administration).

CONTRAINDICATIONS

Prozac is contraindicated in patients known to be hypersensitive to it.

Monoamine Oxidase Inhibitors—There have been reports of serious, sometimes fatal, reactions (including hyperthermia, rigidity, myoclonus, autonomic instability with possible rapid fluctuations of vital signs, and mental status changes that include extreme agitation progressing to delirium and coma) in patients receiving fluoxetine in combination with a monoamine oxidase inhibitor (MAOI), and in patients who have recently discontinued fluoxetine and are then started on an MAOI. Some cases presented with features resembling neuroleptic malignant syndrome. Therefore, Prozac should not be used in combination with an MAOI, or within a minimum of 14 days of discontining therapy with an MAOI. Since fluoxetine and its major metabolite have very long elimination half-lives, at least 5 weeks (perhaps longer, especially if fluoxetine has been prescribed chronically and/or at higher doses [*See* Accumulation and Slow Elimination *under* Clinical Pharmacology]) should be allowed after stopping Prozac before starting an MAOI.

WARNINGS

Rash and Possibly Allergic Events—In US fluoxetine clinical trials, 7% of 10,782 patients developed various types of rashes and/or urticaria. Among the cases of rash and/or urticaria reported in premarketing clinical trials, almost a third were withdrawn from treatment because of the rash and/or systemic signs or symptoms associated with the rash. Clinical findings reported in association with rash include fever, leukocytosis, arthralgias, edema, carpal tunnel syndrome, respiratory distress, lymphadenopathy, proteinuria, and mild transaminase elevation. Most patients improved promptly with discontinuation of fluoxetine and/or adjunctive treatment with antihistamines or steroids, and all patients experiencing these events were reported to recover completely.

In premarketing clinical trials, 2 patients are known to have developed a serious cutaneous systemic illness. In neither patient was there an unequivocal diagnosis, but 1 was considered to have a leukocytoclastic vasculitis, and the other, a severe disquamating syndrome that was considered variously to be a vasculitis or erythema multiforme. Other patients have had systemic syndromes suggestive of serum sickness.

Since the introduction of Prozac, systemic events, possibly related to vasculitis, have developed in patients with rash. Although these events are rare, they may be serious, involving the lung, kidney, or liver. Death has been reported to occur in association with these systemic events.

Anaphylactoid events, including bronchospasm, angioedema, and urticaria alone and in combination, have been reported.

Pulmonary events, including inflammatory processes of varying histopathology and/or fibrosis, have been reported rarely. These events have occurred with dyspnea as the only preceding symptom.

Whether these systemic events and rash have a common underlying cause or are due to different etiologies or pathogenic processes is not known. Furthermore, a specific underlying immunologic basis for these events has not been identified. Upon the appearance of rash or of other possibly allergic phenomena for which an alternative etiology cannot be identified, Prozac should be discontinued.

PRECAUTIONS

General

Anxiety and Insomnia—In US placebo-controlled clinical trials for depression, 12% to 16% of patients treated with Prozac and 7% to 9% of patients treated with placebo reported anxiety, nervousness, or insomnia.

In US placebo-controlled clinical trials for obsessive-compulsive disorder, insomnia was reported in 28% of patients treated with Prozac and in 22% of patients treated with placebo. Anxiety was reported in 14% of patients treated with Prozac and in 7% of patients treated with placebo.

In US placebo-controlled clinical trials for bulimia nervosa, insomnia was reported in 33% of patients treated with Prozac, 60 mg, and 13% of patients treated with placebo. Anxiety and nervousness were reported respectively in 15% and 11% of patients treated with Prozac, 60 mg, and in 9% and 5% of patients treated with placebo.

Among the most common adverse events associated with discontinuation in US placebo-controlled fluoxetine clinical trials were anxiety (≤2%), insomnia (≤2%) and nervousness (≤1%) (see Table 3, below).

Altered Appetite and Weight—Significant weight loss, especially in underweight depressed or bulimic patients, may be an undesirable result of treatment with Prozac.

In US placebo-controlled clinical trials for depression, 11% of patients treated with Prozac and 2% of patients treated with placebo reported anorexia (decreased appetite). Weight loss was reported in 1.4% of patients treated with Prozac and in 0.5% of patients treated with placebo. However, only rarely have patients discontinued treatment with Prozac because of anorexia or weight loss.

In US placebo-controlled clinical trials for OCD, 17% of patients treated with Prozac and 10% of patients treated with placebo reported anorexia (decreased appetite). One patient discontinued treatment with Prozac because of anorexia.

In US placebo-controlled clinical trials for bulimia nervosa, 8% of patients treated with Prozac, 60 mg, and 4% of patients treated with placebo reported anorexia (decreased appetite). Patients treated with Prozac, 60 mg, on average lost 0.45 kg compared with a gain of 0.16 kg by patients treated with placebo in the 16-week double-blind trial. Weight change should be monitored during therapy.

Activation of Mania/Hypomania—In US placebo-controlled clinical trials for depression, mania/hypomania was reported in 0.1% of patients treated with Prozac and 0.1% of patients treated with placebo. Activation of mania/hypomania has also been reported in a small proportion of patients with Major Affective Disorder treated with marketed antidepressants.

In US placebo-controlled clinical trials for OCD, mania/hypomania was reported in 0.8% of patients treated with Prozac and no patients treated with placebo. No patients reported mania/hypomania in US placebo-controlled clinical trials for bulimia. In all US Prozac clinical trials, 0.7% of 10,782 patients reported mania/hypomania.

Seizures—In US placebo-controlled clinical trials for depression, convulsions (or events described as possibly having been seizures) were reported in 0.1% of patients treated with Prozac and 0.2% of patients treated with placebo. No patients reported convulsions in US placebo-controlled clinical trials for either OCD or bulimia. In all US Prozac clinical trials, 0.2% of 10,782 patients reported convulsions. The percentage appears to be similar to that associated with other marketed antidepressants. Prozac should be introduced with care in patients with a history of seizures.

Suicide—The possibility of a suicide attempt is inherent in depression and may persist until significant remission occurs. Close supervision of high risk patients should accompany initial drug therapy. Prescriptions for Prozac should be written for the smallest quantity of capsules consistent with good patient management, in order to reduce the risk of overdose.

Because of well-established comorbidiy between OCD and depression and bulimia and depression, the same precautions observed when treating patients with depression should be observed when treating patients with OCD or bulimia.

The Long Elimination Half-Lives of Fluoxetine and Its Metabolites—Because of the long elimination half-lives of the parent drug and its major active metabolite, changes in dose will not be fully reflected in plasma for several weeks, affecting both strategies for titration to final dose and withdrawal from treatment (*see* Clinical Pharmacology *and* Dosage and Administration).

Use in Patients With Concomitant Illness—Clinical experience with Prozac in patients with concomitant systemic illness is limited. Caution is advisable in using Prozac in patients with diseases or conditions that could affect metabolism or hemodynamic responses.

Fluoxetine has not been evaluated or used to any appreciable extent in patients with a recent history of myocardial infarction or unstable heart disease. Patients with these diagnoses were systematically excluded from clinical studies during the product's premarket testing. However, the electrocardiograms of 312 patients who received Prozac in double-blind trials were retrospectively evaluated; no conduction abnormalities that resulted in heart block were observed. The mean heart rate was reduced by approximately 3 beats/min.

In subjects with cirrhosis of the liver, the clearances of fluoxetine and its active metabolite, norfluoxetine, were decreased, thus increasing the elimination half-lives of these substances. A lower or less frequent dose should be used in patients with cirrhosis.

Studies in depressed patients on dialysis did not reveal excessive accumulation of fluoxetine or norfluoxetine in plasma (*see* Renal Disease *under* Clinical Pharmacology). Use of a lower or less frequent dose for renally impaired patients is not routinely necessary (*see* Dosage and Administration).

In patients with diabetes, Prozac may alter glycemic control. Hypoglycemia has occurred during therapy with Prozac, and hyperglycemia has developed following discontinuation of the drug. As is true with many other types of medication when taken concurrently by patients with diabetes, insulin and/or oral hypoglycemic dosage may need to be adjusted when therapy with Prozac is instituted or discontinued.

Interference With Cognitive and Motor Performance—Any psychoactive drug may impair judgment, thinking, or motor skills, and patients should be cautioned about operating hazardous machinery, including automobiles, until they are reasonably certain that the drug treatment does not affect them adversely.

Information for Patients—Physicians are advised to discuss the following issues with patients for whom they prescribe Prozac:

- Because Prozac may impair judgment, thinking, or motor skills, patients should be advised to avoid driving a car or operating hazardous machinery until they are reasonably certain that their performance is not affected.
- Patients should be advised to inform their physician if they are taking or plan to take any prescription or over-the-counter drugs or alcohol.
- Patients should be advised to notify their physician if they become pregnant or intend to become pregnant during therapy.
- Patients should be advised to notify their physician if they are breast feeding an infant.
- Patients should be advised to notify their physician if they develop a rash or hives.

Laboratory Tests—There are no specific laboratory tests recommended.

Drug Interactions—As with all drugs, the potential for interaction by a variety of mechanisms (eg, pharmacodynamic, pharmacokinetic drug inhibition or enhancement,

Continued on next page

This product information was prepared in June 1998. Current information on these and other products of Dista Products Company may be obtained by direct inquiry to Lilly Research Laboratories, Lilly Corporate Center, Indianapolis, Indiana 46285, (800) 545-5979.

Prozac—Cont.

etc) is a possibility (*see* Accumulation and Slow Elimination *under* Clinical Pharmacology).

Drugs Metabolized by P450IID6—Approximately 7% of the normal population has a genetic defect that leads to reduced levels of activity of the cytochrome P450 isoenzyme P450IID6. Such individuals have been referred to as "poor metabolizers" of drugs such as debrisoquin, dextromethorphan, and tricyclic antidepressants. Many drugs, such as most antidepressants including fluoxetine and other selective uptake inhibitors of serotonin, are metabolized by this isoenzyme; thus, both the pharmacokinetic properties and relative proportion of metabolites are altered in poor metabolizers. However, for fluoxetine and its metabolite the sum of the plasma concentrations of the 4 active enantiomers is comparable between poor and extensive metabolizers (*see* Variability in Metabolism *under* Clinical Pharmacology).

Fluoxetine, like other agents that are metabolized by P450IID6, inhibits the activity of this isoenzyme, and thus may make normal metabolizers resemble "poor metabolizers." Therapy with medications that are predominantly metabolized by the P450IID6 system and that have a relatively narrow therapeutic index (*see* list below), should be initiated at the low end of the dose range if a patient is receiving fluoxetine concurrently or has taken it in the previous 5 weeks. Thus, his/her dosing requirements resemble those of "poor metabolizers." If fluoxetine is added to the treatment regimen of a patient already receiving a drug metabolized by P450IID6, the need for decreased dose of the original medication should be considered. Drugs with a narrow therapeutic index represent the greatest concern (eg, flecainide, vinblastine, and tricyclic antidepressants).

Drugs Metabolized by Cytochrome P450IIIA4—In an in vivo interaction study involving co-administration of fluoxetine with single doses of terfenadine (a cytochrome P450IIIA4 substrate), no increase in plasma terfenadine concentrations occurred with concomitant fluoxetine. In addition, in vitro studies have shown ketoconazole, a potent inhibitor of P450IIIA4 activity, to be at least 100 times more potent than fluoxetine or norfluoxetine as an inhibitor of the metabolism of several substrates for this enzyme, including astemizole, cisapride, and midazolam. These data indicate that fluoxetine's extent of inhibition of cytochrome P450IIIA4 activity is not likely to be of clinical significance.

CNS Active Drugs—The risk of using Prozac in combination with other CNS active drugs has not been systematically evaluated. Nonetheless, caution is advised if the concomitant administration of Prozac and such drugs is required. In evaluating individual cases, consideration should be given to using lower initial doses of the concomitantly administered drugs, using conservative titration schedules, and monitoring of clinical status (*see* Accumulation and Slow Elimination *under* Clinical Pharmacology).

Anticonvulsants—Patients on stable doses of phenytoin and carbamazepine have developed elevated plasma anticonvulsant concentrations and clinical anticonvulsant toxicity following initiation of concomitant fluoxetine treatment.

Antipsychotics—Some clinical data suggests a possible pharmacodynamic and/or pharmacokinetic interaction between serotonin specific reuptake inhibitors (SSRIs) and antipsychotics. Elevation of blood levels of haloperidol and clozapine has been observed in patients receiving concomitant fluoxetine. A single case report has suggested possible additive effects of primozide and fluoxetine leading to bradycardia.

Benzodiazepines—The half-life of concurrently administered diazepam may be prolonged in some patients (*see* Accumulation and Slow Elimination *under* Clinical Pharmacology). Coadministration of alprazolam and fluoxetine has resulted in increased alprazolam plasma concentrations and in further psychomotor performance decrement due to increased alprazolam levels.

Lithium—There have been reports of both increased and decreased lithium levels when lithium was used concomitantly with fluoxetine. Cases of lithium toxicity and increased serotonergic effects have been reported. Lithium levels should be monitored when these drugs are administered concomitantly.

Tryptophan—Five patients receiving Prozac in combination with tryptophan experienced adverse reactions, including agitation, restlessness, and gastrointestinal distress.

Monoamine Oxidase Inhibitors—*See* Contraindications.

Other Antidepressants—In two studies, previously stable plasma levels of imipramine and desipramine have increased greater than 2 to 10-fold when fluoxetine has been administered in combination. This influence may persist for three weeks or longer after fluoxetine is discontinued. Thus, the dose of tricyclic antidepressant (TCA) may need to be reduced and plasma TCA concentrations may need to be monitored temporarily when fluoxetine is coadministered or has been recently discontinued (*see* Accumulation and Slow Elimination *under* Clinical Pharmacology, and Drugs Metabolized by P450IID6 *under* Drug Interactions).

TABLE 1—MOST COMMON TREATMENT-EMERGENT ADVERSE EVENTS: INCIDENCE IN US DEPRESSION, OCD, AND BULIMIA PLACEBO-CONTROLLED CLINICAL TRIALS

	Percentage of patients reporting event					
	Depression		OCD		Bulimia	
Body System/ Adverse Event	Prozac (N=1728)	Placebo (N=975)	Prozac (N=266)	Placebo (N=89)	Prozac (N=450)	Placebo (N=267)
Body as a Whole						
Asthenia	9	5	15	11	21	9
Flu syndrome	3	4	10	7	8	3
Cardiovascular System						
Vasodilatation	3	2	5	—	2	1
Digestive System						
Nausea	21	9	26	13	29	11
Anorexia	11	2	17	10	8	4
Dry mouth	10	7	12	3	9	6
Dyspepsia	7	5	10	4	10	6
Nervous System						
Insomnia	16	9	28	22	33	13
Anxiety	12	7	14	7	15	9
Nervousness	14	9	14	15	11	5
Somnolence	13	6	17	7	13	5
Tremor	10	3	9	1	13	1
Libido decreased	3	—	11	2	5	1
Abnormal dreams	1	1	5	2	5	3
Respiratory System						
Pharyngitis	3	3	11	9	10	5
Sinusitis	1	4	5	2	6	4
Yawn	—	—	7	—	11	—
Skin and Appendages						
Sweating	8	3	7	—	8	3
Rash	4	3	6	3	4	4
Urogenital System						
Impotence†	2	—	—	—	7	—
Abnormal ejaculation†	—	—	7	—	7	—

†Denominator used was for males only (N=690 Prozac depression; N=410 placebo depression; N=116 Prozac OCD; N=43 placebo OCD; N=14 Prozac bulimia; N=1 placebo bulimia).
—Incidence less than 1%.

Potential Effects of Coadministration of Drugs Tightly Bound to Plasma Proteins—Because fluoxetine is tightly bound to plasma protein, the administration of fluoxetine to a patient taking another drug that is tightly bound to protein (eg, Coumadin, digitoxin) may cause a shift in plasma concentrations potentially resulting in an adverse effect. Conversely, adverse effects may result from displacement of protein bound fluoxetine by other tightly bound drugs (*see* Accumulation and Slow Elimination *under* Clinical Pharmacology).

Warfarin—Altered anti-coagulant effects, including increased bleeding, have been reported when fluoxetine is coadministered with warfarin. Patients receiving warfarin therapy should receive careful coagulation monitoring when fluoxetine is initiated or stopped.

Electroconvulsive Therapy—There are no clinical studies establishing the benefit of the combined use of ECT and fluoxetine. There have been rare reports of prolonged seizures in patients on fluoxetine receiving ECT treatment.

Carcinogenesis, Mutagenesis, Impairment of Fertility—There is no evidence of carcinogenicity, mutagenicity, or impairment of fertility with Prozac.

Carcinogenicity—The dietary administration of fluoxetine to rats and mice for 2 years at doses of up to 10 and 12 mg/kg/day, respectively (approximately 1.2 and 0.7 times, respectively, the maximum recommended human dose [MRHD] of 80 mg on a mg/m^2 basis), produced no evidence of carcinogenicity.

Mutagenicity—Fluoxetine and norfluoxetine have been shown to have no genotoxic effects based on the following assays: bacterial mutation assay, DNA repair assay in cultured rat hepatocytes, mouse lymphoma assay, and in vivo sister chromatid exchange assay in Chinese hamster bone marrow cells.

Impairment of Fertility—Two fertility studies conducted in rats at doses of up to 7.5 and 12.5 mg/kg/day (approximately 0.9 and 1.5 times the MRHD on a mg/m^2 basis), indicated that fluoxetine had no adverse effects on fertility.

Pregnancy—Pregnancy Category C: In embryo-fetal development studies in rats and rabbits, there was no evidence of teratogenicity following administration of up to 12.5 and 15 mg/kg/day, respectively (1.5 and 3.6 times, respectively, the maximum recommended human dose [MRHD] of 80 mg on a mg/m^2 basis) throughout organogenesis. However, in rat reproduction studies, an increase in stillborn pups, a decrease in pup weight, and an increase in pup deaths during the first 7 days postpartum occurred following maternal exposure to 12 mg/kg/day (1.5 times the MRHD on a mg/m^2 basis) during gestation or 7.5 mg/kg/day (0.9 times the MRHD on a mg/m^2 basis) during gestation and lactation. There was no evidence of developmental neurotoxicity in the surviving offspring of rats treated with 12 mg/kg/day during gestation. The no-effect dose for rat pup mortality was 5 mg/kg/day (0.6 times the MRHD on a mg/m^2 basis). Prozac should be used during pregnancy only if the potential benefit justifies the potential risk to the fetus.

Labor and Delivery—The effect of Prozac on labor and delivery in humans is unknown. However, because fluoxetine crosses the placenta and because of the possibility that fluoxetine may have adverse effects on the newborn, fluoxetine should be used during labor and delivery only if the potential benefit justifies the potential risk to the fetus.

Nursing Mothers—Because Prozac is excreted in human milk, nursing while on Prozac is not recommended. In 1 breast milk sample, the concentration of fluoxetine plus norfluoxetine was 70.4 ng/mL. The concentration in the mother's plasma was 295.0 ng/mL. No adverse effects on the infant were reported. In another case, an infant nursed by a mother on Prozac developed crying, sleep disturbance, vomiting, and watery stools. The infant's plasma drug levels were 340 ng/mL of fluoxetine and 208 ng/mL of norfluoxetine on the second day of feeding.

Pediatric Use—Safety and effectiveness in pediatric patients have not been established.

Usage in the Elderly—Evaluation of patients over the age of 60 who received Prozac 20 mg daily revealed no unusual pattern of adverse events relative to the clinical experience in younger patients. However, these data are insufficient to rule out possible age-related differences during chronic use, particularly in elderly patients who have concomitant systemic illnesses or who are receiving concomitant drugs (*see* Age *under* Clinical Pharmacology).

Hyponatremia—Several cases of hyponatremia (some with serum sodium lower than 110 mmol/L) have been reported. The hyponatremia appeared to be reversible when Prozac was discontinued. Although these cases were complex with varying possible etiologies, some were possibly due to the syndrome of inappropriate antidiuretic hormone secretion (SIADH). The majority of these occurrences have been in older patients and in patients taking diuretics or who were otherwise volume depleted. In a placebo-controlled, double-blind trial, 10 of 313 fluoxetine patients and 6 of 320 placebo recipients had a lowering of serum sodium below the reference range; this difference was not statistically significant. The lowest observed concentration was 129 mmol/L. The observed decreases were not clinically significant.

Platelet Function—There have been rare reports of altered platelet function and/or abnormal results from laboratory studies in patients taking fluoxetine. While there have been reports of abnormal bleeding in several patients taking fluoxetine, it is unclear whether fluoxetine had a causative role.

ADVERSE REACTIONS

Multiple doses of Prozac had been administered to 10,782 patients with various diagnoses in US clinical trials as of May 8, 1995. Adverse events were recorded by clinical investigators using descriptive terminology of their own choosing. Consequently, it is not possible to provide a meaningful estimate of the proportion of individuals experiencing adverse events without first grouping similar types of events into a limited (ie, reduced) number of standardized event categories.

In the tables and tabulations that follow, COSTART Dictionary terminology has been used to classify reported adverse events. The stated frequencies represent the proportion of individuals who experienced, at least once, a treatment-emergent adverse event of the type listed. An event was considered treatment-emergent if it occurred for the first time or worsened while receiving therapy following baseline evaluation. It is important to emphasize that events reported during therapy were not necessarily caused by it.

The prescriber should be aware that the figures in the tables and tabulations cannot be used to predict the incidence of side effects in the course of usual medical practice where patient characteristics and other factors differ from those that prevailed in the clinical trials. Similarly, the cited frequencies cannot be compared with figures obtained from other clinical investigations involving different treatments, uses, and investigators. The cited figures, however, do provide the prescribing physician with some basis for estimating the relative contribution of drug and nondrug factors to the side effect incidence rate in the population studied.

Incidence in US Placebo-Controlled Clinical Trials (excluding data from extensions of trials)—Table 1 enumerates the most common treatment-emergent adverse events associated with the use of Prozac (incidence of at least 5% for Prozac and at least twice that for placebo within at least one of the indications) for the treatment of depression, OCD, and bulimia in US controlled clinical trials. Table 2 enumerates treatment-emergent adverse events that occurred in 2% or more patients treated with Prozac and with incidence greater than placebo who participated in US controlled clinical trials comparing Prozac with placebo in the treatment of depression, OCD, or bulimia. Table 2 provides combined data for the pool of studies that are provided separately by indication in Table 1.

[See table 1 at top of previous page]

TABLE 2.
TREATMENT-EMERGENT ADVERSE EVENTS: INCIDENCE IN US DEPRESSION, OCD, AND BULIMIA PLACEBO-CONTROLLED CLINICAL TRIALS

	Percentage of Patients Reporting Event	
	Depression, OCD, and bulimia combined	
Body System/ Adverse Event*	Prozac (N=2444)	Placebo (N=1331)
Body as a Whole		
Headache	21	20
Asthenia	12	6
Flu Syndrome	5	4
Fever	2	1
Cardiovascular System		
Vasodilatation	3	1
Palpitation	2	1
Digestive System		
Nausea	23	10
Diarrhea	12	8
Anorexia	11	3
Dry mouth	10	7
Dyspepsia	8	5
Flatulence	3	2
Vomiting	3	2
Metabolic and Nutritional Disorders		
Weight loss	2	1
Nervous System		
Insomnia	20	11
Anxiety	13	8
Nervousness	13	9
Somnolence	13	6
Dizziness	10	7
Tremor	10	3
Libido decreased	4	—
Respiratory System		
Pharyngitis	5	4
Yawn	3	—
Skin and Appendages		
Sweating	8	3
Rash	4	3
Pruritus	3	2
Special Senses		
Abnormal vision	3	1

TABLE 3—MOST COMMON ADVERSE EVENTS ASSOCIATED WITH DISCONTINUATION IN US DEPRESSION, OCD AND BULIMIA PLACEBO-CONTROLLED CLINICAL TRIALS

Depression, OCD, and bulimia combined	Depression	OCD	Bulimia
—	—	Anxiety (2%)	—
Insomnia (1%)	Insomnia (1%)	—	Insomnia (2%)
—	Nausea (1%)	—	—
Nervousness (1%)	Nervousness (1%)	—	
—	—	Rash (3%)	—

*Included are events reported by at least 2% of patients taking Prozac, except the following events, which had an incidence on placebo ≥Prozac (depression, OCD, and bulimia combined): abdominal pain, abnormal dreams, accidental injury, back pain, chest pain, constipation, cough increased, depression (includes suicidal thoughts), dysmenorrhea, gastrointestinal disorder, infection, myalgia, pain, paresthesia, rhinitis, sinusitis, thinking abnormal.
—Incidence less than 1%.

Associated with Discontinuation in US Placebo-Controlled Clinical Trials (excluding data from extensions of trials)—Table 3 lists the adverse events associated with discontinuation of Prozac treatment (incidence at least twice that for placebo and at least 1% for Prozac in clinical trials) in depression, OCD, and bulimia.

[See table 3 above]

Other Events Observed In All US Clinical Trials—Following is a list of all treatment-emergent adverse events reported at anytime by individuals taking fluoxetine in US clinical trials (10,782 patients) except (1) those listed in the body or footnotes of Table 1 or 2 above or elsewhere in labeling; (2) those for which the COSTART terms were uninformative or misleading; (3) those events for which a causal relationship to Prozac use was considered remote; and (4) events occurring in only 1 patient treated with Prozac and which did not have a substantial probability of being acutely life-threatening.

Events are classified within body system categories using the following definitions: frequent adverse events are defined as those occurring on 1 or more occasions in at least 1/100 patients; infrequent adverse events are those occurring in 1/100 to 1/1,000 patients; rare events are those occurring in less than 1/1,000 patients.

Body as a Whole—*Frequent:* chills; *Infrequent:* chills and fever, face edema, intentional overdose, malaise, pelvic pain, suicide attempt; *Rare:* abdominal syndrome acute, hypothermia, intentional injury, neuroleptic malignant syndrome, photosensitivity reaction.

Cardiovascular System—*Frequent:* hemorrhage, hypertension; *Infrequent:* angina pectoris, arrhythmia, congestive heart failure, hypotension, migraine, myocardial infarct, postural hypotension, syncope, tachycardia, vascular headache; *Rare:* atrial fibrillation, bradycardia, cerebral embolism, cerebral ischemia, cerebrovascular accident, extrasystoles, heart arrest, heart block, pallor, peripheral vascular disorder, phlebitis, shock, thrombophlebitis, thrombosis, vasospasm, ventricular arrhythmia, ventricular extrasystoles, ventricular fibrillation.

Digestive System—*Frequent:* increased appetite, nausea and vomiting; *Infrequent:* aphthous stomatitis, cholelithiasis, colitis, dysphagia, eructation, esophagitis, gastritis, gastroenteritis, glossitis, gum hemmorhage, hyperchlorhydria, increased salivation, liver function tests abnormal, melena, mouth ulceration, nausea/vomiting/diarrhea, stomach ulcer, stomatitis, thirst; *Rare:* biliary pain, bloody diarrhea, cholecystitis, duodenal ulcer, enteritis, esophageal ulcer, fecal incontinence, gastrointestinal hemorrhage, hematemesis, hemorrhage of colon, hepatitis, intestinal obstruction, liver fatty deposit, pancreatitis, peptic ulcer, rectal hemorrhage, salivary gland enlargement, stomach ulcer hemorrhage, tongue edema.

Endocrine System—*Infrequent:* hypothyroidism: *Rare:* diabetic acidosis, diabetes mellitus.

Hemic and Lymphatic System—*Infrequent:* anemia, ecchymosis; *Rare:* blood dyscrasia, hypochromic anemia, leukopenia, lymphedema, lymphocytosis, petechia, purpura, thrombocythemia, thrombocytopenia.

Metabolic and Nutritional—*Frequent:* weight gain; *Infrequent:* dehydration, generalized edema, gout, hypercholesteremia, hyperlipemia, hypokalemia, preipheral edema, *Rare:* alcohol intolerance, alkaline phosphatase increased, BUN increased, creatine phosphokinase increased, hyperkalemia, hyperuricemia, hypocalcemia, iron deficiency anemia, SGPT increased.

Musculoskeletal System—*Infrequent:* arthritis, bone pain, bursitis, leg cramps, tenosynovitis; *Rare:* arthrosis, chondrodystrophy, myasthenia, myopathy, myositis, osteomyelitis, osteoporosis, rheumatoid arthritis.

Nervous System—*Frequent:* agitation, amnesia, confusion, emotional lability, sleep disorder; *Infrequent:* abnormal gait, acute brain syndrome, akathisia, apathy, ataxia, buccoglossal syndrome, CNS depression, CNS stimulation, depersonalization, euphoria, hallucinations, hostility, hyperkinesia, hypertonia, hypesthesia, incoordination, libido increased, myoclonus, nueralgia, neuropathy, neurosis, paranoid reaction, personality disorder†, psychosis, vertigo; *Rare:* abnormal electroencephalogram, antisocial reaction, circumoral paresthesia, coma, delusions, dysarthria, dystonia, extrapyramidal syndrome, foot drop, hyperesthesia, neuritis, paralysis, reflexes decreased, reflexes increased, stupor.

Respiratory System—*Infrequent:* asthma, epistaxis, hiccup, hyperventilation; *Rare:* apnea, atelectasis, cough decreased, emphysema, hemoptysis, hypoventilation, hypoxia, larynx edema, lung edema, pneumothorax, stridor.

Skin and Appendages—*Infrequent:* acne, alopecia, contact dermatitis, eczema, maculopapular rash, skin discoloration, skin ulcer, vesiculobullous rash; *Rare:* furunculosis, herpes zoster, hirsutism, petechial rash, psoriasis, purpuric rash, pustular rash, seborrhea.

Special Senses—*Frequent:* ear pain, taste perversion, tinnitus; *Infrequent:* conjunctivitis, dry eyes, mydriasis, photophobia; *Rare:* blepharitis, deafness, diplopia, exophthalmos, eye hemorrhage, glaucoma, hyperacusis, iritis, parosmia, scleritis, strabismus, taste loss, visual field defect.

Urogenital System—*Frequent:* urinary frequency; *Infrequent:* abortion*, albuminuria, amenorrhea*, anorgasmia, breast enlargement, breast pain, cystitis, dysuria, female lactation*, fibrocystic breast*, hematuria, leukorrhea*, menorrhagia*, metrorrhagia*, nocturia, polyuria, urinary incontinence, urinary retention, urinary urgency, vaginal hemorrhage*; *Rare:* breast engorgement, glycosuria, hypomenorrhea*, kidney pain, oliguria, priapism*, uterine hemorrhage*, uterine fibroids enlarged*.

† Personality disorder is the COSTART term for designating non-aggressive objectionable behavior.
* Adjusted for gender

Postintroduction Reports—Voluntary reports of adverse events temporally associated with Prozac that have been received since market introduction and that may have no causal relationship with the drug include the following: aplastic anemia, atrial fibrillation, cerebral vascular accident, cholestatic jaundice, confusion, dyskinesia (including, for example, a case of buccal-lingual-masticatory syndrome with involuntary tongue protrusion reported to develop in a 77-year-old female after 5 weeks of fluoxetine therapy and which completely resolved over the next few months following drug discontinuation), eosinophilic pneumonia, epidermal necrolysis, erythema nodosum, exfoliative dermatitis, gynecomastia, heart arrest, hepatic failure/necrosis, hyperprolactinemia, immune-related hemolytic anemia, kidney failure, misuse/abuse, movement disorders developing in patients with risk factors including drugs associated with such events and worsening of preexisting movement disorders, neuroleptic malignant syndrome-like events, pancreatitis, pancytopenia, priapism, pulmonary embolism, QT prolongation, Stevens-Johnson syndrome, sudden unexpected death, suicidal ideation, thrombocytopenia, thrombocytopenic purpura, vaginal bleeding after drug withdrawal, and violent behaviors.

DRUG ABUSE AND DEPENDENCE

Controlled Substance Class—Prozac is not a controlled substance.

Physical and Psychological Dependence—Prozac has not been systematically studied, in animals or humans, for its

Continued on next page

This product information was prepared in June 1998. Current information on these and other products of Dista Products Company may be obtained by direct inquiry to Lilly Research Laboratories, Lilly Corporate Center, Indianapolis, Indiana 46285, (800) 545-5979.

Prozac—Cont.

potential for abuse, tolerance or physical dependence. While the premarketing clinical experience with Prozac did not reveal any tendency for a withdrawal syndrome or any drug-seeking behavior, these observations were not systematic and it is not possible to predict on the basis of this limited experience the extent to which a CNS-active drug will be misused, diverted, and/or abused once marketed. Consequently, physicians should carefully evaluate patients for history of drug abuse and follow such patients closely, observing them for signs of misuse or abuse of Prozac (eg, development of tolerance, incrementation of dose, drug-seeking behavior).

OVERDOSAGE

Human Experience—As of December 1987, there were 2 deaths among approximately 38 reports of acute overdose with fluoxetine, either alone or in combination with other drugs and/or alcohol. One death involved a combined overdose with approximately 1,800 mg of fluoxetine and an undetermined amount of maprotiline. Plasma concentrations of fluoxetine and maprotiline were 4.57 mg/L and 4.18 mg/L, respectively. A second death involved 3 drugs yielding plasma concentrations as follows: fluoxetine, 1.93 mg/L; norfluoxetine, 1.10 mg/L; codeine, 1.80 mg/L; temazepam, 3.80 mg/L.

One other patient who reportedly took 3,000 mg of fluoxetine experienced 2 grand mal seizures that remitted spontaneously without specific anticonvulsant treatment (*see* Management of Overdose). The actual amount of drug absorbed may have been less due to vomiting.

Nausea and vomiting were prominent in overdoses involving higher fluoxetine doses. Other prominent symptoms of overdose included agitation, restlessness, hypomania, and other signs of CNS excitation. Except for the 2 deaths noted above, all other overdose cases recovered without residua. Since introduction, reports of death attributed to overdosage of fluoxetine alone have been extremely rare.

Animal Experience—Studies in animals do not provide precise or necessarily valid information about the treatment of human overdose. However, animal experiments can provide useful insights into possible treatment strategies.

The oral median lethal dose in rats and mice was found to be 452 and 248 mg/kg respectively. Acute high oral doses produced hyperirritability and convulsions in several animal species.

Among 6 dogs purposely overdosed with oral fluoxetine, 5 experienced grand mal seizures. Seizures stopped immediately upon the bolus intravenous administration of a standard veterinary dose of diazepam. In this short-term study, the lowest plasma concentration at which a seizure occurred was only twice the maximum plasma concentration seen in humans taking 80 mg/day, chronically.

In a separate single-dose study, the ECG in dogs given high doses did not reveal prolongation of the PR, QRS, or QT intervals. Tachycardia and an increase in blood pressure were observed. Consequently, the value of the ECG in predicting cardiac toxicity is unknown. Nonetheless, the ECG should ordinarily be monitored in cases of human overdose (*see* Management of Overdose).

Management of Overdose—Establish and maintain an airway; ensure adequate oxygenation and ventilation. Activated charcoal, which may be used with sorbitol, may be as or more effective than emesis or lavage, and should be considered in treating overdose.

Cardiac and vital signs monitoring is recommended, along with general symptomatic and supportive measures. Based on experience in animals, which may not be relevant to humans, fluoxetine-induced seizures that fail to remit spontaneously may respond to diazepam.

There are no specific antidotes for Prozac.

Due to the large volume of distribution of Prozac, forced diuresis, dialysis, hemoperfusion, and exchange transfusion are unlikely to be of benefit.

In managing overdosage, consider the possibility of multiple drug involvement. A specific caution involves patients taking or recently having taken fluoxetine who might ingest by accident or intent, excessive quantities of a tricyclic antidepressant. In such a case, accumulation of the parent tricyclic and an active metabolite may increase the possibility of clinically significant sequelae and extend the time needed for close medical observation (*see* Other Antidepressants *under* Precautions).

The physician should consider contacting a poison control center on the treatment of any overdose. Telephone numbers of certified poison control centers are listed in the *Physicians' Desk Reference (PDR)*

DOSAGE AND ADMINISTRATION

Depression—

Initial Treatment—In controlled trials used to support the efficacy of fluoxetine, patients were administered morning doses ranging from 20 mg to 80 mg/day. Studies comparing fluoxetine 20, 40, and 60 mg/day to placebo indicate that 20 mg/day is sufficient to obtain a satisfactory antidepressant

response in most cases. Consequently, a dose of 20 mg/day administered in the morning, is recommended as the initial dose.

A dose increase may be considered after several weeks if no clinical improvement is observed. Doses above 20 mg/day may be administered on a once a day (morning) or b.i.d. schedule (ie, morning and noon) and should not exceed a maximum dose of 80 mg/day.

As with other antidepressants, the full antidepressant effect may be delayed until 4 weeks of treatment or longer.

As with many other medications, a lower or less frequent dosage should be used in patients with hepatic impairment. A lower or less frequent dosage should also be considered for the elderly (*see* Usage in the Elderly *under* Precautions), and for patients with concurrent disease or on multiple concomitant medications. Dosage adjustments for renal impairment are not routinely necessary (*see* Liver Disease and Renal Disease *under* Clinical Pharmacology, *and* Use in Patients with Concomitant Illness *under* Precautions).

Maintenance/Continuation/Extended Treatment—It is generally agreed that acute episodes of depression require several months or longer of sustained pharmacologic therapy. Whether the dose of antidepressant needed to induce remission is identical to the dose needed to maintain and/or sustain euthymia is unknown.

Systematic evaluation of Prozac has shown that its antidepressant efficacy is maintained for periods of up to 38 weeks following 12 weeks of open-label acute treatment (50 weeks total) at a dose of 20 mg/day (*see* Clinical Trials *under* Clinical Pharmacology).

Obsessive-Compulsive Disorder—

Initial Treatment—In the controlled clinical trials of fluoxetine supporting its effectiveness in the treatment of obsessive-compulsive disorder, patients were administered fixed daily doses of 20, 40, or 60 mg of fluoxetine or placebo (*see* Clinical Trials *under* Clinical Pharmacology). In one of these studies, no dose response relationship for effectiveness was demonstrated. Consequently, a dose of 20 mg/day, administered in the morning, is recommended as the initial dose. Since there was a suggestion of a possible dose response relationship for effectiveness in the second study, a dose increase may be considered after several weeks if insufficient clinical improvement is observed. The full therapeutic effect may be delayed until 5 weeks of treatment or longer.

Doses above 20 mg/day may be administered on a once a day (ie, morning) or b.i.d. schedule (ie, morning and noon). A dose range of 20 to 60 mg/day is recommended, however, doses of up to 80 mg/day have been well tolerated in open studies of OCD. The maximum fluoxetine dose should not exceed 80 mg/day.

As with the use of Prozac in depression, a lower or less frequent dosage should be used in patients with hepatic impairment. A lower or less frequent dosage should also be considered for the elderly (*see* Usage in the Elderly *under* Precautions), and for patients with concurrent disease or on multiple concomitant medications. Dosage adjustments for renal impairment are not routinely necessary (*see* Liver Disease and Renal Disease *under* Clinical Pharmacology, *and* Use in Patients with Concomitant Illness *under* Precautions).

Maintenance/Continuation Treatment—While there are no systematic studies that answer the question of how long to continue Prozac, OCD is a chronic condition and it is reasonable to consider continuation for a responding patient. Although the efficacy of Prozac after 13 weeks has not been documented in controlled trials, patients have been continued in therapy under double-blind conditions for up to an additional 6 months without loss of benefit. However, dosage adjustments should be made to maintain the patient on the lowest effective dosage, and patients should be periodically reassessed to determine the need for treatment.

Bulimia Nervosa—

Initial Treatment—In the controlled clinical trials of fluoxetine supporting its effectiveness in the treatment of bulimia nervosa, patients were administered fixed daily fluoxetine doses of 20 or 60 mg, or placebo (*see* Clinical Trials *under* Clinical Pharmacology). Only the 60 mg dose was statistically significantly superior to placebo in reducing the frequency of binge-eating and vomiting. Consequently, the recommended dose is 60 mg/day, administered in the morning. For some patients it may be advisable to titrate up to this target dose over several days. Fluoxetine doses above 60 mg/day have not been systematically studied in patients with bulimia.

As with the use of Prozac in depression and OCD, a lower or less frequent dosage should be used in patients with hepatic impairment. A lower or less frequent dosage should also be considered for the elderly (*see* Usage in the Elderly *under* Precautions), and for patients with concurrent disease or on multiple concomitant medications. Dosage adjustments for renal impairment are not routinely necessary (*see* Liver Disease and Renal Disease *under* Clinical Pharmacology, *and* Use in Patients with Concomitant Illness *under* Precautions).

Maintenance/Continuation Treatment—While there are no systematic studies that answer the question of how long to continue Prozac, bulimia is a chronic condition and it is reasonable to consider continuation for a responding patient. Although the efficacy of Prozac after 16 weeks has not been documented in controlled trials, some patients have been continued in therapy under double-blind conditions for up to an additional 6 months without loss of benefit. However, patients should be periodically reassessed to determine the need for continued treatment.

Switching Patients to a Tricyclic Antidepressant (TCA): Dosage of a TCA may need to be reduced, and plasma TCA concentrations may need to be monitored temporarily when fluoxetine is coadministered or has been recently discontinued (*see* Other Antidepressants *under* Drug Interactions).

Switching Patients to or From a Monoamine Oxidase Inhibitor: At least 14 days should elapse between discontinuation of an MAOI and initiation of therapy with Prozac. In addition, at least 5 weeks, perhaps longer, should be allowed after stopping Prozac before starting an MAOI (*see* Contraindications and Precautions).

HOW SUPPLIED

Prozac® Pulvules®, USP, are available in:

The 10 mg* Pulvule is opaque green and green, imprinted with DISTA 3104 on the cap and Prozac 10 mg on the body:

NDC 0777-3104-02 (PU3104) - Bottles of 100
NDC 0777-3104-07 (PU3104) - Bottles of 2000
NDC 0777-3104-82 (PU3104) - 20 FlexPak§ blister cards of 31

The 20 mg* Pulvule is an opaque green cap and off-white body, imprinted with DISTA 3105 on the cap and Prozac 20 mg on the body:

NDC 0777-3105-30 (PU3105) - Bottles of 30
NDC 0777-3105-02 (PU3105) - Bottles of 100
NDC 0777-3105-07 (PU3105) - Bottles of 2000
NDC 0777-3105-33 (PU3105) - (ID†100) Blisters
NDC 0777-3105-82 (PU3105) - 20 FlexPak§ blister cards of 31

Liquid, Oral Solution is available in:
20 mg* per 5 mL with mint flavor:

NDC 0777-5120-58 (MS-5120‡) - Bottles of 120 mL

---

*Fluoxetine base equivalent.
†Identi-Dose® (unit dose medication, Dista).
‡Dispense in a tight, light-resistant container.
§FlexPak (flexible blister card, Lilly)
Store at controlled room temperature, 59° to 86°F (15° to 30°C).

ANIMAL TOXICOLOGY

Phospholipids are increased in some tissues of mice, rats, and dogs given fluoxetine chronically. This effect is reversible after cessation of fluoxetine treatment. Phospholipid accumulation in animals has been observed with many cationic amphiphilic drugs, including fenfluramine, imipramine, and rantidine. The significance of this effect to humans is unknown.

CAUTION—Federal (USA) law prohibits dispensing without prescription.

Literature revised June 12, 1997
PV 2141 DPP   [061297]
Dista Products Company
Division of Eli Lilly and Company
Indianapolis, Indiana 46285, USA
Shown in Product Identification Guide, page 309

Dow Hickam Pharmaceuticals
**for product information
see Bertek Pharmaceuticals Inc.**

For EMERGENCY telephone numbers,
consult the **Manufacturers' Index.**

DuPont Pharma
WILMINGTON, DE 19805

DUPONT PHARMA
DuPont Merck Plaza, Hickory Run
P.O. Box 80723
Wilmington, DE 19880-0723
(302) 992-5000

Address all product-related inquiries to:
Medical Affairs Department

For Product Information/Adverse Drug Experience Reporting, call
Product Information
(302) 992-4240

COUMADIN® TABLETS ℞
(Warfarin Sodium Tablets, USP) Crystalline
Anticoagulant

COUMADIN® FOR INJECTION ℞
(Warfarin Sodium for Injection, USP)

DESCRIPTION

COUMADIN (crystalline warfarin sodium), is an anticoagulant which acts by inhibiting vitamin K-dependent coagulation factors. Chemically, it is 3-(α-acetonylbenzyl)-4-hydroxycoumarin and is a racemic mixture of the R and S enantiomers. Crystalline warfarin sodium is an isopropanol clathrate. The crystallization of warfarin sodium virtually eliminates trace impurities present in amorphous warfarin. Its empirical formula is $C_{19}H_{15}NaO_4$ and its structural formula may be represented by the following:

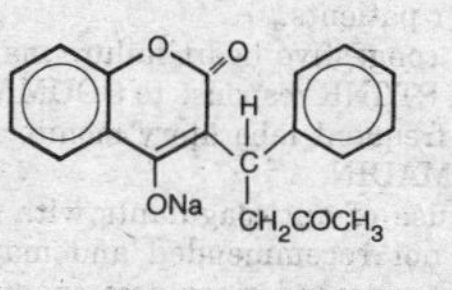

Crystalline warfarin sodium occurs as a white, odorless, crystalline powder, is discolored by light and is very soluble in water; freely soluble in alcohol; very slightly soluble in chloroform and in ether.

COUMADIN Tablets for oral use also contain:

All strengths:	Lactose, starch and magnesium stearate
1 mg:	D&C Red No. 6 Barium Lake
2 mg:	FD&C Blue No. 2 Aluminum Lake and FD&C Red No. 40 Aluminum Lake
2½ mg:	D&C Yellow No. 10 Aluminum Lake and FD&C Blue No. 1 Aluminum Lake
3 mg:	FD&C Yellow No. 6 Aluminum Lake, FD&C Blue No. 2 Aluminum Lake and FD&C Red No. 40 Aluminum Lake
4 mg:	FD&C Blue No. 1 Aluminum Lake
5 mg:	FD&C Yellow No. 6 Aluminum Lake
6 mg:	FD&C Yellow No. 6 Aluminum Lake and FD&C Blue No. 1 Aluminum Lake
7½ mg:	D&C Yellow No. 10 Aluminum Lake and FD&C Yellow No. 6 Aluminum Lake
10 mg:	Dye Free

COUMADIN for Injection is supplied as a sterile, lyophilized powder, which, after reconstitution with 2.7 mL sterile Water for Injection, contains:

Warfarin Sodium	2 mg/mL
Sodium Phosphate, Dibasic, Heptahydrate	4.98 mg/mL
Sodium Phosphate, Monobasic, Monohydrate	0.194 mg/mL
Sodium Chloride	0.1 mg/mL
Mannitol	38.0 mg/mL
Sodium Hydroxide, as needed for pH adjustment to	8.1 to 8.3

CLINICAL PHARMACOLOGY

COUMADIN and other coumarin anticoagulants act by inhibiting the synthesis of vitamin K dependent clotting factors, which include Factors II, VII, IX and X, and the anticoagulant proteins C and S. Half-lives of these clotting factors are as follows: Factor II—60 hours, VII—4-6 hours, IX—24 hours, and X—48-72 hours. The half-lives of proteins C and S are approximately 8 hours and 30 hours, respectively. The resultant *in vivo* effect is a sequential depression of Factors VII, IX, X and II activities. Vitamin K is an essential cofactor for the post ribosomal synthesis of the vitamin K dependent clotting factors. The vitamin promotes the biosynthesis of γ-carboxyglutamic acid residues in the proteins which are essential for biological activity. Warfarin is thought to interfere with clotting factor synthesis by inhibition of the regeneration of vitamin K_1 epoxide. The degree of depression is dependent upon the dosage administered. Therapeutic doses of warfarin decrease the total amount of the active form of each vitamin K dependent clotting factor made by the liver by approximately 30% to 50%.

TABLE 1
CLINICAL STUDIES OF WARFARIN IN NON-RHEUMATIC AF PATIENTS*

Study	N: Warfarin-Treated Patients	N: Control Patients	PT Ratio	INR	Thromboembolism %Risk Reduction	Thromboembolism *p*-value	% Major Bleeding: Warfarin-Treated Patients	% Major Bleeding: Control Patients
AFASAK	335	336	1.5–2.0	2.8–4.2	60	0.027	0.6	0.0
SPAF	210	211	1.3–1.8	2.0–4.5	67	0.01	1.9	1.9
BAATAF	212	208	1.2–1.5	1.5–2.7	86	<0.05	0.9	0.5
CAFA	187	191	1.3–1.6	2.0–3.0	45	0.25	2.7	0.5
SPINAF	260	265	1.2–1.5	1.4–2.8	79	0.001	2.3	1.5

* All study results of warfarin vs. control are based on intention-to-treat analysis and include ischemic stroke and systemic throboembolism, excluding hemorrhage and transient ischemic attacks.

An anticoagulation effect generally occurs within 24 hours after drug administration. However, peak anticoagulant effect may be delayed 72 to 96 hours. The duration of action of a single dose of racemic warfarin is 2 to 5 days. The effects of COUMADIN may become more pronounced as effects of daily maintenance doses overlap. Anticoagulants have no direct effect on an established thrombus, nor do they reverse ischemic tissue damage. However, once a thrombus has occurred, the goal of anticoagulant treatment is to prevent further extension of the formed clot and prevent secondary thromboembolic complications which may result in serious and possibly fatal sequelae.

Pharmacokinetics: COUMADIN is a racemic mixture of the R- and S-enantiomers. The S-enantiomer exhibits 2–5 times more anticoagulant activity than the R-enantiomer in humans, but generally has a more rapid clearance.

Absorption: COUMADIN is essentially completely absorbed after oral administration with peak concentration generally attained within the first 4 hours.

Distribution: There are no differences in the apparent volumes of distribution after intravenous and oral administration of single doses of warfarin solution. Warfarin distributes into a relatively small apparent volume of distribution of about 0.14 liter/kg. A distribution phase lasting 6 to 12 hours is distinguishable after rapid intravenous or oral administration of an aqueous solution. Using a one compartment model, and assuming complete bioavailability, estimates of the volumes of distribution of R- and S-warfarin are similar to each other and to that of the racemate. Concentrations in fetal plasma approach the maternal values, but warfarin has not been found in human milk (see WARNINGS—Lactation). Approximately 99% of the drug is bound to plasma proteins.

Metabolism: The elimination of warfarin is almost entirely by metabolism. COUMADIN is stereoselectively metabolized by hepatic microsomal enzymes (cytochrome P-450) to inactive hydroxylated metabolites (predominant route) and by reductases to reduced metabolites (warfarin alcohols). The warfarin alcohols have minimal anticoagulant activity. The metabolites are principally excreted into the urine; and to a lesser extent into the bile. The metabolites of warfarin that have been identified include dehydrowarfarin, two diastereoisomer alcohols, 4'-, 6-, 7-, 8- and 10-hydroxywarfarin. The Cytochrome P-450 isozymes involved in the metabolism of warfarin include 2C9, 2C19, 2C8, 2C18, 1A2, and 3A4. 2C9 is likely to be the principal form of human liver P-450 which modulates the *in vivo* anticoagulant activity of warfarin.

Excretion: The terminal half-life of warfarin after a single dose is approximately one week; however, the effective half-life ranges from 20 to 60 hours, with a mean of about 40 hours. The clearance of R-warfarin is generally half that of S-warfarin, thus as the volumes of distribution are similar, the half-life of R-warfarin is longer than that of S-warfarin. The half-life of R-warfarin ranges from 37 to 89 hours, while that of S-warfarin ranges from 21 to 43 hours. Studies with radiolabeled drug have demonstrated that up to 92% of the orally administered dose is recovered in urine. Very little warfarin is excreted unchanged in urine. Urinary excretion is in the form of metabolites.

Elderly: There are no significant age-related differences in the pharmacokinetics of racemic warfarin. Limited information suggests that there is no difference in the clearance of S-warfarin in elderly versus young subjects. However, there may be a slight decrease in the clearance of R-warfarin in the elderly compared to the young. Older patients (60 years or older) appear to exhibit greater than expected PT/INR response to the anticoagulant effects of warfarin. As patient age increases, less warfarin is required to produce a therapeutic level of anticoagulation. The cause of this response to warfarin is not known.

Renal Dysfunction: Renal clearance is considered to be a minor determinant of anticoagulant response to warfarin. No dosage adjustment is necessary for patients with renal failure.

Hepatic Dysfunction: Hepatic dysfunction can potentiate the response to warfarin through impaired synthesis of clotting factors and decreased metabolism of warfarin.

The administration of COUMADIN via the intravenous (I.V.) route should provide the patient with the same concentration of an equal oral dose, but maximum plasma concentration will be reached earlier. However, the full anticoagulant effect of a dose of warfarin may not be achieved until 72–96 hours after dosing, indicating that the administration of I.V. COUMADIN should not provide any increased biological effect or earlier onset of action.

Clinical Trials

Atrial Fibrillation (AF): In five prospective randomized controlled clinical trials involving 3711 patients with non-rheumatic AF, warfarin significantly reduced the risk of systemic thromboembolism including stroke (See Table 1). The risk reduction ranged from 60% to 86% in all except one trial (CAFA: 45%) which stopped early due to published positive results from two of these trials. The incidence of major bleeding in these trials ranged from 0.6 to 2.7% (See Table 1). Meta-analysis findings of these studies revealed that the effects of warfarin in reducing thromboembolic events including stroke were similar at either moderately high INR (2.0–4.5) or low INR (1.4–3.0). There was a significant reduction in minor bleeds at the low INR. Similar data from clinical studies in valvular atrial fibrillation patients are not available.

[See table 1 above]

Myocardial Infarction: WARIS (The Warfarin Re-Infarction Study) was a double-blind, randomized study of 1214 patients 2 to 4 weeks post-infarction treated with warfarin to a target INR of 2.8 to 4.8. [(But note that a lower INR was achieved and increased bleeding was associated with INR's above 4.0; see DOSAGE AND ADMINISTRATION.)] The primary endpoint was a combination of total mortality and recurrent infarction. A secondary endpoint of cerebrovascular events was assessed. Mean follow-up of the patients was 37 months. The results for each endpoint separately, including an analysis of vascular death, are provided in the following table:

[See table 2 at top of next page]

Mechanical and Bioprosthetic Heart Valves: In a prospective, randomized, open label, positive-controlled study (Mok et al, 1985) in 254 patients, the thromboembolic-free interval was found to be significantly greater in patients with mechanical prosthetic heart valves treated with warfarin alone compared with dipyridamole-aspirin ($p<0.005$) and pentoxifylline-aspirin ($p<0.05$) treated patients. Rates of thromboembolic events in these groups were 2.2, 8.6, and 7.9/100 patient years, respectively. Major bleeding rates were 2.5, 0.0, and 0.9/100 patient years, respectively.

In a prospective, open label, clinical trial (Saour et al, 1990) comparing moderate (INR 2.65) vs. high intensity (INR 9.0) warfarin therapies in 258 patients with mechanical prosthetic heart valves, thromboembolism occurred with similar frequency in the two groups (4.0 and 3.7 events/100 patient years, respectively). Major bleeding was more common in the high intensity group (2.1 events/100 patient years) vs. 0.95 events/100 patient years in the moderate intensity group.

In a randomized trial (Turpie et al, 1988) in 210 patients comparing two intensities of warfarin therapy (INR 2.0–2.25 vs. INR 2.5–4.0) for a three-month period following tissue heart value replacement, thromboembolism occurred with similar frequency in the two groups (major embolic events 2.0% vs. 1.9%, respectively and minor embolic events 10.8% vs. 10.2%, respectively). Major bleeding complications were more frequent with the higher intensity (major hemorrhages 4.6%) vs. none in the lower intensity.

INDICATIONS AND USAGE

COUMADIN (Warfarin Sodium) is indicated for the prophylaxis and/or treatment of venous thrombosis and its extension, and pulmonary embolism.

Continued on next page

Coumadin—Cont.

COUMADIN is indicated for the prophylaxis and/or treatment of the thromboembolic complications associated with atrial fibrillation and/or cardiac valve replacement.
COUMADIN is indicated to reduce the risk of death, recurrent myocardial infarction, and thromboembolic events such as stroke or systemic embolization after myocardial infarction.

CONTRAINDICATIONS

Anticoagulation is contraindicated in any localized or general physical condition or personal circumstance in which the hazard of hemorrhage might be greater than the potential clinical benefits of anticoagulation, such as:

Pregnancy: COUMADIN is contraindicated in women who are or may become pregnant because the drug passes through the placental barrier and may cause fatal hemorrhage to the fetus *in utero*. Furthermore, there have been reports of birth malformations in children born to mothers who have been treated with warfarin during pregnancy. Embryopathy characterized by nasal hypoplasia with or without stippled epiphyses (chondrodysplasia punctata) has been reported in pregnant women exposed to warfarin during the first trimester. Central nervous system abnormalities also have been reported, including dorsal midline dysplasia characterized by agenesis of the corpus callosum, Dandy-Walker malformation, and midline cerebellar atrophy. Ventral midline dysplasia, characterized by optic atrophy, and eye abnormalities have been observed. Mental retardation, blindness, and other central nervous system abnormalities have been reported in association with second and third trimester exposure. Although rare, teratogenic reports following *in utero* exposure to warfarin include urinary tract anomalies such as single kidney, asplenia, anencephaly, spina bifida, cranial nerve palsy, hydrocephalus, cardiac defects and congenital heart disease, polydactyly, deformities of toes, diaphragmatic hernia, corneal leukoma, cleft palate, cleft lip, schizencephaly, and microcephaly.
Spontaneous abortion and still birth are known to occur and a higher risk of fetal mortality is associated with the use of warfarin. Low birth weight and growth retardation have also been reported.
Women of childbearing potential who are candidates for anticoagulant therapy should be carefully evaluated and the indications critically reviewed with the patient. If the patient becomes pregnant while taking this drug, she should be apprised of the potential risks to the fetus, and the possibility of termination of the pregnancy should be discussed in light of those risks.

Hemorrhagic tendencies or blood dyscrasias.
Recent or contemplated surgery of: (1) central nervous system; (2) eye; (3) traumatic surgery resulting in large open surfaces.
Bleeding tendencies associated with active ulceration or overt bleeding of: (1) gastrointestinal, genitourinary or respiratory tracts; (2) cerebrovascular hemorrhage; (3) aneurysms-cerebral, dissecting aorta; (4) pericarditis and pericardial effusions; (5) bacterial endocarditis.
Threatened abortion, eclampsia and preeclampsia.
Inadequate laboratory facilities.
Unsupervised patients with senility, alcoholism, or psychosis or other lack of patient cooperation.
Spinal puncture and other diagnostic or therapeutic procedures with potential for uncontrollable bleeding.
Miscellaneous: major regional, lumbar block anesthesia, malignant hypertension and known hypersensitivity to warfarin or to any other components of this product.

WARNINGS

The most serious risks associated with anticoagulant therapy with sodium warfarin are hemorrhage in any tissue or organ and, less frequently (<0.1%), necrosis and/or gangrene of skin and other tissues. The risk of hemorrhage is related to the level of intensity and the duration of anticoagulant therapy. Hemorrhage and necrosis have in some cases been reported to result in death or permanent disability. Necrosis appears to be associated with local thrombosis and usually appears within a few days of the start of anticoagulant therapy. In severe cases of necrosis, treatment through debridement or amputation of the affected tissue, limb, breast or penis has been reported. Careful diagnosis is required to determine whether necrosis is caused by an underlying disease. Warfarin therapy should be discontinued when warfarin is suspected to be the cause of developing necrosis and heparin therapy may be considered for anticoagulation. Although various treatments have been attempted, no treatment for necrosis has been considered uniformly effective. See below for information on predisposing conditions. These and other risks associated with anticoagulant therapy must be weighed against the risk of thrombosis or embolization in untreated cases.
It cannot be emphasized too strongly that treatment of each patient is a highly individualized matter. COUMADIN, a narrow therapeutic range (index) drug, may be affected by factors such as other drugs and dietary Vitamin K. Dosage

should be controlled by periodic determinations of prothrombin time (PT)/International Normalized Ratio (INR) or other suitable coagulation tests. Determinations of whole blood clotting and bleeding times are not effective measures for control of therapy. Heparin prolongs the one-stage PT. When heparin and COUMADIN are administered concomitantly, refer below to CONVERSION FROM HEPARIN THERAPY for recommendations.
Caution should be observed when COUMADIN is administered in any situation or in the presence of any predisposing condition and/or gangrene where added risk of hemorrhage or necrosis is present.
Anticoagulation therapy with COUMADIN may enhance the release of atheromatous plaque emboli, thereby increasing the risk of complications from systemic cholesterol microembolization, including the "purple toes syndrome." Discontinuation of COUMADIN therapy is recommended when such phenomena are observed.
Systemic atheroemboli and cholesterol microemboli can present with a variety of signs and symptoms including purple toes syndrome, livedo reticularis, rash, gangrene, abrupt and intense pain in the leg, foot, or toes, foot ulcers, myalgia, penile gangrene, abdominal pain, flank or back pain, hematuria, renal insufficiency, hypertension, cerebral ischemia, spinal cord infarction, pancreatitis, symptoms simulating polyarteritis, or any other sequelae of vascular compromise due to embolic occlusion. The most commonly involved visceral organs are the kidneys followed by the pancreas, spleen, and liver. Some cases have progressed to necrosis or death.
Purple toes syndrome is a complication of oral anticoagulation characterized by a dark, purplish or mottled color of the toes, usually occurring between 3–10 weeks, or later, after the initiation of therapy with warfarin or related compounds. Major features of this syndrome include purple color of plantar surfaces and sides of the toes that blanches on moderate pressure and fades with elevation of the legs; pain and tenderness of the toes; waxing and waning of the color over time. While the purple toes syndrome is reported to be reversible, some cases progress to gangrene or necrosis which may require debridement of the affected area, or may lead to amputation.
Heparin-induced thrombocytopenia: COUMADIN should be used with caution in patients with heparin-induced thrombocytopenia and deep venous thrombosis. Cases of venous limb ischemia, necrosis, and gangrene have occurred in patients with heparin-induced thrombocytopenia and deep venous thrombosis when heparin treatment was discontinued and warfarin therapy was started or continued. In some patients sequelae have included amputation of the involved area and/or death (Warkentin et al, 1997).
A severe elevation (>50 seconds) in activated partial thromboplastin time (aPTT) with a PT/INR in the desired range has been identified as an indication of increased risk of postoperative hemorrhage.
The decision to administer anticoagulants in the following conditions must be based upon clinical judgment in which the risks of anticoagulant therapy are weighed against the benefits:
Lactation: COUMADIN appears in the milk of nursing mothers in an inactive form. Infants nursed by mothers treated with COUMADIN had no change in prothrombin times (PTs). Effects in premature infants have not been evaluated.
Severe to moderate hepatic or renal insufficiency.
Infectious diseases or disturbances of intestinal flora: sprue, antibiotic therapy.
Trauma which may result in internal bleeding.
Surgery or trauma resulting in large exposed raw surfaces.
Indwelling catheters.
Severe to moderate hypertension.
Known or suspected deficiency in protein C mediated anticoagulant response: Hereditary or acquired deficiencies of protein C or its cofactor, protein S, have been associated with tissue necrosis following warfarin administration. Not all patients with these conditions develop necrosis, and tissue necrosis occurs in patients without these deficiencies. Inherited resistance to activated protein C has been de-

scribed in many patients with venous thromboembolic disorders but has not yet been evaluated as a risk factor for tissue necrosis. The risk associated with these conditions, both for recurrent thrombosis and for adverse reactions, is difficult to evaluate since it does not appear to be the same for everyone. Decisions about testing and therapy must be made on an individual basis. It has been reported that concomitant anticoagulation therapy with heparin for 5 to 7 days during initiation of therapy with COUMADIN may minimize the incidence of tissue necrosis. Warfarin therapy should be discontinued when warfarin is suspected to be the cause of developing necrosis and heparin therapy may be considered for anticoagulation.
Miscellaneous: polycythemia vera, vasculitis, and severe diabetes.
Minor and severe allergic/hypersensitivity reactions and anaphylactic reactions have been reported.
In patients with acquired or inherited warfarin resistance, decreased therapeutic responses to COUMADIN have been reported. Exaggerated therapeutic responses have been reported in other patients.
Patients with congestive heart failure may exhibit greater than expected PT/INR response to COUMADIN, thereby requiring more frequent laboratory monitoring, and reduced doses of COUMADIN.
Concomitant use of anticoagulants with streptokinase or urokinase is not recommended and may be hazardous. (Please note recommendations accompanying these preparations.)

PRECAUTIONS

Periodic determination of PT/INR or other suitable coagulation test is essential.
Numerous factors, alone or in combination, including travel, changes in diet, environment, physical state and medication may influence response of the patient to anticoagulants. It is generally good practice to monitor the patient's response with additional PT/INR determinations in the period immediately after discharge from the hospital, and whenever other medications are initiated, discontinued or taken irregularly. The following factors are listed for reference; however, other factors may also affect the anticoagulant response.
Drugs may interact with COUMADIN through pharmacodynamic or pharmacokinetic mechanisms. Pharmacodynamic mechanisms for drug interactions with COUMADIN are synergism (impaired hemostasis, reduced clotting factor synthesis), competitive antagonism (vitamin K), and altered physiologic control loop for vitamin K metabolism (hereditary resistance). Pharmacokinetic mechanisms for drug interactions with COUMADIN are mainly enzyme induction, enzyme inhibition, and reduced plasma protein binding. It is important to note that some drugs may interact by more than one mechanism.
The following factors, alone or in combination, may be responsible for INCREASED PT/INR response:

ENDOGENOUS FACTORS:
blood dyscrasias—see CONTRAINDICATIONS
cancer
collagen vascular disease
congestive heart failure
diarrhea
elevated temperature
hepatic disorders
   infectious hepatitis
   jaundice
hyperthyroidism
poor nutritional state
steatorrhea
vitamin K deficiency

EXOGENOUS FACTORS:
Potential drug interactions with COUMADIN are listed below by drug class and by specific drugs.
Classes of Drugs
5-lipoxygenase Inhibitor
Adrenergic Stimulants, Central
Alcohol Abuse Reduction Preparations
Analgesics

TABLE 2

Event	Warfarin (N=607)	Placebo (N=607)	RR (95%CI)	% Risk Reduction (p-value)
Total Patient Years of Follow-up	2018	1944		
Total Mortality	94 (4.7/100 py)	123 (6.3/100 py)	0.76 (0.60, 0.97)	24 (p=0.030)
Vascular Death	82 (4.1/100 py)	105 (5.4/100 py)	0.78 (0.60, 1.02)	22 (p=0.068)
Recurrent MI	82 (4.1/100 py)	124 (6.4/100 py)	0.66 (0.51, 0.85)	34 (p=0.001)
Cerebrovascular Event	20 (1.0/100 py)	44 (2.3/100 py)	0.46 (0.28, 0.75)	54 (p=0.002)

RR=Relative risk; Risk reduction=(I–RR); CI=Confidence interval; MI=Myocardial infarction; py=patient years

Anesthetics, Inhalation
Antiandrogen
Antiarrhythmics†
Antibiotics†
    Aminoglycosides (oral)
    Cephalosporins, parenteral
    Macrolides
    Miscellaneous
    Penicillins, intravenous, high dose
    Quinolones (fluoroquinolones)
    Sulfonamides, long acting
    Tetracyclines
Anticoagulants
Anticonvulsants†
Antidepressants†
Antimalarial Agents
Antineoplastics†
Antiparasitic/Antimicrobials
Antiplatelet Drugs/Effects
Antithyroid Drugs†
Beta-Adrenergic Blockers
Bromelains
Cholelitholytic Agents
Diabetes Agents, Oral
Diuretics†
Fungal Medications, Systemic†
Gastric Acidity and Peptic Ulcer Agents†
Gastrointestinal, Ulcerative Colitis Agents
Gout Treatment Agents
Hemorrheologic Agents
Hepatotoxic Drugs
Hyperglycemic Agents
Hypertensive Emergency Agents
Hypnotics†
Hypolipidemics†
Leukotriene Receptor Antagonist
Monoamine Oxidase Inhibitors
Narcotics, prolonged
Nonsteroidal Anti-Inflammatory Agents
Psychostimulants
Pyrazolones
Salicylates
Selective Serotonin Reuptake Inhibitors
Steroids, Adrenocortical†
Steroids, Anabolic (17-Alkyl Testosterone Derivatives)
Thrombolytics
Thyroid Drugs
Tuberculosis Agents†
Uricosuric Agents
Vaccines
Vitamins†

Specific Drugs Reported
acetaminophen
alcohol†
allopurinol
aminosalicylic acid
amiodarone HCl
aspirin
azithromycin
cefamandole
cefazolin
cefoperazone
cefotetan
cefoxitin
ceftriaxone
chenodiol
chloramphenicol
chloral hydrate†
chlorpropamide
cholestyramine†
cimetidine
ciprofloxacin
clarithromycin
clofibrate
COUMADIN overdose
cyclophosphamide†
danazol
dextran
dextrothyroxine
diazoxide
diclofenac
dicumarol
diflunisal
disulfiram
doxycycline
erythromycin
ethacrynic acid
fenoprofen
fluconazole
fluorouracil
fluoxetine
flutamide
fluvoxamine
glucagon
halothane

heparin
ibuprofen
ifosfamide
indomethacin
influenza virus vaccine
itraconazole
ketoprofen
ketorolac
levamisole
levothyroxine
liothyronine
lovastatin
mefenamic acid
methimazole†
methyldopa
methylphenidate
methylsalicylate ointment (topical)
metronidazole
miconazole
moricizine hydrochloride†
nalidixic acid
naproxen
neomycin
norfloxacin
ofloxacin
olsalazine
omeprazole
oxaprozin
oxymetholone
paroxetine
penicillin G, intravenous
pentoxifylline
phenylbutazone
phenytoin†
piperacillin
piroxicam
prednisone†
propafenone
propoxyphene
propranolol
propylthiouracil†
quinidine
quinine
ranitidine†
sertraline
simvastatin
stanozolol
streptokinase
sulfamethizole
sulfamethoxazole
sulfinpyrazone
sulfisoxazole
sulindac
tamoxifen
tetracycline
thyroid
ticarcillin
ticlopidine
tissue plasminogen activator (t-PA)
tolbutamide
trimethoprim/sulfamethoxazole
urokinase
valproate
vitamin E
zafirlukast
zileuton
also: other medications affecting blood elements which may
        modify hemostasis
        dietary deficiencies
        prolonged hot weather
        unreliable PT/INR determinations
†Increased and decreased PT/INR responses have been reported.

**The following factors, alone or in combination, may be re-
sponsible for DECREASED PT/INR response:**

ENDOGENOUS FACTORS:
edema
hereditary coumarin resistance
hyperlipemia
hypothyroidism
nephrotic syndrome

EXOGENOUS FACTORS:
**Potential drug interactions with COUMADIN are listed be-
low by drug class and by specific drugs.**
Classes of Drugs
Adrenal Cortical Steroid Inhibitors
Antacids
Antianxiety Agents
Antiarrhythmics†
Antibiotics†
Anticonvulsants†
Antidepressants†
Antihistamines
Antineoplastics†
Antipsychotic Medications

Antithyroid Drugs†
Barbiturates
Diuretics†
Enteral Nutritional Supplements
Fungal Medications, Systemic†
Gastric Acidity and Peptic Ulcer
    Agents†
Hypnotics†
Hypolipidemics†
Immunosuppressives
Oral Contraceptives, Estrogen Containing
Steroids, Adrenocortical†
Tuberculosis Agents†
Vitamins†

Specific Drugs Reported
alcohol†
aminoglutethimide
amobarbital
azathioprine
butabarbital
butalbital
carbamazepine
chloral hydrate†
chlordiazepoxide
chlorthalidone
cholestyramine†
corticotropin
cortisone
COUMADIN underdosage
cyclophosphamide†
dicloxacillin
ethchlorvynol
glutethimide
griseofulvin
haloperidol
meprobamate
6-mercaptopurine
methimazole†
moricizine hydrochloride†
nafcillin
paraldehyde
pentobarbital
phenobarbital
phenytoin†
prednisone†
primidone
propylthiouracil†
ranitidine†
rifampin
secobarbital
spironolactone
sucralfate
trazodone
vitamin C (high dose)
vitamin K
also: diet high in vitamin K
            unreliable PT/INR determinations
†Increased and decreased PT/INR responses have been reported.

Because a patient may be exposed to a combination of the
above factors, the net effect of COUMADIN on PT/INR response may be unpredictable. More frequent PT/INR monitoring is therefore advisable. Medications of unknown interaction with coumarins are best regarded with caution.
When these medications are started or stopped, more frequent PT/INR monitoring is advisable.
It has been reported that concomitant administration of
warfarin and ticlopidine may be associated with cholestatic
hepatitis.

Effect on Other Drugs: Coumarins may also affect the action of other drugs. Hypoglycemic agents (chlorpropamide
and tolbutamide) and anticonvulsants (phenytoin and phenobarbital) may accumulate in the body as a result of interference with either their metabolism or excretion.

Special Risk Patients: COUMADIN is a narrow therapeutic range (index) drug, and caution should be observed when
warfarin sodium is administered to certain patients such as
the elderly or debilitated or when administered in any situation or physical condition where added risk of hemorrhage
is present.
Intramuscular (I.M.) injections of concomitant medications
should be confined to the upper extremities which permits
easy access for manual compression, inspections for bleeding and use of pressure bandages.
Caution should be observed when COUMADIN (or warfarin) is administered concomitantly with nonsteroidal anti-
inflammatory drugs (NSAIDs), including aspirin, to be certain that no change in anticoagulation dosage is required.
In addition to specific drug interactions that might affect
PT/INR, NSAIDs, including aspirin, can inhibit platelet aggregation, and can cause gastrointestinal bleeding, peptic
ulceration and/or perforation.

Continued on next page

Coumadin—Cont.

Acquired or inherited warfarin resistance should be suspected if large daily doses of COUMADIN are required to maintain a patient's PT/INR within a normal therapeutic range.

Information for Patients: The objective of anticoagulant therapy is to decrease the clotting ability of the blood so that thrombosis is prevented, while avoiding spontaneous bleeding. Effective therapeutic levels with minimal complications are in part dependent upon cooperative and well-instructed patients who communicate effectively with their physician. Patients should be advised: Strict adherence to prescribed dosage schedule is necessary. Do not take or discontinue any other medication, including salicylates (e.g., aspirin and topical analgesics) and other over-the-counter medications except on advice of the physician. Avoid alcohol consumption. Do not take COUMADIN during pregnancy and do not become pregnant while taking it (see CONTRAINDICATIONS). Avoid any activity or sport that may result in traumatic injury. Prothrombin time tests and regular visits to physician or clinic are needed to monitor therapy. Carry identification stating that COUMADIN is being taken. If the prescribed dose of COUMADIN is forgotten, notify the physician immediately. Take the dose as soon as possible on the same day but do not take a double dose of COUMADIN the next day to make up for missed doses. The amount of vitamin K in food may affect therapy with COUMADIN. Eat a normal, balanced diet maintaining a consistent amount of vitamin K. Avoid drastic changes in dietary habits, such as eating large amounts of green leafy vegetables. Contact physician to report any illness, such as diarrhea, infection or fever. Notify physician immediately if any unusual bleeding or symptoms occur. Signs and symptoms of bleeding include: pain, swelling or discomfort, prolonged bleeding from cuts, increased menstrual flow or vaginal bleeding, nosebleeds, bleeding of gums from brushing, unusual bleeding or bruising, red or dark brown urine, red or tar black stools, headache, dizziness, or weakness. If therapy with COUMADIN is discontinued, patients should be cautioned that the anticoagulant effects of COUMADIN may persist for about 2 to 5 days. **Patients should be informed that all warfarin sodium, USP, products represent the same medication, and should not be taken concomitantly, as overdosage may result.**

Carcinogenesis, Mutagenesis, Impairment of Fertility: Carcinogenicity and mutagenicity studies have not been performed with COUMADIN. The reproductive effects of COUMADIN have not been evaluated.

Use in Pregnancy: Pregnancy Category X—See CONTRAINDICATIONS.

Pediatric Use: Safety and effectiveness in pediatric patients below the age of 18 have not been established, in randomized, controlled clinical trials. However, the use of COUMADIN in pediatric patients is well-documented for the prevention and treatment of thromboembolic events. Difficulty achieving and maintaining therapeutic PT/INR ranges in the pediatric patient has been reported. More frequent PT/INR determinations are recommended because of possible changing warfarin requirements.

ADVERSE REACTIONS

Potential adverse reactions to COUMADIN may include:

- Fatal or nonfatal hemorrhage from any tissue or organ. This is a consequence of the anticoagulant effect. The signs, symptoms, and severity will vary according to the location and degree or extent of the bleeding. Hemorrhagic complications may present as paralysis; paresthesia; headache, chest, abdomen, joint, muscle or other pain; dizziness; shortness of breath, difficult breathing or swallowing; unexplained swelling; weakness; hypotension; or unexplained shock. Therefore, the possibility of hemorrhage should be considered in evaluating the condition of any anticoagulated patient with complaints which do not indicate an obvious diagnosis. Bleeding during anticoagulant therapy does not always correlate with PT/INR. (See OVERDOSAGE—Treatment.)

- Bleeding which occurs when the PT/INR is within the therapeutic range warrants diagnostic investigation since it may unmask a previously unsuspected lesion, e.g., tumor, ulcer, etc.

- Necrosis of skin and other tissues. (See WARNINGS.)

- Adverse reactions reported infrequently include: hypersensitivity/allergic reactions, systemic cholesterol microembolization, purple toes syndrome, hepatitis, cholestatic hepatic injury, jaundice, elevated liver enzymes, vasculitis, edema, fever, rash, dermatitis, including bullous eruptions, urticaria, abdominal pain including cramping, flatulence/bloating, fatigue, lethargy, malaise, asthenia, nausea, vomiting, diarrhea, pain, headache, dizziness, taste perversion, pruritus, alopecia, cold intolerance, and paresthesia including feeling cold and chills.

Rare events of tracheal or tracheobronchial calcification have been reported in association with long-term warfarin therapy. The clinical significance of this event is unknown.

Priapism has been associated with anticoagulant administration, however, a causal relationship has not been established.

OVERDOSAGE

Signs and Symptoms: Suspected or overt abnormal bleeding (e.g., appearance of blood in stools or urine, hematuria, excessive menstrual bleeding, melena, petechiae, excessive bruising or persistent oozing from superficial injuries) are early manifestations of anticoagulation beyond a safe and satisfactory level.

Treatment: Excessive anticoagulation, with or without bleeding, may be controlled by discontinuing COUMADIN therapy and if necessary, by administration of oral or parenteral vitamin K_1. (Please see recommendations accompanying vitamin K_1 preparations prior to use.)

Such use of vitamin K_1 reduces response to subsequent COUMADIN therapy. Patients may return to a pretreatment thrombotic status following the rapid reversal of a prolonged PT/INR. Resumption of COUMADIN administration reverses the effect of vitamin K, and a therapeutic PT/INR can again be obtained by careful dosage adjustment. If rapid anticoagulation is indicated, heparin may be preferable for initial therapy.

If minor bleeding progresses to major bleeding, give 5 to 25 mg (rarely up to 50 mg) parenteral vitamin K_1. In emergency situations of severe hemorrhage, clotting factors can be returned to normal by administering 200 to 500 mL of fresh whole blood or fresh frozen plasma, or by giving commercial Factor IX complex.

A risk of hepatitis and other viral diseases is associated with the use of these blood products; Factor IX complex is also associated with an increased risk of thrombosis. Therefore, these preparations should be used only in exceptional or life-threatening bleeding episodes secondary to COUMADIN overdosage.

Purified Factor IX preparations should not be used because they cannot increase the levels of prothrombin, Factor VII and Factor X which are also depressed along with the levels of Factor IX as a result of COUMADIN (Warfarin Sodium) treatment. Packed red blood cells may also be given if significant blood loss has occurred. Infusions of blood or plasma should be monitored carefully to avoid precipitating pulmonary edema in elderly patients or patients with heart disease.

DOSAGE AND ADMINISTRATION

The dosage and administration of COUMADIN must be individualized for each patient according to the particular patient's PT/INR response to the drug. The dosage should be adjusted based upon the patient's PT/INR. (See LABORATORY CONTROL below for full discussion on INR.)

Venous Thromboembolism (including pulmonary embolism): Available clinical evidence indicates that an INR of 2.0–3.0 is sufficient for prophylaxis and treatment of venous thromboembolism and minimizes the risk of hemorrhage associated with higher INRs. In patients with risk factors for recurrent venous thromboembolism including venous insufficiency, inherited thrombophilia, idiopathic venous thromboembolism, and a history of thrombotic events, consideration should be given to longer term therapy (Schulman et al, 1995 and Schulman et al, 1997).

Atrial Fibrillation: Five recent clinical trials evaluated the effects of warfarin in patients with non-valvular atrial fibrillation (AF). Meta-analysis findings of these studies revealed that the effects of warfarin in reducing thromboembolic events including stroke were similar at either moderately high INR (2.0–4.5) or low INR (1.4–3.0). There was a significant reduction in minor bleeds at the low INR. Similar data from clinical studies in valvular atrial fibrillation patients are not available. The trials in non-valvular atrial fibrillation support the American College of Chest Physicians' (ACCP) recommendation that an INR of 2.0–3.0 be used for long term warfarin therapy in appropriate AF patients.

Post-Myocardial Infarction: In post-myocardial infarction patients, COUMADIN therapy should be initiated early (2–4 weeks post-infarction) and dosage should be adjusted to maintain an INR of 2.5–3.5 long-term. The recommendation is based on the results of the WARIS study in which treatment was initiated 2 to 4 weeks after the infarction. In patients thought to be at an increased risk of bleeding complications or on aspirin therapy, maintenance of COUMADIN therapy at the lower end of this INR range is recommended.

Mechanical and Bioprosthetic Heart Valves: In patients with mechanical heart valve(s), long term prophylaxis with warfarin to an INR of 2.5–3.5 is recommended. In patients with bioprosthetic heart valve(s), based on limited data, the American College of Chest Physicians recommends warfarin therapy to an INR of 2.0–3.0 for 12 weeks after valve insertion. In patients with additional risk factors such as atrial fibrillation or prior thromboembolism, consideration should be given for longer term therapy.

Recurrent Systemic Embolism: In cases where the risk of thromboembolism is great, such as in patients with recurrent systemic embolism, a higher INR may be required.

An INR of greater than 4.0 appears to provide no additional therapeutic benefit in most patients and is associated with a higher risk of bleeding.

Initial Dosage: The dosing of COUMADIN must be individualized according to patient's sensitivity to the drug as indicated by the PT/INR. Use of a large loading dose may increase the incidence of hemorrhagic and other complications, does not offer more rapid protection against thrombi formation, and is not recommended. Low initiation doses are recommended for elderly and/or debilitated patients and patients with potential to exhibit greater than expected PT/INR response to COUMADIN (see PRECAUTIONS). It is recommended that COUMADIN therapy be initiated with a dose of 2 to 5 mg per day with dosage adjustments based on the results of PT/INR determinations.

Maintenance: Most patients are satisfactorily maintained at a dose of 2 to 10 mg daily. Flexibility of dosage is provided by breaking scored tablets in half. The individual dose and interval should be gauged by the patient's prothrombin response.

Duration of Therapy: The duration of therapy in each patient should be individualized. In general, anticoagulant therapy should be continued until the danger of thrombosis and embolism has passed.

Missed Dose: The anticoagulant effect of COUMADIN persists beyond 24 hours. If the patient forgets to take the prescribed dose of COUMADIN at the scheduled time, the dose should be taken as soon as possible on the same day. The patient should not take the missed dose by doubling the daily dose to make up for missed doses, but should refer back to his or her physician.

Intravenous Route of Administration: COUMADIN for Injection provides an alternate administration route for patients who cannot receive oral drugs. The I.V. dosages would be the same as those that would be used orally if the patient could take the drug by the oral route. COUMADIN for Injection should be administered as a slow bolus injection over 1 to 2 minutes into a peripheral vein. It is not recommended for intramuscular administration. The vial should be reconstituted with 2.7 mL of sterile Water for Injection and inspected for particulate matter and discoloration immediately prior to use. Do not use if either particulate matter and/or discoloration is noted. After reconstitution, COUMADIN for Injection is chemically and physically stable for 4 hours at room temperature. It does not contain any antimicrobial preservative and, thus, care must be taken to assure the sterility of the prepared solution. The vial is not recommended for multiple use and unused solution should be discarded.

LABORATORY CONTROL The PT reflects the depression of vitamin K dependent Factors VII, X and II. There are several modifications of the one-stage PT and the physician should become familiar with the specific method used in his laboratory. The degree of anticoagulation indicated by any range of PTs may be altered by the type of thromboplastin used; the appropriate therapeutic range must be based on the experience of each laboratory. The PT should be determined daily after the administration of the initial dose until PT/INR results stabilize in the therapeutic range. Intervals between subsequent PT/INR determinations should be based upon the physician's judgment of the patient's reliability and response to COUMADIN in order to maintain the individual within the therapeutic range. Acceptable intervals for PT/INR determinations are normally within the range of one to four weeks after a stable dosage has been determined. To ensure adequate control, it is recommended that additional PT tests are done when other warfarin products are interchanged with COUMADIN and also if other medications are coadministered with COUMADIN (see PRECAUTIONS). To ensure adequate control, it is recommended that additional PT tests are done when other warfarin products are interchanged with warfarin sodium tablets, USP, as well as whenever other medications are initiated, discontinued, or taken irregularly (see PRECAUTIONS).

Different thromboplastin reagents vary substantially in their sensitivity to sodium warfarin-induced effects on PT. To define the appropriate therapeutic regimen it is important to be familiar with the sensitivity of the thromboplastin reagent used in the laboratory and its relationship to the International Reference Preparation (IRP), a sensitive thromboplastin reagent prepared from human brain.

A system of standardizing the PT in oral anticoagulant control was introduced by the World Health Organization in 1983. It is based upon the determination of an International Normalized Ratio (INR) which provides a common basis for communication of PT results and interpretations of therapeutic ranges. The INR system of reporting is based on a logarithmic relationship between the PT ratios of the test and reference preparation. The INR is the PT ratio that would be obtained if the International Reference Preparation (IRP), which has an ISI of 1.0, were used to perform the test. Early clinical studies of oral anticoagulants, which formed the basis for recommended therapeutic ranges of 1.5 to 2.5 times control mean normal PT, used sensitive human brain thromboplastin. When using the less sensitive rabbit

TABLE 3
Relationship Between INR and PT Ratios
For Thromboplastins With Different ISI Values (Sensitivities)

	PT RATIOS				
	ISI 1.0	ISI 1.4	ISI 1.8	ISI 2.3	ISI 2.8
INR=2.0–3.0	2.0–3.0	1.6–2.2	1.5–1.8	1.4–1.6	1.3–1.5
INR=2.5–3.5	2.5–3.5	1.9–2.4	1.7–2.0	1.5–1.7	1.4–1.6

	30's	100's	1000's	Hospital Unit-Dose blister package of 100
1 mg pink		NDC 0056-0169-70	NDC 0056-0169-90	NDC 0056-0169-75
2 mg lavender	NDC 0056-0170-30	NDC 0056-0170-70	NDC 0056-0170-90	NDC 0056-0170-75
2½ mg green	NDC 0056-0176-30	NDC 0056-0176-70	NDC 0056-0176-90	NDC 0056-0176-75
3 mg tan		NDC 0056-0188-70	NDC 0056-0188-90	NDC 0056-0188-75
4 mg blue		NDC 0056-0168-70	NDC 0056-0168-90	NDC 0056-0168-75
5 mg peach	NDC 0056-0172-30	NDC 0056-0172-70	NDC 0056-0172-90	NDC 0056-0172-75
6 mg teal		NDC 0056-0189-70	NDC 0056-0189-90	NDC 0056-0189-75
7½ mg yellow		NDC 0056-0173-70		NDC 0056-0173-75
10 mg white (Dye Free)		NDC 0056-0174-70		NDC 0056-0174-75

brain thromboplastins commonly employed in PT assays today, adjustments must be made to the targeted PT range that reflect this decrease in sensitivity.

The INR can be calculated as:
$$INR = (observed\ PT\ ratio)^{ISI}$$
where the ISI (International Sensitivity Index) is the correction factor in the equation that relates the PT ratio of the local reagent to the reference preparation and is a measure of the sensitivity of a given thromboplastin to reduction of vitamin K-dependent coagulation factors; the lower the ISI, the more "sensitive" the reagent and the closer the derived INR will be to the observed PT ratio.[1]

The proceedings and recommendations of the 1992 National Conference on Antithrombotic Therapy[2–4] review and evaluate issues related to oral anticoagulant therapy and the sensitivity of thromboplastin reagents and provide additional guidelines for defining the appropriate therapeutic regimen.

The conversion of the INR to PT ratios for the less-intense (INR 2.0–3.0) and more intense (INR 2.5–3.5) therapeutic range recommended by the ACCP for thromboplastins over a range of ISI values is shown in Table 3.[5]
[See table 3 above]

TREATMENT DURING DENTISTRY AND SURGERY The management of patients who undergo dental and surgical procedures requires close liaison between attending physicians, surgeons and dentists. PT/INR determination is recommended just prior to any dental or surgical procedure. In patients undergoing minimal invasive procedures who must be anticoagulated prior to, during, or immediately following these procedures, adjusting the dosage of COUMADIN to maintain the PT/INR at the low end of the therapeutic range may safely allow for continued anticoagulation. The operative site should be sufficiently limited and accessible to permit the effective use of local procedures for hemostasis. Under these conditions, dental and minor surgical procedures may be performed without undue risk of hemorrhage. Some dental or surgical procedures may necessitate the interruption of COUMADIN therapy. When discontinuing COUMADIN even for a short period of time, the benefits and risks should be strongly considered.

CONVERSION FROM HEPARIN THERAPY Since the anticoagulant effect of COUMADIN is delayed, heparin is preferred initially for rapid anticoagulation. Conversion to COUMADIN may begin concomitantly with heparin therapy or may be delayed 3 to 6 days. To ensure continuous anticoagulation, it is advisable to continue full dose heparin therapy and that COUMADIN therapy be overlapped with heparin for 4 to 5 days, until COUMADIN has produced the desired therapeutic response as determined by PT/INR. When COUMADIN has produced the desired PT/INR or prothrombin activity, heparin may be discontinued.

COUMADIN may increase the aPTT test, even in the absence of heparin. During initial therapy with COUMADIN, the interference with heparin anticoagulation is of minimal clinical significance.

As heparin may affect the PT/INR, patients receiving both heparin and COUMADIN should have blood for PT/INR determination drawn at least:
• 5 hours after the last IV bolus dose of heparin, or
• 4 hours after cessation of a continuous IV infusion of heparin, or
• 24 hours after the last subcutaneous heparin injection.

HOW SUPPLIED
Tablets: For oral use, single scored, imprinted numerically and packaged in bottles with potencies and colors as follows:
[See second table from top of page]
COUMADIN oral tablet is available in 1, 2, 2-1/2, 3, 4, 5, 6, 7-1/2 and 10 mg of warfarin sodium with one face inscribed with the word COUMADIN, single scored and imprinted

numerically with the 1, 2, 2-1/2, 3, 4, 5, 6, 7-1/2 or 10 superimposed, and on the other face inscribed with the word "DuPont."

Protect from light. Store in carton until contents have been used. Store at controlled room temperature (59°–86°F, 15°–30°C). Dispense in a tight, light-resistant container as defined in the USP.

Injection: Available for intravenous use only. Not recommended for intramuscular administration. Reconstitute with 2.7 mL of sterile Water for Injection to yield 2 mg/mL. Net contents 5.4 mg lyophilized powder. Maximum yield 2.5 mL.

5 mg vial (box of 6)   NDC 0590-0324-35
Protect from light. Keep vial in box until used. Store at controlled room temperature (59°–86°F, 15°–30°C).
After reconstitution, store at controlled room temperature (59°–86°F, 15°–30°C) and use within 4 hours. Do not refrigerate. Discard any unused solution.
CAUTION: Federal law prohibits dispensing without a prescription.

REFERENCES
1. Poller, L.: Laboratory Control of Anticoagulant Therapy. Seminars in Thrombosis and Hemostasis, Vol. 12, No. 1, pp. 13-19, 1986.
2. Hirsh, J.: Is the Dose of Warfarin Prescribed by American Physicians Unnecessarily High? *Arch Int Med,* Vol. 147, pp. 769-771, 1987.
3. Cook, D.J., Guyatt, H.G., Laupacis, A., Sackett, D.L.: Rules of Evidence and Clinical Recommendations on the Use of Antithrombotic Agents. Chest ACCP Consensus Conference on Antithrombotic Therapy. *Chest,* Vol. 102(Suppl), pp. 305S-311S, 1992.
4. Hirsh, J., Dalen, J., Deykin, D., Poller, L: Oral Anticoagulants Mechanism of Action, Clinical Effectiveness, and Optimal Therapeutic Range. Chest ACCP Consensus Conference on Antithrombotic Therapy. *Chest,* Vol. 102(Suppl), pp. 312S-326S, 1992.
5. Hirsh, J., M.D., F.C.C.P.: Hamilton Civic Hospitals Research Center, Hamilton, Ontario, Personal Communication.

DuPont Pharma
Wilmington, Delaware 19880
COUMADIN® and the color and configuration of COUMADIN tablets are trademarks of The DuPont Merck Pharmaceutical Company. Any unlicensed use of these trademarks is expressly prohibited under the U.S. Trademark Act.
Printed in U.S.A.
Copyright © DuPont Pharma 1998
6466-01/Rev. April 1998   CU-31864-02
Shown in Product Identification Guide, page 309

HESPAN®   ℞
[hes' pan]
(6% hetastarch in
0.9% sodium chloride injection)

DESCRIPTION
HESPAN (6% hetastarch in 0.9% sodium chloride injection) is a sterile, nonpyrogenic solution. The composition of each 100 mL is as follows:
Hetastarch .... 6.0 g
Sodium Chloride, USP .... 0.9 g
Water for Injection, USP .... qs
pH adjusted with Sodium Hydroxide NF
Concentration of Electrolytes (mEq/liter): Sodium 154, Chloride 154
pH: 3.5-7.0; Calc. Osmolarity: 310 mOsM/liter

Hetastarch is an artificial colloid derived from a waxy starch composed almost entirely of amylopectin. Hydroxyethyl ether groups are introduced into the glucose units of the starch and the resultant material is hydrolyzed to yield a product with a molecular weight suitable for use as a plasma volume expander and erythrocyte sedimenting agent. Hetastarch is characterized by its molar substitution, and also by its molecular weight. The molar substitution is 0.7 which means hetastarch has 7 hydroxyethyl groups for every 10 glucose units. The weight average molecular weight is approximately 480,000 with a range of 400,000 to 550,000 and with 80% of the polymers falling between the range of 30,000 and 2,400,000. Hydroxyethyl groups are attached by ether linkage primarily at C-2 of the glucose unit and to a lesser extent at C-3 and C-6. The polymer resembles glycogen, and the polymerized glucose units are joined primarily by 1-4 linkages with occasional 1-6 branching linkages. The degree of branching is approximately 1:20 which means that there is one 1-6 branch for every 20 glucose monomer units.
The chemical name for hetastarch is hydroxyethyl starch. The structural formula is as follows:

Amylopectin derivative in which R_2, R_3, and R_6 are H or CH_2CH_2OH, or R_6 is a branching point in the starch polymer connected through a 1-6 linkage to additional α-D-glucopyranosyl units.
HESPAN is a clear, pale yellow to amber solution. Exposure to prolonged adverse storage conditions may result in a change to a turbid deep brown or the formation of a crystalline precipitate. Do not use the solution if these conditions are evident.
The plastic container is made from a multi-layered film specifically developed for parenteral drugs. It contains no plasticizers and exhibits virtually no leachables. The solution contact layer is a rubberized copolymer of ethylene and propylene. The container is nontoxic and biologically inert. The container-solution unit is a closed system and is not dependent upon entry of external air during administration. The container is overwrapped to provide protection from the physical environment and to provide an additional moisture barrier when necessary.
The closure system has two ports; the one for the administration set has a tamper evident plastic protector.

CLINICAL PHARMACOLOGY
The plasma volume expansion produced by HESPAN approximate those of 5% human albumin. Intravenous infusion of HESPAN results in expansion of plasma volume that decreases over the succeeding 24 to 36 hours. The degree of plasma volume expansion and improvement in hemodynamic state depend upon the patient's intravascular status. Hetastarch molecules below 50,000 molecular weight are rapidly eliminated by renal excretion. A single dose of approximately 500 mL of HESPAN (approximately 30 g) results in elimination in the urine of approximately 33% of the dose within 24 hours. This is a variable process but generally results in an intravascular hetastarch concentration of less than 10% of the total dose injected by two weeks. A study of the biliary excretion of HESPAN in 10 healthy males accounted for less than 1% of the dose over a 14-day period. The hydroxyethyl group is not cleaved by the body, but remains intact and attached to glucose units when excreted. Significant quantities of glucose are not produced as hydroxyethylation prevents complete metabolism of the smaller polymers.
The addition of HESPAN to whole blood increases the erythrocyte sedimentation rate. Therefore, HESPAN is used to improve the efficiency of granulocyte collection by centrifugal means.

INDICATIONS AND USAGE
HESPAN® (6% hetastarch in 0.9% sodium chloride injection) is indicated in the treatment of hypovolemia when plasma volume expansion is desired. It is not a substitute for blood or plasma.
The adjunctive use of HESPAN in leukapheresis has also been shown to be safe and efficacious in improving the harvesting and increasing the yield of granulocytes by centrifugal means.

CONTRAINDICATIONS
HESPAN is contraindicated in patients with known hypersensitivity to hydroxyethyl starch, or with bleeding disorders, or with congestive heart failure where volume over-

Continued on next page

Hespan—Cont.

load is a potential problem. HESPAN should not be used in renal disease with oliguria or anuria not related to hypovolemia.

WARNINGS

Life threatening anaphylactic/anaphylactoid reactions have been rarely reported with HESPAN; death has occurred, but a causal relationship has not been established. Patients who develop severe anaphylactic/anaphylactoid reactions may need continued supportive care until symptoms have resolved.

Hypersensitivity reactions can occur even after HESPAN has been discontinued.

Usage in Plasma Volume Expansion

Large volumes of HESPAN may transiently alter the coagulation mechanism due to hemodilution and a mild direct inhibitory action on Factor VIII. In addition, administration of HESPAN may result in transient prolongation of prothrombin time, activated partial thromboplastin, clotting, and bleeding times.

Hematocrit may be decreased and plasma proteins diluted excessively by administration of large volumes of HESPAN. Administration of packed red cells, platelets, and fresh frozen plasma should be considered if excessive dilution occurs.

In randomized, controlled, comparative studies of HESPAN (n=92) and albumin (n=85) in surgical patients, no patient in either treatment group had a bleeding complication and no significant difference was found in the amount of blood loss between the treatment groups.[1-4]

Use over extended periods: HESPAN has not been adequately evaluated to establish its safety in situations other than leukapheresis that require frequent use of colloidal solutions over extended periods. In some cases, HESPAN has been associated with coagulation abnormalities in conjunction with an acquired, reversible von Willebrand's-like syndrome and/or Factor VIII deficiency when used over a period of days. Replacement therapy should be considered if a severe Factor VIII deficiency is identified. If a coagulopathy develops, it may take several days to resolve. Certain conditions may affect the safe use of HESPAN on a chronic basis. For example, in patients with subarachnoid hemorrhage where HESPAN is used repeatedly over a period of days for the prevention of cerebral vasospasm, significant clinical bleeding may occur. Intracranial bleeding resulting in death has been reported.[5]

Usage in Leukapheresis

Slight declines in platelet counts and hemoglobin levels have been observed in donors undergoing repeated leukapheresis procedures using HESPAN due to the volume expanding effects of HESPAN and to the collection of platelets and erythrocytes. Hemoglobin levels usually return to normal within 24 hours. Hemodilution by HESPAN and saline may also result in 24 hour declines of total protein, albumin, calcium and fibrinogen values. None of these decreases are to a degree recognized to be clinically significant risks to healthy donors.

PRECAUTIONS

General

Regular and frequent clinical evaluation and complete blood counts (CBC) are necessary for proper monitoring of HESPAN use during leukapheresis. If the frequency of leukapheresis is to exceed the guidelines for whole blood donation, you may wish to consider the following additional studies: total leukocyte and platelet counts, leukocyte differential count, hemoglobin and hematocrit, prothrombin time (PT), and partial thromboplastin time (PTT) tests.

The possibility of circulatory overload should be kept in mind. Caution should be used when the risk of pulmonary edema and/or congestive heart failure is increased. Special care should be exercised in patients who have impaired renal clearance since this is the principal way in which hetastarch is eliminated.

Indirect bilirubin levels of 8.3 mg/L (normal 0.0-7.0 mg/L) have been reported in 2 out of 20 normal subjects who received multiple HESPAN infusions. Total bilirubin was within normal limits at all times; indirect bilirubin returned to normal by 96 hours following the final infusion. The significance, if any, of these elevations is not known; however, caution should be observed before administering HESPAN to patients with a history of liver disease.

If a hypersensitivity effect occurs, administration of the drug should be discontinued and appropriate treatment and supportive measures should be undertaken (see WARNINGS).

Caution should be used when administering HESPAN to patients allergic to corn because such patients can also be allergic to HESPAN.

The EXCEL® Container has a natural gum rubber/latex-containing injection port. Unless medication addition occurs, a diaphragm prevents the latex from coming in contact with the HESPAN solution. In patients with latex hypersensitivity, caution should be exercised when adding medication through the port of the EXCEL container.

Elevated serum amylase levels may be observed temporarily following administration of HESPAN®, (6% hetastarch in 0.9% sodium chloride injection) although no association with pancreatitis has been demonstrated. Serum amylase levels cannot be used to assess or to evaluate for pancreatitis for 3-5 days after administration of HESPAN. Elevated serum amylase levels persist for longer periods of time in patients with renal impairment. HESPAN has not been shown to increase serum lipase.

One report suggests that in the presence of renal glomerular damage, larger molecules of HESPAN can leak into the urine and elevate the specific gravity. The elevation of specific gravity can obscure the diagnosis of renal failure. HESPAN is not eliminated by hemodialysis. The utility of other extracorporeal elimination techniques has not been evaluated.

If administration is by pressure infusion, all air should be withdrawn or expelled from the bag through the medication port prior to infusion.

Carcinogenesis, Mutagenesis, Impairment of Fertility

Long-term studies of animals have not been performed to evaluate the carcinogenic potential of hetastarch.

Teratogenic Effects

Pregnancy Category C. HESPAN has been shown to have an embryocidal effect on New Zealand rabbits when given intravenously over the entire organogenesis period in a daily dose $1/2$ times the maximum recommended therapeutic human dose (1500 mL), and on BD rats when given intraperitoneally, from the 16th to the 21st day of pregnancy, in a daily dose 2.3 times the maximum recommended therapeutic human dose. When HESPAN was administered to New Zealand rabbits, BD rats and swiss mice with intravenous daily doses of 2 times, $1/3$ times and 1 time the maximum recommended therapeutic human dose respectively over several days during the period of gestation, no evidence of teratogenicity was evident. There are no adequate and well controlled studies in pregnant women. HESPAN should be used during pregnancy only if the potential benefit justifies the potential risk to the fetus.

Nursing Mothers

It is not known whether hetastarch is excreted in human milk. Because many drugs are excreted in human milk, caution should be exercised when HESPAN is administered to a nursing woman.

Pediatric Use

The safety and effectiveness of HESPAN in pediatric patients have not been established. Adequate, well-controlled clinical trials to establish the safety and effectiveness of HESPAN in pediatric patients have not been conducted. However, in one small double-blind study, 47 infants, children, and adolescents (Ages 1 year to 15.5 years) scheduled for repair of congenital heart disease with moderate hypothermia were randomized to receive either 6% hetastarch or albumin as a postoperative volume expander during the first 24 hours after surgery. Thirty-eight children required colloid replacement therapy, of which 20 children received 6% hetastarch. No differences were found in the coagulation parameters or in the amount of replacement fluids required in the children receiving 20 mL/kg or less of either colloid replacement therapy. In children who received greater than 20 mL/kg of 6% hetastarch, an increase in prothrombin time was demonstrated (p = 0.006).[6] There were no neonates included in this study.

ADVERSE REACTIONS

Reported adverse reactions associated with HESPAN include:

General

Hypersensitivity (see WARNINGS).

Death, life-threatening anaphylactic/anaphylactoid reactions, cardiac arrest, ventricular fibrillation, severe hypotension, non-cardiac pulmonary edema, laryngeal edema, bronchospasm, angioedema, wheezing, restlessness, tachypnea, stridor, fever, chest pain, bradycardia, tachycardia, shortness of breath, chills, urticaria, pruritus, facial and periorbital edema, coughing, sneezing, flushing, erythema multiforme and rash.

Cardiovascular

Circulatory overload, congestive heart failure, and pulmonary edema (see PRECAUTIONS).

Hematologic

Intracranial bleeding, bleeding and/or anemia due to hemodilution (see WARNINGS) and/or Factor VIII deficiency, acquired von Willebrand's-like syndrome, and coagulopathy including rare cases of disseminated intravascular coagulopathy and hemolysis.

Metabolic

Metabolic acidosis.

Other

Vomiting, peripheral edema of the lower extremities, submaxillary and parotid glandular enlargement, mild influenza-like symptoms, headaches and muscle pains.

Hydroxyethyl-starch-associated pruritus has been reported in some patients with deposits of hydroxyethyl starch in peripheral nerves.

DOSAGE AND ADMINISTRATION

Dosage for Acute Use in Plasma Volume Expansion

HESPAN is administered by intravenous infusion only. Total dosage and rate of infusion depend upon the amount of blood or plasma lost and the resultant hemoconcentration.

Adults: The amount usually administered is 500 to 1000 mL. Doses of more than 1500 mL per day for the typical 70 kg patient (approximately 20 mL per kg of body weight) are usually not required, although higher doses have been reported in postoperative and trauma patients where severe blood loss has occurred.

Pediatric Patients: Adequate, well-controlled clinical trials to establish the safety and effectiveness of HESPAN® (6% hetastarch in 0.9% sodium chloride injection) in pediatric patients have not been conducted (see PRECAUTIONS, Pediatric Use).

Dosage in Leukapheresis

250 to 700 mL of HESPAN to which citrate anticoagulant has been added is typically administered by aseptic addition to the input line of the centrifugation apparatus at a ratio of 1:8 to 1:13 to venous whole blood. The HESPAN and citrate should be thoroughly mixed to assure effective anticoagulation of blood as it flows through the leukapheresis machine. When stored at room temperature, HESPAN admixtures of 500-560 mL with citrate concentrations up to 2.5% were compatible for 24 hours. The safety and compatibility of additives other than citrate have not been established.

General Recommendations

Do not use plastic container in series connection.

If administration is controlled by a pumping device, care must be taken to discontinue pumping action before the container runs dry or air embolism may result.

This solution is intended for intravenous administration using sterile equipment. It is recommended that intravenous administration apparatus be replaced at least once every 24 hours.

Use only if solution is clear and container and seals are intact.

Parenteral drug products should be inspected visually for particulate matter and discoloration prior to administration whenever solution and container permit.

If administration is by pressure infusion, all air should be withdrawn or expelled from the bag through the medication port prior to infusion.

CAUTION: Before administering to the patient, review these directions:

To Open

Do not remove the plastic infusion container from its overwrap until immediately before use. To open, tear overwrap down at notch and remove solution container. Check for minute leaks by squeezing solution container firmly. If leaks are found, discard solution as sterility may be impaired.

Invert container and carefully inspect the solution in good light for cloudiness, haze, or particulate matter. Any container which is suspect should not be used.

Preparation for Administration (Use aseptic technique)

1. Close flow control clamp of administration set.
2. Twist off plug from port designated "Infusion Set Port".
3. Insert spike of infusion set into port with a twisting motion until the set is firmly seated.
4. Suspend container from hanger.
5. Follow manufacturer's recommended procedures for the administration set.
6. Discontinue administration and notify physician immediately if patient exhibits signs of adverse reactions.

HOW SUPPLIED

HESPAN (6% hetastarch in 0.9% sodium chloride injection) is supplied sterile and nonpyrogenic in 500 mL and 250 mL EXCEL® Containers.

NDC	Size
HESPAN (6% hetastarch in 0.9% sodium chloride injection)	
0056-0037-46	500 mL (12 per case)
0056-0037-42	250 mL (24 per case)

Exposure of pharmaceutical products to heat should be minimized. Avoid excessive heat. Protect from freezing. It is recommended that the product be stored at room temperature (25°C); however, brief exposure up to 40°C does not adversely affect the product.

CAUTION: Federal (USA) law prohibits dispensing without prescription.

REFERENCES

1. Diehl J., et al. Clinical Comparison of Hetastarch and Albumin in Postoperative Cardiac Patients. The Annals of Thoracic Surgery. 1982;34(6):674-679.
2. Gold M., et al. Comparison of Hetastarch to Albumin for Perioperative Bleeding in Patients Undergoing Abdominal Aortic Aneurysm Surgery, Annals of Surgery, 1990;211(4):482-485.
3. Kirklin J., et al. Hydroxyethyl Starch versus Albumin for Colloid Infusion Following Cardiopulmonary Bypass in Patients Undergoing Myocardial Revascularization, The Annals of Thoracic Surgery, 1984;37(1):40-46.

4. Moggio RA., et al. Hemodynamic Comparison of Albumin and Hydroxyethyl Starch in Postoperative Cardiac Surgery Patients, *Critical Care Medicine,* 1983;11(12):943-945.
5. Damon L., Intracranial Bleeding During Treatment with Hydroxyethyl Starch, *New England Journal of Medicine,* 1987;317(15):964-965.
6. Brutocao D., et al. Comparison of Hetastarch with Albumin for Postoperative Volume Expansion in Children After Cardiopulmonary Bypass, *Journal of Cardiothoracic and Vascular Anesthesia,* 1996;10(3):348–351.

Marketed and Distributed by:
DuPont Pharma
Wilmington, Delaware 19880
Distributed and Manufactured by:
McGaw, Inc.
Irvine, CA USA 92614-5895
6253-4/Rev. October 1997
U.S. Patent No. 4,803,102
EXCEL® is a registered trademark of McGaw, Inc.
HESPAN® is a registered trademark of The DuPont Merck Pharmaceutical Co.

PENTASPAN® ℞
(10% pentastarch in 0.9% sodium chloride injection)

DESCRIPTION

PENTASPAN (10% pentastarch in 0.9% sodium chloride injection) is a sterile, nonpyrogenic solution. The composition of each 100 mL is as follows:

Pentastarch .... 10.0 g
Sodium Chloride USP .... 0.9 g
Water for Injection, USP .... qs
pH adjusted with Sodium Hydroxide NF
Concentration of Electrolytes (mEq/liter): Sodium 154; Chloride 154
pH: Approx. 4.8 (3.5-7.0); Calculated Osmolarity: Approx. 326 mOsM

Pentastarch is an artificial colloid derived from a waxy starch composed almost entirely of amylopectin. Hydroxyethyl ether groups are introduced into the glucose units of the starch and the resultant material is hydrolyzed to yield a product with a molecular weight suitable for use as an erythrocyte sedimenting agent. Pentastarch is characterized by its molar substitution, and also by its molecular weight. The degree of substitution is 0.45 which means pentastarch has 45 hydroxyethyl groups for every 100 glucose units. The weight average molecular weight of pentastarch is approximately 264,000 with a range of 150,000 to 350,000 and with 80% of the polymers falling between 10,000 and 2,000,000. Hydroxyethyl groups are attached by an ether linkage primarily at C-2 of the glucose unit and to a lesser extent at C-3 and C-6. The polymer resembles glycogen, and the polymerized glucose units are joined primarily by 1–4 linkages with occasional 1–6 branching linkages. The degree of branching is approximately 1:20 which means that there is one 1–6 branch for every 20 glucose monomer units.

The chemical name for pentastarch is hydroxyethyl starch. The structural formula is as follows:

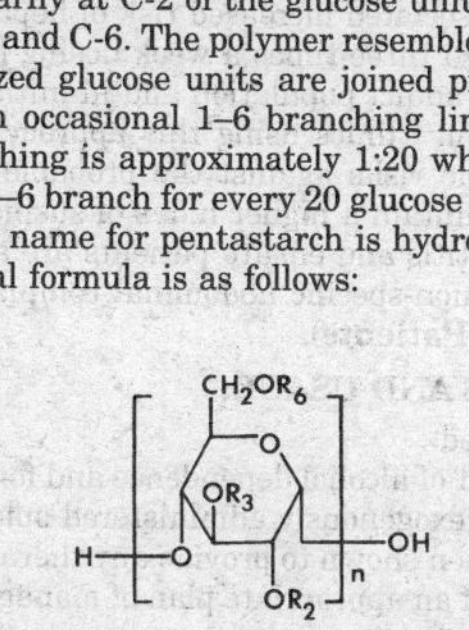

Amylopectin derivative in which R_2, R_3, and R_6 are H or CH_2CH_2OH, or R_6 is a branching point in the starch polymer connected through a 1–6 linkage to additional α-D-glucopyranosyl units.

PENTASPAN is a clear, pale yellow to amber solution. Exposure to prolonged adverse storage conditions may result in a change to a turbid deep brown or the formation of a crystalline precipitate. Do not use the solution if these conditions are evident.

CLINICAL PHARMACOLOGY

The addition of PENTASPAN to whole blood increases the erythrocyte sedimentation rate. Therefore, 10% pentastarch in 0.9% sodium chloride injection is used to improve the efficiency of leukocyte collection by centrifugal means.

Pentastarch molecules below 50,000 molecular weight are rapidly eliminated by renal excretion. A single dose of approximately 500 mL of PENTASPAN (approximately 50 g) results in elimination in the urine of approximately 70% of the dose within 24 hours, and approximately 80% of the dose within one week. An additional 5–6% of the pentastarch dose is recovered in the leukapheresis collection bag. The remaining 12–15% (approximately 6.8 g) of an administered dose is presumed to undergo slower elimination. This is a variable process but generally results in an intravascular pentastarch concentration below the level of detection by one week. The hydroxyethyl group is not cleaved by the body, but remains intact and attached to glucose units when excreted.

The colloidal properties of the related product HESPAN® (6% hetastarch in 0.9% sodium chloride injection) approximate those of 5% human albumin. Intravenous infusion of HESPAN results in expansion of plasma volume that decreases over the succeeding 24 to 36 hours. Similar, although reduced duration, volume expansion may be expected to occur following use of PENTASPAN® (10% pentastarch in 0.9% sodium chloride injection) in leukapheresis procedures.

INDICATIONS AND USAGE

PENTASPAN is indicated as an adjunct in leukapheresis, to improve the harvesting and increase the yield of leukocytes by centrifugal means.

CONTRAINDICATIONS

PENTASPAN is contraindicated in donors with known hypersensitivity to hydroxyethyl starch, or with bleeding disorders, or with congestive heart failure where volume overload is a potential problem. PENTASPAN should not be used in renal disease with oliguria or anuria.

WARNINGS

Slight declines in platelet counts and hemoglobin levels have been observed in donors undergoing repeated leukapheresis procedures using HESPAN due to the volume expanding effects of HESPAN and to the collection of platelets and erythrocytes. Hemoglobin levels usually return to normal within 24 hours. Similar effects may be expected with PENTASPAN. Hemodilution by PENTASPAN and saline may also result in 24 hour declines of total protein, albumin, calcium and fibrinogen values. None of these decreases are to a degree recognized to be clinically significant risks to healthy donors.

Large volumes of PENTASPAN may slightly alter the coagulation mechanism; *i.e.,* transient prolongation of prothrombin, partial thromboplastin and clotting times. The physician should also be alert to the possibility of transient prolongation of bleeding time.

PRECAUTIONS

General

Regular and frequent clinical evaluation and complete blood counts (CBC) are necessary for proper monitoring of PENTASPAN use during leukapheresis. If the frequency of leukapheresis is to exceed the guidelines for whole blood donation, you may wish to consider the following additional studies: total leukocyte and platelet counts, leukocyte differential count, hemoglobin and hematocrit, prothrombin time (PT), and partial thromboplastin time (PTT) tests.

The possibility of circulatory overload should be kept in mind. Caution should be used when the risk of pulmonary edema and/or congestive heart failure is increased. Special care should be exercised in patients who have impaired renal clearance since this is the principal way in which pentastarch is eliminated.

The serum chemistries of sixteen normal volunteers who were given 500 to 2000 mL infusions of PENTASPAN were essentially unchanged pre- and post-infusion, except for dilutional effects. However, indirect bilirubin levels of 8.3 mg/L (normal 0–7 mg/L) have been reported in 2 out of 20 normal subjects who received multiple HESPAN infusions. Total bilirubin was within normal limits at all times; indirect bilirubin returned to normal by 96 hours following the final infusion. The significance, if any, of these elevations is not known; however, caution should be observed before administering PENTASPAN to patients with a history of liver disease.

PENTASPAN has been reported to produce hypersensitivity reactions such as wheezing, urticaria and hypotension. Anaphylactic/anaphylactoid reactions have been rarely reported with PENTASPAN; however, a causal relationship has not been established. If hypersensitivity effects occur, discontinue the drug and, if necessary, administer appropriate therapy.

Caution should be exercised when administering PENTASPAN (10% pentastarch in 0.9% sodium chloride injection) to patients allergic to corn because such patients can also be allergic to PENTASPAN.

Elevated serum amylase levels may be observed temporarily following administration of PENTASPAN, although no association with pancreatitis has been demonstrated. HESPAN® (6% hetastarch in 0.9% sodium chloride injection) has not been shown to increase serum lipase. Similar effects may be expected with PENTASPAN.

Carcinogenesis, Mutagenesis, Impairment of Fertility

Long-term studies in animals have not been performed to evaluate the carcinogenic potential of pentastarch.

Teratogenic Effects

Pregnancy Category C. PENTASPAN has been shown to be embryocidal in New Zealand rabbits and in Swiss Mice when given in doses 5 times the human dose. PENTASPAN was administered to mated New Zealand rabbits and Swiss Mice with intravenous doses of 10, 20, and 40 mL/kg/day during the period of gestation. The results demonstrated that at 10 and 20 mL/kg/day pentastarch produced no higher incidence of teratogenicity or embryotoxicity in either species than normal saline did in control animals. At 40 mL/kg/day, however, pentastarch increased the number of resorptions and minor visceral anomalies (diffuse edema of the trunk and extremities and diffuse whitish color of the heart, lungs, liver, and kidneys) in rabbits and reduced nidation in the mouse. There are no adequate and well-controlled clinical studies using pentastarch in pregnant women. PENTASPAN should be used during pregnancy only if the potential benefits justify the potential risk to the fetus.

Nursing Mothers

It is not known whether pentastarch is excreted in human milk. Because many drugs are excreted in human milk, caution should be exercised when PENTASPAN is administered to a nursing woman.

Pediatric Use

The safety and effectiveness of PENTASPAN in pediatric patients have not been established.

ADVERSE REACTIONS

PENTASPAN has been reported to produce hypersensitivity reactions such as wheezing, urticaria, and hypotension. Anaphylactic/anaphylactoid reactions have been reported with PENTASPAN. A causal relationship has not been established (see **PRECAUTIONS**).

The following have been reported in association with the use of PENTASPAN in leukapheresis: headache, diarrhea, nausea, weakness, temporary weight gain, insomnia, fatigue, fever, edema, paresthesia, acne, malaise, shakiness, dizziness, chest pain, chills, nasal congestion, anxiety, and increased heart rate. It is uncertain whether they are attributable to the drug, the procedure, additional adjunctive medication, or some combination of these factors.

DOSAGE AND ADMINISTRATION

250 to 700 mL of PENTASPAN to which citrate anticoagulant has been added is typically administered by aseptic addition to the input line of the centrifugation apparatus at a ratio of 1:8 to 1:13 to venous whole blood. The bottle containing PENTASPAN and citrate should be thoroughly mixed to assure effective anticoagulation of blood as it flows through the leukapheresis machine.

Parenteral drug products should be inspected visually for particulate matter and discoloration prior to administration whenever solution and container permit.

When stored at room temperature, PENTASPAN® (10% pentastarch in 0.9% sodium chloride injection) admixtures of 500–560 mL with citrate up to 2.5% were compatible for 24 hours. The safety and compatibility of other additives have not been established.

General Recommendations

This solution is intended for intravenous administration using sterile equipment. It is recommended that intravenous administration apparatus be replaced at least once every 24 hours.

Use only if solution is clear and container and seals are intact.

Directions for Use

Caution: Before administering to patient, perform the following checks:

1. Each container should be inspected before use. Read the label. Insure solution is the one ordered, is within the expiration date, and that label name agrees with the abbreviated name stamped on closure. Check the security of bail and band.
2. Invert container and carefully inspect the solution in good light for cloudiness, haze, or particulate matter; check the bottle for cracks or other damage. In checking for cracks, do not be confused by normal surface mold marks and seams on bottom and sides of bottle. These are not flaws. Look instead for bright reflections that have depth and penetrate into the wall of the bottle. Reject any such bottle.
3. Check for vacuum, first by confirming the presence of depressions in the latex disk and then by audible hiss when the disk is removed. Reject any container that does not meet these criteria.
4. After admixtures and during administration, reinspect solution as frequently as possible. If any evidence of solution contamination or instability is found or if the patient exhibits any signs of fever or chills or other reaction not readily explainable, discontinue administration immediately and notify physician.

HOW SUPPLIED

NDC 0056-0081-95: PENTASPAN® (10% pentastarch in 0.9% sodium chloride injection) is supplied sterile and nonpyrogenic in 500 mL intravenous infusion bottles packaged 12 per case.

Exposure of pharmaceutical products to heat should be minimized. Avoid excessive heat. Protect from freezing. It is rec-

Continued on next page

Pentaspan—Cont.

ommended that the product be stored at room temperature (25°C); however, brief exposure up to 40°C does not adversely affect the product.
Caution: Federal (USA) law prohibits dispensing without prescription.
Distributed by:
DuPont Pharma
Wilmington, Delaware 19880
Manufactured by:
McGaw, Inc.
Irvine, CA USA 92614-5895
6270-3/Rev. November, 1997
PENTASPAN® and HESPAN® are registered trademarks of
The DuPont Merck Pharmaceutical Co.

REVIA® ℞

[reh "vēē 'uh "]
(naltrexone hydrochloride tablets)

DESCRIPTION:

REVIA (naltrexone hydrochloride), an opioid antagonist, is a synthetic congener of oxymorphone with no opioid agonist properties. Naltrexone differs in structure from oxymorphone in that the methyl group on the nitrogen atom is replaced by a cyclopropylmethyl group. REVIA is also related to the potent opioid antagonist, naloxone, or n-allylnoroxymorphone [NARCAN® (naloxone hydrochloride)].

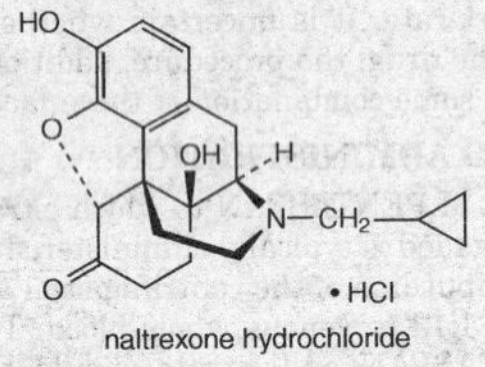

naltrexone hydrochloride

REVIA is a white, crystalline compound. The hydrochloride salt is soluble in water to the extent of about 100 mg/mL. REVIA is available in scored film-coated tablets containing 50 mg of naltrexone hydrochloride.
REVIA Tablets also contain: lactose, microcrystalline cellulose, crospovidone, colloidal silicon dioxide, magnesium stearate, hydroxypropyl methylcellulose, titanium dioxide, polyethylene glycol, polysorbate 80, yellow iron oxide and red iron oxide.

CLINICAL PHARMACOLOGY:

Pharmacodynamic Actions: REVIA is a pure opioid antagonist. It markedly attenuates or completely blocks, reversibly, the subjective effects of intravenously administered opioids.
When co-administered with morphine, on a chronic basis, REVIA blocks the physical dependence to morphine, heroin and other opioids.
REVIA has few, if any, intrinsic actions besides its opioid blocking properties. However, it does produce some pupillary constriction, by an unknown mechanism.
The administration of REVIA is not associated with the development of tolerance or dependence. In subjects physically dependent on opioids, REVIA will precipitate withdrawal symptomatology.
Clinical studies indicate that 50 mg of REVIA will block the pharmacologic effects of 25 mg of intravenously administered heroin for periods as long as 24 hours. Other data suggest that doubling the dose of REVIA provides blockade for 48 hours, and tripling the dose of REVIA provides blockade for about 72 hours.
REVIA blocks the effects of opioids by competitive binding (i.e., analogous to competitive inhibition of enzymes) at opioid receptors. This makes the blockade produced potentially surmountable, but overcoming full naltrexone blockade by administration of very high doses of opiates has resulted in excessive symptoms of histamine release in experimental subjects.
The mechanism of action of REVIA in alcoholism is not understood; however, involvement of the endogenous opioid system is suggested by preclinical data. REVIA, an opioid receptor antagonist, competitively binds to such receptors and may block the effects of endogenous opioids. Opioid antagonists have been shown to reduce alcohol consumption by animals, and REVIA has been shown to reduce alcohol consumption in clinical studies.
REVIA is not aversive therapy and does not cause a disulfiram-like reaction either as a result of opiate use or ethanol ingestion.

Pharmacokinetics
REVIA is a pure opioid receptor antagonist. Although well absorbed orally, naltrexone is subject to significant first pass metabolism with oral bioavailability estimates ranging from 5 to 40%. The activity of naltrexone is believed to be due to both parent and the 6-β-naltrexol metabolite. Both parent drug and metabolites are excreted primarily by the kidney (53% to 79% of the dose), however, urinary excretion of unchanged naltrexone accounts for less than 2% of an oral dose and fecal excretion is a minor elimination pathway. The mean elimination half-life (T-1/2) values for naltrexone and 6-β-naltrexol are 4 hours and 13 hours, respectively. Naltrexone and 6-β-naltrexol are dose proportional in terms of AUC and C_{max} over the range of 50 to 200 mg and do not accumulate after 100 mg daily doses.

Absorption
Following oral administration, naltrexone undergoes rapid and nearly complete absorption with approximately 96% of the dose absorbed from the gastrointestinal tract. Peak plasma levels of both naltrexone and 6-β-naltrexol occur within one hour of dosing.

Distribution
The volume of distribution for naltrexone following intravenous administration is estimated to be 1350 liters. *In vitro* tests with human plasma show naltrexone to be 21% bound to plasma proteins over the therapeutic dose range.

Metabolism
The systemic clearance (after intravenous administration) of naltrexone is ~3.5 L/min, which exceeds liver blood flow (~1.2 L/min). This suggests both that naltrexone is a highly extracted drug (>98% metabolized) and that extra-hepatic sites of drug metabolism exist. The major metabolite of naltrexone is 6-β-naltrexol. Two other minor metabolites are 2-hydroxy-3-methoxy-6-β-naltrexol and 2-hydroxy-3-methyl-naltrexone. Naltrexone and its metabolites are also conjugated to form additional metabolic products.

Elimination
The renal clearance for naltrexone ranges from 30-127 mL/min and suggests that renal elimination is primarily by glomerular filtration. In comparison, the renal clearance for 6-β-naltrexol ranges from 230-369 mL/min, suggesting an additional renal tubular secretory mechanism. The urinary excretion of unchanged naltrexone accounts for less than 2% of an oral dose; urinary excretion of unchanged and conjugated 6-β-naltrexol accounts for 43% of an oral dose. The pharmacokinetic profile of naltrexone suggests that naltrexone and its metabolites may undergo enterohepatic recycling.

Hepatic and Renal Impairment
Naltrexone appears to have extra-hepatic sites of drug metabolism and its major metabolite undergoes active tubular secretion (see **Metabolism** above). Adequate studies of naltrexone in patients with severe hepatic or renal impairment have not been conducted (see **PRECAUTIONS: Special Risk Patients**).

Clinical Trials:
Alcoholism:
The efficacy of REVIA as an aid to the treatment of alcoholism was tested in placebo-controlled, outpatient, double blind trials. These studies used a dose of REVIA 50 mg once daily for 12 weeks as an adjunct to social and psychotherapeutic methods when given under conditions that enhanced patient compliance. Patients with psychosis, dementia, and secondary psychiatric diagnoses were excluded from these studies.
In one of these studies, 104 alcohol-dependent patients were randomized to receive either REVIA 50 mg once daily or placebo. In this study, REVIA proved superior to placebo in measures of drinking including abstention rates (51% vs. 23%), number of drinking days, and relapse (31% vs. 60%). In a second study with 82 alcohol-dependent patients, the group of patients receiving REVIA were shown to have lower relapse rates (21% vs. 41%), less alcohol craving, and fewer drinking days compared with patients who received placebo, but these results depended on the specific analysis used.
The clinical use of REVIA as adjunctive pharmacotherapy for the treatment of alcoholism was also evaluated in a multicenter safety study. This study of 865 individuals with alcoholism included patients with comorbid psychiatric conditions, concomitant medications, polysubstance abuse and HIV disease. Results of this study demonstrated that the side effect profile of REVIA appears to be similar in both alcoholic and opioid dependent populations, and that serious side effects are uncommon.
In the clinical studies, treatment with REVIA supported abstinence, prevented relapse and decreased alcohol consumption. In the uncontrolled study, the patterns of abstinence and relapse were similar to those observed in the controlled studies. REVIA was not uniformly helpful to all patients, and the expected effect of the drug is a modest improvement in the outcome of conventional treatment.

Treatment of Opioid Addiction:
REVIA has been shown to produce complete blockade of the euphoric effects of opioids in both volunteer and addict populations. When administered by means that enforce compliance, it will produce an effective opioid blockade, but has not been shown to affect the use of cocaine or other non-opioid drugs of abuse.
There are no data that demonstrate an unequivocally beneficial effect of REVIA on rates of recidivism among detoxified, formerly opioid-dependent individuals who self-administer the drug. The failure of the drug in this setting appears to be due to poor medication compliance.
The drug is reported to be of greatest use in good prognosis opioid addicts who take the drug as part of a comprehensive occupational rehabilitative program, behavioral contract, or other compliance-enhancing protocol. REVIA, unlike methadone or LAAM (levo-alpha-acetylmethadol), does not reinforce medication compliance and is expected to have a therapeutic effect only when given under external conditions that support continued use of the medication.

Individualization of Dosage:
DO NOT ATTEMPT TREATMENT WITH REVIA UNLESS, IN THE MEDICAL JUDGEMENT OF THE PRESCRIBING PHYSICIAN, THERE IS NO REASONABLE POSSIBILITY OF OPIOID USE WITHIN THE PAST 7-10 DAYS. IF THERE IS ANY QUESTION OF OCCULT OPIOID DEPENDENCE, PERFORM A NARCAN CHALLENGE TEST.

Treatment of Alcoholism:
The placebo-controlled studies that demonstrated the efficacy of REVIA as an adjunctive treatment of alcoholism used a dose regimen of REVIA (naltrexone hydrochloride) 50 mg once daily for up to 12 weeks. Other dose regimens or durations of therapy were not studied in these trials.
Physicians are advised that 5-15% of patients taking REVIA for alcoholism will complain of non-specific side effects, chiefly gastrointestinal upset. Prescribing physicians have tried using an initial 25 mg dose, splitting the daily dose, and adjusting the time of dosing with limited success. No dose or pattern of dosing has been shown to be more effective than any other in reducing these complaints for all patients.

Treatment of Opioid Dependence:
Once the patient has been started on REVIA, 50 mg once a day will produce adequate clinical blockade of the actions of parenterally administered opioids. As with many non-agonist treatments for addiction, REVIA is of proven value only when given as part of a comprehensive plan of management that includes some measure to ensure the patient takes the medication.
A flexible approach to a dosing regimen may be employed to enhance compliance. Thus, patients may receive 50 mg of REVIA every weekday with a 100 mg dose on Saturday or patients may receive 100 mg every other day, or 150 mg every third day. Several of the clinical studies reported in the literature have employed the following dosing regimen: 100 mg on Monday, 100 mg on Wednesday, and 150 mg on Friday. This dosing schedule appeared to be acceptable to many REVIA patients successfully maintaining their opioid-free state.
Experience with the supervised administration of a number of potentially hepatotoxic agents suggests that supervised administration and single doses of REVIA higher than 50 mg may have an associated increased risk of hepatocellular injury, even though three-times a week dosing has been well tolerated in the addict population and in initial clinical trials in alcoholism. Clinics using this approach should balance the possible risks against the probable benefits and may wish to maintain a higher index of suspicion for drug-associated hepatitis and ensure patients are advised of the need to report non-specific abdominal complaints (see **Information for Patients**).

INDICATIONS AND USAGE:

REVIA is indicated :
In the treatment of alcohol dependence and for the blockade of the effects of exogenously administered opioids.
REVIA has not been shown to provide any therapeutic benefit except as part of an appropriate plan of management for the addictions.

CONTRAINDICATIONS:

REVIA is contraindicated in:
1) Patients receiving opioid analgesics.
2) Patients currently dependent on opioids.
3) Patients in acute opioid withdrawal (see **WARNINGS**).
4) Any individual who has failed the NARCAN challenge test or who has a positive urine screen for opioids.
5) Any individual with a history of sensitivity to REVIA or any other components of this product. It is not known if there is any cross-sensitivity with naloxone or the phenanthrene containing opioids.
6) Any individual with acute hepatitis or liver failure.

WARNINGS:

Hepatotoxicity:

REVIA has the capacity to cause hepatocellular injury when given in excessive doses.
REVIA is contraindicated in acute hepatitis or liver failure, and its use in patients with active liver disease must be carefully considered in light of its hepatotoxic effects.
The margin of separation between the apparently safe dose of REVIA and the dose causing hepatic injury ap-

pears to be only five-fold or less. REVIA does not appear to be a hepatotoxin at the recommended doses. Patients should be warned of the risk of hepatic injury and advised to stop the use of REVIA and seek medical attention if they experience symptoms of acute hepatitis.

Evidence of the hepatotoxic potential of REVIA is derived primarily from a placebo controlled study in which REVIA was administered to obese subjects at a dose approximately five-fold that recommended for the blockade of opiate receptors (300 mg per day). In that study, 5 of 26 REVIA recipients developed elevations of serum transaminases (i.e., peak ALT values ranging from a low of 121 to a high of 532; or 3 to 19 times their baseline values) after three to eight weeks of treatment. Although the patients involved were generally clinically asymptomatic and the transaminase levels of all patients on whom follow-up was obtained returned to (or toward) baseline values in a matter of weeks, the lack of any transaminase elevations of similar magnitude in any of the 24 placebo patients in the same study is persuasive evidence that REVIA is a direct (i.e., not idiosyncratic) hepatotoxin.

This conclusion is also supported by evidence from other placebo controlled studies in which exposure to REVIA at doses above the amount recommended for the treatment of alcoholism or opiate blockade (50 mg/day) consistently produced more numerous and more significant elevations of serum transaminases than did placebo. Transaminase elevations in 3 of 9 patients with Alzheimer's Disease who received REVIA (at doses up to 300 mg/day) for 5 to 8 weeks in an open clinical trial have been reported.

Although no cases of hepatic failure due to REVIA administration have ever been reported, physicians are advised to consider this as a possible risk of treatment and to use the same care in prescribing REVIA as they would other drugs with the potential for causing hepatic injury.

Unintended Precipitation of Abstinence:

To prevent occurrence of an acute abstinence syndrome, or exacerbation of a pre-existing subclinical abstinence syndrome, patients must be opioid-free for a minimum of 7-10 days before starting REVIA. Since the absence of an opioid drug in the urine is often not sufficient proof that a patient is opioid-free, a NARCAN challenge should be employed if the prescribing physician feels there is a risk of precipitating a withdrawal reaction following administration of REVIA. The NARCAN challenge test is described in the DOSAGE AND ADMINISTRATION section.

Attempt to Overcome Blockade:

While REVIA is a potent antagonist with a prolonged pharmacologic effect (24 to 72 hours), the blockade produced by REVIA is surmountable. This is useful in patients who may require analgesia, but poses a potential risk to individuals who attempt, on their own, to overcome the blockade by administering large amounts of exogenous opioids. Indeed, any attempt by a patient to overcome the antagonism by taking opioids is very dangerous and may lead to a fatal overdose. Injury may arise because the plasma concentration of exogenous opioids attained immediately following their acute administration may be sufficient to overcome the competitive receptor blockade. As a consequence, the patient may be in immediate danger of suffering life endangering opioid intoxication (e.g., respiratory arrest, circulatory collapse). Patients should be told of the serious consequences of trying to overcome the opiate blockade (See Information for Patients).

There is also the possibility that a patient who had been treated with naltrexone will respond to lower doses of opioids than previously used, particularly if taken in such a manner that high plasma concentrations remain in the body beyond the time that naltrexone exerts its therapeutic effects. This could result in potentially life-threatening opioid intoxication (respiratory compromise or arrest, circulatory collapse, etc.). Patients should be aware that they may be more sensitive to lower doses of opioids after naltrexone treatment is discontinued.

Ultra Rapid Opioid Withdrawal:

Safe use of REVIA in ultra rapid opiate detoxification programs has not been established (see **ADVERSE REACTIONS**).

PRECAUTIONS: General

When Reversal of REVIA Blockade is Required: In an emergency situation in patients receiving fully blocking doses of REVIA, a suggested plan of management is regional analgesia, conscious sedation with a benzodiazepine, use of nonopioid analgesics or general anesthesia.

In a situation requiring opioid analgesia, the amount of opioid required may be greater than usual, and the resulting respiratory depression may be deeper and more prolonged.

A rapidly acting opioid analgesic which minimizes the duration of respiratory depression is preferred. The amount of analgesic administered should be titrated to the needs of the patient. Non-receptor mediated actions may occur and

should be expected (e.g., facial swelling, itching, generalized erythema, or bronchoconstriction) presumably due to histamine release.

Irrespective of the drug chosen to reverse REVIA blockade, the patient should be monitored closely by appropriately trained personnel in a setting equipped and staffed for cardiopulmonary resuscitation.

Accidentally Precipitated Withdrawal: Severe opioid withdrawal syndromes precipitated by the accidental ingestion of REVIA have been reported in opioid-dependent individuals. Symptoms of withdrawal have usually appeared within five minutes of ingestion of REVIA and have lasted for up to 48 hours. Mental status changes including confusion, somnolence and visual hallucinations have occurred. Significant fluid losses from vomiting and diarrhea have required intravenous fluid administration. In all cases patients were closely monitored and therapy with non-opioid medications was tailored to meet individual requirements.

Use of REVIA does not eliminate or diminish withdrawl symptoms. If REVIA is initiated early in the abstinence process, it will not preclude the patient's experience of the full range of signs and symptoms that would be experienced if REVIA had not been started. Numerous adverse events are known to be associated with withdrawal.

Special Risk Patients:

Renal Impairment: REVIA and its primary metabolite are excreted primarily in the urine, and caution is recommended in administering the drug to patients with renal impairment.

Hepatic Impairment: Cautions should be exercised when naltrexone hydrochloride is administered to patients with liver disease. An increase in naltrexone AUC of approximately 5- and 10-fold in patients with compensated and decompensated liver cirrhosis, respectively, compared with subjects with normal liver function has been reported. These data also suggest that alterations in naltrexone bioavailability are related to liver disease severity.

Suicide: The risk of suicide is known to be increased in patients with substance abuse with or without concomitant depression. This risk is not abated by treatment with REVIA (see **ADVERSE REACTIONS**).

Information for Patients: It is recommended that the prescribing physician relate the following information to patients being treated with REVIA:

You have been prescribed REVIA as part of the comprehensive treatment for your alcoholism or drug dependence. You should carry identification to alert medical personnel to the fact that you are taking REVIA (naltrexone hydrochloride). A REVIA medication card may be obtained from your physician and can be used for this purpose. Carrying the identification card should help to ensure that you can obtain adequate treatment in an emergency. If you require medical treatment, be sure to tell the treating physician that you are receiving REVIA therapy.

You should take REVIA as directed by your physician. If you attempt to self-administer heroin or any other opiate drug, in small doses while on REVIA, you will not perceive any effect. Most important, however, if you attempt to self-administer large doses of heroin or any other opioid while on REVIA, you may die or sustain serious injury, including coma. REVIA is well-tolerated in the recommended doses, but may cause liver injury when taken in excess or in people who develop liver disease from other causes. If you develop abdominal pain lasting more than a few days, white bowel movements, dark urine, or yellowing of your eyes, you should stop taking REVIA immediately and see your doctor as soon as possible.

Laboratory Tests: A high index of suspicion for drug-related hepatic injury is critical if the occurrence of liver damage induced by REVIA is to be detected at the earliest possible time. Evaluations, using appropriate batteries of tests to detect liver injury are recommended at a frequency appropriate to the clinical situation and the dose of REVIA. REVIA does not interfere with thin-layer, gas-liquid, and high pressure liquid chromatographic methods which may be used for the separation and detection of morphine, methadone or quinine in the urine. REVIA may or may not interfere with enzymatic methods for the detection of opioids depending on the specificity of the test. Please consult the test manufacturer for specific details.

Drug Interactions: Studies to evaluate possible interactions between REVIA and drugs other than opiates have not been performed. Consequently, caution is advised if the concomitant administration of REVIA and other drugs is required.

The safety and efficacy of concomitant use of REVIA and disulfiram is unknown, and the concomitant use of two potentially hepatotoxic medications is not ordinarily recommended unless the probable benefits outweigh the known risks.

Lethargy and somnolence have been reported following doses of REVIA and thioridazine.

Patients taking REVIA may not benefit from opioid containing medicines, such as cough and cold preparations, antidiarrheal preparations, and opioid analgesics. In an emergency situation when opioid analgesia must be adminis-

tered to a patient receiving REVIA, the amount of opioid required may be greater than usual, and the resulting respiratory depression may be deeper and more prolonged (see **PRECAUTIONS**).

Carcinogenesis, Mutagenesis and Impairment of Fertility: Carcinogenicity studies in rats and mice were conducted at doses as high as 100 times the human dose. There was no statistically significant increase in the incidence of any tumors and, except for vascular tumors in the REVIA-treated female rats, the incidence of tumors observed in the studies were within ranges seen in historical control groups. REVIA was negative in bacterial and cultured mammalian cell mutation, *in vitro* chromosome aberration, and *in vivo* micronucleus, chromosome aberration, and heritable translocation assays. It was weakly positive in the *Drosophila melanogaster* recessive lethal test and gave equivocal responses in *E. coli* DNA repair and in *in vitro* mammalian cell mutation and anaphase chromosome assays. Overall, the study results indicate that the genotoxic potential of REVIA is low. REVIA (100 mg/kg, approximately 100 times the human therapeutic dose) caused an increase in pseudopregnancy and a decrease in the pregnancy rates of female rats. The relevance to these observations to human fertility is not known.

Pregnancy: Category C. REVIA has been shown to have embryocidal and fetotoxic effects in rats and rabbits when given in dosages 30 and 60 times, respectively, the human dose.

There are no adequate and well-controlled studies in pregnant women. REVIA should be used in pregnancy only when the potential benefit justifies the potential risk to the fetus.

Labor and Delivery: Whether or not REVIA affects the duration of labor and delivery is unknown.

Nursing Mothers: Whether or not REVIA is excreted in human milk is unknown. Because many drugs are excreted in human milk, caution should be exercised when REVIA is administered to a nursing woman.

Pediatric Use: The safe use of REVIA in pediatric patients younger than 18 years old has not been established.

ADVERSE REACTIONS:

During two randomized, double-blind placebo-controlled 12 week trials to evaluate the efficacy of REVIA as an adjunctive treatment of alcohol dependence, most patients tolerated REVIA well. In these studies, a total of 93 patients received REVIA at a dose of 50 mg once daily. Five of these patients discontinued REVIA because of nausea. No serious adverse events were reported during these two trials.

While extensive clinical studies evaluating the use of REVIA in detoxified, formerly opioid-dependent individuals failed to identify any single, serious untoward risk of REVIA use, placebo controlled studies employing up to five-fold higher doses of REVIA (up to 300 mg per day) than that recommended for use in opiate receptor blockade have shown that REVIA causes hepatocellular injury in a substantial proportion of patients exposed at higher doses (see **WARNINGS** and **PRECAUTIONS: Laboratory Tests**).

Aside from this finding, and the risk of precipitated opioid withdrawal, available evidence does not incriminate REVIA, used at any dose, as a cause of any other serious adverse reaction for the patient who is "opioid free." It is critical to recognize that REVIA can precipitate or exacerbate abstinence signs and symptoms in any individual who is not completely free of exogenous opioids.

Patients with addictive disorders, especially opioid addiction, are at risk for multiple numerous adverse events and abnormal laboratory findings, including liver function abnormalities. Data from both controlled and observational studies suggest that these abnormalities, other than the dose-related hepatotoxicity described above, are not related to the use of REVIA.

Among opioid free individuals, REVIA administration at the recommended dose has not been associated with a predictable profile of serious adverse or untoward events. However, as mentioned above, among individuals using opioids, REVIA may cause serious withdrawal reactions (see **CONTRAINDICATIONS, WARNINGS, DOSAGE AND ADMINISTRATION**).

Reported Adverse Events

REVIA has not been shown to cause significant increases in complaints in placebo-controlled trials in patients known to be free of opioids for more than 7-10 days. Studies in alcoholic populations and in volunteers in clinical pharmacology studies have suggested that a small fraction of patients may experience an opioid withdrawal-like symptom complex consisting of tearfulness, mild nausea, abdominal cramps, restlessness, bone or joint pain, myalgia, and nasal symptoms. This may represent the unmasking of occult opioid use, or it may represent symptoms attributable to naltrexone. A number of alternative dosing patterns have been recommended to try to reduce the frequency of these complaints (see **Individualization of Dosage**).

Alcoholism:

In an open label safety study with approximately 570 individuals with alcoholism receiving REVIA, the following new-

Continued on next page

ReVia—Cont.

onset adverse reactions occurred in 2% or more of the patients: nausea (10%), headache (7%), dizziness (4%), nervousness (4%), fatigue (4%), insomnia (3%), vomiting (3%), anxiety (2%) and somnolence (2%).

Depression, suicidal ideation, and suicidal attempts have been reported in all groups when comparing naltrexone, placebo, or controls undergoing treatment for alcoholism.

RATE RANGES OF NEW ONSET EVENTS

	Naltrexone	Placebo
Depression	0–15%	0–17%
Suicide Attempt/ Ideation	0–1%	0–3%

Although no causal relationship with REVIA is suspected, physicians should be aware that treatment with REVIA does not reduce the risk of suicide in these patients (see **PRECAUTIONS**).

Opioid Addiction:
The following adverse reactions have been reported both at baseline and during the REVIA clinical trials in opioid addiction at an incidence rate of more than 10%:

Difficulty sleeping, anxiety, nervousness, abdominal pain/cramps, nausea and/or vomiting, low energy, joint and muscle pain, and headache.

The incidence was less than 10% for:

Loss of appetite, diarrhea, constipation, increased thirst, increased energy, feeling down, irritability, dizziness, skin rash, delayed ejaculation, decreased potency, and chills.

The following events occurred in less than 1% of subjects:

Respiratory: nasal congestion, itching, rhinorrhea, sneezing, sore throat, excess mucus or phlegm, sinus trouble, heavy breathing, hoarseness, cough, shortness of breath.

Cardiovascular: nose bleeds, phlebitis, edema, increased blood pressure, non-specific ECG changes, palpitations, tachycardia.

Gastrointestinal: excessive gas, hemorrhoids, diarrhea, ulcer.

Musculoskeletal: painful shoulders, legs or knees; tremors, twitching.

Genitourinary: increased frequency of, or discomfort during, urination; increased or decreased sexual interest.

Dermatologic: oily skin, pruritus, acne, athlete's foot, cold sores, alopecia.

Psychiatric: depression, paranoia, fatigue, restlessness, confusion, disorientation, hallucinations, nightmares, bad dreams.

Special senses: eyes—blurred, burning, light sensitive, swollen, aching, strained; ears—"clogged", aching, tinnitus.

General: increased appetite, weight loss, weight gain, yawning, somnolence, fever, dry mouth, head "pounding", inguinal pain, swollen glands, "side" pains, cold feet, "hot spells."

Post-Marketing Experience: Data collected from post-marketing use of REVIA show that most events usually occur early in the course of drug therapy and are transient. It is not always possible to distinguish these occurences from those signs and symptoms that may result from a withdrawal syndrome. Events that have been reported include anorexia, asthenia, chest pain, fatigue, headache, hot flushes, malaise, changes in blood pressure, agitation, dizziness, hyperkinesia, nausea, vomiting, tremor, abdominal pain, diarrhea, elevations in liver enzymes or bilirubin, hepatic function abnormalities or hepatitis, palpitations, myalgia, anxiety, confusion, emphoria, hallucinations, insomnia, nervousness, somnolence, abnormal thinking, dyspnea, rash, increased sweating, and vision abnormalities.

Depression, suicide, attempted suicide and suicidal ideation have been reported in the post-marketing experience with REVIA used in the treatment of opioid dependence. No causal relationship has been demonstrated. In the literature, endogenous opioids have been theorized to contribute to a variety of conditions. In some individuals the use of opioid antagonists has been associated with a change in baseline levels of some hypothalamic, pituitary, adrenal, or gonadal hormones. The clinical significance of such changes is not fully understood.

Adverse events, including withdrawal symptoms and death, have been reported with the use of REVIA (naltrexone hydrochloride) in ultra rapid opiate detoxification programs. No causal relationship between REVIA and these deaths has been established (see **WARNINGS**).

Laboratory tests: With the exception of liver test abnormalities (see **WARNINGS** and **PRECAUTIONS**), results of laboratory tests, like adverse reaction reports, have not shown consistent patterns of abnormalities that can be attributed to treatment with REVIA.

Idiopathic thrombocytopenic purpura was reported in one patient who may have been sensitized to REVIA in a previous course of treatment with REVIA. The condition cleared without sequelae after discontinuation of REVIA and corticosteroid treatment.

DRUG ABUSE AND DEPENDENCE:

REVIA is a pure opioid antagonist. It does not lead to physical or psychological dependence. Tolerance to the opioid antagonist effect is not known to occur.

OVERDOSAGE:

There is limited clinical experience with REVIA overdosage in humans. In one study, subjects who received 800 mg daily REVIA for up to one week showed no evidence of toxicity.

In the mouse, rat and guinea pig, the oral LD50s were 1,100–1,550 mg/kg; 1,450 mg/kg; and 1,490 mg/kg; respectively. High doses of REVIA (generally ≥ 1,000 mg/kg) produced salivation, depression/reduced activity, tremors, and convulsions. Mortalities in animals due to high-dose REVIA administration usually were due to clonic-tonic convulsions and/or respiratory failure.

Treatment Of Overdosage: In view of the lack of actual experience in the treatment of REVIA overdose, patients should be treated symptomatically in a closely supervised environment. Physicians should contact a poison control center for the most up-to-date information.

DOSAGE AND ADMINISTRATION:

IF THERE IS ANY QUESTION OF OCCULT OPIOID DEPENDENCE, PERFORM A NARCAN CHALLENGE TEST AND DO NOT INITIATE REVIA THERAPY UNTIL THE NARCAN CHALLENGE IS NEGATIVE.

Treatment of Alcoholism:
A dose of 50 mg once daily is recommended for most patients (see **Individualization of Dosage**). The placebo-controlled studies that demonstrated the efficacy of REVIA as an adjunctive treatment of alcoholism used a dose regimen of REVIA 50 mg once daily for up to 12 weeks. Other dose regimens or durations of therapy were not evaluated in these trials.

A patient is a candidate for treatment with REVIA if:

- The patient is willing to take a medicine to help with alcohol dependence
- The patient is opioid free for 7–10 days
- The patient does not have severe or active liver or kidney problems
  (Typical guidelines suggest liver function tests no greater than 3 times the upper limits of normal, and bilirubin normal.)
- The patient is not allergic to REVIA , and no other contraindications are present

Refer to **CONTRAINDICATIONS**, **WARNINGS**, and **PRECAUTIONS** Sections for additional information.

REVIA should be considered as only one of many factors determining the success of treatment of alcoholism. Factors associated with a good outcome in the clinical trials with REVIA were the type, intensity, and duration of treatment; appropriate management of comorbid conditions; use of community-based support groups; and good medication compliance. To achieve the best possible treatment outcome, appropriate compliance-enhancing techniques should be implemented for all components of the treatment program, especially medication compliance.

Treatment of Opioid Dependence:
Initiate treatment with REVIA using the following guidelines:

1. Treatment should not be attempted unless the patient has remained opioid-free for at least 7–10 days. Self-reporting of abstinence from opioids in opioid addicts should be verified by analysis of the patient's urine for absence of opioids. The patient should not be manifesting withdrawal signs or reporting withdrawal symptoms.
2. If there is any question of occult opioid dependence, perform a NARCAN challenge test. If signs of opioid withdrawal are still observed following NARCAN challenge, treatment with REVIA should not be attempted. The NARCAN challenge can be repeated in 24 hours.
3. Treatment should be initiated carefully, with an initial dose of 25 mg of REVIA. If no withdrawal signs occur, the patient may be started on 50 mg a day thereafter.

NARCAN Challenge Test: The NARCAN challenge test should not be performed in a patient showing clinical signs or symptoms of opioid withdrawal, or in a patient whose urine contains opioids. The NARCAN challenge test may be administered by either the intravenous or subcutaneous routes.

Intravenous:
Inject 0.2 mg NARCAN.

Observe for 30 seconds for signs or symptoms of withdrawal.

If no evidence of withdrawal, inject 0.6 mg of NARCAN.

Observe for an additional 20 minutes.

Subcutaneous:
Administer 0.8 mg NARCAN.

Observe for 20 minutes for signs or symptoms of withdrawal.

Note: Individual patients, especially those with opioid dependence, may respond to lower doses of NARCAN. In some cases, 0.1 mg IV NARCAN has produced a diagnostic response.

Interpretation of the Challenge: Monitor vital signs and observe the patient for signs and symptoms of opioid withdrawal. These may include, but are not limited to: nausea, vomiting, dysphoria, yawning, sweating, tearing, rhinorrhea, stuffy nose, craving for opioids, poor appetite, abdominal cramps, sense of fear, skin erythema, disrupted sleep patterns, fidgeting, uneasiness, poor ability to focus, mental lapses, muscle aches or cramps, pupillary dilation, piloerection, fever, changes in blood pressure, pulse or temperature, anxiety, depression, irritability, back ache, bone or joint pains, tremors, sensations of skin crawling or fasciculations. If signs or symptoms of withdrawal appear, the test is positive and no additional NARCAN should be administered.

Warning: If the test is positive, do NOT initiate REVIA Therapy. Repeat the challenge in 24 hours. If the test is negative, REVIA therapy may be started if no other contraindictions are present. If there is any doubt about the result of the test, hold REVIA and repeat the challenge in 24 hours.

Alternative Dosing Schedules:
Once the patient has been started on REVIA, 50 mg every 24 hours will produce adequate clinical blockade of the actions of parenterally administered opioids (i.e., this dose will block the effects of a 25 mg intravenous heroin challenge). A flexible approach to a dosing regimen may need to be employed in cases of supervised administration. Thus, patients may receive 50 mg of REVIA every weekday with a 100 mg dose on Saturday, 100 mg every other day, or 150 mg every third day. The degree of blockade produced by REVIA may be reduced by these extended dosing intervals.

There may be a higher risk of hepatocellular injury with single doses above 50 mg, and use of higher doses and extended dosing intervals should balance the possible risks against the probable benefits (see **WARNINGS** and **Individualization of Dosage**).

Patient Compliance: REVIA should be considered as only one of many factors determining the success of treatment. To achieve the best possible treatment outcome, appropriate compliance-enhancing techniques should be implemented for all components of the treatment program, including medication compliance.

HOW SUPPLIED

REVIA (naltrexone hydrochloride) tablets are available in pale yellow 50 mg capsule-shaped film-coated tablets, scored and imprinted with "DuPont" on one side and "11" on the other, as follows:

Bottles of 30 Tablets	NDC 0056-0011-30
Bottles of 100 Tablets	NDC 0056-0011-70

Store at controlled room temperature (59°–86°F, 15°–30°C).

Dispense in a tight container as defined the USP.

Rx only

DuPont Pharma
Wilmington, Delaware 19880

NARCAN® is a Registered U.S. Trademark of DuPont Pharmaceuticals Co.

RIVIA® is a Registered U.S. Trademark of DuPont Pharmaceuticals Co.

Copyright© DuPont Pharma 1998.

6430–2/Rev. July, 1998

Shown in Product Identification Guide, page 309

SINEMET® (CARBIDOPA-LEVODOPA) TABLETS ℞

DESCRIPTION

SINEMET* (Carbidopa-Levodopa) is a combination of carbidopa and levodopa for the treatment of Parkinson's disease and syndrome.

Carbidopa, an inhibitor of aromatic amino acid decarboxylation, is a white, crystalline compound, slightly soluble in water, with a molecular weight of 244.3. It is designated chemically as (—)-L-α-hydrazino-α-methyl-β-(3,4-dihydroxybenzene) propanoic acid monohydrate. Its empirical formula is $C_{10}H_{14}N_2O_4 \cdot H_2O$, and its structural formula is:

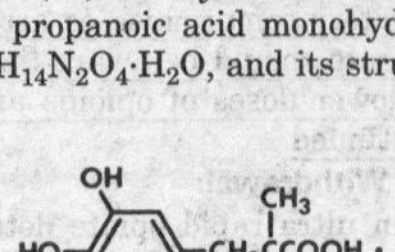
OH
CH3
HO
CH2CCOOH · H2O
NHNH2

Tablet content is expressed in terms of anhydrous carbidopa which has a molecular weight of 226.3.

Levodopa, an aromatic amino acid, is a white, crystalline compound, slightly soluble in water, with a molecular weight of 197.2. It is designated chemically as (—)-L-α-amino-β-(3,4-dihydroxybenzene) propanoic acid. Its empirical formula is $C_9H_{11}NO_4$, and its structural formula is:

[See chemical structure at top of next column]

SINEMET is supplied as tablets in three strengths:

SINEMET 25-100, containing 25 mg of carbidopa and 100 mg of levodopa.

SINEMET 10-100, containing 10 mg of carbidopa and 100 mg of levodopa.

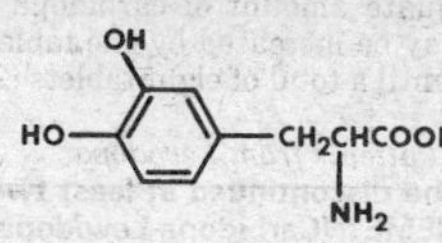

SINEMET 25-250, containing 25 mg of carbidopa and 250 mg of levodopa.
Inactive ingredients are cellulose, magnesium stearate, and starch. Tablets SINEMET 10-100 and 25-250 also contain FD&C Blue 2. Tablets SINEMET 25-100 also contain D&C Yellow 10 and FD&C Yellow 6.

CLINICAL PHARMACOLOGY

Parkinson's disease is a progressive, neurodegenerative disorder of the extrapyramidal nervous system affecting the mobility and control of the skeletal muscular system. Its characteristic features include resting tremor, rigidity, and bradykinetic moments. Symptomatic treatments, such as levodopa therapies, may permit the patient better mobility.

Mechanism of Action

Current evidence indicates that symptoms of Parkinson's disease are related to depletion of dopamine in the corpus striatum. Administration of dopamine is ineffective in the treatment of Parkinson's disease apparently because it does not cross the blood-brain barrier. However, levodopa, the metabolic precursor of dopamine. does cross the blood-brain barrier, and presumably is converted to dopamine in the brain. This is thought to be the mechanism whereby levodopa relieves symptoms of Parkinson's disease.

Pharmacodynamics

When levodopa is administered orally it is rapidly decarboxylated to dopamine in extracerebral tissues so that only a small portion of a given dose is transported unchanged to the central nervous system. For this reason, large doses of levodopa are required for adequate therapeutic effect and these may often be accompanied by nausea and other adverse reactions, some of which are attributable to dopamine formed in extracerebral tissues.

Since levodopa competes with certain amino acids for transport across the gut wall, the absorption of levodopa may be impaired in some patients on a high protein diet.

Carbidopa inhibits decarboxylation of peripheral levodopa. It does not cross the blood-brain barrier and does not affect the metabolism of levodopa within the central nervous system.

The incidence of levodopa-induced nausea and vomiting is less with SINEMET than with levodopa. In many patients, this reduction in nausea and vomiting will permit more rapid dosage titration.

Since its decarboxylase inhibiting activity is limited to extracerebral tissues, administration of carbidopa with levodopa makes more levodopa available for transport to the brain.

Pharmacokinetics

Carbidopa reduces the amount of levodopa required to produce a given response by about 75 percent and, when administered with levodopa, increases both plasma levels and the plasma half-life of levodopa, and decreases plasma and urinary dopamine and homovanillic acid.

The plasma half-life of levodopa is about 50 minutes, without carbidopa. When carbidopa and levodopa are administered together, the half-life of levodopa is increased to about 1.5 hours. The bioavailablity of carbidopa from SINEMET tablets is approximately 99%.

In clinical pharmacologic studies, simultaneous administration of carbidopa and levodopa produced greater urinary excretion of levodopa in proportion to the excretion of dopamine than administration of the two drugs at separate times.

Pyridoxine hydrochloride (vitamin B_6), in oral doses of 10 mg to 25 mg, may reverse the effects of levodopa by increasing the rate of aromatic amino acid decarboxylation. Carbidopa inhibits this action of pyridoxine; therefore, SINEMET can be given to patients receiving supplemental pyridoxine (vitamin B_6).

INDICATIONS AND USAGE

SINEMET is indicated in the treatment of the symptoms of idiopathic Parkinson's disease (paralysis agitans), postencephalitic parkinsonism, and symptomatic parkinsonism which may follow injury to the nervous system by carbon monoxide intoxication and/or manganese intoxication. SINEMET is indicated in these conditions to permit the administration of lower doses of levodopa with reduced nausea and vomiting, with more rapid dosage titration, with a somewhat smoother response, and with supplemental pyridoxine (vitamin B_6).

In some patients a somewhat smoother antiparkinsonian effect results from therapy with SINEMET than with levodopa. However, patients with markedly irregular ("on-off") responses to levodopa have not been shown to benefit from SINEMET.

Although the administration of carbidopa permits control of parkinsonism and Parkinson's disease with much lower doses of levodopa, there is no conclusive evidence at present that this is beneficial other than in reducing nausea and vomiting, permitting more rapid titration, and providing a somewhat smoother response to levodopa.

Certain patients who responded poorly to levodopa have improved when SINEMET was substituted. This is most likely due to decreased peripheral decarboxylation of levodopa which results from administration of carbidopa rather than to a primary effect of carbidopa on the nervous system. Carbidopa has not been shown to enhance the intrinsic efficacy of levodopa in parkinsonian syndromes.

In considering whether to give SINEMET to patients already on levodopa who have nausea and/or vomiting, the practitioner should be aware that, while many patients may be expected to improve, some do not. Since one cannot predict which patients are likely to improve, this can only be determined by a trial of therapy. It should be further noted that in controlled trials comparing SINEMET with levodopa, about half of the patients with nausea and/or vomiting on levodopa improved spontaneously despite being retained on the same dose of levodopa during the controlled portion of the trial.

CONTRAINDICATIONS

Nonselective monoamine oxidase (MAO) inhibitors are contraindicated for use with SINEMET. These inhibitors must be discontinued at least two weeks prior to initiating therapy with SINEMET. SINEMET may be administered concomitantly with the manufacturer's recommended dose of an MAO inhibitor with selectivity for MAO type B (e.g., selegiline HCl).

SINEMET is contraindicated in patients with known hypersensitivity to any component of this drug, and in narrow-angle glaucoma.

Because levodopa may activate a malignant melanoma, SINEMET should not be used in patients with suspicious, undiagnosed skin lesions or a history of melanoma.

WARNINGS

When SINEMET (Carbidopa-Levodopa) is to be given to patients who are being treated with levodopa, levodopa must be discontinued at least twelve hours before therapy with SINEMET (Carbidopa-Levodopa) is started. In order to reduce adverse reactions, it is necessary to individualize therapy. See DOSAGE AND ADMINISTRATION section before initiating therapy.

The addition of carbidopa with levodopa in the form of SINEMET reduces the peripheral effects (nausea, vomiting) due to decarboxylation of levodopa; however, carbidopa does not decrease the adverse reactions due to the central effects of levodopa. Because carbidopa permits more levodopa to reach the brain and more dopamine to be formed, certain adverse CNS effects, e.g., dyskinesias (involuntary movements), may occur at lower dosages and sooner with SINEMET than with levodopa alone.

Levodopa alone, as well as SINEMET, is associated with dyskinesias. The occurrence of dyskinesias may require dosage reduction.

As with levodopa, SINEMET may cause mental disturbances. These reactions are thought to be due to increased brain dopamine following administration of levodopa. All patients should be observed carefully for the development of depression with concomitant suicidal tendencies. Patients with past or current psychoses should be treated with caution.

SINEMET should be administered cautiously to patients with severe cardiovascular or pulmonary disease, bronchial asthma, renal, hepatic or endocrine disease.

As with levodopa, care should be exercised in administering SINEMET to patients with a history of myocardial infarction who have residual atrial, nodal, or ventricular arrhythmias. In such patients, cardiac function should be monitored with particular care during the period of initial dosage adjustment, in a facility with provisions for intensive cardiac care.

As with levodopa, treatment with SINEMET may increase the possibility of upper gastrointestinal hemorrhage in patients with a history of peptic ulcer.

Neuroleptic Malignant Syndrome (NMS): Sporadic cases of a symptom complex resembling NMS have been reported in association with dose reduction or withdrawal of therapy with SINEMET. Therefore, patients should be observed carefully when the dosage of SINEMET is reduced abruptly or discontinued, especially if the patient is receiving neuroleptics.

NMS is an uncommon but life-threatening syndrome characterized by fever or hyperthermia. Neurological findings, including muscle rigidity, involuntary movements, altered consciousness, mental status changes; other disturbances, such as autonomic dysfunction, tachycardia, tachypnea, sweating, hyper- or hypotension; laboratory findings, such as creatine phosphokinase elevation, leukocytosis, myoglobinuria, and increased serum myoglobin, have been reported.

The early diagnosis of this condition is important for the appropriate management of these patients. Considering NMS as a possible diagnosis and ruling out other acute illnesses (e.g., pneumonia, systemic infection, etc.) is essential. This may be especially complex if the clinical presentation includes both serious medical illness and untreated or inadequately treated extrapyramidal signs and symptoms (EPS). Other important considerations in the differential diagnosis include central anticholinergic toxicity, heat stroke, drug fever, and primary central nervous system (CNS) pathology.

The management of NMS should include: 1) intensive symptomatic treatment and medical monitoring and 2) treatment of any concomitant serious medical problems for which specific treatments are available. Dopamine agonists, such as bromocriptine, and muscle relaxants, such as dantrolene, are often used in the treatment of NMS, however, their effectiveness has not been demonstrated in controlled studies.

PRECAUTIONS

General

As with levodopa, periodic evaluations of hepatic, hematopoietic, cardiovascular, and renal function are recommended during extended therapy.

Patients with chronic wide-angle glaucoma may be treated cautiously with SINEMET provided the intraocular pressure is well controlled and the patient is monitored carefully for changes in intraocular pressure during therapy.

Information for Patients

The patient should be informed that SINEMET is an immediate-release formulation of carbidopa-levodopa that is designed to begin release of ingredients within 30 minutes. It is important that SINEMET be taken at regular intervals according to the schedule outlined by the physician. The patient should be cautioned not to change the prescribed dosage regimen and not to add any additional antiparkinson medications, including other carbidopa-levodopa preparations, without first consulting the physician.

Patients should be advised that sometimes a 'wearing-off' effect may occur at the end of the dosing interval. The physician should be notified if such response poses a problem to life-style.

Patients should be advised that occasionally, dark color (red, brown, or black) may appear in saliva, urine, or sweat after ingestion of SINEMET. Although the color appears to be clinically insignificant, garments may become discolored.

The patients should be advised that a change in diet to foods that are high in protein may delay the absorption of levodopa and may reduce the amount taken up in the circulation. Excessive acidity also delays stomach emptying, thus delaying the absorption of levodopa. Iron salts (such as in multi-vitamin tablets) may also reduce the amount of levodopa available to the body. The above factors may reduce the clinical effectiveness of the levodopa or carbidopa-levodopa therapy.

NOTE: The suggested advice to patients being treated with SINEMET is intended to aid in the safe and effective use of this medication. It is not a disclosure of all possible adverse or intended effects.

Laboratory Tests

Abnormalities in laboratory tests may include elevations of liver function tests such as alkaline phosphatase, SGOT (AST), SGPT (ALT), lactic dehydrogenase, and bilirubin. Abnormalities in blood urea nitrogen and positive Coombs test have also been reported. Commonly, levels of blood urea nitrogen, creatinine, and uric acid are lower during administration of SINEMET than with levodopa.

SINEMET may cause a false-positive reaction for urinary ketone bodies when a test tape is used for determination of ketonuria. This reaction will not be altered by boiling the urine specimen. False-negative tests may result with the use of glucose-oxidase methods of testing for glucosuria.

Cases of falsely diagnosed pheochromocytoma in patients on carbidopa-levodopa therapy have been reported very rarely. Caution should be exercised when interpreting the plasma and urine levels of catecholamines and their metabolites in patients on levodopa or carbidopa-levodopa therapy.

Drug Interactions

Caution should be exercised when the following drugs are administered concomitantly with SINEMET (Carbidopa-Levodopa).

Symptomatic postural hypotension has occurred when SINEMET is added to the treatment of a patient receiving antihypertensive drugs. Therefore, when therapy with SINEMET is started, dosage adjustment of the antihypertensive drug may be required. For patients receiving MAO inhibitors (Type A or B), see CONTRAINDICATIONS.

There have been rare reports of adverse reactions, including hypertension and dyskinesia, resulting from the concomitant use of tricyclic antidepressants and SINEMET.

Phenothiazines, butyrophenones and isoniazid may reduce the therapeutic effects of levodopa. In addition, the beneficial effects of levodopa in Parkinson's disease have been reported to be reversed by phenytoin and papaverine. Patients taking these drugs with SINEMET should be carefully observed for loss of therapeutic response.

Continued on next page

Sinemet—Cont.

Iron salts may reduce the bioavailability of levodopa and carbidopa. The clinical relevance is unclear.

Although metoclopramide may increase the bioavailability of levodopa by increasing gastric emptying, metoclopramide may also adversely affect disease control by its dopamine receptor antagonistic properties.

Carcinogenesis, Mutagenesis, Impairment of Fertility

In a two-year bioassay of SINEMET, no evidence of carcinogenicity was found in rats receiving doses of approximately two times the maximum daily human dose of carbidopa and four times the maximum daily human dose of levodopa.

In reproduction studies with SINEMET, no effects on fertility were found in rats receiving doses of approximately two times the maximum daily human dose of carbidopa and four times the maximum daily human dose of levodopa.

Pregnancy

Pregnancy Category C. No teratogenic effects were observed in a study in mice receiving up to 20 times the maximum recommended human dose of SINEMET. There was a decrease in the number of live pups delivered by rats receiving approximately two times the maximum recommended human dose of carbidopa and approximately five times the maximum recommended human dose of levodopa during organogenesis. SINEMET caused both visceral and skeletal malformations in rabbits at all doses and ratios of carbidopa/levodopa tested, which ranged from 10 times/5 times the maximum recommended human dose of carbidopa/levodopa to 20 times/10 times the maximum recommended human dose of carbidopa/levodopa.

There are no adequate or well-controlled studies in pregnant women. It has been reported from individual cases that levodopa crosses the human placental barrier, enters the fetus, and is metabolized. Carbidopa concentrations in fetal tissue appeared to be minimal. Use of SINEMET in women of child-bearing potential requires that the anticipated benefits of the drug be weighed against possible hazards to mother and child.

Nursing Mothers

It is not known whether this drug is excreted in human milk. Because many drugs are excreted in human milk, caution should be exercised when SINEMET is administered to a nursing woman.

Pediatric Use

Safety and effectiveness in pediatric patients have not been established. Use of the drug in patients below the age of 18 is not recommended.

ADVERSE REACTIONS

The most common adverse reactions reported with SINEMET have included dyskenesias, such as choreiform, dystonic, and other involuntary movements and nausea. Other adverse reactions have included mental changes including paranoid ideation and psychotic episodes, depression with or without development of suicidal tendencies, and dementia. Convulsions also have occurred; however, a causal relationship with SINEMET has not been established.

The following other adverse reactions have been reported with SINEMET:

Body as a Whole: chest pain, asthenia.

Cardiovascular: cardiac irregularities, hypotension including orthostatic hypotension, hypertension, syncope, phlebitis, palpitation.

Digestive: gastrointestinal bleeding, development of duodenal ulcer, anorexia, vomiting, diarrhea, constipation, dyspepsia, dry mouth, taste alterations.

Hematologic: agranulocytosis, hemolytic and non-hemolytic anemia, thrombocytopenia, leukopenia.

Musculoskeletal: back pain, shoulder pain, muscle cramps.

Nervous System/Psychiatric: hallucinations, bradykinetic episodes ("on-off" phenomenon), confusion, agitation, dizziness, somnolence, dream abnormalities including nightmares, insomnia, paresthesia, headache.

Respiratory: dyspnea, upper respiratory infection.

Skin: rash, pruritus, increased sweating, alopecia.

Urogenital: urinary tract infection, urinary frequency.

Laboratory Tests: decreased hemoglobin and hematocrit; abnormalities in alkaline phosphatase, SGOT (AST), SGPT (ALT), lactic dehydrogenase, bilirubin, blood urea nitrogen (BUN), Coombs test; elevated serum glucose; white blood cells, bacteria, and blood in the urine.

Other adverse reactions that have been reported with levodopa alone and with various carbidopa-levodopa formulations, and may occur with SINEMET are:

Nervous System/Psychiatric: ataxia, extrapyramidal disorder, falling, anxiety, gait abnormalities, nervousness, decreased mental acuity, memory impairment, disorientation, delusions, euphoria, blepharospasm (which may be taken as an early sign of excess dosage; consideration of dosage reduction may be made at this time), trismus, increased tremor, numbness, muscle twitching, activation of latent Horner's syndrome, peripheral neuropathy.

Body as a Whole: abdominal pain and distress, fatigue.

Cardiovascular: myocardial infarction.

Digestive: gastrointestinal pain, dysphagia, sialorrhea, flatulence, dark saliva, bruxism, burning sensation of the tongue, heartburn, hiccups.

Metabolic: edema, weight gain, weight loss.

Musculoskeletal: leg pain.

Respiratory: pharyngeal pain, cough.

Skin: malignant melanoma (see also CONTRAINDICATIONS), flushing, dark sweat.

Special Senses: oculogyric crises, diplopia, blurred vision, dilated pupils.

Urogenital: urinary retention, dark urine, urinary incontinence, priapism.

Miscellaneous: neuroleptic malignant syndrome, bizarre breathing patterns, faintness, hoarseness, malaise, hot flashes, sense of stimulation.

Laboratory Tests: decreased white blood cell count and serum potassium; increased serum creatinine and uric acid; protein and glucose in urine.

Other adverse reactions that have been reported with levodopa alone and with various carbidopa-levodopa formulations, and may occur with SINEMET are:

Nervous System/Psychiatric: ataxia, extrapyramidal disorder, falling, anxiety, gait abnormalities, nervousness, decreased mental acuity, memory impairment, disorientation, delusions, euphoria, blepharospasm (which may be taken as an early sign of excess dosage; consideration of dosage reduction may be made at this time), trismus, increased tremor, numbness, muscle twitching, activation of latent Horner's syndrome, peripheral neuropathy.

Body as a Whole: abdominal pain and distress, fatigue.

Cardiovascular: myocardial infarction.

Digestive: gastrointestinal pain, dysphagia, sialorrhea, flatulence, dark saliva, bruxism, burning sensation of the tongue, heartburn, hiccups.

Metabolic: edema, weight gain, weight loss.

Musculoskeletal: leg pain.

Respiratory: pharyngeal pain, cough.

Skin: malignant melanoma (see also CONTRAINDICATIONS), flushing, dark sweat.

Special Senses: oculogyric crises, diplopia, blurred vision, dilated pupils.

Urogenital: urinary retention, dark urine, urinary incontinence, priapism.

Miscellaneous: neuroleptic malignant syndrome, bizarre breathing patterns, faintness, hoarseness, malaise, hot flashes, sense of stimulation.

Laboratory Tests: decreased white blood cell count and serum potassium; increased serum creatinine and uric acid; protein and glucose in urine.

OVERDOSAGE

Management of acute overdosage with SINEMET is the same as management of acute overdosage with levodopa. Pyridoxine is not effective in reversing the actions of SINEMET.

General supportive measures should be employed, along with immediate gastric lavage. Intravenous fluids should be administered judiciously and an adequate airway maintained. Electrocardiographic monitoring should be instituted and the patient carefully observed for the development of arrhythmias; if required, appropriate anti-arrhythmic therapy should be given. The possibility that the patient may have taken other drugs as well as SINEMET should be taken into consideration. To date, no experience has been reported with dialysis; hence, its value in overdosage is not known.

Based on studies in which high doses of levodopa and/or carbidopa were administered, a significant proportion of rats and mice given single oral doses of levodopa of approximately 1500–2000 mg/kg are expected to die. A significant proportion of infant rats of both sexes are expected to die at a dose of 800 mg/kg. A significant proportion of rats are expected to die after treatment with similar doses of carbidopa. The addition of carbidopa in a 1:10 ratio with levodopa increases the dose at which a significant proportion of mice are expected to die to 3360 mg/kg.

DOSAGE AND ADMINISTRATION

The optimum daily dosage of SINEMET must be determined by careful titration in each patient. SINEMET tablets are available in a 1:4 ratio of carbidopa to levodopa (SINEMET 25-100) as well as 1:10 ratio (SINEMET 25-250 and SINEMET 10-100). Tablets of the two ratios may be given separately or combined as needed to provide the optimum dosage.

Studies show that peripheral dopa decarboxylase is saturated by carbidopa at approximately 70 to 100 mg a day. Patients receiving less than this amount of carbidopa are more likely to experience nausea and vomiting.

Usual Initial Dosage

Dosage is best initiated with one tablet of SINEMET 25-100 three times a day. This dosage schedule provides 75 mg of carbidopa per day. Dosage may be increased by one tablet every day or every other day, as necessary, until a dosage of eight tablets of SINEMET 25-100 a day is reached.

If SINEMET 10-100 is used, dosage may be initiated with one tablet three or four times a day. However, this will not provide an adequate amount of carbidopa for many patients. Dosage may be increased by one tablet every day or every other day until a total of eight tablets (2 tablets q.i.d.) is reached.

How to Transfer Patients from Levodopa

Levodopa must be discontinued at least twelve hours before starting SINEMET (Carbidopa-Levodopa). A daily dosage of SINEMET should be chosen that will provide approximately 25 percent of the previous levodopa dosage. Patients who are taking less than 1500 mg of levodopa a day should be started on one tablet of SINEMET 25-100 three or four times a day. The suggested starting dosage for most patients taking more than 1500 mg of levodopa is one tablet of SINEMET 25-250 three or four times a day.

Maintenance

Therapy should be individualized and adjusted according to the desired therapeutic response. At least 70 to 100 mg of carbidopa per day should be provided. When a greater proportion of carbidopa is required, one tablet of SINEMET 25-100 may be substituted for each tablet of SINEMET 10-100. When more levodopa is required, SINEMET 25-250 should be substituted for SINEMET 25-100 or SINEMET 10-100. If necessary, the dosage of SINEMET 25-250 may be increased by one-half or one tablet every day or every other day to a maximum of eight tablets a day. Experience with total daily dosages of carbidopa greater than 200 mg is limited.

Because both therapeutic and adverse responses occur more rapidly with SINEMET than with levodopa alone, patients should be monitored closely during the dose adjustment period. Specifically, involuntary movements will occur more rapidly with SINEMET than with levodopa. The occurrence of involuntary movements may require dosage reduction. Blepharospasm may be a useful early sign of excess dosage in some patients.

Addition of Other Antiparkinsonian Medications

Standard drugs for Parkinson's disease, other than levodopa without a decarboxylase inhibitor, may be used concomitantly while SINEMET is being administered, although dosage adjustments may be required.

Interruption of Therapy

Sporadic cases of a symptom complex resembling Neuroleptic Malignant Syndrome (NMS) have been associated with dose reductions and withdrawal of SINEMET. Patients should be observed carefully if abrupt reduction or discontinuation of SINEMET is required, especially if the patient is receiving neuroleptics. (See WARNINGS.)

If general anesthesia is required, SINEMET may be continued as long as the patient is permitted to take fluids and medication by mouth. If therapy is interrupted temporarily, the patient should be observed for symptoms resembling NMS, and the usual daily dosage may be administered as soon as the patient is able to take oral medication.

HOW SUPPLIED

Tablets SINEMET 25-100 are yellow, oval, uncoated tablets, that are scored and coded 650 on one side and SINEMET on the other side. They are supplied as follows:

NDC 0056-0650-68 bottles of 100

NDC 0056-0650-28 unit dose packages of 100.

Tablets SINEMET 10-100 are dark dapple-blue, oval, uncoated tablets, that are scored and coded 647 on one side and SINEMET on the other side. They are supplied as follows:

NDC 0056-0647-68 bottles of 100

NDC 0056-0647-28 unit dose packages of 100.

Tablets SINEMET 25-250 are light dapple-blue, oval, uncoated tablets, that are scored and coded 654 on one side and SINEMET on the other side. They are supplied as follows:

NDC 0056-0654-68 bottles of 100

NDC 0056-0654-28 unit dose packages of 100.

Storage

Tablets SINEMET 10-100 and Tablets SINEMET 25-250 must be protected from light.

Manufactured by:

MERCK & CO., INC.

WEST POINT, PA 19486, USA

For:

DuPont Pharma

Wilmington, Delaware 19880

6350-3/November 1997

Shown in Product Identification Guide, page 309

*Registered trademark of MERCK & CO., INC.

COPYRIGHT © MERCK & CO., INC. 1996.

All rights reserved

SINEMET® CR   ℞

(CARBIDOPA-LEVODOPA)

SUSTAINED-RELEASE TABLETS

DESCRIPTION

SINEMET* CR (Carbidopa-Levodopa) is a sustained-release combination of carbidopa and levodopa for the treatment of Parkinson's disease and syndrome.

Carbidopa, an inhibitor of aromatic amino acid decarboxylation, is a white, crystalline compound, slightly soluble in water, with a molecular weight of 244.3. It is designated chemically as (-)-*L*-α-hydrazino-α-methyl-β-(3,4-dihydroxybenzene) propanoic acid monohydrate. Its empirical formula is $C_{10}H_{14}N_2O_4 \cdot H_2O$ and its structural formula is:

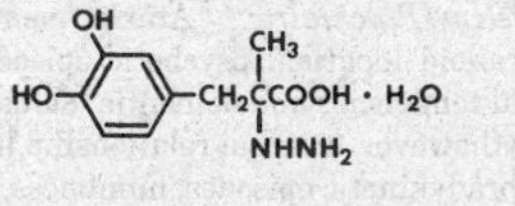

Tablet content is expressed in terms of anhydrous carbidopa, which has a molecular weight of 226.3.

Levodopa, an aromatic amino acid, is a white, crystalline compound, slightly soluble in water, with a molecular weight of 197.2. It is designated chemically as (-)-*L*-α-amino-β-(3,4-dihydroxybenzene) propanoic acid. Its empirical formula is $C_9H_{11}NO_4$ and its structural formula is:

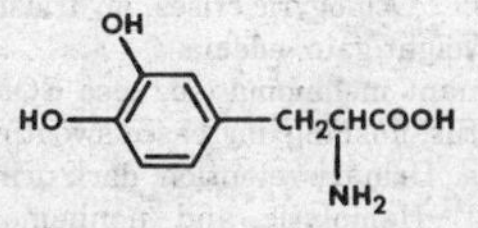

SINEMET CR is supplied as sustained-release tablets containing either 50 mg of carbidopa and 200 mg of levodopa, or 25 mg of carbidopa and 100 mg of levodopa. Inactive ingredients: hydroxypropyl cellulose, polyvinylacetate-crotonic acid copolymer, magnesium stearate and red ferric oxide. SINEMET CR 50–200 also contains D&C Yellow 10.

The 50–200 tablet is supplied as an oval, scored, biconvex, compressed tablet that is peach colored. The 25–100 tablet is supplied as an oval, biconvex, compressed tablet that is pink colored. The SINEMET CR tablet is a polymeric-based drug delivery system that controls the release of carbidopa and levodopa as it slowly erodes. SINEMET CR 25–100 is available to facilitate titration and as an alternative to the half-tablet of SINEMET CR 50–200.

CLINICAL PHARMACOLOGY

Mechanism of Action

Parkinson's disease is a progressive, neurodegenerative disorder of the extrapyramidal nervous system affecting the mobility and control of the skeletal muscular system. Its characteristic features include resting tremor, rigidity, and bradykinetic movements. Symptomatic treatments, such as levodopa therapies, may permit the patient better mobility.

Current evidence indicates that symptoms of Parkinson's disease are related to depletion of dopamine in the corpus striatum. Administration of dopamine is ineffective in the treatment of Parkinson's disease apparently because it does not cross the blood-brain barrier. However, levodopa, the metabolic precursor of dopamine, does cross the blood-brain barrier, and presumably is converted to dopamine in the brain. This is thought to be the mechanism whereby levodopa relieves symptoms of Parkinson's disease.

Pharmacodynamics

When levodopa is administered orally it is rapidly decarboxylated to dopamine in extracerebral tissues so that only a small portion of a given dose is transported unchanged to the central nervous system. For this reason, large doses of levodopa are required for adequate therapeutic effect and these may often be accompanied by nausea and other adverse reactions, some of which are attributable to dopamine formed in extracerebral tissues.

Since levodopa competes with certain amino acids for transport across the gut wall, the absorption of levodopa may be impaired in some patients on a high protein diet.

Carbidopa inhibits decarboxylation of peripheral levodopa. It does not cross the blood-brain barrier and does not affect the metabolism of levodopa within the central nervous system.

Since its decarboxylase inhibiting activity is limited to extracerebral tissues, administration of carbidopa with levodopa makes more levodopa available for transport to the brain.

Patients treated with levodopa therapy for Parkinson's disease may develop motor fluctuations characterized by end-of-dose failure, peak dose dyskinesia, and akinesia. The advanced form of motor fluctuations ('on-off' phenomenon) is characterized by unpredictable swings from mobility to immobility. Although the causes of the motor fluctuations are not completely understood, in some patients they may be attenuated by treatment regimens that produce steady plasma levels of levodopa.

SINEMET CR contains either 50 mg of carbidopa and 200 mg of levodopa, or 25 mg of carbidopa and 100 mg of levodopa in a sustained-release dosage form designed to release these ingredients over a 4- to 6-hour period. With SINEMET CR there is less variation in plasma levodopa levels than with SINEMET* (Carbidopa-Levodopa), the conventional formulation. *However, SINEMET CR (Carbidopa-Levodopa, Sustained-Release) is less systemically bioavailable than SINEMET (Carbidopa-Levodopa) and may require increased daily doses to achieve the same level of symptomatic relief as provided by SINEMET (Carbidopa-Levodopa).*

In clinical trials, patients with moderate to severe motor fluctuations who received SINEMET CR *did not experience quantitatively significant reductions* in 'off' time when compared to SINEMET (Carbidopa-Levodopa). However, global ratings of improvement as assessed by both patient and physician were better during therapy with SINEMET CR than with SINEMET (Carbidopa-Levodopa). In patients without motor fluctuations, SINEMET CR, under controlled conditions, provided the same therapeutic benefit with less frequent dosing when compared to SINEMET (Carbidopa-Levodopa).

Pharmacokinetics

Carbidopa reduces the amount of levodopa required to produce a given response by about 75 percent and, when administered with levodopa, increases both plasma levels and the plasma half-life of levodopa, and decreases plasma and urinary dopamine and homovanillic acid.

Elimination half-life of levodopa in the presence of carbidopa is about 1.5 hours. Following SINEMET CR, the apparent half-life of levodopa may be prolonged because of continuous absorption.

In healthy elderly subjects (56–67 years old) the mean time to peak concentration of levodopa after a single dose of SINEMET CR 50–200 was about 2 hours as compared to 0.5 hours after standard SINEMET (Carbidopa-Levodopa). The maximum concentration of levodopa after a single dose of SINEMET CR was about 35% of the standard SINEMET (Carbidopa-Levodopa) (1151 vs 3256 ng/mL). The extent of availability of levodopa from SINEMET CR was about 70–75% relative to intravenous levodopa or standard SINEMET (Carbidopa-Levodopa) in the elderly. The absolute bioavailability of levodopa from SINEMET CR (relative to I.V.) in young subjects was shown to be only about 44%. The extent of availability and the peak concentrations of levodopa were comparable in the elderly after a single dose and at steady state after t.i.d. administration of SINEMET CR 50–200. In elderly subjects, the average trough levels of levodopa at steady state after the CR tablet were about 2 fold higher than after the standard SINEMET (Carbidopa-Levodopa) (163 vs 74 ng/mL).

In these studies, using similar total daily doses of levodopa, plasma levodopa concentrations with SINEMET CR fluctuated in a narrower range than with SINEMET (Carbidopa-Levodopa). Because the bioavailability of levodopa from SINEMET CR relative to SINEMET (Carbidopa-Levodopa) is approximately 70–75%, the daily dosage of levodopa necessary to produce a given clinical response with the sustained-release formulation will usually be higher.

The extent of availability and peak concentrations of levodopa after a single dose of SINEMET CR 50–200 increased by about 50% and 25%, respectively, when administered with food.

Pyridoxine hydrochloride (vitamin B_6), in oral doses of 10 mg to 25 mg, may reverse the effects of levodopa by increasing the rate of aromatic amino acid decarboxylation. Carbidopa inhibits this action of pyridoxine.

INDICATIONS AND USAGE

SINEMET CR is indicated in the treatment of the symptoms of idiopathic Parkinson's disease (paralysis agitans), postencephalitic parkinsonism, and symptomatic parkinsonism which may follow injury to the nervous system by carbon monoxide intoxication and/or manganese intoxication.

CONTRAINDICATIONS

Nonselective MAO inhibitors are contraindicated for use with SINEMET CR. These inhibitors must be discontinued at least two weeks prior to initiating therapy with SINEMET CR. SINEMET CR may be administered concomitantly with the manufacturer's recommended dose of an MAO inhibitor with selectivity for MAO type B (e.g., selegiline HCl).

SINEMET CR is contraindicated in patients with known hypersensitivity to any component of this drug and in patients with narrow-angle glaucoma.

Because levodopa may activate a malignant melanoma, SINEMET CR should not be used in patients with suspicious, undiagnosed skin lesions or a history of melanoma.

WARNINGS

When patients are receiving levodopa without a decarboxylase inhibitor, levodopa must be discontinued at least twelve hours before SINEMET CR is started. In order to reduce adverse reactions, it is necessary to individualize therapy. SINEMET CR should be substituted at a dosage that will provide approximately 25 percent of the previous levodopa dosage (see DOSAGE AND ADMINISTRATION).

Carbidopa does not decrease adverse reactions due to central effects of levodopa. By permitting more levodopa to reach the brain, particularly when nausea and vomiting is not a dose-limiting factor, certain adverse CNS effects, e.g., dyskinesias, will occur at lower dosages and sooner during therapy with SINEMET CR (Carbidopa-Levodopa. Sustained-Release) than with levodopa alone.

Patients receiving SINEMET CR may develop increased dyskinesias compared to SINEMET (Carbidopa-Levodopa). Dyskinesias are a common side effect of carbidopa-levodopa treatment. The occurrence of dyskinesias may require dosage reduction.

As with levodopa, SINEMET CR may cause mental disturbances. These reactions are thought to be due to increased brain dopamine following administration of levodopa. All patients should be observed carefully for the development of depression with concomitant suicidal tendencies. Patients with past or current psychoses should be treated with caution.

SINEMET CR should be administered cautiously to patients with severe cardiovascular or pulmonary disease, bronchial asthma, renal, hepatic or endocrine disease.

As with levodopa, care should be exercised in administering SINEMET CR to patients with a history of myocardial infarction who have residual atrial, nodal, or ventricular arrhythmias. In such patients, cardiac function should be monitored with particular care during the period of initial dosage adjustment, in a facility with provisions for intensive cardiac care.

As with levodopa, treatment with SINEMET CR may increase the possibility of upper gastrointestinal hemorrhage in patients with a history of peptic ulcer.

Neuroleptic Malignant Syndrome (NMS): Sporadic cases of a symptom complex resembling NMS have been reported in association with dose reductions or withdrawal of SINEMET and SINEMET CR.

Therefore, patients should be observed carefully when the dosage of SINEMET CR is reduced abruptly or discontinued, especially if the patient is receiving neuroleptics.

NMS is an uncommon but life-threatening syndrome characterized by fever or hyperthermia. Neurological findings, including muscle rigidity, involuntary movements, altered consciousness, mental status changes; other disturbances, such as autonomic dysfunction, tachycardia, tachypnea, sweating, hyper- or hypotension; laboratory findings, such as creatine phosphokinase elevation, leukocytosis, myoglobinuria, and increased serum myoglobin have been reported.

The early diagnosis of this condition is important for the appropriate management of these patients. Considering NMS as a possible diagnosis and ruling out other acute illnesses (e.g., pneumonia, systemic infection, etc.) is essential. This may be especially complex if the clinical presentation includes both serious medical illness and untreated or inadequately treated extrapyramidal signs and symptoms (EPS). Other important considerations in the differential diagnosis include central anticholinergic toxicity, heat stroke, drug fever, and primary central nervous system (CNS) pathology.

The management of NMS should include: 1) intensive symptomatic treatment and medical monitoring and 2) treatment of any concomitant serious medical problems for which specific treatments are available. Dopamine agonists, such as bromocriptine, and muscle relaxants, such as dantrolene, are often used in the treatment of NMS; however, their effectiveness has not been demonstrated in controlled studies.

PRECAUTIONS

General

As with levodopa, periodic evaluations of hepatic, hematopoietic, cardiovascular, and renal function are recommended during extended therapy.

Patients with chronic wide-angle glaucoma may be treated cautiously with SINEMET CR provided the intraocular pressure is well controlled and the patient is monitored carefully for changes in intraocular pressure during therapy.

Information for Patients

The patient should be informed that SINEMET CR is a sustained-release formulation of carbidopa-levodopa which releases these ingredients over a 4- to 6-hour period. It is important that SINEMET CR be taken at regular intervals according to the schedule outlined by the physician. The patient should be cautioned not to change the prescribed dosage regimen and not to add any additional antiparkinson medications, including other carbidopa-levodopa preparations, without first consulting the physician.

If abnormal involuntary movements appear or get worse during treatment with SINEMET CR, the physician should be notified, as dosage adjustment may be necessary.

Patients should be advised that sometimes the onset of effect of the first morning dose of SINEMET CR may be delayed for up to 1 hour compared with the response usually obtained from the first morning dose of SINEMET (Carbidopa-Levodopa). The physician should be notified if such delayed responses pose a problem in treatment.

Patients should be advised that, occasionally, dark color (red, brown, or black) may appear in saliva, urine, or sweat after ingestion of SINEMET CR. Although the color appears to be clinically insignificant, garments may become discolored.

The patient should be informed that a change in diet to foods that are high in protein may delay the absorption of

Continued on next page

Sinemet CR—Cont.

levodopa and may reduce the amount taken up in circulation. Excessive acidity also delays stomach emptying, thus delaying the absorption of levodopa. Iron salts (such as in multi-vitamin tablets) may also reduce the amount of levodopa available to the body. The above factors may reduce the clinical effectiveness of the levodopa or carbidopa-levodopa therapy.

Patients must be advised that the whole or half tablet should be swallowed without chewing or crushing.

NOTE: The suggested advice to patients being treated with SINEMET CR is intended to aid in the safe and effective use of this medication. It is not a disclosure of all possible adverse or intended effects.

Laboratory Tests

Abnormalities in laboratory tests may include elevations of liver function tests such as alkaline phosphatase, SGOT (AST), SGPT (ALT), lactic dehydrogenase, and bilirubin. Abnormalities in blood urea nitrogen and positive Coombs test have also been reported. Commonly, levels of blood urea nitrogen, creatinine, and uric acid are lower during administration of carbidopa-levodopa preparations than with levodopa.

Carbidopa-levodopa preparations, such as SINEMET (Carbidopa-Levodopa) and SINEMET CR, may cause a false-positive reaction for urinary ketone bodies when a test tape is used for determination of ketonuria. This reaction will not be altered by boiling the urine specimen. False-negative tests may result with the use of glucose-oxidase methods of testing for glucosuria.

Cases of falsely diagnosed pheochromocytoma in patients on carbidopa-levodopa therapy have been reported very rarely. Caution should be exercised when interpreting the plasma and urine levels of catecholamines and their metabolites in patients on levodopa or carbidopa-levodopa therapy.

Drug Interactions

Caution should be exercised when the following drugs are administered concomitantly with SINEMET CR (Carbidopa-Levodopa, Sustained-Release).

Symptomatic postural hypotension has occurred when carbidopa-levodopa preparations were added to the treatment of patients receiving some antihypertensive drugs. Therefore, when therapy with SINEMET CR is started, dosage adjustment of the antihypertensive drug may be required.

For patients receiving monoamine oxidase (MAO) inhibitors (Type A or B), see CONTRAINDICATIONS.

There have been rare reports of adverse reactions, including hypertension and dyskinesia, resulting from the concomitant use of tricyclic antidepressants and carbidopa-levodopa preparations.

Phenothiazines, butyrophenones and isoniazid may reduce the therapeutic effects of levodopa. In addition, the beneficial effects of levodopa in Parkinson's disease have been reported to be reversed by phenytoin and papaverine. Patients taking these drugs with SINEMET CR should be carefully observed for loss of therapeutic response.

Iron salts may reduce the bioavailability of levodopa and carbidopa. The clinical relevance is unclear.

Although metoclopramide may increase the bioavailability of levodopa by increasing gastric emptying, metoclopramide may also adversely affect disease control by its dopamine receptor antagonistic properties.

Carcinogenesis, Mutagenesis, Impairment of Fertility

In a two-year bioassay of SINEMET (Carbidopa-Levodopa), no evidence of carcinogenicity was found in rats receiving doses of approximately two times the maximum daily human dose of carbidopa and four times the maximum daily human dose of levodopa (equivalent to 8 SINEMET CR tablets).

In reproduction studies with SINEMET (Carbidopa-Levodopa), no effects on fertility were found in rats receiving doses of approximately two times the maximum daily human dose of carbidopa and four times the maximum daily human dose of levodopa (equivalent to 8 SINEMET CR tablets).

Pregnancy

Pregnancy Category C. No teratogenic effects were observed in a study in mice receiving up to 20 times the maximum recommended human dose of SINEMET (Carbidopa-Levodopa). There was a decrease in the number of live pups delivered by rats receiving approximately two times the maximum recommended human dose of carbidopa and approximately five times the maximum recommended human dose of levodopa during organogenesis. SINEMET (Carbidopa-Levodopa) caused both visceral and skeletal malformations in rabbits at all doses and ratios of carbidopa/levodopa tested, which ranged from 10 times/5 times the maximum recommended human dose of carbidopa/levodopa to 20 times/10 times the maximum recommended human dose of carbidopa/levodopa.

There are no adequate or well-controlled studies in pregnant women. It has been reported from individual cases that levodopa crosses the human placental barrier, enters the fetus, and is metabolized. Carbidopa concentrations in fetal tissue appeared to be minimal. Use of SINEMET CR in women of childbearing potential requires that the anticipated benefits of the drug be weighed against possible hazards to mother and child.

Nursing Mothers

It is not known whether this drug is excreted in human milk. Because many drugs are excreted in human milk, caution should be exercised when SINEMET CR is administered to a nursing woman.

Pediatric Use

Safety and effectiveness in pediatric patients have not been established. Use of the drug in patients below the age of 18 is not recommended.

ADVERSE REACTIONS

In controlled clinical trials, patients predominantly with moderate to severe motor fluctuations while on SINEMET (Carbidopa-Levodopa) were randomized to therapy with either SINEMET (Carbidopa-Levodopa) or SINEMET CR. The adverse experience frequency profile of SINEMET CR did not differ substantially from that of SINEMET (Carbidopa-Levodopa), as shown in Table I.

Table I.
Clinical Adverse Experiences Occurring in 1% or Greater of Patients

Adverse Experience	SINEMET CR n=491 %	SINEMET (Carbidopa-Levodopa) n=524 %
Dyskinesia	16.5	12.2
Nausea	5.5	5.7
Hallucinations	3.9	3.2
Confusion	3.7	2.3
Dizziness	2.9	2.3
Depression	2.2	1.3
Urinary tract infection	2.2	2.3
Headache	2.0	1.9
Dream abnormalities	1.8	0.8
Dystonia	1.8	0.8
Vomiting	1.8	1.9
Upper respiratory infection	1.8	1.0
Dyspnea	1.6	0.4
'On-Off' phenomena	1.6	1.1
Back pain	1.6	0.6
Dry mouth	1.4	1.1
Anorexia	1.2	1.1
Diarrhea	1.2	0.6
Insomnia	1.2	1.0
Orthostatic hypotension	1.0	1.1
Shoulder pain	1.0	0.6
Chest pain	1.0	0.8
Muscle cramps	0.8	1.0
Paresthesia	0.8	1.1
Urinary frequency	0.8	1.1
Dyspepsia	0.6	1.1
Constipation	0.2	1.5

Abnormal laboratory findings occurring at a frequency of 1% or greater in approximately 443 patients who received SINEMET CR and 475 who received SINEMET (Carbidopa-Levodopa) during controlled clinical trials included: decreased hemoglobin and hematocrit; elevated serum glucose; white blood cells, bacteria and blood in the urine.

The adverse experiences observed in patients in uncontrolled studies were similar to those seen in controlled clinical studies.

Other adverse experiences reported overall in clinical trials in 748 patients treated with SINEMET CR, listed by body system in order of decreasing frequency, include:

Nervous System / Psychiatric: Chorea, somnolence, falling, anxiety disorder, disorientation, decreased mental acuity, gait abnormalities, extrapyramidal disorder, agitation, nervousness, sleep disorders, memory impairment.

Body as a Whole: Asthenia, fatigue, abdominal pain, orthostatic effects.

Digestive: Gastrointestinal pain, dysphagia, heartburn.

Cardiovascular: Palpitation, essential hypertension, hypotension, myocardial infarction.

Special Senses: Blurred vision.

Metabolic: Weight loss.

Skin: Rash.

Respiratory: Cough, pharyngeal pain, common cold.

Urogenital: Urinary incontinence.

Musculoskeletal: Leg pain.

Laboratory Tests: Decreased white blood cell count and serum potassium; increased BUN, serum creatinine and serum LDH; protein and glucose in the urine.

The following other adverse experiences have been reported with SINEMET CR:

Cardiovascular: Cardiac irregularities, syncope.

Nervous System / Psychiatric: Increased tremor, peripheral neuropathy.

Gastrointestinal: Taste alterations.

Skin: Alopecia.

Other adverse reactions that have been reported with levodopa alone and with various carbidopa-levodopa formulations and may occur with SINEMET CR are:

Nervous System / Psychiatric: Ataxia, mental changes including paranoid ideation, psychotic episodes, depression with suicidal tendencies and dementia; delusions, euphoria, convulsions (however, a causal relationship has not been established); bradykinetic episodes, numbness, muscle twitching, blepharospasm (which may be taken as an early sign of excess dosage; consideration of dosage reduction may be made at this time), trismus, activation of latent Horner's syndrome, nightmares.

Gastrointestinal: Gastrointestinal bleeding, development of duodenal ulcer, dark saliva, sialorrhea, bruxism, hiccups, flatulence, burning sensation of tongue.

Cardiovascular: Phlebitis

Special Senses: Oculogyric crises, mydriasis, diplopia.

Metabolic: Weight gain, edema.

Skin: Malignant melanoma (see also CONTRAINDICATIONS), pruritus, flushing, increased sweating, dark sweat.

Genitourinary: Urinary retention, dark urine, priapism.

Hematologic: Hemolytic and nonhemolytic anemia, thrombocytopenia, leukopenia, agranulocytosis.

Hypersensitivity: Henoch-Schonlein purpura.

Laboratory Tests: Abnormalities in alkaline phophatase, SGOT (AST), SGPT (ALT), bilirubin, Coombs test.

Miscellaneous: Faintness, hoarseness, malaise, hot flashes, sense of stimulation, bizarre breathing patterns, neuroleptic malignant syndrome.

OVERDOSAGE

Management of acute overdosage with SINEMET CR is the same as with levodopa. Pyridoxine is not effective in reversing the actions of SINEMET CR.

General supportive measures should be employed, along with immediate gastric lavage. Intravenous fluids should be administered judiciously and an adequate airway maintained. Electrocardiographic monitoring should be instituted and the patient carefully observed for the development of arrhythmias; if required, appropriate antiarrhythmic therapy should be given. The possibility that the patient may have taken other drugs as well as SINEMET CR should be taken into consideration. To date, no experience has been reported with dialysis; hence, its value in overdosage is not known.

Based on studies in which high doses of levodopa and/or carbidopa were administered, a significant proportion of rats and mice given single oral doses of levodopa of approximately 1500–2000 mg/kg are expected to die. A significant proportion of infant rats of both sexes are expected to die at a dose of 800 mg/kg. A significant proportion of rats are expected to die after treatment with similar doses of carbidopa. The addition of carbidopa in a 1:10 ratio with levodopa increases the dose at which a significant proportion of mice are expected to die to 3360 mg/kg.

DOSAGE AND ADMINISTRATION

SINEMET CR contains carbidopa and levodopa in a 1:4 ratio as either the 50–200 tablet or the 25–100 tablet. The daily dosage of SINEMET CR must be determined by careful titration. Patients should be monitored closely during the dose adjustment period, particularly with regard to appearance or worsening of involuntary movements, dyskinesias or nausea. SINEMET CR 50–200 may be administered as whole or as half-tablets which should not be chewed or crushed. SINEMET CR 25–100 may be used in combination with SINEMET CR 50–200 to titrate to the optimum dosage, or as an alternative to the 50–200 half tablet.

Standard drugs for Parkinson's disease, other than levodopa without a decarboxylase inhibitor, may be used concomitantly while SINEMET CR is being administered, although their dosage may have to be adjusted.

Since carbidopa prevents the reversal of levodopa effects caused by pyridoxine, SINEMET CR can be given to patients receiving supplemental pyridoxine (vitamin B_6).

Initial Dosage

Patients currently treated with conventional carbidopa-levodopa preparations: Dosage with SINEMET CR should be substituted at an amount that provides approximately 10% more levodopa per day, although this may need to be increased to a dosage that provides up to 30% more levodopa per day depending on clinical response (see DOSAGE AND ADMINISTRATION, *Titration*). The interval between doses of SINEMET CR should be 4–8 hours during the waking day. (See CLINICAL PHARMACOLOGY, *Pharmacodynamics.*)

A guideline for initiation of SINEMET CR is shown in Table II.

Table II.
Guidelines for Initial Conversion
from SINEMET (Carbidopa-Levodopa) to SINEMET CR

SINEMET (Carbidopa-Levodopa) Total Daily Dose* Levodopa (mg)	SINEMET CR Suggested Dosage Regimen
300–400	200 mg b.i.d.
500–600	300 mg b.i.d. or 200 mg t.i.d.
700–800	A total of 800 mg in 3 or more divided doses (e.g., 300 mg a.m., 300 mg early p.m. and 200 mg later p.m.)
900–1000	A total of 1000 mg in 3 or more divided doses (e.g., 400 mg a.m., 400 mg early p.m., and 200 mg later p.m.)

* For dosing ranges not shown in the table see DOSAGE AND ADMINISTRATION, *Initial Dosage—Patients currently treated with conventional carbidopa-levodopa preparations.*

Patients currently treated with levodopa without a decarboxylase inhibitor: Levodopa must be discontinued at least twelve hours before therapy with SINEMET CR is started. SINEMET CR should be substituted at a dosage that will provide approximately 25% of the previous levodopa dosage. In patients with mild to moderate disease, the initial dose is usually 1 tablet of SINEMET CR 50–200 b.i.d.
Patients not receiving levodopa: In patients with mild to moderate disease, the initial recommended dose is 1 tablet of SINEMET CR 50-200 b.i.d. Initial dosage should not be given at intervals of less than 6 hours.
Titration with SINEMET CR
Following initiation of therapy, doses and dosing intervals may be increased or decreased depending upon therapeutic response. Most patients have been adequately treated with doses of SINEMET CR that provide 400 to 1600 mg of levodopa per day, administered as divided doses at intervals ranging from 4 to 8 hours during the waking day. Higher doses of SINEMET CR (2400 mg or more of levodopa per day) and shorter intervals (less than 4 hours) have been used, but are not usually recommended.
When doses of SINEMET CR are given at intervals of less than 4 hours, and/or if the divided doses are not equal, it is recommended that the smaller doses be given at the end of the day.
An interval of at least 3 days between dosage adjustments is recommended.
Maintenance
Because Parkinson's disease is progressive, periodic clinical evaluations are recommended; adjustment of the dosage regimen of SINEMET CR may be required.
Addition of Other Antiparkinson Medications
Anticholinergic agents, dopamine agonists, and amantadine can be given with SINEMET CR. Dosage adjustment of SINEMET CR may be necessary when these agents are added.
A dose of SINEMET (Carbidopa-Levodopa) 25–100 or 10–100 (one half or a whole tablet) can be added to the dosage regimen of SINEMET CR in selected patients with advanced disease who need additional immediate-release levodopa for a brief time during daytime hours.
Interruption of Therapy
Sporadic cases of a symptom complex resembling Neuroleptic Malignant Syndrome (NMS) have been associated with dose reductions and withdrawal of SINEMET (Carbidopa-Levodopa) or SINEMET CR.
Patients should be observed carefully if abrupt reduction or discontinuation of SINEMET CR is required, especially if the patient is receiving neuroleptics. (See WARNINGS).
If general anesthesia is required, SINEMET CR may be continued as long as the patient is permitted to take oral medication. If therapy is interrupted temporarily, the patient should be observed for symptoms resembling NMS, and the usual dosage should be administered as soon as the patient is able to take oral medication.

HOW SUPPLIED

SINEMET CR 50–200 (Carbidopa-Levodopa) SUSTAINED-RELEASE TABLETS containing 50 mg of carbidopa and 200 mg of levodopa, are peach colored, oval, biconvex, compressed tablets, that are scored and coded 521 on one side and SINEMET CR on the other side. They are supplied as follows:
NDC 0056-0521-68 bottles of 100
(6505-01-343-3482, 100's)
NDC 0056-0521-28 unit dose package of 100.
(6505-01-343-3483, individually sealed 100's).
SINEMET CR 25–100 (Carbidopa-Levodopa) SUSTAINED-RELEASE TABLETS containing 25 mg carbidopa and 100 mg of levodopa, are pink colored, oval, biconvex, compressed

tablets, that are coded 601 (with bar) on one side and SINEMET CR on the other side. They are supplied as follows:
NDC 0056-0601-68 bottles of 100
NDC 0056-0601-28 unit dose packages of 100.
Storage
Avoid temperatures above 30°C (86°F). Store in a tightly closed container.
Manufactured by:
MERCK & CO., INC.
WEST POINT, PA 19486, USA
For:
DuPont Pharma
Wilmington, Delaware 19880
6351-3   Issued November 1997
Shown in Product Identification Guide, page 309

---

* Registered trademark of MERCK & CO., INC.
COPYRIGHT © MERCK & CO INC. 18916
All rights reserved

The following material is provided as an educational service to all healthcare professionals:

EDUCATIONAL MATERIAL

COUMADIN® (Warfarin Sodium Tablets, USP) Crystalline

Books/Booklets/Brochures
"COUMADIN® Patient Aid". This booklet explains key points of anticoagulation therapy, how it affects the patient's lifestyle, warning signs, and Vitamin K information. It also includes a COUMADIN® ID card and a dosage calendar. Available in English and Spanish.
"Multilingual Patient Support". Important facts about COUMADIN® therapy are translated into 50 languages in this booklet. Key points include: reporting problems, having blood tested and following the prescribed weekly schedule.
"Atrial Fibriwhat ? Brochure". This easy-to-read patient brochure outlines what atrial fibrillation is, the risks associated with the disorder, and treatment plans available in English and Spanish.

Video/Audio
"COUMADIN® Therapy and You". This 11 minute, $\frac{1}{2}$-inch VHS video is designed to be shown by the physician to his/her patients on COUMADIN® in order to increase patient commitment and understanding of COUMADIN® therapy. An audiocassette of the same program, "COUMADIN® Therapy and You," is available for patients to take home.

Both items are available in English and Spanish.

Charts
"COUMADIN® Patient Anticoagulation Flow Sheet". This laminated 8-$\frac{1}{2}$" × 11" chart provides a convenient way to record patient prothrombin times and COUMADIN® doses.
"COUMADIN® Patient Education Easel Flip Chart". An easel that allows the physician or nurse to educate the patient about COUMADIN® therapy in a practical question-and-answer format. Available in English and Spanish.

All of the above material is available at no charge to physicians, pharmacists, and other healthcare professionals involved with the management of patients on COUMADIN® therapy by calling 1-800-COUMADIN.

SINEMET®
(Carbidopa-Levodopa)
SINEMET® CR
(Carbidopa-Levodopa)
Sustained-Release Tablets

Booklets
"A Patient's Guide to Parkinson's Disease and Sinemet® CR (Carbidopa-Levopoda) Sustained Release" (CR-31412-2)
"Tips on taking Sinemet® CR" (CR-31414-02)
Available at no charge. Write DuPont Pharma and ask for materials by CR # or call (302) 992-4240.

REVIA® (naltrexone HCl tablets)
Booklets/Brochures
"REVIA® Patient Q & A". This booklet answers the most commonly asked questions about REVIA®.
"REVIA® Counselor Q & A". Answers most commonly asked question in a more detailed level for counselors. Provides information needed on how to use REVIA®.
"REVIA® Counselor Brochure". A practical implementation piece on what a counselor should see when using REVIA®. Effectively and completely communicates the features and benefits of REVIA®.

Dura Pharmaceuticals, Inc.
7475 LUSK BOULEVARD
SAN DIEGO, CA 92121

Direct Inquiries and
For Medical Information Contact:
Medical Affairs Department
(888) 859-8583
FAX: (619) 657-0977

For Sales Representatives requests Contact:
800-859-8586

CAPASTAT® SULFATE   Rx
STERILE CAPREOMYCIN SULFATE, USP
For Intramuscular and Intravenous Infusion Only

Not for Pediatric Use

WARNINGS
The use of Capastat® Sulfate (Sterile Capreomycin Sulfate, USP) in patients with renal insufficiency or preexisting auditory impairment must be undertaken with great caution, and the risk of additional cranial nerve VIII impairment or renal injury should be weighed against the benefits to be derived from therapy.
Refer to ANIMAL PHARMACOLOGY for additional information.
Since other parenteral antituberculosis agents (streptomycin, viomycin) also have similar and sometimes irreversible toxic effects, particularly on cranial nerve VIII and renal function, simultaneous administration of these agents with Capastat Sulfate is not recommended. Use with nonantituberculosis drugs (polymyxin A sulfate, colistin sulfate, amikacin, gentamicin, tobramycin, vancomycin, kanamycin, and neomycin) having ototoxic or nephrotoxic potential should be undertaken only with great caution.
Usage in Pregnancy: The safety of the use of Capastat Sulfate in pregnancy has not been determined.
Pediatric Usage: Safety and effectiveness in pediatric patients have not been established.

DESCRIPTION

Capastat Sulfate is a polypeptide antibiotic isolated from *Streptomyces capreolus*. It is a complex of 4 microbiologically active components which have been characterized in part; however, complete structural determination of all the components has not been established.
Capreomycin is supplied as the disulfate salt and is soluble in water. In complete solution, it is almost colorless.
Each vial contains the equivalent of 1 g capreomycin activity.
The structural formula is as follows:

	R	
Capreomycin IA	OH	$C_{25}H_{44}N_{14}O_8$
Capreomycin IB	H	$C_{25}H_{44}N_{14}O_7$

CLINICAL PHARMACOLOGY

Human Pharmacology: Capreomycin is not absorbed in significant quantities from the gastrointestinal tract and must be administered parenterally. In 2 studies of 10 patients each, peak serum concentrations following 1 g of capreomycin given intramuscularly were achieved 1 to 2 hours after administration, and average peak levels reached were 28 and 32 µg/mL respectively (range, 20 to 47 µg/mL). Low serum concentrations were present at 24 hours. However, 1 g of capreomycin daily for 30 days or more produced no significant accumulation in subjects with normal renal function. Two patients with marked reduction of renal function had high serum concentrations 24 hours after administra-

Continued on next page

Capastat Sulfate—Cont.

tion of the drug. When a 1-g dose of capreomycin was given intramuscularly to normal volunteers, 52% was excreted in the urine within 12 hours.

Lehmann, et al, examined the pharmacokinetics of single dose capreomycin (1.0 g) administered intramuscularly and by intravenous infusion (1 hour) in 6 healthy volunteers. The area under the serum concentration versus time curve was similar for the two routes of administration. Capreomycin peak concentrations after intravenous infusion were 30 ± 47% higher than after intramuscular administration.[1,2] Paper chromatographic studies indicated that capreomycin is excreted essentially unaltered. Urine concentrations averaged 1.68 µg/mL (average urine volume, 228 mL) during the 6 hours following a 1-g dose.

Microbiology: Capreomycin is active against strains of *Mycobacterium tuberculosis* found in humans.

Susceptibility Tests: The in vitro susceptibility of strains of *M. tuberculosis* to capreomycin varies with the media and techniques employed. In general, the minimum inhibitory concentrations for *M. tuberculosis* are lowest in liquid media that are free of egg protein (7H10 or Dubos) and range from 1 to 5 µg/mL when the indirect method is used. Comparable inhibitory concentrations are obtained when 7H10 agar is used for direct susceptibility testing. When indirect susceptibility tests are performed on standard tube slants with 7H10 media, susceptible strains are inhibited by 10 to 25 µg/mL capreomycin. Egg-containing media, such as Löwenstein-Jensen or ATS, require concentrations of 25 to 50 µg/mL to inhibit susceptible strains.

Cross-Resistance: Frequent cross-resistance occurs between capreomycin and viomycin. Varying degrees of cross-resistance between capreomycin and kanamycin and neomycin have been reported. No cross-resistance has been observed between capreomycin and isoniazid, aminosalicylic acid, cycloserine, streptomycin, ethionamide, or ethambutol.

INDICATIONS AND USAGE

Capastat Sulfate, which is to be used concomitantly with other appropriate antituberculosis agents, is indicated in pulmonary infections caused by capreomycin-susceptible strains of *M. tuberculosis* when the primary agents (isoniazid, rifampin, ethambutol, aminosalicylic acid, and streptomycin) have been ineffective or cannot be used because of toxicity or the presence of resistant tubercle bacilli.

Susceptibility studies should be performed to determine the presence of a capreomycin-susceptible strain of *M. tuberculosis*.

CONTRAINDICATION

Capastat Sulfate is contraindicated in patients who are hypersensitive to capreomycin.

PRECAUTIONS

General: Audiometric measurements and assessment of vestibular function should be performed prior to initiation of therapy with Capastat Sulfate and at regular intervals during treatment.

Renal injury, with tubular necrosis, elevation of the blood urea nitrogen (BUN) or serum creatinine, and abnormal urinary sediment, has been noted. Slight elevation of the BUN and serum creatinine has been observed in a significant number of patients receiving prolonged therapy. The appearance of casts, red cells, and white cells in the urine has been noted in a high percentage of these cases. Elevation of the BUN above 30 mg/100 mL or any other evidence of decreasing renal function with or without a rise in BUN levels calls for careful evaluation of the patient, and the dosage should be reduced or the drug completely withdrawn. The clinical significance of abnormal urine sediment and slight elevation in the BUN (or serum creatinine) observed during long-term therapy with Capastat Sulfate has not been established.

The peripheral neuromuscular blocking action that has been attributed to other polypeptide antibiotics (colistin sulfate, polymyxin A sulfate, paromomycin, and viomycin) and to aminoglycoside antibiotics (streptomycin, dihydrostreptomycin, neomycin, and kanamycin) has been studied with Capastat Sulfate. A partial neuromuscular blockade was demonstrated after large intravenous doses of Capastat Sulfate. This action was enhanced by ether anesthesia (as has been reported for neomycin) and was antagonized by neostigmine.

Caution should be exercised in the administration of antibiotics, including Capastat Sulfate, to any patient who has demonstrated some form of allergy, particularly to drugs.

Laboratory Tests: Regular tests of renal function should be made throughout the period of treatment, and reduced dosage should be employed in patients with known or suspected renal impairment.

Renal function studies should be made both before therapy with Capastat Sulfate is started and on a weekly basis during treatment.

Since hypokalemia may occur during therapy, serum potassium levels should be determined frequently.

Drug Interactions: For neuromuscular blocking action of this drug, *see* PRECAUTIONS, GENERAL.

Carcinogenesis, Mutagenesis, Impairment of Fertility: Studies have not been performed to determine potential for carcinogenicity, mutagenicity, or impairment of fertility.

Usage in Pregnancy—Pregnancy Category C: Capastat Sulfate has been shown to be teratogenic in rats when given in doses 3 1/2 times the human dose. There are no adequate and well-controlled studies in pregnant women. Capastat Sulfate should be used during pregnancy only if the potential benefit justifies the potential risk to the fetus (*see boxed* WARNINGS *and* ANIMAL PHARMACOLOGY).

Nursing Mothers: It is not known whether this drug is excreted in human milk. Because many drugs are excreted in human milk, caution should be exercised when Capastat Sulfate is administered to a nursing woman.

Pediatric Use: Safety and effectiveness in pediatric patients have not been established (*see boxed* WARNINGS).

ADVERSE REACTIONS

Nephrotoxicity: In 36% of 722 patients treated with Capastat Sulfate, elevation of the BUN above 20 mg/100 mL has been observed. In many instances, there was also depression of PSP excretion and abnormal urine sediment. In 10% of this series, the BUN elevation exceeded 30 mg/100 mL. Toxic nephritis was reported in 1 patient with tuberculosis and portal cirrhosis who was treated with Capastat Sulfate (1 g) and aminosalicylic acid daily for 1 month. This patient developed renal insufficiency and oliguria and died. Autopsy showed subsiding acute tubular necrosis.

Electrolyte disturbances resembling Bartter's syndrome have been reported in 1 patient.

Ototoxicity: Subclinical auditory loss was noted in approximately 11% of 722 patients undergoing treatment with Capastat Sulfate. This was a 5- to 10-decibel loss in the 4,000- to 8,000-CPS range. Clinically apparent hearing loss occurred in 3% of the 722 subjects. Some audiometric changes were reversible. Other cases with permanent loss were not progressive following withdrawal of Capastat Sulfate.

Tinnitus and vertigo have occurred.

Liver: Serial tests of liver function have demonstrated a decrease in BSP excretion without change in AST (SGOT) or ALT (SGPT) in the presence of preexisting liver disease. Abnormal results in liver function tests have occurred in many persons receiving Capastat Sulfate in combination with other antituberculosis agents that also are known to cause changes in hepatic function. The role of Capastat Sulfate in producing these abnormalities is not clear; however, periodic determinations of liver function are recommended.

Blood: Leukocytosis and leukopenia have been observed. The majority of patients treated have had eosinophilia exceeding 5% while receiving daily injections of Capastat Sulfate. This has subsided with reduction of the Capastat Sulfate dosage to 2 or 3 g weekly.

Pain and induration at the injection site have been observed. Excessive bleeding at the injection site has been reported. Sterile abscesses have been noted. Rare cases of thrombocytopenia have been reported.

Hypersensitivity: Urticaria and maculopapular skin rashes associated in some cases with febrile reactions have been reported when Capastat Sulfate and other antituberculosis drugs were given concomitantly.

OVERDOSAGE

Signs and Symptoms: Nephrotoxicity following the parenteral administration of Capastat Sulfate is most closely related to the area under the curve of the serum concentration versus time graph. The elderly patient, patients with abnormal renal function or dehydration, and patients receiving other nephrotoxic drugs are at much greater risk for developing acute tubular necrosis.

Damage to the auditory and vestibular divisions of cranial nerve VIII has been associated with Capastat Sulfate given to patients with abnormal renal function or dehydration and in those receiving medications with additive auditory toxicities. These patients often experience dizziness, tinnitus, vertigo, and a loss of high-tone acuity.

Neuromuscular blockage or respiratory paralysis may occur following rapid intravenous infusion.

If capreomycin is ingested, toxicity would be unlikely because it is poorly absorbed (less than 1%) from an intact gastrointestinal system.

Hypokalemia, hypocalcemia, hypomagnesemia, and an electrolyte disturbance resembling Bartter's syndrome have been reported to occur in patients with capreomycin toxicity. The subcutaneous median lethal dose in mice was 514 mg/kg.

Treatment: To obtain up-to-date information about the treatment of overdose, a good resource is your certified Regional Poison Control Center. Telephone numbers of certified poison control centers are listed in the *Physicians' Desk Reference (PDR)*. In managing overdosage, consider the possibility of multiple drug overdoses, interaction among drugs, and unusual drug kinetics in your patient.

Protect the patient's airway and support ventilation and perfusion. Meticulously monitor and maintain, within ac-

ceptable limits, the patient's vital signs, blood gases, serum electrolytes, etc. Absorption of drugs from the gastrointestinal tract may be decreased by giving activated charcoal, which, in many cases, is more effective than emesis or lavage; consider charcoal instead of or in addition to gastric emptying. Repeated doses of charcoal over time may hasten elimination of some drugs that have been absorbed. Safeguard the patient's airway when employing gastric emptying or charcoal.

Patients who have received an overdose of capreomycin and have normal renal function should be carefully hydrated to maintain a urine output of 3 to 5 mL/kg/h. Fluid balance, electrolytes, and creatinine clearance should be carefully monitored.

Hemodialysis may be effectively used to remove capreomycin in patients with significant renal disease.

DOSAGE AND ADMINISTRATION

Capastat Sulfate may be administered intramuscularly or intravenously following reconstitution. Reconstitution is achieved by dissolving the vial contents (1 g) in 2 mL of 0.9% Sodium Chloride Injection or Sterile Water for Injection. Two to 3 minutes should be allowed for complete dissolution.

Intravenously—For intravenous infusion, reconstituted Capastat Sulfate should be diluted in 100 mL of 0.9% Sodium Chloride Injection and administered over 60 minutes.

Intramuscularly—Reconstituted Capastat Sulfate should be given by deep intramuscular injection into a large muscle mass, since superficial injection may be associated with increased pain and the development of sterile abscesses.

For administration of a 1-g dose, the entire contents of the vial should be given. For doses lower than 1 g, the following dilution table may be used.

DILUTION TABLE

Diluent Added to 1-g, 10-mL Vial	Volume of Capastat Sulfate Solution	Concentration (Approx)
2.15 mL	2.85 mL	350 mg*/mL
2.63 mL	3.33 mL	300 mg*/mL
3.3 mL	4 mL	250 mg*/mL
4.3 mL	5 mL	200 mg*/mL

*Equivalent to capreomycin activity.

The solution may acquire a pale straw color and darken with time, but this is not associated with loss of potency or the development of toxicity. After reconstitution, all solutions of Capastat Sulfate may be stored for up to 24 hours under refrigeration.

Capreomycin is always administered in combination with at least 1 other antituberculosis agent to which the patient's strain of tubercle bacilli is susceptible. The usual dose is 1 g daily (not to exceed 20 mg/kg/day) given intramuscularly or intravenously for 60 to 120 days, followed by 1 g by either route 2 or 3 times weekly. (*Note*—Therapy for tuberculosis should be maintained for 12 to 24 months. If facilities for administering injectable medication are not available, a change to appropriate oral therapy is indicated on the patient's release from the hospital.)

Patients with reduced renal function should have dosage reduction based on creatinine clearance using the guidelines included in Table 1. These dosages are designed to achieve a mean steady-state capreomycin level of 10 µg/mL.

Table 1. Estimated Dosages to Attain Mean Steady-State Serum Capreomycin Concentration of 10 µg/mL (Based on Creatinine Clearance)

CrCl (mL/min)	Capreomycin Clearance (L/kg/h × 10⁻²)	Half-life (hours)	Doseᵃ (mg/kg) for the Following Dosing Intervals 24 h	48 h	72 h
0	0.54	55.5	1.29	2.58	3.87
10	1.01	29.4	2.43	4.87	7.30
20	1.49	20.0	3.58	7.16	10.7
30	1.97	15.1	4.72	9.45	14.2
40	2.45	12.2	5.87	11.7	
50	2.92	10.2	7.01	14.0	
60	3.40	8.8	8.16		
80	4.35	6.8	10.4ᵇ		
100	5.31	5.6	12.7ᵇ		
110	5.78	5.2	13.9ᵇ		

a. For patients with renal impairment, initial maintenance dose estimates are given for optional dosing intervals; longer dosing intervals are expected to provide greater peak and lower trough serum capreomycin levels than shorter dosing intervals.

b. The usual dosage for patients with *normal* renal function is 1,000 mg daily, not to exceed 20 mg/kg/day, for 60 to 120 days, then 1,000 mg 2 to 3 times weekly.

Parenteral drug products should be inspected visually for particulate matter and discoloration prior to administration, whenever solution and container permit.

HOW SUPPLIED

Capastat® Sulfate, Sterile Capreomycin Sulfate, USP, is available in:

Vials: 1 g*/10 mL size (UC5001) (1s) NDC 51479-018-01

---

*Equivalent to capreomycin activity.

Store at controlled room temperature 59° to 86°F (15° to 30°C) prior to reconstitution.

ANIMAL PHARMACOLOGY

In addition to renal and cranial nerve VIII toxicity demonstrated in animal toxicology studies, cataracts developed in 2 dogs on doses of 62 mg/kg and 100 mg/kg for prolonged periods.

In teratology studies, a low incidence of "wavy ribs" was noted in litters of female rats treated with daily doses of 50 mg/kg or more of capreomycin.

REFERENCES

1. Lehmann CR, Garrett LE, Winn RE, Springberg PD, Vicks S, Porter DK, Pierson WP, Wolny JD, Brier GL, Black HR. Capreomycin kinetics in renal impairment and clearance by hemodialysis. *Am Rev Respir Dis* 1988;138/5:1312-3.
2. Unpublished data on file at Lilly.

CAUTION: Federal (USA) law prohibits dispensing without prescription.

Literature revised April 1, 1997

Dura
PHARMACEUTICALS
Manufactured by: Eli Lilly and Company
Indianapolis, IN 46285
Distributed by: DURA Pharmaceuticals, Inc.
San Diego, CA 92121
PA 7953 UCP   CSV003D0297

CECLOR® CD
(cefaclor extended release tablets)   ℞

DESCRIPTION

Cefaclor, USP, the active ingredient in Ceclor® CD (cefaclor extended release tablets), is a semisynthetic cephalosporin antibiotic for oral administration. Cefaclor, USP, is chemically designated as 3-chloro-7-D-(2-phenylglycinamido)-3-cephem-4-carboxylic acid monohydrate. The Ceclor CD formulation of cefaclor differs pharmacokinetically from the Ceclor® formulation of cefaclor. (See **CLINICAL PHARMACOLOGY**.) Cefaclor monohydrate has a molecular formula of $C_{15}H_{14}ClN_3O_4S \cdot H_2O$ and a molecular weight of 385.82.

Each Ceclor CD tablet contains cefaclor monohydrate equivalent to 375 mg (1.02 mmol) or 500 mg (1.36 mmol) anhydrous cefaclor. In addition, each extended release tablet contains the following inactive ingredients: celluloses; FD&C Blue No. 2; magnesium stearate; mannitol; methacrylic acid copolymer type C; propylene glycol; stearic acid; titanium dioxide; polyethylene glycol; talc; and edible black ink.

CLINICAL PHARMACOLOGY

Pharmacokinetics: The Ceclor CD formulation of cefaclor is pharmacokinetically different from the Ceclor® Pulvules® formulation. (See Table 1.) No direct comparisons with the suspension formulation of cefaclor have been conducted; therefore, there are no data with which to compare the pharmacokinetic properties of the CD formulation and the suspension formulation. Until further data are available, the pharmacokinetic equivalence of the CD and the suspension formulations should NOT be assumed.

Absorption and Metabolism: The extent of absorption (AUC) and the maximum plasma concentration (C_{max}) of cefaclor from Ceclor CD are greater when the extended release tablet is taken with food.

[NOTE: The extent of absorption (AUC) of cefaclor from Ceclor Pulvules is unaffected by food intake; however, when Ceclor Pulvules are taken with food, the C_{max} is decreased.] There is no evidence of metabolism of cefaclor in humans.

Comparative Serum Pharmacokinetics—Serum pharmacokinetic parameters for Ceclor CD and Ceclor Pulvules are shown in the following table.

[See table 1 above]

Table 1
COMPARATIVE PHARMACOKINETICS OF CECLOR PULVULES VS CECLOR CD IN FASTING AND FED STATES

Parameter	Ceclor CD		Ceclor CD		Ceclor Pulvules	
	375 mg		500 mg		2 × 250 mg	
	fed	fast	fed	fast	fed	fast
	n = 10		n = 16	n = 16	n = 15	n = 16
C_{max}	3.7 (1.1)	NA	8.2 (4.2)	5.4 (1.6)	9.3 (2.7)	16.8 (4.7)
T_{max}	2.7 (1.0)	NA	2.5 (0.8)	1.5 (0.7)	1.5 (0.6)	0.9 (0.4)
AUC	9.9 (2.2)	NA	18.1 (4.2)	14.8 (4.0)	20.5 (2.8)	19.2 (5.0)

(± 1 standard deviation)
NA = data not available

No drug accumulation was noted when Ceclor CD was given twice daily.

The plasma half-life in healthy subjects is independent of dosage form and averages approximately 1 hour.

Food Effect on Pharmacokinetics: When Ceclor CD is taken with food, the AUC is 10% lower while the C_{max} is 12% lower and occurs 1 hour later compared to Ceclor Pulvules. In contrast, when Ceclor CD is taken without food, the AUC is 23% lower while the C_{max} is 67% lower and occurs 0.6 hours later, using an equivalent milligram dose of Ceclor Pulvules as a reference. **Therefore, Ceclor CD should be taken with food.**

Special Populations:

Renal Insufficiency—In patients with reduced renal function, the serum half-life of cefaclor is slightly prolonged. In those with complete absence of renal function, the plasma half-life of the intact molecule is 2.3 to 2.8 hours. Excretion pathways in patients with markedly impaired renal function have not been determined. Hemodialysis shortens the half-life by 25% to 30%.

Geriatric Patients—In elderly subjects (over age 65) with normal serum creatinine values, higher peak plasma concentrations and AUCs have been observed. This is considered to be primarily a result of an age-related decrement in renal function, and has no apparent clinical significance. Therefore, dosage adjustment is not necessary in elderly subjects with normal serum creatinine values.

Microbiology:

Cefaclor has *in vitro* activity against a broad range of gram-positive and gram-negative bacteria. The bactericidal action of cefaclor results from inhibition of cell-wall synthesis. Cefaclor is stable in the presence of some bacterial β-lactamases; consequently, some β-lactamase-producing organisms may be susceptible to cefaclor.

Ceclor CD has been shown to be active against most strains of the following microorganisms both *in vitro* and in clinical infections as described in the **INDICATIONS AND USAGE** section:

Gram-positive aerobes:
Staphylococcus aureus
Streptococcus pneumoniae
Streptococcus pyogenes

NOTE: Cefaclor is inactive against methicillin-resistant staphylococci.

Gram-negative aerobes:
Haemophilus influenzae (non-β-lactamase-producing strains only)
Moraxella catarrhalis (including β-lactamase-producing strains)

The following *in vitro* data are available, **but their clinical significance is unknown**. Cefaclor exhibits *in vitro* minimum inhibitory concentrations (MICs) of 8 µg/mL or less (systemic susceptibility breakpoint) against most (≥90%) strains of the following microorganisms; however, the safety and effectiveness of Ceclor CD in treating clinical infections due to these microorganisms have not been established in adequate and well-controlled trials.

Gram-positive aerobes:
Staphylococcus epidermidis

Gram-negative aerobes:
Haemophilus parainfluenzae
Klebsiella pneumoniae

Anaerobic bacteria:
Peptococcus niger
Peptostreptococci
Propionibacterium acnes

NOTE: *Acinetobacter calcoaceticus*, *Enterobacter* spp., *Enterococcus* spp., *Morganella morganii*, *Proteus vulgaris*, *Providencia* spp., *Pseudomonas* spp., and *Serratia* spp. are resistant to cefaclor.

Susceptibility Testing:Dilution Techniques—Quantitative methods are used to determine antimicrobial minimum inhibitory concentrations (MICs). These MICs provide estimates of the susceptibility of bacteria to antimicrobial compounds. The MICs should be determined using a standardized procedure. Standardized procedures are based on a dilution method[1] (broth, agar, or microdilution) or equivalent with standardized inoculum concentrations and standardized amounts of cefaclor powder. The MIC values should be interpreted according to the following criteria:

MIC (µg/mL)	Interpretation
≤8	Susceptible (S)
16	Intermediate (I)
≥32	Resistant (R)

A report of "Susceptible" indicates that the pathogen is likely to be inhibited if the antimicrobial compound in blood reaches the concentrations usually achievable. A report of "Intermediate" indicates that the result should be considered equivocal, and, if the microorganism is not fully susceptible to alternative, clinically feasible drugs, the test should be repeated. This category implies possible clinical applicability in body sites where the drug is physiologically concentrated or in situations where high dosage of drug can be used. This category also provides a buffer zone which prevents small uncontrolled technical factors from causing major discrepancies in interpretation. A report of "Resistant" indicates that the pathogen is not likely to be inhibited if the antimicrobial compound in the blood reaches the concentrations usually achievable; other therapy should be selected.

Standardized susceptibility test procedures require the use of laboratory control microorganisms to control the technical aspects of the laboratory procedures. Standard cefaclor powder should provide the following MIC values:

Microorganism		MIC range (µg/mL)
E. coli	ATCC 25922	1–4
E. faecalis	ATCC 29212	>32
S. aureus	ATCC 29213	1–4
H. influenzae	ATCC 49766*	1–4

*Broth microdilution tests performed using Haemophilus Test Medium (HTM)[1]

Diffusion Techniques: Quantitative methods that require measurement of zone diameters also provide reproducible estimates of the susceptibility of bacteria to antimicrobial compounds. One such standardized procedure[2] requires the use of standardized inoculum concentrations. This procedure uses paper disks impregnated with 30-µg cefaclor to test the susceptibility of microorganisms to cefaclor.

Reports from the laboratory providing results of the standard single-disk susceptibility test with a 30-µg cefaclor disk should be interpreted according to the following criteria:

Zone diameter (mm)	Interpretation
≥18	Susceptible (S)
15–17	Intermediate (I)
≤14	Resistant (R)

When testing* *H. Influenzae*, the following interpretive criteria should be used:

Zone diameter (mm)	Interpretation
≥20	Susceptible (S)
17–19	Intermediate (I)
≤16	Resistant (R)

*Disk susceptibility tests performed using Haemophilus Test Medium (HTM)[2]

Interpretation should be as stated above for results using dilution techniques. Interpretation involves correlation of the diameter obtained in the disk test with the MIC for cefaclor.

As with standardized dilution techniques, diffusion methods require the use of laboratory control microorganisms that

Continued on next page

Ceclor CD—Cont.

are used to control the technical aspects of the laboratory procedures. For the diffusion technique, the 30-µg cefaclor disk should provide the following zone diameters in these laboratory test quality control strains:

Microorganisms		Zone Diameter (mm)
E. coli	ATCC 25922	23–27
S. aureus	ATCC 25923	27–31
H. influenzae*	ATCC 49766	25–31

---

*Disk susceptibility tests performed using Haemophilus Test Medium (HTM)[2]

INDICATIONS AND USAGE

The safety and effectiveness of Ceclor CD in treating some of the indications and pathogens for which other formulations of cefaclor are approved have NOT been established. When administered at the recommended dosages and durations of therapy, Ceclor CD is indicated for the treatment of patients with the following mild to moderate infections when caused by susceptible strains of the designated organisms. (*See* **DOSAGE AND ADMINISTRATION** and **CLINICAL STUDIES** sections.)

Acute bacterial exacerbations of chronic bronchitis due to *Haemophilus influenzae* (non-β-lactamase-producing strains only), *Moraxella catarrhalis* (including β-lactamase-producing strains) or *Streptococcus pneumoniae.*

NOTE: In view of the insufficient numbers of isolates of β-lactamase-producing strains of *Haemophilus influenzae* that were obtained from clinical trials with Ceclor CD for patients with acute bacterial exacerbations of chronic bronchitis or secondary bacterial infections of acute bronchitis, it was not possible to adequately evaluate the effectiveness of Ceclor CD for bronchitis known, suspected, or considered potentially to be caused by β-lactamase-producing *H. influenzae.*

Secondary bacterial infections of acute bronchitis due to *Haemophilus influenzae* (non-β-lactamase-producing strains only), *Moraxella catarrhalis* (including β-lactamase-producing strains), or *Streptococcus pneumoniae.* (See above NOTE.)

Pharyngitis and tonsillitis due to *Streptococcus pyogenes.*

NOTE: Only penicillin by the intramuscular route of administration has been shown to be effective in the prophylaxis of rheumatic fever. Ceclor CD is generally effective in the eradication of *S. pyogenes* from the oropharynx; however, data establishing the efficacy of Ceclor CD for the prophylaxis of subsequent rheumatic fever are not available.

Uncomplicated skin and skin and structure infections due to *Staphylococcus aureus* (methicillin-susceptible).

NOTE: In view of the insufficient numbers of isolates of *Streptococcus pyogenes* that were obtained from clinical trials with Ceclor CD for patients with uncomplicated skin and skin structure infections, it was not possible to adequately evaluate the effectiveness of Ceclor CD for skin infections known, suspected, or considered potentially to be caused by *S. pyogenes.*

CONTRAINDICATIONS

Ceclor CD is contraindicated in patients with known hypersensitivity to cefaclor and other cephalosporins.

WARNINGS

BEFORE THERAPY WITH CECLOR CD IS INSTITUTED, CAREFUL INQUIRY SHOULD BE MADE TO DETERMINE WHETHER THE PATIENT HAS HAD PREVIOUS HYPERSENSITIVITY REACTIONS TO CEFACLOR, CEPHALOSPORINS, PENICILLINS, OR OTHER DRUGS. IF THIS PRODUCT IS TO BE GIVEN TO PENICILLIN-SENSITIVE PATIENTS, CAUTION SHOULD BE EXERCISED BECAUSE CROSS-SENSITIVITY AMONG BETA-LACTAM ANTIBIOTICS HAS BEEN CLEARLY DOCUMENTED AND MAY OCCUR IN UP TO 10% OF PATIENTS WITH A HISTORY OF PENICILLIN ALLERGY. IF AN ALLERGIC REACTION TO CECLOR CD OCCURS, DISCONTINUE THE DRUG. SERIOUS ACUTE HYPERSENSITIVITY REACTIONS MAY REQUIRE TREATMENT WITH EPINEPHRINE AND OTHER EMERGENCY MEASURES, INCLUDING OXYGEN, INTRAVENOUS FLUIDS, INTRAVENOUS ANTIHISTAMINES, CORTICOSTEROIDS, PRESSOR AMINES, AND AIRWAY MANAGEMENT, AS CLINICALLY INDICATED.

Pseudomembranous colitis has been reported with nearly all antibacterial agents, including cefaclor, and may range from mild to life-threatening. Therefore, it is important to consider this diagnosis in patients who present with diarrhea subsequent to the administration of antibacterial agents.

Treatment with antibacterial agents alters the normal flora of the colon and may permit overgrowth by clostridia. Studies indicate that a toxin produced by *Clostridium difficile* is a primary cause of "antibiotic-associated colitis."

After the diagnosis of pseudomembranous colitis has been established, therapeutic measures should be initiated. Mild cases of pseudomembranous colitis usually respond to discontinuation of the drug alone. In moderate to severe cases, consideration should be given to management with fluids and electrolytes, protein supplementation and treatment with an antibacterial drug clinically effective against *Clostridium difficile.*

PRECAUTIONS

General: Superinfection (overgrowth by non-susceptible organisms) should always be considered a possibility in a patient being treated with a broad-spectrum antimicrobial. Careful observation of the patient is essential. If superinfection occurs during therapy, appropriate measures should be taken.

Drug Interactions:

Antacids—The extent of absorption of Ceclor CD is diminished if magnesium or aluminum hydroxide-containing antacids are taken within 1 hour of administration; H_2 blockers do not alter either the rate or the extent of absorption of Ceclor CD.

Probenecid—The renal excretion of cefaclor is inhibited by probenecid.

Warfarin—There have been rare reports of increased prothrombin time with or without clinical bleeding in patients receiving cefaclor and warfarin concomitantly. No specific studies have been performed to rule in or rule out this potential drug/drug interaction.

Laboratory Test Interactions: Administration of Ceclor CD may result in a false-positive reaction for glucose in the urine. This phenomenon has been seen in patients taking cephalosporin antibiotics when the test is performed using Benedict's and Fehling's solutions and also with Clinitest®tablets.

Carcinogenesis, Mutagenesis, Impairment of Fertility: Studies in animals have not been performed to evaluate the carinogenic or mutagenic potential for cefaclor. Reproduction studies have revealed no evidence of impaired fertility.

Usage in Pregnancy—Teratogenic Effect: Pregnancy Category B: Reproduction studies using cefaclor have been performed in mice, rats, and ferrets at doses up to 3–5 times the maximum human dose (1500 mg/day) based on mg/m[2]. These studies have revealed no harm to the fetus due to cefaclor. There are, however, no adequate and well-controlled studies in pregnant women. Because animal reproduction studies are not always predictive of human response. Ceclor CD should be used during pregnancy only if clearly needed.

Labor and Delivery: Ceclor CD has not been studied for use during labor and delivery. Treatment should be given only if clearly needed.

Nursing Mothers: No studies in lactating women have been performed with Ceclor CD. Small amounts of cefaclor (≤0.21 µg/mL) have been detected in human milk following administration of single 500-mg doses of Ceclor. The effect on nursing infants is not known. Caution should be exercised when Ceclor CD is administered to a nursing woman.

Pediatric Use: Safety and effectiveness of Ceclor CD in pediatric patients less than 16 years of age have not been established.

Geriatric Use: Healthy geriatric volunteers (≥65 years old) who received a single 750-mg dose of Ceclor CD had 40%–50% higher AUC and 20% lower renal clearance values when compared to healthy adult volunteers less than 45 years of age. These differences are considered to be primarily a result of age-related decreases in renal function. In clinical studies when geriatric patients received the usual recommended adult doses, clinical efficacy and safety were comparable to results in non-geriatric adult patients. No dosage changes are recommended for healthy geriatric patients.

ADVERSE REACTIONS

Clinical Trials: There were 3272 patients treated with multiple doses of Ceclor CD in controlled clinical trials and an additional 211 subjects in pharmacology studies. There were no deaths in these trials thought to be related to toxicity from Ceclor CD. Treatment was discontinued in 1.7% of patients due to adverse events thought to be possibly or probably drug-related.

The following adverse clinical and laboratory events were reported during the Ceclor CD clinical trials conducted in North America at doses of 375 mg or 500 mg BID; however, relatedness of the adverse events to the drug was not assigned by clinical investigations during the trials (See Tables 2 and 3).

[See table 2 above]

Adverse reactions occurring during the clinical trials with cefaclor extended release tablets with an incidence of less than 1% but greater than 0.1% included the following (listed alphabetically):

Accidental injury, anorexia, anxiety, arthralgia, asthma, bronchitis, chest pain, chills, congestive heart failure, conjunctivitis, constipation, dizziness, dysmenorrhea, dyspep-

Table 2
ADVERSE CLINICAL EVENTS
CECLOR CD MULTIPLE DOSE DOSING REGIMENS
CLINICAL TRIALS—NORTH AMERICA
(n = 1400)

	EVENT	INCIDENCE
	Headache	4.9%
	Rhinitis	3.9%
	Diarrhea	3.8%
Incidence Equal	Nausea	3.4%
to or Greater	Vaginitis*	2.4%
Than 1%	Vaginal Moniliasis*	2.2%
	Abdominal Pain	1.6%
	Cough Increased	1.5%
	Pharyngitis	1.4%
	Pruritus	1.4%
	Back Pain	1.0%

*n=934 for these events (subset of female participants).

Table 3
ADVERSE CLINICAL LABORATORY EVENTS
CECLOR CD MULTIPLE DOSE DOSING REGIMENS
CLINICAL TRIALS—NORTH AMERICA

	EVENT	INCIDENCE
	Albumin decreased	0.3%
	Alkaline phosphatase increased	0.3%
	ALT/SGPT increased	0.3%
	Bilirubin total increased	0.3%
	Blood urea nitrogen (BUN) increased	0.2%
	Calcium decreased	0.7%
	Creatine phosphokinase increased	0.7%
Incidence Less	Creatinine increased	0.5%
Than 1%, But	Eosinophils increased	0.3%
Greater Than	Erythrocyte count decreased	0.3%
0.1%	GGT increased	0.2%
	Hemoglobin decreased	0.2%
	Lymphocytes decreased	0.3%
	Mean Cell Volume (MCV) increased	0.7%
	Neutrophils segmented decreased	0.3%
	Phosphorus increased	0.7%
	Platelet count decreased	0.3%
	Potassium increased	0.4%
	Sodium decreased	0.3%
	Sodium increased	0.4%

sia, dysuria, ear pain, edema, fever, flatulence, flu syndrome, gastritis, infection, insomnia, leukorrhea, lung disorder, maculopapular rash, malaise, menstrual disorder, myalgia, nausea and vomiting, neck pain, nervousness, nocturia, otitis media, pain, palpitation, peripheral edema, rash, respiratory disorder, sinusitis, somnolence, surgical procedure, sweating, tremor, urticaria, vomiting.

NOTE: One case of **serum-sickness-like** reaction was reported among the 3272 adult patients treated with Ceclor CD during the controlled clinical trials. These reactions have also been reported with the use of cefaclor in other oral formulations and are seen more frequently in pediatric patients than in adults. These reactions are characterized by findings of erythema multiforme, rash, and other skin manifestations accompanied by arthritis/arthralgia, with or without fever, and differ from classic serum sickness in that there is infrequently associated lymphadenopathy and proteinuria, no circulating immune complexes and no evidence to date of sequelae of the reaction. While further investigation is ongoing, **serum-sickness-like** reactions appear to be due to hypersensitivity and more often occur during or following a second (or subsequent) course of therapy with cefaclor. Such reactions have been reported with overall occurrence ranging from 1 in 200 (0.5%) in one focused trial; to 2 in 8346 (0.024%) in overall clinical trials (with an incidence in pediatric patients in clinical trials of 0.055%); to 1 in 38,000 (0.003%) in spontaneous event reports. Signs and symptoms usually occur a few days after initiation of therapy and subside within a few days after cessation of therapy. Occasionally these reactions have resulted in hospitalization, usually of short duration (median hospitalization = 2 to 3 days, based on postmarketing surveillance studies). In those patients requiring hospitalization, the symptoms have ranged from mild to severe at the time of admission with more of the severe reactions occurring in pediatric patients.

[See table 3 on previous page]

In Postmarketing Experience: In addition to the events reported during clinical trials with Ceclor CD, the following adverse experiences are among those that have been reported during worldwide postmarketing surveillance: allergic reaction, anaphylactoid reaction, angioedema, face edema, hypotension, Stevens-Johnson syndrome, syncope, paresthesia, vasodilatation, and vertigo.

Other Adverse Reactions Associated With Other Formulations of Cefaclor: In addition to the above, the following other adverse reactions and altered laboratory tests have been associated with cefaclor in other oral formulations:

Clinical: Severe hypersensitivity reactions, including Stevens-Johnson syndrome, toxic epidermal necrolysis, and anaphylaxis, have been reported rarely. Anaphylactoid events may be manifested by solitary symptoms, including angioedema, edema (including face and limbs), parasthesias, syncope, or vasodilatation. Anaphylaxis may be more common in patients with a history of penicillin allergy. Rarely, hypersensitivity symptoms may persist for several months.

Symptoms of pseudomembranous colitis may appear either during or after antibiotic treatment. (*See* **WARNINGS**.)

Laboratory: Abnormal urinalysis, eosinophilia, leukopenia, neutropenia, transient elevations in AST, and transient thrombocytopenia have been reported.

Cephalosporin-Class Reactions: In addition to the adverse reactions listed above, the following adverse reactions and altered laboratory tests have been reported for cephalosporin-class antibiotics:

Clinical: Confusion, erythema multiforme, genital pruritus, hepatic dysfunction including cholestasis, hemolytic anemia, reversible hyperactivity, hypertonia, and reversible interstitial nephritis.

Laboratory—Positive direct Coombs' test.

OVERDOSAGE

The toxic symptoms following an overdose of cefaclor may include nausea, vomiting, epigastric distress, and diarrhea. The severity of the epigastric distress and the diarrhea are dose-related.

Absorption of drugs from the gastrointestinal tract may be decreased by giving activated charcoal, which, in many cases, is more effective than emesis or lavage. Consider charcoal instead of or in addition to gastric emptying. Repeated doses of charcoal over time may hasten elimination of some drugs that have been absorbed.

Although cefaclor is considered dialyzable, neither forced diuresis, peritoneal dialysis, hemodialysis, nor charcoal hemoperfusion have been demonstrated to be beneficial in an overdose of cefaclor.

DOSAGE AND ADMINISTRATION

The absorption of Ceclor CD is enhanced when it is administered with food. (*See* **CLINICAL PHARMACOLOGY**.) Therefore, **Ceclor CD should be administered with meals (i.e., at least within one hour of eating)**. The extended release tablets should not be cut, crushed, or chewed.

See INDICATIONS AND USAGE for information about patients for whom Ceclor CD is indicated.

Adults (age 16 years and older): Type of Infection (as qualified in the INDICATIONS AND USAGE section of this labeling)	Total Daily Dose	Dose and Frequency	Duration
Acute Bacterial Exacerbations of Chronic Bronchitis due to *H. influenzae* (non-β-lactamase-producing strains only), *Moraxella catarrhalis* (including β-lactamase-producing strains), or *Streptococcus pneumoniae* (See **INDICATIONS and USAGE**.)	1000 mg	500 mg q12 hours	7 days
Secondary Bacterial Infections of Acute Bronchitis due to *H. influenzae* (non-β-lactamase-producing strains only), *M. catarrhalis* (including β-lactamase-producing strains), or *S. pneumoniae* (See **INDICATIONS and USAGE**.)	1000 mg	500 mg q12 hours	7 days
Pharyngitis and/or tonsillitis *due to S. pyogenes*	750 mg	375 mg q12 hours	10 days
Uncomplicated Skin and Skin Structure infections due to *S. aureus* (methicillin-susceptible strains) (See **INDICATIONS and USAGE**.)	750 mg	375 mg q12 hours	7–10 days

NOTE: 500 mg BID of Ceclor CD is clinically equivalent to 250 mg TID of cefaclor as a pulvule in those indications listed in the **INDICATIONS AND USAGE** section of this label. **500 mg BID of Ceclor CD is NOT equivalent to 500 mg TID of other cefaclor formulations.**

[See table above]

Elderly patients with normal renal function do not require dosage adjustments.

HOW SUPPLIED

Tablets (extended release):
375 mg, blue (UC 5391)—(60s) NDC 51479-036-60
500 mg, blue (UC 5392)—(60s) NDC 51479-035-60

Store at controlled room temperature, 15° to 30°C (59° to 86°F).

CLINICAL STUDIES:

ACUTE BACTERIAL EXACERBATIONS OF CHRONIC BRONCHITIS AND SECONDARY BACTERIAL INFECTIONS OF ACUTE BRONCHITIS: In adequate and well-controlled clinical trials of Ceclor CD in the treatment of acute bacterial exacerbations of chronic bronchitis (ABECB) and secondary bacterial infections of acute bronchitis (SBIAB), only 4 evaluable patients with ABECB and no evaluable patients with SBIAB had infections caused by β-lactamase-producing *H. influenzae*. Four patients do not provide adequate data upon which to judge clinical efficacy of Ceclor CD against β-lactamase-producing *H. influenzae*.

UNCOMPLICATED SKIN AND SKIN STRUCTURE INFECTIONS: Ceclor CD (375 mg Q12H) (n=115) was compared to Ceclor Pulvules (250 mg TID) (n=106) for the treatment of patients with uncomplicated skin and skin structure infections, including cellulitis, pyoderma, abscess, and impetigo. Patients were treated for 7 to 10 days and were evaluated for clinical resolution and bacterial eradication approximately one week after completing therapy. To be evaluable, all patients had to have a recognized pathogen isolated from the skin infection just prior to the initiation of therapy. The results of this randomized, double-blinded, U.S. trial demonstrated:

(1) overall clinical cure rates were 72% (83 of 115 patients) and 75% (80 of 106 patients), respectively, for Ceclor CD and Ceclor Pulvules [95% CI around 3% difference = −16% to +9%], and

(2) overall bacteriologic eradication rates against *Straphylococcus aureus* were comparable (see Table 4).

Table 4
CLINICAL RESPONSE* IN PATIENTS WITH SKIN AND SKIN STRUCTURE INFECTIONS

Outcome by Pathogen	CECLOR CD		CECLOR Pulvules	
Staphylococcus aureus	67/95	(71%)	58/81	(71%)
Streptococcus pyogenes	10/16	(63%)	8/9	(89%)
Other streptococci	7/11	(64%)	5/6	(83%)
Total	84/122	(69%)	71/96	(74%)

* Cure plus improvement

REFERENCES

1. National Committee for Clinical Laboratory Standards. Methods for Dilution Antimicrobial Susceptibility Tests for Bacteria that Grow Aerobically—Third edition; Approved Standard NCCLS Document M7-A3, Vol 13, No 25, NCCLS, Villanova, PA, December 1993

2. National Committee for Clinical Laboratory Standards. Performance Standards for Antimicrobial Disk Susceptibility Tests—Fifth edition; Approved Standard NCCLS Document M2-A5, Vol 13, No 24, NCCLS, Villanova, PA, December 1993

PV 2741 AMP   [082096]

CAUTION—Federal (USA) law prohibits dispensing without prescription.

DURA PHARMACEUTICALS
Literature issued July 28, 1997

Manufactured by
Eli Lilly and Company
Indianapolis, IN 46285, USA
Distributed by DURA Pharmaceuticals, Inc.
San Diego, CA 92121
PV 2740 UCP   CC D001A0497

D.A. CHEWABLE™ Tablets   ℞

DESCRIPTION

Each D.A. CHEWABLE TABLET for oral administration contains:

chlorpheniramine maleate .... 2 mg
phenylephrine HCl .... 10 mg
methscopolamine nitrate .... 1.25 mg

in an orange-flavored and orange-colored chewable tablet.

Chlorpheniramine maleate is an antihistamine having the chemical name: 2-Pyridinepropanamine, γ-(4chlorophenyl)-N,N-dimethyl-,(Z)-2-butenedioate(1:1)

Phenylephrine HCl is a decongestant having the chemical name:
Benzenemethanol, 3-hydroxy-α[(methylamino) methyl]-,hydrochloride.

Methscopolamine nitrate is an anticholinergic having the chemical name: 3-Oxa-9-azoniatricyclo[3.3.1.0^{2,4}] nonane, 7-(3-hydroxy-1-oxo-2-phenylpropoxy)-9,9-dimethyl-, nitrate, [7(S)-(1 α, 2 β, 4 β, 5 α, 7 β)]-

Inactive ingredients: artificial orange flavor, aspartame, colloidal silicon dioxide, croscarmellose sodium, FD&C yellow #6 (aluminum lake), magnesium stearate, malic acid, mannitol, microcrystalline cellulose, vanillin.

HOW SUPPLIED

D.A. CHEWABLE Tablets are available as orange flavored and orange colored scored tablets imprinted with *DURA* on one side and *CHEW* on the other.
Bottles of 100 (NDC 51479-013-01).
Store at room temperature, 15°–25°C (59°–77°F).
Dispense in a tight, light-resistant container (USP/NF) with a child-resistant closure.

Rx only

Manufactured for:
Dura Pharmaceuticals, Inc.
San Diego, CA 92121

Continued on next page

D.A. Chewable—Cont.

Manufactured by
Anabolic, Inc.
Irvine, CA 92614
Revised June 1998
DACT005J98

DURA–GEST® ℞
DECONGESTANT/EXPECTORANT CAPSULE

DESCRIPTION
Each Dura-Gest gray and white capsule for oral administration contains:

phenylephrine hydrochloride	5 mg
phenylpropanolamine hydrochloride	45 mg
guaifenesin	200 mg

HOW SUPPLIED
DURA-GEST gray and white capsules are imprinted with "DURA-GEST" and "51479005".
Bottles of 100 (NDC 51479-005-01).
Bottles of 500 (NDC 51479-005-05).
Dispense in a tight, light-resistant container (USP/NF) with a child-resistant closure. Store at controlled room temperature 15°–25°C (59°–77°F).
Rx only
Manufactured for Dura Pharmaceuticals, Inc. San Diego, CA 92121
Manufactured by Anabolic, Inc. Irvine, CA 92614
Revised June 1998　　　　　　　　　DG003F98

DURA-TAP/PD® ℞
Antihistamine/Decongestant

DESCRIPTION
Each Dura-Tap/PD opaque blue and clear capsule containing white beads for oral administration contains:

chlorpheniramine maleate	4 mg
pseudoephedrine hydrochloride	60 mg

in a specially-prepared base to provide a prolonged therapeutic effect.

HOW SUPPLIED
Dura-Tap/PD is available as an opaque blue and clear capsule coded with the imprints 51479 and 007. Bottles of 100 (NDC 51479-007-01).
Store at room temperature, 15°–23°C (59°–73°F).
Dispense in a tight, light-resistant container (USP/NF) with a child-resistant closure.
Rx only
Manufactured for
Dura Pharmaceuticals, Inc.
San Diego, CA 92121
Manufactured by
Schwarz Pharma Mfg., Inc.
Seymour, IN 47274
Revised June 1998
DTPD002H98

DURA-VENT® ℞
DECONGESTANT/EXPECTORANT TABLET

DESCRIPTION
Each DURA-VENT white, scored tablet for oral administration contains:

Phenylpropanolamine hydrochloride	75 mg
Guaifenesin	600 mg

in a special base to provide a prolonged therapeutic effect.
Phenylpropanolamine hydrochloride is a decongestant having the chemical name:
Benzenemethanol, α-(1-aminoethyl)-, hydrochloride, (R^*, S^*)-,(±).
Guaifenesin is an expectorant having the chemical name: 1,2-Propanediol, 3-(2-methoxyphenoxy)-.
Inactive ingredients: dicalcium phosphate, hydrogenated cottonseed oil, magnesium stearate, methylcellulose, microcrystalline cellulose, silicon dioxide, stearic acid, tricalcium phosphate.

CLINICAL PHARMACOLOGY
Phenylpropanolamine hydrochloride is a sympathomimetic amine that causes vasoconstriction via the activation of post-junctional α-adrenergic receptors located on the precapillary and post-capillary blood vessels of the nasal mucosa. Activation of these receptors occurs directly by binding of phenylpropanolamine or indirectly by binding of norepinephrine released from sympathomimetic nerve endings in response to phenylpropanolamine. The resulting vasoconstriction decreases blood flow through the nasal mucosa and results in a shrinkage of this tissue. Phenylpropanolamine

also has beta adrenergic effects. This increases heart rate, force of contraction, cardiac output, and excitability. Phenylpropanolamine causes CNS stimulation and reportedly has an anorexigenic effect.
Guaifenesin promotes lower respiratory tract drainage by thinning bronchial secretions, and facilitates removal of viscous, inspissated mucus. By reducing the viscosity of secretions, guaifenesin increases the efficiency of the cough reflex and of the ciliary action in removing accumulated secretions from the trachea and bronchi.

INDICATIONS AND USAGE
DURA-VENT is indicated for the temporary symptomatic relief of sinusitis, bronchitis, pharyngitis, and the common cold when these conditions are associated with nasal congestion and viscous mucus in the lower respiratory tract.

CONTRAINDICATIONS
Patients with hypersensitivity or idiosyncrasy to any of its ingredients. Sympathomimetic amines are contraindicated in patients with severe hypertension, severe coronary artery disease and patients on monoamine oxidase (MAO) inhibitor therapy.

WARNINGS
Sympathomimetic amines should be used cautiously in patients with hypertension, diabetes mellitus, ischemic heart disease, hyperthyroidism, increased intraocular pressure and prostatic hypertrophy. **See Contraindications**. Sympathomimetic amines may produce CNS stimulation and convulsions or cardiovascular collapse with accompanying hypotension. The elderly (60 years and older) are more likely to exhibit adverse reactions. Do not exceed recommended dosage. Also, this produce should not be taken simultaneously with other products containing phenylpropanolamine, phenylephrine, pseudoephedrine, ephedrine, or amphetamines.

PRECAUTIONS
General: Should be used with caution in patients with diabetes mellitus, hypertension, cardiovascular disease and hyperreactivity to sympathomimetic amines.
Information for Patients: Do not crush or chew DURA-VENT tablets prior to swallowing.
Drug Interactions: Monoamine oxidase (MAO) inhibitors and beta-adrenergic blockers increase the effect of sympathomimetic amines. Sympathomimetic amines may reduce the antihypertensive effects of methyldopa, mecamylamine and reserpine.
Drug/Laboratory Test Interactions: Guaifenesin has been reported to interfere with clinical laboratory determinations of urinary 5-hydroxyindoleacetic acid (5-HIAA) and urinary vanillymandelic acid (VMA).
Pregnancy Category C: Animal reproduction studies have not been conducted with DURA-VENT. It is also not known whether DURA-VENT can cause fetal harm when administered to a pregnant woman or can affect reproduction capacity. DURA-VENT should be given to a pregnant woman only if clearly needed.
Nursing Mothers: It is not known whether the drugs in DURA-VENT are excreted in human milk. Because many drugs are excreted in human milk and because of the potential for serious adverse reactions in nursing infants, a decision should be made whether to discontinue nursing or discontinue the product, taking into account the importance of the drug to the mother.
Pediatric Use: Safety and effectiveness of DURA-VENT in pediatric patients below the age of 6 years have not been established.

ADVERSE REACTIONS
Sympathomimetic amines may cause tachycardia, palpitations, nervousness, insomnia, restlessness, headache, gastric irritation, and irritability. Sympathomimetic amines have been associated with certain untoward reactions including fear, anxiety, tenseness, restlessness, tremor, weakness, pallor, respiratory difficulty, dysuria, insomnia, hallucinations, convulsions, CNS depression, arrhythmias and cardiovascular collapse with hypotension. Urinary retention may occur in patients with prostatic hypertrophy. Guaifenesin may cause nausea, vomiting, diarrhea, and gastric irritation.

OVERDOSAGE
The treatment of overdosage should provide symptomatic and supportive care. Induction of emesis and gastric lavage may be performed if the patient is alert and seen within early hours after ingestion. Drug remaining in the stomach may be absorbed by the administration of activated charcoal. Stimulants should not be used because they may precipitate convulsions. If convulsions or marked CNS excitement occur, treatment with appropriate measures is indicated. Since the effects of DURA-VENT may last up to 12 hours, the patient should be monitored for at least that length of time and treated as necessary.

DOSAGE AND ADMINISTRATION
Adults and adolescents 12 years of age and older: one tablet twice daily (every 12 hours). **Children 6 to under 12**

years: one-half (¹/₂) tablet twice daily (every 12 hours). DURA-VENT is not recommended for pediatric patients under 6 years of age. Tablets may be broken in half for ease of administration without affecting release of medication, but should not be crushed or chewed prior to swallowing.

HOW SUPPLIED
DURA-VENT is available as a white, scored tablet imprinted with 7.5/7.5 on one side and DURA on the other.
Bottles of 100 (NDC 51479–006–01).
Bottles of 600 (NDC 51479–006–06).
Store at room temperature, 15°–25°C (59°–77°F).
Dispense in a tight, light-resistant container (USP/NF) with a child-resistant closure.
Rx only.
Manufactured by
Anabolic, Inc.
Irvine, CA 92614
Revised June, 1998
DV001H98

DURA-VENT®/A ℞
Decongestant/Antihistamine

DESCRIPTION
Each Dura-Vent/A clear capsule for oral administration contains:

phenylpropanolamine hydrochloride	75 mg
chlorpheniramine maleate	10 mg

Phenylpropanolamine hydrochloride is a decongestant having the chemical name:
Benzenemethanol, α-(1-amino-ethyl)-, hydrochloride, (R^*,S^*)-,(±).
Chlorpheniramine maleate is an antihistamine having the chemical name:
2-Pyridinepropanamine, γ-(4-chlorophenyl)-N,N-dimethyl-, (Z)-2-butenedioate (1:1)
Inactive ingredients: benzyl alcohol, butylparaben, corn starch, edetate calcium disodium, gelatin, methylparaben, pharmaceutical glaze, propylparaben, sodium lauryl sulfate, sodium propionate, sucrose, and other proprietary ingredients.

HOW SUPPLIED
Dura-Vent/A clear capsules are imprinted with DURA-VENT/A and 51479002.
Bottles of 100 (NDC 51479-002-01).
Store at room temperature, 15°–23°C (59°–73°F).
Dispense in a tight, light-resistant container (USP/NF) with a child-resistant closure.
Rx only.
Manufactured for Dura Pharmaceuticals, Inc.
San Diego, CA 92121
Manufactured by Schwarz Pharma Manufacturing, Inc.
Seymour, IN 47274
©1996 Dura Pharmaceuticals, Inc.
Revised June 1998　　　　　　　　　DVA002H98

D.A. II® Tablet ℞
Dura-Vent®/DA Tablet

DESCRIPTION
Antihistamine/decongestant/anticholinergic combination tablets for oral use.

D.A. II™ Tablet

Each white, capsule-shaped tablet contains:

chlorpheniramine maleate	4 mg
phenylephrine HCl	10 mg
methscopolamine nitrate	1.25 mg

In a specially prepared base to provide a prolonged therapeutic effect.
Inactive ingredients: dicalcium phosphate, hydrogenated cottonseed oil, magnesium stearate, methylcellulose, stearic acid, microcrystalline cellulose, and silicon dioxide.

Dura-Vent®/DA Tablet

Each light brown, scored tablet contains:

chlorpheniramine maleate	8 mg
phenylephrine HCl	20 mg
methscopolamine nitrate	2.5 mg

In a specially prepared base to provide a prolonged therapeutic effect.
Inactive ingredients: D&C yellow #10 (aluminum lake), dicalcium phosphate, FD&C blue #1 (aluminum lake), FD&C red #40 (aluminum lake), hydrogenated cottonseed oil, magnesium stearate, methylcellulose, silica gel, and stearic acid.

Chlorpheniramine maleate is an antihistamine having the chemical name: 2-Pyridinepropanamine, γ-(4-chlorophenyl)-N,N-dimethyl-, (Z)-2-butenedioate(1:1).

Phenylephrine HCl is a decongestant having the chemical name: Benzenemethanol, 3-hydroxy-α-[(methylamino) methyl]-, hydrochloride.

Methscopolamine nitrate is an anticholinergic having the chemical name: 3-Oxa-9-azonlatricyclo [3.3.1.0² ⁴] nonane, 7-(3-hydroxy-1-oxo-2-phenylpropoxy)-9,9-dimethyl-,nitrate, [7(S)-(1α, 2β, 4β, 5α, 7β)]-.

CLINICAL PHARMACOLOGY

Chlorpheniramine maleate is an alkylamine-type antihistamine with anticholinergic and sedative effects. Antihistamines competitively antagonize histamine at the H₁ receptor site. This prevents histamine mediated increased vascular permeability, increased mucus production, pruritis and sneezing.

Phenylephrine HCl is a sympathomimetic amine that causes vasoconstriction via the activation of post-junctional α-adrenergic receptors located on the pre-capillary and post-capillary blood vessels of the nasal mucosa. Activation of these receptors occur directly by binding of phenylephrine or indirectly by binding of norepinephrine released from sympathomimetic nerve endings in response to phenylephrine. The resulting vasoconstriction decreases blood flow through the nasal mucosa and results in a shrinkage of this tissue.

Methscopolamine nitrate is a quaternary ammonium derivative of the anticholinergic scopolamine, which possesses the peripheral actions of the belladonna alkaloids, but does not exhibit the central actions because of its lack of ability to cross the blood-brain barrier. Its antimuscarinic effect causes drying of mucous secretions.

INDICATIONS AND USAGE

For the temporary relief of symptoms associated with allergic rhinitis, vasomotor rhinitis, sinusitis and the common cold.

CONTRAINDICATIONS

Patients with hypersensitivity or idiosyncrasy to any of its ingredients. Sympathomimetic amines are contraindicated in patients with severe hypertension, severe coronary artery disease and patients on monoamine oxidase (MAO) inhibitor therapy. Antihistamines and anticholinergics are contraindicated in patients with narrow-angle glaucoma, urinary retention, peptic ulcer disease and during an asthma attack.

WARNINGS

Sympathomimetic amines should be used cautiously in patients with hypertension, diabetes mellitus, ischemic heart disease, hyperthyroidism, increased intraocular pressure and prostatic hypertrophy. See Contraindications. Sympathomimetic amines may produce CNS stimulation and convulsions or cardiovascular collapse with accompanying hypotension. The elderly (60 years and older) are more likely to exhibit adverse reactions. Antihistamines may cause excitability, especially in children. At dosages higher than the recommended dose, nervousness, dizziness or sleepiness may occur. Do not exceed recommended dose.

PRECAUTIONS

General: Should be used with caution in patients with diabetes mellitus, hypertension, cardiovascular disease and hyperreactivity to sympathomimetic amines. Antihistamines may cause drowsiness and ambulatory patients who operate machinery or motor vehicles should be cautioned accordingly.

Information for Patients: Antihistamines may impair mental and physical abilities required for the performance of potentially hazardous tasks, such as driving a vehicle or operating machinery. Do not crush or chew D.A. II or Dura-Vent/DA prior to swallowing. The antihistamine in this product may have additive effects with alcohol and other central nervous system depressants (hypnotics, sedatives, tranquilizers).

Drug Interactions: Monoamine oxidase (MAO) inhibitors and beta-adrenergic blockers increase the effect of sympathomimetic amines. Sympathomimetic amines may reduce the antihypertensive effects of methyldopa, mecamylamine and reserpine. Concomitant use of antihistamines with alcohol, tricyclic antidepressants, barbiturates and other CNS depressants may have an additive effect.

Pregnancy Category C: Animal reproduction studies have not been conducted with these products. It is also not known whether these products can cause fetal harm when administered to a pregnant woman or can affect reproductive capacity. Give to pregnant women only if clearly needed.

Nursing Mothers: It is not known whether the drugs in these products are excreted in human milk. Because many drugs are excreted in human milk and because of the potential for serious adverse reactions in nursing infants, a decision should be made whether to discontinue nursing or discontinue the product, taking into account the importance of the drug to the mother.

Pediatric Usage: Safety and effectiveness in pediatric patients below the age of 6 have not been established.

ADVERSE REACTIONS

Sympathomimetic amines may cause tachycardia, palpitations, nervousness, insomnia, restlessness, headache, gastric irritation, and irritability. Sympathomimetic amines have been associated with certain untoward reactions including fear, anxiety, tenseness, restlessness, tremor, weakness, pallor, respiratory difficulty, dysuria, insomnia, hallucinations, convulsions, CNS depression, arrhythmias, and cardiovascular collapse with hypotension. Urinary retention may occur in patients with prostatic hypertrophy. Antihistamines and anticholinergics may cause drowsiness, dizziness, blurred vision and excessive dryness of the nose, throat and mouth.

OVERDOSAGE

The treatment of overdosage should provide symptomatic and supportive care. Induction of emesis and gastric lavage may be performed if the patient is alert and seen within early hours after ingestion. Drug remaining in the stomach may be absorbed by the administration of activated charcoal. Stimulants should not be used because they may precipitate convulsions. If convulsions or marked CNS excitement occurs, treatment with appropriate measures is indicated. Since the effects of D.A. II and Dura-Vent/DA may last up to 12 hours, the patient should be monitored for at least that length of time and treated as necessary.

DOSAGE AND ADMINISTRATION

D.A. II Tablet

Adults and adolescents 12 years of age and older: two tablets twice daily (every 12 hours). Children 6 to 12 years of age: one tablet twice daily (every 12 hours). D.A. II is not recommended for pediatric patients under 6 years of age. Do not crush or chew tablets prior to swallowing.

Dura-Vent/DA Tablet

Adults and adolescents 12 years of age and older: one tablet twice daily (every 12 hours). Children 6 to 12 years of age: one-half (¹/₂) tablet twice daily (every 12 hours). Dura-Vent/DA is not recommended for pediatric patients under 6 years of age. Tablets may be broken in half for ease of administration without affecting release of medication, but should not be crushed or chewed prior to swallowing.

HOW SUPPLIED

D.A. II is available as a white, capsule-shaped tablet imprinted with *DURA* on one side and *DA II* on the other. Bottles of 100 (NDC 51479-028-01).

Dura-Vent/DA is available as a light brown, scored tablet imprinted with *DURA* on one side and *DA* on the other. Bottles of 100 (NDC 51479-008-01).

Store at room temperature 15°–25°C (59°–77°F). Dispense in a tight, light-resistant container (USP/NF) with a child-resistant closure.

Rx only.

Manufactured for
DURA Pharmaceuticals, Inc.
San Diego, CA 92121
Manufactured by
Anabolic, Inc.
Irvine, CA 92614
Revised June 1998   DURA197C98

ENTEX® capsules   ℞

[n 'tex]
(phenylephrine hydrochloride/
phenylpropanolamine
hydrochloride/guaifenesin)

DESCRIPTION

Each Entex orange and white capsule for oral administration contains

phenylephrine hydrochloride	5 mg
phenylpropanolamine hydrochloride	45 mg
guaifenesin	200 mg

This product contains ingredients of the following therapeutic classes: decongestant and expectorant.

HOW SUPPLIED

Orange and White Entex Capsules are imprinted "ENTEX" and "5147 9030".

NDC 51479-030-01 Bottles of 100
NDC 51479-030-05 Bottles of 500
Store below 77°F (25°C).
Rx only.

Manufactured by
WelPharm, Inc., Irvine, CA 92614
Manufactured for
DURA Pharmaceuticals, Inc.
San Diego, CA 92121
REVISED June, 1998   EC003C98

ENTEX® LIQUID   ℞

[n 'tex]
(phenylephrine hydrochloride/
phenylpropanolamine
hydrochloride/guaifenesin)

DESCRIPTION

Each 5 mL (one teaspoonful) for oral administration contains

phenylephrine hydrochloride	5 mg
phenylpropanolamine hydrochloride	20 mg
guaifenesin	100 mg
alcohol	5%

HOW SUPPLIED

Entex Liquid is available as an orange-colored, pleasant-tasting liquid.
NDC 51479-031-48 1 Pint (470 mL) bottle.
Store below 77°F (25°C). DO NOT REFRIGERATE.
Rx only.
Manufactured by
Schwarz Pharma Mfg., Inc.
Seymour, In 47274
Manufactured for
DURA Pharmaceuticals, Inc.
San Diego, CA 92121
Revised June, 1998   EL002C98

ENTEX® LA   ℞

[n 'tex]
(phenylpropanolamine
hydrochloride/guaifenesin)

DESCRIPTION

Each Entex LA orange, scored, long-acting tablet for oral administration contains

phenylpropanolamine hydrochloride	75 mg
guaifenesin	400 mg

in a special base to provide a prolonged therapeutic effect. This product contains ingredients of the following therapeutic classes: decongestant and expectorant.

Phenylpropanolamine hydrochloride is a decongestant having the chemical name, benzenemethanol, α-(1-aminoethyl)-, hydrochloride (R*, S*), (±), with the following structure:

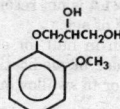

Guaifenesin is an expectorant having the chemical name, 1,2-propanediol, 3-(2-methoxyphenoxy)-, with the following structure:

Inactive Ingredients: Each tablet contains carbomer 934 P, compressible sugar, docusate sodium, FD&C Yellow No. 6 Aluminum Lake, hydroxypropyl cellulose, hydroxypropyl methylcellulose, polyethylene glycol, silicon dioxide, stearic acid, titanium dioxide, and zinc stearate.

CLINICAL PHARMACOLOGY

Phenylpropanolamine hydrochloride is an α-adrenergic receptor agonist (sympathomimetic) which produces vasoconstriction by stimulating α-receptors within the mucosa of the respiratory tract. Clinically, phenylpropanolamine shrinks swollen mucous membranes, reduces tissue hyperemia, edema, and nasal congestion, and increases nasal airway patency. Guaifenesin promotes lower respiratory tract drainage by thinning bronchial secretions, lubricates irritated respiratory tract membranes through increased mucous flow, and facilitates removal of viscous, inspissated mucus. As a result of these drugs, sinus and bronchial drainage is improved, and dry, nonproductive coughs become more productive and less frequent.

INDICATIONS AND USAGE

Entex LA is indicated for the symptomatic relief of sinusitis, bronchitis, pharyngitis, and coryza when these conditions are associated with nasal congestion and viscous mucus in the lower respiratory tract.

CONTRAINDICATIONS

Entex LA is contraindicated in individuals with known hypersensitivity to sympathomimetics, severe hypertension, or in patients receiving monoamine oxidase inhibitors.

Continued on next page

Entex LA—Cont.

WARNINGS

Sympathomimetic amines should be used with caution in patients with hypertension, diabetes mellitus, heart disease, peripheral vascular disease, increased intraocular pressure, hyperthyroidism, or prostatic hypertrophy.

PRECAUTIONS

Information for Patients: Do not crush or chew **Entex LA** tablets prior to swallowing.
Drug Interactions: **Entex LA** should not be used in patients taking monoamine oxidase inhibitors or other sympathomimetics.
Drug/Laboratory Test Interactions: Guaifenesin has been reported to interfere with clinical laboratory determinations of urinary 5-hydroxyindoleacetic acid (5-HIAA) and urinary vanillylmandelic acid (VMA).
Pregnancy: Pregnancy Category C. Animal reproduction studies have not been conducted with **Entex LA**. It is also not known whether **Entex LA** can cause fetal harm when administered to a pregnant woman or can affect reproduction capacity. **Entex LA** should be given to a pregnant woman only if clearly needed.
Nursing Mothers: It is not known whether the drugs in **Entex LA** are excreted in human milk. Because many drugs are excreted in human milk and because of the potential for serious adverse reactions in nursing infants, a decision should be made whether to discontinue nursing or to discontinue the product, taking into account the importance of the drug to the mother.
Pediatric Use: Safety and effectiveness of **Entex LA** tablets in pediatric patients below the age of 6 have not been established.

ADVERSE REACTIONS

Possible adverse reactions include nervousness, insomnia, restlessness, headache, nausea, or gastric irritation. These reactions seldom, if ever, require discontinuation of therapy. Urinary retention may occur in patients with prostatic hypertrophy.

OVERDOSAGE

The treatment of overdosage should provide symptomatic and supportive care. If the amount ingested is considered dangerous or excessive, induce vomiting with ipecac syrup unless the patient is convulsing, comatose, or has lost the gag reflex, in which case perform gastric lavage using a large-bore tube. If indicated, follow with activated charcoal and a saline cathartic. Since the effects of **Entex LA** may last up to 12 hours, treatment should be continued for at least that length of time.

DOSAGE AND ADMINISTRATION

Adults and adolescents 12 years of age and older: one tablet twice daily (every 12 hours).
Children 6 to under 12 years: one-half ($^1/_2$) tablet twice daily (every 12 hours). **Entex LA** is not recommended for pediatric patients under 6 years of age.
Tablets may be broken in half for ease of administration without affecting release of medication but should not be crushed or chewed prior to swallowing.

HOW SUPPLIED

Entex LA is available as an orange, scored tablet coded with "ENTEX LA" on one side and "033 033" on the scored side.
NDC 51479-033-01 bottles of 100
NDC 51479-033-05 bottles of 500
Dispense in tight, light-resistant containers as defined in USP.
Store below 77°F (25°C).
Rx only.
Manufactured by
WelPharm, Inc.
Irvine, CA 92614
Manufactured for
DURA Pharmaceuticals, Inc.
San Diego, CA 92121
REVISED June, 1998　　　　　　　　　　ELA 004C98

ENTEX® PSE　　　　　℞

[n 'tex P-S-E]
(pseudoephedrine hydrochloride/guaifenesin)

DESCRIPTION

Each **Entex PSE** yellow coated, scored, long-acting tablet for oral administration contains
pseudoephedrine hydrochloride .... 120 mg
guaifenesin .... 600 mg
in a special base to provide a prolonged therapeutic effect. This product contains ingredients of the following therapeutic classes: decongestant and expectorant.
Pseudoephedrine hydrochloride is a decongestant having the chemical name, benzenemethanol,α-[1-(methylamino)

ethyl]-[S-(R*, R*)]-, hydrochloride, with the following structure:

Guaifenesin is an expectorant having the chemical name, 1,2-propanediol, 3-(2-methoxyphenoxy)-, with the following structure:

Inactive Ingredients: Each tablet contains compressible sugar, D&C Yellow No. 10 Aluminum Lake, dioctyl sodium sulfosuccinate, FD&C Yellow No. 6 Aluminum Lake, hydroxypropyl cellulose, hydroxypropyl methylcellulose, magnesium stearate, polyethylene glycol, purified water, silicon dioxide, sodium citrate, stearic acid, and titanium dioxide.

CLINICAL PHARMACOLOGY

Pseudoephedrine hydrochloride is an α-adrenergic receptor agonist (sympathomimetic) which produces vasoconstriction by stimulating α-receptors within the mucosa of the respiratory tract. Clinically, pseudoephedrine shrinks swollen mucous membranes, reduces tissue hyperemia, edema, and nasal congestion, and increases nasal airway patency. Guaifenesin promotes lower respiratory tract drainage by thinning bronchial secretions, lubricates irritated respiratory tract membranes through increased mucous flow, and facilitates removal of viscous, inspissated mucus. As a result of these drugs, sinus and bronchial drainage is improved, and dry, nonproductive coughs become more productive and less frequent.

INDICATIONS AND USAGE

Entex PSE tablets are indicated for the relief of nasal congestion due to the common cold, hay fever or other upper respiratory allergies, and nasal congestion associated with sinusitis. To promote nasal or sinus drainage; for the symptomatic relief of respiratory conditions characterized by dry nonproductive cough and in the presence of tenacious mucus and/or mucous plugs in the respiratory tract.

CONTRAINDICATIONS

Entex PSE tablets are contraindicated in patients with a known hypersensitivity to any of its ingredients, in nursing mothers, or in patients with severe hypertension, severe coronary artery disease, prostatic hypertrophy, or in patients on MAO inhibitor therapy.

WARNINGS

Sympathomimetic amines should be used with caution in patients with hypertension, diabetes mellitus, heart disease, peripheral vascular disease, increased intraocular pressure, hyperthyroidism, or prostatic hypertrophy.

PRECAUTIONS

General: Hypertensive patients should use **Entex PSE** tablets only with medical advice, as they may experience a change in blood pressure due to added vasoconstriction.
Information for Patients: Persistent cough may indicate a serious condition. If cough persists for more than one week, tends to recur, or is accompanied by a high fever, rash, or persistent headache, consult a physician.
Drug Interactions: MAO inhibitors and beta adrenergic blockers increase effects of sympathomimetics. Sympathomimetics may reduce the antihypertensive effects if methyldopa, guanethidine, mecamylamine, reserpine and veratrum alkaloids.
Drug/Laboratory Test Interactions: Guaifenesin has been reported to interfere with clinical laboratory determinations of urinary 5-hydroxyindoleacetic acid (5-HIAA) and urinary vanillylmandelic acid (VMA).
Pregnancy: Pregnancy Category C. Animal reproduction studies have not been conducted with **Entex PSE** tablets. It is also not known whether **Entex PSE** tablets can cause fetal harm when administered to a pregnant woman or can affect reproduction capacity. **Entex PSE** tablets should be given to a pregnant woman only if clearly needed.
Nursing Mothers: **Entex PSE** tablets are contraindicated in the nursing mother because of the higher than usual risks to infants from sympathomimetic agents.
Usage in Elderly: Patients 60 years and older are more likely to experience adverse reactions to sympathomimetics. Overdose may cause hallucinations, convulsions, CNS depression and death. Demonstrate safe use of a short-acting sympathomimetic before use of a sustained action formulation in elderly patients.

Pediatric Use: Safety and effectiveness of **Entex PSE** tablets in pediatric patients below the age of 6 have not been established.

ADVERSE REACTIONS

Gastrointestinal: nausea and vomiting.
Central Nervous System: nervousness, dizziness, sleeplessness, lightheadedness, tremor, hallucinations, convulsions, CNS depression, fear, anxiety, headache, increased irritability or excitement.
Cardiovascular: palpitations, tachycardia, cardiovascular collapse and death.
General: weakness.
Respiratory: respiratory difficulties.

OVERDOSAGE

Symptoms: Overdose may cause hallucinations, convulsions, CNS depression, cardiovascular collapse and death.
Treatment: Treatment of overdosage should provide symptomatic care. If the amount ingested is considered dangerous or excessive, induce vomiting with ipecac syrup unless the patient is convulsing, comatose, or has lost the gag reflex, in which case, perform gastric lavage using a large-bore tube. If indicated, follow with activated charcoal and a saline cathartic. Since the effects of **Entex PSE** tablets may last up to 12 hours, treatment should be continued for at least that length of time.

DOSAGE AND ADMINISTRATION

Adults and adolescents 12 years of age and older: one tablet twice daily (every 12 hours).
Children 6 to under 12 years: one-half ($^1/_2$) tablet twice daily (every 12 hours). **Entex PSE** tablets are not recommended for pediatric patients under 6 years of age.
Tablets may be broken in half for ease of administration without affecting release of medication but should not be crushed or chewed prior to swallowing.

HOW SUPPLIED

Entex PSE tablets are coated yellow, scored and coded with "Entex PSE" on one side and "032 032" on the scored side.
NDC 51479-032-01 bottles of 100
Store at controlled room temperature (59°–77°F or 15°–25°C).
Dispense in tight, light-resistant containers as defined in USP.
Rx only.
Manufactured by
WelPharm, Inc.
Irvine, CA 92614
Manufactured for
DURA Pharmaceuticals, Inc.
San Diego, CA 92121
REVISED June, 1998
EPSE003C98

FENESIN™　　　　　℞
ORAL EXPECTORANT TABLET

DESCRIPTION

Each light blue, scored, sustained-release tablet provides 600 mg guaifenesin in a specially-prepared base to provide a prolonged therapeutic effect. Guaifenesin is an expectorant having the chemical name: 1,2-Propanediol, 3-(2-methoxy phenoxy)-.
Inactive Ingredients: colloidal silicon dioxide, FD&C Blue #1, partially hydrogenated cottonseed oil, dicalcium phosphate, hydroxypropyl methylcellulose, magnesium stearate, stearic acid.

HOW SUPPLIED

Fenesin is available as a light blue, scored tablet embossed with DURA on one side and 009 on the other.
Bottles of 100 (NDC 51479-009-01)
Bottles of 600 (NDC 51479-009-06)
Store at room temperature, 15°–25°C (59°–77°F).
Dispense in a tight, light-resistant container (USP/NF) with a child-resistant closure.
Rx only
Manufactured for Dura Pharmaceuticals, Inc., San Diego, CA 92121
Manufactured by Anabolic, Inc., Irvine, CA 92614
Revised June, 1998　　　　　　　　　　F001I98

FENESIN™ DM　　　　　℞
ANTITUSSIVE/EXPECTORANT TABLET

DESCRIPTION

Each dark blue, scored tablet for oral administration contains:
dextromethorphan
　hydrobromide .... 30 mg
guaifenesin .... 600 mg
in a special base to provide a prolonged therapeutic effect.

HOW SUPPLIED

Fenesin DM is available as a dark blue, scored tablet embossed with *Dura* on one side and *FDM 014* on the other. Bottles of 100 (NDC 51479-014-01).
Store at controlled room temperature 15°–25°C (59°–77°F).
Dispense in a tight, light-resistant container (USP/NF) with a child-resistant closure.
Rx only
Manufactured for Dura Pharmaceuticals, Inc., San Diego, CA 92121
Manufactured by Anabolic, Inc., Irvine, CA 92614
Revised June, 1998 FDM003E98

FURADANTIN® ℞
(nitrofurantoin)
Oral Suspension

DESCRIPTION

Furadantin (nitrofurantoin) a synthetic chemical, is a stable, yellow, crystalline compound. **Furadantin** is an antibacterial agent for specific urinary tract infections. **Furadantin** is available in 25 mg/5 mL liquid suspension for oral administration.

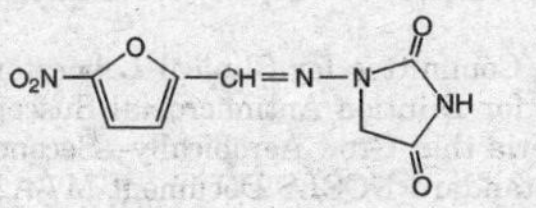

1-[[(5-nitro-2-furanyl)methylene]amino]-2,
4-imidazolidinedione

Inactive Ingredients: Furadantin Oral Suspension contains carboxymethylcellulose sodium, citric acid, flavors, glycerin, magnesium aluminum silicate, methylparaben, propylparaben, purified water, saccharin, sodium citrate, and sorbitol.

CLINICAL PHARMACOLOGY

Orally administered **Furadantin** is readily absorbed and rapidly excreted in urine. Blood concentrations at therapeutic dosage are usually low. It is highly soluble in urine, to which it may impart a brown color.
Following a dose regimen of 100 mg q.i.d. for 7 days, average urinary drug recoveries (0–24 hours) on day 1 and day 7 were 42.7% and 43.6%.
Unlike many drugs, the presence of food or agents delaying gastric emptying can increase the bioavailability of **Furadantin**, presumably by allowing better dissolution in gastric juices.
Microbiology: Nitrofurantoin is bactericidal in urine at therapeutic doses. The mechanism of the antimicrobial action of nitrofurantoin is unusual among antibacterials. Nitrofurantoin is reduced by bacterial flavoproteins to reactive intermediates which inactivate or alter bacterial ribosomal proteins and other macromolecules. As a result of such inactivations, the vital biochemical processes of protein synthesis, aerobic energy metabolism, DNA synthesis, RNA synthesis, and cell wall synthesis are inhibited. The broad-based nature of this mode of action may explain the lack of acquired bacterial resistance to nitrofurantoin, as the necessary multiple and simultaneous mutations of the target macromolecules would likely be lethal to the bacteria. Development of resistance to nitrofurantoin has not been a significant problem since its introduction in 1953. Cross-resistance with antibiotics and sulfonamides has not been observed, and transferable resistance is, at most, a very rare phenomenon.
Nitrofurantoin, in the form of **Furadantin**, has been shown to be active against most strains of the following bacteria both *in vitro* and in clinical infections: (See INDICATIONS AND USAGE.)

Gram-Positive Aerobes
Staphylococcus aureus
Enterococci (e.g., *Enterococcus faecalis*)
Gram-Negative Aerobes
Escherichia coli

NOTE: Some strains of *Enterobacter* species and *Klebsiella* species are resistant to nitrofurantoin.
Nitrofurantoin also demonstrates *in vitro* activity against the following microorganisms, although the clinical significance of these data with respect to treatment with **Furadantin** is unkown:

Gram-Positive Aerobes
Coagulase-negative staphylococci (including *Staphylococcus epidermidis* and *Staphylococcus saprophyticus*)
Streptococcus agalactiae
Group D streptococci)
Viridans group streptococci
Gram-Negative Aerobes
Citrobacter amalonaticus
Citrobacter diversus
Citrobacter freundii
Klebsiella oxytoca
Klebsiella ozaenae

Nitrofurantoin is not active against most strains of *Proteus* species or *Serratia* species. It has no activity against *Pseudomonas* species.
Antagonism has been demonstrated *in vitro* between nitrofurantoin and quinolone antimicrobial agents. The clinical significance of this finding is unknown.
Susceptibility Tests:
Diffusion Techniques:
Quantitative methods that require measurement of zone diameters give the most precise estimate of the susceptibility of bacteria to antimicrobial agents. One such standard procedure,[1] which has been recommended for use with disks to test susceptibility of organisms to nitrofurantoin, uses the 300-mcg nitrofurantoin disk. Interpretation involves the correlation of the diameter obtained in the disk test with the minimum inhibitory concentration (MIC) for nitrofurantoin.
Reports from the laboratory giving results of the standard single-disk susceptibility test with a 300-mcg nitrofurantoin disk should be interpreted according to the following criteria:

Zone Diameter (mm)	Interpretation
≥17	Susceptible
15-16	Intermediate
≤14	Resistant

A report of "susceptible" indicates that the pathogen is likely to be inhibited by generally achievable urinary levels. A report of "intermediate" indicates that the result be considered equivocal and, if the organism is not fully susceptible to alternative clinically feasible drugs, the test should be repeated. This category provides a buffer zone which prevents small uncontrolled technical factors from causing major discrepancies in interpretations. A report of "resistant" indicates that achievable concentrations are unlikely to be inhibitory, and other therapy should be selected.
Standardized procedures require the use of laboratory control organisms. The 300-mcg nitrofurantoin disk should give the following zone diameters:

Organism	Zone Diameter (mm)
E. coli ATCC 25922	20-25
S. aureas ATCC 25923	18-22

Dilution Techniques:
Use a standardized dilution method[2] (broth, agar, microdilution) or equivalent with nitrofurantoin powder. The MIC values obtained should be interpreted according to the following criteria:

MIC (mcg/mL)	Interpretation
≤32	Susceptible
64	Intermediate
≥128	Resistant

As with standard diffusion techniques, dilution methods require the use of laboratory control organisms. Standard nitrofurantoin powder should provide the following MIC values:

Organism	MIC (mcg/mL)
E. coli ATCC 25922	4-16
S. aureus ATCC 29213	8-32
E. faecalis ATCC 29212	4-16

INDICATIONS AND USAGE

Furadantin is specifically indicated for the treatment of urinary tract infections when due to susceptible strains of *Escherichia coli*, enterococci, *Staphylococcus aureus*, and certain susceptible strains of *Klebsiella* and *Enterobacter* species.
Nitrofurantoin is not indicated for the treatment of pyelonephritis or perinephric abscesses.
Nitrofurantoins lack the broader tissue distribution of other therapeutic agents approved for urinary tract infections. Consequently, many patients who are treated with **Furadantin** are predisposed to persistence or reappearance of bacteriuria. Urine specimens for culture and susceptibility testing should be obtained before and after completion of therapy. If persistence or reappearance of bacteriuria occurs after treatment with **Furadantin**, other therapeutic agents with broader tissue distribution should be selected. In considering the use of **Furadantin**, lower eradication rates should be balanced against the increased potential for systemic toxicity and for the development of antimicrobial resistance when agents with broader tissue distribution are utilized.

CONTRAINDICATIONS

Anuria, oliguria, or significant impairment of renal function (creatinine clearance under 60 mL per minute or clinically significant elevated serum creatinine) are contraindications. Treatment of this type of patient carries an increased risk of toxicity because of impaired excretion of the drug.
Because of the possibility of hemolytic anemia due to immature erythrocyte enzyme systems (glutathione instability), the drug is contraindicated in pregnant patients at term (38–42 weeks gestation), during labor and delivery, or when the onset of labor is imminent. For the same reason, the drug is contraindicated in neonates under one month of age. **Furadantin** is also contraindicated in those patients with known hypersensitivity to nitrofurantoin.

WARNINGS

ACUTE, SUBACUTE, OR CHRONIC PULMONARY REACTIONS HAVE BEEN OBSERVED IN PATIENTS TREATED WITH NITROFURANTOIN. IF THESE REACTIONS OCCUR, FURADANTIN SHOULD BE DISCONTINUED AND APPROPRIATE MEASURES TAKEN. REPORTS HAVE CITED PULMONARY REACTIONS AS A CONTRIBUTING CAUSE OF DEATH.
CHRONIC PULMONARY REACTIONS (DIFFUSE INTERSTITIAL PNEUMONITIS OR PULMONARY FIBROSIS, OR BOTH) CAN DEVELOP INSIDIOUSLY. THESE REACTIONS OCCUR RARELY AND GENERALLY IN PATIENTS RECEIVING THERAPY FOR SIX MONTHS OR LONGER. CLOSE MONITORING OF THE PULMONARY CONDITION OF PATIENTS RECEIVING LONG-TERM THERAPY IS WARRANTED AND REQUIRES THAT THE BENEFITS OF THERAPY BE WEIGHED AGAINST POTENTIAL RISKS. (SEE RESPIRATORY REACTIONS.)
Hepatic reactions, including hepatitis, cholestatic jaundice, chronic active hepatitis, and hepatic necrosis, occur rarely. Fatalities have been reported. The onset of chronic active hepatitis may be insidious, and patients should be monitored periodically for changes in liver function. If hepatitis occurs, the drug should be withdrawn immediately and appropriate measures should be taken.
Peripheral neuropathy, which may become severe or irreversible, has occurred. Fatalities have been reported. Conditions such as renal impairment (creatinine clearance under 60 mL per minute or clinically significant elevated serum creatinine), anemia, diabetes mellitus, electrolyte imbalance, vitamin B deficiency, and debilitating disease may enhance the occurrence of peripheral neuropathy. Patients receiving long-term therapy should be monitored periodically for changes in renal function. Optic neuritis has been reported rarely in postmarketing experience with nitrofurantoin formulations.
Cases of hemolytic anemia of the primaquine-sensitivity type have been induced by nitrofurantoin. Hemolysis appears to be linked to a glucose-6-phosphate dehydrogenase deficiency in the red blood cells of the affected patients. This deficiency is found in 10 percent of Blacks and a small percentage of ethnic groups of Mediterranean and Near-Eastern origin. Hemolysis is an indication for discontinuing **Furadantin**; hemolysis ceases when the drug is withdrawn.
Pseudomembranous colitis has been reported with nearly all antibacterial agents, including nitrofurantoin, and may range from mild to life threatening. Therefore, it is important to consider this diagnosis in patients with diarrhea subsequent to the administration of antibacterial agents.
Treatment with antibacterial agents alters the normal flora of the colon and may permit overgrowth of clostridia. Studies indicate that a toxin produced by *Clostridium difficile* is one primary cause of antibiotic-associated colitis.
After the diagnosis of pseudomembranous colitis has been established, appropriate therapeutic measures should be initiated. Mild cases of pseudomembranous colitis usually respond to drug discontinuation alone. In moderate to severe cases, consideration should be given to management with fluids and electrolytes, protein supplementation, and treatment with an antibacterial drug clinically effective against *Clostridium difficile* colitis.

PRECAUTIONS

Information for Patients: Patients should be advised to take **Furadantin** with food to further enhance tolerance and improve drug absorption. Patients should be instructed to complete the full course of therapy; however, they should be advised to contact their physician if any unusual symptoms occur during therapy.
Patients should be advised not to use antacid preparations containing magnesium trisilicate while taking **Furadantin**.
Drug Interactions: Antacids containing magnesium trisilicate, when administered concomitantly with nitrofurantoin, reduce both the rate and extent of absorption. The mechanism for this interaction probably is adsorption of nitrourantoin onto the surface of magnesium trisilicate.
Uricosuric drugs, such as probenecid and sulfinpyrazone, can inhibit renal tubular secretion of nitrofurantoin. The resulting increase in nitrofurantoin serum levels may increase toxicity, and the decreased urinary levels could lessen its efficacy as a urinary tract antibacterial.
Drug/Laboratory Test Interactions: As a result of the presence of nitrofurantoin, a false-positive reaction for glucose in the urine may occur. This has been observed with Benedict's and Fehling's solutions but not with the glucose enzymatic test.

Continued on next page

Furadantin—Cont.

Carcinogenesis, Mutagenesis, Impairment of Fertility: Nitrofurantoin was not carcinogenic when fed to female Holtzman rats for 44.5 weeks or to female Sprague-Dawley rats for 75 weeks. Two chronic rodent bioassays utilizing male and female Sprague-Dawley rats and two chronic bioassays in Swiss mice and in BDF, mice revealed no evidence of carcinogenicity.

Nitrofuratoin presented evidence of carcinogenic activity in female B6C3F$_1$ mice as shown by increased incidences of tubular adenomas, benign mixed tumors, and granulosa cell tumors of the ovary. In male F344/N rats, there were increased incidences of uncommon kidney tubular cell neoplasms, osteosarcomas of the bone, and neoplasms of the subcutaneous tissue. In one study involving subcutaneous administration of 75 mg/kg nitrofurantoin to pregnant female mice, lung papillary adenomas of unknown significance were observed in the F1 generation.

Nitrofurantoin has been shown to induce point mutations in certain strains of *Salmonella typhimurium* and forward mutations in L5178Y mouse lymphoma cells. Nitrofurantoin induced increased numbers of sister chromatid exchanges and chromosomal aberrations in Chinese hamster ovary cells but not in human cells in culture. Results of the sex-linked recessive lethal assay in Drosophila were negative after administration of nitrofurantoin by feeding or by injection. Nitrofurantoin did not induce heritable mutation in the rodent models examined.

The significance of the carcinogenicity and mutagenicity findings relative to the therapeutic use of nitrofurantoin in humans is unknown.

The administration of high doses of nitrofurantoin to rats causes temporary spermatogenic arrest; this is reversible on discontinuing the drug. Doses of 10 mg/kg/day or greater in healthy humans males may, in certain unpredictable instances, produce a slight to moderate spermatogenic arrest with a decrease in sperm count.

Pregnancy:

Teratogenic effects: Pregnancy Category B.

Pregnancy Category B. Several reproduction studies have been performed in rabbits and rats at doses up to six times the human dose and have revealed no evidence of impaired fertility or harm to the fetus due to nitrofurantoin. In a single published study conducted in mice at 68 times the human dose (based on mg/kg administered to the dam), growth retardation and a low incidence of minor and common malformations were observed. However, at 25 times the human dose, fetal malformations were not observed: the relevance of these findings to humans is uncertain. There are, however, no adequate and well-controlled studies in pregnant women. Because animal reproduction studies are not always predictive of human response, this drug should be used during pregnancy only if clearly needed.

Non-teratogenic effects: Nitrofurantoin has been shown in one published transplacental carcinogenicity study to induce lung papillary adenomas in the F1 generation mice at doses 19 times the human dose on a mg/kg basis. The relationship of this finding, to potential human carcinogenesis is presently unknown. Because of the uncertainty regarding the human implications of these animal data, this drug should be used during pregnancy only if clearly needed.

Labor and Delivery: See CONTRAINDICATIONS.

Nursing Mothers: Nitrofurantoin has been detected in human breast milk in trace amounts. Because of the potential for serious adverse reactions from nitrofurantoin in nursing infants under one month of age, a decision should be made whether to discontinue nursing or to discontinue the drug, taking into account the importance of the drug to the mother. (See CONTRAINDICATIONS.)

Pediatric Use: Safety and effectiveness of **Furadantin** in neonates below the age of one month have not been established. (See CONTRAINDICATIONS.)

ADVERSE REACTIONS

Respiratory:

CHRONIC, SUBACUTE, OR ACUTE PULMONARY HYPERSENSITIVITY REACTIONS MAY OCCUR.

CHRONIC PULMONARY REACTIONS OCCUR GENERALLY IN PATIENTS WHO HAVE RECEIVED CONTINUOUS TREATMENT FOR SIX MONTHS OR LONGER. MALAISE, DYSPNEA ON EXERTION, COUGH, AND ALTERED PULMONARY FUNCTION ARE COMMON MANIFESTATIONS WHICH CAN OCCUR INSIDIOUSLY. RADIOLOGIC AND HISTOLOGIC FINDINGS OF DIFFUSE INTERSTITIAL PNEUMONITIS OR FIBROSIS, OR BOTH, ARE ALSO COMMON MANIFESTATIONS OF THE CHRONIC PULMONARY REACTION. FEVER IS RARELY PROMINENT.

THE SEVERITY OF CHRONIC PULMONARY REACTIONS AND THEIR DEGREE OF RESOLUTION APPEAR TO BE RELATED TO THE DURATION OF THERAPY AFTER THE FIRST CLINICAL SIGNS APPEAR. PULMONARY FUNCTION MAY BE IMPAIRED PERMANENTLY, EVEN AFTER CESSATION OF THERAPY. THE RISK IS GREATER WHEN CHRONIC PULMONARY REACTIONS ARE NOT RECOGNIZED EARLY.

In subacute pulmonary reactions, fever and eosinophilia occur less often than in the acute form. Upon cessation of therapy, recovery may require several months. If the symptoms are not recognized as being drug-related and nitrofurantoin therapy is not stopped, the symptoms may become more severe.

Acute pulmonary reactions are commonly manifested by fever, chills, cough, chest pain, dyspnea, pulmonary infiltration with consolidation or pleural effusion on x-ray, and eosinophilia. Acute reactions usually occur within the first week of treatment and are reversible with cessation of therapy. Resolution often is dramatic. (See **WARNINGS**.)

Changes in EKG (eg, non-specific ST/T wave changes, bundle branch block) have been reported in association with pulmonary reactions.

Cyanosis has been reported rarely.

Hepatic: Hepatic reactions, including hepatitis, cholestatic jaundice, chronic active hepatitis, and hepatic necrosis, occur rarely. (See **WARNINGS**.)

Neurologic: Peripheral neuropathy, which may become severe or irreversible, has occurred. Fatalities have been reported. Conditions such as renal impairment (creatinine clearance under 60 mL per minute or clinically significant elevated serum creatinine), anemia, diabetes mellitus, electrolyte imbalance, vitamin B deficiency, and debilitating diseases may increase the possibility of peripheral neuropathy. (See **WARNINGS**.)

Asthenia, vertigo, nystagmus, dizziness, headache, and drowsiness have also been reported with the use of nitrofurantoin.

Benign intracranial hypertension (pseudotumor cerebri), confusion, depression, optic neuritis, and psychotic reactions have been reported rarely. Bulging fontanels, as a sign of benign intracranial hypertension in infants, have been reported rarely.

Dermatologic: Exfoliative dermatitis and erythema multiform (including Stevens-Johnson syndrome) have been reported rarely. Transient alopecia also has been reported.

Allergic: A lupus-like syndrome associated with pulmonary reactions to nitrofurantoin has been reported. Also, angioedema; maculopapular, erythematous, or eczematous eruptions; pruritus; urticaria; anaphylaxis; arthralgia; myalgia; drug fever; and chills have been reported.

Gastrointestinal: Nausea, emesis, and anorexia occur most often. Abdominal pain and diarrhea are less common gastrointestinal reactions. These dose-related reactions can be minimized by reduction of dosage. Sialadenitis and pancreatitis have been reported. There have been sporadic reports of pseudomembranous colitis with the use of nitrofurantoin. The onset of pseudomembranous colitis symptoms may occur during or after antimicrobial treatment. (See **WARNINGS**.)

Hematologic: Cyanosis secondary to methemoglobinemia has been reported rarely.

Miscellaneous: As with other antimicrobial agents, superinfections caused by resistant organisms, eg, *Pseudomonas* species or *Candida* species, can occur.

Laboratory Adverse Events: The following laboratory adverse events have been reported with the use of nitrofurantoin: increased AST (SGOT), increased ALT (SGPT), decreased hemoglobin, increased serum phosphorus, eosinophilia, glucose-6-phosphate dehydrogenase deficiency anemia (see **WARNINGS**), agranulocytosis, leukopenia, granulocytopenia, hemolytic anemia, thrombocytopenia, megaloblastic anemia. In most cases, these hematologic abnormalities resolved following cessation of therapy. Aplastic anemia has been reported rarely.

OVERDOSAGE

Occasional incidents of acute overdosage of **Furadantin** have not resulted in any specific symptoms other than vomiting. Induction of emesis is recommended. There is no specific antidote, but a high fluid intake should be maintained to promote urinary excretion of the drug. It is dialyzable.

DOSAGE AND ADMINISTRATION

Furadantin should be given with food to improve drug absorption and, in some patients, tolerance.

Adults: 50–100 mg four times a day — the lower dosage level is recommended for uncomplicated urinary tract infections.

Children: 5–7 mg/kg of body weight per 24 hours given in four divided doses (contraindicated under one month of age).

The following table is based on an average weight in each range receiving 5 to 6 mg/kg of body weight per 24 hours, given in four divided doses. It can be used to calculate an average dose of **Furadantin** Oral Suspension (25 mg/5 mL) for children (one 5-mL teaspoon of **Furadantin** Oral Suspension contains 25 mg of **Furadantin**):

Body Weight		No. Teaspoonfuls
Pounds	Kilograms	4 Times Daily
15 to 26	7 to 11	1/2 (2.5 mL)
27 to 46	12 to 21	1 (5 mL)
47 to 68	22 to 30	1-1/2 (7.5 mL)
69 to 91	31 to 41	2 (10 mL)

Therapy should be continued for one week or for at least 3 days after sterility of the urine is obtained. Continued infection indicates the need for reevaluation.

For long-term suppressive therapy in adults, a reduction of dosage to 50-100 mg at bedtime may be adequate. For long-term suppressive therapy in children, dose as low as 1 mg/kg per 24 hours, given in a single dose or in two divided doses may be adequate. **SEE WARNINGS SECTION REGARDING RISKS ASSOCIATED WITH LONG-TERM THERAPY.**

HOW SUPPLIED

Furadantin Oral Suspension is available in:

NDC 51479-029-06	glass amber bottle of 60 mL
NDC 51479-029-47	glass amber bottle of 470 mL

Avoid exposure to strong light which may darken the drug. It is stable when stored between 20°–25°C (68°–77°F); protect from freezing. It should be dispensed in glass amber bottles.

CAUTION: Federal law prohibits dispensing without prescription.

REFERENCES

1. National Committee for Clinical Laboratory Standards. Performance Standards for Antimicrobial Disk Susceptibility Tests—Fourth Edition. Approved Standard NCCLS Document M2-A4, Vol. 10, No. 7, NCCLS, Villanova, PA, 1990.
2. National Committee for Clinical Laboratory Standards. Methods for Dilution Antimicrobial Susceptibility Tests for Bacteria that Grow Aerobically—Second Edition. Approved Standard NCCLS Document M7-A2, Vol. 10, No. 8, NCCLS, Villanova, PA, 1990.

Manufactured by
Procter & Gamble Pharmaceuticals
Cincinnati, Ohio 45202
Manufactured for
Dura Pharmaceuticals, Inc.
San Diego, California 92121
REVISED February, 1998
FOS001C0298

GUAI-VENT™ /PSE ℞
DECONGESTANT/EXPECTORANT

DESCRIPTION

Each Guai-Vent/PSE white, uncoated, scored, sustained-release tablet for oral administration contains:

pseudoephedrine hydrochloride	120 mg
guaifenesin	600 mg

in a special base to provide a prolonged therapeutic effect.

HOW SUPPLIED

Guai-Vent/PSE tablets are white, uncoated, scored and coated with *"015"* on one side and *"DURA"* on the scored side.

Bottles of 100 (NDC 51479-015-01).

Store at controlled room temperature (59°–77°F or 15°–25°C). Dispense in a tight, light-resistant container as defined in USP/NF with a child-resistant closure.

Rx only.

Manufactured for Dura Pharmaceuticals, Inc. San Diego, CA 92121
Manufactured by Anabolic, Inc., Irvine, CA 92614
Revised June, 1998 GPSE001D98

KEFTAB® ℞
[*kĕf 'tăb*]
cephalexin hydrochloride, USP

DESCRIPTION

Keftab is a semisynthetic cephalosporin antibiotic intended for oral administration. Chemically, it is designated 7-(D-2-Amino-2-phenylacetamido)-3-methyl-3-cephem-4-carboxylic acid hydrochloride monohydrate, and the chemical formula is $C_{16}H_{17}N_3O_4S \cdot HCl \cdot H_2O$. The molecular weight is 401.87, and it has the following structural formula:

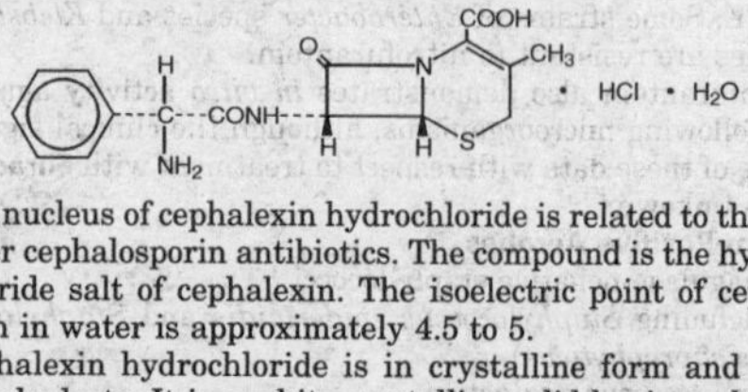

The nucleus of cephalexin hydrochloride is related to that of other cephalosporin antibiotics. The compound is the hydrochloride salt of cephalexin. The isoelectric point of cephalexin in water is approximately 4.5 to 5.

Cephalexin hydrochloride is in crystalline form and is a monohydrate. It is a white crystalline solid having a bitter taste. Solubility in water is high at room temperature; greater than 10 mg/mL may be dissolved readily.

The cephalosporins differ from penicillins in the structure of the bicyclic ring system. Cephalexin has a D-phenylglycyl group as substituent at the 7-amino position and an unsubstituted methyl group at the 3-position.

Each tablet contains cephalexin hydrochloride equivalent to 500 mg (1.439 μmol) cephalexin. The tablets also contain D & C Yellow No. 10, F D & C Blue No. 1, F D & C Red No. 40, magnesium stearate, silicon dioxide, stearic acid, sucrose, titanium dioxide, and other inactive ingredients.

CLINICAL PHARMACOLOGY

Human Pharmacology—Keftab is acid stable and may be given without regard to meals. It is rapidly absorbed after oral administration. Following doses of 250 mg and 500 mg, average peak serum levels of approximately 9 and 18 μg/mL respectively were obtained at 1 hour and declined to 1.6 and 3.4 μg/mL respectively at 3 hours. Measurable levels were present 6 hours after administration. Cephalexin is excreted in the urine by glomerular filtration and tubular secretion. Studies showed that approximately 70% of the drug was excreted unchanged in the urine within 12 hours. During the first 6 hours, average urine concentrations following the 250-mg and 500-mg doses were approximately 200 μg/mL (range, 54 to 663) and 500 μg/mL (range, 137 to 1,306) respectively. The average serum half-life is 1.1 hours.

Microbiology—In vitro tests demonstrate that the cephalosporins are bactericidal because of their inhibition of cell-wall synthesis. Keftab is active against the following organisms in vitro:

β-hemolytic streptococci

Staphylococcus aureus, including penicillinase-producing strains

Streptococcus pneumoniae

Escherichia coli

Proteus mirabilis

Klebsiella spp.

Haemophilus influenzae

Moraxella (Branhamella) catarrhalis

Note—Most strains of enterococci (*Enterococcus faecalis* [formerly *Streptococcus faecalis*]) and a few strains of staphylococci are resistant to Keftab. When tested by in vitro methods, staphylococci exhibit cross-resistance between Keftab and methicillin-type antibiotics. Keftab is not active against most strains of *Enterobacter* spp., *Morganella morganii* (formerly *Proteus morganii*), *Serratia* spp., and *Proteus vulgaris*. It has no activity against *Pseudomonas* or *Acinetobacter* spp.

Disk Susceptibility Tests—Quantitative methods that require measurement of zone diameters give the most precise estimates of antibiotic susceptibility. One such procedure[1] has been recommended for use with cephalosporin class (cephalothin) disks for testing susceptibility to cephalexin. The currently accepted zone diameter interpretation for the cephalothin disks' is appropriate for determining susceptibility to cephalexin. Interpretations correlate zone diameters of the disk test with MIC values for cephalexin. With this procedure, a report from the laboratory of "resistant" indicates a zone diameter of 14 mm or less and suggests that the infecting organism is not likely to respond to therapy. A report of "susceptibility" indicates a zone diameter of 18 mm or greater. A report of "intermediate susceptibility" indicates zone diameters between 15 and 17 mm and suggests that the organism would be susceptible if the infection is confined to the urine, in which high antibiotic levels can be obtained, or if high dosage is used in other types of infection.

Standardized procedures require use of control organisms.[1] The 30-μg cephalothin disk should give zone diameters between 18 and 23 mm and 25 and 37 mm for the reference strains *E. coli* ATCC 25922 and *S. aureus* ATCC 25923 respectively.

INDICATIONS AND USAGE

Keftab is indicated for the treatment of the following infections when caused by susceptible strains of the designated microorganisms:

Respiratory tract infections caused by *S. pneumoniae* and group A β-hemolytic streptococci (Penicillin is the usual drug of choice in the treatment and prevention of streptococcal infections, including the prophylaxis of rheumatic fever. Keftab is generally effective in the eradication of streptococci from the nasopharynx; however, substantial data establishing the efficacy of Keftab in the subsequent prevention of rheumatic fever are not available at present.)

Skin and skin structure infections caused by *S. aureus* and/or β-hemolytic streptococci.

Bone infections caused by *S. aureus* and/or *P. mirabilis*.

Genitourinary tract infections, including acute prostatitis, caused by *E. coli*, *P. mirabilis*, and *Klebsiella* spp.

Note—Culture and susceptibility tests should be initiated prior to and during therapy. Renal function studies should be performed when indicated.

CONTRAINDICATIONS

Keftab is contraindicated in patients with known allergy to the cephalosporin group of antibiotics.

WARNINGS

BEFORE CEPHALEXIN THERAPY IS INSTITUTED, CAREFUL INQUIRY SHOULD BE MADE CONCERNING PREVIOUS HYPERSENSITIVITY REACTIONS TO CEPHALOSPORINS AND PENICILLIN. CEPHALOSPORIN C DERIVATIVES SHOULD BE GIVEN CAUTIOUSLY TO PENICILLIN-SENSITIVE PATIENTS. SERIOUS ACUTE HYPERSENSITIVITY REACTIONS MAY REQUIRE EPINEPHRINE AND OTHER EMERGENCY MEASURES.

There is some clinical and laboratory evidence of partial cross-allergenicity of the penicillins and the cephalosporins. Patients have been reported to have had severe reactions (including anaphylaxis) to both drugs.

Any patient who has demonstrated some form of allergy, particularly to drugs, should receive antibiotics cautiously. No exception should be made with regard to Keftab.

Pseudomembranous colitis has been reported with virtually all broad-spectrum antibiotics (including macrolides, semisynthetic penicillins, and cephalosporins); therefore, it is important to consider its diagnosis in patients who develop diarrhea in association with the use of antibiotics. Such colitis may range in severity from mild to life threatening.

Treatment with broad-spectrum antibiotics alters the normal flora of the colon and may permit overgrowth of clostridia. Studies indicate that a toxin produced by *Clostridium difficile* is a primary cause of antibiotic-associated colitis.

Mild cases of pseudomembranous colitis usually respond to drug discontinuance alone. In moderate to severe cases, management should include sigmoidoscopy, appropriate bacteriologic studies, and fluid, electrolyte, and protein supplementation. When the colitis does not improve after the drug has been discontinued or when it is severe, treatment with an oral antibacterial drug effective against *C. difficile* is recommended. Other causes of colitis should be ruled out.

PRECAUTIONS

General—Patients should be followed carefully so that any side effects or unusual manifestations of drug idiosyncrasy may be detected. If an allergic reaction to Keftab occurs, the drug should be discontinued and the patient treated with the usual agents (eg, epinephrine or other pressor amines, antihistamines, or corticosteroids).

Prolonged use of Keftab may result in the overgrowth of nonsusceptible organisms. Careful observation of the patient is essential. If superinfection occurs during therapy, appropriate measures should be taken.

Positive direct Coombs' tests have been reported during treatment with the cephalosporin antibiotics. In hematologic studies or in transfusion cross-matching procedures when antiglobulin tests are performed on the minor side or in Coombs' testing of newborns whose mothers have received cephalosporin antibiotics before parturition, it should be recognized that a positive Coombs' test may be due to the drug.

Keftab should be administered with caution in the presence of markedly impaired renal function. Under such conditions, careful clinical observation and laboratory studies should be made because safe dosage may be lower than that usually recommended.

As a result of administration of Keftab, a false-positive reaction for glucose in the urine may occur. This has been observed with Benedict's and Fehling's solutions and also with Clinitest® tablets.

Broad-spectrum antibiotics should be prescribed with caution in individuals with a history of gastrointestinal disease, particularly colitis.

Pregnancy—Pregnancy Category B—Reproduction studies have been performed on rats in doses of 250 or 500 mg/kg/day and have revealed no evidence of impaired fertility or harm to the fetus due to cephalexin. There are, however, no adequate and well-controlled studies in pregnant women. Because animal reproduction studies are not always predictive of human response, this drug should be used during pregnancy only if clearly needed.

Nursing Mothers—The excretion of cephalexin in the milk increased up to 4 hours after a 500-mg dose; the drug reached a maximum level of 4 μg/mL, then decreased gradually, and had disappeared 8 hours after administration. A decision should be considered to discontinue nursing temporarily during therapy with Keftab.

Pediatric Use—Safety and effectiveness in pediatric patients have not been established.

ADVERSE REACTIONS

Gastrointestinal—Symptoms of pseudomembranous colitis may appear either during or after antibiotic treatment. Nausea and vomiting have been reported rarely. The most frequent side effect has been diarrhea. It was very rarely severe enough to warrant cessation of therapy. Abdominal pain, gastritis, and dyspepsia have also occurred. As with some penicillins and some other cephalosporins, transient hepatitis and cholestatic jaundice have been reported rarely.

Hypersensitivity—Allergic reactions in the form of rash, urticaria, angioedema, and, rarely, erythema multiforme, Ste-

vens-Johnson syndrome, or toxic epidermal necrolysis have been observed. These reactions usually subsided upon discontinuation of the drug. In some of these reactions, supportive therapy may be necessary. Anaphylaxis has also been reported.

Other reactions have included genital and anal pruritus, genital moniliasis, vaginitis and vaginal discharge, dizziness, fatigue, headache, agitation, confusion, hallucinations, arthralgia, arthritis, and joint disorder. Reversible interstitial nephritis has been reported rarely. Eosinophilia, neutropenia, thrombocytopenia, slight elevations in aspartate aminotransferase (AST) and alanine aminotransferase (ALT), and elevated creatinine and BUN have been reported.

In addition to the adverse reactions listed above that have been observed in patients treated with Keftab, the following adverse reactions and altered laboratory tests have been reported for cephalosporin class antibiotics:

Adverse Reactions—Allergic reactions, including fever, colitis, renal dysfunction, toxic nephropathy, and hepatic dysfunction, including cholestasis.

Several cephalosporins have been implicated in triggering seizures, particularly in patients with renal impairment when the dosage was not reduced (see Indications and Usage *and* Precautions, General). If seizures associated with drug therapy should occur, the drug should be discontinued. Anticonvulsant therapy can be given if clinically indicated.

Altered Laboratory Tests—Increased prothrombin time, increased alkaline phosphatase, and leukopenia.

OVERDOSAGE

Signs and Symptoms—Symptoms of oral overdose may include nausea, vomiting, epigastric distress, diarrhea, and hematuria. If other symptoms are present, it is probably secondary to an underlying disease state, an allergic reaction, or toxicity due to ingestion of a second medication.

Treatment—To obtain up-to-date information about the treatment of overdose, a good resource is your certified Regional Poison Control Center. Telephone numbers of certified poison control centers are listed in the *Physicians' Desk Reference (PDR)*. In managing overdosage, consider the possibility of multiple drug overdoses, interaction among drugs, and unusual drug kinetics in your patient.

Unless 5 to 10 times the normal dose of cephalexin has been ingested, gastrointestinal decontamination should not be necessary.

Protect the patient's airway and support ventilation and perfusion. Meticulously monitor and maintain, within acceptable limits, the patient's vital signs, blood gases, serum electrolytes, etc. Absorption of drugs from the gastrointestinal tract may be decreased by giving activated charcoal, which, in many cases, is more effective than emesis or lavage; consider charcoal instead of or in addition to gastric emptying. Repeated doses of charcoal over time may hasten elimination of some drugs that have been absorbed. Safeguard the patient's airway when employing gastric emptying or charcoal.

Forced diuresis, peritoneal dialysis, hemodialysis, or charcoal hemoperfusion have not been established as beneficial for an overdose of cephalexin; however, it should be extremely unlikely that one of these procedures would be indicated.

The oral median lethal dose of cephalexin in rats is 5,000 mg/kg.

DOSAGE AND ADMINISTRATION

Keftab is administered orally.

The adult dosage ranges from 1 to 4 g daily in divided doses. For the following infections, a dosage of 500 mg may be administered every 12 hours: streptococcal pharyngitis, skin and skin structure infections, and uncomplicated cystitis. Cystitis therapy should be continued for 7 to 14 days. For other infections, the usual dosing is every 6 hours. For more severe infections or those caused by less susceptible organisms, larger doses may be needed. If daily doses of Keftab greater than 4 g are required, parenteral cephalosporins, in appropriate doses, should be considered.

HOW SUPPLIED

Tablets (elliptical-shaped):

500 mg* (dark-green) (UC5395)—(100s) NDC 51479-034-01

Store at controlled room temperature, 59° to 86°F (15° to 30°C).

*Equivalent to cephalexin

CAUTION—Federal (USA) law prohibits dispensing without prescription.

Literature revised Oct. 1, 1997

PV 2061 UCP

KEF010B0997

1. 21 CFR 460.1 *Federal Register* 1987; 838-842.

DURA PHARMACEUTICALS

Manufactured by

Eli Lilly and Company

Indianapolis, IN, USA 46285

Continued on next page

Keftab—Cont.

Distributed by DURA Pharmaceuticals, Inc.
San Diego, CA 92121

NASALIDE® ℞
[na 'ză-lide]
(flunisolide)
Nasal Solution
0.025%

DESCRIPTION

NASALIDE® (flunisolide) nasal solution is intended for administration as a spray to the nasal mucosa. Flunisolide, the active component of NASALIDE nasal solution, is an anti-inflammatory steroid with the chemical name: 6α-fluoro-11β,16α,17,21-tetrahydroxypregna-1,4-diene-3,20-dione cyclic 16,17-acetal with acetone (USAN).
It has the following chemical structure:

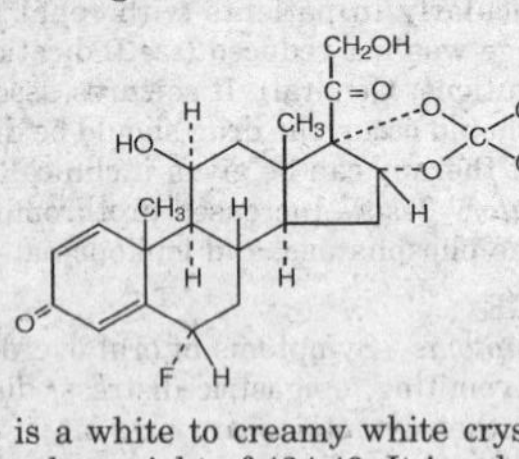

Flunisolide is a white to creamy white crystalline powder with a molecular weight of 434.49. It is soluble in acetone, sparingly soluble in chloroform, slightly soluble in methanol, and practically insoluble in water. It has a melting point of about 245°C.
Each 25 mL spray bottle contains flunisolide 6.25 mg (0.25 mg/mL) in a solution of propylene glycol, polyethylene glycol 3350, citric acid, sodium citrate, butylated hydroxyanisole, edetate disodium, benzalkonium chloride and purified water, with NaOH and/or HCl added to adjust the pH to approximately 5.3. It contains no fluorocarbons.
After priming the delivery system for NASALIDE, each actuation of the unit delivers a metered droplet spray containing approximately 25 mcg of flunisolide. The size of the droplets produced by the unit is in excess of 8 microns to facilitate deposition on the nasal mucosa. The contents of one nasal spray bottle deliver at least 200 sprays.

CLINICAL PHARMACOLOGY

NASALIDE has demonstrated potent glucocorticoid and weak mineralocorticoid activity in classical animal test systems. As a glucocorticoid it is several hundred times more potent than the cortisol standard. Clinical studies with flunisolide have shown therapeutic activity on nasal mucous membranes with minimal evidence of systemic activity at the recommended doses.
A study in approximately 100 patients that compared the recommended dose of flunisolide nasal solution with an oral dose providing equivalent systemic amounts of flunisolide has shown that the clinical effectiveness of NASALIDE, when used topically as recommended, is due to its direct local effect and not to an indirect effect through systemic absorption.
Following administration of flunisolide to man, approximately half of the administered dose is recovered in the urine and half in the stool; 65% to 70% of the dose recovered in urine is the primary metabolite, which has undergone loss of the 6α fluorine and addition of a 6β hydroxy group. Flunisolide is well absorbed but is rapidly converted by the liver to the much less active primary metabolite and to glucuronate and/or sulfate conjugates. Because of first-pass liver metabolism, only 20% of the flunisolide reaches the systemic circulation when it is given orally whereas 50% of the flunisolide administered intranasally reaches the systemic circulation unmetabolized. The plasma half-life of flunisolide is 1 to 2 hours.
The effects of flunisolide on hypothalamic-pituitary-adrenal (HPA) axis function have been studied in adult volunteers. NASALIDE was administered intranasally as a spray in total doses over 7 times the recommended dose (2200 mcg, equivalent to 88 sprays/day) in 2 subjects for 4 days, about 3 times the recommended dose (800 mcg, equivalent to 32 sprays/day) in 4 subjects for 4 days, and over twice the recommended dose (700 mcg, equivalent to 28 sprays/day) in 6 subjects for 10 days. Early morning plasma cortisol concentrations and 24-hour urinary 17-ketogenic steroids were measured daily. There was evidence of decreased endogenous cortisol production at all three doses.
In controlled studies, NASALIDE was found to be effective in reducing symptoms of stuffy nose, runny nose and sneezing in most patients. These controlled clinical studies have been conducted in 488 adult patients at doses ranging from 8 to 16 sprays (200–400 mcg) per day and 127 pediatric patients at doses ranging from 6 to 8 sprays (150 to 200 mcg) per day for periods as long as 3 months. In 170 patients who had cortisol levels evaluated at baseline and after 3 months or more of flunisolide treatment, there was no unequivocal flunisolide-related depression of plasma cortisol levels.
The mechanisms responsible for the anti-inflammatory action of corticosteroids and for the activity of the aerosolized drug on the nasal mucosa are unknown.

INDICATIONS

NASALIDE is indicated for the topical treatment of the symptoms of seasonal or perennial rhinitis when effectiveness of or tolerance to conventional treatment is unsatisfactory.
Clinical studies have shown that improvement is based on a local effect rather than systemic absorption and is usually apparent within a few days after starting NASALIDE. However, symptomatic relief may not occur in some patients for as long as 2 weeks. Although systemic effects are minimal at recommended doses, NASALIDE should not be continued beyond 3 weeks in the absence of significant symptomatic improvement.
NASALIDE should not be used in the presence of untreated localized infection involving nasal mucosa.

CONTRAINDICATIONS

Hypersensitivity to any of the ingredients.

WARNINGS

The replacement of a systemic corticosteroid with a topical corticoid can be accompanied by signs of adrenal insufficiency, and in addition some patients may experience symptoms of withdrawal, eg, joint and/or muscular pain, lassitude and depression. Patients previously treated for prolonged periods with systemic corticosteroids and transferred to NASALIDE should be carefully monitored to avoid acute adrenal insufficiency in response to stress.
When transferred to NASALIDE, careful attention must be given to patients previously treated for prolonged periods with systemic corticosteroids. This is particularly important in those patients who have associated asthma or other clinical conditions, where too rapid a decrease in systemic corticosteroids may cause a severe exacerbation of their symptoms.
The use of NASALIDE with alternate-day prednisone systemic treatment could increase the likelihood of HPA suppression compared to a therapeutic dose of either one alone. Therefore, NASALIDE treatment should be used with caution in patients already on alternate-day prednisone regimens for any disease.
Persons who are on drugs that suppress the immune system are more susceptible to infections than healthy individuals. Chicken pox and measles, for example, can have a more serious or even fatal course in nonimmune pediatric patients or adults on corticosteroids. In such pediatric patients or adults who have not had these diseases, particular care should be taken to avoid exposure. How the dose, route and duration of corticosteroid administration affects the risk of developing a disseminated infection is not known. The contribution of the underlying disease and/or prior corticosteroid treatment to the risk is also not known. If exposed to chicken pox, prophylaxis with varicella zoster immune globulin (VZIG) may be indicated. If exposed to measles, prophylaxis with pooled intramuscular immunoglobulin (IG) may be indicated. (See the respective package insert for complete VZIG and IG prescribing information.) If chicken pox develops, treatment with antiviral agents may be considered.

PRECAUTIONS

General: In clinical studies with flunisolide administered intranasally, the development of localized infections of the nose and pharynx with *Candida albicans* has occurred only rarely. When such an infection develops it may require treatment with appropriate local therapy or discontinuance of treatment with NASALIDE.
Flunisolide is absorbed into the circulation. Use of excessive doses of NASALIDE may suppress hypothalamic-pituitary-adrenal function.
Flunisolide should be used with caution, if at all in patients with active or quiescent tuberculosis infections of the respiratory tract or in untreated fungal, bacterial or systemic viral infections or ocular herpes simplex.
Because of the inhibitory effect of corticosteroids on wound healing, in patients who have experienced recent nasal septal ulcers, recurrent epistaxis, nasal surgery or trauma, a nasal corticosteroids should be used with caution until healing has occurred.
Although systemic effects have been minimal with recommended doses, this potential increases with excessive dosages. Therefore, larger than recommended doses should be avoided.
Information for Patients: Patients should use NASALIDE at regular intervals since its effectiveness depends on its regular use. The patient should take the medication as directed. It is not acutely effective and the prescribed dosage should not be increased. Instead, nasal vasoconstrictors or oral antihistamines may be needed until the effects of NASALIDE are fully manifested. One to 2 weeks may pass before full relief is obtained. The patient should contact the physician if symptoms do not improve, or if the condition worsens, or if sneezing or nasal irritation occurs.
Person who are on immunosuppressant doses of corticosteroids should be warned to avoid exposure to chicken pox or measles. Patients should also be advised that if they are exposed, medical advice should be sought without delay.
For the proper use of this unit and to attain maximum improvement, the patient should read and follow the accompanying Patient Instructions carefully.
Carcinogenesis: Long-term studies were conducted in mice and rats using oral administration to evaluate the carcinogenic potential of the drug. There was an increase in the incidence of pulmonary adenomas in mice but not in rats. Female rats receiving the highest oral dose had an increased incidence of mammary adenocarcinoma compared to control rats. An increased incidence of this tumor type has been reported for other corticosteroids.
Impairment of Fertility: Female rats receiving high doses of flunisolide (200 mcg/kg/day) showed some evidence of impaired fertility. Reproductive performance in the low (8 mcg/kg/day) and mid-dose (40 mcg/kg/day) groups was comparable to controls.
Pregnancy: Teratogenic Effects: Pregnancy Category C. As with other corticosteroids, flunisolide has been shown to be teratogenic in rabbits and rats at doses of 40 and 200 mcg/kg/day respectively. It was also fetotoxic in these animal reproductive studies. There are no adequate and well-controlled studies in pregnant women. Flunisolide should be used during pregnancy only if the potential benefit justifies the potential risk to the fetus.
Nursing Mothers: It is not known whether this drug is excreted in human milk. Because other corticosteroids are excreted in human milk, caution should be exercised when flunisolide is administered to nursing women.
Pediatric Use: NASALIDE is not recommended for use in pediatric patients less than 6 years of age as safety and efficacy, including possible adverse effects on growth, have not been assessed in this age group.

ADVERSE REACTIONS

Adverse reactions reported in controlled clinical trials and long-term open studies in 595 patients treated with NASALIDE are described below. Of these patients, 409 were treated for 3 months or longer, 323 for 6 months or longer, 259 for 1 year or longer and 91 for 2 years or longer.
In general, side effects elicited in the clinical studies have been primarily associated with the nasal mucous membranes. The most frequent complaints were those of mild transient nasal burning and stinging, which were reported in approximately 45% of the patients treated with NASALIDE in placebo-controlled and long-term studies. These complaints do not usually interfere with treatment; in only 3% of patients was it necessary to decrease dosage or stop treatment because of these symptoms. Approximately the same incidence of mild transient nasal burning and stinging was reported in patients on placebo as was reported in patients treated with NASALIDE in controlled studies, implying that these complaints may be related to the vehicle or the delivery system. The incidence of complaints of nasal burning and stinging decreased with increasing duration of treatment.
Other side effects reported at a frequency of 5% or less were: nasal congestion, sneezing, epistaxis and/or bloody mucus, nasal irritation, watery eyes, sore throat, nausea and/or vomiting and headaches. As with other nasally inhaled corticosteroids, nasal septal perforations have been reported in rare instances with the use of flunisolide nasal solutions. Temporary or permanent loss of the sense of smell and taste have also been reported with the use of flunisolide nasal solutions.
Systemic corticosteroid side effects were not reported during the controlled clinical trials. If recommended doses are exceeded, or if individuals are particularly sensitive, symptoms of hypercorticism, ie, Cushing's syndrome, could occur.

OVERDOSAGE

IV flunisolide in animals at doses up to 4 mg/kg showed no effect. One spray bottle contains 6.25 mg of NASALIDE; therefore acute overdosage is unlikely.

DOSAGE AND ADMINISTRATION

The therapeutic effects of corticosteroids, unlike those of decongestants, are not immediate. This should be explained to the patient in advance in order to ensure cooperation and continuation of treatment with the prescribed dosage regimen. Full therapeutic benefit requires regular use and is usually evident within a few days. However, a longer period of therapy may be required for some patients to achieve maximum benefit (up to 3 weeks). If no improvement is evident by that time, NASALIDE should not be continued.
Patients with blocked nasal passages should be encouraged to use a decongestant just before NASALIDE administration to ensure adequate penetration of the spray. Patients should also be advised to clear their nasal passages of secretions prior to use.

Adults: The recommended starting dose of NASALIDE is 2 sprays (50 mcg) in each nostril 2 times a day (total dose 200 mcg/day). If needed, this dose may be increased to 2 sprays in each nostril times a day (total dose 300 mcg/day).

Pediatric Patients 6 to 14 years: The recommended starting dose of NASALIDE is 1 spray (25 mcg) in each nostril 3 times a day or 2 sprays (50 mcg) in each nostril 2 times a day (total dose 150 to 200 mcg/day). NASALIDE is not recommended for use in pediatric patients less than 6 years of age as safety and efficacy studies, including possible adverse effects on growth, have not been conducted.

Maximum total daily doses should not exceed 8 sprays in each nostril for adults (total dose 400 mcg/day) and 4 sprays in each nostril for pediatric patients under 14 years of age (total dose 200 mcg/day). Since there is no evidence that exceeding the maximum recommended dosage is more effective and increased systemic absorption would occur, higher doses should be avoided.

After the desired clinical effect is obtained, the maintenance dose should be reduced to the smallest amount necessary to control the symptoms. Approximately 15% of patients with perennial rhinitis may be maintained on as little as 1 spray in each nostril per day.

HOW SUPPLIED

Each 25 mL NASALIDE nasal solution spray bottle (NDC 51479-038-25) contains 6.25 mg (0.25 mg/mL) of flunisolide and is supplied in a nasal pump dispenser with dust cover and with a patient leaflet of instructions.

Store at 15°–30°C (59°–86°F).

Revised: March 1977

Manufactured for:
Dura Pharmaceuticals, Inc.
San Diego, CA 92121
Manufactured by:
Oread, Inc.
Palo Alto, CA 94304 NIDE001A0397

NASAREL® ℞

[*Nā 'ză ril*]
(flunisolide)
Nasal Solution 0.025%

DESCRIPTION

Flunisolide, the active component of NASAREL nasal solution, is an anti-inflammatory glucocorticosteroid with the chemical name: 6α-fluoro-11β,16α,17,21 tetrahydroxypregna-1,4-diene-3,20-dione cyclic 16, 17-acetal with acetone, hemihydrate.

It has the following chemical structure:

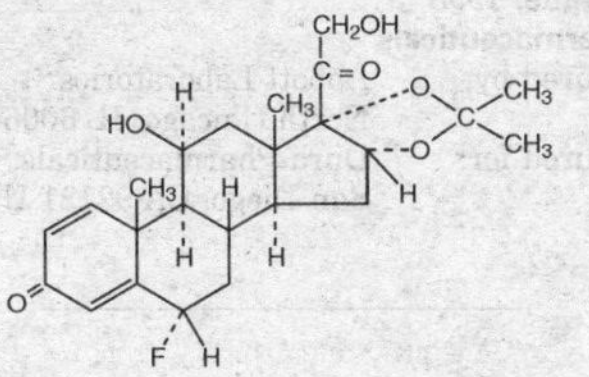

Flunisolide is a white to creamy white crystalline powder with a molecular weight of 443.51. It is soluble in acetone, sparingly soluble in chloroform, slightly soluble in methanol, and practically insoluble in water. It has a melting point of about 245°C. The octanol:water partition coefficient is 2.17 at neutral pH.

NASAREL is a metered dose manual pump spray unit containing 0.025% w/w flunisolide in an aqueous medium containing benzalkonium chloride, butylated hydroxytoluene, citric acid, edetate disodium, polyethylene glycol 400, polysorbate 20, propylene glycol, sodium citrate dihydrate, sorbitol, and purified water. Sodium hydroxide and/or hydrochloric acid may be added to adjust the pH to approximately 5.2. It contains no fluorocarbons. Each 25 mL spray bottle contains 6.25 mg of flunisolide.

After initial priming (5 to 6 actuations), each actuation of the pump spray unit delivers a metered spray containing approximately 25 mcg of flunisolide. The size of 99.5% of the droplets produced by the unit is greater than 8 microns. The contents of one nasal spray bottle deliver 200 sprays in addition to the priming sprays.

CLINICAL PHARMACOLOGY

General Pharmacology: Flunisolide nasal solution has demonstrated potent glucocorticoid and weak mineralocorticoid activity in classical animal test systems. As a glucocorticoid it was 180 times more potent than the cortisol standard in a rat anti-granuloma assay.

Pharmacokinetics: Flunisolide is well absorbed and is rapidly converted by the liver to the much less active primary metabolite and to glucuronide and sulfate conjugates. The primary metabolite results from the loss of the 6-alpha fluorine and addition of a 6-beta hydroxy group. Following administration of radiolabeled flunisolide to man, approximately half of the label is recovered in the urine and half in the stool. The primary metabolite accounts for 65% to 70% of the amount recovered in the urine. Due to first-pass liver metabolism, only 20% of an oral flunisolide dose reaches the systemic circulation unmetabolized as compared to 50% of an intranasal dose. The plasma half-life of flunisolide is 1 to 2 hours.

In a pharmacokinetic study comparing NASAREL with NASALIDE®, the original formulation, the two formulations were not bioequivalent. The total absorption of NASAREL was 25% less than that of NASALIDE, and the peak plasma concentration was 30% lower. The clinical significance of these differences is likely to be small, particularly since clinical efficacy is attributable to a local effect on the nasal mucosa. (see *Pharmacodynamics.*)

Pharmacodynamics: A study in approximately 100 patients compared control of hay fever symptoms by the recommended dose of flunisolide as NASALIDE (200 mcg/day) with control by an oral dose of flunisolide providing equivalent plasma levels. The results demonstrated that the clinical effectiveness was due to the direct topical effect of flunisolide and not to an indirect effect through systemic absorption.

The effects of flunisolide on hypothalamic-pituitary-adrenal (HPA) axis function have been studied in adult volunteers. Flunisolide as NASALIDE, the original nasal formulation, was administered to 20 subjects intranasally in average total daily doses ranging from approximately 350 mcg to 2200 mcg (equivalent to about 14 to 88 sprays per day) for 4 to 10 days. Early morning plasma cortisol concentrations and 24-hour urinary 17-ketogenic steroids were measured daily. There was no consistent effect on endogenous cortisol production, although evidence of mild adrenal suppression was seen in some subjects.

Controlled studies evaluated adult patients receiving average total daily doses ranging from approximately 50 to 400 mcg (equivalent to about 2 to 16 sprays per day) of NASALIDE, the original flunisolide nasal solution, for periods as long as 3 months. Three hundred and thirty-nine patients from these studies were entered into a long-term open label study. Morning plasma cortisol levels were available for 182 patients at baseline, 129 after 6 months, and 36 after 12 months of continuous treatment with flunisolide. No effect of flunisolide on cortisol production was detected.

The mechanisms responsible for the anti-inflammatory action of corticosteroids and for their effect on the nasal mucosa are not completely understood.

CLINICAL TRIALS

The effectiveness of NASAREL was tested in 289 patients for up to 6 weeks at doses up to 300 mcg per day. NASAREL was shown to be effective in treating the symptoms of allergic rhinitis, including rhinorrhea, nasal congestion and sneezing.

A pivotal, 3-center trial involved 196 patients with seasonal allergic rhinitis randomized to NASALIDE, the vehicle of NASALIDE, NASAREL and the vehicle of NASAREL. Both active treatments were statistically significantly more effective than the vehicles. There was not statistically significant difference in efficacy between NASALIDE and NASAREL.

The two formulations do differ in the nature and incidence of adverse complaints. There were more reports of nasal burning and stinging with NASALIDE and more problems related to taste, such as aftertaste, with NASAREL, owing to the differences in their respective vehicles. Some patients may prefer one formulation to the other.

INDIVIDUALIZATION OF DOSAGE

The therapeutic effects of corticosteroid nasal sprays, unlike those of decongestants, are not immediate. This should be explained to the patient in advance in order to ensure cooperation and continuation of treatment with the prescribed dosage regimen. Full therapeutic benefit requires regular use and is usually evident within a few days. A longer period of therapy may be required for some patients. However, NASAREL should not be continued beyond 3 weeks in the absence of significant symptomatic improvement (see PRECAUTIONS, WARNINGS, *Information For Patients* and ADVERSE REACTIONS sections).

A starting dose of 2 sprays in each nostril twice daily is recommended. If greater control of symptoms is needed, the dose may be increased to 2 sprays in each nostril 3 times a day. For adults, maximum total daily doses should not exceed 8 sprays in each nostril per day (400 mcg/day).

After the desired clinical effect is obtained, the maintenance dose should be reduced to the smallest amount necessary to control the symptoms. Some patients with perennial rhinitis may be maintained on as little as 1 spray in each nostril per day. It is always desirable to titrate an individual patient to the minimum effective dose to reduce the possibility of side effects.

NASAREL and NASALIDE should not be considered to be identical. Physicians should consider the observed differences in the mean responses in terms of side effects (see ADVERSE REACTIONS) and flunisolide absorption (see *Pharmacokinetics*) in treating individual patients.

For pediatric patients 6 to 14 years of age, the recommended starting dose of NASAREL is one spray (25 mcg) in each nostril 3 times a day (total dose 150 mcg/day) or 2 sprays (50 mcg) in each nostril 2 times a day (total dose 200 mcg/day). Maximum daily doses should not exceed 4 sprays in each nostril per day (total dose 200 mcg/day) as the safety and efficacy of higher doses have not been established. NASAREL is not recommended for use in pediatric patients less than 6 years of age as the safety and efficacy have not been assessed in this age-group.

INDICATIONS AND USAGE

NASAREL is indicated for the management of the symptoms of seasonal or perennial rhinitis.

CONTRAINDICATIONS

Hypersensitivity to any of the ingredients.

NASAREL should not be used in the presence of untreated localized infection involving the nasal mucosa.

WARNINGS

The replacement of a systemic corticosteroid with a topical corticoid can be accompanied by signs of adrenal insufficiency, and in addition some patients may experience symptoms of withdrawal, e.g., joint and/or muscular pain, lassitude and depression. Patients previously treated for prolonged periods with systemic corticosteroids and transferred to NASAREL should be carefully monitored to avoid acute adrenal insufficiency in response to stress.

Careful attention must also be given to patients who have associated asthma or other clinical conditions where too rapid a decrease in systemic corticosteroids may exacerbate their symptoms.

The use of NASAREL with systemic prednisone as alternate day therapy or with daily doses of less than 7.5 mg could increase the likelihood of hypothalamic-pituitary-adrenal axis suppression compared to a therapeutic dose of either one alone. Therefore, NASAREL treatment should be used with caution in patients already on prednisone regimens for any disease.

Persons who are on drugs which suppress the immune system are more susceptible to infections than healthy individuals. Chicken pox and measles, for example, can have a more serious or even fatal course in non-immune children or adults on corticosteroids. In such children or adults who have not had these diseases, particular care should be taken to avoid exposure. How the dose, route and duration of corticosteroid administration affects the risk of developing a disseminated infection is not known. The contribution of the underlying disease and/or prior corticosteroid treatment to the risk is also not known. If exposed to chicken pox, prophylaxis with varicella zoster immune globulin (VZIG) may be indicated. If exposed to measles, prophylaxis with pooled intramuscular immunoglobulin (IG) may be indicated. (See the respective package insert for complete VZIG and IG prescribing information). If chicken pox develops, treatment with antiviral agents may be considered.

PRECAUTIONS

General: In clinical studies with flunisolide administered intranasally, the development of localized infections of the nose and pharynx with *Candida albicans* has occurred only rarely. When such an infection develops it may require treatment with appropriate local therapy or discontinuance of treatment with NASAREL.

Since there is no evidence that exceeding the maximum recommended dose of NASAREL is more effective, higher doses should be avoided.

Patients should be advised to clear their nasal passages of secretions prior to use. NASAREL should not be used in the presence of untreated local infection involving the nasal mucosa.

Flunisolide should be used with caution, if at all, in patients with active or quiescent tuberculosis infections, fungal, bacterial or systemic viral infections or ocular herpes simplex.

As with other nasally inhaled corticosteroids, nasal septal perforations have been reported in rare instances with the use of flunisolide nasal solutions. Temporary or permanent loss of the sense of smell and taste have also been reported with the use of flunisolide nasal solutions.

Because of the inhibitory effect of corticosteroids on wound healing, a nasal corticosteroid should be used with caution in patients who have experienced recent nasal septal ulcers, recurrent epistaxis, nasal surgery or trauma, until healing has occurred.

Although systemic corticoid effects typical of Cushing's syndrome are minimal with recommended doses of topical steroids, this potential increases with excessive doses. If recommended doses are exceeded with long-term use, or if individuals are particularly sensitive, symptoms of hypercorticism could occur including suppression of hypothalamic-pituitary-adrenal function and/or retardation of growth in children or teenagers. Therefore, larger than recommended doses of NASAREL should be avoided.

Continued on next page

Nasarel—Cont.

Information for Patients: Patients should use NASAREL at regular intervals since its effectiveness depends on its regular use. Patients should take the medication as directed and should not exceed the prescribed dose. A decrease in symptoms can be expected to occur within a few days of initiating therapy in allergic rhinitis patients. Patients should contact their physician if the condition worsens, if sneezing or nasal irritation occurs, or if symptoms do not improve by three weeks.

Persons taking immunosuppressant doses of corticosteroids should be warned to avoid exposure to chicken pox or measles. Patients should also be advised that if they are exposed, medical advice should be sought without delay.

For the proper use of this unit and to attain maximum improvement, the patient should read and follow the accompanying Patient Instructions carefully.

Carcinogenesis: Long-term studies were conducted in mice and rats using oral administration to evaluate the carcinogenic potential of the drug. Flunisolide was administered to mice at doses of 5, 50 and 500 µg/kg/day (15, 150, and 1500 µg/m^2 respectively) and to rats at doses of 0.5, 1 and 2.5 µg/kg/day (3.0, 5.9 and 14.8 µg/m^2 respectively). There was an increase in the incidence of benign pulmonary adenomas in mice, but not in rats.

Female rats receiving the highest oral dose had an increased incidence of mammary adenocarcinoma compared to control rats. An increased incidence of this tumor type has been reported for other corticosteroids.

Impairment of Fertility: Female rats receiving high doses of flunisolide (200 µg/kg/day or 1180 µg/m^2 body surface area) showed some evidence of impaired fertility. Reproductive performance in the low (8 µg/kg/day or 47.2 µg/m^2) and mid-dose (40 µg/kg/day or 236 µg/m^2) groups was comparable to controls.

Pregnancy: Teratogenic effects: Pregnancy Category C. As with other corticosteroids, flunisolide has been shown to be teratogenic in rabbits and rats at doses of 40 and 200 mcg/kg/day (480 µg/m^2 and 1180 µg/m^2) respectively. It was also fetotoxic in these animals reproductive studies. There are no adequate and well-controlled studies in pregnant women. Flunisolide should be used during pregnancy only if the potential benefit justifies the potential risk to the fetus.

Nursing Mothers: It is not known whether this drug is excreted in human milk. Because other corticosteroids are excreted in human milk, caution should be exercised when flunisolide is administered to nursing women.

Pediatric Use: **NASAREL** is not recommended for use in pediatric patients less than 6 years of age as safety and efficacy, including possible adverse effects on growth, have not been assessed in this age group. For pediatric patients 6 years of age and over, recommended maximum daily doses should not be exceeded in order to minimize the risk of systemic corticoid effects, including potential growth retardation. (See INDIVIDUALIZATION OF DOSAGE and DOSAGE AND ADMINISTRATION.)

ADVERSE REACTIONS

The adverse event rates listed below are based on symptoms spontaneously reported in multidose controlled clinical trials in comparing NASAREL and NASALIDE for treatment of allergic rhinitis. In patients receiving NASAREL the most common adverse events were transient aftertaste (17%) and transient nasal burning and stinging (13%). These symptoms did not usually interfere with treatment.

Adverse Event Rates for NASAREL:

Incidence Greater than 1% (probably causally related)

Respiratory: Nasal burning/stinging (13%), epistaxis*, nasal dryness, pharyngitis, cough increased

Gastrointestinal: Nausea

Special Senses: Aftertaste (17%)

Incidence 1% or Less (probably causally related)

Respiratory: Hoarseness

Special Senses: Abnormal sense of smell

Incidence 1% or less (causal relationship unknown)†

Respiratory: Sinusitis

Adverse Event Rates for NASALIDE:

Incidence Greater than 1% (probably causally related)

Respiratory: Nasal burning/stinging (44%), epistaxis*, nasal dryness*, pharyngitis*, cough increased

Gastrointestinal: Nausea

Special Senses: Aftertaste (8%)

Incidence 1% or Less (probably causally related)

Respiratory: Hoarseness, nasal ulcer

Incidence 1% or Less (causal relationship unknown)†

Respiratory: Sinusitis

*Incidence of reported reaction between 3% and 9%. Those reactions occurring in less than 3% of the patients are unmarked.

†Reactions occurred under circumstances where the causal relationship has not been clearly established; they are presented as alerting information for physicians.

OVERDOSAGE

In mice, rats and dogs, intravenous flunisolide at doses up to 4 mg/kg showed no effect. One spray bottle contains 6.25 mg of flunisolide; therefore acute overdosage is unlikely.

DOSAGE AND ADMINISTRATION

For adults, the recommended starting dose of NASAREL is 2 sprays (50 mcg) in each nostril 2 times a day (total dose 200 mcg/day): the effect should be assessed in 4 to 7 days (See INDIVIDUALIZATION OF DOSAGE section). Some relief can be expected in approximately two-thirds of patients within that time. This dose may be increased to 2 sprays in each nostril 3 times a day (total dose 300 mcg/day) if greater effect is needed. For adults, maximum total daily doses should not exceed 8 sprays in each nostril per day (400 mcg/day). After the desired clinical effect is obtained, the maintenance dose should be reduced to the smallest amount necessary to control the symptoms (See INDIVIDUALIZATION OF DOSAGE section).

For pediatric patients 6 to 14 years of age, the recommended starting dose of NASAREL is 1 spray (25 mcg) in each nostril 3 times a day (total dose 150 mcg/day) or 2 sprays (50 mcg) in each nostril 2 times a day (total dose 200 mcg/day). For pediatric patients 6 to 14 years of age, maximum daily doses should not exceed 4 sprays in each nostril per day (total dose 200 mcg/day) as the safety and efficacy of higher doses have not been established.

NASAREL is not recommended for use in pediatric patients less than 6 years of age as safety and efficacy, including possible adverse effects on growth, have not been assessed in this age group.

NASAREL and NASALIDE should not be considered to be identical products. Physicians should consider the observed differences in the mean responses in terms of side effects (see ADVERSE REACTIONS) and flunisolide absorption (see *Pharmacokinetics*) in treating individual patients.

HOW SUPPLIED

Each 25 mL of NASAREL 0.025% nasal solution (6.25 mg flunisolide) is supplied in a spray bottle fitted with a meter pump, nasal adapter and a white protective cap (NDC 51479-037-25). The unit contains 200 metered sprays and comes with a patient instruction leaflet.

Store at 15°–30°C (59°–86°F).

CONTENTS MADE IN CANADA

Revised: August, 1997

Manufactured for:
Dura Pharmaceuticals, Inc.
San Diego, CA 92121
Manufactured by:
Patheon, Inc.
Mississauga, Ontatio L5N 7K9

NREL001B0897

RONDEC® Chewable Tablets ℞
with brompheniramine

DESCRIPTION

A scored, pink-colored, strawberry-tasting chewable tablet. Each tablet contains:

Brompheniramine maleate	4 mg
Pseudoephedrine hydrochloride	60 mg

Rondec® Chewable Tablets with brompheniramine contain ingredients of the following therapeutic classes: antihistamine and nasal decongestant.

HOW SUPPLIED

Bottles of 100 NDC 51479-017-01. Each tablet is coded *"DURA"* on one side and *"017"* on the reverse side.

Dispense in a tight, light-resistant container as defined in USP/NF with a child-resistant closure. Store between 15°–23°C (59°–73°F).

Rx only

Manufactured for Dura Pharmaceuticals, Inc.
San Diego, CA 92121
Manufactured by Schwarz Pharma Mfg, Inc.
Seymour, IN 47274
Revised June, 1998
RC002E98

RONDEC® Oral Drops ℞
RONDEC® Syrup ℞
RONDEC® Tablet ℞
RONDEC-TR® Tablet ℞

DESCRIPTION

Antihistamine/Decongestant for oral use

For infants (1–18 months)
RONDEC® Oral Drops ℞
Each dropperful (1 mL) contains carbinoxamine maleate, 2 mg; pseudoephedrine hydrochloride, 25 mg.

Inactive Ingredients: Citric acid, DC Red No. 33, FDC Yellow No. 6, glycerin, methylparaben, propylparaben, purified water, sodium benzoate, sodium citrate, sorbitol and artificial flavoring.

For pediatric patients (over 18 months)
RONDEC® Syrup ℞
Each teaspoonful (5 mL) contains carbinoxamine maleate, 4 mg; pseudoephedrine hydrochloride, 60 mg.

Inactive Ingredients: Citric acid, DC Red No. 33, FDC Yellow No. 6, glycerin, methylparaben, propylparaben, purified water, sodium benzoate, sodium citrate, sorbitol and artificial flavoring.

For adults and pediatric patients (6 yrs. and over)
RONDEC® Tablet ℞
Each tablet contains carbinoxamine maleate, 4 mg; pseudoephedrine hydrochloride, 60 mg.

Inactive Ingredients: Cellulosic polymers, FDC Yellow No. 6, hydrogenated vegetable oil wax, lactose, magnesium stearate, microcrystalline cellulose, polyethylene glycol, povidone, propylene glycol, silicon dioxide, sodium starch glycolate, sorbitan monooleate, titanium dioxide and vanillin.

For adults and adolescents (12 yrs. and over)
RONDEC-TR® Tablet ℞
Each timed-release tablet contains carbinoxamine maleate, 8 mg; pseudoephedrine hydrochloride, 120 mg.

Inactive Ingredients: Castor oil, cellulosic polymers, confectioner's sugar, cornstarch, FDC Blue No. 1, lactose, magnesium stearate, methyl acrylate-methyl methacrylate copolymer, microcrystalline cellulose, povidone, propylene glycol, sorbitan monooleate and titanium dioxide.

HOW SUPPLIED

Rondec Oral Drops, berry-flavored, in 30-mL bottles for dropper dosage, **NDC** 51479-020-30. Calibrated shatterproof dropper enclosed in each carton. Container meets safety closure requirements.

Rondec Syrup, berry-flavored, in 16-fl-oz (1-pint) bottles, **NDC** 51479-021-48; and 4-fl-oz bottles, **NDC** 51479-021-12. Dispense in USP tight glass container.

Rondec Tablet, in bottles of 100, **NDC** 51479-022-01; and bottles of 500, **NDC** 51479-022-05. Each orange-colored tablet marked with and the number 5726 for professional identification. Dispense in USP tight container.

Rondec-TR Tablet, in bottles of 100, **NDC** 51479-025-01. Each blue-colored tablet marked with and the number 6240 for professional identification. Dispense in USP tight container.

Recommended storage: Store below 86°F (30°C).

Rx only

Revised: June, 1998

DURA Pharmaceuticals

Manufactured by:	Abbott Laboratories North Chicago, IL 60064 U.S.A.
Manufactured for:	Dura Pharmaceuticals, Inc. San Diego, CA 92121 U.S.A.

R002D98

RONDEC®-DM Syrup ℞
RONDEC®-DM Oral Drops ℞

DESCRIPTION

Antihistamine/Decongestant/ Antitussive for oral use

for adults and pediatric patients (18 months and over)
RONDEC®-DM Syrup ℞
Each teaspoonful (5 mL) contains:

carbinoxamine maleate	4 mg
pseudoephedrine hydrochloride	60 mg
dextromethorphan hydrobromide	15 mg

Inactive Ingredients: Citric acid, DC Red No. 33, FDC Blue No. 1, glycerin, menthol, purified water, sodium benzoate, sodium citrate, sorbitol, natural and artificial flavoring and other ingredients.

for infants (1–18 months)
RONDEC®-DM Oral Drops ℞
Each dropperful (1 mL) contains:

carbinoxamine maleate	2 mg
pseudoephedrine hydrochloride	25 mg
dextromethorphan hydrobromide	4 mg

Inactive Ingredients: Citric acid, DC Red No. 33, FDC Blue No. 1, glycerin, menthol, purified water, sodium benzoate, sodium citrate, sorbitol, natural and artificial flavoring and other ingredients.

HOW SUPPLIED

Rondec-DM Syrup, grape-flavored, in 16-fl-oz (1-pint) bottles, **NDC** 51479-024-48; and 4-fl-oz bottles, **NDC** 51479-024-12. Dispense in USP tight, light-resistant, glass container. Avoid exposure to excessive heat.

Rondec-DM Oral Drops, grape-flavored, in 30-mL bottles for dropper dosage. Calibrated, shatterproof dropper enclosed in each carton. Container meets safety closure requirements **NDC** 51479-023-03. Avoid exposure to excessive heat.

Rx only

Revised June, 1998

DURA PHARMACEUTICALS

Manufactured by:	Abbott Laboratories North Chicago, IL 60064 U.S.A.
Manufactured for:	DURA Pharmaceuticals, Inc. San Diego, CA 92121 U.S.A.

RDM001C98

SEROMYCIN® ℞
CYCLOSERINE CAPSULES, USP

DESCRIPTION

Seromycin® (Cycloserine Capsules, USP), 3-isoxazolidinone, 4-amino-, (R)- is a broad-spectrum antibiotic that is produced by a strain of *Streptomyces orchidaceus* and has also been synthesized. Cycloserine is a white to off-white powder that is soluble in water and stable in alkaline solution. It is rapidly destroyed at a neutral or acid pH.

Cycloserine has a pH between 5.5 and 6.5 in a solution containing 100 mg/mL. The molecular weight of cycloserine is 102.09, and it has an empirical formula of $C_3H_6N_2O_2$. The structural formula of cycloserine is as follows:

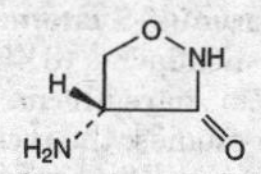

Each capsule contains cycloserine, 250 mg (2.45 mmol); D & C Yellow No. 10, F D & C Blue No. 1, F D & C Red No. 3, F D & C Yellow No. 6, gelatin, iron oxide, talc, titanium dioxide, and other inactive ingredients.

CLINICAL PHARMACOLOGY

After oral administration, cycloserine is readily absorbed from the gastrointestinal tract, with peak blood levels occurring in 4 to 8 hours. Blood levels of 25 to 30 µg/mL can generally be maintained with the usual dosage of 250 mg twice a day, although the relationship of plasma levels to dosage is not always consistent. Concentrations in the cerebrospinal fluid, pleural fluid, fetal blood, and mother's milk approach those found in the serum. Detectable amounts are found in ascitic fluid, bile, sputum, amniotic fluid, and lung and lymph tissues. Approximately 65% of a single dose of cycloserine can be recovered in the urine within 72 hours ofter oral administration. The remaining 35% is apparently metabolized to unknown substances. The maximum excretion rate occurs 2 to 6 hours after administration, with 50% of the drug eliminated in 12 hours.

Microbiology: Cycloserine inhibits cell-wall synthesis in susceptible strains of gram-positive and gram-negative bacteria and in *Mycobacterium tuberculosis*.

Susceptibility Tests: Cycloserine clinical laboratory standard powder is available for both direct and indirect methods[1] of determining the susceptibility of strains of mycobacteria. Cycloserine MICs for susceptible strains are 25 µg/mL or lower.

INDICATIONS AND USAGE

Seromycin is indicated in the treatment of active pulmonary and extrapulmonary tuberculosis (including renal disease) when the causative organisms are susceptible to this drug and when treatment with the primary medications (streptomycin, isoniazid, rifampin, and ethambutol) has proved inadequate. Like all antituberculosis drugs, Seromycin should be administered in conjuction with other effective chemotherapy and not as the sole therapeutic agent.

Seromycin may be effective in the treatment of acute urinary tract infections caused by susceptible strains of gram-positive and gram-negative bacteria, especially *Enterobacter* sp. and *Escherichia coli*. It is generally no more and is usually less effective than other antimicrobial agents in the treatment of urinary tract infections caused by bacteria other than mycobacteria. Use of Seromycin in these infections should be considered only when more conventional therapy has failed and when the organism has been demonstrated to be susceptible to the drug.

CONTRAINDICATIONS

Administration is contraindicated in patients with any of the following:

- Hypersensitivity to cycloserine
- Epilepsy
- Depression, severe anxiety, or psychosis
- Severe renal insufficiency
- Excessive concurrent use of alcohol

WARNINGS

Administration of Seromycin should be discontinued or the dosage reduced if the patient develops allergic dermatitis or symptoms of CNS toxicity, such as convulsions, psychosis, somnolence, depression, confusion, hyperreflexia, headache, tremor, vertigo, paresis, or dysarthria.

The toxicity of Seromycin is closely related to excessive blood levels (above 30 µg/mL), as determined by high dosage or inadequate renal clearance. The ratio of toxic dose to effective dose in tuberculosis is small.

The risk of convulsions is increased in chronic alcoholics. Patients should be monitored by hematologic, renal excretion, blood level, and liver function studies.

PRECAUTIONS

General: Before treatment with Seromycin is initiated, cultures should be taken and the organism's susceptibility to the drug should be established. In tuberculous infections, the organism's susceptibility to the other antituberculosis agents in the regimen should also be demonstrated.

Anticonvulsant drugs or sedatives may be effective in controlling symptoms of CNS toxicity, such as convulsions, anxiety, and tremor. Patients receiving more than 500 mg of Seromycin daily should be closely observed for such symptoms. The value of pyridoxine in preventing CNS toxicity from Seromycin has not been proved.

Administration of Seromycin and other antituberculosis drugs has been associated in a few instances with vitamin B_{12} and/or folic-acid deficiency, megaloblastic anemia, and sideroblastic anemia. If evidence of anemia develops during treatment, appropriate studies and therapy should be instituted.

Laboratory Tests: Blood levels should be determined at least weekly for patients with reduced renal function, for individuals receiving a daily dosage of more than 500 mg, and for those showing signs and symptoms suggestive of toxicity. The dosage should be adjusted to keep the blood level below 30 µg/mL.

Drug Interactions: Concurrent administration of ethionamide has been reported to potentiate neurotoxic side effects.

Alcohol and Seromycin are incompatible, especially during a regimen calling for large doses of the latter. Alcohol increases the possibility and risk of epileptic episodes.

Concurrent administration of isoniazid may result in increased incidence of CNS effects, such as dizziness or drowsiness. Dosage adjustments may be necessary and patients should be monitored closely for signs of CNS toxicity.

Carcinogenesis, Mutagenicity, and Impairment of Fertility: Studies have not been performed to determine potential for carcinogenicity. The Ames test and unscheduled DNA repair test were negative. A study in 2 generations of rats showed no impairment of fertility relative to controls for the first mating but somewhat lower fertility in the second mating.

Pregnancy Category C: A study in 2 generations of rats given doses up to 100 mg/kg/day demonstrated no teratogenic effect in offspring. It is not known whether Seromycin can cause fetal harm when administered to a pregnant woman or can affect reproduction capacity. Seromycin should be given to a pregnant woman only if clearly needed.

Nursing Mothers: Because of the potential for serious adverse reactions in nursing infants from Seromycin, a decision should be made to whether to discontinue nursing or to discontinue the drug, taking into account the importance of the drug to the mother.

Usage in Pediatric Patients: Safety and effectiveness in pediatric patients have not been established.

ADVERSE REACTIONS

Most adverse reactions occurring during therapy with Seromycin involve the nervous system or are manifestations of drug hypersensitivity. The following side effects have been observed in patients receivng Seromycin:

Nervous system symptoms (which appear to be related to higher dosages of the drug, ie, more than 500 mg daily)

Convulsions
Drowsiness and somnolence
Headache
Tremor
Dysarthria
Vertigo
Confusion and disorientation with loss of memory
Psychoses, possibly with suicidal tendencies
Character changes
Hyperirritability
Aggression
Paresis
Hyperreflexia
Paresthesia
Major and minor (localized) clonic seizures
Coma

Cardiovascular

Sudden development of congestive heart failure in patients receiving 1 to 1.5 g of Seromycin daily has been reported

Allergy (apparently not related to dosage)

Skin Rash

Miscellaneous

Elevated serum transaminase, especially in patients with preexisting liver disease

OVERDOSAGE

Signs and Symptoms: Acute toxicity from cycloserine can occur if more than 1 g is ingested by an adult. Chronic toxicity from cycloserine is dose related and can occur if more than 500 mg is administered daily. Patients with renal impairment will accumulate cycloserine and may develop toxicity if the dosing regimen is not modified. Patients with severe renal impairment should not receive the drug. The central nervous system is the most common organ system involved with toxicity. Toxic effects may include headache, vertigo, confusion, drowsiness, hyperirritability, paresthesias, dysarthria, and psychosis. Following larger ingestions, paresis, convulsions, and coma often occur. Ethyl alcohol may increase the risk of seizures in patients receiving cycloserine.

The oral median lethal dose in mice is 5,290 mg/kg.

Treatment: To obtain up-to-date information about the treatment of overdose, a good resource is your certified Regional Poison Control Center. Telephone numbers of certified poison control centers are listed in the *Physicians' Desk Reference (PDR)*. In managing overdosage, consider the possibility of multiple drug overdoses, interaction among drugs, and unusual drug kinetics in your patient.

Overdoses of cycloserine have been reported rarely. The following is provided to serve as a guide should such an overdose be encountered.

Protect the patient's airway and support ventilation and perfusion. Meticulously monitor and maintain, within acceptable limits, the patient's vital signs, blood gases, serum electrolytes, etc. Absorption of drugs from the gastrointestinal tract may be decreased by giving activated charcoal, which, in many cases, is more effective than emesis or lavage; consider charcoal instead of or in addition to gastric emptying. Repeated doses of charcoal over time may hasten elimination of some drugs that have been absorbed. Safeguard the patient's airway when employing gastric emptying or charcoal.

In adults, many of the neurotoxic effects of cycloserine can be both treated and prevented with the administration of 200 to 300 mg of pyridoxine daily.

The use of hemodialysis has been shown to remove cycloserine from the bloodstream. This procedure should be reserved for patients with life-threatening toxicity that is unresponsive to less invasive therapy.

DOSAGE AND ADMINISTRATION

Seromycin is effective orally and is currently administered only by this route. The usual dosage is 500 mg to 1 g daily in divided doses monitored by blood levels.[2] The initial adult dosage most frequently given is 250 mg twice daily at 12-hour intervals for the first 2 weeks. A daily dosage of 1 g should not be exceeded.

HOW SUPPLIED

Seromycin® is available as a red and gray capsule coded with the imprints 51479-019 on each half.

Bottles of 40 (UC5000) NDC 51479-019-01.

Store at controlled room temperature, 59° to 86°F (15° to 30°C).

REFERENCES

1. Kubica GP, Dye WE: Laboratory methods for clinical and public health—mycobacteriology. US Department of Health, Education and Welfare, Public Health Service, 1967, pp 47-55, 66-70.
2. Jones LR: Colorimetric determination of cycloserine, a new antibiotic. *Anal Chem* 1956;28:39.

CAUTION—Federal (USA) law prohibits dispensing without prescription.

DURA PHARMACEUTICALS

Literature revised May 7, 1996

Manufactured by: Eli Lilly and Company
Indianapolis, IN 46285

Distributed by: DURA Pharmaceuticals, Inc.
San Diego, CA 92121

PV 0681 UCP

SC002B0496

TORNALATE® ℞
(bitolterol mesylate)
Solution for Inhalation, 0.2%

DESCRIPTION

Tornalate (bitolterol mesylate) is the di-p-toluate ester of the β-adrenergic agonist bronchodilator *N*-t-butylarterenol (colterol). It has a molecular weight of 557.7 and the molecular formula is $C_{25}H_{31}NO \cdot CH_3SO_3H$. Bitolterol mesylate is known chemically as 4-[2-[(1,1-dimethylethyl) amino]-1-hydroxyethyl]-1,2-phenylene 4-methylbenzoate (ester)

Continued on next page

Tornalate Solution—Cont.

methanesulfonate (salt) and has the following structural formula:

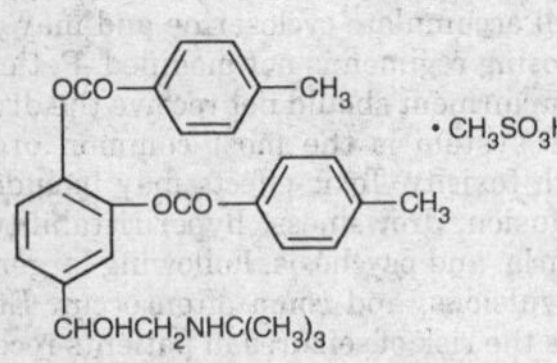

Tornalate Solution for Inhalation contains 0.2% bitolterol mesylate in an aqueous vehicle containing alcohol 25% (v/v), citric acid, propylene glycol, and sodium hydroxide. Tornalate's pH range is 3.0–3.4

Each mL of Tornalate Solution for Inhalation, 0.2% contains 2.0 mg of bitolterol mesylate.

CLINICAL PHARMACOLOGY

Tornalate is administered as a pro-drug which is hydrolyzed by esterases in tissue and blood to the active moiety colterol. Tornalate administered by nebulization has a rapid onset of activity (2 to 3 minutes) after administration in most patients based on interpolation between baseline and 5 minutes. The duration of action with Tornalate administered by nebulization is 6 hours or more in most patients and 8 hours in 40% of patients based on 15% or greater increase in forced expiratory volume in one second (FEV_1), as demonstrated in 3-month isoproterenol controlled multicenter trials in nonsteroid dependent patients. Based on mid-maximal expiratory flow (MMEF) measurements, the duration of action is 7.5 to 8 hours in most patients. Median duration of effect in steroid-dependent asthmatic patients ranged from 4.3 to 7.1 hours based on 15% or greater increase in FEV_1. The mean maximum increase in FEV_1 over baseline in patients during the three-month studies was 49% to 55% and occurred by 30 to 60 minutes in most patients.

In vitro studies and in vivo pharmacologic studies have demonstrated that Tornalate has a preferential effect on beta-2 adrenergic receptors compared with isoproterenol. While it is recognized that beta-2 adrenergic receptors are the prominent receptors in bronchial smooth muscle, recent data indicate that there are between 10% to 50% beta-2 receptors in the human heart. The precise function of these, however, is not yet established. Tornalate has been shown in most controlled clinical trials to have more effect on the respiratory tract, in the form of bronchial smooth muscle relaxation than isoproterenol at comparable doses, while producing fewer cardiovascular effects. Controlled clinical studies and other clinical experience have shown the inhaled Tornalate, like other beta-adrenergic agonists, can produce a significant cardiovascular effect in some patients, as measured by pulse rate, blood pressure, symptoms and/or ECG changes.

The incidence of cardiovascular side effects such as tachycardia and palpitation was less in patients treated with bitolterol mesylate as compared with patients treated with isoproterenol hydrochloride. The incidence of tachycardia and palpitation was 3.7% and 3.1%, respectively, in patients treated with bitolterol mesylate as compared with an incidence of 12.3% and 12.6% for tachycardia and palpitation for patients treated with isoproterenol.

Blood levels of colterol formed by gradual release from the pro-drug (bitolterol) in the lungs are too low to be measured by currently available assay methods and the bioavailability, pharmacokinetics and metabolism of bitolterol following administration as a solution for inhalation are not known. Data on disposition are available from oral studies in man. Following oral administration of 5.9 mg tritiated bitolterol to man, radioactivity measurements indicated mean maximum colterol concentration in blood of approximately 2.1 μg/mL one hour after medication. Urinary excretion data indicate that 83% of the radioactivity of this oral dose was excreted within the first 24 hours. By 72 hours, 85.6% of the tritium had been excreted in the urine and 8.1% in the feces. Most of the radioactivity was excreted as conjugated colterol; free colterol accounted for 2.1% to 3.7% of the total radioactivity excreted in the urine. No intact bitolterol was detected in urine.

The pharmacologic effects of β-adrenergic agonist drugs, including bitolterol mesylate, are at least in part attributable to stimulation through beta adrenergic receptors of intracellular adenyl cyclase, the enzyme which catalyzes the conversion of adenosine triphosphate (ATP) to cyclic-3′, 5′-adenosine monophosphate (c-AMP). Increased c-AMP levels are associated with relaxation of bronchial smooth muscle and inhibition of release of mediators of immediate hypersensitivity from cells, especially from mast cells.

In repetitive dosing studies, continued effectiveness was demonstrated throughout the three-month period of treatment in the majority of patients. In steroid-dependent asthmatics, the median duration of bronchodilator activity as measured by FEV_1 was greater on the first test day as compared with later test days, but patient response remained constant throughout the balance of the three-month period. Recent studies in laboratory animals (minipigs, rodents, and dogs) recorded the occurrence of cardiac arrhythmias and sudden death (with histologic evidence of myocardial necrosis) when beta agonists and methylxanthines were administered concurrently. The significance of these findings when applied to humans is currently unknown.

INDICATIONS AND USAGE

Tornalate Solution for Inhalation, 0.2% is indicated for both prophylaxis and treatment of asthma or other conditions characterized by reversible bronchospasm. It may be used with or without concurrent theophylline and/or steroid therapy.

CONTRAINDICATIONS

Tornalate Solution for Inhalation, 0.2% is contraindicated in patients who are hypersensitive to bitolterol mesylate or any other ingredients of the formulation.

WARNINGS

As with other β-adrenergic agents, bitolterol mesylate should not be used in excess. Fatalities have been reported in association with excessive use of inhaled sympathomimetic drugs. The exact cause of death is unknown.Use of β-adrenergic drugs may have a deleterious cardiac effect. Paradoxical bronchoconstriction (which can be life-threatening) has been reported with administration of β-adrenergic agents. Immediate hypersensitivity reactions can occur after the administration of sympathomimetic agents. In such instances, the drug should be discontinued immediately and alternative therapy instituted.

In controlled clinical studies, clinically significant increases in pulse rate, increases and decreases in systolic and diastolic blood pressure have been demonstrated in individual patients after administration of Tornalate. Therefore, caution should be exercised when administering bitolterol mesylate to patients with underlying cardiovascular disease. Even though the changes may be significant in a small number of patients, these changes occur within a short period of time after administration and have not been shown to be persistent.

If an unusual smell or taste is noted with use of this product, the patient should discontinue use in consultation with his/her physician.

PRECAUTIONS

General As with all β-adrenergic stimulating agents, caution should be used when administering Tornalate to patients with cardiovascular disease such as ischemic heart disease or hypertension. Caution is also advised in patients with hyperthyroidism, diabetes mellitus, cardiac arrhythmias, convulsive disorders or unusual responsiveness to β-adrenergic agonists. Use of any β-adrenergic bronchodilator may produce significant changes in systolic and diastolic blood pressure in some patients.

Information for Patients The effects of Tornalate may last up to eight hours or longer. It should not be used more often than recommended and the patient should not increase the number of treatments or dose without first consulting with the physician. If symptoms of asthma get worse, adverse reactions occur, or the patient does not respond to the usual dose, the patient should be instructed to contact the physician immediately. Drug stability and safety of Tornalate when mixed with other drugs in a nebulizer have not been established. The patient should be advised as to the proper use of the equipment used for nebulization and to see the Illustrated Patient's Instructions for Use.

Drug Interactions Other sympathomimetic bronchodilators or epinephrine should not be used concomitantly with Tornalate because they may have additive effects.

Tornalate should be administered with caution to patients being treated with monoamine oxidase inhibitors or tricyclic antidepressants, since the action of bitolterol on the vascular system may be potentiated.

Carcinogenesis, Mutagenesis, and Impairment of Fertility No tumorigenicity (and specifically no increase in leiomyomas) was observed in a two-year oral study in Sprague-Dawley CD rats at doses of Tornalate corresponding to 12 or 62 times the maximal total daily human inhalational dose (8.0 mg bitolterol mesylate per day). Tornalate was not tumorigenic in an 18-month oral study in Swiss-Webster mice at doses up to 312 times the maximal daily human inhalational dose. Ames Salmonella and mouse lymphoma mutation assays in vitro revealed no mutagenesis due to Tornalate. Reproductive studies in male and female rats revealed no significant effects on fertility at doses of Tornalate up to 241 times the maximal daily human inhalational dose.

Teratogenic Effects—Pregnancy Category C No teratogenic effects were seen in rats and rabbits after oral doses of Tornalate up to 361 times the maximal daily human inhalational dose and in mice after oral doses up to 188 times the maximal daily human inhalational dose.

When Tornalate (as base) was injected subcutaneously into mice in doses of 2 mg/kg, 10 mg/kg, and 20 mg/kg (corresponding to 15, 75, and 151 times the maximal daily human inhalational dose) the incidence of cleft palate was 5.7%, 3.8%, and 3.3%, respectively. Occurrence of cleft palate with isoproterenol (as base) at 10 mg/kg subcutaneously was 10.7%. Since no well-controlled studies in pregnant women are available, Tornalate should be used during pregnancy only if the potential benefit justifies the potential risk to the fetus.

Nursing Mothers It is not known whether Tornalate is excreted in human milk. Because many drugs are excreted in human milk, caution should be exercised when Tornalate is administered to a nursing woman.

Pediatric Use Safety and effectiveness of Tornalate in children 12 years of age or younger has not been established.

ADVERSE REACTIONS

The adverse reactions observed with Tornalate are consistent with those seen with other beta-adrenergic agonists. The frequency of most cardiovascular effects was less after bitolterol mesylate than after isoproterenol in 3-month repetitive dose studies.

Like the findings noted after the administration of other beta-adrenergic agonist drugs, infrequent laboratory abnormalities with undetermined clinical significance were noted after administration of Tornalate. These include decreases in hemoglobin and hematocrit, decreases in WBC, elevation of liver enzymes, increases in blood sugar, decreases in serum potassium and abnormal urinalysis. In addition, one patient in a Tornalate controlled clinical trial had increased liver function tests and documented hepatomegaly.

The results of all clinical trials with Tornalate (323 patients) showed the following side effects:

Central/Peripheral Nervous System: Tremors (26.6%), nervousness (11.1%), headache (8.4%), lightheadedness (6.8%), dizziness (4.0%), paresthesia (1.5%), somnolence (1.2%). In three-month studies, the incidence of tremors decreased from 22% during the first month to 9% during the third month.

Cardiovascular: Tachycardia (3.7%), palpitation (3.1%), irregular pulse (1.2%).

Respiratory: Coughing (2.5%), bronchospasm (1.5%), chest discomfort (1.5%), rhinitis (1.5%).

Oro-Pharyngeal: Throat irritation (2.5%), mouth irritation (1.9%).

Gastrointestinal: Nausea (1.9%).

Other: Fatigue (1.5%).

The incidence of the following adverse reactions was less than one percent:

CNS: Vertigo, insomnia, euphoria, incoordination, hyperkinesia, hypoesthesia, anxiety.

Cardiovascular: Transient ECG changes (ventricular premature contractions, atrial arrhythmia, inverted T waves, junctional rhythm), chest discomfort, increase in blood pressure, chills, heart rate decrease, flushing.

Respiratory: Dyspnea, sputum increase.

Gastrointestinal: Vomiting, hepatomegalia.

Others: Pruritus, urticaria, asthenia, arthralgia, eye irritation, facial discomfort, taste loss.

Clinical relevance or relationship to administration of Tornalate and rarely reported elevations of SGOT, SGPT, LDH are not known.

OVERDOSAGE

Overdosage with Tornalate may be expected to result in exaggeration of those drug effects listed in the ADVERSE REACTIONS section. In such cases therapy with Tornalate and all β-adrenergic stimulating drugs should be stopped, supportive therapy provided, and judicious use of a cardioselective β-adrenergic blocking agent should be considered bearing in mind the possibility that such agents can produce profound bronchospasm. As with all sympathomimetic aerosol medications, cardiac arrest and even death may be associated with abuse.

The oral LD_{50} of Tornalate in rats was 5,650 mg/kg and in mice it was 6,575 mg/kg.

DOSAGE AND ADMINISTRATION

Tornalate Solution for Inhalation, 0.2% can be administered by nebulization to adults and children over 12 years of age. As with all medications, the physician should begin therapy with the lowest effective dose according to the individual patient's requirements following manufacturer's dosage recommendation. Tornalate should be administered during a ten to fifteen-minute period. The treatment period can be adjusted by varying the amount of diluent (normal saline solution) placed in the nebulizer with the medication. The total volume (medication plus diluent) is usually adjusted to 2.0 mL to 4.0 mL. Safety of the treatment should be monitored by measuring blood pressure and pulse.

Clinical studies were conducted with two types of nebulizer systems.

Intermittent Aerosol Flow (Patient-Activated Nebulizer) This nebulizer is operated by a patient-activated valve to permit the release of aerosol mist only during inspiration.

Continuous Aerosol Flow Nebulizer This nebulizer generates a continuous flow of mist while the patient inhales and exhales through the nebulizer resulting in the loss of some medication through an exhaust port.

When using these types of nebulizer systems the following dosing regimens are recommended:

Tornalate Solution for Inhalation, 0.2%

Doses	Continuous Flow Nebulization Volume	Continuous Flow Nebulization Tornalate	Intermittent Flow Nebulization Volume	Intermittent Flow Nebulization Tornalate
Usual Dose	**1.25 mL**	**2.5 mg**	0.5 mL	1.0 mg
Decreased Dose	0.75 mL	1.5 mg	0.25 mL	0.5 mg
Increased Dose	1.75 mL	3.5 mg	0.75 mL	1.5 mg

Up to 1.0 mL of Tornalate Solution for Inhalation, 0.2% (2.0 mg Tornalate) can be administered with the intermittent flow system to severely-obstructed patients.
The usual frequency of treatments is three times a day. Treatments may be increased up to four times daily, however the interval between treatments should not be less than four hours. For some patients two treatments a day may be adequate. If a previously effective dosage regimen fails to provide the usual relief, the patient should be advised to seek medical advice immediately as this is often a sign of seriously-worsening asthma that would require reassessment of therapy.
The maximum daily dose should not exceed 8.0 mg Tornalate with an intermittent flow nebulization system or 14.0 mg Tornalate with a continuous flow nebulization system.
Tornalate Solution for Inhalation, 0.2% should be added to the nebulizer just prior to use and should not be left in the nebulizer.
Drug stability and safety of Tornalate (bitolterol mesylate) Solution for Inhalation, 0.2% when mixed with other drugs in a nebulizer have not been established. Tornalate Solution for Inhalation, 0.2% should not be mixed with other drugs such as cromolyn sodium or acetylcysteine at clinically-recommended doses due to chemical and/or physical incompatibilities.

HOW SUPPLIED

Amber Glass Bottle of 10 mL with .75 cc dropper (NDC 51479-011-01)
Amber Glass Bottle of 30 mL with 1.25 cc dropper (NDC 51479-011-03)
Amber Glass Bottle of 60 mL with 1.25 cc dropper (NDC 51479-011-06)
Included in each carton is an overwrapped graduated medicine dropper for use with Tornalate Solution for Inhalation, 0.2%.
Do not use the solution if it is discolored or contains a precipitate.
Store at controlled room temperature between 15°C–30°C (59°F–86°F).
CAUTION: Federal law prohibits dispensing without a prescription.
Distributed by DURA Pharmaceuticals, Inc., San Diego, CA 92121
Manufactured by Nycomed Puerto Rico Inc., Barceloneta, Puerto Rico 00617
Copyright, Sanofi Winthrop, Inc. 1991
DURA PHARMACEUTICALS
Revised December 1994
TS007D1294

TORNALATE® ℞

(bitolterol mesylate)
Metered Dose Inhaler
Bronchodilator for Oral Inhalation

DESCRIPTION

Tornalate (bitolterol mesylate) is the di-p -toluate ester of the β-adrenergic agonist bronchodilator *N-t* -butylarterenol (colterol). It has a molecular weight of 557.7. Bitolterol mesylate is known chemically as 4-[2-[(1,1-dimethylethyl) amino]-1-hydroxyethyl]-1,2-phenylene 4-methylbenzoate (ester) methanesulfonate (salt) and has the following structural formula:

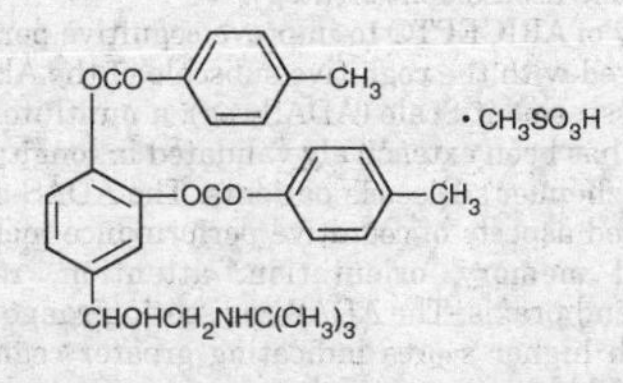

Tornalate (bitolterol mesylate), Metered Dose Inhaler is a complete aerosol unit for oral inhalation. It consists of a plastic-coated bottle of ready-to-use aerosol solution and a detachable plastic mouthpiece with built-in nebulizer. The bottle contains 16.4 g (15 mL) of 0.8% bitolterol mesylate in a vehicle containing 38% alcohol (w/w), inert propellants (dichlorodifluoromethane and dichlorotetrafluoroethane), ascorbic acid, saccharin, and menthol.
Each bottle provides at least 300 actuations. Each actuation delivers a measured dose of 0.37 mg of bitolterol mesylate as a fine, even mist.

CLINICAL PHARMACOLOGY

Tornalate (bitolterol mesylate) is administered as a prodrug which is hydrolyzed by esterases in tissue and blood to the active moiety colterol. Tornalate administered as an inhaled aerosol has a rapid (3 to 4 minutes) onset of bronchodilator activity. The duration of action with Tornalate is at least 5 hours in most patients and 8 or more hours in 25% to 35% of patients, based on 15% or greater increase in forced expiratory volume in one second (FEV_1), as demonstrated in 3-month isoproterenol controlled multicenter trials. Based on mean maximal expiratory flow (MMEF) measurements, the duration of action is 6 to 7 hours. The duration of bronchodilator action with Tornalate in these trials is longer than that seen with isoproterenol, especially in steroid-dependent patients. Duration of effect was reduced over time in steroid-dependent asthmatic patients where the duration was 3.5 to 5 hours for FEV_1. The mean maximum increase in FEV_1 over baseline in the majority of patients was 39% to 42% and occurred by 30 to 60 minutes, similar to that seen in the isoproterenol group.
Tornalate is a beta-adrenergic agonist which has been shown by in vitro and in vivo pharmacological studies in animals to exert a preferential effect on $beta_2$ adrenergic receptors, such as those located in bronchial smooth muscle. However, controlled clinical trials in patients who were administered the drug have not revealed a preferential $beta_2$ adrenergic effect. At doses that produced long duration of bronchodilator activity (up to 8 hours in some patients) with a mean maximum bronchodilating effect of approximately 40% increase in FEV_1 (forced expiratory volume in one second), a less than 10 beat per minute mean maximum increase in heart rate was seen. The effect on the heart rate was transient and similar to the increases seen in the isoproterenol treated patients in these studies.
Although blood levels of colterol formed by gradual release from the pro-drug (bitolterol) in the lungs are too low to be measured by currently available assay methods, data on disposition are available from oral studies in man. Following oral administration of 5.9 mg tritiated bitolterol mesylate to man, radioactivity measurements indicated mean maximum colterol concentration in blood of approximately 2.1 μg/mL one hour after medication. Urinary excretion data indicate that 83 percent of the radioactivity of this oral dose was excreted within the first 24 hours. By 72 hours, 85.6 percent of the tritium had been excreted in the urine and 8.1 percent in the feces. Most of the radioactivity was excreted as conjugated colterol; free colterol accounted for 2.1 to 3.7 percent of the total radioactivity excreted in the urine. No intact bitolterol was detected in urine.
The pharmacologic effects of β-adrenergic drugs including Tornalate (bitolterol mesylate) are attributable to stimulation of adenyl cyclase, the enzyme which catalyzes the conversion of adenosine triphosphate (ATP) to cyclic-3′, 5′-adenosine monophosphate (c-AMP). Increased c-AMP levels are associated with relaxation of bronchial smooth muscle and with inhibition of release of mediators of immediate hypersensitivity from cells, especially from mast cells.
In a six-week clinical trial in which 24 asthmatic patients received Tornalate and theophylline concurrently, improvement in pulmonary function was enhanced over that seen with either drug alone. No potentiation of side effects was observed, and 24-hour ECG recordings (Holter monitoring) indicated no greater degree of cardiac toxicity with Tornalate alone or in combination with theophylline than that which occurred with theophylline alone.
Tornalate did not adversely affect arterial oxygen tension in a blood-gas study in 24 asthmatic patients. However, a decrease in arterial oxygen tension has been reported with other adrenergic bronchodilators and could be anticipated to occur with Tornalate as well.
In repetitive dosing studies, continued effectiveness was demonstrated throughout the 3-month period of treatment in the majority of patients. However, some overall decrease was observed in steroid-dependent asthmatics.

INDICATIONS AND USAGE

Tornalate (bitolterol mesylate) is indicated for both prophylactic and therapeutic use as a bronchodilator for bronchial asthma and for reversible bronchospasm. It may be used with or without concurrent theophylline and/or steroid therapy.

CONTRAINDICATIONS

Tornalate (bitolterol mesylate) is contraindicated in patients who are hypersensitive to any of its ingredients.

WARNINGS

As with other β-adrenergic aerosols, Tornalate (bitolterol mesylate) should not be used in excess. Fatalities have been reported in association with excessive use of inhaled sympathomimetic drugs. The exact cause of death is unknown. Use of aerosolized β-adrenergic drugs may have a deleterious cardiac effect. Paradoxical bronchoconstriction (which can be life-threatening) has been reported with administration of β-adrenergic agents. Immediate hypersensitivity (allergic) reactions can occur after the administration of Tornalate. In such instances, the drug should be discontinued immediately and alternative therapy instituted.
The contents of Tornalate Metered Dose Inhaler are under pressure. Do not puncture. Do not use or store near heat or open flame. Exposure to temperatures above 120°F may cause bursting. Never throw container into fire or incinerator. Keep out of reach of children.
If an unusual smell or taste is noted with the use of this product, the patient should discontinue use in consultation with his/her physician.

PRECAUTIONS

General As with all β-adrenergic stimulating agents, caution should be used when administering Tornalate (bitolterol mesylate) to patients with cardiovascular disease such as ischemic heart disease or hypertension. Caution is also advised in patients with hyperthyroidism, diabetes mellitus, cardiac arrhythmias, convulsive disorders or unusual responsiveness to β-adrenergic agonists. Significant changes in systolic and diastolic blood pressure have been seen in individual patients and could be expected to occur in some patients after use of any β-adrenergic aerosol bronchodilator.
Information for Patients The effects of Tornalate may last up to eight hours or longer. It should not be used more often than recommended and the patient should not increase the number of inhalations or frequency of use without first asking the physician. If symptoms of asthma get worse, adverse reactions occur, or the patient does not respond to the usual dose, the patient should be instructed to contact the physician immediately. The patient should be advised to see the illustrated Patients Instructions for Use.
Drug Interactions Other sympathomimetic aerosol bronchodilators should not be used concomitantly with Tornalate. If additional adrenergic drugs are to be administered by any route, they should be used with caution to avoid deleterious cardiovascular effects.
Carcinogenesis, Mutagenesis, and Impairment of Fertility No tumorigenicity (and specifically no increase in leiomyomas) was observed in a two-year oral study in Sprague-Dawley CD rats at doses of Tornalate corresponding to 23 or 114 times the maximal daily human inhalational dose. Tornalate was not tumorigenic in an 18-month oral study in Swiss-Webster mice at doses up to 568 times the maximal daily human inhalational dose.
Ames Salmonella and mouse lymphoma mutation assays in vitro revealed no mutagenesis due to Tornalate. Reproductive studies in male and female rats revealed no significant effects on fertility at doses of Tornalate up to 364 times the maximal daily human inhalational dose.
Teratogenic Effects—Pregnancy Category C No teratogenic effects were seen in rats and rabbits after oral doses of Tornalate up to 557 times the maximal daily human inhalational dose and in mice after oral doses up to 284 times the maximal daily human inhalational dose.
When Tornalate was injected subcutaneously into mice at doses of 2 mg/kg, 10 mg/kg, and 20 mg/kg (corresponding to 23, 114, and 227 times the maximal daily human inhalational dose) cleft palate incidences of 5.7 percent, 3.8 percent, and 3.3 percent (compared with 0.9 percent in controls) were found. Cleft palate induction with isoproterenol at 10 mg/kg SC as the positive control was 10.7 percent. Since no well-controlled studies in pregnant women are available, Tornalate should be used during pregnancy only if the potential benefit justifies the potential risk to the fetus.
Nursing Mothers It is not known whether Tornalate is excreted in human milk. Because many drugs are excreted in human milk, caution should be exercised when Tornalate is administered to a nursing woman.
Pediatric Use Safety and effectiveness of Tornalate in pediatric patients 12 years of age or younger has not been established.

ADVERSE REACTIONS

The results of all clinical trials with Tornalate (bitolterol mesylate) in 492 patients showed the following side effects:
CNS: Tremors (14%), nervousness (5%), headache (4%), dizziness (3%), lightheadedness (3%), insomnia (<1%), hyperkinesia (<1%).
Gastrointestinal: Nausea (3%).
Oro-Pharyngeal: Throat irritation (5%).
Cardiovascular: The overall incidence of cardiovascular effects was approximately 5% of patients and these effects included palpitations (approximately 3%), and chest discomfort (approximately 1%). Tachycardia was seen in less than 1%. Premature ventricular contractions and flushing were rarely seen.

Continued on next page

Tornalate Inhaler—Cont.

Respiratory: Coughing (4%), bronchospasm (<1%), dyspnea (<1%), chest tightness (<1%).

Clinical relevance or relationship to Tornalate administration of rarely reported elevations of SGOT, decrease in platelets, decrease in WBC levels or proteinuria are not known.

In comparing the adverse reactions for bitolterol mesylate treated patients to those of isoproterenol treated patients, during three-month clinical trials involving approximately 400 patients, the following moderate to severe reactions, as judged by the investigators, were reported for both steroid and non-steroid dependent patients. The table does not include mild reactions or those occurring only with the first dose.

PERCENT INCIDENCE OF MODERATE TO SEVERE ADVERSE REACTIONS

Reaction	Bitolterol N=197	Isoproterenol N=194
Central Nervous System		
Tremors	9.1%	1.5%
Nervousness	1.5%	1.0%
Headache	3.5%	6.1%
Dizziness	1.0%	1.5%
Insomnia	0.5%	0%
Cardiovascular		
Palpitations	1.5%	0%
PVC—Transient		
Increase	0.5%	0%
Chest Discomfort	0.5%	0%
Respiratory		
Cough	4.1%	1.0%
Bronchospasm	1.0%	0%
Dyspnea	1.0%	0%
Oro-Pharyngeal		
Throat Irritation	3.0%	3.1%
Gastrointestinal		
Nausea (Dyspepsia)	0.5%	0.5%

NOTE: In most patients, the total isoproterenol dosage was divided into three equally dosed inhalations, administered at three-minute intervals. This procedure may have reduced the incidence of adverse reactions observed with isoproterenol.

OVERDOSAGE

Overdosage with Tornalate (bitolterol mesylate) may be expected to result in exaggeration of those drug effects listed in the ADVERSE REACTIONS section. In such cases therapy with Tornalate and all β-adrenergic stimulating drugs should be stopped, supportive therapy provided, and judicious use of a cardioselective β-adrenergic blocking agent should be considered bearing in mind the possibility that such agents can produce profound bronchospasm. As with all sympathomimetic aerosol medications, cardiac arrest and even death may be associated with abuse.

The oral LD$_{50}$ of Tornalate in rats was greater than 5,000 mg/kg and in mice greater than 6,000 mg/kg.

DOSAGE AND ADMINISTRATION

The usual dose to relieve bronchospasm for adults and adolescents over 12 years of age is two inhalations at an interval of at least one to three minutes followed by a third inhalation if needed. For prevention of bronchospasm, the usual dose is two inhalations every 8 hours. The dose of Tornalate (bitolterol mesylate) should never exceed 3 inhalations every 6 hours or 2 inhalations every 4 hours. If a previously effective dosage regimen fails to provide the usual relief, the patient should be advised to seek medical advice immediately as this is often a sign of seriously worsening asthma that would require reassessment of therapy.

HOW SUPPLIED

Tornalate (bitolterol mesylate) Metered Dose Inhaler is supplied in 16.4 g (15mL) self-contained aerosol units (NDC 51479-012-01).

Note The indented statement below is required by the Federal government's Clean Air Act for all products containing or manufactured with chlorofluorocarbons (CFC's).

> **WARNING Contains dichlorodifluoromethane and dichlorotetrafluoroethane, substances which harm public health and environment by destroying ozone in the upper atmosphere.**

A notice similar to the above WARNING has been placed in the information for the patient of this product pursuant to EPA regulations.

Store at controlled room temperature between 15°C and 30°C (59°F and 86°F). Use of the product outside this temperature range may result in improper dosing.

Rx only.

DURA
PHARMACEUTICALS

Distributed by DURA Pharmaceuticals, Inc., San Diego, CA 92121

Manufactured by Nycomed Puerto Rico Inc., Barceloneta, Puerto Rico 00617

Revised July, 1998 TM009G98

ECR Pharmaceuticals

**Distributor of ECR, &
Wm. P. Poythress Products
3981 DEEP ROCK ROAD
P. O. BOX 71600
RICHMOND, VA 23255**

Direct Inquiries to:
Professional Services Department
(804) 527-1950
FAX: (804) 527-1959

For Medical Information Contact:
In Emergencies:
Professional Services Department
(804) 527-1950
FAX: (804) 527-1959

NDC 0095	Product	
—0131	**Anaplex DM Cough Syrup** Each teaspoon (5 ml) contains: Dextromethrophan Hydrobromide, 30 mg. Brompheniramine Maleate, 4 mg. Pseudoephedrine HCl, 60 mg.	Rx
—0130	**Anaplex HD Cough Syrup** Each teaspoon (5 ml) contains: Hydrocodone Bitartrate, 1.7 mg; Phenylephrine HCl, 5 mg; Chlorpheniramine Maleate, 2 mg. Sugar Free. Alcohol Free.	Rx Ⓒ
—0240	**Bupap Tablets** (Butalbital, 50 mg; Acetaminophen, 650 mg)	Rx
—0016	**Bensulfoid Cream** (Sulfur, 8%; Resorcinol 2%; Alcohol, 10%)	OTC
—6004	**Lodrane Liquid** Each teaspoon (5 ml) contains: Brompheniramine Maleate, 4 mg; Pseudoephedrine HCl, 60 mg. Sugar Free. Alcohol Free. Dye Free.	Rx
—0006	**Lodrane Allergy Capsules** (Brompheniramine Maleate, 6 mg.) Sustained Release, Dye Free	Rx
—6006	**Lodrane LD Capsules** (Brompheniramine Maleate, 6 mg; Pseudoephedrine HCl, 60 mg) Sustained Release, Dye Free	Rx
—0225	**Nasatab LA Tablets** (Guaifenesin, 500 mg; Pseudoephedrine HCl, 120 mg) Sustained Release, Dye Free	Rx
—0021	**Panalgesic Gold Cream** (Methyl Salicylate, 35%; Menthol, 4%)	OTC
—0120	**Panalgesic Gold Liniment** (Methyl Salicylate, 55%; Camphor, 3%; Menthol, 1%)	OTC
—0600	**Pneumomist Tablets** (Guaifenesin, 600 mg) Sustained Release, Dye Free	Rx
—0065	**Pneumotussin HC Cough Syrup** Each teaspoon (5 ml) contains: (Guaifenesin, 100 mg; Hydrocodone Bitartrate, 5 mg)	Rx Ⓒ

Eisai Inc.
**500 FRANK W. BURR BOULEVARD
TEANECK, NJ 07666**

Direct Inquiries to:
Eisai Medical Services
1 (888) 274-2378 (888-Aricept)
FAX: (201) 287-9744
Medical Emergency Contact:
Medical Emergencies:
24 hours/day, 7 days/week
1 (888) 274-2378 (888-Aricept)

ARICEPT® ℞
(Donepezil Hydrochloride Tablets)

DESCRIPTION

ARICEPT® (donepezil hydrochloride) is a reversible inhibitor of the enzyme acetylcholinesterase, known chemically as (±)-2,3-dihydro-5,6-dimethoxy- 2-[[1-(phenylmethyl) -4-piperidinyl]methyl]-1H-inden-1-one hydrochloride. Donepezil hydrochloride is commonly referred to in the pharmacological literature as E2020. It has an empirical formula of $C_{24}H_{29}NO_3HCl$ and a molecular weight of 415.96. Donepezil hydrochloride is a white crystalline powder and is freely soluble in chloroform, soluble in water and in glacial acetic acid, slightly soluble in ethanol and in acetonitrile and practically insoluble in ethyl acetate and in n-hexane.

ARICEPT® is available for oral administration in film-coated tablets containing 5 or 10 mg of donepezil hydrochloride. Inactive ingredients are lactose monohydrate, corn starch, microcrystalline cellulose, hydroxypropyl cellulose, and magnesium stearate. The film coating contains talc, polyethylene glycol, hydroxypropyl methylcellulose and titanium dioxide. Additionally, the 10 mg tablet contains yellow iron oxide (synthetic) as a coloring agent.

CLINICAL PHARMACOLOGY

Current theories on the pathogenesis of the cognitive signs and symptoms of Alzheimer's Disease attribute some of them to a deficiency of cholinergic neurotransmission. Donepezil hydrochloride is postulated to exert its therapeutic effect by enhancing cholinergic function. This is accomplished by increasing the concentration of acetylcholine through reversible inhibition of its hydrolysis by acetylcholinesterase. If this proposed mechanism of action is correct, donepezil's effect may lessen as the disease process advances and fewer cholinergic neurons remain functionally intact. There is no evidence that donepezil alters the course of the underlying dementing process.

Clinical Trial Data

The effectiveness of ARICEPT® as a treatment for Alzheimer's Disease is demonstrated by the results of two randomized, double-blind, placebo-controlled clinical investigations in patients with Alzheimer's Disease (diagnosed by NINCDS and DSM III-R criteria, Mini-Mental State Examination ≥10 and ≤26 and Clinical Dementia Rating of 1 or 2). The mean age of patients participating in ARICEPT® trials was 73 years with a range of 50 to 94. Approximately 62% of patients were women and 38% were men. The racial distribution was white 95%, black 3% and other races 2%.

Study Outcome Measures: In each study, the effectiveness of treatment with ARICEPT® was evaluated using a dual outcome assessment strategy.

The ability of ARICEPT® to improve cognitive performance was assessed with the cognitive subscale of the Alzheimer's Disease Assessment Scale (ADAS-cog), a multi-item instrument that has been extensively validated in longitudinal cohorts of Alzheimer's Disease patients. The ADAS-cog examines selected aspects of cognitive performance including elements of memory, orientation, attention, reasoning, language and praxis. The ADAS-cog scoring range is from 0 to 70, with higher scores indicating greater cognitive impairment. Elderly normal adults may score as low as 0 or 1, but it is not unusual for non-demented adults to score slightly higher.

The patients recruited as participants in each study had mean scores on the Alzheimer's Disease Assessment Scale (ADAS-cog) of approximately 26 units, with a range from 4

to 61. Experience gained in longitudinal studies of ambulatory patients with mild to moderate Alzheimer's Disease suggest that they gain 6 to 12 units a year on the ADAS-cog. However, lesser degrees of change are seen in patients with very mild or very advanced disease because the ADAS-cog is not uniformly sensitive to change over the course of the disease. The annualized rate of decline in the placebo patients participating in ARICEPT® trials was approximately 2 to 4 units per year.

The ability of ARICEPT® to produce an overall clinical effect was assessed using a Clinician's Interview Based Impression of Change that required the use of caregiver information, the CIBIC plus. The CIBIC plus is not a single instrument and is not a standardized instrument like the ADAS-cog. Clinical trials for investigational drugs have used a variety of CIBIC formats, each different in terms of depth and structure. As such, results from a CIBIC plus reflect clinical experience from the trial or trials in which it was used and cannot be compared directly with the results of CIBIC plus evaluations from other clinical trials. The CIBIC plus used in ARICEPT® trials was a semi-structured instrument that was intended to examine four major areas of patient function: General, Cognitive, Behavioral and Activities of Daily Living. It represents the assessment of a skilled clinician based upon his/her observations at an interview with the patient, in combination with information supplied by a caregiver familiar with the behavior of the patient over the interval rated. The CIBIC plus is scored as a seven point categorical rating, ranging from a score of 1, indicating "markedly improved," to a score of 4, indicating "no change" to a score of 7, indicating "markedly worse." The CIBIC plus has not been systematically compared directly to assessments not using information from caregivers (CIBIC) or other global methods.

Thirty-Week Study

In a study of 30 weeks duration, 473 patients were randomized to receive single daily doses of placebo, 5 mg/day or 10 mg/day of ARICEPT®. The 30-week study was divided into a 24-week double-blind active treatment phase followed by a 6-week single-blind placebo washout period. The study was designed to compare 5 mg/day or 10 mg/day fixed doses of ARICEPT® to placebo. However, to reduce the likelihood of cholinergic effects, the 10 mg/day treatment was started following an initial 7-day treatment with 5 mg/day doses.

Effects of the ADAS-cog:

Figure 1 illustrates the time course for the change from baseline in ADAS-cog scores for all three dose groups over the 30 weeks of the study. After 24 weeks of treatment, the mean differences in the ADAS-cog change scores for ARICEPT® treated patients compared to the patients on placebo were 2.8 and 3.1 units for the 5 mg/day and 10 mg/day treatments, respectively. These differences were statistically significant. While the treatment effect size may appear to be slightly greater for the 10 mg/day treatment, there was no statistically significant difference between the two active treatments.

Following 6 weeks of placebo washout, scores on the ADAS-cog for both the ARICEPT® treatment groups were indistinguishable from those patients who had received only placebo for 30 weeks. This suggests that the beneficial effects of ARICEPT® abate over 6 weeks following discontinuation of treatment and do not represent a change in the underlying disease. There was no evidence of a rebound effect 6 weeks after abrupt discontinuation of therapy.

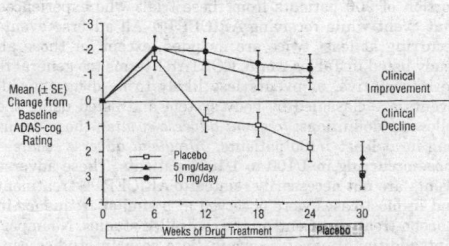

Figure 1. Time-course of the Change from Baseline in ADAS-cog Score for Patients Completing 24 Weeks of Treatment.

Figure 2 illustrates the cumulative percentages of patients from each of the three treatment groups who had attained the measure of improvement in ADAS-cog score shown on the X axis. Three change scores, (7-point and 4-point reductions from baseline or no change in score) have been identified for illustrative purposes and the percent of patients in each group achieving that result is shown in the inset table. The curves demonstrate that both patients assigned to placebo and ARICEPT® have a wide range of responses, but that the active treatment groups are more likely to show the greater improvements. A curve for an effective treatment would be shifted to the left of the curve for placebo, while an ineffective or deleterious treatment would be superimposed upon or shifted to the right of the curve for placebo, respectively.

[See figure 2 at top of next column]

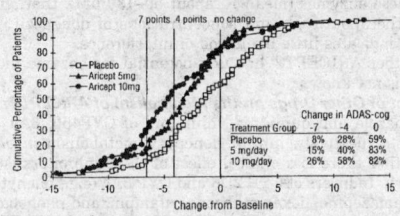

Figure 2. Cumulative Percentage of Patients Completing 24 Weeks of Double-blind Treatment with Specified Changes from Baseline ADAS-cog Scores. The Percentages of Randomized Patients who Completed the Study were: Placebo 80%, 5 mg/day 85% and 10 mg/day 68%.

Effects on the CIBIC plus:

Figure 3 is a histogram of the frequency distribution of CIBIC plus scores attained by patients assigned to each of the three treatment groups who completed 24 weeks of treatment. The mean drug-placebo differences for these groups of patients were 0.35 units and 0.39 units for 5 mg/day and 10 mg/day of ARICEPT®, respectively. These differences were statistically significant. There was no statistically significant difference between the two active treatments.

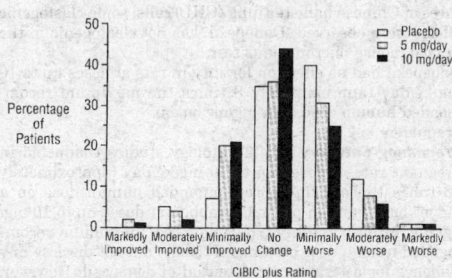

Figure 3. Frequency Distribution of CIBIC plus Scores at Week 24

Fifteen-Week Study

In a study of 15 weeks duration, patients were randomized to receive single daily doses of placebo or either 5 mg/day or 10 mg/day of ARICEPT® for 12 weeks, followed by a 3-week placebo washout period. As in the 30-week study, to avoid acute cholinergic effects, the 10 mg/day treatment followed an initial 7-day treatment with 5 mg/day doses.

Effects on the ADAS-Cog:

Figure 4 illustrates the time course of the change from baseline in ADAS-scores for all three dose groups over the 15 weeks of the study. After 12 weeks of treatment, the differences in mean ADAS-cog change scores for the ARICEPT® treated patients compared to the patients on placebo were 2.7 and 3.0 units each, for the 5 and 10 mg/day ARICEPT® treatment groups respectively. These differences were statistically significant. The effect size for the 10 mg/day group may appear to be slightly larger than that for 5 mg/day. However, the differences between active treatments were not statistically significant.

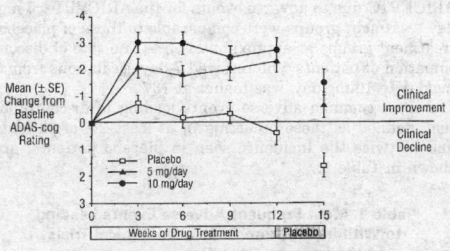

Figure 4. Time-course of the Change from Baseline in ADAS-cog Score for Patients Completing the 15-week Study.

Following 3 weeks of placebo washout, scores on the ADAS-cog for both the ARICEPT® treatment groups increased, indicating that discontinuation of ARICEPT® resulted in a loss of its treatment effect. The duration of this placebo washout period was not sufficient to characterize the rate of loss of the treatment effect, but, the 30-week study (see above) demonstrated that treatment effects associated with the use of ARICEPT® abate within 6 weeks of treatment discontinuation.

Figure 5 illustrates the cumulative percentages of patients from each of the three treatment groups who attained the measure of improvement in ADAS-cog score shown on the X axis. The same three change scores, (7-point and 4-point reductions from baseline or no change in score) as selected for the 30-week study have been used for this illustration. The percentages of patients achieving those results are shown in the inset table.

As observed in the 30-week study, the curves demonstrate that patients assigned to either placebo or to ARICEPT® have a wide range of responses, but that the ARICEPT®

treated patients are more likely to show the greater improvements in cognitive performance.

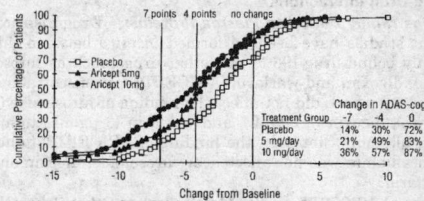

Figure 5. Cumulative Percentage of Patients with Specified Changes from Baseline ADAS-cog Scores. The Percentages of Randomized Patients Within Each Treatment Group Who Completed the Study Were: Placebo 93%, 5 mg/day 90% and 10 mg/day 82%.

Effects on the CIBIC plus:

Figure 6 is a histogram of the frequency distribution of CIBIC plus scores attained by patients assigned to each of the three treatment groups who completed 12 weeks of treatment. The differences in mean scores for ARICEPT® treated patients compared to the patients on placebo at Week 12 were 0.36 and 0.38 units for the 5 mg/day and 10 mg/day treatment groups, respectively. These differences were statistically significant.

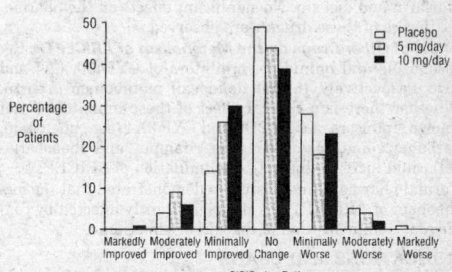

Figure 6. Frequency Distribution of CIBIC plus Scores at Week 12

In both studies, patient age, sex and race were not found to predict the clinical outcome of ARICEPT® treatment.

Clinical Pharmacokinetics

Donepezil is well absorbed with a relative oral bioavailability of 100% and reaches peak plasma concentrations in 3 to 4 hours. Pharmacokinetics are linear over a dose range of 1–10 mg given once daily. Neither food nor time of administration (morning vs. evening dose) influences the rate or extent of absorption. The elimination half life of donepezil is about 70 hours and the mean apparent plasma clearance (Cl/F) is 0.13 L/hr/kg. Following multiple dose administration, donepezil accumulates in plasma by 4–7 fold and steady state is reached within 15 days. The steady state volume of distribution is 12 L/kg. Donepezil is approximately 96% bound to human plasma proteins, mainly to albumins (about 75%) and alpha$_1$-acid glycoprotein (about 21%) over the concentration range of 2-1000 ng/mL.

Donepezil is both excreted in the urine intact and extensively metabolized to four major metabolites, two of which are known to be active, and a number of minor metabolites, not all of which have been identified. Donepezil is metabolized by CYP 450 isoenzymes 2D6 and 3A4 and undergoes glucuronidation. Following administration of ^{14}C-labeled donepezil, plasma radioactivity, expressed as a percent of the administered dose, was present primarily as intact donepezil (53%) and as 6-0-desmethyl donepezil (11%), which has been reported to inhibit AChE to the same extent as donepezil in vitro and was found in plasma at concentrations equal to about 20% of donepezil. Approximately 57% and 15% of the total radioactivity was recovered in urine and feces, respectively, over a period of 10 days, while 28% remained unrecovered, with about 17% of the donepezil dose recovered in the urine as unchanged drug.

Special Populations:

Hepatic Disease: In a study of 10 patients with stable alcoholic cirrhosis, the clearance of ARICEPT® was decreased by 20% relative to 10 healthy age and sex matched subjects.

Renal Disease: In a study of 4 patients with moderate to severe renal impairment (Cl$_{Cr}$ <22 mL/min/1.73 m^2) the clearance of ARICEPT® did not differ from 4 age and sex matched healthy subjects.

Age: No formal pharmacokinetic study was conducted to examine age related differences in the pharmacokinetics of ARICEPT®. However, mean plasma ARICEPT® concentrations measured during therapeutic drug monitoring of elderly patients with Alzheimer's Disease are comparable to those observed in young healthy volunteers.

Gender and Race: No specific pharmacokinetic study was conducted to investigate the effects of gender and race on the disposition of ARICEPT®. However, retrospective pharmacokinetic analysis indicates that gender and race (Japanese and Caucasians) did not affect the clearance of ARICEPT®.

Continued on next page

Aricept—Cont.

Drug-Drug Interactions

Drugs Highly Bound to Plasma Proteins: Drug displacement studies have been performed *in vitro* between this highly bound drug (96%) and other drugs such as furosemide, digoxin, and warfarin. ARICEPT® at concentrations of 0.3–10 µg/mL did not affect the binding of furosemide (5 µg/mL), digoxin (2 ng/mL), and warfarin (3 µg/mL) to human albumin. Similarly, the binding of ARICEPT® to human albumin was not affected by furosemide, digoxin and warfarin.

Effect of ARICEPT® on the Metabolism of Other Drugs: No *in vivo* clinical trials have investigated the effect of ARICEPT® on the clearance of drugs metabolized by CYP 3A4 (e.g. cisapride, terfenadine) or by CYP 2D6 (e.g. imipramine). However, *in vitro* studies show a low rate of binding to these enzymes (mean K_i about 50–130 µM), that, given the therapeutic plasma concentrations of donepezil (164 nM), indicates little likelihood of interference.

Whether ARICEPT® has any potential for enzyme induction is not known.

Formal pharmacokinetic studies evaluated the potential of ARICEPT® for interaction with theophylline, cimetidine, warfarin and digoxin. No significant effects on the pharmacokinetics of these drugs were observed.

Effect of Other Drugs on the Metabolism of ARICEPT®: Ketoconazole and quinidine, inhibitors of CYP450, 3A4 and 2D6, respectively, inhibit donepezil metabolism *in vitro*. Whether there is a clinical effect of these inhibitors is not known. Inducers of CYP 2D6 and CYP 3A4 (e.g., phenytoin, carbamazepine, dexamethasone, rifampin, and phenobarbital) could increase the rate of elimination of ARICEPT®.

Formal pharmacokinetic studies demonstrated that the metabolism of ARICEPT® is not significantly affected by concurrent administration of digoxin or cimetidine.

INDICATIONS AND USAGE

ARICEPT® is indicated for the treatment of mild to moderate dementia of the Alzheimer's type.

CONTRAINDICATIONS

ARICEPT® in contraindicated in patients with known hypersensitivity to donepezil hydrochloride or to piperidine derivatives.

WARNINGS

Anesthesia: ARICEPT®, as a cholinesterase inhibitor, is likely to exaggerate succinylcholine-type muscle relaxation during anesthesia.

Cardiovascular Conditions: Because of their pharmacological action, cholinesterase inhibitors may have vagotonic effects on heart rate (e.g., bradycardia). The potential for this action may be particularly important to patients with "sick sinus syndrome" or other supraventricular cardiac conduction conditions. Syncopal episodes have been reported in association with the use of ARICEPT®.

Gastrointestinal Conditions: Through their primary action, cholinesterase inhibitors may be expected to increase gastric acid secretion due to increased cholinergic activity. Therefore, patients should be monitored closely for symptoms of active or occult gastrointestinal bleeding, especially those at increased risk for developing ulcers, e.g., those with a history of ulcer disease or those receiving concurrent nonsteroidal anti-inflammatory drugs (NSAIDS). Clinical studies of ARICEPT® have shown no increase, relative to placebo, in the incidence of either peptic ulcer disease or gastrointestinal bleeding.

ARICEPT®, as a predictable consequence of its pharmacological properties, has been shown to produce diarrhea, nausea and vomiting. These effects, when they occur, appear more frequently with the 10 mg/day dose than with the 5 mg/day dose. In most cases, these effects have been mild and transient, sometimes lasting one to three weeks, and have resolved during continued use of ARICEPT®.

Genitourinary: Although not observed in clinical trials of ARICEPT®, cholinomimetics may cause bladder outflow obstruction.

Neurological Conditions: Seizures: Cholinomimetics are believed to have some potential to cause generalized convulsions. However, seizure activity also may be a manifestation of Alzheimer's Disease.

Pulmonary Conditions: Because of their cholinomimetic actions, cholinesterase inhibitors should be prescribed with care to patients with a history of asthma or obstructive pulmonary disease.

PRECAUTIONS

Drug-Drug Interactions (see Clinical Pharmacology: Clinical Pharmacokinetics: Drug-drug Interactions)

Effect of ARICEPT® on the Metabolism of Other Drugs: No *in vivo* clinical trials have investigated the effect of ARICEPT® on the clearance of drugs metabolized by CYP 3A4 (e.g. cisapride, terfenadine) or by CYP 2D6 (e.g. imipramine). However, *in vitro* studies show a low rate of binding to these enzymes (mean K_i about 50–130 µM), that, given the therapeutic plasma concentrations of donepezil (164 nM), indicates little likelihood of interference.

Whether ARICEPT® has any potential for enzyme induction is not known.

Effect of Other Drugs on the Metabolism of ARICEPT®: Ketoconazole and quinidine, inhibitors of CYP450, 3A4 and 2D6, respectively, inhibit donepezil metabolism *in vitro*. Whether there is a clinical effect of these inhibitors is not known. Inducers of CYP 2D6 and CYP 3A4 (e.g., phenytoin, carbamazepine, dexamethasone, rifampin, and phenobarbital) could increase the rate of elimination of ARICEPT®.

Used with Anticholinergics: Because of their mechanism of action, cholinesterase inhibitors have the potential to interfere with the activity of anticholinergic medications.

Use with Cholinomimetics and Other Cholinesterase Inhibitors: A synergistic effect may be expected when cholinesterase inhibitors are given concurrently with succinylcholine, similar neuromuscular blocking agents or cholinergic agonists such as bethanechol.

Carcinogenesis, Mutagenesis, Impairment of Fertility

Carcinogenicity studies of donepezil have not been completed.

Donepezil was not mutagenic in the Ames reverse mutation assay in bacteria. In the chromosome aberration test in cultures of Chinese hamster lung (CHL) cells, some clastogenic effects were observed. Donepezil was not clastogenic in the *in vivo* mouse micronucleus test.

Donepezil had no effect on fertility in rats at doses up to 10 mg/kg/day (approximately 8 times the maximum recommended human dose on a mg/m^2 basis).

Pregnancy

Pregnancy Category C: Teratology studies conducted in pregnant rats at doses up to 16 mg/kg/day (approximately 13 times the maximum recommended human dose on a mg/m^2 basis) and in pregnant rabbits at doses up to 10 mg/kg/day (approximately 16 times the maximum recommended human dose on a mg/m^2 basis) did not disclose any evidence for a teratogenic potential of donepezil. However, in a study in which pregnant rats were given up to 10 mg/kg/day (approximately 8 times the maximum recommended human dose on a mg/m^2 basis) from day 17 of gestation through day 20 postpartum, there was a slight increase in still births and a slight decrease in pup survival through day 4 postpartum at this dose; the next lower dose tested was 3 mg/kg/day. There are no adequate or well-controlled studies in pregnant women. ARICEPT® should be used during pregnancy only if the potential benefit justifies the potential risk to the fetus.

Nursing Mothers

It is not known whether donepezil is excreted in human breast milk. ARICEPT® has no indication for use in nursing mothers.

Pediatric Use

There are no adequate and well-controlled trials to document the safety and efficacy of ARICEPT® in any illness occurring in children.

ADVERSE REACTIONS

Adverse Events Leading to Discontinuation

The rates of discontinuation from controlled clinical trials of ARICEPT® due to adverse events for the ARICEPT® 5 mg/day treatment groups were comparable to those of placebo-treatment groups at approximately 5%. The rate of discontinuation of patients who received 7-day escalations from 5 mg/day to 10 mg/day, was higher at 13%.

The most common adverse events leading to discontinuation, defined as those occurring in at least 2% of patients and at twice the incidence seen in placebo patients, are shown in Table 1.

Table 1. Most Frequent Adverse Events Leading to Withdrawal from Controlled Clinical Trials by Dose Group

Dose Group	Placebo	5 mg/day ARICEPT®	10 mg/day ARICEPT®
Patients Randomized	355	350	315
Event/% Discontinuing			
Nausea	1%	1%	3%
Diarrhea	0%	<1%	3%
Vomiting	<1%	<1%	2%

Most Frequent Adverse Clinical Events Seen in Association with the Use of ARICEPT®

The most common adverse events, defined as those occurring at a frequency of at least 5% in patients receiving 10 mg/day and twice the placebo rate, are largely predicted by ARICEPT®'s cholinomimetic effects. These include nausea, diarrhea, insomnia, vomiting, muscle cramp, fatigue and anorexia. These adverse events were often of mild intensity and transient, resolving during continued ARICEPT® treatment without the need for dose modification.

There is evidence to suggest that the frequency of these common adverse events may be affected by the rate of titration. An open-label study was conducted with 269 patients who received placebo in the 15 and 30-week studies. These patients were titrated to a dose of 10 mg/day over a 6-week period. The rates of common adverse events were lower than those seen in patients titrated to 10 mg/day over one week in the controlled clinical trials and were comparable to those seen in patients on 5 mg/day.

See Table 2 for a comparison of the most common adverse events following one and six week titration regimens.

Table 2. Comparison of rates of adverse events in patients titrated to 10 mg/day over 1 and 6 weeks

	No titration		One week titration	Six week titration
Adverse Event	**Placebo (n=315)**	**5 mg/day (n=311)**	**10 mg/day (n=315)**	**10 mg/day (n=269)**
Nausea	6%	5%	19%	6%
Diarrhea	5%	8%	15%	9%
Insomnia	6%	6%	14%	6%
Fatigue	3%	4%	8%	3%
Vomiting	3%	3%	8%	5%
Muscle Cramps	2%	6%	8%	3%
Anorexia	2%	3%	7%	3%

Adverse Events Reported in Controlled Trials

The events cited reflect experience gained under closely monitored conditions of clinical trials in a highly selected patient population. In actual clinical practice or in other clinical trials, these frequency estimates may not apply, as the conditions of use, reporting behavior, and the kinds of patients treated may differ. Table 3 lists treatment emergent signs and symptoms that were reported in at least 2% of patients in placebo-controlled trials who received ARICEPT® and for which the rate of occurrence was greater for ARICEPT® assigned than placebo assigned patients. In general, adverse events occurred more frequently in female patients and with advancing age.

[See table 3 at bottom of next page]

Other Adverse Events Observed During Clinical Trials

ARICEPT® has been administered to over 1700 individuals during clinical trials worldwide. Approximately 1200 of these patients have been treated for at least 3 months and more than 1000 patients have been treated for at least 6 months. Controlled and uncontrolled trials in the United States included approximately 900 patients. In regards to the highest dose of 10 mg/day, this population includes 650 patients treated for 3 months, 475 patients treated for 6 months and 116 patients treated for over 1 year. The range of patient exposure is from 1 to 1214 days.

Treatment emergent signs and symptoms that occurred during 3 controlled clinical trials and two open-label trials in the United States were recorded as adverse events by the clinical investigators using terminology of their own choosing. To provide an overall estimate of the proportion of individuals having similar types of events, the events were grouped into a smaller number of standardized categories using a modified COSTART dictionary and event frequencies were calculated across all studies. These categories are used in the listing below. The frequencies represent the proportion of 900 patients from these trials who experienced that event while receiving ARICEPT®. All adverse events occurring at least twice are included, except for those already listed in Tables 2 or 3, COSTART terms too general to be informative, or events less likely to be drug caused. Events are classified by body system and listed using the following definitions: *frequent adverse events*—those occurring in at least 1/100 patients; *infrequent adverse events*—those occurring in 1/100 to 1/1000 patients. These adverse events are not necessarily related to ARICEPT® treatment and in most cases were observed at a similar frequency in placebo-treated patients in the controlled studies. No important additional adverse events were seen in studies conducted outside the United States.

Body as a Whole: *Frequent:* influenza, chest pain, toothache; *Infrequent:* fever, edema face, periorbital edema, hernia hiatal, abscess, cellulitis, chills, generalized coldness, head fullness, listlessness.

Cardiovascular System: *Frequent:* hypertension, vasodilation, atrial fibrillation, hot flashes, hypotension; *Infrequent:* angina pectoris, postural hypotension, myocardial infarction, AV block (first degree), congestive heart failure, arteritis, bradycardia, peripheral vascular disease, supraventricular tachycardia, deep vein thrombosis.

Digestive System: *Frequent:* fecal incontinence, gastrointestinal bleeding, bloating, epigastric pain; *Infrequent:* eructation, gingivitis, increased appetite, flatulence, periodontal abscess, cholelithiasis, diverticulitis, drooling, dry mouth, fever sore, gastritis, irritable colon, tongue edema, epigastric distress, gastroenteritis, increased transaminases, hemorrhoids, ileus, increased thirst, jaundice, melena, polydypsia, duodenal ulcer, stomach ulcer.

Endocrine System: *Infrequent:* diabetes mellitus, goiter.

Hemic and Lymphatic System: *Infrequent:* anemia, thrombocythemia, thrombocytopenia, eosinophilia, erythrocytopenia.

Metabolic and Nutritional Disorders: *Frequent:* dehydration; *Infrequent:* gout, hypokalemia, increased creatine kinase, hyperglycemia, weight increase, increased lactate dehydrogenase.

Musculoskeletal System: *Frequent:* bone fracture; *Infrequent:* muscle weakness, muscle fasciculation.

Nervous System: *Frequent:* delusions, tremor, irritability, paresthesia, aggression, vertigo, ataxia, increased libido, restlessness, abnormal crying, nervousness, aphasia; *Infrequent:* cerebrovascular accident, intracranial hemorrhage, transient ischemic attack, emotional lability, neuralgia, coldness (localized), muscle spasm, dysphoria, gait abnormality, hypertonia, hypokinesia, neurodermatitis, numbness (localized), paranoia, dysarthria, dysphasia, hostility, decreased libido, melancholia, emotional withdrawal, nystagmus, pacing.

Respiratory System: *Frequent:* dyspnea, sore throat, bronchitis; *Infrequent:* epistaxis, post nasal drip, pneumonia, hyperventilation, pulmonary congestion, wheezing, hypoxia, pharyngitis, pleurisy, pulmonary collapse, sleep apnea, snoring.

Skin and Appendages: *Frequent:* pruritus, diaphoresis, urticaria; *Infrequent:* dermatitis, erythema, skin discoloration, hyperkeratosis, alopecia, fungal dermatitis, herpes zoster, hirsutism, skin striae, night sweats, skin ulcer.

Special Senses: *Frequent:* cataract, eye irritation, vision blurred; *Infrequent:* dry eyes, glaucoma, earache, tinnitus, blepharitis, decreased hearing, retinal hemorrhage, otitis externa, otitis media, bad taste, conjunctival hemorrhage, ear buzzing, motion sickness, spots before eyes.

Urogenital System: *Frequent:* urinary incontinence, nocturia; *Infrequent:* dysuria, hematuria, urinary urgency, metrorrhagia, cystitis, enuresis, prostate hypertrophy, pyelonephritis, inability to empty bladder, breast fibroadenosis, fibrocystic breast, mastitis, pyuria, renal failure, vaginitis.

Postintroduction Reports

Voluntary reports of adverse events temporally associated with ARICEPT® that have been received since market introduction that are not listed above, and that there is inadequate data to determine the causal relationship with the drug include the following: abdominal pain, agitation, cholecystitis, confusion, convulsions, hallucinations, hemolytic anemia, pancreatitis, and rash.

OVERDOSAGE

Because strategies for the management of overdose are continually evolving, it is advisable to contact a Poison Control Center to determine the latest recommendations for the management of an overdose of any drug.

As in any case of overdose, general supportive measures should be utilized. Overdosage with cholinesterase inhibitors can result in cholinergic crisis characterized by severe nausea, vomiting, salivation, sweating, bradycardia, hypotension, respiratory depression, collapse and convulsions. Increasing muscle weakness is a possibility and may result in death if respiratory muscles are involved. Tertiary anticholinergics such as atropine may be used as an antidote for ARICEPT® overdosage. Intravenous atropine sulfate titrated to effect is recommended: an initial dose of 1.0 to 2.0 mg IV with subsequent doses based upon clinical response. Atypical responses in blood pressure and heart rate have been reported with other cholinomimetics when co-administered with quaternary anticholinergics such as glycopyrrolate. It is not known whether ARICEPT® and/or its metabolites can be removed by dialysis (hemodialysis, peritoneal dialysis, or hemofiltration).

Dose-related signs of toxicity in animals included reduced spontaneous movement, prone position, staggering gait, lacrimation, clonic convulsions, depressed respiration, salivation, miosis, tremors, fasciculation and lower body surface temperature.

DOSAGE AND ADMINISTRATION

The dosages of ARICEPT® shown to be effective in controlled clinical trials are 5 mg and 10 mg administered once per day.

The higher dose of 10 mg did not provide a statistically significantly greater clinical benefit than 5 mg. There is a suggestion, however, based upon order of group mean scores and dose trend analyses of data from these clinical trials, that a daily dose of 10 mg of ARICEPT® might provide additional benefit for some patients. Accordingly, whether or not to employ a dose of 10 mg is a matter of prescriber and patient preference.

Evidence from the controlled trials indicates that the 10 mg dose, with a one week titration, is likely to be associated with a higher incidence of cholinergic adverse events than the 5 mg dose. In open label trials using a 6 week titration, the frequency of these same adverse events was similar between the 5 mg and 10 mg dose groups. Therefore, because steady state is not achieved for 15 days and because the incidence of untoward effects may be influenced by the rate of dose escalation, treatment with a dose of 10 mg should not be contemplated until patients have been on a daily dose of 5 mg for 4 to 6 weeks.

ARICEPT® should be taken in the evening, just prior to retiring. ARICEPT® can be taken with or without food.

HOW SUPPLIED

ARICEPT® is supplied as film-coated, round tablets containing either 5 mg or 10 mg of donepezil hydrochloride.

The 5 mg tablets are white. The strength, in mg (5), is debossed on one side and the medication code number (E 245) is debossed on the other side.

The 10 mg tablets are yellow and have the strength debossed on one side (10) and the medication code (E 246) on the other side.

5 mg (White) Bottles of 30 (NDC# 62856-245-30)
              Unit Dose Blister Package 100 (10×10)
              (NDC# 62856-245-41)
10 mg (Yellow) Bottles of 30 (NDC# 62856-246-30)
              Unit Dose Blister Package 100 (10×10)
              (NDC# 62856-246-41)

Storage: Store at controlled room temperature, 15°C to 30°C (59°F to 86°F).

Table 3. Adverse Events Reported in Controlled Clinical Trials in at Least 2% of Patients Receiving ARICEPT® and at a Higher Frequency than Placebo-treated Patients

Body System/Adverse Event	Placebo (n=355)	ARICEPT® (n=747)
Percent of Patients with any Adverse Event	72	74
Body as a Whole		
Headache	9	10
Pain, various locations	8	9
Accident	6	7
Fatigue	3	5
Cardiovascular System		
Syncope	1	2
Digestive System		
Nausea	6	11
Diarrhea	5	10
Vomiting	3	5
Anorexia	2	4
Hemic and Lymphatic System		
Ecchymosis	3	4
Metabolic and Nutritional Systems		
Weight Decrease	1	3
Musculoskeletal System		
Muscle Cramps	2	6
Arthritis	1	2
Nervous System		
Insomnia	6	9
Dizziness	6	8
Depression	<1	3
Abnormal Dreams	0	3
Somnolence	<1	2
Urogenital System		
Frequent Urination	1	2

ARICEPT® is a registered trademark of Eisai Co., Ltd., Tokyo, Japan
Marketed by Eisai Inc., Teaneck, NJ 07666
Manufactured and Distributed/Marketed by
Roerig Division of Pfizer Inc, New York, NY 10017
©1998 Eisai Inc.
69-5210-00-3   Revised April, 1998
Shown in Product Identification Guide, page 309

Available to physicians through Eisai Medical Sales Specialists, free of charge. All are available in spanish also.

Understanding Alzheimers Disease Brochure
Managing Alzheimers Disease Brochure
(both are disease specific brochures)

Know your Medicine Brochure
(for patients on Aricept)

12 week patient diary
(also for patients on Aricept)

Elkins-Sinn, Inc.
2 ESTERBROOK LANE
CHERRY HILL, NJ 08003-4099

Direct Inquiries to:
Professional Service
(610) 688-4400

For Emergency Medical Information Contact:
Day: (800) 934–5556 8:30 AM to 4:30 PM
       (Eastern Standard Time), Weekdays only
Night: (610) 688-4400 (Emergencies only; non-emergencies should wait until the next day)

For Medical/Pharmacy Inquiries on Marketed Products Call:
(800) 934-5556 8:30 AM to 4:30 PM
(Eastern Standard Time), Weekdays only

Elkins-Sinn's DOSETTE® line offers a broad spectrum of injectable products in a variety of unit-of-use containers—DOSETTE® vials, DOSETTE® ampuls, DOSETTE® syringes, and DOSETTE® cartridge-needle units. Easily adaptable to any hospital pharmacy set-up, the DOSETTE® system combines easily identifiable, clearly printed product labeling with space-conserving packaging. Each DOSETTE® container is characterized by product name and strength in large, bold-faced type, important usage and storage data, lot identification number, and expiration date. Elkins-Sinn also produces a vast number of multiple dose vials. Listed below are the major ESI products. For prescribing information on products listed, write to Professional Service, Wyeth-Ayerst Laboratories, P.O. Box 8299, Philadelphia, PA 19101, or contact your local Wyeth-Ayerst representative.

AMIKACIN SULFATE INJECTION, USP
250 mg/mL	2 mL Dosette Vial
250 mg/mL	4 mL Vial

AMINOCAPROIC ACID INJECTION, USP
250 mg/mL	20 mL Multiple Dose Vial

ATROPINE SULFATE INJECTION, USP
400 mcg/mL	1 mL Dosette Vial
(0.4 mg, 1/150 gr)	
400 mcg/mL	1 mL Dosette Ampul
(0.4 mg, 1/150 gr)	
400 mcg/mL	20 mL Multiple Dose Vial
(0.4 mg, 1/150 gr)	
1 mg (1/60 gr)	1 mL Dosette Vial

CHLORPROMAZINE HYDROCHLORIDE INJECTION, USP
25 mg/mL	1 mL Dosette Ampul
50 mg/2 mL	2 mL Dosette Ampul

CYANOCOBALAMIN INJECTION, USP
1 mg/mL (1000 mcg)	1 mL Dosette Vial
1 mg/mL (1000 mcg)	10 mL Multiple Dose Vial
1 mg/mL (1000 mcg)	30 mL Multiple Dose Vial

DEXAMETHASONE SODIUM PHOSPHATE INJECTION, USP
4 mg/mL	1 mL Dosette Vial
4 mg/mL	5 mL Multiple Dose Vial
10 mg/mL	1 mL Dosette Vial
10 mg/mL	10 mL Multiple Dose Vial

DIAZEPAM INJECTION, USP Ⓘⓥ
5 mg/mL	1 mL Dosette Vial
5 mg/mL	10 mL Multiple Dose Vial
5 mg/mL	1 mL Dosette Syringe
10 mg/2 mL	2 mL Dosette Ampul
10 mg/2 mL	2 mL Dosette Ampul
10 mg/2 mL	2 mL Dosette Syringe

Continued on next page

Product Info. - Elkins-Sinn—Cont.

DIAZEPAM INJECTION, USP (CIV)
DOSETTE CARTRIDGE NEEDLE UNITS
5 mg/mL — 1 mL Dosette Cartridge
10 mg/2 mL — 2 mL Dosette Cartridge

DIGOXIN INJECTION, USP
500 mcg/2 mL (0.5 mg) — 2 mL Dosette Ampul

DIPHENHYDRAMINE HYDROCHLORIDE INJECTION, USP
50 mg/mL — 1 mL Dosette Vial

DOPAMINE HYDROCHLORIDE INJECTION, USP
200 mg/5 mL — 5 mL Dosette Ampul
200 mg/5 mL — 5 mL Single Use Vial
400 mg/5 mL — 5 mL Dosette Ampul
400 mg/5 mL — 5 mL Single Use Vial

DURAMORPH® (Morphine Sulfate Injection, USP) (CII) (Preservative-Free for Epidural & Intrathecal Administration)
5 mg/10 mL (0.5 mg/mL) — 10 mL Dosette Ampul
10 mg/10 mL (1 mg/mL) — 10 mL Dosette Ampul

EPINEPHRINE INJECTION, USP
1 mg/mL (1:1000) — 1 mL Dosette Ampul

FENTANYL CITRATE INJECTION, USP (Preservative-Free) (CII)
100 mcg/2 mL (0.05 mg/mL) — 2 mL Dosette Ampul
250 mcg/5 mL (0.05 mg/mL) — 5 mL Dosette Ampul
500 mcg/10 mL (0.05 mg/mL) — 10 mL Dosette Ampul
1000 mcg/20 mL (0.05 mg/mL) — 20 mL Dosette Ampul
1500 mcg/30 mL — Single Dose Vial
2500 mcg/50 mL — Single Dose Vial

FUROSEMIDE INJECTION, USP (Preservative-Free)
20 mg/2 mL — 2 mL Dosette Ampul
40 mg/4 mL — 4 mL Dosette Ampul
40 mg/4 mL — 4 mL Single Use Vial
100 mg/10 mL — 10 mL Single Use Vial

GENTAMICIN SULFATE INJECTION, USP
20 mg/2 mL (10 mg/mL—Pediatric) — 2 mL Dosette Vial
80 mg/2 mL (40 mg/mL) — 2 mL Dosette Vial
800 mg/20 mL (40 mg/mL) — 20 mL Multiple Dose Vial

GENTAMICIN SULFATE INJECTION, USP
DOSETTE CARTRIDGE NEEDLE UNITS
60 mg/1.5 mL — 1.5 mL Dosette Cartridge
80 mg/2 mL — 2 mL Dosette Cartridge

HEPARIN SODIUM INJECTION, USP (Porcine Derived)
1,000 Units/mL — 1 mL Dosette Vial
5,000 Units/mL — 1 mL Dosette Vial
5,000 Units/mL — 10 mL Multiple Dose Vial
10,000 Units/mL — 1 mL Dosette Vial

HEPARIN SODIUM INJECTION, USP (Porcine Derived)
DOSETTE CARTRIDGE NEEDLE UNITS
5,000 Units/0.5 mL — 0.5 mL Dosette Cartridge
5,000 Units/1 mL — 1 mL Dosette Cartridge
10,000 Units/1 mL — 1 mL Dosette Cartridge

HEP-LOCK® (Heparin Lock Flush Solution, USP)
10 Units/mL — 1 mL Dosette Vial
10 Units/mL — 2 mL Dosette Vial
10 Units/mL — 10 mL Multiple Dose Vial
10 Units/mL — 30 mL Multiple Dose Vial
100 Units/mL — 1 mL Dosette Vial
100 Units/mL — 2 mL Dosette Vial
100 Units/mL — 10 mL Multiple Dose Vial
100 Units/mL — 30 mL Multiple Dose Vial

HEP-LOCK® (Heparin Lock Flush Solution, USP)
DOSETTE CARTRIDGE NEEDLE UNITS
10 Units/1 mL — 1 mL Dosette Cartridge
25 Units/2.5 mL — 2.5 mL Dosette Cartridge
100 Units/1 mL — 1 mL Dosette Cartridge
250 Units/2.5 mL — 2.5 mL Dosette Cartridge

HEP-LOCK® (Preservative-Free Heparin Lock Flush Solution, USP)
10 Units/mL — 1 mL Dosette Vial
100 Units/mL — 1 mL Dosette Vial

HYDROMORPHONE HYDROCHLORIDE INJECTION, USP (CII)
2 mg/mL — 1 mL Dosette Vial
2 mg/mL — 20 mL Multiple Dose Vial

HYDROXYZINE HYDROCHLORIDE I.M. INJECTION, USP
25 mg/mL — 1 mL Dosette Vial
50 mg/mL — 1 mL Dosette Vial
100 mg/2 mL — 2 mL Dosette Vial
50 mg/mL — 10 mL Multiple Dose Vial

INFUMORPH® 200
(Preservative-free Morphine Sulfate Sterile Solution) (CII)
For Use in Continuous Microinfusion Devices
200 mg/20 mL (10 mg/mL) — 20 mL Dosette Ampul

INFUMORPH® 500
(Preservative-free Morphine Sulfate Sterile Solution) (CII)
For Use in Continuous Microinfusion Devices
500 mg/20 mL (25 mg/mL) — 20 mL Dosette Ampul

ISOPROTERENOL HYDROCHLORIDE INJECTION, USP (Refrigeration not required)
0.2 mg/mL (1:5000) — 5 mL Dosette Ampul

LEUCOVORIN CALCIUM FOR INJECTION (Lyophilized)
50 mg — Single Use Vial
100 mg — Single Use Vial

LIDOCAINE HYDROCHLORIDE INJECTION, USP (Preserved)
1% (10 mg/mL) — 30 mL Multiple Dose Vial
1% (10 mg/mL) — 50 mL Multiple Dose Vial
2% (20 mg/mL) — 30 mL Multiple Dose Vial
2% (20 mg/mL) — 50 mL Multiple Dose Vial

LIDOCAINE HYDROCHLORIDE INJECTION, USP (Preservative-Free, Single Use)
1% (10 mg/mL) — 5 mL Single Use Vial
2% (20 mg/mL) — 5 mL Single Use Vial

LIDOCAINE HYDROCHLORIDE AND EPINEPHRINE INJECTION, USP (1:100,000) (Refrigeration not required)
1% (10 mg/mL) — 30 mL Multiple Dose Vial
2% (20 mg/mL) — 30 mL Multiple Dose Vial

MEPERIDINE HYDROCHLORIDE INJECTION, USP (CII)
25 mg/mL — 1 mL Dosette Vial
25 mg/mL — 1 mL Dosette Ampul
50 mg/mL — 1 mL Dosette Vial
50 mg/mL — 1 mL Dosette Ampul
75 mg/mL — 1 mL Dosette Vial
75 mg/mL — 1 mL Dosette Ampul
100 mg/mL — 1 mL Dosette Vial
100 mg/mL — 1 mL Dosette Ampul

MORPHINE SULFATE INJECTION, USP (CII)
1 mg/mL — 60 mL Single Use Vial
5 mg/mL (1/12 gr) — 1 mL Dosette Vial
8 mg/mL (1/8 gr) — 1 mL Dosette Vial
8 mg/mL (1/8 gr) — 1 mL Dosette Ampul
10 mg/mL (1/6 gr) — 1 mL Dosette Vial
10 mg/mL (1/6 gr) — 1 mL Dosette Ampul
10 mg/mL (1/6 gr) — 10 mL Multiple Dose Vial
15 mg/mL (1/4 gr) — 1 mL Dosette Vial
15 mg/mL (1/4 gr) — 1 mL Dosette Ampul
15 mg/mL (1/4 gr) — 20 mL Multiple Dose Vial

NALOXONE HYDROCHLORIDE INJECTION, USP
400 mcg/mL (0.4 mg/mL) — 1 mL Dosette Vial
400 mcg/mL (0.4 mg/mL) — 1 mL Dosette Ampul
400 mcg/mL (0.4 mg/mL) — 10 mL Multiple Dose Vial

NEOSTIGMINE METHYLSULFATE INJECTION, USP
1:1000 (1 mg/mL) — 10 mL Multiple Dose Vial
1:2000 (0.5 mg/mL) — 10 mL Multiple Dose Vial

PANCURONIUM BROMIDE INJECTION
1 mg/mL — 10 mL Multiple Dose Vial
2 mg/mL — 2 mL Dosette Vial
2 mg/mL — 2 mL Dosette Ampul
2 mg/mL — 5 mL Dosette Ampul
2 mg/mL — 5 mL Single Use Vial

PHENOBARBITAL SODIUM INJECTION, USP (CIV)
65 mg/mL (1 gr) — 1 mL Dosette Vial
130 mg/mL (2 gr) — 1 mL Dosette Vial

PHENYLEPHRINE HYDROCHLORIDE INJECTION, USP
10 mg/mL — 1 mL Dosette Vial

PHENYTOIN SODIUM INJECTION, USP
100 mg/2 mL (50 mg/mL) — 2 mL Dosette Vial
100 mg/2 mL (50 mg/mL) — 2 mL Dosette Ampul
250 mg/5 mL (50 mg/mL) — 5 mL Single Use Vial

PROCAINAMIDE HYDROCHLORIDE INJECTION, USP
100 mg/mL (1 gram/10 mL) — 10 mL Multiple Dose Vial
500 mg/mL (1 gram/2 mL) — 2 mL Multiple Dose Vial

PROCHLORPERAZINE EDISYLATE INJECTION, USP
10 mg/2 mL — 2 mL Dosette Vial

PROMETHAZINE HYDROCHLORIDE INJECTION, USP
25 mg/mL — 1 mL Dosette Ampul
50 mg/mL — 1 mL Dosette Ampul

PROTAMINE SULFATE INJECTION, USP (Preservative-Free) (Refrigeration not required)
50 mg/5 mL — 5 mL Dosette Ampul
250 mg/25 mL — 25 mL Single Use Vial

SODIUM CHLORIDE INJECTION, USP (Preservative-Free, Single Use)
0.9% — 2 mL Dosette Vial
0.9% — 5 mL Dosette Ampul
0.9% — 10 mL Dosette Ampul

SODIUM CHLORIDE INJECTION, BACTERIOSTATIC, USP (Preserved with 0.9% Benzyl Alcohol)
0.9% — 30 mL Multiple Dose Vial
0.9% — 2 mL Dosette Cartridge

SOTRADECOL® (Sodium Tetradecyl Sulfate Injection)
1% — 2 mL Dosette Ampul
3% — 2 mL Dosette Ampul

SUFENTANIL CITRATE INJECTION, USP
500 mcg/mL — 1 mL Dosette Ampul
100 mcg/2 mL — 2 mL Dosette Ampul
250 mcg/5 mL — 5 mL Dosette Ampul

SULFAMETHOXAZOLE & TRIMETHOPRIM CONCENTRATE FOR INJECTION, USP
80 mg/mL Sulfamethoxazole with 16 mg/mL Trimethoprim — 5 mL Dosette Ampul
80 mg/mL Sulfamethoxazole with 16 mg/mL Trimethoprim — 5 mL Single Use Vial
80 mg/mL Sulfamethoxazole with 16 mg/mL Trimethoprim — 10 mL Single Use Vial
80 mg/mL Sulfamethoxazole with 16 mg/mL Trimethoprim — 30 mL Multiple Dose Vial

THIAMINE HYDROCHLORIDE INJECTION, USP
100 mg/mL — 1 mL Dosette Vial

WATER FOR INJECTION, BACTERIOSTATIC, USP (Preserved with 0.9% Benzyl Alcohol)
30 mL Multiple Dose Vial

AMIKACIN ℞
[ă 'mĭ-că-sĭn]
SULFATE INJECTION, USP

WARNINGS

Patients treated with parenteral aminoglycosides should be under close clinical observation because of the potential ototoxicity and nephrotoxicity associated with their use. Safety for treatment periods which are longer than 14 days has not been established.

Neurotoxicity, manifested as vestibular and permanent bilateral auditory ototoxicity, can occur in patients with preexisting renal damage and in patients with normal renal function treated at higher doses and/or for periods longer than those recommended. The risk of aminoglycoside-induced ototoxicity is greater in patients with renal damage. High frequency deafness usually occurs first and can be detected only by audiometric testing. Vertigo may occur and may be evidence of vestibular injury. Other manifestations of neurotoxicity may include numbness, skin tingling, muscle twitching and convulsions. The risk of hearing loss due to aminoglycosides increases with the degree of exposure to either high peak or high trough serum concentrations. Patients developing cochlear damage may not have symptoms during therapy to warn them of developing eighth-nerve toxicity, and total or partial irreversible bilateral deafness may occur after the drug has been discontinued. Aminoglycoside-induced ototoxicity is usually irreversible.

Aminoglycosides are potentially nephrotoxic. The risk of nephrotoxicity is greater in patients with impaired renal function and in those who receive high doses or prolonged therapy.

Neuromuscular blockade and respiratory paralysis have been reported following parenteral injection, topical instillation (as in orthopedic and abdominal irrigation or in local treatment of empyema) and following oral use of aminoglycosides. The possibility of these phenomena should be considered if aminoglycosides are administered by any route, especially in patients receiving anesthetics; neuromuscular blocking agents such as tubocurarine, succinylcholine, decamethonium; or in patients receiving massive transfusions of citrate-anticoagulated blood. If blockage occurs, calcium salts may reverse these phenomena, but mechanical respiratory assistance may be necessary.

Renal and eighth-nerve function should be closely monitored especially in patients with known or suspected renal impairment at the onset of therapy and also in those whose renal function is initially normal but who develop signs of renal dysfunction during therapy. Serum concentrations of amikacin should be monitored when feasible to assure adequate levels and to avoid potentially toxic levels and prolonged peak concentrations above 35 micrograms per mL. Urine should be examined for decreased specific gravity, increased excretion of proteins and the presence of cells or casts. Blood urea nitrogen, serum creatinine or creatinine clearance should be measured periodically. Serial audiograms should be obtained where feasible in patients old enough to be tested, particularly high risk patients. Evidence of ototoxicity (dizziness, vertigo, tinnitus, roaring in the ears and hearing loss) or nephrotoxicity requires discontinuation of the drug or dosage adjustment.

Concurrent and/or sequential systemic, oral or topical use of other neurotoxic or nephrotoxic products, particularly bacitracin, cisplatin, amphotericin B, cephaloridine, paromomycin, viomycin, polymyxin B, colistin, vancomycin or other aminoglycosides should be avoided. Other factors that may increase risk of toxicity are advanced age and dehydration.

The concurrent use of amikacin with potent diuretics (ethacrynic acid or furosemide) should be avoided since diuretics by themselves may cause ototoxicity. In addi-

tion, when administered intravenously, diuretics may enhance aminoglycoside toxicity by altering antibiotic concentrations in serum and tissue.

DESCRIPTION

Amikacin sulfate, a semi-synthetic aminoglycoside antibiotic derived from kanamycin, has the following structural formula:

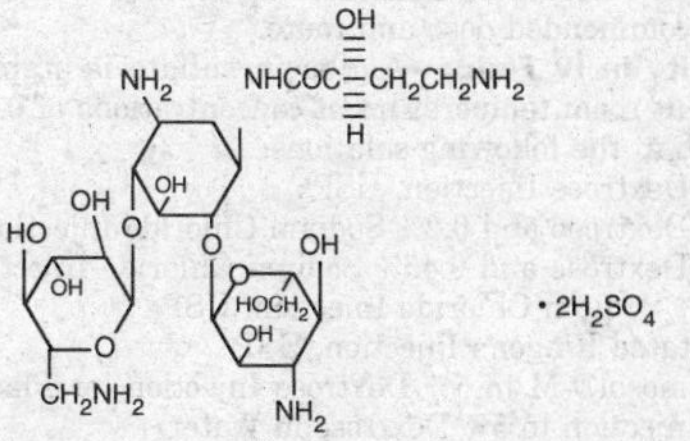

D-Streptamine, *O*-3-amino-3-deoxy-α-D-glucopyranosyl-(1→6)-*O* - [6-amino-6-deoxy-α-D-glucopyranosyl-(1→4)] - N^1-(4-amino-2-hydroxy-1-oxobutyl)-2-deoxy-, (*S*)-, sulfate (1:2) (salt)

$C_{22}H_{43}N_5O_{13} \cdot 2H_2SO_4$ Molecular weight 781.75

The dosage form is supplied as a sterile, colorless to light straw-colored solution for IM or IV use.

Each mL contains 250 mg amikacin as the sulfate, sodium citrate (dihydrate) 28.5 mg and sodium metabisulfite 6.6 mg in Water for Injection. pH 3.5–5.5; sodium hydroxide and/or sulfuric acid added, if needed, for pH adjustment. Sealed under nitrogen.

CLINICAL PHARMACOLOGY

INTRAMUSCULAR ADMINISTRATION

Amikacin is rapidly absorbed after intramuscular administration. In normal adult volunteers, average peak serum concentrations of about 12, 16 and 21 mcg/mL are obtained 1 hour after intramuscular administration of 250 mg (3.7 mg/kg), 375 mg (5 mg/kg), 500 mg (7.5 mg/kg), single doses, respectively. At 10 hours, serum levels are about 0.3 mcg/mL, 1.2 mcg/mL and 2.1 mcg/mL, respectively.

Tolerance studies in normal volunteers reveal that amikacin is well tolerated locally following repeated intramuscular dosing, and when given at maximally recommended doses, no ototoxicity or nephrotoxicity has been reported. There is no evidence of drug accumulation with repeated dosing for 10 days when administered according to recommended doses.

With normal renal function, about 91.9% of an intramuscular dose is excreted unchanged in the urine in the first 8 hours and 98.2% within 24 hours. Mean urine concentrations for 6 hours are 563 mcg/mL following a 250 mg dose, 697 mcg/mL following a 375 mg dose and 832 mcg/mL following a 500 mg dose.

Preliminary intramuscular studies in newborns of different weights (less than 1.5 kg, 1.5 to 2 kg, over 2 kg) at a dose of 7.5 mg/kg revealed that, like other aminoglycosides, serum half-life values were correlated inversely with post-natal age and renal clearances of amikacin. The volume of distribution indicates that amikacin, like other aminoglycosides, remains primarily in the extracellular fluid space of neonates. Repeated dosing every 12 hours in all the above groups did not demonstrate accumulation after 5 days.

INTRAVENOUS ADMINISTRATION

Single doses of 500 mg (7.5 mg/kg) administered to normal adults as an infusion over a period of 30 minutes produced a mean peak serum concentration of 38 mcg/mL at the end of the infusion and levels of 24 mcg/mL, 18 mcg/mL and 0.75 mcg/mL at 30 minutes, 1 hour and 10 hours post-infusion, respectively. Eighty-four percent of the administered dose was excreted in the urine in 9 hours and about 94% within 24 hours.

Repeat infusions of 7.5 mg/kg every 12 hours in normal adults were well tolerated and caused no drug accumulation.

GENERAL

Pharmacokinetic studies in normal adult subjects reveal the mean serum half-life to be slightly over 2 hours with a mean total apparent volume of distribution of 24 liters (28% of the body weight). By the ultrafiltration technique, reports of serum protein binding range from 0 to 11%. The mean serum clearance rate is about 100 mL/min and the renal clearance rate is 94 mL/min in subjects with normal renal function.

Amikacin is excreted primarily by glomerular filtration. Patients with impaired renal function or diminished glomerular filtration pressure excrete the drug much more slowly (effectively prolonging the serum half-life). Therefore, renal function should be monitored carefully and dosage adjusted accordingly (see suggested dosage schedule under **DOSAGE AND ADMINISTRATION).**

Following administration at the recommended dose, therapeutic levels are found in bone, heart, gallbladder and lung tissue in addition to significant concentrations in urine; bile; sputum; bronchial secretions; interstitial, pleural and synovial fluids.

Spinal fluid levels in normal infants are approximately 10 to 20% of the serum concentrations and may reach 50% when the meninges are inflamed. Amikacin has been demonstrated to cross the placental barrier and yield significant concentrations in amniotic fluid. The peak fetal serum concentration is about 16% of the peak maternal serum concentration and maternal and fetal serum half-life values are about 2 and 3.7 hours, respectively.

MICROBIOLOGY

Gram-negative—Amikacin is active *in vitro* against *Pseudomonas* species, *Escherichia coli, Proteus* species (indole-positive and indole-negative), *Providencia* species, *Klebsiella-Enterobacter-Serratia* species, *Acinetobacter* (formerly *Mima-Herellea*) species and *Citrobacter freundii*.

When strains of the above organisms are found to be resistant to other aminoglycosides, including gentamicin, tobramycin and kanamycin, many are susceptible to amikacin *in vitro*.

Gram-positive—Amikacin is active *in vitro* against penicillinase and non-penicillinase-producing *Staphylococcus* species, including methicillin-resistant strains. However, aminoglycosides in general have a low order of activity against other gram-positive organisms, viz., *Streptococcus pyogenes*, enterococci and *Streptococcus pneumoniae* (formerly *Diplococcus pneumoniae).*

Amikacin resists degradation by most aminoglycoside inactivating enzymes known to affect gentamicin, tobramycin and kanamycin.

In vitro studies have shown that amikacin sulfate combined with a beta-lactam antibiotic acts synergistically against many clinically significant gram-negative organisms.

Disc Susceptibility Tests—Quantitative methods that require measurement of zone diameters give the most precise estimates of antibiotic susceptibility. One such procedure* has been recommended for use with discs to test susceptibility to amikacin. Interpretation involves correlation of the diameters obtained in the disc test with MIC values for amikacin. When the causative organism is tested by the Kirby-Bauer method of disc susceptibility, a 30 mcg amikacin disc should give a zone of 17 mm or greater to indicate susceptibility. Zone sizes of 14 mm or less indicate resistance. Zone sizes of 15 to 16 mm indicate intermediate susceptibility. With this procedure, a report from the laboratory of "susceptible" indicates that the infecting organism is likely to respond to therapy. A report of "resistant" indicates that the infecting organism is not likely to respond to therapy. A report of "intermediate susceptibility" suggests that the organism would be susceptible if the infection is confined to tissues and fluids (e.g., urine) in which high antibiotic levels are attained.

INDICATIONS AND USAGE

Amikacin Sulfate Injection is indicated in the short-term treatment of serious infections due to susceptible strains of gram-negative bacteria, including *Pseudomonas* species, *Escherichia coli,* species of indole-positive and indole-negative *Proteus, Providencia* species, *Klebsiella-Enterobacter-Serratia* species and *Acinetobacter (Mima-Herellea)* species.

Clinical studies have shown Amikacin Sulfate Injection to be effective in bacterial septicemia (including neonatal sepsis); in serious infections of the respiratory tract, bones and joints, central nervous system (including meningitis) and skin and soft tissue; intra-abdominal infections (including peritonitis); and in burns and post-operative infections (including post-vascular surgery). Clinical studies have shown amikacin also to be effective in serious complicated and recurrent urinary tract infections due to these organisms. Aminoglycosides, including amikacin, are not indicated in uncomplicated initial episodes of urinary tract infections unless the causative organisms are not susceptible to antibiotics having less potential toxicity.

Bacteriologic studies should be performed to identify causative organisms and their susceptibilities to amikacin. Amikacin may be considered as initial therapy in suspected gram-negative infections, and therapy may be instituted before obtaining the results of susceptibility testing. Clinical trials demonstrated that amikacin was effective in infections caused by gentamicin- and/or tobramycin-resistant strains of gram-negative organisms, particularly *Proteus rettgeri, Providencia stuartii, Serratia marcescens* and *Pseudomonas aeruginosa.* The decision to continue therapy with the drug should be based on results of the susceptibility tests, the severity of the infection and the response of the patient, as well as important additional considerations (see **WARNINGS** box).

Amikacin has also been shown to be effective in staphylococcal infections and may be considered as initial therapy under certain conditions in the treatment of known or suspected staphylococcal disease such as severe infections where the causative organism may be either a gram-negative bacterium or a staphylococcus, infections due to susceptible strains of staphylococci in patients allergic to other antibiotics and in mixed staphylococcal/gram-negative infections.

In certain severe infections such as neonatal sepsis, concomitant therapy with a penicillin-type drug may be indicated because of the possibility of infections due to gram-positive organisms such as streptococci or pneumococci.

CONTRAINDICATIONS

A history of hypersensitivity to amikacin is a contraindication for its use. A history of hypersensitivity or serious toxic reactions to aminoglycosides may contraindicate the use of any other aminoglycoside because of the known cross-sensitivities of patients to drugs in this class.

WARNINGS

See **WARNINGS** box above.

Aminoglycosides can cause fetal harm when administered to a pregnant woman. Aminoglycosides cross the placenta and there have been several reports of total irreversible, bilateral congenital deafness in children whose mothers received streptomycin during pregnancy. Although serious side effects to the fetus or newborns have not been reported in the treatment of pregnant women with other aminoglycosides, the potential for harm exists. Reproduction studies of amikacin have been performed in rats and mice and revealed no evidence of impaired fertility or harm to the fetus due to amikacin. There are no well-controlled studies in pregnant women, but investigational experience does not include any positive evidence of adverse effects to the fetus. If this drug is used during pregnancy, or if the patient becomes pregnant while taking this drug, the patient should be apprised of the potential hazard to the fetus.

Contains sodium metabisulfite, a sulfite that may cause allergic-type reactions including anaphylactic symptoms and life-threatening or less severe asthmatic episodes in certain susceptible people. The overall prevalence of sulfite sensitivity in the general population is unknown and probably low. Sulfite sensitivity is seen more frequently in asthmatic than nonasthmatic people.

PRECAUTIONS

Aminoglycosides are quickly and almost totally absorbed when they are applied topically, except to the urinary bladder, in association with surgical procedures. Irreversible deafness, renal failure and death due to neuromuscular blockade have been reported following irrigation of both small and large surgical fields with an aminoglycoside preparation.

Amikacin Sulfate Injection is potentially nephrotoxic, ototoxic and neurotoxic. The concurrent or serial use of other ototoxic or nephrotoxic agents should be avoided either systemically or topically because of the potential for additive effects. Increased nephrotoxicity has been reported following concomitant parenteral administration of aminoglycoside antibiotics and cephalosporins. Concomitant cephalosporins may spuriously elevate creatinine determinations. Since amikacin is present in high concentrations in the renal excretory system, patients should be well-hydrated to minimize chemical irritation of the renal tubules. Kidney function should be assessed by the usual methods prior to starting therapy and daily during the course of treatment. If signs of renal irritation appear (casts, white or red cells or albumin), hydration should be increased. A reduction in dosage (see **DOSAGE AND ADMINISTRATION**) may be desirable if other evidence of renal dysfunction occurs such as decreased creatinine clearance; decreased urine specific gravity; increased BUN, creatinine or oliguria. If azotemia increases or if a progressive decrease in urinary output occurs, treatment should be stopped.

Note: When patients are well hydrated and kidney function is normal, the risk of nephrotoxic reactions with amikacin is low if the dosage recommendations (see **DOSAGE AND ADMINISTRATION**) are not exceeded.

Elderly patients may have reduced renal function which may not be evident in routine screening tests such as BUN or serum creatinine. A creatinine clearance determination may be more useful. Monitoring of renal function during treatment with aminoglycosides is particularly important.

Aminoglycosides should be used with caution in patients with muscular disorders such as myasthenia gravis or parkinsonism since these drugs may aggravate muscle weakness because of their potential curare-like effect on the neuromuscular junction.

In vitro mixing of aminoglycosides with beta-lactam antibiotics (penicillin or cephalosporins) may result in a significant mutual inactivation. A reduction in serum half-life or serum level may occur when an aminoglycoside or penicillin-type drug is administered by separate routes. Inactivation of the aminoglycoside is clinically significant only in patients with severely impaired renal function. Inactivation may continue in specimens of body fluids collected for assay, resulting in inaccurate aminoglycoside readings. Such specimens should be properly handled (assayed promptly, frozen or treated with beta-lactamase).

Continued on next page

Amikacin—Cont.

Cross-allergenicity among aminoglycosides has been demonstrated.
As with other antibiotics, the use of amikacin may result in overgrowth of non-susceptible organisms. If this occurs, appropriate therapy should be instituted.
Aminoglycosides should not be given concurrently with potent diuretics (see **WARNINGS** box).

CARCINOGENESIS, MUTAGENESIS, IMPAIRMENT OF FERTILITY
Studies in humans have not been performed with the aminoglycosides to determine their effect on carcinogenesis, mutagenesis or impairment of fertility.

PREGNANCY
Pregnancy Category D (see **WARNINGS** section).

NURSING MOTHERS
It is not known whether this drug is excreted in human milk. As a general rule, nursing should not be undertaken while a patient is on a drug since many drugs are excreted in human milk.

PEDIATRIC USE
Aminoglycosides should be used with caution in premature and neonatal infants because of the renal immaturity of these patients and the resulting prolongation of serum half-life of these drugs.

ADVERSE REACTIONS

All aminoglycosides have the potential to induce auditory, vestibular and renal toxicity and neuromuscular blockade (see **WARNINGS** box). They occur more frequently in patients with present or past history of renal impairment, of treatment with other ototoxic or nephrotoxic drugs and in patients treated for longer periods and/or with higher doses than recommended.
Neurotoxicity-Ototoxicity—Toxic effects on the eighth cranial nerve can result in hearing loss, loss of balance or both. Amikacin primarily affects auditory function. Cochlear damage includes high frequency deafness and usually occurs before clinical hearing loss can be detected.
Neurotoxicity-Neuromuscular Blockage—Acute muscular paralysis and apnea can occur following treatment with aminoglycoside drugs.
Nephrotoxicity—Elevation of serum creatinine, albuminuria, presence of red and white cells, casts, azotemia and oliguria have been reported. Renal function changes are usually reversible when the drug is discontinued.
Other—In addition to those described above, other adverse reactions which have been reported on rare occasions are skin rash, drug fever, headache, paresthesia, tremor, nausea and vomiting, eosinophilia, arthralgia, anemia and hypotension.

OVERDOSAGE

In the event of overdosage or toxic reaction, peritoneal dialysis or hemodialysis will aid in the removal of amikacin from the blood. In the newborn infant, exchange transfusion may also be considered.

DOSAGE AND ADMINISTRATION

The patient's pretreatment body weight should be obtained for calculation of correct dosage. Amikacin Sulfate Injection may be given intramuscularly or intravenously.
The status of renal function should be estimated by measurement of the serum creatinine concentration or calculation of the endogenous creatinine clearance rate. The blood urea nitrogen (BUN) is much less reliable for this purpose. Reassessment of renal function should be made periodically during therapy.
Whenever possible, amikacin concentrations in serum should be measured to assure adequate but not excessive levels. It is desirable to measure both peak and trough serum concentrations intermittently during therapy. Peak concentrations (30–90 minutes after injection) above 35 micrograms per mL and trough concentrations (just prior to the next dose) above 10 micrograms per mL should be avoided. Dosage should be adjusted as indicated.

INTRAMUSCULAR ADMINISTRATION FOR PATIENTS WITH NORMAL RENAL FUNCTION
The recommended dosage for adults, children and older infants (see **WARNINGS** box) with normal renal function is 15 mg/kg/day divided into 2 or 3 equal doses administered at equally divided intervals, i.e., 7.5 mg/kg q12h or 5 mg/kg q8h. Treatment of patients in the heavier weight classes should not exceed 1.5 gram/day.
When amikacin is indicated in newborns (see **WARNINGS** box), it is recommended that a loading dose of 10 mg/kg be administered initially to be followed with 7.5 mg/kg every 12 hours.
The usual duration of treatment is 7 to 10 days. It is desirable to limit the duration of treatment to short-term whenever feasible. The total daily dose by all routes of administration should not exceed 15 mg/kg/day. In difficult and complicated infections where treatment beyond 10 days is considered, the use of amikacin should be reevaluated. If continued, amikacin serum levels and renal, auditory and vestibular functions should be monitored. At the recommended dosage level, uncomplicated infections due to amikacin-sensitive organisms should respond in 24 to 48 hours. If definite clinical response does not occur within 3 to 5 days, therapy should be stopped and the antibiotic susceptibility pattern of the invading organism should be rechecked. Failure of the infection to respond may be due to resistance of the organism or to the presence of septic foci requiring surgical drainage.
When amikacin is indicated in uncomplicated urinary tract infections, a dose of 250 mg twice daily may be used.

DOSAGE GUIDELINES
ADULTS AND CHILDREN WITH NORMAL RENAL FUNCTION

Patient Weight		Dosage		
lbs	kg	7.5 mg/kg q12h	OR	5 mg/kg q8h
99	45	337.5 mg		225 mg
110	50	375 mg		250 mg
121	55	412.5 mg		275 mg
132	60	450 mg		300 mg
143	65	487.5 mg		325 mg
154	70	525 mg		350 mg
165	75	562.5 mg		375 mg
176	80	600 mg		400 mg
187	85	637.5 mg		425 mg
198	90	675 mg		450 mg
209	95	712.5 mg		475 mg
220	100	750 mg		500 mg

INTRAMUSCULAR ADMINISTRATION FOR PATIENTS WITH IMPAIRED RENAL FUNCTION
Whenever possible, serum amikacin concentrations should be monitored by appropriate assay procedures. Doses may be adjusted in patients with impaired renal function either by administering normal doses at prolonged intervals or by administering reduced doses at a fixed interval.
Both methods are based on the patient's creatinine clearance or serum creatinine values since these have been found to correlate with aminoglycoside half-lives in patients with diminished renal function. These dosage schedules must be used in conjunction with careful clinical and laboratory observations of the patient and should be modified as necessary. Neither method should be used when dialysis is being performed.
Normal Dosage at Prolonged Intervals—If the creatinine clearance rate is not available and the patient's condition is stable, a dosage interval in hours for the normal dose can be calculated by multiplying the patient's serum creatinine by 9, e.g., if the serum creatinine concentration is 2 mg/100 mL, the recommended single dose (7.5 mg/kg) should be administered every 18 hours.
Reduced Dosage at Fixed Time Intervals—When renal function is impaired and it is desirable to administer amikacin at a fixed time interval, dosage must be reduced. In these patients, serum amikacin concentrations should be measured to assure accurate administration of amikacin and to avoid concentrations above 35 mcg/mL. If serum assay determinations are not available and the patient's condition is stable, serum creatinine and creatinine clearance values are the most readily available indicators of the degree of renal impairment to use as a guide for dosage.
First, initiate therapy by administering a normal dose, 7.5 mg/kg, as a loading dose. This loading dose is the same as the normally recommended dose which would be calculated for a patient with a normal renal function as described above.
To determine the size of maintenance doses administered every 12 hours, the loading dose should be reduced in proportion to the reduction in the patient's creatinine clearance rate:

$$\text{Maintenance Dose Every 12 hours} = \frac{\text{observed CC in mL/min}}{\text{normal CC in mL/min}} \times \text{calculated loading dose in mg}$$

(CC—creatinine clearance rate)
An alternate rough guide for determining reduced dosage at 12-hour intervals (for patients whose steady state serum creatinine values are known) is to divide the normally recommended dose by the patient's serum creatinine.
The above dosage schedules are not intended to be rigid recommendations but are provided as guides to dosage when the measurement of amikacin serum levels is not feasible.

INTRAVENOUS ADMINISTRATION

The individual dose, the total daily dose and the total cumulative dose of amikacin sulfate are identical to the dose recommended for intramuscular administration. The solution for intravenous use is prepared by adding the contents of a 500 mg vial to 100–200 mL of sterile diluent such as Normal Saline or 5% Dextrose in Water or any other compatible solution.
The solution is administered to adults over a 30 to 60 minute period. The total daily dose should not exceed 15 mg/kg/day and may be divided into either 2 or 3 equally divided doses at equally divided intervals.
In pediatric patients, the amount of fluid used will depend on the amount ordered for the patient. It should be a sufficient amount to infuse the amikacin over a 30 to 60 minute period. Infants should receive a 1 to 2 hour infusion.
Amikacin should not be physically premixed with other drugs but should be administered separately according to the recommended dose and route.
Stability in IV Fluids—Amikacin sulfate is stable for 24 hours at room temperature at concentrations of 0.25 and 5 mg/mL in the following solutions:
- 5% Dextrose Injection, USP
- 5% Dextrose and 0.2% Sodium Chloride Injection, USP
- 5% Dextrose and 0.45% Sodium Chloride Injection, USP
- 0.9% Sodium Chloride Injection, USP
- Lactated Ringer's Injection, USP
- Normosol® M in 5% Dextrose Injection (or Plasma-Lyte 56 Injection in 5% Dextrose in Water)
- Normosol® R in 5% Dextrose Injection (or Plasma-Lyte 148 Injection in 5% Dextrose in Water)

Aminoglycosides administered by any of the above routes should not be physically premixed with other drugs but should be administered separately.
Because of the potential toxicity of aminoglycosides, "fixed dosage" recommendations which are not based upon body weight are not advised. Rather, it is essential to calculate the dosage to fit the needs of each patient.
Parenteral drug products should be inspected visually for particulate matter and discoloration prior to administration whenever the solution and container permit.

HOW SUPPLIED

Amikacin Sulfate Injection, USP is available in the following packages:
250 mg/mL
- 2 mL (500 mg) DOSETTE® vials packaged in 10s (*NDC* 0641-0123-23)
- 4 mL (1 gram) vials packaged in 10s (*NDC* 0641-2357-43)

STORAGE
Amikacin Sulfate Injection, USP is supplied as a colorless solution which requires no refrigeration. Store at controlled room temperature 15°–30°C (59°–86°F).
Store solutions for intravenous use as directed in **DOSAGE AND ADMINISTRATION.**
At times, the solution may become a very pale yellow; this does not indicate a decrease in potency.

*Bauer, AW; Kirby, WMM; Sherris, JC and Turck, M: Antibiotic Testing by a Standardized Single Disc Method, AM J CLIN PATHOL, 45:493, 1966; Standardized Disc Susceptibility Test, *FEDERAL REGISTER*, 37:20527-29, 1972.

Manufactured by
ELKINS-SINN, INC.
Cherry Hill, NJ 08003-4099
A subsidiary of A.H. Robins Company

DURAMORPH® Ⓒ II
[*dūr "a 'mŏrf*]
(morphine sulfate injection, USP)
Preservative-Free

Warning: May be habit forming.

DESCRIPTION

Morphine is the most important alkaloid of opium and is a phenanthrene derivative. It is available as the sulfate salt, having the following structural formula:

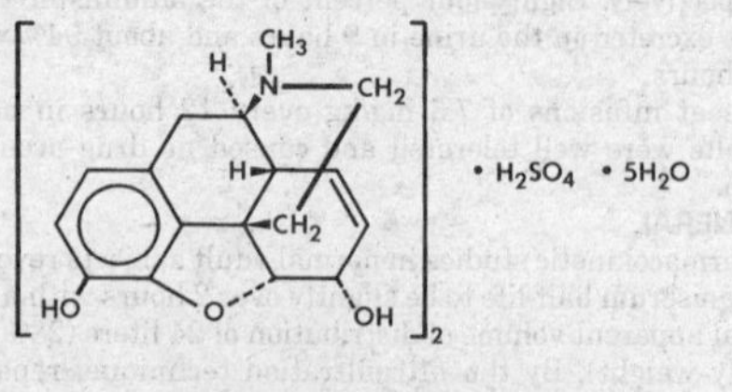

7,8 Didehydro-4,5-epoxy-17-methyl-(5α,6α)-morphinan-3,6-diol sulfate (2:1) (salt), pentahydrate

$(C_{17}H_{19}NO_3)_2 \cdot H_2SO_4 \cdot 5H_2O$ Molecular weight is 758.83

Preservative-free DURAMORPH® (Morphine Sulfate Injection, USP) is a sterile, nonpyrogenic, isobaric solution of morphine sulfate, free of antioxidants, preservatives or other potentially neurotoxic additives and is intended for intravenous, epidural or intrathecal administration as a narcotic analgesic. Each milliliter contains morphine sulfate 0.5 mg or 1 mg and sodium chloride 9 mg in Water for Injection. pH range is 2.5–6.5. Ampuls are sealed under nitro-

gen. Each Dosette® ampul of DURAMORPH® is intended for **SINGLE USE ONLY.** *Discard any unused portion.* DO NOT HEAT-STERILIZE.

CLINICAL PHARMACOLOGY

Morphine produces a wide spectrum of pharmacologic effects including analgesia, dysphoria, euphoria, somnolence, respiratory depression, diminished gastrointestinal motility and physical dependence. Opiate analgesia involves at least three anatomical areas of the central nervous system: the periaqueductal-periventricular gray matter, the ventromedial medulla and the spinal cord. A systemically administered opiate may produce analgesia by acting at any, all or some combination of these distinct regions. Morphine interacts predominantly with the μ-receptor. The μ-binding sites of opioids are very discretely distributed in the human brain, with high densities of sites found in the posterior amygdala, hypothalamus, thalamus, nucleus caudatus, putamen and certain cortical areas. They are also found on the terminal axons of primary afferents within laminae I and II (substantia gelatinosa) of the spinal cord and in the spinal nucleus of the trigeminal nerve.

Morphine has an apparent volume of distribution ranging from 1.0 to 4.7 L/kg after *intravenous* dosage. Protein binding is low, about 36%, and muscle tissue binding is reported as 54%. A blood-brain barrier exists, and when morphine is introduced outside of the CNS (e.g. *intravenously*), plasma concentrations of morphine remain higher than the corresponding CSF morphine levels. Conversely, when morphine is injected into the *intrathecal space*, it diffuses out into the systemic circulation slowly, accounting for the long duration of action of morphine administered by this route. Morphine has a total plasma clearance which ranges from 0.9 to 1.2 L/kg/h (liters/kilogram/hour) in postoperative patients, but shows considerable interindividual variation. The major pathway of clearance is hepatic glucuronidation to morphine-3-glucuronide, which is pharmacologically inactive. The major excretion path of the conjugate is through the kidneys, with about 10% in the feces. Morphine is also eliminated by the kidneys, 2 to 12% being excreted unchanged in the urine. Terminal half-life is commonly reported to vary from 1.5 to 4.5 hours, although the longer half-lives were obtained when morphine levels were monitored over protracted periods with very sensitive radioimmunoassay methods. The accepted elimination half-life in normal subject is 1.5 to 2 hours.

"Selective" blockade of pain sensation is possible by neuraxial application of morphine. In addition, duration of analgesia may be much longer by this route compared to systemic administration. However, CNS effects, associated with systemic administration, are still seen. These include respiratory depression, sedation, nausea and vomiting, pruritus and urinary retention. In particular, both early and late respiratory depression (up to 24 hours post dosing) have been reported following neuraxial administration. Circulation of the spinal fluid may also result in high concentrations of morphine reaching the brain stem directly.

The incidence of unwanted CNS effects, including delayed respiratory depression, associated with neuraxial application of morphine, is related to the circulatory dynamics of the epidural venous plexus and the spinal fluid. The lipid solubility and degree of ionization of morphine plays an important part in both the onset and duration of analgesia and the CNS effects. Morphine has a pK_a 7.9, with an octanol/water partition coefficient of 1.42 at pH 7.4. At this pH, the tertiary amino group in each of the opioids is mostly ionized, making the molecule water soluble. Morphine, with additional hydroxyl groups on the molecule, is significantly more water soluble than any other opioid in clinical use.

Morphine, injected into the *epidural space*, is rapidly absorbed into the general circulation. Absorption is so rapid that the plasma concentration-time profiles closely resemble those obtained after intravenous or intramuscular administration. Peak plasma concentrations averaging 33–40 ng/mL (range 5–62 ng/mL) are achieved within 10 to 15 minutes after administration of 3 mg of morphine. Plasma concentrations decline in a multiexponential fashion. The terminal half-life is reported to range from 39 to 249 minutes (mean of 90±34.3 min) and, though somewhat shorter, is similar in magnitude as values reported after intravenous and intramuscular administration (1.5–4.5 h). CSF concentrations of morphine, after epidural doses of 2 to 6 mg in postoperative patients, have been reported to be 50 to 250 times higher than corresponding plasma concentrations. The CSF levels of morphine exceed those in plasma after only 15 minutes and are detectable for as long as 20 hours after the injection of 2 mg of epidural morphine. Approximately 4% of the dose injected epidurally reaches the CSF. This corresponds to the relative minimum effective epidural and intrathecal doses of 5 mg and 0.25 mg, respectively. The disposition of morphine in the CSF follows a biphasic pattern, with an early half-life of 1.5 h and a late phase half-life of about 6 h. Morphine crosses the dura slowly, with an absorption half-life across the dura averaging 22 minutes. Maximum CSF concentrations are seen 60–90 minutes after injection. Minimum effective CSF concentrations for postoperative analgesia average 150 ng/mL (range <1–380 ng/mL).

The *intrathecal route* of administration circumvents meningeal diffusion barriers and, therefore, lower doses of morphine produce comparable analgesia to that induced by the epidural route. After intrathecal bolus injection of morphine, there is a rapid initial distribution phase lasting 15–30 minutes and a half-life in the CSF of 42–136 min (mean 90±16 min). Derived from limited data, it appears that the disposition of morphine in the CSF, from 15 minutes postintrathecal administration to the end of a six-hour observation period, represents a combination of the distribution and elimination phases. Morphine concentrations in the CSF averaged 332±137 ng/mL at 6 hours, following a bolus dose of 0.3 mg of morphine. The apparent volume of distribution of morphine in the intrathecal space is about 22±8 mL.

Time-to-peak plasma concentrations, however, are similar (5–10 min) after either epidural or intrathecal bolus administration of morphine. Maximum plasma morphine concentrations after 0.3 mg intrathecal morphine have been reported from <1 to 7.8 ng/mL. The minimum analgesic morphine plasma concentration during Patient-Controlled Analgesia (PCA) has been reported as 20–40 ng/mL, suggesting that any analgesic contribution from systemic redistribution would be minimal after the first 30–60 minutes with epidural administration and virtually absent with intrathecal administration of morphine.

INDICATIONS AND USAGE

DURAMORPH® is a systemic narcotic analgesic for administration by the intravenous, epidural or intrathecal routes. It is used for the management of pain not responsive to non-narcotic analgesics. DURAMORPH®, administered epidurally or intrathecally, provides pain relief for extended periods without attendant loss of motor, sensory or sympathetic function.

CONTRAINDICATIONS

DURAMORPH® is contraindicated in those medical conditions which would preclude the administration of opioids by the intravenous route—allergy to morphine or other opiates, acute bronchial asthma, upper airway obstruction.

WARNINGS

Morphine sulfate may be habit forming. (See DRUG ABUSE AND DEPENDENCE.)

DURAMORPH® administration should be limited to use by those familiar with the management of respiratory depression. Rapid intravenous administration may result in chest wall rigidity.

Prior to any epidural or intrathecal drug administration, the physician should be familiar with patient conditions (such as infection at the injection site, bleeding diathesis, anticoagulant therapy, etc.) which call for special evaluation of the benefit versus risk potential.

In the case of epidural or intrathecal administration, DURAMORPH® should be administered by or under the direction of a physician experienced in the techniques and familiar with the patient management problems associated with epidural or intrathecal drug administration. Because epidural administration has been associated with less potential for immediate or late adverse effects than intrathecal administration, the epidural route should be used whenever possible.

SEVERE RESPIRATORY DEPRESSION UP TO 24 HOURS FOLLOWING EPIDURAL OR INTRATHECAL ADMINISTRATION HAS BEEN REPORTED.

BECAUSE OF THE RISK OF SEVERE ADVERSE EFFECTS WHEN THE EPIDURAL OR INTRATHECAL ROUTE OF ADMINISTRATION IS EMPLOYED, PATIENTS MUST BE OBSERVED IN A FULLY EQUIPPED AND STAFFED ENVIRONMENT FOR AT LEAST 24 HOURS AFTER THE INITIAL DOSE.

THE FACILITY MUST BE EQUIPPED TO RESUSCITATE PATIENTS WITH SEVERE OPIATE OVERDOSAGE, AND THE PERSONNEL MUST BE FAMILIAR WITH THE USE AND LIMITATIONS OF SPECIFIC NARCOTIC ANTAGONISTS (NALOXONE, NALTREXONE) IN SUCH CASES.

TOLERANCE AND MYOCLONIC ACTIVITY

PATIENTS SOMETIMES MANIFEST UNUSUAL ACCELERATION OF NEURAXIAL MORPHINE REQUIREMENTS, WHICH MAY CAUSE CONCERN REGARDING SYSTEMIC ABSORPTION AND THE HAZARDS OF LARGE DOSES; THESE PATIENTS MAY BENEFIT FROM HOSPITALIZATION AND DETOXIFICATION. TWO CASES OF MYOCLONIC-LIKE SPASM OF THE LOWER EXTREMITIES HAVE BEEN REPORTED IN PATIENTS RECEIVING MORE THAN 20 MG/DAY OF INTRATHECAL MORPHINE. AFTER DETOXIFICATION, IT MIGHT BE POSSIBLE TO RESUME TREATMENT AT LOWER DOSES, AND SOME PATIENTS HAVE BEEN SUCCESSFULLY CHANGED FROM CONTINUOUS EPIDURAL MORPHINE TO CONTINUOUS INTRATHECAL MORPHINE. REPEAT DETOXIFICATION MAY BE INDICATED AT A LATER DATE. THE UPPER DAILY DOSAGE LIMIT FOR EACH PATIENT DURING CONTINUING TREATMENT MUST BE INDIVIDUALIZED.

PRECAUTIONS

GENERAL

Control of pain by neuraxial opiate delivery is always accompanied by considerable risk to the patients and requires a high level of skill to be successfully accomplished. The task of treating these patients must be undertaken by experienced clinical teams, well-versed in patient selection, evolving technology and emerging standards of care. For safety reasons, it is recommended that administration of DURAMORPH® by the epidural or intrathecal routes be limited to the lumbar area. Intrathecal use has been associated with a higher incidence of respiratory depression than epidural use.

Seizures may result from high doses. Patients with known seizure disorders should be carefully observed for evidence of morphine-induced seizure activity.

USE IN PATIENTS WITH INCREASED INTRACRANIAL PRESSURE OR HEAD INJURY

DURAMORPH® should be used with extreme caution in patients with head injury or increased intracranial pressure. Pupillary changes (miosis) from morphine may obscure the existence, extent and course of intracranial pathology. High doses of neuraxial morphine may produce myoclonic events (see WARNINGS and ADVERSE REACTIONS). Clinicians should maintain a high index of suspicion for adverse drug reactions when evaluating altered mental status or movement abnormalities in patients receiving this modality of treatment.

USE IN CHRONIC PULMONARY DISEASE

Care is urged in using this drug in patients who have a decreased respiratory reserve (e.g., emphysema, severe obesity, kyphoscoliosis or paralysis of the phrenic nerve). DURAMORPH® should not be given in cases of chronic asthma, upper airway obstruction or in any other chronic pulmonary disorder without due consideration of the known risk of acute respiratory failure following morphine administration in such patients.

USE IN HEPATIC OR RENAL DISEASE

The elimination half-life of morphine may be prolonged in patients with reduced metabolic rates and with hepatic and/or renal dysfunction. Hence, care should be exercised in administering DURAMORPH® epidurally to patients with these conditions, since high blood morphine levels, due to reduced clearance, may take several days to develop.

USE IN BILIARY SURGERY OR DISORDERS OF THE BILIARY TRACT

As significant morphine is released into the systemic circulation from neuraxial administration, the ensuring smooth muscle hypertonicity may result in biliary colic.

USE WITH DISORDERS OF THE URINARY SYSTEM

Initiation of neuraxial opiate analgesia is frequently associated with disturbances of micturition, especially in males with prostatic enlargement. Early recognition of difficulty in urination and prompt intervention in cases of urinary retention is indicated.

USE IN AMBULATORY PATIENTS

Patients with reduced circulating blood volume, impaired myocardial function or on sympatholytic drugs should be monitored for the possible occurrence of orthostatic hypotension, a frequent complication in single-dose neuraxial morphine analgesia.

USE WITH OTHER CENTRAL NERVOUS SYSTEM DEPRESSANTS

The depressant effects of morphine are potentiated by the presence of other CNS depressants such as alcohol, sedatives, antihistaminics or psychotropic drugs. Use of neuroleptics in conjunction with neuraxial morphine may increase the risk of respiratory depression.

CARCINOGENESIS, MUTAGENESIS, IMPAIRMENT OF FERTILITY

Morphine is without known carcinogenic or mutagenic effects and is not known to impair fertility at non-narcotic doses in animals, but studies of the carcinogenic and mutagenic potential or the effect on fertility of DURAMORPH® have not been conducted.

PREGNANCY

Teratogenic Effects—Pregnancy Category C. Morphine sulfate is not teratogenic in rats at 35 mg/kg/day (thirty-five times the usual human dose) but does result in increased pup mortality and growth retardation at doses that narcotize the animal (>10 mg/kg/day, ten times the usual human dose). DURAMORPH® should only be given to pregnant women when no other method of controlling pain is available and means are at hand to manage the delivery and perinatal care of the opiate-dependent infant.

Nonteratogenic Effects. Infants born to mothers who have been taking morphine chronically may exhibit withdrawal symptoms.

Continued on next page

Duramorph—Cont.

LABOR AND DELIVERY
Intravenous morphine readily passes into the fetal circulation and may result in respiratory depression in the neonate. Naloxone and resuscitative equipment should be available for reversal of narcotic-induced respiratory depression in the neonate. In addition, intravenous morphine may reduce the strength, duration and frequency of uterine contraction resulting in prolonged labor.
Epidurally and intrathecally administered morphine readily passes into the fetal circulation and may result in respiratory depression of the neonate. Controlled clinical studies have shown that *epidural* administration has little or no effect on the relief of labor pain.
NURSING MOTHERS
Morphine is excreted in maternal milk. Effects on the nursing infant are not known.
PEDIATRIC USE
Adequate studies, to establish the safty and effectiveness of spinal morphine in children, have not been performed, and usage in this population is not recommended.
USE IN THE AGED
The pharmacodynamic effects of neuraxial morphine in the aged are more variable than in the younger population. Patients will vary widely in the effective initial dose, rate of development of tolerance and the frequency and magnitude of associated adverse effects as the dose is increased. Initial doses should be based on careful clinical obsrvation following "test doses", after making due allowances for the effects of the patient's age and infirmity on his/her ability to clear the drug, particularly in patients receiving epidural morphine.

ADVERSE REACTIONS
The most serious adverse experience encountered during administration of DURAMORPH® is respiratory depression. This depression may be severe and could require intervention. (See WARNINGS AND OVERDOSAGE.) Because of delay in maximum CNS effect with intravenously administered drug (30 min), rapid administration may result in overdosing. Single-dose neuraxial administration may result in acute or delayed respiratory depression for periods at least as long as 24 hours.
Tolerance and myoclonus: See **WARNINGS** for discussion of these and related hazards.
While low doses of intravenously administered morphine have little effect on cardiovascular stability, high doses are excitatory, resulting from **sympathetic hyperactivity** and increase in circulating catecholamines. Excitation of the central nervous system, resulting in **convulsions**, may accompany high doses of morphine given intravenously. **Dysphoric reactions** may occur after any size dose and **toxic psychoses** have been reported.
Pruritus: Single-dose epidural or intrathecal administration is accompanied by a high incidence of *pruritus* that is dose-related but not confined to the site of administration. Pruritus, following continuous infusion of epidural or intrathecal morphine, is occasionally reported in the literature; these reactions are poorly understood as to their cause.
Urinary retention: Urinary retention, which may persist 10 to 20 hours following single epidural or intrathecal administration, is a frequent side effect and must be anticipated primarily in male patients, with a somewhat lower incidence in females. Also frequently reported in the literature is the occurrence of urinary retention during the first several days of hospitalization for the initiation of continuous intrathecal or epidural morphine therapy. Patients who develop urinary retention have responded to cholinomimetic treatment and/or judicious use of catheters (see PRECAUTIONS).
Constipation: Constipation is frequently encountered during continuous infusion of morphine; this can usually be managed by conventional therapy.
Headache: Lumbar puncture-type headache is encountered in a significant minority of cases for several days following intrathecal catheter implantation; this, generally, responds to bed rest and/or other conventional therapy.
Other: Other adverse experiences reported following morphine therapy include—**Dizziness, euphoria, anxiety, depression of cough reflex, interference with thermal regulation and oliguria.** Evidence of histamine release such as **urticaria, wheals** and/or **local tissue irritation** may occur. **Nausea** and **vomiting** are frequently seen in patients following morphine administration.
Pruritus, nausea/vomiting and urinary retention, if associated with continuous infusion therapy, may respond to intravenous administration of a low dose of naloxone (0.2 mg). The risks of using narcotic antagonists in patients chronically receiving narcotic therapy should be considered.
In general, side effects are amenable to reversal by narcotic antagonists.

NALOXONE INJECTION AND RESUSCITATIVE EQUIPMENT SHOULD BE IMMEDIATELY AVAILABLE FOR ADMINISTRATION IN CASE OF LIFE-THREATENING OR INTOLERABLE SIDE EFFECTS AND WHENEVER DURAMORPH® THERAPY IS BEING INITIATED.

DRUG ABUSE AND DEPENDENCE
CONTROLLED SUBSTANCE
Morphine sulfate is a Schedule II narcotic under the United States Controlled Substance Act (21 U.S.C. 801–886).
Morphine is the most commonly cited prototype for narcotic substances that possess an addiction-forming or addiction-sustaining liability. A patient may be at risk for developing a dependence to morphine if used improperly or for overly long periods of time. As with all potent opioids which are μ-agonists, tolerance as well as psychological and physicial dependence to morphine may develop irrespective of the route of administration (intravenous, intramuscular, intrathecal, epidural or oral). Individuals with a prior history of opioid or other substance abuse or dependence, being more apt to respond to the euphorogenic and reinforcing properties of morphine, would be considered to be at greater risk. Care must be taken to avert withdrawal in those patients who have been maintained on parenteral/oral narcotics when epidural or intrathecal administration is considered. Withdrawal symptoms may occur when morphine is discontinued abruptly or upon administration of a narcotic antagonist.

OVERDOSAGE
PARENTERAL ADMINISTRATION OF NARCOTICS IN PATIENTS RECEIVING EPIDURAL OR INTRATHECAL MORPHINE MAY RESULT IN OVERDOSAGE.
Overdosage of morphine is characterized by respiratory depression, with or without concomitant CNS depression. Since respiratory arrest may result either through direct depression of the respiratory center or as the result of hypoxia, primary attention should be given to the establishment of adequate respiratory exchange through provision of a patent airway and institution of assisted, or controlled, ventilation. The narcotic antagonist, naloxone, is a specific antidote. An initial dose of 0.4 to 2 mg of naloxone should be administered intravenously, simultaneously with respiratory resuscitation. If the desired degree of counteraction and improvement in respiratory function is not obtained, naloxone may be repeated at 2- to 3-minute intervals. If no response is observed after 10 mg of naloxone has been administered, the diagnosis of narcotic-induced, or partial narcotic-induced, toxicity should be questioned. Intramuscular or subcutaneous administration may be used if the intravenous route is not available.
As the duration of effect of naloxone is considerably shorter than that of epidural or intrathecal morphine, repeated administration may be necessary. Patients should be closely observed for evidence of renarcotization.

DOSAGE AND ADMINISTRATION
DURAMORPH® is intended for intravenous, epidural or intrathecal administration.
INTRAVENOUS ADMINISTRATION
Dosage: The initial dose of morphine should be 2 mg to 10 mg/70 kg of body weight. No information is available regarding the use of DURAMORPH® in patients under the age of 18.
EPIDURAL ADMINISTRATION
DURAMORPH® SHOULD BE ADMINISTERED EPIDURALLY BY OR UNDER THE DIRECTION OF A PHYSICIAN EXPERIENCED IN THE TECHNIQUE OF EPIDURAL ADMINISTRATION AND WHO IS THOROUGHLY FAMILIAR WITH THE LABELING. IT SHOULD BE ADMINISTERED ONLY IN SETTINGS WHERE ADEQUATE PATIENT MONITORING IS POSSIBLE. RESUSCITATIVE EQUIPMENT AND A SPECIFIC ANTAGONIST (NALOXONE INJECTION) SHOULD BE IMMEDIATELY AVAILABLE FOR THE MANAGEMENT OF RESPIRATORY DEPRESSION AS WELL AS COMPLICATIONS WHICH MIGHT RESULT FROM INADVERTENT INTRATHECAL OR INTRAVASCULAR INJECTION. (NOTE: INTRATHECAL DOSAGE IS USUALLY $^1/_{10}$ THAT OF EPIDURAL DOSAGE.) **PATIENT MONITORING SHOULD BE CONTINUED FOR AT LEAST 24 HOURS AFTER EACH DOSE, SINCE DELAYED RESPIRATORY DEPRESSION MAY OCCUR.**
Proper placement of a needle or catheter in the epidural space should be verified before DURAMORPH® is injected. Acceptable techniques for verifying proper placement include: a) aspiration to check for absence of blood or cerebrospinal fluid, or b) administration of 5 mL (3 mL in obstetric patients) of 1.5% PRESERVATIVE-FREE Lidocaine and Epinephrine (1:200,000) Injection and then observe the patient for lack of tachycardia (this indicates that vascular injection has *not* been made) and lack of sudden onset of segmental anesthesia (this indicates that intrathecal injection has *not* been made).
Epidural Adult Dosage: Initial injection of 5 mg in the lumbar region may provide satisfactory pain relief for up to 24 hours. If adequate pain relief is not achieved within one hour, careful administration of incremental doses of 1 to 2 mg at intervals sufficient to assess effectiveness may be given. No more than 10 mg/24 hr should be administered.
Thoracic administration has been shown to dramatically increase the incidence of early and late respiratory depression even at doses of 1 to 2 mg.
For continuous infusion, an initial dose of 2 to 4 mg/24 hours is recommended. Further doses of 1 to 2 mg may be given if pain relief is not achieved initially.
Aged patients—Administer with extreme caution. (See PRECAUTIONS.)
Epidural Pediatric Use: No information on use in pediatric patients is available. (See PRECAUTIONS.)
INTRATHECAL ADMINISTRATION

NOTE: INTRATHECAL DOSAGE IS USUALLY 1/10 THAT OF EPIDURAL DOSAGE.

DURAMORPH® SHOULD BE ADMINISTERED INTRATHECALLY BY OR UNDER THE DIRECTION OF A PHYSICIAN EXPERIENCED IN THE TECHNIQUE OF INTRATHECAL ADMINISTRATION AND WHO IS THOROUGHLY FAMILIAR WITH THE LABELING. IT SHOULD BE ADMINISTERED ONLY IN SETTINGS WHERE ADEQUATE PATIENT MONITORING IS POSSIBLE. RESUSCITATIVE EQUIPMENT AND A SPECIFIC ANTAGONIST (NALOXONE INJECTION) SHOULD BE IMMEDIATELY AVAILABLE FOR THE MANAGEMENT OF RESPIRATORY DEPRESSION AS WELL AS COMPLICATIONS WHICH MIGHT RESULT FROM INADVERTENT INTRAVASCULAR INJECTION. **PATIENT MONITORING SHOULD BE CONTINUED FOR AT LEAST 24 HOURS AFTER EACH DOSE, SINCE DELAYED RESPIRATORY DEPRESSION MAY OCCUR.** RESPIRATORY DEPRESSION (BOTH EARLY AND LATE ONSET) HAS OCCURRED MORE FREQUENTLY FOLLOWING INTRATHECAL ADMINISTRATION THAN EPIDURAL ADMINISTRATION.
Intrathecal Adult Dosage: A single injection of 0.2 to 1 mg may provide satisfactory pain relief for up to 24 hours. (CAUTION: THIS IS ONLY 0.4 TO 2 ML OF THE 5 MG/10 ML AMPUL OR 0.2 TO 1 ML OF THE 10 MG/10 ML AMPUL OF DURAMORPH®). DO NOT INJECT INTRATHECALLY MORE THAN 2 ML OF THE 5 MG/10 ML AMPUL OR 1 ML OF THE 10 MG/10 ML AMPUL. USE IN THE LUMBAR AREA ONLY IS RECOMMENDED. Repeated intrathecal injections of DURAMORPH® are not recommended. A constant intravenous infusion of naloxone, 0.6 mg/hr, for 24 hours after intrathecal injection may be used to reduce the incidence of potential side effects.
Aged patients—Administer with extreme caution. (See PRECAUTIONS.)
Repeat Dosage: If pain recurs, alternative routes of administration should be considered, since experience with repeated doses of morphine by the intrathecal route is limited.
Intrathecal Pediatric Use: No information on use in pediatric patients is available. (See PRECAUTIONS.)
SAFETY AND HANDLING INSTRUCTIONS

DURAMORPH® is supplied in sealed ampuls. Accidental dermal exposure should be treated by the removal of any contaminated clothing and rinsing the affected area with water.
Each ampul of DURAMORPH® contains a potent narcotic which has been associated with abuse and dependence among health care providers. **Due to the limited indications for this product, the risk of overdosage and the risk of its diversion and abuse, it is recommended that special measures be taken to control this product within the hospital or clinic. DURAMORPH® should be subject to rigid accounting, rigorous control of wastage and restricted access.**
Parenteral drug products should be inspected for particulate matter and discoloration prior to administration, whenever solution and container permit. DO NOT USE IF COLOR IS DARKER THAN PALE YELLOW, IF IT IS DISCOLORED IN ANY OTHER WAY OR IF IT CONTAINS A PRECIPITATE.

HOW SUPPLIED
Preservative-free DURAMORPH® (Morphine Sulfate Injection, USP) is available in amber DOSETTE® ampuls for intravenous, epidural or intrathecal administration:
5 mg/10 mL (0.5 mg/mL) packaged in 10s (NDC 0641-1112-33)
10 mg/10 mL (1 mg/1 mL) packaged in 10s (NDC 0641-1114-33)
Also available from Elkins-Sinn: INFUMORPH® (Preservative-free Morphine Sulfate Sterile Solution) 200 mg/20 mL (10 mg/mL) and 500 mg/20 mL (25 mg/mL) for epidural and intrathecal administration via a continuous microinfusion device. See insert J-1131.

STORAGE

Protect from light. Store in carton at controlled room temperature, 15° to 30°C (59° to 86°F) until ready to use. DO NOT FREEZE.

DURAMORPH® contains no preservative or antioxidant. DISCARD ANY UNUSED PORTION. DO NOT HEAT-STERILIZE.

* * * *

Manufactured by
ELKINS-SINN, INC., Cherry Hill, NJ 08003-4099
A division of A.H. Robins Company

INFUMORPH® 200 Ⓒ
INFUMORPH® 500 Ⓒ

(Preservative-free Morphine Sulfate Sterile Solution)
WARNING: May be habit forming.
For Use in Continuous Microinfusion Devices

DESCRIPTION

Morphine is the most important alkaloid of opium and is a phenanthrene derivative. It is available as the sulfate salt, having the following structural formula:

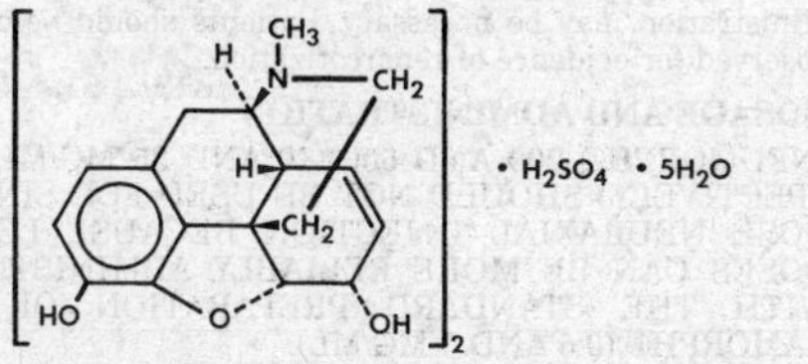

7,8-Didehydro-4,5-epoxy-17-methyl-(5α,6α)-morphinan-3,6-diol sulfate (2:1) (salt), pentahydrate
$(C_{17}H_{19}NO_3)_2 \cdot H_2SO_4 \cdot 5H_2O$ **MW 758.83.**

INFUMORPH® is a sterile, nonpyrogenic, isobaric, **high potency solution of morphine sulfate,** free of antioxidants, preservatives or other potentially neurotoxic additives. **INFUMORPH® is intended for use in continuous microinfusion devices for intraspinal administration in the management of pain.**

Each 20 mL ampul of **INFUMORPH® 200** contains morphine sulfate, USP 200 mg or 10 mg/mL and sodium chloride 8 mg/mL in Water for Injection, USP. Each 20 mL ampul of **INFUMORPH® 500** contains morphine sulfate, USP 500 mg or 25 mg/mL and sodium chloride 6.25 mg/mL in Water for Injection, USP. If needed, sodium hydroxide and/or sulfuric acid are added for pH adjustment to 4.5. Ampuls are sealed under nitrogen. Each 20 mL DOSETTE® ampul of **INFUMORPH®** is intended for **single use only.** *Discard any unused portion.* DO NO HEAT-STERILIZE.

CLINICAL PHARMACOLOGY

Morphine produces a wide spectrum of pharmacologic effects including analgesia, dysphoria, euphoria, somnolence, respiratory depression, diminished gastrointestinal motility and physical dependence. Opiate analgesia involves at least three anatomical areas of the central nervous system: the periaqueductal-periventricular gray matter, the ventromedial medulla and the spinal cord. A systemically administered opiate may produce analgesia by acting at any, all or some combination of these distinct regions. Morphine interacts predominantly with the μ-receptor. The μ-binding sites of opioids are very discretely distributed in the human brain, with high densities of sites found in the posterior amygdala, hypothalamus, thalamus, nucleus caudatus, putamen and certain cortical areas. They are also found on the terminal axons of primary afferents within laminae I and II (substantia gelatinosa) of the spinal cord and in the spinal nucleus of the trigeminal nerve.

Morphine has an apparent volume of distribution ranging from 1.0 to 4.7 L/kg after *intravenous* dosage. Protein binding is low, about 36%, and muscle tissue binding is reported as 54%. A blood-brain barrier exists, and when morphine is introduced outside of the CNS (e.g., *intravenously*), plasma concentrations of morphine remain higher than the corresponding CSF morphine levels. Conversely, when morphine is injected into the *intrathecal space,* it diffuses out into the systemic circulation slowly, accounting for the long duration of action of morphine administered by this route.

Morphine has a total plasma clearance which ranges from 0.9 to 1.2 L/kg/h (liters/kilogram/hour) in postoperative patients, but shows considerable interindividual variation. The major pathway of clearance is hepatic glucuronidation to morphine-3-glucuronide, which is pharmacologically inactive. The major excretion path of the conjugate is through the kidneys, with about 10% in the feces. Morphine is also eliminated by the kidneys, 2 to 12% being excreted unchanged in the urine. Terminal half-life is commonly reported to vary from 1.5 to 4.5 hours, although the longer half-lives were obtained when morphine levels were monitored over protracted periods with very sensitive radioimmunoassay methods. The accepted elimination half-life in normal subjects is 1.5 to 2 hours.

"Selective" blockade of pain sensation is possible by neuraxial application of morphine. In addition, duration of analgesia may be much longer by this route compared to systemic administration. However, CNS effects, associated with systemic administration, are still seen. These include respiratory depression, sedation, nausea and vomiting, pruritis and urinary retention. In particular, both early and late respiratory depression (up to 24 hours post dosing) have been reported following neuraxial administration. Circulation of the spinal fluid may also result in high concentrations of morphine reaching the brain stem directly.

The incidence of unwanted CNS effects, including delayed respiratory depression, associated with neuraxial application of morphine, is related to the circulatory dynamics of the epidural venous plexus and the spinal fluid. The lipid solubility and degree of ionization of morphine plays an important part in both the onset and duration of analgesia and the CNS effects. Morphine has a pK_a 7.9, with an octanol/water partition coefficient of 1.42 at pH 7.4. At this pH, the tertiary amino group in each of the opioids is mostly ionized, making the molecule water soluble. Morphine, with additional hydroxyl groups on the molecule, is significantly more water soluble than any other opioid in clinical use.

Morphine, injected into the *epidural space,* is rapidly absorbed into the general circulation. Absorption is so rapid that the plasma concentration-time profiles closely resembled those obtained after intravenous or intramuscular administration. Peak plasma concentrations averaging 33–40 ng/mL (range 5–62 ng/mL) are achieved within 10 to 15 minutes after administration of 3 mg of morphine. Plasma concentrations decline in a multiexponential fashion. The terminal half-life is reported to range from 39 to 249 minutes (mean of 90 ± 34.3 min) and, though somewhat shorter, is similar in magnitude as values reported after intravenous and intramuscular administration (1.5–4.5 h). CSF concentrations of morphine, after epidural doses of 2 to 6 mg in postoperative patients, have been reported to be 50 to 250 times higher than corresponding plasma concentrations. The CSF levels of morphine exceed those in plasma after only 15 minutes and are detectable for as long as 20 hours after the injection of 2 mg of epidural morphine. Approximately 4% of the dose injected epidurally reaches the CSF. This corresponds to the relative minimum effective epidural and intrathecal doses of 5 mg and 0.25 mg, respectively. The disposition of morphine in the CSF follows a biphasic pattern, with an early half-life of 1.5 h and a late phase half-life of about 6 h. Morphine crosses the dura slowly, with an absorption half-life across the dura averaging 22 minutes. Maximum CSF concentrations are seen 60–90 minutes after injection. Minimum effective CSF concentrations for postoperative analgesia average 150 ng/mL (range <1–380 ng/mL).

The *intrathecal route* of administration circumvents meningeal diffusion barriers and, therefore, lower doses of morphine produce comparable analgesia to that induced by the epidural route. After intrathecal bolus injection of morphine, there is a rapid initial distribution phase lasting 15–30 minutes and a half-life in the CSF of 42–136 min (mean 90 ± 16 min). Derived from limited data, it appears that the disposition of morphine in the CSF, from 15 minutes postintrathecal administration to the end of a six-hour observation period, represents a combination of the distribution and elimination phases. Morphine concentrations in the CSF averaged 332 ± 137 ng/mL at 6 hours, following a bolus dose of 0.3 mg of morphine. The apparent volume of distribution of morphine in the intrathecal space is about 22 ± 8 mL.

Time-to-peak plasma concentrations, however, is similar (5–10 min) after either epidural or intrathecal bolus administration of morphine. Maximum plasma morphine concentrations after 0.3 mg intrathecal morphine have been reported from <1 to 7.8 ng/mL. The minimum analgesic morphine plasma concentration during Patient-Controlled Analgesia (PCA) has been reported as 20–40 ng/mL, suggesting that any analgesic contribution from systemic redistribution would be minimal after the first 30–60 minutes with epidural administration and virtually absent with intrathecal administration of morphine.

INDICATION AND USAGE

INFUMORPH® (Preservative-free Morphine Sulfate Sterile Solution) is indicated only for intrathecal or epidural infusion in the treatment of intractable chronic pain. It was developed for use in continuous microinfusion devices and may require dilution before use as dictated by the characteristics of the device and the dosage requirements of the individual patient.

INFUMORPH® IS NOT RECOMMENDED FOR SINGLE-DOSE INTRAVENOUS, INTRAMUSCULAR OR SUBCUTANEOUS ADMINISTRATION DUE TO THE VERY LARGE AMOUNT OF MORPHINE IN THE AMPUL AND THE ASSOCIATED RISK OF OVERDOSAGE.

CONTRAINDICATIONS

The only absolute contraindication to the use of INFUMORPH® is known allergy to morphine. Contraindications to the use of neuraxial analgesia include: the presence of infection at the injection microinfusion site, concomitant anticoagulant therapy, uncontrolled bleeding diathesis and the presence of any other concomitant therapy or medical condition which would render epidural or intrathecal administration of medication especially hazardous.

WARNINGS

THIS PRODUCT WAS DEVELOPED FOR USE (AFTER APPROPRIATE DILUTION, IF NECESSARY) IN CONTINUOUS MICROINFUSION DEVICES FOR INTRATHECAL OR EPIDURAL INFUSION OF NARCOTICS TO CONTROL SEVERE CANCER PAIN. CHRONIC NEURAXIAL OPIOID ANALGESIA IS APPROPRIATE ONLY WHEN LESS INVASIVE MEANS OF CONTROLLING PAIN HAVE FAILED AND SHOULD ONLY BE UNDERTAKEN BY THOSE WHO ARE EXPERIENCED IN APPLYING THE TREATMENT IN A SETTING WHERE ITS COMPLICATIONS CAN BE ADEQUATELY MANAGED.

BECAUSE OF THE RISK OF SEVERE ADVERSE EFFECTS, PATIENTS MUST BE OBSERVED IN A FULLY EQUIPPED AND STAFFED ENVIRONMENT FOR AT LEAST 24 HOURS AFTER THE INITIAL (SINGLE) TEST DOSE AND, AS APPROPRIATE, FOR THE FIRST SEVERAL DAYS AFTER CATHETER IMPLANTATION.

THE FACILITY MUST BE EQUIPPED TO RESUSCITATE PATIENTS WITH SEVERE OPIATE OVERDOSAGE, AND THE PERSONNEL MUST BE FAMILIAR WITH THE USE AND LIMITATIONS OF SPECIFIC NARCOTIC ANTAGONISTS (NALOXONE, NALTREXONE) IN SUCH CASES.

RESERVOIR FILLING MUST BE PERFORMED BY FULLY TRAINED AND QUALIFIED PERSONNEL, FOLLOWING THE DIRECTIONS PROVIDED BY THE DEVICE MANUFACTURER. CARE SHOULD BE TAKEN IN SELECTING THE PROPER REFILL FREQUENCY TO PREVENT DEPLETION OF THE RESERVOIR, WHICH WOULD RESULT IN EXACERBATION OF SEVERE PAIN AND/OR REFLUX OF CSF INTO SOME DEVICES. STRICT ASEPTIC TECHNIQUE IN FILLING IS REQUIRED TO AVOID BACTERIAL CONTAMINATION AND SERIOUS INFECTION. **EXTREME CARE MUST BE TAKEN TO ENSURE THAT THE NEEDLE IS PROPERLY IN THE FILLING PORT OF THE DEVICE BEFORE ATTEMPTING TO REFILL THE RESERVOIR. INJECTING THE SOLUTION INTO THE TISSUE AROUND THE DEVICE OR (IN THE CASE OF DEVICES THAT HAVE MORE THAN ONE PORT) ATTEMPTING TO INJECT THE REFILL DOSE INTO THE DIRECT INJECTION PORT WILL RESULT IN A LARGE, CLINICALLY SIGNIFICANT, OVERDOSAGE TO THE PATIENT.**

A PERIOD OF OBSERVATION APPROPRIATE TO THE CLINICAL SITUATION SHOULD FOLLOW EACH REFILL OR MANIPULATION OF THE DRUG RESERVOIR. BEFORE DISCHARGE, THE PATIENT AND ATTENDANT(S) SHOULD RECEIVE INSTRUCTION IN THE PROPER HOME CARE OF THE DEVICE AND INSERTION SITE AND IN THE RECOGNITION AND PRACTICAL TREATMENT OF AN OVERDOSE OF NEURAXIAL MORPHINE.

TOLERANCE AND MYOCLONIC ACTIVITY

PATIENTS SOMETIMES MANIFEST UNUSUAL ACCELERATION OF NEURAXIAL MORPHINE REQUIREMENTS, WHICH MAY CAUSE CONCERN REGARDING SYSTEMIC ABSORPTION AND THE HAZARDS OF LARGE DOSES; THESE PATIENTS MAY BENEFIT FROM HOSPITALIZATION AND DETOXIFICATION. TWO CASES OF MYOCLONIC-LIKE SPASM OF THE LOWER EXTREMITIES HAVE BEEN REPORTED IN PATIENTS RECEIVING MORE THAN 20 MG/DAY OF INTRATHECAL MORPHINE. AFTER DETOXIFICATION, IT MIGHT BE POSSIBLE TO RESUME TREATMENT AT LOWER DOSES, AND SOME PATIENTS HAVE BEEN SUCCESSFULLY CHANGED FROM CONTINUOUS EPIDURAL MORPHINE TO CONTINUOUS INTRATHECAL MORPHINE. REPEAT DETOXIFICATION MAY BE INDICATED AT A LATER DATE. THE UPPER DAILY DOSAGE LIMIT FOR EACH PATIENT DURING CONTINUING TREATMENT MUST BE INDIVIDUALIZED.

PRECAUTIONS

Control of pain by neuraxial opiate delivery, using a continuous microinfusion device, is always accompanied by considerable risk to the patients and requires a high level of skill to be successfully accomplished. The task of treating these patients must be undertaken by experienced clinical teams, well-versed in patient selection, evolving technology and emerging standards of care. For reasons of safety, it is

Continued on next page

Infumorph—Cont.

recommended that administration of INFUMORPH® 200 and 500 (10 and 25 mg/mL, respectively) by the intrathecal route be limited to the lumbar area.

USE IN PATIENTS WITH INCREASED INTRACRANIAL PRESSURE OR HEAD INJURY

INFUMORPH® (Preservative-free Morphine Sulfate Sterile Solution) should be used with extreme caution in patients with head injury or increased intracranial pressure. Pupillary changes (miosis) from morphine may obscure the existence, extent and course of intracranial pathology. High doses of neuraxial morphine may produce myoclonic events (see WARNINGS and ADVERSE REACTIONS). Clinicians should maintain a high index of suspicion for adverse drug reactions when evaluating altered mental status or movement abnormalities in patients receiving this modality of treatment.

USE IN CHRONIC PULMONARY DISEASE

Care is urged in using this drug in patients who have a decreased respiratory reserve (e.g., emphysema, severe obesity, kyphoscoliosis or paralysis of the phrenic nerve). INFUMORPH® should not be given in cases of chronic asthma, upper airway obstruction or in any other chronic pulmonary disorder without due consideration of the known risk of acute respiratory failure following morphine administration in such patients.

USE IN HEPATIC OR RENAL DISEASE

The elimination half-life of morphine may be prolonged in patients with reduced metabolic rate and with hepatic and/or renal dysfunction. Hence, care should be exercised in administering INFUMORPH® epidurally to patients with these conditions, since high blood morphine levels, due to reduced clearance, may take several days to develop.

USE IN BILIARY SURGERY OR DISORDERS OF THE BILIARY TRACT

As significant morphine is released into the systemic circulation from neuraxial administration, the ensuing smooth muscle hypertonicity may result in biliary colic.

USE WITH DISORDERS OF THE URINARY SYSTEM

Initiation of neuraxial opiate analgesia is frequently associated with disturbances of micturition, especially in males with prostatic enlargement. Early recognition of difficulty in urination and prompt intervention in cases of urinary retention is indicated.

USE IN AMBULATORY PATIENTS

Patients with reduced circulating blood volume, impaired myocardial function or on sympatholytic drugs should be monitored for the possible occurrence of orthostatic hypotension, a frequent complication in single-dose neuraxial morphine analgesia.

USE WITH OTHER CENTRAL NERVOUS SYSTEM DEPRESSANTS

The depressant effects of morphine are potentiated by the presence of other CNS depressants such as alcohol, sedatives, antihistaminics or psychotropic drugs. Use of neuroleptics in conjunction with neuraxial morphine may increase the risk of respiratory depression.

CARCINOGENESIS, MUTAGENESIS, IMPAIRMENT OF FERTILITY

Morphine is without known carcinogenic or mutagenic effects and is not known to impair fertility at non-narcotic doses in animals, but studies of the carcinogenic and mutagenic potential or the effect on fertility of INFUMORPH® have not been conducted.

PREGNANCY CATEGORY C

Morphine sulfate is not teratogenic in rats at 35 mg/kg/day (thirty-five times the usual human dose) but does result in increased pup mortality and growth retardation at doses that narcotize the animal (>10 mg/kg/day, ten times the usual human dose). INFUMORPH® should only be given to pregnant women when no other method of controlling pain is available and means are at hand to manage the delivery and perinatal care of the opiate-dependent infant.

LABOR AND DELIVERY

INFUMORPH® 200 and 500 (10 and 25 mg/mL, respectively) are too highly concentrated for routine use in obstetric neuraxial analgesia.

NURSING MOTHERS

Morphine is excreted in maternal milk. Effects on the nursing infant are not known.

PEDIATRIC USE

Adequate studies, to establish the safety and effectiveness of spinal morphine in children, have not been performed, and usage in this population is not recommended.

USE IN THE AGED

The pharmacodynamic effects of neuraxial morphine in the aged are more variable than in the younger population. Patients will vary widely in the effective initial dose, rate of development of tolerance and the frequency and magnitude of associated adverse effects as the dose is increased. Initial doses should be based on careful clinical observation following "test doses", after making due allowances for the effects of the patient's age and infirmity on their ability to clear the drug, particularly in patients receiving epidural morphine.

ADVERSE REACTIONS

IMPROPER OR ERRONEOUS SUBSTITUTION OF INFUMORPH® 200 or 500 (10 or 25 mg/mL, respectively) FOR REGULAR DURAMORPH® (0.5 or 1 mg/mL) IS LIKELY TO RESULT IN SERIOUS OVERDOSAGE, LEADING TO SEIZURES, RESPIRATORY DEPRESSION AND, POSSIBLY, FATAL OUTCOME.

The most serious adverse experiences encountered during continuous intrathecal or epidural infusion of INFUMORPH® are respiratory depression and myoclonus.

1. Single-dose neuraxial administration may result in acute or delayed respiratory depression for periods at least as long as 24 hours. **Severe respiratory depression, potentially life-threatening, can result from technical errors during refill, e.g., injection of INFUMORPH® outside the filling port, unintentional injection into the direct by-pass-dosing port featured on some devices or local infiltration.**
2. **Tolerance and myoclonus:** See **WARNINGS** for discussion of these and related hazards.

While low doses of intravenously administered morphine have little effect on cardiovascular stability, high doses are excitatory, resulting from **sympathetic hyperactivity** and increase in circulatory catecholamines. Excitation of the central nervous system, resulting in **convulsions,** may accompany high doses of morphine given intravenously.

Dysphoric reactions may occur after any size dose and **toxic psychoses** have been reported.

Pruritus: Single-dose epidural or intrathecal administration is accompanied by a high incidence of **pruritus** that is dose-related but not confined to the site of administration. Pruritus, following continuous infusion of epidural or intrathecal morphine, is occasionally reported in the literature; these reactions are poorly understood as to their cause.

Urinary retention: Urinary retention, which may persist 10 to 20 hours following single epidural or intrathecal administration, is a frequent side effect and must be anticipated primarily in male patients, with a somewhat lower incidence in females. Also frequently reported in the literature is the occurrence of urinary retention during the first several days of hospitalization for the initiation of continuous intrathecal or epidural morphine therapy. Patients who develop urinary retention have responded to cholinomimetic treatment and/or judicious use of catheters (see PRECAUTIONS).

Constipation: Constipation is frequently encountered during continuous infusion of morphine; this can usually be managed by conventional therapy.

Headache: Lumbar puncture-type headache is encountered in a significant minority of cases for several days following intrathecal catheter implantation; this, generally, responds to bed rest and/or other conventional therapy.

Peripheral edema: There are several reports of peripheral edema, including unexplained genital swelling in male patients, following infusion-device implant surgery.

Other: Other adverse experiences reported following morphine therapy include—**Dizziness, euphoria, anxiety, depression of cough reflex, interference with thermal regulation** and **oliguria.** Evidence of histamine release such as **urticaria, wheals** and/or **local tissue irritation** may occur.

Pruritus, nausea/vomiting and urinary retention, if associated with continuous infusion therapy, may respond to intravenous administration of a low dose of naloxone (0.2 mg). The risks of using narcotic antagonists in patients chronically receiving narcotic therapy should be considered.

NALOXONE INJECTION AND RESUSCITATIVE EQUIPMENT SHOULD BE IMMEDIATELY AVAILABLE FOR USE IN CASE OF LIFE-THREATENING OR INTOLERABLE SIDE EFFECTS AND WHENEVER INFUMORPH® THERAPY IS BEING INITIATED, THE RESERVOIR IS BEING REFILLED OR ANY MANIPULATION OF THE RESERVOIR SYSTEM IS TAKING PLACE.

DRUG ABUSE AND DEPENDENCE

CONTROLLED SUBSTANCE

Morphine sulfate is a Schedule II narcotic under the United States Controlled Substance Act (21 U.S.C. 801–886).

Morphine is the most commonly cited prototype for narcotic substances that possess an addiction-forming or addiction-sustaining liability. A patient may be at risk for developing a dependence to morphine if used improperly or for overly long periods of time. As with all potent opioids which are μ-agonists, tolerance as well as psychological and physical dependence to morphine may develop irrespective of the route of administration (intravenous, intramuscular, intrathecal, epidural or oral). Individuals with a prior history of opioid or other substance abuse or dependence, being more apt to respond to the euphorogenic and reinforcing properties of morphine, would be considered to be a greater risk. Care must be taken to avert withdrawal in patients who have been maintained on parenteral/oral narcotics when epidural or intrathecal administration is considered. Withdrawal symptoms may occur when morphine is discontinued abruptly or upon administration of a narcotic antagonist.

OVERDOSAGE

PARENTERAL ADMINISTRATION OF NARCOTICS IN PATIENTS RECEIVING EPIDURAL OR INTRATHECAL MORPHINE MAY RESULT IN OVERDOSAGE.

Overdosage of morphine is characterized by respiratory depression, with or without concomitant CNS depression. Since respiratory arrest may result either through direct depression of the respiratory center, or as the result of hypoxia, primary attention should be given to the establishment of adequate respiratory exchange through provision of a patent airway and institution of assisted, or controlled, ventilation. The narcotic antagonist, naloxone, is a specific antidote. An initial dose of 0.4 to 2 mg of naloxone should be administered intravenously, simultaneously with respiratory resuscitation. If the desired degree of counteraction and improvement in respiratory function is not obtained, naloxone may be repeated at 2- to 3-minute intervals. If no response is observed after 10 mg of naloxone has been administered, the diagnosis of narcotic-induced, or partial narcotic-induced, toxicity should be questioned. Intramuscular or subcutaneous administration may be used if the intravenous route is not available.

As the duration of effect of naloxone is considerably shorter than that of epidural or intrathecal morphine, repeated administration may be necessary. Patients should be closely observed for evidence of renarcotization.

DOSAGE AND ADMINISTRATION

INFUMORPH® 200 AND 500 (10 AND 25 MG/ML, RESPECTIVELY) SHOULD NOT BE USED FOR SINGLE-DOSE NEURAXIAL INJECTION BECAUSE LOWER DOSES CAN BE MORE RELIABLY ADMINISTERED WITH THE STANDARD PREPARATION OF DURAMORPH® (0.5 AND 1 MG/ML).

CANDIDATES FOR NEURAXIAL ADMINISTRATION OF INFUMORPH® IN A CONTINUOUS MICROINFUSION DEVICE SHOULD BE HOSPITALIZED TO PROVIDE FOR ADEQUATE PATIENT MONITORING DURING ASSESSMENT OF RESPONSE TO SINGLE DOSES OF INTRATHECAL OR EPIDURAL MORPHINE. HOSPITALIZATION SHOULD BE MAINTAINED FOR SEVERAL DAYS AFTER SURGERY INVOLVING THE INFUSION DEVICE FOR ADDITIONAL MONITORING AND ADJUSTMENT OF DAILY DOSAGE. THE FACILITY MUST BE EQUIPPED WITH RESUSCITATIVE EQUIPMENT, OXYGEN, NALOXONE INJECTION AND OTHER RESUSCITATIVE DRUGS. BECAUSE OF THE RISK OF DELAYED RESPIRATORY DEPRESSION, PATIENTS SHOULD BE OBSERVED IN A FULLY EQUIPPED AND STAFFED ENVIRONMENT FOR AT LEAST 24 HOURS AFTER EACH TEST DOSE AND, AS INDICATED, FOR THE FIRST SEVERAL DAYS AFTER SURGERY.

Familiarization with the continuous microinfusion device is essential. The desired amount of morphine should be withdrawn from the ampul through a microfilter. **To minimize risk from glass or other particles, the product must be filtered through a 5 μ (or smaller) microfilter before injecting into the microinfusion device.** If dilution is required, 0.9% Sodium Chloride Injection is recommended.

Intrathecal Dosage: The starting dose must be individualized, based upon in-hospital evaluation of the response to serial single-dose intrathecal bolus injections of regular DURAMORPH® (Morphine Sulfate Injection, USP) 0.5 mg/mL or 1 mg/mL, with close observation of the analgesic efficacy and adverse effects *prior* to surgery involving the continuous microinfusion device.

The recommended initial lumbar intrathecal dose range in patients with no tolerance to opioids is 0.2 to 1 mg/day. The published range of doses for individuals who have some degree of opioid tolerance varies from 1 to 10 mg/day. The upper daily dosage limit for each patient must be individualized.

Limited experience with continuous intrathecal infusion of morphine has shown that the daily doses have to be increased over time. Although the rate of increase, over time, in the dose required to sustain analgesia is highly variable, an estimate of the expected rate of increase is shown in the following Figure.

[See figure at top of next column]

Doses above 20 mg/day should be employed with caution since they may be associated with a higher likelihood of serious side effects (see WARNINGS concerning potential neurological hazards and ADVERSE REACTIONS).

Epidural Dosage: The starting dose must be individualized, based upon in-hospital evaluation of the response to serial single-dose epidural bolus injections of regular DURAMORPH® (Morphine Sulfate Injection, USP) 0.5 mg/mL or 1 mg/mL, with dose observation for analgesic efficacy and adverse effects *prior* to surgery involving the continuous microinfusion device.

The recommended initial epidural dose in patients who are not tolerant to opioids ranges from 3.5 to 7.5 mg/day. The usual starting dose for continuous epidural infusion, based upon limited data in patients who have some degree of opioid tolerance, is 4.5 to 10 mg/day. The dose requirements may increase significantly during treatment,

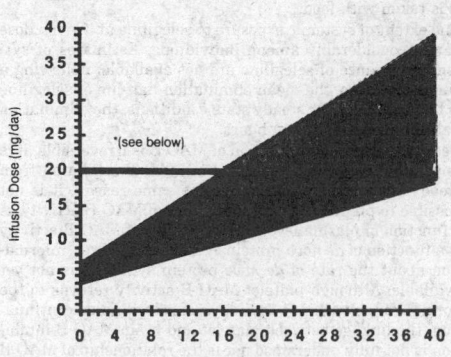

Figure: Dose Trend in Continuous Infusions of Intrathecal Morphine (Mean and 95% Confidence Intervals)

*20 mg/day is the lowest dose for which regional myoclonus has been reported.
The rate of occurrence cannot be estimated.

frequently to 20–30 mg/day. The upper daily limit for each patient must be individualized.

SAFETY AND HANDLING INFORMATION

INFUMORPH® is supplied in sealed ampuls. Accidental dermal exposure should be treated by the removal of any contaminated clothing and rinsing the affected area with water.

Each ampul of INFUMORPH® contains a large amount of potent narcotic which has been associated with abuse and dependence among health care providers. **Due to the limited indications for this product, the risk of overdosage and the risk of its diversion and abuse, it is recommended that special measures be taken to control this product within the hospital or clinic. INFUMORPH® should be subject to rigid accounting, rigorous control of wastage and restricted access.**

This parenteral drug product must be inspected for particulate matter before opening the amber ampul and again for color after removing contents from the ampul. Do not use if the solution in the unopened ampul contains a precipitate which does not disappear upon shaking. After removal, do not use unless the solution is colorless or pale yellow.

HOW SUPPLIED

Amber DOSETTE® ampuls for epidural or intrathecal administration via a continuous microinfusion device.
INFUMORPH® 200 (Preservative-free Morphine Sulfate Sterile Solution) 200 mg/20 mL (10 mg/mL) packaged individually (NDC 0641-1131-31)
INFUMORPH® 500 (Preservative-free Morphine Sulfate Sterile Solution) 500 mg/20 mL (25 mg/mL) packaged individually (NDC 0641-1132-31)
Also available from Elkins-Sinn, Inc. DURAMORPH® (Morphine Sulfate Injection, USP) 5 mg/10 mL (0.5 mg/mL) and 10 mg/10 mL (1 mg/mL). See insert J-1113.
STORAGE
Protect from light. Store in carton at controlled room temperature 15°–30°C (59°–86°F) until ready to use. DO NOT FREEZE. INFUMORPH® contains no preservative or antioxidant. DISCARD ANY UNUSED PORTION. DO NOT HEAT-STERILIZE.

＊　＊　＊　＊　＊
Manufactured by
ELKINS-SINN, INC. Cherry Hill, NJ 08003-4099
A subsidiary of A.H. Robins Company

SOTRADECOL® ℞
[sō 'trah "de 'kol "]
(Sodium Tetradecyl Sulfate Injection)
For Intravenous Use Only

DESCRIPTION

Sodium tetradecyl sulfate is an anionic surfactant which occurs as a white, waxy solid. The structural formula is as follows:

$$CH_3(CH_2)_3CH(CH_2)_2CHOSONa$$
with $CH_2CH(CH_3)_2$ and C_2H_5 groups

$C_{14}H_{29}NaSO_4$
7-Ethyl-2-methyl-4-hendecanol sulfate sodium salt
M.W. 316.44

Sotradecol® (Sodium Tetradecyl Sulfate Injection) is a sterile nonpyrogenic solution for intravenous use as a sclerosing agent. Each mL contains sodium tetradecyl sulfate 10 mg or 30 mg, benzyl alcohol 0.02 mL and dibasic sodium phosphate, anhydrous 0.72 mg in Water for Injection. pH 7.9; monobasic sodium phosphate and/or sodium hydroxide added, if needed, for pH adjustment.

CLINICAL PHARMACOLOGY

Sotradecol® (Sodium Tetradecyl Sulfate Injection) is a mild sclerosing agent. Intravenous injection causes intima inflammation and thrombus formation. This usually occludes the injected vein. Subsequent formation of fibrous tissue results in partial or complete vein obliteration.

INDICATIONS AND USAGE

Indicated in the treatment of small uncomplicated varicose veins of the lower extremities that show simple dilation with competent valves. The benefit-to-risk ratio should be considered in selected patients who are great surgical risks.

CONTRAINDICATIONS

Contraindicated in previous hypersensitivity reactions to the drug; in acute superficial thrombophlebitis; significant valvular or deep vein incompetence; huge superficial veins with wide open communications to deeper veins; phlebitis migrans; acute cellulitis; allergic conditions; acute infections; varicosities caused by abdominal and pelvic tumors unless the tumor has been removed; bedridden patients; such uncontrolled systemic diseases as diabetes, toxic hyperthyroidism, tuberculosis, asthma, neoplasm, sepsis, blood dyscrasias and acute respiratory or skin diseases.

WARNINGS

Since severe adverse local effects, including tissue necrosis, may occur following extravasation, Sotradecol® (Sodium Tetradecyl Sulfate Injection), should be administered only by a physician familiar with proper injection technique. Extreme care in needle placement and using the minimal effective volume at each injection site are, therefore, important.
Allergic reactions, including anaphylaxis, have been reported that led to death. Therefore, as a precaution against anaphylactic shock, it is recommended that 0.5 mL of Sotradecol® be injected into a varicosity, followed by observation of the patient for several hours before administration of a second or larger dose. The possibility of an anaphylactic reaction should be kept in mind, and the physician should be prepared to treat it appropriately. In extreme emergencies, 0.25 mL of 1:1000 Epinephrine Injection (0.25 mg) intravenously should be used and side reactions controlled with antihistamines.

PRECAUTIONS

GENERAL

The drug should only be administered by physicians who are familiar with an acceptable injection technique. Because of the danger of thrombosis extension into the deep venous system, thorough preinjection evaluation for valvular competency should be carried out and slow injections with a small amount (not over 2 mL) of the preparation should be injected into the varicosity. In particular, deep venous patency must be determined by angiography and/or the Perthes test before sclerotherapy is undertaken. Venous sclerotherapy should not be undertaken if tests, such as the Trendelenberg and Perthes, and angiography show significant valvular or deep venous incompetence. The physician should bear in mind that injection necrosis is likely to result from extravascular injection of sclerosing agents.
Extreme caution must be exercised in the presence of underlying arterial disease such as marked peripheral arteriosclerosis or thromboangiitis obliterans (Buerger's Disease). Embolism may occur as long as four weeks after injection of sodium tetradecyl sulfate. The incidence of recurrence is low if the patient wears elastic stockings.

DRUG INTERACTIONS

No well-controlled studies have been performed on patients taking antiovulatory agents. The physician must use judgment and evaluate any patient taking antiovulatory drugs prior to initiating treatment with Sotradecol®. (See ADVERSE REACTIONS.)
Heparin should not be included in the same syringe as Sotradecol®, since the two are incompatible.

CARCINOGENESIS, MUTAGENESIS, IMPAIRMENT OF FERTILITY

When tested in the L5178YTK⁺/⁻ mouse lymphoma assay, sodium tetradecyl sulfate did not induce a dose-related increase in the frequency of thymidine kinase-deficient mutants and, therefore, was judged to be nonmutagenic in this system. However, no long-term animal carcinogenicity studies with sodium tetradecyl sulfate have been performed.

PREGNANCY

Teratogenic Effects—Pregnancy Category C. Animal reproduction studies have not been conducted with Sotradecol®. It is also not known whether Sotradecol® can cause fetal harm when administered to a pregnant woman or can affect reproduction capacity. Sotradecol® should be given to a pregnant woman only if clearly needed.

NURSING MOTHERS

It is not known whether this drug is excreted in human milk. Because many drugs are excreted in human milk, caution should be exercised when Sotradecol® is administered to a nursing woman.

PEDIATRIC USE

Safety and effectiveness in pediatric patients have not been established.

ADVERSE REACTIONS

Local reactions consisting of pain, urticaria or ulceration may occur at the site of injection. A permanent discoloration, usually small and hardly noticeable but which may be objectionable from a cosmetic viewpoint, may remain along the path of the sclerosed vein segment. Sloughing and necrosis of tissue may occur following extravasation of the drug.
Allergic reactions such as hives, asthma, hayfever and anaphylactic shock have been reported. Mild systemic reactions that have been reported include headache, nausea and vomiting. (See WARNINGS.)
Four deaths have been reported with the use of Sotradecol®. One death has been reported in a patient who received Sotradecol® and who had been receiving an antiovulatory agent. Another death (fatal pulmonary embolism) has been reported in a 36-year-old female treated with sodium tetradecyl acetate and who was **not** taking oral contraceptives. Two cases of anaphylactic shock leading to death have been reported in patients who received Sotradecol®. One of the patients reported a medical history of asthma, a contraindication to the administration of Sotradecol®.

DOSAGE AND ADMINISTRATION

For intravenous use only. Do not use if precipitated or discolored. The strength of solution required depends on the size and degree of varicosity. In general, the 1% solution will be found most useful with the 3% solution preferred for larger varicosities. The dosage should be kept small, using 0.5 to 2 mL (preferably 1 mL maximum) for each injection, and the maximum single treatment should not exceed 10 mL.
Parenteral drug products should be inspected visually for particulate matter and discoloration prior to administration, whenever solution and container permit.

HOW SUPPLIED

Sotradecol® (Sodium Tetradecyl Sulfate Injection)
1%—2 mL DOSETTE® ampuls packaged in 5s (NDC 0641-1514-34)
3%—2 mL DOSETTE® ampuls packaged in 5s (NDC 0641-1516-34)
STORAGE
Store at controlled room temperature 15°–30°C (59°–86°F).

ANIMAL TOXICOLOGY

The intravenous LD_{50} of sodium tetradecyl sulfate in mice was reported to be 90 ± 5 mg/kg.
In the rat, the acute intravenous LD_{50} of sodium tetradecyl sulfate was estimated to be between 72 mg/kg and 108 mg/kg.
Purified sodium tetradecyl sulfate was found to have an LD_{50} of 2 g/kg when administered orally by stomach tube as a 25% aqueous solution to rats. In rats given 0.15 g/kg in drinking water for 30 days, no appreciable toxicity was seen, although some growth inhibition was discernible.

＊　＊　＊　＊
Manufactured by
ELKINS-SINN, INC., Cherry Hill, NJ 08003-4099
A division of A.H. Robins Company

ENDO PHARMACEUTICALS INC.

223 Wilmington West Chester Pike
Chadds Ford, PA 19317
Endo Laboratories
Endo Generic Products

Direct Inquiries to:
Customer Service:
(800) 462-3636
Fax: (302) 992-3006
For Medical Information/Adverse Drug Experience Reporting Contact:
(800) 462-3636

Other Products Available:

Amantadine HCl Syrup, USP
Amiloride HCl and HCTZ Tablets, USP
Captopril Tablets, USP
Captopril/HCTZ Tablets, USP
Carbidopa and Levodopa Tablets, USP

Continued on next page

Product Listing - Endo—Cont.

Cimetidine Tablets, USP
Cimetidine HCl Injection
Cimetidine HCl Oral Solution
Cyclobenzaprine HCl Tablets, USP
Dicyclomine HCl Capsules, USP
Dicyclomine HCl Tablets, USP
Diflunisal Tablets, USP
Endocet Tablets, USP CII
Endodan Tablets, USP CII
Etodolac Capsules
Etodolac Tablets
Glipizide Tablets, USP
Hydrochlorothiazide Tablets, USP
Hydrocodone Bitartrate/APAP Tablets, USP CIII
Hydromorphone HCl Tablets, USP CII
Indomethacin Extended-Release Capsules, USP
Methyldopa Tablets, USP
Methyldopa/HCTZ Tablets, USP
Selegiline HCl Tablets, USP
Sulindac Tablets, USP
Timolol Maleate Tablets, USP

CARBEX® ℞

[*căr-bĕx*]
(selegiline hydrochloride) Tablets, USP

DESCRIPTION

CARBEX (selegiline hydrochloride) is a levorotatory acetylenic derivative of phenethylamine. It is commonly referred to in the clinical and pharmacological literature as L-deprenyl.
The chemical name is: (R)-(-)-N,2-dimethyl-N-2-propynylphenethylamine hydrochloride. It is a white to near white crystalline powder, freely soluble in water, chloroform, and methanol. The molecular formula is $C_{13}H_{17}N \bullet HCl$; and the molecular weight is 223.75. The structural formula is as follows:

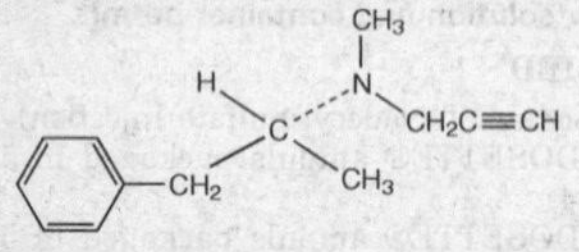

Each tablet, for oral administration, contains selegiline hydrochloride, 5 mg and the following inactive ingredients: corn starch, lactose monohydrate, magnesium stearate, povidone, and talc.

CLINICAL PHARMACOLOGY

The mechanisms accounting for selegiline's beneficial adjunctive action in the treatment of Parkinson's disease are not fully understood. Inhibition of monoamine oxidase, type B, activity is generally considered to be of primary importance; in addition, there is evidence that selegiline may act through other mechanisms to increase dopaminergic activity.
Selegiline is best known as an irreversible inhibitor of monoamine oxidase (MAO), an intracellular enzyme associated with the outer membrane of mitochondria. Selegiline inhibits MAO by acting as a 'suicide' substrate for the enzyme; that is, it is converted by MAO to an active moiety which combines irreversibly with the active site and/or the enzyme's essential FAD cofactor. Because selegiline has greater affinity for type B rather than for type A active sites, it can serve as a selective inhibitor of MAO type B if it is administered at the recommended dose.
MAOs are widely distributed throughout the body; their concentration is especially high in liver, kidney, stomach, intestinal wall, and brain. MAOs are currently subclassified into two types, A and B, which differ in their substrate specificity and tissue distribution. In humans, intestinal MAO is predominantly type A, while most of that in brain is type B. In CNS neurons, MAO plays an important role in the catabolism of catecholamines (dopamine, norepinephrine and epinephrine) and serotonin. MAOs are also important in the catabolism of various exogenous amines found in a variety of foods and drugs. MAO in the GI tract and liver (primarily type A), for example, is thought to provide vital protection from exogenous amines (e.g., tyramine) that have the capacity, if absorbed intact, to cause a 'hypertensive crisis', the so-called 'cheese reaction'. (If large amounts of certain exogenous amines gain access to the systemic circulation – e.g., from fermented cheese, red wine, herring, over-the-counter cough/cold medications, etc. – they are taken up by adrenergic neurons and displace norepinephrine from storage sites within membrane bound vesicles. Subsequent release of the displaced norepinephrine causes the rise in systemic blood pressure, etc.)
In theory, since MAO A of the gut is not inhibited, patients treated with selegiline at a dose of 10 mg a day should be able to take medications containing pharmacologically active amines and consume tyramine-containing foods without risk of uncontrolled hypertension. Although rare, a few reports of hypertensive reactions have occurred in patients receiving selegiline at the recommended dose, with tyramine-containing foods. In addition, one case of hypertensive crisis has been reported in a patient taking the recommended dose of selegiline and a sympathomimetic medication, ephedrine. The pathophysiology of the 'cheese reaction' is complicated and, in addition to its ability to inhibit MAO B selectively, selegiline's relative freedom from this reaction has been attributed to an ability to prevent tyramine and other indirect acting sympathomimetics from displacing norepinephrine from adrenergic neurons. However, until the pathophysiology of the cheese reaction is more completely understood, it seems prudent to assume that selegiline can ordinarily only be used safely without dietary restrictions at doses where it presumably selectively inhibits its MAO B (e.g., 10 mg/day).
In short, attention to the dose dependent nature of selegiline's selectivity is critical if it is to be used without elaborate restrictions being placed on diet and concomitant drug use although, as noted above, a few cases of hypertensive reactions have been reported at the recommended dose. (See WARNINGS and PRECAUTIONS.)
It is important to be aware that selegiline may have pharmacological effects unrelated to MAO B inhibition. As noted above, there is some evidence that it may increase dopaminergic activity by other mechanisms, including interfering with dopamine re-uptake at the synapse. Effects resulting from selegiline administration may also be mediated through its metabolites. Two of its three principle metabolites, amphetamine and methamphetamine, have pharmacological actions of their own; they interfere with neuronal uptake and enhance release of several neurotransmitters (e.g., norepinephrine, dopamine, serotonin). However, the extent to whcih these metabolites contribute to the effects of selegiline are unknown.

Rationale for the Use of a Selective Monoamine Oxidase Type B Inhibitor in Parkinson's Disease:
Many of the prominent symptoms of Parkinson's disease are due to a deficiency of striatal dopamine that is the consequence of a progressive degeneration and loss of a population of dopaminergic neurons which originate in the substantia nigra of the midbrain and project to the basal ganglia or striatum. Early in the course of Parkinson's disease, the deficit in the capacity of these neurons to synthesize dopamine can be overcome by administration of exogenous levodopa, usually given in combination with a peripheral decarboxylase inhibitor (carbidopa).
With the passage of time, due to the progression of the disease and/or the effect of sustained treatment, the efficacy and quality of the therapeutic response to levodopa diminishes. Thus, after several years of levodopa treatment, the response, for a given dose of levodopa, is shorter, has less predictable onset and offset (i.e., there is 'wearing off'), and is often accompanied by side effects (e.g., dyskinesia, akinesias, on-off phenomena, freezing, etc.).
This deteriorating response is currently interpreted as a manifestation of the inability of the ever decreasing population of intact nigrostriatal neurons to synthesize and release adequate amounts of dopamine.
MAO B inhibition may be useful in this setting because, by blocking the catabolism of dopamine, it would increase the net amount of dopamine available (i.e., it would increase the pool of dopamine). Whether or not this mechanism or an alternative one actually accounts for the observed beneficial effects of adjunctive selegiline is unknown.
Selegiline's benefit in Parkinson's disease has only been documented as an adjunct to levodopa/carbidopa. Whether or not it might be effective as a sole treatment is unknown, but past attempts to treat Parkinson's disease with non-selective MAOI monotherapy are reported to have been unsuccessful. It is important to note that attempts to treat Parkinsonian patients with combinations of levodopa and currently marketed non-selective MAO inhibitors were abondoned because of multiple side effects including hypertension, increase in involuntary movement, and toxic delirium.

Pharmacokinetic Information (Absorption, Distribution, Metabolism and Elimination – ADME):
The absolute bioavailability of selegiline following oral dosing is not known; however, selegiline undergoes extensive metabolism (presumably attributable to presystemic clearance in gut and liver). The major plasma metabolites are N-desmethylselegiline, L-amphetamine and L-methamphetamine. Only N-desmethylselegiline has MAO B inhibiting activity. The peak plasma levels of these metabolites following a single oral dose of 10 mg are from 4 to almost 20 times greater than that of the maximum plasma concentration of selegiline (1 ng/mL). The maximum concentrations of amphetamine and methamphetamine, however, are far below those ordinarily expected to produce clinically important effects.
Single oral dose studies do not predict multiple dose kinetics, however. At steady state, the peak plasma level of selegiline is 4 fold that obtained following a single dose. Metabolite concentrations increase to a lesser extent, averaging 2 fold that seen after a single dose.
The bioavailability of selegiline is increased 3 to 4 fold when it is taken with food.
The extent of systemic exposure to selegiline at a given dose varies considerably among individuals. Estimates of systemic clearance of selegiline are not available. Following a single oral dose, the mean elimination half-life of selegiline is two hours. Under steady state conditions, the elimination half-life increases to ten hours.
Because selegiline's inhibition of MAO B is irreversible, it is impossible to predict the extent of MAO B inhibition from steady state plasma levels. For the same reason, it is not possible to predict the rate of recovery of MAO B activity as a function of plasma levels. The recovery of MAO B activity is a function of *de novo* protein synthesis; however, information about the rate of *de novo* protein synthesis is not yet available. Although platelet MAO B activity returns to the normal range within 5 to 7 days of selegiline discontinuation, the linkage between platelet and brain MAO B inhibition is not fully understood nor is the relationship of MAO B inhibition to the clinical effect established (see **CLINICAL PHARMACOLOGY**).

Special Populations:

Renal Impairment:
No pharmacokinetic information is available on selegiline or its matabolites in renally impaired subjects.

Hepatic Impairment:
No pharmacokinetic information is available on selegiline or its metabolites in hepatically impaired subjects.

Age:
Although a general conclusion about the effects of age on the pharmacokinetics of selegiline is not warranted because of the size of the sample evaluated (12 subjects greater than 60 years of age, 12 subjects between the ages of 18 to 30), systemic exposure was about twice as great in older as compared to a younger population given a single oral dose of 10 mg.

Gender:
No information is available on the effects of gender on the pharmacokinetics of selegiline.

INDICATIONS AND USAGE

CARBEX (selegiline hydrochloride) is indicated as an adjunct in the management of Parkinsonian patients being treated with levodopa/carbidopa who exhibit deterioration in the quality of their response to this therapy. There is no evidence from controlled studies that selegiline has any beneficial effect in the absence of concurrent levodopa therapy.
Evidence supporting this claim was obtained in randomized controlled clinical investigations that compared the effects of added selegiline or placebo in patients receiving levodopa/carbidopa. Selegiline was significantly superior to placebo on all three principal outcome measures employed: change from baseline in daily levodopa/carbidopa dose, the amount of 'off' time, and patient self-rating of treatment success. Beneficial effects were also observed on other measures of treatment success (e.g., measures of reduced end of dose akinesia, decreased tremor and sialorrhea, improved speech and dressing ability and improved overall disability as assessed by walking and comparison to prevoious state).

CONTRAINDICATIONS

CARBEX is contraindicated in patients with a known hypersensitivity to this drug.
CARBEX is contraindicated for use with meperidine. This contraindication is often extended to other opioids. (See **Drug Interactions.**)

WARNINGS

Selegiline should not be used at daily doses exceeding those recommended (10 mg/day) because of the risks associated with non-selective inhibition of MAO. (See CLINICAL PHARMACOLOGY.)
The selectivity of selegiline for MAO B may be absolute even at the recommended daily dose of 10 mg a day. Rare cases of hypertensive reactions associated with ingestion of tyramine-containing foods have been reported in patients taking the recommended daily dose of selegiline. The selectivity is further diminished with increasing daily doses. The precise dose at which selegiline becomes a non-selective inhibitor of all MAO is unknown, but may be in the range of 30 to 40 mg a day.
Severe CNS toxicity associated with hyperpyrexia and death have been reported with the combination of tricyclic antidepressants and non-selective MAOIs (Phenelzine, Tranylcypromine). A similar reaction has been reported for a patient on amitriptyline and selegiline. Another patient receiving protriptyline and selegiline developed tremors, agitation, and restlessness followed by unresponsiveness and death two weeks after selegiline was added. Related adverse events including hypertension, syncope, asystole, diaphoresis, seizures, changes in behavioral and mental status,

and muscular rigidity have also been reported in some patients receiving selegiline and various tricyclic antidepressants.

Serious, sometimes fatal, reactions with signs and symptoms that may include hyperthermia, rigidity, myoclonus, autonomic instability with rapid fluctuations of the vital signs, and mental status changes that include extreme agitation progressing to delirium and coma have been reported with patients receiving a combination of fluoxetine hydrochloride and non-selective MAOIs. Similar signs have been reported in some patients on the combination of selegiline (10 mg a day) and selective serotonin reuptake inhibitors including fluoxetine, sertraline and paroxetine.

Since the mechanisms of these reactions are not fully understood, it seems prudent, in general, to avoid this combination of selegiline and tricyclic antidepressants as well as selegiline and selective serotonin reuptake inhibitors. At least 14 days should elapse between discontinuation of selegiline and initiation of treatment with a tricyclic antidepressant or selective serotonin reuptake inhibitors. Because of the long half-lives or fluoxetine and its active metabolite, at least five weeks (perhaps longer, especially if fluoxetine has been prescribed chronically and/or at higher doses) should elapse between discontinuation of fluoxetine and initiation of treatment with selegiline.

PRECAUTIONS

General:

Some patients given selegiline may experience an exacerbation of levodopa associated side effects, presumably due to the increased amounts of dopamine reaction with super sensitive post-synaptic receptors. These effects may often be mitigated by reducing the dose of levodopa/carbidopa by approximately 10 to 30%.

The decision to prescribe selegiline should take into consideration that the MAO system of enzymes is complex and incompletely understood and there is only a limited amount of carefully documented clinical experience with selegiline. Consequently, the full spectrum of possible responses to selegiline may not have been observed in pre-marketing evaluation of the drug. It is advisable, therefore, to observe patients closely for atypical responses.

Information for Patients:

Patients should be advised of the possible need to reduce levodopa dosage after the initiation of CARBEX therapy. Patients (or their families if the patient is incompetent) should be advised not to exceed the daily recommended dose of 10 mg. The risk of using higher daily doses of selegiline should be explained, and a brief description of the 'cheese reaction' provided. Rare hypertensive reactions with selegiline at recommended doses associated with dietary influences have been reported.

Consequently, it may be useful to inform patients (or their families) about the signs and symptoms associated with MAOI induced hypertensive reactions. In particular, patients should be urged to report, immediately, any severe headache or other atypical or unusual symptoms not previously experienced.

Laboratory Tests:

No specific laboratoy tests are deemed essential for the management of patients on CARBEX. Periodic routine evaluation of all patients, however, is appropriate.

Drug Interactions:

The occurrence of stupor, muscular rigidity, severe agitation, and elevated temperature has been reported in some patients receiving the combination of selegiline and meperidine. Symptoms usually resolve over days when the combination is discontinued. This is typical of the interaction of meperidine and MAOIs. Other serious reactions (including severe agitation, hallucinations, and death) have been reported in patients receiving this combination (see **CONTRAINDICATIONS**). Severe toxicity has also been reported in patients receiving the combination of tricyclic antidepressants and selegiline and selective serotonin reuptake inhibitors and selegiline. (See **WARNINGS** for details.) One case of hypertensive crisis has been reported in a patient taking the recommended doses of selegiline and a sympathomimetic medication (ephedrine).

Carcinogenesis, Mutagenesis, and Impairment of Fertility:

Assessment of the carcinogenic potential of selegiline in mice and rats is ongoing.

Selegiline did not induce mutations or chromosomal damage when tested in the bacterial mutation assay in *Salmonella typhimurium* and an *in vivo* chromosomal aberration assay. While these studies provide some reassurance that selegiline is not mutagenic or clastogenic, they are not definitive because of methodological limitations. No definitive *in vitro* chromosomal aberration or *in vitro* mammalian gene mutation assays have been performed.

The effect of selegiline on fertility has not been adequately assessed.

Pregnancy:

Pregnancy, Teratogenic Effects, Pregnancy Category C. No teratogenic effects were observed in a study of embryo-fetal development in Sprague-Dawley rats at oral doses of 4, 12, and 36 mg/kg or 4, 12 and 35 times the human therapeutic

dose of a mg/m² basis. No teratogenic effects were observed in a study of embryo-fetal development in New Zealand White rabbits at oral doses of 5, 25, and 50 mg/kg or 10, 48, and 95 times the human therapeutic dose on a mg/m² basis; however, in this study, the number of litters produced at the two higher doses was less than recommended for assessing teratogenic potential. In the rat study, there was a decrease in fetal body weight at the highest dose tested. In the rabbit study, increases in total resorptions and % post-implantation loss, and a decrease in the number of live fetuses per dam occurred at the highest dose tested. In a peri- and postnatal development study in Sprague-Dawley rats (oral doses of 4, 16, and 64 mg/kg or 4, 15, and 62 times the human therapeutic dose on a mg/m² basis), an increase in the number of stillbirths and decreases in the number of pups per dam, pup survival, and pup body weight (at birth and throughout the lactation period) were observed at the two highest doses. At the highest dose tested, no pups born alive survived to Day 4 postpartum. Postnatal development at the highest dose tested in dams could not be evaluated because of the lack of surviving pups. The reproductive performance of the untreated offspring was not assessed.

There are no adequate and well-controlled studies in pregnant women. Selegiline should be used during pregnancy only if the potential benefit justifies the potential risk to the fetus.

Nursing Mothers:

It is not known whether selegiline hydrochloride is excreted in human milk. Because many drugs are excreted in human milk, consideration should be given to discontinuing the use of all but absolutely essential drug treatments in nursing women.

Pediatric Use:

The effects of selegiline hydrochloride in pediatric patients have not been evaluated.

ADVERSE REACTIONS

Introduction:

The number of patients who received selegiline in prospectively monitored pre-marketing studies is limited. While other sources of information about the use of selegiline are available (e.g., literature reports, foreign post-marketing reports, etc.) they do not provide the kind of information necessary to estimate the incidence of adverse events. Thus, overall incidence figures for adverse reactions associated with the use of selegiline cannot be provided. Many of the adverse reactions seen have also been reported as symptoms of dopamine excess.

Moreover, the importance and severity of various reactions reported often cannot be ascertained. One index of relative importance, however, is whether or not a reaction caused treatment discontinuation. In prospective pre-marketing studies, the following events led, in decreasing order of frequency, to discontinuation of treatment with selegiline: nausea, hallucinations, confusion, depression, loss of balance, insomnia, orthostatic hypotension, increased akinetic involuntary movements, agitation, arrhythmia, bradykinesia, chorea, delusions, hypertension, new or increased angina pectoris and syncope. Events reported only once as a cause of discontinuation are ankle edema, anxiety, burning lips/mouth, constipation, drowsiness/lethargy, dystonia, excess perspiration, increased freezing, gastrointestinal bleeding, hair loss, increased tremor, nervousness, weakness and weight loss.

Experience with selegiline hydrochloride obtained in parallel, placebo controlled, randomized studies provides only a limited basis for estimates of adverse reaction rates. The following reactions that occurred with greater frequency among the 49 patients assigned to selegiline as compared to the 50 patients assigned to placebo in the only parallel, placebo controlled trial performed in patients with Parkinson's disease are shown in the following Table. None of these adverse reactions led to a discontinuation of treatment.

INCIDENCE OF TREATMENT-EMERGENT ADVERSE EXPERIENCES IN THE PLACEBO-CONTROLLED CLINICAL TRIAL

Adverse Event	Number of Patients Reporting Events	
	selegiline hydrochloride N=49	placebo N=50
Nausea	10	3
Dizziness/Lightheaded/ Fainting	7	1
Abdominal Pain	4	2
Confusion	3	0
Hallucinations	3	1
Dry mouth	3	1
Vivid Dreams	2	0
Dyskinesias	2	5
Headache	2	1

The following events were reported once in either or both groups:

Ache, generalized	1	0
Anxiety/Tension	1	1
Anemia	0	1
Diarrhea	1	0
Hair Loss	0	1
Insomnia	1	1
Lethargy	1	0
Leg Pain	1	0
Low back pain	1	0
Malaise	0	1
Palpitations	1	0
Urinary Retention	1	0
Weight Loss	1	0

In all prospectively monitored clinical investigations, enrolling approximately 920 patients, the following adverse events, classified by body system, were reported.

Central Nervous System:

Motor/Coordination/Extrapyramidal:

increased tremor, chorea, loss of balance, restlessness, blepharospasm, increased bradykinesia, facial grimace, falling down, heavy leg, muscle twitch*, myoclonic jerks*, stiff neck, tardive dyskinesia, dystonic symptoms, dyskinesia, involuntary movements, freezing, festination, increased apraxia, muscle cramps.

Mental Status/Behavioral/Psychiatric:

hallucinations, dizziness, confusion, anxiety, depression, drowsiness, behavior/mood change, dreams/nightmares, tiredness, delusions, disorientation, lightheadedness, impaired memory*, increased energy*, transient high*, hollow feeling, lethargy/malaise, apathy, overstimulation, vertigo, personality change, sleep disturbance, restlessness, weakness, transient irritability.

Pain/Altered Sensation:

headache, back pain, leg pain, tinnitus, migraine, supraorbital pain, throat burning, generalized ache, chills, numbness of toes/fingers, taste disturbance.

Autonomic Nervous System:

dry mouth, blurred vision, sexual dysfunction.

Cardiovascular:

orthostatic hypotension, hypertension, arrhythmia, palpitations, new or increased angina pectoris, hypotension, tachycardia, peripheral edema, sinus bradycardia, syncope.

Gastrointestinal:

nausea/vomiting, constipation, weight loss, anorexia, poor appetite, dysphagia, diarrhea, heartburn, rectal bleeding, bruxism*, gastrointestinal bleeding (exacerbation of preexisting ulcer disease).

Genitourinary/Gynecologic/Endocrine:

slow urination, transient anorgasmia*, nocturia, prostatic hypertrophy, urinary hesitancy, urinary retention, decreased penile sensation*, urinary frequency.

Skin and Appendages:

increased sweating, diaphoresis, facial hair, hair loss, hematoma, rash, photosensitivity.

Miscellaneous:

asthma, diplopia, shortness of breath, speech affected.

Postmarketing Reports:

The following experiences were described in spontaneous post-marketing reports. These reports do not provide sufficient information to establish a clear causal relationship with the use of CARBEX (selegiline hydrochloride).

CNS:

Seizure in dialyzed chronic renal failure patient on concomitant medications.

---

*indicates events reported only at doses greater than 10 mg/day.

OVERDOSAGE

Selegiline:

No specific information is available about clinically significant overdoses with CARBEX. However, experience gained during selegiline's development reveals that some individuals exposed to doses of 600 mg of d,l-selegiline suffered severe hypotension and psychomotor agitation.

Since the selective inhibition of MAO B by selegiline hydrochloride is achieved only at doses in the range recommended for the treatment of Parkinson's disease (e.g., 10 mg/day), overdoses are likely to cause significant inhibition of both MAO A and MAO B. Consequently, the signs and symptoms of overdose may resemble those observed with marketed non-selective MAO inhibitors (e.g., tranylcypromine, isocarboxazide, and phenelzine).

Overdose with Non-Selective MAO Inhibition:

NOTE: This section is provided for reference; it does not describe events that have actually been observed with selegiline in overdose.

Characteristically, signs and symptoms of non-selective MAOI overdose may not appear immediately. Delays of up to 12 hours between ingestion of drug and the appearance of

Continued on next page

Carbex—Cont.

signs may occur. Importantly, the peak intensity of the syndrome may not be reached for upwards of a day following the overdose. Death has been reported following overdosage. Therefore, immediate hospitalization, with continuous patient observation and monitoring for a period of at least two days following the ingestion of such drugs in overdose, is strongly recommended.

The clinical picture of MAOI overdose varies considerably; its severity may be a function of the amount of drug consumed. The central nervous and cardiovascular systems are prominently involved.

Signs and symptoms of overdosage may include, alone or in combination, any of the following: drowsiness, dizziness, faintness, irritability, hyperactivity, agitation, severe headache, hallucinations, trismus, opisthotonos, convulsions, and coma; rapid and irregular pulse, hypertension, hypotension and vascular collapse; precordial pain, respiratory depression and failure, hyperpyrexia, diaphoresis, and cool, clammy skin.

Treatment Suggestions For Overdose:
NOTE: Because there is no recorded experience with selegiline overdose, the following suggestions are offered based upon the assumption that selegiline overdose may be modeled by non-selective MAOI poisoning. In any case, up-to-date information about the treatment of overdose can often be obtained from a certified Regional Poison Control Center. Telephone numbers of certified Poison Control Centers are listed in the Physicians' Desk Reference (PDR). Treatment of overdose with non-selective MAOIs is symptomatic and supportive. Induction of emesis or gastric lavage with instillation of charcoal slurry may be helpful in early poisoning, provided the airway has been protected against aspiration. Signs and symptoms of central nervous system stimulation, including convulsions, should be treated with diazepam, given slowly intravenously. Phenothiazine derivatives and central nervous system stimulants should be avoided. Hypotension and vascular collapse should be treated with intravenous fluids and, if necessary, blood pressure titration with an intravenous infusion of a dilute pressor agent. It should be noted that adrenergic agents may produce a markedly increased pressor response. Respiration should be supported by appropriate measures, including management of the airway, use of supplemental oxygen, and mechanical ventilatory assistance, as required. Body temperature should be monitored closely. Intensive management of hyperpyrexia may be required. Maintenance of fluid and electrolyte balance is essential.

DOSAGE AND ADMINISTRATION

CARBEX (selegiline hydrochloride) is intended for administration to Parkinsonian patients receiving levodopa/carbidopa therapy who demonstrate a deteriorating response to this treatment. The recomended regimen for the administration of CARBEX is 10 mg per day administered as divided doses of 5 mg each taken at breakfast and lunch. There is no evidence that additional benefit will be obtained from the administration of higher doses. Moreover, higher doses should ordinarily be avoided because of the increased risk of side effects.

After two or three days of selegiline treatment, an attempt may be made to reduce the dose of levodopa/carbidopa. A reduction of 10 to 30% was achieved with the typical participant in the domestic placebo controlled trials who was assigned to selegiline treatment. Further reductions of levodopa/carbidopa may be possible during continued selegiline therapy.

HOW SUPPLIED

CARBEX (selegiline hydrochloride) Tablets, USP are supplied as follows:
5 mg – white, oval tablets; debossed with "CARBEX" on one side and plain on the other.

   Bottles of 60   NDC 63481-408-60
Store at controlled room temperature, 15°–30°C (59°–86°F). Dispense in a tight, light-resistant container, as defined in the USP, with a child-resistant closure (as required).
Rx only
CARBEX® is a registered trademark of Endo Pharmaceuticals Inc.
Copyright © Endo Pharmaceuticals Inc. 1998
                    6493-01/Rev. May, 1998
Shown in Product Identification Guide, page 309

HYCODAN®   Ⓒ
[hī-kō-dan]
(hydrocodone bitartrate and homatropine methylbromide)
Tablets and Syrup
Antitussive

DESCRIPTION

HYCODAN contains hydrocodone (dihydrocodeinone) bitartrate, a semisynthetic centrally-acting narcotic antitussive. Homatropine methylbromide is included in a subtherapeutic amount to discourage deliberate overdosage.

Each HYCODAN tablet or teaspoonful (5 mL) contains:
Hydrocodone bitartrate, USP   5 mg
WARNING: May be habit forming.
Homatropine methylbromide, USP   1.5 mg
HYCODAN tablets also contain: calcium phosphate dibasic, colloidal silicon dioxide, lactose, magnesium stearate, starch and stearic acid.
HYCODAN syrup: caramel coloring, FD&C Red 40, liquid sugar, methylparaben, propylparaben, sorbitol solution and wild cherry imitation flavor.
The hydrocodone component is 4,5α-epoxy-3-methoxy-17-methylmorphinan-6-one tartrate (1:1) hydrate (2:5), a fine white crystal or crystalline powder, which is derived from the opium alkaloid, thebaine, has a molecular weight of (494.50) and may be represented by the following structural formula.

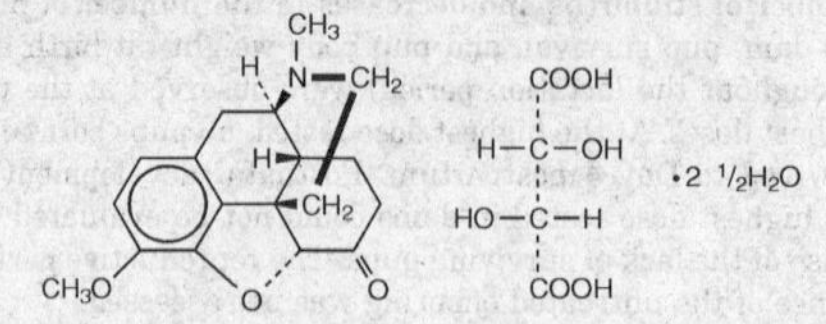

$C_{18}H_{21}NO_3 \cdot C_4H_6O_6 \cdot 2 \; ^1/_2 H_2O$
HYDROCODONE BITARTRATE

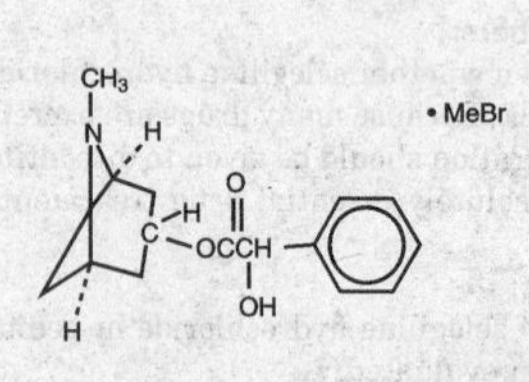

$C_{17}H_{24}BrNO_3$
HOMATROPINE METHYLBROMIDE

Homatropine methylbromide is 8-Azoniabicyclo[3.2.1] octane, 3- [(hydroxyphenylacetyl) oxy] -8, 8-dimethyl-, bromide, endo-; a white crystal or fine white crystalline powder, with a molecular weight of (370.29).

CLINICAL PHARMACOLOGY

Hydrocodone is a semisynthetic narcotic antitussive and analgesic with multiple actions qualitatively similar to those of codeine. The precise mechanism of action of hydrocodone and other opiates is not known; however, hydrocodone is believed to act directly on the cough center. In excessive doses, hydrocodone, like other opium derivatives, will depress respiration. The effects of hydrocodone in therapeutic doses on the cardiovascular system are insignificant. Hydrocodone can produce miosis, euphoria, physical and physiological dependence.

Following a 10 mg oral dose of hydrocodone administered to five adult male subjects, the mean peak concentration was 23.6 ± 5.2 ng/mL. Maximum serum levels were achieved at 1.3 ± 0.3 hours and the half-life was determined to be 3.8 ± 0.3 hours. Hydrocodone exhibits a complex pattern of metabolism including O-demethylation, N-demethylation and 6-keto reduction to the corresponding 6-α-and 6-β-hydroxymetabolites.

INDICATIONS AND USAGE

HYCODAN (hydrocodone bitartrate and homatropine methylbromide) is indicated for the symptomatic relief of cough.

CONTRAINDICATIONS

HYCODAN should not be administered to patients who are hypersensitive to hydrocodone or homatropine methylbromide.

WARNINGS

May be habit forming. Hydrocodone can produce drug dependence of the morphine type and, therefore, has the potential for being abused. Psychic dependence, physical dependence and tolerance may develop upon repeated administration of HYCODAN and it should be prescribed and administered with the same degree of caution appropriate to the use of other narcotic drugs (see DRUG ABUSE AND DEPENDENCE).

Respiratory Depression: HYCODAN produces dose-related respiratory depression by directly acting on brain stem respiratory centers. If respiratory depression occurs, it may be antagonized by the use of naloxone hydrochloride and other supportive measures when indicated.

Head Injury And Increased Intracranial Pressure: The respiratory depression properties of narcotics and their capacity to elevate cerebrospinal fluid pressure may be markedly exaggerated in the presence of head injury, other intracranial lesions or a pre-existing increase in intracranial pressure. Furthermore, narcotics produce adverse reactions which may obscure the clinical course of patients with head injuries.

Acute Abdominal Conditions: The administration of HYCODAN or other narcotics may obscure the diagnosis or clinical course of patients with acute abdominal conditions.

Pediatric Use: In young children, as well as adults, the respiratory center is sensitive to the depressant action of narcotic cough suppressants in a dose-dependent manner. Benefit to risk ratio should be carefully considered especially in children with respiratory embarrassment (e.g., croup).

PRECAUTIONS

General: Before prescribing medication to suppress or modify cough, it is important to ascertain that the underlying cause of cough is identified, that modification of cough does not increase the risk of clinical or physiological complications, and that appropriate therapy for the primary disease is provided.

Special Risk Patients: HYCODAN should be given with caution to certain patients such as the elderly or debilitated, and those with severe impairment of hepatic or renal functions, hypothyroidism, Addison's disease, prostatic hypertrophy or urethral stricture, asthma, and narrow-angle glaucoma.

Information For Patients: Hydrocodone may impair the mental and/or physical abilities required for the performance of potentially hazardous tasks such as driving a car or operating machinery. The patient using HYCODAN should be cautioned accordingly.

Drug Interactions: Patients receiving narcotics, antihistamines, antipsychotics, antianxiety agents or other CNS depressants (including alcohol) concomitantly with HYCODAN (hydrocodone bitartrate and homatropine methylbromide) may exhibit an additive CNS depression. When combined therapy is contemplated, the dose of one or both agents should be reduced. The use of MAO inhibitors or tricyclic antidepressants with hydrocodone preparations may increase the effect of either the antidepressant or hydrocodone.

Carcinogenesis, Mutagenesis, Impairment Of Fertility: Studies of HYCODAN in animals to evaluate the carcinogenic and mutagenic potential and the effect on fertility have not been conducted.

PREGNANCY

Teratogenic Effects: Pregnancy Category C; Animal reproduction studies have not been conducted with HYCODAN. It is also not known whether HYCODAN can cause fetal harm when administered to a pregnant woman or can affect reproduction capacity. HYCODAN should be given to a pregnant woman only if clearly needed.

Nonteratogenic Effects: Babies born to mothers who have been taking opioids regularly prior to delivery will be physically dependent. The withdrawal signs include irritability and excessive crying, tremors, hyperactive reflexes, increased respiratory rate, increased stools, sneezing, yawning, vomiting and fever. The intensity of the syndrome does not always correlate with the duration of maternal opioid use or dose.

Labor and Delivery: As with all narcotics, administration of HYCODAN to the mother shortly before delivery may result in some degree of respiratory depression in the newborn, especially if higher doses are used.

Nursing Mothers: It is not known whether this drug is excreted in human milk. Because many drugs are excreted in human milk and because of the potential for serious adverse reactions in nursing infants from HYCODAN, a decision should be made whether to discontinue nursing or to discontinue the drug, taking into account the importance of the drug to the mother.

Pediatric Use: Safety and effectiveness of HYCODAN in pediatric patients under six have not been established.

ADVERSE REACTIONS

Central Nervous System: Sedation, drowsiness, mental clouding, lethargy, impairment of mental and physical performance, anxiety, fear, dysphoria, dizziness, psychic dependence, mood changes.

Gastrointestinal System: Nausea and vomiting may occur; they are more frequent in ambulatory than in recumbent patients. Prolonged administration of HYCODAN may produce constipation.

Genitourinary System: Ureteral spasm, spasm of vesicle sphincters and urinary retention have been reported with opiates.

Respiratory Depression: HYCODAN may produce dose-related respiratory depression by acting directly on brain stem respiratory centers (see OVERDOSAGE).

Dermatological: Skin rash, pruritus.

DRUG ABUSE AND DEPENDENCE

HYCODAN is a Schedule III narcotic. Psychic dependence, physical dependence and tolerance may develop upon repeated administration of narcotics; therefore, HYCODAN should be prescribed and administered with caution. However, psychic dependence is unlikely to develop when HYCODAN is used for a short time for the treatment of cough. Physical dependence, the condition in which continued administration of the drug is required to prevent the appearance of a withdrawal syndrome, assumes clinically significant proportions only after several weeks of continued oral narcotic use, although some mild degree of physical dependence may develop after a few days of narcotic therapy.

OVERDOSAGE

Signs and Symptoms: Serious overdosage with hydrocodone is characterized by respiratory depression (a decrease in respiratory rate and/or tidal volume, Cheyne-Stokes respiration, cyanosis), extreme somnolence progressing to stupor or coma, skeletal muscle flaccidity, cold and clammy skin, and sometimes bradycardia and hypotension. In severe overdosage, apnea, circulatory collapse, cardiac arrest and death may occur. The ingestion of very large amounts of HYCODAN (hydrocodone bitartrate and homatropine methylbromide) may, in addition, result in acute homatropine intoxication.

Treatment: Primary attention should be given to the reestablishment of adequate respiratory exchange through provision of a patent airway and the institution of assisted or controlled ventilation. The narcotic antagonist naloxone hydrochloride is a specific antidote for respiratory depression which may result from overdosage or unusual sensitivity to narcotics including hydrocodone. Therefore, an appropriate dose of naloxone hydrochloride should be administered, preferably by the intravenous route, simultaneously with efforts at respiratory resuscitation. For further information, see full prescribing information for naloxone hydrochloride. An antagonist should not be administered in the absence of clinically significant respiratory depression. Oxygen, intravenous fluids, vasopressors and other supportive measures should be employed as indicated. Gastric emptying may be useful in removing unabsorbed drug.

DOSAGE AND ADMINISTRATION

Adults: One (1) tablet or one (1) teaspoonful (5 mL) of the syrup every 4 to 6 hours as needed; do not exceed six (6) tablets or six (6) teaspoonfuls in 24 hours.

Children 6 to 12 years of age: One-half ($^1/_2$) tablet or one-half ($^1/_2$) teaspoonful (2.5 mL) of the syrup every 4 to 6 hours as needed; do not exceed three (3) tablets or three (3) teaspoonfuls in 24 hours.

HOW SUPPLIED

As white tablets with one face scored and inscribed HY-CODAN, and the other face plain and is available in:

Bottles of 100	NDC 63481-042-70
Bottles of 500	NDC 63481-042-85

As a clear red colored, wild cherry flavored syrup in:

Bottles of one pint	NDC 63481-234-16

Store at controlled room temperature (59°–86°F, 15°–30°C). Oral prescription where permitted by State law.
HYCODAN® is a Registered Trademark of Endo Pharmaceuticals Inc.

6445/March, 1996

Shown in Product Identification Guide, page 309

HYCOMINE® COMPOUND
[hĭ-ko-mēn kom 'pound]

DESCRIPTION

HYCOMINE Compound tablets contain hydrocodone (dihydrocodeinone) bitartrate, a semi-synthetic centrally-acting narcotic antitussive; chlorpheniramine maleate, an antihistamine; phenylephrine hydrochloride, a sympathomimetic amine decongestant; acetaminophen, an analgesic/antipyretic; and caffeine, a centrally-acting stimulant, for oral administration.

HYDROCODONE BITARTRATE

CHLORPHENIRAMINE MALEATE

PHENYLEPHRINE HYDROCHLORIDE

ACETAMINOPHEN

CAFFEINE

Each HYCOMINE Compound tablet contains:

Hydrocodone bitartrate, USP	5 mg
WARNING: May be habit forming	
Chlorpheniramine maleate, USP	2 mg
Phenylephrine hydrochloride, USP	10 mg
Acetaminophen, USP	250 mg
Caffeine, anhydrous, USP	30 mg

HYCOMINE Compound tablets also contain: cherry flavor, colloidal silicon dioxide, FD&C Red 40, magnesium stearate, microcrystalline cellulose, povidone and starch.

CLINICAL PHARMACOLOGY

Clinical trials have proven hydrocodone bitartrate to be an effective antitussive agent which is pharmacologically 2 to 8 times as potent as codeine. At equi-effective doses, its sedative action is greater than codeine. The precise mechanism of action of hydrocodone and other opiates is not known, however, hydrocodone is believed to act by directly depressing the cough center. In excessive doses hydrocodone, like other opium derivatives, will depress respiration. The effects of hydrocodone in therapeutic doses on the cardiovascular system is insignificant. The constipation effects of hydrocodone are much weaker than that of morphine and no stronger than that of codeine. Hydrocodone can produce miosis, euphoria, physical and psychological dependence. At therapeutic antitussive doses, it does exert analgesic effects. Following a 10 mg oral dose of hydrocodone administered to five adult male human subjects, the mean peak concentration was 23.6 ± 5.2 ng/mL. Maximum serum levels were achieved at 1.3 ± 0.3 hours and the half-life was determined to be 3.8 ± 0.3 hours. Hydrocodone exhibits a complex pattern of metabolism including O-demethylation, N-demethylation and 6-keto reduction to the corresponding 6-α- and 6-β-hydroxymetabolites.

Chlorpheniramine maleate is a competitive H_1-receptor histamine blocking drug, thereby counteracting the effects of histamine release associated with allergic manifestations of upper respiratory tract inflammatory disorders. H_1-blocking drugs inhibit the actions of histamine on smooth muscle, capillary permeability, and can both stimulate and depress the central nervous system. Phenylephrine hydrochloride effects its vasoconstrictor activity by releasing noradrenaline from sympathetic nerve endings, and from direct stimulation of α-adrenoreceptors in blood vessels. Acetaminophen is an antipyretic and peripherally acting analgesic. Caffeine is a central nervous system stimulant.

INDICATIONS AND USAGE

HYCOMINE Compound is indicated for the symptomatic relief of cough, nasal congestion, and discomfort associated with upper respiratory tract infections.

CONTRAINDICATIONS

HYCOMINE Compound is contraindicated in patients hypersensitive to any component of the drug, and concurrent MAO inhibitor therapy. Patients known to be hypersensitive to other opioids, antihistamines, or sympathomimetic amines may exhibit cross sensitivity with HYCOMINE Compound. Phenylephrine is contraindicated in patients with heart disease, hypertension, diabetes or hyperthyroidism. Hydrocodone is contraindicated in the presence of an intracranial lesion associated with increased intracranial pressure, and whenever ventilatory function is depressed.

WARNINGS

May be habit forming. Hydrocodone can produce drug dependence of the morphine type and therefore has the potential for being abused. Psychic dependence, physical dependence and tolerance may develop upon repeated administration of HYCOMINE Compound and it should be prescribed and administered with the same degree of caution appropriate to the use of other narcotic drugs. (See DRUG ABUSE AND DEPENDENCE.)

Respiratory Depression: HYCOMINE Compound produces dose-related respiratory depression by directly acting on brain stem respiratory centers. If respiratory depression occurs, it may be antagonized by the use of NARCAN® (naloxone hydrochloride) and other supportive measures when indicated.

Head Injury and Increased Intracranial Pressure: The respiratory depressant properties of narcotics and their capacity to elevate cerebrospinal fluid pressure may be markedly exaggerated in the presence of head injury, other intracranial lesions or a pre-existing increase in intracranial pressure. Furthermore, narcotics produce adverse reactions which may obscure the clinical course of patients with head injuries.

Acute Abdominal Conditions: The administration of HYCOMINE Compound or other narcotics may obscure the diagnosis or clinical course of patients with acute abdominal conditions.

Phenylephrine: Hypertensive crises can occur with concurrent use of phenylephrine and monoamine oxidase (MAO) inhibitors, indomethacin or with beta-blockers and methyldopa.

If a hypertensive crisis occurs these drugs should be discontinued immediately and therapy to lower blood pressure should be instituted immediately. Fever should be managed by means of external cooling.

Chlorpheniramine: Antihistamines may produce drowsiness or excitation, particularly in children and elderly patients.

PRECAUTIONS

Before prescribing medication to suppress or modify cough, it is important to ascertain that the underlying cause of cough is identified, that modification of cough does not increase the risk of clinical or physiologic complications, and that appropriate therapy for the primary disease is provided.

Usage in Ambulatory Patients: Hydrocodone, like all narcotics, and antihistamines such as chlorpheniramine maleate, may impair the mental and/or physical abilities required for the performance of potentially hazardous tasks such as driving a car or operating machinery; phenylephrine may produce a rapid pulse, dizziness or palpitations; patients should be cautioned accordingly.

Drug Interactions: Patients receiving other narcotic analgesics, general anesthetics, phenothiazines, other tranquilizers, sedative-hypnotics or other CNS depressants (including alcohol) concomitantly with hydrocodone may exhibit an additive CNS depression. When such combined therapy is contemplated, the dose of one or both agents should be reduced. The use of phenylephrine with other sympathomimetic amines and MAO inhibitors may produce an additive elevation of blood pressure. MAO inhibitors may prolong the anticholinergic effects of antihistamines. (See WARNINGS.)

Carcinogenesis, Mutagenesis, Impairment of Fertility: Carcinogenicity, mutagenicity, and reproduction studies have not been conducted with HYCOMINE Compound.

Usage in Pregnancy: Pregnancy Category C. Animal reproduction studies have not been conducted with HYCOMINE Compound. It is also not known whether HYCOMINE Compound can cause fetal harm when administered to a pregnant woman or can affect reproductive capacity. HYCOMINE Compound should be given to a pregnant woman only if clearly needed.

Nonteratogenic Effects: Babies born to mothers who have been taking opioids regularly prior to delivery will be physically dependent. The withdrawal signs include irritability and excessive crying, tremors, hyperactive reflexes, increased respiratory rate, increased stools, sneezing, yawning, vomiting and fever. The intensity of the syndrome does not always correlate with the duration of maternal opioid use or dose. Chlorpromazine 0.7–1.0 mg/kg q 6 h, phenobarbital 2 mg/kg q 6 h, and paregoric 2–4 drops/kg q 4 h, have been used to treat withdrawal symptoms in infants. The duration of therapy is 4 to 28 days, with the dosages decreased as tolerated.

Nursing Mothers: It is not known whether this drug is excreted in human milk. Because many drugs are excreted in human milk and because of the potential for serious adverse reactions in nursing infants from HYCOMINE Compound, a decision should be made whether to discontinue nursing or discontinue the drug, taking into account the importance of the drug to the mother.

Pediatric Use: Safety and effectiveness in pediatric patients below the age of 2 years have not been established.

ADVERSE REACTIONS

Respiratory System: Hydrocodone produces dose-related respiratory depression by acting directly on brain stem respiratory centers.

Cardiovascular System: Hypertension, postural hypotension, tachycardia and palpitations.

Genitourinary System: Ureteral spasm, spasm of vesical sphincters and urinary retention have been reported with opiates.

Central Nervous System: Sedation, drowsiness, mental clouding, lethargy, impairment of mental and physical performance, anxiety, fear, dysphoria, dizziness, psychic dependence, mood changes, and blurred vision.

Gastrointestinal System: Nausea and vomiting occur more frequently in ambulatory than in recumbent patients.

Continued on next page

Hycomine Compound—Cont.

DRUG ABUSE AND DEPENDENCE

Special care should be exercised in prescribing hydrocodone for emotionally unstable patients and for those with a history of drug misuse. Such patients should be closely supervised when long-term therapy is contemplated.

HYCOMINE Compound is a Schedule III narcotic. Psychic dependence, physical dependence, and tolerance may develop upon repeated administration of narcotics; therefore, HYCOMINE Compound should always be prescribed and administered with caution. Physical dependence is the condition in which continued administration of the drug is required to prevent the appearance of a withdrawal syndrome.

Patients physically dependent on opioids will develop an abstinence syndrome upon abrupt discontinuation of the opioid or following the administration of a narcotic antagonist. The character and severity of the withdrawal symptoms are related to the degree of physical dependence. Manifestations of opioid withdrawal are similar to but milder than that of morphine and include lacrimation, rhinorrhea, yawning, sweating, restlessness, dilated pupils, anorexia, gooseflesh, irritability and tremor. In more severe forms, nausea, vomiting, intestinal spasm and diarrhea, increased heart rate and blood pressure, chills, and pains in bones and muscles of the back and extremities may occur. Peak effects will usually be apparent at 48 to 72 hours.

Treatment of withdrawal is usually managed by providing sufficient quantities of an opioid to suppress **severe** withdrawal symptoms and then gradually reducing the dose of opioid over a period of several days.

OVERDOSAGE

The signs and symptoms of overdosage of the individual components of HYCOMINE Compound may be modified in varying degrees by the presence of other active ingredients. Overdosage with phenylephrine alone may result in tremor, restlessness, increased motor activity, agitation and hallucinations.

Acetaminophen

Signs and Symptoms: In acute acetaminophen overdosage, dose-dependent, potentially fatal hepatic necrosis is the most serious adverse effect. Renal tubular necrosis, hypoglycemic coma and thrombocytopenia may also occur.

Acetaminophen in massive overdosage may cause hepatic toxicity in some patients. In cases of suspected overdose, you may wish to call your regional poison center for assistance in diagnosis and for directions in the use of N-acetylcysteine as an antidote.

In adults, hepatic toxicity has rarely been reported with acute overdoses of less than 10 grams and fatalities with less than 15 grams. Importantly, young children seem to be more resistant than adults to the hepatotoxic effect of an acetaminophen overdose. Despite this, the measures outlined below should be initiated in any adult or child suspected of having ingested an acetaminophen overdose.

Early symptoms following a potentially hepatotoxic overdose may include nausea, vomiting, diaphoresis and general malaise. Clinical and laboratory evidence of hepatic toxicity may not be apparent until 48 to 72 hours post-ingestion.

Treatment: The stomach should be emptied promptly by lavage or by induction of emesis with syrup of ipecac. Patient's estimates of the quantity of a drug ingested are notoriously unreliable. Therefore, if an acetaminophen overdose is suspected, a serum acetaminophen assay should be obtained as early as possible, but no sooner than four hours following ingestion. Liver function studies should be obtained initially and repeated at 24-hour intervals.

The antidote, N-acetylcysteine should be administered as early as possible, preferably within 16 hours of the overdose ingestions for optimal results, but in any case, within 24 hours. Following recovery, there are no residual structural or functional hepatic abnormalities.

Hydrocodone

Signs and Symptoms: Serious overdosage with hydrocodone is characterized by respiratory depression (a decrease in respiratory rate and/or tidal volume, Cheyne-Stokes respiration, cyanosis), extreme somnolence progressing to stupor or coma, skeletal muscle flaccidity, cold and clammy skin, and sometimes bradycardia and hypotension. In severe overdosage, apnea, circulatory collapse, cardiac arrest and death may occur.

Treatment: Primary attention should be given to the reestablishment of adequate respiratory exchange through provision of a patent airway and the institution of assisted or controlled ventilation. The narcotic antagonist naloxone hydrochloride is a specific antidote for respiratory depression which may result from overdosage or unusual sensitivity to narcotics including hydrocodone. Therefore, an appropriate dose of naloxone hydrochloride should be administered, preferably by the intravenous route, simultaneously with efforts at respiratory resuscitation. For further information, see full prescribing information for naloxone hydrochloride. An antagonist should not be administered in the absence of clinically significant respiratory depression. Oxygen, intravenous fluids, vasopressors and other supportive measures should be employed as indicated. Gastric emptying may be useful in removing unabsorbed drug. Activated charcoal may be of benefit.

DOSAGE AND ADMINISTRATION

Usual dosage, not less than 4 hours apart:
Adults: 1 tablet 4 times a day
Children: 6 to 12 years: 1/2 tablet 4 times a day

HOW SUPPLIED

HYCOMINE® Compound is available as a coral pink, scored tablet in bottles as follows:

Bottles of 100	NDC 63481-048-70
Bottles of 500	NDC 63481-048-85

Store at controlled room temperature 15°–30°C (59°–86°F)
Oral prescription where permitted by State Law.
Dispense in a tight, light-resistant container defined in the USP.
HYCOMINE® is a Registered Trademark of Endo Pharmaceuticals Inc.
NARCAN® is a Registered Trademark of Endo Pharmaceuticals Inc.

6491-00/November, 1997

Shown in Product Identification Guide, page 309

HYCOMINE® Ⓒ III
(hydrocodone bitartrate and phenylpropanolamine hydrochloride)
Pediatric Syrup

HYCOMINE® Ⓒ III
(hydrocodone bitartrate and phenylpropanolamine hydrochloride)
Syrup

DESCRIPTION

HYCOMINE contains hydrocodone (dihydrocodeinone) bitartrate, a semi-synthetic centrally-acting narcotic antitussive and phenylpropanolamine hydrochloride, a sympathomimetic amine decongestant for oral administration.

The pH of HYCOMINE and HYCOMINE Pediatric Syrup is 3.2–4.2. The hydrocodone component is (5α)-4,5-epoxy-3-methoxy-17-methylmorphinan-6-one [R-(R*,R*)]-2,3-dihydroxybutanedioate (1:1) hydrate (2:5), a fine white crystal or crystalline powder, which is derived from the opium alkaloid, thebaine, and has a molecular weight of 494.50. The phenylpropanolamine component is (±)-(R*,S*)-α-(1-aminoethyl) benzenemethanol hydrochloride and has a molecular weight of 187.67. These may be represented by the following structural formulas:

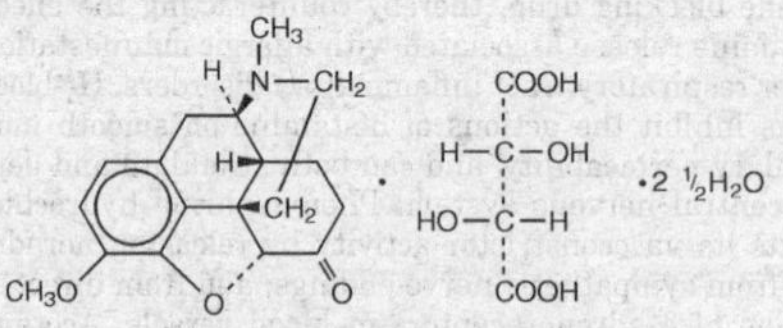

HYDROCODONE BITARTRATE

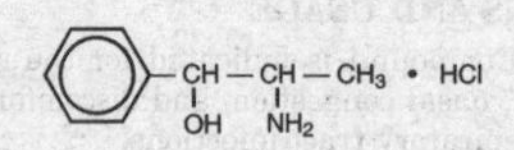

PHENYLPROPANOLAMINE HYDROCHLORIDE

HYCOMINE
Pediatric Syrup
Each teaspoonful (5 mL) contains:

Hydrocodone bitartrate, USP	2.5 mg
WARNING: May be habit forming	
Phenylpropanolamine hydrochloride, USP	12.5 mg

HYCOMINE Syrup
Each teaspoonful (5 mL) contains:

Hydrocodone bitartrate, USP	5 mg
WARNING: May be habit forming	
Phenylpropanolamine hydrochloride, USP	25 mg

Also, HYCOMINE, both strengths, contain: artificial cherry flavor, glycerin, methylparaben, propylparaben, saccharin sodium, and sorbitol solution. HYCOMINE Pediatric Syrup contains: D&C Yellow 10 and FD&C Green 3. HYCOMINE Syrup: FD&C Red 40 and FD&C Yellow 6.

CLINICAL PHARMACOLOGY

Hydrocodone is a semisynthetic narcotic antitussive and analgesic with multiple actions qualitatively similar to those of codeine. The precise mechanism of action of hydrocodone and other opiates is not known; however, hydrocodone is believed to act directly on the cough center. In excessive doses, hydrocodone, like other opium derivatives, will depress respiration. The effects of hydrocodone in therapeutic doses on the cardiovascular system are insignificant. Hydrocodone can produce miosis, euphoria, physical and physiological dependence.

Following a 10 mg oral dose of hydrocodone administered to five adult male subjects, the mean peak concentration was 23.6 ± 5.2 ng/mL. Maximum serum levels were achieved at 1.3 ± 0.3 hours and the half-life was determined to be 3.8 ± 0.3 hours. Hydrocodone exhibits a complex pattern of metabolism including O-demethylation, N-demethylation and 6-keto reduction to the corresponding 6-α- and 6-β-hydroxymetabolites.

Phenylpropanolamine effects its vasoconstrictor activity by releasing noradrenaline from sympathetic nerve endings, and from direct stimulation of α-adrenoreceptors of blood vessels.

INDICATIONS AND USAGE

HYCOMINE is indicated for the symptomatic relief of cough and nasal congestion.

CONTRAINDICATIONS

HYCOMINE (hydrocodone bitartrate and phenylpropanolamine hydrochloride) is contraindicated in patients hypersensitive to hydrocodone or phenylpropanolamine, and in patients on concurrent MAO inhibitor therapy. Patients known to be hypersensitive to other opioids or sympathomimetic amines may exhibit cross sensitivity to HYCOMINE. Phenylpropanolamine is contraindicated in patients with heart disease, hypertension, diabetes or hyperthyroidism. Hydrocodone is contraindicated in the presence of an intracranial lesion associated with increased intracranial pressure; and whenever ventilatory function is depressed.

WARNINGS

May be habit forming. Hydrocodone can produce drug dependence of the morphine type and, therefore, has the potential for being abused. Psychic dependence, physical dependence and tolerance may develop upon repeated administration of HYCOMINE and it should be prescribed and administered with the same degree of caution appropriate to the use of other narcotic drugs (see DRUG ABUSE AND DEPENDENCE).

Respiratory Depression: HYCOMINE produces dose-related respiratory depression by directly acting on brain stem respiratory centers. If respiratory depression occurs, it may be antagonized by the use of naloxone hydrochloride and other supportive measures when indicated.

Head Injury and Increased Intracranial Pressure: The respiratory depression properties of narcotics and their capacity to elevate cerebrospinal fluid pressure may be markedly exaggerated in the presence of head injury, other intracranial lesions or a preexisting increase in intracranial pressure. Furthermore, narcotics produce adverse reactions which may obscure the clinical course of patients with head injuries.

Acute Abdominal Conditions: The administration of HYCOMINE or other narcotics may obscure the diagnosis or clinical course of patients with acute abdominal conditions.

Pediatric Use: In young children, as well as adults, the respiratory center is sensitive to the depressant action of narcotic cough suppressants in a dose-dependent manner. Benefit to risk ratio should be carefully considered especially in children with respiratory embarrassment (e.g., croup).

Phenylpropanolamine: Hypertensive crises can occur with concurrent use of phenylpropanolamine and monoamine oxidase (MAO) inhibitors, indomethacin or with beta-blockers and methyldopa.

If a hypertensive crisis occurs, these drugs should be discontinued immediately and therapy to lower blood pressure should be instituted immediately. Fever should be managed by means of external cooling.

PRECAUTIONS

General: Before prescribing medication to suppress or modify cough, it is important to ascertain that the underlying cause of cough is identified, that modification of cough does not increase the risk of clinical or physiologic complications, and that appropriate therapy for the primary disease is provided.

Special Risk Patients: HYCOMINE should be given with caution to certain patients such as the elderly or debilitated, and those with severe impairment of hepatic or renal functions, hypothyroidism, Addison's disease, prostatic hypertrophy or urethral stricture, asthma, narrow-angle glaucoma, and uncontrolled hypertension.

Information for Patients: Hydrocodone may impair the mental and/or physical abilities required for the performance of potentially hazardous tasks such as driving a car or operating machinery; phenylpropanolamine may produce a rapid pulse, dizziness or palpitations. The patient using HYCOMINE (hydrocodone bitartrate and phenylpropanolamine hydrochloride) should be cautioned accordingly.

Drug Interactions: Patients receiving other narcotic analgesics, general anesthetics, phenothiazines, other tranquilizers, sedative-hypnotics or other CNS depressants (including alcohol) concomitantly with hydrocodone may exhibit an

additive CNS depression. When such combined therapy is contemplated, the dose of one or both agents should be reduced. The use of phenylpropanolamine with other sympathomimetic amines and MAO inhibitors may produce an additive elevation of blood pressure (see WARNINGS).

Carcinogenesis, Mutagenesis, Impairment of Fertility: Carcinogenicity, mutagenicity and reproduction studies have not been conducted with HYCOMINE.

Pregnancy: Teratogenic Effects: Pregnancy Category C: Animal reproduction studies have not been conducted with HYCOMINE. It is also not known whether HYCOMINE can cause fetal harm when administered to a pregnant woman or can affect reproductive capacity. HYCOMINE should be given to a pregnant woman only if clearly needed.

Nonteratogenic Effects: Babies born to mothers who have been taking opioids regularly prior to delivery will be physically dependent. The withdrawal signs include irritability and excessive crying, tremors, hyperactive reflexes, increased respiratory rate, increased stools, sneezing, yawning, vomiting and fever. The intensity of the syndrome does not always correlate with the duration of maternal opioid use or dose.

Labor and Delivery: As with all narcotics, administration of HYCOMINE to the mother shortly before delivery may result in some degree of respiratory depression in the newborn, especially if higher doses are used.

Nursing Mothers: It is not known whether this drug is excreted in human milk. Because many drugs are excreted in human milk and because of the potential for serious adverse reactions in nursing infants from HYCOMINE, a decision should be made whether to discontinue nursing or discontinue the drug, taking into account the importance of the drug to the mother.

Pediatric Use: Safety and effectiveness of HYCOMINE in pediatric patients under six have not been established.

ADVERSE REACTIONS

Respiratory System: Hydrocodone produces dose-related respiratory depression by acting directly on brain stem respiratory centers. (See OVERDOSAGE).

Cardiovascular System: Hypertension, postural hypotension, tachycardia and palpitations.

Genitourinary System: Ureteral spasm, spasm of vesical sphincters and urinary retention have been reported with opiates.

Central Nervous System: Sedation, drowsiness, mental clouding, lethargy, impairment of mental and physical performance, anxiety, fear, dysphoria, dizziness, psychic dependence, mood changes and blurred vision.

Gastrointestinal System: Nausea and vomiting occur more frequently in ambulatory than in recumbent patients. Prolonged administration of HYCOMINE may produce constipation.

Dermatological: Skin rash, pruritus.

DRUG ABUSE AND DEPENDENCE

Hycomine is a Schedule III narcotic. Psychic dependence, physical dependence, and tolerance may develop upon repeated administration of narcotics; therefore, HYCOMINE should be prescribed and administered with caution. However, psychic dependence is unlikely to develop when HYCOMINE is used for a short time for the treatment of cough. Physical dependence, the condition in which continued administration of the drug is required to prevent the appearance of a withdrawal syndrome, assumes clinically significant proportions only after several weeks of continued oral narcotic use, although some mild degree of physical dependence may develop after a few days of narcotic therapy.

OVERDOSAGE

Signs and Symptoms: Serious overdosage with HYCOMINE is characterized by respiratory depression (a decrease in respiratory rate and/or tidal volume, Cheyne-Stokes respiration, cyanosis), extreme somnolence progressing to stupor or coma, skeletal muscle flaccidity, cold and clammy skin, and sometimes bradycardia and hypotension. In severe overdosage, apnea, circulatory collapse, cardiac arrest, and death may occur.

The signs and symptoms of overdosage of the individual components of HYCOMINE (hydrocodone bitartrate and phenylpropanolamine hydrochloride) may be modified in varying degrees by the presence of other active ingredients. Overdosage with phenylpropanolamine alone may result in tremor, restlessness, increased motor activity, agitation and hallucinations.

Treatment: Primary attention should be given to the reestablishment of adequate respiratory exchange through provision of a patent airway and the institution of assisted or controlled ventilation. The narcotic antagonist naloxone hydrochloride is a specific antidote for respiratory depression which may result from overdosage or unusual sensitivity to narcotics including hydrocodone. Therefore, an appropriate dose of naloxone hydrochloride should be administered preferably by the intravenous route, simultaneously with efforts at respiratory resuscitation.

For further information, see full prescribing information for naloxone hydrochloride. An antagonist should not be admin-

istered in the absence of clinically significant respiratory depression. Oxygen, intravenous fluids, vasopressors, and other supportive measures should be employed as indicated. Gastric emptying may be useful in removing unabsorbed drug.

DOSAGE AND ADMINISTRATION

Adults: The usual dose for adults is one teaspoonful HYCOMINE Syrup (hydrocodone bitartrate 5 mg and phenylpropanolamine hydrochloride 25 mg/5 cc) every four hours as needed, not to exceed six teaspoonfuls in a 24 hour period.

Children 6 to 12 years of age: The usual dose for children 6 to 12 years of age is one teaspoonful HYCOMINE Pediatric Syrup (hydrocodone bitartrate 2.5 mg and phenylpropanolamine hydrochloride 12.5 mg/5 cc) every four hours as needed, not to exceed six teaspoonfuls in a 24 hour period.

HOW SUPPLIED

HYCOMINE Syrup (5 mg hydrocodone bitartrate, USP and 25 mg phenylpropanolamine hydrochloride, USP—per 5 mL teaspoonful) is available as an orange-colored, cherry-flavored syrup in bottles as follows:

One Pint (473.2 mL):   NDC 63481-246-16

HYCOMINE Pediatric Syrup (2.5 mg hydrocodone bitartrate, USP and 12.5 mg phenylpropanolamine hydrochloride, USP—per 5 mL teaspoonful) is available as a green-colored, cherry-flavored syrup in bottles as follows:

One Pint (473.2 mL):   NDC 63481-247-16

Store at controlled room temperature 15°–30°C (59°–86°F). Oral prescription where permitted by State law.

HYCOMINE® is a Registered Trademark of Endo Pharmaceuticals Inc.

Copyright © Endo Pharmaceuticals Inc. 1997

6480/August, 1997

HYCOTUSS®   Ⓒ
[hī-kō-tus]
Expectorant

DESCRIPTION

HYCOTUSS Expectorant Syrup contains hydrocodone (dihydrocodeinone) bitartrate, a semi-synthetic centrally-acting narcotic antitussive and guaifenesin, an expectorant for oral administration.

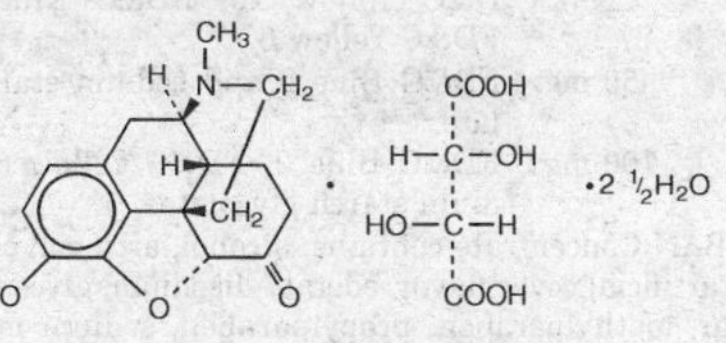

HYDROCODONE BITARTRATE

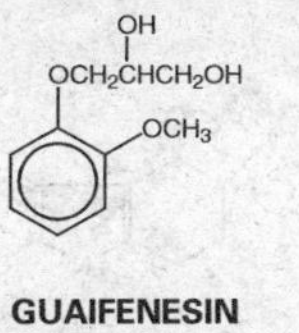

GUAIFENESIN

Each teaspoonful (5 mL) contains:

Hydrocodone bitartrate, USP .... 5 mg
    WARNING: May be habit forming
Guaifenesin, USP .... 100 mg
Alcohol, USP .... 10% v/v

HYCOTUSS Expectorant Syrup also contains: artificial butterscotch flavor, FD&C Red 40, FD&C Yellow 6, glycerin, liquid sugar, methylparaben, propylparaben, saccharin sodium, and sorbitol solution.

CLINICAL PHARMACOLOGY

Clinical trials have proven hydrocodone bitartrate to be an effective antitussive agent which is pharmacologically 2 to 8 times as potent as codeine. At equi-effective doses, its sedative action is greater than codeine. The precise mechanism of action of hydrocodone and other opiates is not known, however, hydrocodone is believed to act by directly depressing the cough center. In excessive doses hydrocodone, like other opium derivatives, can depress respiration. The effects of hydrocodone in therapeutic doses on the cardiovascular system is insignificant. The constipation effects of hydrocodone are much weaker than that of morphine and no stronger than that of codeine. Hydrocodone can produce miosis, euphoria, physical and psychological dependence. At therapeutic antitussive doses, it does exert analgesic effects. Following a 10 mg oral dose of hydrocodone administered to five male human subjects, the mean peak concentration was 23.6 ± 5.2 ng/mL. Maximum serum levels were achieved at 1.3 ± 0.3 hours and half-life was determined to be 3.8 ± 0.3 hours. Hydrocodone exhibits a complex pattern of metabo-

lism including O-demethylation, N-demethylation and 6-keto reduction to the corresponding 6-α- and 6-β-hydroxymetabolites.

The exact mechanism of action is not established but guaifenesin is believed to act by stimulating receptors in the gastric mucosa that initiates a reflex secretion of respiratory tract fluid, thereby increasing the volume and decreasing the viscosity of bronchial secretions. Studies with guaifenesin indicate that it is rapidly absorbed from the gastrointestinal tract and has a half-life of one hour.

INDICATIONS AND USAGE

HYCOTUSS (hydrocodone bitartrate and guaifenesin) Expectorant is indicated for the symptomatic relief of irritating non-productive cough associated with upper and lower respiratory tract congestion.

CONTRAINDICATIONS

HYCOTUSS Expectorant is contraindicated in patients hypersensitive to hydrocodone or guaifenesin. Patients known to be hypersensitive to other opioids may exhibit cross sensitivity to HYCOTUSS Expectorant. Hydrocodone is contraindicated in the presence of an intracranial lesion associated with increased intracranial pressure; and whenever ventilatory function is depressed.

WARNINGS

May be habit forming. Hydrocodone can produce drug dependence of the morphine type and therefore has the potential for being abused. Psychic dependence, physical dependence and tolerance may develop upon repeated administration of HYCOTUSS Expectorant and it should be prescribed and administered with the same degree of caution appropriate to the use of other narcotic drugs (see DRUG ABUSE AND DEPENDENCE).

Respiratory Depression: HYCOTUSS Expectorant produces dose-related respiratory depression by directly acting on the brain stem respiratory centers. If respiratory depression occurs, it may be antagonized by the use of NARCAN® (naloxone hydrochloride) and other supportive measures when indicated.

Head Injury and Increased Intracranial Pressure: The respiratory depressant properties of narcotics and their capacity to elevate cerebrospinal fluid pressure may be markedly exaggerated in the presence of head injury, other intracranial lesions or a pre-existing increase in intracranial pressure. Furthermore, narcotics produce adverse reactions which may obscure the clinical course of patients with head injuries.

Acute Abdominal Conditions: The administration of HYCOTUSS Expectorant or other opioids may obscure the diagnosis or clinical course of patients with acute abdominal conditions.

PRECAUTIONS

Before prescribing medication to suppress or modify cough, it is important to ascertain that the underlying cause of cough is identified, that modification of cough does not increase the risk of clinical or physiologic complications, and that appropriate therapy for the primary disease is provided.

Usage in Ambulatory Patients: Hydrocodone, like all narcotics, may impair the mental and/or physical abilities required for the performance of potentially hazardous tasks such as driving a car or operating machinery, and patients should be warned accordingly.

Drug Interactions: Patients receiving other narcotics, analgesics, general anesthetics, phenothiazines, other tranquilizers, sedative hypnotics or other CNS depressants (including alcohol) concomitantly with hydrocodone may exhibit an additive CNS depression. When such combined therapy is contemplated, the dose of one or both agents should be reduced (see WARNINGS).

Laboratory Interactions: The metabolite of guaifenesin has been found to produce an apparent increase in urinary 5-hydroxyindoleacetic acid, and guaifenesin therefore may interfere with the interpretation of this test for the diagnosis of carcinoid syndrome. Guaifenesin administration should be discontinued 24 hours prior to the collection of urine specimens for the determination of 5-hydroxyindoleacetic acid.

Carcinogenesis, Mutagenesis, Impairment of Fertility: Carcinogenicity, mutagenicity and reproduction studies have not been conducted with HYCOTUSS (hydrocodone bitartrate and guaifenesin) Expectorant.

Usage in Pregnancy: Pregnancy Category C. Animal reproduction studies have not been conducted with HYCOTUSS Expectorant. It is also not known whether HYCOTUSS Expectorant can cause fetal harm when administered to a pregnant woman or can affect reproductive capacity. HYCOTUSS Expectorant should be given to a pregnant woman only if clearly needed.

Nonteratogenic Effects: Babies born to mothers who have been taking opioids regularly prior to delivery will be physically dependent. The withdrawal signs include irritability

Continued on next page

Hycotuss—Cont.

and excessive crying, tremors, hyperactive reflexes, increased respiratory rate, increased stools, sneezing, yawning, vomiting and fever. The intensity of the syndrome does not always correlate with the duration of maternal opioid use or dose. There is no consensus on the best method of managing withdrawal. Chlorpromazine 0.7–1.0 mg/kg q 6 h, phenobarbital 2 mg/kg q 6 h, and paregoric 2–4 drops/kg q 4 h, have been used to treat withdrawal symptoms in infants. The duration of therapy is 4 to 28 days, with the dosages decreased as tolerated.

Nursing Mothers: It is not known whether this drug is excreted in human milk. Because many drugs are excreted in human milk and because of the potential for serious adverse reactions in nursing infants from HYCOTUSS Expectorant, a decision should be made whether to discontinue nursing or discontinue the drug, taking into account the importance of the drug to the mother.

ADVERSE REACTIONS

Respiratory System: Hydrocodone produces dose-related respiratory depression by acting directly on brain stem respiratory centers.

Cardiovascular System: Hypertension, postural hypotension and palpitations.

Genitourinary System: Ureteral spasm, spasm of vesical sphincters and urinary retention have been reported with opiates.

Central Nervous System: Sedation, drowsiness, mental clouding, lethargy, impairment of mental and physical performance, anxiety, fear, dysphoria, dizziness, psychic dependence, mood changes and blurred vision.

Gastrointestinal System: Nausea and vomiting occur more frequently in ambulatory than in recumbent patients.

DRUG ABUSE AND DEPENDENCE

Special care should be exercised in prescribing hydrocodone for emotionally unstable patients and for those with a history of drug misuse. Such patients should be closely supervised when long-term therapy is contemplated.

HYCOTUSS Expectorant is a Schedule III narcotic. Psychic dependence, physical dependence and tolerance may develop upon repeated administration of narcotics; therefore, HYCOTUSS Expectorant should always be prescribed and administered with caution. Physical dependence is the condition in which continued administration of the drug is required to prevent the appearance of a withdrawal syndrome.

Patients physically dependent on opioids will develop an abstinence syndrome upon abrupt discontinuation of the opioid or following the administration of a narcotic antagonist. The character and severity of the withdrawal symptoms are related to the degree of physical dependence. Manifestations of opioid withdrawal are similar to but milder than that of morphine and include lacrimation, rhinorrhea, yawning, sweating, restlessness, dilated pupils, anorexia, gooseflesh, irritability and tremor. In more severe forms, nausea, vomiting, intestinal spasm and diarrhea, increased heart rate and blood pressure, chills, and pains in bones and muscles of the back and extremities may occur. Peak effects will usually be apparent at 48 to 72 hours. Treatment of withdrawal is usually managed by providing sufficient quantities of an opioid to suppress **severe** withdrawal symptoms and then gradually reducing the dose of opioid over a period of several days.

OVERDOSAGE

Signs and Symptoms: Serious overdosage with HYCOTUSS (hydrocodone bitartrate and guaifenesin) Expectorant is characterized by respiratory depression (a decrease in respiratory rate and/or tidal volume, Cheyne-Stokes respiration, cyanosis), extreme somnolence progressing to stupor or coma, skeletal muscle flaccidity, cold and clammy skin, and sometimes bradycardia and hypotension. In severe overdosage, apnea, circulatory collapse, cardiac arrest, and death may occur.

Treatment: Primary attention should be given to the reestablishment of adequate respiratory exchange through provision of a patent airway and the institution of assisted or controlled ventilation. The narcotic antagonist naloxone hydrochloride is a specific antidote for respiratory depression which may result from overdosage or unusual sensitivity to narcotics including hydrocodone. Therefore, an appropriate dose of naloxone hydrochloride should be administered, preferably by the intravenous route, simultaneously with efforts at respiratory resuscitation. For further information, see full prescribing information for naloxone hydrochloride. An antagonist should not be administered in the absence of clinically significant respiratory depression. Oxygen, intravenous fluids, vasopressors and other supportive measures should be employed as indicated. Gastric emptying may be useful in removing unabsorbed drug. Activated charcoal may be of benefit.

DOSAGE AND ADMINISTRATION

Usual Adult Dose: One teaspoonful (5 mL) after meals and at bedtime, not less than 4 hours apart (not to exceed 6 tea-

spoonful in a 24 hour period). Treatment should be initiated with one teaspoonful and subsequent doses, up to a maximum single dose of 3 teaspoonsful, adjusted if required.

Usual Children's Dose:

Over 12 years: Initial dose 1 teaspoonful; maximum single dose, 2 teaspoonsful.

6 to 12 years: Initial dose ½ teaspoonful; maximum single dose, 1 teaspoonful.

HOW SUPPLIED

HYCOTUSS Expectorant is available as an orange-colored, butterscotch flavored syrup in bottles as follows:

One pint: NDC 63481-235-16

Store at controlled room temperature 15°–30°C (59°–86°F).

Oral prescription where permitted by State Law.

HYCOTUSS® is a Registered Trademark of Endo Pharmaceuticals Inc.

NARCAN® is a Registered Trademark of Endo Pharmaceuticals Inc.

Copyright © Endo Pharmaceuticals Inc. 1997

6481-00/November, 1997

MOBAN®

[mō 'ban]

(molindone hydrochloride)

℞

DESCRIPTION

MOBAN (molindone hydrochloride) is a dihydroindolone compound which is not structurally related to the phenothiazines, the butyrophenones or the thioxanthenes.

MOBAN is 3-ethyl-6, 7-dihydro-2-methyl-5-(morpholinomethyl) indol-4 (5H)-one hydrochloride. It is a white to off-white crystalline powder, freely soluble in water and alcohol and has a molecular weight of 312.67.

MOBAN Tablets also contain:

All strengths:	calcium sulfate, lactose, magnesium stearate, microcrystalline cellulose and povidone.
5 mg:	alginic acid, colloidal silicon dioxide and FD&C Yellow 6.
10 mg:	alginic acid, colloidal silicon dioxide, FD&C Blue 2 and FD&C Red 40.
25 mg:	alginic acid, colloidal silicon dioxide, D&C Yellow 10, FD&C Blue 2, and FD&C Yellow 6.
50 mg:	FD&C Blue 2 and sodium starch glycolate.
100 mg:	FD&C Blue 2, FD&C Yellow 6 and sodium starch glycolate.

MOBAN Concentrate contains: alcohol, artificial cherry flavor, artificial cover flavor, edetate disodium, glycerin, liquid sugar, methylparaben, propylparaben, sodium metabisulfite, sorbitol solution, and hydrochloric acid reagent grade for pH adjustment.

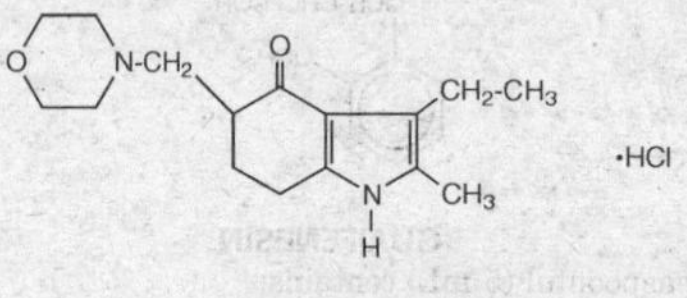

MOLINDONE HYDROCHLORIDE

ACTIONS

MOBAN has a pharmacological profile in laboratory animals which predominantly resembles that of major tranquilizers causing reduction of spontaneous locomotion and aggressiveness, suppression of a conditioned response and antagonism of the bizarre stereotyped behavior and hyperactivity induced by amphetamines. In addition, MOBAN antagonizes the depression caused by the tranquilizing agent tetrabenazine.

In human clinical studies tranquilization is achieved in the absence of muscle relaxing or incoordinating effects. Based on EEG studies, MOBAN exerts its effect on the ascending reticular activating system.

Human metabolic studies show MOBAN to be rapidly absorbed and metabolized when given orally. Unmetabolized drug reached a peak blood level at 1.5 hours. Pharmacological effect from a single oral dose persists for 24–36 hours. There are 36 recognized metabolites with less than 2–3% unmetabolized MOBAN being excreted in urine and feces.

INDICATIONS

MOBAN is indicated for the management of the manifestations of psychotic disorders. The antipsychotic efficacy of MOBAN was established in clinical studies which enrolled newly hospitalized and chronically hospitalized, acutely ill, schizophrenic patients as subjects.

CONTRAINDICATIONS

MOBAN is contraindicated in severe central nervous system depression (alcohol, barbiturates, narcotics, etc.) or comatose states, and in patients with known hypersensitivity to the drug.

WARNINGS

Tardive Dyskinesia

Tardive dyskinesia, a syndrome consisting of potentially irreversible, involuntary, dyskinetic movements may develop in patients treated with neuroleptic (antipsychotic) drugs. Although the prevalence of the syndrome appears to be highest among the elderly, especially elderly women, it is impossible to rely upon prevalence estimates to predict, at the inception of neuroleptic treatment, which patients are likely to develop the syndrome. Whether neuroleptic drug products differ in their potential to cause tardive dyskinesia is unknown.

Both the risk of developing the syndrome and the likelihood that it will become irreversible are believed to increase as the duration of treatment and the total cumulative dose of neuroleptic drugs administered to the patient increase. However, the syndrome can develop, although much less commonly, after relatively brief treatment periods at low doses.

There is no known treatment for established cases of tardive dyskinesia, although the syndrome may remit, partially or completely, if neuroleptic treatment is withdrawn. Neuroleptic treatment, itself, however, may suppress (or partially suppress) the signs and symptoms of the syndrome and thereby may possibly mask the underlying disease process. The effect that symptomatic suppression has upon the long-term course of the syndrome is unknown.

Given these considerations, neuroleptics should be prescribed in a manner that is most likely to minimize the occurrence of tardive dyskinesia. Chronic neuroleptic treatment should generally be reserved for patients who suffer from a chronic illness that, 1) is known to respond to neuroleptic drugs, and 2) for whom alternative, equally effective, but potentially less harmful treatments are not available or appropriate. In patients who do require chronic treatment, the smallest dose and the shortest duration of treatment producing a satisfactory clinical response should be sought. The need for continued treatment should be reassessed periodically.

If signs and symptoms of tardive dyskinesia appear in a patient on neuroleptics, drug discontinuation should be considered. However, some patients may require treatment despite the presence of the syndrome.

(For further information about the description of tardive dyskinesia and its clinical detection, please refer to the section on Adverse Reactions.)

Neuroleptic Malignant Syndrome (NMS)

A potentially fatal symptom complex sometimes referred to as Neuroleptic Malignant Syndrome (NMS) has been reported in association with antipsychotic drugs. Clinical manifestations of NMS are hyperpyrexia, muscle rigidity, altered mental status and evidence of autonomic instability (irregular pulse or blood pressure, tachycardia, diaphoresis, and cardiac dysrhythmias).

The diagnostic evaluation of patients with this syndrome is complicated. In arriving at a diagnosis, it is important to identify cases where the clinical presentation includes both serious medical illness (e.g., pneumonia, systemic infection, etc.) and untreated or inadequately treated extrapyramidal signs and symptoms (EPS). Other important considerations in the differential diagnosis include central anticholinergic toxicity, heat stroke, drug fever and primary central nervous system (CNS) pathology.

The management of NMS should include, 1) immediate discontinuation of antipsychotic drugs and other drugs not essential to concurrent therapy, 2) intensive symptomatic treatment and medical monitoring, and 3) treatment of any concomitant serious medical problems for which specific treatments are available. There is no general agreement about specific pharmacological treatment regimens for uncomplicated NMS.

If a patient requires antipsychotic drug treatment after recovery from NMS, the potential reintroduction of drug therapy should be carefully considered. The patient should be carefully monitored, since recurrences of NMS have been reported.

Usage in Pregnancy: Studies in pregnant patients have not been carried out. Reproduction studies have been performed in the following animals:

Pregnant Rats oral dose—	
no adverse effect	20 mg/kg/day—10 days
no adverse effect	40 mg/kg/day—10 days
Pregnant Mice oral dose—	
slight increase resorptions	20 mg/kg/day—10 days
slight increase resorptions	40 mg/kg/day—10 days
Pregnant Rabbits oral dose—	
no adverse effect	5 mg/kg/day—12 days
no adverse effect	10 mg/kg/day—12 days
no adverse effect	20 mg/kg/day—12 days

Animal reproductive studies have not demonstrated a teratogenic potential. The anticipated benefits must be weighed against the unknown risks to the fetus if used in pregnant patients.

Nursing Mothers: Data are not available on the content of MOBAN (molindone hydrochloride) in the milk of nursing mothers.

Pediatric use: Use of MOBAN (molindone hydrochloride) in pediatric patients below the age of twelve years is not recommended because safe and effective conditions for its usage have not been established.

MOBAN has not been shown effective in the management of behavioral complications in patients with mental retardation.

Sulfites Sensitivity: MOBAN Concentrate contains sodium metabisulfite, a sulfite that may cause allergic-type reactions including anaphylactic symptoms and life-threatening or less severe asthmatic episodes in certain susceptible people. The overall prevalence of sulfite sensitivity in the general population is unknown and probably low. Sulfite sensitivity is seen more frequently in asthmatic than in nonasthmatic people.

PRECAUTIONS

Some patients receiving MOBAN may note drowsiness initially and they should be advised against activities requiring mental alertness until their response to the drug has been established.

Increased activity has been noted in patients receiving MOBAN. Caution should be exercised where increased activity may be harmful.

MOBAN does not lower the seizure threshold in experimental animals to the degree noted with more sedating antipsychotic drugs. However, in humans convulsive seizures have been reported in a few instances.

The physician should be aware that this tablet preparation contains calcium sulfate as an excipient and that calcium ions may interfere with the absorption of preparations containing phenytoin sodium and tetracyclines.

MOBAN has an antiemetic effect in animals. A similar effect may occur in humans and may obscure signs of intestinal obstruction or brain tumor.

Neuroleptic drugs elevate prolactin levels; the elevation persists during chronic administration. Tissue culture experiments indicate that approximately one-third of human breast cancers are prolactin dependent *in vitro*, a factor of potential importance if the prescription of these drugs is contemplated in a patient with a previously detected breast cancer. Although disturbances such as galactorrhea, amenorrhea, gynecomastia, and impotence have been reported, the clinical significance of elevated serum prolactin levels is unknown for most patients. An increase in mammary neoplasms has been found in rodents after chronic administration of neuroleptic drugs. Neither clinical studies nor epidemiologic studies conducted to date, however, have shown an association between chronic administration of these drugs and mammary tumorigenesis; the available evidence is considered too limited to be conclusive at this time.

ADVERSE REACTIONS
CNS EFFECTS
The most frequently occurring effect is initial drowsiness that generally subsides with continued usage of the drug or lowering of the dose.

Noted less frequently were depression, hyperactivity and euphoria.
Neurological
Extrapyramidal Reactions
Extrapyramidal reactions noted below may occur in susceptible individuals and are usually reversible with appropriate management.
Akathisia
Motor restlessness may occur early.
Parkinson Syndrome
Akinesia, characterized by rigidity, immobility and reduction of voluntary movements and tremor, have been observed. Occurrence is less frequent than akathisia.
Dystonic Syndrome
Prolonged abnormal contractions of muscle groups occur infrequently. These symptoms may be managed by the addition of a synthetic antiparkinson agent (other than L-dopa), small doses of sedative drugs, and/or reduction in dosage.
Tardive Dyskinesia
Neuroleptic drugs are known to cause a syndrome of dyskinetic movements commonly referred to as tardive dyskinesia. The movements may appear during treatment or upon withdrawal of treatment and may be either reversible or irreversible (i.e., persistent) upon cessation of further neuroleptic administration.

The syndrome is known to have a variable latency for development and the duration of the latency cannot be determined reliably. It is thus wise to assume that any neuroleptic agent has the capacity to induce the syndrome and act accordingly until sufficient data has been collected to settle the issue definitively for a specific drug product. In the case of neuroleptics known to produce the irreversible syndrome, the following has been observed:

Tardive dyskinesia has appeared in some patients on long-term therapy and has also appeared after drug therapy has been discontinued. The risk appears to be greater in elderly patients on high-dose therapy, especially females. The symptoms are persistent and in some patients appear to be irreversible. The syndrome is characterized by rhythmical involuntary movements of the tongue, face, mouth or jaw (e.g., protrusion of tongue, puffing of cheeks, puckering of mouth, chewing movements). There may be involuntary movements of extremities.

There is no known effective treatment of tardive dyskinesia; antiparkinsonism agents usually do not alleviate the symptoms of this syndrome. It is suggested that all antipsychotic agents be discontinued if these symptoms appear. Should it be necessary to reinstitute treatment, or increase the dosage of the agent, or switch to a different antipsychotic agent, the syndrome may be masked. It has been reported that fine vermicular movements of the tongue may be an early sign of the syndrome and if the medication is stopped at that time the syndrome may not develop (See WARNINGS).
Autonomic Nervous System
Occasionally blurring of vision, tachycardia, nausea, dry mouth and salivation have been reported. Urinary retention and constipation may occur particularly if anticholinergic drugs are used to treat extrapyramidal symptoms. One patient being treated with MOBAN (molindone hydrochloride) experienced priapism which required surgical intervention, apparently resulting in residual impairment of erectile function.
Laboratory Tests
There have been rare reports of leucopenia and leucocytosis. If such reactions occur, treatment with MOBAN may continue if clinical symptoms are absent. Alterations of blood glucose, B.U.N., and red blood cells have not been considered clinically significant.
Metabolic and Endocrine Effects
Alteration of thyroid function has not been significant. Amenorrhea has been reported infrequently. Resumption of menses in previously amenorrheic women has been reported. Initially heavy menses may occur. Galactorrhea and gynecomastia have been reported infrequently. Increase in libido has been noted in some patients. Impotence has not been reported. Although both weight gain and weight loss have been in the direction of normal or ideal weight, excessive weight gain has not occurred with MOBAN.
Hepatic Effects
There have been rare reports of clinically significant alterations in liver function in association with MOBAN use.
Cardiovascular
Rare, transient, non-specific T wave changes have been reported on E.K.G. Association with a clinical syndrome has not been established. Rarely has significant hypotension been reported.
Ophthalmological
Lens opacities and pigmentary retinopathy have not been reported where patients have received MOBAN. In some patients, phenothiazine induced lenticular opacities have resolved following discontinuation of the phenothiazine while continuing therapy with MOBAN.
Skin
Early, non-specific skin rash, probably of allergic origin, has occasionally been reported. Skin pigmentation has not been seen with MOBAN usage alone.

MOBAN has certain pharmacological similarities to other antipsychotic agents. Because adverse reactions are often extensions of the pharmacological activity of a drug, all of the known pharmacological effects associated with other antipsychotic drugs should be kept in mind when MOBAN is used. Upon abrupt withdrawal after prolonged high dosage an abstinence syndrome has not been noted.

DOSAGE AND ADMINISTRATION
Initial and maintenance doses of MOBAN (molindone hydrochloride) should be individualized.
Initial Dosage Schedule
The usual starting dosage is 50–75 mg/day.
 — Increase to 100 mg/day in 3 or 4 days.
 — Based on severity of symptomatology, dosage may be titrated up or down depending on individual patient response.
 — An increase to 225 mg/day may be required in patients with severe symptomatology.
Elderly and debilitated patients should be started on lower dosage.

Strength	Description	NDC
5 mg	Orange, round, biconvex tablet, one face inscribed with "Moban 5", and the other face plain.	NDC 63481-072-70
10 mg	Lavender, round, biconvex tablet, one face inscribed with "Moban 10", and the other face plain.	NDC 63481-073-70
25 mg	Green, round, biconvex tablet, one face scored and inscribed with "Moban 25", and the other face plain with partial bisect.	NDC 63481-074-70
50 mg	Blue, round, biconvex tablet, one face scored and inscribed with "Moban 50", and the other face plain.	NDC 63481-076-70
100 mg	Tan, round, biconvex tablet, one face scored and inscribed with "Moban 100", and the other face plain.	NDC 63481-077-70

Maintenance Dosage Schedule
1. Mild-5 mg-15 mg three or four times a day.
2. Moderate-10 mg-25 mg three or four times a day.
3. Severe-225 mg/day may be required.

DRUG INTERACTIONS
Potentiation of drugs administered concurrently with MOBAN has not been reported. Additionally, animal studies have not shown increased toxicity when MOBAN is given concurrently with representative members of three classes of drugs (i.e., barbiturates, chloral hydrate and antiparkinson drugs).

MANAGEMENT OF OVERDOSAGE
Symptomatic, supportive therapy should be the rule.
Gastric lavage is indicated for the reduction of absorption of MOBAN which is freely soluble in water.
Since the adsorption of MOBAN by activated charcoal has not been determined, the use of this antidote must be considered of theoretical value.
Emesis in a comatose patient is contraindicated. Additionally, while the emetic effect of apomorphine is blocked by MOBAN in animals, this blocking effect has not been determined in humans.
A significant increase in the rate of removal of unmetabolized MOBAN from the body by forced diuresis, peritoneal or renal dialysis would not be expected. (Only 2% of a single ingested dose of MOBAN is excreted unmetabolized in the urine). However, poor response of the patient may justify use of these procedures.
While the use of laxatives or enemas might be based on general principles, the amount of unmetabolized MOBAN in feces is less than 1%. Extrapyramidal symptoms have responded to the use of diphenhydramine (Benadryl*), Amantadine HCl (Symmetrel®*) and the synthetic anticholinergic antiparkinson agents, (i.e., Artane*, Cogentin*, Akineton*).

HOW SUPPLIED
As tablets in bottles of 100 with potencies and colors as follows:
[See table above]
As a concentrate (clear, colorless to straw-yellow syrup) containing 20 mg molindone hydrochloride per mL in 4 oz. (120 mL) bottles, NDC 63481-460-04.
Store at controlled room temperature 15°–30°C (59°–86°F). Protect from light.
*Benadryl-Trademark, Parke Davis and Co.
*Artane-Trademark, Lederle Laboratories
*Cogentin-Trademark, Merck Sharp & Dohme
*Akineton-Trademark, Knoll Pharmaceutical Co.
*Symmetrel-Trademark, Endo Pharmaceuticals Inc.
MOBAN® is a Registered Trademark of Endo Pharmaceuticals Inc.
Copyright © Endo Pharmaceuticals Inc. 1998
6500-00/January, 1998
Shown in Product Identification Guide, page 310

NARCAN®   ℞
[nar'kan]
(naloxone hydrochloride injection, USP)
Opioid Antagonist

DESCRIPTION
NARCAN (naloxone hydrochloride injection, USP), an opioid antagonist, is a synthetic congener of oxymorphone. In structure it differs from oxymorphone in that the methyl group on the nitrogen atom is replaced by an allyl group.

NALOXONE HYDROCHLORIDE
(-)-17-Allyl-4, 5α-epoxy-3, 14 - dihydroxy
morphinan-6-one hydrochloride

Continued on next page

Narcan—Cont.

Naloxone hydrochloride occurs as a white to slightly off-white powder, and is soluble in water, in dilute acids, and in strong alkali; slightly soluble in alcohol; practically insoluble in ether and in chloroform.

NARCAN injection is available as a sterile solution for intravenous, intramuscular and subcutaneous administration in three concentrations: 0.02 mg, 0.4 mg and 1.0 mg of naloxone hydrochloride per mL. One mL of the 0.02 mg and 0.4 mg strengths contains 8.6 mg of sodium chloride. One mL of the 1.0 mg strength contains 8.35 mg of sodium chloride. In the 10 mL multiple dose vial, one mL of the 0.4 mg and 1.0 mg strengths also contains 2.0 mg of methylparaben and propylparaben as preservatives in a ratio of 9 to 1. pH is adjusted to 3.5 ± 0.5 with hydrochloric acid.

NARCAN injection is also available in a paraben-free formulation in three concentrations: 0.02 mg. 0.4 mg and 1.0 mg of naloxone hydrochloride per mL. One mL of each strength contains 9.0 mg of sodium chloride. pH is adjusted to 3.5 ± 0.5 with hydrochloric acid.

CLINICAL PHARMACOLOGY

Complete or Partial Reversal of Opioid Depression NARCAN prevents or reverses the effects of opioids including respiratory depression, sedation and hypotension. Also, it can reverse the psychotomimetic and dysphoric effects of agonist-antagonists such as pentazocine.

NARCAN is an essentially pure opioid antagonist, i.e., it does not possess the "agonistic" or morphine-like properties characteristic of other opioid antagonists; NARCAN does not produce respiratory depression, psychotomimetic effects or pupillary constriction. In the absence of opioids or agonistic effects of other opioid antagonists, it exhibits essentially no pharmacologic activity.

NARCAN has not been shown to produce tolerance or cause physical or psychological dependence.

In the presence of physical dependence on opioids NARCAN will produce withdrawal symptoms.

While the mechanism of action of NARCAN is not fully understood, the preponderance of evidence suggests that NARCAN antagonizes opioid effects by competing for the same receptor sites.

When NARCAN is administered intravenously, the onset of action is generally apparent within two minutes; the onset of action is only slightly less rapid when it is administered subcutaneously or intramuscularly. The duration of action is dependent upon the dose and route of administration of NARCAN. Intramuscular administration produces a more prolonged effect than intravenous administration. The requirement for repeat doses of NARCAN, however, will also be dependent upon the amount, type and route of administration of the opioid being antagonized.

Following parenteral administration, NARCAN is rapidly distributed in the body. It is metabolized in the liver, primarily by glucuronide conjugation and excreted in urine. In one study the serum half-life in adults ranged from 30 to 81 minutes (mean 64 ± 12 minutes). In a neonatal study the mean plasma half-life was observed to be 3.1 ± 0.5 hours.

Adjunctive Use in Septic Shock Although the mechanism of action is not completely understood, NARCAN appears to block endorphin-mediated hypotension in septic shock patients.

NARCAN has been shown in some cases of septic shock to produce a rise in blood pressure that may last up to several hours; however, this pressor response has not been demonstrated to improve patient survival.

Patients who have responded to NARCAN received the drug early in the course of treatment of septic shock. Because of the limited number of patients who have been treated, optimal dosage and treatment regimens have not been established. Published reports demonstrating a pressor effect have evaluated single bolus injections of 0.4 mg over three (3) to five (5) minutes, which have been repeated for 3–5 doses depending on the response. Bolus infusion doses ranging from 0.03 mg/kg to 0.2 mg/kg over five (5) minutes have also been reported. If a response was elicited, treatment was continued by intravenous infusion of concentrations of 0.03 mg/kg/hour to 0.3 mg/kg/hour for 1–24 hours or more depending upon the clinical response.

INDICATIONS AND USAGE

NARCAN is indicated for the complete or partial reversal of opioid depression, including respiratory depression, induced by natural and synthetic opioids, including propoxyphene, methadone and certain mixed agonist-antagonist analgesics: nalbuphine, pentazocine and butorphanol. NARCAN is also indicated for the diagnosis of suspected opioid tolerance or acute opioid overdosage.

NARCAN may be useful as an adjunctive agent to increase blood pressure in the management of septic shock (see **CLINICAL PHARMACOLOGY; Adjunctive Use in Septic Shock**).

CONTRAINDICATIONS

NARCAN is contraindicated in patients known to be hypersensitive to naloxone hydrochloride or to any of the other ingredients in NARCAN.

WARNINGS

NARCAN should be administered cautiously to persons including newborns of mothers who are known or suspected to be physically dependent on opioids. In such cases an abrupt and complete reversal of opioid effects may precipitate an acute withdrawal syndrome.

The signs and symptoms of opioid withdrawal in a patient physically dependent on opioids may include, but are not limited to, the following: body aches, diarrhea, tachycardia, fever, runny nose, sneezing, piloerection, sweating, yawning, nausea or vomiting, nervousness, restlessness or irritability, shivering or trembling, abdominal cramps, weakness, and increased blood pressure. In the neonate, opioid withdrawal may also include: convulsions, excessive crying, and hyperactive reflexes.

The patient who has satisfactorily responded to NARCAN should be kept under continued surveillance and repeated doses of NARCAN should be administered, as necessary, since the duration of action of some opioids may exceed that of NARCAN.

NARCAN is not effective against respiratory depression due to non-opioid drugs. Reversal of buprenorphine-induced respiratory depression may be incomplete. If an incomplete response occurs, respirations should be mechanically assisted.

PRECAUTIONS

General In addition to NARCAN, other resuscitative measures such as maintenance of a free airway, artificial ventilation, cardiac massage, and vasopressor agents should be available and employed when necessary to counteract acute opioid poisoning.

Abrupt postoperative reversal of opioid depression may result in nausea, vomiting, sweating, tremulousness, tachycardia, increased blood pressure, seizures, ventricular tachycardia and fibrillation, pulmonary edema, and cardiac arrest which may result in death.

Several instances of hypotension, hypertension, ventricular tachycardia and fibrillation, pulmonary edema, and cardiac arrest have been reported in postoperative patients. Death, coma, and encephalopathy have been reported as sequelae of these events. These have occurred in patients most of whom had pre-existing cardiovascular disorders or received other drugs which may have similar adverse cardiovascular effects. Although a direct cause and effect relationship has not been established, NARCAN should be used with caution in patients with pre-existing cardiac disease or patients who have received medications with potential adverse cardiovascular effects, such as hypotension, ventricular tachycardia or fibrillation, and pulmonary edema. It has been suggested that the pathogenesis of pulmonary edema associated with the use of NARCAN is similar to neurogenic pulmonary edema, i.e., a centrally mediated massive catecholamine response leading to a dramatic shift of blood volume into the pulmonary vascular bed resulting in increased hydrostatic pressures.

Carcinogenesis, Mutagenesis, Impairment of Fertility Studies in animals to assess the carcinogenic potential of NARCAN have not been conducted. NARCAN was weakly positive in the Ames mutagenicity and *in vitro* human lymphocyte chromosome aberration tests and was negative in the *in vitro* Chinese hamster V79 cell HGPRT mutagenicity assay and in an *in vivo* rat bone marrow chromosome aberration study. Reproduction studies conducted in mice and rats at doses as high as 50 times the usual human dose (10 mg/day) demonstrated no impairment of fertility.

Use in Pregnancy

Teratogenic Effects Pregnancy Category B: Reproduction studies performed in mice and rats at doses as high as 50 times the usual human dose (10 mg/day), revealed no evidence of impaired fertility or harm to the fetus due to NARCAN. There are however, no adequate and well controlled studies in pregnant women. Because animal reproduction studies are not always predictive of human response, NARCAN should be used during pregnancy only if clearly needed.

Non-teratogenic Effects Risk-benefit must be considered before NARCAN is administered to a pregnant woman who is known or suspected to be opioid-dependent since maternal dependence may often be accompanied by fetal dependence. Naloxone crosses the placenta and may precipitate withdrawal in the fetus as well as in the mother.

Use in Labor and Delivery It is not known if NARCAN affects the duration of labor and/or delivery.

Nursing Mothers It is not known whether NARCAN is excreted in human milk. Because many drugs are excreted in human milk, caution should be exercised when NARCAN is administered to a nursing woman.

Usage in Pediatric Patients and Neonates for Septic Shock The safety and effectiveness of NARCAN in the treatment of hypotension in pediatric patients and neonates with septic shock have not been established.

Renal Insufficiency/Failure The safety and effectiveness of NARCAN in patients with renal insufficiency/failure have not been established in well-controlled clinical trials. Caution should be exercised when NARCAN is administered to this patient population.

Liver Disease The safety and effectiveness of NARCAN in patients with liver disease have not been established in well-controlled clinical trials. In one small study in patients with liver cirrhosis, plasma naloxone concentrations were approximately six times higher than in patients without liver disease. NARCAN was well tolerated and no adverse events were reported. Caution should be exercised when NARCAN is administered to patients with liver disease.

ADVERSE REACTIONS

Postoperative The following adverse events have been associated with the use of NARCAN in postoperative patients: hypotension, hypertension, ventricular tachycardia and fibrillation, dyspnea, pulmonary edema, and cardiac arrest. Death, coma, and encephalopathy have been reported as sequelae of these events. Excessive doses of NARCAN in postoperative patients may result in significant reversal of analgesia and may cause agitation (see **PRECAUTIONS** and **DOSAGE AND ADMINISTRATION; Usage in Adults; Postoperative Opioid Depression**).

Opioid Depression Abrupt reversal of opioid depression may result in nausea, vomiting, sweating, tachycardia, increased blood pressure, tremulousness, seizures, ventricular tachycardia and fibrillation, pulmonary edema, and cardiac arrest which may result in death (see **PRECAUTIONS**).

Opioid Dependence Abrupt reversal of opioid effects in persons who are physically dependent on opioids may precipitate an acute withdrawal syndrome which may include, but is not limited to, the following signs and symptoms: body aches, fever, sweating, runny nose, sneezing, piloerection, yawning, weakness, shivering or trembling, nervousness, restlessness or irritability, diarrhea, nausea or vomiting, abdominal cramps, increased blood pressure, tachycardia. In the neonate, opioid withdrawal may also include: convulsions; excessive crying; hyperactive reflexes (see **WARNINGS**).

Agitation and paresthesias have been infrequently reported with the use of NARCAN (naloxone hydrochloride injection, USP).

DRUG ABUSE AND DEPENDENCE

NARCAN is an opioid antagonist. Physical dependence associated with the use of NARCAN has not been reported. Tolerance to the opioid antagonist effect of NARCAN is not known to occur.

OVERDOSAGE

There is limited clinical experience with NARCAN overdosage in humans.

Adult Patients In one study, volunteers and morphine-dependent subjects who received 24 mg/70 kg did not demonstrate toxicity.

In another study, 36 patients with acute stroke received a loading dose of 4 mg/kg (10 mg/m^2/min) of NARCAN followed immediately by 2 mg/kg/hr for 24 hours. There were a few reports of serious adverse events: seizures (2 patients), severe hypertension (1), and hypotension and/or bradycardia(3).

At doses of 2 mg/kg in normal subjects, memory impairment has been reported.

Pediatric Patients Up to 11 doses of 0.2 mg of naloxone (2.2 mg) have been administered to children following overdose of diphenoxylate hydrochloride with atropine sulfate. Pediatric reports include a 2-1/2 year old child who inadvertently received a dose of 20 mg of naloxone and a 4-1/2 year-old who received 11 doses during a 12-hour period, both of whom had no adverse sequelae.

Patient Management Patients who experience a NARCAN overdose should be treated symptomatically in a closely-supervised environment. Physicians should contact a poison control center for the most up-to-date patient management information.

Animal Data The intravenous single-dose LD_{50} (95% confidence limits) in rats and mice is 150 (135–165) mg/kg and 109 (97–121) mg/kg, respectively. In newborn rats, the subcutaneous single-dose LD_{50} (95% confidence limits) is 260 (228–296) mg/kg. Subcutaneous injection in rats at 100 mg/kg/day for three weeks produced only transiently increased salivation and partial ptosis; no drug-related effects were seen at 10 mg/kg/day for three weeks.

Some chemical impurities in naloxone, i.e., noroxymorphone and bisnaloxone, have been shown to produce emesis in dogs when administered alone at i.v. doses equivalent to impurity levels present in naloxone at 60 times the usual human dose (10 mg/day).

DOSAGE AND ADMINISTRATION

NARCAN may be administered intravenously, intramuscularly, or subcutaneously. The most rapid onset of action is achieved by intravenous administration, which is recommended in emergency situations.

Since the duration of action of some opioids may exceed that of NARCAN, the patient should be kept under continued surveillance. Repeated doses of NARCAN should be administered, as necessary.

Intravenous Infusion NARCAN may be diluted for intravenous infusion in normal saline or 5% dextrose solutions.

0.4 mg/mL	10 mL multiple dose vial-box of 1	NDC 63481-365-05
0.4 mg/mL (paraben-free)	1 mL ampul-box of 10	NDC 63481-358-10
1.0 mg/mL	10 mL multiple dose vial-box of 1	NDC 63481-368-05
1.0 mg/mL (paraben-free)	2 mL ampul-box of 10	NDC 63481-377-10
0.02 mg/mL (paraben-free)	2 mL ampul-box of 10	NDC 63481-359-10

The addition of 2 mg of NARCAN in 500 mL of either solution provides a concentration of 0.004 mg/mL. Mixtures should be used within 24 hours. After 24 hours, the remaining unused mixture must be discarded. The rate of administration should be titrated in accordance with the patient's response.

NARCAN should not be mixed with preparations containing bisulfite, metabisulfite, long-chain or high molecular weight anions, or any solution having an alkaline pH. No drug or chemical agent should be added to NARCAN unless its effect on the chemical and physical stability of the solution has first been established.

General Parenteral drug products should be inspected visually for particulate matter and discoloration prior to administration whenever solution and container permit.

Usage in Adults

Opioid Overdose - Known or Suspected An initial dose of 0.4 mg to 2 mg of NARCAN may be administered intravenously. If the desired degree of counteraction and improvement in respiratory functions are not obtained, it may be repeated at two- to three-minute intervals. If no response is observed after 10 mg of NARCAN have been administered, the diagnosis of opioid-induced or partial opioid-induced toxicity should be questioned. Intramuscular or subcutaneous administration may be necessary if the intravenous route is not available.

Postoperative Opioid Depression For the partial reversal of opioid depression following the use of opioids during surgery, smaller doses of NARCAN are usually sufficient. The dose of NARCAN should be titrated according to the patient's response. For the initial reversal of respiratory depression, NARCAN should be injected in increments of 0.1 to 0.2 mg intravenously at two- to three-minute intervals to the desired degree of reversal i.e., adequate ventilation and alertness without significant pain or discomfort. Larger than necessary dosage of NARCAN may result in significant reversal of analgesia and increase in blood pressure. Similarly, too rapid reversal may induce nausea, vomiting, sweating or circulatory stress.

Repeat doses of NARCAN may be required within one- to two-hour intervals depending upon the amount, type (i.e., short or long acting) and time interval since last administration of an opioid. Supplemental intramuscular doses have been shown to produce a longer lasting effect.

NARCAN Challenge Test Used for the diagnosis of suspected opioid tolerance or acute opioid overdosage. The NARCAN challenge test should not be performed in a patient showing clinical signs or symptoms of opioid withdrawal, or in a patient whose urine contains opioids. The NARCAN challenge test may be administered by either the intravenous or subcutaneous routes.

Intravenous:
Inject 0.2 mg NARCAN.
Observe for 30 seconds for signs or symptoms of withdrawal.
If no evidence of withdrawal, inject 0.6 mg NARCAN.
Observe for an additional 20 minutes.

Subcutaneous:
Administer 0.8 mg NARCAN.
Observe for 20 minutes for signs or symptoms of withdrawal.

Note: Individual patients, especially those with opioid dependence, may respond to lower doses of NARCAN. In some cases, 0.1 mg I.V. NARCAN has produced a diagnostic response.

Interpretation of the Challenge Monitor vital signs and observe the patient for signs and symptoms of opioid withdrawal. These may include, but are not limited to: nausea, vomiting, dysphoria, yawning, sweating, tearing, rhinorrhea, stuffy nose, craving for opioid, poor appetite, abdominal cramps, sense of fear, skin erythema, disrupted sleep patterns, fidgeting, uneasiness, poor ability to focus, mental lapses, muscle aches or cramps, pupillary dilation, piloerection, fever, changes in blood pressure, pulse or temperature, anxiety, depression, irritability, back ache, bone or joint pains, tremors, sensations of skin crawling or fasciculations. If signs or symptoms of withdrawal appear, the test is positive and no additional NARCAN should be administered.

Septic Shock The optimal dosage of NARCAN or duration of therapy for the treatment of hypotension in septic shock patients has not been established (see **CLINICAL PHARMACOLOGY**).

Usage in Children

Opioid Overdose - Known or Suspected The usual initial dose in children is 0.01 mg/kg body weight given I.V. If this dose does not result in the desired degree of clinical improvement, a subsequent dose of 0.1 mg/kg body weight may

be administered. If an I.V. route of administration is not available, NARCAN may be administered I.M. or S.C. in divided doses. If necessary, NARCAN can be diluted with sterile water for injection.

Postoperative Opioid Depression Follow the recommendations and cautions under **Adult Postoperative Depression**. For the initial reversal of respiratory depression, NARCAN should be injected in increments of 0.005 mg to 0.01 mg intravenously at two- to three-minute intervals to the desired degree of reversal.

Usage in Neonates

Opioid-induced Depression The usual initial dose is 0.01 mg/kg body weight administered I.V., I.M., or S.C. This dose may be repeated in accordance with adult administration guidelines for postoperative opioid depression.

HOW SUPPLIED

NARCAN (naloxone hydrochloride injection, USP) for intravenous, intramuscular and subcutaneous administration is available as:
[See table above]

Store at controlled room temperature 15°–30°C (59°–86°F). Protect from excessive light.

Store in carton until contents have been used.

CAUTION: Federal (USA) law prohibits dispensing without prescription.

NARCAN® is a Registered Trademark of Endo Pharmaceuticals Inc.

Copyright © Endo Pharmaceuticals Inc. 1998

6487-00/January, 1998

NUBAIN®
[nū 'bān]
(nalbuphine hydrochloride)

℞

DESCRIPTION

NUBAIN (nalbuphine hydrochloride) is a synthetic narcotic agonist-antagonist analgesic of the phenanthrene series. It is chemically related to both the widely used narcotic antagonist, naloxone, and the potent narcotic analgesic, oxymorphone.

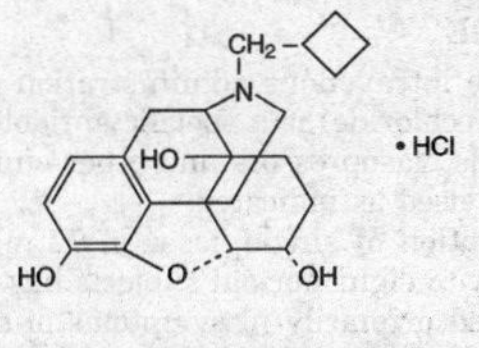

NALBUPHINE HYDROCHLORIDE

(-)-17-(cyclobutylmethyl)-4, 5α-
epoxymorphinan-3, 6α, 14-triol, hydrochloride

NUBAIN is a sterile solution suitable for subcutaneous, intramuscular, or intravenous injection. NUBAIN is available in two concentrations, 10 mg and 20 mg of nalbuphine hydrochloride per mL. Both strengths in 10 mL vials contain 0.94% sodium citrate hydrous, 1.26% citric acid anhydrous, and 0.2% of a 9:1 mixture of methylparaben and propylparaben as preservatives; pH is adjusted, if necessary, to 3.5 to 3.7 with hydrochloric acid. The 10 mg/mL strength contains 0.2% sodium chloride.

NUBAIN is also available in ampuls in a sterile, paraben-free formulation in two concentrations, 10 mg and 20 mg of nalbuphine hydrochloride per mL. One mL of each strength contains 0.94% sodium citrate hydrous, and 1.26% citric acid anhydrous; pH is adjusted, if necessary, to 3.5 to 3.7 with hydrochloric acid. The 10 mg/mL strength contains 0.2% sodium chloride.

CLINICAL PHARMACOLOGY

NUBAIN is a potent analgesic. Its analgesic potency is essentially equivalent to that of morphine on a milligram basis. Receptor studies show that NUBAIN binds to mu, kappa, and delta receptors, but not to sigma receptors. NUBAIN is primarily a kappa agonist/partial mu antagonist analgesic.

The onset of action of NUBAIN occurs within 2 to 3 minutes after intravenous administration, and in less than 15 minutes following subcutaneous or intramuscular injection. The plasma half-life of nalbuphine is 5 hours, and in clinical studies the duration of analgesic activity has been reported to range from 3 to 6 hours.

The narcotic antagonist activity of NUBAIN is one-fourth as potent as nalorphine and 10 times that of pentazocine.

NUBAIN may produce the same degree of respiratory depression as equianalgesic doses of morphine. However, NUBAIN exhibits a ceiling effect such that increases in dose greater than 30 mg do not produce further respiratory depression.

NUBAIN by itself has potent narcotic antagonist activity at doses equal to or lower than its analgesic dose. When administered following or concurrent with mu agonist opioid analgesics (e.g., morphine, oxymorphone, fentanyl), NUBAIN may partially reverse or block narcotic-induced respiratory depression from the mu agonist analgesic. NUBAIN may precipitate withdrawal in patients dependent on opioid narcotic drugs. NUBAIN should be used with caution in patients who have been receiving mu opioid analgesics on a regular basis.

INDICATIONS AND USAGE

NUBAIN is indicated for the relief of moderate to severe pain. NUBAIN can also be used as a supplement to balanced anesthesia, for preoperative and postoperative analgesia, and for obstetrical analgesia during labor and delivery.

CONTRAINDICATIONS

NUBAIN should not be administered to patients who are hypersensitive to nalbuphine hydrochloride, or to any of the other ingredients in NUBAIN.

WARNINGS

NUBAIN should be administered as a supplement to general anesthesia only by persons specifically trained in the use of intravenous anesthetics and management of the respiratory effects of potent opioids.

Naloxone, resuscitative and intubation equipment and oxygen should be readily available.

Drug Abuse Caution should be observed in prescribing NUBAIN for emotionally unstable patients, or for individuals with a history of narcotic abuse. Such patients should be closely supervised when long-term therapy is contemplated (see **DRUG ABUSE AND DEPENDENCE**).

Use in Ambulatory Patients NUBAIN may impair the mental or physical abilities required for the performance of potentially dangerous tasks such as driving a car or operating machinery. Therefore, NUBAIN should be administered with caution to ambulatory patients who should be warned to avoid such hazards.

Use in Emergency Procedures Maintain patient under observation until recovered from NUBAIN effects that would affect driving or other potentially dangerous tasks.

Use in Pregnancy (other than labor) Safe use of NUBAIN in pregnancy has not been established. Although animal reproductive studies have not revealed teratogenic or embryotoxic effects, nalbuphine should be administered to pregnant women only if clearly needed.

Use During Labor and Delivery The placental transfer of nalbuphine is high, rapid, and variable with a maternal to fetal ratio ranging from 1:0.37 to 1:1.6. Fetal and neonatal adverse effects that have been reported following the administration of nalbuphine to the mother during labor include fetal bradycardia, respiratory depression at birth, apnea, cyanosis and hypotonia. Maternal administration of naloxone during labor has normalized these effects in some cases. Severe and prolonged fetal bradycardia has been reported. Permanent neurological damage attributed to fetal bradycardia has occurred. A sinusoidal fetal heart rate pattern associated with the use of nalbuphine has also been reported. NUBAIN should be used with caution in women during during labor and delivery, and newborns should be monitored for respiratory depression, apnea, bradycardia, and arrhythmias if NUBAIN has been used.

Head Injury and Intracranial Pressure The possible respiratory depressant effects and the potential of potent analgesics to elevate cerebrospinal fluid pressure (resulting from vasodilation following CO_2 retention) may be markedly exaggerated in the presence of head injury, intracranial lesions or a pre-existing increase in intracranial pressure. Furthermore, potent analgesics can produce effects which may obscure the clinical course of patients with head injuries. Therefore, NUBAIN should be used in these circumstances only when essential, and then should be administered with extreme caution.

Interaction With Other Central Nervous System Depressants Although NUBAIN possesses narcotic antagonist activity, there is evidence that in nondependent patients it will not antagonize a narcotic analgesic administered just before, concurrently, or just after an injection of NUBAIN. Therefore, patients receiving a narcotic analgesic, general

Continued on next page

Nubain—Cont.

anesthetics phenothiazines, or other tranquilizers, sedatives, hypnotics, or other CNS depressants (including alcohol) concomitantly with NUBAIN may exhibit an additive effect. When such combined therapy is contemplated, the dose of one or both agents should be reduced.

PRECAUTIONS

General

Impaired Respiration At the usual adult dose of 10mg/70kg, NUBAIN causes some respiratory depression approximately equal to that produced by equal doses of morphine. However, in contrast to morphine, respiratory depression is not appreciably increased with higher doses of NUBAIN. Respiratory depression induced by NUBAIN can be reversed by NARCAN® (naloxone hydrochloride) when indicated. NUBAIN should be administered with caution at low doses to patients with impaired respiration (e.g., from other medication, uremia, bronchial asthma, severe infection, cyanosis, or respiratory obstructions).

Impaired Renal or Hepatic Function Because NUBAIN is metabolized in the liver and excreted by the kidneys, NUBAIN should be used with caution in patients with renal or liver dysfunction and administered in reduced amounts.

Myocardial Infarction As with all potent analgesics, NUBAIN should be used with caution in patients with myocardial infarction who have nausea or vomiting.

Biliary Tract Surgery As with all narcotic analgesics, NUBAIN should be used with caution in patients about to undergo surgery of the biliary tract since it may cause spasm of the sphincter of Oddi.

Cardiovascular System During evaluation of NUBAIN in anesthesia, a higher incidence of bradycardia has been reported in patients who did not receive antropine pre-operatively.

Information for Patients

Patients should be advised of the following information:

— NUBAIN is associated with sedation and may impair mental and physical abilities required for the performance of potentially dangerous tasks such as driving a car or operating machinery.
— NUBAIN is to be used as prescribed by a physician. Dose or frequency should not be increased without first consulting with a physician since NUBAIN may cause psychological or physical dependence.
— The use of NUBAIN with other narcotics can cause signs and symptoms of withdrawal.
— Abrupt discontinuation of NUBAIN after prolonged usage may cause signs and symptoms or withdrawal.

Laboratory Tests

NUBAIN (nalbuphine hydrochloride) may interfere with enzymatic methods for the detection of opioids depending on the specificity/sensitivity of the test. Please consult the test manufacturer for specific details.

Carcinogenesis, Mutagenesis, Impairment of Fertility

No evidence of carcinogenicity was found in a 24-month carcinogenicity study in rats and an 18-month carcinogenicity study in mice at oral doses as high as the equivalent of approximately three times the maximum recommended therapeutic dose.

No evidence of mutagenic/genotoxic potential to NUBAIN was found in the Ames, Chinese Hamster Ovary HGPRT, and Sister Chromatid Exchange, mouse micronucleus, and rat bone marrow cytogenicity assays. Nalbuphine induced an increased frequency of mutation in mouse lymphoma cells.

Usage in Pregnancy

Teratogenic Effects

Pregnancy Category B—Reproduction studies have been performed in rats and in rabbits at dosages as high as approximately 14 and 31 times respectively the maximum recommended daily dose and revealed no evidence of impaired fertility or harm to the fetus due to NUBAIN. There are, however, no adequate and well-controlled studies in pregnant women. Because animal reproduction studies are not always predictive of human response, this drug should be used during pregnancy only if clearly needed (see **WARNINGS**).

Non-teratogenic Effects

Neonatal body weight and survival was reduced when NUBAIN was subcutaneously administered to female rats prior to mating and throughout gestation and lactation or to pregnant rats during the last third of gestation and throughout lactation at doses approximately 8 to 17 times the maximum recommended therapeutic dose. The clinical significance of this effect is unknown.

Use During Labor and Delivery

See **WARNINGS**.

Nursing Mothers

Limited data suggest that NUBAIN is excreted in maternal milk but only in a small amount (less than 1% of the administered dose) and with a clinically insignificant effect. Caution should be exercised when NUBAIN is administered to a nursing woman.

Pediatric Use

Safety and effectiveness in pediatric patients below the age of 18 years have not been established.

ADVERSE REACTIONS

The most frequent adverse reaction in 1066 patients treated in clinical studies with NUBAIN was sedation 381 (36%).

Less frequent reactions were: sweaty/clammy 99 (9%), nausea/vomiting 68 (6%), dizziness/vertigo 58 (5%), dry mouth 44 (4%), and headache 27 (3%).

Other adverse reactions which occurred (reported incidence of 1% or less) were:

CNS Effects Nervousness, depression, restlessness, crying, euphoria, floating, hostility, unusual dreams, confusion, faintness, hallucinations, dysphoria, feeling of heaviness, numbness, tingling, unreality. The incidence of psychotomimetic effects, such as unreality, depersonalization, delusions, dysphoria and hallucinations has been shown to be less than that which occurs with pentazocine.

Cardiovascular Hypertension, hypotension, bradycardia, tachycardia.

Gastrointestinal Cramps, dyspepsia, bitter taste.

Respiratory Depression, dyspnea, asthma.

Dermatologic Itching, burning, urticaria.

Miscellaneous Speech difficulty, urinary urgency, blurred vision, flushing and warmth.

Allergic Reactions Anaphylactic/anaphylactoid and other serious hypersensitivity reactions have been reported following the use of nalbuphine and may require immediate, supportive medical treatment. These reactions may include shock, respiratory distress, respiratory arrest, bradycardia, cardiac arrest, hypotension, or laryngeal edema. Other allergic-type reactions reported include stridor, bronchospasm, wheezing, edema, rash, pruritus, nausea, vomiting, diaphoresis, weakness, and shakiness.

Post-marketing Other reports include pulmonary edema, agitation and injection site reactions such as pain, swelling, redness, burning, and hot sensations.

DRUG ABUSE AND DEPENDENCE

NUBAIN has been shown to have a low abuse potential. When compared with drugs which are not mixed agonist-antagonists, it has been reported that nalbuphrine's potential for abuse would be less than that of codeine and propoxyphene. Drug abuse has been reported infrequently. Psychological and physical dependence and tolerance may follow the abuse or misuse of nalbuphine (see **WARNINGS**).

Care should be taken to avoid increases in dosage or frequency of administration which in susceptible individuals might result in physical dependence.

Abrupt discontinuation of NUBAIN following prolonged use has been followed by symptoms of narcotic withdrawal i.e., abdominal cramps, nausea and vomiting, rhinorrhea, lacrimation, restlessness, anxiety, elevated temperature and piloerection.

OVERDOSAGE

The immediate intravenous administration of NARCAN® (naloxone hydrochloride) is a specific antidote. Oxygen, intravenous fluids, vasopressors and other supportive measures should be used as indicated.

The administration of single doses of 72 mg of NUBAIN subcutaneously to eight normal subjects has been reported to have resulted primarily in symptoms of sleepiness and mild dysphoria.

DOSAGE AND ADMINISTRATION

The usual recommended adult dose is 10 mg for a 70 kg individual, administered subcutaneously, intramuscularly or intravenously; this dose may be repeated every 3 to 6 hours as necessary. Dosage should be adjusted according to the severity of the pain, physical status of the patient, and other medications which the patient may be receiving. (See **Interaction with Other Central Nervous System Depressants** under **WARNINGS**). In non-tolerant individuals, the recommended single maximum dose is 20 mg, with a maximum total daily dose of 160 mg.

The use of NUBAIN as a supplement to balanced anesthesia requires larger doses than those recommended for analgesia. Induction doses of NUBAIN range from 0.3 mg/kg to 3 mg/kg intravenously to be administered over a 10 to 15 minute period with maintenance doses of 0.25 to 0.5 mg/kg in single intravenous administrations as required. The use of NUBAIN may be followed by respiratory depression which can be reversed with the narcotic antagonist NARCAN® (naloxone hydrochloride).

NUBAIN is physically incompatible with nafcillin and ketorolac.

Patients Dependent on Narcotics Patients who have been taking narcotics chronically may experience withdrawal symptoms upon the administration of NUBAIN. If unduly troublesome, narcotic withdrawal symptoms can be controlled by the slow intravenous administration of small increments of morphine, until relief occurs. If the previous analgesic was morphine, meperidine, codeine, or other narcotic with similar duration of activity, one-fourth of the anticipated dose of NUBAIN can be administered initially and the patient observed for signs of withdrawal, i.e., abdominal cramps, nausea, and vomiting, lacrimation, rhinorrhea, anxiety, restlessness, elevation of temperature or piloerection. If untoward symptoms do not occur, progressively larger doses may be tried at appropriate intervals until the desired level of analgesia is obtained with NUBAIN.

HOW SUPPLIED

NUBAIN® (nalbuphine hydrochloride) injection for intramuscular, subcutaneous, or intravenous use is a sterile solution available in:

NDC 63481-432-10	(sulfite-free) 10 mg/mL, 10 mL multiple dose vials (box of 1)
NDC 63481-508-01	(sulfite/paraben-free) 10 mg/mL, 1 mL ampuls (box of 10)
NDC 63481-433-10	(sulfite-free) 20 mg/mL, 10 mL multiple dose vials (box of 1)
NDC 63481-509-01	(sulfite/paraben-free) 20 mg/mL, 1 mL ampuls (box of 10)

Store at controlled room temperature (59°–86°F, 15°–30°C). Protect from excessive light. Store in carton until contents have been used.

Parenteral drug products should be inspected visually for particulate matter and discoloration prior to administration whenever solution and container permit.

CAUTION Federal law prohibits dispensing without prescription.

6436-1/Rev. April, 1996

NUMORPHAN® Ⓒ II

[*nū-mor 'fan*]

Oxymorphone Hydrochloride Injection, USP
Oxymorphone Hydrochloride Suppositories, USP
Opioid Analgesic

DESCRIPTION

NUMORPHAN (oxymorphone hydrochloride, USP), a semi-synthetic opioid substitute for morphine, is a potent analgesic.

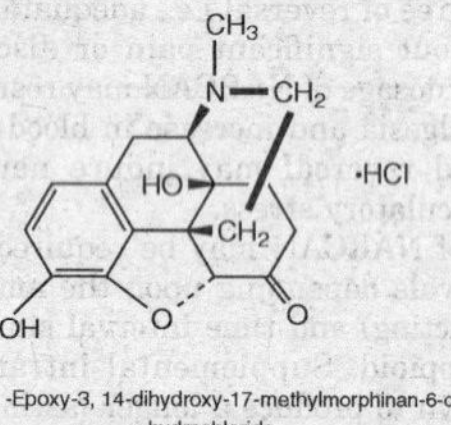

4.5α -Epoxy-3, 14-dihydroxy-17-methylmorphinan-6-one hydrochloride

Oxymorphone hydrochloride is a white or slightly off-white, odorless powder, which is sparingly soluble in alcohol and ether, but freely soluble in water. The molecular weight of oxymorphone hydrochloride is 337.80. The pK_{a1} and pK_{a2} of oxymorphone at 37°C are 8.17 and 9.54, respectively. The octanol/aqueous partition coefficient at 37°C and pH 7.4 is 0.98.

NUMORPHAN Injection is available in two concentrations, 1 mg/mL, 1 mL ampul and 1.5 mg/mL, 10 mL vial of oxymorphone hydrochloride. In addition, each 1 mg/mL ampul contains 8.0 mg/mL sodium chloride. Each 1.5mg/mL vial contains 8.0 mg/mL sodium chloride, 1.8 mg/mL methylparaben and 0.2 mg/mL propylparaben. pH for both the ampul and vial is adjusted with hydrochloric acid.

The NUMORPHAN Rectal Suppository is available in a concentration of 5 mg of oxymorphone hydrochloride in a base consisting of polyethylene glycol 1000 and polyethylene glycol 3350.

CLINICAL PHARMACOLOGY

NUMORPHAN is a potent opioid analgesic. Administered parenterally, 1 mg of NUMORPHAN is approximately equivalent in analgesic activity to 10 mg of morphine sulfate.

Many of the effects described below are common to the class of opioid analgesics, including NUMORPHAN.

Central Nervous System (CNS): Opioid analgesics exert their principal pharmacologic effects on the CNS and the gastrointestinal tract. The principal actions of therapeutic value are analgesia and sedation. The precise mechanism of the analgesic action is unknown. However, specific CNS opiate receptors have been identified and likely play a role in the expression of analgesic effects.

Opioids produce respiratory depression by direct action on brain stem respiratory centers. The mechanism of respiratory depression involves a reduction in the responsiveness of the brain stem respiratory centers to increases in carbon dioxide tension and to electrical stimulation. Opioids depress the cough reflex by direct action on the cough center in the medulla. Opioids cause miosis. Pinpoint pupils are a common sign of opioid overdose but are not pathognomonic. Marked mydriasis may be seen with worsening hypoxia.

Gastrointestinal Tract and Other Smooth Muscle: Opioids decrease gastric, biliary, and pancreatic secretions. These drugs cause a reduction in motility associated with an increase in tone in the antrum of the stomach and duodenum. Digestion of food in the small intestine is delayed and propulsive contractions are decreased. Propulsive peristaltic waves in the colon are decreased while tone is increased to the point of spasm. The end result is constipation. Opioids can cause a marked increase in biliary tract pressure as a result of spasm of the sphincter of Oddi.
Opioids increase smooth muscle tone in the urinary tract and can induce spasms. Urinary urgency and difficulty with urination may result. These effects, in conjunction with the central effect of these drugs on release of vasopressin, may produce oliguria.

Pharmacokinetics
The onset of action of parenterally administered NUMORPHAN is rapid; initial effects are usually perceived within 5 to 10 minutes. Its duration of action is approximately 3 to 6 hours.
Distribution: After an IV dose, the steady state volume of distribution was 3.08 ± 1.14 L/kg in healthy male and female subjects.
Metabolism: Oxymorphone undergoes extensive hepatic metabolism in humans. After a 10 mg oral dose, 49% was excreted over a five-day period in the urine. Of this, 82% was excreted in the first 24 hours after administration. The recovered drug-related products contained the oxymorphone (1.9%), the conjugate of oxymorphone (44.1%), the 6β-carbinol produced by 6-keto reduction of oxymorphone (0.3%), and the conjugates of 6β-carbinol (2.6%) and 6α-carbinol (0.1%).
Elimination: In healthy subjects, the mean terminal half-life of oxymorphone was 1.3 ± 0.7 hours. The mean systemic clearance was 2.0 ± 0.5 L/min.

INDICATIONS AND USAGE

NUMORPHAN Suppository is indicated for the relief of moderate to severe pain.
NUMORPHAN Injection is indicated for the relief of moderate to severe pain. It is also indicated for preoperative medication, for support of anesthesia, for obstetrical analgesia, and for relief of anxiety in patients with dyspnea associated with pulmonary edema secondary to acute left ventricular dysfunction.

CONTRAINDICATIONS

NUMORPHAN should not be administered to patients who are hypersensitive to oxymorphone hydrochloride or to any of the other ingredients in NUMORPHAN, or hypersensitive to morphine analogs.
NUMORPHAN should not be administered to individuals during an acute asthmatic attack or to patients with severe respiratory depression, upper airway obstruction, or any patient who has or is suspected of having a paralytic ileus.
NUMORPHAN should not be used in the treatment of pulmonary edema secondary to a chemical respiratory irritant. Opioid analgesics cause pooling of blood in the extremities by decreasing peripheral vascular resistance. This effect results in decreases in venous return, cardiac work, and pulmonary venous pressure, and blood is shifted from the central to peripheral circulation which would not be beneficial in the treatment of pulmonary edema secondary to a chemical respiratory irritant.

WARNINGS

Interactions with other central nervous system depressants: Patients receiving other opioid analgesics, general anesthetics, phenothiazines, other tranquilizers, sedatives, hypnotics or other CNS depressants (including alcohol) concomitantly with NUMORPHAN may exhibit an additive CNS depression (See PRECAUTIONS; Drug Interactions).
Respiratory depression: NUMORPHAN should be administered with extreme caution to patients with conditions accompanied by hypoxia, hypercapnia or decreased respiratory reserve such as: asthma, chronic obstructive pulmonary disease or cor pulmonale, severe obesity, sleep apnea syndrome, myxedema, kyphoscoliosis, CNS depression or coma.
Head injury and increased intracranial pressure: The possible respiratory depressant effects of potent analgesics and their potential to elevate cerebrospinal fluid pressure (resulting from vasodilation following CO_2 retention) may be markedly exaggerated in the presence of head injury, intracranial lesions or a preexisting increase in intracranial pressure. Furthermore, potent analgesics can produce effects which may obscure the clinical course of patients with head injuries. Therefore, NUMORPHAN should be used in these circumstances only when essential, and then should be administered with extreme caution.
Acute abdominal conditions: The administration of opioids may obscure the diagnosis or clinical course of patients with acute abdominal conditions.
Drug dependence: NUMORPHAN, as with other opioid drugs, can produce tolerance, psychological dependence, and physical dependence and has the potential for being abused (See DRUG ABUSE AND DEPENDENCE).
Pregnancy: Safe use in pregnancy has not been established (relative to possible adverse effects on fetal development). As with other analgesics, the use of NUMORPHAN in pregnancy, in nursing mothers, or in women of child-bearing potential requires that the possible benefits of the drug be weighed against the possible hazards to the mother and the child (See PRECAUTIONS).

PRECAUTIONS

General
Special risk patients: NUMORPHAN should be used with caution in elderly and debilitated patients and in patients who are known to be sensitive to central nervous system depressants, such as those with cardiovascular, pulmonary, renal or hepatic disease. Caution should also be exercised in patients with hypothyroidism, acute alcoholism, delirium tremens, convulsive disorders, Addison's disease, gallbladder disease or gallstones, prostatic hypertrophy or urethral stricture, recent gastrointestinal or genitourinary tract surgery, inflammatory bowel disease, diarrhea secondary to poisoning until the toxin is eliminated, diarrhea secondary to pseudomembranous colitis, cardiac arrhythmias, increased ocular pressure, and toxic psychosis. Debilitated and elderly patients and those with severe liver disease should receive smaller doses of NUMORPHAN.
Hypotensive effect: Opioid analgesics may cause severe hypotension in patients whose ability to maintain blood pressure has been compromised by a depleted blood volume or coadministration of drugs such as phenothiazines or general anesthetics. Administer with caution to patients in circulatory shock, since vasodilatation produced by the drug may further reduce cardiac output and blood pressure. Orthostatic hypotension may occur in ambulatory patients.

Information for Patients
Patients should be cautioned regarding the following:
Drowsiness, dizziness, or lightheadedness related to the use of this medication may impair mental and/or physical abilities required for the performance of potentially hazardous tasks, such as driving a car, operating machinery, etc.
This medication, like other opioid analgesics, will add to the effect of alcohol and other CNS depressants [such as antihistamines, sedatives, hypnotics, tranquilizers, general anesthetics, phenothiazines, other opioids, tricyclic antidepressants, and monoamine oxidase (MAO) inhibitors]. Alcohol should not be consumed while taking NUMORPHAN.
Withdrawal side effects may be precipitated by suddenly stopping this drug after prolonged use (regular use for several weeks or more). The medication should be gradually reduced before completely discontinuing use.
Elderly patients are more sensitive to opioid analgesics, especially the respiratory depressant effects and opioid induced urinary retention. Lower doses or longer dosing intervals may be required.
Orthostatic hypotension may occur with the use of this medication, especially in ambulatory patients. Patients should get up slowly from a lying or sitting position.
NUMORPHAN may be habit forming and has the potential for being abused. Tolerance, psychological and physical dependence can occur.
Safe use in pregnancy has not been established. Prolonged use of opioid analgesics during pregnancy may cause fetal-neonatal physical dependence, and neonatal withdrawal may occur.

Laboratory Tests
Opioids may increase biliary tract pressure with resultant increases in plasma amylase or lipase.

Drug Interactions
The concomitant use of other CNS depressants including sedatives, hypnotics, tranquilizers, general anesthetics, phenothiazines, other opioids, tricyclic antidepressants, monoamine oxidase (MAO) inhibitors, and alcohol may produce additive CNS depressant effects. When such combined therapy is contemplated, the dose of one or both agents should be reduced (See WARNINGS).
Anticholinergics or other medications with anticholinergic activity when used concurrently with opioid analgesics may result in increased risk of urinary retention and/or severe constipation, which may lead to paralytic ileus.
It has been reported that the incidence of bradycardia was increased when oxymorphone was combined with propofol for induction of anesthesia.
In addition, CNS toxicity has been reported (confusion, disorientation, respiratory depression, apnea, seizures) following coadministration of cimetidine with opioid analgesics; no clear-cut cause and effect relationship was established.

Carcinogenesis, Mutagenesis, Impairment of Fertility
Long-term studies have not been performed in animals to evaluate the carcinogenic potential of NUMORPHAN (oxymorphone hydrochloride, USP). Studies to evaluate the mutagenic potential of NUMORPHAN have not been conducted. There have been no studies to evaluate the effect of NUMORPHAN on fertility.

Usage in Pregnancy
Teratogenic Effects
Pregnancy Category C - NUMORPHAN was reported to produce malformations in offspring of hamsters that received 1,500 times the recommended human dose on Day 8 of gestation. There have been no adequate and well-controlled studies of reproductive toxicity in other laboratory animals or in pregnant women. It is not known whether NUMORPHAN can cause fetal harm when administered to a pregnant woman or can affect reproductive capacity. As with other opioid analgesics, the use of NUMORPHAN in pregnancy or in women of child-bearing potential requires that the possible benefits of the drug be weighed against the possible hazards to the mother and the child.
Non-teratogenic Effects - Prolonged use of opioid analgesics during pregnancy may cause fetal-neonatal physical dependence. Neonatal withdrawal may occur. Symptoms usually appear during the first days of life and may include convulsions, irritability, excessive crying, tremors, hyperactive reflexes, fever, vomiting, diarrhea, sneezing, yawning, and increased respiratory rate.

Labor and Delivery
NUMORPHAN should be used with caution during labor. Sinusoidal fetal heart rate patterns may occur with the use of opioid analgesics.
Opioid analgesics in therapeutic doses may prolong labor. Generally, the effect of opioids on the pregnant uterus appears to depend on the time of administration; administration of the drugs during the latent phase of the first stage of labor, or before cervical dilation of 4–5 cm has occurred, may hamper the progress of labor.
Opioid analgesics, including NUMORPHAN, may cause respiratory depression in the newborn. The effect of NUMORPHAN, if any, on the later growth, development, and functional maturation of the child is unknown.

Nursing Mothers
It is not known whether NUMORPHAN is excreted in human milk. Because many drugs, including some opiods, are excreted in human milk, caution should be exercised when NUMORPHAN is administered to a nursing woman.

Pediatric Use
Safety and effectiveness of NUMORPHAN in pediatric patients below the age of 18 years have not been established.

ADVERSE REACTIONS

As with all potent opioid analgesics, possible side effects when using NUMORPHAN include:
Central Nervous System: Drowsiness, sedation, lightheadedness, unusual tiredness or weakness, headache, dysphoria, euphoria, miosis, diplopia, blurred vision, nervousness, restlessness, confusion, mental clouding, trouble sleeping, paradoxical CNS stimulation, hallucinations, mental depression.
Gastrointestinal System: Nausea, vomiting, dry mouth, constipation, biliary tract spasm, cramps or pain, loss of appetite, paralytic ileus or toxic megacolon in patients with inflammatory bowel disease.
Cardiovascular System: Hypotension, orthostatic hypotension particularly in ambulatory patients, tachycardia, bradycardia, palpitations, flushing.
Respiratory System: Respiratory depression, atelectasis, allergic bronchospastic reaction, allergic laryngeal edema, allergic laryngospasm.
Genitourinary System: Ureteral spasm, urinary hesitancy or retention, antidiuretic effect.
Dermatologic: Itching, sweating, injection site reaction, allergic reaction (such as skin rash, hives, and/or itching, swelling of the face).

DRUG ABUSE AND DEPENDENCE

NUMORPHAN is a Schedule II opioid and is subject to the Federal Controlled Substances Act.
NUMORPHAN, as with other opioid drugs, can produce tolerance, psychological dependence, and physical dependence and has the potential for being abused. The addiction potential of the drug appears to be about the same as for morphine.
Withdrawal symptoms may occur when opioids are abruptly discontinued after prolonged use. Withdrawal symptoms may be characterized by some or all of the following: restlessness, lacrimation, rhinorrhea, yawning, perspiration, gooseflesh, restless sleep, and mydriasis during the first 24 hours. These symptoms often increase in severity and over the next 72 hours may be accompanied by increasing irritability, anxiety, weakness, twitching, and spasms of muscles; kicking movements; severe backaches; abdominal and leg pains; abdominal and muscle cramps; hot and cold flashes; insomnia; nausea, anorexia, vomiting, intestinal spasm, diarrhea, coryza, and repetitive sneezing; increase in body temperature, blood pressure, respiratory rate and heart rate. Because of excessive loss of fluids through sweating, vomiting and diarrhea, there is usually marked weight loss, dehydration, ketosis, and disturbances in acid-base balance. Cardiovascular collapse can occur. Without treatment most observable symptoms disappear in 5–14 days; however, there appears to be a phase of secondary or chronic abstinence which may last for 2–6 months characterized by decreasing insomnia, irritability, and muscular aches. In ad-

Continued on next page

Numorphan —Cont.

dition, the patient may have miosis and a slight lowering of blood pressure, pulse rate, and body temperature; respiratory centers exhibit a decreased response to the stimulatory effects of carbon dioxide.

The dose of NUMORPHAN should be gradually reduced before discontinuation in those patients who require treatment for physical dependence.

Infants born to mothers physically dependent on opioids will also be physically dependent and may exhibit respiratory difficulties and withdrawal symptoms (See PRECAUTIONS; Usage in Pregnancy).

OVERDOSAGE

Signs and Symptoms: Serious overdosage with NUMORPHAN is characterized by respiratory depression, (a decrease in respiratory rate and/or tidal volume, Cheyne-Stokes respiration, cyanosis), extreme somnolence progressing to stupor or coma, skeletal muscle flaccidity, cold and clammy skin, and sometimes bradycardia and hypotension. In severe overdosage, apnea, circulatory collapse, cardiac arrest and death may occur.

Treatment: Primary attention should be given to the reestablishment of adequate respiratory exchange through provision of a patent airway and the institution of assisted or controlled ventilation. The opioid antagonist naloxone hydrochloride (NARCAN®) is a specific antidote against respiratory depression which may result from overdosage or unusual sensitivity to opioids including oxymorphone. Therefore, an appropriate dose of naloxone hydrochloride should be administered (usual initial adult dose 0.4 mg-2 mg) preferably by the intravenous route and simultaneously with efforts at respiratory resuscitation. Since the duration of action of oxymorphone may exceed that of the antagonist, the patient should be kept under continued surveillance and repeated doses of the antagonist should be administered as needed to maintain adequate respiration.

Naloxone hydrochloride should not be administered in the absence of clinically significant respiratory or cardiovascular depression. In addition, it should be considered that the use of an opioid antagonist in patients physically dependent on opioids may precepitate an acute withdrawal syndrome that cannot be readily suppressed while the action of the antagonist persists. If respiratory depression is associated with muscular rigidity, administration of a neuromuscular blocking agent may be necessary to facilitate assisted or controlled ventilation. Muscular rigidity may also respond to opioid antagonist therapy.

Oxygen, intravenous fluids, vasopressors and other supportive measures should be employed as indicated.

DOSAGE AND ADMINISTRATION

Smaller doses of NUMORPHAN than those recommended below should be used for debilitated and elderly patients and those with severe liver disease.

Usual Adult Dosage of NUMORPHAN Injection: Subcutaneous or intramuscular administration: initially 1 mg to 1.5 mg, repeated every 4 to 6 hours as needed. Intravenous: 0.5 mg initially. In nondebilitated patients the dose can be cautiously increased until satisfactory pain relief is obtained.

For analgesia during labor 0.5 mg to 1 mg intramuscularly is recommended.

Parenteral drug products should be inspected visually for particulate matter and discoloration prior to administration whenever solution and container permit.

Usual Adult Dosage of NUMORPHAN Rectal Suppositories: One suppository, 5 mg, every 4 to 6 hours. In nondebilitated patients the dose can be cautiously increased until satisfactory pain relief is obtained.

HOW SUPPLIED

For Injection: DEA Order Form Required
1 mg/mL 1 mL ampuls (paraben/sodium dithionite-free) (box of 10)   NDC 63481-444-10
1.5 mg/mL 10 mL multiple dose vials (sodium dithionite-free) (box of 1)   NDC 63481-445-01
Store at controlled room temperature 15°–30°C (59°–86°F). Protect from light.

For Rectal Suppositories: DEA Order Form Required
5 mg Wrapped in gold foil (box of 6) NDC 63481-761-06
Store under refrigeration 2°–8°C (36°–46°F).

CAUTION: Federal (USA) law prohibits dispensing without prescription.

NUMORPHAN® is a Registered Trademark of Endo Pharmaceuticals Inc.

NARCAN® is a Registered Trademark of Endo Pharmaceuticals Inc.

Copyright © Endo Pharmaceuticals Inc. 1998
    6477-00/January, 1998

2620 PERCOCET®
[perk 'o-set]
(oxycodone and acetaminophen tablets, USP)

DESCRIPTION

Each tablet of PERCOCET contains:
Oxycodone hydrochloride .... 5 mg*
    WARNING: May be habit forming

Acetaminophen, USP .... 325 mg
*5 mg oxycodone HCl is equivalent to 4.4815 mg of oxycodone.

PERCOCET Tablets also contain: microcrystalline cellulose, povidone, pregelatinized starch, stearic acid and other ingredients.

Acetaminophen occurs as a white, odorless, crystalline powder, possessing a slightly bitter taste.

The oxycodone component is 14-hydroxydihydrocodeinone, a white, odorless, crystalline powder having a saline, bitter taste. It is derived from the opium alkaloid thebaine, and may be represented by the following structural formula:

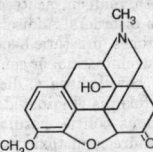

CLINICAL PHARMACOLOGY

The principal ingredient, oxycodone, is a semisynthetic narcotic analgesic with multiple actions qualitatively similar to those of morphine; the most prominent of these involve the central nervous system and organs composed of smooth muscle. The principal actions of therapeutic value of the oxycodone in PERCOCET are analgesia and sedation.

Oxycodone is similar to codeine and methadone in that it retains at least one-half of its analgesic activity when administered orally.

Acetaminophen is a non-opiate, non-salicylate analgesic and antipyretic.

INDICATIONS AND USAGE

PERCOCET is indicated for the relief of moderate to moderately severe pain.

CONTRAINDICATIONS

PERCOCET should not be administered to patients who are hypersensitive to oxycodone or acetaminophen.

WARNINGS

Drug Dependence: Oxycodone can produce drug dependence of the morphine type and, therefore, has the potential for being abused. Psychic dependence, physical dependence and tolerance may develop upon repeated administration of PERCOCET, and it should be prescribed and administered with the same degree of caution appropriate to the use of other oral narcotic-containing medications. Like other narcotic-containing medications, PERCOCET is subject to the Federal Controlled Substances Act (Schedule II).

PRECAUTIONS

General
Head Injury and Increased Intracranial Pressure: The respiratory depressant effects of narcotics and their capacity to elevate cerebrospinal fluid pressure may be markedly exaggerated in the presence of head injury, other intracranial lesions or a pre-existing increase in intracranial pressure. Furthermore, narcotics produce adverse reactions which may obscure the clinical course of patients with head injuries.

Acute Abdominal Conditions: The administration of PERCOCET or other narcotics may obscure the diagnosis or clinical course in patients with acute abdominal conditions.

Special Risk Patients: PERCOCET should be given with caution to certain patients such as the elderly or debilitated, and those with severe impairment of hepatic or renal function, hypothyroidism, Addison's disease, and prostatic hypertrophy or urethral stricture.

Information for Patients
Oxycodone may impair the mental and/or physical abilities required for the performance of potentially hazardous tasks such as driving a car or operating machinery. The patient using PERCOCET should be cautioned accordingly.

Drug Interactions
Patients receiving other narcotic analgesics, general anesthetics, phenothiazines, other tranquilizers, sedative-hypnotics or other CNS depressants (including alcohol) concomitantly with PERCOCET may exhibit an additive CNS depression. When such combined therapy is contemplated, the dose of one or both agents should be reduced.

The use of MAO inhibitors or tricyclic antidepressants with oxycodone preparations may increase the effect of either the antidepressant or oxycodone.

The concurrent use of anticholinergics with narcotics may produce paralytic ileus.

Usage in Pregnancy
Pregnancy Category C: Animal reproductive studies have not been conducted with PERCOCET. It is also not known whether PERCOCET can cause fetal harm when administered to a pregnant woman or can affect reproductive capac-

ity. PERCOCET should not be given to a pregnant woman unless in the judgment of the physician, the potential benefits outweigh the possible hazards.

Nonteratogenic Effects: Use of narcotics during pregnancy may produce physical dependence in the neonate.

Labor and Delivery: As with all narcotics, administration of PERCOCET to the mother shortly before delivery may result in some degree of respiratory depression in the newborn and the mother, especially if higher doses are used.

Nursing Mothers
It is not known whether PERCOCET is excreted in human milk. Because many drugs are excreted in human milk, caution should be exercised when PERCOCET is administered to a nursing woman.

Pediatric Use
Safety and effectiveness in children have not been established.

ADVERSE REACTIONS

The most frequently observed adverse reactions include lightheadedness, dizziness, sedation, nausea and vomiting. These effects seem to be more prominent in ambulatory than in nonambulatory patients, and some of these adverse reactions may be alleviated if the patient lies down.

Other adverse reactions include euphoria, dysphoria, constipation, skin rash and pruritus. At higher doses, oxycodone has most of the disadvantages of morphine including respiratory depression.

DRUG ABUSE AND DEPENDENCE

PERCOCET (oxycodone and acetaminophen) Tablets are a Schedule II controlled substance.

Oxycodone can produce drug dependence and has the potential for being abused. (See WARNINGS.)

OVERDOSAGE

Acetaminophen
Signs and Symptoms: In acute acetaminophen overdosage, dose-dependent, potentially fatal hepatic necrosis is the most serious adverse effect. Renal tubular necrosis, hypoglycemic coma and thrombocytopenia may also occur.

In adults, hepatic toxicity has rarely been reported with acute overdoses of less than 10 grams and fatalities with less than 15 grams. Importantly, young children seem to be more resistant than adults to the hepatotoxic effect of an acetaminophen overdose. Despite this, the measures outlined below should be initiated in any adult or child suspected of having ingested an acetaminophen overdose.

Early symptoms following a potentially hepatotoxic overdose may include: nausea, vomiting, diaphoresis and general malaise. Clinical and laboratory evidence of hepatic toxicity may not be apparent until 48 to 72 hours postingestion.

Treatment: The stomach should be emptied promptly by lavage or by induction of emesis with syrup of ipecac. Patient's estimates of the quantity of a drug ingested are notoriously unreliable. Therefore, if an acetaminophen overdose is suspected, a serum acetaminophen assay should be obtained as early as possible, but no sooner than four hours following ingestion. Liver function studies should be obtained initially and repeated at 24-hour intervals.

The antidote, N-acetylcysteine, should be administered as early as possible, preferably within 16 hours of the overdose ingestion for optimal results, but in any case, within 24 hours. Following recovery, there are no residual, structural, or functional hepatic abnormalities.

Oxycodone
Signs and Symptoms: Serious overdosage with oxycodone is characterized by respiratory depression (a decrease in respiratory rate and/or tidal volume, Cheyne-Stokes respiration, cyanosis), extreme somnolence progressing to stupor or coma, skeletal muscle flaccidity, cold and clammy skin, and sometimes bradycardia and hypotension. In severe overdosage, apnea, circulatory collapse, cardiac arrest and death may occur.

Treatment: Primary attention should be given to the reestablishment of adequate respiratory exchange through provision of a patent airway and the institution of assisted or controlled ventilation. The narcotic antagonist naloxone hydrochloride (Narcan®) is a specific antidote against respiratory depression which may result from overdosage or unusual sensitivity to narcotics, including oxycodone. Therefore, an appropriate dose of naloxone hydrochloride (usual initial adult dose 0.4 mg to 2 mg) should be administered preferably by the intravenous route, and simultaneously with efforts at respiratory resuscitation (see package insert). Since the duration of action of oxycodone may exceed that of the antagonist, the patient should be kept under continued surveillance and repeated doses of the antagonist should be administered as needed to maintain adequate respiration.

An antagonist should not be administered in the absence of clinically significant respiratory or cardiovascular depression. Oxygen, intravenous fluids, vasopressors and other supportive measures should be employed as indicated.

Gastric emptying may be useful in removing unabsorbed drug.

DOSAGE AND ADMINISTRATION

Dosage should be adjusted according to the severity of the pain and the response of the patient. It may occasionally be necessary to exceed the usual dosage recommended below in cases of more severe pain or in those patients who have become tolerant to the analgesic effect of narcotics. PERCOCET is given orally. The usual adult dosage is one tablet every 6 hours as needed for pain.

HOW SUPPLIED

PERCOCET (5 mg oxycodone hydrochloride and 325 mg acetaminophen tablets, USP), supplied as a white tablet, with one face scored and inscribed PERCOCET, and the other imprinted with "5" is available in:

Bottles of 100	NDC 63481-127-70
Bottles of 500	NDC 63481-127-85
Hospital Blister Pack of 25	NDC 63481-127-75
(in units of 100)	

Store at controlled room temperature 15°–30°C (59°–86°F).
DEA Order Form Required
PERCOCET® is a Registered Trademark of Endo Pharmaceuticals Inc.
NARCAN® is a Registered Trademark of Endo Pharmaceuticals Inc.
Copyright © Endo Pharmaceuticals Inc.

6482/September, 1997

Shown in Product Identification Guide, page 310

PERCODAN®   Ⅱ
[perk 'o-dan]
(oxycodone and aspirin tablets, USP)

DESCRIPTION

Each tablet of PERCODAN contains:

Oxycodone hydrochloride .... 4.50 mg*
   WARNING: May be habit forming
Oxycodone terephthalate .... 0.38 mg**
   WARNING: May be habit forming
Aspirin, USP .... 325 mg
  *4.50 mg oxycodone HCl is equivalent to 4.0338 mg of oxycodone.
  **0.38 mg oxycodone terephthalate is equivalent to 0.3008 mg of oxycodone.

PERCODAN Tablets also contain: D&C Yellow 10, FD&C Yellow 6, microcrystalline cellulose and starch.
The oxycodone component is 14-hydroxydihydrocodeinone, a white odorless crystalline powder which is derived from the opium alkaloid, thebaine, and may be represented by the following structural formula:

ACTIONS

The principal ingredient, oxycodone, is a semisynthetic narcotic analgesic with multiple actions qualitatively similar to those of morphine; the most prominent of these involve the central nervous system and organs composed of smooth muscle. The principal actions of therapeutic value of the oxycodone in PERCODAN are analgesia and sedation.
Oxycodone is similar to codeine and methadone in that it retains at least one-half of its analgesic activity when administered orally.
PERCODAN also contains the non-narcotic antipyretic-analgesic, aspirin.

INDICATIONS

For the relief of moderate to moderately severe pain.

CONTRAINDICATIONS

Hypersensitivity to oxycodone or aspirin.

WARNINGS

Drug Dependence: Oxycodone can produce drug dependence of the morphine type and, therefore, has the potential for being abused. Psychic dependence, physical dependence and tolerance may develop upon repeated administration of PERCODAN, and it should be prescribed and administered with the same degree of caution appropriate to the use of other oral narcotic-containing medications. Like other narcotic-containing medications, PERCODAN is subject to the Federal Controlled Substances Act.
Usage in ambulatory patients: Oxycodone may impair the mental and/or physical abilities required for the performance of potentially hazardous tasks such as driving a car or operating machinery. The patient using PERCODAN should be cautioned accordingly.
Interaction with other central nervous system depressants: Patients receiving other narcotic analgesics, general anes-

thetics, phenothiazines, other tranquilizers, sedative-hypnotics or other CNS depressants (including alcohol) concomitantly with PERCODAN may exhibit an additive CNS depression. When such combined therapy is contemplated, the dose of one or both agents should be reduced.
Usage in pregnancy: Safe use in pregnancy has not been established relative to possible adverse effects on fetal development. Therefore, PERCODAN should not be used in pregnant women unless, in the judgment of the physician, the potential benefits outweigh the possible hazards.
Pediatric Use: PERCODAN should not be administered to pediatric patients. PERCODAN®-Demi, containing half the amount of oxycodone, can be considered. (See product prescribing information for PERCODAN-Demi).
Reye Syndrome is a rare but serious disease which can follow flu or chicken pox in children and teenagers. While the cause of Reye Syndrome is unknown, some reports claim aspirin (or salicylates) may increase the risk of developing this disease.
Salicylates should be used with caution in the presence of peptic ulcer or coagulation abnormalities.

PRECAUTIONS

Head injury and increased intracranial pressure: The respiratory depressant effects of narcotics and their capacity to elevate cerebrospinal fluid pressure may be markedly exaggerated in the presence of head injury, other intracranial lesions or a pre-existing increase in intracranial pressure. Furthermore, narcotics produce adverse reactions which may obscure the clinical course of patients with head injuries.
Acute abdominal conditions: The administration of PERCODAN (oxycodone and aspirin) or other narcotics may obscure the diagnosis or clinical course in patients with acute abdominal conditions.
Special risk patients: PERCODAN should be given with caution to certain patients such as the elderly or debilitated, and those with severe impairment of hepatic or renal function, hypothyroidism, Addison's disease, and prostatic hypertrophy or urethral stricture.

ADVERSE REACTIONS

The most frequently observed adverse reactions include light-headedness, dizziness, sedation, nausea and vomiting. These effects seem to be more prominent in ambulatory than in nonambulatory patients, and some of these adverse reactions may be alleviated if the patient lies down.
Other adverse reactions include euphoria, dysphoria, constipation and pruritus.

DRUG ABUSE AND DEPENDENCE

PERCODAN tablets are a Schedule II controlled substance. Oxycodone can produce drug dependence and has the potential for being abused. (See WARNINGS.)

DOSAGE AND ADMINISTRATION

Dosage should be adjusted according to the severity of the pain and the response of the patient. It may occasionally be necessary to exceed the usual dosage recommended below in cases of more severe pain or in those patients who have become tolerant to the analgesic effect of narcotics. PERCODAN is given orally. The usual adult dose is one tablet every 6 hours as needed for pain.

DRUG INTERACTIONS

The CNS depressant effects of PERCODAN may be additive with that of other CNS depressants. (See WARNINGS.)
Aspirin may enhance the effect of anticoagulants and inhibit the uricosuric effects of uricosuric agents.

MANAGEMENT OF OVERDOSAGE

Signs and Symptoms: Serious overdose with PERCODAN is characterized by respiratory depression (a decrease in respiratory rate and/or tidal volume, Cheyne-Stokes respiration, cyanosis), extreme somnolence progressing to stupor or coma, skeletal muscle flaccidity, cold and clammy skin, and sometimes bradycardia and hypotension. In severe overdosage, apnea, circulatory collapse, cardiac arrest and death may occur. The ingestion of very large amounts of PERCODAN may, in addition, result in acute salicylate intoxication.
Treatment: Primary attention should be given to the reestablishment of adequate respiratory exchange through provision of a patent airway and the institution of assisted or controlled ventilation. The narcotic antagonist naloxone hydrochloride (NARCAN®) is a specific antidote against respiratory depression which may result from overdosage or unusual sensitivity to narcotics including oxycodone. Therefore, an appropriate dose of naloxone hydrochloride should be administered (usual initial adult dose: 0.4 mg–2 mg) preferably by the intravenous route, simultaneously with efforts at respiratory resuscitation. Since the duration of action of oxycodone may exceed that of the antagonist, the patient should be kept under continued surveillance and repeated doses of the antagonist should be administered as needed to maintain adequate respiration.
Oxygen, intravenous fluids, vasopressors and other supportive measures should be employed as indicated.

Gastric emptying may be useful in removing unabsorbed drug.

HOW SUPPLIED

PERCODAN (4.50 mg oxycodone hydrochloride, 0.38 mg oxycodone terephthalate, 325 mg Aspirin, USP), supplied as a yellow tablet, with one face scored and inscribed PERCODAN and plain on the other side is available in:

Bottles of 100	NDC 63481-135-70
Bottles of 500	NDC 63481-135-85
Hospital blister pack of 25	NDC 63481-135-75
(in units of 100 tablets)	

Store at controlled room temperature 15°–30°C (59°–86°F).
DEA Order Form Required.
PERCODAN® is a Registered Trademark of Endo Pharmaceuticals Inc.
NARCAN® is a Registered Trademark of Endo Pharmaceuticals Inc.
Copyright © Endo Pharmaceuticals Inc. 1997

6483/September, 1997

Shown in Product Identification Guide, page 310

PERCODAN®-DEMI   Ⅱ
[perk 'o-dan]
(oxycodone and aspirin)

DESCRIPTION

Each tablet of PERCODAN-Demi contains:

Oxycodone hydrochloride .... 2.25 mg*
WARNING: May be habit forming
Oxycodone terephthalate .... 0.19 mg**
WARNING: May be habit forming
Aspirin, USP .... 325 mg
  *2.25 mg oxycodone HCl is equivalent to 2.0169 mg of oxycodone.
  **0.19 mg oxycodone terephthalate is equivalent to 0.1504 mg of oxycodone.

PERCODAN-Demi Tablets also contain: microcrystalline cellulose and starch.
The oxycodone component is 14-hydroxydihydrocodeinone, a white odorless crystalline powder which is derived from the opium alkaloid, thebaine, and may be represented by the following structural formula:

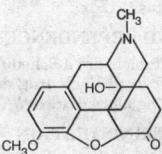

ACTIONS

The principal ingredient, oxycodone, is a semisynthetic narcotic analgesic with multiple actions qualitatively similar to those of morphine; the most prominent of these involve the central nervous system and organs composed of smooth muscle. The principal actions of therapeutic value of the oxycodone in PERCODAN-Demi are analgesia and sedation.
Oxycodone is similar to codeine and methadone in that it retains at least one half of its analgesic activity when administered orally.
PERCODAN-Demi also contains the non-narcotic antipyretic-analgesic, aspirin.

INDICATIONS

For the relief of moderate to moderately severe pain.

CONTRAINDICATIONS

Hypersensitivity to oxycodone or aspirin.

WARNINGS

Drug Dependence: Oxycodone can produce drug dependence of the morphine type and, therefore, has the potential for being abused. Psychic dependence, physical dependence and tolerance may develop upon repeated administration of PERCODAN-Demi, and it should be prescribed and administered with the same degree of caution appropriate to the use of other oral narcotic-containing medications. Like other narcotic-containing medications, PERCODAN-Demi is subject to the Federal Controlled Substances Act.
Usage in ambulatory patients: Oxycodone may impair the mental and/or physical abilities required for the performance of potentially hazardous tasks such as driving a car or operating machinery. The patient using PERCODAN-Demi should be cautioned accordingly.
Interaction with other central nervous system depressants: Patients receiving other narcotic analgesics, general anesthetics, phenothiazines, other tranquilizers, sedative-hypnotics or other CNS depressants (including alcohol) concom-

Continued on next page

Percodan-Demi—Cont.

itantly with PERCODAN-Demi may exhibit an additive CNS depression. When such combined therapy is contemplated, the dose of one or both agents should be reduced.

Usage in pregnancy: Safe use in pregnancy has not been established relative to possible adverse effects on fetal development. Therefore, PERCODAN-Demi should not be used in pregnant women unless, in the judgement of the physician, the potential benefits outweigh the possible hazards.

Reye Syndrome is a rare but serious disease which can follow flu or chicken pox in children and teenagers. While the cause of Reye Syndrome is unknown, some reports claim aspirin (or salicylates) may increase the risk of developing this disease.

Salicylates should be used with caution in the presence of peptic ulcer or coagulation abnormalities.

PRECAUTIONS

Head Injury and Increased Intracranial pressure: The respiratory depressant effects of narcotics and their capacity to elevate cerebrospinal fluid pressure may be markedly exaggerated in the presence of head injury, other intracranial lesions or a pre-existing increase in intracranial pressure. Furthermore, narcotics produce adverse reactions which may obscure the clinical course of patients with head injuries.

Acute abdominal conditions: The administration of PERCODAN-Demi or other narcotics may obscure the diagnosis or clinical course in patients with acute abdominal conditions.

Special risk patients: PERCODAN-Demi (oxycodone and aspirin) should be given with caution to certain patients such as the elderly or debilitated, and those with severe impairment of hepatic or renal function, hypothyroidism, Addison's disease, and prostatic hypertrophy or urethral stricture.

ADVERSE REACTIONS

The most frequently observed adverse reactions include lightheadedness, dizziness, sedation, nausea and vomiting. These effects seem to be more prominent in ambulatory than in non-ambulatory patients, and some of these adverse reactions may be alleviated if the patient lies down.

Other adverse reactions include euphoria, dysphoria, constipation and pruritus.

DRUG ABUSE AND DEPENDENCE

PERCODAN-Demi tablets are a Schedule II controlled substance. Oxycodone can produce drug dependence and has the potential for being abused. (See WARNINGS)

DOSAGE AND ADMINISTRATION

Dosage should be adjusted according to the severity of the pain and the response of the patient. It may occasionally be necessary to exceed the usual dosage recommended below in cases of more severe pain or in those patients who have become tolerant to the analgesic effect of narcotics. PERCODAN-Demi is given orally.

Dosage: Adults—One or two tablets every six hours.

Children 12 years and older—One-half tablet every six hours.

Children 6 to 12 years—One-quarter tablet every six hours. PERCODAN-Demi is not indicated for children under 6 years of age.

DRUG INTERACTIONS

The CNS depressant effects of PERCODAN-Demi may be additive with that of other CNS depressants. (See WARNINGS)

Aspirin may enhance the effect of anticoagulants and inhibit the uricosuric effect of uricosuric agents.

MANAGEMENT OF OVERDOSAGE

Signs and Symptoms: Serious overdose with PERCODAN-Demi is characterized by respiratory depression (a decrease in respiratory rate and/or tidal volume, Cheyne-Stokes respiration, cyanosis), extreme somnolence progressing to stupor or coma, skeletal muscle flaccidity, cold and clammy skin, and sometimes bradycardia and hypotension. In severe overdosage, apnea, circulatory collapse, cardiac arrest and death may occur. The ingestion of very large amounts of PERCODAN-Demi may, in addition, result in acute salicylate intoxication.

Treatment: Primary attention should be given to the reestablishment of adequate respiratory exchange through provision of a patent airway and the institution of assisted or controlled ventilation. The narcotic antagonist naloxone hydrochloride (NARCAN®) is a specific antidote against respiratory depression which may result from overdosage or unusual sensitivity to narcotics including oxycodone. Therefore, an appropriate dose of naloxone hydrochloride should be administered (usual initial adult dose 0.4 mg–2 mg) preferably by the intravenous route, simultaneously with efforts at respiratory resuscitation. Since the duration of action of oxycodone may exceed that of the antagonist, the patient

should be kept under continued surveillance and repeated doses of the antagonist should be administered as needed to maintain adequate respiration.

Oxygen, intravenous fluids, vasopressors and other supportive measures should be employed as indicated.

Gastric emptying may be useful in removing unabsorbed drug.

HOW SUPPLIED

As white, scored tablets available in:
Bottles of 100 NDC 63481-166-70
Store at controlled room temperature (59°–86°F, 15°–30°C).
DEA Order Form Required.

6234-2/Rev. June, 1993

Shown in Product Identification Guide, page 310

PERCOLONE™ Ⅱ
[perk 'ŏ-lōne]
(oxycodone hydrochloride)
Tablets, USP

DESCRIPTION

Each PERCOLONE tablet contains:
Oxycodone Hydrochloride, USP .... 5 mg*
(WARNING: May be habit forming)

*5 mg oxycodone HCl is equivalent to 4.4815 mg of oxycodone.

Inactive ingredients: Microcrystalline cellulose and stearic acid.

Oxycodone is 14-hydroxydihydrocodeinone, a white odorless crystalline powder which is derived from the opium alkaloid, thebaine, and may be represented by the following structural formula:

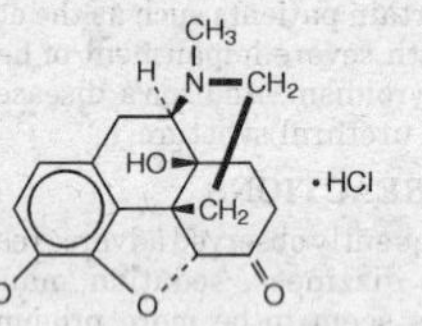

ACTIONS

The analgesic ingredient, oxycodone, is a semisynthetic narcotic with multiple actions qualitatively similar to those of morphine; the most prominent of these involve the central nervous system and organs composed of smooth muscle. The principal actions of therapeutic value of PERCOLONE are analgesia and sedation.

PERCOLONE is similar to codeine and methadone in that it retains at least one half of its analgesic activity when administered orally.

INDICATIONS

For the relief of moderate to moderately severe pain.

CONTRAINDICATIONS

Hypersensitivity to PERCOLONE.

WARNINGS

Drug Dependence: PERCOLONE can produce drug dependence of the morphine type and, therefore, has the potential for being abused. Psychic dependence, physical dependence and tolerance may develop upon repeated administration of this drug, and it should be prescribed and administered with the same degree of caution appropriate to the use of other oral narcotic-containing medications. Like other narcotic-containing medications, this drug is subject to the Federal Controlled Substances Act.

Usage in Ambulatory Patients: PERCOLONE may impair the mental and/or physical abilities required for the performance of potentially hazardous tasks such as driving a car or operating machinery. The patient using this drug should be cautioned accordingly.

Interaction with Other Central Nervous System Depressants: Patients receiving other narcotic analgesics, general anesthetics, phenothiazines, other tranquilizers, sedative-hypnotics or other CNS depressants (including alcohol) concomitantly with PERCOLONE may exhibit an additive CNS depression. When such combined therapy is contemplated, the dose of one or both agents should be reduced.

Usage in Pregnancy: Safe use in pregnancy has not been established relative to possible adverse effects on fetal development. Therefore, this drug should not be used in pregnant women unless, in the judgment of the physician, the potential benefits outweigh the possible hazards.

Pediatric Use: This drug should not be administered to pediatric patients.

PRECAUTIONS

Head Injury and Increased Intracranial Pressure: The respiratory depressant effects of narcotics and their capacity to elevate cerebrospinal fluid pressure may be markedly exaggerated in the presence of head injury, other intracranial lesions or a pre-existing increase in intracranial pressure.

Furthermore, narcotics produce adverse reactions which may obscure the clinical course of patients with head injuries.

Acute Abdominal Conditions: The administration of this drug or other narcotics may obscure the diagnosis or clinical course in patients with acute abdominal conditions.

Special Risk Patients: This drug should be given with caution to certain patients such as the elderly, or debilitated, and those with severe impairment of hepatic or renal function, hypothyroidism, Addison's disease and prostatic hypertrophy or urethral stricture.

ADVERSE REACTIONS

The most frequently observed adverse reactions include lightheadedness, dizziness, sedation, nausea and vomiting. These effects seem to be more prominent in ambulatory than in nonambulatory patients, and some of these adverse reactions may be alleviated if the patient lies down.

Other adverse reactions include euphoria, dysphoria, constipation, skin rash and pruritus.

DOSAGE AND ADMINISTRATION

The usual adult oral dose is 10 to 30 mg every 4 hours as needed for pain or as directed by physician. The does must be individually adjusted according to severity of pain, patient response and patient size. More severe pain may require 30 mg or more every 4 hours. If the pain increases in severity, analgesia is not adequate or tolerance occurs, a gradual increase in dosage may be required.

For control of severe, chronic pain in patients with certain terminal diseases, this drug should be administered on a regularly scheduled basis, every 4 hours, at the lowest dosage level that will achieve adequate analgesia.

DRUG INTERACTIONS

The CNS depressant effects of PERCOLONE (oxycodone hydrochloride) may be additive with that of other CNS depressants. See WARNINGS.

MANAGEMENT OF OVERDOSAGE

Signs and Symptoms: Serious overdose of PERCOLONE is characterized by respiratory depression (a decrease in respiratory rate and/or tidal volume, Cheyne-Stokes respiration, cyanosis), extreme somnolence progressing to stupor or coma, skeletal muscle flaccidity, cold and clammy skin, and sometimes bradycardia and hypotension. In severe overdosage, apnea, circulatory collapse, cardiac arrest and death may occur.

Treatment: Primary attention should be given to the reestablishment of adequate respiratory exchange through provision of a patent airway and the institution of assisted or controlled ventilation. The narcotic antagonist naloxone is a specific antidote against respiratory depression which may result from overdosage or unusual sensitivity to narcotics, including PERCOLONE. Therefore, an appropriate dose of naloxone (usual initial adult dose: 0.4 mg) should be administered, preferably by the intravenous route, simultaneously with efforts at respiratory resuscitation. Since the duration of action of PERCOLONE may exceed that of the antagonist, the patient should be kept under continued surveillance and repeated doses of the antagonist should be administered as needed to maintain adequate respiration.

An antagonist should not be administered in the absence of clinically significant respiratory or cardiovascular depression.

Oxygen, intravenous fluids, vasopressors and other supportive measures should be employed as indicated.

Gastric emptying may be useful in removing unabsorbed drug.

HOW SUPPLIED

PERCOLONE is supplied as 5 mg white, round, biconvex tablets, bisected and debossed with "EPI" over "132" on one side and debossed with "5" on the other side as follows:

Bottles of 100   NDC 63481-132-70
Blister Packs of 25   NDC 63481-132-75
(in units of 100)

DEA Order Form Required.

Dispense in a well-closed container as defined in the USP/NF. Protect from moisture. Store at controlled room temperature, 15°–30°C (59°–86°F).

Caution: Federal (USA) law prohibits dispensing without prescription.

PERCOLONE™ is a trademark of Endo Pharmaceuticals Inc.

Copyright © Endo Pharmaceuticals Inc. 1997
6450-01/Rev. September, 1997

Shown in Product Identification Guide, page 310

SYMMETREL® ℞
[sim 'e-trel]
(amantadine hydrochloride)
Tablets and Syrup, USP

DESCRIPTION

SYMMETREL is designated generically as amantadine hydrochloride and chemically as 1-adamantanamine hydrochloride.

[See chemical structure at top of next column]

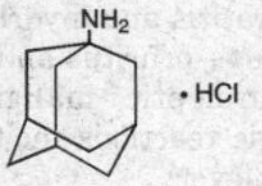

Amantadine hydrochloride is a stable white or nearly white crystalline powder, freely soluble in water and soluble in alcohol and in chloroform.
Amantadine hydrochloride has pharmacological actions as both an anti-Parkinson and an antiviral drug.
SYMMETREL is available in tablets and syrup.
Each tablet intended for oral administration contains 100 mg amantadine hydrochloride and has the following inactive ingredients: hydroxypropyl methylcellulose, magnesium stearate, microcrystalline cellulose, sodium starch glycolate, FD&C Yellow No. 6.
SYMMETREL syrup contains 50 mg of amantadine hydrochloride per 5 mL and has the following inactive ingredients: artficial raspberry flavor, citric acid, methylparaben, propylparaben, and sorbitol solution.

CLINICAL PHARMACOLOGY

Pharmacodynamics

Mechanism of Action: Antiviral The mechanism by which amantadine exerts its antiviral activity is not clearly understood. It appears to mainly prevent the release of infectious viral nucleic acid into the host cell by interfering with the function of the transmembrane domain of the viral M2 protein. In certain cases, amantadine is also known to prevent virus assembly during virus replication. It does not appear to interfere with the immunogenicity of inactivated influenza A virus vaccine.
Antiviral Activity: Amantadine inhibits the replication of influenza A virus isolates from each of the subtypes, i.e., H1N1, H2N2 and H3N2. It has very little or no activity against influenza B virus isolates. A quantitative relationship between the *in vitro* susceptibility of influenza A virus to amantadine and the clinical response to therapy has not been established in man. Sensitivity test results, expressed as the concentration of amantadine required to inhibit by 50% the growth of virus (ED_{50}) in tissue culture vary greatly (from 0.1 µg/mL to 25.0 µg/mL) depending upon the assay protocol used, size of virus inoculum, isolates of influenza A virus strains tested, and the cell type used. Host cells in tissue culture readily tolerated amantadine up to a concentration of 100 µg/mL.
Drug Resistance: Influenza A variants with reduced *in vitro* sensitivity to amantadine have been isolated from epidemic strains in areas where adamantane derivatives are being used. Influenza viruses with reduced *in vitro* sensitivity have been shown to be transmissible and to cause typical influenza illness. The quantitative relationship between the *in vitro* sensitivity of influenza A variants to amantadine and the clinical response to therapy has not been established.
Mechanism of Action: Parkinson's Disease The mechanism of action of amantadine in the treatment of Parkinson's disease and drug-induced extrapyramidal reactions is not known. Data from animal studies have either shown or suggested SYMMETREL:
(a) To enhance extracellular concentrations of dopamine by increasing dopamine release or decreasing reuptake of dopamine into presynaptic neurons;
(b) To stimulate the dopamine receptor itself or drive the post synaptic dopaminergic system to a more dopamine sensitive status.
However, doses employed in the animal studies were often of a magnitude greater than the clinically therapeutic doses. More recent work using doses in the low clinically therapeutic range (low µM) showed amantadine to inhibit the N-methyl-D-aspartic acid (NMDA) receptor-mediated stimulation of acetylcholine release from rat striatum, most likely at the MK-801 site. Although amantadine does not possess anticholinergic activity in dogs at doses of 31.5 mg/kg, equivalent to an approximate human dose of 15.8 mg/kg (based on body surface area conversions), clinically, it exhibits anticholinergic-like side effects such as dry mouth, urinary retention, and constipation.
Pharmacokinetics: SYMMETREL is well absorbed orally. Maximum plasma concentrations are directly related to dose for doses up to 200 mg/day. Doses above 200 mg/day may result in a greater than proportional increase in maximum plasma concentrations. It is primarily excreted unchanged in the urine by glomerular filtration and tubular secretion. Eight metabolites of amantadine have been identified in human urine. One metabolite, an N-acetylated compound, was quantified in human urine and accounted for 5–15% of the administered dose. Plasma acetylamantadine accounted for up to 80% of the concurrent amantadine plasma concentration in 5 of 12 healthy volunteers following the ingestion of a 200 mg dose of amantadine. Acetylamantadine was not detected in the plasma of the remaining seven volunteers. The contribution of this metabolite to efficacy or toxicity is not known.
There appears to be a relationship between plasma amantadine concentrations and toxicity. As concentration increases, toxicity seems to be more prevalent, however, absolute values of amantadine concentrations associated with adverse effects have not been fully defined.
Amantadine pharmacokinetics were determined in 24 normal adult male volunteers after the oral administration of a single amantadine hydrochloride 100 mg soft gel capsule. The mean ± SD maximum plasma concentration was 0.22 ± 0.03 µg/mL (range: 0.18 to 0.32 µg/mL). The time to peak concentration was 3.3 ± 1.5 hours (range: 1.5 to 8.0 hours). The apparent oral clearance was 0.28 ± 0.11 L/hr/kg (range: 0.14 to 0.62 L/hr/kg). The half-life was 17 ± 4 hours (range: 10 to 25 hours). Across other studies, amantadine plasma half-life has averaged 16 ± 6 hours (range: 9 to 31 hours) in 19 healthy volunteers.
After oral administration of a single dose of 100 mg amantadine syrup to five healthy volunteers, the mean ± SD maximum plasma concentration C_{max} was 0.24 ± 0.04 µg/mL and ranged from 0.18 to 0.28 µg/mL. After 15 days of amantadine 100 mg b.i.d., the C_{max} was 0.47 ± 0.11 µg/mL in four of the five volunteers. The administration of amantadine tablets as a 200 mg single dose to 6 healthy subjects resulted in a C_{max} of 0.51 ± 0.14 µg/mL. Across studies, the time to C_{max} (T_{max}) averaged about 2 to 4 hours.
Plasma amantadine clearance ranged from 0.2 to 0.3 L/hr/kg after the administration of 5 mg to 25 mg intravenous doses of amantadine to 15 healthy volunteers.
In six healthy volunteers, the ratio of amantadine renal clearance to apparent oral plasma clearance was 0.79 ± 0.17 (mean ± SD).
The volume of distribution determined after the intravenous administration of amantadine to 15 healthy subjects was 3 to 8 L/kg, suggesting tissue binding. Amantadine, after single oral 200 mg doses to 6 healthy young subjects and to 6 healthy elderly subjects has been found in nasal mucus at mean ± SD concentrations of 0.15 ± 0.16, 0.28 ± 0.26, and 0.39 ± 0.34 µg/g at 1, 4, and 8 hours after dosing, respectively. These concentrations represented 31 ± 33%, 59 ± 61%, and 95 ± 86% of the corresponding plasma amantadine concentrations. Amantadine is approximately 67% bound to plasma proteins over a concentration range of 0.1 to 2.0 µg/mL. Following the administration of amantadine 100 mg as a single dose, the mean ± SD red blood cell to plasma ratio ranged from 2.7 ± 0.5 in 6 healthy subjects to 1.4 ± 0.2 in 8 patients with renal insufficiency.
The apparent oral plasma clearance of amantadine is reduced and the plasma half-life and plasma concentrations are increased in healthy elderly individuals age 60 and older. After single dose administration of 25 to 75 mg to 7 healthy, elderly male volunteers, the apparent plasma clearance of amantadine was 0.10 ± 0.04 L/hr/kg (range 0.06 to 0.17 L/hr/kg) and the half-life was 29 ± 7 hours (range 20 to 41 hours). Whether these changes are due to decline in renal function or other age related factors is not known.
In a study of young healthy subjects (n=20), mean renal clearance of amantadine, normalized for body mass index, was significantly higher in males compared to females ($p<0.032$).
Compared with otherwise healthy adult individuals, the clearance of amantadine is significantly reduced in adult patients with renal insufficiency. The elimination half-life increases two to three fold or greater when creatinine clearance is less than 40 mL/min/1.73 m^2 and averages eight days in patients on chronic maintenance hemodialysis. Amantadine is removed in negligible amounts by hemodialysis.
The pH of the urine has been reported to influence the excretion rate of SYMMETREL. Since the excretion rate of SYMMETREL increases rapidly when the urine is acidic, the administration of urine acidifying drugs may increase the elimination of the drug from the body.

INDICATIONS AND USAGE

SYMMETREL is indicated for the prophylaxis and treatment of signs and symptoms of infection caused by various strains of influenza A virus. SYMMETREL (amantadine hydrochloride) is also indicated in the treatment of parkinsonism and drug-induced extrapyramidal reactions.
Influenza A Prophylaxis: SYMMETREL is indicated for chemoprophylaxis against signs and symptoms of influenza A virus infection when early vaccination is not feasible or when the vaccine is contraindicated or not available. In the prophylaxis of influenza, early vaccination on an annual basis as recommended by the Centers for Disease Control's Immunization Practices Advisory Committee is the method of choice. Because SYMMETREL does not completely prevent the host immune response to influenza A infection, individuals who take this drug may still develop immune responses to natural disease or vaccination and may be protected when later exposed to antigenically related viruses. Following vaccination during an influenza A outbreak, SYMMETREL prophylaxis should be considered for the 2- to 4-week time period required to develop an antibody response.
Influenza A Treatment: SYMMETREL is also indicated in the treatment of uncomplicated respiratory tract illness caused by influenza A virus strains especially when administered early in the course of illness. There are no well-controlled clinical studies demonstrating that treatment with SYMMETREL will avoid the development of influenza A virus pneumonitis or other complications in high risk patients.
There is no clinical evidence indicating that SYMMETREL is effective in the prophylaxis or treatment of viral respiratory tract illnesses other than those caused by influenza A virus strains.
Parkinson's Disease/Syndrome: SYMMETREL is indicated in the treatment of idiopathic Parkinson's disease (Paralysis Agitans), postencephalitic parkinsonism, and symptomatic parkinsonism which may follow injury to the nervous system by carbon monoxide intoxication. It is indicated in those elderly patients believed to develop parkinsonism in association with cerebral arteriosclerosis. In the treatment of Parkinson's disease, SYMMETREL is less effective than levodopa, (-)-3-(3,4-dihydroxyphenyl)-L-alanine, and its efficacy in comparison with the anticholinergic antiparkinson drugs has not yet been established.
Drug-Induced Extrapyramidal Reactions: SYMMETREL is indicated in the treatment of drug-induced extrapyramidal reactions. Although anticholinergic-type side effects have been noted with SYMMETREL when used in patients with drug-induced extrapyramidal reactions, there is a lower incidence of these side effects than that observed with the anticholinergic antiparkinson drugs.

CONTRAINDICATIONS

SYMMETREL is contraindicated in patients with known hypersensitivity to amantadine hydrochloride or to any of the other ingredients in SYMMETREL.

WARNINGS

Deaths: Deaths have been reported from overdose with SYMMETREL. The lowest reported acute lethal dose was 2 grams. Acute toxicity may be attributable to the anticholinergic effects of amantadine. Drug overdose has resulted in cardiac, respiratory, renal or central nervous system toxicity. Cardiac dysfunction includes arrhythmia, tachycardia and hypertension (see OVERDOSAGE).
Suicide Attempts: Suicide attempts, some of which have been fatal, have been reported in patients treated with SYMMETREL, many of whom received short courses for influenza treatment or prophylaxis. The incidence of suicide attempts is not known and the pathophysiologic mechanism is not understood. Suicide attempts and suicidal ideation have been reported in patients with and without prior history of psychiatric illness. SYMMETREL can exacerbate mental problems in patients with a history of psychiatric disorders or substance abuse. Patients who attempt suicide may exhibit abnormal mental states which include disorientation, confusion, depression, personality changes, agitation, aggressive behavior, hallucinations, paranoia, other psychotic reactions, and somnolence or insomnia. Because of the possibility of serious adverse effects, caution should be observed when prescribing SYMMETREL to patients being treated with drugs having CNS effects, or for whom the potential risks outweigh the benefit of treatment.
CNS Effects: Patients with a history of epilepsy or other "seizures" should be observed closely for possible increased seizure activity.
Patients receiving SYMMETREL who note central nervous system effects or blurring of vision should be cautioned against driving or working in situations where alertness and adequate motor coordination are important.
Other: Patients with a history of congestive heart failure or peripheral edema should be followed closely as there are patients who developed congestive heart failure while receiving SYMMETREL.
Patients with Parkinson's disease improving on SYMMETREL should resume normal activities gradually and cautiously, consistent with other medical considerations, such as the presence of osteoporosis or phlebothrombosis.
Because SYMMETREL has anticholinergic effects and may cause mydriasis, it should not be given to patients with untreated angle closure glaucoma.

PRECAUTIONS

SYMMETREL should not be discontinued abruptly in patients with Parkinson's disease since a few patients have experienced a parkinsonian crisis, i.e., a sudden marked clinical deterioration, when this medication was suddenly stopped. The dose of anticholinergic drugs or of SYMMETREL should be reduced if atropine-like effects appear when these drugs are used concurrently.
Neuroleptic Malignant Syndrome (NMS): Sporadic cases of possible Neuroleptic Malignant Syndrome (NMS) have been reported in association with dose reduction or withdrawal of SYMMETREL therapy. Therefore, patients

Continued on next page

Symmetrel —Cont.

should be observed carefully when the dosage of SYMMETREL is reduced abruptly or discontinued, especially if the patient is receiving neuroleptics.

NMS is an uncommon but life-threatening syndrome characterized by fever or hyperthermia; neurologic findings including muscle rigidity, involuntary movements, altered consciousness; mental status changes; other disturbances such as autonomic dysfunction, tachycardia, tachypnea, hyper- or hypotension; laboratory findings such as creatine phosphokinase elevation, leukocytosis, myoglobinuria, and increased serum myoglobin.

The early diagnosis of this condition is important for the appropriate management of these patients. Considering NMS as a possible diagnosis and ruling out other acute illnesses (e.g., pneumonia, systemic infection, etc.) is essential. This may be especially complex if the clinical presentation includes both serious medical illness and untreated or inadequately treated extrapyramidal signs and symptoms (EPS). Other important considerations in the differential diagnosis include central anticholinergic toxicity, heat stroke, drug fever and primary central nervous system (CNS) pathology.

The management of NMS should include: 1) intensive symptomatic treatment and medical monitoring, and 2) treatment of any concomitant serious medical problems for which specific treatments are available. Dopamine agonists, such as bromocriptine, and muscle relaxants, such as dantrolene are often used in the treatment of NMS, however, their effectiveness has not been demonstrated in controlled studies.

Renal disease: Because SYMMETREL is mainly excreted in the urine, it accumulates in the plasma and in the body when renal function declines. Thus, the dose of SYMMETREL should be reduced in patients with renal impairment and in individuals who are 65 years of age or older. Hemodialysis does not remove significant amounts of SYMMETREL; in patients with renal failure, a 4-hour hemodialysis removed 7 to 15 mg after a single 300 mg oral dose[1] (see DOSAGE AND ADMINISTRATION; Dosage for Impaired Renal Function).

Liver disease: Care should be exercised when administering SYMMETREL to patients with liver disease. Rare instances of reversible elevation of liver enzymes have been reported in patients receiving SYMMETREL, though a specific relationship between the drug and such changes has not been established.

Other: The dose of SYMMETREL may need careful adjustment in patients with congestive heart failure, peripheral edema, or orthostatic hypotension. Care should be exercised when administering SYMMETREL to patients with a history of recurrent eczematoid rash, or to patients with psychosis or severe psychoneurosis not controlled by chemotherapeutic agents.

Information for Patients:

Patients should be advised of the following information:

Blurry vision and/or impaired mental acuity may occur.

Gradually increase physicial activity as the symptoms of Parksinson's disease improve.

Avoid excessive alcohol usage, since it may increase the potential for CNS effects such as dizziness, confusion, lightheadedness and orthostatic hypotension.

Avoid getting up suddenly from a sitting or lying position. If dizziness or lightheadedness occurs, notify physician.

Notify physician if mood/mental changes, swelling of extremities, difficulty urinating and/or shortness of breath occur.

Do not take more medication than prescribed because of the risk of overdose. If there is no improvement in a few days, or if medication appears less effective after a few weeks, discuss with a physician.

Consult physician before discontinuing medication.

Seek medical attention immediately if it is suspected that an overdose of medication has been taken.

Drug Interactions: Careful observation is required when SYMMETREL is administered concurrently with central nervous system stimulants.

Agents with anticholinergic properties may potentiate the anticholinergic-like side effects of amantadine.

Coadministration of thioridazine has been reported to worsen the tremor in elderly patients with Parkinson's disease, however, it is not known if other phenothiazines produce a similar response.

Coadministration of Dyazide (triamterene/hydrochlorothiazide) resulted in a higher plasma amantadine concentration in a 61-year-old man receiving SYMMETREL (amantadine hydrochloride) 100 mg TID for Parkinson's disease.[2] It is not known which of the components of Dyazide contributed to the observation or if related drugs produce a similar response.

Coadministration of trimethoprim-sulfamethoxazole may impair renal clearance of amantadine resulting in higher plasma concentrations.

Coadministration of quinine or quinidine with amantadine was shown to reduce the renal clearance of amantadine.

Carcinogenesis and Mutagenesis: Long-term *in vivo* animal studies designed to evaluate the carcinogenic potential of SYMMETREL have not been performed. In several *in vitro* assays for gene mutation, SYMMETREL did not increase the number of spontaneously observed mutations in four strains of *Salmonella typhimurium* (Ames Test) or in a mammalian cell line (Chinese Hamster Ovary cells) when incubations were performed either with or without a liver metabolic activation extract. Further, there was no evidence of chromosome damage observed in an *in vitro* test using freshly derived and stimulated human peripheral blood lymphocytes (with and without metabolic activation) or in an *in vivo* mouse bone marrow micronucleus test (140–550 mg/kg; estimated human equivalent doses of 11.7–45.8 mg/kg based on body surface area conversion).

Impairment of Fertility: In a three litter reproduction study in rats, SYMMETREL at a dose of 32 mg/kg/day (estimated human equivalent dose of 4.5 mg/kg/day, based on body surface area conversions) administered to both males and females slightly impaired fertility. There were no effects on fertility at a dose level of 10 mg/kg/day (estimated human equivalent dose of 1.4 mg/kg/day); intermediate doses were not tested.

Failed fertility has been reported during human *in vitro* fertilization (IVF) when the sperm donor ingested amantadine 2 weeks prior to, and during the IVF cycle.

Pregnancy Category C: SYMMETREL has been reported to be teratogenic in rats at 50 mg/kg/day and embryotoxic at 100 mg/kg/day (estimated human equivalent dose of 7.1 mg/kg/day and 14.2 mg/kg/day, respectively, based on body surface area conversion). A dose of 37 mg/kg/day (estimated human equivalent dose of 5.3 mg/kg/day) did not produce a teratogenic or embryotoxic effect in the rat. Embryotoxic and teratogenic effects were not seen in rabbits that received 32 mg/kg/day (estimated human equivalent dose of 9.6 mg/kg/day, based on body surface area conversion). There are no adequate and well-controlled studies in pregnant women. Human data regarding teratogenicity after maternal use of amantadine is scarce. Tetralogy of Fallot and tibial hemimelia (normal karyotype) occurred in an infant exposed to amantadine during the first trimester of pregnancy (100 mg P.O. for 7 days during the 6th and 7th week of gestation). Cardiovascular maldevelopment (single ventricle with pulmonary atresia) was associated with maternal exposure to amantadine (100 mg/d) administered during the first 2 weeks of pregnancy. SYMMETREL should be used during pregnancy only if the potential benefit justifies the potential risk to the embryo or fetus.

Nursing Mothers: SYMMETREL is excreted in human milk. Use is not recommended in nursing mothers.

Pediatric Use: The safety and efficacy of SYMMETREL in newborn infants and infants below the age of 1 year have not been established.

Usage in the Elderly: Because SYMMETREL is primarily excreted in the urine, it accumulates in the plasma and in the body when renal function declines. Thus, the dose of SYMMETREL should be reduced in patients with renal impairment and in individuals who are 65 years of age or older. The dose of SYMMETREL may need reduction in patients with congestive heart failure, peripheral edema, or orthostatic hypotension (see DOSAGE AND ADMINISTRATION).

ADVERSE REACTIONS

The adverse reactions reported most frequently at the recommended dose of SYMMETREL (5–10%) are: nausea, dizziness (lightheadedness), and insomnia.

Less frequently (1–5%) reported adverse reactions are: depression, anxiety and irritability, hallucinations, confusion, anorexia, dry mouth, constipation, ataxia, livedo reticularis, peripheral edema, orthostatic hypotension, headache, somnolence, nervousness, dream abnormality, agitation, dry nose, diarrhea and fatigue.

Infrequently (0.1–1%) occurring adverse reactions are: congestive heart failure, psychosis, urinary retention, dyspnea, skin rash, vomiting, weakness, slurred speech, euphoria, thinking abnormality, amnesia, hyperkinesia, hypertension, decreased libido, and visual disturbance, including punctate subepithelial or other corneal opacity, corneal edema, decreased visual acuity, sensitivity to light, and optic nerve palsy.

Rare (less than 0.1%) occurring adverse reactions are: instances of convulsion, leukopenia, neutropenia, eczematoid dermatitis, oculogyric episodes, suicidal attempt, suicide, and suicidal ideation (see WARNINGS).

Other adverse reactions reported during postmarketing experience with SYMMETREL usage include:

Nervous System/Psychiatric—coma, stupor, delirium, hypokinesia, hypertonia, delusions, aggressive behavior, paranoid reaction, manic reaction, involuntary muscle contractions, gait abnormalities, paresthesia, EEG changes, and tremor;

Cardiovascular—cardiac arrest, arrhythmias including malignant arrhythmias, hypotension, and tachycardia;

Respiratory—acute respiratory failure, pulmonary edema, and tachypnea;

Gastrointestinal—dysphagia;

Hematologic—leukocytosis;

Special Senses—keratitis and mydriasis;

Skin and Appendages—pruritus and diaphoresis;

Miscellaneous—neuroleptic malignant syndrome (see WARNINGS), allergic reactions including anaphylactic reactions, edema, and fever;

Laboratory Test—elevated: CPK, BUN, serum creatinine, alkaline phosphatase, LDH, bilirubin, GGT, SGOT, and SGPT.

OVERDOSAGE

Deaths have been reported from overdose with SYMMETREL. The lowest reported acute lethal dose was 2 grams. Because some patients have attempted suicide by overdosing with amantadine, prescriptions should be written for the smallest quantity consistent with good patient management.

Acute toxicity may be attributable to the anticholinergic effects of amantadine. Drug overdose has resulted in cardiac, respiratory, renal or central nervous system toxicity. Cardiac dysfunction includes arrhythmia, tachycardia and hypertension. Pulmonary edema and respiratory distress (including adult respiratory distress syndrome—ARDS) have been reported; renal dysfunction including increased BUN, decreased creatinine clearance and renal insufficiency can occur. Central nervous system effects that have been reported include insomnia, anxiety, agitation, aggressive behavior, hypertonia, hyperkinesia, ataxia, gait abnormality, tremor, confusion, disorientation, depersonalization, fear, delirium, hallucinations, psychotic reactions, lethargy, somnolence and coma. Seizures may be exacerbated in patients with prior history of seizure disorders. Hyperthermia has also been observed in cases where a drug overdose has occurred.

There is no specific antidote for an overdose of SYMMETREL. However, slowly administered intravenous physostigmine in 1 and 2 mg doses in an adult[3] at 1- to 2-hour intervals and 0.5 mg doses in a child[4] at 5- to 10-minute intervals up to a maximum of 2 mg/hour have been reported to be effective in the control of central nervous system toxicity caused by amantadine hydrochloride. For acute overdosing, general supportive measures should be employed along with immediate gastric lavage or induction of emesis. Fluids should be forced, and if necessary, given intravenously. Hemodialysis does not remove significant amounts of SYMMETREL; in patients with renal failure, a 4-hour hemodialysis removed 7 to 15 mg after a single 300 mg oral dose.[1] The pH of the urine has been reported to influence the excretion rate of SYMMETREL. Since the excretion rate of SYMMETREL increases rapidly when the urine is acidic, the administration of urine acidifying drugs may increase the elimination of the drug from the body. The blood pressure, pulse, respiration and temperature should be monitored. The patient should be observed for hyperactivity and convulsions; if required, sedation, and anticonvulsant therapy should be administered. The patient should be observed for the possible development of arrhythmias and hypotension; if required, appropriate antiarrhythmic and antihypotensive therapy should be given. Electrocardiographic monitoring may be required after ingestion, since malignant tachyarrhythmias can appear after overdose.

Care should be exercised when administering adrenergic agents, such as isoproterenol, to patients with a SYMMETREL overdose, since the dopaminergic activity of SYMMETREL has been reported to induce malignant arrhythmias. The blood electrolytes, urine pH and urinary output should be monitored. If there is no record of recent voiding, catheterization should be done.

DOSAGE AND ADMINISTRATION

The dose of SYMMETREL may need reduction in patients with congestive heart failure, peripheral edema, orthostatic hypotension, or impaired renal function (see Dosage for Impaired Renal Function).

Dosage for Prophylaxis and Treatment of Uncomplicated Influenza A Virus Illness:

Adult: The adult daily dosage of SYMMETREL (amantadine hydrochloride) is 200 mg; two 100 mg tablets (or four teasponfuls of syrup as a single daily dose. The daily dosage may be split into one tablet of 100 mg (or two teaspoonfuls of syrup) twice a day. If central nervous system effects develop in once-a-day dosage, a split dosage schedule may reduce such complaints. In persons 65 years of age or older, the daily dosage of SYMMETREL is 100 mg.

A 100 mg daily dose has also been shown in experimental challenge studies to be effective as prophylaxis in healthy adults who are not at high risk for influenza-related complications. However, it has not been demonstrated that a 100 mg daily dose is as effective as a 200 mg daily dose for prophylaxis, nor has the 100 mg daily dose been studied in the treatment of acute influenza illness. In recent clinical trials, the incidence of central nervous system (CNS) side effects associated with the 100 mg daily dose was at or near the level of placebo. The 100 mg dose is recommended for persons who have demonstrated intolerance to 200 mg of SYMMETREL daily because of CNS or other toxicities.

Pediatric Patients: 1 yr.–9 yrs. of age: The total daily dose should be calculated on the basis of 2 to 4 mg/lb/day (4.4 to 8.8 mg/kg/day), but not to exceed 150 mg per day.

9 yrs.–12 yrs. of age: The total daily dose is 200 mg given as one tablet of 100 mg (or two teaspoonfuls of syrup) twice a day. The 100 mg daily dose has not been studied in this pediatric population. Therefore, there are no data which demonstrate that this dose is as effective as or is safer than the 200 mg daily dose in this patient population.

Prophylactic dosing should be started in anticipation of an influenza A outbreak and before or after contact with individuals with influenza A virus respiratory tract illness. SYMMETREL should be continued daily for at least 10 days following a known exposure. If SYMMETREL is used chemoprophylactically in conjunction with inactivated influenza A virus vaccine until protective antibody responses develop, then it should be administered for 2 to 4 weeks after the vaccine has been given. When inactivated influenza A virus vaccine is unavailable or contraindicated, SYMMETREL should be administered for the duration of known influenza A in the community because of repeated and unknown exposure.

Treatment of influenza A virus illness should be started as soon as possible, preferably within 24 to 48 hours after onset of signs and symptoms, and should be continued for 24 to 48 hours after the disappearance of signs and symptoms.

Dosage for Parkinsonism:

Adult: The usual dose of SYMMETREL is 100 mg twice a day when used alone. SYMMETREL has an onset of action usually within 48 hours.

The initial dose of SYMMETREL is 100 mg daily for patients with serious associated medical illnesses or who are receiving high doses of other antiparkinson drugs. After one to several weeks at 100 mg once daily, the dose may be increased to 100 mg twice daily, if necessary.

Occasionally, patients whose responses are not optimal with SYMMETREL at 200 mg daily may benefit from an increase up to 400 mg daily in divided doses. However, such patients should be supervised closely by their physicians.

Patients initially deriving benefit from SYMMETREL not uncommonly experience a fall-off of effectiveness after a few months. Benefit may be regained by increasing the dose to 300 mg daily. Alternatively, temporary discontinuation of SYMMETREL for several weeks, followed by reinitiation of the drug, may result in regaining benefit in some patients. A decision to use other antiparkinson drugs may be necessary.

Dosage for Concomitant Therapy: Some patients who do not respond to anticholinergic antiparkinson drugs may respond to SYMMETREL. When SYMMETREL or anticholinergic antiparkinson drugs are each used with marginal benefit, concomitant use may produce additional benefit.

When SYMMETREL and levodopa are initiated concurrently, the patient can exhibit rapid therapeutic benefits. SYMMETREL should be held constant at 100 mg daily or twice daily while the daily dose of levodopa is gradually increased to optimal benefit.

When SYMMETREL is added to optimal well-tolerated doses of levodopa, additional benefit may result, including smoothing out the fluctuations in improvement which sometimes occur in patients on levodopa alone. Patients who require a reduction in their usual dose of levodopa because of development of side effects may possibly regain lost benefit with the addition of SYMMETREL.

Dosage for Drug-Induced Extrapyramidal Reactions:

Adult: The usual dose of SYMMETREL is 100 mg twice a day. Occasionally, patients whose responses are not optimal with SYMMETREL at 200 mg daily may benefit from an increase up to 300 mg daily in divided doses.

Dosage for Impaired Renal Function:

Depending upon creatinine clearance, the following dosage adjustments are recommended:

CREATININE CLEARANCE (mL/min/1.73m²)	SYMMETREL DOSAGE
30–50	200 mg 1st day and 100 mg each day thereafter
15–29	200 mg 1st day followed by 100 mg on alternate days
<15	200 mg every 7 days

The recommended dosage for patients on hemodialysis is 200 mg every 7 days.

HOW SUPPLIED

SYMMETREL is available in light orange, convex curved, triangular shaped 100 mg tablets with "SYMMETREL" debossed on one side and plain on the other side as follows:

Bottles of 100   NDC 63481-108-70
Bottles of 500   NDC 63481-108-85

As a clear, colorless syrup [each 5 mL (1 teaspoonful) contains 50 mg amantadine hydrochloride] in:

16 oz. (480 mL) bottles   NDC 63481-205-16

Store at controlled room temperature 15°–30°C (59°–86°F). Dispense in a tight container as defined in the USP.

REFERENCES

1. V.W. Horadam, et al., *Ann. Intern. Med.* 94:454, 1981.
2. W.W. Wilson and A.H. Rajput, Amantadine-Dyazide Interaction, *Can. Med. Assoc. J.* 129:974–975, 1983.
3. D.F. Casey, *N. Engl. J. Med.* 298:516, 1978.
4. C.D. Berkowitz, *J. Pediatr.* 95:144, 1979.

Caution: Federal (USA) law prohibits dispensing without prescription.

SYMMETREL® is a Registered Trademark of Endo Pharmaceuticals Inc.

Copyright © Endo Pharmaceuticals Inc., 1998

6486-01/Rev. February, 1998

Shown in Product Identification Guide, page 310

ZYDONE®

[zī "dōn ']

(Hydrocodone Bitartrate and Acetaminophen) Capsules

DESCRIPTION

ZYDONE is supplied in capsule form for oral administration.

Hydrocodone bitartrate is an opioid analgesic and antitussive and occurs as fine, white crystals or as a crystalline powder. It is affected by light. The chemical name is: 4,5α-epoxy-3-methoxy-17-methylmorphinan-6-one tartrate (1:1) hydrate (2:5). It has the following structural formula:

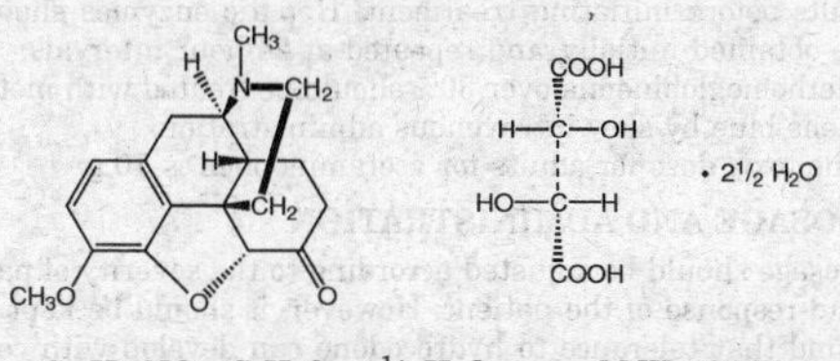

$$C_{18}H_{21}NO_3 \cdot C_4H_6O_6 \cdot 2\frac{1}{2} H_2O \qquad M.W. \; 494.50$$

Acetaminophen, 4'-hydroxyacetanilide, a slightly bitter, white, odorless, crystalline powder, is a non-opiate, non-salicylate analgesic and antipyretic. It has the following structural formula:

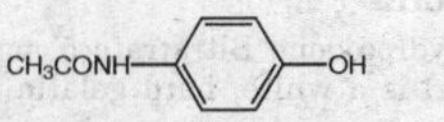

$$C_8H_9NO_2 \qquad M.W. \; 151.16$$

Each ZYDONE capsule contains:
  Hydrocodone Bitartrate   5 mg
    (Warning: May be habit forming)
  Acetaminophen   500 mg

In addition each capsule contains the following inactive ingredients: FD&C Red 7, FD&C Yellow 6, gelatin, pharmaceutical glaze, silicon dioxide, sodium lauryl sulfate and titanium dioxide.

CLINICAL PHARMACOLOGY

Hydrocodone is a semisynthetic narcotic analgesic and antitussive with multiple actions qualitatively similar to those of codeine. Most of these involve the central nervous system and smooth muscle. The precise mechanism of action of hydrocodone and other opiates is not known, although it is believed to relate to the existence of opiate receptors in the central nervous system. In addition to analgesia, narcotics may produce drowsiness, changes in mood and mental clouding.

The analgesic action of acetaminophen involves peripheral influences, but the specific mechanism is as yet undetermined. Antipyretic activity is mediated through hypothalamic heat regulating centers. Acetaminophen inhibits prostaglandin synthetase. Therapeutic doses of acetaminophen have negligible effects on the cardiovascular or respiratory systems; however, toxic doses may cause circulatory failure and rapid, shallow breathing.

Pharmacokinetics: The behavior of the individual components is described below:

Hydrocodone: Following a 10 mg oral dose of hydrocodone administered to five adult male subjects, the mean peak concentration was 23.6 ± 5.2 ng/mL. Maximum serum levels were achieved at 1.3 ± 0.3 hours and the half-life was determined to be 3.8 ± 0.3 hours. Hydrocodone exhibits a complex pattern of metabolism including O-demethylation, N-demethylation and 6-keto reduction to the corresponding 6-α- and 6-β-hydroxymetabolites.

See OVERDOSAGE for toxicity information.

Acetaminophen: Acetaminophen is rapidly absorbed from the gastrointestinal tract and is distributed throughout most body tissues. The plasma half-life is 1.25 to 3 hours, but may be increased by liver damage and following overdosage. Elimination of acetaminophen is principally by liver metabolism (conjugation) and subsequent renal excretion of metabolites. Approximately 85% of an oral dose appears in the urine within 24 hours of administration, most as the glucuronide conjugate, with small amounts of other conjugates and unchanged drug.

See OVERDOSAGE for toxicity information.

INDICATIONS AND USAGE

ZYDONE capsules are indicated for the relief of moderate to moderately severe pain.

CONTRAINDICATIONS

This product should not be administered to patients who have previously exhibited hypersensitivity to hydrocodone or acetaminophen.

WARNINGS

Respiratory Depression: At high doses or in sensitive patients, hydrocodone may produce dose-related respiratory depression by acting directly on the brain stem respiratory center. Hydrocodone also affects the center that controls respiratory rhythm, and may produce irregular and periodic breathing.

Head Injury and Increased Intracranial Pressure: The respiratory depressant effects of narcotics and their capacity to elevate cerebrospinal fluid pressure may be markedly exaggerated in the presence of head injury, other intracranial lesions or a preexisting increase in intracranial pressure. Furthermore, narcotics produce adverse reactions which may obscure the clinical course of patients with head injuries.

Acute Abdominal Conditions: The administration of narcotics may obscure the diagnosis or clinical course of patients with acute abdominal conditions.

PRECAUTIONS

General: Special Risk Patients: As with any narcotic analgesic agent, hydrocodone bitartrate and acetaminophen capsules should be used with caution in elderly or debilitated patients and those with severe impairment of hepatic or renal function, hypothyroidism, Addison's disease, prostatic hypertrophy or urethral stricture. The usual precautions should be observed and the possibility of respiratory depression should be kept in mind.

Cough reflex: Hydrocodone suppresses the cough reflex; as with all narcotics, caution should be exercised when hydrocodone bitartrate and acetaminophen capsules are used postoperatively and in patients with pulmonary disease.

Information for Patients: Hydrocodone, like all narcotics, may impair mental and/or physical abilities required for the performance of potentially hazardous tasks such as driving a car or operating machinery; patients should be cautioned accordingly.

Alcohol and other CNS depressants may produce an additive CNS depression, when taken with this combination product, and should be avoided.

Hydrocodone may be habit-forming. Patients should take the drug only for as long as it is prescribed, in the amounts prescribed, and no more frequently than prescribed.

Laboratory Tests: In patients with severe hepatic or renal disease, effects of therapy should be monitored with serial liver and/or renal function tests.

Drug Interactions: Patients receiving narcotics, antipsychotics, antianxiety agents, or other CNS depressants (including alcohol) concomitantly with hydrocodone bitartrate and acetaminophen capsules may exhibit an additive CNS depression. When combined therapy is contemplated, the dose of one or both agents should be reduced.

The use of MAO inhibitors or tricyclic antidepressants with hydrocodone preparations may increase the effect of either the antidepressant or hydrocodone.

Drug/Laboratory Test Interactions: Acetaminophen may produce false-positive test results for urinary 5-hydroxyindoleacetic acid.

Carcinogenesis, Mutagenesis, Impairment of Fertility: No adequate studies have been conducted in animals to determine whether hydrocodone or acetaminophen have a potential for carcinogenesis, mutagenesis, or impairment of fertility.

Pregnancy:

Teratogenic Effects: Pregnancy Category C: There are no adequate and well-controlled studies in pregnant women. ZYDONE (Hydrocodone Bitartrate and Acetaminophen) capsules should be used during pregnancy only if the potential benefit justifies the potential risk to the fetus.

Nonteratogenic Effects: Babies born to mothers who have been taking opioids regularly prior to delivery will be physically dependent. The withdrawal signs include irritability and excessive crying, tremors, hyperactive reflexes, increased respiratory rate, increased stools, sneezing, yawning, vomiting, and fever. The intensity of the syndrome does not always correlate with the duration of maternal opioid use or dose. There is no consensus on the best method of managing withdrawal.

Labor and Delivery: As with all narcotics, administration of this product to the mother shortly before delivery may result in some degree of respiratory depression in the newborn, especially if higher doses are used.

Nursing Mothers: Acetaminophen is excreted in breast milk in small amounts, but the significance of its effects on nursing infants is not known. It is not known whether hydrocodone is excreted in human milk. Because many drugs

Continued on next page

Zydone—Cont.

are excreted in human milk and because of the potential for serious adverse reactions in nursing infants from hydrocodone and acetaminophen, a decision should be made whether to discontinue nursing or to discontinue the drug, taking into account the importance of the drug to the mother.

Pediatric Use: Safety and effectiveness in pediatric patients have not been established.

ADVERSE REACTIONS

The most frequently reported adverse reactions are lightheadedness, dizziness, sedation, nausea and vomiting. These effects seem to be more prominent in ambulatory than in nonambulatory patients, and some of these adverse reactions may be alleviated if the patient lies down.

Other adverse reactions include:

Central Nervous System: Drowsiness, mental clouding, lethargy, impairment of mental and physical performance, anxiety, fear, dysphoria, psychic dependence, mood changes.

Gastrointestinal System: Prolonged administration of hydrocodone bibartrate and acetaminophen capsules may produce constipation.

Genitourinary System: Ureteral spasm, spasm of vesical sphincters and urinary retention have been reported with opiates.

Respiratory Depression: Hydrocodone bitartrate may produce dose-related respiratory depression by acting directly on brain stem respiratory centers. (see OVERDOSAGE).

Dermatological: Skin rash, pruritus.

The following adverse drug events may be borne in mind as potential effects of acetaminophen: allergic reactions, rash, thrombocytopenia, agranulocytosis.

Potential effects of high dosage are listed in the OVERDOSAGE section.

DRUG ABUSE AND DEPENDENCE

Controlled Substance: ZYDONE (Hydrocodone Bitartrate and Acetaminophen) Capsules are classified as a Schedule III controlled substance.

Abuse and Dependence: Psychic dependence, physical dependence, and tolerance may develop upon repeated administration of narcotics; therefore, this product should be prescribed and administered with caution. However, psychic dependence is unlikely to develop when hydrocodone bitartrate and acetaminophen capsules are used for a short time for the treatment of pain.

Psychical dependence, the condition in which continued administration of the drug is required to prevent the appearance of a withdrawal syndrome, assumes clinically significant proportions only after several weeks of continued narcotic use, although some mild degree of physical dependence may develop after a few days of narcotic therapy. Tolerance, in which increasingly large doses are required in order to produce the same degree of analgesia, is manifested initially by a shortened duration of analgesic effect, and subsequently by decreases in the intensity of analgesia. The rate of development of tolerance varies among patients.

OVERDOSAGE

Following an acute overdosage, toxicity may result from hydrocodone or acetaminophen.

Signs and Symptoms:

Hydrocodone: Serious overdose with hydrocodone is characterized by respiratory depression (a decrease in respiratory rate and/or tidal volume, Cheyne-Stokes respiration, cyanosis) extreme somnolence progressing to stupor or coma, sketetal muscle flaccidity, cold and clammy skin, and sometimes bradycardia and hypotension. In severe overdosage, apnea, circulatory collapse, cardiac arrest and death may occur.

Acetaminophen: In acetaminophen overdosage: dose-dependent, potentially fatal hepatic necrosis is the most serious adverse effect. Renal tubular necrosis, hypoglycemic coma and thrombocytopenia may also occur.

Early symptoms following a potentially hepatotoxic overdose may include: nausea, vomiting, diaphoresis and general malaise. Clinical and laboratory evidence of hepatic toxicity may not be apparent until 48 to 72 hours post-ingestion.

In adults, hepatic toxicity has rarely been reported with acute overdoses of less than 10 grams, or fatalities with less than 15 grams.

Treatment: A single or multiple overdose with hydrocodone and acetaminophen is a potentially lethal polydrug overdose, and consultation with a regional poison control center is recommended.

Immediate treatment includes support of cardiorespiratory function and measures to reduce drug absorption. Vomiting should be induced mechanically, or with syrup of ipecac, if the patient is alert (adequate pharyngeal and laryngeal reflexes). Oral activated charcoal (1 g/kg) should follow gastic emptying. The first dose should be accompanied by an appropriate cathartic. If repeated doses are used, the cathartic might be included with altermate doses as required. Hypotension is usually hypovolemic and should respond to fluids. Vasopressors and other supportive measures should be employed as indicated. A cuffed endo-tracheal tube should be inserted before gastric lavage of the unconscious patient and, when necessary, to provide assisted respiration.

Meticulous attention should be given to maintaining adequate pulmonary ventilation. In severe cases of intoxication, pertitoneal dialysis, or preferably hemodialysis may be considered. If hypoprothrombinemia occurs due to acetaminophen overdose, vitamin K should be asministered intravenously.

Naloxone, a narcotic antagonist, can reverse respiratory depression and coma associated with opioid overdose. Naloxone hydrochloride 0.4 mg to 2 mg is given parenterally. Since the duration of action of hydrocodone may exceed that of the naloxone, the patient should be kept under continuous surveillance and repeated doses of the antagonist should be administered as needed to maintain adequate respiration. A narcotic antagonist should not be administered in the absence of clinically significant respiratory or cardiovascular depression.

If the dose of acetaminophen may have exceeded 140 mg/kg, acetylcysteine should be administered as early as possible. Serum acetaminophen levels should be obtained, since levels four or more hours following ingestion help predict acetaminophen toxicity. Do not await acetaminophen assay results before initiating treatment. Hepatic enzymes should be obtained initially, and repeated at 24-hour intervals.

Methemoglobinemia over 30% should be treated with methylene blue by slow intravenous administration.

The toxic dose for adults for acetaminophen is 10 g.

DOSAGE AND ADMINISTRATION

Dosage should be adjusted according to the severity of pain and response of the patient. However, it should be kept in mind that tolerance to hydrocodone can develop with continued use and that the incidence of untoward effects is dose related.

The usual adult dosage is one or two capsules every four to six hours as needed for pain. The total daily dosage should not exceed 8 capsules.

HOW SUPPLIED

ZYDONE (Hydrocodone Bitratrate 5 mg and Acetaminophen 500 mg) is a white, hard gelatin capsule with red band.

Bottles of 100: NDC 63481-091-70

Storage: Store at controlled room temperature 15°-30°C (59°-86°F).

CAUTION: Federal law prohibits dispensing without prescription.

Manufactured by
D.M. Graham Laboratories, Inc.,
Hobart, New York 13788

6173-8/Rev. Feb., 1996

Enzon, Inc.

**20 KINGSBRIDGE RD.
PISCATAWAY, NJ 08854**

Direct Inquiries to:
Toni L. Klich
(732) 980-4619
FAX: (732) 980-5911

For Medical Information Contact:
In Emergencies:
Anna T. Viau, Ph.D.
(732) 980-4677
FAX: (732) 980-9642

ADAGEN® ℞

[ad-a-jen]
(pegademase bovine) Injection

PRODUCT OVERVIEW

KEY FACTS

ADAGEN® (pegademase bovine) Injection is a modified enzyme used to provide direct and specific replacement of adenosine deaminase (ADA), an enzyme that is deficient in some patients with severe combined immunodeficiency disease (SCID). While regular administration of the compound can improve immune function and reduce the incidence of opportunistic infections in patients with ADA-deficient SCID, it is of no value in patients with immunodeficiency due to other causes. Further, it is not intended as a replacement for HLA-identical bone marrow transplant therapy.

MAJOR USES

ADAGEN® is to be used as enzyme replacement therapy in patients who have SCID associated with a deficiency of ADA, and who are not suitable candidates for-or who have failed-bone marrow transplantation. ADAGEN® should be used in infants from birth or in children of any age at the time of diagnosis.

SAFETY INFORMATION

ADAGEN® should be administered with caution to patients with thrombocytopenia and should not be given if thrombocytopenia is severe.

PRESCRIBING INFORMATION

ADAGEN® ℞

[ad-a-jen]
(pegademase bovine) Injection

DESCRIPTION

ADAGEN® (pegademase bovine) Injection is a modified enzyme used for enzyme replacement therapy for the treatment of severe combined immunodeficiency disease (SCID) associated with a deficiency of adenosine deaminase.

ADAGEN® (pegademase bovine) Injection is supplied in an isotonic, pyrogen free, sterile solution, pH 7.2–7.4, for intramuscular injection only. The solution is clear and colorless. It is supplied in 1.5 mL single-dose vials.

The chemical name for **ADAGEN®** (pegademase bovine) Injection is (monomethoxypolyethylene glycol succinimidyl)$_{11-17}$-adenosine deaminase. It is a conjugate of numerous strands of monomethoxypolyethylene glycol (PEG), molecular weight 5,000, covalently attached to the enzyme adenosine deaminase (ADA). ADA (adenosine deaminase EC 3.5.4.4) used in the manufacture of **ADAGEN®** (pegademase bovine) Injection is derived from bovine intestine.

The structural formula of **ADAGEN®** (pegademase bovine) Injection is:

$$[CH_3-(OCH_2CH_2)_x-O-\underset{\displaystyle O}{\overset{\|}{C}}-CH_2CH_2-\underset{\displaystyle O}{\overset{\|}{C}}-NH]_y-\text{adenosine deaminase}$$

x = 114 oxyethylene groups per PEG strand.
y = 11–17 primary amino groups of lysine onto which succinyl PEG is attached.

Each milliliter of **ADAGEN®** (pegademase bovine) Injection contains:

Pegademase bovine	250 units*
Monobasic sodium phosphate, USP	1.20 mg
Dibasic sodium phosphate, USP	5.58 mg
Sodium Chloride, USP	8.50 mg
Water for Injection, USP	q.s. to 1.0 mL

*One unit of activity is defined as the amount of ADA that converts 1 µM of adenosine to inosine per minute at 25°C and pH 7.3.

CLINICAL PHARMACOLOGY

Severe Combined Immunodeficiency Disease Associated with ADA Deficiency

Severe combined immunodeficiency disease (SCID) associated with a deficiency of ADA is a rare, inherited, and often fatal disease. In the absence of the ADA enzyme, the purine substrates adenosine and 2′-deoxyadenosine accumulate, causing metabolic abnormalities that are directly toxic to lymphocytes.

The immune deficiency can be cured by bone marrow transplantation. When a suitable bone marrow donor is unavailable or when bone marrow transplantation fails, non-selective replacement of the ADA enzyme has been provided by periodic irradiated red blood cell transfusions. However, transmission of viral infections and iron overload are serious risks associated with irradiated red blood cell transfusions, and relatively few ADA deficient patients have benefitted from chronic transfusion therapy.

ADAGEN® (pegademase bovine) Injection provides specific and direct replacement of the deficient enzyme, but will not benefit patients with immunodeficiency due to other causes. In patients with ADA deficiency, rigorous adherence to a schedule of **ADAGEN®** (pegademase bovine) Injection administration can eliminate the toxic metabolites of ADA deficiency and result in improved immune function. It is imperative that treatment with **ADAGEN®** (pegademase bovine) Injection be carefully monitored by measurement of the level of ADA activity in plasma. Monitoring of the level of deoxyadenosine triphosphate (dATP) in erythrocytes is also helpful in determining that the dose of **ADAGEN®** (pegademase bovine) Injection is adequate.

Actions

ADAGEN® (pegademase bovine) Injection provides specific replacement of the deficient enzyme.

In the absence of the enzyme ADA, the purine substrates adenosine, 2′-deoxyadenosine and their metabolites are toxic to lymphocytes. The direct action of **ADAGEN®** (pegademase bovine) Injection is the correction of these metabolic abnormalities. Improvement in immune function and diminished frequency of opportunistic infections compared

with the natural history of combined immunodeficiency due to ADA deficiency only occurs after metabolic abnormalities are corrected. There is a lag between the correction of the metabolic abnormalities and improved immune function. This period of time is variable, and has been reported to be from a few weeks to as long as 6 months. In contrast to the natural history of combined immunodeficiency disease due to ADA deficiency, a trend toward diminished frequency of opportunistic infections and fewer complications of infections has occurred in patients receiving **ADAGEN®** (pegademase bovine) Injection.

Pharmacokinetics

The pharmacokinetics and biochemical effects of **ADAGEN®** (pegademase bovine) Injection have been studied in six children ranging in age from 6 weeks to 12 years with SCID associated with ADA deficiency.

After the intramuscular injection of **ADAGEN®** (pegademase bovine) Injection, peak plasma levels of ADA activity were reached 2 to 3 days following administration. The plasma elimination half-life of ADA following the administration of **ADAGEN®** (pegademase bovine) Injection was variable, even for the same child. The range was 3 to >6 days. Following weekly injections of **ADAGEN®** (pegademase bovine) Injection at 15 U/kg, the average trough level of ADA activity in plasma was between 20 and 25 µmol/hr/mL.

Biochemical Effects

The changes in red blood cell deoxyadenosine nucleotide (dATP) and S-adenosylhomocysteine hydrolase (SAHase) have been evaluated. In patients with ADA deficiency, inadequate elimination of 2′-deoxyadenosine caused a marked elevation in dATP and a decrease in SAHase level in red blood cells. Prior to treatment with **ADAGEN®** (pegademase bovine) Injection, the levels of dATP in the red blood cells ranged from 0.056 to 0.899 µmol/mL of erythrocytes. After 2 months of maintenance treatment with **ADAGEN®** (pegademase bovine) Injection, the levels decreased to a range of 0.007 to 0.015 µmol/mL. The normal value of dATP is below 0.001 µmol/mL. In the same period of time, the levels of SAHase increased from the pretreatment range of 0.09 to 0.22 nmol/hr/mg protein to a range of 2.37 to 5.16 nmol/hr/mg protein. The normal value for SAHase is 4.18± 1.9 nmol/hr/mg protein.

The optimal dosage and schedule of administration of **ADAGEN®** (pegademase bovine) Injection should be established for each patient, based on monitoring of plasma ADA activity levels (trough levels before maintenance injection), biochemical markers of ADA deficiency (primarily red cell dATP content), and parameters of immune function. Since improvement in immune function follows correction of metabolic abnormalities, maintenance dosage in individual patients should be aimed at achieving the following biochemical goals: 1) maintain plasma ADA activity (trough levels) in the range of 15–35 µmol/hr/mL (assayed at 37°C); and 2) decline in erythrocyte dATP to ≤ 0.005–0.015 µmol/mL packed erythrocytes, or ≤ 1% of the total erythrocyte adenine nucleotide (ATP + dATP) content, with a normal ATP level, as measured in a pre-injection sample.

In vitro immunologic data (lymphocyte response to mitogens and lymphocyte surface antigens) were obtained, but their clinical significance is unknown. Prior to treatment with **ADAGEN®** (pegademase bovine) Injection, immune status was significantly below normal, as indicated by <10% of normal mitogen responses and circulating mononuclear cells bearing T-cell surface antigens. These parameters improved, though not always to normal, within 2 to 6 months of therapy.

INDICATIONS AND USAGE

ADAGEN® (pegademase bovine) Injection is indicated for enzyme replacement therapy for adenosine deaminase (ADA) deficiency in patients with severe combined immunodeficiency disease (SCID) who are not suitable candidates for—or who have failed—bone marrow transplantation. **ADAGEN®** (pegademase bovine) Injection is recommended for use in infants from birth or in children of any age at the time of diagnosis. **ADAGEN®** (pegademase bovine) Injection is not intended as a replacement for HLA indentical bone marrow transplant therapy. **ADAGEN®** (pegademase bovine) Injection is also not intended to replace continued close medical supervision and the initiation of appropriate diagnostic tests and therapy (e.g., antibiotics, nutrition, oxygen, gammaglobulin) as indicated for intercurrent illnesses.

CONTRAINDICATIONS

There is no evidence to support the safety and efficacy of **ADAGEN®** (pegademase bovine) Injection as preparatory or support therapy for bone marrow transplantation. Since **ADAGEN®** (pegademase bovine) Injection is administered by intramuscular injection, it should be used with caution in patients with thrombocytopenia and should not be used if thrombocytopenia is severe.

PRECAUTIONS

Warnings

At present, testing prior to distribution may not assure the initial and continuing potency of each new lot of **ADAGEN®** (pegademase bovine) Injection. Any laboratory or clinical indication of a decrease in potency of **ADAGEN®** (pegademase bovine) Injection should be reported immediately by telephone to ENZON, Inc. Telephone 732-980-4500. Fax 732-980-5911.

General

There have been no reports of hypersensitivity reactions in patients who have been treated with **ADAGEN®** (pegademase bovine) Injection.

One of 12 patients showed an enhanced rate of clearance of plasma ADA activity after 5 months of therapy at 15 U/kg/week. Enhanced clearance was correlated with the appearance of an antibody that directly inhibited both unmodified ADA and **ADAGEN®** (pegademase bovine) Injection. Subsequently, the patient was treated with twice weekly intramuscular injections at an increased dose of 20 U/kg, or a total weekly dose of 40 U/kg. No adverse effects were observed at the higher dose and effective levels of plasma ADA were restored. After 4 months, the patient returned to a weekly dosage schedule of 20 U/kg and effective plasma levels have been maintained.

Appropriate care to protect immune deficient patients should be maintained until improvement in immune function has been documented. The degree of immune function improvement may vary from patient to patient and, therefore, each patient will require appropriate care consistent with immunologic status.

Laboratory Tests

The treatment of SCID associated with ADA deficiency with **ADAGEN®]** (pegademase bovine) Injection should be monitored by measuring plasma ADA activity and red blood cell dATP levels.

Plasma ADA activity and red cell dATP should be determined prior to treatment. Once treatment with **ADAGEN®** (pegademase bovine) Injection has been initiated, a desirable range of plasma ADA activity (trough level before maintenance injection) should be 15–35 µmol/hr/mL. This minimum trough level will ensure that plasma ADA activity from injection to injection is maintained above the level of total erythrocyte ADA activity in the blood of normal individuals.

Plasma ADA activity (pre-injection) should be determined every 1–2 weeks during the first 8–12 weeks of treatment in order to establish an effective dose of **ADAGEN®** (pegademase bovine) Injection. After two months of maintenance treatment with **ADAGEN®** (pegademase bovine) Injection, red cell dATP levels should decrease to a range of ≤0.005 to 0.015 µmol/mL. The normal value of dATP is below 0.001 µmol/mL. Once the level of dATP has fallen adequately, it should be measured 2–4 times a year during the remainder of the first year and 2–3 times a year thereafter, assuming no interruption in therapy.

Between 3 and 9 months, plasma ADA should be determined twice a month, then monthly until after 18–24 months of treatment with **ADAGEN®** (pegademase bovine) Injection.

Patients who have successfully been maintained on therapy for two years should continue to have plasma ADA measured every 2–4 months and red cell dATP measured twice yearly. More frequent monitoring would be necessary if therapy were interrupted or if an enhanced rate of clearance of plasma ADA activity develops.

Once effective ADA plasma levels have been established, should a patient's plasma ADA activity level fall below 10 µmol/hr/mL (which cannot be attributed to improper dosing, sample handling or antibody development) then all patients receiving this lot of **ADAGEN®** (pegademase bovine) Injection will be required to have a blood sample for plasma ADA determination taken prior to their next injection of **ADAGEN®** (pegademase bovine) Injection. The index patient will require re-testing for determination of plasma ADA activity prior to his/her next injection of **ADAGEN®** (pegademase bovine) Injection. If this value, as well as the value from one of the other patients from a different site, is less than 10 µmol/hr/mL then the lot in use will be recalled and replaced with a new clinical lot by ENZON, Inc.

Immune function, including the ability to produce antibodies, generally improves after 2–6 months of therapy, and matures over a longer period. Compared with the natural history of combined immunodeficiency disease due to ADA deficiency, a trend toward diminished frequency of opportunistic infections and fewer complications of infections has occurred in patients receiving **ADAGEN®** (pegademase bovine) Injection. However, the lag between the correction of the metabolic abnormalities and improved immune function with a trend toward diminished frequency of infections and complications of infection is variable, and has ranged from a few weeks to approximately 6 months. Improvement in the general clinical status of the patient may be gradual (as evidenced by improvement in various clinical parameters) but should be apparent by the end of the first year of therapy.

Antibody to **ADAGEN®** (pegademase bovine) Injection may develop in patients and may result in more rapid clearance of **ADAGEN®** (pegademase bovine) Injection. Antibody to **ADAGEN®** (pegademase bovine) Injection should be suspected if a persistent fall in pre-injection levels of plasma ADA to ≤10 µmol/hr/mL occurs. If other causes for a decline in plasma ADA levels can be ruled out [such as improper storage of **ADAGEN®** (pegademase bovine) Injection vials (freezing or prolonged storage at temperatures above 8°C), or improper handling of plasma samples (e.g., repeated freezing and thawing during transport to laboratory)], then a specific assay for antibody to ADA and **ADAGEN®** (pegademase bovine) Injection (ELISA, enzyme inhibition) should be performed.

In patients undergoing treatment with **ADAGEN®** (pegademase bovine) Injection, a decline in immune function, with increased risk of opportunistic infections and complications of infection, will result from failure to maintain adequate levels of plasma ADA activity [whether due to the development of antibody to **ADAGEN®** (pegademase bovine) Injection, to improper calculation of **ADAGEN®** (pegademase bovine) Injection dosage, to interruption of treatment or to improper storage of **ADAGEN®** (pegademase bovine) Injection with subsequent loss of activity]. If a persistent decline in plasma ADA activity occurs, immune function and clinical status should be monitored closely and precautions should be taken to minimize the risk of infection. If antibody to ADA or **ADAGEN®** (pegademase bovine) Injection is found to be the cause of a persistent fall in plasma ADA activity, then adjustment in the dosage of **ADAGEN®** (pegademase bovine) Injection and other measures may be taken to induce tolerance and restore adequate ADA activity.

Drug Interactions

There are no known drug interactions with **ADAGEN®** (pegademase bovine) Injection. However, Vidarabine is a substrate for ADA and 2′-deoxycoformycin is a potent inhibitor of ADA. Thus, the activities of these drugs and **ADAGEN®** (pegademase bovine) Injection could be substantially altered if they are used in combination with one another.

Carcinogenesis, Mutagenesis, Impairment of Fertility

Long-term carcinogenic studies in animals have not been performed with **ADAGEN®** (pegademase bovine) Injection nor have studies been performed on impairment of fertility. **ADAGEN®** (pegademase bovine) Injection did not exhibit a mutagenic effect when tested against Salmonella typhimurium strains in the Ames assay.

Pregnancy

Pregnancy Category C. Animal reproduction studies have not been conducted with **ADAGEN®** (pegademase bovine) Injection. It is also not known whether **ADAGEN®** (pegademase bovine) Injection can cause fetal harm when administered to a pregnant woman or can affect reproduction capacity. **ADAGEN®** (pegademase bovine) Injection should be given to a pregnant woman only if clearly needed.

Nursing Mothers

It is not known whether **ADAGEN®** (pegademase bovine) Injection is excreted in human milk. Because many drugs are excreted in human milk, caution should be exercised when **ADAGEN®** (pegademase bovine) Injection is administered to a nursing woman.

ADVERSE REACTIONS

Clinical experience with **ADAGEN®** (pegademase bovine) Injection has been limited. The following adverse reactions have been reported: headache in one patient and pain at the injection site in two patients.

OVERDOSAGE

There is no documented experience with **ADAGEN®** (pegademase bovine) Injection overdosage. An intraperitoneal dose of 50,000 U/kg of **ADAGEN®** (pegademase bovine) Injection in mice resulted in weight loss up to 9%.

DOSAGE AND ADMINISTRATION

Before prescribing **ADAGEN®** (pegademase bovine) Injection the physician should be thoroughly familiar with the details of this prescribing information. For further information concerning the essential monitoring of **ADAGEN®** (pegademase bovine) Injection therapy, the prescribing physician should contact ENZON, Inc., 20 Kingsbridge Road, Piscataway, NJ 08854. Telephone 732-980-4500. Fax 732-980-5911.

ADAGEN® (pegademase bovine) Injection is recommended for use in infants from birth or in children of any age at the time of diagnosis.

Parenteral drug products should be inspected visually for particulate matter and discoloration prior to administration, whenever solution and container permits.

ADAGEN® (pegademase bovine) Injection should not be diluted nor mixed with any other drug prior to administration.

ADAGEN® (pegademase bovine) Injection should be administered every 7 days as an intramuscular injection. The dosage of **ADAGEN®** (pegademase bovine) Injection should be individualized. The recommended dosing schedule is 10 U/kg for the first dose, 15 U/kg for the second dose, and 20 U/kg for the third dose. The usual maintenance dose is 20 U/kg per week. Further increases of 5 U/kg/week may be necessary, but a maximum single dose of 30 U/kg should not be exceeded. Plasma levels of ADA more than twice the up-

Continued on next page

Adagen—Cont.

per limit of 35 μmol/hr/mL have occurred on occasion in several patients, and have been maintained for several weeks in one patient who received twice weekly injections (20 U/kg per dose) of **ADAGEN®** (pegademase bovine) Injection. No adverse effects have been observed at these higher levels; there is no evidence that maintaining pre-injection plasma ADA above 35 μmol/hr/mL produces any additional clinical benefits.

Dose proportionality has not been established and patients should be closely monitored when the dosage is increased. **ADAGEN®** (pegademase bovine) Injection is not recommended for intravenous administration. The optimal dosage and schedule of administration should be established for each patient based on monitoring of plasma ADA activity levels (trough levels before maintenance injection) and biochemical markers of ADA deficiency (primarily red cell dATP content). Since improvement in immune function follows correction of metabolic abnormalities, maintenance dosage in individual patients should be aimed at achieving the following biochemical goals: 1) maintain plasma ADA activity (trough levels before maintenance injection) in the range of 15–35 μmol/hr/mL (assayed at 37°C); and 2) decline in erythrocyte dATP to ≤0.005–0.015 μmol/mL packed erythrocytes, or ≤1% of the total erythrocyte adenine nucleotide (ATP + dATP) content, with a normal ATP level, as measured in a pre-injection sample. In addition, continued monitoring of immune function and clinical status is essential in any patient with a primary immunodeficiency disease and should be continued in patients undergoing treatment with **ADAGEN®** (pegademase bovine) Injection.

HOW SUPPLIED

ADAGEN® (pegademase bovine) Injection is a clear, colorless solution for intramuscular injection. Each vial contains 250 units/mL and is supplied as a 1.5 mL single-use vial, in boxes of 4 vials (NDC-57665-001-01).

Refrigerate. Store between +2°C and +8°C (36°F and 46°F). DO NOT FREEZE. **ADAGEN®** (pegademase bovine) Injection should not be stored at room temperature. This product should not be used if there are any indications that it may have been frozen.

REFERENCES

1. Hershfield MS, Buckley RH, Greenberg ML, et al. Treatment of adenosine deaminase deficiency with polyethylene glycol-modified adenosine deaminase. N Engl J Med 1987; 316:589–96.
2. Levy Y, Hershfield MS, Fernandez-Mejia C, Polmar ST, Scudiery D, Berger M, Sorensen RU. Adenosine deaminase deficiency with late onset of recurrent infections: response to treatment with polyethylene glycol-modified adenosine deaminase. J. Pediatr 1988; 113:312–17.
3. Kredich NM, Hershfield MS. Immunodeficiency diseases caused by adenosine deaminase deficiency and purine nucleoside phosphorylase deficiency. 6th ed. In: Scriver CR, Beaudet AL, Sly WS, Valle D, eds. The metabolic basis of inherited disease. New York: McGraw Hill, 1989; 1045–75.
4. Hirschhorn R. Inherited enzyme deficiencies and immunodeficiency: adenosine deaminase (ADA) and purine nucleoside phosphorylase (PNP) deficiencies. Clin Immunol Immunopathol 1986; 40:157–65.
5. Hirschhorn R, Roegner-Maniscalco V, Kuritsky L, Rosen FS. Bone marrow transplantation only partially restores purine metabolites to normal adenosine deaminase-deficient patients. J Clin Invest 1981; 68:1387–93.
6. Polmar AH, Stern RC, Schwartz AL, Wetzler EM, Chase PA, Hirschhorn R. Enzyme replacement therapy for adenosine deaminase deficiency and severe combined immunodeficiency. N Engl J Med 1976; 295:1337–43.
7. Rubinstein A, Hirschhorn R, Sicklick M, Murphy RA. In vivo and in vitro effects of thymosin and adenosine deaminase on adenosine-deaminase-deficient lymphocytes. N Engl J Med 1979; 300:387–92.
8. Hirschhorn R, Papageorgiou PS, Kesarwala HH, Taft LT. Amelioration of neurologic abnormalities after "enzyme replacement" in adenosine deaminase deficiency. N Engl J Med 1980; 303:377–80.
9. Hirshhorn R, Ratech H, Rubinstein A, et al. Increased excretion of modified adenine nucleosides by children with adenosine deaminase deficiency. Pediatr Res 1982; 16:362–9.
10. Polmar SH. Enzyme replacement and other biochemical approaches to the therapy of adenosine deaminase deficiency. In: Elliott K, Whelan J, eds. Enzyme defects and immune dysfunction. Amsterdam: Excerpta Medica, 1979; 213–30.

ESI Lederle Inc.
P.O. BOX 41502
PHILADELPHIA, PA 19101

Direct Inquiries to:
Professional Service
(610) 688-4400

For Emergency Medical Information Contact:
Day: (800) 934–5556 8:30 AM to 4:30 PM
(Eastern Standard Time), Weekdays only
Night: (610) 688-4400 (Emergencies only; non-emergencies should wait until the next day)
For Medical/Pharmacy Inquiries on Marketed Products Call:
(800) 934–5556 8:30 AM to 4:30 PM
(Eastern Standard Time), Weekdays only

ESI Lederle Inc. was formerly known as ESI Pharma, Inc. Products previously listed under the ESI Pharma, Inc. heading are now products of ESI Lederle Inc. and are described below.

AYGESTIN®　　　　　　　　　　　　　　℞
[ā-jĕs 'tĭn]
(norethindrone acetate tablets, USP)

Caution: Federal law prohibits dispensing without prescription.

> **WARNING:**
> THE USE OF Aygestin DURING THE FIRST FOUR MONTHS OF PREGNANCY IS NOT RECOMMENDED.
> Progestational agents have been used beginning with the first trimester of pregnancy in an attempt to prevent habitual abortion. There is no adequate evidence that such use is effective when such drugs are given during the first four months of pregnancy. Furthermore, in the vast majority of women, the cause of abortion is a defective ovum which progestational agents could not be expected to influence. In addition, the use of progestational agents, with their uterine-relaxant properties, in patients with fertilized defective ova may cause a delay in spontaneous abortion. Therefore, the use of such drugs during the first four months of pregnancy is not recommended.
> Several reports suggest an association between intrauterine exposure to progestational drugs in the first trimester of pregnancy and genital abnormalities in male and female fetuses. The risk of hypospadias, 5 to 8 per 1,000 male births in the general population, may be approximately doubled with exposure to these drugs. There are insufficient data to quantify the risk to exposed female fetuses, but insofar as some of these drugs induce mild virilization of the external genitalia of the female fetus, and because of the increased association of hypospadias in the male fetus, it is prudent to avoid the use of these drugs during the first trimester of pregnancy.
> If the patient is exposed to Aygestin (norethindrone acetate tablets, USP) during the first four months of pregnancy or if she becomes pregnant while taking this drug, she should be apprised of the potential risks to the fetus.

DESCRIPTION
Aygestin (norethindrone acetate tablets, USP)—5 mg oral tablets.
Aygestin, (17-hydroxy-19-nor-17α-pregn-4-en-20-yn-3-one acetate), a synthetic, orally active progestin, is the acetic acid ester of norethindrone. It is a white, or creamy white, crystalline powder.

Aygestin Tablets contain the following inactive ingredients: lactose, magnesium stearate, and microcrystalline cellulose.

CLINICAL PHARMACOLOGY
Norethindrone acetate induces secretory changes in an estrogen-primed endometrium. It acts to inhibit the secretion of pituitary gonadotropins which, in turn, prevent follicular maturation and ovulation. On a weight basis, it is twice as potent as norethindrone.

INDICATIONS AND USAGE
Aygestin is indicated for the treatment of secondary amenorrhea, endometriosis, and abnormal uterine bleeding due to hormonal imbalance in the absence of organic pathology, such as submucous fibroids or uterine cancer.

CONTRAINDICATIONS
Thrombophlebitis, thromboembolic disorders, cerebral apoplexy, or a past history of these conditions.
Markedly impaired liver function or liver disease.
Known or suspected carcinoma of the breast.
Undiagnosed vaginal bleeding.
Missed abortion.
As a diagnostic test for pregnancy.

WARNINGS
1. Discontinue medication pending examination if there is a sudden partial or complete loss of vision or if there is sudden onset of proptosis, diplopia, or migraine. If examination reveals papilledema or retinal vascular lesions, medication should be withdrawn.
2. Because of the occasional occurrence of thrombophlebitis and pulmonary embolism in patients taking progestogens, the physician should be alert to the earliest manifestations of the disease.
3. Masculinization of the female fetus has occurred when progestogens have been used in pregnant women.

PRECAUTIONS
GENERAL PRECAUTIONS.
1. The pretreatment physical examination should include special reference to breasts and pelvic organs, as well as a Papanicolaou smear.
2. Because this drug may cause some degree of fluid retention, conditions which might be influenced by this factor, such as epilepsy, migraine, asthma, cardiac or renal dysfunctions, require careful observation.
3. In cases of breakthrough bleeding, as in all cases of irregular bleeding per vaginam, nonfunctional causes should be borne in mind. In cases of undiagnosed vaginal bleeding, adequate diagnostic measures are indicated.
4. Patients who have a history of psychic depression should be carefully observed and the drug discontinued if the depression recurs to a serious degree.
5. Any possible influence of prolonged progestogen therapy on pituitary, ovarian, adrenal, hepatic, or uterine functions awaits further study.
6. Concomitant Use in Estrogen Replacement Therapy: In postmenopausal estrogen replacement therapy, studies of the addition of a progestin for 7 or more days of a cycle of estrogen administration have reported a lowered incidence of endometrial hyperplasia. Morphological and biochemical studies of the endometrium suggest that 10 to 13 days of progestin are needed to provide maximal maturation of the endometrium and to eliminate any hyperplastic changes. Whether this will provide protection from endometrial carcinoma has not been clearly established. There are possible additional risks which may be associated with the inclusion of progestin in estrogen replacement regimens. Progestin therapy may have an adverse effect on lipid metabolism.
7. A decrease in glucose tolerance has been observed in a small percentage of patients on estrogen-progestogen combination drugs. The mechanism of this decrease is obscure. For this reason, diabetic patients should be carefully observed while receiving progestogen therapy.
8. The age of the patient constitutes no absolute limiting factor, although treatment with progestogens may mask the onset of the climacteric.
9. The pathologist should be advised of progestogen therapy when relevant specimens are submitted.
INFORMATION FOR THE PATIENT.
See text which appears at the end of this insert.
CARCINOGENESIS, MUTAGENESIS, AND IMPAIRMENT OF FERTILITY.
Some beagle dogs treated with medroxyprogesterone acetate developed mammary nodules. Although nodules occasionally appeared in control animals, they were intermittent in nature, whereas nodules in treated animals were larger and more numerous, and persisted. There is no general agreement as to whether the nodules are benign or malignant. Their significance with respect to humans has not been established.
PREGNANCY CATEGORY X.
See Boxed Warning.
NURSING MOTHERS.
Detectable amounts of progestogens have been identified in the milk of mothers receiving them. The effect of this on the nursing infant has not been determined.
PEDIATRIC USE.
Safety and effectiveness in pediatric patients have not been established.

ADVERSE REACTIONS
The following adverse reactions have been observed in women taking progestins:
Breakthrough bleeding.
Spotting.

Change in menstrual flow.
Amenorrhea.
Edema.
Changes in weight (decreases, increases).
Changes in cervical erosion and cervical secretions.
Cholestatic jaundice.
Rash (allergic) with and without pruritus.
Melasma or chloasma.
Mental depression.
Progestins may alter the result of pregnanediol determinations. The following laboratory results may be altered by the concomitant use of estrogens with progestins:
Hepatic function.
Coagulation tests—increase in prothrombin, factors VII, VIII, IX, and X.
Increase in PBI, BEI, and a decrease in T^3 uptake.
Reduced response to metyrapone test.
A statistically significant association has been demonstrated between use of estrogen-progestogen combination drugs and the following serious adverse reactions: thrombophlebitis, pulmonary embolism, and cerebral thrombosis and embolism. For this reason, patients on progestogen therapy should be carefully observed. Although available evidence is suggestive of an association, such a relationship has been neither confirmed nor refuted for the following serious adverse reactions:
Neuro-ocular lesions, *e.g.*, retinal thrombosis and optic neuritis.
The following adverse reactions have been observed in patients receiving estrogen-progestogen combination drugs:
1. Rise in blood pressure in susceptible individuals.
2. Premenstrual-like syndrome.
3. Changes in libido.
4. Changes in appetite.
5. Cystitis-like syndrome.
6. Headache.
7. Nervousness.
8. Dizziness.
9. Fatigue.
10. Backache.
11. Hirsutism.
12. Loss of scalp hair.
13. Erythema multiforme.
14. Erythema nodosum.
15. Hemorrhagic eruption.
16. Itching.

In view of these observations, patients on progestogen therapy should be carefully observed.

DOSAGE AND ADMINISTRATION

Therapy with Aygestin must be adapted to the specific indications and therapeutic response of the individual patient. This dosage schedule assumes the interval between menses to be 28 days.
Secondary amenorrhea, abnormal uterine bleeding due to hormonal imbalance in the absence of organic pathology: 2.5 to 10 mg Aygestin may be given daily for 5 to 10 days during the second half of the theoretical menstrual cycle to produce an optimum secretory transformation of an endometrium that has been adequately primed with either endogenous or exogenous estrogen.
Progestin withdrawal bleeding usually occurs within three to seven days after discontinuing Aygestin therapy. Patients with a past history of recurrent episodes of abnormal uterine bleeding may benefit from planned menstrual cycling with Aygestin.
Endometriosis: Initial daily dosage of 5 mg Aygestin for two weeks. Dosage should be increased by 2.5 mg per day every two weeks until 15 mg per day of Aygestin is reached. Therapy may be held at this level for six to nine months or until annoying breakthrough bleeding demands temporary termination.

HOW SUPPLIED

Each white, scored Aygestin® Tablet contains 5 mg norethindrone acetate, USP, in bottles of 50 (NDC 59911-5894-1).
Store at room temperature (approximately 25° C)
Dispense in a well-closed container as defined in the USP

INFORMATION FOR THE PATIENT

Your doctor has prescribed Aygestin (norethindrone acetate tablets, USP), a progestin, for you. Aygestin is similar to the progesterone hormones naturally produced by the body. Progestins are used to treat menstrual disorders and to test if the body is producing certain hormones.
Warning
Progesterone or progesterone-like drugs have been used to prevent miscarriage in the first few months of pregnancy. No adequate evidence is available to show that they are effective for this purpose. Furthermore, most cases of early miscarriage are due to causes which could not be helped by these drugs.
There is an increased risk of minor birth defects in children whose mothers take this drug during the first four months of pregnancy. Several reports suggest an association between mothers who take these drugs in the first trimester of pregnancy and genital abnormalities in male and female babies. The risk to the male baby is the possibility of being born with a condition in which the opening of the penis is on the underside rather than the tip of the penis (hypospadias). Hypospadias occurs in about 5 to 8 per 1,000 male births and is about doubled with exposure to these drugs. There is not enough information to quantify the risk to exposed female fetuses, but enlargement of the clitoris and fusion of the labia may occur, although rarely.
Therefore, since drugs of this type may induce mild masculinization of the external genitalia of the female fetus, as well as hypospadias in the male fetus, it is wise to avoid using the drug during the first trimester of pregnancy.
These drugs have been used as a test for pregnancy but such use is no longer considered safe because of possible damage to a developing baby. Also, more rapid methods for testing for pregnancy are now available.
If you take Aygestin (norethindrone acetate tablets, USP) and later find you were pregnant when you took it, be sure to discuss this with your doctor as soon as possible.

HOW SUPPLIED

Aygestin® (norethindrone acetate tablets, USP)—white, scored 5 mg tablets, in bottles of 50, for oral administration.
ESI Lederle Inc.
Philadelphia, PA 19101
Shown in Product Identification Guide, page 310

CYCRIN® ℞
[*sic 'crĭn*]
(medroxyprogesterone acetate tablets, USP)

WARNING
THE USE OF CYCRIN DURING THE FIRST FOUR MONTHS OF PREGNANCY IS NOT RECOMMENDED.
Progestational agents have been used, beginning with the first trimester of pregnancy, in an attempt to prevent habitual abortion. There is no adequate evidence that such use is effective when such drugs are given during the first 4 months of pregnancy. Furthermore, in the vast majority of women, the cause of abortion is a defective ovum, which progestational agents could not be expected to influence. In addition, the use of progestational agents with their uterine-relaxant properties, in patients with fertilized defective ova, may cause a delay in spontaneous abortion. Therefore, the use of such drugs during the first 4 months of pregnancy is not recommended.
Several reports suggest an association between intrauterine exposure to progestational drugs in the first trimester of pregnancy and genital abnormalities in male and female fetuses. The risk of hypospadias, 5 to 8 per 1,000 male births in the general population, may be approximately doubled with exposure to these drugs. There are insufficient data to quantify the risk to exposed female fetuses, but insofar as some of these drugs induce mild virilization of the external genitalia of the female fetus, and because of the increased association of hypospadias in the male fetus, it is prudent to avoid the use of these drugs during the first trimester of pregnancy.
If the patient is exposed to Cycrin (medroxyprogesterone acetate) during the first 4 months of pregnancy, or if she becomes pregnant while taking this drug, she should be apprised of the potential risks to the fetus.

DESCRIPTION

Cycrin tablets contain medroxyprogesterone acetate, which is a derivative of progesterone. It is a white to off-white, odorless, crystalline powder, stable in air, melting between 200°C and 210°C. It is freely soluble in chloroform, soluble in acetone and in dioxane, sparingly soluble in alcohol and in methanol, slightly soluble in ether, and insoluble in water.
The chemical name for medroxyprogesterone acetate is pregn-4-ene-3,20-dione, 17-(acetyloxy)-6-methyl-, (6α)-.
Its structural formula is:

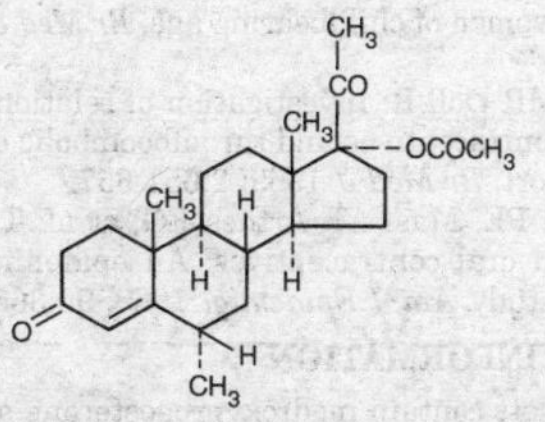

Cycrin is available in tablet form for oral administration. Each tablet contains 2.5 mg, 5 mg, or 10 mg of medroxyprogesterone acetate and the following inactive ingredients: lactose, magnesium stearate, methylcellulose, and microcrystalline cellulose. Each dosage strength also contains the following:
5 mg—D&C Red #30 and FD&C Blue #1;
10 mg—D&C Red #30 and D&C Yellow #10.

CLINICAL PHARMACOLOGY

Medroxyprogesterone acetate, administered orally or parenterally in the recommended doses to women with adequate endogenous estrogen, transforms proliferative into secretory endometrium. Androgenic and anabolic effects have been noted, but the drug is apparently devoid of significant estrogenic activity. While parenterally administered medroxyprogesterone acetate inhibits gonadotropin production, which in turn prevents follicular maturation and ovulation, available data indicate that this does not occur when the usually recommended oral dosage is given as single daily doses.

INDICATIONS AND USAGE

Secondary amenorrhea; abnormal uterine bleeding due to hormonal imbalance in the absence of organic pathology, such as fibroids or uterine cancer.

CONTRAINDICATIONS

1. Thrombophlebitis, thromboembolic disorders, cerebral apoplexy, or patients with a past history of these conditions.
2. Liver dysfunction or disease.
3. Known or suspected malignancy of breast or genital organs.
4. Undiagnosed vaginal bleeding.
5. Missed abortion.
6. As a diagnostic test for pregnancy.
7. Known sensitivity to medroxyprogesterone acetate.

WARNINGS

1. The physician should be alert to the earliest manifestations of thrombotic disorders (thrombophlebitis, cerebrovascular disorders, pulmonary embolism, and retinal thrombosis). Should any of these occur or be suspected, the drug should be discontinued immediately.
2. Beagle dogs treated with medroxyprogesterone acetate developed mammary nodules, some of which were malignant. Although nodules occasionally appeared in control animals, they were intermittent in nature, whereas the nodules in the drug-treated animals were larger, more numerous, persistent, and there were some breast malignancies with metastases. Their significance with respect to humans has not been established.
3. Discontinue medication pending examination if there is sudden partial or complete loss of vision, or if there is a sudden onset of proptosis, diplopia, or migraine. If examination reveals papilledema or retinal vascular lesions, medication should be withdrawn.
4. Detectable amounts of progestin have been identified in the milk of mothers receiving the drug. The effect of this on the nursing infant has not been determined.
5. Usage in pregnancy is not recommended (see Boxed Warning).
6. Retrospective studies of morbidity and mortality in Great Britain and studies of morbidity in the United States have shown a statistically significant association between thrombophlebitis, pulmonary embolism, and cerebral thrombosis and embolism and the use of oral contraceptives.[1-4] The estimate of the relative risk of thromboembolism in the study by Vessey and Doll[3] was about sevenfold, while Sartwell and associates[4] in the United States found a relative risk of 4.4, meaning that the users are several times as likely to undergo thromboembolic disease without evident cause as nonusers. The American study also indicated that the risk did not persist after discontinuation of administration, and that it was not enhanced by long, continued administration. The American study was not designed to evaluate a difference between products.

PRECAUTIONS

1. The pretreatment physical examination should include special reference to breasts and pelvic organs, as well as Papanicolaou smear.
2. Because progestogens may cause some degree of fluid retention, conditions which might be influenced by this factor, such as epilepsy, migraine, asthma, cardiac or renal dysfunction, require careful observation.
3. In cases of breakthrough bleeding, as in all cases of irregular bleeding per vaginum, nonfunctional causes should be borne in mind. In cases of undiagnosed vaginal bleeding, adequate diagnostic measures are indicated.
4. Patients who have a history of psychic depression should be carefully observed and the drug discontinued if the depression recurs to a serious degree.
5. Any possible influence of prolonged progestin therapy on pituitary, ovarian, adrenal, hepatic, or uterine functions awaits further study.

Continued on next page

Cycrin—Cont.

6. A decrease in glucose tolerance has been observed in a small percentage of patients on estrogen-progestin combination drugs. The mechanism of this decrease is obscure. For this reason, diabetic patients should be carefully observed while receiving progestin therapy.

7. The age of the patient constitutes no absolute limiting factor, although treatment with progestins may mask the onset of the climacteric.

8. The pathologist should be advised of progestin therapy when relevant specimens are submitted.

9. Because of the occasional occurrence of thrombotic disorders (thrombophlebitis, pulmonary embolism, retinal thrombosis, and cerebrovascular disorders) in patients taking estrogen-progestin combinations, and since the mechanism is obscure, the physician should be alert to the earliest manifestation of these disorders.

10. CONCOMITANT USE IN ESTROGEN REPLACEMENT THERAPY: Studies of the addition of a progestin product to an estrogen replacement regimen for 7 or more days of a cycle of estrogen administration have reported a lowered incidence of endometrial hyperplasia. Morphological and biochemical studies of the endometrium suggest that 10 to 13 days of a progestin are needed to provide maximal maturation of the endometrium and to eliminate any hyperplastic changes. Whether this will provide protection from endometrial carcinoma has not been clearly established. There are possible additional risks which may be associated with the inclusion of progestin in estrogen replacement regimens. The potential risks include adverse effects on carbohydrate and lipid metabolism. The dosage used may be important in minimizing these adverse effects.

11. Aminoglutethimide administered concomitantly with Cycrin may significantly depress the bioavailability of Cycrin.

CARCINOGENESIS, MUTAGENESIS, IMPAIRMENT OF FERTILITY

Long-term intramuscular administration of medroxyprogesterone acetate has been shown to produce mammary tumors in beagle dogs (see "Warnings" above). There was no evidence of a carcinogenic effect associated with the oral administration of medroxyprogesterone acetate to rats and mice. Medroxyprogesterone acetate was not mutagenic in a battery of *in vitro* or *in vivo* genetic toxicity assays.

Medroxyprogesterone acetate at high doses is an antifertility drug and high doses would be expected to impair fertility until the cessation of treatment.

INFORMATION FOR THE PATIENT
See Patient Information at the end of insert.

ADVERSE REACTIONS
PREGNANCY: (See Boxed Warning for possible adverse effects on the fetus.)
BREAST: Breast tenderness or galactorrhea has been reported rarely.
SKIN: Sensitivity reactions consisting of urticaria, pruritus, edema, and generalized rash have occurred in an occasional patient. Acne, alopecia, and hirsutism have been reported in a few cases.
THROMBOEMBOLIC PHENOMENA: Thromboembolic phenomena, including thrombophlebitis and pulmonary embolism, have been reported.
The following adverse reactions have been observed in women taking progestins, including Cycrin (medroxyprogesterone acetate tablets):
  breakthrough bleeding
  spotting
  change in menstrual flow
  amenorrhea
  edema
  change in weight (increase or decrease)
  change in cervical erosion and cervical
    secretions
  cholestatic jaundice
  anaphylactoid reactions and anaphylaxis
  rash (allergic) with and without pruritus
  mental depression
  pyrexia
  insomnia
  nausea
  somnolence
A statistically significant association has been demonstrated between use of estrogen-progestin combination drugs and the following serious adverse reactions: thrombophlebitis; pulmonary embolism; and cerebral thrombosis and embolism. For this reason patients on progestin therapy should be carefully observed.
Although available evidence is suggestive of an association, such a relationship has been neither confirmed nor refuted for the following serious adverse reactions: neuro-ocular lesions, e.g., retinal thrombosis and optic neuritis.
The following adverse reactions have been observed in patients receiving estrogen-progestin combination drugs:

  rise in blood pressure in susceptible individuals
  premenstrual-like syndrome
  changes in libido
  changes in appetite
  cystitis-like syndrome
  headache
  nervousness
  dizziness
  fatigue
  backache
  hirsutism
  loss of scalp hair
  erythema multiforme
  erythema nodosum
  hemorrhagic eruption
  itching
In view of these observations, patients on progestin therapy should be carefully observed.
The following laboratory results may be altered by the use of estrogen-progestin combination drugs:
Increased sulfobromophthalein retention and other hepatic-function tests.
Coagulation tests: increase in prothrombin factors VII, VIII, IX, and X.
Metyrapone test.
Pregnanediol determination
Thyroid function: increase in PBI, and butanol extractable protein bound iodine and decrease in T_3 uptake values.

DOSAGE AND ADMINISTRATION

SECONDARY AMENORRHEA: Cycrin (medroxyprogesterone acetate tablets) may be given in dosages of 5 mg to 10 mg daily for from 5 to 10 days. A dose for inducing an optimum secretory transformation of an endometrium that has been adequately primed with either endogenous or exogenous estrogen is 10 mg of Cycrin daily for 10 days. In cases of secondary amenorrhea, therapy may be started at any time. Progestin withdrawal bleeding usually occurs within 3 to 7 days after discontinuing Cycrin therapy.
ABNORMAL UTERINE BLEEDING DUE TO HORMONAL IMBALANCE IN THE ABSENCE OF ORGANIC PATHOLOGY: Beginning on the calculated 16th or 21st day of the menstrual cycle, 5 to 10 mg of medroxyprogesterone acetate may be given daily for from 5 to 10 days. To produce an optimum secretory transformation of an endometrium that has been adequately primed with either endogenous or exogenous estrogen, 10 mg of medroxyprogesterone acetate daily for 10 days beginning on the 16th day of the cycle is suggested. Progestin withdrawal bleeding usually occurs within three to seven days after discontinuing therapy with Cycrin. Patients with a past history of recurrent episodes of abnormal uterine bleeding may benefit from planned menstrual cycling with Cycrin.

HOW SUPPLIED

Cycrin® (medroxyprogesterone acetate tablets, USP) is available for oral administration in the following dosage strengths:
2.5 mg, white, oval tablet with a score debossed on one side and opposing "C"s debossed on the reverse, in bottles of 100 (NDC 59911-5898-1) and bottles of 1,000 (NDC 59911-5898-3).
5 mg, light-purple, oval tablet with "CYCRIN" and a score debossed on one side and opposing "C"s debossed on the reverse, in bottles of 100 (NDC 59911-5897-1) and bottles of 1,000 (NDC 59911-5897-3).
10 mg, peach, oval tablet with "CYCRIN" and a score debossed on one side and opposing "C"s debossed on the reverse, in bottles of 100 (NDC 59911-5896-1) and bottles of 1,000 (NDC 59911-5896-3).
The appearance of these tablets is a registered trademark.
Store at controlled room temperature, 20°–25° C (68°–77° F).
Dispense in a well-closed container as defined in the USP.
Caution: Federal law prohibits dispensing without prescription.

REFERENCES

1. Royal College of General Practitioners: Oral contraception and thromboembolic disease. *J Coll Gen Pract* 1967; 13:267-279.
2. Inman WHW, Vessey MP: Investigation of deaths from pulmonary, coronary, and cerebral thrombosis and embolism in women of childbearing age. *Br Med J* 1968; 2:193-199.
3. Vessey MP, Doll R: Investigation of relation between use of oral contraceptives and thromboembolic disease. A further report. *Br Med J* 1969; 2:651-657.
4. Sartwell PE, Masi AT, Arthes FG, et al: Thromboembolism and oral contraceptives: An epidemiological case-control study. *Am J Epidemiol* 1969; 90:365-380.

PATIENT INFORMATION

Cycrin tablets contain medroxyprogesterone acetate, a progesterone. The information below is that which the U.S. Food and Drug Administration requires be provided for all patients taking progesterones. The information below relates only to the risk to the unborn child associated with use of progesterone during pregnancy. For further information on the use, side effects, and other risks associated with this product, ask your doctor.

Warning For Women

Progesterone or progesterone-like drugs have been used to prevent miscarriage in the first few months of pregnancy. No adequate evidence is available to show that they are effective for this purpose. Furthermore, most cases of early miscarriage are due to causes which could not be helped by these drugs.

There is an increased risk of minor birth defects in children whose mothers take this drug during the first four months of pregnancy. Several reports suggest an association between mothers who take these drugs in the first trimester of pregnancy and genital abnormalities in male and female babies. The risk to the male baby is the possibility of being born with a condition in which the opening of the penis is on the underside rather than the tip of the penis (hypospadias). Hypospadias occurs in about 5 to 8 per 1,000 male births and is about doubled with exposure to these drugs. There is not enough information to quantify the risk to exposed female fetuses, but enlargement of the clitoris and fusion of the labia may occur, although rarely.

Therefore, since drugs of this type may induce mild masculinization of the external genitalia of the female fetus, as well as hypospadias in the male fetus, it is wise to avoid using the drug during the first trimester of pregnancy.

These drugs have been used as a test for pregnancy, but such use is no longer considered safe because of possible damage to a developing baby. Also, more rapid methods for testing for pregnancy are now available.

If you take Cycrin (medroxyprogesterone acetate tablets, USP) and later find you were pregnant when you took it, be sure to discuss this with your doctor as soon as possible.

ESI Lederle Inc.
Philadelphia, PA 19101
Shown in Product Identification Guide, page 310

ESI Pharma, Inc.

**P.O. BOX 41502
PHILADELPHIA, PA 19101**

The name ESI Pharma, Inc. has been changed to ESI Lederle Inc. All products listed under the ESI Pharma company heading can now be found under ESI Lederle Inc. Please turn to page 992 of this 1999 PDR.

Everett Laboratories, Inc.

**29 SPRING STREET
WEST ORANGE, NEW JERSEY 07052**

Direct Inquiries to:
Professional Service Department
Phone: (973) 324-0200
Fax: (973) 324-0795

CORTIC ear drops ℞

Each 1 ml contains:

Chloroxylenol	1 mg
Pramoxine HCl	10 mg
Hydrocortisone	10 mg

SUPPLIED
Plastic dropper vials of 10 ml.

STROVITE FORTE CAPLETS ℞
Sugar, Sodium and Yeast Free

Vitamin A (beta carotene & acetate)	4000 IU
Vitamin E (dl-alpha tocopheryl acetate)	60 IU
Vitamin D3	400 IU
Vitamin C (ascorbic acid)	500 MG
Vitamin B1 (thiamine mononitrate)	20 MG
Vitamin B2 (riboflavin)	20 MG
Vitamin B6 (pyridoxine HCL)	25 MG
Vitamin B12 (cyanocobalamin)	50 MCG
Niacin (as niacinamide)	100 MG
Biotin	0.15 MG
Pathothenic Acid (calcium pantothenate)	25 MG
Folic Acid	1 MG
Iron (ferrous fumarate)	10 MG

Chromium (chromium chloride)	0.1 MG
Magnesium (magnesium oxide)	50 MG
Molybdenum (sodium molybdate)	25 MCG
Copper (cupric oxide)	3 MG
Selenium (sodium selenate)	50 MCG
Zinc (zinc oxide)	15 MG

SUPPLIED

Bottle of 100—imprinted EV 0204

STROVITE FORTE SYRUP   ℞
Vitamin Mineral Supplement
Sugar, Sodium, and Yeast Free

SUPPLIED

Bottle 16 Oz.—Unit Dose 15 ml

TUSSAFED-HC   Ⓒ

Each 5 ml Contains:

Hydrocodone Bitarate	2.5 mg
Phenylephrine HCL	7.5 mg
Guaifenesin	50 mg

SUPPLIED

Bottle 16 Oz.

VITAFOL Caplets   ℞
Vitamins, Minerals, Iron, Folic Acid Supplement
Sugar Free

SUPPLIED

Boxes of 100 (10×10) Unit Dose Pack
Imprinted EV-0072

VITAFOL-PN (Prenatal) Caplets ℞
Sugar, Sodium and Yeast Free

Vitamin A (beta carotene & acetate)	1700 IU
Vitamin D3	400 IU
Vitamin E (dl-alpha-tocopheryl acetate)	30 IU
Vitamin C (ascorbic acid)	60 MG
Folic Acid	1 MG
Vitamin B1 (thiamine mononitrate)	1.6 MG
Vitamin B2 (riboflavin)	1.8 MG
Vitamin B6 (pyridoxine hydrochloride)	2.5 MG
Vitamin B12 (cyanocobalamin)	5 MCG
Niacin (as niacinamide)	15 MG
Calcium (calcium carbonate)	125 MG
Elemental Iron (ferrous fumarate)	65 MG
Magnesium (magnesium oxide)	25 MG
Zinc (zinc gluconate)	15 MG

Supplied: Boxes of 100 (10×10) Unit Dose Pack
   Imprinted EV0078

VITAFOL Syrup   ℞
Vitamins, Minerals, Iron, Folic Acid Supplement
Sodium, Alcohol, and Yeast Free

SUPPLIED

Bottles of 16 oz.

Faulding Laboratories
5511 CAPITAL CENTER DRIVE
SUITE P116
RALEIGH, NC 27606

(919) 233-5788
Direct Inquiries to:
Customer Service
(800) 432-8534

KADIAN®   Ⓒ ℞
Morphine Sulfate Sustained Release
KADIAN® 20 mg Capsules
KADIAN® 50 mg Capsules
KADIAN® 100 mg Capsules

WARNING: May be habit forming

DESCRIPTION
KADIAN® capsules 20, 50 and 100 mg contain identical polymer coated sustained release pellets of morphine sulfate for oral administration.

Chemically, morphine sulfate is 7,8-didehydro-4,5 α- epoxy-17-methyl-morphinan-3,6 α- diol sulfate (2:1) (salt) pentahydrate and has the following structural formula:

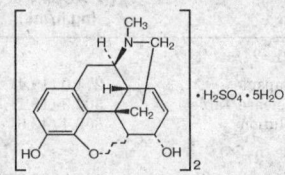

Morphine sulfate is an odorless, white, crystalline powder with a bitter taste and a molecular weight of 758 (as the sulfate). It has a solubility of 1 in 21 parts of water and 1 in 1000 parts of alcohol, but is practically insoluble in chloroform or ether. The octanol: water partition coefficient of morphine is 1.42 at physiologic pH and the pK_b is 7.9 for the tertiary nitrogen (mostly ionized at pH 7.4).

Each KADIAN® sustained release capsule contains either 20, 50 or 100 mg of Morphine Sulfate USP and the following inactive ingredients common to all strengths: Hydroxypropyl Methylcellulose, Ethylcellulose, Methacrylic Acid Copolymer, Polyethylene Glycol, Diethyl Phthalate, Talc, Black Ink SW-9009, Corn Starch and Sucrose.

CLINICAL PHARMACOLOGY
Morphine is a natural product that is the prototype for the class of natural and synthetic opioid analgesics. Opioids produce a wide spectrum of pharmacologic effects including analgesia, dysphoria, euphoria, somnolence, respiratory depression, diminished gastrointestinal motility, altered circulatory dynamics, histamine release and physical dependence.

Morphine produces both its therapeutic and its adverse effects by interaction with one or more classes of specific opioid receptors located throughout the body. Morphine acts as a pure agonist, binding with and activating opioid receptors at sites in the peri-aqueducal and peri-ventricular grey matter, the ventro-medial medulla and the spinal cord to produce analgesia.

Effects on the Central Nervous System
The principal therapeutic actions of morphine are analgesia, sedation and alterations of mood. Opioids of this class do not usually eliminate pain, but they do reduce the perception of pain by the central nervous system.

Morphine produces respiratory depression by reducing the responsiveness of the brain stem respiratory centers to increases in carbon dioxide tension (or to direct electrical stimulation).

Morphine depresses the cough reflex by direct effect on the cough center in the medulla. Antitussive effects may occur with doses lower than those usually required for analgesia. Morphine causes miosis, even in total darkness, and little tolerance develops to this effect. Pinpoint pupils are a sign of opioid overdose but are not pathognomonic (e.g. pontine lesions of hemorrhagic or ischemic origins may produce similar findings). Marked mydriasis rather than miosis may be seen due to severe hypoxia in overdose situations.

Effects on the Gastrointestinal Tract
Gastric, biliary and pancreatic secretions are decreased by morphine. Morphine causes a reduction in motility associated with an increase in tone in the antrum of the stomach and duodenum. Digestion of food in the small intestine is delayed and propulsive contractions are decreased. Propulsive peristaltic waves in the colon are decreased, while tone is increased to the point of spasm. The end result is constipation. Morphine can cause a marked increase in biliary tract pressure as a result of spasm of the sphincter of Oddi.

Effects on the Cardiovascular System
Morphine produces peripheral vasodilation which may result in orthostatic hypotension or syncope. Release of histamine may be induced by morphine and can contribute to opioid-induced hypotension. Manifestations of histamine release and/or peripheral vasodilation may include pruritus, flushing, red eyes and sweating.

Pharmacodynamics
The relationship between the blood level of morphine and the analgesic response will depend on the patient's age, state of health, medical condition, and the extent of previous opioid treatment.

A minimum effective concentration (MEC) of morphine for pain relief has been reported as 27.2 ± 14.5 ng/mL (mean ± SD) in cancer patients treated with morphine solution. These results compare with the MEC for plasma morphine reported as 14.7 ± 4.8 ng/mL (mean ± SD) in patients with postoperative pain. The high degree of variation is of clinical significance as it may result in either under-dosing or over-dosing if the dosage is not adjusted to the patient's clinical status and analgesic response (see **PRECAUTIONS** and **DOSAGE AND ADMINISTRATION**).

For opioid-tolerant patients the situation is much more complex. Some patients will become rapidly tolerant to the analgesic effects of morphine, and will require high daily oral morphine doses for adequate pain control. Since the de-

velopment of tolerance to both the therapeutic and adverse effects of opioids is highly individualized, the dose of morphine should be individualized to the patient's condition and should not be based on an arbitrary choice of a dose or blood level to be achieved.

Pharmacokinetics
KADIAN® capsules contain polymer coated sustained release pellets of morphine sulfate that release morphine significantly more slowly than from morphine sulfate tablets and shorter-acting controlled-release oral morphine sulfate preparations. KADIAN® activity is primarily due to morphine. One metabolite, morphine-6-glucuronide, has been shown to have analgesic activity, but poorly crosses the blood-brain barrier.

Following oral administration, the extent of absorption is essentially the same for immediate or sustained release formulations, although the time to peak blood level (T_{max}) will be longer and the C_{max} will be lower for formulations that delay the release of the morphine in the gastrointestinal tract. Elimination of morphine is primarily via hepatic metabolism to glucuronide metabolites (55 to 65%) which are then renally excreted. The terminal half-life of morphine is 2 to 4 hours, however, a longer term half-life of about 15 hours has been reported in studies where blood has been sampled up to 48 hours.

The single-dose pharmacokinetics of KADIAN® are linear over the dosage range of 30 to 100 mg. The single dose and multiple dose pharmacokinetic parameters of KADIAN® in normal volunteers are summarized in Table 1.
[See table at top of next page]

Absorption
Following the administration of oral morphine solution, approximately 50% of the morphine absorbed reaches the systemic circulation within 30 minutes. However, following the administration of an equal amount of KADIAN® to healthy volunteers, this occurs, on average, after 8 hours. As with most forms of oral morphine, because of pre-systemic elimination, only about 20 to 40% of the administered dose reaches the systemic circulation.

Food Effects: While concurrent administration of food slows the rate of absorption of KADIAN®, the extent of absorption is not affected and KADIAN® can be administered without regard to meals.

Steady State: When KADIAN® is given on a fixed dosing regimen to patients with chronic pain due to malignancy, steady state is achieved in about two days. At steady state, KADIAN® will have a significantly lower C_{max} and a higher C_{min} than equivalent doses of oral morphine solution and some other controlled-release preparations (see Graph 1).

Graph 1 (Study # MOR-1/90):
Mean steady state plasma morphine concentrations for KADIAN® (twice a day), controlled-release morphine tablet (twice a day) and oral morphine solution (every 4 hours); plasma concentrations are normalized to 100 mg every 24 hours. (n=24).

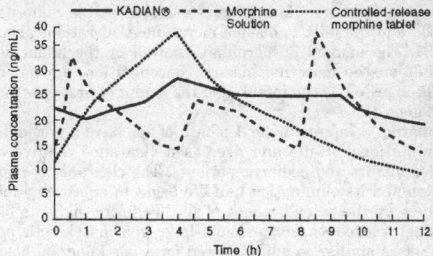

When given once-daily (every 24 hours) to 24 patients with malignancy, KADIAN® had a similar C_{max} and higher C_{min} at steady state in clinical use, when compared to twice-daily (every 12 hours) controlled-release morphine tablets (MS Contin®), given at an equivalent total daily dosage (see Graph 2 and Table 1). Drug-disease interactions are frequently seen in the older and more gravely ill patients, and may result in both altered absorption and reduced clearance as compared to normal volunteers (see **Geriatric, Hepatic Failure,** and **Renal Insufficiency** sections).

Graph 2 (Study # MOR-9/92):
Dose normalized mean steady state plasma morphine concentrations for KADIAN® (once a day), and an equivalent dose of a 12-hour, controlled-release morphine tablet given twice a day. Plasma concentrations are normalized to 100 mg every 24 hours. (n=24).

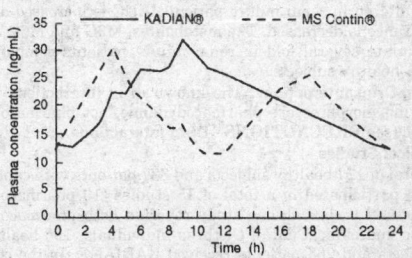

Continued on next page

Kadian—Cont.

Distribution
Once absorbed, morphine is distributed to skeletal muscle, kidneys, liver, intestinal tract, lungs, spleen and brain.
The volume of distribution of morphine is approximately 3 to 4 L/kg. Morphine is 30 to 35% reversibly bound to plasma proteins.
Although the primary site of action of morphine is in the CNS, only small quantities pass the blood-brain barrier. Morphine also crosses the placental membranes (see **PRECAUTIONS - Pregnancy**) and has been found in breast milk (see **PRECAUTIONS - Nursing Mothers**).

Metabolism
The major pathway of the detoxification of morphine is conjugation, either with D-glucuronic acid in the liver to produce glucuronides or with sulfuric acid to give morphine-3-ethereal sulfate. Although a small fraction (less than 5%) of morphine is demethylated, for all practical purposes, virtually all morphine is converted to glucuronide metabolites including morphine-3-glucuronide, M3G (about 50%) and morphine-6-glucuronide, M6G (about 5 to 15%). Studies in healthy subjects and cancer patients have shown that the glucuronide metabolite to morphine mean molar ratios (based on AUC) are similar after both single doses and at steady state for KADIAN®, 12-hour controlled-release morphine sulfate tablets and morphine sulfate solution.
M3G has no significant analgesic activity. M6G has been shown to have opioid agonist and analgesic activity in humans.

Excretion
Approximately 10% of morphine dose is excreted unchanged in the urine. Most of the dose is excreted in the urine as M3G and M6G. A small amount of the glucuronide metabolites is excreted in the bile and there is some minor enterohepatic cycling. Seven to 10% of administered morphine is excreted in the feces.
The mean adult plasma clearance is about 20-30 mL/minute/kg. The effective terminal half-life of morphine after IV administration is reported to be approximately 2.0 hours. Longer plasma sampling in some studies suggests a longer terminal half-life of morphine of about 15 hours.

Special Populations
Geriatric: The elderly may have increased sensitivity to morphine and may achieve higher and more variable serum levels than younger patients. In adults, the duration of analgesia increases progressively with age, though the degree of analgesia remains unchanged. KADIAN® pharmacokinetics have not been investigated in elderly patients (>65 years) although such patients were included in the clinical studies.
Nursing Mothers: Morphine is excreted in the maternal milk, and the milk to plasma morphine AUC ratio is about 2.5:1. The amount of morphine received by the infant depends on the maternal plasma concentration, amount of milk ingested by the infant, and the extent of first pass metabolism.
Pediatric: Infants under 1 month of age have a prolonged elimination half-life and decreased clearance relative to older infants and pediatric patients. The clearance of morphine and its elimination half-life begin to approach adult values by the second month of life. Pediatric patients old enough to take capsules should have pharmacokinetic parameters similar to adults, dosed on a per kilogram basis (see **PRECAUTIONS - Pediatric Use**).
Gender: No meaningful differences between male and female patients were demonstrated in the analysis of the pharmacokinetic data from clinical studies.
Race: Pharmacokinetic differences due to race may exist. Chinese subjects given intravenous morphine in one study had a higher clearance when compared to caucasian subjects (1852 ± 116 mL/min versus 1495 ± 80 mL/min).
Hepatic Failure: The pharmacokinetics of morphine were found to be significantly altered in individuals with alcoholic cirrhosis. The clearance was found to decrease with a corresponding increase in half-life. The M3G and M6G to morphine plasma AUC ratios also decreased in these patients indicating a decrease in metabolic activity.
Renal Insufficiency: The pharmacokinetics of morphine are altered in renal failure patients. AUC is increased and clearance is decreased. The metabolites, M3G and M6G accumulate several fold in renal failure patients compared with healthy subjects.
Drug-Drug Interactions: The known drug interactions involving morphine are pharmacodynamic, not pharmacokinetic (see **PRECAUTIONS - Drug Interactions**).

Clinical Studies
A total of 177 healthy subjects and 337 patients with cancer pain participated in a total of 15 studies (10 pharmacokinetic and 6 clinical; one study reported both pharmacokinetic and clinical data). Of these individuals, 158 healthy subjects and 268 patients received KADIAN®. In the controlled clinical studies patients were followed for a median duration of 7 days and in the open label studies patients were followed for up to 12-24 months. KADIAN® was compared to oral morphine solution and to either MS Contin® or to a 12-hour controlled-release morphine tablet bioequivalent to MS Contin® using trial designs that followed the clinical and pharmacokinetic performance of each treatment in cancer patients receiving chronic opioid therapy.
In two controlled studies, patients with moderate to severe cancer pain were titrated with immediate-release morphine (IRM) solution or tablets to a stable total daily dose of morphine for at least three consecutive days, then randomized to KADIAN® or 12-hour controlled-release morphine for seven days of observation. KADIAN® given once a day proved similar to the same total dose of morphine given in divided doses in a 12-hour dosage form, with respect to pain relief, use of rescue medication, patient and investigator global assessment, and quality of sleep. Individual patient differences in the pattern of pain control emphasize the need to individualize both dose and dosing interval (see **DOSAGE AND ADMINISTRATION**).

Table 1: Mean pharmacokinetic parameters (% coefficient variation) resulting from a fasting single dose study in normal volunteers and a multiple dose study in patients with cancer pain.

Regimen/ Dosage Form	AUC#,+ (ng.h/mL)	C_{max}+ (ng/mL)	T_{max} (h)	C_{min}+ (ng/mL)	Fluctuation*
Single Dose (n=24)					
KADIAN® Capsule	271.0 (19.4)	15.6 (24.4)	8.6 (41.1)	na^	na
Controlled-Release Tablet	304.3 (19.1)	30.5 (32.1)	2.5 (52.6)	na	na
Morphine Solution	362.4 (42.6)	64.4 (38.2)	0.9 (55.8)	na	na
Multiple Dose (n=24)					
KADIAN® Capsule q24h	500.9 (38.6)	37.3 (37.7)	10.3 (32.2)	9.9 (52.3)	3.0 (45.5)
Controlled-Release Tablet q12h	457.3 (40.2)	36.9 (42.0)	4.4 (53.0)	7.6 (60.3)	4.1 (51.5)

For single dose AUC = $AUC_{0\text{-}48h}$, for multiple dose AUC = $AUC_{0\text{-}24h}$ at steady state
+ For single dose parameter normalized to 100 mg, for multiple dose parameter normalized to 100 mg per 24 hours
* Steady-state fluctuation in plasma concentrations = C_{max}–C_{min}/C_{min}
^ Not applicable

INDICATIONS AND USAGE
KADIAN® is indicated for the management of moderate to severe pain where treatment with an opioid analgesic is indicated for more than a few days (see **CLINICAL PHARMACOLOGY; Clinical Studies**).
KADIAN® was developed for use in patients with chronic pain who require repeated dosing with a potent opioid analgesic, and has been tested in patients with pain due to malignant conditions. KADIAN® has not been tested as an analgesic for the treatment of acute pain or in the postoperative setting and is not recommended for such use.

CONTRAINDICATIONS
KADIAN® is contraindicated in patients with a known hypersensitivity to morphine, morphine salts or any of the capsule components.
KADIAN® is contraindicated in patients with respiratory depression in the absence of resuscitative equipment, and in patients with acute or severe bronchial asthma.
KADIAN® is contraindicated in any patient who has or is suspected of having paralytic ileus.

WARNINGS (See also CLINICAL PHARMACOLOGY)
Impaired Respiration
Respiratory depression is the chief hazard of all morphine preparations. Respiratory depression occurs more frequently in elderly and debilitated patients, and those suffering from conditions accompanied by hypoxia, hypercapnia, or upper airway obstruction (when even moderate therapeutic doses may significantly decrease pulmonary ventilation).
Morphine should be used with extreme caution in patients with chronic obstructive pulmonary disease or cor pulmonale, and in patients having a substantially decreased respiratory reserve (e.g. severe kyphoscoliosis), hypoxia, hypercapnia, or pre-existing respiratory depression. In such patients, even usual therapeutic doses of morphine may increase airway resistance and decrease respiratory drive to the point of apnea.

Head Injury and Increased Intracranial Pressure
The respiratory depressant effects of morphine with carbon dioxide retention and secondary elevation of cerebrospinal fluid pressure may be markedly exaggerated in the presence of head injury, other intracranial lesions, or a pre-existing increase in intracranial pressure. Morphine produces effects which may obscure neurologic signs of further increases in pressure in patients with head injuries. Morphine should only be administered under such circumstances when considered essential and then with extreme care.

Hypotensive Effect
KADIAN®, like all opioid analgesics, may cause severe hypotension in an individual whose ability to maintain blood pressure has already been compromised by a reduced blood volume, or a concurrent administration of drugs such as phenothiazines or general anesthetics. (see also **PRECAUTIONS - Drug Interactions**). KADIAN® may produce orthostatic hypotension and syncope in ambulatory patients.
KADIAN®, like all opioid analgesics, should be administered with caution to patients in circulatory shock, as vasodilation produced by the drug may further reduce cardiac output and blood pressure.

Gastrointestinal Obstruction
KADIAN® should not be given to patients with gastrointestinal obstruction, particularly paralytic ileus, as there is a risk of the product remaining in the stomach for an extended period and the subsequent release of a bolus of morphine when normal gut motility is restored. As with other solid morphine formulations diarrhea may reduce morphine absorption.

PRECAUTIONS (See also CLINICAL PHARMACOLOGY)
General
KADIAN® is intended for use in patients who require continuous treatment with a potent opioid analgesic. As with any potent opioid, it is critical to adjust the dosing regimen for KADIAN® for each patient, taking into account the patient's prior analgesic treatment experience. Although it is clearly impossible to enumerate every consideration that is important to the selection of the initial dose of KADIAN®, attention should be given to the points under **DOSAGE AND ADMINISTRATION.**

Cordotomy
Patients taking KADIAN® who are scheduled for cordotomy or other interruption of pain transmission pathways should have KADIAN® ceased 24 hours prior to the procedure and the pain controlled by parenteral short-acting opioids. In addition, the post-procedure titration of analgesics for such patients should be individualized to avoid either oversedation or withdrawal syndromes.

Use in Pancreatic/Biliary Tract Disease
KADIAN® may cause spasm of the sphincter of Oddi and should be used with caution in patients with biliary tract disease, including acute pancreatitis. Opioids may cause increases in the serum amylase level.

Special risk groups
KADIAN® should be administered with caution, and in reduced dosages in elderly or debilitated patients; patients with severe renal or hepatic insufficiency; patients with Addison's disease; myxedema; hypothyroidism; prostatic hypertrophy or urethral stricture.
Caution should also be exercised in the administration of KADIAN® to patients with CNS depression, toxic psychosis, acute alcoholism and delirium tremens, and convulsive disorders.

Driving and operating machinery
Morphine may impair the mental and/or physical abilities needed to perform potentially hazardous activities such as driving a car or operating machinery. Patients must be cautioned accordingly. Patients should also be warned about the potential combined effects of morphine with other CNS depressants, including other opioids, phenothiazines, sedative/hypnotics and alcohol (see **Drug Interactions**).

Information for Patients
If clinically advisable, patients receiving KADIAN® should be given the following instructions by the physician:
1. KADIAN® capsules should be swallowed whole (not chewed, crushed, or dissolved). Alternatively, KADIAN® capsules may be opened and the entire contents sprinkled on a small amount of applesauce immediately prior to ingestion. The pellets should NOT be chewed, crushed, or dissolved due to risk of overdose. When prescribing KADIAN® by the sprinkle method, details of proper technique should be explained to the patient. (also see **DOSAGE AND ADMINISTRATION**)
2. The dose of KADIAN® should not be adjusted without consulting the physician.
3. Morphine may impair mental and/or physical ability required for the performance of potentially hazardous tasks (e.g. driving, operating machinery). Patients started on KADIAN® or whose dose has been changed should refrain from dangerous activity until it is established that they are not adversely affected.

4. Morphine should not be taken with alcohol or other CNS depressants (sleeping medication, tranquilizers) because additive effects including CNS depression may occur. A physician should be consulted if other medications are currently being used or are prescribed for future use.

5. Women of childbearing potential who become or are planning to become pregnant, should consult a physician.

6. Upon completion of therapy, it may be appropriate to taper the morphine dose, rather than abruptly discontinuing it.

7. While psychological dependence ("addiction") to morphine used in the treatment of pain is very rare, morphine is one of a class of drugs known to be abused and should be handled accordingly.

8. As with other opioids, patients taking KADIAN® should be advised that severe constipation could occur and appropriate laxatives, stool softeners and other appropriate treatments should be initiated from the beginning of opioid therapy.

Drug Interactions

CNS Depressants: Morphine should be used with great caution and in reduced dosage in patients who are concurrently receiving other central nervous system (CNS) depressants including sedatives, hypnotics, general anesthetics, antiemetics, phenothiazines, other tranquilizers and alcohol because of the risk of respiratory depression, hypotension and profound sedation or coma. When such combined therapy is contemplated, the initial dose of one or both agents should be reduced by at least 50%.

Muscle Relaxants: Morphine may enhance the neuromuscular blocking action of skeletal relaxants and produce an increased degree of respiratory depression.

Mixed Agonist/Antagonist Opioid Analgesics: From a theoretical perspective, mixed agonist/antagonist analgesics (i.e. pentazocine, nalbuphine and butorphanol) should NOT be administered to patients who have received or are receiving a course of therapy with a pure opioid agonist analgesic. In these patients, mixed agonist/antagonist analgesics may reduce the analgesic effect and/or may precipitate withdrawal symptoms.

Monoamine Oxidase Inhibitors (MAOIs): MAOIs have been reported to intensify the effects of at least one opioid drug causing anxiety, confusion and significant depression of respiration or coma. We do not recommend the use of KADIAN® in patients taking MAOIs or within 14 days of stopping such treatment.

Cimetidine: There is an isolated report of confusion and severe respiratory depression when a hemodialysis patient was concurrently administered morphine and cimetidine.

Diuretics: Morphine can reduce the efficacy of diuretics by inducing the release of antidiuretic hormone. Morphine may also lead to acute retention of urine by causing spasm of the sphincter of the bladder, particularly in men with prostatism.

Food: KADIAN® capsules should be swallowed whole (not chewed, crushed, or dissolved). Alternatively, KADIAN® capsules may be opened and the entire contents sprinkled on a small amount of applesauce immediately prior to ingestion. The pellets in KADIAN® should NOT be chewed, crushed, or dissolved due to risk of overdose. (see **DOSAGE AND ADMINISTRATION,** and **INFORMATION FOR PATIENTS**)

Carcinogenicity/Mutagenicity/Impairment of Fertility

Long-term studies in animals to evaluate the carcinogenic potential of morphine have not been conducted. There are no reports of carcinogenic effects in humans.

In vitro studies have reported that morphine is non-mutagenic in the Ames test with Salmonella, and induces chromosomal aberrations in human leukocytes and lethal mutation induction in Drosophila. Morphine was found to be mutagenic in vitro in human T-cells, increasing the DNA fragmentation. In vivo, morphine was mutagenic in the mouse micronucleus test and induced chromosomal aberrations in spermatids and murine lymphocytes.

Chronic opioid abusers (e.g., heroin abusers) and their offspring display higher rates of chromosomal damage. However, the rates of chromosomal abnormalities were similar in nonexposed individuals and in heroin users enrolled in long term opioid maintenance programs.

Pregnancy

Teratogenic effects (Pregnancy Category C)

Teratogenic effects of morphine have been reported in the animal literature. High parental doses during the second trimester were teratogenic in neurological, soft and skeletal tissue. The abnormalities included encephalopathy and axial skeletal fusions. These doses were often maternally toxic and were 0.3 to 3-fold the maximum recommended human dose (MRHD) on a mg/m² basis. The relative contribution of morphine-induced maternal hypoxia and malnutrition, each of which can be teratogenic, has not been clearly defined. Treatment of male rats with approximately 3-fold the MRHD for 10 days prior to mating decreased litter size and viability.

Nonteratogenic effects

Morphine given subcutaneously, at non-maternally toxic doses, to rats during the third trimester with approximately 0.15-fold the MRHD caused reversible reductions in brain and spinal cord volume, and testes size and body weight in the offspring, and decreased fertility in female offspring. The offspring of rats and hamsters treated orally or intraperitoneally throughout pregnancy with 0.04- to 0.3-fold the MRHD of morphine have demonstrated delayed growth, motor and sexual maturation and decreased male fertility. Chronic morphine exposure of fetal animals resulted in mild withdrawal, altered reflex and motor skill development, and altered responsiveness to morphine that persisted into adulthood.

There are no well-controlled studies of chronic in utero exposure to morphine sulfate in human subjects. However, uncontrolled retrospective studies of human neonates chronically exposed to other opioids in utero, demonstrated reduced brain volume which normalized over the first month of life. Infants born to opioid-abusing mothers are more often small for gestational age, have a decreased ventilatory response to CO_2 and increased risk of sudden infant death syndrome.

Morphine should only be used during pregnancy if the need for strong opioid analgesia justifies the potential risk to the fetus.

Labor and Delivery

KADIAN® is not recommended for use in women during and immediately prior to labor, where shorter acting analgesics or other analgesic techniques are more appropriate. Occasionally, opioid analgesics may prolong labor through actions which temporarily reduce the strength, duration and frequency of uterine contractions. However, this effect is not consistent and may be offset by an increased rate of cervical dilatation which tends to shorten labor.

Neonates whose mothers received opioid analgesics during labor should be observed closely for signs of respiratory depression. A specific opioid antagonist, such as naloxone or nalmefene, should be available for reversal of opioid-induced respiratory depression in the neonate.

Neonatal Withdrawal Syndrome

Chronic maternal use of opiates or opioids during pregnancy coexposes the fetus. The newborn may experience subsequent neonatal withdrawal syndrome (NWS). Manifestations of NWS include irritability, hyperactivity, abnormal sleep pattern, high-pitched cry, tremor, vomiting, diarrhea, weight loss, and failure to gain weight. The onset, duration, and severity of the disorder differ based on such factors as the addictive drug used, time and amount of mother's last dose, and rate of elimination of the drug from the newborn. Approaches to the treatment of this syndrome have included supportive care and, when indicated, drugs such as paragoric or phenobarbital.

Nursing Mothers

Low levels of morphine sulfate have been detected in human milk. Withdrawal symptoms can occur in breast-feeding infants when maternal administration of morphine sulfate is stopped. Because of the potential for adverse reactions in nursing infants from KADIAN®, a decision should be made whether to discontinue nursing or discontinue the drug, taking into account the importance of the drug to the mother.

Pediatric Use

There are studies from the literature reporting the safe and effective use of both immediate and sustained release oral morphine preparations for analgesia in pediatric patients who were dosed on a per kilogram basis. However, the safety of KADIAN®, both the entire capsule and the pellets sprinkled on applesauce, have not been directly investigated in pediatric patients below the age of 18 years. The range of doses available is not suitable for the treatment of very young pediatric patients or those who are not old enough to take capsules safely. The applesauce sprinkling method is not an appropriate alternative for these patients.

ADVERSE REACTIONS

Serious adverse reactions that may be associated with KADIAN® therapy in clinical use are those observed with other opioid analgesics and include: respiratory depression, respiratory arrest, circulatory depression, cardiac arrest, hypotension, and/or shock (see **OVERDOSAGE, WARNINGS**).

The less severe adverse events seen on initiation of therapy with KADIAN® are also typical opioid side effects. These events are dose dependent, and their frequency depends on the clinical setting, the patient's level of opioid tolerance, and host factors specific to the individual. They should be expected and managed as a part of opioid analgesia. The most frequent of these include drowsiness, dizziness, constipation and nausea. In many cases, the frequency of these events during initiation of therapy may be minimized by careful individualization of starting dosage, slow titration, and the avoidance of large rapid swings in plasma concentrations of the opioid. Many of these adverse events, will cease or decrease as KADIAN® therapy is continued and some degree of tolerance is developed, but others may be expected to remain troublesome throughout therapy.

Management of Excessive Drowsiness

Most patients receiving morphine will experience initial drowsiness. This usually disappears within 3–5 days and is not a cause of concern unless it is excessive, or accompanied by unsteadiness or confusion. Dizziness and unsteadiness may be associated with postural hypotension, particularly in elderly or debilitated patients, and has been associated with syncope and falls in non-tolerant patients started on opioids.

Excessive or persistent sedation should be investigated. Factors to be considered should include: concurrent sedative medications, the presence of hepatic or renal insufficiency, hypoxia or hypercapnia due to exacerbated respiratory failure, intolerance to the dose used (especially in older patients), disease severity and the patient's general condition. The dosage should be adjusted according to individual needs, but additional care should be used in the selection of initial doses for the elderly patient, the cachectic or gravely ill patient, or in patients not already familiar with opioid analgesic medications to prevent excessive sedation at the onset of treatment.

Management of Nausea and Vomiting

Nausea and vomiting are common after single doses of morphine or as an early undesirable effect of chronic opioid therapy. The prescription of a suitable antiemetic should be considered, with the awareness that sedation may result (see **Drug Interactions**). The frequency of nausea and vomiting usually decreases within a week or so but may persist due to opioid-induced gastric stasis. Metoclopramide is often useful in such patients.

Management of Constipation

Virtually all patients suffer from constipation while taking opioids on a chronic basis. Some patients, particularly elderly, debilitated or bedridden patients may become impacted. Tolerance does not usually develop for the constipating effects of opioids. Patients must be cautioned accordingly and laxatives, softeners and other appropriate treatments should be used prophylactically from the beginning of opioid therapy.

Adverse Events Probably Related to KADIAN® Administration

In controlled clinical trials in patients with chronic cancer pain the most common adverse events reported by patients at least once during therapy were drowsiness (9%), constipation (9%), nausea (7%), dizziness (6%), and anxiety (6%). Other less common side effects expected from morphine or seen in less than 3% of patients in the clinical trials were:

Body as a Whole: Asthenia, accidental injury, fever, pain, chest pain, headache, diaphoresis, chills, flu syndrome, back pain, malaise, withdrawal syndrome

Cardiovascular: Tachycardia, atrial fibrillation, hypotension, hypertension, pallor, facial flushing, palpitations, bradycardia, syncope

Central Nervous System: Confusion, dry mouth, anxiety, abnormal thinking, abnormal dreams, lethargy, depression, tremor, loss of concentration, insomnia, amnesia, paresthesia, agitation, vertigo, foot drop, ataxia, hypesthesia, slurred speech, hallucinations, vasodilation, euphoria, apathy, seizures, myoclonus

Endocrine: Hyponatremia due to inappropriate ADH secretion, gynecomastia

Gastrointestinal: Vomiting, anorexia, dysphagia, dyspepsia, diarrhea, abdominal pain, stomach atony disorder, gastro-esophageal reflux, delayed gastric emptying, biliary colic

Hemic & Lymphatic: Anemia, leukopenia, thrombocytopenia

Metabolic & Nutritional: Peripheral edema, hyponatremia, edema

Musculoskeletal: Back pain, bone pain, arthralgia

Respiratory: Hiccup, rhinitis, atelectasis, asthma, hypoxia, dyspnea, respiratory insufficiency, voice alteration, depressed cough reflex, non-cardiogenic pulmonary edema

Skin and Appendages: Rash, decubitus ulcer, pruritus, skin flush

Special Senses: Amblyopia, conjunctivitis, miosis, blurred vision, nystagmus, diplopia

Urogenital: Urinary abnormality, amenorrhea, urinary retention, urinary hesitancy, reduced libido, reduced potency, prolonged labor

DRUG ABUSE AND DEPENDENCE

Morphine is the prototype of opioid agonist drugs, and may be subject to misuse, abuse and addiction. Addiction to opioids prescribed for pain management is rare, but requests for opioids from patients addicted to opioids are common and physicians should take appropriate care in prescribing this controlled substance.

Opioid analgesics may cause physical dependence. Physical dependence results in withdrawal symptoms in patients who abruptly discontinue the drug. Withdrawal also may be precipitated through the administration of drugs with opioid antagonist activity, e.g. naloxone, nalmefene, or mixed agonist/antagonist analgesics (pentazocine, butorphanol, nalbuphine), (see also **OVERDOSAGE**).

Physical dependence usually does not occur to a clinically significant degree until after several weeks of continued opioid usage. Tolerance, in which increasingly large doses

Continued on next page

Kadian—Cont.

are required in order to produce the same degree of analgesia, is initially manifested by a shortened duration of analgesic effect, and subsequently, by decreases in the intensity of analgesia.

In chronic pain patients, and in opioid-tolerant cancer patients, the administration of KADIAN® should be guided by the degree of tolerance manifested. Physical dependence, per se, is not ordinarily a concern when one is dealing with a patient in pain, and fear of tolerance should not deter using adequate doses to adequately relieve pain.

If morphine is abruptly discontinued an abstinence syndrome may occur. This is usually mild and is characterized by rhinitis, myalgia, abdominal cramping and occasional diarrhea. Most observable symptoms disappear in 5–14 days without treatment; however, there may be a phase of secondary or chronic abstinence which may last for 2–6 months characterized by insomnia, irritability and muscular aches. If treatment of physical dependence of patients taking morphine is necessary, the patient may be detoxified by gradual reduction of the dose. Gastrointestinal disturbances or dehydration should be treated with supportive care.

KADIAN® has no role in the management of opioid addiction.

OVERDOSAGE

Symptoms

Acute overdosage with morphine is manifested by respiratory depression, somnolence progressing to stupor or coma, skeletal muscle flaccidity, cold and clammy skin, constricted pupils, and, sometimes, pulmonary edema, bradycardia, hypotension and death. Marked mydriasis rather than miosis may be seen due to severe hypoxia in overdose situations.

Treatment

Primary attention should be given to the re-establishment of a patent airway and institution of assisted or controlled ventilation. Gastric contents may need to be emptied to remove unabsorbed drug when a sustained release formulation such as KADIAN® has been taken. Care should be taken to secure the airway before attempting treatment by gastric emptying or activated charcoal.

The pure opioid antagonists, naloxone or nalmefene, are specific antidotes to respiratory depression which results from opioid overdose. Since the duration of reversal would be expected to be less than the duration of action of KADIAN®, the patient must be carefully monitored until spontaneous respiration is reliably re-established. KADIAN® will continue to release and add to the morphine load for up to 24 hours after administration and the management of an overdose should be monitored accordingly. If the response to opioid antagonists is suboptimal or not sustained, additional antagonist should be given as directed by the manufacturer of the product.

Opioid antagonists should not be administered in the absence of clinically significant respiratory or circulatory depression secondary to morphine overdose. Such agents should be administered cautiously to persons who are known, or suspected to be physically dependent on KADIAN®. In such cases, an abrupt or complete reversal of opioid effects may precipitate an acute abstinence syndrome.

Opioid Tolerant Individuals: In an individual physically dependent on opioids, administration of the usual dose of the antagonist will precipitate an acute withdrawal. The severity of the withdrawal produced will depend on the degree of physical dependence and the dose of the antagonist administered. Use of an opioid antagonist should be reserved for cases where such treatment is clearly needed. If it is necessary to treat serious respiratory depression in the physically dependent patient, administration of the antagonist should be begun with care and by titration with smaller than usual doses.

Supportive measures (including oxygen, vasopressors) should be employed in the management of circulatory shock and pulmonary edema as indicated. Cardiac arrest or arrhythmias may require cardiac massage or defibrillation.

DOSAGE AND ADMINISTRATION

KADIAN® CAPSULES SHOULD BE SWALLOWED WHOLE (NOT CHEWED, CRUSHED, OR DISSOLVED).

ALTERNATIVELY, KADIAN® CAPSULES MAY BE OPENED AND THE ENTIRE CONTENTS SPRINKLED ON A SMALL AMOUNT OF APPLESAUCE IMMEDIATELY PRIOR TO INGESTION. THE PELLETS IN KADIAN® CAPSULES SHOULD NOT BE CHEWED, CRUSHED, OR DISSOLVED DUE TO RISK OF OVERDOSE.

TAKING CHEWED OR CRUSHED KADIAN® CAPSULES OR PELLETS WILL LEAD TO THE RAPID RELEASE AND ABSORPTION OF A POTENTIALLY TOXIC DOSE OF MORPHINE.

The sustained release nature of KADIAN® allows it to be administered on **either** a once-a-day or twice-a-day schedule. KADIAN® produces analgesia similar to that produced by conventional immediate-release and controlled-release formulations for the same total daily dose of morphine.

However, peak and trough blood levels depend on the release characteristics of each specific formulation, and other oral morphines may not be therapeutically equivalent to KADIAN® for an individual patient.

KADIAN® capsules have the same extent of absorption (AUC) as immediate-release oral formulations and controlled-release oral formulations of morphine sulfate. However, key pharmacokinetic parameters (e.g. C_{max}, T_{max}) for KADIAN® are significantly different from other controlled-release oral formulations.

As with any potent opioid drug product, it is critical to adjust the dosing regimen for each patient individually, taking into account the patient's prior analgesic treatment experience. In the selection of the initial dose of KADIAN®, attention should be given to:

1) the total daily dose, potency and kind of opioid the patient has been taking previously;
2) the reliability of the relative potency estimate used to calculate the equivalent dose of morphine needed;
3) the patient's degree of opioid tolerance;
4) the general condition and medical status of the patient;
5) concurrent medication;
6) the type and severity of the patient's pain.

The following dosing recommendations, therefore, can only be considered suggested approaches to what is actually a series of clinical decisions over time in the management of the pain of an individual patient.

Conversion from Other Oral Morphine Formulations to KADIAN®

Patients on other oral morphine formulations may be converted to KADIAN® by administering one-half of the patient's total daily oral morphine dose as KADIAN® capsules every 12 hours (twice-a-day) or by administering the total daily oral morphine dose as KADIAN® capsules every 24 hours (once-a-day). KADIAN® should not be given more frequently than every 12 hours.

Conversion from Parenteral Morphine or Other Parenteral or Oral Opioids to KADIAN®

KADIAN® can be administered to patients previously receiving treatment with parenteral morphine or other opioids. While there are useful tables of oral and parenteral equivalents in cancer analgesia, there is substantial interpatient variation in the relative potency of different opioid drugs and formulations. For these reasons, it is better to underestimate the patient's 24 hour oral morphine requirement and provide rescue medication, than to overestimate and manage an adverse event. The following general points should be considered:

Parenteral to oral morphine ratio: It may take anywhere from 2–6 mg of oral morphine to provide analgesia equivalent to 1 mg of parenteral morphine. A dose of oral morphine three times the daily parenteral morphine requirement may be sufficient in chronic use settings.

Other parenteral or oral opioids to oral morphine sulfate: Physicians are advised to refer to published relative potency data, keeping in mind that such ratios are only approximate. In general, it is safest to give half of the estimated daily morphine demand as the initial dose, and to manage inadequate analgesia by supplementation with immediate-release morphine. (See discussion which follows.)

The first dose of KADIAN® may be taken with the last dose of any immediate-release (short-acting) opioid medication due to the long delay until the peak effect after administration of KADIAN®.

Use of KADIAN® as the First Opioid Analgesic

There has been no evaluation of KADIAN® as an initial opioid analgesic in the management of pain. Because it may be more difficult to titrate a patient to adequate analgesia using a sustained release morphine, it is ordinarily advisable to begin treatment using an immediate-release morphine formulation.

Individualization of Dosage

The best use of opioid analgesics in the management of chronic malignant and non-malignant pain is challenging, and is well described in materials published by the World Health Organization and the Agency for Health Care Policy and Research which are available from Faulding Laboratories upon request. KADIAN® is a third step drug which is most useful when the patient requires a constant level of opioid analgesia as a "floor" or "platform" from which to manage breakthrough pain. When a patient has reached the point where comfort cannot be provided with a combination of non-opioid medications (NSAIDs and acetaminophen) and intermittent use of moderate or strong opioids, the patient's total opioid therapy should be converted into a 24 hour oral morphine equivalent.

KADIAN® should be started by administering one-half of the estimated total daily oral morphine dose every 12 hours (twice-a-day) or by administering the total daily oral morphine dose every 24 hours (once-a-day). The dose should be titrated no more frequently than every-other-day to allow the patients to stabilize before escalating the dose. If breakthrough pain occurs, the dose may be supplemented with a small dose (less than 20% of the total daily dose) of a short-acting analgesic. Patients who are excessively sedated after

a once-a-day dose or who regularly experience inadequate analgesia before the next dose should be switched to twice-a-day dosing.

Patients who do not have a proven tolerance to opioids should preferably be titrated to clinical response using an immediate-release morphine formulation and then converted to a long-acting product. However, if KADIAN® is chosen as initial opioid, patients should be started on either 20 mg every 12 hours or 40 mg once-a-day. If necessary, the dose of KADIAN® should be increased conservatively in opioid-naive patients and it is recommended that increments of not greater than 40 mg total daily dose are given every-other-day.

Most patients will rapidly develop some degree of tolerance, requiring dosage adjustment until they have achieved their individual best balance between baseline analgesia and opioid side effects such as confusion, sedation and constipation. No guidance can be given as to the recommended maximal dose, especially in patients with chronic pain of malignancy. In such cases the total dose of KADIAN® should be advanced until the desired therapeutic endpoint is reached or clinically significant opioid-related adverse reactions intervene.

Alternative Methods of Administration

In a study of healthy volunteers, KADIAN® pellets sprinkled over applesauce were found to be bioequivalent to KADIAN® capsules swallowed whole with applesauce under fasting conditions. Other foods have not been tested. Patients who have difficulty swallowing whole capsules or tablets may benefit from this alternative method of administration.

1) Sprinkle the pellets onto a small amount of applesauce. Applesauce should be room temperature or cooler.
2) Use immediately.
3) Rinse mouth to ensure all pellets have been swallowed.
4) Patients should consume entire portion and should not divide applesauce into separate doses.

Considerations in the Adjustment of Dosing Regimens

If signs of excessive opioid effects are observed early in the dosing interval, the next dose should be reduced. If this adjustment leads to inadequate analgesia, that is, if breakthrough pain occurs when KADIAN® is administered on an every 24 hours dosing regimen, consideration should be given to dosing every 12 hours. If breakthough pain occurs on a 12 hour dosing regimen a supplemental dose of short-acting analgesic may be given. As experience is gained, adjustments in both dose and dosing interval can be made to obtain an appropriate balance between pain relief and opioid side effects. To avoid accumulation the dosing interval of KADIAN® should not be reduced below 12 hours.

Conversion from KADIAN® to Other Controlled-Release Oral Morphine Formulations

KADIAN® is not bioequivalent to other controlled-release morphine preparations. Although for a given dose the same total amount of morphine is available from KADIAN® as from morphine solution or controlled-release morphine tablets, the slower release of morphine from KADIAN® results in reduced maximum and increased minimum plasma morphine concentrations than with shorter acting morphine products. Conversion from KADIAN® to the same total daily dose of controlled-release morphine preparations may lead to either excessive sedation at peak or inadequate analgesia at trough and close observation and appropriate dosage adjustments are recommended.

Conversion from KADIAN® to Parenteral Opioids

When converting a patient from KADIAN® to parenteral opioids, it is best to calculate an equivalent parenteral dose, and then initiate treatment at half of this calculated value. For example, to estimate the required 24 hour dose of parenteral morphine for a patient taking KADIAN®, one would take the 24 hour KADIAN® dose, divide by an oral to parenteral conversion ratio of 3, divide the estimated 24 hour parenteral dose into six divided doses (for a four hour dosing interval), then halve this dose as an initial trial.

For example, to estimate the required parenteral morphine dose for a patient taking 360 mg of KADIAN® a day, divide the 360 mg daily oral morphine dose by a conversion ratio of 1 mg of parenteral morphine for every 3 mg of oral morphine. The estimated 120 mg daily parenteral requirement is then divided into six 20 mg doses, and half of this, or 10 mg, is then given every 4 hours as an initial trial dose.

This approach is likely to require a dosage increase in the first 24 hours for many patients, but is recommended because it is less likely to cause overdose than trying to establish an equivalent dose without titration.

Opioid analgesic agents may not effectively relieve dysesthetic pain, post-herpetic neuralgia, stabbing pains, activity-related pain, and some forms of headache. This does not mean that patients suffering from these types of pain should not be given an adequate trial of opioid analgesics. However, such patients may need to be promptly evaluated for other types of pain therapy.

Safety and Handling

KADIAN® consists of closed hard gelatin capsules containing polymer coated morphine sulfate pellets that pose no known handling risk to health care workers. Oral morphine

products are not known to be associated with a high risk of diversion, but all strong opioids are liable to diversion and misuse both by the general public and health care workers, and should be handled accordingly.

HOW SUPPLIED

KADIAN® capsules contain white to off-white or tan colored polymer coated sustained release pellets of morphine sulfate and are available in three dose strengths:
20 mg size 4 capsule, clear cap imprinted KADIAN and clear body imprinted with 20 mg. Capsules are supplied in bottles of 60 (NDC 63857-322-06).
50 mg size 2 capsule, clear cap imprinted KADIAN and clear body imprinted with 50 mg. Capsules are supplied in bottles of 60 (NDC 63857-323-06).
100 mg size 0 capsule, clear cap imprinted KADIAN and clear body imprinted with 100 mg. Capsules are supplied in bottles of 60 (NDC 63857-324-06).
Store at controlled room temperature between 15°–30°C (59°–86°F). Protect from light and moisture.
Dispense in a sealed, tamper-evident, childproof, light-resistant container.

CAUTION

DEA Order Form Required.

Federal law prohibits dispensing without prescription.

KADIAN® is a registered trademark of F H Faulding & Co Limited

MS Contin® is a registered trademark of The Purdue Frederick Company

Manufactured for: **FAULDING LABORATORIES**
(A Division of Faulding Pharmaceutical Co.)
5511 Capital Center Drive, Raleigh, NC 27606
by: Purepac Pharmaceutical Co.
Elizabeth, NJ 07207 USA
40-8827   Revised—January 1998
Shown in Product Identification Guide, page 310

Ferndale Laboratories, Inc.
780 W. EIGHT MILE ROAD
FERNDALE, MI 48220

Direct Inquiries to:
Mr. Thayer McMillan
(248) 548-0900
FAX: (248) 548-8427

For Medical Information Contact:
In Emergencies:
Mr. Pravin M. Patel
(248) 548-0900
FAX: (248) 548-0708

ANALPRAM–HC® CREAM   ℞
Rectal Cream
ANALPRAM–HC® LOTION 2.5%   ℞

DESCRIPTION

ANALPRAM-HC® CREAM: Contains Hydrocortisone Acetate 1% or 2.5% and Pramoxine HCl 1% in a hydrophilic cream base containing stearic acid, cetyl alcohol, aquaphor, isopropylpalmitate, polyoxyl-40 stearate, potassium sorbate, sorbic acid, triethanolamine lauryl sulfate and water.

ANALPRAM-HC® LOTION 2.5%: Contains Hydrocortisone Acetate 2.5% and Pramoxine Hydrochloride 1% in a hydrophilic lotion base containing stearic acid, cetyl alcohol, forlan-L, glycerin, triethanolamine, polyoxyl 40 stearate, diisopropyl adipate, povidone, silicone, potassium sorbate, sorbic acid, and purified water.

Topical corticosteroids are anti-inflammatory and antipruritic agents. The structural formula, the chemical name, molecular formula and molecular weight for active ingredients are presented below.

Hydrocortisone acetate
(Pregn-4-ene-3,20-dione,21 - (acetyloxy)-11, 17-dihydroxy-,(11 β)-).
$C_{23}H_{32}O_6$; mol wt: 404.50

Pramoxine hydrochloride
(4-(3-(p-butoxyphenoxy)propyl)morpholine hydrochloride)
$C_{17}H_{27}NO_3$.HCl; mol wt: 329.87

CLINICAL PHARMACOLOGY

Topical corticosteroids share anti-inflammatory, anti-pruritic and vasoconstrictive actions.

The mechanism of anti-inflammatory activity of the topical corticosteroids is unclear. Various laboratory methods, including vasoconstrictor assays, are used to compare and predict potencies and/or clinical efficacies of the topical corticosteroids. There is some evidence to suggest that a recognizable correlation exists between vasoconstrictor potency and therapeutic efficacy in man.

Pramoxine hydrochloride is a topical anesthetic agent which provides temporary relief from itching and pain. It acts by stabilizing the neuronal membrane of nerve endings with which it comes into contact.

Pharmacokinetics: The extent of percutaneous absorption of topical corticosteroids is determined by many factors including the vehicle, the integrity of the epidermal barrier, and the use of occlusive dressings.

Topical corticosteroids can be absorbed from normal intact skin. Inflammation and/or other disease processes in the skin increase percutaneous absorption. Occlusive dressings substantially increase the percutaneous absorption of topical corticosteroids. Thus, occlusive dressings may be a valuable therapeutic adjunct for treatment of resistant dermatoses (See DOSAGE AND ADMINISTRATION).

Once absorbed through the skin, topical corticosteroids are handled through pharmacokinetic pathways similar to systemically administered corticosteroids. Corticosteroids are bound to plasma proteins in varying degrees. Corticosteroids are metabolized primarily in the liver and are then excreted by the kidneys. Some of the topical corticosteroids and their metabolites are also excreted into the bile.

INDICATIONS AND USAGE

Topical corticosteroids are indicated for the relief of the inflammatory and pruritic manifestations of corticosteroid-responsive dermatoses of the anal region.

CONTRAINDICATIONS

Topical corticosteroids are contraindicated in those patients with a history of hypersensitivity to any of the components of the preparation.

PRECAUTIONS

General: Systemic absorption of topical corticosteroids has produced reversible hypothalamic-pituitary-adrenal (HPA) axis suppression, manifestations of Cushing's syndrome, hyperglycemia, and glucosuria in some patients.

Conditions which augment systemic absorption include the application of the more potent steroids, use over large surface areas, prolonged use, and the addition of occlusive dressings.

Therefore, patients receiving a large dose of a potent topical steroid applied to a large surface area and under an occlusive dressing should be evaluated periodically for evidence of HPA axis suppression by using the urinary free cortisol and ACTH stimulation tests. If HPA axis suppression is noted, an attempt should be made to withdraw the drug, to reduce the frequency of application, or to substitute a less potent steroid.

Recovery of HPA axis function is generally prompt and complete upon discontinuation of the drug. Infrequently, signs and symptoms of steroid withdrawal may occur, requiring supplemental systemic corticosteroids.

Children may absorb proportionally larger amounts of topical corticosteroids and thus be more susceptible to systemic toxicity. (See PRECAUTIONS—Pediatric Use).

If irritation develops, topical corticosteroids should be discontinued and appropriate therapy instituted.

In the presence of dermatological infections, the use of an appropriate antifungal or antibacterial agent should be instituted. If a favorable response does not occur promptly, the corticosteroid should be discontinued until the infection has been adequately controlled.

Information for the Patient: Patients using topical corticosteroids should receive the following information and instructions:
1. This medication is to be used as directed by the physician. It is for external use only. Avoid contact with the eyes.
2. Patients should be advised not to use this medication for any disorder other than for which it was prescribed.
3. The treated skin area should not be bandaged or otherwise covered or wrapped as to be occlusive unless directed by the physician.
4. Patients should report any signs of local adverse reactions especially under occlusive dressing.
5. Parents of pediatric patients should be advised not to use tightfitting diapers or plastic pants on a child being treated in the diaper area, as these garments may constitute occlusive dressings.

Laboratory Tests: The following tests may be helpful in evaluating the HPA axis suppression:
Urinary free cortisol test
ACTH stimulation test

Carcinogenesis, Mutagenesis, and Impairment of Fertility: Long-term animal studies have not been performed to evaluate the carcinogenic potential or the effect on fertility of topical corticosteroids.

Studies to determine mutagenicity with prednisolone and hydrocortisone have revealed negative results.

Pregnancy Category C: Corticosteroids are generally teratogenic in laboratory animals when administered systemically at relatively low dosage levels. The more potent corticosteroids have been shown to be teratogenic after dermal application in laboratory animals. There are no adequate and well-controlled studies in pregnant women on teratogenic effects from topically applied corticosteroids. Therefore, topical corticosteroids should be used during pregnancy only if the potential benefit justifies the potential risk to the fetus. Drugs of this class should not be used extensively on pregnant patients, in large amounts, or for prolonged periods of time.

Nursing Mothers: It is not known whether topical administration of corticosteroids could result in sufficient systemic absorption to produce detectable amounts in breast milk. Systemically administered corticosteroids are secreted into breast milk in quantities NOT likely to have a deleterious effect on the infant. Nevertheless, caution should be exercised when topical corticosteroids are administered to a nursing woman.

Pediatric Use: PEDIATRIC PATIENTS MAY DEMONSTRATE GREATER SUSCEPTIBILITY TO TOPICAL CORTICOSTEROID-INDUCED HPA AXIS SUPPRESSION AND CUSHING'S SYNDROME THAN MATURE PATIENTS BECAUSE OF A LARGER SKIN SURFACE AREA TO BODY WEIGHT RATIO.

Hypothalamic-pituitary-adrenal (HPA) axis suppression, Cushing's syndrome, and intracranial hypertension have been reported in children receiving topical corticosteroids. Manifestations of adrenal suppression in children include linear growth retardation, delayed weight gain, low plasma cortisol levels, and absence of response to ACTH stimulation. Manifestations of intracranial hypertension include bulging fontanelles, headaches, and bilateral papilledema. Administration of topical corticosteroids to children should be limited to the least amount compatible with an effective therapeutic regimen. Chronic corticosteroid therapy may interfere with the growth and development of children.

ADVERSE REACTIONS

The following local adverse reactions are reported infrequently with topical corticosteroids, but may occur more frequently with the use of occlusive dressings. These reactions are listed in an approximate decreasing order of occurrence:

Burning	Hypopigmentation
Itching	Perioral dermatitis
Irritation	Allergic contact dermatitis
Dryness	Maceration of the skin
Folliculitis	Secondary infection
Hypertrichosis	Skin Atrophy
Acneiform eruptions	Striae
	Miliaria

OVERDOSAGE

Topically applied corticosteroids can be absorbed in sufficient amounts to produce systemic effects (See PRECAUTIONS).

DOSAGE AND ADMINISTRATION

Topical corticosteroids are generally applied to the affected area as a thin film three or four times daily depending on the severity of the condition.

Occlusive dressings may be used for the management of psoriasis or recalcitrant conditions. If an infection develops, the use of occlusive dressings should be discontinued and appropriate antimicrobial therapy instituted.

For cleansing of anogenital area, spread Analpram HC® Lotion 2.5% on cotton or tissue and wipe affected area.

HOW SUPPLIED

ANALPRAM-HC® CREAM 1% is supplied in 1 oz tube with rectal applicator. NDC 0496–0778–04
ANALPRAM-HC® CREAM 2.5% is supplied in 1 oz tube with rectal applicator. NDC 0496-0800-04
ANALPRAM-HC® LOTION 2.5% is supplied in 2 fl oz bottle. NDC 0496–0829–04
Dispense in a tight container as defined in the official compendium.

Store at controlled room temperature 15°– 30°C (59°– 86°F).

DECUBITENE™ Oxygenated Oil   OTC
[dĕ-cū-bĭ-tēne]

Decubitene is a specially formulated preparation consisting of 99% oxygenated triglycerides of corn oil origin designed

Continued on next page

Decubitene—Cont.

specifically as a first response to dermal warning lesions (Stage I pressure ulcers) on mobility restricted patients.

HOW SUPPLIED

Decubitene™ is supplied in spray bottles containing 20 ml UPC 7-34118-0845-2-1

DERMAMIST™ OTC

[*dĕrm-a-mĭst*]

Dermamist™ is a skin protectant spray designed to prevent the loss of vital moisture after showering.

HOW SUPPLIED

Dermamist™ is supplied in aerosol cans containing 125 ml NDC 0496-0847-04

ELA-*Max*™
Topical Anesthetic Cream ℞

[*elă-măx*]

(lidocaine 4%)

DESCRIPTION

ELA-Max™ Cream (lidocaine 4%) is a topical anesthetic cream. Lidocaine is chemically designated as acetamide, 2-(diethylamino)-N-(2,6–dimethylphenyl), has an octanol: water partition ratio of 43 at pH 7.4, and has the following structure:

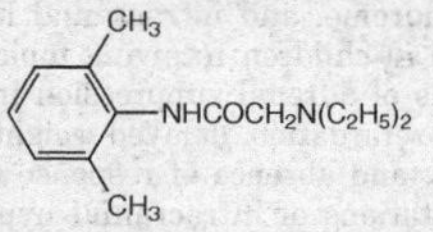

CH3
NHCOCH2N(C2H5)2
CH3

$C_{14}H_{22}N_2O$ Mol. wt. 234.33

Each gram of ELA-Max Cream contains lidocaine 40 mg, lecithin, propylene glycol, benzyl alcohol, vitamin E acetate, cholesterol, carbomer 940, triethanolamine, polysorbate 80, purified water.

CLINICAL PHARMACOLOGY

Mechanism of Action: ELA-Max Cream (lidocaine 4%) applied to intact skin provides dermal analgesia by a release of lidocaine from the cream into the epidermal and dermal layers of the skin, and by the accumulation of lidocaine in the vicinity of pain receptors and nerve endings. Lidocaine is an amide-type local anesthetic agent which stabilizes neuronal membranes by inhibiting the ionic fluxes required for the initiation and conduction of impulses, thereby effecting local anesthetic action. The onset, depth and duration of dermal analgesia provided by ELA-Max Cream depends primarily on the duration of application.

Dermal application of ELA-Max Cream may cause a transient, local blanching followed by a transient, local redness or erythemia.

Pharmacokinetics: The amount of lidocaine systemically absorbed from ELA-Max Cream is directly related to both the duration of application and to the area over which it is applied.

It is not known if lidocaine is metabolized into the skin. Lidocaine is metabolized rapidly by the liver to a number of metabolites including monoethylglycinexylidide (MEGX) and glycinexylidide (GX), both of which have pharmacologic activity similar to, but less potent to that of lidocaine. The metabolite, 2,6–xylidine, has unknown pharmacologic activity but is carcinogenic in rats (see Carcinogenesis subsection of PRECAUTIONS).

Following intravenous administration, MEGX and GX concentrations in serum range from 11 to 36% and from 5 to 11% of lidocaine concentrations, respectively.

The half-life of lidocaine elimination from the plasma following IV administration is approximately 65 to 150 minutes (mean 110,±24 SD, n = 13). This half-life may be increased in cardiac or hepatic dysfunction. More than 98% of an absorbed dose of lidocaine can be recovered in the urine as metabolites or parent drug. The systemic clearance is 10 to 20 mL/min/kg (mean 13,±3 SD, n = 13).

INDICATION AND USAGE

ELA-Max Cream (lidocaine 4%) is indicated for the temporary relief of pain associated with minor cuts and abrasions of the skin, minor burns, including sumburn, minor skin irritation and insect bites.

ELA-Max Cream is not recommended on mucous membranes because limited studies show greater absorption of lidocaine than through intact skin. Safe dosing recommendations for use on mucous membranes cannot be made because it has not been studied adequately. ELA-Max Cream is not recommended in any clinical situation in which penetration or migration beyond the tympanic membrane into the middle ear is possible because of ototoxic effects observed in animal studies (see WARNINGS).

CONTRAINDICATIONS

ELA-Max Cream (lidocaine 4%) is contra-indicated in patients with a known history of sensitivity to local anesthetics of the amide type or to any other component of the product.

WARNINGS

For external use only. Avoid contact with eyes. Do not apply to irritated skin or if excessive irritation develops. If condition worsens, or if symptoms persist unaltered for more than seven days or clear up and occur again within only a few days, discontinue use of this product and consult a doctor. Do not use in large quantities, particularly over raw or blistered areas. As with any drug, if you are pregnant or nursing a baby, seek the advice of a health professional before using this product. In case of accidental ingestion, seek professional help or contact a poison control center immediately. Keep this and all medicines out of the reach of children.

Application of ELA-Max Cream to larger areas of for longer times than those recommended could result in sufficient absorption of lidocaine resulting in serious adverse effects (see DOSAGE AND ADMINISTRATION).

Studies in laboratory animals (guinea pigs) have shown that lidocaine cream has an ototoxic effect when instilled into the middle ear. In these same studies, animals exposed to lidocaine cream in the external auditory canal only showed no abnormality. ELA-Max Cream should not be used in any clinical situation in which its penetration or migration beyond the tympanic membrane into the middle ear is possible.

PRECAUTIONS

General: Repeated doese of ELA-Max Cream may increase blood levels of lidocaine. ELA-Max Cream should be used with caution in patients who may be more sensitive to the systemic effects of lidocaine including acutely ill, debilitated, or elderly patients.

ELA-Max Cream coming in contact with the eye should be avoided because animal studies have demonstrated severe eye irritation. Also the loss of protective reflexes can permit corneal irritation and potential abrasion. Absorption of lidocaine cream in conjunctival tissues has not been determined. If eye contact occurs, immediately wash out the eye with water or saline and protect the eye until sensation returns.

Patients allergic to para-aminobenzoic acid derivitives (procaine, tetracaine, benzocaine, etc.) have not shown cross sensitivity to lidocaine; however, ELA-Max Cream should be used with caution in patients with a history of drug sensitivities, especially if the etiologic agent is uncertain. Patients with severe hepatic disease, because of their inability to metabolize local anesthetics normally, are at greater risk of developing toxic plasma concentrations of lidocaine.

Information for Patients: When ELA-Max Cream is used, the patient should be aware that the production of dermal analgesia may be accompanied by the block of all sensations in the treated skin. For this reason, the patient should avoid inadvertant trauma to the treated area by scratching, rubbing, or exposure to extreme hot or cold temperatures until complete sensation has returned.

Drug Interactions: ELA-Max™ Cream should be used with caution in patients receiving Class 1 antiarrhythmic drugs (such as tocainide and mexiletine) since the toxic effects are additive and generally synergistic.

Carcinogenesis, Mutagenesis, Impairment of Fertility:

Carcinogenesis: Metabolites of lidocaine have been shown to be carcinogenic in laboratory animals.

Mutagenesis: The mutagenic potential of lidocaine HCl has been tested in the Ames Salmonella/mammalian microsome test and by analysis of structural chromosome aberrations in human lymphocytes *in vitro*, and by mouse micronucleus test *in vivo*. There was no indication in these tests of any mutagenic effects.

The mutagenicity of 2,6-xylidine, a metabolite of lidocaine, has been studied in different tests with mixed results. The compound was found to be weakly mutagenic in the Ames test only under metabolic activation conditions. In addition, 2,6-xylidine was observed to be mutagenic at the thymidine kinase locus, with or without activation, and induced chromosome aberrations and sister chromatic exchanges at concentrations at which the drug precipitated out of the solution (1.2 mg/mL). No evidence of genotoxicity was found in the *in vivo* assays measuring unscheduled DNA synthesis in rat hepatocytes, chromosome damage in polychromatic erythrocytes or preferential killing of DNA repair-deficient bacteria in liver, lung, kidney, testes and blood extracts from mice. However, covalent binding studies of DNA from liver and ethmoid turbinates in rats indicate that 2,6-xylidine may be genotoxic under certain conditions *in vivo*.

Impairment of Fertility: See Use in Pregnancy

Use in Pregnancy:

Teratogenic Effects: Pregnancy Catagory B: There are no adequate and well-controlled studies in pregnant women. Because animal reproduction studies are not always predictive of human response, ELA-Max Cream should be used during pregnancy only if clearly needed.

Labor and Delivery: Lidocaine is not contraindicated in labor and delivery. Should ELA-Max Cream be used concomitantly with other products containing lidocaine, total doses contributed by all formulations must be considered.

Nursing Mothers:

Lidocaine is excreted in human milk. Therefore, caution should be exercised when ELA-Max Cream is administered to a nursing mother since the milk:plasma ration of lidocaine is 0.4.

Pediatric Use:

Consult a doctor prior to use on children under 2 years of age. When using ELA-Max Cream in young children, care must be taken to insure that application of the cream is limited to the intended site (See DOSAGE AND ADMINISTRATION). Accidental ingestion may lead to dose related toxicity.

ADVERSE REACTIONS

Localized reactions: During or immediately after treatment with ELA-Max Cream, the skin at the site of treatment may develop erythema or edema or may be the locus of abnormal sensation.

Allergic Reactions: Allergic and anaphylactoid reactions associated with lidocaine can occur. They are characterized by urticaria, angioedema, bronchospasm, and shock. If they occur they should be managed by conventional means. The detection of sensitivity by skin testing is of doubtful value.

System (Dose Related) Reactions:

Systemic adverse reactions following appropriate use of ELA-Max Cream are unlikely due to the small dose absorbed. Systemic adverse reactions of lidocaine are similar in nature to those observed with other amide local anesthetic agents including CNS excitation and/or depression (light-headedness, nervousness, apprehension, euphoria, confusion, dizziness, drowsiness, tinnitus, blurred or double vision, vomiting, sensations of heat, cold or numbness, twitching, tremors, convulsions, unconsciousness, respiratory depression and arrest). Excitatory CNS reactions may be brief or not occur at all, in which case the first manifestation may be drowsiness merging into unconsciousness. Cardiovascular manifestations may include bradycardia, hypotension, and cardiovascular collapse leading to arrest.

OVERDOSAGE

Peak blood levels following a 60g application to 400 cm^2 for 3 hours are 0.05 to 0.16 µg/mL for lidocaine. Toxic levels of lidocaine (>5 µg/mL) cause decreases in cardiac output, total peripheral resistance and mean arterial pressure. These changes may be attributable to direct depressant effects of these local anesthetic agents on the cardiovascular system. In the absence of massive topical overdose or oral ingestion, evaluation should include other etiologies for the clinical effects of overdosage from other sources of lidocaine or other local anesthetics.

DOSAGE AND ADMINISTRATION

A thick layer of ELA-Max Cream is applied to intact skin. A single application of ELA-Max Cream in a child weighing less than 10 kg should not be applied over an area larger than 100 cm^2. A single application of ELA-Max Cream in children weighing between 10 kg and 20 kg should not be applied over an area larger than 100 cm^2.

When applying ELA-Max Cream to young children, care must be taken to maintain careful observation of the child to prevent accidental ingestion of ELA-Max Cream.

When ELA-Max Cream (lidocaine 4%) is used concomitantly with other products containing local anesthetic agents, the amount absorbed from all formulations must be considered. The amount absorbed in the case of ELA-Max Cream is determined by the area over which it is applied and the duration of application. Although the incidence of systemic adverse reactions with ELA-Max Cream is very low, caution should be exercised, particularly when applying it over large areas and leaving it on for longer than 2 hours. The incidence of systemic adverse reactions can be expected to be directly proportional to the area and time of exposure.

HOW SUPPLIED

ELA-Max Cream is available as the following:

NDC 0496-0823-06 5 gram tube, box of 5
NDC 0496-0823-30 30 gram tube

Store between 15° and 30°C (59° – 86°F).

Caution: Federal Law Prohibits Dispensing Without Prescription.

NOT FOR OPHTHALMIC USE.

KEEP CONTAINER TIGHTLY CLOSED AT ALL TIMES WHEN NOT IS USE.

Manufactured Jointly by:
Ferndale Laboratories, Inc.
Ferndale, MI 48220 and
BioZone Laboratories, Inc.
Pittsburg, CA 94565

ELA-MAX is a trademark of
Ferndale Laboratories, Inc.
©Ferndale Laboratories, Inc.
MG #13350 Iss: 09/97

ELA-Max™5 Anorectal Cream ℞

[*elă 'măx-five*]
(lidocaine 5%)

DESCRIPTION

ELA-Max™5 Anorectal Cream (lidocaine 5%) is a topical anesthetic cream. Lidocaine is chemically designated as acetamide, 2-(diethylamino)-N-(2,6-dimethylphenyl), has an octanol:water partition ratio of 43 at pH 7.4, and has the following structure:

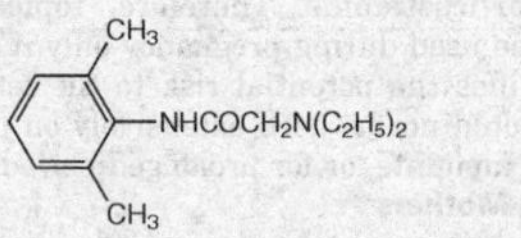

$C_{14}H_{22}N_2O$ Mol. wt. 234.33

Each gram of ELA-Max5 Anorectal Cream contains lidocaine 50 mg, lecithin, propylene glycol, benzyl alcohol, vitamin E acetate, cholesterol, isopropyl myristate, carbomer 940, triethanolamine, polysorbate 80, purified water.

CLINICAL PHARMACOLOGY

Mechanism of Action: ELA-Max5 Anorectal Cream (lidocaine 5%) applied to intact skin provides dermal analgesia by a release of lidocaine from the cream into the epidermal and dermal layers of the skin, and by the accumulation of lidocaine in the vicinity of pain receptors and nerve endings. Lidocaine is an amide-type local anesthetic agent which stablizes neuronal membranes by inhibiting the ionic fluxes required for the initiation and conduction of impulses, thereby effecting local anesthetic action. The onset, depth and duration of dermal analgesia provided by ELA-Max5 Anorectal Cream depends primarily on the duration of application.

Dermal application of ELA-Max5 Anorectal Cream may cause a transient, local blanching followed by a transient, local redness or erythemia.

Pharmacokinetics: The amount of lidocaine systemically absorbed from ELA-Max5 Anorectal Cream is directly related to both the duration of application and to the area over which it is applied.

It is not known if lidocaine is metabolized into the skin. Lidocaine is metabolized rapidly by the liver to a number of metabolites including monoethylglycinexylidide (MEGX) and glycinexylidide (GX), both of which have pharmacologic activity similar to, but less potent to that of lidocaine. The metabolite, 2,6-xylidine, has unknown pharmacologic activity but is carcinogenic in rats (see Carcinogenesis subsection of PRECAUTIONS). Following intravenous administration, MEGX and GX concentrations in serum range from 11 to 36% and from 5 to 11% of lidocaine concentrations, respectively.

The half-life of lidocaine elimination from the plasma following IV administration is approximately 65 to 150 minutes (mean 110, ±24 SD, n=13). This half-life may be increased in cardiac or hepatic dysfunction. More than 98% of an absorbed dose of lidocaine can be recovered in the urine as metabolites or parent drug. The systemic clearance is 10 to 20 mL/min/kg (mean 13, ±3 SD, n=13).

INDICATION AND USAGE

ELA-Max5 Anorectal Cream (lidocaine 5%) is indicated for the temporary relief of local discomfort, including pain and itching, soreness or burning associated with anorectal disorders. ELA-Max5 Anorectal Cream is not recommended on mucous membranes because limited studies show greater absorption of lidocaine than through intact skin. Safe dosing recommendations for use on mucous membranes cannot be made because it has not been studied adequately.

ELA-Max5 Anorectal Cream is not recommended in any clinical situation in which penetration or migration beyond the tympanic membrane into the middle ear is possible because of ototoxic effects observed in animal studies (see WARNINGS).

CONTRAINDICATIONS

ELA-Max5 Anorectal Cream (lidocaine 5%) is contra-indicated in patients with a known history of sensitivity to local anesthetics of the amide type or to any other component of the product.

WARNINGS

For external use only. Avoid contact with eyes. Do not apply to irritated skin or if excessive irritation develops. If condition worsens, or if symptoms persist unaltered for seven days, or clear up and occur again within only a few days, discontinue use of this product and consult a doctor. Do not exceed the recommended daily dosage unless directed by a doctor. Do not apply to raw or blistered areas. In case of bleeding, consult a doctor promptly. Do not put this product into the rectum using fingers or any mechanical device or applicator. Certain persons can develop allergic reactions to ingredients in this product. If redness, irritation, swelling, pain or other symptoms develop or increase, discontinue use and consult a doctor. As with any drug, if you are pregnant or nursing a baby, seek the advice of a health professional before using this product. In case of accidental ingestion, seek professional help or contact a poison control center immediately. Keep this and all medicines out of the reach of children.

Application of ELA-Max5 Anorectal Cream to larger areas or for longer times than those recommended could result in sufficient absorption of lidocaine resulting in serious adverse effects (see DOSAGE AND ADMINISTRATION). Studies in laboratory animals (guinea pigs) have shown that lidocaine cream has an ototoxic effect when instilled into the middle ear. In these same studies, animals exposed to lidocaine cream in the external auditory canal only showed no abnormality.

ELA-Max5 Anorectal Cream should not be used in any clinical situation in which its penetration or migration beyond the tympanic membrane into the middle ear is possible.

PRECAUTIONS

General: Repeated doses of ELA-Max5 Anorectal Cream may increase blood levels of lidocaine.

ELA-Max5 Anorectal Cream should be used with caution in patients who may be more sensitive to the systemic effects of lidocaine including acutely ill, debilitated, or elderly patients.

ELA-Max5 Anorectal Cream coming in contact with the eye should be avoided because animal studies have demonstrated severe eye irritation. Also the loss of protective reflexes can permit corneal irritation and potential abrasion. Absorption of lidocaine cream in conjunctival tissues has not been determined. If eye contact occurs, immediately wash out the eye with water or saline and protect the eye until sensation returns. Patients allergic to para-aminobenzoic acid derivatives (procaine, tetracaine, benzocaine, etc.) have not shown cross-sensitivity to lidocaine; however, ELA-Max5 Anorectal Cream should be used with caution in patients with a history of drug sensitivities, especially if the etiologic agent is uncertain. Patients with severe hepatic disease, because of their inability to metabolize local anesthetics normally, are at greater risk of developing toxic plasma concentrations of lidocaine.

Information for Patients: When **ELA-Max™5** Anorectal Cream is used, the patient should be aware that the production of dermal analgesia may be accompanied by the block of all sensations in the treated skin. For this reason, the patient should avoid inadvertant trauma to the treated area by scratching, rubbing, or exposure to extreme hot or cold temperatures until complete sensation has returned.

Drug Interactions: ELA-Max5 Anorectal Cream should be used with caution in patients receiving Class I antiarrhythmic drugs (such as tocainide and mexiletine) since the toxic effects are additive and generally synergistic.

Carcinogenesis, Mutagenesis, Impairment of Fertility:

Carcinogenesis: Metabolites of lidocaine have been shown to be carcinogenic in laboratory animals.

Mutagenesis: The mutagenic potential of lidocaine HCl has been tested in the Ames Salmonella/mammalian microsome test and by analysis of structural chromosome aberrations in human lymphocytes *in vitro,* and by mouse micronucleus test *in vivo.* There was no indication in these tests of any mutagenic effects. The mutagenicity of 2,6-xylidine, a metabolite of lidocaine, has been studied in different tests with mixed results. The compound was found to be weakly mutagenic in the Ames test only under metabolic activation conditions. In addition, 2,6-xylidine was observed to be mutagenic at the thymidine kinase locus, with or without activation, and induced chromosome aberrations and sister chromatic exchanges at concentrations at which the drug precipitated out of the solution (1.2 mg/mL). No evidence of genotoxicity was found in the *in vivo* assays measuring unscheduled DNA synthesis in rat hepatocytes, chromosome damage in polychromatic erythrocytes or preferential killing of DNA repair-deficient bacteria in liver, lung, kidney, testes and blood extracts from mice. However, covalent binding studies of DNA from liver and ethmoid turbinates in rats indicate that 2,6-xylidine may be genotoxic under certain conditions *in vivo.*

Impairment of Fertility: See Use in Pregnancy

Use in Pregnancy:

Teratogenic Effects: Pregnancy Category B. There are no adequate and well-controlled studies in pregnant women. Because animal reproduction studies are not always predictive of human response, ELA-Max5 Anorectal Cream should be used during pregnancy only if clearly needed.

Labor and Delivery: Lidocaine is not contraindicated in labor and delivery. Should ELA-Max5 Anorectal Cream be used concomitantly with other products containing lidocaine, total doses contributed by all formulations must be considered.

Nursing Mothers: Lidocaine is excreted in human milk. Therefore, caution should be exercised when ELA-Max5 Anorectal Cream is administered to a nursing mother since the milk:plasma ratio of lidocaine is 0.4.

Pediatric Use: Consult a doctor prior to use on children under 12 years of age. When using ELA-Max5 Anorectal Cream in young children, care must be taken to insure that application of the cream is limited to the intended site (see DOSAGE AND ADMINISTRATION). Accidental ingestion may lead to dose related toxicity.

ADVERSE REACTIONS

Localized reactions: During or immediately after treatment with ELA-Max5 Anorectal Cream, the skin at the site of treatment may develop erythema or edema or may be the locus of abnormal sensation.

Allergic Reactions: Allergic and anaphylactoid reactions associated with lidocaine can occur. They are characterized by urticaria, angioedema, bronchospasm, and shock. If they occur they should be managed by conventional means. The detection of sensitivity by skin testing is of doubtful value.

System (Dose Related) Reactions: Systemic adverse reactions following appropriate use of ELA-Max5 Anorectal Cream are unlikely due to the small dose absorbed. Systemic adverse reactions of lidocaine are similar in nature to those observed with other amide local anesthetic agents including CNS excitation and/or depression (light-headedness, nervousness, apprehension, euphoria, confusion, dizziness, drowsiness, tinnitus, blurred or double vision, vomiting, sensations of heat, cold or numbness, twitching, tremors, convulsions, unconsciousness, respiratory depression and arrest). Excitatory CNS reactions may be brief or not occur at all, in which case the first manifestation may be drowsiness merging into unconsciousness. Cardiovascular manifestations may include bradycardia, hypotension, and cardiovascular collapse leading to arrest.

OVERDOSAGE

Peak blood levels following a 60g application to 400 cm^2 for 3 hours are 0.05 to 0.16 µg/mL for lidocaine. Toxic levels of lidocaine (>5 µg/mL) cause decreases in cardiac output, total peripheral resistance and mean arterial pressure. These changes may be attributable to direct depressant effects of these local anesthetic agents on the cardiovascular system. In the absence of massive topical overdose or oral ingestion, evaluation should include other etiologies for the clinical effects of overdosage from other sources of lidocaine or other local anesthetics.

DOSAGE AND ADMINISTRATION

A thick layer of ELA-Max5 Anorectal Cream is applied to intact skin. A single application of ELA-Max5 Anorectal Cream in a child weighing less than 10 kg should not be applied over an area larger than 100 cm^2 A single application of ELA-Max5 Anorectal Cream in children weighing between 10 kg and 20 kg should not be applied over an area larger than 100 cm^2.

When applying ELA-Max5 Anorectal Cream to young children, care must be taken to maintain careful observation of the child to prevent accidental ingestion of ELA-Max5 Anorectal Cream.

When ELA-Max5 Anorectal Cream (lidocaine 5%) is used concomitantly with other products containing local anesthetic agents, the amount absorbed from all formulations must be considered. The amount absorbed in the case of ELA-Max5 Anorectal Cream is determined by the area over which it is applied and the duration of application. Although the incidence of systemic adverse reactions with ELA-Max5 Anorectal Cream is very low, caution should be exercised, particularly when applying it over large areas and leaving it on for longer than 2 hours. The incidence of systemic adverse reactions can be expected to be directly proportional to the area and time of exposure.

HOW SUPPLIED

ELA-Max5 Anorectal Cream is available as the following:
NDC 0496-0824-30 30 gram tube

Store between 15° and 30°C (59°–86°F).

Caution: Federal Law Prohibits Dispensing Without Prescription.

NOT FOR OPHTHALMIC USE.

KEEP CONTAINER TIGHTLY CLOSED AT ALL TIMES WHEN NOT IN USE.

Manufactured Jointly by:
Ferndale Laboratories, Inc.
Ferndale, MI 48220 and
BioZone Laboratories, Inc.
Pittsburg, CA 94565
ELA-MAX is a trademark of
Ferndale Laboratories, Inc.
©Ferndale Laboratories, Inc.
MG #13351 Iss: 09/97

Continued on next page

KRONOFED–A® Kronocaps ℞
KRONOFED–A–JR® Kronocaps ℞

Each sustained release Kronofed A®, white and clear capsule contains:

Pseudoephedrine HCl .... 120 mg
Chlorpheniramine Maleate .... 8 mg
Each sustained release Kronofed-A-Jr®, white and clear capsule contains:
Pseudoephedrine HCl .... 60 mg
Chlorpheniramine Maleate .... 4 mg

INDICATIONS

For temporary relief of upper respiratory and nasal congestion associated with the common cold, hay fever and allergies, sinusitis and vasomotor and allergic rhinitis.

CONTRAINDICATIONS

Severe hypertension or severe cardiac disease. Sensitivity to antihistamines or sympathomimetic agents.

PRECAUTIONS

Use with caution in patients with hyperthyroidism. Patients susceptible to the soporific effects of chlorpheniramine should be warned against driving or operating of machinery which requires complete mental alertness.

PREGNANCY

Pregnancy Category C: Animal reproduction studies have not been conducted with **KRONOFED-A®** medications. It is also not known whether **KRONOFED-A®** medications can cause fetal harm when administered to a pregnant woman or can affect reproduction capacity. **KRONOFED-A®** medications should be given to a pregnant woman only if clearly needed.

Nursing Mothers: Due to the possible passage of pseudoephedrine and chlorpheniramine into breast milk, and, because of the higher than usual risk for infants from sympathomimetic amines and antihistamines, the benefit to the mother vs. the potential risk should be considered and a decision should be made whether to discontinue nursing or to discontinue the drug.

CAUTION

Federal law prohibits dispensing without prescription.

DOSAGE

Kronofed-A® Capsules: Adults and children over 12 years of age—1 capsule every 12 hours. **Kronofed-A-JR®** Capsules: Children 6–12 years of age—1 capsule every 12 hours. Adults 1 or 2 capsules every 12 hours.

HOW SUPPLIED

Kronofed-A® Kronocaps
Bottles of 100 NDC 0496–0382–02
Bottles of 500 NDC 0496–0382–10

Kronofed-A-Jr® Kronocaps
Bottles of 100 NDC 0496–0434–02
Bottles of 500 NDC 0496–0434–10

LOCOID® ℞
(hydrocortisone butyrate)
Cream 0.1%
Ointment 0.1%
Topical Solution 0.1%

CAUTION: Federal law prohibits dispensing without prescription.

DESCRIPTION

LOCOID® cream, ointment and topical solution contain the topical corticosteroid, hydrocortisone butyrate, a non-fluorinated hydrocortisone ester. It has the chemical name: pregn-4-ene-3, 20-dione, 11, 21-dihydroxy-17-[(1-oxobutyl)oxy-,(11β)-; the molecular formula: $C_{25}H_{36}O_6$; the molecular weight: 432.54; and the CAS registry number: 13609-67-1. Its structural formula is:

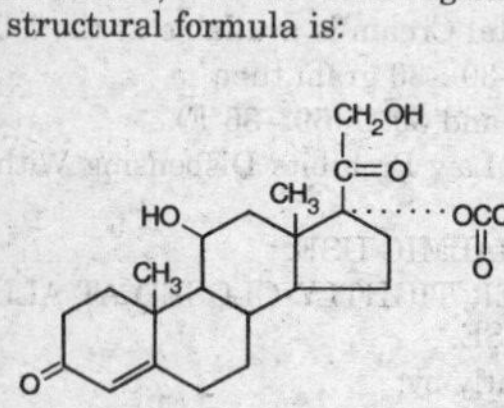

LOCOID® Cream 0.1%
Each gram of LOCOID® cream contains 1 mg of hydrocortisone butyrate in a hydrophilic base consisting of cetostearyl alcohol, ceteth-20, mineral oil, white petrolatum, citric acid, sodium citrate, propylparaben and butylparaben (preservatives) and purified water.

LOCOID® Ointment 0.1%
Each gram of LOCOID® ointment contains 1 mg of hydrocortisone butyrate in a base consisting of mineral oil and polyethylene.

LOCOID® Solution 0.1%
Each mL of LOCOID® solution contains 1 mg of hydrocortisone butyrate in a vehicle consisting of isopropyl alcohol (50%), glycerin, povidone, citric acid, sodium citrate and purified water.

CLINICAL PHARMACOLOGY

Topical corticosteroids share anti-inflammatory, anti-pruritic and vasoconstrictive actions.

The mechanism of anti-inflammatory activity of the topical corticosteroids is unclear. Various laboratory methods, including vasoconstrictor assays, are used to compare and predict potencies and/or clinical efficacies of the topical corticosteroids. There is some evidence to suggest that a recognizable correlation exists between vasoconstrictor potency and therapeutic efficacy in man.

Pharmacokinetics
The extent of percutaneous absorption of topical corticosteroids is determined by many factors including the vehicle, the integrity of the epidermal barrier, and the use of occlusive dressings.

Topical corticosteroids can be absorbed from normal intact skin. Inflammation and/or other disease processes in the skin increase percutaneous absorption. Occlusive dressings substantially increase the percutaneous absorption of topical corticosteroids. Thus, occlusive dressings may be a valuable therapeutic adjunct for treatment of resistant dermatoses. (See DOSAGE AND ADMINISTRATION.)

Once absorbed through the skin, topical corticosteroids are handled through pharmacokinetic pathways similar to systemically administered corticosteroids. Corticosteroids are bound to plasma proteins in varying degrees. Corticosteroids are metabolized primarily in the liver and are then excreted by the kidneys. Some of the topical corticosteroids and their metabolites are also excreted into the bile.

INDICATIONS AND USAGE

LOCOID® cream 0.1% and ointment 0.1% (hydrocortisone butyrate) are indicated for the relief of the inflammatory and pruritic manifestations of corticosteroid-responsive dermatoses.

LOCOID® solution 0.1% (hydrocortisone butyrate) is indicated for the relief of the inflammatory and pruritic manifestations of seborrheic dermatitis.

CONTRAINDICATIONS

Topical corticosteroids are contraindicated in those patients with a history of hypersensitivity to any of the components of the preparation.

PRECAUTIONS

General: Systemic absorption of topical corticosteroids has produced reversible hypothalamic-pituitary-adrenal (HPA) axis suppression, manifestations of Cushing's syndrome, hyperglycemia, and glucosuria in some patients. Conditions which augment systemic absorption include the application of the more potent steroids, use over large surface areas, prolonged use, and the addition of occlusive dressings.

Therefore, patients receiving a large dose of a potent topical steroid applied to a large surface area or under an occlusive dressing should be evaluated periodically for evidence of HPA axis suppression by using the urinary free cortisol and ACTH stimulation tests. If HPA axis suppression is noted, an attempt should be made to withdraw the drug, to reduce the frequency of application, or to substitute a less potent steroid.

Recovery of HPA axis function is generally prompt and complete upon discontinuation of the drug. Infrequently, signs and symptoms of steroid withdrawal may occur, requiring supplemental systemic corticosteroids.

Children may absorb proportionally larger amounts of topical corticosteroids and thus be more susceptible to systemic toxicity (See PRECAUTIONS—PEDIATRIC USE.)

If irritation develops, topical corticosteroids should be discontinued and appropriate therapy instituted. In the presence of dermatological infections, the use of an appropriate antifungal or antibacterial agent should be instituted. If a favorable response does not occur promptly, the corticosteroid should be discontinued until the infection has been adequately controlled.

Information for the patient
Patients using topical corticosteroids should receive the following information and instructions:

1. This medication is to be used as directed by the physician. It is for external use only. Avoid contact with the eyes.
2. Patients should be advised not to use this medication for any disorder other than for which it was prescribed.
3. The treated skin area should not be bandaged or otherwise covered or wrapped as to be occlusive unless directed by the physician.
4. Patients should report any signs of local adverse reactions especially under occlusive dressing.
5. Parents of pediatric patients should be advised not to use tight-fitting diapers or plastic pants on a child being treated in the diaper area, as these garments may constitute occlusive dressings.

Laboratory tests
The following tests may be helpful in evaluating the HPA axis suppression:
Urinary free cortisol test
ACTH stimulation test

Carcinogenesis, Mutagenesis, and Impairment of Fertility
Long-term animal studies have not been performed to evaluate the carcinogenic potential or the effect on fertility of topical corticosteroids.

Studies to determine mutagenicity with prednisolone and hydrocortisone have revealed negative results.

Pregnancy Category C
Corticosteroids are generally teratogenic in laboratory animals when administered systemically at relatively low dosage levels. The more potent corticosteroids have been shown to be teratogenic after dermal application in laboratory animals. There are no adequate and well-controlled studies in pregnant women on teratogenic effects from topically applied corticosteroids. Therefore, topical corticosteroids should be used during pregnancy only if the potential benefit justifies the potential risk to the fetus. Drugs of this class should not be used extensively on pregnant patients, in large amounts, or for prolonged periods of time.

Nursing Mothers
It is not known whether topical administration of corticosteroids could result in sufficient systemic absorption to produce detectable quantities in breast milk. Systemically administered corticosteroids are secreted into breast milk, in quantities not likely to have a deleterious effect on the infant. Nevertheless, caution should be exercised when topical corticosteroids are administered to a nursing woman.

Pediatric Use
Pediatric patients may demonstrate greater susceptibility to topical corticosteroid-induced HPA axis suppression and Cushing's syndrome than mature patients because of a larger skin surface area to body weight ratio.

Hypothalamic-pituitary-adrenal (HPA) axis suppression, Cushing's syndrome, and intracranial hypertension have been reported in children receiving topical corticosteroids. Manifestations of adrenal suppression in children include linear growth retardation, delayed weight gain, low plasma cortisol levels, and absence of response to ACTH stimulation. Manifestations of intracranial hypertension include bulging fontanelles, headaches, and bilateral papilledema.

Administration of topical corticosteroids to children should be limited to the least amount compatible with an effective therapeutic regimen. Chronic corticosteroid therapy may interfere with the growth and development of children.

ADVERSE REACTIONS

The following local adverse reactions are reported infrequently with topical corticosteroids, but may occur more frequently with the use of occlusive dressings. These reactions are listed in an approximate decreasing order of occurrence: burning, itching, irritation, dryness, folliculitis, hypertrichosis, acneiform eruptions, hypopigmentation, perioral dermatitis, allergic contact dermatitis, maceration of the skin, secondary infection, skin atrophy, striae, miliaria.

OVERDOSAGE

Topically applied corticosteroids can be absorbed in sufficient amounts to produce systemic effects. (See PRECAUTIONS.)

DOSAGE AND ADMINISTRATION

LOCOID® cream 0.1% or LOCOID® ointment 0.1% (hydrocortisone butyrate) should be applied to the affected area as a thin film two to three times daily depending on the severity of the condition.

Occlusive dressings may be used for the management of psoriasis or recalcitrant conditions.

If an infection develops, the use of occlusive dressings should be discontinued and appropriate antimicrobial therapy instituted.

LOCOID® solution 0.1% (hydrocortisone butyrate) should be applied to the affected area as a thin film from two to three times daily depending on the severity of the condition.

HOW SUPPLIED

LOCOID® cream 0.1% (hydrocortisone butyrate) is supplied in tubes containing:
15 g NDC 0496-0802-15
45 g NDC 0496-0802-45

LOCOID® ointment 0.1% (hydrocortisone butyrate) is supplied in tubes containing:
15 g NDC 0496-0803-15
45 g NDC 0496-0803-45

LOCOID® solution 0.1% (hydrocortisone butyrate) is supplied in polyethylene bottles:
30 mL NDC 0496-0804-30
60 mL NDC 0496-0804-60

STORAGE

LOCOID® cream 0.1%: Store between 59° and 77°F (15° and 25°C).

LOCOID® ointment 0.1%: Store between 36°and 86°F (2°and 30°C).

LOCOID® solution 0.1%: Store between 41°and 77°F (5°and 25°C).

MARKETED BY:
FERNDALE LABORATORIES, INC.
FERNDALE, MICHIGAN 48220
MANUFACTURED BY:
Yamanouchi Europe bv
Leiderdorp/Netherlands
Revised: October 1996

LOCOID LIPOCREAM® CREAM ℞
[lō'coĭd lĭpō'-cream]
(hydrocortisone butyrate cream)

For Dermatological Use Only

DESCRIPTION
LOCOID Lipocream® Cream contains the topical corticosteroid hydrocortisone butyrate, a hydrocortisone ester. It has the chemical name: (11β)-11,21-dihydroxy-17-[(1-oxobutyl)oxy]-pregn-4-ene-3,20-dione; the molecular formula: $C_{25}H_{36}O_6$; the molecular weight: 432.54; and the CAS registry number: 13609-67-1. The structural formula is:

LOCOID Lipocream® Cream, 0.1%
Each gram of LOCOID Lipocream® Cream contains 1 mg of hydrocortisone butyrate in a hydrophilic base consisting of cetostearyl alcohol, ceteth-20, mineral oil, white petrolatum, citric acid, sodium citrate, propyl paraben and butyl paraben (preservatives) and purified water.

CLINICAL PHARMACOLOGY
Topical corticosteroids share anti-inflammatory, anti-pruritic and vasoconstrictive actions. The mechanism of anti-inflammatory activity of the topical corticosteroids is unclear. Various laboratory methods, including vasoconstrictor assays, are used to compare and predict potencies and/or clinical efficacies of the topical corticosteroids. There is some evidence to suggest that a recognizable correlation exists between vasoconstrictor potency and therapeutic efficacy in man.

PHARMACOKINETICS
The extent of percutaneous absorption of topical corticosteroids is determined by many factors including the vehicle, the integrity of the epidermal barrier, and the use of occlusive dressings.
Topical corticosteroids can be absorbed from normal intact skin. Inflammation and/or other disease processes in the skin increase percutaneous absorption. Occlusive dressings or widespread application may increase the possibility of hypothalamic-pituitary-adrenal (HPA) axis suppression.
The vasoconstrictor assay showed that LOCOID Lipocream® Cream has a more pronounced skin blanching effect than LOCOID® Cream, suggesting greater percutaneous absorption from the former. At the present time, no adequate HPA axis suppression studies have been conducted for LOCOID Lipocream® Cream. Once absorbed through the skin, topical corticosteroids are handled through pharmacokinetic pathways similar to systemically administered corticosteroids. Corticosteroids are bound to plasma proteins in varying degrees.
Corticosteroids are metabolized primarily in the liver and are then excreted by the kidneys. Some of the topical corticosteroids and their metabolites are also excreted in the bile.

INDICATIONS AND USAGE
LOCOID Lipocream® Cream 0.1% (hydrocortisone butyrate cream) is indicated for the relief of the inflammatory and pruritic manifestations of corticosteroid-responsive dermatoses.

CONTRAINDICATIONS
Topical corticosteroids are contraindicated in those patients with a history of hypersensitivity to any of the components of the preparation.

PRECAUTIONS
General
Systemic absorption of topical corticosteroids has produced reversible HPA axis suppression, manifestations of Cushing's syndrome, hyperglycemia, and glucosuria in some patients.
Conditions which increase the risk of systemic toxicity include the application of the more potent steroids, use over large surface areas, prolonged use, and the addition of occlusive dressings.

Children may absorb proportionally larger amounts of topical corticosteroids and thus be more susceptible to systemic toxicity. (See PRECAUTIONS — PEDIATRIC USE).
If irritation develops, topical corticosteroids should be discontinued and appropriate therapy instituted. In the presence of dermatological infections, the use of an appropriate antifungal or antibacterial agent should be instituted. If a favorable response does not occur promptly, the corticosteroid should be discontinued until the infection has been adequately controlled.

Information for the Patient
Patients using topical corticosteroids should receive the following information and instructions:
1. This medication is to be used as directed by the physician. It is for external use only. Avoid contact with the eyes.
2. Patients should be advised not to use this medication for any disorder other than for which it was prescribed.
3. The treated skin area should not be bandaged or otherwise covered or wrapped as to be occlusive.
4. Patients should report any signs of local adverse reactions.
5. Parents of pediatric patients should be advised not to use tight-fitting diapers or plastic pants on a child being treated in the diaper area, as these garments may constitute occlusive dressings.

Laboratory Tests
The following tests may be helpful in evaluating the HPA axis suppression:
Urinary free cortisol test
ACTH stimulation test

Carcinogenesis, Mutagenesis, and Impairment of Fertility
Long-term animal studies have not been performed to evaluate the carcinogenic potential or the effect on fertility of topical corticosteroids.
Studies to determine mutagenicity in *Salmonella ryphimurium* strains TA98, TA100, and TA92 with prednisolone and hydrocortisone have revealed negative results.

Pregnancy: Teratogenic Effects:
Pregnancy Category C:
Corticosteroids are generally teratogenic in laboratory animals when administered systemically at relatively low dosage levels. Some corticosteroids have been shown to be teratogenic after dermal application in laboratory animals. In teratogenicity studies, topical administration of 1% or 10% hydrocortisone butyrate in a ointment to pregnant Wistar rats (gestational days 6–15) or New Zealand white rabbits (gestational days 6–18) resulted in no teratogenic findings. However, a dose-dependent increase in fetal resorptions was reported in rabbits, and fetal resorptions were observed in rats treated with 10% hydrocortisone butyrate.
The doses given to rats are approximately 8 to 80 times the human topical dose based on a body surface area comparison (assuming 100% absorption). For rabbits, the doses given were approximately 0.2 and 2 times the human topical dose. Increased resorptions were also noted in Wistar rats given subcutaneous administrations of hydrocortisone butyrate (9mg/kg/day; 3 times the human topical dose) on gestational days 9 through 15. In CS mice given subcutaneously administrations of 1mg/kg/day (0.2 times the human topical dose), an increased number of cervical ribs and one fetus with clubbed legs was reported. There are no adequate and well-controlled studies in pregnant women on teratogenic effects from topically applied corticosteroids. Therefore, topical corticosteroids should be used during pregnancy only if the potential benefit justifies the potential risk to the fetus. LOCOID Lipocream® Cream 0.1% (hydrocortisone butyrate cream) should not be used extensively on pregnant patients, in large amounts, or for longer than two weeks.

Nursing Mothers
It is not known whether topical administration of corticosteroids could result in sufficient systemic absorption to produce detectable quantities in breast milk.
Systemically administered corticosteroids are secreted into breast milk in quantities *not* likely to have a deleterious effect on the infant. Nevertheless, caution should be exercised when topical corticosteroids are administered to a nursing woman.

Pediatric Use
Safety and effectiveness in pediatric patients have not been established.
Pediatric patients may demonstrate greater susceptibility to topical corticosteroid-induced HPA axis suppression and Cushing's syndrome than mature patients because of a larger skin surface area to body weight ratio.
HPA axis suppression, Cushing's syndrome, and intracranial hypertension have been reported in children receiving topical corticosteroids.
Manifestations of adrenal suppression in children include linear growth retardation, delayed weight gain, low plasma cortisol levels, and absence of response to ACTH stimulation. Manifestations of intracranial hypertension include bulging fontanelles, headaches, and bilateral papilledema. Chronic corticosteroid therapy may interfere with the growth and development of children.

ADVERSE REACTIONS
The following local adverse reactions are reported infrequently with topical corticosteroids but may occur more frequently with the use of occlusive dressings. These reactions are listed in an approximate decreasing order of occurrence: burning, itching, irritation, dryness, folliculitis, hypertrichosis, acneiform eruptions, hypopigmentation, perioral dermatitis, allergic contact dermatitis, maceration of the skin, secondary infection, skin atrophy, striae and miliaria.

OVERDOSAGE
Topically applied corticosteroids can be absorbed in sufficient amounts to produce systemic effects. (See PRECAUTIONS).

DOSAGE AND ADMINISTRATION
LOCOID Lipocream® Cream 0.1% (hydrocortisone butyrate cream) should be applied to the affected area as a thin film two or three times daily (depending on the severity of the condition) and for no longer than two weeks.
If an infection develops, appropriate antimicrobial therapy should be instituted.

HOW SUPPLIED
LOCOID Lipocream® Cream 0.1% (hydrocortisone butyrate cream) is supplied in tubes containing:
15 g NDC 0496-0821-15
45 g NDC 0496-0821-45

STORAGE
Store at controlled room temperature between 59° and 77°F (15° and 25°C).

CAUTION
Federal law prohibits dispensing without prescription.

Marketed by:
FERNDALE LABORATORIES, INC.
Ferndale, Michigan 48220 USA
U.S. Patent No. 5,635,497
Manufactured by:
Yamanouchi Europe B.V.
Leiderdorp/The Netherlands

12143004/1
(010997)

PRAMOSONE® CREAM, LOTION AND OINTMENT ℞

DESCRIPTION
Pramosone® Cream: Contains Hydrocortisone acetate 1% or 2.5% and Pramoxine HCl 1% in a hydrophilic base containing stearic acid, cetyl alcohol, aquaphor, isopropyl palmitate, polyoxyl 40 stearate, propylene glycol, potassium sorbate, sorbic acid, triethanolamine lauryl sulfate and water.
Pramosone® Lotion: Contains Hydrocortisone acetate 1% or 2.5% and Pramoxine HCl 1% in a base containing forlan-L, cetyl alcohol, stearic acid, di-isopropyl adipate, polyoxyl 40 stearate, silicone, triethanolamine, glycerine, polyvinylpyrolidone, potassium sorbate, sorbic acid and water.
Pramosone® Ointment: Contains Hydrocortisone acetate 1% or 2.5% and Pramoxine HCl 1% in an emollient ointment base containing Sorbitan sesquioleate, Water, Aquaphor and White petrolatum.
Topical corticosteroids are anti-inflammatory and antipruritic agents. The structural formula, the chemical name, molecular formula and molecular weight for active ingredients are presented below.

Hydrocortisone acetate
(Pregn-4-ene-3,20-dione,21-(acetyloxy)-11, 17-dihydroxy-,(11 β)-.)
$C_{23}H_{32}O_6$; mol wt: 404.50

Pramoxine hydrochloride
(4-(3-(p-butoxyphenoxy)propyl)morpholine hydrochloride)
$C_{17}H_{27}NO_3 \cdot HCl$; mol wt: 329.87

CLINICAL PHARMACOLOGY
Topical corticosteroids share anti-inflammatory, anti-pruritic and vasoconstrictive actions.

Continued on next page

Pramosone—Cont.

The mechanism of anti-inflammatory activity of the topical corticosteroids is unclear. Various laboratory methods, including vasoconstrictor assays, are used to compare and predict potencies and/or clinical efficacies of the topical corticosteroids. There is some evidence to suggest that a recognizable correlation exists between vasoconstrictor potency and therapeutic efficacy in man.

Pramoxine hydrochloride is a topical anesthetic agent which provides temporary relief from itching and pain. It acts by stabilizing the neuronal membrane of nerve endings with which it comes into contact.

Pharmacokinetics: The extent of percutaneous absorption of topical corticosteroids is determined by many factors including the vehicle, the integrity of the epidermal barrier, and the use of occlusive dressings.

Topical corticosteroids can be absorbed from normal intact skin. Inflammation and/or other disease processes in the skin increase percutaneous absorption. Occlusive dressings substantially increase the percutaneous absorption of topical corticosteroids. Thus, occlusive dressings may be a valuable therapeutic adjunct for treatment of resistant dermatoses (See DOSAGE AND ADMINISTRATION).

Once absorbed through the skin, topical corticosteroids are handled through pharmacokinetic pathways similar to systemically administered corticosteroids. Corticosteroids are bound to plasma proteins in varying degrees. Corticosteroids are metabolized primarily in the liver and are then excreted by the kidneys. Some of the topical corticosteroids and their metabolites are also excreted into the bile.

INDICATIONS AND USAGE

Topical corticosteroids are indicated for the relief of the inflammatory and pruritic manifestations of corticosteroid-responsive dermatoses.

CONTRAINDICATIONS

Topical corticosteroids are contraindicated in those patients with a history of hypersensitivity to any of the components of the preparation.

PRECAUTIONS

General: Systemic absorption of topical corticosteroids has produced reversible hypothalamic-pituitary-adrenal (HPA) axis suppression, manifestations of Cushing's syndrome, hyperglycemia, and glucosuria in some patients.

Conditions which augment systemic absorption include the application of the more potent steroids, use over large surface areas, prolonged use, and the addition of occlusive dressings.

Therefore, patients receiving a large dose of a potent topical steroid applied to a large surface area and under an occlusive dressing should be evaluated periodically for evidence of HPA axis suppression by using the urinary free cortisol and ACTH stimulation tests. If HPA axis suppression is noted, an attempt should be made to withdraw the drug, to reduce the frequency of application, or to substitute a less potent steroid.

Recovery of HPA axis function is generally prompt and complete upon discontinuation of the drug. Infrequently, signs and symptoms of steroid withdrawal may occur, requiring supplemental systemic corticosteroids.

Children may absorb proportionally larger amounts of topical corticosteroids and thus be more susceptible to systemic toxicity. (See PRECAUTIONS—Pediatric Use).

If irritation develops, topical corticosteroids should be discontinued and appropriate therapy instituted.

In the presence of dermatological infections, the use of an appropriate antifungal or antibacterial agent should be instituted. If a favorable response does not occur promptly, the corticosteroid should be discontinued until the infection has been adequately controlled.

Information for the Patient: Patients using topical corticosteroids should receive the following information and instructions:

1. This medication is to be used as directed by the physician. It is for external use only. Avoid contact with the eyes.
2. Patients should be advised not to use this medication for any disorder other than for which it was prescribed.
3. The treated skin area should not be bandaged or otherwise covered or wrapped as to be occlusive unless directed by the physician.
4. Patients should report any signs of local adverse reactions especially under occlusive dressing.
5. Parents of pediatric patients should be advised not to use tightfitting diapers or plastic pants on a child being treated in the diaper area, as these garments may constitute occlusive dressings.

Laboratory Tests: The following tests may be helpful in evaluating the HPA axis suppression:

Urinary free cortisol test
ACTH stimulation test

Carcinogenesis, Mutagenesis, and Impairment of Fertility: Long-term animal studies have not been performed to evaluate the carcinogenic potential or the effect on fertility of topical corticosteroids.

Studies to determine mutagenicity with prednisolone and hydrocortisone have revealed negative results.

Pregnancy Category C: Corticosteroids are generally teratogenic in laboratory animals when administered systemically at relatively low dosage levels. The more potent corticosteroids have been shown to be teratogenic after dermal application in laboratory animals. There are no adequate and well-controlled studies in pregnant women on teratogenic effects from topically applied corticosteroids. Therefore, topical corticosteroids should be used during pregnancy only if the potential benefit justifies the potential risk to the fetus. Drugs of this class should not be used extensively on pregnant patients, in large amounts, or for prolonged periods of time.

Nursing Mothers: It is not known whether topical administration of corticosteroids could result in sufficient systemic absorption to produce detectable amounts in breast milk. Systemically administered corticosteroids are secreted into breast milk in quantities NOT likely to have a deleterious effect on the infant. Nevertheless, caution should be exercised when topical corticosteroids are administered to a nursing woman.

Pediatric Use: PEDIATRIC PATIENTS MAY DEMONSTRATE GREATER SUSCEPTIBILITY TO TOPICAL CORTICOSTEROID-INDUCED HPA AXIS SUPPRESSION AND CUSHING'S SYNDROME THAN MATURE PATIENTS BECAUSE OF A LARGER SKIN SURFACE AREA TO BODY WEIGHT RATIO.

Hypothalamic-pituitary-adrenal (HPA) axis suppression, Cushing's syndrome, and intracranial hypertension have been reported in children receiving topical corticosteroids. Manifestations of adrenal suppression in children include linear growth retardation, delayed weight gain, low plasma cortisol levels, and absence of response to ACTH stimulation. Manifestations of intracranial hypertension include bulging fontanelles, headaches, and bilateral papilledema. Administration of topical corticosteroids to children should be limited to the least amount compatible with an effective therapeutic regimen. Chronic corticosteroid therapy may interfere with the growth and development of children.

ADVERSE REACTIONS

The following local adverse reactions are reported infrequently with topical corticosteroids, but may occur more frequently with the use of occlusive dressings. These reactions are listed in an approximate decreasing order of occurrence:

Burning	Hypopigmentation
Itching	Perioral dermatitis
Irritation	Allergic contact dermatitis
Dryness	Maceration of the skin
Folliculitis	Secondary infection
Hypertrichosis	Skin Atrophy
Acneiform eruptions	Striae
	Miliaria

OVERDOSAGE

Topically applied corticosteroids can be absorbed in sufficient amounts to produce systemic effects (See PRECAUTIONS).

DOSAGE AND ADMINISTRATION

Topical corticosteroids are generally applied to the affected area as a thin film three or four times daily depending on the severity of the condition.

Occlusive dressings may be used for the management of psoriasis or recalcitrant conditions. If an infection develops, the use of occlusive dressings should be discontinued and appropriate antimicrobial therapy instituted.

HOW SUPPLIED

CREAM:	1%	1 oz Tube	NDC 0496-0716-04
		2 oz Tube	NDC 0496-0716-03
	2.5%	1 oz Tube	NDC 0496-0717-04
		2 oz Tube	NDC 0496-0717-03
LOTION:	1%	2 fl oz	NDC 0496-0729-06
		4 fl oz	NDC 0496-0729-04
		8 fl oz	NDC 0496-0729-03
	2.5%	2 fl oz	NDC 0496-0726-06
		4 fl oz	NDC 0496-0726-04
OINTMENT:	1%	1 oz Tube	NDC 0496-0763-04
	2.5%	1 oz Tube	NDC 0496-0777-04

Dispense in a tight container as defined in the official compendium.

Store at controlled room temperature 15°–30°C (59°–86°F).

PRAX® LOTION* OTC
(Pramoxine HCl 1% in an emollient hydrophilic base)

HOW SUPPLIED

Prax® Lotion is supplied in dispenser bottles containing
4 fl oz NDC 0496-0748-04
8 fl oz NDC 0496-0748-03

*Additional information available upon request.

PRO-Q™ Skin Protectant OTC

Pro-Q™ is a revolutionary topical preparation designed to fortify the skin's natural capacity to protect the body from the destructive effects of external irritants and sensitizers.

HOW SUPPLIED

Pro-Q™ is supplied in canisters containing
35 ml NDC 0496-0842-01
75 ml NDC 0496-0842-02
161 ml NDC 0496-0842-05

SBR-LIPOCREAM™ OTC

SBR-Lipocream™ is specially designed to help repair and maintain the body's natural skin barrier function. SBR-Lipocream™ is for patients with sensitive skin or skin that is predisposed to chronic skin disease and irritation.

HOW SUPPLIED

SBR-Lipocream™ is supplied in tubes containing
100 g NDC 0496-0819-01

Ferring Pharmaceuticals Inc.
120 WHITE PLAINS ROAD, SUITE #400
TARRYTOWN, NY 10591

Direct Inquiries to:
Ferring Pharmaceuticals Inc.
Customer Service Department
120 White Plains Road, Suite #400
Tarrytown, NY 10591
1-(888)-FERRING (337-7464)

For Medical Information Contact:
In Emergencies:
Ferring Pharmaceuticals Inc.
Professional Services Department
120 White Plains Road, Suite #400
Tarrytown, NY 10591
(800) 822-8214

ACTHREL® ℞
(corticorelin ovine triflutate for injection)
For intravenous injection only
DIAGNOSTIC USE ONLY

DESCRIPTION

ACTHREL® (corticorelin ovine triflutate for injection) is a sterile, nonpyrogenic, lyophilized white cake powder, containing corticorelin ovine triflutate, a trifluoroacetate salt of a synthetic peptide that is used for the determination of pituitary corticotroph responsiveness. Corticorelin ovine has an amino acid sequence identical to ovine corticotropin-releasing hormone (oCRH). Corticorelin ovine is an analogue of the naturally occurring human CRH (hCRH) peptide. Both peptides are potent stimulators of adrenocorticotropic hormone (ACTH) release from the anterior pituitary. ACTH stimulates cortisol production from the adrenal cortex. The structural formula for corticorelin ovine triflutate is described below:

Ser-Gln-Glu-Pro-Pro-Ile-Ser-Leu-Asp-Leu-Thr-Phe-His-Leu-Leu-Arg-Glu-Val-Leu-Glu-Met-Thr-Lys-Ala-Asp-Gln-Leu-Ala-Gln-Gln-Ala-His-Ser-Asn-Arg-Lys-Leu-Leu-Asp-Ile-Ala-NH_2 • xCF_3COOH

whereas x= 4–8.

The empirical formula of corticorelin ovine is $C_{205}H_{339}N_{59}O_{63}S$ with a molecular weight of 4670.35 Daltons.

ACTHREL® for Injection is available in vials containing 100 mcg corticorelin ovine (as the trifluoroacetate), 0.88 mg ascorbic acid, 10 mg lactose, and 26 mg cysteine hydrochloride monohydrate. Trace amounts of chloride ion may be present from the manufacturing process. The preparation is intended for intravenous administration.

CLINICAL PHARMACOLOGY

Pharmacodynamics: In normal subjects, intravenous administration of corticorelin results in a rapid and sustained increase of plasma ACTH levels and a near parallel increase of plasma cortisol. In addition, intravenous administration of corticorelin to normal subjects causes a concomitant and prolonged release of the related proopiomelanocortin pep-

tides β- and γ-lipotropins (β- and γ-LPH) and β-endorphin (β-END). A number of dose-response studies have been performed on normal subjects using a range of corticorelin doses. In one study, doses of corticorelin ranging from 0.001 to 30 mcg/kg body weight were administered to 29 healthy volunteers. Blood samples were taken over a 2-hour period for determination of plasma ACTH and cortisol concentrations. There was a direct dose-dependent relationship that was more pronounced for ACTH than for cortisol. The threshold dose was 0.03 mcg/kg, the half-maximal dose was 0.3–1.0 mcg/kg and the maximally effective dose was 3–10 mcg/kg.

Plasma ACTH levels in normal subjects increased 2 minutes after injection of corticorelin doses of ≥0.3 mcg/kg and reached peak levels after 10–15 minutes. Plasma cortisol levels increased within 10 minutes and reached peak levels at 30 to 60 minutes. As the dose of corticorelin was increased, the rises in plasma ACTH and cortisol were more sustained, showing a biphasic response with a second lower peak at 2–3 hours after injection. Similar results were found in another study using 0.3, 3.0, and 30 mcg/kg doses. The duration of mean plasma ACTH increase after injection of 0.3, 3.0, and 30 mcg/kg was 4, 7, and 8 hours, respectively. The effect on plasma cortisol was similar, but more prolonged. Because there are differences in basal levels and peak response levels following a.m. or p.m. administration, it is recommended that subsequent evaluations in the same patient using the corticorelin stimulation test be carried out at the same time of day as the original evaluation.

Baseline ACTH and cortisol levels are usually higher in the morning. Pooled ACTH values from normal unstressed subjects (n=119) were 25 ± 7 pg/mL in the a.m. and 10 ± 3 in the p.m.; similar pooled cortisol values (n=170) were 11 ± 3 mcg/dL in the a.m. and 4 ± 2 mcg/dL in the p.m. The normal unstressed person has about seven to ten secretory episodes of ACTH each day. Most of them occur in the early morning hours and are responsible for the morning plasma cortisol surge. The following figure shows the daily circadian rhythm of ACTH and cortisol secretions in a normal unstressed person. Insulin, plasma renin activity, prolactin, and growth hormone release are not affected by corticorelin administration in humans.

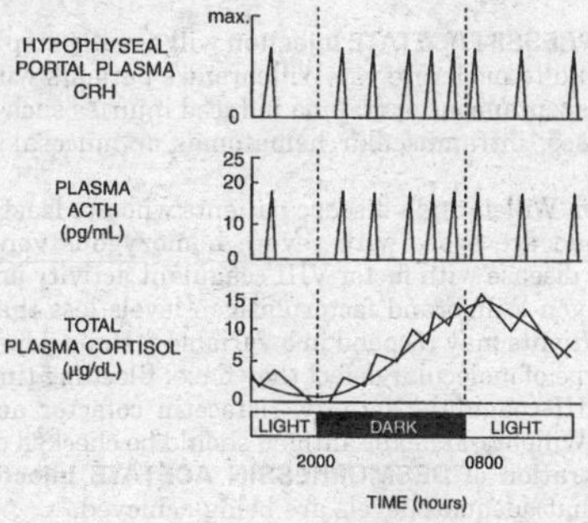

Continuous 24-hour infusion of corticorelin (0.5, 1.0, and 3.0 mcg/kg/hr) increased plasma ACTH concentrations to a plateau of 15–20 pg/mL by the third hour and urinary-free cortisol reaches 173 ± 43 mcg/dL by 24 hours, comparable to those levels observed in patients with major depression, but less than levels noted in Cushing's disease. Continuous infusion did not abolish the circadian rhythm of plasma ACTH and cortisol, but did appear to desensitize the corticotroph. Intermittent doses of corticorelin (25 mcg every 4 hours for 72 hours), however, continued to elicit the expected ACTH and cortisol responses.

Intravenous administration of 1 mcg/kg corticorelin in combination with 10 pressor units intramuscular vasopressin had a synergistic effect on ACTH and a less marked synergistic effect on cortisol secretion.

The basal and peak response levels of ACTH and cortisol to a 1 mcg/kg or 100 mcg dose of corticorelin administered to normal volunteers in the morning and the evening are given below. These values were obtained by combining the results from 9 clinical trials conducted in the a.m. and 4 clinical trials conducted in the p.m.

The following table is to be used only as a general guide.

[See table at top of page]

Pharmacokinetics: Following a single intravenous injection of 1 mcg/kg of corticorelin to normal men, the disappearance of immunoreactive corticorelin (IR-corticorelin) from plasma follows a biexponential decay curve. Plasma half-lives for IR-corticorelin are 11.6 ± 1.5 minutes (mean ± SE) for the fast component and 73 ± 8 minutes for the slow component. The mean volume of distribution for IR-corticorelin is 6.2 ± 0.5 L with an approximate metabolic clearance rate of 95 ± 11 L/m^2/day. Graded intravenous doses of corticorelin (0.01, 0.03, 0.1, 0.3, 1, 3, 10, 30 mcg/kg) produced a linear increase in plasma IR-corticorelin. Corticorelin does not appear to be bound specifically by a circulating plasma protein.

Basal Concentrations and Peak Responses of ACTH and Cortisol in Normal Subjects after 1 mcg/kg or 100 mcg of ACTHREL®

Time of Day	No. of Subjects	ACTH Concentration mean (range) pg/mL		Cortisol Concentration mean (range) mcg/dL	
		Basal	Peak	Basal	Peak
a.m.	143	28 (16-65)	68 (39-114)	11 (8-13)	21 (17-25)
p.m.	70	9 (8-13)	30 (25-42)	4 (2-6)	16 (15-18)

INDICATIONS AND USAGE

ACTHREL® is indicated for use in differentiating pituitary and ectopic production of ACTH in patients with ACTH-dependent Cushing's syndrome.

Differential Diagnosis: There are two forms of Cushing's syndrome:

(a) ACTH-dependent (83%), in which hypercortisolism is due either to pituitary hypersecretion of ACTH (Cushing's disease) resulting from an adenoma (40%, usually microadenomas) or nonadenomatous hyperplasia, possibly of hypothalamic origin (28%), or to hypercortisolism that is secondary to ectopic secretion of ACTH (15%) and,

(b) ACTH-independent (17%), in which hypercortisolism is due to autonomous cortisol secretion by an adrenal tumor (9% adenomas, 8% carcinomas).

After the establishment of hypercortisolism consistent with the presence of Cushing's syndrome, and following the elimination of autonomous adrenal hyperfunction as its cause, the corticorelin test is used to aid in establishing the source of excessive ACTH secretion.

The corticorelin stimulation test helps to differentiate between the etiologies of ACTH-dependent hypercortisolism as follows:

1. High basal plasma ACTH plus high basal plasma cortisol (20–40 mcg/dL).
   ACTHREL® injection (1 mcg/kg) results in:
   a. Increased plasma ACTH levels
   b. Increased plasma cortisol levels
   Diagnosis: Cushing's disease (ACTH of pituitary origin)
2. High basal plasma ACTH (may be very high) plus high basal plasma cortisol (20–40 mcg/dL).
   ACTHREL® injection (1 mcg/kg) results in:
   a. Little or no response of plasma ACTH levels
   b. Little or no response of plasma cortisol levels
   Diagnosis: Ectopic ACTH syndrome

Test Methodology: To evaluate the status of the pituitary-adrenal axis in the differentiation of a pituitary source from an ectopic source of excessive ACTH secretion, a corticorelin test procedure requires a minimum of five blood samples.

Procedure

1. Venous blood samples should be drawn 15 minutes before and immediately prior to ACTHREL® administration. The ACTH baseline is obtained by averaging the values of the two samples.
2. Administer ACTHREL® as an intravenous infusion over a 30- to 60- second interval at a dose of 1 mcg/kg body weight. Higher dosages are not recommended (see **PRECAUTIONS** and **ADVERSE REACTIONS**).
3. Draw venous blood samples at 15, 30, and 60 minutes after administration.
4. Blood samples should be handled as recommended by the laboratory that will determine their ACTH content. It is extremely important to recognize that the reliability of the ACTHREL® test is directly related to the inter-assay and intra-assay variability of the laboratory performing the assay.

Cortisol determinations may be performed on the same blood samples for the same time points as outlined above. The blood sample handling precautions noted for ACTH should be followed for cortisol.

Interpretation of Test Results: The interpretation of the ACTH and cortisol responses following ACTHREL® administration requires a knowledge of the clinical status of the individual patient, understanding of hypothalamic-pituitary-adrenal physiology, and familiarity with the normal hormonal ranges and the standards used by the laboratory that performs the ACTH and cortisol assays.

Cushing's Disease

The results of challenge with corticorelin injection have been reported in approximately 300 patients with Cushing's disease. Although the ACTH and cortisol responses were variable, a hyper-response to corticorelin was seen in a majority of patients, despite high basal cortisol levels. This response pattern indicates an impairment of the negative feedback of cortisol on the pituitary. Patients with pituitary-dependent Cushing's disease tested with corticorelin do not show the negative correlation between basal and stimulated levels of ACTH and cortisol that is found in normal subjects.

A positive correlation between basal ACTH levels and maximum ACTH increments after corticorelin administration has been found in Cushing's disease patients.

Ectopic ACTH Secretion

Patients with Cushing's syndrome due to ectopic ACTH secretion (N=32) were found to have very high basal levels of ACTH and cortisol, which were not further stimulated by corticorelin. However, there have been rare instances of patients with ectopic sources of ACTH that have responded to the corticorelin test.

SUMMARY OF ACTH RESPONSES IN PATIENTS WITH HIGH BASAL CORTISOL

	High ACTH Response	Low ACTH Response
High Basal ACTH	Cushing's Disease	Ectopic ACTH Secretion

CUSHING'S DISEASE ACTH RESPONSES
(mean of 181 patients)
Basal ACTH 63 ± 72 pg/mL (mean ± SD)
Peak ACTH 189 ± 262 pg/mL (mean ± SD)
Mean of individual change from baseline +227%

ECTOPIC ACTH SECRETION RESPONSES
(mean for 31 patients)
Basal ACTH 266 ± 464 pg/mL (mean ± SD)
Peak ACTH 276 ± 466 pg/mL (mean ± SD)
Mean of individual change from baseline +15%

False negative responses to the corticorelin test in Cushing's disease patients occur approximately 5 to 10% of the time, which may lead the clinician to an incorrect diagnosis of ectopic production of ACTH at that frequency. (See **INDICATIONS AND USAGE, Differential Diagnosis**)

PRECAUTIONS

General: The severity of adverse effects to a corticorelin injection appear to be dose-dependent. Dosages above 1 mcg/kg are not recommended. While few adverse effects have been observed at the 1 mcg/kg or 100 mcg dose, higher doses have been associated with transient tachycardia, decreased blood pressure, loss of consciousness, and asystole (see **ADVERSE REACTIONS**). These symptoms can be substantially reduced by administering the drug as a 30-second intravenous infusion instead of a bolus injection. At a dose of 200 mcg corticorelin, 4 of 60 volunteers and patients with disturbances of the hypothalamic-pituitary-adrenal (HPA) axis were reported to have had decreased blood pressures. One patient had a severe hypotensive reaction with asystole. Three other patients had an "absence-like" loss of consciousness lasting approximately 5 minutes. In subsequent investigations by the same researchers over a 3-year period using 100 mcg of corticorelin, one patient in approximately 150 to 200 experienced a severe drop in blood pressure and loss of sinus rhythm after receiving 55 mcg of corticorelin, which may have been due to interaction with heparin. (See **Drug Interactions**)

Drug Interactions: The plasma ACTH response to corticorelin injection is inhibited or blunted in normal subjects pretreated with dexamethasone. The use of a heparin solution to maintain i.v. cannula patency during the corticorelin test is not recommended. A possible interaction between corticorelin and heparin may have been responsible for a major hypotensive reaction that occurred after corticorelin administration. (See **ADVERSE REACTIONS**)

Carcinogenesis, Mutagenesis, Impairment of Fertility: Animal studies have not been conducted with corticorelin to evaluate carcinogenic potential, mutagenicity, or effect on fertility.

Pregnancy (Pregnancy Category C): Animal reproduction studies have not been conducted with corticorelin. It is also not known whether corticorelin can cause fetal harm when administered to a pregnant woman or can affect reproductive capacity. ACTHREL® should be given to a pregnant woman only if clearly needed.

Nursing Mothers: It is not known whether corticorelin is secreted in human milk. Because many drugs are excreted

Continued on next page

Acthrel—Cont.

in human milk, caution should be exercised when ACTHREL® is administered to a nursing woman.

PEDIATRIC USE

Only a few tests have been performed on children. Dosages were 1 mcg/kg body weight. Patient studies have involved only children with multiple hypothalamic and/or pituitary hormone deficiencies, or tumors. Only two studies with normal pediatric subjects have been conducted. No differences in response to the corticorelin test have been reported in the children studied.

ADVERSE REACTIONS

Adverse effects reported with 1 mcg/kg or 100 mcg/patient include flushing of the face, neck, and upper chest (16%; 45/276), beginning almost immediately and lasting 3 to 5 minutes. Recipients have also reported an urge to take a deep breath (6%; 3/49), which occurs with a timing similar to, but less frequently than, that of flushing. Higher doses (≥3 mcg/kg) are associated with more prolonged flushing, tachycardia, hypotension, dyspnea, and "chest compression" or tightness. In addition, at doses of ≥5 mcg/kg, significant increases in heart rate and decreases in blood pressure were observed. The cardiovascular effects occurred 2–3 minutes after injection and lasted for 30–60 minutes. The facial flushing was more prolonged, lasting up to 4 hours in some subjects. All signs and symptoms could be reduced by administering the drug as a 30-second infusion instead of by bolus injection.

Total doses of up to 200 mcg of corticorelin were administered as a bolus injection to 60 men and women, including both healthy normal subjects and patients with endocrine disorders. In most cases, only minor adverse effects, such as transient flushing and feelings of dyspnea, were noted. However, a few patients with disorders of the pituitary-adrenal axis had major symptoms. One patient had a precipitous fall in blood pressure and pulse rate and developed asystole, which required resuscitation. In two patients with Cushing's disease and in one with secondary adrenal insufficiency, an "absence-like" loss of consciousness occurred, which started within a few seconds after injection of corticorelin and lasted from 10 seconds to 5 minutes. This was accompanied by a slight fall in blood pressure. One patient with a well documented seizure diathesis experienced a grand mal epileptic seizure following ACTHREL® administration. The patient had discontinued anti-convulsant therapy the day of the procedure. (See **PRECAUTIONS** and **Drug Interactions**)

OVERDOSAGE

Symptoms of overdose include severe facial flushing, cardiovascular changes, and dyspnea. In the event of toxic overdose (see **ADVERSE REACTIONS**), adverse effects should be treated symptomatically.

DOSAGE AND ADMINISTRATION

Dosage: A single intravenous dose of ACTHREL® at 1 mcg/kg is recommended for the testing of pituitary corticotrophin function. A dose of 1 mcg/kg is the lowest dose that produces maximal cortisol responses and significant (though apparently sub-maximal) ACTH responses. Doses above 1 mcg/kg are not recommended. (See **PRECAUTIONS** and **ADVERSE REACTIONS**)

At a dose of 1 mcg/kg, the ACTH and cortisol responses to ACTHREL® are prolonged and remain elevated for up to 2 hours. The maximum increment in plasma ACTH occurs between 15 and 60 minutes after ACTHREL® administration, whereas the maximum increment in plasma cortisol occurs between 30 and 120 minutes. In a clinical study of 30 normal healthy men, the peak plasma ACTH and cortisol responses to ACTHREL® administration in the early afternoon occurred at 42 ± 29 minutes and 65 ± 26 minutes (average ± SD), respectively. **If a repeat evaluation using the corticorelin stimulation test with ACTHREL® is needed, it is recommended that the repeat test be carried out at the same time of day as the original test because there are differences in basal levels and peak response levels following a.m. or p.m. administration to normal humans.**

Administration: ACTHREL® is to be reconstituted aseptically with 2 mL of Sodium Chloride Injection, USP (0.9% sodium chloride), at the time of use by injecting 2 mL of the saline diluent into the lyophilized drug product cake. To avoid bubble formation, DO NOT SHAKE the vial; instead, roll the vial to dissolve the drug product. The sterile solution containing 50 mcg corticorelin/mL is then ready for injection by the intravenous route. The dosage to be administered is determined by the patient's weight (1 mcg corticorelin/kg). Some of the adverse effects can be reduced by administering the drug as an infusion over 30 seconds instead of as a bolus injection.

Parenteral drug products should be inspected visually for particulate matter and discoloration prior to administration, whenever solution and container permit.

HOW SUPPLIED

ACTHREL® is supplied as a sterile, nonpyrogenic, lyophilized, white cake containing 100 mcg corticorelin ovine (as

the trifluoroacetate), 0.88 mg ascorbic acid, 10 mg lactose, and 26 mg cysteine hydrochloride monohydrate. Trace amounts of chloride ion may be present from the manufacturing process. The package provides a single-dose, rubber-capped, 5-mL, brown-glass vial (NDC 55566-0302-1) containing 100 mcg corticorelin ovine (as the trifluoroacetate). ACTHREL® is stable in the lyophilized form when stored refrigerated at 2°C to 8°C (36°F to 45°F) and protected from light. The reconstituted solution is stable up to 8 hours under refrigerated conditions. Discard unused reconstituted solution.

Manufactured for:
Ferring Pharmaceuticals Inc.
Tarrytown, New York 10591
By:
Ben Venue Laboratories, Inc.
Bedford, OH 44146

Caution: Federal law prohibits dispensing without a prescription

©1997 FERRING PHARMACEUTICALS INC.
01/97   OIDC171

DESMOPRESSIN ACETATE Injection ℞

DESCRIPTION

DESMOPRESSIN ACETATE Injection is an antidiuretic hormone affecting renal water conservation and is a synthetic analogue of 8-arginine vasopressin. It is chemically defined as follows:

Mol. Wt. 1183.2
Empirical Formula: $C_{48}H_{74}N_{14}O_{17}S_2$

$$SCH_2CH_2CO\text{-}Tyr\text{-}Phe\text{-}Gln\text{-}Asn\text{-}Cys\text{-}Pro\text{-}D\text{-}Arg\text{-}Gly\text{-}NH_2 \cdot C_2H_4O_2 \cdot 3H_2O$$

1-(3-mercaptopropionic acid)-8-D-arginine vasopressin monoacetate (salt) trihydrate.

DESMOPRESSIN ACETATE Injection is provided as a sterile, aqueous solution for injection.

Each mL provides: Desmopressin acetate   4.0 mcg
                   Sodium chloride   9.0 mg
                   Hydrochloric acid to adjust pH to 4.0

The 10 mL vial contains chlorobutanol as a preservative (5.0 mg/mL).

CLINICAL PHARMACOLOGY

DESMOPRESSIN ACETATE Injection contains as active substance, 1-(3-mercaptopropionic acid)-8-D-arginine vasopressin, a synthetic analogue of the natural hormone arginine vasopressin. One mL (4 mcg) of desmopressin acetate solution has an antidiuretic activity of about 16 IU; 1 mcg of desmopressin acetate solution is equivalent to 4 IU.

Desmopressin acetate has been shown to be more potent than arginine vasopressin in increasing plasma levels of factor VIII activity in patients with hemophilia and von Willebrand's disease Type I.

Dose-response studies were performed in healthy persons, using doses of 0.1 to 0.4 mcg/kg body weight, infused over a 10-minute period. Maximal dose response occurred at 0.3 to 0.4 mcg/kg. The response to **DESMOPRESSIN ACETATE Injection** of factor VIII activity and plasminogen activator is dose-related, with maximal plasma levels of 300 to 400 percent of initial concentrations obtained after infusion of 0.4 mcg/kg body weight. The increase is rapid and evident within 30 minutes, reaching a maximum at a point ranging from 90 minutes to two hours. The factor VIII related antigen and ristocetin cofactor activity were also increased to a smaller degree, but still are dose-dependent.

1. The biphasic half-lives of desmopressin acetate were 7.8 and 75.5 minutes for the fast and slow phases, respectively, compared with 2.5 and 14.5 minutes for lysine vasopressin, another form of the hormone. As a result, **DESMOPRESSIN ACETATE Injection** provides a prompt onset of antidiuretic action with a long duration after each administration.

2. The change in structure of arginine vasopressin to desmopressin acetate has resulted in a decreased vasopressor action and decreased actions on visceral smooth muscle relative to the enhanced antidiuretic activity, so that clinically effective antidiuretic doses are usually below threshold levels for effects on vascular or visceral smooth muscle.

3. When administered by injection, desmopressin acetate has an antidiuretic effect about ten times that of an equivalent dose administered intranasally.

4. The bioavailability of the subcutaneous route of administration was determined qualitatively using urine output data. The exact fraction of drug absorbed by that route of administration has not been quantitatively determined.

5. The percentage increase of factor VIII levels in patients with mild hemophilia A and von Willebrand's disease was

not significantly different from that observed in normal healthy individuals when treated with 0.3 mcg/kg of desmopressin acetate infused over 10 minutes.

6. Plasminogen activator activity increases rapidly after desmopressin acetate infusion, but there has been no clinically significant fibrinolysis in patients treated with **DESMOPRESSIN ACETATE Injection**.

7. The effect of repeated DESMOPRESSIN ACETATE administration when doses were given every 12 to 24 hours has generally shown a gradual diminution of the factor VIII activity increase noted with a single dose. The initial response is reproducible in any particular patient if there are 2 or 3 days between administrations.

INDICATION AND USAGE

HEMOPHILIA A

DESMOPRESSIN ACETATE Injection is indicated for patients with hemophilia A with factor VIII coagulant activity levels greater than 5%.

DESMOPRESSIN ACETATE Injection will often maintain hemostasis in patients with hemophilia A during surgical procedures and postoperatively when administered 30 minutes prior to scheduled procedure.

DESMOPRESSIN ACETATE Injection will also stop bleeding in hemophilia A patients with episodes of spontaneous or trauma-induced injuries such as hemarthroses, intramuscular hematomas or mucosal bleeding.

DESMOPRESSIN ACETATE Injection is not indicated for the treatment of hemophilia A with factor VIII coagulant activity levels equal to or less than 5%, or for the treatment of hemophilia B, or in patients who have factor VIII antibodies.

In certain clinical situations, it may be justified to try **DESMOPRESSIN ACETATE Injection** in patients with factor VIII levels between 2%-5%; however, these patients should be carefully monitored.

von Willebrand's Disease (Type I)

DESMOPRESSIN ACETATE Injection is indicated for patients with mild to moderate classic von Willebrand's disease (Type I) with factor VIII levels greater than 5%. **DESMOPRESSIN ACETATE Injection** will often maintain hemostasis in patients with mild to moderate von Willebrand's disease during surgical procedures and postoperatively when administered 30 minutes prior to the scheduled procedure.

DESMOPRESSIN ACETATE Injection will usually stop bleeding in mild to moderate von Willebrand's patients with episodes of spontaneous or trauma induced injuries such as hemarthroses, intramuscular hematomas or mucosal bleeding.

Those von Willebrand's disease patients who are least likely to respond are those with severe homozygous von Willebrand's disease with factor VIII coagulant activity and factor VIII von Willebrand factor antigen levels less than 1%. Other patients may respond in a variable fashion depending on the type of molecular defect they have. Bleeding time and factor VIII coagulant activity, ristocetin cofactor activity, and von Willebrand factor antigen should be checked during administration of **DESMOPRESSIN ACETATE Injection** to ensure that adequate levels are being achieved.

DESMOPRESSIN ACETATE Injection is not indicated for the treatment of severe classic von Willebrand's disease (Type I) and when there is evidence of an abnormal molecular form of factor VIII antigen. See Warning.

Diabetes Insipidus

DESMOPRESSIN ACETATE Injection is indicated as antidiuretic replacement therapy in the management of central (cranial) diabetes insipidus and for the management of the temporary polyuria and polydipsia following head trauma or surgery in the pituitary region. **DESMOPRESSIN ACETATE Injection** is ineffective for the treatment of nephrogenic diabetes insipidus.

Desmopressin acetate is also available as an intranasal preparation. However, this means of delivery can be compromised by a variety of factors that can make nasal insufflation ineffective or inappropriate. These include poor intranasal absorption, nasal congestion and blockage, nasal discharge, atrophy of nasal mucosa, and severe atrophic rhinitis. Intranasal delivery may be inappropriate where there is an impaired level of consciousness. In addition, cranial surgical procedures, such as transsphenoidal hypophysectomy, create situations where an alternative route of administration is needed as in cases of nasal packing or recovery from surgery.

CONTRAINDICATION

Known hypersensitivity to desmopressin acetate.

WARNINGS

Patients who do not have need of antidiuretic hormone for its antidiuretic effect, in particular those who are young or elderly, should be cautioned to ingest only enough fluid to satisfy thirst, in order to decrease the potential occurrence of water intoxication and hyponatremia.

Fluid intake should be adjusted downward, particularly in very young and elderly patients, in order to decrease the potential occurrence of water intoxication and hyponatremia.

Particular attention should be paid to the possibility of the rare occurrence of an extreme decrease in plasma osmolality that may result in seizures which could lead to coma. Desmopressin acetate should not be used to treat patients with Type IIB von Willebrand's disease since platelet aggregation may be induced.

PRECAUTIONS

GENERAL: For injection use only.
DESMOPRESSIN ACETATE Injection has infrequently produced changes in blood pressure causing either a slight elevation in blood pressure or a transient fall in blood pressure and a compensatory increase in heart rate. The drug should be used with caution in patients with coronary artery insufficiency and/or hypertensive cardiovascular disease.

DESMOPRESSIN ACETATE Injection should be used with caution in patients with conditions associated with fluid and electrolyte imbalance, such as cystic fibrosis, because these patients are prone to hyponatremia.

There have been rare reports of thrombotic events following **DESMOPRESSIN ACETATE** Injection in patients predisposed to thrombus formation. No causality has been determined, however, the drug should be used with caution in these patients.

Severe allergic reactions have been reported rarely. Fatal anaphylaxis has been reported in one patient who received intravenous desmopressin acetate. It is not known whether antibodies to **DESMOPRESSIN ACETATE** Injection are produced after repeated injections.

Hemophilia A
Laboratory tests for assessing patient status include levels of factor VIII coagulant, factor VIII antigen and factor VIII ristocetin cofactor (von Willebrand factor) as well as activated partial thromboplastin time. Factor VIII coagulant activity should be determined before giving desmopressin acetate for hemostasis. If factor VIII coagulant activity is present at less than 5% of normal, desmopressin acetate should not be relied on.

von Willebrand's Disease
Laboratory tests for assessing patient status include levels of factor VIII coagulant activity, factor VIII ristocetin cofactor activity, and factor VIII von Willebrand factor antigen. The skin bleeding time may be helpful in following these patients.

Diabetes Insipidus
Laboratory tests for monitoring the patient include urine volume and osmolality. In some cases, plasma osmolality may be required.

DRUG INTERACTIONS: Although the pressor activity of desmopressin acetate is very low compared with the antidiuretic activity, use of doses as large as 0.3 mcg/kg of DESMOPRESSIN ACETATE with other pressor agents should be done only with careful patient monitoring.
Desmopressin acetate has been used with epsilon aminocaproic acid without adverse effects.

CARCINOGENICITY, MUTAGENICITY, IMPAIRMENT OF FERTILITY: Teratology studies in rats have shown no abnormalities. No further data are available.

PREGNANCY CATEGORY B: Reproduction studies performed in rats and rabbits with subcutaneous doses up to 12.5 times the human dose when used for factor VIII stimulation and 125 times the human dose when used in diabetes insipidus have revealed no evidence of harm to the fetus due to desmopressin acetate. There are several publications of management of diabetes insipidus in pregnant women with no harm to the fetus reported; however, there are no adequate and well-controlled studies in pregnant woman. Published reports stress that, as opposed to preparations containing the natural hormones, desmopressin acetate in antidiuretic doses has no uterotonic action, but the physician will have to weight possible therapeutic advantages against possible danger in each case.

NURSING MOTHERS: It is not known whether this drug is excreted in human milk. Because many drugs are excreted in human milk, caution should be exercised when desmopressin acetate is administered to a nursing woman.

PEDIATRIC USE: Use in infants and children will require careful fluid intake restriction to prevent possible hyponatremia and water intoxication. *DESMOPRESSIN ACETATE Injection should not be used in infants younger than three months* in the treatment of hemophilia A or von Willebrand's disease; safety and effectiveness in children under 12 years of age with diabetes insipidus have not been established.

ADVERSE REACTIONS

Infrequently, desmopressin acetate has produced transient headache, nausea, mild abdominal cramps and vulval pain. These symptoms disappeared with reduction in dosage. Occasionally, injection of desmopressin acetate has produced local erythema, swelling or burning pain. Occasional facial flushing has been reported with the administration of desmopressin acetate.

DESMOPRESSIN ACETATE Injection has infrequently produced changes in blood pressure causing either a slight elevation or a transient fall and a compensatory increase in heart rate. Severe allergic reactions including anaphylaxis have been reported rarely with **DESMOPRESSIN ACETATE** Injection.

See WARNING for the possibility of water intoxication and hyponatremia.

There have been rare reports of thrombotic events (acute cerebrovascular thrombosis, acute myocardial infarction) following **DESMOPRESSIN ACETATE** Injection in patients predisposed to thrombus formation.

OVERDOSAGE

See ADVERSE REACTIONS above. In case of overdosage, the dosage should be reduced, frequency of administration decreased, or the drug withdrawn according to the severity of the condition.

There is no known specific antidote for desmopressin acetate.

An oral LD_{50} has not been established. An intravenous dose of 2 mg/kg in mice demonstrated no effect.

DOSAGE AND ADMINISTRATION

Hemophilia A and von Willebrand's Disease (Type I)
DESMOPRESSIN ACETATE Injection is administered as an intravenous infusion at a dose of 0.3 mcg desmopressin acetate/kg body weight diluted in sterile physiological saline and infused slowly over 15 to 30 minutes. In adults and children weighing more than 10 kg, 50 mL of diluent is used; in children weighing 10 kg or less, 10 mL of diluent is used. Blood pressure and pulse should be monitored during infusion. If **DESMOPRESSIN ACETATE** Injection is used preoperatively, it should be administered 30 minutes prior to the scheduled procedure.

The necessity for repeat administration of desmopressin acetate or use of any blood products for hemostasis should be determined by laboratory response as well as the clinical condition of the patient. The tendency toward tachyphylaxis (lessening of response) with repeated administration given more frequently than every 48 hours should be considered in treating each patient.

Diabetes Insipidus
This formulation is administered subcutaneously or by direct intravenous injection. **DESMOPRESSIN ACETATE Injection** dosage must be determined for each patient and adjusted according to the pattern of response. Response should be estimated by two parameters: adequate duration of sleep and adequate, not excessive, water turnover.

The usual dosage range in adults is 0.5 mL (2.0 mcg) to 1 mL (4.0 mcg) daily, administered intravenously or subcutaneously, usually in two divided doses. The morning and evening doses should be separately adjusted for an adequate diurnal rhythm of water turnover. For patients who have been controlled on intranasal desmopressin acetate and who must be switched to the injection form, either because of poor intranasal absorption or because of the need for surgery, the comparable antidiuretic dose of the injection is about one-tenth the intranasal dose.

Parenteral drug products should be inspected visually for particulate matter and discoloration prior to administration whenever solution and container permit.

HOW SUPPLIED

DESMOPRESSIN ACETATE Injection is available as a sterile solution in cartons of ten 1 mL single-dose ampules (NDC 55566-5030-1) and in 10 mL multiple-dose vials (NDC 55566-5040-1) each containing 4.0 mcg desmopressin acetate per mL. Keep refrigerated at about 4°C (39°F).

Caution: Federal (U.S.A.) law prohibits dispensing without prescription.
Rev. 1/96   DC-140A
Manufactured for
FERRING PHARMACEUTICALS INC.
120 White Plains Rd., Suite 400
Tarrytown, NY 10591
By Ferring Pharmaceuticals, Malmö, Sweden   41 38 51

DESMOPRESSIN   ℞
ACETATE
RHINAL TUBE

DESCRIPTION

Desmopressin Acetate Rhinal Tube is an antidiuretic hormone affecting renal water conservation and a synthetic analogue of 8-arginine vasopressin. It is chemically defined as follows:

Mol.wt. 1183.2
Empirical formula: $C_{48}H_{74}N_{14}O_{17}S_2$

SCH2CH2CO-Tyr-Phe-Gln-Asn-Cys-Pro-D-Arg-Gly-NH2 • C2H4O2 • 3H2O

1-(3-mercaptopropionic acid)-8-D-arginine vasopressin monoacetate (salt) trihydrate.

Desmopressin Acetate Rhinal Tube is provided as a sterile, aqueous solution for intranasal use. Each mL contains:

Desmopressin acetate	0.1 mg
Chlorobutanol	5.0 mg
Sodium Chloride	9.0 mg
Hydrochloric acid to adjust pH to approximately 4	

CLINICAL PHARMACOLOGY

Desmopressin Acetate Rhinal Tube contains as active substance 1-(3-mercaptopropionic acid)-8-D-arginine vasopressin, which is a synthetic analogue of the natural hormone arginine vasopressin. One mL (0.1 mg) of Desmopressin Acetate Rhinal Tube has an antidiuretic activity of about 400 IU; 10 mcg of desmopressin acetate is equivalent to 40 IU.

1. The biphasic half-lives for Desmopressin Acetate Rhinal Tube were 7.8 and 75.5 minutes for the fast and slow phases, compared with 2.5 and 14.5 minutes for lysine vasopressin, another form of the hormone used in this condition. As a result, Desmopressin Acetate Rhinal Tube provides a prompt onset of antidiuretic action with a long duration after each administration.

2. The change in structure of arginine vasopressin to Desmopressin Acetate Rhinal Tube has resulted in a decreased vasopressor action and decreased actions on visceral smooth muscle relative to the enhanced antidiuretic activity, so that clinically effective antidiuretic doses are usually below threshold levels for effects on vascular or visceral smooth muscle.

3. Desmopressin Acetate Rhinal Tube administered intranasally has an antidiuretic effect about one-tenth that of an equivalent dose administered by injection.

INDICATIONS AND USAGE

Primary Nocturnal Enuresis: Desmopressin Acetate Rhinal Tube is indicated for the management of primary nocturnal enuresis. It may be used alone or adjunctive to behavioral conditioning or other non-pharmacological intervention. It has been shown to be effective in some cases that are refractory to conventional therapies.

Central Cranial Diabetes Insipidus: Desmopressin Acetate Rhinal Tube is indicated as antidiuretic replacement therapy in the management of central cranial diabetes insipidus and for management of the temporary polyuria and polydipsia following head trauma or surgery in the pituitary region. It is ineffective for the treatment of nephrogenic diabetes insipidus.

The use of Desmopressin Acetate Rhinal Tube in patients with an established diagnosis will result in a reduction in urinary output with increase in urine osmolality and a decrease in plasma osmolality. This will allow the resumption of a more normal life-style with a decrease in urinary frequency and nocturia.

There are reports of an occasional change in response with time, usually greater than 6 months. Some patients may show a decreased responsiveness, others a shortened duration of effect. There is no evidence this effect is due to the development of binding antibodies but may be due to a local inactivation of the peptide.

Patients are selected for therapy by establishing the diagnosis by means of the water deprivation test, the hypertonic saline infusion test, and/or the response to antidiuretic hormone. Continued response to Desmopressin Acetate Rhinal Tube can be monitored by urine volume and osmolality.

Desmopressin Acetate is also available as a solution for injection when the intranasal route may be compromised. These situations include nasal congestion and blockage, nasal discharge, atrophy of nasal mucosa, and severe atrophic rhinitis. Intranasal delivery may also be inappropriate where there is an impaired level of consciousness. In addition, cranial surgical procedures, such as transphenoidal hypophysectomy create situations where an alternative route of administration is needed as in cases of nasal packing or recovery from surgery.

CONTRAINDICATION

Known hypersensitivity to Desmopressin Acetate Rhinal Tube.

WARNINGS

1. For intranasal use only.

2. In very young and elderly patients in particular, fluid intake should be adjusted in order to decrease the potential occurrence of water intoxication and hyponatremia. Particular attention should be paid to the possibility of the rare occurrence of an extreme decrease in plasma osmolality and resulting seizures.

PRECAUTIONS

General: Desmopressin Acetate Rhinal Tube at high dosage has infrequently produced a slight elevation of blood pressure, which disappeared with a reduction in dosage. The drug should be used with caution in patients with coronary artery insufficiency and/or hypertensive cardiovascular disease because of possible rise in blood pressure.

Continued on next page

Desmopressin Acetate—Cont.

Desmopressin Acetate Rhinal Tube should be used with caution in patients with conditions associated with fluid and electrolyte imbalance, such as cystic fibrosis, because these patients are prone to hyponatremia.

Central Cranial Diabetes Insipidus: Since Desmopressin Acetate Rhinal Tube is used intranasally, changes in the nasal mucosa such as scarring, edema, or other disease may cause erratic, unreliable absorption in which case Desmopressin Acetate Rhinal Tube should not be used. For such situations, Desmopressin Acetate Injection should be considered.

Primary Nocturnal Enuresis: If changes in the nasal mucosa have occurred, unreliable absorption may result. Desmopressin Acetate Rhinal Tube should be discontinued until the nasal problems resolve.

Laboratory Tests:

Laboratory tests for following the patient with central cranial diabetes insipidus or post-surgical or head trauma-related polyuria and polydipsia include urine volume and osmolality. In some cases plasma osmolality may be required. For the healthy patient with primary nocturnal enuresis, serum electrolytes should be checked at least once if therapy is continued beyond 7 days.

Drug Interactions: Although the pressor activity of Desmopressin Acetate Rhinal Tube is very low compared to the antidiuretic activity, use of large doses of Desmopressin Acetate Rhinal Tube with other pressor agents should only be done with careful patient monitoring.

Carcinogenesis, Mutagenesis, Impairment of Fertility: Teratology studies in rats have shown no abnormalities. No further information is available.

Pregnancy—Category B: Reproduction studies performed in rats and rabbits with doses up to 12.5 times the human intranasal dose (i.e. about 125 times the total adult human dose given systemically) have revealed no evidence of harm to the fetus due to desmopressin acetate. There are several publications of management of diabetes insipidus in pregnant women with no harm to the fetus reported; however, no controlled studies in pregnant women have been carried out. Published reports stress that, as opposed to preparations containing the natural hormones, Desmopressin Acetate Rhinal Tube in antidiuretic doses has no uterotonic action, but the physician will have to weigh possible therapeutic advantages against possible dangers in each individual case.

Nursing Mothers: There have been no controlled studies in nursing mothers. A single study in a post-partum woman demonstrated a marked change in plasma, but little if any change in assayable Desmopressin Acetate Rhinal Tube in breast milk following an intranasal dose of 10 mcg.

Pediatric Use

Primary Nocturnal Enuresis: Desmopressin Acetate Rhinal Tube has been used in childhood nocturnal enuresis. Short-term (4–8 weeks) Desmopressin Acetate Rhinal Tube administration has been shown to be safe and modestly effective in children aged 6 years or older with severe childhood nocturnal enuresis. Adequately controlled studies with Desmopressin Acetate Rhinal Tube in primary nocturnal enuresis have not been conducted beyond 4–8 weeks. The dose should be individually adjusted to achieve the best results.

Central Cranial Diabetes Insipidus: Desmopressin Acetate Rhinal Tube has been used in children with diabetes insipidus. Use in infants and children will require careful fluid intake restriction to prevent possible hyponatremia and water intoxication. The dose must be individually adjusted to the patient with attention in the very young to the danger of an extreme decrease in plasma osmolality with resulting convulsions. Dose should start at 0.05 mL or less. There are reports of an occasional change in response with time, usually greater than 6 months. Some patients may show a decreased responsiveness, others a shortened duration of effect. There is no evidence this effect is due to the development of binding antibodies but may be due to a local inactivation of the peptide.

ADVERSE REACTIONS

Infrequently, high dosages have produced transient headache and nausea. Nasal congestion, rhinitis and flushing have also been reported occasionally along with mild abdominal cramps. These symptoms disappeared with reduction in dosage. Nosebleed, sore throat, cough and upper respiratory infections have also been reported.

The following table lists the percent of patients having adverse experiences without regard to relationship to study drug from the pooled pivotal study data for nocturnal enuresis.

ADVERSE REACTION	PLACEBO (N=59) %	DESMOPRESSIN 20 mcg (N=60) %	DESMOPRESSIN 40 mcg (N=61) %
BODY AS A WHOLE			
Abdominal Pain	0	2	2
Asthenia	0	0	2
Chills	0	0	2
Headache	0	2	5
Throat Pain	2	0	0
NERVOUS SYSTEM			
Depression	2	0	0
Dizziness	0	0	3
RESPIRATORY SYSTEM			
Epistaxis	2	3	0
Nostril Pain	0	2	0
Respiratory Infection	2	0	0
Rhinitis	2	8	3
CARDIOVASCULAR SYSTEM			
Vasodilation	2	0	0
DIGESTIVE SYSTEM			
Gastrointestinal Disorder	0	2	0
Nausea	0	0	2
SKIN & APPENDAGES			
Leg Rash	0	2	0
Rash	2	0	0
SPECIAL SENSES			
Conjunctivitis	0	2	0
Edema Eyes	0	2	0
Lachrymation Disorder	0	0	2

OVERDOSAGE

See adverse reactions above. In case of overdosage, the dose should be reduced, frequency of administration decreased, or the drug withdrawn according to the severity of the condition. There is no known specific antidote for Desmopressin Acetate Rhinal Tube.

An oral LD$_{50}$ has not been established. An intravenous dose of 2 mg/kg in mice demonstrated no effect.

DOSAGE AND ADMINISTRATION

Primary Nocturnal Enuresis: Dosage should be adjusted according to the individual. The recommended initial dose for those 6 years of age and older is 20 mcg or 0.2 mL solution intranasally at bedtime. Adjustment up to 40 mcg is suggested if the patient does not respond. Some patients may respond to 10 mcg and adjustment to that lower dose may be done if the patient has shown a response to 20 mcg. It is recommended that one-half of the dose be administered per nostril. Adequately controlled studies with Desmopressin Acetate Rhinal Tube in primary nocturnal enuresis have not been conducted beyond 4–8 weeks.

Central Cranial Diabetes Insipidus: This drug is administered into the nose through a soft, flexible plastic rhinal tube which has four graduation marks on it that measure 0.2, 0.15, 0.1 and 0.05 mL. Desmopressin Acetate Rhinal Tube dosage must be determined for each individual patient and adjusted according to the diurnal pattern of response. Response should be estimated by two parameters: adequate duration of sleep and adequate, not excessive, water turnover. Patients with nasal congestion and blockage have often responded well to Desmopressin Acetate Rhinal Tube. The usual dosage range in adults is 0.1 to 0.4 mL daily, either as a single dose or divided into two or three doses. Most adults require 0.2 mL daily in two divided doses. The morning and evening doses should be separately adjusted for an adequate diurnal rhythm of water turnover. For children aged 3 months to 12 years, the usual dosage range is 0.05 to 0.3 mL daily, either as a single dose or divided into two doses.

About $^{1}/_{4}$ to $^{1}/_{3}$ of patients can be controlled by a single daily dose.

HOW SUPPLIED

2.5 mL per vial, packaged with two rhinal tube applicators per carton (NDC 55566-5020-1). Also available in shelf packs of 10 × 2.5 mL cartons (NDC 55566-5020-2).

KEEP REFRIGERATED AT ABOUT 4°C (39°F).

When traveling—controlled room temperature 22°C (72°F) closed sterile bottles will maintain stability for 3 weeks.

Caution: Federal (U.S.A.) law prohibits dispensing without prescription.

Manufactured for

FERRING PHARMACEUTICALS INC.
120 White Plains Rd., Suite 400
Tarrytown, NY 10591
By Ferring Pharmaceuticals, Malmö, Sweden
DC-135
10/93

PATIENT INSTRUCTION GUIDE
DESMOPRESSIN
acetate
RHINAL TUBE

1. Pull plastic tag on neck of bottle.

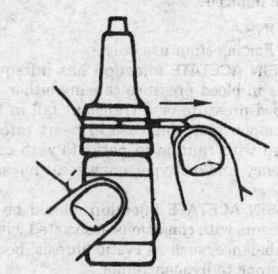

2. Break security seal and remove plastic cap.

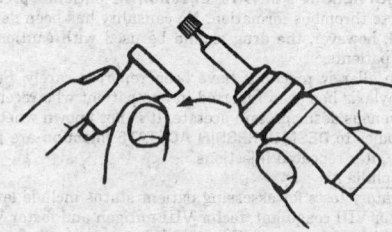

3. Twist off the small knurled seal from the dropper. Use the same seal reversed to prevent subsequent leakage, especially if the bottle is not stored upright.

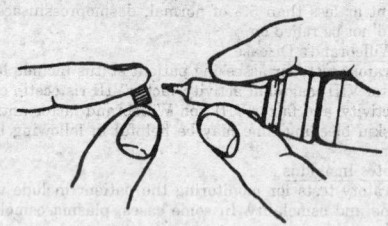

4. The drug is administered by a soft, flexible, plastic rhinal tube which has dose marks at 0.2, 0.15, 0.1 and 0.05 mL. Take the arrow-marked part of the tube in one hand and place the fingers of the other hand around the cylindrical part of the closure. Insert the top of the dropper in a downward position into the arrow-marked end of the tube and squeeze the dropper until the solution has reached the desired calibration mark. The dose is measured from the arrow-marked end of the tube to the appropriate calibration. Disconnect the tube from the bottle by withdrawing the bottle quickly downwards. In order to prevent air bubbles from forming in the tube, maintain constant pressure on the dropper. If difficulty is experienced in filling the tube, a diabetic or tuberculin syringe may be used to draw up the dose and load the tube.

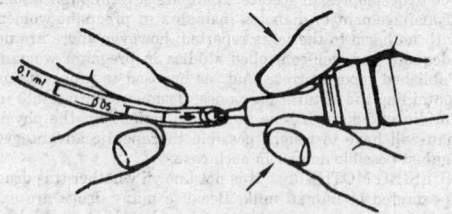

5. Hold the tube with the fingers approximately $^{3}/_{4}$ inch from the end and insert into a nostril until the tips of the fingers reach the nostril.

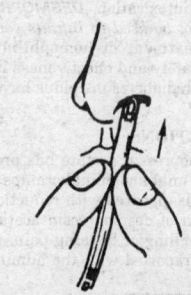

6. Put the other end of the tube into the mouth. Hold the breath, tilt the head back and then blow with a short strong

puff through the tube so that the solution reaches the right place in the nasal cavity. Through this procedure, medication is limited to the nasal cavity and the preparation does not pass down into the throat.

In very young patients, it may be necessary for an adult to blow the solution into the child's nose. In such cases, the tube will not need to be put into the nose as far as in the older child or adult. The tube should be placed in the nose gently just far enough so that the solution does not run out. A baby must be held firmly and securely.

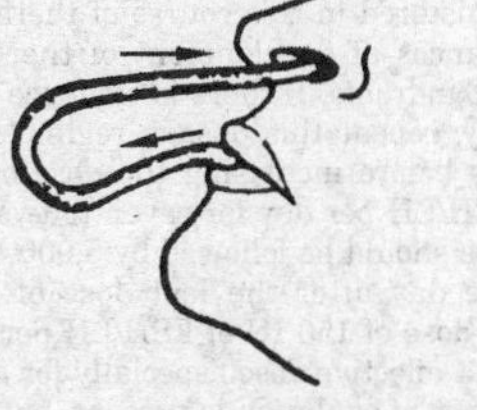

7. After use, reseal dropper tip and close the bottle with the plastic cap. Wash the tube in water and shake thoroughly, until no more water is left. The tube can then be used for the next application.

IMPORTANT:
Replace Knurled Seal

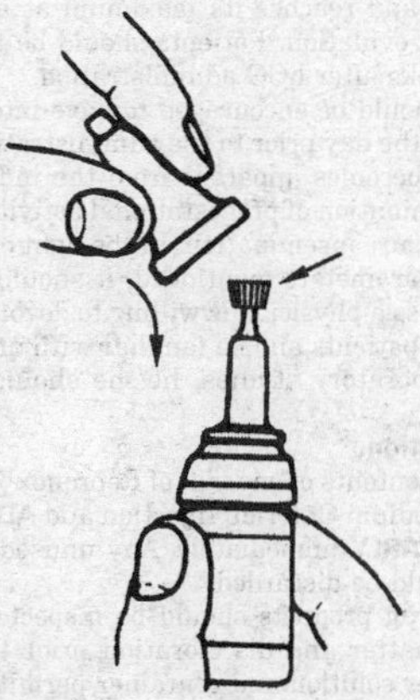

KEEP REFRIGERATED AT ABOUT 4°C(39°F).

When traveling—controlled room temperature 22°C(72°F) closed sterile bottles will maintain stability for 3 weeks.

Manufactured for
FERRING PHARMACEUTICALS INC.
120 White Plains Rd., Suite 400
Tarrytown, NY 10591
By Ferring Pharmaceuticals, Malmö, Sweden
DC-150
10/93 41 21 81

REPRONEX™ ℞
(MENOTROPINS FOR INJECTION, USP)
FOR INTRAMUSCULAR INJECTION

DESCRIPTION

Repronex™ (menotropins for injection, USP) is a purified preparation of gonadotropins extracted from the urine of postmenopausal women. Each vial of Repronex™ contains 75 International Units (IU) or 150 IU of follicle-stimulating hormone (FSH) activity and 75 IU or 150 IU of luteinizing hormone (LH) activity, respectively, plus 20 mg lactose monohydrate in a sterile, lyophilized form. Human Chorionic Gonadotropin (hCG), a naturally occurring hormone in postmenopausal urine, is detected in Repronex™. Repronex™ is administered by intramuscular injection.

Repronex™ is biologically standardized for FSH and LH (ICSH) gonadotropin activities in terms of the Second International Reference Preparation for Human Menopausal Gonadotropins established in September, 1964 by the Expert Committee on Biological Standards of the World Health Organization.

Both FSH and LH are glycoproteins that are acidic and water soluble. Therapeutic class: Infertility.

CLINICAL PHARMACOLOGY

Women:

Menotropins administered for seven to twelve days produces ovarian follicular growth in women who do not have primary ovarian failure. Treatment with menotropins in most instances results only in follicular growth and maturation. In order to effect ovulation, human chorionic gonadotropin (hCG) must be given following the administration of menotropins when clinical assessment of the patient indicates that sufficient follicular maturation has occurred.

Men:

Menotropins administered concomitantly with human chorionic gonadotropin (hCG) for at least three months induces spermatogenesis in men with primary or secondary pituitary hypofunction who have achieved adequate masculinization with prior hCG therapy.

INDICATIONS AND USAGE

Women:

Menotropins and hCG given in a sequential manner are indicated for the induction of ovulation and pregnancy in the anovulatory infertile patient, in whom the cause of anovulation is functional and is not due to primary ovarian failure.

Menotropins and hCG may also be used to stimulate the development of multiple follicles in ovulatory patients participating in an *in vitro* fertilization program.

Men:

Menotropins with concomitant hCG is indicated for the stimulation of spermatogenesis in men who have primary or secondary hypogonadotropic hypogonadism.

Menotropins with concomitant hCG has proven effective in inducing spermatogenesis in men with primary hypogonadotropic hypogonadism due to a congenital factor or prepubertal hypophysectomy and in men with secondary hypogonadotropic hypogonadism due to hypophysectomy, craniopharyngioma, cerebral aneurysm or chromophobe adenoma.

SELECTION OF PATIENTS

Women:

1. Before treatment with Repronex™ is instituted, a thorough gynecologic and endocrinologic evaluation must be performed. Except for those patients enrolled in an *in vitro* fertilization program, this should include a hysterosalpingogram (to rule out uterine and tubal pathology) and documentation of anovulation by means of basal body temperature, serial vaginal smears, examination of cervical mucus, determination of serum (or urine) progesterone, urinary pregnanediol and endometrial biopsy. Patients with tubal pathology should receive menotropins only if enrolled in an *in vitro* fertilization program.
2. Primary ovarian failure should be excluded by the determination of gonadotropin levels.
3. Careful examination should be made to rule out the presence of an early pregnancy.
4. Patients in late reproductive life have a greater predilection to endometrial carcinoma as well as a higher incidence of anovulatory disorders. Cervical dilation and curettage should always be done for diagnosis before starting Repronex™ therapy in such patients who demonstrate abnormal uterine bleeding or other signs of endometrial abnormalities.
5. Evaluation of the husband's fertility potential should be included in the workup.

Men:

Patient selection should be made based on a documented lack of pituitary function. Prior to hormonal therapy, these patients will have low testosterone levels and low or absent gonadotropin levels. Patients with primary hypogonadotropic hypogonadism will have a subnormal development of masculinization, and those with secondary hypogonadotropic hypogonadism will have decreased masculinization.

CONTRAINDICATIONS

Women:

Repronex™ is contraindicated in women who have:
1. A high FSH level indicating primary ovarian failure.
2. Uncontrolled thyroid and adrenal dysfunction.
3. An organic intracranial lesion such as a pituitary tumor.
4. The presence of any cause of infertility other than anovulation unless they are candidates for *in vitro* fertilization.
5. Abnormal bleeding of undetermined origin.
6. Ovarian cysts or enlargement not due to polycystic ovary syndrome.
7. Prior hypersensitivity to menotropins.
8. Repronex™ is contraindicated in women who are pregnant and may cause fetal harm when administered to a pregnant woman. There are limited human data on the effects of menotropins when administered during pregnancy.

Men:

Repronex™ is contraindicated in men who have:
1. Normal gonadotropin levels indicating normal pituitary function.
2. Elevated gonadotropin levels indicating primary testicular failure.
3. Infertility disorders other than hypogonadotropic hypogonadism.

WARNINGS

Repronex™ is a drug that should only be used by physicians who are thoroughly familiar with infertility problems. It is a potent gonadotropic substance capable of causing mild to severe adverse reactions in women. Gonadotropin therapy requires a certain time commitment by physicians and supportive health professionals, and its use requires the availability of appropriate monitoring facilities (see "PRECAUTIONS—Laboratory Tests"). In female patients it must be used with a great deal of care.

Overstimulation of the Ovary During Repronex™ Therapy

Ovarian Enlargement: Mild to moderate uncomplicated ovarian enlargement which may be accompanied by abdominal distension and/or abdominal pain occurs in approximately 20% of those treated with menotropins and hCG, and generally regresses without treatment within two or three weeks.

In order to minimize the hazard associated with the occasional abnormal ovarian enlargement which may occur with Repronex™-hCG therapy, the lowest dose consistent with expectation of good results, should be used. Careful monitoring of ovarian response can further minimize the risk of overstimulation.

If the ovaries are abnormally enlarged on the last day of Repronex™ therapy, hCG should not be administered in this course of therapy; this will reduce the chances of development of the Ovarian Hyperstimulation Syndrome.

The Ovarian Hyperstimulation Syndrome (OHSS): OHSS is a medical event distinct from uncomplicated ovarian enlargement. OHSS may progress rapidly to become a serious medical event. It is characterized by an apparent dramatic increase in vascular permeability which can result in a rapid accumulation of fluid in the peritoneal cavity, thorax, and potentially, the pericardium. The early warning signs of development of OHSS are severe pelvic pain, nausea, vomiting, and weight gain. The following symptomatology has been seen with cases of OHSS: abdominal pain, abdominal distension, gastrointestinal symptoms including nausea, vomiting and diarrhea, severe ovarian enlargement, weight gain, dyspnea, and oliguria. Clinical evaluation may reveal hypovolemia, hemoconcentration, electrolyte imbalances, ascites, hemoperitoneum, pleural effusions, hydrothorax, acute pulmonary distress, and thromboembolic events (see "Pulmonary and Vascular Complications" below). Transient liver function test abnormalities suggestive of hepatic dysfunction, which may be accompanied by morphologic changes on liver biopsy, have been reported in association with the Ovarian Hyperstimulation Syndrome (OHSS).

OHSS occurs in approximately 0.4% of patients when the recommended dose is administered and in 1.3% of patients when higher than recommended doses are administered. Cases of OHSS are more common, more severe and more protracted if pregnancy occurs. OHSS develops rapidly; therefore patients should be followed for at least two weeks after hCG administration. Most often, OHSS occurs after treatment has been discontinued and reaches its maximum at about seven to ten days following treatment. Usually, OHSS resolves spontaneously with the onset of menses. If there is evidence that OHSS may be developing prior to hCG administration (see "PRECAUTIONS—Laboratory Tests"), the hCG should be withheld.

If OHSS occurs, treatment should be stopped and the patient hospitalized. Treatment is primarily symptomatic, consisting of bed rest, fluid and electrolyte management, and analgesics if needed. The phenomenon of hemoconcentration associated with fluid loss into the peritoneal cavity, pleural cavity, and the pericardial cavity has been seen to occur and should be thoroughly assessed in the following manner: 1) fluid intake and output, 2) weight, 3) hematocrit, 4) serum and urinary electrolytes, 5) urine specific gravity, 6) BUN and creatinine, and 7) abdominal girth. These determinations are to be performed daily or more often if the need arises.

With OHSS there is an increased risk of injury to the ovary. The ascitic, pleural, and pericardial fluid should not be removed unless absolutely necessary to relieve symptoms such as pulmonary distress or cardiac tamponade. Pelvic examination may cause rupture of an ovarian cyst, which may result in hemoperitoneum, and should therefore be avoided. If this does occur, and if bleeding becomes such that surgery is required, the surgical treatment should be designed to control bleeding and to retain as much ovarian tissue as possible. Intercourse should be prohibited in those patients in whom significant ovarian enlargement occurs after ovulation because of the danger of hemoperitoneum resulting from ruptured ovarian cysts.

The management of OHSS may be divided into three phases: the acute, the chronic, and the resolution phases. Because the use of diuretics can accentuate the diminished intravascular volume, diuretics should be avoided except in the late phase of resolution as described below.

Acute Phase: Management during the acute phase should be designed to prevent hemoconcentration due to loss of intravascular volume to the third space and to minimize the risk of thromboembolic phenomena and kidney damage. Treatment is designed to normalize electrolytes while maintaining an acceptable but somewhat reduced intravascular

Continued on next page

Repronex—Cont.

volume. Full correction of the intravascular volume deficit may lead to an unacceptable increase in the amount of third space fluid accumulation. Management includes administration of limited intravenous fluids, electrolytes, and human serum albumin. Monitoring for the development of hyperkalemia is recommended.

Chronic Phase: After stabilizing the patient during the acute phase, excessive fluid accumulation in the third space should be limited by instituting severe potassium, sodium, and fluid restriction.

Resolution Phase: A fall in hematocrit and an increasing urinary output without an increased intake are observed due to the return of third space fluid to the intravascular compartment. Peripheral and/or pulmonary edema may result if the kidneys are unable to excrete third space fluid as rapidly as it is mobilized. Diuretics may be indicated during the resolution phase if necessary to combat pulmonary edema.

Pulmonary and Vascular Complications
Serious pulmonary conditions (e.g., atelectasis, acute respiratory distress syndrome) have been reported. In addition, thromboembolic events both in association with, and separate from, the Ovarian Hyperstimulation Syndrome have been reported following menotropins therapy. Intravascular thrombosis and embolism, which may originate in venous or arterial vessels, can result in reduced blood flow to critical organs or the extremities. Sequelae of such events have included venous thrombophlebitis, pulmonary embolism, pulmonary infarction, cerebral vascular occlusion (stroke), and arterial occlusion resulting in loss of limb. In rare cases, pulmonary complications and/or thromboembolic events have resulted in death.

Multiple Births
Data from a clinical trial revealed the following results regarding multiple births: Of the pregnancies following therapy with menotropins and hCG, 80% resulted in single births, 15% in twins, and 5% of the total pregnancies resulted in three or more concepti. The patient and her husband should be advised of the frequency and potential hazards of multiple gestation before starting treatment.

Hypersensitivity/Anaphylactic Reactions
Hypersensitivity/anaphylactic reactions associated with menotropins administration have been reported in some patients. These reactions presented as generalized urticaria, facial edema, angioneurotic edema, and/or dyspnea suggestive of laryngeal edema. The relationship of these symptoms to uncharacterized urinary proteins is uncertain.

PRECAUTIONS
General
Careful attention should be given to diagnosis in the selection of candidates for menotropins therapy (see "INDICATIONS AND USAGE—SELECTION OF PATIENTS").

Information for Patients
Prior to therapy with Repronex™ patients should be informed of the duration of treatment and the monitoring of their condition that will be required. Possible adverse reactions (see "ADVERSE REACTIONS" section) and the risk of multiple births should also be discussed.

Laboratory Tests
Women:
Treatment for Induction of Ovulation
In most instances, treatment with menotropins results only in follicular growth and maturation. In order to effect ovulation, hCG must be given following the administration of Repronex™ when clinical assessment of the patient indicates that sufficient follicular maturation has occurred. This may be directly estimated by measuring serum (or urinary) estrogen levels and sonographic visualization of the ovaries. The combination of both estradiol levels and ultrasonography are useful for monitoring the growth and development of follicles, timing hCG administration, as well as minimizing the risk of the Ovarian Hyperstimulation Syndrome and multiple gestation.

Other clinical parameters which may have potential use for monitoring menotropins therapy include:
a) Changes in the vaginal cytology;
b) Appearance and volume of the cervical mucus;
c) Spinnbarkeit; and
d) Ferning of the cervical mucus.
The above clinical indices provide an indirect estimate of the estrogenic effect upon the target organs, and therefore should only be used adjunctively with more direct estimates of follicular development, i.e., serum estradiol and ultrasonography.

The clinical confirmation of ovulation, with the exception of pregnancy, is obtained by direct and indirect indices of progesterone production. The indices most generally used are as follows:
a) A rise in basal body temperature;
b) Increase in serum progesterone; and
c) Menstruation following the shift in basal body temperature.

When used in conjunction with indices of progesterone production, sonographic visualization of the ovaries will assist in determining if ovulation has occurred. Sonographic evidence of ovulation may include the following:
a) Fluid in the cul-de-sac;
b) Ovarian stigmata; and
c) Collapsed follicle.
Because of the subjectivity of the various tests for the determination of follicular maturation and ovulation, it cannot be overemphasized that the physician should choose tests with which he/she is thoroughly familiar.

Drug Interactions
No clinically significant drug/drug or drug/food adverse interactions have been reported during menotropins therapy.

Carcinogenesis and Mutagenesis
Long-term toxicity studies in animals have not been performed to evaluate the carcinogenic potential of menotropins.

Pregnancy
Pregnancy Category X: See "CONTRAINDICATIONS" section.

Nursing Mothers
It is not known whether this drug is excreted in human milk. Because many drugs are excreted in human milk, caution should be exercised if menotropins is administered to a nursing woman.

ADVERSE REACTIONS
Women:
The following adverse reactions, reported during menotropins therapy, are listed in decreasing order of potential severity:
1. Pulmonary and vascular complications (see "WARNINGS")
2. Ovarian Hyperstimulation Syndrome (see "WARNINGS")
3. Hemoperitoneum
4. Adnexal torsion (as a complication of ovarian enlargement)
5. Mild to moderate ovarian enlargement
6. Ovarian cysts
7. Abdominal pain
8. Sensitivity to menotropins. (Febrile reactions suggestive of allergic response have been reported following the administration of menotropins. Reports of flu-like symptoms including fever, chills, musculoskeletal aches, joint pains, nausea, headaches, and malaise have also been reported).
9. Gastrointestinal symptoms (nausea, vomiting, diarrhea, abdominal cramps, bloating)
10. Pain, rash, swelling and/or irritation at the site of injection
11. Body rashes
12. Dizziness, tachycardia, dyspnea, tachypnea
The following medical events have been reported subsequent to pregnancies resulting from menotropins therapy:
1. Ectopic pregnancy
2. Congenital abnormalities
From a study of 287 completed pregnancies following menotropins-hCG therapy, five incidents of birth defects were reported (1.7%). One infant had multiple congenital anomalies consisting of imperforate anus, aplasia of the sigmoid colon, third degree hypospadias, cecovesicle fistula, bifid scrotum, meningocele, bilateral internal tibial torsion, and right metatarsus adductus. Another infant was born with an imperforate anus and possible congenital heart lesions; another had a supermumerary digit; another was born with hypospadias and exstrophy of the bladder; and the fifth child had Down's syndrome. None of the investigators felt that these defects were drug-related. Subsequently one report of an infant death due to hydrocephalus and cardiac anomalies has been received.
There have been infrequent reports of ovarian neoplasms, both benign and malignant, in women who have undergone multiple drug regimens for ovulation induction; however, a causal relationship has not been established.
Men:
1. Gynecomastia may occur occasionally during menotropins-hCG therapy. This is a known effect of the hCG treatment.
2. Erythrocytosis (hct 50%, hgb 17.8g%) was recorded in one patient.

DRUG ABUSE AND DEPENDENCE
There have been no reports of abuse or dependence with menotropins.

OVERDOSAGE
Aside from possible ovarian hyperstimulation (see "WARNINGS"), little is known concerning the consequences of acute overdosage with menotropins.

DOSAGE AND ADMINISTRATION
Women:
1. Dosage:
The dose of Repronex™ to produce maturation of the follicle must be individualized for each patient. It is recommended

that the initial dose to any patient should be 75 IU of FSH/LH per day, **ADMINISTERED INTRAMUSCULARLY**, for seven to twelve days followed by hCG, 5,000 U to 10,000 U, one day after the last dose of Repronex™. Administration of Repronex™ should not exceed 12 days in a single course of therapy. The patient should be treated until indices of estrogenic activity, as indicated under "PRECAUTIONS" above, are equivalent to or greater than those of the normal individual. If serum or urinary estradiol determinations or ultrasonographic visualizations are available, they may be useful as a guide to therapy. If the ovaries are abnormally enlarged on the last day of Repronex™ therapy, hCG should not be administered in this course of therapy; this will reduce the chances of development of the Ovarian Hyperstimulation Syndrome. If there is evidence of ovulation but no pregnancy, repeat this dosage regime for at least two more courses before increasing the dose of Repronex™ to 150 IU of FSH/LH per day for seven to twelve days. As before, this dose should be followed by 5,000 U to 10,000 U of the hCG one day after the last dose of menotropins. A menotropins dose of 150 IU of FSH/LH per day has proven to be the most effective dose especially for *in vitro* fertilization. If evidence of ovulation is present, but pregnancy does not ensue, repeat the same dose for two more courses. Doses larger than this are not routinely recommended.

During treatment with both Repronex™ and hCG and during a two-week post-treatment period, patients should be examined at least every other day for signs of excessive ovarian stimulation. It is recommended that Repronex™ administration be stopped if the ovaries become abnormally enlarged or abdominal pain occurs. Most of the Ovarian Hyperstimulation Syndrome occurs after treatment has been discontinued and reaches its maximum at about seven to ten days post-ovulation. Patients should be followed for at least two weeks after hCG administration.

The couple should be encouraged to have intercourse daily, beginning on the day prior to the administration of hCG until ovulation becomes apparent from the indices employed for the determination of progestational activity. Care should be taken to insure insemination. In the light of the foregoing indices and parameters mentioned, it should become obvious that, unless a physician is willing to devote considerable time to these patients and be familiar with and conduct the necessary laboratory studies, he/she should not use Repronex™.

2. Administration:
Dissolve the contents of one vial of Repronex™ in one to two mL of 0.9% Sodium Chloride Injection and **ADMINISTER INTRAMUSCULARLY** immediately. Any unused reconstituted material should be discarded.
Parenteral drug products should be inspected visually for particulate matter and discoloration prior to administration, whenever solution and container permit.
Men:
1. Dosage:
Prior to concomitant therapy with Repronex™ and hCG, pretreatment with hCG alone (5,000 U three times a week) is required. Treatment should continue for a period sufficient to achieve serum testosterone levels within the normal range and masculinization as judged by the appearance of secondary sex characteristics. Such pretreatment may require four to six months, then the recommended dose of Repronex™ is 75 IU FSH/LH **ADMINISTERED INTRAMUSCULARLY**, three times a week and the recommended dose of hCG is 2,000 U twice a week. Therapy should be carried on for a minimum of four more months to insure detecting spermatozoa in the ejaculate, as it takes 74 ± 4 days in the human male for germ cells to reach the spermatozoa stage. If the patient has not responded with evidence of increased spermatogenesis at the end of four months of therapy, treatment may continue with 75 IU FSH/LH three times a week, or the dose can be increased to 150 IU FSH/LH three times a week, with the hCG dose unchanged.

2. Administration:
Dissolve the contents of one vial of Repronex™ in one to two mL of 0.9% Sodium Chloride Injection and **ADMINISTER INTRAMUSCULARLY** immediately. Any unused reconstituted material should be discarded.
Parenteral drug products should be inspected visually for particulate matter and discoloration prior to administration, whenever solution and container permit.

HOW SUPPLIED
Repronex™ is available in vials as a sterile, lyophilized, white to off-white powder or pellet.
75 IU FSH and 75 IU of LH activity, supplied as:
    NDC 55566-7175-1—Box of 1 vial
    NDC 55566-7175-2—Box of 5 vials
150 IU FSH and 150 IU of LH activity, supplied as:
    NDC 55566-7115-1—Box of 1 vial
By biological assay, one IU of LH for the Second International Reference Preparation (2nd-IRP) for hMG is biologically equivalent to approximately 0.5 U of hCG.
Lyophilized powder may be stored refrigerated or at room temperature 3°-25°C (37°-77°F). Protect from light. Use immediately after reconstitution. Discard unused material.

	% Pts. Ovul.	% Pts. Preg.	% Abort.	% Multi Preg.	% Twins	% 3 or more Concepti	% Hyperstim. Syndr.
Primary Amenorrhea	62	22	14	25	25	0	0
Secondary Amenorrhea	61	28	24	28	18	10	1.9
Secondary Amenorrhea w/Galactorrhea	77	42	21	41	31	10	1.2
Polycystic Ovaries	76	26	39	17	17	0	1.1
Anovulatory Cycles	77	24	15	14	9	5	2
Miscellaneous	83	20	36	2	2	0	0.1

CLINICAL STUDIES

Women:
The results of the clinical experience and effectiveness of the administration of menotropins to 1,286 patients in 3,002 courses of therapy are summarized below. The values include patients who were treated with other than the recommended dosage regime. The values for the presently recommended dosage regime are essentially the same.

	%
Patients ovulating	75
Patients pregnant	25
Patients aborting	25*
Multiple pregnancies	20**
Twins	15**
Three or more concepti	5**
Fetal abnormalities	1.7**
Hyperstimulation syndrome	1.3

*Based on total pregnancies
**Based on total deliveries

Results by diagnosis group are summarized below (these values include patients who were treated with other than the present recommended dosage regime):
[See table above]

Men:
Clinical results of the treatment of men with primary or secondary hypogonadotropic hypogonadism are as follows:
In a Cooperative study, with an adequate treatment period of 3 to 8 months, 60 of 70 men with primary hypogonadotropic hypogonadism and 8 of 11 men with secondary hypogonadotropic hypogonadism responded with mean increases in their sperm counts from less than 5 to 24 million spermatozoa per milliliter of ejaculate. Forty-one wives of 54 men with primary hypogonadotropic hypogonadism desiring offspring and 7 wives of men with secondary hypogonadotropic hypogonadism conceived. Patients treated with menotropins and hCG for less than 3 months or with menotropins alone did not respond to therapy.
A world-wide data search revealed that of 160 recorded pregnancies as the result of use of menotropins-hCG in men, there were 7 spontaneous abortions, one ectopic pregnancy and 3 congenital anomalies at birth (esophageal atresia in a female infant which was later corrected by surgery, unilateral cryptorchidism, inguinal hernia).
Caution: Federal law prohibits dispensing without prescription.
Manufactured for:
FERRING PHARMACEUTICALS INC.
TARRYTOWN, NY 10591
By: LEDERLE PARENTERALS, INC.
Carolina, Puerto Rico 00986
4/97
02dc162.doc

SECRETIN–FERRING   ℞
[si-krē'tin]

HOW SUPPLIED
Secretin-Ferring is supplied as a lyophilized sterile powder in 10 mL vials (NDC 55566-1075-1) containing 75 CU. The unreconstituted product should be stored at −20° C (freezer). However, the biological activity of Secretin-Ferring will not be significantly decreased by storage at temperatures up to 25° C for up to 3 weeks. Expiration date is marked on the label.
Please see full prescribing information in the Diagnostic Product Information section.

THYREL® TRH   ℞
(protirelin)
Injection
FOR INTRAVENOUS ADMINISTRATION

HOW SUPPLIED
As 1 mL ampuls—boxes of 5 (NDC 55566-0081-5). Each mL contains Thyrel TRH 0.50 mg (500 μg), sodium chloride 9.0 mg for isotonicity, hydrochloric acid and sodium hydroxide as needed to adjust pH.

Store at controlled room temperature (59° to 86°F).
Please see full prescribing information in the Diagnostic Product Information section.

The Fielding Company
112 WELDON PARKWAY
MARYLAND HEIGHTS, MO 63043

Direct Inquires to:
Professional Services Department
(314) 567-5462
For Medical Information Contact:
In Emergencies:
(314) 567-5462

GERIMED® Tablets   OTC

DESCRIPTION
A multivitamin-multimineral supplement useful as adjunctive therapy in osteoporosis. Provides a balanced ratio of calcium and phosphorus (2.8 to 1) with adequate Vitamin D for proper absorption.
Each tablet contains:

Dibasic Calcium Phosphate*	600	mg.
Calcium Carbonate*	200	mg.
Vitamin A	5000	I. U.
Vitamin D₂	400	I. U.
Vitamin E	30	I. U.
Vitamin C	120	mg.
Thiamine B₁	3	mg.
Riboflavin B₂	3	mg.
Niacinamide	25	mg.
Pyridoxine B₆	2	mg.
Vitamin B₁₂	6	mcg.
Zinc	15	mg.

*Total Calcium	370	mg.
*Total Phosphorus	130	mg.
Calcium/Phosphorus ratio 2.8 - 1		

DOSAGE
One tablet daily, or as prescribed by the physician.
HOW SUPPLIED
Bottle of 60 tablets.
NDC 0421-0080-60

IROSPAN® Tablets/Capsules   OTC
Each tablet or capsule contains:

Iron	65 mg.
(Ferrous Sulfate-Exsic. 200 mg.)	
Ascorbic Acid	150 mg.

DESCRIPTION
Irospan is a unique presentation of extended release exsiccated ferrous sulfate and ascorbic acid. Irospan is of particular value during pregnancy and lactation providing excellent tolerance and absorption.
DOSAGE
One tablet or capsule daily or as prescribed by the physician.
HOW SUPPLIED
Irospan Tablets—bottles of 100.   NDC 0421-0360-01
Irospan Capsules—bottles of 60.   NDC 0421-0361-60

LURLINE® PMS Tablets   OTC
Each tablet contains:

Acetaminophen	500 mg.
Pamabrom	25 mg.
Pyridoxine	50 mg.

DESCRIPTION
Lurline PMS is a safe and effective approach for relief of the multi-symptom complex of premenstrual syndrome. The medication combines an analgesic, a mild diuretic and pyridoxine, representing a safe first line treatment.
Lurline PMS contains no hormones, no sedatives and is aspirin free.

DOSAGE
Start Lurline PMS at the first sign of pain or discomfort, usually 7 to 10 days before menses. Usual dosage is one tablet 3 or 4 times daily. Do not exceed the maximum dose of 8 tablets a day.

HOW SUPPLIED
Lurline PMS—bottles of 24. NDC 0421-8787-24
Lurline PMS—bottles of 50. NDC 0421-8787-50
Physician samples and literature available.

NESTABS® CBF Tablets   ℞
Prenatal Tablets

DESCRIPTION
Each tablet contains:

Vitamin A (from beta carotene)	4,000 IU
Vitamin D	400 IU
Vitamin E	30 IU
Vitamin C	120 mg.
Folic Acid	1 mg.
Thiamine	3 mg.
Riboflavin	3 mg.
Niacinamide	20 mg.
Pyridoxine	3 mg.
Vitamin B₁₂	8 mcg.
Calcium (from 500mg. calcium carbonate)	200 mg.
Iodine	150 mcg.
Zinc	15 mg.
Iron (from carbonyl iron)	50 mg.

A comprehensive vitamin-mineral supplement expressly formulated for use during pregnancy and lactation.

DOSAGE
One tablet daily, or as prescribed by the physician.

PRECAUTION
Folic acid may obscure pernicious anemia in that hematologic remission can occur while neurological manifestations remain progressive.

> WARNING: Accidental overdose of iron-containing products is a leading cause of fatal poisoning in children under 6. Keep this product out of reach of children. In case of accidental overdose, call a doctor or poison control center immediately.

HOW SUPPLIED
Bottles of 100 tablets.
NDC 0421-1594-01

C. B. Fleet Co., Inc.
4615 MURRAY PL.
LYNCHBURG, VA 24506-1349

Direct Inquiries to:
David Vaughan
Director of Quality Assurance:
(804) 528-4000

FLEET® BISACODYL LAXATIVES, ENEMA, SUPPOSITORIES, AND TABLETS   OTC
(bisacodyl U.S.P.)

COMPOSITION
FLEET® Laxative Tablets - Enteric coated 5 mg bisacodyl tablets
FLEET® Laxative Suppositories - 10 mg bisacodyl suppositories
Latex free FLEET® Ready-to-Use Bisacodyl Enema - 10 mg bisacodyl enema solution in 37 ml disposable squeeze bottle with a 2-inch, pre-lubricated Comfortip®.

Continued on next page

Fleet Bisacodyl—Cont.

ACTION AND USES

FLEET® Bisacodyl is a stimulant laxative, given either orally or rectally, acting directly on the colonic mucosa where it stimulates sensory nerve endings to produce parasympathetic reflexes resulting in increased peristaltic contractions of the colon. The contact action of the drug is restricted to the colon and motility in the small intestine is not appreciably influenced. FLEET® Laxative Tablets usually work within 6–12 hours. FLEET® Laxative Suppositories produce a bowel movement within 15 minutes to 1 hour and the latex free FLEET® Bisacodyl Enema produces a bowel movement within 15–20 minutes. It is useful as a laxative for occasional relief of constipation, in bowel cleansing in preparation for X-ray and endoscopic examination. May be used as a laxative in postoperative, antepartum, or postpartum care or in preparation for delivery.

GENERAL LAXATIVE WARNINGS

Do not use a laxative product when nausea, vomiting, or abdominal pain is present unless directed by a physician. If you have noticed a sudden change in bowel habits that persists over a period of 2 weeks, consult a physician before using a laxative. Rectal bleeding or failure to have a bowel movement after use of a laxative may indicate a serious condition. Discontinue use and consult a physician. Laxative products should not be used longer than 1 week unless directed by a physician. This product may cause abdominal discomfort, faintness, rectal burning, and mild cramps. Keep this and all drugs out of the reach of children. In case of accidental ingestion, seek professional assistance or contact a Poison Control Center immediately.

DOSAGE AND ADMINISTRATION

Enema
SHAKE BEFORE USING.
REMOVE PROTECTIVE SHIELD FROM TIP BEFORE ADMINISTERING.
Adults and children 12 years of age and over: 1 unit (30 mL) in a single daily dose.
Children under 12 years of age — DO NOT USE.
Administration: Preferred position—Lying on left side with left knee slightly bent and the right leg drawn up, or knee-chest position. Diaphragm at base of tube prevents accidental leakage and assures controlled flow of the enema solution. May be used at room temperature.
Tablets
Adults and children 12 years of age and over: Take 2 tablets in a single dose once daily.
Children 6 to under 12 years of age: Take 1 tablet once daily. Expect results in 6–12 hours if taken at bedtime or within 6 hours if taken before breakfast. Do not chew or crush tablets. Do not administer tablets within 1 hour after taking an antacid, milk, or milk products.
Children under 6 years of age: Consult your physician.
Suppositories
Adults and children 12 years of age and over: Use 1 suppository once daily. Remove foil wrapper. Lie on your side and, with pointed end first, push suppository high into the rectum so it will not slip out. Retain it for 15 to 20 minutes. If you feel the suppository must come out immediately, it was not inserted high enough and should be pushed higher.
Children 6 to under 12 years of age: One half of one 10 mg suppository once daily.
Children under 6 years of age: Consult your physician.

PROFESSIONAL ADMINISTRATION

See FLEET® Ready-to-Use Enema and FLEET® Prep Kits.

FLEET® ENEMA, A SALINE LAXATIVE   OTC
FLEET® ENEMA FOR CHILDREN, A SALINE LAXATIVE

COMPOSITION

FLEET® ENEMA: Each 118 mL. (delivered dose) contains 19 g. monobasic sodium phosphate monohydrate and 7 g. dibasic sodium phosphate heptahydrate. The latex free FLEET® Enema unit, with a 2-inch, pre-lubricated Comfortip®, contains 4.5 fl. oz. (133 mL) of enema solution in a hand-size plastic squeeze bottle. FLEET® ENEMA FOR CHILDREN: Each 59 mL (delivered dose) contains 9.5 g. monobasic sodium phosphate monohydrate and 3.5 g. dibasic sodium phosphate heptahydrate. The latex free FLEET® Enema for Children unit, with a 2-inch, pre-lubricated Comfortip® contains 2.25 fl. oz. (66 mL) of enema solution in a hand-size plastic squeeze bottle. Designed for quick, convenient administration by nurse or patient according to instructions. Disposable after single use.
ELEMENTAL & ELECTROLYTIC CONTENT
mEq Phosphate (PO_4) per ml 4.15
mEq Sodium (NA) per ml 1.61

ACTION AND USES

FLEET® Enema is useful as a laxative in the relief of occasional constipation, and as part of a bowel cleansing regimen in preparing the patient for surgery or for preparing the colon for x-ray and endoscopic examination. Used as directed, FLEET® Enema provides thorough yet safe cleansing action and induces complete emptying of the left colon usually within 2 to 5 minutes without pain or spasm. Also used for general postoperative care and to help relieve fecal or barium impaction.

GENERAL LAXATIVE WARNINGS

Do not use laxative products when nausea, vomiting, or abdominal pain is present unless directed by a physician. If you notice a sudden change in bowel habits that persists over a period of 2 weeks, consult a physician. Rectal bleeding or failure to have a bowel movement after use of a laxative may indicate a serious condition. Discontinue use and consult a physician. Laxative products should not be used longer than 1 week unless directed by a physician. As with any drug, if you are pregnant or nursing a baby, seek the advice of a health professional before using this product. Keep this and all drugs out of the reach of children. In case of accidental ingestion or overdose, seek professional assistance or contact a Poison Control Center immediately.

PROFESSIONAL USE WARNINGS

Do not use in patients with congenital megacolon, bowel obstruction, imperforate anus or congestive heart failure.
Use with caution in patients with impaired renal function, pre-existing electrolyte disturbances or in patients on diuretics or other medications which may affect electrolyte levels—or where colostomy exists.
Since FLEET® Enema contains sodium phosphates, there is a risk of elevated serum levels of sodium and phosphate and decreased levels of calcium and potassium and consequent hypocalcemia, hyperphosphatemia, hypernatremia, and acidosis may occur. This is of particular concern in children with megacolon or any other condition where there is retention of enema solution.
Additional fluids by mouth are recommended with all bowel cleansing dosages.
SINCE FLEET® BRAND ENEMAS ARE AVAILABLE IN ADULT AND CHILDREN'S SIZES, PRESCRIBE CAREFULLY.

PRECAUTIONS

DO NOT ADMINISTER 4.5 OZ. ADULT SIZE TO CHILDREN UNDER 12 YEARS OF AGE. DO NOT ADMINISTER 2.25 OZ. CHILDREN'S SIZE TO CHILDREN UNDER 2 YEARS OF AGE. IF AFTER THE ENEMA SOLUTION IS ADMINISTERED THERE IS NO RETURN OF LIQUID, CONTACT A PHYSICIAN IMMEDIATELY AS DEHYDRATION COULD OCCUR.

OVERDOSAGE

Overdosage or retention of FLEET® Enema may cause hypocalcemia, hyperphosphatemia, hypernatremia, hypernatremic dehydration and acidosis.
Hypocalcemia, hyperphosphatemia, hypernatremia and acidosis
Calcium, Phosphate, Potassium and Sodium levels should be carefully monitored. Immediate corrective action should be taken to restore electrolyte balance with appropriate fluid replacements. Prompt parenteral administration of fluids with lower concentrations of Sodium and Chloride than extracellular fluid (40–50 mEq/liter) and moderate concentration of Potassium (20–30 mEq/liter) administered at a rate of 3,000 to 4,000 cc/sq. m of body surface during the first 12 to 24 hours dependent on the severity of dehydration and the clinical response.

ADMINISTRATION AND DOSAGE

REMOVE PROTECTIVE SHIELD FROM TIP BEFORE ADMINISTERING.
Preferred position: Lying on left side with left knee slightly bent and the right leg drawn up, or knee-chest position. Dosage: Adults, 4.5 fl. oz. in a single daily dose. Child, 2.25 fl. oz. in a single daily dose. Diaphragm at base of tube prevents accidental leakage and assures controlled flow of the enema solution. May be used at room temperature. Adult, each 118 mL (delivered dose) contains 4.4 g. (191 mEq) sodium. Child, each 59 mL (delivered dose) contains 2.2 g (95.5 mEq) sodium.

PROFESSIONAL DOSAGE AND ADMINISTRATION

FLEET® Ready-To-Use 4.5 oz. Adult Size Enema should not be used in children under 12 years of age. In those cases where complications are reported, infants and young children are often involved. FLEET® Ready-To-Use Enema for Children should be used with caution in children of any age. Careful consideration of the use of enemas in general in children is recommended. The adult size enema should not be used in children under 12 years of age. For children 2 to under 12 years of age, use FLEET® Ready-To-Use Enema for Children, which contains a dosage of one-half the adult size enema. For children less than 2 years of age, FLEET® Glycerin Suppositories for Children should be used.

Proper and safe use of FLEET® Ready-To-Use Enema also requires that the product be administered according to the Directions for Use. Health care professionals should remember, when administering the product, to gently insert the enema into the rectum with the tip pointing toward the navel. Insertion may be made easier by having the patient bear down as they would in having a bowel movement. Care during insertion is necessary due to lack of sensory innervation of the rectum and due to possibility of bowel perforation. Once inserted, squeeze the bottle until nearly all the liquid is expelled. If resistance is encountered on insertion of the nozzle or in administering the solution, the procedure should be discontinued. Forcing the enema can result in perforation and/or abrasion of the rectum.
If an enema containing phosphate or sodium is not advised, use FLEET® Bisacodyl Enema.

HOW SUPPLIED

FLEET® Enema is supplied in a 4.5 fl. oz. (133 mL) ready-to-use squeeze bottle. Children's size, 2.25 fl. oz. (66 mL) IMPORTANT: FLEET® Enema, Adult and Child size, ARE NOT INTENDED FOR ORAL CONSUMPTION, in any dosage size.

IS THIS PRODUCT OTC?

Yes.

FLEET® MINERAL OIL ENEMA   OTC
A LUBRICANT LAXATIVE

COMPOSITION

The latex free FLEET® Mineral Oil Enema unit, with a 2-inch, prelubricated Comfortip®, delivers 118 mL of mineral oil USP in a hand-size plastic squeeze bottle. FLEET® Mineral Oil Enema is sodium free.

ACTION AND INDICATIONS

Serves to soften and lubricate hard stools, easing their passage without irritating the mucosa. Results approximate a normal bowel movement in that only the rectum, sigmoid, and part or all of the descending colon are evacuated. Indicated for relief of fecal impaction; valuable in relief of occasional constipation when straining must be avoided (in hypertension, coronary occlusion, proctologic procedures, postoperative care); for removal of barium sulfate residues from the colon after barium administration for GI series or outlining the left atrium; to obtain the laxative benefits of mineral oil while avoiding possible untoward effects of oral administration such as (1) interference with intestinal absorption of fat-soluble vitamins A, D, E and K and other nutrients (2) danger of systemic absorption (3) possible risk of lipid pneumonia due to aspiration. Generally effective in 2 to 15 minutes.

WARNINGS

Do not use laxative products when nausea, vomiting, or abdominal pain is present unless directed by a physician. If you have noticed a sudden change in bowel habits that persists over a period of 2 weeks, consult a physician. Rectal bleeding or failure to have a bowel movement after use of a laxative may indicate a serious condition. Discontinue use and consult a physician. Laxative products should not be used longer than 1 week unless directed by a physician. As with any drug, if you are pregnant or nursing a baby, seek the advice of a health professional before using this product. Keep this and all drugs out of the reach of children. In case of accidental ingestion, seek professional assistance or contact a Poison Control Center immediately.

PRECAUTIONS

DO NOT ADMINISTER TO CHILDREN UNDER 2 YEARS OF AGE.

ADMINISTRATION AND DOSAGE

REMOVE PROTECTIVE SHIELD FROM TIP BEFORE ADMINISTERING.
Preferred position: Lying on left side with left knee slightly bent and the right leg drawn up, or knee-chest position. Dosage: Adults and children 12 years of age and over: one bottle (118 ml delivered dose) in a single daily dose. Children 2 to under 12 years of age: $^1/_2$ bottle (59 ml delivered dose) in a single daily dose. Diaphragm at base of tube prevents accidental leakage and assures controlled flow of the enema solution. May be used at room temperature. Follow with regular FLEET® Enema according to dosage instructions contained in PDR for more thorough cleansing.

PROFESSIONAL DOSAGE AND ADMINISTRATION

FLEET® Ready-To-Use Mineral Oil Enema should not be used in children under 2 years of age. FLEET® Ready-To-Use Mineral Oil Enema should be used with caution in children of any age. Careful consideration of the use of enemas in general in children is recommended.
Proper and safe use of FLEET® Ready-To-Use Mineral Oil Enema also requires that the product be administered ac-

cording to the Directions for Use. Health care professionals should remember, when administering the product, to gently insert the enema into the rectum with the tip pointing toward the naval. Insertion may be made easier by having the patient bear down as they would in having a bowel movement. Care during insertion is necessary due to lack of sensory innervation of the rectum and due to possibility of bowel perforation. Once inserted, squeeze the bottle until nearly all the liquid is expelled. If resistance is encountered on insertion of the nozzle or in administering the solution, the procedure should be discontinued. Forcing the enema can result in perforation and/or abrasion of the rectum.

HOW SUPPLIED

FLEET® Mineral Oil Enema is supplied in 4.5 fl.oz. (133 mL) ready-to-use squeeze bottle.

IS THIS PRODUCT OTC?

Yes.

FLEET® PHOSPHO®-SODA   OTC
A BUFFERED ORAL SALINE LAXATIVE

COMPOSITION

Each 5 mL of regular or flavored FLEET® Phospho-soda contains 2.4 g. Monobasic Sodium Phosphate Monohydrate and 0.9 g. Dibasic Sodium Phosphate Heptahydrate in a stable, buffered aqueous solution.
Elemental and Electrolytic Content
mEq Phosphate (PO_4) per ml   12.45
mEq Sodium (Na) per ml   4.82

INDICATIONS

As a laxative, for the relief of occasional constipation. As a purgative, for use as part of a bowel cleansing regimen in preparing the patient for surgery or for preparing the colon for x-ray or endoscopic examination.

ACTION AND USES

Versatile in action as a gentle laxative or purgative, according to dosage. This product produces a bowel movement in $\frac{1}{2}$ to 6 hours, depending on dosage. Especially useful as a bowel prep for colonoscopy, surgery, and radiology procedures. See DOSAGE AND ADMINISTRATION. Patient instruction pads available upon request.

CONTRAINDICATIONS

DO NOT USE THIS PRODUCT IF YOU HAVE KIDNEY DISEASE OR ARE ON A SODIUM RESTRICTED DIET UNLESS DIRECTED BY A PHYSICIAN. EACH TEASPOONFUL (5 mL) CONTAINS 556 MG (24.17 MILLIEQUIVALENTS) SODIUM.

PROFESSIONAL USE WARNINGS

Do not use in patients with congenital megacolon, bowel obstruction, ascites or congestive heart failure.
Use with caution in patients with impaired renal function, pre-existing electrolyte imbalances or with debilitated patients.
Since FLEET® Phospho-soda contains sodium phosphates, there is a risk of elevated serum levels of sodium and phosphate and decreased levels of calcium and potassium and consequent hypocalcemia, hyperphosphatemia, hypernatremia, and acidosis may occur.
Additional fluids by mouth are recommended with all bowel cleansing dosages.

WARNINGS

TAKING MORE THAN THE RECOMMENDED DOSE IN 24 HOURS CAN BE HARMFUL. IF THERE IS NO BOWEL MOVEMENT AFTER MAXIMUM DOSAGE, CONTACT A PHYSICIAN AS DEHYDRATION COULD OCCUR.
SINCE FLEET® PHOSPHO-SODA IS AVAILABLE IN TWO SIZES, PRESCRIBE BY VOLUMES. DO NOT PRESCRIBE "BY THE BOTTLE" AS SERIOUS SIDE EFFECTS FROM OVERDOSAGE MAY OCCUR.
Ask a doctor before using this product if you are on a sodium restricted diet, have a kidney disease or are pregnant or nursing a baby. Ask a doctor before using any laxative if you have nausea, vomiting, abdominal pain, have a sudden change in bowel habits lasting more than 2 weeks or have already used a laxative for more than 1 week. Stop using this product and consult a doctor if you have rectal bleeding or have no bowel movement after use as dehydration may occur. These symptoms may indicate a serious condition. Keep this and all drugs out of the reach of children. In case of overdose or accidental ingestion, seek professional assistance or contact a Poison Control Center immediately.

OVERDOSAGE

Overdosage or retention of FLEET® Phospho-soda may cause hypocalcemia, hyperphosphatemia, hypernatremia, hypernatremic dehydration and acidosis.
Hypocalcemia, hyperphosphatemia, hypernatremia and acidosis

Calcium, Phosphate, Potassium and Sodium levels should be carefully monitored. Immediate corrective action should be taken to restore electrolyte balance with appropriate fluid replacements. Prompt parenteral administration of fluids with lower concentrations of Sodium and Chloride than extracellular fluid (40–50 mEq./liter) and moderate concentration of Potassium (20–30 mEq./liter) administered at a rate of 3,000 to 4,000 cc/sq. m of body surface during the first 12 to 24 hours dependent on the severity of dehydration and the clinical response.

DOSAGE AND ADMINISTRATION

For best results, take on an empty stomach. Most effective when taken upon rising, at least 30 minutes before a meal, or at bedtime for overnight action. **Dilute recommended dosage with one-half glass (4 fl. oz.) cool water. Drink, then follow with one glass (8 fl. oz.) cool water.**
DOSAGE: SINCE FLEET® PHOSPHO-SODA IS AVAILABLE IN TWO SIZES, PRESCRIBE BY VOLUMES; DO NOT PRESCRIBE "BY THE BOTTLE". DO NOT EXCEED RECOMMENDED DOSAGE AS SERIOUS SIDE EFFECTS MAY OCCUR.
SINGLE DAILY DOSAGE: DO NOT TAKE MORE UNLESS DIRECTED BY A DOCTOR. SEE WARNINGS.

Adults and children 12 years and older	20 to 45 mL* (4 to 9 teaspoons*)
Children 10 and 11 years	10 to 20 mL* (2 to 4 teaspoons*)
Children 5 to 9 years	5 to 10 mL* (1 to 2 teaspoons*)
Children under 5 years	Ask a doctor

* DO NOT TAKE MORE THAN THIS AMOUNT IN A 24-HOUR PERIOD.

HOW SUPPLIED

Regular or flavored, in bottles of $1\frac{1}{2}$, and 3 fl. oz. FLEET® Phospho-soda should not be confused with FLEET® Enema, a sodium phosphates disposable ready-to-use enema. FLEET® Enema, Adult and Child size, ARE NOT INTENDED FOR ORAL CONSUMPTION, in any dosage size.

IS THIS PRODUCT OTC?

Yes.

FLEET® PREP KITS   OTC
Bowel Evacuant

DESCRIPTION

FLEET® Prep Kit No. 1 contains:
1. FLEET® Phospho-soda—$1\frac{1}{2}$ fl. oz. (45 mL) Ingredients: Each teaspoonful (5 mL) contains : Active Ingredients: Monobasic Sodium Phosphate Monohydrate 2.4 g and Dibasic Sodium Phosphate Hepatohydrate 0.9 g.
2. FLEET® Bisacodyl—4 laxative tablets. Ingredients: Each enteric-coated tablet contains Bisacodyl, USP, 5 mg.
3. FLEET® Bisacodyl—1 laxative suppository. Ingredients: Bisacodyl, USP, 10 mg.
4. 1 Patient Instruction Sheet.
FLEET® Prep Kit No. 2 contains:
1. FLEET® Phospho-soda—$1\frac{1}{2}$ fl. oz. (45 mL).
2. FLEET® Bisacodyl—4 tablets.
3. FLEET® Bagenema—1.
4. 1 Patient Instruction Sheet.
FLEET® Prep Kit No. 3 contains:
1. FLEET® Phospho-soda—1 $\frac{1}{2}$ fl. oz. (45 mL)
2. FLEET® Bisacodyl—4 tablets.
3. FLEET® Bisacodyl Enema 1 $\frac{1}{4}$ fl. oz. (37 mL)—1 laxative enema. Ingredients: 1–30 mL. dose containing 10 mg. of Bisacodyl, USP.
4. 1 Patient Instruction Sheet.

ACTIONS

Bowel Cleansing System

INDICATIONS

For use as part of a bowel cleansing regimen in preparation of the colon for radiology (prior to barium enemas or I.V.P.'s), surgery, and many endoscopic and colonoscopic procedures.

WARNINGS

DO NOT EXCEED RECOMMENDED DOSE UNLESS DIRECTED BY A PHYSICIAN. SERIOUS SIDE EFFECTS MAY OCCUR FROM EXCESS DOSAGE.
Each recommended dose ($1\frac{1}{2}$ fl. oz.) (45 mL) of Phospho-soda contains 5004 mg sodium. **Persons on a sodium restricted diet or with kidney disease should consult a health professional before use.**
Bisacodyl products may cause abdominal discomfort, faintness, rectal burning, and mild cramps.

WARNINGS

Do not chew tablets or give to persons who cannot swallow without chewing unless directed by a physician. Do not take tablets within 1 hour after taking antacids, milk, or milk products.
Keep this and all drugs out of the reach of children. In case of accidental overdose or ingestion, seek professional assistance or contact a Poison Control Center immediately.

PROFESSIONAL USE WARNINGS

Do not use in patients with congenital megacolon, bowel obstruction, ascites or congestive heart failure.
Use with caution in patients with impaired renal function, pre-existing electrolyte imbalances or with debilitated patients.
Since FLEET® Phospho-soda contains sodium phosphates, there is a risk of elevated serum levels of sodium and phosphate and decreased levels of calcium and potassium and consequent hypocalcemia, hyperphosphatemia, hypernatremia, and acidosis may occur.
Additional fluids by mouth are recommended with all bowel cleansing dosages.
If any of these complications occur following administration of FLEET® Phospho-soda, immediate corrective action should be taken to restore electrolyte balance with appropriate fluid replacements. Calcium, magnesium, and phosphorus levels should be carefully monitored. **See individual listings FLEET® Phospho-soda, and FLEET® Bisacodyl Enema for additional warnings.**
THESE KITS SHOULD NOT BE USED BY PATIENTS UNDER 12 YEARS OF AGE.

PRECAUTIONS

DO NOT EXCEED RECOMMENDED DOSE UNLESS DIRECTED BY A PHYSICIAN, AS SERIOUS SIDE EFFECTS MAY OCCUR. IF THERE IS NO BOWEL MOVEMENT AFTER MAXIMUM DOSAGE, CONTACT A PHYSICIAN AS DEHYDRATION COULD OCCUR.

DOSAGE AND ADMINISTRATION

SEE PATIENT INSTRUCTION SHEET FOR 18, 24, AND 48 HOUR PREPARATION SCHEDULE IN EACH KIT.

HOW SUPPLIED

See "Description" for contents of each kit.
Shipping Unit: 48 FLEET® Prep Kits per carton.
For full prescribing information on specific products, see individual listings (FLEET® Phospho-soda, FLEET® Bisacodyl Enema).

IS THIS PRODUCT OTC?

Yes.

Fleming & Company
1600 FENPARK DR.
FENTON, MO 63026

Direct Inquiries to:
H.C. Mansmann, Jr. MD
314-343-8200

AEROLATE SR & JR & III Capsules   ℞
(theophylline, anhydrous T.D.)

AEROLATE LIQUID
(theophylline, anhydrous)

COMPOSITION

Contains theophylline 4 grs. (260 mg) as SR, 2 grs (130 mg) as JR, 1 gr. as III (65 mg), in red/clear capsules. Liquid has 150 mg theophylline/15cc in a non-sugar, non-alcoholic, non-saccharin tangerine flavored base.

ACTION AND USES

Timed action pellets by-pass stomach to prevent gastric upset. Bronchodilation is achieved through bowel absorption only. Liquid is for the acute attack primarily.

ADMINISTRATION AND DOSAGE

One capsule every 12 hours. Every 8 hours in severe attacks. Liquid—adults—40 ml (2.5 tablespoonfuls) for acute attack. Children—0.25 ml/lb. Maintainance therapy—adults—for the first 6 doses, 25 ml (1.5 tablespoonfuls) before breakfast, at 3 p.m., at bedtime. Then 15 ml doses at above times. Children—0.15 ml/lb at these times, then 0.1 ml/lb per dose.

SIDE EFFECTS

Nausea, vomiting, epigastric or substernal pain, palpitation, headache, dizziness may occur.

Continued on next page

Aerolate—Cont.

HOW SUPPLIED

Capsules in bottles of 100.
Liquid in pints.

CHLOR–3　　　　　OTC

DESCRIPTION

Medical condiment containing sodium chloride 50%; potassium chloride 30%; magnesium chloride 20%.

INDICATIONS AND USAGE

To reduce sodium intake for patients on diuretics; for potential hypertensives and cardiacs.
To encourage physicians to recommend a condiment to replace "table salt" for family use and gourmet cooking.

HOW SUPPLIED

Shaker 8 oz. plastic bottles.

CONGESS SR & JR Capsules　　　Rx
Expectorant/Decongestant T.D.

COMPOSITION

Contains guaifenesin 250 mgs/pseudoephedrine 120 mgs as SR; guaifenesin 125 mgs/pseudoephedrine 60 mgs as JR in blue/pink capsules.

ACTION AND USES

To loosen mucus plugs in upper respiratory tract and congestion in acute pulmonary disorders, and in coughing. Nasal decongestion and alleviation of bronchospasm is also achieved up to 12 hrs. that accompany most coughs, especially during the nocturnal period.

INDICATIONS

Nasal congestion, sinusitis, acute aerotitis media, bronchial asthma, serous otitis media, and symptoms of the common cold.

DOSAGE

Adults and children over 12 yrs. one SR capsule every 12 hrs. Under 12 yrs. one JR capsule as prescribed by physician.

PRECAUTION AND SIDE EFFECTS

Use with care in severe hypertension, heart disease, hyperthyroidism, diabetes. Low grade sensitivity to drugs may be experienced.

CONTRAINDICATIONS

Prostatic hypertrophy, patients receiving MAO inhibitors.

HOW SUPPLIED

Plastic bottles of 100.

EXTENDRYL　　　　　Rx
T.D. Capsules SR & JR, Syrup and Tablets

Each timed action SR capsule contains phenylephrine HCl 20 mg; methscopolamine nitrate 2.5 mg; chlorpheniramine maleate 8 mg. The JR potency is exactly half-strength. Green/red color for both. Each 5 cc of root beer flavored syrup and tablet contains: phenylephrine HCl 10 mg;methscopolamine nitrate 1.25 mg; chlorpheniramine maleate 2 mg.

ACTION AND USES

Antihistaminic-decongestant for relief of respiratory congestion; allergic rhinitis; allergic skin reactions of urticaria and angioedema.

ADMINISTRATION AND DOSAGE

Capsules—one every 12 hrs of the SR for adults; one JR every 12 hrs for children 6–12 yrs. Syrup-two teaspoonfuls every 4 hrs for adults; children 1 teaspoonful every 4 hrs. Tablets—adults two and children one every 4 hrs. Do not exceed 4 doses in 24 hrs.
Children under 6 yrs. as recommended by a physician.

PRECAUTIONS

Withdraw therapy if drowsiness occurs. Patients are cautioned against driving or operating mechanical devices.

CONTRAINDICATIONS

Glaucoma, cardiac disease, hyperthyroidism and hypertension.

HOW SUPPLIED

Capsules and tablets in bottles of 100. Syrup in pints and gallons.

IMPREGON Concentrate　　　OTC

ACTIVE INGREDIENT

Tetrachlorosalicylanilide 2%

INDICATIONS

Diaper Rash Relief, 'Staph' control, Mold inhibitor.

ACTIONS

This is a bacteriostatic/fungistatic agent for home usage and hospital usage.

WARNINGS

Impregon should not be exposed to direct sunlight for long periods after applications.

PRECAUTION

Addition of bleach prior to diaper treatment negates application effects.

DOSAGE AND ADMINISTRATION

One capful (5ml) per gallon of water to impregnate diapers in the diaper pail. Dilutions for many home areas accompany the full package.

NOTE

For disposable-type diapers, add one teaspoonful to 8 oz of water to a 'Windex-type' sprayer. Spray middle half area of diapers until damp, and allow to dry before using, to prevent rashes.

HOW SUPPLIED

Four ounce black plastic bottles.

MAGONATE TABLETS　　　OTC
MAGONATE LIQUID
Magnesium Gluconate (Dihydrate)

ACTIVE INGREDIENTS

Each tablet contains magnesium gluconate (dihydrate) 500mg (27mg of Mg^{++}). Each 5cc of Magonate Liquid contains magnesium gluconate (dihydrate) 1000mg (54mg of Mg^{++}).

INDICATIONS

For all patients in negative magnesium balance.

PRECAUTION

Excessive dosage may cause loose stools.

DOSAGE AND ADMINISTRATION

Magonate is recommended during and for three weeks after a course in chemotherapy, then monitored regularly.
Adults and children over 12 yrs.—one or two tablets or $1/2$ to 1 teaspoon of liquid t.i.d. Under 12 yrs.—one tablet or $1/2$ teaspoon of liquid t.i.d. Dosage may be increased in severe cases.

HOW SUPPLIED

Magonate Tablets are supplied in bottles of 100 and 1000 tablets. Magonate Liquid is supplied in pints.

MARBLEN　　　　　OTC
(calcium and magnesium carbonates)
ANTACID SUSPENSION AND TABLET

(See PDR For Nonprescription Drugs.)

NEPHROCAPS　　　　Rx
Dialysis Vitamin Supplement

DESCRIPTION

Each black oval gelatin 'liquid' capsule provides:
Thiamin 1.5 mg; Riboflavin 1.7 mg; Niacin 20 mg; Pantothenic acid 5 mg; Biotin 150 mcg; Cyanocobalamin 6 mcg; Pyridoxin 10 mg; Ascorbic acid 100 mg and Folic acid 1.0 mg.

INDICATIONS

The wasting syndrome in chronic renal failure; uremia; impaired metabolic functions of the kidney.

DOSAGE

One capsule daily. On dialysis days, one Nephrocap must be taken after treatment.

SUPPLIED

Plastic bottles of 100 only.

NEPHROX SUSPENSION　　　OTC
(aluminum hydroxide)
Antacid Suspension

(See PDR For Nonprescription Drugs.)

NICOTINEX Elixir　　　　OTC
nicotinic acid

(See PDR For Nonprescription Drugs.)

OCEAN MIST　　　　OTC
(buffered isotonic saline)

(See PDR For Nonprescription Drugs.)

PIMA Syrup　　　　　Rx
(potassium iodide)

COMPOSITION

Contains KI 5 grs./tsp., in a black raspberry flavored base.

ACTION AND USES

An expectorant in the symptomatic treatment of chronic pulmonary diseases where tenacious mucus complicates the problem, including bronchial asthma, bronchitis and pulmonary emphysema.

ADMINISTRATION AND DOSAGE

Children—one half to one tsp. and adults one or two tsp. every 4-6 hours.

SIDE EFFECTS

May include gastrointestinal upset, metallic taste, minor skin eruptions, nausea, vomiting and epigastric pain. Therapy should be withdrawn.

PRECAUTIONS

In patients sensitive to iodides, in hyperthyroidism, and in rare cases iodine-induced goiter may occur.

HOW SUPPLIED

Plastic pints.

PURGE　　　　　OTC
(flavored castor oil)

(See PDR For Nonprescription Drugs.)

RUM–K　　　　　Rx
(potassium chloride 15% conc.)

DESCRIPTION

Each 10 ml. contains 1.5 Gm. potassium chloride (20 mEq) in a butter/rum synthetic flavored base that is alcohol and sugar free.

INDICATIONS

Hypokalemic-hypochloremic alkalosis; digitalis toxicity; hypokalemia prevention secondary to corticosteroid or diuretic administration.

CONTRAINDICATIONS

Impaired renal function, untreated Addison's Disease, acute dehydration, heat cramps, hyperkalemia.

PRECAUTIONS

Do not use in patients with low urinary output or renal decompensation. Potassium replacements vary and should be individualized. Patients should be checked frequently, ECG and plasma K^+ levels should be made. High serum concentrations of K^+ cause death thru cardiac depression, arrhythmias or arrest. Use with caution in cardiac disease.

ADVERSE REACTIONS

Vomiting, nausea, abdominal discomfort, diarrhea may occur. Symptoms and signs of potassium overdose include paresthesias of extremities, flaccid paralysis, listlessness, fall in blood pressure, weakness and heaviness of the legs, cardiac arrhythmias and heart block. Hyperkalemia may cause ECG changes as disappearance of the P wave, widening and slurring of QRS complex, changes of the S-T segment, tall peaked T waves.

DOSAGE AND ADMINISTRATION

Adults—two teaspoonsful (10ml) in 4–6 oz water 2 to 4 times daily after meals to supply 40–80 mEq of elemental potassium and chloride. Larger doses may be required and administered under close supervision due to possible potassium intoxication or saline laxative effect.

HOW SUPPLIED

Pints.

Forest Pharmaceuticals, Inc.

(Subsidiary of Forest Laboratories, Inc.)
13622 LAKEFRONT DRIVE
ST LOUIS, MO 63045

Direct Inquiries to:
Professional Affairs Department
13622 Lakefront Drive
St. Louis, MO 63045
(800) 678-1605

AEROBID® ℞

AEROBID®-M
(flunisolide)
Inhaler System
For oral inhalation only

DESCRIPTION

Flunisolide, the active component of **AEROBID** Inhaler System, is an anti-inflammatory steroid having the chemical name 6α-fluoro-11β, 16α, 17, 21-tetrahydroxypregna-1, 4-diene-3, 20-dione cyclic-16, 17-acetal with acetone.
It has the following structure:

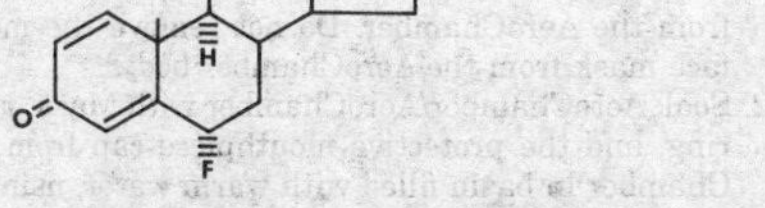

Flunisolide is a white to creamy white crystalline powder with a molecular weight of 434.49. It is soluble in acetone, sparingly soluble in chloroform, slightly soluble in methanol, and practically insoluble in water. It has a melting point of about 245°C.
AEROBID Inhaler is delivered in a metered-dose aerosol system containing a microcrystalline suspension of flunisolide as the hemihydrate in propellants (trichloromonofluoromethane, dichlorodifluoromethane and dichlorotetrafluoroethane) with sorbitan trioleate as a dispersing agent. **AEROBID-M** also contains menthol as a flavoring agent. Each activation delivers approximately 250 mcg of flunisolide to the patient. One **AEROBID** Inhaler System is designed to deliver at least 100 metered inhalations.

CLINICAL PHARMACOLOGY

Flunisolide has demonstrated marked anti-inflammatory and anti-allergic activity in classical test systems. It is a corticosteroid that is several hundred times more potent in animal anti-inflammatory assays than the cortisol standard. The molar dose of each activation of flunisolide in this preparation is approximately 2.5 to 7 times that of comparable inhaled corticosteroid products marketed for the same indication. The dose of flunisolide delivered per activation in this preparation is 10 times that per activation of Nasalide® (flunisolide) nasal solution. Clinical studies have shown therapeutic activity on bronchial mucosa with minimal evidence of systemic activity at recommended doses.
After oral inhalation of 1 mg flunisolide, total systemic availability was 40%. The flunisolide that is swallowed is rapidly and extensively converted to the 6β-OH metabolite and to water-soluble conjugates during the first pass through the liver. This offers a metabolic explanation for the low systemic activity of oral flunisolide itself since the metabolite has the low corticosteroid potency (on the order of the cortisol standard). The inhaled flunisolide absorbed through the bronchial tree is converted to the same metabolites. Repeated inhalation of 2.0 mg of flunisolide per day (the maximum recommended dose) for 14 days did not show accumulation of the drug in plasma. The plasma half-life of flunisolide is approximately 1.8 hours.
The following observations relevant to systemic absorption were made in clinical studies. In one uncontrolled study a statistically significant decrease in responsiveness to metyrapone was noted in 15 adult steroid-independent patients treated with 2.0 mg of flunisolide per day (the maximum recommended dose) for 3 months. A small but statistically significant drop in eosinophils from 11.5% to 7.4% of total circulating leucocytes was noted in another study in children who were not taking oral corticosteroids simultaneously. A 5% incidence of menstrual disturbances was reported during open studies, in which there were no control groups for comparison.
Aerosol administration of flunisolide 2.0 mg twice daily for one week to 6 healthy male subjects revealed neither suppression of adrenal function as measured by early morning cortisol levels nor impairment of HPA axis function as determined by insulin hypoglycemia tests.
Controlled clinical studies have included over 500 patients with asthma, among them 150 children age 6 and over. More than 120 patients have been treated in open trials for two years or more. No significant adrenal suppression attributed to flunisolide was seen in these studies.
Significant decreases of systemic steroid dosages have been possible in flunisolide-treated patients. Recommended doses of flunisolide appear to be the therapeutic equivalent of an average of 10 mg/day of oral prednisone. Asthma patients have had further symptomatic improvement with flunisolide treatment even while reducing concomitant medication.

INDICATIONS AND USAGE

AEROBID (flunisolide) Inhaler is indicated in the maintenance treatment of asthma as prophylactic therapy.
AEROBID is also indicated for asthma patients who require systemic corticosteroid administration, where adding **AEROBID** may reduce or eliminate the need for the systemic corticosteroids.
AEROBID Inhaler is NOT indicated for the relief of acute bronchospasm.

CONTRAINDICATIONS

AEROBID (flunisolide) Inhaler is contraindicated in the primary treatment of status asthmaticus or other acute episodes of asthma where intensive measures are required.
Hypersensitivity to any of the ingredients of this preparation contraindicates its use.

WARNINGS
Particular care is needed in patients who are transferred from systemically active corticosteroids to **AEROBID** Inhaler because deaths due to adrenal insufficiency have occurred in asthmatic patients during and after transfer from systemic corticosteroids to aerosol corticosteroids. After withdrawal from systemic corticosteroids, a number of months are required for recovery of hypothalamic-pituitary-adrenal (HPA) function. During this period of HPA suppression, patients may exhibit signs and symptoms of adrenal insufficiency when exposed to trauma, surgery or infections, particularly gastroenteritis. Although **AEROBID** Inhaler may provide control of asthmatic symptoms during these episodes, it does NOT provide the systemic steroid that is necessary for coping with these emergencies. During periods of stress or a severe asthmatic attack, patients who have been withdrawn from systemic corticosteroids should be instructed to resume systemic steroids (in large doses) immediately and to contact their physician for further instruction. These patients should also be instructed to carry a warning card indicating that they may need supplementary systemic steroids during periods of stress or a severe asthma attack. To assess the risk of adrenal insufficiency in emergency situations, routine tests of adrenal cortical function, including measurement of early morning resting cortisol levels, should be performed periodically in all patients. An early morning resting cortisol level may be accepted as normal if it falls at or near the normal mean level.

Localized infections with *Candida albicans* or *Aspergillus niger* have occurred in the mouth and pharynx and occasionally in the larynx. Positive cultures for oral *Candida* may be present in up to 34% of patients. Although the frequency of clinically apparent infection is considerably lower, these infections may require treatment with appropriate antifungal therapy or discontinuance of treatment with **AEROBID** Inhaler.
AEROBID Inhaler is not to be regarded as a bronchodilator and is not indicated for rapid relief of bronchospasm.
Patients should be instructed to contact their physician immediately when episodes of asthma that are not responsive to bronchodilators occur during the course of treatment. During such episodes, patients may require therapy with systemic corticosteroids. Theoretically, the use of inhaled corticosteroids with alternate day prednisone systemic treatment should be accompanied by more HPA suppression than a therapeutically equivalent regimen of either alone.
Transfer of patients from systemic steroid therapy to **AEROBID** Inhaler may unmask allergic conditions previously suppressed by the systemic steroid therapy, e.g. rhinitis, conjunctivitis, and eczema.
Persons who are on drugs which suppress the immune system are more susceptible to infections than healthy individuals. Chicken pox and measles, for example, can have a more serious or even fatal course in non-immune children or adults on corticosteroids. In such children or adults who have not had these diseases, particular care should be taken to avoid exposure. How the dose, route and duration of corticosteriod administration affects the risk of developing a disseminated infection is not known. The contribution of the underlying disease and/or prior corticosteroid treatment to the risk is also not known. If exposed to chicken pox, prophylaxis with varicella zoster immune globulin (VZIG) may be indicated. If exposed to measles, prophylaxis with pooled intramuscular immunoglobulin (IG) may be indicated. (See the respective package inserts for complete VZIG and IG prescribing information). If chicken pox develops, treatment with antiviral agents may be considered.

PRECAUTIONS

General: Because of the relatively high molar dose of flunisolide per activation in this preparation, and because of the evidence suggesting higher levels of systemic absorption with flunisolide than with other comparable inhaled corticosteroids (see CLINICAL PHARMACOLOGY section), patients treated with **AEROBID** (flunisolide) should be observed carefully for any evidence of systemic corticosteroid effect, including suppression of bone growth in children. Particular care should be taken in observing patients postoperatively or during periods of stress for evidence of a decrease in adrenal function. During withdrawal from oral steroids, some patients may experience symptoms of systemically active steroid withdrawal, e.g., joint and/or muscular pain, lassitude and depression, despite maintenance or even improvement of respiratory function. (See DOSAGE AND ADMINISTRATION for details.)
In responsive patients, flunisolide may permit control of asthmatic symptoms without suppression of HPA function. Since flunisolide is absorbed into the circulation and can be systemically active, the beneficial effects of **AEROBID** Inhaler in minimizing or preventing HPA dysfunction may be expected only when recommended dosages are not exceeded. The long-term local and systemic effects of **AEROBID** (flunisolide) in human subjects are still not fully known. In particular, the effects resulting from chronic use of **AEROBID** on developmental or immunologic processes in the mouth, pharynx, trachea, and lung are unknown.
Inhaled corticosteroids should be used with caution, if at all, in patients with active or quiescent tuberculosis infection of the respiratory tract; untreated systemic fungal, bacterial, parasitic or viral infections; or ocular herpes simplex.
Pulmonary infiltrates with eosinophilia may occur in patients on **AEROBID** Inhaler therapy. Although it is possible that in some patients this state may become manifest because of systemic steroid withdrawal when inhalational steroids are administered, a causative role for the drug and/or its vehicle cannot be ruled out.

Information for Patients:
Since the relief from **AEROBID** Inhaler depends on its regular use and on proper inhalation technique, patients must be instructed to take inhalations at regular intervals. They should also be instructed in the correct method of use (See Patient Instruction Leaflet).
Patients whose systemic corticosteroids have been reduced or withdrawn should be instructed to carry a warning card indicating that they may need supplemental systemic steroids during periods of stress or a severe asthmatic attack that is not responsive to bronchodilators.
Persons who are on immunosuppressant doses of corticosteroids should be warned to avoid exposure to chicken pox or measles. Patients should also be advised that if they are exposed, medical advice should be sought without delay.
An illustrated leaflet of patient instructions for proper use accompanies each **AEROBID** Inhaler System.
CONTENTS UNDER PRESSURE
Do not puncture. Do not use or store near heat or open flame. Exposure to temperatures above 120°F (49°C) may cause container to explode. Never throw container into fire or incinerator. Keep out of reach of children.
Carcinogenesis: Long-term studies were conducted in mice and rats using oral administration to evaluate the carcinogenic potential of the drug. There was an increase in the incidence of pulmonary adenomas in mice, but not in rats. Female rats receiving the highest oral dose had an increased incidence of mammary adenocarcinoma compared to control rats. An increased incidence of this tumor type has been reported for other corticosteroids.
Impairment of Fertility: Female rats receiving high doses of flunisolide (200 mcg/kg/day) showed some evidence of impaired fertility. Reproductive performance in the low-(8 mcg/kg/day) and mid-dose (40 mcg/kg/day) groups was comparable to controls.
Pregnancy: Pregnancy Category C. As with other corticosteroids, flunisolide has been shown to be teratogenic in rabbits and rats at doses of 40 and 200 mcg/kg/day respectively. It was also fetotoxic in these animal reproductive studies. There are no adequate and well-controlled studies in pregnant women. Flunisolide should be used during pregnancy only if the potential benefit justifies the potential risk to the fetus.
Nursing Mothers: It is not known whether this drug is excreted in human milk. Because other corticosteroids are excreted in human milk, caution should be exercised when flunisolide is administered to nursing women.
Pediatric Use: Safety and effectiveness have not been established in children below the age of 6. Oral corticoids have been shown to cause growth suppression in children and adolescents, particularly with higher doses over extended

Continued on next page

Aerobid—Cont.

periods. If a child or adolescent on any corticoid appears to have growth suppression, the possibility that they are particularly sensitive to this effect of steroids should be considered.

ADVERSE REACTIONS

Adverse events reported in controlled clinical trials and long-term open studies in 514 patients treated with **AEROBID** (flunisolide) are described below. Of those patients, 463 were treated for 3 months or longer, 407 for 6 months or longer, 287 for 1 year or longer, and 122 for 2 years or longer.

Musculoskeletal reactions were reported in 35% of steroid-dependent patients in whom the dose of oral steroid was being tapered. This is a well-known effect of steroid withdrawal.

Incidence 10% or greater:

Gastrointestinal: diarrhea (10%), nausea and/or vomiting (25%), upset stomach (10%)
General: flu (10%)
Mouth and Throat: sore throat (20%)
Nervous System: headache (25%)
Respiratory: cold symptoms (15%), nasal congestion (15%), upper respiratory infection (25%)
Special Senses: unpleasant taste (10%)

Incidence 3–9%

Cardiovascular: palpitations
Gastrointestinal: abdominal pain, heartburn
General: chest pain, decreased appetite, edema, fever
Mouth and Throat: *Candida* infection
Nervous System: dizziness, irritability, nervousness, shakiness
Reproductive: menstrual disturbances
Respiratory: chest congestion, cough*, hoarseness, rhinitis, runny nose, sinus congestion, sinus drainage, sinus infection, sinusitis, sneezing, sputum, wheezing*
Skin: eczema, itching (pruritus), rash
Special Senses: ear infection, loss of smell or taste

Incidence 1–3%

General: chills, increased appetite and weight gain, malaise, peripheral edema, sweating, weakness
Cardiovascular: hypertension, tachycardia
Gastrointestinal: constipation, dyspepsia, gas
Hemic/Lymph: capillary fragility, enlarged lymph nodes
Mouth and Throat: dry throat, glossitis, mouth irritation, pharyngitis, phlegm, throat irritation
Nervous System: anxiety, depression, faintness, fatigue, hyperactivity, hypoactivity, insomnia, moodiness, numbness, vertigo
Respiratory: bronchitis, chest tightness*, dyspnea, epistaxis, head stuffiness, laryngitis, nasal irritation, pleurisy, pneumonia, sinus discomfort
Skin: acne, hives or urticaria
Special Senses: blurred vision, earache, eye discomfort, eye infection

Incidence less than 1%, judged by investigators as possibly or probably drug related: abdominal fullness, shortness of breath.

---

*The incidences as shown of cough, wheezing, and chest tightness were judged by investigators to be possibly or probably drug-related. In placebo-controlled trials, the *overall* incidences of these adverse events (regardless of investigators' judgment of drug relationship) were similar for drug and placebo-treated groups. They may be related to the vehicle or delivery system.

DOSAGE AND ADMINISTRATION

The **AEROBID** (flunisolide) Inhaler System is for oral inhalation only.

Adults: The recommended starting dose is 2 inhalations twice daily, morning and evening, for a total daily dose of 1 mg. The maximum daily dose should not exceed 4 inhalations twice a day for a total daily dose of 2 mg. When the drug is used chronically at 2 mg/day, patients should be monitored periodically for effects on the hypothalamic-pituitary-adrenal (HPA) axis.

Pediatric Patients: For children and adolescents 6–15 years of age, two inhalations may be administered twice daily for a total daily dose of 1 mg. Higher doses have not been studied. Insufficient information is available to warrant use in children under age 6. With chronic use, pediatric patients should be monitored for growth as well as for effects on the HPA axis.

Rinsing the mouth after inhalation is advised.

Different considerations must be given to the following groups of patients in order to obtain the full therapeutic benefit of **AEROBID** (flunisolide) Inhaler.

Patients Not Receiving Systemic Corticosteroids:
Patients who require maintenance therapy of their asthma may benefit from treatment with **AEROBID** at the doses recommended above. In patients who respond to **AEROBID**, improvement in pulmonary function is usually apparent within one to four weeks after the start of therapy. Once the desired effect is achieved, consideration should be given to tapering to the lowest effective dose.

Patients Maintained on Systemic Corticosteroids:
Clinical studies have shown that **AEROBID** may be effective in the management of asthmatics dependent or maintained on systemic corticosteroids and may permit replacement or significant reduction in the dosage of systemic corticosteroids.

The patient's asthma should be reasonably stable before treatment with **AEROBID** is started. Initially, **AEROBID** should be used concurrently with the patient's usual maintenance dose of systemic corticosteroid. After approximately one week, gradual withdrawal of the systemic corticosteroid is started by reducing the daily or alternate daily dose. Reductions may be made after an interval of one or two weeks, depending on the response of the patient. A slow rate of withdrawal is strongly recommended. Generally, these decrements should not exceed 2.5 mg of prednisone or its equivalent. During withdrawal, some patients may experience symptoms of systemic corticosteroid withdrawal; e.g., joint and/or muscular pain, lassitude and depression, despite maintenance or even improvement of pulmonary function. Such patients should be encouraged to continue with the inhaler but should be monitored for objective signs of adrenal insufficiency. If evidence of adrenal insufficiency occurs, the systemic corticosteroid doses should be increased temporarily and thereafter withdrawal should continue more slowly. During periods of stress or a severe asthma attack, transfer patients may require supplementary treatment with systemic corticosteroids.

HOW SUPPLIED

AEROBID (flunisolide) Inhaler Systems are available in canisters of 100 metered inhalations.

NDC 0456-0672-99 **AEROBID**
NDC 0456-0670-99 **AEROBID-M**

"Note: The indented statement below is required by the Federal government's Clean Air Act for all products containing or manufactured with chlorofluorocarbons (CFC's)."

> WARNING: Contains trichloromonofluoromethane, dichlorodifluoromethane and dichlorotetrafluoroethane, substances which harm public health and environment by destroying ozone in the upper atmosphere.

"A notice similar to the above WARNING has been placed in the information for the patient of this product pursuant to EPA regulations."

Caution: Federal Law prohibits dispensing without prescription.

Revised 4/96

mfd for
FOREST PHARMACEUTICALS, INC.
St. Louis, MO 63045
mfd by
3M Pharmaceuticals
St. Paul, MN

16053

Shown in Product Identification Guide, page 310

AeroChamber® ℞
AeroChamber® with *Mask—Small*
AeroChamber® with *Mask*
AeroChamber® with *Mask—Large*

Valved Aerosol Holding Chamber/Aerosol Holding Chamber with *Mask* for Use With Metered Dose Inhalers.

Before using AeroChamber/AeroChamber with *Mask*, it is important to read these instructions very carefully, including the CAUTION sections that follow:

CAUTION

1. When cleaning, the only part of the AeroChamber/AeroChamber with Mask to be removed is the rubber-like ring that holds the Metered Dose Inhaler and the protective mouthpiece cap from the AeroChamber. Do not remove the mouthpiece/face mask from the AeroChamber body.
2. Except as stated in 1 above, do not disassemble the AeroChamber/AeroChamber with Mask, as the overall reliability and safety of the product may be affected.
3. Replace AeroChamber/AeroChamber with Mask at once and do not use if the one-way valve becomes dislodged (partially or fully) or begins to harden or curl.
4. Running water through the AeroChamber/AeroChamber with Mask at high pressure may harm the valve. Examine AeroChamber/AeroChamber with Mask visually before and after cleaning to make sure the one-way valve and other parts are properly secured.
5. Disassembly may loosen or dislodge the one-way valve. Examine the AeroChamber/AeroChamber with Mask visually before and after use to make sure the one-way valve and other parts are properly secured.
6. Do not allow children to play with the AeroChamber/AeroChamber with Mask—allowing them to do so may alter its function and/or overall reliability. The mask membrane, the one-way valve, and the exhalation valve (Mask-Small) can be damaged as a result of pulling or poking.
7. As indicated, your AeroChamber/AeroChamber with Mask should be inspected visually before and after daily use and may need to be replaced after 6 to 12 months of use.

INTRODUCTION

The AeroChamber/AeroChamber with Mask line is a family of valved aerosol holding chambers available from Forest Pharmaceuticals, Inc., designed to be used with virtually all Metered Dose Inhalers [MDI's]. When you release a puff of aerosol into the AeroChamber/AeroChamber with Mask, the puff will be held there for a few seconds. The valved holding chamber selectively removes most large aerosol-drug particles that normally deposit in the mouth and throat, while allowing the smaller, therapeutic particles to pass through the patented one-way valve into the lungs. This provides effective treatment and helps to reduce unwanted side effects. In addition, the AeroChamber/AeroChamber with Mask is designed to make Metered Dose Inhalers easier to use.

CLEANING INSTRUCTIONS

The AeroChamber/AeroChamber with Mask is made of durable plastic materials and has one or two moving parts; the one-way valve and, in the AeroChamber with Mask-Small, an exhalation valve. With repeated use, residue may accumulate inside the AeroChamber/AeroChamber with Mask and around the one-way valve. This may eventually interfere with effective use. We suggest cleaning the Metered Dose Inhaler as instructed by the manufacturer and AeroChamber/AeroChamber with Mask about once a week or more often depending on your usage of the product.

To clean the AeroChamber/AeroChamber with Mask:

1. Remove the rubber-like ring from the end that holds the Metered Dose Inhaler and the protective mouthpiece cap from the AeroChamber. Do not remove the mouthpiece/face mask from the AeroChamber body.
2. Soak AeroChamber/AeroChamber with Mask, rubber-like ring, and the protective mouthpiece cap from the AeroChamber in basin filled with warm water, using mild detergent to dislodge or loosen any residue.
3. Rinse AeroChamber/AeroChamber with Mask, rubber-like ring, and the protective mouthpiece cap from the AeroChamber in basin filled with clean warm water, using a gentle motion.
4. Lightly shake away excess water droplets and leave on clean surface to air-dry.
5. Be sure the AeroChamber/AeroChamber with Mask is completely dry before use.
6. Replace the rubber-like ring on the AeroChamber/AeroChamber with Mask.

TECHNICAL INFORMATION

This apparently simple device is a product of considerable medical research and engineering. It was developed in a leading medical center.

The valved holding chamber selectively removes large aerosol particles that normally deposit in the mouth and throat, while allowing the smaller treatment particles to pass into the lungs. This provides effective treatment and helps reduce unwanted side effects.

AeroChamber

INSTRUCTIONS FOR USE

Please discuss the use of the AeroChamber with your physician, pharmacist, or other healthcare professional.

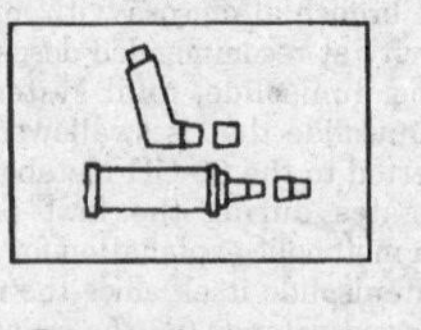

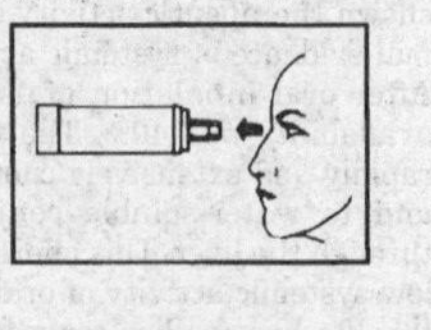

1. Remove the protective cap from Metered-Dose Inhaler [MDI]. Remove the protective cap from the mouthpiece of AeroChamber.

2. Visually check the AeroChamber for foreign objects. Ensure that all parts are secure, including the one-way valve.

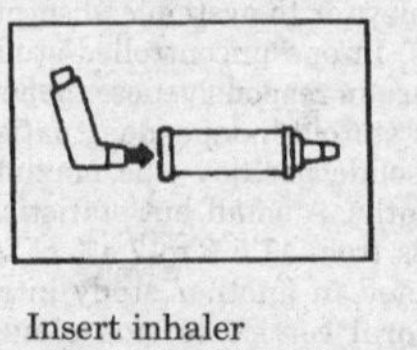

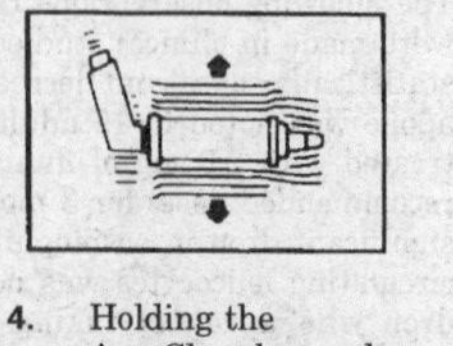

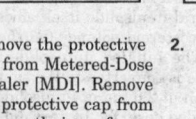

3. Insert inhaler mouth-piece into the round opening in the rubber-like ring at the end of the AeroChamber.

4. Holding the AeroChamber and Inhaler [MDI] firmly, shake vigorously 3 or 4 times.

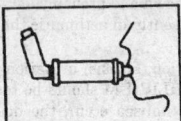
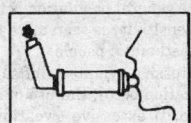

5. Exhale normally. Place the AeroChamber mouthpiece in mouth and close lips.

6. Spray only one puff from the inhaler [MDI] into the AeroChamber per inhalation maneuver. Spraying more than one puff into the AeroChamber before or during an inhalation maneuver will result in delivery of improper dose of medication.

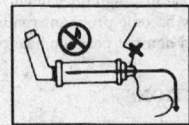

7. Breathe in slowly and deeply through mouth until you have taken a full breath. Do not breathe in so fast as to activate the flow signal whistle. A whistling sound from the flow signal indicates that you are breathing in too quickly.

8. Hold breath for 5 to 10 seconds.

9. Repeat steps 4 to 8 as prescribed by your physician.

10. Remove inhaler and examine the AeroChamber to make certain that the one-way valve is properly secured.

11. Replace protective cap on AeroChamber and MDI.

HELPFUL HINTS:

1. In order to obtain the maximum benefit from your Metered Dose Inhaler, it is extremely important to fill your lungs during inhalation by taking a *slow*, deep breath. If the flow signal makes a whistling sound, it is an indication that you are breathing in too quickly.

2. The one-way valve allows you to inhale at your own rate so that coordination of inhalation with the actuation of the inhaler is not a problem.

3. If you have trouble inhaling through your mouth, with the AeroChamber mouthpiece between your lips, it may be necessary to gently pinch your nose while inhaling the medication.

4. For the elderly and small children who may have difficulty using the AeroChamber, there is also an AeroChamber available with Mask which allows another person to assist with coordination.

5. When using the AeroChamber with a corticosteroid Metered Dose Inhaler, it is recommended by the manufacturer of these drugs to rinse your mouth with water to remove any medication residue.

IMPORTANT INFORMATION

Package insert dosing instructions should be consulted for all Metered Dose Inhalers [MDIs] when used with AeroChamber. Dosage and administration recommendations vary for different MDIs, and the limitations and conditions of use for each product should be considered before utilizing this device, particularly for younger and older patients.

This device helps deliver aerosol medication to the lungs more reliably. Should you have any problem using the AeroChamber please contact your doctor.

CAUTION: Federal law restricts this device to sale by, or on the order of, a physician.

Manufactured by Monaghan Medical Corporation, Plattsburgh, NY 12901

Assembled in USA of Canadian Components covered by one or more of the following patent numbers: 4,470,412; 5,042,467; 5,012,803; 4,809,692; 4,832,015; 5,012,804

AeroChamber with *Mask—Small*

INSTRUCTIONS FOR USE

Please discuss the use of the AeroChamber with Mask-Small with your physician, pharmacist, or other healthcare professional.

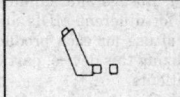
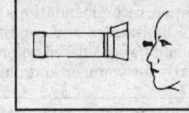

1. Remove the protective cap from Metered Dose Inhaler [MDI].

2. Visually check the AeroChamber with Mask-Small for foreign objects. Ensure that all parts are secure.

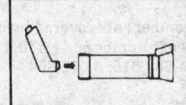
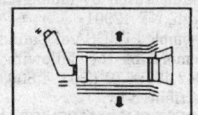

3. Insert inhaler mouthpiece into the round opening in the rubber-like end of the AeroChamber with Mask-Small.

4. Holding the AeroChamber with Mask-Small and inhaler firmly, shake vigorously 3 or 4 times.

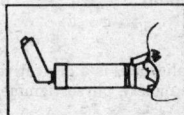
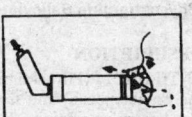

5. Place the soft mask gently to the face so that the mouth and nose are covered. Be certain to create a good seal; leaks will inhibit the delivery of the medication. The exhalation valve allows the patient to exhale comfortably while the mask is held firmly around their mouth and nose.

6. While the patient is exhaling, spray only one puff from the inhaler into the AeroChamber with Mask-Small. Spraying more than one puff into the AeroChamber with Mask-Small before or during an inhalation maneuver will result in delivery of improper dose of medication.

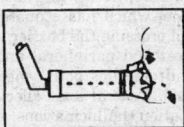

7. Hold the mask firmly to the patient's face for at least six (6) breaths.

8. Repeat steps 4 to 7 as prescribed by your physician, waiting at least 30 seconds between puffs.

9. Remove inhaler and replace its protective cap.

AeroChamber with *Mask*

INSTRUCTIONS FOR USE

Please discuss the use of the AeroChamber with Mask with your physician, pharmacist, or other healthcare professional.

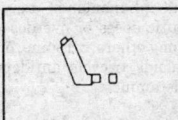
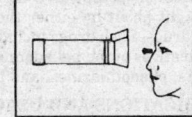

1. Remove the protective cap from Metered Dose Inhaler (MDI).

2. Visually check the AeroChamber with Mask for foreign objects. Ensure that all parts are secure.

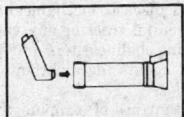
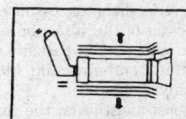

3. Insert inhaler mouthpiece into the opening in the soft rubber-like end of the AeroChamber with Mask.

4. Holding the AeroChamber with Mask and inhaler firmly, shake vigorously 3 or 4 times.

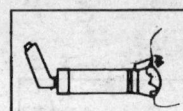
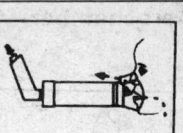

5. Place the soft mask gently to the face so that the mouth and nose are covered. Be certain to create a good seal: leaks will inhibit the delivery of the medication. The exhalation valve allows the patient to exhale comfortably while the mask is held firmly around their mouth and nose.

6. While the patient is exhaling, spray only one puff from the inhaler into the AeroChamber with Mask. Spraying more than one puff into the AeroChamber with Mask before or during an inhalation maneuver will result in delivery of improper dose of medication.

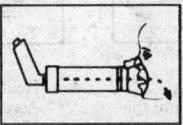

7. Hold the mask firmly to the patient's face for at least six (6) breaths.

8. Repeat steps 4 to 7 as prescribed by your physician, waiting at least 30 seconds between puffs.

9. Remove inhaler and replace its protective cap.

HELPFUL HINTS

1. Some children may resist their treatment by grabbing at the mask. Place the child on your lap and wrap one arm around the child to simplify placing the mask on the child's face.

2. In the case of a smaller child it may be more comfortable to lay the child on a bed while administering the medication.

3. If the child seems frightened by the AeroChamber with Mask-Small or AeroChamber with Mask, familiarize the child with the device by stroking his or her cheek with the soft mask. If the child cries during treatment with the AeroChamber with Mask-Small or AeroChamber with Mask, the medication will still be delivered as long as there is a good seal between the mask and the child's face. Remember, the child will inhale after crying or screaming.

4. When using the AeroChamber with Mask-Small or AeroChamber with Mask with a corticosteroid Metered Dose Inhaler, it is recommended that the patient's face be cleaned with soap and water to remove any medication residue.

IMPORTANT INFORMATION:

Package insert dosing instructions should be consulted for all Metered Dose Inhalers [MDIs] when used with AeroChamber with Mask-Small or AeroChamber with Mask. Dosage and administration recommendations vary for different MDIs, and the limitations and conditions of use for each product should be considered before utilizing this device, particularly for younger and older patients.

This device helps deliver aerosol medication to the lungs more reliably. Should you have any problem using the AeroChamber with Mask-Small or AeroChamber with Mask, please contact your doctor.

CAUTION: Federal law restricts this device to sale by, or on the order of, a physician.

Manufactured by Monaghan Medical corporation, Plattsburgh, NY 12901

Assembled in USA of Canadian components covered by one or more of the following patent numbers: 4,470,412; 5,042,467; 5,012,803; 4,809,692; 4,832,015; 5,012,804

AeroChamber with *Mask—Large*

INSTRUCTIONS FOR USE:

Please discuss the use of the AeroChamber with Mask-Large with your physician, pharmacist, or other healthcare professional.

Continued on next page

Aerochamber—Cont.

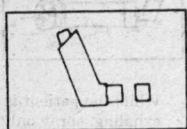 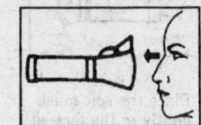

1. Remove the protective cap from Metered Dose Inhaler [MDI].

2. Visually check the AeroChamber with Mask-Large for foreign objects. Ensure that all parts are secure, including the one-way valve.

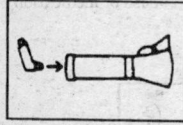 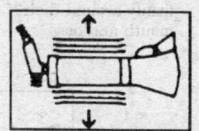

3. Insert inhaler mouthpiece into the round opening in the rubber-like ring at the end of the AeroChamber with Mask-Large.

4. Holding the AeroChamber with Mask-Large and inhaler [MDI] firmly, shake vigorously 3 or 4 times.

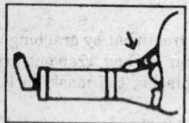 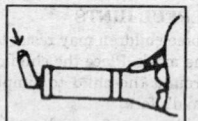

5. Place the soft mask gently to the face so that the mouth and nose are covered. Be certain to create a good seal. Leaks will inhibit the delivery of the medication. Seeing the diaphragm move is a helpful indication of a good seal.

6. Spray only one puff from the inhaler [MDI] into the AeroChamber with Mask-Large per inhalation maneuver. Spraying more than one puff into the AeroChamber with Mask-Large before or during an inhalation maneuver will result in delivery of improper dose of medication.

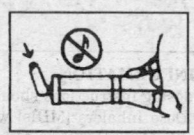

7. Breathe in slowly and deeply until you have taken a full breath. Do not breathe in so fast as to activate the flow signal whistle. A whistle sound from the flow signal indicates that you are breathing in too quickly.

8. Repeat steps 4 to 7 as prescribed by your physician.

9. Remove inhaler and examine the AeroChamber with Mask-Large to make certain that the one-way valve is properly secured.

HELPFUL HINTS

1. In order to obtain the maximum benefit from your Metered Dose Inhaler, it is extremely important to fill your lungs during inhalation by taking a *slow*, deep breath. If the flow signal makes a whistling sound, it is an indication that you are breathing in too quickly.

2. The one-way valve allows you to inhale at your own rate so that coordination of inhalation with the actuation of the inhaler is not a problem.

3. When using the AeroChamber with Mask-Large with a corticosteroid Metered Dose Inhaler, it is recommended that the patient's face be cleaned with soap and water to remove any medication residue.

IMPORTANT INFORMATION

Package insert dosing instructions should be consulted for all Metered Dose Inhalers [MDIs] when used with AeroChamber with Mask-Large. Dosage and administration recommendations vary for different MDIs and the limitations and conditions of use for each product should be considered before utilizing this device, particularly for younger and older patients.

This device helps deliver aerosol medication to the lungs more reliably. Should you have any problem using the AeroChamber with Mask-Large, please contact your doctor.

CAUTION: Federal law restricts this device to sale by, or on the order of, a physician.

Manufactured by Monaghan Medical Corporation, Plattsburgh, NY 12901

Assembled in USA of Canadian components covered by one or more of the following patent numbers: 4,470,412; 5,042,467; 5,012,803; 4,809,692; 4,832,015; 5,012,804

Distributed by:

FOREST PHARMACEUTICALS, INC.
UAD LABORATORIES
St. Louis, Missouri 63045
REV 7/96 ACL

Shown in Product Identification Guide, page 310

ANTILIRIUM® ℞
(Physostigmine Salicylate Injection)

DESCRIPTION

ANTILIRIUM (Physostigmine Salicylate) is a derivative of the Calabar bean, and its active moiety, physostigmine, is also known as eserine.

It is soluble in water and a 0.5% aqueous solution has a pH of 5.8.

ANTILIRIUM Injection is available in 2 ml ampuls, each ml containing 1 mg of Physostigmine Salicylate in a vehicle composed of sodium bisulfite 0.1%, benzyl alcohol 2.0% as a preservative in water for injection.

CLINICAL PHARMACOLOGY

ANTILIRIUM is a reversible anticholinesterase which effectively increases the concentration of acetylcholine at the sites of cholinergic transmission. The action of acetylcholine is normally very transient because of its hydrolysis by the enzyme, acetylcholinesterase. ANTILIRIUM inhibits the destructive action of acetylcholinesterase and thereby prolongs and exaggerates the effect of the acetylcholine.

ANTILIRIUM contains a tertiary amine and easily penetrates the blood brain barrier, while an anticholinesterase, such as neostigmine, which has a quaternary ammonium ion is not capable of crossing the barrier. ANTILIRIUM can reverse both central and peripheral anticholinergia. The anticholinergic syndrome has both central and peripheral signs and symptoms. Central toxic effects include anxiety, delirium, disorientation, hallucinations, hyper-activity and seizures. Severe poisoning may produce coma, medullary paralysis and death. Peripheral toxicity is characterized by tachycardia, hyperpyrexia, mydriasis, vasodilatation, urinary retention, diminution of gastrointestinal motility, decrease of secretion in salivary and sweat glands, and loss of secretions in the pharynx, bronchi, and nasal passages.

Dramatic reversal of the effects of anticholinergic symptoms can be expected in minutes after the intravenous administration of ANTILIRIUM, if the diagnosis is correct and the patient has not suffered anoxia or other insult. The duration of action of ANTILIRIUM is relatively short, approx. 45 to 60 minutes.

Numerous drugs and some plants produce the anticholinergic syndrome either directly or as a side effect; this undesirable or potentially dangerous phenomenon may be brought about by either therapeutic doses or overdoses of the drugs. Such drugs include among others, atropine, other derivatives of the belladonna alkaloids, tricyclic antidepressants, phenothiazines, and antihistamines.

INDICATIONS AND USAGES

To reverse the effect upon the central nervous system, caused by clinical or toxic dosages of drugs capable of producing the anticholinergic syndrome.

CONTRAINDICATIONS

ANTILIRIUM should not be used in the presence of asthma, gangrene, diabetes, cardiovascular disease, mechanical obstruction of the intestine or urogenital tract or any vagotonic state, and in patients receiving choline esters or depolarizing neuromuscular blocking agents (decamethonium succinylcholine).

For post-anesthesia, the concomitant use of atropine with the physostigmine salicylate is not recommended, since the atropine antagonizes the action of physostigmine.

WARNINGS

Contains sodium bisulfite, a sulfite that may cause allergic-type reactions including anaphylactic symptoms and life-threatening or less severe asthmatic episodes in certain susceptible people. The overall prevalence of sulfite sensitivity in the general population is unknown and probably low. Sulfite sensitivity is seen more frequently in asthmatic than in non-asthmatic people.

If excessive symptoms of salivation, emesis, urination and defecation occur, the use of ANTILIRIUM should be terminated. If excessive sweating or nausea occur, the dosage should be reduced.

Intravenous administration should be a slow, controlled rate, no more than 1 mg per minute (see dosage). Rapid administration can cause bradycardia, hypersalivation leading to respiratory difficulties and possible convulsions.

An overdosage of ANTILIRIUM can cause a cholinergic crisis.

PRECAUTIONS

Because of the possibility of hypersensitivity in an occasional patient, atropine sulfate injection should always be at hand since it is an antagonist and antidote for physostigmine.

USAGE IN PREGNANCY

Safe use in pregnancy and lactation has not been established; therefore, use in pregnant women, nursing mothers or women who may become pregnant requires that possible benefits be weighed against possible hazards to mother and child.

ADVERSE REACTIONS

Nausea, vomiting and salivation, can be offset by reducing dosage. Bradycardia and convulsions, if intravenous administration is too rapid. See DOSAGE AND ADMINISTRATION.

OVERDOSAGE

Can cause a cholinergic crisis. Appropriate antidote is atropine sulfate.

DOSAGE AND ADMINISTRATION

Post Anesthesia Care: 0.5 to 1.0 mg intramuscularly or intravenously. INTRAVENOUS ADMINISTRATION SHOULD BE AT A SLOW CONTROLLED RATE OF NO MORE THAN 1 MG PER MINUTE. Dosage may be repeated at intervals of 10 to 30 minutes if desired patient response is not obtained.

Overdosages of Drugs That Cause Anticholinergia: 2.0 mg intramuscularly or INTRAVENOUSLY AT SLOW CONTROLLED RATE (SEE ABOVE). Dosage may be repeated if life threatening signs, such as arrhythmia, convulsions or coma occurs.

Pediatric Dosage: Recommended dosage is 0.02 mg/kg, intramuscularly or by slow intravenous injection, no more than 0.5 mg per minute. If the toxic effects persist, and there is no sign of cholinergic effects, the dosage may be repeated at 5 to 10 minute intervals until a therapeutic effect is obtained or a maximum dose of 2 mg is attained.

IN ALL CASES OF POISONING, THE USUAL SUPPORTIVE MEASURES SHOULD BE UNDERTAKEN.

HOW SUPPLIED

Ampuls, 2 ml packed 12 per box, 1 mg per ml NDC-0456-1037-12.

Store at controlled room temperature 15°–30°C (59°–86°F).

CAUTION

Federal law prohibits dispensing without prescription.

SOME DRUGS WHICH PRODUCE THE ANTICHOLINERGIC SYNDROME:

Amitriptyline, Amoxapine, Anisotropine, Atropine, Benztropine, Biperiden, Carbinoxamine, Clidinium, Cyclobenzaprine, Desipramine, Doxepin, Homatropine, Hyoscine, Hyoscyamine, Hyoscyamus, Imipramine, Lorazepam, Maprotiline, Mepenzolate, Nortriptyline, Propantheline, Protriptyline, Scopolamine, Trimipramine.

SOME PLANTS THAT PRODUCE THE ANTICHOLINERGIC SYNDROME:

Black Henbane, Deadly Night Shade, Devil's Apple, Jimson Weed, Loco Seeds or Weeds, Matrimony Vine, Night Blooming Jessamine, Stinkweed.

ARMOUR® THYROID Tablets ℞
[thī 'roid]
(THYROID TABLETS, U.S.P.)

DESCRIPTION

Armour Thyroid Tablets (Thyroid Tablets, USP) for oral use are natural preparations derived from porcine thyroid glands. (T_3 liothyronine is approximately four times as potent as T_4 levothyroxine on a microgram for microgram ba-

sis.) They provide 38 mcg levothyroxine (T_4) and 9 mcg liothyronine (T_3) per grain of thyroid. The inactive ingredients are calcium stearate, dextrose and mineral oil.

HOW SUPPLIED

Armour Thyroid Tablets (thyroid tablets, USP) are supplied as follows:

Size	Available in	NDC No.
15 mg (1/4 gr)	Bottles of 100	0456-0457-01
30 mg (1/2 gr)	Bottles of 100	0456-0458-01
	Bottles of 1000	0456-0458-00
	Drums of 50,000	0456-0458-69
	Unit dose cartons of 100	0456-0458-63
60 mg (1 gr)	Bottles of 100	0456-0459-01
	Bottles of 1000	0456-0459-00
	Bottles of 5000	0456-0459-51
	Drums of 50,000	0456-0459-69
	Unit dose cartons of 100	0456-0459-63
90 mg (1 1/2 gr)	Bottles of 100	0456-0460-01
120 mg (2 gr)	Bottles of 100	0456-0461-01
	Bottles of 1000	0456-0461-00
	Drums of 50,000	0456-0461-69
180 mg (3 gr)	Bottles of 100	0456-0462-01
	Bottles of 1000	0456-0462-00
240 mg (4 gr)	Bottles of 100	0456-0463-01
300 mg (5 gr)	Bottles of 100	0456-0464-01

The bottles of 100 are special dispensing bottles with child-resistant closures.

Note: (T_3 liothyronine is approximately four times as potent as T_4 levothyroxine on a microgram-for-microgram basis.)

Tablets should be stored at controlled room temperature, 59°–86°F (15°–30°C), in capped bottles or unbroken plastic strip packing.

Forest Pharmaceuticals, Inc.
A Subsidiary of Forest Laboratories, Inc.
St. Louis, MO 63045
REV 8/95 81640895

Shown in Product Identification Guide, page 310

CERVIDIL® ℞

Brand of dinoprostone vaginal insert

DESCRIPTION

Dinoprostone vaginal insert is a thin, flat, polymeric slab which is rectangular in shape with rounded corners contained within the pouch of a knitted polyester retrieval system, an integral part of which is a long tape. Each slab is buff colored, semitransparent and contains 10 mg of dinoprostone. The hydrogel insert is contained within the pouch of an off-white knitted polyester retrieval system designed to aid retrieval at the end of the dosing interval. The finished product is a controlled release formulation which has been found to release dinoprostone *in vivo* at a rate of approximately 0.3 mg/hr.

The chemical name for dinoprostone (commonly known as prostaglandin E_2 or PGE_2) is 11α, 15S-dihydroxy-9-oxo-prosta-5Z, 13E-dien-1-oic acid and the structural formula is represented below:

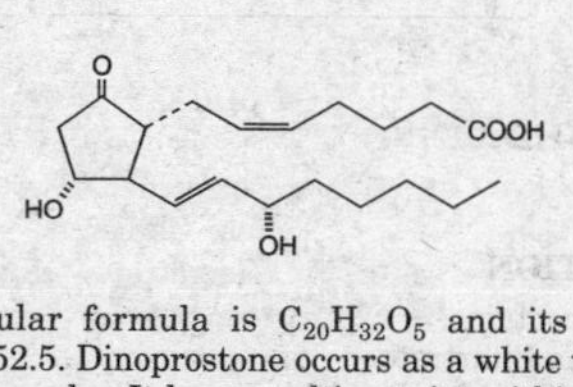

The molecular formula is $C_{20}H_{32}O_5$ and its molecular weight is 352.5. Dinoprostone occurs as a white to off-white crystalline powder. It has a melting point within the range of 65° to 69°C. Dinoprostone is soluble in ethanol and in 25% ethanol in water. Each insert contains 10 mg of dinoprostone in 236 mg of a cross-linked polyethylene oxide/urethane polymer which is a semi-opaque, beige colored, flat rectangular slab measuring 29 mm by 9.5 mm and 0.8 mm in thickness. The insert and its retrieval system, made of polyester yarn, are non-toxic and when placed in a moist environment, absorb water, swell, and release dinoprostone.

CLINICAL PHARMACOLOGY

Dinoprostone (PGE_2) is a naturally-occurring biomolecule. It is found in low concentrations in most tissues of the body and functions as a local hormone (1–3). As with any local hormone, it is very rapidly metabolized in the tissues of synthesis (the half-life estimated to be 2.5–5 minutes). The rate limiting step for inactivation is regulated by the enzyme 15-hydroxyprostaglandin dehydrogenase (PGDH) (1,4). Any PGE_2 that escapes local inactivation is rapidly cleared to the extent of 95% on the first pass through the pulmonary circulation (1,2).

Table 1
Total Cervidil-Treated Drug Related Adverse Events

	Controlled Studies[1]		STUDY 101–801[2]	
	Active	Placebo	Active	Placebo
Uterine hyperstimulation with fetal distress	2.8%	0.3%	2.9%	0%
Uterine hyperstimulation without fetal distress	4.7%	0%	2.0%	0%
Fetal Distress without uterine hyperstimulation	3.8%	1.2%	2.9%	1.0%
N	320	338	102	104

[1] Controlled Studies (with and without retrieval system)
[2] Controlled Study (with retrieval system)

In pregnancy, PGE_2 is secreted continuously by the fetal membranes and placenta and plays an important role in the final events leading to the initiation of labor (1,2). It is known that PGE_2 stimulates the production of $PGF_{2}\alpha$ which in turn sensitizes the myometrium to endogenous or exogenously administrated oxytocin. Although PGE_2 is capable of initiating uterine contractions and may interact with oxytocin to increase uterine contractility, the available evidence indicates that, in the concentrations found during the early part of labor, PGE_2 plays an important role in cervical ripening without affecting uterine contractions (5–7). This distinction serves as the basis for considering cervical ripening and induction of labor, usually by the use of oxytocin (8–10), as two separate processes.

PGE_2 plays an important role in the complex set of biochemical and structural alterations involved in cervical ripening. Cervical ripening involves a marked relaxation of the cervical smooth muscle fibers of the uterine cervix which must be transformed from a rigid structure to a softened, yielding and dilated configuration to allow passage of the fetus through the birth canal (11–13). This process involves activation of the enzyme collagenase, which is responsible for digestion of some of the structural collagen network of the cervix (1,14). This is associated with a concomitant increase in the amount of hydrophilic glycosaminoglycan, hyaluronic acid, and a decrease in dermatan sulfate (1). Failure of the cervix to undergo these natural physiologic changes, usually assessed by the method described by Bishop (15,16), prior to the onset of effective uterine contractions, results in an unfavorable outcome for successful vaginal delivery and may result in fetal compromise. It is estimated that in approximately 5% of pregnancies the cervix does not ripen normally (17). In an additional 10–11% of pregnancies, labor must be induced for medical or obstetric reasons prior to the time of cervical ripening (17).

The delivery rate of PGE_2 *in vivo* is about 0.3 mg/hour over a period of 12 hours. The controlled release of PGE_2 from the hydrogel insert is an attempt to provide sufficient quantities of PGE_2 to the local receptors to satisfy hormonal requirements. In the majority of patients, these local effects are manifested by changes in the consistency, dilatation and effacement of the cervix as measured by the Bishop score. Although some patients experience uterine hyperstimulation as a result of direct PGE_2- or $PGF_{2}\alpha$-mediated sensitization of the myometrium to oxytocin, systemic effects of PGE_2 are rarely encountered. The insert is fitted with a biocompatible retrieval system which facilitates removal at the conclusion of therapy or in the event of an adverse reaction.

No correlation could be established between PGE_2 release and plasma concentrations of PGE_m. The relative contributions of endogenously and exogenously released PGE_2 to the plasma levels of the metabolite PGE_m could not be determined. Moreover, it is uncertain as to whether the measured concentrations of PGE_m reflect the natural progression of PGE_m concentrations in blood as birth approaches or to what extent the measured concentrations following PGE_2 administration represent an increase over basal levels that might be measured in control patients.

INDICATIONS AND USAGE

Cervidil Vaginal Insert (dinoprostone, 10 mg) is indicated for the initiation and/or continuation of cervical ripening in patients at or near term in whom there is a medical or obstetrical indication for the induction of labor.

CONTRAINDICATIONS

Cervidil is contraindicated in:

- Patients with known hypersensitivity to prostaglandins.
- Patients in whom there is clinical suspicion or definite evidence of fetal distress where delivery is not imminent.
- Patients with unexplained vaginal bleeding during this pregnancy.
- Patients in whom there is evidence or strong suspicion of marked cephalopelvic disproportion.
- Patients in whom oxytocic drugs are contraindicated or when prolonged contraction of the uterus may be detrimental to fetal safety or uterine integrity (previous cesarean section or major uterine surgery).
- Patients already receiving intravenous oxytocic drugs.
- Multipara with 6 or more previous term pregnancies.

WARNINGS

For hospital use only

Cervidil should be administered only by trained obstetrical personnel in a hospital setting with appropriate obstetrical care facilities.

PRECAUTIONS

1. General Precautions: Since prostaglandins potentiate the effect of oxytocin, Cervidil must be removed before oxytocin administration is initiated and the patient's uterine activity carefully monitored for uterine hyperstimulation. If uterine hyperstimulation is encountered or if labor commences, the vaginal insert should be removed. Cervidil should also be removed prior to amniotomy.

Caution should be exercised in the administration of Cervidil for cervical ripening in patients with ruptured membranes, in cases of non-vertex, or non-singleton presentation, and in patients with a history of previous uterine hypertony, glaucoma, or a history of childhood asthma, even though there have been no asthma attacks in adulthood.

Uterine activity, fetal status and the progression of cervical dilatation and effacement should be carefully monitored whenever the dinoprostone vaginal insert is in place. Any evidence of uterine hyperstimulation, sustained uterine contractions, fetal distress, or other fetal or maternal adverse reactions, should be a cause for consideration of removal of the insert.

2. Drug Interactions: Cervidil may augment the activity of oxytocic agents and their concomitant use is not recommended. A dosing interval of at least 30 minutes is recommended for the sequential use of oxytocin following the removal of the dinoprostone vaginal insert. No other drug interactions have been identified.

3. Carcinogenesis, Mutagenesis, Impairment of Fertility: Long-term carcinogenicity and fertility studies have not been conducted with Cervidil (dinoprostone) Vaginal Insert. No evidence of mutagenicity has been observed with prostaglandin E_2 in the Unscheduled DNA Synthesis Assay, the Micronucleus Test, or Ames Assay.

4. Pregnancy, Teratogenic Effects:
Pregnancy Category C:

Prostaglandin E_2 has produced an increase in skeletal anomalies in rats and rabbits. No effect would be expected clinically, when used as indicated, since Cervidil (dinoprostone) Vaginal Insert is administered after the period of organogenesis. Prostaglandin E_2 has been shown to be embryotoxic in rats and rabbits, and any dose that produces sustained increased uterine tone could put the embryo or fetus at risk.

ADVERSE REACTIONS

Cervidil is well tolerated. In placebo-controlled trials in which 658 women were entered and 320 received active therapy (218 without retrieval system, 102 with retrieval system), the following events were reported.

[See table above]

Drug related fever, nausea, vomiting, diarrhea, and abdominal pain were noted in less than 1% of patients who received Cervidil.

In study 101–801 (with the retrieval system) cases of hyperstimulation reversed within 2 to 13 minutes of removal of the product. Tocolytics were required in one of the five cases.

In cases of fetal distress, when product removal was thought advisable there was a return to normal rhythm and no neonatal sequelae.

Five minute Apgar scores were 7 or above in 98.2% (646/658) of studied neonates whose mothers received Cervidil. In a report of a 3 year pediatric follow-up study in 121 infants, 51 of whose mothers received Cervidil, there were no deleterious effects on physical examination or psychomotor evaluation (18).

DRUG ABUSE AND DEPENDENCE

No drug abuse or dependence has been seen with the use of Cervidil.

Continued on next page

Cervidil—Cont.

OVERDOSAGE

Cervidil is used as a single dosage in a single application. Overdosage is usually manifested by uterine hyperstimulation which may be accompanied by fetal distress and is responsive to removal of the insert. Other treatment must be symptomatic since, to date, clinical experience with prostaglandin antagonists is insufficient.

The use of beta-adrenergic agents should be considered in the event of undesirable increased uterine activity.

DOSAGE AND ADMINISTRATION

The dosage of dinoprostone in the vaginal insert is 10 mg designed to be released at approximately 0.3 mg/hour over a 12 hour period. Cervidil should be removed upon onset of active labor or 12 hours after insertion.

One Cervidil is placed transversely in the posterior fornix of the vagina immediately after removal from its foil package. The insertion of the vaginal insert does not require sterile conditions. The vaginal insert must not be used without its retrieval system. There is no need for previous warming of the product. A minimal amount of K-Y® jelly (or other water-miscible lubricant) may be used to assist in insertion of Cervidil. Care should be taken not to permit excess contact or coating with the lubricant and thus prevent optimal swelling and release of dinoprostone from the vaginal insert. Patients should remain in the supine position for 2 hours following insertion, but thereafter may be ambulatory.

HOW SUPPLIED

Cervidil (NDC 0456-4123-63) contains 10 mg dinoprostone. The product is wound and enclosed in an aluminum sleeve which is contained in an aluminum/polyethylene pack.

Store in a freezer: between −20°C and −10°C (−4°F and 14°F). Cervidil is packed in foil and is stable when stored in a freezer for a period of three years. Vaginal inserts exposed to high humidity will absorb moisture from the air and thereby alter the release characteristics of dinoprostone. Once used, the vaginal insert should be discarded.

Rx only

CLINICAL STUDIES

[See table below]

REFERENCES

1. Physiology of Labor. In: Williams Obstetrics. Eds. Pritchard, J.A., MacDonald, P.C., and Gant, N.F. Appleton-Century-Crofts, Conn, Pp 295-321, (1985).
2. Rall, T.W. and Schliefer, L.S. Oxytocin, prostaglandin, ergot alkaloids, and other drugs; tocolytics agents, In: The Pharmacological Basis of Therapeutics. Eds. Gilman, A.G., Goodman, L.S., Rall, T.W., and Murad, F. MacMillan Publ. Co., New York, Pp 926-945, (1985).
3. Casey, M.L. and MacDonald, P.C. The initiation of labor in women: Regulation of phospholipid and arachidonic acid metabolism and of prostaglandin production. Semin. Perinat. 10: 270-275, (1986).
4. Casey, M.L., MacDonald, P.C. and Mitchell, M.D. Stimulation of prostaglandin E_2 production in amnion cells in culture by a substance(s) in human fetal urine. Biochem. Biophys. Res. Comm. 114:1056, (1983).
5. Olson, C.M., Lye, S.J., Skinner, K., and Challis, J.R.G. Prostanoid concentrations in maternal/fetal plasma and amniotic fluid and intrauterine tissue prostanoid output in relation to myometrial contractility during the onset of Endocrinology. 116: 389-397, (1985).
6. Ledger, W.L., Ellwood, D.A., and Taylor, M.J. Cervical softening in late pregnant sheep by infusion of prostaglandin E-2 into cervical artery. J. Reprod. Fert. 69, 511-515, (1983).
7. Olson, D.M., Lye, S.J., Skinner, K., and Challis, J.R.G. Early changes in prostaglandin concentrations in ovine maternal and fetal plasma, amniotic fluid and from dispersed cells of intrauterine tissues before the onset of ACTH-induced pre-term labor. J. Reprod. Fert. 71: 45-55, (1984).
8. Caldero-Garcia, R. and Posiero, J. Oxytocin and the contractility of the human uterus, Ann, N.Y. Acad. Sci. 75: 813, (1959).
9. Posiero, J. and Noriega-Guerra, L. Dose-response relationships in uterine effects of oxytocin infusion. Oxytocin. Eds., Caldero-Garcia, R. and Heller, J. Pergamon Press, New York, (1961).
10. Cibils, L. Enhancement of induction of labor. In: Risks in the Practice of Modern Obstetrics. Aldjem, S. Ed. Mosby Publishing, St. Louis, (1972).
11. Bryman, I., Lindblom, B., and Norstrom, A. Extreme sensitivity of cervical musculature to prostaglandin E_2 in early pregnancy. Lancet, 2:1471, (1982).
12. Thiery, M. Induction of labor with prostaglandins. In: Human Parturition. Eds. Keirse, M.J.N.C., Anderson, A.B.M.; and Gravenhorst, J.B. Martinus Nijhoff Publ., Boston, 155-164, (1979).
13. Thiery, M. and Amy, J.J. Induction of labor with prostaglandins. In: Advances in Prostaglandin Research. Prostaglandin and Reproduction. Karim, S.M.M., Ed., MTP, Lancaster, Pp. 149-228, (1975).
14. MacLennan, A.H., Katz, M., and Creasey, R. The morphologic characteristics of cervical ripening induced by the hormones relaxin and prostaglandin F_2 in a rabbit model. Am. J. Obstet. Gynecol, 152: 910696, (1985).
15. Bishop, E. Elective induction of labor. Obstet. & Gynecol. 5: 519-527, (1955).
16. Bishop, E. Pelvic scoring for elective induction. Obstet. & Gynecol. 24: 266-268. (1969).
17. Thiery, M. Preinduction cervical ripening. In: Obstetrics and Gynecology Annual, Vol. 12 Ed. Wynn, R.M. Appleton-Century-Crofts, New York, Pp. 103-146, (1983).
18. MacKenzie, I.; Information on File: Controlled Therapeutics (Scotland).

Mfg by:
Controlled Therapeutics
East Kilbride, Scotland G74 5PB

Made in the U.K.

Distributed by:
FOREST PHARMACEUTICALS, INC.
Subsidiary of Forest Laboratories, Inc.
St. Louis, MO 63045 USA

RMS 311
SAP 226
Rev. 5/98

Shown in Product Identification Guide, page 310

DALALONE D.P.® ℞
(Sterile Dexamethasone Acetate Suspension, USP)
Equivalent to Dexamethasone 16 mg/mL

PRESCRIBING INFORMATION

DALALONE D.P. ℞
(Sterile Dexamethasone Acetate Suspension, USP)
Equivalent to Dexamethasone 16 mg/mL

**NOT FOR INTRAVENOUS OR INTRALESIONAL USE
FOR INTRAMUSCULAR, INTRA-ARTICULAR AND
SOFT TISSUE USE**

DESCRIPTION

Dexamethasone acetate, a synthetic adrenocortical steroid, is a white to practically white, odorless powder. It is a practically insoluble ester of dexamethasone. The structural formula is

Dexamethasone acetate is present in sterile dexamethasone acetate suspension as the monohydrate, with the molecular formula, $C_{24}H_{31}FO_6 \cdot H_2O$, and molecular weight, 452.52. Dexamethasone acetate is designated chemically as 21-(acetyloxy)-9-fluoro-11β,17-dihydroxy-16α-methylpregna-1,4-diene-3,20-dione.
Sterile Dexamethasone Acetate suspension is a sterile white suspension (pH 5.0 to 7.5) that settles on standing, but is easily resuspended by mild shaking.
Each ml. contains: Dexamethasone Acetate equivalent to Dexamethasone 16 mg.
6.67 mg Sodium Chloride
5 mg Creatinine
0.5 mg Edetate Disodium
5 mg Carboxymethylcellulose Sodium
0.75 mg Polysorbate 80
1 mg Sodium Bisulfite
9 mg Benzyl Alcohol
as preservatives in Water for Injection q.s., Sodium Hydroxide may have been used to adjust pH.

HOW SUPPLIED

Sterile dexamethasone acetate suspension, equivalent to dexamethasone 16 mg/mL is available in:
1 mL vials, individually boxed;
5 mL multiple dose vials, individually boxed.
NDC 0456-1097-41
NDC 0456-1097-05
STORE AT CONTROLLED ROOM TEMPERATURE 15°–30° C (59°–86° F). DO NOT PERMIT TO FREEZE. SENSITIVE TO HEAT—DO NOT AUTOCLAVE. SHAKE WELL BEFORE USING.
PROTECT FROM LIGHT. Store in carton until contents are used.

CAUTION

Federal law prohibits dispensing without prescription.
Literature Revised: August 1994
Product No. 0669-01, 0669-05.
Manufactured by
Steris Laboratories, Inc.
Phoenix, AZ 85043
Mfd. for
FOREST PHARMACEUTICALS, INC.
SUBSIDIARY OF FOREST LABORATORIES, INC.
ST. LOUIS, MISSOURI 63045

ENDAL™-HD ℃ ℞
[ĕn dăl-HD]

DESCRIPTION

Each 5mL contains:
Hydrocodone Bitartrate	1.67 mg
(WARNING: May Be Habit Forming)	
Phenylephrine Hydrochloride	5 mg
Chlorpheniramine Maleate	2 mg

HOW SUPPLIED

Endal-HD is supplied in bottles of one pint (473 mL) NDC# 0785-6200-16.

ESGIC® Capsules ℞
[es 'jik]
(Butalbital, Acetaminophen and Caffeine Capsules, USP)
50 mg/325 mg/40 mg

Shown in Product Identification Guide, page 310

ESGIC® Tablets ℞
(Butalbital, Acetaminophen and Caffeine Tablets, USP)
50 mg/325 mg/40 mg

Table 2
Efficacy of Cervidil in Double Blind Studies

Parameter	Study #	Primip/Nullip		Multip		P-Value
		Cervidil	Placebo	Cervidil	Placebo	
Treatment	101–103 (N=81)	65%	28%	87%	29%	<0.001
Success*	101–003 (N=371)	68%	24%	77%	24%	<0.001
	101–801 (N=206)	72%	48%	55%	41%	0.003
Time to Delivery (hours)						
Average	101–103 (N=81)	33.7	48.6	14.0	28.6	
Median		25.7	34.5	12.3	24.6	0.001
Average	101–801 (N=206)	31.1	51.8	52.3	45.9	
Median		25.5	37.2	20.8	27.4	<0.001
Time to Onset of Labor (hours)						
Average	101–103 (N=81)	19.9	39.4	6.8	22.4	
Median		12.0	19.2	6.9	18.3	<0.001

---

* Treatment success was defined as Bishop score increase at 12 hours of ≥3, vaginal delivery within 12 hours or Bishop score at 12 hours ≥6. These studies were not designed with the power to show differences in cesarean section rates between Cervidil and placebo groups and none were noted.

ESGIC-PLUS™ Tablets ℞
(Butalbital, Acetaminophen and Caffeine Tablets, USP)
50 mg/500 mg/40 mg

DESCRIPTION
Esgic-Plus is supplied in tablet form for oral administration. Butalbital (5-allyl-5-isobutylbarbituric acid), a slightly bitter, white, odorless, crystalline powder, is a short to intermediate-acting barbiturate. It has the following structural formula:

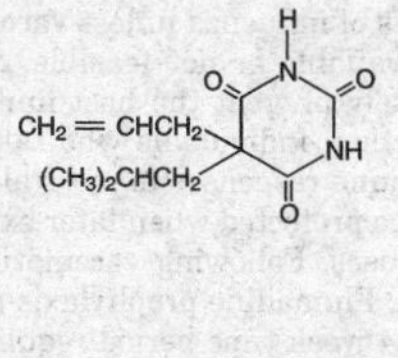

$C_{11}H_{16}N_2O_3$ MW=224.26

Acetaminophen (4'-hydroxyacetanilide), a slightly bitter, white, odorless, crystalline powder, is a non-opiate, non-salicylate analgesic and antipyretic. It has the following structural formula:

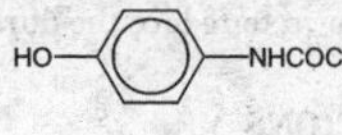

$C_8H_9NO_2$ MW=151.17

Caffeine (1,3,7-trimethylxanthine), a bitter, white powder or white-glistening needles, is a central nervous system stimulant. It has the following structural formula:

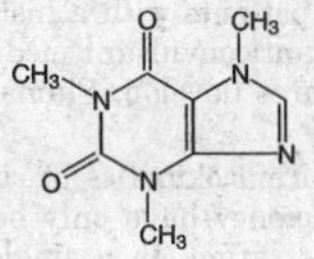

$C_8H_{10}N_4O_2$ MW=194.19

Each Esgic-Plus Tablet contains:

Butalbital*	50 mg
(*Warning: May be habit forming)	
Acetaminophen	500 mg
Caffeine	40 mg

In addition, each tablet contains the following inactive ingredients: colloidal silicon dioxide, croscarmellose sodium, microcrystalline cellulose, and stearic acid.

CLINICAL PHARMACOLOGY
This combination drug product is intended as a treatment for tension headache.
It consists of a fixed combination of butalbital, acetaminophen and caffeine. The role each component plays in the relief of the complex of symptoms known as tension headache is incompletely understood.
Pharmacokinetics: The behavior of the individual components is described below.
Butalbital: Butalbital is well absorbed from the gastrointestinal tract and is expected to distribute to most tissues in the body. Barbiturates in general may appear in breast milk and readily cross the placental barrier. They are bound to plasma and tissue proteins to a varying degree and binding increases directly as a function of lipid solubility.
Elimination of butalbital is primarily via the kidney (59% to 88% of the dose) as unchanged drug or metabolites. The plasma half-life is about 35 hours. Urinary excretion products include parent drug (about 3.6% of the dose), 5-isobutyl-5-(2,3-dihydroxypropyl) barbituric acid (about 24% of the dose), 5-allyl-5 (3-hydroxy-2-methyl-1-propyl) barbituric acid (about 4.8% of the dose), products with the barbituric acid ring hydrolyzed with excretion of urea (about 14% of the dose), as well as unidentified materials. Of the material excreted in the urine, 32% is conjugated.
See **OVERDOSAGE** for toxicity information.
Acetaminophen: Acetaminophen is rapidly absorbed from the gastrointestinal tract and is distributed throughout most body tissues. The plasma half-life is 1.25 to 3 hours, but may be increased by liver damage and following overdosage. Elimination of acetaminophen is principally by liver metabolism (conjugation) and subsequent renal excretion of metabolites. Approximately 85% of an oral dose appears in the urine within 24 hours of administration, most as the glucuronide conjugate, with small amounts of other conjugates and unchanged drug.
See **OVERDOSAGE** for toxicity information.
Caffeine: Like most xanthines, caffeine is rapidly absorbed and distributed in all body tissues and fluids, including the CNS, fetal tissues, and breast milk.
Caffeine is cleared through metabolism and excretion in the urine. The plasma half-life is about 3 hours. Hepatic biotransformation prior to excretion, results in about equal amounts of 1-methylxanthine and 1-methyluric acid. Of the 70% of the dose that is recovered in the urine, only 3% is unchanged drug.
See **OVERDOSAGE** for toxicity information.

INDICATIONS AND USAGE
Esgic-Plus (butalbital, acetaminophen and caffeine) Tablets are indicated for the relief of the symptom complex of tension (or muscle contraction) headache.
Evidence supporting the efficacy and safety of this combination product in the treatment of multiple recurrent headaches is unavailable. Caution in this regard is required because butalbital is habit-forming and potentially abusable.

CONTRAINDICATIONS
This product is contraindicated under the following conditions:
- Hypersensitivity or intolerance to any component of this product.
- Patients with porphyria.

WARNINGS
Butalbital is habit-forming and potentially abusable. Consequently, the extended use of this product is not recommended.

PRECAUTIONS
General: Esgic-Plus Tablets should be prescribed with caution in certain special-risk patients, such as the elderly or debilitated, and those with severe impairment of renal or hepatic function, or acute abdominal conditions.
Information for Patients: This product may impair mental and/or physical abilities required for the performance of potentially hazardous tasks such as driving a car or operating machinery. Such tasks should be avoided while taking this product.
Alcohol and other CNS depressants may produce an additive CNS depression, when taken with this combination product, and should be avoided.
Butalbital may be habit-forming. Patients should take the drug only for as long as it is prescribed, in the amounts prescribed, and no more frequently than prescribed.
Laboratory Tests: In patients with severe hepatic or renal disease, effects of therapy should be monitored with serial liver and/or renal function tests.
Drug Interactions: The CNS effects of butalbital may be enhanced by monoamine oxidase (MAO) inhibitors.
Butalbital, acetaminophen and caffeine may enhance the effects of: other narcotic analgesics, alcohol, general anesthetics, tranquilizers such as chlordiazepoxide, sedative-hypnotics, or other CNS depressants, causing increased CNS depression.
Drug/Laboratory Test Interactions: Acetaminophen may produce false-positive test results for urinary 5-hydroxyindoleacetic acid.
Carcinogenesis, Mutagenesis, Impairment of Fertility. No adequate studies have been conducted in animals to determine whether acetaminophen or butalbital have a potential for carcinogenesis, mutagenesis or impairment of fertility.
Pregnancy: *Teratogenic Effects:* Pregnancy Category C. Animal reproduction studies have not been conducted with this combination product. It is also not known whether butalbital, acetaminophen and caffeine can cause fetal harm when administered to a pregnant woman or can affect reproduction capacity. This product should be given to a pregnant woman only when clearly needed.
Nonteratogenic Effects: Withdrawal seizures were reported in a two-day-old male infant whose mother had taken a butalbital-containing drug during the last two months of pregnancy. Butalbital was found in the infant's serum. The infant was given phenobarbital 5 mg/kg, which was tapered without further seizure or other withdrawal symptoms.
Nursing Mothers: Caffeine, barbiturates and acetaminophen are excreted in breast milk in small amounts, but the significance of their effects on nursing infants is not known. Because of potential for serious adverse reactions in nursing infants from butalbital, acetaminophen and caffeine, a decision should be made whether to discontinue nursing or to discontinue drug, taking into account the importance of the drug to the mother.
Pediatric Use: Safety and effectiveness in pediatric patients below the age of 12 have not been established.

ADVERSE REACTIONS
Frequently Observed: The most frequently reported adverse reactions are drowsiness, lightheadedness, dizziness, sedation, shortness of breath, nausea, vomiting, abdominal pain, and intoxicated feeling.
Infrequently Observed: All adverse events tabulated below are classified as infrequent.
Central Nervous: headache, shaky feeling, tingling, agitation, fainting, fatigue, heavy eyelids, high energy, hot spells, numbness, sluggishness, seizure. Mental confusion, excitement or depression can also occur due to intolerance, particularly in elderly or debilitated patients, or due to overdosage of butalbital.
Autonomic Nervous: dry mouth, hyperhidrosis.
Gastrointestinal: difficulty swallowing, heartburn, flatulence.
Cardiovascular: tachycardia.
Musculoskeletal: leg pain, muscle fatigue.
Genitourinary: diuresis.
Miscellaneous: pruritus, fever, earache, nasal congestion, tinnitus, euphoria, allergic reactions.
Several cases of dermatological reactions, including toxic epidermal necrolysis and erythema multiforme, have been reported.
The following adverse drug events may be borne in mind as potential effects of the components of this product. Potential effects of high dosage are listed in the OVERDOSAGE section.
Acetaminophen: allergic reactions, rash, thrombocytopenia, agranulocytosis.
Caffeine: cardiac stimulation, irritability, tremor, dependence, nephrotoxicity, hyperglycemia.

DRUG ABUSE AND DEPENDENCE
Abuse and Dependence: Butalbital: *Barbiturates may be habit-forming:* Tolerance, psychological dependence, and physical dependence may occur especially following prolonged use of high doses of barbiturates. The average daily dose for the barbiturate addict is usually about 1500 mg. As tolerance to barbiturates develops, the amount needed to maintain the same level of intoxication increases; tolerance to a fatal dosage, however, does not increase more than two-fold. As this occurs, the margin between an intoxication dosage and fatal dosage becomes smaller. The lethal dose of a barbiturate is far less if alcohol is also ingested. Major withdrawal symptoms (convulsions and delirium) may occur within 16 hours and last up to 5 days after abrupt cessation of these drugs. Intensity of withdrawal symptoms gradually declines over a period of approximately 15 days. Treatment of barbiturate dependence consists of cautious and gradual withdrawal of the drug. Barbiturate-dependent patients can be withdrawn by using a number of different withdrawal regimens. One method involves initiating treatment at the patient's regular dosage level and gradually decreasing the daily dosage as tolerated by the patient.

OVERDOSAGE
Following an acute overdosage of butalbital, acetaminophen and caffeine, toxicity may result from the barbiturate or the acetaminophen. Toxicity due to caffeine is less likely, due to the relatively small amounts in this formulation.
Signs and Symptoms: Toxicity from barbiturate poisoning include drowsiness, confusion, and coma; respiratory depression; hypotension; and hypovolemic shock.
In acetaminophen overdosage, dose-dependent, potentially fatal hepatic necrosis is the most serious adverse effect. Renal tubular necroses, hypoglycemic coma and thrombocytopenia may also occur. Early symptoms following a potentially hepatotoxic overdose may include: nausea, vomiting, diaphoresis and general malaise. Clinical and laboratory evidence of hepatic toxicity may not be apparent until 48 to 72 hours post-ingestion. In adults, hepatic toxicity has rarely been reported with acute overdoses of less than 10 grams, or fatalities with less than 15 grams.
Acute caffeine poisoning may cause insomnia, restlessness, tremor, delirium, tachycardia and extrasystoles.
Treatment: A single or multiple overdose with this combination product is a potentially lethal polydrug overdose, and consultation with a regional poison control center is recommended.
Immediate treatment includes support of cardiorespiratory function and measures to reduce drug absorption. Vomiting should be induced mechanically, or with syrup of ipecac, if the patient is alert (adequate pharyngeal and laryngeal reflexes). Oral activated charcoal (1 g/kg) should follow gastric emptying. The first dose should be accompanied by an appropriate cathartic. If repeated doses are used, the cathartic might be included with alternate doses as required.
Hypotension is usually hypovolemic and should respond to fluids. Pressors should be avoided. A cuffed endotracheal tube should be inserted before gastric lavage of the unconscious patient and, when necessary, to provide assisted respiration. If renal function is normal, forced diuresis may aid in the elimination of the barbiturate. Alkalinization of the urine increases renal excretion of some barbiturates, especially phenobarbital.
Meticulous attention should be given to maintaining adequate pulmonary ventilation. In severe cases of intoxication, peritoneal dialysis, or preferably hemodialysis may be

Continued on next page

Esgic-Plus—Cont.

considered. If hypoprothrombinemia occurs due to acetaminophen overdose, vitamin K should be administered intravenously.

If the dose of acetaminophen may have exceeded 140 mg/kg, acetylcysteine should be administered as early as possible. Serum acetaminophen levels should be obtained, since levels four or more hours following ingestion help predict acetaminophen toxicity. Do not await acetaminophen assay results before initiating treatment. Hepatic enzymes should be obtained initially, and repeated at 24-hour intervals.

Methemoglobinemia over 30% should be treated with methylene blue by slow intravenous administration.

Toxic Doses (for adults):
Butalbital:
toxic dose 1 g (20 tablets)
Acetaminophen:
toxic dose 10 g (20 tablets)
Caffeine:
toxic dose 1 g (25 tablets)

DOSAGE AND ADMINISTRATION

One tablet every four hours. Total daily dosage should not exceed 6 tablets.

Extended and repeated use of this product is not recommended because of the potential for physical dependence.

HOW SUPPLIED

Esgic-Plus Tablets, containing butalbital* 50 mg (*Warning: May be habit forming), acetaminophen 500 mg and caffeine 40 mg, are white, capsule-shaped, single-scored, and are debossed "FOREST" on the upper side and "678" on one side of the score on the lower side. They are supplied in bottles of 100, NDC 0456-0678-01, and in bottles of 500, NDC 0456-0678-02.

Storage: Store at controlled room temperature 15°–30°C (59°–86°F).

Dispense in a tight, light-resistant container with a child-resistant closure.

CAUTION: Federal law prohibits dispensing without prescription.

Manufactured by:
MIKART, INC.
Atlanta, GA 30318
Distributed by:
FOREST PHARMACEUTICALS, INC.
Subsidiary of
Forest Laboratories, Inc.
St. Louis, Missouri 63045
Rev. 7/97 Code 374A00

Shown in Product Identification Guide, page 310

FLUMADINE® TABLETS ℞
(rimantadine hydrochloride tablets)

FLUMADINE® SYRUP ℞
(rimantadine hydrochloride syrup)

DESCRIPTION

Flumadine (rimantadine hydrochloride) is a synthetic antiviral drug available as a 100 mg film-coated tablet and as a syrup for oral administration. Each film-coated tablet contains 100 mg of rimantadine hydrochloride plus hydroxypropyl methylcellulose, magnesium stearate, microcrystalline cellulose, sodium starch glycolate, FD&C Yellow No. 6 Lake and FD&C Yellow No. 6. The film coat contains hydroxypropyl methylcellulose and polyethylene glycol. Each teaspoonful (5 mL) of the syrup contains 50 mg of rimantadine hydrochloride in an aqueous solution containing citric acid, parabens (methyl and propyl), saccharin sodium, sorbitol, D&C Red No. 33 and flavors.

Rimantadine hydrochloride is a white to off-white crystalline powder which is freely soluble in water (50 mg/mL at 20°C). Chemically, rimantadine hydrochloride is alpha-methyltricyclo-[3.3.1.1/3.7]decane-1-methanamine hydrochloride, with an empirical formula of $C_{12}H_{21}N{\cdot}HCl$, a molecular weight of 215.77 and the following structural formula:

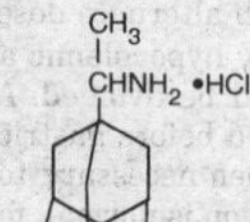

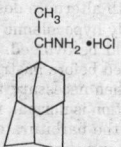

CLINICAL PHARMACOLOGY

Mechanism of Action: The mechanism of action of rimantadine is not fully understood. Rimantadine appears to exert its inhibitory effect early in the viral replicative cycle, possibly inhibiting the uncoating of the virus. Genetic studies suggest that a virus protein specified by the virion M_2 gene plays an important role in the susceptibility of influenza A virus to inhibition by rimantadine.

Microbiology: Rimantadine is inhibitory to the *in vitro* replication of influenza A virus isolates from each of the three antigenic subtypes, i.e., H1N1, H2N2 and H3N2, that have been isolated from man. Rimantadine has little or no activity against influenza B virus (Ref. 1,2). Rimantadine does not appear to interfere with the immunogenicity of inactivated influenza A vaccine.

A quantitative relationship between the *in vitro* susceptibility of influenza A virus to rimantadine and clinical response to therapy has not been established.

Susceptibility test results, expressed as the concentration of the drug required to inhibit virus replication by 50% or more in a cell culture system, vary greatly (from 4 ng/mL to 20 µg/mL) depending upon the assay protocol used, size of the virus inoculum, isolates of the influenza A virus strains tested, and the cell type used (Ref. 2).

Rimantadine-resistant strains of influenza A virus have emerged among freshly isolated epidemic strains in closed settings where rimantadine has been used. Resistant viruses have been shown to be transmissible and to cause typical influenza illness (Ref. 3).

Pharmacokinetics: Although the pharmacokinetic profile of Flumadine has been described, no pharmacodynamic data establishing a correlation between plasma concentration and its antiviral effect are available.

The tablet and syrup formulations of Flumadine are equally absorbed after oral administration. The mean ± SD peak plasma concentration after a single 100 mg dose of Flumadine was 74 ± 22 ng/mL (range: 45 to 138 ng/mL). The time to peak concentration was 6 ± 1 hours in healthy adults (age 20 to 44 years). The single dose elimination half-life in this population was 25.4 ± 6.3 hours (range: 13 to 65 hours). The single dose elimination half-life in a group of healthy 71 to 79 year-old subjects was 32 ± 16 hours (range: 20 to 65 hours).

After the administration of rimantadine 100 mg twice daily to healthy volunteers (age 18 to 70 years) for 10 days, area under the curve (AUC) values were approximately 30% greater than predicted from a single dose. Plasma trough levels at steady state ranged between 118 and 468 ng/mL. In these patients no age-related differences in pharmacokinetics were detected. However, in a comparison of three groups of healthy older subjects (age 50-60, 61-70 and 71-79 years), the 71 to 79 year-old group had average AUC values, peak concentrations and elimination half-life values at steady state that were 20 to 30% higher than the other two groups. Steady-state concentrations in elderly nursing home patients (age 68 to 102 years) were 2- to 4-fold higher than those seen in healthy young and elderly adults.

The pharmacokinetic profile of rimantadine in children has not been established. In a group (n=10) of children 4 to 8 years old who were given a single dose (6.6 mg/kg) of Flumadine syrup, plasma concentrations of rimantadine ranged from 446 to 988 ng/mL at 5 to 6 hours and from 170 to 424 ng/mL at 24 hours. In some children drug was detected in plasma 72 hours after the last dose.

Following oral administration, rimantadine is extensively metabolized in the liver with less than 25% of the dose excreted in the urine as unchanged drug. Three hydroxylated metabolites have been found in plasma. These metabolites, an additional conjugated metabolite and parent drug account for 74 ± 10% (n=4) of a single 200 mg dose of rimantadine excreted in urine over 72 hours.

In a group (n=14) of patients with chronic liver disease, the majority of whom were stabilized cirrhotics, the pharmacokinetics of rimantadine were not appreciably altered following a single 200 mg oral dose compared to 6 healthy subjects who were sex, age and weight matched to 6 of the patients with liver disease. After administration of a single 200 mg dose to patients (n=10) with severe hepatic dysfunction, AUC was approximately 3-fold larger, elimination half-life was approximately 2-fold longer and apparent clearance was about 50% lower when compared to historic data from healthy subjects.

Studies of the effects of renal insufficiency on the pharmacokinetics of rimantadine have given inconsistent results. Following administration of a single 200 mg oral dose of rimantadine to 8 patients with a creatinine clearance (CrCl) of 31–50 mL/min and 6 patients with a CrCl of 11–30 mL/min, the apparent clearance was 37% and 16% lower, respectively, and plasma metabolite concentrations were higher when compared to weight-, age-, and sex-matched healthy subjects (n=9, CrCl >50 mL/min). After a single 200 mg oral dose of rimantadine was given to 8 hemodialysis patients (CrCl 0–10 mL/min), there was a 1.6-fold increase in the elimination half-life and a 40% decrease in apparent clearance compared to age-matched healthy subjects. Hemodialysis did not contribute to the clearance of rimantadine.

The *in vitro* human plasma protein binding of rimantadine is about 40% over typical plasma concentrations. Albumin is the major binding protein.

INDICATIONS AND USAGE

Flumadine is indicated for the prophylaxis and treatment of illness caused by various strains of influenza A virus in adults.

Flumadine is indicated for prophylaxis against influenza A virus in children.

Prophylaxis: In controlled studies of children over the age of 1 year, healthy adults and elderly patients, Flumadine has been shown to be safe and effective in preventing signs and symptoms of infection caused by various strains of influenza A virus. Early vaccination on an annual basis as recommended by the Centers for Disease Control's Immunization Practices Advisory Committee is the method of choice in the prophylaxis of influenza unless vaccination is contraindicated, not available or not feasible. Since Flumadine does not completely prevent the host immune response to influenza A infection, individuals who take this drug may still develop immune responses to natural disease or vaccination and may be protected when later exposed to antigenically-related viruses. Following vaccination during an influenza outbreak, Flumadine prophylaxis should be considered for the 2 to 4 week time period required to develop an antibody response. However, the safety and effectiveness of Flumadine prophylaxis have not been demonstrated for longer than 6 weeks.

Treatment: Flumadine therapy should be considered for adults who develop an influenza-like illness during known or suspected influenza A infection in the community. When administered within 48 hours after onset of signs and symptoms of infection caused by influenza A virus strains, Flumadine has been shown to reduce the duration of fever and systemic symptoms.

CONTRAINDICATIONS

Flumadine is contraindicated in patients with known hypersensitivity to drugs of the adamantane class, including rimantadine and amantadine.

PRECAUTIONS

General: An increased incidence of seizures has been reported in patients with a history of epilepsy who received the related drug amantadine. In clinical trials of Flumadine, the occurrence of seizure-like activity was observed in a small number of patients with a history of seizures who were not receiving anticonvulsant medication while taking Flumadine. If seizures develop, Flumadine should be discontinued.

The safety and pharmacokinetics of rimantadine in renal and hepatic insufficiency have only been evaluated after single-dose administration. In a single-dose study of patients with anuric renal failure, the apparent clearance of rimantadine was approximately 40% lower and the elimination half-life was 1.6-fold greater than that in healthy age-matched controls. In a study of 14 persons with chronic liver disease (mostly stabilized cirrhotics), no alterations in the pharmacokinetics were observed after the administration of a single dose of rimantadine. However, the apparent clearance of rimantadine following a single dose to 10 patients with severe liver dysfunction was 50% lower than reported for healthy subjects. Because of the potential for accumulation of rimantadine and its metabolites in plasma, caution should be exercised when patients with renal or hepatic insufficiency are treated with rimantadine.

Transmission of rimantadine resistant virus should be considered when treating patients whose contacts are at high risk for influenza A illness. Influenza A virus strains resistant to rimantadine can emerge during treatment and such resistant strains have been shown to be transmissible and to cause typical influenza illness (Ref. 3). Although the frequency, rapidity, and clinical significance of the emergence of drug-resistant virus are not yet established, several small studies have demonstrated that 10% to 30% of patients with initially sensitive virus, upon treatment with rimantadine, shed rimantadine resistant virus (Ref. 3, 4, 5, 6).

Clinical response to rimantadine, although slower in those patients who subsequently shed resistant virus, was not significantly different from those who did not shed resistant virus (Ref. 3). No data are available in humans that address the activity or effectiveness of rimantadine therapy in subjects infected with resistant virus.

Drug Interactions: Cimetidine: The effects of chronic cimetidine use on the metabolism of rimantadine are not known. When a single 100 mg dose of Flumadine was administered one hour after the initiation of cimetidine (300 mg four times a day), the apparent total rimantadine clearance of this single dose in normal healthy adults was reduced by 18% (compared to the apparent total rimantadine clearance in the same subjects in the absence of cimetidine).

Acetaminophen: Flumadine, 100 mg, was given twice daily for 13 days to 12 healthy volunteers. On day 11, acetaminophen (650 mg four times daily) was started and continued for 8 days. The pharmacokinetics of rimantadine were assessed on days 11 and 13. Coadministration with acetaminophen reduced the peak concentration and AUC values for rimantadine by approximately 11%.

Aspirin: Flumadine, 100 mg, was given twice daily for 13 days to 12 healthy volunteers. On day 11, aspirin (650 mg, four times daily) was started and continued for 8 days. The pharmacokinetics of rimantadine were assessed on days 11 and 13. Peak plasma concentrations and AUC of rimantadine were reduced approximately 10% in the presence of aspirin.

Carcinogenesis, Mutagenesis, and Impairment of Fertility:
Carcinogenesis: Carcinogenicity studies in animals have not been performed.

Mutagenesis: No mutagenic effects were seen when rimantadine was evaluated in several standard assays for mutagenicity.

Impairment of Fertility: A reproduction study in male and female rats did not show detectable impairment of fertility at dosages up to 60 mg/kg/day (3 times the maximum human dose based on body surface area comparisons).

Pregnancy: *Teratogenic Effects:* Pregnancy Category C. There are no adequate and well-controlled studies in pregnant women. Rimantadine is reported to cross the placenta in mice. Rimantadine has been shown to be embryotoxic in rats when given at a dose of 200 mg/kg/day (11 times the recommended human dose based on body surface area comparisons). At this dose the embryotoxic effect consisted of increased fetal resorption in rats, this dose also produced a variety of maternal effects including ataxia, tremors, convulsions and significantly reduced weight gain. No embryotoxicity was observed when rabbits were given doses up to 50 mg/kg/day (5 times the recommended human dose based on body surface area comparisons). However, there was evidence of a developmental abnormality in the form of a change in the ratio of fetuses with 12 to 13 ribs. This ratio is normally about 50:50 in a litter but was 80:20 after rimantadine treatment.

Nonteratogenic Effects: Rimantadine was administered to pregnant rats in a peri- and postnatal reproduction toxicity study at doses of 30, 60 and 120 mg/kg/day (1.7, 3.4 and 6.8 times the recommended human dose based on body surface area comparisons). Maternal toxicity during gestation was noted at the two higher doses of rimantadine, and at the highest dose, 120 mg/kg/day, there was an increase in pup mortality during the first 2 to 4 days postpartum. Decreased fertility of the F1 generation was also noted for the two higher doses.

For these reasons, Flumadine should be used during pregnancy only if the potential benefit justifies the risk to the fetus.

Nursing Mothers: Flumadine should not be administered to nursing mothers because of the adverse effects noted in offspring of rats treated with rimantadine during the nursing period. Rimantadine is concentrated in rat milk in a dose-related manner: 2 to 3 hours following administration of rimantadine, rat breast milk levels were approximately twice those observed in the serum.

Pediatric Use: In children, Flumadine is recommended for the prophylaxis of influenza A. The safety and effectiveness of Flumadine in the treatment of symptomatic influenza infection in children have not been established. Prophylaxis studies with Flumadine have not been performed in children below the age of 1 year.

ADVERSE REACTIONS

In 1,027 patients treated with Flumadine in controlled clinical trials at the recommended dose of 200 mg daily, the most frequently reported adverse events involved the gastrointestinal and nervous systems.

Incidence >1%: Adverse events reported most frequently (1-3%) at the recommended dose in controlled clinical trials are shown in the table below.

	Rimantadine (n=1027)	Control (n=986)
Nervous System		
Insomnia	2.1%	0.9%
Dizziness	1.9%	1.1%
Headache	1.4%	1.3%
Nervousness	1.3%	0.6%
Fatigue	1.0%	0.9%
Gastrointestinal System		
Nausea	2.8%	1.6%
Vomiting	1.7%	0.6%
Anorexia	1.6%	0.8%
Dry mouth	1.5%	0.6%
Abdominal Pain	1.4%	0.8%
Body as a Whole		
Asthenia	1.4%	0.5%

Less frequent adverse events (0.3 to 1%) at the recommended dose in controlled clinical trials were: *Gastrointestinal System:* diarrhea, dyspepsia; *Nervous System:* impairment of concentration, ataxia, somnolence, agitation, depression; *Skin and Appendages:* rash; *Hearing and Vestibular:* tinnitus; *Respiratory:* dyspena.

Additional adverse events (less than 0.3%) reported at recommended doses in controlled clinical trials were: Nervous System: gait abnormality, euphoria, hyperkinesia, tremor, hallucination, confusion, convulsions; *Respiratory:* bronchospasm, cough; *Cardiovascular:* pallor, palpitation, hypertension, cerebrovascular disorder, cardiac failure, pedal edema, heart block, tachycardia, syncope; *Reproduction:* non-puerperal lactation; *Special Senses;* taste loss/change, parosmia.

Rates of adverse events, particularly those involving the gastrointestinal and nervous systems, increased significantly in controlled studies using higher than recommended doses of Flumadine. In most cases, symptoms resolved rapidly with discontinuation of treatment. In addition to the adverse events reported above, the following were also reported at higher than recommended doses: increased lacrimation, increased micturition frequency, fever, rigors, agitation, constipation, diaphoresis, dysphagia, stomatitis, hypesthesia and eye pain.

Adverse Reactions in Trials of Rimantadine and Amantadine: In a six-week prophylaxis study of 436 healthy adults comparing rimantadine with amantadine and placebo, the following adverse reactions were reported with an incidence >1%.

	Rimantadine 200 mg/day (n=145)	Placebo (n=143)	Amantadine 200 mg/day (n=148)
Nervous System			
Insomnia	3.4%	0.7%	7.0%
Nervousness	2.1%	0.7%	2.8%
Impaired Concentration	2.1%	1.4%	2.1%
Dizziness	0.7%	0.0%	2.1%
Depression	0.7%	0.7%	3.5%
Total % of subjects with adverse reactions	6.9%	4.1%	14.7%
Total % of subjects withdrawn due to adverse reactions	6.9%	3.4%	14.0%

Usage in the Elderly: In general, the incidence of adverse events in controlled clinical trials in the elderly was higher in both the Flumadine and placebo-treated groups compared to younger adults and children. In a placebo-controlled study of 83 nursing home patients with influenza, 10.6% of those treated with Flumadine compared with 8.3% in the placebo group experienced events related to the central nervous system. The profile of these events was similar to that for the most frequent adverse events reported in other controlled trials (see list above).

Pooled data from controlled studies of prophylaxis and treatment of influenza with Flumadine in persons over 65 years of age showed an increase in adverse clinical events associated with the recommended dose of Flumadine (100 mg twice a day) compared to controls as follows: central and peripheral nervous systems, 12.5% for Flumadine versus 8.7% for control patients; gastrointestinal system, 17.0% for Flumadine versus 11.3% for controls.

OVERDOSAGE

As with any overdose, supportive therapy should be administered as indicated. Overdoses of a related drug, Amantadine, have been reported with adverse reactions consisting of agitation, hallucinations, cardiac arrhythmia and death. The administration of intravenous physostigmine (a cholinergic agent) at doses of 1 to 2 mg in adults (Ref. 7) and 0.5 mg in children (Ref. 8) repeated as needed as long as the dose did not exceed 2 mg/hour has been reported anecdotally to be beneficial in patients with central nervous system effects from overdoses of Amantadine.

DOSAGE AND ADMINISTRATION

FOR PROPHYLAXIS IN ADULTS AND CHILDREN:
Adults: The recommended adult dose of Flumadine is 100 mg twice a day. In patients with severe hepatic dysfunction, renal failure (CrCl≤10 mL/min.) and elderly nursing home patients, a dose reduction to 100 mg daily is recommended. There are currently no data available regarding the safety of rimantadine during multiple dosing in subjects with renal or hepatic impairment. Because of the potential for accumulation of rimantadine metabolites during multiple dosing, patients with any degree of renal insufficiency should be monitored for adverse effects, with dosage adjustments being made as necessary.

Children: In children less than 10 years of age, Flumadine should be administered once a day, at a dose of 5 mg/kg but not exceeding 150 mg. For children 10 years of age or older, use the adult dose.

FOR TREATMENT IN ADULTS: The recommended adult dose of Flumadine is 100 mg twice a day. In patients with severe hepatic dysfunction, renal failure (CrCl≤10 mL/min) and elderly nursing home patients, a dose reduction to 100 mg daily is recommended. There are currently no data available regarding the safety of rimantadine during multiple dosing in subjects with renal or hepatic impairment. Because of the potential for accumulation of rimantadine metabolites during multiple dosing, patients with any degree of renal insufficiency should be monitored for adverse effects, with dosage adjustments being made as necessary.

Flumadine therapy should be initiated as soon as possible, preferably within 48 hours after onset of signs and symptoms of influenza A infection. Therapy should be continued for approximately seven days from the initial onset of symptoms.

HOW SUPPLIED

Flumadine tablets (rimantadine hydrochloride tablets) are supplied as 100 mg tablets (orange, oval-shaped, film-coated) in bottles of 100 (NDC 0456-0521-01). Imprint on tablets: (Front) FLUMADINE 100; (Back) FOREST.

Flumadine syrup (rimantadine hydrochloride syrup) containing 50 mg of rimantadine hydrochloride per teaspoonful (5 mL) (purplish-red, raspberry-flavored) is supplied in bottles of 8 oz (NDC 0456-0527-08).

Tablets and syrup should be stored at 15°– 30°C (59°– 86°F).

CAUTION: Federal (U.S.A.) law prohibits dispensing without prescription.

REFERENCES

1. Belshe, R.B., Burk, B., Newman, F., Cerruti, R.L. and Sim, I.S. (1989) J. Infect. Dis. 159, 430–435.
2. Sim, I.S., Cerruti, R.L. and Connell, E.V., (1989) J. Resp. Dis. (Suppl.), S46–S51.
3. Hayden, F.G., Belshe, R.B, Clover, R.D. et al (1989) N. Engl. J. Med. 321 (25), 1696–1702.
4. Hall, C.B., Dolin, R., Gala, C.L., et al (1987) Pediatrics 80, 275–282.
5. Thompson, J., Fleet, W., Lawrence, E. et al (1987) J. Med. Vir. 21, 249–255.
6. Belshe, R.B., Smith, M.H., Hall, C.B., et al (1988) J. Virol. 62, 1508–1512.
7. Casey, D.F.N. Engl. J. Med. 1978:298:516.
8. Berkowitz, C.D. J. Pediatrics. 1979:95:144

Rev. 1/97
MG#9040 (04)

FOREST PHARMACEUTICALS, INC.
Subsidiary of Forest Laboratories, Inc.
St. Louis, MO 63045

Shown in Product Identification Guide, page 310

INFASURF® for Neonatal RDS ℞

[in' 'fă-surf]
(calfactant)
Intratracheal Suspension
Sterile Suspension for Intratracheal Use Only

Rx only

DESCRIPTION

Infasurf® (calfactant) Intratracheal Suspension is a sterile, non-pyrogenic lung surfactant intended for intratracheal instillation only. It is an extract of natural surfactant from calf lungs which includes phospholipids, neutral lipids, and hydrophobic surfactant-associated proteins B and C (SP-B and SP-C). It contains no preservatives.

Infasurf is an off-white suspension of calfactant in 0.9% aqueous sodium chloride solution. It has a pH of 5.0 – 6.0. Each milliliter of Infasurf contains 35 mg total phospholipids (including 26 mg phosphatidylcholine of which 16 mg is disaturated phosphatidylcholine) and 0.65 mg proteins including 0.26 mg of SP-B.

CLINICAL PHARMACOLOGY

Endogenous lung surfactant is essential for effective ventilation because it modifies alveolar surface tension thereby stabilizing the alveoli. Lung surfactant deficiency is the cause of Respiratory Distress Syndrome (RDS) in premature infants. Infasurf restores surface activity to the lungs of these infants.

Activity: Infasurf adsorbs rapidly to the surface of the air-liquid interface and modifies surface tension similarly to natural lung surfactant. A minimum surface tension of ≤ 3 mN/m is produced *in vitro* by Infasurf as measured on a pulsating bubble surfactometer. *Ex vivo*, Infasurf restores the pressure volume mechanics and compliance of surfactant-deficient rat lungs. *In vivo*, Infasurf improves lung compliance, respiratory gas exchange, and survival in preterm lambs with profound surfactant deficiency.

Animal Metabolism: Infasurf is administered directly to the lung lumen surface, its site of action. No human studies of absorption, biotransformation or excretion of Infasurf have been performed. The administration of Infasurf with radiolabeled phospholipids into the lungs of adult rabbits results in the persistence of 50% of radioactivity in the lung alveolar lining and 25% of radioactivity in the lung tissue 24 hours later. Less than 5% of the radioactivity is found in other organs. In premature lambs with lethal surfactant deficiency, less than 30% of instilled Infasurf is present in the lung lining after 24 hours.

Clinical Studies: The efficacy of infasurf was demonstrated in two multiple-dose controlled clinical trials involving approximately 2,000 infants treated with Infasurf (approximately 100 mg phospholipid/kg) or Exosurf Neonatal®. In addition, two controlled trials on Infasurf versus Sur-

Continued on next page

Infasurf—Cont.

vanta®, and four uncontrolled trials were conducted that involved approximately 15,500 patients treated with Infasurf.

Infasurf versus Exosurf Neonatal®

Treatment Trial

A total of 1,126 infants ≤ 72 hours of age with RDS who required endotracheal intubation and had an a/A PO_2 < 0.22 were enrolled into a multiple-dose, randomized, double-blind treatment trial comparing Infasurf (3 mL/kg) and Exosurf Neonatal® (5 mL/kg). Patients were given an initial dose and one repeat dose 12 hours later if intubation was still required. The dose was instilled in two aliquots through a side-port adapter into the proximal end of the endotracheal tube. Each aliquot was given in small bursts over 20–30 inspiratory cycles. After each aliquot was instilled, the infant was positioned with either the right or the left side dependent. Results for efficacy parameters evaluated at 28 days or to discharge for all treated patients from this treatment trial are shown in Table 1.

Table 1 — Infasurf vs Exosurf Neonatal® Treatment Trial:

Efficacy Parameter	Infasurf (N=570) %	Exosurf Neonatal® (N=556) %	p-value
Incidence of air leaks[a]	11	22	≥0.001
Death due to RDS	4	4	0.95
Any death to 28 day	8	10	0.21
Any death before discharge	9	12	0.07
BPD[b]	5	6	0.41
Crossover to other surfactant[c]	4	4	1

[a] Pneumothorax and/or pulmonary interstitial emphysema.
[b] BPD is bronchopulmonary dysplasia, diagnosed by positive X-ray and oxygen dependence at 28 days.
[c] Protocol permitted use of comparator surfactant in patients who failed to respond to therapy with the initial randomized surfactant if the infant was < 96 hours of age, had received a full course of the randomized surfactant, and had an a/A PO_2 ratio < 0.10

Prophylaxis Trial

A total of 853 infants < 29 weeks gestation were enrolled into a multiple-dose, randomized, double-blind prophylaxis trial comparing Infasurf (3 mL/kg) and Exosurf Neonatal® (5 mL/kg). The initial dose was administered within 30 minutes of birth. Repeat doses were administered at 12 and 24 hours if the patient remained intubated. Each dose was administered divided in 2 equal aliquots, and given through a side port adapter into the proximal end of the endotracheal tube. Each aliquot was given in small bursts over 20–30 inspiratory cycles. After each aliquot was instilled, the infant was positioned with either the right or the left side dependent. Results for efficacy parameters evaluated to day 28 or to discharge for all treated patients from this prophylaxis trial are shown in Table 2.

Table 2 — Infasurf vs Exosurf Neonatal® Prophylaxis Trial:

Efficacy Parameter	Infasurf (N=431) %	Exosurf Neonatal® (N=422) %	p-value
Incidence of RDS	15	47	≤0.001
Incidence of air leaks[a]	10	15	0.01
Death due to RDS	2	5	≤0.01
Any death to 28 days	12	16	0.10
Any death before discharge	18	19	0.56
BPD[b]	16	17	0.60
Crossover to other surfactant[c]	0.2	3	≤0.001

[a] Pneumothorax and/or pulmonary interstitial emphysema.
[b] BPD is bronchopulmonary dysplasia, diagnosed by positive X-ray and oxygen dependence at 28 days.
[c] Protocol permitted use of comparator surfactant in patients who failed to respond to therapy with the initial randomized surfactant if the infant was < 72 hours of age, had received a full course of the randomized surfactant, and had an a/A PO_2 ratio was < 0.10

Infasurf versus Survanta®

Treatment Trial

A total of 662 infants with RDS who required endotracheal intubation and had an a/A PO_2 < 0.22 were enrolled into a multiple-dose, randomized, double-blind treatment trial comparing Infasurf (4 mL/kg of a formulation that contained 25 mg of phospholipids/mL rather than the 35 mg/mL in the marketed formulation) and Survanta® (4 mL/kg). Repeat doses were allowed ≥ 6 hours following the previous treatment (for up to three doses before 96 hours of age) if the patient required ≥ 30% oxygen. The surfactant was given through a 5 French feeding catheter inserted into the endotracheal tube. The total dose was instilled in four equal aliquots with the catheter removed between each of the instillations and mechanical ventilation resumed for 0.5 to 2 minutes. Each of the aliquots was administered with the patient in one of four different positions (prone, supine, right, and left lateral) to facilitate even distribution of the surfactant. Results for the major efficacy parameters evaluated at 28 days or to discharge (incidence of air leaks, death due to respiratory causes or to any cause, BPD, or treatment failure) for all treated patients from this treatment trial were not significantly different between Infasurf and Survanta®.

Prophylaxis Trial

A total of 457 infants ≤ 30 weeks gestation and < 1251 grams birth weight were enrolled into a multiple-dose, randomized, double-blind trial comparing Infasurf (4 mL/kg of a formulation that contained 25 mg of phospholipids/mL rather than the 35 mg/mL in the marketed formulation) and Survanta® (4 mL/kg). The initial dose was administered within 15 minutes of birth and repeat doses were allowed ≥ 6 hours following the previous treatment (for up to three doses before 96 hours of age) if the patient required ≥ 30% oxygen. The surfactant was given through a 5 French feeding catheter inserted into the endotracheal tube. The total dose was instilled in four equal aliquots with the catheter removed between each of the instillations and mechanical ventilation resumed for 0.5 to 2 minutes. Each of the aliquots was administered with the patient in one of four different positions: prone, supine, right, and left lateral.

Results for efficacy endpoints evaluated at 28 days or to discharge for all treated patients from this prophylaxis trial showed an increase in mortality from any cause at 28 days (p=0.03) and in death due to respiratory causes (p=0.005) in Infasurf-treated infants. For evaluable patients (patients who met the protocol-defined entry criteria), mortality from any cause and mortality due to respiratory causes were also higher in the Infasurf group (p=0.07 and 0.03, respectively). However, these observations have not been replicated in other adequate and well-controlled trials and their relevance to the intended population is unknown. All other efficacy outcomes (incidence of RDS, air leaks, BPD, and treatment failure) were not significantly different between Infasurf and Survanta® when analyzed for all treated patients and for evaluable patients.

Acute Clinical Effects: As with other surfactants, marked improvements in oxygenation and lung compliance may occur shortly after the administration of Infasurf. All controlled clinical trials with Infasurf demonstrated significant improvements in fraction of inspired oxygen (F_iO_2) and mean airway pressure (MAP) during the first 24 to 48 hours following initiation of Infasurf therapy.

INDICATIONS AND USAGE

Infasurf is indicated for the prevention of Respiratory Distress Syndrome (RDS) in premature infants at high risk for RDS and for the treatment ("rescue") of premature infants who develop RDS. Infasurf decreases the incidence of RDS, mortality due to RDS, and air leaks associated with RDS.

Prophylaxis

Prophylaxis therapy at birth with Infasurf is indicated for premature infants < 29 weeks of gestational age at significant risk for RDS. Infasurf prophylaxis should be administered as soon as possible, preferably within 30 minutes after birth.

Treatment

Infasurf therapy is indicated for infants ≤ 72 hours of age with RDS (confirmed by clinical and radiologic findings) and requiring endotracheal intubation.

WARNINGS

Infasurf is intended for intratracheal use only.
THE ADMINISTRATION OF EXOGENOUS SURFACTANTS, INCLUDING INFASURF, OFTEN RAPIDLY IMPROVES OXYGENATION AND LUNG COMPLIANCE. Following administration of Infasurf, patients should be carefully monitored so that oxygen therapy and ventilatory support can be modified in response to changes in respiratory status.
Infasurf therapy is not a substitute for neonatal intensive care. Optimal care of premature infants at risk for RDS and newborn infants with RDS who need endotracheal intubation requires an acute care unit organized, staffed, equipped, and experienced with intubation, ventilator management, and general care of these patients.
TRANSIENT EPISODES OF REFLUX OF INFASURF INTO THE ENDOTRACHEAL TUBE, CYANOSIS, BRADYCARDIA, OR AIRWAY OBSTRUCTION HAVE OCCURRED DURING THE DOSING PROCEDURES. These events require stopping Infasurf administration and taking appropriate measures to alleviate the condition. After the patient is stable, dosing can proceed with appropriate monitoring.

PRECAUTIONS

When repeat dosing was given at fixed 12-hour intervals in the Infasurf vs. Exosurf Neonatal® trials, transient episodes of cyanosis, bradycardia, reflux of surfactant into the endotracheal tube, and airway obstruction were observed more frequently among infants in the Infasurf-treated group.
An increased proportion of patients with both intraventricular hemorrhage (IVH) and periventricular leukomalacia (PVL) was observed in Infasurf-treated infants in the Infasurf-Exosurf Neonatal® controlled trials. These observations were not associated with increased mortality.
No data are available on the use of Infasurf in conjunction with experimental therapies of RDS, e.g., high-frequency ventilation.
Data from controlled trials on the efficacy of Infasurf are limited to doses of approximately 100 mg phospholipid/kg body weight and up to a total of 4 doses.

Carcinogenesis, Mutagenesis, Impairment of Fertility
Carcinogenesis studies and animal reproduction studies have not been performed with Infasurf. A single mutagenicity study (Ames assay) was negative.

ADVERSE REACTIONS

The most common adverse reactions associated with Infasurf dosing procedures in the controlled trials were: cyanosis (65%), airway obstruction (39%), bradycardia (34%), reflux of surfactant into the endotracheal tube (21%), requirement for manual ventilation (16%), and reintubation (3%). These events were generally transient and not associated with serious complications or death.
The incidence of common complications of prematurity and RDS in the four controlled Infasurf trials are presented in Table 3. Prophylaxis and treatment study results for each surfactant are combined.
[See table below]

Follow-up Evaluations
Two year follow-up data of neurodevelopmental outcomes in 415 infants enrolled in 5 centers that participated in the Infasurf vs. Exosurf Neonatal® controlled trials demonstrated significant developmental delays in equal percentages of Infasurf and Exosurf Neonatal® patients.

OVERDOSAGE

There have been no reports of overdosage with Infasurf. While there are no known adverse effects of excess lung sur-

Table 3 — Common Complications of Prematurity and RDS in Controlled Trials:

Complication	Infasurf (N=1001) %	Exosurf Neonatal® (N=978) %	Infasurf (N=553) %	Survanta® (N=566) %
Apnea	61	61	76	76
Patient ductus arteriosus	47	48	45	48
Intracranial hemorrhage	29	31	36	36
Severe intracranial hemorrhage[a]	12	10	9	7
IVH and PVL[b]	7	3	5	5
Sepsis	20	22	28	27
Pulmonary air leaks	12	22	15	15
Pulmonary interstitial emphysema	7	17	10	10
Pulmonary hemorrhage	7	7	7	6
Necrotizing enterocolitis	5	5	17	18

[a] Grade III and IV by the method of Papile.
[b] Combined incidence of intraventricular hemorrhage and periventricular leukomalacia.

factant, overdosage would result in overloading the lungs with an isotonic solution. Ventilation should be supported until clearance of the liquid is accomplished.

DOSAGE AND ADMINISTRATION

FOR INTRATRACHEAL ADMINISTRATION ONLY

Infasurf should be administered under the supervision of clinicians experienced in the acute care of newborn infants with respiratory failure who require intubation.

Rapid and substantial increases in blood oxygenation and improved lung compliance often follow Infasurf instillation. Close clinical monitoring and surveillance following administration may be needed to adjust oxygen therapy and ventilator pressures appropriately.

Dosage

Each dose of Infasurf is 3 mL/kg body weight at birth. Infasurf has been administered every 12 hours for a total of up to 3 doses.

Directions for Use

Infasurf is a suspension which settles during storage. Gentle swirling or agitation of the vial is often necessary for redispersion. DO NOT SHAKE. Visible flecks in the suspension and foaming at the surface are normal for Infasurf.

Infasurf should be stored at refrigerated temperature 2°–8°C (36° to 46°F). Warning of Infasurf before administration is not necessary.

Unopened, unused vials of Infasurf that have warmed to room temperature can be returned to refrigerated storage within 24 hours for future use. Repeated warming to room temperature should be avoided. Each single-use vial should be entered only once and the vial with any unused material should be discarded after the initial entry.

INFASURF DOES NOT REQUIRE RECONSTITUTION. DO NOT DILUTE OR SONICATE.

Dosing Procedures

General

Infasurf should only be administered intratracheally through an endotracheal tube. The dose of Infasurf is 3 mL/kg birth weight. The dose is drawn into a syringe from the single-use vial using a 20-gauge or larger needle with care taken to avoid excessive foaming. Administration is made by instillation of the Infasurf suspension into the endotracheal tube.

Administration for Treatment of RDS

Initial Dose

Infasurf should be administered intratracheally through a side-port adapter into the endotracheal tube. Two attendants, one to instill the Infasurf, the other to monitor the patient and assist in positioning, facilitate the dosing. The dose (3 mL/kg) sould be administered in two aliquots of 1.5 mL/kg each. After each aliquot is instilled, the infant should be positioned with either the right or the left side dependent. Administration is made while ventilation is continued over 20–30 breaths for each aliquot, with small bursts timed only during the inspiratory cycles. A pause followed by evaluation of the respiratory status and repositioning should separate the two aliquots.

Repeat Doses

Repeat doses of 3 mL/kg of birth weight, up to a total of 3 doses 12 hours apart, have been given in the Infasurf controlled clinical trials if the patient was still intubated.

In the Infasurf versus Survanta® trials, Infasurf was administered through a 5 French feeding catheter inserted into the endotracheal tube. The total dose was instilled in four equal aliquots with the catheter removed between each of the instillations and mechanical ventilation resumed for 0.5 to 2 minutes. Each of the aliquots was administered with the patient in one of four different positions (prone, supine, right, and left lateral) to facilitate even distribution of the surfactant. Repeat doses were administered as early as 6 hours after the previous dose for a total of up to 4 doses if the infant was still intubated and required at least 30% inspired oxygen to maintain a $P_aO_2 \leq 80$ torr.

Administration for Prophylaxis of RDS at Birth

The amount of a prophylaxis dose of Infasurf should be based on the infant's birth weight. Administration of Infasurf should be given as soon as possible after birth. Usually the immediate care and stabilization of the premature infant born with hypoxemia and/or bradycardia should precede Infasurf prophylaxis.

The dosing procedures are described under Administration for Treatment of RDS.

Dosing Precautions

During administration of Infasurf liquid suspension into the airway, infants often experience bradycardia, reflux of Infasurf into the endotracheal tube, airway obstruction, cyanosis, dislodgement of the endotracheal tube, or hypoventilation. If any of these events occur, the administration should be interrupted and the infant's condition should be stabilized using appropriate interventions before the administration of Infasurf is resumed. Endotracheal suctioning or reintubation is sometimes needed when there are signs of airway obstruction during the administration of the surfactant.

HOW SUPPLIED

Infasurf (calfactant) Intratracheal Suspension is supplied sterile in single-use, rubber-stoppered glass vials containing 6 mL off-white suspension (NDC 0456-4600-06).

Store Infasurf (calfactant) Intratracheal Suspension at refrigerated temperature 2° to 8°C (36° to 46°F) and protect from light. Vials are for single use only. After opening, discard unused drug.

Manufactured for:
FOREST PHARMACEUTICALS, INC.
Subsidiary of Forest Laboratories, Inc.
St. Louis, MO 63045
Manufactured by:
ONY, Inc.
Amherst, NY 14228
RMC 235 Rev. 07/98

Shown in Product Identification Guide, page 310

LEVOTHROID® Tablets ℞

[*lēv 'o-throid "*]
(levothyroxine sodium tablets, USP)

Dist. by
FOREST PHARMACEUTICALS, INC.
A Subsidiary of Forest Laboratories, Inc.
St. Louis, MO 63045

DESCRIPTION

LEVOTHROID TABLETS (levothyroxine sodium tablets, USP) provide crystalline sodium levothyroxine (T_4), a potent thyroid hormone, in twelve different strengths to permit easy, convenient dosage adjustment.

The structural formula for sodium levothyroxine as contained in Levothroid Tablets is:

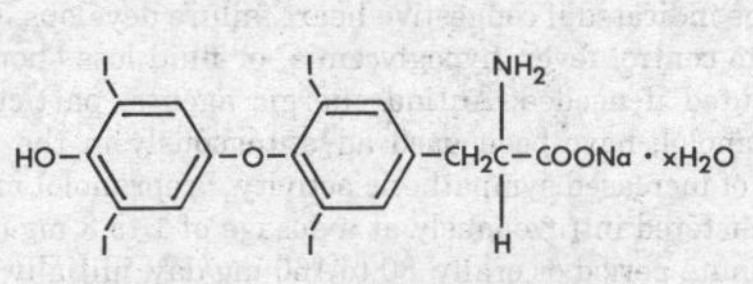

Sodium L-3, 3′, 5, 5′-tetraiodothyronine

CLINICAL PHARMACOLOGY

The major thyroid hormones are L-thyroxine (T_4) and L-triiodothyronine (T_3). The amounts of T_4 and T_3 released into the circulation from the normally functioning thyroid gland are regulated by the amount of thyrotropin (TSH) secreted from the anterior pituitary gland. TSH secretion is in turn regulated by the levels of circulating T_4 and T_3 and by secretion of thyrotropin releasing factor (TRH) from the hypothalamus. Recognition of this complex feedback system is important in the diagnosis and treatment of thyroid dysfunction.

The principal effect of exogenous thyroid hormone is to increase the metabolic rate of body tissues.

The thyroid hormones are also concerned with growth and differentiation of tissues. In deficiency states in the young there is retardation of growth and failure of maturation of the skeletal and other body systems, especially in failure of ossification in the epiphyses and in the growth and development of the brain.

The precise mechanism of action by which thyroid hormones affect thermogenesis and cellular growth and differentiation is not known. It is recognized that these physiologic effects are mediated at the cellular level primarily by T_3, a large part of which is derived from T_4 by deiodination in the peripheral tissues. Thyroxine (T_4) is the major component of normal secretions of the thyroid gland and is thus the primary determinant of normal thyroid function.

Depending on other factors, absorption has varied from 48 to 79 percent of the administered dose. Fasting increases absorption. Malabsorption syndromes, as well as dietary factors, (children's soybean formula, concomitant use of anionic exchange resins such as cholestyramine) cause excessive fecal loss.

More than 99 percent of circulating hormones are bound to serum proteins, including thyroid-binding globulin (TBg), thyroid-binding prealbumin (TBPA), and albumin (TBa), whose capacities and affinities vary for the hormones. L-thyroxine displays greater binding affinity than L-triiodothyronine, both in the circulation and at the cellular level, which explains its longer duration of action. The half-life of T_4 in normal plasma is 6–7 days while that of T_3 is about 1 day. The plasma half-lives of T_4 and T_3 are decreased in hyperthyroidism and increased in hypothyroidism.

INDICATIONS AND USAGE

Levothroid Tablets (levothyroxine sodium tablets, USP) are indicated as replacement or substitution therapy for diminished or absent thyroid function (e.g., cretinism, myxedema, non-toxic goiter or hypothyroidism generally, including the hypothyroid state in children, in pregnancy and in the elderly) resulting from functional deficiency, primary atrophy, from partial or complete absence of the gland or from the effects of surgery, radiation or antithyroid agents. Therapy must be maintained continuously to control the symptoms of hypothyroidism.

It may also be used to suppress the secretion of thyrotropin (TSH), action which may be beneficial in simple nonendemic goiter and in chronic lymphocytic thyroiditis. This may cause a reduction in the goiter size.

Thyroid hormone drugs are indicated as a diagnostic agent in suppression tests to differentiate suspected mild hyperthyroidism or thyroid gland autonomy.

Thyroid hormones may also be used with antithyroid drugs to treat thyrotoxicosis. This combination has been used to prevent goitrogenesis and hypothyroidism.

CONTRAINDICATIONS

Levothroid Tablets administration is contraindicated in untreated thyrotoxicosis and in acute myocardial infarction. Levothroid Tablets are contraindicated in the presence of uncorrected adrenal insufficiency because it increases the tissue demands for adrenocortical hormones and may cause an acute adrenal crisis in such patients. (See PRECAUTIONS).

WARNINGS

> Drugs with thyroid hormone activity, alone or together with other therapeutic agents, have been used for the treatment of obesity. In euthyroid patients, doses within the range of daily hormonal requirements are ineffective for weight reduction. Larger doses may produce serious or even life-threatening manifestations of toxicity, particularly when given in association with sympathomimetic amines such as those used for their anorectic effects.

The use of thyroid hormones in the therapy of obesity, alone or combined with other drugs, is unjustified and has been shown to be ineffective. Neither is their use justified for the treatment of male or female infertility unless this condition is accompanied by hypothyroidism.

PRECAUTIONS

GENERAL—Levothroid Tablets should be used with caution in patients with cardiovascular disease, including hypertension. The development of chest pain or other aggravation of cardiovascular disease will require a decrease in dosage.

Thyroid hormone therapy in patients with concomitant diabetes mellitus or diabetes insipidus or adrenal cortical insufficiency aggravates the intensity of their symptoms. Appropriate adjustments of the various therapeutic measures directed at these concomitant endocrine diseases are required. The therapy of myxedema coma requires simultaneous administration of glucocorticoids. (See DOSAGE AND ADMINISTRATION).

In infants, excessive doses of thyroid hormone preparations may produce craniosynostosis.

INFORMATION FOR THE PATIENT—Patients on thyroid preparations and parents of children on thyroid therapy should be informed that:

1. Replacement therapy is to be taken essentially for life, with the exception of cases of transient hypothyroidism, usually associated with thyroiditis, and in those patients receiving a therapeutic trial of the drug.
2. They should immediately report during the course of therapy any signs or symptoms of thyroid hormone toxicity, e.g., chest pain, increased pulse rate, palpitations, excessive sweating, heat intolerance, nervousness, or any other unusual event.
3. In case of concomitant diabetes mellitus, the daily dosage of antidiabetic medication may need readjustment as thyroid hormone replacement is achieved. If thyroid medication is stopped, a downward readjustment of the dosage of insulin or oral hypoglycemic agent may be necessary to avoid hypoglycemia. At all times, close monitoring of urinary glucose levels is mandatory in such patients.
4. In case of concomitant oral anticoagulant therapy, the prothrombin time should be measured frequently to determine if the dosage of oral anticoagulants is to be readjusted.
5. Partial loss of hair may be experienced by children in the first few months of thyroid therapy, but this is usually a transient phenomenon and later recovery is usually the rule.

LABORATORY TESTS—The patient's response to thyroid replacement may be followed by laboratory tests such as serum thyroxine (T_4), serum triiodothyronine (T_3), free thyroxine index and thyroid stimulating hormone (TSH) blood levels.

DRUG INTERACTIONS—In patients with diabetes mellitus, addition of thyroid hormone therapy may cause an increase in the required dosage of insulin or oral hypoglycemic agents. Conversely, decreasing the dose of thyroid hormone

Continued on next page

Levothroid—Cont.

may possibly cause hypoglycemic reactions if the dosage of insulin or oral hypoglycemic agents is not adjusted.

Thyroid replacement may potentiate anticoagulant effects with agents such as warfarin or bishydroxycoumarin and reduction of one-third in anticoagulant dosage should be undertaken upon initiation of Levothroid Tablets therapy. Subsequent anticoagulant dosage adjustment should be made on the basis of frequent prothrombin determinations.

Injection of epinephrine in patients with coronary artery disease may precipitate an episode of coronary insufficiency. This may be enhanced in patients receiving thyroid preparations. Careful observation is required if catecholamines are administered to patients in this category.

Cholestyramine or colestipol binds both T_4 and T_3 in the intestine, thus impairing absorption of these thyroid hormones. *In vitro* studies indicate that the binding is not easily removed. Therefore, four to five hours should elapse between administration of cholestyramine or colestipol and thyroid hormones.

Estrogens tend to increase serum thyroxine-binding globulin (TBg). In a patient with a non-functioning thyroid gland who is receiving thyroid replacement therapy, free levothyroxine may be decreased when estrogens are started thus increasing thyroid requirements. However, if the patient's thyroid gland has sufficient function the decreased free thyroxine will result in a compensatory increase in thyroxine output by the thyroid. Therefore, patients without a functioning thyroid gland who are on thyroid replacement therapy may need to increase their thyroid dose if estrogens or estrogen-containing oral contraceptives are given.

DRUG/LABORATORY TEST INTERACTIONS—The following drugs or moieties are known to interfere with laboratory tests performed in patients on thyroid hormone therapy: androgens, corticosteroids, estrogens, oral contraceptives containing estrogens, iodine-containing preparations, and the numerous preparations containing salicylates.

1. Changes in TBg concentration should be taken into consideration in the interpretation of T_4 and T_3 values. In such cases, the unbound (free) hormone should be measured. Pregnancy, estrogens, and estrogen-containing oral contraceptives increase TBg concentrations. TBg may also be increased during infectious hepatitis. Decreases in TBg concentrations are observed in nephrosis, acromegaly, and after androgen or corticosteroid therapy. Familial hyper- or hypothyroxine-binding-globulinemias have been described. The incidence of TBg deficiency approximates 1 in 9000. The binding of thyroxine by thyroid-binding prealbumin (TBPA) is inhibited by salicylates.

2. Medical or dietary iodine interferes with all *in vivo* tests of radioiodine uptake, producing low uptakes which may not be reflective of a true decrease in hormone synthesis.

3. The persistence of clinical and laboratory evidence of hypothyroidism in spite of adequate dosage replacement indicates either poor patient compliance, poor absorption, excessive fecal loss, or inactivity of the preparation. Intracellular resistance to thyroid hormone is quite rare.

CARCINOGENESIS, MUTAGENESIS, AND IMPAIRMENT OF FERTILITY—A reportedly apparent association between prolonged thyroid therapy and breast cancer has not been confirmed and patients on thyroid for established indications should not discontinue therapy. No confirmatory long-term studies in animals have been performed to evaluate carcinogenic potential, mutagenicity, or impairment of fertility in either males or females.

PREGNANCY-CATEGORY A—Thyroid hormones do not readily cross the placental barrier. The clinical experience to date does not indicate any adverse effect on fetuses when thyroid hormones are administered to pregnant women. On the basis of current knowledge, thyroid replacement therapy to hypothyroid women should not be discontinued during pregnancy.

NURSING MOTHERS—Minimal amounts of thyroid hormones are excreted in human milk. Thyroid is not associated with serious adverse reactions and does not have a known tumorigenic potential. However, caution should be exercised when thyroid is administered to a nursing woman.

PEDIATRIC USE—The diagnosis and institution of therapy for cretinism should be done as soon after birth as feasible to prevent developmental deficiency. Screening tests for serum T_4 and TSH will identify this group of newborn patients.

ADVERSE REACTIONS

Patients who are sensitive to lactose may show intolerance to Levothroid Tablets since this substance is used in the manufacture of the product.

Adverse reactions other than those indicative of hyperthyroidism because of therapeutic overdosage, either initially or during the maintenance period, are rare. (See OVERDOSAGE).

OVERDOSAGE

Excessive dosage of thyroid medication may result in symptoms of hyperthyroidism. Since, however, the effects do not appear at once the symptoms may not appear for one to three weeks after the dosage regimen is begun. The most common signs and symptoms of overdosage are weight loss, palpitation, nervousness, diarrhea or abdominal cramps, sweating, tachycardia, cardiac arrhythmias, angina pectoris, tremors, headache, insomnia, intolerance to heat and fever. If symptoms of overdosage appear, discontinue medication for several days and reinstitute treatment at a lower dosage level.

Laboratory tests such as serum T_4, and serum T_3 and the free thyroxine index will be elevated during the period of overdosage.

Complications as a result of the induced hypermetabolic state may include cardiac failure and death due to arrhythmia or failure.

TREATMENT OF OVERDOSAGE—Dosage should be reduced or therapy temporarily discontinued if signs and symptoms of overdosage appear. Treatment may be reinstituted at a lower dosage. In normal individuals, normal hypothalamic-pituitary-thyroid axis function is restored in 6 to 8 weeks after thyroid suppression.

Treatment of acute massive thyroid hormone overdosage is aimed at reducing gastrointestinal absorption of the drugs and counteracting central and peripheral effects, mainly those of increased sympathetic activity. Vomiting may be induced initially if further gastrointestinal absorption can reasonably be prevented and barring contraindications such as coma, convulsions, or loss of the gagging reflex. Treatment is symptomatic and supportive. Oxygen may be administered and ventilation maintained. Cardiac glycosides may be indicated if congestive heart failure develops. Measures to control fever, hypoglycemia, or fluid loss should be instituted if needed. Antiadrenergic agents, particularly propranolol, have been used advantageously in the treatment of increased sympathetic activity. Propranolol may be administered intravenously at a dosage of 1 to 3 mg over a 10-minute period or orally, 80 to 160 mg/day, initially, especially when no contraindications exist for its use. Other adjunctive measures may include administration of cholestyramine to interfere with thyroxine absorption, and glucocorticoids to inhibit conversion of T_4 to T_3.

DOSAGE AND ADMINISTRATION

The goal of therapy should be the restoration of euthyroidism as judged by clinical response and confirmed by appropriate laboratory values. In adults with no complicating endocrine or cardiovascular disease, the predicted full maintenance dose may be achieved immediately with adjustments made as indicated by clinical evaluation. The usual maintenance dose of Levothroid Tablets is 100 to 200 mcg.

In patients with known complications or in case of doubt, individual dose titration at 2- to 4-week intervals is recommended. The usual starting dose is 50 mcg with increases of 50 mcg at 2- to 4-week intervals until the patient is euthyroid or symptoms ensue which preclude further dose increase.

In adult myxedema or hypothyroid patients with angina, the starting dose should be 25 mcg with increases at 2- to 4-week intervals of 25 to 50 mcg as determined by clinical response.

Myxedema coma is usually precipitated in the hypothyroid patient of long-standing by intercurrent illness or drugs such as sedatives and anesthetics and should be considered a medical emergency. Therapy should be directed at the correction of electrolyte disturbances and possible infection besides the administration of thyroid hormones. Corticosteroids should be administered routinely. T_4 and T_3 may be administered via a nasogastric tube, but the preferred route of administration of both hormones is intravenous. Sodium levothyroxine (T_4) is given at a starting dose of 200–500 mcg (100 mcg/mL given rapidly), and is usually well tolerated, even in the elderly. This initial dose is followed by daily supplements of 100 to 200 mcg given IV. Normal T_4 levels are achieved in 24 hours followed in 3 days by threefold increase of T_3. Oral therapy with Levothroid Tablets should be resumed as soon as the clinical situation has been stabilized and the patient is able to take oral medication.

Pediatric dosage should follow the recommendations summarized in Table I. In infants with congenital hypothyroidism, therapy with full doses should be instituted as soon as the diagnosis has been made. Levothroid Tablets may be given to infants and children who cannot swallow intact tablets by crushing the proper dose tablet and suspending the **freshly crushed** tablet in a small amount of water or formula. The suspension can be given by spoon or dropper. DO NOT STORE THE SUSPENSION FOR ANY PERIOD OF TIME. The crushed tablet may also be sprinkled over a small amount of food, such as cooked cereal or apple sauce.

TABLE I
Recommended Pediatric Dosage For Congenital Hypothyroidism*

LEVOTHROID TABLETS
(levothyroxine sodium tablets, USP)

Age	Dose per day	Daily dose per kg of body weight
0–6 mos	25–50 mcg	8–10 mcg
6–12 mos	50–75 mcg	6–8 mcg
1–5 yrs	75–100 mcg	5–6 mcg
6–12 yrs	100–150 mcg	4–5 mcg

* To be adjusted on the basis of clinical response and laboratory tests (See **Laboratory Tests**).

HOW SUPPLIED

Strength	Package Size	NDC Number
25 mcg	bottle of 100	0456-0320-01
50 mcg	bottle of 100	0456-0321-01
50 mcg	bottle of 1000	0456-0321-00
50 mcg	bottle of 5000	0456-0321-51
50 mcg	unit dose carton of 100	0456-0321-63
75 mcg	bottle of 100	0456-0322-01
88 mcg	bottle of 100	0456-0329-01
100 mcg	bottle of 100	0456-0323-01
100 mcg	bottle of 1000	0456-0323-00
100 mcg	bottle of 5000	0456-0323-51
100 mcg	unit dose carton of 100	0456-0323-63
112 mcg	bottle of 100	0456-0330-01
125 mcg	bottle of 100	0456-0324-01
125 mcg	unit dose carton of 100	0456-0324-63
137 mcg	bottle of 100	0456-0331-01
150 mcg	bottle of 100	0456-0325-01
150 mcg	bottle of 1000	0456-0325-00
150 mcg	bottle of 5000	0456-0325-51
150 mcg	unit dose carton of 100	0456-0325-63
175 mcg	bottle of 100	0456-0326-01
200 mcg	bottle of 100	0456-0327-01
200 mcg	bottle of 1000	0456-0327-00
200 mcg	bottle of 5000	0456-0327-51
200 mcg	unit dose carton of 100	0456-0327-63
300 mcg	bottle of 100	0456-0328-01
300 mcg	unit dose carton of 100	0456-0328-63

Strength	Tablet Color	Markings
25 mcg	Orange	25
50 mcg	White	50
75 mcg	Grey	75
88 mcg	Mint Green	88
100 mcg	Yellow	100
112 mcg	Rose	112
125 mcg	Purple	125
137 mcg	Blue	137
150 mcg	Light Blue	150
175 mcg	Turquoise	175
200 mcg	Pink	200
300 mcg	Lime Green	300

Tablets should be stored at controlled room temperature, 59°–86°F (15°–30°C) in capped bottles or unbroken plastic strip packing.

CAUTION: Federal law prohibits dispensing without prescription.

Rev. 1/96 03690196

Shown in Product Identification Guide, page 310

LORCET®-HD Ⓒ℞

[*lōr-sét h d*]

DESCRIPTION

Each Lorcet-HD capsule contains 5 mg Hydrocodone* Bitartrate *(WARNING: May be habit forming) and 500 mg Acetaminophen.

HOW SUPPLIED

Lorcet-HD capsules are opaque maroon capsules imprinted with the UAD logo; 1120 and are supplied in bottles of 100 capsules. Each capsule contains Hydrocodone* Bitartrate, 5mg *(WARNING: May Be Habit Forming) and Acetaminophen (APAP), 500 mg. NDC# 0785-1120-01.

Mfd. by:
Mallinckrodt
Hobart, NY 13788

Mfd. for:
UAD Laboratories
Division of
Forest Pharmaceuticals, Inc.
St. Louis, MO 63045

LORCET® PLUS Ⓒ ℞
[lōr-sét plus]
**Hydrocodone Bitartrate and
Acetaminophen Tablets USP
7.5 mg/650 mg**

DESCRIPTION
Each Lorcet Plus tablet contains:
Hydrocodone* Bitartrate .... 7.5 mg
       *(WARNING: May be habit forming)
Acetaminophen .... 650 mg

HOW SUPPLIED
Lorcet Plus, Hydrocodone Bitartrate and Acetaminophen Tablets USP, each tablet of which contains hydrocodone* bitartrate 7.5 mg *(WARNING: May be habit forming) and acetaminophen 650 mg, are white, capsule-shaped, scored tablets, debossed "U" on one side and "201" on the other side, and are supplied in containers of 100 tablets, NDC #0785-1122-01, containers of 500 tablets, NDC #0785-1122-50, and in unit-dose cartons of 100 tablets (4 cards of 25 tablets per card), NDC #0785-1122-63.

Shown in Product Identification Guide, page 310

LORCET® 10/650 Ⓒ ℞
[lōr sēt]
**HYDROCODONE* BITARTRATE
AND ACETAMINOPHEN TABLETS USP
10 mg/650 mg**

DESCRIPTION
Hydrocodone bitartrate and acetaminophen is supplied in tablet form for oral administration.

Hydrocodone bitartrate is an opioid analgesic and antitussive and occurs as fine, white crystals or as a crystalline powder. It is affected by light. The chemical name is: 4, 5α-epoxy-3-methoxy-17-methylmorphinan-6-one tartrate (1:1) hydrate (2:5). It has the following structural formula:

$C_{18}H_{21}NO_3 \cdot C_4H_6O_6 \cdot 2^1/_2\ H_2O$ M.W. 494.50

Acetaminophen, 4'-hydroxyacetanilide, a slightly bitter, white, odorless, crystalline powder, is a nonopiate, non-salicylate analgesic and antipyretic. It has the following structural formula:

$C_8H_9NO_2$ M.W. 151.17

Each Lorcet 10/650 tablet contains:
   Hydrocodone
   Bitartrate .... 10 mg
*(WARNING: May be habit forming)
   Acetaminophen .... 650 mg
In addition, each tablet contains the following inactive ingredients: colloidal silicon dioxide, croscarmellose sodium, crospovidone, microcrystalline cellulose, povidone, pregelatinized starch, stearic acid and FD&C Blue #1 Lake.

HOW SUPPLIED
Lorcet 10/650, Hydrocodone* Bitartrate and Acetaminophen Tablets, each tablet of which contains hydrocodone* bitartrate 10 mg *(WARNING: May be habit forming) and acetaminophen 650 mg, are light-blue, capsule-shaped, scored tablets, debossed "UAD" on one side and "63 50" on the other side, and are supplied in containers of 100 tablets, NDC 0785-6350-01 and in containers of 500 tablets, NDC 0785-6350-50, and in containers of unit dose (4 × 25's), NDC 0785-6350-63.

Shown in Product Identification Guide, page 310

MONUROL® ℞
[mon ' ur ol]
**(fosfomycin tromethamine)
SACHET**

DESCRIPTION
MONUROL (fosfomycin tromethamine) sachet contains fosfomycin tromethamine, a synthetic, broad-spectrum, bactericidal antibiotic for oral administration. It is available as a single-dose sachet which contains white granules consisting of 5.631 grams of fosfomycin tromethamine (equivalent to 3 grams of fosfomycin), and the following inactive ingredients: mandarin flavor, orange flavor, saccharin, and sucrose. The contents of the sachet must be dissolved in water. Fosfomycin tromethamine, a phosphonic acid derivative, is available as (1R, 2S)-(1,2-epoxypropyl)phosphonic acid, compound with 2-amino-2-(hydroxymethyl)-1,3-propanediol (1:1). It is a white granular compound with a molecular weight of 259.2. Its empirical formula is $C_3H_7O_4P \bullet C_4H_{11}NO_3$, and its chemical structure is as follows:

CLINICAL PHARMACOLOGY
Absorption: Fosfomycin tromethamine is rapidly absorbed following oral administration and converted to the free acid, fosfomycin. Absolute oral bioavailability under fasting conditions is 37%. After a single 3-gm dose of MONUROL, the mean ($\pm$ 1 SD) maximum serum concentration (C_{max}) achieved was 26.1 ($\pm$ 9.1) µg/mL within 2 hours. The oral bioavailability of fosfomycin is reduced to 30% under fed conditions. Following a single 3-gm oral dose of MONUROL with a high-fat meal, the mean C_{max} achieved was 17.6 ($\pm$ 4.4) µg/mL within 4 hours.

Cimetidine does not affect the pharmacokinetics of fosfomycin when coadministered with MONUROL. Metoclopramide lowers the serum concentrations and urinary excretion of fosfomycin when coadministered with MONUROL. (See **PRECAUTIONS, Drug Interactions**.)

Distribution: The mean apparent steady-state volume of distribution (V_{ss}) is 136.1 ($\pm$ 44.1) L following oral administration of MONUROL. Fosfomycin is not bound to plasma proteins.

Fosfomycin is distributed to the kidneys, bladder wall, prostate, and seminal vesicles. Following a 50 mg/kg dose of fosfomycin to patients undergoing urological surgery for bladder carcinoma, the mean concentration of fosfomycin in the bladder, taken at a distance from the neoplastic site, was 18.0 µg per gram of tissue at 3 hours after dosing. Fosfomycin has been shown to cross the placental barrier in animals and man.

Excretion: Fosfomycin is excreted unchanged in both urine and feces. Following oral administration of MONUROL, the mean total body clearance (CL_{TB}) and mean renal clearance (CL_R) of fosfomycin were 16.9 ($\pm$ 3.5) L/hr and 6.3 ($\pm$ 1.7) L/hr, respectively. Approximately 38% of a 3-gm dose of MONUROL is recovered from urine, and 18% is recovered from feces. Following intravenous administration, the mean CL_{TB} and mean CL_R of fosfomycin were 6.1 ($\pm$ 1.0) L/hr and 5.5 ($\pm$ 1.2) L/hr, respectively.

A mean urine fosfomycin concentration of 706 ($\pm$ 466) µg/mL was attained within 2–4 hours after a single oral 3-gm dose of MONUROL under fasting conditions. The mean urinary concentration of fosfomycin was 10 µg/mL in samples collected 72–84 hours following a single oral dose of MONUROL.

Following a 3-gm dose of MONUROL administered with a high-fat meal, a mean urine fosfomycin concentration of 537 ($\pm$ 252) µg/mL was attained within 6–8 hours. Although the rate of urinary excretion of fosfomycin was reduced under fed conditions, the cumulative amount of fosfomycin excreted in the urine was the same, 1118 ($\pm$ 201) mg (fed) vs. 1140 ($\pm$ 238) mg (fasting). Further, urinary concentrations equal to or greater than 100 µg/mL were maintained for the same duration, 26 hours, indicating that MONUROL can be taken without regard to food.

Following oral administration of MONUROL, the mean half-life for elimination ($t_{1/2}$) is 5.7 ($\pm$ 2.8) hours.

Special Populations:
Geriatric: Based on limited data regarding 24-hour urinary drug concentrations, no differences in urinary excretion of fosfomycin have been observed in elderly subjects. No dosage adjustment is necessary in the elderly.

Gender: There are no gender differences in the pharmacokinetics of fosfomycin.

Renal Insufficiency: In 5 anuric patients undergoing hemodialysis, the $t_{1/2}$ of fosfomycin during hemodialysis was 40 hours. In patients with varying degrees of renal impairment (creatinine clearances varying from 54 mL/min to 7 mL/min), the $t_{1/2}$ of fosfomycin increased from 11 hours to 50 hours. The percent of fosfomycin recovered in urine decreased from 32% to 11% indicating that renal impairment significantly decreases the excretion of fosfomycin.

Microbiology
Fosfomycin (the active component of fosfomycin tromethamine) has *in vitro* activity against a broad range of gram-positive and gram-negative aerobic microorganisms which are associated with uncomplicated urinary tract infections. Fosfomycin is bactericidal in urine at therapeutic doses. The bactericidal action of fosfomycin is due to its inactivation of the enzyme enolpyruvyl transferase, thereby irreversibly blocking the condensation of uridine diphosphate-N-acetylglucosamine with p-enolpyruvate, one of the first steps in bacterial cell wall synthesis. It also reduces adherence of bacteria to uroepithelial cells.

There is generally no cross-resistance between fosfomycin and other classes of antibacterial agents such as beta-lactams and aminoglycosides.

Fosfomycin has been shown to be active against most strains of the following microorganisms, both *in vitro* and in clinical infections as described in the **INDICATIONS AND USAGE** section:
Aerobic gram-positive microorganisms
Enterococcus faecalis
Aerobic gram-negative microorganisms
Escherichia coli
The following *in vitro* data are available, **but their clinical significance is unknown.**

Fosfomycin exhibits *in vitro* minimum inhibitory concentrations (MICs) of 64 µg/mL or less against most ($\geq$ 90%) strains of the following microorganisms; however, the safety and effectiveness of fosfomycin in treating clinical infections due to these microorganisms has not been established in adequate and well-controlled clinical trials:
Aerobic gram-positive microorganisms
Enterococcus faecium
Aerobic gram-negative microorganisms
Citrobacter diversus
Citrobacter freundii
Enterobacter aerogenes
Klebsiella oxytoca
Klebsiella pneumoniae
Proteus mirabilis
Proteus vulgaris
Serratia marcescens

SUSCEPTIBILITY TESTING
Dilution Techniques:
Quantitative methods are used to determine minimum inhibitory concentrations (MICs). These MICs provide estimates of the susceptibility of bacteria to antimicrobial compounds. One such standardized procedure uses a standardized agar dilution method[1] or equivalent with standardized inoculum concentrations and standardized concentrations of fosfomycin tromethamine (in terms of fosfomycin base content) powder supplemented with 25 µg/mL of glucose-6-phosphate. **BROTH DILUTION METHODS SHOULD NOT BE USED TO TEST SUSCEPTIBILITY TO FOSFOMYCIN.** The MIC values obtained should be interpreted according to the following criteria:

MIC (µg/mL)	Interpretation
$\leq$64	Susceptible (S)
128	Intermediate (I)
$\geq$256	Resistant (R)

A report of "susceptible" indicates that the pathogen is likely to be inhibited by usually achievable concentrations of the antimicrobial compound in the urine. A report of "intermediate" indicates that the result should be considered equivocal, and, if the microorganism is not fully susceptible to alternative, clinically feasible drugs, the test should be repeated. This category provides a buffer zone that prevents small uncontrolled technical factors from causing major discrepancies in interpretation. A report of "resistant" indicates that usually achievable concentrations of the antimicrobial compound in the urine are unlikely to be inhibitory and that other therapy should be selected.

Standardized susceptibility test procedures require the use of laboratory control microorganisms. Standard fosfomycin tromethamine powder should provide the following MIC values for agar dilution testing in media containing 25 µg/mL of glucose-6-phosphate. **[Broth dilution testing should not be performed].**

Microorganism	MIC (µg/mL)
Enterococcus faecalis ATCC 29212	32–128
Escherichia coli ATCC 25922	0.5–2
Pseudomonas aeruginosa ATCC 27853	2–8
Staphylococcus aureus ATCC 29213	0.5–4

Diffusion Techniques:
Quantitative methods that require measurement of zone diameters also provide reproducible estimates of the susceptibility of bacteria to antimicrobial agents. One such standardized procedure[2] requires the use of standardized inoculum concentrations. This procedure uses paper disks impregnated with 200-µg fosfomycin and 50-µg of glucose-6-phosphate to test the susceptibility of microorganisms to fosfomycin.

Reports from the laboratory providing results of the standard single-disk susceptibility test with disks containing

Continued on next page

Monurol—Cont.

200 µg of fosfomycin and 50 µg of glucose-6-phosphate should be interpreted according to the following criteria:

Zone Diameter (mm)	Interpretation
≥16	Susceptible (S)
13–15	Intermediate (I)
≤12	Resistant (R)

Interpretation should be stated as above for results using dilution techniques. Interpretation involves correlation of the diameter obtained in the disk test with the MIC for fosfomycin.

As with standardized dilution techniques, diffusion methods require use of laboratory control microorganisms that are used to control the technical aspects of the laboratory procedures. For the diffusion technique, the 200-µg fosfomycin disk with the 50-µg of glucose-6-phosphate should provide the following zone diameters in these laboratory quality control strains:

Microorganism	Zone Diameter (mm)
Escherichia coli ATCC 25922	22–29
Staphylococcus aureus ATCC 25923	25–33

INDICATIONS AND USAGE
MONUROL is indicated only for the treatment of uncomplicated urinary tract infections (acute cystitis) in women due to susceptible strains of *Escherichia coli* and *Enterococcus faecalis*. MONUROL is not indicated for the treatment of pyelonephritis or perinephric abscess.
If persistence or reappearance of bacteriuria occurs after treatment with MONUROL, other therapeutic agents should be selected. (See **PRECAUTIONS** and **CLINICAL STUDIES** section.)

CONTRAINDICATIONS
MONUROL is contraindicated in patients with known hypersensitivity to the drug.

PRECAUTIONS
General
Do not use more than one single dose of MONUROL to treat a single episode of acute cystitis. Repeated daily doses of MONUROL did not improve the clinical success or microbiological eradication rates compared to single dose therapy, but did increase the incidence of adverse events.
Urine specimens for culture and susceptibility testing should be obtained before and after completion of therapy.
Information for Patients
Patients should be informed:
• That MONUROL (fosfomycin tromethamine) can be taken with or without food.

• That their symptoms should improve in two to three days after taking MONUROL; if not improved, the patient should contact her health care provider.
Drug Interactions
Metoclopramide: When coadministered with MONUROL, metoclopramide, a drug which increases gastrointestinal motility, lowers the serum concentration and urinary excretion of fosfomycin. Other drugs that increase gastrointestinal motility may produce similar effects.
Cimetidine: Cimetidine does not affect the pharmacokinetics of fosfomycin when coadministered with MONUROL.
Carcinogenesis, Mutagenesis, Impairment of Fertility
Long-term carcinogenicity studies in rodents have not been conducted because MONUROL is intended for single dose treatment in humans. MONUROL was not mutagenic or genotoxic in the *in vitro* Ames' bacterial reversion test, in cultured human lymphocytes, in Chinese hamster V79 cells, and the *in vivo* mouse micronucleus assay. MONUROL did not affect fertility or reproductive performance in male and female rats.
Pregnancy: Teratogenic Effects
Pregnancy Category B
When administered intramuscularly as the sodium salt at a dose of 1 gm to pregnant women, fosfomycin crosses the placental barrier. MONUROL crosses the placental barrier of rats; it does not produce teratogenic effects in pregnant rats at dosages as high as 1000 mg/kg/day (approximately 9 and 1.4 times the human dose based on body weight and mg/m², respectively). When administered to pregnant female rabbits at dosages as high as 1000 mg/kg/day (approximately 9 and 2.7 times the human dose based on body weight and mg/m², respectively), fetotoxicities were observed. However, these toxicities were seen at maternally toxic doses and were considered to be due to the sensitivity of the rabbit to changes in the intestinal microflora resulting from the antibiotic administration. There are, however, no adequate and well-controlled studies in pregnant women. Because animal reproduction studies are not always predictive of human response, this drug should be used during pregnancy only if clearly needed.
Nursing Mothers
It is not known whether fosfomycin tromethamine is excreted in human milk. Because many drugs are excreted in human milk and because of the potential for serious adverse reactions in nursing infants from MONUROL, a decision should be made whether to discontinue nursing or not to administer the drug, taking into account the importance of the drug to the mother.
Pediatric Use
Safety and effectiveness in children age 12 years and under have not been established in adequate and well-controlled studies.

Use in the Elderly
There were no clinically significant differences in the bacteriological effectiveness or safety profiles of MONUROL for women 65 years of age or younger compared to women over 65 years of age.

ADVERSE REACTIONS
Clinical Trials:
In clinical studies, drug-related adverse events which were reported in greater than 1% of the fosfomycin-treated study population are listed below:
[See first table below]
In clinical trials, the most frequently reported adverse events occurring in > 1% of the study population regardless of drug relationship, were: diarrhea 10.4%, headache 10.3%, vaginitis 7.6%, nausea 5.2%, rhinitis 4.5%, back pain 3.0%, dysmenorrhea 2.6%, pharyngitis 2.5%, dizziness 2.3%, abdominal pain 2.2%, pain 2.2%, dyspepsia 1.8%, asthenia 1.7%, and rash 1.4%.
The following adverse events occurred in clinical trials at a rate of less than 1%, regardless of drug relationship: abnormal stools, anorexia, constipation, dry mouth, dysuria, ear disorder, fever, flatulence, flu syndrome, hematuria, infection, insomnia, lymphadenopathy, menstrual disorder, migraine, myalgia, nervousness, paresthesia, pruritus, SGPT increase, skin disorder, somnolence and vomiting.
One patient developed unilateral optic neuritis, an event considered possibly related to MONUROL therapy.
Post-marketing Experience:
Serious adverse events from the marketing experience with MONUROL outside of the United States have been rarely reported and include: angioedema, aplastic anemia, asthma (exacerbation), cholestatic jaundice, hepatic necrosis, and toxic megacolon.
Laboratory Changes:
Significant laboratory changes reported in U.S. clinical trials of MONUROL without regard to drug relationship include: increased eosinophil count, increased or decreased WBC count, increased bilirubin, increased SGPT, increased SGOT, increased alkaline phosphatase, decreased hematocrit, decreased hemoglobin, increased and decreased platelet count. The changes were generally transient and were not clinically significant.

OVERDOSAGE
In acute toxicology studies, oral administration of high doses of MONUROL up to 5 gm/kg were well-tolerated in mice and rats, produced transient and minor incidences of watery stool in rabbits, and produced diarrhea with anorexia in dogs occurring 2–3 days after single dose administration. These doses represent 50–125 times the human therapeutic dose.
There have been no reported cases of overdosage. In the event of overdosage, treatment should be symptomatic and supportive.

DOSAGE AND ADMINISTRATION
The recommended dosage for women 18 years of age and older for uncomplicated urinary tract infection (acute cystitis) is one sachet of MONUROL. MONUROL may be taken with or without food.
MONUROL should not be taken in its dry form. Always mix MONUROL with water before ingesting. (See PREPARATION section.)
PREPARATION
MONUROL should be taken orally. Pour the entire contents of a single-dose sachet of MONUROL into 3 to 4 ounces of water (¹/₂ cup) and stir to dissolve. Do not use hot water. MONUROL should be taken immediately after dissolving in water.

HOW SUPPLIED
MONUROL is available as a single-dose sachet containing the equivalent of 3 grams of fosfomycin.
NDC # 0456-4300-08
Store at controlled room temperature 15° to 30°C (59° to 86°F).
Caution: Federal law prohibits dispensing without prescription.
Keep this and all drugs out of the reach of children.
Manufactured by:
Inpharzam S.A.
Division of Zambon Group, SpA
Via Industria
6814 Cadempino, Switzerland
Made in Switzerland
Distributed by:
Forest Pharmaceuticals, Inc.
Subsidiary of Forest Laboratories, Inc.
St. Louis, MO 63045

REFERENCES
1. National Committee for Clinical Laboratory Standards, Methods for Dilution. Antimicrobial Susceptibility Tests for Bacteria that Grow Aerobically - Third Edition; Approved Standard NCCLS Document M7-A3, Vol. 13, No. 25 NCCLS, Villanova, PA, December, 1993.
2. National Committee for Clinical Laboratory Standards, Performance Standard for Antimicrobial Disk Susceptibility

Drug-Related Adverse Events (%) in Fosfomycin and Comparator Populations

Adverse Events	Fosfomcyin N = 1233	Nitrofurantoin N = 374	Trimethoprim/ sulfamethoxazole N = 428	Ciprofloxacin N = 445
Diarrhea	9.0	6.4	2.3	3.1
Vaginitis	5.5	5.3	4.7	6.3
Nausea	4.1	7.2	8.6	3.4
Headache	3.9	5.9	5.4	3.4
Dizziness	1.3	1.9	2.3	2.2
Asthenia	1.1	0.3	0.5	0.0
Dyspepsia	1.1	2.1	0.7	1.1

Treatment Arm	Treatment Duration (days)	Microbiologic Eradication Rate		Clinical Success Rate	Outcome (based on difference in microbiologic eradication rates at 5–11 days post therapy)
		5–11 days post therapy	Study day 12–21		
Fosfomycin	1	630/771 (82%)	591/771 (77%)	542/771 (70%)	
Ciprofloxacin	7	219/222 (98%)	219/222 (98%)	213/222 (96%)	Fosfomycin inferior to ciprofloxacin
Trimethoprim/ sulfamethoxazole	10	194/197 (98%)	194/197 (98%)	186/197 (94%)	Fosfomycin inferior to trimethoprim/ sulfamethoxazole
Nitrofurantoin	7	180/238 (76%)	180/238 (76%)	183/238 (77%)	Fosfomycin equivalent to nitrofurantoin

Pathogen	Fosfomycin 3 gm single dose	Ciprofloxacin 250 mg bid × 7d	Trimethoprim/ sulfamethoxazole 160 mg/800 mg bid × 10d	Nitrofurantoin 100 mg bid ×7d
E. coli	509/644 (79%)	184/187 (98%)	171/174 (98%)	146/187 (78%)
E. faecalis	10/10 (100%)	0/0	4/4 (100%)	1/2 (50%)

Tests - Fifth Edition; Approved Standard NCCLS Document M2-A5, Vol. 13, No. 24 NCCLS, Villanova, PA, December, 1993.

CLINICAL STUDIES

In controlled, double-blind studies of acute cystitis performed in the United States, a single-dose of MONUROL was compared to three other oral antibiotics (See table below). The study population consisted of patients with symptoms and signs of acute cystitis of less than 4 days duration, no manifestations of upper tract infection (e.g., flank pain, chills, fever), no history of recurrent urinary tract infections (20% of patients in the clinical studies had a prior episode of acute cystitis within the preceding year), no known structural abnormalities, and no clinical or laboratory evidence of hepatic dysfunction, and no known or suspected CNS disorders, such as epilepsy, or other factors which would predispose to seizures. In these studies, the following clinical success (resolution of symptoms) and microbiologic eradication rates were obtained:

[See table at bottom of previous page]

FOREST PHARMACEUTICALS, INC.
Subsidiary of Forest Laboratories, Inc.
St. Louis, Missouri 63045
Rev. 5/97

Shown in Product Identification Guide, page 310

SUS-PHRINE®   ℞

[sŭs 'frĭn "]
(epinephrine 5 mg/ml)
1:200
Injectable Suspension
For Subcutaneous Injection only

DESCRIPTION

Each mL of SUS-PHRINE (epinephrine) contains 5 mg epinephrine in a sterile, non-pyrogenic aqueous vehicle containing ascorbic acid 10 mg and thioglycolic acid 6.6 mg (as sodium salts) phenol 5 mg and glycerin (USP) 325 mg. Sodium hydroxide is added to adjust the pH. Approximately 80% of the total epinephrine is in suspension. SUS-PHRINE is sulfite-free.

$C_9H_{13}NO_3$ M.W. 183.21

Epinephrine is a white to off-white, odorless, microcrystalline powder or granules. It is affected by light. The chemical name is:
(R)-4-[1-hydroxy-2-(methylamino)ethyl]-1,2-benzenediol

CLINICAL PHARMACOLOGY

SUS-PHRINE (epinephrine) acts at both the alpha and beta receptor sites. Beta stimulation provides bronchodilator action by relaxing bronchial muscle. Alpha stimulation increases vital capacity by relieving congestion of the bronchial mucosa and by constricting pulmonary vessels.

Recent studies in laboratory animals (minipigs, rodents, and dogs) recorded the occurrence of cardiac arrhythmias and sudden death (with histologic evidence of myocardial necrosis) when beta agonists and methylxanthines were administered concurrently. The significance of these findings when applied to humans is currently unknown.

SUS-PHRINE (epinephrine) provides both rapid and sustained epinephrine activity. The rapid action is due to the epinephrine in solution, while the sustained activity is due to the crystalline epinephrine-free base in suspension.

INDICATIONS AND USAGE

For the symptomatic treatment of bronchial asthma, and reversible bronchospasm associated with chronic bronchitis and emphysema.

CONTRAINDICATIONS

Hypersensitivity to any of the components.
Narrow angle glaucoma, shock, cerebral arteriosclerosis and organic heart disease. Epinephrine is also contraindicated during general anesthesia with halogenated hydrocarbons or cyclopropane, and in local anesthesia of certain areas, e.g., fingers, toes, because of the danger of vasoconstriction producing sloughing of tissue, and in labor because the drug may delay the second stage.

WARNINGS

SUS-PHRINE (epinephrine) SHOULD NOT BE EMPLOYED TO CORRECT DRUG-INDUCED HYPOTENSION.
Administer with caution to elderly people; those with cardiovascular disease, diabetes, hypertension or hyperthyroidism; in psychoneurotic individuals and in pregnancy. Administer with extreme caution to patients with long-standing bronchial asthma and emphysema who have developed degenerative heart disease.

Cardiac arrhythmias may follow administration of epinephrine.
Anginal pain may be induced when coronary insufficiency is present.

PRECAUTIONS

Parenteral drug products should be inspected visually for foreign particulate matter and discoloration before administration whenever container permits.
DO NOT USE IF PRODUCT IS DISCOLORED. Discoloration indicates the oxidation of epinephrine and possible loss of potency.
Use of SUS-PHRINE (epinephrine) with digitalis, mercurial diuretics or other drugs that sensitize the heart to arrhythmias is not recommended.
Patients should be instructed to contact a physician immediately if severe pain at the site of injection develops.
SUS-PHRINE (epinephrine) should not be administered concomitantly with other sympathomimetic agents, since their combined effects on the cardiovascular system may be deleterious to the patient.
The effects of epinephrine may be potentiated by tricyclic antidepressants; sodium L-thyroxine, and certain antihistamines (e.g., diphenhydramine, tripelennamine or chlorpheniramine).

ADVERSE REACTIONS

In some individuals, restlessness, anxiety, headache, tremor, weakness, dizziness, pallor, respiratory difficulties, palpitation, nausea and vomiting may occur. These reactions may be exaggerated in hyperthyroidism. Occlusion of the central retinal artery, clostridial myonecrosis and shock have also been reported.
Also, urticaria, wheal and hemorrhage at the site of injection may occur. Repeated injections at the same site may result in necrosis from vascular constriction.
Tolerance to epinephrine may occur with prolonged use.

OVERDOSAGE

Overdosage or inadvertent intravenous injection may cause cerebrovascular hemorrhage resulting from the sharp rise in blood pressure. Fatalities may also result from pulmonary edema because of peripheral constriction and cardiac stimulation produced. Rapidly acting vasodilators such as nitrites, or alpha blocking agents may counteract the marked pressor effects. Cardiac arrhythmias may be countered by administering rapidly acting antiarrhythmic or beta blocking agents.

DOSAGE AND ADMINISTRATION
NOTE: INJECT SUBCUTANEOUSLY.

As with all sterile products, failure to follow aseptic procedures may result in microbial contamination causing adverse consequences which could lead to life threatening illness.
It is suggested that SUS-PHRINE (epinephrine) be administered with a tuberculin syringe and a 26 gauge, $^1/_2$ inch needle.
A small initial test dose may be administered subcutaneously as a possible aid in determining patient sensitivity to epinephrine.
Site of injection should be varied to avoid necrosis at the site of injection.
Each time before withdrawing SUS-PHRINE (epinephrine) into syringe, **SHAKE VIAL OR AMPUL THOROUGHLY** to disperse particles and obtain a uniform suspension. Inject promptly subcutaneously to avoid settling of suspension in the syringe.
ADULTS:
Adult dosage range is 0.1 to 0.3 mL depending on patient response.
Subsequent doses should be administered only when necessary and not more frequently than every six hours.
Infants 1 month to 2 years and Children 2 to 12 years:
Pediatric dose is 0.005 mL/kg (2.2 lb) body weight injected subcutaneously.
FOR CHILDREN 30 kg OR LESS MAXIMUM SINGLE DOSE IS 0.15 mL
Subsequent doses should be administered only when necessary and not more frequently than every six hours.

CLINICAL STUDIES

Controlled studies comparing the effectiveness of SUS-PHRINE (epinephrine) 1:200 and an aqueous solution of epinephrine 1:1000 were conducted in both pediatric and adult asthmatics. The studies demonstrated rapid bronchodilator activity following administration of either SUS-PHRINE (epinephrine) or epinephrine 1:1000; however during the 6 hour study period, a greater improvement in FEV_1 and $FEF_{25-75\%}$ was observed 4 to 6 hours subsequent to SUS-PHRINE (epinephrine) administration. Improvement in Wright Peak Expiratory Flow Rate was greater for SUS-PHRINE (epinephrine) than epinephrine 1:1000 3 to 8 hours following administration (10 hour study duration).

HOW SUPPLIED

In boxes of:
10 × 0.3 mL colorless glass ampuls ..... NDC 0456-0664-39

25 × 0.3 mL colorless glass ampuls ..... NDC 0456-0664-34
5.0 mL multiple dose colorless glass vial .... NDC 0456-0664-05
Store under refrigeration between 2° and 8°C (36° and 46°F). Do not freeze.
Caution Statement:
Federal Law Prohibits Dispensing without a prescription.
Revised 6/94
mfd by
Steris Laboratories, Inc.
Phoenix, AZ 85043
mfd for
Forest Pharmaceuticals, Inc.
Subsidiary of Forest Laboratories, Inc.
St. Louis, Missouri 63045

TESSALON®   ℞
(benzonatate USP)

DESCRIPTION

TESSALON, a non-narcotic oral antitussive agent, is 2, 5, 8, 11, 14, 17, 20, 23, 26-nonaoxaoctacosan-28-yl p-(butylamino) benzoate; with a molecular weight of 603.7.

$$CH_3(CH_2)_2CH_2NH \underset{C_{30}H_{53}NO_{11}}{} COOCH_2CH_2(OCH_2CH_2)_nOCH_3$$

Each TESSALON Perle contains:
Benzonatate, USP   100 mg
TESSALON Perles also contain: D&C Yellow 10, gelatin, glycerin, methylparaben and propylparaben.

CLINICAL PHARMACOLOGY

TESSALON acts peripherally by anesthetizing the stretch receptors located in the respiratory passages, lungs, and pleura by dampening their activity and thereby reducing the cough reflex at its source. It begins to act within 15 to 20 minutes and its effect lasts for 3 to 8 hours. TESSALON has no inhibitory effect on the respiratory center in recommended dosage.

INDICATIONS AND USAGE

TESSALON is indicated for the symptomatic relief of cough.

CONTRAINDICATIONS

Hypersensitivity to benzonatate or related compounds.

WARNINGS

Severe hypersensitivity reactions (including bronchospasm, laryngospasm and cardiovascular collapse) have been reported which are possibly related to local anesthesia from sucking or chewing the perle instead of swallowing it. Severe reactions have required intervention with vasopressor agents and supportive measures.
Isolated instances of bizarre behavior, including mental confusion and visual hallucinations, have also been reported in patients taking TESSALON in combination with other prescribed drugs.

PRECAUTIONS

Benzonatate is chemically related to anesthetic agents of the para-amino-benzoic acid class (e.g., procaine; tetracaine) and has been associated with adverse CNS effects possibly related to a prior sensitivity to related agents or interaction with concomitant medication.
Information for Patients: Release of TESSALON from the perle in the mouth can produce a temporary local anesthesia of the oral mucosa and choking could occur. Therefore, the perles should be swallowed without chewing.
Usage in Pregnancy: Pregnancy Category C. Animal reproduction studies have not been conducted with TESSALON. It is also not known whether TESSALON can cause fetal harm when administered to a pregnant woman or can affect reproduction capacity. TESSALON should be given to a pregnant woman only if clearly needed.
Nursing Mothers: It is not known whether this drug is excreted in human milk. Because many drugs are excreted in human milk caution should be exercised when TESSALON is administered to a nursing woman.
Carcinogenesis, Mutagenesis, Impairment of Fertility: Carcinogenicity, mutagenicity, and reproduction studies have not been conducted with TESSALON.
Pediatric Use: Safety and effectiveness in children below the age of 10 has not been established.

ADVERSE REACTIONS

Potential Adverse Reactions to TESSALON may include:
Hypersensitivity reactions including bronchospasm, laryngospasm, cardiovascular collapse possibly related to local anesthesia from chewing or sucking the perle.

Continued on next page

Tessalon—Cont.

CNS: sedation; headache; dizziness; mental confusion; visual hallucinations.
GI: constipation, nausea, GI upset.
Dermatologic: pruritus; skin eruptions.
Other: nasal congestion; sensation of burning in the eyes; vague "chilly" sensation; numbness of the chest; hypersensitivity.
Rare instances of deliberate or accidental overdose have resulted in death.

OVERDOSAGE

Overdose may result in death.
The drug is chemically related to tetracaine and other topical anesthetics and shares various aspects of their pharmacology and toxicology. Drugs of this type are generally well absorbed after ingestion.
Signs and Symptoms:
If perles are chewed or dissolved in the mouth, oropharyngeal anesthesia will develop rapidly. CNS stimulation may cause restlessness and tremors which may proceed to clonic convulsions followed by profound CNS depression.
Treatment:
Evacuate gastric contents and administer copious amounts of activated charcoal slurry. Even in the conscious patient, cough and gag reflexes may be so depressed as to necessitate special attention to protection against aspiration of gastric contents and orally administered materials. Convulsions should be treated with a short-acting barbiturate given intravenously and carefully titrated for the smallest effective dosage. Intensive support of respiration and cardiovascular-renal function is an essential feature of the treatment of severe intoxication from overdosage.
Do not use CNS stimulants.

DOSAGE AND ADMINISTRATION

Adults and Children over 10: Usual dose is one 100 mg perle t.i.d. as required. If necessary, up to 6 perles daily may be given.

HOW SUPPLIED

Perles, 100 mg (yellow); bottles of 100   NDC 0456-0688-01
Perles, 100 mg (yellow); bottles of 500   NDC 0456-0688-02
Store at controlled room temperature 15°–30°C (59°–86°F).

Rev. 9/95
MG #11385

Mfd by
R.P. Scherer-North America
St. Petersburg, Florida 33716

for

**FOREST PHARMACEUTICALS, INC.
SUBSIDIARY OF FOREST LABORATORIES, INC.
ST. LOUIS, MISSOURI 63045**
Shown in Product Identification Guide, page 310

THYROLAR® Tablets   ℞
[thī-rō-lär]
(Liotrix Tablets, USP)

DESCRIPTION

Thyrolar Tablets (Liotrix Tablets, USP) contain triiodothyronine (T_3 liothyronine) sodium and tetraiodothyronine (T_4 levothyroxine) sodium in the amounts listed in the "How Supplied" section. (T_3 liothyronine sodium is approximately four times as potent at T_4 thyroxine on a microgram for microgram basis.)
The inactive ingredients are calcium phosphate, colloidal silicon dioxide, cornstarch, lactose, and magnesium stearate. The tablets also contain the following dyes: Thyrolar $^1/_4$-FD&C Blue #1 and FD&C Red #40; Thyrolar $^1/_2$-FD&C Red #40 and D&C Yellow #10; Thyrolar 1-FD&C Red #40; Thyrolar 2-FD&C Blue #1, FD&C Red #40, and D&C Yellow #10; Thyrolar 3-FD&C Red #40 and D&C Yellow #10.

STRUCTURAL FORMULAS

[See Chemical Structures at top of next column]

HOW SUPPLIED

Thyrolar Tablets (Liotrix Tablets, USP) are available in five potencies, coded as follows:
[See table below]
Supplied in bottles of 100, two-layered compressed tablets.

Liothyronine (T₃) Sodium

Levothyroxine (T₄) Sodium

Tablets should be stored at cold temperature, between 36° and 46°F (2° and 8°C) in a tight, light-resistant container.
Note: (T_3) liothyronine sodium is approximately four times as potent as T_4 thyroxine on a microgram-for-microgram basis.)
Rev. 06/96   14360696
FOREST PHARMACEUTICALS, INC.
A Subsidiary of Forest Laboratories, Inc.
St. Louis, MO 63045
Shown in Product Identification Guide, page 310

TIAZAC®   ℞
**(diltiazem hydrochloride)
Extended Release Capsules**

DESCRIPTION

Tiazac (diltiazem hydrochloride) is a calcium ion cellular influx inhibitor (slow channel blocker). Chemically, diltiazem hydrochloride is 1,5-Benzothiazepin-4(5H)-one,3-(acetyloxy)-5[2-(dimethylamino)ethyl]-2,-3-dihydro-2(4-methoxyphenyl)-, monohydrochloride, (+)-cis. The chemical structure is:

Diltiazem hydrochloride is a white to off-white crystalline powder with a bitter taste. It is soluble in water, methanol and chloroform and has a molecular weight of 450.98. Tiazac capsules contain diltiazem hydrochloride in extended release beads at doses of 120, 180, 240, 300 and 360 mg. Tiazac also contains: Microcrystalline Cellulose NF, Sucrose Stearate, Eudragit, Povidone USP, Talc USP, Magnesium Stearate NF, Hydroxypropylmethylcellulose USP, Titanium Dioxide USP, Polysorbate NF, Simethicone USP, Gelatin NF, FD&C Blue #1, FD&C Red #40, D&C Red #28, FD&C Green #3, Black Iron Oxide USP, and other solids.
For oral administration.

CLINICAL PHARMACOLOGY

The therapeutic effects of diltiazem hydrochloride are believed to be related to its ability to inhibit the cellular influx of calcium ions during membrane depolarization of cardiac and vascular smooth muscle.
Mechanisms of Action.
Hypertension: Diltiazem produces its antihypertensive effect primarily by relaxation of vascular smooth muscle and the resultant decrease in peripheral vascular resistance. The magnitude of blood pressure reduction is related to the degree of hypertension: thus hypertensive individuals experience an antihypertensive effect, whereas there is only a modest fall in blood pressure in normotensives.
Angina: Diltiazem HCl has been shown to produce increases in exercise tolerance, probably due to its ability to reduce myocardial oxygen demand. This is accomplished via reductions in heart rate and systemic blood pressure at submaximal and maximal work loads.

Diltiazem has been shown to be a potent dilator of coronary arteries, both epicardial and subendocardial. Spontaneous and ergonovine-induced coronary artery spasm are inhibited by diltiazem.
In animal models, diltiazem interferes with the slow inward (depolarizing) current in excitable tissue. It causes excitation-contraction uncoupling in various myocardial tissues without changes in the configuration of the action potential. Diltiazem produces relaxation of the coronary vascular smooth muscle and dilation of both large and small coronary vascular smooth muscle and dilation of both large and small coronary arteries at drug levels which cause little or no negative inotropic effect. The resultant increases in coronary blood flow (epicardial and subendocardial) occur in ischemic and nonischemic models and are accompanied by dose-dependent decreases in systemic blood pressure and decreases in peripheral resistance.
Hemodynamic and Electrophysiologic Effects. Like other calcium channel antagonists, diltiazem decreases sinoatrial and atrioventricular conduction in isolated tissues and has a negative inotropic effect in isolated preparations. In the intact animal, prolongation of the AH interval can be seen at higher doses.
In man, diltiazem prevents spontaneous and ergonovine-provoked coronary artery spasm. It causes a decrease in peripheral vascular resistance and a modest fall in blood pressure in normotensive individuals and, in exercise tolerance studies in patients with ischemic heart disease, reduces the heart rate-blood pressure product for any given work load. Studies to date, primarily in patients with good ventricular function, have not revealed evidence of a negative inotropic effect; cardiac output, ejection fraction, and left ventricular end diastolic pressure have not been affected. Such data have no predictive value with respect to effects in patients with poor ventricular function, and increased heart failure has been reported in patients with preexisting impairment of ventricular function. There are as yet few data on the interaction of diltiazem and beta-blockers in patients with poor ventricular function. Resting heart rate is usually slightly reduced by diltiazem.
Tiazac produces antihypertensive effects both in the supine and standing positions. Postural hypotension is infrequently noted upon suddenly assuming an upright position. No reflex tachycardia is associated with the chronic antihypertensive effects.
Diltiazem hydrochloride decreases vascular resistance, increases cardiac output (by increasing stroke volume), and produces a slight decrease or no change in heart rate. During dynamic exercise, increases in diastolic pressure are inhibited while maximum achievable systolic pressure is usually reduced. Chronic therapy with diltiazem hydrochloride produces no change or an increase in plasma catecholamines. No increased activity of the renin-angiotensin-aldosterone axis has been observed. Diltiazem hydrochloride reduces the renal and peripheral effects of angiotensin II. Hypertensive animal models respond to diltiazem with reductions in blood pressure and increased urinary output and natriuresis without a change in urinary sodium/potassium ratio. In man, transient natriuresis and kaliuresis have been reported, but only in high intravenous doses of 0.5 mg/kg of body weight.
Diltiazem-associated prolongation of the AH interval is not more pronounced in patients with first degree heart block.
In patients with sick sinus syndrome, diltiazem significantly prolongs sinus cycle length (up to 50% in some cases). Intravenous diltiazem in doses of 20 mg prolongs AH conduction time and AV node functional and effective refractory periods by approximately 20%.
In two short-term, double-blind, placebo-controlled studies in 256 hypertensive patients with doses up to 540 mg/day, Tiazac showed a clinically unimportant but statistically significant, dose-related increase in PR interval (0.008 seconds). There were no instances of greater than first-degree AV block in any of the clinical trials (see WARNINGS).
Pharmacodynamics.
Hypertension: In short-term, double-blind, placebo-controlled clinical trials Tiazac demonstrated a dose-related antihypertensive response among patients with mild to moderate hypertension. In one parallel-group study of 198 patients Tiazac was given for four weeks. The changes in diastolic blood pressure measured at trough (24 hours after the dose) for placebo, 90mg, 180mg, 360mg and 540mg were -5.4, -6.3, -6.2, -8.2, and -11.8mm Hg, respectively. Supine diastolic blood pressure as well as standing diastolic and systolic blood pressures also showed statistically significant linear dose response effects.
In another clinical trial that followed a dose-escalation design, Tiazac also reduced blood pressure in a linear dose-related manner. Supine diastolic blood pressure measured following two week intervals of treatment was reduced by -3.7mm Hg with 120 mg/day versus -2.0mm Hg with placebo, by -7.6mm Hg after escalation to 240 mg/day versus -2.3mm Hg with placebo, by -8.1mm Hg after escalation to 360 mg/day versus -0.9mm Hg with placebo, and by -10.8mm Hg after escalation to 480/540 mg/day versus -2.2mm Hg with placebo.
Angina: In a double-blind, parallel-group, placebo-controlled trial (approximately 50 patients/group, in patients with chronic stable angina), Tiazac at doses of 120–540/day increased exercise tolerance time. At trough, 24 hours after

THYROLAR® Tablets

Name	Composition (T_3/T_4 per tablet)	Color	Armacode®
Thyrolar—$^1/_4$(0456–0040–01)	3.1 mcg/12.5 mcg	Violet/White	YC
Thyrolar—$^1/_2$(0456–0045–01)	6.25 mcg/25 mcg	Peach/White	YD
Thyrolar—1 (0456–0050–01)	12.5 mcg/50 mcg	Pink/White	YE
Thyrolar—2 (0456–0055–01)	25 mcg/100 mcg	Green/White	YF
Thyrolar—3 (0456–0060–01)	37.5 mcg/150 mcg	Yellow/White	YH

dosing, exercise tolerance times using a Bruce exercise protocol, increased by 14, 26, 41, 33 and 32 seconds over baseline for placebo and the 120 mg, 240 mg, 360 mg, and 540 mg/day treated patient groups, respectively. At peak, 8 hours after dosing, exercise tolerance times relative to baseline were statistically significantly increased by 13, 38, 64, 55 and 42 seconds for placebo and 120 mg, 240 mg, 360 mg, and 540 mg/day Tiazac treated patients, respectively. Compared to baseline, Tiazac treated patients experienced statistically significant reductions in anginal attacks and decreased nitroglycerin requirements when compared to placebo treated patients.

Pharmacokinetics and Metabolism. Diltiazem is well absorbed from the gastrointestinal tract but undergoes substantial hepatic first-pass effect. The absolute bioavailability of an oral dose of an immediate release formulation (compared to intravenous administration) is approximately 40%. Only 2% to 4% of unchanged diltiazem appears in the urine. The plasma elimination half-life of diltiazem is approximately 3.0–4.5 h. Drugs which induce or inhibit hepatic microsomal enzymes may alter diltiazem disposition. Therapeutic blood levels of diltiazem appear to be in the range of 40–200 ng/mL. There is a departure from linearity when dose strengths are increased; the half-life is slightly increased with dose.

The two primary metabolites of diltiazem are desacetyldiltiazem and desmethyldiltiazem. The desacetyl metabolite is approximately 25% to 50% as potent a coronary vasodilator as diltiazem and is present in plasma at concentrations of 10% to 20% of parent diltiazem. However, recent studies employing sensitive and specific analytical methods have confirmed the existence of several sequential metabolic pathways of diltiazem. As many as nine diltiazem metabolites have been identified in the urine of humans. Total radioactivity measurements following single intravenous dose administration in healthy volunteers suggest the presence of other unidentified metabolites. These metabolites are more slowly excreted, (with a half-life of total radioactivity of approximately 20 hours) and attain concentrations in excess of diltiazem.

In vitro binding studies show diltiazem HCl is 70% to 80% bound to plasma proteins. Competitive *in vitro* ligand binding studies have also shown diltiazem HCl binding is not altered by therapeutic concentrations of digoxin, hydrochlorothiazide, phenylbutazone, propranolol, salicylic acid, or warfarin. A study that compared patients with normal hepatic function to patients with cirrhosis who received immediate release diltiazem found an increase in diltiazem elimination half-life and a 69% increase in bioavailability in the hepatically impaired patients. Patients with severely impaired renal function (creatinine clearance <50 mL/min) who received immediate release diltiazem had modestly increased diltiazem concentrations compared to patients with normal renal function.

Tiazac® Capsules. When compared to a regimen of immediate-release tablets at steady-state, approximately 93% of drug is absorbed from the Tiazac formulation. When Tiazac was coadministered with a high fat content breakfast, the extent of diltiazem absorption was not affected; T_{max}, however, occurred slightly earlier. The apparent elimination half-life after single or multiple dosing is 4 to 9.5 hours (mean 6.5 hours).

Tiazac demonstrates non-linear pharmacokinetics. As the daily dose of Tiazac capsules is increased from 120 to 540 mg, there was a more than proportional increase in diltiazem plasma concentrations as evidenced by an increase of AUC, C_{max} and C_{min} of 6,8, 6 and 8.6 times, respectively, for a 4.5 times increase in dose.

INDICATIONS AND USAGE

Hypertension:

Tiazac is indicated for the treatment of hypertension. It may be used alone or in combination with other antihypertensive medications.

Chronic Stable Angina:

Tiazac is indicated for the treatment of chronic stable angina.

CONTRAINDICATIONS

Diltiazem is contraindicated in (1) patients with sick sinus syndrome except in the presence of a functioning ventricular pacemaker, (2) patients with second- or third-degree AV block except in the presence of a functioning ventricular pacemaker, (3) patients with severe hypotension (less than 90 mm Hg systolic), (4) patients who have demonstrated hypersensitivity to the drug, and (5) patients with acute myocardial infarction and pulmonary congestion documented by x-ray on admission.

WARNINGS

1. Cardiac Conduction. Diltiazem hydrochloride prolongs AV node refractory periods without significantly prolonging sinus node recovery time, except in patients with sick sinus syndrome. This effect may rarely result in abnormally slow heart rates (particularly in patients with sick sinus syndrome) or second- or third-degree AV block (13 of 3007 patients or 0.43%). Concomitant use of diltiazem with beta-blockers or digitalis may result in additive effects on cardiac conduction. A patient with Prinzmetal's angina developed periods of asystole (2 to 5 seconds) after a single dose of 60 mg of diltiazem.

2. Congestive Heart Failure. Although diltiazem has a negative inotropic effect in isolated animal tissue preparations, hemodynamic studies in humans with normal ventricular function have not shown a reduction in cardiac index nor consistent negative effects on contractility (dp/dt). An acute study of oral diltiazem in patients with impaired ventricular function (ejection fraction 24% ± 6%) showed improvement in indices of ventricular function without significant decrease in contractile function (dp/dt). Worsening of congestive heart failure has been reported in patients with preexisting impairment of ventricular function. Experience with the use of diltiazem hydrochloride in combination with beta-blockers in patients with impaired ventricular function is limited. Caution should be exercised when using this combination.

3. Hypotension. Decreases in blood pressure associated with diltiazem hydrochloride therapy may occasionally result in symptomatic hypotension.

4. Acute Hepatic Injury. Mild elevations of transaminases with and without concomitant elevation in alkaline phosphatase and bilirubin have been observed in clinical studies. Such elevations were usually transient and frequently resolved even with continued diltiazem treatment. In rare instances, significant elevations in enzymes such as alkaline phosphatase, LDH, SGOT, and SGPT, and other phenomena consistent with acute hepatic injury have been noted. These reactions tended to occur early after therapy initiation (1 to 8 weeks) and have been reversible upon discontinuation of drug therapy. The relationship to diltiazem hydrochloride is uncertain in some cases, but probable in some (see PRECAUTIONS).

PRECAUTIONS

General. Diltiazem hydrochloride is extensively metabolized by the liver and excreted by the kidneys and in bile. As with any drug given over prolonged periods, laboratory parameters of renal and hepatic function should be monitored at regular intervals. The drug should be used with caution in patients with impaired renal or hepatic function. In subacute and chronic dog and rat studies designed to produce toxicity, high doses of diltiazem were associated with hepatic damage. In special subacute hepatic studies, oral doses of 125 mg/kg and higher in rats were associated with histological changes in the liver which were reversible when the drug was discontinued. In dogs, doses of 20 mg/kg were also associated with hepatic changes; however, these changes were reversible with continued dosing.

Dermatological events (see ADVERSE REACTIONS section) may be transient and may disappear despite continued use of diltiazem hydrochloride. However, skin eruptions progressing to erythema multiforme and/or exfoliative dermatitis have also been infrequently reported. Should a dermatologic reaction persist, the drug should be discontinued.

Drug Interactions. Due to the potential for additive effects, caution and careful titration are warranted in patients receiving diltiazem hydrochloride concomitantly with other agents known to affect cardiac contractility and/or conduction (see WARNINGS). Pharmacologic studies indicate that there may be additive effects in prolonging AV conduction when using beta-blockers or digitalis concomitantly with Tiazac (see WARNINGS). As with all drugs, care should be exercised when treating patients with multiple medications. Diltiazem hydrochloride undergoes biotransformation by cytochrome P-450 mixed function oxidase. Coadministration of diltiazem hydrochloride with other agents which follow the same route of biotransformation may result in the competitive inhibition of metabolism. Dosages of similarly metabolized drugs such as cyclosporin, particularly those of low therapeutic ratio or in patients with renal and/or hepatic impairment, may require adjustment when starting or stopping concomitantly administered diltiazem hydrochloride to maintain optimum therapeutic blood levels.

Beta Blockers. Controlled and uncontrolled domestic studies suggest that concomitant use of diltiazem hydrochloride and beta-blockers is usually well tolerated, but available data are not sufficient to predict the effects of concomitant treatment in patients with left ventricular dysfunction or cardiac conduction abnormalities. Administration of diltiazem hydrochloride concomitantly with propranolol in five normal volunteers resulted in increased propranolol levels in all subjects and bioavailability of propranolol was increased approximately 50%. *In vitro*, propranolol appears to be displaced from its binding sites by diltiazem. If combination therapy is initiated or withdrawn in conjunction with propranolol, an adjustment in the propranolol dose may be warranted (see WARNINGS).

Cimetidine. A study in six healthy volunteers has shown a significant increase in peak diltiazem plasma levels (58%) and area-under-the-curve (53%) after a 1-week course of cimetidine 1200 mg per day and a single dose of diltiazem 60 mg. Ranitidine produced smaller, nonsignificant increases. The effect may be mediated by cimetidine's known inhibition of hepatic cytochrome P-450, the enzyme system responsible for the first-pass metabolism of diltiazem. Patients currently receiving diltiazem therapy should be carefully monitored for a change in pharmacological effect when initiating and discontinuing therapy with cimetidine. An adjustment in the diltiazem dose may be warranted.

Digitalis. Administration of diltiazem hydrochloride with digoxin in 24 healthy male subjects increased plasma digoxin concentrations approximately 20%. Another investigator found no increase in digoxin levels in 12 patients with coronary artery disease. Since there have been conflicting results regarding the effect of digoxin levels, it is recommended that digoxin levels be monitored when initiating, adjusting, and discontinuing diltiazem hydrochloride therapy to avoid possible over- or under-digitalization (see WARNINGS).

Anesthetics. The depression of cardiac contractility, conductivity, and automaticity as well as the vascular dilation associated with anesthetics may be potentiated by calcium channel blockers. When used concomitantly, anesthetics and calcium blockers should be titrated carefully.

Cyclosporine. A pharmacokinetic interaction between diltiazem and cyclosporine has been observed during studies involving renal and cardiac transplant patients. In renal and cardiac transplant recipients, a reduction of cyclosporine dose ranging from 15% to 48% was necessary to maintain cyclosporine trough concentrations similar to those seen prior to the addition of diltiazem. If these agents are to be administered concurrently, cyclosporine concentrations should be monitored, especially when diltiazem therapy is initiated, adjusted, or discontinued.

The effect of cyclosporine on diltiazem plasma concentrations has not been evaluated.

Carbamazepine. Concomitant administration of diltiazem with carbamazepine has been reported to result in elevated serum levels of carbamazepine (40% to 72% increase), resulting in toxicity in some cases. Patients receiving these drugs concurrently should be monitored for a potential drug interaction.

Carcinogenesis, Mutagenesis, Impairment of Fertility. A 24-month study in rats at oral dosage levels of up to 100 mg/kg/day and a 21-month study in mice at oral dosage levels of up to 30 mg/kg/day showed no evidence of carcinogenicity. There was also no mutagenic response *in vitro* or *in vivo* in mammalian cell assays or *in vitro* in bacteria. No evidence of impaired fertility was observed in a study performed in male and female rats at oral dosages of up to 100 mg/kg/day.

Pregnancy. Category C. Reproduction studies have been conducted in mice, rats, and rabbits. Administration of doses ranging from 4 to 6 times (depending on species) the upper limit of the optimum dosage range in clinical trials (480 mg q.d. or 8 mg/kg q.d. for a 60 kg patient) resulted in embryo and fetal lethality. These studies revealed, in one species or another, a propensity to cause abnormalities of the skeleton, heart, retina, and tongue. Also observed were reductions in early individual pup weights and pup survival, prolonged delivery and increased incidence of stillbirths. There are no well-controlled studies in pregnant women; therefore, use diltiazem hydrochloride in pregnant women only if the potential benefit justifies the potential risk to the fetus.

Nursing Mothers. Diltiazem is excreted in human milk. One report suggests that concentrations in breast milk may approximate serum levels. If use of Tiazac is deemed essential, an alternative method of infant feeding should be instituted.

Pediatric Use. Safety and effectiveness in children have not been established.

ADVERSE REACTIONS

Serious adverse reactions have been rare in studies with Tiazac, as well as with other diltiazem formulations. It should be recognized that patients with impaired ventricular function and cardiac conduction abnormalities have usually been excluded from these studies. A total of 256 hypertensives were treated for between 4 and 8 weeks; a total of 207 patients with chronic stable angina were treated for 3 weeks with doses of Tiazac ranging from 120–540 mg once daily. Two patients experienced first-degree AV block at 540 mg dose. The following table presents the most common adverse reactions, whether or not drug-related, reported in placebo-controlled trials in patients receiving Tiazac up to 360 mg and up to 540 mg with rates in placebo patients shown for comparison.

[See first table at top of next page]

[See second table at top of next page]

In addition, the following events have been reported infrequently (less than 2%) in clinical trials with other diltiazem products:

Cardiovascular. Angina, arrhythmia, AV block (second- or third-degree), bundle branch block, congestive heart failure, ECG abnormalities, hypotension, palpitations, syncope, tachycardia, ventricular extrasystoles.

Continued on next page

Tiazac—Cont.

Nervous System. Abnormal dreams, amnesia, depression, gait abnormality, hallucinations, insomnia, nervousness, paresthesia, personality change, somnolence, tinnitus, tremor.

Gastrointestinal. Anorexia, constipation, diarrhea, dry mouth, dysgeusia, mild elevations of SGOT, SGPT, LDH, and alkaline phosphatase (see hepatic warnings), nausea, thirst, vomiting, weight increase.

Dermatological. Petechiae, photosensitivity, pruritus.

Other. Albuminuria, allergic reaction, amblyopia, asthenia, CPK increase, crystalluria, dyspnea, edema, epistaxis, eye irritation, headache, hyperglycemia, hyperuricemia, impotence, muscle cramps, nasal congestion, neck rigidity, nocturia, osteoarticular pain, pain, polyuria, rhinitis, sexual difficulties, gynecomastia.

In addition, the following postmarketing events have been reported infrequently in patients receiving diltiazem hydrochloride: alopecia, erythema multiforme, exfoliative dermatitis, Stevens-Johnson syndrome, toxic epidermal necrolysis, extrapyramidal symptoms, gingival hyperplasia, hemolytic anemia, increased bleeding time, leukopenia, purpura, retinopathy, and thrombocytopenia. In addition, events such as myocardial infarction have been observed which are not readily distinguishable from the natural history of the disease in these patients. A number of well-documented cases of generalized rash, characterized as leukocytoclastic vasculitis, have been reported. However, a definitive cause and effect relationship between these events and diltiazem hydrochloride therapy is yet to be established.

OVERDOSAGE

The oral LD50's in mice and rats range from 415 to 740 mg/kg and from 560 to 810 mg/kg, respectively. The intravenous LD50's in these species were 60 and 38 mg/kg, respectively. The oral LD50 in dogs is considered to be in excess of 50 mg/kg, while lethality was seen in monkeys at 360 mg/kg.

The toxic dose in man is not known. Due to extensive metabolism, blood levels after a standard dose of diltiazem can vary over tenfold, limiting the usefulness of blood levels in overdose cases. There have been 29 reports of diltiazem overdose in doses ranging from less than 1 gm to 10.8 gm. Sixteen of these reports involved multiple drug ingestions. Twenty-two reports indicated patients had recovered from diltiazem overdose ranging from less than 1 gm to 10.8 gm. There were seven reports with a fatal outcome; although the amount of diltiazem ingested was unknown, multiple drug ingestions were confirmed in six of the seven reports.

Events observed following diltiazem overdose included bradycardia, hypotension, heart block, and cardiac failure. Most reports of overdose described some supportive medical measure and/or drug treatment. Bradycardia frequently responded favorably to atropine as did heart block, although cardiac pacing was also frequently utilized to treat heart block. Fluids and vasopressors were used to maintain blood pressure, and in cases of cardiac failure, inotropic agents were administered. In addition, some patients received treatment with ventilatory support, activated charcoal, and/or intravenous calcium. Evidence of the effectiveness of intravenous calcium administration to reverse the pharmacological effects of diltiazem overdose was conflicting.

In the event of overdose or exaggerated response, appropriate supportive measures should be employed in addition to gastrointestinal decontamination. Diltiazem does not appear to be removed by peritoneal or hemodialysis. Based on the known pharmacological effects of diltiazem and/or reported clinical experiences, the following measures may be considered:

Bradycardia: Administer atropine (0.60 to 1.0 mg). If there is no response to vagal blockage, administer isoproterenol cautiously.

High-Degree AV Block: Treat as for bradycardia above. Fixed high-degree AV block should be treated with cardiac pacing.

Cardiac Failure: Administer inotropic agents (isoproterenol, dopamine, or dobutamine) and diuretics.

Hypotension: Vasopressors (e.g., dopamine or levarterenol bitartrate). Actual treatment and dosage should depend on the severity of the clinical situation and the judgment and experience of the treating physician.

In a few reported cases, overdose with calcium channel blockers has been associated with hypotension and bradycardia, initially refractory to atropine but becoming more responsive to this treatment when the patients received large doses (close to 1 gram/hour for more than 24 hours) of calcium chloride.

Due to extensive metabolism, plasma concentrations after a standard dose of diltiazem can vary over tenfold, which significantly limits their value in evaluation cases of overdosage.

Charcoal hemoperfusion has been used successfully as an adjunct therapy to hasten drug elimination. Overdoses with as much as 10.8 gm of oral diltiazem have been successfully treated using appropriate supportive care.

DOSAGE AND ADMINISTRATION

Hypertension: Dosage needs to be adjusted by titration to individual patient needs. When used as monotherapy, usual starting doses are 120 to 240 mg once daily. Maximum antihypertensive effect is usually observed by 14 days of chronic therapy; therefore, dosage adjustments should be scheduled accordingly. The usual dosage range studied in clinical trials was 120 to 540 mg once daily. Current clinical experience with 540 mg dose is limited; however, the dose may be increased to 540 mg once daily.

Angina: Dosages for the treatment of angina should be adjusted to each patient's needs, starting with a dose of 120 mg to 180 mg once daily. Individual patients may respond to higher doses of up to 540 mg once daily. When necessary, titration should be carried out over 7 to 14 days.

Concomitant use with Other Cardiovascular Agents.

1. Sublingual Nitroglycerin may be taken as required to abort acute anginal attacks during diltiazem hydrochloride therapy.

2. Prophylactic Nitrate Therapy — Diltiazem hydrochloride may be safely co-administered with short- and long-acting nitrates.

3. Beta-blockers. (See WARNINGS and PRECAUTIONS.)

4. Antihypertensives — Diltiazem hydrochloride has an additive antihypertensive effect when used with other antihypertensive agents. Therefore, the dosage of diltiazem hydrochloride or the concomitant antihypertensives may need to be adjusted when adding one to the other.

Hypertensive or anginal patients who are treated with other formulations of diltiazem can safely be switched to Tiazac capsules at the nearest equivalent total daily dose. Subsequent titration to higher or lower doses may, however, be necessary and should be initiated as clinically indicated.

HOW SUPPLIED

Tiazac (diltiazem hydrochloride) Extended-Release Capsules

[See table below]

Storage conditions: Store at controlled room temperature 20°–25°C (68°–77°F). Avoid excessive humidity.

CAUTION: Federal (U.S.A.) Law prohibits dispensing without prescription.

Manufactured by:
Biovail Laboratories Inc., Carolina, Puerto Rico
Encapsulated and Made in Canada

Manufactured for:
Forest Pharmaceuticals, Inc.
Subsidiary of Forest Laboratories, Inc.
St. Louis, Missouri 63045

Rev: 01/98   LB-0001-04

Shown in Product Identification Guide, page 310

MOST COMMON ADVERSE EVENTS IN DOUBLE-BLIND PLACEBO-CONTROLLED HYPERTENSION TRIALS*

Adverse Events (COSTART Term)	Placebo n = 57 # pts(%)	Tiazac® Up to 360 mg n = 149 # pts(%)	Tiazac® 480–540 mg n = 48 # pts(%)	Adverse Events (COSTART Term)	Placebo n = 57 # pts(%)	Tiazac® Up to 360 mg n = 149 # pts(%)	Tiazac® 480–540 mg n = 48 # pts(%)
edema, peripheral	1 (2)	8 (5)	7 (15)	rash	0 (0)	3 (2)	0 (0)
dizziness	4 (7)	6 (4)	2 (4)	infection	2 (4)	2 (1)	3 (6)
vasodilation	1 (2)	5 (3)	1 (2)	diarrhea	0 (0)	2 (1)	1 (2)
dyspepsia	0 (0)	7 (5)	0 (0)	palpitations	0 (0)	2 (1)	1 (2)
pharyngitis	2 (4)	3 (2)	3 (6)	nervousness	0 (0)	3 (2)	0 (0)

MOST COMMON ADVERSE EVENTS IN DOUBLE-BLIND PLACEBO-CONTROLLED ANGINA TRIALS*

Adverse Events (COSTART Term)	Placebo n = 50 # pts(%)	Tiazac® Up to 360 mg n = 158 # pts(%)	Tiazac® 540 mg n = 49 # pts(%)	Adverse Events (COSTART Term)	Placebo n = 50 # pts(%)	Tiazac® Up to 360 mg n = 158 # pts(%)	Tiazac® 540 mg n = 49 # pts(%)
headache	1 (2)	13 (8)	4 (8)	flu syndrome	0 (0)	0 (0)	1 (2)
edema, peripheral	1 (2)	3 (2)	5 (10)	cough increase	0 (0)	2 (1)	1 (2)
pain	1 (2)	10 (6)	3 (6)	extrasystoles	0 (0)	0 (0)	1 (2)
dizziness	0 (0)	5 (3)	5 (10)	gout	0 (0)	2 (1)	1 (2)
asthenia	0 (0)	1 (1)	2 (4)	myalgia	0 (0)	0 (0)	1 (2)
dyspepsia	0 (0)	2 (1)	3 (6)	impotence	0 (0)	0 (0)	1 (2)
dyspnea	0 (0)	1 (1)	3 (6)	conjunctivitis	0 (0)	0 (0)	1 (2)
bronchitis	0 (0)	1 (1)	2 (4)	rash	0 (0)	2 (1)	1 (2)
AV block	0 (0)	0 (0)	2 (4)	abdominal enlargement	0 (0)	0 (0)	1 (2)
infection	0 (0)	2 (1)	1 (2)				

* Adverse events occurring in treated patients at 2% or more than placebo-treated patients.

Strength	Description	Quantity	NDC#
120 mg	#3 lavender/lavender capsule imprinted: Tiazac 120	30's	0456-2612-30
		90's	0456-2612-90
		1000's	0456-2612-00
		HUD's	0456-2612-63
180 mg	#2 white/blue-green capsule imprinted: Tiazac 180	30's	0456-2613-30
		90's	0456-2613-90
		1000's	0456-2613-00
		HUD's	0456-2613-63
240 mg	#1 blue-green/lavender capsule imprinted: Tiazac 240	30's	0456-2614-30
		90's	0456-2614-90
		1000's	0456-2614-00
		HUD's	0456-2614-63
300 mg	#0 white/lavender capsule imprinted: Tiazac 300	30's	0456-2615-30
		90's	0456-2615-90
		1000's	0456-2615-00
		HUD's	0456-2615-63
360 mg	#0 blue-green/blue-green capsule imprinted: Tiazac 360	30's	0456-2616-30
		90's	0456-2616-90
		1000's	0456-2616-00
		HUD's	0456-2616-63

Fujisawa Healthcare, Inc.

PARKWAY NORTH CENTER
3 PARKWAY NORTH
DEERFIELD, IL 60015-2548

For Medical Information Contact:
Generally:
Medical and Scientific Information
(800) 727-7003
In Emergencies:
Medical and Scientific Information
(800) 727-7003

ADENOCARD® IV ℞
(adenosine)
For Rapid Bolus Intravenous Use

DESCRIPTION

Adenosine is an endogenous nucleoside occurring in all cells of the body. It is chemically 6-amino-9-β-D-ribofuranosyl-9-H-purine and has the following structural formula:

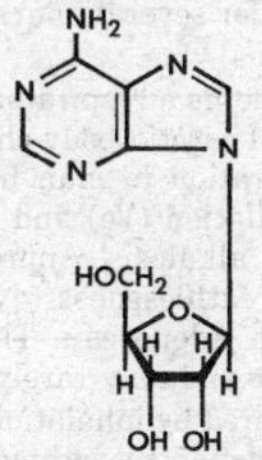

$C_{10}H_{13}N_5O_4$ **267.24**

Adenosine is a white crystalline powder. It is soluble in water and practically insoluble in alcohol. Solubility increases by warming and lowering the pH. Adenosine is not chemically related to other antiarrhythmic drugs. Adenocard® (adenosine) is a sterile solution for rapid bolus intravenous injection. Each mL contains 3 mg adenosine and 9 mg sodium chloride in Water for Injection. The pH of the solution is between 5.5 and 7.5.

CLINICAL PHARMACOLOGY

Mechanism of Action

Adenocard (adenosine) slows conduction time through the A-V node, can interrupt the reentry pathways through the A-V node, and can restore normal sinus rhythm in patients with paroxysmal supraventricular tachycardia (PSVT), including PSVT associated with Wolff-Parkinson-White Syndrome.

Adenocard is antagonized competitively by methylxanthines such as caffeine and theophylline, and potentiated by blockers of nucleoside transport such as dipyridamole. Adenocard is not blocked by atropine.

Hemodynamics

The usual intravenous bolus dose of 6 or 12 mg Adenocard (adenosine) will have no systemic hemodynamic effects. When larger doses are given by infusion, adenosine decreases blood pressure by decreasing peripheral resistance.

Pharmacokinetics

Intravenously administered adenosine is rapidly cleared from the circulation via cellular uptake, primarily by erythrocytes and vascular endothelial cells. This process involves a specific transmembrane nucleoside carrier system that is reversible, nonconcentrative, and bidirectionally symmetrical. Intracellular adenosine is rapidly metabolized either via phosphorlation to adenosine monophosphate by adenosine kinase, or via deamination to inosine by adenosine deaminase in the cytosol. Since adenosine kinase has a lower K_m and V_{max} than adenosine deaminase, deamination plays a significant role only when cytosolic adenosine saturates the phosphorylation pathway. Inosine formed by deamination of adenosine can leave the cell intact or can be degraded to hypoxanthine, xanthine, and ultimately uric acid. Adenosine monophosphate formed by phosphorylation of adenosine is incorporated into the high-energy phosphate pool. While extracellular adenosine is primarily cleared by cellular uptake with a half-life of less than 10 seconds in whole blood, excessive amounts may be deaminated by an ecto-form of adenosine deaminase. As Adenocard requires no hepatic or renal function for its activation or inactivation, hepatic and renal failure would not be expected to alter its effectiveness or tolerability.

Clinical Trial Results

In controlled studies in the United States, bolus doses of 3, 6, 9, and 12 mg were studied. A cumulative 60% of patients with paroxysmal supraventricular tachycardia had converted to normal sinus rhythm within one minute after an intravenous bolus dose of 6 mg Adenocard (some converted on 3 mg and failures were given 6 mg), and a cumulative 92% converted after a bolus dose of 12 mg. Seven to sixteen percent of patients converted after 1–4 placebo bolus injections. Similar responses were seen in a variety of patient subsets, including those using or not using digoxin, those with Wolff-Parkinson-White Syndrome, males, females, blacks, Caucasians, and Hispanics.

Adenosine is not effective in converting rhythms other than PSVT, such as atrial flutter, atrial fibrillation, or ventricular tachycardia, to normal sinus rhythm. To date, such patients have not had adverse consequences following administration of adenosine.

INDICATIONS AND USAGE

Intravenous Adenocard (adenosine) is indicated for the following.

Conversion to sinus rhythm of paroxysmal supraventricular tachycardia (PSVT), including that associated with accessory bypass tracts (Wolff-Parkinson-White Syndrome). When clinically advisable, appropriate vagal maneuvers (e.g., Valsalva maneuver), should be attempted prior to Adenocard administration.

It is important to be sure the Adenocard solution actually reaches the systemic circulation (see **DOSAGE AND ADMINISTRATION**).

Adenocard does not convert atrial flutter, atrial fibrillation, or ventricular tachycardia to normal sinus rhythm. In the presence of atrial flutter or atrial fibrillation, a transient modest slowing of ventricular response may occur immediately following Adenocard administration.

CONTRAINDICATIONS

Intravenous Adenocard (adenosine) is contraindicated in:

1. Second- or third-degree A-V block (except in patients with a functioning artificial pacemaker).
2. Sinus node disease, such as sick sinus syndrome or symptomatic bradycardia (except in patients with a functioning artificial pacemaker).
3. Known hypersensitivity to adenosine.

WARNINGS

Heart Block

Adenocard (adenosine) exerts its effect by decreasing conduction through the A-V node and may produce a short lasting first-, second- or third-degree heart block. In extreme cases, transient asystole may result (one case has been reported in a patient with atrial flutter who was receiving carbamazepine). Appropriate therapy should be instituted as needed. Patients who develop high-level block on one dose of Adenocard should not be given additional doses. Because of the very short half-life of adenosine, these effects are generally self-limiting.

Rarely, ventricular fibrillation has been reported following Adenocard administration, including both resuscitated and fatal events. In most instances, these cases were associated with the concomitant use of digoxin and, less frequently with digoxin and verapamil. Although no causal relationship or drug-drug interaction has been established, Adenocard should be used with caution in patients receiving digoxin or digoxin and verapamil in combination. Appropriate resuscitative measures should be available.

Arrhythmias at Time of Conversion

At the time of conversion to normal sinus rhythm, a variety of new rhythms may appear on the electrocardiogram. They generally last only a few seconds without intervention, and may take the form of premature ventricular contractions, atrial premature contractions, sinus bradycardia, sinus tachycardia, skipped beats, and varying degrees of A-V nodal block. Such findings were seen in 55% of patients.

Bronchoconstriction

Adenocard (adenosine) is a respiratory stimulant (probably through activation of carotid body chemoreceptors) and intravenous administration in man has been shown to increase minute ventilation (Ve) and reduce arterial PCO_2 causing respiratory alkalosis.

Adenosine administered by inhalation has been reported to cause bronchoconstriction in asthmatic patients, presumably due to mast cell degranulation and histamine release. These effects have not been observed in normal subjects. Adenocard has been administered to a limited number of patients with asthma and mild to moderate exacerbation of their symptoms has been reported. Respiratory compromise has occurred during adenosine infusion in patients with obstructive pulmonary disease. Adenocard should be used with caution in patients with obstructive lung disease not associated with bronchoconstriction (e.g., emphysema, bronchitis, etc.) and should be avoided in patients with bronchoconstriction or bronchospasm (e.g., asthma). Adenocard should be discontinued in any patient who develops severe respiratory difficulties.

PRECAUTIONS

Drug Interactions

Intravenous Adenocard (adenosine) has been effectively administered in the presence of other cardioactive drugs, such as quinidine, beta-adrenergic blocking agents, calcium channel blocking agents, and angiotensin converting enzyme inhibitors, without any change in the adverse reaction profile. Digoxin and verapamil use may be rarely associated with ventricular fibrillation when combined with Adenocard (see **WARNINGS**). Because of the potential for additive or synergistic depressant effects on the SA and AV nodes, however, Adenocard should be used with caution in the presence of these agents. The use of Adenocard in patients receiving digitalis may be rarely associated with ventricular fibrillation (see **WARNINGS**).

The effects of adenosine are antagonized by methylxanthines such as caffeine and theophylline. In the presence of these methylxanthines, larger doses of adenosine may be required or adenosine may not be effective. Adenosine effects are potentiated by dipyridamole. Thus, smaller doses of adenosine may be effective in the presence of dipyridamole. Carbamazepine has been reported to increase the degree of heart block produced by other agents. As the primary effect of adenosine is to decrease conduction through the A-V node, higher degrees of heart block may be produced in the presence of carbamazepine.

Carcinogenesis, Mutagenesis, Impairment of Fertility

Studies in animals have not been performed to evaluate the carcinogenic potential of Adenocard (adenosine). Adenosine was negative for genotoxic potential in the Salmonella (Ames Test) and Mammalian Microsome Assay.

Adenosine, however, like other nucleosides at millimolar concentrations present for several doubling times of cells in culture, is known to produce a variety of chromosomal alterations. In rats and mice, adenosine administered intraperitoneally once a day for five days at 50, 100, and 150 mg/kg [10–30 (rats) and 5–15 (mice) times human dosage on a mg/M² basis] caused decreased spermatogenesis and increased numbers of abnormal sperm, a reflection of the ability of adenosine to produce chromosomal damage.

Pregnancy Category C

Animal reproduction studies have not been conducted with adenosine; nor have studies been performed in pregnant women. As adenosine is a naturally occurring material, widely dispersed throughout the body, no fetal effects would be anticipated. However, since it is not known whether Adenocard can cause fetal harm when administered to pregnant women, Adenocard should be used during pregnancy only if clearly needed.

Pediatrics

No controlled studies have been conducted in pediatric patients.

ADVERSE REACTIONS

The following reactions were reported with intravenous Adenocard (adenosine) used in controlled U.S. clinical trials. The placebo group had a less than 1% rate of all of these reactions.

Cardiovascular	Facial flushing, (18%), headache (2%), sweating, palpitations, chest pain, hypotension (less than 1%).
Respiratory	Shortness of breath/ dyspnea (12%), chest pressure (7%), hyperventilation, head pressure (less than 1%).
Central Nervous System	Lightheadedness (2%), dizziness, tingling in arms, numbness (1%), apprehension, blurred vision, burning sensation, heaviness in arms, neck and back pain (less than 1%).
Gastrointestinal	Nausea (3%), metallic taste, tightness in throat, pressure in groin (less than 1%).

In post-market clinical experience with Adenocard, cases of prolonged asystole, ventricular tachycardia, ventricular fibrillation, transient increase in blood pressure, bradycardia, hypotension, atrial fibrillation, and bronchospasm, in association with Adenocard use, have been reported.

OVERDOSAGE

The half-life of Adenocard (adenosine) is less than 10 seconds. Thus, adverse effects are generally rapidly self-limiting. Treatment of any prolonged adverse effects should be individualized and be directed toward the specific effect. Methylxanthines, such as caffeine and theophylline, are competitive antagonists of adenosine.

DOSAGE AND ADMINISTRATION

For rapid bolus intravenous use only.

Adenocard (adenosine) Injection should be given as a rapid bolus by the peripheral intravenous route. To be certain the solution reaches the systemic circulation, it should be administered either directly into a vein or, if given into an IV line, it should be given as close to the patient as possible and followed by a rapid saline flush.

The dose recommendation is based on clinical studies with peripheral venous bolus dosing. Central venous (CVP or other) administration of Adenocard has not been systematically studied.

Continued on next page

Adenocard—Cont.

The recommended intravenous doses for adults are as follows:

Initial dose: 6 mg given as a rapid intravenous bolus (administered over a 1–2 second period).

Repeat administration: If the first dose does not result in elimination of the supraventricular tachycardia within 1–2 minutes, 12 mg should be given as a rapid intravenous bolus. This 12 mg dose may be repeated a second time if required.

Doses greater than 12 mg are not recommended.

NOTE: Parenteral drug products should be inspected visually for particulate matter and discoloration prior to administration.

HOW SUPPLIED

Adenocard® (adenosine) Injection is supplied as a sterile solution in normal saline.

NDC 0469-0872-02 Product Code 87102 6 mg/2 mL (3mg/mL) in 2 mL flip-top vials, packaged in 10's

NDC 0469-7234-12 Product Code 723412 6 mg/2 mL (3mg/mL) in 2 mL disposable syringe, in a package of five.

NDC 0469-7234-14 Product Code 723414 12 mg/4 mL (3mg/mL) in a 5 mL disposable syringe, in a package of five.

Store at controlled room temperature 15°–30°C (59°–86°F).

DO NOT REFRIGERATE as crystallization may occur. If crystallization has occurred, dissolve crystals by warming to room temperature. The solution must be clear at the time of use.

Contains no preservatives. Discard unused portion.

CAUTION: Federal law prohibits dispensing without prescription.

Fujisawa USA, Inc., Deerfield IL 60015
Under license from Medco Research, Inc.
Research Triangle Park, NC 27709
45514H
Revised: July 1996

ADENOSCAN® ℞

adenosine
For Intravenous Infusion Only

DESCRIPTION

Adenosine is an endogenous nucleoside occurring in all cells of the body. It is chemically 6-amino-9-beta-D-ribofuranosyl-9-H-purine and has the following structural formula:

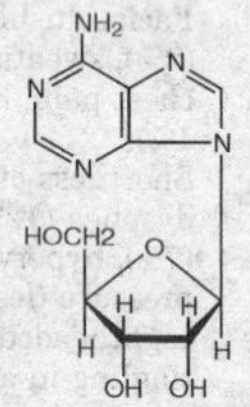

$C_{10}H_{13}N_5O_4$ **267.24**

Adenosine is a white crystalline powder. It is soluble in water and practically insoluble in alcohol. Solubility increases by warming and lowering the pH of the solution.

Each Adenoscan vial contains a sterile, nonpyrogenic solution of adenosine 3 mg/mL and sodium chloride 9 mg/mL in Water for Injection, q.s. The pH of the solution is between 4.5 and 7.5.

CLINICAL PHARMACOLOGY

Mechanism of Action

Adenosine is a potent vasodilator in most vascular beds, except in renal afferent arterioles and hepatic veins where it produces vasoconstriction. Adenosine is thought to exert its pharmacological effects through activation of purine receptors (cell-surface A_1 and A_2 adenosine receptors). Although the exact mechanism by which adenosine receptor activation relaxes vascular smooth muscle is not known, there is evidence to support both inhibition of the slow inward calcium current reducing calcium uptake, and activation of adenylate cyclase through A_2 receptors in smooth muscle cells. Adenosine may also lessen vascular tone by modulating sympathetic neurotransmission. The intracellular uptake of adenosine is mediated by a specific transmembrane nucleoside transport system. Once inside the cell, adenosine is rapidly phosphorylated by adenosine kinase to adenosine monophosphate, or deaminated by adenosine deaminase to inosine. These intracellular metabolites of adenosine are not vasoactive.

Myocardial uptake of thallium-201 is directly proportional to coronary blood flow. Since Adenoscan significantly increases blood flow in normal coronary arteries with little or no increase in stenotic arteries, Adenoscan causes relatively less thallium-201 uptake in vascular territories supplied by stenotic coronary arteries i.e., a greater difference is seen after Adenoscan between areas served by normal and areas served by stenotic vessels than is seen prior to Adenoscan.

Hemodynamics

Adenosine produces a direct negative chronotropic, dromotropic and inotropic effect on the heart, presumably due to A_1-receptor agonism, and produces peripheral vasodilation, presumably due to A_2-receptor agonism. The net effect of Adenoscan in humans is typically a mild to moderate reduction in systolic, diastolic and mean arterial blood pressure associated with a reflex increase in heart rate. Rarely, significant hypotension and tachycardia have been observed.

Pharmacokinetics

Intravenously administered adenosine is rapidly cleared from the circulation via cellular uptake, primarily by erythrocytes and vascular endothelial cells. This process involves a specific transmembrane nucleoside carrier system that is reversible, nonconcentrative, and bidirectionally symmetrical. Intracellular adenosine is rapidly metabolized either via phosphorylation to adenosine monophosphate by adenosine kinase, or via deamination to inosine by adenosine deaminase in the cytosol. Since adenosine kinase has a lower K_m and V_{max} than adenosine deaminase, deamination plays a significant role only when cytosolic adenosine saturates the phosphorylation pathway. Inosine formed by deamination of adenosine can leave the cell intact or can be degraded to hypoxanthine, xanthine, and ultimately uric acid. Adenosine monophosphate formed by phosphorylation of adenosine is incorporated into the high-energy phosphate pool. While extracellular adenosine is primarily cleared by cellular uptake with a half-life of less than 10 seconds in whole blood, excessive amounts may be deaminated by an ectoform of adenosine deaminase. As Adenoscan requires no hepatic or renal function for its activation or inactivation, hepatic and renal failure would not be expected to alter its effectiveness or tolerability.

Clinical Trials

In two crossover comparative studies involving 319 subjects who could exercise (including 106 healthy volunteers and 213 patients with known or suspected coronary disease), Adenoscan and exercise thallium images were compared by blinded observers. The images were concordant for the presence of perfusion defects in 85.5% of cases by global analysis (patient by patient) and up to 93% of cases based on vascular territories. In these two studies, 193 patients also had recent coronary arteriography for comparison (healthy volunteers were not catheterized). The sensitivity (true positive Adenoscan divided by the number of patients with positive (abnormal) angiography) for detecting angiographically significant disease (≥50% reduction in the luminal diameter of at least one major vessel) was 64% for Adenoscan and 64% for exercise testing, while the specificity (true negative divided by the number of patients with negative angiograms) was 54% for Adenoscan and 65% for exercise testing. The 95% confidence limits for Adenoscan sensitivity were 56% to 78% and for specificity were 37% to 71%.

Intracoronary Doppler flow catheter studies have demonstrated that a dose of intravenous Adenoscan of 140 mcg/kg/min produces maximum coronary hyperemia (relative to intracoronary papaverine) in approximately 95% of cases within two to three minutes of the onset of the infusion. Coronary blood flow velocity returns to basal levels within one to two minutes of discontinuing the Adenoscan infusion.

INDICATIONS AND USAGE

Intravenous Adenoscan is indicated as an adjunct to thallium-201 myocardial perfusion scintigraphy in patients unable to exercise adequately. (See **WARNINGS**).

CONTRAINDICATIONS

Intravenous Adenoscan (adenosine) should not be administered to individuals with:

1. Second- or third-degree AV block (except in patients with a functioning artificial pacemaker).
2. Sinus node disease, such as sick sinus syndrome or symptomatic bradycardia (except in patients with a functioning artificial pacemaker).
3. Known or suspected bronchoconstrictive or bronchospastic lung disease (e.g., asthma).
4. Known hypersensitivity to adenosine.

WARNINGS

Fatal Cardiac Arrest, Life Threatening Ventricular Arrhythmias, and Myocardial Infarction.

Fatal cardiac arrest, sustained ventricular tachycardia (requiring resuscitation), and nonfatal myocardial infarction have been reported coincident with Adenoscan infusion. Patients with unstable angina may be at greater risk. Appropriate resuscitative measures should be available.

Sinoatrial and Atrioventricular Nodal Block

Adenoscan (adenosine) exerts a direct depressant effect on the SA and AV nodes and has the potential to cause first-, second- or third-degree AV block, or sinus bradycardia. Approximately 6.3% of patients develop AV block with Adenoscan, including first-degree (2.9%), second-degree (2.6%) and third-degree (0.8%) heart block. All episodes of AV block have been asymptomatic, transient, and did not require intervention. Adenoscan can cause sinus bradycardia. Adenoscan should be used with caution in patients with preexisting first-degree AV block or bundle branch block and should be avoided in patients with high-grade AV block or sinus node dysfunction (except in patients with a functioning artificial pacemaker). Adenoscan should be discontinued in any patient who develops persistent or symptomatic high-grade AV block. Sinus pause has been rarely observed with adenosine infusions.

Hypotension

Adenoscan (adenosine) is a potent peripheral vasodilator and can cause significant hypotension. Patients with an intact baroreceptor reflux mechanism are able to maintain blood pressure and tissue perfusion in response to Adenoscan by increasing heart rate and cardiac output. However, Adenoscan should be used with caution in patients with autonomic dysfunction, stenotic valvular heart disease, pericarditis or pericardial effusions, stenotic carotid artery disease with cerebrovascular insufficiency, or uncorrected hypovolemia, due to the risk of hypotensive complications in these patients. Adenoscan should be discontinued in any patient who develops persistent or symptomatic hypotension.

Hypertension

Increases in systolic and diastolic pressure have been observed (as great as 140 mm Hg systolic in one case) concomitant with Adenoscan infusion; most increases resolved spontaneously within several minutes, but in some cases, hypertension lasted for several hours.

Bronchoconstriction

Adenoscan (adenosine) is a respiratory stimulant (probably through activation of carotid body chemoreceptors) and intravenous administration in man has been shown to increase minute ventilation (Ve) and reduce arterial PCO_2 causing respiratory alkalosis. Approximately 28% of patients experience breathlessness (dyspnea) or an urge to breathe deeply with Adenoscan. These respiratory complaints are transient and only rarely require intervention.

Adenosine administered by inhalation has been reported to cause bronchoconstriction in asthmatic patients, presumably due to mast cell degranulation and histamine release. These effects have not been observed in normal subjects. Adenoscan has been administered to a limited number of patients with asthma and mild to moderate exacerbation of their symptoms has been reported. Respiratory compromise has occurred during adenosine infusion in patients with obstructive pulmonary disease. Adenoscan should be used with caution in patients with obstructive lung disease not associated with bronchoconstriction (e.g., emphysema, bronchitis, etc.) and should be avoided in patients with bronchoconstriction or bronchospasm (e.g., asthma). Adenoscan should be discontinued in any patient who develops severe respiratory difficulties.

PRECAUTIONS

Drug Interactions

Intravenous Adenoscan (adenosine) has been given with other cardioactive drugs (such as beta adrenergic blocking agents, cardiac glycosides, and calcium channel blockers) without apparent adverse interactions, but its effectiveness with these agents has not been systematically evaluated. Because of the potential for additive or synergistic depressant effects on the SA and AV nodes, however, Adenoscan should be used with caution in the presence of these agents. The vasoactive effects of the Adenoscan are inhibited by adenosine receptor antagonists, such as alkylxanthines (e.g., caffeine and theophylline). The safety and efficacy of Adenoscan in the presence of these agents has not been systematically evaluated.

The vasoactive effects of Adenoscan are potentiated by nucleoside transport inhibitors, such as dipyridamole. The safety and efficacy of Adenoscan in the presence of dipyridamole has not been systematically evaluated.

Whenever possible, drugs that might inhibit or augment the effects of adenosine should be withheld for at least five half-lives prior to the use of Adenoscan.

Carcinogenesis, Mutagenesis, Impairment of Fertility

Studies in animals have not been performed to evaluate the carcinogenic potential of Adenoscan (adenosine). Adenosine was negative for genotoxic potential in the Salmonella (Ames Test) and Mammalian Microsome Assay.

Adenosine, however, like other nucleosides at millimolar concentrations present for several doubling times of cells in culture, is known to produce a variety of chromosomal alterations. In rats and mice, adenosine administered intraperitoneally once a day for five days at 50, 100, and 150 mg/kg [10-30 (rats) and 5-15 (mice) times human dosage on a mg/M^2 basis] caused decreased spermatogenesis and increased numbers of abnormal sperm, a reflection of the ability of adenosine to produce chromosomal damage.

Pregnancy Category C

Animal reproduction studies have not been conducted with adenosine; nor have studies been performed in pregnant women. Because it is not known whether Adenoscan can cause fetal harm when administered to pregnant women, Adenoscan should be used during pregnancy only if clearly needed.

Pediatric Use
The safety and effectiveness of Adenoscan in patients less than 18 years of age have not been established.

ADVERSE REACTIONS
The following reactions with an incidence of at least 1% were reported with intravenous Adenoscan among 1421 patients enrolled in controlled and uncontrolled U.S. clinical trials. Despite the short half-life of adenosine, 10.6% of the side effects occurred not with the infusion of Adenoscan but several hours after the infusion terminated. Also, 8.4% of the side effects that began coincident with the infusion persisted for up to 24 hours after the infusion was complete. In many cases, it is not possible to know whether these late adverse events are the result of Adenoscan infusion.

Flushing	44%
Chest discomfort	40%
Dyspnea or urge to breathe deeply	28%
Headache	18%
Throat, neck or jaw discomfort	15%
Gastrointestinal discomfort	13%
Lightheadedness/dizziness	12%
Upper extremity discomfort	4%
ST segment depression	3%
First-degree AV block	3%
Second-degree AV block	3%
Paresthesia	2%
Hypotension	2%
Nervousness	2%
Arrhythmias	1%

Adverse experiences of any severity reported in less than 1% of patients include:
Body as a Whole: back discomfort; lower extremity discomfort; weakness.
Cardiovascular System: nonfatal myocardial infarction; life-threatening ventricular arrhythmia; third-degree AV block; bradycardia; palpitation; sinus exit block; sinus pause; sweating; T-wave changes, hypertension (systolic blood pressure >200 mm Hg).
Central Nervous System: drowsiness; emotional instability; tremors.
Genital/Urinary System: vaginal pressure; urgency.
Respiratory System: cough.
Special Senses: blurred vision; dry mouth; ear discomfort; metallic taste; nasal congestion; scotomas; tongue discomfort.

OVERDOSAGE
The half-life of adenosine is less than 10 seconds and side effects of Adenoscan (when they occur) usually resolve quickly when the infusion is discontinued, although delayed or persistent effects have been observed. Methylxanthines, such as caffeine and theophylline, are competitive adenosine receptor antagonists and theophylline has been used to effectively terminate persistent side effects. In controlled U.S. clinical trials, theophylline (50-125 mg slow intravenous injection) was needed to abort Adenoscan side effects in less than 2% of patients.

DOSAGE AND ADMINISTRATION
For intravenous infusion only.
Adenoscan should be given as a continuous peripheral intravenous infusion.
The recommended intravenous dose for adults is 140 mcg/kg/min infused for six minutes (total dose of 0.84 mg/kg).
The required dose of thallium-201 should be injected at the midpoint of the Adenoscan infusion (i.e., after the first three minutes of Adenoscan). Thallium-201 is physically compatible with Adenoscan and may be injected directly into the Adenoscan infusion set.
The injection should be as close to the venous access as possible to prevent an inadvertent increase in the dose of Adenoscan (the contents of the IV tubing) being administered. There are no data on the safety or efficacy of alternative Adenoscan infusion protocols.
The safety and efficacy of Adenoscan administered by the intracoronary route have not been established.
The following Adenoscan infusion nomogram may be used to determine the appropriate infusion rate corrected for total body weight:

Patient Weight		Infusion Rate
kg	lbs	mL/min
45	99	2.1
50	110	2.3
55	121	2.6
60	132	2.8
65	143	3.0
70	154	3.3
75	165	3.5
80	176	3.8
85	187	4.0
90	198	4.2

This nomogram was derived from the following general formula:

$$\frac{0.140 \text{ (mg/kg/min)} \times \text{total body weight (kg)}}{\text{Adenoscan concentration (3 mg/mL)}} = \frac{\text{infusion rate}}{\text{(mL/min)}}$$

Note: Parenteral drug products should be inspected visually for particulate matter and discoloration prior to administration.

HOW SUPPLIED
Adenoscan (adenosine) is supplied as 20 mL and 30 mL vials of sterile nonpyrogenic solution in normal saline.

Product Code	NDC No.	
87120	0469-0871-20	60 mg/20 mL (3 mg/mL) in a 20 mL single-dose, flip-top glass vial, packaged individually and in packages of ten.
87130	0469-0871-30	90 mg/30 mL (3mg/mL) in a 30 mL single-dose, flip-top glass vial, packaged individually and in packages of ten.

Store at controlled room temperature 15°-30°C (59°-86°F). Do not refrigerate as crystallization may occur. If crystallization has occurred, dissolve crystals by warming to room temperature. The solution must be clear at the time of use. Contains no preservative. Discard unused portion.
CAUTION: Federal law prohibits dispensing without a prescription.
Fujisawa USA, Inc.
Deerfield, IL 60015
Under license from Medco Research, Inc.
Research Triangle Park, NC 27709
45558E/Revised: August 1997

AMBISOME®   ℞
[ăm-bĭ-sōme]
(amphotericin B) liposome for injection

DESCRIPTION
AmBisome for injection is a sterile, non-pyrogenic lyophilized product for intravenous infusion. Each vial contains 50 mg of amphotericin B, USP, intercalated into a liposomal membrane consisting of approximately 213 mg hydrogenated soy phosphatidylcholine; 52 mg cholesterol, NF; 84 mg distearoylphosphatidylglycerol; 0.64 mg alpha tocopherol, USP; together with 900 mg sucrose, NF; and 27 mg disodium succinate hexhydrate as buffer. Following reconstitution with Sterile Water for Injection, USP, the resulting pH of the suspension is between 5.0–6.0.
AmBisome is a true single bilayer liposomal drug delivery system. Liposomes are closed, spherical vesicles created by mixing specific proportions of amphophilic substances such as phospholipids and cholesterol so that they arrange themselves into multiple concentric bilayer membranes when hydrated in aqueous solutions. Single bilayer liposomes are then formed by microemulsification of multilamellar vesicles using a homogenizer. AmBisome consists of these unilamellar bilayer liposomes with amphotericin B intercalated within the membrane. Due to the nature and quantity of amphophilic substances used, and the lipophilic moiety in the amphotericin B molecule, the drug is an integral part of the overall structure of the AmBisome liposomes. AmBisome contains true liposomes that are less than 100 nm in diameter. A schematic depiction of the liposome is presented below.

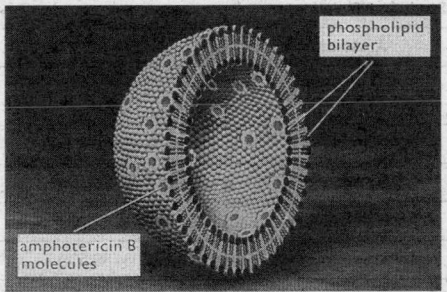

Cross-Sectional View of AmBisome Liposome

Note: Liposomal encapsulation or incorporation into a lipid complex can substantially affect a drug's functional properties relative to those of the unencapsulated drug or non-lipid associated drug. In addition, different liposomal or lipid-complex products with a common active ingredient may vary from one another in the chemical composition and physical form of the lipid component. Such differences may affect the functional properties of these drug products.

Amphotericin B is a macrocyclic, polyene, antifungal antibiotic produced from a strain of *Streptomyces nodosus.*
Amphotericin B is designated chemically as:
[1R-(1R*,3S*,5R*,6R*,9R*,11R*,15S*,16R*,17R*,18S*,19E, 21E,23E,25E,27E,29E,31E,33R*,35S*,36R*,37S*,)]-33-[(3-Amino-3,6-dideoxy-β-D-mannopyranosyl)-oxy]-1,3,5,6,9,11, 17,37-octahydroxy-15,16,18-trimethyl-13-oxo-14,39-dioxabicyclo[33.3.1]nonatriaconta-19,21,23,25,27,29,31-heptaene-36-carboxylic acid (CAS No. 1397-89-3).
Amphotericin B has a molecular formula of $C_{47}H_{73}NO_{17}$ and a molecular weight of 924.09.
The structure of amphotericin B is shown below:

MICROBIOLOGY
Mechanism of Action
Amphotericin B, the active ingredient of AmBisome, acts by binding to the sterol component of a cell membrane leading to alterations in cell permeability and cell death. While amphotericin B has a higher affinity for the ergosterol component of the fungal cell membrane, it can also bind to the cholesterol component of the mammalian cell leading to cytotoxicity. AmBisome, the liposomal preparation of amphotericin B, has been shown to penetrate the cell wall of both extracellular and intracellular forms of susceptible fungi.
Activity *In Vitro* and *In Vivo*
AmBisome has shown *in vitro* activity comparable to amphotericin B against the following organisms: *Aspergillus* species (*A. fumigatus, A. flavus*), *Candida* species (*C. albicans, C. krusei, C. lusitaniae, C. parapsilosis, C. tropicalis*), *Cryptococcus neoformans,* and *Blastomyces dermatitidis.* However, standardized techniques for susceptibility testing of antifungal agents have not been established and results of such studies do not necessarily correlate with clinical outcome.
AmBisome is active in animal models against *Aspergillus fumigatus, Candida albicans, Candida krusei, Candida lusitaniae, Cryptococcus neoformans, Blastomyces dermatitidis, Coccidioides immitis, Histoplasma capsulatum, Paracoccidioides brasiliensis, Leishmania donovani* and *Leishmania infatum.* The administration of AmBisome in these animal models demonstrated prolonged survival of infected animals, reduction of microorganisms from target organs, or a decrease in lung weight.
Drug Resistance
Mutants with decreased susceptibility to amphotericin B have been isolated from several fungal species after serial passage in culture media containing the drug, and from some patients receiving prolonged therapy. Drug combination studies *in vitro* and *in vivo* suggest that imidazoles may induce resistance to amphotericin B. However, the clinical relevance to drug resistance has not been established.

CLINICAL PHARMACOLOGY
Pharmacokinetics
The assay used to measure amphotericin B in the serum after administration of AmBisome does not distinguish amphotericin B that is complexed with the phospholipids of AmBisome from amphotericin B that is uncomplexed. The pharmacokinetic profile of amphotericin B after administration of AmBisome is based upon total serum concentrations of amphotericin B. The pharmacokinetic profile of amphotericin B was determined in febrile neutropenic cancer and bone marrow transplant patients who received 1–2 hour infusions of 1.0 to 5.0 mg/kg/day AmBisome for 3 to 20 days. The pharmacokinetics of amphotericin B after administration of AmBisome are nonlinear such that there is a greater than proportional increase in serum concentrations with an increase in dose from 1.0 to 5.0 mg/kg/day. The pharmacokinetic parameters of total amphotericin B (mean ± SD) after the first dose and at steady state are shown in the table below.
[See table at top of next page]
Distribution
Based on total amphotericin B concentrations measured within a dosing interval (24 hours) after administration of AmBisome, the mean half-life was 7–10 hours. However, based on total amphotericin B concentration measured up to 49 days after dosing AmBisome, the mean half-life was 100–153 hours. The long terminal elimination half-life is probably a slow redistribution from tissues. Steady state concentrations were generally achieved within 4 days of dosing.

Continued on next page

Ambisome—Cont.

Although variable, mean trough concentrations of amphotericin B remained relatively constant with repeated administration of the same dose over the range of 1.0 to 5.0 mg/kg/day, indicating no significant drug accumulation in the serum.

Metabolism
The metabolic pathways of AmBisome are not known.

Excretion
The mean clearance at steady state was independent of dose. The excretion of amphotericin B after administration of AmBisome has not been studied.

Pharmacokinetics in Special Populations

Renal Impairment
The effect of renal impairment on the disposition of AmBisome has not been studied. However, AmBisome has been successfully administered to patients with pre-existing renal impairment (see **DESCRIPTION OF CLINICAL STUDIES**).

Hepatic Impairment
The effect of hepatic impairment on the disposition of AmBisome is not known.

Pediatric and Elderly Patients
The pharmacokinetics of amphotericin B after administration of AmBisome in pediatric and elderly patients have not been studied; however, AmBisome has been used in pediatric and elderly patients (see **DESCRIPTION OF CLINICAL STUDIES**).

Gender and Ethnicity
The effect of gender or ethnicity on the pharmacokinetics of amphotericin B after administration of AmBisome is not known.

INDICATIONS AND USAGE

AmBisome is indicated for the following:

• Empirical therapy for presumed fungal infection in febrile, neutropenic patients.

• Treatment of patients with *Aspergillus* species, *Candida* species and/or *Cryptococcus* species infections refractory to amphotericin B deoxycholate, or in patients where renal impairment or unacceptable toxicity precludes the use of amphotericin B deoxycholate.

• Treatment of visceral leishmaniasis. In immunocompromised patients treated with AmBisome, relapse rates were high following initial clearance of parasites (see **DESCRIPTION OF CLINICAL STUDIES**).

See **DOSAGE AND ADMINISTRATION** for recommended doses by indication.

DESCRIPTION OF CLINICAL STUDIES

Nine clinical studies supporting the efficacy and safety of AmBisome were conducted. This clinical program included both controlled and uncontrolled clinical studies. These studies, which involved 1654 patients, included patients with confirmed systemic mycoses, empirical therapy, and visceral leishmaniasis.

Fifteen hundred and six episodes were evaluable for efficacy, of which 979 (273 patients and 706 adults) were treated with AmBisome.

Three controlled empirical therapy trials compared the efficacy and safety of AmBisome to amphotericin B. One of these studies was conducted in a pediatric population, one in adults, and one in patients aged 2–80 years.

One compassionate use study enrolled patients who had failed amphotericin B deoxycholate therapy or who were unable to receive amphotericin B deoxycholate because of renal insufficiency.

Empirical Therapy in Febrile Neutropenic Patients
Study 94-0-002, a randomized, double-blind, comparative multi-center trial, evaluated the efficacy of AmBisome (1.5–6.0 mg/kg/day) compared with amphotericin B deoxycholate (0.3–1.2 mg/kg/day) in the empirical treatment of 687 adult and pediatric neutropenic patients who were febrile despite

having received at least 96 hours of broad spectrum antibacterial therapy. Therapeutic success required (a) resolution of fever during the neutropenic period, (b) absence of an emergent fungal infection, (c) patient survival for at least 7 days post therapy, (d) no discontinuation of therapy due to toxicity or lack of efficacy, and (e) resolution of any study-entry fungal infection.

The overall therapeutic success rates for AmBisome and amphotericin B deoxycholate were equivalent. Results are summarized in the following table. Note: The categories presented below are not mutually exclusive.

[See table below]

This therapeutic equivalence had no apparent relationship to the use of prestudy antifungal prophylaxis or concomitant granulocytic colony stimulating factors.

The incidence of mycologically confirmed and clinically diagnosed, emergent fungal infections are presented in the following table. AmBisome and amphotericin B were found to be equivalent with respect to the total number of emergent fungal infections.

[See first table at bottom of next page]

Mycologically confirmed fungal infections at study-entry were cured in 8 of 11 patients in the AmBisome group and 7 of 10 in the amphotericin B group.

Two supportive prospective randomized, open label, comparative multi-center studies examined the efficacy of two dosages of AmBisome (1 and 3 mg/kg/day) compared to amphotericin B deoxycholate (1 mg/kg/day) in the treatment of neutropenic patients with presumed fungal infections. These patients were undergoing chemotherapy as part of a bone marrow transplant or had hematological disease. Study 104–10 enrolled adult patients (n=134). Study 104–14 enrolled pediatric patients (n=214). Both studies support the efficacy equivalence of AmBisome and amphotericin B as empirical therapy in febrile neutropenic patients.

Treatment of Patients with *Aspergillus* Species, *Candida* Species and/or *Cryptococcus* Species Infections Refractory to Amphotericin B Deoxycholate, or in Patients Where Renal Impairment or Unacceptable Toxicity Precludes the Use of Amphotericin B Deoxycholate

AmBisome was evaluated in a compassionate use study in hospitalized patients with systemic fungal infections. These patients either had fungal infections refractory to amphotericin B deoxycholate, were intolerant to the use of amphotericin B deoxycholate, or had pre-existing renal insufficiency. Patient recruitment involved 140 infectious episodes in 133 patients, with 53 episodes evaluable for mycological response and 91 episodes evaluable for clinical outcome.

Clinical success and mycological eradication occurred in some patients with documented aspergillosis, candidiasis, and cryptococcus.

Treatment of Visceral Leishmaniasis
AmBisome was studied in patients with visceral leishmaniasis who were infected in the Mediterranean basin with documented or presumed *Leishmaniasis infantum*. Clinical studies have not provided conclusive data regarding efficacy against *L. donovani* and *L. chagasi*.

AmBisome achieved high rates of acute parasite clearance in immunocompetent patients when total doses of 12–30 mg/kg were administered. Most of these immunocompetent patients remained relapse-free during follow-up periods of 6 months or longer. While acute parasite clearance was achieved in most of the immunocompromised patients who received total doses of 30–40 mg/kg, the majority of these patients were observed to relapse in the 6 months following the completion of therapy. Of the 21 immunocompromised patients studied, 17 were coinfected with HIV, approximately half of the HIV infected patients had AIDS. The following table presents a comparison of efficacy rates among immunocompetent and immunocompromised patients infected in the Mediterranean basin who had no prior treatment or remote prior treatment for visceral leishmaniasis. Efficacy is expressed as both acute parasite clearance at the end of therapy (EOT) and as overall success (clearance with no relapse) during the follow-up period (F/U) of greater than 6 months for immunocompromised patients:

[See table at bottom of next page]

When followed for 6 months or more after treatment, the overall success rates among immunocompetent patients was 96.5% and the overall success rate among immunocompromised patients was 11.8% due to relapse in the majority of patients. While case reports have suggested there may be a role for long-term therapy to prevent relapses in HIV coinfected patients (Lopez-Dupla, et al. *J. Antimicrob Chemother* 1993;32:657-659), there were no data to date documenting the efficacy or safety of repeat courses of AmBisome or of maintenance therapy with this drug among immunocompromised patients.

CONTRAINDICATIONS

AmBisome is contraindicated in those patients who have demonstrated or have known hypersensitivity to amphotericin B deoxycholate or any other constituents of the product unless, in the opinion of the treating physician, the benefit of therapy outweighs the risk.

WARNINGS

Anaphylaxis has been reported with amphotericin B deoxycholate and other amphotericin B-containing drugs, including AmBisome. If a severe anaphylactic reaction occurs, the infusion should be immediately discontinued and the patient should not receive further infusions of AmBisome.

PRECAUTIONS

General
As with any amphotericin B-containing product the drug should be administered by medically trained personnel. During the initial dosing period, patients should be under close clinical observation. AmBisome has been shown to be significantly less toxic than amphotericin B deoxycholate; however, adverse events may still occur.

Laboratory Tests
Patient management should include laboratory evaluation of renal, hepatic and hematopoietic function, and serum electrolytes (particularly magnesium and potassium).

Drug Interactions
No formal clinical studies of drug interactions have been conducted with AmBisome. However, the following drugs are known to interact with amphotericin B and may interact with AmBisome.

Pharmacokinetic Parameters of AmBisome

Dose (mg/kg(day)):	1.0		2.5		5.0	
Day	1 n = 8	Last n = 7	1 n = 7	Last n = 7	1 n = 12	Last n = 9
Parameters						
C_{max} (mcg/mL)	7.3 ± 3.8	12.2 ± 4.9	17.2 ± 7.1	31.4 ± 17.8	57.6 ± 21.0	83.0 ± 35.2
AUC_{0-24} (mcg•hr/mL)	27 ± 14	60 ± 20	65 ± 33	197 ± 183	269 ± 96	555 ± 311
$t_{1/2}$(hr)	10.7 ± 6.4	7.0 ± 2.1	8.1 ± 2.3	6.3 ± 2.0	6.4 ± 2.1	6.8 ± 2.1
V_{ss}(L/kg)	0.44 ± 0.27	0.14 ± 0.05	0.40 ± 0.37	0.16 ± 0.09	0.16 ± 0.10	0.10 ± 0.07
Cl (mL/hr/kg)	39 ± 22	17 ± 6	51 ± 44	22 ± 15	21 ± 14	11 ± 6

Empirical Therapy in Febrile Neutropenic Patients: Randomized, Double-Blind Study in 687 Patients

	AmBisome	Amphotericin B
Number of Patients receiving at least one dose of study drug	343	344
Overall Success	171 (49.9%)	169 (49.1%)
Fever resolution during neutropenic period	199 (58.0%)	200 (58.1%)
No treatment emergent fungal infection	300 (87.5%)	301 (87.7%)
Survival through 7 days post study drug	318 (92.7%)	308 (89.5%)
Study drug not prematurely discontinued due to toxicity or lack of efficacy*	294 (85.7%)	280 (81.4%)

* 8 and 10 patients, respectively, were treated as failures due to premature discontinuation alone.

Antineoplastic agents: Concurrent use of antineoplastic agents may enhance the potential for renal toxicity, bronchospasm, and hypotension. Antineoplastic agents should be given concomitantly with caution.

Corticosteroids and corticotropin (ACTH): Concurrent use of corticosteroids and ACTH may potentiate hypokalemia which could predipose the patient to cardiac dysfunction. If used concomitantly, serum electrolytes and cardiac function should be closely monitored.

Digitalis glycosides: Concurrent use may induce hypokalemia and may potentiate digitalis toxicity. When administered concomitantly, serum potassium levels should be closely monitored.

Flucytosine: Concurrent use of flucytosine may increase the toxicity of flucytosine by possibly increasing its cellular uptake and/or impairing its renal excretion.

Azoles (e.g. ketoconazole, miconazole, clotrimazole, fluconazole, etc.): In vitro and in vivo animal studies of the combination of amphotericin B and imidazoles suggest that imidazoles may induce fungal resistance to amphotericin B. Combination therapy should be administered with caution, especially in immunocompromised patients.

Leukocyte transfusions: Acute pulmonary toxicity has been reported in patients simultaneously receiving intravenous amphotericin B and leukocyte transfusions.

Other nephrotoxic medications: Concurrent use of amphotericin B and other nephrotoxic medications may enhance the potential for drug-induced renal toxicity. Intensive monitoring of renal function is recommended in patients requiring any combination of nephrotoxic medications.

Skeletal muscle relaxants: Amphotericin B-induced hypokalemia may enhance the curariform effect of skeletal muscle relaxants (e.g. tubocurarine) due to hypokalemia. When administered concomitantly, serum potassium levels should be closely monitored.

Carcinogenesis, Mutagenesis, Impairment of Fertility

No long term studies in animals have been performed to evaluate carcinogenic potential of AmBisome. AmBisome has not been tested to determine its mutagenic potential. A Segment I Reproductive Study in rats found an abnormal estrous cycle (prolonged diestrus) and decreased number of corpora lutea in the high dose groups (10 and 15 mg/kg, doses equivalent to human doses of 1.6 and 2.4 mg/kg based on body surface area considerations). AmBisome did not affect fertility or days to copulation. There were no effects on male reproductive function.

Pregnancy Category B

There have been no adequate and well-controlled studies of AmBisome in pregnant women. Systemic fungal infections have been successfully treated in pregnant women with amphotericin B deoxycholate, but the number of cases reported has been small.

Segment II studies in both rats and rabbits have concluded that AmBisome had no teratogenic potential in these species. In rats the maternal non-toxic dose of AmBisome was estimated to be 5 mg/kg (equivalent to 0.16 to 0.8 times the recommended human clinical dose range of 1 to 5 mg/kg) and in rabbits, 3 mg/kg (equivalent to 0.2 to 1 times the recommended human clinical dose range), based on body surface area correction. Rabbits receiving the higher doses,

(equivalent to 0.5 to 2 times the recommended human dose) of AmBisome experienced a higher rate of spontaneous abortions than did the control groups. AmBisome should only be used during pregnancy if the possible benefits to be derived outweigh the potential risks involved.

Nursing Mothers

Many drugs are excreted in human milk. However, it is not known whether AmBisome is excreted in human milk. Due to the potential for serious adverse reactions in breast-fed infants, a decision should be made whether to discontinue nursing or whether to discontinue the drug, taking into account the importance of the drug to the mother.

Pediatric Use

Pediatric patients, age 1 month to 16 years, with presumed fungal infection (empirical therapy), confirmed systemic fungal infections or with visceral leishmaniasis have been successfully treated with AmBisome. In studies which included 273 pediatric patients administered AmBisome and 111 administered amphotericin B, there was no evidence of any differences in efficacy or safety of AmBisome compared to adults. Since pediatric patients have received AmBisome at doses comparable to those used in adults on a per kilogram body weight basis, no dosage adjustment is required in this population. Safety and effectiveness in pediatric patients below the age of one month has not been established. See **DESCRIPTION OF CLINICAL STUDIES—Empirical Therapy in Febrile Neutropenic Patients** and **DOSAGE AND ADMINISTRATION**.

Elderly Patients

Experience with AmBisome in the elderly (65 years or older) comprised 71 patients. It has not been necessary to alter the dose of AmBisome for this population. As with most other drugs, elderly patients receiving AmBisome should be carefully monitored.

ADVERSE REACTIONS

The following adverse events are based on the experience of 592 adult patients (295 treated with AmBisome and 297 treated with amphotericin B deoxycholate) and 95 pediatric patients (48 treated with AmBisome and 47 treated with amphotericin B deoxycholate) in Study 94-0-002, a randomized, double-blind, multi-center study in febrile, neutropenic patients. AmBisome and amphotericin B were infused over two hours.

The incidence of common adverse events (incidence of 10% or greater) occurring with AmBisome compared to amphotericin B deoxycholate, regardless of relationship to study drug, is in the following table:

[See table at top of next page]

AmBisome was well tolerated. AmBisome had a lower incidence of chills, hypertension, hypotension, tachycardia, hypoxia, hypokalemia, and various events related to decreased kidney function as compared to amphotericin B deoxycholate.

In pediatric patients (16 years of age or less) in this double-blind study, AmBisome compared to amphotericin B deoxycholate had a lower incidence of hypokalemia (37% versus 55%), chills (29% versus 68%), vomiting (27% versus 55%), and hypertension (10% versus 21%). Similar trends, although with a somewhat lower incidence, were observed in

open-label, randomized Study 104-14 involving 205 febrile neutropenic pediatric patients (141 treated with AmBisome and 64 treated with amphotericin B deoxycholate). Pediatric patients appear to have more tolerance than older individuals for the nephrotoxic effects of amphotericin B deoxycholate.

Infusion Related Reactions

In Study 94-0-002, the large, double-blind study of pediatric and adult febrile neutropenic patients, no premedication to prevent infusion related reaction was administered prior to the first dose of study drug (Day 1). AmBisome-treated patients had a lower incidence of infusion related fever (17% versus 44%), chills/rigor (18% versus 54%), and vomiting (6% versus 8%) on Day 1 as compared to amphotericin B deoxycholate-treated patients.

The incidence of infusion related reactions on Day 1 in pediatric and adult patients is summarized in the following table:

[See table at top of page 1039]

Cardiorespiratory events, except for vasodilation (flushing), during all study drug infusions were more frequent in amphotericin B-treated patients as summarized in the following table:

Incidence of Infusion Related Cardiorespiratory Events

Event	AmBisome n=343	Amphotericin B n=344
Hypotension	12 (3.5%)	28 (8.1%)
Tachycardia	8 (2.3%)	43 (12.5%)
Hypertension	8 (2.3%)	39 (11.3%)
Vasodilatation	18 (5.2%)	2 (0.6%)
Dyspnea	16 (4.7%)	25 (7.3%)
Hyperventilation	4 (1.2%)	17 (4.9%)
Hypoxia	1 (0.3%)	22 (6.4%)

The percentage of patients who received drugs either for the treatment or prevention of infusion related reactions (e.g., acetaminophen, diphenhydramine, meperidine and hydrocortisone) was lower in AmBisome-treated patients compared with amphotericin B deoxycholate-treated patients. There have been reports of flushing, back pain with or without chest tightness, and chest pain associated with AmBisome administration; on occasion this has been severe. Where these symptoms were noted, the reaction developed within a few minutes after the start of infusion and disappeared rapidly when the infusion was stopped. The symptoms do not occur with every dose and usually do not recur on subsequent administrations when the infusion rate is slowed.

Toxicity and Discontinuation of Dosing

In Study 94-0-002, a significantly lower incidence of grade 3 or 4 toxicity was observed in the AmBisome group compared with the amphotericin B group. In addition, nearly three times as many patients administered amphotericin B required a reduction in dose due to toxicity or discontinuation of study drug due to an infusion related reaction compared with those administered AmBisome.

Less Common Adverse Events

The following adverse events also have been reported in 2% to 10% of AmBisome-treated patients receiving chemotherapy or bone marrow transplantation in four comparative, clinical trials:

Body as a Whole—abdomen enlarged, allergic reaction, cellulitis, cell mediated immunological reaction, face edema, graft versus host disease, malaise, and neck pain.

Cardiovascular System—arrhythmia, atrial fibrillation, bradycardia, cardiac arrest, cardiomegaly, hemorrhage, postural hypotension, valvular heart disease, vascular disorder, and vasodilatation (flushing).

Digestive System—anorexia, constipation, dry mouth/nose, dyspepsia, dysphagia, eructation, fecal incontinence, flatulence, gastrointestinal hemorrhage, hemorrhoids, gum/oral hemorrhage, hematemesis, hepatocellular damage, hepatomegaly, liver function test abnormal, mucositis, rectal disorder, stomatitis, ulcerative stomatitis, and veno-occlusive liver disease.

Hemic & Lymphatic System—anemia, coagulation disorder, ecchymosis, fluid overload, petechia, prothrombin decreased, prothrombin increased, and thrombocytopenia.

Metabolic & Nutritional Disorders—acidosis, amylase increased, hyperchloremia, hyperkalemia, hypermagnesemia, hyperphosphatemia, hyponatremia, hypophosphatemia, hypoproteinemia, lactate dehydrogenase increased, nonprotein nitrogen (NPN) increased, and respiratory alkalosis.

Musculoskeletal System—arthralgia, bone pain, dystonia, myalgia, and rigors.

Empirical Therapy in Febrile Neutropenic Patients: Emergent Fungal Infections

	AmBisome	Amphotericin B
Number of Patients receiving at least one dose of study drug	343	344
Mycologically confirmed fungal infection	11 (3.2%)	27 (7.8%)
Clinically diagnosed fungal infection	32 (9.3%)	16 (4.7%)
Total emergent fungal infections	43 (12.5%)	43 (12.5%)

AmBisome Efficacy in Visceral Leishmaniasis

Immunocompetent Patients

No. of Patients	Parasite (%) Clearance at EOT	Overall Success (%) at FU
87	86/87 (98.9)	83/86 (96.5)

Immunocompromised Patients

Regimen	Total Dose	Parasite (%) Clearance at EOT	Overall Success (%) at FU
100 mg/day X 21 days	29.0-38.9 mg/kg	10/10 (100)	2/10 (20.0)
4 mg/kg/day, days 1-5,			
and 10, 17, 24, 31, 38	40 mg/kg	8/9 (88.9)	0/7 (0.0)
TOTAL		18/19 (94.7)	2/17 (11.8)

Continued on next page

Ambisome—Cont.

Nervous System—agitation, coma, convulsion, cough, depression, dysesthesia, dizziness, hallucinations, nervousness, paresthesia, somnolence, thinking abnormality, and tremor.

Respiratory System—asthma, atelectasis, hemoptysis, hiccup, hyperventilation, influenza-like symptoms, lung edema, pharyngitis, pneumonia, respiratory insufficiency, respiratory failure, and sinusitis.

Skin & Appendages—alopecia, dry skin, herpes simplex, injection site inflammation, purpura, skin discoloration, skin disorder, skin ulcer, urticaria, and vesiculobullous rash.

Special Senses—conjunctivitis, dry eyes, and eye hemorrhage.

Urogenital System—abnormal renal function, acute kidney failure, acute renal failure, dysuria, kidney failure, toxic nephropathy, urinary incontinence, and vaginal hemorrhage.

The following infrequent adverse experience have been reported in post-marketing surveillance, in addition to those mentioned above: angioedema, erythema, urticaria, cyanosis/hypoventilation, pulmonary edema, agranulocytosis, hemorrhagic cystitis.

Clinical Laboratory Values

The effect of AmBisome on renal and hepatic function and on serum electrolytes was assessed from laboratory values measured repeatedly in Study 94-0-002. The frequency and magnitude of hepatic test abnormalities were similar in the AmBisome and amphotericin B groups. Nephrotoxicity was defined as creatinine values increasing 100% or more over pretreatment levels in pediatric patients, and creatinine values increasing 100% or more over pretreatment levels in adult patients provided the peak creatinine concentration was >1.2 mg/dL. Hypokalemia was defined as potassium levels ≤2.5 mmol/L any time during treatment.

Incidence of nephrotoxicity, mean peak serum creatinine concentration, mean change from baseline in serum creatinine, and, incidence of hypokalemia in the double-blind randomized study were lower in the AmBisome group as summarized in the following table:

Study 94-0-002 Laboratory Evidence of Nephrotoxicity

	AmBisome	Amphotericin B
Total number of patients receiving at least one dose of study drug	343	344
Nephrotoxicity	64 (18.7%)	116 (33.7%)
Mean peak creatinine	1.24 mg/dL	1.52 mg/dL
Mean change from baseline in creatinine	0.48 mg/dL	0.77 mg/dL
Hypokalemia	23 (6.7%)	40 (11.6%)

The effect of AmBisome (3 mg/kg/day) vs. amphotericin B (0.6 mg/kg/day) on renal function in adult patients enrolled in this study is illustrated in the following figure:

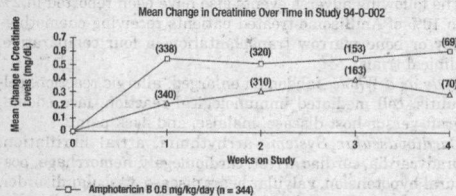

Mean Change in Creatinine Over Time in Study 94-0-002

—□— Amphotericin B 0.6 mg/kg/day (n = 344)
—△— AmBisome 3 mg/kg/day (n = 343)

The following graph shows the average serum creatinine concentrations in the compassionate use study and shows that there is a drop from pretreatment concentrations for all patients, especially those with elevated (greater than 1.7 mg/dL) pretreatment creatinine concentrations.
[See figure in next column]

OVERDOSAGE

The toxicity of AmBisome due to overdose has not been defined. Repeated daily doses up to 7.5 mg/kg have been administered in clinical trials with no reported dose-related toxicity.

Management—If overdosage should occur, cease administration immediately. Symptomatic supportive measures should be instituted. Particular attention should be given to monitoring renal function.

Empirical Therapy Study 94-0-002 Common Adverse Events

Adverse Event by Body System	AmBisome n=343 %	Amphotericin B n=344 %
Body as a Whole		
Abdominal pain	19.8	21.8
Asthenia	13.1	10.8
Back pain	12.0	7.3
Blood product transfusion react.	18.4	18.6
Chills	47.5	75.9
Infection	11.1	9.3
Pain	14.0	12.8
Sepsis	14.0	11.3
Cardiovascular System		
Chest pain	12.0	11.6
Hypertension	7.9	16.3
Hypotension	14.3	21.5
Tachycardia	13.4	20.9
Digestive System		
Diarrhea	30.3	27.3
Gastrointestinal hemorrhage	9.9	11.3
Nausea	39.7	38.7
Vomiting	31.8	43.9
Metabolic and Nutritional Disorders		
Alkaline phosphatase increased	22.2	19.2
ALT (SGPT) increased	14.6	14.0
AST (SGOT) increased	12.8	12.8
Bilirubinemia	18.1	19.2
BUN increased	21.0	31.1
Creatinine increased	22.4	42.2
Edema	14.3	14.8
Hyperglycemia	23.0	27.9
Hypernatremia	4.1	11.0
Hypervolemia	12.2	15.4
Hypocalcemia	18.4	20.9
Hypokalemia	42.9	50.6
Hypomagnesemia	20.4	25.6
Peripheral edema	14.6	17.2
Nervous System		
Anxiety	13.7	11.0
Confusion	11.4	13.4
Headache	19.8	20.9
Insomnia	17.2	14.2
Respiratory System		
Cough increased	17.8	21.8
Dyspnea	23.0	29.1
Epistaxis	14.9	20.1
Hypoxia	7.6	14.8
Lung disorder	17.8	17.4
Pleural effusion	12.5	9.6
Rhinitis	11.1	11.0
Skin and Appendages		
Pruritus	10.8	10.2
Rash	24.8	24.4
Sweating	7.0	10.8
Urogenital System		
Hematuria	14.0	14.0

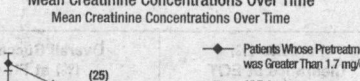

Mean Creatinine Concentrations Over Time

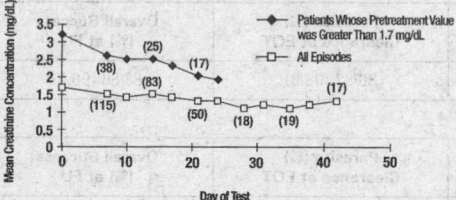

Mean Creatinine Concentrations Over Time

◆ Patients Whose Pretreatment Value was Greater Than 1.7 mg/dL
□ All Episodes

DOSAGE AND ADMINISTRATION

AmBisome should be administered by intravenous infusion, using a controlled infusion device, over a period of approximately 120 minutes. Infusion time may be reduced to approximately 60 minutes in patients in whom the treatment is well-tolerated. If the patient experiences discomfort during infusion, the duration of infusion may be increased. The recommended initial dose of AmBisome for each indication for adult and pediatric patients is as follows:

Indication	Dose (mg/kg/day)
Empirical therapy	3.0
Systemic fungal infections:	3.0-5.0
Aspergillus	
Candida	
Cryptococcus	

Incidence of Day 1 Infusion Related Reactions (IRR) By Patient Age

	Pediatric Patients (≤ 16 years of age)		Adult Patients (> 16 years of age)	
	AmBisome	Amphotericin B	AmBisome	Amphotericin B
Total number of patients receiving at least one dose of study drug	48	47	295	297
Patients with fever† Increase ≥ 1.0°C	6 (13%)	22 (47%)	52 (18%)	128 (43%)
Patients with chills/rigors	4 (8%)	22 (47%)	59 (20%)	165 (56%)
Patients with nausea	4 (8%)	4 (9%)	38 (13%)	31 (10%)
Patients with vomiting	2 (4%)	7 (15%)	19 (6%)	21 (7%)
Patients with other reactions	10 (21%)	13 (28%)	47 (16%)	69 (23%)

†Day 1 body temperature increased above the temperature taken within 1 hour prior to infusion (preinfusion temperature) or above the lowest infusion value (no preinfusion temperature recorded).

Dosing and rate of infusion should be individualized to the needs of the specific patient to ensure maximum efficacy while minimizing systemic toxicities or adverse events. Doses recommended for visceral leishmaniasis are presented below:

Visceral Leishmaniasis	Dose (mg/kg/day)
Immunocompetent patients	3.0 (days 1-5) and 3.0 on days 14, 21
Immunocompromised patients	4.0 (days 1-5) and 4.0 on days 10, 17, 24, 31, 38

For immunocompetent patients who do not achieve parasitic clearance with the recommended dose, a repeat course of therapy may be useful.
For immunocompromised patients who do not clear parasites or who experience relapses, expert advice regarding further treatment is recommended. For additional information see **DESCRIPTION OF CLINICAL STUDIES.**
Directions for Reconstitution, Filtration and Dilution
Read This Entire Section Carefully Before Beginning Reconstitution
AmBisome **must** be reconstituted using Sterile Water for Injection, USP (without a bacteriostatic agent). Vials of AmBisome containing 50 mg of amphotericin B are prepared as follows:
Reconstitution
1. Aseptically add 12 mL of Sterile Water for Injection, USP to each AmBisome vial to yield a preparation containing 4 mg amphotericin B/mL.
CAUTION: DO NOT RECONSTITUTE WITH SALINE OR ADD SALINE TO THE RECONSTITUTED CONCENTRATION, OR MIX WITH OTHER DRUGS. The use of any solution other than those recommended, or the presence of a bacteriostatic agent in the solution, may cause precipitation of AmBisome.
2. **Immediately after the addition of water, SHAKE THE VIAL VIGOROUSLY** for 30 seconds to completely disperse the AmBisome. AmBisome forms a yellow, translucent suspension. Visually inspect the vial for particulate matter and continue shaking until completely dispersed.
Filtration and Dilution
3. Calculate the amount of reconstituted (4 mg/mL) AmBisome to be further diluted.
4. Withdraw this amount of reconstituted AmBisome into a sterile syringe.
5. Attach a 5-micron filter, provided, to the syringe. Inject the syringe contents through the filter, into the appropriate amount of 5% Dextrose Injection. (Use only one filter per vial of AmBisome.)
6. AmBisome must be diluted with 5% Dextrose Injection to a final concentration of 1.0 to 2.0 mg/mL prior to administration. Lower concentrations (0.2 to 0.5 mg/mL) may be appropriate for infants and small children to provide sufficient volume for infusion. **DISCARD PARTIALLY USED VIALS.**
STORAGE OF AMBISOME
Unopened vials of lyophilized material must be stored under refrigeration at 2°–8° C (36°–46° F).
Storage of Reconstituted Product Concentrate
The reconstituted product concentrate may be stored for up to 24 hours at 2°–8° C (36°–46° F) following reconstitution with Sterile Water for Injection, USP. Do not freeze.
Storage for Diluted Product
Injection of AmBisome should commence within 6 hours of dilution with 5% Dextrose Injection.
As with all parenteral drug products, the reconstituted AmBisome should be inspected visually for particulate matter and discoloration prior to administration, whenever solution and container permit. Do not use material if there is any evidence of precipitation or foreign matter. Aseptic tech-

nique must be strictly observed in all handling since no preservative or bacteriostatic agent is present in AmBisome or in the materials specified for reconstitution and dilution.
An in-line membrane filter may be used for the intravenous infusion of AmBisome; provided, **THE MEAN PORE DIAMETER OF THE FILTER SHOULD BE LESS THAN 1.0 MICRON.**
NOTE: An existing intravenous line must be flushed with 5% Dextrose Injection prior to infusion of AmBisome. If this is not feasible, AmBisome should be administered through a separate line.
HOW SUPPLIED
AmBisome for Injection is available as single 50 mg vial cartons and in packs of ten individual vial cartons (NDC 0469-3051-30).
Each carton contains one pre-packaged, disposable sterile 5 micron filter.
CAUTION:
Federal law prohibits dispensing without prescription.
Manufactured for:
Fujisawa USA, Inc.
Deerfield, IL 60015-2548
http://www.AmBisome.com
by:
NEXSTAR
Pharmaceuticals, Inc.
San Dimas, CA 91773
AmBisome® is a registered trademark of NeXstar Pharmaceuticals, Inc.
002   Revised January 1998

ARISTOCORT®   ℞
[*a-ris-tō-cort*]
Sterile Triamcinolone Diacetate
Suspension
25 mg/mL
INTRALESIONAL
NOT FOR INTRAVENOUS USE

DESCRIPTION
ARISTOCORT triamcinolone diacetate possesses glucocorticoid properties while being essentially devoid of mineralocorticoid activity thus causing little or no sodium retention. Supplied as a sterile suspension of 25 mg/mL micronized triamcinolone diacetate in the following vehicle:

Polysorbate 80	0.20%
Polyethylene Glycol 3350	3%
Sodium Chloride	0.85%
Benzyl Alcohol (preservative)	0.90%
Water for Injection q.s.	100%

Hydrochloric acid and/or sodium hydroxide may be used during manufacture to adjust pH of suspension to approximately 6.
Chemically triamcinolone diacetate is 9-Fluoro-11β,16α, 17,21-tetrahydroxypregna-1,4-diene-3,20-dione 16,21-diacetate.
Molecular weight is 478.51. Its structural formula is:

HOW SUPPLIED
ARISTOCORT® (sterile triamcinolone diacetate) suspension, 25 mg/mL, Intralesional, NOT FOR INTRAVENOUS USE.
NDC 0469-5117-05   Product Code 511705
5 mL Vial
Store at Controlled Room Temperature 15°–30°C (59°–86°F).
DO NOT FREEZE.
Manufactured for Fujisawa USA, Inc., Deerfield, IL 60015, by
Lederle Parenterals, Inc.,
Carolina, Puerto Rico 00987
41207-94/Issued April 1994
FP4

ARISTOCORT A®   ℞
[*a-ris-tō-cort*]
(triamcinolone acetonide)
0.025% CREAM
with AQUATAIN™ hydrophilic base

DESCRIPTION
0.025% TOPICAL CREAM
Each gram of ARISTOCORT A Topical Cream contains 0.25 mg of the highly active steroid Triamcinolone Acetonide (a derivative of triamcinolone) in AQUATAIN, a specially formulated cream base composed of Emulsifying Wax, Isopropyl Palmitate, Glycerin, Sorbitol Solution, Lactic Acid, 2% Benzyl Alcohol and Purified Water. AQUATAIN is non-staining, water-washable, paraben-free, spermaceti-free and has a light texture and consistency.
Triamcinolone acetonide is (11β, 16α)-9-Fluoro-11, 21-dihydroxy-16,17-[(1-methylethylidene)bis(oxy)]pregna-1, 4-diene-3,20-dione. Its structural formula is:

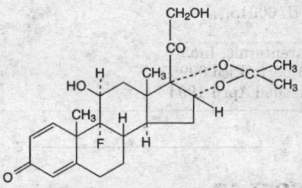

Molecular Weight 434.50 $C_{24}H_{31}FO_6$

The topical corticosteroids constitute a class of primarily synthetic steroids used as anti-inflammatory and antipruritic agents.

HOW SUPPLIED
ARISTOCORT A® (triamcinolone acetonide) Cream 0.025% (0.25 mg/g) with AQUATAIN™ hydrophilic base.
NDC 0469-5101-15   Product Code 510115
15 g tube
NDC 0469-5101-60   Product Code 510160
60 g tube
Store at Controlled Room Temperature 15°–30°C (59°–86°F).
DO NOT FREEZE.
Manufactured for Fujisawa USA, Inc., Deerfield, IL 60015, by
Lederle Laboratories Division,
American Cyanamid Company,
Pearl River, NY 10965
CI 4546-1   Issued November 13, 1995

ARISTOCORT® Forte   ℞
[*a-ris-tō-cort*]
(sterile triamcinolone diacetate)
Suspension 40 mg/mL
Parenteral
NOT FOR INTRAVENOUS USE

DESCRIPTION
A sterile suspension of 40 mg/mL of triamcinolone diacetate (micronized) suspended in a vehicle consisting of:

Polysorbate 80	0.20%
Polyethylene Glycol 3350	3%
Sodium Chloride	0.85%
Benzyl Alcohol (preservative)	0.90%
Water for injection q.s.	100%

Hydrochloric acid and/or sodium hydroxide may be used during manufacture to adjust pH of suspension to approximately 6.

Continued on next page

Aristocort Forte—Cont.

This preparation is a slightly soluble suspension suitable for parenteral administration through a 24-gauge needle (or larger), but NOT suitable for intravenous use. It may be administered by the intramuscular, intra-articular, or intrasynovial routes, depending upon the situation. The response to each glucocorticoid varies considerably with each type of disease indication and each corticosteroid prescribed. Irreversible clumping occurs when product is frozen.

Chemically triamcinolone diacetate is 9-Fluoro-11β, 16α, 17,21-tetrahydroxypregna-1,4-diene-3,20-dione 16,21-diacetate.

Molecular weight is 478.51. Its structural formula is:

HOW SUPPLIED

ARISTOCORT® FORTE (sterile triamcinolone diacetate) suspension, 40 mg/mL, Parenteral, NOT FOR INTRAVENOUS USE.
NDC 0469-5116-01   Product Code 511601
1 mL Vial
NDC 0469-5116-05   Product Code 511605
5 mL Vial
Store at Controlled Room Temperature 15°–30°C (59°–86°F).
DO NOT FREEZE.
Irreversible clumping occurs when product is frozen.
Manufactured for Fujisawa USA, Inc.,
Deerfield, IL 60015,
by
Lederle Parenterals, Inc.,
Carolina, Puerto Rico 00987
41233-94/Issued April 1994
FP5

ARISTOCORT A® ℞
[a-ris-tō-cort]
(triamcinolone acetonide)
0.1% OINTMENT
with PROPYLENE GLYCOL

DESCRIPTION

0.1% TOPICAL OINTMENT
Each gram of ARISTOCORT Topical Ointment contains 1 mg of the highly active steroid Triamcinolone Acetonide (a derivative of triamcinolone) in a specially formulated ointment base composed of White Petrolatum, Propylene Glycol, Emulsifying Wax, Tenox II (butylated hydroxanisole, propyl gallate, citric acid, propylene glycol) and Lactic Acid.
Triamcinolone acetonide is (11β,16α)-9-Fluoro-11,21-dihydroxy -16,17- [(1-methylethylidene) bis (oxy)] pregna-1,4 - diene-3,20-dione.
Chemically triamcinolone acetonide is:

Molecular Weight 434.50 $C_{24}H_{31}FO_6$

The topical corticosteroids constitute a class of primarily synthetic steroids used as anti-inflammatory and anti-pruritic agents.

HOW SUPPLIED

ARISTOCORT A® (triamcinolone acetonide) Ointment 0.1% (1 mg/mL) with Propylene Glycol
NDC 0469-5105-15   Product Code 510515
15 g tube
NDC 0469-5105-60   Product Code 510560
60 g tube
Store at Controlled Room Temperature 15°–30°C (59°–86°F).
Manufactured for Fujisawa USA, Inc., Deerfield, IL 60015, by
Lederle Laboratories Division,

American Cyanamid Company,
Pearl River, NY 10965
CI 4564–1   Issued November 13, 1995

ARISTOCORT A® ℞
[a-ris-tō-cort]
(triamcinolone acetonide)
0.1% CREAM
with AQUATAIN™ hydrophilic base

DESCRIPTION

0.1% TOPICAL CREAM
Each gram of ARISTOCORT A Topical Cream contains 1 mg of the highly active steroid Triamcinolone Acetonide (a derivative of triamcinolone) in AQUATAIN, a specially formulated cream base composed of Emulsifying Wax, Isopropyl Palmitate, Glycerin, Sorbitol Solution, Lactic Acid, 2% Benzyl Alcohol and Purified Water. AQUATAIN is non-staining, water-washable, paraben-free, spermaceti-free and has a light texture and consistency.
Triamcinolone acetonide is (11β,16α)-9-Fluoro-11,21-dihydroxy-16,17- [(1-methylethylidene)bis(oxy)]pregna-1,4-diene3,20-dione. Its structural formula is:

Molecular Weight 434.50 $C_{24}H_{31}FO_6$

The topical corticosteroids constitute a class of primarily synthetic steroids used as anti-inflammatory and antipruritic agents.

HOW SUPPLIED

ARISTOCORT A® (triamcinolone acetonide) Cream 0.1% (1 mg/g) with AQUATAIN™ hydrophilic base
NDC 0469-5102-15   Product Code 510215
15 g tube
NDC 0469-5102-60   Product Code 510260
60 g tube
NDC 0469-5102-24   Product Code 510324
240 g jar
Store at Controlled Room Temperature 15°–30°C (59°–86°F). DO NOT FREEZE.
Manufactured for Fujisawa USA, Inc., Deerfield, IL 60015, by
Lederle Laboratories Division,
American Cyanamid Company,
Pearl River, NY 10965
CI 4428–1   Issued November 2, 1995

ARISTOCORT A® ℞
[a-ris-tō-cort]
(triamcinolone acetonide)
0.5% CREAM with AQUATAIN™ hydrophilic base

DESCRIPTION

0.5% TOPICAL CREAM
Each gram of ARISTOCORT A Topical Cream contains 5 mg of the highly active steroid Triamcinolone Acetonide (a derivative of triamcinolone) in AQUATAIN, a specially formulated cream base composed of Emulsifying Wax, Isopropyl Palmitate, Glycerin, Sorbitol Solution, Lactic Acid, 2% Benzyl Alcohol and Purified Water. AQUATAIN is non-staining, water-washable, paraben-free, spermaceti-free and has a light texture and consistency.
Triamcinolone acetonide is (11β, 16α)-9-Fluoro-11,21-dihydroxy-16, 17-[(1-methylethylidene)bis(oxy)]pregna-1,4-diene-3,20-dione. Its structural formula is:

Molecular Weight 434.50 $C_{24}H_{31}FO_6$

The topical corticosteroids constitute a class of primarily synthetic steroids used as anti-inflammatory and antipruritic agents.

HOW SUPPLIED

ARISTOCORT A® (triamcinolone acetonide) Cream 0.5% (5 mg/g) with AQUATAIN™ hydrophilic base
NDC 0469-5104-15   Product Code 510415
15 g tube
Store at Controlled Room Temperature 15°–30°C (59°–86°F).
DO NOT FREEZE.
Manufactured by Fujisawa USA, Inc., Deerfield, IL 60015, by
Lederle Laboratories Division,
American Cyanamid Company,
Pearl River, NY 10965
CI 4425–1   Issued November 13, 1995

ARISTOSPAN® ℞
[a-ris-tō-span]
(sterile triamcinolone hexacetonide)
Suspension 5 mg/mL
Parenteral For Intralesional Use
NOT FOR INTRAVENOUS USE

DESCRIPTION

A sterile suspension containing 5 mg/mL of micronized triamcinolone hexacetonide in the following inactive ingredients:

Polysorbate 80	0.20%
Sorbitol Solution	50%
Benzyl Alcohol (preservative)	0.90%
Water for Injection q.s.	100%

Hydrochloric Acid and Sodium Hydroxide, if required, to adjust pH to 4.5–6.5.
The hexacetonide ester of the potent glucocorticoid triamcinolone is relatively insoluble (0.0002% at 25°C in water). When injected intralesionally or sublesionally, it can be expected to be absorbed slowly from the injection site.
Chemically triamcinolone hexacetonide is 9-Fluoro-11β, 16α, 17,21-tetrahydroxypregna-1,4-diene-3,20-dionecyclic 16,17-acetal with acetone 21-(3,3-dimethylbutyrate). Molecular weight is 532.65. The structural formula is:

HOW SUPPLIED

ARISTOSPAN® (sterile triamcinolone hexacetonide) suspension, 5 mg/mL, for Intralesional Use. NOT FOR INTRAVENOUS USE.
NDC 0469-5118-05   Product Code 511805
5 mL Vial
Store at Controlled Room Temperature 15–30°C (59–86°F).
DO NOT FREEZE.
Manufactured for Fujisawa USA, Inc., Deerfield, IL 60015, by
Lederle Parenterals, Inc.,
Carolina, Puerto Rico 00987
41209-94/Issued April 1994
FP5

ARISTOSPAN® ℞
[a-ris-tō-span]
(sterile triamcinolone hexacetonide)
Suspension 20 mg/mL
Parenteral For Intra-articular Use
NOT FOR INTRAVENOUS USE

DESCRIPTION

A sterile suspension containing 20 mg/mL of micronized triamcinolone hexacetonide in the following inactive ingredients:

Polysorbate 80	0.40%
Sorbitol Solution	50%
Benzyl Alcohol (preservative)	0.90%
Water for Injection qs	100%

Hydrochloric Acid and Sodium Hydroxide, if required, to adjust pH to 4.5–6.5.
The hexacetonide ester of the potent glucocorticoid triamcinolone is relatively insoluble (0.0002% at 25°C in water). When injected intra-articularly, it can be expected to be absorbed slowly from the injection site.

Chemically triamcinolone hexacetonide is 9-Fluoro-11β, 16α, 17,21-tetrahydroxypregna-1,4-diene-3,20-dionecyclic 16,17-acetal with acetone 21-(3,3-dimethylbutyrate). Molecular weight is 532.65. The structural formula is:

HOW SUPPLIED

ARISTOSPAN® (sterile triamcinolone hexacetonide) suspension 20 mg/mL, for Intra-articular Use. NOT FOR INTRAVENOUS USE.

NDC 0469-5119-01   Product Code 511901
1 mL Vial
NDC 0469-5119-05   Product Code 511905
5 mL vial
Store at Controlled Room Temperature 15–30°C (59–86°F). DO NOT FREEZE.
Manufactured for Fujisawa USA, Inc.,
Deerfield, IL 60015,
by
Lederle Parenterals, Inc.,
Carolina, Puerto Rico 00987
41232-94/Issued April 1994
FP5

CEFIZOX®
(sterile ceftizoxime sodium)
For Intramuscular or Intravenous Use

℞

DESCRIPTION

Cefizox® (sterile ceftizoxime sodium) is a sterile, semisynthetic, broad-spectrum, beta-lactamase resistant cephalosporin antibiotic for parenteral (I.V., I.M.) administration. It is the sodium salt of [6R-[6a, 7β(Z)]]-7-[[(2,3-dihydro-2-imino-4-thiazolyl) (methoxyimino) acetyl] amino]-8-oxo-5-thia-1-azabicyclo [4.2.0] oct-2-ene-2-carboxylic acid. Its sodium content is approximately 60 mg (2.6 mEq) per gram of ceftizoxime activity.

It has the following structural formula:

$C_{13}H_{12}N_5NaO_5S_2$ 405.38

Sterile ceftizoxime sodium is a white to pale yellow crystalline powder.
Cefizox is supplied in vials equivalent to 500 mg, 1 gram or 2 grams of ceftizoxime, and in "Piggyback" Vials for intravenous admixture equivalent to 1 gram or 2 grams of ceftizoxime.

CLINICAL PHARMACOLOGY

The table below demonstrates the serum levels and duration of Cefizox (sterile ceftizoxime sodium) following intramuscular administration of 500 mg and 1 gram doses, respectively, to normal volunteers.

Serum Concentrations After Intramuscular Administration
Serum Concentration (mcg/mL)

Dose	½ hr	1 hr	2 hr	4 hr	6 hr	8 hr
500 mg	13.3	13.7	9.2	4.8	1.9	0.7
1 gm	36.0	39.0	31.0	15.0	6.0	3.0

Following intravenous administration of 1, 2, and 3 gram doses of Cefizox to normal volunteers, the following serum levels were obtained.

Serum Concentrations After Intravenous Administration
Serum Concentration (mcg/mL)

Dose	5 min	10 min	30 min	1 hr	2 hr	4 hr	8 hr
1 gram	ND	ND	60.5	38.9	21.5	8.4	1.4
2 grams	131.8	110.9	77.5	53.6	33.1	12.1	2.0
3 grams	221.1	174.0	112.7	83.9	47.4	26.2	4.8

ND=Not Done

A serum half-life of approximately 1.7 hours was observed after intravenous or intramuscular administration.
Cefizox is 30% protein bound.
Cefizox is not metabolized, and is excreted virtually unchanged by the kidneys in 24 hours. This provides a high urinary concentration. Concentrations greater than 6000 mcg/mL have been achieved in the urine by 2 hours after a 1 gram dose of Cefizox intravenously. Probenecid slows tubular secretion and produces even higher serum levels, increasing the duration of measurable serum concentrations. Cefizox achieves therapeutic levels in various body fluids, e.g., cerebrospinal fluid (in patients with inflamed meninges), bile, surgical wound fluid, pleural fluid, aqueous humor, ascitic fluid, peritoneal fluid, prostatic fluid and saliva, and in the following body tissues: heart, gallbladder, bone, biliary, peritoneal, prostatic, and uterine.
In clinical experience to date, no disulfiram-like reactions have been reported with Cefizox.

Microbiology

The bactericidal action of Cefizox (sterile ceftizoxime sodium) results from inhibition of cell-wall synthesis. Cefizox is highly resistant to a broad spectrum of beta-lactamases (penicillinase and cephalosporinase), including Richmond types I, II, III, TEM, and IV, produced by both aerobic and anaerobic gram-positive and gram-negative organisms. Cefizox is active against a wide range of gram-positive and gram-negative organisms, and is usually active against the following organisms in vitro and in clinical situations (see Indications and Usage.)

Gram-Positive Aerobes

Staphylococcus aureus (including penicillinase- and non-penicillinase-producing strains)
NOTE: Methicillin-resistant staphylococci are resistant to cephalosporins, including ceftizoxime.
Staphylococcus epidermidis (including penicillinase- and nonpenicillinase-producing strains)
Streptococcus agalactiae
Streptococcus pneumoniae
Streptococcus pyogenes
NOTE: Ceftizoxime is usually inactive against most strains of Enterococcus faecalis (formerly S. faecalis).

Gram-Negative Aerobes

Acinetobacter spp.
Enterobacter spp.
Escherichia coli
Haemophilus influenzae (including ampicillin-resistant strains)
Klebsiella pneumoniae
Morganella morganii (formerly Proteus morganii)
Neisseria gonorrhoeae
Proteus mirabilis
Proteus vulgaris
Providencia rettgeri (formerly Proteus rettgeri)
Pseudomonas aeruginosa
Serratia marcescens

Anaerobes

Bacteroides spp.
Peptococcus spp.
Peptostreptococcus spp.

Ceftizoxime is usually active against the following organisms in vitro, but the clinical significance of these data is unknown.

Gram-Positive Aerobes

Corynebacterium diphtheriae

Gram-Negative Aerobes

Aeromonas hydrophila
Citrobacter spp.
Moraxella spp.
Neisseria meningitidis
Pasteurella multocida
Providencia stuartii
Salmonella spp.
Shigella spp.
Yersinia enterocolitica

Anaerobes

Actinomyces spp.
Bifidobacterium spp.
Clostridium spp.
NOTE: Most strains of Clostridium difficile are resistant.
Eubacterium spp.
Fusobacterium spp.
Propionibacterium spp.
Veillonella spp.

Susceptibility Testing: Diffusion Techniques

Quantitative methods that require measurement of zone diameters give the most precise estimate of the susceptibility of bacteria to antimicrobial agents. One such standard procedure[1] has been recommended for use with disks to test susceptibility of organisms to ceftizoxime. Interpretation involves the correlation of the diameters obtained in the disk test with the minimum inhibitory concentration (MIC) for ceftizoxime.

Organisms should be tested with the ceftizoxime disk, since ceftizoxime has been shown by in vitro tests to be active against certain strains found resistant when other beta-lactam disks are used.
Reports from the laboratory giving results of the standard single-disk susceptibility test with a 30 mcg ceftizoxime disk should be interpreted according to the following criteria (with the exception of Pseudomonas aeruginosa).

Zone Diameter (mm)	Interpretation
≥20	(S) Susceptible
15–19	(MS) Moderately Susceptible
≤14	(R) Resistant

A report of "Susceptible" indicates that the pathogen is likely to be inhibited by generally achievable blood levels. A report of "Moderately Susceptible" suggests that the organism would be susceptible if high dosage is used or if the infection is confined to tissue and fluids (e.g., urine) in which high antibiotic levels are attained. A report of "Resistant" indicates that achievable concentrations of the antibiotic are unlikely to be inhibitory and other therapy should be selected.
Standardized procedures require the use of laboratory control organisms. The 30 mcg ceftizoxime disk should give the following zone diameters.

Organism	ATCC	Zone Diameter (mm)
Escherichia coli	25922	30–36
Pseudomonas aeruginosa	27853	12–17
Staphylococcus aureus	25923	27–35

Susceptibility Testing for Pseudomonas in Urinary Tract Infections

Most strains of Pseudomonas aeruginosa are moderately susceptible to ceftizoxime. Ceftizoxime achieves high levels in the urine (greater than 6000 mcg/mL at 2 hours with 1 gram I.V.) and, therefore, the following zone sizes should be used when testing ceftizoxime for treatment of urinary tract infections caused by Pseudomonas aeruginosa.

Susceptible organisms produce zones of 20 mm or greater, indicating that the test organism is likely to respond to therapy.
Organisms that produce zones of 11 to 19 mm are expected to be susceptible when the infection is confined to the urinary tract (in which high antibiotic levels are attained).
Resistant organisms produce zones of 10 mm or less, indicating that other therapy should be selected.

Susceptibility Testing: Dilution Techniques

When using the NCCLS agar dilution or broth dilution (including microdilution) method[2] or equivalent, the following MIC data should be used for interpretation.

MIC (mcg/mL)	Interpretation
≤8	(S) Susceptible
16–32	(MS) Moderately Susceptible
≥64	(R) Resistant

As with standard disk diffusion methods, dilution procedures require the use of laboratory control organisms. Standard ceftizoxime powder should give MIC values in the following ranges.

Organism	ATCC	MIC (mcg/mL)
Escherichia coli	25922	0.03–0.12
Pseudomonas aeruginosa	27853	16–64
Staphylococcus aureus	29213	2–8

INDICATIONS AND USAGE

Cefizox (sterile ceftizoxime sodium) is indicated in the treatment of infections due to susceptible strains of the microorganisms listed below.
Lower Respiratory Tract Infections caused by Klebsiella spp.; Proteus mirabilis; Escherichia coli; Haemophilus influenzae including ampicillin-resistant strains; Staphylococcus aureus (penicillinase- and nonpenicillinase-producing); Serratia spp.; Enterobacter spp.; Bacteroides spp.; and Streptococcus spp. including S. pneumoniae, but excluding enterococci.
Urinary Tract Infections caused by Staphylococcus aureus (penicillinase- and nonpenicillinase-producing); Escherichia coli; Pseudomonas spp. including P. aeruginosa; Proteus mirabilis; P. vulgaris; Providencia rettgeri (formerly Proteus rettgeri) and Morganella morganii (formerly Proteus morganii); Klebsiella spp.; Serratia spp. including S. marcescens; and Enterobacter spp.
Gonorrhea including uncomplicated cervical and urethral gonorrhea caused by Neisseria gonorrhoeae.

Continued on next page

Cefizox for IM/IV Use—Cont.

Pelvic Inflammatory Disease caused by *Neisseria gonorrhoeae*, *Escherichia coli* or *Streptococcus agalactiae*.
NOTE: Ceftizoxime, like other cephalosporins, has no activity against *Chlamydia trachomatis*. Therefore, when cephalosporins are used in the treatment of patients with pelvic inflammatory disease and *C. trachomatis* is one of the suspected pathogens, appropriate antichlamydial coverage should be added.
Intra-Abdominal Infections caused by *Escherichia coli*; *Staphylococcus epidermidis*; *Streptococcus* spp. (excluding enterococci); *Enterobacter* spp.; *Klebsiella* spp.; *Bacteroides* spp. including *B. fragilis*; and anaerobic cocci, including *Peptococcus* spp. and *Peptostreptococcus* spp.
Septicemia caused by *Streptococcus* spp. including *S. pneumoniae* (but excluding enterococci); *Staphylococcus aureus* (penicillinase- and nonpenicillinase-producing); *Escherichia coli*; *Bacteroides* spp. including *B. fragilis*; *Klebsiella* spp.; and *Serratia* spp.
Skin and Skin Structure Infections caused by *Staphylococcus aureus* (penicillinase- and nonpenicillinase-producing); *Staphylococcus epidermidis*; *Escherichia coli*; *Klebsiella* spp.; *Streptococcus* spp. including *Streptococcus pyogenes* (but excluding enterococci); *Proteus mirabilis*; *Serratia* spp.; *Enterobacter* spp.; *Bacteroides* spp. including *B. fragilis*; and anaerobic cocci, including *Peptococcus* spp. and *Peptostreptococcus* spp.
Bone and Joint Infections caused by *Staphylococcus aureus* (penicillinase- and nonpenicillinase-producing); *Streptococcus* spp. (excluding enterococci); *Proteus mirabilis*; *Bacteroides* spp.; and anaerobic cocci, including *Peptococcus* spp. and *Peptostreptococcus* spp.
Meningitis caused by *Haemophilus influenzae*. Cefizox has also been used successfully in the treatment of a limited number of pediatric and adult cases of meningitis caused by *Streptococcus pneumoniae*.
Cefizox has been effective in the treatment of seriously ill, compromised patients, including those who were debilitated, immunosuppressed, or neutropenic.
Infections caused by aerobic gram-negative and by mixtures of organisms resistant to other cephalosporins, aminoglycosides, or penicillins have responded to treatment with Cefizox.
Because of the serious nature of some urinary tract infections due to *P. aeruginosa* and because many strains of *Pseudomonas* species are only moderately susceptible to Cefizox, higher dosage is recommended. Other therapy should be instituted if the response is not prompt.
Susceptibility studies on specimens obtained prior to therapy should be used to determine the response of causative organisms to Cefizox. Therapy with Cefizox may be initiated pending results of the studies; however, treatment should be adjusted according to study findings. In serious infections, Cefizox has been used concomitantly with aminoglycosides (see Precautions). Before using Cefizox concomitantly with other antibiotics, the prescribing information for those agents should be reviewed for contraindications, warnings, precautions, and adverse reactions. Renal function should be carefully monitored.

CONTRAINDICATIONS

Cefizox (sterile ceftizoxime sodium) is contraindicated in patients who have known allergy to the drug.

WARNINGS

BEFORE THERAPY WITH CEFIZOX IS INSTITUTED, CAREFUL INQUIRY SHOULD BE MADE TO DETERMINE WHETHER THE PATIENT HAS HAD PREVIOUS HYPERSENSITIVITY REACTIONS TO CEFIZOX, OTHER CEPHALOSPORINS, PENICILLINS, OR OTHER DRUGS. IF THIS PRODUCT IS TO BE GIVEN TO PENICILLIN-SENSITIVE PATIENTS, CAUTION SHOULD BE EXERCISED BECAUSE CROSS HYPERSENSITIVITY AMONG BETA–LACTAM ANTIBIOTICS HAS BEEN CLEARLY DOCUMENTED AND MAY OCCUR IN UP TO 10% OF PATIENTS WITH A HISTORY OF PENICILLIN ALLERGY. IF AN ALLERGIC REACTION TO CEFIZOX OCCURS, DISCONTINUE THE DRUG. SERIOUS ACUTE HYPERSENSITIVITY REACTIONS MAY REQUIRE TREATMENT WITH EPINEPHRINE AND OTHER EMERGENCY MEASURES, INCLUDING OXYGEN, INTRAVENOUS FLUIDS, INTRAVENOUS ANTIHISTAMINES, CORTICOSTEROIDS, PRESSOR AMINES, AND AIRWAY MANAGEMENT, AS CLINICALLY INDICATED.

Pseudomembranous colitis has been reported with nearly all antibacterial agents, including ceftizoxime, and may range in severity from mild to life threatening. Therefore, it is important to consider this diagnosis in patients who present with diarrhea subsequent to the administration of antibacterial agents.
Treatment with antibacterial agents alters the normal flora of the colon and may permit overgrowth of clostridia. Studies indicate that a toxin produced by *Clostridium difficile* is a primary cause of "antibiotic-associated" colitis.
After the diagnosis of pseudomembranous colitis has been established, appropriate therapeutic measures should be initiated. Mild cases of pseudomembranous colitis usually respond to drug discontinuation alone. In moderate to severe cases, consideration should be given to management with fluids and electrolytes, protein supplementation, and treatment with an antibacterial drug clinically effective against *Clostridium difficile* colitis.

PRECAUTIONS

General
As with all broad-spectrum antibiotics, Cefizox (sterile ceftizoxime sodium) should be prescribed with caution in individuals with a history of gastrointestinal disease, particularly colitis.
Although Cefizox has not been shown to produce an alteration in renal function, renal status should be evaluated, especially in seriously ill patients receiving maximum dose therapy. As with any antibiotic, prolonged use may result in overgrowth of nonsusceptible organisms. Careful observation is essential; appropriate measures should be taken if superinfection occurs.

Drug Interactions
Although the occurrence has not been reported with Cefizox, nephrotoxicity has been reported following concomitant administration of other cephalosporins and aminoglycosides.

Carcinogenesis, Mutagenesis, Impairment of Fertility
Long term studies in animals to evaluate the carcinogenic potential of ceftizoxime have not been conducted.
In an *in vitro* bacterial cell assay (i.e., Ames test), there was no evidence of mutagenicity at ceftizoxime concentrations of 0.001–0.5 mcg/plate. Ceftizoxime did not produce increases in micronuclei in the *in vivo* mouse micronucleus test when given to animals at doses up to 7500 mg/kg, approximately six times greater than the maximum human daily dose on a mg/M^2 basis.
Ceftizoxime had no effect on fertility when administered subcutaneously to rats at daily doses of up to 1000 mg/kg/day, approximately two times the maximum human daily dose on a mg/M^2 basis. Ceftizoxime produced no histological changes in the sexual organs of male and female dogs when given intravenously for thirteen weeks at a dose of 1000 mg/kg/day, approximately five times greater than the maximum human daily dose on a mg/M^2 basis.

Pregnancy: Teratogenic Effects: Pregnancy Category B.
Reproduction studies performed in rats and rabbits have revealed no evidence of impaired fertility or harm to the fetus due to Cefizox. There are, however, no adequate and well-controlled studies in pregnant women. Because animal reproduction studies are not always predictive of human effects, this drug should be used during pregnancy only if clearly needed.

Labor and Delivery
Safety of Cefizox use during labor and delivery has not been established.

Nursing Mothers
Cefizox is excreted in human milk in low concentrations. Caution should be exercised when Cefizox is administered to a nursing woman.

Pediatric Use
Safety and efficacy in pediatric patients from birth to six months of age have not been established. In pediatric patients six months of age and older, treatment with Cefizox has been associated with transient elevated levels of eosinophils, AST (SGOT), ALT (SGPT), and CPK (creatine phosphokinase). The CPK elevation may be related to I.M. administration.
The potential for the toxic effect in pediatric patients from chemicals that may leach from the single-dose I.V. preparation in plastic has not been determined.

ADVERSE REACTIONS

Cefizox® (sterile ceftizoxime sodium) is generally well tolerated. The *most* frequent adverse reactions (*greater* than 1% but *less* than 5%) are:
Hypersensitivity—Rash, pruritus, fever.
Hepatic—Transient elevation in AST (SGOT), ALT (SGPT), and alkaline phosphatase.
Hematologic—Transient eosinophilia, thrombocytosis. Some individuals have developed a positive Coombs test.
Local—Injection site—Burning, cellulitis, phlebitis with I.V. administration, pain, induration, tenderness, paresthesia.
The *less* frequent adverse reactions (*less* than 1%) are:
Hypersensitivity—Numbness and anaphylaxis have been reported rarely.
Hepatic—Elevation of bilirubin has been reported rarely.
Renal—Transient elevations of BUN and creatinine have been occasionally observed with Cefizox.
Hematologic—Anemia, including hemolytic anemia with occasional fatal outcome, leukopenia, neutropenia, and thrombocytopenia have been reported rarely.
Urogenital—Vaginitis has occurred rarely.
Gastrointestinal—Diarrhea; nausea and vomiting have been reported occasionally.
Symptoms of pseudomembranous colitis can appear during or after antibiotic treatment (see Warnings).

In addition to the adverse reactions listed above which have been observed in patients treated with ceftizoxime, the following adverse reactions and altered laboratory tests have been reported for cephalosporin-class antibiotics:
Stevens-Johnson syndrome, erythema multiforme, toxic epidermal necrolysis, serum-sickness like reaction, toxic nephropathy, aplastic anemia, hemorrhage, prolonged prothrombin time, elevated LDH, pancytopenia, and agranulocytosis.
Several cephalosporins have been implicated in triggering seizures, particularly in patients with renal impairment, when the dosage was not reduced. (See DOSAGE AND ADMINISTRATION.) If seizures associated with drug therapy occur, the drug should be discontinued. Anticonvulsant therapy can be given if clinically indicated.

DOSAGE AND ADMINISTRATION

The usual adult dosage is 1 or 2 grams of Cefizox (sterile ceftizoxime sodium) every 8 to 12 hours. Proper dosage and route of administration should be determined by the condition of the patient, severity of the infection, and susceptibility of the causative organisms.

General Guidelines for Dosage of Cefizox

Type of Infection	Daily Dose (Grams)	Frequency and Route
Uncomplicated Urinary Tract	1	500 mg q12h I.M. or I.V.
Other Sites	2–3	1 gram q8–12h I.M. or I.V.
Severe or Refractory	3–6	1 gram q8h I.M. or I.V. 2 grams q8–12h I.M.[a] or I.V.
PID[b]	6	2 grams q8h I.V.
Life-Threatening[c]	9–12	3–4 grams q8h I.V.

a) When administering 2 gram I.M. doses, the dose should be divided and given in different large muscle masses.
b) If *C. trachomatis* is a suspected pathogen, appropriate anti-chlamydial coverage should be added, because ceftizoxime has no activity against this organism.
c) In life-threatening infections, dosages up to 2 grams every 4 hours have been given.

Because of the serious nature of urinary tract infections due to *P. aeruginosa* and because many strains of *Pseudomonas* species are only moderately susceptible to Cefizox, higher dosage is recommended. Other therapy should be instituted if the response is not prompt.
A single, 1 gram I.M. dose is the usual dose for treatment of uncomplicated gonorrhea.
The intravenous route may be preferable for patients with bacterial septicemia, localized parenchymal abscesses (such as intra-abdominal abscess), peritonitis, or other severe or life-threatening infections.
In those with normal renal function, the intravenous dosage for such infections is 2 to 12 grams of Cefizox (sterile ceftizoxime sodium) daily. In conditions such as bacterial septicemia, 6 to 12 grams/day may be given initially by the intravenous route for several days, and the dosage may then be gradually reduced according to clinical response and laboratory findings.

Pediatric Dosage Schedule

	Unit Dose	Frequency
Pediatric patients 6 months and older	50 mg/kg	q6-8h

Dosage may be increased to a total daily dose of 200 mg/kg (not to exceed the maximum adult dose for serious infection).

Impaired Renal Function
Modification of Cefizox dosage is necessary in patients with impaired renal function. Following an initial loading dose of 500 mg–1 gram I.M. or I.V., the maintenance dosing schedule shown below should be followed. Further dosing should be determined by therapeutic monitoring, severity of the infection, and susceptibility of the causative organisms.
When only the serum creatinine level is available, creatinine clearance may be calculated from the following formula. The serum creatinine level should represent current renal function at the steady state.

Males

$$Clcr = \frac{Weight\ (kg) \times (140 - age)}{72 \times serum\ creatinine\ (mg/100\ mL)}$$

Females are 0.85 of the calculated clearance values for males.
In patients undergoing hemodialysis, no additional supplemental dosing is required following hemodialysis; however, dosing should be timed so that the patient receives the dose (according to the table below) at the end of the dialysis.

Dosage in Adults with Reduced Renal Function

Creatinine Clearance mL/min	Renal Function	Less Severe Infections	Life-Threatening Infections
79–50	Mild impairment	500 mg q8h	0.75–1.5 grams q8h
49–5	Moderate to severe impairment	250–500 mg q12h	0.5–1 gram q12h
4–0	Dialysis patients	500 mg q48h or 250 mg q24h	0.5–1 gram q48h or 0.5 gram q24h

Preparation of Parenteral Solution
RECONSTITUTION

I.M. Administration: Reconstitute with Sterile Water for Injection. SHAKE WELL.

Vial Size	Diluent to Be Added	Approx. Avail. Vol.	Approx. Avg. Concentration	Room Temp. Stability
500 mg	1.5 mL	1.8 mL	280 mg/mL	16 hours
1 gram	3.0 mL	3.7 mL	270 mg/mL	16 hours
2 grams*	6.0 mL	7.4 mL	270 mg/mL	16 hours

*When administering 2 gram I.M. doses, the dose should be divided and given in different large muscle masses.

I.V. Administration: Reconstitute with Sterile Water for Injection. SHAKE WELL.

Vial Size	Diluent to Be Added	Approx. Avail. Vol.	Approx. Avg. Concentration
500 mg	5 mL	5.3 mL	95 mg/mL
1 gram	10 mL	10.7 mL	95 mg/mL
2 grams	20 mL	21.4 mL	95 mg/mL

These solutions of Cefizox are stable 24 hours at room temperature or 96 hours if refrigerated (5°C).

Parenteral drug products should be inspected visually for particulate matter prior to administration. If particulate matter is evident in reconstituted fluids, then the drug solution should be discarded. Reconstituted solutions may range from yellow to amber without changes in potency.

"Piggyback" Vials: Reconstitute with 50 to 100 mL of Sodium Chloride Injection or any other I.V. solution listed below.

SHAKE WELL

Administer with primary I.V. fluids, as a single dose. These Piggyback vial solutions of Cefizox are stable 24 hours at room temperature or 96 hours if refrigerated (5°C).

A solution of 1 gram Cefizox in 13 mL Sterile Water for Injection is isotonic.

I.M. Injection
Inject well within the body of a relatively large muscle. Aspiration is necessary to avoid inadvertent injection into a blood vessel. When administering 2 gram I.M. doses, the dose should be divided and given in different large muscle masses.

I.V. Administration
Direct (bolus) injection, slowly over 3 to 5 minutes, directly or through tubing for patients receiving parenteral fluids (see list below). Intermittent or continuous infusion, dilute reconstituted Cefizox in 50 to 100 mL of one of the following solutions:
- Sodium Chloride Injection
- 5% or 10% Dextrose Injection
- 5% Dextrose and 0.9%, 0.45%, or 0.2% Sodium Chloride Injection
- Ringer's Injection
- Lactated Ringer's Injection
- Invert Sugar 10% in Sterile Water for Injection
- 5% Sodium Bicarbonate in Sterile Water for Injection
- 5% Dextrose in Lactated Ringer's Injection (only when reconstituted with 4% Sodium Bicarbonate Injection)

In these fluids, Cefizox is stable 24 hours at room temperature or 96 hours if refrigerated (5°C).

HOW SUPPLIED
Cefizox® (sterile ceftizoxime sodium)

NDC 0469-7250-01   Product No. 725001
   Equivalent to 500 mg ceftizoxime in 10 mL, single-dose, flip-top vials, individually packaged

NDC 0469-7251-01   Product No. 725101
   Equivalent to 1 gram ceftizoxime in 20 mL, single-dose, flip-top vials, individually packaged

NDC 0469-7252-01   Product No. 725201
   Equivalent to 1 gram ceftizoxime in 100 mL, single-dose, Piggyback, flip-top vials, packaged in tens

NDC 0469-7253-02   Product No. 725302
   Equivalent to 2 grams ceftizoxime in 20 mL, single-dose, flip-top vials, individually packaged

NDC 0469-7254-02   Product No. 725402
   Equivalent to 2 grams ceftizoxime in 100 mL, single-dose, Piggyback, flip-top vials, packaged in tens

Unreconstituted Cefizox should be protected from excessive light, and stored at controlled room temperature (59°–86°F) in the original package until used.
Product of Japan

REFERENCES
1. National Committee for Clinical Laboratory Standards, Approved Standard. *Performance Standards for Antimicrobial Disk Susceptibility Test*, 4th Edition, Vol 10 (7): M2-A4. Villanova, PA, April 1990.
2. National Committee for Clinical Laboratory Standards, Approved Standard. *Methods for Dilution Antimicrobial Susceptibility Tests for Bacteria that Grow Aerobically*, 2nd Edition, Vol 10 (8):M7-A2. Villanova, PA, April 1990.

Revised October 1997

CEFIZOX®   ℞
(sterile ceftizoxime sodium)
For Intramuscular or Intravenous Use
PHARMACY BULK PACKAGE—NOT FOR DIRECT INFUSION

DESCRIPTION
Cefizox® (sterile ceftizoxime sodium) pharmacy bulk vial is a sterile dosage form which contains many single doses for use in a pharmacy admixture program in the preparation of parenteral fluids. Cefizox is a sterile, semi-synthetic, broad-spectrum, beta-lactamase resistant cephalosporin antibiotic for parenteral (I.V., I.M.) administration. It is the sodium salt of [6R-[6a, 7β(Z)]]7-[[(2,3-dihydro-2-imino-4-thiazolyl) (methoxyimino) acetyl] amino]-8-oxo-5-thia-1-azabicyclo [4.2.0] oct-2-ene-2-carboxylic acid. Its sodium content is approximately 60 mg (2.6 mEq) per gram of ceftizoxime activity.

It has the following structural formula:

$C_{13}H_{12}N_5NaO_5S_2$ 405.38

Sterile ceftizoxime sodium is a white to pale yellow crystalline powder. Cefizox is supplied in vials equivalent to 10 grams of ceftizoxime in pharmacy bulk packaging.

HOW SUPPLIED
Cefizox® (sterile ceftizoxime sodium)

NDC 0469-7255-10   Product No. 725510
   Equivalent to 10 grams ceftizoxime in 100 mL, Pharmacy Bulk Package, packaged in tens

Unreconstituted Cefizox should be protected from excessive light, and stored at controlled room temperature (59°–86°F) in the original package until used.
Product of Japan

Revised October 1997

CEFIZOX®   ℞
(ceftizoxime for injection, USP)
For Intravenous Infusion

DESCRIPTION
Cefizox® (ceftizoxime for injection, USP) is a sterile, semi-synthetic, broad-spectrum, beta-lactamase resistant cephalosporin antibiotic for parenteral (I.V., I.M.) administration. It is the sodium salt of [6R-[6a, 7β(Z)]]-7-[[(2,3-dihydro-2-imino-4-thiazolyl) (methoxyimino) acetyl] amino]-8-oxo-5-thia-1-azabicyclo [4.2.0] oct-2-ene-2-carboxylic acid. Its sodium content is approximately 60 mg (2.6 mEq) per gram of ceftizoxime activity.

It has the following structural formula:

$C_{13}H_{12}N_5NaO_5S_2$ 405.38

Ceftizoxime for injection is a white to pale yellow crystalline powder.

Cefizox is supplied in ADD-Vantage® vials as ceftizoxime sodium equivalent to 1 gram and 2 grams of ceftizoxime.

HOW SUPPLIED
Cefizox® (ceftizoxime for injection, USP) in ADD-Vantage® Vials

NDC 0469-7271-01   Product No. 727101
   equivalent to 1 gram ceftizoxime, packaged in tens

NDC 0469-7272-02   Product No. 727202
   equivalent to 2 grams ceftizoxime, packaged in tens

Unreconstituted Cefizox should be protected from excessive light, and stored at controlled room temperature 15°–30°C (59°–86°F) in the original package until used.

ADD-Vantage® is a registered trademark of Abbott Laboratories.
Product of Japan
U.S. Patent 4,427,674
Manufactured for Fujisawa USA, Inc., Deerfield, IL 60015, by SmithKline Beecham, Philadelphia, PA 19101.

CF:L4AV   Revised Apr. 1998

CEFIZOX®   ℞
(ceftizoxime injection)
in Galaxy® Plastic Container (PL 2040)
For Intravenous Use

DESCRIPTION
Cefizox® (ceftizoxime injection) in the Galaxy® plastic container (PL 2040) contains ceftizoxime as ceftizoxime sodium. It is a sterile, semisynthetic, broad spectrum, cephalosporin antibiotic for intravenous administration.

Chemically, it is the sodium (6R,7R)-7-[2-(2-imino-4-thiazolin-4-yl), glyoxylamido]-8-oxo-5-thia-1-azabicyclo [4.2.0]oct-2-ene-2-carboxylate 7²-(Z)-(O—methyloxime). The molecular formula is $C_{13}H_{12}N_5NaO_5S_2$ and the molecular weight is 405.38. The structural formula of ceftizoxime sodium is as follows:

Cefizox (ceftizoxime injection) in the Galaxy® plastic container is a frozen iso-osmotic, sterile, nonpyrogenic premixed 50 mL solution containing 1 g or 2 g of ceftizoxime as ceftizoxime sodium. Dextrose, USP has been added to these dosages to adjust osmolality (approximately 1.9 g and 950 mg to the 1 g and 2 g dosages as dextrose hydrous, respectively). Thawed solutions range from very pale yellow to yellow. The pH of thawed solutions range from 5.5 to 8.0. After thawing to room temperature, the solution is intended for intravenous use only.

The Galaxy® container is fabricated from a specially designed multilayer plastic (PL 2040). Solutions are in contact with the polyethylene layer of this container and can leach out certain chemical components of the plastic in very small amounts within the expiration dating period. The suitability of the plastic has been confirmed in tests in animals according to the USP biological tests for plastic containers, as well as by tissue culture toxicity studies.

HOW SUPPLIED
Cefizox® (ceftizoxime injection) is supplied as a frozen, sio-osmotic, sterile, nonpyrogenic solution in 50 mL single dose Galaxy® plastic containers (PL2040) as follows:

NDC 0469-7220-01   Product No. 722001
   1 g ceftizoxime/50 mL container

NDC 0469-7221-02   Product No. 722102
   2 g ceftizoxime/50 mL container

Store at or below −20°C/−4°F.

See DIRECTIONS FOR USE OF CEFIZOX® (ceftizoxime injection) IN GALAXY® PLASTIC CONTAINER (PL 2040).

Galaxy® is a registered trademark of Baxter International Inc.

Ceftizoxime sodium is a product of Japan.

Manufactured for Fujisawa USA, Inc.
Deerfield, IL 60015 by
Baxter Healthcare Corporation, Deerfield, IL 60015,
45621E/Revised January 1998

Continued on next page

CYCLOCORT® ℞
[amcinonide]

DESCRIPTION

The topical corticosteroids constitute a class of primarily synthetic steroids used as anti-inflammatory and antipruritic agents.

TOPICAL LOTION 0.1%

Each gram of CYCLOCORT (amcinonide) topical Lotion contains 1 mg of the active steroid amcinonide in AQUATAIN,* a white, smooth, homogeneous, opaque emulsion composed of Benzyl Alcohol 1% (wt/wt) as preservative, Emulsifying Wax, Glycerin, Isopropyl Palmitate, Lactic Acid, Purified Water, and Sorbitol Solution. In addition, contains Polyethylene Glycol 400.

Sodium hydroxide may be used to adjust pH to approximately 4.4 during manufacture.

TOPICAL CREAM 0.1%

Each gram of CYCLOCORT (amcinonide) topical Cream contains 1 mg of the active steroid amcinonide in AQUATAIN,* a white, smooth, homogeneous, opaque emulsion composed of Benzyl Alcohol 2% (wt/wt) as preservative, Emulsifying Wax, Glycerin, Isopropyl Palmitate, Lactic Acid, Purified Water, and Sorbitol Solution.

*AQUATAIN™ is non-staining, water-washable, paraben-free, spermaceti-free, and has a light texture and consistency.

TOPICAL OINTMENT 0.1%

Each gram of CYCLOCORT (amcinonide) topical Ointment contains 1 mg of the active steroid amcinonide in a specially formulated base composed of Benzyl Alcohol 2% as preservative, White Petrolatum, Emulsifying Wax, and Tenox II (Butylated Hydroxyanisole, Propyl Gallate, Citric Acid, Propylene Glycol).

Chemically, amcinonide is:

Molecular Weight 502.58 $C_{28}H_{35}FO_7$

Pregna-1,4-diene-3,20-dione, 21-(acetyloxy)-16,17-[cyclopentylidenebis(oxy)]-9-fluoro-11-hydroxy-, (11β, 16α).

HOW SUPPLIED

CYCLOCORT® (amcinonide) Topical Lotion 0.1% (1 mg/g) with AQUATAIN™ hydrophilic base

| NDC 0469-7404-20 | Product Code 740420 |
20 mL (19.6 g) Bottle
| NDC 0469-7404-60 | Product Code 740460 |
60 mL (58.8 g) Bottle

CYCLOCORT® (amcinonide) Topical Cream 0.1% (1 mg/g) with AQUATAIN™ hydrophilic base

| NDC 0469-7054-15 | Product Code 705415 |
15 gram Tube
| NDC 0469-7054-30 | Product Code 705430 |
30 gram Tube
| NDC 0469-7054-60 | Product Code 705460 |
60 gram Tube

CYCLOCORT® (amcinonide) Topical Ointment 0.1% (1 mg/g)

| NDC 0469-7115-15 | Product Code 711515 |
15 gram Tube
| NDC 0469-7115-30 | Product Code 711530 |
30 gram Tube
| NDC 0469-7115-60 | Product Code 711560 |
60 gram Tube

Store at controlled room temperature 15°–30°C (59°–86°F). DO NOT FREEZE.

Manufactured for Fujisawa USA, Inc., Deerfield, IL 60015 by

Lederle Laboratories Division,
American Cyanamid Company,
Pearl River, NY 10965
CI 4432–1   Issued November 20, 1995

PROGRAF® ℞
tacrolimus capsules
tacrolimus injection (for intravenous infusion only)

DESCRIPTION

Prograf is available for oral administration as capsules (tacrolimus capsules) containing the equivalent of 1 mg or 5 mg of anhydrous tacrolimus. Inactive ingredients include lactose, hydroxypropyl methylcellulose, croscarmellose sodium, and magnesium stearate. The 1 mg capsule shell contains gelatin and titanium dioxide, and the 5 mg capsule shell contains gelatin, titanium dioxide and ferric oxide.

Prograf is also available as a sterile solution (tacrolimus injection) containing the equivalent of 5 mg anhydrous tacrolimus in 1 mL for administration by intravenous infusion only. Each mL contains polyoxyl 60 hydrogenated castor oil (HCO-60), 200 mg, and dehydrated alcohol, USP, 80.0% v/v. Prograf injection must be diluted with 0.9% Sodium Chloride Injection or 5% Dextrose Injection before use.

Tacrolimus, previously known as FK506, is the active ingredient in Prograf. Tacrolimus is a macrolide immunosuppressant produced by *Streptomyces tsukubaensis*. Chemically, tacrolimus is designated as [3S–[3R*[E(1S*,3S*,4S*)], 4S*,5R*,8S*,9E,12R*,14R*,15S*,16R*,18S*,19S*,26aR*]]-5,6,8,11,12,13,14,15,16,17,18,19,24,25,26,26a-hexadecahydro-5,19-dihydroxy-3-[2-(4-hydroxy-3-methoxycyclohexyl)-1-methylethenyl]-14,16-dimethoxy-4,10,12,18-tetramethyl-8-(2-propenyl)-15,19-epoxy-3H-pyrido[2,1-c][1,4] oxaazacyclotricosine-1,7,20,21(4H,23H)-tetrone, monohydrate. The chemical structure of tacrolimus is:

Tacrolimus has an empirical formula of $C_{44}H_{69}NO_{12} \cdot H_2O$ and a formula weight of 822.05. Tacrolimus appears as white crystals or crystalline powder. It is practically insoluble in water, freely soluble in ethanol, and very soluble in methanol and chloroform.

CLINICAL PHARMACOLOGY

Mechanism of Action

Tacrolimus prolongs the survival of the host and transplanted graft in animal transplant models of liver, kidney, heart, bone marrow, small bowel and pancreas, lung and trachea, skin, cornea, and limb.

In animals, tacrolimus has been demonstrated to suppress some humoral immunity and, to a greater extent, cell-mediated reactions such as allograft rejection, delayed type hypersensitivity, collagen-induced arthritis, experimental allergic encephalomyelitis, and graft versus host disease. Tacrolimus inhibits T-lymphocyte activation, although the exact mechanism of action is not known. Experimental evidence suggests that tacrolimus binds to an intracellular protein, FKBP-12. A complex of tacrolimus-FKBP-12, calcium, calmodulin, and calcineurin is then formed and the phosphatase activity of calcineurin inhibited. This effect may prevent the dephosphorylation and translocation of nuclear factor of activated T-cells (NF-AT), a nuclear component thought to initiate gene transcription for the formation of lymphokines (such as interleukin-2, gamma interferon). The net result is the inhibition of T-lymphocyte activation (i.e., immunosuppression).

Pharmacokinetics

Tacrolimus activity is primarily due to the parent drug. The pharmacokinetic parameters (means ± S.D.) of tacrolimus have been determined following intravenous (IV) and oral (PO) administration in healthy volunteers, liver transplant and kidney transplant patients. (See table below.)

Due to intersubject variability in tacrolimus pharmacokinetics, individualization of dosing regimen is necessary for optimal therapy. (See DOSAGE AND ADMINISTRATION). Pharmacokinetic data indicate that whole blood concentrations rather than plasma concentrations serve as the more appropriate sampling compartment to describe tacrolimus pharmacokinetics.

Absorption

Absorption of tacrolimus from the gastrointestinal tract after oral administration is incomplete and variable. The absolute bioavailability of tacrolimus was 17 ± 10% in adult kidney transplant patients (N = 26), 22 ± 6% in adult liver transplant patients (N = 17), and 18 ± 5% in healthy volunteers (N = 16).

A single dose study conducted in 32 healthy volunteers established the bioequivalence of the 1 mg and 5 mg capsules. Tacrolimus maximum blood concentration (C_{max}) and area under the curve (AUC) appeared to increase in a dose-proportional fashion in 18 fasted healthy volunteers receiving a single oral dose of 3, 7 and 10 mg.

In 18 kidney transplant patients, tacrolimus trough concentrations from 3 to 30 ng/mL measured at 10–12 hours postdose (C_{min}) correlated well with the AUC (correlation coefficient 0.93). In 24 liver transplant patients over a concentration range of 10 to 60 ng/mL, the correlation coefficient was 0.94.

Food Effects: The rate and extent of tacrolimus absorption were greatest under fasted conditions. The presence and composition of food decreased both the rate and extent of tacrolimus absorption when administered to 15 healthy volunteers.

The effect was most pronounced with a high-fat meal (848 kcal, 46% fat): mean AUC and C_{max} were decreased 37% and 77%, respectively; T_{max} was lengthened 5-fold. A high-carbohydrate meal (668 kcal, 85% carbohydrate) decreased mean AUC and mean C_{max} by 28% and 65%, respectively.

In healthy volunteers (N = 16), the time of the meal also affected tacrolimus bioavailability. When given immediately following the meal, mean C_{max} was reduced 71%, and mean AUC was reduced 39%, relative to the fasted condition.

Population	N	Route (Dose)	C_{max} (ng/mL)	T_{max} (hr)	AUC (ng·hr/mL)	$t_{1/2}$ (hr)	Cl (L/hr/kg)	V (L/kg)
					Parameters			
Healthy Volunteers	8	IV (0.025 mg/kg/4hr)	—	—	598* ± 125	34.2 ± 7.7	0.040 ± 0.009	1.91 ± 0.31
	16	PO (5 mg)	29.7 ± 7.2	1.6 ± 0.7	243** ± 73	34.8 ± 11.4	0.041† ± 0.008	1.94† ± 0.53
Kidney Transplant Pts	26	IV (0.02 mg/kg/12hr)	—	—	294*** ± 262	18.8 ± 16.7	0.083 ± 0.050	1.41 ± 0.66
		PO (0.2 mg/kg/day)	19.2 ± 10.3	3.0	203*** ± 42	#	#	#
		PO (0.3 mg/kg/day)	24.2 ± 15.8	1.5	288*** ± 93	#	#	#
Liver Transplant Pts	17	IV (0.05 mg/kg/12 hr)	—	—	3300*** ± 2130	11.7 ± 3.9	0.053 ± 0.017	0.85 ± 0.30
		PO (0.3 mg/kg/day)	68.5 ± 30.0	2.3 ± 1.5	519*** ± 179	#	#	#

† Corrected for individual bioavailability
* AUC_{0-120}
** AUC_{0-72}
*** AUC_{0-inf}
— not applicable
not available

When administered 1.5 hours following the meal, mean C_{max} was reduced 63%, and mean AUC was reduced 39%, relative to the fasted condition.

In 11 liver transplant patients, Prograf administered 15 minutes after a high fat (400 kcal, 34% fat) breakfast, resulted in decreased AUC (27 ± 18%) and C_{max} (50 ± 19%), as compared to a fasted state.

Distribution
The plasma protein binding of tacrolimus is approximately 99% and is independent of concentration over a range of 5–50 ng/mL. Tacrolimus is bound mainly to albumin and alpha-1-acid glycoprotein, and has a high level of association with erythrocytes. The distribution of tacrolimus between whole blood and plasma depends on several factors, such as hematocrit, temperature at the time of plasma separation, drug concentration, and plasma protein concentration. In a U.S. study, the ratio of whole blood concentration to plasma concentration averaged 35 (range 12 to 67).

Metabolism
Tacrolimus is extensively metabolized by the mixed-function oxidase system, primarily the cytochrome P-450 system (CYP3A). A metabolic pathway leading to the formation of 8 possible metabolites has been proposed. Demethylation and hydroxylation were identified as the primary mechanisms of biotransformation in vitro. The major metabolite identified in incubations with human liver microsomes is 13-demethyl tacrolimus. In in vitro studies, a 31-demethyl metabolite has been reported to have the same activity as tacrolimus.

Excretion
The mean clearance following IV administration of tacrolimus is 0.040, 0.083 and 0.053 L/hr/kg in healthy volunteers, adult kidney transplant patients and adult liver transplant patients, respectively. In man, less than 1% of the dose administered is excreted unchanged in urine.

In a mass balance study of IV administered radiolabeled tacrolimus to 6 healthy volunteers, the mean recovery of radiolabel was 77.8 ± 12.7%. Fecal elimination accounted for 92.4 ± 1.0% and the elimination half-life based on radioactivity was 48.1 ± 15.9 hours whereas it was 43.5 ± 11.6 hours based on tacrolimus concentrations. The mean clearance of radiolabel was 0.029 ± 0.015 L/hr/kg and clearance of tacrolimus was 0.029 ± 0.009 L/hr/kg.

When administered PO, the mean recovery of the radiolabel was 94.9 ± 30.7%. Fecal elimination accounted for 92.6 ± 30.7%, urinary elimination accounted for 2.3 ± 1.1% and the elimination half-life based on radioactivity was 31.9 ± 10.5 hours whereas it was 48.4 ± 12.3 hours based on tacrolimus concentrations. The mean clearance of radiolabel was 0.226 ± 0.116 L/hr/kg and clearance of tacrolimus 0.172 ± 0.088 L/hr/kg.

Special Populations
Pediatric
Pharmacokinetics of tacrolimus have been studied in liver transplantation patients, 0.7 to 13.2 years of age. Following IV administration of a 0.037 mg/kg/day dose to 12 pediatric patients, mean terminal half-life, volume of distribution and clearance were 11.5 ± 3.8 hours, 2.6 ± 2.1 L/kg and 0.138 ± 0.071 L/hr/kg, respectively. Following oral administration to 9 patients, mean AUC and C_{max} were 337 ± 167 ng·hr/mL and 43.4 ± 27.9 ng/mL, respectively. The absolute bioavailability was 31 ± 21%.

Whole blood trough concentrations from 31 patients less than 12 years old showed that pediatric patients needed higher doses than adults to achieve similar tacrolimus trough concentrations. (See **DOSAGE AND ADMINISTRATION**).

Renal and Hepatic Insufficiency
The mean pharmacokinetic parameters for tacrolimus following single administrations to patients with renal and hepatic impairment are given in the following table.
[See table above]

Renal Insufficiency:
Tacrolimus pharmacokinetics following a single IV administration were determined in 12 patients (7 not on dialysis and 5 on dialysis, serum creatinine of 3.9 ± 1.6 and 12.0 ± 2.4 mg/dL, respectively) prior to their kidney transplant. The pharmacokinetic parameters obtained were similar for both groups.

The mean clearance of tacrolimus in patients with renal dysfunction was similar to that in normal volunteers (see previous table).

Hepatic Insufficiency:
Tacrolimus pharmacokinetics have been determined in six patients with mild hepatic dysfunction (mean Pugh score: 6.2) following single IV and oral administrations. The mean clearance of tacrolimus in patients with mild hepatic dysfunction was not substantially different from that in normal volunteers (see previous table).

Race
A formal study to evaluate the pharmacokinetic disposition of tacrolimus in Black transplant patients has not been conducted. However, a retrospective comparison of Black and Caucasian kidney transplant patients indicated that Black patients required higher tacrolimus doses to attain similar trough concentrations. (See **DOSAGE AND ADMINISTRATION**).

Population (No. of Patients)	Dose	AUC_{0-t} (ng·hr/mL)	$t_{1/2}$ (hr)	V (L/kg)	Cl (L/hr/kg)
Renal Impairment (n=12)	0.02 mg/kg/4hr IV	393±123*	26.3±9.2	1.07 ±0.20	0.038 ±0.014
Mild Hepatic Impairment (n=6)	0.02 mg/kg/4hr IV	367±107**	60.6±43.8 Range: 27.8–141	3.1 ±1.6	0.042 ±0.02
	7.7 mg PO	488±320**	66.1±44.8 Range: 29.5–138	3.7 ±4.7***	0.034 ±0.019***

* 0–60 hr.
** 0–72 hr.
*** corrected for bioavailability

Gender
The effect of gender on tacrolimus pharmacokinetics has not been evaluated, however, there was no difference in dosing by gender in the kidney transplant trial.

Clinical Studies
Liver Transplantation
The safety and efficacy of Prograf-based immunosuppression following orthotopic liver transplantation were assessed in two prospective, randomized, non-blinded multicenter studies. The active control groups were treated with a cyclosporine-based immunosuppressive regimen. Both studies used concomitant adrenal corticosteroids as part of the immunosuppressive regimens. These studies were designed to evaluate whether the two regimens were therapeutically equivalent, with patient and graft survival at 12 months following transplantation as the primary endpoints. The Prograf-based immunosuppressive regimen was found to be equivalent to the cyclosporine-based immunosuppressive regimens.

In one trial, 529 patients were enrolled at 12 clinical sites in the United States; prior to surgery, 263 were randomized to the Prograf-based immunosuppressive regimen and 266 to a cyclosporine-based immunosuppressive regimen (CBIR). In 10 of the 12 sites, the same CBIR protocol was used, while 2 sites used different control protocols. This trial excluded patients with renal dysfunction, fulminant hepatic failure with Stage IV encephalopathy, and cancers; pediatric patients (≤ 12 years old) were allowed.

In the second trial, 545 patients were enrolled at 8 clinical sites in Europe; prior to surgery, 270 were randomized to the Prograf-based immunosuppressive regimen and 275 to CBIR. In this study, each center used its local standard CBIR protocol in the active-control arm. This trial excluded pediatric patients, but did allow enrollment of subjects with renal dysfunction, fulminant hepatic failure in Stage IV encephalopathy, and cancers other than primary hepatic with metastases.

One-year patient survival and graft survival in the Prograf-based treatment groups were equivalent to those in the CBIR treatment groups in both studies. The overall one-year patient survival (CBIR and Prograf-based treatment groups combined) was 88% in the U.S. study and 78% in the European study. The overall one-year graft survival (CBIR and Prograf-based treatment groups combined) was 81% in the U.S. study and 73% in the European study. In both studies, the median time to convert from IV to oral Prograf dosing was 2 days.

Because of the nature of the study design, comparisons of differences in secondary endpoints, such as incidence of acute rejection, refractory rejection or use of OKT®3 for steroid-resistant rejection, could not be reliably made.

Kidney Transplantation
Prograf-based immunosuppression following kidney transplantation was assessed in a randomized, multicenter, non-blinded, prospective study. There were 412 kidney transplant patients enrolled at 19 clinical sites in the United States. Study therapy was initiated when renal function was stable as indicated by a serum creatinine ≤ 4 mg/dL (median of 4 days after transplantation, range 1 to 14 days). Patients less than 6 years of age were excluded.

There were 205 patients randomized to Prograf-based immunosuppression and 207 patients were randomized to cyclosporine-based immunosuppression. All patients received prophylactic induction therapy consisting of an antilymphocyte antibody preparation, corticosteroids and azathioprine. Overall one year patient and graft survival was 96.1% and 89.6%, respectively and was equivalent between treatment arms.

Because of the nature of the study design, comparisons of differences in secondary endpoints, such as incidence of acute rejection, refractory rejection or use of OKT®3 for steroid-resistant rejection, could not be reliably made.

INDICATIONS AND USAGE
Prograf is indicated for the prophylaxis of organ rejection in patients receiving allogeneic liver or kidney transplants. It is recommended that Prograf be used concomitantly with adrenal corticosteroids. Because of the risk of anaphylaxis, Prograf injection should be reserved for patients unable to take Prograf capsules orally.

CONTRAINDICATIONS
Prograf is contraindicated in patients with a hypersensitivity to tacrolimus. Prograf injection is contraindicated in patients with a hypersensitivity to HCO-60 (polyoxyl 60 hydrogenated castor oil).

WARNINGS
(See boxed **WARNING**.)

Insulin-dependent post-transplant diabetes mellitus (PTDM) was reported in 20% of Prograf-treated kidney transplant patients (See Table). The median time to onset of PTDM was 68 days. Insulin dependence was reversible in 15% of these patients at one year and in 50% at two years post transplant. Black and Hispanic kidney transplant patients were at an increased risk of development of PTDM.

Incidence of Post Transplant Diabetes Mellitus (PTDM)* and Insulin Use at 24 Months in Kidney Transplant Recipients

	Prograf	CBIR
Patients without pretransplant history of diabetes mellitus	151	151
New onset PTDM*, 1st Year	30/151 (20%)	6/151 (4%)
Still insulin dependent at one year in those without prior history of diabetes	25/151 (17%)	5/151 (3%)
New onset PTDM* post 1 year	1	0
Patients with PTDM* at 24 months	16/151 (11%)	5/151 (3%)

---

* use of insulin for 30 or more consecutive days, with < 5 day gap, without a prior history of insulin dependent diabetes mellitus or non insulin dependent diabetes mellitus.

[See first table at top of next page]

Insulin-dependent post-transplant diabetes mellitus was reported in 18% and 11% of Prograf-treated liver transplant patients and was reversible in 45% and 31% of these patients at one year post transplant, in the U.S. and European randomized studies, respectively (See Table below). Hyperglycemia was associated with the use of Prograf in 47% and 33% of liver transplant recipients in the U.S. and European randomized studies, respectively, and may require treatment (see **ADVERSE REACTIONS**).

[See second table at top of next page]

Prograf can cause neurotoxicity and nephrotoxicity, particularly when used in high doses. Nephrotoxicity was reported in approximately 52% of kidney transplantation patients and in 40% and 36% of liver transplantation patients receiving Prograf in the U.S. and European randomized trials, respectively (see **ADVERSE REACTIONS**). More overt nephrotoxicity is seen early after transplantation, characterized by increasing serum creatinine and a decrease in urine output. Patients with impaired renal function should be monitored closely as the dosage of Prograf may need to be reduced. In patients with persistent elevations of serum creatinine who are unresponsive to dosage adjustments, consideration should be given to changing to another immunosuppressive therapy. Care should be taken in using tacrolimus with other nephrotoxic drugs. **In particular, to avoid excess nephrotoxicity, Prograf should not be used simultaneously with cyclosporine. Prograf or cyclosporine should be discontinued at least 24 hours prior to initiating the other. In the presence of elevated Prograf or cyclosporine concentrations, dosing with the other drug usually should be further delayed.**

Mild to severe hyperkalemia was reported in 31% of kidney transplant receipients and in 45% and 13% of liver transplant recipients treated with Prograf in the U.S. and European randomized trials, respectively, and may require treatment (see **ADVERSE REACTIONS**). **Serum potassium levels should be monitored and potassium-sparing diuretics should not be used during Prograf therapy (see PRECAUTIONS).**

Continued on next page

Prograf—Cont.

Neurotoxicity, including tremor, headache, and other changes in motor function, mental status, and sensory function were reported in approximately 55% of liver transplant recipients in the two randomized studies. Tremor occurred more often in Prograf-treated kidney transplant patients (54%) compared to cyclosporine-treated patients. The incidence of other neurological events in kidney transplant patients was similar in the two treatment groups (see **ADVERSE REACTIONS**). Tremor and headache have been associated with high whole-blood concentrations of tacrolimus and may respond to dosage adjustment. Seizures have occurred in adult and pediatric patients receiving Prograf (see **ADVERSE REACTIONS**). Coma and delirium also have been associated with high plasma concentrations of tacrolimus.

As in patients receiving other immunosuppressants, patients receiving Prograf are at increased risk of developing lymphomas and other malignancies, particularly of the skin. The risk appears to be related to the intensity and duration of immunosuppression rather than to the use of any specific agent. A lymphoproliferative disorder (LPD) related to Epstein-Barr Virus (EBV) infection has been reported in immunosuppressed organ transplant recipients. The risk of LPD appears greatest in young children who are at risk for primary EBV infection while immunosuppressed or who are switched to Prograf following long-term immunosuppression therapy. Because of the danger of oversuppression of the immune system which can increase susceptibility to infection, combination immunosuppressant therapy should be used with caution.

A few patients receiving Prograf injection have experienced anaphylactic reactions. Although the exact cause of these reactions is not known, other drugs with castor oil derivatives in the formulation have been associated with anaphylaxis in a small percentage of patients. Because of this potential risk of anaphylaxis, Prograf injection should be reserved for patients who are unable to take Prograf capsules. **Patients receiving Prograf injection should be under continuous observation for at least the first 30 minutes following the start of the infusion and at frequent intervals thereafter. If signs or symptoms of anaphylaxis occur, the infusion should be stopped. An aqueous solution of epinephrine should be available at the bedside as well as a source of oxygen.**

PRECAUTIONS

General

Hypertension is a common adverse effect of Prograf therapy (see **ADVERSE REACTIONS**). Mild or moderate hypertension is more frequently reported than severe hypertension. Antihypertensive therapy may be required; the control of blood pressure can be accomplished with any of the common antihypertensive agents. Since tacrolimus may cause hyperkalemia, potassium-sparing diuretics should be avoided. While calcium-channel blocking agents can be effective in treating Prograf-associated hypertension, care should be taken since interference with tacrolimus metabolism may require a dosage reduction (see ***Drug Interactions***).

Renally and Hepatically Impaired Patients

For patients with renal insufficiency some evidence suggests that lower doses should be used (see **DOSAGE AND ADMINISTRATION**).

The use of Prograf in liver transplant recipients experiencing post-transplant hepatic impairment may be associated with increased risk of developing renal insufficiency related to high whole-blood levels of tacrolimus. These patients should be monitored closely and dosage adjustments should be considered. Some evidence suggests that lower doses should be used in these patients (see **DOSAGE AND ADMINISTRATION**).

Myocardial Hypertrophy

Myocardial hypertrophy has been reported in association with the administration of Prograf, and is generally manifested by echocardiographically demonstrated concentric increases in left ventricular posterior wall and interventricular septum thickness. Hypertrophy has been observed in infants, children and adults. This condition appears reversible in most cases following dose reduction or discontinuance of therapy. In a group of 20 patients with pre- and post-treatment echocardiograms who showed evidence of myocardial hypertrophy, mean tacrolimus whole blood concentrations during the period prior to diagnosis of myocardial hypertrophy ranged from 11 to 53 ng/mL in infants (N = 10, age 0.4 to 2 years), 4 to 46 ng/mL in children (N = 7, age 2 to 15 years) and 11 to 24 ng/mL in adults (N = 3, age 37 to 53 years).

In patients who develop renal failure or clinical manifestations of ventricular dysfunction while receiving Prograf therapy, echocardiographic evaluation should be considered. If myocardial hypertrophy is diagnosed, dosage reduction or discontinuation of Prograf should be considered.

Information for Patients

Patients should be informed of the need for repeated appropriate laboratory tests while they are receiving Prograf.

Development of Post Transplant Diabetes Mellitus (PTDM) by Race and by Treatment Group during First Year Post Kidney Transplantation

Patient Race	Prograf: No. of Patients at Risk	Prograf: Patients Who Developed PTDM*	CBIR: No. of Patients at Risk	CBIR: Patients Who Developed PTDM*
Black	41	15 (37%)	36	3 (8%)
Hispanic	17	5 (29%)	18	1 (6%)
Caucasian	82	10 (12%)	87	1 (1%)
Other	11	0 (0%)	10	1 (10%)
Total	151	30 (20%)	151	6 (4%)

* use of insulin for 30 or more consecutive days, with < 5 day gap, without a prior history of insulin dependent diabetes mellitus or non insulin dependent diabetes mellitus.

Incidence of Post Transplant Diabetes Mellitus (PTDM)* and Insulin Use at One Year in Liver Transplant Recipients

Status of PTDM*	US Study: Prograf	US Study: CBIR	European Study: Prograf	European Study: CBIR
Patients at risk**	239	236	239	249
New Onset PTDM*	42 (18%)	30 (13%)	26 (11%)	12 (5%)
Patients still on insulin at 1 year	23 (10%)	19 (8%)	18 (8%)	6 (2%)

*use of insulin for 30 or more consecutive days, with < 5 day gap, without a prior history of insulin dependent diabetes mellitus or non insulin dependent diabetes mellitus.

**Patients without pretransplant history of diabetes mellitus.

They should be given complete dosage instructions, advised of the potential risks during pregnancy, and informed of the increased risk of neoplasia. Patients should be informed that changes in dosage should not be undertaken without first consulting their physician.

Patients should be informed that Prograf can cause diabetes mellitus and should be advised of the need to see their physician if they develop frequent urination, increased thirst or hunger.

Laboratory Tests

Serum creatinine, potassium, and fasting glucose should be assessed regularly. Routine monitoring of metabolic and hematologic systems should be performed as clinically warranted.

Drug Interactions

Drug interaction studies with tacrolimus have not been conducted. Due to the potential for additive or synergistic impairment of renal function, care should be taken when administering Prograf with drugs that may be associated with renal dysfunction. These include, but are not limited to, aminoglycosides, amphotericin B, and cisplatin. Initial clinical experience with the co-administration of Prograf and cyclosporine resulted in additive/synergistic nephrotoxicity. Patients switched from cyclosporine to Prograf should receive the first Prograf dose no sooner than 24 hours after the last cyclosporine dose. Dosing may be further delayed in the presence of elevated cyclosporine levels.

Drugs that May Alter Tacrolimus Concentrations

Since tacrolimus is metabolized mainly by the CYP3A enzyme systems, substances known to inhibit these enzymes may decrease the metabolism of tacrolimus with resultant increases in whole blood or plasma concentrations. Drugs known to induce these enzyme systems may result in an increased metabolism of tacrolimus and decreased whole blood or plasma concentrations. Monitoring of blood concentrations and appropriate dosage adjustments are essential when such drugs are used concomitantly.

[See table below]

Interaction studies with drugs used in HIV therapy have not been conducted. However, care should be exercised when drugs that are nephrotoxic (e.g., ganciclovir) or that are metabolized by CYP3A (e.g., ritonavir) are administered concomitantly with tacrolimus. Grapefruit juice affects CYP3A-mediated metabolism and should be avoided **(See DOSAGE AND ADMINISTRATION)**.

Other Drug Interactions

Immunosuppressants may affect vaccination. Therefore, during treatment with Prograf, vaccination may be less effective. The use of live vaccines should be avoided; live vaccines may include, but are not limited to measles, mumps, rubella, oral polio, BCG, yellow fever, and TY21a typhoid.[1]

Carcinogenesis, Mutagenesis and Impairment of Fertility

An increased incidence of malignancy is a recognized complication of immunosuppression in recipients of organ transplants. The most common forms of neoplasms are non-Hodgkin's lymphomas and carcinomas of the skin. As with other immunosuppressive therapies, the risk of malignancies in Prograf recipients may be higher than in the normal, healthy population. Lymphoproliferative disorders associated with Epstein-Barr Virus infection have been seen. It has been reported that reduction or discontinuation of immunosuppression may cause the lesions to regress.

No evidence of genotoxicity was seen in bacterial (Salmonella and E. coli) or mammalian (Chinese hamster lung-derived cells) *in vitro* assays of mutagenicity, the *in vitro* CHO/HGPRT assay of mutagenicity, or *in vivo*, clastogenicity assays performed in mice; tacrolimus did not cause unscheduled DNA synthesis in rodent hepatocytes.

Carcinogenicity studies were carried out in male and female rats and mice. In the 80-week mouse study and in the 104-week rat study no relationship of tumor incidence to tacrolimus dosage was found. The highest doses used in the mouse and rat studies were 0.8–2.5 times (mice) and 3.5–7.1 times (rats) the recommended clinical dose range of 0.1–0.2 mg/kg/day when corrected for body surface area.

No impairment of fertility was demonstrated in studies of male and female rats. Tacrolimus, given orally at 1.0 mg/kg (0.7–1.4× the recommended clinical dose range of 0.1–0.2 mg/kg/day based on body surface area corrections) to male and female rats, prior to and during mating, as well as to dams during gestation and lactation, was associated with embryolethality and with adverse effects on female reproduction. Effects on female reproductive function (parturition) and embryolethal effects were indicated by a higher rate of pre-implantation loss and increased numbers of undelivered and nonviable pups. When given at 3.2 mg/kg (2.3–4.6× the recommended clinical dose range based on body surface area correction), tacrolimus was associated with maternal and paternal toxicity as well as reproductive toxicity including marked adverse effects on estrus cycles, parturition, pup viability, and pup malformations.

Pregnancy: Category C

In reproduction studies in rats and rabbits, adverse effects on the fetus were observed mainly at dose levels that were toxic to dams. Tacrolimus at oral doses of 0.32 and 1.0 mg/kg during organogenesis in rabbits was associated with maternal toxicity as well as an increase in incidence of abortions; these doses are equivalent to 0.5–1× and 1.6–3.3× the recommended clinical dose range (0.1–0.2 mg/kg) based on body surface area corrections. At the higher dose only, an increased incidence of malformations and developmental variations was also seen. Tacrolimus, at oral doses of 3.2

****Drugs That May Increase Tacrolimus Blood Concentrations:***

Calcium Channel Blockers	Antifungal Agents	Macrolide Antibiotics	Gastrointestinal Prokinetic Agents	Other Drugs
diltiazem	clotrimazole	clarithromycin	cisapride	bromocriptine
nicardipine	fluconazole	erythromycin	metoclopramide	cimetidine
nifedipine	itraconazole	troleandomycin		cyclosporine
verapamil	ketoconazole			danazol
				methylprednisolone
				protease inhibitors

****Drugs That May Decrease Tacrolimus Blood Concentrations:***

Anticonvulsants	Antibiotics
carbamazepine	rifabutin
phenobarbital	rifampin
phenytoin	

*This table is not all inclusive

mg/kg during organogenesis in rats, was associated with maternal toxicity and caused an increase in late resorptions, decreased numbers of live births, and decreased pup weight and viability. Tacrolimus, given orally at 1.0 and 3.2 mg/kg (equivalent to 0.7–1.4× and 2.3–4.6× the recommended clinical dose range based on body surface area corrections) to pregnant rats after organogenesis and during lactation, was associated with reduced pup weights.

No reduction in male or female fertility was evident.

There are no adequate and well-controlled studies in pregnant women. Tacrolimus is transferred across the placenta. The use of tacrolimus during pregnancy has been associated with neonatal hyperkalemia and renal dysfunction. Prograf should be used during pregnancy only if the potential benefit to the mother justifies potential risk to the fetus.

Nursing Mothers

Since tacrolimus is excreted in human milk, nursing should be avoided.

Pediatric Patients

Experience with Prograf in pediatric kidney transplant patients is limited. Successful liver transplants have been performed in pediatric patients (ages up to 16 years) using Prograf. The two randomized active-controlled trials of Prograf in primary liver transplantation included 56 pediatric patients. Thirty-one patients were randomized to Prograf-based and 25 to cyclosporine-based therapies. Additionally, a minimum of 122 pediatric patients were studied in an uncontrolled trial of tacrolimus in living related donor liver transplantation. Pediatric patients generally required higher doses of Prograf to maintain blood trough concentrations of tacrolimus similar to adult patients (see **DOSAGE AND ADMINISTRATION**).

ADVERSE REACTIONS

Liver Transplantation

The principal adverse reactions of Prograf are tremor, headache, diarrhea, hypertension, nausea, and renal dysfunction. These occur with oral and IV administration of Prograf and may respond to a reduction in dosing. Diarrhea was sometimes associated with other gastrointestinal complaints such as nausea and vomiting.

Hyperkalemia and hypomagnesemia have occurred in patients receiving Prograf therapy. Hyperglycemia has been noted in many patients; some may require insulin therapy (see **WARNINGS**).

The incidence of adverse events was determined in two randomized comparative liver transplant trials among 514 patients receiving tacrolimus and steroids and 515 patients receiving a cyclosporine-based regimen (CBIR). The proportion of patients reporting more than one adverse event was 99.8% in the tacrolimus group and 99.6% in the CBIR group. Precautions must be taken when comparing the incidence of adverse events in the U.S. study to that in the European study. The 12–month posttransplant information from the U.S. study and from the European study is presented below. The two studies also included different patient populations and patients were treated with immunosuppressive regimens of differing intensities. Adverse events reported in ≥ 15% in tacrolimus patients (combined study results) are presented below for the two controlled trials in liver transplantation:

[See first table above]

LIVER TRANSPLANTATION: ADVERSE EVENTS OCCURRING IN ≥ 15% OF PROGRAF-TREATED PATIENTS

	U.S. STUDY (%)		EUROPEAN STUDY (%)	
	Prograf (N=250)	CBIR (N=250)	Prograf (N=264)	CBIR (N=265)
Nervous System				
Headache (See WARNINGS)	64	60	37	26
Tremor (See WARNINGS)	56	46	48	32
Insomnia	64	68	32	23
Paresthesia	40	30	17	17
Gastrointestinal				
Diarrhea	72	47	37	27
Nausea	46	37	32	27
Constipation	24	27	23	21
LFT Abnormal	36	30	6	5
Anorexia	34	24	7	5
Vomiting	27	15	14	11
Cardiovascular				
Hypertension (See PRECAUTIONS)	47	56	38	43
Urogenital				
Kidney Function Abnormal (See WARNINGS)	40	27	36	23
Creatinine Increased (See WARNINGS)	39	25	24	19
BUN Increased (See WARNINGS)	30	22	12	9
Urinary Tract Infection	16	18	21	19
Oliguria	18	15	19	12
Metabolic and Nutritional				
Hyperkalemia (See WARNINGS)	45	26	13	9
Hypokalemia	29	34	13	16
Hyperglycemia (See WARNINGS)	47	38	33	22
Hypomagnesemia	48	45	16	9
Hemic and Lymphatic				
Anemia	47	38	5	1
Leukocytosis	32	26	8	8
Thrombocytopenia	24	20	14	19
Miscellaneous				
Abdominal Pain	59	54	29	22
Pain	63	57	24	22
Fever	48	56	19	22
Asthenia	52	48	11	7
Back Pain	30	29	17	17
Ascites	27	22	7	8
Peripheral Edema	26	26	12	14
Respiratory System				
Pleural Effusion	30	32	36	35
Atelectasis	28	30	5	4
Dyspnea	29	23	5	4
Skin and Appendages				
Pruritus	36	20	15	7
Rash	24	19	10	4

Less frequently observed adverse reactions in both liver transplantation and kidney transplantation patients are described under the subsection. **Less Frequently Reported Adverse Reactions** shown below.

Kidney Transplantation

The most common adverse reactions reported were infection, tremor, hypertension, decreased renal function, constipation, diarrhea, headache, abdominal pain and insomnia.

Adverse events that occurred in ≥ 15% of Prograf-treated kidney transplant patients are presented below:

Less frequently observed adverse reactions in both liver transplantation and kidney transplantation patients are described under the subsection. Less Frequently Reported Adverse Reactions shown below.

[See second table above]

KIDNEY TRANSPLANTATION: ADVERSE EVENTS OCCURRING IN ≥ 15% OF PROGRAF-TREATED PATIENTS

	Prograf (N=205)	CBIR (N=207)
Nervous System		
Tremor (See WARNINGS)	54	34
Headache (See WARNINGS)	44	38
Insomnia	32	30
Paresthesia	23	16
Dizziness	19	16
Gastrointestinal		
Diarrhea	44	41
Nausea	38	36
Constipation	35	43
Vomiting	29	23
Dyspepsia	28	20
Cardiovascular		
Hypertension (See PRECAUTIONS)	50	52
Chest pain	19	13
Urogenital		
Creatinine increased (See WARNINGS)	45	42
Urinary tract infection	34	35
Metabolic and Nutritional		
Hypophosphatemia	49	53
Hypomagnesemia	34	17
Hyperlipemia	31	38
Hyperkalemia (See WARNINGS)	31	32
Diabetes mellitus (See WARNINGS)	24	9
Hypokalemia	22	25
Hyperglycemia (See WARNINGS)	22	16
Edema	18	19
Hemic and Lymphatic		
Anemia	30	24
Leukopenia	15	17
Miscellaneous		
Infection	45	49
Peripheral edema	36	48
Asthenia	34	30
Abdominal pain	33	31
Pain	32	30
Fever	29	29
Back pain	24	20
Respiratory System		
Dyspnea	22	18
Cough increased	18	15
Musculoskeletal		
Arthralgia	25	24
Skin		
Rash	17	12
Pruritus	15	7

Less Frequently Reported Adverse Reactions

The following adverse events were reported in the range of 3% to less than 15% incidence in either liver or kidney transplant recipients who were treated with tacrolimus in the Phase 3 comparative trials.

NERVOUS SYSTEM: (see **WARNINGS**) abnormal dreams, agitation, amnesia, anxiety, confusion, convulsion, depression, dizziness, emotional lability, encephalopathy, hallucinations, hypertonia, incoordination, myoclonus, nervousness, neuropathy, psychosis, somnolence, thinking abnormal; SPECIAL SENSES: abnormal vision, amblyopia, ear pain, otitis media, tinnitus; GASTROINTESTINAL: anorexia, cholangitis, cholestatic jaundice, dyspepsia, dysphagia, esophagitis, flatulence, gastritis, gastrointestinal hemorrhage, GGT increase, GI perforation, hepatitis, ileus, increased appetite, jaundice, liver damage, liver function test abnormal, oral moniliasis, rectal disorder, stomatitis; CARDIOVASCULAR: angina pectoris, chest pain, deep thrombophlebitis, abnormal ECG, hemorrhage, hypotension, postural hypotension, peripheral vascular disorder, phlebitis, tachycardia, thrombosis, vasodilatation; UROGENITAL: (see **WARNINGS**) albuminuria, cystitis, dysuria, hematuria, hydronephrosis, kidney failure, kidney tubular necrosis, nocturia, pyuria, toxic nephropathy, oliguria, urinary frequency, urinary incontinence, vaginitis; METABOLIC/NUTRITIONAL: acidosis, alkaline phosphatase increased, alkalosis, ALT (SGPT) increased, AST (SGOT) increased, bicarbonate decreased, bilirubinemia, BUN increased, dehydration, GGT increased, healing abnormal, hypercalcemia, hypercholesterolemia, hyperlipemia, hyperphosphatemia, hyperuricemia, hypervolemia, hypocalcemia, hypoglycemia, hyponatremia, hypophosphatemia, hypoproteinemia, lactic dehydrogenase increase, weight gain; ENDOCRINE: (see **PRECAUTIONS**) Cushing's syndrome, diabetes mellitus; HEMIC/LYMPHATIC: coagulation disorder, ecchymosis, hypochromic anemia, leukocytosis, leukopenia, polycythemia, prothrombin decreased, serum iron decreased, thrombocytopenia; MISCELLANEOUS: abdomen enlarged, abscess, accidental injury, allergic reaction, cellulitis, chills, flu syndrome, generalized edema, hernia, peritonitis, photosensitivity reaction, sepsis; MUSCULOSKELETAL: arthralgia, cramps, generalized spasm, joint disorder, leg cramps, myalgia, myasthenia, osteoporosis; RESPIRATORY: asthma, bronchitis, cough increased, lung disorder, pneumothorax, pulmonary edema, pharyngitis, pneumonia, respiratory disorder, rhinitis, sinusitis, voice alteration; SKIN: acne, alopecia, exfoliative dermatitis, fungal dermatitis, herpes simplex, hirsutism, skin discoloration, skin disorder, skin ulcer, sweating.

There have been rare spontaneous reports of myocardial hypertrophy associated with clinically manifested ventricular dysfunction in patients receiving Prograf therapy (see **PRECAUTIONS-Myocardial Hypertrophy**).

OVERDOSAGE

Limited overdosage experience is available. Acute overdosages of up to 30 times the intended dose have been reported. Almost all cases have been asymptomatic and all patients recovered with no sequelae. Occasionally, acute overdosage has been followed by adverse reactions consistent with those listed in the **ADVERSE REACTIONS** section except in one case where transient urticaria and lethargy were observed. Based on the poor aqueous solubility and extensive erythrocyte and plasma protein binding, it is anticipated that tacrolimus is not dialyzable to any significant extent; there is no experience with charcoal hemoperfusion. The oral use of activated charcoal has been reported in treating acute overdoses, but experience has not been sufficient to warrant recommending its use. General supportive measures and treatment of specific symptoms should be followed in all cases of overdosage.

In acute oral and IV toxicity studies, mortalities were seen at or above the following doses: in adult rats, 52X the recommended human oral dose; in immature rats, 16X the recommended oral dose; and in adult rats, 16X the recommended human IV dose (all based on body surface area corrections).

DOSAGE AND ADMINISTRATION

Prograf Injection (tacrolimus injection)

For IV Infusion Only

NOTE: Anaphylactic reactions have occurred with injectables containing castor oil derivatives. See WARNINGS.

In patients unable to take oral Prograf capsules, therapy may be initiated with Prograf injection. The initial dose of Prograf should be administered no sooner than 6 hours af-

Continued on next page

Prograf—Cont.

ter transplantation. The recommended starting dose of Prograf injection is 0.03–0.05 mg/kg/day as a continuous IV infusion. Adult patients should receive doses at the lower end of the dosing range. Concomitant adrenal corticosteroid therapy is recommended early post-transplantation. Continuous IV infusion of Prograf injection should be continued only until the patient can tolerate oral administration of Prograf capsules.

Preparation for Administration/Stability

Prograf injection must be diluted with 0.9% Sodium Chloride Injection or 5% Dextrose Injection to a concentration between 0.004 mg/mL and 0.02 mg/mL prior to use. Diluted infusion solution should be stored in glass or polyethylene containers and should be discarded after 24 hours. The diluted infusion solution should not be stored in a PVC container due to decreased stability and the potential for extraction of phthalates. In situations where more dilute solutions are utilized (e.g., pediatric dosing, etc.), PVC-free tubing should likewise be used to minimize the potential for significant drug adsorption onto the tubing. Parenteral drug products should be inspected visually for particulate matter and discoloration prior to administration, whenever solution and container permit. Due to the chemical instability of tacrolimus in alkaline media, Prograf injection should not be mixed or co-infused with solutions of pH 9 or greater (e.g., ganciclovir or acyclovir).

Prograf capsules (tacrolimus capsules)-

[See first table below]

Liver Transplantation

It is recommended that patients initiate oral therapy with Prograf capsules if possible. If IV therapy is necessary, conversion from IV to oral Prograf is recommended as soon as oral therapy can be tolerated. This usually occurs within 2–3 days. The initial dose of Prograf should be administered no sooner than 6 hours after transplantation. In a patient receiving an IV infusion, the first dose of oral therapy should be given 8–12 hours after discontinuing the IV infusion. The recommended starting oral dose of Prograf capsules is 0.10–0.15 mg/kg/day administered in two divided daily doses every 12 hours. Co-administered grapefruit juice has been reported to increase tacrolimus blood trough concentrations in liver transplant patients. (See **Drugs that May Alter Tacrolimus Concentrations**).

Dosing should be titrated based on clinical assessments of rejection and tolerability. Lower Prograf dosages may be sufficient as maintenance therapy. Adjunct therapy with adrenal corticosteroids is recommended early post transplant.

Dosage and typical tacrolimus whole blood trough concentrations are shown in the table above; blood concentration details are described in **Blood Concentration Monitoring: Liver Transplantation** below.

Kidney Transplantation

The recommended starting oral dose of Prograf is 0.2 mg/kg/day administered every 12 hours in two divided doses. The initial dose of Prograf may be administered within 24 hours of transplantation, but should be delayed until renal function has recovered (as indicated for example by a serum creatinine ≤ 4 mg/dL). Black patients may require higher doses to achieve comparable blood concentrations. Dosage and typical tacrolimus whole blood trough concentrations are shown in the table above; blood concentration details are described in **Blood Concentration Monitoring: Kidney Transplantation** below.

The data in kidney transplant patients indicate that the Black patients required a higher dose to attain comparable trough concentrations compared to Caucasian patients.

[See second table below]

Pediatric Patients

Pediatric liver transplantation patients without pre-existing renal or hepatic dysfunction have required and tolerated

higher doses than adults to achieve similar blood concentrations. Therefore, it is recommended that therapy be initiated in pediatric patients at a starting IV dose of 0.03–0.05 mg/kg/day and a starting oral dose of 0.15–0.20 mg/kg/day. Dose adjustments may be required. Experience in pediatric kidney transplantation patients is limited.

Patients with Hepatic or Renal Dysfunction

Due to the potential for nephrotoxicity, patients with renal or hepatic impairment should receive doses at the lowest value of the recommended IV and oral dosing ranges. Further reductions in dose below these ranges may be required. Prograf therapy usually should be delayed up to 48 hours or longer in patients with post-operative oliguria.

Conversion from One Immunosuppressive Regimen to Another

Prograf should not be used simultaneously with cyclosporine. Prograf or cyclosporine should be discontinued at least 24 hours before initiating the other. In the presence of elevated Prograf or cyclosporine concentrations, dosing with the other drug usually should be further delayed.

Blood Concentration Monitoring

Monitoring of tacrolimus blood concentrations in conjunction with other laboratory and clinical parameters is considered an essential aid to patient management for the evaluation of rejection, toxicity, dose adjustments and compliance. Factors influencing frequency of monitoring include but are not limited to hepatic or renal dysfunction, the addition or discontinuation of potentially interacting drugs and the posttransplant time. Blood concentration monitoring is not a replacement for renal and liver function monitoring and tissue biopsies.

Two methods have been used for the assay of tacrolimus, a microparticle enzyme immunoassay (MEIA) and an ELISA. Both methods have the same monoclonal antibody for tacrolimus. Comparison of the concentrations in published literature to patient concentrations using the current assays must be made with detailed knowledge of the assay methods and biological matrices employed. Whole blood is the matrix of choice and specimens should be collected into tubes containing ethylene diamine tetraacetic acid (EDTA) anti-coagulant. Heparin anti-coagulation is not recommended because of the tendency to form clots on sotrage. Samples which are not analyzed immediately should be stored at room temperature or in a refrigerator and assayed within 7 days; if samples are to be kept longer they should be deep frozen at −20°C for up to 12 months.

Liver Transplantation

Although there is a lack of direct correlation between tacrolimus concentrations and drug efficacy, data from Phase II and III studies of liver transplant patients have shown an increasing incidence of adverse events with increasing trough blood concentrations. Most patients are stable when trough whole blood concentrations are maintained between 5 to 20 ng/mL. Long term posttransplant patients often are maintained at the low end of this target range.

Data from the U.S. clinical trial show that tacrolimus whole blood concentrations, as measured by ELISA, were most variable during the first week post-transplantation. After this early period, the median trough blood concentrations, measured at intervals from the second week to one year post-transplantation, ranged from 9.8 ng/mL to 19.4 ng/mL. *Therapeutic Drug Monitoring*, 1995, Volume 17, Number 6 contains a consensus document and several position papers regarding the therapeutic monitoring of tacrolimus from the 1995 International Consensus Conference on Immunosuppressive Drugs. Refer to these manuscripts for further discussions of tacrolimus monitoring.

Kidney Transplantation

Data from the U.S. study indicates that trough concentrations of tacrolimus in whole blood, as measured by IMx®, were most variable during the first week of dosing. During the first three months, 80% of the patients maintained trough concentrations between 7–20 ng/mL, and then between 5–15 ng/mL, through one-year.

The relative risk of toxicity is increased with higher trough concentrations. Therefore, monitoring of whole blood trough concentrations is recommended to assist in the clinical evaluation of toxicity.

HOW SUPPLIED

Prograf capsules (tacrolimus capsules) 1 mg

Oblong, white, branded with red "1 mg" on the capsule cap and "☐617" on the capsule body, supplied in 100–count bottles (NDC 0469-0617-71) and 10 blister cards of 10 capsules (NDC 0469-0617-10), containing the equivalent of 1 mg anhydrous tacrolimus.

Prograf capsules (tacrolimus capsules) 5 mg

Oblong, grayish/red, branded with white "5 mg" on the capsule cap and "☐657" on the capsule body, supplied in 100–count bottles (NDC 0469-0657-71) and 10 blister cards of 10 capsules (NDC 0469-0657-10), containing the equivalent of 5 mg anhydrous tacrolimus.

Store and Dispense

Store at controlled room temperature, 15°C–30°C (59°F–86°F).

Prograf injection (tacrolimus injection) 5 mg (for IV infusion only)

Supplied as a sterile solution in 1 mL ampules containing the equivalent of 5 mg of anhydrous tacrolimus per mL, in boxes of 10 ampules (NDC 0469-3016-01).

Store and Dispense

Store between 5°C and 25°C (41°F and 77°F).

CAUTION: Federal law prohibits dispensing without prescription.

Made in Ireland
for Fujisawa USA, Inc.
Deerfield, IL 60015–2548
by Fujisawa Ireland, Ltd.
Killorglin, Co. Kerry, Ireland

REFERENCE

1. CDC: Recommendations of the Advisory Committee on Immunization Practices: Use of vaccines and immune globulins in persons with altered immunocompetence. MMWR 1993;42(RR-4):1–18.

Shown in Product Identification Guide, page 310

Galderma Laboratories, Inc.
P.O. BOX 331329
FT. WORTH, TX 76163

Direct Inquiries to:
(888) 898–DERM (3376)
8:00 am—5:00 pm Central
Monday through Friday

BENZAC AC® 2¹⁄₂, 5 & 10 ℞
(benzoyl peroxide gel)

BENZAC AC® Wash 2¹⁄₂, 5 & 10 ℞
(benzoyl peroxide)

BENZAC W® 2¹⁄₂, 5 & 10 Water Base Gel ℞

BENZAC W® WASH 5 & 10 ℞
(benzoyl peroxide)

BENZAC® 5 & 10 Gel ℞
(benzoyl peroxide)

DESCRIPTION

Benzac AC® 2¹⁄₂, 5 and 10 (benzoyl peroxide gel), Benzac AC® Wash 2¹⁄₂, 5 and 10 (benzoyl peroxide), Benzac W® 2¹⁄₂, 5 and 10, (benzoyl peroxide) and Benzac W® Wash 5 and 10, are topical, water-base, benzoyl peroxide containing preparations for use in the treatment of acne vulgaris. Benzac (benzoyl peroxide) 5 and 10 are topical alcohol-base preparations. Benzoyl peroxide is an oxidizing agent which possesses antibacterial properties and is classified as a keratolytic. Benzoyl peroxide ($C_{14}H_{10}O_4$) is represented by the following chemical structure:

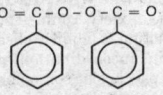

Benzac AC® 2¹⁄₂, Benzac AC® 5, and Benzac AC® 10 contain, respectively, benzoyl peroxide 2¹⁄₂%, 5% and 10% as the active ingredient in a gel base containing docusate sodium, edetate disodium, poloxamer 182, carbomer 940, propylene glycol, acrylates copolymer, glycerin, silicon dioxide, sodium hydroxide and purified water. May contain citric acid to adjust pH.

Summary of Initial Oral Dosage Recommendations and Typical Whole Blood Trough Concentrations

Patient Population	Recommended Initial Oral Dose*	Typical Whole Blood Trough Concentrations
Adult kidney transplant patients	0.2 mg/kg/day	month 1–3 : 7–20 ng/mL month 4–12 : 5–15 ng/mL
Adult liver transplant patients	0.10–0.15 mg/kg/day	month 1–12 : 5–20 ng/mL
Pediatric liver transplant patients	0.15–0.20 mg/kg/day	month 1–12 : 5–20 ng/mL

*Note: two divided doses, q12h

Time After Transplant	Caucasian n = 114		Black n = 56	
	Dose (mg/kg)	Trough Concentrations (ng/mL)	Dose (mg/kg)	Trough Concentrations (ng/mL)
Day 7	0.18	12.0	0.23	10.9
Month 1	0.17	12.8	0.26	12.9
Month 6	0.14	11.8	0.24	11.5
Month 12	0.13	10.1	0.19	11.0

Benzac AC® Wash 2^1/$_2$, Benzac AC® Wash 5 and Benzac AC® Wash 10 contain, respectively, benzoyl peroxide 2^1/$_2$%, 5% and 10% as the active ingredient in a vehicle consisting of purified water, sodium C14–16 olefin sulfonate, acrylates copolymer, glycerin, sodium hydroxide, and carbomer 940. May contain citric acid to adjust pH.

Benzac® 5 and Benzac® 10 contain, respectively, benzoyl peroxide 5% and 10% as the active ingredient in a gel base containing alcohol 12% (w/w), laureth 4, dimethicone, carbomer 940, sodium hydroxide, fragrance and purified water. May contain citric acid to adjust pH.

Benzac W® 2^1/$_2$, Benzac W® 5 and Benzac W® 10 contain, respectively, benzoyl peroxide 2^1/$_2$%, 5% and 10% as the active ingredient in a gel base containing docusate sodium, edetate disodium, poloxamer 182, carbomer 940, propylene glycol, silicon dioxide, sodium hydroxide and purified water. May contain citric acid to adjust pH.

Benzac W® Wash 5 and Benzac W® Wash 10 contain, respectively, benzoyl peroxide 5% and 10% as the active ingredient in a vehicle consisting of sodium C14–16 olefin sulfonate, carbomer 940, and purified water. May contain citric acid to adjust pH.

CLINICAL PHARMACOLOGY

The mechanism of action of benzoyl peroxide is not totally understood but its antibacterial activity against *Propionibacterium acnes* is thought to be a major mode of action. In addition, patients treated with benzoyl peroxide show a reduction in lipids and free fatty acids and mild desquamation (drying and peeling activity) with a simultaneous reduction in comedones and acne lesions.

Little is known about the percutaneous penetration, metabolism, and excretion of benzoyl peroxide, although it has been shown that benzoyl peroxide absorbed by the skin is metabolized to benzoic acid and then excreted as benzoate in the urine. There is no evidence of systemic toxicity caused by benzoyl peroxide in humans.

INDICATIONS AND USAGE

Benzac® 5 and 10 and Benzac W® 2^1/$_2$, 5 and 10 are indicated for the topical treatment of acne vulgaris. Benzac W® Wash 5 and 10 are indicated for the topical treatment of mild to moderate acne vulgaris. In severe, complicated acne, Benzac W® Wash 5 and 10 may be used as an adjunct to other therapeutic regimens.
Benzac AC 2^1/$_2$, 5 and 10 and Benzac AC® Wash 2^1/$_2$, 5 and 10 are indicated for the topical treatment of acne vulgaris.

CONTRAINDICATIONS

These preparations are contraindicated in patients with a history of hypersensitivity to any of their components.

PRECAUTIONS

General: For external use only. If severe irritation develops, discontinue use and institute appropriate therapy. After the reaction clears, treatment may often be resumed with less frequent application. These preparations should not be used in or near the eyes or on mucous membranes.
Information for patients: Avoid contact with eyes, eyelids, lips and mucous membranes. If accidental contact occurs, rinse with water. Contact with any colored material (including hair and fabric) may result in bleaching or discoloration. If excessive irritation develops, discontinue use and consult your physician.
Carcinogenesis, Mutagenesis, Impairment of Fertility: Data from several studies employing a strain of mice that are highly susceptible to developing cancer suggest that benzoyl peroxide acts as a tumor promotor. The clinical significance of these findings to humans is unknown. Benzoyl peroxide has not been found to be mutagenic (Ames Test) and there are no published data indicating it impairs fertility.
Pregnancy: Teratogenic Effects: *Pregnancy Category C:* Animal reproduction studies have not been conducted with benzoyl peroxide. It is not known whether benzoyl peroxide can cause fetal harm when administered to a pregnant woman or can affect reproduction capacity. Benzoyl peroxide should be used by a pregnant woman only if clearly needed. There are no available data on the effect of benzoyl peroxide on the later growth, development and functional maturation of the unborn child.
Nursing Mothers: It is not known whether this drug is excreted in human milk. Because many drugs are excreted in human milk, caution should be exercised when benzoyl peroxide is administered to a nursing woman.
Pediatric Use: Safety and effectiveness in children have not been established.

ADVERSE REACTIONS

Allergic contact dermatitis and dryness have been reported with topical benzoyl peroxide therapy.

OVERDOSAGE

If excessive scaling, erythema or edema occur, the use of this preparation should be discontinued. To hasten resolution of the adverse effects, cool compresses may be used. After symptoms and signs subside, a reduced dosage schedule may be cautiously tried if the reaction is judged to be due to excessive use and not allergenicity.

DOSAGE AND ADMINISTRATION

Benzac AC 2^1/$_2$, 5 or 10 should be applied once or twice daily to cover affected areas after washing with a mild cleanser and water.
Benzac AC Wash 2^1/$_2$, 5 or 10. Wash once or twice daily avoiding contact with the eyes and mucous membranes. Wet the area of application. Apply Benzac AC Wash 2^1/$_2$, 5 or 10 to the hands and wash the affected areas. Rinse with water and pat dry.
Benzac 5 or 10 or Benzac W 2^1/$_2$, 5 or 10 should be applied once or twice daily to cover affected areas after washing with a mild cleanser and water. Wash with Benzac W Wash 5 or 10 once or twice daily, avoiding contact with eyes and mucous membranes. Wet the area of application. Apply Benzac W Wash 5 or 10 to the hands and wash the affected areas. Rinse with water and dry. The degree of drying and peeling can be adjusted by modification of the dosage schedule.

HOW SUPPLIED

Benzac AC® 2^1/$_2$ Water Base Gel
60 g tubes—**NDC 0299-3620-60**
90 g tubes—**NDC 0299-3620-90**
Benzac AC® 5 Water Base Gel
60 g tubes—**NDC 0299-3625-60**
90 g tubes—**NDC 0299-3625-90**
Benzac AC® 10 Water Base Gel
60 g tubes—**NDC 0299-3630-60**
90 g tubes—**NDC 0299-3630-90**
Benzac AC® Wash 2^1/$_2$
8 oz plastic bottles—**NDC 0299-3635-08**
Benzac AC® Wash 5
8 oz plastic bottles—**NDC 0299-3640-08**
Benzac AC® Wash 10
8 oz plastic bottles—**NDC 0299-3645-08**
Benzac® 5 Gel
60 g tubes—**NDC 0299-3655-01**
Benzac® 10 Gel
60 g tubes—**NDC 0299-3665-01**
Benzac W® 2^1/$_2$ Water Base Gel
60 g tubes—**NDC 0299-3590-60**
90 g tubes—**NDC 0299-3590-90**
Benzac W® 5 Water Base Gel
60 g tubes—**NDC 0299-3600-01**
90 g tubes—**NDC 0299-3600-09**
Benzac W® 10 Water Base Gel
60 g tubes—**NDC 0299-3610-01**
90 g tubes—**NDC 0299-3610-09**
Benzac W® Wash 5
4 oz plastic bottles—**NDC 0299-3670-04**
8 oz plastic bottles—**NDC 0299-3670-08**
Benzac W® Wash 10
8 oz plastic bottles—**NDC 0299-3672-08**

STORAGE

Store **Benzac AC®** and **Benzac AC® Wash** at controlled room temperature (59°–86°F).
Store **Benzac W®** and **Benzac W® Wash** at controlled room temperature (59°–86°F). Store **Benzac®** below 75°F.

CAUTION

Federal law prohibits dispensing without prescription.
Marketed by:
Galderma Laboratories, Inc.
Fort Worth, Texas 76133
Mfd. by: DPT Laboratories, Ltd.
San Antonio, Texas 78215
Revised: March 1994

CETAPHIL®   OTC
[cē'-ta-phil]
Gentle Skin Cleanser—Soap Substitute

CETAPHIL®
Oily Skin Cleanser

COMPOSITION

Cetaphil® Gentle Skin Cleanser contains water, cetyl alcohol, propylene glycol, sodium lauryl sulfate, stearyl alcohol, methylparaben, propylparaben and butylparaben.
Cetaphil® Oily Skin Cleanser contains purified water, peg-200 hydrogenated glyceryl palmate (and) peg-7 glyceryl cocoate, sodium lauroyl sarcosinate, acrylates/steareth-20 methacrylate copolymer, glycerin, sodium laureth sulfate, butylene glycol phenoxyethanol, masking fragrance, panthenol, peg-60 hydrogenated castor oil, disodium edta, methylparaben.

ACTION AND USES

Cetaphil® Gentle Skin Cleanser was formulated for dermatologists as a gentle, non-irritating cleanser for dry, sensitive skin.
Cetaphil Gentle Skin Cleanser is completely non-alkaline, non-comedogenic, fragrance free, and mild enough for all skin types.

Cetaphil Gentle Skin Cleanser soothes and softens as it cleanses, helping the skin retain needed moisture. **Cetaphil** Gentle Skin Cleanser is also an excellent cleanser for the delicate skin of babies.
Cetaphil® Oily Skin Cleanser was formulated for dermatologists as a gentle, non-irritating cleanser for oily or combination skin.
Cetaphil® Oily Skin Cleanser removes surface oils, dirt and makeup without leaving skin tight or overly dry.
Cetaphil® Oily Skin Cleanser non-comedogenic, so it won't clog pores.
Cetaphil® Oily Skin Cleanser rinses clean without leaving any irritating residue.

ADMINISTRATION AND DOSAGE

Cetaphil® Gentle Skin Cleanser can be used with or without water.
Without water: Apply a liberal amount to the skin and rub gently. The unique, low lathering formula allows gentle, yet thorough cleansing. Remove excess with a soft cloth, leaving a thin film of **Cetaphil** on the skin. The emollient quality will leave the skin soft and moist.
With water: Apply to the skin and rub gently. Rinse.
Cetaphil® Oily Skin Cleanser: Massage a small amount onto wet skin. Rinse.

HOW SUPPLIED

Cetaphil® Gentle Skin Cleanser 4 fl oz (UPC 0299-3921-40)
Cetaphil® Gentle Skin Cleanser 8 fl oz (UPC 0299-3921-08);
Cetaphil® Gentle Skin Cleanser 16 fl oz (UPC 0299-3921-16).
Cetaphil® Oily Skin Cleanser 2 fl oz (UPC 0299-3927-02).

CETAPHIL®   OTC
[cē'-ta-phil]
Gentle Cleansing Bar and Cetaphil® antibacterial gentle cleansing bar

COMPOSITION

Contains sodium cocoyl isethionate, stearic acid, sodium tallowate, water, sodium stearate, sodium dodecylbenzene sulfonate, sodium cocoate, PEG-20, sodium chloride, masking fragrance, sodium isethionate, petrolatum, sodium isostearoyl lactylate, sucrose laurate, titanium dioxide, pentasodium pentetate, tetrasodium etidronate. May also contain sodium palm kernelate. **Cetaphil®** antibacterial bar also contains the active ingredient: triclosan.

ACTION AND USES

Cetaphil® gentle cleansing bar's non-soap formulation is designed for cleansing dry, sensitive skin.
Cetaphil® antibacterial bar provides gentle cleansing of dry, sensitive skin with the added benefit of antibacterial activity.

ADMINISTRATION AND DOSAGE

Cetaphil gentle cleansing bar and **Cetaphil®** antibacterial bar are ideal for bath or shower. **Cetaphil®** gentle cleansing bar and **Cetaphil®** antibacterial bar are non-comedogenic and contain no harsh detergents that might dry or irritate the skin.

HOW SUPPLIED

Cetaphil® gentle cleansing bar net wt. 4.5 oz (UPC 0299-3923-04)
Cetaphil® antibacterial gentle cleansing bar net wt. 4.5 oz. (UPC 0299-3925-04)

CETAPHIL®   OTC
[cē'-ta-phil]
Moisturizing Cream

COMPOSITION

Contains purified water, polyglycerylmethacrylate (and) propylene glycol, petrolatum, dicaprylyl ether, PEG-5 glyceryl stearate, glycerin, dimethicone (and) dimethiconol, cetyl alcohol, sweet almond oil, acrylates/C10–30 alkyl acrylate crosspolymer, tocopheryl acetate, phenoxyethanol, benzyl alcohol, disodium EDTA, sodium hydroxide, lactic acid.

ACTION AND USES

Cetaphil® Moisturizing Cream was formulated specifically for chronic dry, sensitive skin. Contains a superior system of extra-strength emollients and humectants, clinically proven to bind water to the skin and prevent moisture loss. Provides long-lasting relief to even severe dry skin. Free of lanolins, parabens and fragrances that can irritate sensitive skin. Non-comedogenic.

ADMINISTRATION AND DOSAGE

Apply liberally as often as needed, or as directed by physician.

Continued on next page

Cetaphil Cream—Cont.

HOW SUPPLIED

Cetaphil® Moisturizing Cream 16 oz (UPC 0299-3917-16)
Cetaphil® Moisturizing Cream 3 oz tube (UPC 0299-3917-02)

CETAPHIL® OTC

[*cē '-ta-phil*]
Moisturizing Lotion

COMPOSITION

Contains purified water, glycerin, hydrogenated polyisobutene, cetearyl alcohol (and) ceteareth-20, macadamia nut oil, dimethicone, tocopheryl acetate, stearoxytrimethylsilane (and) stearyl alcohol. panthenol, farnesol, benzyl alcohol, phenoxyethanol, acrylates/C10–30 alkyl acrylate crosspolymer, sodium hydroxide, citric acid.

ACTION AND USES

Cetaphil® Moisturizing Lotion was formulated specifically for chronic dry, sensitive skin. Contains a superior system of extra-strength emollients and humectants, clinically proven to bind water to the skin and prevent moisture loss. Provides long-lasting relief to even severe dry skin. Free of lanolins, parabens and fragrances that can irritate sensitive skin. Non-comedogenic.

ADMINISTRATION AND DOSAGE

Apply daily to dry skin as needed or as directed by physician.

HOW SUPPLIED

Cetaphil® Moisturizing Lotion 16 fl oz (UPC 0299-3918-16)

DESOWEN® ℞

(desonide cream, ointment and lotion)
Cream 0.05%
Ointment 0.05%
and Lotion 0.05%

For Dermatologic Use Only–
Not for Ophthalmic Use–

DESCRIPTION

DesOwen® Cream 0.05%, Ointment 0.05%, and Lotion 0.05% contain desonide (Pregna-1,4-diene-3,20-dione,11, 21-dihydroxy-16,17-[(1-methylethylidene)bis(oxy)]-,(11β, 16α-) a synthetic nonfluorinated corticosteroid for topical dermatologic use. The corticosteroids constitute a class of primarily synthetic steroids used topically as anti-inflammatory and anti-pruritic agents.
Chemically, desonide is $C_{24}H_{32}O_6$. It has the following structural formula:

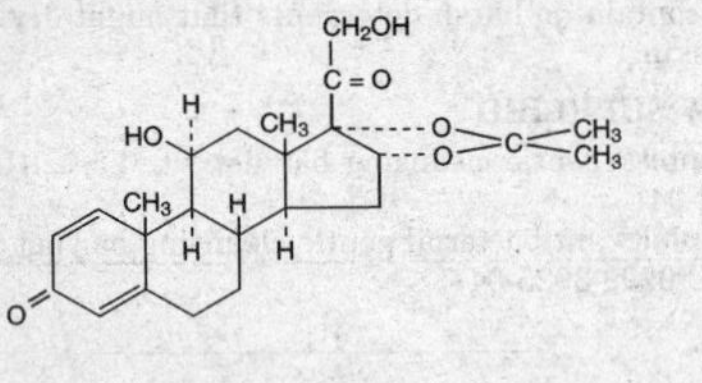

Desonide has the molecular weight of 416.51. It is a white to off white odorless powder which is soluble in methanol and practically insoluble in water.
Each gram of **DesOwen®** Cream contains 0.5 mg of desonide in a base of purified water, emulsifying wax, propylene glycol, stearic acid, isopropyl palmitate, synthetic beeswax, polysorbate 60, potassium sorbate, sorbic acid, propyl gallate, citric acid, and sodium hydroxide.
Each gram of **DesOwen®** Ointment contains 0.5 mg of desonide in a base of mineral oil and polyethylene.
Each gram of **DesOwen®** Lotion contains 0.5 mg of desonide in a base of sodium lauryl sulfate, light mineral oil, cetyl alcohol, stearyl alcohol, propylene glycol, methylparaben, propylparaben, sorbitan monostearate, glyceryl stearate SE, edetate sodium and purified water. May contain citric acid and/or sodium hydroxide for pH adjustment.

CLINICAL PHARMACOLOGY

Like other topical corticosteroids, desonide has anti-inflammatory, antipruritic and vasoconstrictive properties. The mechanism of the anti-inflammatory activity of the topical steroids, in general, is unclear. However corticosteroids are thought to act by the induction of phospholipase A_2 inhibitory proteins, collectively called lipocortins. It is postulated that these proteins control the biosynthesis of potent mediators of inflammation such as prostaglandins and leukotrienes by inhibiting the release of their common precursor arachidonic acid. Arachidonic acid is released from membrane phospholipids by phospholipase A_2.
Pharmacokinetics: The extent of percutaneous absorption of topical corticosteroids is determined by many factors including the vehicle and the integrity of the epidermal barrier. Occlusive dressings with hydrocortisone for up to 24 hours have not been demonstrated to increase penetration; however, occlusion of hydrocortisone for 96 hours markedly enhances penetration. Topical corticosteroids can be absorbed from normal intact skin. Inflammation and/or other disease processes in the skin may increase percutaneous absorption.
Studies performed with **DesOwen®** (desonide cream, ointment and lotion) Cream, Ointment, and Lotion indicate that they are in the low to medium range of potency as compared with other topical corticosteroids.

INDICATION AND USAGE

DesOwen® Cream, Ointment and Lotion are low to medium potency corticosteroids indicated for the relief of the inflammatory and pruritic manifestations of corticosteroid responsive dermatoses.

CONTRAINDICATIONS

DesOwen® Cream, Ointment and Lotion are contraindicated in those patients with a history of hypersensitivity to any of the components of the preparations.

PRECAUTIONS

General: Systemic absorption of topical corticosteroids can produce reversible hypothalamic-pituitary-adrenal (HPA) axis suppression with the potential for glucocorticosteroid insufficiency after withdrawal of treatment. Manifestations of Cushing's syndrome, hyperglycemia, and glucosuria can also be produced in some patients by systemic absorption of topical corticosteroids while on treatment.
Patients applying a topical steroid to a large surface area or to areas under occlusion should be evaluated periodically for evidence of HPA axis suppression. This may be done by using the ACTH stimulation, A.M. plasma cortisol, and urinary free cortisol tests. Patients receiving superpotent corticosteroids should not be treated for more than 2 weeks at a time and only small areas should be treated at any one time due to the increased risk of HPA axis suppression.
If HPA axis suppression is noted, an attempt should be made to withdraw the drug, to reduce the frequency of application, or to substitute a less potent corticosteroid. Recovery of HPA axis function is generally prompt and complete upon discontinuation of topical corticosteroids. Infrequently, signs and symptoms of glucocorticosteroid insufficiency may occur requiring supplemental systemic corticosteroids. For information on systemic supplementation, see prescribing information for those products.
Pediatric patients may be more susceptible to systemic toxicity from equivalent doses due to their larger skin surface to body mass ratios. (See PRECAUTIONS—Pediatric use).
If irritation develops, **DesOwen®** Cream, Ointment or Lotion should be discontinued and appropriate therapy instituted. Allergic contact dermatitis with corticosteroids is usually diagnosed by observing *failure to heal* rather than noting a clinical exacerbation as with most topical products not containing corticosteroids. Such an observation should be corroborated with appropriate diagnostic patch testing.
If concomitant skin infections are present or develop, an appropriate antifungal or antibacterial agent should be used. If a favorable response does not occur promptly, use of **DesOwen®** (desonide cream, ointment and lotion) Cream, Ointment or Lotion should be discontinued until the infection has been adequately controlled.
Information for patients: Patients using topical corticosteroids should receive the following information and instructions:

1. This medication is to be used as directed by the physician. It is for external use only. Avoid contact with the eyes.
2. This medication should not be used for any disorder other than that for which it was prescribed.
3. The treated skin area should not be bandaged or otherwise covered or wrapped so as to be occlusive unless directed by the physician.
4. Patients should report to their physician any signs of local adverse reactions.

Laboratory tests: The following tests may be helpful in evaluating patients for HPA axis suppression:
ACTH stimulation test
A.M. plasma cortisol test
Urinary free cortisol test
Carcinogenesis, mutagenesis, and impairment of fertility: Long-term animal studies have not been performed to evaluate the carcinogenic potential or the effect on reproduction with the use of **DesOwen®** Cream, Ointment, and Lotion.
Pregnancy: *Teratogenic effects: Pregnancy category C:* Corticosteroids have been shown to be teratogenic in laboratory animals when administered systemically at relatively low dosage levels. Some corticosteroids have been shown to be teratogenic after dermal application in laboratory animals. Animal reproduction studies have not been conducted with **DesOwen®** Cream, Ointment or Lotion. It is also not known whether **DesOwen®** Cream, Ointment or Lotion can cause fetal harm when administered to a pregnant woman or can affect reproduction capacity. **DesOwen®** Cream, Ointment and Lotion should be given to a pregnant woman only if clearly needed.
Nursing mothers: Systemically administered corticosteroids appear in human milk and could suppress growth, interfere with endogenous corticosteroid production, or cause other untoward effects. It is not known whether topical administration of corticosteroids could result in sufficient systemic absorption to produce detectable quantities in human milk. Because many drugs are excreted in human milk, caution should be exercised when **DesOwen®** Cream, Ointment or Lotion is administered to a nursing woman.
Pediatric use: Safety and effectiveness in pediatric patients have not been established. Because of a higher ratio of skin surface area to body mass, pediatric patients are at a greater risk than adults of HPA axis suppression when they are treated with topical corticosteroids. They are therefore also at greater risk of glucocorticosteroid insufficiency after withdrawal of treatment and of Cushing's syndrome while on treatment. Adverse effects including striae have been reported with inappropriate use of topical corticosteroids in infants and children.
HPA axis suppression, Cushing's syndrome, linear growth retardation, delayed weight gain and intracranial hypertension have been reported in children receiving topical corticosteroids. Manifestations of adrenal suppression in children include low plasma cortisol levels, and absence of response to ACTH stimulation. Manifestations of intracranial hypertension include bulging fontanelles, headaches, and bilateral papilledema.

ADVERSE REACTIONS

In controlled clinical trials, the total incidence of adverse reactions associated with the use of desonide was approximately 8%. These were: stinging and burning approximately 3%, irritation, contact dermatitis, condition worsened, peeling of skin, itching, intense transient erythema, and dryness/scaliness, each less than 2%.
The following additional local adverse reactions have been reported infrequently with other topical corticosteroids, and they may occur more frequently with the use of occlusive dressings, especially with higher potency corticosteroids. These reactions are listed in an approximate decreasing order of occurrence: folliculitis, acneiform eruptions, hypopigmentation, perioral dermatitis, secondary infection, skin atrophy, striae, and miliaria.

OVERDOSAGE

Topically applied **DesOwen®** (desonide cream, ointment, and lotion) Cream, Ointment and Lotion can be absorbed in sufficient amounts to produce systemic effects (See PRECAUTIONS).

DOSAGE AND ADMINISTRATION

DesOwen® Cream, Ointment or Lotion should be applied to the affected areas as a thin film two or three times daily depending on the severity of the condition. SHAKE LOTION WELL BEFORE USING.
As with other corticosteroids, therapy should be discontinued when control is achieved. If no improvement is seen within 2 weeks, reassessment of diagnosis may be necessary.
DesOwen® Cream, Ointment and Lotion should not be used with occlusive dressings.

HOW SUPPLIED

DesOwen® (desonide cream) Cream 0.05% is supplied in tubes containing:
15 g **NDC** 0299-5770-15
60 g **NDC** 0299-5770-60
DesOwen® (desonide ointment) Ointment 0.05% is supplied in tubes containing:
15 g **NDC** 0299-5775-15
60 g **NDC** 0299-5775-60
DesOwen® (desonide lotion) Lotion 0.05% is supplied in bottles containing:
2 fl oz **NDC** 0299-5765-02
4 fl oz **NDC** 0299-5765-04
Storage Conditions: Store between 2° and 30°C (36° and 86°F).
CAUTION: Federal law prohibits dispensing without prescription.
Marketed by:
Galderma Laboratories, Inc.
Fort Worth, Texas 76133, USA
Mfd. by: DPT Laboratories, Ltd.
San Antonio, Texas 78215, USA
225025-0395 Revised: March 1995

DIFFERIN® ℞

(adapalene gel)
Gel, 0.1%

DESCRIPTION

Differin® Gel, containing adapalene, is used for the topical treatment of acne vulgaris. Each gram of **Differin®** Gel con-

tains adapalene 0.1% (1mg) in a vehicle consisting of propylene glycol, carbomer 940, poloxamer 182, edetate disodium, methylparaben, sodium hydroxide, and purified water. May contain hydrochloric acid to adjust pH.
The chemical name of adapalene is 6-[3-(1-adamantyl)-4-methoxyphenyl]-2-naphthoic acid. Adapalene is a white to off-white powder which is soluble in tetrahydrofuran, sparingly soluble in ethanol, and practically insoluble in water. The molecular formula is $C_{28}H_{28}O_3$ and molecular weight is 412.52. Adapalene is represented by the following structural formula:

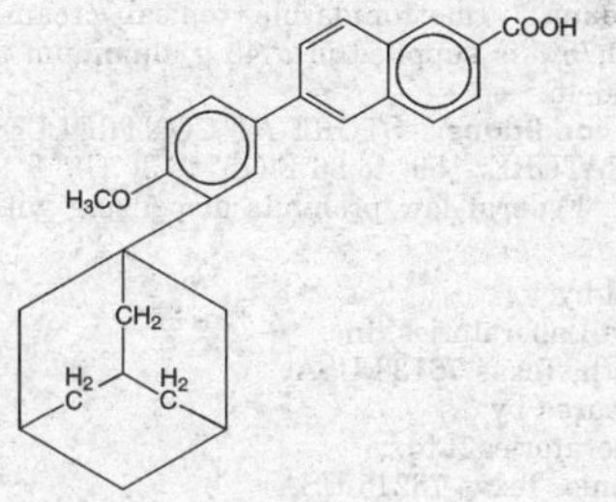

CLINICAL PHARMACOLOGY

Adapalene is a chemically stable, retinoid-like compound. Biochemical and pharmacological profile studies have demonstrated that adapalene is a modulator of cellular differentiation, keratinization, and inflammatory processes all of which represent important features in the pathology of acne vulgaris.
Mechanistically, adapalene binds to specific retinoic acid nuclear receptors but does not bind to the cytosolic receptor protein. Although the exact mode of action of adapalene is unknown, it is suggested that topical adapalene may normalize the differentiation of follicular epithelial cells resulting in decreased microcomedone formation.
Pharmacokinetics: Absorption of adapalene through human skin is low. Only trace amounts (<0.25 ng/mL) of parent substance have been found in the plasma of acne patients following chronic topical application of adapalene in controlled clinical trials. Excretion appears to be primarily by the biliary route.

INDICATIONS AND USAGE

Differin® Gel is indicated for the topical treatment of acne vulgaris.

CONTRAINDICATIONS

Differin® Gel should not be administered to individuals who are hypersensitive to adapalene or any of the components in the vehicle gel.

WARNINGS

Use of **Differin®** Gel should be discontinued if hypersensitivity to any of the ingredients is noted. Patients with sunburn should be advised not to use the product until fully recovered.

PRECAUTIONS

General: If a reaction suggesting sensitivity or chemical irritation occurs, use of the medication should be discontinued. Exposure to sunlight, including sunlamps, should be minimized during the use of adapalene. Patients who normally experience high levels of sun exposure, and those with inherent sensitivity to sun, should be warned to exercise caution. Use of sunscreen products and protective clothing over treated areas is recommended when exposure cannot be avoided. Weather extremes, such as wind or cold, also may be irritating to patients under treatment with adapalene.
Avoid contact with the eyes, lips, angles of the nose, and mucous membranes. The product should not be applied to cuts, abrasions, eczematous skin, or sunburned skin.
Certain cutaneous signs and symptoms such as erythema, dryness, scaling, burning, or pruritus may be experienced during treatment. These are most likely to occur during the first two to four weeks and will usually lessen with continued use of the medication. Depending upon the severity of adverse events, patients should be instructed to reduce the frequency of application or discontinue use.
Drug Interactions: As **Differin®** Gel has the potential to produce local irritation in some patients, concomitant use of other potentially irritating topical products (medicated or abrasive soaps and cleansers, soaps and cosmetics that have a strong drying effect, and products with high concentrations of alcohol, astringents, spices, or lime) should be approached with caution. Particular caution should be exercised in using preparations containing sulfur, resorcinol, or salicylic acid in combination with **Differin®** Gel. If these preparations have been used, it is advisable not to start therapy with **Differin®** Gel until the effects of such preparations in the skin have subsided.
Carcinogenesis, Mutagenesis, Impairment of Fertility: Carcinogenicity studies with adapalene have been conducted in mice at topical doses of 0.3, 0.9, and 2.6 mg/kg/day and in rats at oral doses of 0.15, 0.5, and 1.5 mg/kg/day, approximately 4–75 times the maximal daily human topical dose. In the oral study, positive linear trends were observed in the incidence of follicular cell adenomas and carcinomas in the thyroid glands of female rats, and in the incidence of benign and malignant pheochromocytomas in the adrenal medullas of male rats.
No photocarcinogenicity studies were conducted. Animal studies have shown an increased tumorigenic risk with the use of pharmacologically similar drugs (e.g., retinoids) when exposed to UV irradiation in the laboratory or to sunlight. Although the significance of these studies to human use is not clear, patients should be advised to avoid or minimize exposure to either sunlight or artificial UV irradiation sources.
In a series of *in vivo* and *in vitro* studies, adapalene did not exhibit mutagenic or genotoxic activities.
Pregnancy: Teratogenic effects. Pregnancy Category C. No teratogenic effects were seen in rats at oral doses of adapalene 0.15 to 5.0 mg/kg/day, up to 120 times the maximal daily human topical dose. Cutaneous route teratology studies conducted in rats and rabbits at doses of 0.6, 2.0, and 6.0 mg/kg/day, up to 150 times the maximal daily human topical dose exhibited no fetotoxicity and only minimal increases in supernumerary ribs in rats. There are no adequate and well-controlled studies in pregnant women. Adapalene should be used during pregnancy only if the potential benefit justifies the potential risk to the fetus.
Nursing Mothers: It is not known whether this drug is excreted in human milk. Because many drugs are excreted in human milk, caution should be exercised when **Differin®** Gel is administered to a nursing woman.
Pediatric Use: Safety and effectiveness in pediatric patients below the age of 12 have not been established.

ADVERSE REACTIONS

Some adverse effects such as erythema, scaling, dryness, pruritus, and burning will occur in 10–40% of patients. Pruritus or burning immediately after application also occurs in approximately 20% of patients. The following additional adverse experiences were reported in approximately 1% or less of patients: skin irritation, burning/stinging, erythema, sunburn, and acne flares. These are most commonly seen during the first month of therapy and decrease in frequency and severity thereafter. All adverse effects with use of **Differin®** Gel during clinical trials were reversible upon discontinuation of therapy.

OVERDOSAGE

Differin® Gel is intended for cutaneous use only. If the medication is applied excessively, no more rapid or better results will be obtained and marked redness, peeling, or discomfort may occur. The acute oral toxicity of **Differin®** Gel in mice and rats is greater than 10 mL/kg. Chronic ingestion of the drug may lead to the same side effects as those associated with excessive oral intake of Vitamin A.

DOSAGE AND ADMINISTRATION

Differin® Gel should be applied once a day to affected areas after washing in the evening before retiring. A thin film of the gel should be applied, avoiding eyes, lips, and mucous membranes.
During the early weeks of therapy, an apparent exacerbation of acne may occur. This is due to the action of the medication on previously unseen lesions and should not be considered a reason to discontinue therapy. Therapeutic results should be noticed after eight to twelve weeks of treatment.

HOW SUPPLIED

Differin® (adapalene gel) Gel, 0.1% is supplied in the following sizes:
15 g laminate tube-**NDC** 0299-5910-15
45 g laminate tube-**NDC** 0299-5910-45
Storage: Store at controlled room temperature 20°–25°C (68°–77°F).
CAUTION: Federal law prohibits dispensing without prescription.
Marketed by:
Galderma Laboratories, Inc.
Fort Worth, Texas 76133 USA
Mfd. by:
DPT Laboratories, Ltd.
San Antonio, Texas 78215 USA
225022-0596
Revised: May 1996

DIFFERIN® ℞
(adapalene solution)
Solution, 0.1%

DESCRIPTION

DIFFERIN® Solution, containing adapalene, is used for the topical treatment of acne vulgaris. Each mL of DIFFERIN® Solution contains adapalene 0.1% (1 mg) in a vehicle consisting of polyethylene glycol 400 and SD alcohol 40-B, 30% (w/v).
The chemical name of adapalene is 6-[3-(1-adamantyl)-4-methoxyphenyl]-2-naphthoic acid. Adapalene is a white to off-white powder which is soluble in tetrahydrofuran, sparingly soluble in ethanol, and practically insoluble in water. The molecular formula is $C_{28}H_{28}O_3$ and molecular weight is 412.52. Adapalene is represented by the following structural formula:

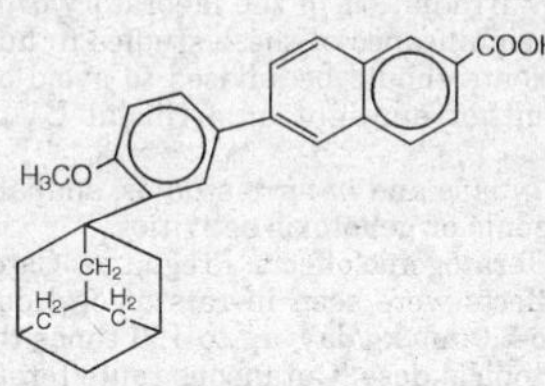

CLINICAL PHARMACOLOGY

Adapalene is a chemically stable, retinoid-like compound. Biochemical and pharmacological profile studies have demonstrated that adapalene is a modulator of cellular differentiation, keratinization, and inflammatory processes all of which represent important features in the pathology of acne vulgaris. Mechanistically, adapalene binds to specific retinoic acid nuclear receptors but does not bind to the cytosolic receptor protein. Although the exact mode of action of adapalene is unknown, it is suggested that topical adapalene may normalize the differentiation of follicular epithelial cells resulting in decreased microcomedone formation.
Pharmacokinetics: Absorption of adapalene through human skin is low. Only trace amounts (< 0.25 ng/mL) of parent substance have been found in the plasma of acne patients following chronic topical application of adapalene in controlled clinical trials. Excretion appears to be primarily by the biliary route.

INDICATIONS AND USAGE

DIFFERIN® Solution is indicated for the topical treatment of acne vulgaris.

CONTRAINDICATIONS

DIFFERIN® Solution should not be administered to individuals who are hypersensitive to adapalene or any of the components in the vehicle solution.

WARNINGS

Use of DIFFERIN® Solution should be discontinued if hypersensitivity to any of the ingredients is noted. Patients with sunburn should be advised not to use the product until fully recovered.

PRECAUTIONS

General: If a reaction suggesting sensitivity or chemical irritation occurs, use of the medication should be discontinued. Exposure to sunlight, including sunlamps, should be minimized during the use of adapalene. Patients who normally experience high levels of sun exposure, and those with inherent sensitivity to sun, should be warned to exercise caution. Use of sunscreen products and protective clothing over treated areas is recommended when exposure cannot be avoided. Weather extremes, such as wind or cold, also may be irritating to patients under treatment with adapalene.
Avoid contact with the eyes, lips, angles of the nose, and mucous membranes. The product should not be applied to cuts, abrasions, eczematous skin, or sunburned skin.
Certain cutaneous signs and symptoms such as erythema, dryness, scaling, burning, or pruritus may be experienced during treatment. These are most likely to occur during the first two to four weeks and will usually lessen with continued use of the medication. Depending upon the severity of adverse events, patients should be instructed to reduce the frequency of application or discontinue use.
Drug Interactions: As DIFFERIN® Solution has the potential to produce local irritation in some patients, concomitant use of other potentially irritating topical products (medicated or abrasive soaps and cleansers, soaps and cosmetics that have a strong drying effect, and products with high concentrations of alcohol, astringents, spices, or lime) should be approached with caution. Particular caution should be exercised in using preparations containing sulfur, resorcinol, or salicylic acid in combination with DIFFERIN® Solution. If these preparations have been used, it is advisable not to start therapy with DIFFERIN® Solution until the effects of such preparations in the skin have subsided.
Carcinogenesis, Mutagenesis, Impairment of Fertility: Carcinogenicity studies with adapalene have been conducted in mice at topical doses of 0.3, 0.9, and 2.6 mg/kg/day and in rats at oral doses of 0.15, 0.5, and 1.5 mg/kg/day, approximately 4–75 times the maximal daily human topical dose.

Continued on next page

Differin Solution—Cont.

In the oral study, positive linear trends were observed in the incidence of follicular cell adenomas and carcinomas in the thyroid glands of female rats, and in the incidence of benign and malignant pheochromocytomas in the adrenal medullas of male rats.
No photocarcinogenicity studies were conducted. Animal studies have shown an increased tumorigenic risk with the use of pharmacologically similar drugs (e.g., retinoids) when exposed to UV irradiation in the laboratory or to sunlight. Although the significance of these studies to human use is not clear, patients should be advised to avoid or minimize exposure to either sunlight or artificial UV irradiation sources.
In a series of *in vivo* and *in vitro* studies, adapalene did not exhibit mutagenic or genotoxic activities.
Pregnancy: Teratogenic effects. Pregnancy Category C. No teratogenic effects were seen in rats at oral doses of adapalene 0.15 to 5.0 mg/kg/day, up to 120 times the maximal daily human topical dose. Cutaneous route teratology studies conducted in rats and rabbits at doses of 0.6, 2.0, and 6.0 mg/kg/day, up to 150 times the maximal daily human topical dose exhibited no fetotoxicity and only minimal increases in supernumerary ribs in rats. There are no adequate and well-controlled studies in pregnant women. Adapalene should be used during pregnancy only if the potential benefit justifies the potential risk to the fetus.
Nursing Mothers: It is not known whether this drug is excreted in human milk. Because many drugs are excreted in human milk, caution should be exercised when DIFFERIN® Solution is administered to a nursing woman.
Pediatric Use: Safety and effectiveness in pediatric patients below the age of 12 have not been established.

ADVERSE REACTIONS

Some adverse effects such as erythema, scaling, dryness, pruritus, and burning will occur in 30–60% of patients. Pruritus or burning immediately after application also occurs in approximately 30% of patients. The following additional adverse experiences were reported in approximately 1% or less of patients: skin irritation, burning/stinging, erythema, sunburn, and acne flares. These are most commonly seen during the first month of therapy and decrease in frequency and severity thereafter. All adverse effects with use of DIFFERIN® Solution during clinical trials were reversible upon discontinuation of therapy.

OVERDOSAGE

DIFFERIN® Solution is intended for cutaneous use only. If the medication is applied excessively, no more rapid or better results will be obtained and marked redness, peeling, or discomfort may occur. The acute oral toxicity of DIFFERIN® Solution in mice and rats is greater than 10 mL/kg. Chronic ingestion of the drug may lead to the same side effects as those associated with excessive oral intake of Vitamin A.

DOSAGE AND ADMINISTRATION

DIFFERIN® Solution should be applied once a day to affected areas after washing in the evening before retiring. A thin film of the solution should be applied, avoiding eyes, lips and mucous membranes.
During the early weeks of therapy, an apparent exacerbation of acne may occur. This is due to the action of the medication on previously unseen lesions and should not be considered a reason to discontinue therapy. Therapeutic results should be noticed after eight to twelve weeks of treatment.

HOW SUPPLIED

DIFFERIN® (adapalene solution) Solution, 0.1% is supplied in the following size:
30 mL glass bottle with applicator – **NDC** 0299-5905-30
The applicator is designed so that the solution may be applied directly to the involved skin.
Storage: Store at controlled room temperature 20° – 25°C (68° – 77°F). Keep container tightly closed and store upright.
CAUTION: Federal law prohibits dispensing without prescription.
Marketed by:
GALDERMA LABORATORIES, INC.
Fort Worth, Texas 76133 USA
Mfd. by:
DPT Laboratories, Ltd.
San Antonio, Texas 78215 USA
325031-0797
Revised: July 1997

METROCREAM™ ℞
(metronidazole topical cream)
Topical Cream, 0.75%
FOR TOPICAL USE ONLY
(NOT FOR OPHTHALMIC USE)

DESCRIPTION

MetroCream™ Topical Cream contains metronidazole, USP, at a concentration of 7.5 mg per gram (0.75%) in an emollient cream consisting of emulsifying wax, sorbitol solution, glycerin, isopropyl palmitate, benzyl alcohol, lactic acid and/or sodium hydroxide to adjust pH, and purified water. Metronidazole is a member of the imidazole class of antibacterial agents and is classified therapeutically as an antiprotozoal and antibacterial agent. Chemically, metronidazole is 2-methyl-5-nitro-1*H*-imidazole-1-ethanol. The molecular formula is $C_6H_9N_3O_3$ and molecular weight is 171.16. Metronidazole is represented by the following structural formula:

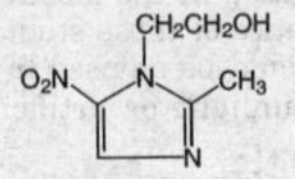

CLINICAL PHARMACOLOGY

The mechanisms by which metronidazole acts in the treatment of rosacea are unknown, but appear to include an anti-inflammatory effect.

INDICATIONS AND USAGE

MetroCream™ (metronidazole topical cream) Topical Cream is indicated for topical application in the treatment of inflammatory papules and pustules of rosacea.

CONTRAINDICATIONS

MetroCream™ (metronidazole topical cream) Topical Cream is contraindicated in individuals with a history of hypersensitivity to metronidazole, or other ingredients of the formulation.

PRECAUTIONS

General: Topical metronidazole has been reported to cause tearing of the eyes. Therefore, contact with the eyes should be avoided. If a reaction suggesting local irritation occurs, patients should be directed to use the medication less frequently or discontinue use. Metronidazole is a nitroimidazole and should be used with care in patients with evidence of, or history of blood dyscrasia.
Information for patients: This medication is to be used as directed by the physician. It is for external use only. Avoid contact with the eyes.
Drug Interactions: Oral metronidazole has been reported to potentiate the anticoagulant effect of warfarin and coumarin anticoagulants, resulting in a prolongation of prothrombin time. The effect of topical metronidazole on prothrombin time is not known.
Carcinogenesis, mutagenesis, impairment of fertility: Metronidazole has shown evidence of carcinogenic activity in a number of studies involving chronic, oral administration in mice and rats but not in studies involving hamsters.
Metronidazole has shown evidence of mutagenic activity in several *in vitro* bacterial assay systems. In addition, a dose-response increase in the frequency of micronuclei was observed in mice after intraperitoneal injections and an increase in chromosome aberrations have been reported in patients with Crohn's disease who were treated with 200-1200 mg/day of metronidazole for 1 to 24 months. However, no excess chromosomal aberrations in circulating human lymphocytes have been observed in patients treated for 8 months.
Pregnancy: *Teratogenic effects: Pregnancy category B:* There are no adequate and well-controlled studies with the use of **MetroCream™** (metronidazole topical cream) Topical Cream in pregnant women. Metronidazole crosses the placental barrier and enters the fetal circulation rapidly. No fetotoxicity was observed after oral metronidazole in rats or mice. However, because animal reproduction studies are not always predictive of human response and since oral metronidazole has been shown to be a carcinogen in some rodents, this drug should be used during pregnancy only if clearly needed.
Nursing Mothers: After oral administration, metronidazole is secreted in breast milk in concentrations similar to those found in the plasma. Even though blood levels are significantly lower with topically applied metronidazole than those achieved after oral administration of metronidazole, a decision should be made whether to discontinue nursing or to discontinue the drug, taking into account the importance of the drug to the mother.
Pediatric Use: Safety and effectiveness in pediatric patients have not been established.

ADVERSE REACTIONS

In controlled clinical trials, the total incidence of adverse reactions associated with the use of **MetroCream™** Topical Cream was approximately 10%. Skin discomfort (burning and stinging) was the most frequently reported event followed by erythema, skin irritation, pruritus and worsening of rosacea. All individual events occurred in less than 3% of patients.
The following additional adverse experiences have been reported with the topical use of metronidazole: dryness, transient redness, metallic taste, tingling or numbness of extremities and nausea.

DOSAGE AND ADMINISTRATION

Apply and rub in a thin layer of **MetroCream™** (metronidazole topical cream) Topical Cream twice daily, morning and evening, to entire affected areas after washing.
Areas to be treated should be washed with a mild cleanser before application. Patients may use cosmetics after application of **MetroCream™** Topical Cream.

HOW SUPPLIED

MetroCream™ (metronidazole topical cream) Topical Cream, 0.75% is supplied in a 45 g aluminum tube–**NDC** 0299-3836-45.
Storage conditions: STORE AT CONTROLLED ROOM TEMPERATURE: 59° to 86°F (15° to 30°C).
Caution: Federal law prohibits dispensing without prescription.
Marketed by:
Galderma Laboratories, Inc.
Fort Worth, Texas 76133 USA
Manufactured by:
DPT Laboratories, Ltd.
San Antonio, Texas 78215 USA
225029-0695
Revised: June 1995

METROGEL® ℞
(metronidazole topical gel)
Topical Gel, 0.75%
FOR TOPICAL USE ONLY
(NOT FOR OPHTHALMIC USE)

DESCRIPTION

MetroGel® Topical Gel contains metronidazole, USP, at a concentration of 7.5 mg per gram (0.75%) in a gel consisting of purified water, methylparaben, propylparaben, propylene glycol, carbomer 940, sodium hydroxide, and edetate disodium. Metronidazole is classified therapeutically as an antiprotozoal and antibacterial agent. Chemically, metronidazole is named 2-methyl-5-nitro-1*H* -imidazole-1-ethanol and has the following structure:

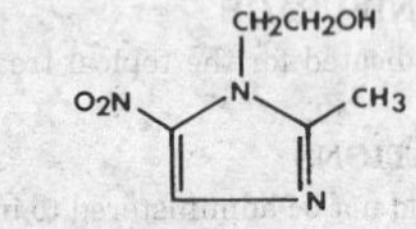

CLINICAL PHARMACOLOGY

Bioavailability studies on the topical administration of 1 gram of **MetroGel®** Topical Gel (7.5 mg of metronidazole) to the face of 10 rosacea patients showed a maximum serum concentration of 66 nanograms per milliliter in one patient. This concentration is approximately 100 times less than concentrations afforded by a single 250 mg oral tablet. The serum metronidazole concentrations were below the detectable limits of the assay at the majority of time points in all patients. Three of the patients had no detectable serum concentrations of metronidazole at any time point. The mean dose of gel applied during clinical studies was 600 mg which represents 4.5 mg of metronidazole per application. Therefore, under normal usage levels, the formulation affords minimal serum concentrations of metronidazole. The mechanisms by which **MetroGel®** (metronidazole topical gel) Topical Gel acts in the treatment of rosacea are unknown, but appear to include an anti-inflammatory effect.

INDICATIONS AND USAGE

MetroGel® Topical Gel is indicated for topical application in the treatment of inflammatory papules and pustules of rosacea.

CONTRAINDICATIONS

MetroGel® Topical Gel is contraindicated in individuals with a history of hypersensitivity to metronidazole, parabens, or other ingredients of the formulation.

PRECAUTIONS

General: MetroGel® Topical Gel has been reported to cause tearing of the eyes. Therefore, contact with the eyes should be avoided. If a reaction suggesting local irritation occurs, patients should be directed to use the medication less frequently or discontinue use. Metronidazole is a nitroimidazole and should be used with care in patients with evidence of, or history of blood dyscrasia.
Information for patients: This medication is to be used as directed by the physician. It is for external use only. Avoid contact with the eyes.
Drug Interactions: Oral metronidazole has been reported to potentiate the anticoagulant effect of coumarin and war-

farin resulting in a prolongation of prothrombin time. The effect of topical metronidazole on prothrombin time is not known.

Carcinogenesis, mutagenesis, impairment of fertility: Metronidazole has shown evidence of carcinogenic activity in a number of studies involving chronic, oral administration in mice and rats but not in studies involving hamsters.

Metronidazole has shown evidence of mutagenic activity in several *in vitro* bacterial assay systems. In addition, a dose-response increase in the frequency of micronuclei was observed in mice after intraperitoneal injections and an increase in chromosome aberrations have been reported in patients with Crohn's disease who were treated with 200–1200 mg/day of metronidazole for 1 to 24 months. However, no excess chromosomal aberrations in circulating human lymphocytes have been observed in patients treated for 8 months.

Pregnancy: ***Teratogenic effects: Pregnancy category B:*** There has been no experience to date with the use of **MetroGel®** (metronidazole topical gel) Topical Gel in pregnant patients. Metronidazole crosses the placental barrier and enters the fetal circulation rapidly. No fetotoxicity was observed after oral metronidazole in rats or mice. However, because animal reproduction studies are not always predictive of human response and since oral metronidazole has been shown to be a carcinogen in some rodents, this drug should be used during pregnancy only if clearly needed.

Nursing mothers: After oral administration, metronidazole is secreted in breast milk in concentrations similar to those found in the plasma. Even though **MetroGel®** Topical Gel blood levels are significantly lower than those achieved after oral metronidazole, a decision should be made whether to discontinue nursing or to discontinue the drug, taking into account the importance of the drug to the mother.

Pediatric use: Safety and effectiveness in pediatric patients have not been established.

ADVERSE REACTIONS

The following adverse experiences have been reported with the topical use of metronidazole: burning, skin irritation, dryness, transient redness, metallic taste, tingling or numbness of extremities and nausea.

DOSAGE AND ADMINISTRATION

Apply and rub in a thin film of METROGEL Topical Gel twice daily, morning and evening, to entire affected areas after washing.

Areas to be treated should be cleansed before application of **MetroGel®** (metronidazole topical gel) Topical Gel. Patients may use cosmetics after application of **MetroGel®** Topical Gel.

HOW SUPPLIED

MetroGel® (metronidazole topical gel) Topical Gel is supplied in a 1 oz (28.4 g) aluminum tube—**NDC** 0299-3835-28 and a 45 g aluminum tube—**NDC** 0299-3835-45.

Storage conditions: STORE AT CONTROLLED ROOM TEMPERATURE: 59° to 86°F (15° to 30°C).

Caution: Federal law prohibits dispensing without prescription.

GALDERMA

Marketed by:

Galderma Laboratories, Inc., Fort Worth, Texas 76133 USA

Manufactured by: DPT Laboratories, Ltd.

San Antonio, Texas 78215 USA

225032-0895

Revised: August 1995

GATE Pharmaceuticals

Div. of TEVA Pharmaceuticals USA
650 CATHILL ROAD
SELLERSVILLE, PA 18960

Direct Inquiries to:

650 Cathill Road
Sellersville, PA 18960
(800) 292–4283

ADIPEX-P® Ⓒ℞
(phentermine HCl 37.5 mg)

DESCRIPTION

Phentermine hydrochloride USP has the chemical name of α,α-Dimethylphenethylamine hydrochloride. The structural formula is as follows:

[See chemical structure at top of next column]

Phentermine hydrochloride is a white, odorless, hygroscopic, crystalline powder which is soluble in water and lower alcohols, slightly soluble in chloroform and insoluble in ether.

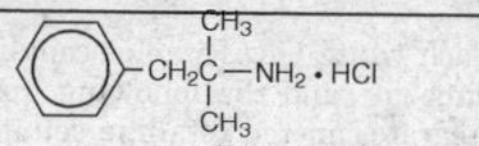

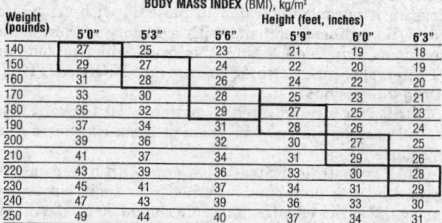

$C_{10}H_{15}N \cdot HCl$ M.W. 185.7

ADIPEX-P®, an anorectic agent for oral administration, is available as a capsule or tablet containing 37.5 mg of phentermine hydrochloride (equivalent to 30 mg of phentermine base).

ADIPEX-P® Capsules contain the inactive ingredients Corn Starch, Gelatin, Lactose Monohydrate, Magnesium Stearate, Titanium Dioxide, Black Iron Oxide, FD&C Blue #1, FD&C Red #40 and D&C Red #33.

ADIPEX-P® Tablets contain the inactive ingredients Acacia, Anhydrous Lactose, Confectioner's Sugar, Corn Starch, Lactose Monohydrate, Magnesium Stearate, Pregelatinized Starch, Stearic Acid, and FD&C Blue #1.

CLINICAL PHARMACOLOGY

ADIPEX-P® is a sympathomimetic amine with pharmacologic activity similar to the prototype drugs of this class used in obesity, the amphetamines. Actions include central nervous system stimulation and elevation of blood pressure. Tachyphylaxis and tolerance have been demonstrated with all drugs of this class in which these phenomena have been looked for.

Drugs of this class used in obesity are commonly known as "anorectics" or "anorexigenics." It has not been established that the action of such drugs in treating obesity is primarily one of appetite suppression. Other central nervous system actions, or metabolic effects, may be involved, for example. Adult obese subjects instructed in dietary management and treated with "anorectic" drugs lose more weight on the average than those treated with placebo and diet, as determined in relatively short-term clinical trials.

The magnitude of increased weight loss of drug-treated patients over placebo-treated patients is only a fraction of a pound a week. The rate of weight loss is greatest in the first weeks of therapy for both drug and placebo subjects and tends to decrease in succeeding weeks. The possible origins of the increased weight loss due to the various drug effects are not established. The amount of weight loss associated with the use of an "anorectic" drug varies from trial to trial, and the increased weight loss appears to be related in part to variables other than the drugs prescribed, such as the physician-investigator, the population treated and the diet prescribed. Studies do not permit conclusions as to the relative importance of the drug and non-drug factors on weight loss.

The natural history of obesity is measured in years, whereas the studies cited are restricted to a few weeks' duration; thus, the total impact of drug-induced weight loss over that of diet alone must be considered clinically limited.

INDICATIONS AND USAGE

ADIPEX-P® (phentermine hydrochloride) is indicated as a short-term (a few weeks) adjunct in a regimen of weight reduction based on exercise, behavioral modification and caloric restriction in the management of exogenous obesity for patients with an initial body mass index $\geq$30 kg/m^2, or $\geq$27 kg/m^2 in the presence of other risk factors (e.g., hypertension, diabetes, hyperlipidemia).

Below is a chart of Body Mass Index (BMI) based on various heights and weights.

BMI is calculated by taking the patient's weight, in kilograms (kg), divided by the patient's height, in meters (m), squared. Metric conversions are as follows: pounds ÷ 2.2 = kg; inches × 0.0254 = meters.

BODY MASS INDEX (BMI), kg/m^2

Weight (pounds)	Height (feet, inches) 5'0"	5'3"	5'6"	5'9"	6'0"	6'3"
140	27	25	23	21	19	18
150	29	27	24	22	20	19
160	31	28	26	24	22	20
170	33	30	28	25	23	21
180	35	32	29	27	25	23
190	37	34	31	28	26	24
200	39	36	32	30	27	25
210	41	37	34	31	29	26
220	43	39	36	33	30	28
230	45	41	37	34	31	29
240	47	43	39	36	33	30
250	49	44	40	37	34	31

The limited usefulness of agents of this class (see **CLINICAL PHARMACOLOGY**) should be measured against possible risk factors inherent in their use such as those described below.

CONTRAINDICATIONS

Advanced arteriosclerosis, cardiovascular disease, moderate to severe hypertension, hyperthyroidism, known hypersensitivity or idiosyncrasy to the sympathomimetic amines, glaucoma.

Agitated states.

Patients with a history of drug abuse.

During or within 14 days following the administration of monoamine oxidase inhibitors (hypertensive crises may result).

WARNINGS

ADIPEX-P® is indicated only as short-term monotherapy for the management of exogenous obesity. The safety and efficacy of combination therapy with phentermine and any other drug products for weight loss, including selective serotonin reuptake inhibitors (e.g., fluoxetine, sertraline, fluvoxamine, paroxetine), have not been established. Therefore, coadministration of these drug products for weight loss is not recommended.

Primary Pulmonary Hypertension (PPH) – a rare, frequently fatal disease of the lungs – has been reported to occur in patients receiving a combination of phentermine with fenfluramine or dexfenfluramine. The possibility of an association between PPH and the use of phentermine alone cannot be ruled out; there have been rare cases of PPH in patients who reportedly have taken phentermine alone. The initial symptoms of PPH is usually dyspnea. Other initial symptoms include: angina pectoris, syncope or lower extremity edema. Patients should be advised to report immediately any deterioration in exercise tolerance. Treatment should be discontinued in patients who develop new, unexplained symptoms of dyspnea, angina pectoris, syncope or lower extremity edema.

Valvular Heart Disease: Serious regurgitant cardiac valvular disease, primarily affecting the mitral, aortic and/or tricuspid valves, has been reported in otherwise healthy persons who had taken a combination of phentermine with fenfluramine or dexfenfluramine for weight loss. The etiology of these valvulopathies has not been established and their course in individuals after the drugs are stopped is not known. There have been no reported cases to date of this valvular condition occurring with the use of phentermine alone.

Tolerance to the anorectic effect usually develops within a few weeks. When this occurs, the recommended dose should not be exceeded in an attempt to increase the effect; rather, the drug should be discontinued.

ADIPEX-P® may impair the ability of the patient to engage in potentially hazardous activities such as operating machinery or driving a motor vehicle; the patient should therefore be cautioned accordingly.

DRUG ABUSE AND DEPENDENCE

ADIPEX-P® is related chemically and pharmacologically to the amphetamines. Amphetamines and related stimulant drugs have been extensively abused, and the possibility of abuse of ADIPEX-P® should be kept in mind when evaluating the desirability of including a drug as part of a weight reduction program. Abuse of amphetamines and related drugs may be associated with intense psychological dependence and severe social dysfunction. There are reports of patients who have increased the dosage to many times that recommended. Abrupt cessation following prolonged high dosage administration results in extreme fatigue and mental depression; changes are also noted on the sleep EEG. Manifestations of chronic intoxication with anorectic drugs include severe dermatoses, marked insomnia, irritability, hyperactivity and personality changes. The most severe manifestation of chronic intoxications is psychosis, often clinically indistinguishable from schizophrenia.

Usage with Alcohol: Concomitant use of alcohol with ADIPEX-P® may result in an adverse drug interaction.

PRECAUTIONS

General

Caution is to be exercised in prescribing ADIPEX-P® (phentermine hydrochloride) for patients with even mild hypertension.

Insulin requirements in diabetes mellitus may be altered in association with the use of ADIPEX-P® and the concomitant dietary regimen.

ADIPEX-P® may decrease the hypotensive effect of guanethidine.

The least amount feasible should be prescribed or dispensed at one time in order to minimize the possibility of overdosage.

Carcinogenesis, Mutagenesis, Impairment of Fertility: Studies have not been performed with ADIPEX-P® (phentermine hydrochloride) to determine the potential for carcinogenesis, mutagenesis or impairment of fertility.

Pregnancy–Teratogenic Effects: Pregnancy Category C. Animal reproduction studies have not been conducted with ADIPEX-P®. It is also not known whether ADIPEX-P® can cause fetal harm when administered to a pregnant woman or can affect reproductive capacity. ADIPEX-P® should be given to a pregnant woman only if clearly needed.

Nursing Mothers

Because of the potential for serious adverse reactions in nursing infants, a decision should be made whether to discontinue nursing or to discontinue the drug, taking into account the importance of the drug to the mother.

Pediatric Use

Safety and effectiveness in pediatric patients have not been established.

Continued on next page

Adipex-P—Cont.

ADVERSE REACTIONS

Cardiovascular: Primary pulmonary hypertension and/or regurgitant cardiac valvular disease (see **WARNINGS**), palpitation, tachycardia, elevation of blood pressure.
Central Nervous System: Overstimulation, restlessness, dizziness, insomnia, euphoria, dysphoria, tremor, headache; rarely psychotic episodes at recommended doses.
Gastrointestinal: Dryness of the mouth, unpleasant taste, diarrhea, constipation, other gastrointestinal disturbances.
Allergic: Urticaria.
Endocrine: Impotence, changes in libido.

OVERDOSAGE

Manifestations of acute overdosage with phentermine include restlessness, tremor, hyperreflexia, rapid respiration, confusion, assaultiveness, hallucinations, panic states. Fatigue and depression usually follow the central stimulation. Cardiovascular effects include arrhythmia, hypertension or hypotension, and circulatory collapse. Gastrointestinal symptoms include nausea, vomiting, diarrhea and abdominal cramps. Fatal poisoning usually terminates in convulsions and coma.
Management of acute phentermine intoxication is largely symptomatic and includes lavage and sedation with a barbiturate. Experience with hemodialysis or peritoneal dialysis is inadequate to permit recommendations in this regard. Acidification of the urine increases phentermine excretion. Intravenous phentolamine (Regitine®, CIBA) has been suggested for possible acute, severe hypertension, if this complicates phentermine overdosage.

DOSAGE AND ADMINISTRATION

Exogenous Obesity: Dosage should be individualized to obtain an adequate response with the lowest effective dose. The usual adult dose is one capsule or tablet (37.5 mg) daily, administered before breakfast or 1–2 hours after breakfast. For tablets, the dosage may be adjusted to the patient's need. For some patients ½ tablet (18.75 mg) daily may be adequate, while in some cases it may be desirable to give ½ tablet (18.75 mg) two times a day.
Late evening medication should be avoided because of the possibility of resulting insomnia.
Phentermine is not recommended for use in patients sixteen (16) years of age and under.

HOW SUPPLIED

Available in tablets and capsules containing 37.5 mg phentermine hydrochloride (equivalent to 30 mg phentermine base). Each blue and white, oblong, scored tablet is debossed with "LEMMON" and "9"-"9". The #3 capsule has an opaque white body and an opaque light blue cap. Each capsule is imprinted with "ADIPEX-P"-"37.5" on the cap and two stripes on the body using dark blue ink.
Tablets are packaged in bottles of 100 (NDC 57844-009-01); 400 (NDC 57844-009-26); and 1000 (NDC 57844-009-10).
Capsules are packaged in bottles of 100 (NDC 57844-019-01).
Store at controlled room temperature 15°–30°C (59°–86°F).
Dispense in a tight container as defined in the USP, with a child-resistant closure (as required).

Manufactured for:
GATE PHARMACEUTICALS
Div. of Teva Pharmaceuticals USA
Sellersville, PA 18960

Manufactured by:
TEVA PHARMACEUTICALS USA
Sellersville, PA 18960

Printed in USA
Rev. L 1/98

Shown in Product Identification Guide, page 310

ORAP® (Pimozide) ℞
Tablets

DESCRIPTION

ORAP® (pimozide) is an orally active antipsychotic agent of the diphenyl-butylpiperidine series. The structural formula of pimozide, 1-[1-[4,4-bis(4-fluorophenyl)butyl]-4-piperidinyl]-1,3-dihydro-2*H*-benzimidazole-2-one is:

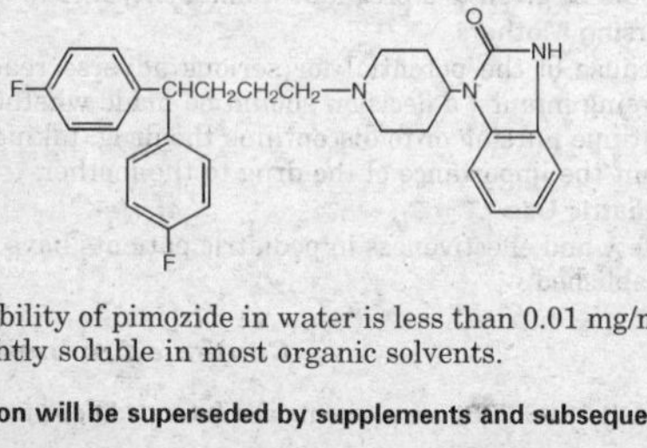

The solubility of pimozide in water is less than 0.01 mg/mL; it is slightly soluble in most organic solvents.
Each white ORAP tablet contains either 1 mg or 2 mg of pimozide and the following inactive ingredients: calcium stearate, microcrystalline cellulose, lactose anhydrous and corn starch.

CLINICAL PHARMACOLOGY

Pharmacodynamic Actions
ORAP (pimozide) is an orally active antipsychotic drug product which shares with other antipsychotics the ability to blockade dopaminergic receptors on neurons in the central nervous system. Although its exact mode of action has not been established, the ability of pimozide to suppress motor and phonic tics in Tourette's Disorder is thought to be a function of its dopaminergic blocking activity. However, receptor blockade is often accompanied by a series of secondary alterations in central dopamine metabolism and function which may contribute to both pimozide's therapeutic and untoward effects. In addition, pimozide, in common with other antipsychotic drugs, has various effects on other central nervous system receptor systems which are not fully characterized.
Metabolism and Pharmacokinetics
More than 50% of a dose of pimozide is absorbed after oral administration. Based on the pharmacokinetic and metabolic profile, pimozide appears to undergo significant first pass metabolism. Peak serum levels occur generally six to eight hours (range 4–12 hours) after dosing.
Pimozide is extensively metabolized, primarily by N-dealkylation in the liver. Two major metabolites have been identified, 1-(4-piperidyl)-2-benzimidazolinone and 4,4-bis(4-fluorophenyl) butyric acid. The antipsychotic activity of these metabolites is undetermined. The major route of elimination of pimozide and its metabolites is through the kidney.
The mean serum elimination half-life of pimozide in schizophrenic patients was approximately 55 hours. There was 13-fold interindividual difference in the area under the serum pimozide level-time curve and an equivalent degree of variation in peak serum levels among patients studied. The significance of this is unclear since there are few correlations between plasma levels and clinical findings.
Effects of food, disease or concomitant medication upon the absorption, distribution, metabolism and elimination of pimozide are not known.

INDICATIONS AND USAGE

ORAP (pimozide) is indicated for the suppression of motor and phonic tics in patients with Tourette's Disorder who have failed to respond satisfactorily to standard treatment. ORAP is not intended as a treatment of first choice nor is it intended for the treatment of tics that are merely annoying or cosmetically troublesome. ORAP should be reserved for use in Tourette's Disorder patients whose development and/or daily life function is severely compromised by the presence of motor and phonic tics.
Evidence supporting approval of pimozide for use in Tourette's Disorder was obtained in two controlled clinical investigations which enrolled patients between the ages of 8 and 53 years. Most subjects in the two trials were 12 or older.

CONTRAINDICATIONS

1. ORAP (pimozide) is contraindicated in the treatment of simple tics or tics other than those associated with Tourette's Disorder.
2. ORAP should not be used in patients taking drugs tha may, themselves, cause motor and phonic tics (e.g., pemoline, methylphenidate and amphetamines) until such patients have been withdrawn from these drugs to determine whether or not the drug, rather than Tourette's Disorder, are responsible for the tics.
3. Because ORAP prolongs the QT interval of the electrocardiogram it is contraindicated in patients with congenital long QT syndrome, patients with a history of cardiac arrhythmias, or patients taking other drugs which prolong the QT interval of the electrocardiogram (see **PRECAUTIONS - Drug Interactions**).
4. ORAP is contraindicated in patients with severe toxic central nervous system depression or comatose states from any cause.
5. ORAP is contraindicated in patients with hypersensitivity to it. As it is not known whether cross-sensitivity exists among the antipsychotics, pimozide should be used with appropriate caution in patients who have demonstrated hypersensitivity to other antipsychotic drugs.
6. Ventricular arrhythmias have been rarely associated with the use of macrolide antibiotics in patients with prolonged QT intervals, as might be produced by ORAP. Specifically, two sudden deaths have been reported when clarithromycin was added to ongoing pimozide therapy. Furthermore, some evidence suggests that pimozide is metabolized partly by the enzyme system cytochrome P450 3A (CYP 3A). Macrolide antibiotics are inhibitors of CYP 3A, and thus could potentially impede pimozide metabolism. For these reasons, ORAP is contraindicated in patients receiving the macrolide antibiotics clarithromycin, erythromycin, azithromycin, and dirithromycin.
Because azole antifungal agents are also inhibitors of the CYP 3A enzymes and thus may likewise impair pimozide metabolism, ORAP is contraindicated in patients receiving the azole antifungal agents itraconazole and ketoconazole. Similarly, protease inhibitor drugs are also inhibitors of CYP 3A, and thus ORAP is contraindicated in patients receiving protease inhibitors such as ritonavir, saquinovir, indinavir, and nelfinavir.

WARNINGS

The use of ORAP (pimozide) in the treatment of Tourette's Disorder involves different risk/benefit considerations than when antipsychotic drugs are used to treat other conditions. Consequently, a decision to use ORAP should take into consideration the following (see also **PRECAUTIONS - Information for Patients**).
Tardive Dyskinesia
A syndrome consisting of potentially irreversible, involuntary, dyskinetic movements may develop in patients treated with antipsychotic drugs. Although the prevalence of the syndrome appears to be highest among the elderly, especially elderly women, it is impossible to rely upon prevalence estimates to predict, at the inception of antipsychotic treatment, which patients are likely to develop the syndrome. Whether antipsychotic drug products differ in their potential to cause tardive dyskinesia is unknown.
Both the risk of developing tardive dyskinesia and the likelihood that it will become irreversible are believed to increase as the duration of treatment and the total cumulative dose of antipsychotic drugs administered to the patient increase. However, the syndrome can develop, although much less commonly, after relatively brief treatment periods at low doses.
There is no known treatment for established cases of tardive dyskinesia, although the syndrome may remit, partially or completely, if antipsychotic treatment is withdrawn. Antipsychotic treatment itself, however, may suppress (or partially suppress) the signs and symptoms of the syndrome and thereby may possibly mask the underlying process. The effect that symptomatic suppression has upon the long-term course of the syndrome is unknown.
Given these considerations, antipsychotic drugs should be prescribed in a manner that is most likely to minimize the occurrence of tardive dyskinesia. Chronic antipsychotic treatment should generally be reserved for patients who suffer from a chronic illness that, 1) is known to respond to antipsychotic drugs, and, 2) for whom alternative, equally effective, but potentially less harmful treatments are not available or appropriate. In patients who do require chronic treatment, the smallest dose and the shortest duration of treatment producing a satisfactory clinical response should be sought. The need for continued treatment should be reassessed periodically.
If signs and symptoms of tardive dyskinesia appear in a patient on antipsychotics, drug discontinuation should be considered. However, some patients may require treatment despite the presence of the syndrome.
(For further information about the description of tardive dyskinesia and its clinical detection, please refer to **ADVERSE REACTIONS** and **PRECAUTIONS - Information for Patients.**)
Neuroleptic Malignant Syndrome (NMS)
A potentially fatal symptom complex sometimes referred to as Neuroleptic Malignant Syndrome (NMS) has been reported in association with antipsychotic drugs. Clinical manifestations of NMS are hyperpyrexia, muscle rigidity, altered mental status (including catatonic signs) and evidence of autonomic instability (irregular pulse or blood pressure, tachycardia, diaphoresis, and cardiac dysrhythmias). Additional signs may include elevated creatine phosphokinase, myoglobinuria (rhabdomyolysis) and acute renal failure.
The diagnostic evaluation of patients with this syndrome is complicated. In arriving at a diagnosis, it is important to identify cases where the clinical presentation includes both serious medical illness (e.g., pneumonia, systemic infection, etc.) and untreated or inadequately treated extrapyramidal signs and symptoms (EPS). Other important considerations in the differential diagnosis include central anticholinergic toxicity, heat stroke, drug fever and primary central nervous system (CNS) pathology.
The management of NMS should include 1) immediate discontinuation of antipsychotic drugs and other drugs not essential to concurrent therapy, 2) intensive symptomatic treatment and medical monitoring, and 3) treatment of any concomitant serious medical problems for which specific treatment are available. There is no general agreement about specific pharmacological treatment regimens for uncomplicated NMS.
If a patient requires antipsychotic drug treatment after recovery from NMS, the potential reintroduction of drug therapy should be carefully considered. The patient should be carefully monitored, since recurrences of NMS have been reported.
Hyperpyrexia, not associated with the above symptom complex, has been reported with other antipsychotic drugs.
Other
Sudden, unexpected deaths have occurred in experimental studies of conditions other than Tourette's Disorder. These

deaths occurred while patients were receiving dosages in the range of 1 mg per kg. One possible mechanism for such deaths is prolongation of the QT interval predisposing patients to ventricular arrhythmia. An electrocardiogram should be performed before ORAP treatment is initiated and periodically thereafter, especially during the period of dose adjustment.

ORAP may have a tumorigenic potential. Based on studies conducted in mice, it is known that pimozide can produce a dose-related increase in pituitary tumors. The full significance of this finding is not known, but should be taken into consideration in the physician's and patient's decisions to use this drug product. This finding should be given special consideration when the patient is young and chronic use of pimozide is anticipated (see **PRECAUTIONS - Carcinogenesis, Mutagenesis, Impairment of Fertility**).

PRECAUTIONS

General

ORAP (pimozide) may impair the mental and/or physical abilities required for the performance of potentially hazardous tasks, such as driving a car or operating machinery, especially during the first few days of therapy.

ORAP produces anticholinergic side effects and should be used with caution in individuals whose conditions may be aggravated by anticholinergic activity.

ORAP should be administered cautiously to patients with impairment of liver or kidney function, because it is metabolized by the liver and excreted by the kidneys.

Antipsychotics should be administered with caution to patients receiving anticonvulsant medication, with a history of seizures, or with EEG abnormalities, because they may lower the convulsive threshold. If indicated, adequate anticonvulsant therapy should be maintained concomitantly.

Information for Patients

Treatment with ORAP exposes the patient to serious risks. A decision to use ORAP chronically in Tourette's Disorder is one that deserves full consideration by the patient (or patient's family) as well as by the treating physician. Because the goal of treatment is symptomatic improvement, the patient's view of the need for treatment and assessment of response are critical in evaluating the impact of therapy and weighing its benefits against the risks. Since the physician is the primary source of information about the use of a drug in any disease, it is recommended that the following information be discussed with patients and/or their families.

ORAP is intended only for use in patients with Tourette's Disorder whose symptoms are severe and who cannot tolerate, or who do not respond to HALDOL® (haloperidol).

Given the likelihood that a proportion of patients exposed chronically to antipsychotics will develop tardive dyskinesia, it is advised that all patients in whom chronic use is contemplated be given, if possible, full information about this risk. The decision to inform patients and/or their guardians must obviously take into account the clinical circumstances and the competency of the patient to understand the information provided.

There is limited information available on the use of ORAP in children under 12 years of age.

The information available on ORAP from foreign marketing experience and from U.S. clinical trials indicates that ORAP has a side effect profile similar to that of other antipsychotic drugs. Patients should be informed that all types of side effects associated with the use of antipsychotics may be associated with the use of ORAP.

In addition, sudden, unexpected deaths have occurred in patients taking high doses of ORAP for conditions other than Tourette's Disorder. These deaths may have been the result of an effect of ORAP upon the heart. Therefore, patients should be instructed not to exceed the prescribed dose of ORAP and they should realize the need for the initial ECG and for follow-up ECGs during treatment.

Also, pimozide, at a dose about 15 times that given humans, caused an increase in the number of benign tumors of the pituitary gland in female mice. It is not possible to say how important this is. Similar tumors were not seen in rats given pimozide, nor at lower doses in mice, which is reassuring. However, any such finding must be considered to suggest a possible risk of long term use of the drug.

Laboratory Tests

An ECG should be done at baseline and periodically thereafter throughout the period of dose adjustment. Any indication of prolongation of QTc interval beyond an absolute limit of 0.47 seconds (children) or 0.52 seconds (adults), or more than 25% above the patient's original baseline should be considered a basis for stopping further dose increase (see **CONTRAINDICATIONS**) and considering a lower dose.

Since hypokalemia has been associated with ventricular arrhythmias, potassium insufficiency, secondary to diuretics, diarrhea, or other cause, should be corrected before ORAP therapy is initiated and normal potassium maintained during therapy.

Drug Interactions

Because ORAP prolongs the QT interval of the electrocardiogram, an additive effect on QT interval would be anticipated if administered with other drugs, such as phenothiazines, tricyclic antidepressants or antiarrhythmic agents, which prolong the QT interval. Also, the use of macrolide antibiotics in patients with prolonged QT intervals has been rarely associated with ventricular arrhythmias. Such concomitant administration should not be undertaken (see **CONTRAINDICATIONS**).

ORAP may be capable of potentiating CNS depressants, including analgesics, sedatives, anxiolytics, and alcohol.

Carcinogenesis, Mutagenesis, Impairment of Fertility

Carcinogenicity studies were conducted in mice and rats. In mice, pimozide causes a dose-related increase in pituitary and mammary tumors.

When mice were treated for up to 18 months with pimozide, pituitary gland changes developed in females only. These changes were characterized as hyperplasia at doses approximating the human dose and adenoma at doses about fifteen times the maximum recommended human dose on a mg per kg basis. The mechanism for the induction of pituitary tumors in mice is not known.

Mammary gland tumors in female mice were also increased, but these tumors are expected in rodents treated with antipsychotic drugs which elevate prolactin levels. Chronic administration of an antipsychotic also causes elevated prolactin levels in humans. Tissue culture experiments indicate that approximately one-third of human breast cancers are prolactin-dependent *in vitro*, a factor of potential importance if the prescription of these drugs is contemplated in a patient with a previously detected breast cancer. Although disturbances such as galactorrhea, amenorrhea, gynecomastia, and impotence have been reported with antipsychotic drugs, the clinical significance of elevated serum prolactin levels is unknown for most patients. Neither clinical studies nor epidemiologic studies conducted to date have shown an association between chronic administration of these drugs and mammary tumorigenesis. The available evidence, however, is considered too limited to be conclusive at this time.

In a 24-month carcinogenicity study in rats, animals received up to 50 times the maximum recommended human dose. No increased incidence of overall tumors or tumors at any site was observed in either sex. Because of the limited number of animals surviving this study, the meaning of these results is unclear.

Pimozide did not have mutagenic activity in the Ames test with four bacterial test strains, in the mouse dominant lethal test or in the micronucleus test in rats.

Reproduction studies in animals were not adequate to assess all aspects of fertility. Nevertheless, female rats administered pimozide had prolonged estrus cycles, an effect also produced by other antipsychotic drugs.

Pregnancy

Category C. Reproduction studies performed in rats and rabbits at oral doses up to 8 times the maximum human dose did not reveal evidence of teratogenicity. In the rat, however, this multiple of the human dose resulted in decreased pregnancies and in the retarded development of fetuses. These effects are thought to be due to an inhibition or delay in implantation which is also observed in rodents administered other antipsychotic drugs. In the rabbit, maternal toxicity, mortality, decreased weight gain, and embryotoxicity including increased resorptions were dose-related. Because animal reproduction studies are not always predictive of human response, pimozide should be given to a pregnant woman only if the potential benefits of treatment clearly outweigh the potential risks.

Labor and Delivery

This drug has no recognized use in labor or delivery.

Nursing Mothers

It is not known whether pimozide is excreted in human milk. Because many drugs are excreted in human milk and because of the potential for tumorigenicity and unknown cardiovascular effects in the infant, a decision should be made whether to discontinue nursing or to discontinue the drug, taking into account the importance of the drug to the mother.

Pediatric Use

Although Tourette's Disorder most often has its onset between the ages of 2 and 15 years, information on the use and efficacy of ORAP in patients less than 12 years of age is limited. A 24-week open label study in 36 children between the ages of 2 and 12 demonstrated that pimozide has a similar safety profile in this age group as in older patients and there were no safety findings that would preclude its use in this age group.

Because its use and safety have not been evaluated in other childhood disorders, ORAP is not recommended for use in any condition other than Tourette's Disorder.

ADVERSE REACTIONS

General

Extrapyramidal Reactions: Neuromuscular (extrapyramidal) reactions during the administration of ORAP (pimozide) have been reported frequently, often during the first few days of treatment. In most patients, these reactions involved Parkinson-like symptoms which, when first observed, were usually mild to moderately severe and usually reversible.

Other types of neuromuscular reactions (motor restlessness, dystonia, akathisia, hyperreflexia, opisthotonos, oculogyric crises) have been reported far less frequently. Severe extrapyramidal reactions have been reported to occur at relatively low doses. Generally the occurrence and severity of most extrapyramidal symptoms are dose-related since they occur at relatively high doses and have been shown to disappear or become less severe when the dose is reduced. Administration of antiparkinson drugs such as benztropine mesylate or trihexyphenidyl hydrochloride may be required for control of such reactions. It should be noted that persistent extrapyramidal reactions have been reported and that the drug may have to be discontinued in such cases.

Withdrawal Emergent Neurological Signs: Generally, patients receiving short term therapy experience no problems with abrupt discontinuation of antipsychotic drugs. However, some patients on maintenance treatment experience transient dyskinetic signs after abrupt withdrawal. In certain of these cases the dyskinetic movements are indistinguishable from the syndrome described below under "Tardive Dyskinesia" except for duration. It is not known whether gradual withdrawal of antipsychotic drugs will reduce the rate of occurrence of withdrawal emergent neurological signs, but until further evidence becomes available, it seems reasonable to gradually withdraw use of ORAP®.

Tardive Dyskinesia: ORAP may be associated with persistent dyskinesias. Tardive dyskinesia, a syndrome consisting of potentially irreversible, involuntary, dyskinetic movements, may appear in some patients on long-term therapy or may occur after drug therapy has been discontinued. The risk appears to be greater in elderly patients on high-dose therapy, especially females. The symptoms are persistent and in some patients appear irreversible. The syndrome is characterized by rhythmical involuntary movements of tongue, face, mouth or jaw (e.g., protrusion of tongue, puffing of cheeks, puckering of mouth, chewing movements). Sometimes these may be accompanied by involuntary movements of extremities and the trunk.

There is no known effective treatment for tardive dyskinesia; antiparkinson agents usually do not alleviate the symptoms of this syndrome. It is suggested that all antipsychotic agents be discontinued if these symptoms appear. Should it be necessary to reinstitute treatment, or increase the dosage of the agent, or switch to a different antipsychotic agent, this syndrome may be masked.

It has been reported that fine vermicular movement of the tongue may be an early sign of tardive dyskinesia and if the medication is stopped at that time the syndrome may not develop.

Electrocardiographic Changes: Electrocardiographic changes have been observed in clinical trials of ORAP in Tourette's Disorder and schizophrenia. These have included prolongation of the QT interval, flattening, notching and inversion of the T wave and the appearance of U wave. Sudden, unexpected deaths and grand mal seizure have occurred at doses above 20 mg/day.

Neuroleptic Malignant Syndrome: Neuroleptic malignant syndrome (NMS) has been reported with ORAP. (See **WARNINGS** for further information concerning NMS.)

Hyperpyrexia: Hyperpyrexia has been reported with other antipsychotic drugs.

Clinical Trials

The following adverse reaction tabulation was derived from 20 patients in a 6-week long placebo-controlled clinical trial of ORAP in Tourette's Disorder.

Body System/ Adverse Reaction	Pimozide (N = 20)	Placebo (N = 20)
Body as a Whole		
Headache	1	2
Gastrointestinal		
Dry mouth	5	1
Diarrhea	1	0
Nausea	0	2
Vomiting	0	1
Constipation	4	2
Eructations	0	1
Thirsty	1	0
Appetite increase	1	0
Endocrine		
Menstrual disorder	0	1
Breast secretions	0	1

Continued on next page

Orap—Cont.

Musculoskeletal

Muscle cramps	0	1
Muscle tightness	3	0
Stooped posture	2	0

CNS

Drowsiness	7	3
Sedation	14	5
Insomnia	2	2
Dizziness	0	1
Akathisia	8	0
Rigidity	2	0
Speech disorder	2	0
Handwriting change	1	0
Akinesia	8	0

Psychiatric

Depression	2	3
Excitement	0	1
Nervous	1	0
Adverse behavior effect	5	0

Special Senses

Visual disturbance	4	0
Taste change	1	0
Sensitivity of eyes to light	1	0
Decreased accommodation	4	1
Spots before eyes	0	1

Urogenital

Impotence	3	0

The following adverse event tabulation was derived from 36 children (age 2 to 12) in a 24-week open trial of ORAP in Tourette's Disorder.

Body System/ Adverse Reaction	Number of Patients Experiencing Each Event (%)	
	All Events	Drug-Related Events
	(N=36)	(N=36)
Body as a Whole		
Asthenia	9 (25.0)	5 (13.8)
Headache	8 (22.2)	1 (2.7)
Gastrointestinal		
Dysphagia	1 (2.7)	1 (2.7)
Increased Salivation	5 (13.8)	2 (5.5)
Musculoskeletal		
Myalgia	1 (2.7)	1 (2.7)
Central Nervous System		
Dreaming Abnormal	1 (2.7)	1 (2.7)
Hyperkinesia	2 (5.5)	1 (2.7)
Somnolence	10 (27.7)	9 (25.0)
Torticollis	1 (2.7)	1 (2.7)
Tremor, Limbs	1 (2.7)	1 (2.7)
Psychiatric		
Adverse Behavior Effect	10 (27.7)	8 (22.2)
Nervous	3 (8.3)	2 (5.5)
Skin		
Rash	3 (8.3)	1 (2.7)
Special Senses		
Visual Disturbance	2 (5.5)	1 (2.7)
Cardiovascular		
ECG	1 (2.7)	1 (2.7)

Because clinical investigational experience with ORAP in Tourette's Disorder is limited, uncommon adverse reactions may not have been detected. The physician should consider that other adverse reactions associated with antipsychotics may occur.

Other Adverse Reactions
In addition to the adverse reactions listed above, those listed below have been reported in U.S. clinical trials of ORAP in conditions other than Tourette's Disorder.
Body as a Whole: Asthenia, chest pain, periorbital edema

Cardiovascular / Respiratory: Postural hypotension, hypertension, tachycardia, palpitations
Gastrointestinal: Increased salivation, nausea, vomiting, anorexia, GI distress
Endocrine: Loss of libido
Metabolic / Nutritional: Weight gain, weight loss
Central Nervous System: Dizziness, tremor, parkinsonism, fainting, dyskinesia
Psychiatric: Excitement
Skin: Rash, sweating, skin irritation
Special Senses: Blurred vision, cataracts
Urogenital: Nocturia, urinary frequency

Postmarketing Reports
The following experiences were described in spontaneous postmarketing reports. These reports do not provide sufficient information to establish a clear causal relationship with the use of ORAP.
Gastrointestinal: Gingival hyperplasia in one patient
Hematologic: Hemolytic anemia
Metabolic / Nutritional: Hyponatremia
Other: Seizure

OVERDOSAGE
In general, the signs and symptoms of overdosage with ORAP (pimozide) would be an exaggeration of known pharmacologic effects and adverse reactions, the most prominent of which would be: 1) electrocardiographic abnormalities, 2) severe extrapyramidal reactions, 3) hypotension, 4) a comatose state with respiratory depression.
In the event of overdosage, gastric lavage, establishment of a patent airway and, if necessary, mechanically-assisted respiration are advised. Electrocardiographic monitoring should commence immediately and continue until the ECG parameters are within the normal range. Hypotension and circulatory collapse may be counteracted by use of intravenous fluids, plasma, or concentrated albumin, and vasopressor agents such as metaraminol, phenylephrine and norepinephrine. Epinephrine should not be used. In case of severe extrapyramidal reactions, antiparkinson medication should be administered. Because of the long half-life of pimozide, patients who take an overdose should be observed for at least 4 days. As with all drugs, the physician should consider contacting a poison control center for additional information on the treatment of overdose.

DOSAGE AND ADMINISTRATION
General
The suppression of tics by ORAP requires a slow and gradual introduction of the drug. The patient's dose should be carefully adjusted to a point where the suppression of tics and the relief afforded is balanced against the untoward side effects of the drug.
An ECG should be done at baseline and periodically thereafter, especially during the period of dose adjustment (see **WARNINGS** and **PRECAUTIONS - Laboratory Tests**). Periodic attempts should be made to reduce the dosage of ORAP to see whether or not tics persist at the level and extent first identified. In attempts to reduce the dosage of ORAP, consideration should be given to the possibility that increases of tic intensity and frequency may represent a transient, withdrawal-related phenomenon rather than a return of disease symptoms. Specifically, one to two weeks should be allowed to elapse before one concludes that an increase in tic manifestations is a function of the underlying disease syndrome rather than a response to drug withdrawal. A gradual withdrawal is recommended in any case.
Children
Reliable dose response data for the effects of ORAP (pimozide) on tic manifestation in Tourette's Disorder patients below the age of twelve are not available.
Treatment should be initiated at a dose of 0.5 mg/kg preferably taken once at bedtime. The dose may be increased every third day to a maximum of 0.2 mg/kg not to exceed 10 mg/day.
Adults
In general, treatment with ORAP should be initiated with a dose of 1 to 2 mg a day in divided doses. The dose may be increased thereafter every other day. Most patients are maintained at less than 0.2 mg/kg per day, or 10 mg/day, whichever is less. Doses greater than 0.2 mg/kg/day or 10 mg/day are not recommended.

ANIMAL PHARMACOLOGY
A chronic study in dogs indicated that pimozide caused gingival hyperplasia when administered for several months at about 5 times the maximum recommended human dose. This condition was reversible after withdrawal.

HOW SUPPLIED
ORAP® (pimozide) 1 mg tablets are white, oval, scored tablets, debossed "ORAP 1". They are available in bottles of 100 (NDC 57844-151-01).
ORAP® (pimozide) 2 mg tablets are white, oval, scored tablets, debossed "LEMON" on one side and "ORAP 2" on the other. They are available in bottles of 100 (NDC 57844-187-01).
Store at controlled room temperature 15°–30°C (59°–86°F).

Dispense in a tight, light-resistant container as defined in the official compendium.
Pharmacist: Dispense in child-resistant container.
CAUTION: Federal law prohibits dispensing without prescription.

Manufactured for:
GATE PHARMACEUTICALS
Div. of Teva Pharmaceuticals USA
Sellersville, PA 18960
Manufactured by:
TEVA PHARMACEUTICALS USA
Sellersville, PA 18960

Printed in USA
Rev. H 12/97
Shown in Product Identification Guide, page 311

Gebauer Company
9410 ST. CATHERINE AVE.
CLEVELAND, OH 44104

Direct Inquiries to:
(800) 321-9348
(216) 271-5252
www.gebauerco.com
For Medical Information Contact:
In Emergencies:
(800) 321-9348
(216) 271-5252
After Hours and Weekend Emergencies:
Chemtrac:
(800) 424-9300

ETHYL CHLORIDE, U.S.P.
(Chloroethane)   ℞

INDICATIONS AND USAGE
Ethyl Chloride is a vapocoolant intended for topical application to control pain associated with minor surgical procedures (such as lancing boils, or incision and drainage of small abscesses), athletic injuries, injections, and for treatment of myofascial pain, restricted motion, and muscle spasm.

PRECAUTIONS
Inhalation of Ethyl Chloride should be avoided as it may produce narcotic and general anesthetic effects, and may produce deep anesthesia or fatal coma with respiratory or cardiac arrest. Ethyl Chloride is **FLAMMABLE** and should never be used in the presence of an open flame, or electrical cautery equipment. When used to produce local freezing of tissues, adjacent skin areas should be protected by application of petrolatum. The thawing process may be painful, and freezing may lower local resistance to infection and delay healing.

ADVERSE REACTIONS
Cutaneous sensitization may occur, but appears to be extremely rare. Freezing can occasionally alter pigmentation.

CONTRAINDICATIONS
Ethyl Chloride is contraindicated in individuals with a history of hypersensitivity to it.

WARNINGS
For external use only.
Skin absorption of Ethyl Chloride can occur; no cases of chronic poisoning have been reported. Ethyl Chloride is known as a liver and kidney toxin; long term exposure may cause liver or kidney damage.
Contents under pressure. Store in a cool place. Do not store above 120°F. Do not store on or near high frequency ultrasound equipment. Store upright only.

DOSAGE AND ADMINISTRATION
To apply Ethyl Chloride from amber bottle with dispenseal valve, invert over the treatment area approximately 12 inches (30 cm.) away from site of application. Open dispenseal spring valve completely allowing Ethyl Chloride to flow in a stream from the bottle.
1. TOPICAL ANESTHESIA IN MINOR SURGERY
The operative site should be cleansed with a suitable antiseptic. Apply petrolatum to protect the adjacent area. Spray Ethyl Chloride for a few seconds until the tissue becomes white. Avoid prolonged spraying of skin beyond this state. The anesthetic action of Ethyl Chloride rarely lasts more than a few seconds to a minute. Quickly swab operative site with antiseptic and promptly make incision. Reapply as needed.
2. SPORTS INJURIES
The pain of bruises, contusions, abrasions, swelling, and minor sprains may be controlled with Ethyl Chloride.

The amount of cooling depends on the dosage. Dosage varies with duration of application. The smallest dose needed to produce the desired effect should be used. The anesthetic effect of Ethyl Chloride rarely lasts more than a few seconds to a minute. This time interval is usually sufficient to help reduce or relieve the initial trauma of the injury.
Determine the extent of injury (fracture, sprain, etc.). Spray the affected area from a distance of approximately 12 inches (with dispenseal valve bottle) continuously for 3 to 5 seconds until the skin begins to turn white; do not frost skin. Use as you would ice.

3. FOR PRE-INJECTION ANESTHESIA

Prepare syringe and have it ready. Spray skin with Ethyl Chloride from a distance of about 12 inches (30 cm.) continuously for 3 to 5 seconds; do not frost skin. Swab skin with antiseptic and quickly introduce needle with skin taut.

4. SPRAY and STRETCH for MYOFASCIAL PAIN

Ethyl Chloride may be used as a counterirritant in the management of myofascial pain, restricted motion, and muscle spasm. Clinical conditions that may respond to Ethyl Chloride include low back pain (due to muscle spasm), acute stiff neck, torticollis, acute bursitis of the shoulder, muscle spasm associated with osteoarthritis, tight hamstring, sprained ankle, masseter muscle spasm, certain types of headache, and referred pain due to irritated trigger point. Relief of pain facilitates early mobilization in restoration of muscle function. The Spray and Stretch technique is a therapeutic system which involves three stages: EVALUATION, SPRAYING, and STRETCHING.
The therapeutic value of Spray and Stretch becomes most effective when the practitioner has mastered all stages and applies them in the proper sequence.

I. EVALUATION

During the evaluation phase the cause of pain is determined as local spasm or an irritated trigger point. The method of applying the spray to a muscle spasm differs slightly from application to a trigger point. A trigger point is a deep hypersensitive localized spot in a muscle which causes a referred pain pattern. With trigger points the source of pain is seldom the site of the pain. A trigger point may be detected by a snapping palpation over the muscle, causing the muscle in which the irritated trigger point is situated to "jump".

II. SPRAYING

A. Patient should assume a comfortable position.
B. Take precautions to cover the patient's eyes, nose, mouth, if spraying near face.
C. Hold bottle in an upside down position 12 to 18 inches (30 to 45 cm.) away from the treatment surface allowing the jet stream of vapocoolant to meet the skin at an acute angle to lessen the shock of impact.
D. The spray is directed in parallel sweeps .6 to .8 inches (1.5 to 2 cm.) apart. The rate of spraying is approximately 4 inches/sec. (10 cm/sec.) and is continued until the entire muscle has been covered. The number of sweeps is determined by the size of the muscle. In the case of trigger point, the spray should be applied over the trigger point, through and over the reference zone. In case of muscle spasm, the spray should be applied from origin to insertion.

III. STRETCHING

During application of the spray, the muscle is passively stretched. Force is gradually increased with successive sweeps, and the slack is smoothly taken up as the muscle relaxes, establishing a new stretch length.
Reaching the full normal length of the muscle is necessary to completely inactivate trigger points and relieve pain.
After rewarming, the procedure may be repeated as necessary. Moist heat should be applied for 10 to 15 minutes following treatment. For lasting benefit, any factors that perpetuate the trigger mechanism must be eliminated.

HOW SUPPLIED

3.5 ounce amber glass bottle:
Fine Spray .... (NDC 0386-0001-04)
Medium Spray .... (NDC 0386-0001-03)
3.0 ounce amber glass bottle:
"Spra Pak" Mist Spray .... (NDC 0386-0001-01)

CAUTION

Federal law restricts this device to sale by or on the order of a physician or other practitioner licensed by state law to use or order the use of the device.

©1994, Gebauer Company

For information on over-the-counter drugs, consult **PDR For Nonprescription Drugs**.

Genentech, Inc.

1 DNA Way
SOUTH SAN FRANCISCO, CA 94080-4990

For Medical Information Contact:
Medical Information or Drug Experience Departments (24 hours):
(800) 821-8590
(650) 225-1000
Or write:
Medical Information or Drug Experience Departments
Genetech, Inc.
1 DNA Way
South San Francisco, CA 94080-4990

ACTIVASE® ℞
Alteplase
recombinant

DESCRIPTION

Activase®, Alteplase, is a tissue plasminogen activator produced by recombinant DNA technology. It is a sterile, purified glycoprotein of 527 amino acids. It is synthesized using the complementary DNA (cDNA) for natural human tissue-type plasminogen activator obtained from a human melanoma cell line. The manufacturing process involves the secretion of the enzyme alteplase into the culture medium by an established mammalian cell line (Chinese Hamster Ovary cells) into which the cDNA for alteplase has been genetically inserted. Fermentation is carried out in a nutrient medium containing the antibiotic gentamycin, 100 mg/L. However, the presence of the antibiotic is not detectable in the final product.
Phosphoric acid and/or sodium hydroxide may be used prior to lyophilization for pH adjustment.
Activase is a sterile, white to off-white, lyophilized powder for intravenous administration after reconstitution with Sterile Water for Injection, USP.
[See table below]

Quantitative Composition of the Lyophilized Product

	100 mg Vial	50 mg Vial
Alteplase	100 mg (58 million IU)	50 mg (29 million IU)
L-Arginine	3.5 g	1.7 g
Phosphoric Acid	1 g	0.5 g
Polysorbate 80	less than or equal to 11 mg	less than or equal to 4 mg
Vacuum	No	Yes

Biological potency is determined by an in vitro clot lysis assay and is expressed in International Units as tested against the WHO standard. The specific activity of Activase is 580,000 IU/mg.

CLINICAL PHARMACOLOGY

Activase is an enzyme (serine protease) which has the property of fibrin-enhanced conversion of plasminogen to plasmin. It produces limited conversion of plasminogen in the absence of fibrin. When introduced into the systemic circulation at pharmacologic concentration, Activase binds to fibrin in a thrombus and converts the entrapped plasminogen to plasmin. This initiates local fibrinolysis with limited systemic proteolysis. Following administration of 100 mg Activase, there is a decrease (16%–36%) in circulating fibrinogen.[1,2] In a controlled trial, 8 of 73 patients (11%) receiving Activase (1.25 mg/kg body weight over 3 hours) experienced a decrease in fibrinogen to below 100 mg/dL.[2]
The clearance of Alteplase in AMI patients has shown that it is rapidly cleared from the plasma with an initial half-life of less than 5 minutes. There is no difference in the dominant initial plasma half-life between the 3-Hour and accelerated regimens for AMI. The plasma clearance of Alteplase is 380–570 mL/min.[3,4] The clearance is mediated primarily by the liver. The initial volume of distribution approximates plasma volume.

Acute Myocardial Infarction (AMI) Patients

Coronary occlusion due to a thrombus is present in the infarct-related coronary artery in approximately 80% of patients experiencing a transmural myocardial infarction evaluated within 4 hours of onset of symptoms.[5,6]
Two Activase dose regimens have been studied in patients experiencing acute myocardial infarction. (Please see DOSAGE AND ADMINISTRATION.) The comparative efficacy of these two regimens has not been evaluated.

Accelerated Infusion in AMI Patients

Accelerated infusion of Activase was studied in an international, multi-center trial (GUSTO) that randomized 41,021 patients with acute myocardial infarction to four thrombolytic regimens. Entry criteria included onset of chest pain within 6 hours of treatment and ST segment elevation of ECG. The regimens included accelerated infusion of Activase (≤100 mg over 90 minutes, see DOSAGE AND ADMINISTRATION) plus intravenous (IV) heparin (accelerated infusion of Alteplase, n=10,396), or the Kabikinase brand of Streptokinase (1.5 million units over 60 minutes) plus IV heparin (SK [IV], n=10,410), or Streptokinase (as above) plus subcutaneous (SQ) heparin (SK [SQ], n=9841). A fourth regimen combined Alteplase and Streptokinase. Aspirin and heparin use was directed by the GUSTO study protocol as follows: All patients were to receive 160 mg chewable aspirin administered as soon as possible, followed by 160–325 mg daily. IV heparin was directed to be a 5000 U IV bolus initiated as soon as possible, followed by a 1000 U/hour continuous IV infusion for at least 48 hours; subsequent heparin therapy was at the discretion of the attending physician. SQ heparin was directed to be 12,500 U administered 4 hours after initiation of SK therapy, followed by 12,500 U twice daily for 7 days or until discharge, whichever came first. Many of the patients randomized to receive SQ heparin received some IV heparin, usually in response to recurrent chest pain and/or the need for a medical procedure. Some received IV heparin on arrival to the emergency room prior to enrollment and randomization.
Results for the primary endpoint of the study, 30-day mortality, are shown in Table 1. The incidence of 30-day mortality for accelerated infusion of Alteplase was 1.0% lower than for SK (IV) and 1.0% lower than for SK (SQ). The secondary endpoints of combined 30-day mortality or nonfatal stroke, and 24-hour mortality, as well as the safety endpoints of total stroke and intracerebral hemorrhage are also shown in Table 1. The incidence of combined 30-day mortality or nonfatal stroke for the Alteplase accelerated infusion was 1.0% lower than for SK (IV) and 0.8% lower than for SK (SQ).
[See table 1 at top of next page]
Subgroup analysis of patients by age, infarct location, time from symptom onset to thrombolytic treatment, and treatment in the U.S. or elsewhere showed consistently lower 30-day mortality for the Alteplase accelerated infusion group. For patients who were over 75 years of age, a predefined subgroup consisting of 12% of patients enrolled, the incidence of stroke was 4.0% for the Alteplase accelerated infusion group, 2.8% for SK (IV), and 3.2% for SK (SQ); the incidence of combined 30-day mortality or nonfatal stroke was 20.6% for accelerated infusion of Alteplase, 21.5% for SK (IV), and 22.0% for SK (SQ).
An angiographic substudy of the GUSTO trial provided data on infarct-related artery patency. Table 2 presents 90-minute, 180-minute, 24 hour, and 5–7 day patency values by TIMI flow grade for the three treatment regimens. Reocclusion rates were similar for all three treatment regimens.
[See table 2 at top of next page]
The safety and efficacy of the accelerated infusion of Alteplase have not been evaluated using antithrombotic or antiplatelet regimens other than those used in the GUSTO trial.

3-Hour Infusion in AMI Patients

In patients studied in a controlled trial with coronary angiography at 90 and 120 minutes following infusion of Activase, infarct artery patency was observed in 71% and 85% of patients (n=85), respectively.[2] In a second study, where patients received coronary angiography prior to and following infusion of Activase within 6 hours of the onset of symptoms, reperfusion of the obstructed vessel occurred within 90 minutes after the commencement of therapy in 71% of 83 patients.[1]
In a double-blind, randomized trial (138 patients) comparing Activase to placebo, patients infused with Activase within 4 hours of onset of symptoms experienced improved left ventricular function at day 10 compared to the placebo group, when ejection fraction was measured by gated blood pool scan (53.2% vs 46.4%, p=0.018). Relative to baseline (day 1) values, the net changes in ejection fraction were +3.6% and −4.7% for the treated and placebo groups, respectively (p=0.0001). Also documented was a reduced incidence of clinical congestive heart failure in the treated group (14%) compared to the placebo group (33%) (p=0.009).[7]
In a double-blind, randomized trial (145 patients) comparing Activase to placebo, patients infused with Activase within 2.5 hours of onset of symptoms experienced improved left ventricular function at a mean of 21 days compared to the placebo group, when ejection fraction was measured by gated blood pool scan (52% vs 48%, p=0.08) and by contrast ventriculogram (61% vs 54%, p=0.006).

Continued on next page

Activase—Cont.

Although the contribution of Activase alone is unclear, the incidence of nonischemic cardiac complications when taken as a group (i.e., congestive heart failure, pericarditis, atrial fibrillation, and conduction disturbance) was reduced when compared to those patients treated with placebo (p <0.01).[8]
In a double-blind, randomized trial (5013 patients) comparing Activase to placebo (ASSET study), patients infused with Activase within 5 hours of the onset of symptoms of acute myocardial infarction experienced improved 30-day survival compared to those treated with placebo. At 1 month, the overall mortality rates were 7.2% for the Activase-treated group and 9.8% for the placebo-treated group (p=0.001).[9,10] This benefit was maintained at 6 months for Activase-treated patients (10.4%) compared to those treated with placebo (13.1%, p=0.008).[10]
In a double-blind, randomized trial (721 patients) comparing Activase to placebo, patients infused with Activase within 5 hours of the onset of symptoms experienced improved ventricular function 10–22 days after treatment compared to the placebo group, when global ejection fraction was measured by contrast ventriculography (50.7% vs 48.5%, p=0.01). Patients treated with Activase had a 19% reduction in infarct size, as measured by cumulative release of HBDH (α-hydroxybutyrate dehydrogenase) activity compared to placebo-treated patients (p=0.001). Patients treated with Activase had significantly fewer episodes of cardiogenic shock (p=0.02), ventricular fibrillation (p<0.04) and pericarditis (p=0.01) compared to patients treated with placebo. Mortality at 21 days in Activase-treated patients was reduced to 3.7% compared to 6.3% in placebo-treated patients (1-sided p=0.05).[11] Although these data do not demonstrate unequivocally a significant reduction in mortality for this study, they do indicate a trend that is supported by the results of the ASSET study.

Acute Ischemic Stroke Patients

Two placebo-controlled, double-blind trials (The NINDS t-PA Stroke Trial, Part 1 and Part 2) have been conducted in patients with acute ischemic stroke.[12] Both studies enrolled patients with measurable neurological deficit who could complete screening and begin study treatment within 3 hours from symptom onset. A cranial computerized tomography (CT) scan was performed prior to treatment to rule out the presence of intracranial hemorrhage (ICH). Patients were also excluded for the presence of conditions related to risks of bleeding (see CONTRAINDICATIONS), for minor neurological deficit, for rapidly improving symptoms prior to initiating study treatment, or for blood glucose of <50 or >400 mg/dL.
Patients were randomized to receive either 0.9 mg/kg Activase (maximum of 90 mg), or placebo. Activase was administered as a 10% initial bolus over 1 minute followed by continuous intravenous infusion of the remainder over 60 minutes (see DOSAGE AND ADMINISTRATION). In patients without recent use of oral anticoagulants or heparin, study treatment was initiated prior to the availability of coagulation study results. However, the infusion was discontinued if either a pre-treatment prothrombin time (PT) >15 seconds or an elevated activated partial thromboplastin time (aPTT) was identified. Although patients with or without prior aspirin use were enrolled, administration of anticoagulants and antiplatelet agents was prohibited for the first 24 hours following symptom onset.
The initial study (NINDS-Part 1, n=291) evaluated neurological improvement at 24 hours after stroke onset. The primary endpoint, the proportion of patients with a 4 or more point improvement in the National Institutes of Health Stroke Scale (NIHSS) score or complete recovery (NIHSS score=0), was not significantly different between treatment groups. A secondary analysis suggested improved 3-month outcome associated with Activase treatment using the following stroke assessment scales: Barthel Index, Modified Rankin Scale, Glasgow Outcome Scale, and the NIHSS.
A second study (NINDS-Part 2, n=333) assessed clinical outcome at 3 months as the primary outcome. A favorable outcome was defined as minimal or no disability using the four stroke assessment scales: Barthel Index (score ≥95), Modified Rankin Scale (score ≤1), Glasgow Outcome Scale (score=1), and NIHSS (score ≤1). The results comparing Activase- and placebo-treated patients for the four outcome scales together (Generalized Estimating Equations) and individually are presented in Table 3. In this study, depending upon the scale, the favorable outcome of minimal or no disability occurred in at least 11 per 100 more patients treated with Activase than those receiving placebo. Secondary analyses demonstrated consistent functional and neurological improvement within all four stroke scales as indicated by median scores. These results were highly consistent with the 3-month outcome treatment effects observed in the Part 1 study.
[See table 3 at right]
The incidences of all-cause 90-day mortality, ICH, and new ischemic stroke following Activase treatment compared to placebo are presented in Table 4 as a combined safety analysis (n=624) for Parts 1 and 2. These data indicated a significant increase in ICH following Activase treatment, particularly symptomatic ICH within 36 hours. In Activase-treated patients, there were no increases compared to placebo in the incidences of 90-day mortality or severe disability.
[See table 4 at bottom of next page]
In a prespecified subgroup analysis in patients receiving aspirin prior to onset of stroke symptoms, there was preserved favorable outcome for Activase-treated patients.
Exploratory, multivariate analyses of both studies combined (n=624) to investigate potential predictors of ICH and treatment effect modifiers were performed. In Activase-treated patients presenting with severe neurological deficit (e.g., NIHSS >22) or of advanced age (e.g., >77 years of age), the trends toward increased risk for symptomatic ICH within the first 36 hours were more prominent. Similar trends were also seen for total ICH and for all-cause 90-day mortality in these patients. When risk was assessed by the combination of death and severe disability in these patients, there was no difference between placebo and Activase groups. Analyses for efficacy suggested a reduced but still favorable clinical outcome for Activase-treated patients with severe neurological deficit or advanced age at presentation.

Pulmonary Embolism Patients

In a comparative randomized trial (n=45),[13] 59% of patients (n=22) treated with Activase (100 mg over 2 hours) experienced moderate or marked lysis of pulmonary emboli when assessed by pulmonary angiography 2 hours after treatment initiation. Activase-treated patients also experienced a significant reduction in pulmonary embolism-induced pulmonary hypertension within 2 hours of treatment (p=0.003). Pulmonary perfusion at 24 hours, as assessed by radionuclide scan, was significantly improved (p=0.002).

INDICATIONS AND USAGE

Acute Myocardial Infarction

Activase is indicated for use in the management of acute myocardial infarction in adults for the improvement of ventricular function following AMI, the reduction of the incidence of congestive heart failure, and the reduction of mortality associated with AMI. Treatment should be initiated as soon as possible after the onset of AMI symptoms (see CLINICAL PHARMACOLOGY).

Acute Ischemic Stroke

Activase is indicated for the management of acute ischemic stroke in adults for improving neurological recovery and reducing the incidence of disability. Treatment should only be initiated within 3 hours after the onset of stroke symptoms, and after exclusion of intracranial hemorrhage by a cranial computerized tomography (CT) scan or other diagnostic imaging method sensitive for the presence of hemorrhage (see CONTRAINDICATIONS).

Pulmonary Embolism

Activase is indicated in the management of acute massive pulmonary embolism (PE) in adults for:
the lysis of acute pulmonary emboli, defined as obstruction of blood flow to a lobe or multiple segments of the lungs, and
the lysis of pulmonary emboli accompanied by unstable hemodynamics, e.g., failure to maintain blood pressure without supportive measures.
The diagnosis should be confirmed by objective means, such as pulmonary angiography or noninvasive procedures such as lung scanning.

CONTRAINDICATIONS

Acute Myocardial Infarction or Pulmonary Embolism

Activase therapy in patients with acute myocardial infarction or pulmonary embolism is contraindicated in the following situations because of an increased risk of bleeding:
- Active internal bleeding
- History of cerebrovascular accident
- Recent intracranial or intraspinal surgery or trauma (see WARNINGS)
- Intracranial neoplasm, arteriovenous malformation, or aneurysm
- Known bleeding diathesis
- Severe uncontrolled hypertension

Acute Ischemic Stroke

Activase therapy in patients with acute ischemic stroke is contraindicated in the following situations because of an increased risk of bleeding, which could result in significant disability or death:
- Evidence of intracranial hemorrhage on pretreatment evaluation
- Suspicion of subarachnoid hemorrhage
- Recent intracranial surgery or serious head trauma or recent previous stroke
- History of intracranial hemorrhage

Table 1

Event	Accelerated Activase	SK (IV)	p-Value[1]	SK (SQ)	p-Value[1]
30-Day Mortality	6.3%	7.3%	0.003	7.3%	0.007
30-Day Mortality or Nonfatal Stroke	7.2%	8.2%	0.006	8.0%	0.036
24-Hour Mortality	2.4%	2.9%	0.009	2.8%	0.029
Any Stroke	1.6%	1.4%	0.32	1.2%	0.03
Intracerebral Hemorrhage	0.7%	0.6%	0.22	0.5%	0.02

[1] Two-tailed p-value is for comparison of Accelerated Activase®, Alteplase, recombinant to the respective SK control arm.

Table 2

Patency (TIMI 2 or 3)	Accelerated Activase	SK (IV)	p-Value	SK (SQ)	p-Value
90-Minute	n=272	n=261		n=260	
	81.3%	59.0%	<0.0001	53.5%	<0.0001
180-Minute	n=80	n=76		n=95	
	76.3%	72.4%	0.58	71.6%	0.48
24 Hour	n=81	n=72		n=67	
	88.9%	87.5%	0.24	82.1%	0.79
5–7 Day	n=72	n=77		n=75	
	83.3%	90.9%	0.47	78.7%	0.17

Table 3
The NINDS t-PA Stroke Trial, Part 2
3-Month Efficacy Outcomes

Analysis	Frequency of Favorable Outcome[1]				
	Placebo (n=165)	Activase (n=168)	Absolute Difference (95% CI)	Relative Frequency[2] (95% CI)	p-Value[3]
Generalized Estimating Equations (Multivariate)	—	—		1.34 (1.05, 1.72)	0.02
Barthel Index	37.6%	50.0%	12.4% (3.0, 21.9)	1.33 (1.04, 1.71)	0.02
Modified Rankin Scale	26.1%	38.7%	12.6% (3.7, 21.6)	1.48 (1.08, 2.04)	0.02
Glasgow Outcome Scale	31.5%	44.0%	12.5% (3.3, 21.8)	1.40 (1.05, 1.85)	0.02
NIHSS	20.0%	31.0%	11.0% (2.6, 19.3)	1.55 (1.06, 2.26)	0.02

[1] Favorable Outcome is defined as recovery with minimal or no disability.
[2] Value >1 indicates frequency of recovery in favor of Activase treatment.
[3] p-Value for Relative Frequency is from Generalized Estimating Equations with log link.

- Uncontrolled hypertension at time of treatment (e.g., >185 mm Hg systolic or >110 mm Hg diastolic)
- Seizure at the onset of stroke
- Active internal bleeding
- Intracranial neoplasm, arteriovenous malformation, or aneurysm
- Known bleeding diathesis including but not limited to:
  —Current use of oral anticoagulants (e.g., warfarin sodium) with prothrombin time (PT) >15 seconds
  —Administration of heparin within 48 hours preceding the onset of stroke and have an elevated activated partial thromboplastin time (aPTT) at presentation
  —Platelet count <100,000/mm³

WARNINGS

Bleeding

The most common complication encountered during Activase®, Alteplase, recombinant therapy is bleeding. The type of bleeding associated with thrombolytic therapy can be divided into two broad categories:

- Internal bleeding, involving intracranial and retroperitoneal sites, or the gastrointestinal, genitourinary, or respiratory tracts.
- Superficial or surface bleeding, observed mainly at invaded or disturbed sites (e.g., venous cutdowns, arterial punctures, sites of recent surgical intervention).

The concomitant use of heparin anticoagulation may contribute to bleeding. Some of the hemorrhage episodes occurred 1 or more days after the effects of Activase had dissipated, but while heparin therapy was continuing.

As fibrin is lysed during Activase therapy, bleeding from recent puncture sites may occur. Therefore, thrombolytic therapy requires careful attention to all potential bleeding sites (including catheter insertion sites, arterial and venous puncture sites, cutdown sites, and needle puncture sites). Intramuscular injections and nonessential handling of the patient should be avoided during treatment with Activase. Venipunctures should be performed carefully and only as required.

Should an arterial puncture be necessary during an infusion of Activase, it is preferable to use an upper extremity vessel that is accessible to manual compression. Pressure should be applied for at least 30 minutes, a pressure dressing applied, and the puncture site checked frequently for evidence of bleeding.

Should serious bleeding (not controllable by local pressure) occur, the infusion of Activase and any concomitant heparin should be terminated immediately.

Each patient being considered for therapy with Activase should be carefully evaluated and anticipated benefits weighed against potential risks associated with therapy.

In the following conditions, the risks of Activase therapy for all approved indications may be increased and should be weighed against the anticipated benefits:

- Recent major surgery, e.g., coronary artery bypass graft, obstetrical delivery, organ biopsy, previous puncture of noncompressible vessels
- Cerebrovascular disease
- Recent gastrointestinal or genitourinary bleeding
- Recent trauma
- Hypertension: systolic BP ≥180 mm Hg and/or diastolic BP ≥110 mm Hg
- High likelihood of left heart thrombus, e.g., mitral stenosis with atrial fibrillation
- Acute pericarditis
- Subacute bacterial endocarditis
- Hemostatic defects including those secondary to severe hepatic or renal disease
- Significant hepatic dysfunction
- Pregnancy
- Diabetic hemorrhagic retinopathy, or other hemorrhagic ophthalmic conditions
- Septic thrombophlebitis or occluded AV cannula at seriously infected site
- Advanced age, (e.g., over 75 years old)

- Patients currently receiving oral anticoagulants, e.g., warfarin sodium
- Any other condition in which bleeding constitutes a significant hazard or would be particularly difficult to manage because of its location

Cholesterol Embolization

Cholesterol embolism has been reported rarely in patients treated with all types of thrombolytic agents; the true incidence is unknown. This serious condition, which can be lethal, is also associated with invasive vascular procedures (e.g., cardiac catheterization, angiography, vascular surgery) and/or anticoagulant therapy. Clinical features of cholesterol embolism may include livedo reticularis, "purple toe" syndrome, acute renal failure, gangrenous digits, hypertension, pancreatitis, myocardial infarction, cerebral infarction, spinal cord infarction, retinal artery occlusion, bowel infarction, and rhabdomyolysis.

Arrhythmias

Coronary thrombolysis may result in arrhythmias associated with reperfusion. These arrhythmias (such as sinus bradycardia, accelerated idioventricular rhythm, ventricular premature depolarizations, ventricular tachycardia) are not different from those often seen in the ordinary course of acute myocardial infarction and may be managed with standard antiarrhythmic measures. It is recommended that antiarrhythmic therapy for bradycardia and/or ventricular irritability be available when infusions of Activase®, Alteplase, recombinant are administered.

Use in Acute Ischemic Stroke

In addition to the previously listed conditions, the risks of Activase therapy to treat acute ischemic stroke may be increased in the following conditions and should be weighed against the anticipated benefits:

- Patients with severe neurological deficit (e.g., NIHSS >22) at presentation. There is an increased risk of intracranial hemorrhage in these patients.
- Patients with major early infarct signs on a computerized cranial tomography (CT) scan (e.g., substantial edema, mass effect, or midline shift).

In patients without recent use of oral anticoagulants or heparin, Activase treatment can be initiated prior to the availability of coagulation study results. However, infusion should be discontinued if either a pre-treatment prothrombin time (PT) >15 seconds or an elevated activate partial thromboplastin time (aPTT) is identified.

Treatment should be limited to facilities that can provide appropriate evaluation and management of ICH.

In acute ischemic stroke, neither the incidence of intracranial hemorrhage nor the benefits of therapy are known in patients treated with Activase more than 3 hours after the onset of symptoms. **Therefore, treatment of patients with acute ischemic stroke more than 3 hours after symptom onset is not recommended.**

The safety and efficacy of treatment with Activase in patients with minor neurological deficit or with rapidly improving symptoms prior to the start of Activase administration has not been evaluated.

Use in Pulmonary Embolism

It should be recognized that the treatment of pulmonary embolism with Activase has not been shown to constitute adequate clinical treatment of underlying deep vein thrombosis. Furthermore, the possible risk of reembolization due to the lysis of underlying deep venous thrombi should be considered.

PRECAUTIONS

General

Standard management of myocardial infarction or pulmonary embolism should be implemented concomitantly with Activase treatment. Noncompressible arterial puncture must be avoided and internal jugular and subclavian venous punctures should be avoided to minimize bleeding from noncompressible sites. Arterial and venous punctures

should be minimized. In the event of serious bleeding, Activase and heparin should be discontinued immediately. Heparin effects can be reversed by protamine.

Readministration

There is no experience with readministration of Activase. If an anaphylactoid reaction occurs, the infusion should be discontinued immediately and appropriate therapy initiated.

Although sustained antibody formation in patients receiving one dose of Activase has not been documented, readministration should be undertaken with caution. Detectable levels of antibody (a single point measurement) were reported in one patient, but subsequent antibody test results were negative.

Drug-Laboratory Test Interactions

During Activase therapy, if coagulation tests and/or measures of fibrinolytic activity are performed, the results may be unreliable unless specific precautions are taken to prevent in vitro artifacts. Activase is an enzyme that when present in blood in pharmacologic concentrations remains active under in vitro conditions. This can lead to degradation of fibrinogen in blood samples removed for analysis. Collection of blood samples in the presence of aprotinin (150–200 units/mL) can to some extent mitigate this phenomenon.

Drug Interactions

The interaction of Activase with other cardioactive or cerebroactive drugs has not been studied. In addition to bleeding associated with heparin and vitamin K antagonists, drugs that alter platelet function (such as acetylsalicylic acid, dipyridamole and Abciximab) may increase the risk of bleeding if administered prior to, during, or after Activase therapy.

Use of Antithrombotics

Aspirin and heparin have been administered concomitantly with and following infusions of Activase in the management of acute myocardial infarction or pulmonary embolism. Because heparin, aspirin, or Activase may cause bleeding complications, careful monitoring for bleeding is advised, especially at arterial puncture sites.

The concomitant use of heparin or aspirin during the first 24 hours following symptom onset were prohibited in The NINDS t-PA Stroke Trial. The safety of such concomitant use with Activase for the management of acute ischemic stroke is unknown.

Blood Pressure Control

Blood pressure should be monitored frequently and controlled during and following Activase administration in the management of acute ischemic stroke. In The NINDS t-PA Stroke Trial, blood pressure was monitored for 24 hours and was actively controlled (≤185/110 mm Hg) during this period with appropriate medication.

Carcinogenesis, Mutagenesis, Impairment of Fertility

Long-term studies in animals have not been performed to evaluate the carcinogenic potential or the effect on fertility. Short-term studies, which evaluated tumorigenicity of Activase and effect on tumor metastases in rodents, were negative.

Studies to determine mutagenicity (Ames test) and chromosomal aberration assays in human lymphocytes were negative at all concentrations tested. Cytotoxicity, as reflected by a decrease in mitotic index, was evidenced only after prolonged exposure and only at the highest concentrations tested.

Pregnancy (Category C)

Animal reproduction studies have not been conducted with Activase. It is also not known whether Activase can cause fetal harm when administered to a pregnant woman or can affect reproduction capacity. Activase should be given to a pregnant woman only if clearly needed.

Nursing Mothers

It is not known whether Activase is excreted in human milk. Because many drugs are excreted in human milk, caution should be exercised when Activase is administered to a nursing woman.

Pediatric Use

Safety and effectiveness of Activase in pediatric patients have not been established.

ADVERSE REACTIONS

Bleeding

The most frequent adverse reaction associated with Activase in all approved indications is bleeding (see WARNINGS[14,15]).

Should serious bleeding in a critical location (intracranial, gastrointestinal, retroperitoneal, pericardial) occur, Activase therapy should be discontinued immediately, along with any concomitant therapy with heparin. Death and permanent disability are not uncommonly reported in patients that have experienced stroke (including intracranial bleeding) and other serious bleeding episodes.

In the GUSTO trial for the treatment of acute myocardial infarction, using the accelerated infusion regimen the incidence of all strokes for the Activase-treated patients was 1.6%, while the incidence of nonfatal stroke was 0.9%. The

Table 4
The NINDS t-PA Stroke Trial
Safety Outcome

	Part 1 and Part 2 Combined		
	Placebo (n=312)	Activase (n=312)	p-Value[2]
All-Cause 90-day Mortality	64 (20.5%)	54 (17.3%)	0.36
Total ICH[1]	20 (6.4%)	48 (15.4%)	<0.01
Symptomatic	4 (1.3%)	25 (8.0%)	<0.01
Asymptomatic	16 (5.1%)	23 (7.4%)	0.32
Symptomatic ICH within 36 hours	2 (0.6%)	20 (6.4%)	<0.01
New Ischemic Stroke (3-months)	17 (5.4%)	18 (5.8%)	1.00

[1] Within trial follow-up period. Symptomatic ICH was defined as the occurrence of sudden clinical worsening followed by subsequent verification of ICH on CT scan. Asymptomatic ICH was defined as ICH detected on a routine repeat CT scan without preceding clinical worsening.
[2] Fisher's Exact Test

Continued on next page

Activase—Cont.

incidence of hemorrhagic stroke was 0.7%, not all of which were fatal. The incidence of all strokes, as well as that for hemorrhagic stroke, increased with increasing age (see CLINICAL PHARMACOLOGY: Accelerated Infusion in AMI Patients). Data from previous trials utilizing a 3-hour infusion of ≤100 mg indicated that the incidence of total stroke in six randomized double-blind placebo controlled trials[2,7-11,16] was 1.2% (37/3161) in Alteplase-treated patients compared with 0.9% (27/3092) in placebo-treated patients.

For the 3-hour infusion regimen, the incidence of significant internal bleeding (estimated as >250 cc blood loss) has been reported in studies in over 800 patients. These data do not include patients treated with the Alteplase accelerated infusion:

	Total Dose ≤100 mg
gastrointestinal	5%
genitourinary	4%
ecchymosis	1%
retroperitoneal	<1%
epistaxis	<1%
gingival	<1%

The incidence of intracranial hemorrhage (ICH) in acute myocardial infarction patients treated with Activase is as follows:

Dose	Number of Patients	ICH (%)
100 mg, 3-hours	3272	0.4
≤100 mg, accelerated	10,396	0.7
150 mg	1779	1.3
1–1.4 mg/kg	237	0.4

These data indicate that a dose of 150 mg of Activase should not be used in the treatment of AMI because it has been associated with an increase in intracranial bleeding[17].

For acute massive pulmonary embolism, bleeding events were consistent with the general safety profile observed with Activase in acute myocardial infarction patients receiving the 3-hour infusion regimen.

The incidence of ICH, especially symptomatic ICH, in patients with acute ischemic stroke was higher in Activase-treated patients than placebo patients (see CLINICAL PHARMACOLOGY).

A study of another alteplase product, Actilyse, in acute ischemic stroke, suggested that doses greater than 0.9 mg/kg may be associated with an increased incidence of ICH[18]. **Doses greater than 0.9 mg/kg (maximum 90 mg) should not be used in the management of acute schemic stroke.**

Bleeding events other than ICH were noted in the studies of acute ischemic stroke and were consistent with the general safety profile of Activase. In The NINDS t-PA Stroke Trial (Parts 1 and 2), the frequency of bleeding requiring red blood cell transfusions was 6.4% for Activase-treated patients compared to 3.8% for placebo (p=0.19, using Mantel-Haenszel Chi-Square).

Fibrin which is part of the hemostatic plug formed at needle puncture sites will be lysed during Activase therapy. Therefore, Activase therapy requires careful attention to potential bleeding sites, e.g., catheter insertion sites, and arterial puncture sites.

Allergic Reactions

Allergic-type reactions, e.g., anaphylactoid reaction, laryngeal edema, rash, and urticaria have been reported very rarely (<0.02%). A cause and effect relationship to Activase therapy has not been established. When such reactions occur, they usually respond to conventional therapy.

Other Adverse Reactions

Patients with myocardial infarction or pulmonary embolism can experience disease-related events such as cardiogenic shock, arrhythmias, pulmonary edema, heart failure, cardiac arrest, recurrent ischemia, reinfarction, myocardial rupture, mitral regurgitation, pericardial effusion, pericarditis, cardiac tamponade, venous thrombosis and embolism, and electromechanical dissociation. These events can be life-threatening and may lead to death. Other adverse reactions have been reported, principally nausea and/or vomiting, hypotension, and fever. These reactions are frequent sequelae of myocardial infarction and may or may not be attributable to Activase therapy.

DOSAGE AND ADMINISTRATION

Activase®, Alteplase, recombinant is for intravenous administration only. Extravasation of Activase infusion can cause ecchymosis and/or inflammation. Management consists of terminating the infusion at that IV site and application of local therapy.

Acute Myocardial Infarction

Administer Activase as soon as possible after the onset of symptoms.

There are two Activase dose regimens for use in the management of acute myocardial infarction; controlled studies to compare clinical outcomes with these regimens have not been conducted.

A DOSE OF 150 mg OF ACTIVASE SHOULD NOT BE USED FOR THE TREATMENT OF ACUTE MYOCARDIAL INFARCTION BECAUSE IT HAS BEEN ASSOCIATED WITH AN INCREASE IN INTRACRANIAL BLEEDING.

Accelerated Infusion

The recommended total dose is based upon patient weight, not to exceed 100 mg. For patients weighing >67 kg, the recommended dose administered is 100 mg as a 15 mg intravenous bolus, followed by 50 mg infused over the next 30 minutes, and then 35 mg infused over the next 60 minutes. For patients weighing ≤67 kg, the recommended dose is administered as a 15 mg intravenous bolus, followed by 0.75 mg/kg infused over the next 30 minutes not to exceed 50 mg, and then 0.50 mg/kg over the next 60 minutes not to exceed 35 mg.

The safety and efficacy of this accelerated infusion of Alteplase regimen has only been investigated with concomitant administration of heparin and aspirin as described in CLINICAL PHARMACOLOGY.

a. The bolus dose may be prepared in one of the following ways:
  1. By removing 15 mL from the vial of reconstituted (1 mg/mL) Activase using a syringe and needle. If this method is used with the 50 mg vials, the syringe should not be primed with air and the needle should be inserted into the Activase vial stopper. If the 100 mg vial is used, the syringe should not be primed with air and the needle should be inserted away from the puncture mark made by the transfer device.
  2. By removing 15 mL from a port (second injection site) on the infusion line after the infusion set is primed.
  3. By programming an infusion pump to deliver a 15 mL (1 mg/mL) bolus at the initiation of the infusion.
b. The remainder of the Activase®, Alteplase, recombinant dose may be administered as follows:
  50 mg vials—administer using either a polyvinyl chloride bag or glass vial and infusion set
  100 mg vial—insert the spike end of an infusion set through the same puncture site created by the transfer device in the stopper of the vial of reconstituted Activase. Hang the Activase vial from the plastic molded capping attached to the bottom of the vial.

3-Hour Infusion

The recommended dose is 100 mg administered as 60 mg (34.8 million IU) in the first hour (of which 6 to 10 mg is administered as a bolus), 20 mg (11.6 million IU) over the second hour, and 20 mg (11.6 million IU) over the third hour. For smaller patients (<65 kg), a dose of 1.25 mg/kg administered over 3 hours, as described above, may be used[14].

Although the value of the use of anticoagulants during and following administration of Activase has not been fully studied, heparin has been administered concomitantly for 24 hours or longer in more than 90% of patients.

Aspirin and/or dipyridamole have been given to patients receiving Alteplase during and/or following heparin treatment.

a. The bolus dose may be prepared in one of the following ways:
  1. By removing 6 to 10 mL from the vial of reconstituted (1 mg/mL) Activase using a syringe and needle. If this method is used with the 50 mg vials, the syringe should not be primed with air and the needle should be inserted into the Activase vial stopper. If the 100 mg vial is used, the syringe should not be primed with air and the needle should be inserted away from the puncture mark made by the transfer device.
  2. By removing 6 to 10 mL from a port (second injection site) on the infusion line after the infusion set is primed.
  3. By programming an infusion pump to deliver a 6 to 10 mL (1 mg/mL) bolus at the initiation of the infusion.
b. The remainder of the Activase dose may be administered as follows:
  50 mg vials—administer using either a polyvinyl chloride bag or glass vial and infusion set
  100 mg vial—insert the spike end of an infusion set through the same puncture site created by the transfer device in the stopper of the vial of reconstituted Activase. Hang the Activase vial from the plastic molded capping attached to the bottom of the vial.

Acute Ischemic Stroke

The recommended dose is 0.9 mg/kg (maximum of 90 mg) infused over 60 minutes with 10% of the total dose administered as an initial intravenous bolus over 1 minute.

The safety and efficacy of this regimen with concomitant administration of heparin and aspirin during the first 24 hours after symptom onset has not been investigated.

THE DOSE FOR TREATMENT OF ACUTE ISCHEMIC STROKE SHOULD NOT EXCEED 90 mg.

a. The bolus dose may be prepared in one of the following ways:

1. By removing the appropriate volume from the vial of reconstituted (1 mg/mL) Activase using a syringe and needle. If this method is used with the 50 mg vials, the syringe should not be primed with air and the needle should be inserted into the Activase vial stopper. If the 100 mg vial is used, the syringe should not be primed with air and the needle should be inserted away from the puncture mark made by the transfer device.
2. By removing the appropriate volume from a port (second injection site) on the infusion line after the infusion set is primed.
3. By programming an infusion pump to deliver the appropriate volume as a bolus at the initiation of the infusion.
b. The remainder of the Activase dose may be administered as follows:
  50 mg vials—administer using either a polyvinyl chloride bag or glass vial and infusion set
  100 mg vial—remove from the vial any quantity of drug in excess of that specified for patient treatment. Insert the spike end of an infusion set through the same puncture site created by the transfer device in the stopper of the vial of reconstituted Activase. Hang the Activase vial from the plastic molded capping attached to the bottom of the vial.

Pulmonary Embolism

The recommended dose is 100 mg administered by intravenous infusion over 2 hours. Heparin therapy should be instituted or reinstituted near the end of or immediately following the Activase infusion when the partial thromboplastin time or thrombin time returns to twice normal or less. The Activase dose may be administered as follows:

50 mg vials—administer using either a polyvinyl chloride bag or glass vial and infusion set
100 mg vial—insert the spike end of an infusion set through the same puncture site created by the transfer device in the stopper of the vial of reconstituted Activase. Hang the Activase vial from the plastic molded capping attached to the bottom of the vial.

Reconstitution and Dilution

Activase should be reconstituted by aseptically adding the appropriate volume of the accompanying Sterile Water for Injection, USP to the vial. It is important that Activase be reconstituted only with Sterile Water for Injection, USP, without preservatives. Do not use Bacteriostatic Water for Injection, USP. The reconstituted preparation results in a colorless to pale yellow transparent solution containing Activase 1 mg/mL at approximately pH 7.3. The osmolality of this solution is approximately 215 mOsm/kg.

Because Activase contains no antibacterial preservatives, it should be reconstituted immediately before use. The solution may be used for intravenous administration within 8 hours following reconstitution when stored between 2–30°C (36–86°F). Before further dilution or administration, the product should be visually inspected for particulate matter and discoloration prior to administration whenever solution and container permit.

Activase may be administered as reconstituted at 1 mg/mL. As an alternative, the reconstituted solution may be diluted further immediately before administration in an equal volume of 0.9% Sodium Chloride Injection, USP or 5% Dextrose Injection, USP to yield a concentration of 0.5 mg/mL. Either polyvinyl chloride bags or glass vials are acceptable. Activase is stable for up to 8 hours in these solutions at room temperature. Exposure to light has no effect on the stability of these solutions. Excessive agitation during dilution should be avoided; mixing should be accomplished with gentle swirling and/or slow inversion. Do not use other infusion solutions, e.g., Sterile Water for Injection, USP or preservative-containing solutions for further dilution.

50 mg Vials

Reconstitution should be carried out using a large bore needle (e.g.,18 gauge) and a syringe, directing the stream of Sterile Water for Injection, USP into the lyophilized cake. DO NOT USE IF VACUUM IS NOT PRESENT. Slight foaming upon reconstitution is not unusual; standing undisturbed for several minutes is usually sufficient to allow dissipation of any large bubbles.

No other medication should be added to infusion solutions containing Activase®, Alteplase. Any unused infusion solution should be discarded.

100 mg Vial

Reconstitution should be carried out using the transfer device provided, adding the contents of the accompanying 100 mL vial of Sterile Water for Injection, USP to the contents of the 100 mg vial of Activase powder. Slight foaming upon reconstitution is not unusual; standing undisturbed for several minutes is usually sufficient to allow dissipation of any large bubbles. Please refer to the accompanying Instructions for Reconstitution and Administration. **100 mg VIALS DO NOT CONTAIN VACUUM.**

100 mg VIAL RECONSTITUTION

1. Use aseptic technique throughout.
2. Remove the protective flip-caps from one vial of Activase and one vial of Sterile Water for Injection, USP (SWFI).

3. Open the package containing the transfer device by peeling the paper label off the package.

4. Remove the protective cap from one end of the transfer device and keeping the vial of SWFI upright, insert the piercing pin vertically into the center of the stopper of the vial of SWFI.

5. Remove the protective cap from the other end of the transfer device. **DO NOT INVERT THE VIAL OF SWFI.**

6. Holding the vial of Activase®, Alteplase, recombinant upside-down, position it so that the center of the stopper is directly over the exposed piercing pin of the transfer device.

7. Push the vial of Activase down so that the piercing pin is inserted through the center of the Activase vial stopper.

8. Invert the two vials so that the vial of Activase is on the bottom (upright) and the vial of SWFI is upside-down, allowing the SWFI to flow down through the transfer device. Allow the entire contents of the vial of SWFI to flow into the Activase vial (approximately 0.5 cc of SWFI will remain in the diluent vial). Approximately 2 minutes are required for this procedure.

9. Remove the transfer device and the empty SWFI vial from the Activase vial. Safely discard both the transfer device and the empty diluent vial according to institutional procedures.

10. Swirl gently to dissolve the Activase powder. **DO NOT SHAKE.**

No other medication should be added to infusion solutions containing Activase®, Alteplase. Any unused infusion solution should be discarded.

HOW SUPPLIED

Activase is supplied as a sterile, lyophilized powder in 50 mg vials containing vacuum and in 100 mg vials without vacuum.

Each 50 mg Activase vial (29 million IU) is packaged with diluent for reconstitution (50 mL Sterile Water for Injection, USP): NDC 50242-044-13..

Each 100 mg Activase vial (58 million IU) is packaged with diluent for reconstitution (100 mL Sterile Water for Injection, USP), and one transfer device: NDC 50242-085-27.

Storage

Store lyophilized Activase at controlled room temperature not to exceed 30°C (86°F), or under refrigeration (2–8°C/36–46°F). Protect the lyophilized material during extended storage from excessive exposure to light.

Do not use beyond the expiration date stamped on the vial.

REFERENCES

1. Mueller H, Rao AK, Forman SA, et al. Thrombolysis in myocardial infarction (TIMI): comparative studies of coronary reperfusion and systemic fibrinogenolysis with two forms of recombinant tissue-type plasminogen activator. J Am Coll Cardiol. 1987;10:479–90.

2. Topol EJ, Morriss DC, Smalling RW, et al. A multicenter, randomized, placebo-controlled trial of a new form of intravenous recombinant tissue-type plasminogen activator (Activase®) in acute myocardial infarction. J Am Coll Cardiol. 1987;9:1205–13.

3. Seifried E, Tanswell P, Ellbrück D, et al. Pharmacokinetics and haemostatic status during consecutive infusions of recombinant tissue-type plasminogen activator in patients with acute myocardial infarction. Thromb Haemostas. 1989;61:497–501.

4. Tanswell P, Tebbe U, Neuhaus K-L, et al. Pharmacokinetics and fibrin specificity of Alteplase during accelerated infusions in acute myocardial infarction. J Am Coll Cardiol. 1992;19:1071–5.

5. De Wood MA, Spores J, Notske R, et al. Prevalence of total coronary occlusion during the early hours of transmural myocardial infarction. New Engl J Med. 1980;303:897–902.

6. Chesebro JH, Knatterud G, Roberts R, et al. Thrombolysis in myocardial infarction (TIMI) trial, Phase I: a comparison between intravenous tissue plasminogen activator and intravenous streptokinase. Circulation. 1987;76(1):142–54.

7. Guerci AD, Gerstenblith G, Brinker JA, et al. A randomized trial of intravenous tissue plasminogen activator for acute myocardial infarction with subsequent randomization to elective coronary angioplasty. New Engl J Med. 1987;317:1613–18.

8. O'Rourke M, Baron D, Keogh A, et al. Limitation of myocardial infarction by early infusion of recombinant tissue-plasminogen activator. Circulation. 1988;77:1311–15.

9. Wilcox RG, von der Lippe G, Olsson CG, et al. Trial of tissue plasminogen activator for mortality reduction in acute myocardial infarction: ASSET. Lancet. 1988;2:525–30.

10. Hampton JR, The University of Nottingham. Personal communication.

11. Van de Werf F, Arnold AER, et al. Effect of intravenous tissue-plasminogen activator on infarct size, left ventricular function and survival in patients with acute myocardial infarction. Br Med J. 1988;297:1374–9.

12. The National Institute of Neurological Disorders and Stroke t-PA Stroke Study Group. Tissue plasminogen activator for acute ischemic stroke. New Engl J Med. 1995;333:1581–7.

13. Goldhaber SZ, Kessler CM, Heit J, et al. A randomized controlled trial of recombinant tissue plasminogen activator versus urokinase in the treatment of acute pulmonary embolism. Lancet. 1988;2:293–8.

14. Califf RM, Topol EJ, George BS, et al. Hemorrhagic complications associated with the use of intravenous tissue plasminogen activator in treatment of acute myocardial infarction. Am J Med. 1988;85:353–9.

15. Bovill EG, Terrin ML, Stump DC, et al. Hemorrhagic events during therapy with recombinant tissue-type plasminogen activator, heparin, and aspirin for acute myocardial infarction: results from the thrombolysis in myocardial infarction (TIMI), Phase II trial. Ann Int Med. 1991;115(4):256–65.

16. National Heart Foundation of Australia Coronary Thrombolysis Group. Coronary thrombolysis and myocardial infarction salvage by tissue plasminogen activator given up to 4 hours after onset of myocardial infarction. Lancet. 1988;1:203–7.

17. Gore JM, Sloan M, Price TR, et al. and the TIMI Investigators. Intracerebral hemorrhage, cerebral infarction, and subdural hematoma after acute myocardial infarction and thrombolytic therapy in the thrombolysis in myocardial infarction study. Circulation. 1991;83:448–59.

18. Hacke W, Kaste M, Fieschi C, Toni D, Lesaffre E, von Kummer R, et al. for the ECASS Study Group. Intravenous thrombolysis with recombinant tissue plasminogen activator for acute hemispheric stroke. The European Cooperative Acute Stroke Study (ECASS). JAMA. 1995;274:1017–25.

Activase®, Alteplase, recombinant   G48005-R9
Manufactured by
GENENTECH, INC.
460 Point San Bruno Boulevard   Revised June 1996
South San Francisco, CA 94080-4990

© 1996 Genentech, Inc.

Shown in Product Identification Guide, page 311

NUTROPIN®   ℞
[somatropin (rDNA origin) for injection]

DESCRIPTION

Nutropin® [somatropin (rDNA origin) for injection] is a human growth hormone (hGH) produced by recombinant DNA technology. Nutropin has 191 amino acid residues and a molecular weight of 22,125 daltons. The amino acid sequence of the product is identical to that of pituitary-derived human growth hormone. The protein is synthesized by a specific laboratory strain of *E. coli* as a precursor consisting of the rhGH molecule preceded by the secretion signal from an *E. coli* protein. This precursor is directed to the plasma membrane of the cell. The signal sequence is removed and the native protein is secreted into the periplasm so that the protein is folded appropriately as it is synthesized.

Nutropin is a highly purified preparation. Biological potency is determined by measuring the increase in body weight induced in hypophysectomized rats.

Nutropin is a sterile, white, lyophilized powder intended for subcutaneous administration after reconstitution with Bacteriostatic Water for Injection, USP (benzyl alcohol preserved). The reconstituted product is nearly isotonic at a concentration of 5 mg/mL growth hormone (GH) and has a pH of approximately 7.4.

Each 5 mg Nutropin vial contains 5 mg (approximately 15 IU) somatropin, lyophilized with 45 mg mannitol, 1.7 mg sodium phosphates (0.4 mg sodium phosphate monobasic and 1.3 mg sodium phosphate dibasic), and 1.7 mg glycine.

Each 10 mg Nutropin vial contains 10 mg (approximately 30 IU) somatropin, lyophilized with 90 mg mannitol, 3.4 mg sodium phosphates (0.8 mg sodium phosphate monobasic and 2.6 mg sodium phosphate dibasic), and 3.4 mg glycine. Bacteriostatic Water for Injection, USP is sterile water containing 0.9 percent benzyl alcohol per mL as an antimicrobial preservative packaged in a multidose vial. The diluent pH is 4.5–7.0.

CLINICAL PHARMACOLOGY

General

In vitro and in vivo preclinical and clinical testing have demonstrated that Nutropin is therapeutically equivalent to pituitary-derived human GH (hGH). Pediatric patients who lack adequate endogenous GH secretion, patients with chronic renal insufficiency, and patients with Turner syndrome that were treated with Nutropin resulted in an increase in growth rate and an increase in insulin-like growth factor-I (IGF-I) levels similar to that seen with pituitary-derived hGH.

Actions that have been demonstrated for Nutropin, somatrem, and/or pituitary-derived hGH include:

A. Tissue Growth—1) Skeletal Growth: GH stimulates skeletal growth in pediatric patients with growth failure due to a lack of adequate secretion of endogenous GH or secondary to chronic renal insufficiency and in patients with Turner syndrome. Skeletal growth is accomplished at the epiphyseal plates at the ends of a growing bone. Growth and metabolism of epiphyseal plate cells are directly stimulated by GH and one of its mediators, IGF-I. Serum levels of IGF-I are low in children and adolescents who are GH deficient, but increase during treatment with GH. In pediatric patients, new bone is formed at the epiphyses in response to GH and IGF-I. This results in linear growth until these growth plates fuse at the end of puberty. 2) Cell Growth: Treatment with hGH results in an increase in both the number and the size of skeletal muscle cells. 3) Organ Growth: GH influences the size of internal organs, including kidneys, and increases red cell mass. Treatment of hypophysectomized or genetic dwarf rats with GH results in organ growth that is proportional to the overall body growth. In normal rats subjected to nephrectomy-induced uremia, GH promoted skeletal and body growth.

B. Protein Metabolism—Linear growth is facilitated in part by GH-stimulated protein synthesis. This is reflected by nitrogen retention as demonstrated by a decline in urinary nitrogen excretion and blood urea nitrogen during GH therapy.

C. Carbohydrate Metabolism—GH is a modulator of carbohydrate metabolism. For example, patients with inadequate secretion of GH sometimes experience fasting hypoglycemia that is improved by treatment with GH. GH therapy may decrease insulin sensitivity. Untreated patients with chronic renal insufficiency and Turner syndrome have an increased incidence of glucose intolerance. Administration of hGH to adults or children resulted in increases in serum fasting and postprandial insulin levels, more commonly in overweight or obese individuals. In addition, mean fasting and postprandial glucose and hemoglobin A_{1c} levels remained in the normal range.

D. Lipid Metabolism—In GH-deficient patients, administration of GH resulted in lipid mobilization, reduction in body fat stores, increased plasma fatty acids, and decreased plasma cholesterol levels.

E. Mineral Metabolism—The retention of total body potassium in response to GH administration apparently results from cellular growth. Serum levels of inorganic phosphorus may increase slightly in patients with inadequate secretion of endogenous GH, chronic renal insufficiency, or patients with Turner syndrome during GH therapy due to metabolic activity associated with bone growth as well as increased tubular reabsorption of phosphate by the kidney. Serum calcium is not significantly altered in these patients. Sodium retention also occurs. Adults with childhood-onset GH deficiency show low bone mineral density (BMD). (See PRECAUTIONS: Laboratory Tests.)

F. Connective Tissue Metabolism—GH stimulates the synthesis of chondroitin sulfate and collagen as well as the urinary excretion of hydroxyproline.

Pharmacokinetics

Subcutaneous Absorption—The absolute bioavailability of recombinant human growth hormone (rhGH) after subcutaneous administration in healthy adult males has been determined to be 81±20%. The mean terminal $t_{1/2}$ after subcutaneous administration is significantly longer than that seen after intravenous administration (2.1±0.43 hr vs. 19.5±3.1 min) indicating that the subcutaneous absorption of the compound is slow and rate-limiting.

Distribution—Animal studies with rhGH showed that GH localizes to highly perfused organs, particularly the liver and kidney. The volume of distribution at steady state for rhGH in healthy adult males is about 50 mL/kg body weight, approximating the serum volume.

Metabolism—Both the liver and kidney have been shown to be important metabolizing organs for GH. Animal studies suggest that the kidney is the dominant organ of clearance. GH is filtered at the glomerulus and reabsorbed in the proximal tubules. It is then cleaved within renal cells into its constituent amino acids, which return to the systemic circulation.

Elimination—The mean terminal $t_{1/2}$ after intravenous administration of rhGH in healthy adult males is estimated to be 19.5±3.1 minutes. Clearance of rhGH after intravenous administration in healthy adults and children is reported to be in the range of 116–174 mL/hr/kg.

Bioequivalence of Formulations—Nutropin has been determined to be bioequivalent to Nutropin AQ® [somatropin (rDNA origin) injection] based on the statistical evaluation of AUC and C_{max}.

Special Populations

Pediatric—Available literature data suggest that rhGH clearances are similar in adults and children.

Gender—No data are available for exogenously administered rhGH. Available data for methionyl recombinant GH, pituitary-derived GH, and endogenous GH suggest no consistent gender-based differences in GH clearance.

Continued on next page

Nutropin—Cont.

Geriatrics—Limited published data suggest that the plasma clearance and average steady-state plasma concentration of rhGH may not be different between young and elderly patients.

Race—Reported values for half-lives for endogenous GH in normal adult black males are not different from observed values for normal adult white males. No data for other races are available.

Growth Hormone Deficiency (GHD)—Reported values for clearance of rhGH in adults and children with GHD range from 138–245 mL/hr/kg and are similar to those observed in healthy adults and children. Mean terminal $t_{1/2}$ values following intravenous and subcutaneous administration in adult and pediatric GHD patients are also similar to those observed in healthy adult males.

Renal Insufficiency—Children and adults with chronic renal failure (CRF) and end-stage renal disease (ESRD) tend to have decreased clearance compared to normals. Endogenous GH production may also increase in some individuals with ESRD. However, no rhGH accumulation has been reported in children with CRF or ESRD dosed with current regimens.

Turner Syndrome—No pharmacokinetic data are available for exogenously administered rhGH. However, reported half-lives, absorption, and elimination rates for endogenous GH in this population are similar to the ranges observed for normal subjects and GHD populations.

Hepatic Insufficiency—A reduction in rhGH clearance has been noted in patients with severe liver dysfunction. The clinical significance of this decrease is unknown.

Summary of Nutropin Pharmacokinetic Parameters in Healthy Adult Males
0.1 mg (approximately 0.3 IU[a])/kg SC

	C_{max} (μg/L)	T_{max} (hr)	$t_{1/2}$ (hr)	$AUC_{0-\infty}$ (μg•hr/L)	CL/F_{SC} (mL/[hr•kg])
MEAN[b]	67.2	6.2	2.1	643	158
CV%	29	37	20	12	12

Abbreviations: C_{max}=maximum concentration; $t_{1/2}$ =half life; $AUC_{0-\infty}$=area under the curve; CL/F_{SC}=systemic clearance; F_{SC}=subcutaneous bioavailability (not determined); CV%=coefficient of variation in %; SC=subcutaneous

[a]Based on current International Standard of 3 IU=1 mg
[b]n=36

Single Dose Mean Growth Hormone Concentrations in Healthy Adult Males

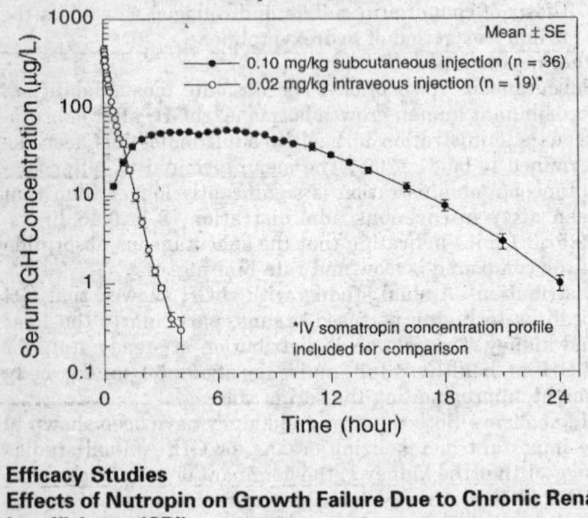
Mean ± SE
0.10 mg/kg subcutaneous injection (n = 36)
0.02 mg/kg intraveous injection (n = 19)*
Serum GH Concentration (μg/L)
1000
100
10
1
0.1
0
6
12
18
24
Time (hour)
*IV somatropin concentration profile included for comparison

Efficacy Studies

Effects of Nutropin on Growth Failure Due to Chronic Renal Insufficiency (CRI)

Two multicenter, randomized, controlled clinical trials were conducted to determine whether treatment with Nutropin prior to renal transplantation in patients with chronic renal insufficiency could improve their growth rates and height deficits. One study was a double-blind, placebo-controlled trial and the other was an open-label, randomized trial. The dose of Nutropin in both controlled studies was 0.05 mg/kg/day (0.35 mg/kg/wk) administered daily by subcutaneous injection. Combining the data from those patients completing two years in the two controlled studies results in 62 patients treated with Nutropin and 28 patients in the control groups (either placebo-treated or untreated). The mean first year growth rate was 10.8 cm/yr for Nutropin-treated patients, compared with a mean growth rate of 6.5 cm/yr for placebo/untreated controls ($p<0.00005$). The mean second year growth rate was 7.8 cm/yr for the Nutropin-treated group, compared with 5.5 cm/yr for controls ($p<0.00005$). There was a significant increase in mean height standard deviation (SD) score in the Nutropin group (–2.9 at baseline to –1.5 at Month 24, n=62) but no significant change in the controls (–2.8 at baseline to –2.9 at Month 24, n=28). The mean third year growth rate of 7.6 cm/yr in the Nutropin-treated patients (n=27) suggests that Nutropin stimulates growth beyond two years. However, there are no control data for the third year because control patients crossed over to Nutropin treatment after two years of participation. The gains in height were accompanied by appropriate advancement of skeletal age. These data demonstrate that Nutropin therapy improves growth rate and corrects the acquired height deficit associated with chronic renal insufficiency. Currently there are insufficient data regarding the benefit of treatment beyond three years. Although predicted final height was improved during Nutropin therapy, the effect of Nutropin on final adult height remains to be determined.

Post-Transplant Growth

The North American Pediatric Renal Transplant Cooperative Study (NAPRTCS) has reported data for growth post-transplant in children who did not receive GH. The average change in height SD score during the initial two years post-transplant was 0.18 (n=300, J Pediatr. 1993;122:397–402). Controlled studies of GH treatment for the short stature associated with CRI were not designed to compare the growth of treated or untreated patients after they received renal transplants. However, growth data are available from a small number of patients who have been followed for at least 11 months. Of the 7 control patients, 4 increased their height SD score and 3 had either no significant change or a decrease in height SD score. The 13 patients treated with Nutropin prior to transplant had either no significant change or an increase in height SD score after transplantation, indicating that the individual gains achieved with GH therapy prior to transplant were maintained after transplantation. The differences in the height deficit narrowed between the treated and untreated groups in the post-transplant period.

Turner Syndrome

One long-term, randomized, open-label, multicenter, concurrently controlled study, two long-term, open-label, multicenter, historically controlled studies and one long-term, randomized, dose-response study were conducted to evaluate the efficacy of GH for the treatment of girls with short stature due to Turner syndrome.

In the randomized study GDCT, comparing GH-treated patients to a concurrent control group who received no GH, the GH-treated patients who received a dose of 0.3 mg/kg/week given 6 times per week from a mean age of 11.7 years for a mean duration of 4.7 years attained a mean near final height of 146.0 cm (n=27) as compared to the control group who attained a near final height of 142.1 cm (n=19). By analysis of covariance, the effect of GH therapy was a mean height increase of 5.4 cm (p=0.001).

In two of the studies (85-023 and 85-044), the effect of long-term GH treatment (0.375 mg/kg/week given either 3 times per week or daily) on adult height was determined by comparing adult heights in the treated patients with those of age-matched historical controls with Turner syndrome who never received any growth-promoting therapy. In Study 85-023, estrogen treatment was delayed until patients were at least age 14. GH therapy resulted in a mean adult height gain of 7.4 cm (mean duration of GH therapy of 7.6 years) vs. matched historical controls by analysis of covariance.

In Study 85-044, patients treated with early GH therapy were randomized to receive estrogen replacement therapy (conjugated estrogens, 0.3 mg escalating to 0.625 mg daily) at either age 12 or 15 years. Compared with matched historical controls, early GH therapy (mean duration of GH therapy 5.6 years) combined with estrogen replacement at age 12 years resulted in an adult height gain of 5.9 cm (n=26), whereas girls who initiated estrogen at age 15 years (mean duration of GH therapy 6.1 years) had a mean adult height gain of 8.3 cm (n=29). Patients who initiated GH therapy after age 11 (mean age 12.7 years; mean duration of GH therapy 3.8 years) had a mean adult height gain of 5.0 cm (n=51).

Thus, in both studies, 85-023 and 85-044, the greatest improvement in adult height was observed in patients who received early GH treatment and estrogen after age 14 years.

In a randomized, blinded, dose-response study, GDCI, patients were treated from a mean age of 11.1 years for a mean duration of 5.3 years with a weekly dose of either 0.27 mg/kg or 0.36 mg/kg administered 3 or 6 times weekly. The mean near final height of patients receiving growth hormone was 148.7 cm (n=31). This represents a mean gain in adult height of approximately 5 cm compared with previous observations of untreated Turner syndrome girls.

In these studies, Turner syndrome patients (n=181) treated to final adult height achieved statistically significant average estimated adult height gains ranging from 5.0–8.3 cm. [See table below]

Adult Growth Hormone Deficiency (GHD)

Two multicenter, double-blind, placebo-controlled clinical trials were conducted using Nutropin in GH-deficient adults. One study was conducted in subjects with adult-onset GHD, mean age 48.3 years, n=166, at doses of 0.0125 or 0.00625 mg/kg/day; doses of 0.025 mg/kg/day were not tolerated in these subjects. A second study was conducted in previously treated subjects with childhood-onset GHD, mean age 23.8 years, n=64, at randomly assigned doses of 0.025 or 0.0125 mg/kg/day. The studies were designed to assess the effects of replacement therapy with GH on body composition.

Significant changes from baseline to Month 12 of treatment in body composition (i.e., total body % fat mass, trunk % fat mass, and total body % lean mass by DEXA scan) were seen in all Nutropin groups in both studies ($p<0.0001$ for change from baseline and vs. placebo), whereas no statistically significant changes were seen in either of the placebo groups. In the adult-onset study, the Nutropin group improved mean total body fat from 35.0% to 31.5%, mean trunk fat from 33.9% to 29.5%, and mean lean body mass from 62.2% to 65.7%, whereas the placebo group had mean changes of 0.2% or less (p=not significant). Due to the possible effect of GH-induced fluid retention on DEXA measurements of lean body mass, DEXA scans were repeated approximately 3 weeks after completion of therapy; mean % lean body mass in the Nutropin group was 65.0%, a change of 2.8% from baseline, compared with a change of 0.4% in the placebo group ($p<0.0001$ between groups).

In the childhood-onset study, the high-dose Nutropin group improved mean total body fat from 38.4% to 32.1%, mean trunk fat from 36.7% to 29.0%, and mean lean body mass from 59.1% to 65.5%; the low-dose Nutropin group improved mean total body fat from 37.1% to 31.3%, mean trunk fat from 37.9% to 30.6%, and mean lean body mass from 60.0% to 66.0%; the placebo group had mean changes of 0.6% or less (p=not significant).

[See table at top of next page]

In the adult-onset study, significant decreases from baseline to Month 12 in LDL cholesterol and LDL:HDL ratio were seen in the Nutropin group compared to the placebo group, $p<0.02$; there were no statistically significant between-group differences in change from baseline to Month 12 in total cholesterol, HDL cholesterol, or triglycerides. In the childhood-onset study, significant decreases from baseline to Month 12 in total cholesterol, LDL cholesterol, and LDL:HDL ratio were seen in the high-dose Nutropin group only, compared to the placebo group, $p<0.05$. There were no statistically significant between-group differences in HDL cholesterol or triglycerides from baseline to Month 12.

Muscle strength, physical endurance, and quality of life measurements were not markedly abnormal at baseline, and no statistically significant effects of Nutropin therapy were observed in the two studies.

INDICATIONS AND USAGE

Pediatric Patients

Nutropin® [somatropin (rDNA origin) for injection] is indicated for the long-term treatment of growth failure due to a lack of adequate endogenous GH secretion.

Nutropin® [somatropin (rDNA origin) for injection] is also indicated for the treatment of growth failure associated with chronic renal insufficiency up to the time of renal transplantation. Nutropin therapy should be used in conjunction with optimal management of chronic renal insufficiency.

Nutropin® [somatropin (rDNA origin) for injection] is also indicated for the long-term treatment of short stature associated with Turner syndrome.

Study/Group	Study Design[a]	N at Adult Height	GH Age (yr)	Estrogen Age (yr)	GH Duration (yr)	Adult Height Gain (cm)[b]
GDCT	RCT	27	11.7	13	4.7	5.4
85-023	MHT	17	9.1	15.2	7.6	7.4
85-044: A*	MHT	29	9.4	15.0	6.1	8.3
B*		26	9.6	12.3	5.6	5.9
C*		51	12.7	13.7	3.8	5.0
GDCI	RDT	31	11.1	8–13.5	5.3	~5[c]

[a] RCT: randomized controlled trial; MHT: matched historical controlled trial; RDT: randomized dose-response trial.
[b] Analysis of covariance vs. controls
[c] Compared with historical data
*A: GH age <11 yr, estrogen age 15 yr
B: GH age <11 yr, estrogen age 12 yr
C: GH age >11 yr, estrogen at Month 12

Mean Changes from Baseline to Month 12 in Proportion of Fat and Lean by DEXA for Studies M0431g and M0381g (Adult-onset and Childhood-onset GHD, respectively)

	M0431g			M0381g		
Proportion	Placebo (n=62)	Nutropin (n=63)	Between-groups t-test p-value	Placebo (n=13)	Nutropin 0.0125 mg/kg/day (n=15)	Nutropin 0.025 mg/kg/day (n=15)
Total body percent fat						
Baseline	36.8	35.0	0.38	35.0	37.1	38.4
Month 12	36.8	31.5		35.2	31.3	32.1
Baseline to Month 12 change	**−0.1**	**−3.6**	<0.0001	**+0.2**	**−5.8**	**−6.3**
Post-washout	36.4	32.2		N/A	N/A	N/A
Baseline to post-washout change	**−0.4**	**−2.8**	<0.0001	N/A	N/A	N/A
Trunk percent fat						
Baseline	35.3	33.9	0.50	32.5	37.9	36.7
Month 12	35.4	29.5		33.1	30.6	29.0
Baseline to Month 12 change	**0.0**	**−4.3**	<0.0001	**+0.6**	**−7.3**	**−7.6**
Post-washout	34.9	30.5		N/A	N/A	N/A
Baseline to post-washout change	**−0.3**	**−3.4**		N/A	N/A	N/A
Total body percent lean						
Baseline	60.4	62.2	0.37	62.0	60.0	59.1
Month 12	60.5	65.7		61.8	66.0	65.5
Baseline to Month 12 change	**+0.2**	**+3.6**	<0.0001	**−0.2**	**+6.0**	**+6.4**
Post-washout	60.9	65.0		N/A	N/A	N/A
Baseline to post-washout change	**+0.4**	**+2.8**	<0.0001	N/A	N/A	N/A

Adult Patients

Nutropin® [somatropin (rDNA origin) for injection] is indicated for the replacement of endogenous GH in patients with adult GH deficiency who meet both of the following two criteria:

1. Biochemical diagnosis of adult GH deficiency by means of a subnormal response to a standard growth hormone stimulation test (peak GH≤5 μg/L), and

2. Adult-onset: Patients who have adult GH deficiency either alone or with multiple hormone deficiencies (hypopituitarism) as a result of pituitary disease, hypothalamic disease, surgery, radiation therapy, or trauma; or

Childhood-onset: Patients who were GH deficient during childhood, confirmed as an adult before replacement therapy with Nutropin is started.

CONTRAINDICATIONS

Nutropin should not be used for growth promotion in pediatric patients with closed epiphyses.

Nutropin should not be used in patients with active neoplasia. GH therapy should be discontinued if evidence of neoplasia develops.

Nutropin, when reconstituted with Bacteriostatic Water for Injection, USP (benzyl alcohol preserved) should not be used in patients with a known sensitivity to benzyl alcohol.

WARNINGS

Benzyl alcohol as a preservative in Bacteriostatic Water for Injection, USP has been associated with toxicity in newborns. When administering Nutropin to newborns, reconstitute with Sterile Water for Injection, USP. USE ONLY ONE DOSE PER NUTROPIN VIAL AND DISCARD THE UNUSED PORTION.

PRECAUTIONS

General: Nutropin should be prescribed by physicians experienced in the diagnosis and management of patients with GH deficiency, Turner syndrome, or chronic renal insufficiency. No studies have been completed of Nutropin therapy in patients who have received renal transplants. Currently, treatment of patients with functioning renal allografts is not indicated.

Experience with prolonged rhGH treatment in adults is limited.

Patients with epiphyseal closure who were treated with GH replacement therapy in childhood should be re-evaluated according to the criteria in the INDICATIONS AND USAGE SECTION before continuation of GH therapy at the reduced dose level recommended for GH-deficient adults.

Because Nutropin may reduce insulin sensitivity, patients should be monitored for evidence of glucose intolerance.

For patients with diabetes mellitus, the insulin dose may require adjustment when GH therapy is instituted. Because GH may reduce insulin sensitivity, particularly in obese individuals, patients should be observed for evidence of glucose intolerance. Patients with diabetes or glucose intolerance should be monitored closely during GH therapy.

Nutropin therapy in adults with GHD of adult onset was associated with an increase of median fasting insulin in the Nutropin 0.0125 mg/kg/day group from 9.0 μU/mL at baseline to 13.0 μU/mL at month 12 with a return to the baseline median after a 3-week post-washout period off GH therapy. In the placebo group there was no change from 8.0 μU/mL at baseline to month 12, and after the post-washout the median was 9.0 μU/mL. The between-treatment-groups difference in change from baseline to month 12 was significant, $p<0.0001$. In childhood-onset subjects there was a change of median fasting insulin in the Nutropin 0.025 mg/kg/day group from 11.0 μU/mL at baseline to 20.0 μU/mL at month 12, in the Nutropin 0.0125 mg/kg/day group from 8.5 μU/mL to 11.0 μU/mL, and in the placebo group from 7.0 μU/mL to 8.0 μU/mL. The between-treatment-groups difference for these changes was significant, $p=0.0007$.

In subjects with adult-onset GHD there was no between-treatment-group difference in changes from baseline to month 12 in mean HbA1c, $p=0.08$. In childhood-onset mean HbA1c increased in the Nutropin 0.025 mg/kg/day group from 5.2% at baseline to 5.5% at month 12, and did not change in the Nutropin 0.0125 mg/kg/day group from 5.1% at baseline or in the placebo group from 5.3% at baseline. The between-treatment-groups difference was significant, $p=0.009$.

Patients with a history of an intracranial lesion should be examined frequently for progression or recurrence of the lesion. In pediatric patients, clinical literature has demonstrated no relationship between GH replacement therapy and CNS tumor recurrence or new extracranial tumors. In adults, it is unknown whether there is any relationship between GH replacement therapy and CNS tumor recurrence.

Patients with growth failure secondary to chronic renal insufficiency should be examined periodically for evidence of progression of renal osteodystrophy. Slipped capital femoral epiphysis or avascular necrosis of the femoral head may be seen in children with advanced renal osteodystrophy, and it is uncertain whether these problems are affected by GH therapy. X-rays of the hip should be obtained prior to initiating GH therapy for CRI patients. Physicians and parents should be alert to the development of a limp or complaints of hip or knee pain in patients treated with Nutropin.

Slipped capital femoral epiphysis may occur more frequently in patients with endocrine disorders or in patients undergoing rapid growth.

Progression of scoliosis can occur in patients who experience rapid growth. Because GH increases growth rate, patients with a history of scoliosis who are treated with GH should be monitored for progression of scoliosis. GH has not been shown to increase the incidence of scoliosis. Skeletal abnormalities including scoliosis are commonly seen in untreated Turner syndrome patients. Physicians should be alert to these abnormalities, which may manifest during GH therapy.

Patients with Turner syndrome should be evaluated carefully for otitis media and other ear disorders since these patients have an increased risk of ear or hearing disorders. In a randomized-controlled trial, there was a statistically significant increase, as compared to untreated controls, in otitis media (43% vs. 26%) and ear disorders (18% vs. 5%) in patients receiving GH. In addition, patients with Turner syndrome should be monitored closely for cardiovascular disorders (e.g., stroke, aortic aneurysm, hypertension) as these patients are also at risk for these conditions.

Intracranial hypertension (IH) with papilledema, visual changes, headache, nausea, and/or vomiting has been reported in a small number of patients treated with GH products. Symptoms usually occurred within the first eight (8) weeks of the initiation of GH therapy. In all reported cases, IH-associated signs and symptoms resolved after termination of therapy or a reduction of the GH dose. Funduscopic examination of patients is recommended at the initiation and periodically during the course of GH therapy. Patients with CRI and Turner syndrome may be at increased risk for development of IH.

See WARNINGS for use of Bacteriostatic Water for Injection, USP (benzyl alcohol preserved) in newborns.

As with any protein, local or systemic allergic reactions may occur. Parents/Patient should be informed that such reactions are possible and that prompt medical attention should be sought if allergic reactions occur.

Laboratory Tests: Serum levels of inorganic phosphorus, alkaline phosphatase, and parathyroid hormone (PTH) may increase with Nutropin therapy.

Untreated hypothyroidism prevents optimal response to Nutropin. Patients with Turner syndrome have an inherently increased risk of developing autoimmune thyroid disease. Changes in thyroid hormone laboratory measurements may develop during Nutropin treatment. Therefore, patients should have periodic thyroid function tests and should be treated with thyroid hormone when indicated.

Drug Interaction: Excessive glucocorticoid therapy will inhibit the growth-promoting effect of human GH. Patients with ACTH deficiency should have their glucocorticoid replacement dose carefully adjusted to avoid an inhibitory effect on growth.

The use of Nutropin in patients with chronic renal insufficiency receiving glucocorticoid therapy has not been evaluated. Concomitant glucocorticoid therapy may inhibit the growth-promoting effect of Nutropin. If glucocorticoid replacement is required, the glucocorticoid dose should be carefully adjusted.

There was no evidence in the controlled studies of Nutropin's interaction with drugs commonly used in chronic renal insufficiency patients. Limited published data indicate that GH treatment increases cytochrome P450 (CP450) mediated antipyrine clearance in man. These data suggest that GH administration may alter the clearance of compounds known to be metabolized by CP450 liver enzymes (e.g., corticosteroids, sex steroids, anticonvulsants, cyclosporin). Careful monitoring is advisable when GH is administered in combination with other drugs known to be metabolized by CP450 liver enzymes.

Carcinogenesis, Mutagenesis, Impairment of Fertility: Carcinogenicity, mutagenicity, and reproduction studies have not been conducted with Nutropin.

Pregnancy: Pregnancy (Category C). Animal reproduction studies have not been conducted with Nutropin. It is also not known whether Nutropin can cause fetal harm when administered to a pregnant woman or can affect reproduction capacity. Nutropin should be given to a pregnant woman only if clearly needed.

Nursing Mothers: It is not known whether Nutropin is excreted in human milk. Because many drugs are excreted in human milk, caution should be exercised when Nutropin is administered to a nursing mother.

Information for Patients: Patients being treated with GH and/or their parents should be informed of the potential benefits and risks associated with treatment. If home use is determined to be desirable by the physician, instructions on appropriate use should be given, including a review of the contents of the Patient Information Insert. This information is intended to aid in the safe and effective administration of the medication. It is not a disclosure of all possible adverse or intended effects.

If home use is prescribed, a puncture-resistant container for the disposal of used syringes and needles should be recommended to the patient. Patients and/or parents should be thoroughly instructed in the importance of proper disposal and cautioned against any reuse of needles and syringes (see Patient Information Insert).

ADVERSE REACTIONS

As with all protein pharmaceuticals, a small percentage of patients may develop antibodies to the protein. GH antibody binding capacities below 2 mg/L have not been associated with growth attenuation. In some cases when binding capacity exceeds 2 mg/L, growth attenuation has been observed. In clinical studies of pediatric patients that were treated with Nutropin for the first time, 0/107 growth hormone-deficient (GHD) patients, 0/125 CRI patients, and 0/112 Turner syndrome patients screened for antibody production developed antibodies with binding capacities ≥2 mg/L at six months.

Additional short-term immunologic and renal function studies were carried out in a group of patients with chronic renal insufficiency after approximately one year of treatment to detect other potential adverse effects of antibodies to GH. Testing included measurements of C1q, C3, C4, rheumatoid factor, creatinine, creatinine clearance, and BUN. No adverse effects of GH antibodies were noted.

In addition to an evaluation of compliance with the prescribed treatment program and thyroid status, testing for antibodies to GH should be carried out in any patient who fails to respond to therapy.

In studies in patients treated with Nutropin, injection site pain was reported infrequently.

Leukemia has been reported in a small number of GHD patients treated with GH. It is uncertain whether this increased risk is related to the pathology of GH deficiency itself, GH therapy, or other associated treatments such as radiation therapy for intracranial tumors. On the basis of current evidence, experts cannot conclude that GH therapy is responsible for these occurrences. The risk to GHD, CRI, or Turner syndrome patients, if any, remains to be established.

Continued on next page

Nutropin—Cont.

Other adverse drug reactions that have been reported in GH-treated patients include the following: 1) Metabolic: Mild, transient peripheral edema. In GHD adults, edema or peripheral edema was reported in 41% of GH-treated patients and 25% of placebo-treated patients. 2) Musculoskeletal: Arthralgias; carpal tunnel syndrome. In GHD adults, arthralgias and other joint disorders were reported in 27% of GH-treated patients and 15% of placebo-treated patients. 3) Skin: Rare increased growth of pre-existing nevi; patients should be monitored for malignant transformation. 4) Endocrine: Gynecomastia. Rare pancreatitis.

OVERDOSAGE

Acute overdosage could lead to hyperglycemia. Long-term overdosage could result in signs and symptoms of gigantism and/or acromegaly consistent with the known effects of excess GH. (See recommended and maximal dosage instructions given below.)

DOSAGE AND ADMINISTRATION

The Nutropin dosage and administration schedule should be individualized for each patient. Response to growth hormone therapy in pediatric patients tends to decrease with time. However, in pediatric patients failure to increase growth rate, particularly during the first year of therapy, suggests the need for close assessment of compliance and evaluation of other causes of growth failure, such as hypothyroidism, under-nutrition, and advanced bone age.

Dosage

Pediatric Growth Hormone Deficiency (GHD)

A weekly dosage of up to 0.30 mg/kg of body weight divided into daily subcutaneous injection is recommended.

Adult Growth Hormone Deficiency (GHD)

The recommended dosage at the start of therapy is not more than 0.006 mg/kg given as a daily subcutaneous injection. The dose may be increased according to individual patient requirements to a maximum of 0.025 mg/kg daily in patients under 35 years and to a maximum of 0.0125 mg/kg daily in patients over 35 years.

To minimize the occurrence of adverse events in older or overweight patients, lower doses may be necessary. During therapy, dosage should be decreased if required by the occurrence of side effects or excessive IGF-I levels.

Chronic Renal Insufficiency (CRI)

A weekly dosage of up to 0.35 mg/kg of body weight divided into daily subcutaneous injection is recommended.

Nutropin therapy may be continued up to the time of renal transplantation.

In order to optimize therapy for patients who require dialysis, the following guidelines for injection schedule are recommended:

1. Hemodialysis patients should receive their injection at night just prior to going to sleep or at least 3–4 hours after their hemodialysis to prevent hematoma formation due to the heparin.
2. Chronic Cycling Peritoneal Dialysis (CCPD) patients should receive their injection in the morning after they have completed dialysis.
3. Chronic Ambulatory Peritoneal Dialysis (CAPD) patients should receive their injection in the evening at the time of the overnight exchange.

Turner Syndrome

A weekly dosage of up to 0.375 mg/kg of body weight divided into equal doses 3 to 7 times per week by subcutaneous injection is recommended.

Administration

After the dose has been determined, reconstitute as follows: each 5 mg vial should be reconstituted with 1–5 mL of Bacteriostatic Water for Injection, USP (benzyl alcohol preserved); or each 10 mg vial should be reconstituted with 1–10 mL of Bacteriostatic Water for Injection, USP (benzyl alcohol preserved) only. For use in newborns see WARNINGS. The pH of Nutropin after reconstitution with Bacteriostatic Water for Injection, USP (benzyl alcohol preserved) is approximately 7.4.

To prepare the Nutropin solution, inject the Bacteriostatic Water for Injection, USP (benzyl alcohol preserved) into the Nutropin vial, aiming the stream of liquid against the glass wall. Then swirl the product vial with a **GENTLE** rotary motion until the contents are completely dissolved. **DO NOT SHAKE.** Because Nutropin is a protein, shaking can result in a cloudy solution. The Nutropin solution should be clear immediately after reconstitution. Occasionally, after refrigeration, you may notice that small colorless particles of protein are present in the Nutropin solution. This is not unusual for solutions containing proteins. If the solution is cloudy immediately after reconstitution or refrigeration, the contents **MUST NOT** be injected.

Before needle insertion, wipe the septum of both the Nutropin and diluent vials with rubbing alcohol or an antiseptic solution to prevent contamination of the contents by microorganisms that may be introduced by repeated needle insertions. It is recommended that Nutropin be administered

using sterile, disposable syringes and needles. The syringes should be of small enough volume that the prescribed dose can be drawn from the vial with reasonable accuracy.

STABILITY AND STORAGE

Before Reconstitution—Nutropin® [somatropin (rDNA origin) for injection] and Bacteriostatic Water for Injection, USP (benzyl alcohol preserved) must be stored at 2°C–8°C/36°F–46°F (under refrigeration). **Avoid freezing the vials of Nutropin and Bacteriostatic Water for Injection, USP (benzyl alcohol preserved).** Expiration dates are stated on the labels.

After Reconstitution—Vial contents are stable for 14 days when reconstituted with Bacteriostatic Water for Injection, USP (benzyl alcohol preserved) and stored at 2°C–8°C/36°F–46°F (under refrigeration). Store the unused portion of Bacteriostatic Water for Injection, USP (benzyl alcohol preserved) at 2°C–8°C/36°F–46°F (under refrigeration). **Avoid freezing the reconstituted vial of Nutropin and the Bacteriostatic Water for Injection, USP (benzyl alcohol preserved).**

HOW SUPPLIED

Nutropin is supplied as 5 mg (approximately 15 IU) or 10 mg (approximately 30 IU) of lyophilized, sterile somatropin per vial.

Each 5 mg carton contains two vials of Nutropin® [somatropin (rDNA origin) for injection] (5 mg per vial) and one 10 mL multiple dose vial of Bacteriostatic Water for Injection, USP (benzyl alcohol preserved). NDC 50242-072-02

Each 10 mg carton contains two vials of Nutropin® [somatropin (rDNA origin) for injection] (10 mg per vial) and two 10 mL multiple dose vials of Bacteriostatic Water for Injection, USP (benzyl alcohol preserved).

NDC 50242-018-20

Nutropin® [somatropin (rDNA origin) for injection] manufactured by:

Genentech, Inc.
1 DNA Way
South San Francisco, CA 94080-4990
Bacteriostatic Water for Injection, USP (benzyl alcohol preserved) manufactured for:
Genentech, Inc.

4808604

©1997 Genentech, Inc.　　　Revised December 1997
Shown in Product Identification Guide, page 311

NUTROPIN AQ®　　　　　　　　　　　Ŗ
[somatropin (rDNA origin) injection]

DESCRIPTION

Nutropin AQ® [somatropin (rDNA origin) injection] is a human growth hormone (hGH) produced by recombinant DNA technology. Nutropin AQ has 191 amino acid residues and a molecular weight of 22,125 daltons. The amino acid sequence of the product is identical to that of pituitary-derived human growth hormone. The protein is synthesized by a specific laboratory strain of *E. coli* as a precursor consisting of the rhGH molecule preceded by the secretion signal from an *E. coli* protein. This precursor is directed to the plasma membrane of the cell. The signal sequence is removed and the native protein is secreted into the periplasm so that the protein is folded appropriately as it is synthesized.

Nutropin AQ is a highly purified preparation. Biological potency is determined by measuring the increase in body weight induced in hypophysectomized rats. Nutropin AQ may contain not more than fifteen percent deamidated growth hormone (GH) at expiration. The deamidated form of GH has been extensively characterized and has been shown to be safe and fully active.

Nutropin AQ is a sterile liquid intended for subcutaneous administration. The product is nearly isotonic at a concentration of 5 mg of GH per mL and has a pH of approximately 6.0.

Each 2 mL vial contains 10 mg (approximately 30 IU) somatropin, formulated in 17.4 mg sodium chloride, 5 mg phenol, 4 mg polysorbate 20, and 10 mM sodium citrate.

CLINICAL PHARMACOLOGY
General

In vitro and in vivo preclinical and clinical testing have demonstrated that Nutropin AQ is therapeutically equivalent to pituitary-derived human GH (hGH). Pediatric patients who lack adequate endogenous GH secretion, patients with chronic renal insufficiency, and patients with Turner syndrome that were treated with Nutropin AQ or Nutropin® [somatropin (rDNA origin) for injection] resulted in an increase in growth rate and an increase in insulin-like growth factor-I (IGF-I) levels similar to that seen with pituitary-derived hGH.

Actions that have been demonstrated for Nutropin AQ, somatropin, somatrem, and/or pituitary-derived hGH include:

A. Tissue Growth—1) Skeletal Growth: GH stimulates skeletal growth in pediatric patients with growth failure due to a lack of adequate secretion of endogenous GH or sec-

ondary to chronic renal insufficiency and in patients with Turner syndrome. Skeletal growth is accomplished at the epiphyseal plates at the ends of a growing bone. Growth and metabolism of epiphyseal plate cells are directly stimulated by GH and one of its mediators, IGF-I. Serum levels of IGF-I are low in children and adolescents who are GH deficient, but increase during treatment with GH. In pediatric patients, new bone is formed at the epiphyses in response to GH and IGF-I. This results in linear growth until these growth plates fuse at the end of puberty. 2) Cell Growth: Treatment with hGH results in an increase in both the number and the size of skeletal muscle cells. 3) Organ Growth: GH influences the size of internal organs, including kidneys, and increases red cell mass. Treatment of hypophysectomized or genetic dwarf rats with GH results in organ growth that is proportional to the overall body growth. In normal rats subjected to nephrectomy-induced uremia, GH promoted skeletal and body growth.

B. Protein Metabolism—Linear growth is facilitated in part by GH-stimulated protein synthesis. This is reflected by nitrogen retention as demonstrated by a decline in urinary nitrogen excretion and blood urea nitrogen during GH therapy.

C. Carbohydrate Metabolism—GH is a modulator of carbohydrate metabolism. For example, patients with inadequate secretion of GH sometimes experience fasting hypoglycemia that is improved by treatment with GH. GH therapy may decrease insulin sensitivity. Untreated patients with chronic renal insufficiency and Turner syndrome have an increased incidence of glucose intolerance. Administration of hGH to adults or children resulted in increases in serum fasting and postprandial insulin levels, more commonly in overweight or obese individuals. In addition, mean fasting and postprandial glucose and hemoglobin A_{1c} levels remained in the normal range.

D. Lipid Metabolism—In GH–deficient patients, administration of GH resulted in lipid mobilization, reduction in body fat stores, increased plasma fatty acids, and decreased plasma cholesterol levels.

E. Mineral Metabolism—The retention of total body potassium in response to GH administration apparently results from cellular growth. Serum levels of inorganic phosphorus may increase slightly in patients with inadequate secretion of endogenous GH, chronic renal insufficiency, or patients with Turner syndrome during GH therapy due to metabolic activity associated with bone growth as well as increased tubular reabsorption of phosphate by the kidney. Serum calcium is not significantly altered in these patients. Sodium retention also occurs. Adults with childhood-onset GH deficiency show low bone mineral density (BMD). (See PRECAUTIONS: Laboratory Tests.)

F. Connective Tissue Metabolism—GH stimulates the synthesis of chondroitin sulfate and collagen as well as the urinary excretion of hydroxyproline.

Pharmacokinetics

Subcutaneous Absorption—The absolute bioavailability of recombinant human growth hormone (rhGH) after subcutaneous administration in healthy adult males has been determined to be 81±20%. The mean terminal $t_{1/2}$ after subcutaneous administration is significantly longer than that seen after intravenous administration (2.1±0.43 hr vs. 19.5±3.1 min) indicating that the subcutaneous absorption of the compound is slow and rate-limiting.

Distribution—Animal studies with rhGH showed that GH localizes to highly perfused organs, particularly the liver and kidney. The volume of distribution at steady state for rhGH in healthy adult males is about 50 mL/kg body weight, approximating the serum volume.

Metabolism—Both the liver and kidney have been shown to be important metabolizing organs for GH. Animal studies suggest that the kidney is the dominant organ of clearance. GH is filtered at the glomerulus and reabsorbed in the proximal tubules. It is then cleaved within renal cells into its constituent amino acids, which return to the systemic circulation.

Elimination—The mean terminal $t_{1/2}$ after intravenous administration of rhGH in healthy adult males is estimated to be 19.5±3.1 minutes. Clearance of rhGH after intravenous administration in healthy adults and children is reported to be in the range of 116–174 mL/hr/kg.

Bioequivalence of Formulations—Nutropin AQ® [somatropin (rDNA origin) injection] has been determined to be bioequivalent to Nutropin® [somatropin (rDNA origin) for injection] based on the statistical evaluation of AUC and C_{max}.

Special Populations

Pediatric—Available literature data suggest that rhGH clearances are similar in adults and children.

Gender—No data are available for exogenously administered rhGH. Available data for methionyl recombinant GH, pituitary-derived GH, and endogenous GH suggest no consistent gender-based differences in GH clearance.

Summary of Nutropin AQ Pharmacokinetic Parameters in Healthy Adult Males 0.1 mg (approximately 0.3 IU[a])/kg SC

	C_{max} (µg/L)	T_{max} (hr)	$t_{1/2}$ (hr)	$AUC_{0-\infty}$ (µg•hr/L)	CL/F_{sc} (mL/[hr•kg])
MEAN[b]	71.1	3.9	2.3	677	150
CV%	17	56	18	13	13

Abbreviations: C_{max}=maximum concentration; $t_{1/2}$=half-life; $AUC_{0-\infty}$=area under the curve; CL/F_{sc}=systemic clearance; F_{sc}=subcutaneous bioavailability (not determined); CV%=coefficient of variation in %; SC=subcutaneous

[a] Based on current International Standard of 3 IU=1 mg
[b] n=36

Geriatrics—Limited published data suggest that the plasma clearance and average steady-state plasma concentration of rhGH may not be different between young and elderly patients.

Race—Reported values for half-lives for endogenous GH in normal adult black males are not different from observed values for normal adult white males. No data for other races are available.

Growth Hormone Deficiency (GHD)—Reported values for clearance of rhGH in adults and children with GHD range from 138–245 mL/hr/kg and are similar to those observed in healthy adults and children. Mean terminal $t_{1/2}$ values following intravenous and subcutaneous administration in adult and pediatric GHD patients are also similar to those observed in healthy adult males.

Renal Insufficiency—Children and adults with chronic renal failure (CRF) and end-stage renal disease (ESRD) tend to have decreased clearance compared to normals. Endogenous GH production may also increase in some individuals with ESRD. However, no rhGH accumulation has been reported in children with CRF or ESRD dosed with current regimens.

Turner Syndrome—No pharmacokinetic data are available for exogenously administered rhGH. However, reported half-lives, absorption, and elimination rates for endogenous GH in this population are similar to the ranges observed for normal subjects and GHD populations.

Hepatic Insufficiency—A reduction in rhGH clearance has been noted in patients with severe liver dysfunction. The clinical significance of this decrease is unknown.

[See table above]

Single Dose Mean Growth Hormone Concentrations in Healthy Adult Males

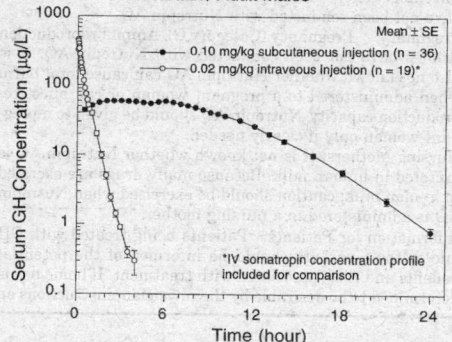

Efficacy Studies

Effects of Nutropin® [somatropin (rDNA origin) for injection] on Growth Failure Due to Chronic Renal Insufficiency (CRI)

Two multicenter, randomized, controlled clinical trials were conducted to determine whether treatment with Nutropin prior to renal transplantation in patients with chronic renal insufficiency could improve their growth rates and height deficits. One study was a double-blind, placebo-controlled trial and the other was an open-label, randomized trial. The dose of Nutropin in both controlled studies was 0.05 mg/kg/day (0.35 mg/kg/wk) administered daily by subcutaneous injection. Combining the data from those patients completing two years in the two controlled studies results in 62 patients treated with Nutropin and 28 patients in the control groups (either placebo-treated or untreated). The mean first year growth rate was 10.8 cm/yr for Nutropin-treated patients, compared with a mean growth rate of 6.5 cm/yr for placebo/untreated controls (p<0.00005). The mean second year growth rate was 7.8 cm/yr for the Nutropin-treated group, compared with 5.5 cm/yr for controls (p<0.00005). There was a significant increase in mean height standard deviation (SD) score in the Nutropin group (−2.9 at baseline to −1.5 at Month 24, n=62) but no significant change in the controls (−2.8 at baseline to −2.9 at Month 24, n=28). The mean third year growth rate of 7.6 cm/yr in the Nutropin-treated patients (n=27) suggests that Nutropin stimulates growth beyond two years. However, there are no control data for the third year because control patients crossed over to Nutropin treatment after two years of participation. The gains in height were accompanied by appropriate advancement of skeletal age. These data demonstrate that Nutropin therapy improves growth rate and corrects the acquired height deficit associated with chronic renal insufficiency. Currently there are insufficient data regarding the benefit of treatment beyond three years. Although predicted final height was improved during Nutropin therapy, the effect of Nutropin on final adult height remains to be determined.

Post-Transplant Growth

The North American Pediatric Renal Transplant Cooperative Study (NAPRTCS) has reported data for growth post-transplant in children who did not receive GH. The average change in height SD score during the initial two years post-transplant was 0.18 (n=300, J Pediatr. 1993;122:397–402). Controlled studies of GH treatment for the short stature associated with CRI were not designed to compare the growth of treated or untreated patients after they received renal transplants. However, growth data are available from a small number of patients who have been followed for at least 11 months. Of the 7 control patients, 4 increased their height SD score and 3 had either no significant change or a decrease in height SD score. The 13 patients treated with Nutropin® [somatropin (rDNA origin) for injection] prior to transplant had either no significant change or an increase in height SD score after transplantation, indicating that the individual gains achieved with GH therapy prior to transplant were maintained after transplantation. The differences in the height deficit narrowed between the treated and untreated groups in the post-transplant period.

Turner Syndrome

One long-term, randomized, open-label, multicenter, concurrently controlled study, two long-term, open-label, multicenter, historically controlled studies and one long-term, randomized, dose-response study were conducted to evaluate the efficacy of GH for the treatment of girls with short stature due to Turner syndrome.

In the randomized study GDCT, comparing GH–treated patients to a concurrent control group who received no GH, the GH–treated patients who received a dose of 0.3 mg/kg/week given 6 times per week from a mean age of 11.7 years for a mean duration of 4.7 years attained a mean near final height of 146.0 cm (n=27) as compared to the control group who attained a near final height of 142.1 cm (n=19). By analysis of covariance, the effect of GH therapy was a mean height increase of 5.4 cm (p=0.001).

In two of the studies (85-023 and 85-044), the effect of long-term GH treatment (0.375 mg/kg/week given either 3 times per week or daily) on adult height was determined by comparing adult heights in the treated patients with those of age-matched historical controls with Turner syndrome who never received any growth-promoting therapy. In Study 85-023, estrogen treatment was delayed until patients were at least age 14. GH therapy resulted in a mean adult height gain of 7.4 cm (mean duration of GH therapy of 7.6 years) vs. matched historical controls by analysis of covariance.

In Study 85-044, patients treated with early GH therapy were randomized to receive estrogen replacement therapy (conjugated estrogens, 0.3 mg escalating to 0.625 mg daily) at either age 12 or 15 years. Compared with matched historical controls, early GH therapy (mean duration of GH therapy 5.6 years) combined with estrogen replacement at age 12 years resulted in an adult height gain of 5.9 cm (n=26), whereas girls who initiated estrogen at age 15 years (mean duration of GH therapy 6.1 years) had a mean adult height gain of 8.3 cm (n=29). Patients who initiated GH therapy after age 11 (mean age 12.7 years; mean duration of GH therapy 3.8 years) had a mean adult height gain of 5.0 cm (n=51).

Thus, in both studies, 85-023 and 85-044, the greatest improvement in adult height was observed in patients who received early GH treatment and estrogen after age 14 years. In a randomized, blinded, dose-response study, GDCI, patients were treated from a mean age of 11.1 years for a mean duration of 5.3 years with a weekly dose of either 0.27 mg/kg or 0.36 mg/kg administered 3 or 6 times weekly. The mean near final height of patients receiving growth hormone was 148.7 cm (n=31). This represents a mean gain in adult height of approximately 5 cm compared with previous observations of untreated Turner syndrome girls.

In these studies, Turner syndrome patients (n=181) treated to final adult height achieved statistically significant average estimated adult height gains ranging from 5.0–8.3 cm. [See table below]

Adult Growth Hormone Deficiency (GHD)

Two multicenter, double-blind, placebo-controlled clinical trials were conducted using Nutropin® [somatropin (rDNA origin) for injection] in GH–deficient adults. One study was conducted in subjects with adult-onset GHD, mean age 48.3 years, n=166, at doses of 0.0125 or 0.00625 mg/kg/day; doses of 0.025 mg/kg/day were not tolerated in these subjects. A second study was conducted in previously treated subjects with childhood-onset GHD, mean age 23.8 years, n=64, at randomly assigned doses of 0.025 or 0.0125 mg/kg/day. The studies were designed to assess the effects of replacement therapy with GH on body composition.

Significant changes from baseline to Month 12 of treatment in body composition (i.e., total body % fat mass, trunk % fat mass, and total body % lean mass by DEXA scan) were seen in all Nutropin groups in both studies (p<0.0001 for change from baseline and vs. placebo), whereas no statistically significant changes were seen in either of the placebo groups. In the adult-onset study, the Nutropin group improved mean total body fat from 35.0% to 31.5%, mean trunk fat from 33.9% to 29.5%, and mean lean body mass from 62.2% to 65.7%, whereas the placebo group had mean changes of 0.2% or less (p=not significant). Due to the possible effect of GH-induced fluid retention on DEXA measurements of lean body mass, DEXA scans were repeated approximately 3 weeks after completion of therapy; mean % lean body mass in the Nutropin group was 65.0%, a change of 2.8% from baseline, compared with a change of 0.4% in the placebo group (p<0.0001 between groups).

In the childhood-onset study, the high-dose Nutropin group improved mean total body fat from 38.4% to 32.1%, mean trunk fat from 36.7% to 29.0%, and mean lean body mass from 59.1% to 65.5%; the low-dose Nutropin group improved mean total body fat from 37.1% to 31.3%, mean trunk fat from 37.9% to 30.6%, and mean lean body mass from 60.0% to 66.0%; the placebo group had mean changes of 0.6% or less (p=not significant).

[See table at bottom of next page]

In the adult-onset study, significant decreases from baseline to Month 12 in LDL cholesterol and LDL:HDL ratio were seen in the Nutropin group compared to the placebo group, p<0.02; there were no statistically significant between-group differences in change from baseline to Month 12 in total cholesterol, HDL cholesterol, or triglycerides. In the childhood-onset study, significant decreases from baseline to Month 12 in total cholesterol, LDL cholesterol, and LDL:HDL ratio were seen in the high-dose Nutropin group only, compared to the placebo group, p<0.05. There were no statistically significant between-group differences in HDL cholesterol or triglycerides from baseline to Month 12.

Muscle strength, physical endurance, and quality of life measurements were not markedly abnormal at baseline, and no statistically significant effects of Nutropin therapy were observed in the two studies.

Continued on next page

Study/ Group	Study Design[a]	N at Adult Height	GH Age (yr)	Estrogen Age (yr)	GH Duration (yr)	Adult Height Gain (cm)[b]
GDCT	RCT	27	11.7	13	4.7	5.4
85-023	MHT	17	9.1	15.2	7.6	7.4
85-044: A*	MHT	29	9.4	15.0	6.1	8.3
B*		26	9.6	12.3	5.6	5.9
C*		51	12.7	13.7	3.8	5.0
GDCI	RDT	31	11.1	8–13.5	5.3	~5[c]

[a] RCT: randomized controlled trial; MHT: matched historical controlled trial; RDT: randomized dose-response trial;
[b] Analysis of convariance vs. controls
[c] Compared with historical data
* A: GH age <11 yr, estrogen age 15 yr
  B: GH age <11 yr, estrogen age 12 yr
  C: GH age >11 yr, estrogen at Month 12

Nutropin AQ—Cont.

INDICATIONS AND USAGE

Pediatric Patients

Nutropin AQ® [somatropin (rDNA origin) injection] is indicated for the long-term treatment of growth failure due to a lack of adequate endogenous GH secretion.

Nutropin AQ® [somatropin (rDNA origin) injection] is also indicated for the treatment of growth failure associated with chronic renal insufficiency up to the time of renal transplantation. Nutropin AQ therapy should be used in conjunction with optimal management of chronic renal insufficiency.

Nutropin AQ® [somatropin (rDNA origin) injection] is also indicated for the long-term treatment of short stature associated with Turner syndrome.

Adult Patients

Nutropin AQ® [somatropin (rDNA origin) injection] is indicated for the replacement of endogenous GH in patients with adult GH deficiency who meet both of the following two criteria:

1. Biochemical diagnosis of adult GH deficiency by means of a subnormal response to a standard growth hormone stimulation test (peak GH≤5 µg/L), and

2. Adult-onset: Patients who have adult GH deficiency either alone or with multiple hormone deficiencies (hypopituitarism) as a result of pituitary disease, hypothalamic disease, surgery, radiation therapy, or trauma; or

Childhood-onset: Patients who were GH deficient during childhood, confirmed as an adult before replacement therapy with Nutropin AQ is started.

CONTRAINDICATIONS

Nutropin AQ should not be used for growth promotion in pediatric patients with closed epiphyses.

Nutropin AQ should not be used in patients with active neoplasia. GH therapy should be discontinued if evidence of neoplasia develops.

WARNINGS

None.

PRECAUTIONS

General: Nutropin AQ should be prescribed by physicians experienced in the diagnosis and management of patients with GH deficiency, Turner syndrome, or chronic renal insufficiency. No studies have been completed of Nutropin AQ therapy in patients who have received renal transplants. Currently, treatment of patients with functioning renal allografts is not indicated.

Experience with prolonged rhGH treatment in adults is limited.

Patients with epiphyseal closure who were treated with GH replacement therapy in childhood should be re-evaluated according to the criteria in the INDICATIONS AND USAGE SECTION before continuation of GH therapy at the reduced dose level recommended for GH-deficient adults.

Because Nutropin AQ may reduce insulin sensitivity, patients should be monitored for evidence of glucose intolerance.

For patients with diabetes mellitus, the insulin dose may require adjustment when GH therapy is instituted. Because GH may reduce insulin sensitivity, particularly in obese individuals, patients should be observed for evidence of glucose intolerance. Patients with diabetes or glucose intolerance should be monitored closely during GH therapy.

Nutropin therapy in adults with GH deficiency of adult onset was associated with an increase of median fasting insulin in the Nutropin 0.0125 mg/kg/day group from 9.0 µU/mL at baseline to 13.0 µU/mL at month 12 with a return to the baseline median after a 3-week post-washout period off GH therapy. In the placebo group there was no change from 8.0 µU/mL at baseline to month 12, and after the post-washout the median was 9.0 µU/mL. The between-treatment-groups difference in change from baseline to month 12 was significant, $p<0.0001$. In childhood-onset subjects there was a change of median fasting insulin in the Nutropin 0.025 mg/kg/day group from 11.0 µU/mL at baseline to 20.0 µU/mL at month 12, in the Nutropin 0.0125 mg/kg/day group from 8.5 µU/mL to 11.0 µU/mL, and in the placebo group from 7.0 µU/mL to 8.0 µU/mL. The between-treatment-groups difference for these changes was significant, $p=0.0007$.

In subjects with adult-onset GH deficiency there was no between-treatment- group difference in changes from baseline to month 12 in mean HbA1c, $p=0.08$. In childhood-onset mean HbA1c increased in the Nutropin 0.025 mg/kg/day group from 5.2% to 5.5% at month 12, and did not change in the Nutropin 0.0125 mg/kg/day group from 5.1% at baseline or in the placebo group from 5.3% at baseline. The between-treatment-groups difference was significant, $p=0.009$.

Patients with a history of an intracranial lesion should be examined frequently for progression or recurrence of the lesion. In pediatric patients, clinical literature has demonstrated no relationship between GH replacement therapy and CNS tumor recurrence or new extracranial tumors. In adults, it is unknown whether there is any relationship between GH replacement therapy and CNS tumor recurrence. Patients with growth failure secondary to chronic renal insufficiency should be examined periodically for evidence of progression of renal osteodystrophy. Slipped capital femoral epiphysis or avascular necrosis of the femoral head may be seen in children with advanced renal osteodystrophy, and it is uncertain whether these problems are affected by GH therapy. X-rays of the hip should be obtained prior to initiating GH therapy for CRI patients. Physicians and parents should be alert to the development of a limp or complaints of hip or knee pain in patients treated with Nutropin AQ.

Slipped capital femoral epiphysis may occur more frequently in patients with endocrine disorders or in patients undergoing rapid growth.

Progression of scoliosis can occur in patients who experience rapid growth. Because GH increases growth rate, patients with a history of scoliosis who are treated with GH should be monitored for progression of scoliosis. GH has not been shown to increase the incidence of scoliosis. Skeletal abnormalities including scoliosis are commonly seen in untreated Turner syndrome patients. Physicians should be alert to these abnormalities, which may manifest during GH therapy.

Patients with Turner syndrome should be evaluated carefully for otitis media and other ear disorders since these patients have an increased risk of ear or hearing disorders. In a randomized-controlled trial, there was a statistically significant increase, as compared to untreated controls, in otitis media (43% vs. 26%) and ear disorders (18% vs. 5%) in patients receiving GH. In addition, patients with Turner syndrome should be monitored closely for cardiovascular disorders (e.g., stroke, aortic aneurysm, hypertension) as these patients are also at risk for these conditions.

Intracranial hypertension (IH) with papilledema, visual changes, headache, nausea, and/or vomiting has been reported in a small number of patients treated with GH products. Symptoms usually occurred within the first eight (8) weeks of the initiation of GH therapy. In all reported cases, IH-associated signs and symptoms resolved after termination of therapy or a reduction of the GH dose. Funduscopic examination of patients is recommended at the initiation and periodically during the course of GH therapy. Patients with CRI and Turner syndrome may be at increased risk for development of IH.

As with any protein, local or systemic allergic reactions may occur. Parents/Patient should be informed that such reactions are possible and that prompt medical attention should be sought if allergic reactions occur.

Laboratory Tests: Serum levels of inorganic phosphorus, alkaline phosphatase, and parathyroid hormone (PTH) may increase with Nutropin AQ therapy.

Untreated hypothyroidism prevents optimal response to Nutropin AQ. Patients with Turner syndrome have an inherently increased risk of developing autoimmune thyroid disease. Changes in thyroid hormone laboratory measurements may develop during Nutropin AQ treatment. Therefore, patients should have periodic thyroid function tests and should be treated with thyroid hormone when indicated.

Drug Interaction: Excessive glucocorticoid therapy will inhibit the growth-promoting effect of human GH. Patients with ACTH deficiency should have their glucocorticoid replacement dose carefully adjusted to avoid an inhibitory effect on growth.

The use of Nutropin AQ in patients with chronic renal insufficiency receiving glucocorticoid therapy has not been evaluated. Concomitant glucocorticoid therapy may inhibit the growth-promoting effect of Nutropin AQ. If glucocorticoid replacement is required, the glucocorticoid dose should be carefully adjusted.

There was no evidence in the controlled studies of GH's interaction with drugs commonly used in chronic renal insufficiency patients. Limited published data indicate that GH treatment increases cytochrome P450 (CP450) mediated antipyrine clearance in man. These data suggest that GH administration may alter the clearance of compounds known to be metabolized by CP450 liver enzymes (e.g., corticosteroids, sex steroids, anticonvulsants, cyclosporin). Careful monitoring is advisable when GH is administered in combination with other drugs known to be metabolized by CP450 liver enzymes.

Carcinogenesis, Mutagenesis, Impairment of Fertility: Carcinogenicity, mutagenicity, and reproduction studies have not been conducted with Nutropin AQ.

Pregnancy: Pregnancy (Category C). Animal reproduction studies have not been conducted with Nutropin AQ. It is also not known whether Nutropin AQ can cause fetal harm when administered to a pregnant woman or can affect reproduction capacity. Nutropin AQ should be given to a pregnant woman only if clearly needed.

Nursing Mothers: It is not known whether Nutropin AQ is excreted in human milk. Because many drugs are excreted in human milk, caution should be exercised when Nutropin AQ is administered to a nursing mother.

Information for Patients: Patients being treated with GH and/or their parents should be informed of the potential benefits and risks associated with treatment. If home use is determined to be desirable by the physician, instructions on

Mean Changes from Baseline to Month 12 in Proportion of Fat and Lean by DEXA for Studies M0431g and M0381g (Adult-onset and Childhood-onset GHD, Respectively)

Proportion	M0431g			M0381g			
	Placebo (n=62)	Nutropin (n=63)	Between-groups t-test p-value	Placebo (n=13)	Nutropin 0.0125 mg/kg/day (n=15)	Nutropin 0.025 mg/kg/day (n=15)	Placebo vs. pooled Nutropin t-test p-value
Total body percent fat							
Baseline	36.8	35.0	0.38	35.0	37.1	38.4	0.45
Month 12	36.8	31.5		35.2	31.3	32.1	
Baseline to Month 12 change	−0.1	−3.6	<0.0001	+0.2	−5.8	−6.3	<0.0001
Post-washout	36.4	32.2		N/A	N/A	N/A	
Baseline to post-washout change	−0.4	−2.8	<0.0001	N/A	N/A	N/A	
Trunk percent fat							
Baseline	35.3	33.9	0.50	32.5	37.9	36.7	0.23
Month 12	35.4	29.5		33.1	30.6	29.0	
Baseline to Month 12 change	0.0	−4.3	<0.0001	+0.6	−7.3	−7.6	<0.0001
Post-washout	34.9	30.5		N/A	N/A	N/A	
Baseline to post-washout change	−0.3	−3.4		N/A	N/A	N/A	
Total body percent lean							
Baseline	60.4	62.2	0.37	62.0	60.0	59.1	0.48
Month 12	60.5	65.7		61.8	66.0	65.5	
Baseline to Month 12 change	+0.2	+3.6	<0.0001	−0.2	+6.0	+6.4	<0.0001
Post-washout	60.9	65.0		N/A	N/A	N/A	
Baseline to post-washout change	+0.4	+2.8	<0.0001	N/A	N/A	N/A	

appropriate use should be given, including a review of the contents of the Patient Information Insert. This information is intended to aid in the safe and effective administration of the medication. It is not a disclosure of all possible adverse or intended effects.

If home use is prescribed, a puncture-resistant container for the disposal of used syringes and needles should be recommended to the patient. Patients and/or parents should be thoroughly instructed in the importance of proper disposal and cautioned against any reuse of needles and syringes (see Patient Information Insert).

ADVERSE REACTIONS

As with all protein pharmaceuticals, a small percentage of patients may develop antibodies to the protein. GH antibody binding capacities below 2 mg/L have not been associated with growth attenuation. In some cases when binding capacity exceeds 2 mg/L, growth attenuation has been observed. In clinical studies of pediatric patients that were treated with Nutropin® [somatropin (rDNA origin) for injection] for the first time, 0/107 growth hormone-deficient (GHD) patients, 0/125 CRI patients, and 0/112 Turner syndrome patients screened for antibody production developed antibodies with binding capacities ≥2 mg/L at six months. In a clinical study of patients that were treated with Nutropin AQ® [somatropin (rDNA origin) injection] for the first time, 0/38 GHD patients screened for antibody production, for up to 15 months, developed antibodies with binding capacities ≥2 mg/L.

Additional short-term immunologic and renal function studies were carried out in a group of patients with chronic renal insufficiency after approximately one year of treatment to detect other potential adverse effects of antibodies to GH. Testing included measurements of C1q, C3, C4, rheumatoid factor, creatinine, creatinine clearance, and BUN. No adverse effects of GH antibodies were noted.

In addition to an evaluation of compliance with the prescribed treatment program and thyroid status, testing for antibodies to GH should be carried out in any patient who fails to respond to therapy.

Injection site discomfort has been reported. This is more commonly observed in children switched from another GH product to Nutropin AQ. Experience with Nutropin AQ in adults is limited.

Leukemia has been reported in a small number of GHD patients treated with GH. It is uncertain whether this increased risk is related to the pathology of GH deficiency itself, GH therapy, or other associated treatments such as radiation therapy for intracranial tumors. On the basis of current evidence, experts cannot conclude that GH therapy is responsible for these occurrences. The risk to GHD, CRI, or Turner syndrome patients, if any, remains to be established.

Other adverse drug reactions that have been reported in GH-treated patients include the following: 1) Metabolic: Mild, transient peripheral edema. In GHD adults, edema or peripheral edema was reported in 41% of GH-treated patients and 25% of placebo-treated patients. 2) Musculoskeletal: Arthralgias; carpal tunnel syndrome. In GHD adults, arthralgias and other joint disorders were reported in 27% of GH-treated patients and 15% of placebo-treated patients. 3) Skin: Rare increased growth of pre-existing nevi; patients should be monitored for malignant transformation. 4) Endocrine: Gynecomastia. Rare pancreatitis.

OVERDOSAGE

Acute overdosage could lead to hyperglycemia. Long-term overdosage could result in signs and symptoms of gigantism and/or acromegaly consistent with the known effects of excess GH. (See recommended and maximal dosage instructions given below.)

DOSAGE AND ADMINISTRATION

The Nutropin AQ dosage and administration schedule should be individualized for each patient. Response to GH therapy in pediatric patients tends to decrease with time. However, in pediatric patients failure to increase growth rate, particularly during the first year of therapy, suggests the need for close assessment of compliance and evaluation of other causes of growth failure, such as hypothyroidism, under-nutrition, and advanced bone age.

Dosage

Pediatric Growth Hormone Deficiency (GHD)

A weekly dosage of up to 0.30 mg/kg of body weight divided into daily subcutaneous injection is recommended.

Adult Growth Hormone Deficiency (GHD)

The recommended dosage at the start of therapy is not more than 0.006 mg/kg given as a daily subcutaneous injection. The dose may be increased according to individual patient requirements to a maximum of 0.025 mg/kg daily in patients under 35 years and to a maximum of 0.0125 mg/kg daily in patients over 35 years.

To minimize the occurrence of adverse events in older or overweight patients, lower doses may be necessary. During therapy, dosage should be decreased if required by the occurrence of side effects or excessive IGF-I levels.

Chronic Renal Insufficiency (CRI)

A weekly dosage of up to 0.35 mg/kg of body weight divided into daily subcutaneous injection is recommended.

Nutropin AQ therapy may be continued up to the time of renal transplantation.

In order to optimize therapy for patients who require dialysis, the following guidelines for injection schedule are recommended:

1. Hemodialysis patients should receive their injection at night just prior to going to sleep or at least 3–4 hours after their hemodialysis to prevent hematoma formation due to the heparin.
2. Chronic Cycling Peritoneal Dialysis (CCPD) patients should receive their injection in the morning after they have completed dialysis.
3. Chronic Ambulatory Peritoneal Dialysis (CAPD) patients should receive their injection in the evening at the time of the overnight exchange.

Turner Syndrome

A weekly dosage of up to 0.375 mg/kg of body weight divided into equal doses 3 to 7 times per week by subcutaneous injection is recommended.

Administration

The solution should be clear immediately after removal from the refrigerator. Occasionally, after refrigeration, you may notice that small colorless particles of protein are present in the solution. This is not unusual for solutions containing proteins. Allow the vial to come to room temperature and gently swirl. If the solution is cloudy, the contents **MUST NOT** be injected.

Before needle insertion, wipe the septum of the Nutropin AQ vial with rubbing alcohol or an antiseptic solution to prevent contamination of the contents by microorganisms that may be introduced by repeated needle insertions. It is recommended that Nutropin AQ be administered using sterile, disposable syringes and needles. The syringes should be of small enough volume that the prescribed dose can be drawn from the vial with reasonable accuracy.

STABILITY AND STORAGE

Vial contents are stable for 28 days after initial use when stored at 2–8°C/36–46°F (under refrigeration). **Avoid freezing the vial of Nutropin AQ.**

HOW SUPPLIED

Nutropin AQ is supplied as 10 mg (approximately 30 IU) of sterile liquid somatropin per vial.

Each carton contains six single vial cartons containing one 2 mL vial of Nutropin AQ® [somatropin (rDNA origin) injection] (5 mg/mL). NDC 50242-114-11.

Nutropin AQ® [somatropin (rDNA origin) injection]   4810902

Manufactured by   Revised December 1997
Genentech, Inc.   © 1997 Genentech, Inc.
1 DNA Way
South San Francisco, CA 94080-4990

Shown in Product Identification Guide, page 311

PROTROPIN®   ℞
(somatrem for injection)

DESCRIPTION

Protropin® (somatrem for injection), is a polypeptide hormone produced by recombinant DNA technology. Protropin has 192 amino acid residues and a molecular weight of about 22,000 daltons. The product contains the identical sequence of 191 amino acids constituting pituitary-derived human growth hormone plus an additional amino acid, methionine, on the N-terminus of the molecule. Protropin is synthesized in a special laboratory strain of *E. coli* bacteria which has been modified by the addition of the gene for human growth hormone production.

Protropin is a highly purified preparation. Biological potency is determined by measuring the increase in body weight induced in hypophysectomized rats.

Protropin is a sterile, white, lyophilized powder intended for intramuscular or subcutaneous administration after reconstitution with Bacteriostatic Water for Injection, USP (benzyl alcohol preserved).

Each 5 mg Protropin vial 5 mg (approximately 15 IU) somatrem, lyophilized with 40 mg mannitol, and 1.7 mg sodium phosphates (0.1 mg sodium phosphate monobasic and 1.6 mg sodium phosphate dibasic).

Each 10 mg Protropin vial contains 10 mg (approximately 30 IU) somatrem, lyophilized with 80 mg mannitol, and 3.4 mg sodium phosphates (0.2 mg sodium phosphate monobasic and 3.2 mg sodium phosphate dibasic).

Phosphoric acid may be used for pH adjustment.

Bacteriostatic Water for Injection, USP is a sterile water containing 0.9 percent benzyl alcohol per mL as an antimicrobial preservative packaged in a multi-dose vial. The diluent pH is 4.5–7.0.

CLINICAL PHARMACOLOGY

General

In vitro and in vivo preclinical, and clinical testing have demonstrated that Protropin is therapeutically equivalent to pituitary-derived human growth hormone. Treatment of children who lack adequate endogenous growth hormone secretion with Protropin resulted in an increase in growth rate and an increase in insulin-like growth factor-l levels similar to that seen with pituitary-derived human growth hormone.

Actions that have been demonstrated for Protropin, somatropin and/or pituitary-derived human growth hormone include:

A. **Tissue Growth**—1) Skeletal Growth: Protropin stimulates skeletal growth in children with growth failure due to a lack of adequate secretion of endogenous growth hormone. Skeletal growth is accomplished at the epiphyseal plates at the ends of a growing bone. Growth and metabolism of epiphyseal plate cells are directly stimulated by growth hormone and one of its mediators, insulin-like growth factor-l. Serum levels of insulin-like growth factor-l are low in children and adolescents who are growth hormone deficient, but increase during treatment with Protropin. New bone is formed at the epiphyses in response to growth hormone. This results in linear growth until these growth plates fuse at the end of puberty. 2) Cell Growth: Treatment with pituitary-derived human growth hormone results in an increase in both the number and the size of skeletal muscle cells. 3) Organ Growth: Growth hormone of human pituitary origin influences the size of internal organs, including kidneys, and increases red cell mass. Treatment of hypophysectomized or genetic dwarf rats with somatropin results in organ growth that is proportional to the overall body growth.

B. **Protein Metabolism**—Linear growth is facilitated in part by growth hormone-stimulated protein synthesis. This is reflected by nitrogen retention as demonstrated by a decline in urinary nitrogen excretion and blood urea nitrogen during growth hormone therapy.

C. **Carbohydrate Metabolism**—Growth hormone is a modulator of carbohydrate metabolism. For example, children with inadequate secretion of growth hormone sometimes experience fasting hypoglycemia that is improved by treatment with growth hormone. Protropin therapy may decrease glucose tolerance. Administration of Protropin to normal adults and patients who lacked adequate secretion of endogenous growth hormone resulted in increases in mean serum fasting and postprandial insulin levels. However, mean glucose and hemoglobin A$_{1C}$ levels remained in the normal range.

D. **Lipid Metabolism**—Acute administration of pituitary-derived human growth hormone to humans resulted in lipid mobilization. Nonesterified fatty acids increased in plasma within two hours of pituitary-derived human growth hormone administration. In growth hormone deficient patients, long-term growth hormone administration often decreases body fat. Mean cholesterol levels decreased in patients treated with growth hormone.

E. **Mineral Metabolism**—The retention of total body potassium in response to growth hormone administration apparently results from cellular growth. Serum levels of inorganic phosphorus may increase slightly in patients with inadequate secretion of endogenous growth hormone after growth hormone therapy due to metabolic activity associated with bone growth as well as increased tubular reabsorption of phosphate by the kidney. Serum calcium is not significantly altered in these patients. Sodium retention also occurs. (See PRECAUTIONS: Laboratory Tests.)

F. **Connective Tissue Metabolism**—Growth hormone stimulates the synthesis of chondroitin sulfate and collagen as well as the urinary excretion of hydroxyproline.

INDICATIONS AND USAGE

Protropin® (somatrem for injection) is indicated only for the long-term treatment of children who have growth failure due to a lack of adequate endogenous growth hormone secretion. Other etiologies of short stature should be excluded.

CONTRAINDICATIONS

Protropin should not be used in subjects with closed epiphyses.

Protropin should not be used in patients with active neoplasia. Growth hormone therapy should be discontinued if evidence of neoplasia develops.

Protropin, when reconstituted with Bacteriostatic Water for Injection, USP (benzyl alcohol preserved) should not be used in patients with a known sensitivity to benzyl alcohol.

WARNINGS

Benzyl alcohol as a preservative in Bacteriostatic Water for Injection, USP has been associated with toxicity in newborns. When administering Protropin to newborns, reconstitute with Sterile Water for Injection, USP. USE ONLY ONE DOSE PER PROTROPIN VIAL AND DISCARD THE UNUSED PORTION.

PRECAUTIONS

General: Protropin should be prescribed by physicians experienced in the diagnosis and management of patients with growth failure.

Continued on next page

Protropin—Cont.

Because Protropin may induce a state of insulin resistance, patients should be observed for evidence of glucose intolerance.

Patients with a history of an intracranial lesion should be examined frequently for progression or recurrence of the lesion.

Slipped capital femoral epiphysis may occur more frequently in patients with endocrine disorders or in patients undergoing rapid growth. Physicians and parents should be alert to the development of a limp or complaints of hip or knee pain in Protropin-treated patients.

Progression of scoliosis can occur in children who experience rapid growth. Because growth hormone increases growth rate, patients with a history of scoliosis who are treated with growth hormone should be monitored for progression of scoliosis. Growth hormone has not been shown to increase the incidence of scoliosis.

Intracranial hypertension (IH) with papilledema, visual changes, headache, nausea and/or vomiting has been reported in a small number of patients treated with growth hormone products. Symptoms usually occurred within the first eight (8) weeks of the initiation of growth hormone therapy. In all reported cases, IH-associated signs and symptoms resolved after termination of therapy or a reduction of the growth hormone dose. Funduscopic examination of patients is recommended at the initiation and periodically during the course of growth hormone therapy.

See WARNINGS for use of Bacteriostatic Water for Injection, USP (benzyl alcohol preserved) in newborns.

As with any protein, local or systemic allergic reactions may occur. Parents/Patient should be informed that such reactions are possible and that prompt medical attention should be sought if allergic reactions occur.

Laboratory Tests: Serum levels of inorganic phosphorus, alkaline phosphatase, and parathyroid hormone (PTH) may increase with Protropin therapy. Changes in thyroid hormone laboratory measurements may develop during Protropin treatment of children who lack adequate endogenous growth hormone secretion. Untreated hypothyroidism prevents optimal response to Protropin. Therefore, patients should have periodic thyroid function tests and should be treated with thyroid hormone when indicated.

Drug Interactions: Concomitant glucocorticoid therapy may inhibit the growth promoting effect of Protropin. If glucocorticoid replacement is required, the dose should be carefully adjusted.

Carcinogenesis, Mutagenesis, Impairment of Fertility: Carcinogenicity, mutagenicity and reproduction studies have not been conducted with Protropin.

Pregnancy: Pregnancy (Category C). Animal reproduction studies have not been conducted with Protropin. It is also not known whether Protropin can cause fetal harm when administered to a pregnant woman or can affect reproduction capacity. Protropin should be given to a pregnant woman only if clearly needed.

Nursing Mothers: It is not known whether this drug is excreted in human milk. Because many drugs are excreted in human milk, caution should be exercised when Proptropin is administered to a nursing mother.

Information for Patients: Patients being treated with growth hormone and/or their parents should be informed of the potential benefits and risks associated with treatment. If home use is determined to be desirable by the physician, instructions on appropriate use should be given, including a review of the contents of the Patient Information Insert. This information is intended to aid in the safe and effective administration of the medication. It is not a disclosure of all possible adverse or intended effects.

If home use is prescribed, a puncture resistant container for the disposal of used syringes and needles should be recommended to the patient. Patients and/or parents should be thoroughly instructed in the importance of proper disposal and cautioned against any reuse of needles and syringes (see Patient Information Insert).

ADVERSE REACTIONS

As with all protein pharmaceuticals, a small percentage of patients may develop antibodies to the protein. Growth hormone antibody binding capacities below 2 mg/L have not been associated with growth attenuation. In some cases when binding capacity exceeds 2 mg/L, growth attenuation has been observed. In clinical studies and postmarketing experience of patients treated with Protropin, approximately 0.4 percent of patients screened for antibody productin developed antibodies with binding capacities > 2 mg/L at six months. Out of approximately 26,000 patients who have been treated with Protropin, 5 patients have had growth deceleration associated with binding capacities > 2 mg/L. If growth deceleration is observed that is not attributable to another cause, the patient should be tested for antibodies to growth hormone. Although no evidence exists to indicate that the methionine on the N-terminus of somatrem causes antibodies to growth hormone, the physician should con-

sider transferring the patient to somatropin (rDNA origin) for injection, if a patient has antibody binding capacity > 2 mg/L, and has exhibited growth attenuation.

In addition to an evaluation of compliance with the prescribed treatment program and thyroid status, testing for antibodies to human growth hormone should be carried out in any patient who fails to respond to therapy.

Additional short-term immunologic and renal function studies were carried out in a group of patients after approximately two years of treatment to detect other potential adverse effects of antibodies to growth hormone. The antibody was determined to be of the IgG class; no antibodies to growth hormone of the IgE class were detected. Testing included immune complex determination, measurement of total hemolytic complement and specific complement components, and immunochemical analyses. No adverse effects of growth hormone antibody formation were observed.

These findings are supported by a toxicity study conducted in a primate model in which a similar antibody response to growth was observed. Protropin, administered to monkeys by intramuscular injection at doses of 125 and 625 ug/kg TIW, was compared to pituitary-human growth hormone at the same doses and with placebo over a period of 90 days. Most monkeys treated with high-dose Protropin developed persistent antibodies at week four. There were no biologically significant drug related changes in standard laboratory variables. Histopathologic examination of the kidney and other selected organs (pituitary, lungs, liver and pancreas) showed no treatment related toxicity. There was no evidence of immune complexes or immune complex toxicity when the kidney was also examined for the presence of immune complexes and possible toxic effects of immune complexes by immunohistochemistry and electron microscopy.

In studies in children treated with Protropin, injection site pain was reported infrequently.

Leukemia has been reported in a small number of growth hormone deficient patients treated with growth hormone. It is uncertain whether this increased risk is related to the pathology of growth hormone deficiency itself, growth hormone therapy, or other associated treatments such as radiation therapy for intracranial tumors. On the basis of current evidence, experts cannot conclude that growth hormone therapy is responsible for these occurrences. The risk to an individual patient, if any, remains to be established.

Other adverse drug reactions that have been reported in growth hormone-treated patients include the following: 1) Metabolic: Infrequent, mild and transient peripheral edema. 2) Musculoskeletal: Rare carpal tunnel syndrome. 3) Skin: Rare increased growth of pre-existing nevi. Malignant nevi transformation has not been reported. 4) Endocrine: Rare gynecomastia. Rare pancreatitis.

OVERDOSAGE

The recommended dosage of up to 0.30 mg/kg (approximately 0.90 IU/kg) of body weight weekly should not be exceeded due to the potential risk of known effects of excess human growth hormone.

DOSAGE AND ADMINISTRATION

A weekly dosage of 0.30 mg/kg (approximately 0.90 IU/kg) of body weight administered by daily intramuscular or subcutaneous injection is recommended.

The Protropin dosage and administration schedule should be individualized for each patient. Therapy should not be continued if final height is achieved or epiphyseal fusion occurs.

Patients who fail to respond adequately while on Protropin therapy should be evaluated to determine the cause of unresponsiveness.

After the dose has been determined, reconstitute as follows: each 5 mg vial should be reconstituted with 1–5 mL of Bacteriostatic Water for Injection, USP (benzyl alcohol preserved); or each 10 mg vial should be reconstituted with 1–10 mL Bacteriostatic Water for Injection, USP (benzyl alcohol preserved) only. For use in newborns see WARNINGS. The pH of Protropin after reconstitution with Bacteriostatic Water for Injection, USP (benzyl alcohol preserved) is approximately 7.8.

To prepare the Protropin solution, inject the Bacteriostatic Water for Injection, USP (benzyl alcohol preserved) into the Protropin vial, aiming the stream of liquid against the glass wall. Then swirl the product vial with a GENTLE rotary motion until the contents are completely dissolved. DO NOT SHAKE. Because Protropin is a protein, shaking can result in a cloudy solution. The Protropin solution should be clear immediately after reconstitution. Occasionally, after refrigeration, you may notice that small colorless particles of protein are present in the Protropin solution. This is not unusual for solutions containing proteins. If the solution is cloudy immediately after reconstitution or refrigeration, the contents MUST NOT be injected.

Before needle insertion, wipe the septum of both the Protropin and diluent vials with rubbing alcohol or an antiseptic solution to prevent contamination of the contents by microorganisms that may be introduced by repeated needle insertions. It is recommended that Protropin be administered us-

ing sterile, disposable syringes and needles. The syringes should be of small enough volume that the prescribed dose can be drawn from the vial with reasonable accuracy.

STABILITY AND STORAGE

Before Reconstitution—Protropin® (somatrem for injection), and Bacteriostatic Water for Injection, USP (benzyl alcohol preserved), must be stored at 2–8°C/36–46°F (under refrigeration). Avoid freezing the vials of Protropin and Bacteriostatic Water for Injection, USP (benzyl alcohol preserved). Expiration dates are stated on the labels.

After Reconstitution—Vial contents are stable for 14 days when reconstituted with Bacteriostatic Water for Injection, USP (benzyl alcohol preserved) at 2–8°C/36–46°F (under refrigeration). Store the unused portion of Bacteriostatic Water for Injection, USP (benzyl alcohol preserved) at 2–8°C/36–46°F (under refrigeration). Avoid freezing the vials of Protropin and Bacteriostatic Water for Injection, USP (benzyl alcohol preserved).

HOW SUPPLIED

Protropin® (somatrem for injection) is supplied as 5 mg (approximately 15 IU) or 10 mg (approximately 30 IU) of lyophilized, sterile, somatrem per vial.

Each 5 mg carton contains two vials of Protropin (somatrem for injection) (5 mg per vial) and one 10 mL multiple dose vial of Bacteriostatic Water for Injection, USP (benzyl alcohol preserved). NDC 50242-015-02

Each 10 mg carton contains two vials of Protropin (somatrem for injection) (10 mg per vial) and two 10 mL multiple dose vials of Bacteriostatic Water for Injection, USP (benzyl alcohol preserved). NDC 50242-016-20

Protropin® (somatrem for injection) Manufactured by:

Genetech, Inc.
460 Point San Bruno Boulevard
South San Francisco, CA 94080-4990
Bacteriostatic Water for Injection, USP (benzyl alcohol preserved)

Manufactured for:
Genentech, Inc.
Protropin®
(somatrem for injection)

From Genentech, Inc.   G40053-R9
©1995 Genentech, Inc.   Revised July, 1995
Shown in Product Identification Guide, page 311

PULMOZYME®   ℞
(dornase alfa)
recombinant
INHALATION SOLUTION

DESCRIPTION

PULMOZYME® (dornase alfa) Inhalation Solution is a sterile, clear, colorless, highly purified solution of recombinant human deoxyribonuclease I (rhDNase), an enzyme which selectively cleaves DNA. The protein is produced by genetically engineered Chinese Hamster Ovary (CHO) cells containing DNA encoding for the native human protein, deoxyribonuclease I (DNase). Fermentation is carried out in a nutrient medium containing the antibiotic gentamicin, 100-200 mg/L. However, the presence of the antibiotic is not detectable in the final product. The product is purified by tangential flow filtration and column chromatography. The purified glycoprotein contains 260 amino acids with an approximate molecular weight of 37,000 daltons (1). The primary amino acid sequence is identical to that of the native human enzyme.

PULMOZYME is administered by inhalation of an aerosol mist produced by a compressed air driven nebulizer system (see Clinical Experience; DOSAGE AND ADMINISTRATION). Each PULMOZYME single-use ampule will deliver 2.5 mL of the solution to the nebulizer bowl. The aqueous solution contains 1.0 mg/mL dornase alfa, 0.15 mg/mL calcium chloride dihydrate and 8.77 mg/mL sodium chloride. The solution contains no preservative. The nominal pH of the solution is 6.3.

CLINICAL PHARMACOLOGY
General

In cystic fibrosis (CF) patients, retention of viscous purulent secretions in the airways contributes both to reduced pulmonary function and to exacerbations of infection (2,3).

Purulent pulmonary secretions contain very high concentrations of extracellular DNA released by degenerating leukocytes that accumulate in response to infection (4). In vitro, PULMOZYME hydrolyzes the DNA in sputum of CF patients and reduces sputum viscoelasticity (1).

Pharmacokinetics

When 2.5 mg PULMOZYME was administered by inhalation to eighteen CF patients, mean sputum concentrations of 3 µg/mL DNase were measurable within 15 minutes. Mean sputum concentrations declined to an average of 0.6 µg/mL two hours following inhalation. Inhalation of up to 10 mg TID of PULMOZYME by 4 CF patients for six consecutive days, did not result in a significant elevation of

serum concentrations of DNase above normal endogenous levels (5,6). After administration of up to 2.5 mg of PULMOZYME twice daily for six months to 321 CF patients, no accumulation of serum DNase was noted.

PULMOZYME, 2.5 mg by inhalation, was administered daily to 98 patients aged 3 months to ≤10 years, and bronchoalveolar lavage (BAL) fluid was obtained within 90 minutes of the first dose. BAL DNase concentrations were detectable in all patients but showed a broad range, from 0.007 to 1.8 mcg/mL. Over an average of 14 days of exposure, serum DNase concentrations (mean ± s.d.) increased by 1.3 ± 1.3 ng/mL for the 3 months to <5 year age group and by 0.8 ± 1.2 ng/mL for the 5 to ≤10 year age group. The relationship between BAL or serum DNase concentration and adverse experiences and clinical outcomes is unknown.

Clinical Experience

PULMOZYME has been evaluated in a randomized, placebo-controlled trial of clinically stable cystic fibrosis patients, 5 years of age and older, with baseline forced vital capacity (FVC) greater than or equal to 40% of predicted and receiving standard therapies for cystic fibrosis (7). Patients were treated with placebo (325 patients), 2.5 mg of PULMOZYME once a day (322 patients), or 2.5 mg of PULMOZYME twice a day (321 patients) for six months administered via a Hudson T Up-draft II nebulizer with a Pulmo-Aide compressor.

Both doses of PULMOZYME resulted in significant reductions when compared with the placebo group in the number of patients experiencing respiratory tract infections requiring use of parenteral antibiotics. Administration of PULMOZYME reduced the relative risk of developing a respiratory tract infection by 27% and 29% for the 2.5 mg daily dose and the 2.5 mg twice daily dose, respectively (see Table 1). The data suggest that the effects of PULMOZYME on respiratory tract infections in older patients (>21 years) may be smaller than in younger patients, and that twice daily dosing may be required in the older patients. Patients with baseline FVC>85% may also benefit from twice a day dosing (see Table 1). The reduced risk of respiratory infection observed in PULMOZYME treated patients did not directly correlate with improvement in FEV_1 during the initial two weeks of therapy.

Within 8 days of the start of treatment with PULMOZYME, mean FEV_1 increased 7.9% in those treated once a day and 9.0% in those treated twice a day compared to the baseline values. The overall mean FEV_1 during long-term therapy increased 5.8% from baseline at the 2.5 mg daily dose level and 5.6% from baseline at the 2.5 mg twice daily dose level. Placebo recipients did not show significant mean changes in pulmonary function testing (see Figure 1).

For patients 5 years of age or older, with baseline FVC greater than or equal to 40%, administration of PULMOZYME decreased the incidence of occurrence of first respiratory tract infection requiring parenteral antibiotics, and improved mean FEV_1, regardless of age or baseline FVC.

[See table 1 above]

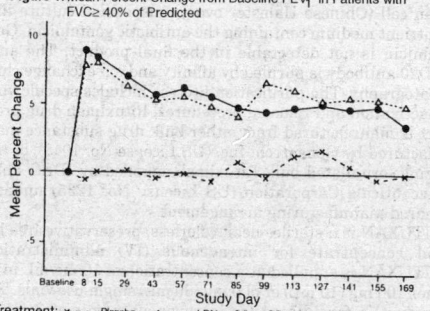

Figure 1: Mean Percent Change from Baseline FEV_1 in Patients with FVC≥ 40% of Predicted

Treatment: ✕ - - - Placebo   △····· rhDNase 2.5 mg QD   ●—— rhDNase 2.5 mg BID

PULMOZYME has also been evaluated in a second randomized, placebo-controlled study in clinically stable patients with baseline FVC <40% of predicted (8). Patients were enrolled and treated with placebo (162 patients) or PULMOZYME 2.5 mg QD (158 patients) for twelve weeks. In patients who received PULMOZYME, there was an increase in mean change (as percent of baseline) compared to placebo in FEV_1 (9.4% vs. 2.1%, p< 0.001) and in FVC (12.4% vs. 7.3% p<0.01). PULMOZYME did not significantly reduce the risk of developing a respiratory tract infection requiring parenteral antibiotics (54% of PULMOZYME patients vs 55% of placebo patients had experienced a respiratory tract infection by 12 weeks, relative risk =.93, p=0.62).

Other Studies

Clinical trials have indicated that PULMOZYME therapy can be continued or initiated during an acute respiratory exacerbation.

Short-term dose ranging studies demonstrated that doses in excess of 2.5 mg BID did not provide further improvement in FEV_1. Patients who have received drug on a cyclical regimen (ie, administration of PULMOZYME 10 mg BID for 14 days, followed by a 14 day wash out period) showed rapid improvement in FEV_1 with the initiation of each cycle and a return to baseline with each PULMOZYME withdrawal.

INDICATIONS AND USAGE

Daily administration of PULMOZYME in conjunction with standard therapies is indicated in the management of cystic fibrosis patients to improve pulmonary function. In patients with an FVC ≥40% of predicted, daily administration of PULMOZYME has also been shown to reduce the risk of respiratory tract infections requiring parenteral antibiotics. Safety and efficacy of daily administration have not been demonstrated in patients for longer than twelve months.

CONTRAINDICATIONS

PULMOZYME is contraindicated in patients with known hypersensitivity to dornase alfa, Chinese Hamster Ovary cell products, or any component of the product.

WARNINGS

None.

PRECAUTIONS

General

PULMOZYME should be used in conjunction with standard therapies for CF.

Information for Patients

PULMOZYME must be stored in the refrigerator at 2–8°C (36–46°F) and protected from strong light. It should be kept refrigerated during transport and should not be exposed to room temperatures for a total time of 24 hours. The solution should be discarded if it is cloudy or discolored. PULMOZYME contains no preservative and, once opened, the entire contents of the ampule must be used or discarded. Patients should be instructed in the proper use and maintenance of the nebulizer and compressor system used in its delivery.

PULMOZYME should not be diluted or mixed with other drugs in the nebulizer. Mixing of PULMOZYME with other drugs could lead to adverse physicochemical and/or functional changes in PULMOZYME or the admixed compound.

Drug Interactions

Clinical trials have indicated that PULMOZYME can be effectively and safely used in conjunction with standard cystic fibrosis therapies including oral, inhaled and/or parenteral antibiotics, bronchodilators, enzyme supplements, vitamins, oral or inhaled corticosteroids, and analgesics. No formal drug interaction studies have been performed.

Carcinogenesis, Mutagenesis, Impairment of Fertility

Carcinogenesis: Lifetime studies in Sprague Dawley rats showed no carcinogenic effect when PULMOZYME was administered at doses up to 246 µg/kg body weight per day. PULMOZYME was administered to rats as an aerosol for up to 30 minutes per day, daily for two years, with resulting lower respiratory tract doses of up to 246 µg/kg per day, which represents up to a 28.8-fold multiple of the clinical dose. There was no increase in the development of benign or malignant neoplasms and no occurrence of unusual tumor types in rats after a lifetime exposure.

Mutagenesis: Ames tests using six different tester strains of bacteria (4 of S. typhimurium and 2 of E. coli) at concentrations up to 5000 µg/plate, a cytogenetic assay using human peripheral blood lymphocytes at concentrations up to 2000 µg/plate, and a mouse lymphoma assay at concentrations up to 1000 µg/plate, with and without metabolic activation, revealed no evidence of mutagenesis potential. PULMOZYME was tested in a micronucleus (in vivo) assay for its potential to produce chromosome damage in bone marrow cells of mice following a bolus intravenous dose of 10 mg/kg on two consecutive days. No evidence of chromosomal damage was noted.

Impairment of Fertility: In studies with rats receiving up to 10 mg/kg/day, a dose representing systemic exposures greater than 600 times that expected following the recommended human dose, fertility and reproductive performance of both males and females was not affected.

Pregnancy (Category B)

Reproduction studies have been performed in rats and rabbits with intravenous doses up to 10 mg/kg/day, representing systemic exposures greater than 600 times that expected following the recommended human dose. These studies have revealed no evidence of impaired fertility, harm to the fetus, or effects on development due to PULMOZYME. There are, however, no adequate and well-controlled studies in pregnant women. Because animal reproductive studies are not always predictive of the human response, this drug should be used during pregnancy only if clearly needed.

Nursing Mothers

It is not known whether PULMOZYME is excreted in human milk. Small amounts of dornase alfa were detected in maternal milk of cynomolgus monkeys when administered a bolus dose (100 µg/kg) of dornase alfa followed by a six hour intravenous infusion (80 µg/kg/hr). Little or no measurable dornase alfa would be expected in human milk after chronic aerosol administration of recommended doses. Because many drugs are excreted in human milk, caution should still be exercised when PULMOZYME is administered to a nursing woman.

Pediatric Use

Because of the limited experience with the administration of Pulmozyme to patients younger than 5 years of age, its use should be considered only for those patients in whom there is a potential for benefit in pulmonary function or in risk of respiratory tract infection.

ADVERSE REACTIONS

Patients have been exposed to PULMOZYME for up to 12 months in clinical trials.

In a randomized, placebo-controlled clinical trial in patients with FVC ≥40% of predicted, over 600 patients received PULMOZYME once or twice daily for six months; most adverse events were not more common on PULMOZYME than on placebo and probably reflected the sequelae of the underlying lung disease. In most cases events that were increased were mild, transient in nature, and did not require alterations in dosing. Few patients experienced adverse events resulting in permanent discontinuation from PULMOZYME, and the discontinuation rate was similar for placebo (2%) and PULMOZYME (3%). Events that were more frequent (greater than 3%) in PULMOZYME treated patients than in placebo-treated patients are listed in Table 2.

In a randomized, placebo-controlled trial of patients with advanced disease (FVC <40% of predicted) the safety profile for most adverse events was similar to that reported for the trial in patients with mild to moderate disease. For this study, adverse events that were reported with a higher frequency (greater than 3%) in the PULMOZYME treated patients, are also listed in Table 2.

[See table 2 at top of next page]

Events Observed at Similar Rates in PULMOZYME® (dornase alfa) Inhalation Solution and Placebo Treated Patients with FVC ≥40% of predicted

Body as a Whole   Abdominal pain, Asthenia, Fever, Flu syndrome, Malaise, Sepsis

Continued on next page

Table 1
Incidence of First Respiratory Tract Infection Requiring Parenteral Antibiotics in Patients with FVC ≥40% of Predicted

	Placebo N=325	2.5 mg QD N=322	2.5 mg BID N=321
Percent of Patients Infected	43%	34%	33%
Relative Risk (vs placebo)		0.73	0.71
p-value (vs placebo)		0.015	0.007
Subgroup by Age and Baseline FVC	Placebo (N)	2.5 mg QD (N)	2.5 mg BID (N)
Age			
5–20 years	42% (201)	25% (199)	28% (184)
21 years and older	44% (124)	48% (123)	39% (137)
Baseline FVC			
40–85% Predicted	54% (194)	41% (201)	44% (203)
>85% Predicted	27% (131)	21% (121)	14% (118)

Pulmozyme—Cont.

Digestive System	Intestinal Obstruction, Gall Bladder disease, Liver disease, Pancreatic disease
Metabolic Nutritional System	Diabetes Mellitus, Hypoxia, Weight Loss
Respiratory System	Apnea, Bronchiectasis, Bronchitis, Change in Sputum, Cough Increase, Dyspnea, Hemoptysis, Lung Function Decrease, Nasal Polyps, Pneumonia, Pneumothorax, Rhinitis, Sinusitis, Sputum Increase, Wheeze

Mortality rates observed in controlled trials were similar for the placebo and PULMOZYME treated patients. Causes of death were consistent with progression of cystic fibrosis and included apnea, cardiac arrest, cardiopulmonary arrest, cor pulmonale, heart failure, massive hemoptysis, pneumonia, pneumothorax, and respiratory failure.

The safety of Pulmozyme, 2.5 mg by inhalation, was studied with 2 weeks of daily administration in 98 patients with cystic fibrosis (65 aged 3 months to <5 years, 33 aged 5 to ≤10 years). The PARI BABY™ reusable nebulizer (which uses a facemask instead of a mouthpiece) was utilized in patients unable to demonstrate the ability to inhale or exhale orally throughout the entire treatment period (54/65, 83% of the younger and 2/33, 6% of the older patients). The number of patients reporting cough was higher in the younger age group as compared to the older age group (29/65, 45% compared to 10/33, 30%) as was the number reporting moderate to severe cough (24/65, 37% as compared to 6/33, 18%). Other events tended to be of mild to moderate severity. The number of patients reporting rhinitis was higher in the younger age group as compared to the older age group (23/65, 35% compared to 9/33, 27%) as was the number reporting rash (4/65, 6% as compared to 0/33). The nature of adverse events was similar to that seen in the larger trials of Pulmozyme.

Allergic Reactions

There have been no reports of anaphylaxis attributed to the administration of PULMOZYME to date. Skin rash and urticaria have been observed, and were mild and transient in nature. Within all of the studies, a small percentage (average of 2-4%) of patients treated with PULMOZYME developed serum antibodies to PULMOZYME. None of these patients developed anaphylaxis, and the clinical significance of serum antibodies to PULMOZYME is unknown.

OVERDOSAGE

Single-dose inhalation studies in rats and monkeys at doses up to 180-times higher than doses routinely used in clinical studies are well tolerated. Single dose oral administration of PULMOZYME in doses up to 200 mg/kg are also well tolerated by rats.

Cystic fibrosis patients have received up to 20 mg BID for up to 6 days and 10 mg BID intermittently (2 weeks on/2 weeks off drug) for 168 days. These doses were well tolerated.

DOSAGE AND ADMINISTRATION

The recommended dose for use in most cystic fibrosis patients is one 2.5 mg single-use ampule inhaled once daily using a recommended nebulizer. Some patients may benefit from twice daily administration (see Clinical Experience, Table 1). Clinical trials have been performed with the following nebulizers and compressors: the disposable jet nebulizer Hudson T Up-draft II and disposable jet nebulizer Marquest Acorn II in conjunction with a Pulmo-Aide compressor, and the reusable PARI LC Jet⁺ nebulizer, in conjunction with the PARI PRONEB compressor. Safety and efficacy have been demonstrated only with these recommended nebulizer systems.

In the two-week trial of deposition and safety in patients 3 months to ≤10 years of age, those patients who were unable to demonstrate the ability to inhale or exhale orally throughout the entire treatment period used the PARI BABY™ reusable nebulizer. The PARI BABY™ nebulizer is identical to the PARI LC Jet⁺ system except that the mouthpiece is replaced by a tight fitting facemask connected to an elbow piece.

No clinical data are currently available that support the safety and efficacy of administration of PULMOZYME with other nebulizer systems. The patient should follow the manufacturer's instructions on the use and maintenance of the equipment.

PULMOZYME should not be diluted or mixed with other drugs in the nebulizer. Mixing of PULMOZYME with other drugs could lead to adverse physicochemical and/or functional changes in PULMOZYME or the admixed compound.

HOW SUPPLIED

PULMOZYME® (dornase alfa) Inhalation Solution is supplied in single-use ampules. Each ampule delivers 2.5 mL of a sterile, clear, colorless, aqueous solution containing

Table 2
Adverse Events Increased 3% or More in PULMOZYME Treated Patients Over Placebo in CF Clinical Trials

Adverse Event (of any severity or seriousness)	Trial in Mild to Moderate CF Patients (FVC ≥40% of predicted) treated for 24 weeks			Trial in Advanced CF Patients (FVC <40% of predicted) treated for 12 weeks	
	Placebo	PULMOZYME QD	PULMOZYME BID	Placebo	PULMOZYME QD
	n=325	n=322	n=321	n=159	n=161
Voice alteration	7%	12%	16%	6%	18%
Pharyngitis	33%	36%	40%	28%	32%
Rash	7%	10%	12%	1%	3%
Laryngitis	1%	3%	4%	1%	3%
Chest Pain	16%	18%	21%	23%	25%
Conjunctivitis	2%	4%	5%	0%	1%
Rhinitis				24%	30%
FVC decrease of ≥10% of predicted°	Differences were less than 3% for these adverse events in the Trial in mild to moderate CF patients			17%	22%
Fever				28%	32%
Dyspepsia				0%	3%
Dyspnea (when reported as serious)	Difference was less than 3% for this adverse event in the Trial in mild to moderate CF patients			12%†	17%†

°Single measurement only, does not reflect overall FVC changes
†Total reports of dyspnea (regardless of severity or seriousness) had a difference of less than 3% for the Trial in advanced CF patients

1.0 mg/mL dornase alfa, 0.15 mg/mL calcium chloride dihydrate and 8.77 mg/mL sodium chloride with no preservative. The nominal pH of the solution is 6.3.
PULMOZYME is supplied in:
- 14 unit cartons, containing 14 single-use ampules in single-unit foil pouches: NDC 50242-100-38
- 30 unit cartons containing 5 foil pouches of 6 single-use ampules: NDC 50242-100-40.

Storage

PULMOZYME® (dornase alfa) Inhalation Solution should be stored under refrigeration (2–8°C/36–46°F). Ampules should be protected from strong light. Do not use beyond the expiration date stamped on the ampule. Unused ampules should be stored in their protective foil pouch under refrigeration.

REFERENCES

1. Shak S, Capon DJ, Hellmiss R, Marsters SA, Baker CL. Recombinant human DNase I reduces the viscosity of cystic fibrosis sputum. Proc Natl Acad Sci USA 1990;87: 9188–92.
2. Boat TF. Cystic Fibrosis. In: Murray JF, Nadel JA, editors. Textbook of respiratory medicine. Philadelphia: Saunders WB, 1988;1:1126-52.
3. Collins FS. Cystic Fibrosis: molecular biology and therapeutic implications. Science 1992;256:774–9.
4. Potter JL, Spector S, Matthews LW, Lemm J. Studies of pulmonary secretions. Am Rev of Respir Dis 1969;99: 909–15.
5. Hubbard RC, McElvaney NG, Birrer P, Shak S, Robinson WW, Jolley C, et al. A preliminary study of aerosolized recombinant human deoxyribonuclease I in the treatment of cystic fibrosis. N Eng J Med 1992;326: 812–5.
6. Aitken ML, Burke W, McDonald G, Shak S, Montgomery AB, Smith A. Recombinant human DNase inhalation in normal subjects and patients with cystic fibrosis. JAMA 1992;267(14):1947–51.
7. Fuchs HJ, Borowitz DS, Christiansen DH, Morris EM, Nash ML, Ramsey BW, et al. Effect of aerosolized recombinant human DNase on exacerbations of respiratory symptoms and on pulmonary function in patients with cystic fibrosis. N Engl J Med 1994;331:637-42.
8. McCoy K, Hamilton S, Johnson C. Effects of 12-week administration of dornase alfa in patients with advanced cystic fibrosis lung disease. Chest 1996;110:889-95.

PULMOZYME®   4812403
(dornase alfa)   Revised February 1998
recombinant   © 1998 Genentech, Inc.
INHALATION SOLUTION
Manufactured by
GENENTECH, Inc.
1 DNA Way
South San Francisco, CA 94080-4990
Shown in Product Identification Guide, page 311

RITUXAN™   ℞
[rī-tʌks-ān]
Rituximab

DESCRIPTION

The RITUXAN (Rituximab) antibody is a genetically engineered chimeric murine/human monoclonal antibody directed against the CD20 antigen found on the surface of normal and malignant B lymphocytes. The antibody is an IgG₁ kappa immunoglobulin containing murine light- and heavy-chain variable region sequences and human constant region sequences. Rituximab is composed of two heavy chains of 451 amino acids and two light chains of 213 amino acids (based on cDNA analysis) and has an approximate molecular weight of 145 kD. Rituximab has a binding affinity for the CD20 antigen of approximately 8.0 nM.

The chimeric anti-CD20 antibody is produced by mammalian cell (Chinese Hamster Ovary) suspension culture in a nutrient medium containing the antibiotic gentamicin. Gentamicin is not detectable in the final product. The anti-CD20 antibody is purified by affinity and ion exchange chromatography. The purification process includes specific viral inactivation and removal procedures. Rituximab drug product is manufactured from either bulk drug substance manufactured by Genentech, Inc. (US License No. 1048), or utilizing formulated bulk Rituximab supplied by IDEC Pharmaceuticals Corporation (US License No. 1235) under a shared manufacturing arrangement.

RITUXAN is a sterile, clear, colorless, preservative-free liquid concentrate for intravenous (IV) administration. RITUXAN is supplied at a concentration of 10 mg/mL in either 100 mg (10 mL) or 500 mg (50 mL) single-use vials. The product is formulated for intravenous administration in 9.0 mg/mL sodium chloride, 7.35 mg/mL sodium citrate dihydrate, 0.7 mg/mL polysorbate 80, and Sterile Water for Injection. The pH is adjusted to 6.5.

CLINICAL PHARMACOLOGY
General

Rituximab binds specifically to the antigen CD20 (human B-lymphocyte-restricted differentiation antigen, Bp35), a hydrophobic transmembrane protein with a molecular weight of approximately 35 kD located on pre-B and mature B lymphocytes.[1,2] The antigen is also expressed on >90% of B-cell non-Hodgkin's lymphomas (NHL)[3] but is not found on hematopoietic stem cells, pro-B cells, normal plasma cells or other normal tissues.[4] CD20 regulates an early step(s) in the activation process for cell cycle initiation and differentiation,[4] and possibly functions as a calcium ion channel.[5] CD20 is not shed from the cell surface and does not internalize upon antibody binding.[6] Free CD20 antigen is not found in the circulation.[2]

Pre-clinical Pharmacology and Toxicology
Mechanism of Action: The Fab domain of Rituximab binds to the CD20 antigen on B-lymphocytes and the Fc domain

recruits immune effector functions to mediate B-cell lysis *in vitro*. Possible mechanisms of cell lysis include complement-dependent cytotoxicity (CDC)[7] and antibody-dependent cell mediated cytotoxicity (ADCC). The antibody has been shown to induce apoptosis in the DHL-4 human B-cell lymphoma line.[8]

Normal Tissue Cross-reactivity: Rituximab binding was observed on lymphoid cells in the thymus, the white pulp of the spleen, and a majority of B-lymphocytes in peripheral blood and lymph nodes. Little or no binding was observed in non-lymphoid tissues examined.

Human Pharmacokinetics/Pharmacodynamics

In patients given single doses at 10, 50, 100, 250 or 500 mg/m[2] as an IV infusion, serum levels and the half-life of Rituximab were proportional to dose. In 9 patients given 375 mg/m[2] as an IV infusion for four doses, the mean serum half-life was 59.8 hours (range 11.1 to 104.6 hours) after the first infusion and 174 hours (range 26 to 442 hours) after the fourth infusion. The wide range of half-lives may reflect the variable tumor burden among patients and the changes in CD20 positive (normal and malignant) B-cell populations upon repeated administrations.

Rituximab at a dose of 375 mg/m[2] was administered as an IV infusion at weekly intervals for four doses to 166 patients. The peak and trough serum levels of Rituximab were inversely correlated with baseline values for the number of circulating CD20 positive B cells and measures of disease burden. Median steady-state serum levels were higher for responders compared to nonresponders; however, no difference was found in the rate of elimination as measured by serum half-life. Serum levels were higher in patients with International Working Formulation (IWF) subtypes B, C, and D as compared to those with subtype A. Rituximab was detectable in the serum of patients three to six months after completion of treatment.

The pharmacokinetic profile of Rituximab when administered as six infusions of 375 mg/m[2] in combination with six cycles of CHOP chemotherapy was similar to that seen with Rituximab alone.

Administration of RITUXAN resulted in a rapid and sustained depletion of circulating and tissue-based B cells. Lymph node biopsies performed 14 days after therapy showed a decrease in the percentage of B-cells in seven of eight patients who had received single doses of Rituximab ≥100 mg/m[2].[9] Among the 166 patients in the pivotal study, circulating B-cells (measured as CD19 positive cells) were depleted within the first three doses with sustained depletion for up to 6 to 9 months post-treatment in 83% of patients. One of the responding patients (1%), failed to show significant depletion of CD19 positive cells after the third infusion of Rituximab as compared to 19% of the nonresponding patients. B-cell recovery began at approximately six months following completion of treatment. Median B-cell levels returned to normal by twelve months following completion of treatment.

There were sustained and statistically significant reductions in both IgM and IgG serum levels observed from 5 through 11 months following Rituximab administration. However, only 14% of patients had reductions in IgG and/or IgM serum levels, resulting in values below the normal range.

CLINICAL STUDIES

A multicenter, open-label, single-arm study was conducted in 166 patients with relapsed or refractory low-grade or follicular B-cell NHL who received 375 mg/m[2] of RITUXAN given as an IV infusion weekly for four doses. Patients with tumor masses >10 cm or with >5,000 lymphocytes/µL in the peripheral blood were excluded from the study. The overall response rate (ORR) was 48% (80/166) with a 6% (10/166) complete response (CR) and a 42% (70/166) partial response (PR) rate. Disease-related signs and symptoms (including B-symptoms) were present in 23% (39/166) of patients at study entry and resolved in 64% (25/39) of those patients. The median time to onset of response was 50 days and the median duration of response is projected to be 10 to 12 months.

In a multivariate analysis, the ORR was higher in patients with IWF B, C, and D histologic subtypes as compared to IWF A subtype (58% vs. 12%), higher in patients whose largest lesion was <5 cm vs. >7 cm in greatest diameter (53% vs. 38%), and higher in patients with chemosensitive relapse as compared to chemoresistant (defined as duration of response <3 months) relapse (53% vs. 36%). ORR in patients previously treated with autologous bone marrow transplant was 78% (18/23). The following factors were not associated with a lower response rate: age ≥60 years, extranodal disease, prior anthracycline therapy, and bone marrow involvement.

In a second multicenter, multiple-dose study, 37 patients with relapsed or refractory B-cell NHL received 375 mg/m[2] of RITUXAN as an IV infusion once weekly for four doses.[10,11] The ORR was 46% with a median duration of response of 8.6 months (range 2.6 to 26.2+). Single doses of up to 500 mg/m[2] were well-tolerated.[9]

Twenty patients have received two courses and one patient has received three courses of RITUXAN as 4 weekly infusions of 375 mg/m[2] per infusion. The percentage of patients reporting adverse events upon retreatment was similar to that reported following the first course, although the incidence of specific adverse events differed (see ADVERSE EVENTS). All patients had obtained an objective clinical response (CR or PR) to the first course of RITUXAN; upon retreatment, 6 of 12 patients evaluable for response obtained a complete or partial remission.

Twenty-nine patients with relapsed or refractory, bulky (single lesion of >10 cm in diameter), low grade NHL received 375 mg/m[2] of RITUXAN as four weekly infusions. The overall incidence of adverse events and the incidence of Grade 3 and 4 adverse events was higher in patients with bulky disease than in patients with non-bulky disease (see ADVERSE EVENTS). Ten of 21 patients evaluable for response have obtained a complete or partial remission.

INDICATIONS AND USAGE

RITUXAN is indicated for the treatment of patients with relapsed or refractory low-grade or follicular, CD20 positive, B-cell non-Hodgkin's lymphoma.

CONTRAINDICATIONS

RITUXAN is contraindicated in patients with known Type I hypersensitivity or anaphylactic reactions to murine proteins or to any component of this product. (See WARNINGS.)

WARNINGS

RITUXAN rapidly decreases CD20 positive cells that are both benign and malignant. Tumor lysis syndrome has been reported to occur within 12 to 24 hours after the first RITUXAN infusion in patients with high numbers of circulating malignant lymphocytes. Other patients with high tumor burden may also be at risk. Consideration should be given to prophylactic treatment of tumor lysis syndrome in patients who are considered to be at high risk.

RITUXAN is associated with hypersensitivity reactions which may respond to adjustments in the infusion rate. Hypotension, bronchospasm, and angioedema have occurred in association with RITUXAN infusion as part of an infusion-related symptom complex. RITUXAN infusion should be interrupted for severe reactions and can be resumed at a 50% reduction in rate (e.g., from 100 mg/hr to 50 mg/hr) when symptoms have completely resolved. Treatment of these symptoms with diphenhydramine and acetaminophen is recommended; additional treatment with bronchodilators or IV saline may be indicated. In most cases, patients who have experienced non-life-threatening reactions have been able to complete the full course of therapy. (See DOSAGE and ADMINISTRATION.) Medications for the treatment of hypersensitivity reactions, e.g., epinephrine, antihistamines and corticosteroids should be available for immediate use in the event of a reaction during administration.

Infusions should be discontinued in the event of serious or life-threatening cardiac arrhythmias. Patients who develop clinically significant arrhythmias should undergo cardiac monitoring during and after subsequent infusions of RITUXAN. Patients with preexisting cardiac conditions including arrhythmias and angina have had recurrences of these events during RITUXAN therapy and should be monitored throughout the infusion and immediate post-infusion period.

PRECAUTIONS

Laboratory Monitoring: Complete blood counts (CBC) and platelet counts should be obtained at regular intervals during RITUXAN therapy and more frequently in patients who develop cytopenias (see ADVERSE EVENTS). In patients who appear to be at risk for developing tumor lysis syndrome, appropriate laboratory studies should be monitored and prophylactic treatment used (see WARNINGS).

Drug/Laboratory Interactions: There have been no formal drug interaction studies performed with RITUXAN.

HAMA/HACA Formation: Human anti-murine antibody (HAMA) was not detected in 67 patients evaluated. Less than 1.0% (3/355) of patients evaluated for human antichimeric antibody (HACA) were positive. Patients who develop HAMA/HACA titers may have allergic or hypersensitivity reactions when treated with this or other murine or chimeric monoclonal antibodies.

Immunization: The safety of immunization with any vaccine, particularly live viral vaccines, following RITUXAN therapy has not been studied. The ability to generate a primary or anamnestic humoral response to any vaccine has also not been studied.

Carcinogenesis, Mutagenesis, Impairment of Fertility: No long-term animal studies have been performed to establish the carcinogenic or mutagenic potential of RITUXAN, or to determine its effects on fertility in males or females. Individuals of childbearing potential should use effective contraceptive methods during treatment and for up to 12 months following RITUXAN therapy.

Pregnancy Category C: Animal reproduction studies have not been conducted with RITUXAN. It is not known whether RITUXAN can cause fetal harm when administered to a pregnant woman or whether it can affect reproductive capacity. Human IgG is known to pass the placental barrier, and thus may potentially cause fetal B-cell depletion; therefore, RITUXAN should be given to a pregnant woman only if clearly needed.

Nursing Mothers: It is not known whether RITUXAN is excreted in human milk. Because human IgG is excreted in human milk and the potential for absorption and immunosuppression in the infant is unknown, women should be advised to discontinue nursing until circulating drug levels are no longer detectable. (See CLINICAL PHARMACOLOGY.)

Pediatric Use: The safety and effectiveness of RITUXAN in children have not been established.

ADVERSE REACTIONS

Safety data are based on 315 patients treated in five single-agent studies of RITUXAN. This includes patients with bulky disease (lesions >10 cm), those who have received more than one course of RITUXAN, and patients receiving 375 mg/m[2] for eight doses.

Infusion-Related Events: An infusion-related symptom complex consisting of fever and chills/rigors occurred in the majority of patients during the first RITUXAN infusion. Other frequent infusion-related symptoms included nausea, urticaria, fatigue, headache, pruritus, bronchospasm, dyspnea, sensation of tongue or throat swelling (angioedema), rhinitis, vomiting, hypotension, flushing, and pain at disease sites. These reactions generally occurred within 30 minutes to 2 hours of beginning the first infusion, and resolved with slowing or interruption of the RITUXAN infusion and with supportive care (IV saline, diphenhydramine, and acetaminophen). The incidence of infusion-related events decreased from 80% (7% Grade 3/4) during the first infusion to approximately 40% (5% to 10% Grade 3/4) with subsequent infusions. Mild to moderate hypotension requiring interruption of RITUXAN infusion with or without the administration of IV saline occurred in 32 (10%) patients. Isolated occurrences of severe reactions requiring epinephrine have been reported in patients receiving RITUXAN for other indications. Angioedema was reported in 41 (13%) patients and was serious in one patient. Bronchospasm occurred in 24 (8%) patients; one-quarter of these patients were treated with bronchodilators. A single report of bronchiolitis obliterans was noted.

Immunologic Events: RITUXAN induced B-cell depletion in 70 to 80% of patients and was associated with decreased serum immunoglobulins in a minority of patients. The incidence of infection did not appear to be increased. During the treatment period, 50 patients in the pivotal trial developed 68 infectious events; 6 (9%) were Grade 3 in severity and none were Grade 4 events. Of the 6 serious infectious events, none were associated with neutropenia. The serious bacterial events included sepsis due to Listeria (n=1), Staphylococcal bacteremia (n=1) and polymicrobial sepsis (n=1). In the post-treatment period (30 days to 11 months following the last dose), bacterial infections included sepsis (n=1); significant viral infections included herpes simplex infections (n=2) and herpes zoster (n=3).

Retreatment Events: Twenty-one patients have received more than one course of RITUXAN. The percentage of patients reporting any adverse event upon retreatment was similar to the percentage of patients reporting adverse events upon initial exposure. The following adverse events were reported more frequently in retreated subjects: asthenia, throat irritation, flushing, tachycardia, anorexia, leukopenia, thrombocytopenia, anemia, peripheral edema, dizziness, depression, respiratory symptoms, night sweats, and pruritus.

Hematologic Events: During the treatment period (up to 30 days following last dose) severe thrombocytopenia occurred in 1.3% of patients, severe neutropenia occurred in 1.9% of patients, and severe anemia occurred in 1.0% of patients. A single occurrence of transient aplastic anemia (pure red cell aplasia) and two occurrences of hemolytic anemia following RITUXAN therapy were reported.

Cardiac Events: Four patients developed arrhythmias during RITUXAN infusion. One of the four discontinued treatment because of ventricular tachycardia and supraventricular tachycardias. The other three patients experienced trigeminy (1) and irregular pulse (2) and did not require discontinuation of therapy. Angina was reported during infusion and myocardial infarction occurred 4 days post-infusion in one subject with a prior history of myocardial infarction.

[See table 1 at top of next page]

Severe and life-threatening (Grade 3 and 4) events were reported in 10% (32/315) of patients. The following Grade 3 and 4 adverse events were reported: neutropenia (1.9%), chills (1.6%), leukopenia and thrombocytopenia (1.3% for each), hypotension, anemia, bronchospasm, and urticaria

Continued on next page

Rituxan—Cont.

(1.0% for each), headache, abdominal pain, arrhythmia (0.6% for each), and asthenia, hypertension, nausea, vomiting, coagulation disorder, angioedema, arthralgia, pain, rhinitis, increased cough, dyspnea, bronchiolitis obliterans, hypoxia, asthma, pruritus, and rash (one patient each, 0.3%).

The following adverse events occurred in ≥1.0% but <5.0% of patients, in order of decreasing incidence: flushing, arthralgia, diarrhea, anemia, cough increase, hypertension, lacrimation disorder, pain, hyperglycemia, back pain, peripheral edema, paresthesia, dyspepsia, chest pain, anorexia, anxiety, malaise, tachycardia, agitation, insomnia, sinusitis, conjunctivitis, abdominal enlargement, postural hypotension, LDH increase, hypocalcemia, hypesthesia, respiratory disorder, tumor pain, pain at injection site, bradycardia, hypertonia, nervousness, bronchitis, and taste perversion.

The proportion of patients reporting any adverse event was similar in patients with bulky disease and those with lesions <10 cm in diameter. However, the incidence of dizziness, neutropenia, thrombocytopenia, myalgia, anemia and chest pain was higher in patients with lesions >10 cm. The incidence of any Grade 3 and 4 event was higher (31% vs. 13%) and the incidence of Grade 3 or 4 neutropenia, anemia, hypotension, and dyspnea was also higher in patients with bulky disease compared with patients with lesions <10 cm.

OVERDOSAGE

There has been no experience with overdosage in human clinical trials. Single doses higher than 500 mg/m² have not been tested.

DOSAGE AND ADMINISTRATION

Usual Dose:

The recommended dosage of RITUXAN is 375 mg/m² given as an IV infusion once weekly for four doses (days 1, 8, 15, and 22). RITUXAN may be administered in an outpatient setting. **DO NOT ADMINISTER AS AN INTRAVENOUS PUSH OR BOLUS. (See Administration.)**

Instructions for Administration

Preparation for Administration: Use appropriate aseptic technique. Withdraw the necessary amount of RITUXAN and dilute to a final concentration of 1 to 4 mg/mL into an infusion bag containing either 0.9% Sodium Chloride USP or 5% Dextrose in Water USP. Gently invert the bag to mix the solution. Discard any unused portion left in the vial. Parenteral drug products should be inspected visually for particulate matter and discoloration prior to administration.

RITUXAN solutions for infusion are stable at 2° to 8° C (36° to 46° F) for 24 hours and at room temperature for an additional 12 hours. No incompatibilities between RITUXAN and polyvinylchloride or polyethylene bags have been observed.

Administration: **DO NOT ADMINISTER AS AN INTRAVENOUS PUSH OR BOLUS.** Hypersensitivity reactions may occur (see WARNINGS). Premedication, consisting of acetaminophen and diphenhydramine, should be considered before each infusion of RITUXAN. Premedication may attenuate infusion-related events. Since transient hypotension may occur during RITUXAN infusion, consideration should be given to withholding anti-hypertensive medications 12 hours prior to RITUXAN infusion.

First Infusion: The RITUXAN solution for infusion should be administered intravenously at an initial rate of 50 mg/hr. RITUXAN should not be mixed or diluted with other drugs. If hypersensitivity or infusion-related events do not occur, escalate the infusion rate in 50 mg/hr increments every 30 minutes, to a maximum of 400 mg/hr. If hypersensitivity or an infusion-related event develops, the infusion should be temporarily slowed or interrupted (see WARNINGS). The infusion can continue at one-half the previous rate upon improvement of patient symptoms.

Subsequent Infusions: Subsequent RITUXAN infusions can be administered at an initial rate of 100 mg/hr, and increased by 100 mg/hr increments at 30-minute intervals, to a maximum of 400 mg/hr as tolerated.

Stability and Storage: RITUXAN vials are stable at 2° to 8° C (36° to 46° F). Do not use beyond expiration date stamped on carton. RITUXAN vials should be protected from direct sunlight.

HOW SUPPLIED

RITUXAN is supplied as 100 mg and 500 mg of sterile, preservative-free, single-use vials.

Single unit 100 mg carton: Contains one 10 mL vial of RITUXAN (10 mg/mL). NDC 50242-051-21

Single unit 500 mg carton: Contains one 50 mL vial of RITUXAN (10 mg/mL). NDC 50242-053-06

REFERENCES

1. Valentine MA, Meier KE, Rossie S, et al. Phosphorylation of the CD20 phosphoprotein in resting B lymphocytes. J. Biol. Chem. 1989 264(19): 11282–11287.
2. Einfeld DA, Brown JP, Valentine MA, et al. Molecular cloning of the human B cell CD20 receptor predicts a hydrophobic protein with multiple transmembrane domains. EMBO J. 1988 7(3):711–717.
3. Anderson KC, Bates MP, Slaughenhoupt BL, et al. Expression of human B cell-associated antigens on leukemias and lymphomas: A model of human B cell differentiation. Blood 1984 63(6):1424–1433.
4. Tedder TF, Boyd AW, Freedman AS, et al. The B cell surface molecule B1 is functionally linked with B cell activation and differentiation. J. Immunol. 1985 135(2): 973–979.
5. Tedder TF, Zhou LJ, Bell PD, et al. The CD20 surface molecule of B lymphocytes functions as a calcium channel. J. Cell. Biochem. 1990 14D:195.
6. Press OW, Applebaum F, Ledbetter JA, Martin PJ, Zarling J, Kidd P, et al. Monoclonal antibody 1F5 (anti-CD20) serotherapy of human B-cell lymphomas. Blood 1987 69(2):584–591.
7. Reff ME, Carner C, Chambers KS, Chinn PC, Leonard JE, Raab R, et al. Depletion of B cells in vivo by a chimeric mouse human monoclonal antibody to CD20. Blood 1994 83(2):435–445.
8. Demidem A, Lam T, Alas S, Hariharan K, Hanna N, and Bonavida B. Chimeric anti-CD20 (IDEC-C2B8) monoclonal antibody sensitizes a B cell lymphoma cell line to cell killing by cytotoxic drugs. Cancer Chemotherapy & Radiopharmaceuticals 1997 12(3):177–186.
9. Maloney DG, Liles TM, Czerwinski C, Waldichuk J, Rosenberg J, Grillo-López A, et al. Phase I clinical trial using escalating single-dose infusion of chimeric anti-CD20 monoclonal antibody (IDEC-C2B8) in patients with recurrent B-cell lymphoma. Blood 1994 84(8):2457–2466.
10. Maloney DG, Grillo-López AJ, Bodkin D, White CA, Liles T-M, Royston I, et al. IDEC-C2B8: Results of a phase I multiple-dose trial in patients with relapsed non-Hodgkin's lymphoma. J. Clin. Oncol. 1997 15(10): 3266–3274.
11. Maloney DG, Grillo-López AJ, White CA, Bodkin D, Schilder RJ, Neidhart JA, et al. IDEC-C2B8 (Rituximab) anti-CD20 monoclonal antibody therapy in patients with relapsed low-grade non-Hodgkin's lymphoma. Blood 1997 90(6):2188–2195.

Jointly Marketed by:

IDEC Pharmaceuticals Corporation
11011 Torreyana Road
San Diego, CA 92121

Genentech, Inc.
1 DNA Way

South San Francisco, CA 94080-4990

© 1998 IDEC Pharmaceuticals Corporation and Genentech, Inc.

4809702

Revised July, 1998

Shown in Product Identification Guide, page 311

Table 1.
Adverse Events ≥5% of Patients (N=315)

	Incidence All Grades	
	N	%
Any Adverse Event	275	87
Body As A Whole		
Fever	154	49
Chills	102	32
Asthenia	49	16
Headache	43	14
Throat Irritation	19	6
Abdominal Pain	18	6
Cardiovascular System		
Hypotension	32	10
Digestive System		
Nausea	55	18
Vomiting	23	7
Hemic and Lymphatic System		
Leukopenia	33	11
Thrombocytopenia	25	8
Neutropenia	21	7
Metabolic and Nutritional System		
Angioedema	41	13
Musculo-Skeletal System		
Myalgia	21	7
Nervous System		
Dizziness	23	7
Respiratory System		
Rhinitis	25	8
Bronchospasm	24	8
Skin and Appendages		
Pruritus	32	10
Rash	31	10
Urticaria	24	8

Genetics Institute
87 CAMBRIDGE PARK DRIVE
CAMBRIDGE, MA 02140

Direct Inquiries to:
1-888-NEUMEGA
1-888-638-6342

NEUMEGA®
℞
[*nĕu-mĕga*]
(Oprelvekin)

DESCRIPTION

Interleukin eleven (IL-11) is a thrombopoietic growth factor that directly stimulates the proliferation of hematopoietic stem cells and megakaryocyte progenitor cells and induces megakaryocyte maturation resulting in increased platelet production. IL-11 is a member of a family of human growth factors which includes human growth hormone, granulocyte colony-stimulating factor (G-CSF), and other growth factors.
Oprelvekin, the active ingredient in Neumega, is produced in *Escherichia coli* (*E. coli*) by recombinant DNA methods. The protein has a molecular mass of approximately 19,000 daltons, and is non-glycosylated. The polypeptide is 177 amino acids in length and differs from the 178 amino acid length of native IL-11 only in lacking the amino-terminal proline residue. This alteration has not resulted in measurable differences in bioactivity either *in vitro* or *in vivo*.
Neumega is available for subcutaneous administration in single-use vials containing 5 mg of Oprelvekin (specific activity approximately 8×10^6 Units/mg) as a sterile, lyophilized powder with 23 mg Glycine, USP, 1.6 mg Dibasic Sodium Phosphate Heptahydrate, USP, and 0.55 mg Monobasic Sodium Phosphate Monohydrate, USP. When reconstituted with 1 mL of Sterile Water for Injection, USP, the resulting solution has a pH of 7.0 and a concentration of 5 mg/mL.

CLINICAL PHARMACOLOGY

The primary hematopoietic activity of Neumega is stimulation of megakaryocytopoiesis and thrombopoiesis. Neumega has shown potent thrombopoietic activity in animal models of compromised hematopoiesis, including moderately to severely myelosuppressed mice and nonhuman primates. In these models, Neumega improved platelet nadirs and accelerated platelet recoveries compared to controls.
Preclinical studies have shown that mature megakaryocytes which develop during *in vivo* treatment with Neumega are ultrastructurally normal. Platelets produced in response to Neumega were morphologically and functionally normal and possessed a normal life-span.
IL-11 has also been shown to have non-hematopoietic activities in animals including: the regulation of intestinal epithelium growth (enhanced healing of gastrointestinal lesions), the inhibition of adipogenesis, the induction of acute phase protein synthesis, inhibition of pro-inflammatory cytokine production by macrophages, and the stimulation of osteoclastogenesis and neurogenesis.
IL-11 is produced by bone marrow stromal cells and is part of the cytokine family that shares the gp130 signal transducer. Primary osteoblasts and mature osteoclasts express mRNAs for both IL-11 receptor (IL-11R alpha) and gp130. Both bone-forming and bone-resorbing cells are potential targets of IL-11. (1)

Pharmacokinetics

The pharmacokinetics of Neumega have been evaluated in studies in healthy, adult subjects and oncology patients receiving chemotherapy. In a study in which a single 50 μg/kg subcutaneous dose was administered to eighteen men, the peak serum concentration (Cmax) of 17.4±5.4 ng/mL (mean ± S.D.) was reached at 3.2±2.4 hrs (Tmax) following dosing. The terminal half life was 6.9±1.7 hrs. In a second study in which single 75 μg/kg subcutaneous and intravenous doses were administered to twenty-four healthy subjects, the pharmacokinetic profiles were similar between men and women. The absolute bioavailability of Neumega was >80%. In a study in which multiple, subcutaneous doses of both 25 and 50 μg/kg were administered to cancer patients receiving chemotherapy, Neumega did not accumulate and clearance of Neumega was not impaired following multiple doses.
Neumega was also administered to twenty-eight infants, children, and adolescents receiving ICE (ifosfamide, carboplatin, etoposide) chemotherapy. Analysis of data from twenty-three pediatric patients showed that Cmax and Tmax were comparable to the adult population. The mean ± S.D. area under the concentration-time curve (AUC) for pediatric patients (8 months to 17 years), receiving 50 μg/kg or 100 μg/kg was 137±56 ng*hr/mL or 237±20 ng*hr/mL, respectively, compared with 189±41 ng*hr/mL in adults receiving 50 μg/kg. Available data suggest that clearance of IL-11 decreases with patient age, and that clearance in infants and children (8 months to 11 years) is approximately 1.2 to 1.6 fold higher than adults and adolescents (ages 12 and over).
In preclinical studies in rats, radiolabeled Neumega was rapidly cleared from the serum and distributed to highly perfused organs. The kidney was the primary route of elimination. The amount if intact Neumega in urine was low, indicating that the molecule was metabolized before excretion. In a clinical study, a single dose of Neumega was administered to subjects with severely impaired renal function (creatinine clearance < 15 mL/min). The mean ± S.D. values for Cmax and AUC were 30.8 ± 8.6 ng/mL and 373 ± 106 ng*hr/mL, respectively. When compared with control subjects in this study with normal renal function, the mean Cmax was 2.2 fold higher and the mean AUC was 2.6 fold (95% confidence interval 1.7–3.8) higher in the subjects with severe renal impairment. In the subjects with severe renal impairment, clearance was approximately 40% of the value seen in subjects with normal renal function. The average terminal half-life was similar in subjects with severe renal impairment and those with normal renal function.

Pharmacodynamics

In a study in which Neumega was administered to non-myelosuppressed cancer patients, daily subcutaneous dosing for 14 days with Neumega increased the platelet count in a dose-dependent manner. Platelet counts began to increase relative to baseline between 5 and 9 days after the start of dosing with Neumega. After cessation of treatment, platelet counts continued to increase for up to 7 days then returned toward baseline within 14 days. No change in platelet reactivity as measured by platelet activation in response to ADP, and platelet aggregation in response to ADP, epinephrine, collagen, ristocetin and arachidonic acid has been observed in association with Neumega treatment.
In a randomized, double-blind, placebo-controlled study in normal volunteers, subjects receiving Neumega had a mean increase in plasma volume of >20%, and all subjects receiving Neumega had at least a 10% increase in plasma volume. Red blood cell volume decreased similarly (due to repeated phlebotomy) in the Neumega and placebo groups. As a result, whole blood volume increased approximately 10% and hemoglobin concentration decreased approximately 10% in subjects receiving Neumega compared with subjects receiving placebo. Mean 24 hour sodium excretion decreased, and potassium excretion did not increase, in subjects receiving Neumega compared with subjects receiving placebo.

CLINICAL STUDIES

Two randomized, double-blind, placebo-controlled trials studied Neumega for the prevention of severe thrombocytopenia following single or repeated sequential cycles of various myelosuppressive chemotherapy regimens.
One study evaluated the effectiveness of Neumega in eliminating the need for platelet transfusions in patients who had recovered from an episode of severe chemotherapy-induced thrombocytopenia (defined as a platelet count ≤20,000/μL), and were to receive one additional cycle of the same chemotherapy without dose reduction. Patients had various underlying non-myeloid malignancies, and were undergoing dose-intensive chemotherapy with a variety of regimens. Patients were randomized to receive Neumega at a dose of 25 μg/kg or 50 μg/kg, or placebo. The primary endpoint was whether the patient required one or more platelet transfusions in the subsequent chemotherapy cycle. Ninety-three patients were randomized. Five patients withdrew from the study prior to receiving study drug. As a result, eighty-eight patients were included in a modified intent-to-treat analysis. The results for the Neumega 50 μg/kg and placebo groups are summarized in Table 1. The placebo group includes one patient who underwent chemotherapy dose reduction and who avoided platelet transfusions.
[See table above]

TABLE 1
STUDY RESULTS

	Placebo n=30	Neumega 50 μg/kg n=29
Number (%) of patients avoiding platelet transfusion	2 (7%)	8 (28%)
Number (%) of patients requiring platelet transfusion	28 (93%)	21 (72%)
Median (mean) number of platelet transfusion events	2.5 (3.3)	1 (2.2)

In the primary efficacy analysis, more patients avoided platelet transfusion in the Neumega 50 μg/kg arm than in the placebo arm (p=0.04, Fisher's Exact test, 2-tailed). The difference in the proportion of patients avoiding platelet transfusions in the Neumega 50 μg/kg and placebo groups was 21% (95% confidence interval 2 to 40%). The results observed in patients receiving 25 μg/kg of Neumega were intermediate between those of the placebo and the 50 μg/kg groups.
A second study evaluated the effectiveness of Neumega in eliminating platelet transfusions over two dose-intensive chemotherapy cycles in breast cancer patients who had not previously experienced severe chemotherapy-induced thrombocytopenia. All patients received the same chemotherapy regimen (cyclophosphamide 3,200 mg/m^2 and doxorubicin 75 mg/m^2). All patients received concomitant Filgrastim (G-CSF) in all cycles. The patients were stratified by whether or not they had received prior chemotherapy, and randomized to receive Neumega 50 μg/kg or placebo. The primary endpoint was whether or not a patient required one or more platelet transfusions in the two study cycles. Seventy-seven patients were randomized. Thirteen patients failed to complete both study cycles—eight of these had insufficient data to be evaluated for the primary endpoint. The results of this trial are summarized in Table 2.
[See table at top of next page]
This study showed a trend in favor of Neumega, particularly in the subgroup of patients with prior chemotherapy. Open-label treatment with Neumega has been continued for up to four consecutive chemotherapy cycles without evidence of any adverse effect on the rate of neutrophil recovery or red blood cell transfusion requirements. Some patients continued to maintain platelet nadirs >20,000 cells/μL for at least four sequential cycles of chemotherapy without the need for transfusions, chemotherapy dose reduction, or changes in treatment schedules.
Platelet activation studies done on a limited number of patients showed no evidence of abnormal spontaneous platelet activation, or an abnormal response to ADP. In an unblinded, retrospective analysis of the two placebo-controlled studies, 19 of 69 patients (28%) receiving Neumega 50 μg/kg and 34 of 67 patients (51%) receiving placebo reported at least one hemorrhagic adverse event which involved bleeding.
In a randomized, double-blind, placebo-controlled, phase 2 study conducted in patients who received autologous bone marrow transplantation following myeloablative chemotherapy, the incidence of platelet transfusions and time to neutrophil and platelet engraftment were similar in the Neumega and placebo-treated arms.
In long term follow-up of patients, the distribution of survival and progression-free survival times was similar between patients randomized to Neumega therapy and those randomized to receive placebo.

INDICATIONS AND USAGE

Neumega is indicated for the prevention of severe thrombocytopenia and the reduction of the need for platelet transfusions following myelosuppressive chemotherapy in patients with nonmyeloid malignancies who are at high risk of severe thrombocytopenia. Efficacy was demonstrated in patients who had experienced severe thrombocytopenia following the previous chemotherapy cycle. Neumega is not indicated following myeloablative chemotherapy.

CONTRAINDICATIONS

Neumega is contraindicated in patients with a history of hypersensitivity to Neumega or any component of the product.

WARNINGS

Neumega is known to cause fluid retention (see CLINICAL PHARMACOLOGY: Pharmacodynamics), and it should be used with caution in patients with clinically evident congestive heart failure, patients who may be susceptible to developing congestive heart failure, and patients with a history of heart failure who are well-compensated and receiving appropriate medical therapy (see PRECAUTIONS: Fluid Retention).
Close monitoring of fluid and electrolyte status should be performed in patients receiving chronic diuretic therapy. Sudden deaths have occurred in Oprelvekin-treated patients receiving chronic diuretic therapy and ifosfamide who developed severe hypokalemia (see ADVERSE REACTIONS).

PRECAUTIONS

General

Dosing with Neumega should begin 6 to 24 hours following the completion of chemotherapy dosing. The safety and efficacy of Neumega given immediately prior to or concurrently with cytotoxic chemotherapy have not been established (see DOSAGE AND ADMINISTRATION).

Continued on next page

Neumega—Cont.

Neumega has not been evaluated in patients receiving chemotherapy regimens of greater than 5 days duration or regimens associated with delayed myelosuppression (e.g., nitrosoureas, mitomycin-C).

The parenteral administration of Neumega should be attended by appropriate precautions in case allergic reactions occur (see CONTRAINDICATIONS).

Fluid Retention

Patients receiving Neumega have commonly experienced mild to moderate fluid retention as indicated by peripheral edema or dyspnea on exertion. Weight gain has been uncommon. The fluid retention is reversible within several days following discontinuation of Neumega. In some patients, preexisting pleural effusions have increased during administration of Neumega. Preexisting fluid collections, including pericardial effusions or ascites, should be monitored. Drainage should be considered if medically indicated. Capillary leak syndrome has not been observed following treatment with Neumega.

Moderate decreases in hemoglobin concentration, hematocrit, and red blood cell count (~10–15%) without a decrease in red blood cell mass have been observed. These changes are predominantly due to an increase in plasma volume (dilutional anemia) that is primarily related to renal sodium and water retention. The decrease in hemoglobin concentration typically begins within 3–5 days of the initiation of Neumega, and is reversible over approximately a week following discontinuation of Neumega.

During dosing with Neumega, fluid balance should be monitored and appropriate medical management is advised. If a diuretic is used, fluid and electrolyte balance should be carefully monitored. Neumega should be used with caution in patients who may develop fluid retention as a result of associated medical conditions or whose medical condition may be exacerbated by fluid retention.

Cardiovascular Events

Neumega should be used with caution in patients with a history of atrial arrhythmia, and only after consideration of the potential risks in relation to anticipated benefit. Transient atrial arrhythmias (atrial fibrillation or atrial flutter) have occurred in approximately 10% of patients following treatment with Neumega. In some patients this may be due to increased plasma volume associated with fluid retention (See PRECAUTIONS: Fluid Retention); Neumega has been shown not to be directly arrhythmogenic. Arrhythmias have usually been brief in duration and usually without clinical sequelae; however sequelae including stroke have been observed in patients receiving Neumega who experienced atrial arrhythmias. Conversion to sinus rhythm typically occurred spontaneously or after rate-control drug therapy. Most patients have continued to receive Neumega without recurrence of atrial arrhythmia. A retrospective analysis of data from clinical studies of Neumega suggests that advancing age and other conditions associated with an increased risk of atrial arrhythmias such as use of cardiac medications and a history of doxorubicin exposure are risk factors for the development of atrial fibrillation or atrial flutter in patients receiving Neumega. Ventricular arrhythmias have not been attributed to the use of Neumega.

Ophthalmologic Events

Transient, mild visual blurring has occasionally been reported by patients treated with Neumega. Papilledema has been reported in approximately 1.5% of patients treated with Neumega following repeated cycles of exposure. Nonhuman primates treated with Neumega at a dose of 1,000 µg/kg SC once daily for 4 to 13 weeks developed papilledema which was not associated with inflammation or any other histologic abnormality and was reversible after dosing was discontinued. Neumega should be used with caution in patients with preexisting papilledema, or with tumors involving the central nervous system since it is possible that papilledema could worsen or develop during treatment.

Antibody Formation/Allergic Reactions

A small proportion (1%) of patients receiving Neumega in clinical studies developed antibodies to Oprelvekin and transient rashes were occasionally observed at the injection site following Neumega administration. The presence of these antibodies or injection site reactions have not been correlated with clinical symptoms such as anaphylactoid reactions or a loss of clinical response to Neumega. No anaphylactoid or other severe adverse allergic reactions were reported in clinical studies following single or repeated doses of Neumega.

Chronic Administration

Neumega has been administered safely using the recommended dosing schedule (see DOSAGE AND ADMINISTRATION) for up to 6 cycles following chemotherapy. The safety and efficacy of chronic administration of Neumega have not been established. Continuous dosing (2–13 weeks) in nonhuman primates produced joint capsule and tendon fibrosis and periosteal hyperostosis (see PRECAUTIONS: Pediatric Use). The relevance of these findings to humans is unclear.

TABLE 2
STUDY RESULTS

	Overall n=77		No Prior Chemotherapy n=54		Prior Chemotherapy n=23	
	Placebo n=37	Neumega n=40	Placebo n=27	Neumega n=27	Placebo n=10	Neumega n=13
Number (%) of patients avoiding platelet transfusion	15 (41%)	26 (65%)	14 (52%)	19 (70%)	1 (10%)	7 (54%)
Number (%) of patients requiring platelet transfusion	16 (43%)	12 (30%)	9 (33%)	7 (26%)	7 (70%)	5 (38%)
Number (%) of patients not evaluable	6 (16%)	2 (5%)	4 (15%)	1 (4%)	2 (20%)	1 (8%)

Information for Patients

In situations when the physician determines that Neumega may be used outside of the hospital or office setting, persons who will be administering Neumega should be instructed as to the proper dose, and the method for reconstituting and administering Neumega (See DOSAGE AND ADMINISTRATION and Patient Information at the end of this insert). If home use is prescribed, patients should be instructed in the importance of proper disposal and cautioned against the reuse of needles, syringes, drug product, and diluent. A puncture resistant container should be used by the patient for the disposal of used needles.

Patients should be informed of the most common adverse reactions associated with Neumega administration, including those symptoms related to fluid retention (see ADVERSE REACTIONS and PRECAUTIONS). Mild to moderate peripheral edema and shortness of breath on exertion can occur within the first week of treatment and may continue for the duration of administration of Neumega. Patients who have preexisting pleural or other effusions or a history of congestive heart failure should be advised to contact their physician for worsening of dyspnea. Most patients who receive Neumega develop some anemia. Patients who are older or who have other risk factors for the development of atrial arrhythmias should be cautioned to contact their physician if symptoms attributable to atrial arrhythmia develop and are not transient. Female patients of childbearing potential should be advised of the possible risks to the fetus of Neumega (see PRECAUTIONS: Pregnancy).

Laboratory Monitoring

A complete blood count should be obtained prior to chemotherapy and at regular intervals during Neumega therapy (see DOSAGE AND ADMINISTRATION). Platelet counts should be monitored during the time of the expected nadir and until adequate recovery has occurred (post-nadir counts ≥50,000).

Drug Interactions

Most patients in trials evaluating Neumega were treated concomitantly with Filgrastim (granulocyte colony-stimulating factor[G-CSF]) with no adverse effect of Neumega on the activity of G-CSF. No information is available on the clinical use of Sargramostim (granulocyte-macrophage colony-stimulating factor [GM-CSF]) with Neumega. However, in a study in nonhuman primates in which Neumega and GM-CSF were coadministered, there were no adverse interactions between Neumega and GM-CSF and no apparent difference in the pharmacokinetic profile of Neumega.

Drug interactions between Neumega and other drugs have not been fully evaluated. Based on in vitro and nonclinical in vivo evaluations of Neumega, drug-drug interactions with known substrates of P450 enzymes would not be predicted.

Carcinogenesis, Mutagenesis, Impairment of Fertility

No studies have been performed to assess the carcinogenic potential of Neumega. In vitro, Neumega did not stimulate the growth of tumor colony-forming cells harvested from patients with a variety of human malignancies. Neumega has been shown to be non-genotoxic in in vitro studies. These data suggest that Neumega is not mutagenic. Although prolonged estrus cycles have been noted at 2 to 20 times the human dose, no effects on fertility have been observed in rats treated with Neumega at doses up to 1000 µg/kg/day.

Pregnancy Category C

Neumega has been shown to have embryocidal effects in pregnant rats and rabbits when given in doses of 0.2 to 20 times the human dose. There are no adequate and well-controlled studies of Neumega in pregnant women. Neumega should be used during pregnancy only if the potential benefit justifies the potential risk to the fetus.

Neumega has been tested in studies of fertility and early embryonic development in rats and in studies of organogenesis (teratogenicity) in rats and rabbits. Parental toxicity has been observed when Neumega is given at doses of 2 to 20 times the human dose (≥100 µg/kg/day) in the rat and when given in doses of 0.02 to 2.0 times the human dose (≥1 µg/kg/day) in the rabbit. Findings in the rat consisted of transient hypoactivity and dyspnea after administration, as well as prolonged estrus cycle, increased early embryonic deaths and decreased numbers of live fetuses. In addition, low fetal body weights and a reduced number of ossified sacral and caudal vertebrae (i.e., retarded fetal development) occurred in rats at 20 times the human dose, but no long-term behavioral or developmental abnormalities were evident. Findings in the rabbits consisted of decreased (fecal/urine) eliminations (the only toxicity noted at 1 µg/kg/day) as well as decreased food consumption, body weight loss, abortion, increased embryonic and fetal deaths, and decreased numbers of live fetuses. There have been no teratogenic effects of Neumega observed in rabbits.

Nursing Mothers

It is not known if Neumega is excreted in human milk. Because many drugs are excreted in human milk and because of the potential for serious adverse reactions in nursing infants from Neumega, a decision should be made whether to discontinue nursing or to discontinue the drug, taking into account the importance of the drug to the mother.

Pediatric Use

Efficacy trials have not been conducted in a pediatric population. Preliminary data are available from an ongoing pharmacokinetic study in twenty-eight patients ages 8 months to 17 years who have been treated with Neumega at doses of 25 to 100 µg/kg following ICE (ifosfamide, etoposide, carboplatin) chemotherapy. Neumega treatment was given once daily for a maximum of 28 days in up to eight cycles. Based upon this study, a dose of 75 to 100 µg/kg in the pediatric population will produce plasma levels consistent with those obtained in adults given 50 µg/kg (see CLINICAL PHARAMACOLOGY: Pharmacokinetics).

Adverse events in this pediatric open-label, non-comparative study were generally similar to those observed using Neumega at a dose of 50 µg/kg in the randomized chemotherapy studies in adults. Most adverse events that were associated with Neumega in adults occurred either with similar or lower frequency in the pediatric study compared with adults. The incidences of tachycardia (46% [13/28]) and conjunctival injection (50% [14/28]) in the pediatric study were higher than in adults (see ADVERSE REACTIONS). There was no evidence of a dose-response relationship for any of the Neumega-associated adverse events among the pediatric patients.

No studies have been performed to assess the long-term effects of Neumega on growth and development. In growing rodents treated with 100, 300, or 1000 µg/kg/day for a minimum of 28 days, thickening of femoral and tibial growth plates was noted, which did not completely resolve after a 28-day non-treatment period. In a nonhuman primate toxicology study of Neumega, animals treated for 2 to 13 weeks at doses of 10 to 1000 µg/kg showed partially reversible joint capsule and tendon fibrosis and periosteal hyperostosis. The clinical significance of these findings is not known. An asymptomatic, laminated periosteal reaction in the diaphyses of the femur, tibia and fibula has been observed in one patient during pediatric trials involving multiple courses of Neumega treatment. The relationship of these findings to treatment with Neumega is unclear.

Use in Patients with Renal Impairment

Neumega is eliminated primarily by the kidneys. The pharmacokinetics of Neumega have not been studied in patients with mild or moderate renal impairment (creatinine clearance ≥ 15 mL/min). Fluid retention associated with Neumega treatment has not been studied in patients with renal impairment, but fluid balance should be carefully monitored in these patients (See PRECAUTIONS: Fluid Retention).

ADVERSE REACTIONS

Three hundred eight subjects, with ages ranging from 8 months to 75 years, have been exposed to Neumega treatment. Subjects have received up to six (eight in pediatric patients) sequential courses of Neumega treatment, with each course lasting from 1 to 28 days. Apart from the sequelae of the underlying malignancy or cytotoxic chemotherapy, most adverse events were mild or moderate in severity and reversible after discontinuation of Neumega dosing.

In general, the incidence and type of adverse events were similar between Neumega 50 µg/kg and placebo groups. The following adverse events, occurring in ≥10% of patients, were observed at equal or greater frequency in placebo-treated patients: asthenia, pain, chills, abdominal pain, infection, anorexia, constipation, dyspepsia, ecchymosis, my-

TABLE 3
SELECTED ADVERSE EVENTS

Body System Adverse Event	Placebo n=67	(%)	50 µg/kg n=69	(%)
Body as a Whole				
Edema*	10	(15)	41	(59)
Neutropenic fever	28	(42)	33	(48)
Headache	24	(36)	28	(41)
Fever	19	(28)	25	(36)
Cardiovascular System				
Tachycardia*	2	(3)	14	(20)
Vasodilatation	6	(9)	13	(19)
Palpitations*	2	(3)	10	(14)
Syncope	4	(6)	9	(13)
Atrial fibrillation/flutter*	1	(1)	8	(12)
Digestive System				
Nausea/vomiting	47	(70)	53	(77)
Mucositis	25	(37)	30	(43)
Diarrhea	22	(33)	30	(43)
Oral moniliasis*	1	(1)	10	(14)
Nervous System				
Dizziness	19	(28)	26	(38)
Insomnia	18	(27)	23	(33)
Respiratory System				
Dyspnea*	15	(22)	33	(48)
Rhinitis	21	(31)	29	(42)
Cough increased	15	(22)	20	(29)
Pharyngitis	11	(16)	17	(25)
Pleural effusions*	0	(0)	7	(10)
Skin and Appendages				
Rash	11	(16)	17	(25)
Special Senses				
Conjunctival injection*	2	(3)	13	(19)

*Occurred in significantly more Neumega-treated patients than in placebo-treated patients.

algia, bone pain, nervousness, and alopecia. Selected adverse events that occurred in Neumega-treated patients are listed in Table 3.

[See table above]

The following adverse events also occurred more frequently in cancer patients receiving Neumega than in those receiving placebo: amblyopia, paresthesia, dehydration, skin discoloration, exfoliative dermatitis, and eye hemorrhage; a statistically significant association of Neumega to these events has not been established. Other than a higher incidence of severe asthenia in Neumega treated patients (10 [14%] in Neumega patients versus 2 [3%] in placebo patients), the incidence of severe or life-threatening adverse events was comparable in the Neumega and placebo treatment groups.

The incidence of fever, neutropenic fever, flu-like symptoms, thrombocytosis, thrombotic events, the average number of units of red blood cells transfused per patient, and the duration of neutropenia <500 cells/µL were similar in the Neumega 50 µg/kg and placebo groups.

Two patients with cancer treated with Neumega experienced sudden death which the investigator considered possibly or probably related to Neumega. Both deaths occurred in patients with severe hypokalemia (<3.0 mEq/L) who had received high doses of ifosfamide and were receiving daily doses of a diuretic. The relationship of these deaths to Neumega remains unclear.

Abnormal Laboratory Values

The most common laboratory abnormality reported in patients in clinical trials was a decrease in hemoglobin concentration predominantly as a result of expansion of the plasma volume (see PRECAUTIONS: Fluid Retention). The increase in plasma volume is also associated with a decrease in the serum concentration of albumin and several other proteins (e.g., transferrin and gamma globulins). A parallel decrease in calcium without clinical effects has been documented.

After daily SC injections, treatment with Neumega resulted in a two-fold increase in plasma fibrinogen. Other acute-phase proteins also increased. These protein levels returned to normal after dosing with Neumega was discontinued. Von Willebrand factor (vWF) concentrations increased with a normal multimer pattern in healthy subjects receiving Neumega.

OVERDOSAGE

Doses of Neumega above 100 µg/kg have not been administered to humans. While clinical experience is limited, doses of Neumega greater than 50 µg/kg may be associated with an increased incidence of cardiovascular events in adult patients (see PRECAUTIONS: Fluid Retention/Cardiovascular). If an overdose of Neumega is administered. Neumega should be discontinued, and the patient should be closely observed for signs of toxicity (see PRECAUTIONS and ADVERSE REACTIONS). Reinstitution of Neumega therapy should be based upon individual patient factors (e.g., evidence of toxicity, continued need for therapy).

DOSAGE AND ADMINISTRATION

The recommended dose of Neumega in adults is 50 µg/kg given once daily. Neumega should be administered subcutaneously as a single injection in either the abdomen, thigh, or hip (or upper arm if not self-injecting). Based upon a pharmacokinetic study, a dose of 75 to 100 µg/kg in the pediatric population will produce plasma levels consistent with those obtained in adults given 50 µg/kg (see CLINICAL PHARMACOLOGY: Pharmacokinetics).

Dosing should be initiated 6 to 24 hours after the completion of chemotherapy. Platelet counts should be monitored periodically to assess the optimal duration of therapy. Dosing should be continued until the post-nadir platelet count is ≥50,000 cells/µL. In controlled clinical studies, doses were administered in courses of 10 to 21 days. Dosing beyond 21 days per treatment course is not recommended. Treatment with Neumega should be discontinued at least 2 days before starting the next planned cycle of chemotherapy.

Preparation of Neumega

1. Neumega is a sterile, white, preservative-free, lyophilized powder for subcutaneous injection upon reconstitution. Neumega (5 mg vials) should be reconstituted aseptically with 1.0 mL of Sterile Water for Injection, USP (without preservative). The reconstituted Neumega solution is clear, colorless, isotonic, with a pH of 7.0, and contains 5 mg/mL of Neumega. The single-use vial should not be re-entered or reused. Any unused portion of either reconstituted Neumega solution or Sterile Water for Injection, USP should be discarded.

2. During reconstitution, the Sterile Water for Injection, USP should be directed at the side of the vial and the contents gently swirled. EXCESSIVE OR VIGOROUS AGITATION SHOULD BE AVOIDED.

3. Parenteral drug products should be inspected visually for particulate matter and discoloration prior to administration, whenever solution and container permit. If particulate matter is present or the solution is discolored, the vial should not be used.

4. Because neither Neumega powder for injection nor its accompanying diluent, Sterile Water for Injection, USP contains a preservative, Neumega should be used as soon as possible following reconstitution. Neumega may be used within 3 hours of reconstitution when stored either at 2 to 8°C (36 to 46°F) or at room temperature up to 25°C (77°F). DO NOT FREEZE OR SHAKE THE RECONSTITUTED SOLUTION.

HOW SUPPLIED

Neumega is supplied as a sterile, white, preservative-free, lyophilize powder in vials containing 5 mg Oprelvekin. Neumega is available in boxes containing one single-dose Neumega vial and one 5-mL vial of diluent for Neumega (Sterile Water for Injection, USP) – NDC 58394-004-01; and boxes containing seven single-dose Neumega vials and seven 5-mL vials of diluent for Neumega (Sterile Water for Injection, USP) – NDC 58394-004-02.

Storage

Lyophilized Neumega and diluent should be stored in a refrigerator at 2 to 8°C (36 to 46°F). DO NOT FREEZE. Reconstituted Neumega must be used within 3 hours of reconstitution and can be stored in the vial either at 2 to 8°C (36 to 46°F) or at room temperature up to 25°C (77°F).

REFERENCES

(1) Du, X, and Williams, D., Interleukin 11: Review of Molecular, Cell Biology and Clinical Use. Blood. 89(11): 3897-3908, 1997.

GENETICS INSTITUTE

Genetics Institute, Inc.
Cambridge, MA 02140-2387, USA
US License Number 1163
Telephone: 1-888-446-3344
IL1131.00 Rev. 12/97

NEUMEGA®

(Oprelvekin)

PATIENT INFORMATION

General Information

Neumega is intended for use under the guidance and supervision of a health care professional. If, however, your physician recommends self-injection, you should be instructed in the preparation of Neumega, the proper method for self-injection, and the correct dose to use. You should not try self-administration until you are certain that you understand your health care professional's instructions. Each dose should be given at about the same time each day. If you miss a dose, continue with the next scheduled dose.

Possible Side Effects

As with any medication, use of Neumega may be associated with side effects. In clinical studies, these effects were generally mild or moderate and stopped after treatment. The most common side effects seen in studies of Neumega were edema (swelling) of the arms and/or legs, shortness of breath when moving about, and anemia. These side effects are probably related to water retention. Edema and shortness of breath on exertion can occur within the first week of treatment and may continue for the duration of administration of Neumega. It is also possible that you may experience irregular heartbeats. If you experience chest pain, shortness of breath, fatigue, blurred vision, or an irregular pulse that persists, contact your physician. If you have any other problems, whether or not you think they are related to Neumega, you should tell your doctor.

If you are a woman of child-bearing potential, you should be aware that use of Neumega poses possible risks of the fetus. If you become pregnant or wish to become pregnant during treatment with Neumega, consult your physician about continuing to use Neumega.

Dosage and Administration

The Neumega vial contains a powder which must be reconstituted prior to injection in 1 mL of Sterile Water for Injection, USP provided with Neumega. Powdered Neumega and Sterile Water for Injection, USP should be stored in a refrigerator at 2 to 8°C (36 to 46°F). DO NOT FREEZE.

A new vial of Neumega and Sterile Water for Injection, USP should be used to prepare each dose. Do not use Neumega or Sterile Water for Injection, USP beyond the expiration date printed on the vial. Any unused portion of reconstituted Neumega medication or Sterile Water for Injection, USP remaining in the vial should be discarded. Because neither Neumega powder for injection nor its accompanying Sterile Water for Injection, USP contain a preservative, the single-use vials should not be reentered or reused.

Neumega should be used as soon as possible following reconstitution and must be used within 3 hours of reconstitution. The reconstituted Neumega solution can be stored in the vial for up to 3 hours either at room temperature up to 25°C (77°F), or in the refrigerator at 2 to 8°C (36 to 46°F) THE RECONSTITUTED SOLUTION SHOULD NOT BE STORED IN A SYRINGE.

NOTE: Follow aseptic technique in reconstitution and administration as demonstrated by the health care professional.

Reconstituting Neumega

1. Have all supplies (four sterile alcohol swabs, syringe, needle, Neumega vial, and "Sterile Water for Injection, USP") available before starting procedure. Wash hands thoroughly with soap and water before preparing the medication.

2. Flip off the protective cap from the vial labeled "Sterile Water for Injection, USP" and the vial labeled "Neumega." Wipe the top of each vial with a sterile alcohol swab, using a different swab for each vial. Leave the swabs on top of the vials.

3. Remove syringe and needle from sterile packaging. Attach needle to syringe (if needle is not already attached). Remove protective cover from the tip of the syringe. Do not touch the needle with your hand or allow it to come in contact with other surfaces.

Continued on next page

Neumega—Cont.

4. Pull the plunger of the syringe back to the 1.2 mL mark.
5. Remove the alcohol swab from the top of vial labeled "Sterile Water for Injection, USP." Keep the vial upright and push the needle through the center of the rubber stopper. Inject the air from the syringe into the vial.

6. Keep the needle in the vial and gently turn the vial with the needle in it upside down. Withdraw 1.0 mL of Sterile Water for Injection, USP by slowly pulling back on the plunger. Make sure that the tip of the needle remains in the fluid at all times.

7. Remove syringe from the vial of Sterile Water for Injection, USP. Discard used vial. Remove the alcohol swab from the Neumega vial. Keep the vial of Neumega upright and push the needle of the syringe containing Sterile Water for Injection, USP through the center of the rubber stopper. Press the plunger of the syringe SLOWLY. Direct the stream of Sterile Water down the inside wall of the vial.

Without removing the syringe, **GENTLY** swirl the vial until the powder is dissolved.

DO NOT SHAKE THE VIAL. (Shaking will cause foaming.) Once mixed, the solution should be colorless and clear of any particles. **DO NOT** inject if any cloudiness or particles are seen.

8. Turn the vial and syringe upside down. Keep needle tip in the solution and slowly pull back on the plunger to fill the syringe to the mark specified for the dosage being administered. If bubbles appear in the syringe, push bubbles back into the vial. Withdraw additional medication to specified mark.

9. Withdraw needle from vial. Hold syringe and needle straight up and lightly tap the side of the syringe to bring any air bubbles to the top.
10. Hold syringe upright and press plunger slightly to push air out through the needle. A small amount of solution may exit the syringe. This will ensure that all air is removed from the syringe.

Injecting Neumega

1. Identify the area on the abdomen, thigh, or hip (or upper arm if not self-injecting). Select a different site each time Neumega is injected. This will help avoid soreness in one area.

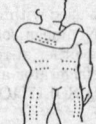

2. Cleanse the skin where the injection is to be made with an alcohol swab. Hold the syringe "like a dart" between the thumb and first finger close to the syringe/needle connection.
3. With the other hand, pinch about an inch of skin between thumb and forefinger, forming a bulge in the skin at the injection site.
4. Insert the needle quickly into the skin at a 45 degree angle. Release pinched skin.

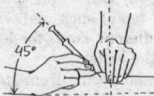

5. GENTLY pull back on the syringe plunger. If blood comes into the syringe, do not inject. Withdraw the needle from skin and inject at a different cleaned site.
6. Inject Neumega by slowly pushing the plunger all the way down in one continuous motion.

---

7. Hold a new alcohol swab near the needle and pull the needle straight out of the skin. Press the alcohol swab over the injection site for several seconds. DO NOT RUB SITE.
8. DO NOT RECAP NEEDLE. Immediately after use discard used syringe and needle into "Sharps Container."
Genetics Institute, Inc.
Rev. 12/97   Cambridge, MA 02140-2387, USA
Shown in Product Identification Guide, page 311

Geneva Pharmaceuticals, Inc.
2655 WEST MIDWAY BLVD.
P.O. BOX 446
BROOMFIELD, CO 80038-0446

Direct Inquiries to:
Customer Support Department
(800) 525-8747
(303) 466-2400
FAX: (303) 469-6467

GENEVA PHARMACEUTICALS

NDC # 00781-	Product/Strength	Rx	OTC
1671	Albuterol Tablets USP 2mg	Rx	
1672	Albuterol Tablets USP 4mg	Rx	
1061	Alprazolam Tablets USP .25mg	Rx Cᴵⱽ	
1077	Alprazolam Tablets USP .50mg	Rx Cᴵⱽ	
1079	Alprazolam Tablets USP 1.0mg	Rx Cᴵⱽ	
1089	Alprazolam Tablets USP 2.0 mg	Rx Cᴵⱽ	
1486	Amitriptyline HCl Tablets USP 10mg	Rx	
1487	Amitriptyline HCl Tablets USP 25mg	Rx	
1488	Amitriptyline HCl Tablets USP 50mg	Rx	
1489	Amitriptyline HCl Tablets USP 75mg	Rx	
1490	Amitriptyline HCl Tablets USP 100mg	Rx	
1491	Amitriptyline HCl Tablets USP 150mg	Rx	
1844	Amoxapine Tablets USP 25mg	Rx	
1845	Amoxapine Tablets USP 50mg	Rx	
1846	Amoxapine Tablets USP 100mg	Rx	
1847	Amoxapine Tablets USP 150mg	Rx	
1078	Atenolol Tablets USP 25mg	Rx	
1506	Atenolol Tablets USP 50mg	Rx	
1507	Atenolol Tablets USP 100mg	Rx	
1817	Bromocriptine Mesylate Tablets USP 2.5mg		
1828	Captopril Tablets USP 12.5mg	Rx	
1829	Captopril Tablets USP 25mg	Rx	
1838	Captopril Tablets USP 50mg	Rx	
1839	Captopril Tablets USP 100mg	Rx	
1050	Carisoprodol Tablets USP 350mg	Rx	
1715	Chlorpromazine HCl Tablets USP 10mg	Rx	
1716	Chlorpromazine HCl Tablets USP 25mg	Rx	
1717	Chlorpromazine HCl Tablets USP 50mg	Rx	
1718	Chlorpromazine HCl Tablets USP 100mg	Rx	
1719	Chlorpromazine HCl Tablets USP 200mg	Rx	
1447	Cimetidine Tablets USP 200mg	Rx	
1448	Cimetidine Tablets USP 300mg	Rx	
1449	Cimetidine Tablets USP 400mg	Rx	
1444	Cimetidine Tablets USP 800mg	Rx	
1358	Clemastine Fumarate Tablets USP 1.34mg		OTC
1359	Clemastine Fumarate Tablets USP 2.68mg	Rx	
6131	Clemastine Fumarate Syrup .5mg/5ml	Rx	
2027	Clomipramine HCl Capsules 25mg	Rx	
2037	Clomipramine HCl Capsules 50mg	Rx	
2047	Clomipramine HCl Capsules 75mg	Rx	
1324	Cyclobenzaprine HCl Tablets USP 10mg	Rx	
1971	Desipramine HCl Tablets USP 10mg	Rx	
1972	Desipramine HCl Tablets USP 25mg	Rx	
1973	Desipramine HCl Tablets USP 50mg	Rx	
1974	Desipramine HCl Tablets USP 75mg	Rx	
1975	Desipramine HCl Tablets USP 100mg	Rx	
1976	Desipramine HCl Tablets USP 150mg	Rx	
1785	Diclofenac Sodium Delayed-Release Tablets 25mg		
1787	Diclofenac Sodium Delayed-Release Tablets 50mg	Rx	
1789	Diclofenac Sodium Delayed-Release Tablets 75mg		
1600	Disobrom®	Rx	
2800	Doxepin HCl Capsules USP 10mg	Rx	
2801	Doxepin HCl Capsules USP 25mg	Rx	
1995	Ercaf (Ergotamine Tartrate and Caffeine Tablets USP)	Rx	
1234	Etodolac Tablets 400mg	Rx	
1918	Fiorpap Tablets (Butalbital/APAP/ Caffeine) Tablets USP 50/325/40mg	Rx Cᴵᴵᴵ	
2120	Fiortal (Butalbital/Aspirin/Caffeine Capsules USP 50/325/40mg)	Rx Cᴵᴵᴵ	
2221	Fiortal with Codeine (Butalbital/Aspirin/caffeine/Codeine) Capsules USP 50/325/40/30mg	Rx Cᴵᴵᴵ	

NDC # 00781-	Product/Strength	Rx	OTC
1129	Flurbiprofen Tablets 100mg	Rx	
1436	Fluphenazine HCl Tablets USP 1mg	Rx	
1437	Fluphenazine HCl Tablets USP 2.5mg	Rx	
1438	Fluphenazine HCl Tablets USP 5mg	Rx	
1439	Fluphenazine HCl Tablets USP 10mg	Rx	
1818	Furosemide Tablets USP 20mg	Rx	
1966	Furosemide Tablets USP 40mg	Rx	
1446	Furosemide Tablets USP 80mg	Rx	
1452	Glipizide Tablets USP 5mg	Rx	
1453	Glipizide Tablets USP 10mg	Rx	
1391	Haloperidol Tablets USP 0.5mg	Rx	
1392	Haloperidol Tablets USP 1mg	Rx	
1393	Haloperidol Tablets USP 2mg	Rx	
1396	Haloperidol Tablets USP 5mg	Rx	
1397	Haloperidol Tablets USP 10mg	Rx	
1398	Haloperidol Tablets USP 20mg	Rx	
1407	Hydroxychloroquine Sulfate Tablets USP 200mg	Rx	
1762	Imipramine HCl Tablets USP 10mg	Rx	
1764	Imipramine HCl Tablets USP 25mg	Rx	
1766	Imipramine HCl Tablets USP 50mg	Rx	
2325	Indomethacin Capsules USP 25mg	Rx	
2350	Indomethacin Capsules USP 50mg	Rx	
1635	Isosorbide Dinitrate Tablets USP 5mg	Rx	
1556	Isosorbide Dinitrate Tablets USP 10mg	Rx	
1695	Isosorbide Dinitrate Tablets USP 20mg	Rx	
1840	Isoxsuprine HCl Tablets USP 10mg	Rx	
1842	Isoxsuprine HCl Tablets USP 20mg	Rx	
2410	Ketoprofen Capsules 50mg	Rx	
1262	Lonox Tablets 2.5mg/0.025mg (Diphenoxylate HCl and Atropine Sulfate Tablets USP)	Rx Cᵛ	
2761	Loperamide HCl Capsules USP 2mg	Rx Cᵛ	
1403	Lorazepam Tablets USP 0.5mg	Rx Cᴵⱽ	
1404	Lorazepam Tablets USP 1.0mg	Rx Cᴵⱽ	
1405	Lorazepam Tablets USP 2.0mg	Rx Cᴵⱽ	
1345	Meclizine HCl Tablets USP 12.5mg		OTC
1375	Meclizine HCl Tablets USP 25mg		OTC
1542	Meclizine HCl Tablets USP 12.5mg	Rx	
1544	Meclizine HCl Tablets USP 25mg	Rx	
1072	Methazolamide Tablets USP 25mg	Rx	
1071	Methazolamide Tablets USP 50mg	Rx	
1760	Methocarbamol Tablets USP 500mg	Rx	
1750	Methocarbamol Tablets USP 750mg	Rx	
1223	Metoprolol Tartrate Tablets USP 50mg	Rx	
1228	Metoprolol Tartrate Tablets USP 100mg	Rx	
2130	Mexiletine HCl Capsules USP 150mg	Rx	
2131	Mexiletine HCl Capsules USP 200mg	Rx	
2132	Mexiletine HCl Capsules USP 250mg	Rx	
1163	Naproxen Tablets USP 250mg	Rx	
1164	Naproxen Tablets USP 375mg	Rx	
1165	Naproxen Tablets USP 500mg	Rx	
1187	Naproxen Sodium Tablets USP 275mg	Rx	
1188	Naproxen Sodium Tablets USP 550mg	Rx	
2630	Nortriptyline HCl Capsules USP 10mg	Rx	
2631	Nortriptyline HCl Capsules USP 25mg	Rx	
2632	Nortriptyline HCl Capsules USP 50mg	Rx	
2633	Nortriptyline HCl Capsules USP 75mg	Rx	
2809	Oxazepam Capsules USP 10mg	Rx Cᴵⱽ	
2810	Oxazepam Capsules USP 15mg	Rx Cᴵⱽ	
2811	Oxazepam Capsules USP 30mg	Rx Cᴵⱽ	
1265	Perphenazine and Amitriptyline HCl Tablets USP 2mg/10mg	Rx	
1266	Perphenazine and Amitriptyline HCl Tablets USP 4mg/10mg	Rx	
1267	Perphenazine and Amitriptyline HCl Tablets USP 4mg/25mg	Rx	
1268	Perphenazine and Amitriptyline HCl Tablets USP 4mg/50mg	Rx	
1273	Perphenazine and Amitriptyline HCl Tablets USP 2mg/25mg	Rx	
1046	Perphenazine Tablets USP 2mg	Rx	
1047	Perphenazine Tablets USP 4mg	Rx	
1048	Perphenazine Tablets USP 8mg	Rx	
1049	Perphenazine Tablets USP 16mg	Rx	
1168	Pindolol Tablets 5mg USP	Rx	
1169	Pindolol Tablets 10mg USP	Rx	
1830	Promethazine HCl Tablets USP 25mg	Rx	
1832	Promethazine HCl Tablets USP 50mg	Rx	
1378	Propoxyphene HCl and Acetaminophen Tablets USP 65mg/650mg	Rx Cᴵⱽ	
1720	Propoxyphene Napsylate and Acetaminophen Tablets USP 100mg/650mg	Rx Cᴵⱽ	
1533	Pseudoephedrine HCl Tablets USP 30mg		OTC
1535	Pseudoephedrine HCl Tablets USP 60mg		OTC
1804	Quinidine Gluconate Extended-Release Tablets USP 324mg	Rx	
1883	Ranitidine HCl Tablets USP 150mg	Rx	
1884	Ranitidine HCl Tablets USP 300mg	Rx	
2855	Ranitidine HCl Capsules USP 150mg	Rx	
2865	Ranitidine HCl Capsules USP 300mg	Rx	
2018	Rimactane® Capsules 300mg	Rx	
1599	Spironolactone Tablets USP 25mg	Rx	
1811	Sulindac Tablets USP 150mg	Rx	
1812	Sulindac Tablets USP 200mg	Rx	
2209	Temazepam Capsules USP 7.5mg	Rx Cᴵⱽ	

2201	Temazepam Capsules USP 15mg	℞ C-IV
2202	Temazepam Capsules USP 30mg	℞ C-IV
1604	Thioridazine HCl Tablets USP 10mg	℞
1614	Thioridazine HCl Tablets USP 15mg	℞
1624	Thioridazine HCl Tablets USP 25mg	℞
1634	Thioridazine HCl Tablets USP 50mg	℞
1644	Thioridazine HCl Tablets USP 100mg	℞
1664	Thioridazine HCl Tablets USP 150mg	℞
1674	Thioridazine HCl Tablets USP 200mg	℞
2226	Thiothixene Capsules USP 1mg	℞
2227	Thiothixene Capsules USP 2mg	℞
2228	Thiothixene Capsules USP 5mg	℞
2229	Thiothixene Capsules USP 10mg	℞
1807	Trazodone HCl Tablets USP 50mg	℞
1808	Trazodone HCl Tablets USP 100mg	℞
1123	Triamterene and Hydrochlorothiazide Tablets USP 37.5mg/25mg	℞
2074	Triamterene and Hydrochlorothiazide Capsules USP 37.5mg/25mg	℞
2715	Triamterene and Hydrochlorothiazide Red Capsules USP 50mg/25mg	℞
2540	Triamterene and Hydrochlorothiazide White Capsules USP 50mg/25mg	℞
1008	Triamterene and Hydrochlorothiazide Tablets USP 75mg/50mg	℞
1030	Trifluoperazine HCl Tablets USP 1mg	℞
1032	Trifluoperazine HCl Tablets USP 2mg	℞
1034	Trifluoperazine HCl Tablets USP 5mg	℞
1036	Trifluoperazine HCl Tablets USP 10mg	℞
1014	Verapamil HCl Tablets USP 40mg	℞
1016	Verapamil HCl Tablets USP 80mg	℞
1017	Verapamil HCl Tablets USP 120mg	℞

Genzyme Corporation

ONE KENDALL SQUARE
CAMBRIDGE, MA 02139

Direct Inquiries to:
Clinical Services
(800) 745-4447
FAX: (617) 252-7700

For Medical Information Contact:
In Emergencies:
(800) 745-4447

CEREDASE ℞
[*sĕr 'ĕ-dāse*]
(alglucerase injection)

PRESCRIBING INFORMATION

DESCRIPTION

Ceredase® (alglucerase injection) is a modified form of the enzyme, β-glucocerebrosidase (β-D-glucosyl-N-acylsphingosine glucohydrolase, EC 3.2.1.45). Alglucerase is a monomeric glycoprotein of 497 amino acids with carbohydrates making up approximately 6% of the molecule (M_r = 59,300 as determined by SDS-PAGE). The unmodified enzyme (β-glucocerebrosidase) also contains 497 amino acids and contains approximately 12% carbohydrate (M_r = 67,000). The carbohydrates on the unmodified enzyme consist of N-linked carbohydrate chains of the complex and high mannose type. Glucocerebrosidase and alglucerase catalyze the hydrolysis of the glycolipid, glucocerebroside, within the lysosomes of the reticuloendothelial system.

Alglucerase is prepared by modification of the oligosaccharide chains of human β-glucocerebrosidase. The modification alters the sugar residues at the non-reducing ends of the oligosaccharide chains of the glycoprotein so that they are predominantly terminated with mannose residues which are specifically recognized by carbohydrate receptors on macrophage cells. **Ceredase®** is supplied as a clear sterile non-pyrogenic solution of alglucerase in a citrate buffered solution (53 mM citrate, 143 mM sodium) containing 1% albumin human USP. The enzyme is supplied in two concentrations, 400 units per bottle (80 units/mL) and 50 units per bottle (10 units/mL) with a fill volume of 5 mL per bottle. An enzyme unit (U) is defined as the amount of enzyme required to hydrolyze in one minute one micromole of the synthetic substrate, p-nitrophenyl-β-D-glucopyranoside.

Ceredase® is purified from a large pool of human placental tissue collected from selected donors. Steps have been introduced into the manufacturing process to reduce further the risk of viral contamination. However, no procedure has been shown to be totally effective in removing viral infectivity. (See PRECAUTIONS). Each lot of product has been tested and found negative for hepatitis B surface antigen (HBsAg) and for human immunodeficiency virus antigen (HIV-1) and antibody (HIV-1/2).

Human chorionic gonadotropin (hCG), is a naturally occurring hormone in human placenta. It is likely the hCG is partially deglycosylated. *In vitro* studies have previously demonstrated biological activity of approximately 3 units of hCG activity per unit **Ceredase®**, as determined by an *in vitro* cell based assay. New process steps have since been introduced into the manufacturing process that significantly reduce the amount of hCG present in the **Ceredase®** product. Initial manufacturing data indicate that the resulting level of hCG in the product is less than 1 µg hCG per mg **Ceredase®** protein, as determined by the ELISA assay. This data indicates that the level of hCG in the product has been reduced about 15 fold as a result of the new process steps.

CLINICAL PHARMACOLOGY

Ceredase® (alglucerase injection) catalyzes the hydrolysis of the glycolipid, glucocerebroside, to glucose and ceramide as part of the normal degradation pathway for membrane lipids. Glucocerebroside is primarily derived from hematologic cell turnover. Gaucher disease is characterized by a functional deficiency in β-glucocerebrosidase enzymatic activity and the resultant accumulation of lipid glucocerebroside in tissue macrophages which become engorged and are termed Gaucher cells. Gaucher cells are typically found in liver, spleen and bone marrow and occasionally, as well, in lung, kidney and intestine. Secondary hematologic sequelae include severe anemia and thrombocytopenia in addition to the characteristic progressive hepatosplenomegaly. Skeletal complications, including osteonecrosis and osteopenia with secondary pathological fractures, are a common feature of Gaucher disease.

Pharmacokinetics

Following an intravenous infusion of different doses (between 0.6 and 234 units/kg) of **Ceredase®** (alglucerase injection) over a 4-hour period, steady-state enzymatic activity was achieved by 60 minutes. Individual steady-state enzymatic activity and area under the curve of the activity increased linearly with the infused dose (0.6 to 121 units/kg). Following infusion termination, plasma enzymatic activity declined rapidly with elimination half-life ranging between 3.6 and 10.4 minutes. Plasma clearance of **Ceredase®**, calculated from its plasma enzymatic activity, was variable and ranged between 6.34 and 25.39 mL/min/kg, whereas the volume of distribution ranged from 49.4 to 282.1 mL/kg. Within the dosage range of 0.6 and 121 units/kg, elimination half-life, plasma clearance, and volume of distribution values appear to be independent of the infused dose.

Pharmacologic Actions

Chronic administration of **Ceredase®** (alglucerase injection) in 13 patients with Type 1 Gaucher disease from initial studies induced the following effects:

1. **Splenomegaly and hepatomegaly** were significantly reduced, presumably by disruption of the lysosomal storage sites and metabolism of glucocerebroside in Gaucher cells. This effect was demonstrated within 6 months of initiation of therapy.
2. **Hematologic deficiencies** in hemoglobin, hematocrit, erythrocyte and platelet counts were significantly improved. In most patients a change in hemoglobin was the first observable effect. In some patients hemoglobin levels were normalized after 6 months of therapy.
3. **Improved mineralization** of bone, as revealed by plain radiographs of long bones, occurred in three patients after prolonged treatment as a result of a reduction in the osteolytic actions of lipid-laden Gaucher cells in the marrow.
4. **Cachexia and wasting** in children were reduced.

INDICATIONS AND USAGE

Ceredase® (alglucerase injection) is indicated for use as long-term enzyme replacement therapy for patients with a confirmed diagnosis of Type 1 Gaucher disease who exhibit signs and symptoms that are severe enough to result in one or more of the following conditions:

a) moderate-to-severe anemia;
b) thrombocytopenia with bleeding tendency;
c) bone disease;
d) significant hepatomegaly or splenomegaly.

CONTRAINDICATIONS

There are no known contraindications to the use of **Ceredase®** (alglucerase injection).

WARNINGS

Approximately 13% of patients treated clinically and tested to date have developed IgG antibody to **Ceredase®** during the first year of therapy. It appears that patients who will develop IgG antibody are most likely to do so within 6 months of treatment and will rarely develop antibodies to **Ceredase®** after 12 months of therapy. Approximately 25% of patients with detectable IgG antibodies experienced symptoms of hypersensitivity.

Thus, patients with antibody to **Ceredase®** have a higher risk of hypersensitivity reaction. Conversely, not all patients with symptoms of hypersensitivity have detectable antibody and further evaluation of their antibody isotypes and mechanisms is continuing. It is suggested that patients be monitored periodically for IgG antibody formation.

At present, should a patient experience a reaction with symptoms suggestive of hypersensitivity, it is recommended that a serum sample for tryptase levels and complement activation be drawn within two hours of the event after appropriate treatment of the symptoms. Subsequent serum for testing antibody to **Ceredase®** would be helpful. Decreased efficacy has been noted in less than 0.5% of treated patients due to antibodies to **Ceredase®**.

PRECAUTIONS

General

Therapy with **Ceredase®** (alglucerase injection) should be directed by physicians knowledgeable in the management of patients with Gaucher disease. Treatment with **Ceredase®** should be approached with caution in patients who have exhibited symptoms of hypersensitivity to the product. Pretreatment with antihistamines has allowed continued use of **Ceredase®** in some patients (See **ADVERSE REACTIONS**). As hCG has been detected in **Ceredase®** physicians should be alert for signs of early virilization in males under the age of ten. One case or precocious puberty has been reported to date, however due to the recent introduction of manufacturing steps designed to reduce the level of hCG in **Ceredase®**, the likelihood of this occurrence is reduced. **Ceredase®** should also be used with caution in patients with androgen sensitive malignancies e.g. prostate cancer and patients with known prior allergies to hCG.

Ceredase® is prepared from pooled human placental tissue that may contain the causative agents of some viral diseases. Manufacturing steps have been designed to reduce the risk of transmitting viral infectious agents. These steps have demonstrated *in vitro* inactivation of a panel of model viruses, including human immunodeficiency virus (HIV-1). The risk of contamination from slowly acting or latent viruses, including the Creutzfeldt-Jacob disease agent, is believed to be remote but has not been tested. Accordingly, the benefits and the risks of treatment with this product should be assessed prior to use.

Carcinogenesis, Mutagenesis, Impairment of Fertility

Studies have not been conducted to assess the potential effects of **Ceredase®** on carcinogenesis or mutagenesis. Histopathology studies using hCG-reduced **Ceredase®** to detect effects on spermatogenesis in rats have revealed no testicular changes.

Pregnancy Category C

Animal reproductive studies have not been conducted with **Ceredase®**. It is also not known whether **Ceredase®** can cause fetal harm when administered to a pregnant woman, or can affect reproductive capacity. **Ceredase®** should be given to a pregnant woman only if clearly needed.

Nursing Mothers

Since **Ceredase®** may be excreted in human milk, caution should be exercised when **Ceredase®**is administered to a nursing woman.

ADVERSE REACTIONS

Experience in over 1000 patients treated with **Ceredase®** has revealed a small number of adverse events. Some of these events were related to the route of administration including discomfort, pruritus, burning and swelling or sterile abscess at the site of venipuncture. The remaining experiences consisted of slight fever, chills, abdominal discomfort, nausea or vomiting. None of these events were judged to require medical intervention.

Symptoms suggestive of hypersensitivity have been noted in a limited number of patients. Onset of such symptoms has occurred during or shortly after infusions; these symptoms have included pruritus, flushing, urticaria/angioedema (a small number of patients have had upper airway involvement), chest discomfort, respiratory symptoms, nausea and abdominal cramping. Hypotension has been reported to occur during a few of these events (see **WARNINGS**).

Pre-treatment with antihistamines and reduced rate of infusion has allowed continued use of **Ceredase®** in most patients. Additional adverse symptoms which have been reported include: fatigue, vasomotor irritability or hot flash, weakness, headache, light headedness, dysosmia, oral ulcerations, backache and transient peripheral edema, and diarrhea. Menstrual abnormalities and false positive pregnancy tests have previously been reported, but due to the introduction of manufacturing steps designed to reduce the level of hCG in **Ceredase®**, the likelihood of these occurrences is reduced.

OVERDOSE

No obvious toxicity was detected after single doses up to 234 units/kg. There is no experience with larger doses.

DOSAGE AND ADMINISTRATION

Ceredase® (alglucerase injection) is administered by intravenous infusion over 1–2 hours. Dosage should be individualized for each patient. Initial dosage may be as little as 2.5 units/kg of body weight 3 times a week up to as much as 60 units/kg administered as frequently as once a week or as infrequently as every 4 weeks. 60 units/kg every 2 weeks is the dose for which the most data is available. Disease severity may dictate that the drug be initiated with relatively high doses or relatively frequent administration. After patient response is well-established, a reduction in dosage

Continued on next page

Ceredase—Cont.

may be attempted for maintenance therapy. Progressive reductions can be made at intervals of 3–6 months while carefully monitoring response parameters.

Ceredase® should not be shaken. Each bottle should be inspected visually for particulate matter and discoloration before use. Any bottles exhibiting particulate matter or discoloration should not be used. DO NOT USE **Ceredase®** after the expiration date on the bottle.

On the day of use, the appropriate amount of **Ceredase®** for each patient is diluted with 0.9% sodium chloride IV solution to a final volume not to exceed 200 mL. Aseptic techniques should be used when diluting the dose. **Ceredase®**, when diluted to 100 to 200 mL, has been shown to be stable for up to 18 hours when stored at 2–8°C. The use of an in-line particulate filter is recommended for the infusion apparatus. Since **Ceredase®** does not contain any preservative, after opening, bottles should not be stored for subsequent use.

Relatively low toxicity, combined with the extended time course of response, allows small dosage adjustments to be made occasionally to avoid discarding partially used bottles. Thus, the dosage administered in individual infusions may be slightly increased or decreased to utilize fully each bottle as long as the monthly administered dosage remains substantially unaltered.

HOW SUPPLIED

Ceredase® (alglucerase injection) is supplied as a clear sterile citrate buffered solution (53 mM citrate, 143 mM sodium) containing 1% albumin human USP. The following packages are available:

–The 400 unit bottle contains 5 mL in a 10 mL glass bottle. NDC 58468-1060-1.

–The 50 unit bottle contains 5 mL in a 6 mL glass bottle. NDC 58468-1781-1.

Store at 2–8°C.

CAUTION! FEDERAL (U.S.A.) LAW PROHIBITS DISPENSING WITHOUT A PRESCRIPTION.

Ceredase® (alglucerase injection) is manufactured by:
Genzyme Corporation
One Kendall Square
Cambridge, MA 02139

Certain manufacturing operations have been performed by other firms.

1811 REV 7 (8/96).

CEREZYME ℞

[*sĕr 'ĕ-zīm*]

imiglucerase for injection

PRESCRIBING INFORMATION

DESCRIPTION

Cerezyme® (imiglucerase for injection) is an analogue of the human enzyme, β-glucocerebrosidase produced by recombinant DNA technology. β-Glucocerebrosidase (β-D-glucosyl-N-acylsphingosine glucohydrolase, E.C. 3.2.1.45) is a lysosomal glycoprotein enzyme which catalyzes the hydrolysis of the glycolipid glucocerebroside to glucose and ceramide.

Cerezyme® is produced by recombinant DNA technology using mammalian cell culture (Chinese hamster ovary). Purified imiglucerase is a monomeric glycoprotein of 497 amino acids, containing 4 N-linked glycosylation sites (Mr = 60,430). Imiglucerase differs from placental glucocerebrosidase by one amino acid at position 495 where histidine is substituted for arginine. The oligosaccharide chains at the glycosylation sites have been modified to terminate in mannose sugars. The modified carbohydrate structures on imiglucerase are somewhat different from those on placental glucocerebrosidase. These mannose-terminated oligosaccharide chains of imiglucerase are specifically recognized by endocytic carbohydrate receptors on macrophages, the cells that accumulate lipid in Gaucher disease.

Cerezyme® is supplied as a sterile, non-pyrogenic, white to off-white lyophilized product. The quantitative composition of the lyophilized drug per vial is:

Imiglucerase 212 units (total amount)*
Mannitol 155 mg
Sodium Citrates 70 mg
(Trisodium Citrate 52 mg and Disodium Hydrogen Citrate 18 mg)
Polysorbate 80, NF 0.53 mg
Citric Acid and/or Sodium Hydroxide may have been added at the time of manufacture to adjust pH.

*This provides a withdrawal dose of 200 units of imiglucerase.

An enzyme unit (U) is defined as the amount of enzyme that catalyzes the hydrolysis of one micromole of the synthetic substrate para-nitrophenyl β-D-glucopyranoside (pNP-Glc) per minute at 37°C. The product is stored at 2–8°C (36–46°F.) After reconstitution with 5.1 mL of Sterile Water for Injection, USP, the imiglucerase concentration is 40 U/mL in a final volume of 5.3 mL which provides a withdrawal volume of 5.0 mL (200 enzyme units). Reconstituted solutions have a pH of approximately 6.1.

In addition, Haemaccel® (cross-linked gelatin polypeptides), which is used as a stabilizing agent during the manufacturing process, may also be present in very small amounts in the final product.

CLINICAL PHARMACOLOGY

Mechanism of Action/Pharmacodynamics

Gaucher disease is characterized by a deficiency of β-glucocerebrosidase activity, resulting in accumulation of glucocerebroside in tissue macrophages which become engorged and are typically found in the liver, spleen, and bone marrow and occasionally in lung, kidney, and intestine. Secondary hematologic sequelae include severe anemia and thrombocytopenia in addition to the characteristic progressive hepatosplenomegaly, skeletal complications, including osteonecrosis and osteopenia with secondary pathological fractures. **Cerezyme®** (imiglucerase for injection) catalyzes the hydrolysis of glucocerebroside to glucose and ceramide. In clinical trials, **Cerezyme®** improved anemia and thrombocytopenia, reduced spleen and liver size, and decreased cachexia to a degree similar to that observed with Ceredase®.

Pharmacokinetics

During one hour intravenous infusions of four doses (7.5, 15, 30, 60 U/Kg) of **Cerezyme®** (imiglucerase for injection) steady-state enzymatic activity was achieved by 30 minutes. Following infusion, plasma enzymatic activity declined rapidly with a half-life ranging from 3.6 to 10.4 minutes. Plasma clearance ranged from 9.8 to 20.3 mL/min/Kg, (mean ± S.D, 14.5 ± 4.0 mL/min/kg). The volume of distribution corrected for weight ranged from 0.09 to 0.15 L/Kg (0.12 ± 0.02 L/kg). These variables do not appear to be influenced by dose or duration of infusion. However, only one or two patients were studied at each dose level and infusion rate. The pharmacokinetics of **Cerezyme®** do not appear to be different from placental-derived alglucerase (Ceredase®).

In patients who developed IgG antibody to **Cerezyme®**, an apparent effect on serum enzyme levels resulted in diminished volume of distribution and clearance and increased elimination half-life compared to patients without antibody (see **WARNINGS**).

INDICATIONS AND USAGE

Cerezyme® (imiglucerase for injection) is indicated for long-term enzyme replacement therapy for patients with a confirmed diagnosis of Type 1 Gaucher disease that results in one or more of the following conditions:

a. anemia
b. thrombocytopenia
c. bone disease
d. hepatomegaly or splenomegaly

CONTRAINDICATIONS

There are no known contraindications to the use of **Cerezyme®** (imiglucerase for injection). Treatment with **Cerezyme®** should be carefully re-evaluated if there is significant clinical evidence of hypersensitivity to the product.

WARNINGS

Approximately 15% of 85 patients treated and tested to date have developed IgG antibody to **Cerezyme®** during the first year of therapy. Patients who developed IgG antibody largely did so within 6 months of treatment and rarely developed antibodies to **Cerezyme®** after 12 months of therapy. Approximately 46% of patients with detectable IgG antibodies experienced symptoms of hypersensitivity.

Patients with antibody to **Cerezyme®** have a higher risk of hypersensitivity reaction. Conversely, not all patients with symptoms of hypersensitivity have detectable IgG antibody. It is suggested that patients be monitored periodically for IgG antibody formation during the first year of treatment.

Treatment with **Cerezyme®** should be approached with caution in patients who have exhibited symptoms of hypersensitivity to the product.

PRECAUTIONS

General

Therapy with **Cerezyme®** (imiglucerase for injection) should be directed by physicians knowledgeable in the management of patients with Gaucher disease.

Caution may be advisable in administration of **Cerezyme®** to patients previously treated with Ceredase® and who have developed antibody to Ceredase® or who have exhibited symptoms of hypersensitivity to Ceredase®.

Carcinogenesis, Mutagenesis, Impairment of Fertility

Studies have not been conducted in either animals or humans to assess the potential effects of **Cerezyme®** (imiglucerase for injection) on carcinogenesis, mutagenesis, or impairment of fertility.

Teratogenic Effects: Pregnancy Category C

Animal reproduction studies have not been conducted with **Cerezyme®** (imiglucerase for injection). It is also not known whether **Cerezyme®** can cause fetal harm when administered to a pregnant woman, or can affect reproductive capacity. **Cerezyme®** should not be administered during pregnancy except when the indication and need are clear and the potential benefit is judged by the physician to substantially justify the risk.

Nursing Mothers

It is not known whether this drug is excreted in human milk. Because many drugs are excreted in human milk, caution should be exercised when **Cerezyme®** (imiglucerase for injection) is administered to a nursing woman.

ADVERSE REACTIONS

Experience in over 200 patients treated with **Cerezyme®** to date has revealed a small number of adverse events. Some of the adverse events were related to the route of administration. These include discomfort, pruritis, burning, swelling or sterile abscess at the site of venipuncture.

Symptoms suggestive of hypersensitivity have been noted in a limited number of patients. Onset of such symptoms has occurred during or shortly after infusions; these symptoms include pruritus, flushing, urticaria/angioedema (a small number of patients have had upper airway involvement), chest discomfort, and respiratory symptoms. Hypotension has been reported to occur during a few of these events. (See **WARNINGS**).

Pre-treatment with antihistamines and reduced rate of infusion has allowed continued use of **Cerezyme®** in most patients.

Additional adverse reactions that have been reported in a limited number of patients treated with **Cerezyme®** include nausea, abdominal cramping, diarrhea, rash, fatigue, headache, fever, and dizziness.

In addition to the adverse reactions that have been observed in patients treated with **Cerezyme®**, the following adverse reactions have been reported for this therapeutic class of drug: backache and transient peripheral edema, chills, abdominal discomfort, or vomiting. None of these events were judged to be serious.

OVERDOSE

Effects of dosages exceeding 120 U/kg per four weeks have not been studied and therefore dosages above 120 U/kg are not recommended.

DOSAGE AND ADMINISTRATION

Cerezyme® (imiglucerase for injection) is administered by intravenous infusion over 1–2 hours. Dosage should be individualized to each patient. Initial dosage may be as little as 2.5 units/kg of body weight 3 times a week up to as much as 60 U/kg administered as frequently as once a week or as infrequently as every 4 weeks. 60 units/kg every 2 weeks is the dosage for which the most data are available. Disease severity may dictate that treatment be initiated at a relatively high dose or relatively frequent administration. After patient response is well established, a reduction in dosage may be attempted for maintenance therapy. Progressive reductions can be made at intervals of 3–6 months while carefully monitoring response parameters.

Cerezyme® should be stored at 2–8°C (36–46°F). Each vial, after reconstitution with 5.1 mL Sterile Water for Injection, USP, should be inspected visually for particulate matter and discoloration before use. Any vials exhibiting particulate matter or discoloration should not be used. DO NOT USE **Cerezyme®** after the expiration date on the vial.

On the day of use, after the correct amount of **Cerezyme®** to be administered to the patient has been determined, the appropriate number of vials are each reconstituted with 5.1 mL of Sterile Water for Injection, USP, to give a reconstituted volume of 5.3 mL. A nominal 5.0 mL volume is then withdrawn from each vial. The appropriate amount of **Cerezyme®** for each patient is diluted with 0.9% Sodium Chloride Injection, USP, to a final volume of 100 to 200 mL. **Cerezyme®** is administered by intravenous infusion over 1 to 2 hours. Alternatively, the appropriate dose of **Cerezyme®** may be administered such that a rate of no greater than 1 unit per kg body weight per minute is infused. Aseptic techniques should be used when diluting the dose. Since **Cerezyme®** does not contain any preservative, after reconstitution, vials should be promptly diluted and not stored for subsequent use. **Cerezyme®**, after reconstitution, has been shown to be stable for up to 12 hours when stored at room temperature (25°C). **Cerezyme®**, when diluted to 50 mL has been shown to be stable for up to 24 hours when stored at 2–8°C (36–46°F).

Relatively low toxicity, combined with the extended time course of response, allows small dosage adjustments to be made occasionally to avoid discarding partially used bottles. Thus, the dosage administered in individual infusions may be slightly increased or decreased to utilize fully each vial as long as the monthly administered dosage remains substantially unaltered.

HOW SUPPLIED

Cerezyme® (imiglucerase for injection) is supplied as a sterile, non-pyrogenic, lyophilized product. It is available as follows:

200 Units per Vial
NDC 58468–1983–1
Store at 2–8°C (36–46°F).

CAUTION: FEDERAL (U.S.A.) LAW PROHIBITS DISPENSING WITHOUT A PRESCRIPTION.
Cerezyme® (imiglucerase for injection) is manufactured by:
Genzyme Corporation
One Kendall Square
Cambridge, MA 02139
Certain manufacturing operations may have been performed by other firms.
4336 (10/96)

Gilead Sciences

333 LAKESIDE DRIVE
FOSTER CITY, CA 94404

Direct Inquiries To:
Customer Service
(800) GILEAD5

Medical Emergency Contact:
Director, Medical Information
(800) GILEAD5
FAX: (650) 577-5477

VISTIDE®   Rx
(cidofovir injection)
FOR INTRAVENOUS INFUSION ONLY.
NOT FOR INTRAOCULAR INJECTION.

WARNING:
RENAL IMPAIRMENT IS THE MAJOR TOXICITY OF VISTIDE. TO MINIMIZE POSSIBLE NEPHROTOXICITY, INTRAVENOUS PREHYDRATION WITH NORMAL SALINE AND ADMINISTRATION OF PROBENECID MUST BE USED WITH EACH VISTIDE INFUSION. RENAL FUNCTION (SERUM CREATININE AND URINE PROTEIN) MUST BE MONITORED WITHIN 48 HOURS PRIOR TO EACH DOSE OF VISTIDE AND THE DOSE OF VISTIDE MODIFIED FOR CHANGES IN RENAL FUNCTION AS APPROPRIATE (SEE DOSAGE AND ADMINISTRATION). VISTIDE IS CONTRAINDICATED IN PATIENTS WHO ARE RECEIVING OTHER NEPHROTOXIC AGENTS.
GRANULOCYTOPENIA HAS BEEN OBSERVED IN ASSOCIATION WITH VISTIDE TREATMENT AND NEUTROPHIL COUNTS SHOULD BE MONITORED DURING VISTIDE THERAPY.
VISTIDE IS INDICATED ONLY FOR THE TREATMENT OF CMV RETINITIS IN PATIENTS WITH ACQUIRED IMMUNODEFICIENCY SYNDROME.
IN ANIMAL STUDIES CIDOFOVIR WAS CARCINOGENIC, TERATOGENIC AND CAUSED HYPOSPERMIA (SEE CARCINOGENESIS, MUTAGENESIS, & IMPAIRMENT OF FERTILITY).

DESCRIPTION

VISTIDE® is the brand name for cidofovir injection. The chemical name of cidofovir is 1-[(S)-3-hydroxy-2-(phosphonomethoxy)propyl]cytosine dihydrate (HPMPC), with the molecular formula of $C_8H_{14}N_3O_6P \cdot 2H_2O$ and a molecular weight of 315.22 (279.19 for anhydrous). The chemical structure is:

Cidofovir is a white crystalline powder with an aqueous solubility of ≥170 mg/mL at pH 6-8 and a log P (octanol/aqueous buffer, pH 7.1) value of -3.3.
VISTIDE is a sterile, hypertonic aqueous solution for intravenous infusion only. The solution is clear and colorless. It is supplied in clear glass vials, each containing 375 mg of anhydrous cidofovir in 5 mL aqueous solution at a concentration of 75 mg/mL. The formulation is pH-adjusted to 7.4 with sodium hydroxide and/or hydrochloric acid and contains no preservatives. The appropriate volume of VISTIDE must be removed from the single-use vial and diluted prior to administration (see DOSAGE AND ADMINISTRATION).

MICROBIOLOGY

Mechanism of Action: Cidofovir suppresses cytomegalovirus (CMV) replication by selective inhibition of viral DNA synthesis. Biochemical data support selective inhibition of CMV DNA polymerase by cidofovir diphosphate, the active intracellular metabolite of cidofovir. Cidofovir diphosphate inhibits herpesvirus polymerases at concentrations that are 8- to 600-fold lower than those needed to inhibit human cellular DNA polymerases alpha, beta, and gamma[1, 2, 3]. Incorporation of cidofovir into the growing viral DNA chain results in reductions in the rate of viral DNA synthesis.
In Vitro Susceptibility: Cidofovir is active *in vitro* against a variety of laboratory and clinical isolates of CMV and other herpesviruses (Table 1). Controlled clinical studies of efficacy have been limited to patients with AIDS and CMV retinitis.

Table 1. Cidofovir Inhibition of Virus Multiplication in Cell Culture

Virus	IC_{50} (µM)
Wild-type CMV Isolates	0.5–2.8
HSV-1, HSV-2	12.7–31.7
VZV*	0.79
EBV	0.03
HHV-6	<6.3

* mean result for 4 human VZV strains

Resistance: CMV isolates with reduced susceptibility to cidofovir have been selected *in vitro* in the presence of high concentrations of cidofovir[4]. IC_{50} values for selected resistant isolates ranged from 7–15 µM.
There are insufficient data at this time to assess the frequency or the clinical significance of the development of resistant isolates following VISTIDE administration to patients.
Cross Resistance: Cidofovir-resistant isolates selected *in vitro* following exposure to increasing concentrations of cidofovir were assessed for susceptibility to ganciclovir and foscarnet[4]. All were cross resistant to ganciclovir, but remained susceptible to foscarnet. Ganciclovir- or ganciclovir/foscarnet-resistant isolates that are cross resistant to cidofovir have been obtained from drug naive patients and from patients following ganciclovir or ganciclovir/foscarnet therapy. To date, the majority of ganciclovir-resistant isolates are UL97 gene product (phosphokinase) mutants and remain susceptible to cidofovir[5]. Reduced susceptibility to cidofovir, however, has been reported for DNA polymerase mutants of CMV which are resistant to ganciclovir[6-8]. To date, all clinical isolates which exhibit high level resistance to ganciclovir, due to mutations in the DNA polymerase gene, have been shown to be cross resistant to cidofovir. Cidofovir is active against some, but not all, CMV isolates which are resistant to foscarnet[9-11]. The incidence of foscarnet-resistant isolates that are resistant to cidofovir is not known.
A few triple-drug resistant isolates have been described. Genotypic analysis of two of these triple-resistant isolates revealed several point mutations in the CMV DNA polymerase gene. The clinical significance of the development of these cross-resistant isolates is not known.

CLINICAL PHARMACOLOGY

PHARMACOKINETICS

VISTIDE must be administered with probenecid. The pharmacokinetics of cidofovir, administered both without and with probenecid, are described below.
The pharmacokinetics of cidofovir without probenecid were evaluated in 27 HIV-infected patients with or without asymptomatic CMV infection. Dose-independent pharmacokinetics were demonstrated after one hr infusions of 1.0 (n = 5), 3.0 (n = 10), 5.0 (n = 2) and 10.0 (n = 8) mg/kg (See Table 2 for pharmacokinetic parameters). There was no evidence of cidofovir accumulation after 4 weeks of repeated administration of 3 mg/kg/week (n = 5) without probenecid. In pa-

Table 2. Cidofovir Pharmacokinetic Parameters Following 3.0 and 5.0 mg/kg Infusions, Without and With Probenecid*

PARAMETERS	VISTIDE ADMINISTERED WITHOUT PROBENECID		VISTIDE ADMINISTERED WITH PROBENECID	
	3 mg/kg (n = 10)	5 mg/kg (n = 2)	3 mg/kg (n = 12)	5 mg/kg (n = 6)
AUC (µg·hr/mL)	20.0 ± 2.3	28.3	25.7 ± 8.5	40.8 ± 9.0
Cmax (end of infusion) (µg/mL)	7.3 ± 1.4	11.5	9.8 ± 3.7	19.6 ± 7.2
Vdss (mL/kg)	537 ± 126 (n = 12)		410 ± 102 (n = 18)	
Clearance (mL/min/1.73 m²)	179 ± 23.1 (n = 12)		148 ± 38.8 (n = 18)	
Renal Clearance (mL/min/1.73 m²)	150 ± 26.9 (n = 12)		98.6 ± 27.9 (n = 11)	

* See DOSAGE AND ADMINISTRATION

tients with normal renal function, approximately 80 to 100% of the VISTIDE dose was recovered unchanged in urine within 24 hr (n = 27). The renal clearance of cidofovir was greater than creatinine clearance, indicating renal tubular secretion contributes to the elimination of cidofovir.
The pharmacokinetics of cidofovir administered with probenecid were evaluated in 12 HIV-infected patients with or without asymptomatic CMV infection and 10 patients with relapsing CMV retinitis. Dose-independent pharmacokinetics were observed for cidofovir, administered with probenecid, after one hr infusions of 3.0 (n = 12), 5.0 (n = 6), and 7.5 (n = 4) mg/kg (See Table 2). Approximately 70 to 85% of the VISTIDE dose administered with concomitant probenecid was excreted as unchanged drug within 24 hr. When VISTIDE was administered with probenecid, the renal clearance of cidofovir was reduced to a level consistent with creatinine clearance, suggesting that probenecid blocks active renal tubular secretion of cidofovir.
[See table above]
In vitro, cidofovir was less than 6% bound to plasma or serum proteins over the cidofovir concentration range 0.25 to 25 µg/mL. CSF concentrations of cidofovir following intravenous infusion of VISTIDE 5 mg/kg with concomitant probenecid and intravenous hydration were undetectable (< 0.1 µg/mL, assay detection threshold) at 15 minutes after the end of a 1 hr infusion in one patient whose corresponding serum concentration was 8.7 µg/mL.

DRUG-DRUG INTERACTIONS

Zidovudine
The pharmacokinetics of zidovudine were evaluated in 10 patients receiving zidovudine alone or with intravenous cidofovir (without probenecid). There was no evidence of an effect of cidofovir on the pharmacokinetics of zidovudine.

SPECIAL POPULATIONS

Renal Insufficiency
Cidofovir pharmacokinetics have not been investigated in patients with renal insufficiency. No data are currently available on the pharmacokinetics of cidofovir in patients with creatinine clearance values below 55 mL/min. The effect of dialysis on cidofovir pharmacokinetics is not known.

Geriatric/Gender/Race
The effects of age, gender, and race on cidofovir pharmacokinetics have not been investigated.

INDICATION AND USAGE

VISTIDE is indicated for the treatment of CMV retinitis in patients with acquired immunodeficiency syndrome (AIDS). THE SAFETY AND EFFICACY OF VISTIDE HAVE NOT BEEN ESTABLISHED FOR TREATMENT OF OTHER CMV INFECTIONS (SUCH AS PNEUMONITIS OR GASTROENTERITIS), CONGENITAL OR NEONATAL CMV DISEASE, OR CMV DISEASE IN NON-HIV-INFECTED INDIVIDUALS.

DESCRIPTION OF CLINICAL TRIALS

Two phase 2/3 controlled trials of VISTIDE have been conducted in HIV-infected patients with CMV retinitis.
Delayed Versus Immediate Therapy (Study 106): In an open-label trial, 48 previously untreated patients with peripheral CMV retinitis were randomized to either immediate treatment with VISTIDE (5 mg/kg once a week for 2 weeks, then 5 mg/kg every other week), or to have VISTIDE delayed until progression of CMV retinitis. Patient baseline characteristics and disposition are shown in Table 3. Of 25 and 23 patients in the immediate and delayed groups respectively, 23 and 21 were evaluable for retinitis progression as determined by retinal photography. Based on masked readings of retinal photographs, the median [95% confidence interval (CI)] times to retinitis progression were 120 days (40, 134) and 22 days (10, 27) for the immediate and delayed therapy groups, respectively.

Continued on next page

Vistide—Cont.

This difference was statistically significant. However, because of the limited number of patients remaining on treatment over time (3 of 25 patients received VISTIDE for 120 days or longer), the median time to progression for the immediate therapy group was difficult to precisely estimate. Median (95% CI) times to the alternative endpoint of retinitis progression or study drug discontinuation (including adverse events, withdrawn consent, and systemic CMV disease) were 52 days (37, 85) and 22 days (13, 27) for the immediate and delayed therapy groups, respectively. This difference was statistically significant. Time to progression estimates from this study may not be directly comparable to estimates reported for other therapies.

Table 3. Patient Characteristics and Disposition (Study 106)

	Immediate Therapy (n = 25)	Delayed Therapy (n = 23)
Baseline Characteristics		
Age (years)	38	38
Sex (M/F)	24/1	22/1
Median CD4 Cell Count	6	9
Endpoints		
CMV Retinitis Progression	10	18
Discontinued Due to Adverse Event	6	0
Withdrew Consent	3[a]	1
Discontinued Due to Intercurrent Illness	2[b]	1[b]
Discontinued Based on Ophthalmological Examination	1[c]	1[c]
No Progression at Study Completion	1	0
Not Evaluable at Baseline	2	2

[a] One patient died 2 weeks after withdrawing consent.
[b] Two patients on immediate therapy were diagnosed with CMV disease and discontinued from study. One patient on delayed therapy was diagnosed with CMV gastrointestinal disease.
[c] CMV retinitis progression not confirmed by retinal photography.

Dose-response study of VISTIDE (Study 107): In an open-label trial, 100 patients with relapsing CMV retinitis were randomized to receive 5 mg/kg once a week for 2 weeks and then either 5 mg/kg (n = 49) or 3 mg/kg (n = 51) every other week. Enrolled patients had been diagnosed with CMV retinitis approximately 1 year prior to randomization and had received a median of 4 prior courses of systemic CMV therapy. Eighty-four of the 100 patients were considered evaluable for progression by serial retinal photographs (43 randomized to 5 mg/kg and 41 randomized to 3 mg/kg). Twenty-three and 20 patients discontinued therapy due to either an adverse event, intercurrent illness, excluded medication, or withdrawn consent in the 5 mg/kg and 3 mg/kg groups, respectively. Based on masked readings of retinal photographs, the median (95% CI) times to retinitis progression for the 5 mg/kg and 3 mg/kg groups were 115 days (70, not reached) and 49 days (35, 52), respectively. This difference was statistically significant. Similar to Study 106, the median time to retinitis progression for the 5 mg/kg group was difficult to precisely estimate due to the limited number of patients remaining on treatment over time (4 of the 49 patients in the 5 mg/kg group were treated for 115 days or longer). Median (95% CI) times to the alternative endpoint of retinitis progression or study drug discontinuation were 49 days (38, 63) and 35 days (27, 39) for the 5 mg/kg and 3 mg/kg groups, respectively. This difference was statistically significant.

CONTRAINDICATIONS

Initiation of therapy with VISTIDE is contraindicated in patients with a serum creatinine > 1.5 mg/dL, a calculated creatinine clearance ≤ 55 mL/min, or a urine protein ≥ 100 mg/dL (equivalent to ≥ 2+ proteinuria).
VISTIDE is contraindicated in patients receiving agents with nephrotoxic potential. Such agents must be discontinued at least seven days prior to starting therapy with VISTIDE.
VISTIDE is contraindicated in patients with hypersensitivity to cidofovir.
VISTIDE is contraindicated in patients with a history of clinically severe hypersensitivity to probenecid or other sulfa-containing medications.
Direct intraocular injection of VISTIDE is contraindicated; direct injection of cidofovir has been associated with iritis, ocular hypotony, and permanent impairment of vision.

WARNINGS

Nephrotoxicity: Dose-dependent nephrotoxicity is the major dose-limiting toxicity related to VISTIDE administration. Renal function (serum creatinine and urine protein) must be monitored within 48 hours prior to each dose of VISTIDE. Dose adjustment or discontinuation is required for changes in renal function (serum creatinine and/or urine protein) while on therapy. Proteinuria, as measured by urinalysis in a clinical laboratory, may be an early indicator of VISTIDE-related nephrotoxicity. Continued administration of VISTIDE may lead to additional proximal tubular cell injury, which may result in glycosuria, decreases in serum phosphate, uric acid, and bicarbonate, elevations in serum creatinine, and/or acute renal failure, in some cases, resulting in the need for dialysis. Patients with these adverse events occurring concurrently and meeting a criteria of Fanconi's syndrome have been reported. Renal function that did not return to baseline after drug discontinuation has been observed in clinical studies of VISTIDE.
Intravenous normal saline hydration and oral probenecid must accompany each VISTIDE infusion. Probenecid is known to interact with the metabolism or renal tubular excretion of many drugs (see PRECAUTIONS). The safety of VISTIDE has not been evaluated in patients receiving other known potentially nephrotoxic agents, such as intravenous aminoglycosides (e.g., tobramycin, gentamicin, and amikacin), amphotericin B, foscarnet, intravenous pentamidine, vancomycin, and non-steroidal anti-inflammatory agents (see DOSAGE AND ADMINISTRATION).
Preexisting Renal Impairment: Initiation of therapy with VISTIDE is contraindicated in patients with a baseline serum creatinine > 1.5 mg/dL, a creatinine clearance ≤ 55 mL/min, or a urine protein ≥ 100 mg/dL (equivalent to ≥ 2+ proteinuria).
Hematological Toxicity: Neutropenia may occur during VISTIDE therapy. Neutrophil count should be monitored while receiving VISTIDE therapy.
Metabolic Acidosis: Fanconi's syndrome and decreases in serum bicarbonate associated with evidence of renal tubular damage have been reported in patients receiving VISTIDE (see ADVERSE EVENTS). Serious metabolic acidosis, in association with liver failure, pancreatitis, mucormycosis, aspegillus, disseminated mycobacterial infection, and progression to death occurred in 1 patient (< 1%) receiving VISTIDE.

PRECAUTIONS

General
Due to the potential for increased nephrotoxicity, doses greater than the recommended dose must not be administered and the frequency or rate of administration must not be exceeded (see DOSAGE AND ADMINISTRATION).
VISTIDE is formulated for intravenous infusion only and must not be administered by intraocular injection. Administration of VISTIDE by infusion must be accompanied by oral probenecid and intravenous saline prehydration (see DOSAGE AND ADMINISTRATION).
Information for Patients
Patients should be advised that VISTIDE is not a cure for CMV retinitis, and that they may continue to experience progression of retinitis during and following treatment. Patients receiving VISTIDE should be advised to have regular follow-up ophthalmologic examinations. Patients may also experience other manifestations of CMV disease despite VISTIDE therapy.
HIV-infected patients may continue taking antiretroviral therapy, but those taking zidovudine should be advised to temporarily discontinue zidovudine administration or decrease their zidovudine dose by 50%, on days of VISTIDE administration only, because probenecid reduces metabolic clearance of zidovudine.
Patients should be informed of the major toxicity of VISTIDE, namely renal impairment, and that dose modification, including reduction, interruption, and possibly discontinuation, may be required. Close monitoring of renal function (routine urinalysis and serum creatinine) while on therapy should be emphasized.
The importance of completing a full course of probenecid with each VISTIDE dose should be emphasized. Patients should be warned of potential adverse events caused by probenecid (e.g., headache, nausea, vomiting, and hypersensitivity reactions). Hypersensitivity/allergic reactions may include rash, fever, chills and anaphylaxis. Administration of probenecid after a meal or use of antiemetics may decrease the nausea. Prophylactic or therapeutic antihistamines and/or acetaminophen can be used to ameliorate hypersensitivity reactions.
Patients should be advised that cidofovir causes tumors, primarily mammary adenocarcinomas, in rats. VISTIDE should be considered a potential carcinogen in humans (See Carcinogenesis, Mutagenesis, & Impairment of Fertility).
Women should be advised of the limited enrollment of women in clinical trials of VISTIDE.
Patients should be advised that VISTIDE caused reduced testes weight and hypospermia in animals. Such changes may occur in humans and cause infertility. Women of childbearing potential should be advised that cidofovir is embryotoxic in animals and should not be used during pregnancy. Women of childbearing potential should be advised to use effective contraception during and for 1 month following treatment with VISTIDE. Men should be advised to practice barrier contraceptive methods during and for 3 months after treatment with VISTIDE.

Drug Interactions
Probenecid: Probenecid is known to interact with the metabolism or renal tubular excretion of many drugs (e.g., acetaminophen, acyclovir, angiotensin-converting enzyme inhibitors, aminosalicylic acid, barbiturates, benzodiazepines, bumetanide, clofibrate, methotrexate, famotidine, furosemide, nonsteroidal anti-inflammatory agents, theophylline, and zidovudine). Concomitant medications should be carefully assessed.
Nephrotoxic agents: Concomitant administration of VISTIDE and agents with nephrotoxic potential [e.g., intravenous aminoglycosides (e.g., tobramycin, gentamicin, and amikacin), amphotericin B, foscarnet, intravenous pentamidine, vancomycin, and non-steroidal anti-inflammatory agents] is contraindicated. Such agents must be discontinued at least seven days prior to starting therapy with VISTIDE.
Carcinogenesis, Mutagenesis, & Impairment of Fertility
Chronic, two-year carcinogenicity studies in rats and mice have not been carried out to evaluate the carcinogenic potential of cidofovir. However, a 26-week toxicology study evaluating once weekly subscapular subcutaneous injections of cidofovir in rats was terminated at 19 weeks because of the induction, in females, of palpable masses, the first of which was detected after six doses. The masses were diagnosed as mammary adenocarcinomas which developed at doses as low as 0.6 mg/kg/week, equivalent to 0.04 times the human systemic exposure at the recommended intravenous VISTIDE dose based on AUC comparisons.
In a 26-week intravenous toxicology study in which rats received 0.6, 3, or 15 mg/kg cidofovir once weekly, a significant increase in mammary adenocarcinomas in female rats as well as a significant incidence of Zymbal's gland carcinomas in male and female rats were seen at the high dose but not at the lower two doses. The high dose was equivalent to 1.1 times the human systemic exposure at the recommended dose of VISTIDE, based on comparisons of AUC measurements. In light of the results of these studies, cidofovir should be considered to be a carcinogen in rats as well as a potential carcinogen in humans.
Cynomolgus monkeys received intravenous cidofovir, alone and in conjunction with concomitant oral probenecid, intravenously once weekly for 52 weeks at doses resulting in exposures of approximately 0.7 times the human systemic exposure at the recommended dose of VISTIDE. No tumors were detected. However, the study was not designed as a carcinogenicity study due to the small number of animals at each dose and the short duration of treatment.
No mutagenic response was observed in microbial mutagenicity assays involving *Salmonella typhimurium* (Ames) and *Escherichia coli* in the presence and absence of metabolic activation. An increase in micronucleated polychromatic erythrocytes *in vivo* was seen in mice receiving ≥ 2000 mg/kg, a dosage approximately 65-fold higher than the maximum recommended clinical intravenous VISTIDE dose based on body surface area estimations. Cidofovir induced chromosomal aberrations in human peripheral blood lymphocytes *in vitro* without metabolic activation. At the 4 cidofovir levels tested, the percentage of damaged metaphases and number of aberrations per cell increased in a concentration-dependent manner.
Studies showed that cidofovir caused inhibition of spermatogenesis in rats and monkeys. However, no adverse effects on fertility or reproduction were seen following once weekly intravenous injections of cidofovir in male rats for 13 consecutive weeks at doses up to 15 mg/kg/week (equivalent to 1.1 times the recommended human dose based on AUC comparisons). Female rats dosed intravenously once weekly at 1.2 mg/kg/week (equivalent to 0.09 times the recommended human dose based on AUC) or higher, for up to 6 weeks prior to mating and for 2 weeks post mating had decreased litter sizes and live births per litter and increased early resorptions per litter. Peri- and post-natal development studies in which female rats received subcutaneous injections of cidofovir once daily at doses up to 1.0 mg/kg/day from day 7 of gestation through day 21 postpartum (approximately 5 weeks) resulted in no adverse effects on viability, growth, behavior, sexual maturation or reproductive capacity in the offspring.
Pregnancy: Category C
Cidofovir was embryotoxic (reduced fetal body weights) in rats at 1.5 mg/kg/day and in rabbits at 1.0 mg/kg/day, doses which were also maternally toxic, following daily intravenous dosing during the period of organogenesis. The no-observable-effect levels for embryotoxicity in rats (0.5 mg/kg/day) and in rabbits (0.25 mg/kg/day) were approximately 0.04 and 0.05 times the clinical dose (5 mg/kg every other week) based on AUC, respectively. An increased incidence of fetal external, soft tissue and skeletal anomalies (meningocele, short snout, and short maxillary bones) occurred in rabbits at the high dose (1.0 mg/kg/day) which was also maternally toxic. There are no adequate and well-controlled studies in pregnant women. VISTIDE should be used during pregnancy only if the potential benefit justifies the potential risk to the fetus.

Nursing Mothers

It is not known whether cidofovir is excreted in human milk. Since many drugs are excreted in human milk and because of the potential for adverse reactions as well as the potential for tumorigenicity shown for cidofovir in animal studies, VISTIDE should not be administered to nursing mothers. The U.S. Public Health Service Centers for Disease Control and Prevention advises HIV-infected women not to breast-feed to avoid postnatal transmission of HIV to a child who may not yet be infected.

Pediatric Use

Safety and effectiveness in children have not been studied. The use of VISTIDE in children with AIDS warrants extreme caution due to the risk of long-term carcinogenicity and reproductive toxicity. Administration of VISTIDE to children should be undertaken only after careful evaluation and only if the potential benefits of treatment outweigh the risks.

Use in Elderly Patients

No studies of the safety or efficacy of VISTIDE in patients over the age of 60 have been conducted. Since elderly individuals frequently have reduced glomerular filtration, particular attention should be paid to assessing renal function before and during VISTIDE administration (see DOSAGE AND ADMINISTRATION).

ADVERSE REACTIONS

1. ***Nephrotoxicity***: Renal toxicity, as manifested by >1+ proteinuria, serum creatinine elevations of ≥ 0.4 mg/dL, or decreased creatinine clearance ≤ 55 mL/min, occurred in 47 of 89 (53%) patients receiving VISTIDE at a maintenance dose of 5 mg/kg every other week. Maintenance dose reductions from 5 mg/kg to 3 mg/kg due to proteinuria or serum creatinine elevations were made for 12 of 41 (29%) patients who had not received prior therapy for CMV retinitis (Study 106) and 11 of 48 (23%) patients who had received prior therapy for CMV retinitis (Study 107). Prior foscarnet use has been associated with an increased risk of nephrotoxicity, therefore such patients must be monitored closely.
2. ***Neutropenia***: In clinical trials, at the 5 mg/kg maintenance dose, neutropenia to ≤ 500 cells/mm^3 occurred in 20% of patients. Granulocyte colony stimulating factor (GCSF) was used in 34% of patients.
3. ***Ocular hypotony***: Among the subset of patients monitored for intraocular pressure changes, ocular hypotony (≥ 50% decrease from baseline) was reported in 5 patients. Hypotony was reported in 1 patient with concomitant diabetes mellitus. Risk of ocular hypotony may be increased in patients with preexisting diabetes.
4. ***Metabolic Acidosis***: A diagnosis of Fanconi's syndrome, as manifested by multiple abnormalities of proximal tubule function, was reported in 2% of patients. Decreases in serum bicarbonate to ≤ 16 mEq/L associated with evidence of renal tubular damage occurred in approximately 9% of patients. Serious metabolic acidosis, in association with liver failure, pancreatitis, mucormycosis, aspergillus, disseminated mycobacterial infection, and progression to death occurred in 1 patient (< 1%) receiving VISTIDE.

In clinical trials, VISTIDE was withdrawn due to adverse events in approximately 25% of patients treated with 5 mg/kg every other week as maintenance therapy.

The incidence of adverse reactions reported as serious in two controlled clinical studies in patients with CMV retinitis, regardless of presumed relationship to drug, is listed in Table 4.

Table 4. Serious Clinical Adverse Events or Laboratory Abnormalities Occurring in >5% of Patients

	N = 89[a]	%
Proteinuria (≥100 mg/dL)	42	48
Neutropenia (≤500 cells/mm^3)	18	20
Creatinine Elevation	13	15
Fever	13	15
Infection	11	12
Dyspnea	9	10
Pneumonia	8	9
Decreased Serum Bicarbonate (≤16 mEq/L)	8	9
Creatinine Elevation (to ≥2.0 mg/dL)	7	8
Nausea with Vomiting	7	8
Diarrhea	6	7
Asthenia	6	7
Ocular Hypotony[b]	5	12

[a] Patients receiving 5 mg/kg maintenance regimen in Studies 106 and 107.

[b] Incidence based on 42 patients receiving 5 mg/kg maintenance regimen in Studies 106 and 107 with pretreatment baseline intraocular pressure reading and follow-up evaluation ≤50% of baseline.

The most frequently reported adverse events regardless of relationship to study drugs (cidofovir or probenecid) or severity are shown in Table 5.

$$\text{Creatinine clearance for males} = \frac{[140\text{-age (years)}] \times [\text{body wt (kg)}]}{72 \times [\text{serum creatinine (mg/dL)}]}$$

$$\text{Creatinine clearance for females} = \frac{[140\text{-age (years)}] \times [\text{body wt (kg)}] \times 0.85}{72 \times [\text{serum creatinine (mg/dL)}]}$$

The following additional list of adverse events/intercurrent illnesses have been observed in clinical studies of VISTIDE and are listed below regardless of causal relationship to VISTIDE.

Body as a Whole: allergic reaction, face edema, malaise, back pain, chest pain, neck pain, sarcoma, sepsis

Cardiovascular System: hypotension, postural hypotension, pallor, syncope, tachycardia

Digestive System: colitis, constipation, tongue discoloration, dyspepsia, dysphagia, flatulence, gastritis, hepatomegaly, abnormal liver function tests, melena, oral candidiasis, rectal disorder, stomatitis, aphthous stomatitis, mouth ulceration

Hemic & Lymphatic System: thrombocytopenia

Metabolic & Nutritional System: edema, dehydration, hyperglycemia, hyperlipemia, hypocalcemia, hypokalemia, increased alkaline phosphatase, increased SGOT, increased SGPT, weight loss

Musculoskeletal System: arthralgia, myasthenia, myalgia

Nervous System: amnesia, anxiety, confusion, convulsion, depression, dizziness, dry mouth, abnormal gait, hallucinations, insomnia, neuropathy, paresthesia, somnolence, vasodilatation

Respiratory System: asthma, bronchitis, coughing, dyspnea, hiccup, increased sputum, lung disorder, pharyngitis, pneumonia, rhinitis, sinusitis

Skin & Appendages: alopecia, acne, skin discoloration, dry skin, herpes simplex, pruritus, rash, sweating, urticaria

Special Senses: amblyopia, conjunctivitis, eye disorder, hypotony, iritis, retinal detachment, taste perversion, uveitis, abnormal vision

Urogenital System: decreased creatinine clearance, glycosuria, hematuria, urinary incontinence, urinary tract infection

Table 5. All Clinical Adverse Events, Laboratory Abnormalities or Intercurrent Illnesses Regardless of Severity Occurring in >15% of Patients

	N = 89[a]	%
Any Adverse Event	89	100
Proteinuria	71	80
Nausea +/− Vomiting	58	65
Fever	51	57
Asthenia	41	46
Neutropenia (<750/mm^3)	28	31
Rash	27	30
Headache	24	27
Diarrhea	24	27
Alopecia	22	25
Infections	22	25
Chills	21	24
Anorexia	20	22
Dyspnea	20	22
Anemia	18	20
Creatinine Elevation (to >1.5 mg/dL)	16	18
Abdominal Pain	15	17

[a] Patients receiving 5 mg/kg maintenance regimen in Studies 106 and 107.

Reporting of Adverse Reactions

Malignancies or serious adverse reactions that occur in patients who have received VISTIDE should be reported to Gilead in writing to the Director of Clinical Research, Gilead Sciences, Inc., 353 Lakeside Drive, Foster City, CA 94404 or by calling 1-800-GILEAD-5 (445-3235), or to FDA MedWatch 1-800-FDA-1088/fax 1-800-FDA-0178.

OVERDOSAGE

Two cases of cidofovir overdose have been reported. These patients received single doses of VISTIDE at 16.3 mg/kg and 17.4 mg/kg, respectively, with concomitant oral probenecid and intravenous hydration. In both cases, the patients were hospitalized and received oral probenecid (one gram three times daily) and vigorous intravenous hydration with normal saline for 3 to 5 days. Significant changes in renal function were not observed in either patient.

DOSAGE AND ADMINISTRATION

VISTIDE MUST NOT BE ADMINISTERED BY INTRAOCULAR INJECTION.

Dosage

THE RECOMMENDED DOSAGE, FREQUENCY, OR INFUSION RATE MUST NOT BE EXCEEDED. VISTIDE MUST BE DILUTED IN 100 MILLILITERS 0.9% (NORMAL) SALINE PRIOR TO ADMINISTRATION. TO MINIMIZE POTENTIAL NEPHROTOXICITY, PROBENECID AND INTRAVENOUS SALINE PREHYDRATION MUST BE ADMINISTERED WITH EACH VISTIDE INFUSION.

Induction Treatment The recommended induction dose of VISTIDE for patients with a serum creatinine of ≤ 1.5 mg/dL, a calculated creatinine clearance > 55 mL/min, and a urine protein < 100 mg/dL (equivalent to < 2+ proteinuria) is 5 mg/kg body weight (given as an intravenous infusion at a constant rate over 1 hr) administered once weekly for two consecutive weeks. Because serum creatinine in patients with advanced AIDS and CMV retinitis may not provide a complete picture of your patient's underlying renal status, it is important to utilize the Cockcroft-Gault formula to more precisely estimate creatinine clearance (CrCl). As creatinine clearance is dependent on serum creatinine and patient weight, it is necessary to calculate clearance prior to initiation of VISTIDE. CrCl (mL/min) should be calculated according to the following formula:

[See table above]

Maintenance Treatment The recommended maintenance dose of VISTIDE is 5 mg/kg body weight (given as an intravenous infusion at a constant rate over 1 hr) administered once every two weeks.

Dose Adjustment

Changes in Renal Function During VISTIDE Therapy: The dose of VISTIDE must be reduced from 5 mg/kg to 3 mg/kg for an increase in serum creatinine of 0.3–0.4 mg/dL above baseline. VISTIDE therapy must be discontinued for an increase in serum creatinine of ≥ 0.5 mg/dL above baseline or development of ≥ 3+ proteinuria.

Preexisting Renal Impairment: VISTIDE is contraindicated in patients with a serum creatinine concentration > 1.5 mg/dL, a calculated creatinine clearance ≤ 55 mL/min, or a urine protein ≥ 100 mg/dL (equivalent to ≥ 2+ proteinuria).

Probenecid Probenecid must be administered orally with each VISTIDE dose. Two grams must be administered 3 hr prior to the VISTIDE dose and one gram administered at 2 and again at 8 hr after completion of the 1 hr VISTIDE infusion (for a total of 4 grams).

Ingestion of food prior to each dose of probenecid may reduce drug-related nausea and vomiting. Administration of an antiemetic may reduce the potential for nausea associated with probenecid ingestion. In patients who develop allergic or hypersensitivity symptoms to probenecid, the use of an appropriate prophylactic or therapeutic antihistamine and/or acetaminophen should be considered (see CONTRAINDICATIONS).

Hydration Patients must receive at least one liter of 0.9% (normal) saline solution intravenously with each infusion of VISTIDE. The saline solution should be infused over a 1–2 hr period immediately before the VISTIDE infusion. Patients who can tolerate the additional fluid load should receive a second liter. If administered, the second liter of saline should be initiated either at the start of the VISTIDE infusion or immediately afterwards, and infused over a 1 to 3 hr period.

Method of Preparation and Administration

Inspect vials visually for particulate matter and discoloration prior to administration. If particulate matter or discoloration is observed, the vial should not be used.

With a syringe, extract the appropriate volume of VISTIDE from the vial and transfer the dose to an infusion bag containing 100 mL 0.9% (normal) saline solution. Infuse the entire volume intravenously into the patient at a constant rate over a 1 hr period. Use of a standard infusion pump for administration is recommended.

It is recommended that VISTIDE infusion admixtures be administered within 24 hr of preparation and that refrigerator or freezer storage not be used to extend this 24 hr limit. If admixtures are not intended for immediate use, they may be stored under refrigeration (2–8°C) for no more than 24 hr. Refrigerated admixtures should be allowed to equilibrate to room temperature prior to use.

The chemical stability of VISTIDE admixtures was demonstrated in polyvinyl chloride composition and ethylene/propylene copolymer composition commercial infusion bags, and in glass bottles. **No data are available to support the addition of other drugs or supplements to the cidofovir admixture for concurrent administration.**

VISTIDE is supplied in single-use vials. Partially used vials should be discarded (see Handling and Disposal).

Compatibility with Ringer's solution, Lactated Ringer's solution or bacteriostatic infusion fluids has not been evaluated.

Handling and Disposal

Due to the mutagenic properties of cidofovir, adequate precautions including the use of appropriate safety equipment are recommended for the preparation, administration, and disposal of VISTIDE. The National Institutes of Health presently recommends that the preparation of such agents be prepared in a Class II laminar flow biological safety cabinet and that personnel preparing drugs of this class wear surgical gloves and a closed front surgical-type gown with knit cuffs. If VISTIDE contacts the skin, wash membranes

Continued on next page

Vistide—Cont.

and flush thoroughly with water. Excess VISTIDE and all other materials used in the admixture preparation and administration should be placed in a leak-proof, puncture-proof container. The recommended method of disposal is high temperature incineration.

Patient Monitoring

Serum creatinine and urine protein must be monitored within 48 hours prior to each dose. White blood cell counts with differential should be monitored prior to each dose. In patients with proteinuria, intravenous hydration should be administered and the test repeated. Intraocular pressure, visual acuity and ocular symptoms should be monitored periodically.

HOW SUPPLIED

VISTIDE (cidofovir injection) 75 mg/mL for intravenous infusion, is supplied as a non-preserved solution in single-use clear glass vials as follows:

NDC 61958-0101-1   375 mg in a 5 mL vial in a single-unit carton

VISTIDE should be stored at controlled room temperature 20°–25°C (68°–77°F).

CAUTION: Federal law prohibits dispensing without prescription.

Manufactured by:
Ben Venue Laboratories, Inc.
Bedford, OH 44146-0568

Manufactured for and distributed by:
Gilead Sciences, Inc.
353 Lakeside Drive
Foster City, CA 94404

VISTIDE® (cidofovir injection) is covered by U.S. Patent No. 5,142,051 and its foreign counterparts. Other patents pending.

REFERENCES

1. Ho HT, Woods KL, Bronson JJ, De Boeck H, Martin JC and Hitchcock MJM. Intracellular Metabolism of the Antiherpesvirus Agent (S)-1-[3-hydroxy-2-(phosphonyl-methoxy)propyl]cytosine. *Mol Pharmacol*, **41**:197-202, 1992.
2. Cherrington JM, Allen SJW, McKee BH, and Chen MS. Kinetic Analysis of the Interaction Between the Diphosphate of (S)-1-(3-hydroxy-2-phosphonylmethoxypropyl)-cytosine, zalcitabineTP, zidovudineTP, and FIAUTP with Human DNA Polymerases β and γ. *Biochem Pharmacol*, **48**:1986-1988, 1994.
3. Xiong X, Kim C, Huang E, Smith JL, and Chen MS. Kinetic Analysis of the Interaction of Cidofovir Diphosphate with Human Cytomegalovirus DNA Polymerase. *Biochem Pharmacol*, **51**:1563-1567, 1996.
4. Cherrington JM, Mulato AS, Fuller MD, Chen MS. *In Vitro* Selection of a Human Cytomegalovirus (HCMV) that is Resistant to Cidofovir. 35th International Conference on Antimicrobial Agents and Chemotherapy (ICAAC), San Francisco, CA. Abstract H117, 1995.
5. Stanat SC, Reardon JE, Erice A, Jordan MC, Drew WL, and Biron KK. Ganciclovir-Resistant Cytomegalovirus Clinical Isolates: Mode of Resistance to Ganciclovir. *Antimicrob Agents Chemother*, **35**:2191-2197, 1991.
6. Sullivan V, Biron KK, Talarico C, Stanat SC, Davis M, Pozzi M, and Coen DM. A Point Mutation in the Human Cytomegalovirus DNA Polymerase Gene Confers Resistance to Ganciclovir and phosphonylmethoxyalkyl Derivatives. *Antimicrob Agents Chemother*, **37**:19-25, 1993.
7. Tatarowicz WA, Lurain NS, and Thompson KD. A Ganciclovir-Resistant Clinical Isolate of Human Cytomegalovirus Exhibiting Cross-Resistance to other DNA Polymerase Inhibitors. *J Infect Dis*, **166**:904-907, 1992.
8. Lurain NS, Thompson KD, Holmes EW, and Read GS. Point Mutations in the DNA Polymerase Gene of Human Cytomegalovirus that Result in Resistance to Antiviral Agents. *J Virol*, **66**:7146-7152, 1992.
9. Sullivan V and Coen DM. Isolation of Foscarnet-Resistant Human Cytomegalovirus Patterns of Resistance and Sensitivity to Other Antiviral Drugs. *J Infect Dis*, **164**:781-784, 1991.
10. Snoeck R, Andrei G, and De Clercq E. Human Cytomegalovirus (HCMV) Strains Selected Under Selective Pressure of Phosphonoformate (PFA) and phosphonylmethoxyethyl (PME) Derivatives *In Vitro*. *Antiviral Res*, **26**, Abstract 177, 1995.
11. Baldanti F, Underwood MR, Stanat SC, Biron KK, Chou S, Sarasini A, Silini E, and Gerna G. Single Amino Acid Changes in the DNA Polymerase Confer Foscarnet Resistance and Slow-Growth Phenotype, While Mutations in the UL97-Encoded Phosphotransferase Confer Ganciclovir Resistance in Three Double-Resistant Human Cytomegalovirus Strains Recovered from Patients with AIDS. *J Virol*, **70**:1390-1395, 1996.

© Gilead Sciences, Inc., 1996; all rights reserved.

Part Number: RM-1117   September 1996

Glaxo Wellcome Inc.
FIVE MOORE DRIVE
RESEARCH TRIANGLE PARK, NC 27709

For Medical Information for Healthcare Professionals Contact:
1-888-Talk-2 GW or direct 1-919-315-3272
Medical Information Department: 1-800-334-0089

In Emergencies:
Medical Information Department: 1-800-334-0089

For Consumer inquiries Contact:
1-888-Talk-2 GW

ACLOVATE®   ℞
[a'klō-vāt'']
(alclometasone dipropionate cream)
Cream, 0.05%

ACLOVATE®   ℞
(alclometasone dipropionate ointment)
Ointment, 0.05%

For Dermatologic Use Only—
Not for Ophthalmic Use.

DESCRIPTION

ACLOVATE Cream and Ointment contain alclometasone dipropionate (7α-chloro- 11β,17,21-trihydroxy -16α- methyl-pregna-1,4-diene-3,20-dione 17,21-dipropionate), a synthetic corticosteroid for topical dermatologic use. The corticosteroids constitute a class of primarily synthetic steroids used topically as anti-inflammatory and antipruritic agents. Chemically, alclometasone dipropionate is $C_{28}H_{37}ClO_7$. Alclometasone dipropionate has the molecular weight of 521. It is a white powder, insoluble in water, slightly soluble in propylene glycol, and moderately soluble in hexylene glycol.

Each gram of ACLOVATE Cream contains 0.5 mg of alclometasone dipropionate in a hydrophilic, emollient cream base of propylene glycol, white petrolatum, cetearyl alcohol, glyceryl stearate, PEG 100 stearate, Ceteth-20, monobasic sodium phosphate, chlorocresol, phosphoric acid, and purified water.

Each gram of ACLOVATE Ointment contains 0.5 mg of alclometasone dipropionate in an ointment base of hexylene glycol, white wax, propylene glycol stearate, and white petrolatum.

CLINICAL PHARMACOLOGY

Like other topical corticosteroids, alclometasone dipropionate has anti-inflammatory, antipruritic, and vasoconstrictive properties. The mechanism of the anti-inflammatory activity of the topical steroids, in general, is unclear. However, corticosteroids are thought to act by the induction of phospholipase A_2 inhibitory proteins, collectively called lipocortins. It is postulated that these proteins control the biosynthesis of potent mediators of inflammation such as prostaglandins and leukotrienes by inhibiting the release of their common precursor, arachidonic acid. Arachidonic acid is released from membrane phospholipids by phospholipase A_2.

Pharmacokinetics: The extent of percutaneous absorption of topical corticosteroids is determined by many factors, including the vehicle and the integrity of the epidermal barrier. Occlusive dressings with hydrocortisone for up to 24 hours have not been demonstrated to increase penetration; however, occlusion of hydrocortisone for 96 hours markedly enhances penetration. Topical corticosteroids can be absorbed from normal intact skin. Inflammation and/or other disease processes in the skin may increase percutaneous absorption. A study utilizing a radiolabeled alclometasone dipropionate ointment formulation was performed to measure systemic absorption and excretion. Results indicated that approximately 3% of the steroid was absorbed during 8 hours of contact with intact skin of normal volunteers. Studies performed with ACLOVATE Cream and Ointment indicate that these products are in the low to medium range of potency as compared with other topical corticosteroids.

INDICATIONS AND USAGE

ACLOVATE Cream and Ointment are low to medium potency corticosteroids indicated for the relief of the inflammatory and pruritic manifestations of corticosteroid-responsive dermatoses. ACLOVATE Cream and Ointment may be used in pediatric patients 1 year of age or older, although the safety and efficacy of drug use for longer than 3 weeks have not been established (see PRECAUTIONS: Pediatric Use). Since the safety and efficacy of ACLOVATE Cream and Ointment have not been established in pediatric patients below 1 year of age, their use in this age-group is not recommended.

CONTRAINDICATIONS

ACLOVATE Cream and Ointment are contraindicated in those patients with a history of hypersensitivity to any of the components in these preparations.

PRECAUTIONS

General: Systemic absorption of topical corticosteroids can produce reversible hypothalamic-pituitary-adrenal (HPA) axis suppression with the potential for glucocorticosteroid insufficiency after withdrawal of treatment. Manifestations of Cushing's syndrome, hyperglycemia, and glucosuria can also be produced in some patients by systemic absorption of topical corticosteroids while on treatment.

Patients applying a topical steroid to a large surface area or to areas under occlusion should be evaluated periodically for evidence of HPA axis suppression. This may be done by using the ACTH stimulation, A.M. plasma cortisol, and urinary free cortisol tests.

The effects of ACLOVATE Cream and Ointment on the HPA axis have been evaluated. In one study, ACLOVATE Cream and Ointment were applied to 30% of the body twice daily for 7 days, and occlusive dressings were used in selected patients either 12 hours or 24 hours daily. In another study, ACLOVATE Cream was applied to 80% of the body surface of normal subjects twice daily for 21 days with daily 12-hour periods of whole body occlusion. Average plasma and urinary free cortisol levels and urinary levels of 17-hydroxy-steroids were decreased (about 10%), suggesting suppression of the HPA axis under these conditions. Plasma cortisol levels have also been demonstrated to decrease in pediatric patients treated twice daily for 3 weeks without occlusion. If HPA axis suppression is noted, an attempt should be made to withdraw the drug, to reduce the frequency of application, or to substitute a less potent corticosteroid. Recovery of HPA axis function is generally prompt upon discontinuation of topical corticosteroids. Infrequently, signs and symptoms of glucocorticosteroid insufficiency may occur, requiring supplemental systemic corticosteroids. For information on systemic supplementation, see prescribing information for those products.

Pediatric patients may be more susceptible to systemic toxicity from equivalent doses due to their larger skin surface area to body mass ratios (see PRECAUTIONS: Pediatric Use).

If irritation develops, ACLOVATE Cream or Ointment should be discontinued and appropriate therapy instituted. Allergic contact dermatitis with corticosteroids is usually diagnosed by observing *a failure to heal* rather than noting a clinical exacerbation, as with most topical products not containing corticosteroids. Such an observation should be corroborated with appropriate diagnostic patch testing.

If concomitant skin infections are present or develop, an appropriate antifungal or antibacterial agent should be used. If a favorable response does not occur promptly, use of ACLOVATE Cream or Ointment should be discontinued until the infection has been adequately controlled.

Information for Patients: Patients using topical corticosteroids should receive the following information and instructions:

1. This medication is to be used as directed by the physician. It is for external use only. Avoid contact with the eyes.
2. This medication should not be used for any disorder other than that for which it was prescribed.
3. The treated skin area should not be bandaged, otherwise covered or wrapped so as to be occlusive, unless directed by the physician.
4. Patients should report to their physician any signs of local adverse reactions.
5. Parents of pediatric patients should be advised not to use ACLOVATE Cream or Ointment in the treatment of diaper dermatitis. ACLOVATE Cream or Ointment should not be applied in the diaper area as diapers or plastic pants may constitute occlusive dressing (see DOSAGE AND ADMINISTRATION).
6. This medication should not be used on the face, underarms, or groin areas unless directed by the physician.
7. As with other corticosteroids, therapy should be discontinued when control is achieved. If no improvement is seen within 2 weeks, contact the physician.

Laboratory Tests: The following tests may be helpful in evaluating patients for HPA axis suppression:
ACTH stimulation test
A.M. plasma cortisol test
Urinary free cortisol test

Carcinogenesis, Mutagenesis, Impairment of Fertility: Long-term animal studies have not been performed to evaluate the carcinogenic potential or the effect on fertility of topical corticosteroids.

Pregnancy: *Teratogenic Effects: Pregnancy Category C:* Corticosteroids have been shown to be teratogenic in laboratory animals when administered systemically at relatively low dosage levels. Some corticosteroids have been shown to be teratogenic after dermal application in laboratory animals. There are no adequate and well-controlled

studies in pregnant women. ACLOVATE Cream or Ointment should be used during pregnancy only if the potential benefit justifies the potential risk to the fetus.

Nursing Mothers: Systemically administered corticosteroids appear in human milk and could suppress growth, interfere with endogenous corticosteroid production, or cause other untoward effects. It is not known whether topical administration of topical corticosteroids could result in sufficient systemic absorption to produce detectable quantities in human milk. Because many drugs are excreted in human milk, caution should be exercised when ACLOVATE Cream or Ointment is administered to a nursing woman.

Pediatric Use: ACLOVATE Cream and Ointment may be used with caution in pediatric patients 1 year of age or older, although the safety and efficacy of drug use for longer than 3 weeks have not been established. Use of ACLOVATE Cream and Ointment is supported by results from adequate and well-controlled studies in pediatric patients with corticosteroid-responsive dermatoses. Since the safety and efficacy of ACLOVATE Cream and Ointment have not been established in pediatric patients below 1 year of age, its use in this age-group is not recommended. Because of a higher ratio of skin surface area to body mass, pediatric patients are at a greater risk than adults of HPA axis suppression and Cushing's syndrome when they are treated with topical corticosteroids. They are therefore also at greater risk of adrenal insufficiency during and/or after withdrawal of treatment. Adverse effects, including striae, have been reported with use of topical corticosteroids in infants and children. Pediatric patients applying ACLOVATE Cream or Ointment to >20% of the body surface area are at higher risk for HPA axis suppression.

HPA axis suppression, Cushing's syndrome, linear growth retardation, delayed weight gain, and intracranial hypertension have been reported in pediatric patients receiving topical corticosteroids. Manifestations of adrenal suppression in pediatric patients include low plasma cortisol levels and absence of response to ACTH stimulation. Manifestations of intracranial hypertension include bulging fontanelles, headaches, and bilateral papilledema.

ACLOVATE Cream or Ointment should not be used in the treatment of diaper dermatitis.

ADVERSE REACTIONS

The following local adverse reactions have been reported with ACLOVATE Cream in approximately 2% of patients: itching and burning, erythema, dryness, irritation, and papular rashes.

The following local adverse reactions have been reported with ACLOVATE Ointment in approximately 1% of patients: itching, burning, and erythema.

The following additional local adverse reactions have been reported infrequently with topical corticosteroids, but may occur more frequently with the use of occlusive dressings. These reactions are listed in approximate decreasing order of occurrence: folliculitis, acneiform eruptions, hypopigmentation, perioral dermatitis, allergic contact dermatitis, secondary infection, skin atrophy, striae, and miliaria.

OVERDOSAGE

Topically applied ACLOVATE Cream and Ointment can be absorbed in sufficient amounts to produce systemic effects (see PRECAUTIONS).

DOSAGE AND ADMINISTRATION

Apply a thin film of ACLOVATE Cream or Ointment to the affected skin areas two or three times daily; massage gently until the medication disappears.

ACLOVATE Cream and Ointment may be used in pediatric patients 1 year of age or older. Safety and effectiveness of ACLOVATE Cream or Ointment in pediatric patients for more than 3 weeks of use have not been established. Use in pediatric patients under 1 year of age is not recommended. As with other corticosteroids, therapy should be discontinued when control is achieved. If no improvement is seen within 2 weeks, reassessment of diagnosis may be necessary.

ACLOVATE Cream or Ointment should not be used with occlusive dressings unless directed by a physician.

ACLOVATE Cream or Ointment should not be applied in the diaper area if the child still requires diapers or plastic pants as these garments may constitute occlusive dressing.

HOW SUPPLIED

ACLOVATE Cream, 0.05% is supplied in 15-g (NDC 0173-0401-00), 45-g (NDC 0173-0401-01), and 60-g (NDC 0173-0401-06) tubes.

ACLOVATE Ointment, 0.05% is supplied in 15-g (NDC 0173-0402-00), 45-g (NDC 0173-0402-01), and 60-g (NDC 0173-0402-06) tubes.

Store between 2° and 30°C (36° and 86°F).

April 1996/RL-217

Shown in Product Identification Guide, page 311

ALKERAN® ℞
[ăl 'kur-ăn]
(melphalan hydrochloride)
for Injection

> **WARNING:** Melphalan should be administered under the supervision of a qualified physician experienced in the use of cancer chemotherapeutic agents. Severe bone marrow suppression with resulting infection or bleeding may occur. Controlled trials comparing intravenous (IV) to oral melphalan have shown more myelosuppression with the IV formulation. Hypersensitivity reactions, including anaphylaxis, have occurred in approximately 2% of patients who received the IV formulation. Melphalan is leukemogenic in humans. Melphalan produces chromosomal aberrations in vitro and in vivo and, therefore, should be considered potentially mutagenic in humans.

DESCRIPTION

Melphalan, also known as L-phenylalanine mustard, phenylalanine mustard, L-PAM, or L-sarcolysin, is a phenylalanine derivative of nitrogen mustard. Melphalan is a bifunctional alkylating agent that is active against selected human neoplastic diseases. It is known chemically as 4-[bis(2-chloroethyl)amino]-L-phenylalanine. The molecular formula is $C_{13}H_{18}Cl_2N_2O_2$ and the molecular weight is 305.20.

Melphalan is the active L-isomer of the compound and was first synthesized in 1953 by Bergel and Stock; the D-isomer, known as medphalan, is less active against certain animal tumors, and the dose needed to produce effects on chromosomes is larger than that required with the L-isomer. The racemic (DL-) form is known as merphalan or sarcolysin. Melphalan is practically insoluble in water and has a pKa_1 of ~2.5.

ALKERAN for Injection is supplied as a sterile, non-pyrogenic, freeze-dried powder. Each single-use vial contains melphalan hydrochloride equivalent to 50 mg melphalan and 20 mg povidone. ALKERAN for Injection is reconstituted using the sterile diluent provided. Each vial of sterile diluent contains sodium citrate 0.2 g, propylene glycol 6.0 mL, ethanol (96%) 0.52 mL, and Water for Injection to a total of 10 mL. ALKERAN for Injection is administered intravenously.

CLINICAL PHARMACOLOGY

Melphalan is an alkylating agent of the bischloroethylamine type. As a result, its cytotoxicity appears to be related to the extent of its interstrand cross-linking with DNA, probably by binding at the N^7 position of guanine. Like other bifunctional alkylating agents, it is active against both resting and rapidly dividing tumor cells.

Pharmacokinetics: The pharmacokinetics of melphalan after IV administration has been extensively studied in adult patients. Following injection, drug plasma concentrations declined rapidly in a biexponential manner with distribution phase and terminal elimination phase half-lives of approximately 10 and 75 minutes, respectively. Estimates of average total body clearance varied among studies, but typical values of approximately 7 to 9 mL/min per kg (250 to 325 mL/min/m²) were observed. One study has reported that on repeat dosing of 0.5 mg/kg every 6 weeks, the clearance of melphalan decreased from 8.1 mL/min per kg after the first course, to 5.5 mL/min per kg after the third course, but did not decrease appreciably after the third course. Mean (±SD) peak melphalan plasma concentrations in myeloma patients given IV melphalan at doses of 10 or 20 mg/m² were 1.2±0.4 and 2.8±1.9 ng/mL, respectively.

The steady-state volume of distribution of melphalan is 0.5 L/kg. Penetration into cerebrospinal fluid (CSF) is low. The extent of melphalan binding to plasma proteins ranges from 60% to 90%. Serum albumin is the major binding protein, while α_1-acid glycoprotein appears to account for about 20% of the plasma protein binding. Approximately 30% of the drug is (covalently) irreversibly bound to plasma proteins. Interactions with immunoglobulins have been found to be negligible.

Melphalan is eliminated from plasma primarily by chemical hydrolysis to monohydroxymelphalan and dihydroxymelphalan. Aside from these hydrolysis products, no other melphalan metabolites have been observed in humans. Although the contribution of renal elimination to melphalan clearance appears to be low, one study noted an increase in the occurrence of severe leukopenia in patients with elevated BUN after 10 weeks of therapy.

Clinical Trial: A randomized trial compared prednisone plus IV melphalan to prednisone plus oral melphalan in the treatment of myeloma. As discussed below, overall response rates at week 22 were comparable; however, because of changes in trial design, conclusions as to the relative activity of the two formulations after week 22 are impossible to make.

Both arms received oral prednisone starting at 0.8 mg/kg per day with doses tapered over 6 weeks. Melphalan doses in each arm were:

Arm 1   Oral melphalan 0.15 mg/kg per day × 7 followed by 0.05 mg/kg per day when WBC began to rise.

Arm 2   IV melphalan 16 mg/m² q 2 weeks × 4 (over 6 weeks) followed by the same dose every 4 weeks.

Doses of melphalan were adjusted according to the following criteria:

WBC/mm³	Platelets	Percent of Full Dose
≥4000	≥100000	100
≥3000	≥75000	75
≥2000	≥50000	50
<2000	<50000	0

One hundred seven patients were randomized to the oral melphalan arm and 203 patients to the IV melphalan arm. More patients had a poor-risk classification (58% versus 44%) and high tumor load (51% versus 34%) on the oral compared to the IV arm ($P<0.04$). Response rates at week 22 are shown in the following table:

Initial Arm	Evaluable Patients	Responders n (%)	P
Oral melphalan	100	44 (44%)	P>0.2
IV melphalan	195	74 (38%)	

Because of changes in protocol design after week 22, other efficacy parameters such as response duration and survival can not be compared.

Severe myelotoxicity (WBC ≤1000 and/or platelets ≤25000) was more common in the IV melphalan arm (28%) than in the oral melphalan arm (11%).

An association was noted between poor renal function and myelosuppression; consequently, an amendment to the protocol required a 50% reduction in IV melphalan dose if the BUN was ≥30 mg/dL. The rate of severe leukopenia in the IV arm in the patients with BUN over 30 mg/dL decreased from 50% (8/16) before protocol amendment to 11% (3/28) ($P = .01$) after the amendment.

Before the dosing amendment, there was a 10% (8/77) incidence of drug-related death in the IV arm. After the dosing amendment, this incidence was 3% (3/108). This compares to an overall 1% (1/100) incidence of drug-related death in the oral arm.

INDICATIONS AND USAGE

ALKERAN for Injection is indicated for the palliative treatment of patients with multiple myeloma for whom oral therapy is not appropriate.

CONTRAINDICATIONS

Melphalan should not be used in patients whose disease has demonstrated prior resistance to this agent. Patients who have demonstrated hypersensitivity to melphalan should not be given the drug.

WARNINGS

Melphalan should be administered in carefully adjusted dosage by or under the supervision of experienced physicians who are familiar with the drug's actions and the possible complications of its use.

As with other nitrogen mustard drugs, excessive dosage will produce marked bone marrow suppression. Bone marrow suppression is the most significant toxicity associated with ALKERAN for Injection in most patients. Therefore, the following tests should be performed at the start of therapy and prior to each subsequent dose of ALKERAN: platelet count, hemoglobin, white blood cell count, and differential. Thrombocytopenia and/or leukopenia are indications to withhold further therapy until the blood counts have sufficiently recovered. Frequent blood counts are essential to determine optimal dosage and to avoid toxicity. Dose adjustment on the basis of blood counts at the nadir and day of treatment should be considered.

Hypersensitivity reactions including anaphylaxis have occurred in approximately 2% of patients who received the IV

Continued on next page

This product information is based on labeling in effect on June 1, 1998. For further information, contact via direct mail, phone, or web site Medical Information: Glaxo Wellcome Inc., PO Box 13398, Research Triangle Park, NC 27709. Healthcare Professionals (Medical Information): 800-334-0089 Patients (Customer Response Center): 888-TALK2GW (1-888-825-5249) Glaxo Wellcome Corporate Web Site: www.glaxowellcome.com

Alkeran for Injection—Cont.

formulation (see ADVERSE REACTIONS). These reactions usually occur after multiple courses of treatment. Treatment is symptomatic. The infusion should be terminated immediately, followed by the administration of volume expanders, pressor agents, corticosteroids, or antihistamines at the discretion of the physician. If a hypersensitivity reaction occurs, IV or oral melphalan should not be readministered since hypersensitivity reactions have also been reported with oral melphalan.

Carcinogenesis: Secondary malignancies, including acute nonlymphocytic leukemia, myeloproliferative syndrome, and carcinoma, have been reported in patients with cancer treated with alkylating agents (including melphalan). Some patients also received other chemotherapeutic agents or radiation therapy. Precise quantitation of the risk of acute leukemia, myeloproliferative syndrome, or carcinoma is not possible. Published reports of leukemia in patients who have received melphalan (and other alkylating agents) suggest that the risk of leukemogenesis increases with chronicity of treatment and with cumulative dose. In one study, the 10-year cumulative risk of developing acute leukemia or myeloproliferative syndrome after oral melphalan therapy was 19.5% for cumulative doses ranging from 730 to 9652 mg. In this same study, as well as in an additional study, the 10-year cumulative risk of developing acute leukemia or myeloproliferative syndrome after oral melphalan therapy was less than 2% for cumulative doses under 600 mg. This does not mean that there is a cumulative dose below which there is no risk of the induction of secondary malignancy. The potential benefits from melphalan therapy must be weighed on an individual basis against the possible risk of the induction of a second malignancy.

Adequate and well-controlled carcinogenicity studies have not been conducted in animals. However, intraperitoneal (IP) administration of melphalan in rats (5.4 to 10.8 mg/m^2) and in mice (2.25 to 4.5 mg/m^2) three times per week for 6 months followed by 12 months post-dose observation produced peritoneal sarcoma and lung tumors, respectively.

Mutagenesis: Melphalan has been shown to cause chromatid or chromosome damage in humans. Intramuscular administration of melphalan at 6 and 60 mg/m^2 produced structural aberrations of the chromatid and chromosomes in bone marrow cells of Wistar rats.

Impairment of Fertility: Melphalan causes suppression of ovarian function in premenopausal women, resulting in amenorrhea in a significant number of patients. Reversible and irreversible testicular suppression have also been reported.

Pregnancy: Pregnancy Category D. Melphalan may cause fetal harm when administered to a pregnant woman. While adequate animal studies have not been conducted with IV melphalan, oral (6 to 18 mg/m^2 per day for 10 days) and IP (18 mg/m^2 per kg single dose) administration in rats was embryolethal and teratogenic. Malformations resulting from melphalan included alterations of the brain (underdevelopment, deformation, meningocele, and encephalocele) and eye (anophthalmia and microphthalmos), reduction of the mandible and tail, as well as hepatocele (exomphaly). There are no adequate and well-controlled studies in pregnant women. If this drug is used during pregnancy, or if the patient becomes pregnant while taking this drug, the patient should be apprised of the potential hazard to the fetus. Women of childbearing potential should be advised to avoid becoming pregnant.

PRECAUTIONS

General: In all instances where the use of ALKERAN for Injection is considered for chemotherapy, the physician must evaluate the need and usefulness of the drug against the risk of adverse events. Melphalan should be used with extreme caution in patients whose bone marrow reserve may have been compromised by prior irradiation or chemotherapy or whose marrow function is recovering from previous cytotoxic therapy.

Dose reduction should be considered in patients with renal insufficiency receiving IV melphalan. In one trial, increased bone marrow suppression was observed in patients with BUN levels ≥30 mg/dL. A 50% reduction in the IV melphalan dose decreased the incidence of severe bone marrow suppression in the latter portion of this study.

Information for Patients: Patients should be informed that the major acute toxicities of melphalan are related to bone marrow suppression, hypersensitivity reactions, gastrointestinal toxicity, and pulmonary toxicity. The major long-term toxicities are related to infertility and secondary malignancies. Patients should never be allowed to take the drug without close medical supervision and should be advised to consult their physicians if they experience skin rash, signs or symptoms of vasculitis, bleeding, fever, persistent cough, nausea, vomiting, amenorrhea, weight loss, or unusual lumps/masses. Women of childbearing potential should be advised to avoid becoming pregnant.

Laboratory Tests: Periodic complete blood counts with differentials should be performed during the course of treat-

ment with melphalan. At least one determination should be obtained prior to each dose. Patients should be observed closely for consequences of bone marrow suppression, which include severe infections, bleeding, and symptomatic anemia (see WARNINGS).

Drug Interactions: The development of severe renal failure has been reported in patients treated with a single dose of IV melphalan followed by standard oral doses of cyclosporine. Cisplatin may affect melphalan kinetics by inducing renal dysfunction and subsequently altering melphalan clearance. IV melphalan may also reduce the threshold for BCNU lung toxicity. When nalidixic acid and IV melphalan are given simultaneously, the incidence of severe hemorrhagic necrotic enterocolitis has been reported to increase in pediatric patients.

Carcinogenesis, Mutagenesis, Impairment of Fertility: See WARNINGS section.

Pregnancy: *Teratogenic Effects:* Pregnancy Category D: See WARNINGS section.

Nursing Mothers: It is not known whether this drug is excreted in human milk. IV melphalan should not be given to nursing mothers.

Pediatric Use: The safety and effectiveness in pediatric patients have not been established.

Geriatric Use: Clinical experience with ALKERAN has not identified differences in responses between the elderly and younger patients. In general, dose selection for an elderly patient should be cautious, reflecting the greater frequency of decreased hepatic, renal, or cardiac function, and of concomitant disease or other drug therapy.

ADVERSE REACTIONS (see OVERDOSAGE)

The following information on adverse reactions is based on data from both oral and IV administration of melphalan as a single agent, using several different dose schedules for treatment of a wide variety of malignancies.

Hematologic: The most common side effect is bone marrow suppression. White blood cell count and platelet count nadirs usually occur 2 to 3 weeks after treatment, with recovery in 4 to 5 weeks after treatment. Irreversible bone marrow failure has been reported.

Gastrointestinal: Gastrointestinal disturbances such as nausea and vomiting, diarrhea, and oral ulceration occur infrequently. Hepatic toxicity, including veno-occlusive disease, has been reported.

Hypersensitivity: Acute hypersensitivity reactions including anaphylaxis were reported in 2.4% of 425 patients receiving ALKERAN for Injection for myeloma (see WARNINGS). These reactions were characterized by urticaria, pruritus, edema, and in some patients, tachycardia, bronchospasm, dyspnea, and hypotension. These patients appeared to respond to antihistamine and corticosteroid therapy. If a hypersensitivity reaction occurs, IV or oral melphalan should not be readministered since hypersensitivity reactions have also been reported with oral melphalan.

Miscellaneous: Other reported adverse reactions include skin hypersensitivity, skin ulceration at injection site, skin necrosis rarely requiring skin grafting, vasculitis, alopecia, hemolytic anemia, allergic reaction, pulmonary fibrosis, and interstitial pneumonitis.

OVERDOSAGE

Overdoses resulting in death have been reported. Overdoses, including doses up to 290 mg/m^2, have produced the following symptoms: severe nausea and vomiting, decreased consciousness, convulsions, muscular paralysis, and cholinomimetic effects. Severe mucositis, stomatitis, colitis, diarrhea, and hemorrhage of the gastrointestinal tract occur at high doses (>100 mg/m^2). Elevations in liver enzymes and veno-occlusive disease occur infrequently. Significant hyponatremia caused by an associated inappropriate secretion of ADH syndrome has been observed. Nephrotoxicity and adult respiratory distress syndrome have been reported rarely. The principal toxic effect is bone marrow suppression. Hematologic parameters should be closely followed for 3 to 6 weeks. An uncontrolled study suggests that administration of autologous bone marrow or hematopoietic growth factors (i.e., sargramostim, filgrastim) may shorten the period of pancytopenia. General supportive measures together with appropriate blood transfusions and antibiotics should be instituted as deemed necessary by the physician. This drug is not removed from plasma to any significant degree by hemodialysis or hemoperfusion. A pediatric patient survived a 254-mg/m^2 overdose treated with standard supportive care.

DOSAGE AND ADMINISTRATION

The usual IV dose is 16 mg/m^2. Dosage reduction of up to 50% should be considered in patients with renal insufficiency (BUN ≥30 mg/dL) (see PRECAUTIONS: General). The drug is administered as a single infusion over 15 to 20 minutes. Melphalan is administered at 2-week intervals for four doses, then, after adequate recovery from toxicity, at 4-week intervals. Available evidence suggests about one third to one half of the patients with multiple myeloma show a favorable response to the drug. Experience with oral melphalan suggests that repeated courses should be given

since improvement may continue slowly over many months, and the maximum benefit may be missed if treatment is abandoned prematurely. Dose adjustment on the basis of blood cell counts at the nadir and day of treatment should be considered.

Administration Precautions: As with other toxic compounds, caution should be exercised in handling and preparing the solution of ALKERAN. Skin reactions associated with accidental exposure may occur. The use of gloves is recommended. If the solution of ALKERAN contacts the skin or mucosa, immediately wash the skin or mucosa thoroughly with soap and water.

Procedures for proper handling and disposal of anticancer drugs should be considered. Several guidelines on this subject have been published.[1–7] There is no general agreement that all of the procedures recommended in the guidelines are necessary or appropriate.

Parenteral drug products should be visually inspected for particulate matter and discoloration prior to administration whenever solution and container permit. If either occurs, do not use this product.

Preparation for Administration/Stability:

1. ALKERAN for Injection must be reconstituted by rapidly injecting 10 mL of the supplied diluent directly into the vial of lyophilized powder using a sterile needle (20-gauge or larger needle diameter) and syringe. Immediately shake vial vigorously until a clear solution is obtained. This provides a 5-mg/mL solution of melphalan. Rapid addition of the diluent followed by immediate vigorous shaking is important for proper dissolution.

2. **Immediately** dilute the dose to be administered in 0.9% Sodium Chloride Injection, USP, to a concentration not greater than 0.45 mg/mL.

3. Administer the diluted product over a minimum of 15 minutes.

4. Complete administration within 60 minutes of reconstitution.

The time between reconstitution/dilution and administration of ALKERAN should be kept to a minimum because reconstituted and diluted solutions of ALKERAN are unstable. Over as short a time as 30 minutes, a citrate derivative of melphalan has been detected in reconstituted material from the reaction of ALKERAN with Sterile Diluent for ALKERAN. Upon further dilution with saline, nearly 1% label strength of melphalan hydrolyzes every 10 minutes. A precipitate forms if the reconstituted solution is stored at 5°C. DO NOT REFRIGERATE THE RECONSTITUTED PRODUCT.

HOW SUPPLIED

ALKERAN for Injection is supplied in a carton containing one single-use clear glass vial of freeze-dried melphalan hydrochloride equivalent to 50 mg melphalan and one 10 mL clear glass vial of sterile diluent (NDC 0173-0130-93).

Store at controlled room temperature 15° to 30°C (59° to 86°F) and protect from light.

REFERENCES

1. Recommendations for the safe handling of parenteral antineoplastic drugs. Washington, DC: Division of Safety, National Institutes of Health; 1983. US Dept of Health and Human Services, Public Health Service publication NIH 83-2621.

2. AMA Council on Scientific Affairs. Guidelines for handling parenteral antineoplastics. *JAMA.* 1985; 253:1590-1591.

3. National Study Commission on Cytotoxic Exposure. Recommendations for handling cytotoxic agents. 1987. Available from Louis P. Jeffrey, Chairman, National Study Commission on Cytotoxic Exposure. Massachusetts College of Pharmacy and Allied Health Sciences, 179 Longwood Avenue, Boston, MA 02115.

4. Clinical Oncological Society of Australia. Guidelines and recommendations for safe handling of antineoplastic agents. *Med J Australia.* 1983;1:426-428.

5. Jones RB, Frank R, Mass T. Safe handling of chemotherapeutic agents: a report from the Mount Sinai Medical Center. *CA-A Cancer J for Clin.* 1983;33:258-263.

6. American Society of Hospital Pharmacists. ASHP technical assistance bulletin on handling cytotoxic and hazardous drugs. *Am J Hosp Pharm.* 1990;47:1033-1049.

7. Yodaiken RE, Bennett D. OSHA work-practice guidelines for personnel dealing with cytotoxic (antineoplastic) drugs. *Am J Hosp Pharm.* 1986;43:1193-1204.

U.S. Patent No. 4,997,651
©Copyright 1996 Glaxo Wellcome Inc.
All rights reserved.
August 1997/RL-451

Shown in Product Identification Guide, page 311

ALKERAN® ℞
[ăl-kur 'ăn]
(melphalan)
2-mg Scored Tablets

> **WARNING:** ALKERAN (melphalan) should be administered under the supervision of a qualified physician experienced in the use of cancer chemotherapeutic agents. Severe bone marrow suppression with resulting infection or bleeding may occur. Melphalan is leukemogenic in humans.
> Melphalan produces chromosomal aberrations in vitro and in vivo and, therefore, should be considered potentially mutagenic in humans.

DESCRIPTION

ALKERAN (melphalan), also known as L-phenylalanine mustard, phenylalanine mustard, L-PAM, or L-sarcolysin, is a phenylalanine derivative of nitrogen mustard. Melphalan is a bifunctional alkylating agent which is active against selective human neoplastic diseases. It is known chemically as 4-[bis(2-chloroethyl)amino]-L-phenylalanine. The molecular formula is $C_{13}H_{18}Cl_2N_2O_2$ and the molecular weight is 305.20.

Melphalan is the active L-isomer of the compound and was first synthesized in 1953 by Bergel and Stock; the D-isomer, known as medphalan, is less active against certain animal tumors, and the dose needed to produce effects on chromosomes is larger than that required with the L-isomer. The racemic (DL–) form is known as merphalan or sarcolysin. Melphalan is practically insoluble in water and has a pKa_1 of ~2.5.

ALKERAN (melphalan) is available in tablet form for oral administration. Each scored tablet contains 2 mg melphalan and the inactive ingredients lactose, magnesium stearate, potato starch, povidone, and sucrose.

CLINICAL PHARMACOLOGY

Melphalan is an alkylating agent of the bischloroethylamine type. As a result, its cytotoxicity appears to be related to the extent of its interstrand cross-linking with DNA, probably by binding at the N^7 position of guanine. Like other bifunctional alkylating agents, it is active against both resting and rapidly dividing tumor cells.

Pharmacokinetics: The pharmacokinetics of ALKERAN after oral administration has been extensively studied in adult patients. Plasma melphalan levels are highly variable after oral dosing, both with respect to the time of the first appearance of melphalan in plasma (range 0 to 336 minutes) and to the peak plasma concentration (range 0.166 to 3.741 mcg/mL) achieved. These results may be due to incomplete intestinal absorption, a variable "first pass" hepatic metabolism, or to rapid hydrolysis. Five patients were studied after both oral and intravenous (IV) dosing with 0.6 mg/kg as a single bolus dose by each route. The areas under the plasma concentration-time curves after oral administration averaged 61% ± 26% (± standard deviation; range 25% to 89%) of those following IV administration. In 18 patients given a single oral dose of 0.6 mg/kg of ALKERAN, the terminal plasma half-disappearance time of parent drug was 89.5 ± 50 minutes. The 24-hour urinary excretion of parent drug in these patients was 10% ± 4.5%, suggesting that renal clearance is not a major route of elimination of parent drug.

One study using universally labeled ^{14}C-melphalan, found substantially less radioactivity in the urine of patients given the drug by mouth (30% of administered dose in 9 days) than in the urine of those given it intravenously (35% to 65% in 7 days). Following either oral or IV administration, the pattern of label recovery was similar, with the majority being recovered in the first 24 hours. Following oral administration, peak radioactivity occurred in plasma at 2 hours and then disappeared with a half-life of approximately 160 hours. In one patient where parent drug (rather than just radiolabel) was determined, the melphalan half-disappearance time was 67 minutes.

The steady-state volume of distribution of melphalan is 0.5 L/kg. Penetration into cerebrospinal fluid (CSF) is low. The extent of melphalan binding to plasma proteins ranges from 60% to 90%. Serum albumin is the major binding protein, while α_1-acid glycoprotein appears to account for about 20% of the plasma protein binding. Approximately 30% of melphalan is (covalently) irreversibly bound to plasma proteins. Interactions with immunoglobulins have been found to be negligible.

Melphalan is eliminated from plasma primarily by chemical hydrolysis to monohydroxymelphalan and dihydroxymelphalan. Aside from these hydrolysis products, no other melphalan metabolites have been observed in humans. Although the contribution of renal elimination to melphalan clearance appears to be low, one pharmacokinetic study showed a significant positive correlation between the elimination rate constant for melphalan and renal function and a significant negative correlation between renal function and the area under the plasma melphalan concentration/time curve.

INDICATIONS AND USAGE

ALKERAN Tablets are indicated for the palliative treatment of multiple myeloma and for the palliation of nonresectable epithelial carcinoma of the ovary.

CONTRAINDICATIONS

ALKERAN should not be used in patients whose disease has demonstrated a prior resistance to this agent. Patients who have demonstrated hypersensitivity to melphalan should not be given the drug.

WARNINGS

ALKERAN should be administered in carefully adjusted dosage by or under the supervision of experienced physicians who are familiar with the drug's actions and the possible complications of its use.

As with other nitrogen mustard drugs, excessive dosage will produce marked bone marrow suppression. Bone marrow suppression is the most significant toxicity associated with ALKERAN in most patients. Therefore, the following tests should be performed at the start of therapy and prior to each subsequent course of ALKERAN: platelet count, hemoglobin, white blood cell count, and differential. Thrombocytopenia and/or leukopenia are indications to withhold further therapy until the blood counts have sufficiently recovered. Frequent blood counts are essential to determine optimal dosage and to avoid toxicity (see PRECAUTIONS: Laboratory Tests). Dose adjustment on the basis of blood counts at the nadir and day of treatment should be considered.

Hypersensitivity reactions, including anaphylaxis, have occurred rarely (see ADVERSE REACTIONS). These reactions have occurred after multiple courses of treatment and have recurred in patients who experienced a hypersensitivity reaction to IV ALKERAN. If a hypersensitivity reaction occurs, oral or IV ALKERAN should not be readministered.

Carcinogenesis: Secondary malignancies, including acute nonlymphocytic leukemia, myeloproliferative syndrome, and carcinoma have been reported in patients with cancer treated with alkylating agents (including melphalan). Some patients also received other chemotherapeutic agents or radiation therapy. Precise quantitation of the risk of acute leukemia, myeloproliferative syndrome, or carcinoma is not possible. Published reports of leukemia in patients who have received melphalan (and other alkylating agents) suggest that the risk of leukemogenesis increases with chronicity of treatment and with cumulative dose. In one study, the 10-year cumulative risk of developing acute leukemia or myeloproliferative syndrome after melphalan therapy was 19.5% for cumulative doses ranging from 730 mg to 9652 mg. In this same study, as well as in an additional study, the 10-year cumulative risk of developing acute leukemia or myeloproliferative syndrome after melphalan therapy was less than 2% for cumulative doses under 600 mg. This does not mean that there is a cumulative dose below which there is no risk of the induction of secondary malignancy. The potential benefits from melphalan therapy must be weighed on an individual basis against the possible risk of the induction of a second malignancy.

Adequate and well-controlled carcinogenicity studies have not been conducted in animals. However, i.p. administration of melphalan in rats (5.4 to 10.8 mg/m²) and in mice (2.25 to 4.5 mg/m²) three times per week for 6 months followed by 12 months post-dose observation produced peritoneal sarcoma and lung tumors, respectively.

Mutagenesis: ALKERAN has been shown to cause chromatid or chromosome damage in humans. Intramuscular administration of ALKERAN at 6 and 60 mg/m² produced structural aberrations of the chromatid and chromosomes in bone marrow cells of Wistar rats.

Impairment of Fertility: ALKERAN causes suppression of ovarian function in premenopausal women, resulting in amenorrhea in a significant number of patients. Reversible and irreversible testicular suppression have also been reported.

Pregnancy: Pregnancy Category D. ALKERAN may cause fetal harm when administered to a pregnant woman. Melphalan was embryolethal and teratogenic in rats following oral (6 to 18 mg/m² per day for 10 days) and intraperitoneal (18 mg/m² per kg single dose) administration. Malformations resulting from melphalan included alterations of the brain (underdevelopment, deformation, meningocele, and encephalocele) and eye (anophthalmia and microphthalmos), reduction of the mandible and tail, as well as hepatocele (exomphaly).

There are no adequate and well-controlled studies in pregnant women. If this drug is used during pregnancy, or if the patient becomes pregnant while taking this drug, the patient should be apprised of the potential hazard to the fetus. Women of childbearing potential should be advised to avoid becoming pregnant.

PRECAUTIONS

General: In all instances where the use of ALKERAN is considered for chemotherapy, the physician must evaluate the need and usefulness of the drug against the risk of adverse events. ALKERAN should be used with extreme caution in patients whose bone marrow reserve may have been compromised by prior irradiation or chemotherapy, or whose marrow function is recovering from previous cytotoxic therapy. If the leukocyte count falls below 3,000 cells/mcL, or the platelet count below 100,000 cells/mcL, ALKERAN should be discontinued until the peripheral blood cell counts have recovered.

A recommendation as to whether or not dosage reduction should be made routinely in patients with renal insufficiency cannot be made because:

(a) There is considerable inherent patient-to-patient variability in the systemic availability of melphalan in patients with normal renal function.

(b) Only a small amount of the administered dose appears as parent drug in the urine of patients with normal renal function.

Patients with azotemia should be closely observed, however, in order to make dosage reductions, if required, at the earliest possible time.

Information for Patients: Patients should be informed that the major toxicities of ALKERAN are related to bone marrow suppression, hypersensitivity reactions, gastrointestinal toxicity, and pulmonary toxicity. The major long-term toxicities are related to infertility and secondary malignancies. Patients should never be allowed to take the drug without close medical supervision and should be advised to consult their physician if they experience skin rash, vasculitis, bleeding, fever, persistent cough, nausea, vomiting, amenorrhea, weight loss, or unusual lumps/masses. Women of childbearing potential should be advised to avoid becoming pregnant.

Laboratory Tests: Periodic complete blood counts with differentials should be performed during the course of treatment with ALKERAN. At least one determination should be obtained prior to each treatment course. Patients should be observed closely for consequences of bone marrow suppression, which include severe infections, bleeding, and symptomatic anemia (see WARNINGS).

Drug Interactions: There are no known drug/drug interactions with oral ALKERAN.

Carcinogenesis, Mutagenesis, Impairment of Fertility: See WARNINGS section.

Pregnancy: *Teratogenic Effects:* Pregnancy Category D: See WARNINGS section.

Nursing Mothers: It is not known whether this drug is excreted in human milk. ALKERAN should not be given to nursing mothers.

Pediatric Use: The safety and effectiveness of ALKERAN in pediatric patients have not been established.

Geriatric Use: Clinical experience with ALKERAN has not identified differences in responses between the elderly and younger patients. In general, dose selection for an elderly patient should be cautious, reflecting the greater frequency of decreased hepatic, renal, or cardiac function, and of concomitant disease or other drug therapy.

ADVERSE REACTIONS

Hematologic: The most common side effect is bone marrow suppression. Although bone marrow suppression frequently occurs, it is usually reversible if melphalan is withdrawn early enough. However, irreversible bone marrow failure has been reported.

Gastrointestinal: Gastrointestinal disturbances such as nausea and vomiting, diarrhea, and oral ulceration occur infrequently. Hepatic toxicity has been reported rarely.

Miscellaneous: Other reported adverse reactions include: pulmonary fibrosis and interstitial pneumonitis, skin hypersensitivity, vasculitis, alopecia, and hemolytic anemia. Allergic reactions, including rare anaphylaxis, have occurred after multiple courses of treatment.

OVERDOSAGE

Overdoses, including doses up to 50 mg/day for 16 days, have been reported. Immediate effects are likely to be vomiting, ulceration of the mouth, diarrhea, and hemorrhage of the gastrointestinal tract. The principal toxic effect is bone marrow suppression. Hematologic parameters should be closely followed for 3 to 6 weeks. An uncontrolled study suggests that administration of autologous bone marrow or hematopoietic growth factors (i.e., sargramostim, filgrastim) may shorten the period of pancytopenia. General supportive measures, together with appropriate blood

Continued on next page

This product information is based on labeling in effect on June 1, 1998. For further information, contact via direct mail, phone, or web site Medical Information: Glaxo Wellcome Inc., PO Box 13398, Research Triangle Park, NC 27709. Healthcare Professionals (Medical Information): 800-334-0089 Patients (Customer Response Center): 888-TALK2GW (1-888-825-5249) Glaxo Wellcome Corporate Web Site: www.glaxowellcome.com

Alkeran Tablets—Cont.

transfusions and antibiotics, should be instituted as deemed necessary by the physician. This drug is not removed from plasma to any significant degree by hemodialysis.[1]

DOSAGE AND ADMINISTRATION

Multiple Myeloma: The usual oral dose is 6 mg (3 tablets) daily. The entire daily dose may be given at one time. The dose is adjusted, as required, on the basis of blood counts done at approximately weekly intervals. After 2 to 3 weeks of treatment, the drug should be discontinued for up to 4 weeks during which time the blood count should be followed carefully. When the white blood cell and platelet counts are rising, a maintenance dose of 2 mg daily may be instituted. Because of the patient-to-patient variation in melphalan plasma levels following oral administration of the drug, several investigators have recommended that the dosage of ALKERAN be cautiously escalated until some myelosuppression is observed in order to assure that potentially therapeutic levels of the drug have been reached.

Other dosage regimens have been used by various investigators. Osserman and Takatsuki have used an initial course of 10 mg/day for 7 to 10 days.[2,3] They report that maximal suppression of the leukocyte and platelet counts occurs within 3 to 5 weeks and recovery within 4 to 8 weeks. Continuous maintenance therapy with 2 mg/day is instituted when the white blood cell count is greater than 4,000 cells/mcL and the platelet count is greater than 100,000 cells/mcL. Dosage is adjusted to between 1 and 3 mg/day depending upon the hematological response. It is desirable to try to maintain a significant degree of bone marrow depression so as to keep the leukocyte count in the range of 3,000 to 3,500 cells/mcL.

Hoogstraten et al have started treatment with 0.15 mg/kg per day for 7 days.[4] This is followed by a rest period of at least 14 days, but it may be as long as 5 to 6 weeks. Maintenance therapy is started when the white blood cell and platelet counts are rising. The maintenance dose is 0.05 mg/kg per day or less and is adjusted according to the blood count.

Available evidence suggests that about one third to one half of the patients with multiple myeloma show a favorable response to oral administration of the drug.

One study by Alexanian et al has shown that the use of ALKERAN in combination with prednisone significantly improves the percentage of patients with multiple myeloma who achieve palliation.[5] One regimen has been to administer courses of ALKERAN at 0.25 mg/kg per day for 4 consecutive days (or, 0.20 mg/kg per day for 5 consecutive days) for a total dose of 1 mg/kg per course. These 4- to 5-day courses are then repeated every 4 to 6 weeks if the granulocyte count and the platelet count have returned to normal levels.

It is to be emphasized that response may be very gradual over many months; it is important that repeated courses or continuous therapy be given since improvement may continue slowly over many months, and the maximum benefit may be missed if treatment is abandoned too soon.

In patients with moderate to severe renal impairment, currently available pharmacokinetic data do not justify an absolute recommendation on dosage reduction to those patients, but it may be prudent to use a reduced dose initially.

Epithelial Ovarian Cancer: One commonly employed regimen for the treatment of ovarian carcinoma has been to administer ALKERAN at a dose of 0.2 mg/kg daily for 5 days as a single course. Courses are repeated every 4 to 5 weeks depending upon hematologic tolerance.[6,7]

Administration Precautions: Procedures for proper handling and disposal of anticancer drugs should be considered. Several guidelines on this subject have been published.[8-14] There is no general agreement that all of the procedures recommended in the guidelines are necessary or appropriate.

HOW SUPPLIED

ALKERAN is supplied as white, scored tablets containing 2 mg melphalan, imprinted with "ALKERAN" and "A2A"; in bottles of 50 (NDC 0173-0045-35).

Store at 15° to 25°C (59° to 77°F) in a dry place, protect from light, and dispense in glass.

REFERENCES

1. Pallante SL, Fenselau C, Mennel RG, et al. Quantitation by gas chromatography-chemical ionization-mass spectrometry of phenylalanine mustard in plasma of patients. *Cancer Res.* 1980;40:2268-2272.
2. Osserman EF. Therapy of plasma cell myeloma with melphalan (1-phenylalanine mustard). *Proc Am Assoc Cancer Res.* 1963;4:50. Abstract.
3. Osserman EF, Takatsuki K. Plasma cell myeloma: gamma globulin synthesis and structure. A review of biochemical and clinical data, with the description of a newly-recognized and related syndrome. "H-gamma-2-chain" (Franklin's) disease. *Medicine* (Balt). 1963;42:357-384.
4. Hoogstraten B, Sheehe PR, Cuttner J, et al. Melphalan in multiple myeloma. *Blood.* 1967;30:74-83.
5. Alexanian R, Haut A, Khan AU, et al. Treatment for multiple myeloma; combination chemotherapy with different melphalan dose regimens. *JAMA.* 1969;208:1680-1685.
6. Smith JP, Rutledge FN: Chemotherapy in advanced ovarian cancer. *Natl Cancer Inst Monogr.* 1975; 42:141-143.
7. Young RC, Chabner BA, Hubbard SP, et al. Advanced ovarian adenocarcinoma: a prospective clinical trial of melphalan (L-PAM) versus combination chemotherapy. *N Engl J Med.* 1978;299:1261-1266.
8. Recommendations for the safe handling of parenteral antineoplastic drugs. Washington, DC: Division of Safety, National Institutes of Health; 1983. US Dept of Health and Human Services, Public Health Service publication NIH 83-2621.
9. AMA Council on Scientific Affairs. Guidelines for handling parenteral antineoplastics. *JAMA.* 1985;253:1590-1591.
10. National Study Commission on Cytotoxic Exposure. Recommendations for handling cytotoxic agents. 1987. Available from Louis P. Jeffrey, Chairman, National Study Commission on Cytotoxic Exposure, Massachusetts College of Pharmacy and Allied Health Sciences, 179 Longwood Avenue, Boston, MA 02115.
11. Clinical Oncological Society of Australia. Guidelines and recommendations for safe handling of antineoplastic agents. *Med J Australia.* 1983;1:426-428.
12. Jones RB, Frank R, Mass T. Safe handling of chemotherapeutic agents: a report from the Mount Sinai Medical Center. *CA-A Cancer J for Clin.* 1983;33:258-263.
13. American Society of Hospital Pharmacists. ASHP technical assistance bulletin on handling cytotoxic and hazardous drugs. *Am J Hosp Pharm.* 1990;47:1033-1049.
14. Yodaiken RE, Bennett D. OSHA work-practice guidelines for personnel dealing with cytotoxic (antineoplastic) drugs. *Am J Hosp Pharm.* 1986;43:1193-1204.

September 1997/RL-467

Shown in Product Identification Guide, page 311

AMERGE™ Tablets ℞

[ə-merge']
(naratriptan hydrochloride)

DESCRIPTION

AMERGE Tablets contain naratriptan as the hydrochloride, which is a selective 5-hydroxytryptamine$_1$ receptor subtype agonist. Naratriptan hydrochloride is chemically designated as N-methyl-3-(1-methyl-4-piperidinyl)-1H-indole-5-ethanesulfonamide monohydrochloride, and it has the following structure:

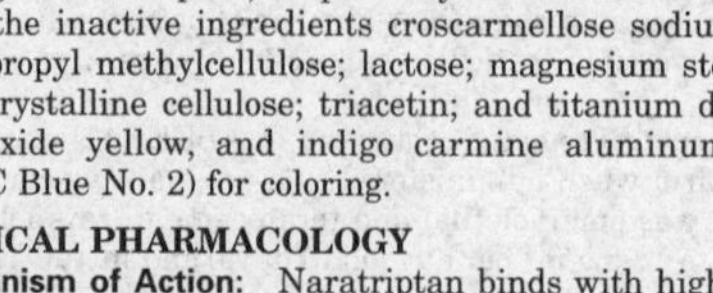

The empirical formula is $C_{17}H_{25}N_3O_2S{\bullet}HCl$, representing a molecular weight of 371.93. Naratriptan hydrochloride is a white to pale yellow powder that is readily soluble in water. Each AMERGE Tablet for oral administration contains 1.11 or 2.78 mg of naratriptan hydrochloride equivalent to 1 or 2.5 mg of naratriptan, respectively. Each tablet also contains the inactive ingredients croscarmellose sodium; hydroxypropyl methylcellulose; lactose; magnesium stearate; microcrystalline cellulose; triacetin; and titanium dioxide, iron oxide yellow, and indigo carmine aluminum lake (FD&C Blue No. 2) for coloring.

CLINICAL PHARMACOLOGY

Mechanism of Action: Naratriptan binds with high affinity to 5-HT_{1D} and 5-HT_{1B} receptors and has no significant affinity or pharmacological activity at 5-HT_{2-4} receptor subtypes or at adrenergic α_1, α_2, or β; dopaminergic D_1 or D_2; muscarinic; or benzodiazepine receptors.

The therapeutic activity of naratriptan in migraine is generally attributed to its agonist activity at 5-$HT_{1D/1B}$ receptors. Two current theories have been proposed to explain the efficacy of 5-$HT_{1D/1B}$ receptor agonists in migraine. One theory suggests that activation of 5-$HT_{1D/1B}$ receptors located on intracranial blood vessels, including those on the arteriovenous anastomoses, leads to vasoconstriction, which is correlated with the relief of migraine headache. The other hypothesis suggests that activation of 5-$HT_{1D/1B}$ receptors on sensory nerve endings in the trigeminal system results in the inhibition of pro-inflammatory neuropeptide release.

In the anesthetized dog, naratriptan has been shown to reduce the carotid arterial blood flow with little or no effect on arterial blood pressure or total peripheral resistance. While the effect on blood flow was selective for the carotid arterial bed, increases in vascular resistance of up to 30% were seen in the coronary arterial bed. Naratriptan has also been shown to inhibit trigeminal nerve activity in rat and cat. In 10 human subjects with suspected coronary artery disease (CAD) undergoing coronary artery catheterization, there was a 1% to 10% reduction in coronary artery diameter following subcutaneous injection of 1.5 mg of naratriptan.

Pharmacokinetics: Naratriptan tablets are well absorbed, with about 70% oral bioavailability. Following administration of a 2.5-mg tablet orally, the peak concentrations are obtained in 2 to 3 hours. After administration of 1- or 2.5-mg tablets, the C_{max} is somewhat (about 50%) higher in women (not corrected for mg/kg dose) than in men. During a migraine attack, absorption was slower, with a t_{max} of 3 to 4 hours. Food does not affect the pharmacokinetics of naratriptan. Naratriptan displays linear kinetics over the therapeutic dose range.

The steady-state volume of distribution of naratriptan is 170 L. Plasma protein binding is 28% to 31% over the concentration range of 50 to 1000 ng/mL.

Naratriptan is predominantly eliminated in urine, with 50% of the dose recovered unchanged and 30% as metabolites in urine. In vitro, naratriptan is metabolized by a wide range of cytochrome P450 isoenzymes into a number of inactive metabolites.

The mean elimination half-life of naratriptan is 6 hours. The systemic clearance of naratriptan is 6.6 mL/min/kg. The renal clearance (220 mL/min) exceeds glomerular filtration rate, indicating active tubular secretion. Repeat administration of naratriptan tablets does not result in drug accumulation.

Special Populations: ***Age:*** A small decrease in clearance (approximately 26%) was observed in healthy elderly subjects (65 to 77 years) compared to younger patients, resulting in slightly higher exposure (see PRECAUTIONS).

Race: The effect of race on the pharmacokinetics of naratriptan has not been examined.

Renal Impairment: Clearance of naratriptan was reduced by 50% in patients with moderate renal impairment (creatinine clearance 18 to 39 mL/min) compared to the normal group. Decrease in clearances resulted in an increase of mean half-life from 6 hours (healthy) to 11 hours (range: 7 to 20 hours). The mean C_{max} increased by approximately 40%. The effects of severe renal impairment (creatinine clearance $\leq$15 mL/min) on the pharmacokinetics of naratriptan has not been assessed. (See CONTRAINDICATIONS and DOSAGE AND ADMINISTRATION.)

Hepatic Impairment: Clearance of naratriptan was decreased by 30% in patients with moderate hepatic impairment (Child-Pugh grade A or B). This resulted in an approximately 40% increase in the half-life (range: 8 to 16 hours). The effects of severe hepatic impairment (Child-Pugh grade C) on the pharmacokinetics of naratriptan have not been assessed. (See CONTRAINDICATIONS and DOSAGE AND ADMINISTRATION.)

Drug Interactions: In normal volunteers, coadministration of single doses of naratriptan tablets and alcohol did not result in substantial modification of naratriptan pharmacokinetic parameters.

From population pharmacokinetic analyses, coadministration of naratriptan and fluoxetine, beta-blockers, or tricyclic antidepressants did not affect the clearance of naratriptan.

Naratriptan does not inhibit monoamine oxidase (MAO) enzymes and is a poor inhibitor of P450; metabolic interactions between naratriptan and drugs metabolized by P450 or MAO are therefore unlikely.

Oral Contraceptives: Oral contraceptives reduced clearance by 32% and volume of distribution by 22%, resulting in slightly higher concentrations of naratriptan. Hormone replacement therapy had no effect on pharmacokinetics in older female patients.

Smoking increased the clearance of naratriptan by 30%.

CLINICAL TRIALS

The efficacy of AMERGE Tablets in the acute treatment of migraine headaches was evaluated in six randomized, double-blind, placebo-controlled studies of which 4 used the recommended dosing regimen and were conducted as outpatient trials. Three of these studies enrolled adult patients who were predominantly female (86%) and Caucasian (96%) with a mean age of 41 (range: 18 to 65). One study enrolled adolescents with a mean age of 14 (range: 12 to 17). In the adolescent study, 54% of the patients were female and 89% were Caucasian. In all studies, patients were instructed to treat at least one moderate to severe headache. Headache response, defined as a reduction in headache severity from moderate or severe pain to mild or no pain, was assessed up to 4 hours after dosing. Associated symptoms such as nausea, vomiting, photophobia, and phonophobia were also assessed. Maintenance of response was assessed for up to 24 hours postdose. A second dose of AMERGE Tablets or other

medication was allowed 4 to 24 hours after the initial treatment for recurrent headache. The frequency and time to use of these additional treatments were also determined.

In all 3 trials in adults utilizing the recommended dosage regimen and outpatient use, the percentage of patients achieving headache response 4 hours after treatment, the primary outcome measure, was significantly greater among patients receiving AMERGE compared to those who received placebo. In all studies, response to 2.5 mg was numerically greater than response to 1 mg and in the largest of the three studies, there was a statistically significant greater percentage of patients with headache response at 4 hours in the 2.5-mg group compared to the 1-mg group. The results are summarized in Table 1.

[See table above]

In the single study in adolescents, there were no statistically significant differences between any of the treatment groups. The headache response rates at 4 hours (n) were 65% (n = 74), 67% (n = 78), and 64% (n = 70) for placebo, 1-mg, and 2.5-mg groups, respectively.

Comparisons of drug performance based upon results obtained in different clinical trials are never reliable. Because studies are conducted at different times, with different samples of patients, by different investigators, employing different criteria and/or different interpretations of the same criteria, under different conditions (dose, dosing regimen, etc.), quantitative estimates of treatment response and the timing of response may be expected to vary considerably from study to study.

The estimated probability of achieving an initial headache response in adults over the 4 hours following treatment is depicted in Figure 1.

Figure 1: Estimated Probability of Achieving Initial Headache Response Within 4 Hours*

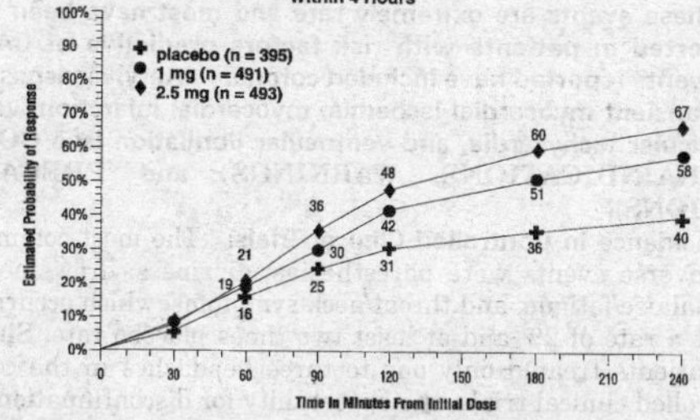

*The figure shows the probability over time of obtaining headache response (no or mild pain) following treatment with naratriptan tablets. The averages displayed are based on pooled data from the three controlled clinical trials providing evidence of efficacy (Studies 1, 2, and 3). In this Kaplan-Meier plot, patients not achieving response within 240 minutes were censored at 240 minutes.

For patients with migraine-associated nausea, photophobia, and phonophobia at baseline, there was a lower incidence of these symptoms 4 hours following administration of 1- and 2.5-mg AMERGE Tablets compared to placebo.

Four to 24 hours following the initial dose of study treatment, patients were allowed to use additional treatment for pain relief in the form of a second dose of study treatment or other medication. The estimated probability of patients taking a second dose or other medication for migraine over the 24 hours following the initial dose of study treatment is summarized in Figure 2.

Figure 2: Estimated Probability of Patients Taking a Second Dose of AMERGE Tablets or Other Medication for Migraine Over the 24 Hours Following the Initial Dose of Study Treatment*

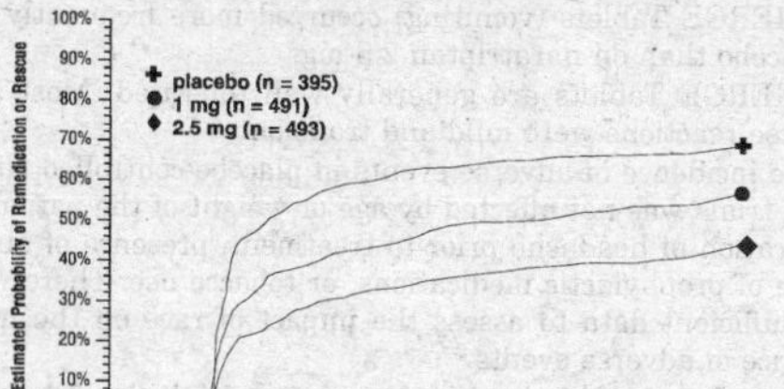

*Kaplan-Meier plot based on data obtained in the three controlled clinical trials (Studies 1, 2, and 3) providing evidence of efficacy with patients not using additional treatments censored at 24 hours. The plot also includes patients who had no response to the initial dose. Remedication was discouraged prior to 4 hours postdose.

There is no evidence that doses of 5 mg provide a greater effect than 2.5 mg. There was no evidence to suggest that treatment with AMERGE was associated with an increase in the severity or frequency of migraine attacks. The efficacy of AMERGE Tablets was unaffected by presence of aura; gender, age, or weight of the patient; oral contraceptive use; or concomitant use of common migraine prophylactic drugs (e.g., beta-blockers, calcium channel blockers, tricyclic antidepressants). There was insufficient data to assess the impact of race on efficacy.

Table 1: Percentage of Adult Patients With Headache Response (Mild or No Headache) 4 Hours Following Treatment

	Placebo	AMERGE 1.0 mg	AMERGE 2.5 mg
Study 1	34% (n = 122)	50%* (n = 117)	60%* (n = 127)
Study 2	27% (n = 104)	52%* (n = 208)	66%*† (n = 199)
Study 3	32% (n = 169)	54%* (n = 166)	65%* (n = 167)

* $P<0.05$ in comparison with placebo.
† $P<0.05$ in comparison with 1 mg.

INDICATIONS AND USAGE

AMERGE Tablets are indicated for the acute treatment of migraine attacks with or without aura in adults.

AMERGE Tablets are not intended for the prophylactic therapy of migraine or for use in the management of hemiplegic or basilar migraine (see CONTRAINDICATIONS). Safety and effectiveness of AMERGE Tablets have not been established for cluster headache, which is present in an older, predominantly male population.

CONTRAINDICATIONS

AMERGE Tablets should not be given to patients with history, symptoms, or signs of ischemic cardiac, cerebrovascular, or peripheral vascular syndromes. In addition, patients with other significant underlying cardiovascular diseases should not receive AMERGE Tablets. Ischemic cardiac syndromes include, but are not limited to, angina pectoris of any type (e.g., stable angina of effort and vasospastic forms of angina such as the Prinzmetal's variant), all forms of myocardial infarction, and silent myocardial ischemia. Cerebrovascular sydromes include, but are not limited to, strokes of any type as well as transient ischemic attacks. Peripheral vascular disease includes, but is not limited to, ischemic bowel disease (see WARNINGS).

Because AMERGE Tablets may increase blood pressure, they should not be given to patients with uncontrolled hypertension (see WARNINGS).

AMERGE Tablets are contraindicated in patients with severe renal impairment (creatinine clearance <15 mL/min) (see CLINICAL PHARMACOLOGY and DOSAGE AND ADMINISTRATION).

AMERGE Tablets are contraindicated in patients with severe hepatic impairment (Child-Pugh grade C) (see CLINICAL PHARMACOLOGY and DOSAGE and ADMINISTRATION).

AMERGE Tablets should not be administered to patients with hemiplegic or basilar migraine.

AMERGE Tablets should not be used within 24 hours of treatment with another 5-HT$_1$ agonist, an ergotamine-containing or ergot-type medication like dihydroergotamine or methysergide.

AMERGE Tablets are contraindicated in patients with hypersensitivity to naratriptan or any of the components.

WARNINGS

AMERGE Tablets should only be used where a clear diagnosis of migraine has been established.

Risk of Myocardial Ischemia and/or Infarction and Other Adverse Cardiac Events: Because of the potential of this class of compounds (5-HT$_{1B/1D}$ agonists) to cause coronary vasospasm, naratriptan should not be given to patients with documented ischemic or vasospastic coronary artery disease (CAD) (see CONTRAINDICATIONS). It is strongly recommended that 5-HT$_1$ agonists (including naratriptan) not be given to patients in whom unrecognized CAD is predicted by the presence of risk factors (e.g., hypertension, hypercholesterolemia, smoker, obesity, diabetes, strong family history of CAD, female with surgical or physiological menopause, or male over 40 years of age) unless a cardiovascular evaluation provides satisfactory clinical evidence that the patient is reasonably free of coronary artery and ischemic myocardial disease or other significant underlying cardiovascular disease. The sensitivity of cardiac diagnostic procedures to detect cardiovascular disease or predisposition to coronary artery vasospasm is modest, at best. If, during the cardiovascular evaluation, the patient's medical history, electrocardiographic, or other investigations reveal findings indicative of, or consistent with, coronary artery vasospasm or myocardial ischemia, naratriptan should not be administered (see CONTRAINDICATIONS).

For patients with risk factors predictive of CAD, who are determined to have a satisfactory cardiovascular evaluation, it is strongly recommended that administration of the first dose of naratriptan take place in the setting of a physician's office or similar medically staffed and equipped facility. Because cardiac ischemia can occur in the absence of clinical symptoms, consideration should be given to obtaining on the first occasion of use an electrocardiogram (ECG) during the interval immediately following administration of AMERGE Tablets, in these patients with risk factors.

It is recommended that patients who are intermittent long-term users of 5-HT$_1$ agonists, including AMERGE Tablets, and who have or acquire risk factors predictive of CAD, as described above, undergo periodic cardiovascular evaluation as they continue to use AMERGE Tablets.

The systematic approach described above is intended to reduce the likelihood that patients with unrecognized cardiovascular disease will be inadvertently exposed to naratriptan.

Cardiac Events and Fatalities Associated With 5-HT$_1$ Agonists: Naratriptan can cause coronary artery vasospasm (see CLINICAL PHARMACOLOGY). Serious adverse cardiac events, including acute myocardial infarction, life-threatening disturbances of cardiac rhythm, and death have been reported within a few hours following the administration of 5-HT$_1$ agonists. Considering the extent of use of 5-HT$_1$ agonists in patients with migraine, the incidence of these events is extremely low.

Premarketing Experience With AMERGE Tablets: Among approximately 3500 patients with migraine who participated in premarketing clinical trials of naratriptan tablets, four patients treated with single oral doses of naratriptan ranging from 1 to 10 mg experienced asymptomatic ischemic ECG changes with at least one, who took 7.5 mg, likely due to coronary vasospasm.

Cerebrovascular Events and Fatalities With 5-HT$_1$ Agonists: Cerebral hemorrhage, subarachnoid hemorrhage, stroke, and other cerebrovascular events have been reported in patients treated with 5-HT$_1$ agonists, and some have resulted in fatalities. In a number of cases, it appears possible that the cerebrovascular events were primary, the agonist having been administered in the incorrect belief that the symptoms experienced were a consequence of migraine, when they were not. It should be noted that patients with migraine may be at increased risk of certain cerebrovascular events (e.g., stroke, hemorrhage, transient ischemic attack).

Other Vasospasm-Related Events: 5-HT$_1$ agonists may cause vasospastic reactions other than coronary artery spasm. Both peripheral vascular ischemia and colonic ischemia with abdominal pain and bloody diarrhea have been reported with 5-HT$_1$ agonists.

Increase in Blood Pressure: In healthy volunteers, dose-related increases in systemic blood pressure have been observed after administration of up to 20 mg of oral naratriptan. At the recommended doses, the elevations are generally small, although an increase of systolic pressure of 32 mmHg was seen in one patient following a single 2.5-mg dose. The effect may be more pronounced in the elderly and hypertensive patients. A patient who was mildly hypertensive (the baseline blood pressure was 150/98) experienced a significant increase in blood pressure to 204/144 mmHg 225 minutes after administration of a 10-mg oral dose. Significant elevation in blood pressure, including hypertensive crisis, has been reported on rare occasions in patients receiving 5-HT$_1$ agonists with and without a history of hypertension. Naratriptan is contraindicated in patients with uncontrolled hypertension (see CONTRAINDICATIONS).

An 18% increase in mean pulmonary artery pressure and an 8% increase in mean aortic pressure was seen following dosing with 1.5 mg of subcutaneous naratriptan in a study evaluating 10 subjects with suspected CAD undergoing cardiac catheterization.

Hypersensitivity: Hypersensitivity (anaphylaxis/anaphylactoid) reactions may occur in patients receiving naratriptan. Such reactions can be life threatening or fatal. In general, hypersensitivity reactions to drugs are more likely to occur in individuals with a history of sensitivity to multiple allergens (see CONTRAINDICATIONS).

PRECAUTIONS

General: Chest discomfort (including pain, pressure, heaviness, tightness) has been reported after administration of 5-HT$_1$ agonists, including AMERGE Tablets. These events have not been associated with arrhythmias or ischemic ECG changes in clinical trials with AMERGE Tab-

Continued on next page

This product information is based on labeling in effect on June 1, 1998. For further information, contact via direct mail, phone, or web site Medical Information: Glaxo Wellcome Inc., PO Box 13398, Research Triangle Park, NC 27709. Healthcare Professionals (Medical Information): 800-334-0089 Patients (Customer Response Center): 888-TALK2GW (1-888-825-5249) Glaxo Wellcome Corporate Web Site: www.glaxowellcome.com

Amerge—Cont.

lets. Because naratriptan may cause coronary artery vasospasm, patients who experience signs or symptoms suggestive of angina following naratriptan should be evaluated for the presence of CAD or a predisposition to Prinzmetal's variant angina before receiving additional doses of naratriptan, and should be monitored electrocardiographically if dosing is resumed and similar symptoms recur. Similarly, patients who experience other symptoms or signs suggestive of decreased arterial flow, such as ischemic bowel syndrome or Raynaud's syndrome following naratriptan administration should be evaluated for atherosclerosis or predisposition to vasospasm (see CONTRAINDICATIONS and WARNINGS).

AMERGE Tablets should also be administered with caution to patients with diseases that may alter the absorption, metabolism, or excretion of drugs, such as impaired renal or hepatic function (see CLINICAL PHARMACOLOGY, CONTRAINDICATIONS, and DOSAGE AND ADMINISTRATION).

Care should be taken to exclude other potentially serious neurological conditions before treating headache in patients not previously diagnosed with migraine or who experience a headache that is atypical for them. There have been rare reports where patients received 5-HT$_1$ agonists for severe headaches that were subsequently shown to have been secondary to an evolving neurologic lesion (see WARNINGS). For a given attack, if a patient has no response to the first dose of naratriptan, the diagnosis of migraine should be reconsidered before administration of a second dose.

Binding to Melanin-Containing Tissues: In rats treated with a single oral dose (10 mg/kg) of radiolabeled naratriptan, the elimination half-life of radioactivity from the eye was 90 days, suggesting that naratriptan and/or its metabolites may bind to the melanin of the eye. Because there could be accumulation in melanin-rich tissues over time, this raises the possibility that naratriptan could cause toxicity in these tissues after extended use. Although no systematic monitoring of ophthalmologic function was undertaken in clinical trials, and no specific recommendations for ophthalmologic monitoring are offered, prescribers should be aware of the possibility of long-term ophthalmologic effects.

Changes in the Precorneal Tear Film: Dogs receiving oral naratriptan showed transient changes in the precorneal tear film. Corneal stippling was seen at the lowest dose tested, 1 mg/kg per day, and occurred intermittently from day 1 throughout the first 2 to 3 weeks of treatment. Although a no-effect dose was not established, the exposure at the lowest dose tested was approximately five times the human exposure after a 5-mg oral dose.

Information for Patients: See PATIENT INFORMATION at the end of this labeling for the text of the separate leaflet provided for patients.

Laboratory Tests: No specific laboratory tests are recommended for monitoring patients prior to and/or after treatment with AMERGE Tablets.

Drug Interactions: Ergot-containing drugs have been reported to cause prolonged vasospastic reactions. Because there is a theoretical basis that these effects may be additive, use of ergotamine-containing or ergot-type medications (like dihydroergotamine or methysergide) and naratriptan within 24 hours is contraindicated (see CONTRAINDICATIONS).

The administration of naratriptan with other 5-HT$_1$ agonists has not been evaluated in migraine patients. Because their vasospastic effects may be additive, coadministration of naratriptan and other 5-HT$_1$ agonists within 24 hours of each other is not recommended (see CONTRAINDICATIONS).

Selective serotonin reuptake inhibitors (SSRIs) (e.g., fluoxetine, fluvoxamine, paroxetine, sertraline) have been reported, rarely, to cause weakness, hyperreflexia, and incoordination when coadministered with 5-HT$_1$ agonists. If concomitant treatment with naratriptan and an SSRI is clinically warranted, appropriate observation of the patient is advised.

Drug/Laboratory Test Interactions: AMERGE Tablets are not known to interfere with commonly employed clinical laboratory tests.

Carcinogenesis, Mutagenesis, Impairment of Fertility: *Carcinogenesis:* Lifetime carcinogenicity studies, 104 weeks in duration, were carried out in mice and rats by oral gavage. There was no evidence of an increase in tumors related to naratriptan administration in mice receiving up to 200 mg/kg/day. That dose was associated with a plasma AUC exposure that was 110 times the exposure in humans receiving the maximum recommended daily dose of 5 mg. Two rat studies were conducted, one using a standard diet and the other a nitrite-supplemented diet (naratriptan can be nitrosated in vitro to form a mutagenic product that has been detected in the stomachs of rats fed a high nitrite diet). Doses of 5, 20, and 90 mg/kg were associated with week 13 AUC exposures that in the standard diet study were 7, 40,

and 236 times, and in the nitrite-supplemented diet study were 7, 29, and 180 times, the exposure attained in humans given the maximum recommended daily dose of 5 mg. In both studies, there was an increase in the incidence of thyroid follicular hyperplasia in high-dose males and females and in thyroid follicular adenomas in high-dose males. In the standard diet study only, there was also an increase in the incidence of benign c-cell adenomas in the thyroid of high-dose males and females. The exposures achieved at the no-effect dose for thyroid tumors were 40 (standard diet) and 29 (nitrite-supplemented diet) times the exposure achieved in humans receiving the maximum recommended daily dose of 5 mg. In the nitrite-supplemented diet study only, the incidence of benign lymphocytic thymoma was increased in all treated groups of females. It was not determined if the nitrosated product is systemically absorbed. However, no changes were seen in the stomachs of rats in that study.

Mutagenesis: Naratriptan was not mutagenic when tested in two gene mutation assays, the Ames test and the in vitro thymidine locus mouse lymphoma assay. It was not clastogenic in two cytogenetics assays, the in vitro human lymphocyte assay and the in vivo mouse micronucleus assay. Naratriptan can be nitrosated in vitro to form a mutagenic product (WHO nitrosation assay) that has been detected in the stomachs of rats fed a nitrite-supplemented diet.

Impairment of Fertility: In a reproductive toxicity study in which male and female rats were dosed prior to and throughout the mating period with 10, 60, 170, or 340 mg/kg/day (plasma exposures [AUC] approximately 11, 70, 230, and 470 times, respectively, the human exposure at the maximum recommended daily dose [MRDD] of 5 mg), there was a treatment-related decrease in the number of females exhibiting normal estrous cycles at doses of 170 mg/kg/day or greater and an increase in preimplantation loss at 60 mg/kg/day or greater. In high-dose group males, testicular/epididymal atrophy accompanied by spermatozoa depletion reduced mating success and may have contributed to the observed preimplantation loss. The exposures achieved at the no-effect doses for preimplantation loss, anestrus, and testicular effects were approximately 11, 70, and 230 times, respectively, the exposures in humans receiving the MRDD.

In a study in which rats were dosed orally with 10, 60, or 340 mg/kg/day for 6 months, changes in the female reproductive tract including atrophic or cystic ovaries and anestrus were seen at the high dose. The exposure at the no-effect dose of 60 mg/kg was approximately 85 times the exposure in humans receiving the MRDD.

Pregnancy: Pregnancy Category C. There are no adequate and well-controlled studies in pregnant women; therefore, naratriptan should be used during pregnancy only if the potential benefit justifies the potential risk to the fetus.

To monitor fetal outcomes of pregnant women exposed to AMERGE, Glaxo Wellcome Inc. maintains a Naratriptan Pregnancy Registry. Health care providers are encouraged to register patients by calling (800) 722-9292, ext. 39441.

In reproductive toxicity studies in rats and rabbits, oral administration of naratriptan was associated with developmental toxicity (embryolethality, fetal abnormalities, pup mortality, offspring growth retardation) at doses producing maternal plasma drug exposures as low as 11 and 2.5 times, respectively, the exposure in humans receiving the maximum recommended daily dose (MRDD) of 5 mg.

When pregnant rats were administered naratriptan during the period of organogenesis at doses of 10, 60, or 340 mg/kg/day, there was a dose-related increase in embryonic death, with a statistically significant difference at the highest dose, and incidences of fetal structural variations (incomplete/irregular ossification of skull bones, sternebrae, ribs) were increased at all doses. The maternal plasma exposures (AUC) at these doses were approximately 11, 70, and 470 times the exposure in humans at the MRDD. The high dose was maternally toxic, as evidenced by decreased maternal body weight gain during gestation. A no-effect dose for developmental toxicity in rats exposed during organogenesis was not established.

When doses of 1, 5, or 30 mg/kg/day were given to pregnant Dutch rabbits throughout organogenesis, the incidence of a specific fetal skeletal malformation (fused sternebrae) was increased at the high dose, and increased incidences of embryonic death and fetal variations (major blood vessel variations, supernumerary ribs, incomplete skeletal ossification) were observed at all doses (4, 20, and 120 times, respectively, the MRDD on a body surface area basis). Maternal toxicity (decreased body weight gain) was evident at the high dose in this study. In a similar study in New Zealand White rabbits (1, 5, or 30 mg/kg/day throughout organogenesis), decreased fetal weights and increased incidences of fetal skeletal variations were observed at all doses (maternal exposures equivalent to 2.5, 19, and 140 times exposure in humans receiving the MRDD), while maternal body weight gain was reduced at 5 mg/kg or greater. A no-effect dose for developmental toxicity in rabbits exposed during organogenesis was not established.

When female rats were treated with 10, 60, or 340 mg/kg/day during late gestation and lactation, offspring behavioral

impairment (tremors) and decreased offspring viability and growth were observed at doses of 60 mg/kg or greater, while maternal toxicity occurred only at the highest dose. Maternal exposures at the no-effect dose for developmental effects in this study were approximately 11 times the exposure in humans receiving the MRDD.

Nursing Mothers: Naratriptan-related material is excreted in the milk of rats. Therefore, caution should be exercised when considering the administration of AMERGE Tablets to a nursing woman.

Pediatric Use: Safety and effectiveness of AMERGE Tablets in pediatric patients (less than 18 years of age) have not been established.

One randomized, placebo-controlled clinical trial evaluating oral naratriptan (0.25 to 2.5 mg) in pediatric patients aged 12 to 17 years evaluated a total of 300 adolescent migraineurs. This study did not establish the efficacy of oral naratriptan compared to placebo in the treatment of migraine in adolescents (see CLINICAL TRIALS). Adverse events observed in this clinical trial were similar in nature to those reported in clinical trials in adults.

Geriatric Use: The use of naratriptan in elderly patients is not recommended.

AMERGE Tablets are known to be substantially excreted by the kidney, and the risk of adverse reactions to this drug may be greater in elderly patients who have reduced renal function. In addition, elderly patients are more likely to have decreased hepatic function; they are at higher risk for CAD; and blood pressure increases may be more pronounced in the elderly. Clinical studies of AMERGE Tablets did not include patients over 65 years of age.

ADVERSE REACTIONS

Serious cardiac events, including some that have been fatal, have occurred following the use of 5-HT$_1$ agonists. These events are extremely rare and most have been reported in patients with risk factors predictive of CAD. Events reported have included coronary artery vasospasm, transient myocardial ischemia, myocardial infarction, ventricular tachycardia, and ventricular fibrillation (see CONTRAINDICATIONS, WARNINGS, and PRECAUTIONS).

Incidence in Controlled Clinical Trials: The most common adverse events were paresthesias, dizziness, drowsiness, malaise/fatigue, and throat/neck symptoms, which occurred at a rate of 2% and at least two times placebo rate. Since patients treated only one to three headaches in the controlled clinical trials, the opportunity for discontinuation of therapy in response to an adverse event was limited. In a long-term, open label study where patients were allowed to treat multiple migraine attacks for up to 1 year, 15 patients (3.6%) discontinued treatment due to adverse events.

Table 2 lists adverse events that occurred in five placebo-controlled clinical trials of approximately 1752 exposures to placebo and AMERGE Tablets in adult migraine patients. The events cited reflect experience gained under closely monitored conditions of clinical trials in a highly selected patient population. In actual clinical practice or in other clinical trials, these frequency estimates may not apply, as the conditions of use, reporting behavior, and the kinds of patients treated may differ. Only events that occurred at a frequency of 2% or more in the AMERGE Tablets 2.5-mg treatment group and were more frequent in that group than in the placebo group are included in Table 2. From this table, it appears that many of these adverse events are dose related.

[See table 2 at bottom of next page]

One event present in more than 1% of patients receiving AMERGE Tablets (vomiting) occurred more frequently on placebo than on naratriptan 2.5 mg.

AMERGE Tablets are generally well tolerated. Most adverse reactions were mild and transient.

The incidence of adverse events in placebo-controlled clinical trials was not affected by age or weight of the patients, duration of headache prior to treatment, presence of aura, use of prophylactic medications, or tobacco use. There was insufficient data to assess the impact of race on the incidence of adverse events.

Other Events Observed in Association With the Administration of AMERGE Tablets: In the paragraphs that follow, the frequencies of less commonly reported adverse clinical events are presented. Because the reports include events observed in open and uncontrolled studies, the role of AMERGE Tablets in their causation cannot be reliably determined. Furthermore, variability associated with adverse event reporting, the terminology used to describe adverse events, etc. limit the value of the quantitative frequency estimates provided. Event frequencies are calculated as the number of patients reporting an event divided by the total number of patients (n = 3557) exposed to oral naratriptan doses up to 10 mg. All reported events are included except those already listed in the previous table, those too general to be informative, and those not reasonably associated with the use of the drug. Events are further classified within body system categories and enumerated in order of decreasing frequency using the following definitions: frequent ad-

verse events are those occurring in at least 1/100 patients, infrequent adverse events are those occurring in 1/100 to 1/1000 patients, and rare adverse events are those occurring in fewer than 1/1000 patients.

Atypical Sensations: Frequent were warm/cold temperature sensations. Infrequent were feeling strange and burning/stinging sensation.

Cardiovascular: Infrequent were palpitations, increased blood pressure, tachyarrhythmias, and abnormal ECG (PR prolongation, QT_c prolongation, ST/T wave abnormalities, premature ventricular contractions, atrial flutter, or atrial fibrillation), and syncope. Rare were bradycardia, varicosities, hypotension, and heart murmurs.

Ear, Nose, and Throat: Frequent were ear, nose, and throat infections. Infrequent were phonophobia, sinusitis, upper respiratory inflammation and tinnitus. Rare were allergic rhinitis; labyrinthitis; ear, nose, and throat hemorrhage; and hearing difficulty.

Endocrine and Metabolic: Infrequent were thirst and polydipsia, dehydration, and fluid retention. Rare were hyperlipidemia, hypercholesterolemia, hypothyroidism, hyperglycemia, glycosuria and ketonuria, and parathyroid neoplasm.

Eye: Frequent was photophobia. Infrequent was blurred vision. Rare were eye pain and discomfort, sensation of eye pressure, eye hemorrhage, dry eyes, difficulty focusing, and scotoma.

Gastrointestinal: Frequent were hyposalivation and vomiting. Infrequent were dyspeptic symptoms, diarrhea, gastrointestinal discomfort and pain, gastroenteritis, and constipation. Rare were abnormal liver function tests, abnormal bilirubin levels, hemorrhoids, gastritis, esophagitis, salivary gland inflammation, oral itching and irritation, regurgitation and reflux, and gastric ulcers.

Hematological Disorders: Infrequent was increased white cells. Rare were thrombocytopenia, quantitative red cell or hemoglobin defects, anemia, and purpura.

Lower Respiratory Tract: Infrequent were bronchitis, cough, and pneumonia. Rare were tracheitis, asthma, pleuritis, and airway constriction and obstruction.

Musculoskeletal: Infrequent were muscle pain, arthralgia and articular rheumatism, muscle cramps and spasms, joint and muscle stiffness, tightness, and rigidity. Rare were bone and skeletal pain.

Neurological: Frequent was vertigo. Infrequent were tremors, cognitive function disorders, sleep disorders, and disorders of equilibrium. Rare were compressed nerve syndromes, confusion, sedation, hyperesthesia, coordination disorders, paralysis of cranial nerves, decreased consciousness, dreams, altered sense of taste, neuralgia, neuritis, aphasia, hypoesthesia, motor retardation, muscle twitching and fasciculation, psychomotor restlessness, and convulsions.

Non-Site Specific: Infrequent were chills and/or fever, descriptions of odor or taste, edema and swelling, allergies, and allergic reactions. Rare were spasms and mobility disorders.

Pain and Pressure Sensations: Frequent were pressure/tightness/heaviness sensations.

Psychiatry: Infrequent were anxiety, depressive disorders, and detachment. Rare were aggression and hostility, agitation, hallucinations, panic, and hyperactivity.

Reproduction: Rare were lumps of female reproductive tract, breast inflammation, inflammation of vagina, inflammation of fallopian tube, breast discharge, endometrium disorders, decreased libido, and lumps of breast.

Skin: Infrequent were sweating, skin rashes, pruritus, and urticaria. Rare were skin erythema, dermatitis and dermatosis, hair loss and alopecia, pruritic skin rashes, acne and folliculitis, allergic skin reactions, macular skin/rashes, skin photosensitivity, photodermatitis, skin flakiness, and dry skin.

Urology: Infrequent were bladder inflammation and polyuria and diuresis. Rare were urinary tract hemorrhage, urinary urgency, pyelitis, and urinary incontinence.

Table 2: Treatment-Emergent Adverse Events Reported by at Least 2% of Patients in Placebo-Controlled Migraine Trials

Adverse Event Type	Placebo (n = 498)	AMERGE 1 mg (n = 627)	AMERGE 2.5 mg (n = 627)
Atypical sensation	1%	2%	4%
Paresthesias (all types)	<1%	1%	2%
Gastrointestinal	5%	6%	7%
Nausea	4%	4%	5%
Neurologial	3%	4%	7%
Dizziness	1%	1%	2%
Drowsiness	<1%	1%	2%
Malaise/fatigue	1%	2%	2%
Pain and pressure sensation	2%	2%	4%
Throat/neck symptoms	1%	1%	2%

DRUG ABUSE AND DEPENDENCE

In one clinical study enrolling 12 subjects, all of whom had experience using oral opiates and other psychoactive drugs, AMERGE Tablets produced less intense subjective responses ordinarily associated with many drugs of abuse than did codeine (30 to 90 mg).

OVERDOSAGE

A patient who was mildly hypertensive experienced a significant increase in blood pressure after administration of a 10-mg dose starting at 30 minutes (baseline value of 150/98 to 204/144 mmHg 225 minutes). This event resolved after treatment with antihypertensive therapy. Oral administration of 25 mg of naratriptan in one healthy young male subject increased blood pressure from 120/67 mmHg pretreatment up to 191/113 mmHg at approximately 6 hours postdose and resulted in adverse events including lightheadedness, tension in the neck, tiredness, and loss of coordination. Blood pressure returned to near baseline by 8 hours after dosing without any pharmacological intervention.

Another subject experienced asymptomatic ischemic ECG changes likely due to coronary artery vasospasm approximately 2 hours following a 7.5-mg oral dose.

The elimination half-life of naratriptan is about 6 hours (see CLINICAL PHARMACOLOGY), and therefore monitoring of patients after overdose with AMERGE Tablets should continue for at least 24 hours or while symptoms or signs persist. There is no specific antidote to naratriptan. Standard supportive treatment should be applied as required. If the patient presents with chest pain or other symptoms consistent with angina pectoris, ECG monitoring should be performed for evidence of ischemia. It is unknown what effect hemodialysis or peritoneal dialysis has on the serum concentrations of naratriptan.

DOSAGE AND ADMINISTRATION

In controlled clinical trials, single doses of 1 and 2.5 mg of AMERGE Tablets taken with fluid were effective for the acute treatment of migraines in adults. A greater proportion of patients had headache response following a 2.5 mg dose than following a 1-mg dose (see CLINICAL TRIALS). Individuals may vary in response to doses of AMERGE Tablets. The choice of dose should therefore be made on an individual basis, weighing the possible benefit of the 2.5-mg dose with the potential for a greater risk of adverse events. If the headache returns or if the patient has only partial response, the dose may be repeated once after 4 hours, for a maximum dose of 5 mg in a 24-hour period. There is evidence that doses of 5 mg do not provide a greater effect than 2.5 mg.

The safety of treating, on average, more than four headaches in a 30-day period has not been established.

Renal Impairment: The use of AMERGE is contraindicated in patients with severe renal impairment (creatinine clearance <15 mL/min) because of decreased clearance of the drug. (See CONTRAINDICATIONS and CLINICAL PHARMACOLOGY.) In patients with mild to moderate renal impairment, the maximum daily dose should not exceed 2.5 mg over a 24-hour period and a lower starting dose should be considered.

Hepatic Impairment: The use of AMERGE is contraindicated in patients with severe hepatic impairment (Child-Pugh grade C) because of decreased clearance (see CONTRAINDICATIONS and CLINICAL PHARMACOLOGY). In patients with mild or moderate hepatic impairment, the maximum daily dose should not exceed 2.5 mg over a 24-hour period and a lower starting dose should be considered (see CLINICAL PHARMACOLOGY).

HOW SUPPLIED

AMERGE Tablets 1 and 2.5 mg of naratriptan (base) as the hydrochloride. AMERGE Tablets, 1 mg, are white, D-shaped, film-coated tablets embossed with "GX CE3" on one side in blister packs of 9 tablets (NDC 0173-0561-00).

AMERGE Tablets, 2.5 mg, are green, D-shaped, film-coated tablets embossed with "GX CE5" on one side in blister packs of 9 tablets (NDC 0173-0562-00).

Store at controlled room temperature, 20° to 25°C (68° to 77°F) (see USP).

PATIENT INFORMATION

The following wording is contained in a separate leaflet provided for patients.

Information for the Patient
AMERGE™ (naratriptan hydrochloride) Tablets

Please read this leaflet carefully before you take AMERGE Tablets. This leaflet provides a summary of the information available about your medicine. Please do not throw away this leaflet until you have finished your medicine. You may need to read this leaflet again. This leaflet does not contain all the information on AMERGE Tablets. For further information or advice, ask your doctor or pharmacist.

Information About Your Medicine:

The name of your medicine is AMERGE (naratriptan hydrochloride) Tablets. It can be obtained only by prescription from your doctor. The decision to use AMERGE Tablets is one that you and your doctor should make jointly, taking into account your individual preferences and medical circumstances. If you have risk factors for heart disease (such as high blood pressure, high cholesterol, obesity, diabetes, smoking, strong family history of heart disease, or you are postmenopausal or a male over 40), you should tell your doctor, who should evaluate you for heart disease in order to determine if AMERGE is appropriate for you. The majority of those who have taken AMERGE Tablets have not experienced any significant side effects. Rarely, deaths and/or serious heart problems have been reported with this class of medicines; in all but a few instances, however, these deaths and/or serious heart problems occurred in people with heart disease and it was not clear whether these medications were a contributing factor.

1. The Purpose of Your Medicine:

AMERGE Tablets are intended to relieve your migraine, but not to prevent or reduce the number of attacks you experience. Use AMERGE Tablets only to treat an actual migraine attack.

2. Important Questions to Consider Before Taking AMERGE Tablets:

If the answer to any of the following questions is **YES** or if you do not know the answer, then please discuss it with your doctor before you use AMERGE Tablets.

- Are you pregnant? Do you think you might be pregnant? Are you trying to become pregnant? Are you not using adequate contraception? Are you breast-feeding?
- Do you have any chest pain, heart disease, shortness of breath, or irregular heartbeats? Have you had a heart attack?
- Do you have risk factors for heart disease (such as high blood pressure, high cholesterol, obesity, diabetes, smoking, strong family history of heart disease, or you are postmenopausal or a male over 40)?
- Have you had a stroke, transient ischemic attacks or "TIAs", or Raynaud syndrome?
- Do you have high blood pressure?
- Have you ever had to stop taking this or any other medication because of an allergy or other problems?
- Are you taking any other migraine medications, including other 5-HT_1 agonists such as IMITREX® (sumatriptan), or medications containing ergotamine, dihydroergotamine, or methysergide?
- Are you taking any medication for depression such as selective serotonin reuptake inhibitors [SSRIs])?
- Have you had, or do you have, any disease of the kidney or liver?
- Is this headache different from your usual migraine attacks?

Remember, if you answered **YES** to any of the above questions, then discuss it with your doctor.

3. The Use of AMERGE Tablets During Pregnancy:

Do not use AMERGE Tablets if you are pregnant, think you might be pregnant, are trying to become pregnant, or are not using adequate contraception, unless you have discussed this with your doctor.

4. How to Use AMERGE Tablets:

For adults, the usual dose is a single tablet taken whole with fluids. It may be given at any time after the headache starts. For an individual attack, if you have no response to the first tablet, do not take a second tablet without first talking to your doctor. If you need more relief due to a par-

Continued on next page

This product information is based on labeling in effect on June 1, 1998. For further information, contact via direct mail, phone, or web site Medical Information: Glaxo Wellcome Inc., PO Box 13398, Research Triangle Park, NC 27709. Healthcare Professionals (Medical Information): 800-334-0089 Patients (Customer Response Center): 888-TALK2GW (1-888-825-5249) Glaxo Wellcome Corporate Web Site: www.glaxowellcome.com

Amerge—Cont.

tial response or return of your headache after the first tablet, a second tablet may be taken but not sooner than 4 hours following the first tablet. Do not take more than a total of two AMERGE Tablets in any 24-hour period. If you have kidney or liver disease, take as directed by your doctor.

5. Side Effects to Watch for:

- Some patients experience pain or tightness in the chest or throat when using AMERGE Tablets. If this happens to you, then discuss it with your doctor before using any more AMERGE Tablets. If the chest pain, tightness, or pressure is severe or does not go away, call your doctor immediately.
- If you have sudden and/or severe abdominal pain following AMERGE Tablets, call your doctor immediately.
- Shortness of breath; wheeziness; heart throbbing, swelling of eyelids, face, or lips; or a skin rash, skin lumps, or hives happens rarely. If it happens to you, then tell your doctor immediately. Do not take any more AMERGE Tablets unless your doctor tells you to do so.
- Some people may have feelings of tingling, heat, flushing (redness of face lasting a short time), heaviness or pressure after treatment with AMERGE Tablets. A few people may feel drowsy, dizzy, tired, or sick. Tell your doctor of these symptoms at your next visit.
- If you feel unwell in any other way or have any symptoms that you do not understand, you should contact your doctor immediately.

6. What to Do if an Overdose is Taken:

If you have taken more medication than you have been told, contact either your doctor, hospital emergency department, or nearest poison control center immediately.

7. Storing Your Medicine:

Keep your medicine in a safe place where children cannot reach it. It may be harmful to children. Store your medication away from heat and light. Do not store at temperatures above 77°F (25°C). If your medication has expired (the expiration date is printed on the treatment pack), throw it away as instructed. If your doctor decides to stop your treatment, do not keep any leftover medicine unless your doctor tells you to. Throw away your medicine as instructed.

US Patent No. 4,997,841

©Copyright 1998 Glaxo Wellcome Inc. All rights reserved.

February 1998/RL-534

Shown in Product Identification Guide, page 311

ANECTINE® ℞

[*ă-nĕk 'tĕn*]

(succinylcholine chloride)

Injection, USP

> **WARNING**
>
> **RISK OF CARDIAC ARREST FROM HYPERKALEMIC RHABDOMYOLYSIS**
>
> There have been rare reports of acute rhabdomyolysis with hyperkalemia followed by ventricular dysrhythmias, cardiac arrest, and death after the administration of succinylcholine to apparently healthy children who were subsequently found to have undiagnosed skeletal muscle myopathy, most frequently Duchenne's muscular dystrophy.
>
> This syndrome often presents as peaked T-waves and sudden cardiac arrest within minutes after the administration of the drug in healthy appearing children (usually, but not exclusively, males, and most frequently 8 years of age or younger). There have also been reports in adolescents.
>
> Therefore, when a healthy appearing infant or child develops cardiac arrest soon after administration of succinylcholine, not felt to be due to inadequate ventilation, oxygenation or anesthetic overdose, immediate treatment for hyperkalemia should be instituted. This should include administration of intravenous calcium, bicarbonate, and glucose with insulin, with hyperventilation. Due to the abrupt onset of this syndrome, routine resuscitative measures are likely to be unsuccessful. However, extraordinary and prolonged resuscitative efforts have resulted in successful resuscitation in some reported cases. In addition, in the presence of signs of malignant hyperthermia, appropriate treatment should be instituted concurrently.
>
> Since there may be no signs or symptoms to alert the practitioner to which patients are at risk, it is recommended that the use of succinylcholine in children should be reserved for emergency intubation or instances where immediate securing of the airway is necessary, e.g., laryngospasm, difficult airway, full stomach, or for intramuscular use when a suitable vein is inaccessible (see PRECAUTIONS: Pediatric Use and DOSAGE AND ADMINISTRATION).

This drug should be used only by individuals familiar with its actions, characteristics, and hazards.

DESCRIPTION

ANECTINE (succinylcholine chloride) is an ultra short-acting depolarizing-type, skeletal muscle relaxant for intravenous (IV) administration.

Succinylcholine chloride is a white, odorless, slightly bitter powder and very soluble in water. The drug is unstable in alkaline solutions but relatively stable in acid solutions, depending upon the concentration of the solution and the storage temperature. Solutions of succinylcholine chloride should be stored under refrigeration to preserve potency.

ANECTINE Injection is a sterile nonpyrogenic solution for IV injection, containing 20 mg succinylcholine chloride in each mL and made isotonic with sodium chloride. The pH is adjusted to 3.5 with hydrochloric acid. Methylparaben (0.1%) is added as a preservative.

The chemical name for succinylcholine chloride is 2,2′-[(1,4-dioxo-1,4-butanediyl)bis(oxy)]bis[*N,N,N* -trimethylethanaminium] dichloride.

CLINICAL PHARMACOLOGY

Succinylcholine is a depolarizing skeletal muscle relaxant. As does acetylcholine, it combines with the cholinergic receptors of the motor end plate to produce depolarization. This depolarization may be observed as fasciculations. Subsequent neuromuscular transmission is inhibited so long as adequate concentration of succinylcholine remains at the receptor site. Onset of flaccid paralysis is rapid (less than one minute after IV administration), and with single administration lasts approximately 4 to 6 minutes.

Succinylcholine is rapidly hydrolyzed by plasma cholinesterase to succinylmonocholine (which possesses clinically insignificant depolarizing muscle relaxant properties) and then more slowly to succinic acid and choline (see PRECAUTIONS). About 10% of the drug is excreted unchanged in the urine. The paralysis following administration of succinylcholine is progressive, with differing sensitivities of different muscles. This initially involves consecutively the levator muscles of the face, muscles of the glottis, and finally, the intercostals and the diaphragm and all other skeletal muscles.

Succinylcholine has no direct action on the uterus or other smooth muscle structures. Because it is highly ionized and has low fat solubility, it does not readily cross the placenta.

Tachyphylaxis occurs with repeated administration (see PRECAUTIONS).

Depending on the dose and duration of succinylcholine administration, the characteristic depolarizing neuromuscular block (Phase I block) may change to a block with characteristics superficially resembling a nondepolarizing block (Phase II block). This may be associated with prolonged respiratory muscle paralysis or weakness in patients who manifest the transition to Phase II block. When this diagnosis is confirmed by peripheral nerve stimulation, it may sometimes be reversed with anticholinesterase drugs such as neostigmine (see PRECAUTIONS). Anticholinesterase drugs may not always be effective. If given before succinylcholine is metabolized by cholinesterase, anticholinesterase drugs may prolong rather than shorten paralysis.

Succinylcholine has no direct effect on the myocardium. Succinylcholine stimulates both autonomic ganglia and muscarinic receptors which may cause changes in cardiac rhythm, including cardiac arrest. Changes in rhythm, including cardiac arrest, may also result from vagal stimulation, which may occur during surgical procedures, or from hyperkalemia, particularly in children (see PRECAUTIONS: Pediatric Use). These effects are enhanced by halogenated anesthetics.

Succinylcholine causes an increase in intraocular pressure immediately after its injection and during the fasciculation phase, and slight increases which may persist after onset of complete paralysis (see WARNINGS).

Succinylcholine may cause slight increases in intracranial pressure immediately after its injection and during the fasciculation phase (see PRECAUTIONS).

As with other neuromuscular blocking agents, the potential for releasing histamine is present following succinylcholine administration. Signs and symptoms of histamine-mediated release such as flushing, hypotension, and bronchoconstriction are, however, uncommon in normal clinical usage.

Succinylcholine has no effect on consciousness, pain threshold, or cerebration. It should be used only with adequate anesthesia (see WARNINGS).

INDICATIONS AND USAGE

Succinylcholine chloride is indicated as an adjunct to general anesthesia, to facilitate tracheal intubation, and to provide skeletal muscle relaxation during surgery or mechanical ventilation.

CONTRAINDICATIONS

Succinylcholine is contraindicated in persons with personal or familial history of malignant hyperthermia, skeletal muscle myopathies, and known hypersensitivity to the drug. It is also contraindicated in patients after the acute phase of injury following major burns, multiple trauma, extensive denervation of skeletal muscle, or upper motor neuron injury, because succinylcholine administered to such individuals may result in severe hyperkalemia which may result in cardiac arrest (see WARNINGS). The risk of hyperkalemia in these patients increases over time and usually peaks at 7 to 10 days after the injury. The risk is dependent on the extent and location of the injury. The precise time of onset and the duration of the risk period are not known.

WARNINGS

SUCCINYLCHOLINE SHOULD BE USED ONLY BY THOSE SKILLED IN THE MANAGEMENT OF ARTIFICIAL RESPIRATION AND ONLY WHEN FACILITIES ARE INSTANTLY AVAILABLE FOR TRACHEAL INTUBATION AND FOR PROVIDING ADEQUATE VENTILATION OF THE PATIENT, INCLUDING THE ADMINISTRATION OF OXYGEN UNDER POSITIVE PRESSURE AND THE ELIMINATION OF CARBON DIOXIDE. THE CLINICIAN MUST BE PREPARED TO ASSIST OR CONTROL RESPIRATION.

TO AVOID DISTRESS TO THE PATIENT, SUCCINYLCHOLINE SHOULD NOT BE ADMINISTERED BEFORE UNCONSCIOUSNESS HAS BEEN INDUCED. IN EMERGENCY SITUATIONS, HOWEVER, IT MAY BE NECESSARY TO ADMINISTER SUCCINYLCHOLINE BEFORE UNCONSCIOUSNESS IS INDUCED.

SUCCINYLCHOLINE IS METABOLIZED BY PLASMA CHOLINESTERASE AND SHOULD BE USED WITH CAUTION, IF AT ALL, IN PATIENTS KNOWN TO BE OR SUSPECTED OF BEING HOMOZYGOUS FOR THE ATYPICAL PLASMA CHOLINESTERASE GENE.

Hyperkalemia: (SEE BOX WARNING) Succinylcholine should be administered with **GREAT CAUTION** to patients suffering from electrolyte abnormalities and those who may have massive digitalis toxicity, because in these circumstances succinylcholine may induce serious cardiac arrhythmias or cardiac arrest due to hyperkalemia.

GREAT CAUTION should be observed if succinylcholine is administered to patients during the acute phase of injury following major burns, multiple trauma, extensive denervation of skeletal muscle, or upper motor neuron injury (see CONTRAINDICATIONS). The risk of hyperkalemia in these patients increases over time and usually peaks at 7 to 10 days after the injury. The risk is dependent on the extent and location of the injury. The precise time of onset and the duration of the risk period are undetermined. Patients with chronic abdominal infection, subarachnoid hemorrhage, or conditions causing degeneration of central and peripheral nervous systems should receive succinylcholine with **GREAT CAUTION** because of the potential for developing severe hyperkalemia.

Malignant Hyperthermia: Succinylcholine administration has been associated with acute onset of malignant hyperthermia, a potentially fatal hypermetabolic state of skeletal muscle. The risk of developing malignant hyperthermia following succinylcholine administration increases with the concomitant administration of volatile anesthetics. Malignant hyperthermia frequently presents as intractable spasm of the jaw muscles (masseter spasm) which may progress to generalized rigidity, increased oxygen demand, tachycardia, tachypnea and profound hyperpyrexia. Successful outcome depends on recognition of early signs, such as jaw muscle spasm, acidosis, or generalized rigidity to initial administration of succinylcholine for tracheal intubation, or failure of tachycardia to respond to deepening anesthesia. Skin mottling, rising temperature, and coagulopathies may occur later in the course of the hypermetabolic process. Recognition of the syndrome is a signal for discontinuance of anesthesia, attention to increased oxygen consumption, correction of acidosis, support of circulation, assurance of adequate urinary output, and institution of measures to control rising temperature. Intravenous dantrolene sodium is recommended as an adjunct to supportive measures in the management of this problem. Consult literature references and the dantrolene prescribing information for additional information about the management of malignant hyperthermic crisis. Continuous monitoring of temperature and expired CO_2 is recommended as an aid to early recognition of malignant hyperthermia.

Other: In both adults and children the incidence of bradycardia, which may progress to asystole, is higher following a second dose of succinylcholine. The incidence and severity of bradycardia is higher in children than in adults. Pretreatment with anticholinergic agents (e.g., atropine) may reduce the occurrence of bradyarrhythmias.

Succinylcholine causes an increase in intraocular pressure. It should not be used in instances in which an increase in intraocular pressure is undesirable (e.g., narrow angle glaucoma, penetrating eye injury) unless the potential benefit of its use outweighs the potential risk.

Succinylcholine is acidic (pH = 3.5) and should not be mixed with alkaline solutions having a pH greater than 8.5 (e.g., barbiturate solutions).

PRECAUTIONS: (SEE BOX WARNING)

General: When succinylcholine is given over a prolonged period of time, the characteristic depolarization block of the

myoneural junction (Phase I block) may change to a block with characteristics superficially resembling a nondepolarizing block (Phase II block). Prolonged respiratory muscle paralysis or weakness may be observed in patients manifesting this transition to Phase II block. The transition from Phase I to Phase II block has been reported in seven of seven patients studied under halothane anesthesia after an accumulated dose of 2 to 4 mg/kg succinylcholine (administered in repeated, divided doses). The onset of Phase II block coincided with the onset of tachyphylaxis and prolongation of spontaneous recovery. In another study, using balanced anesthesia (N_2O/O_2/narcotic-thiopental) and succinylcholine infusion, the transition was less abrupt, with great individual variability in the dose of succinylcholine required to produce Phase II block. Of 32 patients studied, 24 developed Phase II block. Tachyphylaxis was not associated with the transition to Phase II block, and 50% of the patients who developed Phase II block experienced prolonged recovery.

When Phase II block is suspected in cases of prolonged neuromuscular blockade, positive diagnosis should be made by peripheral nerve stimulation prior to administration of any anticholinesterase drug. Reversal of Phase II block is a medical decision which must be made upon the basis of the individual, clinical pharmacology and the experience and judgment of the physician. The presence of Phase II block is indicated by fade of responses to successive stimuli (preferably "train of four"). The use of an anticholinesterase drug to reverse Phase II block should be accompanied by appropriate doses of an anticholinergic drug to prevent disturbances of cardiac rhythm. After adequate reversal of Phase II block with an anticholinesterase agent, the patient should be continually observed for at least 1 hour for signs of return of muscle relaxation. Reversal should not be attempted unless: (1) a peripheral nerve stimulator is used to determine the presence of Phase II block (since anticholinesterase agents will potentiate succinylcholine-induced Phase I block), and (2) spontaneous recovery of muscle twitch has been observed for at least 20 minutes and has reached a plateau with further recovery proceeding slowly; this delay is to ensure complete hydrolysis of succinylcholine by plasma cholinesterase prior to administration of the anticholinesterase agent. Should the type of block be misdiagnosed, depolarization of the type initially induced by succinylcholine (i.e., Phase I block) will be prolonged by an anticholinesterase agent.

Succinylcholine should be employed with caution in patients with fractures or muscle spasm because the initial muscle fasciculations may cause additional trauma.

Succinylcholine may cause a transient increase in intracranial pressure; however, adequate anesthetic induction prior to administration of succinylcholine will minimize this effect.

Succinylcholine may increase intragastric pressure, which could result in regurgitation and possible aspiration of stomach contents.

Neuromuscular blockade may be prolonged in patients with hypokalemia or hypocalcemia.

Reduced Plasma Cholinesterase Activity: Succinylcholine should be used carefully in patients with reduced plasma cholinesterase (pseudocholinesterase) activity. The likelihood of prolonged neuromuscular block following administration of succinylcholine must be considered in such patients (see DOSAGE AND ADMINISTRATION).

Plasma cholinesterase activity may be diminished in the presence of genetic abnormalities of plasma cholinesterase (e.g., patients heterozygous or homozygous for atypical plasma cholinesterase gene), pregnancy, severe liver or kidney disease, malignant tumors, infections, burns, anemia, decompensated heart disease, peptic ulcer, or myxedema. Plasma cholinesterase activity may also be diminished by chronic administration of oral contraceptives, glucocorticoids, or certain monoamine oxidase inhibitors, and by irreversible inhibitors of plasma cholinesterase (e.g., organophosphate insecticides, echothiophate, and certain antineoplastic drugs).

Patients homozygous for atypical plasma cholinesterase gene (1 in 2,500 patients) are extremely sensitive to the neuromuscular blocking effect of succinylcholine. In these patients, a 5- to 10-mg test dose of succinylcholine may be administered to evaluate sensitivity to succinylcholine, or neuromuscular blockade may be produced by the cautious administration of a 1-mg/mL solution of succinylcholine by slow IV infusion. Apnea or prolonged muscle paralysis should be treated with controlled respiration.

Drug Interactions: Drugs which may enhance the neuromuscular blocking action of succinylcholine include: promazine, oxytocin, aprotinin, certain non-penicillin antibiotics, quinidine, β-adrenergic blockers, procainamide, lidocaine, trimethaphan, lithium carbonate, magnesium salts, quinine, chloroquine, diethylether, isoflurane, desflurane, metoclopramide, and terbutaline. The neuromuscular blocking effect of succinylcholine may be enhanced by drugs that reduce plasma cholinesterase activity (e.g., chronically administered oral contraceptives, glucocorticoids, or certain mono-

amine oxidase inhibitors) or by drugs that irreversibly inhibit plasma cholinesterase (see PRECAUTIONS).

If other neuromuscular blocking agents are to be used during the same procedure, the possibility of a synergistic or antagonistic effect should be considered.

Carcinogenesis, Mutagenesis, Impairment of Fertility: There have been no long-term studies performed in animals to evaluate carcinogenic potential.

Pregnancy: *Teratogenic Effects:* Pregnancy Category C. Animal reproduction studies have not been conducted with succinylcholine chloride. It is also not known whether succinylcholine can cause fetal harm when administered to a pregnant woman or can affect reproduction capacity. Succinylcholine should be given to a pregnant woman only if clearly needed.

Nonteratogenic Effects: Plasma cholinesterase levels are decreased by approximately 24% during pregnancy and for several days postpartum. Therefore, a higher proportion of patients may be expected to show increased sensitivity (prolonged apnea) to succinylcholine when pregnant than when nonpregnant.

Labor and Delivery: Succinylcholine is commonly used to provide muscle relaxation during delivery by cesarean section. While small amounts of succinylcholine are known to cross the placental barrier, under normal conditions the quantity of drug that enters fetal circulation after a single dose of 1 mg/kg to the mother should not endanger the fetus. However, since the amount of drug that crosses the placental barrier is dependent on the concentration gradient between the maternal and fetal circulations, residual neuromuscular blockade (apnea and flaccidity) may occur in the newborn after repeated high doses to, or in the presence of atypical plasma cholinesterase in, the mother.

Nursing Mothers: It is not known whether succinylcholine is excreted in human milk. Because many drugs are excreted in human milk, caution should be exercised following succinylcholine administration to a nursing woman.

Pediatric Use: There are rare reports of ventricular dysrhythmias and cardiac arrest secondary to acute rhabdomyolysis with hyperkalemia in apparently healthy children who receive succinylcholine (see BOX WARNING). Many of these children were subsequently found to have a skeletal muscle myopathy such as Duchenne's muscular dystrophy whose clinical signs were not obvious. The syndrome often presents as sudden cardiac arrest within minutes after the administration of succinylcholine. These children are usually, but not exclusively, males, and most frequently 8 years of age or younger. There have also been reports in adolescents. There may be no signs or symptoms to alert the practitioner to which patients are at risk. A careful history and physical may identify developmental delays suggestive of a myopathy. A preoperative creatine kinase could identify some but not all patients at risk. Due to the abrupt onset of this syndrome, routine resuscitative measures are likely to be unsuccessful. Careful monitoring of the electrocardiogram may alert the practitioner to peaked T-waves (an early sign). Administration of IV calcium, bicarbonate, and glucose with insulin, with hyperventilation have resulted in successful resuscitation in some of the reported cases. Extraordinary and prolonged resuscitative efforts have been effective in some cases. In addition, in the presence of signs of malignant hyperthermia, appropriate treatment should be initiated concurrently (see WARNINGS). Since it is difficult to identify which patients are at risk, it is recommended that the use of succinylcholine in children should be reserved for emergency intubation or instances where immediate securing of the airway is necessary, e.g., laryngospasm, difficult airway, full stomach, or for intramuscular use when a suitable vein is inaccessible.

As in adults, the incidence of bradycardia in children is higher following the second dose of succinylcholine. The incidence and severity of bradycardia is higher in children than in adults. Pretreatment with anticholinergic agents, e.g., atropine, may reduce the occurrence of bradyarrhythmias.

ADVERSE REACTIONS

Adverse reactions to succinylcholine consist primarily of an extension of its pharmacological actions. Succinylcholine causes profound muscle relaxation resulting in respiratory depression to the point of apnea; this effect may be prolonged. Hypersensitivity reactions, including anaphylaxis, may occur in rare instances. The following additional adverse reactions have been reported: cardiac arrest, malignant hyperthermia, arrhythmias, bradycardia, tachycardia, hypertension, hypotension, hyperkalemia, prolonged respiratory depression or apnea, increased intraocular pressure, muscle fasciculation, jaw rigidity, postoperative muscle pain, rhabdomyolysis with possible myoglobinuric acute renal failure, excessive salivation, and rash.

OVERDOSAGE

Overdosage with succinylcholine may result in neuromuscular block beyond the time needed for surgery and anesthesia. This may be manifested by skeletal muscle weakness, decreased respiratory reserve, low tidal volume, or apnea. The primary treatment is maintenance of a patent

airway and respiratory support until recovery of normal respiration is assured. Depending on the dose and duration of succinylcholine administration, the characteristic depolarizing neuromuscular block (Phase I) may change to a block with characteristics superficially resembling a nondepolarizing block (Phase II) (see PRECAUTIONS).

DOSAGE AND ADMINISTRATION

The dosage of succinylcholine should be individualized and should always be determined by the clinician after careful assessment of the patient (see WARNINGS).

Parenteral drug products should be inspected visually for particulate matter and discoloration prior to administration whenever solution and container permit. Solutions which are not clear and colorless should not be used.

Adults: *For Short Surgical Procedures:* The average dose required to produce neuromuscular blockade and to facilitate tracheal intubation is 0.6 mg/kg ANECTINE Injection given intravenously. The optimum dose will vary among individuals and may be from 0.3 to 1.1 mg/kg for adults. Following administration of doses in this range, neuromuscular blockade develops in about 1 minute; maximum blockade may persist for about 2 minutes, after which recovery takes place within 4 to 6 minutes. However, very large doses may result in more prolonged blockade. A 5- to 10-mg test dose may be used to determine the sensitivity of the patient and the individual recovery time (see PRECAUTIONS).

For Long Surgical Procedures: The dose of succinylcholine administered by infusion depends upon the duration of the surgical procedure and the need for muscle relaxation. The average rate for an adult ranges between 2.5 and 4.3 mg per minute.

Solutions containing from 1 to 2 mg per mL succinylcholine have commonly been used for continuous infusion. The more dilute solution (1 mg per mL) is probably preferable from the standpoint of ease of control of the rate of administration of the drug and, hence, of relaxation. This IV solution containing 1 mg per mL may be administered at a rate of 0.5 mg (0.5 mL) to 10 mg (10 mL) per minute to obtain the required amount of relaxation. The amount required per minute will depend upon the individual response as well as the degree of relaxation required. Avoid overburdening the circulation with a large volume of fluid. It is recommended that neuromuscular function be carefully monitored with a peripheral nerve stimulator when using succinylcholine by infusion in order to avoid overdose, detect development of Phase II block, follow its rate of recovery, and assess the effects of reversing agents (see PRECAUTIONS).

Intermittent IV injections of succinylcholine may also be used to provide muscle relaxation for long procedures. An IV injection of 0.3 to 1.1 mg/kg may be given initially, followed, at appropriate intervals, by further injections of 0.04 to 0.07 mg/kg to maintain the degree of relaxation required.

Pediatrics: For emergency tracheal intubation or in instances where immediate securing of the airway is necessary, the IV dose of succinylcholine is 2 mg/kg for infants and small children; for older children and adolescents the dose is 1 mg/kg (see BOX WARNING and PRECAUTIONS: Pediatric Use).

Rarely, IV bolus administration of succinylcholine in infants and children may result in malignant ventricular arrythmias and cardiac arrest secondary to acute rhabdomyolysis with hyperkalemia. In such situations, an underlying myopathy should be suspected.

Intravenous bolus administration of succinylcholine in infants or children may result in profound bradycardia or, rarely, asystole. As in adults, the incidence of bradycardia in children is higher following a second dose of succinylcholine. The occurrence of bradyarrhythmias may be reduced by pretreatment with atropine (see PRECAUTIONS: Pediatric Use).

Intramuscular Use: If necessary, succinylcholine may be given intramuscularly to infants, older children, or adults when a suitable vein is inaccessible. A dose of up to 3 to 4 mg/kg may be given, but not more than 150 mg total dose should be administered by this route. The onset of effect of succinylcholine given intramuscularly is usually observed in about 2 to 3 minutes.

Compatibility and Admixtures: Succinylcholine is acidic (pH 3.5) and should not be mixed with alkaline solutions having a pH greater than 8.5 (e.g., barbiturate solutions). Admixtures containing 1 to 2 mg/mL may be prepared by adding 1 g succinylcholine to 1000 or 500 mL sterile solution, such as 5% Dextrose Injection, USP or 0.9% Sodium Chloride Injection, USP. Admixtures of ANECTINE must be

Continued on next page

This product information is based on labeling in effect on June 1, 1998. For further information, contact via direct mail, phone, or web site Medical Information: Glaxo Wellcome Inc., PO Box 13398, Research Triangle Park, NC 27709. Healthcare Professionals (Medical Information): 800-334-0089 Patients (Customer Response Center): 888-TALK2GW (1-888-825-5249) Glaxo Wellcome Corporate Web Site: www.glaxowellcome.com

Anectine—Cont.

used within 24 hours after preparation. Aseptic techniques should be used to prepare the diluted product. Admixtures of ANECTINE should be prepared for single patient use only. The unused portion of diluted ANECTINE should be discarded.

HOW SUPPLIED

For immediate injection of single doses for short procedures: ANECTINE (succinylcholine chloride) Injection, 20 mg in each mL.

Multiple-dose vials of 10 mL, box of 12 vials (NDC 0173-0071-95).

Store in refrigerator at 2° to 8°C (36° to 46°F). The multi-dose vials are stable for up to 14 days at room temperature without significant loss of potency.

©Copyright 1996 Glaxo Wellcome Inc. All rights reserved.
November 1997/RL-496

Shown in Product Identification Guide, page 311

BECLOVENT®

℞

[be 'klō-vent "]
(beclomethasone dipropionate, USP)
Inhalation Aerosol

For Oral Inhalation Only

DESCRIPTION

Beclomethasone dipropionate, USP, the active component of BECLOVENT Inhalation Aerosol, is an anti-inflammatory corticosteroid having the chemical name 9-chloro-11β,17,21-trihydroxy-16β-methylpregna-1,4-diene-3,20-dione 17,21-dipropionate.

Beclomethasone 17,21-dipropionate is a diester of beclomethasone, a synthetic halogenated corticosteroid. Beclomethasone dipropionate is a white to creamy-white, odorless powder with a molecular formula of $C_{28}H_{37}ClO_7$ and a molecular weight of 521.05. It is very slightly soluble in water, very soluble in chloroform, and freely soluble in acetone and in alcohol.

BECLOVENT Inhalation Aerosol is a pressurized metered-dose aerosol unit containing a microcrystalline suspension of beclomethasone dipropionate-trichloromonofluoromethane clathrate in a mixture of propellants (trichloromonofluoromethane and dichlorodifluoromethane) with oleic acid. Each canister contains beclomethasone dipropionate-trichloromonofluoromethane clathrate having a molecular proportion of beclomethasone dipropionate to trichloromonofluoromethane between 3:1 and 3:2. Each actuation delivers a quantity of clathrate equivalent to 42 mcg of beclomethasone dipropionate, USP from the mouthpiece and 50 mcg from the valve. The contents of one 6.7-g canister provide 80 oral inhalations, and the contents of one 16.8-g canister provide 200 oral inhalations.

CLINICAL PHARMACOLOGY

Animal studies show that beclomethasone dipropionate has potent anti-inflammatory activity. When beclomethasone dipropionate was administered systemically to mice, the anti-inflammatory activity was accompanied by other features typical of glucocorticoid action, including thymic involution, liver glycogen deposition, and pituitary-adrenal suppression. After systemic administration of beclomethasone dipropionate to rats, the anti-inflammatory action was associated with little or no effect on other tests of glucocorticoid activity.

Beclomethasone dipropionate is sparingly soluble and is poorly mobilized from subcutaneous or intramuscular injection sites. However, systemic absorption occurs after all routes of administration. When given to animals in the form of an aerosolized suspension of the trichloromonofluoromethane clathrate, the drug is deposited in the mouth and nasal passages, the trachea and principal bronchi, and the lung; a considerable portion of the drug is also swallowed. Absorption occurs rapidly from all respiratory and gastrointestinal tissues, as indicated by the rapid clearance of radioactively labeled drug from local tissues and appearance of tracer in the circulation. There is no evidence of tissue storage of beclomethasone dipropionate or its metabolites. Lung slices can metabolize beclomethasone dipropionate rapidly to beclomethasone 17-monopropionate and more slowly to free beclomethasone (which has very weak anti-inflammatory activity). However, irrespective of the route of administration (injection, oral, or aerosol), the principal route of excretion of the drug and its metabolites is the feces. Less than 10% of the drug and its metabolites is excreted in the urine. In humans, 12% to 15% of an orally administered dose of beclomethasone dipropionate was excreted in the urine as both conjugated and free metabolites of the drug.

The precise mechanisms of glucocorticoid action in asthma are unknown. Inflammation is recognized as an important component in the pathogenesis of asthma. Glucocorticoids

have been shown to inhibit multiple cell types (e.g., mast cells, eosinophils, basophils, lymphocytes, macrophages, and neutrophils) and mediator production or secretion (e.g., histamine, eicosanoids, leukotrienes, and cytokines) involved in the asthmatic response. These anti-inflammatory actions of glucocorticoids may contribute to their efficacy in asthma.

Clinical Trials: The effects of beclomethasone dipropionate on HPA function have been evaluated in adult volunteers. There was no suppression of early morning plasma cortisol concentrations when beclomethasone dipropionate was administered in a dose of 840 mcg/day for 1 month as an aerosol or 1000 mcg/day for 3 days by intramuscular injection. However, partial suppression of plasma cortisol concentration was observed when beclomethasone dipropionate was administered in doses of 2000 mcg/day intramuscularly or 1680 mcg/day by aerosol. Immediate suppression of plasma cortisol concentrations was observed after single doses of 4000 mcg of beclomethasone dipropionate.

In one study the effects of beclomethasone dipropionate on HPA function were examined in patients with asthma. There was no change in basal early morning plasma cortisol concentrations or in the cortisol responses to tetracosactrin (ACTH 1:24) stimulation after daily aerosol administration of 336, 672, or 1008 mcg of beclomethasone dipropionate for 28 days. After daily aerosol administration of 1344 mcg for 28 days, there was slight reduction in basal cortisol concentrations and a statistically significant ($P<.01$) reduction in plasma cortisol responses to tetracosactrin stimulation. Following 52 weeks of aerosol treatment with 840 mcg of beclomethasone dipropionate daily, 7/115 (6%) of patients exhibited a plasma cortisol measurement below the lower limit of normal (150 nmol^{-1}).

Clinical experience has shown that some patients with asthma who require corticosteroid therapy for control of symptoms can be partially or completely withdrawn from systemic corticosteroids if therapy with beclomethasone dipropionate aerosol is substituted. Beclomethasone dipropionate aerosol is not effective for all patients with asthma or at all stages of the disease in a given patient.

INDICATIONS

BECLOVENT Inhalation Aerosol is indicated in the maintenance treatment of asthma as prophylactic therapy. BECLOVENT Inhalation Aerosol is also indicated for asthma patients who require systemic corticosteroid administration, where adding BECLOVENT Inhalation Aerosol may reduce or eliminate the need for the systemic corticosteroids.

BECLOVENT Inhalation Aerosol is NOT indicated for the relief of acute bronchospasm.

CONTRAINDICATIONS

BECLOVENT Inhalation Aerosol is contraindicated in the primary treatment of status asthmaticus or other acute episodes of asthma where intensive measures are required. Hypersensitivity to any of the ingredients of this preparation contraindicates its use.

WARNINGS

Particular care is needed in patients who are transferred from systemically active corticosteroids to BECLOVENT Inhalation Aerosol because deaths due to adrenal insufficiency have occurred in asthmatic patients during and after transfer from systemic corticosteroids to aerosol beclomethasone dipropionate. After withdrawal from systemic corticosteroids, a number of months are required for recovery of hypothalamic-pituitary-adrenal (HPA) function. During this period of HPA suppression, patients may exhibit signs and symptoms of adrenal insufficiency when exposed to trauma, surgery, or infections, particularly gastroenteritis. Although BECLOVENT Inhalation Aerosol may provide control of asthmatic symptoms during these episodes, it does NOT provide the systemic steroid that is necessary for coping with these emergencies.

During periods of stress or a severe asthmatic attack, patients who have been withdrawn from systemic corticosteroids should be instructed to resume systemic steroids (in large doses) immediately and to contact their physician for further instruction. These patients should also be instructed to carry a warning card indicating that they may need supplementary systemic steroids during periods of stress or a severe asthma attack. To assess the risk of adrenal insufficiency in emergency situations, routine tests of adrenal cortical function, including measurement of early morning resting cortisol levels, should be performed periodically in all patients. An early morning resting cortisol level may be accepted as normal only if it falls at or near the normal mean level.

Localized infections with *Candida albicans* or *Aspergillus niger* have occurred in the mouth and pharynx and occasionally in the larynx. Positive cultures for oral *Candida*

may be present in up to 75% of patients. Although the frequency of clinically apparent infection is considerably lower, these infections can develop with any inhaled corticosteroid and may require treatment with appropriate antifungal therapy or discontinuation of treatment with BECLOVENT Inhalation Aerosol.

BECLOVENT Inhalation Aerosol is not a bronchodilator and is not indicated for rapid relief of bronchospasm.

Patients should be instructed to contact their physicians immediately when episodes of asthma that are not responsive to bronchodilators occur during the course of treatment with BECLOVENT Inhalation Aerosol. During such episodes, patients may require therapy with systemic corticosteroids.

Transfer of patients from systemic corticosteroid therapy to BECLOVENT Inhalation Aerosol may unmask allergic conditions previously suppressed by the systemic corticosteroid therapy, e.g., rhinitis, conjunctivitis, and eczema.

Persons who are on drugs that suppress the immune system are more susceptible to infections than healthy individuals. Chickenpox and measles, for example, can have a more serious or even fatal course in nonimmune children or adults on corticosteroids. In such children or adults who have not had these diseases, particular care should be taken to avoid exposure. How the dose, route, and duration of corticosteroid administration affect the risk of developing a disseminated infection is not known. The contribution of the underlying disease and/or prior corticosteroid treatment to the risk is also not known. If exposed to chickenpox, prophylaxis with varicella zoster immune globulin (VZIG) may be indicated. If exposed to measles, prophylaxis with pooled intramuscular immunoglobulin (IG) may be indicated. (See the respective package inserts for complete VZIG and IG prescribing information.) If chickenpox develops, treatment with antiviral agents may be considered.

Avoid spraying in eyes.

PRECAUTIONS

During withdrawal from oral corticosteroids, some patients may experience symptoms of systemically active corticosteroid withdrawal, e.g., joint and/or muscular pain, lassitude, and depression, despite maintenance or even improvement of respiratory function (see DOSAGE AND ADMINISTRATION).

In responsive patients, beclomethasone dipropionate may permit control of asthmatic symptoms without suppression of HPA function, as discussed above (see CLINICAL PHARMACOLOGY). Since beclomethasone dipropionate is absorbed into the circulation and can be systemically active, the beneficial effects of BECLOVENT Inhalation Aerosol in minimizing or preventing HPA dysfunction may be expected only when recommended dosages are not exceeded.

Because of the possibility of systemic absorption of orally inhaled corticosteroids, including beclomethasone, patients should be monitored for symptoms of systemic effects such as mental disturbances, increased bruising, weight gain, cushingoid features, acneiform lesions, and cataracts. Therefore, if such changes occur, BECLOVENT Inhalation Aerosol should be discontinued slowly, consistent with accepted procedures for discontinuing oral steroids.

A reduction of growth velocity in children or teenagers may occur as a result of inadequate control of chronic diseases such as asthma or from use of corticosteroids for treatment. Physicians should closely follow the growth of adolescents taking corticosteroids by any route and weigh the benefits of corticosteroid therapy and asthma control against the possibility of growth suppression if an adolescent's growth appears slowed.

The long-term local and systemic effects of BECLOVENT Inhalation Aerosol in human subjects are still not fully known. In particular, the effects resulting from chronic use of BECLOVENT Inhalation Aerosol on developmental or immunologic processes in the mouth, pharynx, trachea, and lung are unknown.

Inhaled corticosteroids should be used with caution, if at all, in patients with active or quiescent tuberculosis infection of the respiratory tract; untreated systemic fungal, bacterial, parasitic, or viral infections; or ocular herpes simplex.

Pulmonary infiltrates with eosinophilia may occur in patients on BECLOVENT Inhalation Aerosol therapy. Although it is possible that in some patients this state may become manifest because of systemic corticosteroid withdrawal when inhalational corticosteroids are administered, a causative role for beclomethasone dipropionate and/or its vehicle cannot be ruled out.

Information for Patients: Patients being treated with BECLOVENT Inhalation Aerosol should receive the following information and instructions. This information is intended to aid in the safe and effective use of this medication. It is not a disclosure of all possible adverse or intended effects.

Patients should use BECLOVENT Inhalation Aerosol at regular intervals as directed. Results of clinical trials indicated significant improvement may occur within the first day or two of treatment; however, the full benefit may not be achieved until treatment has been administered 1 or 2

weeks or longer. The patient should not increase the prescribed dosage but should contact the physician if symptoms do not improve or if the condition worsens.

Patients should be advised that BECLOVENT Inhalation Aerosol is not intended for use in the treatment of acute asthma. Patients should be made aware of the prophylactic nature of therapy with inhaled beclomethasone dipropionate and that it should be taken regularly even when they are asymptomatic. Patients should be instructed to contact their physicians immediately if there is any deterioration of their asthma.

BECLOVENT Inhalation Aerosol should not be stopped abruptly. If discontinuing use of BECLOVENT Inhalation Aerosol is necessary, the patient's physician should be contacted immediately.

Each patient should be advised to rinse his/her mouth each time after using BECLOVENT Inhalation Aerosol.

Patients should be warned to avoid exposure to chickenpox or measles. Patients should also be advised that if they are exposed, medical advice should be sought without delay.

Carcinogenesis, Mutagenesis, Impairment of Fertility: The carcinogenicity of beclomethasone dipropionate was evaluated in rats that were exposed for a total of 95 weeks, 13 weeks at inhalation doses up to 0.4 mg/kg and the remaining 82 weeks at combined oral and inhalation doses up to 2.4 mg/kg. There was no evidence of carcinogenicity in this study at the highest dose, approximately 20 or 36 times the maximum recommended daily inhalation dose in adults and children, respectively, on a mg/m^2 basis.

Beclomethasone dipropionate did not induce gene mutation in bacterial cells or mammalian Chinese Hamster ovary (CHO) cells in vitro. No significant clastogenic effect was seen in cultured CHO cells in vitro or in the mouse micronucleus test in vivo.

In rats, beclomethasone dipropionate caused decreased conception rates at an oral dose of 16 mg/kg (approximately 130 times the maximum recommended daily inhalation dose in adults on a mg/m^2 basis). Inhibition of the estrous cycle in dogs was observed following oral dosing at 0.5 mg/kg (approximately 15 times the maximum recommended daily inhalation dose in adults on a mg/m^2 basis). No inhibition of the estrous cycle in dogs was seen following 12 months' exposure at an estimated daily inhalation dose of 0.33 mg/kg (approximately 9 times the maximum recommended daily inhalation dose in adults on a mg/m^2 basis).

Pregnancy: Teratogenic Effects: Pregnancy Category C. Like other corticosteroids, beclomethasone dipropionate was teratogenic and embryocidal in the mouse and rabbit at a subcutaneous dose of 0.1 mg/kg in mice or 0.025 mg/kg in rabbits (approximately 1/2 the maximum recommended daily inhalation dose in adults on a mg/m^2 basis). No teratogenicity or embryocidal effects were seen in rats when exposed to an inhalation dose of 0.1 mg/kg plus oral doses of up to 10 mg/kg per day for a combined dose of 10.1 mg/kg (approximately 80 times the maximum recommended daily inhalation dose in adults on a mg/m^2 basis). There are no adequate and well-controlled studies in pregnant women. BECLOVENT Inhalation Aerosol should be used during pregnancy only if the potential benefit justifies the potential risk to the fetus.

Nursing Mothers: Corticosteroids are secreted in human milk. Because of the potential for serious adverse reactions in nursing infants for BECLOVENT Inhalation Aerosol, a decision should be made whether to discontinue nursing or to discontinue the drug, taking into account the importance of the drug to the mother.

Pediatric Use: The safety and effectiveness of BECLOVENT Inhalation Aerosol have been established in children aged 6 years and above. The safety and effectiveness of BECLOVENT Inhalation Aerosol in children below 6 years of age have not been established. Corticosteroids have been shown to cause a reduction in growth velocity in children and teenagers with extended use. If a child or teenager on any corticosteroid appears to have growth suppression, the possibility that they are particularly sensitive to this effect of corticosteroids should be considered (see PRECAUTIONS).

ADVERSE REACTIONS

Deaths due to adrenal insufficiency have occurred in asthmatic patients during and after transfer from systemic corticosteroids to aerosol beclomethasone dipropionate (see WARNINGS).

Suppression of HPA function (reduction of early morning plasma cortisol levels) has been reported in adult patients who received 1344-mcg daily doses of BECLOVENT Inhalation Aerosol for 1 month. A few patients on BECLOVENT Inhalation Aerosol have complained of hoarseness or dry mouth.

In addition, the following adverse events have been reported spontaneously during worldwide postmarketing surveillance. Therefore, the frequency of events and causality cannot be reliably determined. The adverse events reported in association with BECLOVENT Inhalation Aerosol include:

General: Immediate and delayed hypersensitivity reactions including anaphylactic/anaphylactoid reactions, angioedema, bronchospasm, rash, urticaria.

Ear, Nose, and Throat: Dryness and irritation of the nose, throat, and mouth; hoarseness; localized infections with *Candida* or *Aspergillus*; unpleasant taste and smell; loss of taste and smell.

Endocrine and Metabolic: Cushingoid features, growth velocity reduction in children/adolescents, weight gain.

Eye: Cataracts, glaucoma, increased intraocular pressure.

Gastrointestinal: Nausea, vomiting.

Nervous: Dizziness, headache, lightheadedness.

Psychiatry: Agitation, depression, mental disturbances.

Respiratory: Paradoxical bronchospasm, wheezing.

Skin: Acneiform lesions, atrophy, bruising, pruritus, purpura, striae.

OVERDOSAGE

For maximum doses studied in humans, see the Clinical Trials subsection. Chronic overdosage may result in signs/symptoms of hypercorticism (see PRECAUTIONS). No deaths occurred when beclomethasone dipropionate was given as single oral doses of 3000 mg/kg to mice and 2000 mg/kg to rats (approximately 12 000 and 16 000 times, respectively, the maximum recommended human daily inhalation dose on a mg/m^2 basis).

DOSAGE AND ADMINISTRATION

BECLOVENT Inhalation Aerosol should be test sprayed into the air before using for the first time and in cases where the product has not been used for a prolonged period of time.

Adults and Children 12 Years of Age and Older: The usual recommended dosage is two inhalations (84 mcg) given three or four times a day. Alternatively, four inhalations (168 mcg) given twice daily have been shown to be effective in some patients. In patients with severe asthma, it is advisable to start with 12 to 16 inhalations a day (504 to 672 mcg) and adjust the dosage downward according to the response of the patient. The maximal daily intake should not exceed 20 inhalations, 840 mcg (0.84 mg), in adults.

Children 6 to 12 Years of Age: The usual recommended dosage is one or two inhalations (42 to 84 mcg) given three or four times a day according to the response of the patient. Alternatively, four inhalations (168 mcg) given twice daily have been shown to be effective in some patients. The maximal daily intake should not exceed 10 inhalations, 420 mcg (0.42 mg), in children 6 to 12 years of age. Insufficient clinical data exist with respect to the administration of BECLOVENT Inhalation Aerosol in children below the age of 6. Rinsing the mouth after inhalation is advised.

Different considerations must be given to the following groups of patients in order to obtain the full therapeutic benefit of BECLOVENT Inhalation Aerosol.

Patients Not Receiving Systemic Corticosteroids: Patients who require maintenance therapy of their asthma may benefit from treatment with BECLOVENT Inhalation Aerosol at the doses recommended above. In patients who respond to BECLOVENT Inhalation Aerosol, improvement in pulmonary function is usually apparent within 1 to 4 weeks after the start of therapy. Once the desired effect is achieved, consideration should be given to tapering to the lowest effective dose.

Patients Maintained on Systemic Corticosteroids: Clinical studies have shown that BECLOVENT Inhalation Aerosol may be effective in the management of asthmatics dependent or maintained on systemic corticosteroids and may permit replacement or significant reduction in the dosage of systemic corticosteroids.

The patient's asthma should be reasonably stable before treatment with BECLOVENT Inhalation Aerosol is started. Initially, BECLOVENT Inhalation Aerosol should be used concurrently with the patient's usual maintenance dose of systemic corticosteroid. After approximately 1 week, gradual withdrawal of the systemic corticosteroid is started by reducing the daily or alternate-daily dose. Reductions may be made after an interval of 1 or 2 weeks, depending on the response of the patient. Generally, these decrements should not exceed 2.5 mg of prednisone or its equivalent. During withdrawal, some patients may experience symptoms of systemic corticosteroid withdrawal, e.g., joint and/or muscular pain, lassitude, and depression, despite maintenance or even improvement in pulmonary function. Such patients should be encouraged to continue with the inhaler but should be monitored for objective signs of adrenal insufficiency. If evidence of adrenal insufficiency occurs, the systemic corticosteroid doses should be increased temporarily and thereafter withdrawal should continue more slowly. During periods of stress or a severe asthma attack, transfer patients may require supplementary treatment with systemic corticosteroids.

Directions for Use: Illustrated Patient's Instructions for Use accompany each package of BECLOVENT Inhalation Aerosol.

CONTENTS UNDER PRESSURE: Do not puncture. Do not use or store near heat or open flame. Exposure to temperatures above 120°F may cause bursting. Never throw container into fire or incinerator. Keep out of reach of children.

HOW SUPPLIED

BECLOVENT Inhalation Aerosol is supplied in a 6.7-g canister containing 80 metered inhalations with oral adapter and patient's instructions (NDC 0173-0469-00) and in a 16.8-g canister containing 200 metered inhalations with oral adapter and patient's instructions (NDC 0173-0312-88). Also available, BECLOVENT Inhalation Aerosol Refill 16.8-g canister only with patient's instructions (NDC 0173-0312-98). Each actuation delivers a quantity of clathrate equivalent to 42 mcg of beclomethasone dipropionate, USP from the mouthpiece and 50 mcg from the valve.

The BECLOVENT Inhalation Aerosol canister should only be used with the tan BECLOVENT Inhalation Aerosol mouthpiece, and this mouthpiece should not be used with any other inhalation product. A dark brown cap fits over the mouthpiece when not in use.

The correct amount of medication in each inhalation cannot be assured after 80 inhalations from the 6.7-g canister or 200 inhalations from the 16.8-g canister even though the canister is not completely empty. The canister should be discarded when the labeled number of actuations has been used.

Store between 2° and 30°C (36° and 86°F). As with most inhaled medications in aerosol canisters, the therapeutic effect of this medication may decrease when the canister is cold. For optimal results, the canister should be at room temperature before use. Shake well before using.

December 1997/RL-536

Shown in Product Identification Guide, page 311

BECONASE® ℞
[be 'kō-nāz"]
(beclomethasone dipropionate, USP)
Inhalation Aerosol
For Nasal Inhalation Only

DESCRIPTION

Beclomethasone dipropionate, USP, the active component of BECONASE Inhalation Aerosol, is an anti-inflammatory steroid having the chemical name 9-chloro-11β,17,21-trihydroxy-16β-methylpregna-1,4-diene-3,20-dione 17,21-dipropionate.

Beclomethasone dipropionate is a white to creamy-white, odorless powder with a molecular weight of 521.25.

It is very slightly soluble in water, very soluble in chloroform, and freely soluble in acetone and in alcohol.

BECONASE Inhalation Aerosol is a metered-dose aerosol unit containing a microcrystalline suspension of beclomethasone dipropionate-trichloromonofluoromethane clathrate in a mixture of propellants (trichloromonofluoromethane and dichlorodifluoromethane) with oleic acid. Each canister contains beclomethasone dipropionate-trichloromonofluoromethane clathrate having a molecular proportion of beclomethasone dipropionate to trichloromonofluoromethane between 3:1 and 3:2. Each actuation delivers from the compact actuator a quantity of clathrate equivalent to 42 mcg of beclomethasone dipropionate, USP. The contents of one 6.7-g canister provide at least 80 metered doses, and the contents of one 16.8-g canister provide at least 200 metered doses.

CLINICAL PHARMACOLOGY

Beclomethasone 17,21-dipropionate is a diester of beclomethasone, a synthetic halogenated corticosteroid.

Animal studies show that beclomethasone dipropionate has potent glucocorticoid and weak mineralocorticoid activity.

The mechanisms responsible for the anti-inflammatory action of beclomethasone dipropionate are unknown.

The precise mechanism of the aerosolized drug's action in the nose is also unknown. Biopsies of nasal mucosa obtained during clinical studies showed no histopathologic changes when beclomethasone dipropionate was administered intranasally.

The effects of beclomethasone dipropionate on hypothalamic-pituitary-adrenal (HPA) function have been evaluated in adult volunteers by other routes of administration. Studies with beclomethasone dipropionate by the intranasal route may demonstrate that there is more or that there is less absorption by this route of administration. There was no suppression of early morning plasma cortisol concentrations when beclomethasone dipropionate was administered

Continued on next page

This product information is based on labeling in effect on June 1, 1998. For further information, contact via direct mail, phone, or web site Medical Information: Glaxo Wellcome Inc., PO Box 13398, Research Triangle Park, NC 27709. Healthcare Professionals (Medical Information): 800-334-0089 Patients (Customer Response Center): 888-TALK2GW (1-888-825-5249) Glaxo Wellcome Corporate Web Site: www.glaxowellcome.com

Beconase—Cont.

in a dose of 1,000 mcg per day for 1 month as an oral aerosol or for 3 days by intramuscular injection. However, partial suppression of plasma cortisol concentrations was observed when beclomethasone dipropionate was administered in doses of 2,000 mcg per day either by oral aerosol or intramuscular injection. Immediate suppression of plasma cortisol concentrations was observed after single doses of 4,000 mcg of beclomethasone dipropionate. Suppression of HPA function (reduction of early morning plasma cortisol levels) has been reported in adult patients who received 1,600-mcg daily doses of oral beclomethasone dipropionate for 1 month. In clinical studies using beclomethasone dipropionate intranasally, there was no evidence of adrenal insufficiency.

Beclomethasone dipropionate is sparingly soluble. When given by nasal inhalation in the form of an aqueous or aerosolized suspension, the drug is deposited primarily in the nasal passages. A portion of the drug is swallowed. Absorption occurs rapidly from all respiratory and gastrointestinal tissues. There is no evidence of tissue storage of beclomethasone dipropionate or its metabolites. *In vitro* studies have shown that tissue other than the liver (lung slices) can rapidly metabolize beclomethasone dipropionate to beclomethasone 17-monopropionate and more slowly to free beclomethasone (which has very weak anti-inflammatory activity).

However, irrespective of the route of entry, the principal route of excretion of the drug and its metabolites is the feces. In humans, 12% to 15% of an orally administered dose of beclomethasone dipropionate is excreted in the urine as both conjugated and free metabolites of the drug.

Studies have shown that the degree of binding to plasma proteins is 87%.

INDICATIONS AND USAGE

BECONASE Inhalation Aerosol is indicated for the relief of the symptoms of seasonal or perennial rhinitis in those cases poorly responsive to conventional treatment.

BECONASE Inhalation Aerosol is also indicated for the prevention of recurrence of nasal polyps following surgical removal.

Clinical studies in patients with seasonal or perennial rhinitis have shown that improvement is usually apparent within a few days. However, symptomatic relief may not occur in some patients for as long as 2 weeks. Although systemic effects are minimal at recommended doses, BECONASE Inhalation Aerosol should not be continued beyond 3 weeks in the absence of significant symptomatic improvement. BECONASE Inhalation Aerosol should not be used in the presence of untreated localized infection involving the nasal mucosa.

Clinical studies have shown that treatment of the symptoms associated with nasal polyps may have to be continued for several weeks or more before a therapeutic result can be fully assessed. Recurrence of symptoms due to polyps can occur after stopping treatment, depending on the severity of the disease.

CONTRAINDICATIONS

Hypersensitivity to any of the ingredients of this preparation contraindicates its use.

WARNINGS

The replacement of a systemic corticosteroid with BECONASE Inhalation Aerosol can be accompanied by signs of adrenal insufficiency.

Careful attention must be given when patients previously treated for prolonged periods with systemic corticosteroids are transferred to BECONASE Inhalation Aerosol. This is particularly important in those patients who have associated asthma or other clinical conditions where too rapid a decrease in systemic corticosteroids may cause a severe exacerbation of their symptoms.

Studies have shown that the combined administration of alternate-day prednisone systemic treatment and orally inhaled beclomethasone increases the likelihood of HPA suppression compared to a therapeutic dose of either one alone. Therefore, BECONASE Inhalation Aerosol treatment should be used with caution in patients already on alternate-day prednisone regimens for any disease.

If recommended doses of intranasal beclomethasone are exceeded or if individuals are particularly sensitive or predisposed by virtue of recent systemic steroid therapy, symptoms of hypercorticism may occur, including very rare cases of menstrual irregularities, acneiform lesions, cataracts, and cushingoid features. If such changes occur, BECONASE Inhalation Aerosol should be discontinued slowly consistent with accepted procedures for discontinuing oral steroid therapy.

Persons who are on drugs that suppress the immune system are more susceptible to infections than healthy individuals. Chickenpox and measles, for example, can have a more serious or even fatal course in nonimmune children or adults on corticosteroids. In such children or adults who have not

had these diseases, particular care should be taken to avoid exposure. How the dose, route, and duration of corticosteroid administration affects the risk of developing a disseminated infection is not known. The contribution of the underlying disease and/or prior corticosteroid treatment to the risk is also not known. If exposed to chickenpox, prophylaxis with varicella zoster immune globulin (VZIG) may be indicated. If exposed to measles, prophylaxis with pooled intramuscular immunoglobulin (IG) may be indicated. (See the respective package inserts for complete VZIG and IG prescribing information.) If chickenpox develops, treatment with antiviral agents may be considered.

PRECAUTIONS

General: During withdrawal from oral steroids, some patients may experience symptoms of withdrawal, e.g., joint and/or muscular pain, lassitude, and depression.

Rare instances of nasal septum perforation have been spontaneously reported.

Rare instances of wheezing, cataracts, glaucoma, and increased intraocular pressure have been reported following the intranasal use of beclomethasone dipropionate.

In clinical studies with beclomethasone dipropionate administered intranasally, the development of localized infections of the nose and pharynx with *Candida albicans* has occurred only rarely. When such an infection develops, it may require treatment with appropriate local therapy or discontinuation of treatment with BECONASE Inhalation Aerosol.

Beclomethasone dipropionate is absorbed into the circulation. Use of excessive doses of BECONASE Inhalation Aerosol may suppress HPA function.

BECONASE Inhalation Aerosol should be used with caution, if at all, in patients with active or quiescent tuberculous infections of the respiratory tract; untreated fungal, bacterial, or systemic viral infections; or ocular herpes simplex.

For BECONASE Inhalation Aerosol to be effective in the treatment of nasal polyps, the aerosol must be able to enter the nose. Therefore, treatment of nasal polyps with BECONASE Inhalation Aerosol should be considered adjunctive therapy to surgical removal and/or the use of other medications that will permit effective penetration of BECONASE Inhalation Aerosol into the nose. Nasal polyps may recur after any form of treatment.

As with any long-term treatment, patients using BECONASE Inhalation Aerosol over several months or longer should be examined periodically for possible changes in the nasal mucosa.

Because of the inhibitory effect of corticosteroids on wound healing, patients who have experienced recent nasal septum ulcers, nasal surgery, or trauma should not use a nasal corticosteroid until healing has occurred.

Although systemic effects have been minimal with recommended doses, this potential increases with excessive doses. Therefore, larger than recommended doses should be avoided.

Information for Patients: Patients should use BECONASE Inhalation Aerosol at regular intervals since its effectiveness depends on its regular use. The patient should take the medication as directed. It is not acutely effective, and the prescribed dosage should not be increased. Instead, nasal vasoconstrictors or oral antihistamines may be needed until the effects of BECONASE Inhalation Aerosol are fully manifested. One to 2 weeks may pass before full relief is obtained. The patient should contact the physician if symptoms do not improve, if the condition worsens, or if sneezing or nasal irritation occurs. For the proper use of this unit and to attain maximum improvement, the patient should read and follow carefully the patient's instructions section of the package insert.

Persons who are on immunosuppressant doses of corticosteroids should be warned to avoid exposure to chickenpox or measles. Patients should also be advised that if they are exposed, medical advice should be sought without delay.

Carcinogenesis, Mutagenesis, Impairment of Fertility: Treatment of rats for a total of 95 weeks, 13 weeks by inhalation and 82 weeks by the oral route, resulted in no evidence of carcinogenic activity. Mutagenic studies have not been performed.

Impairment of fertility, as evidenced by inhibition of the estrous cycle in dogs, was observed following treatment by the oral route. No inhibition of the estrous cycle in dogs was seen following treatment with beclomethasone dipropionate by the inhalation route.

Pregnancy: *Teratogenic Effects: Pregnancy Category C:* Like other corticoids, parenteral (subcutaneous) beclomethasone dipropionate has been shown to be teratogenic and embryocidal in the mouse and rabbit when given in doses approximately 10 times the human dose. In these studies, beclomethasone was found to produce fetal resorption, cleft palate, agnathia, microstomia, absence of tongue, delayed ossification, and agenesis of the thymus. No teratogenic or embryocidal effects have been seen in the rat when beclomethasone dipropionate was administered by inhalation at 10 times the human dose or orally at 1,000 times the

human dose. There are no adequate and well-controlled studies in pregnant women. Beclomethasone dipropionate should be used during pregnancy only if the potential benefit justifies the potential risk to the fetus.

Nonteratogenic Effects: Hypoadrenalism may occur in infants born of mothers receiving corticosteroids during pregnancy. Such infants should be carefully observed.

Nursing Mothers: It is not known whether beclomethasone dipropionate is excreted in human milk. Because other corticosteroids are excreted in human milk, caution should be exercised when BECONASE Inhalation Aerosol is administered to a nursing woman.

Pediatric Use: Safety and effectiveness in children below 6 years of age have not been established.

ADVERSE REACTIONS

In general, side effects in clinical studies have been primarily associated with the nasal mucous membranes. Adverse reactions reported in controlled clinical trials and long-term open studies in patients treated with BECONASE Inhalation Aerosol are described below.

Sensations of irritation and burning in the nose (11 per 100 patients) following the use of BECONASE Inhalation Aerosol have been reported. Also, occasional sneezing attacks (10 per 100 adult patients) have occurred immediately following the use of the intranasal inhaler. This symptom may be more common in children. Rhinorrhea may occur occasionally (1 per 100 patients).

Localized infections of the nose and pharynx with *Candida albicans* have occurred rarely (see PRECAUTIONS).

Transient episodes of epistaxis have been reported in 2 per 100 patients.

Rare cases of ulceration of the nasal mucosa and instances of nasal septum perforation have been spontaneously reported (see PRECAUTIONS).

Reports of headache, light-headedness, dryness and irritation of the nose and throat, and unpleasant taste and smell have been received. There are rare reports of loss of taste and smell.

Rare instances of wheezing, cataracts, glaucoma, and increased intraocular pressure have been reported following the use of intranasal beclomethasone dipropionate (see PRECAUTIONS).

Rare cases of immediate and delayed hypersensitivity reactions, including urticaria, angioedema, rash, and bronchospasm, have been reported following the oral and intranasal inhalation of beclomethasone.

Systemic corticosteroid side effects were not reported during the controlled clinical trials. If recommended doses are exceeded, however, or if individuals are particularly sensitive, symptoms of hypercorticism, i.e., Cushing's syndrome, could occur.

OVERDOSAGE

When used at excessive doses, systemic corticosteroid effects such as hypercorticism and adrenal suppression may appear. If such changes occur, BECONASE Inhalation Aerosol should be discontinued slowly consistent with accepted procedures for discontinuing oral steroid therapy. The oral LD_{50} of beclomethasone dipropionate is greater than 1g/kg in rodents. One canister of BECONASE Inhalation Aerosol contains 8.4 mg of beclomethasone dipropionate; therefore, acute overdosage is unlikely.

DOSAGE AND ADMINISTRATION

Adults and Children 12 Years of Age and Older: The usual dosage is one inhalation (42 mcg) in each nostril two to four times a day (total dose, 168 to 336 mcg per day). Patients can often be maintained on a maximum dose of one inhalation in each nostril three times a day (252 mcg per day).

Children 6 to 12 Years of Age: The usual dosage is one inhalation in each nostril three times a day (252 mcg per day). BECONASE Inhalation Aerosol is *not* recommended for children below 6 years of age since safety and efficacy studies have not been conducted in this age-group.

In patients who respond to BECONASE Inhalation Aerosol, an improvement of the symptoms of seasonal or perennial rhinitis usually becomes apparent within a few days after the start of BECONASE Inhalation Aerosol therapy. However, symptomatic relief may not occur in some patients for as long as 2 weeks. BECONASE Inhalation Aerosol should not be continued beyond 3 weeks in the absence of significant symptomatic improvement.

The therapeutic effects of corticosteroids, unlike those of decongestants, are not immediate. This should be explained to the patient in advance in order to ensure cooperation and continuation of treatment with the prescribed dosage regimen.

In the presence of excessive nasal mucus secretion or edema of the nasal mucosa, the drug may fail to reach the site of intended action. In such cases it is advisable to use a nasal vasoconstrictor during the first 2 to 3 days of BECONASE Inhalation Aerosol therapy.

Directions for Use: Illustrated Patient's Instructions for Use accompany each package of BECONASE Inhalation Aerosol.

CONTENTS UNDER PRESSURE: Do not puncture. Do not use or store near heat or open flame. Exposure to temperatures above 120°F may cause bursting. Never throw container into fire or incinerator. Keep out of reach of children.

HOW SUPPLIED

BECONASE Inhalation Aerosol is supplied in a 6.7-g canister containing 80 metered doses (NDC 0173-0468-00) and in a 16.8-g canister containing 200 metered doses (NDC 0173-0336-02), each with beige compact actuator and patient's instructions.

Store between 2° and 30°C (36° and 86°F). As with most inhaled medications in aerosol canisters, the therapeutic effect of this medication may decrease when the canister is cold. Shake well before using.

May 1997/RL-424

Shown in Product Identification Guide, page 311

BECONASE AQ® ℞

(beclomethasone dipropionate, monohydrate)
Nasal Spray, 0.042%*
***Calculated on the dried basis.**
For Intranasal Use Only

SHAKE WELL BEFORE USE.

DESCRIPTION

Beclomethasone dipropionate, monohydrate, the active component of BECONASE AQ Nasal Spray, is an anti-inflammatory steroid having the chemical name 9-chloro-11β,17,21-trihydroxy-16β-methylpregna-1,4-diene-3,20-dione 17,21-dipropionate, monohydrate.

Beclomethasone dipropionate, monohydrate is a white to creamy-white, odorless powder with a molecular weight of 539.06. It is very slightly soluble in water, very soluble in chloroform, and freely soluble in acetone and in alcohol.

BECONASE AQ Nasal Spray is a metered-dose, manual pump spray unit containing a microcrystalline suspension of beclomethasone dipropionate, monohydrate equivalent to 0.042% w/w beclomethasone dipropionate, calculated on the dried basis, in an aqueous medium containing microcrystalline cellulose, carboxymethylcellulose sodium, dextrose, benzalkonium chloride, polysorbate 80, and 0.25% v/w phenylethyl alcohol. Hydrochloric acid may be added to adjust pH. The pH is between 4.5 and 7.0.

After initial priming (three to four actuations), each actuation of the pump delivers from the nasal adapter 100 mg of suspension containing beclomethasone dipropionate, monohydrate equivalent to 42 mcg of beclomethasone dipropionate. Each bottle of BECONASE AQ Nasal Spray will provide at least 200 metered doses.

CLINICAL PHARMACOLOGY

Beclomethasone 17,21-dipropionate is a diester of beclomethasone, a synthetic halogenated corticosteroid. Animal studies show that beclomethasone dipropionate has potent glucocorticoid and weak mineralocorticoid activity.

The mechanisms responsible for the anti-inflammatory action of beclomethasone dipropionate are unknown. The precise mechanism of the aerosolized drug's action in the nose is also unknown. Biopsies of nasal mucosa obtained during clinical studies showed no histopathologic changes when beclomethasone dipropionate was administered intranasally.

The effects of beclomethasone dipropionate on hypothalamic-pituitary-adrenal (HPA) function have been evaluated in adult volunteers by other routes of administration. Studies with beclomethasone dipropionate by the intranasal route may demonstrate that there is more or that there is less absorption by this route of administration. There was no suppression of early morning plasma cortisol concentrations when beclomethasone dipropionate was administered in a dose of 1,000 mcg/day for 1 month as an oral aerosol or for 3 days by intramuscular injection. However, partial suppression of plasma cortisol concentrations was observed when beclomethasone dipropionate was administered in doses of 2,000 mcg/day either by oral aerosol or intramuscular injection. Immediate suppression of plasma cortisol concentrations was observed after single doses of 4,000 mcg of beclomethasone dipropionate. Suppression of HPA function (reduction of early morning plasma cortisol levels) has been reported in adult patients who received 1,600-mcg daily doses of oral beclomethasone dipropionate for 1 month. In clinical studies using beclomethasone dipropionate aerosol intranasally, there was no evidence of adrenal insufficiency. The effect of BECONASE AQ Nasal Spray on HPA function was not evaluated but would not be expected to differ from intranasal beclomethasone dipropionate aerosol.

In one study in asthmatic children, the administration of inhaled beclomethasone at recommended daily doses for at least 1 year was associated with a reduction in nocturnal cortisol secretion. The clinical significance of this finding is not clear. It reinforces other evidence, however, that topical beclomethasone may be absorbed in amounts that can have systemic effects and that physicians should be alert for evidence of systemic effects, especially in chronically treated patients (see PRECAUTIONS).

Beclomethasone dipropionate is sparingly soluble. When given by nasal inhalation in the form of an aqueous or aerosolized suspension, the drug is deposited primarily in the nasal passages. A portion of the drug is swallowed. Absorption occurs rapidly from all respiratory and gastrointestinal tissues. There is no evidence of tissue storage of beclomethasone dipropionate or its metabolites. In vitro studies have shown that tissue other than the liver (lung slices) can rapidly metabolize beclomethasone dipropionate to beclomethasone 17-monopropionate and more slowly to free beclomethasone (which has very weak anti-inflammatory activity). However, irrespective of the route of entry, the principal route of excretion of the drug and its metabolites is the feces. In humans, 12% to 15% of an orally administered dose of beclomethasone dipropionate is excreted in the urine as both conjugated and free metabolites of the drug.

Studies have shown that the degree of binding to plasma proteins is 87%.

INDICATIONS AND USAGE

BECONASE AQ Nasal Spray is indicated for the relief of the symptoms of seasonal or perennial allergic and nonallergic (vasomotor) rhinitis.

Results from two clinical trials have shown that significant symptomatic relief was obtained within 3 days. However, symptomatic relief may not occur in some patients for as long as 2 weeks. BECONASE AQ Nasal Spray should not be continued beyond 3 weeks in the absence of significant symptomatic improvement. BECONASE AQ Nasal Spray should not be used in the presence of untreated localized infection involving the nasal mucosa.

BECONASE AQ Nasal Spray is also indicated for the prevention of recurrence of nasal polyps following surgical removal.

Clinical studies have shown that treatment of the symptoms associated with nasal polyps may have to be continued for several weeks or more before a therapeutic result can be fully assessed. Recurrence of symptoms due to polyps can occur after stopping treatment, depending on the severity of the disease.

CONTRAINDICATIONS

Hypersensitivity to any of the ingredients of this preparation contraindicates its use.

WARNINGS

The replacement of a systemic corticosteroid with BECONASE AQ Nasal Spray can be accompanied by signs of adrenal insufficiency.

Careful attention must be given when patients previously treated for prolonged periods with systemic corticosteroids are transferred to BECONASE AQ Nasal Spray. This is particularly important in those patients who have associated asthma or other clinical conditions where too rapid a decrease in systemic corticosteroids may cause a severe exacerbation of their symptoms.

Studies have shown that the combined administration of alternate-day prednisone systemic treatment and orally inhaled beclomethasone increases the likelihood of HPA suppression compared to a therapeutic dose of either one alone. Therefore, BECONASE AQ Nasal Spray treatment should be used with caution in patients already on alternate-day prednisone regimens for any disease.

If recommended doses of intranasal beclomethasone are exceeded or if individuals are particularly sensitive or predisposed by virtue of recent systemic steroid therapy, symptoms of hypercorticism may occur, including very rare cases of menstrual irregularities, acneiform lesions, cataracts, and cushingoid features. If such changes occur, BECONASE AQ Nasal Spray should be discontinued slowly consistent with accepted procedures for discontinuing oral steroid therapy.

Persons who are on drugs that suppress the immune system are more susceptible to infections than healthy individuals. Chickenpox and measles, for example, can have a more serious or even fatal course in nonimmune children or adults on corticosteroids. In such children or adults who have not had these diseases, particular care should be taken to avoid exposure. How the dose, route, and duration of corticosteroid administration affect the risk of developing a disseminated infection is not known. The contribution of the underlying disease and/or prior corticosteroid treatment to the risk is also not known. If exposed to chickenpox, prophylaxis with varicella zoster immune globulin (VZIG) may be indicated. If exposed to measles, prophylaxis with pooled intramuscular immunoglobulin (IG) may be indicated. (See the respective package inserts for complete VZIG and IG prescribing information.) If chickenpox develops, treatment with antiviral agents may be considered.

PRECAUTIONS

General: During withdrawal from oral steroids, some patients may experience symptoms of withdrawal, e.g., joint and/or muscular pain, lassitude, and depression.

Rarely, immediate hypersensitivity reactions may occur after the intranasal administration of beclomethasone (see ADVERSE REACTIONS).

Rare instances of nasal septum perforation have been spontaneously reported.

Rare instances of wheezing, cataracts, glaucoma, and increased intraocular pressure have been reported following the use of intranasal beclomethasone.

In clinical studies with beclomethasone dipropionate administered intranasally, the development of localized infections of the nose and pharynx with *Candida albicans* has occurred only rarely. When such an infection develops, it may require treatment with appropriate local therapy or discontinuation of treatment with BECONASE AQ Nasal Spray.

If persistent nasopharyngeal irritation occurs, it may be an indication for stopping BECONASE AQ Nasal Spray.

Beclomethasone dipropionate is absorbed into the circulation. Use of excessive doses of BECONASE AQ Nasal Spray may suppress HPA function.

BECONASE AQ Nasal Spray should be used with caution, if at all, in patients with active or quiescent tuberculous infections of the respiratory tract; untreated fungal, bacterial, or systemic viral infections; or ocular herpes simplex.

For BECONASE AQ Nasal Spray to be effective in the treatment of nasal polyps, the spray must be able to enter the nose. Therefore, treatment of nasal polyps with BECONASE AQ Nasal Spray should be considered adjunctive therapy to surgical removal and/or the use of other medications that will permit effective penetration of BECONASE AQ Nasal Spray into the nose. Nasal polyps may recur after any form of treatment.

As with any long-term treatment, patients using BECONASE AQ Nasal Spray over several months or longer should be examined periodically for possible changes in the nasal mucosa.

Because of the inhibitory effect of corticosteroids on wound healing, patients who have experienced recent nasal septum ulcers, nasal surgery, or trauma should not use a nasal corticosteroid until healing has occurred.

Although systemic effects have been minimal with recommended doses, this potential increases with excessive doses. Therefore, larger than recommended doses should be avoided.

Information for Patients: Patients being treated with BECONASE AQ Nasal Spray should receive the following information and instructions. This information is intended to aid in the safe and effective use of this medication. It is not a disclosure of all possible adverse or intended effects. Patients should use BECONASE AQ Nasal Spray at regular intervals since its effectiveness depends on its regular use. The patient should take the medication as directed. It is not acutely effective, and the prescribed dosage should not be increased. Instead, nasal vasoconstrictors or oral antihistamines may be needed until the effects of BECONASE AQ Nasal Spray are fully manifested. One to 2 weeks may pass before full relief is obtained. The patient should contact the physician if symptoms do not improve, if the condition worsens, or if sneezing or nasal irritation occurs. For the proper use of the unit and to attain maximum improvement, the patient should read and follow carefully the patient's instructions section of the full prescribing information.

Persons who are on immunosuppressant doses of corticosteroids should be warned to avoid exposure to chickenpox or measles. Patients should also be advised that if they are exposed, medical advice should be sought without delay.

Carcinogenesis, Mutagenesis, Impairment of Fertility: Treatment of rats for a total of 95 weeks, 13 weeks by inhalation and 82 weeks by the oral route, resulted in no evidence of carcinogenic activity. Mutagenic studies have not been performed.

Impairment of fertility, as evidenced by inhibition of the estrous cycle in dogs, was observed following treatment by the oral route. No inhibition of the estrous cycle in dogs was seen following treatment with beclomethasone dipropionate by the inhalation route.

Pregnancy: ***Teratogenic Effects: Pregnancy Category C:*** Like other corticoids, parenteral (subcutaneous) beclomethasone dipropionate has been shown to be teratogenic and embryocidal in the mouse and rabbit when given in doses approximately 10 times the human dose. In these studies, beclomethasone was found to produce fetal resorption, cleft palate, agnathia, microstomia, absence of tongue, delayed ossification, and agenesis of the thymus. No terato-

Continued on next page

This product information is based on labeling in effect on June 1, 1998. For further information, contact via direct mail, phone, or web site Medical Information: Glaxo Wellcome Inc., PO Box 13398, Research Triangle Park, NC 27709. Healthcare Professionals (Medical Information): 800-334-0089 Patients (Customer Response Center): 888-TALK2GW (1-888-825-5249) Glaxo Wellcome Corporate Web Site: www.glaxowellcome.com

Consult 1999 PDR® supplements and future editions for revisions

Beconase AQ—Cont.

genic or embryocidal effects have been seen in the rat when beclomethasone dipropionate was administered by inhalation at 10 times the human dose or orally at 1,000 times the human dose. There are no adequate and well-controlled studies in pregnant women. Beclomethasone dipropionate should be used during pregnancy only if the potential benefit justifies the potential risk to the fetus.

Nonteratogenic Effects: Hypoadrenalism may occur in infants born of mothers receiving corticosteroids during pregnancy. Such infants should be carefully observed.

Nursing Mothers: It is not known whether beclomethasone dipropionate is excreted in human milk. Because other corticosteroids are excreted in human milk, caution should be exercised when BECONASE AQ Nasal Spray is administered to a nursing woman.

Pediatric Use: The safety and effectiveness of BECONASE AQ Nasal Spray have been established in children aged 6 years and above through evidence from extensive clinical use in adult and pediatric patients. The safety and effectiveness of BECONASE AQ Nasal Spray in children below 6 years of age have not been established.

Glucocorticoids have been shown to cause a reduction in growth velocity in children and teenagers with extended use. If a child or teenager on any glucocorticoid appears to have growth suppression, the possibility that they are particularly sensitive to this effect of glucocorticoids should be considered.

ADVERSE REACTIONS

In general, side effects in clinical studies have been primarily associated with irritation of the nasal mucous membranes. Rare cases of immediate and delayed hypersensitivity reactions, including urticaria, angioedema, rash, and bronchospasm, have been reported following the oral and intranasal inhalation of beclomethasone dipropionate.

Adverse reactions reported in controlled clinical trials and open studies in patients treated with BECONASE AQ Nasal Spray are described below.

Mild nasopharyngeal irritation following the use of beclomethasone aqueous nasal spray has been reported in up to 24% of patients treated, including occasional sneezing attacks (about 4%) occurring immediately following use of the spray. In patients experiencing these symptoms, none had to discontinue treatment. The incidence of transient irritation and sneezing was approximately the same in the group of patients who received placebo in these studies, implying that these complaints may be related to vehicle components of the formulation.

Fewer than 5 per 100 patients reported headache, nausea, or lightheadedness following the use of BECONASE AQ Nasal Spray. Fewer than 3 per 100 patients reported nasal stuffiness, nosebleeds, rhinorrhea, or tearing eyes.

Rare cases of ulceration of the nasal mucosa and instances of nasal septum perforation have been spontaneously reported (see PRECAUTIONS).

Reports of dryness and irritation of the nose and throat, and unpleasant taste and smell have been received. There are rare reports of loss of taste and smell.

Rare instances of wheezing, cataracts, glaucoma, and increased intraocular pressure have been reported following the use of intranasal beclomethasone dipropionate (see PRECAUTIONS).

OVERDOSAGE

When used at excessive doses, systemic corticosteroid effects such as hypercorticism and adrenal suppression may appear. If such changes occur, BECONASE AQ Nasal Spray should be discontinued slowly consistent with accepted procedures for discontinuing oral steroid therapy. The oral LD_{50} of beclomethasone dipropionate is greater than 1 g/kg in rodents. One bottle of BECONASE AQ Nasal Spray contains beclomethasone dipropionate, monohydrate equivalent to 10.5 mg of beclomethasone dipropionate; therefore, acute overdosage is unlikely.

DOSAGE AND ADMINISTRATION

Adults and Children 12 Years of Age and Older: The usual dosage is one or two inhalations (42 to 84 mcg) in each nostril twice a day (total dose, 168 to 336 mcg/day).

Children 6 to 12 Years of Age: Patients should be started with one inhalation in each nostril twice a day; patients not adequately responding to 168 mcg or those with more severe symptoms may use 336 mcg (two inhalations in each nostril). BECONASE AQ Nasal Spray is *not* recommended for children below 6 years of age.

In patients who respond to BECONASE AQ Nasal Spray, an improvement of the symptoms of seasonal or perennial rhinitis usually becomes apparent within a few days after the start of BECONASE AQ Nasal Spray therapy. However, symptomatic relief may not occur in some patients for as long as 2 weeks. BECONASE AQ Nasal Spray should not be continued beyond 3 weeks in the absence of significant symptomatic improvement.

The therapeutic effects of corticosteroids, unlike those of decongestants, are not immediate. This should be explained to the patient in advance in order to ensure cooperation and continuation of treatment with the prescribed dosage regimen.

In the presence of excessive nasal mucous secretion or edema of the nasal mucosa, the drug may fail to reach the site of intended action. In such cases it is advisable to use a nasal vasoconstrictor during the first 2 to 3 days of BECONASE AQ Nasal Spray therapy.

Directions for Use: Illustrated Patient's Instructions for Use accompany each package of BECONASE AQ Nasal Spray.

HOW SUPPLIED

BECONASE AQ Nasal Spray, 0.042%* is supplied in an amber glass bottle fitted with a metering atomizing pump and nasal adapter in a box of one (NDC 0173-0388-79) with patient's instructions for use. Each bottle contains 25 g of suspension.

Store between 15° and 30°C (59° and 86°F).

*Calculated on the dried basis.

May 1997/RL-442

Shown in Product Identification Guide, page 311

CEFTIN® Tablets
[*sef 'tin*]
(cefuroxime axetil tablets)

CEFTIN® for Oral Suspension
(cefuroxime axetil powder for oral suspension)

℞

DESCRIPTION

CEFTIN Tablets and CEFTIN for Oral Suspension contain cefuroxime as cefuroxime axetil. CEFTIN is a semisynthetic, broad-spectrum cephalosporin antibiotic for oral administration.

Chemically, cefuroxime axetil, the 1-(acetyloxy) ethyl ester of cefuroxime, is (RS)-1-hydroxyethyl $(6R,7R)$-7-[2-(2-furyl)glyoxylamido]-3-(hydroxymethyl)-8-oxo-5-thia-1-azabicyclo[4.2.0]oct-2-ene-2-carboxylate,7^2-(Z)-$(O$-methyl-oxime), 1-acetate 3-carbamate. Its molecular formula is $C_{20}H_{22}N_4O_{10}S$, and it has a molecular weight of 510.48. Cefuroxime axetil is in the amorphous form.

CEFTIN Tablets are film-coated and contain the equivalent of 125, 250, or 500 mg of cefuroxime as cefuroxime axetil. CEFTIN Tablets contain the inactive ingredients colloidal silicon dioxide, croscarmellose sodium, FD&C Blue No.1 (250- and 500-mg tablets only), hydrogenated vegetable oil, hydroxypropyl methylcellulose, methylparaben, microcrystalline cellulose, propylene glycol, propylparaben, sodium benzoate (125-mg tablets only), sodium lauryl sulfate, and titanium dioxide.

CEFTIN for Oral Suspension, when reconstituted with water, provides the equivalent of 125 mg or 250 mg of cefuroxime (as cefuroxime axetil) per 5 mL of suspension. CEFTIN for Oral Suspension contains the inactive ingredients povidone K30, stearic acid, sucrose, and tutti-frutti flavoring.

CLINICAL PHARMACOLOGY

Absorption and Metabolism: After oral administration, cefuroxime axetil is absorbed from the gastrointestinal tract and rapidly hydrolyzed by nonspecific esterases in the intestinal mucosa and blood to cefuroxime. Cefuroxime is subsequently distributed throughout the extracellular fluids. The axetil moiety is metabolized to acetaldehyde and acetic acid.

Pharmacokinetics: Approximately 50% of serum cefuroxime is bound to protein. Serum pharmacokinetic parameters for CEFTIN Tablets and CEFTIN for Oral Suspension are shown in the tables below.

[See table below]

[See first table at top of next page]

Comparative Pharmacokinetic Properties: A 250 mg/5 mL-dose of CEFTIN Suspension is bioequivalent to two times 125 mg/5 mL-dose of CEFTIN Suspension when administered with food (see table below).

CEFTIN for Oral Suspension was not bioequivalent to CEFTIN Tablets when tested in healthy adults. The tablet and powder for oral suspension formulations are NOT substitutable on a mg/mg basis. The area under the curve for the suspension averaged 91% of that for the tablet, and the peak plasma concentration for the suspension averaged 71%

of the peak plasma concentration of the tablets. Therefore, the safety and effectiveness of both the tablet and oral suspension formulations had to be established in separate clinical trials.

[See second table at top of next page]

Food Effect on Pharmacokinetics: Absorption of the tablet is greater when taken after food (absolute bioavailability of CEFTIN Tablets increases from 37% to 52%). Despite this difference in absorption, the clinical and bacteriologic responses of patients were independent of food intake at the time of tablet administration in two studies where this was assessed.

All pharmacokinetic and clinical effectiveness and safety studies in pediatric patients using the suspension formulation were conducted in the fed state. No data are available on the absorption kinetics of the suspension formulation when administered to fasted pediatric patients.

Renal Excretion: Cefuroxime is excreted unchanged in the urine; in adults, approximately 50% of the administered dose is recovered in the urine within 12 hours. The pharmacokinetics of cefuroxime in the urine of pediatric patients have not been studied at this time. Until further data are available, the renal pharmacokinetic properties of cefuroxime axetil established in adults should not be extrapolated to pediatric patients.

Because cefuroxime is renally excreted, the serum half-life is prolonged in patients with reduced renal function. In a study of 20 elderly patients (mean age = 83.9 years) having a mean creatinine clearance of 34.9 mL/min, the mean serum elimination half-life was 3.5 hours. Despite the lower elimination of cefuroxime in geriatric patients, dosage adjustment based on age is not necessary (see PRECAUTIONS: Geriatric Use).

Microbiology: The *in vivo* bactericidal activity of cefuroxime axetil is due to cefuroxime's binding to essential target proteins and the resultant inhibition of cell-wall synthesis.

Cefuroxime has bactericidal activity against a wide range of common pathogens, including many beta-lactamase–producing strains. Cefuroxime is stable to many bacterial beta-lactamases, especially plasmid-mediated enzymes that are commonly found in enterobacteriaceae.

Cefuroxime has been demonstrated to be active against most strains of the following microorganisms both *in vitro* and in clinical infections as described in the INDICATIONS AND USAGE section (see INDICATIONS AND USAGE section).

Aerobic Gram-positive Microorganisms:

Staphylococcus aureus (including beta-lactamase–producing strains)

Streptococcus pneumoniae

Streptococcus pyogenes

Aerobic Gram-negative Microorganisms:

Escherichia coli

Haemophilus influenzae (including beta-lactamase–producing strains)

Haemophilus parainfluenzae

Klebsiella pneumoniae

Moraxella catarrhalis (including beta-lactamase–producing strains)

Neisseria gonorrhoeae (including beta-lactamase–producing strains)

Spirochetes:

Borrelia burgdorferi

Cefuroxime has been shown to be active *in vitro* against most strains of the following microorganisms; however, the clinical significance of these findings is unknown.

Cefuroxime exhibits *in vitro* minimum inhibitory concentrations (MICs) of 4.0 mcg/mL or less (systemic susceptible breakpoint) against most (≥90%) strains of the following microorganisms; however, the safety and effectiveness of cefuroxime in treating clinical infections due to these microorganisms have not been established in adequate and well-controlled trials.

Aerobic Gram-positive Microorganisms:

Staphylococcus epidermidis

Staphylococcus saprophyticus

Streptococcus agalactiae

Postprandial Pharmacokinetics of Cefuroxime Administered as CEFTIN Tablets to Adults*

Dose† (Cefuroxime Equivalent)	Peak Plasma Concentration (mcg/mL)	Time of Peak Plasma Concentration (h)	Mean Elimination Half-Life (h)	AUC (mcg-h mL)
125 mg	2.1	2.2	1.2	6.7
250 mg	4.1	2.5	1.2	12.9
500 mg	7.0	3.0	1.2	27.4
1,000 mg	13.6	2.5	1.3	50.0

*Mean values of 12 healthy adult volunteers.
†Drug administered immediately after a meal.

Postprandial Pharmacokinetics of Cefuroxime Administered as CEFTIN for Oral Suspension to Pediatric Patients*

Dose† (Cefuroxime Equivalent)	n	Peak Plasma Concentration (mcg/mL)	Time of Peak Plasma Concentration (h)	Mean Elimination Half-Life (h)	AUC (mcg·h·mL)
10 mg/kg	8	3.3	3.6	1.4	12.4
15 mg/kg	12	5.1	2.7	1.9	22.5
20 mg/kg	8	7.0	3.1	1.9	32.8

* Mean age = 23 months.
† Drug administered with milk or milk products.

Pharmacokinetics of Cefuroxime Administered as 250 mg/5 mL or 2 × 125 mg/5 mL CEFTIN for Oral Suspension to Adults* With Food

Dose (Cefuroxime Equivalent)	Peak Plasma Concentration (mcg/mL)	Time of Peak Plasma Concentration (h)	Mean Elimination Half-Life (h)	AUC (mcg·h·mL)
250 mg/5 mL	2.23	3	1.40	8.92
2 × 125 mg/5 mL	2.37	3	1.44	9.75

* Mean values of 18 healthy adult volunteers.

NOTE: Certain strains of enterococci, e.g., *Enterococcus faecalis* (formerly *Streptococcus faecalis*), are resistant to cefuroxime. Methicillin-resistant staphylococci are resistant to cefuroxime.

Aerobic Gram-negative Microorganisms:
Morganella morganii
Proteus inconstans
Proteus mirabilis
Providencia rettgeri
NOTE: *Pseudomonas* spp., *Campylobacter* spp., *Acinetobacter calcoaceticus*, and most strains of *Serratia* spp. and *Proteus vulgaris* are resistant to most first- and second-generation cephalosporins. Some strains of *Morganella morganii*, *Enterobacter cloacae*, and *Citrobacter* spp. have been shown by *in vitro* tests to be resistant to cefuroxime and other cephalosporins.

Anaerobic Microorganisms:
Peptococcus niger
NOTE: Most strains of *Clostridium difficile* and *Bacteroides fragilis* are resistant to cefuroxime.

Susceptibility Tests: *Dilution Techniques:* Quantitative methods that are used to determine MICs provide reproducible estimates of the susceptibility of bacteria to antimicrobial compounds. One such standardized procedure uses a standardized dilution method[1] (broth, agar, or microdilution) or equivalent with cefuroxime powder. The MIC values obtained should be interpreted according to the following criteria:

MIC (mcg/mL)	Interpretation
≤4	(S) Susceptible
8–16	(I) Intermediate
≥32	(R) Resistant

A report of "Susceptible" indicates that the pathogen, if in the blood, is likely to be inhibited by usually achievable concentrations of the antimicrobial compound in blood. A report of "Intermediate" indicates that inhibitory concentrations of the antibiotic may be achieved if high dosage is used or if the infection is confined to tissues or fluids in which high antibiotic concentrations are attained. This category also provides a buffer zone that prevents small, uncontrolled technical factors from causing major discrepancies in interpretation. A report of "Resistant" indicates that usually achievable concentrations of the antimicrobial compound in the blood are unlikely to be inhibitory and that other therapy should be selected.

Standardized susceptibility test procedures require the use of laboratory control microorganisms. Standard cefuroxime powder should give the following MIC values:

Microorganism	MIC (mcg/mL)
Escherichia coli ATCC 25922	2–8
Staphylococcus aureus ATCC 29213	0.5–2

Diffusion Techniques: Quantitative methods that require measurement of zone diameters provide estimates of the susceptibility of bacteria to antimicrobial compounds. One such standardized procedure[2] that has been recommended (for use with disks) to test the susceptibility of microorganisms to cefuroxime uses the 30-mcg cefuroxime disk. Interpretation involves correlation of the diameter obtained in the disk test with the MIC for cefuroxime.

Reports from the laboratory providing results of the standard single-disk susceptibility test with a 30-mcg cefuroxime disk should be interpreted according to the following criteria:

Zone Diameter (mm)	Interpretation
≥23	(S) Susceptible
15–22	(I) Intermediate
≤14	(R) Resistant

Interpretation should be as stated above for results using dilution techniques.

As with standard dilution techniques, diffusion methods require the use of laboratory control microorganisms. The 30-mcg cefuroxime disk provides the following zone diameters in these laboratory test quality control strains:

Microorganism	Zone Diameter (mm)
Escherichia coli ATCC 25922	20–26
Staphylococcus aureus ATCC 25923	27–35

INDICATIONS AND USAGE

NOTE: CEFTIN TABLETS AND CEFTIN FOR ORAL SUSPENSION ARE NOT BIOEQUIVALENT AND ARE NOT SUBSTITUTABLE ON A MG/MG BASIS (SEE CLINICAL PHARMACOLOGY).

CEFTIN Tablets: CEFTIN Tablets are indicated for the treatment of patients with mild to moderate infections caused by susceptible strains of the designated microorganisms in the conditions listed below:

1. **Pharyngitis/Tonsillitis** caused by *Streptococcus pyogenes*.
   NOTE: The usual drug of choice in the treatment and prevention of streptococcal infections, including the prophylaxis of rheumatic fever, is penicillin given by the intramuscular route. CEFTIN Tablets are generally effective in the eradication of streptococci from the nasopharynx; however, substantial data establishing the efficacy of cefuroxime in the subsequent prevention of rheumatic fever are not available. Please also note that in all clinical trials, all isolates had to be sensitive to both penicillin and cefuroxime. There are no data from adequate and well-controlled trials to demonstrate the effectiveness of cefuroxime in the treatment of penicillin-resistant strains of *Streptococcus pyogenes*.

2. **Acute Bacterial Otitis Media** caused by *Streptococcus pneumoniae*, *Haemophilus influenzae* (including beta-lactamase–producing strains), *Moraxella catarrhalis* (including beta-lactamase–producing strains), or *Streptococcus pyogenes*.

3. **Acute Bacterial Maxillary Sinusitis** caused by *Streptococcus pneumoniae* or *Haemophilus influenzae* (non-beta-lactamase–producing strains only). (See CLINICAL STUDIES section.)
   NOTE: In view of the insufficient numbers of isolates of beta-lactamase–producing strains of *Haemophilus influenzae* and *Moraxella catarrhalis* that were obtained from clinical trials with CEFTIN Tablets for patients with acute bacterial maxillary sinusitis, it was not possible to adequately evaluate the effectiveness of CEFTIN Tablets for sinus infections known, suspected, or considered potentially to be caused by beta-lactamase–producing *Haemophilus influenzae* or *Moraxella catarrhalis*.

4. **Acute Bacterial Exacerbations of Chronic Bronchitis and Secondary Bacterial Infections of Acute Bronchitis** caused by *Streptococcus pneumoniae*, *Haemophilus influenzae* (beta-lactamase negative strains), or *Haemophilus parainfluenzae* (beta-lactamase negative strains). (See DOSAGE AND ADMINISTRATION section and CLINICAL STUDIES section).

5. **Uncomplicated Skin and Skin-Structure Infections** caused by *Staphylococcus aureus* (including beta-lactamase–producing strains) or *Streptococcus pyogenes*.

6. **Uncomplicated Urinary Tract Infections** caused by *Escherichia coli* or *Klebsiella pneumoniae*.

7. **Uncomplicated Gonorrhea,** urethral and endocervical, caused by penicillinase-producing and non-penicillinase-producing strains of *Neisseria gonorrhoeae* and uncomplicated gonorrhea, rectal, in females, caused by non-penicillinase–producing strains of *Neisseria gonorrhoeae*.

8. **Early Lyme Disease (erythema migrans)** caused by *Borrelia burgdorferi*.

CEFTIN for Oral Suspension: CEFTIN for Oral Suspension is indicated for the treatment of pediatric patients 3 months to 12 years of age with mild to moderate infections caused by susceptible strains of the designated microorganisms in the conditions listed below. The safety and effectiveness of CEFTIN for Oral Suspension in the treatment of infections other than those specifically listed below have not been established either by adequate and well-controlled trials or by pharmacokinetic data with which to determine an effective and safe dosing regimen.

1. **Pharyngitis/Tonsillitis** caused by *Streptococcus pyogenes*.
   NOTE: The usual drug of choice in the treatment and prevention of streptococcal infections, including the prophylaxis of rheumatic fever, is penicillin given by the intramuscular route. CEFTIN for Oral Suspension is generally effective in the eradication of streptococci from the nasopharynx; however, substantial data establishing the efficacy of cefuroxime in the subsequent prevention of rheumatic fever are not available. Please also note that in all clinical trials, all isolates had to be sensitive to both penicillin and cefuroxime. There are no data from adequate and well-controlled trials to demonstrate the effectiveness of cefuroxime in the treatment of penicillin-resistant strains of *Streptococcus pyogenes*.

2. **Acute Bacterial Otitis Media** caused by *Streptococcus pneumoniae*, *Haemophilus influenzae* (including beta-lactamase–producing strains), *Moraxella catarrhalis* (including beta-lactamase–producing strains), or *Streptococcus pyogenes*.

3. **Impetigo** caused by *Staphylococcus aureus* (including beta-lactamase–producing strains) or *Streptococcus pyogenes*.

Culture and susceptibility testing should be performed when appropriate to determine susceptibility of the causative microorganism(s) to cefuroxime. Therapy may be started while awaiting the results of this testing. Antimicrobial therapy should be appropriately adjusted according to the results of such testing.

CONTRAINDICATIONS

CEFTIN products are contraindicated in patients with known allergy to the cephalosporin group of antibiotics.

WARNINGS

CEFTIN TABLETS AND CEFTIN FOR ORAL SUSPENSION ARE NOT BIOEQUIVALENT AND ARE THEREFORE NOT SUBSTITUTABLE ON A MG/MG BASIS (SEE CLINICAL PHARMACOLOGY).

BEFORE THERAPY WITH CEFTIN PRODUCTS IS INSTITUTED, CAREFUL INQUIRY SHOULD BE MADE TO DETERMINE WHETHER THE PATIENT HAS HAD PREVIOUS HYPERSENSITIVITY REACTIONS TO CEFTIN PRODUCTS, OTHER CEPHALOSPORINS, PENICILLINS, OR OTHER DRUGS. IF THIS PRODUCT IS TO BE GIVEN TO PENICILLIN-SENSITIVE PATIENTS, CAUTION SHOULD BE EXERCISED BECAUSE CROSS-HYPERSENSITIVITY AMONG BETA-LACTAM ANTIBIOTICS HAS BEEN CLEARLY DOCUMENTED AND MAY OCCUR IN UP TO 10% OF PATIENTS WITH A HISTORY OF PENICILLIN ALLERGY. IF A CLINICALLY SIGNIFICANT ALLERGIC REACTION TO CEFTIN PRODUCTS OCCURS, DISCONTINUE THE DRUG AND INSTITUTE APPROPRIATE THERAPY. SERIOUS ACUTE HYPERSENSITIVITY REACTIONS MAY REQUIRE TREATMENT WITH EPINEPHRINE AND OTHER EMERGENCY MEASURES, INCLUDING OXYGEN, INTRAVENOUS FLUIDS, INTRAVENOUS ANTIHISTAMINES, CORTICOSTEROIDS, PRESSOR AMINES, AND AIRWAY MANAGEMENT, AS CLINICALLY INDICATED. Pseudomembranous colitis has been reported with nearly all antibacterial agents, including cefuroxime, and may range from mild to life threatening. Therefore, it is important to consider this diagnosis in patients who present with diarrhea subsequent to the administration of antibacterial agents.

Treatment with antibacterial agents alters normal flora of the colon and may permit overgrowth of clostridia. Studies indicate that a toxin produced by *Clostridium difficile* is one primary cause of antibiotic-associated colitis.

After the diagnosis of pseudomembranous colitis has been established, appropriate therapeutic measures should be initiated. Mild cases of pseudomembranous colitis usually

Continued on next page

This product information is based on labeling in effect on June 1, 1998. For further information, contact via direct mail, phone, or web site Medical Information: Glaxo Wellcome Inc., PO Box 13398, Research Triangle Park, NC 27709. Healthcare Professionals (Medical Information): 800-334-0089 Patients (Customer Response Center): 888-TALK2GW (1-888-825-5249) Glaxo Wellcome Corporate Web Site: www.glaxowellcome.com

Ceftin Tablets/O.S.—Cont.

respond to drug discontinuation alone. In moderate to severe cases, consideration should be given to management with fluids and electrolytes, protein supplementation, and treatment with an antibacterial drug effective against *Clostridium difficile.*

PRECAUTIONS

General: As with other broad-spectrum antibiotics, prolonged administration of cefuroxime axetil may result in overgrowth of nonsusceptible microorganisms. If superinfection occurs during therapy, appropriate measures should be taken.

Cephalosporins, including cefuroxime axetil, should be given with caution to patients receiving concurrent treatment with potent diuretics because these diuretics are suspected of adversely affecting renal function. Cefuroxime axetil, as with other broad-spectrum antibiotics, should be prescribed with caution in individuals with a history of colitis. The safety and effectiveness of cefuroxime axetil have not been established in patients with gastrointestinal malabsorption. Patients with gastrointestinal malabsorption were excluded from participating in clinical trials of cefuroxime axetil.

Information for Patients/Caregivers (Pediatric): 1. During clinical trials, the tablet was tolerated by pediatric patients old enough to swallow the cefuroxime axetil tablet whole. The crushed tablet has a strong, persistent, bitter taste and should not be administered to pediatric patients in this manner. Pediatric patients who cannot swallow the tablet whole should receive the oral suspension.
2. Discontinuation of therapy due to taste and/or problems of administering this drug occurred in 1.4% of pediatric patients given the oral suspension. Complaints about taste (which may impair compliance) occurred in 5% of pediatric patients.

Drug/Laboratory Test Interactions: A false-positive reaction for glucose in the urine may occur with copper reduction tests (Benedict's or Fehling's solution or with CLINITEST® tablets), but not with enzyme-based tests for glycosuria (e.g., CLINISTIX®, TES-TAPE®). As a false-negative result may occur in the ferricyanide test, it is recommended that either the glucose oxidase or hexokinase method be used to determine blood/plasma glucose levels in patients receiving cefuroxime axetil. The presence of cefuroxime does not interfere with the assay of serum and urine creatinine by the alkaline picrate method.

Drug/Drug Interactions: Concomitant administration of probenecid with cefuroxime axetil tablets increases the area under the serum concentration versus time curve by 50%. The peak serum cefuroxime concentration after a 1.5-g single dose is greater when taken with 1 g of probenecid (mean = 14.8 mcg/mL) than without probenecid (mean = 12.2 mcg/mL).

Drugs that reduce gastric acidity may result in a lower bioavailability of CEFTIN compared with that of fasting state and tend to cancel the effect of postprandial absorption.

Carcinogenesis, Mutagenesis, Impairment of Fertility: Although lifetime studies in animals have not been performed to evaluate carcinogenic potential, no mutagenic potential was found for cefuroxime axetil in the micronucleus test and a battery of bacterial mutation tests. Reproduction studies in rats at doses up to 1,000 mg/kg per day (nine times the recommended maximum human dose based on mg/m^2) have revealed no evidence of impaired fertility.

Pregnancy: *Teratogenic Effects: Pregnancy Category B:* Reproduction studies have been performed in rats and mice at doses up to 3,200 mg/kg per day (23 times the recommended maximum human dose based on mg/m^2) and have revealed no evidence of harm to the fetus due to cefuroxime axetil. There are, however, no adequate and well-controlled studies in pregnant women. Because animal reproduction studies are not always predictive of human response, this drug should be used during pregnancy only if clearly needed.

Labor and Delivery: Cefuroxime axetil has not been studied for use during labor and delivery.

Nursing Mothers: Because cefuroxime is excreted in human milk, consideration should be given to discontinuing nursing temporarily during treatment with cefuroxime axetil.

Pediatric Use: In controlled clinical trials, cefuroxime axetil has been administered to pediatric patients ranging in age from 3 months to 12 years (see INDICATIONS AND USAGE and DOSAGE AND ADMINISTRATION sections).

Geriatric Use: In clinical trials when 12- to 64-year-old patients and geriatric patients (65 years of age or older) were treated with usual recommended dosages (i.e., 125 to 500 mg b.i.d., depending on type of infections), no overall differences in effectiveness were observed between the two age-groups. The geriatric patients reported somewhat fewer gastrointestinal events and less frequent vaginal candidiasis compared with patients aged 12 to 64 years old; however, no clinically significant differences were reported between the two age-groups. Therefore, no adjustment of the usual adult dose is necessary based on age alone.

Adverse Reactions
CEFTIN Tablets
Multiple-Dose Dosing Regimens—Clinical Trials

Incidence ≥1%	Diarrhea/loose stools	3.7%
	Nausea/vomiting	3.0%
	Transient elevation in AST	2.0%
	Transient elevation in ALT	1.6%
	Eosinophilia	1.1%
	Transient elevation in LDH	1.0%
Incidence <1% but >0.1%	Abdominal pain	
	Abdominal cramps	
	Flatulence	
	Indigestion	
	Headache	
	Vaginitis	
	Vulvar itch	
	Rash	
	Hives	
	Itch	
	Dysuria	
	Chills	
	Chest pain	
	Shortness of breath	
	Mouth ulcers	
	Swollen tongue	
	Sleepiness	
	Thirst	
	Anorexia	
	Positive Coombs' test	

Adverse Reactions
CEFTIN Tablets
1-g Single-Dose Regimen for Uncomplicated Gonorrhea—Clinical Trials

Incidence ≥1%	Nausea/vomiting	6.8%
	Diarrhea	4.2%
Incidence <1% but >0.1%	Abdominal pain	
	Dyspepsia	
	Erythema	
	Rash	
	Pruritus	
	Vaginal candidiasis	
	Vaginal itch	
	Vaginal discharge	
	Headache	
	Dizziness	
	Somnolence	
	Muscle cramps	
	Muscle stiffness	
	Muscle spasm of neck	
	Tightness/pain in chest	
	Bleeding/pain in urethra	
	Kidney pain	
	Tachycardia	
	Lockjaw-type reaction	

Adverse Reactions
CEFTIN for Oral Suspension
Multiple-Dose Dosing Regimens—Clinical Trials

Incidence ≥1%	Diarrhea/loose stools	8.6%
	Dislike of taste	5.0%
	Diaper rash	3.4%
	Nausea/vomiting	2.6%
Incidence <1% but >0.1%	Abdominal pain	
	Flatulence	
	Gastrointestinal infection	
	Candidiasis	
	Vaginal irritation	
	Rash	
	Hyperactivity	
	Irritable behavior	
	Eosinophilia	
	Positive direct Coombs' test	
	Elevated liver enzymes	
	Viral illness	
	Upper respiratory infection	
	Sinusitis	
	Cough	
	Urinary tract infection	
	Joint swelling	
	Arthralgia	
	Fever	
	Ptyalism	

ADVERSE REACTIONS

CEFTIN TABLETS IN CLINICAL TRIALS: Multiple-Dose Dosing Regimens: *7 to 10 Days Dosing:* Using multiple doses of cefuroxime axetil tablets, 912 patients were treated with the recommended dosages of cefuroxime axetil (125 to 500 mg twice a day). There were no deaths or permanent dis-

CEFTIN Tablets
(May be administered without regard to meals.)

Population/Infection	Dosage	Duration (days)
Adolescents and Adults (13 years and older)		
Pharyngitis/tonsillitis	250 mg b.i.d.	10
Acute bacterial maxillary sinusitis	250 mg b.i.d.	10
Acute bacterial exacerbations of chronic bronchitis	250 or 500 mg b.i.d.	10*
Secondary bacterial infections of acute bronchitis	250 or 500 mg b.i.d.	5–10
Uncomplicated skin and skin-structure infections	250 or 500 mg b.i.d.	10
Uncomplicated urinary tract infections	125 or 250 mg b.i.d.	7–10
Uncomplicated gonorrhea	1,000 mg once	single dose
Early Lyme disease	500 mg b.i.d.	20
Children (who can swallow tablets whole)		
Pharyngitis/tonsillitis	125 mg b.i.d.	10
Acute otitis media	250 mg b.i.d.	10

*The safety and effectiveness of CEFTIN administered for less than 10 days in patients with acute exacerbations of chronic bronchitis have not been established.

CEFTIN for Oral Suspension
(Must be administered with food. Shake well each time before using.)

Population/Infection	Dosage	Daily Maximum Dose	Duration (days)
Infants and children (3 months to 12 years)			
Pharyngitis/tonsillitis	20 mg/kg/day divided b.i.d.	500 mg	10
Acute otitis media	30 mg/kg/day divided b.i.d.	1,000 mg	10
Impetigo	30 mg/kg/day divided b.i.d.	1,000 mg	10

CEFTIN for Oral Suspension	Labeled Volume After Reconstitution	Amount of Water Required for Reconstitution
125 mg/5 mL	50 mL	20 mL
	100 mL	37 mL
	200 mL	74 mL
250 mg/5 mL	50 mL	19 mL
	100 mL	35 mL

abilities thought related to drug toxicity. Twenty (2.2%) patients discontinued medication due to adverse events thought by the investigators to be possibly, probably, or almost certainly related to drug toxicity. Seventeen (85%) of the 20 patients who discontinued therapy did so because of gastrointestinal disturbances, including diarrhea, nausea, vomiting, and abdominal pain. The percentage of cefuroxime axetil tablet-treated patients who discontinued study drug because of adverse events was very similar at daily doses of 1,000, 500, and 250 mg (2.3%, 2.1%, and 2.2%, respectively). However, the incidence of gastrointestinal adverse events increased with the higher recommended doses. The following adverse events were thought by the investigators to be possibly, probably, or almost certainly related to cefuroxime axetil tablets in multiple-dose clinical trials (n = 912 cefuroxime axetil-treated patients).
[See first table at top of previous page]

5-Day Experience (see CLINICAL STUDIES section): In clinical trials using CEFTIN in a dose of 250 mg b.i.d. in the treatment of secondary bacterial infections of acute bronchitis, 399 patients were treated for 5 days and 402 patients were treated for 10 days. No difference in the occurrence of adverse events was found between the two regimens.

In Clinical Trials for Early Lyme Disease With 20 Days Dosing: Two multicenter trials assessed cefuroxime axetil tablets 500 mg twice a day for 20 days. The most common drug-related adverse experiences were diarrhea (10.6% of patients), Jarisch-Herxheimer's reaction (5.6%), and vaginitis (5.4%). Other adverse experiences occurred with frequencies comparable to those reported with 7 to 10 days dosing.

Single-Dose Regimen for Uncomplicated Gonorrhea: In clinical trials using a single dose of cefuroxime axetil tablets, 1,061 patients were treated with the recommended dosage of cefuroxime axetil (1,000 mg) for the treatment of uncomplicated gonorrhea. There were no deaths or permanent disabilities thought related to drug toxicity in these studies.
The following adverse events were thought by the investigators to be possibly, probably, or almost certainly related to cefuroxime axetil in 1,000-mg single-dose clinical trials of cefuroxime axetil tablets in the treatment of uncomplicated gonorrhea conducted in the US.
[See second table at top of previous page]

CEFTIN FOR ORAL SUSPENSION IN CLINICAL TRIALS: In clinical trials using multiple doses of cefuroxime axetil powder for oral suspension, pediatric patients (96.7% of whom were younger than 12 years of age) were treated with the recommended dosages of cefuroxime axetil (20 to 30 mg/kg per day divided twice a day up to a maximum dose of 500 or 1,000 mg/day, respectively). There were no deaths or permanent disabilities in any of the patients in these studies. Eleven US patients (1.2%) discontinued medication due to adverse events thought by the investigators to be possibly, probably, or almost certainly related to drug toxicity. The discontinuations were primarily for gastrointestinal disturbances, usually diarrhea or vomiting. During clinical trials, discontinuation of therapy due to the taste and/or problems with administering this drug occurred in 13 (1.4%) pediatric patients enrolled at centers in the US.
The following adverse events were thought by the investigators to be possibly, probably, or almost certainly related to cefuroxime axetil for oral suspension in multiple-dose clinical trials (n = 931 cefuroxime axetil-treated US patients).
[See third table at top of previous page]

POSTMARKETING EXPERIENCE WITH CEFTIN PRODUCTS
In addition to the adverse events reported during clinical trials, the following adverse events have been observed during clinical practice in patients treated with CEFTIN Tablets or with CEFTIN for Oral Suspension and were reported spontaneously. For some of these events, data are insufficient to allow an estimate of incidence or to establish causation.

General: The following hypersensitivity reactions have been reported: anaphylaxis, angioedema, pruritus, rash, serum sickness-like reaction, and urticaria.
Gastrointestinal: Pseudomembranous colitis (see WARNINGS).
Hematologic: Hemolytic anemia, leukopenia, pancytopenia, and thrombocytopenia.
Hepatic: Jaundice.
Skin: Erythema multiforme, Stevens-Johnson syndrome, and toxic epidermal necrolysis.

CEPHALOSPORIN-CLASS ADVERSE REACTIONS
In addition to the adverse reactions listed above that have been observed in patients treated with cefuroxime axetil, the following adverse reactions and altered laboratory tests have been reported for cephalosporin-class antibiotics: renal dysfunction, toxic nephropathy, hepatic cholestasis, aplastic anemia, hemolytic anemia, hemorrhage, increased prothrombin time, increased BUN, increased creatinine, false-positive test for urinary glucose, increased alkaline phosphatase, neutropenia, thrombocytopenia, leukopenia, elevated bilirubin, pancytopenia, and agranulocytosis.

Several cephalosporins have been implicated in triggering seizures, particularly in patients with renal impairment when the dosage was not reduced (see DOSAGE AND ADMINISTRATION and OVERDOSAGE). If seizures associated with drug therapy occur, the drug should be discontinued. Anticonvulsant therapy can be given if clinically indicated.

OVERDOSAGE
Overdosage of cephalosporins can cause cerebral irritation leading to convulsions. Serum levels of cefuroxime can be reduced by hemodialysis and peritoneal dialysis.

DOSAGE AND ADMINISTRATION
NOTE: CEFTIN TABLETS AND CEFTIN FOR ORAL SUSPENSION ARE NOT BIOEQUIVALENT AND ARE NOT SUBSTITUTABLE ON A MG/MG BASIS (SEE CLINICAL PHARMACOLOGY).
[See first table above]

CEFTIN for Oral Suspension: CEFTIN for Oral Suspension may be administered to infants and children ranging in age from 3 months to 12 years, according to dosages in the following table:
[See second table above]

Patients With Renal Failure: The safety and efficacy of cefuroxime axetil in patients with renal failure have not been established. Since cefuroxime is renally eliminated, its half-life will be prolonged in patients with renal failure.

Directions for Mixing CEFTIN for Oral Suspension: Prepare a suspension at the time of dispensing as follows:
1. Shake the bottle to loosen the powder.
2. Remove the cap.
3. Add the total amount of water for reconstitution (see table below) and replace the cap.
4. Invert the bottle and vigorously rock the bottle from side to side so that water rises through the powder.
5. Once the sound of the powder against the bottle disappears, turn the bottle upright and vigorously shake it in a diagonal direction.
[See third table above]
NOTE: SHAKE THE ORAL SUSPENSION WELL BEFORE EACH USE. Replace cap securely after each opening. The reconstituted suspension should be stored between 2° and 25°C (36° and 77°F) (either in the refrigerator or at room temperature). DISCARD AFTER 10 DAYS.

HOW SUPPLIED
CEFTIN Tablets: CEFTIN Tablets, 125 mg of cefuroxime (as cefuroxime axetil), are white, capsule-shaped, film-coated tablets engraved with "395" on one side and "Glaxo" on the other side as follows:

20 Tablets/Bottle	NDC 0173-0395-00
60 Tablets/Bottle	NDC 0173-0395-01
Unit Dose Packs of 100	NDC 0173-0395-02

CEFTIN Tablets, 250 mg of cefuroxime (as cefuroxime axetil), are light blue, capsule-shaped, film-coated tablets engraved with "387" on one side and "Glaxo" on the other side as follows:

10 Tablets/Bottle	NDC 0173-0387-06
20 Tablets/Bottle	NDC 0173-0387-00
60 Tablets/Bottle	NDC 0173-0387-42
Unit Dose Packs of 100	NDC 0173-0387-01

CEFTIN Tablets, 500 mg of cefuroxime (as cefuroxime axetil), are dark blue, capsule-shaped, film-coated tablets engraved with "394" on one side and "Glaxo" on the other side as follows:

20 Tablets/Bottle	NDC 0173-0394-00
60 Tablets/Bottle	NDC 0173-0394-42
Unit Dose Packs of 50	NDC 0173-0394-01

Store the tablets between 15° and 30°C (59° and 86°F). Replace cap securely after each opening. Protect unit dose packs from excessive moisture.

CEFTIN for Oral Suspension: CEFTIN for Oral Suspension is provided as dry, white to pale yellow, tutti-frutti–flavored powder. When reconstituted as directed, CEFTIN for Oral Suspension provides the equivalent of 125 mg or 250 mg of cefuroxime (as cefuroxime axetil) per 5 mL of suspension. It is supplied in amber glass bottles as follows:

125 mg/5 mL:

50-mL Suspension	NDC 0173-0406-01
100-mL Suspension	NDC 0173-0406-00

250 mg/5 mL:

50-mL Suspension	NDC 0173-0554-00
100-mL Suspension	NDC 0173-0555-00

Before reconstitution, store dry powder between 2° and 30°C (36° and 86°F).

Continued on next page

This product information is based on labeling in effect on June 1, 1998. For further information, contact via direct mail, phone, or web site Medical Information: Glaxo Wellcome Inc., PO Box 13398, Research Triangle Park, NC 27709. Healthcare Professionals (Medical Information): 800-334-0089 Patients (Customer Response Center): 888-TALK2GW (1-888-825-5249) Glaxo Wellcome Corporate Web Site: www.glaxowellcome.com

Ceftin Tablets/O.S.—Cont.

After reconstitution, store suspension between 2° and 25°C (36° and 77°F), in a refrigerator or at room temperature. DISCARD AFTER 10 DAYS.

CLINICAL STUDIES

CEFTIN Tablets: *Acute Bacterial Maxillary Sinusitis:* One adequate and well-controlled study was performed in patients with acute bacterial maxillary sinusitis. In this study each patient had a maxillary sinus aspirate collected by sinus puncture before treatment was initiated for presumptive acute bacterial sinusitis. All patients had to have radiographic and clinical evidence of acute maxillary sinusitis. As shown in the following summary of the study, the general clinical effectiveness of CEFTIN Tablets was comparable to an oral antimicrobial agent that contained a specific beta-lactamase inhibitor in treating acute maxillary sinusitis. However, sufficient microbiology data were obtained to demonstrate the effectiveness of CEFTIN Tablets in treating acute bacterial maxillary sinusitis due only to *Streptococcus pneumoniae* or non-beta-lactamase–producing *Haemophilus influenzae.* An insufficient number of beta-lactamase–producing *Haemophilus influenzae* and *Moraxella catarrhalis* isolates were obtained in this trial to adequately evaluate the effectiveness of CEFTIN Tablets in the treatment of acute bacterial maxillary sinusitis due to these two organisms.

This study enrolled 317 adult patients, 132 patients in the United States and 185 patients in South America. Patients were randomized in a 1:1 ratio to cefuroxime axetil 250 mg b.i.d. or an oral antimicrobial agent that contained a specific beta-lactamase inhibitor. An intent-to-treat analysis of the submitted clinical data yielded the following results:

[See first table below]

In this trial and in a supporting maxillary puncture trial, 15 evaluable patients had non-beta-lactamase–producing *Haemophilus influenzae* as the identified pathogen. Ten (10) of these 15 patients (67%) had their pathogen (non-beta-lactamase–producing *Haemophilus influenzae*) eradicated. Eighteen (18) evaluable patients had *Streptococcus pneumoniae* as the identified pathogen. Fifteen (15) of these 18 patients (83%) had their pathogen (*Streptococcus pneumoniae*) eradicated.

Safety: The incidence of drug-related gastrointestinal adverse events was statistically significantly higher in the control arm (an oral antimicrobial agent that contained a specific beta-lactamase inhibitor) versus the cefuroxime axetil arm (12% versus 1%, respectively; $P<0.001$), particularly drug-related diarrhea (8% versus 1%, respectively; $P=0.001$).

Early Lyme Disease: Two adequate and well-controlled studies were performed in patients with early Lyme disease. In these studies all patients had to present with physician-documented erythema migrans, with or without systemic manifestations of infection. Patients were randomized in a 1:1 ratio to a 20-day course of treatment with cefuroxime axetil 500 mg b.i.d. or doxycycline 100 mg t.i.d. Patients were assessed at 1 month posttreatment for success in treating early Lyme disease (Part I) and at 1 year posttreatment for success in preventing the progression to the sequelae of late Lyme disease (Part II).

A total of 355 adult patients (181 treated with cefuroxime axetil and 174 treated with doxycycline) were enrolled in the two studies. In order to objectively validate the clinical diagnosis of early Lyme disease in these patients, two approaches were used: 1) blinded expert reading of photographs, when available, of the pretreatment erythema migrans skin lesion; and 2) serologic confirmation (using enzyme-linked immunosorbent assay [ELISA] and immunoblot assay ["Western" blot]) of the presence of antibodies specific to *Borrelia burgdorferi,* the etiologic agent of Lyme disease. By these procedures, it was possible to confirm the physician diagnosis of early Lyme disease in 281 (79%) of the 355 study patients. The efficacy data summarized below are specific to this "validated" patient subset, while the safety data summarized below reflect the entire patient population for the two studies.

Analysis of the submitted clinical data for evaluable patients in the "validated" patient subset yielded the following results:

[See second table below]

CEFTIN and doxycycline were effective in prevention of the development of sequelae of late Lyme disease.

Safety: Drug-related adverse events affecting the skin were reported significantly more frequently by patients treated with doxycycline than by patients treated with cefuroxime axetil (12% versus 3%, respectively; $P=0.002$), pri-

marily reflecting the statistically significantly higher incidence of drug-related photosensitivity reactions in the doxycycline arm versus the cefuroxime axetil arm (9% versus 0%, respectively; $P<0.001$). While the incidence of drug-related gastrointestinal adverse events was similar in the two treatment groups (cefuroxime axetil - 13%; doxycycline - 11%), the incidence of drug-related diarrhea in the cefuroxime axetil arm was statistically significantly higher in the cefuroxime axetil arm versus the doxycycline arm (11% versus 3%, respectively; $P=0.005$).

Secondary Bacterial Infections of Acute Bronchitis: Four randomized, controlled clinical studies were performed comparing 5 days versus 10 days of CEFTIN for the treatment of patients with secondary bacterial infections of acute bronchitis. These studies enrolled a total of 1,253 patients (CAE-516 n = 360; CAE-517 n = 177; CAEA4001 n = 362; CAEA4002 n = 354). The protocols for CAE-516 and CAE-517 were identical and compared CEFTIN 250 mg b.i.d. for 5 days, CEFTIN 250 mg b.i.d. for 10 days, and AUGMENTIN® 500 mg t.i.d. for 10 days. These two studies were conducted simultaneously. CAEA4001 and CAEA4002 compared CEFTIN 250 mg b.i.d. for 5 days, CEFTIN 250 mg b.i.d. for 10 days, and CECLOR® 250 mg t.i.d. for 10 days. They were otherwise identical to CAE-516 and CAE-517 and were conducted over the following two years. Patients were required to have polymorphonuclear cells present on the Gram stain of their screening sputum specimen, but isolation of a bacterial pathogen from the sputum culture was not required for inclusion. The following table demonstrates the results of the clinical outcome analysis of the pooled studies CAE-516/CAE-517 and CAEA4001/CAEA4002, respectively:

[See third table below]

The response rates for patients who were both clinically and bacteriologically evaluable were consistent with those reported for the clinically evaluable patients.

Safety: In these clinical trials, 399 patients were treated with CEFTIN for 5 days and 402 patients with CEFTIN for 10 days. No difference in the occurrence of adverse events was observed between the two regimens.

REFERENCES:

1. National Committee for Clinical Laboratory Standards. *Methods for Dilution Antimicrobial Susceptibility Tests for Bacteria that Grow Aerobically.* 3rd ed. Approved Standard NCCLS Document M7-A3, Vol. 13, No. 25. Villanova, Pa: NCCLS; 1993.
2. National Committee for Clinical Laboratory Standards. *Performance Standards for Antimicrobial Disk Susceptibility Tests.* 4th ed. Approved Standard NCCLS Document M2-A4, Vol. 10, No. 7. Villanova, Pa: NCCLS; 1990.

CEFTIN is a registered trademark of Glaxo Wellcome.
CLINITEST and CLINISTIX are registered trademarks of Ames Division, Miles Laboratories, Inc.
TES-TAPE is a registered trademark of Eli Lilly and Company.
U.S. Patents 4,267,320; 4,562,181; 4,865,851; and 4,897,270
©Copyright 1996 Glaxo Wellcome Inc. All rights reserved.
November 1997/RL-511
Shown in Product Identification Guide, pages 311 and 312

Clinical Effectiveness of CEFTIN Tablets Compared to Beta-Lactamase Inhibitor-Containing Control Drug in the Treatment of Acute Bacterial Maxillary Sinusitis

	U.S. Patients*		South American Patients†	
	CEFTIN n = 49	Control n = 43	CEFTIN n = 87	Control n = 89
Clinical success (cure + improvement)	65%	53%	77%	74%
Clinical cure	53%	44%	72%	64%
Clinical improvement	12%	9%	5%	10%

*95% Confidence interval around the success difference [−0.08, +0.32].
†95% Confidence interval around the success difference [−0.10, +0.16].

Clinical Effectiveness of CEFTIN Tablets Compared to Doxycycline in the Treatment of Early Lyme Disease

	Part I (1 Month Posttreatment)*		Part II (1 Year Posttreatment)†	
	CEFTIN n = 125	Doxycycline n = 108	CEFTIN n = 105‡	Doxycycline n = 83‡
Satisfactory clinical outcome§	91%	93%	84%	87%
Clinical cure/success	72%	73%	73%	73%
Clinical improvement	19%	19%	10%	13%

*95% confidence interval around the satisfactory difference for Part I (−0.08, +0.05).
†95% confidence interval around the satisfactory difference for Part II (−0.13, +0.07).
‡n's include patients assessed as unsatisfactory clinical outcomes (failure + recurrence) in Part I (CEFTIN - 11 [5 failure, 6 recurrence]; doxycycline - 8 [6 failure, 2 recurrence]).
§Satisfactory clinical outcome includes cure + improvement (Part I) and success + improvement (Part II).

Clinical Effectiveness of CEFTIN Tablets 250 mg b.i.d. in Secondary Bacterial Infections of Acute Bronchitis: Comparison of 5 Versus 10 Days' Treatment Duration

	CAE-516 and CAE-517*		CAEA4001 and CAEA4002†	
	5 Day (n = 127)	10 Day (n = 139)	5 Day (n = 173)	10 Day (n = 192)
Clinical success (cure + improvement)	80%	87%	84%	82%
Clinical cure	61%	70%	73%	72%
Clinical improvement	19%	17%	11%	10%

*95% Confidence interval around the success difference [−0.164, +0.029].
†95% Confidence interval around the success difference [−0.061, +0.103].

CEPTAZ® ℞

[sĕp ′ tăz]
(ceftazidime for injection)
L-arginine formulation

For Intravenous or Intramuscular Use

DESCRIPTION

Ceftazidime is a semisynthetic, broad-spectrum, beta-lactam antibiotic for parenteral administration. It is the pentahydrate of pyridinium, 1-[[7-[[(2-amino-4-thiazolyl)](1-carboxy-1-methylethoxy) imino]acetyl] amino]-2-carboxy-8-oxo-5-thia-1-azabicyclo[4.2.0]oct-2-en-3-yl]methyl]-, hydroxide, inner salt, [6R-[6α,7β(Z)]].
The empirical formula is $C_{22}H_{32}N_6O_{12}S_2$, representing a molecular weight of 636.6.
CEPTAZ is a sterile, dry mixture of ceftazidime pentahydrate and L-arginine. The L-arginine is at a concentration of 349 mg/g of ceftazidime activity. CEPTAZ dissolves without the evolution of gas. The product contains no sodium ion. Solutions of CEPTAZ range in color from light yellow to amber, depending on the diluent and volume used. The pH of freshly constituted solutions usually ranges from 5 to 7.5.

CLINICAL PHARMACOLOGY

After intravenous (IV) administration of 500-mg and 1-g doses of ceftazidime over 5 minutes to normal adult volunteers, mean peak serum concentrations of 45 and 90 mcg/mL, respectively, were achieved. After IV infusion of 500-mg, 1-g, and 2-g doses of ceftazidime over 20 to 30 minutes to normal adult male volunteers, mean peak serum concentrations of 42, 69, and 170 mcg/mL, respectively,

were achieved. The average serum concentrations following IV infusion of 500-mg, 1-g, and 2-g doses to these volunteers over an 8-hour interval are given in Table 1.

Table 1

Ceftazidime IV Dose	Serum Concentrations (mcg/mL) 0.5 h	1 h	2 h	4 h	8 h
500 mg	42	25	12	6	2
1 g	60	39	23	11	3
2 g	129	75	42	13	5

The absorption and elimination of ceftazidime were directly proportional to the size of the dose. The half-life following IV administration was approximately 1.9 hours. Less than 10% of ceftazidime was protein bound. The degree of protein binding was independent of concentration. There was no evidence of accumulation of ceftazidime in the serum in individuals with normal renal function following multiple IV doses of 1 and 2 g every 8 hours for 10 days.

Following intramuscular (IM) administration of 500-mg and 1-g doses of ceftazidime to normal adult volunteers, the mean peak serum concentrations were 17 and 39 mcg/mL, respectively, at approximately 1 hour. Serum concentrations remained above 4 mcg/mL for 6 and 8 hours after the IM administration of 500-mg and 1-g doses, respectively. The half-life of ceftazidime in these volunteers was approximately 2 hours.

The presence of hepatic dysfunction had no effect on the pharmacokinetics of ceftazidime in individuals administered 2 g intravenously every 8 hours for 5 days. Therefore, a dosage adjustment from the normal recommended dosage is not required for patients with hepatic dysfunction, provided renal function is not impaired.

Approximately 80% to 90% of an IM or IV dose of ceftazidime is excreted unchanged by the kidneys over a 24-hour period. After the IV administration of single 500-mg or 1-g doses, approximately 50% of the dose appeared in the urine in the first 2 hours. An additional 20% was excreted between 2 and 4 hours after dosing, and approximately another 12% of the dose appeared in the urine between 4 and 8 hours later. The elimination of ceftazidime by the kidneys resulted in high therapeutic concentrations in the urine.

The mean renal clearance of ceftazidime was approximately 100 mL/min. The calculated plasma clearance of approximately 115 mL/min indicated nearly complete elimination of ceftazidime by the renal route. Administration of probenecid before dosing had no effect on the elimination kinetics of ceftazidime. This suggested that ceftazidime is eliminated by glomerular filtration and is not actively secreted by renal tubular mechanisms.

Since ceftazidime is eliminated almost solely by the kidneys, its serum half-life is significantly prolonged in patients with impaired renal function. Consequently, dosage adjustments in such patients as described in the DOSAGE AND ADMINISTRATION section are suggested.

Ceftazidime concentrations achieved in specific body tissues and fluids are depicted in Table 2.

[See table 2 above]

Table 2: Ceftazidime Concentrations in Body Tissues and Fluids

Tissue or Fluid	Dose/Route	No. of Patients	Time of Sample Postdose	Average Tissue or Fluid Level (mcg/mL or mcg/g)
Urine	500 mg IM	6	0–2 h	2,100.0
	2 g IV	6	0–2 h	12,000.0
Bile	2 g IV	3	90 min	36.4
Synovial fluid	2 g IV	13	2 h	25.6
Peritoneal fluid	2 g IV	8	2 h	48.6
Sputum	1 g IV	8	1 h	9.0
Cerebrospinal fluid	2 g q8h IV	5	120 min	9.8
(inflamed meninges)	2 g q8h IV	6	180 min	9.4
Aqueous humor	2 g IV	13	1–3 h	11.0
Blister fluid	1 g IV	7	2–3 h	19.7
Lymphatic fluid	1 g IV	7	2–3 h	23.4
Bone	2 g IV	8	0.67 h	31.1
Heart muscle	2 g IV	35	30–280 min	12.7
Skin	2 g IV	22	30–180 min	6.6
Skeletal muscle	2 g IV	35	30–280 min	9.4
Myometrium	2 g IV	31	1–2 h	18.7

Microbiology: Ceftazidime is bactericidal in action, exerting its effect by inhibition of enzymes responsible for cell-wall synthesis. A wide range of gram-negative organisms is susceptible to ceftazidime *in vitro*, including strains resistant to gentamicin and other aminoglycosides. In addition, ceftazidime has been shown to be active against gram-positive organisms. It is highly stable to most clinically important beta-lactamases, plasmid or chromosomal, which are produced by both gram-negative and gram-positive organisms and, consequently, is active against many strains resistant to ampicillin and other cephalosporins.

Ceftazidime has been shown to be active against the following organisms both *in vitro* and in clinical infections (see INDICATIONS AND USAGE).

Aerobes, Gram-negative: *Citrobacter* spp., including *Citrobacter freundii* and *Citrobacter diversus; Enterobacter* spp., including *Enterobacter cloacae* and *Enterobacter aerogenes; Escherichia coli; Haemophilus influenzae,* including ampicillin-resistant strains; *Klebsiella* spp. (including *Klebsiella pneumoniae); Neisseria meningitidis; Proteus mirabilis; Proteus vulgaris; Pseudomonas* spp. (including *Pseudomonas aeruginosa*); and *Serratia* spp.

Aerobes, Gram-positive: *Staphylococcus aureus,* including penicillinase- and non–penicillinase-producing strains; *Streptococcus agalactiae* (group B streptococci); *Streptococcus pneumoniae;* and *Streptococcus pyogenes* (group A beta-hemolytic streptococci).

Anaerobes: *Bacteroides* spp. (NOTE: many strains of *Bacteroides fragilis* are resistant).

Ceftazidime has been shown to be active *in vitro* against most strains of the following organisms; however, the clinical significance of this activity is unknown: *Acinetobacter* spp., *Clostridium* spp. (not including *Clostridium difficile), Haemophilus parainfluenzae, Morganella morganii* (formerly *Proteus morganii), Neisseria gonorrhoeae, Peptococcus* spp., *Peptostreptococcus* spp., *Providencia* spp. (including *Providencia rettgeri,* formerly *Proteus rettgeri*), *Salmonella* spp., *Shigella* spp., *Staphylococcus epidermidis,* and *Yersinia enterocolitica.*

Ceftazidime and the aminoglycosides have been shown to be synergistic *in vitro* against *Pseudomonas aeruginosa* and the enterobacteriaceae. Ceftazidime and carbenicillin have also been shown to be synergistic *in vitro* against *Pseudomonas aeruginosa.*

Ceftazidime is not active *in vitro* against methicillin-resistant staphylococci, *Streptococcus faecalis* and many other enterococci, *Listeria monocytogenes, Campylobacter* spp., or *Clostridium difficile.*

Susceptibility Tests: *Diffusion Techniques:* Quantitative methods that require measurement of zone diameters give an estimate of antibiotic susceptibility. One such procedure[1–3] has been recommended for use with disks to test susceptibility to ceftazidime.

Reports from the laboratory giving results of the standard single-disk susceptibility test with a 30-mcg ceftazidime disk should be interpreted according to the following criteria:

Susceptible organisms produce zones of 18 mm or greater, indicating that the test organism is likely to respond to therapy.

Organisms that produce zones of 15 to 17 mm are expected to be susceptible if high dosage is used or if the infection is confined to tissues and fluids (e.g., urine) in which high antibiotic levels are attained.

Resistant organisms produce zones of 14 mm or less, indicating that other therapy should be selected.

Organisms should be tested with the ceftazidime disk since ceftazidime has been shown by *in vitro* tests to be active against certain strains found resistant when other beta-lactam disks are used.

Standardized procedures require the use of laboratory control organisms. The 30-mcg ceftazidime disk should give zone diameters between 25 and 32 mm for *Escherichia coli* ATCC 25922. For *Pseudomonas aeruginosa* ATCC 27853, the zone diameters should be between 22 and 29 mm. For *Staphylococcus aureus* ATCC 25923, the zone diameters should be between 16 and 20 mm.

Dilution Techniques: In other susceptibility testing procedures, e.g., ICS agar dilution or the equivalent, a bacterial isolate may be considered susceptible if the minimum inhibitory concentration (MIC) value for ceftazidime is not more than 16 mcg/mL. Organisms are considered resistant to ceftazidime if the MIC ≥64 mcg/mL. Organisms having an MIC value of <64 mcg/mL but >16 mcg/mL are expected to be susceptible if high dosage is used or if the infection is confined to tissues and fluids (e.g., urine) in which high antibiotic levels are attained.

As with standard diffusion methods, dilution procedures require the use of laboratory control organisms. Standard ceftazidime powder should give MIC values in the range of 4 to 16 mcg/mL for *Staphylococcus aureus* ATCC 25923. For *Escherichia coli* ATCC 25922, the MIC range should be between 0.125 and 0.5 mcg/mL. For *Pseudomonas aeruginosa* ATCC 27853, the MIC range should be between 0.5 and 2 mcg/mL.

INDICATIONS AND USAGE

CEPTAZ is indicated for the treatment of patients with infections caused by susceptible strains of the designated organisms in the following diseases:

1. **Lower Respiratory Tract Infections,** including pneumonia, caused by *Pseudomonas aeruginosa* and other *Pseudomonas* spp.; *Haemophilus influenzae,* including ampicillin-resistant strains; *Klebsiella* spp.; *Enterobacter* spp.; *Proteus mirabilis; Escherichia coli; Serratia* spp.; *Citrobacter* spp.; *Streptococcus pneumoniae;* and *Staphylococcus aureus* (methicillin-susceptible strains).
2. **Skin and Skin-Structure Infections** caused by *Pseudomonas aeruginosa; Klebsiella* spp.; *Escherichia coli; Proteus* spp., including *Proteus mirabilis* and indole-positive *Proteus; Enterobacter* spp.; *Serratia* spp.; *Staphylococcus aureus* (methicillin-susceptible strains); and *Streptococcus pyogenes* (group A beta-hemolytic streptococci).
3. **Urinary Tract Infections,** both complicated and uncomplicated, caused by *Pseudomonas aeruginosa; Enterobacter* spp.; *Proteus* spp., including *Proteus mirabilis* and indole-positive *Proteus; Klebsiella* spp.; and *Escherichia coli.*
4. **Bacterial Septicemia** caused by *Pseudomonas aeruginosa, Klebsiella* spp., *Haemophilus influenzae, Escherichia coli, Serratia* spp., *Streptococcus pneumoniae,* and *Staphylococcus aureus* (methicillin-susceptible strains).
5. **Bone and Joint Infections** caused by *Pseudomonas aeruginosa, Klebsiella* spp., *Enterobacter* spp., and *Staphylococcus aureus* (methicillin-susceptible strains).
6. **Gynecologic Infections,** including endometritis, pelvic cellulitis, and other infections of the female genital tract caused by *Escherichia coli.*
7. **Intra-abdominal Infections,** including peritonitis caused by *Escherichia coli, Klebsiella* spp., and *Staphylococcus aureus* (methicillin-susceptible strains) and polymicrobial infections caused by aerobic and anaerobic organisms and *Bacteroides* spp. (many strains of *Bacteroides fragilis* are resistant).
8. **Central Nervous System Infections,** including meningitis, caused by *Haemophilus influenzae* and *Neisseria meningitidis.* Ceftazidime has also been used successfully in a limited number of cases of meningitis due to *Pseudomonas aeruginosa* and *Streptococcus pneumoniae.*

Specimens for bacterial cultures should be obtained before therapy in order to isolate and identify causative organisms and to determine their susceptibility to ceftazidime. Therapy may be instituted before results of susceptibility studies are known; however, once these results become available, the antibiotic treatment should be adjusted accordingly.

CEPTAZ may be used alone in cases of confirmed or suspected sepsis. Ceftazidime has been used successfully in clinical trials as empiric therapy in cases where various concomitant therapies with other antibiotics have been used.

CEPTAZ may also be used concomitantly with other antibiotics, such as aminoglycosides, vancomycin, and clindamycin; in severe and life-threatening infections; and in the immunocompromised patient (see COMPATIBILITY AND STABILITY). When such concomitant treatment is appropriate, prescribing information in the labeling for the other antibiotics should be followed. The dosage depends on the severity of the infection and the patient's condition.

CONTRAINDICATIONS

CEPTAZ is contraindicated in patients who have shown hypersensitivity to ceftazidime or the cephalosporin group of antibiotics.

Continued on next page

This product information is based on labeling in effect on June 1, 1998. For further information, contact via direct mail, phone, or web site Medical Information: Glaxo Wellcome Inc., PO Box 13398, Research Triangle Park, NC 27709. Healthcare Professionals (Medical Information): 800-334-0089 Patients (Customer Response Center): 888-TALK2GW (1-888-825-5249) Glaxo Wellcome Corporate Web Site: www.glaxowellcome.com

Ceptaz—Cont.

WARNINGS

BEFORE THERAPY WITH CEPTAZ IS INSTITUTED, CAREFUL INQUIRY SHOULD BE MADE TO DETERMINE WHETHER THE PATIENT HAS HAD PREVIOUS HYPERSENSITIVITY REACTIONS TO CEFTAZIDIME, CEPHALOSPORINS, PENICILLINS, OR OTHER DRUGS. IF THIS PRODUCT IS GIVEN TO PENICILLIN-SENSITIVE PATIENTS, CAUTION SHOULD BE EXERCISED BECAUSE CROSS-HYPERSENSITIVITY AMONG BETA-LACTAM ANTIBIOTICS HAS BEEN CLEARLY DOCUMENTED AND MAY OCCUR IN UP TO 10% OF PATIENTS WITH A HISTORY OF PENICILLIN ALLERGY. IF AN ALLERGIC REACTION TO CEPTAZ OCCURS, DISCONTINUE THE DRUG. SERIOUS ACUTE HYPERSENSITIVITY REACTIONS MAY REQUIRE TREATMENT WITH EPINEPHRINE AND OTHER EMERGENCY MEASURES, INCLUDING OXYGEN, IV FLUIDS, IV ANTIHISTAMINES, CORTICOSTEROIDS, PRESSOR AMINES, AND AIRWAY MANAGEMENT, AS CLINICALLY INDICATED.

Pseudomembranous colitis has been reported with nearly all antibacterial agents, including ceftazidime, and may range from mild to life threatening. Therefore, it is important to consider this diagnosis in patients who present with diarrhea subsequent to the administration of antibacterial agents.

Treatment with antibacterial agents alters the normal flora of the colon and may permit overgrowth of clostridia. Studies indicate that a toxin produced by *Clostridium difficile* is one primary cause of "antibiotic-associated colitis."

After the diagnosis of pseudomembranous colitis has been established, appropriate therapeutic measures should be initiated. Mild cases of pseudomembranous colitis usually respond to drug discontinuation alone. In moderate to severe cases, consideration should be given to management with fluids and electrolytes, protein supplementation, and treatment with an antibacterial drug clinically effective against *Clostridium difficile* colitis.

Elevated levels of ceftazidime in patients with renal insufficiency can lead to seizures, encephalopathy, asterixis, and neuromuscular excitability (see PRECAUTIONS).

PRECAUTIONS

General: Ceftazidime has not been shown to be nephrotoxic; however, high and prolonged serum antibiotic concentrations can occur from usual dosages in patients with transient or persistent reduction of urinary output because of renal insufficiency. The total daily dosage should be reduced when ceftazidime is administered to patients with renal insufficiency (see DOSAGE AND ADMINISTRATION). Elevated levels of ceftazidime in these patients can lead to seizures, encephalopathy, asterixis, and neuromuscular excitability. Continued dosage should be determined by degree of renal impairment, severity of infection, and susceptibility of the causative organisms.

As with other antibiotics, prolonged use of CEPTAZ may result in overgrowth of nonsusceptible organisms. Repeated evaluation of the patient's condition is essential. If superinfection occurs during therapy, appropriate measures should be taken.

Inducible type I beta-lactamase resistance has been noted with some organisms (e.g., *Enterobacter* spp., *Pseudomonas* spp., and *Serratia* spp.). As with other extended-spectrum beta-lactam antibiotics, resistance can develop during therapy, leading to clinical failure in some cases. When treating infections caused by these organisms, periodic susceptibility testing should be performed when clinically appropriate. If patients fail to respond to monotherapy, an aminoglycoside or similar agent should be considered.

Cephalosporins may be associated with a fall in prothrombin activity. Those at risk include patients with renal or hepatic impairment, or poor nutritional state, as well as patients receiving a protracted course of antimicrobial therapy. Prothrombin time should be monitored in patients at risk and exogenous vitamin K administered as indicated. CEPTAZ should be prescribed with caution in individuals with a history of gastrointestinal disease, particularly colitis.

Arginine has been shown to alter glucose metabolism and elevate serum potassium transiently when administered at 50 times the recommended dose. The effect of lower dosing is not known.

Distal necrosis can occur after inadvertent intra-arterial administration of ceftazidime.

Drug Interactions: Nephrotoxicity has been reported following concomitant administration of cephalosporins with aminoglycoside antibiotics or potent diuretics such as furosemide. Renal function should be carefully monitored, especially if higher dosages of the aminoglycosides are to be administered or if therapy is prolonged, because of the potential nephrotoxicity and ototoxicity of aminoglycosidic antibiotics. Nephrotoxicity and ototoxicity were not noted when ceftazidime was given alone in clinical trials.

Chloramphenicol has been shown to be antagonistic to beta-lactam antibiotics, including ceftazidime, based on *in vitro* studies and time kill curves with enteric gram-negative bacilli. Due to the possibility of antagonism *in vivo*, particularly when bactericidal activity is desired, this drug combination should be avoided.

Drug/Laboratory Test Interactions: The administration of ceftazidime may result in a false-positive reaction for glucose in the urine when using CLINITEST® tablets. Benedict's solution, or Fehling's solution. It is recommended that glucose tests based on enzymatic glucose oxidase reactions (such as CLINISTIX® or TES-TAPE®) be used.

Carcinogenesis, Mutagenesis, Impairment of Fertility: Long-term studies in animals have not been performed to evaluate carcinogenic potential. However, a mouse Micronucleus test and an Ames test were both negative for mutagenic effects.

Pregnancy: *Teratogenic Effects: Pregnancy Category B:* Reproduction studies have been performed in mice and rats at doses up to 40 times the human dose and have revealed no evidence of impaired fertility or harm to the fetus due to ceftazidime. CEPTAZ at 23 times the human dose was not teratogenic or embryotoxic in a rat reproduction study. There are, however, no adequate and well-controlled studies in pregnant women. Because animal reproduction studies are not always predictive of human response, this drug should be used during pregnancy only if clearly needed.

Nursing Mothers: Ceftazidime is excreted in human milk in low concentrations. It is not known whether the arginine component of this product is excreted in human milk. Because many drugs are excreted in human milk and because safety of the arginine component of CEPTAZ in nursing infants has not been established, a decision should be made whether to discontinue nursing or to discontinue the drug, taking into account the importance of the drug to the mother.

Pediatric Use: Safety of the arginine component of CEPTAZ in neonates, infants, and children has not been established. This product is for use in patients 12 years and older. If treatment with ceftazidime is indicated for neonates, infants, or children, a sodium carbonate formulation should be used.

ADVERSE REACTIONS

The following adverse effects from clinical trials were considered to be either related to ceftazidime therapy or were of uncertain etiology. The most common were local reactions following IV injection and allergic and gastrointestinal reactions. No disulfiramlike reactions were reported.

Local Effects, reported in fewer than 2% of patients, were phlebitis and inflammation at the site of injection (1 in 69 patients).

Hypersensitivity Reactions, reported in 2% of patients, were pruritus, rash, and fever. Immediate reactions, generally manifested by rash and/or pruritus, occurred in 1 in 285 patients. Toxic epidermal necrolysis, Stevens-Johnson syndrome, and erythema multiforme have also been reported with cephalosporin antibiotics, including ceftazidime. Angioedema and anaphylaxis (bronchospasm and/or hypotension) have been reported very rarely.

Gastrointestinal Symptoms, reported in fewer than 2% of patients, were diarrhea (1 in 78), nausea (1 in 156), vomiting (1 in 500), and abdominal pain (1 in 416). The onset of pseudomembranous colitis symptoms may occur during or after treatment (see WARNINGS).

Central Nervous System Reactions (fewer than 1%) included headache, dizziness, and paresthesia. Seizures have been reported with several cephalosporins, including ceftazidime. In addition, encephalopathy, asterixis, and neuromuscular excitability have been reported in renally impaired patients treated with unadjusted dosing regimens of ceftazidime (see PRECAUTIONS: General).

Less Frequent Adverse Events (fewer than 1%) were candidiasis (including oral thrush) and vaginitis.

Hematologic: Rare cases of hemolytic anemia have been reported.

Laboratory Test Changes noted during ceftazidime clinical trials were transient and included: eosinophilia (1 in 13), positive Coombs' test without hemolysis (1 in 23), thrombocytosis (1 in 45), and slight elevations in one or more of the hepatic enzymes, aspartate aminotransferase (AST, SGOT) (1 in 16), alanine aminotransferase (ALT, SGPT) (1 in 15), LDH (1 in 18), GGT (1 in 19), and alkaline phosphatase (1 in 23). As with some other cephalosporins, transient elevations of blood urea, blood urea nitrogen, and/or serum creatinine were observed occasionally. Transient leukopenia, neutropenia, agranulocytosis, thrombocytopenia, and lymphocytosis were seen very rarely.

In addition to the adverse reactions listed above that have been observed in patients treated with ceftazidime, the following adverse reactions and altered laboratory tests have been reported for cephalosporin-class antibiotics:

Adverse Reactions: Urticaria, colitis, renal dysfunction, toxic nephropathy, hepatic dysfunction including cholestasis, aplastic anemia, hemorrhage.

Altered Laboratory Tests: Prolonged prothrombin time, false-positive test for urinary glucose, elevated bilirubin, pancytopenia.

OVERDOSAGE

Ceftazidime overdosage has occurred in patients with renal failure. Reactions have included seizure activity, encephalopathy, asterixis, and neuromuscular excitability. Patients who receive an acute overdosage should be carefully observed and given supportive treatment. In the presence of renal insufficiency, hemodialysis or peritoneal dialysis may aid in the removal of ceftazidime from the body.

DOSAGE AND ADMINISTRATION

Dosage: The usual adult dosage is 1 gram administered intravenously or intramuscularly every 8 to 12 hours. The dosage and route should be determined by the susceptibility of the causative organisms, the severity of infection, and the condition and renal function of the patient.

The guidelines for dosage of CEPTAZ are listed in Table 3. The following dosage schedule is recommended.
[See table 3 at left]

Impaired Hepatic Function: No adjustment in dosage is required for patients with hepatic dysfunction.

Impaired Renal Function: Ceftazidime is excreted by the kidneys, almost exclusively by glomerular filtration. Therefore, in patients with impaired renal function (glomerular filtration rate [GFR] <50 mL/min), it is recommended that the dosage of ceftazidime be reduced to compensate for its slower excretion. In patients with suspected renal insufficiency, an initial loading dose of 1 gram of CEPTAZ may be given. An estimate of GFR should be made to determine the appropriate maintenance dosage. The recommended dosage is presented in Table 4.

Table 3: Recommended Dosage Schedule

	Dose	Frequency
Patients 12 years and older*		
Usual recommended dosage	1 gram IV or IM	q8–12h
Uncomplicated urinary tract infections	250 mg IV or IM	q12h
Bone and joint infections	2 grams IV	q12h
Complicated urinary tract infections	500 mg IV or IM	q8–12h
Uncomplicated pneumonia; mild skin and skin-structure infections	500 mg–1 gram IV or IM	q8h
Serious gynecologic and intra-abdominal infections	2 grams IV	q8h
Meningitis	2 grams IV	q8h
Very severe life-threatening infections, especially in immunocompromised patients	2 grams IV	q8h
Lung infections caused by *Pseudomonas* spp. in patients with cystic fibrosis with normal renal function†	30–50 mg/kg IV to a maximum of 6 grams per day	q8h

* This product is for use in patients 12 years and older. If treatment with ceftazidime is indicated for patients less than 12 years old, a sodium carbonate formulation should be used.

† Although clinical improvement has been shown, bacteriologic cures cannot be expected in patients with chronic respiratory disease and cystic fibrosis.

Table 4: Recommended Maintenance Dosages of CEPTAZ in Renal Insufficiency
NOTE: IF THE DOSE RECOMMENDED IN TABLE 3 ABOVE IS LOWER THAN THAT RECOMMENDED FOR PATIENTS WITH RENAL INSUFFICIENCY AS OUTLINED IN TABLE 4, THE LOWER DOSE SHOULD BE USED.

Creatinine Clearance (mL/min)	Recommended Unit Dose of CEPTAZ	Frequency of Dosing
50–31	1 gram	q12h
30–16	1 gram	q24h
15–6	500 mg	q24h
<5	500 mg	q48h

When only serum creatinine is available, the following formula (Cockcroft's equation)[4] may be used to estimate creatinine clearance. The serum creatinine should represent a steady state of renal function:

Males:

$$\text{Creatinine clearance (mL/min)} = \frac{\text{Weight (kg)} \times (140-\text{age})}{72 \times \text{serum creatinine (mg/dL)}}$$

Females: 0.85 × male value

In patients with severe infections who would normally receive 6 grams of CEPTAZ daily were it not for renal insufficiency, the unit dose given in the table above may be increased by 50% or the dosing frequency may be increased appropriately. Further dosing should be determined by therapeutic monitoring, severity of the infection, and susceptibility of the causative organism.

In patients undergoing hemodialysis, a loading dose of 1 gram is recommended, followed by 1 gram after each hemodialysis period.

CEPTAZ can also be used in patients undergoing intraperitoneal dialysis and continuous ambulatory peritoneal dialysis. In such patients, a loading dose of 1 gram of CEPTAZ may be given, followed by 500 mg every 24 hours. It is not known whether or not CEPTAZ can be safely incorporated into dialysis fluid.

Note: Generally CEPTAZ should be continued for 2 days after the signs and symptoms of infection have disappeared, but in complicated infections longer therapy may be required.

Administration: CEPTAZ may be given intravenously or by deep IM injection into a large muscle mass such as the upper outer quadrant of the gluteus maximus or lateral part of the thigh. Intra-arterial administration should be avoided (see PRECAUTIONS).

Intramuscular Administration: For IM administration, CEPTAZ should be constituted with one of the following diluents: sterile water for injection, bacteriostatic water for injection, or 0.5% or 1% lidocaine hydrochloride injection. Refer to Table 5.

Intravenous Administration: The IV route is preferable for patients with bacterial septicemia, bacterial meningitis, peritonitis, or other severe or life-threatening infections, or for patients who may be poor risks because of lowered resistance resulting from such debilitating conditions as malnutrition, trauma, surgery, diabetes, heart failure, or malignancy, particularly if shock is present or pending.

For direct intermittent IV administration, constitute CEPTAZ as directed in Table 5 with sterile water for injection, 5% dextrose injection, or 0.9% sodium chloride injection. Slowly inject directly into the vein over a period of 3 to 5 minutes or give through the tubing of an administration set while the patient is also receiving one of the compatible IV fluids (see COMPATIBILITY AND STABILITY).

For IV infusion, constitute the 1- or 2-gram infusion pack with 100 mL of sterile water for injection or one of the compatible IV fluids listed under the COMPATIBILITY AND STABILITY section. Alternatively, constitute the 1- or 2-gram vial and add an appropriate quantity of the resulting solution to an IV container with one of the compatible IV fluids.

Intermittent IV infusion with a Y-type administration set can be accomplished with compatible solutions. However, during infusion of a solution containing ceftazidime, it is desirable to discontinue the other solution.

[See table 5 above]

Solutions of CEPTAZ, like those of most beta-lactam antibiotics, should not be added to solutions of aminoglycoside antibiotics because of potential interaction.

However, if concurrent therapy with CEPTAZ and an aminoglycoside is indicated, each of these antibiotics can be administered separately to the same patient.

Instructions for Constitution: Vials of CEPTAZ as supplied are under a slightly reduced pressure. This may assist entry of the diluent. No gas-relief needle is required when adding the diluent, except for the infusion pack where it is required during the latter stages of addition (in order to preserve product sterility, a gas-relief needle should not be inserted until an overpressure is produced in the vial). No evolution of gas occurs on constitution. When the vial contents are dissolved, vials other than infusion packs may still be under a reduced pressure. This reduced pressure is particularly noticeable for the 10-gram pharmacy bulk package.

Table 5: Preparation of CEPTAZ Solutions

Size	Amount of Diluent to Be Added (mL)	Volume to Be Withdrawn (mL)	Approximate Ceftazidime Concentration (mg/mL)
Intramuscular			
1-gram vial	3.0	Total	250
Intravenous			
1-gram vial	10.0	Total	90
2-gram vial	10.0	Total	170
Infusion pack			
1-gram vial	100	—	10
2-gram vial	100	—	20
Pharmacy bulk package			
10-gram vial	40	Amount needed	200

COMPATIBILITY AND STABILITY

Intramuscular: CEPTAZ , when constituted as directed with sterile water for injection, bacteriostatic water for injection, or 0.5% or 1% lidocaine hydrochloride injection, maintains satisfactory potency for 18 hours at room temperature or for 7 days under refrigeration. Solutions in sterile water for injection that are frozen immediately after constitution in the original container are stable for 6 months when stored at −20°C. Components of the solution may precipitate in the frozen state and will dissolve on reaching room temperature with little or no agitation. Potency is not affected. Frozen solutions should only be thawed at room temperature. Do not force thaw by immersion in water baths or by microwave irradiation. Once thawed, solutions should not be refrozen. Thawed solutions may be stored for up to 12 hours at room temperature or for 7 days in a refrigerator.

Intravenous: ***Ceftazidime concentration greater than 100 mg/mL (2-g vial or 10-g pharmacy bulk package):*** CEPTAZ, when constituted as directed with sterile water for injection. 0.9% sodium chloride injection, or 5% dextrose injection, maintains satisfactory potency for 18 hours at room temperature or for 7 days under refrigeration. Solutions of a similar concentration in sterile water for injection that are frozen immediately after constitution in the original container are stable for 6 months when stored at −20°C. Components of the solution may precipitate in the frozen state and will dissolve on reaching room temperature with little or no agitation. Potency is not affected. Frozen solutions should only be thawed at room temperature. Do not force thaw by immersion in water baths or by microwave irradiation. Once thawed, solutions should not be refrozen. Thawed solutions may be stored for up to 12 hours at room temperature or for 7 days in a refrigerator.

Ceftazidime concentration of 100 mg/mL or less (1-g vial or infusion packs): CEPTAZ, when constituted as directed with sterile water for injection, 0.9% sodium chloride injection, or 5% dextrose injection, maintains satisfactory potency for 24 hours at room temperature or for 7 days under refrigeration. Solutions, prepared by a pharmacist, of the approved arginine formulation of ceftazidime of a similar concentration in sterile water for injection, 0.9% sodium chloride injection, or 5% dextrose injection in the original container or in 0.9% sodium chloride injection in VIAFLEX® (PL 146® Plastic) small-volume containers that are frozen immediately after constitution by the pharmacist are stable for 6 months when stored at −20°C. Solutions in the PL 146 Plastic small-volume containers are in contact with the polyvinyl chloride layer of this container and can leach out certain chemical components of the plastic in very small amounts within the expiration period. The suitability of the plastic has been confirmed in tests in animals according to USP biological tests for plastic containers as well as by tissue culture toxicity studies. Stability of the frozen solution in other containers has not been confirmed. Frozen solutions should only be thawed at room temperature. Do not force thaw by immersion in water baths or by microwave irradiation. For the larger volumes of IV infusion solutions where it may be necessary to warm the frozen product, care should be taken to avoid heating after thawing is complete. Once thawed, solutions should not be refrozen. Thawed solutions may be stored for up to 18 hours at room temperature or for 7 days in a refrigerator.

Components of the solution may precipitate in the frozen state and will dissolve on reaching room temperature with little or no agitation. Potency is not affected. Check for minute leaks in plastic containers by squeezing bag firmly. Discard bag if leaks are found as sterility may be impaired. Do not add supplementary medication to bags. Do not use unless solution is clear and seal is intact.

Use sterile equipment.

Caution: Do not use plastic containers in series connections. Such use could result in air embolism due to residual air being drawn from the primary container before administration of the fluid from the secondary container is complete.

Preparation for Administration:

1. Suspend container from eyelet support.
2. Remove protector from outlet port at bottom of container.
3. Attach administration set. Refer to complete directions accompanying set.

CEPTAZ is compatible with the more commonly used IV infusion fluids. Solutions at concentrations between 1 and 40 mg/mL in 0.9% sodium chloride injection; 1/6 M sodium lactate injection; 5% dextrose injection; 5% dextrose and 0.225% sodium chloride injection; 5% dextrose and 0.45% sodium chloride injection; 5% dextrose and 0.9% sodium chloride injection; 10% dextrose injection; ringer's injection, USP; lactated ringer's injection, USP; 10% invert sugar in sterile water for injection; and NORMOSOL®-M in 5% dextrose injection may be stored for up to 24 hours at room temperature or for 7 days if refrigerated.

CEPTAZ is less stable in sodium bicarbonate injection than in other IV fluids. It is not recommended as a diluent. Solutions of CEPTAZ in 5% dextrose injection and 0.9% sodium chloride injection are stable for at least 6 hours at room temperature in plastic tubing, drip chambers, and volume control devices of common IV infusion sets.

Ceftazidime at a concentration of 4 mg/mL has been found compatible for 24 hours at room temperature or for 7 days under refrigeration in 0.9% sodium chloride injection or 5% dextrose injection when admixed with: cefuroxime sodium (ZINACEF®) 3 mg/mL; heparin sodium in concentrations up to 50 U/mL; or potassium chloride in concentrations up to 40 mEq/L. Ceftazidime may be constituted at a concentration of 20 mg/mL with metronidazole injection 5 mg/mL, and the resultant solution may be stored for 24 hours at room temperature or for 7 days under refrigeration. Ceftazidime at a concentration of 20 mg/mL has been found compatible for 24 hours at room temperature or for 7 days under refrigeration in 0.9% sodium chloride injection or 5% dextrose injection when admixed with 6 mg/mL clindamycin (as clindamycin phosphate).

Vancomycin solution exhibits a physical incompatibility when mixed with a number of drugs, including ceftazidime. The likelihood of precipitation with ceftazidime is dependent on the concentrations of vancomycin and ceftazidime present. It is therefore recommended, when both drugs are to be administered by intermittent IV infusion, that they be given separately, flushing the IV lines (with one of the compatible IV fluids) between the administration of these two agents.

Note: Parenteral drug products should be inspected visually for particulate matter before administration whenever solution and container permit.

As with other cephalosporins, CEPTAZ powder as well as solutions tend to darken, depending on storage conditions; within the stated recommendations, however, product potency is not adversely affected.

Directions for Dispensing: ***Pharmacy Bulk Package—Not for Direct Infusion:*** The pharmacy bulk package is for use in a pharmacy admixture service only under a laminar flow hood. Entry into the vial must be made with a sterile transfer set or other sterile dispensing device, and the contents dispensed in aliquots using aseptic technique. The use of syringe and needle is not recommended as it may cause leakage (see DOSAGE AND ADMINISTRATION). GOOD PHARMACY PRACTICE DICTATES THAT THE CLOSURE BE PENETRATED ONLY ONE TIME AFTER CON-

Continued on next page

This product information is based on labeling in effect on June 1, 1998. For further information, contact via direct mail, phone, or web site Medical Information: Glaxo Wellcome Inc., PO Box 13398, Research Triangle Park, NC 27709. Healthcare Professionals (Medical Information): 800-334-0089 Patients (Customer Response Center): 888-TALK2GW (1-888-825-5249) Glaxo Wellcome Corporate Web Site: www.glaxowellcome.com

Ceptaz—Cont.

STITUTION. AFTER INITIAL PENETRATION OF THE CLOSURE, USE ENTIRE CONTENTS OF VIAL PROMPTLY. ANY UNUSED PORTION MUST BE DISCARDED WITHIN 18 HOURS OF CONSTITUTION.

HOW SUPPLIED

CEPTAZ in the dry state should be stored between 15° and 30°C (59° and 86°F) and protected from light. CEPTAZ is a dry, white to off-white powder supplied in vials and infusion packs as follows:
NDC 0173-0414-00 1-g* Vial (Tray of 25)
NDC 0173-0415-00 2-g* Vial (Tray of 25)
NDC 0173-0416-00 1-g* Infusion Pack (Tray of 10)
NDC 0173-0417-00 2-g* Infusion Pack (Tray of 10)
NDC 0173-0418-00 10-g* Pharmacy Bulk Package (Tray of 6)
*Equivalent to anhydrous ceftazidime.

REFERENCES

1. Bauer AW, Kirby WMM, Sherris JC, Turck M. Antibiotic susceptibility testing by a standardized single disk method. *Am J Clin Pathol.* 1966;45:493-496.
2. National Committee for Clinical Laboratory Standards. *Approved Standard: Performance Standards for Antimicrobial Disc Susceptibility Tests.* (M2-A3). December 1984.
3. Certification procedure for antibiotic sensitivity discs (21 CFR 460.1). *Federal Register.* May 30, 1974;39:19182-19184.
4. Cockcroft DW, Gault MH. Prediction of creatinine clearance from serum creatinine. *Nephron.* 1976;16:31-41.

CEPTAZ and ZINACEF are registered trademarks of Glaxo Wellcome.
CLINITEST and CLINISTIX are registered trademarks of Ames Division, Miles Laboratories, Inc.
TES-TAPE is a registered trademark of Eli Lilly and Company.
VIAFLEX and PL 146 Plastic are registered trademarks of Baxter International Inc.
U.S. Patents 4,258,041; 4,329,453; and 4,582,830
February 1998/RL-544

Shown in Product Identification Guide, page 311

COMBIVIR™ Tablets ℞

[*kom 'bə-vir*]
(lamivudine/zidovudine tablets)

WARNING: ZIDOVUDINE, ONE OF THE TWO ACTIVE INGREDIENTS IN COMBIVIR, HAS BEEN ASSOCIATED WITH HEMATOLOGIC TOXICITY INCLUDING NEUTROPENIA AND SEVERE ANEMIA, PARTICULARLY IN PATIENTS WITH ADVANCED HIV DISEASE (SEE WARNINGS). PROLONGED USE OF ZIDOVUDINE HAS BEEN ASSOCIATED WITH SYMPTOMATIC MYOPATHY.
LACTIC ACIDOSIS AND SEVERE HEPATOMEGALY WITH STEATOSIS, INCLUDING FATAL CASES, HAVE BEEN REPORTED WITH THE USE OF ANTIRETROVIRAL NUCLEOSIDE ANALOGUES ALONE OR IN COMBINATION, INCLUDING ZIDOVUDINE AND LAMIVUDINE (SEE WARNINGS).

DESCRIPTION

COMBIVIR: COMBIVIR Tablets are combination tablets containing lamivudine and zidovudine. Lamivudine (EPIVIR®, 3TC) and zidovudine (RETROVIR®, azidothymidine, AZT, or ZDV) are synthetic nucleoside analogues with activity against human immunodeficiency virus (HIV). COMBIVIR Tablets are for oral administration. Each film-coated tablet contains 150 mg of lamivudine, 300 mg of zidovudine, and the inactive ingredients colloidal silicon dioxide, magnesium stearate, microcrystalline cellulose, and sodium starch glycolate. The film-coating solution contains Opadry YS-1-7706-G White and purified water.

Lamivudine: The chemical name of lamivudine is (2R,cis)-4-amino-1-(2-hydroxymethyl-1,3-oxathiolan-5-yl)-(1H)-pyrimidin-2-one. Lamivudine is the (-)enantiomer of a dideoxy analogue of cytidine. Lamivudine has also been referred to as (-)2',3'-dideoxy, 3'-thiacytidine. It has a molecular formula of $C_8H_{11}N_3O_3S$ and a molecular weight of 229.3. It has the following structural formula:

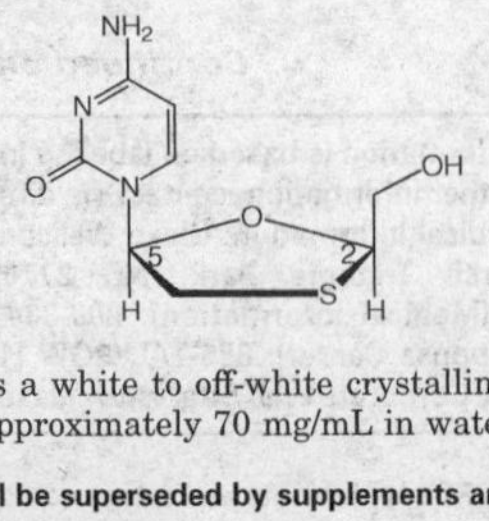

Lamivudine is a white to off-white crystalline solid with a solubility of approximately 70 mg/mL in water at 20°C.

Zidovudine: The chemical name of zidovudine is 3'-azido-3'-deoxythymidine. It has a molecular formula of $C_{10}H_{13}N_5O_4$ and a molecular weight of 267.24. It has the following structural formula:

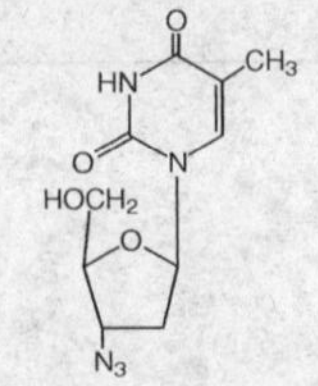

Zidovudine is a white to beige, odorless, crystalline solid with a solubility of 20.1 mg/mL in water at 25°C.

MICROBIOLOGY

Mechanism of Action: ***Lamivudine:*** Lamivudine is a synthetic nucleoside analogue. Intracellularly, lamivudine is phosphorylated to its active 5'-triphosphate metabolite, lamivudine triphosphate (L-TP). The principal mode of action of L-TP is inhibition of reverse transcriptase (RT) via DNA chain termination after incorporation of the nucleoside analogue. L-TP is a weak inhibitor of mammalian DNA polymerases α and β, and mitochondrial DNA polymerase-γ.

Zidovudine: Zidovudine is a synthetic nucleoside analogue. Intracellularly, zidovudine is phosphorylated to its active 5'-triphosphate metabolite, zidovudine triphosphate (ZDV-TP). The principal mode of action of ZDV-TP is inhibition of RT via DNA chain termination after incorporation of the nucleoside analogue. ZDV-TP is a weak inhibitor of the mammalian DNA polymerase-α and mitochondrial DNA polymerase-γ and has been reported to be incorporated into the DNA of cells in culture.

Antiviral Activity In Vitro: The relationship between in vitro susceptibility of HIV to lamivudine or zidovudine and the inhibition of HIV replication in humans has not been established.

Lamivudine Plus Zidovudine: In HIV-1–infected MT-4 cells, lamivudine in combination with zidovudine had synergistic antiretroviral activity. Synergistic activity of lamivudine and zidovudine was also shown in a variable-ratio study.

Lamivudine: In vitro activity of lamivudine against HIV-1 was assessed in a number of cell lines (including monocytes and fresh human peripheral blood lymphocytes). IC_{50} and IC_{90} values (50% and 90% inhibitory concentrations) for lamivudine were 0.0006 mcg/mL to 0.034 mcg/mL and 0.015 to 0.321 mcg/mL, respectively. Lamivudine had anti–HIV-1 activity in all acute virus-cell infections tested.

Zidovudine: In vitro activity of zidovudine against HIV-1 was assessed in a number of cell lines (including monocytes and fresh human peripheral blood lymphocytes). The IC_{50} and IC_{90} values for zidovudine were 0.003 to 0.013 mcg/mL and 0.03 to 0.13 mcg/mL, respectively. Zidovudine had anti–HIV-1 activity in all acute virus-cell infections tested. However, zidovudine activity was substantially less in chronically infected cell lines. In cell culture drug combination studies with zidovudine, interferon-alpha demonstrated additive activity and zalcitabine, didanosine, saquinavir, indinavir, ritonavir, nelfinavir, nevirapine, and delavirdine demonstrated synergistic activity.

Drug Resistance: Lamivudine Plus Zidovudine Administered As Separate Formulations: In patients receiving lamivudine monotherapy or combination therapy with lamivudine plus zidovudine, HIV-1 isolates from most patients became phenotypically and genotypically resistant to lamivudine within 12 weeks. In some patients harboring zidovudine-resistant virus at baseline, phenotypic sensitivity to zidovudine was restored by 12 weeks of treatment with lamivudine and zidovudine. Combination therapy with lamivudine plus zidovudine delayed the emergence of mutations conferring resistance to zidovudine.

HIV-1 strains resistant to both lamivudine and zidovudine have been isolated from patients after prolonged lamivudine/zidovudine therapy. Dual resistance required the presence of multiple mutations, the most essential of which may be at codon 333 (Gly→Glu). The incidence of dual resistance and the duration of combination therapy required before dual resistance occurs are unknown.

Lamivudine: Lamivudine-resistant isolates of HIV-1 have been selected in vitro and have also been recovered from patients treated with lamivudine or lamivudine plus zidovudine. Genotypic analysis of the resistant isolates showed that the resistance was due to mutations in the HIV-1 reverse transcriptase gene at codon 184 from methionine to either isoleucine or valine.

Zidovudine: HIV isolates with reduced susceptibility to zidovudine have been selected in vitro and were also recovered from patients treated with zidovudine. Genotypic analyses of the isolates showed mutations which result in five amino acid substitutions (Met41→Leu, Asp67→Asn, Lys70→Arg, Thr215→Tyr or Phe, and Lys219→Gln) in the HIV-1 reverse transcriptase gene. In general, higher levels of resistance were associated with greater number of mutations.

Cross-Resistance: Cross-resistance among certain reverse transcriptase inhibitors has been recognized.

Lamivudine Plus Zidovudine: Cross-resistance between lamivudine and zidovudine has not been reported. In some patients treated with lamivudine alone or in combination with zidovudine, isolates have emerged with a mutation at codon 184 which confers resistance to lamivudine. In the presence of the 184 mutation, cross-resistance to didanosine and zalcitabine has been seen in some patients; the clinical significance is unknown. In some patients treated with zidovudine plus didanosine or zalcitabine, isolates resistant to multiple drugs, including lamivudine, have emerged (see under Zidovudine below).

Lamivudine: See Lamivudine Plus Zidovudine (above).

Zidovudine: HIV isolates with multidrug resistance to zidovudine, didanosine, zalcitabine, stavudine, and lamivudine were recovered from a small number of patients treated for ≥1 year with zidovudine plus didanosine or zidovudine plus zalcitabine. The pattern of genotypic resistant mutations with such combination therapies was different (Ala62→Val, Val75→Ile, Phe77→Leu, Phe116→Tyr, and Gln151→Met) from the pattern with zidovudine monotherapy, with the 151 mutation being most commonly associated with multidrug resistance. The mutation at codon 151 in combination with the mutations at 62, 75, 77, and 116 results in a virus with reduced susceptibility to zidovudine, didanosine, zalcitabine, stavudine, and lamivudine. Multiple drug resistance has been observed in two of 39 (5%) patients receiving zidovudine and didanosine combination therapy for 2 years.

CLINICAL PHARMACOLOGY

Pharmacokinetics in Adults: ***COMBIVIR:*** One COMBIVIR Tablet was bioequivalent to one EPIVIR Tablet (150 mg) plus one RETROVIR Tablet (300 mg) following single-dose administration to fasting healthy subjects (n = 24).

Lamivudine: The pharmacokinetic properties of lamivudine in fasting patients are summarized in Table 1. Following oral administration, lamivudine is rapidly absorbed and extensively distributed. Binding to plasma protein is low. Approximately 70% of an intravenous dose of lamivudine is recovered as unchanged drug in the urine. Metabolism of lamivudine is a minor route of elimination. In humans, the only known metabolite is the trans-sulfoxide metabolite (approximately 5% of an oral dose after 12 hours).

Zidovudine: The pharmacokinetic properties of zidovudine in fasting patients are summarized in Table 1. Following oral administration, zidovudine is rapidly absorbed and extensively distributed. Binding to plasma protein is low. Zidovudine is eliminated primarily by hepatic metabolism. The major metabolite of zidovudine is 3'-azido-3'-deoxy-5'-*O*-β-*D*-glucopyranuronosylthymidine (GZDV). GZDV area under the curve (AUC) is about three-fold greater than the zidovudine AUC. Urinary recovery of zidovudine and GZDV accounts for 14% and 74% of the dose following oral administration, respectively. A second metabolite, 3'-amino-3'-deoxythymidine (AMT), has been identified in plasma. The AMT AUC was one-fifth of the zidovudine AUC.

[See table 1 at top of next page]

Effect of Food on Absorption of COMBIVIR: COMBIVIR may be administered with or without food. The extent of lamivudine and zidovudine absorption (AUC) following administration of COMBIVIR with food was similar when compared to fasting healthy subjects (n = 24).

Special Populations: ***Impaired Renal Function: COMBIVIR:*** Because lamivudine and zidovudine require dose adjustment in the presence of renal insufficiency, COMBIVIR is not recommended for patients with impaired renal function (see PRECAUTIONS).

Pregnancy: See PRECAUTIONS: Pregnancy.

COMBIVIR: No data are available.

Zidovudine: Zidovudine pharmacokinetics has been studied in a Phase 1 study of eight women during the last trimester of pregnancy. As pregnancy progressed, there was no evidence of drug accumulation. The pharmacokinetics of zidovudine was similar to that of nonpregnant adults. Consistent with passive transmission of the drug across the placenta, zidovudine concentrations in neonatal plasma at birth were essentially equal to those in maternal plasma at delivery. Although data are limited, methadone maintenance therapy in five pregnant women did not appear to alter zidovudine pharmacokinetics. In a nonpregnant adult population, a potential for interaction has been identified (see CLINICAL PHARMACOLOGY: Drug Interactions).

Nursing Mothers: See PRECAUTIONS: Nursing Mothers.

COMBIVIR: No data are available.

Zidovudine: After administration of a single dose of 200 mg zidovudine to 13 HIV-infected women, the mean concentration of zidovudine was similar in human milk and serum.

Pediatric Patients: COMBIVIR: COMBIVIR should not be administered to pediatric patients less than 12 years of age because it is a fixed-dose combination that cannot be adjusted for this patient population.

Table 1: Pharmacokinetic Parameters* for Lamivudine and Zidovudine in Adults

Parameter	Lamivudine		Zidovudine	
Oral bioavailability (%)	86 ± 16	n = 12	64 ± 10	n = 5
Apparent volume of distribution (L/kg)	1.3 ± 0.4	n = 20	1.6 ± 0.6	n = 8
Plasma protein binding (%)	<36		<38	
CSF: plasma ratio**	0.12 [0.04 to 0.47]	n = 38†	0.60 [0.04 to 2.62]	n = 39‡
Systemic clearance (L/h/kg)	0.33 ± 0.06	n = 20	1.6 ± 0.6	n = 6
Renal clearance (L/h/kg)	0.22 ± 0.06	n = 20	0.34 ± 0.05	n = 9
Elimination half-life (h)§	5 to 7		0.5 to 3	

* Data presented as mean ± standard deviation except where noted.
** Median [range].
† Children.
‡ Adults.
§ Approximate range.

Table 2: Effect of Coadministered Drugs on Lamivudine and Zidovudine AUC*

Note: ROUTINE DOSE MODIFICATION OF LAMIVUDINE AND ZIDOVUDINE IS NOT WARRANTED WITH COADMINISTRATION OF THE FOLLOWING DRUGS.

Drugs That May Alter Lamivudine Blood Concentrations

Coadministered Drug and Dose	Lamivudine Dose	n	Lamivudine Concentrations		Concentration of Coadministered
			AUC	Variability	Drug
Nelfinavir 750 mg q 8 hr × 7 to 10 days	single 150 mg	11	↑ AUC 10%	95% CI: 1% to 20%	↔
Trimethoprim 160 mg/ Sulfamethoxazole 800 mg daily × 5 days	single 300 mg	14	↑ AUC 43%	90% CI: 32% to 55%	↔

Drugs That May Alter Zidovudine Blood Concentrations

Coadministered Drug and Dose	Zidovudine Dose	n	Zidovudine Concentrations		Concentration of Coadministered
			AUC	Variability	Drug
Atovaquone 750 mg q 12 h with food	200 mg q 8 h	14	↑ AUC 31%	Range 23% to 78%**	↔
Fluconazole 400 mg daily	200 mg q 8 h	12	↑ AUC 74%	95% CI: 54% to 98%	Not Reported
Methadone 30 to 90 mg daily	200 mg q 4 h	9	↑ AUC 43%	Range 16% to 64%**	↔
Nelfinavir 750 mg q 8 hr × 7 to 10 days	single 200 mg	11	↓ AUC 35%	Range 28% to 41%	↔
Probenecid 500 mg q 6 h × 2 days	2 mg/kg q 8 h × 3 days	3	↑ AUC 106%	Range 100% to 170%**	Not Assessed
Ritonavir 300 mg q 6 h × 4 days	200 mg q 8 h × 4 days	9	↓ AUC 25%	95% CI: 15% to 34%	↔
Valproic acid 250 mg or 500 mg q 8 h × 4 days	100 mg q 8 h × 4 days	6	↑ AUC 80%	Range 64% to 130%**	Not Assessed

↑ = Increase; ↓ = Decrease; ↔ = no significant change; AUC = area under the concentration versus time curve; CI = confidence interval.
* This table is not all inclusive.
** Estimated range of percent difference.

Geriatric Patients: Lamivudine and zidovudine pharmacokinetics have not been studied in patients over 65 years of age.

Gender: COMBIVIR: A pharmacokinetic study in healthy male (n = 12) and female (n = 12) subjects showed no gender differences in zidovudine exposure (AUC∞) or lamivudine AUC∞ normalized for body weight.

Race: Lamivudine: There are no significant racial differences in lamivudine pharmacokinetics.

Drug Interactions: See PRECAUTIONS: Drug Interactions.

COMBIVIR: No drug interaction studies have been conducted using COMBIVIR Tablets.

Lamivudine Plus Zidovudine: No clinically significant alterations in lamivudine or zidovudine pharmacokinetics were observed in 12 asymptomatic HIV-infected adult patients given a single dose of zidovudine (200 mg) in combination with multiple doses of lamivudine (300 mg q 12 h).

[See table 2 above]

INDICATIONS AND USAGE

COMBIVIR is indicated for the treatment of HIV infection.

Description of Clinical Studies: COMBIVIR: There have been no clinical trials conducted with COMBIVIR. See CLINICAL PHARMACOLOGY for information about bioequivalence. One COMBIVIR Tablet given twice a day is an alternative regimen to EPIVIR Tablets 150 mg twice a day plus RETROVIR 600 mg per day in divided doses.

Lamivudine Plus Zidovudine: The NUCB3007 (CAESAR) study was conducted using EPIVIR 150-mg Tablets (150 mg b.i.d.) and RETROVIR 100-mg Capsules (2 × 100 mg t.i.d.). CAESAR was a multicenter, double-blind, placebo-controlled study comparing continued current therapy [zidovudine alone (62% of patients) or zidovudine with didanosine or zalcitabine (38% of patients)] to the addition of EPIVIR or

EPIVIR plus an investigational non-nucleoside reverse transcriptase inhibitor, randomized 1:2:1. A total of 1,816 HIV-infected adults with 25 to 250 (median 122) CD4 cells/mm³ at baseline were enrolled: median age was 36 years, 87% were male, 84% were nucleoside-experienced, and 16% were therapy-naive. The median duration on study was 12 months. Results are summarized in Table 3.
[See table 3 at top of next page]

CONTRAINDICATIONS

COMBIVIR Tablets are contraindicated in patients with previously demonstrated clinically significant hypersensitivity to any of the components of the product.

WARNINGS

COMBIVIR is a fixed-dose combination of lamivudine and zidovudine. Ordinarily, COMBIVIR should not be administered concomitantly with either lamivudine or zidovudine. The complete prescribing information for all agents being considered for use with COMBIVIR should be consulted before combination therapy with COMBIVIR is initiated.

Bone Marrow Suppression: COMBIVIR should be used with caution in patients who have bone marrow compromise evidenced by granulocyte count <1,000 cells/mm³ or hemoglobin <9.5 g/dL (see ADVERSE REACTIONS).

Frequent blood counts are strongly recommended in patients with advanced HIV disease who are treated with COMBIVIR. For HIV-infected individuals and patients with asymptomatic or early HIV disease, periodic blood counts are recommended.

Lactic Acidosis/Severe Hepatomegaly with Steatosis: Lactic acidosis and severe hepatomegaly with steatosis, including fatal cases, have been reported with the use of antiretroviral nucleoside analogues alone or in combination, including zidovudine and lamivudine. A majority of these cases have been in women. Caution should be exercised when administering COMBIVIR to any patient, and particularly to those with known risk factors for liver disease. Treatment with COMBIVIR should be suspended in any patient who develops clinical or laboratory findings suggestive of lactic acidosis or hepatotoxicity.

Myopathy: Myopathy and myositis, with pathological changes similar to that produced by HIV disease, have been associated with prolonged use of zidovudine and therefore may occur with therapy with COMBIVIR.

PRECAUTIONS

General: Reduction of doses of lamivudine is recommended for patients with low body weight (less than 50 kg or 110 lb); therefore patients with low body weight should not receive COMBIVIR.

Patients With HIV and Hepatitis B Virus Coinfection: In clinical trials and postmarketing experience, some patients with HIV infection who have chronic liver disease due to hepatitis B virus infection experienced clinical or laboratory evidence of recurrent hepatitis upon discontinuation of lamivudine. Consequences may be more severe in patients with decompensated liver disease.

Patients With Impaired Renal Function: Reduction of the dosages of lamivudine and zidovudine is recommended for patients with impaired renal function. Patients with creatinine clearance ≤50 mL/min should not receive COMBIVIR.

Information for Patients: COMBIVIR is not a cure for HIV infection and patients may continue to experience illnesses associated with HIV infection, including opportunistic infections. Patients should be advised that the use of COMBIVIR has not been shown to reduce the risk of transmission of HIV to others through sexual contact or blood contamination. Patients should be informed that the major toxicities of COMBIVIR are neutropenia and/or anemia. They should be told of the extreme importance of having their blood counts followed closely while on therapy, especially for patients with advanced HIV disease. Patients should be advised of the importance of taking COMBIVIR as it is prescribed.

Drug Interactions: Coadministration of ganciclovir, interferon-alpha, and other bone marrow suppressive or cytotoxic agents may increase the hematologic toxicity of zidovudine (see CLINICAL PHARMACOLOGY).

Carcinogenesis, Mutagenesis, and Impairment of Fertility:
Carcinogenicity:

Lamivudine: Lamivudine long-term carcinogenicity studies in mice and rats showed no evidence of carcinogenic potential at exposures up to 10 times (mice) and 58 times (rats) those observed in humans at the recommended therapeutic dose.

Continued on next page

This product information is based on labeling in effect on June 1, 1998. For further information, contact via direct mail, phone, or web site Medical Information: Glaxo Wellcome Inc., PO Box 13398, Research Triangle Park, NC 27709. Healthcare Professionals (Medical Information): 800-334-0089 Patients (Customer Response Center): 888-TALK2GW (1-888-825-5249) Glaxo Wellcome Corporate Web Site: www.glaxowellcome.com

Combivir—Cont.

Zidovudine: Zidovudine was administered orally at three dosage levels to separate groups of mice and rats (60 females and 60 males in each group). Initial single daily doses were 30, 60, and 120 mg/kg per day in mice and 80, 220, and 600 mg/kg per day in rats. The doses in mice were reduced to 20, 30, and 40 mg/kg per day after day 90 because of treatment-related anemia, whereas in rats only the high dose was reduced to 450 mg/kg per day on day 91 and then to 300 mg/kg per day on day 279.

In mice, seven late-appearing (after 19 months) vaginal neoplasms (five non-metastasizing squamous cell carcinomas, one squamous cell papilloma, and one squamous polyp) occurred in animals given the highest dose. One late-appearing squamous cell papilloma occurred in the vagina of a middle-dose animal. No vaginal tumors were found at the lowest dose.

In rats, two late-appearing (after 20 months), non-metastasizing vaginal squamous cell carcinomas occurred in animals given the highest dose. No vaginal tumors occurred at the low or middle dose in rats. No other drug-related tumors were observed in either sex of either species.

At doses that produced tumors in mice and rats, the estimated drug exposure (as measured by AUC) was approximately three times (mouse) and 24 times (rat) the estimated human exposure at the recommended therapeutic dose of 100 mg every 4 hours.

Two transplacental carcinogenicity studies were conducted in mice. One study administered zidovudine at doses of 20 mg/kg per day or 40 mg/kg per day from gestation day 10 through parturition and lactation with dosing continuing in offspring for 24 months postnatally. The doses of zidovudine employed in this study produced zidovudine exposures approximately three times the estimated human exposure at recommended doses. After 24 months, at the highest dose, an increase in incidence of vaginal tumors was noted with no increase in tumors in the liver or lung or any other organ in either gender. These findings are consistent with results of the standard oral carcinogenicity study in mice, as described earlier. A second study administered zidovudine at maximum tolerated doses of 12.5 mg/day or 25 mg/day (~1,000 mg/kg nonpregnant body weight or ~450 mg/kg of term body weight) to pregnant mice from days 12 through 18 of gestation. There was an increase in the number of tumors in the lung, liver, and female reproductive tracts in the offspring of mice receiving the higher dose level of zidovudine.

It is not known how predictive the results of rodent carcinogenicity studies may be for humans.

Mutagenicity: Lamivudine: Lamivudine was negative in a microbial mutagenicity screen, in an in vitro cell transformation assay, in a rat micronucleus test, in a rat bone marrow cytogenetic assay, and in an assay for unscheduled DNA synthesis in rat liver. It was mutagenic in a L5178Y/TK$^{+/-}$ mouse lymphoma assay and clastogenic in a cytogenetic assay using cultured human lymphocytes.

Zidovudine: Zidovudine was mutagenic in a L5178Y/TK$^{+/-}$ mouse lymphoma assay, positive in an in vitro cell transformation assay, clastogenic in a cytogenetic assay using cultured human lymphocytes, and positive in mouse and rat micronucleus tests after repeated doses. It was negative in a cytogenetic study in rats given a single dose.

Impairment of Fertility: Lamivudine: In a study of reproductive performance, lamivudine, administered to male and female rats at doses up to 130 times the usual adult dose based on body surface area considerations, revealed no evidence of impaired fertility (judged by conception rates) and no effect on the survival, growth, and development to weaning of the offspring.

Zidovudine: Zidovudine, administered to male and female rats at doses up to 7 times the usual adult dose based on body surface area considerations, had no effect on fertility judged by conception rates.

Pregnancy: Pregnancy Category C.

COMBIVIR: There are no adequate and well-controlled studies of COMBIVIR in pregnant women. Reproduction studies with lamivudine and zidovudine have been performed in animals (see Lamivudine and Zidovudine sections below). COMBIVIR should be used during pregnancy only if the potential benefits outweigh the risks.

Lamivudine: Reproduction studies with orally administered lamivudine have been performed in rats and rabbits at 130 and 60 times, respectively, the usual adult dose (based on relative body surface area) and have revealed no evidence of teratogenicity. Some evidence of early embryolethality was seen in the rabbit at doses similar to those produced by the usual adult dose and higher, but there was no indication of this effect in the rat at orally administered doses up to 130 times the usual adult dose. Studies in pregnant rats and rabbits showed that lamivudine is transferred to the fetus through the placenta.

Zidovudine: Reproduction studies with orally administered zidovudine in the rat and in the rabbit at doses up to 500 mg/kg per day revealed no evidence of teratogenicity with zidovudine. Zidovudine treatment resulted in embryo/fetal toxicity as evidenced by an increase in the incidence of fetal resorptions in rats given 150 or 450 mg/kg per day and rabbits given 500 mg/kg per day. The doses used in the teratology studies resulted in peak zidovudine plasma concentrations (after one-half of the daily dose) in rats 66 to 226 times, and in rabbits 12 to 87 times, mean steady-state peak human plasma concentrations (after one-sixth of the daily dose) achieved with the recommended daily dose (100 mg every 4 hours). In an additional teratology study in rats, a dose of 3,000 mg/kg per day (very near the oral median lethal dose in rats of 3,683 mg/kg) caused marked maternal toxicity and an increase in the incidence of fetal malformations. This dose resulted in peak zidovudine plasma concentrations 350 times peak human plasma concentrations. No evidence of teratogenicity was seen in this experiment at doses of 600 mg/kg per day or less. Two rodent carcinogenicity studies were conducted (see Carcinogenesis, Mutagenesis, Impairment of Fertility).

Antiretroviral Pregnancy Registry: To monitor maternal-fetal outcomes of pregnant women exposed to COMBIVIR and other antiretroviral agents, an Antiretroviral Pregnancy Registry has been established. Physicians are encouraged to register patients by calling (800) 722-9292, ext. 39437.

Nursing Mothers: The Centers for Disease Control and Prevention recommend that HIV-infected mothers not breast-feed their infants to avoid risking postnatal transmission of HIV infection.

COMBIVIR: Zidovudine is excreted in breast milk (see CLINICAL PHARMACOLOGY: Pharmacokinetics: Nursing Mothers); however, no data are available on COMBIVIR or lamivudine. Therefore, there is a potential for adverse effects in nursing infants. **Mothers should be instructed not to breast-feed if they are receiving COMBIVIR.**

Pediatric Use: COMBIVIR should not be administered to pediatric patients less than 12 years of age because it is a fixed-dose combination that cannot be adjusted for this patient population.

ADVERSE REACTIONS

Lamivudine Plus Zidovudine Administered As Separate Formulations: In four randomized, controlled trials of

---

Table 3: Number of Patients (%) With At Least One HIV Disease-Progression Event or Death

Endpoint	Current Therapy (n = 460)	EPIVIR plus Current Therapy (n = 896)	EPIVIR plus a NNRTI* plus Current Therapy (n = 460)
HIV progression or death	90 (19.6%)	86 (9.6%)	41 (8.9%)
Death	27 (5.9%)	23 (2.6%)	14 (3.0%)

*An investigational non-nucleoside reverse transcriptase inhibitor not approved in the United States.

Table 4: Selected Clinical Adverse Events (≥5% Frequency) in Four Controlled Clinical Trials With EPIVIR 300 mg/day and RETROVIR 600 mg/day

Adverse Event	EPIVIR plus RETROVIR (n = 251)
Body as a whole	
Headache	35%
Malaise & fatigue	27%
Fever or chills	10%
Digestive	
Nausea	33%
Diarrhea	18%
Nausea & vomiting	13%
Anorexia and/or decreased appetite	10%
Abdominal pain	9%
Abdominal cramps	6%
Dyspepsia	5%
Nervous system	
Neuropathy	12%
Insomnia & other sleep disorders	11%
Dizziness	10%
Depressive disorders	9%
Respiratory	
Nasal signs & symptoms	20%
Cough	18%
Skin	
Skin rashes	9%
Musculoskeletal	
Musculoskeletal pain	12%
Myalgia	8%
Arthralgia	5%

Table 5: Frequencies of Selected Laboratory Abnormalities Among Adults in Four Controlled Clinical Trials of EPIVIR 300 mg/day plus RETROVIR 600 mg/day*

Test (Abnormal Level)	EPIVIR plus RETROVIR % (n)
Neutropenia (ANC<750/mm^3)	7.2% (237)
Anemia (Hgb<8.0 g/dL)	2.9% (241)
Thrombocytopenia (platelets<50,000/mm^3)	0.4% (240)
ALT (>5.0 × ULN)	3.7% (241)
AST (>5.0 × ULN)	1.7% (241)
Bilirubin (>2.5 × ULN)	0.8% (241)
Amylase (>2.0 × ULN)	4.2% (72)

ULN = Upper limit of normal.
ANC = Absolute neutrophil count.
n = Number of patients assessed.
* Frequencies of these laboratory abnormalities were higher in patients with mild laboratory abnormalities at baseline.

EPIVIR 300 mg per day plus RETROVIR 600 mg per day, the following selected clinical and laboratory adverse events were observed (see Tables 4 and 5).
[See table 4 at top of previous page]
Pancreatitis was observed in three of the 656 adult patients (<0.5%) who received EPIVIR in controlled clinical trials. Selected laboratory abnormalities observed during therapy are listed in Table 5.
[See table 5 at top of previous page]
Observed During Clinical Practice: The following events have been identified during post-approval use of EPIVIR and/or RETROVIR. Because they are reported voluntarily from a population of unknown size, estimates of frequency cannot be made. These events have been chosen for inclusion due to their seriousness, frequency of reporting, causal connection to EPIVIR and/or RETROVIR, or a combination of these factors.
Alopecia, erythema multiforme, hyperglycemia, lactic acidosis and hepatic steatosis (see WARNINGS), pancreatitis, seizures, sensitization reactions (including anaphylaxis), Stevens-Johnson syndrome, urticaria, and vasculitis.

OVERDOSAGE

COMBIVIR: There is no known antidote for COMBIVIR.
Lamivudine: One case of an adult ingesting 6 grams of lamivudine was reported; there were no clinical signs or symptoms noted and hematologic tests remained normal. It is not known whether lamivudine can be removed by peritoneal dialysis or hemodialysis.
Zidovudine: Acute overdoses of zidovudine have been reported in pediatric patients and adults. These involved exposures up to 50 grams. The only consistent findings were nausea and vomiting. Other reported occurrences included headache, dizziness, drowsiness, lethargy, confusion, and one report of a grand mal seizure. Hematologic changes were transient. All patients recovered. Hemodialysis and peritoneal dialysis appear to have a negligible effect on the removal of zidovudine while elimination of its primary metabolite, GZDV, is enhanced.

DOSAGE AND ADMINISTRATION

The recommended oral dose of COMBIVIR for adults and adolescents (at least 12 years of age) is one tablet (containing 150 mg of lamivudine and 300 mg of zidovudine) twice daily.
Dose Adjustment: Because it is a fixed-dose combination, COMBIVIR should not be prescribed for patients requiring dosage adjustment such as those with reduced renal function (creatinine clearance ≤50 mL/min), those with low body weight (<50 kg or 110 lb), or those experiencing dose-limiting adverse events.

HOW SUPPLIED

COMBIVIR Tablets, containing 150 mg lamivudine and 300 mg zidovudine, are white, film-coated, modified-capsule-shaped tablets engraved with "GXFC3" on one side. They are available as follows:
60 Tablets/Bottle (NDC 0173-0595-00)
Store between 2° and 30°C (36° and 86°F).
Unit Dose Pack of 120 (NDC 0173-0595-02)
U.S. Patent Nos. 5,047,407; 4,818,538; 4,828,838; 4,724,232; 4,833,130; and 4,837,208
Store between 2° and 30°C (36° and 86°F).
January 1998/RL-505
Shown in Product Identification Guide, page 312

CUTIVATE® ℞

[kyoot'ə-vāt'']
(fluticasone propionate cream)
Cream, 0.05%

For Dermatologic Use Only—
Not for Ophthalmic Use.

DESCRIPTION

CUTIVATE Cream contains fluticasone propionate [(6α, 11β, 16α, 17α)-6,9,-difluoro-11-hydroxy-16-methyl-3-oxo-17-(1-oxopropoxy)androsta-1,4-diene-17-carbothioic acid, S-fluoromethyl ester], a synthetic fluorinated corticosteroid, for topical dermatologic use. The topical corticosteriods constitute a class of primarily synthetic steroids used as anti-inflammatory and antipruritic agents.
Chemically, fluticasone propionate is $C_{25}H_{31}F_3O_5S$.
Fluticasone propionate has a molecular weight of 500.6. It is a white to off-white powder and is insoluble in water.
Each gram of CUTIVATE Cream contains fluticasone propionate 0.5 mg in a base of propylene glycol, mineral oil, cetostearyl alcohol, Ceteth-20, isopropyl myristate, dibasic sodium phosphate, citric acid, purified water, and imidurea as preservative.

CLINICAL PHARMACOLOGY

Like other topical corticosteroids, fluticasone propionate has anti-inflammatory, antipruritic, and vasoconstrictive properties. The mechanism of the anti-inflammatory activity of the topical steroids, in general, is unclear. However, corticosteroids are thought to act by the induction of phospholipase A_2 inhibitory proteins, collectively called lipocortins. It is postulated that these proteins control the biosynthesis of potent mediators of inflammation such as prostaglandins and leukotrienes by inhibiting the release of their common precursor, arachidonic acid. Arachidonic acid is released from membrane phospholipids by phospholipase A_2.
Fluticasone propionate is lipophilic and has a strong affinity for the glucocorticoid receptor. It has weak affinity for the progesterone receptor, and virtually no affinity for the mineralocorticoid, estrogen, or androgen receptors. The therapeutic potency of glucocorticoids is related to the half-life of the glucocorticoid-receptor complex. Fluticasone propionate binding to the glucocorticoid receptor is rapid. The half-life of the fluticasone propionate-glucocorticoid receptor complex is approximately 10 hours.
Pharmacokinetics: The extent of percutaneous absorption of topical corticosteroids is determined by many factors, including the vehicle and the integrity of the epidermal barrier. Occlusive dressing enhances penetration. Topical corticosteroids can be absorbed from normal intact skin. Inflammation and/or other disease processes in the skin increase percutaneous absorption. Fluticasone propionate absorbed systemically is rapidly metabolized in the liver by esterase-catalyzed hydrolysis to the 17-β-carboxylic acid, which has no significant glucocorticoid or anti-inflammatory activity. Studies performed with CUTIVATE Cream indicate that it is in the medium range of potency as compared with other topical corticosteroids.

INDICATIONS AND USAGE

CUTIVATE Cream is a medium potency corticosteroid indicated for the relief of the inflammatory and pruritic manifestations of corticosteroid-responsive dermatoses.

CONTRAINDICATIONS

CUTIVATE Cream is contraindicated in those patients with a history of hypersensitivity to any of the components of the preparation.

PRECAUTIONS

General: Systemic absorption of topical corticosteroids can produce reversible hypothalamic-pituitary-adrenal (HPA) axis suppression with the potential for glucocorticosteroid insufficiency after withdrawal from treatment. Manifestations of Cushing's syndrome, hypergylcemia, and glucosuria can also be produced in some patients by systemic absorption of topical corticosteroids while on treatment.
Patients applying a potent topical steroid to a large surface area or to areas under occlusion should be evaluated periodically for evidence of HPA axis suppression. This may be done by using the ACTH stimulation, A.M. plasma cortisol, and urinary free cortisol tests.
Fluticasone propionate cream, 0.05% caused depression of A.M. plasma cortisol levels in one of six patients when used daily for 7 days in patients with psoriasis or eczema involving at least 30% of the body surface. After 2 days of treatment, this patient developed a 60% decrease from pretreatment values in the A.M. plasma cortisol level. There was some evidence of corresponding decrease in the 24-hour urinary free cortisol levels. The A.M. plasma cortisol level remained slightly depressed for 48 hours before recovering by day 6 of treatment.
If HPA axis suppression is noted, an attempt should be made to withdraw the drug, to reduce the frequency of application, or to substitute a less potent steroid. Recovery of HPA axis function is generally prompt upon discontinuation of topical corticosteroids. Infrequently, signs and symptoms of glucocorticosteroid insufficiency may occur requiring systemic corticosteroids. For information on systemic supplementation, see prescribing information for those products.
Children may be more susceptible to systemic toxicity from equivalent doses due to their larger skin surface to body mass ratios (see PRECAUTIONS: Pediatric Use).
If irritation develops, CUTIVATE Cream should be discontinued and appropriate therapy instituted. Allergic contact dermatitis with corticosteroids is usually diagnosed by observing failure to heal rather than noting a clinical exacerbation as with most topical products not containing corticosteroids. Such an observation should be corroborated with appropriate patch testing.
If concomitant skin infections are present or develop, an appropriate antifungal or antibacterial agent should be used. If a favorable response does not occur promptly, use of CUTIVATE Cream should be discontinued until the infection has been adequately controlled.
CUTIVATE Cream should not be used in the treatment of preexisting skin atrophy and should not be used where infection is present at the treatment site. CUTIVATE Cream should not be used in the treatment of rosacea and perioral dermatitis.
Information for Patients: Patients using topical corticosteroids should receive the following information and instructions:
1. This medication is to be used as directed by the physician. It is for external use only. Avoid contact with the eyes.
2. This medication should not be used for any disorder other than that for which it was prescribed.
3. The treated skin area should not be bandaged or otherwise covered or wrapped so as to be occlusive unless directed by the physician.
4. Patients should report to their physician any signs of local adverse reactions.
Laboratory Tests: The following tests may be helpful in evaluating patients for HPA axis suppression:
ACTH stimulation test
A.M. plasma cortisol test
Urinary free cortisol test
Carcinogenesis, Mutagenesis, and Impairment of Fertility: Two 18-month studies were performed in mice to evaluate the carcinogenic potential of fluticasone propionate when given topically (as an 0.05% ointment) and orally. No evidence of carcinogenicity was found in either study.
Fluticasone propionate was not mutagenic in the standard Ames test, *E. coli* fluctuation test, *S. cerevisiae* gene conversion test, or Chinese Hamster ovarian cell assay. It was not clastogenic in mouse micronucleus or cultured human lymphocyte tests.
In a fertility and general reproductive performance study in rats, fluticasone propionate administered subcutaneously to females at up to 50 mcg/kg per day and to males up to 100 mcg/kg per day (later reduced to 50 mcg/kg per day) had no effect upon mating performance or fertility. These doses are approximately 15 and 30 times, respectively, the human systemic exposure following use of the recommended human topical dose of fluticasone propionate cream, 0.05%, assuming human percutaneous absorption of approximately 3% and the use in a 70-kg person of 15 g/day.
Pregnancy: ***Teratogenic Effects:*** Pregnancy Category C. Corticosteroids have been shown to be teratogenic in laboratory animals when administered systemically at relatively low dosage levels. Some corticosteroids have been shown to be teratogenic after dermal application in laboratory animals. Teratology studies in the mouse demonstrated fluticasone propionate to be teratogenic (cleft palate) when administered subcutaneously in doses of 45 mcg/kg per day and 150 mcg/kg per day. This dose is approximately 14 and 45 times, respectively, the human topical dose of fluticasone propionate cream, 0.05%. There are no adequate and well-controlled studies in pregnant women. CUTIVATE Cream should be used during pregnancy only if the potential benefit justifies the potential risk to the fetus.
Nursing Mothers: Systemically administered corticosteroids appear in human milk and could suppress growth, interfere with endogenous corticosteroid production, or cause other untoward effects. It is not known whether topical administration of corticosteroids could result in sufficient systemic absorption to produce detectable quantities in human milk. Because many drugs are excreted in human milk, caution should be exercised when CUTIVATE Cream is administered to a nursing woman.
Pediatric Use: Safety and effectiveness in pediatric patients have not been established. Because of a higher ratio of skin surface area to body mass, pediatric patients are at a greater risk than adults of HPA axis suppression when they are treated with topical corticosteroids. They are therefore also at greater risk of glucocorticosteroid insufficiency after withdrawal of treatment and of Cushing's syndrome while on treatment. Adverse effects including striae have been reported with inappropriate use of topical corticosteroids in infants and children.
HPA axis suppression, Cushing's syndrome, linear growth retardation, delayed weight gain, and intracranial hypertension have been reported in children receiving topical corticosteroids. Manifestations of adrenal suppression in children include low plasma cortisol levels and an absence of response to ACTH stimulation. Manifestations of intracranial hypertension include bulging fontanelles, headaches, and bilateral papilledema.

ADVERSE REACTIONS

In controlled clinical trials on b.i.d. administration, the total incidence of adverse reactions associated with the use of CUTIVATE Cream was approximately 4%. These adverse reactions were usually mild, self-limiting, and consisted primarily of pruritus, dryness, numbness of fingers, and burning. These events occurred in 2.9%, 1.2%, 1.0%, and 0.6% of patients, respectively.
The following additional local adverse reactions have been reported infrequently with topical corticosteroids (including fluticasone propionate), and they may occur more frequently with the use of occlusive dressings and higher potency corticosteroids. These reactions are listed in an approximately

Continued on next page

This product information is based on labeling in effect on June 1, 1998. For further information, contact via direct mail, phone, or web site Medical Information: Glaxo Wellcome Inc., PO Box 13398, Research Triangle Park, NC 27709. Healthcare Professionals (Medical Information): 800-334-0089 Patients (Customer Response Center): 888-TALK2GW (1-888-825-5249) Glaxo Wellcome Corporate Web Site: www.glaxowellcome.com

Cutivate Cream—Cont.

decreasing order of occurrence: irritation, folliculitis, acneiform eruptions, hypopigmentation, perioral dermatitis, allergic contact dermatitis, secondary infection, skin atrophy, striae, and miliaria. Also, there are reports of the development of pustular psoriasis from chronic plaque psoriasis following reduction or discontinuation of potent topical corticosteroid products.

In a clinical study that compared q.d. and b.i.d. administration of CUTIVATE Cream, the local adverse events that were considered to be drug related were as follows.

Table 1: Drug-Related Adverse Events—Skin

Adverse Events	Fluticasone q.d.	Fluticasone b.i.d.
Skin infection	1 (0.8%)	0
Infected eczema	1 (0.8%)	2 (1.6%)
Viral warts	0	1 (0.8%)
Herpes simplex	0	1 (0.8%)
Impetigo	1 (0.8%)	0
Atopic dermatitis	1 (0.8%)	0
Eczema	1 (0.8%)	0
Exacerbation of eczema	4 (3.0%)	1 (0.8%)
Erythema	0	2 (1.6%)
Burning	0	2 (1.6%)
Stinging	0	1 (0.8%)
Skin irritation	6 (4.5%)	1 (0.8%)
Pruritus	2 (1.5%)	3 (2.3%)
Exacerbation of pruritus	4 (3.0%)	1 (0.8%)
Folliculitis	1 (0.8%)	1 (0.8%)
Blisters	0	1 (0.8%)
Dryness of skin	1 (0.8%)	1 (0.8%)

OVERDOSAGE

Topically applied CUTIVATE Cream can be absorbed in sufficient amounts to produce systemic effects (see PRECAUTIONS).

DOSAGE AND ADMINISTRATION

Eczema: Apply a thin film of CUTIVATE Cream to the affected skin areas once or twice daily. Rub in gently.

Other Corticosteroid-Responsive Dermatoses: Apply a thin film of CUTIVATE Cream to the affected skin areas twice daily. Rub in gently.

As with other corticosteroids, therapy should be discontinued when control is achieved. If no improvement is seen within 2 weeks, reassessment of diagnosis may be necessary.

CUTIVATE Cream should not be used with occlusive dressings.

HOW SUPPLIED

CUTIVATE Cream is supplied in 15-g (NDC 0173-0430-00), 30-g (NDC 0173-0430-01) and 60-g (NDC 0173-0430-02) tubes.

Store between 2° and 30°C (36° and 86°F).

CLINICAL STUDIES

Psoriasis Studies: In two vehicle-controlled studies, CUTIVATE Cream applied twice daily was significantly more effective than the vehicle in the treatment of moderate to severe psoriasis. The investigator's global evaluation after 28 days of treatment is shown in the following table:

Table 2: Physician's Assessment of Clinical Response

	CUTIVATE Cream		Vehicle	
	Study 1 (n = 59)	Study 2 (n = 74)	Study 1 (n = 66)	Study 2 (n = 75)
Cleared	8%	1%	3%	1%
Excellent	29%	28%	11%	17%
Good	27%	34%	20%	28%
Fair	27%	15%	33%	25%
Poor	7%	22%	24%	27%
Worse	2%	0	9%	1%

The clinical signs of psoriasis were scored on a scale of 0 = absent, 1 = mild, 2 = moderate, and 3 = severe. The mean improvement in the clinical signs at the end of treatment are shown in the following table:

Table 3: Signs and Symptoms: Mean Improvement Over Baseline

	CUTIVATE Cream		Vehicle	
	Study 1	Study 2	Study 1	Study 2
Erythema	1.19	1.07	0.55	0.84
Thickening	1.22	1.17	0.81	0.97
Scaling	1.53	1.39	0.95	1.21

Eczema Studies: In two controlled 28-day studies, CUTIVATE Cream q.d. was equivalent to CUTIVATE Cream b.i.d. in the treatment of moderate to severe eczema. The investigator's global evaluation after 28 days of treatment is shown in the following table:

Table 4: Physician's Assessment of Clinical Response

	CUTIVATE Cream q.d.		CUTIVATE Cream b.i.d.	
	Study 1 (n = 64)	Study 2 (n = 106)	Study 1 (n = 65)	Study 2 (n = 100)
Cleared	30%	20%	48%	21%
Excellent	42%	32%	32%	50%
Good	17%	26%	5%	12%
Fair	3%	14%	6%	10%
Poor	5%	3%	8%	6%
Worse	3%	6%	2%	3%

The clinical signs of eczema were scored on a scale of 0 = absent, 1 = mild, 2 = moderate, and 3 = severe. The mean improvement in the clinical signs at the end of treatment are shown in the following table:

Table 5: Signs and Symptoms: Mean Improvement Over Baseline

	CUTIVATE Cream q.d.		CUTIVATE Cream b.i.d.	
	Study 1	Study 2	Study 1	Study 2
Erythema	1.7	1.5	1.8	1.7
Pruritus	2.1	1.6	2.1	1.7
Thickening	1.6	1.3	1.6	1.5
Lichenification	1.2	1.2	1.2	1.3
Vesiculation	0.5	0.4	0.5	0.5
Crusting	0.6	0.7	0.8	0.8

Caution: Federal (U.S.A.) law prohibits dispensing without prescription.

October 1997/RL-486

Shown in Product Identification Guide, page 312

CUTIVATE® ℞
[kyoot 'ə-vāt ″]
(fluticasone propionate ointment)
Ointment, 0.005%

**For Dermatologic Use Only—
Not for Ophthalmic Use.**

DESCRIPTION

CUTIVATE Ointment, 0.005% contains fluticasone propionate [(6α,11β,16α,17α)-6,9,-difluoro-11-hydroxy-16-methyl-3-oxo-17-(1-oxopropoxy) androsta-1,4-diene-17-carbothioic acid, S-fluoromethyl ester], a synthetic fluorinated corticosteroid, for topical dermatologic use. The topical corticosteroids constitute a class of primarily synthetic steroids used as anti-inflammatory and antipruritic agents.

Chemically, fluticasone propionate is $C_{25}H_{31}F_3O_5S$. Fluticasone propionate has a molecular weight of 500.6. It is a white to off-white powder and is insoluble in water.

Each gram of CUTIVATE Ointment contains fluticasone propionate 0.05 mg in a base of propylene glycol, sorbitan sesquioleate, microcrystalline wax, and liquid paraffin.

CLINICAL PHARMACOLOGY

Like other topical corticosteroids, fluticasone propionate has anti-inflammatory, antipruritic, and vasoconstrictive properties. The mechanism of the anti-inflammatory activity of the topical steroids, in general, is unclear. However, corticosteroids are thought to act by the induction of phospholipase A_2 inhibitory proteins, collectively called lipocortins. It is postulated that these proteins control the biosynthesis of potent mediators of inflammation such as prostaglandins and leukotrienes by inhibiting the release of their common precursor, arachidonic acid. Arachidonic acid is released from membrane phospholipids by phospholipase A_2.

Pharmacokinetics: The extent of percutaneous absorption of topical corticosteroids is determined by many factors, including the vehicle and the integrity of the epidermal barrier. Occlusive dressing with hydrocortisone for up to 24 hours has not been demonstrated to increase penetration; however, occlusion of hydrocortisone for 96 hours markedly enhances penetration. Topical corticosteroids can be absorbed from normal intact skin. Inflammation and/or other disease processes in the skin increase percutaneous absorption.

Studies performed with CUTIVATE Ointment indicate that it is in the medium range of potency as compared with other topical corticosteroids.

INDICATIONS AND USAGE

CUTIVATE Ointment is a medium potency corticosteroid indicated for the relief of the inflammatory and pruritic manifestations of corticosteroid-responsive dermatoses.

CONTRAINDICATIONS

CUTIVATE Ointment is contraindicated in those patients with a history of hypersensitivity to any of the components of the preparation.

PRECAUTIONS

General: Systemic absorption of topical corticosteroids can produce reversible hypothalamic-pituitary-adrenal (HPA) axis suppression with the potential for glucocorticosteroid insufficiency after withdrawal from treatment. Manifestations of Cushing's syndrome, hyperglycemia, and glucosuria can also be produced in some patients by systemic absorption of topical corticosteroids while on treatment.

Patients applying a topical steroid to a large surface area or to areas under occlusion should be evaluated periodically for evidence of HPA axis suppression. This may be done by using the ACTH stimulation, A.M. plasma cortisol, and urinary free cortisol tests.

Fluticasone propionate ointment, 0.05% (a concentration 10 times that of fluticasone propionate ointment, 0.005%) suppressed 24-hour urinary free cortisol levels in two of six patients when used at a dose of 30 g/day for a week in patients with psoriasis or atopic eczema. In a second study, fluticasone propionate ointment, 0.05% caused depression of A.M. plasma cortisol levels in 3 of 12 normal volunteers when applied at doses of 50 g/day for 21 days. Morning plasma levels returned to normal levels within the first week upon discontinuation of fluticasone propionate. In this study there was no corresponding decrease in 24-hour urinary free cortisol levels.

If HPA axis suppression is noted, an attempt should be made to withdraw the drug, to reduce the frequency of application, or to substitute a less potent corticosteroid. Recovery of HPA axis function is generally prompt upon discontinuation of topical corticosteroids. Infrequently, signs and symptoms of glucocorticosteroid insufficiency may occur, requiring supplemental systemic corticosteroids. For information on systemic supplementation, see prescribing information for those products.

Children may be more susceptible to systemic toxicity from equivalent doses due to their larger skin surface to body mass ratios (see PRECAUTIONS: Pediatric Use).

If irritation develops, CUTIVATE Ointment should be discontinued and appropriate therapy instituted. Allergic contact dermatitis with corticosteroids is usually diagnosed by observing failure to heal rather than noting a clinical exacerbation as with most topical products not containing corticosteroids. Such an observation should be corroborated with appropriate diagnostic patch testing.

If concomitant skin infections are present or develop, an appropriate antifungal or antibacterial agent should be used. If a favorable response does not occur promptly, use of CUTIVATE Ointment should be discontinued until the infection has been adequately controlled.

CUTIVATE Ointment should not be used in the treatment of preexisting skin atrophy and should not be used where infection is present at the treatment site. CUTIVATE Ointment should not be used in the treatment of rosacea and perioral dermatitis.

Information for Patients: Patients using topical corticosteroids should receive the following information and instructions:

1. This medication is to be used as directed by the physician. It is for external use only. Avoid contact with the eyes.
2. This medication should not be used for any disorder other than that for which it was prescribed.
3. The treated skin area should not be bandaged or otherwise covered or wrapped so as to be occlusive unless directed by the physician.
4. Patients should report to their physician any signs of local adverse reactions.

Laboratory Tests: The following tests may be helpful in evaluating patients for HPA axis suppression:
ACTH stimulation test
A.M. plasma cortisol test
Urinary free cortisol test

Carcinogenesis, Mutagenesis, and Impairment of Fertility: Two 18-month studies were performed in mice to evaluate the carcinogenic potential of fluticasone propionate when given topically (as an 0.05% ointment) and orally. No evidence of carcinogenicity was found in either study.

Fluticasone propionate was not mutagenic in the standard Ames test, *E. coli* fluctuation test, *S. cerevisiae* gene conversion test, or Chinese Hamster ovarian cell assay. It was not clastogenic in mouse micronucleus or cultured human lymphocyte tests.

In a fertility and general reproductive performance study in rats, fluticasone propionate administered subcutaneously to females at up to 50 µg/kg per day and to males at up to 100 µg/kg per day (later reduced to 50 µg/kg per day) had no effect upon mating performance or fertility. These doses are approximately 150 and 300 times, respectively, the human systemic exposure following use of the recommended human topical dose of fluticasone propionate ointment, 0.005%, assuming human percutaneous absorption of approximately 3% and the use in a 70-kg person of 15 g/day.

Pregnancy: ***Teratogenic Effects: Pregnancy Category C:*** Corticosteroids have been shown to be teratogenic in laboratory animals when administered systemically at relatively low dosage levels. Some corticosteroids have been shown to be teratogenic after dermal application in laboratory animals. Teratology studies in the mouse demonstrated fluticasone propionate to be teratogenic (cleft palate) when administered subcutaneously in doses of 45 µg/kg per day and 150 µg/kg per day. This dose is approximately 140 and 450 times, respectively, the human topical dose of fluticasone propionate ointment, 0.005%. There are no adequate and well-controlled studies in pregnant women. CUTIVATE Ointment should be used during pregnancy only if the potential benefit justifies the potential risk to the fetus.

Nursing Mothers: Systemically administered corticosteroids appear in human milk and could suppress growth, interfere with endogenous corticosteroid production, or cause other untoward effects. It is not known whether topical administration of corticosteroids could result in sufficient systemic absorption to produce detectable quantities in human milk. Because many drugs are excreted in human milk, caution should be exercised when CUTIVATE Ointment is administered to a nursing woman.

Pediatric Use: Safety and effectiveness in pediatric patients have not been established. Because of a higher ratio of skin surface area to body mass, pediatric patients are at a greater risk than adults of HPA axis suppression and Cushing's syndrome when they are treated with topical corticosteroids. They are therefore also at greater risk of adrenal insufficiency during or after withdrawal of treatment. Adverse effects including striae have been reported with inappropriate use of topical corticosteroids in pediatric patients.

HPA axis suppression, Cushing's syndrome, linear growth retardation, delayed weight gain, and intracranial hypertension have been reported in pediatric patients receiving topical corticosteroids. Manifestations of adrenal suppression in pediatric patients include low plasma cortisol levels and an absence of response to ACTH stimulation. Manifestations of intracranial hypertension include bulging fontanelles, headaches, and bilateral papilledema.

ADVERSE REACTIONS

In controlled clinical trials, the total incidence of adverse reactions associated with the use of CUTIVATE Ointment was approximately 4%. These adverse reactions were usually mild, self-limiting, and consisted primarily of pruritus, burning, hypertrichosis, increased erythema, hives, irritation, and lightheadedness. Each of these events occurred individually in less than 1% of patients.

The following additional local adverse reactions have been reported infrequently with topical corticosteroids, including fluticasone propionate, and they may occur more frequently with the use of occlusive dressings and higher potency corticosteroids. These reactions are listed in an approximately decreasing order of occurrence: dryness, folliculitis, acneiform eruptions, hypopigmentation, perioral dermatitis, allergic contact dermatitis, secondary infection, skin atrophy, striae, and miliaria. Also, there are reports of the development of pustular psoriasis from chronic plaque psoriasis following reduction or discontinuation of potent topical corticosteroid products.

OVERDOSAGE

Topically applied CUTIVATE Ointment can be absorbed in sufficient amounts to produce systemic effects (see PRECAUTIONS).

DOSAGE AND ADMINISTRATION

Apply a thin film of CUTIVATE Ointment to the affected skin areas twice daily. Rub in gently.

HOW SUPPLIED

CUTIVATE Ointment, 0.005% is supplied in 15-g (NDC 0173-0431-00), 30-g (NDC 0173-0431-01), and 60-g (NDC 0173-0431-02) tubes.

Store between 2° and 30°C (36° and 86°F).

September 1996/RL-360

Shown in Product Identification Guide, page 312

DARAPRIM® ℞

[*dair 'ah-prĭm "*]

(pyrimethamine)

25 mg Scored Tablets

DESCRIPTION

DARAPRIM (pyrimethamine) is an antiparasitic compound available in tablet form for oral administration.

Each scored tablet contains 25 mg pyrimethamine and the inactive ingredients corn and potato starch, lactose, and magnesium stearate.

Pyrimethamine is known chemically as 5-(4-chlorophenyl)-6-ethyl-2,4-pyrimidinediamine.

CLINICAL PHARMACOLOGY

Pyrimethamine is well absorbed with peak levels occurring between 2 to 6 hours following administration. It is eliminated slowly and has a plasma half-life of approximately 96 hours. Pyrimethamine is 87% bound to human plasma proteins.

Microbiology: Pyrimethamine is a folic acid antagonist and the rationale for its therapeutic action is based on the differential requirement between host and parasite for nucleic acid precursors involved in growth. This activity is highly selective against plasmodia and *Toxoplasma gondii*. Pyrimethamine possesses blood schizonticidal and some tissue schizonticidal activity against malaria parasites of humans. However, the 4-amino-quinoline compounds are more effective against the erythrocytic schizonts. It does not destroy gametocytes, but arrests sporogony in the mosquito.

The action of pyrimethamine against *Toxoplasma gondii* is greatly enhanced when used in conjunction with sulfonamides. This was demonstrated by Eyles and Coleman[1] in the treatment of experimental toxoplasmosis in the mouse. Jacobs et al[2] demonstrated that combination of the two drugs effectively prevented the development of severe uveitis in most rabbits following the inoculation of the anterior chamber of the eye with toxoplasma.

INDICATIONS AND USAGE

Treatment of Toxoplasmosis: DARAPRIM is indicated for the treatment of toxoplasmosis when used conjointly with a sulfonamide, since synergism exists with this combination.

Treatment of Acute Malaria: DARAPRIM is also indicated for the treatment of acute malaria. It should not be used alone to treat acute malaria. Fast-acting schizonticides such as chloroquine or quinine are indicated and preferable for the treatment of acute malaria. However, conjoint use of DARAPRIM with a sulfonamide (e.g., sulfadoxine) will initiate transmission control and suppression of susceptible strains of plasmodia.

Chemoprophylaxis of Malaria: DARAPRIM is indicated for the chemoprophylaxis of malaria due to susceptible strains of plasmodia. However, resistance to pyrimethamine is prevalent worldwide. It is not suitable as a prophylactic agent for travelers to most areas.

CONTRAINDICATIONS

Use of DARAPRIM is contraindicated in patients with known hypersensitivity to pyrimethamine. Use of the drug is also contraindicated in patients with documented megaloblastic anemia due to folate deficiency.

WARNINGS

The dosage of pyrimethamine required for the treatment of toxoplasmosis is 10 to 20 times the recommended antimalaria dosage and approaches the toxic level. If signs of folate deficiency develop (see ADVERSE REACTIONS), reduce the dosage or discontinue the drug according to the response of the patient. Folinic acid (leucovorin) should be administered in a dosage of 5 to 15 mg daily (orally, IV, or IM) until normal hematopoiesis is restored.

Data in two humans indicate that pyrimethamine may be carcinogenic: a 51-year-old female who developed chronic granulocytic leukemia after taking pyrimethamine for 2 years for toxoplasmosis,[3] and a 56-year-old patient who developed reticulum cell sarcoma after 14 months of pyrimethamine for toxoplasmosis.[4] Pyrimethamine has been reported to produce a significant increase in the number of lung tumors in mice when given intraperitoneally at doses of 25 mg/kg.[5]

DARAPRIM should be kept out of the reach of infants and children as they are extremely susceptible to adverse effects from an overdose. Deaths in pediatric patients have been reported after accidental ingestion.

PRECAUTIONS

General: The recommended dosage for chemoprophylaxis of malaria should not be exceeded. A small "starting" dose for toxoplasmosis is recommended in patients with convulsive disorders to avoid the potential nervous system toxicity of pyrimethamine. DARAPRIM should be used with caution in patients with impaired renal or hepatic function or in patients with possible folate deficiency, such as individuals with malabsorption syndrome, alcoholism, or pregnancy, and those receiving therapy, such as phenytoin, affecting folate levels (see Pregnancy subsection).

Information for Patients: Patients should be warned that at the first appearance of a skin rash they should stop use of DARAPRIM and seek medical attention immediately. Patients should also be warned that the appearance of sore throat, pallor, purpura, or glossitis may be early indications of serious disorders which require treatment with DARAPRIM to be stopped and medical treatment to be sought.

Women of childbearing potential who are taking DARAPRIM should be warned against becoming pregnant.

Patients should be warned to keep DARAPRIM out of the reach of children. Patients should be advised not to exceed recommended doses. Patients should be warned that if anorexia and vomiting occur, they may be minimized by taking the drug with meals.

Concurrent administration of folinic acid is strongly recommended when used for the treatment of toxoplasmosis in all patients.

Laboratory Tests: In patients receiving high dosage, as for the treatment of toxoplasmosis, semiweekly blood counts, including platelet counts, should be performed.

Drug Interactions: Pyrimethamine may be used with sulfonamides, quinine and other antimalarials, and with other antibiotics. However, the concomitant use of other antifolic drugs, such as sulfonamides or trimethoprim-sulfamethoxazole combinations, while the patient is receiving pyrimethamine, may increase the risk of bone marrow suppression. If signs of folate deficiency develop, pyrimethamine should be discontinued.

Folinic acid (leucovorin) should be administered until normal hematopoiesis is restored (see WARNINGS). Mild hepatotoxicity has been reported in some patients when lorazepam and pyrimethamine were administered concomitantly.

Carcinogenesis, Mutagenesis, Impairment of Fertility: See WARNINGS section for information on carcinogenesis.

Mutagenesis: Pyrimethamine has been shown to be nonmutagenic in the following in vitro assays: the Ames point mutation assay, the Rec assay, and the *E. coli* WP2 assay. It was positive in the L5178Y/TK +/- mouse lymphoma assay in the absence of exogenous metabolic activation.[6] Human blood lymphocytes cultured in vitro had structural chromosome aberrations induced by pyrimethamine.

In vivo, chromosomes analyzed from the bone marrow of rats dosed with pyrimethamine showed an increased number of structural and numerical aberrations.

Pregnancy: ***Teratogenic Effects:*** Pregnancy Category C. Pyrimethamine has been shown to be teratogenic in rats when given in oral doses 7 times the human dose for chemoprophylaxis of malaria or 2.5 times the human dose for treatment of toxoplasmosis. At these doses in rats, there was a significant increase in abnormalities such as cleft palate, brachygnathia, oligodactyly, and microphthalmia. Pyrimethamine has also been shown to produce terata such as meningocele in hamsters and cleft palate in miniature pigs when given in oral doses 170 and 5 times the human dose, respectively, for chemoprophylaxis of malaria or for treatment of toxoplasmosis.

There are no adequate and well-controlled studies in pregnant women. DARAPRIM should be used during pregnancy only if the potential benefit justifies the potential risk to the fetus.

Concurrent administration of folinic acid is strongly recommended when used for the treatment of toxoplasmosis during pregnancy.

Nursing Mothers: Pyrimethamine is excreted in human milk. Because of the potential for serious adverse reactions in nursing infants from pyrimethamine, a decision should be made whether to discontinue nursing or to discontinue the drug, taking into account the importance of the drug to the mother (see WARNINGS and PRECAUTIONS: Pregnancy).

Pediatric Use: See DOSAGE AND ADMINISTRATION section.

ADVERSE REACTIONS

Hypersensitivity reactions, occasionally severe (such as Stevens-Johnson syndrome, toxic epidermal necrolysis, erythema multiforme, and anaphylaxis), and hyperphenylalaninemia, can occur particularly when pyrimethamine is administered concomitantly with a sulfonamide. With doses of pyrimethamine used for the treatment of toxoplasmosis, anorexia and vomiting may occur. Vomiting may be minimized by giving the medication with meals; it usually disappears promptly upon reduction of dosage. Doses used in toxoplasmosis may produce megaloblastic anemia, leukopenia, thrombocytopenia, pancytopenia, atrophic glossitis, hematuria, and disorders of cardiac rhythm. Hematologic effects, however, may also occur at low doses in certain individuals (see PRECAUTIONS: General).

Pulmonary eosinophilia has been reported rarely.

OVERDOSAGE

Following the ingestion of 300 mg or more of pyrimethamine, gastrointestinal and/or central nervous system signs

Continued on next page

This product information is based on labeling in effect on June 1, 1998. For further information, contact via direct mail, phone, or web site Medical Information: Glaxo Wellcome Inc., PO Box 13398, Research Triangle Park, NC 27709. Healthcare Professionals (Medical Information): 800-334-0089 Patients (Customer Response Center): 888-TALK2GW (1-888-825-5249) Glaxo Wellcome Corporate Web Site: www.glaxowellcome.com

Daraprim—Cont.

may be present, including convulsions. The initial symptoms are usually gastrointestinal and may include abdominal pain, nausea, severe and repeated vomiting, possibly including hematemesis. Central nervous system toxicity may be manifest by initial excitability, generalized and prolonged convulsions which may be followed by respiratory depression, circulatory collapse, and death within a few hours. Neurological symptoms appear rapidly (30 minutes to 2 hours after drug ingestion), suggesting that in gross overdosage pyrimethamine has a direct toxic effect on the central nervous system.

The fatal dose is variable, with the smallest reported fatal single dose being 375 mg. There are, however, reports of pediatric patients who have recovered after taking 375 to 625 mg.

There is no specific antidote to acute pyrimethamine poisoning. In the event of overdosage, symptomatic and supportive measures should be employed. Gastric lavage is recommended and is effective if carried out very soon after drug ingestion. Parenteral diazepam may be used to control convulsions. Folinic acid should also be administered within 2 hours of drug ingestion to be most effective in counteracting the effects on the hematopoietic system (see WARNINGS). Due to the long half-life of pyrimethamine, daily monitoring of peripheral blood counts is recommended for up to several weeks after the overdose until normal hematologic values are restored.

DOSAGE AND ADMINISTRATION

For Treatment of Toxoplasmosis: The dosage of DARAPRIM for the treatment of toxoplasmosis must be carefully adjusted so as to provide maximum therapeutic effect and a minimum of side effects. At the dosage required, there is a marked variation in the tolerance to the drug. Young patients may tolerate higher doses than older individuals. Concurrent administration of folinic acid is strongly recommended in all patients.

The adult *starting* dose is 50 to 75 mg of the drug daily, together with 1 to 4 g daily of a sulfonamide of the sulfapyrimidine type, e.g., sulfadoxine. This dosage is ordinarily continued for 1 to 3 weeks, depending on the response of the patient and tolerance to therapy. The dosage may then be reduced to about one-half that previously given for each drug and continued for an additional 4 to 5 weeks.

The pediatric dosage of DARAPRIM is 1 mg/kg per day divided into two equal daily doses; after 2 to 4 days this dose may be reduced to one-half and continued for approximately 1 month. The usual pediatric sulfonamide dosage is used in conjunction with DARAPRIM.

For Treatment of Acute Malaria: DARAPRIM is NOT recommended alone in the treatment of acute malaria. Fast-acting schizonticides, such as chloroquine or quinine, are indicated for treatment of acute malaria. However, DARAPRIM at a dosage of 25 mg daily for 2 days with a sulfonamide will initiate transmission control and suppression of non-falciparum malaria. DARAPRIM is only recommended for patients infected in areas where susceptible plasmodia exist. Should circumstances arise wherein DARAPRIM must be used alone in semi-immune persons, the adult dosage for acute malaria is 50 mg for 2 days; children 4 through 10 years old may be given 25 mg daily for 2 days. In any event, clinical cure should be followed by the once-weekly regimen described below for chemoprophylaxis. Regimens which include suppression should be extended through any characteristic periods of early recrudescence and late relapse, i.e., for at least 10 weeks in each case.

For Chemoprophylaxis of Malaria:

Adults and pediatric patients over 10 years—25 mg (1 tablet) once weekly

Children 4 through 10 years—12.5 mg (½ tablet) once weekly

Infants and children under 4 years—6.25 mg (¼ tablet) once weekly

HOW SUPPLIED

White, scored tablets containing 25 mg pyrimethamine, imprinted with "DARAPRIM" and "A3A" in bottles of 100 (NDC 0173-0201-55).

Store at 15° to 25°C (59° to 77°F) in a dry place and protect from light.

REFERENCES

1. Eyles DE, Coleman N. Synergistic effect of sulfadiazine and Daraprim against experimental toxoplasmosis in the mouse. *Antibiot Chemother.* 1953;3:483-490.
2. Jacobs L, Melton ML, Kaufman HE. Treatment of experimental ocular toxoplasmosis. *Arch Ophthalmol.* 1964;71:111-118.
3. Jim RTS, Elizaga FV. Development of chronic granulocytic leukemia in a patient treated with pyrimethamine. *Hawaii Med J.* 1977;36:173-176.
4. Sadoff L. Antimalarial drugs and Burkitt's lymphoma. *Lancet.* 1973;2:1262-1263.
5. Bahna L. Pyrimethamine. *LARC Monogr Eval Carcinog Risk Chem.* 1977;13:233-242.
6. Clive D, Johnson KO, Spector JKS, et al. Validation and characterization of the L5178Y/TK +/- mouse lymphoma mutagen assay system. *Mut Res.* 1979;59:61-108.

April 1998/RL-560

Shown in Product Identification Guide, page 312

DIGIBIND® ℞
[*dĭ 'gi-bīnd*]
DIGOXIN IMMUNE FAB (OVINE)

DESCRIPTION

DIGIBIND, Digoxin Immune Fab (Ovine), is a sterile lyophilized powder of antigen binding fragments (Fab) derived from specific antidigoxin antibodies raised in sheep. Production of antibodies specific for digoxin involves conjugation of digoxin as a hapten to human albumin. Sheep are immunized with this material to produce antibodies specific for the antigenic determinants of the digoxin molecule. The antibody is then papain-digested and digoxin-specific Fab fragments of the antibody are isolated and purified by affinity chromatography. These antibody fragments have a molecular weight of approximately 46,200.

Each vial, which will bind approximately 0.5 mg of digoxin (or digitoxin), contains 38 mg of digoxin-specific Fab fragments derived from sheep plus 75 mg of sorbitol as a stabilizer and 28 mg of sodium chloride. The vial contains no preservatives.

DIGIBIND is administered by intravenous injection after reconstitution with Sterile Water for Injection (4 mL per vial).

CLINICAL PHARMACOLOGY

After intravenous injection of Digoxin Immune Fab (Ovine) in the baboon, digoxin-specific Fab fragments are excreted in the urine with a biological half-life of about 9 to 13 hours.[1] In humans with normal renal function the half-life appears to be 15 to 20 hours.[2] Experimental studies in animals indicate that these antibody fragments have a large volume of distribution in the extracellular space, unlike whole antibody which distributes in a space only about twice the plasma volume.[1] Ordinarily, following administration of DIGIBIND, improvement in signs and symptoms of digitalis intoxication begins within one-half hour or less.[2,3,4,5]

The affinity of DIGIBIND for digoxin is in the range of 10^9 to 10^{11} M^{-1}, which is greater than the affinity of digoxin for (sodium, potassium) ATPase, the presumed receptor for its toxic effects. The affinity of DIGIBIND for digitoxin is about 10^8 to 10^9 M^{-1}.

DIGIBIND binds molecules of digoxin, making them unavailable for binding at their site of action on cells in the body. The Fab fragment-digoxin complex accumulates in the blood, from which it is excreted by the kidney. The net effect is to shift the equilibrium away from binding of digoxin to its receptors in the body, thereby reversing its effects.

INDICATIONS AND USAGE

DIGIBIND, Digoxin Immune Fab (Ovine), is indicated for treatment of potentially life-threatening digoxin intoxication.[3] Although designed specifically to treat life-threatening digoxin overdose, it has also been used successfully to treat life-threatening digitoxin overdose.[3] Since human experience is limited and the consequences of repeated exposures are unknown, DIGIBIND is not indicated for milder cases of digitalis toxicity.

Manifestations of life-threatening toxicity include severe ventricular arrhythmias such as ventricular tachycardia or ventricular fibrillation, or progressive bradyarrhythmias such as severe sinus bradycardia or second or third degree heart block not responsive to atropine.

Ingestion of more than 10 mg of digoxin in previously healthy adults or 4 mg of digoxin in previously healthy children, or ingestion causing steady-state serum concentrations greater than 10 ng/mL, often results in cardiac arrest. Digitalis-induced progressive elevation of the serum potassium concentration also suggests imminent cardiac arrest. If the potassium concentration exceeds 5 mEq/L in the setting of severe digitalis intoxication, therapy with DIGIBIND is indicated.

CONTRAINDICATIONS

There are no known contraindications to the use of DIGIBIND.

WARNINGS

Suicidal ingestion often involves more than one drug; thus, toxicity from other drugs should not be overlooked.

One should consider the possibility of anaphylactic, hypersensitivity, or febrile reactions. If an anaphylactoid reaction occurs, the drug infusion should be discontinued and appropriate therapy initiated using aminophylline, oxygen, volume expansion, diphenhydramine, corticosteroids and airway management as indicated. The need for epinephrine should be balanced against its potential risk in the setting of digitalis toxicity.

Since the Fab fragment of the antibody lacks the antigenic determinants of the Fc fragment, it should pose less of an immunogenic threat to patients than does an intact immunoglobulin molecule. Patients with known allergies would be particularly at risk, as would individuals who have previously received antibodies or Fab fragments raised in sheep. Papain is used to cleave the whole antibody into Fab and Fc fragments, and traces of papain or inactivated papain residues may be present in DIGIBIND. Patients with allergies to papain, chymopapain, or other papaya extracts also may be particularly at risk.

Skin testing for allergy was performed during the clinical investigation of DIGIBIND. Only one patient developed erythema at the site of skin testing, with no accompanying wheal reaction; this individual had no adverse reaction to systemic treatment with DIGIBIND. Since allergy testing can delay urgently needed therapy, it is not routinely required before treatment of life-threatening digitalis toxicity with DIGIBIND.

Skin testing may be appropriate for high risk individuals, especially patients with known allergies or those previously treated with Digoxin Immune Fab (Ovine). The intradermal skin test can be performed by: 1. Diluting 0.1 mL of reconstituted DIGIBIND (9.5 mg/mL) in 9.9 mL sterile isotonic saline (1:100 dilution, 95 mcg/mL). 2. Injecting 0.1 mL of the 1:100 dilution (95 mcg) intradermally and observing for an urticarial wheal surrounded by a zone of erythema. The test should be read at 20 minutes.

The scratch test procedure is performed by placing one drop of a 1:100 dilution of DIGIBIND on the skin and then making a ¼-inch scratch through the drop with a sterile needle. The scratch site is inspected at 20 minutes for an urticarial wheal surrounded by erythema.

If skin testing causes a systemic reaction, a tourniquet should be applied above the site of testing and measures to treat anaphylaxis should be instituted. Further administration of DIGIBIND should be avoided unless its use is absolutely essential, in which case the patient should be pretreated with corticosteroids and diphenhydramine. The physician should be prepared to treat anaphylaxis.

PRECAUTIONS

General: Standard therapy for digitalis intoxication includes withdrawal of the drug and correction of factors that may contribute to toxicity, such as electrolyte disturbances, hypoxia, acid-base disturbances and agents such as catecholamines. Also, treatment of arrhythmias may include judicious potassium supplements, lidocaine, phenytoin, procainamide and/or propranolol; treatment of sinus bradycardia or atrioventricular block may involve atropine or pacemaker insertion. Massive digitalis intoxication can cause hyperkalemia; administration of potassium supplements in the setting of massive intoxication may be hazardous (see Laboratory Tests). After treatment with DIGIBIND, the serum potassium concentration may drop rapidly[2] and must be monitored frequently, especially over the first several hours after DIGIBIND is given (see Laboratory Tests).

The elimination half-life in the setting of renal failure has not been clearly defined. Patients with renal dysfunction have been successfully treated with DIGIBIND.[4] There is no evidence to suggest the time-course of therapeutic effect is any different in these patients than in patients with normal renal function, but excretion of the Fab fragment-digoxin complex from the body is probably delayed. In patients who are functionally anephric, one would anticipate failure to clear the Fab fragment-digoxin complex from the blood by glomerular filtration and renal excretion. Whether failure to eliminate the Fab fragment-digoxin complex in severe renal failure can lead to reintoxication following release of newly unbound digoxin into the blood is uncertain. Such patients should be monitored for a prolonged period for possible recurrence of digitalis toxicity.

Patients with intrinsically poor cardiac function may deteriorate from withdrawal of the inotropic action of digoxin. Studies in animals have shown that the reversal of inotropic effect is relatively gradual, occurring over hours. When needed, additional support can be provided by use of intravenous inotropes, such as dopamine or dobutamine, or vasodilators. One must be careful in using catecholamines not to aggravate digitalis toxic rhythm disturbances. Clearly, other types of digitalis glycosides should not be used in this setting.

Redigitalization should be postponed, if possible, until the Fab fragments have been eliminated from the body, which may require several days. Patients with impaired renal function may require a week or longer.

Laboratory Tests: DIGIBIND will interfere with digitalis immunoassay measurements.[6] Thus, the standard serum digoxin concentration measurement can be clinically misleading until the Fab fragment is eliminated from the body.

Serum digoxin or digitoxin concentration should be obtained before administration of DIGIBIND if at all possible. These measurements may be difficult to interpret if drawn soon after the last digitalis dose, since at least 6 to 8 hours are required for equilibration of digoxin between serum and tissue. Patients should be closely monitored, including tem-

TABLE 2: Adult Dose Estimate of DIGIBIND (in # of vials) from Steady-State Serum Digoxin Concentration

Patient Weight (kg)	Serum Digoxin Concentration (ng/mL)						
	1	2	4	8	12	16	20
40	0.5 V	1 V	2 V	3 V	5 V	7 V	8 V
60	0.5 V	1 V	3 V	5 V	7 V	10 V	12 V
70	1 V	2 V	3 V	6 V	9 V	11 V	14 V
80	1 V	2 V	3 V	7 V	10 V	13 V	16 V
100	1 V	2 V	4 V	8 V	12 V	16 V	20 V

V = vials

TABLE 3: Infants and Small Children Dose Estimates of DIGIBIND (in mg) from Steady-State Serum Digoxin Concentration

Patient Weight (kg)	Serum Digoxin Concentration (ng/mL)						
	1	2	4	8	12	16	20
1	0.4* mg	1* mg	1.5* mg	3* mg	5 mg	6 mg	8 mg
3	1* mg	2* mg	5 mg	9 mg	14 mg	18 mg	23 mg
5	2* mg	4 mg	8 mg	15 mg	23 mg	30 mg	38 mg
10	4 mg	8 mg	15 mg	30 mg	46 mg	61 mg	76 mg
20	8 mg	15 mg	30 mg	61 mg	91 mg	122 mg	152 mg

* Dilution of reconstituted vial to 1 mg/mL may be desirable.

TABLE 1: Approximate Dose of DIGIBIND for Reversal of a Single Large Digoxin Overdose

Number of DIGOXIN Tablets or Capsules Ingested*	Dose of DIGIBIND # of Vials
25	10
50	20
75	30
100	40
150	60
200	80

* 0.25 mg tablets with 80% bioavailability or 0.2 mg LANOXICAPS® Capsules with 100% bioavailability.

Calculations Based on Steady-State Serum Digoxin Concentrations: Table 2 gives dosage estimates in number of vials for **adult patients** for whom a steady-state serum digoxin concentration is known. The dose of DIGIBIND (in number of vials) represented in Table 2 can be approximated using the following formula:

Formula 2

$$\text{Dose (in \# of vials)} = \frac{\text{(Serum digoxin concentration in ng/mL) (weight in kg)}}{100}$$

[See table 2 above]

Table 3 gives dosage estimates in milligrams **for infants and small children** based on the steady-state serum digoxin concentration. The dose of DIGIBIND represented in Table 3 can be estimated by multiplying the dose (in number of vials) calculated from Formula 2 by the amount of DIGIBIND contained in a vial (38 mg/vial) (see Formula 3). Since infants and small children can have much smaller dosage requirements, it is recommended that the 38-mg vial be reconstituted as directed and administered with a tuberculin syringe. For very small doses, a reconstituted vial can be diluted with 34 mL of sterile isotonic saline to achieve a concentration of 1 mg/mL.

Formula 3

Dose (in mg) = (Dose [in # of vials]) (38 mg/vial)

[See table 3 above]

Calculation Based on Steady-State Digitoxin Concentration: The DIGIBIND dose for digitoxin toxicity can be approximated using the following formula:

Formula 4

$$\text{Dose (in \# of vials)} = \frac{\text{(Serum digitoxin concentration in ng/mL) (weight in kg)}}{1000}$$

If the dose based on ingested amount differs substantially from that calculated from the serum digoxin or digitoxin concentration, it may be preferable to use the higher dose.

ADMINISTRATION: The contents in each vial to be used should be dissolved with 4 mL of Sterile Water for Injection, by gentle mixing, to give a clear, colorless, approximately isosmotic solution with a protein concentration of 9.5 mg/mL. Reconstituted product should be used promptly. If it is not used immediately, it may be stored under refrigeration at 2 to 8°C (36 to 46°F) for up to 4 hours. The reconstituted product may be diluted with sterile isotonic saline to a convenient volume. Parenteral drug products should be inspected visually for particulate matter and discoloration prior to administration, whenever solution and container permit.

DIGIBIND, Digoxin Immune Fab (Ovine), is administered by the intravenous route over 30 minutes. It is recommended that it be infused through a 0.22 micron membrane filter to ensure no undissolved particulate matter is administered. If cardiac arrest is imminent, it can be given as a bolus injection.

HOW SUPPLIED

Vials containing 38 mg of purified lyophilized digoxin-specific Fab fragments. Box of 1. (NDC 0173-0230-44).

STORAGE

Refrigerate at 2 to 8°C (36 to 46°F). Unreconstituted vials can be stored at up to 30°C (86°F) for a total of 30 days.

Continued on next page

This product information is based on labeling in effect on June 1, 1998. For further information, contact via direct mail, phone, or web site Medical Information: Glaxo Wellcome Inc., PO Box 13398, Research Triangle Park, NC 27709. Healthcare Professionals (Medical Information): 800-334-0089 Patients (Customer Response Center): 888-TALK2GW (1-888-825-5249) Glaxo Wellcome Corporate Web Site: www.glaxowellcome.com

perature, blood pressure, electrocardiogram and potassium concentration, during and after administration of DIGIBIND. The total serum digoxin concentration may rise precipitously following administration of DIGIBIND, but this will be almost entirely bound to the Fab fragment and therefore not able to react with receptors in the body.

Potassium concentrations should be followed carefully. Severe digitalis intoxication can cause life-threatening elevation in serum potassium concentration by shifting potassium from inside to outside the cell. The elevation in serum potassium concentration can lead to increased renal excretion of potassium. Thus, these patients may have hyperkalemia with a total body deficit of potassium. When the effect of digitalis is reversed by DIGIBIND, potassium shifts back inside the cell, with a resulting decline in serum potassium concentration.[4] Hypokalemia may thus develop rapidly. For these reasons, serum potassium concentration should be monitored repeatedly, especially over the first several hours after DIGIBIND is given, and cautiously treated when necessary.

Carcinogenesis, Mutagenesis, Impairment of Fertility: There have been no long-term studies performed in animals to evaluate carcinogenic potential.

Pregnancy: Pregnancy Category C. Animal reproduction studies have not been conducted with DIGIBIND. It is also not known whether DIGIBIND can cause fetal harm when administered to a pregnant woman or can affect reproduction capacity. DIGIBIND should be given to a pregnant woman only if clearly needed.

Nursing Mothers: It is not known whether this drug is excreted in human milk. Because many drugs are excreted in human milk, caution should be exercised when DIGIBIND is administered to a nursing woman.

Pediatric Use: DIGIBIND has been successfully used in infants with no apparent adverse sequelae. As in all other circumstances, use of this drug in infants should be based on careful consideration of the benefits of the drug balanced against the potential risk involved.

ADVERSE REACTIONS

Allergic reactions to DIGIBIND have been reported rarely. Patients with a history of allergy, especially to antibiotics, appear to be at particular risk (see WARNINGS). In a few instances, low cardiac output states and congestive heart failure could have been exacerbated by withdrawal of the inotropic effects of digitalis. Hypokalemia may occur from re-activation of (sodium, potassium) ATPase (see Laboratory Tests). Patients with atrial fibrillation may develop a rapid ventricular response from withdrawal of the effects of digitalis on the atrioventricular node.[4]

DOSAGE AND ADMINISTRATION

GENERAL GUIDELINES:

The dosage of DIGIBIND varies according to the amount of digoxin (or digitoxin) to be neutralized. The average dose used during clinical testing was 10 vials.

Dosage for Acute Ingestion of Unknown Amount: Twenty (20) vials (760 mg) of DIGIBIND is adequate to treat most life-threatening ingestions in both **adults and children**. However, in children it is important to monitor for volume overload. In general, a large dose of DIGIBIND has a faster onset of effect but may enhance the possibility of a febrile reaction. The physician may consider administering 10 vials, observing the patient's response, and following with an additional 10 vials if clinically indicated.

Dosage for Toxicity During Chronic Therapy: For adults, six vials (228 mg) usually is adequate to reverse most cases of toxicity. This dose can be used in patients who are in acute distress or for whom a serum digoxin or digitoxin concentration is not available. In infants and small children (≤ 20 kg) a single vial usually should suffice. Methods for calculating the dose of DIGIBIND required to neutralize the known or estimated amount of digoxin or digitoxin in the body are given below (see DOSAGE CALCULATION section).

When determining the dose for DIGIBIND, the following guidelines should be considered:

— Erroneous calculations may result from inaccurate estimates of the amount of digitalis ingested or absorbed or from nonsteady-state serum digitalis concentrations. Inaccurate serum digitalis concentration measurements are a possible source of error. Most serum digoxin assay kits are designed to measure values less than 5 ng/mL. Dilution of samples is required to obtain accurate measures above 5 ng/mL.

— Dosage calculations are based on a steady-state volume of distribution of approximately 5 L/kg for digoxin (0.5 L/kg for digitoxin) to convert serum digitalis concentration to the amount of digitalis in the body. The conversion is based on the principle that body load equals drug steady-state serum concentration multiplied by volume of distribution. These volumes are population averages and vary widely among individuals. Many patients may require higher doses for complete neutralization. Doses should ordinarily be rounded up to the next whole vial.

— If toxicity has not adequately reversed after several hours or appears to recur, readministration of DIGIBIND at a dose guided by clinical judgment may be required.

— Failure to respond to DIGIBIND raises the possibility that the clinical problem is not caused by digitalis intoxication. If there is no response to an adequate dose of DIGIBIND, the diagnosis of digitalis toxicity should be questioned.

DOSAGE CALCULATION:

Acute Ingestion of Known Amount: Each vial of DIGIBIND contains 38 mg of purified digoxin-specific Fab fragments which will bind approximately 0.5 mg of digoxin (or digitoxin). Thus one can calculate the total number of vials required by dividing the total digitalis body load in mg by 0.5 mg/vial (see Formula 1).

For toxicity from an acute ingestion, total body load in milligrams will be approximately equal to the amount ingested in milligrams for digoxin capsules and digitoxin, or the amount ingested in milligrams multiplied by 0.80 (to account for incomplete absorption) for digoxin tablets.

Table 1 gives dosage estimates in number of vials for **adults and children** who have ingested a single large dose of digoxin and for whom the approximate number of tablets or capsules is known. The dose of DIGIBIND (in number of vials) represented in Table 1 can be approximated using the following formula:

Formula 1

$$\text{Dose (in \# of vials)} = \frac{\text{Total digitalis body load in mg}}{0.5 \text{ mg of digitalis bound/vial}}$$

Digibind—Cont.

REFERENCES

1. Smith TW, Lloyd BL, Spicer N, Haber E. Immunogenicity and kinetics of distribution and elimination of sheep digoxin-specific IgG and Fab fragments in the rabbit and baboon. *Clin Exp Immunol.*1979; 36:384-396.
2. Smith TW, Haber E, Yeatman L, Butler VP Jr. Reversal of advanced digoxin intoxication with Fab fragments of digoxin-specific antibodies. *N Engl J Med.*1976; 294:797-800.
3. Smith TW, Butler VP Jr, Haber E, Fozzard H, Marcus Fl, Bremner WF, Schulman IC, Phillips A. Treatment of life-threatening digitalis intoxication with digoxin-specific Fab antibody fragments: Experience in 26 cases. *N Engl J Med.*1982; 307:1357-1362.
4. Wenger TL, Butler VP Jr, Haber E, Smith TW. Treatment of 63 severely digitalis-toxic patients with digoxin-specific antibody fragments. *J Am Coll Cardiol.*1985; 5:118A-123A.
5. Spiegel A, Marchlinski FE. Time course for reversal of digoxin toxicity with digoxin-specific antibody fragments. *Am Heart J.*1985:109:1397-1399.
6. Gibb I, Adams PC, Parnham AJ, Jennings K. Plasma digoxin: Assay anomalies in Fab-treated patients. *Br J Clin Pharmacol.*1983; 16:445-447.

June 1996/RL-239
Shown in Product Identification Guide, page 312

EMGEL®
(erythromycin) 2%
Topical Gel

For Dermatologic Use Only—
Not for Ophthalmic Use.

℞

DESCRIPTION

EMGEL Topical Gel contains erythromycin. Erythromycin is a macrolide antibiotic obtained from cultures of *Streptomyces erythreus.*
Erythromycin has the empirical formula $C_{37}H_{67}NO_{13}$ and a molecular weight of 733.94.
EMGEL Topical Gel contains erythromycin, USP 2% (20 mg/g) with SD 40-2 alcohol 77%, propylene glycol, and hydroxypropyl cellulose.

CLINICAL PHARMACOLOGY

The exact mechanism by which erythromycin reduces lesions of acne vulgaris is not fully known; however, the effect appears to be due in part to the antibacterial activity of the drug.
Microbiology: Erythromycin appears to inhibit protein synthesis in susceptible organisms by reversibly binding to ribosomal subunits, thereby inhibiting translocation of aminoacyl transfer-RNA and inhibiting polypeptide synthesis. Antagonism has been demonstrated between erythromycin, lincomycin, chloramphenicol, and clindamycin.

INDICATIONS AND USAGE

EMGEL Topical Gel is indicated for the topical treatment of acne vulgaris.

CONTRAINDICATIONS

EMGEL Topical Gel is contraindicated in those individuals who have shown hypersensitivity to any of its components.

PRECAUTIONS

General: For topical use only; not for ophthalmic use. Concomitant topical acne therapy should be used with caution since a possible cumulative irritancy effect may occur, especially with the use of peeling, desquamating, or abrasive agents.
Avoid contact with eyes and all mucous membranes. The use of antibiotic agents may be associated with the overgrowth of antibiotic-resistant organisms. If this occurs, discontinue use and take appropriate measures.
Carcinogenesis, Mutagenesis, Impairment of Fertility: Animal studies to evaluate carcinogenic and mutagenic potential or effects on fertility have not been performed with erythromycin.
Pregnancy Category B: There was no evidence of teratogenicity or any other adverse effect on reproduction in female rats fed erythromycin base (up to 0.25% of diet) before and during mating, during gestation, and through weaning of two successive litters. There are, however, no adequate and well-controlled studies in pregnant women. Because animal reproduction studies are not always predictive of human response, this drug should be used in pregnancy only if clearly needed. Erythromycin has been reported to cross the placental barrier in humans, but fetal plasma levels are generally low.
Nursing Mothers: It is not known whether topically applied erythromycin is excreted in human milk. A decision should be made whether to discontinue nursing or to discontinue the drug, taking into account the importance of the drug to the mother.
Pediatric Use: Safety and effectiveness in children have not been established.

ADVERSE REACTIONS

The most common adverse reaction reported with EMGEL Topical Gel was burning. The following have been reported occasionally: peeling, dryness, itching, erythema, and oiliness. Irritation of the eyes and tenderness of the skin have also been reported with the topical use of erythromycin. A generalized urticarial reaction, which was possibly related to the use of erythromycin and required systemic steroid therapy, has been reported.

DOSAGE AND ADMINISTRATION

Apply sparingly as a thin layer to affected area(s) twice a day, in the morning and the evening, after the skin has been thoroughly washed with soap and water and patted dry. The hands should be washed after application. If there has been no improvement after 6 to 8 weeks, or if the condition becomes worse, treatment should be discontinued, and the physician should be reconsulted. Spread the medication lightly rather than rubbing it in.

HOW SUPPLIED

EMGEL 2% Topical Gel is supplied in plastic bottles containing 27 g (NDC 0173-0440-01) and 50 g (NDC 0173-0440-02).
Note: FLAMMABLE: Keep away from heat and flame. Keep bottle tightly closed. Store at room temperature.
September 1996/RL-358
Shown in Product Identification Guide, page 312

EPIVIR® Tablets
[ep ' ə-vir]
(lamivudine tablets)
EPIVIR® Oral Solution
(lamivudine oral solution)

℞

> **WARNING: LACTIC ACIDOSIS AND SEVERE HEPATOMEGALY WITH STEATOSIS, INCLUDING FATAL CASES, HAVE BEEN REPORTED WITH THE USE OF ANTIRETROVIRAL NUCLEOSIDE ANALOGUES ALONE OR IN COMBINATION, INCLUDING LAMIVUDINE (SEE WARNINGS).**

DESCRIPTION

EPIVIR (formerly known as 3TC) is the brand name for lamivudine, a synthetic nucleoside analogue with activity against HIV. The chemical name of lamivudine is (2R,cis)-4-amino-1-(2-hydroxymethyl-1,3-oxathiolan-5-yl)-(1H)-pyrimidin-2-one. Lamivudine is the (-)enantiomer of a dideoxy analogue of cytidine. Lamivudine has also been referred to as (-)2′,3′-dideoxy, 3′-thiacytidine. It has a molecular formula of $C_8H_{11}N_3O_3S$ and a molecular weight of 229.3. Lamivudine is a white to off-white crystalline solid with a solubility of approximately 70 mg/mL in water at 20°C.
EPIVIR Tablets are for oral administration. Each tablet contains 150 mg of lamivudine and the inactive ingredients magnesium stearate, microcrystalline cellulose, and sodium starch glycolate. Opadry YS-1-7706-G White is the coloring agent in the tablet coating.
EPIVIR Oral Solution is for oral administration. One milliliter (1 mL) of EPIVIR Oral Solution contains 10 mg of lamivudine (10 mg/mL) in an aqueous solution and the inactive ingredients artificial strawberry and banana flavors, citric acid (anhydrous), edetate disodium, ethanol (6% v/v), methylparaben, propylene glycol, propylparaben, and sucrose.

CLINICAL PHARMACOLOGY

Mechanism of Action: Lamivudine is a synthetic nucleoside analogue. *In vitro* studies have shown that, intracellularly, lamivudine is phosphorylated to its active 5′-triphosphate metabolite (L-TP), which has an intracellular half-life of 10.5 to 15.5 hours. The principal mode of action of L-TP is inhibition of HIV reverse transcription via viral DNA chain termination. L-TP also inhibits the RNA- and DNA-dependent DNA polymerase activities of reverse transcriptase (RT). L-TP is a weak inhibitor of mammalian α-, β-, and γ-DNA polymerases.
Microbiology: *Antiviral Activity In Vitro:* The relationship between *in vitro* susceptibility of HIV to lamivudine and the inhibition of HIV replication in humans has not been established. *In vitro* activity of lamivudine against HIV-1 was assessed in a number of cell lines (including monocytes and fresh human peripheral blood lymphocytes) using standard susceptibility assays. IC_{50} values (50% inhibitory concentrations) were in the range of 2 nM to 15 μM. Lamivudine had anti-HIV-1 activity in all acute virus-cell infections tested. In HIV-1–infected MT-4 cells, lamivudine in combination with zidovudine had synergistic antiretroviral activity. Synergistic activity of lamivudine/zidovudine was also shown in a variable-ratio study.
Drug Resistance: Lamivudine-resistant isolates of HIV-1 have been selected *in vitro.* The resistant isolates showed reduced susceptibility to lamivudine and genotypic analysis showed that the resistance was due to specific substitution

mutations in the HIV-1 reverse transcriptase at codon 184 from methionine to either isoleucine or valine. HIV-1 strains resistant to both lamivudine and zidovudine have been isolated.
Susceptibility of clinical isolates to lamivudine and zidovudine was monitored in controlled clinical trials. In patients receiving lamivudine monotherapy or combination therapy with lamivudine plus zidovudine, HIV-1 isolates from most patients became phenotypically and genotypically resistant to lamivudine within 12 weeks. In some patients harboring zidovudine-resistant virus, phenotypic sensitivity to zidovudine by 12 weeks of treatment was restored. Combination therapy with lamivudine plus zidovudine delayed the emergence of mutations conferring resistance to zidovudine.
Pharmacokinetics in Adults: The pharmacokinetic properties of lamivudine have been studied in asymptomatic, HIV-infected adult patients after administration of single intravenous (IV) doses ranging from 0.25 to 8 mg/kg, as well as single and multiple (b.i.d. regimen) oral doses ranging from 0.25 to 10 mg/kg.
Absorption and Bioavailability: Lamivudine was rapidly absorbed after oral administration in HIV-infected patients. Absolute bioavailability in 12 adult patients was 86% ± 16% (mean ± S.D.) for the tablet and 87% ± 13% for the oral solution. After oral administration of 2 mg/kg twice a day to nine adults with HIV, the peak serum lamivudine concentration (C_{max}) was 1.5 ± 0.5 μg/mL (mean ± S.D.). The area under the plasma concentration versus time curve (AUC) and C_{max} increased in proportion to oral dose over the range from 0.25 to 10 mg/kg.
An investigational 25-mg dosage form of lamivudine was administered orally to 12 asymptomatic, HIV-infected patients on two occasions, once in the fasted state and once with food (1,099 kcal; 75 grams fat, 34 grams protein, 72 grams carbohydrate). Absorption of lamivudine was slower in the fed state (T_{max}: 3.2 ± 1.3 hours) compared with the fasted state (T_{max}: 0.9 ± 0.3 hours); C_{max} in the fed state was 40% ± 23% (mean ± S.D.) lower than in the fasted state. There was no significant difference in systemic exposure ($AUC\infty$) in the fed and fasted states; therefore, EPIVIR Tablets and Oral Solution may be administered with or without food.
The accumulation ratio of lamivudine in HIV-positive asymptomatic adults with normal renal function was 1.50 following 15 days of oral administration of 2 mg/kg b.i.d.
Distribution: The apparent volume of distribution after IV administration of lamivudine to 20 patients was 1.3 ± 0.4 L/kg, suggesting that lamivudine distributes into extravascular spaces. Volume of distribution was independent of dose and did not correlate with body weight.
Binding of lamivudine to human plasma proteins is low (<36%). *In vitro* studies showed that, over the concentration range of 0.1 to 100 μg/mL, the amount of lamivudine associated with erythrocytes ranged from 53% to 57% and was independent of concentration.
Metabolism: Metabolism of lamivudine is a minor route of elimination. In man, the only known metabolite of lamivudine is the trans-sulfoxide metabolite. Within 12 hours after a single oral dose of lamivudine in six HIV-infected adults, 5.2% ± 1.4% (mean ± S.D.) of the dose was excreted as the trans-sulfoxide metabolite in the urine. Serum concentrations of this metabolite have not been determined.
Elimination: The majority of lamivudine is eliminated unchanged in urine. In 20 patients given a single IV dose, renal clearance was 0.22 ± 0.06 L/hr*kg (mean ± S.D.), representing 71% ± 16% (mean ± S.D.) of total clearance of lamivudine.
In most single-dose studies in HIV-infected patients with serum sampling for 24 hours after dosing, the observed mean elimination half-life ($T_{1/2}$) ranged from 5 to 7 hours. Total clearance was 0.37 ± 0.05 L/hr*kg (mean ± S.D.). Oral clearance and elimination half-life were independent of dose and body weight over an oral dosing range from 0.25 to 10 mg/kg.
Special Populations: *Adults With Impaired Renal Function:* The pharmacokinetic properties of lamivudine have been determined in a small group of HIV-infected adults with impaired renal function, as summarized in Table 1.

Table 1: Pharmacokinetic Parameters (Mean±S.D.) After a Single 300-mg Oral Dose of Lamivudine in Three Groups of Adults With Varying Degrees of Renal Function (CrCl>60 mL/min, CrCl=10-30 mL/min, and CrCl<10mL/min)

Number of subjects	6	4	6
Creatinine clearance criterion	>60 mL/min	10-30 mL/min	<10 mL/min
Creatinine clearance (mL/min)	111 ± 14	28 ± 8	6 ± 2
C_{max} (μg/mL)	2.6 ± 0.5	3.6 ± 0.8	5.8 ± 1.2
AUC∞ (μg•h/mL)	11.0 ± 1.7	48.0 ± 19	157 ± 74
Cl/F (mL/min)	464 ± 76	114 ± 34	36 ± 11

Exposure (AUC∞), C_{max}, and half-life increased with diminishing renal function (as expressed by creatinine clearance). Apparent total oral clearance (Cl/F) of lamivudine de-

Table 2: Number of Patients (%) With At Least One HIV Disease Progression Event or Death

Endpoint	Current Therapy (n = 460)	EPIVIR plus Current Therapy (n = 896)	EPIVIR plus a NNRTI* plus Current Therapy (n = 460)
HIV progression or death	90 (19.6%)	86 (9.6%)	41 (8.9%)
Death	27 (5.9%)	23 (2.6%)	14 (3.0%)

*An investigational non-nucleoside reverse transcriptase inhibitor not approved in the United States.

creased as creatinine clearance decreased. T_{max} was not significantly affected by renal function. Based on these observations, it is recommended that the dosage of lamivudine be modified in patients with renal impairment (see DOSAGE AND ADMINISTRATION). The effects of renal impairment on lamivudine pharmacokinetics in pediatric patients are not known.

Pediatric Patients: For pharmacokinetic properties of lamivudine in pediatric patients, see PRECAUTIONS: Pediatric Use.

Geriatric Patients: Lamivudine pharmacokinetics have not been specifically studied in patients over 65 years of age.

Gender: The pharmacokinetics of lamivudine with respect to gender have not been evaluated.

Race: The pharmacokinetics of lamivudine with respect to race have not been evaluated.

Drug Interactions: Lamivudine and zidovudine were coadministered to 12 asymptomatic HIV-positive adult patients in a single-center, open-label, randomized, crossover study. No significant differences were observed in AUC∞ or total clearance for lamivudine or zidovudine when the two drugs were administered together. Coadministration of lamivudine with zidovudine resulted in an increase of 39% ± 62% (mean ± S.D.) in C_{max} of zidovudine.

Lamivudine and trimethoprim/sulfamethoxazole (TMP/SMX) were coadministered to 14 HIV-positive patients in a single-center, open-label, randomized, crossover study. Each patient received treatment with a single 300-mg dose of lamivudine and TMP 160 mg/SMX 800 mg once a day for 5 days with concomitant administration of lamivudine 300 mg with the fifth dose in a crossover design.

Coadministration of TMP/SMX with lamivudine resulted in an increase of 44% ± 23% (mean ± S.D.) in lamivudine AUC∞, a decrease of 29% ± 13% in lamivudine oral clearance, and a decrease of 30% ± 36% in lamivudine renal clearance. The pharmacokinetic properties of TMP and SMX were not altered by coadministration with lamivudine.

INDICATIONS AND USAGE

EPIVIR in combination with RETROVIR is indicated for the treatment of HIV infection (see Description of Clinical Studies).

Description of Clinical Studies: Clinical Study: NUCB3007 (CAESAR) was a multicenter, double-blind, placebo-controlled study comparing continued current therapy [zidovudine alone (62% of patients) or zidovudine with didanosine or zalcitabine (38% of patients)] to the addition of EPIVIR or EPIVIR plus an investigational non-nucleoside reverse transcriptase inhibitor, randomized 1:2:1. A total of 1816 HIV-infected adults with 25 to 250 (median = 122 cells/mm³) CD4 cells/mm³ at baseline were enrolled: median age was 36 years, 87% were male, 84% were nucleoside-experienced, and 16% were therapy-naive. The median duration on study was 12 months. Results are summarized in Table 2.
[See table 2 above]

Surrogate Endpoint Studies: Therapy-Naive Adults: A3001 was a randomized, double-blind study comparing EPIVIR 150 mg b.i.d. plus RETROVIR 200 mg b.i.d. plus RETROVIR; EPIVIR 300 mg b.i.d.; and RETROVIR. 366 adults enrolled: male (87%), Caucasian (61%), median age of 34 years, asymptomatic HIV infection (80%), baseline CD4 cell counts of 200 to 500 cells/mm³ (median = 352 cells/mm³), and mean baseline plasma HIV RNA of 4.47 (log 10 copies/mL). B3001 was a randomized, double-blind study comparing EPIVIR 300 mg b.i.d. plus RETROVIR 200 mg t.i.d. versus RETROVIR. 129 adults enrolled: male (74%), Caucasian (82%), median age of 33 years, asymptomatic HIV infection (64%), and baseline CD4 cell counts of 100 to 400 cells/mm³ (median = 260 cells/mm³). Mean changes in CD4 count and HIV RNA through 24 weeks of treatment for study A3001 are summarized in Figures 1 and 2, respectively. Mean change in CD4 count through 24 weeks of treatment for study B3001 is summarized in Figure 3.
[See figures 1-3 in next column]

Therapy-Experienced Adults (≥24 Weeks of Prior Zidovudine Therapy): A3002 was a randomized, double-blind study comparing EPIVIR 150 mg b.i.d. plus RETROVIR 200 mg t.i.d.; EPIVIR 300 mg b.i.d. plus RETROVIR; and RETROVIR plus zalcitabine 0.75 mg t.i.d. 254 adults enrolled: male (83%), Caucasian (63%), median age of 37 years, asymptomatic HIV infection (58%), median duration of prior zidovudine use of 24 months, baseline CD4 cell

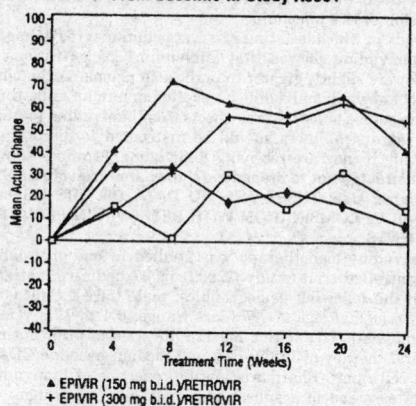

Figure 1: Mean Absolute CD4 Change (cells/mm³) From Baseline in Study A3001

▲ EPIVIR (150 mg b.i.d.)/RETROVIR
+ EPIVIR (300 mg b.i.d.)/RETROVIR
♦ EPIVIR (300 mg b.i.d.)
□ RETROVIR

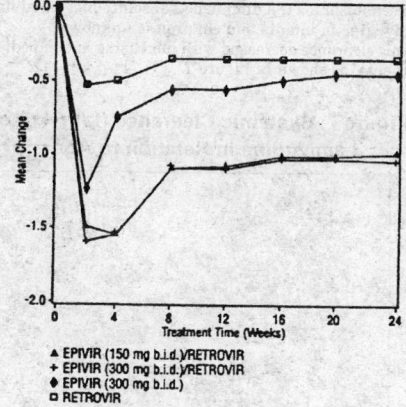

Figure 2: Mean Change From Baseline in Log 10 HIV RNA (copies/mL) in Study A3001

▲ EPIVIR (150 mg b.i.d.)/RETROVIR
+ EPIVIR (300 mg b.i.d.)/RETROVIR
♦ EPIVIR (300 mg b.i.d.)
□ RETROVIR

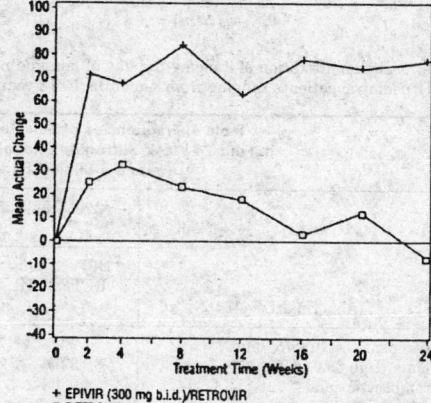

Figure 3: Mean Absolute CD4 Change (cells/mm³) From Baseline in Study B3001

+ EPIVIR (300 mg b.i.d.)/RETROVIR
□ RETROVIR

counts of 100 to 300 cells/mm³ (median = 211 cells/mm³), and mean baseline plasma HIV RNA of 4.60 (log 10 copies/mL). B3002 was a randomized, double-blind study comparing EPIVIR 150 mg b.i.d. plus RETROVIR, EPIVIR 300 mg b.i.d. plus RETROVIR, and RETROVIR. 223 adults enrolled: male (83%), Caucasian (96%), median age of 36 years, asymptomatic HIV infection (53%), median duration of prior zidovudine use of 23 months, and baseline CD4 cell counts of 100 to 400 cells/mm³ (median = 241 cells/mm³).

Mean changes in CD4 count and HIV RNA through 24 weeks of treatment in study A3002 are summarized in Figures 4 and 5, respectively. Mean change in CD4 count through 24 weeks of treatment for study B3002 is summarized in Figure 6.

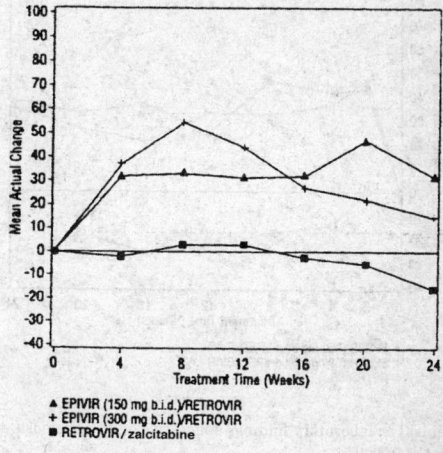

Figure 4: Mean Absolute CD4 Change (cells/mm³) From Baseline in Study A3002

▲ EPIVIR (150 mg b.i.d.)/RETROVIR
+ EPIVIR (300 mg b.i.d.)/RETROVIR
■ RETROVIR/zalcitabine

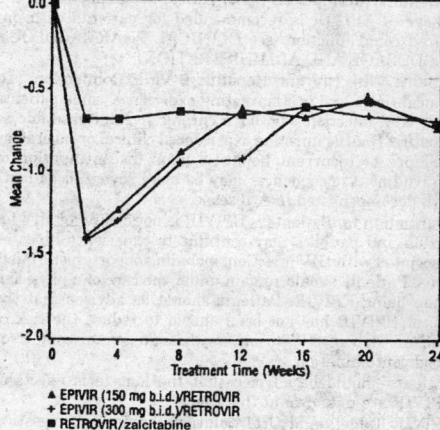

Figure 5: Mean Change From Baseline in Log 10 HIV RNA (copies/mL) in Study A3002

▲ EPIVIR (150 mg b.i.d.)/RETROVIR
+ EPIVIR (300 mg b.i.d.)/RETROVIR
■ RETROVIR/zalcitabine

[See figure 6 at top of next column]

CONTRAINDICATIONS

EPIVIR Tablets and Oral Solution are contraindicated in patients with previously demonstrated clinically significant hypersensitivity to any of the components of the products.

WARNINGS

In pediatric patients with a history of pancreatitis or other significant risk factors for the development of pancreatitis, the combination of EPIVIR and RETROVIR should be used with extreme caution and only if there is no satisfactory alternative therapy. Treatment with EPIVIR should be stopped immediately if clinical signs, symptoms, or laboratory abnormalities suggestive of pancreatitis occur (see ADVERSE REACTIONS).

Lactic Acidosis/Severe Hepatomegaly with Steatosis: Lactic acidosis and severe hepatomegaly with steatosis, including fatal cases, have been reported with the use of antiretroviral nucleoside analogues alone or in combination, including lamivudine. A majority of these cases have been in women. Caution should be exercised when administering EPIVIR to any patient, and particularly to those with known risk factors for liver disease. Treatment with EPIVIR should be suspended in any patient who develops

Continued on next page

This product information is based on labeling in effect on June 1, 1998. For further information, contact via direct mail, phone, or web site Medical Information: Glaxo Wellcome Inc., PO Box 13398, Research Triangle Park, NC 27709. Healthcare Professionals (Medical Information): 800-334-0089 Patients (Customer Response Center): 888-TALK2GW (1-888-825-5249) Glaxo Wellcome Corporate Web Site: www.glaxowellcome.com

Consult 1999 PDR® supplements and future editions for revisions

Epivir—Cont.

Figure 6: Mean Absolute CD4 Change (cells/mm³) From Baseline in Study B3002

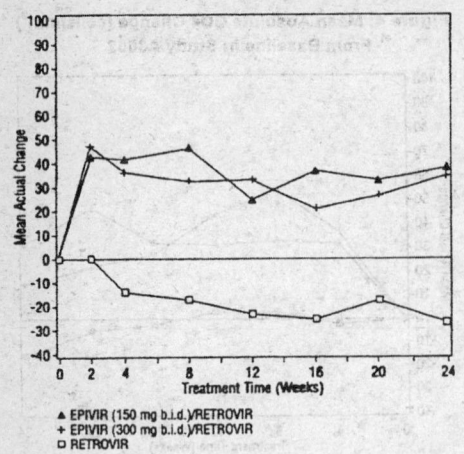

▲ EPIVIR (150 mg b.i.d.)/RETROVIR
+ EPIVIR (300 mg b.i.d.)/RETROVIR
□ RETROVIR

clinical or laboratory findings suggestive of lactic acidosis or hepatotoxicity.

The complete prescribing information for RETROVIR should be consulted before combination therapy with EPIVIR and RETROVIR is initiated.

PRECAUTIONS

Patients With Impaired Renal Function: Reduction of the dosage of EPIVIR is recommended for patients with impaired renal function (see CLINICAL PHARMACOLOGY and DOSAGE AND ADMINISTRATION).

Patients With HIV and Hepatitis B Virus Coinfection: In clinical trials and postmarketing experience, some patients with HIV infection who have chronic liver disease due to hepatitis B virus infection experienced clinical or laboratory evidence of recurrent hepatitis upon discontinuation of lamivudine. Consequences may be more severe in patients with decompensated liver disease.

Information for Patients: EPIVIR is not a cure for HIV infection and patients may continue to experience illnesses associated with HIV infection, including opportunistic infections. Patients should remain under the care of a physician when using EPIVIR. Patients should be advised that the use of EPIVIR has not been shown to reduce the risk of transmission of HIV to others through sexual contact or blood contamination.

Patients should be advised that the long-term effects of EPIVIR are unknown at this time.

EPIVIR Tablets and Oral Solution are for oral ingestion only.

Patients should be advised of the importance of taking EPIVIR exactly as it is prescribed.

Parents or guardians should be advised to monitor pediatric patients for signs and symptoms of pancreatitis.

Drug Interaction: TMP 160 mg/SMX 800 mg once daily has been shown to increase lamivudine exposure (AUC). The effect of higher doses of TMP/SMX on lamivudine pharmacokinetics has not been investigated (see CLINICAL PHARMACOLOGY).

Carcinogenesis, Mutagenesis, and Impairment of Fertility: Lamivudine long-term carcinogenicity studies in mice and rats showed no evidence of carcinogenic potential at exposures up to 10 times (mice) and 58 times (rats) those observed in humans at the recommended therapeutic dose. Lamivudine was not active in a microbial mutagenicity screen or an *in vitro* cell transformation assay, but showed weak *in vitro* mutagenic activity in a cytogenetic assay using cultured human lymphocytes and in the mouse lymphoma assay. However, lamivudine showed no evidence of *in vivo* genotoxic activity in the rat at oral doses of up to 2,000 mg/kg (approximately 65 times the recommended human dose based on body surface area comparisons). In a study of reproductive performance, lamivudine, administered to rats at doses up to 130 times the usual adult dose based on body surface area comparisons, revealed no evidence of impaired fertility and no effect on the survival, growth, and development to weaning of the offspring.

Pregnancy: *Pregnancy Category C:* Reproduction studies have been performed in rats and rabbits at orally administered doses up to approximately 130 and 60 times, respectively, the usual adult dose and have revealed no evidence of harm to the fetus due to lamivudine. Some evidence of early embryolethality was seen in the rabbit at doses similar to those produced by the usual adult dose and higher, but there was no indication of this effect in the rat at orally administered doses up to 130 times the usual adult dose. Stud-

ies in pregnant rats and rabbits showed that lamivudine is transferred to the fetus through the placenta. There are no adequate and well-controlled studies in pregnant women. Because animal reproductive toxicity studies are not always predictive of human response, lamivudine should be used during pregnancy only if the potential benefits outweigh the risks.

Antiretroviral Pregnancy Registry: To monitor maternal-fetal outcomes of pregnant women exposed to EPIVIR, an Antiretroviral Pregnancy Registry has been established. Physicians are encouraged to register patients by calling (800) 722-9292, ext. 39437.

Nursing Mothers: **The Centers for Disease Control and Prevention recommend that HIV-infected mothers not breastfeed their infants to avoid risking postnatal transmission of HIV infection.**

A study in which lactating rats were administered 45 mg/kg of lamivudine showed that lamivudine concentrations in milk were slightly greater than those in plasma. Although it is not known if lamivudine is excreted in human milk, there is the potential for adverse effects from lamivudine in nursing infants. Mothers should be instructed to discontinue nursing if they are receiving lamivudine. **Mothers should be instructed not to breastfeed if they are receiving EPIVIR.**

Pediatric Use: THERE ARE NO DATA ON THE USE OF EPIVIR IN COMBINATION WITH RETROVIR IN PEDIATRIC PATIENTS.

Lamivudine monotherapy was studied in one open-label, uncontrolled trial (study A2002) in 97 pediatric patients with the following demographics: male (56%), Caucasian (57%), median age of 7.7 years (range: 0.4 to 17.3 years), symptomatic HIV (84%), median duration of prior antiretroviral therapy of 148 weeks, and median baseline CD4 of 132 cells/mm³. Pharmacokinetic properties of lamivudine were assessed in a subset of 57 patients (age range: 4.8 months to 16 years, weight range: 5 to 66 kg) after oral and IV administration of 1, 2, 4, 8, 12, and 20 mg/kg per day. In the 9 infants and children receiving 8 mg/kg per day (the usual recommended pediatric dose), absolute bioavailability was 66% ± 26% (mean ± S.D.), which is less than the 86% ± 16% (mean ± S.D.) observed in adolescents and adults. The mechanism for the diminished absolute bioavailability of lamivudine in infants and children is unknown.

Systemic clearance decreased with increasing age in pediatric patients, as shown in Figure 7.

Figure 7: Systemic Clearance (L/hr*kg) of Lamivudine in Relation to Age

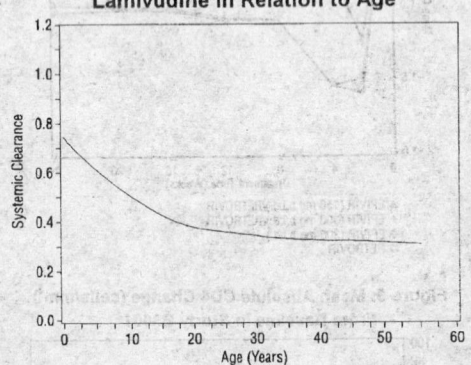

After oral administration of 8 mg/kg per day of lamivudine to 11 pediatric patients ranging from 4 months to 14 years

of age, C_{max} was 1.1 ± 0.6 μg/mL and half-life was 2.0 ± 0.6 hours. (In adults with similar blood sampling, the half-life was 3.7 ± 1 hours.) Total exposure to lamivudine, as reflected by mean AUC values, was comparable between pediatric patients receiving an 8 mg/kg/day dose and adults receiving a 4 mg/kg/day dose.

Distribution of lamivudine into cerebrospinal fluid (CSF) was assessed in 38 pediatric patients after multiple oral dosing with lamivudine. CSF samples were collected between 2 and 4 hours postdose. At the dose of 8 mg/kg/day, CSF lamivudine concentrations in eight patients ranged from 5.6% to 30.9% (mean ± S.D. of 14.2% ± 7.9%) of the concentration in a simultaneous serum sample, with CSF lamivudine concentrations ranging from 0.04 to 0.3 μg/mL. See INDICATIONS AND USAGE: Description of Clinical Studies, WARNINGS, ADVERSE REACTIONS, and DOSAGE AND ADMINISTRATION sections.

ADVERSE REACTIONS

Adults: Selected clinical adverse events with a ≥5% frequency during therapy with EPIVIR 150 mg b.i.d. plus RETROVIR 200 mg t.i.d. compared with zidovudine are listed in Table 3.

Table 3: Selected Clinical Adverse Events (≥5% Frequency) in Four Controlled Clinical Trials (A3001, A3002, B3001, B3002)

Adverse Event	EPIVIR 150 mg b.i.d. plus RETROVIR (n=251)	RETROVIR (n=230)
Body as a Whole		
Headache	35%	27%
Malaise & fatigue	27%	23%
Fever or chills	10%	12%
Digestive		
Nausea	33%	29%
Diarrhea	18%	22%
Nausea & vomiting	13%	12%
Anorexia and/or decreased appetite	10%	7%
Abdominal pain	9%	11%
Abdominal cramps	6%	3%
Dyspepsia	5%	5%
Nervous system		
Neuropathy	12%	10%
Insomnia & other sleep disorders	11%	7%
Dizziness	10%	4%
Depressive disorders	9%	4%
Respiratory		
Nasal signs & symptoms	20%	11%
Cough	18%	13%
Skin		
Skin rashes	9%	6%
Musculoskeletal		
Musculoskeletal pain	12%	10%
Myalgia	8%	6%
Arthralgia	5%	5%

Pancreatitis was observed in 3 of the 656 adult patients (<0.5%) who received EPIVIR in controlled clinical trials.

Table 4: Frequencies of Selected Laboratory Abnormalities in Adults in Four 24-Week Surrogate Endpoint Studies (A3001, A3002, B3001, B3002) and a Clinical Endpoint Study (NUCB3007)

Test (Abnormal Level)	24-Week Surrogate Endpoint Studies		Clinical Endpoint Study*	
	EPIVIR plus RETROVIR %	RETROVIR %	EPIVIR plus Current Therapy	Placebo plus Current Therapy†
Neutropenia (ANC<750/mm³)	7.2%	5.4%	15%	13%
Anemia (Hgb<8.0 g/dL)	2.9%	1.8%	2.2%	3.4%
Thrombocytopenia (platelets<50,000/mm³)	0.4%	1.3%	2.8%	3.8%
ALT (>5.0 × ULN)	3.7%	3.6%	3.8%	1.9%
AST (>5.0 × ULN)	1.7%	1.8%	4.0%	2.1%
Bilirubin (>2.5 × ULN)	0.8%	0.4%	ND	ND
Amylase (>2.0 × ULN)	4.2%	1.5%	2.2%	1.1%

* The median duration on study was 12 months.
† Current therapy was either zidovudine, zidovudine plus didanosine, or zidovudine plus zalcitabine.
ULN = Upper limit of normal.
ANC = Absolute neutrophil count.
ND = Not done.

Selected laboratory abnormalities observed during therapy are listed in Table 4.
[See table 4 at bottom of previous page]
Pediatric Patients: Limited information on the incidence of adverse events in children receiving lamivudine monotherapy is available from one open-label, uncontrolled study (see PRECAUTIONS: Pediatric Use section for description of study A2002). Of 97 pediatric patients, 14 patients (14%) developed pancreatitis while receiving monotherapy with EPIVIR. In a second ongoing study in 47 pediatric patients (age range: 3 months to 18 years) enrolled in an open-label evaluation of EPIVIR/didanosine, EPIVIR/RETROVIR, and EPIVIR/RETROVIR/didanosine, 7 patients (15%) developed pancreatitis (see WARNINGS).
Paresthesias and peripheral neuropathies were reported in 13 patients (13%) in study A2002 and resulted in treatment discontinuation in 3 patients.
Selected laboratory abnormalities during lamivudine therapy in children are listed in Table 5.

Table 5: Frequencies of Selected Laboratory Abnormalities in an Uncontrolled Phase I/II Clinical Trial of EPIVIR in 97 Pediatric Patients

Test (Abnormal Level)	Patients With Normal Baselines % (n)	Patients With Abnormal Baselines % (n)
Neutropenia (ANC<750/mm³)	22% (55)	45% (33)
Anemia (Hgb<8.0 g/dL)	2% (50)	24% (46)
Thrombocytopenia (platelets<40,000/mm³)	0% (68)	25% (12)
ALT (>5.0 × ULN)	4% (51)	29% (42)
AST (>5.0 × ULN)	0% (29)	19% (57)
Amylase (>2.0 ULN)	3% (69)	23% (13)

ULN = Upper limit of normal.
ANC = Absolute neutrophil count.
n = Number of patients assessed.

Observed During Clinical Practice: The following events have been identified during post-approval use of EPIVIR in clinical practice. Because they are reported voluntarily from a population of unknown size, estimates of frequency cannot be made. These events have been chosen for inclusion due to either their seriousness, frequency of reporting, causal connection to EPIVIR, or a combination of these factors.
Alopecia, anaphylaxis, hyperglycemia, lactic acidosis and hepatic steatosis (see WARNINGS), peripheral neuropathy, pruritus, rash, urticaria, and weakness.

OVERDOSAGE

There is no known antidote for EPIVIR. One case of an adult ingesting 6 g of EPIVIR was reported; there were no clinical signs or symptoms noted and hematologic tests remained normal. It is not known whether lamivudine can be removed by peritoneal dialysis or hemodialysis.

DOSAGE AND ADMINISTRATION

Adults and Adolescents (12 to 16 years): The recommended oral dose of EPIVIR for adults and adolescents is 150 mg twice daily administered in combination with RETROVIR. The complete prescribing information for RETROVIR should be consulted for information on its dosage and administration.
For adults with low body weights (less than 50 kg or 110 lb), the recommended oral dose of EPIVIR is 2 mg/kg twice daily administered in combination with RETROVIR. No data are available to support a dosage recommendation for adolescents with low body weight (less than 50 kg).
Pediatric Patients: The recommended oral dose of EPIVIR for pediatric patients 3 months to up to 12 years of age is 4 mg/kg twice daily (up to a maximum of 150 mg twice a day) administered in combination with RETROVIR. The complete prescribing information for RETROVIR should be consulted for information on its dosage and administration.
Dose Adjustment: It is recommended that doses of EPIVIR be adjusted in accordance with renal function in patients older than age 16 years (see Table 6). (See CLINICAL PHARMACOLOGY section.)

Table 6: Adjustment of Dosage of EPIVIR in Accordance With Creatinine Clearance

Creatinine Clearance (mL/min)	Recommended Dosage of EPIVIR
≥50	150 mg twice daily
30-49	150 mg once daily
15-29	150 mg first dose, then 100 mg once daily
5-14	150 mg first dose, then 50 mg once daily
<5	50 mg first dose, then 25 mg once daily

Insufficient data are available to recommend a dosage of EPIVIR in patients undergoing dialysis.

HOW SUPPLIED

EPIVIR Tablets, 150 mg, are white, modified diamond-shaped, film-coated tablets imprinted with "150" on one side and "GX CJ7" on the reverse side. They are available in bottles of 60 tablets (NDC 0173-0470-01) with child-resistant closures. **Store between 2° and 30°C (36° and 86°F) in tightly closed bottles.**
EPIVIR Oral Solution, a clear, colorless to pale yellow, strawberry-banana flavored liquid, contains 10 mg of lamivudine in each 1 mL in plastic bottles of 240 mL (NDC 0173-0471-00) with child-resistant closures. This product does not require reconstitution. **Store between 2° and 25°C (36° and 77°F) in tightly closed bottles.**
U.S. Patent 5,047,407
©Copyright 1996 Glaxo Wellcome Inc. All rights reserved.
December 1997/RL-530

Shown in Product Identification Guide, page 312

EXOSURF NEONATAL®   ℞
[ĕx ′ō-sŭrf nē-ō ′nāt-əl]
(colfosceril palmitate, cetyl alcohol, tyloxapol)
For Intratracheal Suspension

DESCRIPTION

EXOSURF NEONATAL (colfosceril palmitate, cetyl alcohol, tyloxapol) for Intratracheal Suspension is a protein-free synthetic lung surfactant stored under vacuum as a sterile lyophilized powder. EXOSURF NEONATAL is reconstituted with preservative-free Sterile Water for Injection prior to administration by intratracheal instillation. Each 10 mL vial contains 108 mg colfosceril palmitate, commonly known as dipalmitoylphosphatidylcholine (DPPC), 12 mg cetyl alcohol, 8 mg tyloxapol, and 47 mg sodium chloride. Sodium hydroxide or hydrochloric acid may have been added to adjust pH. When reconstituted with 8 mL Sterile Water for Injection, the EXOSURF NEONATAL suspension contains 13.5 mg/mL colfosceril palmitate, 1.5 mg/mL cetyl alcohol, and 1 mg/mL tyloxapol in 0.1 N NaCl. The suspension appears milky white with a pH of 5 to 7 and an osmolality of 185 mOsm/kg.
The chemical names of EXOSURF NEONATAL are colfosceril palmitate (R)-4-hydroxy-N, N, N-trimethyl-10-oxo-7-[(1-oxohexadecyl) oxy]-3,5,9-trioxa-4-phosphapentacosan-1-aminium hydroxide inner salt, 4-oxide; cetyl alcohol (1-hexadecanol); and tyloxapol 4-(1,1,3,3-tetramethylbutyl)phenol polymer with formaldehyde and oxirane.

CLINICAL PHARMACOLOGY

Surfactant deficiency is an important factor in the development of the neonatal respiratory distress syndrome (RDS). Thus, surfactant replacement therapy early in the course of RDS should ameliorate the disease and improve symptoms. Natural surfactant, a combination of lipids and apoproteins, exhibits not only surface tension reducing properties (conferred by the lipids), but also rapid spreading and adsorption (conferred by the apoproteins). The major fraction of the lipid component of natural surfactant is DPPC, which comprises up to 70% of natural surfactant by weight.
Although DPPC reduces surface tension, DPPC alone is ineffective in RDS because DPPC spreads and adsorbs poorly. In EXOSURF NEONATAL, which is protein free, cetyl alcohol acts as the spreading agent for the DPPC on the air-fluid interface. Tyloxapol, a polymeric long-chain repeating alcohol, is a nonionic surfactant which acts to disperse both DPPC and cetyl alcohol. Sodium chloride is added to adjust osmolality.
Pharmacokinetics: EXOSURF NEONATAL is administered directly into the trachea. Human pharmacokinetic studies of the absorption, biotransformation, and excretion of the components of EXOSURF NEONATAL have not been performed. Nonclinical studies, however, have shown that DPPC can be absorbed from the alveolus into lung tissue where it can be catabolized extensively and reutilized for further phospholipid synthesis and secretion. In the developing rabbit, 90% of alveolar phospholipids are recycled. In premature rabbits, the alveolar half-life of intratracheally administered H³-labeled phosphatidylcholine is approximately 12 hours.
Animal Studies: In animal models of RDS, treatment with EXOSURF NEONATAL significantly improved lung volume, compliance, and gas exchange in premature rabbits and lambs. The amount and distribution of lung water were not affected by treatment with EXOSURF NEONATAL of premature rabbit pups. The extent of lung injury in premature rabbit pups undergoing mechanical ventilation was reduced significantly by treatment with EXOSURF NEONATAL. In premature lambs, neither systemic blood flow nor flow through the ductus arteriosus were affected by

treatment with EXOSURF NEONATAL. Survival was significantly better in both premature rabbits and premature lambs treated with EXOSURF NEONATAL.
Clinical Studies: EXOSURF NEONATAL has been studied in the U.S. and Canada in controlled clinical trials involving more than 4400 infants. Over 10,000 infants have received EXOSURF NEONATAL through an open, uncontrolled, North American study designed to provide the drug to premature infants who might benefit and to obtain additional safety information (EXOSURF NEONATAL Treatment IND).
Prophylactic Treatment: The efficacy of a single dose of EXOSURF NEONATAL in prophylactic treatment of infants at risk of developing respiratory distress syndrome (RDS) was examined in three double-blind, placebo-controlled studies, one involving 215 infants weighing 500 to 700 grams, one involving 385 infants weighing 700 to 1100 grams, and one involving 446 infants weighing 700 to 1100 grams. The infants were intubated and placed on mechanical ventilation, and received 5 mL/kg EXOSURF NEONATAL or placebo (air) within 30 minutes of birth.
The efficacy of one versus three doses of EXOSURF NEONATAL in prophylactic treatment of infants at risk of developing RDS was examined in a double-blind, placebo-controlled study of 823 infants weighing 700 to 1100 grams. The infants were intubated and placed on mechanical ventilation, and received a first 5 mL/kg dose of EXOSURF NEONATAL within 30 minutes. Repeat 5 mL/kg doses of EXOSURF NEONATAL or placebo (air) were given to all infants who remained on mechanical ventilation at approximately 12 and 24 hours of age. An initial analysis of 716 infants is available.
The major efficacy parameters from these studies are presented in Table 1.
[See table 1 at bottom of next page]
Rescue Treatment: The efficacy of EXOSURF NEONATAL in the rescue treatment of infants with RDS was examined in two double-blind, placebo-controlled studies. One study enrolled 419 infants weighing 700 to 1350 grams; the second enrolled 1237 infants weighing 1250 grams and above. In the rescue treatment studies, infants received an initial dose (5 mL/kg) of EXOSURF NEONATAL or placebo (air) between 2 and 24 hours of life followed by a second dose (5 mL/kg) approximately 12 hours later to infants who remained on mechanical ventilation. The major efficacy parameters from these studies are presented in Table 2.
[See table 2 at top of next page]
Clinical Results: In these six controlled clinical studies, infants in the group receiving EXOSURF NEONATAL showed significant improvements in FiO₂ and ventilator settings which persisted for at least 7 days. Pulmonary air leaks were significantly reduced in each study. Five of these studies also showed a significant reduction in death from RDS. Further, overall mortality was reduced for all infants weighing >700 grams. The one- versus three-dose prophylactic treatment study in 700 to 1100 gram infants showed a further reduction in overall mortality with two additional doses.
Safety information is presented in Tables 3 and 4 (see ADVERSE REACTIONS). Beneficial effects in the group receiving EXOSURF NEONATAL were observed for some safety assessments. Various forms of pulmonary air leak and use of pancuronium were reduced in infants receiving EXOSURF NEONATAL in all six studies.
Follow-up data at one year adjusted age are available on 1094 of 2470 surviving infants. Growth and development of infants who received EXOSURF NEONATAL in this sample were comparable to infants who received placebo.

INDICATIONS AND USAGE

EXOSURF NEONATAL is indicated for:
1. **Prophylactic** treatment of infants with birth weights of less than 1350 grams who are at risk of developing RDS (see PRECAUTIONS),
2. **Prophylactic** treatment of infants with birth weights greater than 1350 grams who have evidence of pulmonary immaturity, and
3. **Rescue** treatment of infants who have developed RDS.
For **prophylactic** treatment, the first dose of EXOSURF NEONATAL should be administered as soon as possible after birth (see DOSAGE AND ADMINISTRATION: General Guidelines for Administration).
Infants considered as candidates for **rescue** treatment with EXOSURF NEONATAL should be on mechanical ventilation and have a diagnosis of RDS by both of the following criteria:

Continued on next page

This product information is based on labeling in effect on June 1, 1998. For further information, contact via direct mail, phone, or web site Medical Information: Glaxo Wellcome Inc., PO Box 13398, Research Triangle Park, NC 27709. Healthcare Professionals (Medical Information): 800-334-0089 Patients (Customer Response Center): 888-TALK2GW (1-888-825-5249) Glaxo Wellcome Corporate Web Site: www.glaxowellcome.com

Exosurf—Cont.

1. Respiratory distress not attributable to causes other than RDS, based on clinical and laboratory assessments.
2. Chest radiographic findings consistent with the diagnosis of RDS.

During the clinical development of EXOSURF NEONATAL, all infants who received the drug were intubated and on mechanical ventilation. For three-dose prophylactic treatment with EXOSURF NEONATAL, the first dose of drug was administered as soon as possible after birth and repeat doses were given at approximately 12 and 24 hours after birth if infants remained on mechanical ventilation at those times. For rescue treatment, two doses were given; one between 2 and 24 hours of life, and a second approximately 12 hours later if infants remained on mechanical ventilation. Infants who received rescue treatment with EXOSURF NEONATAL had a documented arterial to alveolar oxygen tension ratio (a/A) <0.22.

CONTRAINDICATIONS

There are no known contraindications to treatment with EXOSURF NEONATAL.

WARNINGS

Intratracheal Administration Only: EXOSURF NEONATAL should be administered only by instillation into the trachea (see DOSAGE AND ADMINISTRATION).

General:
The use of EXOSURF NEONATAL requires expert clinical care by experienced neonatologists and other clinicians who are accomplished at neonatal intubation and ventilatory management. Adequate personnel, facilities, equipment, and medications are required to optimize perinatal outcome in premature infants.

Instillation of EXOSURF NEONATAL should be performed **only** by trained medical personnel experienced in airway and clinical management of unstable premature infants. Vigilant clinical attention should be given to all infants prior to, during, and after administration of EXOSURF NEONATAL.

Acute Effects: EXOSURF NEONATAL can rapidly affect oxygenation and lung compliance.

Lung Compliance: If chest expansion improves substantially after dosing, peak ventilator inspiratory pressures should be reduced immediately, without waiting for confirmation of respiratory improvement by blood gas assessment. Failure to reduce inspiratory ventilator pressures rapidly in such instances can result in lung overdistention and fatal pulmonary air leak.

Hyperoxia: If the infant becomes pink and transcutaneous oxygen saturation is in excess of 95%, FiO_2 should be reduced in small but repeated steps (until saturation is 90% to 95%) without waiting for confirmation of elevated arterial pO_2 by blood gas assessment. Failure to reduce FiO_2 in such instances can result in hyperoxia.

Hypocarbia: If arterial or transcutaneous CO_2 measurements are <30 torr, the ventilator rate should be reduced at once. Failure to reduce ventilator rates in such instances can result in marked hypocarbia, which is known to reduce brain blood flow.

Pulmonary Hemorrhage: In the single study conducted in infants weighing <700 grams at birth, the incidence of pulmonary hemorrhage (10% vs 2% in the placebo group) was significantly increased in the group receiving EXOSURF NEONATAL. None of the five studies involving infants with birth weights >700 grams showed a significant increase in pulmonary hemorrhage in the group receiving EXOSURF NEONATAL. In a cross-study analysis of these five studies,

pulmonary hemorrhage was reported for 1% (14/1420) of infants in the placebo group and 2% (27/1411) of infants in the group receiving EXOSURF NEONATAL. Fatal pulmonary hemorrhage occurred in three infants; two in the group receiving EXOSURF NEONATAL and one in the placebo group. Mortality from all causes among infants who developed pulmonary hemorrhage was 43% in the placebo group and 37% in the group receiving EXOSURF NEONATAL. Pulmonary hemorrhage in infants treated with either EXOSURF NEONATAL or placebo was more frequent in infants who were younger, smaller, male, or who had a patent ductus arteriosus. Pulmonary hemorrhage typically occurred in the first 2 days of life in both treatment groups. In more than 7700 infants in the open, uncontrolled study, pulmonary hemorrhage was reported in 4%, but fatal pulmonary hemorrhage was reported rarely (0.4%).

In the controlled clinical studies, infants treated with EXOSURF NEONATAL who received steroids more than 24 hours prior to delivery or indomethacin postnatally had a lower rate of pulmonary hemorrhage than other infants treated with EXOSURF NEONATAL. Attention should be paid to early and aggressive diagnosis and treatment (unless contraindicated) of patent ductus arteriosus during the first 2 days of life (while the ductus arteriosus is often clinically silent). Other potentially protective measures include attempting to decrease FiO_2 preferentially over ventilator pressures during the first 24 to 48 hours after dosing, and attempting to decrease PEEP minimally for at least 48 hours after dosing.

Mucous Plugs: Infants whose ventilation becomes markedly impaired during or shortly after dosing may have mucous plugging of the endotracheal tube, particularly if pulmonary secretions were prominent prior to drug administration. Suctioning of all infants prior to dosing may lessen the chance of mucous plugs obstructing the endotracheal tube. If endotracheal tube obstruction from such plugs is suspected, and suctioning is unsuccessful in removing the obstruction, the blocked endotracheal tube should be replaced immediately.

PRECAUTIONS

General: In the controlled clinical studies, infants known prenatally or postnatally to have major congenital anomalies or who were suspected of having congenital infection were excluded from entry. However, these disorders cannot

be recognized early in life in all cases, and a few infants with these conditions were entered. The benefits of EXOSURF NEONATAL in the affected infants who received drug appeared to be similar to the benefits observed in infants without anomalies or occult infection.

Prophylactic Treatment—Infants <700 Grams: In infants weighing 500 to 700 grams, a single prophylactic dose of EXOSURF NEONATAL significantly: improved FiO_2 and ventilator settings, reduced pneumothorax, and reduced death from RDS, but increased pulmonary hemorrhage (see WARNINGS). Overall mortality did not differ significantly between the group receiving placebo and the group receiving EXOSURF NEONATAL (see Table 1). Data on multiple doses in infants in this weight class are not yet available. Accordingly, clinicians should carefully evaluate the potential risks and benefits of administration of EXOSURF NEONATAL in these infants.

Rescue Treatment—Number of Doses: A small number of infants with RDS have received more than two doses of EXOSURF NEONATAL as rescue treatment. Definitive data on the safety and efficacy of these additional doses are not available.

Carcinogenesis, Mutagenesis, Impairment of Fertility: EXOSURF NEONATAL at concentrations up to 10,000 µg/plate was not mutagenic in the Ames Salmonella assay. Long-term studies have not been performed in animals to evaluate the carcinogenic potential of EXOSURF NEONATAL.

The effects of EXOSURF NEONATAL on fertility have not been studied.

ADVERSE REACTIONS

General: Premature birth is associated with a high incidence of morbidity and mortality. Despite significant reductions in overall mortality associated with EXOSURF NEONATAL, some infants who received EXOSURF NEONATAL developed severe complications and either survived with permanent handicaps or died.

In controlled clinical studies evaluating the safety and efficacy of EXOSURF NEONATAL, numerous safety assessments were made. In infants receiving EXOSURF NEONATAL, pulmonary hemorrhage, apnea, and use of methylxanthines were increased. A number of other adverse events were significantly reduced in the group receiving EXOSURF NEONATAL, particularly various forms of pul-

Table 2. Efficacy Assessments—Rescue Treatment

Number of Doses: Birth Weight Range:	2 Doses 700 to 1350 grams		2 Doses 1250 grams and above	
Treatment Group: Number of Infants:	Placebo (Air) n=213	Exosurf® n=206	Placebo (Air) n=623	Exosurf n=614
	% of Infants		% of Infants	
Death ≤ Day 28[a]	23	11*	7	4†
Death through 1 Year[a]	27	15*	9	6‡
Death from RDS[b]	10	3§	3	1†
Intact Cardiopulmonary Survival[a,c]	62	75§	88	93§
Bronchopulmonary Dysplasia (BPD)[a,d]	18	15	6	3†

[a] "Intent-to-treat" analyses (as randomized)
[b] "As-treated" analyses
[c] Defined by survival through 28 days of life without bronchopulmonary dysplasia
[d] Defined by a combination of clinical and radiographic criteria
* $P<0.001$
† $P<0.05$
‡ $P=0.067$
§ $P<0.01$

Table 1. Efficacy Assessments—Prophylactic Treatment

Number of Doses: Birth Weight Range:	Single Dose 500 to 700 grams		Single Dose 700 to 1350 grams		Single Dose 700 to 1100 grams		1 vs 3 Doses 700 to 1100 grams	
Treatment Group: Number of Infants:	Placebo (Air) n=106	Exosurf® n=109	Placebo (Air) n=185	Exosurf n=176	Placebo (Air) n=222	Exosurf n=224	Exosurf 1 Dose n=356	Exosurf 3 Doses n=360
	% of Infants		% of Infants		% of Infants		% of Infants	
Death ≤Day 28[a]	53	50	11	6	21	15	16	9*
Death through 1 Year[a]	59	60	14	11	30	20†	17	12*
Death from RDS[b]	25	13*	4	3	10	5‡	3	2
Intact Cardiopulmonary Survival[a,c]	29	25	69	78*	65	68	74	78
Bronchopulmonary Dysplasia (BPD)[a,d]	43	44	23	18	19	21	8	12
RDS Incidence[b]	73	81	46	42	55	55	63	68

[a] "Intent-to-treat" analyses (as randomized) except for the 700 to 1350 gram, single-dose study in which infants with congenital infections and anomalies were excluded
[b] "As-treated" analyses
[c] Defined by survival through 28 days of life without bronchopulmonary dysplasia
[d] Defined by a combination of clinical and radiographic criteria
* $P<0.05$
† $P<0.01$
‡ $P=0.051$

Table 3. Safety Assessments[a]—Prophylactic Treatment

Number of Doses: Birth Weight Range:	Single Dose 500 to 700 grams		Single Dose 700 to 1350 grams		Single Dose 700 to 1100 grams		1 vs 3 Doses 700 to 1100 grams	
Treatment Group: Number of Infants:	Placebo (Air) n=108	Exosurf® n=107	Placebo (Air) n=193	Exosurf n=192	Placebo (Air) n=222	Exosurf n=224	Exosurf 1 Dose n=356	Exosurf 3 Doses n=360
	% of Infants		% of Infants		% of Infants		% of Infants	
Intraventricular Hemorrhage (IVH)								
Overall	51	57	31	27	36	36	38	35
Severe IVH	26	25	10	8	13	14	9	9
Pulmonary Air Leak (PAL)								
Overall	52	48	16	11	32	25	29	27
Pneumothorax	23	10*	5	6	19	11*	14	12
Pneumopericardium	1	4	2	0	<1	1	1	1
Pneumomediastinum	2	1	2	3	7	1†	3	2
Pulmonary Interstitial Emphysema	43	44	13	7*	26	20	23	22
Death from PAL	4	6	<1	<1	2	1	2	1
Patent Ductus Arteriosus	49	53	66	70	50	55	59	57
Necrotizing Enterocolitis	2	4	11	13	3	4	6	2*
Pulmonary Hemorrhage	2	10†	2	4	1	4	4	6
Congenital Pneumonia	4	4	2	4	2	2	1	1
Nosocomial Pneumonia	10	10	2	4	4	7	14	15
Non-Pulmonary Infections	33	35	34	39	28	29	35	34
Sepsis	30	34	30	34	23	24	30	27
Death From Sepsis	4	4	3	3	1	2	2	2
Meningitis	4	6	3	1	2	3	1	2
Other Infections	7	4	5	3	6	10	10	11
Major Anomalies	3	1	2	4	7	4	4	4
Hypotension	70	77	52	47	59	62	54	50
Hyperbilirubinemia	22	21	63	61	27	31	20	21
Exchange Transfusion	4	3	1	2	2	2	3	1
Thrombocytopenia[b]	21	25	not available		9	8	12	10
Persistent Fetal Circulation	0	1	1	1	0	2*	1	<1
Seizures	11	8	2	2	11	9	6	5
Apnea	34	33	76	73	55	65*	62	68
Drug Therapy								
Antibiotics	96	99	98	96	98	99	>99	99
Diuretics	55	60	39	37	59	63	64	65
Anticonvulsants	14	18	23	24	20	16	9	8
Inotropes	46	40	20	20	26	20	28	27
Sedatives	62	71	65	64	63	57	52	52
Pancuronium	19	11	22	14*	19	13*	15	11
Methylxanthines	38	43	77	77	61	72*	75	82*

[a] All parameters were examined with "as-treated" analyses.
[b] Thrombocytopenia requiring platelet transfusion.
* $P<0.05$
† $P<0.01$

monary air leak and use of pancuronium (see CLINICAL PHARMACOLOGY: Clinical Results). Tables 3 and 4 summarize the results of the major safety evaluations from the controlled clinical studies.
[See table 3 above]
[See table 4 at bottom of next page]
Pulmonary Hemorrhage: See WARNINGS.
Abnormal Laboratory Values: Abnormal laboratory values are common in critically ill, mechanically ventilated, premature infants. A higher incidence of abnormal laboratory values in the group receiving EXOSURF NEONATAL was not reported.
Events During Dosing: Data on events during dosing are available from more than 8800 infants in the open, uncontrolled clinical study (Table 5).
[See table 5 at bottom of next page]

Reflux: Reflux of EXOSURF NEONATAL into the endotracheal tube during dosing has been observed and may be associated with rapid drug administration. If reflux occurs, drug administration should be halted and, if necessary, peak inspiratory pressure on the ventilator should be increased by 4 to 5 cm H_2O until the endotracheal tube clears.
>20% Drop in Transcutaneous Oxygen Saturation: If transcutaneous oxygen saturation declines during dosing, drug administration should be halted and, if necessary, peak inspiratory pressure on the ventilator should be increased by 4 to 5 cm H_2O for 1 to 2 minutes. In addition, increases of FiO_2 may be required for 1 to 2 minutes.
Mucous Plugs: See WARNINGS.

OVERDOSAGE

There have been no reports of massive overdosage with EXOSURF NEONATAL.

DOSAGE AND ADMINISTRATION

Preparation of Suspension: EXOSURF NEONATAL is best reconstituted immediately before use because it does not contain antibacterial preservatives. However, the reconstituted suspension is chemically and physically stable and remains sterile (when reconstituted using aseptic techniques) when stored at 2° to 30°C (36° to 86°F) for up to 12 hours following reconstitution.

Solutions containing buffers or preservatives should not be used for reconstitution. **Do Not Use Bacteriostatic Water for Injection, USP.** Each vial of EXOSURF NEONATAL should be reconstituted only with **8 mL** of the accompanying diluent (preservative-free Sterile Water for Injection) as follows:
1. Fill a 10 mL or 12 mL syringe with 8 mL preservative-free Sterile Water for Injection using an 18 or 19 gauge needle;
2. Allow the vacuum in the vial to draw the sterile water into the vial;
3. Aspirate as much as possible of the 8 mL out of the vial into the syringe (while maintaining the vacuum), then SUDDENLY release the syringe plunger.
Step 3 should be repeated three or four times to assure adequate mixing of the vial contents. If vacuum is not present, the vial of EXOSURF NEONATAL should not be used.
The appropriate dosage volume for the entire dose (5 mL/kg) should then be drawn into the syringe from **below** the froth in the vial (again maintaining the vacuum). If the infant weighs less than 1600 grams, unused EXOSURF NEONATAL suspension will remain in the vial after the entire dose is drawn into the syringe. If the infant weighs more than 1600 grams, at least two vials will be required for each dose.
Reconstituted EXOSURF NEONATAL is a milky white suspension with a total volume of 8 mL per vial. Each mL of reconstituted EXOSURF NEONATAL contains 13.5 mg colfosceril palmitate, 1.5 mg cetyl alcohol, 1 mg tyloxapol, and sodium chloride to provide a 0.1 N concentration. If the suspension appears to separate, gently shake or swirl the vial to resuspend the preparation. The reconstituted product should be inspected visually for homogeneity immediately before administration; if persistent large flakes or particulates are present, the vial should not be used.
Dosage: Accurate determination of weight at birth is the key to accurate dosing.
Prophylactic Treatment: The first dose of EXOSURF NEONATAL should be administered as a single 5 mL/kg dose as soon as possible after birth. Second and third doses should be administered approximately 12 and 24 hours later to all infants who remain on mechanical ventilation at those times.

Rescue Treatment: EXOSURF NEONATAL should be administered in two 5 mL/kg doses. The initial dose should be administered as soon as possible after the diagnosis of RDS is confirmed. The second dose should be administered approximately 12 hours following the first dose, provided the infant remains on mechanical ventilation. A small number of infants with RDS have received more than two doses of EXOSURF NEONATAL as rescue treatment. Definitive data on the safety and efficacy of these additional doses are not available (see PRECAUTIONS).
Use of Special Endotracheal Tube Adapter: With each vial of EXOSURF NEONATAL for Intratracheal Suspension, five different sized endotracheal tube adapters each with a special right angle Luer®-lock sideport are supplied. The adapters are clean but not sterile. The adapters should be used as follows:
1. Select an adapter size which corresponds to the inside diameter of the endotracheal tube.
2. Insert the adapter into the endotracheal tube with a firm push-twist motion.
3. Connect the breathing circuit wye to the adapter.
4. Remove the cap from the sideport on the adapter. Attach the syringe containing drug to the sideport.
5. After completion of dosing, remove the syringe and RECAP THE SIDEPORT.
Administration: The infant should be suctioned prior to administration of EXOSURF NEONATAL.
EXOSURF NEONATAL suspension is administered via the sideport on the special endotracheal tube adapter **WITHOUT INTERRUPTING MECHANICAL VENTILATION.**

Continued on next page

This product information is based on labeling in effect on June 1, 1998. For further information, contact via direct mail, phone, or web site Medical Information: Glaxo Wellcome Inc., PO Box 13398, Research Triangle Park, NC 27709. Healthcare Professionals (Medical Information): 800-334-0089 Patients (Customer Response Center): 888-TALK2GW (1-888-825-5249) Glaxo Wellcome Corporate Web Site: www.glaxowellcome.com

Exosurf—Cont.

Each dose of EXOSURF NEONATAL is administered in two 2.5 mL/kg half-doses. Each half-dose is instilled slowly over 1 to 2 minutes (30 to 50 mechanical breaths) in small bursts timed with inspiration. After the first 2.5 mL/kg half-dose is administered in the midline position, the infant's head and torso are turned 45° to the **right** for 30 seconds while mechanical ventilation is continued. After the infant is returned to the midline position, the second 2.5 mL/kg half-dose is given in an identical fashion over another 1 to 2 minutes. The infant's head and torso are then turned 45° to the **left** for 30 seconds while mechanical ventilation is continued, and the infant is then turned back to the midline position. These maneuvers allow gravity to assist in the distribution of EXOSURF NEONATAL in the lungs.

During dosing, heart rate, color, chest expansion, facial expressions, the oximeter, and the endotracheal tube patency and position should be monitored. If heart rate slows, the infant becomes dusky or agitated, transcutaneous oxygen saturation falls more than 15%, or EXOSURF NEONATAL backs up in the endotracheal tube, dosing should be slowed or halted and, if necessary, the peak inspiratory pressure, ventilator rate, and/or FiO₂ turned up. On the other hand, rapid improvements in lung function may require immediate reductions in peak inspiratory pressure, ventilator rate, and/or FiO₂. (See WARNINGS and see below for additional information concerning administration.)

Suctioning should not be performed for two hours after EXOSURF NEONATAL is administered, except when dictated by clinical necessity.

General Guidelines for Administration: Administration of EXOSURF NEONATAL should not take precedence over clinical assessment and stabilization of critically ill infants.

Intubation: Prior to dosing with EXOSURF NEONATAL, it is important to ensure that the endotracheal tube tip is in the trachea and not in the esophagus or right or left mainstem bronchus. Brisk and symmetrical chest movement with each mechanical inspiration should be confirmed prior to dosing, as should equal breath sounds in the two axillae. In prophylactic treatment, dosing with EXOSURF NEONATAL need not be delayed for radiographic confirmation of the endotracheal tube tip position. In rescue treatment, bedside confirmation of endotracheal tube tip position is usually sufficient, if at least one chest radiograph subsequent to the last intubation confirmed proper position of the endotracheal tube tip. Some lung areas will remain undosed if the endotracheal tube tip is too low.

Monitoring: Continuous ECG and transcutaneous oxygen saturation monitoring during dosing are essential. In most infants treated prophylactically, it should be possible to initiate such monitoring prior to administration of the first dose of EXOSURF NEONATAL. For subsequent prophylactic and all rescue doses, arterial blood pressure monitoring during dosing is also highly desirable. After both prophylactic and rescue dosing, frequent arterial blood gas sampling is required to prevent post-dosing hyperoxia and hypocarbia (see WARNINGS).

Ventilatory Support During Dosing: The 5 mL/kg dosage volume may cause transient impairment of gas exchange by physical blockage of the airway, particularly in infants on low ventilator settings. As a result, infants may exhibit a drop in oxygen saturation during dosing, especially if they are on low ventilator settings prior to dosing. These transient effects are easily overcome by increasing peak inspiratory pressure on the ventilator by 4 to 5 cm H₂O for 1 to 2 minutes during dosing. FiO₂ can also be increased if necessary. In infants who are particularly fragile or reactive to external stimuli, increasing peak inspiratory pressure by 4 to 5 cm H₂O and/or FiO₂ 20% just prior to dosing may minimize any transient deterioration in oxygenation. However, in virtually all cases it should be possible to return the infant to pre-dose settings within a very short time of dose completion.

Post-Dosing: At the end of dosing, position of the endotracheal tube should be confirmed by listening for equal breath sounds in the two axillae. Attention should be paid to chest expansion, color, transcutaneous saturation, and arterial blood gases. Some infants who receive EXOSURF NEONATAL and other surfactants respond with rapid improvements in pulmonary compliance, minute ventilation, and gas exchange (see WARNINGS). Constant bedside attention of an experienced clinician for at least 30 minutes after dosing is essential. Frequent blood gas sampling also is absolutely essential. Rapid changes in lung function require immediate changes in peak inspiratory pressure, ventilator rate, and/or FiO₂.

Table 4. Safety Assessments[a]—Rescue Treatment

Number of Doses: Birth Weight Range:	2 Doses 700 to 1350 grams		2 Doses 1250 grams and above	
Treatment Group: Number of Infants:	Placebo (Air) n=213	Exosurf® n=206	Placebo (Air) n=622	Exosurf n=615
	% of Infants		% of Infants	
Intraventricular Hemorrhage (IVH)				
Overall	48	52	23	18*
Severe IVH	13	9	5	4
Pulmonary Air Leak (PAL)				
Overall	54	34†	30	18†
Pneumothorax	29	20*	20	10†
Pneumopericardium	4	1	1	2
Pneumomediastinum	8	4	5	2‡
Pulmonary Interstitial Emphysema	48	25 †	24	13†
Death from PAL	7	3	<1	1
Patent Ductus Arteriosus	66	57	54	45*
Necrotizing Enterocolitis	3	3	1	2
Pulmonary Hemorrhage	3	1	<1	1
Congenital Pneumonia	2	3	2	2
Nosocomial Pneumonia	5	7	2	2
Non-Pulmonary Infections	19	22	13	13
Sepsis	15	17	8	8
Death From Sepsis	<1	<1	1	<1
Meningitis	1	<1	1	<1*
Other Infections	5	8	5	6
Major Anomalies	3	3	4	4
Hypotension	62	57	50	39‡
Hyperbilirubinemia	17	19	12	10
Exchange Transfusion	3	4	1	2
Thrombocytopenia[b]	10	11	4	<1‡
Persistent Fetal Circulation	1	1	6	2‡
Seizures	10	10	6	3*
Apnea	48	65 ‡	37	44*
Drug Therapy				
Antibiotics	100	99	98	98
Diuretics	60	65	45	34†
Anticonvulsants	17	17	10	5‡
Inotropes	36	31	27	16†
Sedatives	72	68	76	64†
Pancuronium	34	17 ‡	33	15†
Methylxanthines	62	74 ‡	49	53

[a] All parameters were examined with "as-treated" analyses.
[b] Thrombocytopenia requiring platelet transfusion.
* $P<0.05$
† $P<0.001$
‡ $P<0.01$

Table 5. Events During Dosing in the Open, Uncontrolled Study [a]

Treatment Type: Number of Infants:	Prophylactic Treatment n=1127	Rescue Treatment n=7711
	% of Infants	% of Infants
Reflux of Exosurf Neonatal®	20	31
Drop in O₂ saturation (≥20%)	6	22
Rise in O₂ saturation (≥10%)	5	6
Drop in transcutaneous pO₂ (≥20 mm Hg)	1	8
Rise in transcutaneous pO₂ (≥20 mm Hg)	2	5
Drop in transcutaneous pCO₂ (≥20 mm Hg)	<1	1
Rise in transcutaneous pCO₂ (≥20 mm Hg)	1	3
Bradycardia (<60 beats/min)	1	3
Tachycardia (>200 beats/min)	<1	<1
Gagging	1	5
Mucous Plugs	<1	<1

[a] Infants may have experienced more than one event.
Investigators were prohibited from adjusting FiO₂ and/or ventilator settings during dosing unless significant clinical deterioration occurred.

HOW SUPPLIED

EXOSURF NEONATAL for Intratracheal Suspension is supplied in a carton containing one 10 mL vial of EXOSURF NEONATAL for Intratracheal Suspension, one 10 mL vial of Sterile Water for Injection, and five endotracheal tube adapters (2.5, 3.0, 3.5, 4.0, and 4.5 mm I.D.) (NDC 0173-0207-01)

Store EXOSURF NEONATAL for Intratracheal Suspension at 15° to 30°C (59° to 86°F) in a dry place.

EDUCATIONAL MATERIAL

A videotape on dosing is available from your Glaxo Wellcome Inc. representative. This videotape demonstrates techniques for safe administration of EXOSURF NEONATAL and should be viewed by healthcare professionals who will administer the drug.

Licensed under U.S. Patent Nos. 4312860, 4826821, and 5110806

U.S. Patents No. 5207220 (Method) and 5309903 (Method)

©Copyright 1996 Glaxo Wellcome Inc. All rights reserved.
May 1996/RL-311

Shown in Product Identification Guide, page 312

FLOLAN® ℞
[flō 'lan]
(epoprostenol sodium)
for Injection

DESCRIPTION

FLOLAN (epoprostenol sodium) for Injection is a sterile sodium salt formulated for intravenous (IV) administration. Each vial of FLOLAN contains epoprostenol sodium equivalent to either 0.5 mg (500,000 ng) or 1.5 mg (1,500,000 ng) epoprostenol, 3.76 mg glycine, 2.93 mg sodium chloride, and 50 mg mannitol. Sodium hydroxide may have been added to adjust pH.

Epoprostenol (PGI₂, PGX, prostacyclin), a metabolite of arachidonic acid, is a naturally occurring prostaglandin with potent vasodilatory activity and inhibitory activity of platelet aggregation.

Epoprostenol is $(5Z,9\alpha,11\alpha,13E,15S)$-6,9-epoxy-11,15-dihydroxyprosta-5,13-dien-1-oic acid.

Epoprostenol sodium has a molecular weight of 374.45 and a molecular formula of $C_{20}H_{31}NaO_5$.

FLOLAN is a white to off-white powder that must be reconstituted with STERILE DILUENT for FLOLAN. STERILE DILUENT for FLOLAN is supplied in 50 mL glass vials containing 94 mg glycine, 73.5 mg sodium chloride, sodium hydroxide (added to adjust pH), and Water for Injection, USP. The reconstituted solution of FLOLAN has a pH of 10.2 to 10.8 and is increasingly unstable at a lower pH.

CLINICAL PHARMACOLOGY

General: Epoprostenol has two major pharmacological actions: (1) direct vasodilation of pulmonary and systemic arterial vascular beds, and (2) inhibition of platelet aggregation. In animals, the vasodilatory effects reduce right and left ventricular afterload and increase cardiac output and stroke volume. The effect of epoprostenol on heart rate in animals varies with dose. At low doses, there is vagally mediated bradycardia, but at higher doses, epoprostenol causes reflex tachycardia in response to direct vasodilation and hypotension. No major effects on cardiac conduction have been observed. Additional pharmacologic effects of epoprostenol in animals include bronchodilation, inhibition of gastric acid secretion, and decreased gastric emptying.

Pharmacokinetics: Epoprostenol is rapidly hydrolyzed at neutral pH in blood and is also subject to enzymatic degradation. Animal studies using tritium-labelled epoprostenol have indicated a high clearance (93 mL/min per kg), small volume of distribution (357 mL/kg), and a short half-life (2.7 minutes). During infusions in animals, steady-state plasma concentrations of tritium-labelled epoprostenol were reached within 15 minutes and were proportional to infusion rates.

No available chemical assay is sufficiently sensitive and specific to assess the in vivo human pharmacokinetics of epoprostenol. The in vitro half-life of epoprostenol in human blood at 37°C and pH 7.4 is approximately 6 minutes; the in vivo half-life of epoprostenol in humans is therefore expected to be no greater than 6 minutes. The in vitro pharmacologic half-life of epoprostenol in human plasma, based on inhibition of platelet aggregation, was similar for males (n = 954) and females (n = 1024).

Tritium-labelled epoprostenol has been administered to humans in order to identify the metabolic products of epoprostenol. Epoprostenol is metabolized to two primary metabolites: 6-keto-PGF$_{1\alpha}$ (formed by spontaneous degradation) and 6,15-diketo-13,14-dihydro-PGF$_{1\alpha}$ (enzymatically formed), both of which have pharmacological activity orders of magnitude less than epoprostenol in animal test systems. The recovery of radioactivity in urine and feces over a one-week period was 82% and 4% of the administered dose, respectively. Fourteen additional minor metabolites have been isolated from urine, indicating that epoprostenol is extensively metabolized in humans.

Clinical Trials in Primary Pulmonary Hypertension (PPH):

Hemodynamic Effects: Acute intravenous infusions of FLOLAN for up to 15 minutes in patients with secondary and primary pulmonary hypertension produce dose-related increases in cardiac index (CI) and stroke volume (SV), and dose-related decreases in pulmonary vascular resistance (PVR), total pulmonary resistance (TPR), and mean systemic arterial pressure (SAPm). The effects of FLOLAN on mean pulmonary artery pressure (PAPm) in patients with PPH were variable and minor.

Chronic continuous infusions of FLOLAN in patients with PPH were studied in two prospective, open, randomized trials of 8 and 12 weeks duration comparing FLOLAN plus standard therapy to standard therapy alone. Dosage of FLOLAN was determined as described in DOSAGE AND ADMINISTRATION and averaged 9.2 ng/kg per minute at study end. Standard therapy varied among patients and included some or all of the following: anticoagulants in essentially all patients; oral vasodilators, diuretics, and digoxin in one half to two thirds of patients; and supplemental oxygen in about half the patients. Except for two New York Heart Association (NYHA) functional Class II patients, all patients were either functional Class III or Class IV. As results were similar in the two studies, the pooled results are described. Chronic hemodynamic effects were generally similar to acute effects. CI, SV, and arterial oxygen saturation were increased, and PAPm, right atrial pressure (RAP), TPR, and systemic vascular resistance (SVR) were decreased in patients who received FLOLAN chronically compared to those who did not. Table 1 illustrates the treatment-related hemodynamic changes in these patients after 8 or 12 weeks of treatment.

[See table 1 above]

Table 1
Hemodynamics During Chronic Administration of FLOLAN

Hemodynamic Parameter	Baseline		Mean change from baseline at end of treatment period*	
	FLOLAN® (n = 52)	Standard Therapy (n = 54)	FLOLAN (n = 48)	Standard Therapy (n = 41)
CI (L/min/m^2)	2.0	2.0	0.3**	−0.1
PAPm (mm Hg)	60	60	−5**	1
PVR (Wood U)	16	17	−4**	1
SAPm (mm Hg)	89	91	−4	−3
SV (mL/beat)	44	43	6**	−1
TPR (Wood U)	20	21	−5**	1

*At 8 weeks: FLOLAN n = 10; Standard Therapy n = 11.
At 12 weeks: FLOLAN n = 38; Standard Therapy n = 30.
**Denotes statistically significant change between FLOLAN and Standard Therapy groups.
CI = cardiac index; PAPm = mean pulmonary arterial pressure; PVR = pulmonary vascular resistance; SAPm = mean systemic arterial pressure; SV = stroke volume; TPR = total pulmonary resistance.

These hemodynamic improvements appeared to persist when FLOLAN was administered for at least 36 months in an open, nonrandomized study.

Clinical Effects: Exercise capacity, as measured by the 6-minute walk test, improved significantly in patients receiving continuous intravenous FLOLAN plus standard therapy for 8 or 12 weeks compared to those receiving standard therapy alone. Improvements were apparent as early as the first week of therapy. Increases in exercise capacity were accompanied by significant improvement in dyspnea and fatigue, as measured by the Congestive Heart Failure Questionnaire and the Dyspnea Fatigue Index.

Survival was improved in NYHA functional Class III and Class IV PPH patients treated with FLOLAN for 12 weeks in a multicenter, open, randomized, parallel study. At the end of the treatment period, 8 of 40 patients receiving standard therapy alone died, whereas none of the 41 patients receiving FLOLAN died (*P* = 0.003).

INDICATIONS AND USAGE

FLOLAN is indicated for the long-term intravenous treatment of primary pulmonary hypertension in NYHA Class III and Class IV patients (see CLINICAL PHARMACOLOGY: Clinical Trials).

CONTRAINDICATIONS

A large study evaluating the effect of FLOLAN on survival in NYHA Class III and IV patients with CHF due to severe left ventricular systolic dysfunction was terminated after an interim analysis of 471 patients revealed a higher mortality in patients receiving FLOLAN plus standard therapy than in those receiving standard therapy alone. The chronic use of FLOLAN in patients with CHF due to severe left ventricular systolic dysfunction is therefore contraindicated.

FLOLAN is also contraindicated in patients with known hypersensitivity to the drug or to structurally-related compounds.

WARNINGS

FLOLAN must be reconstituted only as directed using STERILE DILUENT for FLOLAN. FLOLAN must not be reconstituted or mixed with any other parenteral medications or solutions prior to or during administration.

Abrupt Withdrawal: Abrupt withdrawal (including interruptions in drug delivery) or sudden large reductions in dosage of FLOLAN may result in symptoms associated with rebound pulmonary hypertension, including dyspnea, dizziness, and asthenia. In clinical trials, one Class III PPH patient's death was judged attributable to the interruption of FLOLAN. Abrupt withdrawal should be avoided.

Pulmonary Edema: Some patients with primary pulmonary hypertension have developed pulmonary edema during dose-ranging, which may be associated with pulmonary veno-occlusive disease. FLOLAN should not be used chronically in patients who develop pulmonary edema during dose-ranging.

Sepsis: See ADVERSE REACTIONS: Adverse Events Attributable to the Drug Delivery System.

PRECAUTIONS

General: FLOLAN should be used only by clinicians experienced in the diagnosis and treatment of PPH. The diagnosis of PPH should be carefully established by standard clinical tests to exclude secondary causes of pulmonary hypertension.

FLOLAN is a potent pulmonary and systemic vasodilator. Dose-ranging with FLOLAN must be performed in a setting with adequate personnel and equipment for physiologic monitoring and emergency care. Although dose-ranging in clinical trials was performed during right heart catheterization employing a pulmonary artery catheter, in uncontrolled studies utilizing FLOLAN, acute dose-ranging was performed without cardiac catheterization. The risk of cardiac catheterization in patients with PPH should be carefully weighed against the potential benefits. During acute dose-ranging, asymptomatic increases in pulmonary artery pressure coincident with increases in cardiac output occurred rarely. In such cases, dose reduction should be considered, but such an increase does not imply that chronic treatment is contraindicated.

During chronic use, FLOLAN is delivered continuously on an ambulatory basis through a permanent indwelling central venous catheter. Unless contraindicated, anticoagulant therapy should be administered to PPH patients receiving FLOLAN to reduce the risk of pulmonary thromboembolism or systemic embolism through a patent foramen ovale. In order to reduce the risk of infection, aseptic technique must be used in the reconstitution and administration of FLOLAN as well as in routine catheter care. Because FLOLAN is metabolized rapidly, even brief interruptions in the delivery of FLOLAN may result in symptoms associated with rebound pulmonary hypertension including dyspnea, dizziness, and asthenia. The decision to initiate therapy with FLOLAN should be based upon the understanding that there is a high likelihood that intravenous therapy with FLOLAN will be needed for prolonged periods, possibly years, and the patient's ability to accept and care for a permanent intravenous catheter and infusion pump should be carefully considered.

Based on clinical trials, the acute hemodynamic response to FLOLAN did not correlate well with improvement in exercise tolerance or survival during chronic use of FLOLAN. Dosage of FLOLAN during chronic use should be adjusted at the first sign of recurrence or worsening of symptoms attributable to PPH or the occurrence of adverse events associated with FLOLAN (see DOSAGE AND ADMINISTRATION). Following dosage adjustments, standing and supine blood pressure and heart rate should be monitored closely for several hours.

Information for Patients: Patients receiving FLOLAN should receive the following information: **FLOLAN must be reconstituted only with STERILE DILUENT for FLOLAN.** FLOLAN is infused continuously through a permanent indwelling central venous catheter via a small, portable infusion pump. Thus, therapy with FLOLAN requires commitment by the patient to drug reconstitution, drug administration, and care of the permanent central venous catheter. Sterile technique must be adhered to in preparing the drug and in the care of the catheter, and even brief interruptions in the delivery of FLOLAN may result in rapid symptomatic deterioration. The decision to receive FLOLAN for PPH should be based upon the understanding that there is a high likelihood that therapy with FLOLAN will be needed for prolonged periods, possibly years, and the patient's ability to accept and care for a permanent intravenous catheter and infusion pump should be carefully considered.

Drug Interactions: Additional reductions in blood pressure may occur when FLOLAN is administered with diuretics, antihypertensive agents, or other vasodilators. When other antiplatelet agents or anticoagulants are used concomitantly, there is the potential for FLOLAN to increase the risk of bleeding. However, patients receiving infusions of FLOLAN in clinical trials were maintained on anticoagulants without evidence of increased bleeding. In clinical trials, FLOLAN was used with digoxin, diuretics, anticoagulants, oral vasodilators, and supplemental oxygen.

Carcinogenesis, Mutagenesis, Impairment of Fertility: Long-term studies in animals have not been performed to evaluate carcinogenic potential. A micronucleus test in rats revealed no evidence of mutagenicity. The Ames test and DNA elution tests were also negative, although the instability of epoprostenol makes the significance of these tests uncertain. Fertility was not impaired in rats given FLOLAN by subcutaneous injection at doses up to 100 mcg/kg per day [600 mcg/m^2 per day, 2.5 times the recommended human dose (4.6 ng/kg per minute or 245.1 mcg/m^2 per day, IV) based on body surface area].

Continued on next page

This product information is based on labeling in effect on June 1, 1998. For further information, contact via direct mail, phone, or web site Medical Information: Glaxo Wellcome Inc., PO Box 13398, Research Triangle Park, NC 27709. Healthcare Professionals (Medical Information): 800-334-0089 Patients (Customer Response Center): 888-TALK2GW (1-888-825-5249) Glaxo Wellcome Corporate Web Site: www.glaxowellcome.com

Flolan—Cont.

Pregnancy: Pregnancy Category B. Reproductive studies have been performed in pregnant rats and rabbits at doses up to 100 mcg/kg per day (600 mcg/m² per day in rats, 2.5 times the recommended human dose, and 1180 mcg/m² per day in rabbits, 4.8 times the recommended human dose based on body surface area) and have revealed no evidence of impaired fertility or harm to the fetus due to FLOLAN. There are, however, no adequate and well-controlled studies in pregnant women. Because animal reproduction studies are not always predictive of human response, this drug should be used during pregnancy only if clearly needed.

Labor and Delivery: The use of FLOLAN during labor, vaginal delivery, or caesarean section has not been adequately studied in humans.

Nursing Mothers: It is not known whether this drug is excreted in human milk. Because many drugs are excreted in human milk, caution should be exercised when FLOLAN is administered to a nursing woman.

Pediatric Use: Safety and effectiveness in pediatric patients have not been established.

Geriatric Use: Clinical studies of FLOLAN did not include sufficient numbers of patients aged 65 and over to determine whether they respond differently from younger patients. In general, dose selection for an elderly patient should be cautious, reflecting the greater frequency of decreased hepatic, renal, or cardiac function and of concomitant disease or other drug therapy.

ADVERSE REACTIONS

During clinical trials, adverse events were classified as follows: (1) adverse events during acute dose-ranging, (2) adverse events during chronic dosing, and (3) adverse events associated with the drug delivery system.

Adverse Events During Acute Dose-Ranging: During acute dose-ranging, FLOLAN was administered in 2-ng/kg-per-minute increments until the patients developed symptomatic intolerance. The most common adverse events and the adverse events that limited further increases in dose were generally related to the major pharmacologic effect of FLOLAN, vasodilation. The most common dose-limiting adverse events (occurring in ≥1% of patients) were nausea, vomiting, headache, hypotension, and flushing, but also include chest pain, anxiety, dizziness, bradycardia, dyspnea, abdominal pain, musculoskeletal pain, and tachycardia. Table 2 lists the adverse events reported during acute dose-ranging in decreasing order of frequency.

Table 2
Adverse Events During Acute Dose-Ranging

Adverse Events Occurring in ≥1% of Patients	FLOLAN® (% of patients) (n = 391)
Flushing	58
Headache	49
Nausea/Vomiting	32
Hypotension	16
Anxiety, nervousness, agitation	11
Chest pain	11
Dizziness	8
Bradycardia	5
Abdominal pain	5
Musculoskeletal pain	3
Dyspnea	2
Back pain	2
Sweating	1
Dyspepsia	1
Hypesthesia/Paresthesia	1
Tachycardia	1

Adverse Events During Chronic Administration: Interpretation of adverse events is complicated by the clinical features of PPH, which are similar to some of the pharmacologic effects of FLOLAN (e.g., dizziness, syncope). Adverse events probably related to the underlying disease include dyspnea, fatigue, chest pain, right ventricular failure, and pallor. Several adverse events, on the other hand, can clearly be attributed to FLOLAN. These include headache, jaw pain, flushing, diarrhea, nausea and vomiting, flu-like symptoms, and anxiety/nervousness. In an effort to separate the adverse effects of the drug from the adverse effects of the underlying disease, Table 3 lists adverse events that occurred at a rate at least 10% different in the two groups in controlled trials.

Table 3
Adverse Events Regardless of Attribution Occurring with ≥10% Difference Between FLOLAN and Standard Therapy Alone

Adverse Event	FLOLAN® (% of patients) (n = 52)	Standard Therapy (% of patients) (n = 54)
Occurrence More Common with FLOLAN		
GENERAL		
Chills/Fever/Sepsis/ Flu-like symptoms	25	11
CARDIOVASCULAR		
Tachycardia	35	24
Flushing	42	2
GASTROINTESTINAL		
Diarrhea	37	6
Nausea/Vomiting	67	48
MUSCULOSKELETAL		
Jaw Pain	54	0
Myalgia	44	31
Nonspecific musculoskeletal pain	35	15
NEUROLOGICAL		
Anxiety/nervousness/ tremor	21	9
Dizziness	83	70
Headache	83	33
Hypesthesia, Hyperesthesia, Paresthesia	12	2
Occurrence More Common With Standard Therapy		
CARDIOVASCULAR		
Heart Failure	31	52
Syncope	13	24
Shock	0	13
RESPIRATORY		
Hypoxia	25	37

Thrombocytopenia has been reported during uncontrolled clinical trials in patients receiving FLOLAN.

Table 4 lists additional adverse events reported in PPH patients receiving FLOLAN plus standard therapy or standard therapy alone during controlled clinical trials.

Table 4
Adverse Events Regardless of Attribution Occurring with <10% Difference Between FLOLAN and Standard Therapy Alone

Adverse Event	FLOLAN® (% of patients) (n = 52)	Standard Therapy (% of patients) (n = 54)
GENERAL		
Asthenia	87	81
CARDIOVASCULAR		
Angina pectoris	19	20
Arrhythmia	27	20
Bradycardia	15	9
Supraventricular tachycardia	8	0
Pallor	21	30
Cyanosis	31	39
Palpitation	63	61
Cerebrovascular accident	4	0
Hemorrhage	19	11
Hypotension	27	31
Myocardial ischemia	2	6
GASTROINTESTINAL		
Abdominal pain	27	31
Anorexia	25	30
Ascites	12	17
Constipation	6	2
METABOLIC		
Edema	60	63
Hypokalemia	6	4
Weight reduction	27	24
Weight gain	6	4
MUSCULOSKELETAL		
Arthralgia	6	0
Bone pain	0	4
Chest pain	67	65
NEUROLOGICAL		
Confusion	6	11
Convulsion	4	0
Depression	37	44
Insomnia	4	4
RESPIRATORY		
Cough increase	38	46
Dyspnea	90	85
Epistaxis	4	2
Pleural effusion	4	2
DERMATOLOGIC		
Pruritus	4	0
Rash	10	13
Sweating	15	20
SPECIAL SENSES		
Amblyopia	8	4
Vision abnormality	4	0

Adverse Events Attributable to the Drug Delivery System: Chronic infusions of FLOLAN are delivered using a small, portable infusion pump through an indwelling central venous catheter. During controlled trials of up to 12 weeks' duration, 21% of patients reported a local infection and 13% of patients reported pain at the injection site. During long-term follow-up, sepsis was reported at least once in 14% of patients and occurred at a rate of 0.32 infections per patient per year in patients treated with FLOLAN. This rate was higher than reported in patients using chronic indwelling central venous catheters to administer parenteral nutrition, but lower than reported in oncology patients using these catheters. Malfunctions in the delivery system resulting in an inadvertent bolus of or a reduction in FLOLAN were associated with symptoms related to excess or insufficient FLOLAN, respectively (see ADVERSE REACTIONS: Adverse Events During Chronic Administration).

OVERDOSAGE

Signs and symptoms of excessive doses of FLOLAN during clinical trials are the expected dose-limiting pharmacologic effects of FLOLAN, including flushing, headache, hypotension, tachycardia, nausea, vomiting, and diarrhea. Treatment will ordinarily require dose reduction of FLOLAN.

One patient with secondary pulmonary hypertension accidentally received 50 mL of an unspecified concentration of FLOLAN. The patient vomited and became unconscious with an initially unrecordable blood pressure. FLOLAN was discontinued and the patient regained consciousness in seconds. No fatal events have been reported following overdosage of FLOLAN.

Single intravenous doses of FLOLAN at 10 and 50 mg/kg (2,703 and 27,027 times the recommended acute phase human dose based on body surface area) were lethal to mice and rats, respectively. Symptoms of acute toxicity were hypoactivity, ataxia, loss of righting reflex, deep slow breathing, and hypothermia.

DOSAGE AND ADMINISTRATION

Important Note: FLOLAN must be reconstituted only with STERILE DILUENT for FLOLAN. Reconstituted solutions of FLOLAN must not be diluted or administered with other parenteral solutions or medications (see WARNINGS).

Dosage:

Acute Dose-Ranging:
The initial chronic infusion rate of FLOLAN is determined by an acute dose-ranging procedure. During controlled clinical trials, this procedure was performed during cardiac catheterization (see PRECAUTIONS), but in subsequent uncontrolled clinical trials, acute dose-ranging was performed without cardiac catheterization. In either case, the infusion rate is initiated at 2 ng/kg per minute and increased in increments of 2 ng/kg per minute every 15 minutes or longer until dose-limiting pharmacologic effects are elicited. The most common dose-limiting pharmacologic effects (occurring in ≥1% of patients) during dose-ranging are nausea, vomiting, headache, hypotension, and flushing, but also include chest pain, anxiety, dizziness, bradycardia, dyspnea, abdominal pain, musculoskeletal pain, and tachycardia. During acute dose-ranging in clinical trials, the mean maximum dose which did not elicit dose-limiting pharmacologic effects was 8.6 ± 0.3 ng/kg per minute.

Continuous Chronic Infusion:
Chronic continuous infusion of FLOLAN should be administered through a central venous catheter. Temporary peripheral intravenous infusions may be used until central access is established. Chronic infusions of FLOLAN should be initiated at 4 ng/kg per minute less than the maximum-tolerated infusion rate determined during acute dose-ranging. If the maximum-tolerated infusion rate is less than 5 ng/kg per minute, the chronic infusion should be started at one half the maximum-tolerated infusion rate. During clinical trials, the mean initial chronic infusion rate was 5 ng/kg per minute.

Dosage Adjustments: Changes in the chronic infusion rate should be based on persistence, recurrence, or worsening of the patient's symptoms of PPH and the occurrence of adverse events due to excessive doses of FLOLAN. In general, increases in dose from the initial chronic dose should be expected. In the controlled 12-week trial, for example, the dose increased from a mean starting dose of 5.2 ng/kg

Table 5

To make 100 mL of solution with final concentration (ng/mL) of:	Directions:
3,000 ng/mL	Dissolve contents of one 0.5-mg vial with 5 mL of STERILE DILUENT for FLOLAN®. Withdraw 3 mL and add to sufficient STERILE DILUENT for FLOLAN to make a total of 100 mL.
5,000 ng/mL	Dissolve contents of one 0.5-mg vial with 5 mL of STERILE DILUENT for FLOLAN. Withdraw entire vial contents and add sufficient STERILE DILUENT for FLOLAN to make a total of 100 mL.
10,000 ng/mL	Dissolve contents of two 0.5-mg vials each with 5 mL of STERILE DILUENT for FLOLAN. Withdraw entire vial contents and add sufficient STERILE DILUENT for FLOLAN to make a total of 100 mL.
15,000 ng/mL*	Dissolve contents of one 1.5-mg vial with 5 mL of STERILE DILUENT for FLOLAN. Withdraw entire vial contents and add sufficient STERILE DILUENT for FLOLAN to make a total of 100 mL.

* Higher concentrations may be required for patients who receive FLOLAN long-term.

per minute (4 ng/kg per minute less than the new tolerated dose) to 9.2 ng/kg per minute by the end of week 12, just 1.6 ng/kg per minute less than the mean nontolerated dose. Increments in dose should be considered if symptoms of PPH persist or recur after improving. The infusion should be increased by 1- to 2-ng/kg-per-minute increments at intervals sufficient to allow assessment of clinical response; these intervals should be at least 15 minutes. Following establishment of a new chronic infusion rate, the patient should be observed, and standing and supine blood pressure and heart rate monitored for several hours to ensure that the new dose is tolerated.

During chronic infusion, the occurrence of dose-related pharmacological events similar to those observed during acute dose ranging may necessitate a decrease in infusion rate, but the adverse event may occasionally resolve without dosage adjustment. Dosage decreases should be made gradually in 2-ng/kg-per-minute decrements every 15 minutes or longer until the dose-limiting effects resolve. Abrupt withdrawal of FLOLAN or sudden large reductions in infusion rates should be avoided. Except in life-threatening situations (e.g., unconsciousness, collapse, etc.), infusion rates of FLOLAN should be adjusted only under the direction of a physician.

In patients receiving lung transplants, doses of FLOLAN were tapered after the initiation of cardiopulmonary bypass.

Administration: FLOLAN is administered by continuous intravenous infusion via a central venous catheter using an ambulatory infusion pump. During dose-ranging, FLOLAN may be administered peripherally.

The ambulatory infusion pump used to administer FLOLAN should: (1) be small and lightweight, (2) be able to adjust infusion rates in 2-ng/kg-per-minute increments, (3) have occlusion, end of infusion, and low battery alarms, (4) be accurate to ±6% of the programmed rate, and (5) be positive pressure-driven (continuous or pulsatile) with intervals between pulses not exceeding 3 minutes at infusion rates used to deliver FLOLAN. The reservoir should be made of polyvinyl chloride, polypropylene, or glass. Infusion pumps used in clinical trials were the CADD-1 HFX 5100 (Pharmacia Deltec), Walk-Med 410 C (Medfusion, Inc.), and the Auto Syringe AS2F (Baxter Health Care).

To avoid potential interruptions in drug delivery, the patient should have access to a backup infusion pump and intravenous infusion sets. A multi-lumen catheter should be considered if other intravenous therapies are routinely administered.

To facilitate extended use at ambient temperatures exceeding 25°C (77°F), a cold pouch with frozen gel packs was used in clinical trials (see DOSAGE AND ADMINISTRATION: Storage and Stability). The cold pouches and gel packs used in clinical trials were obtained from Palco Labs, Palo Alto, California. Any cold pouch used must be capable of maintaining the temperature of reconstituted FLOLAN between 2° and 8°C for 12 hours.

Reconstitution: FLOLAN is stable only when reconstituted with STERILE DILUENT for FLOLAN. FLOLAN must not be reconstituted or mixed with any other parenteral medications or solutions prior to or during administration.

A concentration for the solution of FLOLAN for acute dose-ranging or chronic therapy should be selected which is compatible with the infusion pump being used with respect to minimum and maximum flow rates, reservoir capacity, and the infusion pump criteria listed above. FLOLAN, when administered chronically, should be prepared in a drug delivery reservoir appropriate for the infusion pump with a total reservoir volume of at least 100 mL. FLOLAN should be prepared using 2 vials of STERILE DILUENT for FLOLAN for use during a 24-hour period. Table 5 gives directions for preparing several different concentrations of FLOLAN:
[See table 5 above]

More than one solution strength may be required to accommodate the range of infusions anticipated during acute dose-ranging. Generally, 3,000 ng/mL and 10,000 ng/mL are

satisfactory concentrations to deliver between 2 to 16 ng/kg per minute in adults. Infusion rates may be calculated using the following formula:

Infusion Rate (mL/hr) =
$$\frac{\text{[Dose (ng/kg/min)} \times \text{Weight (kg)} \times 60 \text{ min/hr]}}{\text{Final Concentration (ng/mL)}}$$

Tables 6 through 9 provide infusion delivery rates for doses up to 16 ng/kg per minute based upon patient weight, drug delivery rate, and concentration of the solution of FLOLAN to be used. These tables may be used to select the most appropriate concentration of FLOLAN that will result in an infusion rate between the minimum and maximum flow rates of the infusion pump and which will allow the desired duration of infusion from a given reservoir volume. Higher infusion rates, and therefore, more concentrated solutions may be necessary with long-term administration of FLOLAN.

Table 6

	Infusion Rates for FLOLAN at a Concentration of 3,000 ng/mL							
Patient Weight	Dose or Drug Delivery Rate (ng/kg/min)							
	2	4	6	8	10	12	14	16
(kg)	Infusion Delivery Rate (mL/hr)							
10	—	—	1.2	1.6	2.0	2.4	2.8	3.2
20	—	1.6	2.4	3.2	4.0	4.8	5.6	6.4
30	1.2	2.4	3.6	4.8	6.0	7.2	8.4	9.6
40	1.6	3.2	4.8	6.4	8.0	9.6	11.2	12.8
50	2.0	4.0	6.0	8.0	10.0	12.0	14.0	16.0
60	2.4	4.8	7.2	9.6	12.0	14.4	16.8	19.2
70	2.8	5.6	8.4	11.2	14.0	16.8	19.6	22.4
80	3.2	6.4	9.6	12.8	16.0	19.2	22.4	25.6
90	3.6	7.2	10.8	14.4	18.0	21.6	25.2	28.8
100	4.0	8.0	12.0	16.0	20.0	24.0	28.0	32.0

Table 7

	Infusion Rates for FLOLAN at a Concentration of 5,000 ng/mL							
Patient Weight	Dose or Drug Delivery Rate (ng/kg/min)							
	2	4	6	8	10	12	14	16
(kg)	Infusion Delivery Rate (mL/hr)							
10	—	—	1.0	1.2	1.4	1.7	1.9
20	—	1.0	1.4	1.9	2.4	2.9	3.4	3.8
30	—	1.4	2.2	2.9	3.6	4.3	5.0	5.8
40	1.0	1.9	2.9	3.8	4.8	5.8	6.7	7.7
50	1.2	2.4	3.6	4.8	6.0	7.2	8.4	9.6
60	1.4	2.9	4.3	5.8	7.2	8.6	10.1	11.5
70	1.7	3.4	5.0	6.7	8.4	10.1	11.8	13.4
80	1.9	3.8	5.8	7.7	9.6	11.5	13.4	15.4
90	2.2	4.3	6.5	8.6	10.8	13.0	15.1	17.3
100	2.4	4.8	7.2	9.6	12.0	14.4	16.8	19.2

Table 8

	Infusion Rates for FLOLAN at a Concentration of 10,000 ng/mL						
Patient Weight	Dose or Drug Delivery Rate (ng/kg/min)						
	4	6	8	10	12	14	16
(kg)	Infusion Delivery Rate (mL/hr)						
20	—	—	1.0	1.2	1.4	1.7	1.9
30	—	1.1	1.4	1.8	2.2	2.5	2.9
40	1.0	1.4	1.9	2.4	2.9	3.4	3.8
50	1.2	1.8	2.4	3.0	3.6	4.2	4.8
60	1.4	2.2	2.9	3.6	4.3	5.0	5.8
70	1.7	2.5	3.4	4.2	5.0	5.9	6.7
80	1.9	2.9	3.8	4.8	5.8	6.7	7.7
90	2.2	3.2	4.3	5.4	6.5	7.6	8.6
100	2.4	3.6	4.8	6.0	7.2	8.4	9.6

Table 9

	Infusion Rates for FLOLAN at a Concentration of 15,000 ng/mL						
Patient Weight	Dose or Drug Delivery Rate (ng/kg/min)						
	4	6	8	10	12	14	16
(kg)	Infusion Delivery Rate (mL/hr)						
30	—	—	1.0	1.2	1.4	1.7	1.9
40	—	1.0	1.3	1.6	1.9	2.2	2.6
50	—	1.2	1.6	2.0	2.4	2.8	3.2
60	1.0	1.4	1.9	2.4	2.9	3.4	3.8
70	1.1	1.7	2.2	2.8	3.4	3.9	4.5
80	1.3	1.9	2.6	3.2	3.8	4.5	5.1
90	1.4	2.2	2.9	3.6	4.3	5.0	5.8
100	1.6	2.4	3.2	4.0	4.8	5.6	6.4

Storage and Stability: Unopened vials of FLOLAN are stable until the date indicated on the package when stored at 15° to 25°C (59° to 77°F) and protected from light in the carton. Unopened vials of STERILE DILUENT for FLOLAN are stable until the date indicated on the package when stored at 15° to 25°C (59° to 77°F).

Prior to use, reconstituted solutions of FLOLAN must be protected from light and must be refrigerated at 2° to 8°C (36° to 46°F) if not used immediately. **Do not freeze reconstituted solutions of FLOLAN. Discard any reconstituted solution that has been frozen. Discard any reconstituted solution if it has been refrigerated for more than 48 hours.** During use, a single reservoir of reconstituted solution of FLOLAN can be administered at room temperature for a total duration of 8 hours, or it can be used with a cold pouch and administered up to 24 hours with the use of two frozen 6-oz gel packs in a cold pouch. When stored or in use, reconstituted FLOLAN must be insulated from temperatures greater than 25°C (77°F) and less than 0°C (32°F), and must not be exposed to direct sunlight.

Use at Room Temperature: Prior to use at room temperature, 15° to 25°C (59° to 77°F), reconstituted solutions of FLOLAN may be stored refrigerated at 2° to 8°C (36° to 46°F) for no longer than 40 hours. When administered at room temperature, reconstituted solutions may be used for no longer than 8 hours. This 48-hour period allows the patient to reconstitute a 2-day supply (200 mL) of FLOLAN. Each 100 mL daily supply may be divided into three equal portions. Two of the portions are stored refrigerated at 2° to 8°C (36° to 46°F) until they are used.

Use with a Cold Pouch: Prior to infusion with the use of a cold pouch, solutions may be stored refrigerated at 2° to 8°C (36° to 46°F) for up to 24 hours. When a cold pouch is employed during the infusion, reconstituted solutions of FLOLAN may be used for no longer than 24 hours. The gel packs should be changed every 12 hours. Reconstituted solutions may be kept at 2° to 8°C (36° to 46°F), either in refrigerated storage or in a cold pouch or a combination of the two, for no more than 48 hours.

Parenteral drug products should be inspected visually for particulate matter and discoloration prior to administration whenever solution and container permit. If either occurs, FLOLAN should not be administered.

HOW SUPPLIED

FLOLAN for Injection is supplied as a sterile freeze-dried powder in 17 mL flint glass vials with gray butyl rubber closures, individually packaged in a carton.

17-mL vial containing epoprostenol sodium equivalent to 0.5 mg (500,000 ng), carton of 1 (NDC 0173-0517-00).

17-mL vial containing epoprostenol sodium equivalent to 1.5 mg (1,500,000 ng), carton of 1 (NDC 0173-0519-00).

Store the vials of FLOLAN at 15° to 25°C (59° to 77°F). Protect from light.

The STERILE DILUENT for FLOLAN is supplied in 50-mL flint glass vials with fluororesin-faced butyl rubber closures. 50-mL vial of STERILE DILUENT for FLOLAN, tray of 4 (NDC 0173-0518-00).

Store the vials of STERILE DILUENT for FLOLAN at 15° to 25°C (59° to 77°F). DO NOT FREEZE.

Caution: Federal law prohibits dispensing without prescription.

Continued on next page

This product information is based on labeling in effect on June 1, 1998. For further information, contact via direct mail, phone, or web site Medical Information: Glaxo Wellcome Inc., PO Box 13398, Research Triangle Park, NC 27709. Healthcare Professionals (Medical Information): 800-334-0089 Patients (Customer Response Center): 888-TALK2GW (1-888-825-5249) Glaxo Wellcome Corporate Web Site: www.glaxowellcome.com

Flolan—Cont.

U.S. Patent Nos. 4,335,139; 4,539,333; and 4,883,812 (Use Patent)
Licensed Under U.S. Patent No. 4,338,325
©Copyright 1996 Glaxo Wellcome Inc. All rights reserved.
October 1997/RL-474
Shown in Product Identification Guide, page 312

FLONASE® ℞

[flō'naz]
(fluticasone propionate)
Nasal Spray, 0.05% w/w (50 mcg/actuation)

For Intranasal Use Only.
SHAKE GENTLY BEFORE USE.

DESCRIPTION

Fluticasone propionate, the active ingredient of FLONASE Nasal Spray, is a synthetic corticosteroid with the chemical name of S-fluoromethyl 6α,9α-difluoro-11β-hydroxy-16α-methyl-3-oxo-17α-propionyloxyandrosta-1,4-diene-17β-carbothioate.

Fluticasone propionate is a white to off-white powder with a molecular weight of 500.6. It is practically insoluble in water, freely soluble in dimethyl sulfoxide and dimethylformamide, and slightly soluble in methanol and 95% ethanol.

FLONASE Nasal Spray 50 mcg is an aqueous suspension of microfine fluticasone propionate for topical administration to the nasal mucosa by means of a metering, atomizing spray pump. FLONASE Nasal Spray also contains microcrystalline cellulose and carboxymethylcellulose sodium, dextrose, 0.02% w/w benzalkonium chloride, polysorbate 80, and 0.25% w/w phenylethyl alcohol, and has a pH between 5 and 7. It is necessary to prime the pump before first use or after a period of non-use (1 week or more). After priming (three to four actuations or until a fine spray appears), each actuation delivers 50 mcg of fluticasone propionate in 100 mg of formulation through the nasal adapter. Each bottle of FLONASE Nasal Spray provides 120 metered sprays. After 120 metered sprays, the amount of fluticasone propionate delivered per actuation may not be consistent and the unit should be discarded.

CLINICAL PHARMACOLOGY

Fluticasone propionate is a synthetic, trifluorinated corticosteroid with anti-inflammatory activity. In-vitro dose response studies on a cloned human glucocorticoid receptor system involving binding and gene expression afforded 50% responses at 1.25 and 0.17 nM concentrations, respectively. Fluticasone propionate was threefold to fivefold more potent than dexamethasone in these assays. Data from the McKenzie vasoconstrictor assay in man also support its potent glucocorticoid activity.

In preclinical studies, fluticasone propionate revealed progesterone-like activity similar to the natural hormone. However, the clinical significance of these findings in relation to the low plasma levels (see Pharmacokinetics) is not known.

The precise mechanism through which fluticasone propionate affects allergic rhinitis symptoms is not known. Corticosteroids have been shown to have a wide range of effects on multiple cell types (e.g., mast cells, eosinophils, neutrophils, macrophages, and lymphocytes) and mediators (e.g., histamine, eicosanoids, leukotrienes, and cytokines) involved in inflammation. In seven trials in adults, FLONASE Nasal Spray has decreased nasal mucosal eosinophils in 66% (35% for placebo) of patients and basophils in 39% (28% for placebo) of patients. The direct relationship of these findings to long-term symptom relief is not known.

FLONASE Nasal Spray, like other corticosteroids, is an agent that does not have an immediate effect on allergic symptoms. A decrease in nasal symptoms has been noted in some patients 12 hours after initial treatment with FLONASE Nasal Spray. Maximum benefit may not be reached for several days. Similarly, when corticosteroids are discontinued, symptoms may not return for several days.

Pharmacokinetics: *Absorption:* The activity of FLONASE Nasal Spray is due to the parent drug, fluticasone propionate. Indirect calculations indicate that fluticasone propionate delivered by the intranasal route has an absolute bioavailability averaging less than 2%. After intranasal treatment of patients with allergic rhinitis for 3 weeks, fluticasone propionate plasma concentrations were above the level of detection (50 pg/mL) only when recommended doses were exceeded and then only in occasional samples at low plasma levels. Due to the low bioavailability by the intranasal route, the majority of the pharmacokinetic data was obtained via other routes of administration. Studies using oral dosing of radiolabeled drug have demonstrated that fluticasone propionate is highly extracted from plasma and absorption is low. Oral bioavailability is negligible, and the majority of the circulating radioactivity is due to an inactive metabolite.

Distribution: Following intravenous administration, the distribution of fluticasone propionate follows a three-compartment open model with an apparent volume of distribution of approximately 3.7 L/kg. The percentage of fluticasone propionate bound to human plasma proteins averaged 91% with no obvious concentration relationship. Fluticasone propionate is weakly and reversibly bound to erythrocytes and freely equilibrates between erythrocytes and plasma. Fluticasone propionate is not significantly bound to human transcortin.

Metabolism: The total blood clearance of fluticasone propionate approximates that of liver blood flow, with renal clearance accounting for less than 1% of total. The only circulating metabolite detected in man is the 17β-carboxylic acid derivative of fluticasone propionate. This metabolite has been shown to have negligible pharmacological activity in animal studies. Other metabolites detected in-vitro using cultured human hepatoma cells have not been detected in man.

In a multiple-dose drug interaction study, coadministration of orally inhaled fluticasone propionate (500 mcg twice daily) and erythromycin (333 mg three times daily) did not affect fluticasone propionate pharmacokinetics.

In a drug interaction study, coadministration of orally inhaled fluticasone propionate (1000 mcg, 5 times the maximum daily intranasal dose) and ketoconazole (200 mg once daily) resulted in increased fluticasone propionate concentrations, a reduction in plasma cortisol AUC, and no effect on urinary excretion of cortisol.

Excretion: Following intravenous dosing, fluticasone propionate had an elimination half-life of approximately 3 hours. Less than 5% of a radiolabeled oral dose was excreted in the urine as metabolites, with the remainder excreted in the feces as parent drug and metabolites.

Special Populations: Fluticasone propionate was not studied in any special populations, and no gender-specific pharmacokinetic data have been obtained.

Pharmacodynamics: In a trial to evaluate the potential systemic and topical effects of FLONASE Nasal Spray on allergic rhinitis symptoms, the benefits of comparable drug blood levels produced by FLONASE Nasal Spray and oral fluticasone propionate were compared. The doses used were 200 mcg of FLONASE Nasal Spray, the nasal spray vehicle (plus oral placebo), and 5 and 10 mg of oral fluticasone propionate (plus nasal spray vehicle) per day for 14 days. Plasma levels were undetectable in the majority of patients after intranasal dosing, but present at low levels in the majority after oral dosing. FLONASE Nasal Spray was significantly more effective in reducing symptoms of allergic rhinitis than either the oral fluticasone propionate or the nasal vehicle. This trial demonstrated that the therapeutic effect of FLONASE Nasal Spray can be attributed to the topical effects of fluticasone propionate.

In another trial, the potential systemic effects of FLONASE Nasal Spray on the hypothalamic-pituitary-adrenal (HPA) axis were also studied in allergic patients. FLONASE Nasal Spray given as 200 mcg once daily or 400 mcg twice daily was compared with placebo or oral prednisone 7.5 or 15 mg given in the morning. FLONASE Nasal Spray at either dose for 4 weeks did not affect the adrenal response to 6-hour cosyntropin stimulation, while both doses of oral prednisone significantly reduced the response to cosyntropin.

Clinical Trials: A total of 13 pivotal, randomized, double-blind, parallel, multicenter, vehicle-controlled clinical trials were conducted in the United States in adults and pediatric patients (4 years of age and older) with seasonal or perennial allergic rhinitis. The trials included 2633 adults (1439 men and 1194 women) with a mean age of 37 years (range, 18 to 79). A total of 440 adolescents (405 boys and 35 girls), mean age of 14 (range, 12 to 17), and 500 children (325 boys and 175 girls), mean age of 9 (range, 4 to 11) were also studied. The overall racial distribution was 89% white, 4% black, and 7% other. These trials evaluated the total nasal symptoms scores (TNSS) that included rhinorrhea, nasal obstruction, sneezing, and nasal itching in known allergic patients who were treated for 2 to 24 weeks. Subjects treated with FLONASE Nasal Spray exhibited significantly greater decreases in TNSS than vehicle placebo-treated patients. Nasal mucosal basophils and eosinophils were also reduced at the end of treatment in adult studies; however, the clinical significance of this decrease is not known.

There were no significant differences between fluticasone propionate regimens whether administered as a single daily dose of 200 mcg (two 50-mcg sprays in each nostril) or as 100 mcg (one 50-mcg spray in each nostril) twice daily in six clinical trials. A clear dose response could not be identified in clinical trials. In one trial, 200 mcg/day was slightly more effective than 50 mcg/day during the first few days of treatment; thereafter, no difference was seen. Doses higher than 200 mcg/day were not more effective.

Individualization of Dosage: Adult patients may be started on a 200-mcg once-a-day regimen (two 50-mcg sprays in each nostril once-a-day). An alternative 200-mcg/day dosage regimen can be given as 100 mcg twice daily (one 50-mcg spray in each nostril twice-a-day). Individual patients will experience a variable time to onset and different degree of

symptom relief. A decrease in nasal symptoms may occur as soon as 12 hours after treatment onset. Maximum effect may take several days. Patients who have responded may be able to be maintained (after 4 to 7 days) on 100 mcg/day (one spray in each nostril once daily).

Pediatric patients (4 years of age and older) should be started with 100 mcg (one spray in each nostril once-a-day). Treatment with 200 mcg (two sprays in each nostril once daily or one spray in each nostril twice daily) should be reserved for pediatric patients not adequately responding to 100 mcg daily. Once adequate control is achieved, the dosage should be decreased to 100 mcg (one spray in each nostril) daily.

Maximum total daily doses should not exceed two sprays in each nostril (total dose, 200 mcg/day). There is no evidence that exceeding the recommended dose is more effective.

INDICATIONS AND USAGE

FLONASE Nasal Spray is indicated for the management of the nasal symptoms of seasonal and perennial allergic rhinitis in adults and pediatric patients 4 years of age and older.

It is not indicated for the treatment of nonallergic rhinitis since efficacy has not been adequately demonstrated in patients with this condition. Safety and effectiveness of FLONASE Nasal Spray in children below 4 years of age have not been adequately established.

CONTRAINDICATIONS

FLONASE Nasal Spray is contraindicated in patients with a hypersensitivity to any of its ingredients.

WARNINGS

The replacement of a systemic corticosteroid with a topical corticosteroid can be accompanied by signs of adrenal insufficiency, and in addition some patients may experience symptoms of withdrawal, e.g., joint and/or muscular pain, lassitude, and depression. Patients previously treated for prolonged periods with systemic corticosteroids and transferred to topical corticosteroids should be carefully monitored for acute adrenal insufficiency in response to stress. In those patients who have asthma or other clinical conditions requiring long-term systemic corticosteroid treatment, too rapid a decrease in systemic corticosteroids may cause a severe exacerbation of their symptoms.

The concomitant use of intranasal corticosteroids with other inhaled corticosteroids could increase the risk of signs or symptoms of hypercorticism and/or suppression of the HPA axis.

Patients who are on immunosuppressant drugs are more susceptible to infections than healthy individuals. Chickenpox and measles, for example, can have a more serious or even fatal course in patients on immunosuppressant doses of corticosteroids. In such patients who have not had these diseases, particular care should be taken to avoid exposure. How the dose, route, and duration of corticosteroid administration affects the risk of developing a disseminated infection is not known. The contribution of the underlying disease and/or prior corticosteroid treatment to the risk is also not known. If exposed to chickenpox, prophylaxis with varicella zoster immune globulin (VZIG) may be indicated. If exposed to measles, prophylaxis with pooled intramuscular immunoglobulin (IG) may be indicated. (See the respective package inserts for complete VZIG and IG prescribing information.) If chickenpox develops, treatment with antiviral agents may be considered.

PRECAUTIONS

General: Rarely, immediate hypersensitivity reactions or contact dermatitis may occur after the administration of FLONASE Nasal Spray. Rare instances of wheezing, nasal septum perforation, cataracts, glaucoma, and increased intraocular pressure have been reported following the intranasal application of corticosteroids, including fluticasone propionate.

Use of excessive doses of corticosteroids may lead to signs or symptoms of hypercorticism, suppression of HPA function, and/or reduction of growth velocity in children or teenagers. Physicians should closely follow the growth of children and adolescents taking corticosteroids, by any route, and weigh the benefits of corticosteroid therapy against the possibility of growth suppression if growth appears slowed.

Although systemic effects have been minimal with recommended doses of FLONASE Nasal Spray, potential risk increases with larger doses. Therefore, larger than recommended doses of FLONASE Nasal Spray should be avoided. When used at higher than recommended doses, or in rare individuals at recommended doses, systemic corticosteroid effects such as hypercorticism and adrenal suppression may appear. If such changes occur, the dosage of FLONASE Nasal Spray should be discontinued slowly consistent with accepted procedures for discontinuing oral corticosteroid therapy.

In clinical studies with fluticasone propionate administered intranasally, the development of localized infections of the nose and pharynx with *Candida albicans* has occurred only rarely. When such an infection develops, it may require treatment with appropriate local therapy and discontinua-

tion of treatment with FLONASE Nasal Spray. Patients using FLONASE Nasal Spray over several months or longer should be examined periodically for evidence of *Candida* infection or other signs of adverse effects on the nasal mucosa.
FLONASE Nasal Spray should be used with caution, if at all, in patients with active or quiescent tuberculous infection; untreated local or systemic fungal or bacterial, or systemic viral infections or parasitic infection; or ocular herpes simplex.
Because of the inhibitory effect of corticosteroids on wound healing, patients who have experienced recent nasal septal ulcers, nasal surgery, or nasal trauma should not use a nasal corticosteroid until healing has occurred.
Information for Patients: Patients being treated with FLONASE Nasal Spray should receive the following information and instructions. This information is intended to aid them in the safe and effective use of this medication. It is not a disclosure of all possible adverse or intended effects.
Patients should be warned to avoid exposure to chickenpox or measles and, if exposed, to consult their physician without delay.
Patients should use FLONASE Nasal Spray at regular intervals as directed since its effectiveness depends on its regular use. A decrease in nasal symptoms may occur as soon as 12 hours after starting therapy with FLONASE Nasal Spray. Results in several clinical trials indicate statistically significant improvement within the first day or two of treatment; however, the full benefit of FLONASE Nasal Spray may not be achieved until treatment has been administered for several days. The patient should not increase the prescribed dosage but should contact the physician if symptoms do not improve or if the condition worsens. For the proper use of the nasal spray and to attain maximum improvement, the patient should read and follow carefully the patient's instructions accompanying the product.
Drug Interactions: In a placebo-controlled, crossover study in eight healthy volunteers, coadministration of a single dose of orally inhaled fluticasone propionate (1000 mcg, 5 times the maximum daily intranasal dose) with multiple doses of ketoconazole (200 mg) to steady state resulted in increased mean fluticasone propionate concentrations, a reduction in plasma cortisol AUC, and no effect on urinary excretion of cortisol. This interaction may be due to an inhibition of the cytochrome P450 3A4 isoenzyme system by ketoconazole, which is also the route of metabolism of fluticasone propionate. No drug interaction studies have been conducted with FLONASE Nasal Spray; however, care should be exercised when fluticasone propionate is coadministered with long-term ketoconazole and other known cytochrome P450 3A4 inhibitors.
Carcinogenesis, Mutagenesis, Impairment of Fertility: Fluticasone propionate demonstrated no tumorigenic potential in mice at oral doses up to 1000 mcg/kg (approximately 20 times the maximum recommended daily intranasal dose in adults and approximately 10 times the maximum recommended daily intranasal dose in children on a mcg/m^2 basis) for 78 weeks or in rats at inhalation doses up to 57 mcg/kg (approximately 2 times the maximum recommended daily intranasal dose in adults and approximately equivalent to the maximum recommended daily intranasal dose in children on a mcg/m^2 basis) for 104 weeks.
Fluticasone propionate did not induce gene mutation in prokaryotic or eukaryotic cells in-vitro. No significant clastogenic effect was seen in cultured human peripheral lymphocytes in-vitro or in the mouse micronucleus test when administered at high doses by the oral or subcutaneous routes. Furthermore, the compound did not delay erythroblast division in bone marrow.
No evidence of impairment of fertility was observed in reproductive studies conducted in male and female rats at subcutaneous doses up to 50 mcg/kg (approximately 2 times the maximum recommended daily intranasal dose in adults on a mcg/m^2 basis). Prostate weight was significantly reduced at a subcutaneous dose of 50 mcg/kg.
Pregnancy: *Teratogenic Effects:* Pregnancy Category C. Subcutaneous studies in the mouse and rat at 45 and 100 mcg/kg, respectively (approximately equivalent to and 4 times the maximum recommended daily intranasal dose in adults on a mcg/m^2 basis, respectively) revealed fetal toxicity characteristic of potent corticosteroid compounds, including embryonic growth retardation, omphalocele, cleft palate, and retarded cranial ossification.
In the rabbit, fetal weight reduction and cleft palate were observed at a subcutaneous dose of 4 mcg/kg (approximately 1/3 the maximum recommended daily intranasal dose in adults on a mcg/m^2 basis).
However, no teratogenic effects were reported at oral doses up to 300 mcg/kg (approximately 25 times the maximum recommended daily intranasal dose in adults on a mcg/m^2 basis) of fluticasone propionate to the rabbit. No fluticasone propionate was detected in the plasma in this study, consistent with the established low bioavailability following oral administration (see CLINICAL PHARMACOLOGY).
Fluticasone propionate crossed the placenta following oral administration of 100 mcg/kg to rats or 300 mcg/kg to rabbits (approximately 4 and 25 times, respectively, the maximum recommended daily intranasal dose in adults on a mcg/m^2 basis).
There are no adequate and well-controlled studies in pregnant women. Fluticasone propionate should be used during pregnancy only if the potential benefit justifies the potential risk to the fetus.
Experience with oral corticosteroids since their introduction in pharmacologic, as opposed to physiologic, doses suggests that rodents are more prone to teratogenic effects from corticosteroids than humans. In addition, because there is a natural increase in corticosteroid production during pregnancy, most women will require a lower exogenous corticosteroid dose and many will not need corticosteroid treatment during pregnancy.
Nursing Mothers: It is not known whether fluticasone propionate is excreted in human breast milk. Subcutaneous administration of tritiated fluticasone propionate to lactating rats (10 mcg/kg, approximately 1/3 the maximum recommended daily intranasal dose in adults on a mcg/m^2 basis) resulted in measurable radioactivity in milk. Because other corticosteroids are excreted in human milk, caution should be exercised when FLONASE Nasal Spray is administered to a nursing woman.
Pediatric Use: Five hundred (500) patients aged 4 to 11 years of age and 440 patients aged 12 to 17 years were studied in US clinical trials with fluticasone propionate nasal spray. The safety and effectiveness of FLONASE Nasal Spray in children below 4 years of age have not been established. Oral and, to a less clear extent, inhaled and intranasal corticosteroids have been shown to have the potential to cause a reduction in growth velocity in children and adolescents with extended use. If a child or adolescent on any corticosteroid appears to have growth suppression, the possibility that they are particularly sensitive to this effect of corticosteroids should be considered (see PRECAUTIONS).
Geriatric Use: A limited number of patients above 60 years of age (n = 132) have been treated with FLONASE Nasal Spray in US and non-US clinical trials. While the number of patients is too small to permit separate analysis of efficacy and safety, the adverse reactions reported in this population were similar to those reported by younger patients.

ADVERSE REACTIONS

In controlled US studies, 2427 patients received treatment with intranasal fluticasone propionate. In general, adverse reactions in clinical studies have been primarily associated with irritation of the nasal mucous membranes, and the adverse reactions were reported with approximately the same frequency by patients treated with the vehicle itself. The complaints did not usually interfere with treatment. Less than 2% of patients in clinical trials discontinued because of adverse events; this rate was similar for vehicle placebo and active comparators.
Systemic corticosteroid side effects were not reported during controlled clinical studies up to 6 months' duration with FLONASE Nasal Spray. If recommended doses are exceeded, however, or if individuals are particularly sensitive, or taking FLONASE Nasal Spray in conjunction with administration of other corticosteroids, symptoms of hypercorticism, e.g., Cushing's syndrome, could occur.
The following incidence of common adverse reactions (>3%, where incidence in fluticasone propionate-treated subjects exceeded placebo) is based upon seven controlled clinical trials in which 536 patients (57 girls and 108 boys aged 4 to 11 years, 137 female and 234 male adolescents and adults) were treated with FLONASE Nasal Spray 200 mcg once daily over 2 to 4 weeks and two controlled clinical trials in which 246 patients (119 female and 127 male adolescents and adults) were treated with FLONASE Nasal Spray 200 mcg once daily over 6 months. Also included in the table are adverse events from two studies in which 167 children (45 girls and 122 boys aged 4 to 11 years) were treated with FLONASE Nasal Spray 100 mcg once daily for 2 to 4 weeks. [See table above]

Overall Adverse Experiences With >3% Incidence on Fluticasone Propionate in Controlled Clinical Trials With FLONASE Nasal Spray in Patients ≥4 Years With Seasonal or Perennial Allergic Rhinitis

	Vehicle Placebo (n = 758) %	FLONASE 100 mcg Once Daily (n = 167) %	FLONASE 200 mcg Once Daily (n = 782) %
Headache	14.6	6.6	16.1
Pharyngitis	7.2	6.0	7.8
Epistaxis	5.4	6.0	6.9
Nasal burning	2.6	2.4	3.2
Nausea/vomiting	2.0	4.8	2.6
Asthma symptoms	2.9	7.2	3.3
Cough	2.8	3.6	3.8

Other adverse events that occurred in ≤3% but ≥1% of patients and that were more common with fluticasone propionate (with uncertain relationship to treatment) included: blood in nasal mucus, runny nose, nasal irritation, abdominal pain, diarrhea, fever, flu-like symptoms, aches and pains, dizziness, bronchitis.
Observed During Clinical Practice: In addition to adverse events reported from clinical trials, the following events have been identified during postapproval use of fluticasone propionate in clinical practice. Because they are reported voluntarily from a population of unknown size, estimates of frequency cannot be made. These events have been chosen for inclusion due to either their seriousness, frequency of reporting, causal connection to fluticasone propionate, occurrence during clinical trials, or a combination of these factors.
General: Hypersensitivity reactions, including angioedema, skin rash, edema of the face and tongue, pruritus, urticaria, bronchospasm, wheezing, dyspnea, and anaphylaxis/anaphylactoid reactions, which in rare instances were severe.
Ear, Nose, and Throat: Alteration or loss of sense of taste and/or smell and, rarely, nasal septal perforation, nasal ulcer, sore throat, throat irritation and dryness, cough, hoarseness, and voice changes.
Eye: Dryness and irritation, conjunctivitis, blurred vision, glaucoma, increased intraocular pressure, and cataracts.

OVERDOSAGE

Chronic overdosage with FLONASE Nasal Spray may result in signs/symptoms of hypercorticism (see PRECAUTIONS). Intranasal administration of 2 mg (10 times the recommended dose) of fluticasone propionate twice daily for 7 days to healthy human volunteers was well tolerated. Single oral doses up to 16 mg have been studied in human volunteers with no acute toxic effects reported. Repeat oral doses up to 80 mg daily for 10 days in volunteers and repeat oral doses up to 10 mg daily for 14 days in patients were well tolerated. Adverse reactions were of mild or moderate severity, and incidences were similar in active and placebo treatment groups. Acute overdosage with this dosage form is unlikely since one bottle of FLONASE Nasal Spray contains approximately 8 mg of fluticasone propionate.
The oral and subcutaneous median lethal doses in mice and rats were >1000 mg/kg (>20000 and >41000 times, respectively, the maximum recommended daily intranasal dose in adults and >10000 and >20000 times, respectively, the maximum recommended daily intranasal dose in children on a mg/m^2 basis).

DOSAGE AND ADMINISTRATION

Patients should use FLONASE Nasal Spray at regular intervals as directed since its effectiveness depends on its regular use.
Adults: The recommended starting dosage in **adults** is two sprays (50 mcg of fluticasone propionate each) in each nostril once-a-day (total daily dose, 200 mcg). The same dosage divided into 100 mcg given twice-a-day (e.g., 8 a.m. and 8 p.m.) is also effective. After the first few days, patients may be able to reduce their dosage to 100 mcg (one spray in each nostril) once daily for maintenance therapy.
Adolescents and Children (4 Years of Age and Older): Patients should be started with 100 mcg (one spray in each nostril once-a-day). Patients not adequately responding to 100 mcg may use 200 mcg (two sprays in each nostril). Once adequate control is achieved, the dosage should be decreased to 100 mcg (one spray in each nostril) daily.
The maximum total daily dosage should not exceed two sprays in each nostril (200 mcg/day). (See Individualization of Dosage and Clinical Trials sections.)

Continued on next page

This product information is based on labeling in effect on June 1, 1998. For further information, contact via direct mail, phone, or web site Medical Information: Glaxo Wellcome Inc., PO Box 13398, Research Triangle Park, NC 27709. Healthcare Professionals (Medical Information): 800-334-0089 Patients (Customer Response Center): 888-TALK2GW (1-888-825-5249) Glaxo Wellcome Corporate Web Site: www.glaxowellcome.com

Flonase—Cont.

FLONASE Nasal Spray is not recommended for children under 4 years of age or for patients with nonallergic rhinitis.

Directions for Use: Illustrated patient's instructions for proper use accompany each package of FLONASE Nasal Spray.

HOW SUPPLIED

FLONASE Nasal Spray 50 mcg is supplied in an amber glass bottle providing 120 actuations, net fill weight 16 g (NDC 0173-0453-01). Each actuation delivers 50 mcg of fluticasone propionate in 100 mg of formulation through the nasal adapter. The bottle should be discarded when the labeled number of actuations have been reached even though the bottle is not completely empty. Each bottle is fitted with a white metering atomizing pump, white nasal adapter, and green dust cover in a box of one with patient's instructions for use.

Store between 4° and 30°C (39° and 86°F).

©Copyright 1997 Glaxo Wellcome Inc. All rights reserved.
U.S. Patent 4,335,121

October 1997/RL-494
Shown in Product Identification Guide, page 312

FLOVENT® 44 mcg
(fluticasone propionate, 44 mcg)
Inhalation Aerosol

FLOVENT® 110 mcg
(fluticasone propionate, 110 mcg)
Inhalation Aerosol

FLOVENT® 220 mcg
(fluticasone propionate, 220 mcg)
Inhalation Aerosol

For Oral Inhalation Only

℞

DESCRIPTION

The active component of FLOVENT 44 mcg Inhalation Aerosol, FLOVENT 110 mcg Inhalation Aerosol, and FLOVENT 220 mcg Inhalation Aerosol is fluticasone propionate, a glucocorticoid having the chemical name S-(fluoromethyl)6α,9-difluoro-11β, 17-dihydroxy-16α-methyl-3-oxoandrosta-1,4-diene-17β-carbothioate, 17-propionate.

Fluticasone propionate is a white to off-white powder with a molecular weight of 500.6. It is practically insoluble in water, freely soluble in dimethyl sulfoxide and dimethylformamide, and slightly soluble in methanol and 95% ethanol.

FLOVENT 44 mcg Inhalation Aerosol, FLOVENT 110 mcg Inhalation Aerosol, and FLOVENT 220 mcg Inhalation Aerosol are pressurized, metered-dose aerosol units intended for oral inhalation only. Each unit contains a microcrystalline suspension of fluticasone propionate (micronized) in a mixture of two chlorofluorocarbon propellants (trichlorofluoromethane and dichlorodifluoromethane) with lecithin. Each actuation of the inhaler delivers 50, 125, or 250 mcg of fluticasone propionate from the valve, and 44, 110, or 220 mcg, respectively, of fluticasone propionate from the actuator.

CLINICAL PHARMACOLOGY

Fluticasone propionate is a synthetic, trifluorinated glucocorticoid with potent anti-inflammatory activity. In vitro assays using human lung cytosol preparations have established fluticasone propionate as a human glucocorticoid receptor agonist with an affinity 18 times greater than dexamethasone, almost twice that of beclomethasone-17-monopropionate (BMP), the active metabolite of beclomethasone dipropionate, and over three times that of budesonide. Data from the McKenzie vasoconstrictor assay in man are consistent with these results.

The precise mechanisms of glucocorticoid action in asthma are unknown. Inflammation is recognized as an important component in the pathogenesis of asthma. Glucocorticoids have been shown to inhibit multiple cell types (e.g., mast cells, eosinophils, basophils, lymphocytes, macrophages, and neutrophils) and mediator production or secretion (e.g., histamine, eicosanoids, leukotrienes, and cytokines) involved in the asthmatic response. These anti-inflammatory actions of glucocorticoids may contribute to their efficacy in asthma.

Though highly effective for the treatment of asthma, glucocorticoids do not affect asthma symptoms immediately. However, improvement following inhaled administration of fluticasone propionate can occur within 24 hours of beginning treatment, although maximum benefit may not be achieved for 1 to 2 weeks or longer after starting treatment. When glucocorticoids are discontinued, asthma stability may persist for several days or longer.

Pharmacokinetics: *Absorption:* The activity of FLOVENT Inhalation Aerosol is due to the parent drug, fluticasone propionate. Studies using oral dosing of labeled and unla-

beled drug have demonstrated that the oral systemic bioavailability of fluticasone propionate is negligible (<1%), primarily due to incomplete absorption and pre-systemic metabolism in the gut and liver. In contrast, the majority of the fluticasone propionate delivered to the lung is systemically absorbed. The systemic bioavailability of fluticasone propionate inhalation aerosol in healthy volunteers averaged about 30% of the dose delivered from the actuator. Peak plasma concentrations after an 800-mcg inhaled dose ranged from 0.1 to 1.0 ng/mL.

Distribution: Following intravenous administration, the initial disposition phase for fluticasone propionate was rapid and consistent with its high lipid solubility and tissue binding. The volume of distribution averaged 4.2 L/kg. The percentage of fluticasone propionate bound to human plasma proteins averaged 91%. Fluticasone propionate is weakly and reversibly bound to erythrocytes. Fluticasone propionate is not significantly bound to human transcortin.

Metabolism: The total clearance of fluticasone propionate is high (average, 1,093 mL/min), with renal clearance accounting for less than 0.02% of the total. The only circulating metabolite detected in man is the 17β-carboxylic acid derivative of fluticasone propionate, which is formed through the cytochrome P450 3A4 pathway. This metabolite had approximately 2,000 times less affinity than the parent drug for the glucocorticoid receptor of human lung cytosol in vitro and negligible pharmacological activity in animal studies. Other metabolites detected in vitro using cultured human hepatoma cells have not been detected in man.

Excretion: Following intravenous dosing, fluticasone propionate showed polyexponential kinetics and had a terminal elimination half-life of approximately 7.8 hours. Less than 5% of a radiolabeled oral dose was excreted in the urine as metabolites, with the remainder excreted in the feces as parent drug and metabolites.

Special Populations: Formal pharmacokinetic studies using fluticasone propionate were not carried out in any special populations. In a clinical study using fluticasone propionate inhalation powder, trough fluticasone propionate plasma concentrations were collected in 76 males and 74 females after inhaled administration of 100 and 500 mcg twice daily. Full pharmacokinetic profiles were obtained from 7 female patients and 13 male patients at these doses, and no overall differences in pharmacokinetic behavior were found.

Pharmacodynamics: To confirm that systemic absorption does not play a role in the clinical response to inhaled fluticasone propionate, a double-blind clinical study comparing inhaled and oral fluticasone propionate was conducted. Doses of 100 and 500 mcg twice daily of fluticasone propionate inhalation powder were compared to oral fluticasone propionate, 20,000 mcg given once daily, and placebo for 6 weeks. Plasma levels of fluticasone propionate were detectable in all three active groups, but the mean values were highest in the oral group. Both doses of inhaled fluticasone propionate were effective in maintaining asthma stability and improving lung function while oral fluticasone propionate and placebo were ineffective. This demonstrates that the clinical effectiveness of inhaled fluticasone propionate is due to its direct local effect and not to an indirect effect through systemic absorption.

The potential systemic effects of inhaled fluticasone propionate on the hypothalamic-pituitary-adrenal (HPA) axis were also studied in asthma patients. Fluticasone propionate given by inhalation aerosol at doses of 220, 440, 660, or 880 mcg twice daily was compared with placebo or oral prednisone 10 mg given once daily for 4 weeks. For most patients, the ability to increase cortisol production in response to stress, as assessed by 6-hour cosyntropin stimulation, remained intact with inhaled fluticasone propionate treatment. No patient had an abnormal response (peak less than 18 mcg/dL) after dosing with placebo or 220 mcg twice daily. Ten percent (10%) to 16% of patients treated with fluticasone propionate at doses of 440 mcg or more twice daily had an abnormal response as compared to 29% of patients treated with prednisone.

Clinical Trials: Double-blind, parallel, placebo-controlled, US clinical trials were conducted in 1,818 adolescent and adult asthma patients to assess the efficacy and/or safety of FLOVENT Inhalation Aerosol in the treatment of asthma. Fixed doses ranging from 22 to 880 mcg twice daily were compared to placebo to provide information about appropriate dosing to cover a range of asthma severity. Asthmatic patients included in these studies were those not adequately controlled with beta-agonists alone, those already maintained on daily inhaled corticosteroids, and those requiring oral corticosteroid therapy. In all efficacy trials, at all doses, measures of pulmonary function (forced expiratory volume in 1 second [FEV$_1$] and morning peak expiratory flow rate [AM PEFR]) were statistically significantly improved as compared with placebo.

In two clinical trials of 660 asthmatic patients inadequately controlled on bronchodilators alone, fluticasone propionate administered by inhalation aerosol was evaluated at doses of 44 and 88 mcg twice daily. Both doses of fluticasone propionate improved asthma control significantly as compared with placebo.

Displayed in the figure below are results of pulmonary function tests for the recommended starting dosage of fluticasone propionate inhalation aerosol (88 mcg twice daily) and placebo from a 12-week trial in asthma patients inadequately controlled on bronchodilators alone. Because this trial used predetermined criteria for lack of efficacy, which caused more patients in the placebo group to be withdrawn, pulmonary function results at Endpoint, which is the last evaluable FEV$_1$ result and includes most patients' lung function data, are also provided. Pulmonary function improved significantly with fluticasone propionate compared with placebo by the second week of treatment, and this improvement was maintained over the duration of the trial.

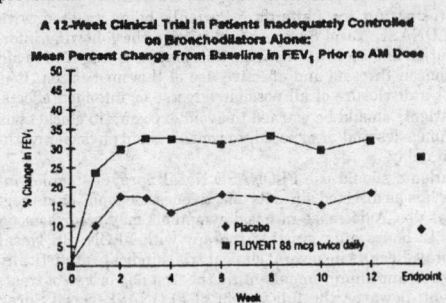

A 12-Week Clinical Trial in Patients Inadequately Controlled on Bronchodilators Alone:
Mean Percent Change From Baseline in FEV$_1$ Prior to AM Dose

In clinical trials of 924 asthmatic patients already receiving daily inhaled corticosteroid therapy (doses of at least 336 mcg/day of beclomethasone dipropionate) in addition to as-needed albuterol and theophylline (46% of all patients), fluticasone propionate inhalation aerosol doses of 22 to 440 mcg twice daily were also evaluated. All doses of fluticasone propionate were efficacious when compared to placebo on major endpoints including lung function and symptom scores. Patients treated with fluticasone propionate were also less likely to discontinue study participation due to asthma deterioration (as defined by predetermined criteria for lack of efficacy including lung function and patient-recorded variables such as AM PEFR, albuterol use, and nighttime awakenings due to asthma).

Displayed in the figure below are results of pulmonary function from a 12-week clinical trial in asthma patients already receiving daily inhaled corticosteroid therapy (beclomethasone dipropionate 336 to 672 mcg/day). The mean percent change from baseline in lung function results for fluticasone propionate inhalation aerosol dosages of 88, 220, and 440 mcg twice daily and placebo are shown over the 12-week trial. Because this trial also used predetermined criteria for lack of efficacy, which caused more patients in the placebo group to be withdrawn, pulmonary function results at Endpoint are included. Pulmonary function improved significantly with fluticasone propionate compared with placebo by the first week of treatment, and the improvement was maintained over the duration of the trial. Analysis of the Endpoint results that adjusted for differential withdrawal rates indicated that pulmonary function significantly improved with fluticasone propionate compared with placebo treatment. Similar improvements in lung function were seen in the other two trials in patients treated with inhaled corticosteroids at baseline.

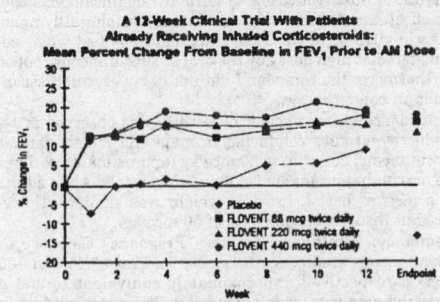

A 12-Week Clinical Trial With Patients Already Receiving Inhaled Corticosteroids:
Mean Percent Change From Baseline in FEV$_1$ Prior to AM Dose

In a clinical trial of 96 severe asthmatic patients requiring chronic oral prednisone therapy (average baseline daily prednisone dose was 10 mg), FLOVENT Inhalation Aerosol doses of 660 and 880 mcg twice daily were evaluated. Both doses enabled a statistically significantly larger percentage of patients to wean successfully from oral prednisone as compared with placebo (69% of the patients on 660 mcg twice daily and 88% of the patients on 880 mcg twice daily as compared with 3% of patients on placebo). Accompanying the reduction in oral corticosteroid use, patients treated with FLOVENT Inhalation Aerosol had significantly improved lung function and fewer asthma symptoms as compared with the placebo group.

[See figure at top of next column]

INDICATIONS AND USAGE

FLOVENT Inhalation Aerosol is indicated for the maintenance treatment of asthma as prophylactic therapy. It is

A 16-Week Clinical Trial in Patients Requiring Chronic Oral Prednisone Therapy: Change in Maintenance Prednisone Dose

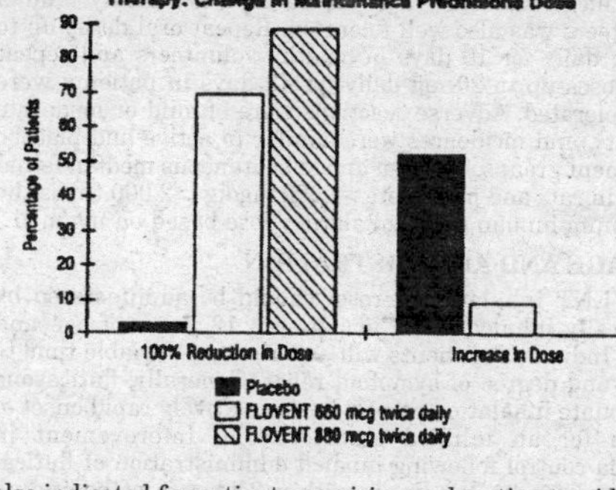
90
80
70
60
50
40
30
20
10
0
Percentage of Patients
100% Reduction in Dose
Increase in Dose
Placebo
FLOVENT 660 mcg twice daily
FLOVENT 880 mcg twice daily

also indicated for patients requiring oral corticosteroid therapy for asthma. Many of these patients may be able to reduce or eliminate their requirement for oral corticosteroids over time.

FLOVENT Inhalation Aerosol is NOT indicated for the relief of acute bronchospasm.

CONTRAINDICATIONS

FLOVENT Inhalation Aerosol is contraindicated in the primary treatment of status asthmaticus or other acute episodes of asthma where intensive measures are required.

Hypersensitivity to any of the ingredients of these preparations contraindicates their use.

WARNINGS

Particular care is needed for patients who are transferred from systemically active corticosteroids to FLOVENT Inhalation Aerosol because deaths due to adrenal insufficiency have occurred in asthmatic patients during and after transfer from systemic corticosteroids to less systemically available inhaled corticosteroids. After withdrawal from systemic corticosteroids, a number of months are required for recovery of HPA function.

Patients who have been previously maintained on 20 mg or more per day of prednisone (or its equivalent) may be most susceptible, particularly when their systemic corticosteroids have been almost completely withdrawn. During this period of HPA suppression, patients may exhibit signs and symptoms of adrenal insufficiency when exposed to trauma, surgery, or infection (particularly gastroenteritis) or other conditions associated with severe electrolyte loss. Although fluticasone propionate inhalation aerosol may provide control of asthma symptoms during these episodes, in recommended doses it supplies less than normal physiological amounts of glucocorticoid systemically and does NOT provide the mineralocorticoid activity that is necessary for coping with these emergencies.

During periods of stress or a severe asthma attack, patients who have been withdrawn from systemic corticosteroids should be instructed to resume oral corticosteroids (in large doses) immediately and to contact their physicians for further instruction. These patients should also be instructed to carry a warning card indicating that they may need supplementary systemic corticosteroids during periods of stress or a severe asthma attack.

Patients requiring oral corticosteroids should be weaned slowly from systemic corticosteroid use after transferring to fluticasone propionate inhalation aerosol. In a trial of 96 patients, prednisone reduction was successfully accomplished by reducing the daily prednisone dose by 2.5 mg on a weekly basis during transfer to inhaled fluticasone propionate. Successive reduction of prednisone dose was allowed only when lung function, symptoms, and as-needed beta-agonist use were better than or comparable to that seen before initiation of prednisone dose reduction. Lung function (FEV_1 or AM PEFR), beta-agonist use, and asthma symptoms should be carefully monitored during withdrawal of oral corticosteroids. In addition to monitoring asthma signs and symptoms, patients should be observed for signs and symptoms of adrenal insufficiency such as fatigue, lassitude, weakness, nausea and vomiting, and hypotension.

Transfer of patients from systemic corticosteroid therapy to fluticasone propionate inhalation aerosol may unmask conditions previously suppressed by the systemic corticosteroid therapy, e.g., rhinitis, conjunctivitis, eczema, and arthritis.

Persons who are on drugs that suppress the immune system are more susceptible to infections than healthy individuals. Chickenpox and measles, for example, can have a more serious or even fatal course in susceptible children or adults on corticosteroids. In such children or adults who have not had these diseases, particular care should be taken to avoid exposure. How the dose, route, and duration of corticosteroid administration affects the risk of developing a disseminated infection is not known. The contribution of the underlying disease and/or prior corticosteroid treatment to the risk is also not known. If exposed to chickenpox, prophylaxis with varicella zoster immune globulin (VZIG) may be indicated. If exposed to measles, prophylaxis with pooled intramuscular immunoglobulin (IG) may be indicated. (See the respective package inserts for complete VZIG and IG prescribing information.) If chickenpox develops, treatment with antiviral agents may be considered.

Fluticasone propionate inhalation aerosol is not to be regarded as a bronchodilator and is not indicated for rapid relief of bronchospasm.

As with other inhaled asthma medications, bronchospasm may occur with an immediate increase in wheezing after dosing. If bronchospasm occurs following dosing with FLOVENT Inhalation Aerosol, it should be treated immediately with a fast-acting inhaled bronchodilator. Treatment with FLOVENT Inhalation Aerosol should be discontinued and alternative therapy instituted.

Patients should be instructed to contact their physicians immediately when episodes of asthma that are not responsive to bronchodilators occur during the course of treatment with fluticasone propionate inhalation aerosol. During such episodes, patients may require therapy with oral corticosteroids.

PRECAUTIONS

General: During withdrawal from oral corticosteroids, some patients may experience symptoms of systemically active corticosteroid withdrawal, e.g., joint and/or muscular pain, lassitude, and depression, despite maintenance or even improvement of respiratory function.

Fluticasone propionate will often permit control of asthma symptoms with less suppression of HPA function than therapeutically equivalent oral doses of prednisone. Since fluticasone propionate is absorbed into the circulation and can be systemically active at higher doses, the beneficial effects of fluticasone propionate inhalation aerosol in minimizing HPA dysfunction may be expected only when recommended dosages are not exceeded and individual patients are titrated to the lowest effective dose. A relationship between plasma levels of fluticasone propionate and inhibitory effects on stimulated cortisol production has been shown after 4 weeks of treatment with fluticasone propionate inhalation aerosol. Since individual sensitivity to effects on cortisol production exists, physicians should consider this information when prescribing fluticasone propionate inhalation aerosol.

Because of the possibility of systemic absorption of inhaled corticosteroids, patients treated with these drugs should be observed carefully for any evidence of systemic corticosteroid effects. Particular care should be taken in observing patients postoperatively or during periods of stress for evidence of inadequate adrenal response.

It is possible that systemic corticosteroid effects such as hypercorticism and adrenal suppression may appear in a small number of patients, particularly at higher doses. If such changes occur, fluticasone propionate inhalation aerosol should be reduced slowly, consistent with accepted procedures for reducing systemic corticosteroids and for management of asthma symptoms.

A reduction of growth velocity in children or teenagers may occur as a result of inadequate control of chronic diseases such as asthma or from use of corticosteroids for treatment. Physicians should closely follow the growth of adolescents taking corticosteroids by any route and weigh the benefits of corticosteroid therapy and asthma control against the possibility of growth suppression if an adolescent's growth appears slowed.

The long-term effects of fluticasone propionate in human subjects are not fully known. In particular, the effects resulting from chronic use of fluticasone propionate on developmental or immunologic processes in the mouth, pharynx, trachea, and lung are unknown. Some patients have received fluticasone propionate inhalation aerosol on a continuous basis for periods of 3 years or longer. In clinical studies with patients treated for nearly 2 years with inhaled fluticasone propionate, no apparent differences in the type or severity of adverse reactions were observed after long- versus short-term treatment.

Rare instances of glaucoma, increased intraocular pressure, and cataracts have been reported following the inhaled administration of corticosteroids, including fluticasone propionate.

In clinical studies with inhaled fluticasone propionate, the development of localized infections of the pharynx with *Candida albicans* has occurred. When such an infection develops, it should be treated with appropriate local or systemic (i.e., oral antifungal) therapy while remaining on treatment with fluticasone propionate inhalation aerosol, but at times therapy with fluticasone propionate may need to be interrupted.

Inhaled corticosteroids should be used with caution, if at all, in patients with active or quiescent tuberculosis infection of the respiratory tract; untreated systemic fungal, bacterial, viral or parasitic infections; or ocular herpes simplex.

Information for Patients: Patients being treated with FLOVENT Inhalation Aerosol should receive the following information and instructions. This information is intended to aid them in the safe and effective use of this medication. It is not a disclosure of all possible adverse or intended effects.

Patients should use FLOVENT Inhalation Aerosol at regular intervals as directed. Results of clinical trials indicated significant improvement may occur within the first day or two of treatment; however, the full benefit may not be achieved until treatment has been administered for 1 to 2 weeks or longer. The patient should not increase the prescribed dosage but should contact the physician if symptoms do not improve or if the condition worsens.

Patients should be warned to avoid exposure to chickenpox or measles and, if they are exposed, to consult their physicians without delay.

For the proper use of FLOVENT Inhalation Aerosol and to attain maximum improvement, the patient should read and follow carefully the Patient's Instructions for Use accompanying the product.

Carcinogenesis, Mutagenesis, Impairment of Fertility: Fluticasone propionate demonstrated no tumorigenic potential in studies of oral doses up to 1,000 mcg/kg (approximately two times the maximum human daily inhalation dose based on mcg/m^2) for 78 weeks in the mouse or inhalation of up to 57 mcg/kg (approximately $^1/_4$ the maximum human daily inhalation dose based on mcg/m^2) for 104 weeks in the rat.

Fluticasone propionate did not induce gene mutation in prokaryotic or eukaryotic cells *in vitro*. No significant clastogenic effect was seen in cultured human peripheral lymphocytes *in vitro* or in the mouse micronucleus test when administered at high doses by the oral or subcutaneous routes. Furthermore, the compound did not delay erythroblast division in bone marrow.

No evidence of impairment of fertilty was observed in reproductive studies conducted in rats dosed subcutaneously with doses up to 50 mcg/kg (approximately $^1/_4$ the maximum human daily inhalation dose based on mcg/m^2) in males and females. However, prostate weight was significantly reduced in rats.

Pregnancy: ***Teratogenic Effects: Pregnancy Category C:*** Subcutaneous studies in the mouse and rat at 45 and 100 mcg/kg, respectively (approximately $^1/_{10}$ and $^1/_2$ the maximum human daily inhalation dose based on mcg/m^2, respectively), revealed fetal toxicity characteristic of potent glucocorticoid compounds, including embryonic growth retardation, omphalocele, cleft palate, and retarded cranial ossification.

In the rabbit, fetal weight reduction and cleft palate were observed following subcutaneous doses of 4 mcg/kg (approximately $^1/_{25}$ the maximum human daily inhalation dose based on mcg/m^2). However, following oral administration of up to 300 mcg/kg (approximately three times the maximum human daily inhalation dose based on mcg/m^2) of fluticasone propionate to the rabbit, there were no maternal effects nor increased incidence of external, visceral, or skeletal fetal defects. No fluticasone propionate was detected in the plasma in this study, consistent with the established low bioavailability following oral administration (see CLINICAL PHARMACOLOGY).

Less than 0.008% of the administered dose crossed the placenta following oral administration of 100 mcg/kg to rats or 300 mcg/kg to rabbits (approximately $^1/_2$ and 3 times the maximum human daily inhalation dose based on mcg/m^2, respectively).

There are no adequate and well-controlled studies in pregnant women. Fluticasone propionate should be used during pregnancy only if the potential benefit justifies the potential risk to the fetus.

Experience with oral glucocorticoids since their introduction in pharmacologic, as opposed to physiologic, doses suggests that rodents are more prone to teratogenic effects from glucocorticoids than humans. In addition, because there is a natural increase in glucocorticoid production during pregnancy, most women will require a lower exogenous glucocorticoid dose and many will not need glucocorticoid treatment during pregnancy.

Nursing Mothers: It is not known whether fluticasone propionate is excreted in human breast milk. Subcutaneous administration of 10 mcg/kg tritiated drug to lactating rats (approximately $^1/_{20}$ the maximum human daily inhalation dose based on mcg/m^2) resulted in measurable radioactivity in both plasma and milk. Because glucocorticoids are ex-

Continued on next page

This product information is based on labeling in effect on June 1, 1998. For further information, contact via direct mail, phone, or web site Medical Information: Glaxo Wellcome Inc., PO Box 13398, Research Triangle Park, NC 27709. Healthcare Professionals (Medical Information): 800-334-0089 Patients (Customer Response Center): 888-TALK2GW (1-888-825-5249) Glaxo Wellcome Corporate Web Site: www.glaxowellcome.com

Flovent—Cont.

creted in human milk, caution should be exercised when fluticasone propionate inhalation aerosol is administered to a nursing woman.

Pediatric Use: One hundred thirty-seven (137) patients between the ages of 12 and 16 years were treated with fluticasone propionate inhalation aerosol in the US pivotal clinical trials. The safety and effectiveness of FLOVENT Inhalation Aerosol in children below 12 years of age have not been established. Oral corticosteroids have been shown to cause a reduction in growth velocity in children and teenagers with extended use. If a child or teenager on any corticosteroid appears to have growth suppression, the possibility that they are particularly sensitive to this effect of corticosteroids should be considered (see PRECAUTIONS).

Geriatric Use: Five hundred seventy-four (574) patients 65 years of age or older have been treated with fluticasone propionate inhalation aerosol in US and non-US clinical trials. There were no differences in adverse reactions compared to those reported by younger patients.

ADVERSE REACTIONS

The following incidence of common adverse experiences is based upon seven placebo-controlled US clinical trials in which 1,243 patients (509 female and 734 male adolescents and adults previously treated with as-needed bronchodilators and/or inhaled corticosteroids) were treated with fluticasone propionate inhalation aerosol (doses of 88 to 440 mcg twice daily for up to 12 weeks) or placebo.

[See first table below]

The table above includes all events (whether considered drug-related or nondrug-related by the investigator) that occurred at a rate of over 3% in the combined fluticasone propionate inhalation aerosol groups and were more common than in the placebo group. In considering these data, differences in average duration of exposure should be taken into account.

These adverse reactions were mostly mild to moderate in severity, with ≤2% of patients discontinuing the studies because of adverse events. Rare cases of immediate and delayed hypersensitivity reactions, including urticaria and rash and other rare events of angioedema and bronchospasm, have been reported.

Systemic glucocorticoid side effects were not reported during controlled clinical trials with fluticasone propionate inhalation aerosol. If recommended doses are exceeded, however, or if individuals are particularly sensitive, symptoms of hypercorticism, e.g., Cushing's syndrome, could occur.

Other adverse events that occurred in these clinical trials using fluticasone propionate inhalation aerosol with an incidence of 1% to 3% and which occurred at a greater incidence than with placebo were:

Ear, Nose, and Throat: Pain in nasal sinus(es), rhinitis.
Eye: Irritation of the eye(s).

Gastrointestinal: Nausea and vomiting, diarrhea, dyspepsia and stomach disorder.
Miscellaneous: Fever.
Mouth and Teeth: Dental problem.
Musculoskeletal: Pain in joint, sprain/strain, aches and pains, pain in limb.
Neurological: Dizziness/giddiness.
Respiratory: Bronchitis, chest congestion.
Skin: Dermatitis, rash/skin eruption.
Urogenital: Dysmenorrhea.

In a 16-week study in asthmatics requiring oral corticosteroids, the effects of fluticasone propionate inhalation aerosol, 660 mcg twice daily (n = 32) and 880 mcg twice daily (n = 32), were compared with placebo. Adverse events (whether considered drug-related or nondrug-related by the investigator) reported by more than three patients in either fluticasone propionate group and which were more common with fluticasone propionate than placebo are shown below:

Ear, Nose, and Throat: Pharyngitis (9% and 25%); nasal congestion (19% and 22%); sinusitis (19% and 22%); nasal discharge (16% and 16%); dysphonia (19% and 9%); pain in nasal sinus(es) (13% and 0%); Candida-like oral lesions (16% and 9%); oropharyngeal candidiasis (25% and 19%).
Respiratory: Upper respiratory infection (31% and 19%); influenza (0% and 13%).
Other: Headache (28% and 34%); pain in joint (19% and 13%); nausea and vomiting (22% and 16%); muscular soreness (22% and 13%); malaise/fatigue (22% and 28%): insomnia (3% and 13%).

Observed During Clinical Practice: In addition to adverse events reported from clinical trials, the following events have been identified during postapproval use of fluticasone propionate in clinical practice. Because they are reported voluntarily from a population of unknown size, estimates of frequency cannot be made. These events have been chosen for inclusion due to either their seriousness, frequency of reporting, causal connection to fluticasone propionate, or a combination of these factors.

Ear, Nose and Throat: Throat soreness and irritation, hoarseness, laryngitis, aphonia.
Endocrine and Metabolic: Cushingoid features, growth velocity reduction in children/adolescents, weight gain, hyperglycemia.
Psychiatry: Restlessness, agitation, aggression, depression.
Respiratory: Immediate bronchospasm, asthma exacerbation, dyspnea, wheeze, chest tightness, bronchospasm, cough.
Skin: Pruritus, contusions, ecchymoses.

OVERDOSAGE

Chronic overdosage may result in signs/symptoms of hypercorticism (see PRECAUTIONS). Inhalation by healthy volunteers of a single dose of 1,760 or 3,520 mcg of fluticasone propionate inhalation aerosol was well tolerated. Flutica-

sone propionate given by inhalation aerosol at doses of 1,320 mcg twice daily for 7 to 15 days to healthy human volunteers was also well tolerated. Repeat oral doses up to 80 mg daily for 10 days in healthy volunteers and repeat oral doses up to 20 mg daily for 42 days in patients were well tolerated. Adverse reactions were of mild or moderate severity, and incidences were similar in active and placebo treatment groups. The oral and subcutaneous median lethal doses in rats and mice were >1,000 mg/kg (>2,000 times the maximum human daily inhalation dose based on mg/m^2).

DOSAGE AND ADMINISTRATION

FLOVENT Inhalation Aerosol should be administered by the orally inhaled route in patients 12 years of age and older. Individual patients will experience a variable time to onset and degree of symptom relief. Generally, fluticasone propionate inhalation aerosol has a relatively rapid onset of action for an inhaled glucocorticoid. Improvement in asthma control following inhaled administration of fluticasone propionate can occur within 24 hours of beginning treatment, although maximum benefit may not be achieved for 1 to 2 weeks or longer after starting treatment.

After asthma stability has been achieved (see below), it is always desirable to titrate to the lowest effective dose to reduce the possibility of side effects. For patients who do not respond adequately to the starting dose after 2 weeks of therapy, higher doses may provide additional asthma control. The safety and efficacy of FLOVENT Inhalation Aerosol when administered in excess of recommended doses has not been established.

Rinsing the mouth after inhalation is advised.

The recommended starting dose and the highest recommended dose of fluticasone propionate inhalation aerosol, based on prior antiasthma therapy, are listed in the following table.

[See second table below]

Geriatric Use: In studies where geriatric patients (65 years of age or older, see PRECAUTIONS) have been treated with fluticasone propionate inhalation aerosol, efficacy and safety did not differ from that in younger patients. Consequently, no dosage adjustment is recommended.

Directions for Use: Illustrated Patient's Instructions for Use accompany each package of FLOVENT Inhalation Aerosol.

HOW SUPPLIED

FLOVENT 44 mcg Inhalation Aerosol is supplied in 7.9-g canisters containing 60 metered inhalations in boxes of one (NDC 0173-0497-00) and in 13-g canisters containing 120 metered inhalations in boxes of one (NDC 0173-0491-00). Each canister is supplied with a dark orange-colored oral actuator with a peach-colored strapcap and patient's instructions. Each actuation of the inhaler delivers 44 mcg of fluticasone propionate from the actuator.

FLOVENT 110 mcg Inhalation Aerosol is supplied in 13-g canisters containing 120 metered inhalations in boxes of one (NDC 0173-0494-00). Each canister is supplied with a dark orange-colored oral actuator with a peach-colored strapcap and patient's instructions. Each actuation of the inhaler delivers 110 mcg of fluticasone propionate from the actuator.

FLOVENT 220 mcg Inhalation Aerosol is supplied in 13-g canisters containing 120 metered inhalations in boxes of one (NDC 0173-0495-00). Each canister is supplied with a dark orange-colored oral actuator with a peach-colored strapcap and patient's instructions. Each actuation of the inhaler delivers 220 mcg of fluticasone propionate from the actuator.

FLOVENT canisters are for use with FLOVENT Inhalation Aerosol actuators only. The actuators should not be used with other aerosol medications.

Store between 2° and 30°C (36° and 86°F). Store canister with nozzle end down. Protect from freezing temperatures and direct sunlight.

Avoid spraying in eyes. Contents under pressure. Do not puncture or incinerate. Do not store at temperatures above 120°F. Keep out of reach of children. For best results, the canister should be at room temperature before use. Shake well before using.

July 1997/RL-439

Shown in Product Identification Guide, page 312

Overall Adverse Experiences With >3% Incidence on Fluticasone Propionate in US Contolled Clinical Trials With MDI in Patients Previously Receiving Bronchodilators and/or Inhaled Corticosteroids

Adverse Event	Placebo (n = 475) %	FLOVENT 88 mcg twice daily (n = 488) %	FLOVENT 220 mcg twice daily (n = 95) %	FLOVENT 440 mcg twice daily (n = 185) %
Ear, nose, and throat				
Pharyngitis	7	10	14	14
Nasal congestion	8	8	16	10
Sinusitis	4	3	6	5
Nasal discharge	3	5	4	4
Dysphonia	1	4	3	8
Allergic rhinitis	4	5	3	3
Oral candidiasis	1	2	3	5
Respiratory				
Upper respiratory infection	12	15	22	16
Influenza	2	3	8	5
Neurological				
Headache	14	17	22	17
Average duration of exposure (days)	44	66	64	59

Previous Therapy	Recommended StartingDose	Highest Recommended Dose
Bronchodilators alone	88 mcg twice daily	440 mcg twice daily
Inhaled corticosteroids	88-220 mcg twice daily*	440 mcg twice daily
Oral corticosteroids†	880 mcg twice daily	880 mcg twice daily

*Starting doses above 88 mcg twice daily may be considered for patients with poorer asthma control or those who have previously required doses of inhaled corticosteroids that are in the higher range for that specific agent.
NOTE: In all patients, it is desirable to titrate to the lowest effective dose once asthma stability is achieved.

†**For Patients Currently Receiving Chronic Oral Corticosteroid Therapy:** Prednisone should be reduced no faster than 2.5 mg/day on a weekly basis, beginning after at least 1 week of therapy with FLOVENT Inhalation Aerosol. Patients should be carefully monitored for signs of asthma instability, including serial objective measures of airflow, and for signs of adrenal insufficiency (see WARNINGS). Once prednisone reduction is complete, the dosage of fluticasone propionate should be reduced to the lowest effective dosage.

FLOVENT® ROTADISK® 50 mcg　　　　　　　　　℞
[flō'věnt rōt 'ə -dĭsk]
(fluticasone propionate inhalation powder, 50 mcg)

FLOVENT® ROTADISK® 100 mcg
(fluticasone propionate inhalation powder, 100 mcg)

FLOVENT® ROTADISK® 250 mcg
(fluticasone propionate inhalation powder, 250 mcg)

For Oral Inhalation Only
For Use With the DISKHALER® Inhalation Device

DESCRIPTION

The active component of FLOVENT ROTADISK 50 mcg, FLOVENT ROTADISK 100 mcg, and FLOVENT

ROTADISK 250 mcg is fluticasone propionate, a corticosteroid having the chemical name S-(fluoromethyl)6α,9-difluoro-11β,17-dihydroxy-16α-methyl-3-oxoandrosta-1,4-diene-17β-carbothioate, 17-propionate and the following chemical structure:

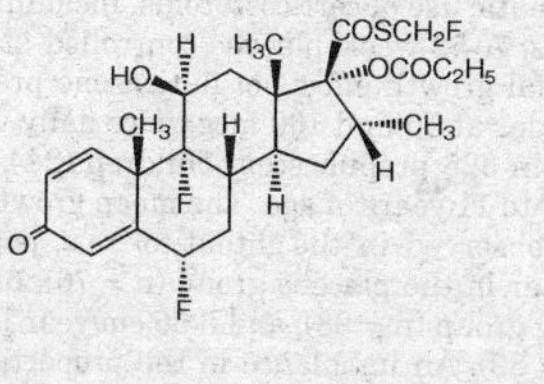

Fluticasone propionate is a white to off-white powder with a molecular weight of 500.6, and the empirical formula is $C_{25}H_{31}F_3O_5S$. It is practically insoluble in water, freely soluble in dimethyl sulfoxide and dimethylformamide, and slightly soluble in methanol and 95% ethanol.

FLOVENT ROTADISK 50 mcg, FLOVENT ROTADISK 100 mcg, and FLOVENT ROTADISK 250 mcg contain a dry powder presentation of fluticasone propionate intended for oral inhalation only. Each double-foil ROTADISK contains four blisters. Each blister contains a mixture of 50, 100, or 250 mcg of microfine fluticasone propionate blended with lactose to a total weight of 25 mg. The contents of each blister are inhaled using a specially designed plastic device for inhaling powder called the DISKHALER. After a fluticasone propionate ROTADISK is loaded into the DISKHALER, a blister containing medication is pierced and the fluticasone propionate is dispersed into the air stream created when the patient inhales through the mouthpiece.

The amount of drug delivered to the lung will depend on patient factors such as inspiratory flow. Under standardized in vitro testing, FLOVENT ROTADISK delivers 44, 88, or 220 mcg of fluticasone propionate from FLOVENT ROTADISK 50 mcg, FLOVENT ROTADISK 100 mcg, or FLOVENT ROTADISK 250 mcg, respectively, when tested at a flow rate of 60 L/min for 3 seconds. In adult and adolescent patients with asthma, mean peak inspiratory flow (PIF) through the DISKHALER was 123 L/min (range, 88 to 159 L/min), and in pediatric patients 4 to 11 years of age with asthma, mean PIF was 110 L/min (range, 43 to 175 L/min).

CLINICAL PHARMACOLOGY

Fluticasone propionate is a synthetic, trifluorinated corticosteroid with potent anti-inflammatory activity. In vitro assays using human lung cytosol preparations have established fluticasone propionate as a human glucocorticoid receptor agonist with an affinity 18 times greater than dexamethasone, almost twice that of beclomethasone-17-monopropionate (BMP), the active metabolite of beclomethasone dipropionate, and over three times that of budesonide. Data from the McKenzie vasoconstrictor assay in man are consistent with these results.

The precise mechanisms of fluticasone propionate action in asthma are unknown. Inflammation is recognized as an important component in the pathogenesis of asthma. Corticosteroids have been shown to inhibit multiple cell types (e.g., mast cells, eosinophils, basophils, lymphocytes, macrophages, and neutrophils) and mediator production or secretion (e.g., histamine, eicosanoids, leukotrienes, and cytokines) involved in the asthmatic response. These anti-inflammatory actions of corticosteroids may contribute to their efficacy in asthma.

Though highly effective for the treatment of asthma, corticosteroids do not affect asthma symptoms immediately. However, improvement following inhaled administration of fluticasone propionate can occur within 24 hours of beginning treatment, although maximum benefit may not be achieved for 1 to 2 weeks or longer after starting treatment. When corticosteroids are discontinued, asthma stability may persist for several days or longer.

Pharmacokinetics: ***Absorption:*** The activity of FLOVENT ROTADISK Inhalation Powder is due to the parent drug, fluticasone propionate. Studies using oral dosing of labeled and unlabeled drug have demonstrated that the oral systemic bioavailability of fluticasone propionate is negligible (<1%), primarily due to incomplete absorption and presystemic metabolism in the gut and liver. In contrast, the majority of the fluticasone propionate delivered to the lung is systemically absorbed. The systemic bioavailability of fluticasone propionate inhalation powder in healthy volunteers averaged about 13.5% of the nominal dose.

Peak plasma concentrations after a 1000-mcg dose of fluticasone propionate inhalation powder ranged from 0.1 to 1.0 ng/mL.

Distribution: Following intravenous administration, the initial disposition phase for fluticasone propionate was rapid and consistent with its high lipid solubility and tissue binding. The volume of distribution averaged 4.2 L/kg. The percentage of fluticasone propionate bound to human plasma proteins averaged 91%.

Fluticasone propionate is weakly and reversibly bound to erythrocytes. Fluticasone propionate is not significantly bound to human transcortin.

Metabolism: The total clearance of fluticasone propionate is high (average, 1093 mL/min), with renal clearance accounting for less than 0.02% of the total. The only circulating metabolite detected in man is the 17β-carboxylic acid derivative of fluticasone propionate, which is formed through the cytochrome P450 3A4 pathway. This metabolite had approximately 2000 times less affinity than the parent drug for the glucocorticoid receptor of human lung cytosol in vitro and negligible pharmacological activity in animal studies. Other metabolites detected in vitro using cultured human hepatoma cells have not been detected in man.

In a multiple-dose drug interaction study, coadministration of fluticasone propionate (500 mcg twice daily) and erythromycin (333 mg three times daily) did not affect fluticasone propionate pharmacokinetics.

In a drug interaction study, coadministration of fluticasone propionate (1000 mcg) and ketoconazole (200 mg once daily) resulted in increased fluticasone propionate concentrations, a reduction in plasma cortisol AUC, and no effect on urinary excretion of cortisol.

Excretion: Following intravenous dosing, fluticasone propionate showed polyexponential kinetics and had a terminal elimination half-life of approximately 7.8 hours. Less than 5% of a radiolabeled oral dose was excreted in the urine as metabolites, with the remainder excreted in the feces as parent drug and metabolites.

Special Populations: Formal pharmacokinetic studies using fluticasone propionate were not carried out in any special populations. In a clinical study using fluticasone propionate inhalation powder, trough fluticasone propionate plasma concentrations were collected in 76 males and 74 females after inhaled administration of 100 and 500 mcg twice daily. Full pharmacokinetic profiles were obtained from 7 female patients and 13 male patients at these doses, and no overall differences in pharmacokinetic behavior were found.

Plasma concentrations of fluticasone propionate were measured 20 and 40 minutes after dosing from 29 children aged 4 to 11 years who were taking either 50 or 100 mcg twice daily of fluticasone propionate inhalation powder. Plasma concentration values ranged from below the limit of quantitation (25 pg/mL) to 117 pg/mL (50-mcg dose) or 154 pg/mL (100-mcg dose). In a study with adults taking the 100-mcg twice-daily dose, the plasma concentrations observed ranged from below the limit of quantitation to 73.1 pg/mL. The median fluticasone propionate plasma concentrations for the 100-mcg dose in children was 58.7 pg/mL; in adults the median plasma concentration was 39.5 pg/mL.

Pharmacodynamics: To confirm that systemic absorption does not play a role in the clinical response to inhaled fluticasone propionate, a double-blind clinical study comparing inhaled and oral fluticasone propionate was conducted. Doses of 100 and 500 mcg twice daily of fluticasone propionate inhalation powder were compared to oral fluticasone propionate, 20 000 mcg given once daily, and placebo for 6 weeks. Plasma levels of fluticasone propionate were detectable in all three active groups, but the mean values were highest in the oral group. Both doses of inhaled fluticasone propionate were effective in maintaining asthma stability and improving lung function while oral fluticasone propionate and placebo were ineffective. This demonstrates that the clinical effectiveness of inhaled fluticasone propionate is due to its direct local effect and not to an indirect effect through systemic absorption.

The potential systemic effects of inhaled fluticasone propionate on the hypothalamic-pituitary-adrenal (HPA) axis were also studied in asthma patients. Fluticasone propionate given by inhalation aerosol at doses of 220, 440, 660, or 880 mcg twice daily was compared with placebo or oral prednisone 10 mg given once daily for 4 weeks. For most patients, the ability to increase cortisol production in response to stress, as assessed by 6-hour cosyntropin stimulation, remained intact with inhaled fluticasone propionate treatment. No patient had an abnormal response (peak serum cortisol <18 mcg/dL) after dosing with placebo or fluticasone propionate 220 mcg twice daily. For patients treated with 440, 660, and 880 mcg twice daily, 10%, 16%, and 12%, respectively, had an abnormal response as compared to 29% of patients treated with prednisone.

In clinical trials with fluticasone propionate inhalation powder, using doses up to and including 250 mcg twice daily, occasional abnormal short cosyntropin tests (peak serum cortisol <18 mcg/dL) were noted in patients receiving fluticasone propionate or placebo. The incidence of abnormal tests at 500 mcg twice daily was greater than placebo. In a 2-year study carried out in 64 patients randomized to fluticasone propionate 500 mcg twice daily or placebo, 1 patient receiving fluticasone propionate (4%) had an abnormal response to 6-hour cosyntropin infusion at 1 year; repeat testing at 18 months and 2 years was normal. Another patient receiving fluticasone propionate (5%) had an abnormal response at 2 years. No patient on placebo had an abnormal response at 1 or 2 years.

Clinical Trials: Double-blind, parallel, placebo-controlled, US clinical trials were conducted in 1197 adolescent and adult asthma patients to assess the efficacy and safety of FLOVENT ROTADISK in the treatment of asthma. Fixed doses of 50, 100, 250, and 500 mcg twice daily were compared to placebo to provide information about appropriate dosing to cover a range of asthma severity. Asthmatic patients included in these studies were those not adequately controlled with beta-agonists alone, and those already maintained on daily inhaled corticosteroids. In these efficacy trials, at all doses, measures of pulmonary function (forced expiratory volume in 1 second [FEV_1] and morning peak expiratory flow rate [AM PEFR]) were statistically significantly improved as compared with placebo. All doses were delivered by inhalation of the contents of one or two blisters from the DISKHALER twice daily.

Displayed in the figure below are results of pulmonary function tests for two recommended dosages of fluticasone propionate inhalation powder (100 and 250 mcg twice daily) and placebo from a 12-week trial in 331 adolescent and adult asthma patients (baseline FEV_1 = 2.63 L/sec) inadequately controlled on bronchodilators alone. Because this trial used predetermined criteria for lack of efficacy, which caused more patients in the placebo group to be withdrawn, pulmonary function results at Endpoint, which is the last evaluable FEV_1 result and includes most patients' lung function data, are also provided. Pulmonary function at both fluticasone propionate dosages improved significantly compared with placebo by the first week of treatment, and this improvement was maintained over the duration of the trial.

A 12-Week Clinical Trial in Patients Inadequately Controlled on Bronchodilators Alone: Mean Percent Change From Baseline in FEV_1 Prior to AM Dose

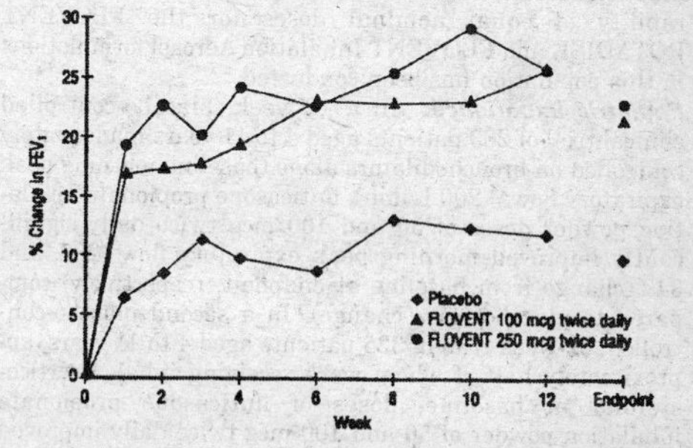

In a second clinical study of 75 patients, 500 mcg twice daily was evaluated in a similar population. In this trial fluticasone propionate significantly improved pulmonary function as compared with placebo.

Displayed in the figure below are results of pulmonary function tests for two recommended dosages of fluticasone propionate inhalation powder (100 and 250 mcg twice daily) and placebo from a 12-week trial in 342 adolescent and adult asthma patients (baseline FEV_1 = 2.49 L/sec) already receiving daily inhaled corticosteroid therapy (≥336 mcg/day of beclomethasone dipropionate or ≥800 mcg/day of triamcinolone acetonide) in addition to as-needed albuterol and theophylline (38% of all patients). Because this trial also used predetermined criteria for lack of efficacy, which caused more patients in the placebo group to be withdrawn, pulmonary function results at Endpoint are included. Pulmonary function at both fluticasone propionate dosages improved significantly compared with placebo by the first week of treatment and the improvement was maintained over the duration of the trial.

[See figure at top of next column]

In a second clinical study of 139 patients, treatment with 500 mcg twice daily was evaluated in a similar patient population. In this trial fluticasone propionate significantly improved pulmonary function as compared with placebo.

In the four trials described above, all dosages of fluticasone propionate were efficacious; however, at higher dosages, patients were less likely to discontinue study participation due to asthma deterioration (as defined by predetermined criteria for lack of efficacy including lung function and patient-recorded variables such as AM PEFR, albuterol use, and nighttime awakenings due to asthma).

In a clinical trial of 96 severe asthmatic patients requiring chronic oral prednisone therapy (average baseline daily

Continued on next page

This product information is based on labeling in effect on June 1, 1998. For further information, contact via direct mail, phone, or web site Medical Information: Glaxo Wellcome Inc., PO Box 13398, Research Triangle Park, NC 27709. Healthcare Professionals (Medical Information): 800-334-0089 Patients (Customer Response Center): 888-TALK2GW (1-888-825-5249) Glaxo Wellcome Corporate Web Site: www.glaxowellcome.com

Flovent Rotadisk—Cont.

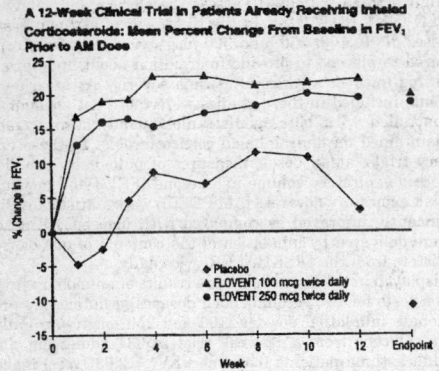

A 12-Week Clinical Trial in Patients Already Receiving Inhaled Corticosteroids: Mean Percent Change From Baseline in FEV₁ Prior to AM Dose

prednisone dose was 10 mg), fluticasone propionate given by inhalation aerosol at doses of 660 and 880 mcg twice daily was evaluated. Both doses enabled a statistically significantly larger percentage of patients to wean successfully from oral prednisone as compared with placebo (69% of the patients on 660 mcg twice daily and 88% of the patients on 880 mcg twice daily as compared with 3% of patients on placebo). Accompanying the reduction in oral corticosteroid use, patients treated with fluticasone propionate had significantly improved lung function and fewer asthma symptoms as compared with the placebo group. These data were obtained from a clinical study using fluticasone propionate inhalation aerosol; no direct assessment of the clinical comparability of equal nominal doses for the FLOVENT ROTADISK and FLOVENT Inhalation Aerosol formulations in this population has been conducted.

Pediatric Experience: In a 12-week, placebo-controlled clinical trial of 263 patients aged 4 to 11 years inadequately controlled on bronchodilators alone (baseline morning peak expiratory flow = 200 L/min), fluticasone propionate inhalation powder doses of 50 and 100 mcg twice daily significantly improved morning peak expiratory flow (28% and 34% change from baseline at endpoint, respectively) compared to placebo (11% change). In a second placebo-controlled, 52-week trial of 325 patients aged 4 to 11 years, approximately half of whom were receiving inhaled corticosteroids at baseline, doses of fluticasone propionate inhalation powder of 50 and 100 mcg twice daily improved lung function by the first week of treatment, and the improvement continued over 1 year compared to placebo. In both studies, patients on active treatment were significantly less likely to discontinue treatment due to lack of efficacy.

INDICATIONS AND USAGE

FLOVENT ROTADISK is indicated for the maintenance treatment of asthma as prophylactic therapy in patients 4 years of age and older. It is also indicated for patients requiring oral corticosteroid therapy for asthma. Many of these patients may be able to reduce or eliminate their requirement for oral corticosteroids over time.

FLOVENT ROTADISK is NOT indicated for the relief of acute bronchospasm.

CONTRAINDICATIONS

FLOVENT ROTADISK is contraindicated in the primary treatment of status asthmaticus or other acute episodes of asthma where intensive measures are required.

Hypersensitivity to any of the ingredients of these preparations contraindicates their use.

WARNINGS

Particular care is needed for patients who are transferred from systemically active corticosteroids to FLOVENT ROTADISK because deaths due to adrenal insufficiency have occurred in asthmatic patients during and after transfer from systemic corticosteroids to less systemically available inhaled corticosteroids. After withdrawal from systemic corticosteroids, a number of months are required for recovery of HPA function.

Patients who have been previously maintained on 20 mg or more per day of prednisone (or its equivalent) may be most susceptible, particularly when their systemic corticosteroids have been almost completely withdrawn. During this period of HPA suppression, patients may exhibit signs and symptoms of adrenal insufficiency when exposed to trauma, surgery, or infection (particularly gastroenteritis) or other conditions associated with severe electrolyte loss. Although fluticasone propionate inhalation powder may provide control of asthma symptoms during these episodes, in recommended doses it supplies less than normal physiological amounts of corticosteroid systemically and does NOT provide the mineralocorticoid activity that is necessary for coping with

these emergencies.

During periods of stress or a severe asthma attack, patients who have been withdrawn from systemic corticosteroids should be instructed to resume oral corticosteroids (in large doses) immediately and to contact their physicians for further instruction. These patients should also be instructed to carry a warning card indicating that they may need supplementary systemic corticosteroids during periods of stress or a severe asthma attack.

Patients requiring oral corticosteroids should be weaned slowly from systemic corticosteroid use after transferring to fluticasone propionate inhalation powder. In a clinical trial of 96 patients, prednisone reduction was successfully accomplished by reducing the daily prednisone dose by 2.5 mg on a weekly basis during transfer to inhaled fluticasone propionate. Successive reduction of prednisone dose was allowed only when lung function, symptoms, and as-needed beta-agonist use were better than or comparable to that seen before initiation of prednisone dose reduction. Lung function (FEV₁ or AM PEFR), beta-agonist use, and asthma symptoms should be carefully monitored during withdrawal of oral corticosteroids. In addition to monitoring asthma signs and symptoms, patients should be observed for signs and symptoms of adrenal insufficiency such as fatigue, lassitude, weakness, nausea and vomiting, and hypotension. Transfer of patients from systemic corticosteroid therapy to fluticasone propionate inhalation powder may unmask conditions previously suppressed by the systemic corticosteroid therapy, e.g., rhinitis, conjunctivitis, eczema, and arthritis. Persons who are on drugs that suppress the immune system are more susceptible to infections than healthy individuals. Chickenpox and measles, for example, can have a more serious or even fatal course in susceptible children or adults on corticosteroids. In such children or adults who have not had these diseases, particular care should be taken to avoid exposure. How the dose, route, and duration of corticosteroid administration affects the risk of developing a disseminated infection is not known. The contribution of the underlying disease and/or prior corticosteroid treatment to the risk is also not known. If exposed to chickenpox, prophylaxis with varicella zoster immune globulin (VZIG) may be indicated. If exposed to measles, prophylaxis with pooled intramuscular immunoglobulin (IG) may be indicated. (See the respective package inserts for complete VZIG and IG prescribing information.) If chickenpox develops, treatment with antiviral agents may be considered.

Fluticasone propionate inhalation powder is not to be regarded as a bronchodilator and is not indicated for rapid relief of bronchospasm.

As with other inhaled asthma medications, bronchospasm may occur with an immediate increase in wheezing after dosing. If bronchospasm occurs following dosing with FLOVENT ROTADISK, it should be treated immediately with a fast-acting inhaled bronchodilator. Treatment with inhaled fluticasone propionate should be discontinued and alternative therapy instituted.

Patients should be instructed to contact their physicians immediately when episodes of asthma that are not responsive to bronchodilators occur during the course of treatment with fluticasone propionate inhalation powder. During such episodes, patients may require therapy with oral corticosteroids.

PRECAUTIONS

General: During withdrawal from oral corticosteroids, some patients may experience symptoms of systemically active corticosteroid withdrawal, e.g., joint and/or muscular pain, lassitude, and depression, despite maintenance or even improvement of respiratory function.

Fluticasone propionate will often permit control of asthma symptoms with less suppression of HPA function than therapeutically equivalent oral doses of prednisone. Since fluticasone propionate is absorbed into the circulation and can be systemically active at higher doses, the beneficial effects of fluticasone propionate inhalation powder in minimizing HPA dysfunction may be expected only when recommended dosages are not exceeded and individual patients are titrated to the lowest effective dose. A relationship between plasma levels of fluticasone propionate and inhibitory effects on stimulated cortisol production has been shown after 4 weeks of treatment with fluticasone propionate inhalation aerosol. Since individual sensitivity to effects on cortisol production exists, physicians should consider this information when prescribing fluticasone propionate inhalation powder.

Because of the possibility of systemic absorption of inhaled corticosteroids, patients treated with these drugs should be observed carefully for any evidence of systemic corticosteroid effects. Particular care should be taken in observing patients postoperatively or during periods of stress for evidence of inadequate adrenal response.

It is possible that systemic corticosteroid effects such as hypercorticism and adrenal suppression may appear in a small number of patients, particularly at higher doses. If

such changes occur, fluticasone propionate inhalation powder should be reduced slowly, consistent with accepted procedures for reducing systemic corticosteroids and for management of asthma symptoms.

A reduction of growth velocity in children or adolescents may occur as a result of poorly controlled asthma or from the therapeutic use of corticosteroids, including inhaled corticosteroids. A 52-week placebo-controlled study to assess the potential growth effects of fluticasone propionate inhalation powder at 50 and 100 mcg twice daily was conducted in the US in 325 prepubescent children (244 males and 81 females), 4 to 11 years of age. The mean growth velocities at 52 weeks observed in the intent-to-treat population were 6.32 cm/year in the placebo group (n = 76), 6.07 cm/year in the 50-mcg group (n = 98), and 5.66 cm/year in the 100-mcg group (n = 89). An imbalance in the proportion of children entering puberty between groups and a higher dropout rate in the placebo group due to poorly controlled asthma may be confounding factors in interpreting these data. A separate subset analysis of children who remained prepubertal during the study revealed growth rates at 52 weeks of 6.10 cm/year in the placebo group (n = 57), 5.91 cm/year in the 50-mcg group (n = 74), and 5.67 cm/year in the 100-mcg group (n = 79). The clinical significance of these growth data is not certain. In children 8.5 years of age, the mean age of children in this study, the range for expected growth velocity is: boys – 3rd percentile = 3.8 cm/year, 50th percentile = 5.4 cm/year, and 97th percentile = 7.0 cm/year; girls – 3rd percentile = 4.2 cm/year, 50th percentile = 5.7 cm/year, and 97th percentile = 7.3 cm/year. The effects of long-term treatment of children with inhaled corticosteroids, including fluticasone propionate, on final adult height are not known. Physicians should closely follow the growth of children and adolescents taking corticosteroids by any route, and weigh the benefits of corticosteroid therapy against the possibility of growth suppression if growth appears slowed. Patients should be maintained on the lowest dose of inhaled corticosteroid that effectively controls their asthma.

The long-term effects of fluticasone propionate in human subjects are not fully known. In particular, the effects resulting from chronic use of fluticasone propionate on developmental or immunologic processes in the mouth, pharynx, trachea, and lung are unknown. Some patients have received inhaled fluticasone propionate on a continuous basis for periods of 3 years or longer. In clinical studies with patients treated for 2 years with inhaled fluticasone propionate, no apparent differences in the type or severity of adverse reactions were observed after long- versus short-term treatment.

Rare instances of glaucoma, increased intraocular pressure, and cataracts have been reported following the inhaled administration of corticosteroids, including fluticasone propionate.

In clinical studies with inhaled fluticasone propionate, the development of localized infections of the pharynx with *Candida albicans* has occurred. When such an infection develops, it should be treated with appropriate local or systemic (i.e., oral antifungal) therapy while remaining on treatment with fluticasone propionate inhalation powder, but at times therapy with fluticasone propionate may need to be interrupted.

Inhaled corticosteroids should be used with caution, if at all, in patients with active or quiescent tuberculous infections of the respiratory tract; untreated systemic fungal, bacterial, viral, or parasitic infections; or ocular herpes simplex.

Information for Patients: Patients being treated with FLOVENT ROTADISK should receive the following information and instructions. This information is intended to aid them in the safe and effective use of this medication. It is not a disclosure of all possible adverse or intended effects. Patients should use FLOVENT ROTADISK at regular intervals as directed. Results of clinical trials indicated significant improvement may occur within the first day or two of treatment; however, the full benefit may not be achieved until treatment has been administered for 1 to 2 weeks or longer. The patient should not increase the prescribed dosage but should contact the physician if symptoms do not improve or if the condition worsens.

Patients should be warned to avoid exposure to chickenpox or measles and, if they are exposed, to consult their physicians without delay.

For the proper use of FLOVENT ROTADISK Inhalation Powder and to attain maximum improvement, the patient should read and follow carefully the Patient's Instructions for Use accompanying the product.

Drug Interactions: In a placebo-controlled, crossover study in eight healthy volunteers, coadministration of a single dose of fluticasone propionate (1000 mcg) with multiple doses of ketoconazole (200 mg) to steady state resulted in increased mean fluticasone propionate concentrations, a reduction in plasma cortisol AUC, and no effect on urinary excretion of cortisol. This interaction may be due to an inhibition of the cytochrome P450 3A4 isoenzyme system by ketoconazole, which is also the route of metabolism of fluticasone propionate. Care should be exercised when

FLOVENT is coadministered with long-term ketoconazole and other known cytochrome P450 3A4 inhibitors.

Carcinogenesis, Mutagenesis, Impairment of Fertility: Fluticasone propionate demonstrated no tumorigenic potential in mice at oral doses up to 1000 mcg/kg (approximately 2 times the maximum recommended daily inhalation dose in adults and approximately 10 times the maximum recommended daily inhalation dose in children on a mcg/m^2 basis) for 78 weeks or in rats at inhalation doses up to 57 mcg/kg (approximately 1/4 the maximum recommended daily inhalation dose in adults and comparable to the maximum recommended daily inhalation dose in children on a mcg/m^2 basis) for 104 weeks.

Fluticasone propionate did not induce gene mutation in prokaryotic or eukaryotic cells in vitro. No significant clastogenic effect was seen in cultured human peripheral lymphocytes in vitro or in the mouse micronucleus test when administered at high doses by the oral or subcutaneous routes. Furthermore, the compound did not delay erythroblast division in bone marrow.

No evidence of impairment of fertility was observed in reproductive studies conducted in male and female rats at subcutaneous doses up to 50 mcg/kg (approximately 1/5 the maximum recommended daily inhalation dose in adults on a mcg/m^2 basis). Prostate weight was significantly reduced at a subcutaneous dose of 50 mcg/kg.

Pregnancy: *Teratogenic Effects:* Pregnancy Category C. Subcutaneous studies in the mouse and rat at 45 and 100 mcg/kg, respectively, (approximately 1/10 and 1/3, respectively, the maximum recommended daily inhalation dose in adults on a mcg/m^2 basis) revealed fetal toxicity characteristic of potent corticosteroid compounds, including embryonic growth retardation, omphalocele, cleft palate, and retarded cranial ossification.

In the rabbit, fetal weight reduction and cleft palate were observed at a subcutaneous dose of 4 mcg/kg (approximately 1/30 the maximum recommended daily inhalation dose in adults on a mcg/m^2 basis). However, no teratogenic effects were reported at oral doses up to 300 mcg/kg (approximately 2 times the maximum recommended daily inhalation dose in adults on a mcg/m^2 basis) of fluticasone propionate. No fluticasone propionate was detected in the plasma in this study, consistent with the established low bioavailability following oral administration (see CLINICAL PHARMACOLOGY).

Fluticasone propionate crossed the placenta following oral administration of 100 mcg/kg to rats or 300 mcg/kg to rabbits (approximately 1/3 and 2 times, respectively, the maximum recommended daily inhalation dose in adults on a mcg/m^2 basis).

There are no adequate and well-controlled studies in pregnant women. Fluticasone propionate should be used during pregnancy only if the potential benefit justifies the potential risk to the fetus.

Experience with oral corticosteroids since their introduction in pharmacologic, as opposed to physiologic, doses suggests that rodents are more prone to teratogenic effects from corticosteroids than humans. In addition, because there is a natural increase in corticosteroid production during pregnancy, most women will require a lower exogenous corticosteroid dose and many will not need corticosteroid treatment during pregnancy.

Nursing Mothers: It is not known whether fluticasone propionate is excreted in human breast milk. Subcutaneous administration to lactating rats of 10 mcg/kg tritiated fluticasone propionate (approximately 1/25 the maximum recommended daily inhalation dose in adults on a mcg/m^2 basis) resulted in measurable radioactivity in milk. Because other corticosteroids are excreted in human milk, caution should be exercised when fluticasone propionate inhalation powder is administered to a nursing woman.

Pediatric Use: Two hundred fourteen (214) patients 4 to 11 years of age and 142 patients 12 to 16 years of age were treated with fluticasone propionate inhalation powder in US clinical trials. The safety and effectiveness of FLOVENT ROTADISK Inhalation Powder in children below 4 years of age have not been established.

Inhaled corticosteroids, including fluticasone propionate, may cause a reduction in growth in children and adolescents (see PRECAUTIONS). If a child or adolescent on any corticosteroid appears to have growth suppression, the possibility that they are particularly sensitive to this effect of corticosteroids should be considered. Patients should be maintained on the lowest dose of inhaled corticosteroid that effectively controls their asthma.

Geriatric Use: One hundred seventy-three (173) patients 65 years of age or older have been treated with fluticasone propionate inhalation powder in US and non-US clinical trials. There were no differences in adverse reactions compared to those reported by younger patients.

ADVERSE REACTIONS

The following incidence of common adverse experiences is based upon six placebo-controlled clinical trials in which 1384 patients ≥4 years of age (520 females and 864 males) previously treated with as-needed bronchodilators and/or

Adverse Event	Placebo (n = 438) %	FLOVENT 50 mcg Twice Daily (n = 255) %	FLOVENT 100 mcg Twice Daily (n = 331) %	FLOVENT 250 mcg Twice Daily (n = 176) %	FLOVENT 500 mcg Twice Daily (n = 184) %
Ear, nose, and throat					
Pharyngitis	7	6	8	8	13
Nasal congestion	5	4	4	7	7
Sinusitis	4	5	4	6	4
Rhinitis	4	4	9	2	3
Dysphonia	0	<1	4	6	4
Oral candidiasis	1	3	3	4	11
Respiratory					
Upper respiratory infection	13	16	17	22	16
Influenza	2	3	3	3	4
Bronchitis	2	4	2	1	2
Other					
Headache	11	11	9	14	15
Diarrhea	1	2	2	0	4
Back problems	<1	<1	1	1	4
Fever	3	4	4	2	2
Average duration of exposure (days)	53	77	68	78	60

Overall Adverse Experiences With >3% Incidence on Fluticasone Propionate in Controlled Clinical Trials With FLOVENT ROTADISK in Patients ≥4 Years Previously Receiving Bronchodilators and/or Inhaled Corticosteroids

Previous Therapy	Recommended Starting Dose	Highest Recommended Dose
Adults and Adolescents		
Bronchodilators alone	100 mcg twice daily	500 mcg twice daily
Inhaled corticosteroids	100-250 mcg twice daily*	500 mcg twice daily
Oral corticosteroids†	1000 mcg twice daily‡	1000 mcg twice daily‡
Children 4 to 11 Years		
Bronchodilators alone	50 mcg twice daily	100 mcg twice daily
Inhaled corticosteroids	50 mcg twice daily	100 mcg twice daily

* Starting doses above 100 mcg twice daily for adults and adolescents and 50 mcg twice daily for children 4 to 11 years of age may be considered for patients with poorer asthma control or those who have previously required doses of inhaled corticosteroids that are in the higher range for that specific agent.
NOTE: In all patients, it is desirable to titrate to the lowest effective dose once asthma stability is achieved.

† **For Patients Currently Receiving Chronic Oral Corticosteroid Therapy:** Prednisone should be reduced no faster than 2.5 mg/day on a weekly basis, beginning after at least 1 week of therapy with FLOVENT. Patients should be carefully monitored for signs of asthma instability, including serial objective measures of airflow, and for signs of adrenal insufficiency (see WARNINGS). Once prednisone reduction is complete, the dosage of fluticasone propionate should be reduced to the lowest effective dosage.

‡ This dosing recommendation is based on clinical data from a study conducted using FLOVENT Inhalation Aerosol. No clinical trials have been conducted in patients on oral corticosteroids using the ROTADISK formulation; no direct assessment of the clinical comparability of equal nominal doses for the FLOVENT ROTADISK and FLOVENT Inhalation Aerosol formulations in this population has been conducted.

inhaled corticosteroids were treated with fluticasone propionate inhalation powder (doses of 50 to 500 mcg twice daily for up to 12 weeks) or placebo.
[See first table above]
The table above includes all events (whether considered drug-related or nondrug-related by the investigator) that occurred at a rate of over 3% in any of the fluticasone propionate inhalation powder groups and were more common than in the placebo group. In considering these data, differences in average duration of exposure should be taken into account.

These adverse reactions were mostly mild to moderate in severity, with <2% of patients discontinuing the studies because of adverse events. Rare cases of immediate and delayed hypersensitivity reactions, including rash and other rare events of angioedema and bronchospasm, have been reported.

Other adverse events that occurred in these clinical trials using fluticasone propionate inhalation powder with an incidence of 1% to 3% and which occurred at a greater incidence than with placebo were:

Ear, Nose, and Throat: Otitis media, tonsillitis, nasal discharge, earache, laryngitis, epistaxis, sneezing.
Eye: Conjunctivitis.
Gastrointestinal: Abdominal pain, viral gastroenteritis, gastroenteritis/colitis, abdominal discomfort.
Miscellaneous: Injury.
Mouth and Teeth: Mouth irritation.
Musculoskeletal: Sprain/strain, pain in joint, disorder/symptoms of neck, muscular soreness, aches and pains.
Neurological: Migraine, nervousness.
Respiratory: Chest congestion, acute nasopharyngitis, dyspnea, irritation due to inhalant.
Skin: Dermatitis, urticaria.
Urogenital: Dysmenorrhea, candidiasis of vagina, pelvic inflammatory disease, vaginitis/vulvovaginitis, irregular menstrual cycle.

There were no clinically relevant differences in the pattern or severity of adverse events in children compared with those reported in adults.

Fluticasone propionate inhalation aerosol (660 or 880 mcg twice daily) was administered for 16 weeks to asthmatics requiring oral corticosteroids. Adverse events reported more frequently in these patients compared to patients not on oral corticosteroids included sinusitis, nasal discharge, oropharyngeal candidiasis, headache, joint pain, nausea and vomiting, muscular soreness, malaise/fatigue, and insomnia.

Observed During Clinical Practice: The following events have been identified during postapproval use of fluticasone propionate in clinical practice. Because they are reported voluntarily from a population of unknown size, estimates of frequency cannot be made. These events have been chosen for inclusion due to either their seriousness, frequency of reporting, causal connection to fluticasone propionate, or a combination of these factors.

Ear, Nose, and Throat: Aphonia, cough, hoarseness, laryngitis, and throat soreness and irritation.
Endocrine and Metabolic: Cushingoid features, growth velocity reduction in children/adolescents, hyperglycemia, and weight gain.
Psychiatry: Agitation, aggression, depression, and restlessness.

Continued on next page

This product information is based on labeling in effect on June 1, 1998. For further information, contact via direct mail, phone, or web site Medical Information: Glaxo Wellcome Inc., PO Box 13398, Research Triangle Park, NC 27709. Healthcare Professionals (Medical Information): 800-334-0089 Patients (Customer Response Center): 888-TALK2GW (1-888-825-5249) Glaxo Wellcome Corporate Web Site: www.glaxowellcome.com

Flovent Rotadisk—Cont.

Respiratory: Asthma exacerbation, bronchospasm, chest tightness, dyspnea, paradoxical bronchospasm, and wheezing.
Skin: Contusions, ecchymoses, and pruritus.

OVERDOSAGE

Chronic overdosage may result in signs/symptoms of hypercorticism (see PRECAUTIONS). Inhalation by healthy volunteers of a single dose of 4000 mcg of fluticasone propionate inhalation powder or single doses of 1760 or 3520 mcg of fluticasone propionate inhalation aerosol was well tolerated. Fluticasone propionate given by inhalation aerosol at doses of 1320 mcg twice daily for 7 to 15 days to healthy human volunteers was also well tolerated. Repeat oral doses up to 80 mg daily for 10 days in healthy volunteers and repeat oral doses up to 20 mg daily for 42 days in patients were well tolerated. Adverse reactions were of mild or moderate severity, and incidences were similar in active and placebo treatment groups. The oral and subcutaneous median lethal doses in mice and rats were >1000 mg/kg (>2000 and >4100 times, respectively, the maximum recommended daily inhalation dose in adults and >9600 and >19 000 times, respectively, the maximum recommended daily inhalation dose in children on a mg/m^2 basis).

DOSAGE AND ADMINISTRATION

FLOVENT ROTADISK should be administered by the orally inhaled route in patients 4 years of age and older. Individual patients will experience a variable time to onset and degree of symptom relief. Generally, fluticasone propionate inhalation powder has a relatively rapid onset of action for an inhaled corticosteroid. Improvement in asthma control following inhaled administration of fluticasone propionate can occur within 24 hours of beginning treatment, although maximum benefit may not be achieved for 1 to 2 weeks or longer after starting treatment.
After asthma stability has been achieved, it is always desirable to titrate to the lowest effective dose to reduce the possibility of side effects. Doses as low as 50 mcg twice daily have been shown to be effective in some patients. For patients who do not respond adequately to the starting dose after 2 weeks of therapy, higher doses may provide additional asthma control. The safety and efficacy of FLOVENT ROTADISK when administered in excess of recommended doses have not been established.
Rinsing the mouth after inhalation is advised.
The recommended starting dose and the highest recommended dose of fluticasone propionate inhalation powder, based on prior anti-asthma therapy, are listed in the following table.
[See second table at top of previous page]
Geriatric Use: In studies where geriatric patients (65 years of age or older, see PRECAUTIONS) have been treated with fluticasone propionate inhalation powder, efficacy and safety did not differ from that in younger patients. Consequently, no dosage adjustment is recommended.
Directions for Use: Illustrated Patient's Instructions for Use accompany each package of FLOVENT ROTADISK.

HOW SUPPLIED

FLOVENT ROTADISK 50 mcg is a circular double-foil pack containing four blisters of the drug. Fifteen (15) ROTADISKS are packaged in a white polypropylene tube, and the tube is packaged in a plastic-coated, moisture-protective foil pouch. A carton contains the foil pouch of 15 ROTADISKS and one dark orange- and peach-colored DISKHALER inhalation device (NDC 0173-0511-00).
FLOVENT ROTADISK 100 mcg is a circular double-foil pack containing four blisters of the drug. Fifteen (15) ROTADISKS are packaged in a white polypropylene tube, and the tube is packaged in a plastic-coated, moisture-protective foil pouch. A carton contains the foil pouch of 15 ROTADISKS and one dark orange- and peach-colored DISKHALER inhalation device (NDC 0173-0509-00).
FLOVENT ROTADISK 250 mcg is a circular double-foil pack containing four blisters of the drug. Fifteen (15) ROTADISKS are packaged in a white polypropylene tube, and the tube is packaged in a plastic-coated, moisture-protective foil pouch. A carton contains the foil pouch of 15 ROTADISKS and one dark orange- and peach-colored DISKHALER inhalation device (NDC 0173-0504-00).
Store at controlled room temperature (see USP), 20° to 25°C (68° to 77°F) in a dry place. Keep out of reach of children. Use the ROTADISK blisters within 2 months after opening of the moisture-protective foil overwrap or before the expiration date, whichever comes first. Do not puncture any fluticasone propionate ROTADISK blister until taking a dose using the DISKHALER.

November 1997/RL-472

Shown in Product Identification Guide, page 312

FORTAZ® ℞
[for ' taz]
(ceftazidime for injection)
FORTAZ® ℞
(ceftazidime sodium injection)

For Intravenous or Intramuscular Use

DESCRIPTION

Ceftazidime is a semisynthetic, broad-spectrum, beta- lactam antibiotic for parenteral administration. It is the pentahydrate of pyridinium, 1-[[7-[[(2-amino-4-thiazolyl)[(1-carboxy-1-methylethoxy) imino]acetyl] amino]-2-carboxy-8-oxo-5-thia-1-azabicyclo[4.2.0]oct-2-en-3-yl]methyl]-, hydroxide, inner salt, [6R-[6α,7β(Z)]].
The empirical formula is $C_{22}H_{32}N_6O_{12}S_2$, representing a molecular weight of 636.6.
FORTAZ is a sterile, dry powdered mixture of ceftazidime pentahydrate and sodium carbonate. The sodium carbonate at a concentration of 118 mg/g of ceftazidime activity has been admixed to facilitate dissolution. The total sodium content of the mixture is approximately 54 mg (2.3 mEq)/g of ceftazidime activity.
FORTAZ in sterile crystalline form is supplied in vials equivalent to 500 mg, 1 g, 2 g, or 6 g of anhydrous ceftazidime and in ADD-Vantage® vials equivalent to 1 or 2 g of anhydrous ceftazidime. Solutions of FORTAZ range in color from light yellow to amber, depending on the diluent and volume used. The pH of freshly constituted solutions usually ranges from 5 to 8.
FORTAZ is available as a frozen, iso-osmotic, sterile, nonpyrogenic solution with 1 or 2 g of ceftazidime as ceftazidime sodium premixed with approximately 2.2 or 1.6 g, respectively, of dextrose hydrous, USP. Dextrose has been added to adjust the osmolality. Sodium hydroxide is used to adjust pH and neutralize ceftazidime pentahydrate free acid to the sodium salt. The pH may have been adjusted with hydrochloric acid. Solutions of premixed FORTAZ range in color from light yellow to amber. The solution is intended for intravenous (IV) use after thawing to room temperature. The osmolality of the solution is approximately 300 mOsmol/kg, and the pH of thawed solutions ranges from 5 to 7.5.
The plastic container for the frozen solution is fabricated from a specially designed multilayer plastic, PL 2040. Solutions are in contact with the polyethylene layer of this container and can leach out certain chemical components of the plastic in very small amounts within the expiration period. The suitability of the plastic has been confirmed in tests in animals according to USP biological tests for plastic containers as well as by tissue culture toxicity studies.

CLINICAL PHARMACOLOGY

After IV administration of 500-mg and 1-g doses of ceftazidime over 5 minutes to normal adult male volunteers, mean peak serum concentrations of 45 and 90 mcg/mL, respectively, were achieved. After IV infusion of 500-mg, 1-g, and 2-g doses of ceftazidime over 20 to 30 minutes to normal adult male volunteers, mean peak serum concentrations of 42, 69, and 170 mcg/mL, respectively, were achieved. The average serum concentrations following IV infusion of 500-mg, 1-g, and 2-g doses to these volunteers over an 8-hour interval are given in Table 1.

Table 1

Ceftazidime	Serum Concentrations (mcg/mL)				
IV Dose	0.5 h	1 h	2 h	4 h	8 h
500 mg	42	25	12	6	2
1 g	60	39	23	11	3
2 g	129	75	42	13	5

The absorption and elimination of ceftazidime were directly proportional to the size of the dose. The half-life following IV administration was approximately 1.9 hours. Less than 10% of ceftazidime was protein bound. The degree of protein binding was independent of concentration. There was no evidence of accumulation of ceftazidime in the serum in individuals with normal renal function following multiple IV doses of 1 and 2 g every 8 hours for 10 days.
Following intramuscular (IM) administration of 500-mg and 1-g doses of ceftazidime to normal adult volunteers, the mean peak serum concentrations were 17 and 39 mcg/mL, respectively, at approximately 1 hour. Serum concentrations remained above 4 mcg/mL for 6 and 8 hours after the IM administration of 500-mg and 1-g doses, respectively. The half-life of ceftazidime in these volunteers was approximately 2 hours.
The presence of hepatic dysfunction had no effect on the pharmacokinetics of ceftazidime in individuals administered 2 g intravenously every 8 hours for 5 days. Therefore, a dosage adjustment from the normal recommended dosage is not required for patients with hepatic dysfunction, provided renal function is not impaired.
Approximately 80% to 90% of an IM or IV dose of ceftazidime is excreted unchanged by the kidneys over a 24-hour period. After the IV administration of single 500-mg or 1-g doses, approximately 50% of the dose appeared in the urine in the first 2 hours. An additional 20% was excreted between 2 and 4 hours after dosing, and approximately another 12% of the dose appeared in the urine between 4 and 8 hours later. The elimination of ceftazidime by the kidneys resulted in high therapeutic concentrations in the urine.
The mean renal clearance of ceftazidime was approximately 100 mL/min. The calculated plasma clearance of approximately 115 mL/min indicated nearly complete elimination of ceftazidime by the renal route. Administration of probenecid before dosing had no effect on the elimination kinetics of ceftazidime. This suggested that ceftazidime is eliminated by glomerular filtration and is not actively secreted by renal tubular mechanisms.
Since ceftazidime is eliminated almost solely by the kidneys, its serum half-life is significantly prolonged in patients with impaired renal function. Consequently, dosage adjustments in such patients as described in the DOSAGE AND ADMINISTRATION section are suggested.
Therapeutic concentrations of ceftazidime are achieved in the following body tissues and fluids.
[See table 2 at top of next page]
Microbiology: Ceftazidime is bactericidal in action, exerting its effect by inhibition of enzymes responsible for cell-wall synthesis. A wide range of gram-negative organisms is susceptible to ceftazidime *in vitro,* including strains resistant to gentamicin and other aminoglycosides. In addition, ceftazidime has been shown to be active against gram-positive organisms. It is highly stable to most clinically important beta-lactamases, plasmid or chromosomal, which are produced by both gram-negative and gram-positive organisms and, consequently, is active against many strains resistant to ampicillin and other cephalosporins.
Ceftazidime has been shown to be active against the following organisms both *in vitro* and in clinical infections (see INDICATIONS AND USAGE).
Aerobes, Gram-negative: *Citrobacter* spp., including *Citrobacter freundii* and *Citrobacter diversus; Enterobacter* spp., including *Enterobacter cloacae* and *Enterobacter aerogenes; Escherichia coli; Haemophilus influenzae,* including ampicillin-resistant strains; *Klebsiella* spp. (including *Klebsiella pneumoniae*); *Neisseria meningitidis; Proteus mirabilis; Proteus vulgaris; Pseudomonas* spp. (including *Pseudomonas aeruginosa*); and *Serratia* spp.
Aerobes, Gram-positive: *Staphylococcus aureus,* including penicillinase- and non–penicillinase-producing strains; *Streptococcus agalactiae* (group B streptococci); *Streptococcus pneumoniae;* and *Streptococcus pyogenes* (group A beta-hemolytic streptococci).
Anaerobes: *Bacteroides* spp. (NOTE: many strains of *Bacteroides fragilis* are resistant).
Ceftazidime has been shown to be active *in vitro* against most strains of the following organisms; however, the clinical significance of these data is unknown: *Acinetobacter* spp., *Clostridium* spp. (not including *Clostridium difficile*), *Haemophilus parainfluenzae, Morganella morganii* (formerly *Proteus morganii*), *Neisseria gonorrhoeae, Peptococcus* spp., *Peptostreptococcus* spp., *Providencia* spp. (including *Providencia rettgeri,* formerly *Proteus rettgeri*), *Salmonella* spp., *Shigella* spp., *Staphylococcus epidermidis,* and *Yersinia enterocolitica.*
Ceftazidime and the aminoglycosides have been shown to be synergistic *in vitro* against *Pseudomonas aeruginosa* and the enterobacteriaceae. Ceftazidime and carbenicillin have also been shown to be synergistic *in vitro* against *Pseudomonas aeruginosa.*
Ceftazidime is not active *in vitro* against methicillin-resistant staphylococci, *Streptococcus faecalis* and many other enterococci, *Listeria monocytogenes, Campylobacter* spp., or *Clostridium difficile.*
Susceptibility Tests: ***Diffusion Techniques:*** Quantitative methods that require measurement of zone diameters give an estimate of antibiotic susceptibility. One such procedure[1–3] has been recommended for use with disks to test susceptibility to ceftazidime.
Reports from the laboratory giving results of the standard single-disk susceptibility test with a 30-mcg ceftazidime disk should be interpreted according to the following criteria:

Susceptible organisms produce zones of 18 mm or greater, indicating that the test organism is likely to respond to therapy.

Organisms that produce zones of 15 to 17 mm are expected to be susceptible if high dosage is used or if the infection is confined to tissues and fluids (e.g., urine) in which high antibiotic levels are attained.

Resistant organisms produce zones of 14 mm or less, indicating that other therapy should be selected.

Organisms should be tested with the ceftazidime disk since ceftazidime has been shown by *in vitro* tests to be active against certain strains found resistant when other beta-lactam disks are used.

Standardized procedures require the use of laboratory control organisms. The 30-mcg ceftazidime disk should give zone diameters between 25 and 32 mm for *Escherichia coli* ATCC 25922. For *Pseudomonas aeruginosa* ATCC 27853, the zone diameters should be between 22 and 29 mm. For *Staphylococcus aureus* ATCC 25923, the zone diameters should be between 16 and 20 mm.

Dilution Techniques: In other susceptibility testing procedures, e.g., ICS agar dilution or the equivalent, a bacterial isolate may be considered susceptible if the minimum inhibitory concentration (MIC) value for ceftazidime is not more than 16 mcg/mL. Organisms are considered resistant to ceftazidime if the MIC is ≥ 64 mcg/mL. Organisms having an MIC value of < 64 mcg/mL but > 16 mcg/mL are expected to be susceptible if high dosage is used or if the infection is confined to tissues and fluids (e.g., urine) in which high antibiotic levels are attained.

As with standard diffusion methods, dilution procedures require the use of laboratory control organisms. Standard ceftazidime powder should give MIC values in the range of 4 to 16 mcg/mL for *Staphylococcus aureus* ATCC 25923. For *Escherichia coli* ATCC 25922, the MIC range should be between 0.125 and 0.5 mcg/mL. For *Pseudomonas aeruginosa* ATCC 27853, the MIC range should be between 0.5 and 2 mcg/mL.

INDICATIONS AND USAGE

FORTAZ is indicated for the treatment of patients with infections caused by susceptible strains of the designated organisms in the following diseases:

1. **Lower Respiratory Tract Infections,** including pneumonia, caused by *Pseudomonas aeruginosa* and other *Pseudomonas* spp.; *Haemophilus influenzae,* including ampicillin-resistant strains; *Klebsiella* spp.; *Enterobacter* spp.; *Proteus mirabilis; Escherichia coli; Serratia* spp.; *Citrobacter* spp.; *Streptococcus pneumoniae;* and *Staphylococcus aureus* (methicillin-susceptible strains).
2. **Skin and Skin-Structure Infections** caused by *Pseudomonas aeruginosa; Klebsiella* spp.; *Escherichia coli; Proteus* spp., including *Proteus mirabilis* and indole-positive *Proteus; Enterobacter* spp.; *Serratia* spp.; *Staphylococcus aureus* (methicillin-susceptible strains); and *Streptococcus pyogenes* (group A beta-hemolytic streptococci).
3. **Urinary Tract Infections,** both complicated and uncomplicated, caused by *Pseudomonas aeruginosa; Enterobacter* spp.; *Proteus* spp., including *Proteus mirabilis* and indole-positive *Proteus; Klebsiella* spp.; and *Escherichia coli.*
4. **Bacterial Septicemia** caused by *Pseudomonas aeruginosa, Klebsiella* spp., *Haemophilus influenzae, Escherichia coli, Serratia* spp., *Streptococcus pneumoniae,* and *Staphylococcus aureus* (methicillin-susceptible strains).
5. **Bone and Joint Infections** caused by *Pseudomonas aeruginosa, Klebsiella* spp., *Enterobacter* spp., and *Staphylococcus aureus* (methicillin-susceptible strains).
6. **Gynecologic Infections,** including endometritis, pelvic cellulitis, and other infections of the female genital tract caused by *Escherichia coli.*
7. **Intra-abdominal Infections,** including peritonitis caused by *Escherichia coli, Klebsiella* spp., and *Staphylococcus aureus* (methicillin-susceptible strains) and polymicrobial infections caused by aerobic and anaerobic organisms and *Bacteroides* spp. (many strains of *Bacteroides fragilis* are resistant).
8. **Central Nervous System Infections,** including meningitis, caused by *Haemophilus influenzae* and *Neisseria meningitidis.* Ceftazidime has also been used successfully in a limited number of cases of meningitis due to *Pseudomonas aeruginosa* and *Streptococcus pneumoniae.*

Specimens for bacterial cultures should be obtained before therapy in order to isolate and identify causative organisms and to determine their susceptibility to ceftazidime. Therapy may be instituted before results of susceptibility studies are known; however, once these results become available, the antibiotic treatment should be adjusted accordingly.

FORTAZ may be used alone in cases of confirmed or suspected sepsis. Ceftazidime has been used successfully in clinical trials as empiric therapy in cases where various concomitant therapies with other antibiotics have been used.

FORTAZ may also be used concomitantly with other antibiotics, such as aminoglycosides, vancomycin, and clindamycin; in severe and life-threatening infections; and in the immunocompromised patient. When such concomitant treatment is appropriate, prescribing information in the labeling for the other antibiotics should be followed. The dose depends on the severity of the infection and the patient's condition.

CONTRAINDICATIONS

FORTAZ is contraindicated in patients who have shown hypersensitivity to ceftazidime or the cephalosporin group of antibiotics.

WARNINGS

BEFORE THERAPY WITH FORTAZ IS INSTITUTED, CAREFUL INQUIRY SHOULD BE MADE TO DETERMINE WHETHER THE PATIENT HAS HAD PREVIOUS HYPERSENSITIVITY REACTIONS TO CEFTAZIDIME, CEPHALOSPORINS, PENICILLINS, OR OTHER DRUGS. IF THIS PRODUCT IS TO BE GIVEN TO PENICILLIN-SENSITIVE PATIENTS, CAUTION SHOULD BE EXERCISED BECAUSE CROSS-HYPERSENSITIVITY AMONG BETA-LACTAM ANTIBIOTICS HAS BEEN CLEARLY DOCUMENTED AND MAY OCCUR IN UP TO 10% OF PATIENTS WITH A HISTORY OF PENICILLIN ALLERGY. IF AN ALLERGIC REACTION TO FORTAZ OCCURS, DISCONTINUE THE DRUG. SERIOUS ACUTE HYPERSENSITIVITY REACTIONS MAY REQUIRE TREATMENT WITH EPINEPHRINE AND OTHER EMERGENCY MEASURES, INCLUDING OXYGEN, IV FLUIDS, IV ANTIHISTAMINES, CORTICOSTEROIDS, PRESSOR AMINES, AND AIRWAY MANAGEMENT, AS CLINICALLY INDICATED.

Pseudomembranous colitis has been reported with nearly all antibacterial agents, including ceftazidime, and may range in severity from mild to life threatening. Therefore, it is important to consider this diagnosis in patients who present with diarrhea subsequent to the administration of antibacterial agents.

Treatment with antibacterial agents alters the normal flora of the colon and may permit overgrowth of clostridia. Studies indicate that a toxin produced by *Clostridium difficile* is one primary cause of "antibiotic-associated colitis."

After the diagnosis of pseudomembranous colitis has been established, appropriate therapeutic measures should be initiated. Mild cases of pseudomembranous colitis usually respond to drug discontinuation alone. In moderate to severe cases, consideration should be given to management with fluids and electrolytes, protein supplementation, and treatment with an antibacterial drug clinically effective against *Clostridium difficile* colitis.

Elevated levels of ceftazidime in patients with renal insufficiency can lead to seizures, encephalopathy, asterixis, and neuromuscular excitability (see PRECAUTIONS).

PRECAUTIONS

General: Ceftazidime has not been shown to be nephrotoxic; however, high and prolonged serum antibiotic concentrations can occur from usual dosages in patients with transient or persistent reduction of urinary output because of renal insufficiency. The total daily dosage should be reduced when ceftazidime is administered to patients with renal insufficiency (see DOSAGE AND ADMINISTRATION). Elevated levels of ceftazidime in these patients can lead to seizures, encephalopathy, asterixis, and neuromuscular excitability. Continued dosage should be determined by degree of renal impairment, severity of infection, and susceptibility of the causative organisms.

As with other antibiotics, prolonged use of FORTAZ may result in overgrowth of nonsusceptible organisms. Repeated evaluation of the patient's condition is essential. If superinfection occurs during therapy, appropriate measures should be taken.

Inducible type I beta-lactamase resistance has been noted with some organisms (e.g., *Enterobacter* spp., *Pseudomonas* spp., and *Serratia* spp.). As with other extended-spectrum beta-lactam antibiotics, resistance can develop during therapy, leading to clinical failure in some cases. When treating infections caused by these organisms, periodic susceptibility testing should be performed when clinically appropriate. If patients fail to respond to monotherapy, an aminoglycoside or similar agent should be considered.

Cephalosporins may be associated with a fall in prothrombin activity. Those at risk include patients with renal and hepatic impairment, or poor nutritional state, as well as patients receiving a protracted course of antimicrobial therapy. Prothrombin time should be monitored in patients at risk and exogenous vitamin K administered as indicated.

FORTAZ should be prescribed with caution in individuals with a history of gastrointestinal disease, particularly colitis.

Distal necrosis can occur after inadvertent intra-arterial administration of ceftazidime.

Drug Interactions: Nephrotoxicity has been reported following concomitant administration of cephalosporins with aminoglycoside antibiotics or potent diuretics such as furosemide. Renal function should be carefully monitored, especially if higher dosages of the aminoglycosides are to be administered or if therapy is prolonged, because of the potential nephrotoxicity and ototoxicity of aminoglycosidic antibiotics. Nephrotoxicity and ototoxicity were not noted when ceftazidime was given alone in clinical trials.

Chloramphenicol has been shown to be antagonistic to beta-lactam antibiotics, including ceftazidime, based on *in vitro* studies and time kill curves with enteric gram-negative bacilli. Due to the possibility of antagonism *in vivo*, particularly when bactericidal activity is desired, this drug combination should be avoided.

Drug/Laboratory Test Interactions: The administration of ceftazidime may result in a false-positive reaction for glucose in the urine using CLINITEST ® tablets, Benedict's solution, or Fehling's solution. It is recommended that glucose tests based on enzymatic glucose oxidase reactions (such as CLINISTIX® or TES-TAPE®) be used.

Carcinogenesis, Mutagenesis, Impairment of Fertility: Long-term studies in animals have not been performed to evaluate carcinogenic potential. However, a mouse Micronucleus test and an Ames test were both negative for mutagenic effects.

Pregnancy: ***Teratogenic Effects: Pregnancy Category B:*** Reproduction studies have been performed in mice and rats at doses up to 40 times the human dose and have revealed no evidence of impaired fertility or harm to the fetus due to FORTAZ. There are, however, no adequate and well-controlled studies in pregnant women. Because animal reproduction studies are not always predictive of human response, this drug should be used during pregnancy only if clearly needed.

Nursing Mothers: Ceftazidime is excreted in human milk in low concentrations. Caution should be exercised when FORTAZ is administered to a nursing woman.

Pediatric Use: (see DOSAGE AND ADMINISTRATION).

ADVERSE REACTIONS

Ceftazidime is generally well tolerated. The incidence of adverse reactions associated with the administration of ceftazidime was low in clinical trials. The most common were local reactions following IV injection and allergic and gastrointestinal reactions. Other adverse reactions were encountered infrequently. No disulfiramlike reactions were reported.

The following adverse effects from clinical trials were considered to be either related to ceftazidime therapy or were of uncertain etiology:

Local Effects, reported in fewer than 2% of patients, were phlebitis and inflammation at the site of injection (1 in 69 patients).

Table 2: Ceftazidime Concentrations in Body Tissues and Fluids

Tissue or Fluid	Dose/ Route	No. of Patients	Time of Sample Postdose	Average Tissue or Fluid Level (mcg/mL or mcg/g)
Urine	500 mg IM	6	0–2 h	2,100.0
	2 g IV	6	0–2 h	12,000.0
Bile	2 g IV	3	90 min	36.4
Synovial fluid	2 g IV	13	2 h	25.6
Peritoneal fluid	2 g IV	8	2 h	48.6
Sputum	1 g IV	8	1 h	9.0
Cerebrospinal fluid	2 g q8h IV	5	120 min	9.8
(inflamed meninges)	2 g q8h IV	6	180 min	9.4
Aqueous humor	2 g IV	13	1–3 h	11.0
Blister fluid	1 g IV	7	2–3 h	19.7
Lymphatic fluid	1 g IV	7	2–3 h	23.4
Bone	2 g IV	8	0.67 h	31.1
Heart muscle	2 g IV	35	30–280 min	12.7
Skin	2 g IV	22	30–180 min	6.6
Skeletal muscle	2 g IV	35	30–280 min	9.4
Myometrium	2 g IV	31	1–2 h	18.7

Continued on next page

This product information is based on labeling in effect on June 1, 1998. For further information, contact via direct mail, phone, or web site Medical Information: Glaxo Wellcome Inc., PO Box 13398, Research Triangle Park, NC 27709. Healthcare Professionals (Medical Information): 800-334-0089 Patients (Customer Response Center): 888-TALK2GW (1-888-825-5249) Glaxo Wellcome Corporate Web Site: www.glaxowellcome.com

Fortaz—Cont.

Hypersensitivity Reactions, reported in 2% of patients, were pruritus, rash, and fever. Immediate reactions, generally manifested by rash and/or pruritus, occurred in 1 in 285 patients. Toxic epidermal necrolysis, Stevens-Johnson syndrome, and erythema multiforme have also been reported with cephalosporin antibiotics, including ceftazidime. Angioedema and anaphylaxis (bronchospasm and/or hypotension) have been reported very rarely.

Gastrointestinal Symptoms, reported in fewer than 2% of patients, were diarrhea (1 in 78), nausea (1 in 156), vomiting (1 in 500), and abdominal pain (1 in 416). The onset of pseudomembranous colitis symptoms may occur during or after treatment (see WARNINGS).

Central Nervous System Reactions (fewer than 1%) included headache, dizziness, and paresthesia. Seizures have been reported with several cephalosporins, including ceftazidime. In addition, encephalopathy, asterixis, and neuromuscular excitability have been reported in renally impaired patients treated with unadjusted dosing regimens of ceftazidime (see PRECAUTIONS: General).

Less Frequent Adverse Events (fewer than 1%) were candidiasis (including oral thrush) and vaginitis.

Hematologic: Rare cases of hemolytic anemia have been reported.

Laboratory Test Changes noted during FORTAZ clinical trials were transient and included: eosinophilia (1 in 13), positive Coombs' test without hemolysis (1 in 23), thrombocytosis (1 in 45), and slight elevations in one or more of the hepatic enzymes, aspartate aminotransferase (AST, SGOT) (1 in 16), alanine aminotransferase (ALT, SGPT) (1 in 15), LDH (1 in 18), GGT (1 in 19), and alkaline phosphatase (1 in 23). As with some other cephalosporins, transient elevations of blood urea, blood urea nitrogen, and/or serum creatinine were observed occasionally. Transient leukopenia, neutropenia, agranulocytosis, thrombocytopenia, and lymphocytosis were seen very rarely.

In addition to the adverse reactions listed above that have been observed in patients treated with ceftazidime, the following adverse reactions and altered laboratory tests have been reported for cephalosporin-class antibiotics:

Adverse Reactions: Urticaria, colitis, renal dysfunction, toxic nephropathy, hepatic dysfunction including cholestasis, aplastic anemia, hemorrhage.

Altered Laboratory Tests: Prolonged prothrombin time, false-positive test for urinary glucose, elevated bilirubin, pancytopenia.

OVERDOSAGE

Ceftazidime overdosage has occurred in patients with renal failure. Reactions have included seizure activity, encephalopathy, asterixis, and neuromuscular excitability. Patients who receive an acute overdosage should be carefully observed and given supportive treatment. In the presence of renal insufficiency, hemodialysis or peritoneal dialysis may aid in the removal of ceftazidime from the body.

DOSAGE AND ADMINISTRATION

Dosage: The usual adult dosage is 1 gram administered intravenously or intramuscularly every 8 to 12 hours. The dosage and route should be determined by the susceptibility of the causative organisms, the severity of infection, and the condition and renal function of the patient.

The guidelines for dosage of FORTAZ are listed in Table 3. The following dosage schedule is recommended.

[See table 3 below]

Impaired Hepatic Function: No adjustment in dosage is required for patients with hepatic dysfunction.

Impaired Renal Function: Ceftazidime is excreted by the kidneys, almost exclusively by glomerular filtration. Therefore, in patients with impaired renal function (glomerular filtration rate [GFR] <50 mL/min), it is recommended that the dosage of ceftazidime be reduced to compensate for its slower excretion. In patients with suspected renal insufficiency, an initial loading dose of 1 gram of FORTAZ may be given. An estimate of GFR should be made to determine the appropriate maintenance dosage. The recommended dosage is presented in Table 4.

Table 4: Recommended Maintenance Dosages of FORTAZ in Renal Insufficiency
NOTE: IF THE DOSE RECOMMENDED IN TABLE 3 ABOVE IS LOWER THAN THAT RECOMMENDED FOR PATIENTS WITH RENAL INSUFFICIENCY AS OUTLINED IN TABLE 4, THE LOWER DOSE SHOULD BE USED.

Creatinine Clearance (mL/min)	Recommended Unit Dose of FORTAZ	Frequency of Dosing
50–31	1 gram	q12h
30–16	1 gram	q24h
15–6	500 mg	q24h
<5	500 mg	q48h

When only serum creatinine is available, the following formula (Cockcroft's equation)[4] may be used to estimate creatinine clearance. The serum creatinine should represent a steady state of renal function:

Males:

$$\text{Creatinine clearance (mL/min)} = \frac{\text{Weight (kg)} \times (140 - \text{age})}{72 \times \text{serum creatinine (mg/dL)}}$$

Females: 0.85 × male value

In patients with severe infections who would normally receive 6 grams of FORTAZ daily were it not for renal insufficiency, the unit dose given in the table above may be increased by 50% or the dosing frequency may be increased appropriately. Further dosing should be determined by therapeutic monitoring, severity of the infection, and susceptibility of the causative organism.

In pediatric patients as for adults, the creatinine clearance should be adjusted for body surface area or lean body mass, and the dosing frequency should be reduced in cases of renal insufficiency.

In patients undergoing hemodialysis, a loading dose of 1 gram is recommended, followed by 1 gram after each hemodialysis period.

FORTAZ can also be used in patients undergoing intraperitoneal dialysis and continuous ambulatory peritoneal dialysis. In such patients, a loading dose of 1 gram of FORTAZ may be given, followed by 500 mg every 24 hours. In addition to IV use, FORTAZ can be incorporated in the dialysis fluid at a concentration of 250 mg for 2 L of dialysis fluid.

Table 3: Recommended Dosage Schedule

	Dose	Frequency
Adults		
Usual recommended dosage	**1 gram IV or IM**	**q8–12h**
Uncomplicated urinary tract infections	250 mg IV or IM	q12h
Bone and joint infections	2 grams IV	q12h
Complicated urinary tract infections	500 mg IV or IM	q8–12h
Uncomplicated pneumonia; mild skin and skin-structure infections	500 mg–1 gram IV or IM	q8h
Serious gynecologic and intra-abdominal infections	2 grams IV	q8h
Meningitis	2 grams IV	q8h
Very severe life-threatening infections, especially in immunocompromised patients	2 grams IV	q8h
Lung infections caused by *Pseudomonas* spp. in patients with cystic fibrosis with normal renal function*	30–50 mg/kg IV to a maximum of 6 grams per day	q8h
Neonates (0–4 weeks)	30 mg/kg IV	q12h
Infants and Children (1 month–12 years)	30–50 mg/kg IV to a maximum of 6 grams per day†	q8h

* Although clinical improvement has been shown, bacteriologic cures cannot be expected in patients with chronic respiratory disease and cystic fibrosis.

† The higher dose should be reserved for immunocompromised pediatric patients or pediatric patients with cystic fibrosis or meningitis.

Note: Generally FORTAZ should be continued for 2 days after the signs and symptoms of infection have disappeared, but in complicated infections longer therapy may be required.

Administration: FORTAZ may be given intravenously or by deep IM injection into a large muscle mass such as the upper outer quadrant of the gluteus maximus or lateral part of the thigh. Intra-arterial administration should be avoided (see PRECAUTIONS).

Intramuscular Administration: For IM administration, FORTAZ should be constituted with one of the following diluents: sterile water for injection, bacteriostatic water for injection, or 0.5% or 1% lidocaine hydrochloride injection. Refer to Table 5.

Intravenous Administration: The IV route is preferable for patients with bacterial septicemia, bacterial meningitis, peritonitis, or other severe or life-threatening infections, or for patients who may be poor risks because of lowered resistance resulting from such debilitating conditions as malnutrition, trauma, surgery, diabetes, heart failure, or malignancy, particularly if shock is present or pending.

For direct intermittent IV administration, constitute FORTAZ as directed in Table 5 with sterile water for injection. Slowly inject directly into the vein over a period of 3 to 5 minutes or give through the tubing of an administration set while the patient is also receiving one of the compatible IV fluids (see COMPATIBILITY AND STABILITY).

For IV infusion, constitute the 1- or 2-gram infusion pack with 100 mL of sterile water for injection or one of the compatible IV fluids listed under the COMPATIBILITY AND STABILITY section. Alternatively, constitute the 500-mg, 1-gram, or 2-gram vial and add an appropriate quantity of the resulting solution to an IV container with one of the compatible IV fluids.

Intermittent IV infusion with a Y-type administration set can be accomplished with compatible solutions. However, during infusion of a solution containing ceftazidime, it is desirable to discontinue the other solution.

ADD-Vantage vials are to be constituted only with 50 or 100 mL of 5% dextrose injection, 0.9% sodium chloride injection, or 0.45% sodium chloride injection in Abbott ADD-Vantage flexible diluent containers (see Instructions for Constitution section of the product package insert). ADD-Vantage vials that have been joined to Abbott ADD-Vantage diluent containers and activated to dissolve the drug are stable for 24 hours at room temperature or for 7 days under refrigeration. Joined vials that have not been activated may be used within a 14-day period; this period corresponds to that for use of Abbott ADD-Vantage containers following removal of the outer packaging (overwrap).

Freezing solutions of FORTAZ in the ADD-Vantage system is not recommended.

[See table 5 at top of next page]

All vials of FORTAZ as supplied are under reduced pressure. When FORTAZ is dissolved, carbon dioxide is released and a positive pressure develops. For ease of use please follow the recommended techniques of constitution described on the detachable Instructions for Constitution section of the product package insert.

Solutions of FORTAZ, like those of most beta-lactam antibiotics, should not be added to solutions of aminoglycoside antibiotics because of potential interaction.

However, if concurrent therapy with FORTAZ and an aminoglycoside is indicated, each of these antibiotics can be administered separately to the same patient.

Directions for Use of FORTAZ Frozen in GALAXY® Plastic Containers: FORTAZ supplied as a frozen, sterile, iso-osmotic, nonpyrogenic solution in plastic containers is to be administered after thawing either as a continuous or intermittent IV infusion. The thawed solution is stable for 24 hours at room temperature or for 7 days if stored under refrigeration. **Do not Refreeze.**

Thaw container at room temperature (25°C) or under refrigeration (5°C). Do not force thaw by immersion in water baths or by microwave irradiation. Components of the solution may precipitate in the frozen state and will dissolve upon reaching room temperature with little or no agitation. Potency is not affected. Mix after solution has reached room temperature. Check for minute leaks by squeezing bag firmly. Discard bag if leaks are found as sterility may be impaired. Do not add supplementary medication. Do not use unless solution is clear and seal is intact.

Use sterile equipment.

Caution: Do not use plastic containers in series connections. Such use could result in air embolism due to residual air being drawn from the primary container before administration of the fluid from the secondary container is complete.

Preparation for Administration:

1. Suspend container from eyelet support.
2. Remove protector from outlet port at bottom of container.
3. Attach administration set. Refer to complete directions accompanying set.

COMPATIBILITY AND STABILITY

Intramuscular: FORTAZ, when constituted as directed with sterile water for injection, bacteriostatic water for in-

Table 5: Preparation of FORTAZ Solutions

Size	Amount of Diluent to be Added (mL)	Approximate Available Volume (mL)	Approximate Ceftazidime Concentration (mg/mL)
Intramuscular			
500-mg vial	1.5	1.8	280
1-gram vial	3.0	3.6	280
Intravenous			
500-mg vial	5.0	5.3	100
1-gram vial	10.0	10.6	100
2-gram vial	10.0	11.5	170
Infusion pack			
1-gram vial	100 *	100	10
2-gram vial	100 *	100	20
Pharmacy bulk package			
6-gram vial	26	30	200

*** Note:** Addition should be in two stages (see Instructions for Constitution accompanying the product package insert).

jection, or 0.5% or 1% lidocaine hydrochloride injection, maintains satisfactory potency for 24 hours at room temperature or for 7 days under refrigeration. Solutions in sterile water for injection that are frozen immediately after constitution in the original container are stable for 3 months when stored at −20°C. Once thawed, solutions should not be refrozen. Thawed solutions may be stored for up to 8 hours at room temperature or for 4 days in a refrigerator.

Intravenous: FORTAZ, when constituted as directed with sterile water for injection, maintains satisfactory potency for 24 hours at room temperature or for 7 days under refrigeration. Solutions in sterile water for injection in the infusion vial or in 0.9% sodium chloride injection in VIAFLEX® small-volume containers that are frozen immediately after constitution are stable for 6 months when stored at −20°C. Do not force thaw by immersion in water baths or by microwave irradiation. Once thawed, solutions should not be refrozen. Thawed solutions may be stored for up to 24 hours at room temperature or for 7 days in a refrigerator. More concentrated solutions in sterile water for injection in the original container that are frozen immediately after constitution are stable for 3 months when stored at −20°C. Once thawed, solutions should not be refrozen. Thawed solutions may be stored for up to 8 hours at room temperature or for 4 days in a refrigerator.

FORTAZ is compatible with the more commonly used IV infusion fluids. Solutions at concentrations between 1 and 40 mg/mL in 0.9% sodium chloride injection; 1/6 M sodium lactate injection; 5% dextrose injection; 5% dextrose and 0.225% sodium chloride injection; 5% dextrose and 0.45% sodium chloride injection; 5% dextrose and 0.9% sodium chloride injection; 10% dextrose injection; ringer's injection, USP; lactated ringer's injection, USP; 10% invert sugar in water for injection; and NORMOSOL®-M in 5% dextrose injection may be stored for up to 24 hours at room temperature or for 7 days if refrigerated.

The 1- and 2-g FORTAZ ADD-Vantage vials, when diluted in 50 or 100 mL of 5% dextrose injection, 0.9% sodium chloride injection, or 0.45% sodium chloride injection, may be stored for up to 24 hours at room temperature or for 7 days under refrigeration.

FORTAZ is less stable in sodium bicarbonate injection than in other IV fluids. It is not recommended as a diluent. Solutions of FORTAZ in 5% dextrose injection and 0.9% sodium chloride injection are stable for at least 6 hours at room temperature in plastic tubing, drip chambers, and volume control devices of common IV infusion sets.

Ceftazidime at a concentration of 4 mg/mL has been found compatible for 24 hours at room temperature or for 7 days under refrigeration in 0.9% sodium chloride injection or 5% dextrose injection when admixed with: cefuroxime sodium (ZINACEF®) 3 mg/mL; heparin 10 or 50 U/mL; or potassium chloride 10 or 40 mEq/L.

Vancomycin solution exhibits a physical incompatibility when mixed with a number of drugs, including ceftazidime. The likelihood of precipitation with ceftazidime is dependent on the concentrations of vancomycin and ceftazidime present. It is therefore recommended, when both drugs are to be administered by intermittent IV infusion, that they be given separately, flushing the IV lines (with one of the compatible IV fluids) between the administration of these two agents.

Note: Parenteral drug products should be inspected visually for particulate matter before administration whenever solution and container permit.

As with other cephalosporins, FORTAZ powder as well as solutions tend to darken, depending on storage conditions; within the stated recommendations, however, product potency is not adversely affected.

HOW SUPPLIED

FORTAZ in the dry state should be stored between 15° and 30°C (59° and 86°F) and protected from light. FORTAZ is a dry, white to off-white powder supplied in vials and infusion packs as follows:

NDC 0173-0377-31 500-mg* Vial (Tray of 25)
NDC 0173-0378-35 1-g* Vial (Tray of 25)
NDC 0173-0379-34 2-g* Vial (Tray of 10)
NDC 0173-0380-32 1-g* Infusion Pack (Tray of 10)
NDC 0173-0381-32 2-g* Infusion Pack (Tray of 10)
NDC 0173-0382-37 6-g* Pharmacy Bulk Package (Tray of 6)
NDC 0173-0434-00 1-g ADD-Vantage® Vial (Tray of 25)
NDC 0173-0435-00 2-g ADD-Vantage® Vial (Tray of 10)
(The above ADD-Vantage vials are to be used only with Abbott ADD-Vantage diluent containers.)

FORTAZ frozen as a premixed solution of ceftazidime sodium should not be stored above −20° C. FORTAZ is supplied frozen in 50-mL, single-dose, plastic containers as follows:

NDC 0173-0412-00 1-g* Plastic Container (Carton of 24)
NDC 0173-0413-00 2-g* Plastic Container (Carton of 24)
*Equivalent to anhydrous ceftazidime.

REFERENCES

1. Bauer AW, Kirby WMM, Sherris JC, Turck M. Antibiotic susceptibility testing by a standardized single disk method. *Am J Clin Pathol.* 1966;45:493–496.
2. National Committee for Clinical Laboratory Standards. *Approved Standard: Performance Standards for Antimicrobial Disc Susceptibility Tests.* (M2-A3). December 1984.
3. Certification procedure for antibiotic sensitivity discs (21 CFR 460.1). *Federal Register.* May 30, 1974;39:19182-19184.
4. Cockcroft DW, Gault MH. Prediction of creatinine clearance from serum creatinine. *Nephron.* 1976;16:31-41.

FORTAZ and ZINACEF are registered trademarks of Glaxo Wellcome.

ADD-Vantage is a registered trademark of Abbott Laboratories.

CLINITEST and CLINISTIX are registered trademarks of Ames Division, Miles Laboratories, Inc.

TES-TAPE is a registered trademark of Eli Lilly and Company.

GALAXY and VIAFLEX are registered trademarks of Baxter International Inc.

US Patents, 4,258,041; 4,329,453; and 4,582,830

February 1998/RL-545

Shown in Product Identification Guide, page 312

IMITREX® ℞

[*ĭm '-ĭ-trĕx "*]
(sumatriptan succinate)
Injection

For Subcutaneous Use Only.

DESCRIPTION

IMITREX (sumatriptan succinate) Injection is a selective 5-hydroxytryptamine$_1$ receptor subtype agonist. Sumatriptan succinate is chemically designated as 3-[2-(dimethylamino)ethyl]-N-methyl-1H-indole-5-methanesulfonamide butane-1,4-dioate(1:1).

The empirical formula is $C_{14}H_{21}N_3O_2S \bullet C_4H_6O_4$, representing a molecular weight of 413.5.

Sumatriptan succinate is a white to off-white powder that is readily soluble in water and in saline.

IMITREX Injection is a clear, colorless to pale yellow, sterile, nonpyrogenic solution for subcutaneous injection. Each 0.5 mL of solution contains 6 mg of sumatriptan (base) as the succinate salt and 3.5 mg of sodium chloride, USP in water for injection, USP. The pH range of the solution is approximately 4.2 to 5.3. The osmolality of the injection is 291 mOsmol.

CLINICAL PHARMACOLOGY

Mechanism of Action: Sumatriptan has been demonstrated to be a selective agonist for a vascular 5-hydroxytryptamine$_1$ receptor subtype (probably a member of the 5-HT_{1D} family) with no significant affinity (as measured using standard radioligand binding assays) or pharmacological activity at 5-HT_2, 5-HT_3 receptor subtypes or at alpha$_1$-, alpha$_2$-, or beta-adrenergic; dopamine$_1$; dopamine$_2$; muscarinic; or benzodiazepine receptors.

The vascular 5-HT_1 receptor subtype to which sumatriptan binds selectively, and through which it presumably exerts its antimigrainous effect, has been shown to be present on cranial arteries in both dog and primate, on the human basilar artery, and in the vasculature of the isolated dura mater of humans. In these tissues, sumatriptan activates this receptor to cause vasoconstriction, an action in humans correlating with the relief of migraine and cluster headache. In the anesthetized dog, sumatriptan selectively reduces the carotid arterial blood flow with little or no effect on arterial blood pressure or total peripheral resistance. In the cat, sumatriptan selectively constricts the carotid arteriovenous anastomoses while having little effect on blood flow or resistance in cerebral or extracerebral tissues.

Corneal Opacities: Dogs receiving oral sumatriptan developed corneal opacities and defects in the corneal epithelium. Corneal opacities were seen at the lowest dosage tested, 2 mg/kg per day, and were present after 1 month of treatment. Defects in the corneal epithelium were noted in a 60-week study. Earlier examinations for these toxicities were not conducted and no-effect doses were not established; however, the relative exposure at the lowest dose tested was approximately five times the human exposure after a 100-mg oral dose or three times the human exposure after a 6-mg subcutaneous dose.

Melanin Binding: In rats with a single subcutaneous dose (0.5 mg/kg) of radiolabeled sumatriptan, the elimination half-life of radioactivity from the eye was 15 days, suggesting that sumatriptan and its metabolites bind to the melanin of the eye. The clinical significance of this binding is unknown.

Pharmacokinetics: Pharmacokinetic parameters following a 6-mg subcutaneous injection into the deltoid area of the arm in nine males (*mean age, 33 years; mean weight, 77 kg*) were systemic clearance: 1,194 ± 149 mL/min (*mean ± S.D.*), distribution half-life: 15 ± 2 minutes, terminal half-life: 115 ± 19 minutes, and volume of distribution central compartment: 50 ± 8 liters. Of this dose, 22% ± 4% was excreted in the urine as unchanged sumatriptan and 38% ± 7% as the indole acetic acid metabolite.

After a single 6-mg subcutaneous manual injection into the deltoid area of the arm in 18 healthy males (*age, 24 ± 6 years; weight, 70 kg*), the maximum serum concentration (C_{max}) was (*mean ± standard deviation*) 74 ± 15 ng/mL and the time to peak concentration (t_{max}) was 12 minutes after injection (*range, 5 to 20 minutes*). In this study, the same dose injected subcutaneously in the thigh gave a C_{max} of 61 ± 15 ng/mL by manual injection versus 52 ± 15 ng/mL by autoinjector techniques. The t_{max} or amount absorbed were not significantly altered by either the site or technique of injection.

The bioavailability of sumatriptan via subcutaneous site injection to 18 healthy male subjects was 97% ± 16% of that obtained following intravenous injection. Protein binding, determined by equilibrium dialysis over the concentration range of 10 to 1,000 ng/mL, is low, approximately 14% to 21%. The effect of sumatriptan on the protein binding of other drugs has not been evaluated.

Special Populations: ***Renal Impairment:*** The effect of renal impairment on the pharmacokinetics of sumatriptan has not been examined, but little clinical effect would be expected as sumatriptan is largely metabolized to an inactive substance.

Hepatic Impairment: The effect of hepatic disease on the pharmacokinetics of subcutaneously and orally administered sumatriptan has been evaluated. There were no statistically significant differences in the pharmacokinetics of subcutaneously administered sumatriptan in hepatically impaired patients compared to healthy controls. However, the liver plays an important role in the presystemic clearance of orally administered sumatriptan. Accordingly, the bioavailability of sumatriptan following oral administration may be markedly increased in patients with liver disease. In one small study of hepatically impaired patients (n = 8) matched for sex, age, and weight with healthy subjects, the hepatically impaired patients had an approximately 70% increase in AUC and C_{max} and a t_{max} 40 minutes earlier compared to the healthy subjects.

Age: The pharmacokinetics of sumatriptan in the elderly (*mean age, 72 years; two males and four females*) and in

Continued on next page

This product information is based on labeling in effect on June 1, 1998. For further information, contact via direct mail, phone, or web site Medical Information: Glaxo Wellcome Inc., PO Box 13398, Research Triangle Park, NC 27709. Healthcare Professionals (Medical Information): 800-334-0089 Patients (Customer Response Center): 888-TALK2GW (1-888-825-5249) Glaxo Wellcome Corporate Web Site: www.glaxowellcome.com

Imitrex Injection—Cont.

patients with migraine (*mean age, 38 years; 25 males and 155 females*) were similar to that in healthy male subjects (*mean age, 30 years).*

Race: The systemic clearance and C_{max} of sumatriptan were similar in black (n = 34) and Caucasian (n = 38) healthy male subjects.

Drug Interactions: *MAO Inhibitors:* In vitro studies with human microsomes suggest that sumatriptan is metabolized by monoamine oxidase (MAO), predominantly the A isoenzyme. In a study of 14 healthy females, pretreatment with MAO-A inhibitor decreased the clearance of sumatriptan. Under the conditions of this experiment, the result was a twofold increase in the area under the sumatriptan plasma concentration × time curve (AUC), corresponding to a 40% increase in elimination half-life. No significant effect was seen with an MAO-B inhibitor.

Pharmacodynamics:

Typical Physiologic Responses:

Blood Pressure: (see WARNINGS)

Peripheral (small) Arteries: In healthy volunteers (n = 18), a study evaluating the effects of sumatriptan on peripheral (small vessel) arterial reactivity failed to detect a clinically significant increase in peripheral resistance.

Heart Rate: Transient increases in blood pressure observed in some patients in clinical studies carried out during sumatriptan's development as a treatment for migraine were not accompanied by any clinically significant changes in heart rate.

Respiratory Rate: Experience gained during the clinical development of sumatriptan as a treatment for migraine failed to detect an effect of the drug on respiratory rate.

Clinical Studies: *Migraine:* In US controlled clinical trials enrolling more than 1,000 patients during migraine attacks who were experiencing moderate or severe pain and one or more of the symptoms enumerated in Table 2 below, onset of relief began as early as 10 minutes following a 6-mg IMITREX Injection. Smaller doses of sumatriptan may also prove effective, although the proportion of patients obtaining adequate relief is decreased and the latency to that relief is greater.

In one well-controlled study where placebo (n = 62) was compared to six different doses of IMITREX Injection (n = 30 each group) in a single-attack, parallel-group design, the dose response relationship was found to be as shown in the following Table 1.

[See table 1 below]

In two US well-controlled clinical trials in 1,104 migraine patients with moderate and severe migraine pain, the onset of relief was rapid (less than 10 minutes). Headache relief, as evidenced by a reduction in pain from severe or moderately severe to mild or no headache, was achieved in 70% of the patients within 1 hour of a single 6-mg subcutaneous dose of IMITREX Injection. Headache relief was achieved in approximately 82% of patients within 2 hours, and 65% of all patients were pain free within 2 hours.

The following table shows the 1- and 2-hour efficacy results.

[See table 2 at bottom of next page]

IMITREX Injection also relieved photophobia, phonophobia (sound sensitivity), nausea, and vomiting associated with migraine attacks. Similar efficacy was seen when patients self-administered IMITREX Injection using an autoinjector.

The efficacy of IMITREX Injection is unaffected by whether or not migraine is associated with aura, duration of attack, gender or age of the patient, or concomitant use of common migraine prophylactic drugs (e.g., beta-blockers).

Cluster Headache: The efficacy of IMITREX Injection in the acute treatment of cluster headache was demonstrated in two randomized, double-blind, placebo-controlled, two-period crossover trials. Patients age 21 to 65 were enrolled and were instructed to treat a moderate to very severe headache within 10 minutes of onset. Headache relief was defined as a reduction in headache severity to mild or no pain. In both trials, the proportion of individuals gaining relief at 10 or 15 minutes was significantly greater among patients receiving 6 mg of IMITREX Injection compared to those who received placebo (see Table 3, below). One study evaluated a 12-mg dose; there was no statistically significant difference in outcome between patients randomized to the 6- and 12-mg doses.

[See table 3 at bottom of next page]

The Kaplan Meier (product limit) Survivorship Plot below (Figure 1) provides an estimate of the cumulative probability of a patient with a cluster headache obtaining relief after being treated with either sumatriptan or placebo.

Figure 1: Time to Relief From Time of Injection*

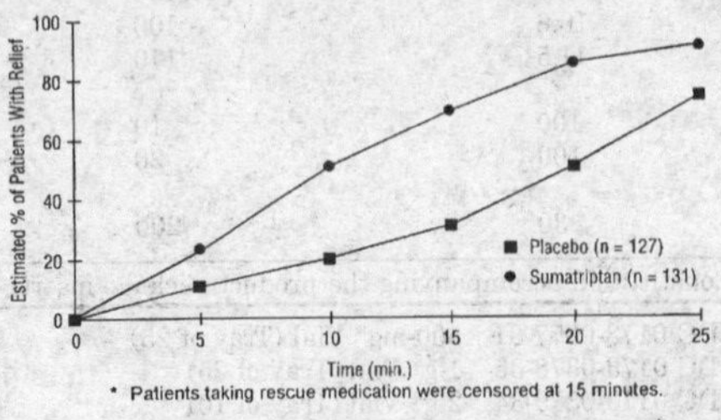

* Patients taking rescue medication were censored at 15 minutes.

The plot was constructed with data from patients who either experienced relief or did not require (request) rescue medication within a period of 2 hours following treatment. As a consequence, the data in the plot are derived from only a subset of the 258 headaches treated (rescue medication was required in 52 of the 127 placebo-treated headaches and 18 of the 131 sumatriptan-treated headaches).

Other data suggest that sumatriptan treatment is not associated with an increase in early recurrence of headache, and that treatment with sumatriptan has little effect on the incidence of latter occurring headaches (i.e., those occurring after 2, but before 18 or 24 hours).

INDICATIONS AND USAGE

IMITREX Injection is indicated for 1) the acute treatment of migraine attacks with or without aura and 2) the acute treatment of cluster headache episodes.

IMITREX Injection is not for use in the management of hemiplegic or basilar migraine (see CONTRAINDICATIONS).

CONTRAINDICATIONS

IMITREX Injection should not be given intravenously because of its potential to cause coronary vasospasm.

IMITREX Injection should not be given subcutaneously to patients with ischemic heart disease (angina pectoris, history of myocardial infarction, or documented silent ischemia) or to patients with Prinzmetal's variant angina.

IMITREX Injection should not be given subcutaneously to patients who are determined to have symptoms or findings consistent with coronary artery vasospasm, ischemic myocardial disease, or other significant underlying cardiovascular disease (see WARNINGS).

Because IMITREX Injection may increase blood pressure, it should not be given to patients with uncontrolled hypertension.

IMITREX Injection should not be used within 24 hours of treatment with an ergotamine-containing or ergot-type medication like dihydroergotamine or methysergide.

IMITREX Injection should not be administered to patients with hemiplegic or basilar migraine.

IMITREX Injection is contraindicated in patients with hypersensitivity to sumatriptan or any of its components.

WARNINGS

IMITREX Injection should only be used where a clear diagnosis of migraine or cluster headache has been established.

Risk of Myocardial Ischemia and/or Infarction and Other Adverse Cardiac Events: It is strongly recommended that sumatriptan not be given to patients in whom unrecognized coronary artery disease (CAD) is predicted by the presence of risk factors (e.g., hypertension, hypercholesterolemia, smoker, obesity, diabetes, strong family history of CAD, female who is surgically or physiologically postmenopausal, or male who is over 40 years of age) unless a cardiovascular evaluation provides satisfactory clinical evidence that the patient is reasonably free of coronary artery and ischemic myocardial disease or other significant underlying cardiovascular disease. The sensitivity of cardiac diagnostic procedures to detect cardiovascular disease or predisposition to coronary artery vasospasm is unknown. In considering this recommendation, it is noted that patients with cluster headache often possess one or more predictive risk factors for CAD. If, during the cardiovascular evaluation, the patient's medical history or electrocardiographic investigations reveal findings indicative of or consistent with coronary artery vasospasm or myocardial ischemia, sumatriptan should not be administered (see CONTRAINDICATIONS).

For patients with risk factors predictive of CAD who are determined to have a satisfactory cardiovascular evaluation, it is strongly recommended that administration of the first dose of sumatriptan injection take place in the setting of a physician's office or similar medically staffed and equipped facility. Because cardiac ischemia can occur in the absence of clinical symptoms, consideration should be given to obtaining on the first occasion of use an electrocardiogram (ECG) during the interval immediately following IMITREX Injection, in these patients with risk factors.

It is recommended that patients who are intermittent long-term users of IMITREX Injection and who have or acquire risk factors predictive of CAD, as described above, undergo periodic interval cardiovascular evaluation as they continue to use IMITREX Injection. In considering this recommendation for periodic cardiovascular evaluation, it is noted that patients with cluster headache are predominantly male and over 40 years of age, which are risk factors for CAD.

The systematic approach described above is intended to reduce the likelihood that patients with unrecognized cardiovascular disease will be inadvertently exposed to sumatriptan.

Drug-Associated Cardiac Events and Fatalities: Serious adverse cardiac events, including acute myocardial infarction, life-threatening disturbances of cardiac rhythm, and death have been reported to have occurred within 1 hour following the administration of IMITREX Injection. Considering the extent of use of sumatriptan in patients with migraine, the incidence of these events is extremely low. The fact that sumatriptan can cause coronary vasospasm gives credence to the possibility that at least some of the cases reported in close temporal association with the use of IMITREX may have been caused by the drug.

Premarketing Experience: Among the more than 1,900 patients with migraine who participated in premarketing controlled clinical trials of sumatriptan, there were eight patients who sustained clinical events during or shortly after receiving subcutaneous sumatriptan that may have reflected coronary artery vasospasm. Six of these eight patients had ECG changes consistent with transient ischemia, but without accompanying clinical symptoms or signs. Of these eight patients, four had either findings suggestive of CAD or risk factors predictive of CAD prior to study enrollment.

Postmarketing Experience: Serious cardiovascular events, some resulting in death, have been reported in association with the use of IMITREX Injection. The uncontrolled nature of postmarketing surveillance, however, makes it impossible to determine definitively the proportion of the reported cases that were actually caused by sumatriptan or to reliably assess causation in individual cases. On clinical grounds, the longer the latency between the administration of IMITREX and the onset of the clinical event, the less likely the association is to be causative. Accordingly, interest has focused on events occurring within 1 hour of the administration of IMITREX.

Cardiac events that have been observed to have onset within 1 hour of sumatriptan administration include: coronary artery vasospasm, transient ischemia, myocardial infarction, ventricular tachycardia and ventricular fibrillation, cardiac arrest, and death.

Some of these events occurred in patients who had no findings of CAD and may represent sequellae of coronary artery vasospasm. However, among domestic cases reported prior to January 1996 involving patients with serious cardiac events within 1 hour of sumatriptan administration, the majority had risk factors predictive of CAD, and use of sumatriptan may have been contraindicated. The presence of significant underlying CAD was established in most of these cases.

Drug-Associated Cerebrovascular Events and Fatalities: Cerebral hemorrhage, subarachnoid hemorrhage, stroke, and other cerebrovascular events have been reported in patients treated with oral and subcutaneous sumatriptan, and some have resulted in fatalities. In a number of cases, it appears possible that the cerebrovascular events were primary, sumatriptan having been administered in the incorrect belief the symptoms experienced were a consequence of migraine when they were not. Accordingly, sumatriptan should not be administered if the headache being experi-

Table 1: Dose Response Relationship For Efficacy

IMITREX® Dose (mg)	% Patients With Relief* at 10 Minutes	% Patients With Relief* at 30 Minutes	% Patients With Relief* at 1 Hour	% Patients With Relief* at 2 Hours	Adverse Events Incidence (%)
placebo	5	15	24	21	55
1	10	40	43	40	63
2	7	23	57	43	63
3	17	47	57	60	77
4	13	37	50	57	80
6	10	63	73	70	83
8	23	57	80	83	93

*Relief is defined as the reduction of moderate or severe pain to no or mild pain after dosing without use of rescue medication.

enced is atypical. In this regard, it should be noted that patients with migraine may be at increased risk of certain cerebrovascular events (e.g., cerebrovascular accident, transient ischemic attack).

Increase in Blood Pressure: Significant elevation in blood pressure, including hypertensive crisis, has been reported on rare occasions in patients with and without a history of hypertension. Sumatriptan in contraindicated in patients with uncontrolled hypertension (see CONTRAINDICATIONS).

Concomitant Drug Use: In patients taking MAO-A inhibitors, sumatriptan plasma levels attained after treatment with recommended doses are nearly double those obtained under other conditions. Accordingly, the co-administration of sumatriptan and an MAO-A inhibitor is not generally recommended. If such therapy is clinically warranted, however, suitable dose adjustment and appropriate observation of the patient is advised (see CLINICAL PHARMACOLOGY).

Use in Women of Childbearing Potential: (see PRECAUTIONS)

Hypersensitivity: Hypersensitivity (anaphylaxis/anaphylactoid) reactions have occurred on rare occasions in patients receiving sumatriptan. Such reactions can be life threatening or fatal. In general, hypersensitivity reactions to drugs are more likely to occur in individuals with a history of sensitivity to multiple allergens (see CONTRAINDICATIONS).

PRECAUTIONS

General: Chest, jaw, or neck tightness is relatively common after administration of IMITREX Injection, but has only rarely been associated with ischemic ECG changes. However, because sumatriptan may cause coronary artery vasospasm, patients who experience signs or symptoms suggestive of angina following sumatriptan should be evaluated for the presence of CAD or a predisposition to Prinzmetal's variant angina before receiving additional doses of sumatriptan (see WARNINGS). Similarly, patients who experience other symptoms or signs suggestive of decreasing arterial flow (such as ischemic abdominal syndromes or Raynaud's syndrome) following sumatriptan should be evaluated for atherosclerosis or predisposition to vasospasm. IMITREX Injection should also be administered with caution to patients with diseases that may alter the absorption, metabolism, or excretion of drugs, such as impaired hepatic or renal function.

There have been rare reports of seizure following administration of sumatriptan.

Care should be taken to exclude other potentially serious neurologic conditions before treating headache in patients not previously diagnosed with migraine or cluster headache or who experience a headache that is atypical for them. There have been rare reports where patients received sumatriptan for severe headaches that were subsequently shown to have been secondary to an evolving neurologic lesion (see WARNINGS). For a given attack, if a patient does not respond to the first dose of sumatriptan, the diagnosis of migraine or cluster headache should be reconsidered before administration of a second dose.

Binding to Melanin-Containing Tissues: Because sumatriptan binds to melanin, it could accumulate in melanin-rich tissues (such as the eye) over time. This raises the possibility that sumatriptan could cause toxicity in these tissues after extended use. However, no effects on the retina related to treatment with sumatriptan were noted in any of the toxicity studies. Although no systematic monitoring of ophthalmologic function was undertaken in clinical trials, and no specific recommendations for ophthalmologic function was undertaken in clinical trials, and no specific recommendations for ophthalmologic monitoring are offered, prescribers should be aware of the possibility of long-term ophthalmologic effects (see CLINICAL PHARMACOLOGY).

Corneal Opacities: Sumatriptan causes corneal opacities and defects in the corneal epithelium in dogs; this raises the possibility that these changes may occur in humans. While patients were not systematically evaluated for these changes in clinical trials, and no specific recommendations for monitoring are being offered, prescribers should be aware of the possibility of these changes (see CLINICAL PHARMACOLOGY).

Patients who are advised to self-administer IMITREX Injection in medically unsupervised situations should receive instruction on the proper use of the product from the physician or other suitably qualified health care professional prior to doing so for the first time.

Information for Patients: With the autoinjector, the needle penetrates approximately 1/4 of an inch (5 to 6 mm). Since the injection is intended to be given subcutaneously, intramuscular or intravascular delivery should be avoided. Patients should be directed to use injection sites with an adequate skin and subcutaneous thickness to accommodate the length of the needle.

See PATIENT INFORMATION at the end of this labeling for the text of the separate leaflet provided for patients.

Laboratory Tests: No specific laboratory tests are recommended for monitoring patients prior to and/or after treatment with IMITREX Injection.

Drug Interactions: There is no evidence that concomitant use of migraine prophylactic medications has any effect on the efficacy or unwanted effects of sumatriptan. In two Phase III trials in the US, a retrospective analysis of 282 patients who had been using prophylactic drugs (verapamil n = 63, amitriptyline n = 57, propranolol n = 94, for 45 other drugs n = 123) were compared to those who had not used prophylaxis (n = 452). There were no differences in relief rates at 60 minutes postdose for IMITREX Injection, whether or not prophylactic medications were used. There were also no differences in overall adverse event rates between the two groups.

Ergot-containing drugs have been reported to cause prolonged vasospastic reactions. Because there is a theoretical basis that these effects may be additive, use of ergotamine-containing or ergot-type medications (like dihydroergotamine or methysergide) and sumatriptan within 24 hours of each other should be avoided (see CONTRAINDICATIONS).

MAO-A inhibitors reduce sumatriptan clearance, significantly increasing systemic exposure. Therefore, the use of sumatriptan in patients receiving MAO-A inhibitors is not ordinarily recommended. If the clinical situation warrants the combined use of sumatriptan and an MAOI, the dose of sumatriptan employed should be reduced (see CLINICAL PHARMACOLOGY and WARNINGS).

There have been rare postmarketing reports describing patients with weakness, hyperreflexia, and incoordination following the use of a selective serotonin reuptake inhibitor (SSRI) and sumatriptan. If concomitant treatment with sumatriptan and an SSRI (e.g., fluoxetine, fluvoxamine, paroxetine, sertraline) is clinically warranted, appropriate observation of the patient is advised.

Drug/Laboratory Test Interactions: IMITREX Injection is not known to interfere with commonly employed clinical laboratory tests.

Carcinogenesis, Mutagenesis, Impairment of Fertility: In carcinogenicity studies, rats and mice were given sumatriptan by oral gavage (rats, 104 weeks) or drinking water (mice, 78 weeks). Average exposures achieved in mice receiving the highest dose were approximately 110 times the exposure attained in humans after the maximum recommended single dose of 6 mg. The highest dose to rats was approximately 260 times the maximum single dose of 6 mg on a mg/m^2 basis. There was no evidence of an increase in tumors in either species related to sumatriptan administration.

Sumatriptan was not mutagenic in the presence or absence of metabolic activation when tested in two gene mutation assays (the Ames test and the in vitro mammalian Chinese hamster V79/HGPRT assay). In two cytogenetics assays (the in vitro human lymphocyte assay and the in vivo rat micronucleus assay) sumatriptan was not associated with clastogenic activity.

A fertility study (Segment I) by the subcutaneous route, during which male and female rats were dosed daily with sumatriptan prior to and throughout the mating period, has shown no evidence of impaired fertility at doses equivalent to approximately 100 times the maximum recommended single human dose of 6 mg on a mg/m^2 basis. However, following oral administration, a treatment-related decrease in fertility, secondary to a decrease in mating, was seen in rats treated with 50 and 500 mg/kg per day. The no-effect dose for this finding was approximately eight times the maximum recommended single human dose of 6 mg on a mg/m^2 basis. It is not clear whether the problem is associated with the treatment of males or females or both.

Pregnancy: Pregnancy Category C. Sumatriptan has been shown to be embryolethal in rabbits when given daily at a dose approximately equivalent to the maximum recommended single human subcutaneous dose of 6 mg on a mg/m^2 basis. There is no evidence that establishes that sumatriptan is a human teratogen; however, there are no adequate and well-controlled studies in pregnant women. IMITREX Injection should be used during pregnancy only if the potential benefit justifies the potential risk to the fetus. In assessing this information, the following additional findings should be considered.

Embryolethality: When given intravenously to pregnant rabbits daily throughout the period of organogenesis, sumatriptan caused embryolethality at doses at or close to

Table 2: Efficacy Data From US Phase III Trials

	Study 1		Study 2	
		IMITREX®		IMITREX
One-Hour Data	Placebo (n = 190)	6 mg (n = 384)	Placebo (n = 180)	6 mg (n = 350)
Patients with pain relief (grade 0/1)	18%	70%*	26%	70%*
Patients with no pain	5%	48%*	13%	49%*
Patients without nausea	48%	73%*	50%	73%*
Patients without photophobia	23%	56%*	25%	58%*
Patients with little or no clinical disability§	34%	76%*	34%	76%*

	Study 1		Study 2	
		IMITREX		IMITREX
Two-Hour Data	Placebo†	6 mg‡	Placebo†	6 mg‡
Patients with pain relief (grade 0/1)	31%	81%*	39%	82%*
Patients with no pain	11%	63%*	19%	65%*
Patients without nausea	56%	82%*	63%	81%*
Patients without photophobia	31%	72%*	35%	71%*
Patients with little or no clinical disability§	42%	85%*	49%	84%*

*$P<0.05$ versus placebo.
†Includes patients that may have received an additional placebo injection 1 hour after the initial injection.
‡Includes patients that may have received an additional 6 mg of IMITREX Injection 1 hour after the initial injection.
§A successful outcome in terms of clinical disability was defined prospectively as ability to work mildly impaired or ability to work and function normally.

Table 3: Efficacy Data From the Pivotal Cluster Headache Studies

	Study 1		Study 2	
		IMITREX®		IMITREX
	Placebo (n=39)	6 mg (n=39)	Placebo (n=88)	6 mg (n=92)
Patients with pain relief (no/mild)				
5 minutes postinjection	8%	21%	7%	23%*
10 minutes postinjection	10%	49%*	25%	49%*
15 minutes postinjection	26%	74%*	35%	75%*

* $P<0.05$.
(n=Number of headaches treated.)

Continued on next page

This product information is based on labeling in effect on June 1, 1998. For further information, contact via direct mail, phone, or web site Medical Information: Glaxo Wellcome Inc., PO Box 13398, Research Triangle Park, NC 27709. Healthcare Professionals (Medical Information): 800-334-0089 Patients (Customer Response Center): 888-TALK2GW (1-888-825-5249) Glaxo Wellcome Corporate Web Site: www.glaxowellcome.com

Imitrex Injection—Cont.

those producing maternal toxicity. The mechanism of the embryolethality is not known. These doses were approximately equivalent to the maximum single human dose of 6 mg on a mg/m^2 basis.

The intravenous administration of sumatriptan to pregnant rats throughout organogenesis at doses that are approximately 20 times a human dose of 6 mg on a mg/m^2 basis, did not cause embryolethality. Additionally, in a study of pregnant rats given subcutaneous sumatriptan daily prior to and throughout pregnancy, there was no evidence of increased embryo/fetal lethality.

Teratogenicity: Term fetuses from Dutch Stride rabbits treated during organogenesis with oral sumatriptan exhibited an increased incidence of cervicothoracic vascular and skeletal abnormalities. The functional significance of these abnormalities is not known. The highest no-effect dose for these effects was 15 mg/kg per day, approximately 50 times the maximum single dose of 6 mg on a mg/m^2 basis.

In a study in rats dosed daily with subcutaneous sumatriptan prior to and throughout pregnancy, there was no evidence of teratogenicity.

To monitor fetal outcomes of pregnant women exposed to IMITREX, Glaxo Wellcome Inc. maintains a Sumatriptan Pregnancy Registry. Physicians are encouraged to register patients by calling (800) 722-9292, ext. 39441.

Nursing Mothers: Sumatriptan is excreted in human breast milk. Therefore, caution should be exercised when considering the administration of IMITREX Injection to a nursing woman.

Pediatric Use: Safety and effectiveness of IMITREX Injection in pediatric patients have not been established.

Use in the Elderly: Although the pharmacokinetic disposition of the drug in elderly is similar to that seen in younger adults, there is no information about the safety and effectiveness of sumatriptan in this population because patients over age 65 were excluded from the controlled clinical trials.

ADVERSE REACTIONS

Serious cardiac events, including some that have been fatal, have occurred following use of IMITREX Injection, but are extremely rare. Events reported have included coronary artery vasospasm, transient myocardial ischemia, myocardial infarction, ventricular tachycardia, and ventricular fibrillation (see CONTRAINDICATIONS, WARNINGS, and PRECAUTIONS).

Significant hypertensive episodes, including hypertensive crises, have been reported on rare occasions in patients with or without a history of hypertension (see WARNINGS).

Among patients in clinical trials of subcutaneous IMITREX Injection (n=6,218), up to 3.5% of patients withdrew for reasons related to adverse events.

Incidence in Controlled Clinical Trials of Migraine Headache: The following Table 4 lists adverse events that occurred in two large US, Phase III, placebo-controlled clinical trials in migraine patients following either a single dose of IMITREX Injection or placebo. Only events that occurred at a frequency of 1% or more in IMITREX Injection treatment groups and were at least as frequent as in the placebo group are included in Table 4.

Table 4: Treatment-Emergent Adverse Experience Incidence in Two Large Placebo-Controlled Migraine Clinical Trials: Events Reported by at Least 1% of IMITREX® Injection Patients

	Percent of Patients Reporting	
Adverse Event Type	IMITREX Injection 6 mg Subcutaneous n = 547	Placebo n = 370
Atypical sensations	42.0	9.2
Tingling	13.5	3.0
Warm/hot sensation	10.8	3.5
Burning sensation	7.5	0.3
Feeling of heaviness	7.3	1.1
Pressure sensation	7.1	1.6
Feeling of tightness	5.1	0.3
Numbness	4.6	2.2
Feeling strange	2.2	0.3
Tight feeling in head	2.2	0.3
Cold sensation	1.1	0.5
Cardiovascular		
Flushing	6.6	2.4
Chest discomfort	4.5	1.4
Tightness in chest	2.7	0.5
Pressure in chest	1.8	0.3
Ear, nose, and throat		
Throat discomfort	3.3	0.5
Discomfort: nasal cavity/ sinuses	2.2	0.3
Eye		
Vision alterations	1.1	0.0
Gastrointestinal		
Abdominal discomfort	1.3	0.8
Dysphagia	1.1	0.0
Injection site reaction	58.7	23.8
Miscellaneous		
Jaw discomfort	1.8	0.0
Mouth and teeth		
Discomfort of mouth/ tongue	4.9	4.6
Musculoskeletal		
Weakness	4.9	0.3
Neck pain/stiffness	4.8	0.5
Myalgia	1.8	0.5
Muscle cramp(s)	1.1	0.0
Neurological		
Dizziness/vertigo	11.9	4.3
Drowsiness/sedation	2.7	2.2
Headache	2.2	0.3
Anxiety	1.1	0.5
Malaise/fatigue	1.1	0.8
Skin		
Sweating	1.6	1.1

The sum of the percentages cited is greater than 100% because patients may experience more than one type of adverse event. Only events that occurred at a frequency of 1% or more in IMITREX Injection treatment groups and were at least as frequent in the placebo groups are included.

The incidence of adverse events in controlled clinical trials was not affected by gender or age of the patients. There was insufficient data to assess the impact of race on the incidence of adverse events.

Incidence in Controlled Trials of Cluster Headache: In the controlled clinical trials assessing sumatriptan's efficacy as a treatment for cluster headache, no new significant adverse events associated with the use of sumatriptan were detected that had not already been identified in association of the drug's use in migraine.

Overall, the frequency of adverse events reported in the studies of cluster headache were generally lower. Exceptions include reports of paresthesia (5% IMITREX, 0% placebo), nausea and vomiting (4% IMITREX, 0% placebo), and bronchospasm (1% IMITREX, 0% placebo).

Other Events Observed in Association With the Administration of IMITREX Injection: In the paragraphs that follow, the frequencies of less commonly reported adverse clinical events are presented. Because the reports cite events observed in open and uncontrolled studies, the role of IMITREX Injection in their causation cannot be reliably determined. Furthermore, variability associated with reporting requirements, the terminology used to describe adverse events, etc., limit the value of the quantitative frequency estimates provided.

Event frequencies are calculated as the number of patients reporting an event divided by the total number of patients (n = 6,218) exposed to subcutaneous IMITREX Injection. Given their imprecision, frequencies for specific adverse event occurrences are defined as follows: "infrequent" indicates a frequency estimated as falling between 1/1,000 and 1/100; "rare," a frequency of less than 1/1,000.

Cardiovascular: Infrequent were hypertension, hypotension, bradycardia, tachycardia, palpitations, pulsating sensations, various transient ECG changes (nonspecific ST or T wave changes, prolongation of PR or QTc intervals, sinus arrhythmia, nonsustained ventricular premature beats, isolated junctional ectopic beats, atrial ectopic beats, delayed activation of the right ventricle), and syncope. Rare were pallor, arrhythmia, abnormal pulse, vasodilatation, and Raynaud's syndrome.

Endocrine and Metabolic: Infrequent was thirst. Rare was polydipsia and dehydration.

Eye: Infrequent was irritation of the eye.

Gastrointestinal: Infrequent were gastroesophageal reflux, diarrhea, and disturbances of liver function tests. Rare were peptic ulcer, retching, flatulence/eructation, and gallstones.

Musculoskeletal: Infrequent were various joint disturbances (pain, stiffness, swelling, ache). Rare were muscle stiffness, need to flex calf muscles, backache, muscle tiredness, and swelling of the extremities.

Neurological: Infrequent were mental confusion, euphoria, agitation, relaxation, chills, sensation of lightness, tremor, shivering, disturbances of taste, prickling sensations, paresthesia, stinging sensations, headaches, facial pain, photophobia, and lacrimation. Rare were transient hemiplegia, hysteria, globus hystericus, intoxication, depression, myoclonia, monoplegia/diplegia, sleep disturbance, difficulties in concentration, disturbances of smell, hyperesthesia, dysesthesia, simultaneous hot and cold sensations, tickling sensations, dysarthria, yawning, reduced appetite, hunger, and dystonia.

Respiratory: Infrequent was dyspnea. Rare were influenza, diseases of the lower respiratory tract, and hiccoughs.

Dermatological: Infrequent were erythema, pruritus, and skin rashes and eruptions. Rare was skin tenderness.

Urogenital: Rare were dysuria, frequency, dysmenorrhea, and renal calculus.

Miscellaneous: Infrequent were miscellaneous laboratory abnormalities, including minor disturbances in liver function tests, "serotonin agonist effect", and hypersensitivity to various agents. Rare was fever.

Postmarketing Experience: The following are spontaneously reported adverse events from postmarketing experience except those events already listed previously in the ADVERSE REACTIONS section or those too general to be informative. Because the reports cite events reported spontaneously from worldwide postmarketing experience, frequency of events and the role of IMITREX Injection in their causation cannot be reliably determined.

Cardiovascular: Cerebrovascular accident, ischemic colitis, Prinzmetal's variant angina, subarachnoid hemorrhage.

Dermatological: Exacerbation of sunburn, photosensitivity. Following subcutaneous administration of sumatriptan, pain, redness, stinging, induration, swelling, contusion, subcutaneous bleeding, and, on rare occasions, lipoatrophy (depression in the skin) or lipohypertrophy (enlargement or thickening of tissue) have been reported.

Hypersensitivity Reactions: Shortness of breath and urticaria. In addition, severe anaphylaxis/anaphylactoid reactions have been reported (see WARNINGS).

Neurological: Dysphasia, seizure.

Non-Site Specific: Death (see WARNINGS). Rarely, lipoatrophy (depression in the skin) or lipohypertrophy (enlargement or thickening of tissue) has been reported following subcutaneous administration of sumatriptan.

Respiratory: Bronchospasm has been reported in patients with and without a history of asthma.

Urogenital: Acute renal failure.

DRUG ABUSE AND DEPENDENCE

The abuse potential of IMITREX Injection cannot be fully delineated in advance of extensive marketing experience. One clinical study enrolling 12 patients with a history of substance abuse failed to induce subjective behavior and/or physiologic response ordinarily associated with drugs that have an established potential for abuse.

OVERDOSAGE

Patients (n = 269) have received single injections of 8 to 12 mg without significant adverse effects. Volunteers (n = 47) have received single subcutaneous doses of up to 16 mg without serious adverse events.

No gross overdoses in clinical practice have been reported. Coronary vasospasm was observed after intravenous administration of IMITREX Injection (see CONTRAINDICATIONS). Overdoses would be expected from animal data (dogs at 0.1 g/kg, rats at 2 g/kg) to possibly cause convulsions, tremor, inactivity, erythema of the extremities, reduced respiratory rate, cyanosis, ataxia, mydriasis, injection site reactions (desquamation, hair loss, and scab formation), and paralysis. The half-life of elimination of sumatriptan is about 2 hours (see CLINICAL PHARMACOLOGY), and therefore monitoring of patients after overdose with IMITREX Injection should continue while symptoms or signs persist, and for at least 10 hours.

It is unknown what effect hemodialysis or peritoneal dialysis has on the serum concentrations of sumatriptan.

DOSAGE AND ADMINISTRATION

The maximum single recommended adult dose of IMITREX Injection is 6 mg injected subcutaneously. Controlled clinical trials have failed to show that clear benefit is associated with the administration of a second 6-mg dose in patients who have failed to respond to a first injection.

The maximum recommended dose that may be given in 24 hours is two 6-mg injections separated by at least 1 hour. Although the recommended dose is 6 mg, if side effects are dose limiting, then lower doses may be used (see CLINICAL PHARMACOLOGY). In patients receiving MAO inhibitors, decreased doses of sumatriptan should be considered (see WARNINGS and CLINICAL PHARMACOLOGY). In patients receiving doses lower than 6 mg, only the single-dose vial dosage form should be used. An autoinjection device is available for use with 6-mg prefilled syringes to facilitate self-administration in patients in whom this dose is deemed necessary. With this device, the needle penetrates approximately 1/4 of an inch (5 to 6 mm). Since the injection is intended to be given subcutaneously, intramuscular or intravascular delivery should be avoided. Patients should be directed to use injection sites with an adequate skin and subcutaneous thickness to accommodate the length of the needle.

Parenteral drug products should be inspected visually for particulate matter and discoloration before administration whenever solution and container permit.

HOW SUPPLIED

IMITREX Injection 6 mg (12 mg/mL) containing sumatriptan (base) as the succinate salt is supplied as a clear, colorless to pale yellow, sterile, nonpyrogenic solution as follows.

(NDC 0173-0479-00) IMITREX® STATdose System® containing two prefilled single-dose syringe cartridges, one IMITREX® STATdose Pen®, and instructions for use
(NDC 0173-0478-00) IMITREX Injection cartridge pack containing two prefilled syringe cartridges for refill of IMITREX STATdose System only.
(NDC 0173-0449-02) 6-mg single-dose vials (0.5 mL in 2 mL) in cartons of five vials
(NDC 0173-0449-01) Unit-of-use syringe (0.5 mL in 1 mL) in cartons of two syringes. Not for use with IMITREX STATdose System.
(NDC 0173-0449-02) 6-mg Single-dose vials (0.5 mL in 2 mL) in cartons of five vials.
Store between 2° and 30°C (36° and 86°F). Protect from light.
Caution: Federal law prohibits dispensing without a prescription.

PATIENT INFORMATION

The following wording is contained in a separate leaflet provided for patients.

Information for the Patient
IMITREX® (sumatriptan succinate) Injection

Please read this leaflet carefully before you take IMITREX Injection. This provides a summary of the information available on your medicine. Please do not throw away this leaflet until you have finished your medicine. You may need to read this leaflet again. This leaflet does not contain all the information on IMITREX Injection. For further information or advice, ask your doctor or pharmacist.

Information About Your Medicine:
The name of your medicine is IMITREX (sumatriptan succinate) Injection. It can be obtained only by prescription from your doctor. The decision to use IMITREX Injection is one that you and your doctor should make jointly, taking into account your individual preferences and medical circumstances. If you have risk factors for heart disease (such as high blood pressure, high cholesterol, obesity, diabetes, smoking, strong family history of heart disease, or you are postmenopausal or a male over 40), you should tell your doctor, who should evaluate you for heart disease in order to determine if IMITREX is appropriate for you. Although the vast majority of those who have taken IMITREX have not experienced any significant side effects, some individuals have experienced problems and, rarely, deaths have been reported. In all but a few instances, however, IMITREX does not appear to have been a contributory factor in these deaths.

1. The Purpose of Your Medicine:
IMITREX Injection is intended to relieve your migraine or cluster headache, but not to prevent or reduce the number of attacks you experience. Use IMITREX Injection only to treat an actual migraine or cluster headache attack.

2. Important Questions to Consider Before Taking IMITREX Injection:
If the answer to any of the following questions is **YES** or if you do not know the answer, then please discuss with your doctor before you use IMITREX Injection.

- Are you pregnant? Do you think you might be pregnant? Are you trying to become pregnant? Are you using inadequate contraception? Are you breast-feeding?
- Do you have any chest pain, heart disease, shortness of breath, or irregular heartbeats? Have you had a heart attack?
- Do you have risk factors for heart disease (such as high blood pressure, high cholesterol, obesity, diabetes, smoking, strong family history of heart disease, or you are postmenopausal or a male over 40)?
- Do you have high blood pressure?
- Have you ever had to stop taking this or any other medication because of an allergy or other problems?
- Are you taking any medications, including migraine medications containing ergotamine, dihydroergotamine, or methysergide?
- Are you taking any medication for depression (monoamine oxidase inhibitors or selective serotonin reuptake inhibitors [SSRIs])?
- Have you had, or do you have, any disease of the liver or kidney?
- Have you had, or do you have, epilepsy or seizures?
- Is this headache different from your usual migraine attacks?

Remember, if you answered **YES** to any of the above questions, then discuss it with your doctor.

3. The Use of IMITREX Injection During Pregnancy:
Do not use IMITREX Injection if you are pregnant, think you might be pregnant, are trying to become pregnant, or are not using adequate contraception, unless you have discussed this with your doctor.

4. How to Use IMITREX Injection:
Before injecting IMITREX, check with your doctor on acceptable injection sites and see the instructions (on or inside the carton) on discarding empty syringes and loading an auotinjector device **Never reuse a syringe.**
For adults, the usual dose is a single injection given just below the skin. It should be given as soon as the symptoms of your migraine appear, but it may be given at any time during an attack. A second injection may be given if your symptoms of migraine come back. If your symptoms do not improve following the first injection, do not give a second injection for the same attack without first consulting with your doctor. Do not have more than two injections in any 24 hours and allow at least 1 hour between each dose.

5. Side Effects to Watch for:

- Some patients experience pain or tightness in the chest or throat when using IMITREX Injection. If this happens to you, then discuss it with your doctor before using any more IMITREX Injection. If the chest pain is severe or does not go away, call your doctor immediately.
- Shortness of breath; wheeziness; heart throbbing; swelling of eyelids, face, or lips; or a skin rash, skin lumps, or hives happens rarely. If it happens to you, then tell your doctor immediately. Do not take any more IMITREX Injection unless your doctor tells you to do so.
- Some people may have feelings of tingling, heat, flushing (redness of face lasting a short time), heaviness or pressure after treatment with IMITREX Injection. A few people may feel drowsy, dizzy, tired, or sick. Tell your doctor of these symptoms at your next visit.
- You may experience pain or redness at the site of injection, but this usually lasts less than an hour.
- If you feel unwell in any other way or have any symptoms that you do not understand, you should contact your doctor immediately.

6. What to Do If an Overdose Is Taken:
If you have taken more medication than you have been told, contact either your doctor, hospital emergency department, or nearest poison control center immediately.

7. Storing Your Medicine:
Keep your medicine in a safe place where children cannot reach it. It may be harmful to children.
Store your medication away from heat and light. Keep your medication in the case provided and do not store at temperatures above 86°F (30°C).
If your medication has expired (the expiration date is printed on the treatment pack), throw it away as instructed. Do not throw away your autoinjector.
If your doctor decides to stop your treatment, do not keep any leftover medicine unless your doctor tells you to. Throw away your medicine as instructed.
U.S. Patent Nos. 4,816,470 and 5,037,845
©Copyright 1996 Glaxo Wellcome Inc. All rights reserved.
December 1997/RL-481
Shown in Product Identification Guide, page 313

IMITREX® ℞
[*ĭm′ ĭ-trĕx″*]
(sumatriptan)
Nasal Spray

DESCRIPTION

IMITREX (sumatriptan) Nasal Spray contains sumatriptan, a selective 5-hydroxytryptamine$_1$ receptor subtype agonist. Sumatriptan is chemically designated as 3-[2-(dimethylamino)ethyl]-N-methyl-1H-indole-5-methanesulfonamide, and it has the following structure:

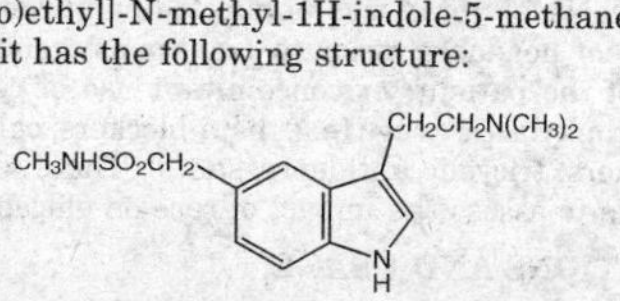
CH2CH2N(CH3)2
CH3NHSO2CH2
N
H

The empirical formula is $C_{14}H_{21}N_3O_2S$, representing a molecular weight of 295.4. Sumatriptan is a white to off-white powder that is readily soluble in water and in saline. Each IMITREX Nasal Spray contains 5 or 20 mg of sumatriptan in a 100-µL unit dose aqueous buffered solution containing monobasic potassium phosphate NF, anhydrous dibasic sodium phosphate USP, sulfuric acid NF, sodium hydroxide NF, and purified water USP. The pH of the solution is approximately 5.5. The osmolality of the solution is 372 or 742 mOsmol for the 5- and 20-mg IMITREX Nasal Spray, respectively.

CLINICAL PHARMACOLOGY

Mechanism of Action: Sumatriptan is an agonist for a vascular 5-hydroxytryptamine$_1$ receptor subtype (probably a member of the 5-HT$_{1D}$ family) having only a weak affinity for 5-HT$_{1A}$, 5-HT$_{5A}$, and 5-HT$_7$ receptors and no significant affinity (as measured using standard radioligand binding assays) or pharmacological activity at 5-HT$_2$, 5-HT$_3$, or 5-HT$_4$ receptor subtypes or at alpha$_1$-, alpha$_2$-, or beta-adrenergic; dopamine$_1$; dopamine$_2$; muscarinic; or benzodiazepine receptors.
The vascular 5-HT$_1$ receptor subtype that sumatriptan activates is present on cranial arteries in both dog and primate, on the human basilar artery, and in the vasculature of human dura mater and mediates vasoconstriction. This action in humans correlates with the relief of migraine headache. In addition to causing vasoconstriction, experimental data from animal studies show that sumatriptan also activates 5-HT$_1$ receptors on peripheral terminals of the trigeminal nerve innervating cranial blood vessels. Such an action may contribute to the antimigrainous effect of sumatriptan in humans.
In the anesthetized dog, sumatriptan selectively reduces the carotid arterial blood flow with little or no effect on arterial blood pressure or total peripheral resistance. In the cat, sumatriptan selectively constricts the carotid arteriovenous anastomoses while having little effect on blood flow or resistance in cerebral or extracerebral tissues.

Pharmacokinetics: In a study of 20 female volunteers, the mean maximum concentration following a 5- and 20-mg intranasal dose was 5 and 16 ng/mL, respectively. The mean C_{max} following a 6-mg subcutaneous injection is 71 ng/mL (range, 49 to 110 ng/mL). The mean C_{max} is 18 ng/mL (range, 7 to 47 ng/mL) following oral dosing with 25 mg and 51 mg/mL (range, 28 to 100 ng/mL) following oral dosing with 100 mg of sumatriptan. In a study of 24 male volunteers, the bioavailability relative to subcutaneous injection was low, approximately 17%, primarily due to presystemic metabolism and partly due to incomplete absorption. Protein binding, determined by equilibrium dialysis over the concentration range of 10 to 1000 ng/mL, is low, approximately 14% to 21%. The effect of sumatriptan on the protein binding of other drugs has not been evaluated, but would be expected to be minor, given the low rate of protein binding. The mean volume of distribution after subcutaneous dosing is 2.7 L/kg and the total plasma clearance is approximately 1200 mL/min.
The elimination half-life of sumatriptan administered as a nasal spray is approximately 2 hours, similar to the half-life seen after subcutaneous injection. Only 3% of the dose is excreted in the urine as unchanged sumatriptan; 42% of the dose is excreted as the major metabolite, the indole acetic acid analogue of sumatriptan.
Clinical and pharmacokinetic data indicate that administration of two 5-mg doses, one dose in each nostril, is equivalent to administration of a single 10-mg dose in one nostril.

Special Populations: ***Renal Impairment:*** The effect of renal impairment on the pharmacokinetics of sumatriptan has not been examined, but little clinical effect would be expected as sumatriptan is largely metabolized to an inactive substance.

Hepatic Impairment: The effect of hepatic disease on the pharmacokinetics of subcutaneously and orally administered sumatriptan has been evaluated, but the intranasal dosage form has not been studied in hepatic impairment. There were no statistically significant differences in the pharmacokinetics of subcutaneously administered sumatriptan in hepatically impaired patients compared to healthy controls. However, the liver plays an important role in the presystemic clearance of orally administered sumatriptan. In one small study involving oral sumatriptan in hepatically impaired patients (n = 8) matched for sex, age, and weight with healthy subjects, the hepatically impaired patients had an approximately 70% increase in AUC and C_{max} and a t_{max} 40 minutes earlier compared to the healthy subjects. The bioavailability of nasally absorbed sumatriptan following intranasal administration, which would not undergo first-pass metabolism, should not be altered in hepatically impaired patients. The bioavailability of the swallowed portion of the intranasal sumatriptan dose has not been determined, but would be increased in these patients. The swallowed intranasal dose is small, however, compared to the usual oral dose, so that its impact should be minimal.

Age: The pharmacokinetics of oral sumatriptan in the elderly (mean age, 72 years; two males and four females) and in patients with migraine (mean age, 38 years; 25 males and 155 females) were similar to that in healthy male subjects (mean age, 30 years). Intranasal sumatriptan has not been evaluated for age differences.

Race: The systemic clearance and C_{max} of sumatriptan were similar in black (n = 34) and Caucasian (n = 38) healthy male subjects. Intranasal sumatriptan has not been evaluated for race differences.

Drug Interactions: ***Monoamine Oxidase Inhibitors (MAOI):*** Treatment with MAOIs generally leads to an increase of sumatriptan plasma levels (see CONTRAINDICATIONS and PRECAUTIONS).
MAOI interaction studies have not been performed with intranasal sumatriptan. Due to gut and hepatic metabolic first-pass effects, the increase of systemic exposure after

Continued on next page

This product information is based on labeling in effect on June 1, 1998. For further information, contact via direct mail, phone, or web site Medical Information: Glaxo Wellcome Inc., PO Box 13398, Research Triangle Park, NC 27709. Healthcare Professionals (Medical Information): 800-334-0089 Patients (Customer Response Center): 888-TALK2GW (1-888-825-5249) Glaxo Wellcome Corporate Web Site: www.glaxowellcome.com

Imitrex Nasal Spray—Cont.

coadministration of an MAO-A inhibitor with oral sumatriptan is greater than after coadministration of the MAOI with subcutaneous sumatriptan. The effects of an MAOI on systemic exposure after intranasal sumatriptan would be expected to be greater than the effect after subcutaneous sumatriptan but smaller than the effect after oral sumatriptan because only swallowed drug would be subject to first-pass effects.

In a study of 14 healthy females, pretreatment with an MAO-A inhibitor decreased the clearance of subcutaneous sumatriptan. Under the conditions of this experiment, the result was a twofold increase in the area under the sumatriptan plasma concentration x time curve (AUC), corresponding to a 40% increase in elimination half-life. This interaction was not evident with an MAO-B inhibitor.

A small study evaluating the effect of pretreatment with an MAO-A inhibitor on the bioavailability from a 25-mg oral sumatriptan tablet resulted in an approximately sevenfold increase in systemic exposure.

Xylometazoline: An in vivo drug interaction study indicated that three drops of xylometazoline (0.1% w/v), a decongestant, administered 15 minutes prior to a 20-mg nasal dose of sumatriptan did not alter the pharmacokinetics of sumatriptan.

CLINICAL TRIALS

The efficacy of IMITREX Nasal Spray in the acute treatment of migraine headaches was demonstrated in eight, randomized, double-blind, placebo-controlled studies, of which five used the recommended dosing regimen and used the marketed formulation. Patients enrolled in these five studies were predominately female (86%) and Caucasian (95%), with a mean age of 41 (range of 18 to 65). Patients were instructed to treat a moderate to severe headache. Headache response, defined as a reduction in headache severity from moderate or severe pain to mild or no pain, was assessed up to 2 hours after dosing. Associated symptoms such as nausea, photophobia, and phonophobia were also assessed. Maintenance of response was assessed for up to 24 hours postdose. A second dose of IMITREX Nasal Spray or other medication was allowed 2 to 24 hours after the initial treatment for recurrent headache. The frequency and time to use of these additional treatments were also determined. In all studies, doses of 10 and 20 mg were compared to placebo in the treatment of one to three migraine attacks. Patients received doses as a single spray into one nostril. In two studies, a 5-mg dose was also evaluated.

In all five trials utilizing the market formulation and recommended dosage regimen, the percentage of patients achieving headache response 2 hours after treatment was significantly greater among patients receiving IMITREX Nasal Spray at all doses (with one exception) compared to those who received placebo. In four of the five studies, there was a statistically significant greater percentage of patients with headache response at 2 hours in the 20-mg group when compared to the lower dose groups (5 and 10 mg). There were no statistically significant differences between the 5- and 10-mg dose groups in any study. The results from the five controlled clinical trials are summarized in Table 1. Note that, in general, comparisons of results obtained in studies conducted under different conditions by different investigators with different samples of patients are ordinarily unreliable for purposes of quantitative comparison.

[See table 1 below]

The estimated probability of achieving an initial headache response over the 2 hours following treatment is depicted in Figure 1.

[See figure at top of next column]

Figure 1: Estimated Probability of Achieving Initial Headache Response Within 120 Minutes*

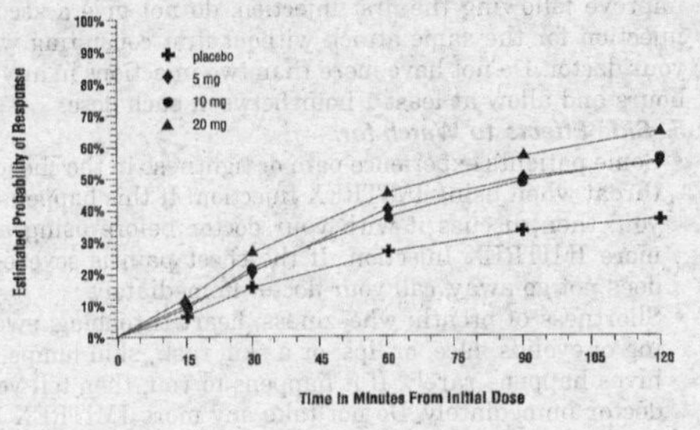

* The figure shows the probability over time of obtaining headache response (no or mild pain) following treatment with intranasal sumatriptan. The averages displayed are based on pooled data from the five clinical controlled trials providing evidence of efficacy. Kaplan-Meier plot with patients not achieving response within 120 minutes censored to 120 minutes.

For patients with migraine-associated nausea, photophobia, and phonophobia at baseline, there was a lower incidence of these symptoms at 2 hours following administration of IMITREX Nasal Spray compared to placebo.

Two to 24 hours following the initial dose of study treatment, patients were allowed to use additional treatment for pain relief in the form of a second dose of study treatment or other medication. The estimated probability of patients taking a second dose or other medication for migraine over the 24 hours following the initial dose of study treatment is summarized in Figure 2.

Figure 2: The Estimated Probability of Patients Taking a Second Dose or Other Medication for Migraine Over the 24 Hours Following the Initial Dose of Study Treatment*

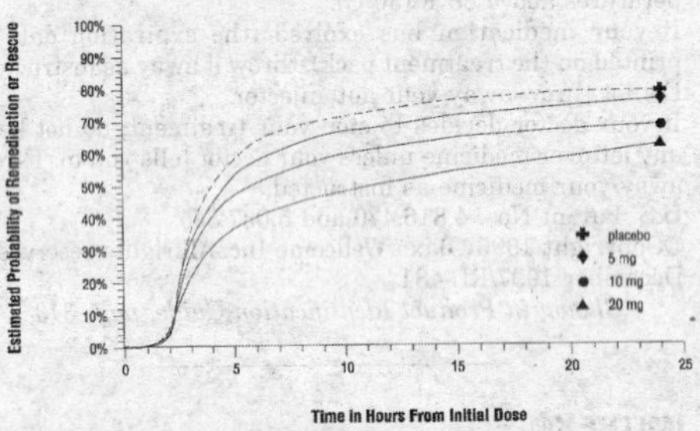

* Kaplan-Meier plot based on data obtained in the three clinical controlled trials providing evidence of efficacy with patients not using additional treatments censored to 24 hours. Plot also includes patients who had no response to the initial dose. No remedication was allowed within 2 hours postdose.

There is evidence that doses above 20 mg do not provide a greater effect than 20 mg. There was no evidence to suggest that treatment with sumatriptan was associated with an increase in the severity of recurrent headaches. The efficacy of IMITREX Nasal Spray was unaffected by presence of aura; duration of headache prior to treatment; gender, age, or weight of the patient; or concomitant use of common migraine prophylactic drugs (e.g., beta-blockers, calcium channel blockers, tricyclic antidepressants). There were insufficient data to assess the impact of race on efficacy.

INDICATIONS AND USAGE

IMITREX Nasal Spray is indicated for the acute treatment of migraine attacks with or without aura in adults.

IMITREX Nasal Spray is not intended for the prophylactic therapy of migraine or for use in the management of hemiplegic or basilar migraine (see CONTRAINDICATIONS). Safety and effectiveness of IMITREX Nasal Spray have not been established for cluster headache, which is present in an older, predominantly male population.

CONTRAINDICATIONS

IMITREX Nasal Spray should not be given to patients with ischemic heart disease (angina pectoris, history of myocardial infarction, or documented silent ischemia) or to patients who have symptoms or findings consistent with ischemic heart disease, coronary artery vasospasm including Prinzmetal's variant angina, or other significant underlying cardiovascular disease (see WARNINGS).

Because IMITREX Nasal Spray may increase blood pressure, it should not be given to patients with uncontrolled hypertension.

IMITREX Nasal Spray should not be used within 24 hours of treatment with an ergotamine-containing or ergot-type medication like dihydroergotamine or methysergide.

Concurrent administration of MAOIs or use of IMITREX Nasal Spray within 2 weeks of discontinuation of MAOI therapy is contraindicated (see CLINICAL PHARMACOLOGY: Drug Interactions and PRECAUTIONS: Drug Interactions).

IMITREX Nasal Spray should not be administered to patients with hemiplegic or basilar migraine.

IMITREX Nasal Spray is contraindicated in patients with hypersensitivity to sumatriptan or any of the components.

WARNINGS

IMITREX Nasal Spray should only be used where a clear diagnosis of migraine headache has been established.

Risk of Myocardial Ischemia and/or Infarction and Other Adverse Cardiac Events: Sumatriptan should not be given to patients with documented ischemic or vasospastic coronary artery disease (see CONTRAINDICATIONS). It is strongly recommended that sumatriptan not be given to patients in whom unrecognized coronary artery disease (CAD) is predicted by the presence of risk factors (e.g., hypertension, hypercholesterolemia, smoker, obesity, diabetes, strong family history of CAD, female with surgical or physiological menopause, or male over 40 years of age) unless a cardiovascular evaluation provides satisfactory clinical evidence that the patient is reasonably free of coronary artery and ischemic myocardial disease or other significant underlying cardiovascular disease. The sensitivity of cardiac diagnostic procedures to detect cardiovascular disease or predisposition to coronary artery vasospasm is modest, at best. If, during the cardiovascular evaluation, the patient's medical history or electrocardiographic investigations reveal findings indicative of, or consistent with, coronary artery vasospasm or myocardial ischemia, sumatriptan should not be administered (see CONTRAINDICATIONS).

For patients with risk factors predictive of CAD, who are determined to have a satisfactory cardiovascular evaluation, it is strongly recommended that administration of the first dose of sumatriptan nasal spray take place in the setting of a physician's office or similar medically staffed and equipped facility unless the patient has previously received sumatriptan. Because cardiac ischemia can occur in the absence of clinical symptoms, consideration should be given to obtaining on the first occasion of use an electrocardiogram (ECG) during the interval immediately following IMITREX Nasal Spray, in these patients with risk factors.

It is recommended that patients who are intermittent long-term users of IMITREX Nasal Spray and who have or acquire risk factors predictive of CAD, as described above, undergo periodic interval cardiovascular evaluation as they continue to use IMITREX Nasal Spray.

The systematic approach described above is intended to reduce the likelihood that patients with unrecognized cardiovascular disease will be inadvertently exposed to sumatriptan.

Drug-Associated Cardiac Events and Fatalities: Serious adverse cardiac events, including acute myocardial infarction, life-threatening disturbances of cardiac rhythm, and death have been reported within a few hours following the administration of IMITREX® (sumatriptan succinate) Injection or IMITREX® (sumatriptan succinate) Tablets. Considering the extent of use of sumatriptan in patients with migraine, the incidence of these events is extremely low. The fact that sumatriptan can cause coronary vasospasm, that some of these events have occurred in patients with no prior cardiac disease history and with documented absence of coronary artery disease, and the close proximity of the events to sumatriptan use support the conclusion that some of these cases were caused by the drug. In many cases, however, where there has been known underlying coronary artery disease, the relationship is uncertain.

Premarketing Experience With Sumatriptan Nasal Spray and Subcutaneous Sumatriptan: Among approximately 4000 patients with migraine who participated in premarketing controlled and uncontrolled clinical trials of sumatriptan nasal spray, one patient experienced an

Table 1: Percentage of Patients With Headache Response (No or Mild Pain) 2 Hours Following Treatment

	Placebo	IMITREX Nasal Spray 5 mg	IMITREX Nasal Spray 10 mg	IMITREX Nasal Spray 20 mg
Study 1	25% (n = 63)	49%* (n = 121)	46%* (n = 112)	64%*†‡ (n = 118)
Study 2	25% (n = 138)	Not applicable	44%* (n = 273)	55%*† (n = 277)
Study 3	35% (n = 100)	Not applicable	54%* (n = 106)	63%* (n = 202)
Study 4	29% (n = 112)	Not applicable	43% (n = 106)	62%*† (n = 215)
Study 5§	36% (n = 198)	45%* (n = 296)	53%* (n = 291)	60%*‡ (n = 286)

* $P<0.05$ in comparison with placebo.
† $P<0.05$ in comparison with 10 mg.
‡ $P<0.05$ in comparison with 5 mg.
§ Data are for attack 1 only of multiattack study for comparison.

asymptomatic subendocardial infarction possibly subsequent to a coronary vasospastic event.

Among the more than 1900 patients with migraine who participated in premarketing controlled clinical trials of subcutaneous sumatriptan, there were eight patients who sustained clinical events during or shortly after receiving sumatriptan that may have reflected coronary artery vasospasm. Six of these eight patients had ECG changes consistent with transient ischemia, but without accompanying clinical symptoms or signs. Of these eight patients, four had either findings suggestive of CAD or risk factors predictive of CAD prior to study enrollment.

Postmarketing Experience With Subcutaneous or Oral Sumatriptan: Serious cardiovascular events, some resulting in death, have been reported in association with the use of IMITREX Injection or IMITREX Tablets. The uncontrolled nature of postmarketing surveillance, however, makes it impossible to determine definitively the proportion of the reported cases that were actually caused by sumatriptan or to reliably assess causation in individual cases. On clinical grounds, the longer the latency between the administration of IMITREX and the onset of the clinical event, the less likely the association is to be causative. Accordingly, interest has focused on events beginning within 1 hour of the administration of IMITREX.

Cardiac events that have been observed to have onset within 1 hour of sumatriptan administration include: coronary artery vasospasm, transient ischemia, myocardial infarction, ventricular tachycardia and ventricular fibrillation, cardiac arrest, and death.

Some of these events occurred in patients who had no findings of CAD and appear to represent consequences of coronary artery vasospasm. However, among domestic reports of serious cardiac events within 1 hour of sumatriptan administration, almost all of the patients had risk factors predictive of CAD and the presence of significant underlying CAD was established in most cases (see CONTRAINDICATIONS).

Drug-Associated Cerebrovascular Events and Fatalities: Cerebral hemorrhage, subarachnoid hemorrhage, stroke, and other cerebrovascular events have been reported in patients treated with oral or subcutaneous sumatriptan, and some have resulted in fatalities. The relationship of sumatriptan to these events is uncertain. In a number of cases, it appears possible that the cerebrovascular events were primary, sumatriptan having been administered in the incorrect belief that the symptoms experienced were a consequence of migraine when they were not. Sumatriptan should not be administered if the headache being experienced is atypical for the patient. It should also be noted that patients with migraine may be at increased risk of certain cerebrovascular events (e.g. cerebrovascular accident, transient ischemic attack).

Other Vasospasm-Related Events: Sumatriptan may cause vasospastic reactions other than coronary artery vasospasm. Both peripheral vascular ischemia and colonic ischemia with abdominal pain and bloody diarrhea have been reported.

Increase in Blood Pressure: Significant elevation in blood pressure, including hypertensive crisis, has been reported on rare occasions in patients with and without a history of hypertension. Sumatriptan is contraindicated in patients with uncontrolled hypertension (see CONTRAINDICATIONS).

Local Irritation: Of the 3378 patients using the nasal spray (5, 10, or 20-mg doses) on one or two occasions in controlled clinical studies, approximately 5% noted irritation in the nose and throat. Irritative symptoms such as burning, numbness, paresthesia, discharge, pain or soreness were noted to be severe in about 1% of patients treated. The symptoms were transient and in approximately 60% of the cases, the symptoms resolved in less than 2 hours. Limited examinations of the nose and throat did not reveal any clinically noticeable injury in these patients. The consequences of extended and repeated use of IMITREX Nasal Spray on the nasal and/or respiratory mucosa have not been systematically evaluated in patients.

No increase in the incidence of local irritation was observed in patients using IMITREX Nasal Spray repeatedly for up to 1 year.

In inhalation studies in rats dosed daily for up to 1 month at exposures as low as one half the maximum daily human exposure (based on dose per surface area of nasal cavity), epithelial hyperplasia (with and without keratinization) and squamous metaplasia were observed in the larynx at all doses tested. These changes were partially reversible after a 2-week drug-free period. When dogs were dosed daily with various formulations by intranasal instillation for up to 13 weeks at exposures of two to four times the maximum daily human exposure (based on dose per surface area of nasal cavity), respiratory and nasal mucosa exhibited evidence of epithelial hyperplasia, focal squamous metaplasia, granulomata, bronchitis, and fibrosing alveolitis. A no-effect dose was not established. The changes observed in both species are not considered to be signs of either preneoplastic or neoplastic transformation.

Local effects on nasal and respiratory tissues after chronic intranasal dosing in animals have not been studied.

Concomitant Drug Use: In patients taking MAO-A inhibitors, sumatriptan plasma levels attained after treatment with recommended doses are twofold (following subcutaneous administration) to sevenfold (following oral administration) higher than those obtained under other conditions. Accordingly, the coadministration of IMITREX Nasal Spray and an MAO-A inhibitor is contraindicated (see CLINICAL PHARMACOLOGY and CONTRAINDICATIONS).

Hypersensitivity: Hypersensitivity (anaphylaxis/anaphylactoid) reactions have occurred on rare occasions in patients receiving sumatriptan. Such reactions can be life threatening or fatal. In general, hypersensitivity reactions to drugs are more likely to occur in individuals with a history of sensitivity to multiple allergens (see CONTRAINDICATIONS).

PRECAUTIONS

General: Chest discomfort, jaw, or neck tightness were infrequent but can occur following administration of IMITREX Nasal Spray. Because sumatriptan may cause coronary artery vasospasm, patients who experience signs or symptoms suggestive of angina following sumatriptan should be evaluated for the presence of CAD or a predisposition to Prinzmetal's variant angina before receiving additional doses of sumatriptan, and should be monitored electrocardiographically if dosing is resumed and similar symptoms recur. Similarly, patients who experience other symptoms or signs suggestive of decreased arterial flow, such as ischemic bowel syndrome or Raynaud's syndrome following sumatriptan should be evaluated for atherosclerosis or predisposition to vasospasm (see WARNINGS).

IMITREX Nasal Spray should also be administered with caution to patients with diseases that may alter the absorption, metabolism, or excretion of drugs, such as impaired hepatic or renal function.

There have been rare reports of seizure following administration of sumatriptan.

Care should be taken to exclude other potentially serious neurologic conditions before treating headache in patients not previously diagnosed with migraine headache or who experience a headache that is atypical for them. There have been rare reports where patients received sumatriptan for severe headaches that were subsequently shown to have been secondary to an evolving neurologic lesion (see WARNINGS).

For a given attack, if a patient does not respond to the first dose of sumatriptan, the diagnosis of migraine headache should be reconsidered before administration of a second dose.

Binding to Melanin-Containing Tissues: In rats treated with a single subcutaneous dose (0.5 mg/kg) or oral dose (2 mg/kg) of radiolabeled sumatriptan, the elimination half-life of radioactivity from the eye was 15 and 23 days, respectively, suggesting that sumatriptan and/or its metabolites bind to the melanin of the eye. Comparable studies were not performed by the intranasal route. Because there could be an accumulation in melanin-rich tissues over time, this raises the possibility that sumatriptan could cause toxicity in these tissues after extended use. However, no effects on the retina related to treatment with sumatriptan were noted in any of the oral or subcutaneous toxicity studies. Although no systematic monitoring of ophthalmologic function was undertaken in clinical trials, and no specific recommendations for ophthalmologic monitoring are offered, prescribers should be aware of the possibility of long-term ophthalmologic effects.

Corneal Opacities: Sumatriptan causes corneal opacities and defects in the corneal epithelium in dogs; this raises the possibility that these changes may occur in humans. While patients were not systematically evaluated for these changes in clinical trials, and no specific recommendations for monitoring are being offered, prescribers should be aware of the possibility of these changes (see ANIMAL TOXICOLOGY).

Information for Patients: See PATIENT INFORMATION at the end of this labeling for the text of the separate leaflet provided for patients.

Laboratory Tests: No specific laboratory tests are recommended for monitoring patients prior to and/or after treatment with IMITREX Nasal Spray.

Drug Interactions: Ergot-containing drugs have been reported to cause prolonged vasospastic reactions. Because there is a theoretical basis that these effects may be additive, use of ergotamine-containing or ergot-type medications (like dihydroergotamine or methysergide) and sumatriptan within 24 hours of each other should be avoided (see CONTRAINDICATIONS).

MAO-A inhibitors reduce sumatriptan clearance, significantly increasing systemic exposure. Therefore, the use of IMITREX Nasal Spray in patients receiving MAO-A inhibitors is contraindicated (see CLINICAL PHARMACOLOGY and CONTRAINDICATIONS).

Selective serotonin reuptake inhibitors (SSRIs) (e.g., fluoxetine, fluvoxamine, paroxetine, sertraline) have been re-

ported, rarely, to cause weakness, hyperreflexia, and incoordination when coadministered with sumatriptan. If concomitant treatment with sumatriptan and an SSRI is clinically warranted, appropriate observation of the patient is advised.

Drug/Laboratory Test Interactions: IMITREX Nasal Spray is not known to interfere with commonly employed clinical laboratory tests.

Carcinogenesis, Mutagenesis, Impairment of Fertility: *Carcinogenesis:* In carcinogenicity studies, rats and mice were given sumatriptan by oral gavage (rats, 104 weeks) or drinking water (mice, 78 weeks). Average exposures achieved in mice receiving the highest dose (target dose of 160 mg/kg per day) were approximately 184 times the exposure attained in humans after the maximum recommended single intranasal dose of 20 mg. The highest dose administered to rats (160 mg/kg per day, reduced from 360 mg/kg per day during week 21) was approximately 78 times the maximum recommended single intranasal dose of 20 mg on a mg/m^2 basis. There was no evidence of an increase in tumors in either species related to sumatriptan administration. Local effects on nasal and respiratory tissue after chronic intranasal dosing in animals have not been evaluated (see WARNINGS).

Mutagenesis: Sumatriptan was not mutagenic in the presence or absence of metabolic activation when tested in two gene mutation assays (the Ames test and the in vitro mammalian Chinese hamster V79/HGPRT assay). In two cytogenetics assays (the in vitro human lymphocyte assay and the in vivo rat micronucleus assay) sumatriptan was not associated with clastogenic activity.

Impairment of Fertility: In a study in which male and female rats were dosed daily with oral sumatriptan prior to and throughout the mating period, there was a treatment-related decrease in fertility secondary to a decrease in mating in animals treated with 50 and 500 mg/kg per day. The highest no-effect dose for this finding was 5 mg/kg per day, or approximately twice the maximum recommended single human intranasal dose of 20 mg on a mg/m^2 basis. It is not clear whether the problem is associated with treatment of the males or females or both combined. In a similar study by the subcutaneous route there was no evidence of impaired fertility at 60 mg/kg per day, the maximum dose tested, which is equivalent to approximately 29 times the maximum recommended single human intranasal dose of 20 mg on a mg/m^2 basis. Fertility studies, in which sumatriptan was administered by the intranasal route were not conducted.

Pregnancy: Pregnancy Category C. In reproductive toxicity studies in rats and rabbits, oral treatment with sumatriptan was associated with embryolethality, fetal abnormalities, and pup mortality. When administered by the intravenous route to rabbits, sumatriptan has been shown to be embryolethal. Reproductive toxicity studies for sumatriptan by the intranasal route have not been conducted. There are no adequate and well-controlled studies in pregnant women. Therefore, IMITREX Nasal Spray should be used during pregnancy only if the potential benefit justifies the potential risk to the fetus. In assessing this information, the following findings should be considered.

Embryolethality: When given orally or intravenously to pregnant rabbits daily throughout the period of organogenesis, sumatriptan caused embryolethality at doses at or close to those producing maternal toxicity. In the oral studies this dose was 100 mg/kg per day and in the intravenous studies this dose was 2.0 mg/kg per day. The mechanism of the embryolethality is not known. The highest no-effect dose for embryolethality by the oral route was 50 mg/kg per day, which is approximately 48 times the maximum single recommended human intranasal dose of 20 mg on a mg/m^2 basis. By the intravenous route, the highest no-effect dose was 0.75 mg/kg per day, or approximately 0.7 times the maximum single recommended human intranasal dose of 20 mg on a mg/m^2 basis.

The intravenous administration of sumatriptan to pregnant rats throughout organogenesis at 12.5 mg/kg per day, the maximum dose tested, did not cause embryolethality. This dose is approximately six times the maximum single recommended human intranasal dose of 20 mg on a mg/m^2 basis. Additionally, in a study in rats given subcutaneous sumatriptan daily, prior to and throughout pregnancy, at 60 mg/kg per day, the maximum dose tested, there was no evidence of increased embryo/fetal lethality. This dose is equivalent to approximately 29 times the maximum recommended single human intranasal dose of 20 mg on a mg/m^2 basis.

Continued on next page

This product information is based on labeling in effect on June 1, 1998. For further information, contact via direct mail, phone, or web site Medical Information: Glaxo Wellcome Inc., PO Box 13398, Research Triangle Park, NC 27709. Healthcare Professionals (Medical Information): 800-334-0089 Patients (Customer Response Center): 888-TALK2GW (1-888-825-5249) Glaxo Wellcome Corporate Web Site: www.glaxowellcome.com

Imitrex Nasal Spray—Cont.

Teratogenicity: Oral treatment of pregnant rats with sumatriptan during the period of organogenesis resulted in an increased incidence of blood vessel abnormalities (cervicothoracic and umbilical) at doses of approximately 250 mg/kg per day or higher. The highest no-effect dose was approximately 60 mg/kg per day, which is approximately 29 times the maximum single recommended human intranasal dose of 20 mg on a mg/m^2 basis. Oral treatment of pregnant rabbits with sumatriptan during the period of organogenesis resulted in an increased incidence of cervicothoracic vascular and skeletal abnormalities. The highest no-effect dose for these effects was 15 mg/kg per day, or approximately 14 times the maximum single recommended human intranasal dose of 20 mg on a mg/m^2 basis.

A study in which rats were dosed daily with oral sumatriptan prior to and throughout gestation demonstrated embryo/fetal toxicity (decreased body weight, decreased ossification, increased incidence of rib variations) and an increased incidence of a syndrome of malformations (short tail/short body and vertebral disorganization) at 500 mg/kg per day. The highest no-effect dose was 50 mg/kg per day, or approximately 24 times the maximum single recommended human intranasal dose of 20 mg on a mg/m^2 basis. In a study in rats dosed daily with subcutaneous sumatriptan prior to and throughout pregnancy, at a dose of 60 mg/kg per day, the maximum dose tested, there was no evidence of teratogenicity. This dose is equivalent to approximately 29 times the maximum recommended single human intranasal dose of 20 mg on a mg/m^2 basis.

Pup Deaths: Oral treatment of pregnant rats with sumatriptan during the period of organogenesis resulted in a decrease in pup survival between birth and postnatal day 4 at doses of approximately 250 mg/kg per day or higher. The highest no-effect dose for this effect was approximately 60 mg/kg per day, or 29 times the maximum single recommended human intranasal dose of 20 mg on a mg/m^2 basis.

Oral treatment of pregnant rats with sumatriptan from gestational day 17 through postnatal day 21 demonstrated a decrease in pup survival measured at postnatal days 2, 4, and 20 at the dose of 1000 mg/kg per day. The highest no-effect dose for this finding was 100 mg/kg per day, approximately 49 times the maximum single recommended human intranasal dose of 20 mg on a mg/m^2 basis. In a similar study in rats by the subcutaneous route there was no increase in pup death at 81 mg/kg per day, the highest dose tested, which is equivalent to 40 times the maximum single recommended human intranasal dose of 20 mg on a mg/m^2 basis.

To monitor fetal outcomes of pregnant women exposed to IMITREX, Glaxo Wellcome Inc. maintains a Sumatriptan Pregnancy Registry. Physicians are encouraged to register patients by calling (800) 722-9292, ext. 39441.

Nursing Mothers: Sumatriptan is excreted in human breast milk. Therefore, caution should be exercised when considering the administration of IMITREX Nasal Spray to a nursing woman.

Pediatric Use: Safety and effectiveness of IMITREX Nasal Spray in pediatric patients have not been established.

Completed placebo-controlled clinical trials evaluating oral sumatriptan (25 to 100 mg) in pediatric patients aged 12 to 17 years have enrolled a total of 701 adolescent migraineurs. These studies did not establish the efficacy of oral sumatriptan compared to placebo in the treatment of migraine in adolescents. Adverse events observed in these clinical trials were similar in nature to those reported in clinical trials in adults. The frequency of all adverse events in these patients appeared to be both dose- and age-dependent, with younger patients reporting events more commonly than older adolescents. Postmarketing experience includes a limited number of reports that describe pediatric patients who have experienced adverse events, some clinically serious, after use of subcutaneous sumatriptan and/or oral sumatriptan. These reports include events similar in nature to those reported rarely in adults. A myocardial infarct has been reported in a 14-year-old male following the use of oral sumatriptan; clinical signs occurred within 1 day of drug administration. Since clinical data to determine the frequency of serious adverse events in pediatric patients who might receive injectable, oral, or intranasal sumatriptan are not presently available, the use of sumatriptan in patients aged younger than 18 years is not recommended.

Use in the Elderly: Although the pharmacokinetic disposition of the drug in the elderly is similar to that seen in younger adults, there is no information about the safety and effectiveness of sumatriptan in this population because patients over age 65 were excluded from the controlled clinical trials.

ADVERSE REACTIONS

Serious cardiac events, including some that have been fatal, have occurred following the use of IMITREX Injection or Tablets. These events are extremely rare and most have been reported in patients with risk factors predictive of CAD. Events reported have included coronary artery vasospasm, transient myocardial ischemia, myocardial infarction, ventricular tachycardia, and ventricular fibrillation (see CONTRAINDICATIONS, WARNINGS, and PRECAUTIONS).

Significant hypertensive episodes, including hypertensive crises, have been reported on rare occasions in patients with or without a history of hypertension (see WARNINGS).

Incidence in Controlled Clinical Trials: Among 3653 patients treated with IMITREX Nasal Spray in active- and placebo-controlled clinical trials, less than 0.4% of patients withdrew for reasons related to adverse events. Table 2 lists adverse events that occurred in worldwide placebo-controlled clinical trials in 3419 migraineurs. The events cited reflect experience gained under closely monitored conditions of clinical trials in a highly selected patient population. In actual clinical practice or in other clinical trials, these frequency estimates may not apply, as the conditions of use, reporting behavior, and the kinds of patients treated may differ.

Only events that occurred at a frequency of 1% or more in the IMITREX Nasal Spray 20-mg treatment group and were more frequent in that group than in the placebo group are included in Table 2.

[See table 2 below]

Phonophobia also occurred in more than 1% of patients but was more frequent on placebo.

IMITREX Nasal Spray is generally well tolerated. Across all doses, most adverse reactions were mild and transient and did not lead to long-lasting effects. The incidence of adverse events in controlled clinical trials was not affected by gender, weight, or age of the patients; use of prophylactic medications; or presence of aura. There was insufficient data to assess the impact of race on the incidence of adverse events.

Other Events Observed in Association With the Administration of IMITREX Nasal Spray: In the paragraphs that follow, the frequencies of less commonly reported adverse clinical events are presented. Because the reports include events observed in open and uncontrolled studies, the role of IMITREX Nasal Spray in their causation cannot be reliably determined. Furthermore, variability associated with adverse event reporting, the terminology used to describe adverse events, etc., limit the value of the quantitative frequency estimates provided. Event frequencies are calculated as the number of patients who used IMITREX Nasal Spray (5, 10, or 20 mg in controlled and uncontrolled trials) and reported an event divided by the total number of patients (n = 3711) exposed to IMITREX Nasal Spray. All reported events are included except those already listed in the previous table, those too general to be informative, and those not reasonably associated with the use of the drug. Events are further classified within body system categories and enumerated in order of decreasing frequency using the following definitions: infrequent adverse events are those occurring in 1/100 to 1/1000 patients and rare adverse events are those occurring in fewer than 1/1000 patients.

Atypical Sensations: Infrequent were tingling, warm/hot sensation, numbness, pressure sensation, feeling strange, feeling of heaviness, feeling of tightness, paresthesia, cold sensation, and tight feeling in head. Rare were dysesthesia and prickling sensation.

Cardiovascular: Infrequent were flushing and hypertension (see WARNINGS), palpitations, tachycardia, changes in ECG, and arrhythmia (see WARNINGS and PRECAUTIONS). Rare were abdominal aortic aneurysm, hypotension, bradycardia, pallor, and phlebitis.

Chest Symptoms: Infrequent were chest tightness, chest discomfort, and chest pressure/heaviness (see PRECAUTIONS: General).

Ear, Nose, and Throat: Infrequent were disturbance of hearing and ear infection. Rare were otalgia and Meniere's disease.

Endocrine and Metabolic: Infrequent was thirst. Rare were galactorrhea, hypothyroidism, and weight loss.

Eye: Infrequent were irritation of eyes and visual disturbance.

Gastrointestinal: Infrequent were abdominal discomfort, diarrhea, dysphagia, and gastroesophageal reflux. Rare were constipation, flatulence/eructation, hematemesis, intestinal obstruction, melena, gastroenteritis, colitis, hemorrhage of gastrointestinal tract, and pancreatitis.

Mouth and Teeth: Infrequent was disorder of mouth and tongue (e.g., burning of tongue, numbness of tongue, dry mouth).

Musculoskeletal: Infrequent were neck pain/stiffness, backache, weakness, joint symptoms, arthritis, and myalgia. Rare were muscle cramps, tetany, intervertebral disc disorder, and muscle stiffness.

Neurological: Infrequent were drowsiness/sedation, anxiety, sleep disturbances, tremors, syncope, shivers, chills, depression, agitation, sensation of lightness, and mental confusion. Rare were difficulty concentrating, hunger, lacrimation, memory disturbances, monoplegia/diplegia, apathy, disturbance of smell, disturbance of emotions, dysarthria, facial pain, intoxication, stress, decreased appetite, difficulty coordinating, euphoria, and neoplasm of pituitary.

Respiratory: Infrequent were dyspnea and lower respiratory tract infection. Rare was asthma.

Skin: Infrequent were rash/skin eruption, pruritus, and erythema. Rare were herpes, swelling of face, sweating, and peeling of skin.

Urogenital: Infrequent were dysuria, disorder of breasts, and dysmenorrhea. Rare were endometriosis and increased urination.

Miscellaneous: Infrequent were cough, edema, and fever. Rare were hypersensitivity, swelling of extremities, voice disturbances, difficulty in walking, and lymphadenopathy.

Postmarketing Experience (Reports for Subcutaneous or Oral Sumatriptan): The following section enumerates potentially important adverse events that have occurred in clinical practice and which have been reported spontaneously to various surveillance systems. The events enumerated represent reports arising from both domestic and nondomestic use of oral or subcutaneous dosage forms of sumatriptan. The events enumerated include all except those already listed in the ADVERSE REACTIONS section above or those too general to be informative. Because the reports cite events reported spontaneously from worldwide postmarketing experience, frequency of events and the role of sumatriptan in their causation cannot be reliably determined. It is assumed, however, that systemic reactions following sumatriptan use are likely to be similar regardless of route of administration.

Blood: Pancytopenia, thrombocytopenia.

Cardiovascular: Cardiomyopathy, colonic ischemia (see WARNINGS), pulmonary embolism, shock.

Dermatological: Exacerbation of sunburn, photosensitivity.

Ear, Nose, and Throat: Deafness.

Eye: Ischemic optic neuropathy, periorbital edema, retinal artery occlusion.

Gastrointestinal: Ischemic colitis with rectal bleeding (see WARNINGS), xerostomia.

Hepatic: Elevated liver function tests.

Hypersensitivity Reactions: Erythema, pruritus, shortness of breath, urticaria. In addition, severe anaphylaxis/anaphylactoid reactions have been reported (see WARNINGS).

Non-Site Specific: Angioneurotic edema, cyanosis, temporal arteritis.

Neurological: Cerebrovascular accident, dysphasia, seizure, subarachnoid hemorrhage.

Respiratory: Bronchospasm in patients with and without a history of asthma.

Psychiatry: Panic disorder.

Urogenital: Acute renal failure.

Table 2: Treatment-Emergent Adverse Events Reported by at Least 1% of Patients in Controlled Migraine Trials

	Percent of Patients Reporting			
Adverse Event Type	Placebo (n = 704)	IMITREX 5 mg (n = 496)	IMITREX 10 mg (n = 1007)	IMITREX 20 mg (n = 1212)
Atypical sensations				
Burning sensation	0.1%	0.4%	0.6%	1.4%
Ear, nose, and throat				
Disorder/discomfort of nasal cavity/sinuse	2.4%	2.8%	2.5%	3.8%
Throat discomfort	0.9%	0.8%	1.8%	2.4%
Gastrointestinal				
Nausea and/or vomiting	11.3%	12.2%	11.0%	13.5%
Neurological				
Bad/unusual taste	1.7%	13.5%	19.3%	24.5%
Dizziness/vertigo	0.9%	1.0%	1.7%	1.4%

DRUG ABUSE AND DEPENDENCE

One clinical study with IMITREX (sumatriptan succinate) Injection enrolling 12 patients with a history of substance abuse failed to induce subjective behavior and/or physiologic response ordinarily associated with drugs that have an established potential for abuse.

OVERDOSAGE

In clinical trials, the highest single doses of IMITREX Nasal Spray administered without significant adverse effects were 40 mg to 12 volunteers and 40 mg to 85 migraine patients, which is twice the highest single recommended dose. In addition, 12 volunteers were administered a total daily dose of 60 mg (20 mg three times daily) for 3.5 days without significant adverse events.

Overdose in animals has been fatal and has been heralded by convulsions, tremor, paralysis, inactivity, ptosis, erythema of the extremities, abnormal respiration, cyanosis, ataxia, mydriasis, salivation, and lacrimation. The elimination half-life of sumatriptan is about 2 hours (see CLINICAL PHARMACOLOGY), and therefore monitoring of patients after overdose with IMITREX Nasal Spray should continue for at least 10 hours or while symptoms or signs persist. It is unknown what effect hemodialysis or peritoneal dialysis has on the serum concentrations of sumatriptan.

DOSAGE AND ADMINISTRATION

In controlled clinical trials, single doses of 5, 10, or 20 mg of IMITREX Nasal Spray administered into one nostril were effective for the acute treatment of migraine in adults. A greater proportion of patients had headache response following a 20-mg dose than following a 5- or 10-mg dose (see CLINICAL TRIALS). Individuals may vary in response to doses of IMITREX Nasal Spray. The choice of dose should therefore be made on an individual basis, weighing the possible benefit of the 20-mg dose with the potential for a greater risk of adverse events. A 10-mg dose may be achieved by the administration of a single 5-mg dose in each nostril. There is evidence that doses above 20 mg do not provide a greater effect than 20 mg.

If the headache returns, the dose may be repeated once after 2 hours, not to exceed a total daily dose of 40 mg. The safety of treating an average of more than four headaches in a 30-day period has not been established.

HOW SUPPLIED

IMITREX Nasal Spray 5 mg (NDC 0173-0524-00) and 20 mg (NDC 0173-0523-00) are each supplied in boxes of 6 nasal spray devices. Each unit dose spray supplies 5 and 20 mg, respectively, of sumatriptan.

Store between 36° and 86°F (2° and 30°C). Protect from light.

Caution: Federal law prohibits dispensing without prescription.

ANIMAL TOXICOLOGY

Corneal Opacities: Dogs receiving oral sumatriptan developed corneal opacities and defects in the corneal epithelium. Corneal opacities were seen at the lowest dosage tested, 2 mg/kg per day, and were present after 1 month of treatment. Defects in the corneal epithelium were noted in a 60-week study. Earlier examinations for these toxicities were not conducted and no-effect doses were not established; however, the relative exposure at the lowest dose tested was approximately five times the human exposure after a 100-mg oral dose or three times the human exposure after a 6-mg subcutaneous dose or 22 times the human exposure after a single 20-mg intranasal dose. There is evidence of alterations in corneal appearance on the first day of intranasal dosing to dogs. Changes were noted at the lowest dose tested, which was approximately two times the maximum single human intranasal dose of 20 mg on a mg/m^2 basis.

PATIENT INFORMATION

The following wording is contained in a separate leaflet provided for patients.

Information for the Patient

IMITREX® (sumatriptan) Nasal Spray

Please read this leaflet carefully before you administer IMITREX Nasal Spray. This provides a summary of the information available on your medicine. Please do not throw away this leaflet until you have finished your medicine. You may need to read this leaflet again. This leaflet does not contain all the information on IMITREX Nasal Spray. For further information or advice, ask your doctor or pharmacist.

Information About Your Medicine:

The name of your medicine is IMITREX (sumatriptan) Nasal Spray. It can be obtained only by prescription from your doctor. The decision to use IMITREX Nasal Spray is one that you and your doctor should make jointly, taking into account your individual preferences and medical circumstances. If you have risk factors for heart disease (such as high blood pressure, high cholesterol, obesity, diabetes, smoking, strong family history of heart disease, or you are postmenopausal or a male over 40), you should tell your doctor, who should evaluate you for heart disease in order to determine if IMITREX is appropriate for you. Although the vast majority of those who have taken IMITREX have not experienced any significant side effects, some individuals have experienced serious heart problems and, rarely, considering the extensiveness of IMITREX use worldwide, deaths have been reported. In all but a few instances, however, serious problems occurred in people with known heart disease and it was not clear whether IMITREX was a contributory factor in these deaths.

1. The Purpose of Your Medicine:

IMITREX Nasal Spray is intended to relieve your migraine, but not to prevent or reduce the number of attacks you experience. Use IMITREX Nasal Spray only to treat an actual migraine attack.

2. Important Questions to Consider Before Using IMITREX Nasal Spray:

If the answer to any of the following questions is **YES** or if you do not know the answer, then please discuss it with your doctor before you use IMITREX Nasal Spray.

- Are you pregnant? Do you think you might be pregnant? Are you trying to become pregnant? Are you using inadequate contraception? Are you breast-feeding?
- Do you have any chest pain, heart disease, shortness of breath, or irregular heartbeats? Have you had a heart attack?
- Do you have risk factors for heart disease (such as high blood pressure, high cholesterol, obesity, diabetes, smoking, strong family history of heart disease, or you are postmenopausal or a male over 40)?
- Do you have high blood pressure?
- Have you ever had to stop taking this or any other medication because of an allergy or other problems?
- Are you taking any other migraine medications, including migraine medications containing ergotamine, dihydroergotamine, or methysergide?
- Are you taking any medication for depression (monoamine oxidase inhibitors or selective serotonin reuptake inhibitors [SSRIs])?
- Have you had, or do you have, any disease of the liver or kidney?
- Have you had, or do you have, epilepsy or seizures?
- Is this headache different from your usual migraine attacks?

Remember, if you answered **YES** to any of the above questions, then discuss it with your doctor.

3. The Use of IMITREX Nasal Spray During Pregnancy:

Do not use IMITREX Nasal Spray if you are pregnant, think you might be pregnant, are trying to become pregnant, or are not using adequate contraception, unless you have discussed this with your doctor.

4. How to Use IMITREX Nasal Spray:

Before using IMITREX Nasal Spray, see the enclosed instruction pamphlet. For adults, the usual dose is a single nasal spray administered into one nostril. If your headache comes back, a second nasal spray may be administered anytime after 2 hours of administering the first spray. For any attack where you have no response to the first nasal spray, do not take a second nasal spray without first consulting with your doctor. Do not administer more than a total of 40 mg of IMITREX Nasal Spray in any 24-hour period. The effects of long-term repeated use of IMITREX Nasal Spray on the surfaces of the nose and throat have not been specifically studied. The safety of treating an average of more than four headaches in a 30-day period has not been established.

5. Side Effects to Watch for:

- Some patients experience pain or tightness in the chest or throat when using IMITREX Nasal Spray. If this happens to you, then discuss it with your doctor before using any more IMITREX Nasal Spray. If the chest pain is severe or does not go away, call your doctor immediately.
- Shortness of breath; wheeziness; heart throbbing; swelling of eyelids, face, or lips; or a skin rash, skin lumps, or hives happens rarely. If it happens to you, then tell your doctor immediately. Do not take any more IMITREX Nasal Spray unless your doctor tells you to do so.
- Some people may have feelings of tingling, heat, flushing (redness of face lasting a short time), heaviness or pressure after treatment with IMITREX Nasal Spray. A few people may feel drowsy, dizzy, tired, sick, or may experience nasal irritation. Tell your doctor of these symptoms at your next visit.
- If you feel unwell in any other way or have any symptoms that you do not understand, you should contact your doctor immediately.

6. What to Do if an Overdose Is Taken:

If you have taken more medication than you have been told, contact either your doctor, hospital emergency department, or nearest poison control center immediately.

7. Storing Your Medicine:

Keep your medicine in a safe place where children cannot reach it. It may be harmful to children. Store your medication away from heat and light. Do not store at temperatures above 86°F (30°C), or below 36°F (2°C). If your medication has expired (the expiration date is printed on the treatment pack), throw it away as instructed. If your doctor decides to stop your treatment, do not keep any leftover medicine unless your doctor tells you to. Throw away your medicine as instructed.

U.S. Patent Nos. 4,816,470; 5,037,845; and 5,554,639

©Copyright 1997 Glaxo Wellcome Inc. All rights reserved.

October 1997/RL-470

Shown in Product Identification Guide, page 313

IMITREX® ℞
[*ĭm ′-ĭ-trĕx* ″]
(sumatriptan succinate)
Tablets

DESCRIPTION

IMITREX Tablets contain sumatriptan (as the succinate), a selective 5-hydroxytryptamine$_1$ receptor subtype agonist. Sumatriptan succinate is chemically designated as 3-[2-(dimethylamino)ethyl]-N-methyl-indole-5-methanesulfonamide succinate (1:1).

The empirical formula is $C_{14}H_{21}N_3O_2S{\bullet}C_4H_6O_4$, representing a molecular weight of 413.5. Sumatriptan succinate is a white to off-white powder that is readily soluble in water and in saline. Each IMITREX Tablet for oral administration contains 35 or 70 mg of sumatriptan succinate equivalent to 25 or 50 mg of sumatriptan, respectively. Each tablet also contains the inactive ingredients croscarmellose sodium, lactose, magnesium stearate, microcrystalline cellulose, and titanium dioxide dye.

CLINICAL PHARMACOLOGY

Mechanism of Action: Sumatriptan is an agonist for a vascular 5-hydroxytryptamine$_1$ receptor subtype (probably a member of the 5-HT$_{1D}$ family) having only a weak affinity for 5-HT$_{1A}$, 5-HT$_{5A}$, and 5-HT$_7$ receptors and no significant affinity (as measured using standard radioligand binding assays) or pharmacological activity at 5-HT$_2$, 5-HT$_3$, or 5-HT$_4$ receptor subtypes or at alpha$_1$-, alpha$_2$-, or beta-adrenergic, dopamine$_1$, dopamine$_2$, muscarinic, or benzodiazepine receptors.

The vascular 5-HT$_1$ receptor subtype that sumatriptan activates is present on cranial arteries in both dog and primate, on the human basilar artery, and in the vasculature of human dura mater and mediates vasoconstriction. This action in humans correlates with the relief of migraine headache. In addition to causing vasoconstriction, experimental data from animal studies show that sumatriptan also activates 5-HT$_1$ receptors on peripheral terminals of the trigeminal nerve innervating cranial blood vessels. Such an action may also contribute to the antimigrainous effect of sumatriptan in humans.

In the anesthetized dog, sumatriptan selectively reduces the carotid arterial blood flow with little or no effect on arterial blood pressure or total peripheral resistance. In the cat, sumatriptan selectively constricts the carotid arteriovenous anastomoses while having little effect on blood flow or resistance in cerebral or extracerebral tissues.

Pharmacokinetics: The mean maximum concentration following oral dosing with 25 mg is 18 ng/mL (range, 7 to 47 ng/mL) and 51 ng/mL (range, 28 to 100 ng/mL) following oral dosing with 100 mg of sumatriptan. This compares with a C_{max} of 5 and 16 ng/mL following dosing with a 5- and 20-mg intranasal dose, respectively. The mean C_{max} following a 6-mg subcutaneous injection is 71 ng/mL (range, 49 to 110 ng/mL). The bioavailability is approximately 15%, primarily due to presystemic metabolism and partly due to incomplete absorption. The C_{max} is similar during a migraine attack and during a migraine-free period, but the t_{max} is slightly later during the attack, approximately 2.5 hours compared to 2.0 hours. When given as a single dose, sumatriptan displays dose proportionality in its extent of absorption (area under the curve [AUC]) over the dose range of 25 to 200 mg, but the C_{max} after 100 mg is approximately 25% less than expected (based on the 25-mg dose).

Food has no significant effect on the bioavailability of sumatriptan, but delays the t_{max} slightly (by about 0.5 hours).

Plasma protein binding is low (14% to 21%). The effect of sumatriptan on the protein binding of other drugs has not been evaluated, but would be expected to be minor, given the low rate of protein binding. The apparent volume of distribution is 2.4 L/kg.

The elimination half-life of sumatriptan is approximately 2.5 hours. Radiolabeled ^{14}C-sumatriptan administered orally is largely renally excreted (about 60%) with about

Continued on next page

This product information is based on labeling in effect on June 1, 1998. For further information, contact via direct mail, phone, or web site Medical Information: Glaxo Wellcome Inc., PO Box 13398, Research Triangle Park, NC 27709. Healthcare Professionals (Medical Information): 800-334-0089 Patients (Customer Response Center): 888-TALK2GW (1-888-825-5249) Glaxo Wellcome Corporate Web Site: www.glaxowellcome.com

Imitrex Tablets—Cont.

40% found in the feces. Most of the radiolabeled compound excreted in the urine is the major metabolite, indole acetic acid (IAA), which is inactive, or the IAA glucuronide. Only 3% of the dose can be recovered as unchanged sumatriptan. In vitro studies with human microsomes suggest that sumatriptan is metabolized by monoamine oxidase (MAO), predominantly the A isoenzyme, and inhibitors of that enzyme may alter sumatriptan pharmacokinetics to increase systemic exposure. No significant effect was seen with an MAO-B inhibitor (see CONTRAINDICATIONS, WARNINGS, and PRECAUTIONS: Drug Interactions).

Special Populations: ***Renal Impairment:*** The effect of renal impairment on the pharmacokinetics of sumatriptan has not been examined, but little clinical effect would be expected as sumatriptan is largely metabolized to an inactive substance.

Hepatic Impairment: The liver plays an important role in the presystemic clearance of orally administered sumatriptan. Accordingly, the bioavailability of sumatriptan following oral administration may be markedly increased in patients with liver disease. In one small study of hepatically impaired patients (n = 8) matched for sex, age, and weight with healthy subjects, the hepatically impaired patients had an approximately 70% increase in AUC and C_{max} and a t_{max} 40 minutes earlier compared to the healthy subjects (see DOSAGE AND ADMINISTRATION).

Age: The pharmacokinetics of oral sumatriptan in the elderly (mean age, 72 years; two males and four females) and in patients with migraine (mean age, 38 years; 25 males and 155 females) were similar to that in healthy male subjects (mean age, 30 years).

Gender: In a study comparing females to males, no pharmacokinetic differences were observed between genders for AUC, C_{max}, t_{max}, and half-life.

Race: The systemic clearance and C_{max} of sumatriptan were similar in black (n = 34) and Caucasian (n = 38) healthy male subjects.

Drug Interactions: *Monoamine Oxidase Inhibitors (MAOI):* Treatment with MAO-A inhibitors generally leads to an increase of sumatriptan plasma levels (see CONTRAINDICATIONS and PRECAUTIONS).

Due to gut and hepatic metabolic first-pass effects, the increase of systemic exposure after coadministration of an MAO-A inhibitor with oral sumatriptan is greater than after coadministration of the MAOI with subcutaneous sumatriptan. In a study of 14 healthy females, pretreatment with an MAO-A inhibitor decreased the clearance of subcutaneous sumatriptan. Under the conditions of this experiment, the result was a twofold increase in the area under the sumatriptan plasma concentration x time curve (AUC), corresponding to a 40% increase in elimination half-life. This interaction was not evident with an MAO-B inhibitor.

A small study evaluating the effect of pretreatment with an MAO-A inhibitor on the bioavailability from a 25-mg oral sumatriptan tablet resulted in an approximately sevenfold increase in systemic exposure.

Alcohol: Alcohol consumed 30 minutes prior to sumatriptan ingestion had no effect on the pharmacokinetics of sumatriptan.

CLINICAL STUDIES

The efficacy of IMITREX Tablets in the acute treatment of migraine headaches was demonstrated in three, randomized, double-blind, placebo-controlled studies. Patients enrolled in these three studies were predominately female (87%) and Caucasian (97%), with a mean age of 40 (range of 18 to 65). Patients were instructed to treat a moderate to severe headache. Headache response, defined as a reduction in headache severity from moderate or severe pain to mild or no pain, was assessed up to 4 hours after dosing. Associated symptoms such as nausea, photophobia, and phonophobia were also assessed. Maintenance of response was assessed for up to 24 hours postdose. A second dose of IMITREX Tablets or other medication was allowed 4 to 24 hours after the initial treatment for recurrent headache. Acetaminophen was offered to patients in Studies 2 and 3 beginning at 2 hours after initial treatment if the migraine pain had not improved or worsened. Additional medications were allowed 4 to 24 hours after the initial treatment for recurrent headache or as rescue in all three studies. The frequency and time to use of these additional treatments were also determined. In all studies, doses of 25, 50, and 100 mg were compared to placebo in the treatment of migraine attacks. In one study, doses of 25, 50, and 100 mg were also compared to each other.

In all three trials, the percentage of patients achieving headache response 2 and 4 hours after treatment was significantly greater among patients receiving IMITREX Tablets at all doses compared to those who received placebo. In one of the three studies, there was a statistically significant greater percentage of patients with headache response at 2 and 4 hours in the 50- or 100-mg group when compared to the 25-mg dose groups. There were no statistically significant differences between the 50- and 100-mg dose groups in any study. The results from the three controlled clinical trials are summarized in Table 1.

Comparisons of drug performance based upon results obtained in different clinical trials are never reliable. Because studies are conducted at different times, with different samples of patients, by different investigators, employing different criteria and/or different interpretations of the same criteria, under different conditions (dose, dosing regimen, etc.), quantitative estimates of treatment response and the timing of response may be expected to vary considerably from study to study.

[See table 1 below]

The estimated probability of achieving an initial headache response over the 4 hours following treatment is depicted in Figure 1.

Figure 1: Estimated Probability of Achieving Initial Headache Response Within 240 Minutes*

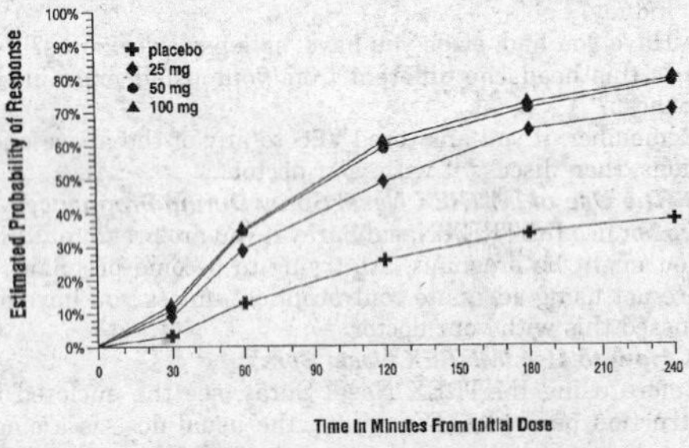

* The figure shows the probability over time of obtaining headache response (no or mild pain) following treatment with sumatriptan. The averages displayed are based on pooled data from the three clinical controlled trials providing evidence of efficacy. Kaplan-Meier plot with patients not achieving response and/or taking rescue within 240 minutes censored to 240 minutes.

For patients with migraine-associated nausea, photophobia, and/or phonophobia at baseline, there was a lower incidence of these symptoms at 2 hours (Study 1) and at 4 hours (Studies 1, 2, and 3) following administration of IMITREX Tablets compared to placebo.

As early as 2 hours in Studies 2 and 3 or 4 hours in Study 1, through 24 hours following the initial dose of study treatment, patients were allowed to use additional treatment for pain relief in the form of a second dose of study treatment or other medication. The estimated probability of patients taking a second dose or other medication for migraine over the 24 hours following the initial dose of study treatment is summarized in Figure 2.

[See figure at top of next column]

There is evidence that doses above 50 mg do not provide a greater effect than 50 mg. There was no evidence to suggest that treatment with sumatriptan was associated with an increase in the severity of recurrent headaches. The efficacy of

Figure 2: The Estimated Probability of Patients Taking a Second Dose or Other Medication for Migraine Over the 24 Hours Following the Initial Dose of Study Treatment*

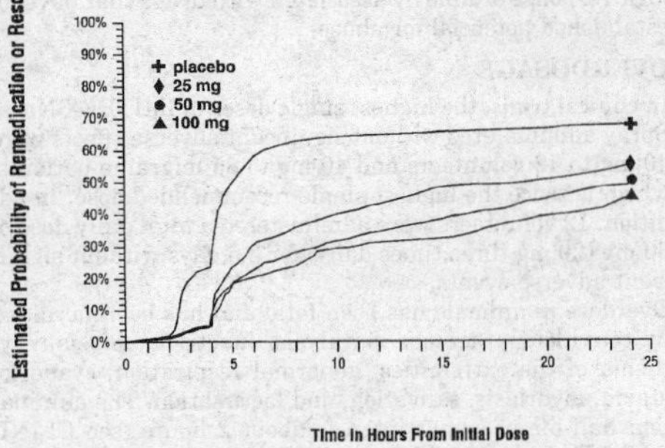

* Kaplan-Meier plot based on data obtained in the three clinical controlled trials providing evidence of efficacy with patients not using additional treatments censored to 24 hours. Plot also includes patients who had no response to the initial dose. No remedication was allowed within 2 hours postdose.

IMITREX Tablets was unaffected by presence of aura; duration of headache prior to treatment; gender, age, or weight of the patient; relationship to menses; or concomitant use of common migraine prophylactic drugs (e.g., beta-blockers, calcium channel blockers, tricyclic antidepressants). There were insufficient data to assess the impact of race on efficacy.

INDICATIONS AND USAGE

IMITREX Tablets are indicated for the acute treatment of migraine attacks with or without aura in adults.

IMITREX Tablets are not intended for the prophylactic therapy of migraine or for use in the management of hemiplegic or basilar migraine (see CONTRAINDICATIONS). Safety and effectiveness of IMITREX Tablets have not been established for cluster headache, which is present in an older, predominantly male population.

CONTRAINDICATIONS

IMITREX Tablets should not be given to patients with history, symptoms, or signs of ischemic cardiac, cerebrovascular, or peripheral vascular syndromes. In addition, patients with other significant underlying cardiovascular diseases should not receive IMITREX Tablets. Ischemic cardiac syndromes include, but are not limited to, angina pectoris of any type (e.g., stable angina of effort and vasospastic forms of angina such as the Prinzmetal's variant), all forms of myocardial infarction, and silent myocardial ischemia. Cerebrovascular sydromes include, but are not limited to, strokes of any type as well as transient ischemic attacks. Peripheral vascular disease includes, but is not limited to, ischemic bowel disease (see WARNINGS).

Because IMITREX Tablets may increase blood pressure, they should not be given to patients with uncontrolled hypertension.

Concurrent administration of MAO-A inhibitors or use within 2 weeks of discontinuation of MAO-A inhibitor therapy is contraindicated (see CLINICAL PHARMACOLOGY: Drug Interactions and PRECAUTIONS: Drug Interactions).

IMITREX Tablets should not be administered to patients with hemiplegic or basilar migraine.

IMITREX Tablets should not be used within 24 hours of treatment with an ergotamine-containing or ergot-type medication like dihydroergotamine or methysergide, or another 5-HT_1 agonist. IMITREX Tablets are contraindicated in patients with hypersensitivity to sumatriptan or any of the ingredients.

WARNINGS

IMITREX Tablets should only be used where a clear diagnosis of migraine headache has been established.

Risk of Myocardial Ischemia and/or Infarction and Other Adverse Cardiac Events: Sumatriptan should not be given to patients with documented ischemic or vasospastic coronary artery disease (CAD) (see CONTRAINDICATIONS). It is strongly recommended that sumatriptan not be given to patients in whom unrecognized CAD is predicted by the presence of risk factors (e.g., hypertension, hypercholesterolemia, smoker, obesity, diabetes, strong family history of CAD, female with surgical or physiological menopause, or male over 40 years of age) unless a cardiovascular evaluation provides satisfactory clinical evidence that the patient is reasonably free of coronary artery and ischemic myocardial disease or other significant underlying cardiovascular disease. The sensitivity of cardiac diagnostic procedures to detect cardiovascular disease or predisposition to coronary artery vasospasm is modest, at best. If, during the cardiovascular evaluation, the patient's medical history or electrocardiographic investigations reveal findings indicative of, or consistent with, coronary artery vasospasm or myocardial ischemia, sumatriptan should not be administered (see CONTRAINDICATIONS).

Table 1: Percentage of Patients With Headache Response (No or Mild Pain) 2 and 4 Hours Following Treatment

	Placebo		IMITREX Tablets 25 mg		IMITREX Tablets 50 mg		IMITREX Tablets 100 mg	
	2 hr	4 hr	2 hr	4 hr	2 hr	4 hr	2 hr	4 hr
Study 1	27%	38%	52%*	67%*	61%*†	78%*†	62%*†	79%*†
	(n = 94)		(n = 298)		(n = 296)		(n = 296)	
Study 2	26%	38%	52%*	70%*	50%*	68%*	56%*	71%*
	(n = 65)		(n = 66)		(n = 62)		(n = 66)	
Study 3	17%	19%	52%*	65%*	54%*	72%*	57%*	78%*
	(n = 47)		(n = 48)		(n = 46)		(n = 46)	

* $P<0.05$ in comparison with placebo.
† $P<0.05$ in comparison with 25 mg.

For patients with risk factors predictive of CAD, who are determined to have a satisfactory cardiovascular evaluation, it is strongly recommended that administration of the first dose of sumatriptan take place in the setting of a physician's office or similar medically staffed and equipped facility unless the patient has previously received sumatriptan. Because cardiac ischemia can occur in the absence of clinical symptoms, consideration should be given to obtaining on the first occasion of use an electrocardiogram (ECG) during the interval immediately following IMITREX Tablets, in these patients with risk factors.

It is recommended that patients who are intermittent long-term users of sumatriptan and who have or acquire risk factors predictive of CAD, as described above, undergo periodic interval cardiovascular evaluation as they continue to use sumatriptan.

The systematic approach described above is intended to reduce the likelihood that patients with unrecognized cardiovascular disease will be inadvertently exposed to sumatriptan.

Drug-Associated Cardiac Events and Fatalities: Serious adverse cardiac events, including acute myocardial infarction, life-threatening disturbances of cardiac rhythm, and death have been reported within a few hours following the administration of IMITREX® (sumatriptan succinate) Injection or IMITREX Tablets. Considering the extent of use of sumatriptan in patients with migraine, the incidence of these events is extremely low. The fact that sumatriptan can cause coronary vasospasm, that some of these events have occurred in patients with no prior cardiac disease history and with documented absence of CAD, and the close proximity of the events to sumatriptan use support the conclusion that some of these cases were caused by the drug. In many cases, however, where there has been known underlying coronary artery disease, the relationship is uncertain.

Premarketing Experience With Oral and Subcutaneous Sumatriptan: Of 6348 patients with migraine who participated in premarketing controlled and uncontrolled clinical trials of oral sumatriptan, two experienced clinical adverse events shortly after receiving oral sumatriptan that may have reflected coronary vasospasm. Neither of these adverse events was associated with a serious clinical outcome.

Among the more than 1900 patients with migraine who participated in premarketing controlled clinical trials of subcutaneous sumatriptan, there were eight patients who sustained clinical events during or shortly after receiving sumatriptan that may have reflected coronary artery vasospasm. Six of these eight patients had ECG changes consistent with transient ischemia, but without accompanying clinical symptoms or signs. Of these eight patients, four had either findings suggestive of CAD or risk factors predictive of CAD prior to study enrollment.

Postmarketing Experience With Subcutaneous or Oral Sumatriptan: Serious cardiovascular events, some resulting in death, have been reported in association with the use of IMITREX Injection or IMITREX Tablets. The uncontrolled nature of postmarketing surveillance, however, makes it impossible to determine definitively the proportion of the reported cases that were actually caused by sumatriptan or to reliably assess causation in individual cases. On clinical grounds, the longer the latency between the administration of IMITREX and the onset of the clinical event, the less likely the association is to be causative. Accordingly, interest has focused on events beginning within 1 hour of the administration of IMITREX.

Cardiac events that have been observed to have onset within 1 hour of sumatriptan administration include: coronary artery vasospasm, transient ischemia, myocardial infarction, ventricular tachycardia and ventricular fibrillation, cardiac arrest, and death.

Some of these events occurred in patients who had no findings of CAD and appear to represent consequences of coronary artery vasospasm. However, among domestic reports of serious cardiac events within 1 hour of sumatriptan administration, almost all of the patients had risk factors predictive of CAD and the presence of significant underlying CAD was established in most cases (see CONTRAINDICATIONS).

Drug-Associated Cerebrovascular Events and Fatalities: Cerebral hemorrhage, subarachnoid hemorrhage, stroke, and other cerebrovascular events have been reported in patients treated with oral or subcutaneous sumatriptan, and some have resulted in fatalities. The relationship of sumatriptan to these events is uncertain. In a number of cases, it appears possible that the cerebrovascular events were primary, sumatriptan having been administered in the incorrect belief that the symptoms experienced were a consequence of migraine when they were not. Sumatriptan should not be administered if the headache being experienced is atypical for the patient. It should also be noted that patients with migraine may be at increased risk of certain cerebrovascular events (e.g. cerebrovascular accident, transient ischemic attack).

Other Vasospasm-Related Events: Sumatriptan may cause vasospastic reactions other than coronary artery vasospasm. Both peripheral vascular ischemia and colonic ischemia with abdominal pain and bloody diarrhea have been reported.

Increase in Blood Pressure: Significant elevation in blood pressure, including hypertensive crisis, has been reported on rare occasions in patients with and without a history of hypertension. Sumatriptan is contraindicated in patients with uncontrolled hypertension (see CONTRAINDICATIONS).

Concomitant Drug Use: In patients taking MAO-A inhibitors, sumatriptan plasma levels attained after treatment with recommended doses are sevenfold higher following oral administration than those obtained under other conditions. Accordingly, the coadministration of IMITREX Tablets and an MAO-A inhibitor is contraindicated (see CLINICAL PHARMACOLOGY and CONTRAINDICATIONS).

Hypersensitivity: Hypersensitivity (anaphylaxis/ anaphylactoid) reactions have occurred on rare occasions in patients receiving sumatriptan. Such reactions can be life threatening or fatal. In general, hypersensitivity reactions to drugs are more likely to occur in individuals with a history of sensitivity to multiple allergens (see CONTRAINDICATIONS).

PRECAUTIONS

General: Chest discomfort, jaw, or neck tightness have been reported following use of IMITREX Tablets and were rarely associated with ischemic ECG changes. Because sumatriptan may cause coronary artery vasospasm, patients who experience signs or symptoms suggestive of angina following sumatriptan should be evaluated for the presence of CAD or a predisposition to Prinzmetal's variant angina before receiving additional doses of sumatriptan, and should be monitored electrocardiographically if dosing is resumed and similar symptoms recur. Similarly, patients who experience other symptoms or signs suggestive of decreased arterial flow, such as ischemic bowel syndrome or Raynaud's syndrome following sumatriptan should be evaluated for atherosclerosis or predisposition to vasospasm (see WARNINGS).

Sumatriptan should also be administered with caution to patients with diseases that may alter the absorption, metabolism, or excretion of drugs, such as impaired hepatic or renal function.

There have been rare reports of seizure following administration of sumatriptan.

Care should be taken to exclude other potentially serious neurologic conditions before treating headache in patients not previously diagnosed with migraine headache or who experience a headache that is atypical for them. There have been rare reports where patients received sumatriptan for severe headaches that were subsequently shown to have been secondary to an evolving neurologic lesion (see WARNINGS).

For a given attack, if a patient does not respond to the first dose of sumatriptan, the diagnosis of migraine should be reconsidered before administration of a second dose.

Binding to Melanin-Containing Tissues: In rats treated with a single subcutaneous dose (0.5 mg/kg) or oral dose (2 mg/kg) of radiolabeled sumatriptan, the elimination half-life of radioactivity from the eye was 15 and 23 days, respectively, suggesting that sumatriptan and/or its metabolites bind to the melanin of the eye. Because there could be an accumulation in melanin-rich tissues over time, this raises the possibility that sumatriptan could cause toxicity in these tissues after extended use. However, no effects on the retina related to treatment with sumatriptan were noted in any of the oral or subcutaneous toxicity studies. Although no systematic monitoring of ophthalmologic function was undertaken in clinical trials, and no specific recommendations for ophthalmologic monitoring are offered, prescribers should be aware of the possibility of long-term ophthalmologic effects.

Corneal Opacities: Sumatriptan causes corneal opacities and defects in the corneal epithelium in dogs; this raises the possibility that these changes may occur in humans. While patients were not systematically evaluated for these changes in clinical trials, and no specific recommendations for monitoring are being offered, prescribers should be aware of the possibility of these changes (see ANIMAL TOXICOLOGY).

Information for Patients: See PATIENT INFORMATION at the end of this labeling for the text of the separate leaflet provided for patients.

Laboratory Tests: No specific laboratory tests are recommended for monitoring patients prior to and/or after treatment with sumatriptan.

Drug Interactions: Ergot-containing drugs have been reported to cause prolonged vasospastic reactions. Because there is a theoretical basis that these effects may be additive, use of ergotamine-containing or ergot-type medications (like dihydroergotamine or methysergide) and sumatriptan within 24 hours of each other should be avoided (see CONTRAINDICATIONS).

MAO-A inhibitors reduce sumatriptan clearance, significantly increasing systemic exposure. Therefore, the use of IMITREX Tablets in patients receiving MAO-A inhibitors is contraindicated (see CLINICAL PHARMACOLOGY and CONTRAINDICATIONS).

Selective serotonin reuptake inhibitors (SSRIs) (e.g., fluoxetine, fluvoxamine, paroxetine, sertraline) have been reported, rarely, to cause weakness, hyperreflexia, and incoordination when coadministered with sumatriptan. If concomitant treatment with sumatriptan and an SSRI is clinically warranted, appropriate observation of the patient is advised.

Drug/Laboratory Test Interactions: IMITREX Tablets are not known to interfere with commonly employed clinical laboratory tests.

Carcinogenesis, Mutagenesis, Impairment of Fertility: ***Carcinogenesis:*** In carcinogenicity studies, rats and mice were given sumatriptan by oral gavage (rats, 104 weeks) or drinking water (mice, 78 weeks). Average exposures achieved in mice receiving the highest dose (target dose of 160 mg/kg per day) were approximately 40 times the exposure attained in humans after the maximum recommended single oral dose of 100 mg. The highest dose administered to rats (160 mg/kg per day, reduced from 360 mg/kg per day during week 21) was approximately 15 times the maximum recommended single human oral dose of 100 mg on a mg/m^2 basis. There was no evidence of an increase in tumors in either species related to sumatriptan administration.

Mutagenesis: Sumatriptan was not mutagenic in the presence or absence of metabolic activation when tested in two gene mutation assays (the Ames test and the in vitro mammalian Chinese hamster V79/HGPRT assay). In two cytogenetics assays (the in vitro human lymphocyte assay and the in vivo rat micronucleus assay) sumatriptan was not associated with clastogenic activity.

Impairment of Fertility: In a study in which male and female rats were dosed daily with oral sumatriptan prior to and throughout the mating period, there was a treatment-related decrease in fertility secondary to a decrease in mating in animals treated with 50 and 500 mg/kg per day. The highest no-effect dose for this finding was 5 mg/kg per day, or approximately one half of the maximum recommended single human oral dose of 100 mg on a mg/m^2 basis. It is not clear whether the problem is associated with treatment of the males or females or both combined. In a similar study by the subcutaneous route there was no evidence of impaired fertility at 60 mg/kg per day, the maximum dose tested, which is equivalent to approximately six times the maximum recommended single human oral dose of 100 mg on a mg/m^2 basis.

Pregnancy: Pregnancy Category C. In reproductive toxicity studies in rats and rabbits, oral treatment with sumatriptan was associated with embryolethality, fetal abnormalities, and pup mortality. When administered by the intravenous route to rabbits, sumatriptan has been shown to be embryolethal. There are no adequate and well-controlled studies in pregnant women. Therefore, IMITREX Tablets should be used during pregnancy only if the potential benefit justifies the potential risk to the fetus. In assessing this information, the following findings should be considered.

Embryolethality: When given orally or intravenously to pregnant rabbits daily throughout the period of organogenesis, sumatriptan caused embryolethality at doses at or close to those producing maternal toxicity. In the oral studies this dose was 100 mg/kg per day and in the intravenous studies this dose was 2.0 mg/kg per day. The mechanism of the embryolethality is not known. The highest no-effect dose for embryolethality by the oral route was 50 mg/kg per day, which is approximately nine times the maximum single recommended human oral dose of 100 mg on a mg/m^2 basis. By the intravenous route, the highest no-effect dose was 0.75 mg/kg per day, or approximately one tenth of the maximum single recommended human oral dose of 100 mg on a mg/m^2 basis.

The intravenous administration of sumatriptan to pregnant rats throughout organogenesis at 12.5 mg/kg per day, the maximum dose tested, did not cause embryolethality. This dose is equivalent to the maximum single recommended human oral dose of 100 mg on a mg/m^2 basis. Additionally, in a study in rats given subcutaneous sumatriptan daily, prior to and throughout pregnancy, at 60 mg/kg per day, the maximum dose tested, there was no evidence of increased embryo/fetal lethality. This dose is equivalent to approximately six times the maximum recommended single human oral dose of 100 mg on a mg/m^2 basis.

Continued on next page

This product information is based on labeling in effect on June 1, 1998. For further information, contact via direct mail, phone, or web site Medical Information: Glaxo Wellcome Inc., PO Box 13398, Research Triangle Park, NC 27709. Healthcare Professionals (Medical Information): 800-334-0089 Patients (Customer Response Center): 888-TALK2GW (1-888-825-5249) Glaxo Wellcome Corporate Web Site: www.glaxowellcome.com

Imitrex Tablets—Cont.

Teratogenicity: Oral treatment of pregnant rats with sumatriptan during the period of organogenesis resulted in an increased incidence of blood vessel abnormalities (cervicothoracic and umbilical) at doses of approximately 250 mg/kg per day or higher. The highest no-effect dose was approximately 60 mg/kg per day, which is approximately six times the maximum single recommended human oral dose of 100 mg on a mg/m^2 basis. Oral treatment of pregnant rabbits with sumatriptan during the period of organogenesis resulted in an increased incidence of cervicothoracic vascular and skeletal abnormalities. The highest no-effect dose for these effects was 15 mg/kg per day, or approximately three times the maximum single recommended human oral dose of 100 mg on a mg/m^2 basis.

A study in which rats were dosed daily with oral sumatriptan prior to and throughout gestation demonstrated embryo/fetal toxicity (decreased body weight, decreased ossification, increased incidence of rib variations) and an increased incidence of a syndrome of malformations (short tail/short body and vertebral disorganization) at 500 mg/kg per day. The highest no-effect dose was 50 mg/kg per day, or approximately five times the maximum single recommended human oral dose of 100 mg on a mg/m^2 basis. In a study in rats dosed daily with subcutaneous sumatriptan prior to and throughout pregnancy, at a dose of 60 mg/kg per day, the maximum dose tested, there was no evidence of teratogenicity. This dose is equivalent to approximately six times the maximum recommended single human oral dose of 100 mg on a mg/m^2 basis.

Pup Deaths: Oral treatment of pregnant rats with sumatriptan during the period of organogenesis resulted in a decrease in pup survival between birth and postnatal day 4 at doses of approximately 250 mg/kg per day or higher. The highest no-effect dose for this effect was approximately 60 mg/kg per day, or six times the maximum single recommended human oral dose of 100 mg on a mg/m^2 basis.

Oral treatment of pregnant rats with sumatriptan from gestational day 17 through postnatal day 21 demonstrated a decrease in pup survival measured at postnatal days 2, 4, and 20 at the dose of 1,000 mg/kg per day. The highest no-effect dose for this finding was 100 mg/kg per day, approximately 10 times the maximum single recommended human oral dose of 100 mg on a mg/m^2 basis. In a similar study in rats by the subcutaneous route there was no increase in pup death at 81 mg/kg per day, the highest dose tested, which is equivalent to eight times the maximum single recommended human oral dose of 100 mg on a mg/m^2 basis.

To monitor fetal outcomes of pregnant women exposed to IMITREX, Glaxo Wellcome Inc. maintains a Sumatriptan Pregnancy Registry. Physicians are encouraged to register patients by calling (800) 722-9292, ext. 39441.

Nursing Mothers: Sumatriptan is excreted in human breast milk. Therefore, caution should be exercised when considering the administration of IMITREX Tablets to a nursing woman.

Pediatric Use: Safety and effectiveness of IMITREX Tablets in pediatric patients have not been established.

Completed placebo-controlled clinical trials evaluating oral sumatriptan (25 to 100 mg) in pediatric patients aged 12 to 17 years have enrolled a total of 701 adolescent migraineurs. These studies did not establish the efficacy of oral sumatriptan compared to placebo in the treatment of migraine in adolescents. Adverse events observed in these clinical trials were similar in nature to those reported in clinical trials in adults. The frequency of all adverse events in these patients appeared to be both dose- and age-dependent, with younger patients reporting events more commonly than older adolescents. Postmarketing experience includes a limited number of reports that describe pediatric patients who have experienced adverse events, some clinically serious, after use of subcutaneous sumatriptan and/or oral sumatriptan. These reports include events similar in nature to those reported rarely in adults. A myocardial infarct has been reported in a 14-year-old male following the use of oral sumatriptan; clinical signs occurred within 1 day of drug administration. Since clinical data to determine the frequency of serious adverse events in pediatric patients who might receive injectable, oral, or intranasal sumatriptan are not presently available, the use of sumatriptan in patients aged younger than 18 years is not recommended.

Use in the Elderly: Although the pharmacokinetic disposition of the drug in the elderly is similar to that seen in younger adults, there is no information about the safety and effectiveness of sumatriptan in this population because patients over age 65 were excluded from the controlled clinical trials.

ADVERSE REACTIONS

Serious cardiac events, including some that have been fatal, have occurred following the use of IMITREX Injection or Tablets. These events are extremely rare and most have been reported in patients with risk factors predictive of CAD. Events reported have included coronary artery vasospasm, transient myocardial ischemia, myocardial infarction, ventricular tachycardia, and ventricular fibrillation (see CONTRAINDICATIONS, WARNINGS, and PRECAUTIONS).

Significant hypertensive episodes, including hypertensive crises, have been reported on rare occasions in patients with or without a history of hypertension (see WARNINGS).

Incidence in Controlled Clinical Trials: Table 2 lists adverse events that occurred in placebo-controlled clinical trials in patients who took at least one dose of study drug. Only events that occurred at a frequency of 2% or more in any IMITREX Tablets treatment group and were more frequent in that group than in the placebo group are included in Table 2. The events cited reflect experience gained under closely monitored conditions of clinical trials in a highly selected patient population. In actual clinical practice or in other clinical trials, these frequency estimates may not apply, as the conditions of use, reporting behavior, and the kinds of patients treated may differ.

[See table 2 below]

Other events that occurred in more than 1% of patients receiving IMITREX Tablets and at least as often on placebo included nausea and/or vomiting, migraine, headache, hyposalivation, dizziness, and drowsiness/sleepiness.

IMITREX Tablets are generally well tolerated. Across all doses, most adverse reactions were mild and transient and did not lead to long-lasting effects. The incidence of adverse events in controlled clinical trials was not affected by gender or age of the patients. There were insufficient data to assess the impact of race on the incidence of adverse events.

Other Events Observed in Association With the Administration of IMITREX Tablets: In the paragraphs that follow, the frequencies of less commonly reported adverse clinical events are presented. Because the reports include events observed in open and uncontrolled studies, the role of IMITREX Tablets in their causation cannot be reliably determined. Furthermore, variability associated with adverse event reporting, the terminology used to describe adverse events, etc., limit the value of quantitative frequency estimates provided. Event frequencies are calculated as the number of patients who used IMITREX Tablets (25, 50, or 100 mg) and reported an event divided by the total number of patients (n = 6348) exposed to IMITREX Tablets. All reported events are included except those already listed in the previous table, those too general to be informative, and those not reasonably associated with the use of the drug. Events are further classified within body system categories and enumerated in order of decreasing frequency using the following definitions: frequent adverse events are defined as those occurring in at least 1/100 patients, infrequent adverse events are those occurring in 1/100 to 1/1000 patients, and rare adverse events are those occurring in fewer than 1/1000 patients.

Atypical Sensations: Frequent were burning sensation and numbness. Infrequent was tight feeling in head. Rare were dysesthesia.

Cardiovascular: Frequent were palpitations, syncope, decreased blood pressure, and increased blood pressure. Infrequent were arrhythmia, changes in ECG, hypertension, hypotension, pallor, pulsating sensations, and tachycardia. Rare were angina, atherosclerosis, bradycardia, cerebral ischemia, cerebrovascular lesion, heart block, peripheral cyanosis, thrombosis, transient myocardial ischemia, and vasodilation.

Ear, Nose, and Throat: Frequent were sinusitis, tinnitus; allergic rhinitis; upper respiratory inflammation; ear, nose, and throat hemorrhage; external otitis; hearing loss; nasal inflammation; and sensitivity to noise. Rare was feeling of fullness in the ear(s).

Endocrine and Metabolic: Infrequent was thirst. Rare were elevated thyrotropin stimulating hormone (TSH) levels; galactorrhea; hyperglycemia; hypoglycemia; hypothyroidism; polydipsia; weight gain; weight loss; endocrine cysts, lumps, and masses; and fluid disturbances.

Eye: Rare were disorders of sclera, mydriasis, blindness and low vision, visual disturbances, eye edema and swelling, eye irritation and itching, accommodation disorders, external ocular muscle disorders, eye hemorrhage, eye pain, and keratitis and conjunctivitis.

Gastrointestinal: Frequent were diarrhea and gastric symptoms. Infrequent were constipation, dysphagia, and gastroesophageal reflux. Rare were gastrointestinal bleeding, hematemesis, melena, peptic ulcer, gastrointestinal pain, dyspeptic symptoms, dental pain, feelings of gastrointestinal pressure, gastroesophageal reflux, gastritis, gastroenteritis, hypersalivation, abdominal distention, oral itching and irritation, salivary gland swelling, and swallowing disorders.

Hematological Disorders: Rare was anemia.

Musculoskeletal: Frequent was myalgia. Infrequent was muscle cramps. Rare were tetany; muscle atrophy, weakness, and tiredness; arthralgia and articular rheumatitis; acquired musculoskeletal deformity; muscle stiffness, tightness, and rigidity; and musculoskeletal inflammation.

Neurological: Frequent were phonophobia and photophobia. Infrequent were confusion, depression, difficulty concentrating, disturbance of smell, dysarthria, euphoria, facial pain, heat sensitivity, incoordination, lacrimation, monoplegia, sleep disturbance, shivering, syncope, and tremor. Rare were aggressiveness, apathy, bradylogia, cluster headache, convulsions, decreased appetite, drug abuse, dystonic reaction, facial paralysis, hallucinations, hunger, hyperesthesia, hysteria, increased alertness, memory disturbance, neuralgia, paralysis, personality change, phobia, radiculopathy, rigidity, suicide, twitching, agitation, anxiety, depressive disorders, detachment, motor dysfunction, neurotic disorders, psychomotor disorders, taste disturbances, and raised intracranial pressure.

Respiratory: Frequent was dyspnea. Infrequent was asthma. Rare were hiccoughs, breathing disorders, cough, and bronchitis.

Skin: Frequent was sweating. Infrequent were erythema, pruritus, rash, and skin tenderness. Rare were dry/scaly skin, tightness of skin, wrinkling of skin, eczema, seborrheic dermatitis, and skin nodules.

Breasts: Infrequent was tenderness. Rare were nipple discharge; breast swelling; cysts, lumps, and masses of breasts; and primary malignant breast neoplasm.

Urogenital: Infrequent were dysmenorrhea, increased urination, and intermenstrual bleeding. Rare were abortion and hematuria, urinary frequency, bladder inflammation, micturition disorders, urethritis, urinary infections, menstruation symptoms, abnormal menstrual cycle, inflammation of fallopian tubes, and menstrual cycle symptoms.

Miscellaneous: Frequent was hypersensitivity. Infrequent were fever, fluid retention, and overdose. Rare were edema, hematoma, lymphadenopathy, speech disturbance, voice disturbances, contusions.

Table 2: Treatment-Emergent Adverse Events Reported by at Least 2% of Patients in Controlled Migraine Trials *

Adverse Event Type	Placebo (n = 309)	Percent of Patients Reporting: IMITREX 25 mg (n = 417)	IMITREX 50 mg (n = 771)	IMITREX 100 mg (n = 437)
ATYPICAL SENSATIONS	4%	5%	6%	6%
Paresthesia (all types)	2%	3%	5%	3%
Sensation warm/cold	2%	3%	2%	3%
PAIN AND OTHER PRESSURE SENSATIONS	4%	6%	6%	8%
Chest - pain/tightness/ pressure and/or heaviness	1%	1%	2%	2%
Neck/throat/jaw - pain/tightness/pressure	<1%	<1%	2%	3%
Pain -location specified	1%	2%	1%	1%
Other - pressure/tightness/ heaviness	2%	1%	1%	3%
NEUROLOGICAL				
Vertigo	<1%	<1%	<1%	2%
OTHER	8%	6%	4%	8%
Malaise/fatigue	<1%	2%	2%	3%

* Events that occurred at a frequency of 2% or more in the IMITREX Tablets group and that occurred more frequently in that group than the placebo group.

Postmarketing Experience (Reports for Subcutaneous or Oral Sumatriptan): The following section enumerates potentially important adverse events that have occurred in clinical practice and which have been reported spontaneously to various surveillance systems. The events enumerated represent reports arising from both domestic and non-domestic use of oral or subcutaneous dosage forms of sumatriptan. The events enumerated include all except those already listed in the ADVERSE REACTIONS section above or those too general to be informative. Because the reports cite events reported spontaneously from worldwide postmarketing experience, frequency of events and the role of sumatriptan in their causation cannot be reliably determined. It is assumed, however, that systemic reactions following sumatriptan use are likely to be similar regardless of route of administration.

Blood: Hemolytic anemia, pancytopenia, thrombocytopenia.

Cardiovascular: Atrial fibrillation, cardiomyopathy, colonic ischemia (see WARNINGS), pulmonary embolism, shock.

Dermatological: Exacerbation of sunburn, photosensitivity.

Ear, Nose, and Throat: Deafness.

Eye: Ischemic optic neuropathy, periorbital edema, retinal artery occlusion.

Gastrointestinal: Ischemic colitis with rectal bleeding (see WARNINGS), xerostomia.

Hepatic: Elevated liver function tests.

Hypersensitivity Reactions: Allergic vasculitis, erythema, pruritus, rash, shortness of breath, urticaria. In addition, severe anaphylaxis/anaphylactoid reactions have been reported (see WARNINGS).

Neurological: Central nervous system vasculitis, dysphasia, seizure, subarachnoid hemorrhage.

Non-Site Specific: Angioneurotic edema, cyanosis, temporal arteritis.

Psychiatry: Panic disorder.

Respiratory: Bronchospasm in patients with and without a history of asthma.

Urogenital: Acute renal failure.

DRUG ABUSE AND DEPENDENCE

One clinical study with IMITREX® (sumatriptan succinate) Injection enrolling 12 patients with a history of substance abuse failed to induce subjective behavior and/or physiologic response ordinarily associated with drugs that have an established potential for abuse.

OVERDOSAGE

Patients (n = 670) have received single oral doses of 140 to 300 mg without significant adverse effects. Volunteers (n = 174) have received single oral doses of 140 to 400 mg without serious adverse events.

Overdose in animals has been fatal and has been heralded by convulsions, tremor, paralysis, inactivity, ptosis, erythema of the extremities, abnormal respiration, cyanosis, ataxia, mydriasis, salivation, and lacrimation. The elimination half-life of sumatriptan is approximately 2.5 hours (see CLINICAL PHARMACOLOGY), and therefore monitoring of patients after overdose with IMITREX Tablets should continue for at least 12 hours or while symptoms or signs persist.

It is unknown what effect hemodialysis or peritoneal dialysis has on the serum concentrations of sumatriptan.

DOSAGE AND ADMINISTRATION

In controlled clinical trials, single doses of 25, 50, or 100 mg of IMITREX TABLETS were effective for the acute treatment of migraine in adults. There is evidence that doses 50 and 100 mg may provide a greater effect than 25 mg (see CLINICAL TRIALS). There is also evidence that doses of 100 mg do not provide a greater effect than 50 mg. Individuals may vary in response to doses of IMITREX TABLETS. The choice of dose should therefore be made on an individual basis, weighing the possible benefit of a higher dose with the potential for a greater risk of adverse events.

If the headache returns or the patient has a partial response to the initial dose, the dose may be repeated after 2 hours, not to exceed a total daily dose of 200 mg. If a headache returns following an initial treatment with IMITREX Injection, additional single IMITREX Tablets (up to 100 mg/day) may be given with an interval of at least 2 hours between tablet doses. The safety of treating an average of more than four headaches in a 30-day period has not been established.

Because of the potential of MAO-A inhibitors to cause unpredictable elevations in the bioavailability of oral sumatriptan, their combined use is contraindicated (see CONTRAINDICATIONS).

Hepatic disease/functional impairment may also cause unpredictable elevations in the bioavailability of orally administered sumatriptan. Consequently, if treatment is deemed advisable in the presence of liver disease, the maximum single dose should in general not exceed 50 mg (see CLINICAL PHARMACOLOGY for the basis of this recommendation).

HOW SUPPLIED

IMITREX Tablets, 25 and 50 mg of sumatriptan (base) as the succinate. IMITREX Tablets, 25 mg are white, round, film-coated tablets embossed with "I" on one side and "25" on the other in blister packs of 9 tablets (NDC 0173-0460-02). IMITREX Tablets, 50 mg are white, capsule-shaped, film-coated tablets embossed with "Imitrex" on one side and "50" on the other in blister packs of 9 tablets (NDC 0173-0459-00).

Store between 36° and 86°F (2° and 30°C).

Caution: Federal law prohibits dispensing without prescription.

ANIMAL TOXICOLOGY

Corneal Opacities: Dogs receiving oral sumatriptan developed corneal opacities and defects in the corneal epithelium. Corneal opacities were seen at the lowest dosage tested, 2 mg/kg per day, and were present after 1 month of treatment. Defects in the corneal epithelium were noted in a 60-week study. Earlier examinations for these toxicities were not conducted and no-effect doses were not established; however, the relative exposure at the lowest dose tested was approximately five times the human exposure after a 100-mg oral dose. There is evidence of alterations in corneal appearance on the first day of intranasal dosing to dogs. Changes were noted at the lowest dose tested, which was approximately one half the maximum single human oral dose of 100 mg on a mg/m² basis.

PATIENT INFORMATION

The following wording is contained in a separate leaflet provided for patients.

Information for the Patient
IMITREX® (sumatriptan succinate) Tablets

Please read this leaflet carefully before you take IMITREX Tablets. This provides a summary of the information available on your medicine. Please do not throw away this leaflet until you have finished your medicine. You may need to read this leaflet again. This leaflet does not contain all the information on IMITREX Tablets. For further information or advice, ask your doctor or pharmacist.

Information About Your Medicine:

The name of your medicine is IMITREX (sumatriptan succinate) Tablets. It can be obtained only by prescription from your doctor. The decision to use IMITREX Tablets is one that you and your doctor should make jointly, taking into account your individual preferences and medical circumstances. If you have risk factors for heart disease (such as high blood pressure, high cholesterol, obesity, diabetes, smoking, strong family history of heart disease, or you are postmenopausal or a male over 40), you should tell your doctor, who should evaluate you for heart disease in order to determine if IMITREX is appropriate for you. Although the vast majority of those who have taken IMITREX have not experienced any significant side effects, some individuals have experienced serious heart problems and, rarely, considering the extensiveness of IMITREX use worldwide, deaths have been reported. In all but a few instances, however, serious problems occurred in people with known heart disease and it was not clear whether IMITREX was a contributory factor in these deaths.

1. The Purpose of Your Medicine:

IMITREX Tablets are intended to relieve your migraine, but not to prevent or reduce the number of attacks you experience. Use IMITREX Tablets only to treat an actual migraine attack.

2. Important Questions to Consider Before Taking IMITREX Tablets:

If the answer to any of the following questions is **YES** or if you do not know the answer, then please discuss it with your doctor before you use IMITREX Tablets.

- Are you pregnant? Do you think you might be pregnant? Are you trying to become pregnant? Are you using inadequate contraception? Are you breast-feeding?
- Do you have any chest pain, heart disease, shortness of breath, or irregular heartbeats? Have you had a heart attack?
- Do you have risk factors for heart disease (such as high blood pressure, high cholesterol, obesity, diabetes, smoking, strong family history of heart disease, or you are postmenopausal or a male over 40)?
- Have you had a stroke, transient ischemic attacks (TIAs), or Raynaud syndrome?
- Do you have high blood pressure?
- Have you ever had to stop taking this or any other medication because of an allergy or other problems?
- Are you taking any other migraine medications, including other 5-HT₁ agonists or any other medications containing ergotamine, dihydroergotamine, or methysergide?
- Are you taking any medication for depression (monoamine oxidase inhibitors or selective serotonin reuptake inhibitors [SSRIs])?
- Have you had, or do you have, any disease of the liver or kidney?
- Have you had, or do you have, epilepsy or seizures?

- Is this headache different from your usual migraine attacks?

Remember, if you answered **YES** to any of the above questions, then discuss it with your doctor.

3. The Use of IMITREX Tablets During Pregnancy:

Do not use IMITREX Tablets if you are pregnant, think you might be pregnant, are trying to become pregnant, or are not using adequate contraception, unless you have discussed this with your doctor.

4. How to Use IMITREX Tablets:

For adults, the usual dose is a single tablet taken whole with fluids. A second tablet may be taken if your symptoms of migraine come back or if you have a partial response to the initial dose, but not sooner than 2 hours following the first tablet. For a given attack, if you have no response to the first tablet, do not take a second tablet without first consulting with your doctor. Do not take more than a total of 200 mg of IMITREX Tablets in any 24-hour period. The safety of treating an average of more than four headaches in a 30-day period has not been established.

5. Side Effects to Watch for:

- Some patients experience pain or tightness in the chest or throat when using IMITREX Tablets. If this happens to you, then discuss it with your doctor before using any more IMITREX Tablets. If the chest pain is severe or does not go away, call your doctor immediately.
- If you have sudden and/or severe abdominal pain following IMITREX Tablets, call your doctor immediately.
- Shortness of breath; wheeziness; heart throbbing; swelling of eyelids, face, or lips; or a skin rash, skin lumps, or hives happens rarely. If it happens to you, then tell your doctor immediately. Do not take any more IMITREX Tablets unless your doctor tells you to do so.
- Some people may have feelings of tingling, heat, flushing (redness of face lasting a short time), heaviness or pressure after treatment with IMITREX Tablets. A few people may feel drowsy, dizzy, tired, or sick. Tell your doctor of these symptoms at your next visit.
- If you feel unwell in any other way or have any symptoms that you do not understand, you should contact your doctor immediately.

6. What to Do if an Overdose is Taken:

If you have taken more medication than you have been told, contact either your doctor, hospital emergency department, or nearest poison control center immediately.

7. Storing Your Medicine:

Keep your medicine in a safe place where children cannot reach it. It may be harmful to children. Store your medication away from heat and light. Do not store at temperatures above 86°F (30°C), or below 36°F (2°C). If your medication has expired (the expiration date is printed on the treatment pack), throw it away as instructed. If your doctor decides to stop your treatment, do not keep any leftover medicine unless your doctor tells you to. Throw away your medicine as instructed.

US Patent Nos. 4,816,470 and 5,037,845
©Copyright 1998 Glaxo Wellcome Inc. All rights reserved.
February 1998/RL-546
Shown in Product Identification Guide, page 313

IMURAN®   ℞
[ĭm´ū-ran˝]
(azathioprine)
50-mg Scored Tablets
100 mg (as the sodium salt) for I.V. injection,
equivalent to 100 mg azathioprine sterile lyophilized
material.

> **WARNING**
> Chronic immunosuppression with this purine antimetabolite increases *risk of neoplasia* in humans. Physicians using this drug should be very familiar with this risk as well as with the mutagenic potential to both men and women and with possible hematologic toxicities. See WARNINGS.

DESCRIPTION

IMURAN (azathioprine), an immunosuppressive antimetabolite, is available in tablet form for oral administration and 100-mg vials for intravenous injection. Each scored tablet contains 50 mg azathioprine and the inactive ingredients lactose, magnesium stearate, potato starch, povidone, and

Continued on next page

This product information is based on labeling in effect on June 1, 1998. For further information, contact via direct mail, phone, or web site Medical Information: Glaxo Wellcome Inc., PO Box 13398, Research Triangle Park, NC 27709. Healthcare Professionals (Medical Information): 800-334-0089 Patients (Customer Response Center): 888-TALK2GW (1-888-825-5249) Glaxo Wellcome Corporate Web Site: www.glaxowellcome.com

Imuran—Cont.

stearic acid. Each 100-mg vial contains azathioprine, as the sodium salt, equivalent to 100 mg azathioprine sterile lyophilized material and sodium hydroxide to adjust pH.
Azathioprine is chemically 6-[(1-methyl-4-nitro-1*H*-imidazol-5-yl)thio]-1*H*-purine. It is an imidazolyl derivative of 6-mercaptopurine (PURINETHOL®) and many of its biological effects are similar to those of the parent compound.
Azathioprine is insoluble in water, but may be dissolved with addition of one molar equivalent of alkali. The sodium salt of azathioprine is sufficiently soluble to make a 10 mg/mL water solution which is stable for 24 hours at 59° to 77°F (15° to 25° C). Azathioprine is stable in solution at neutral or acid pH but hydrolysis to mercaptopurine occurs in excess sodium hydroxide (0.1N), especially on warming. Conversion to mercaptopurine also occurs in the presence of sulfhydryl compounds such as cysteine, glutathione, and hydrogen sulfide.

CLINICAL PHARMACOLOGY

Metabolism:[1] Azathioprine is well absorbed following oral administration. Maximum serum radioactivity occurs at 1 to 2 hours after oral ^{35}S-azathioprine and decays with a half-life of 5 hours. This is not an estimate of the half-life of azathioprine itself, but is the decay rate for all ^{35}S-containing metabolites of the drug. Because of extensive metabolism, only a fraction of the radioactivity is present as azathioprine. Usual doses produce blood levels of azathioprine, and of mercaptopurine derived from it, which are low (<1 mcg/mL). Blood levels are of little predictive value for therapy since the magnitude and duration of clinical effects correlate with thiopurine nucleotide levels in tissues rather than with plasma drug levels. Azathioprine and mercaptopurine are moderately bound to serum proteins (30%) and are partially dialyzable.
Azathioprine is cleaved in vivo to mercaptopurine. Both compounds are rapidly eliminated from blood and are oxidized or methylated in erythrocytes and liver; no azathioprine or mercaptopurine is detectable in urine after 8 hours. Conversion to inactive 6-thiouric acid by xanthine oxidase is an important degradative pathway, and the inhibition of this pathway in patients receiving allopurinol (ZYLOPRIM®) is the basis for the azathioprine dosage reduction required in these patients (see PRECAUTIONS: Drug Interactions). Proportions of metabolites are different in individual patients, and this presumably accounts for variable magnitude and duration of drug effects. Renal clearance is probably not important in predicting biological effectiveness or toxicities, although dose reduction is practiced in patients with poor renal function.
Homograft Survival:[1,2] Summary information from transplant centers and registries indicates relatively universal use of IMURAN with or without other immunosuppressive agents.[3,4,5] Although the use of azathioprine for inhibition of renal homograft rejection is well established, the mechanism(s) for this action are somewhat obscure. The drug suppresses hypersensitivities of the cell-mediated type and causes variable alterations in antibody production. Suppression of T-cell effects, including ablation of T-cell suppression, is dependent on the temporal relationship to antigenic stimulus or engraftment. This agent has little effect on established graft rejections or secondary responses.
Alterations in specific immune responses or immunologic functions in transplant recipients are difficult to relate specifically to immunosuppression by azathioprine. These patients have subnormal responses to vaccines, low numbers of T-cells, and abnormal phagocytosis by peripheral blood cells, but their mitogenic responses, serum immunoglobulins, and secondary antibody responses are usually normal.
Immunoinflammatory Response: Azathioprine suppresses disease manifestations as well as underlying pathology in animal models of autoimmune disease. For example, the severity of adjuvant arthritis is reduced by azathioprine.
The mechanisms whereby azathioprine affects autoimmune diseases are not known. Azathioprine is immunosuppressive, delayed hypersensitivity and cellular cytotoxicity tests being suppressed to a greater degree than are antibody responses. In the rat model of adjuvant arthritis, azathioprine has been shown to inhibit the lymph node hyperplasia which precedes the onset of the signs of the disease. Both the immunosuppressive and therapeutic effects in animal models are dose-related. Azathioprine is considered a slow-acting drug and effects may persist after the drug has been discontinued.

INDICATIONS AND USAGE

IMURAN is indicated as an adjunct for the prevention of rejection in renal homotransplantation. It is also indicated for the management of severe, active rheumatoid arthritis unresponsive to rest, aspirin, or other nonsteroidal anti-inflammatory drugs, or to agents in the class of which gold is an example.
Renal Homotransplantation: IMURAN is indicated as an adjunct for the prevention of rejection in renal homotransplantation. Experience with over 16,000 transplants shows a 5-year patient survival of 35% to 55%, but this is dependent on donor, match for HLA antigens, anti-donor or anti–B-cell alloantigen antibody, and other variables. The effect of IMURAN on these variables has not been tested in controlled trials.
Rheumatoid Arthritis:[6,7] IMURAN is indicated only in adult patients meeting criteria for classic or definite rheumatoid arthritis as specified by the American Rheumatism Association.[8] IMURAN should be restricted to patients with severe, active and erosive disease not responsive to conventional management including rest, aspirin, or other nonsteroidal drugs, or to agents in the class of which gold is an example. Rest, physiotherapy, and salicylates should be continued while IMURAN is given, but it may be possible to reduce the dose of corticosteroids in patients on IMURAN. The combined use of IMURAN with gold, antimalarials, or penicillamine has not been studied for either added benefit or unexpected adverse effects. The use of IMURAN with these agents cannot be recommended.

CONTRAINDICATIONS

IMURAN should not be given to patients who have shown hypersensitivity to the drug.
IMURAN should not be used for treating rheumatoid arthritis in pregnant women.
Patients with rheumatoid arthritis previously treated with alkylating agents (cyclophosphamide, chlorambucil, melphalan, or others) may have a prohibitive risk of neoplasia if treated with IMURAN.[9]

WARNINGS

Severe *leukopenia and/or thrombocytopenia* may occur in patients on IMURAN. Macrocytic anemia and severe bone marrow depression may also occur. Hematologic toxicities are dose-related and may be more severe in renal transplant patients whose homograft is undergoing rejection. It is suggested that patients on IMURAN have complete blood counts, including platelet counts, weekly during the first month, twice monthly for the second and third months of treatment, then monthly or more frequently if dosage alterations or other therapy changes are necessary. Delayed hematologic suppression may occur. Prompt reduction in dosage or temporary withdrawal of the drug may be necessary if there is a rapid fall in or persistently low leukocyte count, or other evidence of bone marrow depression. Leukopenia does not correlate with therapeutic effect; therefore the dose should not be increased intentionally to lower the white blood cell count.
Serious infections are a constant hazard for patients receiving chronic immunosuppression, especially for homograft recipients. Fungal, viral, bacterial, and protozoal infections may be fatal and should be treated vigorously. Reduction of azathioprine dosage and/or use of other drugs should be considered.
IMURAN is mutagenic in animals and humans, carcinogenic in animals, and may increase the patient's *risk of neoplasia.* Renal transplant patients are known to have an increased risk of malignancy, predominantly skin cancer and reticulum cell or lymphomatous tumors.[10] The risk of post-transplant lymphomas may be increased in patients who receive aggressive treatment with immunosuppressive drugs.[11] The degree of immunosuppression is determined, not only by the immunosuppressive regimen, but also by a number of other patient factors. The number of immunosuppressive agents may not necessarily increase the risk of post-transplant lymphomas. However, transplant patients who receive multiple immunosuppressive agents may be at risk for over-immunosuppression; therefore, immunosuppressive drug therapy should be maintained at the lowest effective levels. Information is available on the spontaneous neoplasia risk in rheumatoid arthritis,[12,13] and on neoplasia following immunosuppressive therapy of other autoimmune diseases.[14,15] It has not been possible to define the precise risk of neoplasia due to IMURAN.[16] The data suggest the risk may be elevated in patients with rheumatoid arthritis, though lower than for renal transplant patients.[11,13] However, acute myelogenous leukemia as well as solid tumors have been reported in patients with rheumatoid arthritis who have received azathioprine. Data on neoplasia in patients receiving IMURAN can be found under ADVERSE REACTIONS.
IMURAN has been reported to cause temporary depression in spermatogenesis and reduction in sperm viability and sperm count in mice at doses 10 times the human therapeutic dose;[17] a reduced percentage of fertile matings occurred when animals received 5 mg/kg.[18]
Pregnancy: Pregnancy Category D. IMURAN can cause fetal harm when administered to a pregnant woman. IMURAN should not be given during pregnancy without careful weighing of risk versus benefit. Whenever possible, use of IMURAN in pregnant patients should be avoided. This drug should not be used for treating rheumatoid arthritis in pregnant women.[19]
IMURAN is teratogenic in rabbits and mice when given in doses equivalent to the human dose (5 mg/kg daily). Abnormalities included skeletal malformations and visceral anomalies.[18]
Limited immunologic and other abnormalities have occurred in a few infants born of renal allograft recipients on IMURAN. In a detailed case report,[20] documented lymphopenia, diminished IgG and IgM levels, CMV infection, and a decreased thymic shadow were noted in an infant born to a mother receiving 150 mg azathioprine and 30 mg prednisone daily throughout pregnancy. At 10 weeks most features were normalized. DeWitte et al[21] reported pancytopenia and severe immune deficiency in a preterm infant whose mother received 125 mg azathioprine and 12.5 mg prednisone daily. There have been two published reports of abnormal physical findings. Williamson and Karp[22] described an infant born with preaxial polydactyly whose mother received azathioprine 200 mg daily and prednisone 20 mg every other day during pregnancy. Tallent et al[23] described an infant with a large myelomeningocele in the upper lumbar region, bilateral dislocated hips, and bilateral talipes equinovarus. The father was on long-term azathioprine therapy.
Benefit versus risk must be weighed carefully before use of IMURAN in patients of reproductive potential. There are no adequate and well-controlled studies in pregnant women. If this drug is used during pregnancy or if the patient becomes pregnant while taking this drug, the patient should be apprised of the potential hazard to the fetus. Women of childbearing age should be advised to avoid becoming pregnant.

PRECAUTIONS

General: A gastrointestinal hypersensitivity reaction characterized by severe nausea and vomiting has been reported.[24,25,26] These symptoms may also be accompanied by diarrhea, rash, fever, malaise, myalgias, elevations in liver enzymes, and occasionally, hypotension. Symptoms of gastrointestinal toxicity most often develop within the first several weeks of therapy with IMURAN and are reversible upon discontinuation of the drug. The reaction can recur within hours after rechallenge with a single dose of IMURAN.

Information for Patients:
Patients being started on IMURAN should be informed of the necessity of periodic blood counts while they are receiving the drug and should be encouraged to report any unusual bleeding or bruising to their physician. They should be informed of the danger of infection while receiving IMURAN and asked to report signs and symptoms of infection to their physician. Careful dosage instructions should be given to the patient, especially when IMURAN is being administered in the presence of impaired renal function or concomitantly with allopurinol (see Drug Interactions subsection and DOSAGE AND ADMINISTRATION). Patients should be advised of the potential risks of the use of IMURAN during pregnancy and during the nursing period. The increased risk of neoplasia following therapy with IMURAN should be explained to the patient.
Laboratory Tests: See WARNINGS and ADVERSE REACTIONS sections.
Drug Interactions:
Use with Allopurinol: The principal pathway for detoxification of IMURAN is inhibited by allopurinol. Patients receiving IMURAN and allopurinol concomitantly should have a dose reduction of IMURAN, to approximately $^{1}/_{3}$ to $^{1}/_{4}$ the usual dose.
Use with Other Agents Affecting Myelopoesis: Drugs which may affect leukocyte production, including co-trimoxazole, may lead to exaggerated leukopenia, especially in renal transplant recipients.[27]
Use with Angiotensin-Converting Enzyme Inhibitors: The use of angiotensin-converting enzyme inhibitors to control hypertension in patients on azathioprine has been reported to induce anemia and severe leukopenia.[28]
Use with Warfarin: IMURAN may inhibit the anticoagulant effect of warfarin.
Carcinogenesis, Mutagenesis, Impairment of Fertility: See WARNINGS section.
Pregnancy: ***Teratogenic Effects:*** Pregnancy Category D. See WARNINGS section.
Nursing Mothers: The use of IMURAN in nursing mothers is not recommended. Azathioprine or its metabolites are transferred at low levels, both transplacentally and in breast milk.[29,30,31] Because of the potential for tumorigenicity shown for azathioprine, a decision should be made whether to discontinue nursing or discontinue the drug, taking into account the importance of the drug to the mother.
Pediatric Use: Safety and efficacy of azathioprine in pediatric patients have not been established.

ADVERSE REACTIONS

The principal and potentially serious toxic effects of IMURAN are hematologic and gastrointestinal. The risks of secondary infection and neoplasia are also significant (see WARNINGS). The frequency and severity of adverse reactions depend on the dose and duration of IMURAN as well as on the patient's underlying disease or concomitant therapies. The incidence of hematologic toxicities and neoplasia encountered in groups of renal homograft recipients is sig-

nificantly higher than that in studies employing IMURAN for rheumatoid arthritis. The relative incidences in clinical studies are summarized below:

Toxicity	Renal Homograft	Rheumatoid Arthritis
Leukopenia (any degree)	>50%	28%
<2500 cells/mm³	16%	5.3%
Infections	20%	<1%
Neoplasia		*
Lymphoma	0.5%	
Others	2.8%	

* Data on the rate and risk of neoplasia among persons with rheumatoid arthritis treated with azathioprine are limited. The incidence of lymphoproliferative disease in patients with RA appears to be significantly higher than that in the general population.[12] In one completed study, the rate of lymphoproliferative disease in RA patients receiving higher than recommended doses of azathioprine (5 mg/kg per day) was 1.8 cases per 1000 patient-years of follow-up, compared with 0.8 cases per 1000 patient-years of follow-up in those not receiving azathioprine.[13] However, the proportion of the increased risk attributable to the azathioprine dosage or to other therapies (i.e., alkylating agents) received by patients treated with azathioprine cannot be determined.

Hematologic: Leukopenia and/or thrombocytopenia are dose-dependent and may occur late in the course of therapy with IMURAN. Dose reduction or temporary withdrawal allows reversal of these toxicities. Infection may occur as a secondary manifestation of bone marrow suppression or leukopenia, but the incidence of infection in renal homotransplantation is 30 to 60 times that in rheumatoid arthritis. Macrocytic anemia and/or bleeding have been reported. There are rare individuals with an inherited deficiency of the enzyme thiopurine methyltransferase (TPMT) who may be unusually sensitive to the myelosuppressive effect of azathioprine and prone to developing rapid bone marrow suppression following the initiation of treatment with IMURAN.

Gastrointestinal: Nausea and vomiting may occur within the first few months of therapy with IMURAN, and occurred in approximately 12% of 676 rheumatoid arthritis patients. The frequency of gastric disturbance often can be reduced by administration of the drug in divided doses and/or after meals. However, in some patients, nausea and vomiting may be severe and may be accompanied by symptoms such as diarrhea, fever, malaise, and myalgias (see PRECAUTIONS). Vomiting with abdominal pain may occur rarely with a hypersensitivity pancreatitis. Hepatotoxicity manifest by elevation of serum alkaline phosphatase, bilirubin, and/or serum transaminases is known to occur following azathioprine use, primarily in allograft recipients. Hepatotoxicity has been uncommon (less than 1%) in rheumatoid arthritis patients. Hepatotoxicity following transplantation most often occurs within 6 months of transplantation and is generally reversible after interruption of IMURAN. A rare, but life-threatening hepatic veno-occlusive disease associated with chronic administration of azathioprine has been described in transplant patients and in one patient receiving IMURAN for panuveitis.[32,33,34] Periodic measurement of serum transaminases, alkaline phosphatase, and bilirubin is indicated for early detection of hepatotoxicity. If hepatic veno-occlusive disease is clinically suspected, IMURAN should be permanently withdrawn.

Others: Additional side effects of low frequency have been reported. These include skin rashes, alopecia, fever, arthralgias, diarrhea, steatorrhea, negative nitrogen balance, and reversible interstitial pneumonitis.

OVERDOSAGE

The oral LD$_{50}$s for single doses of IMURAN in mice and rats are 2500 mg/kg and 400 mg/kg, respectively. Very large doses of this antimetabolite may lead to marrow hypoplasia, bleeding, infection, and death. About 30% of IMURAN is bound to serum proteins, but approximately 45% is removed during an 8-hour hemodialysis.[35] A single case has been reported of a renal transplant patient who ingested a single dose of 7500 mg IMURAN. The immediate toxic reactions were nausea, vomiting, and diarrhea, followed by mild leukopenia and mild abnormalities in liver function. The white blood cell count, SGOT, and bilirubin returned to normal 6 days after the overdose.

DOSAGE AND ADMINISTRATION

Renal Homotransplantation: The dose of IMURAN required to prevent rejection and minimize toxicity will vary with individual patients; this necessitates careful management. The initial dose is usually 3 to 5 mg/kg daily, beginning at the time of transplant. IMURAN is usually given as a single daily dose on the day of, and in a minority of cases 1 to 3 days before, transplantation. IMURAN is often initiated with the intravenous administration of the sodium salt, with subsequent use of tablets (at the same dose level) after the postoperative period. Intravenous administration of the sodium salt is indicated only in patients unable to tolerate oral medications. Dose reduction to maintenance levels of 1 to 3 mg/kg daily is usually possible. The dose of IMURAN should not be increased to toxic levels because of threatened rejection. Discontinuation may be necessary for severe hematologic or other toxicity, even if rejection of the homograft may be a consequence of drug withdrawal.

Rheumatoid Arthritis: IMURAN is usually given on a daily basis. The initial dose should be approximately 1.0 mg/kg (50 to 100 mg) given as a single dose or on a twice-daily schedule. The dose may be increased, beginning at 6 to 8 weeks and thereafter by steps at 4-week intervals, if there are no serious toxicities and if initial response is unsatisfactory. Dose increments should be 0.5 mg/kg daily, up to a maximum dose of 2.5 mg/kg per day. Therapeutic response occurs after several weeks of treatment, usually 6 to 8; an adequate trial should be a minimum of 12 weeks. Patients not improved after 12 weeks can be considered refractory. IMURAN may be continued long-term in patients with clinical response, but patients should be monitored carefully, and gradual dosage reduction should be attempted to reduce risk of toxicities.

Maintenance therapy should be at the lowest effective dose, and the dose given can be lowered decrementally with changes of 0.5 mg/kg or approximately 25 mg daily every 4 weeks while other therapy is kept constant. The optimum duration of maintenance IMURAN has not been determined. IMURAN can be discontinued abruptly, but delayed effects are possible.

Use in Renal Dysfunction: Relatively oliguric patients, especially those with tubular necrosis in the immediate postcadaveric transplant period, may have delayed clearance of IMURAN or its metabolites, may be particularly sensitive to this drug, and are usually given lower doses.

Parenteral Administration: Add 10 mL of Sterile Water for Injection, and swirl until a clear solution results. This solution, equivalent to 100 mg azathioprine, is for intravenous use only; it has a pH of approximately 9.6, and it should be used within 24 hours. Further dilution into sterile saline or dextrose is usually made for infusion; the final volume depends on time for the infusion, usually 30 to 60 minutes, but as short as 5 minutes and as long as 8 hours for the daily dose.

Parenteral drug products should be inspected visually for particulate matter and discoloration prior to administration, whenever solution and container permit.

Procedures for proper handling and disposal of this immunosuppressive antimetabolite drug should be considered. Several guidelines on this subject have been published.[36–42] There is no general agreement that all of the procedures recommended in the guidelines are necessary or appropriate.

HOW SUPPLIED

50-mg overlapping circle-shaped, yellow to off-white, scored tablets imprinted with "IMURAN" and "50" on each tablet; bottle of 100 (NDC 0173-0597-55).

Store at 15° to 25°C (59° to 77°F) in a dry place and protect from light.

20-mL vial, each containing the equivalent of 100 mg azathioprine (as the sodium salt) (NDC 0173-0598-71).

Store at 15° to 25°C (59° to 77°F) and protect from light. The sterile, lyophilized sodium salt is yellow, and should be dissolved in Sterile Water for Injection (see DOSAGE AND ADMINISTRATION: Parenteral Administration).

REFERENCES

1. Elion GB, Hitchings GH. Azathioprine. In: Sartorelli AC, Johns DG, eds. *Antineoplastic and Immunosuppressive Agents Pt II.* New York, NY: Springer Verlag; 1975: chap 48.
2. McIntosh J, Hansen P, Ziegler J, et al. Defective immune and phagocytic functions in uraemia and renal transplantation. *Int Arch Allergy Appl Immunol.* 1976;15:544-549.
3. Renal Transplant Registry Advisory Committee. The 12th report of the Human Renal Transplant Registry. *JAMA.* 1975;233:787-796.
4. McGeown M. Immunosuppression for kidney transplantation. *Lancet.* 1973;2:310-312.
5. Simmons RL, Thompson EJ, Yunis EJ, et al. 115 patients with first cadaver kidney transplants followed two to seven and a half years: a multifactorial analysis. *Am J Med.* 1977;62:234-242.
6. Fye K, Talal N. Cytotoxic drugs in the treatment of rheumatoid arthritis. *Ration Drug Ther.* 1975;9:1-5.
7. Davis JD, Muss HB, Turner RA. Cytotoxic agents in the treatment of rheumatoid arthritis. *South Med J.* 1978;71:58-64.
8. McEwen C. The diagnosis and differential diagnosis of rheumatoid arthritis. In: Hollander JL, ed. *Arthritis and Allied Conditions: A Textbook of Rheumatology.* 8th ed. Philadelphia, PA: Lea and Febiger; 1972:403-418.
9. Hoover R, Fraumeni JF. Drug-induced cancer. *Cancer.* 1981;47:1071-1080.
10. Hoover R, Fraumeni JF Jr. Risk of cancer in renal transplant recipients. *Lancet.* 1973;2:55-57.
11. Wilkinson AH, Smith JL, Hunsicker LG, et al. Increased frequency of post-transplant lymphomas in patients treated with cyclosporine, azathioprine, and prednisone. *Transplantation.* 1989;47:293-296.
12. Prior P, Symmons DPM, Hawkins CF, et al. Cancer morbidity in rheumatoid arthritis. *Ann Rheum Dis.* 1984; 43:128-131.
13. Silman AJ, Petrie J, Hazelman B, et al. Lymphoproliferative cancer and other malignancy in patients with rheumatoid arthritis treated with azathioprine: a 20 year follow up study. *Ann Rheum Dis.* 1988; 47:988-992.
14. Louie S, Schwartz RS. Immunodeficiency and pathogenesis of lymphoma and leukemia. *Semin Hematol.* 1978;15:117-138.
15. Wang KK, Czaja AJ, Beaver SJ, et al. Extra hepatic malignancy following long-term immunosuppressive therapy of severe hepatitis B surface antigen-negative chronic active hepatitis. *Hepatology.* 1989; 10:39-43.
16. Sieber SM, Adamson RH. Toxicity of antineoplastic agents in man: chromosomal aberrations, antifertility effects, congenital malformations, and carcinogenic potential. In: Klein G, Weinhouse S, eds. *Advances in Cancer Research.* New York, NY: Academic Press; 1975;22: 57-155.
17. Clark JM. The mutagenicity of azathioprine in mice, *Drosophila Melanogaster and Neurospora Crassa. Mut Res.* 1975; 28:87-99.
18. Data on file, Glaxo Wellcome Inc.
19. Tagatz GE, Simmons RL. Pregnancy after renal transplantation. *Ann Intern Med.* 1975:82:113-114. Editorial Notes.
20. Coté CJ, Meuwissen HJ, Pickering RJ. Effects on the neonate of prednisone and azathioprine administered to the mother during pregnancy. *J Pediatr.* 1974;85:324-328.
21. DeWitte DB, Buick MK, Stephen EC, et al. Neonatal pancytopenia and severe combined immunodeficiency associated with antenatal administration of azathioprine and prednisone. *J Pediatr.* 1984;105:625-628.
22. Williamson RA, Karp LE. Azathioprine teratogenicity: review of the literature and case report. *Obstet Gynecol.* 1981;58:247-250.
23. Tallent MB, Simmons RL, Najarian JS. Birth defects in child of male recipient of kidney transplant. *JAMA.* 1970;211:1854-1855.
24. Assini JF, Hamilton R, Strosberg JM. Adverse reactions to azathioprine mimicking gastroenteritis. *J Rheumatol.* 1986;13:1117-1118.
25. Cochrane D, Adamson AR, Halsey JP. Adverse reactions to azathioprine mimicking gastroenteritis. *J Rheumatol.* 1987;14:1075.
26. Cox J, Daneshmend JK, Hawkey CJ, et al. Devastating diarrhoea caused by azathioprine: management difficulty in inflammatory bowel disease. *Gut.* 1988;29:686-688.
27. Bradley PP, Warden GD, Maxwell JG, et al. Neutropenia and thrombocytopenia in renal allograft recipients treated with trimethoprim-sulfamethoxazole. *Ann Int Med.* 1980;93:560-562.
28. Kirchertz EJ, Grone HJ, Rieger J, et al. Successful low dose captopril rechallenge following drug-induced leucopenia. *Lancet.* 1981;1:1362-1363.
29. Nelson D, Bugge C. Data on file, Glaxo Wellcome Inc.
30. Saarikoski S, Seppälä M. Immunosuppression during pregnancy: transmission of azathioprine and its metabolites from the mother to the fetus. *Am J Obstet Gynecol.* 1973;115:1100-1106.
31. Coulam CB, Moyer TP, Jiang NS, et al. Breast-feeding after renal transplantation. *Transplant Proc.* 1982;14: 605-609.
32. Read AE, Wiesner RH, LaBrecque DR, et al. Hepatic veno-occlusive disease associated with renal transplantation and azathioprine therapy. *Ann Intern Med.* 1986;104:651-655.
33. Katzka DA, Saul SH, Jorkasky D, et al. Azathioprine and hepatic venocclusive disease in renal transplant patients. *Gastroenterology.* 1986;90:446-454.

Continued on next page

This product information is based on labeling in effect on June 1, 1998. For further information, contact via direct mail, phone, or web site Medical Information: Glaxo Wellcome Inc., PO Box 13398, Research Triangle Park, NC 27709. Healthcare Professionals (Medical Information): 800-334-0089 Patients (Customer Response Center): 888-TALK2GW (1-888-825-5249) Glaxo Wellcome Corporate Web Site: www.glaxowellcome.com

Imuran—Cont.

34. Weitz H, Gokel JM, Loeschke K, et al. Veno-occlusive disease of the liver in patients receiving immunosuppressive therapy. *Virchows Arch A.* 1982;395:245-256.
35. Schusziarra V, Ziekursch V, Schlamp R, et al. Pharmacokinetics of azathioprine under haemodialysis. *Int J Clin Pharmacol Biopharm.* 1976;14:298-302.
36. Recommendations for the safe handling of parenteral antineoplastic drugs. Washington, DC: Division of Safety. National Institutes of Health; 1983. US Dept of Health and Human Services, Public Health Service publication NIH 83-2621.
37. AMA Council on Scientific Affairs. Guidelines for handling parenteral antineoplastics. *JAMA.* 1985;253:1590-1591.
38. National Study Commission on Cytotoxic Exposure. Recommendations for handling cytotoxic agents. 1987. Available from Louis P. Jeffrey, Chairman, National Study Commission on Cytotoxic Exposure. Massachusetts College of Pharmacy and Allied Health Sciences, 179 Longwood Avenue, Boston, MA, 02115.
39. Clinical Oncological Society of Australia. Guidelines and recommendations for safe handling of antineoplastic agents. *Med J Australia.* 1983;1:426-428.
40. Jones RB, Frank R, Mass T. Safe handling of chemotherapeutic agents: a report from the Mount Sinai Medical Center. *CA-A Cancer J for Clin.* 1983;33:258-263.
41. American Society of Hospital Pharmacists. ASHP technical assistance bulletin on handling cytotoxic and hazardous drugs. *Am J Hosp Pharm.* 1990;47:1033-1049.
42. Yodaiken RE, Bennett D. OSHA work-practice guidelines for personnel dealing with cytotoxic (antineoplastic) drugs. *Am J Hosp Pharm.* 1986;43:1193-1204.

©Copyright 1996 Glaxo Wellcome Inc. All rights reserved.
November 1997/RL-500

Shown in Product Identification Guide, page 312

LAMICTAL® ℞

[la-mik' tal]
(lamotrigine)
Tablets

SEVERE, POTENTIALLY LIFE-THREATENING RASHES HAVE BEEN REPORTED IN ASSOCIATION WITH THE USE OF LAMICTAL. THESE REPORTS, OCCURRING IN APPROXIMATELY ONE IN EVERY THOUSAND ADULTS, HAVE INCLUDED STEVENS-JOHNSON SYNDROME AND, RARELY, TOXIC EPIDERMAL NECROLYSIS. RARE DEATHS HAVE BEEN REPORTED, BUT THEIR NUMBERS ARE TOO FEW TO PERMIT A PRECISE ESTIMATE OF THE RATE.

THE INCIDENCE OF SEVERE, POTENTIALLY LIFE-THREATENING RASH IN PEDIATRIC PATIENTS, HOWEVER, IS VERY MUCH HIGHER THAN THAT REPORTED IN ADULTS USING LAMICTAL; SPECIFICALLY, REPORTS FROM CLINICAL TRIALS SUGGEST AS MANY AS 1 IN 50 TO 1 IN 100 PEDIATRIC PATIENTS DEVELOP A POTENTIALLY LIFE-THREATENING RASH. IT BEARS EMPHASIS, ACCORDINGLY, THAT LAMICTAL IS NOT APPROVED FOR USE IN PATIENTS BELOW THE AGE OF 16 (SEE INDICATIONS).

OTHER THAN AGE, THERE ARE AS YET NO FACTORS IDENTIFIED THAT ARE KNOWN TO PREDICT THE RISK OF OCCURRENCE OR THE SEVERITY OF RASH ASSOCIATED WITH LAMICTAL. THERE ARE SUGGESTIONS, YET TO BE PROVEN, THAT THE RISK OF RASH MAY ALSO BE INCREASED BY 1) COADMINISTRATION OF LAMICTAL WITH VALPROIC ACID (VPA), 2) EXCEEDING THE RECOMMENDED INITIAL DOSE OF LAMICTAL, OR 3) EXCEEDING THE RECOMMENDED DOSE ESCALATION FOR LAMICTAL. HOWEVER, CASES HAVE BEEN REPORTED IN THE ABSENCE OF THESE FACTORS.

NEARLY ALL CASES OF LIFE-THREATENING RASHES ASSOCIATED WITH LAMICTAL HAVE OCCURRED WITHIN 2 TO 8 WEEKS OF TREATMENT INITIATION. HOWEVER, ISOLATED CASES HAVE BEEN REPORTED AFTER PROLONGED TREATMENT (E.G., 6 MONTHS). ACCORDINGLY, DURATION OF THERAPY CANNOT BE RELIED UPON AS A MEANS TO PREDICT THE POTENTIAL RISK HERALDED BY THE FIRST APPEARANCE OF A RASH.

ALTHOUGH BENIGN RASHES ALSO OCCUR WITH LAMICTAL, IT IS NOT POSSIBLE TO PREDICT RELIABLY WHICH RASHES WILL PROVE TO BE LIFE-THREATENING. ACCORDINGLY, LAMICTAL SHOULD BE DISCONTINUED AT THE FIRST SIGN OF RASH, UNLESS THE RASH IS CLEARLY NOT DRUG RELATED. DISCONTINUATION OF TREATMENT MAY NOT PREVENT A RASH FROM BECOMING LIFE THREATENING OR PERMANENTLY DISABLING OR DISFIGURING.

DESCRIPTION

LAMICTAL (lamotrigine), an antiepileptic drug (AED) of the phenyltriazine class, is chemically unrelated to existing AEDs. Its chemical name is 6-(2,3-dichlorophenyl)-1,2,4-triazine-3,5-diamine, its molecular formula is $C_9H_7Cl_2N_5$, and its molecular weight is 256.09. Lamotrigine is a white to pale cream-colored powder and has a Pka of 5.7. Lamotrigine is very slightly soluble in water (0.17 mg/mL at 25°C) and slightly soluble in 0.1 M HCl (4.1 mg/mL at 25°C).

LAMICTAL is supplied for oral administration as 25-mg (white), 100-mg (peach), 150-mg (cream), and 200-mg (blue) tablets. Each tablet contains the labeled amount of lamotrigine and the following inactive ingredients: lactose; magnesium stearate; microcrystalline cellulose; povidone; sodium starch glycolate; FD&C Yellow No. 6 Lake (100-mg tablet only); ferric oxide, yellow (150-mg tablet only); FD&C Blue No. 2 Lake (200-mg tablet only).

CLINICAL PHARMACOLOGY

Mechanism of Action: The precise mechanism(s) by which lamotrigine exerts its anticonvulsant action are unknown. In animal models designed to detect anticonvulsant activity, lamotrigine was effective in preventing seizure spread in the maximum electroshock (MES) and pentylenetetrazol (scMet) tests, and prevented seizures in the visually and electrically evoked after-discharge (EEAD) tests for antiepileptic activity. The relevance of these models to human epilepsy, however, is not known.

One proposed mechanism of action of LAMICTAL, the relevance of which remains to be established in humans, involves an effect on sodium channels. In vitro pharmacological studies suggest that lamotrigine inhibits voltage-sensitive sodium channels, thereby stabilizing neuronal membranes and consequently modulating presynaptic transmitter release of excitatory amino acids (e.g., glutamate and aspartate).

Pharmacological Properties: Although the relevance for human use is unknown, the following data characterize the performance of LAMICTAL in receptor binding assays. Lamotrigine had a weak inhibitory effect on the serotonin 5-HT_3 receptor (IC_{50} = 18 μM). It does not exhibit high affinity binding (IC_{50}>100 μM) to the following neurotransmitter receptors: adenosine A_1 and A_2, adrenergic α_1, α_2, and β; dopamine D_1 and D_2; γ-aminobutyric acid (GABA) A and B; histamine H_1; kappa opioid; muscarinic acetylcholine; and serotonin 5-HT_2. Studies have failed to detect an effect of lamotrigine on dihydropyridine-sensitive calcium channels. It had weak effects at sigma opioid receptors (IC_{50}= 145 μM). Lamotrigine did not inhibit the uptake of norepinephrine, dopamine, serotonin, or aspartic acid (IC_{50}>100 μM).

Effect of Lamotrigine on NMDA-Mediated Activity: Lamotrigine did not inhibit NMDA-induced depolarizations in rat cortical slices or NMDA-induced cyclic GMP formation in immature rat cerebellum nor did lamotrigine displace compounds that are either competitive or noncompetitive ligands at this glutamate receptor complex (CNQX, CGS, TCHP). The IC_{50} for lamotrigine effects on NMDA-induced currents (in the presence of 3 μM glycine) in cultured hippocampal neurons exceeded 100 μM.

Folate Metabolism: In vitro, lamotrigine was shown to be an inhibitor of dihydrofolate reductase, the enzyme that catalyzes the reduction of dihydrofolate to tetrahydrofolate. Inhibition of this enzyme may interfere with the biosynthesis of nucleic acids and proteins. When oral daily doses of lamotrigine were given to pregnant rats during organogenesis, fetal, placental, and maternal folate concentrations were reduced. Significantly reduced concentrations of folate are associated with teratogenesis (see PRECAUTIONS: Pregnancy). Folate concentrations were also reduced in male rats given repeated oral doses of lamotrigine. Reduced concentrations were partially returned to normal when supplemented with folinic acid.

Accumulation in Kidneys: Lamotrigine was found to accumulate in the kidney of the male rat, causing chronic progressive nephrosis, necrosis, and mineralization. These findings are attributed to α-2 microglobulin, a species- and sex-specific protein that has not been detected in humans or other animal species.

Melanin Binding: Lamotrigine binds to melanin-containing tissues, e.g., in the eye and pigmented skin. It has been found in the uveal tract up to 52 weeks after a single dose in rodents.

Cardiovascular: In dogs, lamotrigine is extensively metabolized to a 2-N-methyl metabolite. This metabolite causes dose-dependent prolongations of the PR interval, widening of the QRS complex, and, at higher doses, complete AV conduction block. Similar cardiovascular effects are not anticipated in humans because only trace amounts of the 2-N-methyl metabolite (<0.6% of lamotrigine dose) have been found in human urine (see *Drug Disposition* below). However, it is conceivable that plasma concentrations of this metabolite could be increased in patients with a reduced capacity to glucuronidate lamotrigine (e.g., in patients with liver disease).

Pharmacokinetics and Drug Metabolism: The pharmacokinetics of lamotrigine have been studied in patients with epilepsy, healthy young and elderly volunteers, and volunteers with chronic renal failure. Lamotrigine pharmacokinetic parameters for adult patients and healthy normal volunteers are summarized in Table 1.

[See table 1 at bottom of next page]

The clearance of lamotrigine is affected by the coadministration of AEDs. Lamotrigine is eliminated more rapidly in patients who have been taking hepatic EIAEDs, including carbamazepine, phenytoin, phenobarbital, and primidone. Most clinical experience is derived from this population.

VPA, however, actually decreases the clearance of lamotrigine (i.e., more than doubles the elimination $T_{1/2}$ of lamotrigine), whether given with or without EIAEDs. Accordingly, if lamotrigine is to be administered to a patient receiving VPA, lamotrigine must be given at a reduced dosage, less than half the dose used in patients not receiving VPA (see DOSAGE AND ADMINISTRATION and PRECAUTIONS: Drug Interactions).

Absorption: Lamotrigine is rapidly and completely absorbed after oral administration with negligible first-pass metabolism (absolute bioavailability is 98%). The bioavailability is not affected by food. Peak plasma concentrations occur anywhere from 1.4 to 4.8 hours following drug administration.

Distribution: Estimates of the mean apparent volume of distribution (Vd/F) of lamotrigine following oral administration ranged from 0.9 to 1.3 L/kg. Vd/F is independent of dose and is similar following single and multiple doses in both patients with epilepsy and in healthy volunteers.

Protein Binding: Data from in vitro studies indicate that lamotrigine is approximately 55% bound to human plasma proteins at plasma lamotrigine concentrations from 1 to 10 mcg/mL (10 mcg/mL is four to six times the trough plasma concentration observed in the controlled efficacy trials.) Because lamotrigine is not highly bound to plasma proteins, clinically significant interactions with other drugs through competition for protein binding sites are unlikely. The binding of lamotrigine to plasma proteins did not change in the presence of therapeutic concentrations of phenytoin, phenobarbital, or VPA. Lamotrigine did not displace other AEDs (carbamazepine, phenytoin, phenobarbital) from protein binding sites.

Drug Disposition: Lamotrigine is metabolized predominantly by glucuronic acid conjugation; the major metabolite is an inactive 2-N-glucuronide conjugate. After oral administration of 240 mg of ^{14}C-lamotrigine (15 μCi) to six healthy volunteers, 94% was recovered in the urine and 2% was recovered in the feces. The radioactivity in the urine consisted of unchanged lamotrigine (10%), the 2-N-glucuronide (76%), a 5-N-glucuronide (10%), a 2-N-methyl metabolite (0.14%), and other unidentified minor metabolites (4%).

Enzyme Induction: The effects of lamotrigine on specific families of mixed-function oxidase isozymes have not been systematically evaluated.

Following multiple administrations (150 mg twice daily) to normal volunteers taking no other medications, lamotrigine induced its own metabolism, resulting in a 25% decrease in $T_{1/2}$ and a 37% increase in CL/F at steady state compared to values obtained in the same volunteers following a single dose. Evidence gathered from other sources suggests that self-induction by LAMICTAL may not occur when LAMICTAL is given as adjunctive therapy in patients receiving EIAEDs.

Dose Proportionality: In healthy volunteers not receiving any other medications and given single doses, the plasma concentrations of lamotrigine increased in direct proportion to the dose administered over the range of 50 to 400 mg. In two small studies (n = 7 and 8) of patients with epilepsy who were maintained on other AEDs, there also was a linear relationship between dose and lamotrigine plasma concentrations at steady state following doses of 50 to 350 mg twice daily.

Elimination: (See Table 1)

Special Populations: Patients With Renal Insufficiency: Twelve volunteers with chronic renal failure (mean creatinine clearance = 13 mL/min; range, 6 to 23) and another six individuals undergoing hemodialysis were each given a single 100-mg dose of LAMICTAL. The mean plasma half-lives determined in the study were 42.9 hours (chronic renal failure), 13.0 hours (during hemodialysis), and 57.4 hours (between hemodialysis) compared to 26.2 hours in healthy volunteers. On average, approximately 20% (range = 5.6 to 35.1) of the amount of lamotrigine present in the body was eliminated during a 4-hour hemodialysis session.

Hepatic Disease: The pharmacokinetic parameters of lamotrigine in patients with impaired liver function have not been studied.

Age: Elderly: In a single-dose study (150 mg of LAMICTAL), the pharmacokinetics of lamotrigine in twelve elderly volunteers between the ages of 65 and 76 years (mean creatinine clearance = 61 mL/min, range = 33 to 108) were similar to those of young healthy volunteers in other studies.

Gender: The clearance of lamotrigine is not affected by gender.

Race: The apparent oral clearance of lamotrigine was 25% lower in non-Caucasians than Caucasians.

Clinical Studies: The effectiveness of LAMICTAL as adjunctive therapy (added to other AEDs) was established in three multicenter, placebo-controlled, double-blind clinical trials in 355 adults with refractory partial seizures. The patients had a history of at least four partial seizures per month in spite of receiving one or more AEDs at therapeutic concentrations and, in two of the studies, were observed on their established AED regimen during baselines that varied between 8 to 12 weeks. In the third, patients were not observed in a prospective baseline. In patients continuing to have at least four seizures per month during the baseline, LAMICTAL or placebo was then added to the existing therapy. In all three studies, change from baseline in seizure frequency was the primary measure of effectiveness. The results given below are for all partial seizures in the intent-to-treat (all patients who received at least one dose of treatment) population in each study, unless otherwise indicated. The median seizure frequency at baseline was 3 per week while the mean at baseline was 6.6 per week for all patients enrolled in efficacy studies.

One study (n = 216) was a double-blind, placebo-controlled, parallel trial consisting of a 24-week treatment period. Patients could not be on more than two other anticonvulsants and VPA was not allowed. Patients were randomized to receive placebo, a target dose of 300 mg/day of LAMICTAL, or a target dose of 500 mg/day of LAMICTAL. The median reductions in the frequency of all partial seizures relative to baseline were 8% in patients receiving placebo, 20% in patients receiving 300 mg/day of LAMICTAL, and 36% in patients receiving 500 mg/day of LAMICTAL. The seizure frequency reduction was statistically significant in the 500-mg/day group compared to the placebo group, but not in the 300-mg/day group.

A second study (n = 98) was a double-blind, placebo-controlled, randomized crossover trial consisting of two 14-week treatment periods (the last 2 weeks of which consisted of dose tapering), separated by a 4-week washout period. Patients could not be on more than two other anticonvulsants and VPA was not allowed. The target dose of LAMICTAL was 400 mg/day. When the first 12 weeks of the treatment periods were analyzed, the median change in seizure frequency was a 25% reduction on LAMICTAL compared to placebo (*P*<0.001).

The third study (n = 41) was a double-blind, placebo-controlled, crossover trial consisting of two 12-week treatment periods, separated by a 4-week washout period. Patients could not be on more than two other anticonvulsants. Thirteen patients were on concomitant VPA; these patients received 150 mg/day of LAMICTAL. The 28 other patients had a target dose of 300 mg/day of LAMICTAL. The median change in seizure frequency was a 26% reduction on LAMICTAL compared to placebo (*P*<0.01).

No differences in efficacy based on age, sex, or race, as measured by change in seizure frequency, were detected.

INDICATIONS AND USAGE

LAMICTAL is indicated as adjunctive therapy in the treatment of partial seizures in adults with epilepsy. Safety and effectiveness in pediatric patients below the age of 16 have not been established (see BOX WARNING).

CONTRAINDICATIONS

LAMICTAL is contraindicated in patients who have demonstrated hypersensitivity to the drug or its ingredients.

WARNINGS

See BOX WARNING REGARDING THE RISK OF SEVERE, POTENTIALLY LIFE-THREATENING RASH ASSOCIATED WITH THE USE OF LAMICTAL.

Rash in the Pediatric Population: The incidence of severe, potentially life-threatening rash in pediatric patients is very much higher than that reported in adults using LAMICTAL. Specifically, reports from clinical trials suggest that as many as 1 in 50 to 1 in 100 pediatric patients develop a potentially life-threatening rash. It bears emphasis, accordingly, that LAMICTAL is not approved for use in patients below the age of 16 (see INDICATIONS).

Hypersensitivity Reactions: Hypersensitivity reactions, some fatal or life threatening, have also occurred. Some of these reactions have included clinical features of multiorgan dysfunction such as hepatic abnormalities and evidence of disseminated intravascular coagulation. It is important to note that early manifestations of hypersensitivity (e.g., fever, lymphadenopathy) may be present even though a rash is not evident. If such signs or symptoms are present, the patient should be evaluated immediately. LAMICTAL should be discontinued if an alternative etiology for the signs or symptoms cannot be established.

Prior to initiation of treatment with LAMICTAL, the patient should be instructed that a rash or other signs or symptoms of hypersensitivity (e.g., fever, lymphadenopathy) may herald a serious medical event and that the patient should report any such occurrence to a physician immediately.

Acute Multiorgan Failure: Fatalities associated with multiorgan failure and various degrees of hepatic failure have been reported in five patients from among 7000 exposed during premarketing development of LAMICTAL. These cases occurred in association with other serious medical events (e.g., status epilepticus, overwhelming sepsis), making it impossible to identify the initiating cause.

Dermatologic Events: In clinical trials, approximately 10% of all patients exposed to LAMICTAL developed a rash. However, in these trials not all cases of rash were attributed to LAMICTAL; 5% of patients exposed to placebo developed a rash. The overall rate of discontinuation due to rash in patients participating in clinical trials (n = 3501) was 3.8%. The incidence of rash appears to be increased among patients being treated with a multidrug regimen that includes both VPA and EIAEDs. When VPA and LAMICTAL have been used as a two-drug combination, the incidence of rash is further increased. NOTE: Dosing recommendations for the use of LAMICTAL and VPA alone cannot be provided because of insufficient experience with that combination (see DOSAGE AND ADMINISTRATION). The incidence of rash also appears to increase with the magnitude of the initial dose and the subsequent rate of dose escalation (see DOSAGE AND ADMINISTRATION).

Rashes associated with LAMICTAL do not appear to have unique identifying features. Typically, rash occurs in the first 2 to 8 weeks following treatment initiation. A benign initial appearance of a rash cannot predict an entirely benign outcome (see BOX WARNING).

Serious Rash Leading to Hospitalization: Rash resulting in hospitalization occurred in 0.3% of the approximately 3400 subjects who participated in premarketing clinical trials. No fatalities occurred among these individuals, but rash has been associated with a fatal outcome in reports from postmarketing experience.

Among the rashes leading to hospitalization were Stevens-Johnson syndrome, toxic epidermal necrolysis, angioedema, and a rash associated with a variable number of the following systemic manifestations: fever, lymphadenopathy, facial swelling, hematologic, and hepatologic abnormalities.

There is evidence that the inclusion of VPA in a multidrug regimen increases the risk of serious, potentially life-threatening rash. Specifically, of 584 patients administered LAMICTAL with VPA in clinical trials, 6 (1%) were hospitalized in association with rash; in contrast, 4 (0.16%) of 2398 clinical trial patients and volunteers administered LAMICTAL in the absence of VPA were hospitalized.

Other examples of serious and potentially life-threatening rash that did not lead to hospitalization also occurred in premarketing development. Among these, one case was reported to be Stevens-Johnson–like.

Pure Red Cell Aplasia (PRCA): A case of PRCA was reported in a 32-year-old male with a history of β-thalassemia. The patient had a microcytic anemia (hemoglobin 11 g/dL) that was stable while he was receiving carbamazepine but had become more severe in the 3 months after LAMICTAL was added. A bone marrow aspirate revealed markedly decreased erythropoiesis but normal granulopoiesis and thrombopoiesis. Erythropoiesis resumed after discontinuation of LAMICTAL and transfusions of packed red cells. Although PRCA is known to occur in patients with hemoglobinopathies, it is not known if β-thalassemia is a specific risk factor for the development of PRCA.

Sudden Unexplained Death in Epilepsy (SUDEP): During the premarketing development of LAMICTAL, 20 sudden and unexplained deaths were recorded among a cohort of 4700 patients with epilepsy (5747 patient-years of exposure).

Some of these could represent seizure-related deaths in which the seizure was not observed, e.g., at night. This represents an incidence of 0.0035 deaths per patient-year. Although this rate exceeds that expected in a healthy population matched for age and sex, it is within the range of estimates for the incidence of sudden unexplained deaths in patients with epilepsy not receiving LAMICTAL (ranging from 0.0005 for the general population of patients with epilepsy, to 0.004 for a recently studied clinical trial population similar to that in the clinical development program for LAMICTAL, to 0.005 for patients with refractory epilepsy). Consequently, whether these figures are reassuring or suggest concern depends on the comparability of the populations reported upon to the cohort receiving LAMICTAL and the accuracy of the estimates provided. Probably most reassuring is the similarity of estimated SUDEP rates in pa-

Continued on next page

Adult Study Population	Number of Subjects	t_max: Time of Maximum Plasma Concentration (h)	T_1/2: Elimination Half-life (h)	CL/F: Plasma Clearance (mL/min/kg)
Table 1: Mean* Pharmacokinetic Parameters in Adult Patients With Epilepsy or Healthy Volunteers				
Patients Taking Enzyme-Inducing Antiepileptic Drugs (EIAEDs)†:				
Single-Dose LAMICTAL	24	2.3 (0.5–5.0)	14.4 (6.4–30.4)	1.10 (0.51–2.22)
Multiple-Dose LAMICTAL	17	2.0 (0.75–5.93)	12.6 (7.5–23.1)	1.21 (0.66–1.82)
Patients Taking EIAEDs + VPA:				
Single-Dose LAMICTAL	25	3.8 (1.0–10.0)	27.2 (11.2–51.6)	0.53 (0.27–1.04)
Patients Taking VPA Only:				
Single-Dose LAMICTAL	4	4.8 (1.8–8.4)	58.8 (30.5–88.8)	0.28 (0.16–0.40)
Healthy Volunteers Taking VPA:				
Single-Dose LAMICTAL	6	1.8 (1.0–4.0)	48.3 (31.5–88.6)	0.30 (0.14–0.42)
Multiple-Dose LAMICTAL	18	1.9 (0.5–3.5)	70.3 (41.9–113.5)	0.18 (0.12–0.33)
Healthy Volunteers Taking No Other Medications:				
Single-Dose LAMICTAL	179	2.2 (0.25–12.0)	32.8 (14.0–103.0)	0.44 (0.12–1.10)
Multiple-Dose LAMICTAL	36	1.7 (0.5–4.0)	25.4 (11.6–61.6)	0.58 (0.24–1.15)

* The majority of parameter means determined in each study had coefficients of variation between 20% and 40% for $T_{1/2}$ and plasma clearance, and between 30% and 70% for t_{max}. The overall mean values were calculated from individual study means that were weighted based on the number of volunteers/patients in each study. The numbers in parentheses below each parameter mean represent the range of individual volunteer/patient values across studies.

† Examples of EIAEDs are carbamazepine, phenobarbital, phenytoin, and primidone.

This product information is based on labeling in effect on June 1, 1998. For further information, contact via direct mail, phone, or web site Medical Information: Glaxo Wellcome Inc., PO Box 13398, Research Triangle Park, NC 27709. Healthcare Professionals (Medical Information): 800-334-0089 Patients (Customer Response Center): 888-TALK2GW (1-888-825-5249) Glaxo Wellcome Corporate Web Site: www.glaxowellcome.com

Lamictal—Cont.

tients receiving LAMICTAL and those receiving another AED that underwent clinical testing in a similar population at about the same time. Importantly, that drug is chemically unrelated to LAMICTAL. This evidence suggests, although it certainly does not prove, that the high SUDEP rates reflect population rates, not a drug effect.

Withdrawal Seizures: As a rule, AEDs should not be abruptly discontinued because of the possibility of increasing seizure frequency. Unless safety concerns require a more rapid withdrawal, the dose of LAMICTAL should be tapered over a period of at least 2 weeks (see DOSAGE AND ADMINISTRATION).

Status Epilepticus: Valid estimates of the incidence of treatment-emergent status epilepticus among patients treated with LAMICTAL are difficult to obtain because reporters participating in clinical trials did not all employ identical rules for identifying cases. At a minimum, 7 of 2343 adult patients had episodes that could unequivocally be described as status. In addition, a number of reports of variably defined episodes of seizure exacerbation (e.g., seizure clusters, seizure flurries, etc.) were made.

PRECAUTIONS

Dermatological Events (see BOX WARNING, WARNINGS): Severe, potentially life-threatening rashes have been reported in association with therapy with LAMICTAL. Rare deaths have been reported, but their numbers are too few to permit a precise estimate of the rate. There are suggestions, yet to be proven, that the risk of rash may also be increased by 1) coadministration of LAMICTAL with VPA, 2) exceeding the recommended dose of LAMICTAL, or 3) exceeding the recommended dose escalation for LAMICTAL. However, cases have been reported in the absence of these factors.

Addition of LAMICTAL to a Multidrug Regimen That Includes VPA: *Dosage Reduction:* Because VPA reduces the clearance of lamotrigine, the dosage of lamotrigine in the presence of VPA is less than half of that required in its absence (see DOSAGE AND ADMINISTRATION).

Use in Patients With Concomitant Illness: Clinical experience with LAMICTAL in patients with concomitant illness is limited. Caution is advised when using LAMICTAL in patients with diseases or conditions that could affect metabolism or elimination of the drug, such as renal, hepatic, or cardiac functional impairment.

Hepatic metabolism to the glucuronide followed by renal excretion is the principal route of elimination of lamotrigine (see CLINICAL PHARMACOLOGY).

A study in individuals with severe chronic renal failure (mean creatinine clearance = 13 mL/min) not receiving other AEDs indicated that the elimination half-life of unchanged lamotrigine is prolonged relative to individuals with normal renal function. Until adequate numbers of patients with severe renal impairment have been evaluated during chronic treatment with LAMICTAL, it should be used with caution in these patients, generally using a reduced maintenance dose for patients with significant impairment.

Because there is no experience with the use of LAMICTAL in patients with impaired liver function, the use in such patients may be associated with as yet unrecognized risks.

Binding in the Eye and Other Melanin-Containing Tissues: Because lamotrigine binds to melanin, it could accumulate in melanin-rich tissues over time. This raises the possibility that lamotrigine may cause toxicity in these tissues after extended use. Although ophthalmological testing was performed in one controlled clinical trial, the testing was inadequate to exclude subtle effects or injury occurring after long-term exposure. Moreover, the capacity of available tests to detect potentially adverse consequences, if any, of lamotrigine's binding to melanin is unknown.

Accordingly, although there are no specific recommendations for periodic ophthalmological monitoring, prescribers should be aware of the possibility of long-term ophthalmologic effects.

Information for Patients: Prior to initiation of treatment with LAMICTAL, the patient should be instructed that a rash or other signs or symptoms of hypersensitivity (e.g., fever, lymphadenopathy) may herald a serious medical event and that the patient should report any such occurrence to a physician immediately. In addition, the patient should notify his physician if worsening of seizure control occurs.

Patients should be advised that LAMICTAL may cause dizziness, somnolence, and other symptoms and signs of central nervous system (CNS) depression. Accordingly, they should be advised neither to drive a car nor to operate other complex machinery until they have gained sufficient experience on LAMICTAL to gauge whether or not it affects their mental and/or motor performance adversely.

Patients should be advised to notify their physicians if they become pregnant or intend to become pregnant during therapy. Patients should be advised to notify their physicians if they intend to breast-feed or are breast-feeding an infant.

Laboratory Tests: The value of monitoring plasma concentrations of LAMICTAL has not been established. Because of the possible pharmacokinetic interactions between LAMICTAL and other AEDs being taken concomitantly (see Table 2), monitoring of the plasma levels of LAMICTAL and concomitant AEDs may be indicated, particularly during dosage adjustments. In general, clinical judgment should be exercised regarding monitoring of plasma levels of LAMICTAL and other antiseizure drugs and whether or not dosage adjustments are necessary.

Drug Interactions: *AEDs:* The use of AEDs in combination is complicated by the potential for pharmacokinetic interactions.

The interaction of lamotrigine with phenytoin, carbamazepine, and VPA has been characterized. With the exception of VPA, the addition of lamotrigine to these AEDs does not affect their steady-state plasma concentrations. The net effects of these various AED combinations on individual AED plasma concentrations are summarized in Table 2.

[See table 2 below]

Specific Effects of Lamotrigine on the Pharmacokinetics of Other AED Products: LAMICTAL Added to Phenytoin: LAMICTAL has no appreciable effect on steady-state phenytoin plasma concentration.

LAMICTAL Added to Carbamazepine: LAMICTAL has no appreciable effect on steady-state carbamazepine plasma concentration. Limited clinical data suggest there is a higher incidence of dizziness, diplopia, ataxia, and blurred vision in patients receiving carbamazepine with LAMICTAL than in patients receiving other EIAEDs with LAMICTAL (see ADVERSE REACTIONS). The mechanism of this interaction is unclear. The effect of lamotrigine on plasma concentrations of carbamazepine-epoxide is unclear. In a small subset of patients (n = 7) studied in a placebo-controlled trial, lamotrigine had no effect on carbamazepine-epoxide plasma concentrations, but in a small uncontrolled study (n = 9), carbamazepine-epoxide levels were seen to increase.

LAMICTAL Added to VPA: When LAMICTAL was administered to healthy volunteers already receiving VPA, the trough steady-state VPA concentrations in plasma decreased by an average of 25% over a 3-week period, and then stabilized.

LAMICTAL Added to VPA + Phenytoin and/or Carbamazepine: Although the effects of LAMICTAL on plasma levels of these AEDs given in combination has not been systematically evaluated, it is expected that the effects would be similar to those when LAMICTAL is added to each independently (e.g., VPA levels decrease, phenytoin and carbamazepine do not change).

Specific Effects of Other AED Products on the Pharmacokinetics of Lamotrigine: Phenytoin Added to LAMICTAL: The addition of phenytoin decreases lamotrigine steady-state concentrations by approximately 45% to 54% depending upon the total daily dose of phenytoin (i.e., from 100 to 400 mg).

Carbamazepine added to LAMICTAL: The addition of carbamazepine decreases lamotrigine steady-state concentrations by approximately 40%.

Phenobarbital or Primidone Added to LAMICTAL: The addition of phenobarbital or primidone decreases lamotrigine steady-state concentrations by approximately 40%.

VPA Added to LAMICTAL: The addition of VPA increases lamotrigine steady-state concentrations in normal volunteers by slightly more than two-fold.

Interactions With Drug Products Other Than Antiepileptics: Folate Inhibitors: Lamotrigine is an inhibitor of dihydrofolate reductase. Prescribers should be aware of this action when prescribing other medications that inhibit folate metabolism.

Drug/Laboratory Test Interactions: None known.

Carcinogenesis, Mutagenesis, Impairment of Fertility: No evidence of carcinogenicity was seen in one mouse study or two rat studies following oral administration of lamotrigine for up to 2 years at maximum tolerated doses (30 mg/kg per day for mice and 10 to 15 mg/kg per day for rats, doses that are equivalent to 90 mg/m^2 and 60 to 90 mg/m^2, respectively). Steady-state plasma concentrations ranged from 1 to 4 mcg/mL in the mouse study and 1 to 10 mcg/mL in the rat study. Plasma concentrations associated with the recommended human doses of 300 to 500 mg/day are generally in the range of 2 to 5 mcg/mL, but concentrations as high as 19 mcg/mL have been recorded.

Lamotrigine was not mutagenic in the presence or absence of metabolic activation when tested in two gene mutation assays (the Ames test and the in vitro mammalian mouse lymphoma assay). In two cytogenetic assays (the in vitro human lymphocyte assay and the in vivo rat bone marrow assay), lamotrigine did not increase the incidence of structural or numerical chromosomal abnormalities.

No evidence of impairment of fertility was detected in rats given oral doses of lamotrigine up to 2.4 times the highest usual human maintenance dose of 8.33 mg/kg per day or 0.4 times the human dose on a mg/m^2 basis. The effect of lamotrigine on human fertility is unknown.

Pregnancy: Pregnancy Category C. No evidence of teratogenicity was found in mice, rats, or rabbits when lamotrigine was orally administered to pregnant animals during the period of organogenesis at doses up to 1.2, 0.5, and 1.1 times, respectively, on a mg/m^2 basis, the highest usual human maintenance dose (i.e., 500 mg/day). However, maternal toxicity and secondary fetal toxicity producing reduced fetal weight and/or delayed ossification were seen in mice and rats, but not in rabbits at these doses. Teratology studies were also conducted using bolus intravenous (IV) administration of the isethionate salt of lamotrigine in rats and rabbits. In rat dams administered an IV dose at 0.6 times the highest usual human maintenance dose, the incidence of intrauterine death without signs of teratogenicity was increased.

A behavioral teratology study was conducted in rats dosed during the period of organogenesis. At day 21, postpartum offspring of dams receiving 5 mg/kg per day or higher displayed a significantly longer latent period for open field exploration and a lower frequency of rearing. In a swimming maze test performed on days 39 to 44 postpartum, time to completion was increased in offspring of dams receiving 25 mg/kg per day. These doses represent 0.1 and 0.5 times the clinical dose on a mg/m^2 basis, respectively.

Lamotrigine did not affect fertility, teratogenesis, or postnatal development when rats were dosed prior to and during mating, and throughout gestation and lactation at doses equivalent to 0.4 times the highest usual human maintenance dose on a mg/m^2 basis.

When pregnant rats were orally dosed at 0.1, 0.14, or 0.3 times the highest human maintenance dose (on a mg/m^2 basis) during the latter part of gestation (days 15 to 20), maternal toxicity and fetal death were seen. In dams, food consumption and weight gain were reduced, and the gestation period was slightly prolonged (22.6 versus 22.0 days in the control group). Stillborn pups were found in all three drug-treated groups with the highest number in the high-dose group. Postnatal death was also seen, but only in the two highest doses, and occurred between day 1 and 20. Some of these deaths appear to be drug-related and not secondary to the maternal toxicity. A no-observed-effect level (NOEL) could not be determined for this study.

Although LAMICTAL was not found to be teratogenic in the above studies, lamotrigine decreases fetal folate concentrations in rats, an effect known to be associated with teratogenesis in animals and humans. There are no adequate and well-controlled studies in pregnant women. Because animal reproduction studies are not always predictive of human response, this drug should be used during pregnancy only if the potential benefit justifies the potential risk to the fetus.

Pregnancy Exposure Registry: To facilitate monitoring fetal outcomes of pregnant women exposed to lamotrigine, physicians are encouraged to register patients in the Antiepileptic Drug Pregnancy Registry by calling (888) 233-2334 (toll free).

Labor and Delivery: The effect of LAMICTAL on labor and delivery in humans is unknown.

Use in Nursing Mothers: Preliminary data indicate that lamotrigine passes into human milk. Because the effects on

Table 2: Summary of AED Interactions With LAMICTAL

AED	AED Plasma Concentration With Adjunctive LAMICTAL*	Lamotrigine Plasma Concentration with Adjunctive AEDs†
Phenytoin (PHT)	↔	↓
Carbamazepine (CBZ)	↔	↓
CBZ epoxide‡	?§	
Valproic Acid (VPA)	↓	↑
VPA + PHT and/or CBZ	NE‖	↔

↔No significant effect.
* From adjunctive clinical trials and volunteer studies.
† Net effects were estimated by comparing the mean clearance values obtained in adjunctive clinical trials and volunteers studies.
‡ Not administered, but an active metabolite of carbamazepine.
§ Conflicting data.
‖ NE = not evaluated.

Table 3: Treatment-Emergent Adverse Event Incidence in Placebo-Controlled Adjunctive Trials*
(Events in at least 1% of patients treated with LAMICTAL
and numerically more frequent than in the placebo group.)

Body System/ Adverse Experience†	Percent of Patients Receiving LAMICTAL (n = 711)	Percent of Patients Receiving Placebo (n = 419)
Body as a whole		
Headache	29.1	19.1
Accidental injury	9.1	8.6
Flu syndrome	7.0	5.5
Fever	5.5	3.6
Abdominal pain	5.2	3.6
Infection	4.4	4.1
Neck pain	2.4	1.2
Malaise	2.3	1.9
Reaction aggravated (seizure exacerbation)	2.3	0.5
Chills	1.3	0.5
Cardiovascular		
Hot Flashes	1.3	0.0
Palpitations	1.0	0.5
Digestive		
Nausea	18.6	9.5
Vomiting	9.4	4.3
Diarrhea	6.3	4.1
Dyspepsia	5.3	2.1
Constipation	4.1	3.1
Tooth disorder	3.2	1.7
Anorexia	1.8	1.4
Dry mouth	1.0	0.2
Musculoskeletal		
Arthralgia	2.0	0.2
Joint disorder	1.3	1.0
Myasthenia	1.3	0.0
Nervous		
Dizziness	38.4	13.4
Ataxia	21.7	5.5
Somnolence	14.2	6.9
Incoordination	6.0	2.1
Insomnia	5.6	1.9
Tremor	4.4	1.4
Depression	4.2	2.6
Anxiety	3.8	2.6
Convulsion	3.2	1.2
Irritability	3.0	1.9
Speech disorder	2.5	0.2
Memory decreased	2.4	1.9
Confusion	1.8	1.7
Concentration disturbance	1.7	0.7
Sleep disorder	1.4	0.5
Emotional lability	1.3	0.2
Vertigo	1.1	0.2
Mind racing	1.0	0.5
Nystagmus	1.0	0.5
Dysarthria	1.0	0.2
Muscle spasm	1.0	0.2
Respiratory		
Rhinitis	13.6	9.3
Pharyngitis	9.8	8.8
Cough increased	7.5	5.7
Dyspnea	1.1	0.2
Skin and appendages		
Rash	10.0	5.0
Pruritus	3.1	1.7
Alopecia	1.3	1.2
Acne	1.3	0.5
Special senses		
Diplopia	27.6	6.7
Blurred vision	15.5	4.5
Vision abnormality	3.4	1.0
Ear pain	1.8	1.7
Tinnitus	1.1	1.0
Urogenital		
Female patients only	(n = 365)	(n = 207)
Dysmenorrhea	6.6	6.3
Vaginitis	4.1	0.5
Amenorrhea	1.9	0.5

* Patients in these adjunctive studies were receiving one to three concomitant enzyme-inducing antiepileptic drugs in addition to LAMICTAL or placebo. Patients may have reported multiple adverse experiences during the study or at discontinuation; thus, patients may be included in more than one category.
† Adverse experiences reported by at least 1% of patients treated with LAMICTAL are included.

the infant exposed to LAMICTAL by this route are unknown, breast-feeding while taking LAMICTAL is not recommended.

Pediatric Use: Safety and effectiveness in pediatric patients below the age of 16 have not been established (see BOX WARNING).

Geriatric Use: Because few patients over the age of 65 (approximately 20) were exposed to LAMICTAL during its premarket evaluation, no specific statements about the safety or effectiveness of LAMICTAL in this age group can be made.

ADVERSE REACTIONS
SEVERE, POTENTIALLY LIFE-THREATENING RASHES, INCLUDING STEVENS-JOHNSON SYNDROME AND TOXIC EPIDERMAL NECROLYSIS, HAVE OCCURRED IN ASSOCIATION WITH THERAPY WITH LAMICTAL. RARE DEATHS HAVE BEEN REPORTED, BUT THEIR NUMBERS ARE TOO FEW TO PERMIT A PRECISE ESTIMATE OF THE RATE (see BOX WARNING).

The most commonly observed adverse experiences associated with the use of LAMICTAL in combination with other AEDs, not seen at an equivalent frequency among placebo-

treated patients, were: dizziness, ataxia, somnolence, headache, diplopia, blurred vision, nausea, vomiting, and rash. Dizziness, diplopia, ataxia, blurred vision, nausea, and vomiting were dose related. Dizziness, diplopia, ataxia, and blurred vision occurred more commonly in patients receiving carbamazepine with LAMICTAL than in patients receiving other EIAEDs with LAMICTAL. Clinical data suggest a higher incidence of rash, including serious rash, in patients receiving concomitant VPA than in patients not receiving VPA (see WARNINGS).

Approximately 10% of the 3501 individuals who received LAMICTAL in premarketing clinical trials discontinued treatment because of an adverse experience. The adverse events most commonly associated with discontinuation were: rash (3.8%), dizziness (1.3%), and headache (1.3%).

In a dose response study, the rate of discontinuation of LAMICTAL for dizziness, ataxia, diplopia, blurred vision, nausea, and vomiting was dose related.

Incidence in Controlled Clinical Studies: Table 3 lists treatment-emergent signs and symptoms that occurred in at least 1% of patients with epilepsy treated with LAMICTAL participating in placebo-controlled trials and were numerically more common in the patients treated with LAMICTAL. In these studies, either LAMICTAL or placebo was added to the patient's current AED therapy. Adverse events were usually mild to moderate in intensity.

The prescriber should be aware that these figures, obtained when LAMICTAL was added to concurrent AED therapy, cannot be used to predict the frequency of adverse experiences in the course of usual medical practice where patient characteristics and other factors may differ from those prevailing during clinical studies. Similarly, the cited frequencies cannot be directly compared with figures obtained from other clinical investigations involving different treatments, uses, or investigators. An inspection of these frequencies, however, does provide the prescriber with one basis to estimate the relative contribution of drug and nondrug factors to the adverse event incidences in the population studied.

[See table 3 above]

In a randomized, parallel study comparing placebo and 300 and 500 mg per day of LAMICTAL, some of the more common drug-related adverse events were dose related (see Table 4).

[See table 4 at top of next page]

Other events that occurred in more than 1% of patients but equally or more frequently in the placebo group included: asthenia, back pain, chest pain, flatulence, menstrual disorder, myalgia, paresthesia, respiratory disorder, and urinary tract infection.

The overall adverse experience profile for LAMICTAL was similar between females and males, and was independent of age. Because the largest non-Caucasian racial subgroup was only 6% of patients exposed to LAMICTAL (46/711) in placebo-controlled trials, there are insufficient data to support a statement regarding the distribution of adverse experience reports by race. Generally, females receiving either adjunctive LAMICTAL or placebo were more likely to report adverse experiences than males. The only adverse experience for which the reports on LAMICTAL were greater than 10% more frequent in females than males (without a corresponding difference by gender on placebo) was dizziness (difference = 16.5%). There was little difference between females and males in the rates of discontinuation of LAMICTAL for individual adverse experiences.

Other Adverse Events Observed During All Clinical Trials:
Other Adverse Events: LAMICTAL has been administered to 3501 individuals during all clinical trials, only some of which were placebo-controlled. During these trials, all adverse events were recorded by the clinical investigators using terminology of their own choosing. To provide a meaningful estimate of the proportion of individuals having adverse events, similar types of events were grouped into a smaller number of standardized categories using modified COSTART dictionary terminology. The frequencies presented represent the proportion of the 3501 individuals exposed to LAMICTAL who experienced an event of the type cited on at least one occasion while receiving LAMICTAL. All reported events are included except those already listed in the previous table, those too general to be informative, and those not reasonably associated with the use of the drug.

Events are further classified within body system categories and enumerated in order of decreasing frequency using the following definitions: *frequent* adverse events are defined as

Continued on next page

This product information is based on labeling in effect on June 1, 1998. For further information, contact via direct mail, phone, or web site Medical Information: Glaxo Wellcome Inc., PO Box 13398, Research Triangle Park, NC 27709. Healthcare Professionals (Medical Information): 800-334-0089 Patients (Customer Response Center): 888-TALK2GW (1-888-825-5249) Glaxo Wellcome Corporate Web Site: www.glaxowellcome.com

Lamictal—Cont.

those occurring in at least 1/100 patients; *infrequent* adverse events are those occurring in 1/100 to 1/1000 patients; *rare* adverse events are those occurring in fewer than 1/1000 patients.

Body as a Whole: ***Infrequent:*** Allergic reaction, face edema, and halitosis. ***Rare:*** Abdomen enlarged, abscess, photosensitivity, and suicide attempt.

Cardiovascular System: ***Infrequent:*** Flushing, migraine, postural hypotension, syncope, tachycardia, and vasodilation. ***Rare:*** Angina pectoris, atrial fibrillation, deep thrombophlebitis, hemorrhage, hypertension, and myocardial infarction.

Dermatological: ***Infrequent:*** Dry skin, eczema, erythema, hirsutism, maculopapular rash, sweating, vesiculobullous rash, and urticaria. ***Rare:*** Angioedema, fungal dermatitis, herpes zoster, leukoderma, petechial rash, pustular rash, seborrhea, skin discoloration, and Stevens-Johnson syndrome.

Digestive System: ***Infrequent:*** Dysphagia, gingivitis, glossitis, gum hyperplasia, increased appetite, increased salivation, liver function tests abnormal, mouth ulceration, stomatitis, and thirst. ***Rare:*** Eructation, gastritis, gastrointestinal hemorrhage, gum hemorrhage, hemorrhagic colitis, hepatitis, melena, stomach ulcer, and tongue edema.

Endocrine System: ***Rare:*** Goiter and hypothyroidism.

Hematologic and Lymphatic System: ***Infrequent:*** Anemia, ecchymosis, eosinophilia, leukocytosis, leukopenia, lymphadenopathy, and petechia. ***Rare:*** Fibrin decrease, fibrinogen decrease, iron deficiency anemia, macrocytic anemia, and thrombocytopenia.

Metabolic and Nutritional Disorders: ***Frequent:*** Weight gain. ***Infrequent:*** Alkaline phosphatase increase, peripheral edema, and weight loss. ***Rare:*** Alcohol intolerance, bilirubinemia, general edema, and hyperglycemia.

Musculoskeletal System: ***Infrequent:*** Twitching. ***Rare:*** Arthritis, bursitis, leg cramps, tendinous contracture, and pathological fracture.

Nervous System: ***Frequent:*** Amnesia, hostility, nervousness, thinking abnormality. ***Infrequent:*** Abnormal dreams, abnormal gait, agitation, akathisia, apathy, aphasia, CNS depression, depersonalization, dyskinesia, dysphoria, euphoria, faintness, hallucinations, hyperkinesia, hypesthesia, myoclonus, panic attack, paranoid reaction, personality disorder, psychosis, and stupor. ***Rare:*** Cerebrovascular accident, cerebellar syndrome, cerebral sinus thrombosis, choreoathetosis, CNS stimulation, delirium, delusions, dystonia, grand mal convulsions, hemiplegia, hyperalgesia, hyperesthesia, hypertonia, hypokinesia, hypomania, hypotonia, libido decreased, libido increased, manic depression reaction, movement disorder, neuralgia, neurosis, paralysis, and suicidal ideation.

Respiratory System: ***Infrequent:*** Epistaxis and hyperventilation. ***Rare:*** Bronchospasm, hiccup, and pneumonia.

Special Senses: ***Infrequent:*** Abnormality of accommodation, conjunctivitis, oscillopsia, photophobia, and taste perversion. ***Rare:*** Deafness, dry eyes, lacrimation disorder, parosmia, ptosis, strabismus, taste loss, and uveitis.

Urogenital System: ***Infrequent:*** Breast pain, female lactation, hematuria, impotence, polyuria, urinary frequency, urinary incontinence, urinary retention, and vaginal moniliasis. ***Rare:*** Abnormal ejaculation, acute kidney failure, breast abscess, cystitis, dysuria, breast neoplasm, creatinine increase, epididymitis, kidney failure, kidney pain, menorrhagia, and urine abnormality.

Postmarketing and Other Experience: In addition to the adverse experiences reported during clinical testing of LAMICTAL, the following adverse experiences have been reported in patients receiving marketed LAMICTAL in other countries and from worldwide noncontrolled investigational use. These adverse experiences have not been listed above and data are insufficient to support an estimate of their incidence or to establish causation. The listing is alphabetized: Aplastic anemia, apnea, disseminated intravascular coagulation, erythema multiforme, esophagitis, hematemesis, hemolytic anemia, hypersensitivity reaction, multiorgan failure, neutropenia, pancreatitis, pancytopenia and progressive immunosuppression.

Table 4: Dose-Related Adverse Events From a Randomized, Placebo-Controlled Trial

Adverse Experience (AE)	Percent of Patients Experiencing AE		
	Placebo (n = 73)	LAMICTAL 300 mg (n = 71)	LAMICTAL 500 mg (n = 72)
Ataxia	10	10	28*†
Blurred vision	10	11	25*†
Diplopia	8	24*	49*†
Dizziness	27	31	54*†
Nausea	11	18	25*
Vomiting	4	11	18*

* Significantly greater than placebo group ($P<0.05$).
† Significantly greater than group receiving LAMICTAL 300 mg ($P<0.05$).

DRUG ABUSE AND DEPENDENCE

The abuse and dependence potential of LAMICTAL have not been evaluated in human studies.

OVERDOSAGE

Human Overdose Experience: Experience with single or daily doses >700 mg is limited. During the clinical development of LAMICTAL, the highest known overdoses were in two women who each ingested doses >4000 mg. The plasma concentration of lamotrigine in one woman was 52 mcg/mL 4 hours after the ingestion (a value more than 10 times greater than that seen in clinical trials). She became comatose and remained comatose for 8 to 12 hours; no electrocardiographic abnormalities were detected. The other patient had dizziness, headache, and somnolence. Both women recovered without sequelae.

Management of Overdose: There are no specific antidotes for LAMICTAL. Following a suspected overdose, hospitalization of the patient is advised. General supportive care is indicated, including frequent monitoring of vital signs and close observation of the patient. If indicated, emesis should be induced or gastric lavage should be performed; usual precautions should be taken to protect the airway. It should be kept in mind that lamotrigine is rapidly absorbed (see CLINICAL PHARMACOLOGY). It is uncertain whether hemodialysis is an effective means of removing lamotrigine from the blood. In six renal failure patients, about 20% of the amount of lamotrigine in the body was removed during 4 hours of hemodialysis. A Poison Control Center should be contacted for information on the management of overdosage of LAMICTAL.

DOSAGE AND ADMINISTRATION

LAMICTAL is recommended as adjunctive therapy in adults. **Safety and effectiveness in pediatric patients below the age of 16 have not been established (see BOX WARNING).**

General Dosing Considerations: The risk of nonserious rash in increased when the recommended initial dose and/or the rate of dose escalation of LAMICTAL is exceeded. There are suggestions, yet to be proven, that the risk of severe, potentially life-threatening rash may be increased by 1) coadministration of LAMICTAL with VPA, 2) exceeding the recommended initial dose of LAMICTAL, or 3) exceeding the recommended dose escalation for LAMICTAL. However, cases have been reported in the absence of these factors (see BOX WARNING). Therefore, it is important that the dosing recommendations be followed closely.

Patients Receiving VPA as One Component of a Combination Regimen Also Including EIAEDs: In patients taking VPA as one component of a combination regimen also including EIAEDs, the initial dose of LAMICTAL is 25 mg every other day for 2 weeks, followed by 25 mg once a day for 2 weeks. Because the clearance of lamotrigine is decreased about 50% in the presence of VPA, the daily dose of LAMICTAL should ordinarily be no more than 150 mg a day, and should be administered on a twice daily schedule. To achieve maintenance, doses may be increased by 25 to 50 mg/day every 1 to 2 weeks (see Table 5).

Note: The efficacy of adjunctive LAMICTAL in patients taking VPA alone has not been evaluated in controlled trials although it has been used in some patients. Consequently, an effective and safe dosing recommendation for the use of LAMICTAL and VPA as a two-drug regimen cannot be offered. If this regimen is nonetheless used, it should be noted that blood concentrations of LAMICTAL appear to be twice those associated with the use of LAMICTAL in a regimen containing both EIAEDs and VPA.

Patients Receiving EIAEDs, But Not VPA: The initial dose of LAMICTAL in patients not taking VPA is 50 mg once a day for 2 weeks, followed by 100 mg/day given in two divided doses for 2 weeks. Thereafter, the usual maintenance dose is 300 to 500 mg/day given in two divided doses. To achieve maintenance, doses may be increased by 100 mg/day every 1 to 2 weeks (see Table 5).

[See table 5 below]

Because of an increased risk of rash, the recommended initial dose and subsequent dose escalations of LAMICTAL should not be exceeded (see BOX WARNING).

The usual maintenance doses identified in the table above are derived from dosing regimens employed in the placebo-controlled adjunctive studies in which the efficacy of LAMICTAL was established. In patients receiving multidrug regimens employing EIAEDs **without VPA**, maintenance doses of LAMICTAL as high as 700 mg/day have been used. In patients receiving multidrug regimens employing EIAEDs **with VPA**, maintenance doses of LAMICTAL as high as 200 mg/day have been used. The advantage of using doses above those recommended in the table above has not been established in controlled trials.

Patients With Renal Functional Impairment: Initial doses of LAMICTAL should be based on patients' AED regimen (see above); reduced maintenance doses may be effective for patients with significant renal functional impairment (see CLINICAL PHARMACOLOGY). Few patients with severe renal impairment have been evaluated during chronic treatment with LAMICTAL. Because there is inadequate experience in this population, LAMICTAL should be used with caution in these patients.

Discontinuation Strategy: For patients receiving LAMICTAL in combination with other AEDs, a reevaluation of all AEDs in the regimen should be considered if a change in seizure control or an appearance or worsening of adverse experiences is observed.

If a decision is made to discontinue therapy with LAMICTAL, a step-wise reduction of dose over at least 2 weeks (approximately 50% per week) is recommended unless safety concerns require a more rapid withdrawal (see PRECAUTIONS).

Discontinuing an EIAED should prolong the half-life of lamotrigine; discontinuing VPA should shorten the half-life of lamotrigine.

Target Plasma Levels: A therapeutic plasma concentration range has not been established for lamotrigine. Dosing of LAMICTAL should be based on therapeutic response.

Table 5: Dose Recommendations for LAMICTAL (mg/day) for Adults (over 16 Years)

	Weeks 1 and 2	Weeks 3 and 4	Usual Maintenance Dose
With EIAEDs* & VPA	25 mg every other day	25 mg (once a day)	100–150 mg/day (two divided doses). To achieve maintenance, doses may be increased by 25–50 mg/day every 1 to 2 weeks.
With EIAEDs & No VPA	50 mg/day (once a day)	100 mg/day (two divided doses)	300 to 500 mg/day (two divided doses). To achieve maintenance, doses may be increased by 100 mg/day every 1 to 2 weeks.

* e.g., Phenytoin, carbamazepine, phenobarbital, and primidone.

HOW SUPPLIED

LAMICTAL Tablets, 25 mg, are white, scored, shield-shaped tablets engraved with "LAMICTAL 25" in bottles of 100 (NDC 0173-0633-02) tablets.

Store at 15° to 25°C (59° to 77°F) in a dry place.

LAMICTAL Tablets, 100 mg, are peach, scored, shield-shaped tablets engraved with "LAMICTAL 100" in bottles of 100 (NDC 0173-0642-55) tablets.

LAMICTAL Tablets, 150 mg, are cream, scored, shield-shaped tablets engraved with "LAMICTAL 150" in bottles of 60 (NDC 0173-0643-60) tablets.

LAMICTAL Tablets, 200 mg, are blue, scored, shield-shaped tablets engraved with "LAMICTAL 200" in bottles of 60 (NDC 0173-0644-60) tablets.

Store at 15° to 25°C (59° to 77°F) in a dry place and protect from light.

Caution: Federal law prohibits dispensing without prescription.

U.S. Patent No. 4,602,017

October 1997/RL-421

Shown in Product Identification Guide, page 313

LANOXICAPS® ℞

[*lă-nŏx 'ĭ-kăps* "]

(digoxin solution in capsules)

50 mcg (0.05 mg) I.D. Imprint A2C (red)
100 mcg (0.1 mg) I.D. Imprint B2C (yellow)
200 mcg (0.2 mg) I.D. Imprint C2C (green)

Table 1: Comparisons of the Systemic Availability and Equivalent Doses for Preparations of LANOXIN

Product	Absolute Bioavailability	Equivalent Doses (mcg)* Among Dosage Forms			
LANOXIN Tablets	60–80%	62.5	125	250	500
LANOXIN Elixir Pediatric	70–85%	62.5	125	250	500
LANOXICAPS®	90–100%	50	100	200	400
LANOXIN Injection/IV	100%	50	100	200	400

* For example, 125 mcg LANOXIN Tablets equivalent to 125 mcg LANOXIN Elixir Pediatric equivalent to 100 mcg LANOXICAPS equivalent to 100 mcg LANOXIN Injection/IV.

DESCRIPTION

LANOXIN (digoxin) is one of the cardiac (or digitalis) glycosides, a closely related group of drugs having in common specific effects on the myocardium. These drugs are found in a number of plants. Digoxin is extracted from the leaves of *Digitalis lanata*. The term "digitalis" is used to designate the whole group of glycosides. The glycosides are composed of two portions: a sugar and a cardenolide (hence "glycosides").

Digoxin is described chemically as (3β,5β,12β)-3-[(*O*-2,6-dideoxy-β-*D*-*ribo*-hexopyranosyl-(1→4)-*O*-2,6-dideoxy-β-*D*-*ribo*-hexopyranosyl-(1→4)-2,6-dideoxy-β-*D*-*ribo*-hexopyranosyl)oxy]-12,14-dihydroxy-card-20(22)-enolide. Its molecular formula is $C_{41}H_{64}O_{14}$, its molecular weight is 780.95.

Digoxin exists as odorless white crystals that melt with decomposition above 230°C. The drug is practically insoluble in water and in ether; slightly soluble in diluted (50%) alcohol and in chloroform; and freely soluble in pyridine.

LANOXICAPS is a stable solution of digoxin enclosed within a soft gelatin capsule for oral use. Each capsule contains the labeled amount of digoxin USP dissolved in a solvent comprised of polyethylene glycol 400 USP, 8 percent ethyl alcohol, propylene glycol USP, and purified water USP. Inactive ingredients in the capsule shell include FD&C Red No. 40 (0.05-mg Capsule), D&C Yellow No. 10 (0.1-mg and 0.2-mg Capsules), FD&C Blue No. 1 (0.2-mg Capsule), gelatin, glycerin, methylparaben and propylparaben (added as preservatives), purified water, and sorbitol. Capsules are printed with edible ink.

CLINICAL PHARMACOLOGY

Mechanism of Action: Digoxin inhibits sodium-potassium ATPase, an enzyme that regulates the quantity of sodium and potassium inside cells. Inhibition of the enzyme leads to an increase in the intracellular concentration of sodium and thus (by stimulation of sodium-calcium exchange) an increase in the intracellular concentration of calcium. The beneficial effects of digoxin result from direct actions on cardiac muscle, as well as indirect actions on the cardiovascular system mediated by effects on the autonomic nervous system. The autonomic effects include: (1) a vagomimetic action, which is responsible for the effects of digoxin on the sinoatrial and atrioventricular (AV) nodes; and (2) baroreceptor sensitization, which results in increased afferent inhibitory activity and reduced activity of the sympathetic nervous system and renin-angiotensin system for any given increment in mean arterial pressure. The pharmacologic consequences of these direct and indirect effects are: (1) an increase in the force and velocity of myocardial systolic contraction (positive inotropic action); (2) a decrease in the degree of activation of the sympathetic nervous system and renin-angiotensin system (neurohormonal deactivating effect); and (3) slowing of the heart rate and decreased conduction velocity through the AV node (vagomimetic effect). The effects of digoxin in heart failure are mediated by its positive inotropic and neurohormonal deactivating effects, whereas the effects of the drug in atrial arrhythmias are related to its vagomimetic actions. In high doses, digoxin increases sympathetic outflow from the central nervous system (CNS). This increase in sympathetic activity may be an important factor in digitalis toxicity.

Pharmacokinetics: ***Absorption:*** Absorption of digoxin from LANOXICAPS Capsules has been demonstrated to be 90% to 100% complete compared to an identical intravenous dose of digoxin (absolute bioavailability). In comparison, the absolute bioavailability of conventional digoxin tablets has been demonstrated to be 60% to 80%. The enhanced absorption from LANOXICAPS compared to digoxin tablets and elixir is associated with reduced between-patient and within-patient variability in steady-state serum concentrations. The peak serum concentrations are higher than those observed after tablets. When digoxin tablets or capsules are taken after meals, the rate of absorption is slowed, but the total amount of digoxin absorbed is usually unchanged. When taken with meals high in bran fiber, however, the amount absorbed from an oral dose may be reduced. Comparisons of the systemic availability and equivalent doses for preparations of LANOXIN are shown in Table 1:

[See table 1 above]

In some patients, orally administered digoxin is converted to inactive reduction products (e.g., dihydrodigoxin) by colonic bacteria in the gut. Data suggest that one in ten patients treated with digoxin tablets will degrade 40% or more of the ingested dose. As a result, certain antibiotics may increase the absorption of digoxin in such patients. Although inactivation of these bacteria by antibiotics is rapid, the serum digoxin concentration will rise at a rate consistent with the elimination half-life of digoxin. The magnitude of rise in serum digoxin concentration relates to the extent of bacterial inactivation, and may be as much as two-fold in some cases. This phenomenon is minimized with LANOXICAPS because they are rapidly absorbed in the upper gastrointestinal tract.

Distribution: Following drug administration, a 6- to 8-hour tissue distribution phase is observed. This is followed by a much more gradual decline in the serum concentration of the drug, which is dependent on the elimination of digoxin from the body. The peak height and slope of the early portion (absorption/distribution phases) of the serum concentration-time curve are dependent upon the route of administration and the absorption characteristics of the formulation. Clinical evidence indicates that the early high serum concentrations (particularly high for digoxin capsules) do not reflect the concentration of digoxin at its site of action, but that with chronic use, the steady-state post-distribution serum levels are in equilibrium with tissue concentrations and correlate with pharmacologic effects. In individual patients, these post-distribution serum concentrations may be useful in evaluating therapeutic and toxic effects (see DOSAGE AND ADMINISTRATION: Serum Digoxin Concentrations).

Digoxin is concentrated in tissues and therefore has a large apparent volume of distribution. Digoxin crosses both the blood-brain barrier and the placenta. At delivery, the serum digoxin concentration in the newborn is similar to the serum concentration in the mother. Approximately 25% of digoxin in the plasma is bound to protein. Serum digoxin concentrations are not significantly altered by large changes in fat tissue weight, so that its distribution space correlates best with lean (i.e., ideal) body weight, not total body weight.

Metabolism: Only a small percentage (16%) of a dose of digoxin is metabolized. The end metabolites, which include 3 β-digoxigenin, 3-keto-digoxigenin, and their glucuronide and sulfate conjugates, are polar in nature and are postulated to be formed via hydrolysis, oxidation, and conjugation. The metabolism of digoxin is not dependent upon the cytochrome P-450 system, and digoxin is not known to induce or inhibit the cytochrome P-450 system.

Excretion: Elimination of digoxin follows first-order kinetics (that is, the quantity of digoxin eliminated at any time is proportional to the total body content). Following intravenous administration to healthy volunteers, 50% to 70% of a digoxin dose is excreted unchanged in the urine. Renal excretion of digoxin is proportional to glomerular filtration rate and is largely independent of urine flow. In healthy volunteers with normal renal function, digoxin has a half-life of 1.5 to 2.0 days. The half-life in anuric patients is prolonged to 3.5 to 5 days. Digoxin is not effectively removed from the body by dialysis, exchange transfusion, or during cardiopulmonary bypass because most of the drug is bound to tissue and does not circulate in the blood.

Special Populations: Race differences in digoxin pharmacokinetics have not been formally studied. Because digoxin is primarily eliminated as unchanged drug via the kidney and because there are no important differences in creatinine clearance among races, pharmacokinetic differences due to race are not expected.

The clearance of digoxin can be primarily correlated with renal function as indicated by creatinine clearance. The Cockcroft and Gault formula for estimation of creatinine clearance includes age, body weight, and gender. A table that provides the usual daily maintenance dose requirements of LANOXICAPS Capsules based on creatinine clearance (per 70kg) is presented in the DOSAGE AND ADMINISTRATION section. Plasma digoxin concentration profiles in patients with acute hepatitis generally fell within the range of profiles in a group of healthy subjects.

Pharmacodynamic and Clinical Effects: The times to onset of pharmacologic effect and to peak effect of preparations of LANOXIN are shown in Table 2:

[See table 2 at top of next page]

Hemodynamic Effects: Digoxin produces hemodynamic improvement in patients with heart failure. Short- and long-term therapy with the drug increases cardiac output and lowers pulmonary artery pressure, pulmonary capillary wedge pressure, and systemic vascular resistance. These hemodynamic effects are accompanied by an increase in the left ventricular ejection fraction and a decrease in end-systolic and end-diastolic dimensions.

Chronic Heart Failure: Two 12-week, double-blind, placebo-controlled studies enrolled 178 (RADIANCE trial) and 88 (PROVED trial) patients with NYHA class II or III heart failure previously treated with digoxin, a diuretic, and an ACE inhibitor (RADIANCE only) and randomized them to placebo or treatment with LANOXIN Tablets. Both trials demonstrated better preservation of exercise capacity in patients randomized to LANOXIN. Continued treatment with LANOXIN reduced the risk of developing worsening heart failure, as evidenced by heart failure-related hospitalizations and emergency care and the need for concomitant heart failure therapy. The larger study also showed treatment-related benefits in NYHA class and patients' global assessment. In the smaller trial, these trended in favor of a treatment benefit.

The Digitalis Investigation Group (DIG) main trial was a multicenter, randomized, double-blind, placebo-controlled mortality study of 6801 patients with heart failure and left ventricular ejection fraction ≤0.45. At randomization, 67% were NYHA class I or II, 71% had heart failure of ischemic etiology, 44% had been receiving digoxin, and most were receiving concomitant ACE inhibitor (94%) and diuretic (82%). Patients were randomized to placebo or LANOXIN Tablets, the dose of which was adjusted for the patient's age, sex, lean body weight, and serum creatinine (see DOSAGE AND ADMINISTRATION), and followed for up to 58 months (median 37 months). The median daily dose prescribed was 0.25 mg. Overall all-cause mortality was 35% with no difference between groups (95% confidence limits for relative risk of 0.91 to 1.07). LANOXIN was associated with a 25% reduction in the number of hospitalizations for heart failure, a 28% reduction in the risk of a patient having at least one hospitalization for heart failure, and a 6.5% reduction in total hospitalizations (for any cause).

Use of LANOXIN was associated with a trend in reduction in time to all-cause death or hospitalization. The trend was evident in subgroups of patients with mild heart failure as well as more severe disease, as shown in Table 3. Although the effect on all-cause death or hospitalization was not statistically significant, much of the apparent benefit derived from effects on mortality and hospitalization attributed to heart failure.

[See table 3 at top of next page]

In situations where there is no statistically significant benefit of treatment evident from a trial's primary endpoint, results pertaining to a secondary endpoint should be interpreted cautiously.

Chronic Atrial Fibrillation: In patients with chronic atrial fibrillation, digoxin slows rapid ventricular response rate in a linear dose-response fashion from 0.25 to 0.75 mg/day. Digoxin should not be used for the treatment of multifocal atrial tachycardia.

INDICATIONS AND USAGE

Heart Failure: LANOXIN is indicated for the treatment of mild to moderate heart failure. LANOXIN increases left ventricular ejection fraction and improves heart failure symptoms as evidenced by exercise capacity and heart failure-related hospitalizations and emergency care, while having no effect on mortality. Where possible, LANOXIN should be used with a diuretic and an angiotensin-converting enzyme inhibitor, but an optimal order for starting these three drugs cannot be specified.

Atrial Fibrillation: LANOXIN is indicated for the control of ventricular response rate in patients with chronic atrial fibrillation.

CONTRAINDICATIONS

Digitalis glycosides are contraindicated in patients with ventricular fibrillation or in patients with a known hyper-

Continued on next page

This product information is based on labeling in effect on June 1, 1998. For further information, contact via direct mail, phone, or web site Medical Information: Glaxo Wellcome Inc., PO Box 13398, Research Triangle Park, NC 27709. Healthcare Professionals (Medical Information): 800-334-0089 Patients (Customer Response Center): 888-TALK2GW (1-888-825-5249) Glaxo Wellcome Corporate Web Site: www.glaxowellcome.com

Lanoxicaps—Cont.

sensitivity to digoxin. A hypersensitivity reaction to other digitalis preparations usually constitutes a contraindication to digoxin.

WARNINGS

Sinus Node Disease and AV Block: Because digoxin slows sinoatrial and AV conduction, the drug commonly prolongs the PR interval. The drug may cause severe sinus bradycardia or sinoatrial block in patients with pre-existing sinus node disease and may cause advanced or complete heart block in patients with pre-existing incomplete AV block. In such patients consideration should be given to the insertion of a pacemaker before treatment with digoxin.

Accessory AV Pathway (Wolff-Parkinson-White Syndrome): After intravenous digoxin therapy, some patients with paroxysmal atrial fibrillation or flutter and a coexisting accessory AV pathway have developed increased antegrade conduction across the accessory pathway bypassing the AV node, leading to a very rapid ventricular response or ventricular fibrillation. Unless conduction down the accessory pathway has been blocked (either pharmacologically or by surgery), digoxin should not be used in such patients. The treatment of paroxysmal supraventricular tachycardia in such patients is usually direct-current cardioversion.

Use in Patients with Preserved Left Ventricular Systolic Function: Patients with certain disorders involving heart failure associated with preserved left ventricular ejection fraction may be particularly susceptible to toxicity of the drug. Such disorders include restrictive cardiomyopathy, constrictive pericarditis, amyloid heart disease, and acute cor pulmonale. Patients with idiopathic hypertrophic subaortic stenosis may have worsening of the outflow obstruction due to the inotropic effects of digoxin.

PRECAUTIONS

Use in Patients with Impaired Renal Function: Digoxin is primarily excreted by the kidneys; therefore, patients with impaired renal function require smaller than usual maintenance doses of digoxin (see DOSAGE AND ADMINISTRATION). Because of the prolonged elimination half-life, a longer period of time is required to achieve an initial or new steady-state serum concentration in patients with renal impairment than in patients with normal renal function. If appropriate care is not taken to reduce the dose of digoxin, such patients are at high risk for toxicity, and toxic effects will last longer in such patients than in patients with normal renal function.

Use in Patients with Electrolyte Disorders: In patients with hypokalemia or hypomagnesemia, toxicity may occur despite serum digoxin concentrations below 2.0 ng/mL, because potassium or magnesium depletion sensitizes the myocardium to digoxin. Therefore, it is desirable to maintain normal serum potassium and magnesium concentrations in patients being treated with digoxin. Deficiencies of these electrolytes may result from malnutrition, diarrhea, or prolonged vomiting, as well as the use of the following drugs or procedures: diuretics, amphotericin B, corticosteroids, antacids, dialysis, and mechanical suction of gastrointestinal secretions.

Hypercalcemia from any cause predisposes the patient to digitalis toxicity. Calcium, particularly when administered rapidly by the intravenous route, may produce serious arrhythmias in digitalized patients. On the other hand, hypocalcemia can nullify the effects of digoxin in humans; thus, digoxin may be ineffective until serum calcium is restored to normal. These interactions are related to the fact that digoxin affects contractility and excitability of the heart in a manner similar to that of calcium.

Use in Thyroid Disorders and Hypermetabolic States: Hypothyroidism may reduce the requirements for digoxin. Heart failure and/or atrial arrhythmias resulting from hypermetabolic or hyperdynamic states (e.g., hyperthyroidism, hypoxia, or arteriovenous shunt) are best treated by addressing the underlying condition. Atrial arrhythmias associated with hypermetabolic states are particularly resistant to digoxin treatment. Care must be taken to avoid toxicity if digoxin is used.

Use in Patients with Acute Myocardial Infarction: Digoxin should be used with caution in patients with acute myocardial infarction. The use of inotropic drugs in some patients in this setting may result in undesirable increases in myocardial oxygen demand and ischemia.

Use During Electrical Cardioversion: It may be desirable to reduce the dose of digoxin for 1 to 2 days prior to electrical cardioversion of atrial fibrillation to avoid the induction of ventricular arrhythmias, but physicians must consider the consequences of increasing the ventricular response if digoxin is withdrawn. If digitalis toxicity is suspected, elective cardioversion should be delayed. If it is not prudent to delay cardioversion, the lowest possible energy level should be selected to avoid provoking ventricular arrhythmias.

Laboratory Test Monitoring: Patients receiving digoxin should have their serum electrolytes and renal function (serum creatinine concentrations) assessed periodically; the

Table 2: Times to Onset of Pharmacologic Effect and to Peak Effect of Preparations of LANOXIN

Product	Time to Onset of Effect*	Time to Peak Effect*
LANOXIN Tablets	0.5–2 hours	2–6 hours
LANOXIN Elixir Pediatric	0.5–2 hours	2–6 hours
LANOXICAPS	0.5–2 hours	2–6 hours
LANOXIN Injection/IV	5–30 minutes†	1–4 hours

* Documented for ventricular response rate in atrial fibrillation, inotropic effects and electrocardiographic changes.
† Depending upon rate of infusion.

Table 3: Subgroup Analyses of Mortality and Hospitalization During the First Two Years Following Randomization

	n	Risk of All-Cause Mortality or All-Cause Hospitalization*			Risk of HF-Related Mortality or HF-Related Hospitalization*		
		Placebo	LANOXIN	Relative risk†	Placebo	LANOXIN	Relative risk†
All patients (EF ≤0.45)	6801	604	593	0.94 (0.88–1.00)	294	217	0.69 (0.63–0.76)
NYHA I/II	4571	549	541	0.96 (0.89–1.04)	242	178	0.70 (0.62–0.80)
EF 0.25–0.45	4543	568	571	0.99 (0.91–1.07)	244	190	0.74 (0.66–0.84)
CTR ≤0.55	4455	561	563	0.98 (0.91–1.06)	239	180	0.71 (0.63–0.81)
NYHA III/IV	2224	719	696	0.88 (0.80–0.97)	402	295	0.65 (0.57–0.75)
EF <0.25	2258	677	637	0.84 (0.76–0.93)	394	270	0.61 (0.53–0.71)
CTR >0.55	2346	687	650	0.85 (0.77–0.94)	398	287	0.65 (0.57–0.75)
EF >0.45‡	987	571	585	1.04 (0.88–1.23)	179	136	0.72 (0.53–0.99)

* Number of patients with an event during the first 2 years per 1000 randomized patients.
† Relative risk (95% confidence interval).
‡ DIG Ancillary Study.

frequency of assessments will depend on the clinical setting. For discussion of serum digoxin concentrations, see DOSAGE AND ADMINISTRATION.

Drug Interactions: Potassium-depleting *diuretics* are a major contributing factor to digitalis toxicity. *Calcium*, particularly if administered rapidly by the intravenous route, may produce serious arrhythmias in digitalized patients. *Quinidine, verapamil, amiodarone, propafenone, indomethacin, itraconazole, alprazolam, and spironolactone* raise the serum digoxin concentration due to a reduction in clearance and/or in volume of distribution of the drug, with the implication that digitalis intoxication may result. *Erythromycin* and *clarithromycin* (and possibly other *macrolide antibiotics*) and *tetracycline* may increase digoxin absorption in patients who inactivate digoxin by bacterial metabolism in the lower intestine, so that digitalis intoxication may result. The risk of this interaction may be reduced if digoxin is given as LANOXICAPS (see CLINICAL PHARMACOLOGY: Absorption). *Propantheline* and *diphenoxylate*, by decreasing gut motility, may increase digoxin absorption. *Antacids, kaolin-pectin, sulfasalazine, neomycin, cholestyramine,* certain *anticancer drugs,* and *metoclopramide* may interfere with intestinal digoxin absorption, resulting in unexpectedly low serum concentrations. *Rifampin* may decrease serum digoxin concentration, especially in patients with renal dysfunction, by increasing the non-renal clearance of digoxin. There have been inconsistent reports regarding the effects of other drugs [e.g., *quinine, penicillamine*] on serum digoxin concentration. *Thyroid* administration to a digitalized, hypothyroid patient may increase the dose requirement of digoxin. Concomitant use of digoxin and *sympathomimetics* increases the risk of cardiac arrhythmias. *Succinylcholine* may cause a sudden extrusion of potassium from muscle cells, and may thereby cause arrhythmias in digitalized patients. Although beta-adrenergic blockers or calcium channel blockers and digoxin may be useful in combination to control atrial fibrillation, their additive effects on AV node conduction can result in advanced or complete heart block.

Due to the considerable variability of these interactions, the dosage of digoxin should be individualized when patients receive these medications concurrently. Furthermore, caution should be exercised when combining digoxin with any drug that may cause a significant deterioration in renal function, since a decline in glomerular filtration or tubular secretion may impair the excretion of digoxin.

Drug/Laboratory Test Interactions: The use of therapeutic doses of digoxin may cause prolongation of the PR interval and depression of the ST segment on the electrocardiogram. Digoxin may produce false positive ST-T changes on the electrocardiogram during exercise testing. These electro-physiologic effects reflect an expected effect of the drug and are not indicative of toxicity.

Carcinogenesis, Mutagenesis, Impairment of Fertility: There have been no long-term studies performed in animals to evaluate carcinogenic potential, nor have studies been conducted to assess the mutagenic potential of digoxin or its potential to affect fertility.

Pregnancy: *Teratogenic Effects:* Pregnancy Category C. Animal reproduction studies have not been conducted with digoxin. It is also not known whether digoxin can cause fetal harm when administered to a pregnant woman or can affect reproduction capacity. Digoxin should be given to a pregnant woman only if clearly needed.

Nursing Mothers: Studies have shown that digoxin concentrations in the mother's serum and milk are similar. However, the estimated exposure of a nursing infant to digoxin via breast feeding will be far below the usual infant maintenance dose. Therefore, this amount should have no pharmacologic effect upon the infant. Nevertheless, caution should be exercised when digoxin is administered to a nursing woman.

Pediatric Use: Newborn infants display considerable variability in their tolerance to digoxin. Premature and immature infants are particularly sensitive to the effects of digoxin, and the dosage of the drug must not only be reduced but must be individualized according to their degree of maturity. Digitalis glycosides can cause poisoning in children due to accidental ingestion.

Geriatric Use: The majority of clinical experience gained with digoxin has been in the elderly population. This experience has not identified differences in response or adverse effects between the elderly and younger patients. However, this drug is known to be substantially excreted by the kidney, and the risk of toxic reactions to this drug may be greater in patients with impaired renal function. Because elderly patients are more likely to have decreased renal function, care should be taken in dose selection, which should be based on renal function, and it may be useful to monitor renal function (see DOSAGE AND ADMINISTRATION).

ADVERSE REACTIONS

In general, the adverse reactions of digoxin are dose-dependent and occur at doses higher than those needed to achieve a therapeutic effect. Hence, adverse reactions are less common when digoxin is used within the recommended dose range or therapeutic serum concentration range and when there is careful attention to concurrent medications and conditions.

Because some patients may be particularly susceptible to side effects with digoxin, the dosage of the drug should al-

ways be selected carefully and adjusted as the clinical condition of the patient warrants. In the past, when high doses of digoxin were used and little attention was paid to clinical status or concurrent medications, adverse reactions to digoxin were more frequent and severe. Cardiac adverse reactions accounted for about one-half, gastrointestinal disturbances for about one-fourth, and CNS and other toxicity for about one-fourth of these adverse reactions. However, available evidence suggests that the incidence and severity of digoxin toxicity has decreased substantially in recent years. In recent controlled clinical trials, in patients with predominantly mild to moderate heart failure, the incidence of adverse experiences was comparable in patients taking digoxin and in those taking placebo. In a large mortality trial, the incidence of hospitalization for suspected digoxin toxicity was 2% in patients taking LANOXIN Tablets compared to 0.9% in patients taking placebo. In this trial, the most common manifestations of digoxin toxicity included gastrointestinal and cardiac disturbances; CNS manifestations were less common.

Adults: ***Cardiac:*** Therapeutic doses of digoxin may cause heart block in patients with pre-existing sinoatrial or AV conduction disorders; heart block can be avoided by adjusting the dose of digoxin. Prophylactic use of a cardiac pacemaker may be considered if the risk of heart block is considered unacceptable. High doses of digoxin may produce a variety of rhythm disturbances, such as first-degree, second-degree (Wenckebach), or third-degree heart block (including asystole); atrial tachycardia with block; AV dissociation; accelerated junctional (nodal) rhythm; unifocal or multiform ventricular premature contractions (especially bigeminy or trigeminy); ventricular tachycardia; and ventricular fibrillation. Digoxin produces PR prolongation and ST segment depression which should not by themselves be considered digoxin toxicity. Cardiac toxicity can also occur at therapeutic doses in patients who have conditions which may alter their sensitivity to digoxin (see WARNINGS and PRECAUTIONS).

Gastrointestinal: Digoxin may cause anorexia, nausea, vomiting, and diarrhea. Rarely, the use of digoxin has been associated with abdominal pain, intestinal ischemia, and hemorrhagic necrosis of the intestines.

CNS: Digoxin can produce visual disturbances (blurred or yellow vision), headache, weakness, dizziness, apathy, confusion, and mental disturbances (such as anxiety, depression, delirium, and hallucination).

Other: Gynecomastia has been occasionally observed following the prolonged use of digoxin.

Thrombocytopenia and maculopapular rash and other skin reactions have been rarely observed.

The following table summarizes the incidence of those adverse experiences listed above for patients treated with LANOXIN Tablets or placebo from two randomized, double-blind, placebo-controlled withdrawal trials. Patients in these trials were also receiving diuretics with or without angiotensin-converting enzyme inhibitors. These patients had been stable on digoxin, and were randomized to digoxin or placebo. The results shown in Table 4 reflect the experience in patients following dosage titration with the use of serum digoxin concentrations and careful follow-up. These adverse experiences are consistent with results from a large, placebo-controlled mortality trial (DIG trial) wherein over half the patients were not receiving digoxin prior to enrollment.

[See table 4 above]

Table 4: Adverse Experiences in Two Parallel, Double-Blind, Placebo-Controlled Withdrawal Trials (Number of Patients Reporting)

Adverse Experience	Digoxin Patients (n = 123)	Placebo Patients (n = 125)
Cardiac		
Palpitation	1	4
Ventricular extrasystole	1	1
Tachycardia	2	1
Heart arrest	1	1
Gastrointestinal		
Anorexia	1	4
Nausea	4	2
Vomiting	2	1
Diarrhea	4	1
Abdominal pain	0	6
CNS		
Headache	4	4
Dizziness	6	5
Mental disturbances	5	1
Other		
Rash	2	1
Death	4	3

Infants and Children: The side effects of digoxin in infants and children differ from those seen in adults in several respects. Although digoxin may produce anorexia, nausea, vomiting, diarrhea, and CNS disturbances in young patients, these are rarely the initial symptoms of overdosage. Rather, the earliest and most frequent manifestation of excessive dosing with digoxin in infants and children is the appearance of cardiac arrhythmias, including sinus bradycardia. In children, the use of digoxin may produce any arrhythmia. The most common are conduction disturbances or supraventricular tachyarrhythmias, such as atrial tachycardia (with or without block) and junctional (nodal) tachycardia. Ventricular arrhythmias are less common. Sinus bradycardia may be a sign of impending digoxin intoxication, especially in infants, even in the absence of first-degree heart block. Any arrhythmia or alteration in cardiac conduction that develops in a child taking digoxin should be assumed to be caused by digoxin, until further evaluation proves otherwise.

OVERDOSAGE

Treatment of Adverse Reactions Produced by Overdosage: Digoxin should be temporarily discontinued until the adverse reaction resolves. Every effort should also be made to correct factors that may contribute to the adverse reaction (such as electrolyte disturbances or concurrent medications). Once the adverse reaction has resolved, therapy with digoxin may be reinstituted, following a careful reassessment of dose. Withdrawal of digoxin may be all that is required to treat the adverse reaction. However, when the primary manifestation of digoxin overdosage is a cardiac arrhythmia, additional therapy may be needed. If the rhythm disturbance is a symptomatic bradyarrhythmia or heart block, consideration should be given to the reversal of toxicity with DIGIBIND® [Digoxin Immune Fab (Ovine)] (see below), the use of atropine, or the insertion of a temporary cardiac pacemaker. However, asymptomatic bradycardia or heart block related to digoxin may require only temporary withdrawal of the drug and cardiac monitoring of the patient. If the rhythm disturbance is a ventricular arrhythmia, consideration should be given to the correction of electrolyte disorders, particularly if hypokalemia (see below) or hypomagnesemia is present. DIGIBIND is a specific antidote for digoxin and may be used to reverse potentially life-threatening ventricular arrhythmias due to digoxin overdosage.

Administration of Potassium: Every effort should be made to maintain the serum potassium concentration between 4.0 and 5.5 mmol/L. Potassium is usually administered orally, but when correction of the arrhythmia is urgent and the serum potassium concentration is low, potassium may be administered cautiously by the intravenous route. The electrocardiogram should be monitored for any evidence of potassium toxicity (e.g., peaking of T waves) and to observe the effect on the arrhythmia. Potassium salts may be dangerous in patients who manifest bradycardia or heart block due to digoxin (unless primarily related to supraventricular tachycardia) and in the setting of massive digitalis overdosage (see Massive Digitalis Overdosage subsection).

Massive Digitalis Overdosage: Manifestations of life-threatening toxicity include ventricular tachycardia or ventricular fibrillation, or progressive bradyarrhythmias, or heart block. The administration of more than 10 mg of digoxin in a previously healthy adult, or more than 4 mg in a previously healthy child, or a steady-state serum concentration greater than 10 ng/mL, often results in cardiac arrest. DIGIBIND should be used to reverse the toxic effects of ingestion of a massive overdose. The decision to administer DIGIBIND to a patient who has ingested a massive dose of digoxin but who has not yet manifested life-threatening toxicity should depend on the likelihood that life-threatening toxicity will occur (see above).

Patients with massive digitalis ingestion should receive large doses of activated charcoal to prevent absorption and bind digoxin in the gut during enteroenteric recirculation. Emesis or gastric lavage may be indicated especially if ingestion has occurred within 30 minutes of the patient's presentation at the hospital. Emesis should not be induced in patients who are obtunded. If a patient presents more than 2 hours after ingestion or already has toxic manifestations, it may be unsafe to induce vomiting or attempt passage of a gastric tube, because such maneuvers may induce an acute vagal episode that can worsen digitalis-related arrhythmias.

Severe digitalis intoxication can cause a massive shift of potassium from inside to outside the cell, leading to life-threatening hyperkalemia. The administration of potassium supplements in the setting of massive intoxication may be hazardous and should be avoided. Hyperkalemia caused by massive digitalis toxicity is best treated with DIGIBIND; initial treatment with glucose and insulin may also be required if hyperkalemia itself is acutely life-threatening.

DOSAGE AND ADMINISTRATION

General: Recommended dosages of digoxin may require considerable modification because of individual sensitivity of the patient to the drug, the presence of associated conditions, or the use of concurrent medications. Due to the more complete absorption of digoxin from soft capsules, recommended oral doses are only 80 percent of those for Tablets and Elixir.

Because the significance of the higher peak serum concentrations associated with once daily capsules is not established, divided daily dosing is presently recommended for:

1. Infants and children under 10 years of age;
2. Patients requiring a daily dose of 300 mcg (0.3mg) or greater;
3. Patients with a previous history of digitalis toxicity;
4. Patients considered likely to become toxic;
5. Patients in whom compliance is not a problem.

Where compliance is considered a problem, single daily dosing may be appropriate.

In selecting a dose of digoxin, the following factors must be considered:

1. The body weight of the patient. Doses should be calculated based upon lean (i.e., ideal) body weight.
2. The patient's renal function, preferably evaluated on the basis of estimated creatinine clearance.
3. The patient's age. Infants and children require different doses of digoxin than adults. Also, advanced age may be indicative of diminished renal function even in patients with normal serum creatinine concentration (i.e., below 1.5 mg/dL).
4. Concomitant disease states, concurrent medications, or other factors likely to alter the pharmacokinetic or pharmacodynamic profile of digoxin (see PRECAUTIONS).

Serum Digoxin Concentrations: In general, the dose of digoxin used should be determined on clinical grounds. However, measurement of serum digoxin concentrations can be helpful to the clinician in determining the adequacy of digoxin therapy and in assigning certain probabilities to the likelihood of digoxin intoxication. About two-thirds of adults considered adequately digitalized (without evidence of toxicity) have serum digoxin concentrations ranging from 0.8 to 2.0 ng/mL. However, digoxin may produce clinical benefits even at serum concentrations below this range. About two-thirds of adult patients with clinical toxicity have serum digoxin concentrations greater than 2.0 ng/mL. However, since one-third of patients with clinical toxicity have concentrations less than 2.0 ng/mL, values below 2.0 ng/mL do not rule out the possibility that a certain sign or symptom is related to digoxin therapy. Rarely, there are patients who are unable to tolerate digoxin at serum concentrations below 0.8 ng/mL. Consequently, the serum concentration of digoxin should always be interpreted in the overall clinical context, and an isolated measurement should not be used alone as the basis for increasing or decreasing the dose of the drug.

To allow adequate time for equilibration of digoxin between serum and tissue, sampling of serum concentrations should be done just before the next scheduled dose of the drug. If this is not possible, sampling should be done at least 6 to 8

Continued on next page

This product information is based on labeling in effect on June 1, 1998. For further information, contact via direct mail, phone, or web site Medical Information: Glaxo Wellcome Inc., PO Box 13398, Research Triangle Park, NC 27709. Healthcare Professionals (Medical Information): 800-334-0089 Patients (Customer Response Center): 888-TALK2GW (1-888-825-5249) Glaxo Wellcome Corporate Web Site: www.glaxowellcome.com

Consult 1999 PDR® supplements and future editions for revisions

Lanoxicaps—Cont.

hours after the last dose, regardless of the route of administration or the formulation used. On a once-daily dosing schedule, the concentration of digoxin will be 10% to 25% lower when sampled at 24 versus 8 hours, depending upon the patient's renal function. On a twice-daily dosing schedule, there will be only minor differences in serum digoxin concentrations whether sampling is done at 8 or 12 hours after a dose.

If a discrepancy exists between the reported serum concentration and the observed clinical response, the clinician should consider the following possibilities:

1. Analytical problems in the assay procedure.
2. Inappropriate serum sampling time.
3. Administration of a digitalis glycoside other than digoxin.
4. Conditions (described in WARNINGS and PRECAUTIONS) causing an alteration in the sensitivity of the patient to digoxin.
5. Serum digoxin concentration may decrease acutely during periods of exercise without any associated change in clinical efficacy due to increased binding of digoxin to skeletal muscle.

Heart Failure: *Adults:* Digitalization may be accomplished by either of two general approaches that vary in dosage and frequency of administration, but reach the same endpoint in terms of total amount of digoxin accumulated in the body.

1. If rapid digitalization is considered medically appropriate, it may be achieved by administering a loading dose based upon projected peak digoxin body stores. Maintenance dose can be calculated as a percentage of the loading dose.
2. More gradual digitalization may be obtained by beginning an appropriate maintenance dose, thus allowing digoxin body stores to accumulate slowly. Steady-state serum digoxin concentrations will be achieved in approximately five half-lives of the drug for the individual patient. Depending upon the patient's renal function, this will take between 1 and 3 weeks.

Rapid Digitalization with a Loading Dose: Peak digoxin body stores of 8 to 12 mcg/kg should provide therapeutic effect with minimum risk of toxicity in most patients with heart failure and normal sinus rhythm. Because of altered digoxin distribution and elimination, projected peak body stores for patients with renal insufficiency should be conservative (i.e., 6 to 10 mcg/kg) [see PRECAUTIONS].

The loading dose should be administered in several portions, with roughly half the total given as the first dose. Additional fractions of this planned total dose may be given at 6- to 8-hour intervals, **with careful assessment of clinical response before each additional dose.**

If the patient's clinical response necessitates a change from the calculated loading dose of digoxin, then calculation of the maintenance dose should be based upon the amount actually given.

A single initial dose of 400 to 600 mcg (0.4 to 0.6 mg) of LANOXICAPS usually produces a detectable effect in 0.5 to 2 hours that becomes maximal in 2 to 6 hours. Additional doses of 100 to 300 mcg (0.1 to 0.3 mg) may be given cautiously at 6- to 8-hour intervals until clinical evidence of an adequate effect is noted. The usual amount of LANOXICAPS that a 70-kg patient requires to achieve 8 to 12 mcg/kg peak body stores is 600 to 1000 mcg (0.6 to 1.0 mg).

LANOXIN Injection is frequently used to achieve rapid digitalization, with conversion to LANOXIN Tablets or LANOXICAPS for maintenance therapy. If patients are switched from intravenous to oral digoxin formulations, allowances must be made for differences in bioavailability when calculating maintenance dosages (see Table 1, CLINICAL PHARMACOLOGY).

Maintenance Dosing: The doses of digoxin tablets used in controlled trials in patients with heart failure have ranged from 125 to 500 mcg (0.125 to 0.5 mg) once daily. In these studies, the digoxin dose has been generally titrated according to the patient's age, lean body weight, and renal function. Therapy is generally initiated at a dose of 250 mcg (0.25 mg) once daily in patients under age 70 with good renal function, at a dose of 125 mcg (0.125 mg) once daily in patients over age 70 or with impaired renal function, and at a dose of 62.5 mcg (0.0625 mg) in patients with marked renal impairment. Doses may be increased every 2 weeks according to clinical response.

In a subset of approximately 1,800 patients enrolled in the DIG trial (wherein dosing was based on an algorithm similar to that in Table 5) the mean ($\pm$SD) serum digoxin concentrations at 1 month and 12 months were 1.01 ± 0.47 ng/mL and 0.97 ± 0.43 ng/mL, respectively.

The maintenance dose should be based upon the percentage of the peak body stores lost each day through elimination. The following formula has had wide clinical use:

Maintenance Dose = Peak Body Stores (i.e., Loading Dose) x % Daily Loss/100

Where: % Daily Loss = 14 + Ccr/5

(Ccr is creatinine clearance, corrected to 70 kg body weight or 1.73 m² body surface area)

Table 5 provides average daily maintenance dose requirements of LANOXICAPS Capsules for patients with heart failure based upon lean body weight and renal function:

[See table 5 below]

Example: Based on the above table, a patient in heart failure with an estimated lean body weight of 70 kg and a Ccr of 60 mL/min, should be given a dose of 200 mcg (0.2 mg)

daily of LANOXICAPS, usually taken as a divided dose of one 100-mcg (0.1-mg) capsule after the morning and evening meals. If no loading dose is administered, steady-state serum concentrations in this patient should be anticipated at approximately 11 days.

Infants and Children: In general, divided daily dosing is recommended for infants and young children (under age 10). In these patients, where dosage adjustment is frequent and outside the fixed dosages available, LANOXICAPS may not be the formulation of choice. In the newborn period, renal clearance of digoxin is diminished and suitable dosage adjustments must be observed. This is especially pronounced in the premature infant. Beyond the immediate newborn period, children generally require proportionally larger doses than adults on the basis of body weight or body surface area. Children over 10 years of age require adult dosages in proportion to their body weight. Some researchers have suggested that infants and young children tolerate slightly higher serum concentrations than do adults.

Daily maintenance doses for each age group are given in Table 6 and should provide therapeutic effects with minimum risk of toxicity in most patients with heart failure and normal sinus rhythm. These recommendations assume the presence of normal renal function:

[See table 6 below]

In children with renal disease, digoxin must be carefully titrated based upon clinical response.

It cannot be overemphasized that both the adult and pediatric dosage guidelines provided are based upon average patient response and substantial individual variation can be expected. Accordingly, ultimate dosage selection must be based upon clinical assessment of the patient.

Atrial Fibrillation: Peak digoxin body stores larger than the 8 to 12 mcg/kg required for most patients with heart failure and normal sinus rhythm have been used for control of ventricular rate in patients with atrial fibrillation. Doses of digoxin used for the treatment of chronic atrial fibrillation should be titrated to the minimum dose that achieves the desired ventricular rate control without causing undesirable side effects. Data are not available to establish the appropriate resting or exercise target rates that should be achieved.

Dosage Adjustment When Changing Preparations: The absolute bioavailability of the capsule formulation is greater than that of the standard tablets and very near that of the intravenous dosage form. As a result, the doses recommended for LANOXICAPS Capsules are the same as those for LANOXIN Injection (see Table 1 in CLINICAL PHARMACOLOGY: Pharmacokinetics). Adjustments in dosage will seldom be necessary when converting a patient from the intravenous formulation to LANOXICAPS. The difference in bioavailability between LANOXIN Injection or LANOXICAPS and LANOXIN Elixir Pediatric or LANOXIN Tablets must be considered when changing patients from one dosage form to another.

Doses of 100 mcg (0.1 mg) and 200 mcg (0.2 mg) of LANOXICAPS are approximately equivalent to 125-mcg (0.125-mg) and 250-mcg (0.25-mg) doses of LANOXIN Tablets and Elixir Pediatric, respectively (see Table 1 in CLINICAL PHARMACOLOGY: Pharmacokinetics).

HOW SUPPLIED

LANOXICAPS (digoxin solution in capsules), 50 mcg (0.05 mg): Bottle of 100 (NDC 0173-0270-55). Imprint A2C (red).

LANOXICAPS (digoxin solution in capsules), 100 mcg (0.1 mg): Bottle of 100 (NDC 0173-0272-55). Imprint B2C (yellow).

LANOXICAPS (digoxin solution in capsules), 200 mcg (0.2 mg): Bottle of 100 (NDC 0173-0274-55). Imprint C2C (green).

Store at 15° to 25°C (59° to 77°F) in a dry place and protect from light.

©Copyright 1996,1998 Glaxo Wellcome Inc. All rights reserved.

May 1998/RL-566

Shown in Product Identification Guide, page 313

Table 5: Usual Daily Maintenance Dose Requirements (mcg) of LANOXICAPS Capsules for Estimated Peak Body Stores of 10 mcg/kg

Corrected Ccr		Lean Body Weight						Number of Days Before Steady State Achieved†
	kg	50	60	70	80	90	100	
(mL/min per 70 kg)*	lb	110	132	154	176	198	220	
0		50‡	100	100	100	150	150	22
10		100	100	100	150	150	150	19
20		100	100	150	150	150	200	16
30		100	150	150	150	200	200	14
40		100	150	150	200	200	250	13
50		150	150	200	200	250	250	12
60		150	150	200	200	250	300	11
70		150	200	200	250	250	300	10
80		150	200	200	250	300	300	9
90		150	200	250	250	300	350	8
100		200	200	250	300	300	350	7

* Ccr is creatinine clearance, corrected to 70 kg body weight or 1.73 m² body surface area. *For adults,* if only serum creatinine concentrations (Scr) are available, a Ccr (corrected to 70 kg body weight) may be estimated in men as (140 - Age)/Scr. For women, this result should be multiplied by 0.85. *Note: This equation cannot be used for estimating creatinine clearance in infants and children.*
† If no loading dose administered.
‡ 50 mcg= 0.05 mg

Table 6: Usual Digitalizing and Maintenance Dosages for LANOXICAPS in Children with Normal Renal Function Based on Lean Body Weight

Age	Digitalizing* Dose (mcg/kg)	**Daily** Maintenance Dose† (mcg/kg)
2 to 5 Years	25 to 35	25% to 35% of the oral or I.V. digitalizing dose‡
5 to 10 Years	15 to 30	
Over 10 Years	8 to 12	

* IV digitalizing doses are the same as digitalizing doses of LANOXICAPS.
† Divided daily dosing is recommended for children under 10 years of age.
‡ Projected or actual digitalizing dose providing desired clinical response.

LANOXIN®   ℞

[lă-nŏx'in″]

(digoxin)

Elixir Pediatric

50 µg (0.05 mg) per mL

DESCRIPTION

LANOXIN (digoxin) is one of the cardiac (or digitalis) glycosides, a closely related group of drugs having in common specific effects on the myocardium. These drugs are found in a number of plants. Digoxin is extracted from the leaves of *Digitalis lanata.* The term "digitalis" is used to designate the whole group of glycosides. The glycosides are composed of two portions: a sugar and a cardenolide (hence "glycosides"). Digoxin is described chemically as (3β,5β, 12β)-3-[(*O*-2,6-dideoxy-β-*D*-ribo-hexopyranosyl-(1→4)-*O*-2,6-di-deoxy-β-*D*-ribo-hexopyranosyl-(1→4)-2,6-dideoxy-β-*D*-ribo-

hexopyranosyl)oxy]-12,14-dihydroxy-card-20(22)-enolide. Its molecular formula is $C_{41}H_{64}O_{14}$, and its molecular weight is 780.95.

Digoxin exists as odorless white crystals that melt with decomposition above 230°C. The drug is practically insoluble in water and in ether; slightly soluble in diluted (50%) alcohol and in chloroform; and freely soluble in pyridine.

LANOXIN Elixir Pediatric is a stable solution of digoxin specially formulated for oral use in infants and children. Each mL contains 50 mcg (0.05 mg) digoxin, USP. The lime-flavored elixir contains the inactive ingredients alcohol 10%, methylparaben 0.1% (added as a preservative), citric acid, D&C Green No. 5 and Yellow No. 10, flavor, propylene glycol, sodium phosphate, and sucrose. Each package is supplied with a specially calibrated dropper to facilitate the administration of accurate dosage even in premature infants. Starting at 0.2 mL, this 1-mL dropper is marked in divisions of 0.1 mL, each corresponding to 5 mcg (0.005 mg) digoxin.

CLINICAL PHARMACOLOGY

Mechanism of Action: Digoxin inhibits sodium-potassium ATPase, an enzyme that regulates the quantity of sodium and potassium inside cells. Inhibition of the enzyme leads to an increase in the intracellular concentration of sodium and thus (by stimulation of sodium-calcium exchange) an increase in the intracellular concentration of calcium. The beneficial effects of digoxin result from direct actions on cardiac muscle, as well as indirect actions on the cardiovascular system mediated by effects on the autonomic nervous system. The autonomic effects include: (1) a vagomimetic action, which is responsible for the effects of digoxin on the sinoatrial and atrioventricular (AV) nodes; and (2) baroreceptor sensitization, which results in increased afferent inhibitory activity and reduced activity of the sympathetic nervous system and renin-angiotensin system for any given increment in mean arterial pressure. The pharmacologic consequences of these direct and indirect effects are: (1) an increase in the force and velocity of myocardial systolic contraction (positive inotropic action); (2) a decrease in the degree of activation of the sympathetic nervous system and renin-angiotensin system (neurohormonal deactivating effect); and (3) slowing of the heart rate and decreased conduction velocity through the AV node (vagomimetic effect). The effects of digoxin in heart failure are mediated by its positive inotropic and neurohormonal deactivating effects, whereas the effects of the drug in atrial arrhythmias are related to its vagomimetic actions. In high doses, digoxin increases sympathetic outflow from the central nervous system (CNS). This increase in sympathetic activity may be an important factor in digitalis toxicity.

Pharmacokinetics: Note: The following data are from studies performed in adults, unless otherwise stated.

Absorption: Absorption of digoxin from LANOXIN Elixir Pediatric formulation has been demonstrated to be 70% to 85% complete compared to an identical intravenous dose of digoxin (absolute bioavailability). When the elixir is taken after meals, the rate of absorption is slowed, but the total amount of digoxin absorbed is usually unchanged. When taken with meals high in bran fiber, however, the amount absorbed from an oral dose may be reduced. Comparisons of the systemic availability and equivalent doses for preparations of LANOXIN are shown in Table 1:

[See table 1 above]

In some patients, orally administered digoxin is converted to inactive reduction products (e.g., dihydrodigoxin) by colonic bacteria in the gut. Data suggest that one in ten patients treated with digoxin tablets will degrade 40% or more of the ingested dose. As a result, certain antibiotics may increase the absorption of digoxin in such patients. Although inactivation of these bacteria by antibiotics is rapid, the serum digoxin concentration will rise at a rate consistent with the elimination half-life of digoxin. The magnitude of rise in serum digoxin concentration relates to the extent of bacterial inactivation, and may be as much as two-fold in some cases.

Distribution: Following drug administration, a 6- to 8-hour tissue distribution phase is observed. This is followed by a much more gradual decline in the serum concentration of the drug, which is dependent on the elimination of digoxin from the body. The peak height and slope of the early portion (absorption/distribution phases) of the serum concentration-time curve are dependent upon the route of administration and the absorption characteristics of the formulation. Clinical evidence indicates that the early high serum concentrations do not reflect the concentration of digoxin at its site of action, but that with chronic use, the steady-state post-distribution serum concentrations are in equilibrium with tissue concentrations and correlate with pharmacologic effects. In individual patients, these post-distribution serum concentrations may be useful in evaluating therapeutic and toxic effects (see DOSAGE AND ADMINISTRATION: Serum Digoxin Concentrations).

Digoxin is concentrated in tissues and therefore has a large apparent volume of distribution. Digoxin crosses both the blood-brain barrier and the placenta. At delivery, the serum

digoxin concentration in the newborn is similar to the serum concentration in the mother. Approximately 25% of digoxin in the plasma is bound to protein. Serum digoxin concentrations are not significantly altered by large changes in fat tissue weight, so that its distribution space correlates best with lean (i.e., ideal) body weight, not total body weight.

Metabolism: Only a small percentage (16%) of a dose of digoxin is metabolized. The end metabolites, which include 3 β-digoxigenin, 3-keto-digoxigenin, and their glucuronide and sulfate conjugates, are polar in nature and are postulated to be formed via hydrolysis, oxidation, and conjugation. The metabolism of digoxin is not dependent upon the cytochrome P-450 system, and digoxin is not known to induce or inhibit the cytochrome P-450 system.

Excretion: Elimination of digoxin follows first-order kinetics (that is, the quantity of digoxin eliminated at any time is proportional to the total body content). Following intravenous administration to healthy volunteers, 50% to 70% of a digoxin dose is excreted unchanged in the urine. Renal excretion of digoxin is proportional to glomerular filtration rate and is largely independent of urine flow. In healthy volunteers with normal renal function, digoxin has a half-life of 1.5 to 2.0 days. The half-life in anuric patients is prolonged to 3.5 to 5 days. Digoxin is not effectively removed from the body by dialysis, exchange transfusion, or during cardiopulmonary bypass because most of the drug is bound to tissue and does not circulate in the blood.

Special Populations: Race differences in digoxin pharmacokinetics have not been formally studied. Because digoxin is primarily eliminated as unchanged drug via the kidney and because there are no important differences in creatinine clearance among races, pharmacokinetic differences due to race are not expected.

The clearance of digoxin can be primarily correlated with renal function as indicated by creatinine clearance. In children with renal disease, digoxin must be carefully titrated based on clinical response.

Plasma digoxin concentration profiles in patients with acute hepatitis generally fell within the range of profiles in a group of healthy subjects.

Pharmacodynamic and Clinical Effects: The times to onset of pharmacologic effect and to peak effect of preparations of LANOXIN are shown in Table 2:

[See table 2 at top of next page]

Hemodynamic Effects: Digoxin produces hemodynamic improvement in patients with heart failure. Short- and long-term therapy with the drug increases cardiac output and lowers pulmonary artery pressure, pulmonary capillary wedge pressure, and systemic vascular resistance. These hemodynamic effects are accompanied by an increase in the left ventricular ejection fraction and a decrease in end-systolic and end-diastolic dimensions.

Chronic Heart Failure: Two 12-week, double-blind, placebo-controlled studies enrolled 178 (RADIANCE trial) and 88 (PROVED trial) adult patients with NYHA class II or III heart failure previously treated with digoxin, a diuretic, and an ACE inhibitor (RADIANCE only) and randomized them to placebo or treatment with LANOXIN Tablets. Both trials demonstrated better preservation of exercise capacity in patients randomized to LANOXIN. Continued treatment with LANOXIN reduced the risk of developing worsening heart failure, as evidenced by heart failure-related hospitalizations and emergency care and the need for concomitant heart failure therapy. The larger study also showed treatment-related benefits in NYHA class and patients' global assessment. In the smaller trial, these trended in favor of a treatment benefit.

The Digitalis Investigation Group (DIG) main trial was a multicenter, randomized, double-blind, placebo-controlled mortality study of 6801 adult patients with heart failure and left ventricular ejection fraction ≤0.45. At randomization, 67% were NYHA class I or II, 71% had heart failure of ischemic etiology, 44% had been receiving digoxin, and most were receiving concomitant ACE inhibitor (94%) and diuretic (82%). Patients were randomized to placebo or LANOXIN Tablets, the dose of which was adjusted for the patient's age, sex, lean body weight, and serum creatinine (see DOSAGE AND ADMINISTRATION), and followed for up to 58 months (median 37 months). The median daily dose prescribed was 0.25 mg.

Overall all-cause mortality was 35% with no difference between groups (95% confidence limits for relative risk of 0.91 to 1.07). LANOXIN was associated with a 25% reduction in the number of hospitalizations for heart failure, a 28% reduction in the risk of a patient having at least one hospitalization for heart failure, and a 6.5% reduction in total hospitalizations (for any cause).

Use of LANOXIN was associated with a trend in reduction in time to all-cause death or hospitalization.

The trend was evident in subgroups of patients with mild heart failure as well as more severe disease, as shown in Table 3. Although the effect on all-cause death or hospitalization was not statistically significant, much of the apparent benefit derived from effects on mortality and hospitalization attributed to heart failure.

[See table 3 at top of next page]

In situations where there is no statistically significant benefit of treatment evident from a trial's primary endpoint, results pertaining to a secondary endpoint should be interpreted cautiously.

Chronic Atrial Fibrillation: In adult patients with chronic atrial fibrillation, digoxin slows rapid ventricular response rate in a linear dose-response fashion from 0.25 to 0.75 mg/day. Digoxin should not be used for the treatment of multifocal atrial tachycardia.

INDICATIONS AND USAGE

Heart Failure: LANOXIN is indicated for the treatment of mild to moderate heart failure. LANOXIN increases left ventricular ejection fraction and improves heart failure symptoms as evidenced by exercise capacity and heart failure-related hospitalizations and emergency care, while having no effect on mortality. Where possible, LANOXIN should be used with a diuretic and an angiotensin-converting enzyme inhibitor, but an optimal order for starting these three drugs cannot be specified.

Atrial Fibrillation: LANOXIN is indicated for the control of ventricular response rate in patients with chronic atrial fibrillation.

CONTRAINDICATIONS

Digitalis glycosides are contraindicated in patients with ventricular fibrillation or in patients with a known hypersensitivity to digoxin. A hypersensitivity reaction to other digitalis preparations usually constitutes a contraindication to digoxin.

WARNINGS

Sinus Node Disease and AV Block: Because digoxin slows sinoatrial and AV conduction, the drug commonly prolongs the PR interval. The drug may cause severe sinus bradycardia or sinoatrial block in patients with pre-existing sinus node disease and may cause advanced or complete heart block in patients with pre-existing incomplete AV block. In such patients consideration should be given to the insertion of a pacemaker before treatment with digoxin.

Accessory AV Pathway (Wolff-Parkinson-White Syndrome): After intravenous digoxin therapy, some patients with paroxysmal atrial fibrillation or flutter and a coexisting accessory AV pathway have developed increased antegrade conduction across the accessory pathway bypassing the AV node, leading to a very rapid ventricular response or ventricular fibrillation. Unless conduction down the accessory pathway has been blocked (either pharmacologically or by surgery), digoxin should not be used in such patients. The treatment of paroxysmal supraventricular tachycardia in such patients is usually direct-current cardioversion.

Use in Patients with Preserved Left Ventricular Systolic Function: Patients with certain disorders involving heart failure associated with preserved left ventricular ejection fraction may be particularly susceptible to toxicity of the drug. Such disorders include restrictive cardiomyopathy, constrictive pericarditis, amyloid heart disease, and acute cor pulmonale. Patients with idiopathic hypertrophic sub-

Continued on next page

Table 1: Comparisons of the Systemic Availability and Equivalent Doses for Preparations of LANOXIN

Product	Absolute Bioavailability	Equivalent Doses (mcg)* Among Dosage Forms			
LANOXIN Tablets	60 – 80%	62.5	125	250	500
LANOXIN Elixir Pediatric	70 – 85%	62.5	125	250	500
LANOXICAPS	90 – 100%	50	100	200	400
LANOXIN Injection/IV	100%	50	100	200	400

*For example, 125 mcg LANOXIN Tablets equivalent to 125 mcg LANOXIN Elixir Pediatric equivalent to 100 mcg LANOXICAPS equivalent to 100 mcg LANOXIN Injection/IV.

Lanoxin Elixir Pediatric—Cont.

aortic stenosis may have worsening of the outflow obstruction due to the inotropic effects of digoxin.

PRECAUTIONS

Use in Patients with Impaired Renal Function: Digoxin is primarily excreted by the kidneys; therefore, patients with impaired renal function require smaller than usual maintenance doses of digoxin (see DOSAGE AND ADMINISTRATION). Because of the prolonged elimination half-life, a longer period of time is required to achieve an initial or new steady-state serum concentration in patients with renal impairment than in patients with normal renal function. If appropriate care is not taken to reduce the dose of digoxin, such patients are at high risk for toxicity, and toxic effects will last longer in such patients than in patients with normal renal function.

Use in Patients with Electrolyte Disorders: In patients with hypokalemia or hypomagnesemia, toxicity may occur despite serum digoxin concentrations below 2.0 ng/mL, because potassium or magnesium depletion sensitizes the myocardium to digoxin. Therefore, it is desirable to maintain normal serum potassium and magnesium concentrations in patients being treated with digoxin. Deficiencies of these electrolytes may result from malnutrition, diarrhea, or prolonged vomiting, as well as the use of the following drugs or procedures: diuretics, amphotericin B, corticosteroids, antacids, dialysis, and mechanical suction of gastrointestinal secretions.

Hypercalcemia from any cause predisposes the patient to digitalis toxicity. Calcium, particularly when administered rapidly by the intravenous route, may produce serious arrhythmias in digitalized patients.

On the other hand, hypocalcemia can nullify the effects of digoxin in humans; thus, digoxin may be ineffective until serum calcium is restored to normal. These interactions are related to the fact that digoxin affects contractility and excitability of the heart in a manner similar to that of calcium.

Use in Thyroid Disorders and Hypermetabolic States: Hypothyroidism may reduce the requirements for digoxin. Heart failure and/or atrial arrhythmias resulting from hypermetabolic or hyperdynamic states (e.g., hyperthyroidism, hypoxia, or arteriovenous shunt) are best treated by addressing the underlying condition. Atrial arrhythmias associated with hypermetabolic states are particularly resistant to digoxin treatment. Care must be taken to avoid toxicity if digoxin is used.

Use in Patients with Acute Myocardial Infarction: Digoxin should be used with caution in patients with acute myocardial infarction. The use of inotropic drugs in some patients in this setting may result in undesirable increases in myocardial oxygen demand and ischemia.

Use During Electrical Cardioversion: It may be desirable to reduce the dose of digoxin for 1 to 2 days prior to electrical cardioversion of atrial fibrillation to avoid the induction of ventricular arrhythmias, but physicians must consider the consequences of increasing the ventricular response if digoxin is withdrawn. If digitalis toxicity is suspected, elective cardioversion should be delayed. If it is not prudent to delay cardioversion, the lowest possible energy level should be selected to avoid provoking ventricular arrhythmias.

Laboratory Test Monitoring: Patients receiving digoxin should have their serum electrolytes and renal function (serum creatinine concentrations) assessed periodically; the frequency of assessments will depend on the clinical setting. For discussion of serum digoxin concentrations, see DOSAGE AND ADMINISTRATION.

Drug Interactions: Potassium-depleting *diuretics* are a major contributing factor to digitalis toxicity. *Calcium*, particularly if administered rapidly by the intravenous route, may produce serious arrhythmias in digitalized patients. *Quinidine, verapamil, amiodarone, propafenone, indomethacin, itraconazole, alprazolam*, and *spironolactone* raise the serum digoxin concentration due to a reduction in clearance and/or in volume of distribution of the drug, with the implication that digitalis intoxication may result. *Erythromycin* and *clarithromycin* (and possibly other *macrolide antibiotics*) and *tetracycline* may increase digoxin absorption in patients who inactivate digoxin by bacterial metabolism in the lower intestine, so that digitalis intoxication may result (see CLINICAL PHARMACOLOGY: Absorption). *Propantheline* and *diphenoxylate*, by decreasing gut motility, may increase digoxin absorption. *Antacids, kaolin-pectin, sulfasalazine, neomycin, cholestyramine, certain anticancer drugs*, and *metoclopramide* may interfere with intestinal digoxin absorption, resulting in unexpectedly low serum concentrations. *Rifampin* may decrease serum digoxin concentration, especially in patients with renal dysfunction, by increasing the non-renal clearance of digoxin. There have been inconsistent reports regarding the effects of other drugs [e.g., *quinine, penicillamine*] on serum digoxin concentration. *Thyroid* administration to a digitalized, hypothyroid patient may increase the dose requirement of digoxin. Concomitant use of digoxin and *sympathomimetics* increases the risk of cardiac arrhythmias. *Succinylcholine* may cause a sudden extrusion of potassium from muscle cells, and may thereby cause arrhythmias in digitalized patients. Although beta-adrenergic blockers or calcium channel blockers and digoxin may be useful in combination to control atrial fibrillation, their additive effects on AV node conduction can result in advanced or complete heart block.

Table 2: Times to Onset of Pharmacologic Effect and to Peak Effect of Preparations of LANOXIN

Product	Time to Onset of Effect*	Time to Peak Effect*
LANOXIN Tablets	0.5 – 2 hours	2 – 6 hours
LANOXIN Elixir Pediatric	0.5 – 2 hours	2 – 6 hours
LANOXICAPS	0.5 – 2 hours	2 – 6 hours
LANOXIN Injection/IV	5 – 30 minutes†	1 – 4 hours

* Documented for ventricular response rate in atrial fibrillation, inotropic effects and electrocardiographic changes.
† Depending upon rate of infusion.

Table 3: Subgroup Analyses of Mortality and Hospitalization During the First Two Years Following Randomization

		Risk of All-Cause Mortality or All-Cause Hospitalization*			Risk of HF-Related Mortality or HF-Related Hospitalization*		
	n	Placebo	LANOXIN	Relative risk†	Placebo	LANOXIN	Relative risk†
All patients (EF ≤0.45)	6801	604	593	0.94 (0.88–1.00)	294	217	0.69 (0.63–0.76)
NYHA I/II	4571	549	541	0.96 (0.89–1.04)	242	178	0.70 (0.62–0.80)
EF 0.25–0.45	4543	568	571	0.99 (0.91–1.07)	244	190	0.74 (0.66–0.84)
CTR ≤0.55	4455	561	563	0.98 (0.91–1.06)	239	180	0.71 (0.63–0.81)
NYHA III/IV	2224	719	696	0.88 (0.80–0.97)	402	295	0.65 (0.57–0.75)
EF <0.25	2258	677	637	0.84 (0.76–0.93)	394	270	0.61 (0.53–0.71)
CTR >0.55	2346	687	650	0.85 (0.77–0.94)	398	287	0.65 (0.57–0.75)
EF >0.45‡	987	571	585	1.04 (0.88–1.23)	179	136	0.72 (0.53–0.99)

*Number of patients with an event during the first 2 years per 1000 randomized patients.
†Relative risk (95% confidence interval).
‡DIG Ancillary Study.

Due to the considerable variability of these interactions, the dosage of digoxin should be individualized when patients receive these medications concurrently. Furthermore, caution should be exercised when combining digoxin with any drug that may cause a significant deterioration in renal function, since a decline in glomerular filtration or tubular secretion may impair the excretion of digoxin.

Drug/Laboratory Test Interactions: The use of therapeutic doses of digoxin may cause prolongation of the PR interval and depression of the ST segment on the electrocardiogram. Digoxin may produce false positive ST-T changes on the electrocardiogram during exercise testing. These electrophysiologic effects reflect an expected effect of the drug and are not indicative of toxicity.

Carcinogenesis, Mutagenesis, Impairment of Fertility: There have been no long-term studies performed in animals to evaluate carcinogenic potential, nor have studies been conducted to assess the mutagenic potential of digoxin or its potential to affect fertility.

Pregnancy: *Teratogenic Effects:* Pregnancy Category C. Animal reproduction studies have not been conducted with digoxin. It is also not known whether digoxin can cause fetal harm when administered to a pregnant woman or can affect reproduction capacity. Digoxin should be given to a pregnant woman only if clearly needed.

Nursing Mothers: Studies have shown that digoxin concentrations in the mother's serum and milk are similar. However, the estimated exposure of a nursing infant to digoxin via breast feeding will be far below the usual infant maintenance dose. Therefore, this amount should have no pharmacologic effect upon the infant. Nevertheless, caution should be exercised when digoxin is administered to a nursing woman.

Pediatric Use: Newborn infants display considerable variability in their tolerance to digoxin. Premature and immature infants are particularly sensitive to the effects of digoxin, and the dosage of the drug must not only be reduced but must be individualized according to their degree of maturity. Digitalis glycosides can cause poisoning in children due to accidental ingestion.

Geriatric Use: The majority of clinical experience gained with digoxin has been in the elderly population. This experience has not identified differences in response or adverse effects between the elderly and younger patients. However, this drug is known to be substantially excreted by the kidney, and the risk of toxic reactions to this drug may be greater in patients with impaired renal function. Because elderly patients are more likely to have decreased renal function, care should be taken in dose selection, which should be based on renal function, and it may be useful to monitor renal function.

ADVERSE REACTIONS

In general, the adverse reactions of digoxin are dose-dependent and occur at doses higher than those needed to achieve a therapeutic effect. Hence, adverse reactions are less common when digoxin is used within the recommended dose range or therapeutic serum concentration range and when there is careful attention to concurrent medications and conditions.

Because some patients may be particularly susceptible to side effects with digoxin, the dosage of the drug should always be selected carefully and adjusted as the clinical condition of the patient warrants. In the past, when high doses of digoxin were used and little attention was paid to clinical status or concurrent medications, adverse reactions to digoxin were more frequent and severe. Cardiac adverse reactions accounted for about one-half, gastrointestinal disturbances for about one-fourth, and CNS and other toxicity for about one-fourth of these adverse reactions. However, available evidence suggests that the incidence and severity of digoxin toxicity has decreased substantially in recent years. In recent controlled clinical trials, in patients with predominantly mild to moderate heart failure, the incidence of adverse experiences was comparable in patients taking digoxin and in those taking placebo. In a large mortality trial, the incidence of hospitalization for suspected digoxin toxicity was 2% in patients taking LANOXIN Tablets compared to 0.9% in patients taking placebo. In this trial, the most common manifestations of digoxin toxicity included gastrointestinal and cardiac disturbances; CNS manifestations were less common.

Adults: *Cardiac:* Therapeutic doses of digoxin may cause heart block in patients with pre-existing sinoatrial or AV conduction disorders; heart block can be avoided by adjusting the dose of digoxin. Prophylactic use of a cardiac pacemaker may be considered if the risk of heart block is considered unacceptable. High doses of digoxin may produce a variety of rhythm disturbances, such as first-degree, second-degree (Wenckebach), or third-degree heart block (including asystole); atrial tachycardia with block; AV dissociation; accelerated junctional (nodal) rhythm; unifocal or multiform ventricular premature contractions (especially bigeminy or trigeminy); ventricular tachycardia; and ventricular fibrillation. Digoxin produces PR prolongation and ST segment depression which should not by themselves be considered digoxin toxicity. Cardiac toxicity can also occur at therapeutic doses in patients who have conditions which may alter their sensitivity to digoxin (see WARNINGS and PRECAUTIONS).

Gastrointestinal: Digoxin may cause anorexia, nausea, vomiting, and diarrhea. Rarely, the use of digoxin has been associated with abdominal pain, intestinal ischemia, and hemorrhagic necrosis of the intestines.

CNS: Digoxin can produce visual disturbances (blurred or yellow vision), headache, weakness, dizziness, apathy, confusion, and mental disturbances (such as anxiety, depression, delirium, and hallucination).

Other: Gynecomastia has been occasionally observed following the prolonged use of digoxin. Thrombocytopenia and maculopapular rash and other skin reactions have been rarely observed. Table 4 summarizes the incidence of those adverse experiences listed above for patients treated with LANOXIN Tablets or placebo from two randomized, double-blind, placebo-controlled withdrawal trials. Patients in these trials were also receiving diuretics with or without angiotensin-converting enzyme inhibitors. These patients had been stable on digoxin, and were randomized to digoxin or placebo. The results shown in Table 4 reflect the experience in patients following dosage titration with the use of serum digoxin concentrations and careful follow-up. These adverse experiences are consistent with results from a large, placebo-controlled mortality trial (DIG trial) wherein over half the patients were not receiving digoxin prior to enrollment. [See table 4 above]

Infants and Children: The side effects of digoxin in infants and children differ from those seen in adults in several respects. Although digoxin may produce anorexia, nausea, vomiting, diarrhea, and CNS disturbances in young patients, these are rarely the initial symptoms of overdosage. Rather, the earliest and most frequent manifestation of excessive dosing with digoxin in infants and children is the appearance of cardiac arrhythmias, including sinus bradycardia. In children, the use of digoxin may produce any arrhythmia. The most common are conduction disturbances or supraventricular tachyarrhythmias, such as atrial tachycardia (with or without block) and junctional (nodal) tachycardia. Ventricular arrhythmias are less common. Sinus bradycardia may be a sign of impending digoxin intoxication, especially in infants, even in the absence of first-degree heart block. Any arrhythmia or alteration in cardiac conduction that develops in a child taking digoxin should be assumed to be caused by digoxin, until further evaluation proves otherwise.

OVERDOSAGE

Treatment of Adverse Reactions Produced by Overdosage: Digoxin should be temporarily discontinued until the adverse reaction resolves. Every effort should also be made to correct factors that may contribute to the adverse reaction (such as electrolyte disturbances or concurrent medications). Once the adverse reaction has resolved, therapy with digoxin may be reinstituted, following a careful reassessment of dose.

Withdrawal of digoxin may be all that is required to treat the adverse reaction. However, when the primary manifestation of digoxin overdosage is a cardiac arrhythmia, additional therapy may be needed. If the rhythm disturbance is a symptomatic bradyarrhythmia or heart block, consideration should be given to the reversal of toxicity with DIGIBIND® [Digoxin Immune Fab (Ovine)] (see below), the use of atropine, or the insertion of a temporary cardiac pacemaker. However, asymptomatic bradycardia or heart block related to digoxin may require only temporary withdrawal of the drug and cardiac monitoring of the patient.

If the rhythm disturbance is a ventricular arrhythmia, consideration should be given to the correction of electrolyte disorders, particularly if hypokalemia (see below) or hypomagnesemia is present. DIGIBIND is a specific antidote for digoxin and may be used to reverse potentially life-threatening ventricular arrhythmias due to digoxin overdosage.

Administration of Potassium: Every effort should be made to maintain the serum potassium concentration between 4.0 and 5.5 mmol/L. Potassium is usually administered orally, but when correction of the arrhythmia is urgent and the serum potassium concentration is low, potassium may be administered cautiously by the intravenous route. The electrocardiogram should be monitored for any evidence of potassium toxicity (e.g., peaking of T waves) and to observe the effect on the arrhythmia. Potassium salts may be dangerous in patients who manifest bradycardia or heart block due to digoxin (unless primarily related to supraventricular tachycardia) and in the setting of massive digitalis overdosage (see Massive Digitalis Overdosage subsection).

Massive Digitalis Overdosage: Manifestations of life-threatening toxicity include ventricular tachycardia or ventricular fibrillation, or progressive bradyarrhythmias, or heart block. The administration of more than 10 mg of digoxin in a previously healthy adult or more than 4 mg in a previously healthy child, or a steady-state serum concentration greater than 10 ng/mL often results in cardiac arrest. DIGIBIND should be used to reverse the toxic effects of ingestion of a massive overdose. The decision to administer DIGIBIND to a patient who has ingested a massive dose of digoxin but who has not yet manifested life-threatening tox-

Table 4: Adverse Experiences In Two Parallel, Double-Blind, Placebo-Controlled Withdrawal Trials (Number of Patients Reporting)

Adverse Experience	Digoxin Patients (n = 123)	Placebo Patients (n = 125)
Cardiac		
Palpitation	1	4
Ventricular extrasystole	1	1
Tachycardia	2	1
Heart arrest	1	1
Gastrointestinal		
Anorexia	1	4
Nausea	4	2
Vomiting	2	1
Diarrhea	4	1
Abdominal pain	0	6
CNS		
Headache	4	4
Dizziness	6	5
Mental disturbances	5	1
Other		
Rash	2	1
Death	4	3

Table 5: Usual Digitalizing and Maintenance Dosages for LANOXIN Elixir Pediatric in Children with Normal Renal Function Based on Lean Body Weight

Age	Oral Digitalizing*Dose (mcg/kg)	**Daily** Maintenance Dose† (mcg/kg)
Premature	20 to 30	20% to 30% of *oral* digitalizing dose‡
Full-Term	25 to 35	
1 to 24 Months	35 to 60	
2 to 5 Years	30 to 40	25% to 35% of *oral* digitalizing dose‡
5 to 10 Years	20 to 35	
Over 10 Years	10 to 15	

*IV digitalizing doses are 80% of oral digitalizing doses.
†Divided daily dosing is recommended for children under 10 years of age.
‡Projected or actual digitalizing dose providing clinical response.

icity should depend on the likelihood that life-threatening toxicity will occur (see above).

Patients with massive digitalis ingestion should receive large doses of activated charcoal to prevent absorption and bind digoxin in the gut during enteroenteric recirculation. Emesis or gastric lavage may be indicated especially if ingestion has occurred within 30 minutes of the patient's presentation at the hospital. Emesis should not be induced in patients who are obtunded. If a patient presents more than 2 hours after ingestion or already has toxic manifestations, it may be unsafe to induce vomiting or attempt passage of a gastric tube, because such maneuvers may induce an acute vagal episode that can worsen digoxin-related arrhythmias.

Severe digitalis intoxication can cause a massive shift of potassium from inside to outside the cell, leading to life-threatening hyperkalemia. The administration of potassium supplements in the setting of massive intoxication may be hazardous and should be avoided. Hyperkalemia caused by massive digitalis toxicity is best treated with DIGIBIND; initial treatment with glucose and insulin may also be required if hyperkalemia itself is acutely life-threatening.

DOSAGE AND ADMINISTRATION

General: Recommended dosages of digoxin may require considerable modification because of individual sensitivity of the patient to the drug, the presence of associated conditions, or the use of concurrent medications. In selecting a dose of digoxin, the following factors must be considered:
1. The body weight of the patient. Doses should be calculated based upon lean (i.e., ideal) body weight.
2. The patient's renal function, preferably evaluated on the basis of estimated creatinine clearance.
3. The patient's age. Infants and children require different doses of digoxin than adults. Also, advanced age may be indicative of diminished renal function even in patients with normal serum creatinine concentration (i.e., below 1.5 mg/dL).
4. Concomitant disease states, concurrent medications, or other factors likely to alter the pharmacokinetic or pharmacodynamic profile of digoxin (see PRECAUTIONS).

Serum Digoxin Concentrations: In general, the dose of digoxin used should be determined on clinical grounds. However, measurement of serum digoxin concentrations can be helpful to the clinician in determining the adequacy of digoxin therapy and in assigning certain probabilities to the likelihood of digoxin intoxication. About two-thirds of adults

considered adequately digitalized (without evidence of toxicity) have serum digoxin concentrations ranging from 0.8 to 2.0 ng/mL. However, digoxin may produce clinical benefits even at serum concentrations below this range. About two-thirds of adult patients with clinical toxicity have serum digoxin concentrations greater than 2.0 ng/mL. However, since one-third of patients with clinical toxicity have concentrations less than 2.0 ng/mL, values below 2.0 ng/mL do not rule out the possibility that a certain sign or symptom is related to digoxin therapy. Rarely, there are patients who are unable to tolerate digoxin at serum concentrations below 0.8 ng/mL. Consequently, the serum concentration of digoxin should always be interpreted in the overall clinical context, and an isolated measurement should not be used alone as the basis for increasing or decreasing the dose of the drug.

To allow adequate time for equilibration of digoxin between serum and tissue, sampling of serum concentrations should be done just before the next scheduled dose of the drug. If this is not possible, sampling should be done at least 6 to 8 hours after the last dose, regardless of the route of administration or the formulation used. On a once-daily dosing schedule, the concentration of digoxin will be 10% to 25% lower when sampled at 24 versus 8 hours, depending upon the patient's renal function. On a twice-daily dosing schedule, there will be only minor differences in serum digoxin concentrations whether sampling is done at 8 or 12 hours after a dose.

If a discrepancy exists between the reported serum concentration and the observed clinical response, the clinician should consider the following possibilities:
1. Analytical problems in the assay procedure.
2. Inappropriate serum sampling time.
3. Administration of a digitalis glycoside other than digoxin.
4. Conditions (described in WARNINGS and PRECAUTIONS) causing an alteration in the sensitivity of the patient to digoxin.

Continued on next page

This product information is based on labeling in effect on June 1, 1998. For further information, contact via direct mail, phone, or web site Medical Information: Glaxo Wellcome Inc., PO Box 13398, Research Triangle Park, NC 27709. Healthcare Professionals (Medical Information): 800-334-0089 Patients (Customer Response Center): 888-TALK2GW (1-888-825-5249) Glaxo Wellcome Corporate Web Site: www.glaxowellcome.com

Lanoxin Elixir Pediatric—Cont.

5. Serum digoxin concentration may decrease acutely during periods of exercise without any associated change in clinical efficacy due to increased binding of digoxin to skeletal muscle.

Heart Failure: Adults: See the LANOXIN Tablets or LANOXICAPS Capsules package insert for specific recommendations.

Infants and Children: In general, divided daily dosing is recommended for infants and young children (under age 10). In the newborn period, renal clearance of digoxin is diminished and suitable dosage adjustments must be observed. This is especially pronounced in the premature infant. Beyond the immediate newborn period, children generally require proportionally larger doses than adults on the basis of body weight or body surface area. Children over 10 years of age require adult dosages in proportion to their body weight. Some researchers have suggested that infants and young children tolerate slightly higher serum concentrations than do adults.

Digitalization may be accomplished by either of two general approaches that vary in dosage and frequency of administration, but reach the same endpoint in terms of total amount of digoxin accumulated in the body.

1. If rapid digitalization is considered medically appropriate, it may be achieved by administering a loading dose based upon projected peak digoxin body stores. Maintenance dose can be calculated as a percentage of the loading dose.
2. More gradual digitalization may be obtained by beginning an appropriate maintenance dose, thus allowing digoxin body stores to accumulate slowly. Steady-state serum digoxin concentrations will be achieved in approximately five half-lives of the drug for the individual patient. Depending upon the patient's renal function, this will take between 1 and 3 weeks.

Rapid Digitalization with a Loading Dose: LANOXIN Injection Pediatric can be used to achieve rapid digitalization, with conversion to an oral formulation of LANOXIN for maintenance therapy. If patients are switched from intravenous to oral digoxin formulations, allowances must be made for differences in bioavailability when calculating maintenance dosages (see Table 1 in CLINICAL PHARMACOLOGY: Pharmacokinetics and dosing Table 5 below).

Peak digoxin body stores of 8 to 12 mcg/kg should provide therapeutic effect with minimum risk of toxicity in most patients with heart failure and normal sinus rhythm. Because of altered digoxin distribution and elimination, projected peak body stores for patients with renal insufficiency should be conservative (i.e., 6 to 10 mcg/kg [see PRECAUTIONS]). Digitalizing and daily maintenance doses for each age group are given in Table 5 and should provide therapeutic effect with minimum risk of toxicity in most patients with heart failure and normal sinus rhythm. These recommendations assume the presence of normal renal function.

The loading dose should be administered in several portions, with roughly half the total given as the first dose. Additional fractions of this planned total dose may be given at 6- to 8-hour intervals, **with careful assessment of clinical response before each additional dose.** If the patient's clinical response necessitates a change from the calculated loading dose of digoxin, then calculation of the maintenance dose should be based upon the amount actually given.

[See table 5 on previous page]

In children with renal disease, digoxin dosing must be carefully titrated based upon desired clinical response.

Gradual Digitalization With A Maintenance Dose: More gradual digitalization can also be accomplished by beginning an appropriate maintenance dose. The range of percentages provided in Table 5 can be used in calculating this dose for patients with normal renal function.

It cannot be overemphasized that these pediatric dosage guidelines are based upon average patient response and substantial individual variation can be expected. Accordingly, ultimate dosage selection must be based upon clinical assessment of the patient.

Atrial Fibrillation: Peak digoxin body stores larger than the 8 to 12 mcg/kg required for most patients with heart failure and normal sinus rhythm have been used for control of ventricular rate in patients with atrial fibrillation. Doses of digoxin used for the treatment of chronic atrial fibrillation should be titrated to the minimum dose that achieves the desired ventricular rate control without causing undesirable side effects. Data are not available to establish the appropriate resting or exercise target rates that should be achieved.

Dosage Adjustment When Changing Preparations: The difference in bioavailability between LANOXIN Injection or LANOXICAPS and LANOXIN Elixir Pediatric or LANOXIN Tablets must be considered when changing patients from one dosage form to another.

Doses of 100 mcg (0.1 mg) and 200 mcg (0.2 mg) of LANOXICAPS are approximately equivalent to 125-mcg (0.125-mg) and 250-mcg (0.25-mg) doses of LANOXIN Tablets and Elixir Pediatric, respectively (see Table 1 in CLINICAL PHARMACOLOGY: Pharmacokinetics).

HOW SUPPLIED

LANOXIN (digoxin) Elixir Pediatric, 50 mcg (0.05 mg) per mL; Bottle of 60 mL with calibrated dropper (NDC 0173-0264-27).

Store at 15° to 25°C (59° to 77°F) and protect from light.

©Copyright 1996, 1998 Glaxo Wellcome Inc. All rights reserved.

April 1998/RL-565

Shown in Product Identification Guide, page 313

LANOXIN® ℞

[lă-nŏx'ĭn"]

(digoxin)

Injection

500 µg (0.5 mg) in 2 mL (250 µg [0.25 mg] per mL)

DESCRIPTION

LANOXIN (digoxin) is one of the cardiac (or digitalis) glycosides, a closely related group of drugs having in common specific effects on the myocardium. These drugs are found in a number of plants. Digoxin is extracted from the leaves of *Digitalis lanata*. The term "digitalis" is used to designate the whole group of glycosides. The glycosides are composed of two portions: a sugar and a cardenolide (hence "glycosides"). Digoxin is described chemically as (3β,5β,12β)-3-[(*O*-2,6-dideoxy-β-*D-ribo*-hexopyranosyl-(1→4)-*O*-2,6-dideoxy-β-*D-ribo*-hexopyranosyl-(1→4)-2,6-dideoxy-β-*D-ribo*-hexopyranosyl)oxy]-12,14-dihydroxy-card-20(22)-enolide. Its molecular formula is $C_{41}H_{64}O_{14}$, and its molecular weight is 780.95.

Digoxin exists as odorless white crystals that melt with decomposition above 230°C. The drug is practically insoluble in water and in ether; slightly soluble in diluted (50%) alcohol and in chloroform; and freely soluble in pyridine.

LANOXIN Injection is a sterile solution of digoxin for intravenous injection. The vehicle contains 40% propylene glycol and 10% alcohol. The injection is buffered to a pH of 6.8 to 7.2 with 0.17% sodium phosphate and 0.08% anhydrous citric acid. Each 2-mL ampul contains 500 mcg (0.5 mg) digoxin (250 mcg [0.25 mg] per mL). Dilution is not required.

CLINICAL PHARMACOLOGY

Mechanism of Action: Digoxin inhibits sodium-potassium ATPase, an enzyme that regulates the quantity of sodium and potassium inside cells. Inhibition of the enzyme leads to an increase in the intracellular concentration of sodium and thus (by stimulation of sodium-calcium exchange) an increase in the intracellular concentration of calcium. The beneficial effects of digoxin result from direct actions on cardiac muscle, as well as indirect actions on the cardiovascular system mediated by effects on the autonomic nervous system. The autonomic effects include: (1) a vagomimetic action, which is responsible for the effects of digoxin on the sinoatrial and atrioventricular (AV) nodes; and (2) baroreceptor sensitization, which results in increased afferent inhibitory activity and reduced activity of the sympathetic nervous system and renin-angiotensin system for any given increment in mean arterial pressure. The pharmacologic consequences of these direct and indirect effects are: (1) an increase in the force and velocity of myocardial systolic contraction (positive inotropic action); (2) a decrease in the degree of activation of the sympathetic nervous system and renin-angiotensin system (neurohormonal deactivating effect); and (3) slowing of the heart rate and decreased conduction velocity through the AV node (vagomimetic effect). The effects of digoxin in heart failure are mediated by its positive inotropic and neurohormonal deactivating effects, whereas the effects of the drug in atrial arrhythmias are related to its vagomimetic actions. In high doses, digoxin increases sympathetic outflow from the central nervous system (CNS). This increase in sympathetic activity may be an important factor in digitalis toxicity.

Pharmacokinetics: Note: the following data are from studies performed in adults, unless otherwise stated.

Absorption: Comparisons of the systemic availability and equivalent doses for preparations of LANOXIN are shown in Table 1:

[See table 1 below]

Distribution: Following drug administration, a 6- to 8-hour tissue distribution phase is observed. This is followed by a much more gradual decline in the serum concentration of the drug, which is dependent on the elimination of digoxin from the body. The peak height and slope of the early portion (absorption/distribution phases) of the serum concentration-time curve are dependent upon the route of administration and the absorption characteristics of the formulation. Clinical evidence indicates that the early high serum concentrations do not reflect the concentration of digoxin at its site of action, but that with chronic use, the steady-state post-distribution serum concentrations are in equilibrium with tissue concentrations and correlate with pharmacologic effects. In individual patients, these post-distribution serum concentrations may be useful in evaluating therapeutic and toxic effects (see DOSAGE AND ADMINISTRATION: Serum Digoxin Concentrations).

Digoxin is concentrated in tissues and therefore has a large apparent volume of distribution. Digoxin crosses both the blood-brain barrier and the placenta. At delivery, the serum digoxin concentration in the newborn is similar to the serum concentration in the mother. Approximately 25% of digoxin in the plasma is bound to protein. Serum digoxin concentrations are not significantly altered by large changes in fat tissue weight, so that its distribution space correlates best with lean (i.e., ideal) body weight, not total body weight.

Metabolism: Only a small percentage (16%) of a dose of digoxin is metabolized. The end metabolites, which include 3 β-digoxigenin, 3-keto-digoxigenin, and their glucuronide and sulfate conjugates, are polar in nature and are postulated to be formed via hydrolysis, oxidation, and conjugation. The metabolism of digoxin is not dependent upon the cytochrome P-450 system, and digoxin is not known to induce or inhibit the cytochrome P-450 system.

Excretion: Elimination of digoxin follows first-order kinetics (that is, the quantity of digoxin eliminated at any time is proportional to the total body content). Following intravenous administration to healthy volunteers, 50% to 70% of a digoxin dose is excreted unchanged in the urine. Renal excretion of digoxin is proportional to glomerular filtration rate and is largely independent of urine flow. In healthy volunteers with normal renal function, digoxin has a half-life of 1.5 to 2.0 days. The half-life in anuric patients is prolonged to 3.5 to 5 days. Digoxin is not effectively removed from the body by dialysis, exchange transfusion, or during cardiopulmonary bypass because most of the drug is bound to tissue and does not circulate in the blood.

Special Populations: Race differences in digoxin pharmacokinetics have not been formally studied. Because digoxin is primarily eliminated as unchanged drug via the kidney and because there are no important differences in creatinine clearance among races, pharmacokinetic differences due to race are not expected.

Table 1: Comparisons of the Systemic Availability and Equivalent Doses for Preparations of LANOXIN

Product	Absolute Bioavailability	Equivalent Doses (mcg)* Among Dosage Forms			
LANOXIN Tablets	60 – 80%	62.5	125	250	500
LANOXIN Elixir Pediatric	70 – 85%	62.5	125	250	500
LANOXICAPS	90 – 100%	50	100	200	400
LANOXIN Injection/IV	100%	50	100	200	400

*For example, 125 mcg LANOXIN Tablets equivalent to 125 mcg LANOXIN Elixir Pediatric equivalent to 100 mcg LANOXICAPS equivalent to 100 mcg LANOXIN Injection/IV.

Table 2: Times to Onset of Pharmacologic Effect and to Peak Effect of Preparations of LANOXIN

Product	Time to Onset of Effect*	Time to Peak Effect*
LANOXIN Tablets	0.5 – 2 hours	2 – 6 hours
LANOXIN Elixir Pediatric	0.5 – 2 hours	2 – 6 hours
LANOXICAPS	0.5 – 2 hours	2 – 6 hours
LANOXIN Injection/IV	5 – 30 minutes†	1 – 4 hours

*Documented for ventricular response rate in atrial fibrillation, inotropic effects and electrocardiographic changes.
†Depending upon rate of infusion.

Table 3: Subgroup Analyses of Mortality and Hospitalization During the First Two Years Following Randomization

	n	Risk of All-Cause Mortality or All-Cause Hospitalization*			Risk of HF-Related Mortality or HF-Related Hospitalization*		
		Placebo	LANOXIN	Relative risk†	Placebo	LANOXIN	Relative risk†
All patients (EF ≤0.45)	6801	604	593	0.94 (0.88–1.00)	294	217	0.69 (0.63–0.76)
NYHA I/II	4571	549	541	0.96 (0.89–1.04)	242	178	0.70 (0.62–0.80)
EF 0.25–0.45	4543	568	571	0.99 (0.91–1.07)	244	190	0.74 (0.66–0.84)
CTR ≤0.55	4455	561	563	0.98 (0.91–1.06)	239	180	0.71 (0.63–0.81)
NYHA III/IV	2224	719	696	0.88 (0.80–0.97)	402	295	0.65 (0.57–0.75)
EF <0.25	2258	677	637	0.84 (0.76–0.93)	394	270	0.61 (0.53–0.71)
CTR >0.55	2346	687	650	0.85 (0.77–0.94)	398	287	0.65 (0.57–0.75)
EF >0.45‡	987	571	585	1.04 (0.88–1.23)	179	136	0.72 (0.53–0.99)

*Number of patients with an event during the first 2 years per 1000 randomized patients.
†Relative risk (95% confidence interval).
‡DIG Ancillary Study.

The clearance of digoxin can be primarily correlated with renal function as indicated by creatinine clearance. The Cockcroft and Gault formula for estimation of creatinine clearance includes age, body weight, and gender. A table that provides the usual daily maintenance dose requirements of LANOXIN Tablets based on creatinine clearance (per 70 kg) is presented in the DOSAGE AND ADMINISTRATION section.

Plasma digoxin concentration profiles in patients with acute hepatitis generally fell within the range of profiles in a group of healthy subjects.

Pharmacodynamic and Clinical Effects: The times to onset of pharmacologic effect and to peak effect of preparations of LANOXIN are shown in Table 2:
[See table 2 at bottom of previous page]

Hemodynamic Effects: Digoxin produces hemodynamic improvement in patients with heart failure. Short- and long-term therapy with the drug increases cardiac output and lowers pulmonary artery pressure, pulmonary capillary wedge pressure, and systemic vascular resistance. These hemodynamic effects are accompanied by an increase in the left ventricular ejection fraction and a decrease in end-systolic and end-diastolic dimensions.

Chronic Heart Failure: Two 12-week, double-blind, placebo-controlled studies enrolled 178 (RADIANCE trial) and 88 (PROVED trial) patients with NYHA class II or III heart failure previously treated with oral digoxin, a diuretic, and an ACE inhibitor (RADIANCE only) and randomized them to placebo or treatment with LANOXIN Tablets. Both trials demonstrated better preservation of exercise capacity in patients randomized to LANOXIN. Continued treatment with LANOXIN reduced the risk of developing worsening heart failure, as evidenced by heart failure-related hospitalizations and emergency care and the need for concomitant heart failure therapy. The larger study also showed treatment-related benefits in NYHA class and patients' global assessment. In the smaller trial, these trended in favor of a treatment benefit.

The Digitalis Investigation Group (DIG) main trial was a multicenter, randomized, double-blind, placebo-controlled mortality study of 6801 patients with heart failure and left ventricular ejection fraction ≤0.45. At randomization, 67% were NYHA class I or II, 71% had heart failure of ischemic etiology, 44% had been receiving digoxin, and most were receiving concomitant ACE inhibitor (94%) and diuretic (82%). Patients were randomized to placebo or LANOXIN Tablets, the dose of which was adjusted for the patient's age, sex, lean body weight, and serum creatinine (see DOSAGE AND ADMINISTRATION), and followed for up to 58 months (median 37 months). The median daily dose prescribed was 0.25 mg. Overall all-cause mortality was 35% with no difference between groups (95% confidence limits for relative risk of 0.91 to 1.07). LANOXIN was associated with a 25% reduction in the number of hospitalizations for heart failure, a 28% reduction in the risk of a patient having at least one hospitalization for heart failure, and a 6.5% reduction in total hospitalizations (for any cause).

Use of LANOXIN was associated with a trend in reduction in time to all-cause death or hospitalization. The trend was evident in subgroups of patients with mild heart failure as well as more severe disease, as shown in Table 3. Although the effect on all-cause death or hospitalization was not sta- tistically significant, much of the apparent benefit derived from effects on mortality and hospitalization attributed to heart failure.
[See table 3 above]
In situations where there is no statistically significant benefit of treatment evident from a trial's primary endpoint, results pertaining to a secondary endpoint should be interpreted cautiously.

Chronic Atrial Fibrillation: In patients with chronic atrial fibrillation, digoxin slows rapid ventricular response rate in a linear dose-response fashion from 0.25 to 0.75 mg/day. Digoxin should not be used for the treatment of multifocal atrial tachycardia.

INDICATIONS AND USAGE

Heart Failure: LANOXIN is indicated for the treatment of mild to moderate heart failure. LANOXIN increases left ventricular ejection fraction and improves heart failure symptoms as evidenced by exercise capacity and heart failure-related hospitalizations and emergency care, while having no effect on mortality. Where possible, LANOXIN should be used with a diuretic and an angiotensin-converting enzyme inhibitor, but an optimal order for starting these three drugs cannot be specified.

Atrial Fibrillation: LANOXIN is indicated for the control of ventricular response rate in patients with chronic atrial fibrillation.

CONTRAINDICATIONS

Digitalis glycosides are contraindicated in patients with ventricular fibrillation or in patients with a known hypersensitivity to digoxin. A hypersensitivity reaction to other digitalis preparations usually constitutes a contraindication to digoxin.

WARNINGS

Sinus Node Disease and AV Block: Because digoxin slows sinoatrial and AV conduction, the drug commonly prolongs the PR interval. The drug may cause severe sinus bradycardia or sinoatrial block in patients with pre-existing sinus node disease and may cause advanced or complete heart block in patients with pre-existing incomplete AV block. In such patients consideration should be given to the insertion of a pacemaker before treatment with digoxin.

Accessory AV Pathway (Wolff-Parkinson-White Syndrome): After intravenous digoxin therapy, some patients with paroxysmal atrial fibrillation or flutter and a coexisting accessory AV pathway have developed increased antegrade conduction across the accessory pathway bypassing the AV node, leading to a very rapid ventricular response or ventricular fibrillation. Unless conduction down the accessory pathway has been blocked (either pharmacologically or by surgery), digoxin should not be used in such patients. The treatment of paroxysmal supraventricular tachycardia in such patients is usually direct-current cardioversion.

Use in Patients with Preserved Left Ventricular Systolic Function: Patients with certain disorders involving heart failure associated with preserved left ventricular ejection fraction may be particularly susceptible to toxicity of the drug. Such disorders include restrictive cardiomyopathy, constrictive pericarditis, amyloid heart disease, and acute cor pulmonale. Patients with idiopathic hypertrophic subaortic stenosis may have worsening of the outflow obstruction due to the inotropic effects of digoxin.

PRECAUTIONS

Use in Patients with Impaired Renal Function: Digoxin is primarily excreted by the kidneys; therefore, patients with impaired renal function require smaller than usual maintenance doses of digoxin (see DOSAGE AND ADMINISTRATION). Because of the prolonged elimination half-life, a longer period of time is required to achieve an initial or new steady-state serum concentration in patients with renal impairment than in patients with normal renal function. If appropriate care is not taken to reduce the dose of digoxin, such patients are at high risk for toxicity, and toxic effects will last longer in such patients than in patients with normal renal function.

Use in Patients with Electrolyte Disorders: In patients with hypokalemia or hypomagnesemia, toxicity may occur despite serum digoxin concentrations below 2.0 ng/mL, because potassium or magnesium depletion sensitizes the myocardium to digoxin. Therefore, it is desirable to maintain normal serum potassium and magnesium concentrations in patients being treated with digoxin. Deficiencies of these electrolytes may result from malnutrition, diarrhea, or prolonged vomiting, as well as the use of the following drugs or procedures: diuretics, amphotericin B, corticosteroids, antacids, dialysis, and mechanical suction of gastrointestinal secretions.

Hypercalcemia from any cause predisposes the patient to digitalis toxicity. Calcium, particularly when administered rapidly by the intravenous route, may produce serious arrhythmias in digitalized patients. On the other hand, hypocalcemia can nullify the effects of digoxin in humans; thus, digoxin may be ineffective until serum calcium is restored to normal. These interactions are related to the fact that digoxin affects contractility and excitability of the heart in a manner similar to that of calcium.

Use in Thyroid Disorders and Hypermetabolic States: Hypothyroidism may reduce the requirements for digoxin. Heart failure and/or atrial arrhythmias resulting from hypermetabolic or hyperdynamic states (e.g., hyperthyroidism, hypoxia, or arteriovenous shunt) are best treated by addressing the underlying condition. Atrial arrhythmias associated with hypermetabolic states are particularly resistant to digoxin treatment. Care must be taken to avoid toxicity if digoxin is used.

Use in Patients with Acute Myocardial Infarction: Digoxin should be used with caution in patients with acute myocardial infarction. The use of inotropic drugs in some patients in this setting may result in undesirable increases in myocardial oxygen demand and ischemia.

Use During Electrical Cardioversion: It may be desirable to reduce the dose of digoxin for 1 to 2 days prior to electrical cardioversion of atrial fibrillation to avoid the induction

Continued on next page

This product information is based on labeling in effect on June 1, 1998. For further information, contact via direct mail, phone, or web site Medical Information: Glaxo Wellcome Inc., PO Box 13398, Research Triangle Park, NC 27709. Healthcare Professionals (Medical Information): 800-334-0089 Patients (Customer Response Center): 888-TALK2GW (1-888-825-5249) Glaxo Wellcome Corporate Web Site: www.glaxowellcome.com

Lanoxin Injection—Cont.

of ventricular arrhythmias, but physicians must consider the consequences of increasing the ventricular response if digoxin is withdrawn. If digitalis toxicity is suspected, elective cardioversion should be delayed. If it is not prudent to delay cardioversion, the lowest possible energy level should be selected to avoid provoking ventricular arrhythmias.

Laboratory Test Monitoring: Patients receiving digoxin should have their serum electrolytes and renal function (serum creatinine concentrations) assessed periodically; the frequency of assessments will depend on the clinical setting. For discussion of serum digoxin concentrations, see DOSAGE AND ADMINISTRATION.

Drug Interactions: Potassium-depleting *diuretics* are a major contributing factor to digitalis toxicity. *Calcium*, particularly if administered rapidly by the intravenous route, may produce serious arrhythmias in digitalized patients. *Quinidine, verapamil, amiodarone, propafenone, indomethacin, itraconazole, alprazolam,* and *spironolactone* raise the serum digoxin concentration due to a reduction in clearance and/or in volume of distribution of the drug, with the implication that digitalis intoxication may result. *Erythromycin* and *clarithromycin* (and possibly other *macrolide antibiotics*) and *tetracycline* may increase digoxin absorption in patients who inactivate digoxin by bacterial metabolism in the lower intestine, so that digitalis intoxication may result. *Propantheline* and *diphenoxylate*, by decreasing gut motility, may increase digoxin absorption. *Antacids, kaolin-pectin, sulfasalazine, neomycin, cholestyramine,* certain *anticancer drugs*, and *metoclopramide* may interfere with intestinal digoxin absorption, resulting in unexpectedly low serum concentrations. *Rifampin* may decrease serum digoxin concentration, especially in patients with renal dysfunction, by increasing the non-renal clearance of digoxin. There have been inconsistent reports regarding the effects of other drugs (e.g., *quinine, penicillamine*) on serum digoxin concentration. *Thyroid* administration to a digitalized, hypothyroid patient may increase the dose requirement of digoxin. Concomitant use of digoxin and *sympathomimetics* increases the risk of cardiac arrhythmias. *Succinylcholine* may cause a sudden extrusion of potassium from muscle cells, and may thereby cause arrhythmias in digitalized patients. Although beta-adrenergic blockers or calcium channel blockers and digoxin may be useful in combination to control atrial fibrillation, their additive effects on AV node conduction can result in advanced or complete heart block.

Due to the considerable variability of these interactions, the dosage of digoxin should be individualized when patients receive these medications concurrently. Furthermore, caution should be exercised when combining digoxin with any drug that may cause a significant deterioration in renal function, since a decline in glomerular filtration or tubular secretion may impair the excretion of digoxin.

Drug/Laboratory Test Interactions: The use of therapeutic doses of digoxin may cause prolongation of the PR interval and depression of the ST segment on the electrocardiogram. Digoxin may produce false positive ST-T changes on the electrocardiogram during exercise testing. These electrophysiologic effects reflect an expected effect of the drug and are not indicative of toxicity.

Carcinogenesis, Mutagenesis, Impairment of Fertility: There have been no long-term studies performed in animals to evaluate carcinogenic potential, nor have studies been conducted to assess the mutagenic potential of digoxin or its potential to affect fertility.

Pregnancy: ***Teratogenic Effects:*** Pregnancy Category C. Animal reproduction studies have not been conducted with digoxin. It is also not known whether digoxin can cause fetal harm when administered to a pregnant woman or can affect reproduction capacity. Digoxin should be given to a pregnant woman only if clearly needed.

Nursing Mothers: Studies have shown that digoxin concentrations in the mother's serum and milk are similar. However, the estimated exposure of a nursing infant to digoxin via breast feeding will be far below the usual infant maintenance dose. Therefore, this amount should have no pharmacologic effect upon the infant. Nevertheless, caution should be exercised when digoxin is administered to a nursing woman.

Pediatric Use: Newborn infants display considerable variability in their tolerance to digoxin. Premature and immature infants are particularly sensitive to the effects of digoxin, and the dosage of the drug must not only be reduced but must be individualized according to their degree of maturity. Digitalis glycosides can cause poisoning in children due to accidental ingestion.

Geriatric Use: The majority of clinical experience gained with digoxin has been in the elderly population. This experience has not identified differences in response or adverse effects between the elderly and younger patients. However, this drug is known to be substantially excreted by the kidney, and the risk of toxic reactions to this drug may be greater in patients with impaired renal function. Because elderly patients are more likely to have decreased renal function, care should be taken in dose selection, which should be based on renal function, and it may be useful to monitor renal function (see DOSAGE AND ADMINISTRATION).

ADVERSE REACTIONS

In general, the adverse reactions of digoxin are dose-dependent and occur at doses higher than those needed to achieve a therapeutic effect. Hence, adverse reactions are less common when digoxin is used within the recommended dose range or therapeutic serum concentration range and when there is careful attention to concurrent medications and conditions.

Because some patients may be particularly susceptible to side effects with digoxin, the dosage of the drug should always be selected carefully and adjusted as the clinical condition of the patient warrants. In the past, when high doses of digoxin were used and little attention was paid to clinical status or concurrent medications, adverse reactions to digoxin were more frequent and severe. Cardiac adverse reactions accounted for about one-half, gastrointestinal disturbances for about one-fourth, and CNS and other toxicity for about one-fourth of these adverse reactions. However, available evidence suggests that the incidence and severity of digoxin toxicity has decreased substantially in recent years. In recent controlled clinical trials, in patients with predominantly mild to moderate heart failure, the incidence of adverse experiences was comparable in patients taking digoxin and in those taking placebo. In a large mortality trial, the incidence of hospitalization for suspected digoxin toxicity was 2% in patients taking LANOXIN Tablets compared to 0.9% in patients taking placebo. In this trial, the most common manifestations of digoxin toxicity included gastrointestinal and cardiac disturbances; CNS manifestations were less common.

Adults: ***Cardiac:*** Therapeutic doses of digoxin may cause heart block in patients with pre-existing sinoatrial or AV conduction disorders; heart block can be avoided by adjusting the dose of digoxin. Prophylactic use of a cardiac pacemaker may be considered if the risk of heart block is considered unacceptable. High doses of digoxin may produce a variety of rhythm disturbances, such as first-degree, second-degree (Wenckebach), or third-degree heart block (including asystole); atrial tachycardia with block; AV dissociation; accelerated junctional (nodal) rhythm; unifocal or multiform ventricular premature contractions (especially bigeminy or trigeminy); ventricular tachycardia; and ventricular fibrillation. Digoxin produces PR prolongation and ST segment depression which should not by themselves be considered digoxin toxicity. Cardiac toxicity can also occur at therapeutic doses in patients who have conditions which may alter their sensitivity to digoxin (see WARNINGS and PRECAUTIONS).

Gastrointestinal: Digoxin may cause anorexia, nausea, vomiting, and diarrhea. Rarely, the use of digoxin has been associated with abdominal pain, intestinal ischemia, and hemorrhagic necrosis of the intestines.

CNS: Digoxin can produce visual disturbances (blurred or yellow vision), headache, weakness, dizziness, apathy, confusion, and mental disturbances (such as anxiety, depression, delirium, and hallucination).

Other: Gynecomastia has been occasionally observed following the prolonged use of digoxin. Thrombocytopenia and maculopapular rash and other skin reactions have been rarely observed. The following table summarizes the incidence of those adverse experiences listed above for patients treated with LANOXIN Tablets or placebo from two randomized, double-blind, placebo-controlled withdrawal trials. Patients in these trials were also receiving diuretics with or without angiotensin-converting enzyme inhibitors. These patients had been stable on digoxin, and were randomized to digoxin or placebo. The results shown in Table 4 reflect the experience in patients following dosage titration with the use of serum digoxin concentrations and careful follow-up. These adverse experiences are consistent with results from a large, placebo-controlled mortality trial (DIG trial) wherein over half the patients were not receiving digoxin prior to enrollment.

]See table 4 below]

Table 4: Adverse Experiences in Two Parallel, Double-Blind, Placebo-Controlled Withdrawal Trials (Number of Patients Reporting)

Adverse Experience	Digoxin Patients (n = 123)	Placebo Patients (n = 125)
Cardiac		
Palpitation	1	4
Ventricular extrasystole	1	1
Tachycardia	2	1
Heart arrest	1	1
Gastrointestinal		
Anorexia	1	4
Nausea	4	2
Vomiting	2	1
Diarrhea	4	1
Abdominal pain	0	6
CNS		
Headache	4	4
Dizziness	6	5
Mental disturbances	5	1
Other		
Rash	2	1
Death	4	3

Infants and Children: The side effects of digoxin in infants and children differ from those seen in adults in several respects. Although digoxin may produce anorexia, nausea, vomiting, diarrhea, and CNS disturbances in young patients, these are rarely the initial symptoms of overdosage. Rather, the earliest and most frequent manifestation of excessive dosing with digoxin in infants and children is the appearance of cardiac arrhythmias, including sinus bradycardia. In children, the use of digoxin may produce any arrhythmia. The most common are conduction disturbances or supraventricular tachyarrhythmias, such as atrial tachycardia (with or without block) and junctional (nodal) tachycardia. Ventricular arrhythmias are less common. Sinus bradycardia may be a sign of impending digoxin intoxication, especially in infants, even in the absence of first-degree heart block. Any arrhythmia or alteration in cardiac conduction that develops in a child taking digoxin should be assumed to be caused by digoxin, until further evaluation proves otherwise.

OVERDOSAGE

Treatment of Adverse Reactions Produced by Overdosage: Digoxin should be temporarily discontinued until the adverse reaction resolves. Every effort should also be made to correct factors that may contribute to the adverse reaction (such as electrolyte disturbances or concurrent medications). Once the adverse reaction has resolved, therapy with digoxin may be reinstituted, following a careful reassessment of dose.

Withdrawal of digoxin may be all that is required to treat the adverse reaction. However, when the primary manifestation of digoxin overdosage is a cardiac arrhythmia, additional therapy may be needed. If the rhythm disturbance is a symptomatic bradyarrhythmia or heart block, consideration should be given to the reversal of toxicity with DIGIBIND® [Digoxin Immune Fab (Ovine)] (see below), the use of atropine, or the insertion of a temporary cardiac pacemaker. However, asymptomatic bradycardia or heart block related to digoxin may require only temporary withdrawal of the drug and cardiac monitoring of the patient.

If the rhythm disturbance is a ventricular arrhythmia, consideration should be given to the correction of electrolyte disorders, particularly if hypokalemia (see below) or hypomagnesemia is present. DIGIBIND is a specific antidote for digoxin and may be used to reverse potentially life-threatening ventricular arrhythmias due to digoxin overdosage.

Administration of Potassium: Every effort should be made to maintain the serum potassium concentration between 4.0 and 5.5 mmol/L. Potassium is usually administered orally, but when correction of the arrhythmia is urgent and the serum potassium concentration is low, potassium may be administered cautiously by the intravenous route. The electrocardiogram should be monitored for any evidence of potassium toxicity (e.g., peaking of T waves) and to observe the effect on the arrhythmia. Potassium salts may be dangerous in patients who manifest bradycardia or heart block

due to digoxin (unless primarily related to supraventricular tachycardia) and in the setting of massive digitalis overdosage (see Massive Digitalis Overdosage subsection).

Massive Digitalis Overdosage: Manifestations of life-threatening toxicity include ventricular tachycardia or ventricular fibrillation, or progressive bradyarrhythmias, or heart block. The administration of more than 10 mg of digoxin in a previously healthy adult, or more than 4 mg in a previously healthy child, or a steady-state serum concentration greater than 10 ng/mL often results in cardiac arrest. DIGIBIND should be used to reverse the toxic effects of ingestion of a massive overdose. The decision to administer DIGIBIND to a patient who has ingested a massive dose of digoxin but who has not yet manifested life-threatening toxicity should depend on the likelihood that life-threatening toxicity will occur (see above).

Patients with massive digitalis ingestion should receive large doses of activated charcoal to prevent absorption and bind digoxin in the gut during enteroenteric recirculation. Emesis or gastric lavage may be indicated especially if ingestion has occurred within 30 minutes of the patient's presentation at the hospital. Emesis should not be induced in patients who are obtunded. If a patient presents more than 2 hours after ingestion or already has toxic manifestations, it may be unsafe to induce vomiting or attempt passage of a gastric tube, because such maneuvers may induce an acute vagal episode that can worsen digitalis-related arrhythmias.

Severe digitalis intoxication can cause a massive shift of potassium from inside to outside the cell, leading to life-threatening hyperkalemia. The administration of potassium supplements in the setting of massive intoxication may be hazardous and should be avoided. Hyperkalemia caused by massive digitalis toxicity is best treated with DIGIBIND; initial treatment with glucose and insulin may also be required if hyperkalemia itself is acutely life-threatening.

DOSAGE AND ADMINISTRATION

General: Recommended dosages of digoxin may require considerable modification because of individual sensitivity of the patient to the drug, the presence of associated conditions, or the use of concurrent medications. Parenteral administration of digoxin should be used only when the need for rapid digitalization is urgent or when the drug cannot be taken orally. Intramuscular injection can lead to severe pain at the injection site, thus intravenous administration is preferred. If the drug must be administered by the intramuscular route, it should be injected deep into the muscle followed by massage. No more than 500 mcg (2 mL) should be injected into a single site.

LANOXIN Injection can be administered undiluted or diluted with a 4-fold or greater volume of Sterile Water for Injection, 0.9% Sodium Chloride Injection, or 5% Dextrose Injection. The use of less than a 4-fold volume of diluent could lead to precipitation of the digoxin. Immediate use of the diluted product is recommended.

If tuberculin syringes are used to measure very small doses, one must be aware of the problem of inadvertent overadministration of digoxin. The syringe should *not* be flushed with the parenteral solution after its contents are expelled into an indwelling vascular catheter.

Slow infusion of LANOXIN Injection is preferable to bolus administration. Rapid infusion of digitalis glycosides has been shown to cause systemic and coronary arteriolar constriction, which may be clinically undesirable. Caution is thus advised and LANOXIN Injection should probably be administered over a period of 5 minutes or longer. Mixing of LANOXIN Injection with other drugs in the same container or simultaneous administration in the same intravenous line is not recommended.

In selecting a dose of digoxin, the following factors must be considered:

1. The body weight of the patient. Doses should be calculated based upon lean (i.e., ideal) body weight.
2. The patient's renal function, preferably evaluated on the basis of estimated creatinine clearance.
3. The patient's age. Infants and children require different doses of digoxin than adults. Also, advanced age may be indicative of diminished renal function even in patients with normal serum creatinine concentration (i.e., below 1.5 mg/dL).
4. Concomitant disease states, concurrent medications, or other factors likely to alter the pharmacokinetic or pharmacodynamic profile of digoxin (see PRECAUTIONS).

Serum Digoxin Concentrations: In general, the dose of digoxin used should be determined on clinical grounds. However, measurement of serum digoxin concentrations can be helpful to the clinician in determining the adequacy of digoxin therapy and in assigning certain probabilities to the likelihood of digoxin intoxication. About two-thirds of adults considered adequately digitalized (without evidence of toxicity) have serum digoxin concentrations ranging from 0.8 to 2.0 ng/mL. However, digoxin may produce clinical benefits even at serum concentrations below this range. About two-thirds of adult patients with clinical toxicity have serum digoxin concentrations greater than 2.0 ng/mL. However, since one-third of patients with clinical toxicity have concentrations less than 2.0 ng/mL, values below 2.0 ng/mL do not rule out the possibility that a certain sign or symptom is related to digoxin therapy. Rarely, there are patients who are unable to tolerate digoxin at serum concentrations below 0.8 ng/mL. Consequently, the serum concentration of digoxin should always be interpreted in the overall clinical context, and an isolated measurement should not be used alone as the basis for increasing or decreasing the dose of the drug.

To allow adequate time for equilibration of digoxin between serum and tissue, sampling of serum concentrations should be done just before the next scheduled dose of the drug. If this is not possible, sampling should be done at least 6 to 8 hours after the last dose, regardless of the route of administration or the formulation used. On a once-daily dosing schedule, the concentration of digoxin will be 10% to 25% lower when sampled at 24 versus 8 hours, depending upon the patient's renal function. On a twice-daily dosing schedule, there will be only minor differences in serum digoxin concentrations whether sampling is done at 8 or 12 hours after a dose.

If a discrepancy exists between the reported serum concentration and the observed clinical response, the clinician should consider the following possibilities:

1. Analytical problems in the assay procedure.
2. Inappropriate serum sampling time.
3. Administration of a digitalis glycoside other than digoxin.
4. Conditions (described in WARNINGS and PRECAUTIONS) causing an alteration in the sensitivity of the patient to digoxin.
5. Serum digoxin concentration may decrease acutely during periods of exercise without any associated change in clinical efficacy due to increased binding of digoxin to skeletal muscle.

Heart Failure: ***Adults:*** Digitalization may be accomplished by either of two general approaches that vary in dosage and frequency of administration, but reach the same endpoint in terms of total amount of digoxin accumulated in the body.

1. If rapid digitalization is considered medically appropriate, it may be achieved by administering a loading dose based upon projected peak digoxin body stores. Maintenance dose can be calculated as a percentage of the loading dose.
2. More gradual digitalization may be obtained by beginning an appropriate maintenance dose, thus allowing digoxin body stores to accumulate slowly. Steady-state serum digoxin concentrations will be achieved in approximately five half-lives of the drug for the individual patient. Depending upon the patient's renal function, this will take between 1 and 3 weeks.

Rapid Digitalization with a Loading Dose: LANOXIN Injection is frequently used to achieve rapid digitalization, with conversion to LANOXIN Tablets or LANOXICAPS for maintenance therapy. If patients are switched from intravenous to oral digoxin formulations, allowances must be made for differences in bioavailability when calculating maintenance dosages (see Table 1, CLINICAL PHARMACOLOGY: Pharmacokinetics and dosing Table 5 below).

Intramuscular injection of digoxin is extremely painful and offers no advantages unless other routes of administration are contraindicated.

Peak digoxin body stores of 8 to 12 mcg/kg should provide therapeutic effect with minimum risk of toxicity in most patients with heart failure and normal sinus rhythm. Because of altered digoxin distribution and elimination, projected peak body stores for patients with renal insufficiency should be conservative (i.e., 6 to 10 mcg/kg) [see PRECAUTIONS]. The loading dose should be administered in several portions, with roughly half the total given as the first dose. Additional fractions of this planned total dose may be given at 6- to 8-hour intervals, **with careful assessment of clinical response before each additional dose.** If the patient's clinical response necessitates a change from the calculated loading dose of digoxin, then calculation of the maintenance dose should be based upon the amount actually given.

A single initial intravenous dose of 400 to 600 mcg (0.4 to 0.6 mg) of LANOXIN Injection usually produces a detectable effect in 5 to 30 minutes that becomes maximal in 1 to 4 hours. Additional doses of 100 to 300 mcg (0.1 to 0.3 mg) may be given cautiously at 6- to 8-hour intervals until clinical evidence of an adequate effect is noted. The usual amount of LANOXIN Injection that a 70-kg patient requires to achieve 8- to 12-mcg/kg peak body stores is 600 to 1,000 mcg (0.6 to 1.0 mg).

Maintenance Dosing: The doses of oral digoxin used in controlled trials in patients with heart failure have ranged from 125 to 500 mcg (0.125 to 0.5 mg) once daily. In these studies, the digoxin dose has been generally titrated according to the patient's age, lean body weight, and renal function. Therapy is generally initiated at a dose of 250 mcg (0.25 mg) once daily in patients under age 70 with good renal function, at a dose of 125 mcg (0.125 mg) once daily in patients over age 70 or with impaired renal function, and at a dose of 62.5 mcg (0.0625 mg) in patients with marked renal impairment. Doses may be increased every 2 weeks according to clinical response.

In a subset of approximately 1,800 patients enrolled in the DIG trial (wherein dosing was based on an algorithm similar to that in Table 5) the mean ($\pm$ SD) serum digoxin concentrations at 1 month and 12 months were 1.01 $\pm$ 0.47 ng/mL and 0.97 $\pm$ 0.43 ng/mL, respectively.

The maintenance dose should be based upon the percentage of the peak body stores lost each day through elimination. The following formula has had wide clinical use:

Maintenance Dose = Peak Body Stores (i.e., Loading Dose) $\times$ % Daily Loss/100

Where: % Daily Loss = 14 + Ccr/5

(Ccr is creatinine clearance, corrected to 70 kg body weight or 1.73 m^2 body surface area.)

Table 5 provides average daily maintenance dose requirements of LANOXIN Injection for patients with heart failure based upon lean body weight and renal function:

[See table 5 above]

Example: Based on the above table, a patient in heart failure with an estimated lean body weight of 70 kg and a Ccr of 60 mL/min should be given a dose of 175 mcg (0.175 mg) daily of LANOXIN Injection. If no loading dose is administered, steady-state serum concentrations in this patient should be anticipated at approximately 11 days.

Table 5: Usual Daily Maintenance Dose Requirements (mcg) of LANOXIN Injection for Estimated Peak Body Stores of 10 mcg/kg*

Corrected Ccr (mL/min per 70 kg)†	Lean Body Weight kg: 50 / lb: 110	60 / 132	70 / 154	80 / 176	90 / 198	100 / 220	Number of Days Before Steady State Achieved‡
0	75§	75	100	100	125	150	22
10	75	100	100	125	150	150	19
20	100	100	125	150	150	175	16
30	100	125	150	150	175	200	14
40	100	125	150	175	200	225	13
50	125	150	175	200	225	250	12
60	125	150	175	200	225	250	11
70	150	175	200	225	250	275	10
80	150	175	200	250	275	300	9
90	150	200	225	250	300	325	8
100	175	200	250	275	300	350	7

*Daily maintenance doses have been rounded to the nearest 25-mcg increment.

†Ccr is creatinine clearance, corrected to 70 mg body weight or 1.73 m^2 body surface area. *For adults,* if only serum creatinine concentrations (Scr) are available, a Ccr (corrected to 70 kg body weight) may be estimated in men as (140 - Age)/Scr. For women, this result should be multiplied by 0.85. *Note: This equation cannot be used for estimating creatinine clearance in infants or children.*

‡If no loading dose administered.

§75 mcg = 0.075 mg

Continued on next page

This product information is based on labeling in effect on June 1, 1998. For further information, contact via direct mail, phone, or web site Medical Information: Glaxo Wellcome Inc., PO Box 13398, Research Triangle Park, NC 27709. Healthcare Professionals (Medical Information): 800-334-0089 Patients (Customer Response Center): 888-TALK2GW (1-888-825-5249) Glaxo Wellcome Corporate Web Site: www.glaxowellcome.com

Lanoxin Injection—Cont.

Infants and Children: See the full prescribing information for LANOXIN Injection Pediatric for specific recommendations.

It cannot be overemphasized that dosage guidelines provided are based upon average patient response and substantial individual variation can be expected. Accordingly, ultimate dosage selection must be based upon clinical assessment of the patient.

Atrial Fibrillation: Peak digoxin body stores larger than the 8 to 12 mcg/kg required for most patients with heart failure and normal sinus rhythm have been used for control of ventricular rate in patients with atrial fibrillation. Doses of digoxin used for the treatment of chronic atrial fibrillation should be titrated to the minimum dose that achieves the desired ventricular rate control without causing undesirable side effects. Data are not available to establish the appropriate resting or exercise target rates that should be achieved.

Dosage Adjustment When Changing Preparations: The difference in bioavailability between LANOXIN Injection or LANOXICAPS and LANOXIN Elixir Pediatric or LANOXIN Tablets must be considered when changing patients from one dosage form to another.

Doses of 100 mcg (0.1 mg) and 200 mcg (0.2 mg) of LANOXICAPS are approximately equivalent to 125-mcg (0.125-mg) and 250-mcg (0.25-mg) doses of LANOXIN Tablets and Elixir Pediatric, respectively (see Table 1 in CLINICAL PHARMACOLOGY: Pharmacokinetics).

HOW SUPPLIED

LANOXIN (digoxin) Injection, 500 mcg (0.5 mg) in 2 mL (250 mcg [0.25 mg] per mL); Boxes of 10 (NDC 0173-0260-10) and 50 ampuls (NDC 0173-0260-35).

Store at 15° to 25°C (59° to 77°F) and protect from light.

©Copyright 1996,1998 Glaxo Wellcome Inc. All rights reserved.

April 1998/RL-563

Shown in Product Identification Guide, page 313

LANOXIN® ℞

[*lă-nŏx ′ĭn* ″]

(digoxin)

Injection Pediatric

100 μg (0.1 mg) in 1 mL

DESCRIPTION

LANOXIN (digoxin) is one of the cardiac (or digitalis) glycosides, a closely related group of drugs having in common specific effects on the myocardium. These drugs are found in a number of plants. Digoxin is extracted from the leaves of *Digitalis lanata*. The term "digitalis" is used to designate the whole group of glycosides. The glycosides are composed of two portions: a sugar and a cardenolide (hence "glycosides"). Digoxin is described chemically as (3β,5β,12β)-3-[(*O*-2,6-dideoxy-β-*D*-*ribo*-hexopyranosyl-(1→4)-*O*-2,6-dideoxy-β-*D*-*ribo*-hexopyranosyl-(1→4)-2,6-dideoxy-β-*D*-*ribo*-hexopyranosyl)oxy]-12,14-dihydroxy-card-20(22)-enolide. Its molecular formula is $C_{41}H_{64}O_{14}$, and its molecular weight is 780.95.

Digoxin exists as odorless white crystals that melt with decomposition above 230°C. The drug is practically insoluble in water and in ether; slightly soluble in diluted (50%) alcohol and in chloroform; and freely soluble in pyridine.

LANOXIN Injection Pediatric is a sterile solution of digoxin for intravenous injection. The vehicle contains 40% propylene glycol and 10% alcohol. The injection is buffered to a pH of 6.8 to 7.2 with 0.17% sodium phosphate and 0.08% anhydrous citric acid. Each 1-mL ampul contains 100 mcg (0.1 mg) digoxin. Dilution is not required.

CLINICAL PHARMACOLOGY

Mechanism of Action: Digoxin inhibits sodium-potassium ATPase, an enzyme that regulates the quantity of sodium and potassium inside cells. Inhibition of the enzyme leads to an increase in the intracellular concentration of sodium and thus (by stimulation of sodium-calcium exchange) an increase in the intracellular concentration of calcium. The beneficial effects of digoxin result from direct actions on cardiac muscle, as well as indirect actions on the cardiovascular system mediated by effects on the autonomic nervous system. The autonomic effects include: (1) a vagomimetic action, which is responsible for the effects of digoxin on the sinoatrial and atrioventricular (AV) nodes; and (2) baroreceptor sensitization, which results in increased afferent inhibitory activity and reduced activity of the sympathetic nervous system and renin-angiotensin system for any given increment in mean arterial pressure. The pharmacologic consequences of these direct and indirect effects are: (1) an increase in the force and velocity of myocardial systolic contraction (positive inotropic action); (2) a decrease in the degree of activation of the sympathetic nervous system and renin-angiotensin system (neurohormonal deactivating effect); and (3) slowing of the heart rate and decreased conduction velocity through the AV node (vagomimetic effect). The effects of digoxin in heart failure are mediated by its positive inotropic and neurohormonal deactivating effects, whereas the effects of the drug in atrial arrhythmias are related to its vagomimetic actions. In high doses, digoxin increases sympathetic outflow from the central nervous system (CNS). This increase in sympathetic activity may be an important factor in digitalis toxicity.

Pharmacokinetics: Note: The following data are from studies performed in adults, unless otherwise stated.

Absorption: Comparisons of the systemic availability and equivalent doses for preparations of digoxin are shown in Table 1:

[See table 1 below]

Distribution: Following drug administration, a 6- to 8-hour tissue distribution phase is observed. This is followed by a much more gradual decline in the serum concentration of the drug, which is dependent on the elimination of digoxin from the body. The peak height and slope of the early portion (absorption/distribution phases) of the serum concentration-time curve are dependent upon the route of administration and the absorption characteristics of the formulation. Clinical evidence indicates that the early high serum concentrations do not reflect the concentration of digoxin at its site of action, but that with chronic use, the steady-state post-distribution serum concentrations are in equilibrium with tissue concentrations and correlate with pharmacologic effects. In individual patients, these post-distribution serum concentrations may be useful in evaluating therapeutic and toxic effects (see DOSAGE AND ADMINISTRATION: Serum Digoxin Concentrations).

Digoxin is concentrated in tissues and therefore has a large apparent volume of distribution. Digoxin crosses both the blood-brain barrier and the placenta. At delivery, the serum digoxin concentration in the newborn is similar to the serum concentration in the mother. Approximately 25% of digoxin in the plasma is bound to protein. Serum digoxin concentrations are not significantly altered by large changes in fat tissue weight, so that its distribution space correlates best with lean (i.e., ideal) body weight, not total body weight.

Metabolism: Only a small percentage (16%) of a dose of digoxin is metabolized. The end metabolites, which include 3 β-digoxigenin, 3-keto-digoxigenin, and their glucuronide and sulfate conjugates, are polar in nature and are postulated to be formed via hydrolysis, oxidation, and conjugation. The metabolism of digoxin is not dependent upon the cytochrome P-450 system, and digoxin is not known to induce or inhibit the cytochrome P-450 system.

Excretion: Elimination of digoxin follows first-order kinetics (that is, the quantity of digoxin eliminated at any time is proportional to the total body content). Following intravenous administration to healthy volunteers, 50% to 70% of a digoxin dose is excreted unchanged in the urine. Renal excretion of digoxin is proportional to glomerular filtration rate and is largely independent of urine flow. In healthy volunteers with normal renal function, digoxin has a half-life of 1.5 to 2.0 days. The half-life in anuric patients is prolonged to 3.5 to 5 days. Digoxin is not effectively removed from the body by dialysis, exchange transfusion, or during cardiopulmonary bypass because most of the drug is bound to tissue and does not circulate in the blood.

Special Populations: Race differences in digoxin pharmacokinetics have not been formally studied. Because digoxin is primarily eliminated as unchanged drug via the kidney and because there are no important differences in creatinine clearance among races, pharmacokinetic differences due to race are not expected.

The clearance of digoxin can be primarily correlated with renal function as indicated by creatinine clearance. In children with renal disease, digoxin must be carefully titrated based upon clinical response. Plasma digoxin concentration profiles in patients with acute hepatitis generally fell within the range of profiles in a group of healthy subjects.

Pharmacodynamic and Clinical Effects:

The times to onset of pharmacologic effect and to peak effect of preparations of LANOXIN are shown in Table 2:

[See table 2 at bottom of next page]

Hemodynamic Effects: Digoxin produces hemodynamic improvement in patients with heart failure. Short- and long-term therapy with the drug increases cardiac output and lowers pulmonary artery pressure, pulmonary capillary wedge pressure, and systemic vascular resistance. These hemodynamic effects are accompanied by an increase in the left ventricular ejection fraction and a decrease in end-systolic and end-diastolic dimensions.

Chronic Heart Failure: Two 12-week, double-blind, placebo-controlled studies enrolled 178 (RADIANCE trial) and 88 (PROVED trial) adult patients with NYHA class II or III heart failure previously treated with oral digoxin, a diuretic, and an ACE inhibitor (RADIANCE only) and randomized them to placebo or treatment with LANOXIN Tablets. Both trials demonstrated better preservation of exercise capacity in patients randomized to LANOXIN. Continued treatment with LANOXIN reduced the risk of developing worsening heart failure, as evidenced by heart failure-related hospitalizations and emergency care and the need for concomitant heart failure therapy. The larger study also showed treatment-related benefits in NYHA class and patients' global assessment. In the smaller trial, these trended in favor of a treatment benefit.

The Digitalis Investigation Group (DIG) main trial was a multicenter, randomized, double-blind, placebo-controlled mortality study of 6801 adult patients with heart failure and left ventricular ejection fraction ≤0.45. At randomization, 67% were NYHA class I or II, 71% had heart failure of ischemic etiology, 44% had been receiving digoxin, and most were receiving concomitant ACE inhibitor (94%) and diuretic (82%). Patients were randomized to placebo or LANOXIN Tablets, the dose of which was adjusted for the patient's age, sex, lean body weight, and serum creatinine (see DOSAGE AND ADMINISTRATION), and followed for up to 58 months (median 37 months). The median daily dose prescribed was 0.25 mg. Overall all-cause mortality was 35% with no difference between groups (95% confidence limits for relative risk of 0.91 to 1.07). LANOXIN was associated with a 25% reduction in the number of hospitalizations for heart failure, a 28% reduction in the risk of a patient having at least one hospitalization for heart failure, and a 6.5% reduction in total hospitalizations (for any cause).

Use of LANOXIN was associated with a trend in reduction in time to all-cause death or hospitalization. The trend was evident in subgroups of patients with mild heart failure as well as more severe disease, as shown in Table 3. Although the effect on all-cause death or hospitalization was not statistically significant, much of the apparent benefit derived from effects on mortality and hospitalization attributed to heart failure.

[See table 3 at bottom of next page]

In situations where there is no statistically significant benefit of treatment evident from a trial's primary endpoint, results pertaining to a secondary endpoint should be interpreted cautiously.

Chronic Atrial Fibrillation: In adult patients with chronic atrial fibrillation, digoxin slows rapid ventricular response rate in a linear dose-response fashion from 0.25 to 0.75 mg/day. Digoxin should not be used for the treatment of multifocal atrial tachycardia.

INDICATIONS AND USAGE

Heart Failure: LANOXIN is indicated for the treatment of mild to moderate heart failure. LANOXIN increases left ventricular ejection fraction and improves heart failure symptoms as evidenced by exercise capacity and heart failure-related hospitalizations and emergency care, while having no effect on mortality. Where possible, LANOXIN should be used with a diuretic and an angiotensin-converting enzyme inhibitor, but an optimal order for starting these three drugs cannot be specified.

Atrial Fibrillation: LANOXIN is indicated for the control of ventricular response rate in patients with chronic atrial fibrillation.

CONTRAINDICATIONS

Digitalis glycosides are contraindicated in patients with ventricular fibrillation or in patients with a known hypersensitivity to digoxin. A hypersensitivity reaction to other digitalis preparations usually constitutes a contraindication to digoxin.

WARNINGS

Sinus Node Disease and AV Block: Because digoxin slows sinoatrial and AV conduction, the drug commonly prolongs the PR interval. The drug may cause severe sinus bradycardia or sinoatrial block in patients with pre-existing sinus

Table 1: Comparisons of the Systemic Availability and Equivalent Doses for Preparations of LANOXIN

Product	Absolute Bioavailability	Equivalent Doses (mcg)* Among Dosage Forms			
LANOXIN Tablets	60 – 80%	62.5	125	250	500
LANOXIN Elixir Pediatric	70 – 85%	62.5	125	250	500
LANOXICAPS	90 – 100%	50	100	200	400
LANOXIN Injection/IV	100%	50	100	200	400

*For example, 125 mcg LANOXIN Tablets equivalent to 125 mcg LANOXIN Elixir Pediatric equivalent to 100 mcg LANOXICAPS equivalent to 100 mcg LANOXIN Injection/IV.

node disease and may cause advanced or complete heart block in patients with pre-existing incomplete AV block. In such patients consideration should be given to the insertion of a pacemaker before treatment with digoxin.

Accessory AV Pathway (Wolff-Parkinson-White Syndrome): After intravenous digoxin therapy, some patients with paroxysmal atrial fibrillation or flutter and a coexisting accessory AV pathway have developed increased antegrade conduction across the accessory pathway bypassing the AV node, leading to a very rapid ventricular response or ventricular fibrillation. Unless conduction down the accessory pathway has been blocked (either pharmacologically or by surgery), digoxin should not be used in such patients. The treatment of paroxysmal supraventricular tachycardia in such patients is usually direct-current cardioversion.

Use in Patients with Preserved Left Ventricular Systolic Function: Patients with certain disorders involving heart failure associated with preserved left ventricular ejection fraction may be particularly susceptible to toxicity of the drug. Such disorders include restrictive cardiomyopathy, constrictive pericarditis, amyloid heart disease, and acute cor pulmonale. Patients with idiopathic hypertrophic subaortic stenosis may have worsening of the outflow obstruction due to the inotropic effects of digoxin.

PRECAUTIONS

Use in Patients with Impaired Renal Function: Digoxin is primarily excreted by the kidneys; therefore, patients with impaired renal function require smaller than usual maintenance doses of digoxin (see DOSAGE AND ADMINISTRATION). Because of the prolonged elimination half-life, a longer period of time is required to achieve an initial or new steady-state serum concentration in patients with renal impairment than in patients with normal renal function. If appropriate care is not taken to reduce the dose of digoxin, such patients are at high risk for toxicity, and toxic effects will last longer in such patients than in patients with normal renal function.

Use in Patients with Electrolyte Disorders: In patients with hypokalemia or hypomagnesemia, toxicity may occur despite serum digoxin concentrations below 2.0 ng/mL, because potassium or magnesium depletion sensitizes the myocardium to digoxin. Therefore, it is desirable to maintain normal serum potassium and magnesium concentrations in patients being treated with digoxin. Deficiencies of these electrolytes may result from malnutrition, diarrhea, or prolonged vomiting, as well as the use of the following drugs or procedures: diuretics, amphotericin B, corticosteroids, antacids, dialysis, and mechanical suction of gastrointestinal secretions.

Hypercalcemia from any cause predisposes the patient to digitalis toxicity. Calcium, particularly when administered rapidly by the intravenous route, may produce serious arrhythmias in digitalized patients. On the other hand, hypocalcemia can nullify the effects of digoxin in humans; thus, digoxin may be ineffective until serum calcium is restored to normal. These interactions are related to the fact that digoxin affects contractility and excitability of the heart in a manner similar to that of calcium.

Use in Thyroid Disorders and Hypermetabolic States: Hypothyroidism may reduce the requirements for digoxin. Heart failure and/or atrial arrhythmias resulting from hypermetabolic or hyperdynamic states (e.g., hyperthyroidism, hypoxia, or arteriovenous shunt) are best treated by addressing the underlying condition. Atrial arrhythmias associated with hypermetabolic states are particularly resistant to digoxin treatment. Care must be taken to avoid toxicity if digoxin is used.

Use in Patients with Acute Myocardial Infarction: Digoxin should be used with caution in patients with acute myocardial infarction. The use of inotropic drugs in some patients in this setting may result in undesirable increases in myocardial oxygen demand and ischemia.

Use During Electrical Cardioversion: It may be desirable to reduce the dose of digoxin for 1 to 2 days prior to electrical cardioversion of atrial fibrillation to avoid the induction of ventricular arrhythmias, but physicians must consider the consequences of increasing the ventricular response if digoxin is withdrawn. If digitalis toxicity is suspected, elective cardioversion should be delayed. If it is not prudent to delay cardioversion, the lowest possible energy level should be selected to avoid provoking ventricular arrhythmias.

Laboratory Test Monitoring: Patients receiving digoxin should have their serum electrolytes and renal function (serum creatinine concentrations) assessed periodically; the frequency of assessments will depend on the clinical setting. For discussion of serum digoxin concentrations, see DOSAGE AND ADMINISTRATION.

Drug Interactions: Potassium-depleting *diuretics* are a major contributing factor to digitalis toxicity. *Calcium*, particularly if administered rapidly by the intravenous route, may produce serious arrhythmias in digitalized patients. *Quinidine, verapamil, amiodarone, propafenone, indomethacin, itraconazole, alprazolam*, and *spironolactone* raise the serum digoxin concentration due to a reduction in clearance and/or volume of distribution of the drug, with the implication that digitalis intoxication may result. *Erythromycin* and *clarithromycin* (and possibly other *macrolide antibiotics*) and *tetracycline* may increase digoxin absorption in patients who inactivate digoxin by bacterial metabolism in the lower intestine, so that digitalis intoxication may result. *Propantheline* and *diphenoxylate*, by decreasing gut motility, may increase digoxin absorption. *Antacids, kaolin-pectin, sulfasalazine, neomycin, cholestyramine*, certain *anticancer drugs*, and *metoclopramide* may interfere with intestinal digoxin absorption, resulting in unexpectedly low serum concentrations. *Rifampin* may decrease serum digoxin concentration, especially in patients with renal dysfunction, by increasing the non-renal clearance of digoxin. There have been inconsistent reports regarding the effects of other drugs [e.g., *quinine, penicillamine*] on serum digoxin concentration. *Thyroid* administration to a digitalized, hypothyroid patient may increase the dose requirement of digoxin. Concomitant use of digoxin and *sympathomimetics* increases the risk of cardiac arrhythmias. *Succinylcholine* may cause a sudden extrusion of potassium from muscle cells, and may thereby cause arrhythmias in digitalized patients. Although beta-adrenergic blockers or calcium channel blockers and digoxin may be useful in combination to control atrial fibrillation, their additive effects on AV node conduction can result in advanced or complete heart block.

Due to the considerable variability of these interactions, dosage of digoxin should be individualized when patients receive these medications concurrently. Furthermore, caution should be exercised when combining digoxin with any drug that may cause a significant deterioration in renal function, since a decline in glomerular filtration or tubular secretion may impair the excretion of digoxin.

Drug/Laboratory Test Interactions: The use of therapeutic doses of digoxin may cause prolongation of the PR interval and depression of the ST segment on the electrocardiogram. Digoxin may produce false positive ST-T changes on the electrocardiogram during exercise testing. These electrophysiologic effects reflect an expected effect of the drug and are not indicative of toxicity.

Carcinogenesis, Mutagenesis, Impairment of Fertility: There have been no long-term studies performed in animals to evaluate carcinogenic potential, nor have studies been conducted to assess the mutagenic potential of digoxin or its potential to affect fertility.

Pregnancy: ***Teratogenic Effects:*** Pregnancy Category C. Animal reproduction studies have not been conducted with digoxin. It is also not known whether digoxin can cause fetal harm when administered to a pregnant woman or can affect reproductive capacity. Digoxin should be given to a pregnant woman only if clearly needed.

Nursing Mothers: Studies have shown that digoxin concentrations in the mother's serum and milk are similar. However, the estimated exposure of a nursing infant to digoxin via breast feeding will be far below the usual infant maintenance dose. Therefore, this amount should have no pharmacologic effect upon the infant. Nevertheless, caution should be exercised when digoxin is administered to a nursing woman.

Pediatric Use: Newborn infants display considerable variability in their tolerance to digoxin. Premature and immature infants are particularly sensitive to the effects of digoxin, and the dosage of the drug must not only be reduced but must be individualized according to their degree of maturity. Digitalis glycosides can cause poisoning in children due to accidental ingestion.

Geriatric Use: The majority of clinical experience gained with digoxin has been in the elderly population. This experience has not identified differences in response or adverse effects between the elderly and younger patients. However, this drug is known to be substantially excreted by the kidney, and the risk of toxic reactions to this drug may be greater in patients with impaired renal function. Because elderly patients are more likely to have decreased renal function, care should be taken in dose selection, which should be based on renal function, and it may be useful to monitor renal function.

ADVERSE REACTIONS

In general, the adverse reactions of digoxin are dose-dependent and occur at doses higher than those needed to achieve a therapeutic effect. Hence, adverse reactions are less common when digoxin is used within the recommended dose range or therapeutic serum concentration range and when there is careful attention to concurrent medications and conditions.

Because some patients may be particularly susceptible to side effects with digoxin, the dosage of the drug should always be selected carefully and adjusted as the clinical condition of the patient warrants. In the past, when high doses of digoxin were used and little attention was paid to clinical status or concurrent medications, adverse reactions to digoxin were more frequent and severe. Cardiac adverse reactions accounted for about one-half, gastrointestinal disturb-

Continued on next page

Table 2: Times to Onset of Pharmacologic Effect and to Peak Effect of Preparations of LANOXIN

Product	Time to Onset of Effect*	Time to Peak Effect*
LANOXIN Tablets	0.5 – 2 hours	2 – 6 hours
LANOXIN Elixir Pediatric	0.5 – 2 hours	2 – 6 hours
LANOXICAPS	0.5 – 2 hours	2 – 6 hours
LANOXIN Injection/IV	5 – 30 minutes†	1 – 4 hours

*Documented for ventricular response rate in atrial fibrillation, inotropic effects and electrocardiographic changes.
†Depending upon rate of infusion.

Table 3: Subgroup Analyses of Mortality and Hospitalization During the First Two Years Following Randomization

		Risk of All-Cause Mortality or All-Cause Hospitalization*			Risk of HF-Related Mortality or HF-Related Hospitalization*		
	n	Placebo	LANOXIN	Relative risk†	Placebo	LANOXIN	Relative risk†
All patients (EF ≤0.45)	6801	604	593	0.94 (0.88–1.00)	294	217	0.69 (0.63–0.76)
NYHA I/II	4571	549	541	0.96 (0.89–1.04)	242	178	0.70 (0.62–0.80)
EF 0.25–0.45	4543	568	571	0.99 (0.91–1.07)	244	190	0.74 (0.66–0.84)
CTR ≤0.55	4455	561	563	0.98 (0.91–1.06)	239	180	0.71 (0.63–0.81)
NYHA III/IV	2224	719	696	0.88 (0.80–0.97)	402	295	0.65 (0.57–0.75)
EF <0.25	2258	677	637	0.84 (0.76–0.93)	394	270	0.61 (0.53–0.71)
CTR >0.55	2346	687	650	0.85 (0.77–0.94)	398	287	0.65 (0.57–0.75)
EF >0.45‡	987	571	585	1.04 (0.88–1.23)	179	136	0.72 (0.53–0.99)

*Number of patients with an event during the first 2 years per 1000 randomized patients.
†Relative risk (95% confidence interval).
‡DIG Ancillary Study.

This product information is based on labeling in effect on June 1, 1998. For further information, contact via direct mail, phone, or web site Medical Information: Glaxo Wellcome Inc., PO Box 13398, Research Triangle Park, NC 27709. Healthcare Professionals (Medical Information): 800-334-0089 Patients (Customer Response Center): 888-TALK2GW (1-888-825-5249) Glaxo Wellcome Corporate Web Site: www.glaxowellcome.com

Lanoxin Injection Pediatric—Cont.

ances for about one-fourth, and CNS and other toxicity for about one-fourth of these adverse reactions. However, available evidence suggests that the incidence and severity of digoxin toxicity has decreased substantially in recent years. In recent controlled clinical trials, in patients with predominantly mild to moderate heart failure, the incidence of adverse experiences was comparable in patients taking digoxin and in those taking placebo. In a large mortality trial, the incidence of hospitalization for suspected digoxin toxicity was 2% in patients taking LANOXIN Tablets compared to 0.9% in patients taking placebo. In this trial, the most common manifestations of digoxin toxicity included gastrointestinal and cardiac disturbances; CNS manifestations were less common.

Adults: *Cardiac:* Therapeutic doses of digoxin may cause heart block in patients with pre-existing sinoatrial or AV conduction disorders; heart block can be avoided by adjusting the dose of digoxin. Prophylactic use of a cardiac pacemaker may be considered if the risk of heart block is considered unacceptable. High doses of digoxin may produce a variety of rhythm disturbances, such as first-degree, second-degree (Wenckebach), or third-degree heart block (including asystole); atrial tachycardia with block; AV dissociation; accelerated junctional (nodal) rhythm; unifocal or multiform ventricular premature contractions (especially bigeminy or trigeminy); ventricular tachycardia; and ventricular fibrillation. Digoxin produces PR prolongation and ST segment depression which should not by themselves be considered digoxin toxicity. Cardiac toxicity can also occur at therapeutic doses in patients who have conditions which may alter their sensitivity to digoxin (see WARNINGS and PRECAUTIONS).

Gastrointestinal: Digoxin may cause anorexia, nausea, vomiting, and diarrhea. Rarely, the use of digoxin has been associated with abdominal pain, intestinal ischemia, and hemorrhagic necrosis of the intestines.

CNS: Digoxin can produce visual disturbances (blurred or yellow vision), headache, weakness, dizziness, apathy, confusion, and mental disturbances (such as anxiety, depression, delirium, and hallucination).

Other: Gynecomastia has been occasionally observed following the prolonged use of digoxin. Thrombocytopenia and maculopapular rash and other skin reactions have been rarely observed. The following table summarizes the incidence of those adverse experiences listed above for patients treated with LANOXIN Tablets or placebo from two randomized, double-blind, placebo-controlled withdrawal trials. Patients in these trials were also receiving diuretics with or without angiotensin-converting enzyme inhibitors. These patients had been stable on digoxin, and were randomized to digoxin or placebo. The results shown in Table 4 reflect the experience in patients following dosage titration with the use of serum digoxin concentrations and careful follow-up. These adverse experiences are consistent with results from a large, placebo-controlled mortality trial (DIG trial) wherein over half the patients were not receiving digoxin prior to enrollment.

[See table 4 below]

Infants and Children: The side effects of digoxin in infants and children differ from those seen in adults in several respects. Although digoxin may produce anorexia, nausea, vomiting, diarrhea, and CNS disturbances in young patients, these are rarely the initial symptoms of overdosage. Rather, the earliest and most frequent manifestation of excessive dosing with digoxin in infants and children is the appearance of cardiac arrhythmias, including sinus bradycardia. In children, the use of digoxin may produce any arrhythmia. The most common are conduction disturbances or supraventricular tachyarrhythmias, such as atrial tachycardia (with or without block) and junctional (nodal) tachycardia. Ventricular arrhythmias are less common. Sinus bradycardia may be a sign of impending digoxin intoxication, especially in infants, even in the absence of first-degree heart block. Any arrhythmia or alteration in cardiac conduction that develops in a child taking digoxin should be assumed to be caused by digoxin, until further evaluation proves otherwise.

OVERDOSAGE

Treatment of Adverse Reactions Produced by Overdosage: Digoxin should be temporarily discontinued until the adverse reaction resolves. Every effort should also be made to correct factors that may contribute to the adverse reaction (such as electrolyte disturbances or concurrent medications). Once the adverse reaction has resolved, therapy with digoxin may be reinstituted, following a careful reassessment of dose.

Withdrawal of digoxin may be all that is required to treat the adverse reaction. However, when the primary manifestation of digoxin overdosage is a cardiac arrhythmia, additional therapy may be needed. If the rhythm disturbance is a symptomatic bradyarrhythmia or heart block, consideration should be given to the reversal of toxicity with DIGIBIND® [Digoxin Immune Fab (Ovine)] (see below), the use of atropine, or the insertion of a temporary cardiac pacemaker. However, asymptomatic bradycardia or heart block related to digoxin may require only temporary withdrawal of the drug and cardiac monitoring of the patient.

If the rhythm disturbance is a ventricular arrhythmia, consideration should be given to the correction of electrolyte disorders, particularly if hypokalemia (see below) or hypomagnesemia is present. DIGIBIND is a specific antidote for digoxin and may be used to reverse potentially life-threatening ventricular arrhythmias due to digoxin overdosage.

Administration of Potassium: Every effort should be made to maintain the serum potassium concentration between 4.0 and 5.5 mmol/L. Potassium is usually administered orally, but when correction of the arrhythmia is urgent and the serum potassium concentration is low, potassium may be administered cautiously by the intravenous route. The electrocardiogram should be monitored for any evidence of potassium toxicity (e.g., peaking of T waves) and to observe the effect on the arrhythmia. Potassium salts may be dangerous in patients who manifest bradycardia or heart block due to digoxin (unless primarily related to supraventricular tachycardia) and in the setting of massive digitalis overdosage (see Massive Digitalis Overdosage subsection).

Massive Digitalis Overdosage: Manifestations of life-threatening toxicity include ventricular tachycardia or ventricular fibrillation, or progressive bradyarrhythmias or heart block. The administration of more than 10 mg of digoxin in a previously healthy adult, or more than 4 mg in a previously healthy child, or a steady-state serum concentration greater than 10 ng/mL often results in cardiac arrest. DIGIBIND should be used to reverse the toxic effects of ingestion of a massive overdose. The decision to administer DIGIBIND to a patient who has ingested a massive dose of digoxin but who has not yet manifested life-threatening toxicity should depend on the likelihood that life-threatening toxicity will occur (see above).

Patients with massive digitalis ingestion should receive large doses of activated charcoal to prevent absorption and bind digoxin in the gut during enteroenteric recirculation.

Emesis or gastric lavage may be indicated especially if ingestion has occurred within 30 minutes of the patient's presentation at the hospital. Emesis should not be induced in patients who are obtunded. If a patient presents more than 2 hours after ingestion or already has toxic manifestations, it may be unsafe to induce vomiting or attempt passage of a gastric tube, because such maneuvers may induce an acute vagal episode that can worsen digitalis-related arrhythmias.

Severe digitalis intoxication can cause a massive shift of potassium from inside to outside the cell, leading to life-threatening hyperkalemia. The administration of potassium supplements in the setting of massive intoxication may be hazardous and should be avoided. Hyperkalemia caused by massive digitalis toxicity is best treated with DIGIBIND; initial treatment with glucose and insulin may also be required if hyperkalemia itself is acutely life-threatening.

DOSAGE AND ADMINISTRATION

General: Recommended dosages of digoxin may require considerable modification because of individual sensitivity of the patient to the drug, the presence of associated conditions, or the use of concurrent medications.

Parenteral administration of digoxin should be used only when the need for rapid digitalization is urgent or when the drug cannot be taken orally. Intramuscular injection can lead to severe pain at the injection site, thus intravenous administration is preferred. If the drug must be administered by the intramuscular route, it should be injected deep into the muscle followed by massage. No more than 200 µg (2 mL) should be injected into a single site.

LANOXIN Injection Pediatric can be administered undiluted or diluted with a 4-fold or greater volume of Sterile Water for Injection, 0.9% Sodium Chloride Injection, or 5% Dextrose Injection. The use of less than a 4-fold volume of diluent could lead to precipitation of the digoxin. Immediate use of the diluted product is recommended.

If tuberculin syringes are used to measure very small doses, one must be aware of the problem of inadvertent overadministration of digoxin. The syringe should *not* be flushed with the parenteral solution after its contents are expelled into an indwelling vascular catheter.

Slow infusion of LANOXIN Injection Pediatric is preferable to bolus administration. Rapid infusion of digitalis glycosides has been shown to cause systemic and coronary arteriolar constriction, which may be clinically undesirable. Caution is thus advised and LANOXIN Injection Pediatric should probably be administered over a period of 5 minutes or longer. Mixing of LANOXIN Injection Pediatric with other drugs in the same container or simultaneous administration in the same intravenous line is not recommended.

In selecting a dose of digoxin, the following factors must be considered:

1. The body weight of the patient. Doses should be calculated based upon lean (i.e., ideal) body weight.
2. The patient's renal function, preferably evaluated on the basis of estimated creatinine clearance.
3. The patient's age. Infants and children require different doses of digoxin than adults. Also, advanced age may be indicative of diminished renal function even in patients with normal serum creatinine concentration (i.e., below 1.5 mg/dL).
4. Concomitant disease states, concurrent medications, or other factors likely to alter the pharmacokinetic or pharmacodynamic profile of digoxin (see PRECAUTIONS).

Serum Digoxin Concentrations: In general, the dose of digoxin used should be determined on clinical grounds. However, measurement of serum digoxin concentrations can be helpful to the clinician in determining the adequacy of digoxin therapy and in assigning certain probabilities to the likelihood of digoxin intoxication. About two-thirds of adults considered adequately digitalized (without evidence of toxicity) have serum digoxin concentrations ranging from 0.8 to 2.0 ng/mL. However, digoxin may produce clinical benefits even at serum concentrations below this range. About two-thirds of adult patients with clinical toxicity have serum digoxin concentrations greater than 2.0 ng/mL. However, since one-third of patients with clinical toxicity have concentrations less than 2.0 ng/mL, values below 2.0 ng/mL do not rule out the possibility that a certain sign or symptom is related to digoxin therapy. Rarely, there are patients who are unable to tolerate digoxin at serum concentrations below 0.8 ng/mL. Consequently, the serum concentration of digoxin should always be interpreted in the overall clinical context, and an isolated measurement should not be used alone as the basis for increasing or decreasing the dose of the drug.

To allow adequate time for equilibration of digoxin between serum and tissue, sampling of serum concentrations should be done just before the next scheduled dose of the drug. If this is not possible, sampling should be done at least 6 to 8 hours after the last dose, regardless of the route of administration or the formulation used. On a once-daily dosing schedule, the concentration of digoxin will be 10% to 25% lower when sampled at 24 versus 8 hours, depending upon

Table 4: Adverse Experiences in Two Parallel, Double-Blind Placebo-Controlled Withdrawal Trials (Number of Patients Reporting)

Adverse Experience	Digoxin Patients (n = 123)	Placebo Patients (n = 125)
Cardiac		
Palpitation	1	4
Ventricular extrasystole	1	1
Tachycardia	2	1
Heart arrest	1	1
Gastrointestinal		
Anorexia	1	4
Nausea	4	2
Vomiting	2	1
Diarrhea	4	1
Abdominal pain	0	6
CNS		
Headache	4	4
Dizziness	6	5
Mental disturbances	5	1
Other		
Rash	2	1
Death	4	3

Table 5: Usual Digitalizing and Maintenance Dosages for LANOXIN Injection Pediatric in Children with Normal Renal Function Based on Lean Body Weight

Age	IV Digitalizing* Dose (mcg/kg)	Daily IV Maintenance Dose† (mcg/kg)
Premature	15 to 25	20% to 30% of the IV digitalizing dose‡
Full-Term	20 to 30	
1 to 24 Months	30 to 50	
2 to 5 Years	25 to 35	25% to 35% of the IV digitalizing dose‡
5 to 10 Years	15 to 30	
Over 10 Years	8 to 12	

* IV digitalizing doses are 80% of oral digitalizing doses.
† Divided daily dosing is recommended for children under 10 years of age.
‡ Projected or actual digitalizing dose providing clinical response.

the patient's renal function. On a twice-daily dosing schedule, there will be only minor differences in serum digoxin concentrations whether sampling is done at 8 or 12 hours after a dose.

If a discrepancy exists between the reported serum concentration and the observed clinical response, the clinician should consider the following possibilities:

1. Analytical problems in the assay procedure.
2. Inappropriate serum sampling time.
3. Administration of a digitalis glycoside other than digoxin.
4. Conditions (described in WARNINGS and PRECAUTIONS) causing an alteration in the sensitivity of the patient to digoxin.
5. Serum digoxin concentration may decrease acutely during periods of exercise without any associated change in clinical efficacy due to increased binding of digoxin to skeletal muscle.

Heart Failure: Adults: See the full prescribing information for LANOXIN Injection for specific recommendations.

Infants and Children: In general, divided daily dosing is recommended for infants and young children (under age 10). In the newborn period, renal clearance of digoxin is diminished and suitable dosage adjustments must be observed. This is especially pronounced in the premature infant. Beyond the immediate newborn period, children generally require proportionally larger doses than adults on the basis of body weight or body surface area. Children over 10 years of age require adult dosages in proportion to their body weight. Some researchers have suggested that infants and young children tolerate slightly higher serum concentrations than do adults.

Digitalization may be accomplished by either of two general approaches that vary in dosage and frequency of administration, but reach the same endpoint in terms of total amount of digoxin accumulated in the body.

1. If rapid digitalization is considered medically appropriate, it may be achieved by administering a loading dose based upon projected peak digoxin body stores. Maintenance dose can be calculated as a percentage of the loading dose.
2. More gradual digitalization may be obtained by beginning an appropriate maintenance dose, thus allowing digoxin body stores to accumulate slowly. Steady-state serum digoxin concentrations will be achieved in approximately five half-lives of the drug for the individual patient. Depending upon the patient's renal function, this will take between 1 and 3 weeks.

Rapid Digitalization with a Loading Dose: LANOXIN Injection Pediatric can be used to achieve rapid digitalization, with conversion to an oral formulation of LANOXIN for maintenance therapy. If patients are switched from intravenous to oral digoxin formulations, allowances must be made for differences in bioavailability when calculating maintenance dosages (see Table 1 in CLINICAL PHARMACOLOGY: Pharmacokinetics and dosing Table 5 below).

Intramuscular injection of digoxin is extremely painful and offers no advantages unless other routes of administration are contraindicated.

Peak digoxin body stores of 8 to 12 mcg/kg should provide therapeutic effect with minimum risk of toxicity in most patients with heart failure and normal sinus rhythm. Because of altered digoxin distribution and elimination, projected peak body stores for patients with renal insufficiency should be conservative (i.e., 6 to 10 mcg/kg) [see PRECAUTIONS].

Digitalizing and daily maintenance doses for each age group are given in Table 5 and should provide therapeutic effect with minimum risk of toxicity in most patients with heart failure and normal sinus rhythm. These recommendations assume the presence of normal renal function.

The loading dose should be administered in several portions, with roughly half the total given as the first dose. Additional fractions of this planned total dose may be given at 4- to 8-hour intervals, **with careful assessment of clinical response before each additional dose.** If the patient's clinical response necessitates a change from the calculated loading dose of digoxin, then calculation of the maintenance dose should be based upon the amount actually given.

[See table 5 above]

In children with renal disease, digoxin dosing must be carefully titrated based on clinical response.

Gradual Digitalization With A Maintenance Dose: More gradual digitalization can also be accomplished by beginning an appropriate maintenance dose. The range of percentages provided in Table 5 can be used in calculating this dose for patients with normal renal function.

It cannot be overemphasized that these pediatric dosage guidelines are based upon average patient response and substantial individual variation can be expected. Accordingly, ultimate dosage selection must be based upon clinical assessment of the patient.

Atrial Fibrillation: Peak digoxin body stores larger than the 8 to 12 mcg/kg required for most patients with heart failure and normal sinus rhythm have been used for control of ventricular rate in patients with atrial fibrillation. Doses of digoxin used for the treatment of chronic atrial fibrillation should be titrated to the minimum dose that achieves the desired ventricular rate control without causing undesirable side effects. Data are not available to establish the appropriate resting or exercise target rates that should be achieved.

Dosage Adjustment When Changing Preparations: The differences in bioavailability between injectable LANOXIN or LANOXICAPS and LANOXIN Elixir Pediatric or LANOXIN Tablets must be considered when changing patients from one dosage form to another.

Doses of 100 mcg (0.1 mg) and 200 mcg (0.2 mg) of LANOXICAPS are approximately equivalent to 125 mcg (0.125 mg) and 250 mcg (0.25 mg) doses of LANOXIN Tablets and Elixir Pediatric, respectively (see Table 1 in CLINICAL PHARMACOLOGY: Pharmacokinetics).

HOW SUPPLIED

LANOXIN (digoxin) Injection Pediatric, 100 mcg (0.1 mg) in 1 mL; box of 10 ampuls (NDC 0173-0262-10).

Store at 15° to 25°C (59° to 77°F) and protect from light.

©Copyright 1996, 1998 Glaxo Wellcome Inc. All rights reserved.

April 1998/RL-564

Shown in Product Identification Guide, page 313

LANOXIN® ℞

[*lă-nŏx ' in*]
(digoxin)
Tablets, USP
125 mcg (0.125 mg) Scored I.D. Imprint Y3B (yellow)
250 mcg (0.25 mg) Scored I.D. Imprint X3A (white)

DESCRIPTION

LANOXIN (digoxin) is one of the cardiac (or digitalis) glycosides, a closely related group of drugs having in common specific effects on the myocardium. These drugs are found in a number of plants. Digoxin is extracted from the leaves of *Digitalis lanata*. The term "digitalis" is used to designate the whole group of glycosides. The glycosides are composed of two portions: a sugar and a cardenolide (hence "glycosides").

Digoxin is described chemically as (3β,5β,12β)-3-[(*O*-2,6-dideoxy-β-*D*-*ribo*-hexopyranosyl-(1→4)-*O*-2,6-dideoxy-β-*D*-*ribo*-hexopyranosyl-(1→4)-2,6-dideoxy-β-*D*-*ribo*-hexopyranosyl)oxy]-12,14-dihydroxy-card-20(22)-enolide. Its molecular formula is $C_{41}H_{64}O_{14}$, and its molecular weight is 780.95.

Digoxin exists as odorless white crystals that melt with decomposition above 230°C. The drug is practically insoluble in water and in ether; slightly soluble in diluted (50%) alcohol and in chloroform; and freely soluble in pyridine.

LANOXIN is supplied as 125-mcg (0.125-mg) or 250-mcg (0.25-mg) tablets for oral administration. Each tablet contains the labeled amount of digoxin USP and the following inactive ingredients: corn and potato starches, lactose, and magnesium stearate. In addition, the dyes used in the 125-mcg (0.125-mg) tablets are D&C Yellow No. 10 and FD&C Yellow No. 6.

CLINICAL PHARMACOLOGY

Mechanism of Action: Digoxin inhibits sodium-potassium ATPase, an enzyme that regulates the quantity of sodium and potassium inside cells. Inhibition of the enzyme leads to an increase in the intracellular concentration of sodium and thus (by stimulation of sodium-calcium exchange) an increase in the intracellular concentration of calcium. The beneficial effects of digoxin result from direct actions on cardiac muscle, as well as indirect actions on the cardiovascular system mediated by effects on the autonomic nervous system. The autonomic effects include: (1) a vagomimetic action, which is responsible for the effects of digoxin on the sinoatrial and atrioventricular (AV) nodes; and (2) baroreceptor sensitization, which results in increased afferent inhibitory activity and reduced activity of the sympathetic nervous system and renin-angiotensin system for any given increment in mean arterial pressure. The pharmacologic consequences of these direct and indirect effects are: (1) an increase in the force and velocity of myocardial systolic contraction (positive inotropic action); (2) a decrease in the degree of activation of the sympathetic nervous system and renin-angiotensin system (neurohormonal deactivating effect); and (3) slowing of the heart rate and decreased conduction velocity through the AV node (vagomimetic effect). The effects of digoxin in heart failure are mediated by its positive inotropic and neurohormonal deactivating effects, whereas the effects of the drug in atrial arrhythmias are related to its vagomimetic actions. In high doses, digoxin increases sympathetic outflow from the central nervous system (CNS). This increase in sympathetic activity may be an important factor in digitalis toxicity.

Pharmacokinetics: ***Absorption:*** Following oral administration, peak serum concentrations of digoxin occur at 1 to 3 hours. Absorption of digoxin from LANOXIN Tablets has been demonstrated to be 60% to 80% complete compared to an identical intravenous dose of digoxin (absolute bioavailability) or LANOXICAPS® (relative bioavailability). When LANOXIN Tablets are taken after meals, the rate of absorption is slowed, but the total amount of digoxin absorbed is usually unchanged. When taken with meals high in bran fiber, however, the amount absorbed from an oral dose may be reduced. Comparisons of the systemic availability and equivalent doses for oral preparations of LANOXIN are shown in Table 1:

[See table 1 at top of next page]

In some patients, orally administered digoxin is converted to inactive reduction products (e.g., dihydrodigoxin) by colonic bacteria in the gut. Data suggest that one in ten patients treated with digoxin tablets will degrade 40% or more of the ingested dose. As a result, certain antibiotics may increase the absorption of digoxin in such patients. Although inactivation of these bacteria by antibiotics is rapid, the serum digoxin concentration will rise at a rate consistent with the elimination half-life of digoxin. The magnitude of rise in serum digoxin concentration relates to the extent of bacterial inactivation, and may be as much as two-fold in some cases.

Distribution: Following drug administration, a 6- to 8-hour tissue distribution phase is observed. This is followed by a much more gradual decline in the serum concentration of the drug, which is dependent on the elimination of digoxin from the body. The peak height and slope of the early portion (absorption/distribution phases) of the serum concentration-time curve are dependent upon the route of administration and the absorption characteristics of the formulation. Clinical evidence indicates that the early high serum concentrations do not reflect the concentration of digoxin at its site of action, but that with chronic use, the steady-state post-distribution serum concentrations are in equilibrium with tissue concentrations and correlate with pharmacologic effects. In individual patients, these post-distribution serum concentrations may be useful in evaluating therapeutic and toxic effects (see DOSAGE AND ADMINISTRATION: Serum Digoxin Concentrations).

Digoxin is concentrated in tissues and therefore has a large apparent volume of distribution. Digoxin crosses both the blood-brain barrier and the placenta. At delivery, the serum digoxin concentration in the newborn is similar to the serum concentration in the mother. Approximately 25% of digoxin in the plasma is bound to protein. Serum digoxin concentrations are not significantly altered by large changes in fat tissue weight, so that its distribution space correlates best with lean (i.e., ideal) body weight, not total body weight.

Metabolism: Only a small percentage (16%) of a dose of digoxin is metabolized. The end metabolites, which include

Continued on next page

This product information is based on labeling in effect on June 1, 1998. For further information, contact via direct mail, phone, or web site Medical Information: Glaxo Wellcome Inc., PO Box 13398, Research Triangle Park, NC 27709. Healthcare Professionals (Medical Information): 800-334-0089 Patients (Customer Response Center): 888-TALK2GW (1-888-825-5249) Glaxo Wellcome Corporate Web Site: www.glaxowellcome.com

Lanoxin Tablets—Cont.

3 β-digoxigenin, 3-keto-digoxigenin, and their glucuronide and sulfate conjugates, are polar in nature and are postulated to be formed via hydrolysis, oxidation, and conjugation. The metabolism of digoxin is not dependent upon the cytochrome P-450 system, and digoxin is not known to induce or inhibit the cytochrome P-450 system.

Excretion: Elimination of digoxin follows first-order kinetics (that is, the quantity of digoxin eliminated at any time is proportional to the total body content). Following intravenous administration to healthy volunteers, 50% to 70% of a digoxin dose is excreted unchanged in the urine. Renal excretion of digoxin is proportional to glomerular filtration rate and is largely independent of urine flow. In healthy volunteers with normal renal function, digoxin has a half-life of 1.5 to 2.0 days. The half-life in anuric patients is prolonged to 3.5 to 5 days. Digoxin is not effectively removed from the body by dialysis, exchange transfusion, or during cardiopulmonary bypass because most of the drug is bound to tissue and does not circulate in the blood.

Special Populations: Race differences in digoxin pharmacokinetics have not been formally studied. Because digoxin is primarily eliminated as unchanged drug via the kidney and because there are no important differences in creatinine clearance among races, pharmacokinetic differences due to race are not expected.

The clearance of digoxin can be primarily correlated with renal function as indicated by creatinine clearance. The Cockcroft and Gault formula for estimation of creatinine clearance includes age, body weight, and gender. A table that provides the usual daily maintenance dose requirements of LANOXIN Tablets based on creatinine clearance (per 70 kg) is presented in the DOSAGE AND ADMINISTRATION section.

Plasma digoxin concentration profiles in patients with acute hepatitis generally fell within the range of profiles in a group of healthy subjects.

Pharmacodynamic and Clinical Effects: The times to onset of pharmacologic effect and to peak effect of preparations of LANOXIN are shown in Table 2:

[See table 2 below]

Hemodynamic Effects: Digoxin produces hemodynamic improvement in patients with heart failure. Short- and long-term therapy with the drug increases cardiac output and lowers pulmonary artery pressure, pulmonary capillary wedge pressure, and systemic vascular resistance. These hemodynamic effects are accompanied by an increase in the left ventricular ejection fraction and a decrease in end-systolic and end-diastolic dimensions.

Chronic Heart Failure: Two 12-week, double-blind, placebo-controlled studies enrolled 178 (RADIANCE trial) and 88 (PROVED trial) patients with NYHA class II or III heart failure previously treated with digoxin, a diuretic, and an ACE inhibitor (RADIANCE only) and randomized them to placebo or treatment with LANOXIN. Both trials demonstrated better preservation of exercise capacity in patients randomized to LANOXIN. Continued treatment with LANOXIN reduced the risk of developing worsening heart failure, as evidenced by heart failure-related hospitalizations and emergency care and the need for concomitant heart failure therapy. The larger study also showed treatment-related benefits in NYHA class and patients' global assessment. In the smaller trial, these trended in favor of a treatment benefit.

The Digitalis Investigation Group (DIG) main trial was a multicenter, randomized, double-blind, placebo-controlled mortality study of 6,801 patients with heart failure and left ventricular ejection fraction ≤0.45. At randomization, 67% were NYHA class I or II, 71% had heart failure of ischemic etiology, 44% had been receiving digoxin, and most were receiving concomitant ACE inhibitor (94%) and diuretic (82%). Patients were randomized to placebo or LANOXIN, the dose of which was adjusted for the patient's age, sex, lean body weight, and serum creatinine (see DOSAGE AND ADMINISTRATION), and followed for up to 58 months (median 37 months). The median daily dose prescribed was 0.25 mg. Overall all-cause mortality was 35% with no difference between groups (95% confidence limits for relative risk of 0.91 to 1.07). LANOXIN was associated with a 25% reduction in the number of hospitalizations for heart failure, a 28% reduction in the risk of a patient having at least one hospitalization for heart failure, and a 6.5% reduction in total hospitalizations (for any cause).

Table 1: Comparisons of the Systemic Availability and Equivalent Doses for Oral Preparations of LANOXIN

Product	Absolute Bioavailability	Equivalent Doses (mcg)* Among Dosage Forms			
LANOXIN Tablets	60 – 80%	62.5	125	250	500
LANOXIN Elixir Pediatric	70 – 85%	62.5	125	250	500
LANOXICAPS®	90 – 100%	50	100	200	400
LANOXIN Injection/IV	100%	50	100	200	400

*For example, 125-mcg LANOXIN Tablets equivalent to 125 mcg LANOXIN Elixir Pediatric equivalent to 100 mcg LANOXICAPS equivalent to 100 mcg LANOXIN Injection/IV.

Use of LANOXIN was associated with a trend in reduction in time to all-cause death or hospitalization. The trend was evident in subgroups of patients with mild heart failure as well as more severe disease, as shown in Table 3. Although the effect on all-cause death or hospitalization was not statistically significant, much of the apparent benefit derived from effects on mortality and hospitalization attributed to heart failure.

[See table 3 at bottom of next page]

In situations where there is no statistically significant benefit of treatment evident from a trial's primary endpoint, results pertaining to a secondary endpoint should be interpreted cautiously.

Chronic Atrial Fibrillation: In patients with chronic atrial fibrillation, digoxin slows rapid ventricular response rate in a linear dose-response fashion from 0.25 to 0.75 mg/day. Digoxin should not be used for the treatment of multifocal atrial tachycardia.

INDICATIONS AND USAGE

Heart Failure: LANOXIN is indicated for the treatment of mild to moderate heart failure. LANOXIN increases left ventricular ejection fraction and improves heart failure symptoms as evidenced by exercise capacity and heart failure-related hospitalizations and emergency care, while having no effect on mortality. Where possible, LANOXIN should be used with a diuretic and an angiotensin-converting enzyme inhibitor, but an optimal order for starting these three drugs cannot be specified.

Atrial Fibrillation: LANOXIN is indicated for the control of ventricular response rate in patients with chronic atrial fibrillation.

CONTRAINDICATIONS

Digitalis glycosides are contraindicated in patients with ventricular fibrillation or in patients with a known hypersensitivity to digoxin. A hypersensitivity reaction to other digitalis preparations usually constitutes a contraindication to digoxin.

WARNINGS

Sinus Node Disease and AV Block: Because digoxin slows sinoatrial and AV conduction, the drug commonly prolongs the PR interval. The drug may cause severe sinus bradycardia or sinoatrial block in patients with pre-existing sinus node disease and may cause advanced or complete heart block in patients with pre-existing incomplete AV block. In such patients consideration should be given to the insertion of a pacemaker before treatment with digoxin.

Accessory AV Pathway (Wolff-Parkinson-White Syndrome): After intravenous digoxin therapy, some patients with paroxysmal atrial fibrillation or flutter and a coexisting accessory AV pathway have developed increased antegrade conduction across the accessory pathway bypassing the AV node, leading to a very rapid ventricular response or ventricular fibrillation. Unless conduction down the accessory pathway has been blocked (either pharmacologically or by surgery), digoxin should not be used in such patients. The treatment of paroxysmal supraventricular tachycardia in such patients is usually direct-current cardioversion.

Use in Patients with Preserved Left Ventricular Systolic Function: Patients with certain disorders involving heart failure associated with preserved left ventricular ejection fraction may be particularly susceptible to toxicity of the drug. Such disorders include restrictive cardiomyopathy, constrictive pericarditis, amyloid heart disease, and acute cor pulmonale. Patients with idiopathic hypertrophic subaortic stenosis may have worsening of the outflow obstruction due to the inotropic effects of digoxin.

PRECAUTIONS

Use in Patients with Impaired Renal Function: Digoxin is primarily excreted by the kidneys; therefore, patients with impaired renal function require smaller than usual maintenance doses of digoxin (see DOSAGE AND ADMINISTRATION). Because of the prolonged elimination half-life, a longer period of time is required to achieve an initial or new steady-state serum concentration in patients with renal impairment than in patients with normal renal function. If appropriate care is not taken to reduce the dose of digoxin, such patients are at high risk for toxicity, and toxic effects will last longer in such patients than in patients with normal renal function.

Use in Patients with Electrolyte Disorders: In patients with hypokalemia or hypomagnesemia, toxicity may occur despite serum digoxin concentrations below 2.0 ng/mL, because potassium or magnesium depletion sensitizes the myocardium to digoxin. Therefore, it is desirable to maintain normal serum potassium and magnesium concentrations in patients being treated with digoxin. Deficiencies of these electrolytes may result from malnutrition, diarrhea, or prolonged vomiting, as well as the use of the following drugs or procedures: diuretics, amphotericin B, corticosteroids, antacids, dialysis, and mechanical suction of gastrointestinal secretions.

Hypercalcemia from any cause predisposes the patient to digitalis toxicity. Calcium, particularly when administered rapidly by the intravenous route, may produce serious arrhythmias in digitalized patients. On the other hand, hypocalcemia can nullify the effects of digoxin in humans; thus, digoxin may be ineffective until serum calcium is restored to normal. These interactions are related to the fact that digoxin affects contractility and excitability of the heart in a manner similar to that of calcium.

Use in Thyroid Disorders and Hypermetabolic States: Hypothyroidism may reduce the requirements for digoxin. Heart failure and/or atrial arrhythmias resulting from hypermetabolic or hyperdynamic states (e.g., hyperthyroidism, hypoxia, or arteriovenous shunt) are best treated by addressing the underlying condition. Atrial arrhythmias associated with hypermetabolic states are particularly resistant to digoxin treatment. Care must be taken to avoid toxicity if digoxin is used.

Use in Patients with Acute Myocardial Infarction: Digoxin should be used with caution in patients with acute myocardial infarction. The use of inotropic drugs in some patients in this setting may result in undesirable increases in myocardial oxygen demand and ischemia.

Use During Electrical Cardioversion: It may be desirable to reduce the dose of digoxin for 1 to 2 days prior to electrical cardioversion of atrial fibrillation to avoid the induction of ventricular arrhythmias, but physicians must consider the consequences of increasing the ventricular response if digoxin is withdrawn. If digitalis toxicity is suspected, elective cardioversion should be delayed. If it is not prudent to delay cardioversion, the lowest possible energy level should be selected to avoid provoking ventricular arrhythmias.

Laboratory Test Monitoring: Patients receiving digoxin should have their serum electrolytes and renal function (serum creatinine concentrations) assessed periodically; the frequency of assessments will depend on the clinical setting. For discussion of serum digoxin concentrations, see DOSAGE AND ADMINISTRATION section.

Drug Interactions: Potassium-depleting *diuretics* are a major contributing factor to digitalis toxicity. *Calcium*, particularly if administered rapidly by the intravenous route, may produce serious arrhythmias in digitalized patients. *Quinidine, verapamil, amiodarone, propafenone, indomethacin, itraconazole, alprazolam*, and *spironolactone* raise the serum digoxin concentration due to a reduction in clearance and/or in volume of distribution of the drug, with the implication that digitalis intoxication may result. *Erythromycin* and *clarithromycin* (and possibly other *macrolide antibiotics*) and *tetracycline* may increase digoxin absorption in patients who inactivate digoxin by bacterial metabolism in the lower intestine, so that digitalis intoxication may result (see CLINICAL PHARMACOLOGY: Absorption). *Propantheline* and *diphenoxylate*, by decreasing gut motility, may increase digoxin absorption. *Antacids, kaolin-pectin, sulfasalazine, neomycin, cholestyramine*, certain *anticancer drugs*, and

Table 2: Times to Onset of Pharmacologic Effect and to Peak Effect of Preparations of LANOXIN

Product	Time to Onset of Effect*	Time to Peak Effect*
LANOXIN Tablets	0.5 – 2 hours	2 – 6 hours
LANOXIN Elixir Pediatric	0.5 – 2 hours	2 – 6 hours
LANOXICAPS	0.5 – 2 hours	2 – 6 hours
LANOXIN Injection/IV	5 – 30 minutes†	1 – 4 hours

* Documented for ventricular response rate in atrial fibrillation, inotropic effects and electrocardiographic changes.
† Depending upon rate of infusion.

metoclopramide may interfere with intestinal digoxin absorption, resulting in unexpectedly low serum concentrations. *Rifampin* may decrease serum digoxin concentration, especially in patients with renal dysfunction, by increasing the non-renal clearance of digoxin. There have been inconsistent reports regarding the effects of other drugs [e.g., *quinine, penicillamine*] on serum digoxin concentration. *Thyroid* administration to a digitalized, hypothyroid patient may increase the dose requirement of digoxin. Concomitant use of digoxin and *sympathomimetics* increases the risk of cardiac arrhythmias. *Succinylcholine* may cause a sudden extrusion of potassium from muscle cells, and may thereby cause arrhythmias in digitalized patients. Although beta-adrenergic blockers or calcium channel blockers and digoxin may be useful in combination to control atrial fibrillation, their additive effects on AV node conduction can result in advanced or complete heart block.

Due to the considerable variability of these interactions, the dosage of digoxin should be individualized when patients receive these medications concurrently. Furthermore, caution should be exercised when combining digoxin with any drug that may cause a significant deterioration in renal function, since a decline in glomerular filtration or tubular secretion may impair the excretion of digoxin.

Drug/Laboratory Test Interactions: The use of therapeutic doses of digoxin may cause prolongation of the PR interval and depression of the ST segment on the electrocardiogram. Digoxin may produce false positive ST-T changes on the electrocardiogram during exercise testing. These electrophysiologic effects reflect an expected effect of the drug and are not indicative of toxicity.

Carcinogenesis, Mutagenesis, Impairment of Fertility: There have been no long-term studies performed in animals to evaluate carcinogenic potential, nor have studies been conducted to assess the mutagenic potential of digoxin or its potential to affect fertility.

Pregnancy: ***Teratogenic Effects:*** Pregnancy Category C. Animal reproduction studies have not been conducted with digoxin. It is also not known whether digoxin can cause fetal harm when administered to a pregnant woman or can affect reproductive capacity. Digoxin should be given to a pregnant woman only if clearly needed.

Nursing Mothers: Studies have shown that digoxin concentrations in the mother's serum and milk are similar. However, the estimated exposure of a nursing infant to digoxin via breast feeding will be far below the usual infant maintenance dose. Therefore, this amount should have no pharmacologic effect upon the infant. Nevertheless, caution should be exercised when digoxin is administered to a nursing woman.

Pediatric Use: Newborn infants display considerable variability in their tolerance to digoxin. Premature and immature infants are particularly sensitive to the effects of digoxin, and the dosage of the drug must not only be reduced but must be individualized according to their degree of maturity. Digitalis glycosides can cause poisoning in children due to accidental ingestion.

Geriatric Use: The majority of clinical experience gained with digoxin has been in the elderly population. This experience has not identified differences in response or adverse effects between the elderly and younger patients. However, this drug is known to be substantially excreted by the kidney, and the risk of toxic reactions to this drug may be greater in patients with impaired renal function. Because elderly patients are more likely to have decreased renal function, care should be taken in dose selection, which should be based on renal function, and it may be useful to monitor renal function (see DOSAGE AND ADMINISTRATION).

ADVERSE REACTIONS

In general, the adverse reactions of digoxin are dose-dependent and occur at doses higher than those needed to achieve a therapeutic effect. Hence, adverse reactions are less common when digoxin is used within the recommended dose range or therapeutic serum concentration range and when there is careful attention to concurrent medications and conditions.

Because some patients may be particularly susceptible to side effects with digoxin, the dosage of the drug should always be selected carefully and adjusted as the clinical condition of the patient warrants. In the past, when high doses of digoxin were used and little attention was paid to clinical status or concurrent medications, adverse reactions to digoxin were more frequent and severe. Cardiac adverse reactions accounted for about one-half, gastrointestinal disturbances for about one-fourth, and CNS and other toxicity for about one-fourth of these adverse reactions. However, available evidence suggests that the incidence and severity of digoxin toxicity has decreased substantially in recent years. In recent controlled clinical trials, in patients with predominantly mild to moderate heart failure, the incidence of adverse experiences was comparable in patients taking digoxin and in those taking placebo. In a large mortality trial, the incidence of hospitalization for suspected digoxin toxicity was 2% in patients taking LANOXIN compared to 0.9% in patients taking placebo. In this trial, the most common manifestations of digoxin toxicity included gastrointestinal and cardiac disturbances; CNS manifestations were less common.

Adults: ***Cardiac:*** Therapeutic doses of digoxin may cause heart block in patients with pre-existing sinoatrial or AV conduction disorders; heart block can be avoided by adjusting the dose of digoxin. Prophylactic use of a cardiac pacemaker may be considered if the risk of heart block is considered unacceptable. High doses of digoxin may produce a variety of rhythm disturbances, such as first-degree, second-degree (Wenckebach), or third-degree heart block (including asystole); atrial tachycardia with block; AV dissociation; accelerated junctional (nodal) rhythm; unifocal or multiform ventricular premature contractions (especially bigeminy or trigeminy); ventricular tachycardia; and ventricular fibrillation. Digoxin produces PR prolongation and ST segment depression which should not by themselves be considered digoxin toxicity. Cardiac toxicity can also occur at therapeutic doses in patients who have conditions which may alter their sensitivity to digoxin (see WARNINGS and PRECAUTIONS).

Gastrointestinal: Digoxin may cause anorexia, nausea, vomiting, and diarrhea. Rarely, the use of digoxin has been associated with abdominal pain, intestinal ischemia, and hemorrhagic necrosis of the intestines.

CNS: Digoxin can produce visual disturbances (blurred or yellow vision), headache, weakness, dizziness, apathy, confusion, and mental disturbances (such as anxiety, depression, delirium, and hallucination).

Other: Gynecomastia has been occasionally observed following the prolonged use of digoxin. Thrombocytopenia and maculopapular rash and other skin reactions have been rarely observed.

Table 3: Subgroup Analyses of Mortality and Hospitalization During the First Two Years Following Randomization

	n	Risk of All-Cause Mortality or All-Cause Hospitalization*			Risk of HF-Related Mortality or HF-Related Hospitalization*		
		Placebo	LANOXIN	Relative risk†	Placebo	LANOXIN	Relative risk†
All patients (EF ≤0.45)	6801	604	593	0.94 (0.88-1.00)	294	217	0.69 (0.63-0.76)
NYHA I / II	4571	549	541	0.96 (0.89-1.04)	242	178	0.70 (0.62-0.80)
EF 0.25-0.45	4543	568	571	0.99 (0.91-1.07)	244	190	0.74 (0.66-0.84)
CTR ≤0.55	4455	561	563	0.98 (0.91-1.06)	239	180	0.71 (0.63-0.81)
NYHA III / IV	2224	719	696	0.88 (0.80-0.97)	402	295	0.65 (0.57-0.75)
EF <0.25	2258	677	637	0.84 (0.76-0.93)	394	270	0.61 (0.53-0.71)
CTR >0.55	2346	687	650	0.85 (0.77-0.94)	398	287	0.65 (0.57-0.75)
EF >0.45‡	987	571	585	1.04 (0.88-1.23)	179	136	0.72 (0.53-0.99)

* Number of patients with an event during the first 2 years per 1000 randomized patients.
† Relative risk (95% confidence interval).
‡ DIG Ancillary Study.

The following table summarizes the incidence of those adverse experiences listed above for patients treated with LANOXIN Tablets or placebo from two randomized, double-blind, placebo-controlled withdrawal trials. Patients in these trials were also receiving diuretics with or without angiotensin-converting enzyme inhibitors. These patients had been stable on digoxin, and were randomized to digoxin or placebo. The results shown in Table 4 reflect the experience in patients following dosage titration with the use of serum digoxin concentrations and careful follow-up. These adverse experiences are consistent with results from a large, placebo-controlled mortality trial (DIG trial) wherein over half the patients were not receiving digoxin prior to enrollment.

Table 4: Adverse Experiences In Two Parallel, Double-Blind, Placebo-Controlled Withdrawal Trials (Number of Patients Reporting)

Adverse Experience	Digoxin Patients (n = 123)	Placebo Patients (n = 125)
Cardiac		
Palpitation	1	4
Ventricular extrasystole	1	1
Tachycardia	2	1
Heart arrest	1	1
Gastrointestinal		
Anorexia	1	4
Nausea	4	2
Vomiting	2	1
Diarrhea	4	1
Abdominal pain	0	6
CNS		
Headache	4	4
Dizziness	6	5
Mental disturbances	5	1
Other		
Rash	2	1
Death	4	3

Infants and Children: The side effects of digoxin in infants and children differ from those seen in adults in several respects. Although digoxin may produce anorexia, nausea, vomiting, diarrhea, and CNS disturbances in young patients, these are rarely the initial symptoms of overdosage. Rather, the earliest and most frequent manifestation of excessive dosing with digoxin in infants and children is the appearance of cardiac arrhythmias, including sinus bradycardia. In children, the use of digoxin may produce any arrhythmia. The most common are conduction disturbances or supraventricular tachyarrhythmias, such as atrial tachycardia (with or without block) and junctional (nodal) tachycardia. Ventricular arrhythmias are less common. Sinus bradycardia may be a sign of impending digoxin intoxication, especially in infants, even in the absence of first-degree heart block. Any arrhythmia or alteration in cardiac conduction that develops in a child taking digoxin should be assumed to be caused by digoxin, until further evaluation proves otherwise.

OVERDOSAGE

Treatment of Adverse Reactions Produced by Overdosage: Digoxin should be temporarily discontinued until the adverse reaction resolves. Every effort should also be made to correct factors that may contribute to the adverse reaction (such as electrolyte disturbances or concurrent medications). Once the adverse reaction has resolved, therapy with digoxin may be reinstituted, following a careful reassessment of dose.

Withdrawal of digoxin may be all that is required to treat the adverse reaction. However, when the primary manifestation of digoxin overdosage is a cardiac arrhythmia, additional therapy may be needed.

If the rhythm disturbance is a symptomatic bradyarrhythmia or heart block, consideration should be given to the reversal of toxicity with DIGIBIND® [Digoxin Immune Fab (Ovine)] (see below), the use of atropine, or the insertion of a temporary cardiac pacemaker. However, asymptomatic bradycardia or heart block related to digoxin may require only temporary withdrawal of the drug and cardiac monitoring of the patient.

If the rhythm disturbance is a ventricular arrhythmia, consideration should be given to the correction of electrolyte disorders, particularly if hypokalemia (see below) or hypo-

Continued on next page

This product information is based on labeling in effect on June 1, 1998. For further information, contact via direct mail, phone, or web site Medical Information: Glaxo Wellcome Inc., PO Box 13398, Research Triangle Park, NC 27709. Healthcare Professionals (Medical Information): 800-334-0089 Patients (Customer Response Center): 888-TALK2GW (1-888-825-5249) Glaxo Wellcome Corporate Web Site: www.glaxowellcome.com

Lanoxin Tablets—Cont.

magnesemia is present. DIGIBIND is a specific antidote for digoxin and may be used to reverse potentially life-threatening ventricular arrhythmias due to digoxin overdosage.

Administration of Potassium: Every effort should be made to maintain the serum potassium concentration between 4.0 and 5.5 mmol/L. Potassium is usually administered orally, but when correction of the arrhythmia is urgent and the serum potassium concentration is low, potassium may be administered cautiously by the intravenous route. The electrocardiogram should be monitored for any evidence of potassium toxicity (e.g., peaking of T waves) and to observe the effect on the arrhythmia. Potassium salts may be dangerous in patients who manifest bradycardia or heart block due to digoxin (unless primarily related to supraventricular tachycardia) and in the setting of massive digitalis overdosage (see Massive Digitalis Overdosage subsection).

Massive Digitalis Overdosage: Manifestations of life-threatening toxicity include ventricular tachycardia or ventricular fibrillation, or progressive bradyarrhythmias, or heart block. The administration of more than 10 mg of digoxin in a previously healthy adult, or more than 4 mg in a previously healthy child, or a steady-state serum concentration greater than 10 ng/mL often results in cardiac arrest. DIGIBIND should be used to reverse the toxic effects of ingestion of a massive overdose. The decision to administer DIGIBIND to a patient who has ingested a massive dose of digoxin but who has not yet manifested life-threatening toxicity should depend on the likelihood that life-threatening toxicity will occur (see above).

Patients with massive digitalis ingestion should receive large doses of activated charcoal to prevent absorption and bind digoxin in the gut during enteroenteric recirculation. Emesis or gastric lavage may be indicated especially if ingestion has occurred within 30 minutes of the patient's presentation at the hospital. Emesis should not be induced in patients who are obtunded. If a patient presents more than 2 hours after ingestion or already has toxic manifestations, it may be unsafe to induce vomiting or attempt passage of a gastric tube, because such maneuvers may induce an acute vagal episode that can worsen digitalis-related arrhythmias.

Severe digitalis intoxication can cause a massive shift of potassium from inside to outside the cell, leading to life-threatening hyperkalemia. The administration of potassium supplements in the setting of massive intoxication may be hazardous and should be avoided. Hyperkalemia caused by massive digitalis toxicity is best treated with DIGIBIND; initial treatment with glucose and insulin may also be required if hyperkalemia itself is acutely life-threatening.

DOSAGE AND ADMINISTRATION

General: Recommended dosages of digoxin may require considerable modification because of individual sensitivity of the patient to the drug, the presence of associated conditions, or the use of concurrent medications. In selecting a dose of digoxin, the following factors must be considered:

1. The body weight of the patient. Doses should be calculated based upon lean (i.e., ideal) body weight.
2. The patient's renal function, preferably evaluated on the basis of estimated creatinine clearance.
3. The patient's age. Infants and children require different doses of digoxin than adults. Also, advanced age may be indicative of diminished renal function even in patients with normal serum creatinine concentration (i.e., below 1.5 mg/dL).
4. Concomitant disease states, concurrent medications, or other factors likely to alter the pharmacokinetic or pharmacodynamic profile of digoxin (see PRECAUTIONS).

Serum Digoxin Concentrations: In general, the dose of digoxin used should be determined on clinical grounds. However, measurement of serum digoxin concentrations can be helpful to the clinician in determining the adequacy of digoxin therapy and in assigning certain probabilities to the likelihood of digoxin intoxication. About two-thirds of adults considered adequately digitalized (without evidence of toxicity) have serum digoxin concentrations ranging from 0.8 to 2.0 ng/mL. However, digoxin may produce clinical benefits even at serum concentrations below this range. About two-thirds of adult patients with clinical toxicity have serum digoxin concentrations greater than 2.0 ng/mL. However, since one-third of patients with clinical toxicity have concentrations less than 2.0 ng/mL, values below 2.0 ng/mL do not rule out the possibility that a certain sign or symptom is related to digoxin therapy. Rarely, there are patients who are unable to tolerate digoxin at serum concentrations below 0.8 ng/mL. Consequently, the serum concentration of digoxin should always be interpreted in the overall clinical context, and an isolated measurement should not be used alone as the basis for increasing or decreasing the dose of the drug.

To allow adequate time for equilibration of digoxin between serum and tissue, sampling of serum concentrations should be done just before the next scheduled dose of the drug. If this is not possible, sampling should be done at least 6 to 8 hours after the last dose, regardless of the route of administration or the formulation used. On a once-daily dosing schedule, the concentration of digoxin will be 10% to 25% lower when sampled at 24 versus 8 hours, depending upon the patient's renal function. On a twice-daily dosing schedule, there will be only minor differences in serum digoxin concentrations whether sampling is done at 8 or 12 hours after a dose.

If a discrepancy exists between the reported serum concentration and the observed clinical response, the clinician should consider the following possibilities:

1. Analytical problems in the assay procedure.
2. Inappropriate serum sampling time.
3. Administration of a digitalis glycoside other than digoxin.
4. Conditions (described in WARNINGS and PRECAUTIONS) causing an alteration in the sensitivity of the patient to digoxin.
5. Serum digoxin concentration may decrease acutely during periods of exercise without any associated change in clinical efficacy due to increased binding of digoxin to skeletal muscle.

Heart Failure: *Adults*: Digitalization may be accomplished by either of two general approaches that vary in dosage and frequency of administration, but reach the same endpoint in terms of total amount of digoxin accumulated in the body.

1. If rapid digitalization is considered medically appropriate, it may be achieved by administering a loading dose based upon projected peak digoxin body stores. Maintenance dose can be calculated as a percentage of the loading dose.
2. More gradual digitalization may be obtained by beginning an appropriate maintenance dose, thus allowing digoxin body stores to accumulate slowly. Steady-state serum digoxin concentrations will be achieved in approximately five half-lives of the drug for the individual patient. Depending upon the patient's renal function, this will take between 1 and 3 weeks.

Rapid Digitalization with a Loading Dose: Peak digoxin body stores of 8 to 12 mcg/kg should provide therapeutic effect with minimum risk of toxicity in most patients with heart failure and normal sinus rhythm. Because of altered digoxin distribution and elimination, projected peak body stores for patients with renal insufficiency should be conservative (i.e., 6 to 10 mcg/kg) [see PRECAUTIONS].

The loading dose should be administered in several portions, with roughly half the total given as the first dose. Additional fractions of this planned total dose may be given at 6- to 8-hour intervals, **with careful assessment of clinical response before each additional dose.** If the patient's clinical response necessitates a change from the calculated loading dose of digoxin, then calculation of the maintenance dose should be based upon the amount actually given.

A single initial dose of 500 to 750 mcg (0.5 to 0.75 mg) of LANOXIN Tablets usually produces a detectable effect in 0.5 to 2 hours that becomes maximal in 2 to 6 hours. Additional doses of 125 to 375 mcg (0.125 to 0.375 mg) may be given cautiously at 6- to 8-hour intervals until clinical evidence of an adequate effect is noted. The usual amount of LANOXIN Tablets that a 70-kg patient requires to achieve 8 to 12 mcg/kg peak body stores is 750 to 1,250 mcg (0.75 to 1.25 mg).

LANOXIN Injection is frequently used to achieve rapid digitalization, with conversion to LANOXIN Tablets or LANOXICAPS for maintenance therapy. If patients are switched from intravenous to oral digoxin formulations, allowances must be made for differences in bioavailability when calculating maintenance dosages (see table, CLINICAL PHARMACOLOGY).

Maintenance Dosing: The doses of digoxin used in controlled trials in patients with heart failure have ranged from 125 to 500 mcg (0.125 to 0.5 mg) once daily. In these studies, the digoxin dose has been generally titrated according to the patient's age, lean body weight, and renal function. Therapy is generally initiated at a dose of 250 mcg (0.25 mg) once daily in patients under age 70 with good renal function, at a dose of 125 mcg (0.125 mg) once daily in patients over age 70 or with impaired renal function, and at a dose of 62.5 mcg (0.0625 mg) in patients with marked renal impairment. Doses may be increased every 2 weeks according to clinical response.

In a subset of approximately 1,800 patients enrolled in the DIG trial (wherein dosing was based on an algorithm similar to that in Table 5) the mean ($\pm$ SD) serum digoxin concentrations at 1 month and 12 months were 1.01 ± 0.47 ng/mL and 0.97 ± 0.43 ng/mL, respectively.

The maintenance dose should be based upon the percentage of the peak body stores lost each day through elimination. The following formula has had wide clinical use:

Maintenance Dose = Peak Body Stores
(i.e., Loading Dose) × % Daily Loss/100

Where: % Daily Loss = 14 + Ccr/5

(Ccr is creatinine clearance, corrected to 70 kg body weight or 1.73 m^2 body surface area)

Table 5 provides average daily maintenance dose requirements of LANOXIN Tablets for patients with heart failure based upon lean body weight and renal function:

[See table 5 below]

Example: Based on the above table, a patient in heart failure with an estimated lean body weight of 70 kg and a Ccr of 60 mL/min should be given a dose of 250 mcg (0.25 mg) daily of LANOXIN Tablets, usually taken after the morning meal. If no loading dose is administered, steady-state serum concentrations in this patient should be anticipated at approximately 11 days.

Infants and Children: In general, divided daily dosing is recommended for infants and young children (under age 10). In the newborn period, renal clearance of digoxin is diminished and suitable dosage adjustments must be observed. This is especially pronounced in the premature infant. Beyond the immediate newborn period, children generally require proportionally larger doses than adults on the basis of body weight or body surface area. Children over 10 years of age require adult dosages in proportion to their body weight. Some researchers have suggested that infants and young children tolerate slightly higher serum concentrations than do adults.

Daily maintenance doses for each age group are given in Table 6 and should provide therapeutic effects with minimum risk of toxicity in most patients with heart failure and normal sinus rhythm. These recommendations assume the presence of normal renal function:

Table 6: Daily Maintenance Doses in Children with Normal Renal Function

Age	Daily Maintenance Dose (mcg/kg)
2 to 5 Years	10 to 15
5 to 10 Years	7 to 10
Over 10 Years	3 to 5

In children with renal disease, digoxin must be carefully titrated based upon clinical response.

Table 5: Usual Daily Maintenance Dose Requirements (mcg) of LANOXIN for Estimated Peak Body Stores of 10 mcg/kg

		Lean Body Weight						
Corrected Ccr	kg	50	60	70	80	90	100	Number of Days Before Steady State Achieved†
(mL/min per 70 kg)*	lb	110	132	154	176	198	220	
0		62.5‡	125	125	125	187.5	187.5	22
10		125	125	125	187.5	187.5	187.5	19
20		125	125	187.5	187.5	187.5	250	16
30		125	187.5	187.5	187.5	250	250	14
40		125	187.5	187.5	250	250	250	13
50		187.5	187.5	250	250	250	250	12
60		187.5	187.5	250	250	250	375	11
70		187.5	250	250	250	250	375	10
80		187.5	250	250	250	375	375	9
90		187.5	250	250	250	375	500	8
100		250	250	250	375	375	500	7

* Ccr is creatinine clearance, corrected to 70 kg body weight or 1.73 m^2 body surface area. *For adults*, if only serum creatinine concentrations (Scr) are available, a Ccr (corrected to 70 kg body weight) may be estimated in men as (140 - Age)/Scr. For women, this result should be multiplied by 0.85. *Note*: This equation cannot be used for estimating creatinine clearance in infants or children.

† If no loading dose administered.

‡ 62.5 mcg = 0.0625 mg

It cannot be overemphasized that both the adult and pediatric dosage guidelines provided are based upon average patient response and substantial individual variation can be expected. Accordingly, ultimate dosage selection must be based upon clinical assessment of the patient.

Atrial Fibrillation: Peak digoxin body stores larger than the 8 to 12 mcg/kg required for most patients with heart failure and normal sinus rhythm have been used for control of ventricular rate in patients with atrial fibrillation. Doses of digoxin used for the treatment of chronic atrial fibrillation should be titrated to the minimum dose that achieves the desired ventricular rate control without causing undesirable side effects. Data are not available to establish the appropriate resting or exercise target rates that should be achieved.

Dosage Adjustment When Changing Preparations: The difference in bioavailability between LANOXIN Injection or LANOXICAPS and LANOXIN Elixir Pediatric or LANOXIN Tablets must be considered when changing patients from one dosage form to another.

Doses of 100 mcg (0.1 mg) and 200 mcg (0.2 mg) of LANOXICAPS are approximately equivalent to 125-mcg (0.125-mg) and 250-mcg (0.25-mg) doses of LANOXIN Tablets and Elixir Pediatric, respectively (see table in CLINICAL PHARMACOLOGY: Pharmacokinetics).

HOW SUPPLIED

LANOXIN (digoxin) Tablets, Scored 125 mcg (0.125 mg): Bottles of 100 with child-resistant cap (NDC 0173-0242-55) and 1000 (NDC 0173-0242-75); unit dose pack of 100 (NDC 0173-0242-56). Imprinted with LANOXIN and Y3B (yellow). **Store at 15° to 25°C (59° to 77°F) in a dry place and protect from light.**

LANOXIN (digoxin) Tablets, Scored 250 mcg (0.25 mg): Bottles of 100 with child-resistant cap (NDC 0173-0249-55), 1000 (NDC 0173-0249-75), and 5000 (NDC 0173-0249-80); carton of 12 bottles of 100 (NDC 0173-0249-01); unit dose pack of 100 (NDC 0173-0249-56). Imprinted with LANOXIN and X3A (white).

Store at 15° to 25°C (59° to 77°F) in a dry place.

September 1997/RL-471

Shown in Product Identification Guide, page 313

LEUKERAN®

℞

[lū 'kŭh-răn]
(chlorambucil)
2-mg Sugar-coated Tablets

> **WARNING:** LEUKERAN (chlorambucil) can severely suppress bone marrow function. Chlorambucil is a carcinogen in humans. Chlorambucil is probably mutagenic and teratogenic in humans. Chlorambucil produces human infertility (see WARNINGS and PRECAUTIONS).

DESCRIPTION

LEUKERAN (chlorambucil) was first synthesized by Everett et al.[1] It is a bifunctional alkylating agent of the nitrogen mustard type that has been found active against selected human neoplastic diseases. Chlorambucil is known chemically as 4-[bis(2-chlorethyl)amino]benzenebutanoic acid. Chlorambucil hydrolyzes in water and has a pKa of 5.8. LEUKERAN (chlorambucil) is available in tablet form for oral administration. Each sugar-coated tablet contains 2 mg chlorambucil and the inactive ingredients acacia, corn and wheat starch, lactose, magnesium stearate, pharmaceutical glaze, polysorbate 60, sucrose, and talc. Printed with edible black ink.

CLINICAL PHARMACOLOGY

Chlorambucil is rapidly and completely absorbed from the gastrointestinal tract. After single oral doses of 0.6 to 1.2 mg/kg, peak plasma chlorambucil levels are reached within 1 hour and the terminal half-life of the parent drug is estimated at 1.5 hours. Chlorambucil undergoes rapid metabolism to phenylacetic acid mustard, the major metabolite, and the combined chlorambucil and phenylacetic acid mustard urinary excretion is extremely low—less than 1% in 24 hours. The peak plasma levels of chlorambucil and phenylacetic acid mustard are similar, approximating 1 mcg/mL; however, the metabolite's half-life is 1.6 times greater than the parent drug.[2,3]

Chlorambucil and its metabolites are extensively bound to plasma and tissue proteins. In vitro, chlorambucil is 99% bound to plasma proteins, specifically albumin.[4] Cerebrospinal fluid levels of chlorambucil have not been determined. Evidence of human teratogenicity suggests that the drug crosses the placenta.[5,6]

Chlorambucil is extensively metabolized in the liver primarily to phenylacetic acid mustard which has antineoplastic activity.[2,3] Chlorambucil and its major metabolite spontaneously degrade in vivo forming monohydroxy and dihydroxy derivatives.[2] After a single dose of radiolabeled chlorambu-

cil (¹⁴C), approximately 15% to 60% of the radioactivity appears in the urine after 24 hours. Again, less than 1% of the urinary radioactivity is in the form of chlorambucil or phenylacetic acid mustard.[2] In summary, the pharmacokinetic data suggest that oral chlorambucil undergoes rapid gastrointestinal absorption and plasma clearance and that it is almost completely metabolized, having extremely low urinary excretion.

INDICATIONS AND USAGE

LEUKERAN (chlorambucil) is indicated in the treatment of chronic lymphatic (lymphocytic) leukemia, malignant lymphomas including lymphosarcoma, giant follicular lymphoma, and Hodgkin's disease. It is not curative in any of these disorders but may produce clinically useful palliation.

CONTRAINDICATIONS

Chlorambucil should not be used in patients whose disease has demonstrated a prior resistance to the agent. Patients who have demonstrated hypersensitivity to chlorambucil should not be given the drug.[7–9] There may be cross-hypersensitivity (skin rash) between chlorambucil and other alkylating agents.[10]

WARNINGS

Because of its carcinogenic properties, chlorambucil should not be given to patients with conditions other than chronic lymphatic leukemia or malignant lymphomas. Convulsions,[11] infertility,[12] leukemia[13,14] and secondary malignancies[15] have been observed when chlorambucil was employed in the therapy of malignant and non-malignant diseases. There are many reports of acute leukemia arising in patients with both malignant[16] and non-malignant[17] diseases following chlorambucil treatment. In many instances, these patients also received other chemotherapeutic agents or some form of radiation therapy. The quantitation of the risk of chlorambucil-induction of leukemia or carcinoma in humans is not possible. Evaluation of published reports of leukemia developing in patients who have received chlorambucil (and other alkylating agents) suggests that the risk of leukemogenesis increases with both chronicity of treatment and large cumulative doses. However, it has proved impossible to define a cumulative dose below which there is no risk of the induction of secondary malignancy. The potential benefits from chlorambucil therapy must be weighed on an individual basis against the possible risk of the induction of a secondary malignancy.

Chlorambucil has been shown to cause chromatid or chromosome damage in humans.[18,19] Both reversible and permanent sterility have been observed in both sexes receiving chlorambucil.

A high incidence of sterility has been documented when chlorambucil is administered to prepubertal and pubertal males.[20] Prolonged or permanent azoospermia has also been observed in adult males.[21] While most reports of gonadal dysfunction secondary to chlorambucil have related to males, the induction of amenorrhea in females with alkylating agents is well documented, and chlorambucil is capable of producing amenorrhea. Autopsy studies of the ovaries from women with malignant lymphoma treated with combination chemotherapy including chlorambucil have shown varying degrees of fibrosis, vasculitis, and depletion of primordial follicles.[22,23]

Rare instances of skin rash progressing to erythema multiforme, toxic epidermal necrolysis, or Stevens-Johnson syndrome have been reported.[8–9] Chlorambucil should be discontinued promptly in patients who develop skin reactions.

Pregnancy: Pregnancy Category D. Chlorambucil can cause fetal harm when administered to a pregnant woman. Unilateral renal agenesis has been observed in two offspring whose mothers received chlorambucil during the first trimester.[5,6] Urogenital malformations, including absence of a kidney, were found in fetuses of rats given chlorambucil.[24] There are no adequate and well-controlled studies in pregnant women. If this drug is used during pregnancy, or if the patient becomes pregnant while taking this drug, the patient should be apprised of the potential hazard to the fetus. Women of childbearing potential should be advised to avoid becoming pregnant.

PRECAUTIONS

General: Many patients develop a slowly progressive lymphopenia during treatment. The lymphocyte count usually rapidly returns to normal levels upon completion of drug therapy. Most patients have some neutropenia after the third week of treatment, and this may continue for up to 10 days after the last dose. Subsequently, the neutrophil count usually rapidly returns to normal. Severe neutropenia appears to be related to dosage and usually occurs only in patients who have received a total dosage of 6.5 mg/kg or more in one course of therapy with continuous dosing. About one quarter of all patients receiving the continuous-dose schedule, and one third of those receiving this dosage in 8 weeks or less may be expected to develop severe neutropenia.[25]

While it is not necessary to discontinue chlorambucil at the first evidence of a fall in neutrophil count, it must be remembered that the fall may continue for 10 days after the

last dose, and that as the total dose approaches 6.5 mg/kg, there is a risk of causing irreversible bone marrow damage. The dose of chlorambucil should be decreased if leukocyte or platelet counts fall below normal values and should be discontinued for more severe depression.

Chlorambucil should **not** be given at full dosages before 4 weeks after a full course of radiation therapy or chemotherapy because of the vulnerability of the bone marrow to damage under these conditions. If the pretherapy leukocyte or platelet counts are depressed from bone marrow disease process prior to institution of therapy, the treatment should be instituted at a reduced dosage.

Persistently low neutrophil and platelet counts or peripheral lymphocytosis suggest bone marrow infiltration. If confirmed by bone marrow examination, the daily dosage of chlorambucil should not exceed 0.1 mg/kg. Chlorambucil appears to be relatively free from gastrointestinal side effects or other evidence of toxicity apart from the bone marrow depressant action. In humans, single oral doses of 20 mg or more may produce nausea and vomiting.

Children with nephrotic syndrome[11] and patients receiving high pulse doses of chlorambucil[26] may have an increased risk of seizures. As with any potentially epileptogenic drug, caution should be exercised when administering chlorambucil to patients with a history of seizure disorder, or head trauma, or who are receiving other potentially epileptogenic drugs.

Information for Patients: Patients should be informed that the major toxicities of chlorambucil are related to hypersensitivity, drug fever, myelosuppression, hepatotoxicity, infertility, seizures, gastrointestinal toxicity, and secondary malignancies. Patients should never be allowed to take the drug without medical supervision and should consult their physician if they experience skin rash, bleeding, fever, jaundice, persistent cough, seizures, nausea, vomiting, amenorrhea, or unusual lumps/masses. Women of childbearing potential should be advised to avoid becoming pregnant.

Laboratory Tests: Patients must be followed carefully to avoid life-endangering damage to the bone marrow during treatment. Weekly examination of the blood should be made to determine hemoglobin levels, total and differential leukocyte counts, and quantitative platelet counts. Also, during the first 3 to 6 weeks of therapy, it is recommended that white blood cell counts be made 3 or 4 days after each of the weekly complete blood counts. Galton et al[25] have suggested that in following patients it is helpful to plot the blood counts on a chart at the same time that body weight, temperature, spleen size, etc., are recorded. It is considered dangerous to allow a patient to go more than 2 weeks without hematological and clinical examination during treatment.

Drug Interactions: There are no known drug/drug interactions with chlorambucil.

Carcinogenesis, Mutagenesis, Impairment of Fertility: See WARNINGS section for information on carcinogenesis, mutagenesis, and impairment of fertility.

Pregnancy: *Teratogenic Effects:* Pregnancy Category D: See WARNINGS section.

Nursing Mothers: It is not known whether this drug is excreted in human milk. Because many drugs are excreted in human milk and because of the potential for serious adverse reactions in nursing infants from chlorambucil, a decision should be made whether to discontinue nursing or to discontinue the drug, taking into account the importance of the drug to the mother.

Pediatric Use: The safety and effectiveness in pediatric patients have not been established.

ADVERSE REACTIONS

Hematologic: The most common side effect is bone marrow suppression.[27] Although bone marrow suppression frequently occurs, it is usually reversible if the chlorambucil is withdrawn early enough. However, irreversible bone marrow failure has been reported.[28,29]

Gastrointestinal: Gastrointestinal disturbances such as nausea and vomiting, diarrhea, and oral ulceration occur infrequently.

CNS: Tremors, muscular twitching, confusion, agitation, ataxia, flaccid paresis, and hallucinations have been reported as rare adverse experiences to chlorambucil which resolve upon discontinuation of drug. Rare, focal and/or generalized seizures have been reported to occur in both children[11,30,31] and adults[26,32–35] at both therapeutic daily doses and pulse-dosing regimens, and in acute overdose (see PRECAUTIONS: General).

Continued on next page

This product information is based on labeling in effect on June 1, 1998. For further information, contact via direct mail, phone, or web site Medical Information: Glaxo Wellcome Inc., PO Box 13398, Research Triangle Park, NC 27709. Healthcare Professionals (Medical Information): 800-334-0089 Patients (Customer Response Center): 888-TALK2GW (1-888-825-5249) Glaxo Wellcome Corporate Web Site: www.glaxowellcome.com

Leukeran—Cont.

Dermatologic: Skin hypersensitivity (including rare reports of skin rash progressing to erythema multiforme,[9] toxic epidermal necrolysis,[8] and Stevens-Johnson syndrome) has been reported (see WARNINGS).

Miscellaneous: Other reported adverse reactions include: pulmonary fibrosis, hepatotoxicity and jaundice, drug fever, peripheral neuropathy, interstitial pneumonia, sterile cystitis, infertility, leukemia, and secondary malignancies (see WARNINGS).

OVERDOSAGE

Reversible pancytopenia was the main finding of inadvertent overdoses of chlorambucil.[36,37] Neurological toxicity ranging from agitated behavior and ataxia to multiple grand mal seizures has also occurred.[30,36] As there is no known antidote, the blood picture should be closely monitored and general supportive measures should be instituted, together with appropriate blood transfusions, if necessary. Chlorambucil is not dialyzable.

Oral LD_{50} single doses in mice are 123 mg/kg. In rats, a single intraperitoneal dose of 12.5 mg/kg of chlorambucil produces typical nitrogen-mustard effects; these include atrophy of the intestinal mucous membrane and lymphoid tissues, severe lymphopenia becoming maximal in 4 days, anemia, and thrombocytopenia. After this dose, the animals begin to recover within 3 days and appear normal in about a week although the bone marrow may not become completely normal for about 3 weeks. An intraperitoneal dose of 18.5 mg/kg kills about 50% of the rats with development of convulsions. As much as 50 mg/kg has been given orally to rats as a single dose, with recovery. Such a dose causes bradycardia, excessive salivation, hematuria, convulsions, and respiratory dysfunction.

DOSAGE AND ADMINISTRATION

The usual oral dosage is 0.1 to 0.2 mg/kg body weight daily for 3 to 6 weeks as required. This usually amounts to 4 to 10 mg per day for the average patient. The entire daily dose may be given at one time. These dosages are for initiation of therapy or for short courses of treatment. The dosage must be carefully adjusted according to the response of the patient and must be reduced as soon as there is an abrupt fall in the white blood cell count. Patients with Hodgkin's disease usually require 0.2 mg/kg daily, whereas patients with other lymphomas or chronic lymphocytic leukemia usually require only 0.1 mg/kg daily. When lymphocytic infiltration of the bone marrow is present, or when the bone marrow is hypoplastic, the daily dose should not exceed 0.1 mg/kg (about 6 mg for the average patient).

Alternate schedules for the treatment of chronic lymphocytic leukemia employing intermittent, biweekly, or once-monthly pulse doses of chlorambucil have been reported.[38,39] Intermittent schedules of chlorambucil begin with an initial single dose of 0.4 mg/kg. Doses are generally increased by 0.1 mg/kg until control of lymphocytosis or toxicity is observed. Subsequent doses are modified to produce mild hematologic toxicity. It is felt that the response rate of chronic lymphocytic leukemia to the biweekly or once-monthly schedule of chlorambucil administration is similar or better to that previously reported with daily administration and that hematologic toxicity was less than or equal to that encountered in studies using daily chlorambucil.

Radiation and cytotoxic drugs render the bone marrow more vulnerable to damage, and chlorambucil should be used with particular caution within 4 weeks of a full course of radiation therapy or chemotherapy. However, small doses of palliative radiation over isolated foci remote from the bone marrow will not usually depress the neutrophil and platelet count. In these cases chlorambucil may be given in the customary dosage.

It is presently felt that short courses of treatment are safer than continuous maintenance therapy, although both methods have been effective. It must be recognized that continuous therapy may give the appearance of "maintenance" in patients who are actually in remission and have no immediate need for further drug. If maintenance dosage is used, it should not exceed 0.1 mg/kg daily and may well be as low as 0.03 mg/kg daily. A typical maintenance dose is 2 mg to 4 mg daily, or less, depending on the status of the blood counts. It may, therefore, be desirable to withdraw the drug after maximal control has been achieved, since intermittent therapy reinstituted at time of relapse may be as effective as continuous treatment.

Procedures for proper handling and disposal of anticancer drugs should be considered. Several guidelines on this subject have been published.[40–46]

There is no general agreement that all of the procedures recommended in the guidelines are necessary or appropriate.

HOW SUPPLIED

White sugar-coated tablet containing 2 mg chlorambucil and printed with "635"; bottle of 50 (NDC 0173-0635-35).

Store at 15° to 25°C (59° to 77°F) in a dry place.

REFERENCES

1. Everett JL, Roberts JJ, Ross WCJ. Aryl-2-halogenoalkylamines. Pt. XII. Some carboxylic derivatives of NN-Di-2-chloroethylaniline. *J Chem Soc.* 1953;3:2386–2392.
2. Alberts DS, Chang SY, Chen H-SG, Larcom BJ, Jones SE. Pharmacokinetics and metabolism of chlorambucil in man. *Cancer Treat Rev.* 1979;6 (suppl):9–17.
3. McLean A, Woods RL, Catovsky D, Farmer P. Pharmacokinetics and metabolism of chlorambucil in patients with malignant disease. *Cancer Treat Rev.* 1979;6(suppl):33–42.
4. Ehrsson H, Lönroth U, Wallin I, Ehrnebo M, Nilsson SO. Degradation of chlorambucil in aqueous solution: influence of human albumin binding. *J Pharm Pharmacol.* 1981;33:313–315. Communications.
5. Shotton D, Monie IW. Possible teratogenic effect of chlorambucil on a human fetus. *JAMA.* 1963;186:74–75.
6. Steege JF, Caldwell DS. Renal agenesis after first trimester exposure to chlorambucil. *South Med J.* 1980;73:1414–1415.
7. Knisley RE, Settipane GA, Albala MM. Unusual reaction to chlorambucil in a patient with chronic lymphocytic leukemia. *Arch Dermatol.* 1971;104:77–79.
8. Pietrantonio F. Moriconi L, Torino F, Romano A, Gangovich A. Unusual reaction to chlorambucil: a case report. *Cancer Lett.* 1990;54:109–111.
9. Hitchins RN, Hocker GA, Thomson DB. Chlorambucil allergy—a series of three cases. *Aust NZ J Med.* 1987;17:600–602.
10. Weiss RB, Bruno S. Hypersensitivity reactions to cancer chemotherapeutic agents. *Ann Intern Med.* 1981; 94:66–72.
11. Williams SA, Makker SP, Grupe WE. Seizures: a significant side effect of chlorambucil therapy in children. *J Pediatr.* 1978;93:516–518.
12. Freckman HA, Fry HL, Mendez FL, Maurer ER. Chlorambucil-prednisolone therapy for disseminated breast carcinoma. *JAMA.* 1964;189:23–26.
13. Aymard JP, Frustin J, Witz F, Colomb JN, Lederlin P, Herbeuval R. Acute leukemia after prolonged chlorambucil treatment for non-malignant disease: a report of a new case and literature survey. *Acta Haematol (Basel).* 1980;63:283–285.
14. Berk PD, Goldberg JD, Silverstein MN, et al. Increased incidence of acute leukemia in polycythemia vera associated with chlorambucil therapy. *N Engl J Med.* 1981;304:441–447.
15. Lerner HJ. Acute myelogenous leukemia in patients receiving chlorambucil as long-term adjuvant chemotherapy for stage II breast cancer. *Cancer Treat Rep.* 1978;62:1135–1138.
16. Zarrabi MH, Grünwald HW, Rosner F. Chronic lymphocytic leukemia terminating in acute leukemia. *Arch Intern Med.* 1977;137:1059–1064.
17. Cameron S: Chlorambucil and leukemia. *N Eng J Med.* 1977;296:1065.
18. Lawler SD, Lele KP. Chromosomal damage induced by chlorambucil in chronic lymphocytic leukemia. *Scand J Haematol.* 1972;9:603–612.
19. Stevenson AC, Patel C. Effects of chlorambucil on human chromosomes. *Mutat Res.* 1973;18:333–351.
20. Guesry P, Lenoir G, Broyer M. Gonadal effects of chlorambucil given to prepubertal and pubertal boys for nephrotic syndrome. *J Pediatr.* 1978;92:299–303.
21. Richter P, Calamera JC, Morgenfeld MC, Kierszenbaum AL, Lavieri JC, Mancini RE. Effect of chlorambucil on spermatogenesis in the human with malignant lymphoma. *Cancer.* 1970;25:1026–1030.
22. Morgenfeld MC, Goldberg V, Parisier H, Bugnard SC, Bur GE. Ovarian lesions due to cytostatic agents during the treatment of Hodgkin's disease. *Surg Gynecol Obstet.* 1972;134:826–828.
23. Sobrinho LG, Levine RA, DeConti RC. Amenorrhea in patients with Hodgkin's disease treated with antineoplastic agents. *Am J Obstet Gynecol.* 1971;109:135–139.
24. Monie IW. Chlorambucil-induced abnormalities of the urogenital system of rat fetuses. *Anat Rec.* 1961;139:145–153.
25. Galton DAG, Israels LG, Nabarro JDN, Till M. Clinical trials of p-(DI-2-chloroethylamino)-phenylbutyric acid (CB 1348) in malignant lymphoma. *Br Med J.* 1955;2:1172–1176.
26. Ciobanu N, Runowicz C, Gucalp R, et al. Reversible central nervous system toxicity associated with high-dose chlorambucil in autologous bone marrow transplantation for ovarian carcinoma. *Cancer Treat Rep.* 1987;71:1324–1325.
27. Moore GE, Bross ID, Ausman R, et al. Effects of chlorambucil (NSC-3088) in 374 patients with advanced cancer. Eastern Clinical Drug Evaluation Program. *Cancer Chemother Rep.* 1968;52(pt 1):661–666.
28. Galton DA, Wiltshaw E, Szur L, Dacie JV. The use of chlorambucil and steroids in the treatment of chronic lymphocytic leukemia. *Br J Haematol.* 1961;7:73–98.
29. Rudd P, Fries JF, Epstein WV. Irreversible bone marrow failure with chlorambucil. *J Rheumatol.* 1975;2:421–429.
30. Wolfson S, Olney MB. Accidental ingestion of a toxic dose of chlorambucil: report of a case in a child. *JAMA.* 1957;165:239–240.
31. Byrne TN, Moseley TAE, Finer MA. Myoclonic seizures following chlorambucil overdose. *Ann Neurol.* 1981;9:191–194.
32. LaDelfa I, Bayer N, Myers R, Hoffstein V. Chlorambucil-induced myoclonic seizures in an adult. *J Clin Oncol.* 1985;3:1691–1692.
33. Naysmith A, Robson RH: Focal fits during chlorambucil therapy. *Postgrad Med J.* 1979;55:806–807.
34. Blank DW, Nanji AA, Schreiber DH, Hudman C, Sanders HD. Acute renal failure and seizures associated with chlorambucil overdose. *J Toxicol Clin Toxicol.* 1983;20:361–365.
35. Ammenti A, Reitter B, Muller-Wiefel DE. Chlorambucil neurotoxicity: report of two cases. *Helv Paediatr Acta.* 1980;35:281–287.
36. Green AA, Naiman JL. Chlorambucil poisoning. *Am J Dis Child.* 1968;116:190–191.
37. Enck RE, Bennett JM. Inadvertent chlorambucil overdose in adults. *NY State J Med.* 1977;77:1480–1481.
38. Knospe WH, Loeb V Jr, Huguley CM. Bi-weekly chlorambucil treatment of chronic lymphocytic leukemia. *Cancer.* 1974;33:555–562.
39. Sawitsky A, Rai KR, Glidewell O, et al. Comparison of daily versus intermittent chlorambucil and prednisone therapy in the treatment of patients with chronic lymphocytic leukemia. *Blood.* 1977;50:1049–1059.
40. Recommendations for the safe handling of parenteral antineoplastic drugs. Washington, DC: Division of Safety; National Institutes of Health; 1983. US Dept of Health and Human Services, Public Health Service publication NIH 83-2621.
41. AMA Council on Scientific Affairs. Guidelines for handling parenteral antineoplastics. *JAMA.* 1985;253:1590–1591.
42. National Study Commission on Cytotoxic Exposure. Recommendations for handling cytotoxic agents. 1987. Available from Louis P. Jeffrey, Chairman, National Study Commission on Cytotoxic Exposure. Massachusetts College of Pharmacy and Allied Health Sciences, 179 Longwood Avenue, Boston, MA, 02115.
43. Clinical Oncological Society of Australia. Guidelines and recommendations for safe handling of antineoplastic agents. *Med J Australia.* 1983;1:426–428.
44. Jones RB, Frank R, Mass T. Safe handling of chemotherapeutic agents: a report from the Mount Sinai Medical Center. *CA-A Cancer J for Clin.* 1983;33:258–263.
45. American Society of Hospital Pharmacists. ASHP technical assistance bulletin on handling cytotoxic and hazardous drugs. *Am J Hosp Pharm.* 1990;47:1033–1049.
46. Yodaiken RE, Bennett D. OSHA work-practice guidelines for personnel dealing with cytotoxic (antineoplastic) drugs. *AM J Hosp Pharm.* 1986;43:1193–1204.

September 1997/RL-468

Shown in Product Identification Guide, page 313

LEUCOVORIN CALCIUM FOR INJECTION ℞
WELLCOVORIN® brand STERILE POWDER
100 mg per vial

DESCRIPTION

WELLCOVORIN brand Leucovorin Calcium For Injection Sterile Powder is one of several active, chemically reduced derivatives of folic acid. It is useful as an antidote to drugs which act as folic acid antagonists.

Also known as folinic acid, Citrovorum factor, or 5-formyl-5,6,7,8-tetrahydrofolic acid, this compound has the chemical designation of Calcium *N*-[4-[[(2-amino-5-formyl-1,4,5,6,7,8-hexahydro-4-oxo-6-pteridinyl)-methyl]amino]benzoyl]-*L*-glutamic acid (1:1). Leucovorin calcium has a molecular weight of 511.51.

Leucovorin Calcium for Injection is a sterile product indicated for intravenous or intramuscular administration and is supplied in 100-mg vials. Each vial of Wellcovorin brand Leucovorin Calcium For Injection Sterile Powder, when reconstituted with 10 mL of sterile diluent, contains leucovorin (as the calcium salt) 10 mg/mL, and the inactive ingredients sodium chloride 80 mg per vial, and sodium hydroxide and/or hydrochloric acid added to adjust the pH to approximately 8.1. The dry product contains no preservative. Reconstitute with Bacteriostatic Water for Injection, USP, which contains benzyl alcohol (see WARNINGS), or with Sterile Water for Injection, USP.

There is 0.004 mEq of calcium per mg of leucovorin

CLINICAL PHARMACOLOGY

Leucovorin is a mixture of the diastereoisomers of the 5-formyl derivative of tetrahydrofolic acid (THF). The biologi-

cally active compound of the mixture is the (-)-*l*-isomer, known as Citrovorum factor or (-)-folinic acid. Leucovorin does not require reduction by the enzyme dihydrofolate reductase in order to participate in reactions utilizing folates as a source of "one-carbon" moieties. *l*-Leucovorin (*l*-5-formyltetrahydrofolate) is rapidly metabolized (via 5,10-methenyltetrahydrofolate then 5,10-methylenetetrahydrofolate) to *l*,5-methyletetrahydrofolate. *l*,5-Methyltetrahydrofolate can in turn be metabolized via other pathways back to 5,10-methylenetetrahydrofolate, which is converted to 5-methyltetrahydrofolate by an irreversible, enzyme catalyzed reduction using the cofactors $FADH_2$ and NAHPH.

Administration of leucovorin can counteract the therapeutic and toxic effects of folic acid antagonists such as methotrexate, which act by inhibiting dihydrofolate reductase.

In contrast, leucovorin can enhance the therapeutic and toxic effects of fluoropyrimidines used in cancer therapy, such as 5-fluorouracil. Concurrent administration of leucovorin does not appear to alter the plasma pharmacokinetics of 5-fluorouracil. 5-Fluorouracil is metabolized to fluorodeoxyuridylic acid, which binds to and inhibits the enzyme thymidylate synthase (an enzyme important in DNA repair and replication).

Leucovorin is readily converted to another reduced folate, 5,10-methylenetetrahydrofolate, which acts to stabilize the binding of fluorodeoxyridylic acid to thymidylate synthase and thereby enhances the inhibition of this enzyme.

The pharmacokinetics after intravenous and intramuscular administration of a 25-mg dose of leucovorin were studied in male volunteers. After intravenous administration, serum total reduced folates (as measured by *Lactobacillus casei* assay) reached a mean peak of 1,259 ng/mL (range 897 to 1,625). The mean time to peak was 10 minutes. This initial rise in total reduced folates was primarily due to the parent compound 5-formyl-THF (measured by *Streptococcus faecalis* assay) which rose to 1,206 ng/mL at 10 minutes. A sharp drop in parent compound followed and coincided with the appearance of the active metabolite 5-methyl-THF which became the predominant circulating form of the drug.

The mean peak of 5-methyl-THF was 258 ng/mL and occurred at 1.3 hours. The terminal half-life for total reduced folates was 6.2 hours. The area under the concentration-versus-time curves (AUCs) for *l*-leucovorin, *d*-leucovorin, and 5-methyltetrahydrofolate were 28.4 ± 3.5, 956 ± 97, and 129 ± 12 (mg.min/L ± SE). When a higher dose of *d, l*-leucovorin (200 mg/m²) was used, similar results were obtained. The *d*-isomer persisted in plasma at concentrations greatly exceeding those of the *l*-isomer.

After intramuscular injection, the mean peak of serum total reduced folates was 436 ng/mL (rage 240 to 725) and occurred at 52 minutes. Similar to IV administration, the initial sharp rise was due to the parent compound. The mean peak of 5-formyl-THF was 360 ng/mL and occurred at 28 minutes. The level of the metabolite 5-methyl-THF increased subsequently over time until at 1.5 hours it represented 50% of the circulating total folates. The mean peak of 5-methyl-THF was 226 ng/mL at 2.8 hours. The terminal half-life of total reduced folates was 6.2 hours. There was no difference of statistical significance between IM and IV administration in the AUC for total reduced folates, 5-formyl-THF, or 5-methyl-THF.

INDICATIONS AND USAGE

Leucovorin calcium rescue is indicated after high-dose methotrexate therapy in osteosarcoma.

Leucovorin calcium is also indicated to diminish the toxicity and counteract the effects of impaired methotrexate elimination and of inadvertent overdosages of folic acid antagonists.

Leucovorin calcium is indicated in the treatment of megaloblastic anemias due to folic acid deficiency when oral therapy is not feasible.

CONTRAINDICATIONS

Leucovorin is improper therapy for pernicious anemia and other megaloblastic anemias secondary to the lack of vitamin B_{12}. A hematologic remission may occur while neurologic manifestations continue to progress.

WARNINGS

In the treatment of accidental overdosages of folic acid antagonists, leucovorin should be administered as promptly as possible. As the time interval between antifolate administration (e.g., methotrexate) and leucovorin rescue increases, leucovorin's effectiveness in counteracting toxicity decreases. Do not administer leucovorin intrathecally.

Monitoring the serum methotrexate concentration is essential in determining the optimal dose and duration of treatment with leucovorin.

Delayed methotrexate excretion may be caused by a third space fluid accumulation (i.e., ascites, pleural effusion), renal insufficiency, or inadequate hydration. Under such circumstances, higher doses of leucovorin or prolonged administration may be indicated. Doses higher than those recommended for oral use must be given intravenously.

There have been rare reports of seizures and/or syncope associated with the use of leucovorin, particularly high doses, in combination with fluorouracil for treatment of malignancies in patients with a history of prior seizures or in patients with central nervous system abnormalities.

Guidelines for Leucovorin Dosage and Administration
DO NOT ADMINISTER LEUCOVORIN INTRATHECALLY

Clinical Situation	Laboratory Findings	Leucovorin Dosage and Duration
Normal Methotrexate Elimination	Serum methotrexate level approximately 10 micromolar at 24 hours after administration, 1 micromolar at 48 hours, and less than 0.2 micromolar at 72 hours.	15 mg PO, IM, or IV q 6 hours for 60 hours (10 doses starting at 24 hours after start of methotrexate infusion).
Delayed Late Methotrexate Elimination	Serum methotrexate level remaining above 0.2 micromolar at 72 hours, and more than 0.05 micromolar at 96 hours after administration	Continue 15 mg PO, IM, or IV q 6 hours, until methotrexate level is less than 0.05 micromolar.
Delayed Early Methotrexate Elimination and/or Evidence of Acute Renal Injury	Serum methotrexate level of 50 micromolar or more at 24 hours, or 5 micromolar or more at 48 hours after administration, OR: a 100% or greater increase in serum creatinine level at 24 hours after methotrexate administration (e.g., an increase from 0.5 mg/dL to a level of 1 mg/dL or more).	150 mg IV q 3 hours, until methotrexate level is less than 1 micromolar; then 15 mg IV q 3 hours until methotrexate level is less than 0.05 micromolar.

The concomitant use of leucovorin with trimethoprim-sulfamethoxazole for the acute treatment of *Pneumocystis carinii* pneumonia in patients with HIV infection was associated with increased rates of treatment failure and morbidity in a placebo-controlled study.

Because of the benzyl alcohol contained in certain diluents used for reconstituting Leucovorin Calcium for Injection, when doses greater than 10 mg/m² are administered, Leucovorin Calcium for Injection should be reconstituted with Sterile Water for Injection, USP, and used immediately (see DOSAGE AND ADMINISTRATION).

Because of the calcium content of the leucovorin solution, no more than 160 mg of leucovorin should be injected intravenously per minute (16 mL of a 10-mg/mL, or 8 mL of a 20-mg/mL solution per minute).

Leucovorin enhances the toxicity of 5-fluorouracil. When these drugs are administered concurrently, the dosage of the 5-fluorouracil must be lower than usually administered. Although the toxicities observed in patients treated with the combination of leucovorin plus 5-fluorouracil are qualitatively similar to those observed in patients treated with 5-fluorouracil alone, gastrointestinal toxicities (particularly stomatitis and diarrhea) are observed more commonly and may be more severe and of prolonged duration in patients treated with the combination.

Therapy with leucovorin and 5-fluorouracil must not be initiated or continued in patients who have symptoms of gastrointestinal toxicity of any severity, until those symptoms have completely resolved.

Patients with diarrhea must be monitored with particular care until the diarrhea has resolved, as rapid clinical deterioration leading to death can occur. In a study utilizing higher weekly doses of 5-fluorouracil and leucovorin, elderly and/or debilitated patients were found to be at greater risk for severe gastrointestinal toxicity.[1]

PRECAUTIONS

General: Parental administration is preferable to oral dosing if there is a possibility that the patient may vomit or not absorb the leucovorin. Leucovorin has no effect on non-hematologic toxicities of methotrexate such as the nephrotoxicity resulting from drug and/or metabolite precipitation in the kidney.

Drug Interactions: Folic acid in large amounts may counteract the anitepileptic effect of phenobarbital, phenytoin, and primidone, and increase the frequency of seizures in susceptible children.

Preliminary animal and human studies have shown that small quantities of systemically administered leucovorin enter the CSF primarily as 5-methyltetrahydrofolate and, in humans, remain one to three orders of magnitude lower than the usual methotrexate concentrations following intrathecal administration. However, high doses of leucovorin may reduce the efficiency of intrathecally administered methotrexate.

Leucovorin may enhance the toxicity of 5-fluorouracil (see WARNINGS).

Pregnancy: ***Teratogenic Effects:*** Pregnancy Category C. Adequate animal reproduction studies have not been conducted with leucovorin. It is also not known whether leucovorin can cause fetal harm when administered to a pregnant woman or can affect reproduction capacity. Leucovorin should be given to a pregnant woman only if clearly needed.

Nursing Mothers: It is not known whether this drug is excreted in human milk. Because many drugs are excreted in human milk, caution should be exercised when leucovorin is administered to a nursing mother.

Pediatric Use: See Drug Interactions

ADVERSE REACTIONS

Allergic sensitization, including anaphylactoid reactions and urticaria, has been reported following administration of both oral and parenteral leucovorin. No other adverse reactions have been attributed to the use of leucovorin *per se*.

OVERDOSAGE

Excessive amounts of leucovorin may nullify the chemotherapeutic effect of folic acid antagonists.

DOSAGE AND ADMINISTRATION

Leucovorin Rescue After High-Dose Methotrexate Therapy: The recommendations for leucovorin rescue are based on a methotrexate dose of 12 to 15 grams/m² administered by intravenous infusion over 4 hours (see methotrexate package insert for full prescribing information).[2]

Leucovorin rescue at a dose of 15 mg (approximately 10 mg/m²) every 6 hours for 10 doses starts 24 hours after the beginning of the methotrexate infusion. In the presence of gastrointestinal toxicity, nausea, or vomiting, leucovorin should be administered parenterally. Do not administer leucovorin intrathecally.

Serum creatinine and methotrexate levels should be determined at least once daily. Leucovorin administration, hydration, and urinary alkalinization (pH of 7.0 or greater) should be continued until the methotrexate level is below 5×10^{-8} M (0.05 micromolar). The leucovorin dose should be adjusted or leucovorin rescue extended based on the following guidelines:

[See table above]

Patients who experience delayed early methotrexate elimination are likely to develop reversible renal failure. In addition to appropriate leucovorin therapy these patients require continuing hydration and urinary alkalinization, and close monitoring of fluid and electrolyte status, until the serum methotrexate level has fallen to below 0.05 micromolar and the renal failure has resolved.

Some patients will have abnormalities in methotrexate elimination or renal function following methotrexate administration, which are significant but less severe than abnormalities described in the table above. These abnormalities may or may not be associated with significant clinical toxicity. If significant clinical toxicity is observed, leucovorin rescue should be extended for an additional 24 hours (total of 14 doses over 84 hours) in subsequent courses of therapy. The possibility that the patient is taking other medications which interact with methotrexate (e.g., medications which may interfere with methotrexate elimination or binding to serum albumin) should always be reconsidered when laboratory abnormalities or clinical toxicities are observed.

Impaired Methotrexate Elimination or Inadvertent Overdosage: Leucovorin rescue should begin as soon as possible after an inadvertent overdosage and within 24 hours of methotrexate administration when there is a delayed excretion (see WARNINGS). Leucovorin 10 mg/m² should be administered IV, IM, or PO every 6 hours until the serum methotrexate level is less than 10^{-8}M. In the presence of gastrointestinal toxicity, nausea, or vomiting, leucovorin

Continued on next page

This product information is based on labeling in effect on June 1, 1998. For further information, contact via direct mail, phone, or web site Medical Information: Glaxo Wellcome Inc., PO Box 13398, Research Triangle Park, NC 27709. Healthcare Professionals (Medical Information): 800-334-0089 Patients (Customer Response Center): 888-TALK2GW (1-888-825-5249) Glaxo Wellcome Corporate Web Site: www.glaxowellcome.com

Leucovorin Calcium for Inj.—Cont.

should be administered parenterally. Do not administer leucovorin intrathecally.

Serum creatinine and methotrexate levels should be determined at 24-hour intervals. If the 24-hour serum creatinine has increased 50% over baseline, or if the 24-hour methotrexate level is greater than 5×10^{-6}M or the 48-hour level is greater than 9×10^{-7}M, the dose of leucovorin should be increased to 100 mg/m^2 IV every 3 hours until the methotrexate level is less than 10^{-8}M.

Hydration (3 L/day) and urinary alkalinization with sodium bicarbonate solution should be employed concomitantly. The bicarbonate dose should be adjusted to maintain the urine pH at 7.0 or greater.

Megaloblastic Anemia Due to Folic Acid Deficiency: Up to 1 mg daily. There is no evidence that doses greater than 1 mg/day have greater efficacy than those of 1 mg; additionally, loss of folate in urine becomes roughly logarithmic as the amount administered exceeds 1 mg.

Preparation: Each 100-mg vial of Wellcovorin brand Leucovorin Calcium for Injection when reconstituted with 10 mL of sterile diluent yields a leucovorin concentration of 10 mg per mL. Leucovorin Calcium for Injection contains no preservative. Reconstitute with Bacteriostatic Water for Injection, USP, which contains benzyl alcohol, or with Sterile Water for Injection, USP. When reconstituted with Bacteriostatic Water for Injection, USP, the resulting solution must be used within 7 days. If the product is reconstituted with Sterile Water for Injection, USP, it must be used immediately.

Because of the benzyl alcohol contained in Bacteriostatic Water for Injection, USP, when doses greater than 10 mg/m^2 are administered, Leucovorin Calcium for Injection should be reconstituted with Sterile Water for Injection, USP, and used immediately.

Because of the calcium content of the leucovorin solution, no more than 160 mg of leucovorin should be injected intravenously per minute (16 mL of a 10-mg/mL, or 8 mL of a 20-mg/mL solution per minute).

Parenteral drug products should be inspected visually for particulate matter and discoloration prior to administration, whenever solution and container permit.

Leucovorin and fluorouracil should not be admixed in the same PVC bag because a precipitate may form.

HOW SUPPLIED

Wellcovorin brand Leucovorin Calcium for Injection is supplied in vials each containing 100 mg/vial, Box of 1 (NDC 0173-0638-93).

Store dry powder and reconstituted solution at controlled room temperature 15° to 30°C (59° to 86°F).

Protect from light.

Caution: Federal Law prohibits dispensing without prescription.

REFERENCES

1. Grem JL, Shoemaker DD, Petrelli NJ, Douglas HO. Severe and fatal toxic effects observed in treatment with high- and low-dose leucovorin plus 5-fluorouracil for colorectal carcinoma. *Cancer Treat Rep.* 1987;71:1122.
2. Link MP, Goorin AH, Miser AW, et al. The effect of adjuvant chemotherapy on relapse-free survival in patients with osteosarcoma of the extremity. *N Engl J Med.* 1986;314:1600–1606.

February 1997/RL-396

Shown in Product Identification Guide, page 313

MEPRON® ℞

[mĕ ′prŏn]
(atovaquone)
Suspension

DESCRIPTION

MEPRON (atovaquone) is an antiprotozoal agent. The chemical name of atovaquone is *trans*-2-[4-(4-chlorophenyl) cyclohexyl]-3-hydroxy-1,4-naphthalenedione. Atovaquone is a yellow crystalline solid that is practically insoluble in water. It has a molecular weight of 366.84 and the molecular formula $C_{22}H_{19}ClO_3$.

MEPRON Suspension is a formulation of micro-fine particles of atovaquone. The atovaquone particles, which were reduced in size to facilitate absorption, are significantly smaller than those in the previously marketed tablet formulation. MEPRON Suspension is for oral administration and is bright yellow with a citrus flavor. Each teaspoonful (5 mL) contains 750 mg of atovaquone and the inactive ingredients benzyl alcohol, flavor, poloxamer 188, purified water, saccharin sodium, and xanthan gum.

CLINICAL PHARMACOLOGY

Mechanism of Action: Atovaquone is a hydroxy-1,4-naphthoquinone, an analog of ubiquinone, with anti-pneumocystis activity. The mechanism of action against *Pneumocystis carinii* has not been fully elucidated. In *Plasmodium* species, the site of action appears to be the cytochrome bc_1 complex (Complex III). Several metabolic enzymes are linked to the mitochondrial electron transport chain via ubiquinone. Inhibition of electron transport by atovaquone will result in indirect inhibition of these enzymes. The ultimate metabolic effects of such blockade may include inhibition of nucleic acid and ATP synthesis.

Microbiology: ***Pneumocystis carinii:*** Several laboratories, using different in vitro methodologies, have shown the IC_{50} (50% Inhibitory Concentration) of atovaquone against rat *P. carinii* to be in the range of 0.1 to 3.0 mcg/mL.

Pharmacokinetics: ***Absorption:*** Atovaquone is a highly lipophilic compound with low aqueous solubility. The bioavailability of atovaquone is highly dependent on formulation and diet. The suspension formulation provides an approximately twofold increase in atovaquone bioavailability in the fasting or fed state compared to the previously marketed tablet formulation. The absolute bioavailability of a 750-mg dose of MEPRON Suspension administered under fed conditions in nine HIV-infected (CD4 >100 cells/mm^3) volunteers was 47% ± 15%. In the same study, the bioavailability of a 750-mg dose of the previously marketed tablet formulation was 23% ± 11%.

Administering atovaquone with food enhances its absorption by approximately two-fold. In one study, 16 healthy volunteers received a single dose of 750 mg MEPRON Suspension after an overnight fast and following a standard breakfast (23 g fat: 610 kCal). The mean (±SD) area under the concentration-time curve (AUC) values were 324 ± 115 and 801 ± 320 hr·mcg/mL under fasting and fed conditions, respectively, representing a 2.6 ± 1.0-fold increase. The effect of food (23 g fat: 400 kCal) on plasma atovaquone concentrations was also evaluated in a multiple-dose, randomized, crossover study in 19 HIV-infected volunteers (CD4< 200 cells/mm^3) receiving daily doses of 500 mg MEPRON Suspension. AUC was 280 ± 114 hr·mcg/mL when atovaquone was administered with food as compared to 169 ± 77 hr·mcg/mL under fasting conditions. Maximum plasma atovaquone concentration (C_{max}) was 15.1 ± 6.1 and 8.8 ± 3.7 mcg/mL when atovaquone was administered with food and under fasting conditions, respectively.

Dose Proportionality: Plasma atovaquone concentrations do not increase proportionally with dose. When MEPRON Suspension was administered with food at dosage regimens of 500 mg once daily, 750 mg once daily, and 1000 mg once daily, average steady-state plasma atovaquone concentrations were 11.7 ± 4.8, 12.5 ± 5.8, and 13.5 ± 5.1 mcg/mL, respectively. The corresponding C_{max} concentrations were 15.1 ± 6.1, 15.3 ± 7.6, and 16.8 ± 6.4 mcg/mL. When MEPRON Suspension was administered to five HIV-infected volunteers at a dose of 750 mg twice daily, the average steady-state plasma atovaquone concentration was 21.0 ± 4.9 mcg/mL and C_{max} was 24.0 ± 5.7 mcg/mL. The minimum plasma atovaquone concentration (C_{min}) associated with the 750-mg twice daily regimen was 16.7 ± 4.6 mcg/mL.

Distribution: Following the intravenous administration of atovaquone, the volume of distribution at steady state (Vd_{ss}) was 0.60 ± 0.17 L/kg (n = 9). Atovaquone is extensively bound to plasma proteins (99.9%) over the concentration range of 1 to 90 mcg/mL. In three HIV-infected children who received 750 mg atovaquone as the tablet formulation four times daily for 2 weeks, the cerebrospinal fluid concentrations of atovaquone were 0.04 mcg, 0.14 mcg, and 0.26 μg/mL, representing less than 1% of the plasma concentration.

Elimination: The plasma clearance of atovaquone following intravenous (IV) administration in nine HIV-infected volunteers was 10.4 ± 5.5 mL/min (0.15 ± 0.09 mL/min per kg). The half-life of atovaquone was 62.5 ± 35.3 hours after IV administration and ranged from 67.0 ± 33.4 to 77.6 ± 23.1 hours across studies following administration of MEPRON Suspension. The half-life of atovaquone is long due to presumed enterohepatic cycling and eventual fecal elimination. In a study where ^{14}C-labelled atovaquone was administered to healthy volunteers, greater than 94% of the dose was recovered as unchanged atovaquone in the feces over 21 days. There was little or no excretion of atovaquone in the urine (less than 0.6%). There is indirect evidence that atovaquone may undergo limited metabolism; however, a specific metabolite has not been identified.

Special Populations: ***Pediatrics:*** Preliminary analysis of an ongoing study of MEPRON Suspension in 15 HIV-infected, asymptomatic infants and children between 1 month and 13 years of age suggests that the pharmacokinetics of atovaquone is age dependent. Those between 2 and 13 years of age achieved average steady-state plasma atovaquone concentrations of 16.8 ± 6.4 mcg and 37.1 ± 10.9 mcg/mL when given doses of 10 and 30 mg/kg, respectively. Those between 3 and 24 months of age achieved average steady-state plasma atovaquone concentrations of 5.7 ± 5.1 mcg and 8.9 ± 3.1 mcg/mL when given doses of 10 and 30 mg/kg, respectively.

Hepatic/Renal Impairment: The pharmacokinetics of atovaquone has not been studied in patients with hepatic or renal impairment.

Drug Interactions: ***Rifampin:*** In a study with 13 HIV-infected volunteers, the oral administration of rifampin 600 mg every 24 hours with MEPRON Suspension 750 mg every 12 hours resulted in a 52% ± 13% decrease in the average steady-state plasma atovaquone concentration and a 37% ± 42% increase in the average steady-state plasma rifampin concentration. The half-life of atovaquone decreased from 82 ± 36 hours when administered without rifampin to 50 ± 16 hours with rifampin.

Rifabutin, another rifamycin, is structurally similar to rifampin and may possibly have some of the same drug interactions as rifampin. No interaction trials have been conducted with MEPRON and rifabutin.

Trimethoprim/Sulfamethoxazole (TMP-SMX): The possible interaction between atovaquone and TMP-SMX was evaluated in six HIV-infected adult volunteers as part of a larger multiple-dose, dose-escalation, and chronic dosing study of MEPRON Suspension. In this cross-over study, MEPRON Suspension 500 mg once daily, or SEPTRA® DS Tablets (160 mg trimethoprim and 800 mg sulfamethoxazole) twice daily, or the combination were administered with food to achieve steady state. No difference was observed in the average steady-state plasma atovaquone concentration after coadministration with TMP-SMX. Coadministration of MEPRON with TMP-SMX resulted in a 17% and 8% decrease in average steady-state concentrations of trimethoprim and sulfamethoxazole in plasma, respectively. This effect is minor and would not be expected to produce clinically significant events.

Zidovudine: Data from 14 HIV-infected volunteers who were given atovaquone tablets 750 mg every 12 hours with zidovudine 200 mg every 8 hours showed a 24% ± 12% decrease in zidovudine apparent oral clearance, leading to a 35% ± 23% increase in plasma zidovudine AUC. The glucuronide metabolite:parent ratio decreased from a mean of 4.5 when zidovudine was administered alone to 3.1 when zidovudine was administered with atovaquone tablets. This effect is minor and would not be expected to produce clinically significant events. Zidovudine had no effect on atovaquone pharmacokinetics.

Relationship Between Plasma Atovaquone Concentration and Clinical Outcome: In a comparative study of atovaquone tablets with trimethoprim-sulfamethoxazole (TMP-SMX) for oral treatment of mild-to-moderate *Pneumocystis carinii* pneumonia (PCP) (see INDICATIONS AND USAGE), where AIDS patients received 750 mg atovaquone tablets three times daily for 21 days, the mean steady-state atovaquone concentration was 13.9 ± 6.9 mcg/mL (n = 133). Analysis of these data established a relationship between plasma atovaquone concentration and successful treatment. This is shown in Table 1.

[See table 1 at top of next page]

A dosing regimen of MEPRON Suspension for the treatment of mild-to-moderate PCP has been selected to achieve average plasma atovaquone concentrations of approximately 20 mcg/mL, because this plasma concentration was previously shown to be well tolerated and associated with the highest treatment success rates (Table 1). In an open-label PCP treatment study with MEPRON Suspension, dosing regimens of 1000 mg once daily, 750 mg twice daily, 1500 mg once daily, and 1000 mg twice daily were explored. The average steady-state plasma atovaquone concentration achieved at the 750 mg twice daily dose given with meals was 22.0 ± 10.1 mcg/mL (n = 18).

INDICATIONS AND USAGE

MEPRON Suspension is indicated for the acute oral treatment of mild-to-moderate *Pneumocystis carinii* pneumonia (PCP) in patients who are intolerant to trimethoprim-sulfamethoxazole (TMP-SMX).

This indication is based on the results of comparative pharmacokinetic studies of the suspension and tablet formulations (see CLINICAL PHARMACOLOGY) and clinical efficacy studies of the tablet formulation which established a relationship between plasma atovaquone concentration and successful treatment. The results of a randomized, double-blind trial comparing MEPRON to TMP-SMX in AIDS patients with mild to moderate PCP (defined in the study protocol as an alveolar-arterial oxygen diffusion gradient [(A-a)DO_2][1]≤45 mm Hg and PaO_2≥60 mm Hg on room air) and a randomized trial comparing MEPRON to IV pentamidine isethionate in patients with mild-to-moderate PCP intolerant to trimethoprim or sulfa-antimicrobials are summarized below:

TMP-SMX Comparative Study: This double-blind, randomized trial initiated in 1990 was designed to compare the safety and efficacy of MEPRON to that of TMP-SMX for the treatment of AIDS patients with histologically confirmed PCP. Only patients with mild-to-moderate PCP were eligible for enrollment.

A total of 408 patients were enrolled into the trial at 37 study centers. Eighty-six patients without histologic confirmation of PCP were excluded from the efficacy analyses. Of the 322 patients with histologically confirmed PCP, 160 were randomized to receive MEPRON and 162 to TMP-SMX.

Study participants randomized to treatment with MEPRON were to receive 750 mg MEPRON (three 250-mg tablets) three times daily for 21 days and those randomized to TMP-SMX were to receive 320 mg TMP plus 1600 mg SMX three times daily for 21 days.

Therapy success was defined as improvement in clinical and respiratory measures persisting at least 4 weeks after cessation of therapy. Therapy failures included lack of response, treatment discontinuation due to an adverse experience, and unevaluable.

There was a significant difference ($P = 0.03$) in mortality rates between the treatment groups. Among the 322 patients with confirmed PCP, 13 of 160 (8%) patients treated with MEPRON and four of 162 (2.5%) patients receiving TMP-SMX died during the 21-day treatment course or 8-week follow-up period. In the intent-to-treat analysis for all 408 randomized patients, there were 16 (8%) deaths in the arm treated with MEPRON and seven (3.4%) deaths in the TMP-SMX arm ($P = 0.051$). Of the 13 patients treated with MEPRON who died, four died of PCP and five died with a combination of bacterial infections and PCP; bacterial infections did not appear to be a factor in any of the four deaths among TMP-SMX-treated patients.

A correlation between plasma atovaquone concentrations and death was demonstrated; in general, patients with lower plasma concentrations were more likely to die. For those patients for whom day 4 plasma atovaquone concentration data are available, five (63%) of the eight patients with concentrations <5 mcg/mL died during participation in the study. However, only one (2.0%) of the 49 patients with day 4 plasma atovaquone concentrations ≥5 mcg/mL died. Sixty-two percent of patients on MEPRON and 64% of patients on TMP-SMX were classified as protocol-defined therapy successes (Table 2).

Table 2: Outcome of Treatment for PCP-Positive Patients Enrolled in the TMP-SMX Comparative Study

Outcome of Therapy*	MEPRON® (n=160)		TMP-SMX (n=162)		P Value
	Number of Patients (% of Total)				
Therapy Success	99	(62%)	103	(64%)	0.75
Therapy Failure					
–Lack of Response	28	(17%)	10	(6%)	<0.01
–Adverse Experience	11	(7%)	33	(20%)	<0.01
–Unevaluable	22	(14%)	16	(10%)	0.28
Required Alternate PCP Therapy During Study	55	(34%)	55	(34%)	0.95

* As defined by the protocol and described in study description above.

The failure rate due to lack of response was significantly larger for patients receiving MEPRON while the failure rate due to adverse experiences was significantly larger for patients receiving TMP-SMX.

There were no significant differences in the effect of either treatment on additional indicators of response (i.e., arterial blood gas measurements, vital signs, serum LDH levels, clinical symptoms, and chest radiographs).

Pentamidine Comparative Study: This unblinded, randomized trial initiated in 1991 was designed to compare the safety and efficacy of MEPRON to that of pentamidine for the treatment of histologically confirmed mild or moderate PCP in AIDS patients. Approximately 80% of the patients either had a history of intolerance to trimethoprim or sulfa-antimicrobials (the primary therapy group) or were experiencing intolerance to TMP-SMX with treatment of an episode of PCP at the time of enrollment in the study (the salvage treatment group).

Patients randomized to MEPRON were to receive 750 mg atovaquone (three 250-mg tablets) three times daily for 21 days and those randomized to pentamidine isethionate were to receive a 3- to 4-mg/kg single IV infusion daily for 21 days.

A total of 174 patients were enrolled into the trial at 22 study centers. Thirty-nine patients without histologic confirmation of PCP were excluded from the efficacy analyses. Of the 135 patients with histologically confirmed PCP, 70 were randomized to receive MEPRON and 65 to pentamidine. One hundred and ten (110) of these were in the primary therapy group and 25 were in the salvage therapy group. One patient in the primary therapy group randomized to receive pentamidine did not receive study medication.

Table 1: Relationship Between Plasma Atovaquone Concentration and Successful Treatment

Steady-State Plasma Atovaquone Concentrations (mcg/mL)	Successful Treatment* (No. Successes/No. In Group) (%)			
	Observed		Predicted †	
0 to <5	0/6	(0%)	1.5/6	(25%)
5 to <10	18/26	(69%)	14.7/26	(57%)
10 to <15	30/38	(79%)	31.9/38	(84%)
15 to <20	18/19	(95%)	18.1/19	(95%)
20 to <25	18/18	(100%)	17.8/18	(99%)
25+	6/6	(100%)	6/6	(100%)

* Successful treatment was defined as improvement in clinical and respiratory measures persisting at least 4 weeks after cessation of therapy. This was based on data from patients for which both outcome and steady-state plasma atovaquone concentration data are available.
† Based on logistic regression analysis.

Table 3: Outcome of Treatment for PCP-Positive Patients Enrolled in the Pentamidine Comparative Study

Outcome of Therapy	Primary Treatment			Salvage Treatment		
	MEPRON® (n = 56)	Pentamidine (n = 53)	P Value	MEPRON (n = 14)	Pentamidine (n = 11)	P Value
Therapy Success	32(57%)	21(40%)	0.09	13(93%)	7(64%)	0.14
Therapy Failure						
—Lack of Response	16(29%)	9(17%)	0.18	0	0	—
—Adverse Experience	2(3.6%)	19(36%)	<0.01	0	3(27%)	0.07
—Unevaluable	6(11%)	4(8%)	0.75	1(7%)	1(9%)	1.00
Required Alternate PCP Therapy During Study	19(34%)	29(55%)	0.04	0	4(36%)	0.03

There was no difference in mortality rates between the treatment groups. Among the 135 patients with confirmed PCP, 10 of 70 (14%) patients randomized to MEPRON and nine of 65 (14%) patients randomized to pentamidine died during the 21-day treatment course or 8-week follow-up period. In the intent-to-treat analysis for all randomized patients, there were 11 (12.5%) deaths in the arm treated with MEPRON and 12 (14%) deaths in the pentamidine arm. For those patients for whom day 4 plasma atovaquone concentrations are available, three of five (60%) patients with concentrations <5 mcg/mL died during participation in the study. However, only two of 21 (9%) patients with day 4 plasma concentrations ≥5 mcg/mL died.

The therapeutic outcomes for the 134 patients who received study medication in this trial are presented in Table 3. [See table 3 above]

Data on Chronic Use: MEPRON has not been systematically evaluated as a chronic suppressive agent to prevent the development of PCP in patients at high risk for *Pneumocystis carinii* disease.

CONTRAINDICATIONS

MEPRON Suspension is contraindicated for patients who develop or have a history of potentially life-threatening allergic reactions to any of the components of the formulation.

WARNINGS

Clinical experience with MEPRON has been limited to patients with mild-to-moderate PCP [(A-a)DO$_2$≤45 mm Hg]. Treatment of more severe episodes of PCP has not been systematically studied with this agent. Also, the efficacy of MEPRON in patients who are failing therapy with TMP-SMX has not been systematically studied. MEPRON has not been evaluated as an agent for PCP prophylaxis.

PRECAUTIONS

General: Absorption of orally administered MEPRON is limited but can be significantly increased when the drug is taken with food. Plasma atovaquone concentrations have been shown to correlate with the likelihood of successful treatment and survival. Therefore, parenteral therapy with other agents should be considered for patients who have difficulty taking MEPRON with food (see CLINICAL PHARMACOLOGY). Gastrointestinal disorders may limit absorption of orally administered drugs. Patients with these disorders also may not achieve plasma concentrations of atovaquone associated with response to therapy in controlled trials.

Based upon the spectrum of in vitro antimicrobial activity, atovaquone is not effective therapy for concurrent pulmonary conditions such as bacterial, viral, or fungal pneumonia or mycobacterial diseases. Clinical deterioration in patients may be due to infections with other pathogens, as well as progressive PCP. All patients with acute PCP should be carefully evaluated for other possible causes of pulmonary disease and treated with additional agents as appropriate.

Information for Patients: The importance of taking the prescribed dose of MEPRON should be stressed. Patients should be instructed to take their daily doses of MEPRON with meals, as the presence of food will significantly improve the absorption of the drug.

Drug Interactions: Atovaquone is highly bound to plasma protein (>99.9%). Therefore, caution should be used when administering MEPRON concurrently with other highly plasma protein-bound drugs with narrow therapeutic indices, as competition for binding sites may occur. The extent of plasma protein binding of atovaquone in human plasma is not affected by the presence of therapeutic concentrations of phenytoin (15 mcg/mL), nor is the binding of phenytoin affected by the presence of atovaquone.

Rifampin: Coadministration of rifampin and MEPRON Suspension results in a significant decrease in average steady-state plasma atovaquone concentration (see CLINICAL PHARMACOLOGY: Drug Interactions). Alternatives to rifampin should be considered during the course of PCP treatment with MEPRON.

Rifabutin, another rifamycin, is structurally similar to rifampin and may possibly have some of the same drug interactions as rifampin. No interaction trials have been conducted with MEPRON and rifabutin.

Drug/Laboratory Test Interactions: It is not known if MEPRON interferes with clinical laboratory test or assay results.

Carcinogenesis, Mutagenesis, Impairment of Fertility: Carcinogenicity studies in rats were negative; 24-month studies in mice showed treatment-related increases in incidence of hepatocellular adenoma and hepatocellular carcinoma at all doses tested which ranged from 1.4 to 3.6 times the average steady-state plasma concentrations in humans during acute treatment of *Pneumocystis carinii* pneumonia. Atovaquone was negative with or without metabolic activation in the Ames *Salmonella* mutagenicity assay, the Mouse Lymphoma mutagenesis assay, and the Cultured Human Lymphocyte cytogenetic assay. No evidence of genotoxicity was observed in the in vivo Mouse Micronucleus assay.

Pregnancy: Pregnancy Category C. Atovaquone was not teratogenic and did not cause reproductive toxicity in rats at plasma concentrations up to two to three times the estimated human exposure. Atovaquone caused maternal toxicity in rabbits at plasma concentrations that were approximately one-half the estimated human exposure. Mean fetal body lengths and weights were decreased and there were higher numbers of early resorption and post-implantation loss per dam. It is not clear whether these effects were caused by atovaquone directly or were secondary to mater-

Continued on next page

This product information is based on labeling in effect on June 1, 1998. For further information, contact via direct mail, phone, or web site Medical Information: Glaxo Wellcome Inc., PO Box 13398, Research Triangle Park, NC 27709. Healthcare Professionals (Medical Information): 800-334-0089 Patients (Customer Response Center): 888-TALK2GW (1-888-825-5249) Glaxo Wellcome Corporate Web Site: www.glaxowellcome.com

Mepron—Cont.

nal toxicity. Concentrations of atovaquone in rabbit fetuses averaged 30% of the concurrent maternal plasma concentrations. In a separate study in rats given a single ^{14}C-radiolabelled dose, concentrations of radiocarbon in rat fetuses were 18% (middle gestation) and 60% (late gestation) of concurrent maternal plasma concentrations. There are no adequate and well-controlled studies in pregnant women. MEPRON should be used during pregnancy only if the potential benefit justifies the potential risk to the fetus.

Nursing Mothers: It is not known whether atovaquone is excreted into human milk. Because many drugs are excreted into human milk, caution should be exercised when MEPRON is administered to a nursing woman. In a rat study, atovaquone concentrations in the milk were 30% of the concurrent atovaquone concentrations in the maternal plasma.

Pediatric Use: Safety and effectiveness in pediatric patients have not been established. Clinical experience with MEPRON Suspension in the pediatric population is limited to a pharmacokinetic study in children who were at risk of developing PCP. Preliminary analysis of a study of MEPRON Suspension in 15 HIV-infected, asymptomatic infants and children between 1 month and 13 years of age suggests that the pharmacokinetics of atovaquone is age-dependent (see CLINICAL PHARMACOLOGY: Special Populations). No treatment-limiting adverse events were observed.

Geriatric Use: MEPRON has not been systematically evaluated in patients greater than 65 years of age. Caution should be exercised when treating elderly patients reflecting the greater frequency of decreased hepatic, renal, and cardiac function in this population.

ADVERSE REACTIONS

Because many patients who participated in clinical trials with MEPRON had complications of advanced HIV disease, it was often difficult to distinguish adverse events caused by MEPRON from those caused by underlying medical conditions. There were no life-threatening or fatal adverse experiences caused by MEPRON.

Table 4 summarizes all the clinical adverse experiences reported by ≥5% of the study population during the TMP-SMX comparative clinical trial of MEPRON (n = 408), regardless of attribution. The incidence of adverse experiences with MEPRON Suspension at the recommended dose was similar to that seen with the tablet formulation of atovaquone.

Table 4: Treatment-Emergent Adverse Experiences in the TMP-SMX Comparative PCP Treatment Study

Treatment-Emergent Adverse Experience	Number of Patients with Treatment-Emergent Adverse Experience (% of Total)			
	MEPRON (n = 203)		TMP-SMX (n = 205)	
Rash (including maculopapular)	47	(23%)	69	(34%)*
Nausea	43	(21%)	90	(44%)*
Diarrhea	39	(19%)*	15	(7%)
Headache	33	(16%)	44	(22%)
Vomiting	29	(14%)	72	(35%)*
Fever	28	(14%)	52	(25%)*
Insomnia	20	(10%)	18	(9%)
Asthenia	17	(8%)	16	(8%)
Pruritus	11	(5%)	18	(9%)
Monilia, Oral	11	(5%)	21	(10%)
Abdominal Pain	9	(4%)	15	(7%)
Constipation	7	(3%)	35	(17%)*
Dizziness	7	(3%)	17	(8%)*
No. Patients Discontinuing Therapy Due to an Adverse Experience	19	(9%)	50	(24%)*
No. Patients Reporting at Least One Adverse Experience	127	(63%)	134	(65%)

* $P<0.05$.

Although an equal percentage of patients receiving MEPRON and TMP-SMX reported at least one adverse experience, more patients receiving TMP-SMX required discontinuation of therapy due to an adverse event. Twenty-four percent of patients receiving TMP-SMX were prematurely discontinued from therapy due to an adverse experience versus 9% of patients receiving MEPRON. Four percent of patients receiving MEPRON had therapy discontinued due to development of rash. The majority of cases of rash among patients receiving MEPRON were mild and did not require the discontinuation of dosing. The only other clinical adverse experience that led to premature discontinuation of dosing of MEPRON by more than one patient was vomiting (<1%). The most common adverse experience requiring discontinuation of dosing in the TMP-SMX group was rash (8%).

Laboratory test abnormalities reported for ≥5% of the study population during the treatment period are summarized in Table 5. Two percent of patients treated with MEPRON and 7% of patients treated with TMP-SMX had therapy prematurely discontinued due to elevations in ALT/AST. In general, patients treated with MEPRON developed fewer abnormalities in measures of hepatocellular function (ALT, AST, alkaline phosphatase) or amylase values than patients treated with TMP-SMX.

Table 5: Treatment-Emergent Laboratory Test Abnormalities in the TMP-SMX Comparative PCP Treatment Study

Laboratory Test Abnormality	Patients Developing a Laboratory Test Abnormality (% of Total)	
	MEPRON	TMP-SMX
Anemia (Hgb<8.0 g/dL)	6%	7%
Neutropenia ANC<750 cells/mm³)	3%	9%
Elevated ALT (>5 × ULN)	6%	16%
Elevated AST (>5 × ULN)	4%	14%
Elevated Alkaline Phosphatase (>2.5 × ULN)	8%	6%
Elevated Amylase (>1.5 × ULN)	7%	12%
Hyponatremia (<0.96 × LLN)	7%	26%

ULN = upper limit of normal range.
LLN = lower limit of normal range.

Table 6 summarizes the clinical adverse experiences reported by ≥5% of the primary therapy study population (n = 144) during the comparative trial of MEPRON and intravenous pentamidine, regardless of attribution. A slightly lower percentage of patients who received MEPRON reported occurrence of adverse events than did those who received pentamidine (63% vs 72%). However, only 7% of patients discontinued treatment with MEPRON due to adverse events, while 41% of patients who received pentamidine discontinued treatment for this reason ($P<0.001$). Of the five patients who discontinued therapy with MEPRON, three reported rash (4%). Rash was not severe in any patient. No other reason for discontinuation of MEPRON was cited more than once. The most frequently cited reasons for discontinuation of pentamidine therapy were hypoglycemia (11%) and vomiting (9%).

Table 6: Treatment-Emergent Adverse Experiences in the Pentamidine Comparative PCP Treatment Study (Primary Therapy Group)

Treatment-Emergent Adverse Experience	Number of Patients with Treatment-Emergent Adverse Experience (% of Total)	
	MEPRON (n = 73)	Pentamidine (n = 71)
Fever	29(40%)	18(25%)
Nausea	16(22%)	26(37%)
Rash	16(22%)	9(13%)
Diarrhea	15(21%)	22(31%)
Insomnia	14(19%)	10(14%)
Headache	13(18%)	20(28%)
Vomiting	10(14%)	12(17%)
Cough	10 (14%)*	1 (1%)
Abdominal Pain	7(10%)	8(11%)
Pain	7(10%)	7(10%)
Sweat	7(10%)	2 (3%)
Monilia, Oral	7(10%)	2 (3%)
Asthenia	6 (8%)	10(14%)
Dizziness	6 (8%)	10(14%)
Anxiety	5 (7%)	7(10%)
Anorexia	5 (7%)	7(10%)
Sinusitis	5 (7%)	4 (6%)
Dyspepsia	4 (5%)	7(10%)
Rhinitis	4 (5%)	5 (7%)
Taste Perversion	2 (3%)	9 (13%)*
Hypoglycemia	1 (1%)	11 (15%)*
Hypotension	1 (1%)	7 (10%)*
No. Patients Discontinuing Therapy Due to an Adverse Experience	5 (7%)	29(41%)†
No. Patients Reporting at Least One Adverse Experience	46(63%)	51(72%)

* $P<0.05$.
† $P<0.001$.

Laboratory test abnormalities reported in ≥5% of patients in the pentamidine comparative study are presented in Table 7. Laboratory abnormality was reported as the reason for discontinuation of treatment in two of 73 patients who received MEPRON. One patient (1%) had elevated creatinine and BUN levels and one patient (1%) had elevated amylase levels. Laboratory abnormalities were the sole or contributing factor in 14 patients who prematurely discontinued pentamidine therapy. In the 71 patients who received pentamidine, laboratory parameters most frequently reported as reasons for discontinuation were hypoglycemia (11%), elevated creatinine levels (6%), and leukopenia (4%).

Table 7: Treatment-Emergent Laboratory Test Abnormalities in the Pentamidine Comparative PCP Treatment Study

Laboratory Test Abnormality	Patients Developing a Laboratory Test Abnormality (% of Total)	
	MEPRON	Pentamidine
Anemia (Hgb<8.0 g/dL)	4%	9%
Neutropenia (ANC<750 cells/mm³)	5%	9%
Hyponatremia (<0.96 × LLN)	10%	10%
Hyperkalemia (>1.18 × ULN)	0%	5%
Alkaline Phosphatase (>2.5 ×ULN)	5%	2%
Hyperglycemia (>1.8 × ULN)	9%	13%
Elevated AST (>5 × ULN)	0%	5%

Elevated Amylase (>1.5 × ULN)	8%	4%
Elevated Creatinine (>1.5 × ULN)	0%	7%

ULN = upper limit of normal range.
LLN = lower limit of normal range.

OVERDOSAGE

There have been no reports of overdosage from the administration of MEPRON.

DOSAGE AND ADMINISTRATION

The recommended oral dose is 750 mg (5 mL) administered with meals twice daily for 21 days (total daily dose 1500 mg). Failure to administer MEPRON Suspension with meals may result in lower plasma atovaquone concentrations and may limit response to therapy (see CLINICAL PHARMACOLOGY and PRECAUTIONS).
SHAKE GENTLY BEFORE USING.

HOW SUPPLIED

MEPRON Suspension (bright yellow, citrus flavored) containing 750 mg atovaquone in each teaspoonful (5 mL).
Bottle of 210 mL with child-resistant cap (NDC 0173-0665-18).
Store at 15° to 25°C (59° to 77°F). DO NOT FREEZE. Dispense in tight container as defined in U.S.P.
[1](A-a)DO$_2$ = [(713 × FiO$_2$) – (PaCO$_2$/0.8)] – PaO$_2$ (mm Hg)
U.S. Patent No. 5,053,432
U.S. Patent No. 4,981,874 (Use Patent)
© Copyright 1996 Glaxo Wellcome Inc. All rights reserved.
September 1997/RL-458
Shown in Product Identification Guide, page 313

MIVACRON® ℞
[mĭv 'ah-krŏn]
**(mivacurium chloride)
Injection
MIVACRON®
(mivacurium chloride)
Premixed Infusion**

This drug should be administered only by adequately trained individuals familiar with its actions, characteristics, and hazards.

DESCRIPTION

MIVACRON (mivacurium chloride) is a short-acting, nondepolarizing skeletal muscle relaxant for intravenous (IV) administration. Mivacurium chloride is [R-[R*,R*-(E)]]-2,2'-[(1,8-dioxo-4-octene-1,8-diyl)bis(oxy-3,1-propanediyl)]-bis[1,2,3,4-tetrahydro-6,7-dimethoxy-2-methyl-1-[(3,4,5-trimethoxyphenyl)methyl]isoquinolinium]dichloride. The molecular formula is $C_{58}H_{80}Cl_2N_2O_{14}$ and the molecular weight is 1100.18.
The partition coefficient of the compound is 0.015 in a 1-octanol/distilled water system at 25°C.
Mivacurium chloride is a mixture of three stereoisomers: (1R, 1'R, 2S, 2'S), the *trans-trans* diester; (1R, 1'R, 2R, 2'S), the *cis-trans* diester; and (1R, 1'R, 2R, 2'R), the *cis-cis* diester. The *trans-trans* and *cis-trans* stereoisomers comprise 92% to 96% of mivacurium chloride and their neuromuscular blocking potencies are not significantly different from each other or from mivacurium chloride. The *cis-cis* diester has been estimated from studies in cats to have one tenth the neuromuscular blocking potency of the other two stereoisomers.
MIVACRON Injection is a sterile, non-pyrogenic solution (pH 3.5 to 5.0) containing mivacurium chloride equivalent to 2 mg/mL mivacurium in Water for Injection. Hydrochloric acid may have been added to adjust pH. Multiple-dose vials contain 0.9% w/v benzyl alcohol. MIVACRON Premixed Infusion is a sterile, non-pyrogenic solution (pH 3.5 to 5.0; 260 mOsmol/L-measured) containing mivacurium chloride equivalent to 0.5 mg/mL mivacurium in 5% Dextrose Injection USP. Hydrochloric acid may have been added to adjust pH.

CLINICAL PHARMACOLOGY

MIVACRON (a mixture of three stereoisomers) binds competitively to cholinergic receptors on the motor end-plate to antagonize the action of acetylcholine, resulting in a block of neuromuscular transmission. This action is antagonized by acetylcholinesterase inhibitors, such as neostigmine.
Pharmacodynamics: The time to maximum neuromuscular block is similar for recommended doses of MIVACRON and intermediate-acting agents (e.g., atracurium), but longer than for the ultra-short-acting agent, succinylcholine. The clinically effective duration of action of the stereoisomers in MIVACRON (a mixture of three stereoisomers) is one third to one half that of intermediate-acting agents and 2 to 2.5 times that of succinylcholine.

Table 1: Pharmacodynamic Dose Response During Opioid/Nitrous Oxide/Oxygen Anesthesia

Initial Dose of MIVACRON* (mg/kg)		Time to Maximum Block[†] (min)	Time to Spontaneous Recovery[†]			
			5% Recovery (min)	25% Recovery[‡] (min)	95% Recovery [§] (min)	T$_4$/T$_1$ Ratio ≥75% [§] (min)
Adults						
0.07 to 0.10	[n=47]	4.9 (2.0-7.6)	11 (7-19)	13 (8-24)	21 (10-36)	21 (10-36)
0.15	[n=50]	3.3 (1.5-8.8)	13 (6-31)	16 (9-38)	26 (16-41)	26 (15-45)
0.20[‖]	[n=50]	2.5 (1.2-6.0)	16 (10-29)	20 (10-36)	31 (15-51)	34 (19-56)
0.25[‖]	[n=48]	2.3 (1.0-4.8)	19 (11-29)	23 (14-38)	34 (22-64)	43 (26-75)
Children 2 to 12 Years						
0.11 to 0.12	[n=17]	2.8 (1.2-4.6)	5 (3-9)	7 (4-10)	—	—
0.20	[n=18]	1.9 (1.3-3.3)	7 (3-12)	10 (6-15)	19 (14-26)	16 (12-23)
0.25	[n=9]	1.6 (1.0-2.2)	7 (4-9)	9 (5-12)	—	—

* Doses administered over 5 to 15 seconds.
† Values shown are medians of means from individual studies (range of individual patient values).
‡ Clinically effective duration of neuromuscular block.
§ Data available for as few as 40% of adults in specific dose groups and for 22% of children in the 0.20-mg/kg dose group due to administration of reversal agents or additional doses of MIVACRON prior to 95% recovery or T$_4$/T$_1$ ratio recovery to ≥75%.
‖ Rapid administration not recommended due to possibility of decreased blood pressure. Administer 0.20 mg/kg over 30 seconds; administer 0.25 mg/kg as divided dose (0.15 mg/kg followed 30 seconds later by 0.10 mg/kg). See DOSAGE AND ADMINISTRATION.

The average ED$_{95}$ (dose required to produce 95% suppression of the adductor pollicis muscle twitch response to ulnar nerve stimulation) of MIVACRON is 0.07 mg/kg (range: 0.06 to 0.09) in adults receiving opioid/nitrous oxide/oxygen anesthesia. The pharmacodynamics of doses of MIVACRON ≥ED$_{95}$ administered over 5 to 15 seconds during opioid/nitrous oxide/oxygen anesthesia are summarized in Table 1. The mean time for spontaneous recovery of the twitch response from 25% to 75% of control amplitude is about 6 minutes (range: 3 to 9, n=32) following an initial dose of 0.15 mg/kg MIVACRON and 7 to 8 minutes (range: 4 to 24, n=85) following initial doses of 0.20 or 0.25 mg/kg MIVACRON.
Volatile anesthetics may decrease the dosing requirement for MIVACRON and prolong the duration of action; the magnitude of these effects may be increased as the concentration of the volatile agent is increased. Isoflurane and enflurane (administered with nitrous oxide/oxygen to achieve 1.25 MAC [Minimum Alveolar Concentration]) may decrease the effective dose of MIVACRON by as much as 25%, and may prolong the clinically effective duration of action and decrease the average infusion requirement by as much as 35% to 40%. At equivalent MAC values, halothane has little or no effect on the ED$_{50}$ of MIVACRON, but may prolong the duration of action and decrease the average infusion requirement by as much as 20% (see CLINICAL PHARMACOLOGY: Individualization of Dosages subsection and PRECAUTIONS: Drug Interactions).
[See table 1 above]
Administration of MIVACRON over 30 to 60 seconds does not alter the time to maximum neuromuscular block or the duration of action. The duration of action of the stereoisomers in MIVACRON may be prolonged in patients with reduced plasma cholinesterase (pseudocholinesterase) activity (see PRECAUTIONS: Reduced Plasma Cholinesterase Activity and CLINICAL PHARMACOLOGY Individualization of Dosages subsection).
Interpatient variability in duration of action occurs with MIVACRON as with other neuromuscular blocking agents. However, analysis of data from 224 patients in clinical studies receiving various doses of MIVACRON during opioid/nitrous oxide/oxygen anesthesia with a variety of premedicants and varying lengths of surgery indicated that approximately 90% of the patients had clinically effective durations of block within 8 minutes of the median duration predicted from the dose-response data shown in Table 1. Variations in plasma cholinesterase activity, including values within the normal range and values as low as 20% below the lower limit of the normal range, were not associated with clinically significant effects on duration. The variability in duration, however, was greater in patients with plasma cholinesterase activity at or slightly below the lower limit of the normal range.
When administered during the induction of adequate anesthesia using thiopental or propofol, nitrous oxide/oxygen, and co-induction agents such as fentanyl and/or midazolam, doses of 0.15 mg/kg (2 × ED$_{95}$) MIVACRON administered over 5 to 15 seconds or 0.20 mg/kg MIVACRON administered over 30 seconds produced generally good-to-excellent tracheal intubation conditions in 2.5 to 3 and 2 to 2.5 minutes, respectively. A dose of 0.25 mg/kg MIVACRON administered as a divided dose (0.15 mg/kg followed 30 seconds later by 0.10 mg/kg) produced generally good-to-excellent intubation conditions in 1.5 to 2 minutes after initiating the dosing regimen.
Repeated administration of maintenance doses or continuous infusion of MIVACRON for up to 2.5 hours is not associated with development of tachyphylaxis or cumulative neuromuscular blocking effects in ASA Physical Status I–II patients. Limited data are available from patients receiving infusions for longer than 2.5 hours. Spontaneous recovery of neuromuscular function after infusion is independent of the duration of infusion and comparable to recovery reported for single doses (Table 1).
The neuromuscular block produced by the stereoisomers in MIVACRON is readily antagonized by anticholinesterase agents. As seen with other nondepolarizing neuromuscular blocking agents, the more profound the neuromuscular block at the time of reversal, the longer the time and the greater the dose of anticholinesterase agent required for recovery of neuromuscular function.
In children (2 to 12 years), MIVACRON has a higher ED$_{95}$ (0.10 mg/kg), faster onset, and shorter duration of action than in adults. The mean time for spontaneous recovery of the twitch response from 25% to 75% of control amplitude is about 5 minutes (n=4) following an initial dose of 0.20 mg/kg MIVACRON. Recovery following reversal is faster in children than in adults (Table 1).
Hemodynamics: Administration of MIVACRON in doses up to and including 0.15 mg/kg (2×ED$_{95}$) over 5 to 15 seconds to ASA Physical Status I–II patients during opioid/nitrous oxide/oxygen anesthesia is associated with minimal changes in mean arterial blood pressure (MAP) or heart rate (HR) (Table 2).

Table 2: Cardiovascular Dose Response During Opioid/Nitrous Oxide/Oxygen Anesthesia

Initial Dose of MIVACRON* (mg/kg)		% of Patients With ≥30% Change			
		MAP		HR	
		Dec	Inc	Dec	Inc
Adults					
0.07 to 0.10	[n=49]	0%	2%	0%	0%
0.15	[n=53]	4%	4%	4%	2%

Continued on next page

This product information is based on labeling in effect on June 1, 1998. For further information, contact via direct mail, phone, or web site Medical Information: Glaxo Wellcome Inc., PO Box 13398, Research Triangle Park, NC 27709. Healthcare Professionals (Medical Information): 800-334-0089 Patients (Customer Response Center): 888-TALK2GW (1-888-825-5249) Glaxo Wellcome Corporate Web Site: www.glaxowellcome.com

Mivacron—Cont.

0.20†	[n=53]	30%	0%	0%	8%
0.25†	[n=44]	39%	2%	0%	14%
Children 2 to 12 years					
0.11 to 0.12	[n=17]	0%	6%	0%	0%
0.20	[n=17]	0%	0%	0%	0%
0.25	[n=8]	13%	0%	0%	0%

* Doses administered over 5 to 15 seconds.
† Rapid administration not recommended due to possibility of decreased blood pressure. Administer 0.20 mg/kg over 30 seconds; administer 0.25 mg/kg as divided dose (0.15 mg/kg followed 30 seconds later by 0.10 mg/kg). See DOSAGE AND ADMINISTRATION.

Higher doses of ≥0.20 mg/kg (≥3×ED_{95}) may be associated with transient decreases in MAP and increases in HR in some patients. These decreases in MAP are usually maximal within 1 to 3 minutes following the dose, typically resolve without treatment in an additional 1 to 3 minutes, and are usually associated with increases in plasma histamine concentration. Decreases in MAP can be minimized by administering MIVACRON over 30 to 60 seconds (see CLINICAL PHARMACOLOGY: Individualization of Dosages subsection and PRECAUTIONS: General).
Analysis of 426 patients in clinical studies receiving initial doses of MIVACRON up to and including 0.30 mg/kg during opioid/nitrous oxide/oxygen anesthesia showed that high initial doses and a rapid rate of injection contributed to a greater probability of experiencing a decrease of ≥30% in MAP after administration of MIVACRON. Obese patients also had a greater probability of experiencing a decrease of ≥30% in MAP when dosed on the basis of actual body weight, thereby receiving a larger dose than if dosed on the basis of ideal body weight (see CLINICAL PHARMACOLOGY: Individualization of Dosages subsection and PRECAUTIONS: General).
Children experience minimal changes in MAP or HR after administration of MIVACRON doses up to and including 0.20 mg/kg over 5 to 15 seconds, but higher doses (≥0.25 mg/kg) may be associated with transient decreases in MAP (Table 2).
Following a dose of 0.15 mg/kg MIVACRON administered over 60 seconds, adult patients with significant cardiovascular disease undergoing coronary artery bypass grafting or valve replacement procedures showed no clinically important changes in MAP or HR. Transient decreases in MAP were observed in some patients after doses of 0.20 to 0.25 mg/kg MIVACRON administered over 60 seconds. The number of patients in whom these decreases in MAP required treatment was small.
Pharmacokinetics: Table 3 describes the results from a study of nine ASA Physical Status I–II adult patients (31 to 48 years) receiving an infusion of MIVACRON at 5 mcg/kg per minute for 60 minutes followed by 10 mcg/kg per minute for 60 minutes. MIVACRON is a mixture of isomers which do not interconvert in vivo. The mivacurium pharmacokinetic parameters presented in Table 3 were determined using a stereospecific assay. The two more potent isomers, *cis-trans* (36% of the mixture) and *trans-trans* (57% of the mixture), have very high clearances that exceed cardiac output, reflecting the extensive metabolism by plasma cholinesterase. The volume of distribution is relatively small, reflecting limited tissue distribution secondary to the polarity and large molecular weight of mivacurium. The combination of high metabolic clearance and low distribution volume results in the short elimination half-life of approximately 2 minutes for the two active isomers. The short elimination half-lives and high metabolic clearances of the active isomers are consistent with the short duration of action of MIVACRON. The steady-state concentrations of the *cis-trans* and *trans-trans* isomers doubled after the infusion rate was increased from 5 to 10 mcg/kg per minute, indicating that their pharmacokinetics is dose-proportional.

Table 3: Stereoisomer Pharmacokinetic Parameters* of MIVACRON in ASA Physical Status I–II Adult Patients† [n=9] During Opioid/Nitrous Oxide/Oxygen Anesthesia

Parameter	*trans-trans* isomer	*cis-trans* isomer
Elimination Half-life ($t_{1/2}$, min)	2.3 (1.4–3.6)	2.1 (0.8–4.8)
Volume of Distribution (L/kg)	0.15 (0.06–0.24)	0.27 (0.08–0.56)
Plasma Clearance (mL/min/kg)	53 (32–105)	99 (52–230)

* Values shown are mean (range).
† Ages 31 to 48 years.

The *cis-cis* isomer (6% of the mixture) has approximately one tenth the neuromuscular blocking potency of the *trans-trans* and *cis-trans* isomers in cats. In the nine patients shown in Table 3, the volume of distribution of the *cis-cis* isomer averaged 0.31 L/kg (range: 0.18 to 0.46), the clearance averaged 4.2 mL/min per kg (range: 2.4 to 5.4), and the half-life averaged 55 minutes (range: 32 to 102). The neuromuscular blocking potency of the *cis-cis* isomer in humans has not been established; however, modeling of clinical pharmacokinetic-pharmacodynamic data suggests that the *cis-cis* isomer produces minimal (<5%) neuromuscular block during a 2-hour infusion. In studies in which infusions of up to 2.5 hours were administered to ASA Physical Status I–II patients, the 25% to 75% recovery times were independent of the duration of infusion, suggesting that the *cis-cis* isomer does not contribute significant neuromuscular block during use for up to 2.5 hours. Limited data are available from infusions of longer duration or from patients with compromised elimination capacities (hepatic or renal failure).
Metabolism and Excretion: Enzymatic hydrolysis by plasma cholinesterase is the primary mechanism for inactivation of mivacurium and yields a quaternary alcohol and a quaternary monoester metabolite. Renal and biliary excretion of unchanged mivacurium are minor elimination pathways; urine and bile are important elimination pathways for the two metabolites. Tests in which these two metabolites were administered to cats and dogs suggest that each metabolite is unlikely to produce clinically significant neuromuscular, autonomic, or cardiovascular effects following administration of MIVACRON.
Special Populations: The pharmacokinetics of mivacurium isomers has not been studied in the elderly or in patients with renal or hepatic disease using a stereospecific assay. The non-stereospecific, total mivacurium assay used in pharmacokinetic-pharmacodynamic studies in these populations provided preliminary evidence that reduced clearance of one or more isomers is responsible for the longer duration of action of MIVACRON seen in patients with end-stage kidney or liver disease. The data did not provide a pharmacokinetic explanation for the 15% to 20% longer duration of block seen in the elderly. Tables 4 and 5 summarize the pharmacodynamic results in these special populations as compared with young adults (ages 18 to 49 years). No data are available from patients with kidney or liver disease not requiring transplantation.

Table 4: Pharmacodynamic Parameters* of MIVACRON in ASA Physical Status I–II Young Adult Patients and Elderly Patients During Isoflurane/Nitrous Oxide/Oxygen Anesthesia

Parameter	Young Adult Patients (18–49 years)		Elderly Patients (68–77 years)
Initial Dose†	0.10 mg/kg [n=9]	0.25 mg/kg‡ [n=9]	0.10 mg/kg [n=8]
Maximum Block (%)	98 (83-100)	100 (100-100)	99 (95-100)
Time to Maximum Block (min)	3.2 (2.0-6.0)	1.7 (1.3-2.5)	4.8 (3.0-7.0)
Clinically Effective Duration of Block§ (min)	17 (9-29)	27 (18-34)	20 (14-28)

* Values shown are mean (range).
† Doses administered over 5 to 15 seconds.
‡ Rapid administration not recommended due to possibility of decreased blood pressure. Administer 0.25 mg/kg as divided dose (0.15 mg/kg followed 30 seconds later by 0.10 mg/kg). See DOSAGE AND ADMINISTRATION.
§ Time from injection to 25% recovery of the control twitch height.

[See table 4 below]
Renal: The clinically effective duration of action of 0.15 mg/kg MIVACRON was about 1.5 times longer in patients with end-stage kidney disease than in healthy patients, presumably due to reduced clearance of one or more isomers.
Hepatic: The clinically effective duration of action of 0.15 mg/kg MIVACRON was three times longer in patients with end-stage liver disease than in healthy patients and is likely related to the markedly decreased plasma cholinesterase activity (30% of healthy patient values) which could decrease the clearance of one or more isomers (see PRECAUTIONS: Reduced Plasma Cholinesterase Activity).
[See table 5 at bottom of next page]
Individualization of Dosages: DOSES OF MIVACRON SHOULD BE INDIVIDUALIZED AND A PERIPHERAL NERVE STIMULATOR SHOULD BE USED TO MEASURE NEUROMUSCULAR FUNCTION DURING MIVACRON ADMINISTRATION IN ORDER TO MONITOR DRUG EFFECT, DETERMINE THE NEED FOR ADDITIONAL DOSES, AND CONFIRM RECOVERY FROM NEUROMUSCULAR BLOCK.
Based on the known actions of MIVACRON (a mixture of three stereoisomers) and other neuromuscular blocking agents, the following factors should be considered when administering MIVACRON:
Renal or Hepatic Impairment: A dose of 0.15 mg/kg MIVACRON is recommended for facilitation of tracheal intubation in patients with renal or hepatic impairment. However, the clinically effective duration of block produced by this dose is about 1.5 times longer in patients with end-stage kidney disease and about 3 times longer in patients with end-stage liver disease than in patients with normal renal and hepatic function. Infusion rates should be decreased by as much as 50% in these patients depending on the degree of renal or hepatic impairment (see PRECAUTIONS: Renal and Hepatic Disease).
Reduced Plasma Cholinesterase Activity: The possibility of prolonged neuromuscular block following administration of MIVACRON must be considered in patients with reduced plasma cholinesterase (pseudocholinesterase) activity. MIVACRON should be used with great caution, if at all, in patients known or suspected of being homozygous for the atypical plasma cholinesterase gene (see WARNINGS). Doses of 0.03 mg/kg produced complete neuromuscular block for 26 to 128 minutes in three such patients; thus initial doses greater than 0.03 mg/kg are not recommended in homozygous patients. Infusions of MIVACRON are not recommended in homozygous patients.
MIVACRON has been used safely in patients heterozygous for the atypical plasma cholinesterase gene and in genotypically normal patients with reduced plasma cholinesterase activity. After an initial dose of 0.15 mg/kg MIVACRON, the clinically effective duration of block in heterozygous patients may be approximately 10 minutes longer than in patients with normal genotype and normal plasma cholinesterase activity. Lower infusion rates of MIVACRON are recommended in these patients (see PRECAUTIONS: Reduced Plasma Cholinesterase Activity).
Drugs or Conditions Causing Potentiation of or Resistance to Neuromuscular Block: As with other neuromuscular blocking agents, MIVACRON may have profound neuromuscular blocking effects in cachectic or debilitated patients, patients with neuromuscular diseases, and patients with carcinomatosis. In these or other patients in whom potentiation of neuromuscular block or difficulty with reversal may be anticipated, the initial dose should be decreased. A test dose of not more than 0.015 to 0.020 mg/kg, which represents the lower end of the dose-response curve for MIVACRON, is recommended in such patients (see PRECAUTIONS: General).
The neuromuscular blocking action of the stereoisomers in MIVACRON is potentiated by isoflurane or enflurane anesthesia. Recommended initial MIVACRON doses (see DOSAGE AND ADMINISTRATION) may be used for intubation prior to the administration of these agents. If MIVACRON is first administered after establishment of stable-state isoflurane or enflurane anesthesia (administered with nitrous oxide/oxygen to achieve 1.25 MAC), the initial dose of MIVACRON should be reduced by as much as 25%, and the infusion rate reduced by as much as 35% to 40%. A greater potentiation of the neuromuscular blocking action of the stereoisomers in MIVACRON may be expected with higher concentrations of enflurane or isoflurane. The use of halothane requires no adjustment of the initial dose of MIVACRON, but may prolong the duration of action and decrease the average infusion rate by as much as 20% (see PRECAUTIONS: Drug Interactions).
When MIVACRON is administered to patients receiving certain antibiotics, magnesium salts, lithium, local anesthetics, procainamide and quinidine, longer durations of neuromuscular block may be expected and infusion requirements may be lower (see PRECAUTIONS: Drug Interactions).
When MIVACRON is administered to patients chronically receiving phenytoin or carbamazepine, slightly shorter durations of neuromuscular block may be anticipated and infusion rate requirements may be higher (see PRECAUTIONS: Drug Interactions).

Severe acid-base and/or electrolyte abnormalities may potentiate or cause resistance to the neuromuscular blocking action of the stereoisomers in MIVACRON. No data are available in such patients and no dosing recommendations can be made (see PRECAUTIONS: General).

Burns: While patients with burns are known to develop resistance to nondepolarizing neuromuscular blocking agents, they may also have reduced plasma cholinesterase activity. Consequently, in these patients, a test dose of not more than 0.015 to 0.020 mg/kg MIVACRON is recommended, followed by additional appropriate dosing guided by the use of a neuromuscular block monitor (see PRECAUTIONS: General).

Cardiovascular Disease: In patients with clinically significant cardiovascular disease, the initial dose of MIVACRON should be 0.15 mg/kg or less, administered over 60 seconds (see CLINICAL PHARMACOLOGY: Hemodynamics subsection and PRECAUTIONS: General).

Obesity: Obese patients (patients weighing ≥30% more than their ideal body weight) dosed on the basis of actual body weight, thereby receiving a larger dose than if dosed on the basis of ideal body weight, had a greater probability of experiencing a decrease of ≥30% in MAP (see CLINICAL PHARMACOLOGY: Hemodynamics subsection and PRECAUTIONS: General). Therefore, in obese patients, the initial dose should be determined using the patient's ideal body weight (IBW), according to the following formulae:

Men: IBW in kg = (106 + [6 × inches in height above 5 feet])/2.2

Women: IBW in kg = (100 + [5 × inches in height above 5 feet])/2.2

Allergy and Sensitivity: In patients with any history suggestive of a greater sensitivity to the release of histamine or related mediators (e.g., asthma), the initial dose of MIVACRON should be 0.15 mg/kg or less, administered over 60 seconds (see PRECAUTIONS: General).

INDICATIONS AND USAGE

MIVACRON is a short-acting neuromuscular blocking agent indicated for inpatients and outpatients, as an adjunct to general anesthesia, to facilitate tracheal intubation and to provide skeletal muscle relaxation during surgery or mechanical ventilation.

CONTRAINDICATIONS

MIVACRON is contraindicated in patients known to have an allergic hypersensitivity to mivacurium chloride or other benzylisoquinolinium agents, as manifested by reactions such as urticaria or severe respiratory distress or hypotension. Use of MIVACRON from multiple-dose vials containing benzyl alcohol as a preservative is contraindicated in patients with a known hypersensitivity to benzyl alcohol.

WARNINGS

MIVACRON SHOULD BE ADMINISTERED IN CAREFULLY ADJUSTED DOSAGE BY OR UNDER THE SUPERVISION OF EXPERIENCED CLINICIANS WHO ARE FAMILIAR WITH THE DRUG'S ACTIONS AND THE POSSIBLE COMPLICATIONS OF ITS USE. THE DRUG SHOULD NOT BE ADMINISTERED UNLESS PERSONNEL AND FACILITIES FOR RESUSCITATION AND LIFE SUPPORT (TRACHEAL INTUBATION, ARTIFICIAL VENTILATION, OXYGEN THERAPY), AND AN ANTAGONIST OF MIVACRON ARE IMMEDIATELY AVAILABLE. IT IS RECOMMENDED THAT A PERIPHERAL NERVE STIMULATOR BE USED TO MEASURE NEUROMUSCULAR FUNCTION DURING THE ADMINISTRATION OF MIVACRON IN ORDER TO MONITOR DRUG EFFECT, DETERMINE THE NEED FOR ADDITIONAL DRUG, AND CONFIRM RECOVERY FROM NEUROMUSCULAR BLOCK.

MIVACRON HAS NO KNOWN EFFECT ON CONSCIOUSNESS, PAIN THRESHOLD, OR CEREBRATION. TO AVOID DISTRESS TO THE PATIENT, NEUROMUSCULAR BLOCK SHOULD NOT BE INDUCED BEFORE UNCONSCIOUSNESS.

MIVACRON IS METABOLIZED BY PLASMA CHOLINESTERASE AND SHOULD BE USED WITH GREAT CAUTION, IF AT ALL, IN PATIENTS KNOWN TO BE OR SUSPECTED OF BEING HOMOZYGOUS FOR THE ATYPICAL PLASMA CHOLINESTERASE GENE.

MIVACRON Injection and MIVACRON Premixed Infusion are acidic (pH 3.5 to 5.0) and may not be compatible with alkaline solutions having a pH greater than 8.5 (e.g., barbiturate solutions).

Multiple-dose vials of MIVACRON contain benzyl alcohol. In newborn infants, benzyl alcohol has been associated with an increased incidence of neurological and other complications which are sometimes fatal. Single-use vials and MIVACRON Premixed Infusion do not contain benzyl alcohol (see PRECAUTIONS: Pediatric Use).

PRECAUTIONS

General: Although MIVACRON (a mixture of three stereoisomers) is not a potent histamine releaser, the possibility of substantial histamine release must be considered. Release of histamine is related to the dose and speed of injection.

Caution should be exercised in administering MIVACRON to patients with clinically significant cardiovascular disease and patients with any history suggesting a greater sensitivity to the release of histamine or related mediators (e.g., asthma). In such patients, the initial dose of MIVACRON should be 0.15 mg/kg or less, administered over 60 seconds; assurance of adequate hydration and careful monitoring of hemodynamic status are important (see CLINICAL PHARMACOLOGY: Hemodynamics and Individualization of Dosages).

Obese patients may be more likely to experience clinically significant transient decreases in MAP than non-obese patients when the dose of MIVACRON is based on actual rather than ideal body weight. Therefore, in obese patients, the initial dose should be determined using the patient's ideal body weight (see CLINICAL PHARMACOLOGY: Hemodynamics and Individualization of Dosages).

Recommended doses of MIVACRON have no clinically significant effects on heart rate; therefore, MIVACRON will not counteract the bradycardia produced by many anesthetic agents or by vagal stimulation.

Neuromuscular blocking agents may have a profound effect in patients with neuromuscular diseases (e.g., myasthenia gravis and the myasthenic syndrome). In these and other conditions in which prolonged neuromuscular block is a possibility (e.g., carcinomatosis), the use of a peripheral nerve stimulator and a dose of not more than 0.015 to 0.020 mg/kg MIVACRON is recommended to assess the level of neuromuscular block and to monitor dosage requirements (see CLINICAL PHARMACOLOGY: Individualization of Dosages).

MIVACRON has not been studied in patients with burns. Resistance to nondepolarizing neuromuscular blocking agents may develop in patients with burns, depending upon the time elapsed since the injury and the size of the burn. Patients with burns may have reduced plasma cholinesterase activity which may offset this resistance (see CLINICAL PHARMACOLOGY: Individualization of Dosages).

Acid-base and/or serum electrolyte abnormalities may potentiate or antagonize the action of neuromuscular blocking agents. The action of neuromuscular blocking agents may be enhanced by magnesium salts administered for the management of toxemia of pregnancy (see CLINICAL PHARMACOLOGY: Individualization of Dosages).

No data are available to support the use of MIVACRON by intramuscular injection.

Renal and Hepatic Disease: The possibility of prolonged neuromuscular block must be considered when MIVACRON is used in patients with renal or hepatic disease (see CLINICAL PHARMACOLOGY: Pharmacokinetics). Most patients with chronic hepatic disease such as hepatitis, liver abscess, and cirrhosis of the liver exhibit a marked reduction in plasma cholinesterase activity. Patients with acute or chronic renal disease may also show a reduction in plasma cholinesterase activity (see CLINICAL PHARMACOLOGY: Individualization of Dosages).

Reduced Plasma Cholinesterase Activity: The possibility of prolonged neuromuscular block following administration of MIVACRON must be considered in patients with reduced plasma cholinesterase (pseudocholinesterase) activity.

Plasma cholinesterase activity may be diminished in the presence of genetic abnormalities of plasma cholinesterase (e.g., patients heterozygous or homozygous for the atypical plasma cholinesterase gene), pregnancy, liver or kidney disease, malignant tumors, infections, burns, anemia, decompensated heart disease, peptic ulcer, or myxedema. Plasma cholinesterase activity may also be diminished by chronic administration of oral contraceptives, glucocorticoids, or certain monoamine oxidase inhibitors and by irreversible inhibitors of plasma cholinesterase (e.g., organophosphate insecticides, echothiophate, and certain antineoplastic drugs).

MIVACRON has been used safely in patients heterozygous for the atypical plasma cholinesterase gene. At doses of 0.10 to 0.20 mg/kg MIVACRON, the clinically effective duration of action was 8 to 11 minutes longer in patients heterozygous for the atypical gene than in genotypically normal patients.

As with succinylcholine, patients homozygous for the atypical plasma cholinesterase gene (one in 2500 patients) are extremely sensitive to the neuromuscular blocking effect of MIVACRON. In three such adult patients, a small dose of 0.03 mg/kg (approximately the ED_{10-20} in genotypically normal patients) produced complete neuromuscular block for 26 to 128 minutes. Once spontaneous recovery had begun, neuromuscular block in these patients was antagonized with conventional doses of neostigmine. One adult patient, who was homozygous for the atypical plasma cholinesterase gene, received a dose of 0.18 mg/kg MIVACRON and exhibited complete neuromuscular block for about 4 hours. Response to post-tetanic stimulation was present after 4 hours, all four responses to train-of-four stimulation were present after 6 hours, and the patient was extubated after 8 hours. Reversal was not attempted in this patient.

Malignant Hyperthermia (MH): In a study of MH-susceptible pigs, MIVACRON did not trigger MH. MIVACRON has not been studied in MH-susceptible patients. Because MH can develop in the absence of established triggering agents, the clinician should be prepared to recognize and treat MH in any patient undergoing general anethesia.

Long-Term Use in the Intensive Care Unit (ICU): No data are available on the long-term use of MIVACRON in patients undergoing mechanical ventilation in the ICU.

Drug Interactions: Although MIVACRON (a mixture of three stereoisomers) has been administered safely following succinylcholine-facilitated tracheal intubation, the interaction between the stereoisomers in MIVACRON and succinylcholine has not been systematically studied. Prior administration of succinylcholine can potentiate the neuromuscular blocking effects of nondepolarizing agents. Evidence of spontaneous recovery from succinylcholine should be observed before the administration of MIVACRON.

The use of MIVACRON before succinylcholine to attenuate some of the side effects of succinylcholine has not been studied.

There are no clinical data on the use of MIVACRON with other nondepolarizing neuromuscular blocking agents.

Isoflurane and enflurane (administered with nitrous oxide/oxygen to achieve 1.25 MAC) decrease the ED_{50} of MIVACRON by as much as 25% (see CLINICAL PHARMACOLOGY: Pharmacodynamics and Individualization of Dosages). These agents may also prolong the clinically effective duration of action and decrease the average infusion requirement of MIVACRON by as much as 35% to 40%. A greater potentiation of the neuromuscular blocking effects of the stereoisomers in MIVACRON may be expected with higher concentrations of enflurane or isoflurane. Halothane has little or no effect on the ED_{50}, but may prolong the duration of action and decrease the average infusion requirement by as much as 20%.

Other drugs which may enhance the neuromuscular blocking action of nondepolarizing agents such as the stereoisomers in MIVACRON include certain antibiotics (e.g., aminoglycosides, tetracyclines, bacitracin, polymyxins, lincomycin, clindamycin, colistin, and sodium colistimethate), magnesium salts, lithium, local anesthetics, procainamide,

Continued on next page

Table 5: Pharmacodynamic Parameters* of MIVACRON in ASA Physical Status I–II Patients and in Patients Undergoing Kidney or Liver Transplantation During Isoflurane/Nitrous Oxide/Oxygen Anesthesia

Parameter	Young Adult Patients	Kidney Transplant Patients	Liver Transplant Patients ‡
Initial Dose	0.15 mg/kg [n=8]	0.15 mg/kg [n=9]	0.15 mg/kg [n=8]
Maximum Block (%)	99.8 (98-100)	100 (100-100)	100 (100-100)
Time to Maximum Block (min)	1.9 (0.8-3.5)	2.6 (1.0-4.5)	2.1 (1.0-4.0)
Clinically Effective Duration of Block† (min)	19 (12-30)	30 (19-58)	57 (29-80)

* Values shown are mean (range).
† Time from injection to 25% recovery of the control twitch height.
‡ Liver transplant patients received isoflurane without nitrous oxide.

This product information is based on labeling in effect on June 1, 1998. For further information, contact via direct mail, phone, or web site Medical Information: Glaxo Wellcome Inc., PO Box 13398, Research Triangle Park, NC 27709. Healthcare Professionals (Medical Information): 800-334-0089 Patients (Customer Response Center): 888-TALK2GW (1-888-825-5249) Glaxo Wellcome Corporate Web Site: www.glaxowellcome.com

Mivacron—Cont.

and quinidine. The neuromuscular blocking effect of MIVACRON may be enhanced by drugs that reduce plasma cholinesterase activity (e.g., chronically administered oral contraceptives, glucocorticoids, or certain monoamine oxidase inhibitors) or by drugs that irreversibly inhibit plasma cholinesterase (see PRECAUTIONS: Reduced Plasma Cholinesterase Activity subsection).

Resistance to the neuromuscular blocking action of nondepolarizing neuromuscular blocking agents has been demonstrated in patients chronically administered phenytoin or carbamazepine. While the effects of chronic phenytoin or carbamazepine therapy on the action of the stereoisomers in MIVACRON are unknown, slightly shorter durations of neuromuscular block may be anticipated and infusion rate requirements may be higher.

Carcinogenesis, Mutagenesis, Impairment of Fertility: Carcinogenesis and fertility studies have not been performed. MIVACRON was evaluated in a battery of four short-term mutagenicity tests. It was non-mutagenic in the Ames Salmonella assay, the mouse lymphoma assay, the human lymphocyte assay, and the in vivo rat bone marrow cytogenetic assay.

Pregnancy: ***Teratogenic Effects:*** Pregnancy Category C. Teratology testing in nonventilated pregnant rats and mice treated subcutaneously with maximum subparalyzing doses of MIVACRON revealed no maternal or fetal toxicity or teratogenic effects. There are no adequate and well-controlled studies of MIVACRON in pregnant women. Because animal studies are not always predictive of human response, and the doses used were subparalyzing, MIVACRON should be used during pregnancy only if the potential benefit justifies the potential risk to the fetus.

Labor and Delivery: The use of MIVACRON during labor, vaginal delivery, or cesarean section has not been studied in humans and it is not known whether MIVACRON administered to the mother has effects on the fetus. Doses of 0.08 and 0.20 mg/kg MIVACRON given to female beagles undergoing cesarean section resulted in negligible levels of the stereoisomers in MIVACRON in umbilical vessel blood of neonates and no deleterious effects on the puppies.

Nursing Mothers: It is not known whether any of the stereoisomers of mivacurium are excreted in human milk. Because many drugs are excreted in human milk, caution should be exercised following administration of MIVACRON to a nursing woman.

Pediatric Use: MIVACRON has not been studied in pediatric patients below the age of 2 years (see CLINICAL PHARMACOLOGY and DOSAGE AND ADMINISTRATION for clinical experience and recommendations for use in children 2 to 12 years of age).

Geriatric Use: MIVACRON was safely administered during clinical trials to 64 elderly (≥65 years) patients, including 31 patients with significant cardiovascular disease (see PRECAUTIONS: General subsection). The duration of neuromuscular block may be slightly longer in elderly patients than in young adult patients (see CLINICAL PHARMACOLOGY).

ADVERSE REACTIONS

Observed in Clinical Trials: MIVACRON (a mixture of three stereoisomers) was well tolerated during extensive clinical trials in inpatients and outpatients. Prolonged neuromuscular block, which is an important adverse experience associated with neuromuscular blocking agents as a class, was reported as an adverse experience in three of 2074 patients administered MIVACRON. The most commonly reported adverse experience following the administration of MIVACRON was transient, dose-dependent cutaneous flushing about the face, neck, and/or chest. Flushing was most frequently noted after the initial dose of MIVACRON and was reported in about 25% of adult patients who received 0.15 mg/kg MIVACRON over 5 to 15 seconds. When present, flushing typically began within 1 to 2 minutes after the dose of MIVACRON and lasted for 3 to 5 minutes. Of 105 patients who experienced flushing after 0.15 mg/kg MIVACRON, two patients also experienced mild hypotension that was not treated, and one patient experienced moderate wheezing that was successfully treated.

Overall, hypotension was infrequently reported as an adverse experience in the clinical trials of MIVACRON. One of 332 (0.3%) healthy adults who received 0.15 mg/kg MIVACRON over 5 to 15 seconds and none of 37 cardiac surgery patients who received 0.15 mg/kg MIVACRON over 60 seconds was treated for a decrease in blood pressure in association with the administration of MIVACRON. One to two percent of healthy adults given ≥0.20 mg/kg MIVACRON over 5 to 15 seconds, 2% to 3% of healthy adults given 0.20 mg/kg over 30 seconds, none of 100 healthy adults given 0.25 mg/kg as a divided dose (0.15 mg/kg followed in 30 seconds by 0.10 mg/kg), and 2% to 4% of cardiac surgery patients given ≥0.20 mg/kg over 60 seconds were treated for a decrease in blood pressure. None of the 63 children who received the recommended dose of 0.20 mg/kg MIVACRON was treated for a decrease in blood pressure in association with the administration of MIVACRON.

The following adverse experiences were reported in patients administered MIVACRON (all events judged by investigators during the clinical trials to have a possible causal relationship):

Incidence Greater Than 1%—

Cardiovascular:	Flushing (16%)

Incidence Less Than 1%—

Cardiovascular:	Hypotension, tachycardia, Bradycardia, cardiac Arrhythmia, phlebitis
Respiratory:	Bronchospasm, wheezing, Hypoxemia
Dermatological:	Rash, urticaria, erythema, Injection site reaction
Nonspecific:	Prolonged drug effect
Neurologic:	Dizziness
Musculoskeletal:	Muscle spasms

Observed in Clinical Practice: Based on initial clinical practice experience in patients who received MIVACRON, spontaneously reported adverse events are uncommon. Some of these events occurred at recommended doses and required treatment. There are insufficient data to establish a causal relationship or to support an estimate of their incidence. Adverse events reported during clinical practice include:

General:	Allergic reactions which, in rare instances, were severe
Musculoskeletal:	Diminished drug effect, Prolonged drug effect
Cardiovascular:	Hypotension (rarely severe), flushing
Respiratory:	Bronchospasm
Integumentary:	Rash

OVERDOSAGE

Overdosage with neuromuscular blocking agents may result in neuromuscular block beyond the time needed for surgery and anesthesia. The primary treatment is maintenance of a patent airway and controlled ventilation until recovery of normal neuromuscular function is assured. Once evidence of recovery from neuromuscular block is observed, further recovery may be facilitated by administration of an anticholinesterase agent (e.g., neostigmine, edrophonium) in conjunction with an appropriate anticholinergic agent (see Antagonism of Neuromuscular Block subsection below). Overdosage may increase the risk of hemodynamic side effects, especially decreases in blood pressure. If needed, cardiovascular support may be provided by proper positioning of the patient, fluid administration, and/or vasopressor agent administration.

Antagonism of Neuromuscular Block: ANTAGONISTS (SUCH AS NEOSTIGMINE) SHOULD NOT BE ADMINISTERED WHEN COMPLETE NEUROMUSCULAR BLOCK IS EVIDENT OR SUSPECTED. THE USE OF A PERIPHERAL NERVE STIMULATOR TO EVALUATE RECOVERY AND ANTAGONISM OF NEUROMUSCULAR BLOCK IS RECOMMENDED.

Administration of 0.030 to 0.064 mg/kg neostigmine or 0.5 mg/kg edrophonium at approximately 10% recovery from neuromuscular block (range: 1 to 15) produced 95% recovery of the muscle twitch response and a T_4/T_1 ratio ≥75% in about 10 minutes. The times from 25% recovery of the muscle twitch response to T_4/T_1 ratio ≥75% following these doses of antagonists averaged about 7 to 9 minutes. In comparison, average times for spontaneous recovery from 25% to T_4/T_1 ≥75% were 12 to 13 minutes.

Patients administered antagonists should be evaluated for adequate clinical evidence of antagonism, e.g., 5-second head lift and grip strength. Ventilation must be supported until no longer required.

Antagonism may be delayed in the presence of debilitation, carcinomatosis, and the concomitant use of certain broad-spectrum antibiotics, or anesthetic agents and other drugs which enhance neuromuscular block or separately cause respiratory depression (see PRECAUTIONS: Drug Interactions). Under such circumstances the management is the same as that of prolonged neuromuscular block (see OVERDOSAGE).

DOSAGE AND ADMINISTRATION

MIVACRON SHOULD ONLY BE ADMINISTERED INTRAVENOUSLY.

The dosage information provided below is intended as a guide only. Doses of MIVACRON should be individualized (see CLINICAL PHARMACOLOGY: Individualization of Dosages). Factors that may warrant dosage adjustment include but may not be limited to: the presence of significant kidney, liver, or cardiovascular disease, obesity (patients weighing ≥30% more than ideal body weight for height), asthma, reduction in plasma cholinesterase activity, and the presence of inhalational anesthetic agents.

When using MIVACRON or other neuromuscular blocking agents to facilitate tracheal intubation, it is important to recognize that the most important factors affecting intubation are the depth of general anesthesia and the level of neuromuscular block. Satisfactory intubating conditions can usually be achieved before complete neuromuscular block is attained if there is adequate anesthesia.

The use of a peripheral nerve stimulator will permit the most advantageous use of MIVACRON, minimize the possibility of overdosage or underdosage, and assist in the evaluation of recovery. When using a stimulator to monitor onset of neuromuscular block, clinical studies have shown that all four twitches of the train-of-four response may be present, with little or no fade, at the times recommended for intubation. Therefore, as with other neuromuscular blocking agents, it is important to use other criteria, such as clinical evaluation of the status of relaxation of jaw muscles and vocal cords, in conjunction with peripheral muscle twitch monitoring, to guide the appropriate time of intubation.

The onset of conditions suitable for tracheal intubation occurs earlier after a conventional intubating dose of succinylcholine than after recommended doses of MIVACRON.

Adults: ***Initial Doses:*** Doses of 0.15 mg/kg administered over 5 to 15 seconds, 0.20 mg/kg administered over 30 seconds, or 0.25 mg/kg administered in divided doses (0.15 mg/kg followed in 30 seconds by 0.10 mg/kg) are recommended for facilitation of tracheal intubation for most patients (see Table 6).

[See table 6 below]

The purpose of slowed or divided dosing of MIVACRON at doses above 0.15 mg/kg is to minimize the transient decreases in blood pressure observed in some patients given these doses over 5 to 15 seconds (see CLINICAL PHARMACOLOGY, PRECAUTIONS, and ADVERSE REACTIONS). The quality of intubation conditions does not significantly differ for the times and doses of MIVACRON recommended in Table 6, but the onset of suitable intubation conditions may be reached earlier with higher doses. The choice of a particular dose and regimen should be based on individual circumstances and patient requirements (see CLINICAL PHARMACOLOGY: Individualization of Dosages).

In patients with clinically significant cardiovascular disease and in patients with any history suggesting a greater sensitivity to the release of histamine or other mediators (e.g., asthma), the dose of MIVACRON should be 0.15 mg/kg or less, administered over 60 seconds (see PRECAUTIONS). No data are available on the use of doses of MIVACRON above 0.15 mg/kg in patients with clinically significant kidney or liver disease.

Clinically effective neuromuscular block may be expected to last for 15 to 20 minutes (range: 9 to 38) and spontaneous recovery may be expected to be 95% complete in 25 to 30 minutes (range: 16 to 41) following 0.15 mg/kg MIVACRON administered to patients receiving opioid/nitrous oxide/oxygen anesthesia. The expected duration of clinically effective block and time to 95% spontaneous recovery following 0.20 mg/kg MIVACRON are approximately 20 and 30 minutes, respectively, and following 0.25 mg/kg MIVACRON are approximately 25 and 35 minutes. Initiation of maintenance dosing during opioid/nitrous oxide/oxygen anesthesia is generally required approximately 15, 20, and 25 minutes following initial doses of 0.15, 0.20, and 0.25 mg/kg MIVACRON, respectively (see Table 1). Maintenance doses of 0.10 mg/kg each provide approximately 15 minutes of ad-

Table 6: Recommended Initial Dosing Regimens for Adults

Dosing Paradigm*	Anesthetic Induction Technique Studied	Time to Generally Good-to-Excellent Intubating Conditions
0.15 mg/kg, IV (over 5 to 15 sec)	Thiopental/opioid/N_2O/O_2 or propofol/opioid	2.5 to 3 min after completion of dose
0.20 mg/kg, IV (over 30 sec)	Thiopental/opioid/N_2O/O_2 or propofol/opioid	2 to 2.5 min after completion of dose
0.25 mg/kg, IV (0.15 mg/kg followed in 30 sec by 0.10 mg/kg)	Propofol/opioid	1.5 to 2 min after completion of 0.15-mg/kg dose

* Dosing instituted after induction of adequate general anesthesia.

Table 8: Infusion Rates for Maintenance of Neuromuscular Block During Opioid/Nitrous Oxide/Oxygen Anesthesia Using MIVACRON Injection (2 mg/mL)

Patient Weight (kg)	Drug Delivery Rate (mcg/kg per minute)									
	4	5	6	7	8	10	14	16	18	20
	Infusion Delivery Rate (mL/hr)									
10	1.2	1.5	1.8	2.1	2.4	3.0	4.2	4.8	5.4	6.0
15	1.8	2.3	2.7	3.2	3.6	4.5	6.3	7.2	8.1	9.0
20	2.4	3.0	3.6	4.2	4.8	6.0	8.4	9.6	10.8	12.0
25	3.0	3.8	4.5	5.3	6.0	7.5	10.5	12.0	13.5	15.0
35	4.2	5.3	6.3	7.4	8.4	10.5	14.7	16.8	18.9	21.0
50	6.0	7.5	9.0	10.5	12.0	15.0	21.0	24.0	27.0	30.0
60	7.2	9.0	10.8	12.6	14.4	18.0	25.2	28.8	32.4	36.0
70	8.4	10.5	12.6	14.7	16.8	21.0	29.4	33.6	37.8	42.0
80	9.6	12.0	14.4	16.8	19.2	24.0	33.6	38.4	43.2	48.0
90	10.8	13.5	16.2	18.9	21.6	27.0	37.8	43.2	48.6	54.0
100	12.0	15.0	18.0	21.0	24.0	30.0	42.0	48.0	54.0	60.0

ditional clinically effective block. For shorter or longer durations of action, smaller or larger maintenance doses may be administered.

The neuromuscular blocking action of MIVACRON is potentiated by isoflurane or enflurane anesthesia. Recommended initial doses of MIVACRON may be used to facilitate tracheal intubation prior to the administration of these agents; however, if MIVACRON is first administered after establishment of stable-state isoflurane or enflurane anesthesia (administered with nitrous oxide/oxygen to achieve 1.25 MAC), the initial dose of MIVACRON may be reduced by as much as 25%. Greater reductions in the dose of MIVACRON may be required with higher concentrations of enflurane or isoflurane. With halothane, which has only a minimal potentiating effect on MIVACRON, a smaller dosage reduction may be considered.

Continuous Infusion: Continuous infusion of MIVACRON may be used to maintain neuromuscular block. Upon early evidence of spontaneous recovery from an initial dose, an initial infusion rate of 9 to 10 mcg/kg per minute is recommended. If continuous infusion is initiated simultaneously with the administration of an initial dose, a lower initial infusion rate should be used (e.g., 4 mcg/kg per minute). In either case, the initial infusion rate should be adjusted according to the response to peripheral nerve stimulation and to clinical criteria. On average, an infusion rate of 6 to 7 mcg/kg per minute (range: 1 to 15) may be expected to maintain neuromuscular block within the range of 89% to 99% for extended periods in adults receiving opioid/nitrous oxide/oxygen anesthesia. Reduction of the infusion rate by up to 35% to 40% should be considered when MIVACRON is administered during stable-state conditions of isoflurane or enflurane anesthesia (administered with nitrous oxide/oxygen to achieve 1.25 MAC). Greater reductions in the infusion rate of MIVACRON may be required with greater concentrations of enflurane or isoflurane. With halothane, smaller reductions in infusion rate may be required.

Children: Initial Doses: Dosage requirements for MIVACRON on a mg/kg basis are higher in children than in adults. Onset and recovery of neuromuscular block occur more rapidly in children than in adults (see CLINICAL PHARMACOLOGY).

The recommended dose of MIVACRON for facilitating tracheal intubation in children 2 to 12 years of age is 0.20 mg/kg administered over 5 to 15 seconds. When administered during stable opioid/nitrous oxide/oxygen anesthesia, 0.20 mg/kg of MIVACRON produces maximum neuromuscular block in an average of 1.9 minutes (range: 1.3 to 3.3) and clinically effective block for 10 minutes (range: 6 to 15). Maintenance doses are generally required more frequently in children than in adults. Administration of doses of MIVACRON above the recommended range (>0.20 mg/kg) is associated with transient decreases in MAP in some children (see CLINICAL PHARMACOLOGY: Hemodynamics). MIVACRON has not been studied in pediatric patients below the age of 2 years.

Continuous Infusion: Children require higher infusion rates of MIVACRON than adults. During opioid/nitrous oxide/oxygen anesthesia the infusion rate required to maintain 89% to 99% neuromuscular block averages 14 mcg/kg per minute (range: 5 to 31). The principles for infusion of MIVACRON in adults are also applicable to children (see above).

Infusion Rate Tables: For adults and children, the amount of infusion solution required per hour depends upon the clinical requirements of the patient, the concentration of MIVACRON in the infusion solution, and the patient's weight. The contribution of the infusion solution to the fluid requirements of the patient must be considered. Tables 7 and 8 provide guidelines for delivery in mL/hr (equivalent to microdrops/min when 60 microdrops/min = 1 mL) of MIVACRON Premixed Infusion (0.5 mg/mL) and of MIVACRON Injection (2 mg/mL).

Table 7: Infusion Rates for Maintenance of Neuromuscular Block During Opioid/Nitrous Oxide/Oxygen Anesthesia Using MIVACRON Premixed Infusion (0.5 mg/mL)

Patient Weight (kg)	Drug Delivery Rate (mcg/kg per minute)								
	4	5	6	7	8	10	14	16	18	20
	Infusion Delivery Rate (mL/hr)								
10	5	6	7	8	10	12	17	19	22	24
15	7	9	11	13	14	18	25	29	32	36
20	10	12	15	17	19	24	34	38	43	48
25	12	15	18	21	24	30	42	48	54	60
35	17	21	26	29	34	42	59	67	76	84
50	24	30	36	42	48	60	84	96	108	120
60	29	36	43	50	58	72	101	115	130	144
70	34	42	50	59	67	84	118	134	151	168
80	39	48	58	67	77	96	134	154	173	192
90	44	54	65	76	86	108	151	173	194	216
100	48	60	72	84	96	120	168	192	216	240

[See table 8 above]

MIVACRON Premixed Infusion in Flexible Plastic Containers:
The flexible plastic container is fabricated from a specially formulated, nonplasticized, thermoplastic co-polyester (CR3). Water can permeate from inside the container into the overwrap but not in amounts sufficient to affect the solution significantly. Solutions inside the plastic container also can leach out certain of the chemical components in very small amounts before the expiration period is attained. However, the safety of the plastic has been confirmed by tests in animals according to USP biological standards for plastic containers.

Instructions for Use:
1. Tear outer wrap at notch and remove solution container. Check for minute leaks by squeezing container firmly. If leaks are found, discard solution as sterility may be impaired.
2. Close flow control clamp of administration set.
3. Remove cover from outlet port at bottom of container.
4. Insert piercing pin of administration set into port with a twisting motion until the pin is firmly seated. NOTE: See full directions on administration set carton.
5. Suspend container from hanger.
6. Squeeze and release drip chamber to establish proper fluid level in chamber during infusion.
7. Open flow control clamp to expel air from set. Close clamp.
8. Attach set to intravenous tubing.
9. Regulate rate of administration with flow control clamp.
Caution: Additives should not be introduced into this solution. Do not administer unless solution is clear and container is undamaged. MIVACRON Premixed Infusion is intended for single patient use only. The unused portion of the solution should be discarded.
Warning: Do not use flexible plastic container in series connections.
MIVACRON Injection Compatibility and Admixtures:
Y-Site Administration: MIVACRON Injection may not be compatible with alkaline solutions having a pH greater than 8.5 (e.g., barbiturate solutions).
Studies have shown that MIVACRON Injection is compatible with:
- 5% Dextrose Injection, USP
- 0.9% Sodium Chloride Injection, USP
- 5% Dextrose and 0.9% Sodium Chloride Injection, USP

- Lactated Ringer's Injection, USP
- 5% Dextrose in Lactated Ringer's Injection
- SUFENTA® (sufentanil citrate) Injection, diluted as directed
- ALFENTA® (alfentanil hydrochloride) Injection, diluted as directed
- SUBLIMAZE® (fentanyl citrate) Injection, diluted as directed
- VERSED® (midazolam hydrochloride) Injection, diluted as directed
- INAPSINE® (droperidol) Injection, diluted as directed
Compatibility studies with other parenteral products have not been conducted.

Dilution Stability: MIVACRON Injection diluted to 0.5 mg mivacurium per mL in 5% Dextrose Injection, USP; 5% Dextrose and 0.9% Sodium Chloride Injection, USP; 0.9% Sodium Chloride Injection, USP; Lactated Ringer's Injection, USP; or 5% Dextrose in Lactated Ringer's Injection is physically and chemically stable when stored in PVC (polyvinyl chloride) bags at 5° to 25°C (41° to 77°F) for up to 24 hours. Aseptic techniques should be used to prepare the diluted product. Admixtures of MIVACRON should be prepared for single patient use only and used within 24 hours of preparation. The unused portion of diluted MIVACRON should be discarded after each case.
NOTE: Parenteral drug products should be inspected visually for particulate matter and discoloration prior to administration whenever solution and container permit. Solutions which are not clear and colorless should not be used.

HOW SUPPLIED: MIVACRON Injection, 2 mg mivacurium in each mL.

5-mL Single-Use Vials. Tray of 10 (NDC 0173-0705-44).
10-mL Single-Use Vials. Tray of 10 (NDC 0173-0705-95).
20-mL Multiple-Dose Vials containing 0.9% w/v benzyl alcohol as a preservative (see WARNINGS concerning newborn infants). Tray of 10 (NDC 0173-0542-00).
50-mL Multiple-Dose Vials containing 0.9% w/v benzyl alcohol as a preservative (see WARNINGS concerning newborn infants). Tray of 3 (NDC 0173-0538-00).
MIVACRON Premixed Infusion in 5% Dextrose Injection USP, 0.5 mg mivacurium in each mL.
50 mL (in a 100 mL unit) Flexible Plastic Containers (NDC 0173-0709-01).
100 mL (in a 100 mL unit) Flexible Plastic Containers (NDC 0173-0709-02).

STORAGE: Store MIVACRON Injection at room temperature of 15° to 25°C (59° to 77°F). Avoid exposure to direct ultraviolet light. DO NOT FREEZE.

Recommended storage for MIVACRON Premixed Infusion is room temperature (15° to 25°C/59° to 77°F). Avoid excessive heat. Avoid exposure to direct ultraviolet light. Protect from freezing.
U.S. Patent No. 4,761,418
©Copyright 1996 Glaxo Wellcome Inc. All rights reserved.
October 1997/RL-469
Shown in Product Identification Guide, page 313

MYLERAN®   ℞
[mĭ 'lə-răn "]
(busulfan)
2 mg Scored Tablets

> **WARNING**
> MYLERAN is a potent drug. It should not be used unless a diagnosis of chronic myelogenous leukemia has been adequately established and the responsible physician is knowledgeable in assessing response to chemotherapy. MYLERAN can induce severe bone marrow hypoplasia. Reduce or discontinue the dosage immediately at the first sign of any unusual depression of bone marrow function as reflected by an abnormal decrease in any of the formed elements of the blood. A bone marrow examination should be performed if the bone marrow status is uncertain.

Continued on next page

This product information is based on labeling in effect on June 1, 1998. For further information, contact via direct mail, phone, or web site Medical Information: Glaxo Wellcome Inc., PO Box 13398, Research Triangle Park, NC 27709. Healthcare Professionals (Medical Information): 800-334-0089 Patients (Customer Response Center): 888-TALK2GW (1-888-825-5249) Glaxo Wellcome Corporate Web Site: www.glaxowellcome.com

Myleran—Cont.

SEE WARNINGS FOR INFORMATION REGARDING BUSULFAN-INDUCED LEUKEMOGENESIS IN HUMANS.

DESCRIPTION

MYLERAN (busulfan) is a bifunctional alkylating agent. Busulfan is known chemically as 1,4-butanediol dimethanesulfonate.

Busulfan is *not* a structural analog of the nitrogen mustards. MYLERAN is available in tablet form for oral administration. Each scored tablet contains 2 mg busulfan and the inactive ingredients magnesium stearate and sodium chloride.

The activity of busulfan in chronic myelogenous leukemia was first reported by D.A.G. Galton in 1953.[1]

CLINICAL PHARMACOLOGY

No analytical method has been found which permits the quantitation of non-radiolabeled busulfan or its metabolites in biological tissues or plasma. All studies of the pharmacokinetics of busulfan in humans have employed radiolabeled drug using either sulfur-35 (labeling the "carrier" portion of the molecule) or carbon-14 or tritium in the alkane portion of the 4-carbon chain (labels in the "alkylating" portion of the molecule).

Studies with ^{35}S-busulfan:[2] Following the intravenous administration of a single therapeutic dose of ^{35}S-busulfan, there was rapid disappearance of radioactivity from the blood; 90% to 95% of the ^{35}S-label disappeared within 3 to 5 minutes after injection. Thereafter, a constant, low level of radioactivity (1% to 3% of the injected dose) was maintained during the subsequent 48-hour period of observation. Following the oral administration of ^{35}S-busulfan, there was a lag period of $^{1}/_{2}$ to 2 hours prior to the detection of radioactivity in the blood. However, at 4 hours the (low) level of circulating radioactivity was comparable to that obtained following intravenous administration.

After either oral or intravenous administration of ^{35}S-busulfan to humans, 45% to 60% of the radioactivity was recovered in the urine in the 48 hours after administration; the majority of the total urinary excretion occurred in the first 24 hours. In humans, over 95% of the urinary sulfur-35 occurs as ^{35}S-methanesulfonic acid.

The fact that urinary recovery of sulfur-35 was equivalent, irrespective of whether the drug was given intravenously or orally, suggests virtually complete absorption by the oral route.

Studies with ^{14}C-busulfan:[2] Oral and intravenous administration of 1,4-^{14}C-busulfan showed the same rapid initial disappearance of plasma radioactivity with a subsequent low-level plateau as observed following the administration of ^{35}S-labeled drug. Cumulative radioactivity in the urine after 48 hours was 25% to 30% of the administered dose (contrasting with 45% to 60% for ^{35}S-busulfan) and suggests a slower excretion of the alkylating portion of the molecule and its metabolites than for the sulfonoxymethyl moieties. Regardless of the route of administration, 1,4-^{14}C-busulfan yielded a complex mixture of at least 12 radiolabeled metabolites in urine; the main metabolite being 3-hydroxytetrahydrothiophene-1, 1-dioxide.

Studies with ^{3}H-busulfan:[3] Human pharmacokinetic studies have been conducted employing busulfan labeled with tritium on the tetramethylene chain. These experiments confirmed a rapid initial clearance of the radioactivity from plasma, irrespective of whether the drug was given orally or intravenously, and showed a gradual accumulation of radioactivity in the plasma after repeated doses. Urinary excretion of less than 50% of the total dose given suggested a slow elimination of the metabolic products from the body. There is no experience with the use of dialysis in an attempt to modify the clinical toxicity of busulfan. One technical difficulty would derive from the extremely poor water solubility of busulfan. Additionally, all studies of the metabolism of busulfan employing radiolabeled materials indicate rapid chemical reactivity of the parent compound with prolonged retention of some of the metabolites (particularly the metabolites arising from the "alkylating" portion of the molecule). The effectiveness of dialysis at removing significant quantities of unreacted drug would be expected to be minimal in such a situation.

No information is available regarding the penetration of busulfan into brain or cerebrospinal fluid.

Biochemical Pharmacology: In aqueous media, busulfan undergoes a wide range of nucleophilic substitution reactions. While this chemical reactivity is relatively non-specific, alkylation of the DNA is felt to be an important biological mechanism for its cytotoxic effect.[4] Coliphage T7 exposed to busulfan was found to have the DNA crosslinked by intrastrand crosslinkages, but no interstrand linkages were found.

The metabolic fate of busulfan has been studied in rats and humans using ^{14}C- and ^{35}S-labeled materials.[2,5,6] In humans,[2] as in the rat,[6] almost all of the radioactivity in ^{35}S-

labeled busulfan is excreted in the urine in the form of ^{35}S-methanesulfonic acid. No unchanged drug was found in human urine,[2] although a small amount has been reported in rat urine.[6] Roberts and Warwick demonstrated that the formation of methanesulfonic acid in vivo in the rat is not due to a simple hydrolysis of busulfan to 1,4-butanediol, since only about 4% of 2,3-^{14}C-busulfan was excreted as carbon dioxide whereas 2,3-^{14}C-1,4-butanediol was converted almost exclusively to carbon dioxide.[5] The predominant reaction of busulfan in the rat is the alkylation of sulfhydryl groups (particularly cysteine and cysteine-containing compounds) to produce a cyclic sulfonium compound which is the precursor of the major urinary metabolite of the 4-carbon portion of the molecule, 3-hydroxytetrahydrothiophene-1, 1-dioxide.[5] This has been termed a "sulfur-stripping" action of busulfan and it may modify the function of certain sulfur-containing amino acids, polypeptides, and proteins; whether this action makes an important contribution to the cytotoxicity of busulfan is unknown.

The biochemical basis for acquired resistance to busulfan is largely a matter of speculation. Although altered transport of busulfan into the cell is one possibility, increased intracellular inactivation of the drug before it reaches the DNA is also possible. Experiments with other alkylating agents have shown that resistance to this class of compounds may reflect an acquired ability of the resistant cell to repair alkylation damage more effectively.[4]

INDICATIONS AND USAGE

MYLERAN (busulfan) is indicated for the palliative treatment of chronic myelogenous (myeloid, myelocytic, granulocytic) leukemia. Although not curative, busulfan reduces the total granulocyte mass, relieves symptoms of the disease, and improves the clinical state of the patient. Approximately 90% of adults with previously untreated chronic myelogenous leukemia will obtain hematologic remission with regression or stabilization of organomegaly following the use of busulfan. It has been shown to be superior to splenic irradiation with respect to survival times and maintenance of hemoglobin levels, and to be equivalent to irradiation at controlling splenomegaly.[7]

It is not clear whether busulfan unequivocally prolongs the survival of responding patients beyond the 31 months experienced by an untreated group of historical controls.[8] Median survival figures of 31 to 42 months have been reported for several groups of patients treated with busulfan, but concurrent control groups of comparable, untreated patients are not available.[7,9,10,11] The median survival figures reported from different studies will be influenced by the percentage of "poor risk" patients initially entered into the particular study. Patients who are alive 2 years following the diagnosis of chronic myelogenous leukemia, and who have been treated during that period with busulfan, are estimated to have a mean annual mortality rate during the second to fifth year which is approximately two-thirds that of patients who received either no treatment, conventional x-ray or ^{32}P-irradiation, or chemotherapy with minimally active drugs.[12]

Busulfan is clearly less effective in patients with chronic myelogenous leukemia who lack the Philadelphia (Ph[1]) chromosome.[13] Also, the so-called "juvenile" type of chronic myelogenous leukemia, typically occurring in young children and associated with the absence of a Philadelphia chromosome, responds poorly to busulfan.[14] The drug is of no benefit in patients whose chronic myelogenous leukemia has entered a "blastic" phase.

CONTRAINDICATIONS

MYLERAN should not be used unless a diagnosis of chronic myelogenous leukemia has been adequately established and the responsible physician is knowledgeable in assessing response to chemotherapy.

MYLERAN should not be used in patients whose chronic myelogenous leukemia has demonstrated prior resistance to this drug.

MYLERAN is of no value in chronic lymphocytic leukemia, acute leukemia, or in the "blastic crisis" of chronic myelogenous leukemia.

WARNINGS

The most frequent, serious side effect of treatment with busulfan is the induction of bone marrow failure (which may or may not be anatomically hypoplastic) resulting in severe pancytopenia. The pancytopenia caused by busulfan may be more prolonged than that induced with other alkylating agents. It is generally felt that the usual cause of busulfan-induced pancytopenia is the failure to stop administration of the drug soon enough; individual idiosyncrasy to the drug does not seem to be an important factor. *MYLERAN should be used with extreme caution and exceptional vigilance in patients whose bone marrow reserve may have been compromised by prior irradiation or chemotherapy, or whose marrow function is recovering from previous cytotoxic therapy.* Although recovery from busulfan-induced pancytopenia may take from 1 month to 2 years, this complication is potentially reversible, and the patient should be vigorously supported through any period of severe pancytopenia.[15]

A rare, important complication of busulfan therapy is the development of bronchopulmonary dysplasia with pulmonary fibrosis.[16] Symptoms have been reported to occur within 8 months to 10 years after initiation of therapy—the average duration of therapy being 4 years. The histologic findings associated with "busulfan lung" mimic those seen following pulmonary irradiation. Clinically, patients have reported the insidious onset of cough, dyspnea, and low-grade fever. Pulmonary function studies have revealed diminished diffusion capacity and decreased pulmonary compliance. It is important to exclude more common conditions (such as opportunistic infections or leukemic infiltration of the lungs) with appropriate diagnostic techniques. If measures such as sputum cultures, virologic studies, and exfoliative cytology fail to establish an etiology for the pulmonary infiltrates, lung biopsy may be necessary to establish the diagnosis. Treatment of established busulfan-induced pulmonary fibrosis is unsatisfactory; in most cases the patients have died within 6 months after the diagnosis was established. There is no specific therapy for this complication other than the immediate discontinuation of busulfan. The administration of corticosteroids has been suggested, but the results have not been impressive or uniformly successful.

Busulfan may cause cellular dysplasia in many organs in addition to the lung. Cytologic abnormalities characterized by giant, hyperchromatic nuclei have been reported in lymph nodes, pancreas, thyroid, adrenal glands, liver, and bone marrow. This cytologic dysplasia may be severe enough to cause difficulty in interpretation of exfoliative cytologic examinations from the lung, bladder, breast, and the uterine cervix.

In addition to the widespread epithelial dysplasia that has been observed during busulfan therapy, chromosome aberrations have been reported in cells from patients receiving busulfan.

Busulfan is mutagenic in mice and, possibly, in humans.

A number of malignant tumors have been reported in patients on busulfan therapy, and this drug may be a human carcinogen. Four cases of acute leukemia occurred among 243 patients treated with busulfan as adjuvant chemotherapy following surgical resection of bronchogenic carcinoma. All four cases were from a subgroup of 19 of these 243 patients who developed pancytopenia while taking busulfan 5 to 8 years before leukemia became clinically apparent. These findings suggest that busulfan is leukemogenic, although its mode of action is uncertain.[17]

Ovarian suppression and amenorrhea with menopausal symptoms commonly occur during busulfan therapy in premenopausal patients. Busulfan interferes with spermatogenesis in experimental animals, and there have been clinical reports of sterility, azoospermia, and testicular atrophy in male patients.

Hepatic veno-occlusive disease, which may be life-threatening, has been reported following the investigational use of very high doses of busulfan in combination with cyclophosphamide or other chemotherapeutic agents prior to bone marrow transplantation.[18-24] Possible risk factors for the development of hepatic veno-occlusive disease include: total busulfan dose exceeding 16 mg/kg based on ideal body weight, and concurrent use of multiple alkylating agents. A clear cause-and-effect relationship with busulfan has not been demonstrated. Periodic measurement of serum transaminases, alkaline phosphatase, and bilirubin is indicated for early detection of hepatotoxicity.

Cardiac tamponade has been reported in a small number of patients with thalassemia (2% in one series) who received high doses of busulfan and cyclophosphamide as the preparatory regimen for bone marrow transplantation. In this series, the cardiac tamponade was often fatal. Abdominal pain and vomiting preceded the tamponade in most patients.

Pregnancy: Pregnancy Category D. Busulfan may cause fetal harm when administered to a pregnant woman. Although there have been a number of cases reported where apparently normal children have been born after busulfan treatment during pregnancy,[25] one case has been cited where a malformed baby was delivered by a mother treated with busulfan. During the pregnancy that resulted in the malformed infant, the mother received x-ray therapy early in the first trimester, mercaptopurine until the third month, then busulfan until delivery.[26] In pregnant rats, busulfan produces sterility in both male and female offspring due to the absence of germinal cells in testes and ovaries.[27] Germinal cell aplasia or sterility in offspring of mothers receiving busulfan during pregnancy has not been reported in humans. There are no adequate and well-controlled studies in pregnant women. If this drug is used during pregnancy, or if the patient becomes pregnant while taking this drug, the patient should be apprised of the potential hazard to the fetus. Women of childbearing potential should be advised to avoid becoming pregnant.

PRECAUTIONS

General: The most consistent, dose-related toxicity is bone marrow suppression. This may be manifest by anemia, leukopenia, thrombocytopenia, or any combination of these. It is imperative that patients be instructed to report promptly the development of fever, sore throat, signs of local infection, bleeding from any site, or symptoms suggestive of anemia. Any one of these findings may indicate busulfan toxicity; however, they may also indicate transformation of the disease to an acute "blastic" form. Since busulfan may have a delayed effect, it is important to withdraw the medication

temporarily at the first sign of an abnormally large or exceptionally rapid fall in any of the formed elements of the blood. *Patients should never be allowed to take the drug without close medical supervision.*

Seizures have been reported in patients receiving very high, investigational doses of busulfan.[18,28-32] As with any potentially epileptogenic drug, caution should be exercised when administering very high doses of busulfan to patients with a history of seizure disorder, head trauma, or receiving other potentially epileptogenic drugs. Some investigators have used prophylactic anticonvulsant therapy in this setting.

Information for Patients: Patients beginning therapy with busulfan should be informed of the importance of having periodic blood counts and to immediately report any unusual fever or bleeding. Aside from the major toxicity of myelosuppression, patients should be instructed to report any difficulty in breathing, persistent cough, or congestion. They should be told that diffuse pulmonary fibrosis is an infrequent, but serious and potentially life-threatening, complication of long-term busulfan therapy. Patients should be alerted to report any signs of abrupt weakness, unusual fatigue, anorexia, weight loss, nausea and vomiting, and melanoderma that could be associated with a syndrome resembling adrenal insufficiency. Patients should never be allowed to take the drug without medical supervision and they should be informed that other encountered toxicities to busulfan include infertility, amenorrhea, skin hyperpigmentation, drug hypersensitivity, dryness of the mucous membranes, and rarely, cataract formation. Women of childbearing potential should be advised to avoid becoming pregnant. The increased risk of a second malignancy should be explained to the patient.

Laboratory Tests: It is recommended that evaluation of the hemoglobin or hematocrit, total white blood cell count and differential count, and quantitative platelet count be obtained weekly while the patient is on busulfan therapy. In cases where the cause of fluctuation in the formed elements of the peripheral blood is obscure, bone marrow examination may be useful for evaluation of marrow status. A decision to increase, decrease, continue, or discontinue a given dose of busulfan must be based not only on the absolute hematologic values, but also on the rapidity with which changes are occurring. The dosage of busulfan may need to be reduced if this agent is combined with other drugs whose primary toxicity is myelosuppression. Occasional patients may be unusually sensitive to busulfan administered at standard dosage and suffer neutropenia or thrombocytopenia after a relatively short exposure to the drug. Busulfan should not be used where facilities for complete blood counts, including quantitative platelet counts, are not available at weekly (or more frequent) intervals.

Drug Interactions: Busulfan may cause additive myelosuppression when used with other myelosuppressive drugs.

In one study, 12 of approximately 330 patients receiving continuous busulfan and thioguanine therapy for treatment of chronic myelogenous leukemia were found to have esophageal varices associated with abnormal liver function tests.[33] Subsequent liver biopsies were performed in four of these patients, all of which showed evidence of nodular regenerative hyperplasia. Duration of combination therapy prior to the appearance of esophageal varices ranged from 6 to 45 months. With the present analysis of the data, no cases of hepatotoxicity have appeared in the busulfan alone arm of the study. Long-term continuous therapy with thioguanine and busulfan should be used with caution.

Carcinogenesis, Mutagenesis, Impairment of Fertility: See WARNINGS section.

Pregnancy: ***Teratogenic effects:*** Pregnancy Category D. See WARNINGS section.

Nonteratogenic Effects: There have been reports in the literature of small infants being born after the mothers received busulfan during pregnancy, in particular, during the third trimester.[34] One case was reported where an infant had mild anemia and neutropenia at birth after busulfan was administered to the mother from the eighth week of pregnancy to term.[25]

Nursing Mothers: It is not known whether this drug is excreted in human milk. Because of the potential for tumorigenicity shown for busulfan in animal and human studies, a decision should be made whether to discontinue nursing or to discontinue the drug, taking into account the importance of the drug to the mother.

Pediatric Use: See INDICATIONS AND USAGE and DOSAGE AND ADMINISTRATION sections.

ADVERSE REACTIONS

Hematological Effects: The most frequent, serious, toxic effect of busulfan is myelosuppression resulting in leukopenia, thrombocytopenia, and anemia. Myelosuppression is most frequently the result of a failure to discontinue dosage in the face of an undetected decrease in leukocyte or platelet counts.[15]

Pulmonary: Interstitial pulmonary fibrosis has been reported rarely, but it is a clinically significant adverse effect when observed and calls for immediate discontinuation of further administration of the drug. The role of corticosteroids in arresting or reversing the fibrosis has been reported to be beneficial in some cases and without effect in others.[16]

Cardiac: Cardiac tamponade has been reported in a small number of patients with thalassemia who received high doses of busulfan and cyclophosphamide as the preparatory regimen for bone marrow transplantation (see WARNINGS).

One case of endocardial fibrosis has been reported in a 79-year-old woman who received a total dose of 7,200 mg of busulfan over a period of 9 years for the management of chronic myelogenous leukemia.[35] At autopsy, she was found to have endocardial fibrosis of the left ventricle in addition to interstitial pulmonary fibrosis.

Ocular: Busulfan is capable of inducing cataracts in rats and there have been several reports indicating that this is a rare complication in humans. In the few cases reported in humans, cataracts have occurred only after prolonged administration of busulfan.[36]

Dermatologic: Hyperpigmentation is the most common adverse skin reaction and occurs in 5% to 10% of patients, particularly those with a dark complexion.

Metabolic: In a few cases, a clinical syndrome closely resembling adrenal insufficiency and characterized by weakness, severe fatigue, anorexia, weight loss, nausea and vomiting, and melanoderma has developed after prolonged busulfan therapy. The symptoms have sometimes been reversible when busulfan was withdrawn. Adrenal responsiveness to exogenously administered ACTH has usually been normal. However, pituitary function testing with metyrapone revealed a blunted urinary 17-hydroxycorticosteroid excretion in two patients.[37] Following the discontinuation of busulfan (which was associated with clinical improvement), rechallenge with metyrapone revealed normal pituitary-adrenal function.

Hyperuricemia and/or hyperuricosuria are not uncommon in patients with chronic myelogenous leukemia. Additional rapid destruction of granulocytes may accompany the initiation of chemotherapy and increase the urate pool. Adverse effects can be minimized by increased hydration, urine alkalinization, and the prophylactic administration of a xanthine oxidase inhibitor such as ZYLOPRIM® (allopurinol).

Hepatic Effects: Esophageal varices have been reported in patients receiving continuous busulfan and thioguanine therapy for treatment of chronic myelogenous leukemia (see PRECAUTIONS: Drug Interactions). Hepatic veno-occlusive disease has been observed in patients receiving higher than recommended doses of busulfan (see WARNINGS).

Miscellaneous: Other reported adverse reactions include: urticaria, erythema multiforme, erythema nodosum, alopecia, porphyria cutanea tarda, excessive dryness and fragility of the skin with anhidrosis, dryness of the oral mucous membranes and cheilosis, gynecomastia, cholestatic jaundice, and myasthenia gravis. Most of these are single case reports, and in many, a clear cause-and-effect relationship with busulfan has not been demonstrated.

Seizures (see PRECAUTIONS: General) have been observed in patients receiving higher than recommended doses of busulfan.

OVERDOSAGE

There is no known antidote to busulfan. The principal toxic effect is on the bone marrow. Survival after a single 140-mg dose has been reported in an 18 kg, 4-year-old child,[38] but hematologic toxicity is likely to be more profound with chronic overdosage. The hematologic status should be closely monitored and vigorous supportive measures instituted if necessary. Induction of vomiting or gastric lavage followed by administration of charcoal would be indicated if ingestion were recent. It is not known whether busulfan is dialyzable (see CLINICAL PHARMACOLOGY).

Oral LD_{50} single doses in mice are 120 mg/kg. Two distinct types of toxic response are seen at median lethal doses given intraperitoneally. Within a matter of hours there are signs of stimulation of the central nervous system with convulsions and death on the first day. Mice are more sensitive to this effect than are rats. With doses at the LD_{50} there is also delayed death due to damage to the bone marrow. At three times the LD_{50}, atrophy of the mucosa of the large intestine is found after a week, whereas that of the small intestine is little affected.[39] After doses in the order of 10 times those used therapeutically were added to the diet of rats, irreversible cataracts were produced after several weeks. Small doses had no such effect.[40]

DOSAGE AND ADMINISTRATION

Busulfan is administered orally. The usual adult dose range for *remission induction* is 4 to 8 mg, total dose, daily. Dosing on a weight basis is the same for both pediatric patients and adults, approximately 60 mcg/kg of body weight or 1.8 mg/m^2 of body surface, daily. Since the rate of fall of the leukocyte count is dose related, daily doses exceeding 4 mg per day should be reserved for patients with the most compelling symptoms; the greater the total daily dose, the greater is the possibility of inducing bone marrow aplasia.

A decrease in the leukocyte count is not usually seen during the first 10 to 15 days of treatment; the leukocyte count may actually increase during this period and it should not be interpreted as resistance to the drug, nor should the dose be increased.[41] Since the leukocyte count may continue to fall for more than 1 month after discontinuing the drug, it is important that busulfan be discontinued *prior* to the total leukocyte count falling into the normal range. When the total leukocyte count has declined to approximately 15,000/mcL the drug should be withheld.

With a constant dose of busulfan, the total leukocyte count declines exponentially; a weekly plot of the leukocyte count on semi-logarithmic graph paper aids in predicting the time when therapy should be discontinued.[42] With the recommended dose of busulfan, a normal leukocyte count is usually achieved in 12 to 20 weeks.

During remission, the patient is examined at monthly intervals and treatment resumed with the induction dosage when the total leukocyte count reaches approximately 50,000/mcL. When remission is shorter than 3 months, maintenance therapy of 1 to 3 mg daily may be advisable in order to keep the hematological status under control and prevent rapid relapse.

Procedures for proper handling and disposal of anticancer drugs should be considered. Several guidelines on this subject have been published.[43-49]

There is no general agreement that all of the procedures recommended in the guidelines are necessary or appropriate.

HOW SUPPLIED

White, scored tablets containing 2 mg busulfan, imprinted with "MYLERAN" and "K2A" on each tablet; bottle of 25 (NDC 0173-0713-25).

Store at 15° to 25°C (59° to 77°F) in a dry place.

REFERENCES

1. Galton DAG. Myleran in chronic myeloid leukemia: results of treatment. *Lancet.* 1953;1:208-213.
2. Nadkarni MV, Trams EG, Smith PK. Preliminary studies on the distribution and fate of TEM, TEPA, and MYLERAN in the human. *Cancer Res.* 1959;19:713-718.
3. Vodopick H, Hamilton HE, Jackson HL, Peng C-T, Sheets RF. Metabolic fate of tritiated busulfan in man. *J Lab Clin Med.* 1969;73:266-276.
4. Fox BW. Mechanism of action of methane sulfonates. In: Sartorelli AC, Johns DG, eds. *Antineoplastic and Immunosuppressive Agents,* Part II. Berlin: Springer Verlag; 1975:35-46.
5. Roberts JJ, Warwick GP. The mode of action of alkylating agents, III: the formation of 3-hydroxytetrahydrothiophene-1:1-dioxide from 1:4-dimethanesulphonyloxybutane (Myleran), S-β-L-alanyltetrahydrothiophenium mesylate, tetrahydrothiophene and tetrahydrothiophene-1:1-dioxide in the rat, rabbit and mouse. *Biochem Pharmacol.* 1961;6:217-227.
6. Peng C-T. Distribution and metabolic fate of S^{35}-labeled Myleran (busulfan) in normal and tumor-bearing rats. *J Pharmacol Exp Ther.* 1957;120:229-238.
7. Medical Research Council's Working Party for Therapeutic Trials in Leukaemia. Chronic granulocytic leukaemia: comparison of radiotherapy and busulfan therapy. *Br Med J.* 1968;1:201-208.
8. Minot GR, Buckman TE, Isaacs R. Chronic myelogenous leukemia: age incidence, duration, and benefit derived from irradiation. *JAMA.* 1924;82:1489-1494.
9. Haut A, Abbott WS, Wintrobe MM, Cartwright GE. Busulfan in the treatment of chronic myelocytic leukemia: the effect of long term intermittent therapy. *Blood.* 1961;17:1-19.
10. Monfardini S, Gee T, Fried J, Clarkson B. Survival in chronic myelogenous leukemia: influence of treatment and extent of disease at diagnosis. *Cancer.* 1973;31:492-501.
11. Conrad FG. Survival in granulocytic leukemia. *Arch Intern Med.* 1973;131:684-685.
12. Sokal JE. Evaluation of survival data for chronic myelocytic leukemia. *Am J Hematol.* 1976;1:493-500.
13. Ezdinli EZ, Sokal JE, Crosswhite L, Sandberg AA. Philadelphia chromosome-positive and -negative chronic myelocytic leukemia. *Ann Intern Med.* 1970;72:175-182.
14. Smith KL, Johnson W. Classification of chronic myelocytic leukemia in children. *Cancer.* 1974; 34:670-679.
15. Stuart JJ, Crocker DL, Roberts HR. Treatment of busulfan-induced pancytopenia. *Arch Intern Med.* 1977;136:1181-1183.
16. Sostman HD, Matthay RA, Putman CE. Cytotoxic drug-induced lung disease. *Am J Med.* 1977;62:608-615.

Continued on next page

This product information is based on labeling in effect on June 1, 1998. For further information, contact via direct mail, phone, or web site Medical Information: Glaxo Wellcome Inc., PO Box 13398, Research Triangle Park, NC 27709. Healthcare Professionals (Medical Information): 800-334-0089 Patients (Customer Response Center): 888-TALK2GW (1-888-825-5249) Glaxo Wellcome Corporate Web Site: www.glaxowellcome.com

Myleran—Cont.

17. Stott H, Fox W, Girling DJ, Stephens RJ, Galton DAG. Acute leukaemia after busulfan. *Br Med J.* 1977;2:1513-1517.
18. Hartmann O, et al. High-dose busulfan and cyclophosphamide with autologous bone marrow transplantation support in advanced malignancies in children: A Phase II study. *J Clin Oncol.* 1986;4:1804-1810.
19. Copelan EA, et al. Marrow transplantation following busulfan and cyclophosphamide for chronic myelogenous leukaemia in accelerated or blastic phase. *Br J Haematol.* 1989; 71:487-491.
20. Kirchner H, et al. Allogeneic and autologous bone marrow transplantation (BMT) after high-dose busulfan and cyclophosphamide treatment. *Blut.* 1988;57:198.. Abstract.
21. Thompson J, et al. Allogeneic bone marrow transplantation (BMT) following transplant preparation with cyclophosphamide (CTX) and busulfan (BU). *Proc ASCO.* 1989; 8:18. Abstract.
22. Geller RB, et al. Allogeneic bone marrow transplantation after high-dose busulfan and cyclophosphamide in patients with acute non-lymphocytic leukemia. *Blood.* 1989; 73:2209-2218.
23. Lu C, et al. Preliminary results of high-dose busulfan and cyclophosphamide with syngeneic or autologous bone marrow rescue. *Cancer Treat Rep.* 1984; 68:711-717.
24. Groshow LB, et al. Pharmacokinetics of busulfan: correlation with veno-occlusive disease in patients undergoing bone marrow transplantation. *Cancer Chemother Pharmacol.* 1989; 25:55-61.
25. Dugdale M, Fort AT. Busulfan treatment of leukemia during pregnancy: case report and review of the literature. *JAMA.* 1967;199:131-133.
26. Diamond I, Anderson MM, McCreadie SR. Transplacental transmission of busulfan (Myleran) in a mother with leukemia: production of fetal malformation and cytomegaly. *Pediatrics.* 1960;25:85-90.
27. Bollag W. Cytostatica in der Schwangerschaft. *Schweiz Med Wochenschr.* 1954;84:393-395.
28. Marcus RE, et al. Convulsions due to high-dose busulfan. *Lancet.* 1984;2:1463. Letter.
29. Martell RW, et al. High-dose busulfan and myoclonic epilepsy. *Ann Intern Med.* 1987; 106:173. Letter.
30. Sureda A, et al. High-dose busulfan and seizures. *Ann Intern Med.* 1989; 111:543-544. Letter.
31. Grigg AP, et al. Busulfan and phenytoin. *Ann Intern Med.* 1989; 111:1049-1050. Letter.
32. Beelen DW, et al. Acute toxicity and first clinical results of intensive post-induction therapy using a modified busulfan and cyclophosphamide regimen with autologous bone marrow rescue in first remission of acute myeloid leukemia. *Blood.* 1989; 74:1507-1516.
33. Key NS, Kelly PMA, Emerson PM, Chapman RWG, Allan NC, McGee JO'D. Oesophageal varices associated with busulfan-thioguanine combination therapy for chronic myeloid leukaemia. *Lancet.* 1987;2:1050-1052.
34. Boros SJ, Reynolds JW. Intrauterine growth retardation following third-trimester exposure to busulfan. *Am J Obstet Gynecol.* 1977;129:111-112.
35. Weinberger A, Pinkhas J, Sandbank U, Shaklai M, deVries A. Endocardial fibrosis following busulfan treatment. *JAMA.* 1975;231:495.
36. Ravindranathan MP, Paul VJ, Kuriakose ET. Cataract after busulfan treatment. *Br Med J.* 1972;1:218-219.
37. Vivacqua RJ, Haurani Fl, Erslev AJ. "Selective" pituitary insufficiency secondary to busulfan. *Ann Intern Med.* 1967;67:380-387.
38. DeOliveira HP, Cruz E, Fonseca A de S, Medeiros M. Accidental ingestion of a toxic dose of Myleran by a child. *Acta Haematol* (Basel). 1963;29:249-255.
39. Sternberg SS, Phillips FS, Scholler J. Pharmacological and pathological effects of alkylating agents. *Ann NY Acad Sci.* 1958;68:811-825.
40. Solomon C, Light AE, deBeer EJ. Cataracts produced in rats by 1,4-dimethane-sulfonoxybutane (MYLERAN). *AMA Arch Ophthal.* 1955;54:850-852.
41. Stryckmans PA: Current concepts in chronic myelogenous leukemia. *Semin Hematol.* 1974;11:101-127.
42. Galton DAG. Chemotherapy of chronic myelocytic leukemia. *Semin Hematol.* 1969;6:323-343.
43. Recommendations for the safe handling of parenteral antineoplastic drugs. Washington, DC: Division of Safety, National Institutes of Health; 1983. US Dept of Health and Human Services, Public Health Service publication NIH 83-2621.
44. AMA Council on Scientific Affairs. Guidelines for handling parenteral antineoplastics. *JAMA.* 1985;253:1590-1591.
45. National Study Commission on Cytotoxic Exposure. Recommendations for handling cytotoxic agents. 1987. Available from Louis P. Jeffrey, Chairman, National Study Commission on Cytotoxic Exposure. Massachusetts College of Pharmacy and Allied Health Sciences, 179 Longwood Avenue, Boston, MA 02115.
46. Clinical Oncological Society of Australia. Guidelines and recommendations for safe handling of antineoplastic agents. *Med J Australia.* 1983;1:426-428.
47. Jones RB, Frank R, Mass T. Safe handling of chemotherapeutic agents: a report from the Mount Sinai Medical Center. *CA-A Cancer J for Clin.* 1983;33:258-263.
48. American Society of Hospital Pharmacists. ASHP technical assistance bulletin on handling cytotoxic and hazardous drugs. *AM J Hosp Pharm.* 1990;47:1033-1049.
49. Yodaiken RE, Bennett D. OSHA work-practice guidelines for personnel dealing with cytotoxic (antineoplastic) drugs. *Am J Hosp Pharm.* 1986;43:1193-1204.

November 1996/RL-375

Shown in Product Identification Guide, page 313

NAVELBINE® ℞

[*na 'vəl-bēn*]
(vinorelbine tartrate)
Injection

> **WARNING:** NAVELBINE (vinorelbine tartrate) Injection should be administered under the supervision of a physician experienced in the use of cancer chemotherapeutic agents. This product is for intraveneous (IV) use only. Intrathecal administration of other vinca alkaloids has resulted in death. Syringes containing this product should be labeled "WARNING—NAVELBINE FOR ITRAVENOUS USE ONLY."
>
> Severe granulocytopenia resulting in increased susceptibility to infection may occur. Granulocyte counts should be ≥1000 cells/mm^3 prior to the administration of NAVELBINE. The dosage should be adjusted according to complete blood counts with differentials obtained on the day of treatment.
>
> Caution—It is extremely important that the intravenous needle or catheter be properly positioned before NAVELBI NE is injected. Administration of NAVELBINE may result in extravasation causing local tissue necrosis and/or thrombophlebitis (see DOSAGE AND ADMINISTRATION: Administration Precautions).

DESCRIPTION

NAVELBINE (vinorelbine tartrate) Injection is for intravenous administration. Each vial contains vinorelbine tartrate equivalent to 10 mg (1-mL vial) or 50 mg (5-mL vial) vinorelbine in Water for Injection. No preservatives or other additives are present. The aqueous solution is sterile and nonpyrogenic.

Vinorelbine tartrate is a semi-synthetic vinca alkaloid with antitumor activity. The chemical name is 3′,4′-didehydro-4′-deoxy-*C*′-norvincaleukoblastine [*R*-(*R**,*R**)-2,3-dihydroxybutanedioate (1:2)(salt)].

Vinorelbine tartrate is a white to yellow or light brown amorphous powder with the molecular formula $C_{45}H_{54}N_4O_8 \cdot 2C_4H_6O_6$ and molecular weight of 1079.12. The aqueous solubility is >1000 mg/mL in distilled water. The pH of NAVELBINE Injection is approximately 3.5.

CLINICAL PHARMACOLOGY

Vinorelbine is a vinca alkaloid that interferes with microtubule assembly. The vinca alkaloids are structurally similar compounds comprised of two multiringed units, vindoline and catharanthine. Unlike other vinca alkaloids, the catharanthine unit is the site of structural modification for vinorelbine. The antitumor activity of vinorelbine is thought to be due primarily to inhibition of mitosis at metaphase through its interaction with tubulin. Like other vinca alkaloids, vinorelbine may also interfere with: 1) amino acid, cyclic AMP, and glutathione metabolism, 2) calmodulin-dependent Ca^{++}-transport ATPase activity, 3) cellular respiration, and 4) nucleic acid and lipid biosynthesis. In intact tectal plates from mouse embryos, vinorelbine, vincristine, and vinblastine inhibited mitotic microtubule formation at the same concentration (2 µM), inducing a blockade of cells at metaphase. Vincristine produced depolymerization of axonal microtubules at 5 µM, but vinblastine and vinorelbine did not have this effect until concentrations of 30 µM and 40 µM, respectively. These data suggest relative selectivity of vinorelbine for mitotic microtubules.

Pharmacokinetics: The pharmacokinetics of vinorelbine were studied in 49 patients who received doses of 30 mg/m^2 in four clinical trials. Doses were administered by 15- to 20-minute constant-rate infusions. Following intravenous administration, vinorelbine concentration in plasma decays in a triphasic manner. The initial rapid decline primarily represents distribution of drug to peripheral compartments followed by metabolism and excretion of the drug during subsequent phases. The prolonged terminal phase is due to relatively slow efflux of vinorelbine from peripheral compartments. The terminal phase half-life averages 27.7 to 43.6 hours and the mean plasma clearance ranges from 0.97 to 1.26 L/hr per kg. Steady-state volume of distribution (V_{SS}) values range from 25.4 to 40.1 L/kg.

Vinorelbine demonstrated high binding to human platelets and lymphocytes. The free fraction was approximately 0.11 in pooled human plasma over a concentration range of 234 to 1169 ng/mL. The binding to plasma constituents in cancer patients ranged from 79.6% to 91.2%. Vinorelbine binding was not altered in the presence of cisplatin, 5-fluorouracil, or doxorubicin.

Vinorelbine undergoes substantial hepatic elimination in humans, with large amounts recovered in feces after intravenous administration to humans. One metabolite, deacetylvinorelbine, has been shown to possess antitumor activity. This metabolite has been detected, but not quantified, in human plasma. The effects of renal or hepatic dysfunction on the disposition of vinorelbine have not been assessed, but based on experience with other anticancer vinca alkaloids, dose adjustments are recommended for patients with impaired hepatic function (see DOSAGE AND ADMINISTRATION).

The disposition of radiolabeled vinorelbine given intravenously was studied in a limited number of patients. Approximately 18% of the administered dose was recovered in the urine and 46% in the feces. Incomplete recovery in humans is consistent with results in animals where recovery is incomplete, even after prolonged sampling times. A separate study of the urinary excretion of vinorelbine using specific chromatographic analytical methodology showed that 10.9% ± 0.7% of a 30-mg/m^2 intravenous dose was excreted unchanged in the urine.

The pharmacokinetics of vinorelbine are not influenced by the concurrent administration of cisplatin with NAVELBINE (see PRECAUTIONS: Drug Interactions).

Clinical Trials: Data from two controlled clinical studies (823 patients), as well as additional data from more than 100 patients enrolled in two uncontrolled clinical trials, support the use of NAVELBINE in patients with advanced non-small cell lung cancer (NSCLC). In a large European clinical trial, 612 patients with Stage III or IV NSCLC, no prior chemotherapy, and WHO Performance Status of 0, 1, or 2 were randomized to treatment with single-agent NAVELBINE (30 mg/m^2 per week), NAVELBINE (30 mg/m^2 per week) plus cisplatin (120 mg/m^2 days 1 and 29, then every 6 weeks), and vindesine (3 mg/m^2 per week for 7 weeks, then every other week) plus cisplatin (120 mg/m^2 days 1 and 29, then every 6 weeks). NAVELBINE plus cisplatin produced longer survival times than vindesine plus cisplatin (median survival 40 weeks versus 32 weeks, P = 0.03). The median survival time for patients receiving single-agent NAVELBINE was similar to that observed with vindesine plus cisplatin (31 weeks versus 32 weeks). The 1-year survival rates were 35% for NAVELBINE plus cisplatin, 27% for vindesine plus cisplatin, and 30% for single-agent NAVELBINE. The overall objective response rate (all partial responses) was significantly higher in the patients treated with NAVELBINE plus cisplatin (28%) than in those treated with vindesine plus cisplatin (19%, P = 0.03) and in those treated with single-agent NAVELBINE (14%, P <0.001). The response rates reported for vindesine plus cisplatin and single-agent NAVELBINE were not significantly different. Significantly less nausea, vomiting, alopecia, and neurotoxicity were observed in patients receiving single-agent NAVELBINE compared to those receiving the combination of vindesine and cisplatin.

Single-agent NAVELBINE was studied in a North American, randomized clinical trial in which patients with Stage IV NSCLC, no prior chemotherapy, and Karnofsky Performance Status ≥70 were treated with NAVELBINE (30 mg/m^2) weekly or 5-fluorouracil (5-FU) (425 mg/m^2 IV bolus) plus leucovorin (LV) (20 mg/m^2 IV bolus) daily for 5 days every 4 weeks. A total of 211 patients were randomized at a 2:1 ratio to NAVELBINE (143) or 5-FU/LV (68). NAVELBINE showed improved survival time compared to 5-FU/LV. In an intent-to-treat analysis, the median survival time for patients receiving NAVELBINE was 30 weeks and for those receiving 5-FU/LV was 22 weeks (P = 0.06). The 1-year survival rates were 24% (±4% SE) for NAVELBINE and 16% (±5% SE) for the 5-FU/LV group, using the Kaplan-Meier product-limit estimates. The median survival time with 5-FU/LV was similar to, or slightly better than, that usually observed in untreated patients with advanced NSCLC, suggesting that the difference was not related to some unknown detrimental effect of 5-FU/LV therapy. The response rates (all partial responses) for NAVELBINE and 5-FU/LV were 12% and 3%, respectively. Quality-of-life (QOL) was also an endpoint in this study. Patients completed a modified Southwest Oncology Group QOL questionnaire which assessed the domains of role functioning, physical functioning, symptom distress, and global QOL. Quality-of-life was not adversely affected by NAVELBINE when compared to control.

A dose-ranging study of NAVELBINE (20, 25, or 30 mg/m^2 per week) plus cisplatin (120 mg/m^2 days 1 and 29, then ev-

ery 6 weeks) in 32 patients with NSCLC demonstrated a median survival of 44 weeks. There were no responses at the lowest dose level; the response rate was 33% in the 21 patients treated at the two highest dose levels.

INDICATIONS AND USAGE

NAVELBINE is indicated as a single agent or in combination with cisplatin for the first-line treatment of ambulatory patients with unresectable, advanced non small cell lung cancer (NSCLC). In patients with Stage IV NSCLC, NAVELBINE is indicated as a single agent or in combination with cisplatin. In Stage III NSCLC, NAVELBINE is indicated in combination with cisplatin.

CONTRAINDICATIONS

Administration of NAVELBINE is contraindicated in patients with pretreatment granulocyte counts <1000 cells/mm³ (see WARNINGS).

WARNINGS

NAVELBINE should be administered in carefully adjusted doses by or under the supervision of a physician experienced in the use of cancer chemotherapeutic agents.
Patients treated with NAVELBINE should be frequently monitored for myelosuppression both during and after therapy. Granulocytopenia is dose-limiting. Granulocyte nadirs occur between 7 and 10 days after dosing with granulocyte count recovery usually within the following 7 to 14 days. Complete blood counts with differentials should be performed and results reviewed prior to administering each dose of NAVELBINE. NAVELBINE should not be administered to patients with granulocyte counts <1000 cells/mm³. Patients developing severe granulocytopenia should be monitored carefully for evidence of infection and/or fever. See DOSAGE AND ADMINISTRATION for recommended dose adjustments for granulocytopenia.
Pregnancy: Pregnancy Category D. NAVELBINE may cause fetal harm if administered to a pregnant woman. A single dose of vinorelbine has been shown to be embryo- and/or fetotoxic in mice and rabbits at doses of 9 mg/m² and 5.5 mg/m², respectively (one third and one sixth the human dose). At nonmaternotoxic doses, fetal weight was reduced and ossification was delayed. There are no studies in pregnant women. If NAVELBINE is used during pregnancy, or if the patient becomes pregnant while receiving this drug, the patient should be apprised of the potential hazard to the fetus. Women of childbearing potential should be advised to avoid becoming pregnant during therapy with NAVELBINE.

PRECAUTIONS

General: Most drug-related adverse events of NAVELBINE are reversible. If severe adverse events occur, NAVELBINE should be reduced in dosage or discontinued and appropriate corrective measures taken. Reinstitution of therapy with NAVELBINE should be carried out with caution and alertness as to possible recurrence of toxicity.
NAVELBINE should be used with extreme caution in patients whose bone marrow reserve may have been compromised by prior irradiation or chemotherapy, or whose marrow function is recovering from the effects of previous chemotherapy (see DOSAGE AND ADMINISTRATION).
Administration of NAVELBINE to patients with prior radiation therapy may result in radiation recall reactions (see ADVERSE REACTIONS and Drug Interactions).
Patients with a prior history or pre-existing neuropathy, regardless of etiology, should be monitored for new or worsening signs and symptoms of neuropathy while receiving NAVELBINE.
Acute shortness of breath and severe bronchospasm have been reported infrequently following the administration of NAVELBINE and other vinca alkaloids, most commonly when the vinca alkaloid was used in combination with mitomycin. These adverse events may require treatment with supplemental oxygen, bronchodilators, and/or corticosteroids, particularly when there is pre-existing pulmonary dysfunction.
Care must be taken to avoid contamination of the eye with concentrations of NAVELBINE used clinically. Severe irritation of the eye has been reported with accidental exposure to another vinca alkaloid. If exposure occurs, the eye should immediately be thoroughly flushed with water.
Information for Patients: Patients should be informed that the major acute toxicities of NAVELBINE are related to bone marrow toxicity, specifically granulocytopenia with increased susceptibility to infection. They should be advised to report fever or chills immediately. Women of childbearing potential should be advised to avoid becoming pregnant during treatment.
Laboratory Tests: Since dose-limiting clinical toxicity is the result of depression of the white blood cell count, it is imperative that complete blood counts with differentials be obtained and reviewed on the day of treatment prior to each dose of NAVELBINE (see ADVERSE REACTIONS: Hematologic).
Hepatic: There is no evidence that the toxicity of NAVELBINE is enhanced in patients with elevated liver en-

zymes. No data are available for patients with severe baseline cholestasis, but the liver plays an important role in the metabolism of NAVELBINE. Because clinical experience in patients with severe liver disease is limited, caution should be exercised when administering NAVELBINE to patients with severe hepatic injury or impairment (see DOSAGE AND ADMINISTRATION).
Drug Interactions: Acute pulmonary reactions have been reported with NAVELBINE and other anticancer vinca alkaloids used in conjunction with mitomycin. Although the pharmacokinetics of vinorelbine are not influenced by the concurrent administration of cisplatin, the incidence of granulocytopenia with NAVELBINE used in combination with cisplatin is significantly higher than with single-agent NAVELBINE. Patients who receive NAVELBINE and paclitaxel, either concomitantly or sequentially, should be monitored for signs and symptoms of neuropathy. Administration of NAVELBINE to patients with prior or concomitant radiation therapy may result in radiosensitizing effects.
Carcinogenesis, Mutagenesis, Impairment of Fertility: The carcinogenic potential of NAVELBINE has not been studied. Vinorelbine has been shown to affect chromosome number and possibly structure in vivo (polyploidy in bone marrow cells from Chinese hamsters and a positive micronucleus test in mice). It was not mutagenic in the Ames test and gave inconclusive results in the mouse lymphoma TK Locus assay. The significance of these or other short-term test results for human risk is unknown. Vinorelbine did not affect fertility to a statistically significant extent when administered to rats on either a once-weekly (9 mg/m², approximately one third the human dose) or alternate-day schedule (4.2 mg/m², approximately one seventh the human dose) prior to and during mating. However, biweekly administration for 13 or 26 weeks in the rat at 2.1 and 7.2 mg/m² (approximately one fifteenth and one fourth the human dose) resulted in decreased spermatogenesis and prostate/seminal vesicle secretion.
Pregnancy: Pregnancy Category D. See WARNINGS section.
Nursing Mothers: It is not known whether the drug is excreted in human milk. Because many drugs are excreted in human milk and because of the potential for serious adverse reactions in nursing infants from NAVELBINE, it is recommended that nursing be discontinued in women who are receiving therapy with NAVELBINE.

Pediatric Use: Safety and effectiveness in pediatric patients have not been established.
Geriatric Use: Of the total number of patients in North American clinical studies of IV NAVELBINE, approximately one third were 65 years of age or greater. No overall differences in effectiveness or safety were observed between these patients and younger patients. Other reported clinical experience has not identified differences in responses between the elderly and younger patients, but greater sensitivity of some older individuals cannot be ruled out.

ADVERSE REACTIONS

Granulocytopenia is the major dose-limiting toxicity with NAVELBINE. Dose adjustments are required for hematologic toxicity and hepatic insufficiency (see DOSAGE AND ADMINISTRATION).
Data in the following table are based on the experience of 365 patients (143 patients with NSCLC; 222 patients with advanced breast cancer) treated with IV NAVELBINE as a single agent in three clinical studies. The dosing schedule in each study was 30 mg/m² NAVELBINE on a weekly basis. [See table 1 above]
Hematologic: Granulocytopenia was the major dose-limiting toxicity with NAVELBINE; it was generally reversible and not cumulative over time. Granulocyte nadirs occurred 7 to 10 days after the dose, with granulocyte recovery usually within the following 7 to 14 days. Granulocytopenia resulted in hospitalizations for fever and/or sepsis in 8% of patients. Septic deaths occurred in approximately 1% of patients. Prophylactic hematologic growth factors have not been routinely used with NAVELBINE. If medically necessary, growth factors may be administered at recommended doses no earlier than 24 hours after the administration of cytotoxic chemotherapy. Growth factors should not be administered in the period 24 hours before the administration of chemotherapy.

Continued on next page

Table 1: Summary of Adverse Events in 365 Patients Receiving Single-Agent NAVELBINE*†

Adverse Event		All Patients (n = 365) (% Incidence)	NSCLC (n = 143) (% Incidence)
Bone Marrow			
Granulocytopenia	<2000 cells/mm³	90	80
	<500 cells/mm³	36	29
Leukopenia	<4000 cells/mm³	92	81
	<1000 cells/mm³	15	12
Thrombocytopenia	<100,000 cells/mm³	5	4
	<50,000 cells/mm³	1	1
Anemia	<11 g/dL	83	77
	<8 g/dL	9	1
Hospitalizations due to granulocytopenic complications		9	8

Adverse Event	All Grades (% Incidence) All Patients	All Grades (% Incidence) NSCLC	Grade 3 (% Incidence) All Patients	Grade 3 (% Incidence) NSCLC	Grade 4 (% Incidence) All Patients	Grade 4 (% Incidence) NSCLC
Clinical Chemistry Elevations						
Total Bilirubin (n = 351)	13	9	4	3	3	2
SGOT (n = 346)	67	54	5	2	1	1
General						
Asthenia	36	27	7	5	0	0
Injection Site Reactions	28	38	2	5	0	0
Injection Site Pain	16	13	2	1	0	0
Phlebitis	7	10	<1	1	0	0
Digestive						
Nausea	44	34	2	1	0	0
Vomiting	20	15	2	1	0	0
Constipation	35	29	3	2	0	0
Diarrhea	17	13	1	1	0	0
Peripheral Neuropathy‡	25	20	1	1	<1	0
Dyspnea	7	3	2	2	1	0
Alopecia	12	12	≤1	1	0	0

* None of the reported toxicities were influenced by age. Grade based on modified criteria from the National Cancer Institute.
† Patients with NSCLC had not received prior chemotherapy. The majority of the remaining patients had received prior chemotherapy.
‡ Incidence of paresthesia plus hypesthesia.

This product information is based on labeling in effect on June 1, 1998. For further information, contact via direct mail, phone, or web site Medical Information: Glaxo Wellcome Inc., PO Box 13398, Research Triangle Park, NC 27709. Healthcare Professionals (Medical Information): 800-334-0089 Patients (Customer Response Center): 888-TALK2GW (1-888-825-5249) Glaxo Wellcome Corporate Web Site: www.glaxowellcome.com

Navelbine—Cont.

Grade 3 or 4 anemia occurred in 1% of patients, although blood products were administered to 18% of patients who received NAVELBINE. Grade 3 or 4 thrombocytopenia was reported in 1% of patients.

Neurologic: Mild to moderate peripheral neuropathy manifested by paresthesia and hypesthesia were the most frequently reported neurologic toxicities. Loss of deep tendon reflexes occurred in less than 5% of patients. The development of severe peripheral neuropathy was infrequent (1%) and generally reversible.

Skin: Alopecia was reported in 12% of patients and was usually mild.

Like other anticancer vinca alkaloids, NAVELBINE is a moderate vesicant. Injection site reactions, including erythema, pain at injection site, and vein discoloration occurred in approximately one-third of patients; 5% were severe. Chemical phlebitis along the vein proximal to the site of injection was reported in 10% of patients.

Gastrointestinal: Mild or moderate nausea occurred in 34% of patients treated with NAVELBINE; severe nausea was infrequent (<2%). Prophylactic administration of antiemetics was not routine in patients treated with single-agent NAVELBINE. Due to the low incidence of severe nausea and vomiting with single-agent NAVELBINE, the use of serotonin antagonists is generally not required. Constipation occurred in 29% of patients, with paralytic ileus occurring in 1%. Vomiting, diarrhea, anorexia, and stomatitis were usually mild or moderate and each occurred in less than 20% of patients.

Hepatic: Transient elevations of liver enzymes were reported without clinical symptoms.

Cardiovascular: Chest pain was reported in 5% of patients. Most reports of chest pain were in patients who had either a history of cardiovascular disease or tumor within the chest. There have been rare reports of myocardial infarction.

Pulmonary: Shortness of breath was reported in 3% of patients; it was severe in 2% (see PRECAUTIONS: General). Interstitial pulmonary changes were documented in a few patients.

Other: Fatigue occurred in 27% of patients. It was usually mild or moderate but tended to increase with cumulative dosing.

Other toxicities that have been reported in less than 5% of patients include jaw pain, myalgia, arthralgia, and rash. Hemorrhagic cystitis and the syndrome of inappropriate ADH secretion were each reported in <1% of patients.

Combination Use: In a randomized study, 206 patients received treatment with NAVELBINE plus cisplatin and 206 patients received single-agent NAVELBINE. The toxicity profile of cisplatin is known (see full prescribing information for cisplatin). The incidence of severe nausea and vomiting was 30% for NAVELBINE/cisplatin compared to <2% for single-agent NAVELBINE. Cisplatin did not appear to increase the incidence of neurotoxicity observed with single-agent NAVELBINE. However, myelosuppression, specifically Grade 3 and 4 granulocytopenia, was greater with the combination of NAVELBINE/cisplatin (79%) than with single-agent NAVELBINE (53%). The incidence of fever and infection may be increased with the combination.

Observed During Clinical Practice: In addition to the adverse events reported from clinical trials, the following events have been identified during post-approval use of NAVELBINE. Because they are reported voluntarily from a population of unknown size, estimates of frequency cannot be made. These events have been chosen for inclusion due to a combination of their seriousness, frequency of reporting, or potential causal connection to NAVELBINE.

Body As A Whole: Systemic allergic reactions reported as anaphylaxis, pruritus, urticaria, and angioedema; flushing; and radiation recall events such as dermatitis and esophagitis (see PRECAUTIONS) have been reported.

Hematologic: Thromboembolic events including pulmonary embolus and deep venous thrombosis have been reported primarily in seriously ill and debilitated patients with known predisposing risk factors for these events.

Neurologic: Peripheral neurotoxicities such as, but not limited to, muscle weakness and disturbance of gait, have been observed in patients with and without prior symptoms. There may be increased potential for neurotoxicity in patients with pre-existing neuropathy, regardless of etiology, who receive NAVELBINE.

Skin: Injection site reactions, including localized rash and urticaria, blister formation, and skin sloughing have been observed in clinical practice. Some of these reactions may be delayed in appearance.

Gastrointestinal: Dysphagia and mucositis have been reported.

Cardiovascular: Hypertension, hypotension, vasodilation, and tachycardia have been reported.

Pulmonary: Pneumonia has been reported.

Musculoskeletal: Headache has been reported, with and without other musculoskeletal aches and pains.

Other: Pain in tumor-containing tissue, back pain, and abdominal pain have been reported. Electrolyte abnormalities, including hyponatremia with or without the syndrome of inappropriate ADH secretion, have been reported in seriously ill and debilitated patients.

Combination Use: Patients with prior exposure to paclitaxel and who have demonstrated neuropathy should be monitored closely for new or worsening neuropathy. Patients who have experienced neuropathy with previous drug regimens should be monitored for symptoms of neuropathy while receiving NAVELBINE. NAVELBINE may result in radiosensitizing effects with prior or concomitant radiation therapy (see PRECAUTIONS).

OVERDOSAGE

There is no known antidote for overdoses of NAVELBINE. The primary anticipated complications of overdosage would consist of bone marrow suppression and peripheral neurotoxicity. If overdosage occurs, general supportive measures together with appropriate blood transfusions and antibiotics should be instituted as deemed necessary by the physician.

DOSAGE AND ADMINISTRATION

The usual initial dose of NAVELBINE is 30 mg/m^2 administered weekly. The recommended method of administration is an intravenous injection over 6 to 10 minutes. In controlled trials, single-agent NAVELBINE was given weekly until progression or dose-limiting toxicity. NAVELBINE was used at the same dose in combination with 120 mg/m^2 of cisplatin, given on days 1 and 29, then every 6 weeks. No dose adjustments are required for renal insufficiency. If moderate or severe neurotoxicity develops, NAVELBINE should be discontinued. The dosage should be adjusted according to hematologic toxicity or hepatic insufficiency, whichever results in the lower dose.

Dose Modifications for Hematologic Toxicity: Granulocyte counts should be ≥1000 cells/mm^3 prior to the administration of NAVELBINE. Adjustments in the dosage of NAVELBINE should be based on granulocyte counts obtained on the day of treatment according to Table 2.

Table 2: Dose Adjustments Based on Granulocyte Counts

Granulocytes (cells/mm^3) on Days of Treatment	Dose of NAVELBINE (mg/m^2)
≥1500	30
1000 to 1499	15
<1000	Do not administer. Repeat granulocyte count in 1 week. If three consecutive weekly doses are held because granulocyte count is <1000 cells/mm^3, discontinue NAVELBINE.

Note: For patients who, during treatment with NAVELBINE, have experienced fever and/or sepsis while granulocytopenic or had two consecutive weekly doses held due to granulocytopenia, subsequent doses of NAVELBINE should be:

22.5 mg/m^2 for granulocytes ≥1500 cells/mm^3
11.25 mg/m^2 for granulocytes 1000 to 1499 cells/mm^3

Dose Modification for Hepatic Insufficiency: NAVELBINE should be administered with caution to patients with hepatic insufficiency. In patients who develop hyperbilirubinemia during treatment with NAVELBINE, the dose should be adjusted for total bilirubin according to Table 3.

Table 3: Dose Modification Based on Total Bilirubin

Total Bilirubin (mg/dL)	Dose of NAVELBINE (mg/m^2)
≤2.0	30
2.1 to 3.0	15
>3.0	7.5

Dose Modification for Concurrent Hematologic Toxicity and Hepatic Insufficiency: In patients with both hematologic toxicity and hepatic insufficiency, the lower of the doses determined from Table 2 and Table 3 should be administered.

Administration Precautions: Caution—NAVELBINE must be administered intravenously. It is extremely important that the intravenous needle or catheter be properly positioned before any NAVELBINE is injected. Leakage into surrounding tissue during intravenous administration of NAVELBINE may cause considerable irritation, local tissue necrosis, and/or thrombophlebitis. If extravasation occurs, the injection should be discontinued immediately, and any

remaining portion of the dose should then be introduced into another vein. Since there are no established guidelines for the treatment of extravasation injuries with NAVELBINE, institutional guidelines may be used. The *ONS Chemotherapy Guidelines* provide additional recommendations for the prevention of extravasation injuries.[1]

As with other toxic compounds, caution should be exercised in handling and preparing the solution of NAVELBINE. Skin reactions may occur with accidental exposure. The use of gloves is recommended. If the solution of NAVELBINE contacts the skin or mucosa, immediately wash the skin or mucosa thoroughly with soap and water. Severe irritation of the eye has been reported with accidental contamination of the eye with another vinca alkaloid. If this happens with NAVELBINE, the eye should be flushed with water immediately and thoroughly.

Procedures for proper handling and disposal of anticancer drugs should be used. Several guidelines on this subject have been published.[2-8] There is no general agreement that all of the procedures recommended in the guidelines are necessary or appropriate.

NAVELBINE Injection is a clear, colorless to pale yellow solution. Parenteral drug products should be visually inspected for particulate matter and discoloration prior to administration whenever solution and container permit. If particulate matter is seen, NAVELBINE should not be administered.

Preparation for Administration: NAVELBINE Injection must be diluted in either a syringe or IV bag using one of the recommended solutions. The diluted NAVELBINE should be administered over 6 to 10 minutes into the side port of a free-flowing IV **closest to the IV bag** followed by flushing with at least 75 to 125 mL of one of the solutions. Diluted NAVELBINE may be used for up to 24 hours under normal room light when stored in polypropylene syringes or polyvinyl chloride bags at 5° to 30°C (41° to 86°F).

Syringe: The calculated dose of NAVELBINE should be diluted to a concentration between 1.5 and 3.0 mg/mL. The following solutions may be used for dilution:

5% Dextrose Injection, USP
0.9% Sodium Chloride Injection, USP

IV Bag: The calculated dose of NAVELBINE should be diluted to a concentration between 0.5 and 2 mg/mL. The following solutions may be used for dilution:

5% Dextrose Injection, USP
0.9% Sodium Chloride Injection, USP
0.45% Sodium Chloride Injection, USP
5% Dextrose and 0.45% Sodium Chloride Injection, USP
Ringer's Injection, USP
Lactated Ringer's Injection, USP

Stability: Unopened vials of NAVELBINE are stable until the date indicated on the package when stored under refrigeration at 2° to 8°C (36° to 46°F) and protected from light in the carton. Unopened vials of NAVELBINE are stable at temperatures up to 25°C (77°F) for up to 72 hours. This product should not be frozen.

HOW SUPPLIED

NAVELBINE Injection is a clear, colorless to pale yellow solution in Water for Injection, containing 10 mg vinorelbine per mL. NAVELBINE Injection is available in single-use, clear glass vials with black elastomeric stoppers and royal blue caps, individually packaged in a carton in the following vial sizes:

10 mg/1 mL Single-Use Vial, Carton of 1 (NDC 0173-0656-01).

50 mg/5 mL Single-Use Vial, Carton of 1 (NDC 0173-0656-44).

Store the vials under refrigeration at 2° to 8°C (36° to 46°F) in the carton. Protect from light. DO NOT FREEZE.

REFERENCES

1. ONS Clinical Practice Committee. Cancer Chemotherapy Guidelines: Recommendations for the management of vesicant extravasation, hypersensitivity, and anaphylaxis. Pittsburgh, Pa: Oncology Nursing Society; 1992: 1-4.
2. Recommendations for the safe handling of parenteral antineoplastic drugs. Washington, DC: Division of Safety, National Institutes of Health; 1983. US Dept of Health and Human Services, Public Health Service publication NIH 83-2621.
3. AMA Council on Scientific Affairs. Guidelines for handling parenteral antineoplastics. *JAMA.* 1985;253:1590-1591.
4. National Study Commission on Cytotoxic Exposure. Recommendations for handling cytotoxic agents. 1987. Available from Louis P. Jeffrey, Chairman, National Study Commission on Cytotoxic Exposure. Massachusetts College of Pharmacy and Allied Health Sciences, 179 Longwood Avenue, Boston, MA 02115.
5. Clinical Oncological Society of Australia. Guidelines and recommendations for safe handling of antineoplastic agents. *Med J Australia.* 1983;1:426-428.
6. Jones RB, Frank R, Mass T. Safe handling of chemotherapeutic agents: a report from the Mount Sinai Medical Center. *CA-A Cancer J for Clin.* 1983;33:258-263.

7. American Society of Hospital Pharmacists. ASHP technical assistance bulletin on handling cytotoxic and hazardous drugs. *Am J Hosp Pharm.* 1990;47:1033-1049.
8. Yodaiken RE, Bennet D. OSHA work-practice guidelines for personnel dealing with cytotoxic (antineoplastic) drugs. *Am J Hosp Pharm.* 1986;43:1193-1204.

U.S. Patent No. 4,307,100
Under license of Pierre Fabre Médicament–Centre National de la Recherche Scientifique-France
©Copyright 1996 Glaxo Wellcome Inc. All rights reserved.
November 1997/RL-512
Shown in Product Identification Guide, page 313

NIMBEX® ℞
[nim 'bex]
(cisatracurium besylate)
Injection

This drug should be administered only by adequately trained individuals familiar with its actions, characteristics, and hazards.

DESCRIPTION

NIMBEX (cisatracurium besylate) is a nondepolarizing skeletal muscle relaxant for intravenous administration. Compared to other neuromuscular blocking agents, it is intermediate in its onset and duration of action. Cisatracurium besylate is one of 10 isomers of atracurium besylate and constitutes approximately 15% of that mixture. Cisatracurium besylate is [1*R*-[1α,2α(1'*R**,2'*R**)]]-2,2'-[1,5-pentanediylbis[oxy(3-oxo-3,1-propanediyl)]]bis[1-[(3,4-dimethoxyphenyl)methyl]-1,2,3,4-tetrahydro-6,7-dimethoxy-2-methylisoquinolinium] dibenzenesulfonate. The molecular formula of the cisatracurium parent bis-cation is $C_{53}H_{72}N_2O_{12}$ and the molecular weight is 929.2. The molecular formula of cisatracurium as the besylate salt is $C_{65}H_{82}N_2O_{18}S_2$ and the molecular weight is 1243.50.

The log of the partition coefficient of cisatracurium besylate is -2.12 in a 1-octanol/distilled water system at 25°C.

NIMBEX Injection is a sterile, non-pyrogenic aqueous solution provided in 5-mL, 10-mL, and 20-mL vials. The pH is adjusted to 3.25 to 3.65 with benzenesulfonic acid. The 5-mL and 10-mL vials each contain cisatracurium besylate, equivalent to 2 mg/mL cisatracurium. The 20-mL vial, **intended for ICU use only,** contains cisatracurium besylate, equivalent to 10 mg/mL cisatracurium. The 10-mL vial, intended for multiple-dose use, contains 0.9% benzyl alcohol as a preservative. The 5-mL and 20-mL vials are single-use vials and do not contain benzyl alcohol.

Cisatracurium besylate slowly loses potency with time at a rate of approximately 5% per *year* under refrigeration (5°C). NIMBEX should be refrigerated at 2° to 8°C (36° to 46°F) in the carton to preserve potency. The rate of loss in potency increases to approximately 5% per *month* at 25°C (77°F). Upon removal from refrigeration to room temperature storage conditions (25°C/77°F), use NIMBEX within 21 days, even if rerefrigerated.

CLINICAL PHARMACOLOGY

NIMBEX binds competitively to cholinergic receptors on the motor end-plate to antagonize the action of acetylcholine, resulting in block of neuromuscular transmission. This action is antagonized by acetylcholinesterase inhibitors such as neostigmine.

Pharmacodynamics: The neuromuscular blocking potency of NIMBEX is approximately threefold that of atracurium besylate. The time to maximum block is up to 2 minutes longer for equipotent doses of NIMBEX compared to atracurium besylate. The clinically effective duration of action and rate of spontaneous recovery from equipotent doses of NIMBEX and atracurium besylate are similar.

The average ED_{95} (dose required to produce 95% suppression of the adductor pollicis muscle twitch response to ulnar nerve stimulation) of cisatracurium is 0.05 mg/kg (range: 0.048 to 0.053) in adults receiving opioid/nitrous oxide/oxygen anesthesia. For comparison, the average ED_{95} for atracurium when also expressed as the parent bis-cation is 0.17 mg/kg under similar anesthetic conditions.

The pharmacodynamics of $2 \times ED_{95}$ to $8 \times ED_{95}$ doses of cisatracurium administered over 5 to 10 seconds during opioid/nitrous oxide/oxygen anesthesia are summarized in Table 1. When the dose is doubled, the clinically effective duration of block increases by approximately 25 minutes. Once recovery begins, the rate of recovery is independent of dose.

Isoflurane or enflurane administered with nitrous oxide/oxygen to achieve 1.25 MAC [Minimum Alveolar Concentration] may prolong the clinically effective duration of action of initial and maintenance doses, and decrease the average infusion rate requirement of NIMBEX. The magnitude of these effects may depend on the duration of administration of the volatile agents. Fifteen to 30 minutes of exposure to 1.25 MAC isoflurane or enflurane had minimal effects on the duration of action of initial doses of NIMBEX and therefore, no adjustment to the initial dose should be necessary when NIMBEX is administered shortly after initiation of volatile agents. In long surgical procedures during enflurane or isoflurane anesthesia, less frequent maintenance dosing, lower maintenance doses, or reduced infusion rates of NIMBEX may be necessary. The average infusion rate requirement may be decreased by as much as 30% to 40%.

The onset, duration of action, and recovery profiles of NIMBEX during propofol/oxygen or propofol/nitrous oxide/oxygen anesthesia are similar to those during opioid/nitrous oxide/oxygen anesthesia.

[See table 1 at bottom of next page]

When administered during the induction of adequate anesthesia using propofol, nitrous oxide/oxygen, and co-induction agents (e.g., fentanyl and midazolam), good or excellent conditions for tracheal intubation occurred in 67/71 (94%) patients in 1.5 to 2.0 minutes following 0.15 mg/kg cisatracurium and in 69/80 (87%) patients in 1.5 minutes following 0.2 mg/kg cisatracurium.

Repeated administration of maintenance doses or a continuous infusion of NIMBEX for up to 3 hours is not associated with development of tachyphylaxis or cumulative neuromuscular blocking effects. The time needed to recover from successive maintenance doses does not change with the number of doses administered as long as partial recovery is allowed to occur between doses. Maintenance doses can therefore be administered at relatively regular intervals with predictable results. The rate of spontaneous recovery of neuromuscular function after infusion is independent of the duration of infusion and comparable to the rate of recovery following initial doses (Table 1).

Long-term infusion (up to 6 days) of NIMBEX during mechanical ventilation in the ICU has been evaluated in two studies. In a randomized, double-blind study using presence of a single twitch during train-of-four (TOF) monitoring to regulate dosage, patients treated with NIMBEX (n = 19) recovered neuromuscular function (T_4:T_1 ratio ≥70%) following termination of infusion in approximately 55 minutes (range: 20 to 270) whereas those treated with vecuronium (n = 12) recovered in 178 minutes (range: 40 minutes to 33 hours). In another study comparing NIMBEX and atracurium, patients recovered neuromuscular function in approximately 50 minutes for both NIMBEX (range: 20 to 175; n = 34) and atracurium (range: 35 to 85; n = 15).

The neuromuscular block produced by NIMBEX is readily antagonized by anticholinesterase agents once recovery has started. As with other nondepolarizing neuromuscular blocking agents, the more profound the neuromuscular block at the time of reversal, the longer the time required for recovery of neuromuscular function.

In children (2 to 12 years) cisatracurium has a lower ED_{95} than in adults (0.04 mg/kg, halothane/nitrous oxide/oxygen anesthesia). At 0.1 mg/kg during opioid anesthesia, cisatracurium had a faster onset and shorter duration of action in children than in adults (Table 1). Recovery following reversal is faster in children than in adults.

Hemodynamics Profile: Cisatracurium has no dose-related effects on mean arterial blood pressure (MAP) or heart rate (HR) following doses ranging from 2 to $8 \times ED_{95}$ (0.1 to 0.4 mg/kg), administered over 5 to 10 seconds, in healthy adult patients (Figure 1).

In patients with serious cardiovascular disease, NIMBEX has no clinically significant effects on MAP or HR following doses up to and including $6 \times ED_{95}$ (0.3 mg/kg), administered over 5 to 10 seconds (Figure 2). In two comparative studies involving patients undergoing coronary artery bypass grafting (CABG), there were no clinically significant differences in the hemodynamic effects following equipotent doses ranging from 0.1 to 0.3 mg/kg cisatracurium or vecuronium. Doses higher than $6 \times ED_{95}$ have not been studied in patients with serious cardiovascular disease.

Unlike atracurium, cisatracurium, at therapeutic doses of $2 \times ED_{95}$ to $8 \times ED_{95}$ (0.1 to 0.4 mg/kg), administered over 5 to 10 seconds, does not cause dose-related elevations in mean plasma histamine concentration. The cardiovascular profile of NIMBEX allows it to be administered by rapid bolus at higher multiples of the ED_{95} than atracurium.

[See figures 1 & 2 at top of next column]

No clinically significant changes in MAP or HR were observed following administration of doses up to 0.1 mg/kg cisatracurium over 5 to 10 seconds in 2- to 12-year-old children receiving either halothane/nitrous oxide/oxygen or opioid/nitrous oxide/oxygen anesthesia.

Pharmacokinetics: ***General:*** The neuromuscular blocking activity of NIMBEX is due to parent drug. Cisatracurium plasma concentration-time data following IV bolus administration are best described by a two-compartment open model (with elimination from both compartments) with an elimination half-life ($t_{1/2}\beta$) of 22 minutes, a plasma clearance (CL) of 4.57 mL/min per kg, and a volume of distribution at steady state (V_{ss}) of 145 mL/kg. Cisatracurium undergoes organ-independent Hofmann elimination (a chemical process dependent on pH and temperature) to form the monoquaternary acrylate metabolite and laudanosine, neither of which has any neuromuscular blocking activity (see Pharmacokinetics: Metabolism section). Following administration of radiolabeled cisatracurium, 95% of the dose was recovered in the urine; less than 10% of the dose was excreted as unchanged parent drug. Laudanosine, a metabolite of cisatracurium (and atracurium) has been noted to cause transient hypotension and, in higher doses, cerebral excitatory effects when administered to several animal species. The relationship between CNS excitation and laudanosine concentrations in humans has not been established (see PRECAUTIONS: Long-term Use in the Intensive Care Unit). Because cisatracurium is three times more potent than atracurium and lower doses are required, the corresponding laudanosine concentrations following cisatracurium are one third of those that would be expected following an equipotent dose of atracurium (see Pharmacokinetics: Special Populations: Intensive Care Unit Patients).

Figure 1

Maximum Percent Change from Preinjection in Heart Rate (HR) and Mean Arterial Pressure (MAP) During First 5 Minutes after Initial 4 x ED_{95} to 8 x ED_{95} Doses of NIMBEX in Healthy Adult Patients Receiving Opioid/Nitrous Oxide/Oxygen Anesthesia (n=44)

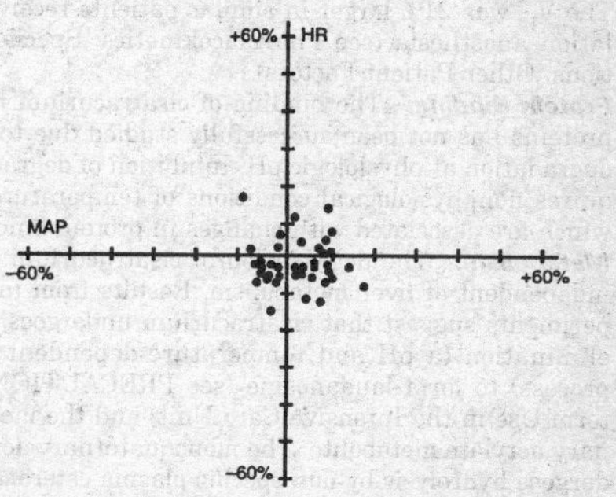

Figure 2

Percent Change from Preinjection in Heart Rate (HR) and Mean Arterial Pressure (MAP) 2 Minutes Following Administration of NIMBEX (2 to 6 x ED_{95}) to Patients Undergoing CABG Surgery Receiving Etomidate/Fentanyl/Midazolam/Oxygen Anesthesia (n=90)

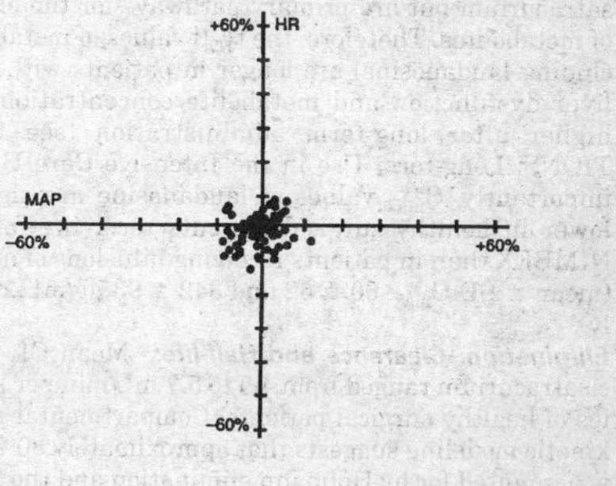

Results from population pharmacokinetic/pharmacodynamic (PK/PD) analyses from 241 healthy surgical patients are summarized in Table 2.

[See table 2 on page 1189]

The magnitude of interpatient variability in CL was low (16%), as expected based on the importance of Hofmann elimination (see Pharmacokinetics: Elimination). The magnitudes of interpatient variability in CL and volume of distribution were low in comparison to those for k_{eo} and EC_{50}. This suggests that any alterations in the time course of cisatracurium-induced block are more likely to be due to variability in the pharmacodynamic parameters than in the pharmacokinetic parameters. Parameter estimates from the population pharmacokinetic analyses were supported by noncompartmental pharmacokinetic analyses on data from healthy patients and from special patient populations.

Conventional pharmacokinetic analyses have shown that the pharmacokinetics of cisatracurium are proportional to dose between 0.1 ($2 \times ED_{95}$) and 0.2 ($4 \times ED_{95}$) mg/kg cisatracurium. In addition, population pharmacokinetic analyses revealed no statistically significant effect of initial dose on CL for doses between 0.1 ($2 \times ED_{95}$) and 0.4 ($8 \times ED_{95}$) mg/kg cisatracurium.

Continued on next page

This product information is based on labeling in effect on June 1, 1998. For further information, contact via direct mail, phone, or web site Medical Information: Glaxo Wellcome Inc., PO Box 13398, Research Triangle Park, NC 27709. Healthcare Professionals (Medical Information): 800-334-0089 Patients (Customer Response Center): 888-TALK2GW (1-888-825-5249) Glaxo Wellcome Corporate Web Site: www.glaxowellcome.com

Nimbex—Cont.

Distribution: The volume of distribution of cisatracurium is limited by its large molecular weight and high polarity. The V_{ss} was equal to 145 mL/kg (Table 2) in healthy 19- to 64-year-old surgical patients receiving opioid anesthesia. The V_{ss} was 21% larger in similar patients receiving inhalation anesthesia (see Pharmacokinetics: Special Populations: Other Patient Factors).

Protein Binding: The binding of cisatracurium to plasma proteins has not been successfully studied due to its rapid degradation at physiologic pH. Inhibition of degradation requires nonphysiological conditions of temperature and pH which are associated with changes in protein binding.

Metabolism: The degradation of cisatracurium is largely independent of liver metabolism. Results from in vitro experiments suggest that cisatracurium undergoes Hofmann elimination (a pH and temperature-dependent chemical process) to form laudanosine (see PRECAUTIONS: Long-term Use in the Intensive Care Unit) and the monoquaternary acrylate metabolite. The monoquaternary acrylate undergoes hydrolysis by non-specific plasma esterases to form the monoquaternary alcohol (MQA) metabolite. The MQA metabolite can also undergo Hofmann elimination but at a much slower rate than cisatracurium. Laudanosine is further metabolized to desmethyl metabolites which are conjugated with glucuronic acid and excreted in the urine.

Organ-independent Hofmann elimination is the predominant pathway for the elimination of cisatracurium. The liver and kidney play a minor role in the elimination of cisatracurium but are primary pathways for the elimination of metabolites. Therefore, the $t_{1/2}\beta$ values of metabolites (including laudanosine) are longer in patients with kidney or liver dysfunction and metabolite concentrations may be higher after long-term administration (see PRECAUTIONS: Long-term Use in the Intensive Care Unit). Most importantly, C_{max} values of laudanosine are significantly lower in healthy surgical patients receiving infusions of NIMBEX than in patients receiving infusions of atracurium (mean ± SD C_{max}: 60 ± 52 and 342 ± 93 ng/mL, respectively).

Elimination: Clearance and Half-life: Mean CL values for cisatracurium ranged from 4.5 to 5.7 mL/min per kg in studies of healthy surgical patients. Compartmental pharmacokinetic modeling suggests that approximately 80% of the CL is accounted for by Hofmann elimination and the remaining 20% by renal and hepatic elimination. These findings are consistent with the low magnitude of interpatient variability in CL (16%) estimated as part of the population PK/PD analyses and with the recovery of parent and metabolites in urine. Following ^{14}C-cisatracurium administration to 6 healthy male patients, 95% of the dose was recovered in the urine (mostly as conjugated metabolites) and 4% in the feces; less than 10% of the dose was excreted as unchanged parent drug in the urine. In 12 healthy surgical patients receiving non-radiolabeled cisatracurium who had Foley catheters placed for surgical management, approximately 15% of the dose was excreted unchanged in the urine.

In studies of healthy surgical patients, mean $t_{1/2}\beta$ values of cisatracurium ranged from 22 to 29 minutes and were consistent with the $t_{1/2}\beta$ of cisatracurium in vitro (29 minutes). The mean ± SD $t_{1/2}\beta$ values of laudanosine were 3.1 ± 0.4 and 3.3 ± 2.1 hours in healthy surgical patients receiving NIMBEX (n = 10) or atracurium (n = 10), respectively. During IV infusions of NIMBEX, peak plasma concentrations (C_{max}) of laudanosine and the MQA metabolite are approximately 6% and 11% of the parent compound, respectively.

Special Populations: Elderly Patients (≥65 years): The results of conventional pharmacokinetic analysis from a study of 12 healthy elderly patients and 12 healthy young adult patients receiving a single IV dose of 0.1 mg/kg NIMBEX are summarized in Table 3. Plasma clearances of cisatracurium were not affected by age; however, the volumes of distribution were slightly larger in elderly patients than in young patients resulting in slightly longer $t_{1/2}\beta$ values for cisatracurium. The rate of equilibration between plasma cisatracurium concentrations and neuromuscular block was slower in elderly patients than in young patients (mean ± SD k_{eo}: 0.071 ± 0.036 and 0.105 ± 0.021 minutes^{-1}, respectively); there was no difference in the patient sensitivity to cisatracurium-induced block, as indicated by EC_{50} values (mean ± SD EC_{50}: 91 ± 22 and 89 ± 23 ng/mL, respectively). These changes were consistent with the 1-minute slower times to maximum block in elderly patients receiving 0.1 mg/kg NIMBEX, when compared to young patients receiving the same dose. The minor differences in PK/PD parameters of cisatracurium between elderly patients and young patients were not associated with clinically significant differences in the recovery profile of NIMBEX.

[See table 3 on next page]

Patients with Hepatic Disease: Table 4 summarizes the conventional pharmacokinetic analysis from a study of NIMBEX in 13 patients with end-stage liver disease undergoing liver transplantation and 11 healthy adult patients undergoing elective surgery. The slightly larger volumes of distribution in liver transplant patients were associated with slightly higher plasma clearances of cisatracurium. The parallel changes in these parameters resulted in no difference in $t_{1/2}\beta$ values. There were no differences in k_{eo} or EC_{50} between patient groups. The times to maximum block were approximately one minute faster in liver transplant patients than in healthy adult patients receiving 0.1 mg/kg NIMBEX. These minor differences in pharmacokinetics were not associated with clinically significant differences in the recovery profile of NIMBEX.

The $t_{1/2}\beta$ values of metabolites are longer in patients with hepatic disease and concentrations may be higher after long-term administration (see Pharmacokinetics: Special Populations: Intensive Care Unit Patients).

[See table 4 on next page]

Patients with Renal Dysfunction: Results from a conventional pharmacokinetic study of NIMBEX in 13 healthy adult patients and 15 patients with end-stage renal disease (ESRD) undergoing elective surgery are summarized in Table 5. The PK/PD parameters of cisatracurium were similar in healthy adult patients and ESRD patients. The times to 90% block were approximately one minute slower in ESRD patients following 0.1 mg/kg NIMBEX. There were no differences in the durations or rates of recovery of NIMBEX between ESRD and healthy adult patients.

The $t_{1/2}\beta$ values of metabolites are longer in patients with renal failure and concentrations may be higher after long-term administration (see Pharmacokinetics: Special Populations: Intensive Care Unit Patients).

[See table 5 on next page]

Population pharmacokinetic analyses revealed that patients with creatinine clearances ≤70 mL/min had a slower rate of equilibration between plasma concentrations and neuromuscular block than patients with normal renal function; this change was associated with a slightly slower (~40 seconds) predicted time to 90% T_1 suppression in patients with renal dysfunction following 0.1 mg/kg NIMBEX. There was no clinically significant alteration in the recovery profile of NIMBEX in patients with renal dysfunction. The recovery profile of NIMBEX is unchanged in the presence of renal or hepatic failure, which is consistent with predominantly organ-independent elimination.

Intensive Care Unit (ICU) Patients: The pharmacokinetics of cisatracurium, atracurium, and their metabolites were determined in six ICU patients receiving NIMBEX and in six ICU patients receiving atracurium and are presented in Table 6. The plasma clearances of cisatracurium and atracurium are similar. The volume of distribution was larger and the $t_{1/2}\beta$ was longer for cisatracurium than for atracurium. The relationships between plasma cisatracurium or atracurium concentrations and neuromuscular block have not been evaluated in ICU patients. The minor differences in pharmacokinetics were not associated with any differences in the recovery profiles of NIMBEX and atracurium in ICU patients.

[See table 6 at top of page 1190]

Plasma metabolite pharmacokinetics are listed in Table 6. Limited pharmacokinetic data are available for patients with liver/kidney dysfunction receiving NIMBEX. Data from studies of atracurium demonstrate that renal/hepatic failure in ICU patients produces little to no effect on its pharmacokinetics, but decreases the biotransformation and elimination of the metabolites. Following atracurium, $t_{1/2}\beta$ values for laudanosine were longer in ICU patients with renal failure than in ICU patients with normal renal function (15 and 6 hours, respectively). The $t_{1/2}\beta$ values of laudanosine were 39 ± 14 hours in ICU patients with liver failure receiving atracurium after an unsuccessful liver

Table 1: Pharmacodynamic Dose Response* of NIMBEX During Opioid/Nitrous Oxide/Oxygen Anesthesia

Initial Dose of NIMBEX (mg/kg)	Time to 90% Block (min)	Time to Maximum Block (min)	Time to Spontaneous Recovery				
			5% Recovery (min)	25% Recovery† (min)	95% Recovery (min)	T_4:T_1 Ratio‡ ≥70% (min)	25%-75% Recovery Index (min)
Adults							
0.1 (2 × ED$_{95}$) (n§ = 98)	3.3 (1.0–8.7)	5.0 (1.2–17.2)	33 (15–51)	42 (22–63)	64 (25–93)	64 (32–91)	13 (5–30)
0.15‖ 3 × ED$_{95}$ (n = 39)	2.6 (1.0–4.4)	3.5 (1.6–6.8)	46 (28–65)	55 (44–74)	76 (60–103)	75 (63–98)	13 (11–16)
0.2 (4 × ED$_{95}$) (n = 30)	2.4 (1.5–4.5)	2.9 (1.9–5.2)	59 (31–103)	65 (43–103)	81 (53–114)	85 (55–114)	12 (2–30)
0.25 (5× ED$_{95}$) (n = 15)	1.6 (0.8–3.3)	2.0 (1.2–3.7)	70 (58–85)	78 (66–86)	91 (76–109)	97 (82–113)	8 (5–12)
0.4 (8× ED$_{95}$) (n = 15)	1.5 (1.3–1.8)	1.9 (1.4–2.3)	83 (37–103)	91 (59–107)	121 (110–134)	126 (115–137)	14 (10–18)
Children (2–12 yr)							
0.08¶ (2× ED$_{95}$) (n = 60)	2.2 (1.2–6.8)	3.3 (1.7–9.7)	22 (11–38)	29 (20–46)	52 (37–64)	50 (37–62)	11 (7–15)
0.1 (n = 16)	1.7 (1.3–2.7)	2.8 (1.8–6.7)	21 (13–31)	28 (21–38)	46 (37–58)	44 (36–58)	10 (7–12)

*Values shown are medians of means from individual studies. Values in parentheses are ranges of individual patient values.
†Clinically effective duration of block.
‡Train-of-four ratio.
§n = the number of patients with Time to Maximum Block data.
‖Propofol anesthesia.
¶Halothane anesthesia.

transplantation and 5 ± 2 hours in similar ICU patients after successful liver transplantation. Therefore, relative to ICU patients with normal renal and hepatic function receiving NIMBEX, metabolite concentrations (plasma and tissues) may be higher in ICU patients with renal or hepatic failure (see Precautions: Long-term Use in the Intensive Care Unit). Consistent with the decreased infusion rate requirements for NIMBEX, metabolite concentrations were lower in patients receiving NIMBEX than in patients receiving atracurium besylate.

Pediatric Patients: The population PK/PD of cisatracurium were described in 20 healthy pediatric patients during halothane anesthesia, using the same model developed for healthy adult patients. The CL was higher in healthy pediatric patients (5.89 mL/min per kg) than in healthy adult patients (4.57 mL/min per kg) during opioid anesthesia. The rate of equilibration between plasma concentrations and neuromuscular block, as indicated by k_{eo}, was faster in healthy pediatric patients receiving halothane anesthesia (0.1330 minutes^{-1}) than in healthy adult patients receiving opioid anesthesia (0.0575 minutes^{-1}). The EC_{50} in healthy pediatric patients (125 ng/mL) was similar to the value in healthy adult patients (141 ng/mL) during opioid anesthesia. The minor differences in the PK/PD parameters of cisatracurium were associated with a faster time to onset and a shorter duration of cisatracurium-induced neuromuscular block in pediatric patients.

Other Patient Factors: Population PK/PD analyses revealed that gender and obesity were associated with statistically significant effects on the pharmacokinetics and/or pharmacodynamics of cisatracurium; these factors were not associated with clinically significant alterations in the predicted onset or recovery profile of NIMBEX. The use of inhalation agents was associated with a 21% larger V_{ss}, a 78% larger k_{eo}, and a 15% lower EC_{50} for cisatracurium. These changes resulted in a slightly faster ($\sim$45 seconds) predicted time to 90% T_1 suppression in patients receiving 0.1mg/kg cisatracurium during inhalation anesthesia than in patients receiving the same dose of cisatracurium during opioid anesthesia; however, there were no clinically significant differences in the predicted recovery profile of NIMBEX between patient groups.

Individualization of Dosages: DOSES OF **NIMBEX** SHOULD BE INDIVIDUALIZED AND A PERIPHERAL NERVE STIMULATOR SHOULD BE USED TO MEASURE NEUROMUSCULAR FUNCTION DURING ADMINISTRATION OF **NIMBEX** IN ORDER TO MONITOR DRUG EFFECT, TO DETERMINE THE NEED FOR ADDITIONAL DOSES, AND TO CONFIRM RECOVERY FROM NEUROMUSCULAR BLOCK.

Based on the known action of NIMBEX and other neuromuscular blocking agents, the following factors should be considered when administering NIMBEX:

Renal and Hepatic Disease: See PRECAUTIONS section.

Long-Term Use in the Intensive Care Unit (ICU): The long-term infusion (up to 6 days) of NIMBEX during mechanical ventilation in the ICU has been evaluated in two studies. Average infusion rates of approximately 3 mcg/kg per minute (range: 0.5 to 10.2) were required to achieve adequate neuromuscular block. As with other neuromuscular blocking agents, these data indicate the presence of wide interpatient variability in dosage requirements. In addition, dosage requirements may increase or decrease with time (see PRECAUTIONS). Use of NIMBEX in the ICU for longer than 6 days has not been studied.

Drugs or Conditions Causing Potentiation of or Resistance to Neuromuscular Block: Persons with certain pre-existing conditions or receiving certain drugs may require individualization of dosing (see PRECAUTIONS).

Burns: Patients with burns have been shown to develop resistance to nondepolarizing neuromuscular blocking agents, and may require individualization of dosing (see PRECAUTIONS).

INDICATIONS AND USAGE

NIMBEX is an intermediate-onset/intermediate-duration neuromuscular blocking agent indicated for inpatients and outpatients as an adjunct to general anesthesia, to facilitate tracheal intubation, and to provide skeletal muscle relaxation during surgery or mechanical ventilation in the ICU.

CONTRAINDICATIONS

NIMBEX is contraindicated in patients known to have an allergic hypersensitivity to NIMBEX or other bis-benzylisoquinolinium agents. Use of NIMBEX from vials containing benzyl alcohol as a preservative is contraindicated in patients with a known hypersensitivity to benzyl alcohol.

WARNINGS

NIMBEX SHOULD BE ADMINISTERED IN CAREFULLY ADJUSTED DOSAGE BY OR UNDER THE SUPERVISION OF EXPERIENCED CLINICIANS WHO ARE FAMILIAR WITH THE DRUG'S ACTIONS AND THE POSSIBLE COMPLICATIONS OF ITS USE. THE DRUG SHOULD NOT BE ADMINISTERED UNLESS PERSONNEL AND FACILITIES FOR RESUSCITATION AND LIFE SUPPORT (TRACHEAL INTUBATION, ARTIFICIAL VENTILATION, OXYGEN THERAPY), AND AN ANTAGONIST OF **NIMBEX** ARE IMMEDIATELY AVAILABLE. IT IS RECOMMENDED THAT A PERIPHERAL NERVE STIMULATOR BE USED TO MEASURE NEUROMUSCULAR FUNCTION DURING THE ADMINISTRATION OF **NIMBEX** IN ORDER TO MONITOR DRUG EFFECT, DETERMINE THE NEED FOR ADDITIONAL DOSES, AND CONFIRM RECOVERY FROM NEUROMUSCULAR BLOCK.

NIMBEX HAS NO KNOWN EFFECT ON CONSCIOUSNESS, PAIN THRESHOLD, OR CEREBRATION. TO AVOID DISTRESS TO THE PATIENT, NEUROMUSCULAR BLOCK SHOULD NOT BE INDUCED BEFORE UNCONSCIOUSNESS.

NIMBEX Injection is acidic (pH 3.25 to 3.65) and may not be compatible with alkaline solutions having a pH greater than 8.5 (e.g., barbiturate solutions).

The 10-mL multiple-dose vials of NIMBEX contain benzyl alcohol. In newborn infants, benzyl alcohol has been associated with an increased incidence of neurological and other complications which are sometimes fatal. Single-use vials (5 mL and 20 mL) of NIMBEX do not contain benzyl alcohol (see PRECAUTIONS: Pediatric Use).

PRECAUTIONS

Because of its intermediate onset of action, NIMBEX is not recommended for rapid sequence endotracheal intubation. Recommended doses of NIMBEX have no clinically significant effects on heart rate; therefore, NIMBEX will not counteract the bradycardia produced by many anesthetic agents or by vagal stimulation.

Neuromuscular blocking agents may have a profound effect in patients with neuromuscular diseases (e.g., myasthenia

---

Table 2: Key Population PK/PD Parameter Estimates for Cisatracurium in Healthy Surgical Patients* Following 0.1 ($2 \times ED_{95}$) to 0.4 mg/kg ($8 \times ED_{95}$) NIMBEX

Parameter	Estimate†	Magnitude of Interpatient Variability (CV)‡
CL (mL/min/kg)	4.57	16%
V_{ss} (mL/kg)§	145	27%
k_{eo} (min^{-1})‖	0.0575	61%
EC_{50} (ng/mL)¶	141	52%

*Healthy male nonobese patients 19–64 years of age with creatinine clearance values greater than 70 mL/min who received cisatracurium during opioid anesthesia and had venous samples collected.
†The percent standard error of the mean (%SEM) ranged from 3% to 12% indicating good precision for the PK/PD estimates.
‡Expressed as a coefficient of variation; the %SEM ranged from 20% to 35% indicating adequate precision for the estimates of interpatient variability.
§V_{ss} is the volume of distribution at steady state estimated using a two-compartment model with elimination from both compartments. V_{ss} is equal to the sum of the volume in the central compartment (V_c) and the volume in the peripheral compartment (V_p); interpatient variability could only be estimated for V_c.
‖Rate constant describing the equilibration between plasma concentrations and neuromuscular block.
¶Concentration required to produce 50% T_1 suppression; an index of patient sensitivity.

Table 3: Pharmacokinetic Parameters* of Cisatracurium in Healthy Elderly and Young Adult Patients Following 0.1 mg/kg ($2 \times ED_{95}$) NIMBEX (Isoflurane/Nitrous Oxide/Oxygen Anesthesia)

Parameter	Healthy Elderly Patients	Healthy Young Adult Patients
Elimination Half-Life ($t_{1/2}\beta$, min)	25.8 ± 3.6†	22.1 ± 2.5
Volume of Distribution at Steady State‡ (mL/kg)	156 ± 17†	133 ± 15
Plasma Clearance (mL/min/kg)	5.7 ± 1.0	5.3 ± 0.9

*Values presented are mean $\pm$ SD.
†P <0.05 for comparisons between healthy elderly and healthy young adult patients.
‡Volume of distribution is underestimated because elimination from the peripheral compartment is ignored.

Table 4: Pharmacokinetic Parameters* of Cisatracurium in Healthy Adult Patients and in Patients Undergoing Liver Transplantation Following 0.1 mg/kg ($2 \times ED_{95}$) NIMBEX (Isoflurane/Nitrous Oxide/Oxygen Anesthesia)

Parameter	Liver Transplant Patients	Healthy Adult Patients
Elimination Half-Life ($t_{1/2}\beta$, min)	24.4 ± 2.9	23.5 ± 3.5
Volume of Distribution at Steady State‡ (mL/kg)	195 ± 38†	161 ± 23
Plasma Clearance (mL/min/kg)	6.6 ± 1.1†	5.7 ± 0.8

*Values presented are mean $\pm$ SD.
†P <0.05 for comparisons between liver transplant patients and healthy adult patients.
‡Volume of distribution is underestimated because elimination from the peripheral compartment is ignored.

Table 5: Pharmacokinetic Parameters* for Cisatracurium in Healthy Adult Patients and in Patients With End-Stage Renal Disease (ESRD) Receiving 0.1 mg/kg ($2 \times ED_{95}$) NIMBEX (Opioid/Nitrous Oxide/Oxygen Anesthesia)

Parameter	Healthy Adult Patients	ESRD Patients
Elimination Half-Life ($t_{1/2}\beta$, min)	29.4 ± 4.1	32.3 ± 6.3
Volume of Distribution at Steady State† (mL/kg)	149 ± 35	160 ± 32
Plasma Clearance (mL/min/kg)	4.66 ± 0.86	4.26 ± 0.62

*Values presented as mean $\pm$ SD.
†Volume of distribution is underestimated because elimination from the peripheral compartment is ignored.

Continued on next page

This product information is based on labeling in effect on June 1, 1998. For further information, contact via direct mail, phone, or web site Medical Information: Glaxo Wellcome Inc., PO Box 13398, Research Triangle Park, NC 27709. Healthcare Professionals (Medical Information): 800-334-0089 Patients (Customer Response Center): 888-TALK2GW (1-888-825-5249) Glaxo Wellcome Corporate Web Site: www.glaxowellcome.com

Nimbex—Cont.

gravis and the myasthenic syndrome). In these and other conditions in which prolonged neuromuscular block is a possibility (e.g., carcinomatosis), the use of a peripheral nerve stimulator and a dose of not more than 0.02 mg/kg NIMBEX is recommended to assess the level of neuromuscular block and to monitor dosage requirements.

Patients with burns have been shown to develop resistance to nondepolarizing neuromuscular blocking agents, including atracurium. The extent of altered response depends upon the size of the burn and the time elapsed since the burn injury. NIMBEX has not been studied in patients with burns; however, based on its structural similarity to atracurium, the possibility of increased dosing requirements and shortened duration of action must be considered if NIMBEX is administered to burn patients.

Patients with hemiparesis or paraparesis also may demonstrate resistance to nondepolarizing muscle relaxants in the affected limbs. To avoid inaccurate dosing, neuromuscular monitoring should be performed on a non-paretic limb.

Acid-base and/or serum electrolyte abnormalities may potentiate or antagonize the action of neuromuscular blocking agents.

No data are available to support the use of NIMBEX by intramuscular injection.

Renal and Hepatic Disease: No clinically significant alterations in the recovery profile were observed in patients with renal dysfunction or in patients with end-stage liver disease following a 0.1-mg/kg dose of cisatracurium. The onset time was approximately 1 minute faster in patients with end-stage liver disease and approximately 1 minute slower in patients with renal dysfunction than in healthy adult control patients.

Malignant Hyperthermia (MH): In a study of MH-susceptible pigs, cisatracurium besylate (highest dose 2000 mcg/kg equivalent to 3 × ED_{95} in pigs and 40 × ED_{95} in humans) did not trigger MH. Cisatracurium besylate has not been studied in MH-susceptible patients. Because MH can develop in the absence of established triggering agents, the clinician should be prepared to recognize and treat MH in any patient undergoing general anesthesia.

Long-Term Use in the Intensive Care Unit (ICU): Long-term infusion (up to 6 days) of NIMBEX during mechanical ventilation in the ICU has been safely used in two studies. Dosage requirements may increase or decrease with time (see CLINICAL PHARMACOLOGY: Individualization of Doses).

Little information is available on the plasma levels and clinical consequences of cisatracurium metabolites that may accumulate during days to weeks of cisatracurium administration in ICU patients. Laudanosine, a major, biologically active metabolite of atracurium and cisatracurium without neuromuscular blocking activity, produces transient hypotension and, in higher doses, cerebral excitatory effects (generalized muscle twitching and seizures) when administered to several species of animals. There have been rare spontaneous reports of seizures in ICU patients who have received atracurium or other agents. These patients usually had predisposing causes (such as cranial trauma, cerebral edema, hypoxic encephalopathy, viral encephalitis, uremia). There are insufficient data to determine whether or not laudanosine contributes to seizures in ICU patients. Consistent with the decreased infusion rate requirements for NIMBEX, laudanosine concentrations were lower in patients receiving NIMBEX than in patients receiving atracurium for up to 48 hours (see Pharmacokinetics: Special Populations: Intensive Care Unit Patients).

In a randomized, double-blind study using train-of-four nerve stimulator monitoring to maintain at least one visible twitch, evaluable patients treated with NIMBEX (n = 19) recovered neuromuscular function (T_4:T_1 ratio ≥70%) following termination of infusion in approximately 55 minutes (range: 20 to 270) whereas evaluable vecuronium-treated patients (n = 12) recovered in 178 minutes (range: 40 minutes to 33 hours). In another study comparing NIMBEX and atracurium, patients recovered neuromuscular function in approximately 50 minutes for both NIMBEX (range: 20 to 175; n = 34) and atracurium (range: 35 to 85; n = 15).

WHENEVER THE USE OF **NIMBEX** OR ANY OTHER NEUROMUSCULAR BLOCKING AGENT IN THE ICU IS CONTEMPLATED, IT IS RECOMMENDED THAT NEUROMUSCULAR FUNCTION BE MONITORED DURING ADMINISTRATION WITH A NERVE STIMULATOR. ADDITIONAL DOSES OF **NIMBEX** OR ANY OTHER NEUROMUSCULAR BLOCKING AGENT SHOULD NOT BE GIVEN BEFORE THERE IS A DEFINITE RESPONSE TO NERVE STIMULATION. IF NO RESPONSE IS ELICITED, INFUSION ADMINISTRATION SHOULD BE DISCONTINUED UNTIL A RESPONSE RETURNS.

The effects of hemofiltration, hemodialysis, and hemoperfusion on plasma levels of NIMBEX and its metabolites are unknown.

Drug Interactions: NIMBEX has been used safely following varying degrees of recovery from succinylcholine-induced neuromuscular block. Administration of 0.1-mg/kg (2 × ED_{95}) NIMBEX at 10% or 95% recovery following an intubating dose of succinylcholine (1 mg/kg) produced ≥95% neuromuscular block. The time to onset of maximum block following NIMBEX is approximately 2 minutes faster with prior administration of succinylcholine. Prior administration of succinylcholine had no effect on the duration of neuromuscular block following initial or maintenance bolus doses of NIMBEX. Infusion requirements of NIMBEX in patients administered succinylcholine prior to infusions of NIMBEX were comparable to or slightly greater than when succinylcholine was not administered.

Table 6: Parameter Estimates* for Cisatracurium, Atracurium, and Metabolites in ICU Patients After Long-Term (24—48 Hour) Administration of NIMBEX or Atracurium Besylate

	Parameter	Cisatracurium (n = 6)	Atracurium (n = 6)
Parent Compound	CL (mL/min/kg)	7.45 ± 1.02	7.49 ± 0.66†
	$t_{1/2}\beta$ (min)	26.8 ± 11.1	16.5 ± 6.0†
	Vβ (mL/kg)‡	280 ± 103	178 ± 71†
Laudanosine	C_{max} (ng/mL)	707 ± 360	2318 ± 1498
	$t_{1/2}\beta$ (hrs)	6.6 ± 4.1	8.4 ± 7.3
MQA metabolite	C_{max} (ng/mL)	152–181§	943 ± 333‖
	$t_{1/2}\beta$ (min)	26–31§	21–58§

*Presented as mean ± standard deviation.
†n = 5.
‡Volume of distribution during the terminal elimination phase, an underestimate because elimination from the peripheral compartment is ignored.
§n = 2, range presented.
‖n = 3.

The use of NIMBEX before succinylcholine to attenuate some of the side effects of succinylcholine has not been studied.

Although not studied systematically in clinical trials, no drug interactions were observed when vecuronium, pancuronium, or atracurium were administered following varying degrees of recovery from single doses or infusions of NIMBEX.

Isoflurane or enflurane administered with nitrous oxide/oxygen to achieve 1.25 MAC (Minimum Alveolar Concentration) may prolong the clinically effective duration of action of initial and maintenance doses of NIMBEX and decrease the required infusion rate of NIMBEX. The magnitude of these effects may depend on the duration of administration of the volatile agents. Fifteen to 30 minutes of exposure to 1.25 MAC isoflurane or enflurane had minimal effects on the duration of action of initial doses of NIMBEX and therefore, no adjustment to the initial dose should be necessary when NIMBEX is administered shortly after initiation of volatile agents. In long surgical procedures during enflurane or isoflurane anesthesia, less frequent maintenance dosing, lower maintenance doses, or reduced infusion rates of NIMBEX may be necessary. The average infusion rate requirement may be decreased by as much as 30% to 40%.

In clinical studies propofol had no effect on the duration of action or dosing requirements for NIMBEX. Other drugs which may enhance the neuromuscular blocking action of nondepolarizing agents such as NIMBEX include certain antibiotics (e.g., aminoglycosides, tetracyclines, bacitracin, polymyxins, lincomycin, clindamycin, colistin, and sodium colistemethate), magnesium salts, lithium, local anesthetics, procainamide, and quinidine.

Resistance to the neuromuscular blocking action of nondepolarizing neuromuscular blocking agents has been demonstrated in patients chronically administered phenytoin or carbamazepine. While the effects of chronic phenytoin or carbamazepine therapy on the action of NIMBEX are unknown, slightly shorter durations of neuromuscular block may be anticipated and infusion rate requirements may be higher.

Drug/Laboratory Test Interactions: None known.

Carcinogenesis, Mutagenesis, Impairment of Fertility: Carcinogenesis and fertility studies have not been performed. Cisatracurium besylate was evaluated in a battery of four short-term mutagenicity tests. It was non-mutagenic in the Ames Salmonella assay, a rat bone marrow cytogenetic assay, and an in vitro human lymphocyte cytogenetics assay. As was the case with atracurium, the mouse lymphoma assay was positive both in the presence and absence of exogenous metabolic activation (rat liver S-9). In the absence of S-9, cisatracurium besylate was positive at in vitro cisatracurium concentrations of 40 mcg/mL and higher. The highest non-mutagenic concentration (30 mcg/mL) and incubation time (4 hours) resulted in an AUC approximately 120 times that noted in clinical studies and approximately 8.5 times the mean peak clinical concentration noted. In the presence of S-9, cisatracurium besylate was positive at a cisatracurium concentration of 300 mcg/mL but not at lower or higher concentrations.

Pregnancy: *Teratogenic Effects:* Pregnancy Category B. Teratology testing in nonventilated pregnant rats treated subcutaneously with maximum subparalyzing doses (4 mg/kg daily; equivalent to 8 × the human ED_{95} following a bolus dose of 0.2 mg/kg IV) and in ventilated rats treated intravenously with paralyzing doses of NIMBEX at 0.5 and 1.0 mg/kg; equivalent to 10 × and 20 × the human ED_{95} dose, respectively, revealed no maternal or fetal toxicity or teratogenic effects. There are no adequate and well-controlled studies of NIMBEX in pregnant women. Because animal studies are not always predictive of human response, NIMBEX should be used during pregnancy only if clearly needed.

Labor and Delivery: The use of NIMBEX during labor, vaginal delivery, or cesarean section has not been studied in humans and it is not known whether NIMBEX administered to the mother has effects on the fetus. Doses of 0.2 or 0.4 mg/kg cisatracurium given to female beagles undergoing cesarean section resulted in negligible levels of cisatracurium in umbilical vessel blood of neonates and no deleterious effects on the puppies. The action of neuromuscular blocking agents may be enhanced by magnesium salts administered for the management of toxemia of pregnancy.

Nursing Mothers: It is not known whether cisatracurium besylate is excreted in human milk. Because many drugs are excreted in human milk, caution should be exercised following administration of NIMBEX to a nursing woman.

Pediatric Use: NIMBEX has not been studied in pediatric patients below the age of 2 years (see CLINICAL PHARMACOLOGY and DOSAGE AND ADMINISTRATION for clinical experience and recommendations for use in children 2 to 12 years of age).

Geriatric Use: NIMBEX was safely administered during clinical trials to 145 elderly (≥65 years) patients, including a subset of patients with significant cardiovascular disease (see CLINICAL PHARMACOLOGY, Elderly Patients and Hemodynamics Profile sections).

Minor differences in the pharmacokinetics of cisatracurium between elderly and young adult patients are not associated with clinically significant differences in the recovery profile of NIMBEX following a single 0.1-mg/kg dose; the time to maximum block is approximately 1 minute slower in elderly patients (see CLINICAL PHARMACOLOGY: Pharmacokinetics).

ADVERSE REACTIONS

Observed in Clinical Trials of Surgical Patients: Adverse experiences were uncommon among the 945 surgical patients who received NIMBEX in conjunction with other drugs in US and European clinical studies in the course of a wide variety of procedures in patients receiving opioid, propofol, or inhalation anesthesia. The following adverse experiences were judged by investigators during the clinical trials to have a possible causal relationship to administration of NIMBEX:

Incidence Greater than 1%: None.

Incidence Less than 1%:

Cardiovascular: Bradycardia (0.4%), hypotension (0.2%), flushing (0.2%).

Respiratory: Bronchospasm (0.2%).

Dermatological: Rash (0.1%).

Observed in Clinical Trials of Intensive Care Unit Patients: Adverse experiences were uncommon among the 68 ICU patients who received NIMBEX in conjunction with other drugs in US and European clinical studies. One patient experienced bronchospasm. In one of the two ICU studies, a randomized and double-blind study of ICU patients using

TOF neuromuscular monitoring, there were two reports of prolonged recovery (167 and 270 minutes) among 28 patients administered NIMBEX and 13 reports of prolonged recovery (range: 90 minutes to 33 hours) among 30 patients administered vecuronium.

Observed During Clinical Practice: In addition to adverse events reported from clinical trials, the following events have been identified during post-approval use of cisatracurium besylate in conjunction with one or more anesthetic agents in clinical practice. Because they are reported voluntarily from a population of unknown size, estimates of frequency cannot be made. These events have been chosen for inclusion due to a combination of their seriousness, frequency of reporting, or potential causal connection to cisatracurium besylate.

General: Hypersensitivity reactions including anaphylactic or anaphylactoid responses which, in rare instances, were severe.

Musculoskeletal: Prolonged neuromuscular block, inadequate neuromuscular block.

OVERDOSAGE

Overdosage with neuromuscular blocking agents may result in neuromuscular block beyond the time needed for surgery and anesthesia. The primary treatment is maintenance of a patent airway and controlled ventilation until recovery of normal neuromuscular function is assured. Once recovery from neuromuscular block begins, further recovery may be facilitated by administration of an anticholinesterase agent (e.g., neostigmine, edrophonium) in conjunction with an appropriate anticholinergic agent (see Antagonism of Neuromuscular Block below).

Antagonism of Neuromuscular Block: ANTAGONISTS (SUCH AS NEOSTIGMINE AND EDROPHONIUM) SHOULD NOT BE ADMINISTERED WHEN COMPLETE NEUROMUSCULAR BLOCK IS EVIDENT OR SUSPECTED. THE USE OF A PERIPHERAL NERVE STIMULATOR TO EVALUATE RECOVERY AND ANTAGONISM OF NEUROMUSCULAR BLOCK IS RECOMMENDED. Administration of 0.04 to 0.07 mg/kg neostigmine at approximately 10% recovery from neuromuscular block (range: 0 to 15%) produced 95% recovery of the muscle twitch response and a $T_4:T_1$ ratio $\geq$70% in an average of 9 to 10 minutes. The times from 25% recovery of the muscle twitch response to a $T_4:T_1$ ratio $\geq$70% following these doses of neostigmine averaged 7 minutes. The mean 25% to 75% recovery index following reversal was 3 to 4 minutes.

Administration of 1.0 mg/kg edrophonium at approximately 25% recovery from neuromuscular block (range: 16% to 30%) produced 95% recovery and a $T_4:T_1$ ratio $\geq$70% in an average of 3 to 5 minutes.

Patients administered antagonists should be evaluated for evidence of adequate clinical recovery (e.g., 5-second head lift and grip strength). Ventilation must be supported until no longer required.

The onset of antagonism may be delayed in the presence of debilitation, cachexia, carcinomatosis, and the concomitant use of certain broad spectrum antibiotics, or anesthetic agents and other drugs which enhance neuromuscular block or separately cause respiratory depression (see PRECAUTIONS: Drug Interactions). Under such circumstances the management is the same as that of prolonged neuromuscular block (see OVERDOSAGE).

DOSAGE AND ADMINISTRATION

NIMBEX SHOULD ONLY BE ADMINISTERED INTRAVENOUSLY.

The dosage information provided below is intended as a guide only. Doses of NIMBEX should be individualized (see CLINICAL PHARMACOLOGY: Individualization of Dosages). The use of a peripheral nerve stimulator will permit the most advantageous use of NIMBEX, minimize the possibility of overdosage or underdosage, and assist in the evaluation of recovery.

Adults: *Initial Doses:* One of two intubating doses of NIMBEX may be chosen, based on the desired time to intubation and the anticipated length of surgery. Doses of 0.15 (3 × ED$_{95}$) and 0.20 (4 × ED$_{95}$) mg/kg NIMBEX, as components of a propofol/nitrous oxide/oxygen induction-intubation technique, may produce generally good or excellent conditions for tracheal intubation in 2.0 and 1.5 minutes, respectively. The clinically effective durations of action for 0.15 and 0.20 mg/kg NIMBEX during propofol anesthesia are 55 minutes (range: 44 to 74 minutes) and 61 minutes (range: 41 to 81 minutes), respectively. Lower doses may result in a longer time for the development of satisfactory intubation conditions. In addition to the dose of the neuromuscular blocking agent, the presence of co-induction agents (e.g., fentanyl and midazolam) and the depth of anesthesia are factors that can influence intubation conditions. Doses up to 8 × ED$_{95}$ NIMBEX have been safely administered to healthy adult patients and the larger doses are associated with longer clinically effective durations of action (see CLINICAL PHARMACOLOGY).

Because slower times to onset of complete neuromuscular block were observed in elderly patients and patients with renal dysfunction, extending the interval between administration of NIMBEX and the intubation attempt for these patients may be required to achieve adequate intubation conditions.

A dose of 0.03 mg/kg NIMBEX is recommended for maintenance of neuromuscular block during prolonged surgical procedures. Maintenance doses of 0.03 mg/kg each sustain neuromuscular block for approximately 20 minutes. Maintenance dosing is generally required 40 to 50 minutes following an initial dose of 0.15 mg/kg NIMBEX and 50 to 60 minutes following an initial dose of 0.20 mg/kg NIMBEX, but the need for maintenance doses should be determined by clinical criteria. For shorter or longer durations of action, smaller or larger maintenance doses may be administered. Isoflurane or enflurane administered with nitrous oxide/oxygen to achieve 1.25 MAC (Minimum Alveolar Concentration) may prolong the clinically effective duration of action of initial and maintenance doses. The magnitude of these effects may depend on the duration of administration of the volatile agents. Fifteen to 30 minutes of exposure to 1.25 MAC isoflurane or enflurane had minimal effects on the duration of action of initial doses of NIMBEX and therefore, no adjustment to the initial dose should be necessary when NIMBEX is administered shortly after initiation of volatile agents. In long surgical procedures during enflurane or isoflurane anesthesia, less frequent maintenance dosing or lower maintenance doses of NIMBEX may be necessary. No adjustments to the initial dose are required when used in patients receiving propofol anesthesia.

Children: *Initial Doses:* The recommended dose of NIMBEX for children 2 to 12 years of age is 0.10 mg/kg administered over 5 to 10 seconds during either halothane or opioid anesthesia. When administered during stable opioid/nitrous oxide/oxygen anesthesia, 0.10 mg/kg NIMBEX produces maximum neuromuscular block in an average of 2.8 minutes (range: 1.8 to 6.7 minutes) and clinically effective block for 28 minutes (range: 21 to 38 minutes). NIMBEX has not been studied in pediatric patients below the age of 2 years.

Use by Continuous Infusion: *Infusion in the Operating Room (OR):* After administration of an initial bolus dose of NIMBEX, a diluted solution of NIMBEX can be administered by continuous infusion to adults and children aged 2 or more years for maintenance of neuromuscular block during extended surgical procedures. Infusion of NIMBEX should be individualized for each patient. The rate of administration should be adjusted according to the patient's response as determined by peripheral nerve stimulation. Accurate dosing is best achieved using a precision infusion device.

Infusion of NIMBEX should be initiated only after early evidence of spontaneous recovery from the initial bolus dose. An initial infusion rate of 3 mcg/kg per minute may be required to rapidly counteract the spontaneous recovery of neuromuscular function. Thereafter, a rate of 1 to 2 mcg/kg per minute should be adequate to maintain continuous neuromuscular block in the range of 89% to 99% in most pediatric and adult patients under opioid/nitrous oxide/oxygen anesthesia.

Reduction of the infusion rate by up to 30% to 40% should be considered when NIMBEX is administered during stable isoflurane or enflurane anesthesia (administered with nitrous oxide/oxygen at the 1.25 MAC level). Greater reductions in the infusion rate of NIMBEX may be required with longer durations of administration of isoflurane or enflurane.

The rate of infusion of atracurium required to maintain adequate surgical relaxation in patients undergoing coronary artery bypass surgery with induced hypothermia (25° to 28°) is approximately half the rate required during normothermia. Based on the structural similarity between NIMBEX and atracurium, a similar effect on the infusion rate of NIMBEX may be expected.

Spontaneous recovery from neuromuscular block following discontinuation of infusion of NIMBEX may be expected to proceed at a rate comparable to that following administration of a single bolus dose.

Infusion in the Intensive Care Unit (ICU): The principles for infusion of NIMBEX in the OR are also applicable to use in the ICU. An infusion rate of approximately 3 mcg/kg per minute (range: 0.5 to 10.2 mcg/kg per minute) should provide adequate neuromuscular block in adult patients in the ICU. There may be wide interpatient variability in dosage requirements and these may increase or decrease with time (see PRECAUTIONS: Long-Term Use in the Intensive Care Unit [ICU]). Following recovery from neuromuscular block, readministration of a bolus dose may be necessary to quickly re-establish neuromuscular block prior to reinstitution of the infusion.

Infusion Rate Tables: The amount of infusion solution required per minute will depend upon the concentration of NIMBEX in the infusion solution, the desired dose of NIMBEX, and the patient's weight. The contribution of the infusion solution to the fluid requirements of the patient also must be considered. Tables 7 and 8 provide guidelines for delivery, in mL/hr (equivalent to microdrops/minute when 60 microdrops = 1 mL), of NIMBEX solutions in concentrations of 0.1 mg/mL (10 mg/100 mL) or 0.4 mg/mL (40 mg/100 mL).

[See tables 7 & 8 above]

NIMBEX Injection Compatibility and Admixtures: *Y-site Administration:* NIMBEX Injection is acidic (pH = 3.25 to 3.65) and may not be compatible with alkaline solution having a pH greater than 8.5 (e.g., barbiturate solutions).
Studies have shown that NIMBEX Injection is compatible with:
• 5% Dextrose Injection, USP
• 0.9% Sodium Chloride Injection, USP

Continued on next page

Table 7: Infusion Rates of NIMBEX for Maintenance of Neuromuscular Block During Opioid/Nitrous Oxide/Oxygen Anesthesia for a Concentration of 0.1 mg/mL

| Patient Weight (kg) | Drug Delivery Rate (mcg/kg per minute) | | | | |
| | 1.0 | 1.5 | 2.0 | 3.0 | 5.0 |
	Infusion Delivery Rate (mL/hr)				
10	6	9	12	18	30
45	27	41	54	81	135
70	42	63	84	126	210
100	60	90	120	180	300

Table 8: Infusion Rates of NIMBEX for Maintenance of Neuromuscular Block During Opioid/Nitrous Oxide/Oxygen Anesthesia for a Concentration of 0.4 mg/mL

| Patient Weight (kg) | Drug Delivery Rate (mcg/kg per minute) | | | | |
| | 1.0 | 1.5 | 2.0 | 3.0 | 5.0 |
	Infusion Delivery Rate (mL/hr)				
10	1.5	2.3	3.0	4.5	7.5
45	6.8	10.1	13.5	20.3	33.8
70	10.5	15.8	21.0	31.5	52.5
100	15.0	22.5	30.0	45.0	75.0

This product information is based on labeling in effect on June 1, 1998. For further information, contact via direct mail, phone, or web site Medical Information: Glaxo Wellcome Inc., PO Box 13398, Research Triangle Park, NC 27709. Healthcare Professionals (Medical Information): 800-334-0089 Patients (Customer Response Center): 888-TALK2GW (1-888-825-5249) Glaxo Wellcome Corporate Web Site: www.glaxowellcome.com

Nimbex—Cont.

- 5% Dextrose and 0.9% Sodium Chloride Injection, USP
- SUFENTA® (sufentanil citrate) Injection, diluted as directed
- ALFENTA® (alfentanil hydrochloride) Injection, diluted as directed
- SUBLIMAZE® (fentanyl citrate) Injection, diluted as directed
- VERSED® (midazolam hydrochloride) Injection, diluted as directed
- Droperidol Injection, diluted as directed

NIMBEX Injection is not compatible with DIPRIVAN® (propofol) Injection or TORADOL® (ketorolac) Injection for Y-site administration. Studies of other parenteral products have not been conducted.

Dilution Stability: NIMBEX Injection diluted in 5% Dextrose Injection, USP; 0.9% Sodium Chloride Injection, USP; or 5% Dextrose and 0.9% Sodium Chloride Injection, USP to 0.1 mg/mL may be stored either under refrigeration or at room temperature for 24 hours without significant loss of potency. Dilutions to 0.1 mg/mL or 0.2 mg/mL in 5% Dextrose and Lactated Ringer's Injection may be stored under refrigeration for 24 hours. NIMBEX Injection should not be diluted in Lactated Ringer's Injection, USP due to chemical instability.

NOTE: Parenteral drug products should be inspected visually for particulate matter and discoloration prior to administration whenever solution and container permit. Solutions which are not clear, or contain visible particulates, should not be used. NIMBEX Injection is a colorless to slightly yellow or greenish-yellow solution.

HOW SUPPLIED

NIMBEX Injection, 2 mg cisatracurium in each mL.
5-mL Single-Use Vials. Package of 10 (NDC 0173-0540-50).
10-mL Multiple-Dose Vials containing 0.9% w/v benzyl alcohol as a preservative (see WARNINGS concerning newborn infants). Package of 10 (NDC 0173-0546-00).
NIMBEX Injection, 10 mg cisatracurium in each mL.
20-mL Single-Use Vials **intended only for use in the ICU.**
Carton of 1 (NDC 0173-0543-01).

STORAGE

NIMBEX Injection should be refrigerated at 2° to 8°C (36° to 46°F) in the carton to preserve potency. Protect from light. DO NOT FREEZE. Upon removal from refrigeration to room temperature storage conditions (25°C/77°F), use NIMBEX Injection within 21 days even if rerefrigerated.

U.S. Patent No. 5,453,510
©1995 Glaxo Wellcome Inc. All rights reserved.
October 1997/RL-475

Shown in Product Identification Guide, page 313

NUROMAX® ℞
[nŏo 'rŏ-măks]
(doxacurium chloride)
Injection

This drug should be administered only by adequately trained individuals familiar with its actions, characteristics, and hazards.

DESCRIPTION

NUROMAX (doxacurium chloride) is a long-acting, nondepolarizing skeletal muscle relaxant for intravenous administration. Doxacurium chloride is [1α,2β(1'S*,2' R*)]-2,2'-[(1,4-dioxo-1,4-butanediyl)bis(oxy-3,1-propanediyl)]bis[1,2,3,4-tetrahydro-6,7,8-trimethoxy-2-methyl-1-[(3,4,5-trimethoxyphyphenyl)methyl]isoquinolinium]dichloride(meso form). The molecular formula is $C_{56}H_{78}Cl_2N_2O_{16}$ and the molecular weight is 1106.14. The compound does not partition into the 1-octanol phase of a distilled water/1-octanol system, i.e., the n-octanol:water partition coefficient is 0. Doxacurium chloride is a mixture of three *trans, trans* stereoisomers, a *dl* pair [(1R, 1' R, 2S, 2' S) and (1S, 1' S, 2R, 2' R)] and a meso form (1R, 1' S, 2S, 2' R).

NUROMAX Injection is a sterile, nonpyrogenic aqueous solution (pH 3.9 to 5.0) containing doxacurium chloride equivalent to 1 mg/mL doxacurium in Water for Injection. Hydrochloric acid may have been added to adjust pH. NUROMAX Injection contains 0.9% w/v benzyl alcohol.

CLINICAL PHARMACOLOGY

NUROMAX binds competitively to cholinergic receptors on the motor end-plate to antagonize the action of acetylcholine, resulting in a block of neuromuscular transmission. This action is antagonized by acetylcholinesterase inhibitors, such as neostigmine.

Pharmacodynamics: NUROMAX is approximately 2.5 to 3 times more potent than pancuronium and 10 to 12 times more potent than metocurine. NUROMAX in doses of 1.5 to 2 x ED_{95} has a clinical duration of action (range and variability) similar to that of equipotent doses of pancuronium and metocurine (historic data and limited comparison). The average ED_{95} (dose required to produce 95% suppression of

the adductor pollicis muscle twitch response to ulnar nerve stimulation) of NUROMAX is 0.025 mg/kg (range: 0.020 to 0.033) in adults receiving balanced anesthesia.

The onset and clinically effective duration (time from injection to 25% recovery) of NUROMAX administered alone or after succinylcholine during stable balanced anesthesia are shown in Table 1.

Table 1: Pharmacodynamic Dose Response* Balanced Anesthesia

	Initial Dose of NUROMAX (mg/kg)		
	0.025† (n=34)	0.05 (n=27)	0.08 (n=9)
Time to Maximum Block (min)	9.3 (5.4-16)	5.2 (2.5-13)	3.5 (2.4-5)
Clinical Duration (min) (Time to 25% Recovery)	55 (9-145)	100 (39-232)	160 (110-338)

* Values shown are means (range).
† NUROMAX administered after 10% to 100% recovery from an intubating dose of succinylcholine.

Initial doses of 0.05 mg/kg (2 x ED_{95}) and 0.08 mg/kg (3 x ED_{95}) NUROMAX administered during the induction of thiopental-narcotic anesthesia produced good-to-excellent conditions for tracheal intubation in 5 minutes (13 of 15 cases studied) and 4 minutes (eight of nine cases studied) (which are before maximum block), respectively.

As with other long-acting agents, the clinical duration of neuromuscular block associated with NUROMAX shows considerable interpatient variability. An analysis of 390 cases in US clinical trials utilizing a variety of premedications, varying lengths of surgery, and various anesthetic agents, indicates that approximately two thirds of the patients had clinical durations within 30 minutes of the duration predicted by dose (based on mg/kg actual body weight). Patients ≥60 years old are approximately twice as likely to experience prolonged clinical duration (30 minutes longer than predicted) than patients <60 years old; thus, care should be used in older patients when prolonged recovery is undesirable (see PRECAUTIONS: Geriatric Use and CLINICAL PHARMACOLOGY: **Individualization of Dosages** subsection). In addition, obese patients (patients weighing ≥30% more than ideal body weight for height) were almost twice as likely to experience prolonged clinical duration than non-obese patients; therefore, dosing should be based on ideal body weight (IBW) for obese patients (see CLINICAL PHARMACOLOGY: **Individualization of Dosages** subsection).

The mean time for spontaneous T_1 recovery from 25% to 50% of control following initial doses of NUROMAX is approximately 26 minutes (range: 7 to 104, n=253) during balanced anesthesia. The mean time for spontaneous T_1 recovery from 25% to 75% is 54 minutes (range: 14 to 184, n=184).

Most patients receiving NUROMAX in clinical trials required pharmacologic reversal prior to full spontaneous recovery from neuromuscular block (see OVERDOSAGE: **Antagonism of Neuromuscular Block**); therefore, relatively few data are available on the time from injection to 95% spontaneous recovery of the twitch response. As with other long-acting neuromuscular blocking agents, NUROMAX

may be associated with prolonged times to full spontaneous recovery. Following an initial dose of 0.025 mg/kg NUROMAX, some patients may require as long as 4 hours to exhibit full spontaneous recovery.

Cumulative neuromuscular blocking effects are not associated with repeated administration of maintenance doses of NUROMAX at 25% T_1 recovery. As with initial doses, however, the duration of action following maintenance doses of NUROMAX may vary considerably among patients.

The NUROMAX ED_{95} for children 2 to 12 years of age receiving halothane anesthesia is approximately 0.03 mg/kg. Children require higher doses of NUROMAX on a mg/kg basis than adults to achieve comparable levels of block. The onset time and duration of block are shorter in children than adults. During halothane anesthesia, doses of 0.03 mg/kg and 0.05 mg/kg NUROMAX produce maximum block in approximately 7 and 4 minutes, respectively. The duration of clinically effective block is approximately 30 minutes after an initial dose of 0.03 mg/kg and approximately 45 minutes after 0.05 mg/kg. NUROMAX has not been studied in pediatric patients below the age of 2 years.

The neuromuscular block produced by NUROMAX may be antagonized by anticholinesterase agents. As with other nondepolarizing neuromuscular blocking agents, the more profound the neuromuscular block at reversal, the longer the time and the greater the dose of anticholinesterase required for recovery of neuromuscular function.

Hemodynamics: Administration of doses of NUROMAX up to and including 0.08 mg/kg (~3 x ED_{95}) over 5 to 15 seconds to healthy adult patients during stable-state balanced anesthesia and to patients with serious cardiovascular disease undergoing coronary artery bypass grafting, cardiac valvular repair, or vascular repair produced no dose-related effects on mean arterial blood pressure (MAP) or heart rate (HR).

No dose-related changes in MAP and HR were observed following administration of up to 0.05 mg/kg NUROMAX over 5 to 15 seconds in 2 - to 12-year-old children receiving halothane anesthesia.

Doses of 0.03 to 0.08 mg/kg (1.2 to 3 x ED_{95}) were not associated with dose-dependent changes in mean plasma histamine concentration. Clinical experience with more than 1000 patients indicates that adverse experiences typically associated with histamine release (e.g., bronchospasm, hypotension, tachycardia, cutaneous flushing, urticaria, etc.) are very rare following the administration of NUROMAX (see ADVERSE REACTIONS).

Pharmacokinetics: Pharmacokinetic and pharmacodynamic results from a study of 24 healthy young adult patients and eight healthy elderly patients are summarized in Table 2. The pharmacokinetics are linear over the dosage range tested (i.e., plasma concentrations are approximately proportional to dose). The pharmacokinetics of NUROMAX are similar in healthy young adult and elderly patients. Some healthy elderly patients tend to be more sensitive to the neuromuscular blocking effects of NUROMAX than healthy young adult patients receiving the same dose. The time to maximum block is longer in elderly patients than in young adult patients (11.2 minutes versus 7.7 minutes at 0.025 mg/kg NUROMAX). In addition, the clinically effective durations of block are more variable and tend to be longer in healthy elderly patients than in healthy young adult patients receiving the same dose.

[See table 2 below]

Table 3 summarizes the pharmacokinetic and pharmacodynamic results from a study of nine healthy young adult patients, eight patients with end-stage kidney disease undergoing kidney transplantation, and seven patients with end-

Table 2: Pharmacokinetic and Pharmacodynamic Parameters* of NUROMAX in Young Adult and Elderly Patients
(Isoflurane Anesthesia)

Parameter	Healthy Young Adult Patients (22 to 49 yrs)			Healthy Elderly Patients (67 to 72 yrs)
	0.025 mg/kg (n=8)	0.05 mg/kg (n=8)	0.08 mg/kg (n=8)	0.025 mg/kg (n=8)
$t_{1/2}$ Elimination (min)	86 (25-171)	123 (61-163)	98 (47-163)	96 (50-114)
Volume of Distribution at Steady State (L/kg)	0.15 (0.10-0.21)	0.24 (0.13-0.30)	0.22 (0.16-0.33)	0.22 (0.14-0.40)
Plasma Clearance (mL/min per kg)	2.22 (1.02-3.95)	2.62 (1.21-5.70)	2.53 (1.88-3.38)	2.47 (1.58-3.60)
Maximum Block (%)	97 (88-100)	100 (100-100)	100 (100-100)	96 (90-100)
Clinically Effective Duration of Block† (min)	68 (35-90)	91 (47-132)	177 (74-268)	97 (36-179)

* Values shown are means (range).
† Time from injection to 25% recovery of the control twitch height.

stage liver disease undergoing liver transplantation. The results suggest that a longer $t_{1/2}$ can be expected in patients with end-stage kidney disease; in addition, these patients may be more sensitive to the neuromuscular blocking effects of NUROMAX. The time to maximum block was slightly longer and the clinically effective duration of block was prolonged in patients with end-stage kidney disease.
[See table 3 at right]

No data are available from patients with liver disease not requiring transplantation. There are no significant alterations in the pharmacokinetics of NUROMAX in liver transplant patients. Sensitivity to the neuromuscular blocking effects of NUROMAX was highly variable in patients undergoing liver transplantation. Three of seven patients developed ≤50% block, indicating that a reduced sensitivity to NUROMAX may occur in such patients. In those patients who developed >50% neuromuscular block, the time to maximum block and the clinically effective duration tended to be longer than in healthy young adult patients (see CLINICAL PHARMACOLOGY: **Individualization of Dosages** subsection).

Consecutively administered maintenance doses of 0.005 mg/kg NUROMAX, each given at 25% T_1 recovery following the preceding dose, do not result in a progressive increase in the plasma concentration of doxacurium or a progressive increase in the depth or duration of block produced by each dose.

NUROMAX is not metabolized in vitro in fresh human plasma. Plasma protein binding of NUROMAX is approximately 30% in human plasma.

In vivo data from humans suggest that NUROMAX is not metabolized and that the major elimination pathway is excretion of unchanged drug in urine and bile. In studies of healthy adult patients, 24% to 38% of an administered dose was recovered as parent drug in urine over 6 to 12 hours after dosing. High bile concentrations of NUROMAX (relative to plasma) have been found 35 to 90 minutes after administration. The overall extent of biliary excretion is unknown. The data derived from analysis of human urine and bile are consistent with data from in vivo studies in the rat, cat, and dog, which indicate that all of an administered dose of NUROMAX is recovered as parent drug in the urine and bile of these species.

Individualization of Dosages: In elderly patients or patients who have impaired renal function, the potential for a prolongation of block may be reduced by decreasing the initial dose of NUROMAX and by titrating the dose to achieve the desired depth of block. In obese patients (patients weighing ≥30% more than ideal body weight for height), the dose of NUROMAX should be determined using the patient's ideal body weight (IBW), according to the following formulae:

Men: IBW in kg = [106 + (6 x inches in height above 5 feet)]/2.2

Women: IBW in kg = [100 + (5 x inches in height above 5 feet)]/2.2

Dosage requirements for patients with severe liver disease are variable; some patients may require a higher than normal initial dose of NUROMAX to achieve clinically effective block. Once adequate block is established, the clinical duration of block may be prolonged in such patients relative to patients with normal liver function.

As with pancuronium, metocurine, and vecuronium, resistance to NUROMAX, manifested by a reduced intensity and/or shortened duration of block, must be considered when NUROMAX is selected for use in patients receiving phenytoin or carbamazepine (see PRECAUTIONS: **Drug Interactions**).

As with other nondepolarizing neuromuscular blocking agents, a reduction in dosage of NUROMAX must be considered in cachectic or debilitated patients; in patients with neuromuscular diseases, severe electrolyte abnormalities, or carcinomatosis; and in other patients in whom potentiation of neuromuscular block or difficulty with reversal is anticipated. Increased doses of NUROMAX may be required in burn patients (see PRECAUTIONS).

INDICATIONS AND USAGE

NUROMAX is a long-acting neuromuscular blocking agent, indicated to provide skeletal muscle relaxation as an adjunct to general anesthesia, for endotracheal intubation or to facilitate mechanical ventilation.

CONTRAINDICATIONS

NUROMAX is contraindicated in patients known to have hypersensitivity to it. Use of NUROMAX from multiple-dose vials containing benzyl alcohol as a preservative is contraindicated in patients with a known hypersensitivity to benzyl alcohol.

WARNINGS

NUROMAX SHOULD BE ADMINISTERED IN CAREFULLY ADJUSTED DOSAGE BY OR UNDER THE SUPERVISION OF EXPERIENCED CLINICIANS WHO ARE FAMILIAR WITH THE DRUG'S ACTIONS AND THE POSSIBLE COMPLICATIONS OF ITS USE. THE DRUG SHOULD NOT BE ADMINISTERED UNLESS FACILITIES FOR INTUBATION, ARTIFICIAL RESPIRATION, OXYGEN THERAPY, AND AN ANTAGONIST ARE WITHIN IMMEDIATE REACH. IT IS RECOMMENDED THAT CLINICIANS ADMINISTERING LONG-ACTING NEUROMUSCULAR BLOCKING AGENTS SUCH AS NUROMAX EMPLOY A PERIPHERAL NERVE STIMULATOR TO MONITOR DRUG RESPONSE, NEED FOR ADDITIONAL RELAXANTS, AND ADEQUACY OF SPONTANEOUS RECOVERY OR ANTAGONISM.

NUROMAX HAS NO KNOWN EFFECT ON CONSCIOUSNESS, PAIN THRESHOLD, OR CEREBRATION. TO AVOID DISTRESS TO THE PATIENT, NEUROMUSCULAR BLOCK SHOULD NOT BE INDUCED BEFORE UNCONSCIOUSNESS.

NUROMAX Injection is acidic (pH 3.9 to 5.0) and may not be compatible with alkaline solutions having a pH greater than 8.5 (e.g., barbiturate solutions).

NUROMAX Injection contains benzyl alcohol. In newborn infants, benzyl alcohol has been associated with an increased incidence of neurological and other complications which are sometimes fatal (see PRECAUTIONS: **Pediatric Use**).

PRECAUTIONS

General: NUROMAX has no clinically significant effects on heart rate; therefore, NUROMAX will not counteract the bradycardia produced by many anesthetic agents or by vagal stimulation.

Neuromuscular blocking agents may have a profound effect in patients with neuromuscular diseases (e.g., myasthenia gravis and the myasthenic syndrome). In these and other conditions in which prolonged neuromuscular block is a possibility (e.g., carcinomatosis), the use of a peripheral nerve stimulator and a small test dose of NUROMAX are recommended to assess the level of neuromuscular block and to monitor dosage requirements. Shorter acting muscle relaxants than NUROMAX may be more suitable for these patients.

Resistance to nondepolarizing neuromuscular blocking agents may develop in patients with burns depending upon the time elapsed since the injury and the size of the burn. NUROMAX has not been studied in patients with burns.

Acid-base and/or serum electrolyte abnormalities may potentiate or antagonize the action of neuromuscular blocking agents. The action of neuromuscular blocking agents may be enhanced by magnesium salts administered for the management of toxemia of pregnancy.

NUROMAX has not been studied in patients with asthma.

No data are available to support the use of NUROMAX by intramuscular injection.

Renal and Hepatic Disease: NUROMAX has been studied in patients with end-stage kidney (n=8) or liver (n=7) disease undergoing transplantation procedures (see CLINICAL PHARMACOLOGY). The possibility of prolonged neuromuscular block in patients undergoing renal transplantation and the possibility of a variable onset and duration of neuromuscular block in patients undergoing liver transplantation must be considered when NUROMAX is used in such patients.

Obesity: Administration of NUROMAX on the basis of actual body weight is associated with a prolonged duration of action in obese patients (patients weighing ≥30% more than ideal body weight for height) (see CLINICAL PHARMACOLOGY). Therefore, the dose of NUROMAX should be based upon ideal body weight in obese patients (see CLINICAL PHARMACOLOGY: **Individualization of Dosages**).

Malignant Hyperthermia (MH): In a study of MH-susceptible pigs, NUROMAX did not trigger MH. NUROMAX has not been studied in MH-susceptible patients. Since MH can develop in the absence of established triggering agents, the clinician should be prepared to recognize and treat MH in any patient scheduled for general anesthesia.

Long-Term Use in the Intensive Care Unit (ICU): Information on the use of NUROMAX in the ICU is limited. In a double-blind, randomized study, 17 patients received NUROMAX by intermittent bolus injection for a mean of 2.7 ± 0.5 days (range: 0.8 to 6.8 days) to facilitate mechanical ventilation. No evidence of tachyphylaxis, accumulation, or prolonged recovery was observed. The adverse experiences in patients receiving NUROMAX were consistent in type, severity, and frequency to those expected in a critically ill patient population. Since many ICU patients have hepatic and/or renal failure, a prolonged duration of block should be anticipated in these patients after administration of NUROMAX.

WHENEVER THE USE OF NUROMAX OR ANY NEUROMUSCULAR BLOCKING AGENT IS CONTEMPLATED IN THE ICU, IT IS RECOMMENDED THAT NEUROMUSCULAR TRANSMISSION BE MONITORED CONTINUOUSLY DURING ADMINISTRATION WITH THE HELP OF A NERVE STIMULATOR. ADDITIONAL DOSES OF NUROMAX OR ANY OTHER NEUROMUSCULAR BLOCKING AGENT SHOULD NOT BE GIVEN BEFORE THERE IS A DEFINITE RESPONSE TO T_1, OR TO THE FIRST TWITCH. IF NO RESPONSE IS ELICITED, BOLUS ADMINISTRATION SHOULD BE DELAYED UNTIL A RESPONSE RETURNS.

Drug Interactions: Prior administration of succinylcholine has no clinically important effect on the neuromuscular blocking action of NUROMAX.

The use of NUROMAX before succinylcholine to attenuate some of the side effects of succinylcholine has not been studied.

There are no clinical data on concomitant use of NUROMAX and other nondepolarizing neuromuscular blocking agents. Isoflurane, enflurane, and halothane decrease the ED_{50} of NUROMAX by 30% to 45%. These agents may also prolong the clinically effective duration of action by up to 25%.

Other drugs which may enhance the neuromuscular blocking action of nondepolarizing agents such as NUROMAX include certain antibiotics (e.g., aminoglycosides, tetracyclines, bacitracin, polymyxins, lincomycin, clindamycin, colistin, and sodium colistimethate), magnesium salts, lithium, local anesthetics, procainamide, and quinidine.

As with some other nondepolarizing neuromuscular blocking agents, the time of onset of neuromuscular block induced by NUROMAX is lengthened and the duration of block is shortened in patients receiving phenytoin or carbamazepine.

Carcinogenesis, Mutagenesis, Impairment of Fertility: Carcinogenesis and fertility studies have not been performed. NUROMAX was evaluated in a battery of four short-term mutagenicity tests. It was nonmutagenic in the Ames Salmonella assay, in the mouse lymphoma assay, and in the human lymphocyte assay. In the in vivo rat bone marrow cytogenetic assay, statistically significant increases in the

Continued on next page

Table 3: Pharmacokinetic and Pharmacodynamic Parameters* of NUROMAX in Healthy Patients and in Patients Undergoing Kidney or Liver Transplantation
(Isoflurane Anesthesia)

Parameter	Healthy Young Adult Patients 0.015 mg/kg (n=9)	Kidney Transplant Patients 0.015 mg/kg (n=8)	Liver Transplant Patients 0.015 mg/kg (n=7)
$t_{1/2}$ Elimination (min)	99 (48-193)	221 (84-592)	115 (69-148)
Volume of Distribution at Steady State (L/kg)	0.22 (0.11-0.43)	0.27 (0.17-0.55)	0.29 (0.17-0.35)
Plasma Clearance (mL/min per kg)	2.66 (1.35-6.66)	1.23 (0.48-2.40)	2.30 (1.96-3.05)
Maximum Block (%)	86 (59-100)	98 (95-100)	70 (0-100)
Clinically Effective Duration of Block (min)	36 (19-80)	80 (29-133)	52 (20-91)

* Values shown are means (range).

This product information is based on labeling in effect on June 1, 1998. For further information, contact via direct mail, phone, or web site Medical Information: Glaxo Wellcome Inc., PO Box 13398, Research Triangle Park, NC 27709. Healthcare Professionals (Medical Information): 800-334-0089 Patients (Customer Response Center): 888-TALK2GW (1-888-825-5249) Glaxo Wellcome Corporate Web Site: www.glaxowellcome.com

Nuromax—Cont.

incidence of structural abnormalities, relative to vehicle controls, were observed in male rats dosed with 0.1 mg/kg (0.625 mg/m^2) NUROMAX and sacrificed at 6 hours, but not at 24 or 48 hours, and in female rats dosed with 0.2 mg/kg (1.25 mg/m^2) NUROMAX and sacrificed at 24 hours, but not at 6 or 48 hours. There was no increase in structural abnormalities in either male or female rats given 0.3 mg/kg (1.875 mg/m^2) NUROMAX and sacrificed at 6, 24, or 48 hours. Thus, the incidence of abnormalities in the in vivo rat bone marrow cytogenetic assay was not dose-dependent and, therefore, the likelihood that the observed abnormalities were treatment-related or clinically significant is low.

Pregnancy: ***Teratogenic Effects:*** Pregnancy Category C. Teratology testing in nonventilated, pregnant rats and mice treated subcutaneously with maximum subparalyzing doses of NUROMAX revealed no maternal or fetal toxicity or teratogenic effects. There are no adequate and well-controlled studies of NUROMAX in pregnant women. Because animal studies are not always predictive of human response and the doses used were subparalyzing, NUROMAX should be used during pregnancy only if the potential benefit justifies the potential risk to the fetus.

Labor and Delivery: The use of NUROMAX during labor, vaginal delivery, or cesarean section has not been studied. It is not known whether NUROMAX administered to the mother has immediate or delayed effects on the fetus. The duration of action of NUROMAX exceeds the usual duration of operative obstetrics (cesarean section). Therefore, NUROMAX is not recommended for use in patients undergoing C-section.

Nursing Mothers: It is not known whether NUROMAX is excreted in human milk. Because many drugs are excreted in human milk, caution should be exercised following administration of NUROMAX to a nursing woman.

Pediatric Use: NUROMAX has not been studied in pediatric patients below the age of 2 years. See CLINICAL PHARMACOLOGY and DOSAGE AND ADMINISTRATION for clinical experience and recommendations for use in children 2 to 12 years of age.

Geriatric Use: NUROMAX has been used in elderly patients, including patients with significant cardiovascular disease. In elderly patients the onset of maximum block is slower and the duration of neuromuscular block produced by NUROMAX is more variable and, in some cases, longer than in young adult patients (see CLINICAL PHARMACOLOGY: **Pharmacodynamics** and **Individualization of Dosages**).

ADVERSE REACTIONS

The most frequent adverse effect of nondepolarizing blocking agents as a class consists of an extension of the pharmacological action beyond the time needed for surgery and anesthesia. This effect may vary from skeletal muscle weakness to profound and prolonged skeletal muscle paralysis resulting in respiratory insufficiency and apnea which require manual or mechanical ventilation until recovery is judged to be clinically adequate (see OVERDOSAGE). Inadequate reversal of neuromuscular block from NUROMAX is possible, as with all nondepolarizing agents. Prolonged neuromuscular block and inadequate reversal may lead to postoperative complications.

Observed in Clinical Trials: Adverse experiences were uncommon among the 1034 surgical patients and volunteers who received NUROMAX and other drugs in US clinical studies in the course of a wide variety of procedures conducted during balanced or inhalational anesthesia. The following adverse experiences were reported in patients administered NUROMAX (all events judged by investigators during the clinical trials to have a possible causal relationship):

Incidence Greater than 1%—None

Incidence Less than 1%—

Cardiovascular:* Hypotension,† flushing,† ventricular fibrillation, myocardial infarction

Respiratory: Bronchospasm, wheezing

Dermatological: Urticaria, injection site reaction

Special Senses: Diplopia

Nonspecific: Difficult neuromuscular block reversal, prolonged drug effect, fever

* Reports of ventricular fibrillation (n=1) and myocardial infarction (n=1) were limited to ASA Class 3-4 patients undergoing cardiac surgery (n=142).

† 0.3% incidence. All other reactions unmarked were ≤0.1%.

OVERDOSAGE

Overdosage with neuromuscular blocking agents may result in neuromuscular block beyond the time needed for surgery and anesthesia. The primary treatment is maintenance of a patent airway and controlled ventilation until recovery of normal neuromuscular function is assured. Once evidence of recovery from neuromuscular block is observed, further recovery may be facilitated by administration of an anticholinesterase agent (e.g., neostigmine, edrophonium) in conjunction with an appropriate anticholinergic agent (see **Antagonism of Neuromuscular Block** below).

Antagonism of Neuromuscular Block: ANTAGONISTS (SUCH AS NEOSTIGMINE) SHOULD NOT BE ADMINISTERED PRIOR TO THE DEMONSTRATION OF SOME SPONTANEOUS RECOVERY FROM NEUROMUSCULAR BLOCK. THE USE OF A NERVE STIMULATOR TO DOCUMENT RECOVERY AND ANTAGONISM OF NEUROMUSCULAR BLOCK IS RECOMMENDED. T_4/T_1 SHOULD BE > ZERO BEFORE ANTAGONISM IS ATTEMPTED.

In an analysis of patients in whom antagonism of neuromuscular block was evaluated following administration of single doses of neostigmine averaging 0.06 mg/kg (range: 0.05 to 0.075) administered at approximately 25% T_1 spontaneous recovery during balanced anesthesia, 71% of patients exhibited $T_4/T_1 \geq 0.7$ before monitoring was discontinued. For these patients, the mean time to $T_4/T_1 \geq 0.7$ was 19 minutes (range: 7 to 55). As with other long-acting nondepolarizing neuromuscular blocking agents, the time for recovery of neuromuscular function following administration of neostigmine is dependent upon the level of residual neuromuscular block at the time of attempted reversal; longer recovery times than those cited above may be anticipated when neostigmine is administered at more profound levels of block (i.e., at <25% T_1 recovery).

Patients should be evaluated for adequate clinical evidence of antagonism, e.g., 5-second head lift, and grip strength. Ventilation must be supported until no longer required. As with other neuromuscular blocking agents, physicians should be alert to the possibility that the action of the drugs used to antagonize neuromuscular block may wear off before the effects of NUROMAX on the neuromuscular junction have declined sufficiently.

Antagonism may be delayed in the presence of debilitation, carcinomatosis, and the concomitant use of certain broad-spectrum antibiotics or anesthetic agents and other drugs which enhance neuromuscular block or separately cause respiratory depression (see PRECAUTIONS: **Drug Interactions**). Under such circumstances the management is the same as that of prolonged neuromuscular block.

In clinical trials, a dose of 1 mg/kg edrophonium was not as effective as a dose of 0.06 mg/kg neostigmine in antagonizing moderate to deep levels of neuromuscular block (i.e., <60% T_1 recovery). Therefore, the use of 1 mg/kg edrophonium is not recommended for reversal from moderate to deep levels of block. The use of pyridostigmine has not been studied.

DOSAGE AND ADMINISTRATION

NUROMAX SHOULD ONLY BE ADMINISTERED INTRAVENOUSLY.

NUROMAX, like other long-acting neuromuscular blocking agents, displays variability in the duration of its effect. The potential for a prolonged clinical duration of neuromuscular block must be considered when NUROMAX is selected for administration. The dosage information provided below is intended as a guide only. Doses should be individualized (see CLINICAL PHARMACOLOGY: **Individualization of Dosages**). Factors that may warrant dosage adjustment include: advancing age, the presence of kidney or liver disease, or obesity (patients weighing ≥30% more than ideal body weight for height). The use of a peripheral nerve stimulator will permit the most advantageous use of NUROMAX, minimize the possibility of overdosage or underdosage, and assist in the evaluation of recovery.

Parenteral drug products should be inspected visually for particulate matter and discoloration prior to administration whenever solution and container permit.

Adults: ***Initial Doses:*** When administered as a component of a thiopental/narcotic induction-intubation paradigm as well as for production of long-duration neuromuscular block during surgery, 0.05 mg/kg (2 x ED_{95}) NUROMAX produces good-to-excellent conditions for tracheal intubation in 5 minutes in approximately 90% of patients. Lower doses of NUROMAX may result in a longer time for development of satisfactory intubation conditions. Clinically effective neuromuscular block may be expected to last approximately 100 minutes on average (range: 39 to 232) following 0.05 mg/kg NUROMAX administered to patients receiving balanced anesthesia.

An initial NUROMAX dose of 0.08 mg/kg (3 x ED_{95}) should be reserved for instances in which a need for very prolonged neuromuscular block is anticipated. In approximately 90% of patients, good-to-excellent intubation conditions may be expected in 4 minutes after this dose; however, clinically effective block may be expected to persist for as long as 160 minutes or more (range: 110 to 338) (see CLINICAL PHARMACOLOGY).

If NUROMAX is administered during steady-state isoflurane, enflurane, or halothane anesthesia, reduction of the dose of NUROMAX by one third should be considered.

When succinylcholine is administered to facilitate tracheal intubation in patients receiving balanced anesthesia, an initial dose of 0.025 mg/kg (ED_{95}) NUROMAX provides about 60 minutes (range: 9 to 145) of clinically effective neuromuscular block for surgery. For a longer duration of action, a larger initial dose may be administered.

Maintenance Doses: Maintenance dosing will generally be required about 60 minutes after an initial dose of 0.025 mg/kg NUROMAX or 100 minutes after an initial dose of 0.05 mg/kg NUROMAX during balanced anesthesia. Repeated maintenance doses administered at 25% T_1 recovery may be expected to be required at relatively regular intervals in each patient. The interval may vary considerably between patients. Maintenance doses of 0.005 and 0.01 mg/kg NUROMAX each provide an average 30 minutes (range: 9 to 57) and 45 minutes (range: 14 to 108), respectively, of additional clinically effective neuromuscular block. For shorter or longer desired durations, smaller or larger maintenance doses may be administered.

Children: When administered during halothane anesthesia, an initial dose of 0.03 mg/kg (ED_{95}) produces maximum neuromuscular block in about 7 minutes (range: 5 to 11) and clinically effective block for an average of 30 minutes (range: 12 to 54). Under halothane anesthesia, 0.05 mg/kg produces maximum block in about 4 minutes (range: 2 to 10) and clinically effective block for 45 minutes (range: 30 to 80). Maintenance doses are generally required more frequently in children than in adults. Because of the potentiating effect of halothane seen in adults, a higher dose of NUROMAX may be required in children receiving balanced anesthesia than in children receiving halothane anesthesia to achieve a comparable onset and duration of neuromuscular block.

NUROMAX has not been studied in pediatric patients below the age of 2 years.

Compatibility: ***Y-site Administration:*** NUROMAX Injection may not be compatible with alkaline solutions with a pH greater than 8.5 (e.g., barbiturate solutions).

NUROMAX is compatible with:

- 5% Dextrose Injection, USP
- 0.9% Sodium Chloride Injection, USP
- 5% Dextrose and 0.9% Sodium Chloride Injection, USP
- Lactated Ringer's Injection, USP
- 5% Dextrose and Lactated Ringer's Injection
- Sufenta® (sufentanil citrate) Injection, diluted as directed
- Alfenta® (alfentanil hydrochloride) Injection, diluted as directed
- Sublimaze® (fentanyl citrate) Injection, diluted as directed

Dilution Stability: NUROMAX diluted up to 1:10 in 5% Dextrose Injection, USP or 0.9% Sodium Chloride Injection, USP has been shown to be physically and chemically stable when stored in polypropylene syringes at 5° to 25°C (41° to 77°F), for up to 24 hours. Since dilution diminishes the preservative effectiveness of benzyl alcohol, aseptic techniques should be used to prepare the diluted product. Immediate use of the diluted product is preferred, and any unused portion of diluted NUROMAX should be discarded after 8 hours.

HOW SUPPLIED

NUROMAX Injection, 1 mg doxacurium in each mL.
5-mL Multiple-dose vials containing 0.9% w/v benzyl alcohol as a preservative (see WARNINGS). Tray of 10 (NDC 0173-0763-44).

STORAGE

Store NUROMAX Injection at room temperature of 15° to 25°C (59° to 77°F). DO NOT FREEZE.

US Patent No. 4,701,460

©Copyright 1996 Glaxo Wellcome Inc. All rights reserved.

December 1997/RL-514

Shown in Product Identification Guide, page 313

OXISTAT® ℞

[äx 'ē-stat"]

(oxiconazole nitrate cream)

Cream, 1%*

OXISTAT®

(oxiconazole nitrate lotion)

Lotion, 1%*

***Potency expressed as oxiconazole**

FOR TOPICAL DERMATOLOGIC USE ONLY—
NOT FOR OPHTHALMIC OR INTRAVAGINAL USE

DESCRIPTION

OXISTAT Cream and Lotion formulations contain the antifungal active compound oxiconazole nitrate. Both formulations are for topical dermatologic use only.

Chemically, oxiconazole nitrate is 2',4'-dichloro-2-imidazol-1-ylacetophenone (*Z*)-[*0*-(2,4-dichlorobenzyl)oxime], mononitrate. The compound has the empirical formula $C_{18}H_{13}ON_3Cl_4 \bullet HNO_3$, and a molecular weight of 492.15.

Oxiconazole nitrate is a nearly white crystalline powder, soluble in methanol; sparingly soluble in ethanol, chloroform, and acetone; and very slightly soluble in water.

OXISTAT Cream contains 10 mg of oxiconazole per gram of cream in a white to off-white, opaque cream base of purified

water USP, white petrolatum USP, stearyl alcohol NF, propylene glycol USP, polysorbate 60 NF, cetyl alcohol NF, and benzoic acid USP 0.2% as a preservative.

OXISTAT Lotion contains 10 mg of oxiconazole per gram of lotion in a white to off-white, opaque lotion base of purified water USP, white petrolatum USP, stearyl alcohol NF, propylene glycol USP, polysorbate 60 NF, cetyl alcohol NF, and benzoic acid USP 0.2% as a preservative.

CLINICAL PHARMACOLOGY

Pharmacokinetics: The penetration of oxiconazole nitrate into different layers of the skin was assessed using an in vitro permeation technique with human skin. Five hours after application of 2.5 mg/cm^2 of oxiconazole nitrate cream onto human skin, the concentration of oxiconazole nitrate was demonstrated to be 16.2 µmol in the epidermis, 3.64 µmol in the upper corium, and 1.29 µmol in the deeper corium. Systemic absorption of oxiconazole nitrate is low. Using radiolabeled drug, less than 0.3% of the applied dose of oxiconazole nitrate was recovered in the urine of volunteer subjects up to 5 days after application of the cream formulation.

Neither in vitro nor in vivo studies have been conducted to establish relative activity between the lotion and cream formulations.

Microbiology: Oxiconazole nitrate is an imidazole derivative whose antifungal activity is derived primarily from the inhibition of ergosterol biosynthesis, which is critical for cellular membrane integrity. It has in vitro activity against a wide range of pathogenic fungi.

Oxiconazole has been shown to be active against most strains of the following organisms both in vitro and in clinical infections at indicated body sites (see INDICATIONS AND USAGE):

Epidermophyton floccosum
Trichophyton mentagrophytes
Trichophyton rubrum
Malassezia furfur

The following in vitro data are available; *however, their clinical significance is unknown.* Oxiconazole exhibits satisfactory in vitro minimum inhibitory concentrations (MICs) against most strains of the following organisms; however, the safety and efficacy of oxiconazole in treating clinical infections due to these organisms have not been established in adequate and well-controlled clinical trials:

Candida albicans
Microsporum audouini
Microsporum canis
Microsporum gypseum
Trichophyton tonsurans
Trichophyton violaceum

INDICATIONS AND USAGE

OXISTAT Cream and Lotion are indicated for the topical treatment of the following dermal infections: tinea pedis, tinea cruris, and tinea corporis due to *Trichophyton rubrum, Trichophyton mentagrophytes,* or *Epidermophyton floccosum.* OXISTAT Cream is indicated for the topical treatment of tinea (pityriasis) versicolor due to *Malassezia furfur* (see DOSAGE AND ADMINISTRATION and CLINICAL STUDIES).

OXISTAT Cream may be used in pediatric patients for tinea corporis, tinea cruris, tinea pedis, and tinea (pityriasis) versicolor; however, these indications for which OXISTAT Cream has been shown to be effective rarely occur in children below the age of 12.

CONTRAINDICATIONS

OXISTAT Cream and Lotion are contraindicated in individuals who have shown hypersensitivity to any of their components.

WARNINGS

OXISTAT Cream and Lotion are not for ophthalmic or intravaginal use.

PRECAUTIONS

General: OXISTAT Cream and Lotion are for external dermal use only. Avoid introduction of OXISTAT Cream or Lotion into the eyes or vagina. If a reaction suggesting sensitivity or chemical irritation should occur with the use of OXISTAT Cream or Lotion, treatment should be discontinued and appropriate therapy instituted. If signs of epidermal irritation should occur, the drug should be discontinued.

Information for Patients: The patient should be instructed to:

1. Use OXISTAT as directed by the physician. The hands should be washed after applying the medication to the affected area(s). Avoid contact with the eyes, nose, mouth, and other mucous membranes. OXISTAT is for external use only.

2. Use the medication for the **full** treatment time recommended by the physician, even though symptoms may have improved. Notify the physician if there is no improvement after 2 to 4 weeks, or sooner if the condition worsens (see below).

3. Inform the physician if the area of application shows signs of increased irritation, itching, burning, blistering, swelling, or oozing.

4. Avoid the use of occlusive dressings unless otherwise directed by the physician.

5. Do not use this medication for any disorder other than that for which it was prescribed.

Drug Interactions: Potential drug interactions between OXISTAT and other drugs have not been systematically evaluated.

Carcinogenesis, Mutagenesis, Impairment of Fertility: Although no long-term studies in animals have been performed to evaluate carcinogenic potential, no evidence of mutagenic effect was found in two mutation assays (Ames test and Chinese hamster V79 in vitro cell mutation assay) or in two cytogenetic assays (human peripheral blood lymphocyte in vitro chromosome aberration assay and in vivo micronucleus assay in mice).

Reproductive studies revealed no impairment of fertility in rats at oral doses of 3 mg/kg per day in females (one time the human dose based on mg/m^2) and 15 mg/kg per day in males (four times the human dose based on mg/m^2). However, at doses above this level, the following effects were observed: a reduction in the fertility parameters of males and females, a reduction in the number of sperm in vaginal smears, extended estrous cycle, and a decrease in mating frequency.

Pregnancy: Teratogenic Effects: *Pregnancy Category B:* Reproduction studies have been performed in rabbits, rats, and mice at oral doses up to 100, 150, and 200 mg/kg per day (57, 40, and 27 times the human dose based on mg/m^2), respectively, and revealed no evidence of harm to the fetus due to oxiconazole nitrate. There are, however, no adequate and well-controlled studies in pregnant women. Because animal reproduction studies are not always predictive of human response, this drug should be used during pregnancy only if clearly needed.

Nursing Mothers: Because oxiconazole is excreted in human milk, caution should be exercised when the drug is administered to a nursing woman.

Pediatric Use: OXISTAT Cream may be used in pediatric patients for tinea corporis, tinea cruris, tinea pedis, and tinea (pityriasis) versicolor; however, these indications for which OXISTAT Cream has been shown to be effective rarely occur in children below the age of 12.

ADVERSE REACTIONS

During clinical trials, of 955 patients treated with oxiconazole nitrate cream, 1%, 41 (4.3%) reported adverse reactions thought to be related to drug therapy. These reactions included pruritus (1.6%); burning (1.4%); irritation and allergic contact dermatitis (0.4% each); folliculitis (0.3%); erythema (0.2%); and papules, fissure, maceration, rash, stinging, and nodules (0.1% each).

In a controlled, multicenter clinical trial of 269 patients treated with oxiconazole nitrate lotion, 1%, 7 (2.6%) reported adverse reactions thought to be related to drug therapy. These reactions included burning and stinging (0.7% each) and pruritus, scaling, tingling, pain, and dyshidrotic eczema (0.4% each).

OVERDOSAGE

When 5% oxiconazole cream (five times the concentration of the marketed product) was applied at a rate of 1 g/kg to approximately 10% of body surface area of a group of 40 male and female rats for 35 days, three deaths and severe dermal inflammation were reported. No overdoses in humans have been reported with use of oxiconazole nitrate cream or lotion.

DOSAGE AND ADMINISTRATION

OXISTAT Cream or Lotion should be applied to affected and immediately surrounding areas once to twice daily in patients with tinea pedis, tinea corporis, or tinea cruris. OXISTAT Cream should be applied once daily in the treatment of tinea (pityriasis) versicolor. Tinea corporis, tinea cruris, and tinea (pityriasis) versicolor should be treated for 2 weeks and tinea pedis for 1 month to reduce the possibility of recurrence. If a patient shows no clinical improvement after the treatment period, the diagnosis should be reviewed.

Note: Tinea (pityriasis) versicolor may give rise to hyperpigmented or hypopigmented patches on the trunk that may extend to the neck, arms, and upper thighs. Treatment of the infection may not immediately result in restoration of pigment to the affected sites. Normalization of pigment following successful therapy is variable and may take months, depending on individual skin type and incidental sun exposure. Although tinea (pityriasis) versicolor is not contagious, it may recur because the organism that causes the disease is part of the normal skin flora.

HOW SUPPLIED

OXISTAT Cream, 1% is supplied in 15-g tubes (NDC 0173-0423-00), 30-g tubes (NDC 0173-0423-01), and 60-g tubes (NDC 0173-0423-04). **Store between 15° and 30°C (59° and**

86°F). OXISTAT Lotion, 1% is supplied in a 30-mL bottle (NDC 0173-0448-01). **Store between 15° and 30°C (59° and 86°F). Shake well before using.**

CLINICAL STUDIES

The following definitions were applied to the clinical and microbiological outcomes in patients enrolled in the clinical trials that form the basis for the approvals of OXISTAT Lotion and OXISTAT Cream.

Definitions:

1. Mycological Cure: No evidence (culture and KOH preparation) of the baseline (original) pathogen in a specimen from the affected area taken at the 2-week post-treatment visit (for tinea [pityriasis] versicolor, mycological cure was limited to KOH only).

2. Treatment Success: Both a global evaluation of ≥90% clinical improvement and a microbiologic eradication (see above) at the 2-week post-treatment visit.

Tinea Pedis: THERE ARE NO HEAD-TO-HEAD COMPARISON TRIALS OF THE OXISTAT CREAM AND LOTION FORMULATIONS IN THE TREATMENT OF TINEA PEDIS.

Lotion Formulation: The clinical trial for the lotion formulation line extension involved 332 evaluable patients with clinically and microbiologically established tinea pedis. Of these evaluable patients, 64% were diagnosed with hyperkeratotic plantar tinea pedis and 28% with interdigital tinea pedis. Seventy-seven percent (77%) had disease secondary to infection with *Trichophyton rubrum*, 18% had disease secondary to infection with *Trichophyton mentagrophytes*, and 4% had disease secondary to infection with *Epidermophyton floccosum*.

The results of this clinical trial at the 2-week post-treatment follow-up visit are shown in the following table:

| | OXISTAT Lotion | | |
Patient Outcome	b.i.d.	q.d.	Vehicle
Mycological cure	67%	64%	28%
Treatment success	41%	34%	10%

In this study, the improvement and cure rates of the b.i.d.- and q.d.-treated groups did not differ significantly (95% confidence interval) from each other but were statistically (95% confidence interval) superior to the vehicle-treated group.

Cream Formulation: The two pivotal trials for the cream formulation involved 281 evaluable patients (total from both trials) with clinically and microbiologically established tinea pedis.

The combined results of these two clinical trials at the 2-week post-treatment follow-up visit are shown in the following table:

| | OXISTAT Lotion | | |
Patient Outcome	b.i.d.	q.d	Vehicle
Mycological cure	77%	79%	33%
Treatment success	52%	43%	14%

All the improvement and cure rates of the b.i.d.- and q.d.-treated groups did not differ significantly (95% confidence interval) from each other but were statistically (95% confidence interval) superior to the vehicle-treated group.

In addition, pediatric data (95 children ages 10 and under) available with the cream formulation indicate that it is safe and effective for use in children when used as directed. Adverse events were reported in two children; one child was reported to have reddening of the skin and one child was reported to have eczema-like skin alterations.

Tinea (pityriasis) Versicolor: Two pivotal clinical trials of OXISTAT Cream in tinea (pityriasis) versicolor involved 219 evaluable patients in the q day OXISTAT and vehicle arms of the trial with clinical and mycological evidence of tinea (pityriasis) versicolor. Patients were treated for 2 weeks with OXISTAT Cream once daily, or with cream vehicle. The combined results of these clinical trials at the 2-week post-treatment follow-up visit are shown in the following table. These results are based on 207 patients (110 in the OXISTAT group and 97 in the vehicle group) with efficacy evaluations at this visit.

Continued on next page

This product information is based on labeling in effect on June 1, 1998. For further information, contact via direct mail, phone, or web site Medical Information: Glaxo Wellcome Inc., PO Box 13398, Research Triangle Park, NC 27709. Healthcare Professionals (Medical Information): 800-334-0089 Patients (Customer Response Center): 888-TALK2GW (1-888-825-5249) Glaxo Wellcome Corporate Web Site: www.glaxowellcome.com

Oxistat—Cont.

	OXISTAT Cream	
Patient Outcome	q.d.	Vehicle
Mycological cure	88%	67%
Treatment success	83%	62%

Only once a day was shown in both studies to be statistically superior to vehicle for all efficacy parameters at 2 weeks and follow-up.

August 1997/RL-457

Shown in Product Identification Guide, page 313

PURINETHOL® ℞
[pur 'in-thawl]
(mercaptopurine)
50-mg Scored Tablets

CAUTION: PURINETHOL (mercaptopurine) is a potent drug. It should not be used unless a diagnosis of acute lymphatic leukemia has been adequately established and the responsible physician is knowledgeable in assessing response to chemotherapy.

DESCRIPTION

PURINETHOL (mercaptopurine) was synthesized and developed by Hitchings, Elion, and associates at the Wellcome Research Laboratories.[1] It is one of a large series of purine analogues which interfere with nucleic acid biosynthesis and has been found active against human leukemias.

Mercaptopurine, known chemically as 1,7-dihydro-6*H*-purine-6-thione monohydrate, is an analogue of the purine bases adenine and hypoxanthine.

PURINETHOL is available in tablet form for oral administration. Each scored tablet contains 50 mg mercaptopurine and the inactive ingredients corn and potato starch, lactose, magnesium stearate, and stearic acid.

CLINICAL PHARMACOLOGY

Clinical studies have shown that the absorption of an oral dose of mercaptopurine in humans is incomplete and variable, averaging approximately 50% of the administered dose.[2] The factors influencing absorption are unknown. Intravenous administration of an investigational preparation of mercaptopurine revealed a plasma half-disappearance time of 21 minutes in pediatric patients and 47 minutes in adults. The volume of distribution usually exceeded that of the total body water.[2]

Following the oral administration of ^{35}S-6-mercaptopurine in one subject, a total of 46% of the dose could be accounted for in the urine (as parent drug and metabolites) in the first 24 hours. Metabolites of mercaptopurine were found in urine within the first 2 hours after administration. Radioactivity (in the form of sulfate) could be found in the urine for weeks afterwards.[3]

There is negligible entry of mercaptopurine into cerebrospinal fluid.

Plasma protein binding averages 19% over the concentration range 10 to 50 mcg/mL (a concentration only achieved by intravenous administration of mercaptopurine at doses exceeding 5 to 10 mg/kg).[2]

Monitoring of plasma levels of mercaptopurine during therapy is of questionable value.[3] There is technical difficulty in determining plasma concentrations which are seldom greater than 1 to 2 mcg/mL after a therapeutic oral dose. More significantly, mercaptopurine enters rapidly into the anabolic and catabolic pathways for purines, and the active intracellular metabolites have appreciably longer half-lives than the parent drug. The biochemical effects of a single dose of mercaptopurine are evident long after the parent drug has disappeared from plasma. Because of this rapid metabolism of mercaptopurine to active intracellular derivatives, hemodialysis would not be expected to appreciably reduce toxicity of the drug. There is no known pharmacologic antagonist to the biochemical actions of mercaptopurine in vivo.

Mercaptopurine competes with hypoxanthine and guanine for the enzyme hypoxanthine-guanine phosphoribosyltransferase (HGPRTase) and is itself converted to thioinosinic acid (TIMP). This intracellular nucleotide inhibits several reactions involving inosinic acid (IMP), including the conversion of IMP to xanthylic acid (XMP) and the conversion of IMP to adenylic acid (AMP) via adenylosuccinate (SAMP). In addition, 6-methylthioinosinate (MTIMP) is formed by the methylation of TIMP. Both TIMP and MTIMP have been reported to inhibit glutamine-5-phosphoribosylpyrophosphate amidotransferase, the first enzyme unique to the de novo pathway for purine ribonucleotide synthesis.[3]

Experiments indicate that radiolabeled mercaptopurine may be recovered from the DNA in the form of deoxythioguanosine.[4] Some mercaptopurine is converted to nucleotide derivatives of 6-thioguanine (6-TG) by the sequential actions of inosinate (IMP) dehydrogenase and xanthylate (XMP) aminase, converting TIMP to thioguanylic acid (TGMP).

Animal tumors that are resistant to mercaptopurine often have lost the ability to convert mercaptopurine to TIMP. However, it is clear that resistance to mercaptopurine may be acquired by other means as well, particularly in human leukemias.

It is not known exactly which of any one or more of the biochemical effects of mercaptopurine and its metabolites are directly or predominantly responsible for cell death.[5]

The catabolism of mercaptopurine and its metabolites is complex. In humans, after oral administration of ^{35}S-6-mercaptopurine, urine contains intact mercaptopurine, thiouric acid (formed by direct oxidation by xanthine oxidase, probably via 6-mercapto-8-hydroxypurine), and a number of 6-methylated thiopurines. The methylthiopurines yield appreciable amounts of inorganic sulfate.[3] The importance of the metabolism by xanthine oxidase relates to the fact that ZYLOPRIM® (allopurinol) inhibits this enzyme and retards the catabolism of mercaptopurine and its active metabolites. A significant reduction in mercaptopurine dosage is mandatory if a potent xanthine oxidase inhibitor and mercaptopurine are used simultaneously in a patient (see PRECAUTIONS).

INDICATIONS AND USAGE

PURINETHOL (mercaptopurine) is indicated for remission induction and maintenance therapy of acute lymphatic leukemia. The response to this agent depends upon the particular subclassification of acute lymphatic leukemia and the age of the patient (pediatric patient or adult).

Acute Lymphatic (Lymphocytic, Lymphoblastic) Leukemia: Given as a single agent for remission induction, PURINETHOL induces complete remission in approximately 25% of pediatric patients and 10% of adults. However, reliance upon PURINETHOL alone is not justified for initial remission induction of acute lymphatic leukemia since combination chemotherapy with vincristine, prednisone, and L-asparaginase results in more frequent complete remission induction than with PURINETHOL alone or in combination. The duration of complete remission induced in acute lymphatic leukemia is so brief without the use of maintenance therapy that some form of drug therapy is considered essential. PURINETHOL, as a single agent, is capable of significantly prolonging complete remission duration; however, combination therapy has produced remission duration longer than that achieved with PURINETHOL alone.

Acute Myelogenous (and Acute Myelomonocytic) Leukemia: As a single agent, PURINETHOL will induce complete remission in approximately 10% of pediatric patients and adults with acute myelogenous leukemia or its subclassifications. These results are inferior to those achieved with combination chemotherapy employing optimum treatment schedules.

Central Nervous System Leukemia: PURINETHOL is not effective for prophylaxis or treatment of central nervous system leukemia.

Other Neoplasms: PURINETHOL is not effective in chronic lymphatic leukemia, the lymphomas (including Hodgkin's Disease), or solid tumors.

CONTRAINDICATIONS

PURINETHOL should not be used unless a diagnosis of acute lymphatic leukemia has been adequately established and the responsible physician is knowledgeable in assessing response to chemotherapy.

PURINETHOL should not be used in patients whose disease has demonstrated prior resistance to this drug. In animals and humans, there is usually complete cross-resistance between mercaptopurine and thioguanine.

WARNINGS

SINCE DRUGS USED IN CANCER CHEMOTHERAPY ARE POTENTIALLY HAZARDOUS, IT IS RECOMMENDED THAT ONLY PHYSICIANS EXPERIENCED WITH THE RISKS OF PURINETHOL AND KNOWLEDGEABLE IN THE NATURAL HISTORY OF ACUTE LEUKEMIAS ADMINISTER THIS DRUG.

Bone Marrow Toxicity: The most consistent, dose-related toxicity is bone marrow suppression. This may be manifest by anemia, leukopenia, thrombocytopenia, or any combination of these. Any of these findings may also reflect progression of the underlying disease. Since mercaptopurine may have a delayed effect, it is important to withdraw the medication temporarily at the first sign of an abnormally large fall in any of the formed elements of the blood.

There are rare individuals with an inherited deficiency of the enzyme thiopurine methyltransferase (TPMT) who may be unusually sensitive to the myelosuppressive effects of mercaptopurine and prone to developing rapid bone marrow suppression following the initiation of treatment.[6,7] Substantial dosage reductions may be required to avoid the development of life-threatening bone marrow suppression in these patients. This toxicity may be more profound in patients treated with concomitant allopurinol (see PRECAUTIONS: Drug Interactions).

Hepatotoxicity: Mercaptopurine is hepatotoxic in animals and humans. A small number of deaths have been reported which may have been attributed to hepatic necrosis due to administration of mercaptopurine. Hepatic injury can occur with any dosage, but seems to occur with more frequency when doses of 2.5 mg/kg/day are exceeded. The histologic pattern of mercaptopurine hepatotoxicity includes features of both intrahepatic cholestasis and parenchymal cell necrosis, either of which may predominate. It is not clear how much of the hepatic damage is due to direct toxicity from the drug and how much may be due to a hypersensitivity reaction. In some patients jaundice has cleared following withdrawal of mercaptopurine and reappeared with its reintroduction.[8]

Published reports have cited widely varying incidences of overt hepatotoxicity. In a large series of patients with various neoplastic diseases, mercaptopurine was administered orally in doses ranging from 2.5 mg/kg to 5.0 mg/kg without any evidence of hepatotoxicity. It was noted by the authors that no definite clinical evidence of liver damage could be ascribed to the drug, although an occasional case of serum hepatitis did occur in patients receiving 6-MP who previously had transfusions.[8] In reports of smaller cohorts of adult and pediatric leukemic patients, the incidence of hepatotoxicity ranged from 0% to 6%.[9-11] In an isolated report by Einhorn and Davidsohn, jaundice was observed more frequently (40%), especially when doses exceeded 2.5 mg/kg.[12] Usually, clinically detectable jaundice appears early in the course of treatment (1 to 2 months). However, jaundice has been reported as early as 1 week and as late as 8 years after the start of treatment with mercaptopurine.[13]

Monitoring of serum transaminase levels, alkaline phosphatase, and bilirubin levels may allow early detection of hepatotoxicity. It is advisable to monitor these liver function tests at weekly intervals when first beginning therapy and at monthly intervals thereafter. Liver function tests may be advisable more frequently in patients who are receiving mercaptopurine with other hepatotoxic drugs or with known pre-existing liver disease.

The concomitant administration of mercaptopurine with other hepatotoxic agents requires especially careful clinical and biochemical monitoring of hepatic function. Combination therapy involving mercaptopurine with other drugs not felt to be hepatotoxic should nevertheless be approached with caution. The combination of mercaptopurine with doxorubicin was reported to be hepatotoxic in 19 of 20 patients undergoing remission-induction therapy for leukemia resistant to previous therapy.[14]

The hepatotoxicity has been associated in some cases with anorexia, diarrhea, jaundice, and ascites. Hepatic encephalopathy has occurred.

The onset of clinical jaundice, hepatomegaly, or anorexia with tenderness in the right hypochondrium are immediate indications for withholding mercaptopurine until the exact etiology can be identified. Likewise, any evidence of deterioration in liver function studies, toxic hepatitis, or biliary stasis should prompt discontinuation of the drug and a search for an etiology of the hepatotoxicity.

Immunosuppression: Mercaptopurine recipients may manifest decreased cellular hypersensitivities and impaired allograft rejection. Induction of immunity to infectious agents or vaccines will be subnormal in these patients; the degree of immunosuppression will depend on antigen dose and temporal relationship to drug. This immunosuppressive effect should be carefully considered with regard to intercurrent infections and risk of subsequent neoplasia.

Pregnancy: Pregnancy Category D. Mercaptopurine can cause fetal harm when administered to a pregnant woman. Women receiving mercaptopurine in the first trimester of pregnancy have an increased incidence of abortion; the risk of malformation in offspring surviving first trimester exposure is not accurately known.[15] In a series of 28 women receiving mercaptopurine after the first trimester of pregnancy, three mothers died undelivered, one delivered a stillborn child, and one aborted; there were no cases of macroscopically abnormal fetuses.[16] Since such experience cannot exclude the possibility of fetal damage, mercaptopurine should be used during pregnancy only if the benefit clearly justifies the possible risk to the fetus, and particular caution should be given to the use of mercaptopurine in the first trimester of pregnancy.

There are no adequate and well-controlled studies in pregnant women. If this drug is used during pregnancy or if the patient becomes pregnant while taking the drug, the patient should be apprised of the potential hazard to the fetus. Women of childbearing potential should be advised to avoid becoming pregnant.

PRECAUTIONS

General: The safe and effective use of PURINETHOL demands a thorough knowledge of the natural history of the condition being treated. After selection of an initial dosage

schedule, therapy will frequently need to be modified depending upon the patient's response and manifestations of toxicity.

The most frequent, serious, toxic effect of PURINETHOL is myelosuppression resulting in leukopenia, thrombocytopenia, and anemia. These toxic effects are often unavoidable during the induction phase of adult acute leukemia. If remission induction is to be successful. Whether or not these manifestations demand modification or cessation of dosage depends both upon the response of the underlying disease and a careful consideration of supportive facilities (granulocyte and platelet transfusions) which may be available. Life-threatening infections and bleeding have been observed as a consequence of mercaptopurine-induced granulocytopenia and thrombocytopenia. Severe hematologic toxicity may require supportive therapy with platelet transfusions for bleeding, and antibiotics and granulocyte transfusions if sepsis is documented.

If it is not the intent to deliberately induce bone marrow hypoplasia, it is important to discontinue the drug temporarily at the first evidence of an abnormally large fall in white blood cell count, platelet count, or hemoglobin concentration. In many patients with severe depression of the formed elements of the blood due to PURINETHOL, the bone marrow appears hypoplastic on aspiration or biopsy, whereas in other cases it may appear normocellular. The qualitative changes in the erythroid elements toward the megaloblastic series, characteristically seen with the folic acid antagonists and some other antimetabolites, are not seen with this drug.

It is probably advisable to start with smaller dosages in patients with impaired renal function, since the latter might result in slower elimination of the drug and metabolites and a greater cumulative effect.

Information for Patients: Patients should be informed that the major toxicities of PURINETHOL are related to myelosuppression, hepatotoxicity, and gastrointestinal toxicity. Patients should never be allowed to take the drug without medical supervision and should be advised to consult their physician if they experience fever, sore throat, jaundice, nausea, vomiting, signs of local infection, bleeding from any site, or symptoms suggestive of anemia. Women of childbearing potential should be advised to avoid becoming pregnant.

Laboratory Tests: It is recommended that evaluation of the hemoglobin or hematocrit, total white blood cell count and differential count, and quantitative platelet count be obtained weekly while the patient is on therapy with PURINETHOL. In cases where the cause of fluctuations in the formed elements in the peripheral blood is obscure, bone marrow examination may be useful for the evaluation of marrow status. The decision to increase, decrease, continue, or discontinue a given dosage of PURINETHOL must be based not only on the absolute hematologic values, but also upon the rapidity with which changes are occurring. In many instances, particularly during the induction phase of acute leukemia, complete blood counts will need to be done more frequently than once weekly in order to evaluate the effect of the therapy.

Drug Interactions: *Interaction with Allopurinol:* When allopurinol and mercaptopurine are administered concomitantly, it is imperative that the dose of mercaptopurine be reduced to one third to one quarter of the usual dose. Failure to observe this dosage reduction will result in a delayed catabolism of mercaptopurine and the strong likelihood of inducing severe toxicity.

There is usually complete cross-resistance between mercaptopurine and thioguanine.

The dosage of mercaptopurine may need to be reduced when this agent is combined with other drugs whose primary or secondary toxicity is myelosuppression. Enhanced marrow suppression has been noted in some patients also receiving trimethoprim-sulfamethoxazole.[17,18]

Carcinogenesis, Mutagenesis, Impairment of Fertility: Mercaptopurine causes chromosomal aberrations in animals and humans and induces dominant-lethal mutations in male mice. In mice, surviving female offspring of mothers who received chronic low doses of mercaptopurine during pregnancy were found sterile, or if they became pregnant, had smaller litters and more dead fetuses as compared to control animals.[19] Carcinogenic potential exists in humans, but the extent of the risk is unknown.

The effect of mercaptopurine on human fertility is unknown for either males or females.

Pregnancy: *Teratogenic Effects:* Pregnancy Category D. See WARNINGS section.

Nursing Mothers: It is not known whether this drug is excreted in human milk. Because many drugs are excreted in human milk, and because of the potential for serious adverse reactions in nursing infants from mercaptopurine, a decision should be made whether to discontinue nursing or to discontinue the drug, taking into account the importance of the drug to the mother.

Pediatric Use: See DOSAGE AND ADMINISTRATION section.

ADVERSE REACTIONS

The principal and potentially serious toxic effects of PURINETHOL are bone marrow toxicity and hepatotoxicity (see WARNINGS).

Hematologic: The most frequent adverse reaction to PURINETHOL is myelosuppression. The induction of complete remission of acute lymphatic leukemia frequently is associated with marrow hypoplasia. Maintenance of remission generally involves multiple-drug regimens whose component agents cause myelosuppression. Anemia, leukopenia, and thrombocytopenia are frequently observed. Dosages and schedules are adjusted to prevent life-threatening cytopenias.

Renal: Hyperuricemia may occur in patients receiving PURINETHOL as a consequence of rapid cell lysis accompanying the antineoplastic effect. Adverse effects can be minimized by increased hydration, urine alkalinization, and the prophylactic administration of a xanthine oxidase inhibitor such as allopurinol. The dosage of PURINETHOL should be reduced to one third to one quarter of the usual dose if allopurinol is given concurrently.

Gastrointestinal: Intestinal ulceration has been reported.[20] Nausea, vomiting, and anorexia are uncommon during initial administration. Mild diarrhea and sprue-like symptoms have been noted occasionally, but it is difficult at present to attribute these to the medication. Oral lesions are rarely seen, and when they occur they resemble thrush rather than antifolic ulcerations.

An increased risk of pancreatitis may be associated with the investigational use of PURINETHOL in inflammatory bowel disease.[21–23]

Miscellaneous: While dermatologic reactions can occur as a consequence of disease, the administration of PURINETHOL has been associated with skin rashes and hyperpigmentation.[24]

Drug fever has been very rarely reported with PURINETHOL. Before attributing fever to PURINETHOL, every attempt should be made to exclude more common causes of pyrexia, such as sepsis, in patients with acute leukemia.

OVERDOSAGE

Signs and symptoms of overdosage may be immediate such as anorexia, nausea, vomiting and diarrhea; or delayed such as myelosuppression, liver dysfunction, and gastroenteritis. Dialysis cannot be expected to clear mercaptopurine. Hemodialysis is thought to be of marginal use due to the rapid intracellular incorporation of mercaptopurine into active metabolites with long persistence. The oral LD_{50} of mercaptopurine was determined to be 480 mg/kg in the mouse and 425 mg/kg in the rat.[25]

There is no known pharmacologic antagonist of mercaptopurine. The drug should be discontinued immediately if unintended toxicity occurs during treatment. If a patient is seen immediately following an accidental overdosage of the drug, it may be useful to induce emesis.

DOSAGE AND ADMINISTRATION

Induction Therapy: PURINETHOL is administered orally. The dosage which will be tolerated and be effective varies from patient to patient, and therefore careful titration is necessary to obtain the optimum therapeutic effect without incurring excessive, unintended toxicity. The usual initial dosage for pediatric patients and adults is 2.5 mg/kg of body weight per day (100 to 200 mg in the average adult and 50 mg in an average 5-year-old child). Pediatric patients with acute leukemia have tolerated this dose without difficulty in most cases; it may be continued daily for several weeks or more in some patients. If, after 4 weeks at this dosage, there is no clinical improvement and no definite evidence of leukocyte or platelet depression, the dosage may be increased up to 5 mg/kg daily. A dosage of 2.5 mg/kg per day may result in a rapid fall in leukocyte count within 1 to 2 weeks in some adults with acute lymphatic leukemia and high total leukocyte counts.

The total daily dosage may be given at one time. It is calculated to the nearest multiple of 25 mg. The dosage of PURINETHOL should be reduced to one third to one quarter of the usual dose if allopurinol is given concurrently. Because the drug may have a delayed action, it should be discontinued at the first sign of an abnormally large or rapid fall in the leukocyte or platelet count. If subsequently the leukocyte count or platelet count remains constant for 2 or 3 days, or rises, treatment may be resumed.

Maintenance Therapy: Once a complete hematologic remission is obtained, maintenance therapy is considered essential. Maintenance doses will vary from patient to patient. A usual daily maintenance dose of PURINETHOL is 1.5 to 2.5 mg/kg per day as a single dose. It is to be emphasized that in pediatric patients with acute lymphatic leukemia in remission, superior results have been obtained when PURINETHOL has been combined with other agents (most frequently with methotrexate) for remission maintenance. PURINETHOL should rarely be relied upon as a single agent for the maintenance of remissions induced in acute leukemia.

Procedures for proper handling and disposal of anticancer drugs should be considered. Several guidelines on this subject have been published.[26–32]

There is no general agreement that all of the procedures recommended in the guidelines are necessary or appropriate.

HOW SUPPLIED

Pale yellow to buff, scored tablets containing 50 mg mercaptopurine, imprinted with "PURINETHOL" and "04A"; bottles of 25 (NDC 0173-0807-25) and 250 (NDC 0173-0807-65).

Store at 15° to 25°C (59°to 77°F) in a dry place.

REFERENCES

1. Hitchings GH, Elion GB. The chemistry and biochemistry of purine analogs. *Ann NY Acad Sci.* 1954; 60:195-199.
2. Loo TL, Luce JK, Sullivan MP, Frei E III. Clinical pharmacologic observations on 6-mercaptopurine and 6-methylthiopurine ribonucleoside. *Clin Pharmacol Ther.* 1968; 9:180-194.
3. Elion GB. Biochemistry and pharmacology of purine analogs. *Fed Proc.* 1967;26:898-904.
4. Scannell JP, Hitchings GH. Thioguanine in deoxyribonucleic acid from tumors of 6-mercaptopurine-treated mice. *Proc Soc Exp Biol Med.* 1966;122:627-629.
5. Paterson ARP, Tidd DM. 6-thiopurines. In Sartorelli AC, Johns DG (eds). *Antineoplastic and Immunosuppressive Agents,* Part II. Berlin, Springer-Verlag; 1975;384-403.
6. Lennard L, Gibson BES, Nicole T, Lilleyman JS. Congenital thiopurine methyltransferase deficiency and 6-mercaptopurine toxicity during treatment for acute lymphoblastic leukemia. *Arch Dis Child.* 1993;69:577-579.
7. Evans WE, Homer M, Chu YQ, Kalwinsky D, Roberts WM. Altered mercaptopurine metabolism, toxic effects, and dosage requirement in a thiopurine methyltransferase-deficient child with acute lymphocytic leukemia. *J Pediatr.* 1991;119:985-989.
8. Burchenal JH, Ellison RR, Murphy ML, et al. Clinical studies on 6-mercaptopurine. *Ann NY Acad Sci.* 1954; 60:359-368.
9. Farber S. Summary of experience with 6-mercaptopurine. *Ann NY Acad Sci.* 1954;60:412-414.
10. Fountain JR. Clinical observations of the treatment of leukemia and allied disorders with 6-mercaptopurine. *Ann NY Acad Sci.* 1954;60:439-446.
11. Hyman GA, Gellhorn A, Wolff JA. The therapeutic effect of mercaptopurine in a variety of human neoplastic diseases. *Ann NY Acad Sci.* 1954;60:430-435.
12. Einhorn M, Davidsohn I. Hepatotoxicity of mercaptopurine. *JAMA.* 1964;188:802-806.
13. Schein PS, Winokur SH. Immunosuppressive and cytotoxic chemotherapy: long-term complications. *Ann Intern Med.* 1975;82:84-95.
14. Stern MH, Minow RA, Casey JH, Luna MA. Hepatotoxicity in patients treated with adriamycin and 6-mercaptopurine for refractory leukemia. *Am J Clin Pathol.* 1975;63:758-759. Abstract.
15. Blatt J, Mulvihill JJ, Ziegler JL, Young RC, Poplack DG. Pregnancy outcome following cancer chemotherapy. *Am J Med.* 1980;69:828-832.
16. Nicholson HO. Cytotoxic drugs in pregnancy: review of reported cases. *J Obstet Gynaecol Br Commonw.* 1968; 75:307-312.
17. Woods WG, Daigle AE, Hutchinson RJ, Robison LL. Myelosuppression associated with cotrimoxazole as a prophylactic antibiotic in the maintenance phase of childhood acute lymphocytic leukemia. *J Pediatr.* 1984; 105:639-644.
18. Rees CA, Lennard L, Lilleyman JS, Maddocks JL. Disturbance of 6-mercaptopurine metabolism by cotrimoxazole in childhood lymphoblastic leukemia. *Cancer Chemother Pharmacol.* 1984;12:87-89.
19. Reimers TJ, Sluss PM. 6-mercaptopurine treatment of pregnant mice: effects on second and third generations. *Science.* 1978;201:65-67.
20. Clark PA, Hsia YE, Huntsman RG. Toxic complications of treatment with 6-mercaptopurine. *Br Med J. [Clin Res].* 1960;1:393-395.
21. Present DH, Meltzer SJ, Wolke A, Korelitz BI. Short and long term toxicity to 6-mercaptopurine in the management of inflammatory bowel disease. *Gastroenterology.* 1985;88:1545. Abstract.

Continued on next page

This product information is based on labeling in effect on June 1, 1998. For further information, contact via direct mail, phone, or web site Medical Information: Glaxo Wellcome Inc., PO Box 13398, Research Triangle Park, NC 27709. Healthcare Professionals (Medical Information): 800-334-0089 Patients (Customer Response Center): 888-TALK2GW (1-888-825-5249) Glaxo Wellcome Corporate Web Site: www.glaxowellcome.com

Purinethol—Cont.

22. Bank L, Wright JP. 6-mercaptopurine-related pancreatitis in 2 patients with inflammatory bowel disease. *Dig Dis Sci.* 1984;29:357-359.
23. Singleton JW, Law DH, Kelley ML Jr, Mekhjian HS, Sturdevant RAL. National cooperative Crohn's disease study: adverse reactions to study drugs. *Gastroenterology.* 1979;77:870-882.
24. Dreizen S, Bodey GP, Rodriguez V, McCredie KB. Cutaneous complications of cancer chemotherapy. *Postgrad Med.* 1975;58:150-158.
25. Unpublished data on file with Glaxo Wellcome Inc.
26. Recommendations for the safe handling of parenteral antineoplastic drugs. Washington, DC: Division of Safety; National Institutes of Health; 1983. US Dept of Health and Human Services. Public Health Service publication NIH 83-2621.
27. AMA Council on Scientific Affairs. Guidelines for handling parenteral antineoplastics. *JAMA.* 1985; 253: 1590-1591.
28. National Study Commission on Cytotoxic Exposure. Recommendations for handling cytotoxic agents. 1987. Available from Louis P. Jeffrey, Chairman, National Study Commission on Cytotoxic Exposure. Massachusetts College of Pharmacy and Allied Health Sciences, 179 Longwood Avenue, Boston, MA 02115.
29. Clinical Oncological Society of Australia. Guidelines and recommendations for safe handling of antineoplastic agents. *Med J Australia.* 1983;1:426-428.
30. Jones RB, Frank R, Mass T. Safe handling of chemotherapeutic agents: a report from the Mount Sinai Medical Center. *CA-A Cancer J for Clinicians.* 1983;33:258-263.
31. American Society of Hospital Pharmacists. ASHP technical assistance bulletin on handling cytotoxic and hazardous drugs. *Am J Hosp Pharm.* 1990;47:1033-1049.
32. Yodaiken RE, Bennett D. OSHA work-practice guidelines for personnel dealing with cytotoxic (antineoplastic) drugs. *Am J Hosp Pharm.* 1986;43:1193-1204.

November 1997/RL-497
Shown in Product Identification Guide, page 313

RAXAR™ Tablets ℞

[răx'ar]
(grepafloxacin hydrochloride tablets)

DESCRIPTION

RAXAR Tablets contain grepafloxacin hydrochloride. RAXAR is a broad-spectrum fluoroquinolone antibiotic for oral administration.
The chemical name for grepafloxacin is (±)-1-cyclopropyl-6-fluoro-1,4-dihydro-5-methyl-7-(3-methyl-1-piperazinyl)-4-oxo-3-quinolinecarboxylic acid monohydrochloride sesquihydrate. Its molecular formula is $C_{19}H_{22}FN_3O_3$ HCl•3/2 H_2O and it has a molecular weight of 422.88. It is soluble in water and very slightly soluble in ethanol. Grepafloxacin has the following structural formula:

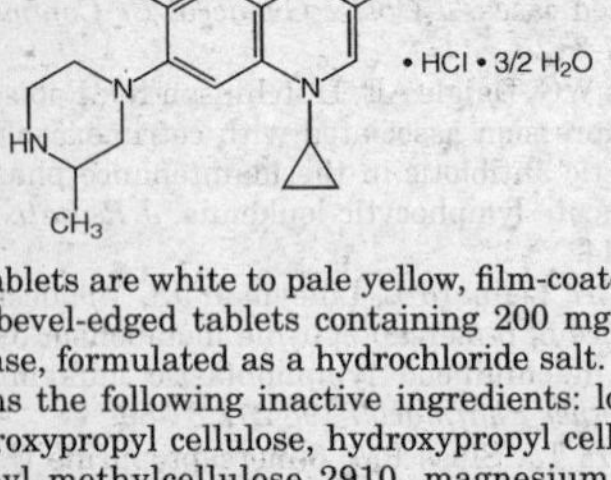

RAXAR Tablets are white to pale yellow, film-coated, round, biconvex, bevel-edged tablets containing 200 mg of grepafloxacin base, formulated as a hydrochloride salt. Each tablet contains the following inactive ingredients: low substituted hydroxypropyl cellulose, hydroxypropyl cellulose, hydroxypropyl methylcellulose 2910, magnesium stearate, microcrystalline cellulose, talc, and titanium dioxide.

CLINICAL PHARMACOLOGY

Absorption: Grepafloxacin is rapidly and extensively absorbed following oral administration of RAXAR Tablets. Bioavailability of the tablet is equivalent to the bioavailability of an oral solution of grepafloxacin. The absolute bioavailability of RAXAR Tablets was estimated by comparing the areas under the plasma grepafloxacin concentration versus time curve (AUC) after intravenous and oral administration of grepafloxacin in separate studies. The absolute bioavailability is approximately 70%.
Single dose and steady-state pharmacokinetic parameters following administration of 400-mg and 600-mg doses to healthy adult males are displayed in Table 1.
[See table 1 below]
On average, the peak plasma drug concentration (C_{max}) is achieved 2 to 3 hours after dosing. Steady-state concentrations of grepafloxacin are achieved within 7 days of once-a-day dosing.
Grepafloxacin pharmacokinetic parameters were determined following administration of 600 mg grepafloxacin immediately following a high fat meal (1,000 kcal, 67 grams fat, 38 grams protein, 63 grams carbohydrates) and administration in the fasted state (n = 29). There was no difference in grepafloxacin pharmacokinetic parameters between the fasted and fed treatments. Milk had no effect on the C_{max}, T_{max}, or AUC of grepafloxacin after oral administration. Neutralization of gastric acidity by intravenous administration of the histamine type-2 receptor antagonist famotidine did not affect the absorption or other pharmacokinetic properties of RAXAR Tablets.
Distribution: The apparent volume of distribution after oral administration of grepafloxacin 400 mg was 5.07 ± 0.95 L/kg, suggesting that grepafloxacin distributes widely into extravascular spaces. Binding of grepafloxacin to human plasma proteins is low (approximately 50%).
Table 2 summarizes the concentrations of grepafloxacin in fluids and tissues compared with serum drug concentration.
[See table 2 at bottom of next page]
Metabolism and Excretion: The plasma elimination half-life of grepafloxacin at steady state was 15.7 ± 4.2 hours. Grepafloxacin is eliminated predominantly through hepatic metabolism and biliary excretion. Less than 10% of an oral dose is excreted as unchanged grepafloxacin in urine. Approximately 88% of an oral dose of radiolabeled grepafloxacin 400 mg was recovered in urine (38%) and feces (50%) over 7 days post dose. Approximately one-half of the AUC in plasma for the 12 hours after dosing was due to unchanged grepafloxacin; 68% of AUC in plasma for 12 hours after dosing was due to unchanged grepafloxacin plus known metabolites. Unchanged grepafloxacin (6% of dose) and several metabolites (in amounts ranging from 0.08% to 5.57% of dose) were recovered in urine. Unchanged grepafloxacin (27% of dose) and several metabolites (in amounts ranging from 1.83% to 3.91% of dose) were recovered in feces. Grepafloxacin metabolites include glucuronide (major metabolite) and sulfate conjugates and oxidative metabolites. The oxidative metabolites are formed mainly by cytochrome P450 1A2 (CYP1A2), while the cytochrome P450 3A4 (CYP3A4) has minor involvement. The nonconjugated metabolites have little antimicrobial activity compared with the parent drug. The conjugated metabolites have no antimicrobial activity.
Special Populations:
Gender: Following administration of RAXAR 600 mg daily for 7 days, C_{max} was approximately 30% to 50% higher and AUC was approximately 20% to 50% higher in females compared to males. The observed differences appear to be due mainly to differences in body weight. Total clearance (per unit body weight), renal clearance (per unit body weight), and half-life did not differ between males and females. The observed differences in pharmacokinetic properties by gender do not necessitate any difference between males and females in dosage and administration.
Geriatric: There are no significant differences in grepafloxacin pharmacokinetics between young and elderly subjects.
Pediatric: Grepafloxacin has not been evaluated in pediatric patients.
Hepatic Insufficiency: Two studies were performed to assess the effect of hepatic failure on grepafloxacin pharmacokinetics. Both studies evaluated subjects with normal hepatic function, with mild (Child-Pugh class A) hepatic failure, or moderate hepatic failure (Child-Pugh class B). In one study, oral clearance was reduced by approximately 50% in patients with mild hepatic failure (n = 5) relative to subjects with normal hepatic function (n = 6). In the second study, oral clearance was reduced by approximately 15% in subjects with mild hepatic failure (n = 5) relative to subjects with normal hepatic function (n = 8). Due to the different results for the two studies, it is not possible to determine an appropriate dose adjustment for subjects with mild hepatic failure. In both studies, oral clearance was decreased by >50% in subjects with moderate hepatic failure (n = 9, n = 3) compared to subjects with normal hepatic function (n = 6, n = 8). RAXAR Tablets are contraindicated for use in patients with hepatic failure. (See **DOSAGE AND ADMINISTRATION.**)
Renal Insufficiency: Renal clearance of grepafloxacin was 0.458 ± 0.04 mL/min/kg in adults with normal renal function. The effect of varying degrees of renal function on the pharmacokinetics of grepafloxacin was assessed in 15 patients with impaired renal function (creatinine clearances ranging from 7.5 to 64 mL/min) compared with five adults with normal renal function. Varying degrees of renal function did not substantially affect the pharmacokinetic properties of grepafloxacin.
Smokers: In a population pharmacokinetics study of grepafloxacin in patients with acute bacterial exacerbations of chronic bronchitis, grepafloxacin clearance was 35% to 43% faster in patients who smoked relative to patients who did not smoke. This observation is consistent with the involvement of CYP1A2 in the metabolism of grepafloxacin and the known induction of this enzyme in smokers. However, in the pivotal clinical trials, smoking did not have an effect on clinical efficacy.
Drug Interactions: (See also **PRECAUTIONS.**)
Antacids: Following administration of 200 mg grepafloxacin with 1 gram aluminum hydroxide, grepafloxacin AUC and C_{max} were both decreased by approximately 60% relative to administration of grepafloxacin alone (n = 6). (See **PRECAUTIONS.**)
Probenecid: Administration of 200 mg grepafloxacin with 500 mg probenecid, followed by 500 mg probenecid every 12 hours for 3 doses, did not alter grepafloxacin pharmacokinetics (n = 6).
Theophylline: Grepafloxacin is a competitive inhibitor of theophylline metabolism. Twelve healthy subjects received an individualized regimen of sustained release theophylline alone for 7 days, followed by coadministration of the theophylline regimen with 600 mg grepafloxacin once daily for 10 days. Following the addition of grepafloxacin, theophylline clearance decreased by approximately 50%, from 0.78 ± 0.25 to 0.40 ± 0.08 mL/min/kg. Steady-state peak theophylline concentration increased from 8.30 ± 1.54 µg/mL to 15.12 ± 3.69 µg/mL. (See **PRECAUTIONS.**)
Warfarin: Fourteen healthy subjects received an individualized regimen of warfarin alone for 14 days, followed by coadministration of the warfarin regimen with 600 mg grepafloxacin once daily for 10 days. Grepafloxacin did not alter the anticoagulant effect of warfarin. Other quinolones have been reported to enhance the anticoagulant effects of warfarin. (See **PRECAUTIONS.**)
Microbiology: Grepafloxacin has *in vitro* activity against a wide range of gram-positive and gram-negative aerobic microorganisms, as well as some atypical microorganisms. Grepafloxacin exerts its antibacterial activity by inhibiting bacterial topoisomerase II (DNA gyrase) and topoisomerase IV, essential enzymes for duplication, transcription, and repair of bacterial DNA. Beta-lactamase production has no effect on grepafloxacin activity and penicillin-resistant *Streptococcus pneumoniae* strains have undiminished *in vitro* susceptibility to grepafloxacin. Grepafloxacin is bactericidal at concentrations equal to or slightly greater than minimum inhibitory concentrations (MIC's).
Resistance to grepafloxacin through spontaneous mutation *in vitro* occurs at a low frequency (10^{-8} to 10^{-10}). As with other fluoroquinolones, the mutation frequency was higher for *Pseudomonas* species and *Stenotrophomonas maltophilia* than for other microorganisms. When resistance develops, it does so through slow stepwise increases in MIC's. In clinical trials, grepafloxacin-resistant mutants were rarely encountered during the treatment of infections caused by susceptible isolates. When they did occur, they were usually *Pseudomonas* species isolates.
Although cross-resistance has been observed between grepafloxacin and some other fluoroquinolones, some organisms resistant to other quinolones are susceptible to grepafloxacin.
Quinolones differ in chemical structure and mode of action from other classes of antimicrobial agents, including beta-lactam antibiotics and aminoglycosides; therefore, microorganisms resistant to these other classes of drugs may be susceptible to grepafloxacin and other quinolones.
In vitro tests show that grepafloxacin has reduced activity against some gram-positive microorganisms when combined with rifampin.
Grepafloxacin has been shown to be active against most strains of the following microorganisms, both *in vitro* and in clinical infections as described in the **INDICATIONS AND USAGE** section:

Table 1: Single-Dose and Steady-State Pharmacokinetic Parameters in Healthy Adult Males

Parameter	Single dose pharmacokinetic parameters		Steady state pharmacokinetic parameters	
	400 mg N = 40	600 mg N = 31	400 mg N = 10	600 mg N = 46
*AUC (µg•h/mL)	12.27 ± 3.81	22.66 ± 5.65	14.08 ± 2.80	27.51 ± 6.95
C_{max} (µg/mL)	1.11 ± 0.34	1.58 ± 0.37	1.35 ± 0.25	2.25 ± 0.48
Trough (µg/mL)	not applicable	not applicable	0.21 ± 0.08	0.55 ± 0.22

*AUC = AUC∞ for single dose; $AUC_{0\text{-}24}$ for steady state.

Aerobic gram-positive microorganisms:
Streptococcus pneumoniae (penicillin-susceptible strains)
Aerobic gram-negative microorganisms:
Haemophilus influenzae
Moraxella catarrhalis
Neisseria gonorrhoeae
Other microorganisms:
Chlamydia trachomatis
Mycoplasma pneumoniae
The following *in vitro* data are available, **but their clinical significance is unknown.**
Grepafloxacin exhibits *in vitro* minimum inhibitory concentrations (MIC's) of 1 µg/mL or less against most (≥90%) strains of the following microorganisms; however, the safety and effectiveness of grepafloxacin in treating clinical infections due to these microorganisms have not been established in adequate and well-controlled clinical trials.
Aerobic gram-positive microorganisms:
Staphylococcus aureus (methicillin-susceptible strains)
Staphylococcus epidermidis (methicillin-susceptible strains)
Streptococcus agalactiae
Streptococcus pneumoniae (penicillin-resistant strains)
Streptococcus pyogenes
Aerobic gram-negative microorganisms:
Citrobacter freundii
Citrobacter (diversus) koseri
Enterobacter aerogenes
Enterobacter cloacae
Escherichia coli
Haemophilus parainfluenzae
Klebsiella oxytoca
Klebsiella pneumoniae
Morganella morganii
Proteus mirabilis
Proteus vulgaris
Susceptibility Tests
Dilution Techniques: Quantitative methods are used to determine antimicrobial minimum inhibitory concentrations (MIC's). These MIC's provide estimates of the susceptibility of bacteria to antimicrobial compounds. The MIC's should be determined using a standardized procedure. Standardized procedures are based on a dilution method[1] (broth or agar) or equivalent with standardized inoculum concentrations and standardized concentrations of grepafloxacin powder. The MIC values should be interpreted according to the following criteria:
For testing aerobic organisms other than *Streptococcus pneumoniae*, *Haemophilus influenzae*, and *Neisseria gonorrhoeae*:

MIC (µg/mL)	Interpretation
≤1	Susceptible (S)
2	Intermediate (I)
≥4	Resistant (R)

For testing *Streptococcus pneumoniae*:[a]

MIC (µg/mL)	Interpretation
≤1	Susceptible (S)

[a] These interpretive standards are applicable only to broth microdilution susceptibility tests using cation-adjusted Mueller-Hinton broth with 2–5% lysed horse blood.
The current absence of data on resistant strains precludes defining any categories other than "Susceptible". Strains yielding MIC results suggestive of a "Nonsusceptible" category should be submitted to a reference laboratory for further testing.
For testing *Haemophilus influenzae*:[b]

MIC (µg/mL)	Interpretation
≤0.25	Susceptible (S)

[b] These interpretive standards are applicable only to broth microdilution susceptibility testing with *Haemophilus influenzae* using *Haemophilus* Test Medium[1].
The current absence of data on resistant strains precludes defining any categories other than "Susceptible". Strains

yielding MIC results suggestive of a "Nonsusceptible" category should be submitted to a reference laboratory for further testing.

For testing *Neisseria gonorrhoeae*:[c]

MIC (µg/mL)	Interpretation
≤0.06	Susceptible (S)

[c] These interpretive standards are applicable only to agar dilution tests with GC agar base and 1% defined growth supplement.
The current absence of data on resistant strains precludes defining any categories other than "Susceptible". Strains yielding MIC results suggestive of a "Nonsusceptible" category should be submitted to a reference laboratory for further testing.
A report of "Susceptible" indicates that the pathogen is likely to be inhibited if the antimicrobial compound in the blood reaches the concentration usually achievable. A report of "Intermediate" indicates that the result should be considered equivocal, and, if the microorganism is not fully susceptible to alternative, clinically feasible drugs, the test should be repeated. This category implies possible clinical applicability in body sites where the drug is physiologically concentrated or in situations where a high dosage of drug can be used. This category also provides a buffer zone which prevents small uncontrolled technical factors from causing major discrepancies in interpretation. A report of "Resistant" indicates that the pathogen is not likely to be inhibited if the antimicrobial compound in the blood reaches the concentration usually achievable; other therapy should be selected.
Standardized susceptibility test procedures require the use of laboratory control microorganisms to control the technical aspects of the laboratory procedures. Standard grepafloxacin powder should provide the following MIC values:

Microorganism	MIC Range (µg/mL)
Escherichia coli ATCC 25922	0.004–0.03
Haemophilus influenzae ATCC 49247[a]	0.002–0.016
Neisseria gonorrhoeae ATCC 49226[b]	0.004–0.03
Staphylococcus aureus ATCC 29213	0.03–0.12
Streptococcus pneumoniae ATCC 49619[c]	0.06–0.5

[a] This quality control range is applicable only to *H. influenzae* ATCC 49247 tested by a broth microdilution procedure using *Haemophilus* Test Medium (HTM)[1].
[b] This quality control range is applicable only to *N. gonorrhoeae* ATCC 49226 tested by agar dilution using GC agar base with 1% defined growth supplement.
[c] This quality control range is applicable only to *S. pneumoniae* ATCC 49619 tested by a broth microdilution procedure using cation-adjusted Mueller-Hinton broth with 2–5% lysed horse blood.

Diffusion Techniques: Quantitative methods that require measurement of zone diameters also provide reproducible estimates of the susceptibility of bacteria to antimicrobial compounds. One such standardized procedure[2] requires the use of standardized inoculum concentrations. This procedure uses paper disks impregnated with 5-µg grepafloxacin to test the susceptibility of microorganisms to grepafloxacin. Reports from the laboratory providing results of the standard single-disk susceptibility test with a 5-µg disk should be interpreted according to the following criteria:
For aerobic organisms other than *Streptococcus pneumoniae*, *Haemophilus influenzae*, and *Neisseria gonorrhoeae*:

Zone Diameter (mm)	Interpretation
≥18	Susceptible (S)
15 – 17	Intermediate (I)
≤14	Resistant (R)

For testing *Streptococcus pneumoniae*:[a]

Zone Diameter (mm)	Interpretation
≥19	Susceptible (S)

[a] These zone diameter standards for *Streptococcus pneumoniae* are applicable only to tests performed using Mueller-Hinton agar supplemented with 5% sheep blood and incubated in 5% CO_2.
The current absence of data on resistant strains precludes defining any categories other than "Susceptible". Strains yielding zone diameter results suggestive of a "Nonsusceptible" category should be submitted to a reference laboratory for further testing.
For testing *Haemophilus influenzae*:[b]

Zone Diameter (mm)	Interpretation
≥24	Susceptible (S)

[b] These zone diameter standards are applicable only to disk diffusion testing with *Haemophilus influenzae* using *Haemophilus* Test Medium (HTM)[2].
The current absence of data on resistant strains precludes defining any categories other than "Susceptible". Strains yielding zone diameter results suggestive of a "Nonsusceptible" category should be submitted to a reference laboratory for further testing.
For testing *Neisseria gonorrhoeae*:[c]

Zone Diameter (mm)	Interpretation
≥37	Susceptible (S)

[c] These zone diameter standards for *Neisseria gonorrhoeae* are applicable only to disk diffusion tests with GC agar base and 1% growth supplement.
The current absence of data on resistant strains precludes defining any categories other than "Susceptible". Strains yielding zone diameter results suggestive of a "Nonsusceptible" category should be submitted to a reference laboratory for further testing.
Interpretation should be as stated above for results using dilution techniques. Interpretation involves correlation of the diameter obtained in the disk test with the MIC for grepafloxacin.
As with standardized dilution techniques, diffusion methods require the use of laboratory control microorganisms that are used to control the technical aspects of the laboratory procedures. For the diffusion technique, the 5-µg grepafloxacin disk should provide the following zone diameters in these laboratory test quality control strains:

Microorganism	Zone Diameter (mm)
Escherichia coli ATCC 25922	28–36
Haemophilus influenzae ATCC 49247[a]	32–39
Neisseria gonorrhoeae ATCC 49226[b]	44–52
Staphylococcus aureus ATCC 25923	26–31
Streptococcus pneumoniae ATCC 49619[c]	21–28

[a] This quality control range is applicable only to *H. influenzae* ATCC 49247 tested by a disk diffusion procedure using *Haemophilus* Test Medium (HTM)[2].
[b] This quality control range is applicable only to *N. gonorrhoeae* ATCC 49226 tested by a disk diffusion procedure using GC agar base with 1% defined growth supplement.
[c] This quality control range is applicable only to *S. pneumoniae* ATCC 49619 tested by a disk diffusion procedure using Mueller-Hinton agar supplemented with 5% sheep blood and incubated in 5% CO_2.

INDICATIONS AND USAGE

RAXAR Tablets are indicated for treatment of adults with mild to moderate infections caused by susceptible strains of the designated microorganisms in the infections listed below:

1. **Acute Bacterial Exacerbations of Chronic Bronchitis** caused by *Haemophilus influenzae*, *Streptococcus pneumoniae*, or *Moraxella catarrhalis*. (See **CLINICAL STUDIES** section.)
2. **Community-acquired Pneumonia** caused by *Haemophilus influenzae*, *Streptococcus pneumoniae*, *Moraxella catarrhalis*, or *Mycoplasma pneumoniae*. (See **CLINICAL STUDIES** section.)
3. **Uncomplicated Gonorrhea (urethral in males and endocervical and rectal in females)** caused by *Neisseria gonorrhoeae*. (See **WARNINGS**.)

Continued on next page

This product information is based on labeling in effect on June 1, 1998. For further information, contact via direct mail, phone, or web site Medical Information: Glaxo Wellcome Inc., PO Box 13398, Research Triangle Park, NC 27709. Healthcare Professionals (Medical Information): 800-334-0089 Patients (Customer Response Center): 888-TALK2GW (1-888-825-5249) Glaxo Wellcome Corporate Web Site: www.glaxowellcome.com

Table 2: Distribution of Grepafloxacin into Tissues and Fluids After Oral Administration
(n = number of subjects)

Tissue or Fluid	Oral Dose (mg)	Hours Post-Dose	n	Concentration (Mean ± SD) Serum (µg/mL)	Concentration (Mean ± SD) Tissue or Fluid (µg/mL or µg/g)	Ratio
Alveolar lining fluid	400	4–5	5	1.76	27.1	15.4
Alveolar macrophages	400	4–5	5	1.76	278	158
Cervix uteri	100	4–5	5	1.23 ± 0.26	3.42 ± 0.65	2.8
Portio vaginalis	100	4–5	5	1.23 ± 0.26	2.58 ± 0.69	2.1
Sputum	200	4	7	0.47 ± 0.11	1.04 ± 0.48	2.2

Raxar—Cont.

4. **Nongonococcal Urethritis and Cervicitis** caused by *Chlamydia trachomatis*. (See **WARNINGS**.)

Appropriate culture and susceptibility testing should be performed to determine susceptibility of the causative microorganism(s) to grepafloxacin. Therapy may be started while awaiting the results of this testing. Antimicrobial therapy should be appropriately adjusted according to the results of such testing.

CONTRAINDICATIONS

RAXAR Tablets are contraindicated in persons with a history of hypersensitivity to grepafloxacin or other members of the quinolone class of antimicrobial agents. RAXAR Tablets are contraindicated in patients with hepatic failure. Because prolongation of the QT_c interval has been observed in healthy volunteers receiving RAXAR, RAXAR Tablets are contraindicated in patients with known QT_c prolongation. RAXAR Tablets are also contraindicated in patients being treated concomitantly with medications known to produce an increase in the QT_c interval and/or torsade de pointes (e.g., terfenadine) unless appropriate cardiac monitoring can be assured (e.g., in hospitalized patients). (See **WARNINGS**.)

WARNINGS

THE SAFETY AND EFFICACY OF GREPAFLOXACIN IN CHILDREN, ADOLESCENTS (LESS THAN 18 YEARS OF AGE), PREGNANT WOMEN, AND LACTATING WOMEN HAVE NOT BEEN ESTABLISHED (SEE PRECAUTIONS - PEDIATRIC USE, PREGNANCY, AND NURSING MOTHERS SUBSECTIONS). Histopathological examination of the weight-bearing joints of juvenile dogs revealed permanent lesions of the cartilage. Related quinolone-class drugs also produce erosions of cartilage of weight-bearing joints and other signs of arthropathy in immature animals of various species. (See **ANIMAL PHARMACOLOGY**.)

Convulsions, increased intracranial pressure, and toxic psychosis have been reported in patients receiving quinolones. Quinolones may also cause central nervous system stimulation which may lead to tremors, restlessness, lightheadedness, confusion, or hallucinations. If these reactions occur in patients receiving grepafloxacin, the drug should be discontinued and appropriate treatment measures instituted. As with other quinolones, RAXAR should be used with caution in patients with known or suspected CNS disorders, such as severe cerebral arteriosclerosis, epilepsy, and other factors that predispose to seizures. (See **ADVERSE REACTIONS**.)

In healthy male and female volunteers who received RAXAR, prolongation of the QT_c interval was observed. Because of a potential risk of cardiac arrhythmias, including torsade de pointes, patients receiving RAXAR should avoid concomitant treatment with medications known to prolong the QT_c interval, e.g., class I antiarrhythmic agents (e.g., quinidine, procainamide), class III antiarrhythmic agents (e.g., amiodarone, sotalol), and bepridil, as well as erythromycin, terfenadine, astemizole, cisapride, pentamidine, tricyclic antidepressants, and some antipsychotics, including phenothiazines, when appropriate cardiac monitoring cannot be assured, e.g., during outpatient therapy. (See **CONTRAINDICATIONS**.) RAXAR is not recommended for use in patients with ongoing pro-arrhythmic conditions (e.g., hypokalemia, significant bradycardia, congestive heart failure, myocardial ischemia, and atrial fibrillation).

Serious and occasionally fatal hypersensitivity (anaphylactoid or anaphylactic) reactions have been reported in patients receiving therapy with quinolones, often following the first dose. Some reactions have been accompanied by cardiovascular collapse, hypotension, shock, seizure, loss of consciousness, tingling, angioedema, (including tongue, laryngeal, throat or facial edema/swelling, etc.), airway obstruction (including bronchospasm, shortness of breath, and acute respiratory distress), dyspnea, urticaria/hives, itching, and other serious skin reactions. Only a few of these patients had a history of prior hypersensitivity reactions. Grepafloxacin should be discontinued if an allergic reaction or any other sign of hypersensitivity appears. Serious acute hypersensitivity reactions require immediate treatment.

Serious and sometimes fatal events of uncertain etiology have been reported in patients receiving therapy with quinolones. Serious events are extremely rare and generally occur following administration of multiple doses. Clinical manifestations of serious adverse events may include one or more of the following: fever, rash or severe dermatologic reactions (e.g., toxic epidermal necrolysis, Stevens-Johnson syndrome, etc.); vasculitis, arthralgia, myalgia, serum sickness; allergic pneumonitis; interstitial nephritis, acute renal insufficiency/failure; hepatitis, jaundice, acute hepatic necrosis/failure; tendon pain, inflammation, or rupture; anemia (including hemolytic and aplastic anemia), thrombocytopenia, including thrombotic thrombocytopenic purpura, leukopenia, agranulocytosis, pancytopenia, and/or other hematologic abnormalities. Grepafloxacin should be discontinued immediately at the first appearance of any such reaction and appropriate intervention should be instituted. (See **PRECAUTIONS: Information for Patients** and **ADVERSE REACTIONS**.)

The efficacy of grepafloxacin for treatment of syphilis is not known. Antimicrobial agents used in high doses for short periods of time to treat gonorrhea may mask or delay the symptoms of incubating syphilis. All patients with gonorrhea should have a serologic test for syphilis at the time of diagnosis. Patients treated with grepafloxacin should have a follow-up serologic test for syphilis 3 months after treatment for gonorrhea.

Pseudomembranous colitis has been reported with nearly all antibacterial agents, including quinolones, and may range in severity from mild to life-threatening. Therefore, it is important to consider this diagnosis in patients who present with diarrhea subsequent to the administration of antibacterial agents.

Treatment with antibacterial agents alters the normal flora of the colon and may permit overgrowth of clostridia. Studies indicate that a toxin produced by *Clostridium difficile* is one primary cause of "antibiotic-associated colitis." After the diagnosis of pseudomembranous colitis has been established, therapeutic measures should be initiated.

Achilles and other tendon ruptures that required surgical repair or resulted in prolonged disability have been reported in patients receiving quinolone antibiotics. Grepafloxacin should be discontinued if the patient experiences pain, inflammation, or rupture of a tendon. (See **PRECAUTIONS: Information for Patients**.)

PRECAUTIONS

General: Phototoxicity reactions have been observed in patients who were exposed to direct sunlight or tanning booths while receiving some quinolones, including grepafloxacin. Excessive sunlight should be avoided. Therapy should be discontinued if phototoxicity occurs.

Information for Patients: Patients should be advised:

- that grepafloxacin may be taken with or without meals.
- that grepafloxacin increases the effects of theophylline, and to advise their physician immediately if they are taking theophylline.
- that multivitamins (containing iron or zinc), antacids (containing magnesium, calcium or aluminum), or sucralfate should not be taken within 4 hours before or 4 hours after taking grepafloxacin. (See **PRECAUTIONS: Drug Interactions**.)
- that grepafloxacin may increase the effects of other drugs metabolized by the liver, and to advise their physician of any of the drugs they are taking.
- to drink fluids liberally.
- that grepafloxacin may increase the effects of caffeine.
- that grepafloxacin may be associated with hypersensitivity reactions, even following a single dose, and to discontinue the drug at the first sign of skin rash, hives, or other skin reactions, a rapid heartbeat, difficulty in swallowing or breathing, or any other symptom of an allergic reaction. (See **WARNINGS**.)
- that grepafloxacin may cause dizziness and lightheadedness; therefore, patients should know how they react to this drug before they operate an automobile or machinery or engage in activities requiring mental alertness and coordination.
- to discontinue treatment; rest and refrain from exercise; and to contact their physician immediately if they experience pain, inflammation, or rupture of a tendon.
- to avoid excessive sunlight or artificial ultraviolet light while taking grepafloxacin and to discontinue therapy if phototoxicity (e.g., sunburn-like reaction or skin eruptions) occurs.

Drug Interactions: (See also **CLINICAL PHARMACOLOGY, Drug Interactions**.)

Antacids, Sucralfate, Metal Cations, Multivitamins: Quinolones form chelates with alkaline earth and transition metal cations. Administration of quinolones with antacids containing aluminum, magnesium, or calcium, with sucralfate, with metal cations such as iron, or with multivitamins containing zinc may substantially interfere with the absorption of quinolones, resulting in systemic concentrations considerably lower than desired. These agents should not be taken within 4 hours before or 4 hours after grepafloxacin administration.

Caffeine, Theobromine: Grepafloxacin, like other quinolones, may inhibit the metabolism of caffeine and theobromine. These stimulants are commonly found in coffee and tea, respectively. In some patients, this may lead to reduced clearance, prolongation of plasma half-life, and enhanced effects of caffeine and theobromine.

Theophylline: Grepafloxacin is a competitive inhibitor of the metabolism of theophylline. Serum theophylline concentrations increase when grepafloxacin is initiated in a patient maintained on theophylline. **When initiating a multi-day course of grepafloxacin in a patient maintained on theophylline, the theophylline maintenance dose should be halved for the period of concurrent use of grepafloxacin and monitoring of serum theophylline concentrations should be initiated as a guide to further dosage adjustments.**

Warfarin: In subjects receiving warfarin, no significant change in clotting time was observed when grepafloxacin was coadministered. However, because some quinolones have been reported to enhance the effects of warfarin or its derivatives, prothrombin time or other suitable anticoagulation test should be monitored closely if a quinolone antimicrobial is administered with warfarin or its derivatives.

Drugs Metabolized by Cytochrome P450 Enzymes: The drug interaction study evaluating the effect of grepafloxacin on theophylline indicates that grepafloxacin inhibits theophylline metabolism, which is mediated by CYP1A2. While no clinical studies have been conducted to evaluate the effect of grepafloxacin on the metabolism of CYP3A4 substrates, *in vitro* data suggest similar effects of grepafloxacin in CYP3A4 mediated metabolism and theophylline metabolism. In addition, other quinolones have been reported to decrease the CYP3A4 mediated metabolism of cyclosporine. Other drugs metabolized by CYP3A4 include terfenadine, astemizole, cisapride, midazolam, and triazolam. The clinical relevance of the potential effect of grepafloxacin on the metabolism of CYP3A4 substrates is not known. Patients receiving concurrent administration of substrates of CYP3A4 were not excluded from clinical trials of grepafloxacin.

Non-steroidal anti-inflammatory drugs: The concomitant administration of a nonsteroidal anti-inflammatory drug with a quinolone may increase the risks of CNS stimulation and convulsions. (See **WARNINGS**.)

Antidiabetic Agents: Disturbances of blood glucose, including hyperglycemia and hypoglycemia, have been reported in patients treated concomitantly with quinolones and an antidiabetic agent. Therefore, careful monitoring of blood glucose is recommended when these agents are coadministered.

Table 3: Drug-Related Adverse Reactions in Grepafloxacin-Treated Patients on Multiple-Dose Dosing Regimens in Clinical Trials

Adverse Reaction	400 mg daily (n = 1,069)	600 mg daily (n = 925)
Nausea	11.1%	15.8%
Taste perversion	9.0%	17.8%
Headache	4.6%	4.9%
Dizziness	4.3%	5.4%
Diarrhea	3.5%	4.2%
Vaginitis	3.3%	1.4%
Abdominal pain	2.2%	2.1%
Vomiting	1.7%	5.7%
Pruritus	1.6%	1.2%
Dyspepsia	1.5%	3.1%
Leukorrhea	1.4%	0.0%
Asthenia	1.4%	2.3%
Infection	1.3%	0.4%
Insomnia	1.3%	2.1%
Rash	1.1%	1.9%
Anorexia	0.8%	1.8%
Somnolence	1.0%	1.5%
Dry mouth	0.8%	1.1%
Photosensitivity reaction	0.7%	1.8%
Constipation	0.7%	2.2%
Pain	0.6%	1.0%
Nervousness	0.6%	1.7%

Carcinogenesis, Mutagenesis, Impairment of Fertility: Long-term studies to determine the carcinogenic potential of grepafloxacin hydrochloride have not been performed. Grepafloxacin was not mutagenic in the Ames test, a forward gene mutation assay, mouse micronucleus assay, and an assay of unscheduled DNA repair (UDS) using rat hepatocytes. Grepafloxacin was mutagenic in a bacterial DNA repair test and in an *in vitro* chromosome aberration test.

In a rat intravenous fertility study, grepafloxacin produced no drug-related changes in the estrous cycle of females; copulation or fertility of males or females.

Pregnancy: Teratogenic Effects: Pregnancy Category C: Grepafloxacin had neither embryolethal nor teratogenic effects in rats when administered orally or intravenously. There was no compound-related effect on maintenance of pregnancy, parturition, implantation of females, ovulation, nursing, or on viability, body weight, or morphology of fetuses. However, a decrease in placental weight and in the number of ossified saccrococcygeal vertebrae were observed in rats at 2.4 times the recommended maximum daily human dose based on mg/m^2 (15 times the recommended maximum daily human dose on a mg/kg basis); this was associated with maternal toxicity (decreased body weight and food consumption). No effect was noted at 420 mg/m^2 per day (equivalent to the human dose).

Grepafloxacin had no embryolethal or teratogenic effects in rabbits. However, fetal body weight was suppressed and there was a tendency for a decrease in placental weight at 60-mg/kg doses. Maternal toxicity was demonstrated by abortion in rabbits at doses of 40 mg/kg or higher, a finding which is common in reproductive studies with antibacterial agents in rabbits.

In a perinatal/postnatal study in rats, death and prolongation of delivery time were observed at 2.4 times the recommended maximum daily human dose based on a mg/m^2 basis (15 times the recommended maximum daily human dose on a mg/kg basis). There was no drug-related effect on delivery index, lactation, or offspring.

Adequate and well-controlled studies have not been conducted in pregnant women. Grepafloxacin should be used during pregnancy only if the potential benefit justifies the potential risk to the fetus. (See **WARNINGS**.)

Nursing Mothers: Grepafloxacin is excreted in human milk. Grepafloxacin was detectable in breast milk of one patient who was studied on the ninth day of treatment at 4 to 5 hours after oral administration of 400 mg of grepafloxacin. Blood and milk concentrations of radioactivity were determined after oral administration of radiolabeled grepafloxacin at a dose of 40 mg/kg in lactating rats at 12 to 13 days post partum. The concentration of radioactivity in milk reached a maximum of 9.03 mcg Eq/mL at 1 hour after administration and decreased to 3.20 mcg Eq/mL at 24 hours after administration. The AUC$_{(0-48\ hr)}$ of radioactivity concentration in milk was 16 times that observed in the blood. It is known that other quinolones are excreted in human milk. Because of the potential for serious adverse experiences from grepafloxacin in nursing infants, a decision should be made to discontinue nursing or discontinue administration of the drug, taking into account the importance of this drug to the mother. (See **WARNINGS**.)

Geriatric Use: Grepafloxacin tablets were administered to 343 elderly adults (age >65 years old) in clinical trials. There was no apparent difference in the frequency, type, or severity of adverse reactions in elderly adults compared with other adults.

The pharmacokinetic properties of grepafloxacin in younger adults and elderly adults did not differ significantly. The same instructions for **DOSAGE AND ADMINISTRATION** apply to elderly adults and younger adults.

Pediatric Use: The safety and effectiveness of grepafloxacin in children and adolescents less than 18 years of age have not been established.

ADVERSE REACTIONS

Adverse reactions were assessed in clinical trials involving approximately 2,500 patients receiving single-dose or multiple-dose regimens of grepafloxacin.

Multiple-Dose Regimens: Most of the adverse reactions reported in clinical trials were transient in nature, mild to moderate in severity, and required no treatment. Twenty of 1,069 patients (1.9%) receiving grepafloxacin 400 mg daily and 50 of 925 patients (5.4%) receiving grepafloxacin 600 mg daily discontinued RAXAR Tablets due to an adverse reaction thought by the investigator to be drug related. Table 3 lists adverse events that occurred with frequencies of 1% or greater. These events were thought by the investigators to be drug-related in patients treated with grepafloxacin in multiple-dose clinical trials.

[See table 3 at bottom of previous page]

Additional drug-related events, occurring in multiple-dose clinical trials at a rate of less than 1%, were:

Body as a whole: back pain, body odor, chest pain, chills, facial edema, fever, malaise, neck rigidity, pelvic pain.

Cardiovascular system: arrhythmia, hypotension, palpitations, peripheral vascular disorder, postural hypotension, syncope, tachycardia, vasodilatation.

Digestive system: abnormal liver function tests, abnormal stools, cheilitis, dysphagia, eructation, flatulence, gastritis, gastrointestinal disorder, gingivitis, glossitis, increased appetite, melena, mouth ulceration, oral moniliasis, rectal disorder, rectal hemorrhage, stomatitis, tenesmus, thirst, tongue discoloration, tongue disorder, tongue edema.

Hemic and lymphatic system: anemia, eosinophilia, hypochromic anemia, leukocytosis, leukopenia, lymphadenopathy, lymphocytosis, lymphoma-like reaction, prothrombin decreased, prothrombin increased, reticuloendothelial hyperplasia, thrombocytopenia, thromboplastin increased.

Metabolic and nutritional system: dehydration, edema, electrolyte abnormality, gout, hyperglycemia, hyperlipidemia, hypernatremia, hyperuricemia, increased alkaline phosphatase, increased BUN, increased creatinine, increased gamma glutamyl transpeptidase, increased SGOT, increased SGPT, peripheral edema, weight loss.

Musculoskeletal system: arthralgia, myalgia.

Nervous system: abnormal dreams, abnormal gait, agitation, anxiety, confusion, depression, emotional lability, hallucinations, hyperkinesia, hypesthesia, hypokinesia, paresthesia, speech disorder, stupor, thinking abnormal, tremor, vertigo.

Respiratory system: asthma, atelectasis, bronchitis, dyspnea, epistaxis, hemoptysis, increased cough, laryngismus, pharyngitis, pleural effusion, rhinitis, sputum increased.

Skin and appendages: acne, alopecia, dry skin, epidermal necrolysis, exfoliative dermatitis, fungal dermatitis, herpes simplex, maculopapular rash, skin disorder, sweating, urticaria, vesiculobullous rash.

Special senses: amblyopia, conjunctivitis, deafness, dry eyes, ear disorder, eye pain, lacrimation disorder, parosmia, photophobia, taste loss, tinnitus.

Urogenital system: albuminuria, balanitis, dysuria, hematuria, impotence, polyuria, urethral pain, uricaciduria, urinary frequency, urinary tract disorder, urination impaired, urine abnormality, vulvovaginal disorder.

Single-Dose Regimens: In clinical trials, patients were treated for uncomplicated gonorrhea using a single dose of RAXAR 400 mg. There were no deaths or permanent disabilities in these studies. Table 4 lists the adverse events which occurred with frequencies of 1% or greater. These events were thought by the investigators to be drug-related in patients treated with RAXAR Tablets in single-dose clinical trials.

Table 4: Drug-Related Adverse Reactions in Grepafloxacin-Treated Patients on a Single-Dose Dosing Regimen in Clinical Trials

Adverse Reaction	400 mg daily (n = 487)
Vaginitis	5.0%
Nausea	3.3%
Dizziness	2.1%
Vomiting	2.1%
Headache	1.8%
Leukorrhea	1.2%
Abdominal pain	1.2%

Continued on next page

This product information is based on labeling in effect on June 1, 1998. For further information, contact via direct mail, phone, or web site Medical Information: Glaxo Wellcome Inc., PO Box 13398, Research Triangle Park, NC 27709. Healthcare Professionals (Medical Information): 800-334-0089 Patients (Customer Response Center): 888-TALK2GW (1-888-825-5249) Glaxo Wellcome Corporate Web Site: www.glaxowellcome.com

Table 5: Recommended Daily Dosages

Infection*	Dose	Frequency	Duration (days)
Acute bacterial exacerbations of chronic bronchitis†	400 or 600 mg	once daily	10
Community-acquired pneumonia	600 mg	once daily	10
Nongonococcal urethritis or cervicitis	400 mg	once daily	7
Uncomplicated gonorrhea	400 mg	single dose	1

*DUE TO THE DESIGNATED PATHOGENS (See INDICATIONS AND USAGE).
†See **CLINICAL STUDIES** section.

Table 6: Clinical Efficacy in Studies of Acute Bacterial Exacerbations of Chronic Bronchitis

Study 106-92-301	End of Treatment (1 – 3 Days Posttreatment)			Follow-up (14 Days Posttreatment)		
	Grepafloxacin 400 mg q.d.	Grepafloxacin 600 mg q.d.	Comparator	Grepafloxacin 400 mg q.d.	Grepafloxacin 600 mg q.d.	Comparator
Overall Efficacy	142/157 (90.4%)	140/150 (93.3%)	152/161 (94.4%)	123/153 (80.4%)	124/149 (83.2%)	137/161 (85.1%)
Efficacy by Individual Organism:						
S. pneumoniae	36/42 (85.7%)	40/41 (97.6%)	43/44 (97.7%)	29/40 (72.5%)	35/41 (85.4%)	38/44 (86.4%)
H. influenzae	63/68 (92.6%)	61/68 (89.7%)	84/90 (93.3%)	55/67 (82.1%)	51/67 (76.1%)	76/90 (84.4%)
M. catarrhalis	41/43 (95.3%)	32/32 (100%)	29/30 (96.7%)	38/42 (90.5%)	31/32 (96.9%)	26/30 (86.7%)

Study 106-92-206	End of Treatment (3 – 5 Days Posttreatment)			Follow-up (14 – 28 Days Posttreatment)		
	Grepafloxacin 400 mg q.d.	Grepafloxacin 600 mg q.d.	Comparator	Grepafloxacin 400 mg q.d.	Grepafloxacin 600 mg q.d.	Comparator
Overall Efficacy	66/72 (91.7%)	66/71 (93.0%)	65/70 (92.9%)	58/71 (81.7%)	61/71 (85.9%)	54/66 (81.8%)
Efficacy by Individual Organism:						
S. pneumoniae	8/8 (100%)	8/9 (88.9%)	3/5 (60%)	7/8 (87.5%)	6/9 (66.7%)	3/5 (60%)
H. influenzae	18/19 (94.7%)	15/16 (93.8%)	17/18 (94.4%)	17/19 (89.5%)	14/16 (87.5%)	15/18 (83.3%)
M. catarrhalis	20/21 (95.2%)	20/21 (95.2%)	18/19 (94.7%)	19/21 (90.5%)	18/21 (85.7%)	15/16 (93.8%)

Raxar—Cont.

Diarrhea	1.2%
Pruritus	1.2%
Taste perversion	1.2%

Additional drug-related events, occurring in single-dose clinical trials at a rate of less than 1%, were:

Body as a whole: asthenia, chest pain, chills, flu-like syndrome, infection, malaise.
Cardiovascular system: syncope, vasodilatation.
Digestive system: anorexia, constipation, increased appetite, tenesmus.
Hemic and lymphatic system: lymphadenopathy.
Nervous system: hyperkinesia, insomnia, nervousness, somnolence.
Respiratory system: rhinitis.
Skin and appendages: acne, rash, sweating.
Urogenital system: balanitis.

OVERDOSAGE

In the event of acute overdosage, the stomach should be emptied by inducing vomiting or by gastric lavage. The patient should be carefully observed and given supportive treatment. As with other quinolones, adequate hydration and electrolyte balance must be maintained. Due to the possibility of prolongation of the QT_c interval and complications including arrhythmias, ECG monitoring is recommended after overdosage with RAXAR. It is not known if grepafloxacin can be efficiently removed by hemodialysis or peritoneal dialysis.

At oral doses of 4500 mg/kg (14,400 mg/m^2) in mice and 3000 mg/kg (21,000 mg/m^2) in rats, significant increases in mortality were noted. These doses were approximately equivalent to 39 (mice) and 57 (rats) times the human dose on a mg/m^2 basis.

DOSAGE AND ADMINISTRATION

RAXAR Tablets may be taken with or without meals. The usual dose for RAXAR is 400 mg or 600 mg orally every 24 hours as described in Table 5.
[See table 5 at top of previous page]
As with other broad-spectrum antimicrobial agents, prolonged use of grepafloxacin may result in overgrowth of non-susceptible organisms. Repeated evaluation of the patient's condition and microbial susceptibility testing is essential. If superinfection occurs during therapy, appropriate measures should be taken.
Patients with Renal Failure: Dosage adjustment is not required in patients with impaired renal function.
Patients with Hepatic Disease: Metabolism and excretion of grepafloxacin are reduced in patients with hepatic failure. RAXAR Tablets are contraindicated in patients with hepatic failure. (See **CLINICAL PHARMACOLOGY.**)

HOW SUPPLIED

RAXAR Tablets (grepafloxacin hydrochloride tablets) are supplied as white to pale yellow, film-coated, round, biconvex, bevel-edged tablets containing 200 mg grepafloxacin base. The tablets are imprinted with "GX CK3" on one side and no printing on the other side.

60 Tablets/Bottle	NDC 0173-0566-03
Unit Dose Packs of 60	NDC 0173-0566-00

Store at controlled room temperature of 20° to 25°C (68° to 77°F) (see United States Pharmacopoeia). Replace cap securely after each opening.

CLINICAL STUDIES

Acute Bacterial Exacerbations of Chronic Bronchitis:
Two separate controlled, randomized trials of grepafloxacin in the treatment of acute bacterial exacerbations of chronic bronchitis yielded overall efficacy rates of grepafloxacin 400 mg and grepafloxacin 600 mg which demonstrated equivalence to comparators. However, these studies suggest that grepafloxacin 400 mg once daily for 10 days may be less effective against *S. pneumoniae* than grepafloxacin 600 mg once daily for 10 days or comparator for 10 days. These studies excluded patients whose respiratory status required the initiation of steroid therapy or an increase in maintenance steroid doses greater than prednisone 10 mg per day (or its equivalent). Clinical success at end of treatment did not always predict clinical success at follow-up. Table 6 presents efficacy data from these two trials at end of treatment (1 to 5 days posttreatment) and at follow-up (14 to 28 days posttreatment).
[See table 6 at top of previous page]
Community-acquired Pneumonia:
The two pivotal clinical trials that assessed the efficacy of grepafloxacin in the treatment of community-acquired pneumonia excluded patients whose respiratory status required the initiation of steroid therapy or an increase in maintenance steroid doses greater than prednisone 10 mg per day (or its equivalent). Study 106-92-302 was a randomized controlled study that assessed the efficacy of grepafloxacin 600 mg once daily for 10 days compared with comparator for 10 days. Study 106-92-205 was an open study

that assessed clinical efficacy of grepafloxacin 600 mg once daily for 10 days. Table 7 presents efficacy results from the two pivotal studies:

Table 7: Clinical Efficacy in Community-Acquired Pneumonia in Two Pivotal Studies

	Grepafloxacin 600 mg q.d.	Comparator
Study 106-92-302		
Success	89/110 (80.9%)	94/117 (80.3%)
Failure	21/110 (19.1%)	23/117 (19.7%)
Study 106-92-205		
Success	116/125 (92.8%)	
Failure	9/125 (7.2%)	

ANIMAL PHARMACOLOGY

Quinolones have been shown to cause arthropathies in juvenile rats and dogs. In addition, these drugs are associated with an increased incidence of osteochondrosis in rats as compared with the incidence in vehicle-treated rats. Grepafloxacin-associated joint toxicity (cavitation with loss of cartilaginous matrix and chondrocytes with cartilage fibrillation) was observed in juvenile dogs receiving 100 mg/kg by intravenous or subcutaneous injection for 1 week. Grepafloxacin-associated joint toxicity (blisters of the articular cartilage) was observed in juvenile dogs given oral doses of 80 mg/kg per day (approximately 4.3 times the recommended maximum daily human dose on a mg/m^2 basis) for 4 weeks. No joint toxicity was observed at lower oral doses of 60 mg/kg per day (approximately 3.2 times the recommended maximum daily human dose on a mg/m^2 basis) for 4 weeks. The clinical relevance of these observations is unknown.
In the dog, oral doses of 30 mg/kg and above ($\geq$1.5 times the maximum human dose on a mg/m^2 basis) caused prolongation of the QT interval, although the results were variable. Intravenous administration of grepafloxacin at 10 mg/kg elicited a moderate hypotension in anesthetized dogs and rabbits. In phototoxicity tests, mice exposed to ultraviolet A radiation (similar to that used in tanning booths; sunlight contains a wider spectrum of UV radiation) after administration of grepafloxacin as a single 200-mg/kg oral dose (1.6 times the highest recommended human dose, based upon body surface area) showed a mild redness on the ears. Phototoxic reactions such as this have been reported with other quinolones.
Lenticular opacities, sometimes observed after long-term, high-dose use with other quinolones, were not observed with grepafloxacin in a 52-week study in monkeys.
Drug interactions resulting in seizures have been reported between some quinolones and nonsteroidal anti-inflammatory drugs (NSAIDs). Grepafloxacin did not induce seizures when administered with a variety of NSAIDs in rats. The NSAIDs studied were fenbufen, flurbiprofen, indomethacin, phenylbutazone, ibuprofen, and diflunisal.

References
1. National Committee for Clinical Laboratory Standards. *Methods for Dilution Antimicrobial Susceptibility Tests for Bacteria that Grow Aerobically*-Fourth Edition. Approved Standard NCCLS Document M7-A4, Volume 17, No. 2, NCCLS, Wayne, PA, January, 1997.
2. National Committee for Clinical Laboratory Standards. *Performance Standards for Antimicrobial Disk Susceptibility Tests*-Sixth Edition. Approved Standard NCCLS Document M2-A6, Volume 17, No. 1. NCCLS, Wayne, PA, January, 1997.

U.S. Patent 5,563,138
©Copyright 1997 Glaxo Wellcome Inc. All rights reserved.
November 1997/RL-498
Shown in Product Identification Guide, page 313

RETROVIR® ℞
[re 'trō-vir]
(zidovudine)
Tablets
RETROVIR® ℞
(zidovudine)
Capsules
RETROVIR® ℞
(zidovudine)
Syrup

WARNING: RETROVIR (ZIDOVUDINE) MAY BE ASSOCIATED WITH HEMATOLOGIC TOXICITY INCLUDING GRANULOCYTOPENIA AND SEVERE ANEMIA PARTICULARLY IN PATIENTS WITH ADVANCED HIV DISEASE (SEE WARNINGS). PROLONGED USE OF RETROVIR HAS BEEN ASSOCIATED WITH SYMPTOMATIC MYOPATHY SIMILAR TO THAT PRODUCED BY HUMAN IMMUNODEFICIENCY VIRUS.
RARE OCCURRENCES OF POTENTIALLY FATAL LACTIC ACIDOSIS IN THE ABSENCE OF HYPOXEMIA, AND SEVERE HEPATOMEGALY WITH STEATOSIS HAVE BEEN REPORTED WITH THE USE OF CERTAIN ANTIRETROVIRAL NUCLEOSIDE ANALOGUES (SEE WARNINGS).

DESCRIPTION

RETROVIR is the brand name for zidovudine (formerly called azidothymidine [AZT]), a pyrimidine nucleoside analogue active against human immunodeficiency virus (HIV).
Tablets: RETROVIR Tablets are for oral administration. Each film-coated tablet contains 300 mg of zidovudine and the inactive ingredients hydroxypropyl methylcellulose, magnesium stearate, microcrystalline cellulose, polyethylene glycol, sodium starch glycolate, and titanium dioxide.
Capsules: RETROVIR Capsules are for oral administration. Each capsule contains 100 mg of zidovudine and the inactive ingredients corn starch, magnesium stearate, microcrystalline cellulose, and sodium starch glycolate. The 100-mg empty hard gelatin capsule, printed with edible black ink, consists of black iron oxide, dimethylpolysiloxane, gelatin, pharmaceutical shellac, soya lecithin, and titanium dioxide. The blue band around the capsule consists of gelatin and FD&C Blue No. 2.
Syrup: RETROVIR Syrup is for oral administration. Each teaspoonful (5 mL) of RETROVIR Syrup contains 50 mg of zidovudine and the inactive ingredients sodium benzoate 0.2% (added as a preservative), citric acid, flavors, glycerin, and liquid sucrose. Sodium hydroxide may be added to adjust pH.
The chemical name of zidovudine is 3'-azido-3'-deoxythymidine.
Zidovudine is a white to beige, odorless, crystalline solid with a molecular weight of 267.24 and a solubility of 20.1 mg/mL in water at 25°C. The molecular formula is $C_{10}H_{13}N_5O_4$.

MICROBIOLOGY

Mechanism of Action: Zidovudine is a synthetic nucleoside analogue of the naturally occurring nucleoside, thymidine, in which the 3'-hydroxy (-OH) group is replaced by an azido (-N_3) group. Within cells, zidovudine is converted to the active metabolite, zidovudine 5'-triphosphate (AztTP), by the sequential action of the cellular enzymes. Zidovudine 5'-triphosphate inhibits the activity of the HIV reverse transcriptase both by competing for utilization with the natural substrate, deoxythymidine 5'-triphosphate (dTTP), and by its incorporation into viral DNA. The lack of a 3'-OH group in the incorporated nucleoside analogue prevents the formation of the 5' to 3' phosphodiester linkage essential for DNA chain elongation and, therefore, the viral DNA growth is terminated. The active metabolite AztTP is also a weak inhibitor of the cellular DNA polymerase-alpha and mitochondrial polymerase-gamma and has been reported to be incorporated into the DNA of cells in culture.
In Vitro HIV Susceptibility: The in vitro anti-HIV activity of zidovudine was assessed by infecting cell lines of lymphoblastic and monocytic origin and peripheral blood lymphocytes with laboratory and clinical isolates of HIV. The IC_{50} and IC_{90} values (50% and 90% inhibitory concentrations) were 0.003 to 0.013 and 0.03 to 0.13 mcg/mL, respectively (1 nM = 0.27 ng/mL). The IC_{50} and IC_{90} values of HIV isolates recovered from 18 untreated AIDS/ARC patients were in the range of 0.003 to 0.013 mcg/mL and 0.03 to 0.3 mcg/mL, respectively. Zidovudine showed antiviral activity in all acutely infected cell lines; however, activity was substantially less in chronically infected cell lines. In drug combination studies with zalcitabine, didanosine, lamivudine, saquinavir, indinavir, ritonavir, nevirapine, delavirdine, or interferon-alpha, zidovudine showed additive to synergistic activity in cell culture. The relationship between the in vitro susceptibility of HIV to reverse transcriptase inhibitors and the inhibition of HIV replication in humans has not been established.
Drug Resistance: HIV isolates with reduced sensitivity to zidovudine have been selected in vitro and were also recovered from patients treated with RETROVIR. Genetic analysis of the isolates showed mutations which result in five amino acid substitutions (Met41→Leu, A67→Asn, Lys70→Arg, Thr215→Tyr or Phe, and Lys219→Gln) in the viral reverse transcriptase. In general, higher levels of resistance were associated with greater number of mutations with 215 mutation being the most significant.
Cross-Resistance: The potential for cross-resistance between HIV reverse transcriptase inhibitors and protease inhibitors is low because of the different enzyme targets involved. Combination therapy with zidovudine plus zalcitabine or didanosine does not appear to prevent the emergence of zidovudine-resistant isolates. Combination therapy with RETROVIR plus EPIVIR® delayed the emergence of mutations conferring resistance to zidovudine. In some patients harboring zidovudine-resistant virus, combination therapy with RETROVIR plus EPIVIR restored phenotypic sensitivity to zidovudine by 12 weeks of treatment. HIV isolates with multidrug resistance to zidovudine, didanosine, zalcitabine, stavudine, and lamivudine were recovered from a small number of patients treated for ≥1 year with the combination of zidovudine and didanosine or zalcitabine. The pattern of resistant mutations in the combination therapy was different (Ala62→Val, Val75→Ile, Phe77→116Tyr, and Gln→151 Met) from monotherapy, with mutation 151 being most significant for multidrug resis-

tance. Site-directed mutagenesis studies showed that these mutations could also result in resistance to zalcitabine, lamivudine, and stavudine.

CLINICAL PHARMACOLOGY

Pharmacokinetics: ***Adults:*** The pharmacokinetics of zidovudine has been evaluated in 22 adult HIV-infected patients in a Phase 1 dose-escalation study. After oral dosing (capsules), zidovudine was rapidly absorbed from the gastrointestinal tract with peak serum concentrations occurring within 0.5 to 1.5 hours. Dose-independent kinetics was observed over the range of 2 mg/kg every 8 hours to 10 mg/kg every 4 hours. The mean zidovudine half-life was approximately 1 hour and ranged from 0.78 to 1.93 hours following oral dosing.

Zidovudine is rapidly metabolized to 3′-azido-3′-deoxy-5′-*O*-β-*D*-glucopyranuronosylthymidine (GZDV) which has an apparent elimination half-life of 1 hour (range 0.61 to 1.73 hours). Following oral administration, urinary recovery of zidovudine and GZDV accounted for 14% and 74% of the dose, respectively, and the total urinary recovery averaged 90% (range 63% to 95%), indicating a high degree of absorption. However, as a result of first-pass metabolism, the average oral capsule bioavailability of zidovudine is 65% (range 52% to 75%). A second metabolite, 3′-amino-3′-deoxythymidine (AMT), has been identified in the plasma following single-dose intravenous (IV) administration of zidovudine. AMT area-under-the-curve (AUC) was one fifth of the AUC of zidovudine and had a half-life of 2.7 ± 0.7 hours. In comparison, GZDV AUC was about threefold greater than the AUC of zidovudine.

Additional pharmacokinetic data following intravenous dosing indicated dose-independent kinetics over the range of 1 to 5 mg/kg with a mean zidovudine half-life of 1.1 hours (range 0.48 to 2.86 hours). Total body clearance averaged 1900 mL/min per 70 kg and the apparent volume of distribution was 1.6 L/kg. Renal clearance is estimated to be 400 mL/min per 70 kg, indicating glomerular filtration and active tubular secretion by the kidneys. Zidovudine plasma protein binding is 34% to 38%, indicating that drug interactions involving binding site displacement are not anticipated.

The zidovudine cerebrospinal fluid (CSF)/plasma concentration ratio was determined in 39 patients receiving chronic therapy with RETROVIR. The median ratio measured in 50 paired samples drawn 1 to 8 hours after the last dose of RETROVIR was 0.6.

Adults with Impaired Renal Function: The pharmacokinetics of zidovudine has been evaluated in patients with impaired renal function following a single 200-mg oral dose. In 14 patients (mean creatinine clearance 18 ± 2 mL/min) the half-life of zidovudine was 1.4 hours compared to 1.0 hour for control subjects with normal renal function; AUC values were approximately twice those of controls. Additionally, GZDV half-life in these patients was 8.0 hours (vs 0.9 hours for control) and AUC was 17 times higher than for control subjects. The pharmacokinetics and tolerance were evaluated in a multiple-dose study in patients undergoing hemodialysis (n = 5) or peritoneal dialysis (n = 6). Patients received escalating doses of zidovudine up to 200 mg five times daily for 8 weeks. Daily doses of 500 mg or less were well tolerated despite significantly elevated plasma levels of GZDV. Apparent oral clearance of zidovudine was approximately 50% of that reported in patients with normal renal function. The plasma concentrations of AMT are not known in patients with renal insufficiency. Daily doses of 300 to 400 mg should be appropriate in HIV-infected patients with severe renal dysfunction (see DOSAGE AND ADMINISTRATION: Dose Adjustment). Hemodialysis and peritoneal dialysis appear to have a negligible effect on the removal of zidovudine, whereas GZDV elimination is enhanced.

Pediatrics: The pharmacokinetics and bioavailability of zidovudine have been evaluated in 21 HIV-infected pediatric patients, aged 6 months through 12 years, following intravenous doses administered over the range of 80 to 160 mg/m^2 every 6 hours, and following oral doses of the IV solution administered over the range of 90 to 240 mg/m^2 every 6 hours. After discontinuation of the IV infusion, zidovudine plasma concentrations decayed biexponentially, consistent with two-compartment pharmacokinetics. Proportional increases in AUC and in zidovudine concentrations were observed with increasing dose, consistent with dose-independent kinetics over the dose range studied. The mean terminal half-life and total body clearance across all dose levels administered were 1.5 hours and 30.9 mL/min per kg, respectively. These values compare to mean half-life and total body clearance in adults of 1.1 hours and 27.1 mL/min per kg.

The mean oral bioavailability of 65% was independent of dose. This value is the same as the bioavailability in adults. Doses of 180 mg/m^2 four times daily in pediatric patients produced similar systemic exposure (24-hour AUC 10.7 hr•mcg/mL) as doses of 200 mg six times daily in adult patients (10.9 hr•mcg/mL).

The pharmacokinetics of zidovudine have been studied in pediatric patients from birth to 3 months of life. In one study of the pharmacokinetics of zidovudine in women during the last trimester of pregnancy, zidovudine elimination was determined immediately after birth in eight neonates who were exposed to zidovudine in utero. The half-life was 13.0 ± 5.8 hours. In another study, the pharmacokinetics of zidovudine was evaluated in pediatric patients (ranging in age of 1 day to 3 months) of normal birth weight for gestational age and with normal renal and hepatic function. In neonates less than or equal to 14 days old, mean ± SD total body clearance was 10.9 ± 4.8 mL/min per kg (n = 18) and half-life was 3.1 ± 1.2 hours (n = 21). In neonates and infants greater than 14 days old, total body clearance was 19.0 ± 4.0 mL/min per kg (n = 16) and half-life was 1.9 ± 0.7 hours (n = 18). Bioavailability was 89% ± 19% (n = 15) in the younger age group and decreased to 61% ± 19% (n = 17) in patients older than 14 days.

Concentrations of zidovudine in cerebrospinal fluid were measured after both intermittent oral and IV drug administration in 21 pediatric patients during Phase 1 and Phase 2 studies. The mean zidovudine CSF/plasma concentration ratio measured at an average time of 2.2 hours postdose at oral doses of 120 to 240 mg/m^2 was 0.52 ± 0.44 (n = 28); after an IV infusion of doses of 80 to 160 mg/m^2 over 1 hour, the mean CSF/plasma concentration ratio was 0.87 ± 0.66 (n = 23) at 3.2 hours after the start of the infusion. During continuous IV infusion, mean steady-state CSF/plasma ratio was 0.26 ± 0.17 (n = 28).

As in adult patients, the major route of elimination in pediatric patients was by metabolism to GZDV. After IV dosing, about 29% of the dose was excreted in the urine unchanged and about 45% of the dose was excreted as GZDV. Overall, the pharmacokinetics of zidovudine in pediatric patients greater than 3 months of age are similar to that of zidovudine in adult patients.

Pregnancy: The pharmacokinetics of zidovudine have been studied in a Phase 1 study of eight women during the last trimester of pregnancy. As pregnancy progressed, there was no evidence of drug accumulation. The pharmacokinetics of zidovudine were similar to that of nonpregnant adults. Consistent with passive transmission of the drug across the placenta, zidovudine concentrations in infant plasma at birth were essentially equal to those in maternal plasma at delivery. Although data are limited, methadone maintenance therapy in five pregnant women did not appear to alter zidovudine pharmacokinetics. However, in another patient population, a potential for interaction has been identified (see PRECAUTIONS).

Nursing Mothers: The U.S. Public Health Service Centers for Disease Control and Prevention advises HIV-infected women not to breastfeed to avoid postnatal transmission of HIV to a child who may not yet be infected. After administration of a single dose of 200 mg zidovudine to 13 HIV-infected women, the mean concentration of zidovudine was similar in human milk and serum (see PRECAUTIONS: Nursing Mothers).

Effect of Food on Absorption: Administration of RETROVIR Capsules with food decreased peak plasma concentrations by greater than 50%; however, bioavailability as determined by AUC may not be affected. The effect of food on the absorption of zidovudine from the tablet formulation is not known.

Tablets: In a single-dose study of 23 healthy volunteers, the mean ± SD relative bioavailability of the RETROVIR 300-mg Tablet relative to three 100-mg RETROVIR Capsules was 110 ± 18%. After administration of the 300-mg RETROVIR Tablet or three 100-mg RETROVIR Capsules, the mean ± SD C_{max} values were 1.81 ± 0.52 and 1.50 ± 0.46 mcg/mL, respectively.

Syrup: In a multiple-dose bioavailability study conducted in 12 HIV-infected adults receiving doses of 100 or 200 mg every 4 hours, RETROVIR Syrup was demonstrated to be bioequivalent to RETROVIR Capsules with respect to area under the zidovudine plasma concentration-time curve (AUC). The rate of absorption of RETROVIR Syrup was greater than that of RETROVIR Capsules, as indicated by mean times to peak concentration of 0.5 and 0.8 hours, respectively. Mean values for steady-state peak concentration (dose-normalized to 200 mg) were 1.5 and 1.2 mcg/mL for syrup and capsules, respectively.

INDICATIONS AND USAGE

RETROVIR is indicated for the treatment of HIV infection when antiretroviral therapy is warranted (see Description of Clinical Studies).

The duration of clinical benefit from antiretroviral therapy may be limited. Alterations in antiretroviral therapy should be considered if disease progression occurs during treatment.

Maternal-Fetal HIV Transmission: RETROVIR is also indicated for the prevention of maternal-fetal HIV transmission as part of a regimen that includes oral RETROVIR beginning between 14 and 34 weeks of gestation, intravenous RETROVIR during labor, and administration of RETROVIR Syrup to the neonate after birth. The efficacy of this regimen for preventing HIV transmission in women who have received RETROVIR for a prolonged period before pregnancy has not been evaluated. The safety of RETROVIR for the mother or fetus during the first trimester of pregnancy has not been assessed (see Description of Clinical Studies).

Description of Clinical Studies: Therapy with RETROVIR has been shown to prolong survival and decrease the incidence of opportunistic infections in patients with advanced HIV disease at the initiation of therapy and to delay disease progression in asymptomatic HIV-infected patients.

Other randomized studies suggest that the duration of the clinical benefit of monotherapy with RETROVIR is time-limited.

Combination Therapy-Adults: ACTG175 was a randomized, double-blind, controlled trial that compared RETROVIR 200 mg t.i.d.; didanosine 200 mg b.i.d.; RETROVIR plus didanosine; and RETROVIR plus zalcitabine 0.75 mg t.i.d. A total of 2467 HIV-infected adults with baseline CD4 counts of 200 to 500 cells/mm^3 (mean = 352) and no prior AIDS-defining event enrolled with the following demographics: male (82%), Caucasian (70%), mean age of 35 years, asymptomatic HIV infection (81%), and prior antiretroviral use (57%, mean duration = 89.5 weeks). The overall median duration of study treatment was 118 weeks. The incidence of AIDS-defining events or death is shown in Table 1.

[See table 1 above]

Table 1
First AIDS-Defining Event or Death and Death Only by Study Arm and Antiretroviral Experience

Treatment Antiretroviral Experience	Event	RETROVIR	Didanosine	RETROVIR plus Didanosine	RETROVIR plus Zalcitabine
Overall	No. of Patients	619	620	613	615
	AIDS/Death	96 (16%)	71 (11%)	66 (11%)	76 (12%)
	Death Only	54 (9%)	29 (5%)	31 (5%)	40 (7%)
Naive	No. of Patients	269	268	263	267
	AIDS/Death	32 (12%)	23 (9%)	20 (8%)	16 (6%)
	Death Only	18 (7%)	11 (4%)	11 (4%)	9 (3%)
Experienced	No. of Patients	350	352	350	348
	AIDS/Death	64 (18%)	48 (14%)	45 (13%)	60 (17%)
	Death Only	36 (10%)	18 (5%)	20 (6%)	31 (9%)

RETROVIR in combination with certain antiretroviral agents has been shown to be superior to monotherapy in one or more of the following: delaying death, delaying development of AIDS, increasing CD4 cell counts, and decreasing plasma HIV RNA. Use of RETROVIR in some combinations is based on surrogate marker data. The complete prescribing information for each drug should be consulted before combination therapy which includes RETROVIR is initiated.

Continued on next page

This product information is based on labeling in effect on June 1, 1998. For further information, contact via direct mail, phone, or web site Medical Information: Glaxo Wellcome Inc., PO Box 13398, Research Triangle Park, NC 27709. Healthcare Professionals (Medical Information): 800-334-0089 Patients (Customer Response Center): 888-TALK2GW (1-888-825-5249) Glaxo Wellcome Corporate Web Site: www.glaxowellcome.com

Retrovir—Cont.

Pregnant Women and Their Neonates: The utility of RETROVIR for the prevention of maternal-fetal HIV transmission was demonstrated in a randomized, double-blind, placebo-controlled trial (ACTG 076) conducted in HIV-infected pregnant women with CD4 cell counts of 200 to 1818 cells/mm^3 (median in the treated group: 560 cells/mm^3) who had little or no previous exposure to RETROVIR. Oral RETROVIR was initiated between 14 and 34 weeks of gestation (median 11 weeks of therapy) followed by IV administration of RETROVIR during labor and delivery. After birth, neonates received oral RETROVIR Syrup for 6 weeks. The study showed a statistically significant difference in the incidence of HIV infection in the neonates (based on viral culture from peripheral blood) between the group receiving RETROVIR and the group receiving placebo. Of 363 neonates evaluated in the study, the estimated risk of HIV infection was 7.8% in the group receiving RETROVIR and 24.9% in the placebo group, a relative reduction in transmission risk of 68.7%. RETROVIR was well tolerated by mothers and infants. There was no difference in pregnancy-related adverse events between the treatment groups.

Dose-Frequency Study: A randomized, double-blind, dose-frequency study of RETROVIR in 320 patients with AIDS or advanced ARC was conducted to assess the safety and tolerability of 600 mg RETROVIR per day given as either 100 mg every 4 hours or as 300 mg every 12 hours for 48 weeks. No significant difference was detected between the two dose frequencies with regard to adverse experiences or hematologic abnormalities. Although this study was not designed to determine efficacy, no differences in the frequency of or time to opportunistic infections, neoplasms, or death were noted between treatment groups. Changes in CD4 cell counts and β_2-microglobulin levels were similar between treatment groups.

CONTRAINDICATIONS

RETROVIR Tablets, Capsules, and Syrup are contraindicated for patients who have potentially life-threatening allergic reactions to any of the components of the formulations.

WARNINGS

Before combination therapy with RETROVIR is initiated, consult the complete prescribing information for each drug. The safety profile of RETROVIR plus other antiretroviral agents reflects the individual safety profiles of each component.

The incidence of adverse reactions appears to increase with disease progression, and patients should be monitored carefully, especially as disease progression occurs.

Bone Marrow Suppression: RETROVIR should be used with caution in patients who have bone marrow compromise evidenced by granulocyte count <1000 cells/mm^3 or hemoglobin <9.5 g/dL. In patients with advanced symptomatic HIV disease, anemia and neutropenia were the most significant adverse events observed (see ADVERSE REACTIONS). There have been reports of pancytopenia associated with the use of RETROVIR, which was reversible in most instances after discontinuance of the drug. However, significant anemia, in many cases requiring dose adjustment, discontinuation of RETROVIR, and/or blood transfusions has occurred during treatment with RETROVIR alone or in combination with other antiretrovirals.

Frequent blood counts are strongly recommended in patients with advanced HIV disease who are treated with RETROVIR. For HIV-infected individuals and patients with asymptomatic or early HIV disease, periodic blood counts are recommended. If anemia or neutropenia develops, dosage adjustments may be necessary (see DOSAGE AND ADMINISTRATION).

Myopathy: Myopathy and myositis with pathological changes, similar to that produced by HIV disease, have been associated with prolonged use of RETROVIR.

Lactic Acidosis/Severe Hepatomegaly with Steatosis: Rare occurrences of potentially fatal lactic acidosis in the absence of hypoxemia, and severe hepatomegaly with steatosis have been reported with the use of certain antiretroviral nucleoside analogues. Lactic acidosis should be considered whenever a patient receiving therapy with RETROVIR develops unexplained tachypnea, dyspnea, or fall in serum bicarbonate level. Under these circumstances, therapy with RETROVIR should be suspended until the diagnosis of lactic acidosis has been excluded. Caution should be exercised when administering RETROVIR to any patient, particularly obese women, with hepatomegaly, hepatitis, or other known risk factor for liver disease. These patients should be followed closely while on therapy with RETROVIR. The significance of elevated aminotransferase levels suggesting hepatic injury in HIV-infected patients prior to starting RETROVIR or while on RETROVIR is unclear. Treatment with RETROVIR should be suspended in the setting of rapidly elevating aminotransferase levels, progressive hepatomegaly, or metabolic/lactic acidosis of unknown etiology.

Other Serious Adverse Reactions: Several serious adverse events have been reported with use of RETROVIR in clinical practice. Reports of pancreatitis, sensitization reactions (including anaphylaxis in one patient), vasculitis, and seizures have been rare. These adverse events, except for sensitization, have also been associated with HIV disease. Changes in skin and nail pigmentation have been associated with the use of RETROVIR.

PRECAUTIONS

General: Zidovudine is eliminated from the body primarily by renal excretion following metabolism in the liver (glucuronidation). In patients with severely impaired renal function, dosage reduction is recommended (see CLINICAL PHARMACOLOGY: Pharmacokinetics and DOSAGE AND ADMINISTRATION). Although very little data are available, patients with severely impaired hepatic function may be at greater risk of toxicity.

Information for Patients: RETROVIR is not a cure for HIV infection, and patients may continue to acquire illnesses associated with HIV infection, including opportunistic infections. Therefore, patients should be advised to seek medical care for any significant change in their health status.

The safety and efficacy of RETROVIR in women, intravenous drug users, and racial minorities is not significantly different than that observed in white males.

Patients should be informed that the major toxicities of RETROVIR are neutropenia and/or anemia. The frequency and severity of these toxicities are greater in patients with more advanced disease and in those who initiate therapy later in the course of their infection. They should be told that if toxicity develops, they may require transfusions or dose modifications including possible discontinuation. They should be told of the extreme importance of having their blood counts followed closely while on therapy, especially for patients with advanced symptomatic HIV disease. They should be cautioned about the use of other medications, including ganciclovir and interferon-alpha, that may exacerbate the toxicity of RETROVIR (see PRECAUTIONS: Drug Interactions). Patients should be informed that other adverse effects of RETROVIR include nausea and vomiting. Patients should also be encouraged to contact their physician if they experience muscle weakness, shortness of breath, symptoms of hepatitis or pancreatitis, or any other unexpected adverse events while being treated with RETROVIR.

RETROVIR Tablets, Capsules, and Syrup are for oral ingestion only. Patients should be told of the importance of taking RETROVIR exactly as prescribed. They should be told not to share medication and not to exceed the recommended dose. Patients should be told that the long-term effects of RETROVIR are unknown at this time.

Pregnant women considering the use of RETROVIR during pregnancy for prevention of HIV-transmission to their infants should be advised that transmission may still occur in some cases despite therapy. The long-term consequences of in utero and infant exposure to RETROVIR are unknown, including the possible risk of cancer.

HIV-infected pregnant women should be advised not to breastfeed to avoid postnatal transmission of HIV to a child who may not yet be infected.

Patients should be advised that therapy with RETROVIR has not been shown to reduce the risk of transmission of HIV to others through sexual contact or blood contamination.

Drug Interactions: Ganciclovir: Use of RETROVIR in combination with ganciclovir increases the risk of hematologic toxicities in some patients with advanced HIV disease. Should the use of this combination become necessary in the treatment of patients with HIV disease, dose reduction or interruption of one or both agents may be necessary to minimize hematologic toxicity. Hematologic parameters, including hemoglobin, hematocrit, and white blood cell count with differential, should be monitored frequently in all patients receiving this combination.

Interferon-alpha: Hematologic toxicities have also been seen when RETROVIR is used concomitantly with interferon-alpha. As with the concomitant use of RETROVIR and ganciclovir, dose reduction or interruption of one or both agents may be necessary, and hematologic parameters should be monitored frequently.

Bone Marrow Suppressive Agents/Cytotoxic Agents: Coadministration of RETROVIR with drugs that are cytotoxic or which interfere with RBC/WBC number or function (e.g., dapsone, flucytosine, vincristine, vinblastine, or adriamycin) may increase the risk of hematologic toxicity.

Probenecid: Limited data suggest that probenecid may increase zidovudine levels by inhibiting glucuronidation and/or by reducing renal excretion of zidovudine. Some patients who have used RETROVIR concomitantly with probenecid have developed flu-like symptoms consisting of myalgia, malaise, and/or fever and maculopapular rash.

Phenytoin: Phenytoin plasma levels have been reported to be low in some patients receiving RETROVIR, while in one case a high level was documented. However, in a pharmacokinetic interaction study in which 12 HIV-positive volun-

teers received a single 300-mg phenytoin dose alone and during steady-state zidovudine conditions (200 mg every 4 hours), no change in phenytoin kinetics was observed. Although not designed to optimally assess the effect of phenytoin on zidovudine kinetics, a 30% decrease in oral zidovudine clearance was observed with phenytoin.

Methadone: In a pharmacokinetic study of nine HIV-positive patients receiving methadone-maintenance (30 to 90 mg daily) concurrent with 200 mg of RETROVIR every 4 hours, no changes were observed in the pharmacokinetics of methadone upon initiation of therapy with RETROVIR and after 14 days of treatment with RETROVIR. No adjustments in methadone-maintenance requirements were reported. For four patients, the mean zidovudine AUC was elevated twofold, while for five patients, the value was equal to that of control patients. The exact mechanism and clinical significance of these data are unknown.

Fluconazole: The coadministration of fluconazole with RETROVIR has been reported to interfere with the oral clearance and metabolism of RETROVIR. In a pharmacokinetic interaction study in which 12 HIV-positive men received RETROVIR 200 mg every 8 hours alone and in combination with fluconazole 400 mg daily, fluconazole increased the zidovudine AUC (74%; range 28% to 173%) and the zidovudine half-life (128%; range -4% to 189%) at steady state. The clinical significance of this interaction is unknown.

Atovaquone: Data from 14 HIV-infected volunteers who were given atovaquone tablets 750 mg every 12 hours with zidovudine 200 mg every 8 hours showed a 24% ± 12% decrease in zidovudine oral clearance, leading to a 35% ± 23% increase in plasma zidovudine AUC. The glucuronide metabolite:parent ratio decreased from a mean of 4.5 when zidovudine was administered alone to 3.1 when zidovudine was administered with atovaquone tablets. Zidovudine had no effect on atovaquone pharmacokinetics.

Valproic Acid: The concomitant administration of valproic acid 250 mg (n = 5) or 500 mg (n = 1) every 8 hours and zidovudine 100 mg orally every 8 hours for 4 days to six HIV-infected, asymptomatic male volunteers resulted in a 79% ± 61% (mean ± SD) increase in the plasma zidovudine AUC and a 22% ± 10% decrease in the plasma GZDV AUC as compared to the administration of zidovudine in the absence of valproic acid. The GZDV/zidovudine urinary excretion ratio decreased 58% ± 12%. Because no change in the zidovudine plasma half-life occurred, these results suggest that valproic acid may increase the oral bioavailability of zidovudine through inhibition of first-pass metabolism. Although the clinical significance of this interaction is unknown, patients should be monitored more closely for a possible increase in zidovudine-related adverse effects. The effect of zidovudine on the pharmacokinetics of valproic acid was not evaluated.

Lamivudine: RETROVIR and lamivudine were coadministered to 12 asymptomatic HIV-positive patients in a single-center, open-label, randomized, crossover study. No significant differences were observed in AUC∞ or total clearance for lamivudine or zidovudine when the two drugs were administered together.

Coadministration of RETROVIR with lamivudine resulted in an increase of 39% ± 62% (mean ± SD) in C_{max} of zidovudine.

Other Agents: Preliminary data from a drug interaction study (n = 10) suggest that coadministration of 200 mg RETROVIR and 600 mg rifampin decreases the area under the plasma concentration curve by an average of 48% ± 34%. However, the effect of once-daily dosing of rifampin on multiple daily doses of RETROVIR is unknown. Some nucleoside analogues affecting DNA replication, such as ribavirin, antagonize the in vitro antiviral activity of RETROVIR against HIV; concomitant use of such drugs should be avoided.

Carcinogenesis, Mutagenesis, Impairment of Fertility: Zidovudine was administered orally at three dosage levels to separate groups of mice and rats (60 females and 60 males in each group). Initial single daily doses were 30, 60, and 120 mg/kg per day in mice and 80, 220, and 600 mg/kg per day in rats. The doses in mice were reduced to 20, 30, and 40 mg/kg per day after day 90 because of treatment-related anemia, whereas in rats only the high dose was reduced to 450 mg/kg per day on day 91 and then to 300 mg/kg per day on day 279.

In mice, seven late-appearing (after 19 months) vaginal neoplasms (five nonmetastasizing squamous cell carcinomas, one squamous cell papilloma, and one squamous polyp) occurred in animals given the highest dose. One late-appearing squamous cell papilloma occurred in the vagina of a middle-dose animal. No vaginal tumors were found at the lowest dose.

In rats, two late-appearing (after 20 months), nonmetastasizing vaginal squamous cell carcinomas occurred in animals given the highest dose. No vaginal tumors occurred at the low or middle dose in rats. No other drug-related tumors were observed in either sex of either species.

At doses that produced tumors in mice and rats, the estimated drug exposure (as measured by AUC) was approxi-

mately three times (mouse) and 24 times (rat) the estimated human exposure at the recommended therapeutic dose of 100 mg every 4 hours.

Two transplacental carcinogenicity studies were conducted in mice. One study administered zidovudine at doses of 20 mg/kg per day or 40 mg/kg per day from gestation day 10 through parturition and lactation with dosing continuing in offspring for 24 months postnatally. The doses of zidovudine employed in this study produced zidovudine exposures approximately three times the estimated human exposure at recommended doses. After 24 months, an increase in incidence of vaginal tumors was noted with no increase in tumors in the liver or lung or any other organ in either gender. These findings are consistent with results of the standard oral carcinogenicity study in mice, as described earlier. A second study administered zidovudine at maximum tolerated doses of 12.5 mg/day or 25 mg/day (~1000 mg/kg nonpregnant body weight or ~450 mg/kg of term body weight) to pregnant mice from days 12 through 18 of gestation. There was an increase in the number of tumors in the lung, liver, and female reproductive tracts in the offspring of mice receiving the higher dose level of zidovudine.

It is not known how predictive the results of rodent carcinogenicity studies may be for humans.

Zidovudine was mutagenic in a $5178Y/TK^{+/-}$ mouse lymphoma assay, positive in an in vitro cell transformation assay, clastogenic in a cytogenetic assay using cultured human lymphocytes, and positive in mouse and rat micronucleus tests after repeated doses. It was negative in a cytogenetic study in rats given a single dose.

Zidovudine, administered to male and female rats at doses up to seven times the usual adult dose based on body surface area considerations, had no effect on fertility judged by conception rates.

Pregnancy: Pregnancy Category C. Oral teratology studies in the rat and in the rabbit at doses up to 500 mg/kg per day revealed no evidence of teratogenicity with zidovudine. Zidovudine treatment resulted in embryo/fetal toxicity as evidenced by an increase in the incidence of fetal resorptions in rats given 150 or 450 mg/kg per day and rabbits given 500 mg/kg per day. The doses used in the teratology studies resulted in peak zidovudine plasma concentrations (after one half of the daily dose) in rats 66 to 226 times, and in rabbits 12 to 87 times, mean steady-state peak human plasma concentrations (after one sixth of the daily dose) achieved with the recommended daily dose (100 mg every 4 hours). In an in vitro experiment with fertilized mouse oocytes, zidovudine exposure resulted in a dose-dependent reduction in blastocyst formation. In an additional teratology study in rats, a dose of 3000 mg/kg per day (very near the oral median lethal dose in rats of 3683 mg/kg) caused marked maternal toxicity and an increase in the incidence of fetal malformations. This dose resulted in peak zidovudine plasma concentrations 350 times peak human plasma concentrations. (Estimated area-under-the-curve [AUC] in rats at this dose level was 300 times the daily AUC in humans given 600 mg per day.) No evidence of teratogenicity was seen in this experiment at doses of 600 mg/kg per day or less.

Two rodent transplacental carcinogenicity studies were conducted (see Carcinogenesis, Mutagenesis, Impairment of Fertility).

A randomized, double-blind, placebo-controlled trial was conducted in HIV-infected pregnant women to determine the utility of RETROVIR for the prevention of maternal-fetal HIV-transmission (see INDICATIONS AND USAGE: Description of Clinical Studies). Congenital abnormalities occurred with similar frequency between neonates born to mothers who received RETROVIR and neonates born to mothers who received placebo. Abnormalities were either problems in embryogenesis (prior to 14 weeks) or were recognized on ultrasound before or immediately after initiation of study drug.

Antiretroviral Pregnancy Registry: To monitor maternal-fetal outcomes of pregnant women exposed to RETROVIR, an Antiretroviral Pregnancy Registry has been established. Physicians are encouraged to register patients by calling 1-800-258-4263.

Nursing Mothers: The U.S. Public Health Service Centers for Disease Control and Prevention advises HIV-infected women not to breastfeed to avoid postnatal transmission of HIV to a child who may not yet be infected. Zidovudine is excreted in human milk (see Pharmacokinetics).

Pediatric Use: RETROVIR has been studied in HIV-infected pediatric patients over 3 months of age who have HIV-related symptoms or who are asymptomatic with abnormal laboratory values indicating significant HIV-related immunosuppression (see ADVERSE REACTIONS, DOSAGE AND ADMINISTRATION, and INDICATIONS AND USAGE: Description of Clinical Studies, and Pharmacokinetics).

ADVERSE REACTIONS

Monotherapy: *Adults:* The frequency and severity of adverse events associated with the use of RETROVIR in adults are greater in patients with more advanced infection

at the time of initiation of therapy. The following table summarizes the relative incidence of hematologic adverse events observed in clinical studies by severity of HIV disease present at the start of treatment:

[See table 2 above]

The anemia reported in patients with advanced HIV disease receiving RETROVIR appeared to be the result of impaired erythrocyte maturation as evidenced by macrocytosis while on drug. Although mean platelet counts in patients receiving RETROVIR were significantly increased compared to mean baseline values, thrombocytopenia did occur in some of these patients with advanced disease. Twelve percent of patients receiving RETROVIR compared to 5% of patients receiving placebo had >50% decreases from baseline platelet count. Mild drug-associated elevations in total bilirubin levels have been reported as an uncommon occurrence in patients treated for asymptomatic HIV infection.

The HIV-infected adults participating in these clinical trials often had baseline symptoms and signs of HIV disease and/or experienced adverse events at some time during study. It was often difficult to distinguish adverse events possibly associated with administration of RETROVIR from

underlying signs of HIV disease or intercurrent illnesses. The following table summarizes clinical adverse events or symptoms which occurred in at least 5% of all patients with advanced HIV disease treated with 1500 mg/day of RETROVIR in the original placebo-controlled study. Of the items listed in the table, only severe headache, nausea, insomnia, and myalgia were reported at a significantly greater rate in patients receiving RETROVIR.

[See table 3 above]

All events of a severe or life-threatening nature were monitored for adults in the placebo-controlled studies in early

Continued on next page

Table 2

Stage of Disease	RETROVIR Daily Dose* (mg)	Granulocytopenia (<750 cells/mm³)	Anemia (Hgb <8.0 g/dL)
Asymptomatic			
ACTG 019	500	1.8%†	1.1%†
Early HIV Disease (CD4 >200 cells/mm³)			
ACTG 016	1200	4%	4%
Advanced HIV Disease (CD4 > 200 cells/mm³)			
BW 02	1500	10%†	3%†‡
(CD4 ≤200 cells/mm³)			
ACTG 002	600	37%	29%
BW 02	1500	47%	29%‡

*The currently recommended dose is 500 to 600 mg daily.
†Not statistically significant compared to placebo.
‡Anemia = Hgb <7.5 g/dL.

Table 3
Percentage (%) of Patients with Clinical Events in Advanced HIV Disease (BW 02)

Adverse Event	RETROVIR 1500 mg/day* (n = 144) %	Placebo (n = 137) %
BODY AS A WHOLE		
Asthenia	19	18
Diaphoresis	5	4
Fever	16	12
Headache	42	37
Malaise	8	7
GASTROINTESTINAL		
Anorexia	11	8
Diarrhea	12	18
Dyspepsia	5	4
GI Pain	20	19
Nausea	46	18
Vomiting	6	3
MUSCULOSKELETAL		
Myalgia	8	2
NERVOUS		
Dizziness	6	4
Insomnia	5	1
Paresthesia	6	3
Somnolence	8	9
RESPIRATORY		
Dyspnea	5	3
SKIN		
Rash	17	15
SPECIAL SENSES		
Taste Perversion	5	8

*The currently recommended dose is 500 to 600 mg daily.

Table 4
Percentage (%) of Patients with Adverse Events in Early HIV Disease (ACTG 016)

Adverse Event	RETROVIR 1200 mg/day* (n = 361) %	Placebo (n = 352) %
BODY AS A WHOLE		
Asthenia	69	62
GASTROINTESTINAL		
Dyspepsia	6	1
Nausea	61	41
Vomiting	25	13

*The currently recommended dose is 500 to 600 mg daily.

This product information is based on labeling in effect on June 1, 1998. For further information, contact via direct mail, phone, or web site Medical Information: Glaxo Wellcome Inc., PO Box 13398, Research Triangle Park, NC 27709. Healthcare Professionals (Medical Information): 800-334-0089 Patients (Customer Response Center): 888-TALK2GW (1-888-825-5249) Glaxo Wellcome Corporate Web Site: www.glaxowellcome.com

Retrovir—Cont.

HIV disease and asymptomatic HIV infection. Data concerning the occurrence of additional signs or symptoms were also collected. No distinction was made in reporting events between those possibly associated with the administration of the study medication and those due to the underlying disease. The following tables summarize all those events reported at a statistically significant greater incidence for patients receiving RETROVIR in these studies:
[See table 4 on previous page]
[See table 5 above]
Several serious adverse events have been reported with the use of RETROVIR in clinical practice. Myopathy and myositis with pathological changes, similar to that produced by HIV disease, have been associated with prolonged use of RETROVIR. Reports of hepatomegaly with steatosis, hepatitis, pancreatitis, lactic acidosis, sensitization reactions (including anaphylaxis in one patient), hyperbilirubinemia, vasculitis, and seizures have been rare. These adverse events, except for sensitization, have also been associated with HIV disease. A single case of macular edema has been reported with the use of RETROVIR.
Additional adverse events reported in clinical trials at a rate not significantly different from placebo are listed below. Selected events from post-marketing clinical experience with RETROVIR are also included. Many of these events may also occur as part of HIV disease. The clinical significance of the association between treatment with RETROVIR and these events is unknown.
Body as a Whole: Abdominal pain, back pain, body odor, chest pain, chills, edema of the lip, fever, flu syndrome, hyperalgesia.
Cardiovascular: Syncope, vasodilation.
Gastrointestinal: Bleeding gums, constipation, diarrhea, dysphagia, edema of the tongue, eructation, flatulence, mouth ulcer, rectal hemorrhage.
Hemic and Lymphatic: Lymphadenopathy.
Musculoskeletal: Arthralgia, muscle spasm, tremor, twitch.
Nervous: Anxiety, confusion, depression, dizziness, emotional lability, loss of mental acuity, nervousness, paresthesia, somnolence, vertigo.
Respiratory: Cough, dyspnea, epistaxis, hoarseness, pharyngitis, rhinitis, sinusitis.
Skin: Acne, changes in skin and nail pigmentation, pruritus, rash, sweat, urticaria.
Special senses: Amblyopia, hearing loss, photophobia, taste perversion.
Urogenital: Dysuria, polyuria, urinary frequency, urinary hesitancy.
Pediatrics: Anemia and granulocytopenia among pediatric patients with advanced HIV disease receiving RETROVIR occurred with similar incidence to that reported for adults with AIDS or advanced ARC (see above). Management of neutropenia and anemia included, in some cases, dose modification and/or blood product transfusions. In the open-label studies, 17% had their dose modified (generally a reduction in dose by 30%) due to anemia and 25% had their dose modified (temporary discontinuation or dose reduction by 30%) for neutropenia. Four pediatric patients had RETROVIR permanently discontinued for neutropenia. The following table summarizes the occurrence of anemia (Hgb <7.5 g/dL) and granulocytopenia (<750 cells/mm^3) among 124 pediatric patients receiving RETROVIR for a mean of 267 days (range 3 to 855 days):

Table 6

Advanced Pediatric HIV Disease (n=124)	Granulocytopenia (<750 cells/mm^3)		Anemia (Hgb <7.5 g/dL)	
	n	%	n	%
	48	39	28*	23

* Twenty-two pediatric patients received one or more transfusions due to a decline in hemoglobin to <7.5 g/dL; an additional 15 pediatric patients were transfused for hemoglobin levels >7.5 g/dL. Fifty-nine percent of the patients transfused had a prestudy history of anemia or transfusion requirement.

Macrocytosis was observed among the majority of pediatric patients enrolled in the studies.
In the open-label studies involving 124 pediatric patients, 16 clinical adverse events were reported by 24 pediatric patients. No event was reported by more than 5.6% of the study populations. Due to the open-label design of the studies, it was difficult to determine possible events related to the use of RETROVIR versus disease-related events. Therefore, all clinical events reported as associated with therapy with RETROVIR or of unknown relationship to therapy with RETROVIR are presented in the following table:

Table 5
Percentage (%) of Patients with Adverse Events* in Asymptomatic HIV Infection (ACTG 019) Disease 016)

Adverse Event	RETROVIR 500 mg/day (n = 453) %	Placebo (n = 428) %
BODY AS A WHOLE		
Asthenia	8.6†	5.8
Headache	62.5	52.6
Malaise	53.2	44.9
GASTROINTESTINAL		
Anorexia	20.1	10.5
Constipation	6.4†	3.5
Nausea	51.4	29.9
Vomiting	17.2	9.8
NERVOUS		
Dizziness	17.9†	15.2

*Reported in ≥5% of study population.
†Not statistically significant versus placebo.

Table 7
Percentage (%) of Pediatric Patients with Clinical Events in Open-Label Studies

Adverse Event	n	%
BODY AS A WHOLE		
Fever	4	3.2
Phlebitis*/Bacteremia	2	1.6
Headache	2	1.6
GASTROINTESTINAL		
Nausea	1	0.8
Vomiting	6	4.8
Abdominal Pain	4	3.2
Diarrhea	1	0.8
Weight Loss	1	0.8
NERVOUS		
Insomnia	3	2.4
Nervousness/Irritability	2	1.6
Decreased Reflexes	7	5.6
Seizure	1	0.8
CARDIOVASCULAR		
Left Ventricular Dilation	1	0.8
Cardiomyopathy	1	0.8
S$_3$ Gallop	1	0.8
Congestive Heart Failure	1	0.8
Generalized Edema	1	0.8
ECG Abnormality	3	2.4
UROGENITAL		
Hematuria/Viral Cystitis	1	0.8

*Peripheral vein IV catheter site.

[See table 7 above]
The clinical adverse events reported among adult recipients of RETROVIR may also occur in pediatric patients.
Use for the Prevention of Maternal-Fetal Transmission of HIV: In a randomized, double-blind, placebo-controlled trial in HIV-infected women and their neonates conducted to determine the utility of RETROVIR for the prevention of maternal-fetal HIV transmission, RETROVIR Syrup at 2 mg/kg was administered every 6 hours for 6 weeks to neonates beginning within 12 hours after birth. The most commonly reported adverse experiences were anemia (hemoglobin <9.0 g/dL) and neutropenia (<1000 cells/mm^3). Anemia occurred in 22% of the neonates who received RETROVIR and in 12% of the neonates who received placebo. The mean difference in hemoglobin values was less than 1.0 g/dL for neonates receiving RETROVIR compared to neonates receiving placebo. No neonates with anemia required transfusion and all hemoglobin values spontaneously returned to normal within 6 weeks after completion of therapy with RETROVIR. Neutropenia was reported with similar frequency in the group that received RETROVIR (21%) and in the group that received placebo (27%). The long-term consequences of in utero and infant exposure to RETROVIR are unknown.

OVERDOSAGE

Cases of acute overdoses in both pediatric patients and adults have been reported with doses up to 50 grams. None were fatal. The only consistent finding in these cases of overdose was spontaneous or induced nausea and vomiting. Hematologic changes were transient and not severe. Some patients experienced nonspecific CNS symptoms such as headache, dizziness, drowsiness, lethargy, and confusion. One report of a grand mal seizure possibly attributable to RETROVIR occurred in a 35-year-old male 3 hours after ingesting 36 grams of RETROVIR. No other cause could be identified. All patients recovered without permanent sequelae. Hemodialysis and peritoneal dialysis appear to have a negligible effect on the removal of zidovudine while elimination of its primary metabolite, GZDV, is enhanced.

DOSAGE AND ADMINISTRATION

Adults: The recommended total oral daily dose of RETROVIR is 600 mg per day in divided doses in combination with other antiretroviral agents and 500 mg (100 mg every 4 hours while awake) or 600 mg per day in divided doses for monotherapy. The effectiveness of this dose compared to higher dosing regimens in improving the neurologic dysfunction associated with HIV disease is unknown. A small randomized study found a greater effect of higher doses of RETROVIR on improvement of neurological symptoms in patients with pre-existing neurological disease.
Pediatrics: The recommended dose in pediatric patients 3 months to 12 years of age is 180 mg/m^2 every 6 hours (720 mg/m^2 per day), not to exceed 200 mg every 6 hours.
Maternal-Fetal HIV Transmission: The recommended dosing regimen for administration to pregnant women (>14 weeks of pregnancy) and their neonates is:
Maternal Dosing: 100 mg orally five times per day until the start of labor (see INDICATIONS AND USAGE: Description of Clinical Studies). During labor and delivery, intravenous RETROVIR should be administered at 2 mg/kg (total body weight) over 1 hour followed by a continuous intravenous infusion of 1 mg/kg per hour (total body weight) until clamping of the umbilical cord.
Neonatal Dosing: 2 mg/kg orally every 6 hours starting within 12 hours after birth and continuing through 6 weeks of age. Neonates unable to receive oral dosing may be administered RETROVIR intravenously at 1.5 mg/kg, infused over 30 minutes, every 6 hours. (See PRECAUTIONS if hepatic disease or renal insufficiency is present.)
Monitoring of Patients: Hematologic toxicities appear to be related to pretreatment bone marrow reserve and to dose and duration of therapy. In patients with poor bone marrow reserve, particularly in patients with advanced symptomatic HIV disease, frequent monitoring of hematologic indices is recommended to detect serious anemia or neutropenia (see WARNINGS). In patients who experience hematologic toxicity, reduction in hemoglobin may occur as early as 2 to 4 weeks, and neutropenia usually occurs after 6 to 8 weeks.
Dose Adjustment: Significant anemia (hemoglobin of <7.5 g/dL or reduction of >25% of baseline) and/or significant neutropenia (granulocyte count of <750 cells/mm^3 or reduction of >50% from baseline) may require a dose interruption

until evidence of marrow recovery is observed (see WARNINGS). For less severe anemia or neutropenia, a reduction in daily dose may be adequate. In patients who develop significant anemia, dose modification does not necessarily eliminate the need for transfusion. If marrow recovery occurs following dose modification, gradual increases in dose may be appropriate depending on hematologic indices and patient tolerance.

In end-stage renal disease patients maintained on hemodialysis or peritoneal dialysis, recommended dosing is 100 mg every 6 to 8 hours (see CLINICAL PHARMACOLOGY: Pharmacokinetics).

There are insufficient data to recommend dose adjustment of RETROVIR in patients with impaired hepatic function.

HOW SUPPLIED

RETROVIR Tablets 300 mg (biconvex, white, round, film-coated) containing 300 mg zidovudine, one side engraved "GX CW3" and "300" on the other side. Bottle of 60 (NDC 0173-0501-00).

Store at 15° to 25°C (59° to 77°F).

RETROVIR Capsules 100 mg (white, opaque cap and body with a dark blue band) containing 100 mg zidovudine and printed with "Wellcome" and unicorn logo on cap and "Y9C" and "100" on body. Bottles of 100 (NDC 0173-0108-55) and Unit Dose Pack of 100 (NDC 0173-0108-56).

Store at 15° to 25°C (59° to 77°F) and protect from moisture.

RETROVIR Syrup (colorless to pale yellow, strawberry-flavored) containing 50 mg zidovudine in each teaspoonful (5 mL). Bottle of 240 mL (NDC 0173-0113-18) with child-resistant cap.

Store at 15° to 25°C (59° to 77°F).

U.S. Patent Nos. 4,818,538 and 4,828,838 (Product Patents); 4,724,232; 4,833,130; and 4,837,208 (Use Patents)

©Copyright 1996 Glaxo Wellcome Inc. All rights reserved.

March 1998/RL-551

Shown in Product Identification Guide, page 313

RETROVIR® ℞

[re 'trō-vir]

(zidovudine)

IV Infusion

FOR INTRAVENOUS INFUSION ONLY

WARNING: RETROVIR (ZIDOVUDINE) MAY BE ASSOCIATED WITH HEMATOLOGIC TOXICITY INCLUDING NEUTROPENIA AND SEVERE ANEMIA PARTICULARLY IN PATIENTS WITH ADVANCED HIV DISEASE (SEE WARNINGS). PROLONGED USE OF RETROVIR HAS BEEN ASSOCIATED WITH SYMPTOMATIC MYOPATHY SIMILAR TO THAT PRODUCED BY HUMAN IMMUNODEFICIENCY VIRUS. RARE OCCURRENCES OF POTENTIALLY FATAL LACTIC ACIDOSIS IN THE ABSENCE OF HYPOXEMIA, AND SEVERE HEPATOMEGALY WITH STEATOSIS HAVE BEEN REPORTED WITH THE USE OF CERTAIN ANTIRETROVIRAL NUCLEOSIDE ANALOGUES (SEE WARNINGS).

DESCRIPTION

RETROVIR is the brand name for zidovudine (formerly called azidothymidine [AZT]), a pyrimidine nucleoside analogue active against human immunodeficiency virus (HIV). RETROVIR IV Infusion is a sterile solution for intravenous infusion only. Each mL contains 10 mg zidovudine in Water for Injection. Hydrochloric acid and/or sodium hydroxide may have been added to adjust the pH to approximately 5.5. RETROVIR IV Infusion contains no preservatives.

The chemical name of zidovudine is 3′-azido-3′-deoxythymidine.

Zidovudine is a white to beige, odorless, crystalline solid with a molecular weight of 267.24 and a solubility of 20.1 mg/mL in water at 25°C. The molecular formula is $C_{10}H_{13}N_5O_4$.

MICROBIOLOGY

Mechanism of Action: Zidovudine is a synthetic nucleoside analogue of the naturally occurring nucleoside, thymidine, in which the 3′-hydroxy (-OH) group is replaced by an azido (-N_3) group. Within cells, zidovudine is converted to the active metabolite, zidovudine 5′-triphosphate (AztTP), by the sequential action of the cellular enzymes. Zidovudine 5′-triphosphate inhibits the activity of the HIV reverse transcriptase both by competing for utilization with the natural substrate, deoxythymidine 5′-triphosphate (dTTP), and by its incorporation into viral DNA. The lack of a 3′- OH group in the incorporated nucleoside analogue prevents the formation of the 5′ to 3′ phosphodiester linkage essential for DNA chain elongation and, therefore, the viral DNA growth is terminated. The active metabolite AztTP is also a weak inhibitor of the cellular DNA polymerase-alpha and mitochondrial polymerase-gamma and has been reported to be incorporated into the DNA of cells in culture.

In Vitro HIV Susceptibility: The in vitro anti-HIV activity of zidovudine was assessed by infecting cell lines of lymphoblastic and monocytic origin and peripheral blood lymphocytes with laboratory and clinical isolates of HIV. The IC_{50} and IC_{90} values (50% and 90% inhibitory concentrations) were 0.003 to 0.013 and 0.03 to 0.13 mcg/mL, respectively (1 nM = 0.27 ng/mL). The IC_{50} and IC_{90} values of HIV isolates recovered from 18 untreated AIDS/ARC patients were in the range of 0.003 to 0.013 mcg/mL and 0.03 to 0.3 mcg/mL, respectively. Zidovudine showed antiviral activity in all acutely infected cell lines; however, activity was substantially less in chronically infected cell lines. In drug combination studies with zalcitabine, didanosine, lamivudine, saquinavir, indinavir, ritonavir, nevirapine, delavirdine, or interferon-alpha, zidovudine showed additive to synergistic activity in cell culture. The relationship between the in vitro susceptibility of HIV to reverse transcriptase inhibitors and the inhibition of HIV replication in humans has not been established.

Drug Resistance: HIV isolates with reduced sensitivity to zidovudine have been selected in vitro and were also recovered from patients treated with RETROVIR. Genetic analysis of the isolates showed mutations which result in five amino acid substitutions (Met41→Leu, A67→Asn, Lys70→Arg, Thr215→Tyr or Phe, and Lys219→Gln) in the viral reverse transcriptase. In general, higher levels of resistance were associated with greater number of mutations with 215 mutation being the most significant.

Cross-Resistance: The potential for cross-resistance between HIV reverse transcriptase inhibitors and protease inhibitors is low because of the different enzyme targets involved. Combination therapy with zidovudine plus zalcitabine or didanosine does not appear to prevent the emergence of zidovudine-resistant isolates. Combination therapy with RETROVIR plus EPIVIR® delayed the emergence of mutations conferring resistance to zidovudine. In some patients harboring zidovudine-resistant virus, combination therapy with RETROVIR plus EPIVIR restored phenotypic sensitivity to zidovudine by 12 weeks of treatment. HIV isolates with multidrug resistance to zidovudine, didanosine, zalcitabine, stavudine, and lamivudine were recovered from a small number of patients treated for ≥1 year with the combination of zidovudine and didanosine or zalcitabine. The pattern of resistant mutations in the combination therapy was different (Ala62→Val, Val75→Ile, Phe77→116Tyr, and Gln→151Met) from monotherapy, with mutation 151 being most significant for multidrug resistance. Site-directed mutagenesis studies showed that these mutations could also result in resistance to zalcitabine, lamivudine, and stavudine.

CLINICAL PHARMACOLOGY

Pharmacokinetics: ***Adults:*** The pharmacokinetics of zidovudine has been evaluated in 22 adult HIV-infected patients in a Phase 1 dose-escalation study. Following intravenous dosing, dose-independent kinetics was observed over the range of 1 to 5 mg/kg with a mean zidovudine half-life of 1.1 hours (range 0.48 to 2.86 hours). Total body clearance averaged 1900 mL/min per 70 kg, and the apparent volume of distribution was 1.6 L/kg. At a dose of 7.5 mg/kg every 4 hours, total body clearance was calculated to be about 1200 mL/min per 70 kg, with no change in half-life. Renal clearance is estimated to be 400 mL/min per 70 kg, indicating glomerular filtration and active tubular secretion by the kidneys. Zidovudine plasma protein binding is 34% to 38%, indicating that drug interactions involving binding site displacement are not anticipated.

The mean steady-state peak and trough concentrations of zidovudine at 2.5 mg/kg every 4 hours were 1.06 and 0.12 mcg/mL, respectively.

The zidovudine cerebrospinal fluid (CSF)/plasma concentration ratio was determined in 39 patients receiving chronic therapy with RETROVIR. The median ratio measured in 50 paired samples drawn 1 to 8 hours after the last dose of RETROVIR was 0.6.

Zidovudine is rapidly metabolized to GZDV which has an apparent elimination half-life of 1 hour (range 0.61 to 1.73 hours). A second metabolite, 3′-amino-3′-deoxythymidine (AMT), has been identified in the plasma following single-dose intravenous administration of zidovudine. AMT area-under-the-curve (AUC) was one fifth of the AUC of zidovudine and had a half-life of 2.7 ± 0.7 hours. In comparison, GZDV AUC was about threefold greater than the AUC of zidovudine. Following intravenous administration, urinary recoveries of zidovudine and GZDV accounted for 18% and 60% of the dose, respectively, and the total urinary recovery averaged 77% (range 64% to 98%).

Adults with Impaired Renal Function: The pharmacokinetics of zidovudine has been evaluated in patients with impaired renal function following a single 200-mg oral dose. In 14 patients (mean creatinine clearance 18 ± 2 mL/min) the half-life of zidovudine was 1.4 hours compared to 1.0 hour for control subjects with normal renal function; AUC values were approximately twice those of controls. Additionally, GZDV half-life in these patients was 8.0 hours (versus 0.9 hours for control) and AUC was 17 times higher than for control subjects. The pharmacokinetics and tolerance were evaluated in a multiple-dose study in patients undergoing hemodialysis (n = 5) or peritoneal dialysis (n = 6). Patients received escalating oral doses of zidovudine up to 200 mg five times daily for 8 weeks. Daily oral doses of 500 mg or less were well tolerated despite significantly elevated plasma levels of GZDV. Apparent oral clearance of zidovudine was approximately 50% of that reported in patients with normal renal function. The plasma concentrations of AMT are not known in patients with renal insufficiency. Daily doses of 300 to 400 mg should be appropriate in HIV-infected patients with severe renal dysfunction (see DOSAGE AND ADMINISTRATION: Dose Adjustment). Hemodialysis and peritoneal dialysis appear to have a negligible effect on the removal of zidovudine, whereas GZDV elimination is enhanced.

Pediatrics: The pharmacokinetics and bioavailability of zidovudine have been evaluated in 21 HIV-infected pediatric patients, aged 6 months through 12 years, following intravenous doses administered over the range of 80 to 160 mg/m^2 every 6 hours, and following oral doses of the intravenous solution administered over the range of 90 to 240 mg/m^2 every 6 hours. After discontinuation of the IV infusion, zidovudine plasma concentrations decayed biexponentially, consistent with two-compartment pharmacokinetics. Proportional increases in AUC and in zidovudine concentrations were observed with increasing dose, consistent with dose-independent kinetics over the dose range studied. The mean terminal half-life and total body clearance across all dose levels administered were 1.5 hours and 30.9 mL/min per kg, respectively. These values compare to mean half-life and total body clearance in adults of 1.1 hours and 27.1 mL/min per kg.

The pharmacokinetics of zidovudine has been studied in pediatric patients from birth to 3 months of life. In one study of the pharmacokinetics of zidovudine in women during the last trimester of pregnancy, zidovudine elimination was determined immediately after birth in eight neonates who were exposed to zidovudine in utero. The half-life was 13.0 ± 5.8 hours. In another study, the pharmacokinetics of zidovudine was evaluated in pediatric patients (ranging in age of 1 day to 3 months) of normal birth weight for gestational age and with normal renal and hepatic function. In neonates less than or equal to 14 days old, mean ± SD total body clearance was 10.9 ± 4.8 mL/min per kg (n = 18) and half-life was 3.1 ± 1.2 hours (n = 21). In neonates and infants greater than 14 days old, total body clearance was 19.0 ± 4.0 mL/min per kg (n = 16) and half-life was 1.9 ± 0.7 hours (n = 18).

Concentrations of zidovudine in cerebrospinal fluid were measured after both intermittent oral and IV drug administration in 21 pediatric patients during Phase 1 and Phase 2 studies. The mean zidovudine CSF/plasma concentration ratio measured at an average time of 2.2 hours postdose at oral doses of 120 to 240 mg/m^2 was 0.52 ± 0.44 (n = 28); after an IV infusion of doses of 80 to 160 mg/m^2 over 1 hour, the mean CSF/plasma concentration ratio was 0.87 ± 0.66 (n = 23) at 3.2 hours after the start of the infusion. During continuous IV infusion, mean steady-state CSF/plasma ratio was 0.26 ± 0.17 (n = 28).

As in adult patients, the major route of elimination in pediatric patients was by metabolism to GZDV. After IV dosing, about 29% of the dose was excreted in the urine unchanged and about 45% of the dose was excreted as GZDV. Overall, the pharmacokinetics of zidovudine in pediatric patients greater than 3 months of age is similar to that of zidovudine in adult patients.

Pregnancy: The pharmacokinetics of zidovudine has been studied in a Phase 1 study of eight women during the last trimester of pregnancy. As pregnancy progressed, there was no evidence of drug accumulation. The pharmacokinetics of zidovudine was similar to that of nonpregnant adults. Consistent with passive transmission of the drug across the placenta, zidovudine concentrations in infant plasma at birth were essentially equal to those in maternal plasma at delivery. Although data are limited, methadone maintenance therapy in five pregnant women did not appear to alter zidovudine pharmacokinetics. However, in another patient population, a potential for interaction has been identified (see PRECAUTIONS).

Nursing Mothers: The US Public Health Service Centers for Disease Control and Prevention advises HIV-infected women not to breastfeed to avoid postnatal transmission of HIV to a child who may not yet be infected. After administration of a single dose of 200 mg zidovudine to 13 HIV-

Continued on next page

This product information is based on labeling in effect on June 1, 1998. For further information, contact via direct mail, phone, or web site Medical Information: Glaxo Wellcome Inc., PO Box 13398, Research Triangle Park, NC 27709. Healthcare Professionals (Medical Information): 800-334-0089 Patients (Customer Response Center): 888-TALK2GW (1-888-825-5249) Glaxo Wellcome Corporate Web Site: www.glaxowellcome.com

Retrovir I.V.—Cont.

infected women, the mean concentration of zidovudine was similar in human milk and serum (see PRECAUTIONS: Nursing Mothers).

INDICATIONS AND USAGE

RETROVIR IV Infusion is indicated for the treatment of HIV infection when antiretroviral therapy is warranted (see Description of Clinical Studies).

The duration of clinical benefit from antiretroviral therapy may be limited. Alterations in antiretroviral therapy should be considered if disease progression occurs during treatment.

Maternal-Fetal HIV Transmission: RETROVIR is also indicated for the prevention of maternal-fetal HIV transmission as part of a regimen that includes oral RETROVIR beginning between 14 and 34 weeks of gestation, intravenous RETROVIR during labor, and administration of RETROVIR Syrup to the neonate after birth. The efficacy of this regimen for preventing HIV transmission in women who have received RETROVIR for a prolonged period before pregnancy has not been evaluated. The safety of RETROVIR for the mother or fetus during the first trimester of pregnancy has not been assessed (see Description of Clinical Studies).

Description of Clinical Studies: RETROVIR has been shown to prolong survival and decrease the incidence of opportunistic infections in patients with advanced HIV disease at the initiation of therapy and to delay disease progression in asymptomatic HIV-infected patients. Other randomized studies suggest that the duration of the clinical benefit of monotherapy with RETROVIR is time-limited.

Pregnant Women and Their Neonates: The utility of RETROVIR for the prevention of maternal-fetal HIV transmission was demonstrated in a randomized, double-blind, placebo-controlled trial (ACTG 076) conducted in HIV-infected pregnant women with CD4 cell counts of 200 to 1818 cells/mm^3 (median in the treated group: 560 cells/mm^3) who had little or no previous exposure to RETROVIR. Oral RETROVIR was initiated between 14 and 34 weeks of gestation (median 11 weeks of therapy) followed by intravenous administration of RETROVIR during labor and delivery. After birth, neonates received oral RETROVIR Syrup for 6 weeks. The study showed a statistically significant difference in the incidence of HIV infection in the neonates (based on viral culture from peripheral blood) between the group receiving RETROVIR and the group receiving placebo. Of 363 neonates evaluated in the study, the estimated risk of HIV infection was 7.8% in the group receiving RETROVIR and 24.9% in the placebo group, a relative reduction in transmission risk of 68.7%. RETROVIR was well tolerated by mothers and infants. There was no difference in pregnancy-related adverse events between the treatment groups.

CONTRAINDICATIONS

RETROVIR IV Infusion is contraindicated for patients who have potentially life-threatening allergic reactions to any of the components of the formulation.

WARNINGS

The incidence of adverse reactions appears to increase with disease progression, and patients should be monitored carefully, especially as disease progression occurs.

Bone Marrow Suppression: RETROVIR should be used with caution in patients who have bone marrow compromise evidenced by granulocyte count <1000 cells/mm^3 or hemoglobin <9.5 g/dL. In patients with advanced symptomatic HIV disease, anemia and neutropenia were the most significant adverse events observed (see ADVERSE REACTIONS). There have been reports of pancytopenia associated with the use of RETROVIR, which was reversible in most instances after discontinuance of the drug. However, significant anemia, in many cases requiring dose adjustment, discontinuation of RETROVIR, and/or blood transfusions has occurred during treatment with RETROVIR alone or in combination with other antiretrovirals.

Frequent blood counts are strongly recommended in patients with advanced HIV disease who are treated with RETROVIR. For HIV-infected individuals and patients with asymptomatic or early HIV disease, periodic blood counts are recommended. If anemia or neutropenia develops, dosage adjustments may be necessary (see DOSAGE AND ADMINISTRATION).

Myopathy: Myopathy and myositis with pathological changes, similar to that produced by HIV disease, have been associated with prolonged use of RETROVIR.

Lactic Acidosis/Severe Hepatomegaly with Steatosis: Rare occurrences of potentially fatal lactic acidosis in the absence of hypoxemia, and severe hepatomegaly with steatosis have been reported with the use of certain antiretroviral nucleoside analogues. Lactic acidosis should be considered whenever a patient receiving therapy with RETROVIR develops unexplained tachypnea, dyspnea, or fall in serum bicarbonate level. Under these circumstances, therapy with RETROVIR should be suspended until the diagnosis of lac-

tic acidosis has been excluded. Caution should be exercised when administering RETROVIR to any patient, particularly obese women, with hepatomegaly, hepatitis, or other known risk factor for liver disease. These patients should be followed closely while on therapy with RETROVIR. The significance of elevated aminotransferase levels suggesting hepatic injury in HIV-infected patients prior to starting RETROVIR or while on RETROVIR is unclear. Treatment with RETROVIR should be suspended in the setting of rapidly elevating aminotransferase levels, progressive hepatomegaly, or metabolic/lactic acidosis of unknown etiology.

Other Serious Adverse Reactions: Several serious adverse events have been reported with use of RETROVIR in clinical practice. Reports of pancreatitis, sensitization reactions (including anaphylaxis in one patient), vasculitis, and seizures have been rare. These adverse events, except for sensitization, have also been associated with HIV disease. Changes in skin and nail pigmentation have been associated with the use of RETROVIR.

PRECAUTIONS

General: Zidovudine is eliminated from the body primarily by renal excretion following metabolism in the liver (glucuronidation). In patients with severely impaired renal function, dosage reduction is recommended (see CLINICAL PHARMACOLOGY: Pharmacokinetics and DOSAGE AND ADMINISTRATION). Although very little data are available, patients with severely impaired hepatic function may be at greater risk of toxicity.

Information for Patients: RETROVIR is not a cure for HIV infection, and patients may continue to acquire illnesses associated with HIV infection, including opportunistic infections. Therefore, patients should be advised to seek medical care for any significant change in their health status.

The safety and efficacy of RETROVIR in treating women, intravenous drug users, and racial minorities is not significantly different than that observed in white males.

Patients should be informed that the major toxicities of RETROVIR are neutropenia and/or anemia. The frequency and severity of these toxicities are greater in patients with more advanced disease and in those who initiate therapy later in the course of their infection. They should be told that if toxicity develops, they may require transfusions or dose modifications including possible discontinuation. They should be told of the extreme importance of having their blood counts followed closely while on therapy, especially for patients with advanced symptomatic HIV disease. They should be cautioned about the use of other medications, including ganciclovir and interferon-alpha, that may exacerbate the toxicity of RETROVIR (see PRECAUTIONS: Drug Interactions). Patients should be informed that other adverse effects of RETROVIR include nausea and vomiting. Patients should also be encouraged to contact their physician if they experience muscle weakness, shortness of breath, symptoms of hepatitis or pancreatitis, or any other unexpected adverse events while being treated with RETROVIR.

Pregnant women considering the use of RETROVIR during pregnancy for prevention of HIV-transmission to their infants should be advised that transmission may still occur in some cases despite therapy. The long-term consequences of in utero and neonatal exposure to RETROVIR are unknown, including the possible risk of cancer.

HIV-infected pregnant women should be advised not to breastfeed to avoid postnatal transmission of HIV to a child who may not yet be infected.

Patients should be advised that therapy with RETROVIR has not been shown to reduce the risk of transmission of HIV to others through sexual contact or blood contamination.

Drug Interactions: Ganciclovir: Use of RETROVIR in combination with ganciclovir increases the risk of hematologic toxicities in some patients with advanced HIV disease. Should the use of this combination become necessary in the treatment of patients with HIV disease, dose reduction or interruption of one or both agents may be necessary to minimize hematologic toxicity. Hematologic parameters, including hemoglobin, hematocrit, and white blood cell count with differential, should be monitored frequently in all patients receiving this combination.

Interferon-alpha: Hematologic toxicities have also been seen when RETROVIR is used concomitantly with interferon-alpha. As with the concomitant use of RETROVIR and ganciclovir, dose reduction or interruption of one or both agents may be necessary, and hematologic parameters should be monitored frequently.

Bone Marrow Suppressive Agents/Cytotoxic Agents: Coadministration of RETROVIR with drugs that are cytotoxic or which interfere with RBC/WBC number or function (e.g., dapsone, flucytosine, vincristine, vinblastine, or adriamycin) may increase the risk of hematologic toxicity.

Probenecid: Limited data suggest that probenecid may increase zidovudine levels by inhibiting glucuronidation and/or by reducing renal excretion of zidovudine. Some patients who have used RETROVIR concomitantly with pro-

benecid have developed flu-like symptoms consisting of myalgia, malaise, and/or fever and maculopapular rash.

Phenytoin: Phenytoin plasma levels have been reported to be low in some patients receiving RETROVIR, while in one case a high level was documented. However, in a pharmacokinetic interaction study in which 12 HIV-positive volunteers received a single 300-mg phenytoin dose alone and during steady-state zidovudine conditions (200 mg every 4 hours), no change in phenytoin kinetics was observed. Although not designed to optimally assess the effect of phenytoin on zidovudine kinetics, a 30% decrease in oral zidovudine clearance was observed with phenytoin.

Methadone: In a pharmacokinetic study of nine HIV-positive patients receiving methadone-maintenance (30 to 90 mg daily) concurrent with 200 mg of RETROVIR every 4 hours, no changes were observed in the pharmacokinetics of methadone upon initiation of therapy with RETROVIR and after 14 days of treatment with RETROVIR. No adjustments in methadone-maintenance requirements were reported. For four patients, the mean zidovudine AUC was elevated twofold, while for five patients, the value was equal to that of control patients. The exact mechanism and clinical significance of these data are unknown.

Fluconazole: The coadministration of fluconazole with RETROVIR has been reported to interfere with the oral clearance and metabolism of RETROVIR. In a pharmacokinetic interaction study in which 12 HIV-positive men received RETROVIR 200 mg every 8 hours alone and in combination with fluconazole 400 mg daily, fluconazole increased the zidovudine AUC (74%; range 28% to 173%) and the zidovudine half-life (128%; range -4% to 189%) at steady state. The clinical significance of this interaction is unknown.

Atovaquone: Data from 14 HIV-infected volunteers who were given atovaquone tablets 750 mg every 12 hours with zidovudine 200 mg every 8 hours showed a 24% ± 12% decrease in zidovudine oral clearance, leading to a 35% ± 23% increase in plasma zidovudine AUC. The glucuronide metabolite:parent ratio decreased from a mean of 4.5 when zidovudine was administered alone to 3.1 when zidovudine was administered with atovaquone tablets. Zidovudine had no effect on atovaquone pharmacokinetics.

Valproic Acid: The concomitant administration of valproic acid 250 mg (n = 5) or 500 mg (n = 1) every 8 hours and zidovudine 100 mg orally every 8 hours for 4 days to six HIV-infected, asymptomatic male volunteers resulted in a 79% ± 61% (mean ± SD) increase in the plasma zidovudine AUC and a 22% ± 10% decrease in the plasma GZDV AUC as compared to the administration of zidovudine in the absence of valproic acid. The GZDV/zidovudine urinary excretion ratio decreased 58% ± 12%. Because no change in the zidovudine plasma half-life occurred, these results suggest that valproic acid may increase the oral bioavailability of zidovudine through inhibition of first-pass metabolism. Although the clinical significance of this interaction is unknown, patients should be monitored more closely for a possible increase in zidovudine-related adverse effects. The effect of zidovudine on the pharmacokinetics of valproic acid was not evaluated.

Lamivudine: RETROVIR and lamivudine were coadministered to 12 asymptomatic HIV-positive patients in a single-center, open-label, randomized, crossover study. No significant differences were observed in AUC∞ or total clearance for lamivudine or zidovudine when the two drugs were administered together. Coadministration of RETROVIR with lamivudine resulted in an increase of 39% ± 62% (mean ± SD) in C_{max} of zidovudine.

Other Agents: Preliminary data from a drug interaction study (n = 10) suggest that coadministration of 200 mg RETROVIR and 600 mg rifampin decreases the area under the plasma concentration curve by an average of 48% ± 34%. However, the effect of once daily dosing of rifampin on multiple daily doses of RETROVIR is unknown. Some nucleoside analogues affecting DNA replication, such as ribavirin, antagonize the in vitro antiviral activity of RETROVIR against HIV; concomitant use of such drugs should be avoided.

Carcinogenesis, Mutagenesis, Impairment of Fertility: Zidovudine was administered orally at three dosage levels to separate groups of mice and rats (60 females and 60 males in each group). Initial single daily doses were 30, 60, and 120 mg/kg per day in mice and 80, 220, and 600 mg/kg per day in rats. The doses in mice were reduced to 20, 30, and 40 mg/kg per day after day 90 because of treatment-related anemia, whereas in rats only the high dose was reduced to 450 mg/kg per day on day 91, and then to 300 mg/kg per day on day 279.

In mice, seven late-appearing (after 19 months) vaginal neoplasms (five nonmetastasizing squamous cell carcinomas, one squamous cell papilloma, and one squamous polyp) occurred in animals given the highest dose. One late-appearing squamous cell papilloma occurred in the vagina of a middle-dose animal. No vaginal tumors were found at the lowest dose.

In rats, two late-appearing (after 20 months), nonmetastasizing vaginal squamous cell carcinomas occurred in ani-

mals given the highest dose. No vaginal tumors occurred at the low or middle dose in rats. No other drug-related tumors were observed in either sex of either species.

At doses that produced tumors in mice and rats, the estimated drug exposure (as measured by AUC) was approximately three times (mouse) and 24 times (rat) the estimated human exposure at the recommended therapeutic dose of 100 mg every 4 hours.

Two transplacental carcinogenicity studies were conducted in mice. One study administered zidovudine at doses of 20 mg/kg per day or 40 mg/kg per day from gestation day 10 through parturition and lactation with dosing continuing in offspring for 24 months postnatally. The doses of zidovudine employed in this study produced zidovudine exposures approximately three times the estimated human exposure at recommended doses. After 24 months, an increase in incidence of vaginal tumors was noted with no increase in tumors in the liver or lung or any other organ in either gender. These findings are consistent with results of the standard oral carcinogenicity study in mice, as described earlier. A second study administered zidovudine at maximum tolerated doses of 12.5 mg/day or 25 mg/day (~1,000 mg/kg nonpregnant body weight or ~450 mg/kg of term body weight) to pregnant mice from days 12 through 18 of gestation. There was an increase in the number of tumors in the lung, liver, and female reproductive tracts in the offspring of mice receiving the higher dose level of zidovudine. It is not known how predictive the results of rodent carcinogenicity studies may be for humans.

Zidovudine was mutagenic in a 5178Y/TK$^{+/-}$ mouse lymphoma assay, positive in an in vitro cell transformation assay, clastogenic in a cytogenetic assay using cultured human lymphocytes, and positive in mouse and rat micronucleus tests after repeated doses. It was negative in a cytogenetic study in rats given a single dose.

Zidovudine, administered to male and female rats at doses up to seven times the usual adult dose based on body surface area considerations, had no effect on fertility judged by conception rates.

Pregnancy: Pregnancy Category C. Oral teratology studies in the rat and in the rabbit at doses up to 500 mg/kg per day revealed no evidence of teratogenicity with zidovudine. Zidovudine treatment resulted in embryo/fetal toxicity as evidenced by an increase in the incidence of fetal resorptions in rats given 150 or 450 mg/kg per day and rabbits given 500 mg/kg per day. The doses used in the teratology studies resulted in peak zidovudine plasma concentrations (after one-half of the daily dose) in rats 66 to 226 times, and in rabbits 12 to 87 times, mean steady-state peak human plasma concentrations (after one-sixth of the daily dose) achieved with the recommended daily dose (100 mg every 4 hours). In an in vitro experiment with fertilized mouse oocytes, zidovudine exposure resulted in a dose-dependent reduction in blastocyst formation. In an additional teratology study in rats, a dose of 3000 mg/kg per day (very near the oral median lethal dose in rats of 3683 mg/kg) caused marked maternal toxicity and an increase in the incidence of fetal malformations. This dose resulted in peak zidovudine plasma concentrations 350 times peak human plasma concentrations. (Estimated area-under-the-curve [AUC] in rats at this dose level was 300 times the daily AUC in humans given 600 mg per day.) No evidence of teratogenicity was seen in this experiment at doses of 600 mg/kg per day or less.

Two rodent transplacental carcinogenicity studies were conducted (see Carcinogenesis, Mutagenesis, Impairment of Fertility).

A randomized, double-blind, placebo-controlled trial was conducted in HIV-infected pregnant women to determine the utility of RETROVIR for the prevention of maternal-fetal HIV-transmission (see INDICATIONS AND USAGE: Description of Clinical Studies). Congenital abnormalities occurred with similar frequency between neonates born to mothers who received RETROVIR and neonates born to mothers who received placebo. Abnormalities were either problems in embryogenesis (prior to 14 weeks) or were recognized on ultrasound before or immediately after initiation of study drug.

Antiretroviral Pregnancy Registry: To monitor maternal-fetal outcomes of pregnant women exposed to RETROVIR, an Antiretroviral Pregnancy Registry has been established. Physicians are encouraged to register patients by calling 1-800-258-4263.

Nursing Mothers: The US Public Health Service Centers for Disease Control and Prevention advises HIV-infected women not to breastfeed to avoid postnatal transmission of HIV to a child who may not yet be infected.

Zidovudine is excreted in human milk (see Pharmacokinetics).

Pediatric Use: RETROVIR has been studied in HIV-infected pediatric patients over 3 months of age who have HIV-related symptoms or who are asymptomatic with abnormal laboratory values indicating significant HIV-related immunosuppression (see ADVERSE REACTIONS, DOSAGE AND ADMINISTRATION, and INDICATIONS AND

Table 1

Stage of Disease	RETROVIR Daily Dose* (mg)	Neutropenia (<750 cells/mm^3)	Anemia (Hgb <8.0 g/dL)
Asymptomatic ACTG 019	500	1.8%†	1.1%†
Early HIV Disease (CD4 >200 cells/mm^3) ACTG 016	1200	4%	4%
Advanced HIV Disease (CD4 >200 cells/mm^3) BW 02	1500	10%†	3%†‡
(CD4 ≤200 cells/mm^3) ACTG 002	600	37%	29%
BW 02	1500	47%	29%‡

* The currently recommended oral dose is 500 to 600 mg daily.
† Not statistically significant compared to placebo.
‡ Anemia = Hgb <7.5 g/dL.

Table 2: Percentage (%) of Patients with Adverse Events in Advanced HIV Disease (BW 02)

Adverse Event	RETROVIR 1500 mg/day* (n = 144) %	Placebo (n = 137) %
BODY AS A WHOLE		
Asthenia	19	18
Diaphoresis	5	4
Fever	16	12
Headache	42	37
Malaise	8	7
GASTROINTESTINAL		
Anorexia	11	8
Diarrhea	12	18
Dyspepsia	5	4
GI Pain	20	19
Nausea	46	18
Vomiting	6	3
MUSCULOSKELETAL		
Myalgia	8	2
NERVOUS		
Dizziness	6	4
Insomnia	5	1
Paresthesia	6	3
Somnolence	8	9
RESPIRATORY		
Dyspnea	5	3
SKIN		
Rash	17	15
SPECIAL SENSES		
Taste Perversion	5	8

*The currently recommended oral dose is 500 to 600 mg daily.

USAGE: Description of Clinical Studies, and Pharmacokinetics).

ADVERSE REACTIONS

The adverse events reported during intravenous administration of RETROVIR IV Infusion are similar to those reported with oral administration; neutropenia and anemia were reported most frequently. Long-term intravenous administration beyond 2 to 4 weeks has not been studied in adults and may enhance hematologic adverse events. Local reaction, pain, and slight irritation during intravenous administration occur infrequently.

Adults: The frequency and severity of adverse events associated with the use of oral RETROVIR in adults are greater in patients with more advanced infection at the time of initiation of therapy. Table 1 summarizes the relative incidence of hematologic adverse events observed in clinical studies by severity of HIV disease present at the start of treatment with oral RETROVIR:

[See table 1 above]

The anemia reported in patients with advanced HIV disease receiving RETROVIR appeared to be the result of impaired erythrocyte maturation as evidenced by macrocytosis while on drug. Although mean platelet counts in patients receiving RETROVIR were significantly increased compared to mean baseline values, thrombocytopenia did occur in some of these patients with advanced disease. Twelve percent of patients receiving RETROVIR compared to 5% of patients receiving placebo had >50% decreases from baseline platelet count. Mild drug-associated elevations in total bilirubin levels have been reported as an uncommon occurrence in patients treated for asymptomatic HIV infection.

The HIV-infected adults participating in these clinical trials often had baseline symptoms and signs of HIV disease and/or experienced adverse events at some time during study. It was often difficult to distinguish adverse events possibly associated with administration of RETROVIR from underlying signs of HIV disease or intercurrent illnesses. Table 2 summarizes clinical adverse events or symptoms which occurred in at least 5% of all patients with advanced HIV disease treated with 1500 mg/day of oral RETROVIR in the original placebo-controlled study. Of the items listed in the table, only severe headache, nausea, insomnia, and myalgia were reported at a significantly greater rate in patients receiving RETROVIR.

[See table 2 above]

All events of a severe or life-threatening nature were monitored for adults in the placebo-controlled studies in early HIV disease and asymptomatic HIV infection. Data concerning the occurrence of additional signs or symptoms were also collected. No distinction was made in reporting events between those possibly associated with the administration of the study medication and those due to the underlying disease. Tables 3 and 4 summarize all those events reported at a statistically significant greater incidence for patients receiving RETROVIR in these studies:

[See table 3 at top of next page]

[See table 4 at top of next page]

Several serious adverse events have been reported with the use of RETROVIR in clinical practice. Myopathy and myositis with pathological changes, similar to that produced by HIV disease, have been associated with prolonged use of RETROVIR. Reports of hepatomegaly with steatosis, hepatitis, pancreatitis, lactic acidosis, sensitization reactions (including anaphylaxis in one patient), hyperbilirubinemia, vasculitis, and seizures have been rare. These adverse

Continued on next page

This product information is based on labeling in effect on June 1, 1998. For further information, contact via direct mail, phone, or web site Medical Information: Glaxo Wellcome Inc., PO Box 13398, Research Triangle Park, NC 27709. Healthcare Professionals (Medical Information): 800-334-0089 Patients (Customer Response Center): 888-TALK2GW (1-888-825-5249) Glaxo Wellcome Corporate Web Site: www.glaxowellcome.com

Retrovir I.V.—Cont.

events, except for sensitization, have also been associated with HIV disease. A single case of macular edema has been reported with the use of RETROVIR.

Additional adverse events reported in clinical trials at a rate not significantly different from placebo are listed below. Selected events from post-marketing clinical experience with RETROVIR are also included. Many of these events may also occur as part of HIV disease. The clinical significance of the association between treatment with RETROVIR and these events is unknown.

Body as a Whole: Abdominal pain, back pain, body odor, chest pain, chills, edema of the lip, fever, flu syndrome, hyperalgesia.

Cardiovascular: Syncope, vasodilation.

Gastrointestinal: Bleeding gums, constipation, diarrhea, dysphagia, edema of the tongue, eructation, flatulence, mouth ulcer, rectal hemorrhage.

Hemic and Lymphatic: Lymphadenopathy.

Musculoskeletal: Arthralgia, muscle spasm, tremor, twitch.

Nervous: Anxiety, confusion, depression, dizziness, emotional lability, loss of mental acuity, nervousness, paresthesia, somnolence, vertigo.

Respiratory: Cough, dyspnea, epistaxis, hoarseness, pharyngitis, rhinitis, sinusitis.

Skin: Acne, changes in skin and nail pigmentation, pruritus, rash, sweat, urticaria.

Special Senses: Amblyopia, hearing loss, photophobia, taste perversion.

Urogenital: Dysuria, polyuria, urinary frequency, urinary hesitancy.

Pediatrics: Anemia and neutropenia among pediatric patients with advanced HIV disease receiving RETROVIR occurred with similar incidence to that reported for adults with AIDS or advanced ARC (see above). Management of neutropenia and anemia included, in some cases, dose modification and/or blood product transfusions. In the open-label studies, 17% had their dose modified (generally a reduction in dose by 30%) due to anemia and 25% had their dose modified (temporary discontinuation or dose reduction by 30%) for neutropenia. Four pediatric patients had RETROVIR permanently discontinued for neutropenia. Table 5 summarizes the occurrence of anemia (Hgb <7.5 g/dL) and neutropenia (<750 cells/mm^3) among 124 pediatric patients receiving oral RETROVIR for a mean of 267 days (range 3 to 855 days):

[See table 5 at right]

Macrocytosis was observed among the majority of pediatric patients enrolled in the studies.

In the open-label studies involving 124 pediatric patients, 16 clinical adverse events were reported by 24 pediatric patients. No event was reported by more than 5.6% of the study populations. Due to the open-label design of the studies, it was difficult to determine possible events related to the use of RETROVIR versus disease-related events. Therefore, all clinical events reported as associated with therapy with RETROVIR or of unknown relationship to therapy with RETROVIR are presented in Table 6:

[See table 6 below]

Table 3: Percentage (%) of Patients with Adverse Events in Early HIV Disease (ACTG 016)

Adverse Event	RETROVIR 1200 mg/day* (n = 361) %	Placebo (n = 352) %
BODY AS A WHOLE		
Asthenia	69	62
GASTROINTESTINAL		
Dyspepsia	6	1
Nausea	61	41
Vomiting	25	13

*The currently recommended oral dose is 500 to 600 mg daily.

Table 4: Percentage (%) of Patients with Adverse Events* in Asymptomatic HIV Infection (ACTG 019)

Adverse Event	RETROVIR 500 mg/day (n = 453) %	Placebo (n = 428) %
BODY AS A WHOLE		
Asthenia	8.6†	5.8
Headache	62.5	52.6
Malaise	53.2	44.9
GASTROINTESTINAL		
Anorexia	20.1	10.5
Constipation	6.4†	3.5
Nausea	51.4	29.9
Vomiting	17.2	9.8
NERVOUS		
Dizziness	17.9†	15.2

* Reported in ≥5% of study population.
† Not statistically significant versus placebo.

Table 5

Advanced Pediatric HIV Disease (n = 124)	Neutropenia (<750 cells/mm^3)		Anemia (Hgb <7.5 g/dL)	
	n	%	n	%
	48	39	28*	23

*Twenty-two pediatric patients received one or more transfusions due to a decline in hemoglobin to <7.5 g/dL; an additional 15 pediatric patients were transfused for hemoglobin levels >7.5 g/dL. Fifty-nine percent of the patients transfused had a prestudy history of anemia or transfusion requirement.

The clinical adverse events reported among adult recipients of RETROVIR may also occur in pediatric patients.

Use for the Prevention of Maternal-Fetal Transmission of HIV: In a randomized, double-blind, placebo-controlled trial in HIV-infected women and their neonates conducted to determine the utility of RETROVIR for the prevention of maternal-fetal HIV transmission, RETROVIR Syrup at 2 mg/kg was administered every 6 hours for 6 weeks to neonates beginning within 12 hours after birth. The most commonly reported adverse experiences were anemia (hemoglobin <9.0 g/dL) and neutropenia (<1000 cells/mm^3). Anemia occurred in 22% of the neonates who received RETROVIR and in 12% of the neonates who received placebo. The mean difference in hemoglobin values was less than 1.0 g/dL for neonates receiving RETROVIR compared to neonates receiving placebo. No neonates with anemia required transfusion, and all hemoglobin values spontaneously returned to normal within 6 weeks after completion of therapy with RETROVIR. Neutropenia was reported with similar frequency in the group that received RETROVIR (21%) and in the group that received placebo (27%). The long-term consequences of in utero and neonatal exposure to RETROVIR are unknown.

OVERDOSAGE

Cases of acute overdoses in both pediatric patients and adults have been reported with doses up to 50 grams. None were fatal. The only consistent finding in these cases of overdose was spontaneous or induced nausea and vomiting. Hematologic changes were transient and not severe. Some patients experienced nonspecific CNS symptoms such as headache, dizziness, drowsiness, lethargy, and confusion. One report of a grand mal seizure possibly attributable to RETROVIR occurred in a 35-year-old male 3 hours after ingesting 36 grams of RETROVIR. No other cause could be identified. All patients recovered without permanent sequelae. Hemodialysis appears to have a negligible effect on the removal of zidovudine while elimination of its primary metabolite, GZDV, is enhanced.

DOSAGE AND ADMINISTRATION

Adults: The recommended intravenous dose is 1 mg/kg infused over 1 hour. This dose should be administered five to six times daily (5 to 6 mg/kg daily). The effectiveness of this dose compared to higher dosing regimens in improving the neurologic dysfunction associated with HIV disease is unknown. A small randomized study found a greater effect of higher doses of RETROVIR on improvement of neurological symptoms in patients with pre-existing neurological disease.

Patients should receive RETROVIR IV Infusion only until oral therapy can be administered. The intravenous dosing regimen equivalent to the oral administration of 100 mg every 4 hours is approximately 1 mg/kg intravenously every 4 hours.

Table 6: Percentage (%) of Pediatric Patients with Clinical Events in Open-Label Studies

Adverse Event	n	%
BODY AS A WHOLE		
Fever	4	3.2
Phlebitis*/Bacteremia	2	1.6
Headache	2	1.6
GASTROINTESTINAL		
Nausea	1	0.8
Vomiting	6	4.8
Abdominal Pain	4	3.2
Diarrhea	1	0.8
Weight Loss	1	0.8
NERVOUS		
Insomnia	3	2.4
Nervousness/Irritability	2	1.6
Decreased Reflexes	7	5.6
Seizure	1	0.8
CARDIOVASCULAR		
Left Ventricular Dilation	1	0.8
Cardiomyopathy	1	0.8
S$_3$ Gallop	1	0.8
Congestive Heart Failure	1	0.8
Generalized Edema	1	0.8
ECG Abnormality	3	2.4
UROGENITAL		
Hematuria/Viral Cystitis	1	0.8

*Peripheral vein IV catheter site.

Maternal-Fetal HIV Transmission: The recommended dosing regimen for administration to pregnant women (>14 weeks of pregnancy) and their neonates is:

Maternal Dosing: 100 mg orally five times per day until the start of labor. During labor and delivery, intravenous RETROVIR should be administered at 2 mg/kg (total body weight) over 1 hour followed by a continuous intravenous infusion of 1 mg/kg per hour (total body weight) until clamping of the umbilical cord.

Neonatal Dosing: 2 mg/kg orally every 6 hours starting within 12 hours after birth and continuing through 6 weeks of age. Neonates unable to receive oral dosing may be administered RETROVIR intravenously at 1.5 mg/kg, infused over 30 minutes, every 6 hours. (See PRECAUTIONS if hepatic disease or renal insufficiency is present.)

Monitoring of Patients: Hematologic toxicities appear to be related to pretreatment bone marrow reserve and to dose and duration of therapy. In patients with poor bone marrow reserve, particularly in patients with advanced symptomatic HIV disease, frequent monitoring of hematologic indices is recommended to detect serious anemia or neutropenia (see WARNINGS). In patients who experience hematologic toxicity, reduction in hemoglobin may occur as early as 2 to 4 weeks, and neutropenia usually occurs after 6 to 8 weeks.

Dose Adjustment: Significant anemia (hemoglobin of <7.5 g/dL or reduction of >25% of baseline) and/or significant neutropenia (granulocyte count of <750 cells/mm³ or reduction of >50% from baseline) may require a dose interruption until some evidence of marrow recovery is observed. For less severe anemia or neutropenia, a reduction in daily dose may be adequate. In patients who develop significant anemia, dose modification does not necessarily eliminate the need for transfusion. If marrow recovery occurs following dose modification, gradual increases in dose may be appropriate depending on hematologic indices and patient tolerance.

In end-stage renal disease patients maintained on hemodialysis or peritoneal dialysis, recommended dosing is 1 mg/kg every 6 to 8 hours (see CLINICAL PHARMACOLOGY: Pharmacokinetics).

There are insufficient data to recommend dose adjustment of zidovudine in patients with impaired hepatic function.

Method of Preparation: RETROVIR IV Infusion must be diluted prior to administration. The calculated dose should be removed from the 20-mL vial and added to 5% Dextrose Injection solution to achieve a concentration no greater than 4 mg/mL. Admixture in biologic or colloidal fluids (e.g., blood products, protein solutions, etc.) is not recommended.

After dilution, the solution is physically and chemically stable for 24 hours at room temperature and 48 hours if refrigerated at 2° to 8°C (36° to 46°F). Care should be taken during admixture to prevent inadvertent contamination. As an additional precaution, the diluted solution should be administered within 8 hours if stored at 25°C (77°F) or 24 hours if refrigerated at 2° to 8°C to minimize potential administration of a microbially contaminated solution.

Parenteral drug products should be inspected visually for particulate matter and discoloration prior to administration whenever solution and container permit. Should either be observed, the solution should be discarded and fresh solution prepared.

Administration: RETROVIR IV Infusion is administered intravenously at a constant rate over one hour. Rapid infusion or bolus injection should be avoided. RETROVIR IV Infusion should not be given intramuscularly.

HOW SUPPLIED

RETROVIR IV Infusion, 10 mg zidovudine in each mL. 20-mL Single-Use Vial, Tray of 10 (NDC 0173-0107-93).

Store vials at 15° to 25°C (59° to 77°F) and protect from light.
US Patent Nos. 4,818,538 (Product Patent)
4,724,232; 4,833,130; and 4,837,208 (Use Patents)
©Copyright 1996 Glaxo Wellcome Inc. All rights reserved.
April 1998/RL-559
Shown in Product Identification Guide, page 313

SEREVENT®   ℞
[ser' a-vent"]
(salmeterol xinafoate)
Inhalation Aerosol

Bronchodilator Aerosol
For Oral Inhalation Only

DESCRIPTION

SEREVENT (salmeterol xinafoate) Inhalation Aerosol contains salmeterol xinafoate as the racemic form of the 1-hydroxy-2-naphthoic acid salt of salmeterol. The active component of the formulation is salmeterol base, a highly selective beta₂-adrenergic bronchodilator. The chemical name of salmeterol xinafoate is 4-hydroxy-α¹-[[[6-(4-phenylbutoxy)hexyl]amino]methyl]-1,3-benzenedimethanol, 1-hydroxy-2-naphthalenecarboxylate.

The molecular weight of salmeterol xinafoate is 603.8, and the empirical formula is $C_{25}H_{37}NO_4 \cdot C_{11}H_8O_3$. Salmeterol

Table 1: Daily Efficacy Measurements In Two Large 12-Week Clinical Trials (Combined Data)

Parameter	Time	Placebo	SEREVENT	Albuterol
No. of randomized subjects		187	184	185
Mean AM peak expiratory flow	baseline	412	409	398
rate (L/min)	12 weeks	414	438*	390
Mean % days with no	baseline	11	11	14
symptoms	12 weeks	17	35*	24
Mean % nights with no	baseline	67	67	65
awakenings	12 weeks	74	87*	74
Rescue medications (mean no.	baseline	4.4	4.1	4.0
of inhalations per day)	12 weeks	3.3	1.3†‡	1.9
Asthma exacerbations		17%	11%	14%

* *P*<0.001 versus albuterol and placebo.
† *P*<0.05 versus albuterol.
‡ *P*<0.001 versus placebo.

xinafoate is a white to off-white powder. It is freely soluble in methanol; slightly soluble in ethanol, chloroform, and isopropanol; and sparingly soluble in water.

SEREVENT Inhalation Aerosol is a pressurized, metered-dose aerosol unit for oral inhalation. It contains a microcrystalline suspension of salmeterol xinafoate in a mixture of two chlorofluorocarbon propellants (trichlorofluoromethane and dichlorodifluoromethane) with lecithin. 36.25 mcg of salmeterol xinafoate is equivalent to 25 mcg of salmeterol base. Each actuation delivers 25 mcg of salmeterol base (as salmeterol xinafoate) from the valve and 21 mcg of salmeterol base (as salmeterol xinafoate) from the actuator. Each 6.5-g canister provides 60 inhalations and each 13-g canister provides 120 inhalations.

CLINICAL PHARMACOLOGY

Mechanism of Action: Salmeterol is a long-acting beta-adrenergic agonist. In vitro studies and in vivo pharmacologic studies demonstrate that salmeterol is selective for beta₂-adrenoceptors compared with isoproterenol, which has approximately equal agonist activity on beta₁- and beta₂-adrenoceptors. In vitro studies show salmeterol to be at least 50 times more selective for beta₂-adrenoceptors than albuterol. Although beta₂-adrenoceptors are the predominant adrenergic receptors in bronchial smooth muscle and beta₁-adrenoceptors are the predominant receptors in the heart, there are also beta₂-adrenoceptors in the human heart comprising 10% to 50% of the total beta-adrenoceptors. The precise function of these is not yet established, but they raise the possibility that even highly selective beta₂-agonists may have cardiac effects.

The pharmacologic effects of beta₂-adrenoceptor agonist drugs, including salmeterol, are at least in part attributable to stimulation of intracellular adenyl cyclase, the enzyme that catalyzes the conversion of adenosine triphosphate (ATP) to cyclic-3',5'-adenosine monophosphate (cyclic AMP). Increased cyclic AMP levels cause relaxation of bronchial smooth muscle and inhibition of release of mediators of immediate hypersensitivity from cells, especially from mast cells.

In vitro tests show that salmeterol is a potent and long-lasting inhibitor of the release of mast cell mediators, such as histamine, leukotrienes, and prostaglandin D₂, from human lung. Salmeterol inhibits histamine-induced plasma protein extravasation and inhibits platelet activating factor-induced eosinophil accumulation in the lungs of guinea pigs when administered by the inhaled route. In humans, single doses of salmeterol attenuate allergen-induced bronchial hyper-responsiveness.

Pharmacokinetics: Salmeterol acts locally in the lung; plasma levels therefore do not predict therapeutic effect. Because of the low therapeutic dose, systemic levels of salmeterol are low or undetectable after inhalation of recommended doses (42 mcg twice daily). Following chronic administration of an inhaled dose of 42 mcg twice daily, salmeterol was detected in plasma within 5 to 10 minutes in six asthmatic patients; plasma concentrations were very low, with peak concentrations of 150 pg/mL and no accumulation with repeated doses. Larger inhaled doses gave approximately proportionally increased blood levels. In these patients, a second peak concentration of 115 pg/mL occurred at about 45 minutes, probably due to absorption of the swallowed portion of the dose (most of the dose delivered by a metered-dose inhaler is swallowed). Oral administration of 1 mg of radiolabeled salmeterol (as salmeterol xinafoate) to two healthy subjects gave peak plasma salmeterol concentrations of about 650 pg/mL at about 45 minutes; the terminal elimination half-life was about 5.5 hours (one volunteer only).

Salmeterol xinafoate, an ionic salt, dissociates in solution so that the salmeterol and 1-hydroxy-2-naphthoic acid (xinafoate) moieties are absorbed, distributed, metabolized, and excreted independently. Salmeterol base is extensively metabolized by hydroxylation, with subsequent elimination predominantly in the feces. In two healthy subjects who received 1 mg of radiolabeled salmeterol (as salmeterol xinafoate) orally, approximately 25% and 60% of the radiola-

beled salmeterol was eliminated in urine and feces, respectively, over a period of 7 days. No significant amount of unchanged salmeterol base was detected in either urine or feces.

Salmeterol is 94% to 98% bound to human plasma proteins in vitro over the concentration range of 8 to 7722 ng of base per milliliter, much higher concentrations than those achieved following therapeutic doses of salmeterol.

The xinafoate moiety has no apparent pharmacologic activity, is highly protein bound (>99%), and has a long elimination half-life of 11 days.

The pharmacokinetics of salmeterol base have not been studied in elderly patients nor in patients with hepatic or renal impairment. Since salmeterol is predominantly cleared by hepatic metabolism, liver function impairment may lead to accumulation of salmeterol in plasma. Therefore, patients with hepatic disease should be closely monitored.

Pharmacodynamics: Inhaled salmeterol, like other beta-adrenergic agonist drugs, can in some patients produce cardiovascular effects (see PRECAUTIONS). The cardiovascular effects (heart rate, blood pressure) associated with salmeterol administration occur with similar frequency, and are of similar type and severity, as those noted following albuterol administration.

The effects of rising inhaled doses of salmeterol and standard inhaled doses of albuterol were studied in volunteers and in patients with asthma. Salmeterol doses up to 84 mcg resulted in heart rate increases of 3 to 16 beats/min, about the same as albuterol dosed at 180 mcg by inhalation aerosol (4 to 10 beats/min). In two double-blind asthma studies, patients receiving either 42 mcg of salmeterol inhalation aerosol twice daily (n = 81) or 180 mcg of albuterol inhalation aerosol four times daily (n = 80) underwent continuous electrocardiographic monitoring during four 24-hour periods; no clinically significant dysrhythmias were noted. Continuous electrocardiographic monitoring was also performed in two double-blind studies in COPD patients (see ADVERSE REACTIONS).

Studies in laboratory animals (minipigs, rodents, and dogs) have demonstrated the occurrence of cardiac arrhythmias and sudden death (with histologic evidence of myocardial necrosis) when beta-agonists and methylxanthines are administered concurrently. The clinical significance of these findings is unknown.

Clinical Trials: Asthma: In placebo- and albuterol-controlled, single-dose clinical trials with SEREVENT Inhalation Aerosol, the time to onset of effective bronchodilatation (>15% improvement in forced expiratory volume in 1 second [FEV₁]) was 10 to 20 minutes after a 42-mcg dose. Maximum improvement in FEV₁ generally occurred within 180 minutes, and clinically significant improvement continued for 12 hours in most patients.

In two large, randomized, double-blind studies, SEREVENT Inhalation Aerosol was compared with albuterol and placebo in patients with mild-to-moderate asthma, including both patients who did and who did not receive concomitant inhaled corticosteroids. The efficacy of SEREVENT Inhalation Aerosol was demonstrated over the 12-week period with no change in effectiveness over this period of time. There were no gender-related differences in safety or efficacy. No development of tachyphylaxis to the bronchodilator effect has been noted in these studies. FEV₁ measurements (percent of predicted) from these two 12-week trials are shown below for both the first and last treatment days.

Continued on next page

This product information is based on labeling in effect on June 1, 1998. For further information, contact via direct mail, phone, or web site Medical Information: Glaxo Wellcome Inc., PO Box 13398, Research Triangle Park, NC 27709. Healthcare Professionals (Medical Information): 800-334-0089 Patients (Customer Response Center): 888-TALK2GW (1-888-825-5249) Glaxo Wellcome Corporate Web Site: www.glaxowellcome.com

Serevent—Cont.

Figure 1: FEV₁, as Percent of Predicted, From Two Large 12-Week Clinical Trials

First Treatment Day

● Salmeterol 42 mcg twice daily (n = 178)
▲ Albuterol 180 mcg four times daily (n = 176)
■ Placebo (n = 181)

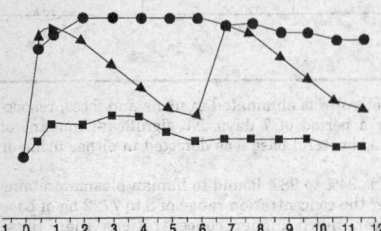

Last Treatment Day (Week 12)

● Salmeterol 42 mcg twice daily (n = 152)
▲ Albuterol 180 mcg four times daily (n = 151)
■ Placebo (n = 150)

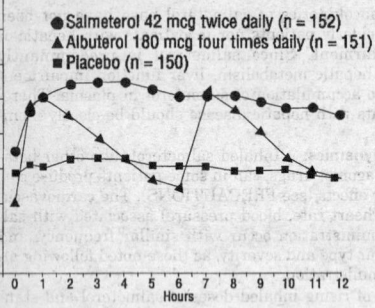

During daily treatment with SEREVENT Inhalation Aerosol for 12 weeks in patients with asthma, the following treatment effects were seen:
[See table 1 at top of previous page]
Safe usage with maintenance of efficacy for periods up to 1 year has been documented.

Exercise-Induced Bronchospasm: Protection against exercise-induced bronchospasm was examined in three controlled studies. Based on median values, patients who received SEREVENT Inhalation Aerosol had consistently less exercise-induced fall in FEV₁ than patients who received placebo, and they were protected for a longer period of time than patients who received albuterol (see table below). There were, however, some patients who were not protected from exercise-induced bronchospasm after SEREVENT administration and others in whom protection against exercise-induced bronchospasm decreased with continued administration over a period of 4 weeks.
[See table 2 below]

Chronic Obstructive Pulmonary Disease (COPD): In two large randomized, double-blind studies, SEREVENT Inha-

lation Aerosol administered twice daily was compared with placebo and ipratropium bromide administered four times daily in patients with COPD (emphysema and chronic bronchitis), including patients who were reversible (≥12% and ≥200 mL increase in baseline FEV₁ after albuterol treatment) and nonreversible to albuterol. After a single 42-mcg dose of SEREVENT, significant improvement in pulmonary function (mean FEV₁ increase of 12% or more) occurred within 30 minutes, reached a peak within 4 hours on average, and persisted for 12 hours with no loss in effectiveness observed over a 12-week treatment period. Serial 12-hour measurements of FEV₁ from these two 12-week trials are shown below for both the first and last treatment days.

Figure 2: FEV₁ From Two Large 12-Week Clinical Trials

First Treatment Day

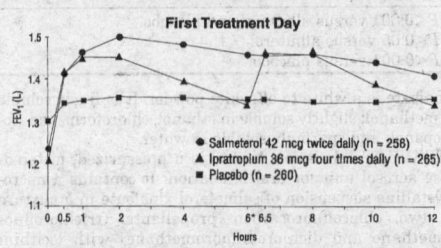

● Salmeterol 42 mcg twice daily (n = 258)
▲ Ipratropium 36 mcg four times daily (n = 265)
■ Placebo (n = 260)

*Ipratropium (or matching placebo) administered immediately following hour 6 assessment.

Last Treatment Day (Week 12)

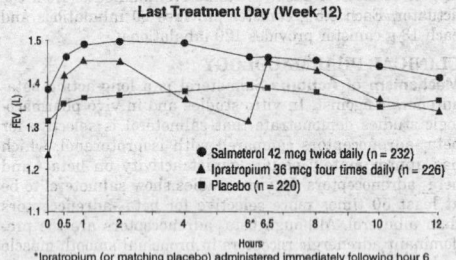

● Salmeterol 42 mcg twice daily (n = 232)
▲ Ipratropium 36 mcg four times daily (n = 226)
■ Placebo (n = 220)

*Ipratropium (or matching placebo) administered immediately following hour 6 assessment.

INDICATIONS AND USAGE

Asthma: SEREVENT Inhalation Aerosol is indicated for long-term, twice-daily (morning and evening) administration in the maintenance treatment of asthma and in the prevention of bronchospasm in patients 12 years of age and older with reversible obstructive airway disease, including patients with symptoms of nocturnal asthma, who require regular treatment with inhaled, short-acting beta₂-agonists. It should not be used in patients whose asthma can be managed by occasional use of inhaled, short-acting beta₂-agonists.
SEREVENT Inhalation Aerosol may be used with or without concurrent inhaled or systemic corticosteroid therapy.
SEREVENT Inhalation Aerosol is also indicated for prevention of exercise-induced bronchospasm in patients 12 years of age and older.

COPD: SEREVENT Inhalation Aerosol is indicated for long-term, twice daily (morning and evening) administration in the maintenance treatment of bronchospasm associated with COPD (including emphysema and chronic bronchitis).

CONTRAINDICATIONS

SEREVENT Inhalation Aerosol is contraindicated in patients with a history of hypersensitivity to salmeterol or any of the components.

WARNINGS

IMPORTANT INFORMATION: SEREVENT INHALATION AEROSOL SHOULD NOT BE INITIATED IN PATIENTS WITH SIGNIFICANTLY WORSENING OR ACUTELY DETERIORATING ASTHMA, WHICH MAY BE A LIFE-THREATENING CONDITION. Serious acute respiratory events, including fatalities, have been reported, both in the United States and worldwide, when SEREVENT Inhalation Aerosol has been initiated in this situation.
Although it is not possible from these reports to determine whether SEREVENT Inhalation Aerosol contributed to these adverse events or simply failed to relieve the deteriorating asthma, the use of SEREVENT Inhalation Aerosol in this setting is inappropriate.
SEREVENT INHALATION AEROSOL SHOULD NOT BE USED TO TREAT ACUTE SYMPTOMS. It is crucial to inform patients of this and prescribe an inhaled, short-acting beta₂-agonist for this purpose as well as warn them that increasing inhaled beta₂-agonist use is a signal of deteriorating asthma.
SEREVENT INHALATION AEROSOL IS NOT A SUBSTITUTE FOR INHALED OR ORAL CORTICOSTEROIDS. Corticosteroids should not be stopped or reduced when SEREVENT Inhalation Aerosol is initiated.
(See PRECAUTIONS: Information for Patients below and the PATIENT'S INSTRUCTIONS FOR USE leaflet.)

1. Do Not Introduce SEREVENT Inhalation Aerosol as a Treatment for Acutely Deteriorating Asthma: SEREVENT Inhalation Aerosol is intended for the maintenance treatment of asthma (see INDICATIONS AND USAGE) and should not be introduced in acutely deteriorating asthma, which is a potentially life-threatening condition. There are no data demonstrating that SEREVENT Inhalation Aerosol provides greater efficacy than or additional efficacy to inhaled, short-acting beta₂-agonists in patients with worsening asthma. Serious acute respiratory events, including fatalities, have been reported, both in the United States and worldwide, in patients receiving SEREVENT Inhalation Aerosol. In most cases, these have occurred in patients with severe asthma (e.g., patients with a history of corticosteroid dependence, low pulmonary function, intubation, mechanical ventilation, frequent hospitalizations, or previous life-threatening acute asthma exacerbations) and/or in some patients in whom asthma has been acutely deteriorating (e.g., unresponsive to usual medications; increasing need for inhaled, short-acting beta₂-agonists; increasing need for systemic corticosteroids; significant increase in symptoms; recent emergency room visits; sudden or progressive deterioration in pulmonary function). However, they have occurred in a few patients with less severe asthma as well. It was not possible from these reports to determine whether SEREVENT Inhalation Aerosol contributed to these events or simply failed to relieve the deteriorating asthma.

2. Do Not Use SEREVENT Inhalation Aerosol to Treat Acute Symptoms: An inhaled, short-acting beta₂-agonist, not SEREVENT Inhalation Aerosol, should be used to relieve acute asthma or COPD symptoms. When prescribing SEREVENT Inhalation Aerosol, the physician must also provide the patient with an inhaled, short-acting beta₂-agonist (e.g., albuterol) for treatment of symptoms that occur acutely, despite regular twice daily (morning and evening) use of SEREVENT Inhalation Aerosol.
When beginning treatment with SEREVENT Inhalation Aerosol, patients who have been taking inhaled, short-acting beta₂-agonists on a regular basis (e.g., four times a day) should be instructed to discontinue the regular use of these drugs and use them only for symptomatic relief of acute asthma or COPD symptoms (see PRECAUTIONS: Information for Patients).

3. Watch for Increasing Use of Inhaled, Short-Acting Beta₂-Agonists, Which Is a Marker of Deteriorating Asthma: Asthma may deteriorate acutely over a period of hours or chronically over several days or longer. If the patient's inhaled, short-acting beta₂-agonist becomes less effective or the patient needs more inhalations than usual, this may be a marker of destabilization of asthma. In this setting, the patient requires immediate reevaluation with reassessment of the treatment regimen, giving special consideration to the possible need for corticosteroids. If the patient uses four or more inhalations per day of an inhaled, short-acting beta₂-agonist for 2 or more consecutive days, or if more than one canister (200 inhalations per canister) of inhaled, short-acting beta₂-agonist is used in an 8-week period in conjunction with SEREVENT Inhalation Aerosol, then the patient should consult the physician for reevaluation. **Increasing the daily dosage of SEREVENT Inhalation Aerosol in this situation is not appropriate. SEREVENT Inhalation Aerosol should not be used more frequently than twice daily (morning and evening) at the recommended dose of two inhalations.**

4. Do Not Use SEREVENT Inhalation Aerosol as a Substitute for Oral or Inhaled Corticosteroids: The use of beta-adrenergic agonist bronchodilators alone may not be adequate to control asthma in many patients. Early consideration should be given to adding anti-inflammatory agents, e.g., corticosteroids. There are no data demonstrating that

---

Table 2: Excercise-Induced Bronchospasm Mean Percentage Fall in Postexercise FEV₁

Clinical Trials/Time After Dose	Treatment		
	Placebo	SEREVENT	Albuterol
Study A: 1st Dose			
6 hours	37	9*	
12 hours	27	16*	
Study A: 4th Week			
6 hours	30	19	
12 hours	24	12	
Study B:			
1 hour	37	0*	2*
6 hours	37	5*†	27
12 hours	34	6*†	33
Study C:			
0.5 hour	43	16*	8*
2.5 hours	33	12*†	30
4.5 hours	—	12†	36
6.0 hours	—	19†	41

* Statistically superior to placebo ($P \leq 0.05$).
† Statistically superior to albuterol ($P \leq 0.05$).

SEREVENT Inhalation Aerosol has a clinical anti-inflammatory effect and could be expected to take the place of, or reduce the dose of, corticosteroids. Patients who already require oral or inhaled corticosteroids for treatment of asthma should be continued on this type of treatment even if they feel better as a result of initiating SEREVENT Inhalation Aerosol. Any change in corticosteroid dosage should be made ONLY after clinical evaluation (see PRECAUTIONS: Information for Patients).

5. Do Not Exceed Recommended Dosage: As with other inhaled beta₂-adrenergic drugs, SEREVENT Inhalation Aerosol should not be used more often or at higher doses than recommended. Fatalities have been reported in association with excessive use of inhaled sympathomimetic drugs. Large doses of inhaled or oral salmeterol (12 to 20 times the recommended dose) have been associated with clinically significant prolongation of the QT_c interval, which has the potential for producing ventricular arrhythmias.

6. Paradoxical Bronchospasm: SEREVENT Inhalation Aerosol can produce paradoxical bronchospasm, which may be life threatening. If paradoxical bronchospasm occurs, SEREVENT Inhalation Aerosol should be discontinued immediately and alternative therapy instituted. It should be recognized that paradoxical bronchospasm, when associated with inhaled formulations, frequently occurs with the first use of a new canister or vial.

7. Immediate Hypersensitivity Reactions: Immediate hypersensitivity reactions may occur after administration of SEREVENT Inhalation Aerosol, as demonstrated by rare cases of urticaria, angioedema, rash, and bronchospasm.

8. Upper Airway Symptoms: Symptoms of laryngeal spasm, irritation, or swelling, such as stridor and choking, have been reported rarely in patients receiving SEREVENT Inhalation Aerosol.

SEREVENT Inhalation Aerosol, like all other beta-adrenergic agonists, can produce a clinically significant cardiovascular effect in some patients as measured by pulse rate, blood pressure, and/or symptoms. Although such effects are uncommon after administration of SEREVENT Inhalation Aerosol at recommended doses, if they occur, the drug may need to be discontinued. In addition, beta-agonists have been reported to produce electrocardiogram (ECG) changes, such as flattening of the T wave, prolongation of the QTc interval, and ST segment depression. The clinical significance of these findings is unknown. Therefore, SEREVENT Inhalation Aerosol, like all sympathomimetic amines, should be used with caution in patients with cardiovascular disorders, especially coronary insufficiency, cardiac arrhythmias, and hypertension.

PRECAUTIONS

General: 1. Use With Spacer or Other Devices: The safety and effectiveness of SEREVENT Inhalation Aerosol when used with a spacer or other devices have not been adequately studied.

2. Cardiovascular and Other Effects: No effect on the cardiovascular system is usually seen after the administration of inhaled salmeterol in recommended doses, but the cardiovascular and central nervous system effects seen with all sympathomimetic drugs (e.g., increased blood pressure, heart rate, excitement) can occur after use of SEREVENT Inhalation Aerosol and may require discontinuation of the drug. Salmeterol, like all sympathomimetic amines, should be used with caution in patients with cardiovascular disorders, especially coronary insufficiency, cardiac arrhythmias, and hypertension; in patients with convulsive disorders or thyrotoxicosis; and in patients who are unusually responsive to sympathomimetic amines.

As has been described with other beta-adrenergic agonist bronchodilators, clinically significant changes in systolic and/or diastolic blood pressure, pulse rate, and electrocardiograms have been seen infrequently in individual patients in controlled clinical studies with salmeterol.

3. Metabolic Effects: Doses of the related beta₂-adrenoceptor agonist albuterol, when administered intravenously, have been reported to aggravate preexisting diabetes mellitus and ketoacidosis. No effects on glucose have been seen with SEREVENT Inhalation Aerosol at recommended doses. Beta-adrenergic agonist medications may produce significant hypokalemia in some patients, possibly through intracellular shunting, which has the potential to produce adverse cardiovascular effects. The decrease is usually transient, not requiring supplementation.

Clinically significant changes in blood glucose and/or serum potassium were seen rarely during clinical studies with long-term administration of SEREVENT Inhalation Aerosol at recommended doses.

Information for Patients: See illustrated Patient's Instructions for Use. SHAKE WELL BEFORE USING.

It is important that patients understand how to use SEREVENT Inhalation Aerosol appropriately and how it should be used in relation to other asthma or COPD medications they are taking. Patients should be given the following information:

1. Shake well before using.

2. The action of SEREVENT Inhalation Aerosol may last up to 12 hours or longer. The recommended dosage (two inhalations twice daily, morning and evening) should not be exceeded.

3. SEREVENT Inhalation Aerosol is not meant to relieve acute asthma or COPD symptoms and extra doses should not be used for that purpose. Acute symptoms should be treated with an inhaled, short-acting beta₂-agonist such as albuterol (the physician should provide the patient with such medication and instruct the patient in how it should be used).

4. Patients should not stop SEREVENT therapy for COPD without physician/provider guidance since symptoms may recur after discontinuation.

5. The physician should be notified immediately if any of the following situations occur, which may be a sign of seriously worsening asthma:

- Decreasing effectiveness of inhaled, short-acting beta₂-agonists
- Need for more inhalations than usual of inhaled, short-acting beta₂-agonists
- Use of four or more inhalations per day of a short-acting beta₂-agonist for 2 or more days consecutively
- Use of more than one canister of an inhaled, short-acting beta₂-agonist in an 8-week period (i.e., canister with 200 inhalations)

6. SEREVENT Inhalation Aerosol should not be used as a substitute for oral or inhaled corticosteroids. The dosage of these medications should not be changed and they should not be stopped without consulting the physician, even if the patient feels better after initiating treatment with SEREVENT Inhalation Aerosol.

7. Patients should be cautioned regarding common adverse cardiovascular effects, such as palpitations, chest pain, rapid heart rate, tremor, or nervousness.

8. In patients receiving SEREVENT Inhalation Aerosol, other inhaled medications should be used only as directed by the physician.

9. When using SEREVENT Inhalation Aerosol to prevent exercise-induced bronchospasm, patients should take the dose at least 30 to 60 minutes before exercise.

10. If you are pregnant or nursing, contact your physician about use of SEREVENT Inhalation Aerosol.

11. Effective and safe use of SEREVENT Inhalation Aerosol includes an understanding of the way that it should be administered.

Drug Interactions: *Short-Acting Beta-Agonists:* In the two 3-month, repetitive-dose clinical asthma trials (n = 184), the mean daily need for additional beta₂-agonist use was 1 to 1½ inhalations per day, but some patients used more. Eight percent of patients used at least eight inhalations per day at least on one occasion. Six percent used 9 to 12 inhalations at least once. There were 15 patients (8%) who averaged over four inhalations per day. Four of these used an average of 8 to 11 inhalations per day. In these 15 patients there was no observed increase in frequency of cardiovascular adverse events. The safety of concomitant use of more than eight inhalations per day of short-acting beta₂-agonists with SEREVENT Inhalation Aerosol has not been established. In 15 patients who experienced worsening of asthma while receiving SEREVENT Inhalation Aerosol, nebulized albuterol (one dose in most) led to improvement in FEV₁ and no increase in occurrence of cardiovascular adverse events.

Monoamine Oxidase Inhibitors and Tricyclic Antidepressants: Salmeterol should be administered with extreme caution to patients being treated with monoamine oxidase inhibitors or tricyclic antidepressants, or within 2 weeks of discontinuation of such agents, because the action of salmeterol on the vascular system may be potentiated by these agents.

Corticosteroids and Cromoglycate: In clinical trials, inhaled corticosteroids and/or inhaled cromolyn sodium did not alter the safety profile of SEREVENT Inhalation Aerosol when administered concurrently.

Methylxanthines: The concurrent use of intravenously or orally administered methylxanthines (e.g., aminophylline, theophylline) by patients receiving SEREVENT Inhalation Aerosol has not been completely evaluated. In one clinical asthma trial, 87 patients receiving SEREVENT Inhalation Aerosol 42 mcg twice daily concurrently with a theophylline product had adverse event rates similar to those in 71 patients receiving SEREVENT Inhalation Aerosol without theophylline. Resting heart rates were slightly higher in the patients on theophylline but were little affected by SEREVENT Inhalation Aerosol therapy.

Beta-adrenergic receptor blocking agents not only block the pulmonary effect of beta-agonists, such as SEREVENT Inhalation Aerosol, but may produce severe bronchospasm in asthmatic patients. Therefore, patients with asthma should not normally be treated with beta-blockers. However, under certain circumstances, e.g., as prophylaxis after myocardial infarction, there may be no acceptable alternatives to the use of beta-adrenergic blocking agents in patients with asthma. In this setting, cardioselective beta-blockers could be considered, although they should be administered with caution.

The ECG changes and/or hypokalemia that may result from the administration of nonpotassium-sparing diuretics (such as loop or thiazide diuretics) can be acutely worsened by beta-agonists, especially when the recommended dose of the beta-agonist is exceeded. Although the clinical significance of these effects is not known, caution is advised in the coadministration of beta-agonists with nonpotassium-sparing diuretics.

Carcinogenesis, Mutagenesis, Impairment of Fertility: In an 18-month oral carcinogenicity study in CD-mice, salmeterol xinafoate at oral doses of 1.4 mg/kg and above (approximately 9 times the maximum recommended daily inhalation dose in adults based on comparison of the area-under-the-plasma concentration versus time curves [AUCs]) caused dose-related increases in the incidence of smooth muscle hyperplasia, cystic glandular hyperplasia, leiomyomas of the uterus, and cysts in the ovaries. The incidence of leiomyosarcomas was not statistically significant. No tumors were seen at 0.2 mg/kg (comparable to the maximum recommended human daily inhalation dose in adults based on comparison of the AUCs).

In a 24-month inhalation and oral carcinogenicity study in Sprague Dawley rats, salmeterol caused dose-related increases in the incidence of mesovarian leiomyomas and ovarian cysts at inhalation and oral doses of 0.68 mg/kg per day and above (approximately 55 times the maximum recommended human daily inhalation dose in adults on a mg/m² basis). No tumors were seen at 0.21 mg/kg per day (approximately 15 times the maximum recommended human daily inhalation dose in adults on a mg/m² basis). These findings in rodents are similar to those reported previously for other beta-adrenergic agonist drugs. The relevance of these findings to human use is unknown.

Salmeterol xinafoate produced no detectable or reproducible increases in microbial and mammalian gene mutation in vitro. No clastogenic activity occurred in vitro in human lymphocytes or in vivo in a rat micronucleus test. No effects on fertility were identified in male and female rats treated orally with salmeterol xinafoate at doses up to 2 mg/kg orally (approximately 160 times the maximum recommended human daily inhalation dose in adults on a mg/m² basis).

Pregnancy: *Teratogenic Effects:* Pregnancy Category C. No teratogenic effects occurred in the rat at oral doses up to 2 mg/kg (approximately 160 times the maximum recommended human daily inhalation dose in adults on a mg/m² basis). In pregnant dutch rabbits administered oral doses of 1 mg/kg and above (approximately 20 times the maximum recommended human daily inhalation dose in adults based on the comparison of the AUCs), salmeterol xinafoate exhibited fetal toxic effects characteristically resulting from beta-adrenoceptor stimulation; these included precocious eyelid openings, cleft palate, sternebral fusion, limb and paw flexures, and delayed ossification of the frontal cranial bones. No significant effects occurred at an oral dose of 0.6 mg/kg (approximately 10 times the maximum recommended human daily inhalation dose in adults based on comparison of the AUCs).

New Zealand White rabbits were less sensitive since only delayed ossification of the frontal bones was seen at oral doses of 10 mg/kg (approximately 1600 times the maximum recommended human daily inhalation dose on a mg/m² basis). Extensive use of other beta-agonists has provided no evidence that these class effects in animals are relevant to use in humans. There are no adequate and well-controlled studies with SEREVENT Inhalation Aerosol in pregnant women. SEREVENT Inhalation Aerosol should be used during pregnancy only if the potential benefit justifies the potential risk to the fetus.

Use in Labor and Delivery: There are no well-controlled human studies that have investigated effects of salmeterol on preterm labor or labor at term. Because of the potential for beta-agonist interference with uterine contractility, use of SEREVENT Inhalation Aerosol for relief of bronchospasm during labor should be restricted to those patients in whom the benefits clearly outweigh the risks.

Nursing Mothers: Plasma levels of salmeterol after inhaled therapeutic doses are very low. In rats, salmeterol xinafoate is excreted in milk. However, since there is no experience with use of SEREVENT Inhalation Aerosol by nursing mothers, a decision should be made whether to discontinue nursing or to discontinue the drug, taking into account the importance of the drug to the mother. Caution should be exercised when salmeterol xinafoate is administered to a nursing woman.

Continued on next page

This product information is based on labeling in effect on June 1, 1998. For further information, contact via direct mail, phone, or web site Medical Information: Glaxo Wellcome Inc., PO Box 13398, Research Triangle Park, NC 27709. Healthcare Professionals (Medical Information): 800-334-0089 Patients (Customer Response Center): 888-TALK2GW (1-888-825-5249) Glaxo Wellcome Corporate Web Site: www.glaxowellcome.com

Serevent—Cont.

Pediatric Use: The safety and effectiveness of SEREVENT Inhalation Aerosol in children younger than 12 years of age have not been established.

Geriatric Use: Of the total number of patients who received SEREVENT Inhalation Aerosol in all asthma clinical studies, 241 were 65 years and older. Geriatric patients (65 years and older) with reversible obstructive airway disease were evaluated in four well-controlled studies of 3 weeks' to 3 months' duration. Two placebo-controlled, crossover studies evaluated twice-daily dosing with salmeterol for 21 to 28 days in 45 patients. An additional 75 geriatric patients were treated with salmeterol for 3 months in two large parallel-group, multicenter studies. These 120 patients experienced increases in AM and PM peak expiratory flow rate and decreases in diurnal variation in peak expiratory flow rate similar to responses seen in the total populations of the two latter studies. The adverse event type and frequency in geriatric patients were not different from those of the total populations studied.

In two large, randomized, double-blind, placebo-controlled 3-month studies involving patients with COPD, 133 patients using SEREVENT Inhalation Aerosol were 65 years and older. These patients experienced similar improvements in FEV_1 as observed for patients younger than 65. No apparent differences in the efficacy and safety of SEREVENT Inhalation Aerosol were observed when geriatric patients were compared with younger patients in asthma and COPD clinical trials. As with other beta$_2$-agonists, however, special caution should be observed when using SEREVENT Inhalation Aerosol in geriatric patients who have concomitant cardiovascular disease that could be adversely affected by this class of drug. Based on available data, no adjustment of salmeterol dosage in geriatric patients is warranted.

ADVERSE REACTIONS

Adverse reactions to salmeterol are similar in nature to reactions to other selective beta$_2$-adrenoceptor agonists, i.e., tachycardia; palpitations; immediate hypersensitivity reactions, including urticaria, angioedema, rash, bronchospasm (see WARNINGS); headache; tremor; nervousness; and paradoxical bronchospasm (see WARNINGS).

Asthma: Two multicenter, 12-week, controlled studies have evaluated twice-daily doses of SEREVENT Inhalation Aerosol in patients 12 years of age and older with asthma. The following table reports the incidence of adverse events in these two studies.

[See table 3 above]

The table above includes all events (whether considered drug related or nondrug related by the investigator) that occurred at a rate of over 3% in the SEREVENT Inhalation Aerosol treatment group and were more common in the SEREVENT Inhalation Aerosol group than in the placebo group.

Pharyngitis, allergic rhinitis, dizziness/giddiness, and influenza occurred at 3% or more but were equally common on placebo. Other events occurring in the SEREVENT Inhalation Aerosol treatment group at a frequency of 1% to 3% were as follows:

Cardiovascular: Tachycardia, palpitations.
Ear, Nose, and Throat: Rhinitis, laryngitis.
Gastrointestinal: Nausea, viral gastroenteritis, nausea and vomiting, diarrhea, abdominal pain.
Hypersensitivity: Urticaria.
Mouth and Teeth: Dental pain.
Musculoskeletal: Pain in joint, back pain, muscle cramp/contraction, myalgia/myositis, muscular soreness.
Neurological: Nervousness, malaise/fatigue.
Respiratory: Tracheitis/bronchitis.
Skin: Rash/skin eruption.
Urogenital: Dysmenorrhea.

Table 3: Adverse Experience Incidence in Two Large 12-Week Asthma Clinical Trials*

Adverse Event Type	Percent of Patients		
	Placebo n = 187	SEREVENT 42 mcg twice daily n = 184	Albuterol 180 mcg four times daily n = 185
Ear, nose, and throat			
Upper respiratory tract infection	13	14	16*
Nasopharyngitis	12	14	11
Disease of nasal cavity/sinus	4	6	1
Sinus headache	2	4	<1
Gastrointestinal			
Stomachache	0	4	0
Neurological			
Headache	23	28	27
Tremor	2	4	3
Respiratory			
Cough	6	7	3
Lower respiratory infection	2	4	2

* The only adverse experience classified as serious was one case of upper respiratory tract infection in a patient treated with albuterol.

In small dose-response studies, tremor, nervousness, and palpitations appeared to be dose related.

COPD: Two multicenter, 12-week, controlled studies have evaluated twice-daily doses of SEREVENT Inhalation Aerosol in patients with COPD. The following table reports the incidence of adverse events in these two studies.

[See table 4 below]

The table above includes all events (whether considered drug related or nondrug related by the investigator) that occurred at a rate of over 3% in the SEREVENT Inhalation Aerosol treatment group and were more common in the SEREVENT Inhalation Aerosol group than in the placebo group.

Common cold, rhinorrhea, bronchitis, cough, exacerbation of chest congestion, chest pain, and dizziness occurred at 3% or more but were equally common on placebo. Other events occurring in the SEREVENT Inhalation Aerosol treatment group at a frequency of 1% to 3% were as follows:

Ear, Nose, and Throat: Cold symptoms, earache, epistaxis, nasal congestion, nasal sinus congestion, sneezing.
Gastrointestinal: Nausea, dyspepsia, gastric pain, gastric upset, abdominal pain, constipation, heartburn, oral candidiasis, xerostomia, vomiting, surgical removal of tooth.
Musculoskeletal: Leg cramps, myalgia, neck pain, pain in arm, shoulder pain, muscle injury of neck.
Neurological: Insomnia, sinus headache.
Non-Site Specific: Fatigue, fever, pain in body, discomfort in chest.
Respiratory: Acute bronchitis, dyspnea, influenza, lower respiratory tract infection, pneumonia, respiratory tract infection, shortness of breath, wheezing.
Urogenital: Urinary tract infection.

Electrocardiographic Monitoring in Patients With COPD: Continuous electrocardiographic (Holter) monitoring was performed on 284 patients in two large COPD clinical trials during five 24-hour periods. No cases of sustained ventricular tachycardia were observed. At baseline, non-sustained, asymptomatic ventricular tachycardia was recorded for 7 (7.1%), 8 (9.4%), and 3 (3.0%) patients in the placebo, SEREVENT, and ipratropium groups, respectively. During treatment, nonsustained, asymptomatic ventricular tachycardia that represented a clinically significant change from baseline was reported for 11 (11.6%), 15 (18.3%), and 20 (20.8%) patients receiving placebo, SEREVENT, and ipratropium, respectively. Four of these cases of ventricular tachycardia were reported as adverse events (1 placebo, 3 SEREVENT) by one investigator based upon review of Holter data. One case of ventricular tachycardia was observed during ECG evaluation of chest pain (ipratropium) and reported as an adverse event.

Observed During Clinical Practice: In extensive US and worldwide postmarketing experience, serious exacerbations of asthma, including some that have been fatal, have been reported. In most cases, these have occurred in patients with severe asthma and/or in some patients in whom asthma has been acutely deteriorating (see WARNINGS no. 1), but they have occurred in a few patients with less severe asthma as well. It was not possible from these reports to determine whether SEREVENT Inhalation Aerosol contributed to these events or simply failed to relieve the deteriorating asthma.

The following events have also been identified during post-approval use of SEREVENT in clinical practice. Because they are reported voluntarily from a population of unknown size, estimates of frequency cannot be made. These events have been chosen for inclusion due to a combination of their seriousness, frequency of reporting, or potential causal connection to SEREVENT.

Respiratory: Rare reports of upper airway symptoms of laryngeal spasm, irritation, or swelling such as stridor or choking.

Cardiovascular: Hypertension, arrhythmias, (including atrial fibrillation, supraventricular tachycardia, extrasystoles).

OVERDOSAGE

The expected symptoms with overdosage are those of excessive beta-adrenergic stimulation and/or occurrence or exaggeration of any of the symptoms listed under ADVERSE REACTIONS, e.g., seizures, angina, hypertension or hypotension, tachycardia with rates up to 200 beats/min, arrhythmias, nervousness, headache, tremor, muscle cramps, dry mouth, palpitation, nausea, dizziness, fatigue, malaise, and insomnia. Overdosage with salmeterol may be expected to result in exaggeration of the pharmacologic adverse effects associated with beta-adrenoceptor agonists, including tachycardia and/or arrhythmia, tremor, headache, and muscle cramps. Overdosage with salmeterol can lead to clinically significant prolongation of the QT_c interval, which can produce ventricular arrhythmias. Other signs of overdosage may include hypokalemia and hyperglycemia.

As with all sympathomimetic aerosol medications, cardiac arrest and even death may be associated with abuse of SEREVENT Inhalation Aerosol.

Treatment consists of discontinuation of SEREVENT Inhalation Aerosol together with appropriate symptomatic therapy. The judicious use of a cardioselective beta-receptor blocker may be considered, bearing in mind that such medication can produce bronchospasm. There is insufficient evidence to determine if dialysis is beneficial for overdosage of SEREVENT Inhalation Aerosol.

No deaths were seen in rats at inhalation doses of 2.9 mg/kg (approximately 240 times the maximum recommended human daily inhalation dose on a mg/m^2 basis) and in dogs at 0.7 mg/kg (approximately 190 times the maximum recommended human daily inhalation dose on a mg/m^2 basis). By the oral route, no deaths occurred in mice at 150 mg/kg (approximately 6100 times the maximum recommended human daily inhalation dose on a mg/m^2 basis) and in rats at 1000 mg/kg (approximately 81 000 times the maximum recommended human daily inhalation dose on a mg/m^2 basis).

DOSAGE AND ADMINISTRATION

SEREVENT Inhalation Aerosol should be administered by the orally inhaled route only (see Patient's Instructions for Use). It is recommended to "test spray" SEREVENT Inha-

Table 4: Adverse Experience Incidence in Two Large 12-Week COPD Clinical Trials

Adverse Event Type	Percent of Patients		
	Placebo n = 278	SEREVENT 42 mcg twice daily n = 267	Ipratropium 36 mcg four times daily n = 271
Ear, nose, and throat			
Upper respiratory tract infection	7	9	9
Sore throat	3	8	6
Nasal sinus infection	1	4	2
Gastrointestinal			
Diarrhea	3	5	4
Musculoskeletal			
Back pain	3	4	3
Neurological			
Headache	10	12	8
Respiratory			
Chest congestion	3	4	3

lation Aerosol into the air four times before using for the first time and in cases where the aerosol has not been used for a prolonged period of time (i.e., more than 4 weeks).

Asthma: For maintenance of bronchodilatation and prevention of symptoms of asthma, including the symptoms of nocturnal asthma, the usual dosage for patients 12 years of age and older is two inhalations (42 mcg) twice daily (morning and evening, approximately 12 hours apart). Adverse effects are more likely to occur with higher doses of salmeterol, and more frequent administration or administration of a larger number of inhalations is not recommended.

To gain full therapeutic benefit, SEREVENT Inhalation Aerosol should be administered twice daily (morning and evening) in the treatment of reversible airway obstruction.

If a previously effective dosage regimen fails to provide the usual response, medical advice should be sought immediately as this is often a sign of destabilization of asthma. Under these circumstances, the therapeutic regimen should be re-evaluated and additional therapeutic options, such as inhaled or systemic corticosteroids, should be considered. If symptoms arise in the period between doses, an inhaled, short-acting $beta_2$-agonist should be taken for immediate relief.

COPD: For maintenance treatment of bronchospasm associated with COPD (including chronic bronchitis and emphysema), the usual dosage for adults is two inhalations (42 mcg) twice daily (morning and evening, approximately 12 hours apart).

Prevention of Exercise-Induced Bronchospasm: Two inhalations at least 30 to 60 minutes before exercise have been shown to protect against exercise-induced bronchospasm in many patients for up to 12 hours. Additional doses of SEREVENT Inhalation Aerosol should not be used for 12 hours after the administration of this drug. Patients who are receiving SEREVENT Inhalation Aerosol twice daily (morning and evening) should not use additional SEREVENT Inhalation Aerosol for prevention of exercise-induced bronchospasm. If this dose is not effective, other appropriate therapy for exercise-induced bronchospasm should be considered.

Geriatric Use: In studies where geriatric patients (65 years of age or older, see PRECAUTIONS) have been treated with SEREVENT Inhalation Aerosol, efficacy and safety of 42 mcg given twice daily (morning and evening) did not differ from that in younger patients. Consequently, no dosage adjustment is recommended.

HOW SUPPLIED

SEREVENT Inhalation Aerosol is supplied in 13-g canisters containing 120 metered actuations in boxes of one. Each actuation delivers 25 mcg of salmeterol base (as salmeterol xinafoate) from the valve and 21 mcg of salmeterol base (as salmeterol xinafoate) from the actuator. Each canister is supplied with a green plastic actuator with a teal-colored strapcap and patient's instructions (NDC 0173-0464-00). Also available, SEREVENT Inhalation Aerosol Refill (NDC 0173-0465-00), a 13-g canister only with patient's instructions.

SEREVENT Inhalation Aerosol is also supplied in a pack that consists of a 6.5-g canister containing 60 metered actuations in boxes of one. Each actuation delivers 25 mcg of salmeterol base (as salmeterol xinafoate) from the valve and 21 mcg of salmeterol base from the actuator (as salmeterol xinafoate). Each canister is supplied with a green plastic actuator with a teal-colored strapcap and patient's instructions (NDC 0173-0467-00).

For use with SEREVENT Inhalation Aerosol actuator only. The green actuator with SEREVENT Inhalation Aerosol should not be used with other aerosol medications, and actuators from other aerosol medications should not be used with a SEREVENT Inhalation Aerosol canister.

The correct amount of medication in each inhalation cannot be assured after 120 actuations from the 13-g canister or 60 actuations from the 6.5-g canister even though the canister is not completely empty. The canister should be discarded when the labeled number of actuations has been used.

Store between 15° and 30°C (59° and 86°F). Store canister with nozzle end down. Protect from freezing temperatures and direct sunlight.

Avoid spraying in eyes. Contents under pressure. Do not puncture or incinerate. Do not store at temperatures above 120°F. Keep out of reach of children. As with most inhaled medications in aerosol canisters, the therapeutic effect of this medication may decrease when the canister is cold; for best results, the canister should be at room temperature before use. Shake well before using.

March 1998/RL-537

Shown in Product Identification Guide, page 314

Table 1: Daily Efficacy Measurements in Two Large 12-Week Clinical Trials (Combined Data)

Parameter	Time	Placebo	SEREVENT	Albuterol
No. of randomized subjects		152	149	148
Mean AM peak expiratory flow rate (L/min)	baseline	394	395	394
	12 weeks	396	427*	394
Mean % days with no asthma symptoms	baseline	14	13	12
	12 weeks	20	33	21
Mean % nights with no awakenings	baseline	70	63	68
	12 weeks	73	85*	71
Rescue medications (mean no. of inhalations per day)	baseline	4.2	4.3	4.3
	12 weeks	3.3	1.6†	2.2
Asthma exacerbations		14%	15%	16%

*Statistically superior to placebo and albuterol ($P<0.001$).
†Statistically superior to placebo ($P<0.001$).

SEREVENT® DISKUS® ℞

[*sĕr′ ə-vent dĭsk′ us*]

(salmeterol xinafoate inhalation powder)

For Oral Inhalation Only

DESCRIPTION

SEREVENT DISKUS (salmeterol xinafoate inhalation powder) contains salmeterol xinafoate as the racemic form of the 1-hydroxy-2-naphthoic acid salt of salmeterol. The active component of the formulation is salmeterol base, a highly selective $beta_2$-adrenergic bronchodilator. The chemical name of salmeterol xinafoate is 4-hydroxy-α^1-[[[6-(4-phenylbutoxy)hexyl]amino]methyl]-1,3-benzenedimethanol, 1-hydroxy-2-naphthalenecarboxylate. Salmeterol xinafoate has the following chemical structure:

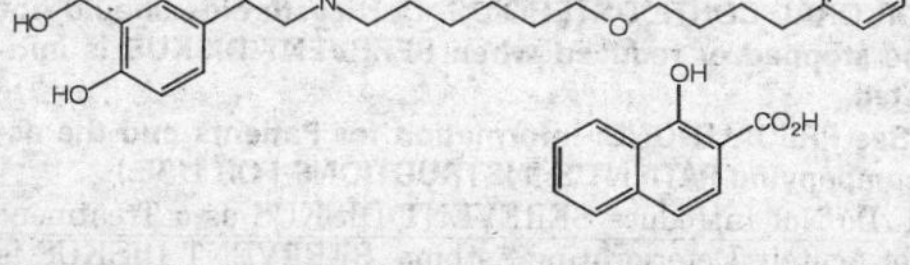

The molecular weight of salmeterol xinafoate is 603.8, and the empirical formula is $C_{25}H_{37}NO_4 \cdot C_{11}H_8O_3$. Salmeterol xinafoate is a white to off-white powder. It is freely soluble in methanol; slightly soluble in ethanol, chloroform, and isopropanol; and sparingly soluble in water.

SEREVENT DISKUS is a specially designed plastic device containing a double-foil blister strip of a powder formulation of salmeterol xinafoate intended for oral inhalation only. Each blister on the double-foil strip within the device contains 50 mcg of salmeterol as the xinafoate in 12.5 mg of formulation containing lactose. When a blister containing medication is opened by activating the device, the medication is dispersed into the air stream created when the patient inhales through the mouthpiece.

The amount of drug delivered to the lung will depend on patient factors such as inspiratory flow. Under standardized in vitro testing, SEREVENT DISKUS delivers 47 mcg when tested at 60 L/min flow rate for 3 seconds. In adult patients with obstructive lung disease and severely compromised lung function (mean FEV_1 0.65 L [range, 0.35 to 0.92 L], 20% to 30% predicted forced expiratory volume in 1 second [$FEV/_1$]), mean peak inspiratory flow (PIF) through SEREVENT DISKUS was 82.4 L/min (range, 46.1 to 115.3 L/min). The emitted dose of salmeterol xinafoate determined in an in vitro experiment modeling these patient-generated flow rates was 46 mcg (range, 45 to 51 mcg).

CLINICAL PHARMACOLOGY

Mechanism of Action: Salmeterol is a long-acting beta-adrenergic agonist. In vitro studies and in vivo pharmacologic studies demonstrate that salmeterol is selective for $beta_2$-adrenoceptors compared with isoproterenol, which has approximately equal agonist activity on $beta_1$- and $beta_2$-adrenoceptors. In vitro studies show salmeterol to be at least 50 times more selective for $beta_2$-adrenoceptors than albuterol. Although $beta_2$-adrenoceptors are the predominant adrenergic receptors in bronchial smooth muscle and $beta_1$-adrenoceptors are the predominant receptors in the heart, there are also $beta_2$-adrenoceptors in the human heart comprising 10% to 50% of the total beta-adrenoceptors. The precise function of these is not yet established, but they raise the possibility that even highly selective $beta_2$-agonists may have cardiac effects.

The pharmacologic effects of $beta_2$-adrenoceptor agonist drugs, including salmeterol, are at least in part attributable to stimulation of intracellular adenyl cyclase, the enzyme that catalyzes the conversion of adenosine triphosphate (ATP) to cyclic-3′,5′-adenosine monophosphate (cyclic AMP). Increased cyclic AMP levels cause relaxation of bronchial smooth muscle and inhibition of release of mediators of immediate hypersensitivity from cells, especially from mast cells.

In vitro tests show that salmeterol is a potent and long-lasting inhibitor of the release of mast cell mediators, such as histamine, leukotrienes, and prostaglandin D_2, from human lung. Salmeterol inhibits histamine-induced plasma protein extravasation and inhibits platelet activating factor-induced eosinophil accumulation in the lungs of guinea pigs when administered by the inhaled route. In humans, single doses of salmeterol administered via inhalation aerosol also attenuate allergen-induced bronchial hyper-responsiveness.

Pharmacokinetics: Salmeterol acts locally in the lung; plasma levels therefore do not predict therapeutic effect. Because of the low therapeutic dose, systemic levels of salmeterol inhalation powder are low or undetectable after inhalation of recommended doses (50 mcg twice daily). Following chronic administration of an inhaled dose of 50 mcg of salmeterol inhalation powder twice daily, salmeterol was detected in plasma within 5 to 45 minutes in seven asthmatic patients; plasma concentrations were very low, with mean peak concentrations of 167 ± 75 pg/mL and no accumulation with repeated doses. Oral administration of 1 mg of radiolabeled salmeterol (as salmeterol xinafoate) to two healthy subjects gave peak plasma salmeterol concentrations of about 650 pg/mL at about 45 minutes; the terminal elimination half-life was about 5.5 hours (one volunteer only).

Salmeterol xinafoate, an ionic salt, dissociates in solution so that the salmeterol and 1-hydroxy-2-naphthoic acid (xinafoate) moieties are absorbed, distributed, metabolized, and excreted independently. Salmeterol base is extensively metabolized by hydroxylation, with subsequent elimination predominantly in the feces. In two healthy subjects who received 1 mg of radiolabeled salmeterol (as salmeterol xinafoate) orally, approximately 25% and 60% of the radiolabeled salmeterol was eliminated in urine and feces, respectively, over a period of 7 days. No significant amount of unchanged salmeterol base was detected in either urine or feces.

Salmeterol is 94% to 98% bound to human plasma proteins in vitro over the concentration range of 8 to 7722 ng of base per milliliter, much higher concentrations than those achieved following therapeutic doses of salmeterol.

The xinafoate moiety has no apparent pharmacologic activity, is highly protein bound (>99%), and has a long elimination half-life of 11 days.

The pharmacokinetics of salmeterol base has not been studied in elderly patients nor in patients with hepatic or renal impairment. Since salmeterol is predominantly cleared by hepatic metabolism, liver function impairment may lead to accumulation of salmeterol in plasma. Therefore, patients with hepatic disease should be closely monitored.

Pharmacodynamics: Inhaled salmeterol, like other beta-adrenergic agonist drugs, can in some patients produce cardiovascular effects (see PRECAUTIONS). The cardiovascular effects (heart rate, blood pressure) associated with salmeterol inhalation aerosol occur with similar frequency, and are of similar type and severity, as those noted following albuterol administration.

The effects of rising doses of salmeterol and standard inhaled doses of albuterol were studied in volunteers and in patients with asthma. Salmeterol doses up to 84 mcg administered as inhalation aerosol resulted in heart rate increases of 3 to 16 beats/min, about the same as albuterol dosed at 180 mcg by inhalation aerosol (4 to 10 beats/min). Patients receiving 50-mcg doses of salmeterol inhalation powder (n = 60) underwent continuous electrocardiographic monitoring during two 12-hour periods after the first dose and after 1 month of therapy, and no clinically significant dysrhythmias were noted.

Studies in laboratory animals (minipigs, rodents, and dogs) have demonstrated the occurrence of cardiac arrhythmias

Continued on next page

This product information is based on labeling in effect on June 1, 1998. For further information, contact via direct mail, phone, or web site Medical Information: Glaxo Wellcome Inc., PO Box 13398, Research Triangle Park, NC 27709. Healthcare Professionals (Medical Information): 800-334-0089 Patients (Customer Response Center): 888-TALK2GW (1-888-825-5249) Glaxo Wellcome Corporate Web Site: www.glaxowellcome.com

Serevent Diskus—Cont.

and sudden death (with histologic evidence of myocardial necrosis) when beta-agonists and methylxanthines are administered concurrently. The clinical significance of these findings is unknown.

Clinical Trials: During the initial treatment day in several multiple-dose clinical trials with salmeterol inhalation powder in patients with asthma, the median time to onset of clinically significant bronchodilatation ($\geq$15% improvement in FEV_1) ranged from 30 to 48 minutes after a 50-mcg dose. One hour after a single dose of 50 mcg of salmeterol inhalation powder, the majority of patients had $\geq$15% improvement in FEV_1. Maximum improvement in FEV_1 generally occurred within 180 minutes, and clinically significant improvement continued for 12 hours in most patients.

In two large, randomized, double-blind studies, salmeterol inhalation powder was compared with albuterol inhalation aerosol and placebo in patients with mild-to-moderate asthma (protocol defined as 50% to 80% predicted FEV_1, actual mean of 67.7% at baseline), including patients who did and who did not receive concurrent inhaled corticosteroids. The efficacy of salmeterol inhalation powder was demonstrated over the 12-week period with no change in effectiveness over this time period. There were no gender- or age-related differences in safety or efficacy. No development of tachyphylaxis to the bronchodilator effect has been noted in these studies. FEV_1 measurements (mean change from baseline) from these two 12-week studies are shown below for both the first and last treatment days.

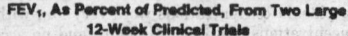

FEV₁, As Percent of Predicted, From Two Large
12-Week Clinical Trials

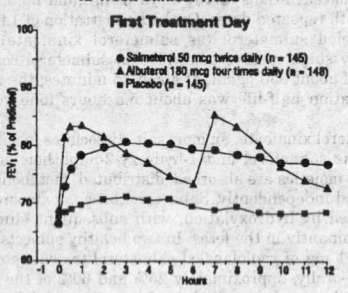

First Treatment Day

- Salmeterol 50 mcg twice daily (n = 145)
- Albuterol 180 mcg four times daily (n = 148)
- Placebo (n = 145)

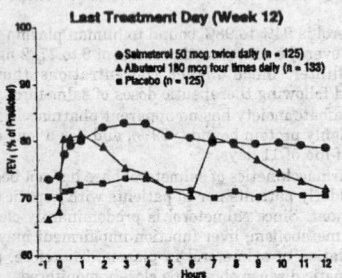

Last Treatment Day (Week 12)

- Salmeterol 50 mcg twice daily (n = 125)
- Albuterol 180 mcg four times daily (n = 133)
- Placebo (n = 125)

During daily treatment with salmeterol inhalation powder for 12 weeks in patients with mild-to-moderate asthma, the following treatment effects were seen:

[See table 1 at top of previous page]

Safe usage with maintenance of efficacy for periods up to 1 year has been documented.

Salmeterol inhalation powder and salmeterol aerosol were compared to placebo in two additional randomized, double-blind clinical trials in adolescent and adult patients with mild-to-moderate asthma. Salmeterol inhalation powder 50 mcg administered via the DISKUS and salmeterol inhalation aerosol 42 mcg, both administered twice daily, produced significant improvements in pulmonary function compared with placebo over the 12-week period. While no statistically significant differences were observed between the active treatments for any of the efficacy assessments or safety evaluations performed, there were some efficacy measures on which the metered-dose inhaler appeared to provide better results. Therefore, while SEREVENT DISKUS was comparable to SEREVENT® (salmeterol xinafoate) Inhalation Aerosol in clinical trials in mild-to-moderate asthmatics, it should not be assumed that the SEREVENT Inhalation Aerosol and SEREVENT DISKUS drug products will produce clinically equivalent outcomes in all patients.

INDICATIONS AND USAGE

SEREVENT DISKUS inhalation powder is indicated for long-term, twice-daily (morning and evening) administration in the maintenance treatment of asthma and in the prevention of bronchospasm in patients 12 years of age and older with reversible obstructive airway disease, including

patients with symptoms of nocturnal asthma, who require regular treatment with inhaled, short-acting beta₂-agonists. It should not be used in patients whose asthma can be managed by occasional use of inhaled, short-acting beta₂-agonists.

SEREVENT DISKUS may be used with or without concurrent inhaled or systemic corticosteroid therapy.

CONTRAINDICATIONS

SEREVENT DISKUS is contraindicated in patients with a history of hypersensitivity to salmeterol or any of its components.

WARNINGS

IMPORTANT INFORMATION: SEREVENT DISKUS SHOULD NOT BE INITIATED IN PATIENTS WITH SIGNIFICANTLY WORSENING OR ACUTELY DETERIORATING ASTHMA, WHICH MAY BE A LIFE-THREATENING CONDITION. Serious acute respiratory events, including fatalities, have been reported, both in the United States and worldwide, when SEREVENT has been initiated in this situation.

Although it is not possible from these reports to determine whether SEREVENT contributed to these adverse events or simply failed to relieve the deteriorating asthma, the use of SEREVENT DISKUS in this setting is inappropriate.

SEREVENT DISKUS SHOULD NOT BE USED TO TREAT ACUTE SYMPTOMS. It is crucial to inform patients of this and prescribe an inhaled, short-acting beta₂-agonist for this purpose as well as warn them that increasing inhaled beta₂-agonist use is a signal of deteriorating asthma.

SEREVENT DISKUS IS NOT A SUBSTITUTE FOR INHALED OR ORAL CORTICOSTEROIDS. Corticosteroids should not be stopped or reduced when SEREVENT DISKUS is initiated.

(See PRECAUTIONS: Information for Patients and the accompanying PATIENT'S INSTRUCTIONS FOR USE.)

1. Do Not Introduce SEREVENT DISKUS as a Treatment for Acutely Deteriorating Asthma: SEREVENT DISKUS is intended for the maintenance treatment of asthma (see INDICATIONS AND USAGE) and should not be introduced in acutely deteriorating asthma, which is a potentially life-threatening condition. There are no data demonstrating that SEREVENT DISKUS provides greater efficacy than or additional efficacy to inhaled, short-acting beta₂-agonists in patients with worsening asthma. Serious acute respiratory events, including fatalities, have been reported, both in the United States and worldwide, in patients receiving SEREVENT. In most cases, these have occurred in patients with severe asthma (e.g., patients with a history of corticosteroid dependence, low pulmonary function, intubation, mechanical ventilation, frequent hospitalizations, or previous life-threatening acute asthma exacerbations) and/or in some patients in whom asthma has been acutely deteriorating (e.g., unresponsive to usual medications; increasing need for inhaled short-acting beta₂-agonists; increasing need for systemic corticosteroids; significant increase in symptoms; recent emergency room visits; sudden or progressive deterioration in pulmonary function). However, they have occurred in a few patients with less severe asthma as well. It was not possible from these reports to determine whether SEREVENT contributed to these events or simply failed to relieve the deteriorating asthma.

2. Do Not Use SEREVENT DISKUS to Treat Acute Symptoms: An inhaled, short-acting beta₂-agonist, not SEREVENT DISKUS, should be used to relieve acute asthma symptoms. When prescribing SEREVENT DISKUS, the physician must also provide the patient with an inhaled, short-acting beta₂-agonist (e.g., albuterol) for treatment of symptoms that occur acutely, despite regular twice-daily (morning and evening) use of SEREVENT DISKUS.

When beginning treatment with SEREVENT DISKUS, patients who have been taking inhaled, short-acting beta₂-agonists on a regular basis (e.g., four times a day) should be instructed to discontinue the regular use of these drugs and use them only for symptomatic relief of acute asthma symptoms (see PRECAUTIONS: Information for Patients).

3. Watch for Increasing Use of Inhaled, Short-Acting Beta₂-Agonists, Which Is a Marker of Deteriorating Asthma: Asthma may deteriorate acutely over a period of hours or chronically over several days or longer. If the patient's inhaled, short-acting beta₂-agonist becomes less effective or the patient needs more inhalations than usual, this may be a marker of destabilization of asthma. In this setting, the patient requires immediate reevaluation with reassessment of the treatment regimen, giving special consideration to the possible need for corticosteroids. If the patient uses four or more inhalations per day of an inhaled, short-acting beta₂-agonist for 2 or more consecutive days, or if more than one canister (200 inhalations per canister) of inhaled, short-acting beta₂-agonist is used in an 8-week period in conjunction with SEREVENT DISKUS, then the patient should consult the physician for reevaluation. **Increasing the daily dosage of SEREVENT DISKUS in this situation is not appropriate. SEREVENT DISKUS should not be used more frequently than twice daily (morning and evening) at the recommended dose of one inhalation.**

4. Do Not Use SEREVENT DISKUS as a Substitute for Oral or Inhaled Corticosteroids: The use of beta-adrenergic agonist bronchodilators alone may not be adequate to control asthma in many patients. Early consideration should be given to adding anti-inflammatory agents, e.g., corticosteroids. There are no data demonstrating that SEREVENT DISKUS has a clinical anti-inflammatory effect and could be expected to take the place of, or reduce the dose of, corticosteroids. Patients who already require oral or inhaled corticosteroids for treatment of asthma should be continued on this type of treatment even if they feel better as a result of initiating SEREVENT DISKUS. Any change in corticosteroid dosage should be made ONLY after clinical evaluation (see PRECAUTIONS: Information for Patients).

5. Do Not Exceed Recommended Dosage: As with other inhaled beta₂-adrenergic drugs, SEREVENT DISKUS should not be used more often or at higher doses than recommended. Fatalities have been reported in association with excessive use of inhaled sympathomimetic drugs. Large doses of inhaled or oral salmeterol (12 to 20 times the recommended dose) have been associated with clinically significant prolongation of the QT_c interval, which has the potential for producing ventricular arrhythmias.

6. Paradoxical Bronchospasm: Inhalation of salmeterol xinafoate can produce paradoxical bronchospasm which may be life threatening. If paradoxical bronchospasm occurs, SEREVENT DISKUS should be discontinued immediately and alternative therapy instituted. It should be recognized that paradoxical bronchospasm, when associated with inhaled formulations, frequently occurs with the first use of a new canister or vial.

7. Immediate Hypersensitivity Reactions: Immediate hypersensitivity reactions may occur after administration of SEREVENT DISKUS, as demonstrated by rare cases of urticaria, angioedema, rash, and bronchospasm.

8. Upper Airway Symptoms: Symptoms of laryngeal spasm, irritation, or swelling, such as stridor and choking, have been reported rarely in patients receiving SEREVENT DISKUS.

SEREVENT DISKUS, like all other beta-adrenergic agonists, can produce a clinically significant cardiovascular effect in some patients as measured by pulse rate, blood pressure, and/or symptoms. Although such effects are uncommon after administration of SEREVENT DISKUS at recommended doses, if they occur, the drug may need to be discontinued. In addition, beta-agonists have been reported to produce electrocardiogram (ECG) changes, such as flattening of the T wave, prolongation of the QT_c interval, and ST segment depression. The clinical significance of these findings is unknown. Therefore, SEREVENT DISKUS, like all sympathomimetic amines, should be used with caution in patients with cardiovascular disorders, especially coronary insufficiency, cardiac arrhythmias, and hypertension.

PRECAUTIONS

General: 1. Cardiovascular and Other Effects: No effect on the cardiovascular system is usually seen after the administration of inhaled salmeterol in recommended doses, but the cardiovascular and central nervous system effects seen with all sympathomimetic drugs (e.g., increased blood pressure, heart rate, excitement) can occur after use of salmeterol and may require discontinuation of the drug. Salmeterol, like all sympathomimetic amines, should be used with caution in patients with cardiovascular disorders, especially coronary insufficiency, cardiac arrhythmias, and hypertension; in patients with convulsive disorders or thyrotoxicosis; and in patients who are unusually responsive to sympathomimetic amines.

As has been described with other beta-adrenergic agonist bronchodilators, clinically significant changes in systolic and/or diastolic blood pressure, pulse rate, and electrocardiograms have been seen infrequently in individual patients in controlled clinical studies with salmeterol.

2. Metabolic Effects: Doses of the related beta₂-adrenoceptor agonist albuterol, when administered intravenously, have been reported to aggravate preexisting diabetes mellitus and ketoacidosis. No effects on glucose have been seen with SEREVENT DISKUS at recommended doses. Beta-adrenergic agonist medications may produce significant hypokalemia in some patients possibly through intracellular shunting, which has the potential to produce adverse cardiovascular effects. The decrease is usually transient, not requiring supplementation.

Clinically significant changes in blood glucose and/or serum potassium were seen rarely during clinical studies with long-term administration of SEREVENT DISKUS at recommended doses.

Information for Patients: See illustrated PATIENT'S INSTRUCTIONS FOR USE provided with the product.

It is important that patients understand how to use the DISKUS inhalation device appropriately and how it should be used in relation to other asthma medications they are taking. Patients should be given the following information:

1. The action of SEREVENT DISKUS may last up to 12 hours or longer. The recommended dosage (one inhalation twice daily, morning and evening) should not be exceeded.

2. SEREVENT DISKUS is not meant to relieve acute asthma symptoms and extra doses should not be used for that purpose. Acute symptoms should be treated with an inhaled, short-acting beta$_2$-agonist such as albuterol (the physician should provide the patient with such medication and instruct the patient in how it should be used).
3. The physician should be notified immediately if any of the following situations occur, which may be a sign of seriously worsening asthma:
- Decreasing effectiveness of inhaled, short-acting beta$_2$-agonists
- Need for more inhalations than usual of inhaled, short-acting beta$_2$-agonists
- Use of four or more inhalations per day of a short-acting beta$_2$-agonist for 2 or more days consecutively
- Use of more than one canister of an inhaled, short-acting beta$_2$-agonist in an 8-week period (i.e., canister with 200 inhalations)

4. SEREVENT DISKUS should not be used as a substitute for oral or inhaled corticosteroids. The dosage of these medications should not be changed and they should not be stopped without consulting the physician, even if the patient feels better after initiating treatment with SEREVENT DISKUS.
5. Patients should be cautioned regarding common adverse cardiovascular effects, such as palpitations, chest pain, rapid heart rate, tremor, or nervousness.
6. In patients receiving SEREVENT DISKUS, other inhaled medications should be used only as directed by the physician.
7. SEREVENT DISKUS should not be used with a spacer.
8. If you are pregnant or nursing, contact your physician about use of SEREVENT DISKUS.
9. Effective and safe use of the DISKUS device includes an understanding of the way that it should be used:
- Never exhale into the DISKUS device.
- Always activate and use the DISKUS device in a level, horizontal position.
- Never wash the mouthpiece or any part of the DISKUS device. KEEP IT DRY.

Drug Interactions: ***Short-Acting Beta-Agonists:*** In the two 12-week, repetitive-dose clinical trials (n = 149), the mean daily need for additional beta$_2$-agonist use in patients using salmeterol inhalation powder was approximately $1^1/_2$ inhalations per day. Twenty-six percent of the patients in these trials used between 8 and 24 inhalations of short-acting beta-agonist per day on one or more occasions. Nine percent of the patients in these trials averaged over 4 inhalations per day over the course of the 12-week trials. No observed increase in frequency of cardiovascular events was noted among the 3 patients who used an average of 8 to 11 inhalations per day; however, the safety of concomitant use of more than 8 inhalations per day of short-acting beta$_2$-agonist with salmeterol inhalation powder has not been established. In 29 patients who experienced worsening of asthma while receiving salmeterol inhalation powder during these trials, albuterol therapy administered via either nebulizer or inhalation aerosol (one dose in most cases) led to improvement in FEV_1 and no increase in occurrence of cardiovascular adverse events.

Monoamine Oxidase Inhibitors and Tricyclic Antidepressants: Salmeterol should be administered with extreme caution to patients being treated with monoamine oxidase inhibitors or tricyclic antidepressants, or within 2 weeks of discontinuation of such agents, because the action of salmeterol on the vascular system may be potentiated by these agents.

Corticosteroids and Cromoglycate: In clinical trials, inhaled corticosteroids and/or inhaled cromolyn sodium did not alter the safety profile of SEREVENT when administered concurrently.

Methylxanthines: The concurrent use of intravenously or orally administered methylxanthines (e.g., aminophylline, theophylline) by patients receiving SEREVENT has not been completely evaluated. In one clinical asthma trial, 87 patients receiving SEREVENT Inhalation Aerosol 42 mcg twice daily concurrently with a theophylline product had adverse event rates similar to those in 71 patients receiving SEREVENT Inhalation Aerosol without theophylline. Resting heart rates were slightly higher in the patients on theophylline but were little affected by therapy with SEREVENT Inhalation Aerosol.

Beta-adrenergic receptor blocking agents not only block the pulmonary effect of beta-agonists, such as SEREVENT DISKUS, but may produce severe bronchospasm in asthmatic patients. Therefore, patients with asthma should not normally be treated with beta-blockers. However, under certain circumstances, e.g., as prophylaxis after myocardial infarction, there may be no acceptable alternatives to the use of beta-adrenergic blocking agents in patients with asthma. In this setting, cardioselective beta-blockers could be considered, although they should be administered with caution.

The ECG changes and/or hypokalemia that may result from the administration of nonpotassium-sparing diuretics (such as loop or thiazide diuretics) can be acutely worsened by beta-agonists, especially when the recommended dose of the beta-agonist is exceeded. Although the clinical significance of these effects is not known, caution is advised in the coadministration of beta-agonists with nonpotassium-sparing diuretics.

Table 2: Adverse Experience Incidence in Two Large 12-Week Clinical Trials

	Percent of Patients		
Adverse Event Type	Placebo n = 152	SEREVENT Inhalation Powder 50 mcg twice daily n = 149	Albuterol Inhalation Aerosol 180 mcg four times daily n = 150
Ear, nose, and throat			
Nasal/sinus congestion, pallor	6	9	8
Rhinitis	4	5	4
Neurological			
Headache	9	13	12
Respiratory			
Asthma	1	3	<1
Tracheitis/bronchitis	4	7	3
Influenza	2	5	5

Carcinogenesis, Mutagenesis, Impairment of Fertility: In an 18-month oral carcinogenicity study in CD-mice, salmeterol xinafoate at oral doses of 1.4 mg/kg and above (approximately nine times the maximum recommended daily inhalation dose in adults based on comparison of the area-under-the plasma-concentration versus time curves [AUCs]) caused dose-related increases in the incidence of smooth muscle hyperplasia, cystic glandular hyperplasia, leiomyomas of the uterus, and cysts in the ovaries. The incidence of leiomyosarcomas was not statistically significant. No tumors were seen at 0.2 mg/kg, comparable to the maximum recommended human daily inhalation dose in adults based on comparison of the AUCs).

In a 24-month inhalation and oral carcinogenicity study in Sprague Dawley rats, salmeterol caused dose-related increases in the incidence of mesovarian leiomyomas and ovarian cysts at inhalation and oral doses of 0.68 mg/kg per day and above (approximately 55 times the maximum recommended human daily inhalation dose in adults on a mg/m^2 basis). No tumors were seen at 0.21 mg/kg per day (approximately 15 times the maximum recommended human daily inhalation dose in adults on a mg/m^2 basis). These findings in rodents are similar to those reported previously for other beta-adrenergic agonist drugs. The relevance of these findings to human use is unknown.

Salmeterol xinafoate produced no detectable or reproducible increases in microbial and mammalian gene mutation in vitro. No clastogenic activity occurred in vitro in human lymphocytes or in vivo in a rat micronucleus test. No effects on fertility were identified in male and female rats treated orally with salmeterol xinatoate at doses up to 2 mg/kg (approximately 160 times the maximum recommended human daily inhalation dose in adults on a mg/m^2 basis).

Pregnancy: ***Teratogenic Effects:*** Pregnancy Category C. No teratogenic effects occurred in the rat at oral doses up to 2 mg/kg per day (approximately 160 times the maximum recommended human daily inhalation dose in adults on a mg/m^2 basis). In pregnant Dutch rabbits administered oral doses of 1 mg/kg and above (approximately 20 times the maximum recommended human daily inhalation dose in adults based on the comparison of the AUCs) salmeterol xinafoate exhibited fetal toxic effects characteristically resulting from beta-adrenoceptor stimulation; these included precocious eyelid openings, cleft palate, sternebral fusion, limb and paw flexures, and delayed ossification of the frontal cranial bones. No significant effects occurred at an oral dose of 0.6 mg/kg (approximately 10 times the maximum recommended human daily inhalation dose in adults based on comparison of the AUCs).

New Zealand White rabbits were less sensitive since only delayed ossification of the frontal cranial bones was seen at oral doses of 10 mg/kg (approximately 1600 times the maximum recommended human daily inhalation dose on a mg/m^2 basis). Extensive use of other beta-agonists has provided no evidence that these class effects in animals are relevant to use in humans. There are no adequate and well-controlled studies with SEREVENT DISKUS in pregnant women. SEREVENT DISKUS should be used during pregnancy only if the potential benefit justifies the potential risk to the fetus.

Use in Labor and Delivery: There are no well-controlled human studies that have investigated effects of salmeterol on preterm labor or labor at term. Because of the potential for beta-agonist interference with uterine contractility, use of SEREVENT DISKUS for prevention of bronchospasm during labor should be restricted to those patients in whom the benefits clearly outweigh the risks.

Nursing Mothers: Plasma levels of salmeterol after inhaled therapeutic doses are very low. In rats, salmeterol xinafoate is excreted in milk. However, since there is no experience with use of SEREVENT DISKUS by nursing mothers, a decision should be made whether to discontinue nursing or to discontinue the drug, taking into account the importance of the drug to the mother. Caution should be exercised when salmeterol xinafoate is administered to a nursing woman.

Pediatric Use: The safety and effectiveness of SEREVENT DISKUS in children younger than 12 years of age have not been established.

Geriatric Use: Of the total number of patients who received salmeterol inhalation powder in adolescent and adult chronic dosing clinical trials, 209 were 65 years of age and older. No apparent differences in the efficacy and safety of SEREVENT inhalation powder were observed when geriatric patients were compared with younger patients in clinical trials. As with other beta$_2$-agonists, however, special caution should be observed when using SEREVENT inhalation powder in geriatric patients who have concomitant cardiovascular disease that could be adversely affected by this class of drug. Based on available data, no adjustment of salmeterol dosage in geriatric patients is warranted.

ADVERSE REACTIONS

Adverse reactions to salmeterol are similar in nature to reactions to other selective beta$_2$-adrenoceptor agonists, i.e., tachycardia; palpitations; immediate hypersensitivity reactions, including urticaria, angioedema, rash, bronchospasm (see WARNINGS); headache; tremor; nervousness; and paradoxical bronchospasm (see WARNINGS).

Two multicenter, 12-week, controlled studies have evaluated twice-daily doses of SEREVENT inhalation powder in patients 12 years of age and older with asthma. The following table reports the incidence of adverse events in these two studies.

[See table 2 above]

The table above includes all events (whether considered drug-related or nondrug-related by the investigator) that occurred at a rate of ≥3% in the SEREVENT inhalation powder treatment group and were more common in the SEREVENT inhalation powder group than in the placebo group.

Pharyngitis, sinusitis, upper respiratory tract infection, and cough occurred at ≥3% but were more common in the placebo group. However, throat irritation has been described at rates exceeding that of placebo in other controlled clinical trials. Other events occurring in the SEREVENT inhalation powder group at a frequency of 1% to 3% and at a greater rate than in placebo were as follows:

Ear, Nose, and Throat: Sinus headache.
Gastrointestinal: Nausea.
Mouth and Teeth: Oral mucosal abnormality.
Musculoskeletal: Pain in joint.
Neurological: Sleep disturbance, paresthesia.
Skin: Contact dermatitis, eczema.
Miscellaneous: Localized aches and pains, pyrexia of unknown origin.

Observed During Clinical Practice: In extensive US and worldwide postmarketing experience with SEREVENT, serious exacerbations of asthma, including some that have been fatal, have been reported. In most cases, these have occurred in patients with severe asthma and/or in some patients in whom asthma has been acutely deteriorating (see WARNINGS no. 1), but they have also occurred in a few patients with less severe asthma as well. It was not possible from these reports to determine whether SEREVENT con-

Continued on next page

This product information is based on labeling in effect on June 1, 1998. For further information, contact via direct mail, phone, or web site Medical Information: Glaxo Wellcome Inc., PO Box 13398, Research Triangle Park, NC 27709. Healthcare Professionals (Medical Information): 800-334-0089 Patients (Customer Response Center): 888-TALK2GW (1-888-825-5249) Glaxo Wellcome Corporate Web Site: www.glaxowellcome.com

Serevent Diskus—Cont.

tributed to these events or simply failed to relieve the deteriorating asthma.

The following events have also been identified during post-approval use of SEREVENT in clinical practice. Because they are reported voluntarily from a population of unknown size, estimates of frequency cannot be made. These events have been chosen for inclusion due to a combination of their seriousness, frequency of reporting, or potential causal connection to SEREVENT.

Respiratory: Rare reports of upper airway symptoms of laryngeal spasm, irritation, or swelling such as stridor or choking.

Cardiovascular: Hypertension, arrhythmias (including atrial fibrillation, supraventricular tachycardia, extrasystoles.

OVERDOSAGE

The expected signs and symptoms with overdosage of SEREVENT DISKUS are those of excessive beta-adrenergic stimulation and/or occurrence or exaggeration of any of the signs and symptoms listed under ADVERSE REACTIONS, e.g., seizures, angina, hypertension or hypotension, tachycardia with rates up to 200 beats/min, arrhythmias, nervousness, headache, tremor, muscle cramps, dry mouth, palpitation, nausea, dizziness, fatigue, malaise, and insomnia. Overdosage with salmeterol may be expected to result in exaggeration of the pharmacologic adverse effects associated with beta-adrenoceptor agonists, including tachycardia and/or arrhythmia, tremor, headache, and muscle cramps. Overdosage with salmeterol can lead to clinically significant prolongation of the QT_c interval, which can produce ventricular arrhythmias. Other signs of overdosage may include hypokalemia and hyperglycemia.

As with all sympathomimetic medications, cardiac arrest and even death may be associated with abuse of SEREVENT DISKUS.

Treatment consists of discontinuation of SEREVENT DISKUS together with appropriate symptomatic therapy. The judicious use of a cardioselective beta-receptor blocker may be considered, bearing in mind that such medication can produce bronchospasm. There is insufficient evidence to determine if dialysis is beneficial for overdosage of SEREVENT DISKUS. Cardiac monitoring is recommended in cases of overdosage.

No deaths were seen in rats at inhalation doses of 2.9 mg/kg (approximately 240 times the maximum recommended human daily inhalation dose on a mg/m² basis) and in dogs at 0.7 mg/kg (approximately 190 times the maximum recommended human daily inhalation dose on a mg/m² basis). By the oral route, no deaths occurred in mice at 150 mg/kg (approximately 6100 times the maximum recommended human daily inhalation dose on a mg/m² basis) and in rats at 1000 mg/kg (approximately 81 000 times the maximum recommended human daily inhalation dose on a mg/m² basis).

DOSAGE AND ADMINISTRATION

SEREVENT DISKUS inhalation powder should be administered by the orally inhaled route only (see PATIENT'S INSTRUCTIONS FOR USE). For maintenance of bronchodilatation and prevention of symptoms of asthma, including the symptoms of nocturnal asthma, the usual dosage for patients 12 years of age and older is one inhalation (50 mcg) twice daily (morning and evening, approximately 12 hours apart). Adverse effects are more likely to occur with higher doses of salmeterol, and more frequent administration or administration of a larger number of inhalations is not recommended.

To gain full therapeutic benefit, SEREVENT DISKUS should be administered twice daily (morning and evening) in the treatment of reversible airway obstruction. The patient must not exhale into the device and the device should only be activated and used in a level, horizontal position.

If a previously effective dosage regimen fails to provide the usual response, medical advice should be sought immediately as this is often a sign of destabilization of asthma. Under these circumstances, the therapeutic regimen should be reevaluated and additional therapeutic options, such as inhaled or systemic corticosteroids, should be considered. If symptoms arise in the period between doses, an inhaled, short-acting beta₂-agonist should be taken for immediate relief.

Geriatric Use: In studies where geriatric patients (65 years of age or older, see PRECAUTIONS) have been treated with SEREVENT inhalation powder, efficacy and safety of 50 mcg given twice daily (morning and evening) did not differ from that in younger patients. Consequently, no dosage adjustment is recommended.

HOW SUPPLIED

SEREVENT DISKUS inhalation powder is supplied as a disposable, teal green colored device containing 60 blisters. The DISKUS inhalation device is packaged within a teal green colored, plastic-coated foil pouch (NDC 0173-0521-00).

SEREVENT DISKUS is also supplied in an institutional pack of one teal green colored, disposable DISKUS inhalation device containing 28 blisters. The DISKUS inhalation device is packaged within a teal green colored, plastic-coated foil pouch (NDC 0173-0520-00).

Store at controlled room temperature, 20° to 25°C (68° to 77°F) in a dry place away from direct heat or sunlight. Keep out of reach of children. The DISKUS inhalation device is not reusable and should be discarded after every blister has been used (when the dose indicator reads "0") or 6 weeks after removal from the moisture-protective foil overwrap pouch, whichever comes first. Do not attempt to take the device apart.

US Patent Nos. 4,992,474; 5,225,445; 5,380,922; 5,590,645; and Des. 5,342,994

May 1998/RL-593

Shown in Product Identification Guide, page 314

TABLOID® brand Thioguanine ℞
[tab 'loid]
40 mg Scored Tablets

CAUTION: TABLOID brand Thioguanine is a potent drug. It should not be used unless a diagnosis of acute nonlymphocytic leukemia has been adequately established and the responsible physician is knowledgeable in assessing response to chemotherapy.

DESCRIPTION

TABLOID brand Thioguanine was synthesized and developed by Hitchings, Elion, and associates at the Wellcome Research Laboratories. It is one of a large series of purine analogues which interfere with nucleic acid biosynthesis, and has been found active against selected human neoplastic diseases.[1]

Thioguanine, known chemically as 2-amino-1,7-dihydro-6H-purine-6-thione, is an analogue of the nucleic acid constituent guanine, and is closely related structurally and functionally to PURINETHOL® (mercaptopurine).

TABLOID brand Thioguanine is available in tablets for oral administration. Each scored tablet contains 40 mg thioguanine and the inactive ingredients gum acacia, lactose, magnesium stearate, potato starch, and stearic acid.

CLINICAL PHARMACOLOGY

Clinical studies have shown that the absorption of an oral dose of thioguanine in humans is incomplete and variable, averaging approximately 30% of the administered dose (range: 14% to 46%).[2,3] Following oral administration of ³⁵S-6-thioguanine, total plasma radioactivity reached a maximum at 8 hours and declined slowly thereafter. Parent drug represented only a very small fraction of the total plasma radioactivity at any time, being virtually undetectable throughout the period of measurements.

The oral administration of radiolabeled thioguanine revealed only trace quantities of parent drug in the urine. However, a methylated metabolite, 2-amino-6-methyl-thiopurine (MTG), appeared very early, rose to a maximum 6 to 8 hours after drug administration, and was still being excreted after 12 to 22 hours. Radiolabeled sulfate appeared somewhat later than MTG but was the principal metabolite after 8 hours. Thiouric acid and some unidentified products were found in the urine in small amounts.[3] Intravenous administration of ³⁵S-6-thioguanine disclosed a median plasma half-disappearance time of 80 minutes (range: 25 to 240 minutes) when the compound was given in single doses of 65 to 300 mg/m². Although initial plasma levels of thioguanine did correlate with the dose level, there was no correlation between the plasma half-disappearance time and the dose.[2]

Thioguanine is incorporated into the DNA and the RNA of human bone marrow cells. Studies with intravenous ³⁵S-6-thioguanine have shown that the amount of thioguanine incorporated into nucleic acids is more than 100 times higher after five daily doses than after a single dose. With the five-dose schedule, from one-half to virtually all of the guanine in the residual DNA was replaced by thioguanine.[2] Tissue distribution studies of ³⁵S-6-thioguanine in mice showed only traces of radioactivity in brain after oral administration. No measurements have been made of thioguanine concentrations in human cerebrospinal fluid (CSF), but observations on tissue distribution in animals, together with the lack of CNS penetration by the closely related compound, mercaptopurine, suggest that thioguanine does not reach therapeutic concentrations in the CSF.

Monitoring of plasma levels of thioguanine during therapy is of questionable value.[3] There is technical difficulty in determining plasma concentrations, which are seldom greater than 1 to 2 mcg/mL after a therapeutic oral dose. More significantly, thioguanine enters rapidly into the anabolic and catabolic pathways for purines, and the active intracellular metabolites have appreciably longer half-lives than the parent drug. The biochemical effects of a single dose of thioguanine are evident long after the parent drug has disappeared

from plasma. Because of this rapid metabolism of thioguanine to active intracellular derivatives, hemodialysis would not be expected to appreciably reduce toxicity of the drug. Thioguanine competes with hypoxanthine and guanine for the enzyme hypoxanthine-guanine phosphoribosyltransferase (HGPRTase) and is itself converted to 6-thioguanylic acid (TGMP). This nucleotide reaches high intracellular concentrations at therapeutic doses. TGMP interferes at several points with the synthesis of guanine nucleotides. It inhibits de novo purine biosynthesis by pseudo-feedback inhibition of glutamine-5-phosphoribosylpyrophosphate amidotransferase—the first enzyme unique to the de novo pathway for purine ribonucleotide synthesis. TGMP also inhibits the conversion of inosinic acid (IMP) to xanthylic acid (XMP) by competition for the enzyme IMP dehydrogenase. At one time TGMP was felt to be a significant inhibitor of ATP:GMP phosphotransferase (guanylate kinase),[4] but recent results have shown this not to be so.[5]

Thioguanylic acid is further converted to the di- and triphosphates, thioguanosine diphosphate (TGDP) and thioguanosine triphosphate (TGTP) (as well as their 2′-deoxyribosyl analogues) by the same enzymes which metabolize guanine nucleotides.[6] Thioguanine nucleotides are incorporated into both the RNA and the DNA by phosphodiester linkages[2] and it has been argued that incorporation of such fraudulent bases contributes to the cytotoxicity of thioguanine.

Thus, thioguanine has multiple metabolic effects and at present it is not possible to designate one major site of action. Its tumor inhibitory properties may be due to one or more of its effects on (a) feedback inhibition of de novo purine synthesis; (b) inhibition of purine nucleotide interconversions; or (c) incorporation into the DNA and the RNA. The net consequence of its actions is a sequential blockade of the synthesis and utilization of the purine nucleotides.[4,6,7]

The catabolism of thioguanine and its metabolites is complex and shows significant differences between humans and the mouse.[2,3] In both humans and mice, after oral administration of ³⁵S-6-thioguanine, urine contains virtually no detectable intact thioguanine. While deamination and subsequent oxidation to thiouric acid occurs only to a small extent in man, it is the main pathway in mice. The product of deamination by guanase, 6-thioxanthine is inactive, having negligible antitumor activity. This pathway of thioguanine inactivation is not dependent on the action of xanthine oxidase, and an inhibitor of that enzyme (such as allopurinol) will not block the detoxification of thioguanine even though the inactive 6-thioxanthine is normally further oxidized by xanthine oxidase to thiouric acid before it is eliminated. In humans, methylation of thioguanine is much more extensive than in the mouse. The product of methylation, 2-amino-6-methylthiopurine, is also substantially less active and less toxic than thioguanine and its formation is likewise unaffected by the presence of allopurinol. Appreciable amounts of inorganic sulfate are also found in both murine and human urine, presumably arising from further metabolism of the methylated derivatives.

In some animal tumors, resistance to the effect of thioguanine correlates with the loss of HGPRTase activity and the resulting inability to convert thioguanine to thioguanylic acid. However, other resistance mechanisms, such as increased catabolism of TGMP by a nonspecific phosphatase, may be operative. Although not invariable, it is usual to find cross-resistance between thioguanine and its close analogue, PURINETHOL (mercaptopurine).

INDICATIONS AND USAGE

a) Acute Nonlymphocytic Leukemias: TABLOID brand Thioguanine is indicated for remission induction, remission consolidation, and maintenance therapy of acute nonlymphocytic leukemias.[8,9] The response to this agent depends upon the age of the patient (younger patients faring better than older) and whether thioguanine is used in previously treated or previously untreated patients. Reliance upon thioguanine alone is seldom justified for initial remission induction of acute nonlymphocytic leukemias because combination chemotherapy including thioguanine results in more frequent remission induction and longer duration of remission than thioguanine alone.

b) Other Neoplasms: TABLOID brand Thioguanine is not effective in chronic lymphocytic leukemia, Hodgkin's lymphoma, multiple myeloma, or solid tumors. Although thioguanine is one of several agents with activity in the treatment of the chronic phase of chronic myelogenous leukemia, more objective responses are observed with MYLERAN® (busulfan), and therefore busulfan is usually regarded as the preferred drug.

CONTRAINDICATIONS

Thioguanine should not be used in patients whose disease has demonstrated prior resistance to this drug. In animals and humans, there is usually complete cross-resistance between PURINETHOL (mercaptopurine) and TABLOID brand Thioguanine.

WARNINGS

SINCE DRUGS USED IN CANCER CHEMOTHERAPY ARE POTENTIALLY HAZARDOUS, IT IS RECOM-

MENDED THAT ONLY PHYSICIANS EXPERIENCED WITH THE RISKS OF THIOGUANINE AND KNOWLEDGEABLE IN THE NATURAL HISTORY OF ACUTE NONLYMPHOCYTIC LEUKEMIAS ADMINISTER THIS DRUG.

The most consistent, dose-related toxicity is bone marrow suppression. This may be manifested by anemia, leukopenia, thrombocytopenia, or any combination of these. Any one of these findings may also reflect progression of the underlying disease. Since thioguanine may have a delayed effect, it is important to withdraw the medication temporarily at the first sign of an abnormally large fall in any of the formed elements of the blood.

It is recommended that evaluation of the hemoglobin concentration or hematocrit, total white blood cell count and differential count, and quantitative platelet count be obtained frequently while the patient is on thioguanine therapy. In cases where the cause of fluctuations in the formed elements in the peripheral blood is obscure, bone marrow examination may be useful for the evaluation of marrow status. The decision to increase, decrease, continue, or discontinue a given dosage of thioguanine must be based not only on the absolute hematologic values, but also upon the rapidity with which changes are occurring. In many instances, particularly during the induction phase of acute leukemia, complete blood counts will need to be done more frequently in order to evaluate the effect of the therapy. The dosage of thioguanine may need to be reduced when this agent is combined with other drugs whose primary toxicity is myelosuppression.

Myelosuppression is often unavoidable during the induction phase of adult acute nonlymphocytic leukemias if remission induction is to be successful. Whether or not this demands modification or cessation of dosage depends both upon the response of the underlying disease and a careful consideration of supportive facilities (granulocyte and platelet transfusions) which may be available. Life-threatening infections and bleeding have been observed as consequences of thioguanine-induced granulocytopenia and thrombocytopenia.

The effect of thioguanine on the immunocompetence of patients is unknown.

Pregnancy: Pregnancy Category D. Drugs such as thioguanine are potential mutagens and teratogens. Thioguanine may cause fetal harm when administered to a pregnant woman. Thioguanine has been shown to be teratogenic in rats when given in doses 5 times the human dose. When given to the rat on the 4th and 5th days of gestation, 13% of surviving placentas did not contain fetuses, and 19% of offspring were malformed or stunted. The malformations noted included generalized edema, cranial defects, and general skeletal hypoplasia, hydrocephalus, ventral hernia, situs inversus, and incomplete development of the limbs.[10]

There are no adequate and well-controlled studies in pregnant women. If this drug is used during pregnancy, or if the patient becomes pregnant while taking the drug, the patient should be apprised of the potential hazard to the fetus. Women of childbearing potential should be advised to avoid becoming pregnant.

PRECAUTIONS

General: Although the primary toxicity of thioguanine is myelosuppression, other toxicities have occasionally been observed, particularly when thioguanine is used in combination with other cancer chemotherapeutic agents.

A few cases of jaundice have been reported in patients with leukemia receiving thioguanine. Among these were two adult male patients and four pediatric patients with acute myelogenous leukemia and an adult male with acute lymphocytic leukemia who developed veno-occlusive hepatic disease while receiving chemotherapy for their leukemia.[11,12] Six patients had received cytarabine prior to treatment with thioguanine, and some were receiving other chemotherapy in addition to thioguanine when they became symptomatic. While veno-occlusive hepatic disease has not been reported in patients treated with thioguanine alone, it is recommended that thioguanine be withheld if there is evidence of toxic hepatitis or biliary stasis, and that appropriate clinical and laboratory investigations be initiated to establish the etiology of the hepatic dysfunction. Deterioration in liver function studies during thioguanine therapy should prompt discontinuation of treatment and a search for an explanation of the hepatotoxicity.

Information for Patients: Patients should be informed that the major toxicities of thioguanine are related to myelosuppression, hepatotoxicity, and gastrointestinal toxicity. Patients should never be allowed to take the drug without medical supervision and should be advised to consult their physician if they experience fever, sore throat, jaundice, nausea, vomiting, signs of local infection, bleeding from any site, or symptoms suggestive of anemia. Women of childbearing potential should be advised to avoid becoming pregnant.

Laboratory Tests: It is advisable to monitor liver function tests (serum transaminases, alkaline phosphatase, bilirubin) at weekly intervals when first beginning therapy and at monthly intervals thereafter. It may be advisable to perform liver function tests more frequently in patients with known pre-existing liver disease or in patients who are receiving thioguanine and other hepatotoxic drugs. Patients should be instructed to discontinue thioguanine immediately if clinical jaundice is detected (see WARNINGS).

Drug Interactions: There is usually complete cross-resistance between PURINETHOL (mercaptopurine) and TABLOID brand Thioguanine.

In one study, 12 of approximately 330 patients receiving continuous busulfan and thioguanine therapy for treatment of chronic myelogenous leukemia were found to have esophageal varices associated with abnormal liver function tests.[13] Subsequent liver biopsies were performed in four of these patients, all of which showed evidence of nodular regenerative hyperplasia. Duration of combination therapy prior to the appearance of esophageal varices ranged from 6 to 45 months. With the present analysis of the data, no cases of hepatotoxicity have appeared in the busulfan-alone arm of the study. Long-term continuous therapy with thioguanine and busulfan should be used with caution.

Carcinogenesis, Mutagenesis, Impairment of Fertility: In view of its action on cellular DNA, thioguanine is potentially mutagenic and carcinogenic, and consideration should be given to the theoretical risk of carcinogenesis when thioguanine is administered (see WARNINGS).

Pregnancy: ***Teratogenic Effects:*** Pregnancy Category D. See WARNINGS section.

Nursing Mothers: It is not known whether this drug is excreted in human milk. Because of the potential for tumorigenicity shown for thioguanine, a decision should be made whether to discontinue nursing or to discontinue the drug, taking into account the importance of the drug to the mother.

Pediatric Use: See DOSAGE AND ADMINISTRATION section.

ADVERSE REACTIONS

The most frequent adverse reaction to thioguanine is myelosuppression. The induction of complete remission of acute myelogenous leukemia usually requires combination chemotherapy in dosages which produce marrow hypoplasia.[14] Since consolidation and maintenance of remission are also effected by multiple-drug regimens whose component agents cause myelosuppression, pancytopenia is observed in nearly all patients. Dosages and schedules must be adjusted to prevent life-threatening cytopenias whenever these adverse reactions are observed.

Hyperuricemia frequently occurs in patients receiving thioguanine as a consequence of rapid cell lysis accompanying the antineoplastic effect. Adverse effects can be minimized by increased hydration, urine alkalinization, and the prophylactic administration of a xanthine oxidase inhibitor such as ZYLOPRIM® (allopurinol). Unlike PURINETHOL (mercaptopurine) and IMURAN® (azathioprine), thioguanine may be continued in the usual dosage when allopurinol is used conjointly to inhibit uric acid formation.

Less frequent adverse reactions include nausea, vomiting, anorexia, and stomatitis. Intestinal necrosis and perforation have been reported in patients who received multiple drug chemotherapy including thioguanine.

Hepatic Effects: Liver enzyme and other liver function studies are occasionally abnormal. If jaundice, hepatomegaly, or anorexia with tenderness in the right hypochondrium occurs, thioguanine should be withheld until the exact etiology can be determined. There have been reports of veno-occlusive liver disease occurring in patients who received combination chemotherapy including thioguanine.[11,12]

Esophageal varices have been reported in patients receiving continuous busulfan and thioguanine therapy for treatment of chronic myelogenous leukemia (see PRECAUTIONS: Drug Interactions).

OVERDOSAGE

Signs and symptoms of overdosage may be immediate, such as nausea, vomiting, malaise, hypertension, and diaphoresis; or delayed, such as myelosuppression and azotemia.[15] It is not known whether thioguanine is dialyzable. Hemodialysis is thought to be of marginal use due to the rapid intracellular incorporation of thioguanine into active metabolites with long persistence. The oral LD_{50} of thioguanine was determined to be 823 mg/kg ± 50.73 mg/kg and 740 mg/kg ± 45.24 mg/kg for male and female rats, respectively.[16] Symptoms of overdosage may occur after a single dose of as little as 2.0 to 3.0 mg/kg thioguanine. As much as 35 mg/kg has been given in a single oral dose with reversible myelosuppression observed. There is no known pharmacologic antagonist of thioguanine. The drug should be discontinued immediately if unintended toxicity occurs during treatment. Severe hematologic toxicity may require supportive therapy with platelet transfusions for bleeding, and granulocyte transfusions and antibiotics if sepsis is documented. If a patient is seen immediately following an accidental overdosage of the drug, it may be useful to induce emesis.

DOSAGE AND ADMINISTRATION

TABLOID brand Thioguanine is administered orally. The dosage which will be tolerated and effective varies according to the stage and type of neoplastic process being treated. Because the usual therapies for adult and pediatric acute nonlymphocytic leukemias involve the use of thioguanine with other agents in combination, physicians responsible for administering these therapies should be experienced in the use of cancer chemotherapy and in the chosen protocol.

Ninety-six (59%) of 163 pediatric patients with previously untreated acute nonlymphocytic leukemia obtained complete remission with a multiple-drug protocol including thioguanine, prednisone, cytarabine, cyclophosphamide, and vincristine. Remission was maintained with daily thioguanine, 4-day pulses of cytarabine and cyclophosphamide, and a single dose of vincristine every 28 days. The median duration of remission was 11.5 months.[8]

Fifty-three percent of previously untreated adults with acute nonlymphocytic leukemias attained remission following use of the combination of thioguanine and cytarabine according to a protocol developed at The Memorial Sloan-Kettering Cancer Center. A median duration of remission of 8.8 months was achieved with the multiple-drug maintenance regimen which included thioguanine.[9]

On those occasions when single-agent chemotherapy with thioguanine may be appropriate, the usual initial dosage for pediatric patients and adults is approximately 2 mg/kg of body weight per day. If, after 4 weeks on this dosage, there is no clinical improvement and no leukocyte or platelet depression, the dosage may be cautiously increased to 3 mg/kg per day. The total daily dose may be given at one time.

The dosage of thioguanine used does not depend on whether or not the patient is receiving ZYLOPRIM (allopurinol); **this is in contradistinction to the dosage reduction which is mandatory when PURINETHOL (mercaptopurine) or IMURAN (azathioprine) is given simultaneously with allopurinol.**

Procedures for proper handling and disposal of anticancer drugs should be considered. Several guidelines on this subject have been published.[17-23]

There is no general agreement that all of the procedures recommended in the guidelines are necessary or appropriate.

HOW SUPPLIED

Greenish-yellow, scored tablets containing 40 mg thioguanine, imprinted with "WELLCOME" and "U3B" on each tablet; in bottle of 25 (NDC 0173-0880-25).

Store at 15° to 25°C (59° to 77°F) in a dry place.

REFERENCES

1. Hitchings GH, Elion GB. The chemistry and biochemistry of purine analogs. *Ann NY Acad Sci.* 1954;60:195-199.
2. LePage GA, Whitecar JP Jr. Pharmacology of 6-thioguanine in man. *Cancer Res.* 1971;31:1627-1631.
3. Elion GB. Biochemistry and pharmacology of purine analogues. *Fed Proc.* 1967;26:898-904.
4. Miech RP, Parks RE Jr, Anderson JH Jr, Sartorelli AC. An hypothesis on the mechanism of action of 6-thioguanine. *Biochem Pharmacol.* 1967;16:2222-2227.
5. Miller RL, Adamczyk DL, Spector T, Agarwal KC, Miech RP, Panks RE Jr. Reassessment of the interactions of guanylate kinase and 6-thioguanine 5′-phosphate. *Biochem Pharmacol.* 1977;26:1573-1576.
6. Paterson ARP, Tidd DN. 6-Thiopurines. In: Sartorelli AC, Johns DG, eds. *Antineoplastic and Immunosuppressive Agents,* Part II. Berlin: Springer Verlag; 1975:384-403.
7. Nelson JA, Carpenter JW, Rose LM, Adamson DJ. Mechanisms of action of 6-thioguanine, 6-mercaptopurine, and 8-azaguanine. *Cancer Res.* 1975;35:2872-2878.
8. Chard RL Jr, Finklestein JZ, Sonley MJ, et al. Increased survival in childhood acute nonlymphocytic leukemia after treatment with prednisone, cytosine arabinoside, 6-thioguanine, cyclophosphamide, and oncovin (PATCO) combination therapy. *Med Ped Oncol.* 1978;4:263-273.
9. Mertelsmann R, Drapkin RL, Gee TS, et al. Treatment of acute nonlymphocytic leukemia in adults: response to 2,2-anhydro-1-B-D-arabinofuranosyl-5-fluorocytosine and thioguanine on the L-12 protocol. *Cancer.* 1981;48:2136-2142.
10. Thiersch JB. Effect of 2-6 diaminopurine (2-6DP): 6 chlorpurine (CIP) and thioguanine (ThG) on rat litter *in utero. Proc Soc Exp Biol Med.* 1957;94:40-43.
11. Griner PF, Elbadawi A, Packman CH. Veno-occlusive disease of the liver after chemotherapy of acute leukemia: report of two cases. *Ann Intern Med.* 1976;85:578-582.

Continued on next page

This product information is based on labeling in effect on June 1, 1998. For further information, contact via direct mail, phone, or web site Medical Information: Glaxo Wellcome Inc., PO Box 13398, Research Triangle Park, NC 27709. Healthcare Professionals (Medical Information): 800-334-0089 Patients (Customer Response Center): 888-TALK2GW (1-888-825-5249) Glaxo Wellcome Corporate Web Site: www.glaxowellcome.com

Thioguanine, Tabloid Brand—Cont.

12. Gill RA, Onstad GR, Cardamone JM, Maneval DC, Sumner HW. Hepatic veno-occlusive disease caused by 6-thioguanine. *Ann Intern Med.* 1982;96:58-60.
13. Key NS, Kelly PMA, Emerson PM, Chapman RWG, Allan NC, McGee JO'D. Oesophageal varices associated with busulfan-thioguanine combination therapy for chronic myeloid leukaemia. *Lancet.* 1987;2:1050-1052.
14. Clarkson BD, Dowling MD, Gee TS, Cunningham IB, Burchenal JH. Treatment of acute leukemia in adults. *Cancer.* 1975;36:775-795.
15. Presant CA, Denes AE, Klein L, Garrett S, Metter GE. Phase I and preliminary phase II observations of high-dose intermittent 6-thioguanine. *Cancer Treat Rep.* 1980;64:1109-1113.
16. Unpublished data on file with Glaxo Wellcome Inc.
17. Recommendations for the safe handling of parenteral antineoplastic drugs. Washington, DC: Division of Safety, National Institutes of Health; 1983. US Dept of Health and Human Services, Public Health Service publication NIH 83-2621.
18. AMA Council on Scientific Affairs. Guidelines for handling parenteral antineoplastics. *JAMA.* 1985;253: 1590-1591.
19. National Study Commission on Cytotoxic Exposure. Recommendations for handling cytotoxic agents. 1987. Available from Louis P. Jeffrey, Chairman, National Study Commission on Cytotoxic Exposure. Massachusetts College of Pharmacy and Allied Health Sciences, 179 Longwood Avenue, Boston, MA 02115.
20. Clinical Oncological Society of Australia. Guidelines and recommendations for safe handling of antineoplastic agents. *Med J Australia.* 1983;1:426-428.
21. Jones RB, Frank R, Mass T. Safe handling of chemotherapeutic agents: a report from the Mount Sinai Medical Center. *CA—A Cancer J for Clin.* 1983;33:258-263.
22. American Society of Hospital Pharmacists. ASHP technical assistance bulletin on handling cytotoxic and hazardous drugs. *Am J Hosp Pharm.* 1990;47:1033-1049.
23. Yodaiken RE, Bennett D. OSHA work-practice guidelines for personnel dealing with cytotoxic (antineoplastic) drugs. *Am. J Hosp Pharm.* 1986;43:1193-1204.

Glaxo Wellcome Inc. All rights reserved.
November 1996/RL-373
Shown in Product Identification Guide, page 314

TEMOVATE®
[tim 'ō-vāt "]
(clobetasol propionate cream)
Cream, 0.05%

TEMOVATE®
(clobetasol propionate ointment)
Ointment, 0.05%

**For Dermatologic Use Only—
Not for Ophthalmic Use.**

DESCRIPTION

TEMOVATE (clobetasol propionate cream and ointment) Cream and Ointment contain the active compound clobetasol propionate, a synthetic corticosteroid, for topical dermatologic use. Clobetasol, an analog of prednisolone, has a high degree of glucocorticoid activity and a slight degree of mineralocorticoid activity.

Chemically, clobetasol propionate is (11β,16β)-21-chloro-9-fluoro-11-hydroxy-16-methyl -17- (1-oxopropoxy)-pregna-1,4-diene-3,20-dione.

Clobetasol propionate has the empirical formula $C_{25}H_{32}ClFO_5$ and a molecular weight of 467. It is a white to cream-colored crystalline powder insoluble in water.

TEMOVATE Cream contains clobetasol propionate 0.5 mg/g in a cream base of propylene glycol, glyceryl monostearate, cetostearyl alcohol, glyceryl stearate, PEG 100 stearate, white wax, chlorocresol, sodium citrate, citric acid monohydrate, and purified water.

TEMOVATE Ointment contains clobetasol propionate 0.5 mg/g in a base of propylene glycol, sorbitan sesquioleate, and white petrolatum.

CLINICAL PHARMACOLOGY

Like other topical corticosteroids, clobetasol propionate has anti-inflammatory, antipruritic, and vasoconstrictive properties. The mechanism of the anti-inflammatory activity of the topical steroids, in general, is unclear. However, corticosteroids are thought to act by the induction of phospholipase A_2 inhibitory proteins, collectively called lipocortins. It is postulated that these proteins control the biosynthesis of potent mediators of inflammation such as prostaglandins and leukotrienes by inhibiting the release of their common precursor, arachidonic acid. Arachidonic acid is released from membrane phospholipids by phospholipase A_2.

Pharmacokinetics: The extent of percutaneous absorption of topical corticosteroids is determined by many factors, including the vehicle and the integrity of the epidermal barrier. Occlusive dressing with hydrocortisone for up to 24 hours has not been demonstrated to increase penetration; however, occlusion of hydrocortisone for 96 hours markedly enhances penetration. Topical corticosteroids can be absorbed from normal intact skin. Inflammation and/or other disease processes in the skin may increase percutaneous absorption.

Studies performed with TEMOVATE Cream and Ointment indicate that they are in the super-high range of potency as compared with other topical corticosteroids.

INDICATIONS AND USAGE

TEMOVATE Cream and Ointment are super-high potency corticosteroid formulations indicated for the relief of the inflammatory and pruritic manifestations of corticosteroid-responsive dermatoses. Treatment beyond 2 consecutive weeks is not recommended, and the total dosage should not exceed 50 g/week because of the potential for the drug to suppress the hypothalamic-pituitary-adrenal (HPA) axis. Use in children under 12 years of age is not recommended. As with other highly active corticosteroids, therapy should be discontinued when control has been achieved. If no improvement is seen within 2 weeks, reassessment of the diagnosis may be necessary.

CONTRAINDICATIONS

TEMOVATE Cream and Ointment are contraindicated in those patients with a history of hypersensitivity to any of the components of the preparations.

PRECAUTIONS

General: TEMOVATE Cream and Ointment should not be used in the treatment of rosacea or perioral dermatitis, and should not be used on the face, groin, or axillae.

Systemic absorption of topical corticosteroids can produce reversible HPA axis suppression with the potential for glucocorticosteroid insufficiency after withdrawal from treatment. Manifestations of Cushing's syndrome, hyperglycemia, and glucosuria can also be produced in some patients by systemic absorption of topical corticosteroids while on therapy.

Patients applying a topical steroid to a large surface area or to areas under occlusion should be evaluated periodically for evidence of HPA axis suppression. This may be done by using the ACTH stimulation, A.M. plasma cortisol, and urinary free cortisol tests. Patients receiving super-potent corticosteroids should not be treated for more than 2 weeks at a time, and only small areas should be treated at any one time due to the increased risk of HPA suppression.

TEMOVATE Cream and Ointment produced HPA axis suppression when used at doses as low as 2 g/day for 1 week in patients with eczema.

If HPA axis suppression is noted, an attempt should be made to withdraw the drug, to reduce the frequency of application, or to substitute a less potent corticosteroid. Recovery of HPA axis function is generally prompt upon discontinuation of topical corticosteroids. Infrequently, signs and symptoms of glucocorticosteroid insufficiency may occur, requiring supplemental systemic corticosteroids. For information on systemic supplementation, see prescribing information for those products.

Pediatric patients may be more susceptible to systemic toxicity from equivalent doses due to their larger skin surface to body mass ratios (see PRECAUTIONS: Pediatric Use).

If irritation develops, TEMOVATE Cream and Ointment should be discontinued and appropriate therapy instituted. Allergic contact dermatitis with corticosteroids is usually diagnosed by observing *failure to heal* rather than noting a clinical exacerbation as with most topical products not containing corticosteroids. Such an observation should be corroborated with appropriate diagnostic patch testing.

If concomitant skin infections are present or develop, an appropriate antifungal or antibacterial agent should be used. If a favorable response does not occur promptly, use of TEMOVATE Cream and Ointment should be discontinued until the infection has been adequately controlled.

Information for Patients: Patients using topical corticosteroids should receive the following information and instructions:

1. This medication is to be used as directed by the physician. It is for external use only. Avoid contact with the eyes.
2. This medication should not be used for any disorder other than that for which it was prescribed.
3. The treated skin area should not be bandaged, otherwise covered, or wrapped so as to be occlusive unless directed by the physician.
4. Patients should report any signs of local adverse reactions to the physician.

Laboratory Tests: The following tests may be helpful in evaluating patients for HPA axis suppression:
ACTH stimulation test
A.M. plasma cortisol test
Urinary free cortisol test

Carcinogenesis, Mutagenesis, Impairment of Fertility: Long-term animal studies have not been performed to evaluate the carcinogenic potential of clobetasol propionate.

Studies in the rat following oral administration at dosage levels up to 50 mg/kg per day revealed that the females exhibited an increase in the number of resorbed embryos and a decrease in the number of living fetuses at the highest dose.

Clobetasol propionate was nonmutagenic in three different test systems: the Ames test, the *Saccharomyces cerevisiae* gene conversion assay, and the *E. coli* B WP2 fluctuation test.

Pregnancy: *Teratogenic Effects: Pregnancy Category C:* Corticosteroids have been shown to be teratogenic in laboratory animals when administered systemically at relatively low dosage levels. Some corticosteroids have been shown to be teratogenic after dermal application to laboratory animals.

Clobetasol propionate has not been tested for teratogenicity when applied topically; however, it is absorbed percutaneously, and when administered subcutaneously it was a significant teratogen in both the rabbit and mouse. Clobetasol propionate has greater teratogenic potential than steroids that are less potent.

Teratogenicity studies in mice using the subcutaneous route resulted in fetotoxicity at the highest dose tested (1 mg/kg) and teratogenicity at all dose levels tested down to 0.03 mg/kg. These doses are approximately 0.33 and 0.01 times, respectively, the human topical dose of TEMOVATE Cream and Ointment. Abnormalities seen included cleft palate and skeletal abnormalities.

In rabbits, clobetasol propionate was teratogenic at doses of 3 and 10 mcg/kg. These doses are approximately 0.001 and 0.003 times, respectively, the human topical dose of TEMOVATE Cream and Ointment. Abnormalities seen included cleft palate, cranioschisis, and other skeletal abnormalities.

There are no adequate and well-controlled studies of the teratogenic potential of clobetasol propionate in pregnant women. TEMOVATE Cream and Ointment should be used during pregnancy only if the potential benefit justifies the potential risk to the fetus.

Nursing Mothers: Systemically administered corticosteroids appear in human milk and could suppress growth, interfere with endogenous corticosteroid production, or cause other untoward effects. It is not known whether topical administration of corticosteroids could result in sufficient systemic absorption to produce detectable quantities in human milk. Because many drugs are excreted in human milk, caution should be exercised when TEMOVATE Cream or Ointment is administered to a nursing woman.

Pediatric Use: Safety and effectiveness of TEMOVATE in pediatric patients have not been established. Use in children under 12 years of age is not recommended. Because of a higher ratio of skin surface area to body mass, pediatric patients are at a greater risk than adults of HPA axis suppression and Cushing's syndrome when they are treated with topical corticosteroids. They are therefore also at greater risk of adrenal insufficiency during or after withdrawal of treatment. Adverse effects including striae have been reported with inappropriate use of topical corticosteroids in infants and children.

HPA axis suppression, Cushing's syndrome, linear growth retardation, delayed weight gain, and intracranial hypertension have been reported in children receiving topical corticosteroids. Manifestations of adrenal suppression in children include low plasma cortisol levels and an absence of response to ACTH stimulation. Manifestations of intracranial hypertension include bulging fontanelles, headaches, and bilateral papilledema.

ADVERSE REACTIONS

In controlled clinical trials, the most frequent adverse reactions reported for TEMOVATE Cream were burning and stinging sensation in 1% of treated patients. Less frequent adverse reactions were itching, skin atrophy, and cracking and fissuring of the skin.

In controlled clinical trials, the most frequent adverse events reported for TEMOVATE Ointment were burning sensation, irritation, and itching in 0.5% of treated patients. Less frequent adverse reactions were stinging, cracking, erythema, folliculitis, numbness of fingers, skin atrophy, and telangiectasia.

Cushing's syndrome has been reported in infants and adults as a result of prolonged use of topical clobetasol propionate formulations.

The following additional local adverse reactions have been reported with topical corticosteroids, and they may occur more frequently with the use of occlusive dressings and higher potency corticosteroids. These reactions are listed in an approximately decreasing order of occurrence: dryness, acneiform eruptions, hypopigmentation, perioral dermatitis, allergic contact dermatitis, secondary infection, irritation, striae, and miliaria.

OVERDOSAGE

Topically applied TEMOVATE Cream and Ointment can be absorbed in sufficient amounts to produce systemic effects (see PRECAUTIONS).

DOSAGE AND ADMINISTRATION

Apply a thin layer of TEMOVATE Cream or Ointment to the affected skin areas twice daily and rub in gently and completely.

TEMOVATE Cream and Ointment are super-high potency topical corticosteroids; therefore, **treatment should be limited to 2 consecutive weeks, and amounts greater than 50 g/week should not be used.**

As with other highly active corticosteroids, therapy should be discontinued when control has been achieved. If no improvement is seen within 2 weeks, reassessment of diagnosis may be necessary.

TEMOVATE Cream and Ointment should not be used with occlusive dressings.

HOW SUPPLIED

TEMOVATE Cream, 0.05% is supplied in 15-g (NDC 0173-0375-73), 30-g (NDC 0173-0375-72), 45-g (NDC 0173-0375-01), and 60-g (NDC 0173-0375-02) tubes.

TEMOVATE Ointment, 0.05% is supplied in 15-g (NDC 0173-0376-73), 30-g (NDC 0173-0376-72), 45-g (NDC 0173-0376-01), and 60-g (NDC 0173-0376-02) tubes.

Store between 15° and 30°C (59° and 86°F). TEMOVATE Cream should not be refrigerated.

September 1996/RL-356

Shown in Product Identification Guide, page 314

TEMOVATE®

[tim´ō-vāt˝]

(clobetasol propionate gel)

Gel, 0.05%

℞

FOR TOPICAL DERMATOLOGIC USE ONLY— NOT FOR OPHTHALMIC, ORAL, OR INTRAVAGINAL USE

DESCRIPTION

TEMOVATE Gel contains the active compound clobetasol propionate, a synthetic corticosteroid, for topical dermatologic use. Clobetasol, an analog of prednisolone, has a high degree of glucocorticoid activity and a slight degree of mineralocorticoid activity.

Chemically, clobetasol propionate is (11β,16β)-21-chloro-9-fluoro-11-hydroxy-16-methyl-17-(1-oxopropoxy)-pregna-1,4-diene-3,20-dione.

Clobetasol propionate has the empirical formula $C_{25}H_{32}ClFO_5$ and a molecular weight of 467. It is a white to cream-colored crystalline powder insoluble in water.

TEMOVATE Gel contains clobetasol propionate 0.5 mg/g in a base of propylene glycol, carbomer 934P, sodium hydroxide, and purified water.

CLINICAL PHARMACOLOGY

Like other topical corticosteroids, clobetasol propionate has anti-inflammatory, antipruritic, and vasoconstrictive properties. The mechanism of the anti-inflammatory activity of the topical steroids, in general, is unclear. However, corticosteroids are thought to act by the induction of phospholipase A_2 inhibitory proteins, collectively called lipocortins. It is postulated that these proteins control the biosynthesis of potent mediators of inflammation such as prostaglandins and leukotrienes by inhibiting the release of their common precursor, arachidonic acid. Arachidonic acid is released from membrane phospholipids by phospholipase A_2.

Pharmacokinetics: The extent of percutaneous absorption of topical corticosteroids is determined by many factors, including the vehicle and the integrity of the epidermal barrier. Occlusive dressing with hydrocortisone for up to 24 hours has not been demonstrated to increase penetration; however, occlusion of hydrocortisone for 96 hours markedly enhances penetration. Topical corticosteroids can be absorbed from normal intact skin, while inflammation and/or other disease processes in the skin may increase percutaneous absorption. Greater absorption was observed for the TEMOVATE gel formulation as compared to the cream formulation in in vitro human skin penetration studies.

Studies performed with TEMOVATE Gel indicate that it is in the super-high range of potency as compared with other topical corticosteroids.

INDICATIONS AND USAGE

TEMOVATE Gel is a super-high potency corticosteroid formulation indicated for the relief of the inflammatory and pruritic manifestations of corticosteroid-responsive dermatoses. Treatment beyond 2 consecutive weeks is not recommended, and the total dosage should not exceed 50 g/week because of the potential for the drug to suppress the hypothalamic-pituitary-adrenal (HPA) axis. Use in children under 12 years of age is not recommended.

CONTRAINDICATIONS

TEMOVATE Gel is contraindicated in those patients with a history of hypersensitivity to any of the components of the preparation.

PRECAUTIONS

General: Clobetasol propionate is a highly potent topical corticosteroid that has been shown to suppress the HPA axis at doses as low as 2 g/day.

Systemic absorption of topical corticosteroids can produce reversible HPA axis suppression with the potential for glucocorticosteroid insufficiency after withdrawal from treatment. Manifestations of Cushing's syndrome, hyperglycemia, and glucosuria can also be produced in some patients by systemic absorption of topical corticosteroids while on therapy.

Patients receiving a large dose applied to a large surface area should be evaluated periodically for evidence of HPA axis suppression. This may be done by using the ACTH stimulation, A.M. plasma cortisol, and urinary free cortisol tests. Patients receiving super-potent corticosteroids should not be treated for more than 2 weeks at a time, and only small areas should be treated at any one time due to the increased risk of HPA suppression.

If HPA axis suppression is noted, an attempt should be made to withdraw the drug, to reduce the frequency of application, or to substitute a less potent corticosteroid. Recovery of HPA axis function is generally prompt and complete upon discontinuation of topical corticosteroids. Infrequently, signs and symptoms of glucocorticosteroid insufficiency may occur that require supplemental systemic corticosteroids. For information on systemic supplementation, see prescribing information for those products.

Children may be more susceptible to systemic toxicity from equivalent doses due to their larger skin surface to body mass ratios (see PRECAUTIONS: Pediatric Use).

If irritation develops, TEMOVATE Gel should be discontinued and appropriate therapy instituted. Allergic contact dermatitis with corticosteroids is usually diagnosed by observing *failure to heal* rather than noting a clinical exacerbation as with most topical products not containing corticosteroids. Such an observation should be corroborated with appropriate diagnostic patch testing.

If concomitant skin infections are present or develop, an appropriate antifungal or antibacterial agent should be used. If a favorable response does not occur promptly, use of TEMOVATE Gel should be discontinued until the infection has been adequately controlled.

TEMOVATE Gel should not be used in the treatment of rosacea or perioral dermatitis, and should not be used on the face, groin, or axillae.

Information for Patients: Patients using topical corticosteroids should receive the following information and instructions:

1. This medication is to be used as directed by the physician. It is for external use only. Avoid contact with the eyes.

2. This medication should not be used for any disorder other than that for which it was prescribed.

3. The treated skin area should not be bandaged or otherwise covered or wrapped so as to be occlusive unless directed by the physician.

4. Patients should report any signs of local adverse reactions to the physician.

5. Patients should inform their physicians that they are using TEMOVATE if surgery is contemplated.

Laboratory Tests: The following tests may be helpful in evaluating patients for HPA axis suppression:

ACTH stimulation test

A.M. plasma cortisol test

Urinary free cortisol test

Carcinogenesis, Mutagenesis, Impairment of Fertility: Long-term animal studies have not been performed to evaluate the carcinogenic potential of clobetasol propionate.

Studies in the rat following oral administration at dosage levels up to 50 mg/kg per day revealed no significant effect on the males. The females exhibited an increase in the number of resorbed embryos and a decrease in the number of living fetuses at the highest dose.

Clobetasol propionate was nonmutagenic in three different test systems: the Ames test, the *Saccharomyces cerevisiae* gene conversion assay, and the *E. coli* B WP2 fluctuation test.

Pregnancy: *Teratogenic Effects: Pregnancy Category C:* Corticosteroids have been shown to be teratogenic in laboratory animals when administered systemically at relatively low dosage levels. Some corticosteroids have been shown to be teratogenic after dermal application to laboratory animals.

Clobetasol propionate has not been tested for teratogenicity by this route; however, it is absorbed percutaneously, and when administered subcutaneously it was a significant teratogen in both the rabbit and mouse. Clobetasol propionate has greater teratogenic potential than steroids that are less potent.

Teratogenicity studies in mice using the subcutaneous route resulted in fetotoxicity at the highest dose tested (1 mg/kg) and teratogenicity at all dose levels tested down to 0.03 mg/kg. These doses are approximately 0.33 and 0.01 times, re-

spectively, the human topical dose of TEMOVATE Gel. Abnormalities seen included cleft palate and skeletal abnormalities.

In rabbits, clobetasol propionate given by the same route was teratogenic at doses of 3 and 10 mcg/kg. These doses are approximately 0.001 and 0.003 times, respectively, the human topical dose of TEMOVATE Gel. Abnormalities seen included cleft palate, cranioschisis, and other skeletal abnormalities.

There are no adequate and well-controlled studies of the teratogenic potential of clobetasol propionate in pregnant women. TEMOVATE Gel should be used during pregnancy only if the potential benefit justifies the potential risk to the fetus.

Nursing Mothers: Systemically administered corticosteroids appear in human milk and could suppress growth, interfere with endogenous corticosteroid production, or cause other untoward effects. It is not known whether topical administration of corticosteroids could result in sufficient systemic absorption to produce detectable quantities in human milk. Because many drugs are excreted in human milk, caution should be exercised when TEMOVATE Gel is administered to a nursing woman.

Pediatric Use: Safety and effectiveness of TEMOVATE Gel in children and infants have not been established; therefore, use in children under 12 years of age is not recommended. Because of a higher ratio of skin surface area to body mass, children are at a greater risk than adults of HPA axis suppression when they are treated with topical corticosteroids. They are therefore also at greater risk of glucocorticosteroid insufficiency after withdrawal of treatment and of Cushing's syndrome while on treatment. Adverse effects including striae have been reported with inappropriate use of topical corticosteroids in infants and children (see PRECAUTIONS).

HPA axis suppression, Cushing's syndrome, and intracranial hypertension have been reported in children receiving topical corticosteroids. Manifestations of adrenal suppression in children include linear growth retardation, delayed weight gain, low plasma cortisol levels, and absence of response to ACTH stimulation. Manifestations of intracranial hypertension include bulging fontanelles, headaches, and bilateral papilledema.

ADVERSE REACTIONS

In a controlled trial with TEMOVATE Gel, the only reported adverse reaction that was considered to be drug related was a report of burning sensation (1.8% of treated patients).

In larger controlled clinical trials with other clobetasol propionate formulations, the most frequently reported adverse reactions have included burning, stinging, irritation, pruritus, erythema, folliculitis, cracking and fissuring of the skin, numbness of fingers, skin atrophy, and telangiectasia (all less than 2%).

Cushing's syndrome has been reported in infants and adults as a result of prolonged use of topical clobetasol propionate formulations.

The following additional local adverse reactions are reported infrequently with topical corticosteroids, but may occur more frequently with super-high potency corticosteroids such as TEMOVATE Gel. These reactions are listed in approximate decreasing order of occurrence: dryness, hypertrichosis, acneiform eruptions, hypopigmentation, perioral dermatitis, allergic contact dermatitis, secondary infection, irritation, striae, and miliaria.

OVERDOSAGE

Topically applied TEMOVATE Gel can be absorbed in sufficient amounts to produce systemic effects (see PRECAUTIONS).

DOSAGE AND ADMINISTRATION

Apply a thin layer of TEMOVATE Gel to the affected skin areas twice daily and rub in gently and completely (see INDICATIONS AND USAGE).

TEMOVATE Gel is a super-high potency topical corticosteroid; therefore, **treatment should be limited to 2 consecutive weeks, and amounts greater than 50 g/week should not be used.**

As with other highly active corticosteroids, therapy should be discontinued when control has been achieved. If no improvement is seen within 2 weeks, reassessment of diagnosis may be necessary.

TEMOVATE Gel should not be used with occlusive dressings.

Continued on next page

This product information is based on labeling in effect on June 1, 1998. For further information, contact via direct mail, phone, or web site Medical Information: Glaxo Wellcome Inc., PO Box 13398, Research Triangle Park, NC 27709. Healthcare Professionals (Medical Information): 800-334-0089 Patients (Customer Response Center): 888-TALK2GW (1-888-825-5249) Glaxo Wellcome Corporate Web Site: www.glaxowellcome.com

Temovate Gel—Cont.

HOW SUPPLIED

TEMOVATE Gel, 0.05% is supplied in 15-g (NDC 0173-0455-01), 30-g (NDC 0173-0455-02), and 60-g (NDC 0173-0455-03) tubes.
Store between 15° and 30°C (59° and 86°F). TEMOVATE Gel should not be refrigerated.
September 1996/RL-357
Shown in Product Identification Guide, page 314

TEMOVATE®   ℞
[*tim 'ō-vāt "*]
(clobetasol propionate scalp application)
Scalp Application, 0.05%

For Dermatologic Use Only—
Not for Ophthalmic Use.

DESCRIPTION

TEMOVATE Scalp Application contains the active compound clobetasol propionate, a synthetic corticosteroid, for topical dermatologic use. Clobetasol, an analog of prednisolone, has a high degree of glucocorticoid activity and a slight degree of mineralocorticoid activity.
Chemically, clobetasol propionate is (11β,16β)-21-chloro-9-fluoro-11-hydroxy-16-methyl-17-(1-oxopropoxy)pregna-1,4-diene-3,20-dione.
Clobetasol propionate has the empirical formula $C_{25}H_{32}ClFO_5$ and a molecular weight of 467. It is a white to cream-colored crystalline powder insoluble in water.
TEMOVATE Scalp Application contains clobetasol propionate 0.5 mg/g in a base composed of purified water, isopropyl alcohol (39.3%), carbomer 934P, and sodium hydroxide.

CLINICAL PHARMACOLOGY

The corticosteroids are a class of compounds comprising steroid hormones secreted by the adrenal cortex and their synthetic analogs. In pharmacologic doses, corticosteroids are used primarily for their anti-inflammatory and/or immunosuppressive effects. Topical corticosteroids such as clobetasol propionate are effective in the treatment of corticosteroid-responsive dermatoses primarily because of their anti-inflammatory, antipruritic, and vasoconstrictive actions. However, while the physiologic, pharmacologic, and clinical effects of the corticosteroids are well known, the exact mechanisms of their actions in each disease are uncertain. Clobetasol propionate, a corticosteroid, has been shown to have topical (dermatologic) and systemic pharmacologic and metabolic effects characteristic of this class of drugs.
Pharmacokinetics: The extent of percutaneous absorption of topical corticosteroids, including clobetasol propionate, is determined by many factors, including the vehicle, the integrity of the epidermal barrier, and the use of occlusive dressings (see DOSAGE AND ADMINISTRATION).
As with all topical corticosteroids, clobetasol propionate can be absorbed from normal intact skin. Inflammation and/or other disease processes in the skin may increase percutaneous absorption. Occlusive dressings substantially increase the percutaneous absorption of topical corticosteroids (see DOSAGE AND ADMINISTRATION).
Once absorbed through the skin, topical corticosteroids enter pharmacokinetic pathways similarly to systemically administered corticosteroids. Corticosteroids are bound to plasma proteins in varying degrees. Corticosteroids are metabolized primarily in the liver and are then excreted by the kidneys. Some of the topical corticosteroids, including clobetasol propionate and its metabolites, are also excreted into the bile.
Following repeated nonocclusive application in the treatment of scalp psoriasis, there is some evidence that TEMOVATE Scalp Application has the potential to depress plasma cortisol levels in some patients. However, hypothalamic-pituitary-adrenal (HPA) axis effects produced by systemically absorbed clobetasol propionate have been shown to be transient and reversible upon completion of a 2-week course of treatment.

INDICATIONS AND USAGE

TEMOVATE Scalp Application is indicated for short-term topical treatment of inflammatory and pruritic manifestations of moderate to severe corticosteroid-responsive dermatoses of the scalp. Treatment beyond 2 consecutive weeks is not recommended, and the total dosage should not exceed 50 mL per week because of the potential for the drug to suppress the HPA axis.
This product is not recommended for use in children under 12 years of age.

CONTRAINDICATIONS

TEMOVATE Scalp Application is contraindicated in patients with primary infections of the scalp, or in patients who are hypersensitive to clobetasol propionate, other corticosteroids, or any ingredient in this preparation.

PRECAUTIONS

General: Clobetasol propionate is a highly potent topical corticosteroid that has been shown to suppress the HPA axis at doses as low as 2 g (of ointment) per day. Systemic absorption of topical corticosteroids has resulted in reversible HPA axis suppression, manifestations of Cushing's syndrome, hyperglycemia, and glucosuria in some patients.
Conditions that augment systemic absorption include the application of the more potent corticosteroids, use over large surface areas, prolonged use, and the addition of occlusive dressings. Therefore, patients receiving a large dose of a potent topical steroid applied to a large surface area should be evaluated periodically for evidence of HPA axis suppression by using the urinary free cortisol and ACTH stimulation tests. If HPA axis suppression is noted, an attempt should be made to withdraw the drug, to reduce the frequency of application, or to substitute a less potent steroid.
Recovery of HPA axis function is generally prompt and complete upon discontinuation of the drug. Infrequently, signs and symptoms of steroid withdrawal may occur, requiring supplemental systemic corticosteroids.
Children may absorb proportionally larger amounts of topical corticosteroids and thus be more susceptible to systemic toxicity (see PRECAUTIONS: Pediatric Use).
If irritation develops, topical corticosteroids should be discontinued and appropriate therapy instituted. Irritation is possible if TEMOVATE Scalp Application contacts the eye. If that should occur, immediate flushing of the eye with a large volume of water is recommended.
If the inflammatory lesion becomes infected, the use of an appropriate antifungal or antibacterial agent should be instituted. If a favorable response does not occur promptly, the corticosteroid should be discontinued until the infection has been adequately controlled.
Although TEMOVATE Scalp Application is intended for the treatment of inflammatory conditions of the scalp, it should be noted that certain areas of the body, such as the face, groin, and axillae, are more prone to atrophic changes than other areas of the body following treatment with corticosteroids. Frequent observation of the patient is important if these areas are to be treated.
As with other potent topical corticosteroids, TEMOVATE Scalp Application should not be used in the treatment of rosacea and perioral dermatitis. Topical corticosteroids in general should not be used in the treatment of acne or as sole therapy in widespread plaque psoriasis.
Information For Patients: Patients using TEMOVATE Scalp Application should receive the following information and instructions:

1. This medication is to be used as directed by the physician and should not be used longer than the prescribed time period. It is for external use only. Avoid contact with the eyes.
2. This medication should not be used for any disorder other than that for which it was prescribed.
3. The treated skin area should not be bandaged or otherwise covered or wrapped so as to be occlusive.
4. Patients should report any signs of local adverse reactions to the physician.

Laboratory Tests: The following tests may be helpful in evaluating HPA axis suppression:
Urinary free cortisol test
ACTH stimulation test
Carcinogenesis, Mutagenesis, Impairment of Fertility: Long-term animal studies have not been performed to evaluate the carcinogenic potential or the effect on fertility of topical corticosteroids.
Studies to determine mutagenicity with prednisolone have revealed negative results.
Pregnancy: *Teratogenic Effects: Pregnancy Category C:* The more potent corticosteroids have been shown to be teratogenic in animals after dermal application. Clobetasol propionate has not been tested for teratogenicity by this route; however, it is absorbed percutaneously, and when administered subcutaneously it was a significant teratogen in both the rabbit and the mouse. Clobetasol propionate has greater teratogenic potential than steroids that are less potent.
There are no adequate and well-controlled studies of the teratogenic effects of topically applied corticosteroids, including clobetasol, in pregnant women. Therefore, clobetasol and other topical corticosteroids should be used during pregnancy only if the potential benefit justifies the potential risk to the fetus, and they should not be used extensively on pregnant patients, in large amounts, or for prolonged periods of time.
Nursing Mothers: It is not known whether topical administration of corticosteroids could result in sufficient systemic absorption to produce detectable quantities in breast milk. Systemically administered corticosteroids are secreted into breast milk in quantities not likely to have a deleterious effect on the infant. Nevertheless, caution should be exercised when topical corticosteroids are prescribed for a nursing woman.

Pediatric Use: Use of TEMOVATE Scalp Application in children under 12 years of age is not recommended.
Pediatric patients may demonstrate greater susceptibility to topical corticosteroid-induced HPA axis suppression and Cushing's syndrome than mature patients because of a larger skin surface area to body weight ratio.
HPA axis suppression, Cushing's syndrome, and intracranial hypertension have been reported in children receiving topical corticosteroids. Manifestations of adrenal suppression in children include linear growth retardation, delayed weight gain, low plasma cortisol levels, and absence of response to ACTH stimulation. Manifestations of intracranial hypertension include bulging fontanelles, headaches, and bilateral papilledema.

ADVERSE REACTIONS

TEMOVATE Scalp Application is generally well tolerated when used for 2-week treatment periods.
The most frequent adverse events reported for TEMOVATE Scalp Application have been local and have included burning and/or stinging sensation, which occurred in 29 of 294 patients; scalp pustules, which occurred in 3 of 294 patients; and tingling and folliculitis, each of which occurred in 2 of 294 patients. Less frequent adverse events were itching and tightness of the scalp, dermatitis, tenderness, headache, hair loss, and eye irritation, each of which occurred in 1 of 294 patients.
The following local adverse reactions are reported infrequently when topical corticosteroids are used as recommended. These reactions are listed in an approximately decreasing order of occurrence: burning, itching, irritation, dryness, folliculitis, hypertrichosis, acneiform eruptions, hypopigmentation, perioral dermatitis, allergic contact dermatitis, maceration of the skin, secondary infection, skin atrophy, striae, and miliaria. Systemic absorption of topical corticosteroids has produced reversible HPA axis suppression, manifestations of Cushing's syndrome, hyperglycemia, and glucosuria in some patients. In rare instances, treatment (or withdrawal of treatment) of psoriasis with corticosteroids is thought to have exacerbated the disease or provoked the pustular form of the disease, so careful patient supervision is recommended.

OVERDOSAGE

Topically applied TEMOVATE Scalp Application can be absorbed in sufficient amounts to produce systemic effects (see PRECAUTIONS).

DOSAGE AND ADMINISTRATION

TEMOVATE Scalp Application should be applied to the affected scalp areas twice daily, once in the morning and once at night.
TEMOVATE Scalp Application is potent; therefore, **treatment must be limited to 2 consecutive weeks, and amounts greater than 50 mL per week should not be used. TEMOVATE Scalp Application is not to be used with occlusive dressings.**

HOW SUPPLIED

TEMOVATE Scalp Application, 0.05% is supplied in plastic squeeze bottles, 25 mL (NDC 0173-0432-00) and 50 mL (NDC 0173-0432-01).
Store between 4° and 25°C (39° and 77°F). Do not use near an open flame.
September 1996/RL-354
Shown in Product Identification Guide, page 314

TEMOVATE E®   ℞
[*tim 'ō-vāt "*]
(clobetasol propionate emollient cream)
Emollient, 0.05%

FOR TOPICAL DERMATOLOGIC USE ONLY—NOT FOR OPHTHALMIC, ORAL, OR INTRAVAGINAL USE

DESCRIPTION

TEMOVATE E Emollient contains the active compound clobetasol propionate, a synthetic corticosteroid, for topical dermatologic use. Clobetasol, an analog of prednisolone, has a high degree of glucocorticoid activity and a slight degree of mineralocorticoid activity.
Chemically, clobetasol propionate is (11β,16β)-21-chloro-9-fluoro-11-hydroxy-16-methyl-17-(1-oxopropoxy)-pregna-1,4-diene-3,20-dione.
Clobetasol propionate has the empirical formula $C_{25}H_{32}ClFO_5$ and a molecular weight of 467. It is a white to cream-colored crystalline powder insoluble in water.
TEMOVATE E Emollient contains clobetasol propionate 0.5 mg/g in an emollient base of cetostearyl alcohol, isopropyl myristate, propylene glycol, cetomacrogol 1000, dimethicone 360, citric acid, sodium citrate, purified water, and imidurea as a preservative.

CLINICAL PHARMACOLOGY

Like other topical corticosteroids, clobetasol propionate has anti-inflammatory, antipruritic, and vasoconstrictive prop-

erties. The mechanism of the anti-inflammatory activity of the topical steroids, in general, is unclear. However, corticosteroids are thought to act by the induction of phospholipase A_2 inhibitory proteins, collectively called lipocortins. It is postulated that these proteins control the biosynthesis of potent mediators of inflammation such as prostaglandins and leukotrienes by inhibiting the release of their common precursor, arachidonic acid. Arachidonic acid is released from membrane phospholipids by phospholipase A_2.

Pharmacokinetics: The extent of percutaneous absorption of topical corticosteroids is determined by many factors, including the vehicle and the integrity of the epidermal barrier. Occlusive dressing with hydrocortisone for up to 24 hours has not been demonstrated to increase penetration; however, occlusion of hydrocortisone for 96 hours markedly enhances penetration. Topical corticosteroids can be absorbed from normal intact skin. Inflammation and/or other disease processes in the skin may increase percutaneous absorption.

Studies performed with TEMOVATE E Emollient indicate that it is in the super-high range of potency as compared with other topical corticosteroids.

INDICATIONS AND USAGE

TEMOVATE E Emollient is a super-high potency corticosteroid formulation indicated for the relief of the inflammatory and pruritic manifestations of corticosteroid-responsive dermatoses. Treatment beyond 2 consecutive weeks is not recommended, and the total dosage should not exceed 50 g/week because of the potential for the drug to suppress the hypothalamic-pituitary-adrenal (HPA) axis. Use in children under 12 years of age is not recommended.

In the treatment of moderate to severe plaque-type psoriasis, TEMOVATE E Emollient applied to 5% to 10% of body surface area can be used up to 4 consecutive weeks. The total dosage should not exceed 50 g/week. When dosing for more than 2 weeks, any additional benefits of extending treatment should be weighed against the risk of HPA suppression. Treatment beyond 4 consecutive weeks is not recommended. Patients should be instructed to use TEMOVATE E Emollient for the minimum amount of time necessary to achieve the desired results (see PRECAUTIONS and INDICATIONS AND USAGE). Use in pediatric patients under 16 years of age has not been studied.

CONTRAINDICATIONS

TEMOVATE E Emollient is contraindicated in those patients with a history of hypersensitivity to any of the components of the preparation.

PRECAUTIONS

General: Clobetasol propionate is a highly potent topical corticosteroid that has been shown to suppress the HPA axis at doses as low as 2 g/day.

Systemic absorption of topical corticosteroids can produce reversible HPA axis suppression with the potential for glucocorticosteroid insufficiency after withdrawal from treatment. Manifestations of Cushing's syndrome, hyperglycemia, and glucosuria can also be produced in some patients by systemic absorption of topical corticosteroids while on therapy.

Patients applying a dose to a large surface area or to areas under occlusion should be evaluated periodically for evidence of HPA axis suppression. This may be done by using the ACTH stimulation, A.M. plasma cortisol, and urinary free cortisol tests. Patients receiving super-potent corticosteroids should not be treated for more than 2 weeks at a time, and only small areas should be treated at any one time due to the increased risk of HPA suppression.

In a controlled clinical trial involving patients with moderate to severe plaque-type psoriasis, TEMOVATE E Emollient applied to 5% to 10% of body surface area resulted in additional benefits in the treatment of patients for 4 consecutive weeks. In this trial, there were no clobetasol-treated patients with clinically significant decreases in morning cortisol levels after 4 weeks of treatment; however, morning cortisol levels may not identify patients with adrenal dysfunction. Therefore, the additional benefits of extending treatment beyond 2 weeks should be weighed against the potential for HPA suppression. Therapy should be discontinued when control has been achieved. Treatment beyound 4 consecutive weeks is not recommended.

If HPA axis suppression is noted, an attempt should be made to withdraw the drug, to reduce the frequency of application, or to substitute a less potent corticosteroid. Recovery of HPA axis function is generally prompt upon discontinuation of topical corticosteroids. Infrequently, signs and symptoms of glucocorticosteroid insufficiency may occur that require supplemental systemic corticosteroids. For information on systemic supplementation, see prescribing information for those products.

Pediatric patients may be more susceptible to systemic toxicity from equivalent doses due to their larger skin surface to body mass ratios (see PRECAUTIONS: Pediatric Use). The use of TEMOVATE E Emollient for 4 consecutive weeks has not been studied in pediatric patients under 16 years of age.

If irritation develops, TEMOVATE E Emollient should be discontinued and appropriate therapy instituted. Allergic contact dermatitis with corticosteroids is usually diagnosed by observing *failure to heal* rather than noting a clinical exacerbation as with most topical products not containing corticosteroids. Such an observation should be corroborated with appropriate diagnostic patch testing.

If concomitant skin infections are present or develop, an appropriate antifungal or antibacterial agent should be used. If a favorable response does not occur promptly, use of TEMOVATE E Emollient should be discontinued until the infection has been adequately controlled.

TEMOVATE E Emollient should not be used in the treatment of rosacea or perioral dermatitis, and should not be used on the face, groin, or axillae.

Information for Patients: Patients using topical corticosteroids should receive the following information and instructions:

1. This medication is to be used as directed by the physician. It is for external use only. Avoid contact with the eyes.
2. This medication should not be used for any disorder other than that for which it was prescribed.
3. The treated skin area should not be bandaged, otherwise covered, or wrapped so as to be occlusive unless directed by the physician.
4. Patients should report any signs of local adverse reactions to the physician.
5. Patients should inform their physicians that they are using TEMOVATE if surgery is contemplated.
6. This medication should not be used on the face, underarms, or groin areas.
7. As with other corticosteroids, therapy should be discontinued when control has been achieved. If no improvement is seen within 2 weeks, contact the physician.

Laboratory Tests: The following tests may be helpful in evaluating patients for HPA axis suppression:

ACTH stimulation test
A.M. plasma cortisol test
Urinary free cortisol test

Carcinogenesis, Mutagenesis, Impairment of Fertility: Long-term animal studies have not been performed to evaluate the carcinogenic potential of clobetasol propionate.

Studies in the rat following oral administration at dosage levels up to 50 mg/kg per day revealed no significant effect on the males. The females exhibited an increase in the number of resorbed embryos and a decrease in the number of living fetuses at the highest dose.

Clobetasol propionate was nonmutagenic in three different test systems: the Ames test, the *Saccharomyces cerevisiae* gene conversion assay, and the *E. coli* B WP2 fluctuation test.

Pregnancy: ***Teratogenic Effects: Pregnancy Category C:*** Corticosteroids have been shown to be teratogenic in laboratory animals when administered systemically at relatively low dosage levels. Some corticosteroids have been shown to be teratogenic after dermal application to laboratory animals.

Clobetasol propionate has not been tested for teratogenicity by this route; however, it is absorbed percutaneously, and when administered subcutaneously it was a significant teratogen in both the rabbit and mouse. Clobetasol propionate has greater teratogenic potential than steroids that are less potent.

Teratogenicity studies in mice using the subcutaneous route resulted in fetotoxicity at the highest dose tested (1 mg/kg) and teratogenicity at all dose levels tested down to 0.03 mg/kg. These doses are approximately 0.33 and 0.01 times, respectively, the human topical dose of TEMOVATE E Emollient. Abnormalities seen included cleft palate and skeletal abnormalities.

In rabbits, clobetasol propionate was teratogenic at doses of 3 and 10 mcg/kg. These doses are approximately 0.001 and 0.003 times, respectively, the human topical dose of TEMOVATE E Emollient. Abnormalities seen included cleft palate, cranioschisis, and other skeletal abnormalities.

There are no adequate and well-controlled studies of the teratogenic potential of clobetasol propionate in pregnant women. TEMOVATE E Emollient should be used during pregnancy only if the potential benefit justifies the potential risk to the fetus.

Nursing Mothers: Systemically administered corticosteroids appear in human milk and could suppress growth, interfere with endogenous corticosteroid production, or cause other untoward effects. It is not known whether topical administration of corticosteroids could result in sufficient systemic absorption to produce detectable quantities in human milk. Because many drugs are excreted in human milk, caution should be exercised when TEMOVATE E Emollient is administered to a nursing woman.

Pediatric Use: Safety and effectiveness of TEMOVATE E Emollient in pediatric patients have not been established, and its use in pediatric patients under 12 years of age is not recommended. For continued use beyond 2 consecutive weeks, the safety of TEMOVATE E Emollient has not been studied. Because of a higher ratio of skin surface area to body mass, pediatric patients are at a greater risk than adults of HPA axis suppression and Cushing's syndrome when they are treated with topical corticosteroids. They are therefore also at greater risk of glucocorticosteroid insufficiency during or after withdrawal of treatment. Adverse effects including striae have been reported with inappropriate use of topical corticosteroids in infants and children.

HPA axis suppression, Cushing's syndrome, linear growth retardation, delayed weight gain, and intracranial hypertension have been reported in children receiving topical corticosteroids. Manifestations of adrenal suppression in children include low plasma cortisol levels and absence of response to ACTH stimulation. Manifestations of intracranial hypertension include bulging fontanelles, headaches, and bilateral papilledema.

ADVERSE REACTIONS

In controlled trials with all clobetasol propionate formulations, the following adverse reactions have been reported: burning/stinging, pruritus, irritation, erythema, folliculitis, cracking and fissuring of the skin, numbness of the fingers, tenderness in the elbow, skin atrophy, and telangiectasia. The incidence of local adverse reactions reported in the trials with TEMOVATE E Emollient was <2% of patients treated with the exception of burning/stinging, which occured in 5% of treated patients.

Cushing's syndrome has been reported in infants and adults as a result of prolonged use of topical clobetasol propionate formulations.

The following additional local adverse reactions are reported infrequently with topical corticosteroids, but may occur more frequently with super-high potency corticosteroids such as TEMOVATE E Emollient. These reactions are listed in an approximately decreasing order of occurrence: dryness, hypertrichosis, acneiform eruptions, hypopigmentation, perioral dermatitis, allergic contact dermatitis, secondary infection, striae, and miliaria.

OVERDOSAGE

Topically applied TEMOVATE E Emollient can be absorbed in sufficient amounts to produce systemic effects.

DOSAGE AND ADMINISTRATION

Apply a thin layer of TEMOVATE E Emollient to the affected skin areas twice daily and rub in gently and completely (see INDICATIONS AND USAGE).

TEMOVATE E Emollient is a super-high potency topical corticosteroid; therefore, **treatment should be limited to 2 consecutive weeks and amounts greater than 50 g/week should not be used.** Use in children under 12 years of age is not recommended.

In moderate to severe plaque-type psoriasis, TEMOVATE E Emollient applied to 5% to 10% of body surface area can be used up to 4 weeks. The total dosage should not exceed 50 g/week. When dosing for more than 2 weeks, any additional benefits of extending treatment should be weighed against the risk of HPA suppression. Therapy should be discontinued when control has been achieved. If no improvement is seen within 2 weeks, reassessment of diagnosis may be necessary. Treatment beyond 4 consecutive weeks is not recommended. Use in pediatric patients under 16 years of age has not been studied.

TEMOVATE E Emollient should not be used with occlusive dressings.

HOW SUPPLIED

TEMOVATE E Emollient, 0.05% is supplied in 15-g (NDC 0173-0454-01), 30-g (NDC 0173-0454-02), and 60-g (NDC 0173-0454-03) tubes.

Store between 15° and 30°C (59° and 86°F). TEMOVATE E Emollient should not be refrigerated.

May 1997/RL-435

Shown in Product Identification Guide, page 314

TRACRIUM® ℞

[*trā ˈkrē ″um*]
(atracurium besylate)
Injection

This drug should be used only by adequately trained individuals familiar with its actions, characteristics, and hazards.

DESCRIPTION

TRACRIUM (atracurium besylate) is an intermediate-duration, nondepolarizing, skeletal muscle relaxant for intrave-

Continued on next page

This product information is based on labeling in effect on June 1, 1998. For further information, contact via direct mail, phone, or web site Medical Information: Glaxo Wellcome Inc., PO Box 13398, Research Triangle Park, NC 27709. Healthcare Professionals (Medical Information): 800-334-0089 Patients (Customer Response Center): 888-TALK2GW (1-888-825-5249) Glaxo Wellcome Corporate Web Site: www.glaxowellcome.com

Tracrium—Cont.

nous administration. Atracurium besylate is designated as 2,2′-[1,5 - pentanediylbis[oxy(3 - oxo-3,1- propanediyl)]]-bis[1-[(3,4 - dimethoxyphenyl)methyl] - 1,2,3,4 -tetrahydro - 6,7-dimethoxy-2-methylisoquinolinium] dibenzenesulfonate. It has a molecular weight of 1243.51, and its molecular formula is $C_{65}H_{82}N_2O_{18}S_2$.
Atracurium besylate is a complex molecule containing four sites at which different stereochemical configurations can occur. The symmetry of the molecule, however, results in only ten, instead of sixteen, possible different isomers. The manufacture of atracurium besylate results in these isomers being produced in unequal amounts but with a consistent ratio. Those molecules in which the methyl group attached to the quaternary nitrogen projects on the opposite side to the adjacent substituted-benzyl moiety predominate by approximately 3:1.
TRACRIUM Injection is a sterile, nonpyrogenic aqueous solution. Each mL contains 10 mg atracurium besylate. The pH is adjusted to 3.25 to 3.65 with benzenesulfonic acid. The multiple-dose vial contains 0.9% benzyl alcohol added as a preservative. TRACRIUM slowly loses potency with time at the rate of approximately 6% per *year* under refrigeration (5°C). TRACRIUM Injection should be refrigerated at 2° to 8°C (36° to 46°F) to preserve potency. Rate of loss in potency increases to approximately 5% per *month* at 25°C (77°F). Upon removal from refrigeration to room temperature storage conditions (25°C/77°F), use TRACRIUM Injection within 14 days even if rerefrigerated.

CLINICAL PHARMACOLOGY

TRACRIUM is a nondepolarizing skeletal muscle relaxant. Nondepolarizing agents antagonize the neurotransmitter action of acetylcholine by binding competitively with cholinergic receptor sites on the motor end-plate. This antagonism is inhibited, and neuromuscular block reversed, by acetylcholinesterase inhibitors such as neostigmine, edrophonium, and pyridostigmine.
TRACRIUM can be used most advantageously if muscle twitch response to peripheral nerve stimulation is monitored to assess degree of muscle relaxation.
The duration of neuromuscular block produced by TRACRIUM is approximately one third to one half the duration of block by d-tubocurarine, metocurine, and pancuronium at initially equipotent doses. As with other nondepolarizing neuromuscular blockers, the time to onset of paralysis decreases and the duration of maximum effect increases with increasing doses of TRACRIUM.
The ED_{95} (dose required to produce 95% suppression of the muscle twitch response with balanced anesthesia) has averaged 0.23 mg/kg (0.11 to 0.26 mg/kg in various studies). An initial dose of TRACRIUM of 0.4 to 0.5 mg/kg generally produces maximum neuromuscular block within 3 to 5 minutes of injection, with good or excellent intubation conditions within 2 to 2.5 minutes in most patients. Recovery from neuromuscular block (under balanced anesthesia) can be expected to begin approximately 20 to 35 minutes after injection. Under balanced anesthesia, recovery to 25% of control is achieved approximately 35 to 45 minutes after injection, and recovery is usually 95% complete approximately 60 to 70 minutes after injection. The neuromuscular blocking action of TRACRIUM is enhanced in the presence of potent inhalation anesthetics. Isoflurane and enflurane increase the potency of TRACRIUM and prolong neuromuscular block by approximately 35%; however, halothane's potentiating effect (approximately 20%) is marginal (see DOSAGE AND ADMINISTRATION).
Repeated administration of maintenance doses of TRACRIUM has no cumulative effect on the duration of neuromuscular block if recovery is allowed to begin prior to repeat dosing. Moreover, the time needed to recover from repeat doses does not change with additional doses. Repeat doses can therefore be administered at relatively regular intervals with predictable results. After an initial dose of 0.4 to 0.5 mg/kg under balanced anesthesia, the first maintenance dose (suggested maintenance dose is 0.08 to 0.10 mg/kg) is generally required within 20 to 45 minutes, and subsequent maintenance doses are usually required at approximately 15- to 25- minute intervals.
Once recovery from the neuromuscular blocking effects of TRACRIUM begins, it proceeds more rapidly than recovery from d-tubocurarine, metocurine, and pancuronium. Regardless of the dose of TRACRIUM, the time from start of recovery (from complete block) to complete (95%) recovery is approximately 30 minutes under balanced anesthesia, and approximately 40 minutes under halothane, enflurane, or isoflurane. Repeated doses have no cumulative effect on recovery rate.
Reversal of neuromuscular block produced by TRACRIUM can be achieved with an anticholinesterase agent such as neostigmine, edrophonium, or pyridostigmine, in conjunction with an anticholinergic agent such as atropine or glycopyrrolate. Under balanced anesthesia, reversal can usually be attempted approximately 20 to 35 minutes after an initial dose of TRACRIUM of 0.4 to 0.5 mg/kg, or approximately 10 to 30 minutes after a 0.08- to 0.10-mg/kg maintenance dose, when recovery of muscle twitch has started. Complete reversal is usually attained within 8 to 10 minutes of the administration of reversing agents. Rare instances of breathing difficulties, possibly related to incomplete reversal, have been reported following attempted pharmacologic antagonism of neuromuscular block induced by TRACRIUM. As with other agents in this class, the tendency for residual neuromuscular block is increased if reversal is attempted at deep levels of block or if inadequate doses of reversal agents are employed.
The pharmacokinetics of TRACRIUM in humans are essentially linear within the 0.3- to 0.6-mg/kg dose range. The elimination half-life is approximately 20 minutes. THE DURATION OF NEUROMUSCULAR BLOCK PRODUCED BY TRACRIUM DOES NOT CORRELATE WITH PLASMA PSEUDOCHOLINESTERASE LEVELS AND IS NOT ALTERED BY THE ABSENCE OF RENAL FUNCTION. This is consistent with the results of in vitro studies which have shown that TRACRIUM is inactivated in plasma via two nonoxidative pathways: ester hydrolysis, catalyzed by nonspecific esterases; and Hofmann elimination, a nonenzymatic chemical process which occurs at physiological pH. Some placental transfer occurs in humans.
Radiolabel studies demonstrated that TRACRIUM undergoes extensive degradation in cats, and that neither kidney nor liver plays a major role in its elimination. Biliary and urinary excretion were the major routes of excretion of radioactivity (totaling >90% of the labeled dose within 7 hours of dosing), of which TRACRIUM represented only a minor fraction. The metabolites in bile and urine were similar, including products of Hofmann elimination and ester hydrolysis.
Elderly patients may have slightly altered pharmacokinetic parameters compared to younger patients, with a slightly decreased total plasma clearance which is offset by a corresponding increase in volume of distribution. The net effect is that there has been no significant difference in clinical duration and recovery from neuromuscular block observed between elderly and younger patients receiving TRACRIUM.
TRACRIUM is a less potent histamine releaser than d-tubocurarine or metocurine. Histamine release is minimal with initial doses of TRACRIUM up to 0.5 mg/kg, and hemodynamic changes are minimal within the recommended dose range. A moderate histamine release and significant falls in blood pressure have been seen following 0.6 mg/kg of TRACRIUM. The histamine and hemodynamic responses were poorly correlated. The effects were generally short-lived and manageable, but the possibility of substantial histamine release in sensitive individuals or in patients in whom substantial histamine release would be especially hazardous (e.g., patients with significant cardiovascular disease) must be considered.
It is not known whether the prior use of other nondepolarizing neuromuscular blocking agents has any effect on the activity of TRACRIUM. The prior use of succinylcholine decreases by approximately 2 to 3 minutes the time to maximum block induced by TRACRIUM, and may increase the depth of block. TRACRIUM should be administered only after a patient recovers from succinylcholine-induced neuromuscular block.

INDICATIONS AND USAGE

TRACRIUM is indicated, as an adjunct to general anesthesia, to facilitate endotracheal intubation and to provide skeletal muscle relaxation during surgery or mechanical ventilation.

CONTRAINDICATIONS

TRACRIUM is contraindicated in patients known to have a hypersensitivity to it. Use of TRACRIUM from multiple-dose vials containing benzyl alcohol as a preservative is contraindicated in patients with a known hypersensitivity to benzyl alcohol.

WARNINGS

TRACRIUM SHOULD BE USED ONLY BY THOSE SKILLED IN AIRWAY MANAGEMENT AND RESPIRATORY SUPPORT. EQUIPMENT AND PERSONNEL MUST BE IMMEDIATELY AVAILABLE FOR ENDOTRACHEAL INTUBATION AND SUPPORT OF VENTILATION, INCLUDING ADMINISTRATION OF POSITIVE PRESSURE OXYGEN. ADEQUACY OF RESPIRATION MUST BE ASSURED THROUGH ASSISTED OR CONTROLLED VENTILATION. ANTICHOLINESTERASE REVERSAL AGENTS SHOULD BE IMMEDIATELY AVAILABLE.
DO NOT GIVE TRACRIUM BY INTRAMUSCULAR ADMINISTRATION.
TRACRIUM has no known effect on consciousness, pain threshold, or cerebration. It should be used only with adequate anesthesia.
TRACRIUM Injection, which has an acid pH, should not be mixed with alkaline solutions (e.g., barbiturate solutions) in the same syringe or administered simultaneously during intravenous infusion through the same needle. Depending on the resultant pH of such mixtures, TRACRIUM may be inactivated and a free acid may be precipitated.
TRACRIUM Injection 10-mL multiple-dose vials contain benzyl alcohol. In neonates, benzyl alcohol has been associated with an increased incidence of neurological and other complications which are sometimes fatal. TRACRIUM Injection 5-mL single-use vials do not contain benzyl alcohol (see PRECAUTIONS: Pediatric Use).

PRECAUTIONS

General: Although TRACRIUM is a less potent histamine releaser than d-tubocurarine or metocurine, the possibility of substantial histamine release in sensitive individuals must be considered. Special caution should be exercised in administering TRACRIUM to patients in whom substantial histamine release would be especially hazardous (e.g., patients with clinically significant cardiovascular disease) and in patients with any history (e.g., severe anaphylactoid reactions or asthma) suggesting a greater risk of histamine release. In these patients, the recommended initial dose of TRACRIUM is lower (0.3 to 0.4 mg/kg) than for other patients and should be administered slowly or in divided doses over 1 minute.
Since TRACRIUM has no clinically significant effects on heart rate in the recommended dosage range, it will not counteract the bradycardia produced by many anesthetic agents or vagal stimulation. As a result, bradycardia during anesthesia may be more common with TRACRIUM than with other muscle relaxants.
TRACRIUM may have profound effects in patients with myasthenia gravis, Eaton-Lambert syndrome, or other neuromuscular diseases in which potentiation of nondepolarizing agents has been noted. The use of a peripheral nerve stimulator is especially important for assessing neuromuscular block in these patients. Similar precautions should be taken in patients with severe electrolyte disorders or carcinomatosis.
Multiple factors in anesthesia practice are suspected of triggering malignant hyperthermia (MH), a potentially fatal hypermetabolic state of skeletal muscle. Halogenated anesthetic agents and succinylcholine are recognized as the principal pharmacologic triggering agents in MH-susceptible patients; however, since MH can develop in the absence of established triggering agents, the clinician should be prepared to recognize and treat MH in any patient scheduled for general anesthesia. Reports of MH have been rare in cases in which TRACRIUM has been used. In studies of MH-susceptible animals (swine) and in a clinical study of MH-susceptible patients, TRACRIUM did not trigger this syndrome.
Resistance to nondepolarizing neuromuscular blocking agents may develop in burn patients. Increased doses of nondepolarizing muscle relaxants may be required in burn patients and are dependent on the time elapsed since the burn injury and the size of the burn.
The safety of TRACRIUM has not been established in patients with bronchial asthma.
Long-Term Use in Intensive Care Unit (ICU): When there is a need for long-term mechanical ventilation, the benefits-to-risk ratio of neuromuscular block must be considered. The long-term (1 to 10 days) infusion of TRACRIUM during mechanical ventilation in the ICU has been evaluated in several studies. Average infusion rates of 11 to 13 mcg/kg per minute (range: 4.5 to 29.5) were required to achieve adequate neuromuscular block. These data suggest that there is wide interpatient variability in dosage requirements. In addition, these studies have shown that dosage requirements may decrease or increase with time. Following discontinuation of infusion of TRACRIUM in these ICU studies, spontaneous recovery of four twitches in a train-of-four occurred in an average of approximately 30 minutes (range: 15 to 75 minutes) and spontaneous recovery to a train-of-four ratio > 75% (the ratio of the height of the fourth to the first twitch in a train-of-four) occurred in an average of approximately 60 minutes (range: 32 to 108 min).
Little information is available on the plasma levels and clinical consequences of atracurium metabolites that may accumulate during days to weeks of atracurium administration in ICU patients. Laudanosine, a major biologically active metabolite of atracurium without neuromuscular blocking activity, produces transient hypotension and, in higher doses, cerebral excitatory effects (generalized muscle twitching and seizures) when administered to several species of animals. There have been rare spontaneous reports of seizures in ICU patients who have received atracurium or other agents. These patients usually had predisposing causes (such as head trauma, cerebral edema, hypoxic encephalopathy, viral encephalitis, uremia). There are insufficient data to determine whether or not laudanosine contributes to seizures in ICU patients.
WHENEVER THE USE OF TRACRIUM OR ANY NEUROMUSCULAR BLOCKING AGENT IS CONTEMPLATED IN THE ICU, IT IS RECOMMENDED THAT NEUROMUSCULAR TRANSMISSION BE MONITORED CONTINUOUSLY DURING ADMINISTRATION WITH THE HELP OF A NERVE STIMULATOR. ADDITIONAL DOSES OF TRACRIUM OR ANY OTHER NEUROMUSCULAR BLOCKING AGENT SHOULD NOT BE GIVEN BEFORE

THERE IS A DEFINITE RESPONSE TO T_1 OR TO THE FIRST TWITCH. IF NO RESPONSE IS ELICITED, INFUSION ADMINISTRATION SHOULD BE DISCONTINUED UNTIL A RESPONSE RETURNS.

Hemofiltration has a minimal effect on plasma levels of atracurium and its metabolites, including laudanosine. The effects of hemodialysis and hemoperfusion on plasma levels of atracurium and its metabolites are unknown.

Drug Interactions: Drugs which may enhance the neuromuscular blocking action of TRACRIUM include: enflurane; isoflurane; halothane; certain antibiotics, especially the aminoglycosides and polymyxins; lithium; magnesium salts; procainamide; and quinidine.

If other muscle relaxants are used during the same procedure, the possibility of a synergistic or antagonist effect should be considered.

The prior administration of succinylcholine does not enhance the duration, but quickens the onset and may increase the depth, of neuromuscular block induced by TRACRIUM. TRACRIUM should not be administered until a patient has recovered from succinylcholine-induced neuromuscular block.

Carcinogenesis, Mutagenesis, Impairment of Fertility: Carcinogenesis and fertility studies have not been performed. Atracurium was evaluated in a battery of three short-term mutagenicity tests. It was nonmutagenic in both the Ames Salmonella assay at concentrations up to 1,000 mcg/plate, and in a rat bone marrow cytogenicity assay at up to paralyzing doses. A positive response was observed in the mouse lymphoma assay under conditions (80 and 100 mcg/mL, in the absence of metabolic activation) which killed over 80% of the treated cells; there was no mutagenicity at 60 mcg/mL and lower, concentrations which killed up to half of the treated cells. A far weaker response was observed in the presence of metabolic activation at concentrations (1,200 mcg/mL and higher) which also killed over 80% of the treated cells.

Mutagenicity testing is intended to simulate chronic (years to lifetime) exposure in an effort to determine potential carcinogenicity. Thus, a single positive mutagenicity response for a drug used infrequently and/or briefly is of questionable clinical relevance.

Pregnancy: ***Teratogenic Effects:*** Pregnancy Category C. TRACRIUM has been shown to be potentially teratogenic in rabbits when given in doses up to approximately one half the human dose. There are no adequate and well-controlled studies in pregnant women. TRACRIUM should be used during pregnancy only if the potential benefit justifies the potential risk to the fetus.

TRACRIUM was administered subcutaneously on days 6 through 18 of gestation to nonventilated Dutch rabbits. Treatment groups were given either 0.15 mg/kg once daily or 0.10 mg/kg twice daily. Lethal respiratory distress occurred in two 0.15-mg/kg animals and in one 0.10-mg/kg animal, with transient respiratory distress or other evidence of neuromuscular block occurring in 10 of 19 and in 4 of 20 of the 0.15-mg/kg and 0.10-mg/kg animals, respectively. There was an increased incidence of certain spontaneously occurring visceral and skeletal anomalies or variations in one or both treated groups when compared to nontreated controls. The percentage of male fetuses was lower (41% vs. 51%) and the post-implantation losses were increased (15% vs. 8%) in the group given 0.15 mg/kg once daily when compared to the controls; the mean numbers of implants (6.5 vs. 4.4) and normal live fetuses (5.4 vs. 3.8) were greater in this group when compared to the control group.

Labor and Delivery: It is not known whether muscle relaxants administered during vaginal delivery have immediate or delayed adverse effects on the fetus or increase the likelihood that resuscitation of the newborn will be necessary. The possibility that forceps delivery will be necessary may increase.

TRACRIUM (0.3 mg/kg) has been administered to 26 pregnant women during delivery by cesarean section. No harmful effects were attributable to TRACRIUM in any of the neonates, although small amounts of TRACRIUM were shown to cross the placental barrier. The possibility of respiratory depression in the neonate should always be considered following cesarean section during which a neuromuscular blocking agent has been administered. In patients receiving magnesium sulfate, the reversal of neuromuscular block may be unsatisfactory and the dose of TRACRIUM should be lowered as indicated.

Nursing Mothers: It is not known whether this drug is excreted in human milk. Because many drugs are excreted in human milk, caution should be exercised when TRACRIUM is administered to a nursing woman.

Pediatric Use: Safety and effectiveness in pediatric patients below the age of 1 month have not been established.

Use in the Elderly: Since marketing in 1983, uncontrolled clinical experience and limited data from controlled trials have not identified differences in effectiveness, safety, or dosage requirements between healthy elderly and younger patients (see CLINICAL PHARMACOLOGY); however, as with other neuromuscular blocking agents, the use of a peripheral nerve stimulator to monitor neuromuscular function is suggested (see DOSAGE AND ADMINISTRATION).

Table 1: Percent Of Patients Reporting Adverse Reactions

Adverse Reaction	Initial Dose of TRACRIUM (mg/kg) 0.00-0.30 (n = 485)	0.31-0.50* (n = 366)	≥0.60 (n = 24)	Total (n = 875)
Skin Flush	1.0%	8.7%	29.2%	5.0%
Erythema	0.6%	0.5%	0%	0.6%
Itching	0.4%	0%	0%	0.2%
Wheezing/Bronchial Secretions	0.2%	0.3%	0%	0.2%
Hives	0.2%	0%	0%	0.1%

*Includes the recommended initial dosage range for most patients.

ADVERSE REACTIONS

Observed in Controlled Clinical Studies: TRACRIUM was well tolerated and produced few adverse reactions during extensive clinical trials. Most adverse reactions were suggestive of histamine release. In studies including 875 patients, TRACRIUM was discontinued in only one patient (who required treatment for bronchial secretions), and six other patients required treatment for adverse reactions attributable to TRACRIUM (wheezing in one, hypotension in five). Of the five patients who required treatment for hypotension, three had a history of significant cardiovascular disease. The overall incidence rate for clinically important adverse reactions, therefore, was 7/875 or 0.8%. Table 1 includes all adverse reactions reported attributable to TRACRIUM during clinical trials with 875 patients.

[See table 1 above]

Most adverse reactions were of little clinical significance unless they were associated with significant hemodynamic changes. Table 2 summarizes the incidences of substantial vital sign changes noted during clinical trials of TRACRIUM with 530 patients, without cardiovascular disease, in whom these parameters were assessed.

[See table 2 at top of next page]

Observed in Clinical Practice: Based on initial clinical practice experience in approximately 3 million patients who received TRACRIUM in the US and in the United Kingdom, spontaneously reported adverse reactions were uncommon (approximately 0.01% to 0.02%). The following adverse reactions are among the most frequently reported, but there are insufficient data to support an estimate of their incidence:

General: Allergic reactions (anaphylactic or anaphylactoid responses) which, in rare instances, were severe (e.g., cardiac arrest).

Musculoskeletal: Inadequate block, prolonged block.

Cardiovascular: Hypotension, vasodilatation (flushing), tachycardia, bradycardia.

Respiratory: Dyspnea, bronchospasm, laryngospasm.

Integumentary: Rash, urticaria, reaction at injection site.

There have been rare spontaneous reports of seizures in ICU patients following long-term infusion of atracurium to support mechanical ventilation. There are insufficient data to define the contribution, if any, of atracurium and/or its metabolite laudanosine. (See PRECAUTIONS: Long-Term Use in Intensive Care Unit [ICU]).

OVERDOSAGE

There has been limited experience with overdosage of TRACRIUM. The possibility of iatrogenic overdosage can be minimized by carefully monitoring muscle twitch response to peripheral nerve stimulation. Excessive doses of TRACRIUM can be expected to produce enhanced pharmacological effects. Overdosage may increase the risk of histamine release and cardiovascular effects, especially hypotension. If cardiovascular support is necessary, this should include proper positioning, fluid administration, and the use of vasopressor agents if necessary. The patient's airway should be assured, with manual or mechanical ventilation maintained as necessary. A longer duration of neuromuscular block may result from overdosage and a peripheral nerve stimulator should be used to monitor recovery. Recovery may be facilitated by administration of an anticholinesterase reversing agent such as neostigmine, edrophonium, or pyridostigmine, in conjunction with an anticholinergic agent such as atropine or glycopyrrolate. The appropriate package inserts should be consulted for prescribing information.

Three pediatric patients (3 weeks, 4 and 5 months of age) unintentionally received doses of 0.8 mg/kg to 1.0 mg/kg of TRACRIUM. The time to 25% recovery (50 to 55 minutes) following these doses, which were 5 to 6 times the ED_{95} dose, was moderately longer than the corresponding time observed following doses 2.0 to 2.5 times the TRACRIUM ED_{95} dose in infants (22 to 36 minutes). Cardiovascular changes were minimal. Nonetheless the possibility of cardiovascular changes must be considered in the case of overdose.

An adult patient (17 years of age) unintentionally received an initial dose of 1.3 mg/kg of TRACRIUM. The time from injection to 25% recovery (83 minutes) was approximately twice that observed following maximum recommended doses in adults (35 to 45 minutes). The patient experienced moderate hemodynamic changes (13% increase in mean arterial pressure and 27% increase in heart rate) which persisted for 40 minutes and did not require treatment.

The intravenous LD_{50}s determined in nonventilated male and female albino mice and male Wistar rats were 1.9, 2.01, and 1.31 mg/kg, respectively. Deaths occurred within 2 minutes and were caused by respiratory paralysis. The subcutaneous LD_{50} determined in nonventilated male Wistar rats was 282.8 mg/kg. Tremors, ptosis, loss of reflexes, and respiratory failure preceded death which occurred 45 to 120 minutes after injection.

DOSAGE AND ADMINISTRATION

To avoid distress to the patient, TRACRIUM should not be administered before unconsciousness has been induced. TRACRIUM should not be mixed in the same syringe, or administered simultaneously through the same needle, with alkaline solutions (e.g., barbiturate solutions).

TRACRIUM should be administered intravenously. DO NOT GIVE TRACRIUM BY INTRAMUSCULAR ADMINISTRATION. Intramuscular administration of TRACRIUM may result in tissue irritation and there are no clinical data to support this route of administration.

As with other neuromuscular blocking agents, the use of a peripheral nerve stimulator will permit the most advantageous use of TRACRIUM, minimizing the possibility of overdosage or underdosage, and assist in the evaluation of recovery.

Parenteral drug products should be inspected visually for particulate matter and discoloration prior to administration, whenever solution and container permit.

Bolus Doses for Intubation and Maintenance of Neuromuscular Block: ***Adults:*** A dose of TRACRIUM of 0.4 to 0.5 mg/kg (1.7 to 2.2 times the ED_{95}), given as an intravenous bolus injection, is the recommended initial dose for most patients. With this dose, good or excellent conditions for nonemergency intubation can be expected in 2 to 2.5 minutes in most patients, with maximum neuromuscular block achieved approximately 3 to 5 minutes after injection. Clinically required neuromuscular block generally lasts 20 to 35 minutes under balanced anesthesia. Under balanced anesthesia, recovery to 25% of control is achieved approximately 35 to 45 minutes after injection, and recovery is usually 95% complete approximately 60 minutes after injection.

TRACRIUM is potentiated by isoflurane or enflurane anesthesia. The same initial dose of TRACRIUM of 0.4 to 0.5 mg/kg may be used for intubation prior to administration of these inhalation agents; however, if TRACRIUM is first administered under steady state of isoflurane or enflurane, the initial dose of TRACRIUM should be reduced by approximately one third, i.e., to 0.25 to 0.35 mg/kg, to adjust for the potentiating effects of these anesthetic agents. With halothane, which has only a marginal (approximately 20%) potentiating effect on TRACRIUM, smaller dosage reductions may be considered.

Doses of TRACRIUM of 0.08 to 0.10 mg/kg are recommended for maintenance of neuromuscular block during prolonged surgical procedures. The first maintenance dose will generally be required 20 to 45 minutes after the initial injection of TRACRIUM, but the need for maintenance doses should be determined by clinical criteria. Because TRACRIUM lacks cumulative effects, maintenance doses may be administered at relatively regular intervals for each patient, ranging approximately from 15 to 25 minutes under balanced anesthesia, slightly longer under isoflurane or enflurane. Higher doses of TRACRIUM (up to 0.2 mg/kg) permit maintenance dosing at longer intervals.

Continued on next page

This product information is based on labeling in effect on June 1, 1998. For further information, contact via direct mail, phone, or web site Medical Information: Glaxo Wellcome Inc., PO Box 13398, Research Triangle Park, NC 27709. Healthcare Professionals (Medical Information): 800-334-0089 Patients (Customer Response Center): 888-TALK2GW (1-888-825-5249) Glaxo Wellcome Corporate Web Site: www.glaxowellcome.com

Tracrium—Cont.

Pediatric Patients: No dosage adjustments of TRACRIUM are required for pediatric patients 2 years of age or older. A dose of TRACRIUM 0.3 to 0.4 mg/kg is recommended as the initial dose for infants (1 month to 2 years of age) under halothane anesthesia. Maintenance doses may be required with slightly greater frequency in infants and children than in adults.

Special Considerations: An initial dose of TRACRIUM of 0.3 to 0.4 mg/kg, given slowly or in divided doses over 1 minute, is recommended for adults, adolescents, children, or infants with significant cardiovascular disease and for adults, adolescents, children, or infants with any history (e.g., severe anaphylactoid reactions or asthma) suggesting a greater risk of histamine release.

Dosage reductions must be considered also in patients with neuromuscular disease, severe electrolyte disorders, or carcinomatosis in which potentiation of neuromuscular block or difficulties with reversal have been demonstrated. There has been no clinical experience with TRACRIUM in these patients, and no specific dosage adjustments can be recommended. No dosage adjustments of TRACRIUM are required for patients with renal disease.

An initial dose of TRACRIUM of 0.3 to 0.4 mg/kg is recommended for adults following the use of succinylcholine for intubation under balanced anesthesia. Further reductions may be desirable with the use of potent inhalation anesthetics. The patient should be permitted to recover from the effects of succinylcholine prior to administration of TRACRIUM. Insufficient data are available for recommendation of a specific initial dose of TRACRIUM for administration following the use of succinylcholine in children and infants.

Use by Continuous Infusion: *Infusion in the Operating Room (OR):* After administration of a recommended initial bolus dose of TRACRIUM (0.3 to 0.5 mg/kg), a diluted solution of TRACRIUM can be administered by continuous infusion to adults and pediatric patients aged 2 or more years for maintenance of neuromuscular block during extended surgical procedures.

Infusion of TRACRIUM should be individualized for each patient. The rate of administration should be adjusted according to the patient's response as determined by peripheral nerve stimulation. Accurate dosing is best achieved using a precision infusion device.

Infusion of TRACRIUM should be initiated only after early evidence of spontaneous recovery from the bolus dose. An initial infusion rate of 9 to 10 mcg/kg per minute may be required to rapidly counteract the spontaneous recovery of neuromuscular function. Thereafter, a rate of 5 to 9 mcg/kg per minute should be adequate to maintain continuous neuromuscular block in the range of 89% to 99% in most pediatric and adult patients under balanced anesthesia. Occasional patients may require infusion rates as low as 2 mcg/kg per minute or as high as 15 mcg/kg per minute.

The neuromuscular blocking effect of TRACRIUM administered by infusion is potentiated by enflurane or isoflurane and, to a lesser extent, by halothane. Reduction in the infusion rate of TRACRIUM should, therefore, be considered for patients receiving inhalation anesthesia. The infusion rate of TRACRIUM should be reduced by approximately one third in the presence of steady-state enflurane or isoflurane anesthesia; smaller reductions should be considered in the presence of halothane.

In patients undergoing cardiopulmonary bypass with induced hypothermia, the rate of infusion of TRACRIUM required to maintain adequate surgical relaxation during hypothermia (25° to 28°C) has been shown to be approximately half the rate required during normothermia.

Spontaneous recovery from neuromuscular block following discontinuation of infusion of TRACRIUM may be expected to proceed at a rate comparable to that following administration of a single bolus dose.

Infusion in the Intensive Care Unit (ICU): The principles for infusion of TRACRIUM in the OR are also applicable to use in the ICU.

An infusion rate of 11 to 13 mcg/kg per minute (range: 4.5 to 29.5) should provide adequate neuromuscular block in adult patients in an ICU. Limited information suggests that infusion rates required for pediatric patients in the ICU may be higher than in adult patients. There may be wide interpatient variability in dosage requirements and these requirements may increase or decrease with time (see PRECAUTIONS: Long-Term Use in Intensive Care Unit [ICU]). Following recovery from neuromuscular block, readministration of a bolus dose may be necessary to quickly re-establish neuromuscular block prior to reinstitution of the infusion.

Infusion Rate Tables: The amount of infusion solution required per minute will depend upon the concentration of TRACRIUM in the infusion solution, the desired dose of TRACRIUM, and the patient's weight. The following tables provide guidelines for delivery, in mL/hr (equivalent to microdrops/min when 60 microdrops = 1 mL), of solutions of TRACRIUM in concentrations of 0.2 mg/mL (20 mg in 100 mL) or 0.5 mg/mL (50 mg in 100 mL) with an infusion pump or a gravity flow device.

Table 2: Percent Of Patients Showing >30% Vital Sign Changes Following Administration Of TRACRIUM

	Initial TRACRIUM Dose (mg/kg)			
Vital Sign Change	0.00-0.30 (n = 365)	0.31-0.50* (n = 144)	≥0.60 (n = 21)	Total (n = 530)
Mean Arterial Pressure				
Increase	1.9%	2.8%	0%	2.1%
Decrease	1.1%	2.1%	14.3%	1.9%
Heart Rate				
Increase	1.6%	2.8%	4.8%	2.1%
Decrease	0.8%	0%	0%	0.6%

*Includes the recommended initial dosage range for most patients.

Table 3: Infusion Rates of TRACRIUM for a Concentration of 0.2 mg/mL

Patient Weight (Kg)	Drug Delivery Rate (mcg/kg per minute) 5	6	7	8	9	10	11	12	13
	Infusion Delivery Rate (mL/hr)								
30	45	54	63	72	81	90	99	108	117
35	53	63	74	84	95	105	116	126	137
40	60	72	84	96	108	120	132	144	156
45	68	81	95	108	122	135	149	162	176
50	75	90	105	120	135	150	165	180	195
55	83	99	116	132	149	165	182	198	215
60	90	108	126	144	162	180	198	216	234
65	98	117	137	156	176	195	215	234	254
70	105	126	147	168	189	210	231	252	273
75	113	135	158	180	203	225	248	270	293
80	120	144	168	192	216	240	264	288	312
90	135	162	189	216	243	270	297	324	351
100	150	180	210	240	270	300	330	360	390

Table 4: Infusion Rates of TRACRIUM for a Concentration of 0.5 mg/mL

Patient Weight (Kg)	Drug Delivery Rate (mcg/kg per minute) 5	6	7	8	9	10	11	12	13
	Infusion Delivery Rate (mL/hr)								
30	18	22	25	29	32	36	40	43	47
35	21	25	29	34	38	42	46	50	55
40	24	29	34	38	43	48	53	58	62
45	27	32	38	43	49	54	59	65	70
50	30	36	42	48	54	60	66	72	78
55	33	40	46	53	59	66	73	79	86
60	36	43	50	58	65	72	79	86	94
65	39	47	55	62	70	78	86	94	101
70	42	50	59	67	76	84	92	101	109
75	45	54	63	72	81	90	99	108	117
80	48	58	67	77	86	96	106	115	125
90	54	65	76	86	97	108	119	130	140
100	60	72	84	96	108	120	132	144	156

Compatibility and Admixtures: Infusion solutions of TRACRIUM may be prepared by admixing TRACRIUM Injection with an appropriate diluent such as 5% Dextrose Injection, USP; 0.9% Sodium Chloride Injection, USP; or 5% Dextrose and 0.9% Sodium Chloride Injection, USP. Infusion solutions should be used within 24 hours of preparation. Unused solutions should be discarded. Solutions containing 0.2 mg/mL or 0.5 mg/mL TRACRIUM in the above diluents may be stored either under refrigeration or at room temperature for 24 hours without significant loss of potency. Care should be taken during admixture to prevent inadvertent contamination. Visually inspect prior to administration.

Spontaneous degradation of TRACRIUM has been demonstrated to occur more rapidly in Lactated Ringer's solution than in 0.9% sodium chloride solution. Therefore, it is recommended that Lactated Ringer's Injection, USP not be used as a diluent in preparing solutions of TRACRIUM for infusion.

HOW SUPPLIED

TRACRIUM Injection, 10 mg atracurium besylate in each mL.

5-mL Single-Use Vial (50 mg atracurium besylate per vial). Tray of 10 (NDC 0173-0940-44).

10-mL Multiple-Dose Vial (100 mg atracurium besylate per vial). Contains benzyl alcohol (see WARNINGS). Tray of 10 (NDC 0173-0545-00).

STORAGE:

TRACRIUM Injection should be refrigerated at 2° to 8°C (36° to 46°F) to preserve potency. DO NOT FREEZE. Upon removal from refrigeration to room temperature storage conditions (25°C/77°F), use TRACRIUM Injection within 14 days even if rerefrigerated.

©Copyright 1996 Glaxo Wellcome Inc. All rights reserved.

November 1997/RL-495

Shown in Product Identification Guide, page 314

TRANDATE® ℞

[trăn 'dāt]

(labetalol hydrochloride)

Injection

DESCRIPTION

TRANDATE Injection is an adrenergic receptor blocking agent that has both selective alpha$_1$-adrenergic and nonselective beta-adrenergic receptor blocking actions in a single substance.

Labetalol hydrochloride (HCl) is a racemate chemically designated as 2-hydroxy-5-[1-hydroxy-2-[(1-methyl-3-phenylpropyl)amino]ethyl]benzamide monohydrochloride.

Labetalol HCl has the empirical formula $C_{19}H_{24}N_2O_3 \cdot HCl$ and a molecular weight of 364.9. It has two asymmetric centers and therefore exists as a molecular complex of two diastereoisomeric pairs. Dilevalol, the R,R' stereoisomer, makes up 25% of racemic labetalol.

Labetalol HCl is a white or off-white crystalline powder, soluble in water.

TRANDATE Injection is a clear, colorless to light yellow, aqueous, sterile, isotonic solution for intravenous (IV) injection. It has a pH range of 3 to 4. Each milliliter contains 5 mg of labetalol HCl, 45 mg of anhydrous dextrose, 0.1 mg of edetate disodium; 0.8 mg of methylparaben and 0.1 mg of propylparaben as preservatives; and citric acid monohydrate and sodium hydroxide, as necessary, to bring the solution into the pH range.

CLINICAL PHARMACOLOGY

Labetalol HCl combines both selective, competitive, alpha$_1$-adrenergic blocking and nonselective, competitive, beta-adrenergic blocking activity in a single substance. In man, the ratios of alpha- to beta-blockade have been estimated to be approximately 1:3 and 1:7 following oral and IV administration, respectively. Beta$_2$-agonist activity has been demonstrated in animals with minimal beta$_1$-agonist (ISA) activity detected. In animals, at doses greater than those required for alpha- or beta-adrenergic blockade, a membrane stabilizing effect has been demonstrated.

Pharmacodynamics: The capacity of labetalol HCl to block alpha receptors in man has been demonstrated by attenuation of the pressor effect of phenylephrine and by a significant reduction of the pressor response caused by immersing the hand in ice-cold water ("cold-pressor test"). Labetalol HCl's beta$_1$-receptor blockade in man was demonstrated by a small decrease in the resting heart rate, attenuation of tachycardia produced by isoproterenol or exercise, and by attenuation of the reflex tachycardia to the hypotension produced by amyl nitrite. Beta$_2$-receptor blockade was demonstrated by inhibition of the isoproterenol-induced fall in diastolic blood pressure. Both the alpha- and beta-blocking actions of orally administered labetalol HCl contribute to a decrease in blood pressure in hypertensive patients. Labetalol HCl consistently, in dose-related fashion, blunted increases in exercise-induced blood pressure and heart rate, and in their double product. The pulmonary circulation during exercise was not affected by labetalol HCl dosing.

Single oral doses of labetalol HCl administered to patients with coronary artery disease had no significant effect on sinus rate, intraventricular conduction, or QRS duration. The atrioventricular (A-V) conduction time was modestly prolonged in two of seven patients. In another study, IV la-

betalol HCl slightly prolonged A-V nodal conduction time and atrial effective refractory period with only small changes in heart rate. The effects on A-V nodal refractoriness were inconsistent.

Labetalol HCl produces dose-related falls in blood pressure without reflex tachycardia and without significant reduction in heart rate, presumably through a mixture of its alpha- and beta-blocking effects. Hemodynamic effects are variable, with small, nonsignificant changes in cardiac output seen in some studies but not others, and small decreases in total peripheral resistance. Elevated plasma renins are reduced.

Doses of labetalol HCl that controlled hypertension did not affect renal function in mildly to severely hypertensive patients with normal renal function.

Due to the $alpha_1$-receptor blocking activity of labetalol HCl, blood pressure is lowered more in the standing than in the supine position, and symptoms of postural hypotension can occur. During dosing with IV labetalol HCl, the contribution of the postural component should be considered when positioning the patient for treatment, and the patient should not be allowed to move to an erect position unmonitored until his ability to do so is established.

In a clinical pharmacologic study in severe hypertensives, an initial 0.25-mg/kg injection of labetalol HCl administered to patients in the supine position decreased blood pressure by an average of 11/7 mmHg. Additional injections of 0.5 mg/kg at 15-minute intervals up to a total cumulative dose of 1.75 mg/kg of labetalol HCl caused further dose-related decreases in blood pressure. Some patients required cumulative doses of up to 3.25 mg/kg. The maximal effect of each dose level occurred within 5 minutes. Following discontinuation of IV treatment with labetalol HCl, the blood pressure rose gradually and progressively, approaching pretreatment baseline values within an average of 16 to 18 hours in the majority of patients.

Similar results were obtained in the treatment of patients with severe hypertension who required urgent blood pressure reduction with an initial dose of 20 mg (which corresponds to 0.25 mg/kg for an 80-kg patient) followed by additional doses of either 40 or 80 mg at 10-minute intervals to achieve the desired effect, or up to a cumulative dose of 300 mg.

Labetalol HCl administered as a continuous IV infusion, with a mean dose of 136 mg (27 to 300 mg) over a period of 2 to 3 hours (mean of 2 hours and 39 minutes), lowered the blood pressure by an average of 60/35 mmHg.

Exacerbation of angina and, in some cases, myocardial infarction and ventricular dysrhythmias have been reported after abrupt discontinuation of therapy with beta-adrenergic blocking agents in patients with coronary artery disease. Abrupt withdrawal of these agents in patients without coronary artery disease has resulted in transient symptoms, including tremulousness, sweating, palpitation, headache, and malaise. Several mechanisms have been proposed to explain these phenomena, among them increased sensitivity to catecholamines because of increased numbers of beta receptors.

Although beta-adrenergic receptor blockade is useful in the treatment of angina and hypertension, there are also situations in which sympathetic stimulation is vital. For example, in patients with severely damaged hearts, adequate ventricular function may depend on sympathetic drive. Beta-adrenergic blockade may worsen A-V block by preventing the necessary facilitating effects of sympathetic activity on conduction. $Beta_2$-adrenergic blockade results in passive bronchial constriction by interfering with endogenous adrenergic bronchodilator activity in patients subject to bronchospasm, and it may also interfere with exogenous bronchodilators in such patients.

Pharmacokinetics and Metabolism: Following IV infusion of labetalol, the elimination half-life is about 5.5 hours and the total body clearance is approximately 33 mL/min per kilogram. The plasma half-life of labetalol following oral administration is about 6 to 8 hours. In patients with decreased hepatic or renal function, the elimination half-life of labetalol is not altered; however, the relative bioavailability in hepatically impaired patients is increased due to decreased "first-pass" metabolism.

The metabolism of labetalol is mainly through conjugation to glucuronide metabolites. The metabolites are present in plasma and are excreted in the urine and, via the bile, into the feces. Approximately 55% to 60% of a dose appears in the urine as conjugates or unchanged labetalol within the first 24 hours of dosing.

Labetalol has been shown to cross the placental barrier in humans. Only negligible amounts of the drug crossed the blood-brain barrier in animal studies. Labetalol is approximately 50% protein bound. Neither hemodialysis nor peritoneal dialysis removes a significant amount of labetalol HCl from the general circulation (<1%).

INDICATIONS AND USAGE

TRANDATE Injection is indicated for control of blood pressure in severe hypertension.

CONTRAINDICATIONS

TRANDATE Injection is contraindicated in bronchial asthma, overt cardiac failure, greater-than-first-degree heart block, cardiogenic shock, severe bradycardia, other conditions associated with severe and prolonged hypotension, and in patients with a history of hypersensitivity to any component of the product (see WARNINGS).

WARNINGS

Hepatic Injury: Severe hepatocellular injury, confirmed by rechallenge in at least one case, occurs rarely with labetalol therapy. The hepatic injury is usually reversible, but hepatic necrosis and death have been reported. Injury has occurred after both short- and long-term treatment and may be slowly progressive despite minimal symptomatology. Similar hepatic events have been reported with a related research compound, dilevalol HCl, including two deaths. Dilevalol HCl is one of the four isomers of labetalol HCl. Thus, for patients taking labetalol, periodic determination of suitable hepatic laboratory tests would be appropriate. Appropriate laboratory testing should be done at the first symptom/sign of liver dysfunction (e.g., pruritus, dark urine, persistent anorexia, jaundice, right upper quadrant tenderness, or unexplained "flulike" symptoms). If the patient has laboratory evidence of liver injury or jaundice, labetalol should be stopped and not restarted.

Cardiac Failure: Sympathetic stimulation is a vital component supporting circulatory function in congestive heart failure. Beta-blockade carries a potential hazard of further depressing myocardial contractility and precipitating more severe failure. Although beta-blockers should be avoided in overt congestive heart failure, if necessary, labetalol HCl can be used with caution in patients with a history of heart failure who are well compensated. Congestive heart failure has been observed in patients receiving labetalol HCl. Labetalol HCl does not abolish the inotropic action of digitalis on heart muscle.

In Patients Without a History of Cardiac Failure: In patients with latent cardiac insufficiency, continued depression of the myocardium with beta-blocking agents over a period of time can, in some cases, lead to cardiac failure. At the first sign or symptom of impending cardiac failure, patients should be fully digitalized and/or be given a diuretic, and the response should be observed closely. If cardiac failure continues despite adequate digitalization and diuretic, therapy with TRANDATE Injection should be withdrawn (gradually, if possible).

Ischemic Heart Disease: Angina pectoris has not been reported upon labetalol HCl discontinuation. However, following abrupt cessation of therapy with some beta-blocking agents in patients with coronary artery disease, exacerbations of angina pectoris and, in some cases, myocardial infarction have been reported. Therefore, such patients should be cautioned against interruption of therapy without the physician's advice. Even in the absence of overt angina pectoris, when discontinuation of TRANDATE Injection is planned, the patient should be carefully observed and should be advised to limit physical activity. If angina markedly worsens or acute coronary insufficiency develops, administration of TRANDATE Injection should be reinstituted promptly, at least temporarily, and other measures appropriate for the management of unstable angina should be taken.

Nonallergic Bronchospasm (e.g., Chronic Bronchitis and Emphysema): Since TRANDATE Injection at the usual IV therapeutic doses has not been studied in patients with nonallergic bronchospastic disease, it should not be used in such patients.

Pheochromocytoma: Intravenous labetalol HCl has been shown to be effective in lowering blood pressure and relieving symptoms in patients with pheochromocytoma; higher than usual doses may be required. However, paradoxical hypertensive responses have been reported in a few patients with this tumor; therefore, use caution when administering labetalol HCl to patients with pheochromocytoma.

Diabetes Mellitus and Hypoglycemia: Beta-adrenergic blockade may prevent the appearance of premonitory signs and symptoms (e.g., tachycardia) of acute hypoglycemia. This is especially important with labile diabetics. Beta-blockade also reduces the release of insulin in response to hyperglycemia; it may therefore be necessary to adjust the dose of antidiabetic drugs.

Major Surgery: The necessity or desirability of withdrawing beta-blocking therapy before major surgery is controversial. Protracted severe hypotension and difficulty in restarting or maintaining a heartbeat have been reported with beta-blockers. The effect of labetalol HCl's alpha-adrenergic activity has not been evaluated in this setting.

A synergism between labetalol HCl and halothane anesthesia has been shown (see PRECAUTIONS: Drug Interactions).

Rapid Decreases of Blood Presure: Caution must be observed when reducing severely elevated blood pressure. Although such findings have not been reported with IV labetalol HCl, a number of adverse reactions, including cerebral infarction, optic nerve infarction, angina, and ischemic changes in the electrocardiogram, have been reported with other agents when severely elevated blood pressure was reduced over time courses of several hours to as long as 1 or 2 days. The desired blood pressure lowering should therefore be achieved over as long a period of time as is compatible with the patient's status.

PRECAUTIONS

General: ***Impaired Hepatic Function:*** TRANDATE Injection should be used with caution in patients with impaired hepatic function since metabolism of the drug may be diminished.

Hypotension: Symptomatic postural hypotension (incidence, 58%) is likely to occur if patients are tilted or allowed to assume the upright position within 3 hours of receiving TRANDATE Injection. Therefore, the patient's ability to tolerate an upright position should be established before permitting any ambulation.

Following Coronary Artery Bypass Surgery: In one uncontrolled study, patients with low cardiac indices and elevated systemic vascular resistance following intravenous labetalol HCl experienced significant declines in cardiac output with little change in systemic vascular resistance. One of these patients developed hypotension following labetalol treatment. Therefore, use of labetalol HCl should be avoided in such patients.

High Dose Labetalol: Administration of up to 3 g/d as an infusion for up to 2 to 3 days has been anecdotally reported; several patients have experienced hypotension or bradycardia.

Jaundice or Hepatic Dysfunction: (see WARNINGS).

Information for Patients: The following information is intended to aid in the safe and effective use of this medication. It is not a disclosure of all possible adverse or intended effects. During and immediately following (for up to 3 hours) TRANDATE Injection, the patient should remain supine. Subsequently, the patient should be advised on how to proceed gradually to become ambulatory and should be observed at the time of first ambulation.

When the patient is started on TRANDATE® (labetalol HCl) Tablets following adequate control of blood pressure with TRANDATE Injection, appropriate directions for titration of dosage should be provided (see DOSAGE AND ADMINISTRATION).

As with all drugs with beta-blocking activity, certain advice to patients being treated with labetalol HCl is warranted. While no incident of the abrupt withdrawal phenomenon (exacerbation of angina pectoris) has been reported with labetalol HCl, dosing with TRANDATE Tablets should not be interrupted or discontinued without a physician's advice. Patients being treated with TRANDATE Tablets should consult a physician at any signs or symptoms of impending cardiac failure or hepatic dysfunction (see WARNINGS). Also, transient scalp tingling may occur, usually when treatment with TRANDATE Tablets is initiated (see ADVERSE REACTIONS).

Laboratory Tests: Routine laboratory tests are ordinarily not required before or after IV labetalol HCl. In patients with concomitant illnesses, such as impaired renal function, appropriate tests should be done to monitor these conditions.

Drug Interactions: Since TRANDATE Injection may be administered to patients already being treated with other medications, including other antihypertensive agents, careful monitoring of these patients is necessary to detect and treat promptly any undesired effect from concomitant administration.

In one survey, 2.3% of patients taking labetalol HCl orally in combination with tricyclic antidepressants experienced tremor as compared to 0.7% reported to occur with labetalol HCl alone. The contribution of each of the treatments to this adverse reaction is unknown, but the possibility of a drug interaction cannot be excluded.

Drugs possessing beta-blocking properties can blunt the bronchodilator effect of beta-receptor agonist drugs in patients with bronchospasm; therefore, doses greater than the normal antiasthmatic dose of beta-agonist bronchodilator drugs may be required.

Cimetidine has been shown to increase the bioavailability of labetalol HCl administered orally. Since this could be explained either by enhanced absorption or by an alteration of hepatic metabolism of labetalol HCl, special care should be used in establishing the dose required for blood pressure control in such patients.

Continued on next page

This product information is based on labeling in effect on June 1, 1998. For further information, contact via direct mail, phone, or web site Medical Information: Glaxo Wellcome Inc., PO Box 13398, Research Triangle Park, NC 27709. Healthcare Professionals (Medical Information): 800-334-0089 Patients (Customer Response Center): 888-TALK2GW (1-888-825-5249) Glaxo Wellcome Corporate Web Site: www.glaxowellcome.com

Trandate Injection—Cont.

Synergism has been shown between halothane anesthesia and intravenously administered labetalol HCl. During controlled hypotensive anesthesia using labetalol HCl in association with halothane, high concentrations (3% or above) of halothane should not be used because the degree of hypotension will be increased and because of the possibility of a large reduction in cardiac output and an increase in central venous pressure. The anesthesiologist should be informed when a patient is receiving labetalol HCl.

Labetalol HCl blunts the reflex tachycardia produced by nitroglycerin without preventing its hypotensive effect. If labetalol HCl is used with nitroglycerin in patients with angina pectoris, additional antihypertensive effects may occur. Care should be taken if labetalol is used concomitantly with calcium antagonists of the verapamil type.

Risk of Anaphylactic Reaction: While taking beta-blockers, patients with a history of severe anaphylactic reaction to a variety of allergens may be more reactive to repeated challenge, either accidental, diagnostic, or therapeutic. Such patients may be unresponsive to the usual doses of epinephrine used to treat allergic reaction.

Drug/Laboratory Test Interactions: The presence of labetalol metabolites in the urine may result in falsely elevated levels of urinary catecholamines, metanephrine, normetanephrine, and vanillylmandelic acid when measured by fluorimetric or photometric methods. In screening patients suspected of having a pheochromocytoma and being treated with labetalol HCl, a specific method, such as a high performance liquid chromatographic assay with solid phase extraction (e.g., *J Chromatogr* 385:241,1987) should be employed in determining levels of catecholamines.

Labetalol HCl has also been reported to produce a false-positive test for amphetamine when screening urine for the presence of drugs using the commercially available assay methods Toxi-Lab A® (thin-layer chromatographic assay) and Emit-d.a.u.® (radioenzymatic assay). When patients being treated with labetalol have a positive urine test for amphetamine using these techniques, confirmation should be made by using more specific methods, such as a gas chromatographic-mass spectrometer technique.

Carcinogenesis, Mutagenesis, Impairment of Fertility: Long-term oral dosing studies with labetalol HCl for 18 months in mice and for 2 years in rats showed no evidence of carcinogenesis. Studies with labetalol HCl using dominant lethal assays in rats and mice and exposing microorganisms according to modified Ames tests showed no evidence of mutagenesis.

Pregnancy: ***Teratogenic Effects: Pregnancy Category C:*** Teratogenic studies were performed with labetalol in rats and rabbits at oral doses up to approximately six and four times the maximum recommended human dose (MRHD), respectively. No reproducible evidence of fetal malformations was observed. Increased fetal resorptions were seen in both species at doses approximating the MRHD. A teratology study performed with labetalol in rabbits at IV doses up to 1.7 times the MRHD revealed no evidence of drug-related harm to the fetus. There are no adequate and well-controlled studies in pregnant women. Labetalol should be used during pregnancy only if the potential benefit justifies the potential risk to the fetus.

Nonteratogenic Effects: Hypotension, bradycardia, hypoglycemia, and respiratory depression have been reported in infants of mothers who were treated with labetalol HCl for hypertension during pregnancy. Oral administration of labetalol to rats during late gestation through weaning at doses of two to four times the MRHD caused a decrease in neonatal survival.

Labor and Delivery: Labetalol HCl given to pregnant women with hypertension did not appear to affect the usual course of labor and delivery.

Nursing Mothers: Small amounts of labetalol (approximately 0.004% of the maternal dose) are excreted in human milk. Caution should be exercised when TRANDATE Injection is administered to a nursing woman.

Pediatric Use: Safety and effectiveness in pediatric patients have not been established.

ADVERSE REACTIONS

TRANDATE Injection is usually well tolerated. Most adverse effects have been mild and transient and, in controlled trials involving 92 patients, did not require labetalol HCl withdrawal. Symptomatic postural hypotension (incidence, 58%) is likely to occur if patients are tilted or allowed to assume the upright position within 3 hours of receiving TRANDATE Injection. Moderate hypotension occurred in 1 of 100 patients while supine. Increased sweating was noted in 4 of 100 patients, and flushing occurred in 1 of 100 patients.

The following also were reported with TRANDATE Injection with the incidence per 100 patients as noted:

Cardiovascular System: Ventricular arrhythmia in 1.

Central and Peripheral Nervous Systems: Dizziness in 9, tingling of the scalp/skin in 7, hypoesthesia (numbness) and vertigo in 1 each.

Gastrointestinal System: Nausea in 13, vomiting in 4, dyspepsia and taste distortion in 1 each.

Metabolic Disorders: Transient increases in blood urea nitrogen and serum creatinine levels occurred in 8 of 100 patients; these were associated with drops in blood pressure, generally in patients with prior renal insufficiency.

Psychiatric Disorders: Somnolence/yawning in 3.

Respiratory System: Wheezing in 1.

Skin: Pruritus in 1.

The incidence of adverse reactions depends upon the dose of labetalol HCl. The largest experience is with oral labetalol HCl (see TRANDATE® [labetalol hydrochloride] Tablets Product Information for details). Certain of the side effects increased with increasing oral dose, as shown in the following table that depicts the entire US therapeutic trials data base for adverse reactions that are clearly or possibly dose related.

[See table below]

In addition, a number of other less common adverse events have been reported:

Cardiovascular: Hypotension, and rarely, syncope, bradycardia, heart block.

Liver and Biliary System: Hepatic necrosis, hepatitis, cholestatic jaundice, elevated liver function tests.

Hypersensitivity: Rare reports of hypersensitivity (e.g., rash, urticaria, pruritus, angioedema, dyspnea) and anaphylactoid reactions.

The oculomucocutaneous syndrome associated with the beta-blocker practolol has not been reported with labetalol HCl during investigational use and extensive foreign marketing experience.

Clinical Laboratory Tests: Among patients dosed with TRANDATE Tablets, there have been reversible increases of serum transaminases in 4% of patients tested and, more rarely, reversible increases in blood urea.

OVERDOSAGE

Overdosage with labetalol HCl causes excessive hypotension that is posture sensitive and, sometimes, excessive bradycardia. Patients should be placed supine and their legs raised if necessary to improve the blood supply to the brain. If overdosage with labetalol HCl follows oral ingestion, gastric lavage or pharmacologically induced emesis (using syrup of ipecac) may be useful for removal of the drug shortly after ingestion. The following additional measures should be employed if necessary: **Excessive bradycardia**—administer atropine or epinephrine. **Cardiac failure**—administer a digitalis glycoside and a diuretic. Dopamine or dobutamine may also be useful. **Hypotension**—administer vasopressors, e.g., norepinephrine. There is pharmacologic evidence that norepinephrine may be the drug of choice. **Bronchospasm**—administer epinephrine and/or an aerosolized beta$_2$-agonist. **Seizures**—administer diazepam.

In severe beta-blocker overdose resulting in hypotension and/or bradycardia, glucagon has been shown to be effective when administered in large doses (5 to 10 mg rapidly over 30 seconds, followed by continuous infusion of 5 mg/h that can be reduced as the patient improves).

Neither hemodialysis nor peritoneal dialysis removes a significant amount of labetalol from the general circulation (<1%).

The oral LD_{50} value of labetalol HCl in the mouse is approximately 600 mg/kg and in the rat is greater than 2 g/kg. The IV LD_{50} in these species is 50 to 60 mg/kg.

DOSAGE AND ADMINISTRATION

TRANDATE Injection is intended for IV use in hospitalized patients. DOSAGE MUST BE INDIVIDUALIZED depending upon the severity of hypertension and the response of the patient during dosing.

Patients should always be kept in a supine position during the period of IV drug administration. A substantial fall in blood pressure on standing should be expected in these patients. The patient's ability to tolerate an upright position should be established before permitting any ambulation, such as using toilet facilities.

Either of two methods of administration of TRANDATE Injection may be used: a) repeated IV injection, or b) slow continuous infusion.

Repeated Intravenous Injection: Initially, TRANDATE Injection should be given in a 20-mg dose (which corresponds to 0.25 mg/kg for an 80-kg patient) by slow IV injection over a 2-minute period.

Immediately before the injection and at 5 and 10 minutes after injection, supine blood pressure should be measured to evaluate response. Additional injections of 40 or 80 mg can be given at 10-minute intervals until a desired supine blood pressure is achieved or a total of 300 mg of labetalol HCl has been injected. The maximum effect usually occurs within 5 minutes of each injection.

Slow Continuous Infusion: TRANDATE Injection is prepared for continuous IV infusion by diluting the vial contents with commonly used IV fluids (see below). Examples of two methods of preparing the infusion solution are:

Add 40 mL of TRANDATE Injection to 160 mL of a commonly used IV fluid such that the resultant 200 mL of solution contains 200 mg of labetalol HCl, 1 mg/mL. The diluted solution should be administered at a rate of 2 mL/min to deliver 2 mg/min.

Alternatively, add 40 mL of TRANDATE Injection to 250 mL of a commonly used IV fluid. The resultant solution will contain 200 mg of labetalol HCl, approximately 2 mg/3 mL. The diluted solution should be administered at a rate of 3 mL/min to deliver approximately 2 mg/min.

The rate of infusion of the diluted solution may be adjusted according to the blood pressure response, at the discretion of the physician. To facilitate a desired rate of infusion, the diluted solution can be infused using a controlled administration mechanism, e.g., graduated burette or mechanically driven infusion pump.

Since the half-life of labetalol is 5 to 8 hours, steady-state blood levels (in the face of a constant rate of infusion) would not be reached during the usual infusion time period. The infusion should be continued until a satisfactory response is obtained and should then be stopped and oral labetalol HCl started (see below). The effective IV dose is usually in the range of 50 to 200 mg. A total dose of up to 300 mg may be required in some patients.

Blood Pressure Monitoring: The blood pressure should be monitored during and after completion of the infusion or IV injection. Rapid or excessive falls in either systolic or diastolic blood pressure during IV treatment should be avoided. In patients with excessive systolic hypertension, the decrease in systolic pressure should be used as an indicator of effectiveness in addition to the response of the diastolic pressure.

Initiation of Dosing With TRANDATE Tablets: Subsequent oral dosing with TRANDATE Tablets should begin when it has been established that the supine diastolic blood pressure has begun to rise. The recommended initial dose is 200 mg, followed in 6 to 12 hours by an additional dose of 200 or 400 mg, depending on the blood pressure response. Thereafter, **inpatient titration with TRANDATE Tablets** may proceed as follows:

Inpatient Titration Instructions

Regimen	Daily Dose*
200 mg b.i.d.	400 mg
400 mg b.i.d.	800 mg
800 mg b.i.d.	1,600 mg
1,200 mg b.i.d.	2,400 mg

*If needed, the total daily dose may be given in three divided doses.

The dosage of TRANDATE Tablets used in the hospital may be increased at 1-day intervals to achieve the desired blood pressure reduction.

For subsequent outpatient titration or maintenance dosing, see DOSAGE AND ADMINISTRATION in the TRANDATE Tablets Product Information for additional recommendations.

Compatibility With Commonly Used Intravenous Fluids: Parenteral drug products should be inspected visually for particulate matter and discoloration before administration whenever solution and container permit.

Labetalol HCl Daily Dose (mg)	200	300	400	600	800	900	1,200	1,600	2,400
Number of patients	522	181	606	608	503	117	411	242	175
Dizziness (%)	2	3	3	3	5	1	9	13	16
Fatigue	2	1	4	4	5	3	7	6	10
Nausea	<1	0	1	2	4	0	7	11	19
Vomiting	0	0	<1	<1	<1	0	1	2	3
Dyspepsia	1	0	2	1	1	0	2	2	4
Paresthesia	2	0	2	2	1	1	2	5	5
Nasal stuffiness	1	1	2	2	2	2	4	5	6
Ejaculation failure	0	2	1	2	3	0	4	3	5
Impotence	1	1	1	1	2	4	3	4	3
Edema	1	0	1	1	1	0	1	2	2

TRANDATE Injection was tested for compatibility with commonly used IV fluids at final concentrations of 1.25 to 3.75 mg of labetalol HCl per milliliter of the mixture.
TRANDATE Injection was found to be compatible with and stable (for 24 hours refrigerated or at room temperature) in mixtures with the following solutions: ringer's injection, USP; lactated ringer's injection, USP; 5% dextrose and ringer's injection; 5% lactated ringer's and 5% dextrose injection; 5% dextrose injection, USP; 0.9% sodium chloride injection, USP; 5% dextrose and 0.2% sodium chloride injection, USP; 2.5% dextrose and 0.45% sodium chloride injection, USP; 5% dextrose and 0.9% sodium chloride injection, USP; and 5% dextrose and 0.33% sodium chloride injection, USP.
TRANDATE Injection was NOT compatible with 5% sodium bicarbonate injection, USP. Care should be taken when administering alkaline drugs, including furosemide, in combination with labetalol. Compatibility should be assured prior to administering these drugs together.

HOW SUPPLIED

TRANDATE Injection, 5 mg/mL, is supplied in 20-mL (100-mg) vials, box of one (NDC 0173-0350-58) and 40-mL (200-mg) vials, box of one (NDC 0173-0350-57).
Store between 2° and 30°C (36° and 86°F). Do not freeze. Protect from light.
May 1997/RL-426
Shown in Product Identification Guide, page 314

TRANDATE® ℞
[*trăn 'dāt*]
(labetalol hydrochloride)
Tablets

DESCRIPTION

TRANDATE Tablets are adrenergic receptor blocking agents that have both selective alpha$_1$-adrenergic and nonselective beta-adrenergic receptor blocking actions in a single substance.
Labetalol hydrochloride (HCl) is a racemate chemically designated as 2-hydroxy-5-[1-hydroxy-2-[(1-methyl-3-phenylpropyl)amino]ethyl]benzamide monohydrochloride.
Labetalol HCl has the empirical formula $C_{19}H_{24}N_2O_3{\cdot}HCl$ and a molecular weight of 364.9. It has two asymmetric centers and therefore exists as a molecular complex of two diastereoisomeric pairs. Dilevalol, the R,R' stereoisomer, makes up 25% of racemic labetalol.
Labetalol HCl is a white or off-white crystalline powder, soluble in water.
TRANDATE Tablets contain 100, 200, or 300 mg of labetalol HCl and are taken orally. The tablets also contain the inactive ingredients corn starch, FD&C Yellow No. 6 (100- and 300-mg tablets only), hydroxypropyl methylcellulose, lactose, magnesium stearate, methylparaben, pregelatinized corn starch, propylparaben, sodium benzoate (200-mg tablet only), talc (100-mg tablet only), and titanium dioxide.

CLINICAL PHARMACOLOGY

Labetalol HCl combines both selective, competitive, alpha$_1$-adrenergic blocking and nonselective, competitive, beta-adrenergic blocking activity in a single substance. In man, the ratios of alpha- to beta-blockade have been estimated to be approximately 1:3 and 1:7 following oral and intravenous (IV) administration, respectively. Beta$_2$-agonist activity has been demonstrated in animals with minimal beta$_1$-agonist (ISA) activity detected. In animals, at doses greater than those required for alpha- or beta-adrenergic blockade, a membrane stabilizing effect has been demonstrated.
Pharmacodynamics: The capacity of labetalol HCl to block alpha receptors in man has been demonstrated by attenuation of the pressor effect of phenylephrine and by a significant reduction of the pressor response caused by immersing the hand in ice-cold water ("cold-pressor test"). Labetalol HCl's beta$_1$-receptor blockade in man was demonstrated by a small decrease in the resting heart rate, attenuation of tachycardia produced by isoproterenol or exercise, and by attenuation of the reflex tachycardia to the hypotension produced by amyl nitrite. Beta$_2$-receptor blockade was demonstrated by inhibition of the isoproterenol-induced fall in diastolic blood pressure. Both the alpha- and beta-blocking actions of orally administered labetalol HCl contribute to a decrease in blood pressure in hypertensive patients. Labetalol HCl consistently, in dose-related fashion, blunted increases in exercise-induced blood pressure and heart rate, and in their double product. The pulmonary circulation during exercise was not affected by labetalol HCl dosing.
Single oral doses of labetalol HCl administered to patients with coronary artery disease had no significant effect on sinus rate, intraventricular conduction, or QRS duration. The atrioventricular (A-V) conduction time was modestly prolonged in two of seven patients. In another study, IV labetalol HCl slightly prolonged A-V nodal conduction time and atrial effective refractory period with only small changes in heart rate. The effects on A-V nodal refractoriness were inconsistent.
Labetalol HCl produces dose-related falls in blood pressure without reflex tachycardia and without significant reduction in heart rate, presumably through a mixture of its alpha- and beta-blocking effects. Hemodynamic effects are variable, with small, nonsignificant changes in cardiac output seen in some studies but not others, and small decreases in total peripheral resistance. Elevated plasma renins are reduced.
Doses of labetalol HCl that controlled hypertension did not affect renal function in mildly to severely hypertensive patients with normal renal function.
Due to the alpha$_1$-receptor blocking activity of labetalol HCl, blood pressure is lowered more in the standing than in the supine position, and symptoms of postural hypotension (2%), including rare instances of syncope, can occur. Following oral administration, when postural hypotension has occurred, it has been transient and is uncommon when the recommended starting dose and titration increments are closely followed (see DOSAGE AND ADMINISTRATION).
Symptomatic postural hypotension is most likely to occur 2 to 4 hours after a dose, especially following the use of large initial doses or upon large changes in dose.
The peak effects of single oral doses of labetalol HCl occur within 2 to 4 hours. The duration of effect depends upon dose, lasting at least 8 hours following single oral doses of 100 mg and more than 12 hours following single oral doses of 300 mg. The maximum, steady-state blood pressure response upon oral, twice-a-day dosing occurs within 24 to 72 hours.
The antihypertensive effect of labetalol has a linear correlation with the logarithm of labetalol plasma concentration, and there is also a linear correlation between the reduction in exercise-induced tachycardia occurring at 2 hours after oral administration of labetalol HCl and the logarithm of the plasma concentration.
About 70% of the maximum beta-blocking effect is present for 5 hours after the administration of a single oral dose of 400 mg with suggestion that about 40% remains at 8 hours.
The antianginal efficacy of labetalol HCl has not been studied. In 37 patients with hypertension and coronary artery disease, labetalol HCl did not increase the incidence or severity of angina attacks.
Exacerbation of angina and, in some cases, myocardial infarction and ventricular dysrhythmias have been reported after abrupt discontinuation of therapy with beta-adrenergic blocking agents in patients with coronary artery disease. Abrupt withdrawal of these agents in patients without coronary artery disease has resulted in transient symptoms, including tremulousness, sweating, palpitation, headache, and malaise. Several mechanisms have been proposed to explain these phenomena, among them increased sensitivity to catecholamines because of increased numbers of beta receptors.
Although beta-adrenergic receptor blockade is useful in the treatment of angina and hypertension, there are also situations in which sympathetic stimulation is vital. For example, in patients with severely damaged hearts, adequate ventricular function may depend on sympathetic drive. Beta-adrenergic blockade may worsen A-V block by preventing the necessary facilitating effects of sympathetic activity on conduction. Beta$_2$-adrenergic blockade results in passive bronchial constriction by interfering with endogenous adrenergic bronchodilator activity in patients subject to bronchospasm, and it may also interfere with exogenous bronchodilators in such patients.
Pharmacokinetics and Metabolism: Labetalol HCl is completely absorbed from the gastrointestinal tract with peak plasma levels occurring 1 to 2 hours after oral administration. The relative bioavailability of labetalol HCl tablets compared to an oral solution is 100%. The absolute bioavailability (fraction of drug reaching systemic circulation) of labetalol when compared to an IV infusion is 25%; this is due to extensive "first-pass" metabolism. Despite "first-pass" metabolism, there is a linear relationship between oral doses of 100 to 3,000 mg and peak plasma levels. The absolute bioavailability of labetalol is increased when administered with food.
The plasma half-life of labetalol following oral administration is about 6 to 8 hours. Steady-state plasma levels of labetalol during repetitive dosing are reached by about the third day of dosing. In patients with decreased hepatic or renal function, the elimination half-life of labetalol is not altered; however, the relative bioavailability in hepatically impaired patients is increased due to decreased "first-pass" metabolism.
The metabolism of labetalol is mainly through conjugation to glucuronide metabolites. These metabolites are present in plasma and are excreted in the urine and, via the bile, into the feces. Approximately 55% to 60% of a dose appears in the urine as conjugates or unchanged labetalol within the first 24 hours of dosing.
Labetalol has been shown to cross the placental barrier in humans. Only negligible amounts of the drug crossed the blood-brain barrier in animal studies. Labetalol is approximately 50% protein bound. Neither hemodialysis nor peritoneal dialysis removes a significant amount of labetalol HCl from the general circulation (<1%).
Elderly Patients: Some pharmacokinetic studies indicate that the elimination of labetalol is reduced in elderly patients. Therefore, although elderly patients may initiate therapy at the currently recommended dosage of 100 mg b.i.d., elderly patients will generally require lower maintenance dosages than nonelderly patients.

INDICATIONS AND USAGE

TRANDATE Tablets are indicated in the management of hypertension. TRANDATE Tablets may be used alone or in combination with other antihypertensive agents, especially thiazide and loop diuretics.

CONTRAINDICATIONS

TRANDATE Tablets are contraindicated in bronchial asthma, overt cardiac failure, greater-than-first-degree heart block, cardiogenic shock, severe bradycardia, other conditions associated with severe and prolonged hypotension, and in patients with a history of hypersensitivity to any component of the product (see WARNINGS).

WARNINGS

Hepatic Injury: Severe hepatocellular injury, confirmed by rechallenge in at least one case, occurs rarely with labetalol therapy. The hepatic injury is usually reversible, but hepatic necrosis and death have been reported. Injury has occurred after both short- and long-term treatment and may be slowly progressive despite minimal symptomatology. Similar hepatic events have been reported with a related research compound, dilevalol HCl, including two deaths. Dilevalol HCl is one of the four isomers of labetalol HCl. Thus, for patients taking labetalol, periodic determination of suitable hepatic laboratory tests would be appropriate. Appropriate laboratory testing should be done at the first symptom/sign of liver dysfunction (e.g., pruritus, dark urine, persistent anorexia, jaundice, right upper quadrant tenderness, or unexplained "flu-like" symptoms). If the patient has laboratory evidence of liver injury or jaundice, labetalol should be stopped and not restarted.
Cardiac Failure: Sympathetic stimulation is a vital component supporting circulatory function in congestive heart failure. Beta-blockade carries a potential hazard of further depressing myocardial contractility and precipitating more severe failure. Although beta-blockers should be avoided in overt congestive heart failure, if necessary, labetalol HCl can be used with caution in patients with a history of heart failure who are well compensated. Congestive heart failure has been observed in patients receiving labetalol HCl. Labetalol HCl does not abolish the inotropic action of digitalis on heart muscle.
In Patients Without a History of Cardiac Failure: In patients with latent cardiac insufficiency, continued depression of the myocardium with beta-blocking agents over a period of time can, in some cases, lead to cardiac failure. At the first sign or symptom of impending cardiac failure, patients should be fully digitalized and/or be given a diuretic, and the response should be observed closely. If cardiac failure continues despite adequate digitalization and diuretic, therapy with TRANDATE Tablets should be withdrawn (gradually, if possible).
Exacerbation of Ischemic Heart Disease Following Abrupt Withdrawal: Angina pectoris has not been reported upon labetalol HCl discontinuation. However, hypersensitivity to catecholamines has been observed in patients withdrawn from beta-blocker therapy; exacerbation of angina and, in some cases, myocardial infarction have occurred after *abrupt* discontinuation of such therapy. When discontinuing chronically administered TRANDATE Tablets, particularly in patients with ischemic heart disease, the dosage should be gradually reduced over a period of 1 to 2 weeks and the patient should be carefully monitored. If angina markedly worsens or acute coronary insufficiency develops, therapy with TRANDATE Tablets should be reinstituted promptly, at least temporarily, and other measures appropriate for the management of unstable angina should be taken. Patients should be warned against interruption or discontinuation of therapy without the physician's advice. Because coronary artery disease is common and may be unrecognized, it may be prudent not to discontinue therapy with TRANDATE Tablets abruptly in patients being treated for hypertension.
Nonallergic Bronchospasm (e.g., Chronic Bronchitis and Emphysema): Patients with bronchospastic disease

Continued on next page

This product information is based on labeling in effect on June 1, 1998. For further information, contact via direct mail, phone, or web site Medical Information: Glaxo Wellcome Inc., PO Box 13398, Research Triangle Park, NC 27709. Healthcare Professionals (Medical Information): 800-334-0089 Patients (Customer Response Center): 888-TALK2GW (1-888-825-5249) Glaxo Wellcome Corporate Web Site: www.glaxowellcome.com

Trandate Tablets—Cont.

should, in general, not receive beta-blockers. TRANDATE Tablets may be used with caution, however, in patients who do not respond to, or cannot tolerate, other antihypertensive agents. It is prudent, if TRANDATE Tablets are used, to use the smallest effective dose, so that inhibition of endogenous or exogenous beta-agonists is minimized.

Pheochromocytoma: Labetalol HCl has been shown to be effective in lowering blood pressure and relieving symptoms in patients with pheochromocytoma. However, paradoxical hypertensive responses have been reported in a few patients with this tumor; therefore, use caution when administering labetalol HCl to patients with pheochromocytoma.

Diabetes Mellitus and Hypoglycemia: Beta-adrenergic blockade may prevent the appearance of premonitory signs and symptoms (e.g., tachycardia) of acute hypoglycemia. This is especially important with labile diabetics. Beta-blockade also reduces the release of insulin in response to hyperglycemia; it may therefore be necessary to adjust the dose of antidiabetic drugs.

Major Surgery: The necessity or desirability of withdrawing beta-blocking therapy before major surgery is controversial. Protracted severe hypotension and difficulty in restarting or maintaining a heartbeat have been reported with beta-blockers. The effect of labetalol HCl's alpha-adrenergic activity has not been evaluated in this setting.

A synergism between labetalol HCl and halothane anesthesia has been shown (see PRECAUTIONS: Drug Interactions).

PRECAUTIONS

General: *Impaired Hepatic Function:* TRANDATE Tablets should be used with caution in patients with impaired hepatic function since metabolism of the drug may be diminished.

Jaundice or Hepatic Dysfunction: (see WARNINGS).

Information for Patients: As with all drugs with beta-blocking activity, certain advice to patients being treated with labetalol HCl is warranted. This information is intended to aid in the safe and effective use of this medication. It is not a disclosure of all possible adverse or intended effects. While no incident of the abrupt withdrawal phenomenon (exacerbation of angina pectoris) has been reported with labetalol HCl, dosing with TRANDATE Tablets should not be interrupted or discontinued without a physician's advice. Patients being treated with TRANDATE Tablets should consult a physician at any signs or symptoms of impending cardiac failure or hepatic dysfunction (see WARNINGS). Also, transient scalp tingling may occur, usually when treatment with TRANDATE Tablets is initiated (see ADVERSE REACTIONS).

Laboratory Tests: As with any new drug given over prolonged periods, laboratory parameters should be observed over regular intervals. In patients with concomitant ill-nesses, such as impaired renal function, appropriate tests should be done to monitor these conditions.

Drug Interactions: In one survey, 2.3% of patients taking labetalol HCl in combination with tricyclic antidepressants experienced tremor, as compared to 0.7% reported to occur with labetalol HCl alone. The contribution of each of the treatments to this adverse reaction is unknown, but the possibility of a drug interaction cannot be excluded.

Drugs possessing beta-blocking properties can blunt the bronchodilator effect of beta-receptor agonist drugs in patients with bronchospasm; therefore, doses greater than the normal antiasthmatic dose of beta-agonist bronchodilator drugs may be required.

Cimetidine has been shown to increase the bioavailability of labetalol HCl. Since this could be explained either by enhanced absorption or by an alteration of hepatic metabolism of labetalol HCl, special care should be used in establishing the dose required for blood pressure control in such patients.

Synergism has been shown between halothane anesthesia and intravenously administered labetalol HCl. During controlled hypotensive anesthesia using labetalol HCl in association with halothane, high concentrations (3% or above) of halothane should not be used because the degree of hypotension will be increased and because of the possibility of a large reduction in cardiac output and an increase in central venous pressure. The anesthesiologist should be informed when a patient is receiving labetalol HCl.

Labetalol HCl blunts the reflex tachycardia produced by nitroglycerin without preventing its hypotensive effect. If labetalol HCl is used with nitroglycerin in patients with angina pectoris, additional antihypertensive effects may occur. Care should be taken if labetalol is used concomitantly with calcium antagonists of the verapamil type.

Risk of Anaphylactic Reaction: While taking beta-blockers, patients with a history of severe anaphylactic reaction to a variety of allergens may be more reactive to repeated challenge, either accidental, diagnostic, or therapeutic. Such patients may be unresponsive to the usual doses of epinephrine used to treat allergic reaction.

Drug/Laboratory Test Interactions: The presence of labetalol metabolites in the urine may result in falsely elevated levels of urinary catecholamines, metanephrine, normetanephrine, and vanillylmandelic acid when measured by fluorimetric or photometric methods. In screening patients suspected of having a pheochromocytoma and being treated with labetalol HCl, a specific method, such as a high performance liquid chromatographic assay with solid phase extraction (e.g., *J Chromatogr* 385:241, 1987) should be employed in determining levels of catecholamines.

Labetalol HCl has also been reported to produce a false-positive test for amphetamine when screening urine for the presence of drugs using the commercially available assay methods Toxi-Lab A® (thin-layer chromatographic assay) and Emit-d.a.u.® (radioenzymatic assay). When patients being treated with labetalol have a positive urine test for amphetamine using these techniques, confirmation should be made by using more specific methods, such as a gas chromatographic-mass spectrometer technique.

Carcinogenesis, Mutagenesis, Impairment of Fertility: Long-term oral dosing studies with labetalol HCl for 18 months in mice and for 2 years in rats showed no evidence of carcinogenesis. Studies with labetalol HCl using dominant lethal assays in rats and mice and exposing microorganisms according to modified Ames tests showed no evidence of mutagenesis.

Pregnancy: *Teratogenic Effects: Pregnancy Category C:* Teratogenic studies were performed with labetalol in rats and rabbits at oral doses up to approximately six and four times the maximum recommended human dose (MRHD), respectively. No reproducible evidence of fetal malformations was observed. Increased fetal resorptions were seen in both species at doses approximating the MRHD. A teratology study performed with labetalol in rabbits at IV doses up to 1.7 times the MRHD revealed no evidence of drug-related harm to the fetus. There are no adequate and well-controlled studies in pregnant women. Labetalol should be used during pregnancy only if the potential benefit justifies the potential risk to the fetus.

Nonteratogenic Effects: Hypotension, bradycardia, hypoglycemia, and respiratory depression have been reported in infants of mothers who were treated with labetalol HCl for hypertension during pregnancy. Oral administration of labetalol to rats during late gestation through weaning at doses of two to four times the MRHD caused a decrease in neonatal survival.

Labor and Delivery: Labetalol HCl given to pregnant women with hypertension did not appear to affect the usual course of labor and delivery.

Nursing Mothers: Small amounts of labetalol (approximately 0.004% of the maternal dose) are excreted in human milk. Caution should be exercised when TRANDATE Tablets are administered to a nursing woman.

Pediatric Use: Safety and effectiveness in pediatric patients have not been established.

Elderly Patients: As in the general population, some elderly patients (60 years of age and older) have experienced orthostatic hypotension, dizziness, or lightheadedness during treatment with labetalol. Because elderly patients are generally more likely than younger patients to experience orthostatic symptoms, they should be cautioned about the possibility of such side effects during treatment with labetalol.

ADVERSE REACTIONS

Most adverse effects are mild and transient and occur early in the course of treatment. In controlled clinical trials of 3 to 4 months' duration, discontinuation of TRANDATE Tablets due to one or more adverse effects was required in 7% of all patients. In these same trials, other agents with solely beta-blocking activity used in the control groups led to discontinuation in 8% to 10% of patients, and a centrally acting alpha-agonist led to discontinuation in 30% of patients.

The incidence rates of adverse reactions listed in the following table were derived from multicenter, controlled clinical trials comparing labetalol HCl, placebo, metoprolol, and propranolol over treatment periods of 3 and 4 months. Where the frequency of adverse effects for labetalol HCl and placebo is similar, causal relationship is uncertain. The rates are based on adverse reactions considered probably drug related by the investigator. If all reports are considered, the rates are somewhat higher (e.g., dizziness, 20%; nausea, 14%; fatigue, 11%), but the overall conclusions are unchanged.

[See table at left]

The adverse effects were reported spontaneously and are representative of the incidence of adverse effects that may be observed in a properly selected hypertensive patient population, i.e., a group excluding patients with bronchospastic disease, overt congestive heart failure, or other contraindications to beta-blocker therapy.

Clinical trials also included studies utilizing daily doses up to 2,400 mg in more severely hypertensive patients. Certain of the side effects increased with increasing dose, as shown in the following table that depicts the entire US therapeutic trials data base for adverse reactions that are clearly or possibly dose related.

[See table at top of next page]

In addition, a number of other less common adverse events have been reported:

Body as a Whole: Fever.

Cardiovascular: Hypotension, and rarely, syncope, bradycardia, heart block.

Central and Peripheral Nervous Systems: Paresthesia, most frequently described as scalp tingling. In most cases, it was mild and transient and usually occurred at the beginning of treatment.

Collagen Disorders: Systemic lupus erythematosus, positive antinuclear factor.

Eyes: Dry eyes.

Immunological System: Antimitochondrial antibodies.

	Labetalol HCl (n = 227) %	Placebo (n = 98) %	Propranolol (n = 84) %	Metoprolol (n = 49) %
Body as a whole				
Fatigue	5	0	12	12
Asthenia	1	1	1	0
Headache	2	1	1	2
Gastrointestinal				
Nausea	6	1	1	2
Vomiting	<1	0	0	0
Dyspepsia	3	1	1	0
Abdominal pain	0	0	1	2
Diarrhea	<1	0	2	0
Taste distortion	1	0	0	0
Central and peripheral nervous systems				
Dizziness	11	3	4	4
Paresthesia	<1	0	0	0
Drowsiness	<1	2	2	2
Autonomic nervous system				
Nasal stuffiness	3	0	0	0
Ejaculation failure	2	0	0	0
Impotence	1	0	1	3
Increased sweating	<1	0	0	0
Cardiovascular				
Edema	1	0	0	0
Postural hypotension	1	0	0	0
Bradycardia	0	0	5	12
Respiratory				
Dyspnea	2	0	1	2
Skin				
Rash	1	0	0	0
Special senses				
Vision abnormality	1	0	0	0
Vertigo	2	0	0	0

Labetalol HCl Daily Dose (mg)	200	300	400	600	800	900	1,200	1,600	2,400
Number of patients	522	181	606	608	503	117	411	242	175
Dizziness (%)	2	3	3	3	5	1	9	13	16
Fatigue	2	1	4	4	5	3	7	6	10
Nausea	<1	0	1	2	4	0	7	11	19
Vomiting	0	0	<1	<1	<1	0	1	2	3
Dyspepsia	1	0	2	1	1	0	2	2	4
Paresthesia	2	0	2	2	1	1	2	5	5
Nasal stuffiness	1	1	2	2	2	2	4	5	6
Ejaculation failure	0	2	1	2	3	0	4	3	5
Impotence	1	1	1	1	2	4	3	4	3
Edema	1	0	1	1	1	0	1	2	2

Liver and Biliary System: Hepatic necrosis, hepatitis, cholestatic jaundice, elevated liver function tests.

Musculoskeletal System: Muscle cramps, toxic myopathy.

Respiratory System: Bronchospasm.

Skin and Appendages: Rashes of various types, such as generalized maculopapular, lichenoid, urticarial, bullous lichen planus, psoriaform, and facial erythema; Peyronie's disease; reversible alopecia.

Urinary System: Difficulty in micturition, including acute urinary bladder retention.

Hypersensitivity: Rare reports of hypersensitivity (e.g., rash, urticaria, pruritus, angioedema, dyspnea) and anaphylactoid reactions.

Following approval for marketing in the United Kingdom, a monitored release survey involving approximately 6,800 patients was conducted for further safety and efficacy evaluation of this product. Results of this survey indicate that the type, severity, and incidence of adverse effects were comparable to those cited above.

Potential Adverse Effects: In addition, other adverse effects not listed above have been reported with other beta-adrenergic blocking agents.

Central Nervous System: Reversible mental depression progressing to catatonia, an acute reversible syndrome characterized by disorientation for time and place, short-term memory loss, emotional lability, slightly clouded sensorium, and decreased performance on psychometrics.

Cardiovascular: Intensification of A-V block (see CONTRAINDICATIONS).

Allergic: Fever combined with aching and sore throat, laryngospasm, respiratory distress.

Hematologic: Agranulocytosis, thrombocytopenic or nonthrombocytopenic purpura.

Gastrointestinal: Mesenteric artery thrombosis, ischemic colitis.

The oculomucocutaneous syndrome associated with the beta-blocker practolol has not been reported with labetalol HCl.

Clinical Laboratory Tests: There have been reversible increases of serum transaminases in 4% of patients treated with labetalol HCl and tested and, more rarely, reversible increases in blood urea.

OVERDOSAGE

Overdosage with labetalol HCl causes excessive hypotension that is posture sensitive and, sometimes, excessive bradycardia. Patients should be placed supine and their legs raised if necessary to improve the blood supply to the brain. If overdosage with labetalol HCl follows oral ingestion, gastric lavage or pharmacologically induced emesis (using syrup of ipecac) may be useful for removal of the drug shortly after ingestion. The following additional measures should be employed if necessary: **Excessive bradycardia**—administer atropine or epinephrine. **Cardiac failure**—administer a digitalis glycoside and a diuretic. Dopamine or dobutamine may also be useful. **Hypotension**—administer vasopressors, e.g., norepinephrine. There is pharmacologic evidence that norepinephrine may be the drug of choice. **Bronchospasm**—administer epinephrine and/or an aerosolized beta$_2$-agonist. **Seizures**—administer diazepam.

In severe beta-blocker overdose resulting in hypotension and/or bradycardia, glucagon has been shown to be effective when administered in large doses (5 to 10 mg rapidly over 30 seconds, followed by continuous infusion of 5 mg per hour that can be reduced as the patient improves).

Neither hemodialysis nor peritoneal dialysis removes a significant amount of labetalol HCl from the general circulation (<1%).

The oral LD$_{50}$ value of labetalol HCl in the mouse is approximately 600 mg/kg and in the rat is >2 g/kg. The IV LD$_{50}$ in these species is 50 to 60 mg/kg.

DOSAGE AND ADMINISTRATION

DOSAGE MUST BE INDIVIDUALIZED. The recommended *initial* dosage is 100 mg *twice* daily whether used alone or added to a diuretic regimen. After 2 or 3 days, using standing blood pressure as an indicator, dosage may be titrated in increments of 100 mg b.i.d. every 2 or 3 days. The usual *maintenance* dosage of labetalol HCl is between 200 and 400 mg *twice* daily.

Since the full antihypertensive effect of labetalol HCl is usually seen within the first 1 to 3 hours of the initial dose or dose increment, the assurance of a lack of an exaggerated hypotensive response can be clinically established in the office setting. The antihypertensive effects of continued dosing can be measured at subsequent visits, approximately 12 hours after a dose, to determine whether further titration is necessary.

Patients with severe hypertension may require from 1,200 to 2,400 mg per day, with or without thiazide diuretics. Should side effects (principally nausea or dizziness) occur with these doses administered twice daily, the same total daily dose administered three times daily may improve tolerability and facilitate further titration. Titration increments should not exceed 200 mg twice daily.

When a diuretic is added, an additive antihypertensive effect can be expected. In some cases this may necessitate a labetalol HCl dosage adjustment. As with most antihypertensive drugs, optimal dosages of TRANDATE Tablets are usually lower in patients also receiving a diuretic.

When transferring patients from other antihypertensive drugs, TRANDATE Tablets should be introduced as recommended and the dosage of the existing therapy progressively decreased.

Elderly Patients: As in the general patient population, labetalol therapy may be initiated at 100 mg twice daily and titrated upwards in increments of 100 mg b.i.d. as required for control of blood pressure. Since some elderly patients eliminate labetalol more slowly, however, adequate control of blood pressure may be achieved at a lower maintenance dosage compared to the general population. The majority of elderly patients will require between 100 and 200 mg b.i.d.

HOW SUPPLIED

TRANDATE Tablets, 100 mg, light orange, round, scored, film-coated tablets engraved on one side with "TRANDATE 100," bottles of 100 (NDC 0173-0346-43) and 500 (NDC 0173-0346-44) and unit dose packs of 100 tablets (NDC 0173-0346-47).

TRANDATE Tablets, 200 mg, white, round, scored, film-coated tablets engraved on one side with "TRANDATE 200," bottles of 100 (NDC 0173-0347-43) and 500 (NDC 0173-0347-44) and unit dose packs of 100 tablets (NDC 0173-0347-47).

TRANDATE Tablets, 300 mg, peach, round, scored, film-coated tablets engraved on one side with "TRANDATE 300," bottles of 100 (NDC 0173-0348-43) and 500 (NDC 0173-0348-44) and unit dose packs of 100 tablets (NDC 0173-0348-47).

TRANDATE Tablets should be stored between 2° and 30°C (36° and 86°F). TRANDATE Tablets in the unit dose boxes should be protected from excessive moisture.

May 1997/RL-423

Shown in Product Identification Guide, page 314

TRITEC® ℞

[*trī 'tĕk*]

(ranitidine bismuth citrate)

Tablets

DESCRIPTION

TRITEC Tablets contain a complex of ranitidine, trivalent bismuth, and citrate. Chemically, ranitidine bismuth citrate is N-2-[5-dimethylaminomethyl-2-furanylmethylthio]ethyl-N′-methyl-2-nitroethenediamine 2-hydroxy-1,2,3-propanetricarboxylate, bismuth (III). Analysis shows that ranitidine bismuth citrate is substoichiometric in ranitidine and citrate.

Ranitidine bismuth citrate is a white to off-white amorphous powder. The approximate molecular formula is $[C_{13}H_{22}N_4O_3S]_{0.84}\cdot Bi\cdot [C_6H_5O_7]_{0.94}$, and the approximate molecular weight is 651. It is readily soluble in water. Each TRITEC Tablet for oral administration contains 400 mg of ranitidine bismuth citrate, equivalent to approximately 162 mg of ranitidine (base), 128 mg of trivalent bismuth, and 110 mg of citrate. Each aqueous film-coated tablet also contains the inactive ingredients FD&C Blue No. 2 Aluminum Lake, magnesium stearate, methylhydroxypropylcellulose, microcrystalline cellulose, Povidone K30, sodium carbonate (anhydrous), titanium dioxide, and triacetin.

CLINICAL PHARMACOLOGY

Pharmacokinetics: Following ingestion, ranitidine bismuth citrate dissociates in intragastric fluid, giving rise to ranitidine and soluble and insoluble forms of bismuth.

Absorption: Following a single oral 400-mg dose of TRITEC to healthy volunteers, mean (±SD) peak ranitidine plasma concentration of 455 (±145.3) ng/mL occurred at 0.5 to 5 hours. The rate and extent of ranitidine absorption derived from TRITEC increased proportionally with increasing doses up to 1600 mg. Ranitidine plasma concentrations showed no evidence of accumulation during a 28-day dosing period.

Oral absorption of bismuth is variable. A mean (±SD) peak bismuth plasma concentration of 3.3 (±2.0) ng/mL occurs at 15 to 60 minutes after a 400-mg dose. The rate and extent of absorption of bismuth from TRITEC do not increase with increasing doses up to 800 mg, but increase more than proportionally with increasing doses above 800 mg. The rate of absorption of bismuth derived from an 800-mg dose of TRITEC is decreased by 50%, and the extent of absorption is decreased by 25% when taken 30 minutes after a meal as compared to 30 minutes before a meal. The absorption of bismuth from an 800-mg dose of TRITEC increased when gastric pH exceeded 6. The increased pH resulted from the administration of an 800-mg dose of TRITEC given 3 hours previously. Mucosal penetration and absorption of bismuth from TRITEC are not affected by the degree of gastritis, the presence of *Helicobacter pylori*, or an active ulcer. Small amounts of bismuth accumulate in plasma during twice-daily dosing with TRITEC. In a 28-day study at 800 mg b.i.d. (twice the recommended daily dose), peak bismuth concentrations did not exceed 20 ng/mL at any time in any patient, with a median peak concentration of 6.3 ng/mL on day 28. Median peak and trough concentrations on day 28 were 105% and 68% of predicted steady-state peak and trough concentrations. In a study at 400 mg b.i.d. for 12 weeks (three times the recommended duration), trough bismuth concentrations did not exceed predicted accumulation in any patient, with a median trough concentration of 2.8 ng/mL at week 12.

Distribution: The volume of distribution for ranitidine is 1.7 L/kg. Serum protein binding of ranitidine averages 15%. Bismuth is 98% bound to human plasma proteins, primarily albumin.

Metabolism: Ranitidine is metabolized to the N-oxide, S-oxide, and N-desmethyl metabolites, accounting for approximately 4%, 1%, and 1% of the dose, respectively. It is not known whether bismuth undergoes any biotransformation.

Excretion: The elimination half-life of ranitidine derived from TRITEC is 2.8 to 3.1 hours. The principal route of elimination for ranitidine is renal, accounting for 30% of the dose. Renal clearance averages 530 mL/min, indicating active tubular secretion. Total clearance is 760 mL/min. Elimination of bismuth is polyexponential, with a terminal elimination half-life of 11 to 28 days. Bismuth has an average renal clearance of 30 to 60 mL/min, indicating net tubular secretion. Less than 1% of bismuth derived from TRITEC is recovered in urine after oral administration. Up to 28% of bismuth was recovered in the feces during a 6-day postdose period. Bismuth also undergoes minor excretion in the bile.

Special Populations: *Geriatric:* Clinically insignificant increases in plasma concentrations of ranitidine were observed in elderly patients. Bismuth concentrations may be elevated in elderly patients as a result of decreased renal elimination.

Pediatric: No information on the pharmacokinetics of ranitidine or bismuth derived from TRITEC was obtained in this population.

Gender: There is no evidence of a difference in the pharmacokinetics of ranitidine between males and females when adjusted for body weight. There is no difference in the extent of absorption of bismuth when adjusted for body weight; significant differences are observed for peak bismuth plasma concentrations in healthy females.

Race: There is no evidence of any racial differences in the pharmacokinetics of bismuth based on trough concentrations observed in clinical studies.

Renal Insufficiency: The renal clearances of ranitidine and bismuth are correlated with renal function (i.e., creatinine clearance), while nonrenal elimination of ranitidine is unaltered by renal impairment. Thus, ranitidine and bismuth concentrations may be elevated in renally impaired patients as a result of decreased renal elimination.

Hepatic Insufficiency: Elimination of either ranitidine or bismuth by the hepatic route is relatively unimportant.

Continued on next page

This product information is based on labeling in effect on June 1, 1998. For further information, contact via direct mail, phone, or web site Medical Information: Glaxo Wellcome Inc., PO Box 13398, Research Triangle Park, NC 27709. Healthcare Professionals (Medical Information): 800-334-0089 Patients (Customer Response Center): 888-TALK2GW (1-888-825-5249) Glaxo Wellcome Corporate Web Site: www.glaxowellcome.com

Tritec—Cont.

Therefore, the pharmacokinetics of ranitidine or bismuth derived from TRITEC were not studied in patients with hepatic insufficiency owing to the minimal impact of this condition.

Pharmacodynamics: ***Antisecretory Activity: 1. Effects on Acid Secretion:*** Ranitidine, derived from TRITEC, inhibits both daytime and nocturnal basal gastric acid secretions as well as gastric acid secretion stimulated by food, betazole, and pentagastrin.

2. Effects on Other Gastrointestinal Secretions:

Plasma Pepsinogen I and II: Ranitidine derived from TRITEC does not alter plasma pepsinogen I and II concentrations or pepsin activity.

Serum Gastrin: Ranitidine derived from TRITEC has little or no effect on fasting or postprandial serum gastrin.

There is no information about the gastric mucosal concentrations of ranitidine, bismuth, clarithromycin, or hydroxyclarithromycin after administration of TRITEC and clarithromycin.

For information on the clinical pharmacology of clarithromycin, refer to the CLINICAL PHARMACOLOGY section of the clarithromycin package insert.

Microbiology: Ranitidine bismuth citrate plus clarithromycin has been shown to be active against most strains of *Helicobacter pylori in vitro* and in clinical infections as described in the INDICATIONS AND USAGE section.

Helicobacter

Helicobacter pylori

Pre-treatment Resistance

Clarithromycin pre-treatment resistance was 12.6% (44/348) in the ranitidine bismuth citrate plus clarithromycin b.i.d. versus t.i.d. clinical study (H2BA3001) conducted in 1996.

[See table 1 below]

Most patients not eradicated of *H pylori* following ranitidine bismuth citrate plus clarithromycin treatment will have clarithromycin resistant *H pylori*. Therefore, for those patients who fail therapy, clarithromycin susceptibility testing should be done when possible. Patients with clarithromycin resistant *H pylori* should not be treated with ranitidine bismuth citrate plus clarithromycin or with regimens which include clarithromycin as the sole antimicrobial agent.

Susceptibility Test for *Helicobacter pylori*

The reference methodology for susceptibility testing of *H pylori* is agar dilution MICs.[1] One to three microliters of an inoculum equivalent to a No.2 McFarland standard (1 x 10^7-1 x 10^8 CFU/mL for *H pylori*) are inoculated directly onto freshly prepared antimicrobial containing Mueller-Hinton agar plates with 5% aged defibrinated sheep blood (≥2 weeks old). The agar dilution plates are incubated at 35°C in a microaerobic environment produced by a gas generating system suitable for campylobacters. After 3 days of incubation, the MICs are recorded as the lowest concentration of antimicrobial agent required to inhibit growth of the organism. The clarithromycin MIC values should be interpreted according to the following criteria:

Clarithromycin MIC (µg/mL)*	Interpretation
≤0.25	Susceptible (S)
0.5-1.0	Intermediate (I)
≥2.0	Resistant (R)

* These are tentative breakpoints for the agar dilution methodology and they should not be used to interpret results obtained using alternative methods.

Standardized susceptibility test procedures require the use of laboratory control microorganisms to control the technical aspects of the laboratory procedures. Standard clarithromycin powder should provide the following MIC values:

Microorganism	Antimicrobial Agent	MIC (µg/mL)*
H pylori ATCC 43504	Clarithromycin	0.015-0.12

*These are quality control ranges for the agar dilution methodology and they should not be used to control test results obtained using alternative methods.

CLINICAL STUDIES

Eradication of *H pylori* Associated With Active Duodenal Ulcer: In a US double-bind, randomized, multicenter, dose comparison trial, TRITEC 400 mg b.i.d. for 4 weeks plus clarithromycin 500 mg b.i.d. for the first 2 weeks was found to have an equivalent *H pylori* eradication rate (based on culture and histology) when compared to TRITEC 400 mg b.i.d. for 4 weeks plus clarithromycin 500 mg t.i.d. for the first 2 weeks. The intent-to-treat and per protocol *H pylori* eradication rates are shown in Table 2.

[See table 2 at top of next page]

H pylori eradication was defined as no positive test at 4 weeks following the end of treatment. Patients must have had two tests performed and these must have been negative to be considered eradicated of *H pylori*. The following patients were excluded from the per-protocol analysis: patients not infected with *H pylori* prestudy, dropouts, patients with major protocol violations, patients with missing *H pylori* tests.

Patients excluded from the intent-to-treat analysis included those not infected with *H pylori* prestudy and those with missing *H pylori* tests prestudy. Patients were assessed for *H pylori* eradication (4 weeks following treatment) regardless of their healing status (at the end of treatment).

The relationship between *H pylori* eradication and duodenal ulcer recurrence was assessed in a combined analysis of six US randomized, double-blind, multicenter, placebo-controlled trials using TRITEC with or without antibiotics. The results from approximately 650 US patients showed that the risk of ulcer recurrence within 6 months of completing treatment was two times less likely in patients whose *H pylori* infection was eradicated compared to patients in whom *H pylori* infection was not eradicated.

INDICATIONS AND USAGE

TRITEC in combination with clarithromycin is indicated for the treatment of patients with an active duodenal ulcer associated with *H pylori* infection. Most patients not eradicated of *H pylori* following TRITEC plus clarithromycin treatment will have clarithromycin resistant *H pylori* isolates. Therefore, for those patients who fail therapy, clarithromycin susceptibility testing should be done when possible. Patients with clarithromycin resistant *H pylori* should not be treated with TRITEC plus clarithromycin or with regimens which include clarithromycin as the sole antimicrobial agent.

The eradication of *H pylori* has been demonstrated to reduce the risk of duodenal ulcer recurrence (see DOSAGE AND ADMINISTRATION and CLINICAL STUDIES).

NOTE: TRITEC should not be prescribed alone for the treatment of active duodenal ulcer.

Table 1: Clarithromycin Susceptibility Test Results and Clinical/Bacteriological Outcomes*

Clarithromycin Pre-treatment Results		Clarithromycin Post-treatment Results				
		H pylori negative-eradicated	*H pylori* positive-not eradicated Post-treatment susceptibility results S†	I†	R†	No MIC
Ranitidine Bismuth Citrate 400 mg B.I.D. plus Clarithromycin 500 mg T.I.D. (H2BA3001)						
Susceptible†	124	98	4		14	8
Intermediate†	3	2				1
Resistant†	17	1			15	1
Ranitidine Bismuth Citrate 400 mg B.I.D. plus Clarithromycin 500 mg B.I.D. (H2BA3001)						
Susceptible†	125	106	1	1	12	5
Intermediate†	2	2				
Resistant†	20	1			19	

*Includes only patients with pre-treatment clarithromycin susceptibility test results.
†Susceptible (S) MIC ≤0.25 µg/mL, Intermediate (I) MIC 0.5–1.0 µg/mL, Resistant (R) MIC ≥2 µg/mL.

CONTRAINDICATIONS

TRITEC is contraindicated in patients known to have hypersensitivity to ranitidine bismuth citrate or any of its ingredients.

For information on clarithromycin contraindications, see clarithromycin package insert.

WARNINGS

The physician should consult the package insert for clarithromycin for information concerning warnings and precautions associated with this drug.

PRECAUTIONS

General: The bismuth derived from TRITEC may cause a temporary and harmless darkening of the tongue and/or stool. Stool darkening should not be confused with melena (blood in the stool).

TRITEC in combination with clarithromycin should not be used in patients with a history of acute porphyria.

This combination therapy is not recommended in patients with creatinine clearance less than 25 mL/min (see DOSAGE AND ADMINISTRATION).

Laboratory Tests: No specific clinical laboratory tests are recommended for monitoring patients prior to and/or after treatment with TRITEC plus clarithromycin. False-positive tests for urine protein with MULTISTIX® may occur during ranitidine therapy, and, therefore, testing with sulfosalicylic acid is recommended.

Drug Interactions: Coadministration of TRITEC with clarithromycin resulted in increased plasma ranitidine concentrations (57%), increased plasma bismuth trough concentrations (48%), and increased 14-hydroxy-clarithromycin plasma concentrations (31%). Coadministration with aspirin results in a slight decrease in the rate of salicylate absorption that is clinically unimportant. Coadministration with a high dose of antacid (170 mEq) results in a 28% decrease in plasma concentrations of ranitidine and may decrease plasma concentrations of bismuth from TRITEC. These effects are clinically insignificant.

For information on drug interactions associated with ranitidine, refer to the ZANTAC® package insert.

Carcinogenesis, Mutagenesis, Impairment of Fertility: In a 24-month oral carcinogenicity study in $B6C3F_1$ mice, ranitidine bismuth citrate at daily doses up to 1000 mg/kg was not carcinogenic. For a 50-kg person of average height (1.46 m^2 body surface area), this dose represents five times the recommended clinical dose of 400 mg b.i.d. (592 mg/m^2). In a 24-month oral carcinogenicity study in Sprague-Dawley rats, ranitidine bismuth citrate at daily doses up to 500 mg/kg, five times the recommended human dose based on body surface area, was not carcinogenic.

Ranitidine bismuth citrate was not genotoxic in the Ames test, the mouse lymphoma cell (L5178Y/TK+/-) forward mutation test, the *ex vivo* rat gastric mucosal unscheduled DNA synthesis (UDS) test, or the *in vivo* rat micronucleus test. It was positive in *in vitro* human lymphocyte chromosomal aberration assay.

Ranitidine bismuth citrate at oral doses up to 1800 mg/kg per day (18 times the recommended human dose based on an average body surface area of 1.46 m^2) was found to have no effect on impairment of fertility and reproductive performance of male and female rats.

Pregnancy: ***Teratogenic Effects:*** Pregnancy Category C. TRITEC used in combination with clarithromycin carries a Pregnancy Category C because clarithromycin carries Pregnancy Category C. (See clarithromycin package insert *Pregnancy* subsection and WARNINGS section.)

Nonteratogenic Effects of Ranitidine Bismuth Citrate: Teratology studies have been performed in pregnant rats at oral doses up to 1800 mg/kg per day (18 times the recommended human dose based on body surface area) and pregnant rabbits at oral doses up to 300 mg/kg per day (6 times the recommended human dose based on body surface area) and have revealed no evidence of harm to the fetus due to ranitidine bismuth citrate.

There are, however, no adequate and well-controlled studies in pregnant women. Because animal reproduction studies are not always predictive of human response, this drug should be used during pregnancy only if clearly needed.

Five patients became pregnant while they were receiving ranitidine bismuth citrate alone at varied doses. Three of these patients had normal pregnancies and newborns, one had a voluntary abortion, and one delivered a baby with postaxial polydactyly. This Caucasian woman had a history of unexplained spontaneous abortions. She had received ranitidine bismuth citrate for 7 days prior to conception and for 20 days after conception. The investigator considered the event unrelated to TRITEC. Postaxial polydactyly is about 10 times more frequent in blacks than in Caucasians. In American whites, incidence figures vary from 1:3300 to 1:630 live births, and in American blacks figures vary from 1:300 to 1:100 live births. (March of Dimes 1996.)

Nursing Mothers: It is not known whether ranitidine bismuth citrate is excreted in human milk. Because many drugs are excreted in human milk, caution should be exer-

Table 2: H pylori Eradication Rates in Study H2BA3001

Analysis	TRITEC 400 mg + Clarithromycin 500 mg B.I.D.	TRITEC 400 mg + Clarithromycin 500 mg T.I.D.	95% CI Rate Difference
ITT	65% (122/188) [58%-72%]	63% (122/195) [55%-69%]	(-8%-12%)
Per Protocol	72% (117/162) [65%-79%]	71% (120/170) [63%-77%]	(-9%-12%)

Table 3: Drug-Related Adverse Reactions During Treatment*

Adverse Reaction	Placebo (n = 469)	TRITEC Tablets 800 mg (n = 903)	Clarithromycin 1,500 mg (n = 120)	TRITEC Tablets 800 mg + Clarithromycin 1,000 mg (n = 196)	TRITEC Tablets 800 mg + Clarithromycin 1,500 mg (n = 329)
Gastrointestinal					
Diarrhea	1%	2%	5%	4%	5%
Nausea & vomiting	1%	<1%	2%	5%	3%
Constipation	<1%	1%	0%	2%	2%
Gas	<1%	<1%	2%	1%	<1%
Neurological					
Headache	<1%	1%	<1%	2%	3%
Dizziness	<1%	<1%	2%	0%	<1%
Miscellaneous					
Disturbance of taste	<1%	<1%	11%	8%	11%
Sleep disorder	<1%	<1%	<1%	<1%	2%
Skin					
Pruritus	0%	<1%	0%	<1%	1%
Rashes	<1%	<1%	0%	2%	<1%
Urogenital					
Gynecological problems†	0% (n = 159)	<1% (n = 267)	6% (n = 32)	1% (n = 69)	2% (n = 125)

*Total daily doses.
†n = number of females.

cised when ranitidine bismuth citrate is administered to a nursing woman. It is known that both ranitidine and bismuth are excreted in rat milk.

Pediatric Use: Safety and effectiveness of ranitidine bismuth citrate plus clarithromycin in pediatric patients have not been established.

Geriatric Use: Ulcer healing and relapse rates in elderly patients (≥65 years of age) were no different from those in younger age-groups. The incidence rates for adverse events and laboratory abnormalities also were not different from those seen in other age-groups. In a pharmacokinetic study, serum levels of ranitidine were increased in elderly patients, but serum bismuth levels were equivalent to those seen in the overall population.

ADVERSE REACTIONS

Placebo-controlled trials in patients with active duodenal ulcer in the United States included 1428 patients given TRITEC alone or in combination with clarithromycin, 120 patients given clarithromycin alone, and 469 patients given placebo.

Incidence of Drug-Related Adverse Reactions in Placebo-Controlled Clinical Trials: The following table lists drug-related adverse reactions that occurred at a frequency of ≥1% among patients treated with TRITEC who participated in US placebo-controlled trials.

[See table 3 above]

Although seen in US clinical trials at a frequency of <1%, the following events may be associated with the use of TRITEC:

Gastrointestinal: Abdominal discomfort, gastric pain.

Hepatic: Transient changes in the liver enzymes SGPT (ALT) and SGOT (AST).

Hypersensitivity: There have been rare reports of hypersensitivity reactions, including skin rash and anaphylaxis.

Central Nervous System: Tremors have been reported rarely in patients receiving TRITEC. The relationship to TRITEC has been unclear.

For information on adverse reactions associated with ranitidine, refer to the ZANTAC® package insert. For information on adverse reactions associated with clarithromycin, refer to the clarithromycin package insert.

OVERDOSAGE

There has been limited experience with overdosage. Adverse events related to overdosage with ranitidine are usually reversible, nonspecific, and non-life threatening and result in no adverse sequelae. Although not seen in clinical trials with TRITEC, bismuth intoxication from prolonged overdosage or deliberate self-poisoning can result in neurotoxicity and nephrotoxicity and possibly other symptoms seen with the use of soluble bismuth compounds. In the event of an overdose or suspected bismuth toxicity, measures should be employed to remove unabsorbed material from the gastro-

intestinal tract, and symptom monitoring and other supportive therapy should be employed, if indicated.

Single oral doses of ranitidine bismuth citrate at 3000 and 4000 mg/kg in male and female mice, respectively (approximately 15 to 20 times the recommended human dose based on body surface area), and at 2000 and 3000 mg/kg in male and female rats, respectively, (approximately 20 to 30 times the recommended human dose based on body surface area) were lethal. Symptoms of acute toxicity were piloerection, tremors, hunched posture, rapid respiration, and decreased activity.

DOSAGE AND ADMINISTRATION

Eradication of H pylori Infection in Patients With an Active Duodenal Ulcer: The recommended dosage of TRITEC is 400 mg b.i.d. for 4 weeks (28 days) in conjunction with clarithromycin 500 mg b.i.d. for the first 2 weeks (14 days). TRITEC and clarithromycin can be taken with or without food.

Days 1–14	Days 15–28
TRITEC 400 mg b.i.d. plus clarithromycin 500 mg t.i.d.	TRITEC 400 mg b.i.d.

An alternative dosage regimen of TRITEC 400 mg b.i.d. for 4 weeks (28 days) in conjunction with clarithromycin 500 mg t.i.d. for the first 2 weeks (14 days) has been shown to be equally effective.

Dosage Adjustment in Elderly Patients: No dosage adjustment is necessary in elderly patients (see PRECAUTIONS: Geriatric Use and clarithromycin package insert).

Dosage Adjustment in Renally Impaired Patients: Because the principal route of excretion is renal, care should be exercised when administering this combination therapy to renally impaired patients. This combination therapy is not recommended in patients with creatinine clearance less than 25 mL/min.

HOW SUPPLIED

TRITEC Tablets 400 mg are blue, aqueous film-coated tablets in an elongated octagonal shape engraved with "TRITEC" on one side and a stomach-shaped logo on the other. They are available in bottles of 60 tablets (NDC 0173-0488-00).

Store between 2° and 30°C (36° and 86°F) in a dry place. Protect from light. Replace cap securely after each opening. For information on clarithromycin, refer to package insert.

REFERENCE

1. National Committee for Clinical Laboratory Standards, Summary Minutes, Subcommittee on Antimicrobial Susceptibility Testing, Tampa, FL, January 11–13, 1998.

US Patent Nos. 5,008,256 and 5,456,925
April 1998/RL-556
Shown in Product Identification Guide, page 314

ULTIVA™ ℞
[ul-tee 'va]
(remifentanil hydrochloride)
for Injection
For IV Use Only

DESCRIPTION

ULTIVA (remifentanil hydrochloride) for Injection is a μ-opioid agonist chemically designated as a 3-[4-methoxycarbonyl-4-[(1-oxopropyl)phenylamino]-1-piperidine] propanoic acid methyl ester, hydrochloride salt, $C_{20}H_{28}N_2O_5 \cdot HCl$, with a molecular weight of 412.91.

ULTIVA is a sterile, nonpyrogenic, preservative-free, white to off-white lyophilized powder for intravenous (IV) administration after reconstitution and dilution. Each vial contains 1, 2, or 5 mg of remifentanil base; 15 mg glycine; and hydrochloric acid to buffer the solutions to a nominal pH of 3 after reconstitution. When reconstituted as directed, solutions of ULTIVA are clear and colorless and contain remifentanil hydrochloride (HCl) equivalent to 1 mg/mL of remifentanil base. The pH of reconstituted solutions of ULTIVA ranges from 2.5 to 3.5. Remifentanil HCl has a pKa of 7.07. Remifentanil HCl has an n-octanol:water partition coefficient of 17.9 at pH 7.3.

CLINICAL PHARMACOLOGY

ULTIVA is a μ-opioid agonist with rapid onset and peak effect, and short duration of action. The μ-opioid activity of ULTIVA is antagonized by opioid antagonists such as naloxone.

Unlike other opioids, ULTIVA is rapidly metabolized by hydrolysis of the propanoic acid-methyl ester linkage by nonspecific blood and tissue esterases. ULTIVA is not a substrate for plasma cholinesterase (pseudocholinesterase) and, therefore, patients with atypical cholinesterase are expected to have a normal duration of action.

Pharmacodynamics: The analgesic effects of ULTIVA are rapid in onset and offset. Its effects and side effects are dose dependent and similar to other μ-opioids. ULTIVA in humans has a rapid blood-brain equilibration half-time of 1 ± 1 minutes (mean ± SD) and a rapid onset of action. The pharmacodynamic effects of ULTIVA closely follow the measured blood concentrations, allowing direct correlation between dose, blood levels, and response. Blood concentration decreases 50% in 3 to 6 minutes after a 1-minute infusion or after prolonged continuous infusion due to rapid distribution and elimination processes and is independent of duration of drug administration. Recovery from the effects of ULTIVA occurs rapidly (within 5 to 10 minutes). New steady-state concentrations occur within 5 to 10 minutes after changes in infusion rate. When used as a component of an anesthetic technique, ULTIVA can be rapidly titrated to the desired depth of anesthesia/analgesia (e.g., as required by varying levels of intraoperative stress) by changing the continuous infusion rate or by administering an IV bolus injection.

Hemodynamics: In premedicated patients undergoing anesthesia, 1-minute infusions of <2 mcg/kg of ULTIVA cause dose-dependent hypotension and bradycardia. While additional doses >2 mcg/kg (up to 30 mcg/kg) do not produce any further decreases in heart rate or blood pressure, the duration of the hemodynamic change is increased in proportion to the blood concentrations achieved. Peak hemodynamic effects occur within 3 to 5 minutes of a single dose of ULTIVA or an infusion rate increase. Glycopyrrolate, atropine, and vagolytic neuromuscular blocking agents attenuate the hemodynamic effects associated with ULTIVA. When appropriate, bradycardia and hypotension can be reversed by reduction of the rate of infusion of ULTIVA, or the dose of concurrent anesthetics, or by the administration of fluids or vasopressors.

Respiration: ULTIVA depresses respiration in a dose-related fashion. Unlike other fentanyl analogs, the duration of action of ULTIVA at a given dose does not increase with increasing duration of administration, due to lack of drug accumulation. When ULTIVA and alfentanil were dosed to equal levels of respiratory depression, recovery of respiratory drive after 3-hour infusions was more rapid and less variable with ULTIVA (see Figure 1).

[See figure at top of next page]

Spontaneous respiration occurs at blood concentrations of 4 to 5 ng/mL in the absence of other anesthetic agents; for example, after discontinuation of a 0.25-mcg/kg/min infusion of remifentanil, these blood concentrations would be

Continued on next page

This product information is based on labeling in effect on June 1, 1998. For further information, contact via direct mail, phone, or web site Medical Information: Glaxo Wellcome Inc., PO Box 13398, Research Triangle Park, NC 27709. Healthcare Professionals (Medical Information): 800-334-0089 Patients (Customer Response Center): 888-TALK2GW (1-888-825-5249) Glaxo Wellcome Corporate Web Site: www.glaxowellcome.com

Ultiva—Cont.

Figure 1: Recovery of Respiratory Drive After Equipotent* Doses of ULTIVA and Alfentanil Using CO_2-Stimulated Minute Ventilation in Volunteers (±1.5 SEM)

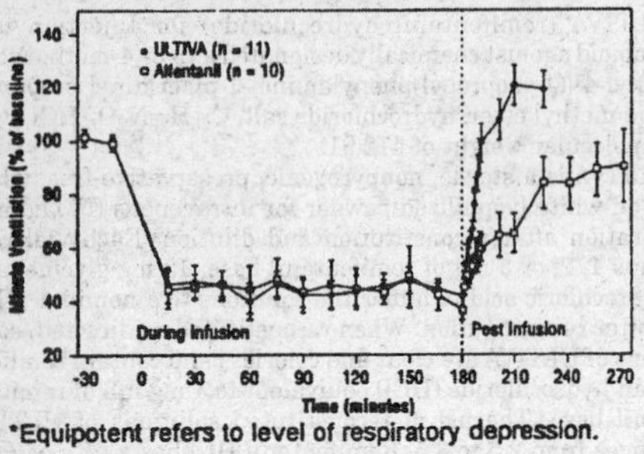

*Equipotent refers to level of respiratory depression.

reached in 2 to 4 minutes. In patients undergoing general anesthesia, the rate of respiratory recovery depends upon the concurrent anesthetic; N_2O < propofol < isoflurane (see CLINICAL TRIALS: Recovery).

Muscle Rigidity: Skeletal muscle rigidity can be caused by ULTIVA and is related to the dose and speed of administration. ULTIVA may cause chest wall rigidity (inability to ventilate) after single doses of >1 mcg/kg administered over 30 to 60 seconds or infusion rates >0.1 mcg/kg/min; peripheral muscle rigidity may occur at lower doses. Administration of doses <1 mcg/kg may cause chest wall rigidity when given concurrently with a continuous infusion of ULTIVA. Prior or concurrent administration of a hypnotic (propofol or thiopental) or a neuromuscular blocking agent may attenuate the development of muscle rigidity. Excessive muscle rigidity can be treated by decreasing the rate or discontinuing the infusion of ULTIVA or by administering a neuromuscular blocking agent.

Histamine Release: Assays of histamine in patients and normal volunteers have shown no elevation in plasma histamine levels after administration of ULTIVA in doses up to 30 mcg/kg over 60 seconds.

Analgesia: Infusions of 0.05 to 0.1 mcg/kg/min, producing blood concentrations of 1 to 3 ng/mL, are typically associated with analgesia with minimal decrease in respiratory rate. Supplemental doses of 0.5 to 1 mcg/kg, incremental increases in infusion rate >0.05 mcg/kg/min, and blood concentrations exceeding 5 ng/mL (typically produced by infusions of 0.2 mcg/kg/min) have been associated with transient and reversible respiratory depression, apnea, and muscle rigidity.

Anesthesia: ULTIVA is synergistic with the activity of hypnotics (propofol and thiopental), inhaled anesthetics, and benzodiazepines (see CLINICAL TRIALS, PRECAUTIONS, and DOSAGE AND ADMINISTRATION).

Age: The pharmacodynamic activity of ULTIVA (as measured by the EC_{50} for development of delta waves on the EEG) increases with increasing age. The EC_{50} of remifentanil for this measure was 50% less in patients over 65 years of age when compared to healthy volunteers (25 years of age) (see DOSAGE AND ADMINISTRATION).

Gender: No differences have been shown in the pharmacodynamic activity (as measured by the EEG) of ULTIVA between men and women.

Drug Interactions: In animals the duration of muscle paralysis from succinylcholine is not prolonged by remifentanil.

Intraocular Pressure: There was no change in intraocular pressure after the administration of ULTIVA prior to ophthalmic surgery under monitored anesthesia care.

Cerebrodynamics: Under isoflurane-nitrous oxide anesthesia ($PaCO_2$ <30 mmHg), a 1-minute infusion of ULTIVA (0.5 or 1.0 mcg/kg) produced no change in intracranial pressure. Mean arterial pressure and cerebral perfusion decreased as expected with opioids. In patients receiving ULTIVA and nitrous oxide anesthesia, cerebrovascular reactivity to carbon dioxide remained intact. In humans, no epileptiform activity was seen on the EEG (n = 44) at remifentanil doses up to 8 mcg/kg/min.

Renal Dysfunction: The pharmacodynamics of ULTIVA (ventilatory response to hypercarbia) are unaltered in patients with end stage renal disease (creatinine clearance <10 mL/min).

Hepatic Dysfunction: The pharmacodynamics of ULTIVA (ventilatory response to hypercarbia) are unaltered in patients with severe hepatic dysfunction awaiting liver transplant.

Pharmacokinetics: After IV doses administered over 60 seconds, the pharmacokinetics of remifentanil fit a three-compartment model with a rapid distribution half-life of 1 minute, a slower distribution half-life of 6 minutes, and a terminal elimination half-life of 10 to 20 minutes. Since the terminal elimination component contributes less than 10% of the overall area under the concentration versus time curve (AUC), the effective biological half-life of ULTIVA is 3 to 10 minutes. This is similar to the 3- to 10-minute half-life measured after termination of prolonged infusions (up to 4 hours; see Figure 2) and correlates with recovery times observed in the clinical setting after infusions up to 12 hours. Concentrations of remifentanil are proportional to the dose administered throughout the recommended dose range. The pharmacokinetics of remifentanil are unaffected by the presence of renal or hepatic impairment.

Distribution: The initial volume of distribution (V_d) of remifentanil is approximately 100 mL/kg and represents distribution throughout the blood and rapidly perfused tissues. Remifentanil subsequently distributes into peripheral tissues with a steady-state volume of distribution of approximately 350 mL/kg. These two distribution volumes generally correlate with total body weight (except in severely obese patients when they correlate better with ideal body weight [IBW]). Remifentanil is approximately 70% bound to plasma proteins of which two-thirds is binding to alpha-1-acid-glycoprotein.

Metabolism: Remifentanil is an esterase-metabolized opioid. A labile ester linkage renders this compound susceptible to hydrolysis by nonspecific esterases in blood and tissues. This hydrolysis results in the production of the carboxylic acid metabolite (3-[4-methoxycarbonyl-4-[(1-oxopropyl)phenylamino]-1-piperidine]propanoic acid), and represents the principal metabolic pathway for remifentanil (>95%). The carboxylic acid metabolite is essentially inactive (1/4,600 as potent as remifentanil in dogs) and is excreted by the kidneys with an elimination half-life of approximately 90 minutes. Remifentanil is not metabolized by plasma cholinesterase (pseudocholinesterase) and is not appreciably metabolized by the liver or lung.

Elimination: The clearance of remifentanil in young, healthy adults is approximately 40 mL/min/kg. Clearance generally correlates with total body weight (except in severely obese patients when it correlates better with IBW). The high clearance of remifentanil combined with a relatively small volume of distribution produces a short elimination half-life of approximately 3 to 10 minutes (see Figure 2). This value is consistent with the time taken for blood or effect site concentrations to fall by 50% (context-sensitive half-times) which is approximately 3 to 6 minutes. Unlike other fentanyl analogs, the duration of action does not increase with prolonged administration.

Figure 2: Mean Concentration (sd) versus Time

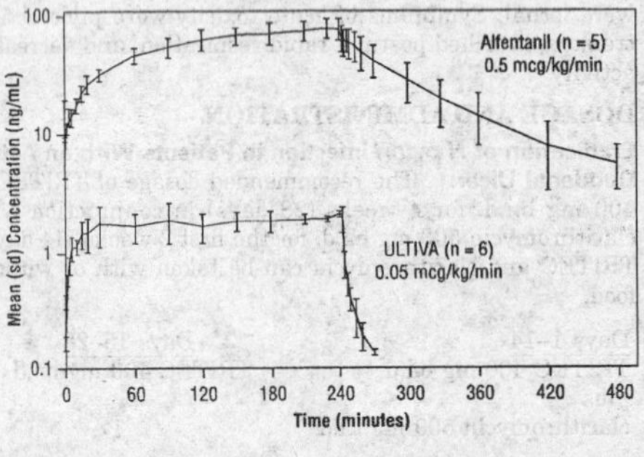

Titration to Effect: The rapid elimination of remifentanil permits the titration of infusion rate without concern for prolonged duration. In general, every 0.1-mcg/kg/min change in the IV infusion rate will lead to a corresponding 2.5-ng/mL change in blood remifentanil concentration within 5 to 10 minutes. In intubated patients only, a more rapid increase (within 3 to 5 minutes) to a new steady state can be achieved with a 1.0-mcg/kg bolus dose in conjunction with an infusion rate increase.

Special Populations: Children: In children 2 to 12 years of age (n = 13), the blood concentrations of remifentanil after a 1-minute infusion of 5.0 mcg/kg were similar to those seen in adults receiving the same dose. The pharmacokinetic parameters of remifentanil in children (volume of distribution, clearance, and half-life) were similar to adults after correcting for differences in weight. The pharmacokinetics of remifentanil have not been studied in patients under 2 years of age.

Renal Impairment: The pharmacokinetic profile of ULTIVA is not changed in patients with end stage renal disease (creatinine clearance <10 mL/min). In anephric patients, the half-life of the carboxylic acid metabolite increases from 90 minutes to 30 hours. The metabolite is removed by hemodialysis with a dialysis extraction ratio of approximately 30%.

Hepatic Impairment: The pharmacokinetics of remifentanil and its carboxylic acid metabolite are unchanged in patients with severe hepatic impairment.

Elderly: The clearance of remifentanil is reduced (approximately 25%) in the elderly (>65 years of age) compared to young adults (average 25 years of age). However, remifentanil blood concentrations fall as rapidly after termination of administration in the elderly as in young adults.

Gender: There is no significant difference in the pharmacokinetics of remifentanil in male and female patients after correcting for differences in weight.

Obesity: There is no difference in the pharmacokinetics of remifentanil in non-obese versus obese (greater than 30% over IBW) patients when normalized to IBW.

Cardiopulmonary Bypass (CPB): Remifentanil clearance is reduced by approximately 20% during hypothermic CPB.

Drug Interactions: Remifentanil clearance is not altered by concomitant administration of thiopental, isoflurane, propofol, or temazepam during anesthesia. *In vitro* studies with atracurium, mivacurium, esmolol, echothiophate, neostigmine, physostigmine, and midazolam revealed no inhibition of remifentanil hydrolysis in whole human blood by these drugs.

CLINICAL TRIALS

ULTIVA was evaluated in 2,808 patients undergoing general anesthesia (n = 2,169) and monitored anesthesia care (n = 639). These patients were evaluated in the following settings: inpatient (n = 1,573) which included cardiovascular (n = 225), and neurosurgical (n = 61), and outpatient (n = 1,235). Three hundred seventy-seven (377) elderly patients (age range 66 to 90 years) and 68 pediatric patients received ULTIVA. Of the general anesthesia patients, 682 also received ULTIVA as an IV analgesic agent during the immediate postoperative period.

Induction and Maintenance of General Anesthesia–Inpatient/Outpatient: The efficacy of ULTIVA was investigated in 1,562 patients in 15 randomized, controlled trials as the analgesic component for the induction and maintenance of general anesthesia. Eight of these studies compared ULTIVA to alfentanil and two studies compared ULTIVA to fentanyl. In these studies, doses of ULTIVA up to the ED_{90} were compared to recommended doses (approximately ED_{50}) of alfentanil or fentanyl. If alfentanil or fentanyl were administered in doses equipotent to the ED_{90} of ULTIVA, an intraoperative profile similar to the results below for ULTIVA could be expected.

Induction of Anesthesia: ULTIVA was administered with isoflurane, propofol, or thiopental for the induction of anesthesia (n = 1,562). The majority of patients (80%) received propofol as the concurrent agent. ULTIVA reduced the propofol and thiopental requirements for loss of consciousness. Compared to alfentanil and fentanyl, a higher relative dose of ULTIVA resulted in fewer responses to intubation (see Table 1). Overall, hypotension occurred in 5% of patients receiving ULTIVA compared to 2% of patients receiving the other opioids.

ULTIVA has been used as a primary agent for the induction of anesthesia; however, it should not be used as a sole agent because loss of consciousness cannot be assured and because of a high incidence of apnea, muscle rigidity, and tachycardia. The administration of an induction dose of propofol or thiopental or a paralyzing dose of a muscle relaxant prior to or concurrently with ULTIVA during the induction of anesthesia markedly decreased the incidence of muscle rigidity from 20% to <1%.

[See table 1 on next page]

Use During Maintenance of Anesthesia: ULTIVA was investigated in 929 patients in seven well-controlled general surgery studies in conjunction with nitrous oxide, isoflurane, or propofol in both inpatient and outpatient settings. These studies demonstrated that ULTIVA could be dosed to high levels of opioid effect and rapidly titrated to optimize analgesia intraoperatively without delaying or prolonging recovery.

Compared to alfentanil and fentanyl, these higher relative doses (ED_{90}) of ULTIVA resulted in fewer responses to intraoperative stimuli (see Table 2) and a higher frequency of hypotension (16% compared to 5% for the other opioids). ULTIVA was infused to the end of surgery, while alfentanil was discontinued 5 to 30 minutes before the end of surgery as recommended. The mean final infusion rates of ULTIVA were between 0.25 and 0.48 mcg/kg/min.

[See table 2 on next page]

In three randomized, controlled studies (n = 407) during general anesthesia, ULTIVA attenuated the signs of light anesthesia within a median time of 3 to 6 minutes after bolus doses of 1 mcg/kg with or without infusion rate increases of 50% to 100% (up to a maximum rate of 2 mcg/kg/min).

In an additional double-blind, randomized study (n = 103), a constant rate (0.25 mcg/kg/min) of ULTIVA was compared to doubling the rate to 0.5 mcg/kg/min approximately 5 minutes before the start of the major surgical stress event. Doubling the rate decreased the incidence of signs of light anesthesia from 67% to 8% in patients undergoing abdominal hysterectomy, and from 19% to 10% in patients undergoing radical prostatectomy. In patients undergoing laminectomy the lower dose was adequate.

Recovery: In 2,169 patients receiving ULTIVA for periods up to 16 hours, recovery from anesthesia was rapid, predictable, and independent of the duration of the infusion of ULTIVA. In the seven controlled, general surgery studies, extubation occurred in a median of 5 minutes (range: -3 to 17 minutes in 95% of patients) in outpatient anesthesia and 10 minutes (range: 0 to 32 minutes in 95% of patients) in inpatient anesthesia. Recovery in studies using nitrous oxide or propofol was faster than in those using isoflurane as

the concurrent anesthetic. There was no case of remifentanil-induced delayed respiratory depression occurring more than 30 minutes after discontinuation of remifentanil (see PRECAUTIONS).

In a double-blind, randomized study, administration of morphine sulfate (0.15 mg/kg) intravenously 20 minutes before the anticipated end of surgery to 98 patients did not delay recovery of respiratory drive in patients undergoing major surgery with remifentanil-propofol total IV anesthesia.

Spontaneous Ventilation Anesthesia: Two randomized, dose-ranging studies (n = 127) examined the administration of ULTIVA to outpatients undergoing general anesthesia with a laryngeal mask. Starting infusion rates of ULTIVA of ≤0.05 mcg/kg/min provided supplemental analgesia while allowing spontaneous ventilation with propofol or isoflurane. **Bolus doses of ULTIVA during spontaneous ventilation lead to transient periods of apnea, respiratory depression, and muscle rigidity.**

Pediatric Anesthesia: ULTIVA has been evaluated in one clinical trial (n = 68) in children 2 to 12 years of age undergoing strabismus surgery. After induction of anesthesia which included the administration of atropine, ULTIVA was administered as an initial infusion of 1 mcg/kg/min with 70% nitrous oxide. The infusion rate required during maintenance of anesthesia was 0.73 to 1.95 mcg/kg/min. Time to extubation and to purposeful movement was a median of 10 minutes (range 1 to 24 minutes).

Coronary Artery Bypass Surgery: In preliminary investigations of cardiac anesthesia, ULTIVA was administered to 217 patients undergoing elective coronary artery bypass graft (CABG) surgery in two dose-finding studies without active comparators. In both studies, patients were preloaded with fluid to PAOP 10 to 15 mmHg and all had preoperative stroke volume >50 mL.

In the total IV anesthesia study (n = 132), patients received diazepam or midazolam preoperatively and randomly received ULTIVA (1, 1.5, or 2 mcg/kg/min) plus propofol (0.5 mg/kg followed by 50 mcg/kg/min) and muscle relaxant for the induction and maintenance of anesthesia. Overall response to sternotomy/maximal sternal spread was 12% with no relationship to dose of ULTIVA. Thirty-nine percent (39%) of patients had treated hypotension reported as an adverse event.

In the other study, ULTIVA (administered at initial doses of 1, 2, 3 mcg/kg/min and then titrated to effect) was administered to 76 patients as a sole agent following a large preoperative dose of lorazepam (40 to 80 mcg/kg). Muscle rigidity at induction occurred in 49% of the patients. Responses at sternotomy occurred in 22% of patients with no relationship to dose of ULTIVA. Most patients (75%) required intermittent isoflurane supplementation for signs of light anesthesia; significantly more patients in the 1-mcg/kg/min group required isoflurane.

In both of these CABG studies, ULTIVA was continued at a rate of 1 mcg/kg/min in the intensive care unit (ICU) for up to 6 hours after surgery. The transition from ULTIVA to other analgesics (IV morphine sulfate; 0.1 to 0.15 mg/kg) was initiated prior to extubation. This transition usually occurred over 30 to 90 minutes with additional morphine, midazolam, and/or propofol administered as needed. Seventy-one percent (71%) of patients were eligible for early (<6 hours after entry into the ICU) extubation. Sixty-two percent (62%) of eligible patients were actually extubated early (range of times to extubation: 1.4 to 5.9 hours). The rate of major adverse cardiac events was 5.1% (myocardial infarction, 3.7%; ventricular failure, 0.5%; and death due to cardiac causes, 0.9%).

Neurosurgery: ULTIVA was administered to 61 patients undergoing craniotomy for removal of a supratentorial mass lesion. In these studies, ventilation was controlled to maintain a predicted $PaCO_2$ of approximately 28 mmHg. In one study (n = 30) with ULTIVA and 66% nitrous oxide, the median time to extubation and to patient response to verbal commands was 5 minutes (range -1 to 19 minutes). Intracranial pressure and cerebrovascular responsiveness to carbon dioxide were normal (see CLINICAL PHARMACOLOGY).

A randomized, controlled study compared ULTIVA (n = 31) to fentanyl (n = 32). ULTIVA (1 mcg/kg/min) and fentanyl (2 mcg/kg/min) were administered after induction with thiopental and pancuronium. A similar number of patients (6%) receiving ULTIVA and fentanyl had hypotension during induction. Anesthesia was maintained with nitrous oxide and ULTIVA at a mean infusion rate of 0.23 mcg/kg/min (range 0.1 to 0.4) compared with a fentanyl mean infusion rate of 0.04 mcg/kg/min (range 0.02 to 0.07). Supplemental isoflurane was administered as needed. The patients receiving ULTIVA required a lower mean isoflurane dose (0.07 MAC-hours) compared with 0.64 MAC-hours for the fentanyl patients (P = 0.04). ULTIVA was discontinued at the end of anesthesia, whereas fentanyl was discontinued at the time of bone flap replacement (a median time of 44 minutes before the end of surgery). Median time to extubation was similar (5 and 3.5 minutes, respectively, with ULTIVA and fentanyl). None of the patients receiving ULTIVA required naloxone compared to seven of the fentanyl patients (P = 0.01). Eighty-one percent (81%) of patients receiving ULTIVA recovered (awake, alert, and oriented) within 30 minutes after surgery compared with 59% of fentanyl patients (P = 0.06). At 45 minutes, recovery rates were similar (81% and 69% respectively for ULTIVA and fentanyl, P = 0.27). Patients receiving ULTIVA required an analgesic for headache sooner than fentanyl patients (median of 35 minutes compared with 136 minutes, respectively [P = 0.04]). No adverse cerebrovascular effects were seen in this study (see CLINICAL PHARMACOLOGY).

Continuation of Analgesic Use into the Immediate Postoperative Period: Analgesia with ULTIVA in the immediate postoperative period (until approximately 30 minutes after extubation) was studied in 401 patients in four dose-finding studies and in 281 patients in two efficacy studies. In the dose-finding studies, the use of bolus doses of ULTIVA and incremental infusion rate increases ≥0.05 mcg/kg/min led to respiratory depression and muscle rigidity. **Bolus doses of ULTIVA to treat postoperative pain are not recommended and incremental infusion rate increases should not exceed 0.025 mcg/kg/min at 5-minute intervals.**

In two efficacy studies, ULTIVA 0.1 mcg/kg/min was started immediately after discontinuing anesthesia. Incremental infusion rate increases of 0.025 mcg/kg/min every 5 minutes were given to treat moderate to severe postoperative pain. In Study 1, 50% decreases in infusion rate were made if respiratory rate decreased below 12 breaths/min and in Study 2, the same decreases were made if respiratory rate was below 8 breaths/min. With this difference in criteria for infusion rate decrease, the incidence of respiratory depression was lower in Study 1 (4%) than in Study 2 (12%). In both studies, ULTIVA provided effective analgesia (no or mild pain with respiratory rate ≥8 breaths/min) in approximately 60% of patients at mean final infusion rates of 0.1 to 0.125 mcg/kg/min.

Study 2 was a double-blind, randomized, controlled study in which patients received either morphine sulfate (0.15 mg/kg administered 20 minutes before the anticipated end of surgery plus 2-mg bolus doses for supplemental analgesia) or ULTIVA (as described above). Emergence from anesthesia was similar between groups; median time to extubation was 5 to 6 minutes for both. ULTIVA provided effective analgesia in 58% of patients compared to 33% of patients who received morphine. Respiratory depression occurred in 12% of patients receiving ULTIVA compared to 4% of morphine patients. For patients who received ULTIVA, morphine sulfate (0.15 mg/kg) was administered in divided doses 5 and 10 minutes before discontinuing ULTIVA. Within 30 minutes after discontinuation of ULTIVA, the percentage of patients with effective analgesia decreased to 34%.

Monitored Anesthesia Care: ULTIVA has been studied in the monitored anesthesia care setting in 609 patients in eight clinical trials. Nearly all patients received supplemental oxygen in these studies. Two early dose-finding studies demonstrated that use of sedation as an endpoint for titration of ULTIVA led to a high incidence of muscle rigidity (69%) and respiratory depression. Subsequent trials titrated ULTIVA to specific clinical endpoints of patient comfort, analgesia, and adequate respiration (respiratory rate >8 breaths/min) with a corresponding lower incidence of muscle rigidity (3%) and respiratory depression. With doses of midazolam >2 mg (4 to 8 mg), the dose of ULTIVA could be decreased by 50%, but the incidence of respiratory depression rose to 32%.

The efficacy of a single dose of ULTIVA (1.0 mcg/kg over 30 seconds) was compared to alfentanil (7 mcg/kg over 30 seconds) in patients undergoing ophthalmic surgery. More patients receiving ULTIVA were pain free at the time of the nerve block (77% versus 44%, P = 0.02) and more experienced nausea (12% versus 4%) than those receiving alfentanil.

In a randomized, controlled study (n = 118), ULTIVA 0.5 mcg/kg over 30 to 60 seconds followed by a continuous infusion of 0.1 mcg/kg/min, was compared to a propofol bolus (500 mcg/kg) followed by a continuous infusion (50 mcg/kg/

Continued on next page

Table 1: Response to Intubation (Propofol/Opioid Induction*)

Opioid Treatment Group/(No. of Patients)	Initial Dose (mcg/kg)	Pre-Intubation Infusion Rate (mcg/kg/min)	No. (%) Muscle Rigidity	No. (%) Hypotension During Induction	No. (%) Response to Intubation
Study 1:					
ULTIVA (35)	1	0.1	1 (3%)	0	27 (77%)
ULTIVA (35)	1	0.4	3 (9%)	0	11 (31%)†
Alfentanil (35)	20	1.0	2 (6%)	0	26 (74%)
Study 2:					
ULTIVA (116)	1	0.5	9 (8%)	5 (4%)	17 (15%)†
Alfentanil (118)	25	1.0	6 (5%)	5 (4%)	33 (28%)
Study 3:					
ULTIVA (134)	1	0.5	2 (1%)	4 (3%)	25 (19%)
Alfentanil (66)	20	2.0	0	0	19 (29%)
Study 4:					
ULTIVA (98)	1	0.2	11 (11%)†	2 (2%)	35 (36%)
ULTIVA (91)	2‡	0.4	11 (12%)†	2 (2%)	12 (13%)†
Fentanyl (97)	3	NA	1 (1%)	1 (1%)	29 (30%)

* Propofol was titrated to loss of consciousness. **Not all doses of ULTIVA were equipotent to the comparator opioid.**
† Differences were statistically significant (P <0.02).
‡ Initial doses greater than 1 mcg/kg are not recommended.

Table 2: Intraoperative Responses*

Opioid Treatment Group/(No. of Patients)	Concurrent Anesthetic	Post-Intubation Infusion Rate (mcg/kg/min)	No. (%) With Intraoperative Hypotension	No. (%) With Response to Skin Incision	No. (%) With Signs of Light Anesthesia	No. (%) With Response to Skin Closure
Study 1:						
ULTIVA (35)		0.1	0	20 (57%)	33 (94%)	6 (17%)
ULTIVA (35)	Nitrous oxide	0.4	0	3 (9%)†	12 (34%)†	2 (6%)†
Alfentanil (35)		1.0	0	24 (69%)	33 (94%)	12 (34%)
Study 2:						
ULTIVA (116)	Isoflurane +	0.25	35 (30%)†	9 (8%)†	66 (57%)†	19 (16%)
Alfentanil (118)	Nitrous oxide	0.5	12 (10%)	20 (17%)	85 (72%)	25 (21%)
Study 3:						
ULTIVA (134)	Propofol	0.5	3 (2%)	14 (11%)†	70 (52%)†	25 (19%)
Alfentanil (66)		2.0	2 (3%)	21 (32%)	47 (71%)	13 (20%)
Study 4:						
ULTIVA (98)		0.2	13 (13%)	12 (12%)†	67 (68%)†	7 (7%)
ULTIVA (91)	Isoflurane	0.4	16 (18%)†	4 (4%)†	44 (48%)†	3 (3%)†
Fentanyl (97)		1.5-3 mcg/kg prn	7 (7%)	32 (33%)	84 (87%)	11 (11%)

* **Not all doses of ULTIVA were equipotent to the comparator opioid.**
† Differences were statistically significant (P<0.05).

This product information is based on labeling in effect on June 1, 1998. For further information, contact via direct mail, phone, or web site Medical Information: Glaxo Wellcome Inc., PO Box 13398, Research Triangle Park, NC 27709. Healthcare Professionals (Medical Information): 800-334-0089 Patients (Customer Response Center): 888-TALK2GW (1-888-825-5249) Glaxo Wellcome Corporate Web Site: www.glaxowellcome.com

Ultiva—Cont.

min) in patients who received a local or regional anesthetic nerve block 5 minutes later. The incidence of moderate or severe pain during placement of the block was similar between groups (2% with ULTIVA and 8% with propofol, $P = 0.2$) and more patients receiving ULTIVA experienced nausea (26% versus 2%, $P < 0.001$). The final mean infusion rate of ULTIVA was 0.08 mcg/kg/min.

In a randomized, double-blind study, ULTIVA with or without midazolam was evaluated in 159 patients undergoing superficial surgical procedures under local anesthesia. ULTIVA was administered without midazolam as a 1-mcg/kg dose over 30 seconds followed by a continuous infusion of 0.1 mcg/kg/min. In the group of patients that received midazolam, ULTIVA was administered as a 0.5-mcg/kg dose over 30 seconds followed by a continuous infusion of 0.05 mcg/kg/min and midazolam 2 mg was administered 5 minutes later. The occurrence of moderate or severe pain during the local anesthetic injection was similar between groups (16% and 20%). Other effects for ULTIVA alone and ULTIVA/midazolam were: respiratory depression with oxygen desaturation ($SPO_2 < 90\%$), 5% and 2%; nausea, 8% and 2%; and pruritus, 23% and 12%. Titration of ULTIVA resulted in prompt resolution of respiratory depression (median 3 minutes, range 0 to 6 minutes). The final mean infusion rate of ULTIVA was 0.12 mcg/kg/min (range 0.03 to 0.3) for the group receiving ULTIVA alone and 0.07 mcg/kg/min (range 0.02 to 0.2) for the group receiving ULTIVA/midazolam.

Because of the risk for hypoventilation, the infusion rate of ULTIVA should be decreased to 0.05 mcg/kg/min following placement of the local or regional block and titrated thereafter in increments of 0.025 mcg/kg/min at 5-minute intervals. Bolus doses of ULTIVA administered simultaneously with a continuous infusion of ULTIVA to spontaneously breathing patients are not recommended.

INDICATIONS AND USAGE

ULTIVA is indicated for IV administration:
1. as an analgesic agent for use during the induction and maintenance of general anesthesia for inpatient and outpatient procedures, and for continuation as an analgesic into the immediate postoperative period under the direct supervision of an anesthesia practitioner in a postoperative anesthesia care unit or intensive care setting.
2. as an analgesic component of monitored anesthesia care.

CONTRAINDICATIONS

Due to the presence of glycine in the formulation, ULTIVA is contraindicated for epidural or intrathecal administration. ULTIVA is also contraindicated in patients with known hypersensitivity to fentanyl analogs.

WARNINGS

Continuous infusions of ULTIVA should be administered only by an infusion device. **IV bolus administration of ULTIVA should be used only during the maintenance of general anesthesia. In nonintubated patients, single doses of ULTIVA should be administered over 30 to 60 seconds. Interruption of an infusion of ULTIVA will result in rapid offset of effect. Rapid clearance and lack of drug accumulation result in rapid dissipation of respiratory depressant and analgesic effects upon discontinuation of ULTIVA at recommended doses. Discontinuation of an infusion of ULTIVA should be preceded by the establishment of adequate postoperative analgesia.**

Injections of ULTIVA should be made into IV tubing at or close to the venous cannula. Upon discontinuation of ULTIVA, the IV tubing should be cleared to prevent the inadvertent administration of ULTIVA at a later point in time. **Failure to adequately clear the IV tubing to remove residual ULTIVA has been associated with the appearance of respiratory depression, apnea, and muscle rigidity upon the administration of additional fluids or medications through the same IV tubing.**

USE OF ULTIVA IS ASSOCIATED WITH APNEA AND RESPIRATORY DEPRESSION. ULTIVA SHOULD BE ADMINISTERED ONLY BY PERSONS SPECIFICALLY TRAINED IN THE USE OF ANESTHETIC DRUGS AND THE MANAGEMENT OF THE RESPIRATORY EFFECTS OF POTENT OPIOIDS, INCLUDING RESPIRATORY AND CARDIAC RESUSCITATION OF PATIENTS IN THE AGE GROUP BEING TREATED. SUCH TRAINING MUST INCLUDE THE ESTABLISHMENT AND MAINTENANCE OF A PATENT AIRWAY AND ASSISTED VENTILATION. ULTIVA SHOULD NOT BE USED IN DIAGNOSTIC OR THERAPEUTIC PROCEDURES OUTSIDE THE MONITORED ANESTHESIA CARE SETTING. PATIENTS RECEIVING MONITORED ANESTHESIA CARE SHOULD BE CONTINUOUSLY MONITORED BY PERSONS NOT INVOLVED IN THE CONDUCT OF THE SURGICAL OR DIAGNOSTIC PROCEDURE. OXYGEN SATURATION SHOULD BE MONITORED ON A CONTINUOUS BASIS. RESUSCITATIVE AND INTUBATION EQUIPMENT, OXYGEN, AND AN OPIOID ANTAGONIST MUST BE READILY AVAILABLE.

Table 3: Adverse Events Reported in ≥1% of Patients in General Anesthesia Studies at the Recommended Doses of ULTIVA*

Adverse Event	Induction/Maintenance ULTIVA (n = 921)	Induction/Maintenance Alfentanil/ Fentanyl (n = 466)	Postoperative Analgesia ULTIVA (n = 281)	Postoperative Analgesia Morphine (n = 98)	After Discontinuation ULTIVA (n=929)	After Discontinuation Alfentanil/ Fentanyl (n = 466)
Nausea	8 (<1%)	0	61 (22%)	15 (15%)	339 (36%)	202 (43%)
Hypotension	178 (19%)	30 (6%)	0	0	16 (2%)	9 (2%)
Vomiting	4 (<1%)	1 (<1%)	22 (8%)	5 (5%)	150 (16%)	91 (20%)
Muscle rigidity	98 (11%)†	37 (8%)	7 (2%)	0	2 (<1%)	1 (<1%)
Bradycardia	62 (7%)	24 (5%)	3 (1%)	3 (3%)	11 (1%)	6 (1%)
Shivering	3 (<1%)	0	15 (5%)	9 (9%)	49 (5%)	10 (2%)
Fever	1 (<1%)	0	2 (<1%)	0	44 (5%)	9 (2%)
Dizziness	0	0	1 (<1%)	0	27 (3%)	9 (2%)
Visual disturbance	0	0	0	0	24 (3%)	14 (3%)
Headache	0	0	1 (<1%)	1 (1%)	21 (2%)	8 (2%)
Respiratory depression	1 (<1%)	0	19 (7%)	4 (4%)	17 (2%)	20 (4%)
Apnea	0	1 (<1%)	9 (3%)	2 (2%)	2 (<1%)	1 (<1%)
Pruritus	2 (<1%)	0	7 (2%)	1 (1%)	22 (2%)	7 (2%)
Tachycardia	6 (<1%)	7 (2%)	0	0	10 (1%)	8 (2%)
Postoperative pain	0	0	7 (2%)	0	4 (<1%)	5 (1%)
Hypertension	10 (1%)	7 (2%)	5 (2%)	3 (3%)	12 (1%)	8 (2%)
Agitation	2 (<1%)	0	3 (1%)	1 (1%)	6 (<1%)	1 (<1%)
Hypoxia	0	0	1 (<1%)	0	10 (1%)	7 (2%)

* See Table 6 for recommended doses. **Not all doses of ULTIVA were equipotent to the comparator opioid. Administration of ULTIVA in excess of the recommended dose (i.e., doses >1 and up to 20 mcg/kg) resulted in a higher incidence of some adverse events: muscle rigidity (37%), bradycardia (12%), hypertension (4%), and tachycardia (4%).**
† Included in the muscle rigidity incidence is chest wall rigidity (5%). The overall muscle rigidity incidence is <1% when remifentanil is administered concurrently or after a hypnotic induction agent.

Table 4: Incidence (%) of Most Common Adverse Events by Gender in General Anesthesia Studies at the Recommended Dose* of ULTIVA

Adverse Event	Induction/Maintenance ULTIVA Male 326	Induction/Maintenance ULTIVA Female 595	Induction/Maintenance Alfentanil/Fentanyl Male 183	Induction/Maintenance Alfentanil/Fentanyl Female 283	Postoperative Analgesia ULTIVA Male 85	Postoperative Analgesia ULTIVA Female 196	Postoperative Analgesia Morphine Male 36	Postoperative Analgesia Morphine Female 62	After Discontinuation ULTIVA Male 332	After Discontinuation ULTIVA Female 597	After Discontinuation Alfentanil/Fentanyl Male 183	After Discontinuation Alfentanil/Fentanyl Female 283
Nausea	2%	<1%	0	0	12%	26%	8%	19%	22%	45%	30%	52%
Hypotension	29%	14%	7%	6%	0	0	0	0	2%	2%	2%	2%
Vomiting	<1%	<1%	0	<1%	4%	10%	0	8%	5%	22%	8%	27%
Muscle rigidity	17%	7%	14%	4%	6%	1%	0	0	<1%	<1%	0	<1%

* See Table 6 for recommended doses. **Not all doses of ULTIVA were equipotent to the comparator opioid.**

Table 5: Adverse Events Reported in ≥1% of Patients in Monitored Anesthesia Care Studies at the Recommended Doses of ULTIVA*

Adverse Event	ULTIVA (n = 159)	ULTIVA +2 mg Midazolam† (n = 103)	Propofol (0.5 mg/kg then 50 mcg/kg/min) (n = 63)
Nausea	70 (44%)	19 (18%)	20 (32%)
Vomiting	35 (22%)	5 (5%)	13 (21%)
Pruritus	28 (18%)	16 (16%)	0
Headache	28 (18%)	12 (12%)	6 (10%)
Sweating	10 (6%)	0	1 (2%)
Shivering	8 (5%)	1 (<1%)	1 (2%)
Dizziness	8 (5%)	5 (5%)	1 (2%)
Hypotension	7 (4%)	0	6 (10%)
Bradycardia	6 (4%)	0	7 (11%)
Respiratory depression	4 (3%)	1 (<1%)*	0
Muscle rigidity	4 (3%)	0	1 (2%)
Chills	2 (1%)	0	2 (3%)
Flushing	2 (1%)	0	0
Warm sensation	2 (1%)	0	0
Pain at study IV site	2 (1%)	0	11 (17%)

* See Table 7 for recommended doses. **Administration of ULTIVA in excess of the recommended infusion rate (i.e., starting doses >0.1 mcg/kg/min) resulted in a higher incidence of some adverse events: nausea (60%), apnea (8%), and muscle rigidity (5%).**
† With higher midazolam doses, higher incidences of respiratory depression and apnea were observed.

Respiratory depression in spontaneously breathing patients is generally managed by decreasing the rate of the infusion of ULTIVA by 50% or by temporarily discontinuing the infusion.

Skeletal muscle rigidity can be caused by ULTIVA and is related to the dose and speed of administration. ULTIVA may cause chest wall rigidity (inability to ventilate) after single doses of >1 mcg/kg administered over 30 to 60 seconds, or after infusion rates >0.1 mcg/kg/min. Single doses <1 mcg/kg may cause chest wall rigidity when given concurrently with a continuous infusion of ULTIVA.

Muscle rigidity induced by ULTIVA should be managed in the context of the patient's clinical condition. Muscle rigidity occurring during the induction of anesthesia should be treated by the administration of a neuromuscular blocking agent and the concurrent induction medications.

Muscle rigidity seen during the use of ULTIVA in spontaneously breathing patients may be treated by stopping or decreasing the rate of administration of ULTIVA. Resolution of muscle rigidity after discontinuing the infusion of ULTIVA occurs within minutes. In the case of life-threatening muscle rigidity, a rapid onset neuromuscular blocker or naloxone may be administered.

ULTIVA should not be administered into the same IV tubing with blood due to potential inactivation by nonspecific esterases in blood products.

Table 6: Dosing Guidelines—General Anesthesia and Continuing as an Analgesic into the Postoperative Care Unit or Intensive Care Setting*

Phase	Continuous IV Infusion of ULTIVA (mcg/kg/min)	Infusion Dose Range of ULTIVA (mcg/kg/min)	Supplemental IV Bolus Dose of ULTIVA (mcg/kg)
Induction of Anesthesia (through intubation)	0.5–1*		
Maintenance of anesthesia with:			
Nitrous oxide (66%)	0.4	0.1–2	1
Isoflurane (0.4 to 1.5 MAC)	0.25	0.05–2	1
Propofol (100 to 200 mcg/kg/min)	0.25	0.05–2	1
Continuation as an analgesic into the immediate postoperative period	0.1	0.025–0.2	not recommended

* An initial dose of 1 mcg/kg may be administered over 30 to 60 seconds.

Table 7: Dosing Guidelines—Monitored Anesthesia Care

Method	Timing	ULTIVA Alone	ULTIVA + 2 mg Midazolam
Single IV Dose	Given 90 seconds before local anesthetic	1 mcg/kg over 30 to 60 seconds	0.5 mcg/kg over 30 to 60 seconds
Continuous IV Infusion	Beginning 5 minutes before local anesthetic	0.1 mcg/kg/min	0.05 mcg/kg/min
	After local anesthetic	0.05 mcg/kg/min (Range: 0.025-0.2 mcg/kg/min)	0.025 mcg/kg/min (Range: 0.025-0.2 mcg/kg/min)

PRECAUTIONS

Vital signs and oxygenation must be continually monitored during the administration of ULTIVA.

General: Bradycardia has been reported with ULTIVA and is responsive to ephedrine or anticholinergic drugs, such as atropine and glycopyrrolate.

Hypotension has been reported with ULTIVA and is responsive to decreases in the administration of ULTIVA or to IV fluids or catecholamine (ephedrine, epinephrine, norepinephrine, etc.) administration.

Intraoperative awareness has been reported in patients under 55 years of age when ULTIVA has been administered with propofol infusion rates of ≤75 mcg/kg/min.

Rapid Offset of Action: WITHIN 5 TO 10 MINUTES AFTER THE DISCONTINUATION OF ULTIVA, NO RESIDUAL ANALGESIC ACTIVITY WILL BE PRESENT. However, respiratory depression may occur in some patients up to 30 minutes after termination of infusion due to residual effects of concomitant anesthetics. Standard monitoring should be maintained in the postoperative period to ensure adequate recovery without stimulation. For patients undergoing surgical procedures where postoperative pain is generally anticipated, other analgesics should be administered prior to the discontinuation of ULTIVA.

Pediatric Use: ULTIVA has not been studied in pediatric patients under 2 years of age. See CLINICAL PHARMACOLOGY and DOSAGE AND ADMINISTRATION for clinical experience and recommendations for use in pediatric patients 2 to 12 years of age.

Use in Elderly Patients: While the effective biological half-life of remifentanil is unchanged, elderly patients have been shown to be twice as sensitive as the younger population to the pharmacodynamic effects of remifentanil. The recommended starting dose of ULTIVA should be decreased by 50% in patients over 65 years of age (see CLINICAL PHARMACOLOGY and DOSAGE AND ADMINISTRATION).

Use in Morbidly Obese Patients: As for all potent opioids, caution is required with use in morbidly obese patients because of alterations in cardiovascular and respiratory physiology (see DOSAGE AND ADMINISTRATION).

Long-term Use in the ICU: No data are available on the long-term (longer than 16 hours) use of ULTIVA as an analgesic in ICU patients.

Carcinogenesis, Mutagenesis, Impairment of Fertility: Animal carcinogenicity studies have not been performed with remifentanil.

Remifentanil did not induce gene mutation in prokaryotic cells *in vitro* and was not genotoxic in the *in vivo* rat hepatocyte unscheduled DNA synthesis assay. No clastogenic effect was seen in cultured Chinese hamster ovary cells or in the *in vivo* mouse micronucleus test. In the *in vitro* mouse lymphoma assay, mutagenicity was seen only with metabolic activation.

Remifentanil has been shown to reduce fertility in male rats when tested after 70+ days of daily IV administration of 0.5 mg/kg, or approximately 40 times the maximum recommended human dose (MRHD) in terms of mg/m² of body surface area. The fertility of female rats was not affected at IV doses as high as 1 mg/kg when administered for at least 15 days before mating.

Pregnancy Category C: Teratogenic effects were not observed following administration of remifentanil at doses up to 5 mg/kg in rats and 0.8 mg/kg in rabbits. These doses are approximately 400 times and 125 times the MRHD, respectively, in terms of mg/m² of body surface area. Administration of radiolabeled remifentanil to pregnant rabbits and rats demonstrated significant placental transfer to fetal tissue. There are no adequate and well-controlled studies in pregnant women. ULTIVA should be used during pregnancy only if the potential benefit justifies the potential risk to the fetus.

Administration of remifentanil to rats throughout late gestation and lactation at IV doses up to 5 mg/kg, or approximately 400 times the MRHD in terms of mg/m² of body surface area, had no significant effect on the survival, development, or reproductive performance of the F₁ generation.

Animal Toxicology: Intrathecal administration of the glycine formulation without remifentanil to dogs caused agitation, pain, hind limb dysfunction, and incoordination. These effects are believed to be caused by the glycine. Glycine is a commonly used excipient in IV products and this finding has no relevance for IV administration of ULTIVA.

Labor and Delivery: Respiratory depression and other opioid effects may occur in newborns whose mothers are given ULTIVA shortly before delivery. The safety of ULTIVA during labor or delivery has not been demonstrated. Placental transfer studies in rats and rabbits showed that pups are exposed to remifentanil and its metabolites. In a human clinical trial, the average maternal remifentanil concentrations were approximately twice those seen in the fetus. In some cases, however, fetal concentrations were similar to those in the mother. The umbilical arterio-venous ratio of remifentanil concentrations was approximately 30% suggesting metabolism of remifentanil in the neonate.

Nursing Mothers: It is not known whether remifentanil is excreted in human milk. After receiving radioactive-labeled remifentanil, the radioactivity was present in the milk of lactating rats. Because fentanyl analogs are excreted in human milk, caution should be exercised when ULTIVA is administered to a nursing woman.

ADVERSE EVENTS

ULTIVA produces adverse events that are characteristic of μ-opioids, such as respiratory depression, bradycardia, hypotension, and skeletal muscle rigidity. These adverse events dissipate within minutes of discontinuing or decreasing the infusion rate of ULTIVA. See CLINICAL PHARMACOLOGY, WARNINGS, and PRECAUTIONS on the management of these events.

Adverse event information is derived from controlled clinical trials that were conducted in a variety of surgical procedures of varying duration, using a variety of premedications and other anesthetics, and in patient populations with diverse characteristics including underlying disease.

Approximately 2,492 patients were exposed to ULTIVA in controlled clinical trials. The frequencies of adverse events during general anesthesia with the recommended doses of ULTIVA are given in Table 3. Each patient was counted once for each type of adverse event.

[See table 3 at top of previous page]

In the elderly population (>65 years), the incidence of hypotension is higher, whereas the incidence of nausea and vomiting is lower.

[See table 4 at top of previous page]

The frequencies of adverse events from the clinical studies at the recommended doses of ULTIVA in monitored anesthesia care are given in Table 5.

[See table 5 at top of previous page]

Other Adverse Events: The frequencies of less commonly reported adverse clinical events from all controlled general anesthesia and monitored anesthesia care studies are presented below.

Event frequencies are calculated as the number of patients who were administered ULTIVA and reported an event divided by the total number of patients exposed to ULTIVA in all controlled studies including cardiac and neurosurgery studies (n = 1,883 general anesthesia, n = 609 monitored anesthesia care).

Incidence Less than 1%:

Digestive: constipation, abdominal discomfort, xerostomia, gastro-esophageal reflux, dysphagia, diarrhea, heartburn, ileus.

Cardiovascular: various atrial and ventricular arrhythmias, heart block, ECG change consistent with myocardial ischemia, elevated CPK-MB level, syncope.

Musculoskeletal: muscle stiffness, musculoskeletal chest pain.

Respiratory: cough, dyspnea, bronchospasm, laryngospasm, rhonchi, stridor, nasal congestion, pharyngitis, pleural effusion, hiccup(s), pulmonary edema, rales, bronchitis, rhinorrhea.

Nervous: anxiety, involuntary movement, prolonged emergence from anesthesia, confusion, awareness under anesthesia without pain, rapid awakening from anesthesia, tremors, disorientation, dysphoria, nightmare(s), hallucinations, paresthesia, nystagmus, twitch, sleep disorder, seizure, amnesia.

Body as a Whole: decreased body temperature, anaphylactic reaction, delayed recovery from neuromuscular block.

Skin: rash, urticaria.

Urogenital: urine retention, oliguria, dysuria, urine incontinence.

Infusion Site Reaction: erythema, pruritus, rash.

Metabolic and Nutrition: abnormal liver function, hyperglycemia, electrolyte disorders, increased CPK level.

Hematologic and Lymphatic: anemia, lymphopenia, leukocytosis, thrombocytopenia.

DRUG ABUSE AND DEPENDENCE

ULTIVA is a Schedule II controlled drug substance that can produce drug dependence of the morphine type and has the potential for being abused.

OVERDOSAGE

As with all potent opioid analgesics, overdosage would be manifested by an extension of the pharmacological actions of ULTIVA. Expected signs and symptoms of overdosage include: apnea, chest-wall rigidity, seizures, hypoxemia, hypotension, and bradycardia.

In case of overdosage or suspected overdosage, discontinue administration of ULTIVA, maintain a patent airway, initiate assisted or controlled ventilation with oxygen, and maintain adequate cardiovascular function. If depressed respiration is associated with muscle rigidity, a neuromuscular blocking agent or a μ-opioid antagonist may be required to facilitate assisted or controlled respiration. Intravenous fluids and vasopressors for the treatment of hypotension and other supportive measures may be employed. Glycopyrrolate or atropine may be useful for the treatment of bradycardia and/or hypotension.

Intravenous administration of an opioid antagonist such as naloxone may be employed as a specific antidote to manage severe respiratory depression or muscle rigidity. Respiratory depression from overdosage with ULTIVA is not expected to last longer than the opioid antagonist, naloxone. Reversal of the opioid effects may lead to acute pain and sympathetic hyperactivity.

DOSAGE AND ADMINISTRATION

ULTIVA is for IV use only. **Continuous infusions of ULTIVA should be administered only by an infusion device. The injection site should be close to the venous cannula and all IV tubing should be cleared at the time of discontinuation of infusion.**

During General Anesthesia: ULTIVA is not recommended as the sole agent in general anesthesia because loss of consciousness cannot be assured and because of a high incidence of apnea, muscle rigidity, and tachycardia. ULTIVA is synergistic with other anesthetics and doses of thiopental, propofol, isoflurane, and midazolam have been reduced by

Continued on next page

This product information is based on labeling in effect on June 1, 1998. For further information, contact via direct mail, phone, or web site Medical Information: Glaxo Wellcome Inc., PO Box 13398, Research Triangle Park, NC 27709. Healthcare Professionals (Medical Information): 800-334-0089 Patients (Customer Response Center): 888-TALK2GW (1-888-825-5249) Glaxo Wellcome Corporate Web Site: www.glaxowellcome.com

Ultiva—Cont.

up to 75% with the coadministration of ULTIVA. The administration of ULTIVA must be individualized based on the patient's response.

Table 6 summarizes the recommended doses in adult patients, predominately ASA physical status I, II, or III. Recommendations for maintenance anesthesia with nitrous oxide also apply to pediatric patients ≥2 years.

[See table 6 at top of previous page]

During Induction of Anesthesia: ULTIVA should be administered at an infusion rate of 0.5 to 1 mcg/kg/min with a hypnotic or volatile agent for the induction of anesthesia. If endotracheal intubation is to occur less than 8 minutes after the start of the infusion of ULTIVA, then an initial dose of 1 mcg/kg may be administered over 30 to 60 seconds.

During Maintenance of Anesthesia: After endotracheal intubation, the infusion rate of ULTIVA should be decreased in accordance with the dosing guidelines in Table 6. Due to the fast onset and short duration of action of ULTIVA, the rate of administration during anesthesia can be titrated upward in 25% to 100% increments or downward in 25% to 50% decrements every 2 to 5 minutes to attain the desired level of μ-opioid effect. In response to light anesthesia or transient episodes of intense surgical stress, supplemental bolus doses of 1 mcg/kg may be administered every 2 to 5 minutes. At infusion rates >1 mcg/kg/min, increases in the concomitant anesthetic agents should be considered to increase the depth of anesthesia.

Continuation as an Analgesic into the Immediate Postoperative Period Under the Direct Supervision of an Anesthesia Practitioner: Infusions of ULTIVA may be continued into the immediate postoperative period for select patients for whom later transition to longer acting analgesics may be desired. The use of bolus injections of ULTIVA to treat pain during the postoperative period is not recommended. When used as an IV analgesic in the immediate postoperative period, ULTIVA should be initially administered by continuous infusion at a rate of 0.1 mcg/kg/min. The infusion rate may be adjusted every 5 minutes in 0.025-mcg/kg/min increments to balance the patient's level of analgesia and respiratory rate. Infusion rates greater than 0.2 mcg/kg/min are associated with respiratory depression (respiratory rate less than 8 breaths/min).

***Guidelines for Discontinuation:* Upon discontinuation of ULTIVA, the IV tubing should be cleared to prevent the inadvertent administration of ULTIVA at a later time.**

Due to the rapid offset of action of ULTIVA, no residual analgesic activity will be present within 5 to 10 minutes after discontinuation. For patients undergoing surgical procedures where postoperative pain is generally anticipated, alternative analgesics should be administered prior to discontinuation of ULTIVA. The choice of analgesic should be appropriate for the patient's surgical procedure and the level of follow-up care (see CLINICAL TRIALS).

Analgesic Component of Monitored Anesthesia Care: It is strongly recommended that supplemental oxygen be supplied to the patient whenever ULTIVA is administered.

Table 7 summarizes the recommended doses for monitored anesthesia care in adult patients, predominately ASA physical status I, II, or III.

[See table 7 on previous page]

Single Dose: A single IV dose of 0.5 to 1 mcg/kg over 30 to 60 seconds of ULTIVA may be given 90 seconds before the placement of the local or regional anesthetic block (see PRECAUTIONS).

Continuous Infusion: When used alone as an IV analgesic component of monitored anesthesia care, ULTIVA should be initially administered by continuous infusion at a rate of 0.1 mcg/kg/min beginning 5 minutes before placement of the local or regional anesthetic block. **Because of the risk for hypoventilation, the infusion rate of ULTIVA should be decreased to 0.05 mcg/kg/min following placement of the block.** Thereafter, rate adjustments of 0.025 mcg/kg/min at 5-minute intervals may be used to balance the patient's level of analgesia and respiratory rate. Rates greater than 0.2 mcg/kg/min are generally associated with respiratory depression (respiratory rates less than 8 breaths/min). **Bolus doses of ULTIVA administered simultaneously with a continuous infusion of ULTIVA to spontaneously breathing patients are not recommended.**

Individualization of Dosage: ***Use in Elderly Patients:*** The starting doses of ULTIVA should be decreased by 50% in elderly patients (>65 years). ULTIVA should then be cautiously titrated to effect.

Use in Pediatric Patients: No data are available on the use of ULTIVA in pediatric patients under 2 years of age. The same doses (per kg) as adults are recommended for pediatric patients 2 years of age and older.

Use in Obese Patients: The starting doses of ULTIVA should be based on ideal body weight (IBW) in obese patients (greater than 30% over their IBW).

Preanesthetic Medication: The need for premedication and the choice of anesthetic agents must be individualized. In clinical studies, patients who received ULTIVA frequently received a benzodiazepine premedication.

Preparation for Administration: To reconstitute solution, add 1 mL of diluent per mg of remifentanil. Shake well to dissolve. When reconstituted as directed, the solution contains approximately 1 mg of remifentanil activity per 1 mL. **ULTIVA should be diluted to a recommended final concentration of 25, 50, or 250 mcg/mL prior to administration (see Table 8). ULTIVA should not be administered without dilution.**

Table 8: Reconstitution and Dilution of ULTIVA

Final Concentration	Amount of ULTIVA in Each Vial	Final Volume After Reconstitution and Dilution
25 mcg/mL	1 mg	40 mL
	2 mg	80 mL
	5 mg	200 mL
50 mcg/mL	1 mg	20 mL
	2 mg	40 mL
	5 mg	100 mL
250 mcg/mL	5 mg	20 mL

Continuous IV infusions of ULTIVA should be administered only by an infusion device. Infusion rates of ULTIVA can be individualized for each patient using Table 9:

Table 9: IV Infusion Rates of ULTIVA (mL/kg/h)

Drug Delivery Rate (mcg/kg/min)	Infusion Delivery Rate (mL/kg/h) 25 mcg/mL	50 mcg/mL	250 mcg/mL
0.0125	0.03	0.015	not recommended
0.025	0.06	0.03	not recommended
0.05	0.12	0.06	0.012
0.075	0.18	0.09	0.018
0.1	0.24	0.12	0.024
0.15	0.36	0.18	0.036
0.2	0.48	0.24	0.048
0.25	0.6	0.3	0.06
0.5	1.2	0.6	0.12
0.75	1.8	0.9	0.18
1.0	2.4	1.2	0.24
1.25	3.0	1.5	0.3
1.5	3.6	1.8	0.36
1.75	4.2	2.1	0.42
2.0	4.8	2.4	0.48

When ULTIVA is used as an analgesic component of monitored analgesia care or for pediatric patients ≥2 years of age, a final concentration of 25 mcg/mL is recommended. Table 10 is a guideline for milliliter-per-hour delivery for a solution of 25 mcg/mL with an infusion device.

[See table 10 below]

Table 11 is a guideline for milliliter-per-hour delivery for a solution of 50 mcg/mL with an infusion device.

Table 10: IV Infusion Rates of ULTIVA (mL/h) for a 25-mcg/mL Solution

Infusion Rate (mcg/kg/min)	Patient Weight (kg) 10	20	30	40	50	60	70	80	90	100
0.0125	0.3	0.6	0.9	1.2	1.5	1.8	2.1	2.4	2.7	3.0
0.025	0.6	1.2	1.8	2.4	3.0	3.6	4.2	4.8	5.4	6.0
0.05	1.2	2.4	3.6	4.8	6.0	7.2	8.4	9.6	10.8	12.0
0.075	1.8	3.6	5.4	7.2	9.0	10.8	12.6	14.4	16.2	18.0
0.1	2.4	4.8	7.2	9.6	12.0	14.4	16.8	19.2	21.6	24.0
0.15	3.6	7.2	10.8	14.4	18.0	21.6	25.2	28.8	32.4	36.0
0.2	4.8	9.6	14.4	19.2	24.0	28.8	33.6	38.4	43.2	48.0

Table 11: IV Infusion Rates of ULTIVA (mL/h) for a 50-mcg/mL Solution

Infusion Rate (mcg/kg/min)	Patient Weight (kg) 30	40	50	60	70	80	90	100
0.025					2.1	2.4	2.7	3.0
0.05		2.4	3.0	3.6	4.2	4.8	5.4	6.0
0.075	2.7	3.6	4.5	5.4	6.3	7.2	8.1	9.0
0.1	3.6	4.8	6.0	7.2	8.4	9.6	10.8	12.0
0.15	5.4	7.2	9.0	10.8	12.6	14.4	16.2	18.0
0.2	7.2	9.6	12.0	14.4	16.8	19.2	21.6	24.0
0.25	9.0	12.0	15.0	18.0	21.0	24.0	27.0	30.0
0.5	18.0	24.0	30.0	36.0	42.0	48.0	54.0	60.0
0.75	27.0	36.0	45.0	54.0	63.0	72.0	81.0	90.0
1.0	36.0	48.0	60.0	72.0	84.0	96.0	108.0	120.0
1.25	45.0	60.0	75.0	90.0	105.0	120.0	135.0	150.0
1.5	54.0	72.0	90.0	108.0	126.0	144.0	162.0	180.0
1.75	63.0	84.0	105.0	126.0	147.0	168.0	189.0	210.0
2.0	72.0	96.0	120.0	144.0	168.0	192.0	216.0	240.0

Table 12 is a guideline for milliliter-per-hour delivery for a solution of 250 mcg/mL with an infusion device.

Table 12: IV Infusion Rates of ULTIVA (mL/h) for a 250-mcg/mL Solution

Infusion Rate (mcg/kg/min)	Patient Weight (kg) 30	40	50	60	70	80	90	100
0.1	0.72	0.96	1.20	1.44	1.68	1.92	2.16	2.40
0.15	1.08	1.44	1.80	2.16	2.52	2.88	3.24	3.60
0.2	1.44	1.92	2.40	2.88	3.36	3.84	4.32	4.80
0.25	1.80	2.40	3.00	3.60	4.20	4.80	5.40	6.00
0.5	3.60	4.80	6.00	7.20	8.40	9.60	10.80	12.00
0.75	5.40	7.20	9.00	10.80	12.60	14.40	16.20	18.00
1.0	7.20	9.60	12.00	14.40	16.80	19.20	21.60	24.00
1.25	9.00	12.00	15.00	18.00	21.00	24.00	27.00	30.00
1.5	10.80	14.40	18.00	21.60	25.20	28.80	32.40	36.00
1.75	12.60	16.80	21.00	25.20	29.40	33.60	37.80	42.00
2.0	14.40	19.20	24.00	28.80	33.60	38.40	43.20	48.00

COMPATIBILITY AND STABILITY

Reconstitution and Dilution Prior to Administration: ULTIVA is stable for 24 hours at room temperature after reconstitution and further dilution to concentrations of 20 to 250 mcg/mL with the IV fluids listed below.

Sterile Water for Injection, USP
5% Dextrose Injection, USP
5% Dextrose and 0.9% Sodium Chloride Injection, USP
0.9% Sodium Chloride Injection, USP
0.45% Sodium Chloride Injection, USP
Lactated Ringer's and 5% Dextrose Injection, USP

ULTIVA is stable for 4 hours at room temperature after reconstitution and further dilution to concentrations of 20 to 250 mcg/mL with Lactated Ringer's Injection, USP.

ULTIVA has been shown to be compatible with these IV fluids when coadministered into a running IV administration set.

Compatibility With Other Therapeutic Agents: ULTIVA has been shown to be compatible with DIPRIVAN® (propofol) Injection when coadministered into a running IV administration set. The compatibility of ULTIVA with other therapeutic agents has not been evaluated.

Incompatibilities: Nonspecific esterases in blood products may lead to the hydrolysis of remifentanil to its carboxylic acid metabolite. Therefore, administration of ULTIVA into the same IV tubing with blood is not recommended.

Note: Parenteral drug products should be inspected visually for particulate matter and discoloration prior to administration whenever solution and container permit. Product should be a clear, colorless liquid after reconstitution and free of visible particulate matter.

ULTIVA does not contain any antimicrobial preservative and thus care must be taken to assure the sterility of prepared solutions.

HOW SUPPLIED

ULTIVA should be stored at 2° to 25°C (36° to 77°F). ULTIVA for IV use is supplied as follows:

NDC 0173-0483-00 1 mg of remifentanil base lyophilized powder, 3-mL Vial (Carton of 10)

NDC 0173-0484-00 2 mg of remifentanil base lyophilized powder, 5-mL Vial (Carton of 10)

NDC 0173-0485-00 5 mg of remifentanil base lyophilized powder, 10-mL Vial (Carton of 10)

DIPRIVAN® is a registered trademark of Zeneca Pharmaceuticals.

©Copyright 1996 Glaxo Wellcome Inc. All rights reserved.

July 1997/RL-446
Shown in Product Identification Guide, page 314

VALTREX® ℞
[*val'trěks*]
(valacyclovir hydrochloride)
Caplets

DESCRIPTION

VALTREX (valacyclovir hydrochloride) is the hydrochloride salt of L-valyl ester of the antiviral drug acyclovir (ZOVIRAX® Brand, Glaxo Wellcome Inc.).

VALTREX Caplets are for oral administration. Each caplet contains valacyclovir hydrochloride equivalent to 500 mg or 1 gram valacyclovir and the inactive ingredients carnauba wax, colloidal silicon dioxide, crospovidone, FD&C Blue No. 2 Lake, hydroxypropyl methylcellulose, magnesium stearate, microcrystalline cellulose, polyethylene glycol, polysorbate 80, povidone, and titanium dioxide. The blue, film-coated caplets are printed with edible white ink.

The chemical name of valacyclovir hydrochloride is *L*-valine, 2-[(2-amino-1,6-dihydro-6-oxo-9*H*-purin-9-yl)methoxy]ethyl ester, monohydrochloride.

Valacyclovir hydrochloride is a white to off-white powder with the molecular formula $C_{13}H_{20}N_6O_4 \bullet HCl$ and a molecular weight of 360.80. The maximum solubility in water at 25°C is 174 mg/mL. The pk_a's for valacyclovir hydrochloride are 1.90, 7.47, and 9.43.

MICROBIOLOGY

Mechanism of Antiviral Action: Valacyclovir hydrochloride is rapidly converted to acyclovir which has demonstrated antiviral activity against herpes simplex virus types 1 (HSV-1) and 2 (HSV-2) and varicella-zoster virus (VZV) both in vitro and in vivo. In cell culture, acyclovir's highest antiviral activity is against HSV-1, followed in decreasing order of potency against HSV-2 and VZV.

The inhibitory activity of acyclovir is highly selective due to its affinity for the enzyme thymidine kinase (TK) encoded by HSV, VZV, and EBV. This viral enzyme converts acyclovir into acyclovir monophosphate, a nucleotide analogue. The monophosphate is further converted into diphosphate by cellular guanylate kinase and into triphosphate by a number of cellular enzymes. In vitro, acyclovir triphosphate stops replication of herpes viral DNA. This is accomplished in three ways: 1) competitive inhibition of viral DNA polymerase, 2) incorporation and termination of the growing viral DNA chain, and 3) inactivation of the viral DNA polymerase. The greater antiviral activity of acyclovir against HSV compared to VZV is due to its more efficient phosphorylation by the viral TK.

Antiviral Activities: The quantitative relationship between the in vitro susceptibility of herpesviruses to antivirals and the clinical response to therapy has not been established in humans, and virus sensitivity testing has not been standardized. Sensitivity testing results, expressed as the concentration of drug required to inhibit by 50% the growth of virus in cell culture (IC_{50}), vary greatly depending upon a number of factors. Using plaque-reduction assays, the IC_{50} against herpes simplex virus isolates ranges from 0.02 to 13.5 mcg/mL for HSV-1 and from 0.01 to 9.9 mcg/mL for HSV-2. The IC_{50} for acyclovir against most laboratory strains and clinical isolates of VZV ranges from 0.12 to 10.8 mcg/mL. Acyclovir also demonstrates activity against the Oka vaccine strain of VZV with a mean IC_{50} of 1.35 mcg/mL.

Drug Resistance: Resistance of VZV to antiviral nucleoside analogues can result from qualitative or quantitative changes in the viral TK or DNA polymerase. Clinical isolates of VZV with reduced susceptibility to acyclovir have been recovered from patients with AIDS. In these cases, TK-deficient mutants of VZV have been recovered.

Resistance of HSV to antiviral nucleoside analogues occurs by the same mechanisms as resistance to VZV. While most of the acyclovir-resistant mutants isolated thus far from immunocompromised patients have been found to be TK-deficient mutants, other mutants involving the viral TK gene (TK partial and TK altered) and DNA polymerase have also been isolated. TK-negative mutants may cause severe disease in immunocompromised patients. The possibility of viral resistance to valacyclovir (and therefore, to acyclovir) should be considered in patients who show poor clinical response during therapy.

CLINICAL PHARMACOLOGY

After oral administration, valacyclovir hydrochloride is rapidly absorbed from the gastrointestinal tract and nearly completely converted to acyclovir and *L*-valine by first-pass intestinal and/or hepatic metabolism.

Pharmacokinetics: The pharmacokinetics of valacyclovir and acyclovir after oral administration of VALTREX have been investigated in 14 volunteer studies involving 283 adults.

Absorption and Bioavailability: The absolute bioavailability of acyclovir after administration of VALTREX is 54.5% ± 9.1% as determined following a 1-gram oral dose of VALTREX and a 350-mg intravenous acyclovir dose to 12 healthy volunteers. Acyclovir bioavailability from the administration of VALTREX is not altered by administration with food (30 minutes after an 873 Kcal breakfast, which included 51 grams of fat).

There was a lack of dose proportionality in acyclovir maximum concentration (C_{max}) and area under the acyclovir concentration-time curve (AUC) after single-dose administration of 100 mg, 250 mg, 500 mg, 750 mg, and 1 gram of VALTREX to eight healthy volunteers. The mean C_{max} (±SD) was 0.83 (± 0.14), 2.15 (± 0.50), 3.28 (± 0.83), 4.17 (± 1.14), and 5.65 (± 2.37) mcg/mL, respectively; and the mean AUC (± SD) was 2.28 (± 0.40), 5.76 (± 0.60), 11.59 (± 1.79), 14.11 (± 3.54), and 19.52 (± 6.04) hr·mcg/mL, respectively.

There was also a lack of dose proportionality in acyclovir C_{max} and AUC after the multiple-dose administration of 250 mg, 500 mg, and 1 gram of VALTREX administered four times daily for 11 days in parallel groups of eight healthy volunteers. The mean C_{max} (± SD) was 2.11 (± 0.33), 3.69 (± 0.87), and 4.96 (± 0.64) mcg/mL, respectively, and the mean AUC (± SD) was 5.66 (± 1.09), 9.88 (± 2.01), and 15.70 (± 2.27) hr·mcg/mL, respectively.

There is no accumulation of acyclovir after the administration of valacyclovir at the recommended dosage regimens in healthy volunteers with normal renal function.

Distribution: The binding of valacyclovir to human plasma proteins ranged from 13.5% to 17.9%.

Metabolism: After oral administration, valacyclovir hydrochloride is rapidly absorbed from the gastrointestinal tract. Valacyclovir is converted to acyclovir and *L*-valine by first-pass intestinal and/or hepatic metabolism. Acyclovir is converted to a small extent to inactive metabolites by aldehyde oxidase and by alcohol and aldehyde dehydrogenase. Neither valacyclovir nor acyclovir metabolism is associated with liver microsomal enzymes. Plasma concentrations of unconverted valacyclovir are low and transient, generally becoming non-quantifiable by 3 hours after administration. Peak plasma valacyclovir concentrations are generally less than 0.5 mcg/mL at all doses. After single-dose administration of 1 gram of VALTREX, average plasma valacyclovir concentrations observed were 0.5, 0.4, and 0.8 mcg/mL in patients with hepatic dysfunction, renal insufficiency, and in healthy volunteers who received concomitant cimetidine and probenecid, respectively.

Elimination: The pharmacokinetic disposition of acyclovir delivered by valacyclovir is consistent with previous experience from intravenous and oral acyclovir. Following the oral administration of a single 1-gram dose of radiolabeled valacyclovir to four healthy subjects, 45.60% and 47.12% of administered radioactivity was recovered in urine and feces over 96 hours, respectively. Acyclovir accounted for 88.60% of the radioactivity excreted in the urine. Renal clearance of acyclovir following the administration of a single 1-gram dose of VALTREX to 12 healthy volunteers was approximately 255 ± 86 mL/min which represents 41.9% of total acyclovir apparent plasma clearance.

The plasma elimination half-life of acyclovir typically averaged 2.5 to 3.3 hours in all studies of VALTREX in volunteers with normal renal function.

End-Stage Renal Disease (ESRD): Following administration of VALTREX to volunteers with ESRD, the average acyclovir half-life is approximately 14 hours. During hemodialysis, the acyclovir half-life is approximately 4 hours. Approximately one-third of acyclovir in the body is removed by dialysis during a 4-hour hemodialysis session. Apparent plasma clearance of acyclovir in dialysis patients was 86.3 ± 21.3 mL/min/1.73 m^2, compared to 679.16 ± 162.76 mL/min/1.73 m^2 in healthy volunteers. Reduction in dosage is recommended in patients with renal impairment (see DOSAGE AND ADMINISTRATION).

Geriatrics: After single-dose administration of 1 gram of VALTREX in healthy geriatric volunteers (n = 9, mean age ± S.D. = 74.0 ± 5.4 years), the half-life of acyclovir was 3.11 ± 0.51 hours, compared to 2.91 ± 0.63 hours in healthy volunteers (n = 33, mean age ± S.D. = 41.2 ± 10.1 years). Dosage modification may be necessary in geriatric patients with reduced renal function (see DOSAGE AND ADMINISTRATION).

Pediatrics: Valacyclovir pharmacokinetics have not been evaluated in pediatric patients.

Liver Disease: Administration of VALTREX to patients with moderate (biopsy-proven cirrhosis) or severe (with and without ascites and biopsy-proven cirrhosis) liver disease indicated that the rate but not the extent of conversion of valacyclovir to acyclovir is reduced, and the acyclovir half-life is not affected. Dosage modification is not recommended for patients with cirrhosis.

HIV Disease: In nine patients with advanced HIV disease (CD4 cell counts <150 cells/mm^3) who received VALTREX at a dosage of 1 gram four times daily for 30 days, the pharmacokinetics of valacyclovir and acyclovir were not different from that observed in healthy volunteers (see WARNINGS).

Drug Interactions: The pharmacokinetics of digoxin was not affected by coadministration of VALTREX 1 gram three times daily, and the pharmacokinetics of acyclovir after a single dose of VALTREX (1 gram) was unchanged by coadministration of digoxin (two doses of 0.75 mg), single doses of antacids (Al^{3+} or Mg^{++}), or multiple doses of thiazide diuretics. Acyclovir C_{max} and AUC following a single dose of VALTREX (1 gram) increased by 8% and 32%, respectively, after a single dose of cimetidine (800 mg), or by 22% and 49%, respectively, after probenecid (1 gram), or by 30% and 78%, respectively, after a combination of cimetidine and probenecid, primarily due to a reduction in renal clearance of acyclovir. These effects are not considered to be of clinical significance in subjects with normal renal function. Therefore, no dosage adjustment is recommended when VALTREX is coadministered with digoxin, antacids, thiazide diuretics, cimetidine, or probenecid in subjects with normal renal function.

Clinical Trials: *Herpes Zoster Infections:* Two randomized double-blind clinical trials in immunocompetent adults with localized herpes zoster were conducted. VALTREX was compared to placebo in patients less than 50 years of age, and to ZOVIRAX in patients greater than 50 years of age. All patients were treated within 72 hours of appearance of zoster rash. In patients less than 50 years of age, the median time to cessation of new lesion formation was 2 days for those treated with VALTREX compared to 3 days for those treated with placebo. In patients greater than 50 years of age, the median time to cessation of new lesions was 3 days in patients treated with either VALTREX or ZOVIRAX. In patients less than 50 years of age, no difference was found with respect to the duration of pain after rash healing (post-herpetic neuralgia) between the recipients of VALTREX and placebo. In patients greater than 50 years of age, among the 83% who reported pain after healing (post-herpetic neuralgia), the median duration of pain after healing [95% confidence interval] in days was: 40 [31, 51], 43 [36, 55], and 59 [41, 77] for 7-day VALTREX, 14-day VALTREX, and 7-day ZOVIRAX, respectively.

Genital Herpes Infections: Initial Episode: Six hundred and forty-three immunocompetent adults with first episode genital herpes who presented within 72 hours of symptom onset were randomized in a double-blind trial to receive 10 days of VALTREX 1 gram b.i.d. (n = 323) or ZOVIRAX 200 mg 5 times a day (n = 320). For both treatment groups: the median time to lesion healing was 9 days, the median time to cessation of pain was 5 days, the median time to cessation of viral shedding was 3 days.

Recurrent Episodes: Two double-blind placebo-controlled trials in immunocompetent adults with recurrent genital herpes were conducted. Patients self-initiated therapy within 24 hours of the first sign or symptom of a recurrent genital herpes episode.

In one study, patients were randomized to receive 5 days of treatment with either VALTREX 500 mg b.i.d. (n = 360) or placebo (n = 259). The median time to lesion healing was 4 days in the group receiving VALTREX 500 mg versus 6 days in the placebo group, and the median time to cessation of viral shedding in patients with at least one positive culture (42% of the overall study population) was 2 days in the group receiving VALTREX 500 mg versus 4 days in the placebo group. The median time to cessation of pain was 3 days in the group receiving VALTREX 500 mg versus 4 days in the placebo group. Results supporting efficacy were replicated in a second trial.

Suppressive Therapy: One thousand, four hundred seventy-nine (1,479) immunocompetent adults with a history of six or more recurrences per year were randomized into a double-blind, placebo-controlled study. Outcomes for the overall study population are shown in Table 1.

[See table 1 at top of next page]

Subjects with nine or fewer recurrences per year showed comparable results with VALTREX 500 mg once daily.

INDICATIONS AND USAGE

Herpes Zoster: VALTREX is indicated for the treatment of herpes zoster (shingles).

Genital Herpes: VALTREX is indicated for the treatment or suppression of genital herpes.

CONTRAINDICATIONS

VALTREX is contraindicated in patients with a known hypersensitivity or intolerance to valacyclovir, acyclovir, or any component of the formulation.

WARNINGS

Thrombotic thrombocytopenic purpura/hemolytic uremic syndrome (TTP/HUS), in some cases resulting in death, has occurred in patients with advanced HIV disease and also in

Continued on next page

This product information is based on labeling in effect on June 1, 1998. For further information, contact via direct mail, phone, or web site Medical Information: Glaxo Wellcome Inc., PO Box 13398, Research Triangle Park, NC 27709. Healthcare Professionals (Medical Information): 800-334-0089 Patients (Customer Response Center): 888-TALK2GW (1-888-825-5249) Glaxo Wellcome Corporate Web Site: www.glaxowellcome.com

Valtrex—Cont.

allogeneic bone marrow transplant and renal transplant recipients participating in clinical trials of VALTREX at doses of 8 grams per day.

PRECAUTIONS

Dosage reduction is recommended when administering VALTREX to patients with renal impairment (see DOSAGE AND ADMINISTRATION). Acute renal failure and central nervous system symptoms have been reported in patients with underlying renal disease who have received inappropriately high doses of VALTREX for their level of renal function. Similar caution should be exercised when administering VALTREX to geriatric patients (see Geriatric Use) and patients receiving potentially nephrotoxic agents.

Precipitation of acyclovir in renal tubules may occur when the solubility (2.5 mg/mL) is exceeded in the intratubular fluid. In the event of acute renal failure and anuria, the patient may benefit from hemodialysis until renal function is restored (see DOSAGE AND ADMINISTRATION).

The efficacy of VALTREX has not been established for the treatment of disseminated herpes zoster or in immunocompromised patients.

Information for Patients: *Herpes Zoster:* There are no data on treatment initiated more than 72 hours after onset of the zoster rash. Patients should be advised to initiate treatment as soon as possible after a diagnosis of herpes zoster.

Genital Herpes: Patients should be informed that VALTREX is not a cure for genital herpes. There are no data evaluating whether VALTREX will prevent transmission of infection to others. Because genital herpes is a sexually transmitted disease, patients should avoid contact with lesions or intercourse when lesions and/or symptoms are present to avoid infecting partners. Genital herpes can also be transmitted in the absence of symptoms through asymptomatic viral shedding. If medical management of a genital herpes recurrence is indicated, patients should be advised to initiate therapy at the first sign or symptom of an episode.

There are no data on the effectiveness of treatment initiated more than 72 hours after the onset of signs and symptoms of a first episode of genital herpes or more than 24 hours of the onset of signs and symptoms of a recurrent episode.

There are no data on the safety or effectiveness of chronic suppressive therapy of more than 1 year's duration.

Drug Interactions: See CLINICAL PHARMACOLOGY: Pharmacokinetics.

Carcinogenesis, Mutagenesis, Impairment of Fertility: The data presented below include references to the steady-state acyclovir AUC observed in humans treated with 1 gram VALTREX given orally three times a day to treat herpes zoster. Plasma drug concentrations in animal studies are expressed as multiples of human exposure to acyclovir (see CLINICAL PHARMACOLOGY: Pharmacokinetics).

Valacyclovir was noncarcinogenic in lifetime carcinogenicity bioassays at single daily doses (gavage) of up to 120 mg/kg/day for mice and 100 mg/kg/day for rats. There was no significant difference in the incidence of tumors between treated and control animals, nor did valacyclovir shorten the latency of tumors. Plasma concentrations of acyclovir were equivalent to human levels in the mouse bioassay and 1.4 to 2.3 times human levels in the rat bioassay.

Valacyclovir was tested in five genetic toxicity assays. An Ames assay was negative in the absence or presence of metabolic activation. Also negative were an in vitro cytogenetic study with human lymphocytes and a rat cytogenetic study at a single oral dose of 3000 mg/kg (8 to 9 times human plasma levels).

In the mouse lymphoma assay, valacyclovir was negative in the absence of metabolic activation. In the presence of metabolic activation (76% to 88% conversion to acyclovir), valacyclovir was weakly mutagenic.

A mouse micronucleus assay was negative at 250 mg/kg but weakly positive at 500 mg/kg (acyclovir concentrations 26 to 51 times human plasma levels).

Valacyclovir did not impair fertility or reproduction in rats at 200 mg/kg per day (6 times human plasma levels).

Pregnancy: *Teratogenic Effects:* Pregnancy Category B. Valacyclovir was not teratogenic in rats or rabbits given 400 mg/kg (which results in exposures of 10 and 7 times human plasma levels, respectively) during the period of major organogenesis. There are no adequate and well-controlled studies of VALTREX or ZOVIRAX in pregnant women. A prospective epidemiologic registry of acyclovir use during pregnancy has been ongoing since 1984. As of June 1996, outcomes of live births have been documented in 494 women exposed to systemic acyclovir during the first trimester of pregnancy. The occurrence rate of birth defects approximates that found in the general population. However, the small size of the registry is insufficient to evaluate the risk for less common defects or to permit reliable and definitive conclusions regarding the safety of acyclovir in pregnant women and their developing fetuses. VALTREX should be used during pregnancy only if the potential benefit justifies the potential risk to the fetus.

Pregnancy Exposure Registry: To monitor maternal-fetal outcomes of pregnant women exposed to VALTREX, Glaxo Wellcome Inc. maintains a Valacyclovir in Pregnancy Registry. Physicians are encouraged to register their patients by calling (800) 722-9292, ext. 39437.

Nursing Mothers: There is no experience with VALTREX. However, acyclovir concentrations have been documented in breast milk in two women following oral administration of ZOVIRAX and ranged from 0.6 to 4.1 times corresponding plasma levels. These concentrations would potentially expose the nursing infant to a dose of acyclovir as high as 0.3 mg/kg/day. VALTREX should be administered to a nursing mother with caution and only when indicated.

Pediatric Use: Safety and effectiveness of VALTREX in pediatric patients have not been established.

Geriatric Use: Of the total number of patients included in clinical studies of VALTREX, 861 were age 65 or older, and 344 were age 75 or older. A total of 34 volunteers age 65 or older completed a pharmacokinetic trial of VALTREX. The pharmacokinetics of acyclovir following single- and multiple-dose oral administration of VALTREX in geriatric volunteers varied with renal function. Dosage reduction may be required in geriatric patients, depending on the underlying renal status of the patient (see CLINICAL PHARMACOLOGY and DOSAGE AND ADMINISTRATION).

ADVERSE REACTIONS

Frequently reported adverse events in clinical trials of VALTREX are listed in Table 2.

[See table 2 above]

Laboratory abnormalities reported in clinical trials of VALTREX are listed in Table 3.

[See table 3 above]

Observed During Clinical Practice: The following events have been identified during post-approval use of VALTREX in clinical practice. Because they are reported voluntarily from a population of unknown size, estimates of frequency cannot be made. These events have been chosen for inclusion due to either their seriousness, frequency of reporting, causal connection to VALTREX, or a combination of these factors.

General: Facial edema, hypertension, tachycardia.

Table 1: Proportions of Patients Recurrence-free at 6 and 12 Months

Treatment Arm	6 Months			12 Months		
	VALTREX 1 gram q.d. (n = 269)	ZOVIRAX 400 mg b.i.d. (n = 267)	Placebo (n = 134)	VALTREX 1 gram q.d. (n = 269)	ZOVIRAX 400 mg b.i.d. (n = 267)	Placebo (n = 134)
Recurrence-free (%)	55	54	7	34	34	4
Recurrences (%)	35	36	83	46	46	85
Unknowns (%)	10	10	10	19	19	10

Table 2: Incidence (%) of Adverse Events in Herpes Zoster and Genital Herpes Study Populations

Adverse Event	Herpes Zoster		Genital Herpes Treatment			Genital Herpes Suppression		
	VALTREX 1 gram t.i.d. (n = 967)	Placebo (n = 195)	VALTREX 1 gram b.i.d. (n = 1,194)	VALTREX 500 mg b.i.d. (n = 359)	Placebo (n = 439)	VALTREX 1 gram q.d. (n = 269)	VALTREX 500 mg q.d. (n = 266)	Placebo (n = 134)
Nausea	15	8	6	6	8	11	11	8
Headache	14	12	16	17	14	35	38	34
Vomiting	6	3	1	1	<1	3	3	2
Dizziness	3	2	3	2	3	4	2	1
Abdominal Pain	3	2	2	3	3	11	9	6
Dysmenorrhea	0	0	<1	1	1	8	5	4
Arthralgia	1	0	<1	1	<1	6	5	4
Depression	1	1	1	0	<1	7	5	5

Table 3: Incidence (%) of Laboratory Abnormalities in Herpes Zoster and Genital Herpes Study Populations

Laboratory Abnormality	Herpes Zoster		Genital Herpes Treatment			Genital Herpes Suppression		
	VALTREX 1 gram t.i.d.	Placebo	VALTREX 1 gram b.i.d.	VALTREX 500 mg b.i.d.	Placebo	VALTREX 1 gram q.d.	VALTREX 500 mg q.d.	Placebo
Anemia	0.8	0	0.3	0.3	0	0	0.8	0.8
Leukopenia	1.3	0.6	0.7	0.8	0.2	0.7	0.8	1.5
Thrombocytopenia	1.0	1.2	0.3	0.6	0.7	0.4	1.1	1.5
AST (SGOT)	1.0	0	1.0	*	0.5	4.1	3.8	3.0
Serum Creatinine	0.2	0	0.7	0	0	0	0	0

* Data were not collected prospectively in this study.

Table 4: Dosages for Patients with Renal Impairment

Indications	Normal Dosage Regimen (Creatinine Clearance ≥50)	Creatinine Clearance (mL/min)		
		30–49	10–29	<10
Herpes zoster	1 gram every 8 hours	1 gram every 12 hours	1 gram every 24 hours	500 mg every 24 hours
Genital herpes				
Initial treatment	1 gram every 12 hours	no reduction	1 gram every 24 hours	500 mg every 24 hours
Recurrent episodes	500 mg every 12 hours	no reduction	500 mg every 24 hours	500 mg every 24 hours
Suppressive therapy	1 gram every 24 hours	no reduction	500 mg every 24 hours	500 mg every 24 hours
Suppressive therapy	500 mg every 24 hours	no reduction	500 mg every 48 hours	500 mg every 48 hours

Allergic: Acute hypersensitivity reactions including anaphylaxis, angioedema, dyspnea, pruritus, rash, and urticaria.

CNS Symptoms: Confusion, agitation, hallucinations (auditory and visual), aggressive behavior, mania.

Gastrointestinal: Diarrhea.

Renal: Elevated creatinine, renal failure.

Hemic: Thrombocytopenia, aplastic anemia.

Skin: Erythema multiforme.

Renal Impairment: Renal failure and CNS symptoms have been reported in patients with renal impairment who received VALTREX or acyclovir at greater than the recommended dose. **Dosage adjustment is recommended in this patient population (see DOSAGE AND ADMINISTRATION).**

OVERDOSAGE

Caution should be exercised to prevent inadvertent overdose (see PRECAUTIONS). Precipitation of acyclovir in renal tubules may occur when the solubility (2.5 mg/mL) is exceeded in the intratubular fluid. In the event of acute renal failure and anuria, the patient may benefit from hemodialysis until renal function is restored (see DOSAGE AND ADMINISTRATION).

DOSAGE AND ADMINISTRATION

VALTREX Caplets may be given without regard to meals.

Herpes Zoster: The recommended dosage of VALTREX for the treatment of herpes zoster is 1 gram orally three times daily for 7 days. Therapy should be initiated at the earliest sign or symptom of herpes zoster and is most effective when started within 48 hours of the onset of zoster rash. No data are available on efficacy of treatment started greater than 72 hours after rash onset.

Genital Herpes: *Initial Episodes:* The recommended dosage of VALTREX for treatment of initial genital herpes is 1 gram twice daily for 10 days.

There are no data on the effectiveness of treatment with VALTREX when initiated more than 72 hours after the onset of signs and symptoms. Therapy was most effective when administered within 48 hours of the onset of signs and symptoms.

Recurrent Episodes: The recommended dosage of VALTREX for the treatment of recurrent genital herpes is 500 mg twice daily for 5 days. If medical management of a genital herpes recurrence is indicated, patients should be advised to initiate therapy at the first sign or symptom of an episode. There are no data on the effectiveness of treatment with VALTREX when initiated more than 24 hours after the onset of signs or symptoms.

Suppressive Therapy: The recommended dosage of VALTREX for chronic suppressive therapy of recurrent genital herpes is 1 gram once daily. In patients with a history of nine or fewer recurrences per year, an alternative dose is 500 mg once daily. The safety and efficacy of therapy with VALTREX beyond 1 year have not been established.

Patients with Acute or Chronic Renal Impairment: In patients with reduced renal function, reduction in dosage is recommended (see Table 4).

[See table 4 on previous page]

Hemodialysis: During hemodialysis, the half-life of acyclovir after administration of VALTREX is approximately 4 hours. About one-third of acyclovir in the body is removed by dialysis during a 4-hour hemodialysis session. Patients requiring hemodialysis should receive the recommended dose of VALTREX after hemodialysis.

Peritoneal Dialysis: There is no information specific to administration of VALTREX in patients receiving peritoneal dialysis. The effect of chronic ambulatory peritoneal dialysis (CAPD) and continuous arteriovenous hemofiltration/dialysis (CAVHD) on acyclovir pharmacokinetics has been studied. The removal of acyclovir after CAPD and CAVHD is less pronounced than with hemodialysis, and the pharmacokinetic parameters closely resemble those observed in patients with ESRD not receiving hemodialysis. Therefore, supplemental doses of VALTREX should not be required following CAPD or CAVHD.

HOW SUPPLIED

VALTREX Caplets (blue, film-coated, capsule-shaped tablets) containing valacyclovir hydrochloride equivalent to 500 mg valacyclovir and printed with "VALTREX 500 mg" - Bottle of 42 (NDC 0173-0933-03) and unit dose pack of 100 (NDC 0173-0933-56).

VALTREX Caplets (blue, film-coated, capsule-shaped tablets) containing valacyclovir hydrochloride equivalent to 1 gram valacyclovir and printed with "VALTREX 1 gram" - Bottle of 20 (NDC 0173-0565-00).

Store at 15° to 25°C (59° to 77°F).

U.S. Patent No. 4,957,924

©Copyright 1996 Glaxo Wellcome Inc. All rights reserved.

September 1997/RL-464

Shown in Product Identification Guide, page 314

VASOXYL®   ℞
[vāz "ox 'ŭl]
(methoxamine hydrochloride)
Injection
20 mg in 1 ml

DESCRIPTION

VASOXYL (methoxamine hydrochloride) Injection is a sterile solution for intravenous (IV) or intramuscular (IM) injection made isotonic with sodium chloride. Each 1-mL ampul contains 20 mg of methoxamine hydrochloride. Citric acid anhydrous 0.3% and sodium citrate 0.3% are added as buffers, and potassium metabisulfite 0.1% is added as an antioxidant.

Methoxamine hydrochloride is a sympathomimetic amine. It has the empirical formula $C_{11}H_{17}NO_3 \cdot HCl$ and a molecular weight of 247.72. The drug is very soluble in water, soluble in ethanol, but practically insoluble in ether, benzene, or chloroform. It is known chemically as α-(1-aminoethyl)-2,5-dimethoxybenzenemethanol hydrochloride.

CLINICAL PHARMACOLOGY

VASOXYL is an alpha-receptor stimulant that produces a prompt and prolonged rise in blood pressure following parenteral administration. It is especially useful for maintaining blood pressure during operations under spinal anesthesia[1-3] and may also be used safely during general anesthesia. VASOXYL does not increase the irritability of the cyclopropane-sensitized heart, making it useful during cyclopropane anesthesia.[4,5] Tachyphylaxis has not been a clinical problem.[1]

The major pharmacological effect of VASOXYL is a potent, prolonged pressor action following parenteral administration. VASOXYL differs from most other sympathomimetic amines both in animals[4,6,7] and in humans[1,8] by having a predominantly peripheral action and lacking inotropic and chronotropic effects. VASOXYL has less arrhythmogenic potential than other sympathomimetic amines and rarely causes ventricular tachycardia, fibrillation, or increased sinoatrial rate.[4] On occasion, a decrease in rate occurs as blood pressure increases,[1,9,10] apparently caused by a carotid sinus reflex. This bradycardia can be abolished by atropine.[9]

The pressor action appears to be due to peripheral vasoconstriction rather than a centrally mediated effect. Evidence for direct action on blood vessels is provided in part by the observation of intense constriction along the course of a vein into which VASOXYL has been injected.[1] VASOXYL also increases venous pressure.[8]

Following IV administration of VASOXYL in dogs[11] and humans,[9,12] the peak pressor effect occurs within 0.5 to 2 minutes. In a group of human surgical patients,[13] the duration of the pressor effect following a single IV dose of 2 to 4 mg of VASOXYL was 10 to 15 minutes. No clinical pharmacology studies are available concerning the onset and duration of action after administration of recommended IM doses (10 to 15 mg). With administration of 10 to 40 mg of VASOXYL intramuscularly to patients, however, the peak effect occurs within 15 to 20 minutes, and the duration of action is approximately 1½ hours.[14]

Data from pharmacokinetic studies of VASOXYL following either IV or IM administration are not available.

INDICATIONS AND USAGE

VASOXYL is intended for supporting, restoring, or maintaining blood pressure during anesthesia (including cyclopropane anesthesia). It can be used to terminate some episodes of supraventricular tachycardia.

CONTRAINDICATIONS

VASOXYL is contraindicated in patients with severe hypertension, or in patients who are hypersensitive to methoxamine.

WARNINGS

The use of VASOXYL in patients receiving monoamine oxidase inhibitors, tricyclic antidepressants, or oxytocic agents such as vasopressin or certain ergot alkaloids may result in potentiation of the pressor effect (see PRECAUTIONS: Drug Interactions).

VASOXYL contains potassium metabisulfite, a sulfite that may cause allergic-type reactions including anaphylactic symptoms and life-threatening or less severe asthmatic episodes in certain susceptible people. The overall prevalence of sulfite sensitivity in the general population is unknown and probably low. Sulfite sensitivity is seen more frequently in asthmatic than in nonasthmatic people.

PRECAUTIONS

General: VASOXYL, like other vasopressor agents, should be used with caution in patients with hyperthyroidism, bradycardia, partial heart block, myocardial disease, or severe arteriosclerosis. Caution should be exercised to avoid overdosage, preventing undesirable high blood pressure and/or bradycardia. Note: Bradycardia may be abolished with atropine (see OVERDOSAGE). Also, caution should be

taken when VASOXYL is used closely following the parenteral injection of ergot alkaloids to avoid an excessive rise in blood pressure.

Drug Interactions: The pressor effect of VASOXYL may be markedly potentiated when VASOXYL is used in conjunction with monoamine oxidase inhibitors, tricyclic antidepressants, vasopressin, or ergot alkaloids such as ergotamine, ergonovine, or methylergonovine. Therefore, when initiating pressor therapy in patients receiving these drugs, the initial dose should be small and given with caution (see WARNINGS).

Drug/Laboratory Test Interactions: VASOXYL may increase plasma cortisol and ACTH levels. Caution should be used when interpreting plasma cortisol and ACTH levels in a patient concurrently receiving VASOXYL.[15,16]

Carcinogenesis, Mutagenesis, Impairment of Fertility: No long-term animal studies have been performed to evaluate the potential of VASOXYL in these areas.

Pregnancy: *Teratogenic Effects:* *Pregnancy Category C:* VASOXYL has been shown to decrease uterine blood flow, decrease fetal heart rate, and adversely affect the fetal acid-base status in pregnant ewes and monkeys at doses comparable to those used in humans. There are no adequate and well-controlled studies in pregnant women. There has been one report of a fetal death; the mother received VASOXYL concomitantly with several other drugs. A direct causal relationship to VASOXYL was not established. VASOXYL should be used during pregnancy only if the potential benefit justifies the potential risk to the fetus.

VASOXYL (2.5 mg IV, one to three times over a 45-minute period) given to seven pregnant ewes showed a significant deterioration in fetal acid-base status as evidenced by hypoxia, hypercarbia, and metabolic acidosis.[17] An inverse relationship between pressor response to VASOXYL and uteroplacental blood flow has been shown in 16 pregnant ewes studied at doses ranging from 0.025 mg/kg to 0.2 mg/kg.[18] Uterine blood flow was decreased at all doses, but no significant change in fetal blood gas or acid-base status was demonstrated. Administration of VASOXYL to four fetuses (50 mcg/kg per minute for 60 minutes) and to four ewes (25 mcg/kg per minute for 30 minutes) was associated with a decrease in fetal heart rate and uterine blood flow.[19] Nine monkeys studied at an average dose of VASOXYL of 1.3 mg/kg administered over 57 minutes showed a decrease in uterine blood flow and a possible association with fetal asphyxia.[20]

Labor and Delivery: If vasopressor drugs are used to correct hypotension or added to the local anesthetic solution during labor and delivery, some oxytocic drugs (vasopressin, ergotamine, ergonovine, methylergonovine) may cause severe persistent hypertension (see WARNINGS and PRECAUTIONS: Drug Interactions).

Note: In pregnant animals, VASOXYL has been shown to decrease uterine blood flow, possibly resulting in fetal asphyxia. Uterine hypertonus and fetal bradycardia may also be produced (see ADVERSE REACTIONS and PRECAUTIONS: Drug Interactions).

Nursing Mothers: It is not known whether this drug is excreted in human milk. Because many drugs are excreted in human milk, caution should be exercised when VASOXYL is administered to a nursing woman.

Pediatric Use: Safety and effectiveness in pediatric patients have not been established.

ADVERSE REACTIONS

The following adverse reactions have been observed, but there are insufficient data to support an estimate of their frequency:

Cardiovascular: Excessive blood pressure elevations particularly with high dosage, ventricular ectopic beats.

Gastrointestinal: Nausea, vomiting (often projectile).

Central Nervous System: Headache (often severe), anxiety.

Integumentary: Sweating, pilomotor response.

Genitourinary: Uterine hypertonus, fetal bradycardia (see PRECAUTIONS: Labor and Delivery), urinary urgency.

OVERDOSAGE

Overdosage of VASOXYL may be manifested as an undesirable elevation in blood pressure and/or bradycardia. Should a clinically significant elevation of blood pressure occur that requires treatment, it may be immediately reversed with an alpha-adrenergic blocking agent (e.g., phentolamine). Bradycardia may be abolished by atropine.

Continued on next page

This product information is based on labeling in effect on June 1, 1998. For further information, contact via direct mail, phone, or web site Medical Information: Glaxo Wellcome Inc., PO Box 13398, Research Triangle Park, NC 27709. Healthcare Professionals (Medical Information): 800-334-0089 Patients (Customer Response Center): 888-TALK2GW (1-888-825-5249) Glaxo Wellcome Corporate Web Site: www.glaxowellcome.com

Vasoxyl—Cont.

DOSAGE AND ADMINISTRATION

Blood volume depletion should always be corrected before any vasopressor is administered. The usual IV dose of VASOXYL for emergencies is 3 to 5 mg, injected slowly. Intravenous injection may be supplemented by IM injections to provide a more prolonged effect. The usual IM dose is 10 to 15 mg given shortly before or at the time of administering spinal anesthesia to prevent a fall in blood pressure. The tendency for the blood pressure to fall is greater with higher levels of spinal anesthesia; hence the dosage may be adjusted accordingly. A dosage of 10 mg may be adequate at lower spinal levels, while 15 to 20 mg may be required at high levels of spinal anesthesia. Repeated doses may be given if necessary, but time should be allowed for the previous dose to act (about 15 minutes, see CLINICAL PHARMACOLOGY). For cases of only moderate hypotension, 5 to 10 mg given intramuscularly may be adequate.

For purposes of correcting a fall in blood pressure, an IM injection of 10 to 15 mg of VASOXYL may be given depending upon the degree of fall. In cases where the systolic pressure falls to 60 mmHg or less, or whenever an emergency exists, an IV injection of 3 to 5 mg of VASOXYL is indicated. This IV dose may be accompanied by 10 to 15 mg given intramuscularly to provide more prolonged effect.

For termination of episodes of supraventricular tachycardia not responsive to other modes of therapy, the usual dose of VASOXYL is 10 mg given intravenously, administered by slow push (i.e., 3 to 5 minutes).

Parenteral drug products should be inspected visually for particulate matter and discoloration prior to administration whenever solution and container permit.

HOW SUPPLIED

1-mL ampuls, containing 20 mg of methoxamine hydrochloride, box of 10 (NDC 0173-0957-10).

Store at 15° to 25°C (59° to 77°F) and protect from light.

REFERENCES

1. King BD, Dripps RD. The use of methoxamine for maintenance of the circulation during spinal anesthesia. *Surg Gynecol Obstet.* 1950;90:659-665.
2. Kistler EM, Ruben JE. Methoxamine in 1 percent procaine as a prophylactic vasopressor in spinal anesthesia. *Arch Surg.* 1951;62:64-69.
3. Poe MF. Use of methoxamine hydrochloride as a pressor agent during spinal analgesia. *Anesthesiology.* 1952;13:89-93.
4. Lahti RE, Brill IC, McCawley EL. The effect of methoxamine hydrochloride (VASOXYL) on cardiac rhythm. *J Pharmacol Exp Ther.* 1955;115:268-274.
5. Stutzman JW, Pettinga FL, Fruggiero EJ. Cardiac effects of methoxamine (β-[2,5-dimethoxy-phenyl]-β-hydroxyisopropylamine HCl) and desoxyephedrine during cyclopropane anesthesia. *J Pharmacol Exp Ther.* 1949;97:385-387.
6. West JW, Faulk AT, Guzman SV. Comparative study of effects of levarterenol and methoxamine in shock associated with acute myocardial ischemia in dogs. *Circ Res.* 1962;10:712-721.
7. Goldberg LI, Cotten M, Darby TD, Howell EV. Comparative heart contractile force effects of equipressor doses of several sympathomimetic amines. *J Pharmacol Exp Ther.* 1953;108:177-185.
8. Aviado DM, Wnuck AL. Mechanisms for cardiac slowing by methoxamine. *J Pharmacol Exp Ther.* 1957;119:99-106.
9. Nathanson MH, Miller H. Clinical observations on a new epinephrin-like compound, methoxamine. *Am J Med Sci.* 1952;223:270-279.
10. Stanfield CA, Yu PN. Hemodynamic effects of methoxamine in mitral valve disease. *Circ Res.* 1960;8:859-864.
11. Imai S, Shigei T, Hashimoto K. Cardiac actions of methoxamine with special reference to its antagonist action to epinephrine. *Circ Res.* 1961;9:552-560.
12. *The Extra Pharmacopoeia, Martindale* 28th Ed., Reynolds, JEF, ed., Pharmaceutical Press (London), pp. 19.
13. Goldberg LI, Bloodwell RD, Braunwald E, et al. The direct effects of norepinephrine, epinephrine, and methoxamine on myocardial contractile force in man. *Circ.* 1960;22:1125-1132.
14. Data on file, Glaxo Wellcome Inc.
15. Laurian L, Oberman Z, Hoerer E, et al. Low cortisol and growth hormone secretion in response to methoxamine administration in obese subjects. *Isr J Med Sci.* 1977;13:477-481.
16. Nakai Y, Imura H, Yoshimi T, Matsukura S. Adrenergic control mechanism for ACTH secretion in man. *Acta Endocrinol.* 1973;74:263-270.
17. Shnider SM, DeLorimier AA, Asling JH, Morishima HO. Vasopressors in obstetrics. II. Fetal hazards of methoxamine administration during obstetric spinal anesthesia. *Am J Obstet Gynecol.* 1970;106:680-686.
18. Ralston DH, Shnider SM, DeLorimier AA. Effects of equipotent ephedrine, metaraminol, mephentermine and methoxamine on uterine blood flow in the pregnant ewe. *Anesthesiology.* 1974;40:354-370.
19. Oakes GK, Ehrenkranz RA, Walker AM, et al. Effect of α-adrenergic agonist and antagonist infusion on the umbilical and uterine circulations of pregnant sheep. *Biol Neonate.* 1980;38:229-237.
20. Eng M, Berges PU, Ueland K, et al. The effects of methoxamine and ephedrine in normotensive pregnant primates. *Anesthesiology.* 1971;35:354-360.

January 1997/RL-391

Shown in Product Identification Guide, page 314

VENTOLIN® ℞

[vent 'ō-lin]

(albuterol, USP)

Inhalation Aerosol

Bronchodilator Aerosol
For Oral Inhalation Only

DESCRIPTION

The active component of VENTOLIN Inhalation Aerosol is albuterol, USP, racemic (α^1-[(*tert*-butylamino)methyl]-4-hydroxy-*m*-xylene-α,α′-diol) and a relatively selective beta$_2$-adrenergic bronchodilator.

Albuterol is the official generic name in the United States. The World Health Organization recommended name for the drug is salbutamol. The molecular weight of albuterol is 239.3, and the empirical formula is $C_{13}H_{21}NO_3$. Albuterol is a white to off-white crystalline solid. It is soluble in ethanol, sparingly soluble in water, and very soluble in chloroform.

VENTOLIN Inhalation Aerosol is a pressurized metered-dose aerosol unit for oral inhalation. It contains a microcrystalline (95%≤10 µm) suspension of albuterol in propellants (trichloromonofluoromethane and dichlorodifluoromethane) with oleic acid. Each actuation delivers 100 mcg of albuterol from the valve and 90 mcg of albuterol from the mouthpiece. Each 6.8-g canister provides 80 inhalations and each 17-g canister provides 200 inhalations.

CLINICAL PHARMACOLOGY

In vitro studies and in vivo pharmacologic studies have demonstrated that albuterol has a preferential effect on beta$_2$-adrenergic receptors compared with isoproterenol. While it is recognized that beta$_2$-adrenergic receptors are the predominant receptors in bronchial smooth muscle, data indicate that there is a population of beta$_2$-receptors in the human heart existing in a concentration between 10% and 50%. The precise function of these receptors has not been established.

The pharmacologic effects of beta-adrenergic agonist drugs, including albuterol, are at least in part attributable to stimulation through beta-adrenergic receptors of intracellular adenyl cyclase, the enzyme that catalyzes the conversion of adenosine triphosphate (ATP) to cyclic-3′,5′-adenosine monophosphate (cyclic AMP). Increased cyclic AMP levels are associated with relaxation of bronchial smooth muscle and inhibition of release of mediators of immediate hypersensitivity from cells, especially from mast cells.

Albuterol has been shown in most controlled clinical trials to have more effect on the respiratory tract, in the form of bronchial smooth muscle relaxation, than isoproterenol at comparable doses while producing fewer cardiovascular effects. Controlled clinical studies and other clinical experience have shown that inhaled albuterol, like other beta-adrenergic agonist drugs, can produce a significant cardiovascular effect in some patients, as measured by pulse rate, blood pressure, symptoms, and/or electrocardiographic changes.

Albuterol is longer acting than isoproterenol in most patients by any route of administration because it is not a substrate for the cellular uptake processes for catecholamines nor for catechol-*O*-methyl transferase.

The effects of rising doses of albuterol and isoproterenol aerosols were studied in volunteers and asthmatic patients. Results in normal volunteers indicated that albuterol is one half to one quarter as active as isoproterenol in producing increases in heart rate. In asthmatic patients similar cardiovascular differentiation between the two drugs was also seen.

Preclinical: Intravenous studies in rats with albuterol sulfate have demonstrated that albuterol crosses the blood-brain barrier and reaches brain concentrations amounting to approximately 5.0% of the plasma concentrations. In structures outside the brain barrier (pineal and pituitary glands), albuterol concentrations were found to be 100 times those in the whole brain.

Studies in laboratory animals (minipigs, rodents, and dogs) have demonstrated the occurrence of cardiac arrhythmias and sudden death (with histologic evidence of myocardial necrosis) when beta-agonists and methylxanthines are administered concurrently. The clinical significance of these findings is unknown.

Pharmacokinetics: Because of its gradual absorption from the bronchi, systemic levels of albuterol are low after inhalation of recommended doses. Studies undertaken with four subjects administered tritiated albuterol resulted in maximum plasma concentrations occurring within 2 to 4 hours. Due to the sensitivity of the assay method, the metabolic rate and half-life of elimination of albuterol in plasma could not be determined. However, urinary excretion provided data indicating that albuterol has an elimination half-life of 3.8 hours. Approximately 72% of the inhaled dose is excreted within 24 hours in the urine, and consists of 28% as unchanged drug and 44% as metabolite.

Clinical Trials: In controlled clinical trials involving adults with asthma, the onset of improvement in pulmonary function was within 15 minutes, as determined by both MMEF (maximum midexpiratory flow rate) and FEV_1 (forced expiratory volume in 1 second). MMEF measurements also showed that near maximum improvement in pulmonary function generally occurs within 60 to 90 minutes following two inhalations of albuterol and that clinically significant improvement generally continues for 3 to 4 hours in most patients. Some patients showed a therapeutic response (defined by maintaining FEV_1 values 15% or more above baseline) that was still apparent at 6 hours. Continued effectiveness of albuterol was demonstrated over a 13-week period in these same trials.

In controlled clinical trials involving children 4 to 12 years of age, FEV_1 measurements showed that maximum improvement in pulmonary function occurs within 30 to 60 minutes. The onset of clinically significant (≥15%) improvement in FEV_1 was observed as soon as 5 minutes following 180 mcg of albuterol in 18 of 30 (60%) children in a controlled dose-ranging study. Clinically significant improvement in FEV_1 continued in the majority of patients for 2 hours and in 33% to 47% for 4 hours among 56 patients receiving inhalation aerosol in one pediatric study. In a second study among 48 patients receiving inhalation aerosol, clinically significant improvement continued in the majority for up to 1 hour and in 23% to 40% for 4 hours. In addition, at least 50% of the patients in both studies achieved an improvement in $FEF_{25\%-75\%}$ (forced expiratory flow rate between 25% and 75% of the forced vital capacity) of at least 20% for 2 to 5 hours. Continued effectiveness of albuterol was demonstrated over the 12-week study period.

In other clinical studies in adults and children, two inhalations of VENTOLIN Inhalation Aerosol taken approximately 15 minutes before exercise prevented exercise-induced bronchospasm, as demonstrated by the maintenance of FEV_1 within 80% of baseline values in the majority of patients. One study in adults also evaluated the duration of the prophylactic effect to repeated exercise challenges, which was evident at 4 hours in the majority of patients and at 6 hours in approximately one third of the patients.

INDICATIONS AND USAGE

VENTOLIN Inhalation Aerosol is indicated for the prevention and relief of bronchospasm in patients 4 years of age and older with reversible obstructive airway disease and for the prevention of exercise-induced bronchospasm in patients 4 years of age and older.

VENTOLIN Inhalation Aerosol can be used with or without concomitant steroid therapy.

CONTRAINDICATIONS

VENTOLIN Inhalation Aerosol is contraindicated in patients with a history of hypersensitivity to albuterol or any of its components.

WARNINGS

Paradoxical Bronchospasm: VENTOLIN Inhalation Aerosol can produce paradoxical bronchospasm, which may be life threatening. If paradoxical bronchospasm occurs, VENTOLIN Inhalation Aerosol should be discontinued immediately and alternative therapy instituted. It should be recognized that paradoxical bronchospasm, when associated with inhaled formulations, frequently occurs with the first use of a new canister or vial.

Cardiovascular Effects: VENTOLIN Inhalation Aerosol, like all other beta-adrenergic agonists, can produce a clinically significant cardiovascular effect in some patients as measured by pulse rate, blood pressure, and/or symptoms. Although such effects are uncommon after administration of VENTOLIN Inhalation Aerosol at recommended doses, if they occur, the drug may need to be discontinued. In addition, beta-agonists have been reported to produce electrocardiogram (ECG) changes, such as flattening of the T wave, prolongation of the QT_c interval, and ST segment depression. The clinical significance of these findings is unknown. Therefore, VENTOLIN Inhalation Aerosol, like all sympathomimetic amines, should be used with caution in patients with cardiovascular disorders, especially coronary insufficiency, cardiac arrhythmias, and hypertension.

Deterioration of Asthma: Asthma may deteriorate acutely over a period of hours or chronically over several days or longer. If the patient needs more doses of VENTOLIN Inhalation Aerosol than usual, this may be a marker of destabilization of asthma and requires reevaluation of the patient

and treatment regimen, giving special consideration to the possible need for anti-inflammatory treatment, e.g., corticosteroids.

Use of Anti-Inflammatory Agents: The use of beta-adrenergic agonist bronchodilators alone may not be adequate to control asthma in many patients. Early consideration should be given to adding anti-inflammatory agents, e.g., corticosteroids.

Immediate Hypersensitivity Reactions: Immediate hypersensitivity reactions may occur after administration of albuterol inhalation aerosol, as demonstrated by rare cases of urticaria, angioedema, rash, bronchospasm, anaphylaxis, and oropharyngeal edema.

The contents of VENTOLIN Inhalation Aerosol are under pressure. Do not puncture. Do not use or store near heat or open flame. Exposure to temperatures above 120°F may cause bursting. Never throw container into fire or incinerator. Keep out of reach of children.

PRECAUTIONS

General: Albuterol, as with all sympathomimetic amines, should be used with caution in patients with cardiovascular disorders, especially coronary insufficiency, cardiac arrhythmias, and hypertension; in patients with convulsive disorders, hyperthyroidism, or diabetes mellitus; and in patients who are unusually responsive to sympathomimetic amines. Clinically significant changes in systolic and diastolic blood pressure have been seen in individual patients and could be expected to occur in some patients after use of any beta-adrenergic bronchodilator.

Large doses of intravenous albuterol have been reported to aggravate preexisting diabetes mellitus and ketoacidosis. As with other beta-agonists, albuterol may produce significant hypokalemia in some patients, possibly through intracellular shunting, which has the potential to produce adverse cardiovascular effects. The decrease is usually transient, not requiring supplementation.

Although there have been no reports concerning the use of VENTOLIN Inhalation Aerosol during labor and delivery, it has been reported that high doses of albuterol administered intravenously inhibit uterine contractions. Although this effect is extremely unlikely as a consequence of aerosol use, it should be kept in mind.

Information for Patients: The action of VENTOLIN Inhalation Aerosol may last up to 6 hours or longer. VENTOLIN Inhalation Aerosol should not be used more frequently than recommended. Do not increase the dose or frequency of VENTOLIN Inhalation Aerosol without consulting your physician. If you find that treatment with VENTOLIN Inhalation Aerosol becomes less effective for symptomatic relief, your symptoms become worse, and/or you need to use the product more frequently than usual, you should seek medical attention immediately. While you are using VENTOLIN Inhalation Aerosol, other inhaled drugs and asthma medications should be taken only as directed by your physician. Common adverse effects include palpitations, chest pain, rapid heart rate, and tremor or nervousness. If you are pregnant or nursing, contact your physician about use of VENTOLIN Inhalation Aerosol. Effective and safe use of VENTOLIN Inhalation Aerosol includes an understanding of the way that it should be administered.

In general, the technique for administering VENTOLIN Inhalation Aerosol to children is similar to that for adults, since children's smaller ventilatory exchange capacity automatically provides proportionally smaller aerosol intake. Children should use VENTOLIN Inhalation Aerosol under adult supervision, as instructed by the patient's physician. See illustrated Patient's Instructions for Use section of the full prescribing information.

Drug Interactions: Other short-acting sympathomimetic aerosol bronchodilators should not be used concomitantly with albuterol. If additional adrenergic drugs are to be administered by any route, they should be used with caution to avoid deleterious cardiovascular effects.

Monoamine Oxidase Inhibitors or Tricyclic Antidepressants: Albuterol should be administered with extreme caution to patients being treated with monoamine oxidase inhibitors or tricyclic antidepressants, or within 2 weeks of discontinuation of such agents, because the action of albuterol on the vascular system may be potentiated.

Beta-Blockers: Beta-adrenergic receptor blocking agents not only block the pulmonary effect of beta-agonists, such as VENTOLIN Inhalation Aerosol, but may produce severe bronchospasm in asthmatic patients. Therefore, patients with asthma should not normally be treated with beta-blockers. However, under certain circumstances, e.g., as prophylaxis after myocardial infarction, there may be no acceptable alternatives to the use of beta-adrenergic blocking agents in patients with asthma. In this setting, cardioselective beta-blockers should be considered, although they should be administered with caution.

Diuretics: The ECG changes and/or hypokalemia that may result from the administration of nonpotassium-sparing diuretics (such as loop or thiazide diuretics) can be acutely worsened by beta-agonists, especially when the recommended dose of the beta-agonist is exceeded. Although the

clinical significance of these effects is not known, caution is advised in the coadministration of beta-agonists with nonpotassium-sparing diuretics.

Digoxin: Mean decreases of 16% to 22% in serum digoxin levels were demonstrated after single-dose intravenous and oral administration of albuterol, respectively, to normal volunteers who had received digoxin for 10 days. The clinical significance of these findings for patients with obstructive airway disease who are receiving albuterol and digoxin on a chronic basis is unclear. Nevertheless, it would be prudent to carefully evaluate the serum digoxin levels in patients who are currently receiving digoxin and albuterol.

Carcinogenesis, Mutagenesis, Impairment of Fertility: In a 2-year study in Sprague-Dawley rats, albuterol sulfate caused a significant dose-related increase in the incidence of benign leiomyomas of the mesovarium at dietary doses of 2.0, 10, and 50 mg/kg (approximately 15, 70, and 340 times, respectively, the maximum recommended daily inhalation dose for adults on a mg/m^2 basis or approximately 6, 30, and 160 times, respectively, the maximum recommended daily inhalation dose for children on a mg/m^2 basis). In another study this effect was blocked by the coadministration of propranolol, a non-selective beta-adrenergic antagonist. In an 18-month study in CD-1 mice, albuterol sulfate showed no evidence of tumorigenicity at dietary doses up to 500 mg/kg (approximately 1700 times the maximum recommended daily inhalation dose for adults on a mg/m^2 basis or approximately 800 times the maximum recommended daily inhalation dose for children on a mg/m^2 basis). In a 22-month study in the Golden hamster albuterol sulfate showed no evidence of tumorigenicity at dietary doses up to 50 mg/kg (approximately 225 times the maximum recommended daily inhalation dose for adults on a mg/m^2 basis or approximately 110 times the maximum recommended daily inhalation dose for children on a mg/m^2 basis).

Albuterol sulfate was not mutagenic in the Ames test with or without metabolic activation using tester strains *S. typhimurium* TA1537, TA1538, and TA98 or *E. coli* WP2, WP2uvrA, and WP67. No forward mutation was seen in yeast strain *S. cerevisiae* S9 nor any mitotic gene conversion in yeast strain *S. cerevisiae* JD1 with or without metabolic activation. Fluctuation assays in *S. typhimurium* TA98 and *E. coli* WP2, both with metabolic activation, were negative. Albuterol sulfate was not clastogenic in a human peripheral lymphocyte assay or in an AH1 strain mouse micronucleus assay at intraperitoneal doses of up to 200 mg/kg.

Reproduction studies in rats demonstrated no evidence of impaired fertility at oral doses up to 50 mg/kg (approximately 340 times the maximum recommended daily inhalation dose for adults on a mg/m^2 basis).

Pregnancy: *Teratogenic Effects:* Pregnancy Category C. Albuterol sulfate has been shown to be teratogenic in mice. A study in CD-1 mice at subcutaneous doses of 0.025, 0.25, and 2.5 mg/kg (approximately 2/25, 1.0, and 8.0 times, respectively, the maximum recommended daily inhalation dose for adults on a mg/m^2 basis), showed cleft palate formation in 5 of 111 (4.5%) fetuses at 0.25 mg/kg and in 10 of 108 (9.3%) fetuses at 2.5 mg/kg. The drug did not induce cleft palate formation at the lowest dose, 0.025 mg/kg. Cleft palate also occurred in 22 of 72 (30.5%) fetuses from females treated with 2.5 mg/kg of isoproterenol (positive control) subcutaneously (approximately 8 times the maximum recommended daily inhalation dose for adults on a mg/m^2 basis).

A reproduction study in Stride Dutch rabbits revealed cranioschisis in 7 of 19 fetuses (37%) fetuses when albuterol sulfate was administered orally at a 50 mg/kg dose (approximately 680 times the maximum recommended daily inhalation dose for adults on a mg/m^2 basis).

There are no adequate and well-controlled studies in pregnant women. Albuterol should be used during pregnancy only if the potential benefit justifies the potential risk to the fetus.

During worldwide marketing experience, various congenital anomalies, including cleft palate and limb defects, have been rarely reported in the offspring of patients being treated with albuterol. Some of the mothers were taking multiple medications during their pregnancies. No consistent pattern of defects can be discerned, and a relationship between albuterol use and congenital anomalies has not been established.

Use in Labor and Delivery: Because of the potential for beta-agonist interference with uterine contractility, use of VENTOLIN Inhalation Aerosol for relief of bronchospasm during labor should be restricted to those patients in whom the benefits clearly outweigh the risk.

Tocolysis: Albuterol has not been approved for the management of preterm labor. The benefit:risk ratio when albuterol is administered for tocolysis has not been established. Serious adverse reactions, including maternal pulmonary edema, have been reported during or following treatment of premature labor with beta$_2$-agonists, including albuterol.

Nursing Mothers: It is not known whether this drug is excreted in human milk. Because of the potential for tumorigenicity shown for albuterol in some animal studies, a deci-

sion should be made whether to discontinue nursing or to discontinue the drug, taking into account the importance of the drug to the mother.

Pediatric Use: Safety and effectiveness in children below 4 years of age have not been established.

ADVERSE REACTIONS

The adverse reactions to albuterol are similar in nature to reactions to other sympathomimetic agents, although the incidence of certain cardiovascular effects is lower with albuterol.

Percent Incidence of Adverse Reactions in Patients ≥12 Years of Age in a 13-Week Clinical Trial*

Reaction	Percent Incidence	
	Albuterol	Isoproterenol
Tremor	<15%	<15%
Nausea	<15%	<15%
Tachycardia	10%	10%
Palpitations	<10%	<15%
Nervousness	<10%	<15%
Increased blood pressure	<5%	<5%
Dizziness	<5%	<5%
Heartburn	<5%	<5%

* A 13-week double-blind study compared albuterol and isoproterenol inhalation aerosols in 147 asthmatic patients.

Percent Incidence of Adverse Reactions in Children 4 to 11 Years of Age in a 12-Week Trial*

Reaction	Percent Incidence
Central nervous system	
Headache	3%
Nervousness	1%
Lightheadedness	<1%
Tremor	<1%
Agitation	1%
Nightmares	1%
Hyperactivity	1%
Aggressive behavior	1%
Gastrointestinal	
Nausea and/or vomiting	6%
Stomachache	3%
Diarrhea	1%
Oropharyngeal	
Throat irritation	6%
Discoloration of teeth	1%
Respiratory	
Epistaxis	3%
Cough	2%
Musculoskeletal	
Muscle cramp	1%

* A 12-week double-blind trial in 104 patients aged 4 to 11 years.

Cases of urticaria, angioedema, rash, bronchospasm, hoarseness, oropharyngeal edema, and arrhythmias (including atrial fibrillation, supraventricular tachycardia, extrasystoles) have been reported after the use of VENTOLIN Inhalation Aerosol.

In addition, albuterol, like other sympathomimetic agents, can cause adverse reactions such as hypertension, angina, vertigo, central nervous system stimulation, sleeplessness, and unusual taste.

OVERDOSAGE

The expected symptoms with overdosage are those of excessive beta-adrenergic stimulation and/or occurrence or exaggeration of any of the symptoms listed under ADVERSE REACTIONS, e.g., seizures, angina, hypertension or hypotension, tachycardia with rates up to 200 beats/min, ar-

Continued on next page

This product information is based on labeling in effect on June 1, 1998. For further information, contact via direct mail, phone, or web site Medical Information: Glaxo Wellcome Inc., PO Box 13398, Research Triangle Park, NC 27709. Healthcare Professionals (Medical Information): 800-334-0089 Patients (Customer Response Center): 888-TALK2GW (1-888-825-5249) Glaxo Wellcome Corporate Web Site: www.glaxowellcome.com

Ventolin Inh. Aero.—Cont.

rhythmias, nervousness, headache, tremor, dry mouth, palpitation, nausea, dizziness, fatigue, malaise, and sleeplessness. Hypokalemia may also occur.

As with all sympathomimetic aerosol medications, cardiac arrest and even death may be associated with abuse of VENTOLIN Inhalation Aerosol. Treatment consists of discontinuation of VENTOLIN Inhalation Aerosol together with appropriate symptomatic therapy. The judicious use of a cardioselective beta-receptor blocker may be considered, bearing in mind that such medication can produce bronchospasm. There is insufficient evidence to determine if dialysis is beneficial for overdosage of VENTOLIN Inhalation Aerosol.

The oral median lethal dose of albuterol sulfate in mice is greater than 2000 mg/kg (approximately 6800 times the maximum recommended daily inhalation dose for adults on a mg/m^2 basis, or, approximately 3200 times the maximum recommended daily inhalation dose for children on a mg/m^2 basis). In mature rats, the subcutaneous median lethal dose of albuterol sulfate is approximately 450 mg/kg (approximately 3000 times the maximum recommended daily inhalation dose for adults on a mg/m^2 basis or approximately 1400 times the maximum recommended daily inhalation dose for children on a mg/m^2 basis). In small young rats, the subcutaneous median lethal dose is approximately 2000 mg/kg (approximately 14 000 times the maximum recommended daily inhalation dose for adults on a mg/m^2 basis or approximately 6400 times the maximum recommended daily inhalation dose for children on a mg/m^2 basis). The inhalation median lethal dose has not been determined in animals.

DOSAGE AND ADMINISTRATION

For treatment of acute episodes of bronchospasm or prevention of asthmatic symptoms, the usual dosage for adults and children 4 years of age and older is two inhalations repeated every 4 to 6 hours; in some patients, one inhalation every 4 hours may be sufficient. More frequent administration or a larger number of inhalations are not recommended. It is recommended to "test spray" VENTOLIN Inhalation Aerosol into the air before using for the first time and in cases where the aerosol has not been used for a prolonged period of time.

The use of VENTOLIN Inhalation Aerosol can be continued as medically indicated to control recurring bouts of bronchospasm. During this time most patients gain optimal benefit from regular use of the inhaler. Safe usage for periods extending over several years has been documented.

If a previously effective dosage regimen fails to provide the usual response, this may be a marker of destabilization of asthma and requires reevaluation of the patient and the treatment regimen, giving special consideration to the possible need for anti-inflammatory treatment, e.g., corticosteroids.

Exercise-Induced Bronchospasm Prevention: The usual dosage for adults and children 4 years and older is two inhalations 15 minutes before exercise.

For treatment, see above.

HOW SUPPLIED

VENTOLIN Inhalation Aerosol is supplied in 6.8-g canisters containing 80 metered inhalations (NDC 0173-0463-00) and in 17-g canisters containing 200 metered inhalations (NDC 0173-0321-88), each in boxes of one. Each actuation delivers 100 mcg of albuterol from the valve and 90 mcg of albuterol from the mouthpiece. Each canister is supplied with a blue oral adapter and patient's instructions. Also available, VENTOLIN Inhalation Aerosol Refill 17-g canister only with patient's instructions (NDC 0173-0321-98).

The blue adapter supplied with VENTOLIN Inhalation Aerosol should not be used with any other product canisters, and adapters from other products should not be used with a VENTOLIN Inhalation Aerosol canister. The correct amount of medication in each canister cannot be assured after 80 actuations from the 6.8-g canister and 200 actuations from the 17.0-g canister, even though the canister is not completely empty. The canister should be discarded when the labeled number of actuations have been used. Store between 15° and 30°C (59° and 86°F). As with most inhaled medications in aerosol canisters, the therapeutic effect of this medication may decrease when the canister is cold; for best results, the canister should be at room temperature before use. Shake well before using.

May 1998/RL-569
Shown in Product Identification Guide, page 314

VENTOLIN®　　　　　　　　　　　　　　　　℞
(albuterol sulfate, USP)
Inhalation Solution, 0.5%*
*Potency expressed as albuterol.

DESCRIPTION

The active component of VENTOLIN Inhalation Solution is albuterol sulfate, USP, the racemic form of albuterol and a

relatively selective beta₂-adrenergic bronchodilator (see CLINICAL PHARMACOLOGY). It has the chemical name α^1-[(tert-butylamino)methyl]-4-hydroxy-m-xylene-α, α′-diol sulfate (2:1)(salt).

Albuterol sulfate has a molecular weight of 576.7, and the empirical formula is $(C_{13}H_{21}NO_3)_2 \cdot H_2SO_4$. Albuterol sulfate is a white crystalline powder, soluble in water and slightly soluble in ethanol.

The World Health Organization recommended name for albuterol base is salbutamol.

VENTOLIN Inhalation Solution, 0.5% is in concentrated form. Dilute the appropriate volume of the solution (see DOSAGE AND ADMINISTRATION) with sterile normal saline solution to a total volume of 3 mL and administer by nebulization.

Each milliliter of VENTOLIN Inhalation Solution contains 5 mg of albuterol (as 6 mg of albuterol sulfate) in an aqueous solution containing benzalkonium chloride; sulfuric acid is used to adjust the pH to between 3 and 5. VENTOLIN Inhalation Solution contains no sulfiting agents. It is supplied in a 20-mL amber glass bottle.

VENTOLIN Inhalation Solution is a clear, colorless to light yellow solution.

CLINICAL PHARMACOLOGY

In vitro studies and in vivo pharmacologic studies have demonstrated that albuterol has a preferential effect on beta₂-adrenergic receptors compared with isoproterenol. While it is recognized that beta₂-adrenergic receptors are the predominant receptors in bronchial smooth muscle, data indicate that there is a population of beta₂-receptors in the human heart existing in a concentration between 10% and 50%. The precise function of these receptors has not been established (see WARNINGS).

The pharmacologic effects of beta-adrenergic agonist drugs, including albuterol, are at least in part attributable to stimulation through beta-adrenergic receptors of intracellular adenyl cyclase, the enzyme that catalyzes the conversion of adenosine triphosphate (ATP) to cyclic-3′,5′-adenosine monophosphate (cyclic AMP). Increased cyclic AMP levels are associated with relaxation of bronchial smooth muscle and inhibition of release of mediators of immediate hypersensitivity from cells, especially from mast cells.

Albuterol has been shown in most controlled clinical trials to have more effect on the respiratory tract, in the form of bronchial smooth muscle relaxation, than isoproterenol at comparable doses while producing fewer cardiovascular effects.

Controlled clinical studies and other clinical experience have shown that inhaled albuterol, like other beta-adrenergic agonist drugs, can produce a significant cardiovascular effect in some patients, as measured by pulse rate, blood pressure, symptoms, and/or electrocardiographic changes. Albuterol is longer acting than isoproterenol in most patients by any route of administration because it is not a substrate for the cellular uptake processes for catecholamines nor for catechol-O-methyl transferase.

Pharmacokinetics: Studies in asthmatic patients have shown that less than 20% of a single albuterol dose was absorbed following either intermittent positive-pressure breathing (IPPB) or nebulizer administration; the remaining amount was recovered from the nebulizer and apparatus and expired air. Most of the absorbed dose was recovered in the urine within 24 hours after drug administration. Following a 3-mg dose of nebulized albuterol in adults, the maximum albuterol plasma levels at 0.5 hours were 2.1 ng/mL (range, 1.4 to 3.2 ng/mL). There was a significant dose-related response in FEV₁ (forced expiratory volume in 1 second) and peak flow rate. It has been demonstrated that following oral administration of 4 mg of albuterol, the elimination half-life was 5 to 6 hours.

Preclinical: Intravenous studies in rats with albuterol sulfate have demonstrated that albuterol crosses the blood-brain barrier and reaches brain concentrations amounting to approximately 5.0% of the plasma concentrations. In structures outside the brain barrier (pineal and pituitary glands), albuterol concentrations were found to be 100 times those in the whole brain.

Studies in laboratory animals (minipigs, rodents, and dogs) have demonstrated the occurrence of cardiac arrhythmias and sudden death (with histologic evidence of myocardial necrosis) when beta-agonists and methylxanthines are administered concurrently. The clinical significance of these findings is unknown.

Clinical Trials: In controlled clinical trials in adults, most patients exhibited an onset of improvement in pulmonary function within 5 minutes as determined by FEV₁. FEV₁ measurements also showed that the maximum average improvement in pulmonary function usually occurred at approximately 1 hour following inhalation of 2.5 mg of albuterol by compressor-nebulizer and remained close to peak for 2 hours. Clinically significant improvement in pulmonary function (defined as maintenance of a 15% or more increase in FEV₁ over baseline values) continued for 3 to 4 hours in most patients, with some patients continuing up to 6 hours.

Published reports of trials in asthmatic children aged 3 years or older have demonstrated significant improvement in either FEV₁ or PEFR within 2 to 20 minutes following single doses of albuterol inhalation solution. An increase of 15% or more in baseline FEV₁ has been observed in children aged 5 to 11 years up to 6 hours after treatment with doses of 0.10 mg/kg or higher of albuterol inhalation solution. Single doses of 3, 4, or 10 mg resulted in improvement in baseline PEFR that was comparable in extent and duration to a 2-mg dose, but doses above 3 mg were associated with heart rate increases of more than 10%.

INDICATIONS AND USAGE

VENTOLIN Inhalation Solution is indicated for the relief of bronchospasm in patients 2 years of age and older with reversible obstructive airway disease and acute attacks of bronchospasm.

CONTRAINDICATIONS

VENTOLIN Inhalation Solution is contraindicated in patients with a history of hypersensitivity to albuterol or any of its components.

WARNINGS

Paradoxical Bronchospasm: VENTOLIN Inhalation Solution can produce paradoxical bronchospasm, which may be life threatening. If paradoxical bronchospasm occurs, VENTOLIN Inhalation Solution should be discontinued immediately and alternative therapy instituted. It should be recognized that paradoxical bronchospasm, when associated with inhaled formulations, frequently occurs with the first use of a new canister or vial.

Fatalities have been reported in association with excessive use of inhaled sympathomimetic drugs and with the home use of nebulizers. It is therefore essential that the physician instruct the patient in the need for further evaluation if his/her asthma becomes worse.

Cardiovascular Effects: VENTOLIN Inhalation Solution, like all other beta-adrenergic agonists, can produce a clinically significant cardiovascular effect in some patients as measured by pulse rate, blood pressure, and/or symptoms. Although such effects are uncommon after administration of VENTOLIN Inhalation Solution at recommended doses, if they occur, the drug may need to be discontinued. In addition, beta-agonists have been reported to produce electrocardiogram (ECG) changes, such as flattening of the T wave, prolongation of the QT$_c$ interval, and ST segment depression. The clinical significance of these findings is unknown. Therefore, VENTOLIN Inhalation Solution, like all sympathomimetic amines, should be used with caution in patients with cardiovascular disorders, especially coronary insufficiency, cardiac arrhythmias, and hypertension.

Deterioration of Asthma: Asthma may deteriorate acutely over a period of hours or chronically over several days or longer. If the patient needs more doses of VENTOLIN Inhalation Solution than usual, this may be a marker of destabilization of asthma and requires reevaluation of the patient and treatment regimen, giving special consideration to the possible need for anti-inflammatory treatment, e.g., corticosteroids.

Immediate Hypersensitivity Reactions: Immediate hypersensitivity reactions may occur after administration of albuterol, as demonstrated by rare cases of urticaria, angioedema, rash, bronchospasm, and oropharyngeal edema.

Use of Anti-Inflammatory Agents: The use of beta-adrenergic agonist bronchodilators alone may not be adequate to control asthma in many patients. Early consideration should be given to adding anti-inflammatory agents, e.g., corticosteroids.

Microbial Contamination: To avoid microbial contamination, proper aseptic technique should be used each time the bottle is opened. Precautions should be taken to prevent contact of the dropper tip of the bottle with any surface, including the nebulizer reservoir and associated ventilatory equipment. In addition, if the solution changes color or becomes cloudy, it should not be used.

PRECAUTIONS

General: Albuterol, as with all sympathomimetic amines, should be used with caution in patients with cardiovascular disorders, especially coronary insufficiency, hypertension, and cardiac arrhythmia; in patients with convulsive disorders, hyperthyroidism, or diabetes mellitus; and in patients who are unusually responsive to sympathomimetic amines. Clinically significant changes in systolic and diastolic blood pressure have been seen in individual patients and could be expected to occur in some patients after use of any beta-adrenergic bronchodilator.

Large doses of intravenous albuterol have been reported to aggravate preexisting diabetes mellitus and ketoacidosis. As with other beta-agonists, albuterol may produce significant hypokalemia in some patients, possibly through intracellular shunting, which has the potential to produce adverse cardiovascular effects. The decrease is usually transient, not requiring supplementation.

Repeated dosing with 0.15 mg/kg of albuterol inhalation solution in children aged 5 to 17 years who were initially normokalemic has been associated with an asymptomatic decline of 20% to 25% in serum potassium levels.

Approximate Weight (kg)	Approximate Weight (lb)	Dose (mg)	Volume of Inhalation Solution
10–15	22–33	1.25	0.25 mL
>15	>33	2.5	0.5 mL

Information for Patients: The action of VENTOLIN Inhalation Solution may last up to 6 hours or longer. VENTOLIN Inhalation Solution should not be used more frequently than recommended. Do not increase the dose or frequency of VENTOLIN Inhalation Solution without consulting your physician. If you find that treatment with VENTOLIN Inhalation Solution becomes less effective for symptomatic relief, your symptoms become worse, and/or you need to use the product more frequently than usual, you should seek medical attention immediately. While you are using VENTOLIN Inhalation Solution, other inhaled drugs and asthma medications should be taken only as directed by your physician. Common adverse effects include palpitations, chest pain, rapid heart rate, and tremor or nervousness. If you are pregnant or nursing, contact your physician about use of VENTOLIN Inhalation Solution. Effective and safe use of VENTOLIN Inhalation Solution includes an understanding of the way that it should be administered.

To avoid microbial contamination, proper aseptic techniques should be used each time the bottle is opened. Precautions should be taken to prevent contact of the dropper tip of the bottle with any surface, including the nebulizer reservoir and associated ventilatory equipment. In addition, if the solution changes color or becomes cloudy, it should not be used.

Drug compatibility (physical and chemical), efficacy, and safety of VENTOLIN Inhalation Solution when mixed with other drugs in a nebulizer have not been established.

See illustrated Patient's Instructions for Use section of the full prescribing information.

Drug Interactions: Other short-acting sympathomimetic aerosol bronchodilators or epinephrine should not be used concomitantly with albuterol. If additional adrenergic drugs are to be administered by any route, they should be used with caution to avoid deleterious cardiovascular effects.

Monoamine Oxidase Inhibitors or Tricyclic Antidepressants: Albuterol should be administered with extreme caution to patients being treated with monoamine oxidase inhibitors or tricyclic antidepressants, or within 2 weeks of discontinuation of such agents, because the action of albuterol on the vascular system may be potentiated.

Beta-Blockers: Beta-adrenergic receptor blocking agents not only block the pulmonary effect of beta-agonists, such as VENTOLIN Inhalation Solution, but may produce severe bronchospasm in asthmatic patients. Therefore, patients with asthma should not normally be treated with beta-blockers. However, under certain circumstances, e.g., as prophylaxis after myocardial infarction, there may be no acceptable alternatives to the use of beta-adrenergic blocking agents in patients with asthma. In this setting, cardioselective beta-blockers could be considered, although they should be administered with caution.

Diuretics: The ECG changes and/or hypokalemia that may result from the administration of nonpotassium-sparing diuretics (such as loop or thiazide diuretics) can be acutely worsened by beta-agonists, especially when the recommended dose of the beta-agonist is exceeded. Although the clinical significance of these effects is not known, caution is advised in the coadministration of beta-agonists with nonpotassium-sparing diuretics.

Digoxin: Mean decreases of 16% to 22% in serum digoxin levels were demonstrated after single-dose intravenous and oral administration of albuterol, respectively, to normal volunteers who had received digoxin for 10 days. The clinical significance of these findings for patients with obstructive airway disease who are receiving albuterol and digoxin on a chronic basis is unclear. Nevertheless, it would be prudent to carefully evaluate the serum digoxin levels in patients who are currently receiving digoxin and albuterol.

Carcinogenesis, Mutagenesis, Impairment of Fertility: In a 2-year study in Sprague-Dawley rats, albuterol sulfate caused a significant dose-related increase in the incidence of benign leiomyomas of the mesovarium at dietary doses of 2.0, 10, and 50 mg/kg (approximately 2, 8, and 40 times, respectively, the maximum recommended daily inhalation dose for adults on a mg/m^2 basis or approximately 3/5, 3, and 15 times, respectively, the maximum recommended daily inhalation dose in children on a mg/m^2 basis). In another study this effect was blocked by the coadministration of propranolol, a non-selective beta-adrenergic antagonist. In an 18-month study in CD-1 mice, albuterol sulfate showed no evidence of tumorigenicity at dietary doses of up to 500 mg/kg (approximately 200 times the maximum recommended daily inhalation dose for adults on a mg/m^2 basis or approximately 75 times the maximum recommended daily inhalation dose for children on a mg/m^2 basis). In a 22-month study in the Golden hamster, albuterol sulfate showed no evidence of tumorigenicity at dietary doses of up to 50 mg/kg (approximately 25 times the maximum recommended daily inhalation dose for adults on a mg/m^2 basis or approximately 10 times the maximum recommended daily inhalation dose for children on a mg/m^2 basis).

Albuterol sulfate was not mutagenic in the Ames test with or without metabolic activation using tester strains *S. typhimurium* TA1537, TA1538, and TA98 or *E. coli* WP2, WP2uvrA, and WP67. No forward mutation was seen in yeast strain *S. cerevisiae* S9 nor any mitotic gene conversion in yeast strain *S. cerevisiae* JD1 with or without metabolic activation. Fluctuation assays in *S. typhimurium* TA98 and *E. coli* WP2, both with metabolic activation, were negative. Albuterol sulfate was not clastogenic in a human peripheral lymphocyte assay or in an AH1 strain mouse micronucleus assay at intraperitoneal doses of up to 200 mg/kg.

Reproduction studies in rats demonstrated no evidence of impaired fertility at oral doses up to 50 mg/kg (approximately 40 times the maximum recommended daily inhalation dose for adults on a mg/m^2 basis).

Pregnancy: *Teratogenic Effects:* Pregnancy Category C. Albuterol has been shown to be teratogenic in mice. A study in CD-1 mice at subcutaneous doses of 0.025, 0.25, and 2.5 mg/kg (approximately 1/100, 1/10, and 1.0 times, respectively, the maximum recommended daily inhalation dose for adults on a mg/m^2 basis) showed cleft palate formation in 5 of 111 (4.5%) fetuses at 0.25 mg/kg and in 10 of 108 (9.3%) fetuses at 2.5 mg/kg. The drug did not induce cleft palate formation at the lowest dose, 0.025 mg/kg. Cleft palate also occurred in 22 of 72 (30.5%) fetuses from females treated with 2.5 mg/kg of isoproterenol (positive control) subcutaneously (aproximately 1.0 time the maximum recommended daily inhalation dose for adults on a mg/m^2 basis).

A reproduction study in Stride Dutch rabbits revealed cranioschisis in 7 of 19 (37%) fetuses when albuterol was administered orally at a 50-mg/kg dose (approximately 80 times the maximum recommended daily inhalation dose for adults on a mg/m^2 basis).

There are no adequate and well-controlled studies in pregnant women. Albuterol should be used during pregnancy only if the potential benefit justifies the potential risk to the fetus.

During worldwide marketing experience, various congenital anomalies, including cleft palate and limb defects, have been rarely reported in the offspring of patients being treated with albuterol. Some of the mothers were taking multiple medications during their pregnancies. No consistent pattern of defects can be discerned, and a relationship between albuterol use and congenital anomalies has not been established.

Use in Labor and Delivery: Because of the potential for beta-agonist interference with uterine contractility, use of VENTOLIN Inhalation Solution for relief of bronchospasm during labor should be restricted to those patients in whom the benefits clearly outweigh the risk.

Tocolysis: Albuterol has not been approved for the management of preterm labor. The benefit:risk ratio when albuterol is administered for tocolysis has not been established. Serious adverse reactions, including maternal pulmonary edema, have been reported during or following treatment of premature labor with beta$_2$-agonists, including albuterol.

Nursing Mothers: It is not known whether this drug is excreted in human milk. Because of the potential for tumorigenicity shown for albuterol in some animal studies, a decision should be made whether to discontinue nursing or to discontinue the drug, taking into account the importance of the drug to the mother.

Pediatric Use: The safety and effectiveness of VENTOLIN Inhalation Solution have been established in children 2 years of age or older. Use of VENTOLIN Inhalation Solution in these age-groups is supported by evidence from adequate and well-controlled studies of VENTOLIN Inhalation Solution in adults; the likelihood that the disease course, pathophysiology, and the drug's effect in pediatric and adult patients are substantially similar; and published reports of trials in pediatric patients 3 years of age or older. The recommended dose for the pediatric population is based upon three published dose comparison studies of efficacy and safety in children 5 to 17 years, and on the safety profile in both adults and pediatric patients at doses equal to or higher than the recommended doses. The safety and effectiveness of VENTOLIN Inhalation Solution in children below 2 years of age have not been established.

ADVERSE REACTIONS

The results of clinical trials with VENTOLIN Inhalation Solution in 135 patients showed the following side effects that were considered probably or possibly drug related:

Percent Incidence of Adverse Reactions

Reaction	Percent Incidence n = 135
Central nervous system	
Tremors	20%
Dizziness	7%
Nervousness	4%
Headache	3%
Sleeplessness	1%
Gastrointestinal	
Nausea	4%
Dyspepsia	1%
Ear, nose, and throat	
Nasal congestion	1%
Pharyngitis	<1%
Cardiovascular	
Tachycardia	1%
Hypertension	1%
Respiratory	
Bronchospasm	8%
Cough	4%
Bronchitis	4%
Wheezing	1%

No clinically relevant laboratory abnormalities related to VENTOLIN Inhalation Solution administration were determined in these studies.

Cases of urticaria, angioedema, rash, bronchospasm, hoarseness, oropharyngeal edema, and arrhythmias (including atrial fibrillation, supraventricular tachycardia, extrasystoles) have been reported after the use of VENTOLIN Inhalation Solution.

OVERDOSAGE

The expected symptoms with overdosage are those of excessive beta-adrenergic stimulation and/or occurrence or exaggeration of any of the symptoms listed under ADVERSE REACTIONS, e.g., seizures, angina, hypertension or hypotension, tachycardia with rates up to 200 beats/min, arrhythmias, nervousness, headache, tremor, dry mouth, palpitation, nausea, dizziness, fatigue, malaise, and sleeplessness. Hypokalemia may also occur. In isolated cases in children 2 to 12 years of age, tachycardia with rates >200 beats/min has been observed.

As with all sympathomimetic medications, cardiac arrest and even death may be associated with abuse of VENTOLIN Inhalation Solution. Treatment consists of discontinuation of VENTOLIN Inhalation Solution together with appropriate symptomatic therapy. The judicious use of a cardioselective beta-receptor blocker may be considered, bearing in mind that such medication can produce bronchospasm. There is insufficient evidence to determine if dialysis is beneficial for overdosage of VENTOLIN Inhalation Solution.

The oral median lethal dose of albuterol sulfate in mice is greater than 2000 mg/kg (approximately 810 times the maximum recommended daily inhalation dose for adults on a mg/m^2 basis or approximately 300 times the maximum recommended daily dose for children on a mg/m^2 basis). In mature rats, the subcutaneous median lethal dose of albuterol sulfate is approximately 450 mg/kg (approximately 365 times the maximum recommended daily inhalation dose for adults on a mg/m^2 basis or approximately 135 times the maximum recommended daily inhalation dose for children on a mg/m^2 basis). In small young rats, the subcutaneous median lethal dose is approximately 2000 mg/kg (approximately 1600 times the maximum recommended daily inhalation dose for adults on a mg/m^2 basis or approximately 600 times the maximum recommended daily inhalation dose for children on a mg/m^2 basis). The inhalational median lethal dose has not been determined in animals.

DOSAGE AND ADMINISTRATION

To avoid microbial contamination, proper aseptic techniques should be used each time the bottle is opened. Precautions should be taken to prevent contact of the dropper tip of the bottle with any surface, including the nebulizer reservoir

Continued on next page

This product information is based on labeling in effect on June 1, 1998. For further information, contact via direct mail, phone, or web site Medical Information: Glaxo Wellcome Inc., PO Box 13398, Research Triangle Park, NC 27709. Healthcare Professionals (Medical Information): 800-334-0089 Patients (Customer Response Center): 888-TALK2GW (1-888-825-5249) Glaxo Wellcome Corporate Web Site: www.glaxowellcome.com

Ventolin Inh. Sol.—Cont.

and associated ventilatory equipment. In addition, if the solution changes color or becomes cloudy, it should not be used.

Children 2 to 12 Years of Age: For children 2 to 12 years of age, initial dosing should be based upon body weight (0.1 to 0.15 mg/kg per dose), with subsequent dosing titrated to achieve the desired clinical response. Dosing should not exceed 2.5 mg three to four times daily by nebulization. The following table outlines approximate dosing according to body weight.

[See table at top left of previous page]

The appropriate volume of the 0.5% inhalation solution should be diluted in sterile normal saline solution to a total volume of 3 mL prior to administration via nebulization.

Adults and Children Over 12 Years of Age: The usual dosage for adults and children 12 years of age and older is 2.5 mg of albuterol administered three to four times daily by nebulization. More frequent administration or higher doses are not recommended. To administer 2.5 mg of albuterol, dilute 0.5 mL of the 0.5% inhalation solution with 2.5 mL of sterile normal saline solution. The flow rate is regulated to suit the particular nebulizer so that VENTOLIN Inhalation Solution will be delivered over approximately 5 to 15 minutes.

The use of VENTOLIN Inhalation Solution can be continued as medically indicated to control recurring bouts of bronchospasm. During this time most patients gain optimal benefit from regular use of the inhalation solution.

If a previously effective dosage regimen fails to provide the usual relief, medical advice should be sought immediately as this is often a sign of seriously worsening asthma that would require reassessment of therapy.

Drug compatibility (physical and chemical), efficacy, and safety of VENTOLIN Inhalation Solution when mixed with other drugs in a nebulizer have not been established.

HOW SUPPLIED

VENTOLIN Inhalation Solution, 0.5% is supplied in amber glass bottles of 20 mL (NDC 0173-0385-58) with accompanying calibrated dropper in boxes of one.

Store between 2° and 25°C (36° and 77°F).

May 1998/RL-570

Shown in Product Identification Guide, page 314

VENTOLIN NEBULES®

[*vent' ō-lin*]

(albuterol sulfate, USP)

Inhalation Solution, 0.083%*

***Potency expressed as albuterol.**

DESCRIPTION

VENTOLIN NEBULES Inhalation Solution is a relatively selective beta$_2$-adrenergic bronchodilator (see CLINICAL PHARMACOLOGY). Albuterol sulfate, USP, the racemic form of albuterol, has the chemical name α^1-[(*tert*-butylamino)methyl]-4-hydroxy-*m*-xylene-α,α'-diol sulfate (2:1)(salt). Albuterol sulfate has a molecular weight of 576.7, and the empirical formula is $(C_{13}H_{21}NO_3)_2 \cdot H_2SO_4$. Albuterol sulfate is a white crystalline powder, soluble in water and slightly soluble in ethanol.

The World Health Organization recommended name for albuterol base is salbutamol.

VENTOLIN NEBULES Inhalation Solution requires no dilution before administration by nebulization.

Each milliliter of VENTOLIN NEBULES Inhalation Solution contains 0.83 mg of albuterol (as 1 mg of albuterol sulfate) in an isotonic, sterile, aqueous solution containing sodium chloride; sulfuric acid is used to adjust the pH to between 3 and 5. VENTOLIN NEBULES Inhalation Solution contains no sulfiting agents or preservatives.

VENTOLIN NEBULES Inhalation Solution is a clear, colorless solution.

CLINICAL PHARMACOLOGY

In vitro studies and in vivo pharmacologic studies have demonstrated that albuterol has a preferential effect on beta$_2$-adrenergic receptors compared with isoproterenol. While it is recognized that beta$_2$-adrenergic receptors are the predominant receptors in bronchial smooth muscle, data indicate that 10% to 50% of the beta-receptors in the human heart may be beta$_2$-receptors. The precise function of these receptors has not been established.

The pharmacologic effects of beta-adrenergic agonist drugs, including albuterol, are at least in part attributable to stimulation through beta-adrenergic receptors of intracellular adenyl cyclase, the enzyme that catalyzes the conversion of adenosine triphosphate (ATP) to cyclic-3',5'-adenosine monophosphate (cyclic AMP). Increased cyclic AMP levels are associated with relaxation of bronchial smooth muscle and inhibition of release of mediators of immediate hypersensitivity from cells, especially from mast cells.

Albuterol has been shown in most controlled clinical trials to have more effect on the respiratory tract, in the form of bronchial smooth muscle relaxation, than isoproterenol at comparable doses while producing fewer cardiovascular effects.

Controlled clinical studies and other clinical experience have shown that inhaled albuterol, like other beta-adrenergic agonist drugs, can produce a significant cardiovascular effect in some patients, as measured by pulse rate, blood pressure, symptoms, and/or electrocardiographic changes. Albuterol is longer acting than isoproterenol in most patients by any route of administration because it is not a substrate for the cellular uptake processes for catecholamines nor for catechol-*O*-methyl transferase.

Pharmacokinetics: Studies in asthmatic patients have shown that less than 20% of a single albuterol dose was absorbed following either IPPB (intermittent positive-pressure breathing) or nebulizer administration; the remaining amount was recovered from the nebulizer and apparatus and expired air. Most of the absorbed dose was recovered in the urine 24 hours after drug administration. Following a 3-mg dose of nebulized albuterol in adults, the maximum albuterol plasma levels at 0.5 hours were 2.1 ng/mL (range, 1.4 to 3.2 ng/mL). There was a significant dose-related response in FEV$_1$ (forced expiratory volume in 1 second) and peak flow rate. It has been demonstrated that following oral administration of 4 mg of albuterol, the elimination half-life was 5 to 6 hours.

Preclinical: Intravenous studies in rats with albuterol sulfate have demonstrated that albuterol crosses the blood-brain barrier and reaches brain concentrations amounting to approximately 5.0% of the plasma concentrations. In structures outside the brain barrier (pineal and pituitary glands), albuterol concentrations were found to be 100 times those in the whole brain.

Studies in laboratory animals (minipigs, rodents, and dogs) have demonstrated the occurrence of cardiac arrhythmias and sudden death (with histologic evidence of myocardial necrosis) when beta-agonists and methylxanthines are administered concurrently. The clinical significance of these findings is unknown.

Clinical Trials: In controlled clinical trials in adults, most patients exhibited an onset of improvement in pulmonary function within 5 minutes as determined by FEV$_1$. FEV$_1$ measurements also showed that the maximum average improvement in pulmonary function usually occurred at approximately 1 hour following inhalation of 2.5 mg of albuterol by compressor-nebulizer and remained close to peak for 2 hours. Clinically significant improvement in pulmonary function (defined as maintenance of a 15% or more increase in FEV$_1$ over baseline values) continued for 3 to 4 hours in most patients, with some patients continuing up to 6 hours.

Published reports of trials in asthmatic children aged 3 years or older have demonstrated significant improvement in either FEV$_1$ or PEFR within 2 to 20 minutes following single doses of albuterol inhalation solution. An increase of 15% or more in baseline FEV$_1$ has been observed in children aged 5 to 11 years up to 6 hours after treatment with doses of 0.10 mg/kg or higher of albuterol inhalation solution. Single doses of 3, 4, or 10 mg resulted in improvement in baseline PEFR that was comparable in extent and duration to a 2-mg dose, but doses above 3 mg were associated with heart rate increases of more than 10%.

INDICATIONS AND USAGE

VENTOLIN NEBULES Inhalation Solution is indicated for the relief of bronchospasm in patients 2 years of age and older with reversible obstructive airway disease and acute attacks of bronchospasm.

CONTRAINDICATIONS

VENTOLIN NEBULES Inhalation Solution is contraindicated in patients with a history of hypersensitivity to albuterol or any of its components.

WARNINGS

Paradoxical Bronchospasm: VENTOLIN NEBULES Inhalation Solution can produce paradoxical bronchospasm, which may be life threatening. If paradoxical bronchospasm occurs, VENTOLIN NEBULES Inhalation Solution should be discontinued immediately and alternative therapy instituted. It should be recognized that paradoxical bronchospasm, when associated with inhaled formulations, frequently occurs with the first use of a new canister or vial.

Cardiovascular Effects: VENTOLIN NEBULES Inhalation Solution, like all other beta-adrenergic agonists, can produce a clinically significant cardiovascular effect in some patients as measured by pulse rate, blood pressure, and/or symptoms. Although such effects are uncommon after administration of VENTOLIN NEBULES Inhalation Solution at recommended doses, if they occur, the drug may need to be discontinued. In addition, beta-agonists have been reported to produce electrocardiogram (ECG) changes, such as flattening of the T wave, prolongation of the QT$_c$ interval, and ST segment depression. The clinical significance of these findings is unknown. Therefore, VENTOLIN

NEBULES Inhalation Solution, like all sympathomimetic amines, should be used with caution in patients with cardiovascular disorders, especially coronary insufficiency, cardiac arrhythmias, and hypertension.

Deterioration of Asthma: Asthma may deteriorate acutely over a period of hours or chronically over several days or longer. If the patient needs more doses of VENTOLIN NEBULES Inhalation Solution than usual, this may be a marker of destabilization of asthma and requires reevaluation of the patient and treatment regimen, giving special consideration to the possible need for anti-inflammatory treatment, e.g., corticosteroids.

Immediate Hypersensitivity Reactions: Immediate hypersensitivity reactions may occur after administration of albuterol, as demonstrated by rare cases of urticaria, angioedema, rash, bronchospasm, and oropharyngeal edema.

Use of Anti-Inflammatory Agents: The use of beta-adrenergic agonist bronchodilators alone may not be adequate to control asthma in many patients. Early consideration should be given to adding anti-inflammatory agents, e.g., corticosteroids.

PRECAUTIONS

General: Albuterol, as with all sympathomimetic amines, should be used with caution in patients with cardiovascular disorders, especially coronary insufficiency, hypertension, and cardiac arrhythmia; in patients with convulsive disorders, hyperthyroidism, or diabetes mellitus; and in patients who are unusually responsive to sympathomimetic amines. Clinically significant changes in systolic and diastolic blood pressure have been seen in individual patients and could be expected to occur in some patients after use of any beta-adrenergic bronchodilator.

Large doses of intravenous albuterol have been reported to aggravate preexisting diabetes mellitus and ketoacidosis. As with other beta-agonists, albuterol may produce significant hypokalemia in some patients, possibly through intracellular shunting, which has the potential to produce adverse cardiovascular effects. The decrease is usually transient, not requiring supplementation.

Repeated dosing with 0.15 mg/kg of albuterol inhalation solution in children aged 5 to 17 years who were initially normokalemic has been associated with an asymptomatic decline of 20% to 25% in serum potassium levels.

Information for Patients: The action of VENTOLIN NEBULES Inhalation Solution may last up to 6 hours or longer. VENTOLIN NEBULES Inhalation Solution should not be used more frequently than recommended. Do not increase the dose or frequency of VENTOLIN NEBULES Inhalation Solution without consulting your physician. If you find that treatment with VENTOLIN NEBULES Inhalation Solution becomes less effective for symptomatic relief, your symptoms become worse, and/or you need to use the product more frequently than usual, you should seek medical attention immediately. While you are using VENTOLIN NEBULES Inhalation Solution, other inhaled drugs and asthma medications should be taken only as directed by your physician. Common adverse effects include palpitations, chest pain, rapid heart rate, and tremor or nervousness. If you are pregnant or nursing, contact your physician about use of VENTOLIN NEBULES Inhalation Solution. Effective and safe use of VENTOLIN NEBULES Inhalation Solution includes an understanding of the way that it should be administered.

Drug compatibility (physical and chemical), efficacy, and safety of VENTOLIN NEBULES Inhalation Solution when mixed with other drugs in a nebulizer have not been established. See illustrated Patient's Instructions for Use section of the full prescribing information.

Drug Interactions: Other short-acting sympathomimetic aerosol bronchodilators or epinephrine should not be used concomitantly with albuterol. If additional adrenergic drugs are to be administered by any route, they should be used with caution to avoid deleterious cardiovascular effects.

Monoamine Oxidase Inhibitors or Tricyclic Antidepressants: Albuterol should be administered with extreme caution to patients being treated with monoamine oxidase inhibitors or tricyclic antidepressants, or within 2 weeks of discontinuation of such agents, because the action of albuterol on the vascular system may be potentiated.

Beta-Blockers: Beta-adrenergic receptor blocking agents not only block the pulmonary effect of beta-agonists, such as VENTOLIN NEBULES Inhalation Solution, but may produce severe bronchospasm in asthmatic patients. Therefore, patients with asthma should not normally be treated with beta-blockers. However, under certain circumstances, e.g., as prophylaxis after myocardial infarction, there may be no acceptable alternatives to the use of beta-adrenergic blocking agents in patients with asthma. In this setting, cardioselective beta-blockers could be considered, although they should be administered with caution.

Diuretics: The ECG changes and/or hypokalemia that may result from the administration of nonpotassium-sparing diuretics (such as loop or thiazide diuretics) can be acutely worsened by beta-agonists, especially when the recommended dose of the beta-agonist is exceeded. Although the clinical significance of these effects is not known, caution is advised in the coadministration of beta-agonists with nonpotassium-sparing diuretics.

Digoxin: Mean decreases of 16% to 22% in serum digoxin levels were demonstrated after single-dose intravenous and oral administration of albuterol, respectively, to normal vol-

unteers who had received digoxin for 10 days. The clinical significance of these findings for patients with obstructive airway disease who are receiving albuterol and digoxin on a chronic basis is unclear. Nevertheless, it would be prudent to carefully evaluate the serum digoxin levels in patients who are currently receiving digoxin and albuterol.

Carcinogenesis, Mutagenesis, Impairment of Fertility: In a 2-year study in Sprague-Dawley rats, albuterol sulfate caused a significant dose-related increase in the incidence of benign leiomyomas of the mesovarium at dietary doses of 2.0, 10, and 50 mg/kg (approximately 2, 8, and 40 times, respectively, the maximum recommended daily inhalation dose for adults on a mg/m^2 basis or approximately 3/5, 3, and 150 times, respectively, the maximum recommended daily inhalation dose in children on a mg/m^2 basis). In another study this effect was blocked by the coadministration of propranolol, a non-selective beta-adrenergic antagonist. In an 18-month study in CD-1 mice, albuterol sulfate showed no evidence of tumorigenicity at dietary doses up to 500 mg/kg (approximately 200 times the maximum recommended daily inhalation dose for adults on a mg/m^2 basis or approximately 75 times the maximum recommended daily inhalation dose for children on a mg/m^2 basis). In a 22-month study in the Golden hamster, albuterol sulfate showed no evidence of tumorigenicity at dietary doses up to 50 mg/kg (approximately 25 times the maximum recommended daily inhalation dose for adults on a mg/m^2 basis or approximately 10 times the maximum recommended daily inhalation dose for children on a mg/m^2 basis).

Albuterol sulfate was not mutagenic in the Ames test with or without metabolic activation using tester strains *S. typhimurium* TA1537, TA1538, and TA98 or *E. coli* WP2, WP2uvrA, and WP67. No forward mutation was seen in yeast strain *S. cerevisiae* S9 nor any mitotic gene conversion in yeast strain *S. cerevisiae* JD1 with or without metabolic activation. Fluctuation assays in *S. typhimurium* TA98 and *E. coli* WP2, both with metabolic activation, were negative. Albuterol sulfate was not clastogenic in a human peripheral lymphocyte assay or in an AH1 strain mouse micronucleus assay at intraperitoneal doses of up to 200 mg/kg.

Reproduction studies in rats demonstrated no evidence of impaired fertility at oral doses up to 50 mg/kg (approximately 40 times the maximum recommended daily inhalation dose for adults on a mg/m^2 basis).

Pregnancy: ***Teratogenic Effects:*** Pregnancy Category C. Albuterol has been shown to be teratogenic in mice. A study in CD-1 mice at subcutaneous doses of 0.025, 0.25, and 2.5 mg/kg (approximately 1/100, 1/10, and 1.0 times, respectively, the maximum recommended daily inhalation dose for adults on a mg/m^2 basis) showed cleft palate formation in 5 of 111 (4.5%) fetuses at 0.25 mg/kg and in 10 of 108 (9.3%) fetuses at 2.5 mg/kg. The drug did not induce cleft palate formation at the lowest dose, 0.025 mg/kg. Cleft palate also occurred in 22 of 72 (30.5%) fetuses from females treated with 2.5 mg/kg of isoproterenol (positive control) subcutaneously (approximately 1.0 time the maximum recommended daily inhalation dose for adults on a mg/m^2 basis).

A reproduction study in Stride Dutch rabbits revealed cranioschisis in 7 of 19 (37%) fetuses when albuterol was administered orally at a 50-mg/kg dose (approximately 80 times the maximum recommended daily inhalation dose for adults on a mg/m^2 basis).

There are no adequate and well-controlled studies in pregnant women. Albuterol should be used during pregnancy only if the potential benefit justifies the potential risk to the fetus.

During worldwide marketing experience, various congenital anomalies, including cleft palate and limb defects, have been rarely reported in the offspring of patients being treated with albuterol. Some of the mothers were taking multiple medications during their pregnancies. No consistent pattern of defects can be discerned, and a relationship between albuterol use and congenital anomalies has not been established.

Use in Labor and Delivery: Because of the potential for beta-agonist interference with uterine contractility, use of VENTOLIN NEBULES Inhalation Solution for relief of bronchospasm during labor should be restricted to those patients in whom the benefits clearly outweigh the risk.

Tocolysis: Albuterol has not been approved for the management of preterm labor. The benefit:risk ratio when albuterol is administered for tocolysis has not been established. Serious adverse reactions, including maternal pulmonary edema, have been reported during or following treatment of premature labor with beta$_2$-agonists, including albuterol.

Nursing Mothers: It is not known whether this drug is excreted in human milk. Because of the potential for tumorigenicity shown for albuterol in some animal studies, a decision should be made whether to discontinue nursing or to discontinue the drug, taking into account the importance of the drug to the mother.

Pediatric Use: The safety and effectiveness of VENTOLIN NEBULES Inhalation Solution have been established in children 2 years of age and older. Use of VENTOLIN NEBULES Inhalation Solution in these age-groups is supported by evidence from adequate and well-controlled studies of VENTOLIN NEBULES Inhalation Solution in adults; the likelihood that the disease course, pathophysiology, and the drug's effect in pediatric and adult patients are substantially similar; and published reports of trials in pediatric patients 3 years of age or older. The recommended dose for the pediatric population is based upon three published dose comparison studies of efficacy and safety in children 5 to 17 years, and on the safety profile in both adults and pediatric patients at doses equal to or higher than the recommended doses. The safety and effectiveness of VENTOLIN NEBULES Inhalation Solution in children below 2 years of age have not been established.

ADVERSE REACTIONS

The results of clinical trials with VENTOLIN® (albuterol sulfate, USP) Inhalation Solution, 0.5% in 135 patients showed the following side effects that were considered probably or possibly drug related:

Percent Incidence of Adverse Reactions

Reaction	Percent Incidence n = 135
Central nervous system	
Tremors	20%
Dizziness	7%
Nervousness	4%
Headache	3%
Sleeplessness	1%
Gastrointestinal	
Nausea	4%
Dyspepsia	1%
Ear, nose, and throat	
Nasal congestion	1%
Pharyngitis	<1%
Cardiovascular	
Tachycardia	1%
Hypertension	1%
Respiratory	
Bronchospasm	8%
Cough	4%
Bronchitis	4%
Wheezing	1%

No clinically relevant laboratory abnormalities related to VENTOLIN Inhalation Solution administration were determined in these studies.

Cases of urticaria, angioedema, rash, bronchospasm, hoarseness, and oropharyngeal edema, and arrhythmias (including atrial fibrillation, supraventricular tachycardia, extrasystoles) have been reported after the use of VENTOLIN NEBULES Inhalation Solution..

OVERDOSAGE

The expected symptoms with overdosage are those of excessive beta-adrenergic stimulation and/or occurrence or exaggeration of any of the symptoms listed under ADVERSE REACTIONS, e.g., seizures, angina, hypertension or hypotension, tachycardia with rates up to 200 beats/min, arrhythmias, nervousness, headache, tremor, dry mouth, palpitation, nausea, dizziness, fatigue, malaise, and sleeplessness. Hypokalemia may also occur. In isolated cases in children 2 to 12 years of age, tachycardia with rates >200 beats/min has been observed.

As with all sympathomimetic medications, cardiac arrest and even death may be associated with abuse of VENTOLIN NEBULES Inhalation Solution. Treatment consists of discontinuation of VENTOLIN NEBULES Inhalation Solution together with appropriate symptomatic therapy. The judicious use of a cardioselective beta-receptor blocker may be considered, bearing in mind that such medication can produce bronchospasm. There is insufficient evidence to determine if dialysis is beneficial for overdosage of VENTOLIN NEBULES Inhalation Solution.

The oral median lethal dose of albuterol sulfate in mice is greater than 2000 mg/kg (approximately 810 times the maximum recommended daily inhalation dose for adults on a mg/m^2 basis or approximately 300 times the maximum recommended daily inhalation dose for children on a mg/m^2 basis). In mature rats, the subcutaneous median lethal dose of albuterol sulfate is approximately 450 mg/kg (approximately 365 times the maximum recommended daily inhalation dose for adults on a mg/m^2 basis or approximately 135 times the maximum recommended daily inhalation dose for children on a mg/m^2 basis). In small young rats, the subcutaneous median lethal dose is approximately 2000 mg/kg (approximately 1600 times the maximum recommended daily inhalation dose for adults on a mg/m^2 basis or approximately 600 times the maximum recommended daily inhalation dose for children on a mg/m^2 basis). The inhalation median lethal dose has not been determined in animals.

DOSAGE AND ADMINISTRATION

Adults and Children 2 to 12 Years of Age: The usual dosage for adults and for children weighing at least 15 kg is 2.5 mg of albuterol (one NEBULE®) administered three to four times daily by nebulization. Children weighing less than 15 kg who require less than 2.5 mg/dose (i.e., less than a full NEBULE) should use VENTOLIN Inhalation Solution instead of VENTOLIN NEBULES Inhalation Solution. More frequent administration or higher doses are not recommended. To administer 2.5 mg of albuterol, administer the entire contents of one sterile unit dose NEBULE (3 mL of 0.083% inhalation solution) by nebulization. The flow rate is regulated to suit the particular nebulizer so that VENTOLIN NEBULES Inhalation Solution will be delivered over approximately 5 to 15 minutes.

The use of VENTOLIN NEBULES Inhalation Solution can be continued as medically indicated to control recurring bouts of bronchospasm. During this time most patients gain optimal benefit from regular use of the inhalation solution.

If a previously effective dosage regimen fails to provide the usual relief, medical advice should be sought immediately as this is often a sign of seriously worsening asthma that would require reassessment of therapy.

Drug compatibility (physical and chemical), efficacy, and safety of VENTOLIN NEBULES Inhalation Solution when mixed with other drugs in a nebulizer have not been established.

HOW SUPPLIED

VENTOLIN NEBULES Inhalation Solution, 0.083% is contained in plastic, sterile, unit dose nebules of 3 mL each supplied in foil pouches in boxes of 25 (NDC 0173-0419-00).

Protect from light. Store in refrigerator between 2° and 8°C (36° and 46°F). VENTOLIN NEBULES Inhalation Solution may be held at room temperature for up to 2 weeks before use. (Nebules must be used within 2 weeks of removal from refrigerator; record date the nebules are removed from the refrigerator in the space provided on the product carton.) Discard if solution becomes discolored. (Note: VENTOLIN NEBULES Inhalation Solution is colorless.)

May 1998/RL-571

Shown in Product Identification Guide, page 314

VENTOLIN ROTACAPS® ℞

[vent'ō-lin]

(albuterol sulfate, USP)

for Inhalation

FOR ORAL INHALATION ONLY

For Use with the ROTAHALER®

Inhalation Device

DESCRIPTION

VENTOLIN ROTACAPS for Inhalation contain a dry powder presentation of albuterol sulfate intended for oral inhalation only. Each light blue and clear, hard gelatin capsule contains a mixture of 200 mcg of microfine (95%≤10 µm) albuterol (as the sulfate) with 25 mg of lactose.

The contents of each capsule are inhaled using a specially designed plastic device for inhaling powder called the ROTAHALER®. When turned, this device opens the capsule and facilitates dispersion of the albuterol sulfate into the airstream created when the patient inhales through the mouthpiece.

VENTOLIN ROTACAPS for Inhalation are an alternative inhalation form of albuterol to the metered-dose pressurized inhaler.

The active component of VENTOLIN ROTACAPS for Inhalation is albuterol sulfate, USP, the racemic form of albuterol and a relatively selective beta$_2$-adrenergic bronchodilator. It has the chemical name α^1-[(*tert*-butylamino)methyl]-4-hydroxy-*m*-xylene-α,α'-diol sulfate (2:1)(salt).

Albuterol sulfate has a molecular weight of 576.7, and the empirical formula is $(C_{13}H_{21}NO_3)_2 \bullet H_2SO_4$. Albuterol sulfate is a white crystalline powder, soluble in water and slightly soluble in ethanol.

The World Health Organization recommended name for albuterol base is salbutamol.

CLINICAL PHARMACOLOGY

In vitro studies and in vivo pharmacologic studies have demonstrated that albuterol has a preferential effect on

Continued on next page

This product information is based on labeling in effect on June 1, 1998. For further information, contact via direct mail, phone, or web site Medical Information: Glaxo Wellcome Inc., PO Box 13398, Research Triangle Park, NC 27709. Healthcare Professionals (Medical Information): 800-334-0089 Patients (Customer Response Center): 888-TALK2GW (1-888-825-5249) Glaxo Wellcome Corporate Web Site: www.glaxowellcome.com

Ventolin Rotacaps—Cont.

beta$_2$-adrenergic receptors compared with isoproterenol. While it is recognized that beta$_2$-adrenergic receptors are the predominant receptors in bronchial smooth muscle, data indicate that there is a population of beta$_2$-receptors in the human heart existing in a concentration between 10% and 50%. The precise function of these receptors has not been established (see WARNINGS).
The pharmacologic effects of beta-adrenergic agonist drugs, including albuterol, are at least in part attributable to stimulation through beta-adrenergic receptors of intracellular adenyl cyclase, the enzyme that catalyzes the conversion of adenosine triphosphate (ATP) to cyclic-3',5'-adenosine monophosphate (cyclic AMP). Increased cyclic AMP levels are associated with relaxation of bronchial smooth muscle and inhibition of release of mediators of immediate hypersensitivity from cells, especially from mast cells.
Albuterol has been shown in most controlled clinical trials to have more effect on the respiratory tract, in the form of bronchial smooth muscle relaxation, than isoproterenol at comparable doses while producing fewer cardiovascular effects. Controlled clinical studies and other clinical experience have shown that inhaled albuterol, like other beta-adrenergic agonist drugs, can produce a significant cardiovascular effect in some patients, as measured by pulse rate, blood pressure, symptoms, and/or electrocardiographic changes.
Albuterol is longer acting than isoproterenol in most patients by any route of administration because it is not a substrate for the normal cellular uptake processes for catecholamines nor for catechol-*O*-methyl transferase.

Pharmacokinetics: Studies undertaken with four subjects administered tritiated albuterol from a metered-dose aerosol inhaler resulted in maximum plasma concentrations occurring within 2 to 4 hours. Due to the sensitivity of the assay method, the metabolic rate and half-life elimination of albuterol in plasma could not be determined. However, urinary excretion provided data indicating that albuterol has an elimination half-life of 3.8 hours. Approximately 72% of the inhaled dose is excreted within 24 hours in the urine, and consists of 28% as unchanged drug and 44% as metabolite.

Preclinical: Intravenous studies in rats with albuterol sulfate have demonstrated that albuterol crosses the blood-brain barrier and reaches brain concentrations amounting to approximately 5.0% of the plasma concentrations. In structures outside the brain barrier (pineal and pituitary glands), albuterol concentrations were found to be 100 times those in the whole brain.
Studies in laboratory animals (minipigs, rodents, and dogs) have demonstrated the occurrence of cardiac arrhythmias and sudden death (with histologic evidence of myocardial necrosis) when beta-agonists and methylxanthines are administered concurrently. The clinical significance of these findings is unknown.

Clinical Trials: In single, dose-range, crossover trials with VENTOLIN ROTACAPS for Inhalation in patients 12 years of age and older, the onset of improvement in pulmonary function was within 5 minutes as determined by a 15% increase in FEV_1 (forced expiratory volume in 1 second) following administration of either a 200- or 400-mcg dose. Maximum increases in FEV_1 occurred within 60 minutes following inhalation of either dose. The duration of effect (defined as an increase in FEV_1 of 15% or greater in a single-dose study) was 1 to 2 hours after the 200-mcg dose and 3 to 4 hours after the 400-mcg dose. In a single-dose study, an increase in forced expiratory flow rate between 25% and 75% of the forced vital capacity ($FEF_{25\%-75\%}$) of 20% or greater continued for 3 to 4 hours after the 200-mcg dose and for 3 to 6 hours following the 400-mcg dose. A therapeutic response continued for 4 hours in the majority of patients and for 6 hours in 38% of the patients following the 400-mcg dose. Twenty-two percent of the patients receiving the 200-mcg dose had a duration of effect of 8 hours.
In 12-week, double-blind, comparative evaluations in patients 12 years of age and older of one 200-mcg VENTOLIN ROTACAPS for Inhalation capsule versus two inhalations of VENTOLIN® (albuterol, USP) Inhalation Aerosol, the two dosage regimens were found to be clinically comparable. Based on a 15% or more increase in FEV_1 determinations, both provided a therapeutic response that persisted for 2 or 3 hours in 50% of 231 patients aged 12 years and older. Similar results were found in two controlled, 12-week clinical trials involving 204 children aged 4 to 11 years. Both formulations produced a therapeutic response (defined as maintenance of mean increase over baseline of at least 15% in FEV_1, or 20% in $FEF_{25\%-75\%}$). Therapeutic improvement of $FEF_{25\%-75\%}$ persisted for 3 to 5 hours in over 50% of the children throughout the study. Continued effectiveness and safety of VENTOLIN ROTACAPS for Inhalation were demonstrated over the 12-week study periods in both adults and children.
In other clinical studies in adults and children, one 200-mcg VENTOLIN ROTACAPS for Inhalation capsule taken approximately 15 minutes before exercise prevented exercise-induced bronchospasm, as demonstrated by the maintenance of FEV_1 within 80% of baseline values in the majority of patients. One study in adults also evaluated the duration of the prophylactic effect to repeated exercise challenges, which was evident at 4 hours in the majority of patients and at 6 hours in approximately one third of the patients.

INDICATIONS AND USAGE

VENTOLIN ROTACAPS for Inhalation are indicated for the prevention and relief of bronchospasm in patients 4 years of age and older with reversible obstructive airway disease and for the prevention of exercise-induced bronchospasm in patients 4 years of age and older. The VENTOLIN ROTACAPS for Inhalation formulation is particularly useful in patients who are unable to properly use the pressurized aerosol form of albuterol or who prefer an alternative formulation. VENTOLIN ROTACAPS for Inhalation can be used with or without concomitant steroid therapy.

CONTRAINDICATIONS

VENTOLIN ROTACAPS for Inhalation are contraindicated in patients with a history of hypersensitivity to albuterol or any of its components.

WARNINGS

Paradoxical Bronchospasm: VENTOLIN ROTACAPS for Inhalation can produce paradoxical bronchospasm, which may be life threatening. If paradoxical bronchospasm occurs, VENTOLIN ROTACAPS for Inhalation should be discontinued immediately and alternative therapy instituted.

Cardiovascular Effects: VENTOLIN ROTACAPS for Inhalation, like all other beta-adrenergic agonists, can produce a clinically significant cardiovascular effect in some patients as measured by pulse rate, blood pressure, and/or symptoms. Although such effects are uncommon after administration of VENTOLIN ROTACAPS for Inhalation at recommended doses, if they occur, the drug may need to be discontinued. In addition, beta-agonists have been reported to produce electrocardiogram (ECG) changes, such as flattening of the T wave, prolongation of the QT_c interval, and ST segment depression. The clinical significance of these findings is unknown. Therefore, VENTOLIN ROTACAPS for Inhalation, like all sympathomimetic amines, should be used with caution in patients with cardiovascular disorders, especially coronary insufficiency, cardiac arrhythmias, and hypertension.

Deterioration of Asthma: Asthma may deteriorate acutely over a period of hours or chronically over several days or longer. If the patient needs more doses of VENTOLIN ROTACAPS for Inhalation than usual, this may be a marker of destabilization of asthma and requires reevaluation of the patient and treatment regimen, giving special consideration to the possible need for anti-inflammatory treatment, e.g., corticosteroids.

Immediate Hypersensitivity Reactions: Immediate hypersensitivity reactions may occur after administration of albuterol, as demonstrated by rare cases of urticaria, angioedema, rash, bronchospasm, anaphylaxis, and oropharyngeal edema.

Use of Anti-Inflammatory Agents: The use of beta-adrenergic agonist bronchodilators alone may not be adequate to control asthma in many patients. Early consideration should be given to adding anti-inflammatory agents, e.g., corticosteroids.
Inhalation of capsule particles may result if damage to the capsule has occurred from handling by the patient.

PRECAUTIONS

General: Albuterol, as with all sympathomimetic amines, should be used with caution in patients with cardiovascular disorders, especially coronary insufficiency, hypertension, and cardiac arrhythmia; in patients with convulsive disorders, hyperthyroidism, or diabetes mellitus; and in patients who are unusually responsive to sympathomimetic amines. Clinically significant changes in systolic and diastolic blood pressure have been seen in individual patients and could be expected to occur in some patients after use of any beta-adrenergic bronchodilator. As with other beta-agonists, albuterol may produce significant hypokalemia in some patients, possibly through intracellular shunting, which has the potential to produce adverse cardiovascular effects. The decrease is usually transient, not requiring supplementation.

Information for Patients: The action of VENTOLIN ROTACAPS for Inhalation may last for up to 6 hours or longer. VENTOLIN ROTACAPS for Inhalation should not be used more frequently than recommended. Do not increase the dose or frequency of VENTOLIN ROTACAPS for Inhalation without consulting your physician. If you find that treatment with VENTOLIN ROTACAPS for Inhalation becomes less effective for symptomatic relief, your symptoms become worse, and/or you need to use the product more frequently than usual, you should seek medical attention immediately. While you are using VENTOLIN ROTACAPS for Inhalation, other inhaled drugs and asthma medications should be taken only as directed by your physician. Common adverse effects include palpitations, chest pain, rapid heart rate, and tremor or nervousness. If you are pregnant or nursing, contact your physician about use of VENTOLIN ROTACAPS for Inhalation. Effective and safe use of VENTOLIN ROTACAPS for Inhalation includes an understanding of the way that it should be administered.
Children should use VENTOLIN ROTACAPS for Inhalation under adult supervision, as instructed by the patient's physician.
See illustrated Patient's Instructions for Use section of the full prescribing information.

Drug Interactions: Other short-acting sympathomimetic aerosol bronchodilators should not be used concomitantly with albuterol. If additional adrenergic drugs are to be administered by any route, they should be used with caution to avoid deleterious cardiovascular effects.

Monoamine Oxidase Inhibitors or Tricyclic Antidepressants: Albuterol should be administered with extreme caution to patients being treated with monoamine oxidase inhibitors or tricyclic antidepressants, or within 2 weeks of discontinuation of such agents, because the action of albuterol on the vascular system may be potentiated.

Beta-Blockers: Beta-adrenergic receptor blocking agents not only block the pulmonary effect of beta-agonists, such as VENTOLIN ROTACAPS for Inhalation, but may produce severe bronchospasm in asthmatic patients. Therefore, patients with asthma should not normally be treated with beta-blockers. However, under certain circumstances, e.g., as prophylaxis after myocardial infarction, there may be no acceptable alternatives to the use of beta-adrenergic blocking agents in patients with asthma. In this setting, cardioselective beta-blockers should be considered, although they could be administered with caution.

Diuretics: The ECG changes and/or hypokalemia that may result from the administration of nonpotassium-sparing diuretics (such as loop or thiazide diuretics) can be acutely worsened by beta-agonists, especially when the recommended dose of the beta-agonist is exceeded. Although the clinical significance of these effects is not known, caution is advised in the coadministration of beta-agonists with nonpotassium-sparing diuretics.

Digoxin: Mean decreases of 16% to 22% in serum digoxin levels were demonstrated after single-dose intravenous and oral administration of albuterol, respectively, to normal volunteers who had received digoxin for 10 days. The clinical significance of these findings for patients with obstructive airway disease who are receiving albuterol and digoxin on a chronic basis is unclear. Nevertheless, it would be prudent to carefully evaluate the serum digoxin levels in patients who are currently receiving digoxin and albuterol.

Carcinogenesis, Mutagenesis, Impairment of Fertility: In a 2-year study in Sprague-Dawley rats, albuterol sulfate caused a significant dose-related increase in the incidence of benign leiomyomas of the mesovarium at dietary doses of 2.0, 10, and 50 mg/kg (approximately 7, 35, and 170 times, respectively, the maximum recommended daily inhalation dose for adults on a mg/m^2 basis or approximately 3, 15, and 80 times, respectively, the maximum recommended daily inhalation dose in children on a mg/m^2 basis). In another study this effect was blocked by the coadministration of propranolol, a non-selective beta-adrenergic antagonist. In an 18-month study in CD-1 mice, albuterol sulfate showed no evidence of tumorigenicity at dietary doses of up to 500 mg/kg (approximately 850 times the maximum recommended daily inhalation dose for adults on a mg/m^2 basis or approximately 400 times the maximum recommended daily inhalation dose for children on a mg/m^2 basis). In a 22-month study in the Golden hamster, albuterol sulfate showed no evidence of tumorigenicity at dietary doses of up to 50 mg/kg (approximately 120 times the maximum recommended daily inhalation dose for adults on a mg/m^2 basis or approximately 55 times the maximum recommended daily inhalation dose for children on a mg/m^2 basis).
Albuterol sulfate was not mutagenic in the Ames test with or without metabolic activation using tester strains *S. typhimurium* TA1537, TA1538, and TA98 or *E. coli* WP2, WP2uvrA, and WP67. No forward mutation was seen in yeast strain *S. cerevisiae* S9 nor any mitotic gene conversion in yeast strain *S. cerevisiae* JD1 with or without metabolic activation. Fluctuation assays in *S. typhimurium* TA98 and *E. coli* WP2, both with metabolic activation, were negative. Albuterol sulfate was not clastogenic in a human peripheral lymphocyte assay or in an AH1 strain mouse micronucleus assay at intraperitoneal doses of up to 200 mg/kg.
Reproduction studies in rats demonstrated no evidence of impaired fertility at oral doses up to 50 mg/kg (approximately 170 times the maximum recommended daily inhalation dose for adults on a mg/m^2 basis.

Pregnancy: ***Teratogenic Effects:*** Pregnancy Category C. Albuterol has been shown to be teratogenic in mice. A study in CD-1 mice at subcutaneous doses of 0.025, 0.25, and 2.5 mg/kg (approximately 1/25, 2/5, and 4 times, respectively, the maximum recommended daily inhalation dose for adults on a mg/m^2 basis) showed cleft palate formation in 5 of 111 (4.5%) fetuses at 0.25 mg/kg and in 10 of 108 (9.3%) fetuses at 2.5 mg/kg. The drug did not induce cleft palate formation at the lowest dose, 0.025 mg/kg. Cleft palate also occurred in

22 of 72 (30.5%) fetuses from females treated with 2.5 mg/kg of isoproterenol (positive control) subcutaneously, approximately four times the maximum recommended daily inhalation dose for adults on a mg/m^2 basis.

A reproduction study in Stride Dutch rabbits revealed cranioschisis in 7 of 19 (37%) fetuses when albuterol was administered orally at a 50-mg/kg dose (approximately 340 times the maximum recommended daily inhalation dose for adults on a mg/m^2 basis).

There are no adequate and well-controlled studies in pregnant women. Albuterol should be used during pregnancy only if the potential benefit justifies the potential risk to the fetus.

During worldwide marketing experience, various congenital anomalies, including cleft palate and limb defects, have been rarely reported in the offspring of patients being treated with albuterol. Some of the mothers were taking multiple medications during their pregnancies. No consistent pattern of defects can be discerned, and a relationship between albuterol use and congenital anomalies has not been established.

Use in Labor and Delivery: Because of the potential for beta-agonist interference with uterine contractility, use of VENTOLIN ROTACAPS for Inhalation for relief of bronchospasm during labor should be restricted to those patients in whom the benefits clearly outweigh the risk.

Tocolysis: Albuterol has not been approved for the management of preterm labor. The benefit:risk ratio when albuterol is administered for tocolysis has not been established. Serious adverse reactions, including maternal pulmonary edema, have been reported during or following treatment of premature labor with beta$_2$-agonists, including albuterol.

Nursing Mothers: It is not known whether this drug is excreted in human milk after inhalation of recommended doses. Because of the potential for tumorigenicity shown for albuterol in some animal studies, a decision should be made whether to discontinue nursing or to discontinue the drug, taking into account the importance of the drug to the mother.

Pediatric Use: Safety and effectiveness in children below 4 years of age have not been established.

ADVERSE REACTIONS

The adverse reactions to albuterol are similar in nature to reactions to other sympathomimetic agents, although the incidence of certain cardiovascular effects is lower with albuterol. Results of clinical trials with VENTOLIN ROTACAPS® for Inhalation 200 mcg in 172 patients aged 12 years and older (adults) and 129 patients aged 4 to 12 years (children) are shown in the following tables:

Percent Incidence of Adverse Reactions in Patients ≥12 Years of Age

Reaction	Percent Incidence
Central nervous system	
Headache	2%
Nervousness	1%
Tremor	1%
Sleeplessness	<1%
Dizziness	<1%
Lightheadedness	<1%
Digestive system	
Throat irritation	2%
Burning in the stomach	<1%
Dry mouth	<1%
Bad taste	<1%
Respiratory system	
Coughing	5%
Bronchospasm	1%

Percent Incidence of Adverse Reactions in Children 4 to 12 Years of Age

Reaction	Percent Incidence
Central nervous system	
Headache	5%
Dizziness	<1%
Hyperactivity	<1%
Gastrointestinal	
Nausea and/or vomiting	4%
Stomachache	2%
Diarrhea	<1%
Respiratory system	
Epistaxis	2%
Hoarseness	2%
Nasal congestion	2%
Cough	2%
Oropharyngeal	
Throat irritation	2%
Unusual taste	2%

Cases of urticaria, angioedema, rash, bronchospasm, hoarseness, oropharyngeal edema, and arrhythmias (including atrial fibrillation, supraventricular tachycardia, extrasystoles) have been reported after the use of VENTOLIN ROTACAPS for Inhalation.

In addition, albuterol, like other sympathomimetic agents, can cause adverse reactions such as hypertension, angina, vertigo, and CNS stimulation.

OVERDOSAGE

The expected symptoms with overdosage are those of excessive beta-adrenergic stimulation and/or occurrence or exaggeration of any of the symptoms listed under ADVERSE REACTIONS, e.g., seizures, angina, hypertension or hypotension, tachycardia with rates up to 200 beats/min, arrhythmias, nervousness, headache, tremor, dry mouth, palpitation, nausea, dizziness, fatigue, malaise, and sleeplessness. Hypokalemia may also occur. As with all sympathomimetic medications, cardiac arrest and even death may be associated with abuse of VENTOLIN ROTACAPS for Inhalation. Treatment consists of discontinuation of VENTOLIN ROTACAPS for Inhalation together with appropriate symptomatic therapy. The judicious use of a cardioselective beta-receptor blocker may be considered, bearing in mind that such medication can produce bronchospasm. There is insufficient evidence to determine if dialysis is beneficial for overdosage of VENTOLIN ROTACAPS for Inhalation.

The oral median lethal dose of albuterol sulfate in mice is greater than 2000 mg/kg (approximately 3400 times the maximum recommended daily inhalation dose for adults on a mg/m^2 basis or approximately 1600 times the maximum recommended daily dose for children on a mg/m^2 basis). In mature rats, the subcutaneous median lethal dose of albuterol sulfate is approximately 450 mg/kg (approximately 1500 times the maximum recommended daily inhalation dose for adults on a mg/m^2 basis or approximately 700 times the maximum recommended daily dose for children on a mg/m^2 basis). In small young rats, the subcutaneous median lethal dose is approximately 2000 mg/kg (approximately 6800 times the maximum recommended daily inhalation dose for adults on a mg/m^2 basis or approximately 3200 times the maximum recommended daily inhalation dose for children on a mg/m^2 basis). The inhalational median lethal dose has not been determined in animals.

Dialysis is not appropriate treatment for overdosage of VENTOLIN ROTACAPS for Inhalation.

DOSAGE AND ADMINISTRATION

The usual dosage of VENTOLIN ROTACAPS for Inhalation for adults and children 4 years of age and older is the contents of one 200-mcg capsule inhaled every 4 to 6 hours using a ROTAHALER inhalation device. In some patients, the contents of two 200-mcg capsules inhaled every 4 to 6 hours may be required. Larger doses or more frequent administration is not recommended.

The use of VENTOLIN ROTACAPS for Inhalation can be continued as medically indicated to control recurring bouts of bronchospasm. During this time most patients gain optimal benefit from regular use of the VENTOLIN ROTACAPS for Inhalation formulation.

If a previously effective dosage regimen fails to provide the usual relief, medical advice should be sought immediately as this is often a sign of seriously worsening asthma that would require reassessment of therapy.

Exercise-Induced Bronchospasm Prevention: The usual dosage of VENTOLIN ROTACAPS for Inhalation for adults and children 4 years of age and older is the contents of one 200-mcg capsule inhaled using a ROTAHALER 15 minutes before exercise.

HOW SUPPLIED

VENTOLIN ROTACAPS for Inhalation, 200 mcg, are light blue and clear, with "VENTOLIN 200" printed on the blue cap and "GLAXO" printed on the clear body.

VENTOLIN ROTACAPS for Inhalation are supplied in a kit containing one white plastic HDPE bottle of 100 capsules and one ROTAHALER inhalation device with patient's instructions (NDC 0173-0389-01). Also available, VENTOLIN ROTACAPS for Inhalation Refill in white plastic HDPE bottle of 100 capsules with patient's instructions (NDC 0173-0389-02).

VENTOLIN ROTACAPS for Inhalation are also supplied in a hospital unit dose kit containing one unit dose double-foil blister pack of 24 capsules and one ROTAHALER inhalation device (NDC 0173-0389-03).

Store between 2° and 30°C (36° and 86°F). Replace cap securely after each opening.

May 1998/RL-572

Shown in Product Identification Guide, page 314

VENTOLIN® ℞
(albuterol sulfate, USP)
Syrup

DESCRIPTION

VENTOLIN Syrup contains albuterol sulfate, USP, the racemic form of albuterol and a relatively selective beta$_2$-adrenergic bronchodilator. Albuterol sulfate has the chemical name α^1-[(*tert*-Butylamino) methyl]-4-hydroxy-*m*-xylene-α,α′-diol sulfate (2:1)(salt).

Albuterol sulfate has a molecular weight of 576.7 and the empirical formula $(C_{13}H_{21}NO_3)_2 \cdot H_2SO_4$. Albuterol sulfate is a white crystalline powder, soluble in water and slightly soluble in ethanol.

The World Health Organization recommended name for albuterol base is salbutamol.

VENTOLIN Syrup contains 2 mg of albuterol as 2.4 mg of albuterol sulfate in each teaspoonful (5 mL).

The inactive ingredients for VENTOLIN Syrup include: citric acid, FD&C Yellow No. 6, flavor, hydroxypropyl methylcellulose, saccharin, sodium benzoate, sodium citrate, and water.

CLINICAL PHARMACOLOGY

The prime action of beta-adrenergic drugs is to stimulate adenyl cyclase, the enzyme which catalyzes the formation of cyclic-3′,5′-adenosine monophosphate (cyclic AMP) from adenosine triphosphate (ATP). The cyclic AMP thus formed mediates the cellular responses. Based on pharmacologic studies in animals, albuterol appears to exert direct and preferential action on beta$_2$-adrenoceptors, including those of the bronchial tree and uterus, and may have less cardiac stimulant effect than isoproterenol when given in the usual recommended dose.

Albuterol is longer acting than isoproterenol in most patients by any route of administration because it is not a substrate for the cellular uptake processes for catecholamines nor for catechol-*O*-methyl transferase.

After oral administration of 10 mL VENTOLIN Syrup (4 mg albuterol) in normal volunteers, albuterol is rapidly absorbed. Maximum plasma albuterol concentrations of about 18 ng/mL are achieved within 2 hours and the drug is eliminated with a half-life of about 5 hours. In other studies, the analysis of urine samples of patients given 8 mg tritiated albuterol orally showed that 76% of the dose was excreted over 3 days, with the majority of the dose being excreted within the first 24 hours. Sixty percent of this radioactivity was shown to be the metabolite. Feces collected over this period contained 4% of the administered dose.

Animal studies show that albuterol does not pass the blood-brain barrier.

INDICATIONS AND USAGE

VENTOLIN Syrup is indicated for the relief of bronchospasm in adults and children 2 years of age and older with reversible obstructive airway disease.

In controlled clinical trials in patients with asthma, the onset of improvement in pulmonary function, as measured by maximal midexpiratory flow rate (MMEF) and forced expiratory volume in one second (FEV$_1$), was within 30 minutes after a dose of VENTOLIN Syrup. Peak improvement of pulmonary function occurred between 2 and 3 hours. In a controlled clinical trial involving 55 children, clinically significant improvement (defined as maintenance of mean values over baseline of 15% to 20% or more in the FEV$_1$ and MMEF, respectively) continued to be recorded up to 6 hours. No decrease in the effectiveness was reported in one uncontrolled study of 32 children who took VENTOLIN Syrup for a 3-month period.

CONTRAINDICATIONS

VENTOLIN Syrup is contraindicated in patients with a history of hypersensitivity to any of its components.

WARNINGS

Immediate hypersensitivity reactions may occur after administration of albuterol, as demonstrated by rare cases of anaphylaxis, angioedema, oropharyngeal edema, bronchospasm, urticaria, and rash.

Rarely, erythema multiforme and Stevens-Johnson syndrome have been associated with the administration of albuterol sulfate syrup in children.

PRECAUTIONS

General: Although albuterol usually has minimal effects on the beta$_1$-adrenoceptors of the cardiovascular system at

Continued on next page

This product information is based on labeling in effect on June 1, 1998. For further information, contact via direct mail, phone, or web site Medical Information: Glaxo Wellcome Inc., PO Box 13398, Research Triangle Park, NC 27709. Healthcare Professionals (Medical Information): 800-334-0089 Patients (Customer Response Center): 888-TALK2GW (1-888-825-5249) Glaxo Wellcome Corporate Web Site: www.glaxowellcome.com

Ventolin Syrup—Cont.

the recommended dosage, occasionally the usual cardiovascular and CNS stimulatory effects common to all sympathomimetic agents have been seen with patients treated with albuterol, necessitating discontinuation. Therefore, albuterol, as with all sympathomimetic amines, should be used with caution in patients with cardiovascular disorders, including coronary insufficiency, cardiac arrhythmias, and hypertension; in patients with convulsive disorders, hyperthyroidism, or diabetes mellitus; and in patients who are unusually responsive to sympathomimetic amines.

Large doses of intravenous albuterol have been reported to aggravate preexisting diabetes mellitus and ketoacidosis. Additionally, albuterol and other beta-agonists, when given intravenously, may cause a decrease in serum potassium, possibly through intracellular shunting. The decrease is usually transient, not requiring supplementation. The relevance of these observations to the use of VENTOLIN Syrup is unknown.

Information for Patients: The action of VENTOLIN Syrup may last up to 6 hours and therefore it should not be taken more frequently than recommended. Do not increase the dose or frequency of medication without medical consultation. If symptoms get worse, medical consultation should be sought promptly. If pregnant or nursing, consult with your physician.

Drug Interactions: The concomitant use of VENTOLIN Syrup and other oral sympathomimetic agents is not recommended since such combined use may lead to deleterious cardiovascular effects. This recommendation does not preclude the judicious use of an aerosol bronchodilator of the adrenergic stimulant type in patients receiving VENTOLIN Syrup. Such concomitant use, however, should be individualized and not given on a routine basis. If regular coadministration is required, then alternative therapy should be considered.

Albuterol should be administered with extreme caution to patients being treated with monoamine oxidase inhibitors or tricyclic antidepressants, since the action of albuterol on the vascular system may be potentiated.

Beta-receptor blocking agents and albuterol inhibit the effect of each other.

Since albuterol may lower serum potassium, care should be taken in patients also using other drugs which lower serum potassium as the effects may be additive.

After single-dose administration of albuterol to normal volunteers who had received digoxin for 10 days, a 16% to 22% decrease in serum digoxin levels was demonstrated. The clinical significance of these findings for patients with obstructive airway disease who are receiving albuterol and digoxin on a chronic basis is unclear. Nevertheless, it would be prudent to carefully evaluate the serum digoxin levels in patients who are concurrently receiving digoxin and albuterol.

Carcinogenesis, Mutagenesis, Impairment of Fertility: Albuterol sulfate, like other agents in its class, caused a significant dose-related increase in the incidence of benign leiomyomas of the mesovarium in a 2-year study in the rat, at doses corresponding to 2, 9, and 46 times the maximum human (child weighing 21 kg) oral dose. In another study this effect was blocked by the coadministration of propranolol. The relevance of these findings to humans is not known. An 18-month study in mice and a lifetime study in hamsters revealed no evidence of tumorigenicity. Studies with albuterol revealed no evidence of mutagenesis. Reproduction studies in rats revealed no evidence of impaired fertility.

Teratogenic Effects-Pregnancy Category C: Albuterol has been shown to be teratogenic in mice when given subcutaneously in doses corresponding to 0.2 times the maximum human (child weighing 21 kg) oral dose. There are no adequate and well-controlled studies in pregnant women. Albuterol should be used during pregnancy only if the potential benefit justifies the potential risk to the fetus. A reproduction study in CD-1 mice with albuterol showed cleft palate formation in 5 of 111 (4.5%) fetuses at 0.25 mg/kg and in 10 of 108 (9.3%) fetuses at 2.5 mg/kg; none was observed at 0.025 mg/kg. Cleft palate also occurred in 22 of 72 (30.5%) fetuses treated with 2.5 mg/kg of isoproterenol (positive control). A reproduction study in Stride Dutch rabbits revealed cranioschisis in 7 of 19 (37%) fetuses at 50 mg/kg, corresponding to 46 times the maximum human (child weighing 21 kg) oral dose of albuterol sulfate. During marketing, various congenital anomalies, including cleft palate and limb defects, have been reported in the offspring of patients being treated with albuterol. Some of the mothers were taking multiple medications during their pregnancies. Because no consistent pattern of defects can be discerned, a relationship between albuterol use and congenital anomalies cannot be established.

Labor and Delivery: Oral albuterol has been shown to delay preterm labor in some reports. There are presently no well-controlled studies which demonstrate that it will stop preterm labor or prevent labor at term. Therefore, cautious use of VENTOLIN Syrup is required in pregnant patients when given for relief of bronchospasm so as to avoid interference with uterine contractibility. Use in such patients should be restricted to those patients in whom the benefits clearly outweigh the risks.

Nursing Mothers: It is not known whether this drug is excreted in human milk. Because of the potential for tumorigenicity shown for albuterol in animal studies, a decision should be made whether to discontinue nursing or to discontinue the drug, taking into account the importance of the drug to the mother.

Pediatric Use: Safety and effectiveness in children below 2 years of age have not yet been adequately demonstrated.

ADVERSE REACTIONS

The adverse reactions to albuterol are similar in nature to those of other sympathomimetic agents. The most frequent adverse reactions to VENTOLIN Syrup in adults and older children were tremor, 10 of 100 patients; nervousness and shakiness, each 9 of 100 patients. Other reported adverse reactions were headache, 4 of 100 patients; dizziness and increased appetite, each 3 of 100 patients; hyperactivity and excitement, each 2 of 100 patients; tachycardia, epistaxis, irritable behavior, and sleeplessness, each 1 of 100 patients. The following adverse effects occurred in less than 1 of 100 patients each: muscle spasm; disturbed sleep; epigastric pain; cough; palpitations; stomach ache; irritable behavior; dilated pupils; sweating; chest pain; weakness.

In young children 2 to 6 years of age, some adverse reactions were noted more frequently than in adults and older children. Excitement was noted in approximately 20% of patients and nervousness in 15%. Hyperkinesia occurred in 4% of patients; insomnia, tachycardia, and gastrointestinal symptoms in 2% each. Anorexia, emotional lability, pallor, fatigue, and conjunctivitis were seen in 1%.

In addition, albuterol, like other sympathomimetic agents, can cause adverse reactions such as hypertension, angina, vomiting, vertigo, central nervous system stimulation, unusual taste, and drying or irritation of the oropharynx.

The reactions are generally transient in nature, and it is usually not necessary to discontinue treatment with VENTOLIN Syrup. In selected cases, however, dosage may be reduced temporarily; after the reaction has subsided, dosage should be increased in small increments to the optimal dosage.

OVERDOSAGE

Manifestations of overdosage include anginal pain, hypertension, hypokalemia, and exaggeration of the effects listed in **ADVERSE REACTIONS**.

The oral LD_{50} in rats and mice was greater than 2,000 mg/kg. Dialysis is not appropriate treatment for overdosage of VENTOLIN Syrup. The judicious use of a cardioselective beta-receptor blocker, such as metoprolol tartrate, is suggested, bearing in mind the danger of inducing an asthmatic attack.

DOSAGE AND ADMINISTRATION

The following dosages of VENTOLIN Syrup are expressed in terms of albuterol base.

Usual Dose The usual starting dosage for adults and children over 14 years of age is 2 mg (1 teaspoonful) or 4 mg (2 teaspoonfuls) three or four times a day.

The usual starting dosage for children 6 to 14 years of age is 2 mg (1 teaspoonful) three or four times a day.

For children 2 to 6 years of age, dosing should be initiated at 0.1 mg/kg of body weight three times a day. This starting dosage should not exceed 2 mg (1 teaspoonful) three times a day.

Dosage Adjustment For adults and children over age 14, a dosage above 4 mg four times a day should be used *only* when the patient fails to respond. If a favorable response does not occur, the dosage may be cautiously increased stepwise, but the dosage should not exceed 8 mg four times a day.

For children from 6 to 14 years of age who fail to respond to the initial starting dosage of 2 mg four times a day, the dosage may be cautiously increased stepwise, but not to exceed 24 mg per day (given in divided doses).

For children 2 to 6 years of age who do not respond satisfactorily to the initial dosage, the dosage may be increased stepwise to 0.2 mg/kg of body weight three times a day, but not to exceed a maximum of 4 mg (2 teaspoonfuls) given three times a day.

For elderly patients and those sensitive to beta-adrenergic stimulation, the initial dosage should be restricted to 2 mg three or four times a day and individually adjusted thereafter.

HOW SUPPLIED

VENTOLIN Syrup, a clear orange-yellow liquid with a strawberry flavor, contains 2 mg albuterol as the sulfate per 5 mL; bottles of 16 fluid ounces (NDC 0173-0351-54).

Store between 2° and 30°C (36° and 86°F).

July 1996/RL-334

Shown in Product Identification Guide, page 314

VENTOLIN® ℞

[vent' ō-lin]

(albuterol sulfate, USP)

Tablets

DESCRIPTION

VENTOLIN Tablets contain albuterol sulfate, USP, the racemic form of albuterol and a relatively selective beta$_2$-adrenergic bronchodilator. Albuterol sulfate has the chemical name (±) α[1]-[(*tert*-butylamino)methyl]-4-hydroxy-*m*-xylene-α,α'-diol sulfate (2:1)(salt).

Albuterol sulfate has a molecular weight of 576.7, and the empirical formula is $(C_{13}H_{21}NO_3)_2 \bullet H_2SO_4$. Albuterol sulfate is a white crystalline powder, soluble in water and slightly soluble in ethanol.

The World Health Organization recommended name for albuterol base is salbutamol.

Each VENTOLIN Tablet contains 2 or 4 mg of albuterol as 2.4 or 4.8 mg, respectively, of albuterol sulfate for oral administration. Each tablet also contains the inactive ingredients corn starch, lactose, and magnesium stearate.

CLINICAL PHARMACOLOGY

In vitro studies and in vivo pharmacologic studies have demonstrated that albuterol has a preferential effect on beta$_2$-adrenergic receptors compared with isoproterenol. While it is recognized that beta$_2$-adrenergic receptors are the predominant receptors in bronchial smooth muscle, data indicate that there is a population of beta$_2$-receptors in the human heart existing in a concentration between 10% and 50%. The precise function of these receptors has not been established (see WARNINGS).

The pharmacologic effects of beta-adrenergic agonist drugs, including albuterol, are at least in part attributable to stimulation through beta-adrenergic receptors of intracellular adenyl cyclase, the enzyme that catalyzes the conversion of adenosine triphosphate (ATP) to cyclic-3',5'-adenosine monophosphate (cyclic AMP). Increased cyclic AMP levels are associated with relaxation of bronchial smooth muscle and inhibition of release of mediators of immediate hypersensitivity from cells, especially from mast cells.

Albuterol has been shown in most controlled clinical trials to have more effect on the respiratory tract, in the form of bronchial smooth muscle relaxation, than isoproterenol at comparable doses while producing fewer cardiovascular effects.

Albuterol is longer acting than isoproterenol in most patients by any route of administration because it is not a substrate for the cellular uptake processes for catecholamines nor for catechol-*O*-methyl transferase.

Preclinical: Intravenous studies in rats with albuterol sulfate have demonstrated that albuterol crosses the blood-brain barrier and reaches brain concentrations amounting to approximately 5.0% of the plasma concentrations. In structures outside the brain barrier (pineal and pituitary glands), albuterol concentrations were found to be 100 times those in the whole brain.

Studies in laboratory animals (minipigs, rodents, and dogs) have demonstrated the occurrence of cardiac arrhythmias and sudden death (with histologic evidence of myocardial necrosis) when beta-agonists and methylxanthines are administered concurrently. The clinical significance of these findings is unknown.

Pharmacokinetics: Albuterol is rapidly absorbed after oral administration of 4-mg VENTOLIN Tablets in normal volunteers. Maximum plasma concentrations of about 18 ng/mL of albuterol are achieved within 2 hours, and the drug is eliminated with a half-life of about 5 hours.

In other studies, the analysis of urine samples of patients given 8 mg of tritiated albuterol orally showed that 76% of the dose was excreted over 3 days, with the majority of the dose being excreted within the first 24 hours. Sixty percent of this radioactivity was shown to be the metabolite. Feces collected over this period contained 4% of the administered dose.

Clinical Trials: In controlled clinical trials in patients with asthma, the onset of improvement in pulmonary function, as measured by maximum midexpiratory flow rate (MMEF), was within 30 minutes after a dose of VENTOLIN Tablets, with peak improvement occurring between 2 and 3 hours. In controlled clinical trials in which measurements were conducted for 6 hours, clinically significant improvement (defined as maintaining a 15% or more increase in forced expiratory volume in 1 second [FEV_1] and a 20% or more increase in MMEF over baseline values) was observed in 60% of patients at 4 hours and in 40% at 6 hours. In other single-dose, controlled clinical trials, clinically significant improvement was observed in at least 40% of the patients at 8 hours. No decrease in the effectiveness of VENTOLIN Tablets was reported in patients who received long-term treatment with the drug in uncontrolled studies for periods up to 6 months.

INDICATIONS AND USAGE

VENTOLIN Tablets are indicated for the relief of bronchospasm in adults and children 6 years of age and older with reversible obstructive airway disease.

CONTRAINDICATIONS

VENTOLIN Tablets are contraindicated in patients with a history of hypersensitivity to albuterol or any of its components.

WARNINGS

Paradoxical Bronchospasm: VENTOLIN Tablets can produce paradoxical bronchospasm, which may be life threatening. If paradoxical bronchospasm occurs, VENTOLIN Tablets should be discontinued immediately and alternative therapy instituted.

Cardiovascular Effects: VENTOLIN Tablets, like all other beta-adrenergic agonists, can produce a clinically significant cardiovascular effect in some patients as measured by pulse rate, blood pressure, and/or symptoms. Although such effects are uncommon after administration of VENTOLIN Tablets at recommended doses, if they occur, the drug may need to be discontinued. In addition, beta-agonists have been reported to produce electrocardiogram (ECG) changes, such as flattening of the T wave, prolongation of the QT_c interval, and ST segment depression. The clinical significance of these findings is unknown. Therefore, VENTOLIN Tablets, like all sympathomimetic amines, should be used with caution in patients with cardiovascular disorders, especially coronary insufficiency, cardiac arrhythmias, and hypertension.

Deterioration of Asthma: Asthma may deteriorate acutely over a period of hours or chronically over several days or longer. If the patient needs more doses of VENTOLIN Tablets than usual, this may be a marker of destabilization of asthma and requires reevaluation of the patient and treatment regimen, giving special consideration to the possible need for anti-inflammatory treatment, e.g., corticosteroids.

Use of Anti-Inflammatory Agents: The use of beta-adrenergic agonist bronchodilators alone may not be adequate to control asthma in many patients. Early consideration should be given to adding anti-inflammatory agents, e.g., corticosteroids.

Immediate Hypersensitivity Reactions: Immediate hypersensitivity reactions may occur after administration of albuterol, as demonstrated by rare cases of urticaria, angioedema, rash, bronchospasm, and oropharyngeal edema. Albuterol, like other beta-adrenergic agonists, can produce a significant cardiovascular effect in some patients, as measured by pulse rate, blood pressure, symptoms, and/or electrocardiographic changes.

Rarely, erythema multiforme and Stevens-Johnson syndrome have been associated with the administration of oral albuterol sulfate in children.

PRECAUTIONS

General: Albuterol, as with all sympathomimetic amines, should be used with caution in patients with cardiovascular disorders, especially coronary insufficiency, hypertension, and cardiac arrhythmia; in patients with convulsive disorders, hyperthyroidism or diabetes mellitus; and in patients who are unusually responsive to sympathomimetic amines. Clinically significant changes in systolic and diastolic blood pressure have been seen in individual patients and could be expected to occur in some patients after use of any beta-adrenergic bronchodilator.

Large doses of intravenous albuterol have been reported to aggravate preexisting diabetes mellitus and ketoacidosis. As with other beta-agonists, albuterol may produce significant hypokalemia in some patients, possibly through intracellular shunting, which has the potential to produce adverse cardiovascular effects. The decrease is usually transient, not requiring supplementation.

Information for Patients: The action of VENTOLIN Tablets may last up to 8 hours or longer. VENTOLIN Tablets should not be taken more frequently than recommended. Do not increase the dose or frequency of VENTOLIN Tablets without consulting your physician. If you find that treatment with VENTOLIN Tablets becomes less effective for symptomatic relief, your symptoms get worse, and/or you need to take the product more frequently than usual, you should seek medical attention immediately. While you are taking VENTOLIN Tablets, other asthma medications and inhaled drugs should be taken only as directed by your physician. Common adverse effects include palpitations, chest pain, rapid heart rate, and tremor or nervousness. If you are pregnant or nursing, contact your physician about use of VENTOLIN Tablets. Effective and safe use of VENTOLIN Tablets includes an understanding of the way that it should be administered.

Drug Interactions: The concomitant use of VENTOLIN Tablets and other oral sympathomimetic agents is not recommended since such combined use may lead to deleterious cardiovascular effects. This recommendation does not preclude the judicious use of an aerosol bronchodilator of the adrenergic stimulant type in patients receiving VENTOLIN Tablets. Such concomitant use, however, should be individualized and not given on a routine basis. If regular coadministration is required, then alternative therapy should be considered.

Monoamine Oxidase Inhibitors or Tricyclic Antidepressants: Albuterol should be administered with extreme caution to patients being treated with monoamine oxidase inhibitors or tricyclic antidepressants, or within 2 weeks of discontinuation of such agents, because the action of albuterol on the vascular system may be potentiated.

Beta-Blockers: Beta-adrenergic receptor blocking agents not only block the pulmonary effect of beta-agonists, such as VENTOLIN Tablets, but may produce severe bronchospasm in asthmatic patients. Therefore, patients with asthma should not normally be treated with beta-blockers. However, under certain circumstances, e.g., as prophylaxis after myocardial infarction, there may be no acceptable alternatives to the use of beta-adrenergic blocking agents in patients with asthma. In this setting, cardioselective beta-blockers could be considered, although they should be administered with caution.

Diuretics: The ECG changes and/or hypokalemia that may result from the administration of nonpotassium-sparing diuretics (such as loop or thiazide diuretics) can be acutely worsened by beta-agonists, especially when the recommended dose of the beta-agonist is exceeded. Although the clinical significance of these effects is not known, caution is advised in the coadministration of beta-agonists with nonpotassium-sparing diuretics.

Digoxin: Mean decreases of 16% to 22% in serum digoxin levels were demonstrated after single-dose intravenous and oral administration of albuterol, respectively, to normal volunteers who had received digoxin for 10 days. The clinical significance of these findings for patients with obstructive airway disease who are receiving albuterol and digoxin on a chronic basis is unclear. Nevertheless, it would be prudent to carefully evaluate the serum digoxin levels in patients who are currently receiving digoxin and albuterol.

Carcinogenesis, Mutagenesis, Impairment of Fertility: In a 2-year study in Sprague-Dawley rats, albuterol sulfate caused a significant dose-related increase in the incidence of benign leiomyomas of the mesovarium at dietary doses of 2.0, 10, and 50 mg/kg (approximately 1/2, 3, and 15 times, respectively, the maximum recommended daily oral dose for adults on a mg/m² basis or 2/5, 2, and 10 times, respectively, the maximum recommended daily oral dose for children on a mg/m² basis). In another study this effect was blocked by the coadministration of propranolol, a non-selective beta-adrenergic antagonist.

In an 18-month study in CD-1 mice, albuterol sulfate showed no evidence of tumorigenicity at dietary doses of up to 500 mg/kg (approximately 65 times the maximum recommended daily oral dose for adults on a mg/m² basis or approximately 50 times the maximum recommended daily oral dose for children on a mg/m² basis). In a 22-month study in the Golden hamster, albuterol sulfate showed no evidence of tumorigenicity at dietary doses of up to 50 mg/kg (approximately 8 times the maximum recommended daily oral dose for adults on a mg/m² basis or approximately 7 times the maximum recommended daily oral dose for children on a mg/m² basis).

Albuterol sulfate was not mutagenic in the Ames test with or without metabolic activation using tester strains *S. typhimurium* TA1537, TA1538, and TA98 or *E. coli* WP2, WP2uvrA, and WP67. No forward mutation was seen in yeast strain *S. cerevisiae* S9 nor any mitotic gene conversion in yeast strain *S. cerevisiae* JD1 with or without metabolic activation. Fluctuation assays in *S. typhimurium* TA98 and *E. coli* WP2, both with metabolic activation, were negative. Albuterol sulfate was not clastogenic in a human peripheral lymphocyte assay or in an AH1 strain mouse micronucleus assay at intraperitoneal doses of up to 200 mg/kg.

Reproduction studies in rats demonstrated no evidence of impaired fertility at oral doses up to 50 mg/kg (approximately 15 times the maximum recommended daily oral dose for adults on a mg/m² basis).

Pregnancy: *Teratogenic Effects:* Pregnancy Category C. Albuterol has been shown to be teratogenic in mice. A study in CD-1 mice at subcutaneous (sc) doses of 0.025, 0.25, and 2.5 mg/kg (approximately 3/1000, 3/100, and 3/10 times, respectively, the maximum recommended daily oral dose for adults on a mg/m² basis) showed cleft palate formation in 5 of 111 (4.5%) fetuses at 0.25 mg/kg and in 10 of 108 (9.3%) fetuses at 2.5 mg/kg. The drug did not induce cleft palate formation at the lowest dose, 0.025 mg/kg. Cleft palate also occurred in 22 of 72 (30.5%) fetuses from females treated with 2.5 mg/kg of isoproterenol (positive control) subcutaneously (approximately 3/10 times the maximum recommended daily oral dose for adults on a mg/m² basis).

A reproduction study in Stride Dutch rabbits revealed cranioschisis in 7 of 19 (37%) fetuses when albuterol was administered orally at a 50-mg/kg dose (approximately 25 times the maximum recommended daily oral dose for adults on a mg/m² basis).

There are no adequate and well-controlled studies in pregnant women. Albuterol should be used during pregnancy only if the potential benefit justifies the potential risk to the fetus.

During worldwide marketing experience, various congenital anomalies, including cleft palate and limb defects, have been rarely reported in the offspring of patients being treated with albuterol. Some of the mothers were taking multiple medications during their pregnancies. No consistent pattern of defects can be discerned, and a relationship between albuterol use and congenital anomalies has not been established.

Use in Labor and Delivery: Because of the potential for beta-agonist interference with uterine contractility, use of VENTOLIN Tablets for relief of bronchospasm during labor should be restricted to those patients in whom the benefits clearly outweigh the risk.

Tocolysis: Albuterol has not been approved for the management of preterm labor. The benefit:risk ratio when albuterol is administered for tocolysis has not been established. Serious adverse reactions, including maternal pulmonary edema, have been reported during or following treatment of premature labor with beta₂-agonists, including albuterol.

Nursing Mothers: It is not known whether this drug is excreted in human milk. Because of the potential for tumorigenicity shown for albuterol in some animal studies, a decision should be made whether to discontinue nursing or to discontinue the drug, taking into account the importance of the drug to the mother.

Pediatric Use: Safety and effectiveness in children below 6 years of age have not been established.

ADVERSE REACTIONS

In clinical trials, the most frequent adverse reactions to VENTOLIN Tablets were:

Percent Incidence of Adverse Reactions

Reaction	Percent Incidence
Central nervous system	
Nervousness	20%
Tremor	20%
Headache	7%
Sleeplessness	2%
Weakness	2%
Dizziness	2%
Drowsiness	<1%
Restlessness	<1%
Irritability	<1%
Cardiovascular	
Tachycardia	5%
Palpitations	5%
Chest discomfort	<1%
Flushing	<1%
Musculoskeletal	
Muscle cramps	3%
Gastrointestinal	
Nausea	2%
Genitourinary	
Difficulty in micturition	<1%

Cases of urticaria, angioedema, rash, bronchospasm, oropharyngeal edema, and arrhythmias (including atrial fibrillation, supraventricular tachycardia, extrasystoles) have been reported after the use of VENTOLIN Tablets.

In addition, albuterol, like other sympathomimetic agents, can cause adverse reactions such as hypertension, angina, vomiting, vertigo, central nervous system stimulation, unusual taste, and drying or irritation of the oropharynx.

The reactions are generally transient in nature, and it is usually not necessary to discontinue treatment with VENTOLIN Tablets. In selected cases, however, dosage may be reduced temporarily; after the reaction has subsided, dosage should be increased in small increments to the optimal dosage.

OVERDOSAGE

The expected symptoms with overdosage are those of excessive beta-adrenergic stimulation and/or occurrence or exaggeration of any of the symptoms listed under ADVERSE REACTIONS, e.g., seizures, angina, hypertension or hypotension, tachycardia with rates up to 200 beats/min, arrhythmias, nervousness, headache, tremor, dry mouth, palpitation, nausea, dizziness, fatigue, malaise, and sleeplessness. Hypokalemia may also occur. As with all sympathomimetic medications, cardiac arrest and even death may be associated with abuse of VENTOLIN Tablets. Treatment consists of discontinuation of VENTOLIN Tablets together with appropriate symptomatic therapy. The judicious use of a cardioselective beta-receptor blocker may be

Continued on next page

This product information is based on labeling in effect on June 1, 1998. For further information, contact via direct mail, phone, or web site Medical Information: Glaxo Wellcome Inc., PO Box 13398, Research Triangle Park, NC 27709. Healthcare Professionals (Medical Information): 800-334-0089 Patients (Customer Response Center): 888-TALK2GW (1-888-825-5249) Glaxo Wellcome Corporate Web Site: www.glaxowellcome.com

Ventolin Tablets—Cont.

considered, bearing in mind that such medication can produce bronchospasm. There is insufficient evidence to determine if dialysis is beneficial for overdosage of VENTOLIN Tablets.

The oral median lethal dose of albuterol sulfate in mice is greater than 2000 mg/kg (approximately 250 times the maximum recommended daily oral dose for adults on a mg/m^2 basis or approximately 200 times the maximum recommended daily oral dose for children on a mg/m^2 basis. In mature rats, the subcutaneous median lethal dose of albuterol sulfate is approximately 450 mg/kg (approximately 110 times the maximum recommended daily oral dose for adults on a mg/m^2 basis or approximately 90 times the maximum recommended daily oral dose for children on a mg/m^2 basis). In small young rats, the subcutaneous median lethal dose is approximately 2000 mg/kg (approximately 500 times the maximum recommended daily oral dose for adults on a mg/m^2 basis or approximately 400 times the maximum recommended daily oral dose for children on a mg/m^2 basis).

DOSAGE AND ADMINISTRATION

The following dosages of VENTOLIN Tablets are expressed in terms of albuterol base.

Usual Dosage: ***Adults and Children Over 12 Years of Age:*** The usual starting dosage for adults and children 12 years and older is 2 or 4 mg three or four times a day.

Children 6 to 12 Years of Age: The usual starting dosage for children 6 to 12 years of age is 2 mg three or four times a day.

Dosage Adjustment: ***Adults and Children Over 12 Years of Age:*** For adults and children 12 years and older, a dosage above 4 mg four times a day should be used *only* when the patient fails to respond. If a favorable response does not occur with the 4-mg initial dosage, it should be cautiously increased stepwise up to a maximum of 8 mg four times a day as tolerated.

Children 6 to 12 Years of Age Who Fail to Respond to the Initial Starting Dosage of 2 mg Four Times a Day: For children from 6 to 12 years of age who fail to respond to the initial starting dosage of 2 mg four times a day, the dosage may be cautiously increased stepwise, but not to exceed 24 mg/day (given in divided doses).

Elderly Patients and Those Sensitive to Beta-adrenergic Stimulators: An initial dosage of 2 mg three or four times a day is recommended for elderly patients and for those with a history of unusual sensitivity to beta-adrenergic stimulators. If adequate bronchodilatation is not obtained, dosage may be increased gradually to as much as 8 mg three or four times a day.

The total daily dose should not exceed 32 mg in adults and children 12 years and older.

HOW SUPPLIED

VENTOLIN Tablets, 2 mg of albuterol as the sulfate, are white, round, compressed tablets impressed with the product name (VENTOLIN) and the number 2 on one side and scored on the other with "GLAXO" impressed on each side of the score in white plastic HDPE bottles of 100 (NDC 0173-0341-43) and 500 (NDC 0173-0341-44).

VENTOLIN Tablets, 4 mg of albuterol as the sulfate, are white, round, compressed tablets impressed with the product name (VENTOLIN) and the number 4 on one side and scored on the other with "GLAXO" impressed on each side of the score in white plastic HDPE bottles of 100 (NDC 0173-0342-43) and 500 (NDC 0173-0342-44).

Store between 2° and 25°C (36° and 77°F). Replace cap securely after each opening.

May 1998/RL-574

Shown in Product Identification Guide, page 314

WELLBUTRIN® ℞

[wel 'byü-trin]

(bupropion hydrochloride)

Tablets

DESCRIPTION

WELLBUTRIN (bupropion hydrochloride), an antidepressant of the aminoketone class, is chemically unrelated to tricyclic, tetracyclic, or other known antidepressant agents. Its structure closely resembles that of diethylpropion; it is related to phenylethylamines. It is designated as (±)-1-(3-chlorophenyl)-2-[(1,1-dimethylethyl)amino]-1-propanone hydrochloride. The molecular weight is 276.2. The empirical formula is $C_{13}H_{18}ClNO \cdot HCl$. Bupropion hydrochloride powder is white, crystalline, and highly soluble in water. It has a bitter taste and produces the sensation of local anesthesia on the oral mucosa.

WELLBUTRIN is supplied for oral administration as 75-mg (yellow-gold) and 100-mg (red) film-coated tablets. Each tablet contains the labeled amount of bupropion hydrochloride and the inactive ingredients: 75-mg tablet—D&C Yellow No. 10 Lake, FD&C Yellow No. 6 Lake, hydroxypropyl cellulose, hydroxypropyl methylcellulose, microcrystalline cellulose, polyethylene glycol, talc, and titanium dioxide; 100-mg tablet—FD&C Red No. 40 Lake, FD&C Yellow No. 6 Lake, hydroxypropyl cellulose, hydroxypropyl methylcellulose, microcrystalline cellulose, polyethylene glycol, talc, and titanium dioxide.

CLINICAL PHARMACOLOGY

Pharmacodynamics and Pharmacological Actions: The neurochemical mechanism of the antidepressant effect of bupropion is not known. Bupropion does not inhibit monoamine oxidase. Compared to classical tricyclic antidepressants, it is a weak blocker of the neuronal uptake of serotonin and norepinephrine; it also inhibits the neuronal reuptake of dopamine to some extent.

Bupropion produces dose-related central nervous system (CNS) stimulant effects in animals, as evidenced by increased locomotor activity, increased rates of responding in various schedule-controlled operant behavior tasks, and, at high doses, induction of mild stereotyped behavior.

Bupropion causes convulsions in rodents and dogs at doses approximately tenfold the dose recommended as the human antidepressant dose.

Absorption, Distribution, Pharmacokinetics, Metabolism, and Elimination: ***Oral Bioavailability and Single-dose Pharmacokinetics:*** In humans, following oral administration of WELLBUTRIN, peak plasma bupropion concentrations are usually achieved within 2 hours, followed by a biphasic decline. The average half-life of the second (postdistributional) phase is approximately 14 hours, with a range of 8 to 24 hours. Six hours after a single dose, plasma bupropion concentrations are approximately 30% of peak concentrations. Plasma bupropion concentrations are dose-proportional following single doses of 100 to 250 mg; however, it is not known if the proportionality between dose and plasma level is maintained in chronic use.

The absolute bioavailability of WELLBUTRIN Tablets in humans has not been determined because an intravenous formulation for human use is not available.

However, it appears likely that only a small proportion of any orally administered dose reaches the systemic circulation intact. For example, the absolute bioavailability of bupropion in animals (rats and dogs) ranges from 5% to 20%.

Metabolism: Following oral administration of 200 mg of ^{14}C-bupropion, 87% and 10% of the radioactive dose were recovered in the urine and feces, respectively. However, the fraction of the oral dose of WELLBUTRIN excreted unchanged was only 0.5%, a finding documenting the extensive metabolism of bupropion.

Several of the known metabolites of bupropion are pharmacologically active, but their potency and toxicity relative to bupropion have not been fully characterized. However, because of their longer elimination half-lives, the plasma concentrations of at least two of the known metabolites can be expected, especially in chronic use, to be very much higher than the plasma concentration of bupropion. This is of potential clinical importance because factors or conditions altering metabolic capacity (e.g., liver disease, congestive heart failure, age, concomitant medications, etc.) or elimination may be expected to influence the degree and extent of accumulation of these active metabolites.

Furthermore, bupropion has been shown to induce its own metabolism in three animal species (mice, rats, and dogs) following subchronic administration. If induction also occurs in humans, the relative contribution of bupropion and its metabolites to the clinical effects of WELLBUTRIN may be changed in chronic use.

Plasma and urinary metabolites so far identified include biotransformation products formed via reduction of the carbonyl group and/or hydroxylation of the *tert*- butyl group of bupropion. Four basic metabolites have been identified. They are the *erythro*- and *threo*- amino alcohols of bupropion, the *erythro*- amino diol of bupropion, and a morpholinol metabolite (formed from hydroxylation of the *tert*- butyl group of bupropion).

The morpholinol metabolite appears in the systemic circulation almost as rapidly as the parent drug following a single oral dose. Its peak level is three times the peak level of the parent drug; it has a half-life on the order of 24 hours; and its AUC 0 to 60 hours is about 15 times that of bupropion.

The *threo*- amino alcohol metabolite has a plasma concentration-time profile similar to that of the morpholinol metabolite. The *erythro*-amino alcohol and the *erythro*- amino diol metabolites generally cannot be detected in the systemic circulation following a single oral dose of the parent drug. The morpholinol and the *threo*- amino alcohol metabolites have been found to be half as potent as bupropion in animal screening tests for antidepressant drugs.

During a chronic dosing study in 14 depressed patients with left ventricular dysfunction, it was found that there was substantial interpatient variability (twofold to fivefold) in the trough steady-state concentrations of bupropion and the morpholinol and *threo*- amino alcohol metabolites. In addition, the steady-state plasma concentrations of these metabolites were 10 to 100 times the steady-state concentrations of the parent drug.

The effect of other disease states and altered organ function on the metabolism and/or elimination of bupropion has not been studied in detail. However, the elimination of the major metabolites of bupropion may be affected by reduced renal or hepatic function because they are moderately polar compounds and are likely to undergo conjugation in the liver prior to urinary excretion. The preliminary results of a comparative single-dose pharmacokinetic study in normal versus cirrhotic patients indicated that half-lives of the metabolites were prolonged by cirrhosis and that the metabolites accumulated to levels two to three times those in normals.

The effect of age on plasma concentrations of bupropion and its metabolites has not been characterized.

In vitro tests show that bupropion is 80% or more bound to human albumin at plasma concentrations up to 800 µmol/L (200 mcg/mL).

INDICATIONS AND USAGE

WELLBUTRIN is indicated for the treatment of depression.

A physician considering WELLBUTRIN for the management of a patient's first episode of depression should be aware that the drug may cause generalized seizures in a dose-dependent manner with an approximate incidence of 0.4% (4/1000). This incidence of seizures may exceed that of other marketed antidepressants by as much as fourfold. This relative risk is only an approximate estimate because no direct comparative studies have been conducted (see WARNINGS) .

The efficacy of WELLBUTRIN has been established in three placebo-controlled trials, including two of approximately 3 weeks' duration in depressed inpatients and one of approximately 6 weeks' duration in depressed outpatients. The depressive disorder of the patients studied corresponds most closely to the Major Depression category of the APA Diagnostic and Statistical Manual III.

Major Depression implies a prominent and relatively persistent depressed or dysphoric mood that usually interferes with daily functioning (nearly every day for at least 2 weeks); it should include at least four of the following eight symptoms: change in appetite, change in sleep, psychomotor agitation or retardation, loss of interest in usual activities or decrease in sexual drive, increased fatigability, feelings of guilt or worthlessness, slowed thinking or impaired concentration, and suicidal ideation or attempts.

Effectiveness of WELLBUTRIN in long-term use, that is, for more than 6 weeks, has not been systematically evaluated in controlled trials. Therefore, the physician who elects to use WELLBUTRIN for extended periods should periodically reevaluate the long-term usefulness of the drug for the individual patient.

CONTRAINDICATIONS

WELLBUTRIN is contraindicated in patients with a seizure disorder. WELLBUTRIN is contraindicated in patients treated with ZYBAN™ (bupropion hydrochloride) Sustained-Release Tablets, or any other medications that contain bupropion because the incidence of seizure is dose dependent. WELLBUTRIN is also contraindicated in patients with a current or prior diagnosis of bulimia or anorexia nervosa because of a higher incidence of seizures noted in such patients treated with WELLBUTRIN. The concurrent administration of WELLBUTRIN and a monoamine oxidase (MAO) inhibitor is contraindicated. At least 14 days should elapse between discontinuation of an MAO inhibitor and initiation of treatment with WELLBUTRIN. WELLBUTRIN is contraindicated in patients who have shown an allergic response to it.

WARNINGS

Patients should be made aware that WELLBUTRIN contains the same active ingredient found in ZYBAN, used as an aid to smoking cessation treatment, and that WELLBUTRIN should not be used in combination with ZYBAN, or any other medications that contain bupropion.

Seizures: Bupropion is associated with seizures in approximately 0.4% (4/1000) of patients treated at doses up to 450 mg/day. This incidence of seizures may exceed that of other marketed antidepressants by as much as fourfold. This relative risk is only an approximate estimate because no direct comparative studies have been conducted. The estimated seizure incidence for WELLBUTRIN increases almost tenfold between 450 and 600 mg/day, which is twice the usually required daily dose (300 mg) and one and one-third the maximum recommended daily dose (450 mg). Given the wide variability among individuals and their capacity to metabolize and eliminate drugs, this disproportionate increase in seizure incidence with dose incrementation calls for caution in dosing.

During the initial development, 25 among approximately 2400 patients treated with WELLBUTRIN experienced seizures. At the time of seizure, seven patients were receiving daily doses of 450 mg or below for an incidence of 0.33% (3/1000) within the recommended dose range. Twelve patients experienced seizures at 600 mg per day (2.3% incidence); six additional patients had seizures at daily doses between 600 and 900 mg (2.8% incidence).

A separate, prospective study was conducted to determine the incidence of seizure during an 8-week treatment exposure in approximately 3200 additional patients who received daily doses of up to 450 mg. Patients were permitted to continue treatment beyond 8 weeks if clinically indicated. Eight seizures occurred during the initial 8-week treatment period and five seizures were reported in patients continuing treatment beyond 8 weeks, resulting in a total seizure incidence of 0.4%.

The risk of seizure appears to be strongly associated with dose. Sudden and large increments in dose may contribute to increased risk. While many seizures occurred early in the course of treatment, some seizures did occur after several weeks at fixed dose.

The risk of seizure is also related to patient factors, clinical situations, and concomitant medications, which must be considered in selection of patients for therapy with WELLBUTRIN.

- **Patient factors:** Predisposing factors that may increase the risk of seizure with bupropion use include history of head trauma or prior seizure, CNS tumor, and concomitant medications that lower seizure threshold.
- **Clinical situations:** Circumstances associated with an increased seizure risk include, among others, excessive use of alcohol; abrupt withdrawal from alcohol or other sedatives; addiction to opiates, cocaine, or stimulants; use of over-the-counter stimulants and anorectics; and diabetes treated with oral hypoglycemics or insulin.
- **Concomitant medications:** Many medications (e.g., antipsychotics, antidepressants, theophylline, systemic steroids) and treatment regimens (e.g., abrupt discontinuation of benzodiazepines) are known to lower seizure threshold.

Recommendations for Reducing the Risk of Seizure: Retrospective analysis of clinical experience gained during the development of WELLBUTRIN suggests that the risk of seizure may be minimized if (1) the total daily dose of WELLBUTRIN does *not* exceed 450 mg, (2) the daily dose is administered three times daily, with each single dose *not* to exceed 150 mg to avoid high peak concentrations of bupropion and/or its metabolites, and (3) the rate of incrementation of dose is very gradual. Extreme caution should be used when WELLBUTRIN is (1) administered to patients with a history of seizure, cranial trauma, or other predisposition(s) toward seizure or (2) prescribed with other agents (e.g., antipsychotics, other antidepressants, theophylline, systemic steroids, etc.) or treatment regimens (e.g., abrupt discontinuation of a benzodiazepine) that lower seizure threshold.

Potential for Hepatotoxicity: In rats receiving large doses of bupropion chronically, there was an increase in incidence of hepatic hyperplastic nodules and hepatocellular hypertrophy. In dogs receiving large doses of bupropion chronically, various histologic changes were seen in the liver, and laboratory tests suggesting mild hepatocellular injury were noted.

PRECAUTIONS

General: *Agitation and Insomnia:* A substantial proportion of patients treated with WELLBUTRIN experience some degree of increased restlessness, agitation, anxiety, and insomnia, especially shortly after initiation of treatment. In clinical studies, these symptoms were sometimes of sufficient magnitude to require treatment with sedative/hypnotic drugs. In approximately 2% of patients, symptoms were sufficiently severe to require discontinuation of treatment with WELLBUTRIN.

Psychosis, Confusion, and Other Neuropsychiatric Phenomena: Patients treated with WELLBUTRIN have been reported to show a variety of neuropsychiatric signs and symptoms including delusions, hallucinations, psychotic episodes, confusion, and paranoia. Because of the uncontrolled nature of many studies, it is impossible to provide a precise estimate of the extent of risk imposed by treatment with WELLBUTRIN. In several cases, neuropsychiatric phenomena abated upon dose reduction and/or withdrawal of treatment.

Activation of Psychosis and/or Mania: Antidepressants can precipitate manic episodes in Bipolar Manic Depressive patients during the depressed phase of their illness and may activate latent psychosis in other susceptible patients. WELLBUTRIN is expected to pose similar risks.

Altered Appetite and Weight: A weight loss of greater than 5 lbs occurred in 28% of patients receiving WELLBUTRIN. This incidence is approximately double that seen in comparable patients treated with tricyclics or placebo. Furthermore, while 34.5% of patients receiving tricyclic antidepressants gained weight, only 9.4% of patients treated with WELLBUTRIN did. Consequently, if weight loss is a major presenting sign of a patient's depressive illness, the anorectic and/or weight reducing potential of WELLBUTRIN should be considered.

Suicide: The possibility of a suicide attempt is inherent in depression and may persist until significant remission occurs. Accordingly, prescriptions for WELLBUTRIN should be written for the smallest number of tablets consistent with good patient management.

Allergic Reactions: Anaphylactoid reactions characterized by symptoms such as pruritus, urticaria, angioedema, and dyspnea requiring medical treatment have been reported in clinical trials with bupropion. In addition, there have been rare spontaneous postmarketing reports of erythema multiforme, Stevens-Johnson syndrome, and anaphylactic shock associated with bupropion.

Use in Patients with Systemic Illness: There is no clinical experience establishing the safety of WELLBUTRIN in patients with a recent history of myocardial infarction or unstable heart disease. Therefore, care should be exercised if it is used in these groups. WELLBUTRIN was well tolerated in patients who had previously developed orthostatic hypotension while receiving tricyclic antidepressants.

Because bupropion HCl and its metabolites are almost completely excreted through the kidney and metabolites are likely to undergo conjugation in the liver prior to urinary excretion, treatment of patients with renal or hepatic impairment should be initiated at reduced dosage as bupropion and its metabolites may accumulate in such patients beyond concentrations expected in patients without renal or hepatic impairment. The patient should be closely monitored for possible toxic effects of elevated blood and tissue levels of drug and metabolites.

Information for Patients: Patients should be made aware that WELLBUTRIN contains the same active ingredient found in ZYBAN, used as an aid to smoking cessation, and that WELLBUTRIN should not be used in combination with ZYBAN or any other medications that contain bupropion hydrochloride.

Physicians are advised to discuss the following issues with patients:

Patients should be instructed to take WELLBUTRIN in equally divided doses three or four times a day to minimize the risk of seizure.

Patients should be told that any CNS-active drug like WELLBUTRIN may impair their ability to perform tasks requiring judgment or motor and cognitive skills. Consequently, until they are reasonably certain that WELLBUTRIN does not adversely affect their performance, they should refrain from driving an automobile or operating complex, hazardous machinery.

Patients should be told that the use and cessation of use of alcohol may alter the seizure threshold, and, therefore, that the consumption of alcohol should be minimized, and, if possible, avoided completely.

Patients should be advised to inform their physician if they are taking or plan to take any prescription or over-the-counter drugs. Concern is warranted because WELLBUTRIN and other drugs may affect each other's metabolism.

Patients should be advised to notify their physicians if they become pregnant or intend to become pregnant during therapy.

Drug Interactions: No systematic data have been collected on the consequences of the concomitant administration of WELLBUTRIN and other drugs.

However, animal data suggest that WELLBUTRIN may be an inducer of drug metabolizing enzymes. This may be of potential clinical importance because the blood levels of co-administered drugs may be altered.

Alternatively, because bupropion is extensively metabolized, the coadministration of other drugs may affect its clinical activity. In particular, care should be exercised when administering drugs known to affect hepatic drug-metabolizing enzyme systems (e.g., carbamazepine, cimetidine, phenobarbital, phenytoin).

Studies in animals demonstrate that the acute toxicity of bupropion is enhanced by the MAO inhibitor phenelzine (see CONTRAINDICATIONS).

Limited clinical data suggest a higher incidence of adverse experiences in patients receiving concurrent administration of WELLBUTRIN and L-dopa. Administration of WELLBUTRIN to patients receiving L-dopa concurrently should be undertaken with caution, using small initial doses and small gradual dose increases.

Concurrent administration of WELLBUTRIN and agents (e.g., antipsychotics, other antidepressants, theophylline, systemic steroids, etc.) or treatment regimens (e.g., abrupt discontinuation of benzodiazepines) that lower seizure threshold should be undertaken only with extreme caution (see WARNINGS). Low initial dosing and small gradual dose increases should be employed.

Carcinogenesis, Mutagenesis, Impairment of Fertility: Lifetime carcinogenicity studies were performed in rats and mice at doses up to 300 and 150 mg/kg/day, respectively. In the rat study there was an increase in nodular proliferative lesions of the liver at doses of 100 to 300 mg/kg per day; lower doses were not tested. The question of whether or not such lesions may be precursors of neoplasms of the liver is currently unresolved. Similar liver lesions were not seen in the mouse study, and no increase in malignant tumors of the liver and other organs was seen in either study.

Bupropion produced a borderline positive response (two to three times control mutation rate) in some strains in the Ames bacterial mutagenicity test, and a high oral dose (300 mg/kg, but not 100 or 200 mg/kg) produced a low incidence of chromosomal aberrations in rats. The relevance of these results in estimating the risk of human exposure to therapeutic doses is unknown.

A fertility study was performed in rats; no evidence of impairment of fertility was encountered at oral doses up to 300 mg/kg per day.

Pregnancy: *Teratogenic Effects:* Pregnancy Category B. Reproduction studies have been performed in rabbits and rats at doses up to 15 to 45 times the human daily dose and have revealed no definitive evidence of impaired fertility or harm to the fetus due to bupropion. (In rabbits, a slightly increased incidence of fetal abnormalities was seen in two studies, but there was no increase in any specific abnormality.) There are no adequate and well-controlled studies in pregnant women. Because animal reproduction studies are not always predictive of human response, this drug should be used during pregnancy only if clearly needed.

To monitor fetal outcomes of pregnant women exposed to WELLBUTRIN, Glaxo Wellcome Inc. maintains a Bupropion Pregnancy Registry. Health care providers are encouraged to register patients by calling (800) 722-9292, ext. 39441.

Labor and Delivery: The effect of WELLBUTRIN on labor and delivery in humans is unknown.

Nursing Mothers: Like many other drugs, bupropion and its metabolites are secreted in human milk. Because of the potential for serious adverse reactions in nursing infants from WELLBUTRIN, a decision should be made whether to discontinue nursing or to discontinue the drug, taking into account the importance of the drug to the mother.

Pediatric Use: The safety and effectiveness of WELLBUTRIN in pediatric patients under 18 years old have not been established.

Use in the Elderly: WELLBUTRIN has not been systematically evaluated in older patients.

ADVERSE REACTIONS

(see also WARNINGS and PRECAUTIONS) Adverse events commonly encountered in patients treated with WELLBUTRIN are agitation, dry mouth, insomnia, headache/migraine, nausea/vomiting, constipation, and tremor. Adverse events were sufficiently troublesome to cause discontinuation of treatment with WELLBUTRIN in approximately ten percent of the 2400 patients and volunteers who participated in clinical trials during the product's initial development. The more common events causing discontinuation include neuropsychiatric disturbances (3.0%), primarily agitation and abnormalities in mental status; gastrointestinal disturbances (2.1%), primarily nausea and vomiting; neurological disturbances (1.7%), primarily seizures, headaches, and sleep disturbances; and dermatologic problems (1.4%), primarily rashes. It is important to note, however, that many of these events occurred at doses that exceed the recommended daily dose.

Accurate estimates of the incidence of adverse events associated with the use of any drug are difficult to obtain. Estimates are influenced by drug dose, detection technique, setting, physician judgments, etc. Consequently, the table below is presented solely to indicate the relative frequency of adverse events reported in representative controlled clinical studies conducted to evaluate the safety and efficacy of WELLBUTRIN under relatively similar conditions of daily dosage (300 to 600 mg), setting, and duration (3 to 4 weeks). The figures cited cannot be used to predict precisely the incidence of untoward events in the course of usual medical practice where patient characteristics and other factors must differ from those which prevailed in the clinical trials. These incidence figures also cannot be compared with those obtained from other clinical studies involving related drug products as each group of drug trials is conducted under a different set of conditions.

Finally, it is important to emphasize that the tabulation does not reflect the relative severity and/or clinical importance of the events. A better perspective on the serious adverse events associated with the use of WELLBUTRIN is provided in WARNINGS and PRECAUTIONS.

[See table at top of next page]

Other Events Observed During the Development of WELLBUTRIN: The conditions and duration of exposure to WELLBUTRIN varied greatly, and a substantial proportion of the experience was gained in open and uncontrolled clinical settings. During this experience, numerous adverse events were reported; however, without appropriate controls, it is impossible to determine with certainty which

Continued on next page

This product information is based on labeling in effect on June 1, 1998. For further information, contact via direct mail, phone, or web site Medical Information: Glaxo Wellcome Inc., PO Box 13398, Research Triangle Park, NC 27709. Healthcare Professionals (Medical Information): 800-334-0089 Patients (Customer Response Center): 888-TALK2GW (1-888-825-5249) Glaxo Wellcome Corporate Web Site: www.glaxowellcome.com

Wellbutrin—Cont.

events were or were not caused by WELLBUTRIN. The following enumeration is organized by organ system and describes events in terms of their relative frequency of reporting in the data base. Events of major clinical importance are also described in WARNINGS and PRECAUTIONS.

The following definitions of frequency are used: Frequent adverse events are defined as those occurring in at least 1/100 patients. Infrequent adverse events are those occurring in 1/100 to 1/1000 patients, while rare events are those occurring in less than 1/1000 patients.

Cardiovascular: Frequent was edema; infrequent were chest pain, electrocardiogram (ECG) abnormalities (premature beats and nonspecific ST-T changes), and shortness of breath/dyspnea; rare were flushing, pallor, phlebitis, and myocardial infarction.

Dermatologic: Frequent were nonspecific rashes; infrequent were alopecia and dry skin; rare were change in hair color, hirsutism, and acne.

Endocrine: Infrequent was gynecomastia; rare were glycosuria and hormone level change.

Gastrointestinal: Infrequent were dysphagia, thirst disturbance, and liver damage/jaundice; rare were rectal complaints, colitis, gastrointestinal bleeding, intestinal perforation, and stomach ulcer.

Genitourinary: Frequent was nocturia; infrequent were vaginal irritation, testicular swelling, urinary tract infection, painful erection, and retarded ejaculation; rare were dysuria, enuresis, urinary incontinence, menopause, ovarian disorder, pelvic infection, cystitis, dyspareunia, and painful ejaculation.

Hematologic/Oncologic: Rare were lymphadenopathy, anemia, and pancytopenia.

Musculoskeletal: Rare was musculosketetal chest pain.

Neurological: (see WARNINGS) Frequent were ataxia/incoordination, seizure, myoclonus, dyskinesia, and dystonia; infrequent were mydriasis, vertigo, and dysarthria; rare were electroencephalogram (EEG) abnormality, abnormal neurological exam, impaired attention, sciatica, and aphasia.

Neuropsychiatric: (see PRECAUTIONS) Frequent were mania/hypomania, increased libido, hallucinations, decrease in sexual function, and depression; infrequent were memory impairment, depersonalization, psychosis, dysphoria, mood instability, paranoia, formal thought disorder, and frigidity; rare was suicidal ideation.

Oral Complaints: Frequent was stomatitis; infrequent were toothache, bruxism, gum irritation, and oral edema; rare was glossitis.

Respiratory: Infrequent were bronchitis and shortness of breath/dyspnea; rare were epistaxis, rate or rhythm disorder, pneumonia, and pulmonary embolism.

Special Senses: Infrequent was visual disturbance; rare was diplopia.

Nonspecific: Frequent were flu-like symptoms; infrequent was nonspecific pain; rare were body odor, surgically related pain, infection, medication reaction, and overdose.

Postintroduction Reports: Voluntary reports of adverse events temporally associated with WELLBUTRIN that have been received since market introduction and which may have no causal relationship with the drug include the following:

Cardiovascular: orthostatic hypotension, third degree heart block

Endocrine: syndrome of inappropriate antidiuretic hormone secretion

Gastrointestinal: esophagitis, hepatitis, liver damage

Hemic and Lymphatic: ecchymosis, leukocytosis, leukopenia

Musculoskeletal: arthralgia, myalgia, muscle rigidity/fever/rhabdomyolysis

Nervous: coma, delirium, dream abnormalities, paresthesia, unmasking of tardive dyskinesia

Skin and Appendages: Stevens-Johnson syndrome, angioedema, exfoliative dermatitis, urticaria

Special Senses: tinnitus

DRUG ABUSE AND DEPENDENCE

Humans: Controlled clinical studies conducted in normal volunteers, in subjects with a history of multiple drug abuse, and in depressed patients showed some increase in motor activity and agitation/excitement.

In a population of individuals experienced with drugs of abuse, a single dose of 400 mg WELLBUTRIN produced mild amphetaminelike activity as compared to placebo on the Morphine-Benzedrine Subscale of the Addiction Research Center Inventories (ARCI) and a score intermediate between placebo and amphetamine on the Liking Scale of the ARCI. These scales measure general feelings of euphoria and drug desirability.

Findings in clinical trials, however, are not known to predict the abuse potential of drugs reliably. Nonetheless, evidence from single-dose studies does suggest that the recommended daily dosage of bupropion when administered in divided doses is not likely to be especially reinforcing to am-

phetamine or stimulant abusers. However, higher doses, which could not be tested because of the risk of seizure, might be modestly attractive to those who abuse stimulant drugs.

Animals: Studies in rodents have shown that bupropion exhibits some pharmacologic actions common to psychostimulants, including increases in locomotor activity and the production of a mild stereotyped behavior and increases in rates of responding in several schedule-controlled behavior paradigms. Drug discrimination studies in rats showed stimulus generalization between bupropion and amphetamine and other psychostimulants. Rhesus monkeys have been shown to self-administer bupropion intravenously.

OVERDOSAGE

Lethal Doses in Animals: In rats, the acute oral LD$_{50}$ values were 607 mg/kg (males) and 482 mg/kg (females). Respective values for mice were 544 mg/kg and 636 mg/kg. Signs of acute toxicity included labored breathing, salivation, arched back, ptosis, ataxia, and convulsions.

Human Overdose Experience: There has been limited clinical experience with overdosage of WELLBUTRIN. Thirteen overdoses occurred during clinical trials. Twelve patients ingested 850 to 4200 mg and recovered without significant sequelae. Another patient who ingested 9000 mg of WELLBUTRIN and 300 mg of tranylcypromine experienced a grand mal seizure and recovered without further sequelae.

Since introduction, overdoses of WELLBUTRIN up to 17500 mg have been reported. Seizure was reported in approximately one third of all cases. Other serious reactions reported with overdoses of WELLBUTRIN alone included hallucinations, loss of consciousness, and tachycardia. Fever, muscle rigidity, rhabdomyolysis, hypotension, stupor, coma, and respiratory failure have been reported when WELLBUTRIN was part of multiple drug overdoses.

Although most patients recovered without sequelae, deaths associated with overdoses of WELLBUTRIN alone have been reported rarely in patients ingesting massive doses of

WELLBUTRIN. Multiple uncontrolled seizures, bradycardia, cardiac failure, and cardiac arrest prior to death were reported in these patients.

Management of Overdose: Following suspected overdose, hospitalization is advised. If the patient is conscious, vomiting should be induced by syrup of ipecac. Activated charcoal also may be administered every 6 hours during the first 12 hours after ingestion. Baseline laboratory values should be obtained. ECG and EEG monitoring also are recommended for the next 48 hours. Adequate fluid intake should be provided.

If the patient is stuporous, comatose, or convulsing, airway intubation is recommended prior to undertaking gastric lavage. Although there is little clinical experience with lavage following an overdose of WELLBUTRIN, it is likely to be of benefit within the first 12 hours after ingestion since absorption of the drug may not yet be complete.

While diuresis, dialysis, or hemoperfusion are sometimes used to treat drug overdosage, there is no experience with their use in the management of overdoses of WELLBUTRIN. Because diffusion of WELLBUTRIN from tissue to plasma may be slow, dialysis may be of minimal benefit several hours after overdose.

Based on studies in animals, it is recommended that seizures be treated with an intravenous benzodiazepine preparation and other supportive measures, as appropriate.

Further information about the treatment of overdoses may be available from a poison control center.

DOSAGE AND ADMINISTRATION

General Dosing Considerations: It is particularly important to administer WELLBUTRIN in a manner most likely to minimize the risk of seizure (see WARNINGS). Increases in dose should not exceed 100 mg/day in a 3-day period. Gradual escalation in dosage is also important if agitation, motor restlessness, and insomnia, often seen during the initial days of treatment, are to be minimized. If necessary, these effects may be managed by temporary reduction of dose or the short-term administration of an intermediate to

Treatment Emergent Adverse Experience Incidence in Placebo-Controlled Clinical Trials* (Percent of Patients Reporting)

Adverse Experience	WELLBUTRIN Patients (n = 323)	Placebo Patients (n = 185)	Adverse Experience	WELLBUTRIN Patients (n = 323)	Placebo Patients (n = 185)
Cardiovascular			Dry mouth	27.6	18.4
Cardiac arrhythmias	5.3	4.3	Excessive sweating	22.3	14.6
Dizziness	22.3	16.2	Headache/migraine	25.7	22.2
Hypertension	4.3	1.6	Impaired sleep quality	4.0	1.6
Hypotension	2.5	2.2	Increased salivary flow	3.4	3.8
Palpitations	3.7	2.2	Insomnia	18.6	15.7
Syncope	1.2	0.5	Muscle spasms	1.9	3.2
Tachycardia	10.8	8.6	Pseudoparkinsonism	1.5	1.6
Dermatologic			Sedation	19.8	19.5
Pruritus	2.2	0.0	Sensory disturbance	4.0	3.2
Rash	8.0	6.5	Tremor	21.1	7.6
Gastrointestinal			Neuropsychiatric		
Anorexia	18.3	18.4	Agitation	31.9	22.2
Appetite increase	3.7	2.2	Anxiety	3.1	1.1
Constipation	26.0	17.3	Confusion	8.4	4.9
Diarrhea	6.8	8.6	Decreased libido	3.1	1.6
Dyspepsia	3.1	2.2	Delusions	1.2	1.1
Nausea/vomiting	22.9	18.9	Disturbed concentration	3.1	3.8
Weight gain	13.6	22.7	Euphoria	1.2	0.5
Weight loss	23.2	23.2	Hostility	5.6	3.8
Genitourinary			Nonspecific		
Impotence	3.4	3.1	Fatigue	5.0	8.6
Menstrual complaints	4.7	1.1	Fever/chills	1.2	0.5
Urinary frequency	2.5	2.2	Respiratory		
Urinary retention	1.9	2.2	Upper respiratory complaints	5.0	11.4
Musculoskeletal			Special Senses		
Arthritis	3.1	2.7	Auditory disturbance	5.3	3.2
Neurological			Blurred vision	14.6	10.3
Akathisia	1.5	1.1	Gustatory disturbance	3.1	1.1
Akinesia/Bradykinesia	8.0	8.6			
Cutaneous temperature disturbance	1.9	1.6			

* Events reported by at least 1% of patients receiving WELLBUTRIN are included.

Dosing Regimen

Treatment Day	Total Daily Dose	Tablet Strength	Number of Tablets		
			Morning	Midday	Evening
1	200 mg	100 mg	1	0	1
4	300 mg	100 mg	1	1	1

long-acting sedative hypnotic. A sedative hypnotic usually is not required beyond the first week of treatment. Insomnia may also be minimized by avoiding bedtime doses. If distressing, untoward effects supervene, dose escalation should be stopped.

No single dose of WELLBUTRIN should exceed 150 mg. WELLBUTRIN should be administered three times daily, preferably with at least 6 hours between successive doses.

Usual Dosage for Adults: The usual adult dose is 300 mg/day, given three times daily. Dosing should begin at 200 mg/day, given as 100 mg twice daily. Based on clinical response, this dose may be increased to 300 mg/day, given as 100 mg three times daily, no sooner than 3 days after beginning therapy (see table below).

[See second table at top of previous page]

Increasing the Dosage Above 300 mg/Day: As with other antidepressants, the full antidepressant effect of WELLBUTRIN may not be evident until 4 weeks of treatment or longer. An increase in dosage, up to a maximum of 450 mg/day, given in divided doses of not more than 150 mg each, may be considered for patients in whom no clinical improvement is noted after several weeks of treatment at 300 mg/day. Dosing above 300 mg/day may be accomplished using the 75 or 100 mg tablets. The 100-mg tablet must be administered four times daily with at least 4 hours between successive doses, in order not to exceed the limit of 150 mg in a single dose. WELLBUTRIN should be discontinued in patients who do not demonstrate an adequate response after an appropriate period of treatment at 450 mg/day.

Elderly Patients: In general, older patients are known to metabolize drugs more slowly and to be more sensitive to the anticholinergic, sedative, and cardiovascular side effects of antidepressant drugs. Clinical trials enrolled several hundred patients 60 years of age and older. The experience with these patients and younger ones was similar.

Maintenance: The lowest dose that maintains remission is recommended. Although it is not known how long the patient should remain on WELLBUTRIN, it is generally recognized that acute episodes of depression require several months or longer of antidepressant drug treatment.

HOW SUPPLIED

WELLBUTRIN Tablets, 75 mg of bupropion hydrochloride, are yellow-gold, round, biconvex tablets printed with "WELLBUTRIN 75" in bottles of 100 (NDC 0173-0177-55).

WELLBUTRIN Tablets, 100 mg of bupropion hydrochloride, are red, round, biconvex tablets printed with "WELLBUTRIN 100" in bottles of 100 (NDC 0173-0178-55).

Store at 15° to 25°C (59° to 77°F). Protect from light and moisture.

©Copyright 1996 Glaxo Wellcome Inc. All rights reserved.

October 1997/RL-477

Shown in Product Identification Guide, page 314

WELLBUTRIN SR® ℞

(bupropion hydrochloride)
Sustained-Release Tablets

DESCRIPTION

WELLBUTRIN SR (bupropion hydrochloride), an antidepressant of the aminoketone class, is chemically unrelated to tricyclic, tetracyclic, selective serotonin re-uptake inhibitor, or other known antidepressant agents. Its structure closely resembles that of diethylpropion; it is related to phenylethylamines. It is (±)-1-(3-chlorophenyl)-2-[(1,1-dimethylethyl)amino]-1-propanone hydrochloride. The molecular weight is 276.2. The molecular formula is $C_{13}H_{18}ClNO{\cdot}HCl$. Bupropion hydrochloride powder is white, crystalline, and highly soluble in water. It has a bitter taste and produces the sensation of local anesthesia on the oral mucosa.

WELLBUTRIN SR Tablets are supplied for oral administration as 100-mg (blue) and 150-mg (purple), film-coated, sustained-release tablets. Each tablet contains the labeled amount of bupropion hydrochloride and the inactive ingredients: carnauba wax, cysteine hydrochloride, hydroxypropyl methylcellulose, magnesium stearate, microcrystalline cellulose, polyethylene glycol, and titanium dioxide and is printed with edible black ink. In addition, the 100-mg tablet contains FD&C Blue No. 1 Lake and polysorbate 80, and the 150-mg tablet contains FD&C Blue No. 2 Lake, FD&C Red No. 40 Lake, and polysorbate 80.

CLINICAL PHARMACOLOGY

Pharmacodynamics: Bupropion is a relatively weak inhibitor of the neuronal uptake of norepinephrine, serotonin, and dopamine, and does not inhibit monoamine oxidase. While the mechanism of action of bupropion, as with other antidepressants, is unknown, it is presumed that this action is mediated by noradrenergic and/or dopaminergic mechanisms.

Pharmacokinetics: Following oral administration of WELLBUTRIN SR Tablets to healthy volunteers, peak plasma concentrations of bupropion are achieved within 3 hours. Food increased C_{max} and AUC of bupropion by 11% and 17%, respectively, indicating that there is no clinically significant food effect.

In vitro tests show that bupropion is 80% or more bound to human albumin at plasma concentrations up to 200 mcg/mL. Plasma protein binding of the major metabolites of bupropion has not been studied.

Following oral administration of 200 mg of ^{14}C-bupropion in humans, 87% and 10% of the radioactive dose were recovered in the urine and feces, respectively. The fraction of the oral dose of bupropion excreted unchanged was only 0.5%, a finding consistent with the extensive metabolism of bupropion.

The mean elimination half-life (±SD) of bupropion after chronic dosing is 21 (±9) hours, and steady-state plasma concentrations of bupropion are reached within 8 days.

Plasma and urinary metabolites so far identified include biotransformation products formed via reduction of the carbonyl group and/or hydroxylation of the *tert*-butyl group of bupropion. Four basic metabolites have been identified. They are the *erythro-* and *threo*-amino alcohols of bupropion, the *erythro*-amino diol of bupropion, and a morpholinol metabolite (formed from hydroxylation of the *tert*-butyl group of bupropion). These metabolites of bupropion are pharmacologically active, but their potency and toxicity relative to bupropion have not been fully characterized. They may be of clinical importance because the plasma concentrations of the metabolites are higher than those of bupropion.

Following a single dose in humans, peak plasma concentrations of the morpholinol metabolite occur approximately 6 hours after administration of WELLBUTRIN SR Tablets. Peak plasma concentrations of the morpholinol metabolite are approximately 10 times the peak level of the parent drug at steady state with WELLBUTRIN SR Tablets. The elimination half-life of the morpholinol metabolite is approximately 20 (±5) hours, and its AUC at steady state is about 17 times that of bupropion.

The times to peak concentrations for the *erythro-* and *threo*-amino alcohol metabolites are similar to that of the morpholinol metabolite. However, their elimination half-lives are longer, 33 (±10) and 37 (±13) hours, respectively, and steady-state AUCs are 1.5 and 7 times that of bupropion.

The *erythro*-amino diol metabolite generally cannot be detected in the systemic circulation following a single oral dose of the parent drug.

In a study comparing chronic dosing with WELLBUTRIN SR Tablets 150 mg twice daily to the immediate-release formulation of bupropion at 100 mg three times daily, peak plasma concentrations of bupropion at steady state for WELLBUTRIN SR Tablets were approximately 85% of those achieved with the immediate-release formulation. There was equivalence for bupropion AUCs, as well as equivalence for both peak plasma concentration and AUCs for all three of the detectable bupropion metabolites. Thus, at steady state, WELLBUTRIN SR Tablets and the immediate-release formulation of bupropion are essentially bioequivalent for both bupropion and the three quantitatively important metabolites.

Bupropion and its metabolites exhibit linear kinetics following chronic administration of 300 to 450 mg/day.

Population Subgroups: Factors or conditions altering metabolic capacity (e.g., liver disease, congestive heart failure, age, concomitant medications, etc.) or elimination may be expected to influence the degree and extent of accumulation of the active metabolites of bupropion. The elimination of the major metabolites of bupropion may be affected by reduced renal or hepatic function because they are moderately polar compounds and are likely to undergo further metabolism or conjugation in the liver prior to urinary excretion.

Hepatic: The disposition of bupropion following a single 200-mg oral dose was compared in eight healthy volunteers and eight weight- and age-matched volunteers with alcoholic liver disease. The half-life of the morpholinol metabolite was significantly prolonged in subjects with alcoholic liver disease (32 hours [±41%] versus 21 hours [±23%]). The differences in half-life for bupropion and the other metabolites in the two patient groups were minimal.

Renal: The effect of renal disease on the pharmacokinetics of bupropion has not been studied. The elimination of the major metabolites of bupropion may be affected by reduced renal function.

Left Ventricular Dysfunction: During a chronic dosing study with bupropion in 14 depressed patients with left ventricular dysfunction (history of congestive heart failure or an enlarged heart on x-ray), there was substantial interpatient variability (twofold to fivefold) in the trough steady-state concentrations of bupropion and the morpholinol and *threo*-amino alcohol metabolites. This variability was in the same range of the variability observed in healthy volunteers (threefold to eightfold). In addition, the steady-state plasma concentrations of these metabolites were 10 to 100 times the steady-state concentrations of the parent drug.

Age: The effects of age on the pharmacokinetics of bupropion and its metabolites have not been fully characterized, but an exploration of steady-state bupropion concentrations from several efficacy studies involving patients dosed in a range of 300 to 750 mg/day, on a three times daily schedule, revealed no relationship between age (18 to 83 years) and plasma concentration of bupropion. These data suggest there is no prominent effect of age on bupropion concentration (see PRECAUTIONS: Use in the Elderly).

Gender: A single-dose study involving 12 healthy male and 12 healthy female volunteers revealed no sex-related differences in the pharmacokinetic parameters of bupropion.

Clinical Trials: The efficacy of the immediate-release formulation of bupropion as a treatment for depression was established in two 4-week, placebo-controlled trials in adult inpatients with depression and in one 6-week, placebo-controlled trial in adult outpatients with depression. In the first study, patients were titrated in a bupropion dose range of 300 to 600 mg/day on a three times daily schedule; 78% of patients received maximum doses of 450 mg/day or less. This trial demonstrated the effectiveness of the immediate-release formulation of bupropion on the Hamilton Depression Rating Scale (HDRS) total score, the depressed mood item (item 1) from that scale, and the Clinical Global Impressions (CGI) severity score. A second study included two fixed doses of the immediate-release formulation of bupropion (300 and 450 mg/day) and placebo. This trial demonstrated the effectiveness of the immediate-release formulation of bupropion, but only at the 450-mg/day dose; the results were positive for the HDRS total score and the CGI severity score, but not for HDRS item 1. In the third study, outpatients received 300 mg/day of the immediate-release formulation of bupropion. This study demonstrated the effectiveness of the immediate-release formulation of bupropion on the HDRS total score, HDRS item 1, the Montgomery-Asberg Depression Rating Scale, the CGI severity score, and the CGI improvement score.

Although there are not as yet independent trials demonstrating the antidepressant effectiveness of the sustained-release formulation of bupropion, studies have demonstrated the bioequivalence of the immediate-release and sustained-release forms of bupropion under steady-state conditions, i.e., bupropion sustained-release 150 mg twice daily was shown to be bioequivalent to 100 mg three times daily of the immediate-release formulation of bupropion, with regard to both rate and extent of absorption, for parent drug and metabolites.

INDICATIONS AND USAGE

WELLBUTRIN SR is indicated for the treatment of depression.

A physician considering WELLBUTRIN SR Tablets for the management of a patient's first episode of depression should be aware that the drug may cause generalized seizures in a dose-dependent manner with an approximate incidence of 0.4% (4/1000) at the upper end of the recommended dose range, i.e., 400 mg/day, and an incidence of 0.1% (1/1000) at a bupropion dose of 300 mg/day. Bupropion's seizure incidence at the 400-mg/day dose may exceed that of other marketed antidepressants and doses of WELLBUTRIN SR Tablets up to 300 mg/day by as much as fourfold. This relative risk is only an approximate estimate because no direct comparative studies have been conducted (see WARNINGS).

The efficacy of bupropion in the treatment of depression was established in two 4-week controlled trials of depressed inpatients and in one 6-week controlled trial of depressed outpatients whose diagnoses corresponded most closely to the Major Depression category of the APA Diagnostic and Statistical Manual (DSM) (see CLINICAL PHARMACOLOGY).

A major depressive episode (DSM-IV) implies the presence of 1) depressed mood or 2) loss of interest or pleasure; in addition, at least five of the following symptoms have been present during the same 2-week period and represent a change from previous functioning: depressed mood, markedly diminished interest or pleasure in usual activities, significant change in weight and/or appetite, insomnia or hypersomnia, psychomotor agitation or retardation, increased fatigue, feelings of guilt or worthlessness, slowed thinking or impaired concentration, a suicide attempt or suicidal ideation.

Effectiveness of bupropion in long-term use (more than 6 weeks) has not been systematically evaluated in controlled trials. Therefore, the physician who elects to use WELLBUTRIN SR Tablets for extended periods should periodically reevaluate the long-term usefulness of the drug for the individual patient.

CONTRAINDICATIONS

WELLBUTRIN SR is contraindicated in patients with a seizure disorder.

Continued on next page

This product information is based on labeling in effect on June 1, 1998. For further information, contact via direct mail, phone, or web site Medical Information: Glaxo Wellcome Inc., PO Box 13398, Research Triangle Park, NC 27709. Healthcare Professionals (Medical Information): 800-334-0089 Patients (Customer Response Center): 888-TALK2GW (1-888-825-5249) Glaxo Wellcome Corporate Web Site: www.glaxowellcome.com

Wellbutrin SR—Cont.

WELLBUTRIN SR is contraindicated in patients treated with ZYBAN™ (bupropion hydrochloride) Sustained-Release Tablets, or any other medications that contain bupropion because the incidence of seizure is dose dependent. WELLBUTRIN SR is contraindicated in patients with a current or prior diagnosis of bulimia or anorexia nervosa because of a higher incidence of seizures noted in such patients treated with the immediate-release formulation of bupropion.

The concurrent administration of WELLBUTRIN SR Tablets and a monoamine oxidase (MAO) inhibitor is contraindicated. At least 14 days should elapse between discontinuation of an MAO inhibitor and initiation of treatment with WELLBUTRIN SR Tablets.

WELLBUTRIN SR is contraindicated in patients who have shown an allergic response to bupropion or the other ingredients that make up WELLBUTRIN SR Tablets.

WARNINGS

Patients should be made aware that WELLBUTRIN SR contains the same active ingredient found in ZYBAN, used as an aid to smoking cessation treatment, and that WELLBUTRIN SR should not be used in combination with ZYBAN, or any other medications that contain bupropion.
Seizures: Bupropion is associated with a dose-related risk of seizures. At doses of WELLBUTRIN SR up to a dose of 300 mg/day, the incidence of seizures is approximately 0.1% (1/1000) but increases to approximately 0.4% (4/1000) at the maximum recommended dose of 400 mg/day. The risk of seizure also appears to be strongly associated with the presence of predisposing factors.

Data for the immediate-release bupropion revealed a seizure incidence of approximately 0.4% (i.e., 13 of 3200 patients followed prospectively) in patients treated at doses in a range of 300 to 450 mg/day. The 450-mg/day upper limit of this dose range is close to the currently recommended maximum dose of 400 mg/day for WELLBUTRIN SR Tablets. This seizure incidence (0.4%) may exceed that of other marketed antidepressants and doses of WELLBUTRIN SR Tablets up to 300 mg/day by as much as fourfold. This relative risk is only an approximate estimate because no direct comparative studies have been conducted.

Additional data accumulated for the immediate-release formulation of bupropion suggested that the estimated seizure incidence increases almost tenfold between 450 and 600 mg/day, which is twice the usual adult target dose and one and one-half the maximum recommended daily dose (400 mg) of WELLBUTRIN SR Tablets. Given the wide variability among individuals and their capacity to metabolize and eliminate drugs, this disproportionate increase in seizure incidence with dose incrementation calls for caution in dosing.

Data for WELLBUTRIN SR Tablets revealed a seizure incidence of approximately 0.1% (i.e., 3 of 3100 patients followed prospectively) in patients treated at doses in a range of 100 to 300 mg/day. It is not possible to know if the lower seizure incidence observed in this study involving the sustained-release formulation of bupropion resulted from the different formulation or the lower dose used. However, as noted above, the immediate-release and sustained-release formulations are bioequivalent regarding both rate and extent of absorption during steady state, the most pertinent condition to estimating seizure incidence since most observed seizures occur under steady-state conditions.

The risk of seizure is also related to patient factors, clinical situations, and concomitant medications, which must be considered in selection of patients for therapy with WELLBUTRIN SR.

• **Patient factors: Predisposing factors that may increase the risk of seizure with bupropion use include history of head trauma or prior seizure, central nervous system (CNS) tumor, and concomitant medications that lower seizure threshold.**
• **Clinical situations: Circumstances associated with an increased seizure risk include, among others, excessive use of alcohol; abrupt withdrawal from alcohol or other sedatives; addiction to opiates, cocaine, or stimulants; use of over-the-counter stimulants and anorectics; and diabetes treated with oral hypoglycemics or insulin.**
• **Concomitant medications: Many medications (e.g., antipsychotics, antidepressants, theophylline, systemic steroids) and treatment regimens (e.g., abrupt discontinuation of benzodiazepines) are known to lower seizure threshold.**

Recommendations for Reducing the Risk of Seizure: Retrospective analysis of clinical experience gained during the development of bupropion suggests that the risk of seizure may be minimized if

• the total daily dose of WELLBUTRIN SR Tablets does *not* exceed 400 mg,
• the daily dose is administered twice daily, and
• the rate of incrementation of dose is gradual.

• No single dose should exceed 200 mg to avoid high peak concentrations of bupropion and/or its metabolites.
• **WELLBUTRIN SR should be administered with extreme caution to patients with a history of seizure, cranial trauma, or other predisposition(s) toward seizure, or patients treated with other agents (e.g., antipsychotics, other antidepressants, theophylline, systemic steroids, etc.) or treatment regimens (e.g., abrupt discontinuation of a benzodiazepine) that lower seizure threshold.**

Potential for Hepatotoxicity: In rats receiving large doses of bupropion chronically, there was an increase in incidence of hepatic hyperplastic nodules and hepatocellular hypertrophy. In dogs receiving large doses of bupropion chronically, various histologic changes were seen in the liver, and laboratory tests suggesting mild hepatocellular injury were noted.

PRECAUTIONS

General: *Agitation and Insomnia:* Patients in placebo-controlled trials with WELLBUTRIN SR Tablets experienced agitation, anxiety, and insomnia as shown in Table 1.

Table 1: Incidence of Agitation, Anxiety, and Insomnia in Placebo-Controlled Trials

Adverse Event Term	WELLBUTRIN SR 300 mg/day (n = 376)	WELLBUTRIN SR 400 mg/day (n = 114)	Placebo (n = 385)
Agitation	3%	9%	2%
Anxiety	5%	6%	3%
Insomnia	11%	16%	6%

In clinical studies, these symptoms were sometimes of sufficient magnitude to require treatment with sedative/hypnotic drugs.
Symptoms were sufficiently severe to require discontinuation of treatment in 1% and 2.6% of patients treated with 300 and 400 mg/day, respectively, of WELLBUTRIN SR Tablets and 0.8% of patients treated with placebo.
Psychosis, Confusion, and Other Neuropsychiatric Phenomena: Patients treated with an immediate-release formulation of bupropion or with WELLBUTRIN SR Tablets have been reported to show a variety of neuropsychiatric signs and symptoms, including delusions, hallucinations, psychosis, concentration disturbance, paranoia, and confusion. In some cases, these symptoms abated upon dose reduction and/or withdrawal of treatment.
Activation of Psychosis and/or Mania: Antidepressants can precipitate manic episodes in bipolar disorder patients during the depressed phase of their illness and may activate latent psychosis in other susceptible patients. WELLBUTRIN SR is expected to pose similar risks.
Altered Appetite and Weight: In placebo-controlled studies, patients experienced weight gain or weight loss as shown in Table 2.

Table 2: Incidence of Weight Gain and Weight Loss in Placebo-Controlled Trials

Weight Change	WELLBUTRIN SR 300 mg/day (n = 339)	WELLBUTRIN SR 400 mg/day (n = 112)	Placebo (n = 347)
Gained >5 lbs	3%	2%	4%
Lost >5 lbs	14%	19%	6%

In studies conducted with the immediate-release formulation of bupropion, 35% of patients receiving tricyclic antidepressants gained weight, compared to 9% of patients treated with the immediate-release formulation of bupropion. If weight loss is a major presenting sign of a patient's depressive illness, the anorectic and/or weight-reducing potential of WELLBUTRIN SR Tablets should be considered.
Suicide: The possibility of a suicide attempt is inherent in depression and may persist until significant remission occurs. Accordingly, prescriptions for WELLBUTRIN SR Tablets should be written for the smallest number of tablets consistent with good patient management.
Allergic Reactions: Anaphylactoid reactions characterized by symptoms such as pruritus, urticaria, angioedema, and dyspnea requiring medical treatment have been reported in clinical trials with bupropion. In addition, there have been rare spontaneous postmarketing reports of erythema multiforme, Stevens-Johnson syndrome, and anaphylactic shock associated with bupropion.
Use in Patients With Systemic Illness: There is no clinical experience establishing the safety of WELLBUTRIN SR Tablets in patients with a recent history of myocardial infarction or unstable heart disease. Therefore, care should be exercised if it is used in these groups. Bupropion was well tolerated in patients who had previously developed orthostatic hypotension while receiving tricyclic antidepressants,

and was also generally well tolerated in a group of 36 depressed inpatients with stable congestive heart failure (CHF). However, bupropion was associated with a rise in supine blood pressure in the study of patients with CHF, resulting in discontinuation of two patients for exacerbation of baseline hypertension.
Because bupropion hydrochloride and its metabolites are almost completely excreted through the kidney and metabolites are likely to undergo conjugation in the liver prior to urinary excretion, treatment of patients with renal or hepatic impairment should be initiated at reduced dosage as bupropion and its metabolites may accumulate in such patients to a greater extent than usual. The patient should be closely monitored for possible toxic effects of elevated blood and tissue levels of drug and metabolites.
Information for Patients: Patients should be made aware that WELLBUTRIN SR contains the same active ingredient found in ZYBAN, used as an aid to smoking cessation, and that WELLBUTRIN SR should not be used in combination with ZYBAN or any other medications that contain bupropion hydrochloride.
Physicians are advised to discuss the following issues with patients:
As dose is increased during initial titration to doses above 150 mg/day, patients should be instructed to take WELLBUTRIN SR Tablets in two divided doses, preferably with at least 8 hours between successive doses, to minimize the risk of seizures.
Patients should be told that any CNS-active drug like WELLBUTRIN SR Tablets may impair their ability to perform tasks requiring judgment or motor and cognitive skills. Consequently, until they are reasonably certain that WELLBUTRIN SR Tablets do not adversely affect their performance, they should refrain from driving an automobile or operating complex, hazardous machinery.
Patients should be told that the use and cessation of use of alcohol may alter the seizure threshold, and, therefore, that the consumption of alcohol should be minimized, and, if possible, avoided completely.
Patients should be advised to inform their physicians if they are taking or plan to take any prescription or over-the-counter drugs. Concern is warranted because WELLBUTRIN SR Tablets and other drugs may affect each other's metabolism.
Patients should be advised to notify their physicians if they become pregnant or intend to become pregnant during therapy.
Patients should be advised to swallow WELLBUTRIN SR Tablets whole so that the release rate is not altered. Do not chew, divide, or crush tablets.
Laboratory Tests: There are no specific laboratory tests recommended.
Drug Interactions: Although no systematic data have been collected on the consequences of the concomitant administration of WELLBUTRIN SR Tablets and other drugs, animal data suggest that bupropion may be an inducer of drug-metabolizing enzymes. This may be of potential clinical importance because the blood levels of coadministered drugs may be altered.
Alternatively, because bupropion is extensively metabolized, the coadministration of other drugs may affect its clinical activity. In particular, certain drugs may induce the metabolism of bupropion (e.g., carbamazepine, phenobarbital, phenytoin), while other drugs may inhibit the metabolism of bupropion (e.g., cimetidine).
In vitro studies indicate that bupropion is primarily metabolized to the morpholinol metabolite by the cytochrome $P_{450}IIB_6$ isoenzyme. Therefore, the potential exists for a drug interaction between WELLBUTRIN SR and drugs that affect the cytochrome $P_{450}IIB_6$ metabolism (e.g., orphenadrine and cyclophosphamide). The *threo*-amino alcohol metabolite of bupropion does not appear to be produced by the cytochrome P_{450} system.
Studies in animals demonstrate that the acute toxicity of bupropion is enhanced by the MAO inhibitor phenelzine (see CONTRAINDICATIONS).
Limited clinical data suggest a higher incidence of adverse experiences in patients receiving concurrent administration of bupropion and levodopa. Administration of WELLBUTRIN SR Tablets to patients receiving levodopa concurrently should be undertaken with caution, using small initial doses and gradual dose increases.
Concurrent administration of WELLBUTRIN SR Tablets and agents (e.g., antipsychotics, other antidepressants, theophylline, systemic steroids, etc.) or treatment regimens (e.g., abrupt discontinuation of benzodiazepines) that lower seizure threshold should be undertaken only with extreme caution (see WARNINGS). Low initial dosing and gradual dose increases should be employed.
Carcinogenesis, Mutagenesis, Impairment of Fertility: Lifetime carcinogenicity studies were performed in rats and mice at doses up to 300 and 150 mg/kg per day, respectively. These doses are approximately seven and two times the maximum recommended human dose (MRHD), respectively, on a mg/m^2 basis. In the rat study there was an increase in nodular proliferative lesions of the liver at doses of 100 to

300 mg/kg per day (approximately two to seven times the MRHD on a mg/m² basis); lower doses were not tested. The question of whether or not such lesions may be precursors of neoplasms of the liver is currently unresolved. Similar liver lesions were not seen in the mouse study, and no increase in malignant tumors of the liver and other organs was seen in either study.

Bupropion produced a positive response (two to three times control mutation rate) in two of five strains in the Ames bacterial mutagenicity test and an increase in chromosomal aberrations in one of three in vivo rat bone marrow cytogenetic studies.

A fertility study in rats at doses up to 300 mg/kg revealed no evidence of impaired fertility.

Pregnancy: *Teratogenic Effects: Pregnancy Category B:* Teratology studies have been performed at doses up to 450 mg/kg in rats, and at doses up to 150 mg/kg in rabbits (approximately 7 to 11 and 7 times the MRHD, respectively, on a mg/m² basis), and have revealed no evidence of harm to the fetus due to bupropion. There are no adequate and well-controlled studies in pregnant women. Because animal reproduction studies are not always predictive of human response, this drug should be used during pregnancy only if clearly needed.

To monitor fetal outcomes of pregnant women exposed to WELLBUTRIN SR, Glaxo Wellcome Inc. maintains a Bupropion Pregnancy Registry. Health care providers are encouraged to register patients by calling (800) 722-9292, ext. 39441.

Labor and Delivery: The effect of WELLBUTRIN SR Tablets on labor and delivery in humans is unknown.

Nursing Mothers: Like many other drugs, bupropion and its metabolites are secreted in human milk. Because of the potential for serious adverse reactions in nursing infants from WELLBUTRIN SR Tablets, a decision should be made whether to discontinue nursing or to discontinue the drug, taking into account the importance of the drug to the mother.

Pediatric Use: The safety and effectiveness of WELLBUTRIN SR Tablets in pediatric patients below 18 years old have not been established.

Use in the Elderly: In general, older patients are known to metabolize drugs more slowly and to be more sensitive to the anticholinergic, sedative, and cardiovascular side effects of antidepressant drugs. A single-dose pharmacokinetic study demonstrated that the disposition of bupropion and its metabolites in elderly subjects was similar to that of younger subjects (see CLINICAL PHARMACOLOGY). Of the approximately 4100 patients who participated in clinical trials with WELLBUTRIN SR Tablets, 204 were 60 to 69 years old and 68 were 70 years of age or older. The experience with patients 60 years of age or older was similar to that in younger patients.

ADVERSE REACTIONS

(See also WARNINGS and PRECAUTIONS)
The information included under the Incidence in Controlled Trials subsection of ADVERSE REACTIONS is based primarily on data from controlled clinical trials with WELLBUTRIN SR Tablets. Information on additional adverse events associated with the sustained-release formulation of bupropion in smoking cessation trials, as well as the immediate-release formulation of bupropion, is included in a separate section (see Other Events Observed During the Clinical Development and Postmarketing Experience of Bupropion).

Incidence in Controlled Trials With WELLBUTRIN SR: *Adverse Events Associated With Discontinuation of Treatment Among Patients Treated With WELLBUTRIN SR Tablets:* In placebo-controlled clinical trials, 9% and 11% of patients treated with 300 and 400 mg/day, respectively, of WELLBUTRIN SR Tablets and 4% of patients treated with placebo discontinued treatment due to adverse events. The specific adverse events in these trials that led to discontinuation in at least 1% of patients treated with either 300 or 400 mg/day of WELLBUTRIN SR Tablets and at a rate at least twice the placebo rate are listed in Table 3.

Table 3: Treatment Discontinuations Due to Adverse Events in Placebo-Controlled Trials

Adverse Event Term	WELLBUTRIN SR 300 mg/day (n = 376)	WELLBUTRIN SR 400 mg/day (n = 114)	Placebo (n = 385)
Rash	2.4%	0.9%	0.0%
Nausea	0.8%	1.8%	0.3%
Agitation	0.3%	1.8%	0.3%
Migraine	0.0%	1.8%	0.3%

Adverse Events Occurring at an Incidence of 1% or More Among Patients Treated With WELLBUTRIN SR Tablets: Table 4 enumerates treatment-emergent adverse events that occurred among patients treated with 300 and 400 mg/day of WELLBUTRIN SR Tablets and with placebo in placebo-controlled trials. Events that occurred in either the 300- or 400-mg/day group at an incidence of 1% or more and were more frequent than in the placebo group are included. Reported adverse events were classified using a COSTART-based Dictionary.

Accurate estimates of the incidence of adverse events associated with the use of any drug are difficult to obtain. Estimates are influenced by drug dose, detection technique, setting, physician judgments, etc. The figures cited cannot be used to predict precisely the incidence of untoward events in the course of usual medical practice where patient characteristics and other factors differ from those that prevailed in the clinical trials. These incidence figures also cannot be compared with those obtained from other clinical studies involving related drug products as each group of drug trials is conducted under a different set of conditions.

Finally, it is important to emphasize that the tabulation does not reflect the relative severity and/or clinical importance of the events. A better perspective on the serious adverse events associated with the use of WELLBUTRIN SR Tablets is provided in the WARNINGS and PRECAUTIONS sections.

Table 4: Treatment-Emergent Adverse Events in Placebo-Controlled Trials*

Body System/ Adverse Event	WELLBUTRIN SR 300 mg/day (n = 376)	WELLBUTRIN SR 400 mg/day (n = 114)	Placebo (n = 385)
Body (General)			
Headache	26%	25%	23%
Infection	8%	9%	6%
Abdominal pain	3%	9%	2%
Asthenia	2%	4%	2%
Chest pain	3%	4%	1%
Pain	2%	3%	2%
Fever	1%	2%	—
Cardiovascular			
Palpitation	2%	6%	2%
Flushing	1%	4%	—
Migraine	1%	4%	1%
Hot flashes	1%	3%	1%
Digestive			
Dry mouth	17%	24%	7%
Nausea	13%	18%	8%
Constipation	10%	5%	7%
Diarrhea	5%	7%	6%
Anorexia	5%	3%	2%
Vomiting	4%	2%	2%
Dysphagia	0%	2%	0%
Musculoskeletal			
Myalgia	2%	6%	3%
Arthralgia	1%	4%	1%
Arthritis	0%	2%	0%
Twitch	1%	2%	—
Nervous system			
Insomnia	11%	16%	6%
Dizziness	7%	11%	5%
Agitation	3%	9%	2%
Anxiety	5%	6%	3%
Tremor	6%	3%	1%
Nervousness	5%	3%	3%
Somnolence	2%	3%	2%
Irritability	3%	2%	2%
Memory decreased	—	3%	1%
Paresthesia	1%	2%	1%
CNS stimulation	2%	1%	1%
Respiratory			
Pharyngitis	3%	11%	2%
Sinusitis	3%	1%	2%
Increased cough	1%	2%	1%
Skin			
Sweating	6%	5%	2%
Rash	5%	4%	1%
Pruritus	2%	4%	2%
Urticaria	2%	1%	0%
Special senses			
Tinnitus	6%	6%	2%
Taste perversion	2%	4%	—
Amblyopia	3%	2%	2%
Urogenital			
Urinary frequency	2%	5%	2%
Urinary urgency	—	2%	0%
Vaginal hemorrhage†	0%	2%	—
Urinary tract infection	1%	0%	—

* Adverse events that occurred in at least 1% of patients treated with either 300 or 400 mg/day of WELLBUTRIN SR Tablets, but equally or more frequently in the placebo group, were: abnormal dreams, accidental injury, acne, appetite increased, back pain, bronchitis, dysmenorrhea, dyspepsia, flatulence, flu syndrome, hypertension, neck pain, respiratory disorder, rhinitis, and tooth disorder.
† Incidence based on the number of female patients.
—Hyphen denotes adverse events occurring in greater than 0 but less than 0.5% of patients.

Incidence of Commonly Observed Adverse Events in Controlled Clinical Trials: Adverse events from Table 4 occurring in at least 5% of patients treated with WELLBUTRIN SR Tablets and at a rate at least twice the placebo rate are listed below for the 300- and 400-mg/day dose groups.
WELLBUTRIN SR 300 mg/day: Anorexia, dry mouth, rash, sweating, tinnitus, and tremor.
WELLBUTRIN SR 400 mg/day: Abdominal pain, agitation, anxiety, dizziness, dry mouth, insomnia, myalgia, nausea, palpitation, pharyngitis, sweating, tinnitus, and urinary frequency.

Other Events Observed During the Clinical Development and Postmarketing Experience of Bupropion: In addition to the adverse events noted above, the following events have been reported in clinical trials with the sustained-release formulation of bupropion in depressed patients and in nondepressed smokers, as well as in clinical trials and postmarketing clinical experience with the immediate-release formulation of bupropion.

Adverse events for which frequencies are provided below occurred in clinical trials with the sustained-release formulation of bupropion. The frequencies represent the proportion of patients who experienced a treatment-emergent adverse event on at least one occasion in placebo-controlled studies for depression (n = 987) or smoking cessation (n = 1013), or patients who experienced an adverse event requiring discontinuation of treatment in an open-label surveillance study with WELLBUTRIN SR Tablets (n = 3100). All treatment-emergent adverse events are included except those listed in Tables 1 through 4, those events listed in other safety-related sections, those adverse events subsumed under COSTART terms that are either overly general or excessively specific so as to be uninformative, those events not reasonably associated with the use of the drug, and those events that were not serious and occurred in fewer than two patients Events of major clinical importance are described in the WARNINGS and PRECAUTIONS sections of the labeling.

Events are further categorized by body system and listed in order of decreasing frequency according to the following definitions of frequency: Frequent adverse events are defined as those occurring in at least 1/100 patients. Infrequent adverse events are those occurring in 1/100 to 1/1000 patients, while rare events are those occurring in less than 1/1000 patients.

Adverse events for which frequencies are not provided occurred in clinical trials or postmarketing experience with the immediate-release formulation of bupropion. Only those adverse events not previously listed for sustained-release bupropion are included. The extent to which these events may be associated with WELLBUTRIN SR is unknown.

Body (General): Infrequent were chills, facial edema, musculoskeletal chest pain, and photosensitivity. Rare was malaise.

Cardiovascular: Infrequent were postural hypotension, stroke, tachycardia, and vasodilation. Rare was syncope. Also observed were complete AV block, extrasystoles, hypotension, myocardial infarction, phlebitis, and pulmonary embolism.

Digestive: Infrequent were abnormal liver function, bruxism, gastric reflux, gingivitis, glossitis, increased salivation, jaundice, mouth ulcers, stomatitis, and thirst. Rare was edema of tongue. Also observed were colitis, esophagitis, gastrointestinal hermorrhage, gum hemorrhage, hepatitis, intestinal perforation, liver damage, pancreatitis, and stomach ulcer.

Endocrine: Also observed was syndrome of inappropriate antidiuretic hormone.

Hemic and Lymphatic: Infrequent was ecchymosis. Also observed were anemia, leukocytosis, leukopenia, lymphadenopathy, and pancytopenia.

Metabolic and Nutritional: Infrequent were edema and peripheral edema. Also observed was glycosuria.

Musculoskeletal: Infrequent were leg cramps. Also observed were muscle rigidity/fever/rhabdomyolysis.

Continued on next page

This product information is based on labeling in effect on June 1, 1998. For further information, contact via direct mail, phone, or web site Medical Information: Glaxo Wellcome Inc., PO Box 13398, Research Triangle Park, NC 27709. Healthcare Professionals (Medical Information): 800-334-0089 Patients (Customer Response Center): 888-TALK2GW (1-888-825-5249) Glaxo Wellcome Corporate Web Site: www.glaxowellcome.com

Wellbutrin SR—Cont.

Nervous System: Infrequent were abnormal coordination, decreased libido, depersonalization, dysphoria, emotional lability, hostility, hyperkinesia, hypertonia, hypesthesia, suicidal ideation, and vertigo. Rare were amnesia, ataxia, derealization, and hypomania. Also observed were abnormal electroencephalogram (EEG), akinesia, aphasia, coma, delirium, dysarthria, dyskinesia, dystonia, euphoria, extrapyramidal syndrome, hypokinesia, increased libido, manic reaction, neuralgia, neuropathy, paranoid reaction, and unmasking tardive dyskinesia.

Respiratory: Rare was bronchospasm. Also observed was pneumonia.

Skin: Rare was maculopapular rash. Also observed were angioedema, exfoliative dermatitis, and hirsutism.

Special Senses: Infrequent were accommodation abnormality and dry eye. Also observed were deafness, diplopia, and mydriasis.

Urogenital: Infrequent were impotence, polyuria, and prostate disorder. Also observed were abnormal ejaculation, cystitis, dyspareunia, dysuria, gynecomastia, menopause, painful erection, salpingitis, urinary incontinence, urinary retention, and vaginitis.

DRUG ABUSE AND DEPENDENCE

Controlled Substance Class: Bupropion is not a controlled substance.

Humans: Controlled clinical studies of bupropion conducted in normal volunteers, in subjects with a history of multiple drug abuse, and in depressed patients showed some increase in motor activity and agitation/excitement.

In a population of individuals experienced with drugs of abuse, a single dose of 400 mg of bupropion produced mild amphetamine-like activity as compared to placebo on the Morphine-Benzedrine Subscale of the Addiction Research Center Inventories (ARCI), and a score intermediate between placebo and amphetamine on the Liking Scale of the ARCI. These scales measure general feelings of euphoria and drug desirability.

Findings in clinical trials, however, are not known to reliably predict the abuse potential of drugs. Nonetheless, evidence from single-dose studies does suggest that the recommended daily dosage of bupropion when administered in divided doses is not likely to be especially reinforcing to amphetamine or stimulant abusers. However, higher doses that could not be tested because of the risk of seizure might be modestly attractive to those who abuse stimulant drugs.

Animals: Studies in rodents have shown that bupropion exhibits some pharmacologic actions common to psychostimulants, including increases in locomotor activity and the production of a mild stereotyped behavior and increases in rates of responding in several schedule-controlled behavior paradigms. Drug discrimination studies in rats showed stimulus generalization between bupropion and amphetamine and other psychostimulants. Rhesus monkeys have been shown to self-administer bupropion intravenously.

OVERDOSAGE

Human Overdose Experience: There has been very limited experience with overdosage of WELLBUTRIN SR Tablets; three cases were reported during clinical trials. One patient ingested 3000 mg of WELLBUTRIN SR Tablets and vomited quickly after the overdose; the patient experienced blurred vision and lightheadedness. A second patient ingested a "handful" of WELLBUTRIN SR Tablets and experienced confusion, lethargy, nausea, jitteriness, and seizure. A third patient ingested 3600 mg of WELLBUTRIN SR Tablets and a bottle of wine; the patient experienced nausea, visual hallucinations, and "grogginess." None of the patients experienced further sequelae.

There has been extensive experience with overdosage of the immediate-release formulation of bupropion. Thirteen overdoses occurred during clinical trials. Twelve patients ingested 850 to 4200 mg and recovered without significant sequelae. Another patient who ingested 9000 mg of the immediate-release formulation of bupropion and 300 mg of tranylcypromine experienced a grand mal seizure and recovered without further sequelae.

Since introduction, overdoses of up to 17500 mg of the immediate-release formulation of bupropion have been reported. Seizure was reported in approximately one third of all cases. Other serious reactions reported with overdoses of the immediate-release formulation of bupropion alone included hallucinations, loss of consciousness, and sinus tachycardia. Fever, muscle rigidity, rhabdomyolysis, hypotension, stupor, coma, and respiratory failure have been reported when the immediate-release formulation of bupropion was part of multiple drug overdoses.

Although most patients recovered without sequelae, deaths associated with overdoses of the immediate-release formulation of bupropion alone have been reported rarely in patients ingesting massive doses of the drug. Multiple uncontrolled seizures, bradycardia, cardiac failure, and cardiac arrest prior to death were reported in these patients.

Management of Overdose: Following suspected overdose, hospitalization is advised. If the patient is conscious, vomiting should be induced by syrup of ipecac. Activated charcoal also may be administered every 6 hours during the first 12 hours after ingestion. Baseline laboratory values should be obtained. Electrocardiogram and EEG monitoring also are recommended for the next 48 hours. Adequate fluid intake should be provided.

If the patient is stuporous, comatose, or convulsing, airway intubation is recommended prior to undertaking gastric lavage. Although there is little clinical experience with lavage following an overdose of the immediate-release formulation of bupropion and none with WELLBUTRIN SR Tablets, it is likely to be of benefit within the first 12 hours after ingestion since absorption of the drug may not yet be complete. Although diuresis, dialysis, or hemoperfusion are sometimes used to treat drug overdosage, there is no experience with their use in the management of overdoses of WELLBUTRIN SR Tablets. Because diffusion of bupropion and its metabolites from tissue to plasma may be slow, dialysis may be of minimal benefit.

Based on studies in animals, it is recommended that seizures be treated with an intravenous benzodiazepine preparation and other supportive measures, as appropriate.

Further information about the treatment of overdoses may be available from a poison control center.

DOSAGE AND ADMINISTRATION

General Dosing Considerations: It is particularly important to administer WELLBUTRIN SR Tablets in a manner most likely to minimize the risk of seizure (see WARNINGS). Gradual escalation in dosage is also important if agitation, motor restlessness, and insomnia, often seen during the initial days of treatment, are to be minimized. If necessary, these effects may be managed by temporary reduction of dose or the short-term administration of an intermediate to long-acting sedative hypnotic. A sedative hypnotic usually is not required beyond the first week of treatment. Insomnia may also be minimized by avoiding bedtime doses. If distressing, untoward effects supervene, dose escalation should be stopped.

Initial Treatment: The usual adult target dose for WELLBUTRIN SR Tablets is 300 mg/day, given as 150 mg twice daily. Dosing with WELLBUTRIN SR Tablets should begin at 150 mg/day given as a single daily dose in the morning. If the 150-mg initial dose is adequately tolerated, an increase to the 300-mg/day target dose, given as 150 mg twice daily, may be made as early as day 4 of dosing. There should be an interval of at least 8 hours between successive doses.

Increasing the Dosage Above 300 mg/day: As with other antidepressants, the full antidepressant effect of WELLBUTRIN SR Tablets may not be evident until 4 weeks of treatment or longer. An increase in dosage to the maximum of 400 mg/day, given as 200 mg twice daily, may be considered for patients in whom no clinical improvement is noted after several weeks of treatment at 300 mg/day.

Maintenance: The lowest dose that maintains remission is recommended. Although it is not known how long the patient should remain on WELLBUTRIN SR Tablets, it is generally recognized that acute episodes of depression require several months or longer of antidepressant drug treatment.

HOW SUPPLIED

WELLBUTRIN SR Sustained-Release Tablets, 100 mg of bupropion hydrochloride, are blue, round, biconvex, film-coated tablets printed with "WELLBUTRIN SR 100" in bottles of 60 (NDC 0173-0947-55).

WELLBUTRIN SR Sustained-Release Tablets, 150 mg of bupropion hydrochloride, are purple, round, biconvex, film-coated tablets printed with "WELLBUTRIN SR 150" in bottles of 60 (NDC 0173-0135-55).

Store at controlled room temperature, 20° to 25°C (68° to 77°F) [see USP]. Dispense in a tight, light-resistant container as defined in the USP.

U.S. Patent Nos. 5,358,970; 5,427,798; and Re. 33,994

October 1997/RL-476

Shown in Product Identification Guide, page 314

ZANTAC® ℞
[zan 'tak]
(ranitidine hydrochloride)
Injection

ZANTAC® ℞
(ranitidine hydrochloride)
Injection Premixed

DESCRIPTION

The active ingredient in ZANTAC Injection and ZANTAC Injection Premixed is ranitidine hydrochloride (HCl), a histamine H_2-receptor antagonist. Chemically it is N[2-[[[5-[(dimethylamino)methyl]-2-furanyl]methyl]thio]ethyl]-N'-methyl-2-nitro-1,1-ethenediamine, hydrochloride.

The empirical formula is $C_{13}H_{22}N_4O_3S \cdot HCl$, representing a molecular weight of 350.87.

Ranitidine HCl is a white to pale yellow, granular substance that is soluble in water.

ZANTAC Injection is a clear, colorless to yellow, nonpyrogenic liquid. The yellow color of the liquid tends to intensify without adversely affecting potency. The pH of the injection solution is 6.7 to 7.3.

Sterile Injection for Intramuscular or Intravenous Administration: Each 1 mL of aqueous solution contains ranitidine 25 mg (as the hydrochloride); phenol 5 mg as preservative; and 0.96 mg of monobasic potassium phosphate and 2.4 mg of dibasic sodium phosphate as buffers.

A pharmacy bulk package is a container of a sterile preparation for parenteral use that contains many single doses. The contents are intended for use in a pharmacy admixture program and are restricted to the preparation of admixtures for intravenous (IV) infusion.

Sterile, Premixed Solution for Intravenous Administration in Single-Dose, Flexible Plastic Containers: Each 50 mL contains ranitidine HCl equivalent to 50 mg of ranitidine, sodium chloride 225 mg, and citric acid 15 mg and dibasic sodium phosphate 90 mg as buffers in water for injection. It contains no preservatives. The osmolarity of this solution is 180 mOsm/L (approx.), and the pH is 6.7 to 7.3.

The flexible plastic container is fabricated from a specially formulated, nonplasticized, thermoplastic co-polyester (CR3). Water can permeate from inside the container into the overwrap but not in amounts sufficient to affect the solution significantly. Solutions inside the plastic container also can leach out certain of the chemical components in very small amounts before the expiration period is attained. However, the safety of the plastic has been confirmed by tests in animals according to USP biological standards for plastic containers.

CLINICAL PHARMACOLOGY

ZANTAC is a competitive, reversible inhibitor of the action of histamine at the histamine H_2-receptors, including receptors on the gastric cells. ZANTAC does not lower serum Ca^{++} in hypercalcemic states. ZANTAC is not an anticholinergic agent.

Antisecretory Activity: 1. Effects on Acid Secretion: ZANTAC Injection inhibits basal gastric acid secretion as well as gastric acid secretion stimulated by betazole and pentagastrin, as shown in the following table:
[See table at top of next page]

In a group of 10 known hypersecretors, ranitidine plasma levels of 71, 180, and 376 ng/mL inhibited basal acid secretion by 76%, 90%, and 99.5%, respectively.

It appears that basal- and betazole-stimulated secretions are most sensitive to inhibition by ZANTAC, while pentagastrin-stimulated secretion is more difficult to suppress.

2. Effects on Other Gastrointestinal Secretions:

Pepsin: ZANTAC does not affect pepsin secretion. Total pepsin output is reduced in proportion to the decrease in volume of gastric juice.

Intrinsic Factor: ZANTAC has no significant effect on pentagastrin-stimulated intrinsic factor secretion.

Serum Gastrin: ZANTAC has little or no effect on fasting or postprandial serum gastrin.

Other Pharmacologic Actions:

a. Gastric bacterial flora—increase in nitrate-reducing organisms, significance not known.

b. Prolactin levels—no effect in recommended oral or IV dosage, but small, transient, dose-related increases in serum prolactin have been reported after IV bolus injections of 100 mg or more.

c. Other pituitary hormones—no effect on serum gonadotropins, TSH, or GH. Possible impairment of vasopressin release.

d. No change in cortisol, aldosterone, androgen, or estrogen levels.

e. No antiandrogenic action.

f. No effect on count, motility, or morphology of sperm.

Pharmacokinetics: Serum concentrations necessary to inhibit 50% of stimulated gastric acid secretion are estimated to be 36 to 94 ng/mL. Following single IV or intramuscular (IM) 50-mg doses, serum concentrations of ZANTAC are in this range for 6 to 8 hours.

Following IV injection, approximately 70% of the dose is recovered in the urine as unchanged drug. Renal clearance averages 530 mL/min, with a total clearance of 760 mL/min. The volume of distribution is 1.4 L/kg, and the elimination half-life is 2 to 2.5 hours.

Four patients with clinically significant renal function impairment (creatinine clearance 25 to 35 mL/min) administered 50 mg of ranitidine intravenously had an average plasma half-life of 4.8 hours, a ranitidine clearance of 29 mL/min, and a volume of distribution of 1.76 L/kg. In general, these parameters appear to be altered in proportion to creatinine clearance (see DOSAGE AND ADMINISTRATION).

ZANTAC is absorbed very rapidly after IM injection. Mean peak levels of 576 ng/mL occur within 15 minutes or less following a 50-mg IM dose. Absorption from IM sites is vir-

tually complete, with a bioavailability of 90% to 100% compared with IV administration. Following oral administration, the relative bioavailability of ZANTAC® (ranitidine HCl) Tablets is 50%.

In humans, the N-oxide is the principal metabolite in the urine; however, this amounts to <4% of the dose. Other metabolites are the S-oxide (1%) and the desmethyl ranitidine (1%). The remainder of the administered dose is found in the stool.

Studies in patients with hepatic dysfunction (compensated cirrhosis) indicate that there are minor, but clinically insignificant, alterations in ranitidine half-life, distribution, clearance, and bioavailability.

Serum protein binding averages 15%.

Clinical Trials: *Active Duodenal Ulcer:* In a multicenter, double-blind, controlled, US study of endoscopically diagnosed duodenal ulcers, earlier healing was seen in the patients treated with oral ZANTAC as shown in the following table:

[See second table at right]

In these studies, patients treated with oral ZANTAC reported a reduction in both daytime and nocturnal pain, and they also consumed less antacid than the placebo-treated patients.

[See third table at right]

Pathological Hypersecretory Conditions (such as Zollinger-Ellison syndrome): ZANTAC inhibits gastric acid secretion and reduces occurrence of diarrhea, anorexia, and pain in patients with pathological hypersecretion associated with Zollinger-Ellison syndrome, systemic mastocytosis, and other pathological hypersecretory conditions (e.g., postoperative, "short-gut" syndrome, idiopathic). Use of oral ZANTAC was followed by healing of ulcers in 8 of 19 (42%) patients who were intractable to previous therapy.

In a retrospective review of 52 Zollinger-Ellison patients given ZANTAC as a continuous IV infusion for up to 15 days, no patients developed complications of acid-peptic disease such as bleeding or perforation. Acid output was controlled to ≤10 mEq/h.

INDICATIONS AND USAGE

ZANTAC Injection and ZANTAC Injection Premixed are indicated in some hospitalized patients with pathological hypersecretory conditions or intractable duodenal ulcers, or as an alternative to the oral dosage form for short-term use in patients who are unable to take oral medication.

CONTRAINDICATIONS

ZANTAC Injection and ZANTAC Injection Premixed are contraindicated for patients known to have hypersensitivity to the drug.

PRECAUTIONS

General: 1. Symptomatic response to ZANTAC therapy does not preclude the presence of gastric malignancy.

2. Since ZANTAC is excreted primarily by the kidney, dosage should be adjusted in patients with impaired renal function (see DOSAGE AND ADMINISTRATION). Caution should be observed in patients with hepatic dysfunction since ZANTAC is metabolized in the liver.

3. In controlled studies in normal volunteers, elevations in SGPT have been observed when H_2-antagonists have been administered intravenously at greater than recommended dosages for 5 days or longer. Therefore, it seems prudent in patients receiving IV ranitidine at dosages ≥100 mg q.i.d. for periods of 5 days or longer to monitor SGPT daily (from day 5) for the remainder of IV therapy.

4. Bradycardia in association with rapid administration of ZANTAC Injection has been reported rarely, usually in patients with factors predisposing to cardiac rhythm disturbances. Recommended rates of administration should not be exceeded (see DOSAGE AND ADMINISTRATION).

5. Rare reports suggest that ZANTAC may precipitate acute porphyria attacks in patients with acute porphyria. ZANTAC should therefore be avoided in patients with a history of acute porphyria.

Laboratory Tests: False-positive tests for urine protein with MULTISTIX® may occur during ZANTAC therapy, and therefore testing with sulfosalicylic acid is recommended.

Drug Interactions: Although ZANTAC has been reported to bind weakly to cytochrome P-450 *in vitro*, recommended doses of the drug do not inhibit the action of the cytochrome P-450–linked oxygenase enzymes in the liver. However, there have been isolated reports of drug interactions that suggest that ZANTAC may affect the bioavailability of certain drugs by some mechanism as yet unidentified (e.g., a pH-dependent effect on absorption or a change in volume of distribution).

Increased or decreased prothrombin times have been reported during concurrent use of ranitidine and warfarin. However, in human pharmacokinetic studies with dosages of ranitidine up to 400 mg/day, no interaction occurred; ranitidine had no effect on warfarin clearance or prothrombin time. The possibility of an interaction with warfarin at dosages of ranitidine higher than 400 mg/day has not been investigated.

Effect of Intravenous ZANTAC® on Gastric Acid Secretion

	Time After Dose, h	% Inhibition of Gastric Acid Output by Intravenous Dose, mg		
		20 mg	60 mg	100 mg
Betazole	Up to 2	93	99	99
Pentagastrin	Up to 3	47	66	77

	Oral ZANTAC*		Oral Placebo*	
	Number Entered	Healed/Evaluable	Number Entered	Healed/Evaluable
Outpatients	195		188	
Week 2		69/182 (38%)†		31/164 (19%)
Week 4		137/187 (73%)†		76/168 (45%)

*All patients were permitted p.r.n. antacids for relief of pain.
†P<0.0001.

Mean Daily Doses of Antacid

	Ulcer Healed	Ulcer Not Healed
Oral ZANTAC	0.06	0.71
Oral placebo	0.71	1.43

As with other agents that lower gastric acidity, ranitidine has been shown to increase the absorption of triazolam resulting in increased plasma concentrations (peak concentration and area under the concentration-time curve) on average 14% to 28%. Ranitidine did not affect the metabolism or elimination of triazolam. The clinical significance of this finding is unknown.

Carcinogenesis, Mutagenesis, Impairment of Fertility: There was no indication of tumorigenic or carcinogenic effects in life-span studies in mice and rats at oral dosages up to 2,000 mg/kg per day.

Ranitidine was not mutagenic in standard bacterial tests (*Salmonella, Escherichia coli*) for mutagenicity at concentrations up to the maximum recommended for these assays. In a dominant lethal assay, a single oral dose of 1,000 mg/kg to male rats was without effect on the outcome of two matings per week for the next 9 weeks.

Pregnancy: *Teratogenic Effects: Pregnancy Category B:* Reproduction studies have been performed in rats and rabbits at oral doses up to 160 times the human oral dose and have revealed no evidence of impaired fertility or harm to the fetus due to ZANTAC. There are, however, no adequate and well-controlled studies in pregnant women. Because animal reproduction studies are not always predictive of human response, this drug should be used during pregnancy only if clearly needed.

Nursing Mothers: ZANTAC is secreted in human milk. Caution should be exercised when ZANTAC is administered to a nursing mother.

Pediatric Use: Safety and effectiveness in pediatric patients have not been established.

Use in Elderly Patients: Ulcer healing rates in elderly patients (65 to 82 years of age) treated with oral ZANTAC were no different than those in younger age-groups. The incidence rates for adverse events and laboratory abnormalities were also not different from those seen in other age-groups.

ADVERSE REACTIONS

Transient pain at the site of IM injection has been reported. Transient local burning or itching has been reported with IV administration of ZANTAC.

The following have been reported as events in clinical trials or in the routine management of patients treated with oral or parenteral ZANTAC. The relationship to ZANTAC therapy has been unclear in many cases. Headache, sometimes severe, seems to be related to ZANTAC administration.

Central Nervous System: Rarely, malaise, dizziness, somnolence, insomnia, and vertigo. Rare cases of reversible mental confusion, agitation, depression, and hallucinations have been reported, predominantly in severely ill elderly patients. Rare cases of reversible blurred vision suggestive of a change in accommodation have been reported. Rare reports of reversible involuntary motor disturbances have been received.

Cardiovascular: As with other H_2-blockers, rare reports of arrhythmias such as tachycardia, bradycardia, asystole, atrioventricular block, and premature ventricular beats.

Gastrointestinal: Constipation, diarrhea, nausea/vomiting, abdominal discomfort/pain, and rare reports of pancreatitis.

Hepatic: In normal volunteers, SGPT values were increased to at least twice the pretreatment levels in 6 of 12 subjects receiving 100 mg q.i.d. intravenously for 7 days, and in 4 of 24 subjects receiving 50 mg q.i.d. intravenously for 5 days. There have been occasional reports of hepatocellular, cholestatic, or mixed hepatitis, with or without jaundice. In such circumstances, ranitidine should be immediately discontinued. These events are usually reversible, but in rare circumstances death has occurred. Rare cases of hepatic failure have also been reported.

Musculoskeletal: Rare reports of arthralgias and myalgias.

Hematologic: Blood count changes (leukopenia, granulocytopenia, and thrombocytopenia) have occurred in a few patients. These were usually reversible. Rare cases of agranulocytosis, pancytopenia, sometimes with marrow hypoplasia, and aplastic anemia and exceedingly rare cases of acquired immune hemolytic anemia have been reported.

Endocrine: Controlled studies in animals and man have shown no stimulation of any pituitary hormone by ZANTAC and no antiandrogenic activity, and cimetidine-induced gynecomastia and impotence in hypersecretory patients have resolved when ZANTAC has been substituted. However, occasional cases of gynecomastia, impotence, and loss of libido have been reported in male patients receiving ZANTAC, but the incidence did not differ from that in the general population.

Integumentary: Rash, including rare cases of erythema multiforme, and, rarely, alopecia.

Other: Rare cases of hypersensitivity reactions (e.g., bronchospasm, fever, rash, eosinophilia), anaphylaxis, angioneurotic edema, and small increases in serum creatinine.

OVERDOSAGE

There has been virtually no experience with overdosage with ZANTAC Injection and limited experience with oral doses of ranitidine. Reported acute ingestions of up to 18 g orally have been associated with transient adverse effects similar to those encountered in normal clinical experience (see ADVERSE REACTIONS). In addition, abnormalities of gait and hypotension have been reported.

When overdosage occurs, clinical monitoring and supportive therapy should be employed.

Studies in dogs receiving dosages of ZANTAC in excess of 225 mg/kg per day have shown muscular tremors, vomiting, and rapid respiration. Single oral doses of 1,000 mg/kg in mice and rats were not lethal. Intravenous LD_{50} values in mice and rats were 77 and 83 mg/kg, respectively.

DOSAGE AND ADMINISTRATION

Parenteral Administration: In some hospitalized patients with pathological hypersecretory conditions or intractable duodenal ulcers, or in patients who are unable to take oral medication, ZANTAC may be administered parenterally according to the following recommendations:

Continued on next page

This product information is based on labeling in effect on June 1, 1998. For further information, contact via direct mail, phone, or web site Medical Information: Glaxo Wellcome Inc., PO Box 13398, Research Triangle Park, NC 27709. Healthcare Professionals (Medical Information): 800-334-0089 Patients (Customer Response Center): 888-TALK2GW (1-888-825-5249) Glaxo Wellcome Corporate Web Site: www.glaxowellcome.com

Zantac Injection—Cont.

Intramuscular Injection: 50 mg (2 mL) every 6 to 8 hours. (No dilution necessary.)

Intermittent Intravenous Injection:

a. Intermittent Bolus: 50 mg (2 mL) every 6 to 8 hours. Dilute ZANTAC Injection, 50 mg, in 0.9% sodium chloride injection or other compatible IV solution (see Stability) to a concentration no greater than 2.5 mg/mL (20 mL). Inject at a rate no greater than 4 mL/min (5 minutes).

b. Intermittent Infusion: 50 mg (2 mL) every 6 to 8 hours. Dilute ZANTAC Injection, 50 mg, in 5% dextrose injection or other compatible IV solution (see Stability) to a concentration no greater than 0.5 mg/mL (100 mL). Infuse at a rate no greater than 5 to 7 mL/min (15 to 20 minutes).

ZANTAC Injection Premixed solution, 50 mg, in 0.45% sodium chloride, 50 mL, requires no dilution and should be infused over 15 to 20 minutes.

In some patients it may be necessary to increase dosage. When this is necessary, the increases should be made by more frequent administration of the dose, but generally should not exceed 400 mg/day.

Continuous Intravenous Infusion: Add ZANTAC Injection to 5% dextrose injection or other compatible IV solution (see Stability). Deliver at a rate of 6.25 mg/h (e.g., 150 mg [6 mL] of ZANTAC Injection in 250 mL of 5% dextrose injection at 10.7 mL/h).

For Zollinger-Ellison patients, dilute ZANTAC Injection in 5% dextrose injection or other compatible IV solution (see Stability) to a concentration no greater than 2.5 mg/mL. Start the infusion at a rate of 1.0 mg/kg per hour. If after 4 hours either a measured gastric acid output is >10 mEq/h or the patient becomes symptomatic, the dose should be adjusted upward in 0.5-mg/kg per hour increments, and the acid output should be remeasured. Dosages up to 2.5 mg/kg per hour and infusion rates as high as 220 mg/h have been used.

ZANTAC Injection Premixed in Flexible Plastic Containers: Instructions for Use: ***To Open:*** Tear outer wrap at notch and remove solution container. Check for minute leaks by squeezing container firmly. If leaks are found, discard unit as sterility may be impaired.

Preparation for Administration: Use aseptic technique.

1. Close flow control clamp of administration set.
2. Remove cover from outlet port at bottom of container.
3. Insert piercing pin of administration set into port with a twisting motion until the pin is firmly seated. NOTE: See full directions on administration set carton.
4. Suspend container from hanger.
5. Squeeze and release drip chamber to establish proper fluid level in chamber during infusion of ZANTAC Injection Premixed.
6. Open flow control clamp to expel air from set. Close clamp.
7. Attach set to venipuncture device. If device is not indwelling, prime and make venipuncture.
8. Perform venipuncture.
9. Regulate rate of administration with flow control clamp.

Caution: ZANTAC Injection Premixed in flexible plastic containers is to be administered by slow IV drip infusion only. **Additives should not be introduced into this solution.** If used with a primary IV fluid system, the primary solution should be discontinued during ZANTAC Injection Premixed infusion.

Do not administer unless solution is clear and container is undamaged.

Warning: Do not use flexible plastic container in series connections.

Dosage Adjustment for Patients With Impaired Renal Function: The administration of ranitidine as a continuous infusion has not been evaluated in patients with impaired renal function. On the basis of experience with a group of subjects with severely impaired renal function treated with ZANTAC, the recommended dosage in patients with a creatinine clearance <50 mL/min is 50 mg every 18 to 24 hours. Should the patient's condition require, the frequency of dosing may be increased to every 12 hours or even further with caution. Hemodialysis reduces the level of circulating ranitidine. Ideally, the dosing schedule should be adjusted so that the timing of a scheduled dose coincides with the end of hemodialysis.

Stability: Undiluted, ZANTAC Injection tends to exhibit a yellow color that may intensify over time without adversely affecting potency. ZANTAC Injection is stable for 48 hours at room temperature when added to or diluted with most commonly used IV solutions, e.g., 0.9% sodium chloride injection, 5% dextrose injection, 10% dextrose injection, lactated ringer's injection, or 5% sodium bicarbonate injection. ZANTAC Injection Premixed in flexible plastic containers is sterile through the expiration date on the label when stored under recommended conditions.

Note: Parenteral drug products should be inspected visually for particulate matter and discoloration before administration whenever solution and container permit.

Directions for Dispensing: ***Pharmacy Bulk Package—Not for Direct Infusion:*** The pharmacy bulk package is for use in a pharmacy admixture service only under a laminar flow hood. The closure should be penetrated only once with a sterile transfer set or other sterile dispensing device, which allows measured distribution of the contents, and the contents dispensed in aliquots using aseptic technique. CONTENTS SHOULD BE USED AS SOON AS POSSIBLE FOLLOWING INITIAL CLOSURE PUNCTURE. DISCARD ANY UNUSED PORTION WITHIN 24 HOURS OF FIRST ENTRY. Following closure puncture, container should be maintained below 30°C (86°F) under a laminar flow hood until contents are dispensed.

HOW SUPPLIED

ZANTAC Injection, 25 mg/mL, containing phenol 0.5% as preservative, is available as follows:

NDC 0173-0362-38 2-mL single-dose vials (Tray of 10)
NDC 0173-0363-01 6-mL multidose vials (Singles)
NDC 0173-0363-00 40-mL pharmacy bulk packages (Singles)

Store between 4° and 30°C (39° and 86°F). Protect from light. Store the 40-mL pharmacy bulk vial in carton until time of use.

ZANTAC Injection Premixed, 50 mg/50 mL, in 0.45% sodium chloride, is available as a sterile, premixed solution for IV administration in single-dose, flexible plastic containers (NDC 0173-0441-00) (case of 24). It contains no preservatives.

Store between 2° and 25°C (36° and 77°F). Protect from light.

Exposure of pharmaceutical products to heat should be minimized. Avoid excessive heat; however, brief exposure up to 40°C does not adversely affect the product. Protect from freezing.

US Patent No. 4,585,790

©Copyright 1996 Glaxo Wellcome Inc. All rights reserved.

December 1997/RL-528

Shown in Product Identification Guide, page 315

ZANTAC® 150 ℞
[*zan 'tak*]
(ranitidine hydrochloride)
Tablets, USP

ZANTAC® 300 ℞
(ranitidine hydrochloride)
Tablets, USP

ZANTAC® 150 ℞
(ranitidine hydrochloride)
GELdose® Capsules

ZANTAC® 300 ℞
(ranitidine hydrochloride)
GELdose® Capsules

ZANTAC® 150 ℞
(ranitidine hydrochloride effervescent)
EFFERdose® Tablets

ZANTAC® 150 ℞
(ranitidine hydrochloride effervescent)
EFFERdose® Granules

ZANTAC® ℞
(ranitidine hydrochloride)
Syrup, USP

DESCRIPTION

The active ingredient in ZANTAC 150 Tablets, ZANTAC 300 Tablets, ZANTAC 150 GELdose Capsules, ZANTAC 300 GELdose Capsules, ZANTAC 150 EFFERdose Tablets, ZANTAC 150 EFFERdose Granules, and ZANTAC Syrup is ranitidine hydrochloride (HCl), USP, a histamine H_2-receptor antagonist. Chemically it is N[2-[[[5-[(dimethylamino) methyl]-2-furanyl]methyl]thio]ethyl]-N′-methyl-2-nitro-1,1-ethenediamine, HCl.

The empirical formula is $C_{13}H_{22}N_4O_3S{\cdot}HCl$, representing a molecular weight of 350.87.

Ranitidine HCl is a white to pale yellow, granular substance that is soluble in water. It has a slightly bitter taste and sulfurlike odor.

Each ZANTAC 150 Tablet for oral administration contains 168 mg of ranitidine HCl equivalent to 150 mg of ranitidine. Each tablet also contains the inactive ingredients FD&C Yellow No. 6 Aluminum Lake, hydroxypropyl methylcellulose, magnesium stearate, microcrystalline cellulose, titanium dioxide, triacetin and yellow iron oxide.

Each ZANTAC 300 Tablet for oral administration contains 336 mg of ranitidine HCl equivalent to 300 mg of ranitidine. Each tablet also contains the inactive ingredients croscarmellose sodium, D&C Yellow No. 10 Aluminum Lake, hydroxypropyl methylcellulose, magnesium stearate, microcrystalline cellulose, titanium dioxide, and triacetin.

ZANTAC 150 GELdose Capsules and ZANTAC 300 GELdose Capsules for oral administration are soft gelatin capsules containing 168 mg of ranitidine HCl equivalent to 150 mg of ranitidine and 336 mg of ranitidine HCl equivalent to 300 mg of ranitidine, respectively, in a nonaqueous matrix of synthetic coconut oil and synthetic triglycerides. The soft gelatin capsule shell contains gelatin, Sorbitol Special™ (sorbitol and sorbitol anhydrides), glycerin, purified water, titanium dioxide, FD&C Yellow No. 6, FD&C Blue No. 1, and FD&C Red No. 40. The capsule shell may also contain mineral oil and soybean lecithin. The capsules are printed with edible ink.

ZANTAC 150 EFFERdose Tablets and ZANTAC 150 EFFERdose Granules for oral administration are effervescent formulations of ranitidine that must be dissolved in water before use. Each individual tablet or the contents of a packet contain 168 mg of ranitidine HCl equivalent to 150 mg of ranitidine and the following inactive ingredients: aspartame, monosodium citrate anhydrous, povidone, and sodium bicarbonate. Each tablet also contains sodium benzoate. The total sodium content of each tablet is 183.12 mg (7.96 mEq) per 150 mg of ranitidine, and the total sodium content of each packet of granules is 173.54 mg (7.55 mEq) per 150 mg of ranitidine.

Each 1 mL of ZANTAC Syrup contains 16.8 mg of ranitidine HCl equivalent to 15 mg of ranitidine. ZANTAC Syrup also contains the inactive ingredients alcohol (7.5%), butylparaben, dibasic sodium phosphate, hydroxypropyl methylcellulose, peppermint flavor, monobasic potassium phosphate, propylparaben, purified water, saccharin sodium, sodium chloride, and sorbitol.

CLINICAL PHARMACOLOGY

ZANTAC is a competitive, reversible inhibitor of the action of histamine at the histamine H_2-receptors, including receptors on the gastric cells. ZANTAC does not lower serum Ca^{++} in hypercalcemic states. ZANTAC is not an anticholinergic agent.

Antisecretory Activity: ***1. Effects on Acid Secretion:*** ZANTAC inhibits both daytime and nocturnal basal gastric acid secretions as well as gastric acid secretion stimulated by food, betazole, and pentagastrin, as shown in the following table:

[See table below]

It appears that basal-, nocturnal-, and betazole-stimulated secretions are most sensitive to inhibition by ZANTAC, responding almost completely to doses of 100 mg or less, while pentagastrin- and food-stimulated secretions are more difficult to suppress.

2. Effects on Other Gastrointestinal Secretions:

Pepsin: Oral ZANTAC does not affect pepsin secretion. Total pepsin output is reduced in proportion to the decrease in volume of gastric juice.

Intrinsic Factor: Oral ZANTAC has no significant effect on pentagastrin-stimulated intrinsic factor secretion.

Serum Gastrin: ZANTAC has little or no effect on fasting or postprandial serum gastrin.

Other Pharmacologic Actions:

a. Gastric bacterial flora—increase in nitrate-reducing organisms, significance not known.

b. Prolactin levels—no effect in recommended oral or intravenous (IV) dosage, but small, transient, dose-related increases in serum prolactin have been reported after IV bolus injections of 100 mg or more.

c. Other pituitary hormones—no effect on serum gonadotropins, TSH, or GH. Possible impairment of vasopressin release.

d. No change in cortisol, aldosterone, androgen, or estrogen levels.

e. No antiandrogenic action.

f. No effect on count, motility, or morphology of sperm.

Pharmacokinetics: ZANTAC is 50% absorbed after oral administration, compared to an IV injection with mean peak levels of 440 to 545 ng/mL occurring at 2 to 3 hours after a 150-mg dose. The syrup, GELdose, and EFFERdose formulations are bioequivalent to the tablets. In a pharmacodynamic comparison of the EFFERdose with the ZANTAC

Effect of Oral ZANTAC on Gastric Acid Secretion

	Time After Dose, h	% Inhibition of Gastric Acid Output by Dose, mg			
		75–80	100	150	200
Basal	Up to 4		99	95	
Nocturnal	Up to 13	95	96	92	
Betazole	Up to 3		97	99	
Pentagastrin	Up to 5	58	72	72	80
Meal	Up to 3		73	79	95

Tablets, during the first hour after administration, the EFFERdose tablet formulation gave a significantly higher intragastric pH, by approximately 1 pH unit, compared to the ZANTAC Tablets. The elimination half-life is 2.5 to 3 hours.

Absorption is not significantly impaired by the administration of food or antacids. Propantheline slightly delays and increases peak blood levels of ZANTAC, probably by delaying gastric emptying and transit time. In one study, simultaneous administration of high-potency antacid (150 mmol) in fasting subjects has been reported to decrease the absorption of ZANTAC.

Serum concentrations necessary to inhibit 50% of stimulated gastric acid secretion are estimated to be 36 to 94 ng/mL. Following a single oral dose of 150 mg, serum concentrations of ZANTAC are in this range up to 12 hours. However, blood levels bear no consistent relationship to dose or degree of acid inhibition.

The principal route of excretion is the urine, with approximately 30% of the orally administered dose collected in the urine as unchanged drug in 24 hours. Renal clearance is about 410 mL/min, indicating active tubular excretion. Four patients with clinically significant renal function impairment (creatinine clearance 25 to 35 mL/min) administered 50 mg of ranitidine intravenously had an average plasma half-life of 4.8 hours, a ranitidine clearance of 29 mL/min, and a volume of distribution of 1.76 L/kg. In general, these parameters appear to be altered in proportion to creatinine clearance (see DOSAGE AND ADMINISTRATION).

In man, the N-oxide is the principal metabolite in the urine; however, this amounts to <4% of the dose. Other metabolites are the S-oxide (1%) and the desmethyl ranitidine (1%). The remainder of the administered dose is found in the stool. Studies in patients with hepatic dysfunction (compensated cirrhosis) indicate that there are minor, but clinically insignificant, alterations in ranitidine half-life, distribution, clearance, and bioavailability.

The volume of distribution is about 1.4 L/kg. Serum protein binding averages 15%.

Clinical Trials: *Active Duodenal Ulcer:* In a multicenter, double-blind, controlled, US study of endoscopically diagnosed duodenal ulcers, earlier healing was seen in the patients treated with ZANTAC as shown in Table I:

[See table I above]

In these studies, patients treated with ZANTAC reported a reduction in both daytime and nocturnal pain, and they also consumed less antacid than the placebo-treated patients.

[See table II at top of next page]

Foreign studies have shown that patients heal equally well with 150 mg b.i.d. and 300 mg h.s. (85% versus 84%, respectively) during a usual 4-week course of therapy. If patients require extended therapy of 8 weeks, the healing rate may be higher for 150 mg b.i.d. as compared to 300 mg h.s. (92% versus 87%, respectively).

Studies have been limited to short-term treatment of acute duodenal ulcer. Patients whose ulcers healed during therapy had recurrences of ulcers at the usual rates.

Maintenance Therapy in Duodenal Ulcer: Ranitidine has been found to be effective as maintenance therapy for patients following healing of acute duodenal ulcers. In two independent, double-blind, multicenter, controlled trials, the number of duodenal ulcers observed was significantly less in patients treated with ZANTAC (150 mg h.s.) than in patients treated with placebo over a 12-month period.

Duodenal Ulcer Prevalence

Double-blind, Multicenter, Placebo-Controlled Trials

Multicenter Trial	Drug	Duodenal Ulcer Prevalence			No. of Patients
		0–4 Months	0–8 Months	0–12 Months	
USA	RAN	20%*	24%*	35%*	138
	PLC	44%	54%	59%	139
Foreign	RAN	12%*	21%*	28%*	174
	PLC	56%	64%	68%	165

% = Life table estimate.
* = P<0.05 (ZANTAC versus comparator).
RAN = ranitidine (ZANTAC).
PLC = placebo.

As with other H₂-antagonists, the factors responsible for the significant reduction in the prevalence of duodenal ulcers include prevention of recurrence of ulcers, more rapid healing of ulcers that may occur during maintenance therapy, or both.

Gastric Ulcer: In a multicenter, double-blind, controlled, US study of endoscopically diagnosed gastric ulcers, earlier

Table I

	ZANTAC*		Placebo*	
	Number Entered	Healed/ Evaluable	Number Entered	Healed/ Evaluable
Outpatients Week 2 Week 4	195	69/182 (38%)† 137/187 (73%)†	188	31/164 (19%) 76/168 (45%)

*All patients were permitted p.r.n. antacids for relief of pain.
†P<0.0001.

healing was seen in the patients treated with ZANTAC as shown in the following table:

	ZANTAC*		Placebo*	
	Number Entered	Healed/ Evaluable	Number Entered	Healed/ Evaluable
Outpatients Week 2 Week 6	92	16/83 (19%) 50/73 (68%)†	94	10/83 (12%) 35/69 (51%)

* All patients were permitted p.r.n. antacids for relief of pain.
† P= 0.009.

In this multicenter trial, significantly more patients treated with ZANTAC became pain free during therapy.

Maintenance of Healing of Gastric Ulcers: In two multicenter, double-blind, randomized, placebo-controlled, 12-month trials conducted in patients whose gastric ulcers had been previously healed, ZANTAC 150 mg h.s. was significantly more effective than placebo in maintaining healing of gastric ulcers.

Pathological Hypersecretory Conditions (such as Zollinger-Ellison syndrome): ZANTAC inhibits gastric acid secretion and reduces occurrence of diarrhea, anorexia, and pain in patients with pathological hypersecretion associated with Zollinger-Ellison syndrome, systemic mastocytosis, and other pathological hypersecretory conditions (e.g., postoperative, "short-gut" syndrome, idiopathic). Use of ZANTAC was followed by healing of ulcers in 8 of 19 (42%) patients who were intractable to previous therapy.

Gastroesophageal Reflux Disease (GERD): In two multicenter, double-blind, placebo-controlled, 6-week trials performed in the United States and Europe, ZANTIC 150 mg b.i.d. was more effective than placebo for the relief of heartburn and other symptoms associated with GERD. Ranitidine-treated patients consumed significantly less antacid than did placebo-treated patients.

The US trial indicated that ZANTAC 150 mg b.i.d. significantly reduced the frequency of heartburn attacks and severity of heartburn pain within 1 to 2 weeks after starting therapy. The improvement was maintained throughout the 6-week trial period. Moreover, patient response rates demonstrated that the effect on heartburn extends through both the day and night time periods.

In two additional US multicenter, double-blind, placebo-controlled, 2-week trials, ZANTAC 150 mg b.i.d. was shown to provide relief of heartburn pain within 24 hours of initiating therapy and a reduction in the frequency of severity of heartburn. In these trials, ZANTAC EFFERdose tablets were shown to provide heartburn relief within 45 minutes of dosing.

Erosive Esophagitis: In two multicenter, double-blind, randomized, placebo-controlled, 12-week trials performed in the United States, ZANTAC 150 mg q.i.d. was significantly more effective than placebo in healing endoscopically diagnosed erosive esophagitis and in relieving associated heartburn. The erosive esophagitis healing rates were as follows:

Erosive Esophagitis Patient Healing Rates

	Healed/Evaluable	
	Placebo* n = 229	ZANTAC 150 mg q.i.d.* n = 215
Week 4	43/198 (22%)	96/206 (47%)†
Week 8	63/176 (36%)	142/200 (71%)†
Week 12	92/159 (58%)	162/192 (84%)†

* All patients were permitted p.r.n. antacids for relief of pain.
† P<0.001 versus placebo.

No additional benefit in healing of esophagitis or in relief of heartburn was seen with a ranitidine dose of 300 mg q.i.d.

Maintenance of Healing of Erosive Esophagitis: In two multicenter, double-blind, randomized, placebo-controlled, 48-week trials conducted in patients whose erosive esophagitis had been previously healed, ZANTAC 150 mg b.i.d. was significantly more effective than placebo in maintaining healing of erosive esophagitis.

INDICATIONS AND USAGE

ZANTAC is indicated in:

1. Short-term treatment of active duodenal ulcer. Most patients heal within 4 weeks. Studies available to date have not assessed the safety of ranitidine in uncomplicated duodenal ulcer for periods of more than 8 weeks.
2. Maintenance therapy for duodenal ulcer patients at reduced dosage after healing of acute ulcers. No placebo-controlled comparative studies have been carried out for periods of longer than 1 year.
3. The treatment of pathological hypersecretory conditions (e.g., Zollinger-Ellison syndrome and systemic mastocytosis).
4. Short-term treatment of active, benign gastric ulcer. Most patients heal within 6 weeks and the usefulness of further treatment has not been demonstrated. Studies available to date have not assessed the safety of ranitidine in uncomplicated, benign gastric ulcer for periods of more than 6 weeks.
5. Maintenance therapy for gastric ulcer patients at reduced dosage after healing of acute ulcers. Placebo-controlled studies have been carried out for 1 year.
6. Treatment of GERD. Symptomatic relief commonly occurs within 24 hours after starting therapy with ZANTAC 150 mg b.i.d.
7. Treatment of endoscopically diagnosed erosive esophagitis. Symptomatic relief of heartburn commonly occurs within 24 hours of therapy initiation with ZANTAC 150 mg q.i.d.
8. Maintenance of healing of erosive esophagitis. Placebo-controlled trials have been carried out for 48 weeks.

Concomitant antacids should be given as needed for pain relief to patients with active duodenal ulcer; active, benign gastric ulcer; hypersecretory states; GERD; and erosive esophagitis.

CONTRAINDICATIONS

ZANTAC is contraindicated for patients known to have hypersensitivity to the drug or any of the ingredients (see PRECAUTIONS).

PRECAUTIONS

General: 1. Symptomatic response to ZANTAC therapy does not preclude the presence of gastric malignancy.

2. Since ZANTAC is excreted primarily by the kidney, dosage should be adjusted in patients with impaired renal function (see DOSAGE AND ADMINISTRATION). Caution should be observed in patients with hepatic dysfunction since ZANTAC is metabolized in the liver.

3. Rare reports suggest that ZANTAC may precipitate acute porphyric attacks in patients with acute porphyria. ZANTAC should therefore be avoided in patients with a history of acute porphyria.

Information for Patients: *Phenylketonurics:* ZANTAC 150 EFFERdose Tablets and ZANTAC 150 EFFERdose Granules contain phenylalanine 16.84 mg per 150 mg of ranitidine.

Laboratory Tests: False-positive tests for urine protein with MULTISTIX® may occur during ZANTAC therapy, and therefore testing with sulfosalicylic acid is recommended.

Drug Interactions: Although ZANTAC has been reported to bind weakly to cytochrome P-450 in vitro, recommended doses of the drug do not inhibit the action of the cytochrome P-450–linked oxygenase enzymes in the liver. However, there have been isolated reports of drug interactions that suggest that ZANTAC may affect the bioavailability of certain drugs by some mechanism as yet unidentified (e.g., a

Continued on next page

This product information is based on labeling in effect on June 1, 1998. For further information, contact via direct mail, phone, or web site Medical Information: Glaxo Wellcome Inc., PO Box 13398, Research Triangle Park, NC 27709. Healthcare Professionals (Medical Information): 800-334-0089 Patients (Customer Response Center): 888-TALK2GW (1-888-825-5249) Glaxo Wellcome Corporate Web Site: www.glaxowellcome.com

Zantac—Cont.

pH-dependent effect on absorption or a change in volume of distribution).

Increased or decreased prothrombin times have been reported during concurrent use of ranitidine and warfarin. However, in human pharmacokinetic studies with dosages of ranitidine up to 400 mg/day, no interaction occurred; ranitidine had no effect on warfarin clearance or prothrombin time. The possibility of an interaction with warfarin at dosages of ranitidine higher than 400 mg/day has not been investigated.

As with other agents that lower gastric acidity, ranitidine has been shown to increase the absorption of triazolam resulting in increased plasma concentrations (peak concentration and area under the concentration-time curve) on average 14% to 28%. Ranitidine did not affect the metabolism or elimination of triazolam. The clinical significance of this finding is unknown.

Carcinogenesis, Mutagenesis, Impairment of Fertility: There was no indication of tumorigenic or carcinogenic effects in life-span studies in mice and rats at dosages up to 2,000 mg/kg per day.

Ranitidine was not mutagenic in standard bacterial tests *(Salmonella, Escherichia coli)* for mutagenicity at concentrations up to the maximum recommended for these assays.

In a dominant lethal assay, a single oral dose of 1,000 mg/kg to male rats was without effect on the outcome of two matings per week for the next 9 weeks.

Pregnancy: ***Teratogenic Effects: Pregnancy Category B:*** Reproduction studies have been performed in rats and rabbits at doses up to 160 times the human dose and have revealed no evidence of impaired fertility or harm to the fetus due to ZANTAC. There are, however, no adequate and well-controlled studies in pregnant women. Because animal reproduction studies are not always predictive of human response, this drug should be used during pregnancy only if clearly needed.

Nursing Mothers: ZANTAC is secreted in human milk. Caution should be exercised when ZANTAC is administered to a nursing mother.

Pediatric Use: Safety and effectiveness in pediatric patients have not been established.

Use in Elderly Patients: Ulcer healing rates in elderly patients (65 to 82 years of age) were no different from those in younger age-groups. The incidence rates for adverse events and laboratory abnormalities were also not different from those seen in other age-groups.

ADVERSE REACTIONS

The following have been reported as events in clinical trials or in the routine management of patients treated with ZANTAC. The relationship to ZANTAC therapy has been unclear in many cases. Headache, sometimes severe, seems to be related to ZANTAC administration.

Central Nervous System: Rarely, malaise, dizziness, somnolence, insomnia, and vertigo. Rare cases of reversible mental confusion, agitation, depression, and hallucinations have been reported, predominantly in severely ill elderly patients. Rare cases of reversible blurred vision suggestive of a change in accommodation have been reported. Rare reports of reversible involuntary motor disturbances have been received.

Cardiovascular: As with other H_2-blockers, rare reports of arrhythmias such as tachycardia, bradycardia, atrioventricular block, and premature ventricular beats.

Gastrointestinal: Constipation, diarrhea, nausea/vomiting, abdominal discomfort/pain, and rare reports of pancreatitis.

Hepatic: There have been occasional reports of hepatocellular, cholestatic, or mixed hepatitis, with or without jaundice. In such circumstances, ranitidine should be immediately discontinued. These events are usually reversible, but in rare circumstances death has occurred. Rare cases of hepatic failure have also been reported. In normal volunteers, SGPT values were increased to at least twice the pretreatment levels in 6 of 12 subjects receiving 100 mg q.i.d. intravenously for 7 days, and in 4 of 24 subjects receiving 50 mg q.i.d. intravenously for 5 days.

Musculoskeletal: Rare reports of arthralgias and myalgias.

Hematologic: Blood count changes (leukopenia, granulocytopenia, and thrombocytopenia) have occurred in a few patients. These were usually reversible. Rare cases of agranulocytosis, pancytopenia, sometimes with marrow hypoplasia, and aplastic anemia and exceedingly rare cases of acquired immune hemolytic anemia have been reported.

Endocrine: Controlled studies in animals and man have shown no stimulation of any pituitary hormone by ZANTAC and no antiandrogenic activity, and cimetidine-induced gynecomastia and impotence in hypersecretory patients have resolved when ZANTAC has been substituted. However, occasional cases of gynecomastia, impotence, and loss of libido have been reported in male patients receiving ZANTAC, but the incidence did not differ from that in the general population.

Table II

Mean Daily Doses of Antacid

	Ulcer Healed	Ulcer Not Healed
ZANTAC	0.06	0.71
Placebo	0.71	1.43

Integumentary: Rash, including rare cases of erythema multiforme, and, rarely, alopecia.

Other: Rare cases of hypersensitivity reactions (e.g.. bronchospasm, fever, rash, eosinophilia), anaphylaxis, angioneurotic edema, and small increases in serum creatinine.

OVERDOSAGE

There has been limited experience with overdosage. Reported acute ingestions of up to 18 g orally have been associated with transient adverse effects similar to those encountered in normal clinical experience (see ADVERSE REACTIONS). In addition, abnormalities of gait and hypotension have been reported.

When overdosage occurs, the usual measures to remove unabsorbed material from the gastrointestinal tract, clinical monitoring, and supportive therapy should be employed.

Studies in dogs receiving dosages of ZANTAC in excess of 225 mg/kg per day have shown muscular tremors, vomiting, and rapid respiration. Single oral doses of 1,000 mg/kg in mice and rats were not lethal. Intravenous LD_{50} values in mice and rats were 77 and 83 mg/kg, respectively.

DOSAGE AND ADMINISTRATION

Active Duodenal Ulcer: The current recommended adult oral dosage of ZANTAC for duodenal ulcer is 150 mg or 10 mL (2 teaspoonfuls equivalent to 150 mg of ranitidine) twice daily. An alternative dosage of 300 mg or 20 mL (4 teaspoonfuls equivalent to 300 mg of ranitidine) once daily after the evening meal or at bedtime can be used for patients in whom dosing convenience is important. The advantages of one treatment regimen compared to the other in a particular patient population have yet to be demonstrated (see Clinical Trials: *Active Duodenal Ulcer*). Smaller doses have been shown to be equally effective in inhibiting gastric acid secretion in US studies, and several foreign trials have shown that 100 mg b.i.d. is as effective as the 150-mg dose. Antacid should be given as needed for relief of pain (see CLINICAL PHARMACOLOGY: Pharmacokinetics).

Maintenance of Healing of Duodenal Ulcers: The current recommended adult oral dosage is 150 mg or 10 mL (2 teaspoonfuls equivalent to 150 mg of ranitidine) at bedtime.

Pathological Hypersecretory Conditions (such as Zollinger-Ellison syndrome): The current recommended adult oral dosage is 150 mg or 10 mL (2 teaspoonfuls equivalent to 150 mg of ranitidine) twice a day. In some patients it may be necessary to administer ZANTAC 150-mg doses more frequently. Dosages should be adjusted to individual patient needs, and should continue as long as clinically indicated. Dosages up to 6 g per day have been employed in patients with severe disease.

Benign Gastric Ulcer: The current recommended adult oral dosage is 150 mg or 10 mL (2 teaspoonfuls equivalent to 150 mg of ranitidine) twice a day.

Maintenance of Healing of Gastric Ulcers: The current recommended adult oral dosage is 150 mg or 10 mL (2 teaspoonfuls equivalent to 150 mg of ranitidine) at bedtime.

GERD: The current recommended adult oral dosage is 150 mg or 10 mL (2 teaspoonfuls equivalent to 150 mg of ranitidine) twice a day.

Erosive Esophagitis: The current recommended adult oral dosage is 150 mg or 10 mL (2 teaspoonfuls equivalent to 150 mg of ranitidine) four times a day.

Maintenance of Healing of Erosive Esophagitis: The current recommended adult oral dosage is 150 mg or 10 mL (2 teaspoonfuls equivalent to 150 mg of ranitidine) twice a day.

Dosage Adjustment for Patients With Impaired Renal Function: On the basis of experience with a group of subjects with severely impaired renal function treated with ZANTAC, the recommended dosage in patients with a creatinine clearance <50 mL/min is 150 mg or 10 mL (2 teaspoonfuls equivalent to 150 mg of ranitidine) every 24 hours. Should the patient's condition require, the frequency of dosing may be increased to every 12 hours or even further with caution. Hemodialysis reduces the level of circulating ranitidine. Ideally, the dosing schedule should be adjusted so that the timing of a scheduled dose coincides with the end of hemodialysis.

Preparation of ZANTAC 150 EFFERdose Tablets and ZANTAC 150 EFFERdose Granules: Dissolve each dose in approximately 6 to 8 oz of water before drinking.

HOW SUPPLIED

ZANTAC 150 Tablets (ranitidine HCl equivalent to 150 mg of ranitidine) are peach, film-coated, five-sided tablets embossed with "ZANTAC 150" on one side and "Glaxo" on the other. They are available in bottles of 60 (NDC 0173-0344-42), 180 (NDC 0173-0344-17), 500 (NDC 0173-0344-14), and 1,000 (NDC 0173-0344-12) tablets and unit dose packs of 100 (NDC 0173-0344-47) tablets.

ZANTAC 300 Tablets (ranitidine HCl equivalent to 300 mg of ranitidine) are yellow, film-coated, capsule-shaped tablets embossed with "ZANTAC 300" on one side and "Glaxo" on the other. They are available in bottles of 30 (NDC 0173-0393-40) and 250 (NDC 0173-0393-06) tablets and unit dose packs of 100 (NDC 0173-0393-47) tablets.

Store between 15° and 30°C (59° and 86°F) in a dry place. Protect from light. Replace cap securely after each opening.

ZANTAC 150 GELdose Capsules (ranitidine HCl equivalent to 150 mg of ranitidine) are beige, soft gelatin capsules imprinted with "ZANTAC 150" on one side and "GLAXO" on the other. They are available in bottles of 60 (NDC 0173-0428-00) capsules and unit dose packs of 60 (NDC 0173-0428-02) capsules.

ZANTAC 300 GELdose Capsules (ranitidine HCl equivalent to 300 mg of ranitidine) are beige, soft gelatin capsules imprinted with "ZANTAC 300" on one side and "GLAXO" on the other. They are available in bottles of 30 (NDC 0173-0429-00) capsules and unit dose packs of 30 (NDC 0173-0429-02) capsules.

Store between 2° and 25°C (36° and 77°F) in a dry place. Protect from light. Replace cap securely after each opening.

ZANTAC 150 EFFERdose Tablets (ranitidine HCl equivalent to 150 mg of ranitidine) are white to pale yellow, round, flat-faced, bevel-edged tablets embossed with "ZANTAC 150" on one side and "427" on the other. They are packaged individually in foil and are available in cartons of 30 (NDC 0173-0427-00) and 60 (NDC 0173-0427-02) tablets.

ZANTAC 150 EFFERdose Granules (ranitidine HCl equivalent to 150 mg of ranitidine) are white to pale yellow granules. Each 150-mg dose of granules (approximately 1.44 g) is packaged in individual foil packets and is available in cartons of 30 (NDC 0173-0451-00) and 60 (NDC 0173-0451-01) packets.

Store between 2° and 30°C (36° and 86°F).

ZANTAC Syrup, a clear, peppermint-flavored liquid, contains 16.8 mg of ranitidine HCl equivalent to 15 mg of ranitidine per 1 mL in bottles of 16 fluid ounces (one pint) (NDC 0173-0383-54).

Store between 4° and 25°C (39° and 77°F). Dispense in tight, light-resistant containers as defined in the USP/NF.

U.S. Patent Nos. 4,585,790 and 5,068,249

December 1997/RL-527

Shown in Product Identification Guide, page 314 & 315

ZINACEF® ℞

[zin 'ah-sef]

(cefuroxime for injection)

ZINACEF® ℞

(cefuroxime injection)

DESCRIPTION

Cefuroxime is a semisynthetic, broad-spectrum, cephalosporin antibiotic for parenteral administration. It is the sodium salt of (6R, 7R)-3-carbamoyloxymethyl-7-[Z-2-methoxyimino-2-(fur-2-yl) acetamido]ceph-3-em-4-carboxylate.

The empirical formula is $C_{16}H_{15}N_4NaO_8S$, representing a molecular weight of 446.4.

ZINACEF contains approximately 54.2 mg (2.4 mEq) of sodium per gram of cefuroxime activity.

ZINACEF in sterile crystalline form is supplied in vials equivalent to 750 mg, 1.5 g, or 7.5 g of cefuroxime as cefuroxime sodium and in ADD-Vantage® vials equivalent to 750 mg or 1.5 g of cefuroxime as cefuroxime sodium. Solutions of ZINACEF range in color from light yellow to amber, depending on the concentration and diluent used. The pH of freshly constituted solutions usually ranges from 6 to 8.5.

ZINACEF is available as a frozen, iso-osmotic, sterile, nonpyrogenic solution with 750 mg or 1.5 g of cefuroxime as cefuroxime sodium. Approximately 1.4 g of Dextrose Hydrous, USP has been added to the 750-mg dose to adjust the osmolality. Sodium Citrate Hydrous, USP has been added as a buffer (300 mg and 600 mg to the 750-mg and 1.5-g doses, respectively). ZINACEF contains approximately 111 mg (4.8 mEq) and 222 mg (9.7 mEq) of sodium in the 750-mg and 1.5-g doses, respectively. The pH has been adjusted with hydrochloric acid and may have been adjusted with sodium hydroxide. Solutions of premixed ZINACEF range in color from light yellow to amber. The solution is intended for intravenous (IV) use after thawing to room temperature. The osmolality of the solution is approximately 300 mOsmol/kg, and the pH of thawed solutions ranges from 5 to 7.5.

The plastic container for the frozen solution is fabricated from a specially designed multilayer plastic, PL 2040. Solu-

tions are in contact with the polyethylene layer of this container and can leach out certain chemical components of the plastic in very small amounts within the expiration period. The suitability of the plastic has been confirmed in tests in animals according to USP biological tests for plastic containers as well as by tissue culture toxicity studies.

CLINICAL PHARMACOLOGY

After intramuscular (IM) injection of a 750-mg dose of cefuroxime to normal volunteers, the mean peak serum concentration was 27 mcg/mL. The peak occurred at approximately 45 minutes (range, 15 to 60 minutes). Following IV doses of 750 mg and 1.5 g, serum concentrations were approximately 50 and 100 mcg/mL, respectively, at 15 minutes. Therapeutic serum concentrations of approximately 2 mcg/mL or more were maintained for 5.3 hours and 8 hours or more, respectively. There was no evidence of accumulation of cefuroxime in the serum following IV administration of 1.5-g doses every 8 hours to normal volunteers. The serum half-life after either IM or IV injections is approximately 80 minutes.

Approximately 89% of a dose of cefuroxime is excreted by the kidneys over an 8-hour period, resulting in high urinary concentrations.

Following the IM administration of a 750-mg single dose, urinary concentrations averaged 1300 mcg/mL during the first 8 hours. Intravenous doses of 750 mg and 1.5 g produced urinary levels averaging 1150 and 2500 mcg/mL, respectively, during the first 8-hour period.

The concomitant oral administration of probenecid with cefuroxime slows tubular secretion, decreases renal clearance by approximately 40%, increases the peak serum level by approximately 30%, and increases the serum half-life by approximately 30%. Cefuroxime is detectable in therapeutic concentrations in pleural fluid, joint fluid, bile, sputum, bone, and aqueous humor.

Cefuroxime is detectable in therapeutic concentrations in cerebrospinal fluid (CSF) of adults and pediatric patients with meningitis. The following table shows the concentrations of cefuroxime achieved in cerebrospinal fluid during multiple dosing of patients with meningitis.

[See table above]

Patients	Dose	Number of Patients	Mean (Range) CSF Cefuroxime Concentrations (mcg/mL) Achieved Within 8 Hours Post Dose
Pediatric patients (4 weeks to 6.5 years)	200 mg/kg/day, divided q 6 hours	5	6.6 (0.9-17.3)
Pediatric patients (7 months to 9 years)	200 to 230 mg/kg/day, divided q 8 hours	6	8.3 (<2-22.5)
Adults	1.5 grams q 8 hours	2	5.2 (2.7-8.9)
Adults	1.5 grams q 6 hours	10	6.0 (1.5-13.5)

Cefuroxime is approximately 50% bound to serum protein.

Microbiology: Cefuroxime has in vitro activity against a wide range of gram-positive and gram-negative organisms, and it is highly stable in the presence of beta-lactamases of certain gram-negative bacteria. The bactericidal action of cefuroxime results from inhibition of cell-wall synthesis.

Cefuroxime is usually active against the following organisms in vitro.

Aerobes, Gram-positive: Staphylococcus aureus, Staphylococcus epidermidis, Streptococcus pneumoniae, and Streptococcus pyogenes (and other streptococci).

NOTE: Most strains of enterococci, e.g., Enterococcus faecalis (formerly Streptococcus faecalis), are resistant to cefuroxime. Methicillin-resistant staphylococci and Listeria monocytogenes are resistant to cefuroxime.

Aerobes, Gram-negative: Citrobacter spp., Enterobacter spp., Escherichia coli, Haemophilus influenzae (including ampicillin-resistant strains), Haemophilus parainfluenzae, Klebsiella spp. (including Klebsiella pneumoniae), Moraxella (Branhamella) catarrhalis (including ampicillin- and cephalothin-resistant strains), Morganella morganii (formerly Proteus morganii), Neisseria gonorrhoeae (including penicillinase- and non–penicillinase-producing strains), Neisseria meningitidis, Proteus mirabilis, Providencia rettgeri (formerly Proteus rettgeri), Salmonella spp., and Shigella spp.

NOTE: Some strains of Morganella morganii, Enterobacter cloacae, and Citrobacter spp. have been shown by in vitro tests to be resistant to cefuroxime and other cephalosporins. Pseudomonas and Campylobacter spp., Acinetobacter calcoaceticus, and most strains of Serratia spp. and Proteus vulgaris are resistant to most first- and second-generation cephalosporins.

Anaerobes: Gram-positive and gram-negative cocci (including Peptococcus and Peptostreptococcus spp.), gram-positive bacilli (including Clostridium spp.), and gram-negative bacilli (including Bacteroides and Fusobacterium spp.).

NOTE: Clostridium difficile and most strains of Bacteroides fragilis are resistant to cefuroxime.

Susceptibility Tests: Diffusion Techniques: Quantitative methods that require measurement of zone diameters give an estimate of antibiotic susceptibility. One such standard procedure[1] that has been recommended for use with disks to test susceptibility of organisms to cefuroxime uses the 30-mcg cefuroxime disk. Interpretation involves the correlation of the diameters obtained in the disk test with the minimum inhibitory concentration (MIC) for cefuroxime.

A report of "Susceptible" indicates that the pathogen is likely to be inhibited by generally achievable blood levels. A report of "Moderately Susceptible" suggests that the organism would be susceptible if high dosage is used or if the infection is confined to tissues and fluids in which high antibiotic levels are attained. A report of "Intermediate" sug-

gests an equivocable or indeterminate result. A report of "Resistant" indicates that achievable concentrations of the antibiotic are unlikely to be inhibitory and other therapy should be selected.

Reports from the laboratory giving results of the standard single-disk susceptibility test for organisms other than Haemophilus spp. and Neisseria gonorrhoeae with a 30-mcg cefuroxime disk should be interpreted according to the following criteria:

Zone Diameter (mm)	Interpretation
≥18	(S) Susceptible
15–17	(MS) Moderately Susceptible
≤14	(R) Resistant

Results for Haemophilus spp. should be interpreted according to the following criteria:

Zone Diameter (mm)	Interpretation
≥24	(S) Susceptible
21–23	(I) Intermediate
≤20	(R) Resistant

Results for Neisseria gonorrhoeae should be interpreted according to the following criteria:

Zone Diameter (mm)	Interpretation
≥31	(S) Susceptible
26–30	(MS) Moderately Susceptible
≤25	(R) Resistant

Organisms should be tested with the cefuroxime disk since cefuroxime has been shown by in vitro tests to be active against certain strains found resistant when other beta-lactam disks are used. The cefuroxime disk should not be used for testing susceptibility to other cephalosporins.

Standardized procedures require the use of laboratory control organisms. The 30-mcg cefuroxime disk should give the following zone diameters.

1. Testing for organisms other than Haemophilus spp. and Neisseria gonorrhoeae:

Organism	Zone Diameter (mm)
Staphylococcus aureus ATCC 25923	27–35
Escherichia coli ATCC 25922	20–26

2. Testing for Haemophilus spp.:

Organism	Zone Diameter (mm)
Haemophilus influenzae ATCC 49766	28–36

3. Testing for Neisseria gonorrhoeae:

Organism	Zone Diameter (mm)
Neisseria gonorrhoeae ATCC 49226	33–41
Staphylococcus aureus ATCC 25923	29–33

Dilution Techniques: Use a standardized dilution method[1] (broth, agar, microdilution) or equivalent with cefuroxime powder. The MIC values obtained for bacterial isolates other than Haemophilus spp. and Neisseria gonorrhoeae should be interpreted according to the following criteria:

MIC (mcg/mL)	Interpretation
≤8	(S) Susceptible
16	(MS) Moderately Susceptible
≥32	(R) Resistant

MIC values obtained for Haemophilus spp. should be interpreted according to the following criteria:

MIC (mcg/mL)	Interpretation
≤4	(S) Susceptible
8	(I) Intermediate
≥16	(R) Resistant

MIC values obtained for Neisseria gonorrhoeae should be interpreted according to the following criteria:

MIC (mcg/mL)	Interpretation
≤1	(S) Susceptible
2	(MS) Moderately Susceptible
≥4	(R) Resistant

As with standard diffusion techniques, dilution methods require the use of laboratory control organisms. Standard cefuroxime powder should provide the following MIC values.

1. For organisms other than Haemophilus spp. and Neisseria gonorrhoeae:

Organism	MIC (mcg/mL)
Staphylococcus aureus ATCC 29213	0.5–2.0
Escherichia coli ATCC 25922	2.0–8.0

2. For Haemophilus spp.:

Organism	MIC (mcg/mL)
Haemophilus influenzae ATCC 49766	0.25–1.0

3. For Neisseria gonorrhoeae:

Organism	MIC (mcg/mL)
Neisseria gonorrhoeae ATCC 49226	0.25–1.0
Staphylococcus aureus ATCC 29213	0.25–1.0

INDICATIONS AND USAGE

ZINACEF is indicated for the treatment of patients with infections caused by susceptible strains of the designated organisms in the following diseases:

1. **Lower Respiratory Tract Infections**, including pneumonia, caused by Streptococcus pneumoniae, Haemophilus influenzae (including ampicillin-resistant strains), Klebsiella spp., Staphylococcus aureus (penicillinase- and non-penicillinase-producing strains), Streptococcus pyogenes, and Escherichia coli.

2. **Urinary Tract Infections** caused by Escherichia coli and Klebsiella spp.

3. **Skin and Skin-Structure Infections** caused by Staphylococcus aureus (penicillinase- and non–penicillinase-producing strains), Streptococcus pyogenes, Escherichia coli, Klebsiella spp., and Enterobacter spp.

4. **Septicemia** caused by Staphylococcus aureus (penicillinase- and non–penicillinase-producing strains), Streptococcus pneumoniae, Escherichia coli, Haemophilus influenzae (including ampicillin-resistant strains), and Klebsiella spp.

5. **Meningitis** caused by Streptococcus pneumoniae, Haemophilus influenzae (including ampicillin-resistant strains), Neisseria meningitidis, and Staphylococcus aureus (penicillinase- and non–penicillinase-producing strains).

6. **Gonorrhea:** Uncomplicated and disseminated gonococcal infections due to Neisseria gonorrhoeae (penicillinase- and non–penicillinase-producing strains) in both males and females.

7. **Bone and Joint Infections** caused by Staphylococcus aureus (penicillinase- and non–penicillinase-producing strains).

Clinical microbiological studies in skin and skin-structure infections frequently reveal the growth of susceptible strains of both aerobic and anaerobic organisms. ZINACEF has been used successfully in these mixed infections in which several organisms have been isolated. Appropriate cultures and susceptibility studies should be performed to determine the susceptibility of the causative organisms to ZINACEF.

Therapy may be started while awaiting the results of these studies; however, once these results become available, the antibiotic treatment should be adjusted accordingly. In certain cases of confirmed or suspected gram-positive or gram-negative sepsis or in patients with other serious infections in which the causative organism has not been identified, ZINACEF may be used concomitantly with an aminoglycoside (see PRECAUTIONS). The recommended doses of both antibiotics may be given depending on the severity of the infection and the patient's condition.

Prevention: The preoperative prophylactic administration of ZINACEF may prevent the growth of susceptible disease-causing bacteria and thereby may reduce the incidence of certain postoperative infections in patients undergoing surgical procedures (e.g., vaginal hysterectomy) that are classified as clean-contaminated or potentially contaminated procedures. Effective prophylactic use of antibiotics in surgery depends on the time of administration. ZINACEF should usually be given one-half to 1 hour before the operation to allow sufficient time to achieve effective antibiotic concentrations in the wound tissues during the procedure. The dose should be repeated intraoperatively if the surgical procedure is lengthy.

Prophylactic administration is usually not required after the surgical procedure ends and should be stopped within 24 hours. In the majority of surgical procedures, continuing

Continued on next page

This product information is based on labeling in effect on June 1, 1998. For further information, contact via direct mail, phone, or web site Medical Information: Glaxo Wellcome Inc., PO Box 13398, Research Triangle Park, NC 27709. Healthcare Professionals (Medical Information): 800-334-0089 Patients (Customer Response Center): 888-TALK2GW (1-888-825-5249) Glaxo Wellcome Corporate Web Site: www.glaxowellcome.com

Zinacef—Cont.

prophylactic administration of any antibiotic does not reduce the incidence of subsequent infections but will increase the possibility of adverse reactions and the development of bacterial resistance.

The perioperative use of ZINACEF has also been effective during open heart surgery for surgical patients in whom infections at the operative site would present a serious risk. For these patients it is recommended that therapy with ZINACEF be continued for at least 48 hours after the surgical procedure ends. If an infection is present, specimens for culture should be obtained for the identification of the causative organism, and appropriate antimicrobial therapy should be instituted.

CONTRAINDICATIONS

ZINACEF is contraindicated in patients with known allergy to the cephalosporin group of antibiotics.

WARNINGS

BEFORE THERAPY WITH ZINACEF IS INSTITUTED, CAREFUL INQUIRY SHOULD BE MADE TO DETERMINE WHETHER THE PATIENT HAS HAD PREVIOUS HYPERSENSITIVITY REACTIONS TO CEPHALOSPORINS, PENICILLINS, OR OTHER DRUGS. THIS PRODUCT SHOULD BE GIVEN CAUTIOUSLY TO PENICILLIN-SENSITIVE PATIENTS. ANTIBIOTICS SHOULD BE ADMINISTERED WITH CAUTION TO ANY PATIENT WHO HAS DEMONSTRATED SOME FORM OF ALLERGY, PARTICULARLY TO DRUGS. IF AN ALLERGIC REACTION TO ZINACEF OCCURS, DISCONTINUE THE DRUG. SERIOUS ACUTE HYPERSENSITIVITY REACTIONS MAY REQUIRE EPINEPHRINE AND OTHER EMERGENCY MEASURES.

Pseudomembranous colitis has been reported with nearly all antibacterial agents, including cefuroxime, and may range in severity from mild to life threatening. Therefore, it is important to consider this diagnosis in patients who present with diarrhea subsequent to the administration of antibacterial agents.

Treatment with antibacterial agents alters the normal flora of the colon and may permit overgrowth of clostridia. Studies indicate that a toxin produced by *Clostridium difficile* is one primary cause of "antibiotic-associated colitis."

After the diagnosis of pseudomembranous colitis has been established, appropriate therapeutic measures should be initiated. Mild cases of pseudomembranous colitis usually respond to drug discontinuation alone. In moderate to severe cases, consideration should be given to management with fluids and electrolytes, protein supplementation, and treatment with an antibacterial drug clinically effective against *Clostridium difficile* colitis.

When the colitis is not relieved by drug discontinuation or when it is severe, oral vancomycin is the treatment of choice for antibiotic-associated pseudomembranous colitis produced by *Clostridium difficile*. Other causes of colitis should also be considered.

PRECAUTIONS

Although ZINACEF rarely produces alterations in kidney function, evaluation of renal status during therapy is recommended, especially in seriously ill patients receiving the maximum doses. Cephalosporins should be given with caution to patients receiving concurrent treatment with potent diuretics as these regimens are suspected of adversely affecting renal function.

The total daily dose of ZINACEF should be reduced in patients with transient or persistent renal insufficiency (see DOSAGE AND ADMINISTRATION), because high and prolonged serum antibiotic concentrations can occur in such individuals from usual doses.

As with other antibiotics, prolonged use of ZINACEF may result in overgrowth of nonsusceptible organisms. Careful observation of the patient is essential. If superinfection occurs during therapy, appropriate measures should be taken. Broad-spectrum antibiotics should be prescribed with caution in individuals with a history of gastrointestinal disease, particularly colitis.

Nephrotoxicity has been reported following concomitant administration of aminoglycoside antibiotics and cephalosporins.

As with other therapeutic regimens used in the treatment of meningitis, mild-to-moderate hearing loss has been reported in a few pediatric patients treated with cefuroxime sodium. Persistence of positive CSF (cerebrospinal fluid) cultures at 18 to 36 hours has also been noted with cefuroxime sodium injection, as well as with other antibiotic therapies; however, the precise relevance of this is unknown.

Drug/Laboratory Test Interactions: A false-positive reaction for glucose in the urine may occur with copper reduction tests (Benedict's or Fehling's solution or with CLINITEST® tablets) but not with enzyme-based tests for glycosuria (e.g., TES-TAPE®). As a false-negative result may occur in the ferricyanide test, it is recommended that either the glucose oxidase or hexokinase method be used to determine blood plasma glucose levels in patients receiving ZINACEF.

Cefuroxime does not interfere with the assay of serum and urine creatinine by the alkaline picrate method.

Carcinogenesis, Mutagenesis, Impairment of Fertility: Although no long-term studies in animals have been performed to evaluate carcinogenic potential, no mutagenic potential of cefuroxime was found in standard laboratory tests.

Reproductive studies revealed no impairment of fertility in animals.

Pregnancy: *Teratogenic Effects:* Pregnancy Category B. Reproduction studies have been performed in mice and rabbits at doses up to 60 times the human dose and have revealed no evidence of impaired fertility or harm to the fetus due to cefuroxime. There are, however, no adequate and well-controlled studies in pregnant women. Because animal reproduction studies are not always predictive of human response, this drug should be used during pregnancy only if clearly needed.

Nursing Mothers: Since cefuroxime is excreted in human milk, caution should be exercised when ZINACEF is administered to a nursing woman.

Pediatric Use: Safety and effectiveness in pediatric patients below 3 months of age have not been established. Accumulation of other members of the cephalosporin class in newborn infants (with resulting prolongation of drug half-life) has been reported.

ADVERSE REACTIONS

ZINACEF is generally well tolerated. The most common adverse effects have been local reactions following IV administration. Other adverse reactions have been encountered only rarely.

Local Reactions: Thrombophlebitis has occurred with IV administration in 1 in 60 patients.

Gastrointestinal: Gastrointestinal symptoms occurred in 1 in 150 patients and included diarrhea (1 in 220 patients) and nausea (1 in 440 patients). The onset of pseudomembranous colitis may occur during or after antibacterial treatment (see WARNINGS).

Hypersensitivity Reactions: Hypersensitivity reactions have been reported in fewer than 1% of the patients treated with ZINACEF and include rash (1 in 125). Pruritus, urticaria, and positive Coombs' test each occurred in fewer than 1 in 250 patients, and, as with other cephalosporins, rare cases of anaphylaxis, drug fever, erythema multiforme, interstitial nephritis, toxic epidermal necrolysis, and Stevens-Johnson syndrome have occurred.

Blood: A decrease in hemoglobin and hematocrit has been observed in 1 in 10 patients and transient eosinophilia in 1 in 14 patients. Less common reactions seen were transient neutropenia (fewer than 1 in 100 patients) and leukopenia (1 in 750 patients). A similar pattern and incidence were seen with other cephalosporins used in controlled studies. As with other cephalosporins, there have been rare reports of thrombocytopenia.

Hepatic: Transient rise in SGOT and SGPT (1 in 25 patients), alkaline phosphatase (1 in 50 patients), LDH (1 in 75 patients), and bilirubin (1 in 500 patients) levels has been noted.

Kidney: Elevations in serum creatinine and/or blood urea nitrogen and a decreased creatinine clearance have been observed, but their relationship to cefuroxime is unknown.

Observed During Clinical Practice: In addition to adverse events reported from clinical trials, the following events have been identified during post-approval use of ZINACEF. Because they are reported voluntarily from a population of unknown size, estimates of frequency cannot be made. These events have been chosen for inclusion due to combination of their seriousness, frequency of reporting, or potential causal connection to ZINACEF.

Neurologic: Seizure.

Non-site specific: Angioedema.

Cephalosporin-class Adverse Reactions: In addition to adverse reactions listed above that have been observed in patients treated with cefuroxime, the following adverse reactions and altered laboratory tests have been reported for cephalosporin-class antibiotics:

Adverse Reactions: Vomiting, abdominal pain, colitis, vaginitis including vaginal candidiasis, toxic nephropathy, hepatic dysfunction including cholestasis, aplastic anemia, hemolytic anemia, hemorrhage.

Several cephalosporins have been implicated in triggering seizures, particularly in patients with renal impairment when the dosage was not reduced (see DOSAGE AND ADMINISTRATION). If seizures associated with drug therapy should occur, the drug should be discontinued. Anticonvulsant therapy can be given if clinically indicated.

Altered Laboratory Tests: Prolonged prothrombin time, pancytopenia, agranulocytosis.

OVERDOSAGE

Overdosage of cephalosporins can cause cerebral irritation leading to convulsions. Serum levels of cefuroxime can be reduced by hemodialysis and peritoneal dialysis.

DOSAGE AND ADMINISTRATION

Dosage: *Adults:* The usual adult dosage range for ZINACEF is 750 mg to 1.5 grams every 8 hours, usually for 5 to 10 days. In uncomplicated urinary tract infections, skin and skin-structure infections, disseminated gonococcal infections, and uncomplicated pneumonia, a 750-mg dose every 8 hours is recommended. In severe or complicated infections, a 1.5-gram dose every 8 hours is recommended.

In bone and joint infections, a 1.5-gram dose every 8 hours is recommended. In clinical trials, surgical intervention was performed when indicated as an adjunct to therapy with ZINACEF. A course of oral antibiotics was administered when appropriate following the completion of parenteral administration of ZINACEF.

In life-threatening infections or infections due to less susceptible organisms, 1.5 grams every 6 hours may be required. In bacterial meningitis, the dosage should not exceed 3 grams every 8 hours. The recommended dosage for uncomplicated gonococcal infection is 1.5 grams given intramuscularly as a single dose at two different sites together with 1 gram of oral probenecid. For preventive use for clean-contaminated or potentially contaminated surgical procedures, a 1.5-gram dose administered intravenously just before surgery (approximately one-half to 1 hour before the initial incision) is recommended. Thereafter, give 750 mg intravenously or intramuscularly every 8 hours when the procedure is prolonged.

For preventive use during open heart surgery, a 1.5-gram dose administered intravenously at the induction of anesthesia and every 12 hours thereafter for a total of 6 grams is recommended.

Impaired Renal Function: A reduced dosage must be employed when renal function is impaired. Dosage should be determined by the degree of renal impairment and the susceptibility of the causative organism (see Table 1).

Table 1: Dosage of ZINACEF in Adults With Reduced Renal Function

Creatinine Clearance (mL/min)	Dose	Frequency
>20	750 mg–1.5 grams	q8h
10–20	750 mg	q12h
<10	750 mg	q24h*

* Since ZINACEF is dialyzable, patients on hemodialysis should be given a further dose at the end of the dialysis.

When only serum creatinine is available, the following formula[2] (based on sex, weight, and age of the patient) may be used to convert this value into creatinine clearance. The serum creatinine should represent a steady state of renal function.

Males: Creatinine clearance (mL/min)=
$$\frac{\text{Weight (kg)} \times (140-\text{age})}{72 \times \text{serum creatinine (mg/dL)}}$$
Females: $0.85 \times$ male value

Note: As with antibiotic therapy in general, administration of ZINACEF should be continued for a minimum of 48 to 72 hours after the patient becomes asymptomatic or after evidence of bacterial eradication has been obtained; a minimum of 10 days of treatment is recommended in infections caused by *Streptococcus pyogenes* in order to guard against the risk of rheumatic fever or glomerulonephritis; frequent bacteriologic and clinical appraisal is necessary during therapy of chronic urinary tract infection and may be required for several months after therapy has been completed; persistent infections may require treatment for several weeks; and doses smaller than those indicated above should not be used. In staphylococcal and other infections involving a collection of pus, surgical drainage should be carried out where indicated.

Pediatric Patients Above 3 Months of Age: Administration of 50 to 100 mg/kg per day in equally divided doses every 6 to 8 hours has been successful for most infections susceptible to cefuroxime. The higher dosage of 100 mg/kg per day (not to exceed the maximum adult dosage) should be used for the more severe or serious infections.

In bone and joint infections, 150 mg/kg per day (not to exceed the maximum adult dosage) is recommended in equally divided doses every 8 hours. In clinical trials, a course of oral antibiotics was administered to pediatric patients following the completion of parenteral administration of ZINACEF.

In cases of bacterial meningitis, a larger dosage of ZINACEF is recommended, 200 to 240 mg/kg per day intravenously in divided doses every 6 to 8 hours.

In pediatric patients with renal insufficiency, the frequency of dosing should be modified consistent with the recommendations for adults.

Preparation of Solution and Suspension: The directions for preparing ZINACEF for both IV and IM use are summarized in Table 2.

For Intramuscular Use: Each 750-mg vial of ZINACEF should be constituted with 3.0 mL of Sterile Water for Injection. Shake gently to disperse and withdraw completely the resulting suspension for injection.

For Intravenous Use: Each 750-mg vial should be constituted with 8.0 mL of Sterile Water for Injection. Withdraw completely the resulting solution for injection.

Each 1.5-gram vial should be constituted with 16.0 mL of Sterile Water for Injection, and the solution should be completely withdrawn for injection.

The 7.5-gram pharmacy bulk vial should be constituted with 77 mL of Sterile Water for Injection; each 8 mL of the resulting solution contains 750 mg of cefuroxime.

Each 750-mg and 1.5-gram infusion pack should be constituted with 100 mL of Sterile Water for Injection, 5% Dextrose Injection, 0.9% Sodium Chloride Injection, or any of the solutions listed under the Intravenous portion of the COMPATIBILITY AND STABILITY section.

[See table 2 above]

Table 2: Preparation of Solution and Suspension

Strength	Amount of Diluent to Be Added (mL)	Volume to Be Withdrawn	Approximate Cefuroxime Concentration (mg/mL)
750-mg Vial	3.0 (IM)	Total*	220
750-mg Vial	8.0 (IV)	Total	90
1.5-gram Vial	16.0 (IV)	Total	90
750-mg Infusion pack	100 (IV)	—	7.5
1.5-gram Infusion pack	100 (IV)	—	15
7.5-gram Pharmacy bulk package	77 (IV)	Amount Needed†	95

***Note:** ZINACEF is a suspension at IM concentrations.

†8 mL of solution contains 750 mg of cefuroxime; 16 mL of solution contains 1.5 grams of cefuroxime.

Administration: After constitution, ZINACEF may be given intravenously or by deep IM injection into a large muscle mass (such as the gluteus or lateral part of the thigh). Before injecting intramuscularly, aspiration is necessary to avoid inadvertent injection into a blood vessel.

Intravenous Administration: The IV route may be preferable for patients with bacterial septicemia or other severe or life-threatening infections or for patients who may be poor risks because of lowered resistance, particularly if shock is present or impending.

For direct intermittent IV administration, slowly inject the solution into a vein over a period of 3 to 5 minutes or give it through the tubing system by which the patient is also receiving other IV solutions.

For intermittent IV infusion with a Y-type administration set, dosing can be accomplished through the tubing system by which the patient may be receiving other IV solutions. However, during infusion of the solution containing ZINACEF, it is advisable to temporarily discontinue administration of any other solutions at the same site.

ADD-Vantage vials are to be constituted only with 50 or 100 mL of 5% Dextrose Injection, 0.9% Sodium Chloride Injection, or 0.45% Sodium Chloride Injection in Abbott ADD-Vantage flexible diluent containers (see Instructions for Constitution section of the product package insert). ADD-Vantage vials that have been joined to Abbott ADD-Vantage diluent containers and activated to dissolve the drug are stable for 24 hours at room temperature or for 7 days under refrigeration. Joined vials that have not been activated may be used within a 14-day period; this period corresponds to that for use of Abbott ADD-Vantage containers following removal of the outer packaging (overwrap).

Freezing solutions of ZINACEF in the ADD-Vantage system is not recommended.

For continuous IV infusion, a solution of ZINACEF may be added to an IV infusion pack containing one of the following fluids: 0.9% Sodium Chloride Injection; 5% Dextrose Injection; 10% Dextrose Injection; 5% Dextrose and 0.9% Sodium Chloride Injection; 5% Dextrose and 0.45% Sodium Chloride Injection; or 1/6 M Sodium Lactate Injection.

Solutions of ZINACEF, like those of most beta-lactam antibiotics, should not be added to solutions of aminoglycoside antibiotics because of potential interaction.

However, if concurrent therapy with ZINACEF and an aminoglycoside is indicated, each of these antibiotics can be administered separately to the same patient.

Directions for Use of ZINACEF Frozen in GALAXY® Plastic Containers: ZINACEF supplied as a frozen, sterile, iso-osmotic, nonpyrogenic solution in plastic containers is to be administered after thawing either as a continuous or intermittent IV infusion. The thawed solution of the premixed product is stable for 28 days if stored under refrigeration (5° C) or for 24 hours if stored at room temperature (25° C). **Do not Refreeze.**

Thaw container at room temperature (25°C) or under refrigeration (5°C). Do not force thaw by immersion in water baths or by microwave irradiation. Components of the solution may precipitate in the frozen state and will dissolve upon reaching room temperature with little or no agitation. Potency is not affected. Mix after solution has reached room temperature. Check for minute leaks by squeezing bag firmly. Discard bag if leaks are found as sterility may be impaired. Do not add supplementary medication. Do not use unless solution is clear and seal is intact.

Use sterile equipment.

Caution: Do not use plastic containers in series connections. Such use could result in air embolism due to residual air being drawn from the primary container before administration of the fluid from the secondary container is complete.

Preparation for Administration:

1. Suspend container from eyelet support.
2. Remove protector from outlet port at bottom of container.
3. Attach administration set. Refer to complete directions accompanying set.

COMPATIBILITY AND STABILITY

Intramuscular: When constituted as directed with Sterile Water for Injection, suspensions of ZINACEF for IM injection maintain satisfactory potency for 24 hours at room temperature and for 48 hours under refrigeration (5°C).

After the periods mentioned above any unused suspensions should be discarded.

Intravenous: When the 750-mg, 1.5-g, and 7.5-g pharmacy bulk vials are constituted as directed with Sterile Water for Injection, the ZINACEF solutions for IV administration maintain satisfactory potency for 24 hours at room temperature and for 48 hours (750-mg and 1.5-g vials) or for 7 days (7.5-g pharmacy bulk vial) under refrigeration (5°C). More dilute solutions, such as 750 mg or 1.5 g plus 100 mL of Sterile Water for Injection, 5% Dextrose Injection, or 0.9% Sodium Chloride Injection, also maintain satisfactory potency for 24 hours at room temperature and for 7 days under refrigeration.

These solutions may be further diluted to concentrations of between 1 and 30 mg/mL in the following solutions and will lose not more than 10% activity for 24 hours at room temperature or for at least 7 days under refrigeration: 0.9% Sodium Chloride Injection; 1/6 M Sodium Lactate Injection; Ringer's Injection, USP; Lactated Ringer's Injection, USP; 5% Dextrose and 0.9% Sodium Chloride Injection; 5% Dextrose Injection; 5% Dextrose and 0.45% Sodium Chloride Injection; 5% Dextrose and 0.225% Sodium Chloride Injection; 10% Dextrose Injection; and 10% Invert Sugar in Water for Injection.

Unused solutions should be discarded after the time periods mentioned above.

ZINACEF has also been found compatible for 24 hours at room temperature when admixed in IV infusion with heparin (10 and 50 U/mL) in 0.9% Sodium Chloride Injection and Potassium Chloride (10 and 40 mEq/L) in 0.9% Sodium Chloride Injection. Sodium Bicarbonate Injection, USP is not recommended for the dilution of ZINACEF.

The 750-mg and 1.5-g ZINACEF ADD-Vantage vials, when diluted in 50 or 100 mL of 5% Dextrose Injection, 0.9% Sodium Chloride Injection, or 0.45% Sodium Chloride Injection, may be stored for up to 24 hours at room temperature or for 7 days under refrigeration.

Frozen Stability: Constitute the 750-mg, 1.5-g, or 7.5-g vial as directed for IV administration in Table 2. Immediately withdraw the total contents of the 750-mg or 1.5-g vial or 8 or 16 mL from the 7.5-g bulk vial and add to a Baxter VIAFLEX® MINI-BAG™ containing 50 or 100 mL of 0.9% Sodium Chloride Injection or 5% Dextrose Injection and freeze. Frozen solutions are stable for 6 months when stored at −20°C. Frozen solutions should be thawed at room temperature and not refrozen. Do not force thaw by immersion in water baths or by microwave irradiation. Thawed solutions may be stored for up to 24 hours at room temperature or for 7 days in a refrigerator.

Note: Parenteral drug products should be inspected visually for particulate matter and discoloration before administration whenever solution and container permit.

As with other cephalosporins, ZINACEF powder as well as solutions and suspensions tend to darken, depending on storage conditions, without adversely affecting product potency.

Directions for Dispensing: *Pharmacy Bulk Package —Not for Direct Infusion:* The pharmacy bulk package is for use in a pharmacy admixture service only under a laminar flow hood. Entry into the vial must be made with a sterile transfer set or other sterile dispensing device, and the contents dispensed in aliquots using aseptic technique. The use of syringe and needle is not recommended as it may cause leakage (see DOSAGE AND ADMINISTRATION). AFTER INITIAL WITHDRAWAL USE ENTIRE CONTENTS OF VIAL PROMPTLY. ANY UNUSED PORTION MUST BE DISCARDED WITHIN 24 HOURS.

HOW SUPPLIED

ZINACEF in the dry state should be stored between 15° and 30°C (59° and 86°F) and protected from light. ZINACEF is a dry, white to off-white powder supplied in vials and infusion packs as follows:

NDC 0173-0352-31 750-mg* Vial (Tray of 25)
NDC 0173-0354-35 1.5-g* Vial (Tray of 25)
NDC 0173-0353-32 750-mg* Infusion Pack (Tray of 10)
NDC 0173-0356-32 1.5-g* Infusion Pack (Tray of 10)
NDC 0173-0400-00 7.5-g* Pharmacy Bulk Package (Tray of 6)
NDC 0173-0436-00 750-mg ADD-Vantage Vial (Tray of 25)
NDC 0173-0437-00 1.5-g ADD-Vantage Vial (Tray of 10)

(The above ADD-Vantage vials are to be used only with Abbott ADD-Vantage diluent containers.)

ZINACEF frozen as a premixed solution of cefuroxime sodium should not be stored above −20° C. ZINACEF is supplied frozen in 50-mL, single-dose, plastic containers as follows:

NDC 0173-0424-00 750-mg* Plastic Container (Carton of 24)
NDC 0173-0425-00 1.5-g* Plastic Container (Carton of 24)

*Equivalent to cefuroxime.

REFERENCES

1. National Committee for Clinical Laboratory Standards. *Performance Standards for Antimicrobial Susceptibility Testing.* Third Informational Supplement. NCCLS Document M100-S3, Vol. 11, No. 17. Villanova, Pa: NCCLS; 1991.
2. Cockcroft DW, Gault MH. Prediction of creatinine clearance from serum creatinine. *Nephron.* 1976;16:31-41.

ZINACEF is a registered trademark of Glaxo Wellcome.

ADD-Vantage is a registered trademark of Abbott Laboratories.

CLINITEST is a registered trademark of Ames Division, Miles Laboratories, Inc.

TES-TAPE is a registered trademark of Eli Lilly and Company.

GALAXY and VIAFLEX are registered trademarks of Baxter International Inc.

April 1998/RL-555

Shown in Product Identification Guide, page 315

ZOFRAN® ℞
[zō 'fran]
(ondansetron hydrochloride)
Injection

ZOFRAN® ℞
(ondansetron hydrochloride)
Injection Premixed

DESCRIPTION

The active ingredient in ZOFRAN Injection and ZOFRAN Injection Premixed is ondansetron hydrochloride (HCl), the racemic form of ondansetron and a selective blocking agent of the serotonin 5-HT_3 receptor type. Chemically it is (±) 1, 2, 3, 9-tetrahydro-9-methyl-3-[(2-methyl-1H-imidazol-1-yl)methyl]-4H-carbazol-4-one, monohydrochloride, dihydrate.

The empirical formula is $C_{18}H_{19}N_3O{\cdot}HCl{\cdot}2H_2O$, representing a molecular weight of 365.9.

Ondansetron HCl is a white to off-white powder that is soluble in water and normal saline.

Sterile Injection for Intravenous (IV) or Intramuscular (IM) Administration: Each 1 mL of aqueous solution in the 2-mL single-dose vial contains 2 mg of ondansetron as the hydrochloride dihydrate; 9.0 mg of sodium chloride, USP; and 0.5 mg citric acid monohydrate, USP and 0.25 mg of sodium citrate dihydrate, USP as buffers in Water for Injection, USP. Each 1 mL of aqueous solution in the 20-mL multidose vial contains 2 mg of ondansetron as the hydrochloride dihydrate; 8.3 mg of sodium chloride, USP; 0.5 mg of citric acid

Continued on next page

This product information is based on labeling in effect on June 1, 1998. For further information, contact via direct mail, phone, or web site Medical Information: Glaxo Wellcome Inc., PO Box 13398, Research Triangle Park, NC 27709. Healthcare Professionals (Medical Information): 800-334-0089 Patients (Customer Response Center): 888-TALK2GW (1-888-825-5249) Glaxo Wellcome Corporate Web Site: www.glaxowellcome.com

Zofran Injection—Cont.

monohydrate, USP and 0.25 mg of sodium citrate dihydrate, USP as buffers; and 1.2 mg of methylparaben, NF and 0.15 mg of propylparaben, NF as preservatives in Water for Injection, USP.

ZOFRAN Injection is a clear, colorless, nonpyrogenic, sterile solution. The pH of the Injection solution is 3.3 to 4.0.

Sterile, Premixed Solution for Intravenous Administration in Single-Dose, Flexible Plastic Containers: Each 50 mL contains ondansetron 32 mg (as the hydrochloride dihydrate); dextrose 2,500 mg; and citric acid 26 mg and sodium citrate 11.5 mg as buffers in Water for Injection, USP. It contains no preservatives. The osmolarity of this solution is 270 mOsm/L (approx.), and the pH is 3.0 to 4.0. The flexible plastic container is fabricated from a specially formulated, nonplasticized, thermoplastic co-polyester (CR3). Water can permeate from inside the container into the overwrap but not in amounts sufficient to affect the solution significantly. Solutions inside the container also can leach out certain of the chemical components in very small amounts before the expiration period is attained. However, the safety of the plastic has been confirmed by tests in animals according to USP biological standards for plastic containers.

CLINICAL PHARMACOLOGY

Pharmacodynamics: Ondansetron is a selective 5-HT$_3$ receptor antagonist. While ondansetron's mechanism of action has not been fully characterized, it is not a dopamine-receptor antagonist. Serotonin receptors of the 5-HT$_3$ type are present both peripherally on vagal nerve terminals and centrally in the chemoreceptor trigger zone of the area postrema. It is not certain whether ondansetron's antiemetic action in chemotherapy-induced emesis is mediated centrally, peripherally, or in both sites. However, cytotoxic chemotherapy appears to be associated with release of serotonin from the enterochromaffin cells of the small intestine. In humans, urinary 5-HIAA (5-hydroxyindoleacetic acid) excretion increases after cisplatin administration in parallel with the onset of emesis. The released serotonin may stimulate the vagal afferents through the 5-HT$_3$ receptors and initiate the vomiting reflex.

In animals, the emetic response to cisplatin can be prevented by pretreatment with an inhibitor of serotonin synthesis, bilateral abdominal vagotomy and greater splanchnic nerve section, or pretreatment with a serotonin 5-HT$_3$ receptor antagonist.

In normal volunteers, single IV doses of 0.15 mg/kg of ondansetron had no effect on esophageal motility, gastric motility, lower esophageal sphincter pressure, or small intestinal transit time. In another study in six normal male volunteers, a 16-mg dose infused over 5 minutes showed no effect of the drug on cardiac output, heart rate, stroke volume, blood pressure, or electrocardiogram (ECG). Multiday administration of ondansetron has been shown to slow colonic transit in normal volunteers. Ondansetron has no effect on plasma prolactin concentrations.

In a gender-balanced pharmacodynamic study (n = 56), ondasetron 4 mg administered intravenously or intramuscularly was dynamically similar in the prevention of emesis and nausea using the ipecacuanha model of emesis. Both treatments were well tolerated.

Ondansetron does not alter the respiratory depressant effects produced by alfentanil or the degree of neuromuscular blockade produced by atracurium. Interactions with general or local anesthetics have not been studied.

Pharmacokinetics: Ondansetron is extensively metabolized in humans, with approximately 5% of a radiolabeled dose recovered as the parent compound from the urine. The primary metabolic pathway is hydroxylation on the indole ring followed by glucuronide or sulfate conjugation.

In normal volunteers, the following mean pharmacokinetic data have been determined following a single 0.15-mg/kg IV dose.

Table 1: Pharmacokinetics in Normal Volunteers

Age-group	n	Peak Plasma Concentration (ng/mL)	Mean Elimination Half-life (h)	Plasma Clearance (L/h/kg)
19-40	11	102	3.5	0.381
61-74	12	106	4.7	0.319
≥75	11	170	5.5	0.262

From a single-dose infusion study, patients with severe hepatic impairment showed a fivefold and those with mild-to-moderate liver impairment a twofold reduction in mean plasma clearance, with increases in the mean apparent volume of distribution of less than twofold, as compared to normals. The mean half-life of 3.6 hours in normals increased to 9.2 hours in patients with mild-to-moderate hepatic impairment and was prolonged to 20.6 hours in patients with severe hepatic insufficiency.

A reduction in clearance and increase in elimination half-life are seen in patients over 75 years old. In clinical trials with patients with cancer, there was neither a difference in safety nor efficacy between patients over 65 years of age and those under 65 years of age; there was an insufficient number of patients over 75 years of age to permit conclusions in that age-group. No adjustment in dosage is recommended in the elderly.

In adult cancer patients, the mean elimination half-life was 4.0 hours, and there was no difference in the multidose pharmacokinetics over a 4-day period. In a study of 21 pediatric cancer patients (aged 4 to 18 years) who received three IV doses of 0.15 mg/kg of ondansetron at 4-hour intervals, patients older than 15 years of age exhibited ondansetron pharmacokinetic parameters similar to those of adults. Patients aged 4 to 12 years generally showed higher clearance and somewhat larger volume of distribution than adults. Most pediatric patients younger than 15 years of age with cancer had a shorter (2.4 hours) ondansetron plasma half-life than patients older than 15 years of age. It is not known whether these differences in ondansetron plasma half-life may result in differences in efficacy between adults and some young pediatric patients (see CLINICAL TRIALS: Pediatric Studies).

In a study of 21 pediatric patients (aged 3 to 12 years) who were undergoing surgery requiring anesthesia for a duration of 45 minutes to 2 hours, a single IV dose of ondansetron, 2 mg (3 to 7 years) or 4 mg (8 to 12 years), was administered immediately prior to anesthesia induction. Mean weight-normalized clearance and volume of distribution values in these pediatric surgical patients were similar to those previously reported for young adults. Mean terminal half-life was slightly reduced in pediatric patients (range, 2.5 to 3 hours) in comparison with adults (range, 3 to 3.5 hours).

In normal volunteers (19 to 39 years old, n = 23), the peak plasma concentration was 264 ng/mL following a single 32-mg dose administered as a 15-minute IV infusion. The mean elimination half-life was 4.1 hours. Systemic exposure to 32 mg of ondansetron was not proportional to dose as measured by comparing dose-normalized AUC values to an 8-mg dose. This is consistent with a small decrease in systemic clearance with increasing plasma concentrations.

A study was performed in normal volunteers (n = 56) to evaluate the pharmacokinetics of a single 4-mg dose administered as a 5-minute infusion compared to a single intramuscular injection. Systemic exposure as measured by mean AUC was equivalent, with values of 156 [95% CI 136, 180] and 161 [95% CI 137, 190] ng•h/mL for IV and IM groups, respectively. Mean peak plasma concentrations were 42.9 [95% CI 33.8, 54.4] ng/mL at 10 minutes after IV infusion and 31.9 [95% CI 26.3, 38.6] ng/mL at 41 minutes after IM injection. The mean elimination half-life was not affected by route of administration.

Table 2: Prevention of Chemotherapy-Induced Nausea and Emesis in Single-Day Cisplatin Therapy*

	ZOFRAN Injection	Placebo	P Value†
Number of patients	14	14	
Treatment response			
0 Emetic episodes	2 (14%)	0 (0%)	
1–2 Emetic episodes	8 (57%)	0 (0%)	
3–5 Emetic episodes	2 (14%)	1 (7%)	
More than 5 emetic episodes/rescued	2 (14%)	13 (93%)	0.001
Median number of emetic episodes	1.5	Undefined‡	
Median time to first emetic episode (h)	11.6	2.8	0.001
Median nausea scores (0–100)§	3	59	0.034
Global satisfaction with control of nausea and vomiting (0–100)‖	96	10.5	0.009

* Chemotherapy was high dose (100 and 120 mg/m²; ZOFRAN Injection n = 6, placebo n = 5) or moderate dose (50 and 80 mg/m²; ZOFRAN Injection n = 8, placebo n = 9). Other chemotherapeutic agents included fluorouracil, doxorubicin, and cyclophosphamide. There was no difference between treatments in the types of chemotherapy that would account for differences in response.
† Efficacy based on "all patients treated" analysis.
‡ Median undefined since at least 50% of the patients were rescued or had more than five emetic episodes.
§ Visual analog scale assessment of nausea: 0 = no nausea, 100 = nausea as bad as it can be.
‖ Visual analog scale assessment of satisfaction: 0 = not at all satisfied, 100 = totally satisfied.

Table 3: Prevention of Emesis Induced by Cisplatin (≥100 mg/m²) Single-Day Therapy*

	ZOFRAN Injection	Metoclopramide	P Value
Dose	0.15 mg/kg × 3	2 mg/kg × 6	
Number of patients in efficacy population	136	138	
Treatment response			
0 Emetic episodes	54 (40%)	41 (30%)	
1–2 Emetic episodes	34 (25%)	30 (22%)	
3–5 Emetic episodes	19 (14%)	18 (13%)	
More than 5 emetic episodes/rescued	29 (21%)	49 (36%)	
Comparison of treatments with respect to			
0 Emetic episodes	54/136	41/138	0.083
More than 5 emetic episodes/rescued	29/136	49/138	0.009
Median number of emetic episodes	1	2	0.005
Median time to first emetic episode (h)	20.5	4.3	<0.001
Global satisfaction with control of nausea and vomiting (0–100)†	85	63	0.001
Acute dystonic reactions	0	8	0.005
Akathisia	0	10	0.002

* In addition to cisplatin, 68% of patients received other chemotherapeutic agents, including cyclophosphamide, etoposide, and fluorouracil. There was no difference between treatments in the types of chemotherapy that would account for differences in response.
† Visual analog scale assessment: 0 = not at all satisfied, 100 = totally satisfied.

Plasma protein binding of ondansetron as measured in vitro was 70% to 76%, with binding constant over the pharmacologic concentration range (10 to 500 ng/mL). Circulating drug also distributes into erythrocytes.

A positive lymphoblast transformation test to ondansetron has been reported, which suggests immunologic sensitivity to ondansetron.

CLINICAL TRIALS

Chemotherapy-Induced Nausea and Vomiting: In a double-blind study of three different dosing regimens of ZOFRAN Injection, 0.015 mg/kg, 0.15 mg/kg, and 0.30 mg/kg, each given three times during the course of cancer chemotherapy, the 0.15-mg/kg dosing regimen was more effective than the 0.015-mg/kg dosing regimen. The 0.30-mg/kg dosing regimen was not shown to be more effective than the 0.15-mg/kg dosing regimen.

Cisplatin-Based Chemotherapy: In a double-blind study in 28 patients, ZOFRAN Injection (three 0.15-mg/kg doses) was significantly more effective than placebo in preventing nausea and vomiting induced by cisplatin-based chemotherapy. Treatment response was as follows:
[See table 2 at top of previous page]

Ondansetron was compared with metoclopramide in a single-blind trial in 307 patients receiving cisplatin ≥ 100 mg/m² with or without other chemotherapeutic agents. Patients received the first dose of ondansetron or metoclopramide 30 minutes before cisplatin. Two additional ondansetron doses were administered 4 and 8 hours later, or five additional metoclopramide doses were administered 2, 4, 7, 10, and 13 hours later. Cisplatin was administered over a period of 3 hours or less. Episodes of vomiting and retching were tabulated over the period of 24 hours after cisplatin. The results of this study are summarized below:
[See table 3 on previous page]

Forty-one of the ondansetron patients were over 65 years of age. The complete response rate (zero emetic episodes) was 41% in this group compared with 40% in those 65 years old or younger.

In a stratified, randomized, double-blind, parallel-group, multicenter study, a single 32-mg dose of ondansetron was compared with three 0.15-mg/kg doses in patients receiving cisplatin doses of either 50 to 70 mg/m² or ≥ 100 mg/m². Patients received the first ondansetron dose 30 minutes before cisplatin. Two additional ondansetron doses were administered 4 and 8 hours later to the group receiving three 0.15-mg/kg doses. In both strata, significantly fewer patients on the single 32-mg dose than those receiving the three-dose regimen failed.
[See table 4 above]

Cyclophosphamide-Based Chemotherapy: In a double-blind, placebo-controlled study of ZOFRAN Injection (three 0.15-mg/kg doses) in 20 patients receiving cyclophosphamide (500 to 600 mg/m²) chemotherapy, ZOFRAN Injection was significantly more effective than placebo in preventing nausea and vomiting. The results are summarized below:
[See table 5 above]

Re-treatment: In uncontrolled trials, 127 patients receiving cisplatin (median dose, 100 mg/m²) and ondansetron who had two or fewer emetic episodes were re-treated with ondansetron and chemotherapy, mainly cisplatin, for a total of 269 re-treatment courses (median, 2; range, 1 to 10). No emetic episodes occurred in 160 (59%), and two or fewer emetic episodes occurred in 217 (81%) re-treatment courses.

Pediatric Studies: Four open-label, noncomparative (one US, three foreign) trials have been performed with 209 pediatric cancer patients aged 4 to 18 years given a variety of cisplatin or noncisplatin regimens. In the three foreign trials, the initial ZOFRAN Injection dose ranged from 0.04 to 0.87 mg/kg for a total dose of 2.16 to 12 mg. This was followed by the oral administration of ondansetron ranging from 4 to 24 mg daily for 3 days. In the US trial, ZOFRAN was administered intravenously (only) in three doses of 0.15 mg/kg each for a total daily dose of 7.2 to 39 mg. In these studies, 58% of the 196 evaluable patients had a complete response (no emetic episodes) on day 1. Thus, prevention of emesis in these pediatric patients was essentially the same as for patients older than 18 years of age. Overall, ZOFRAN Injection was well tolerated in these pediatric patients.

Postoperative Nausea and Vomiting: *Prevention of Postoperative Nausea and Vomiting:* Adult surgical patients who received ondansetron immediately before the induction of general balanced anesthesia (barbiturate: thiopental, methohexital, or thiamylal; opioid: alfentanil or fentanyl; nitrous oxide; neuromuscular blockade: succinylcholine/curare and/or vecuronium or atracurium; and supplemental isoflurane) were evaluated in two double-blind US studies involving 554 patients. ZOFRAN Injection (4 mg) IV given over 2 to 5 minutes was significantly more effective than placebo. The results of these studies are summarized below:
[See table 6 at top of next page]
The study populations in all trials thus far consisted of mainly women undergoing laparoscopic procedures.

While some men were included in some trials with similar results, clearance of the drug is more rapid in men and sufficient numbers of men have not been clinically studied to

Table 4: Prevention of Chemotherapy-Induced Nausea and Emesis in Single-Dose Therapy

	Ondansetron Dose		
	0.15 mg/kg x 3	32 mg x 1	P Value
High-dose cisplatin (≥ 100 mg/m²)			
Number of patients	100	102	
Treatment response			
0 Emetic episodes	41 (41%)	49 (48%)	0.315
1–2 Emetic episodes	19 (19%)	25 (25%)	
3–5 Emetic episodes	4 (4%)	8 (8%)	
More than 5 emetic episodes/rescued	36 (36%)	20 (20%)	0.009
Median time to first emetic episode (h)	21.7	23	0.173
Median nausea scores (0–100)*	28	13	0.004
Medium-dose cisplatin (50–70 mg/m²)			
Number of patients	101	93	
Treatment response			
0 Emetic episodes	62 (61%)	68 (73%)	0.083
1–2 Emetic episodes	11 (11%)	14 (15%)	
3–5 Emetic episodes	6 (6%)	3 (3%)	
More than 5 emetic episodes/rescued	22 (22%)	8 (9%)	0.011
Median time to first emetic episode (h)	Undefined†	Undefined	0.084
Median nausea scores (0–100)*	9	3	0.131

* Visual analog scale assessment: 0 = no nausea, 100 = nausea as bad as it can be.
† Median undefined since at least 50% of patients did not have any emetic episodes.

Table 5: Prevention of Chemotherapy-Induced Nausea and Emesis in Single-Day Cyclophosphamide Therapy*

	ZOFRAN Injection	Placebo	P Value†
Number of patients	10	10	
Treatment response			
0 Emetic episodes	7 (70%)	0 (0%)	0.001
1–2 Emetic episodes	0 (0%)	2 (20%)	
3–5 Emetic episodes	2 (20%)	4 (40%)	
More than 5 emetic episodes/rescued	1 (10%)	4 (40%)	0.131
Median number of emetic episodes	0	4	0.008
Median time to first emetic episode (h)	Undefined‡	8.79	
Median nausea scores (0–100)§	0	60	0.001
Global satisfaction with control of nausea and vomiting (0–100) ‖	100	52	0.008

* Chemotherapy consisted of cyclophosphamide in all patients, plus other agents, including fluorouracil, doxorubicin, methotrexate, and vincristine. There was no difference between treatments in the type of chemotherapy that would account for differences in response.
† Efficacy based on "all patients treated" analysis.
‡ Median undefined since at least 50% of patients did not have any emetic episodes.
§ Visual analog scale assessment of nausea: 0 = no nausea, 100 = nausea as bad as it can be.
‖ Visual analog scale assessment of satisfaction: 0 = not at all satisfied, 100 = totally satisfied.

be certain that efficacy and safety have been established. Few patients undergoing major abdominal surgery have been studied.

Pediatric Studies: Three double-blind, placebo-controlled studies have been performed (one US, two foreign) in 1,049 male and female patients (2 to 12 years of age) undergoing general anesthesia with nitrous oxide. The surgical procedures included tonsillectomy with or without adenoidectomy, strabismus surgery, herniorrhaphy, and orchidopexy. Patients were randomized to either single IV doses of ondansetron (0.1 mg/kg for children weighing 40 kg or less, 4 mg for children weighing more than 40 kg) or placebo. Study drug was administered over at least 30 seconds, immediately prior to or following anesthesia induction. Ondansetron was significantly more effective than placebo in preventing nausea and vomiting. The results of these studies are summarized below:
[See table 7 on next page]

Prevention of Further Postoperative Nausea and Vomiting: Adult surgical patients receiving general balanced anesthesia (barbiturate: thiopental, methohexital, or thiamylal; opioid: alfentanil or fentanyl; nitrous oxide; neuromuscular blockade: succinylcholine/curare and/or vecuronium or atracurium; and supplemental isoflurane) who received no prophylactic antiemetics and who experienced nausea and/or vomiting within 2 hours postoperatively were evaluated in two double-blind US studies involving 441 patients. Patients who experienced an episode of postoperative nausea and/or vomiting were given ZOFRAN Injection (4 mg) IV over 2 to 5 minutes, and this was significantly more effective than placebo. The results of these studies are summarized below:
[See table 8 on next page]
The study populations in all trials thus far consisted of mainly women undergoing laparoscopic procedures.

While some men were included in some trials with similar results, clearance of the drug is more rapid in men and sufficient numbers of men have not been clinically studied to

be certain that efficacy and safety have been established. Few patients undergoing major abdominal surgery have been studied.

Pediatric Studies: One double-blind, placebo-controlled, US study was performed in 351 male and female outpatients (2 to 12 years of age) who received general anesthesia with nitrous oxide and no prophylactic antiemetics. Surgical procedures were unrestricted. Patients who experienced two or more emetic episodes within 2 hours following discontinuation of nitrous oxide were randomized to either single IV dose of ondansetron (0.1 mg/kg for pediatric patients weighing 40 kg or less, 4 mg for children weighing more than 40 kg) or placebo administered over at least 30 seconds. Ondansetron was significantly more effective than placebo in preventing further episodes of nausea and vomiting. The results of the study are summarized below:
[See table 9 at top of page 1269]

INDICATIONS AND USAGE

1. Prevention of nausea and vomiting associated with initial and repeat courses of emetogenic cancer chemotherapy, including high-dose cisplatin. Efficacy of the 32-mg single dose beyond 24 hours in these patients has not been established.

2. Prevention of postoperative nausea and/or vomiting. As with other antiemetics, routine prophylaxis is not recommended for patients in whom there is little expectation that

Continued on next page

This product information is based on labeling in effect on June 1, 1998. For further information, contact via direct mail, phone, or web site Medical Information: Glaxo Wellcome Inc., PO Box 13398, Research Triangle Park, NC 27709. Healthcare Professionals (Medical Information): 800-334-0089 Patients (Customer Response Center): 888-TALK2GW (1-888-825-5249) Glaxo Wellcome Corporate Web Site: www.glaxowellcome.com

Zofran Injection—Cont.

nausea and/or vomiting will occur postoperatively. In patients where nausea and/or vomiting must be avoided postoperatively, ZOFRAN Injection is recommended even where the incidence of postoperative nausea and/or vomiting is low. For patients who have nausea and/or vomiting postoperatively, ZOFRAN Injection may be given to prevent further episodes (see CLINICAL TRIALS).

CONTRAINDICATIONS
ZOFRAN Injection and ZOFRAN Injection Premixed are contraindicated for patients known to have hypersensitivity to the drug.

WARNINGS
Hypersensitivity reactions have been reported in patients who have exhibited hypersensitivity to other selective 5-HT_3 receptor antagonists.

PRECAUTIONS
Ondansetron is not a drug that stimulates gastric or intestinal peristalsis. It should not be used instead of nasogastric suction. The use of ondansetron in patients following abdominal surgery or in patients with chemotherapy-induced nausea and vomiting may mask a progressive ileus and/or gastric distention.

Drug Interactions: Ondansetron does not itself appear to induce or inhibit the cytochrome P-450 drug-metabolizing enzyme system of the liver. Because ondansetron is metabolized by hepatic cytochrome P-450 drug-metabolizing enzymes, inducers or inhibitors of these enzymes may change the clearance and, hence, the half-life of ondansetron. On the basis of limited available data, no dosage adjustment is recommended for patients on these drugs. Tumor response to chemotherapy in the P 388 mouse leukemia model is not affected by ondansetron. In humans, carmustine, etoposide, and cisplatin do not affect the pharmacokinetics of ondansetron.

Carcinogenesis, Mutagenesis, Impairment of Fertility: Carcinogenic effects were not seen in 2-year studies in rats and mice with oral ondansetron doses up to 10 and 30 mg/kg per day, respectively. Ondansetron was not mutagenic in standard tests for mutagenicity. Oral administration of ondansetron up to 15 mg/kg per day did not affect fertility or general reproductive performance of male and female rats.

Pregnancy: *Teratogenic Effects:* Pregnancy Category B. Reproduction studies have been performed in pregnant rats and rabbits at IV doses up to 4 mg/kg per day and have revealed no evidence of impaired fertility or harm to the fetus due to ondansetron. There are, however, no adequate and well-controlled studies in pregnant women. Because animal reproduction studies are not always predictive of human response, this drug should be used during pregnancy only if clearly needed.

Nursing Mothers: Ondansetron is excreted in the breast milk of rats. It is not known whether ondansetron is excreted in human milk. Because many drugs are excreted in human milk, caution should be exercised when ondansetron is administered to a nursing woman.

Pediatric Use: Little information is available about dosage in children under 2 years of age (see DOSAGE AND ADMINISTRATION section for use in pediatric patients 4 to 18 years of age receiving cancer chemotherapy or for use in pediatric patients 2 to 12 years of age receiving general anesthesia).

Use in Elderly Patients: Dosage adjustment is not needed in patients over the age of 65 (see CLINICAL PHARMACOLOGY). Prevention of nausea and vomiting in elderly patients was no different than in younger age-groups.

ADVERSE REACTIONS
Chemotherapy-Induced Nausea and Vomiting: The following adverse events have been reported in individuals receiving ondansetron at a dosage of three 0.15-mg/kg doses or as a single 32-mg dose in clinical trials. These patients were receiving concomitant chemotherapy, primarily cisplatin, and IV fluids. Most were receiving a diuretic.
[See table 10 on next page]
The following have been reported during controlled clinical trials or in the routine management of patients. The percentage figures are based on clinical trial experience.
Gastrointestinal: Constipation has been reported in 11% of chemotherapy patients receiving multiday ondansetron.
Hepatic: In comparative trials in cisplatin chemotherapy patients with normal baseline values of aspartate transaminase (AST) and alanine transaminase (ALT), these enzymes have been reported to exceed twice the upper limit of normal in approximately 5% of patients. The increases were transient and did not appear to be related to dose or duration of therapy. On repeat exposure, similar transient elevations in transaminase values occurred in some courses, but symptomatic hepatic disease did not occur.
There have been reports of liver failure and death in patients with cancer receiving concurrent medications including potentially hepatotoxic cytotoxic chemotherapy and antibiotics. The etiology of the liver failure is unclear.

Table 6: Prevention of Postoperative Nausea and Vomiting

	Ondansetron 4 mg IV	Placebo	P Value
Study 1			
Emetic episodes:			
Number of patients	136	139	
Treatment response over			
24-hr postoperative period			
0 Emetic episodes	103 (76%)	64 (46%)	<0.001
1 Emetic episode	13 (10%)	17 (12%)	
More than 1 emetic episode/rescued	20 (15%)	58 (42%)	
Nausea assessments:			
Number of patients	134	136	
No nausea over 24-h postoperative period	56 (42%)	39 (29%)	
Study 2			
Emetic episodes:			
Number of patients	136	143	
Treatment response over			
24-hr postoperative period			
0 Emetic episodes	85 (63%)	63 (44%)	0.002
1 Emetic episode	16 (12%)	29 (20%)	
More than 1 emetic episode/rescued	35 (26%)	51 (36%)	
Nausea assessments:			
Number of patients	125	133	
No nausea over 24-h postoperative period	48 (38%)	42 (32%)	

Table 7: Prevention of Postoperative Nausea and Vomiting

Treatment Response Over 24 Hours	Ondansetron n (%)	Placebo n (%)	P Value
Study 1			
Number of patients	205	210	
0 Emetic episodes	140 (68%)	82 (39%)	≤0.001
Failure*	65 (32%)	128 (61%)	
Study 2			
Number of patients	112	110	
0 Emetic episodes	68 (61%)	38 (35%)	≤0.001
Failure*	44 (39%)	72 (65%)	
Study 3			
Number of patients	206	206	
0 Emetic episodes	123 (60%)	96 (47%)	≤0.01
Failure*	83 (40%)	110 (53%)	
Nausea assessments†:			
Number of patients	185	191	
None	119 (64%)	99 (52%)	≤0.01

* Failure was one or more emetic episodes, rescued, or withdrawn.
† Nausea measured as none, mild, or severe.

Table 8: Prevention of Further Postoperative Nausea and Vomiting

	Ondansetron 4 mg IV	Placebo	P Value
Study 1			
Emetic episodes:			
Number of patients	104	117	
Treatment response 24 h after study drug			
0 Emetic episodes	49 (47%)	19 (16%)	<0.001
1 Emetic episode	12 (12%)	9 (8%)	
More than 1 emetic episode/rescued	43 (41%)	89 (76%)	
Median time to first emetic episode (min)*	55.0	43.0	
Nausea assessments:			
Number of patients	98	102	
Mean nausea score over 24-h postoperative period†	1.7	3.1	
Study 2			
Emetic episodes:			
Number of patients	112	108	
Treatment response 24 h after study drug			
0 Emetic episodes	49 (44%)	28 (26%)	0.006
1 Emetic episode	14 (13%)	3 (3%)	
More than 1 emetic episode/rescued	49 (44%)	77 (71%)	
Median time to first emetic episode (min)*	60.5	34.0	
Nausea assessments:			
Number of patients	105	85	
Mean nausea score over 24-h postoperative period†	1.9	2.9	

* After administration of study drug.
† Nausea measured on a scale of 0-10 with 0 = no nausea, 10 = nausea as bad as it can be.

Table 9: Prevention of Further Postoperative Nausea and Vomiting

Treatment Response Over 24 Hours	Ondansetron n (%)	Placebo n (%)	P Value
Study 1			
Number of patients	180	171	
0 Emetic episodes	96 (53%)	29 (17%)	≤0.001
Failure*	84 (47%)	142 (83%)	

* Failure was one or more emetic episodes, rescued, or withdrawn.

Table 10: Principal Adverse Events in Comparative Trials

	Number of Patients With Event			
	ZOFRAN Injection 0.15 mg/kg × 3 n = 419	ZOFRAN Injection 32 mg × 1 n = 220	Metoclopramide n = 156	Placebo n = 34
Diarrhea	16%	8%	44%	18%
Headache	17%	25%	7%	15%
Fever	8%	7%	5%	3%
Akathisia	0%	0%	6%	0%
Acute dystonic reactions*	0%	0%	5%	0%

* See Central Nervous System below.

Integumentary: Rash has occurred in approximately 1% of patients receiving ondansetron.

Central Nervous System: There have been rare reports consistent with, but not diagnostic of, extrapyramidal reactions in patients receiving ondansetron.

Cardiovascular: Rare instances of tachycardia, angina (chest pain), bradycardia, hypotension, syncope, and electrocardiographic alterations, including second degree heart block. In many cases the relationship to ZOFRAN Injection was unclear.

Special Senses: Transient blurred vision, in some cases associated with abnormalities of accommodation, and transient dizziness during or shortly after IV infusion.

Local Reactions: Pain, redness, and burning at site of injection.

Other: Rare cases of hypokalemia and grand mal seizures have been reported. The relationship to ZOFRAN Injection was unclear. Rare cases of hypersensitivity reactions, sometimes severe (e.g., anaphylaxis, bronchospasm, shortness of breath, hypotension, shock, angioedema, urticaria), have also been reported.

Postoperative Nausea and Vomiting: The following adverse events have been reported in ≥2% of adults receiving ondansetron at a dosage of 4 mg IV over 2 to 5 minutes in clinical trials. Rates of these events were not significantly different in the ondansetron and placebo groups. These patients were receiving multiple concomitant perioperative and postoperative medications.

Table 11: Adverse Events in ≥2% of Adults Receiving Ondansetron at a Dosage of 4 Mg IV over 2 to 5 Minutes in Clinical Trials

	ZOFRAN Injection 4 mg IV n = 547 patients	Placebo n = 547 patients
Headache	92 (17%)	77 (14%)
Dizziness	67 (12%)	88 (16%)
Musculoskeletal pain	57 (10%)	59 (11%)
Drowsiness/ sedation	44 (8%)	37 (7%)
Shivers	38 (7%)	39 (7%)
Malaise/fatigue	25 (5%)	30 (5%)
Injection site reaction	21 (4%)	18 (3%)
Urinary retention	17 (3%)	15 (3%)
Postoperative CO₂-related pain*	12 (2%)	16 (3%)
Chest pain (unspecified)	12 (2%)	15 (3%)
Anxiety/ agitation	11 (2%)	16 (3%)
Dysuria	11 (2%)	9 (2%)
Hypotension	10 (2%)	12 (2%)
Fever	10 (2%)	6 (1%)
Cold sensation	9 (2%)	8 (1%)
Pruritus	9 (2%)	3 (<1%)
Paresthesia	9 (2%)	2 (<1%)

* Sites of pain included abdomen, stomach, joints, rib cage, shoulder.

Pediatric Use: The following were the most commonly reported adverse events in pediatric patients receiving ondansetron (a single 0.1-mg/kg dose for children weighing 40 kg or less, or 4 mg for pediatric patients weighing more than 40 kg) administered intravenously over at least 30 seconds. Rates of these events were not significantly different in the ondansetron and placebo groups. These patients were receiving multiple concomitant perioperative and postoperative medications.

Table 12: Frequency of Adverse Events From Controlled Studies

Adverse Event	Ondansetron n = 755 Patients	Placebo n = 731 Patients
Wound problem	80 (11%)	86 (12%)
Anxiety/agitation	49 (6%)	47 (6%)
Headache	44 (6%)	43 (6%)
Drowsiness/sedation	41 (5%)	56 (8%)
Pyrexia	32 (4%)	41 (6%)

Drug Abuse and Dependence: Animal studies have shown that ondansetron is not discriminated as a benzodiazepine nor does it substitute for benzodiazepines in direct addiction studies.

OVERDOSAGE

There is no specific antidote for ondansetron overdose. Patients should be managed with appropriate supportive therapy. Individual doses as large as 145 mg and total daily dosages (three doses) as large as 252 mg have been administered intravenously without significant adverse events. These doses are more than 10 times the recommended daily dose.

"Sudden blindness" (amaurosis) of 2 to 3 minutes' duration plus severe constipation occurred in one patient that was administered 72 mg of ondansetron intravenously as a single dose. Hypotension (and faintness) occurred in another patient that took 48 mg of oral ondansetron. Following infusion of 32 mg over only a 4-minute period, a vasovagal episode with transient second degree heart block was observed. In all instances, the events resolved completely.

DOSAGE AND ADMINISTRATION

Prevention of Chemotherapy-Induced Nausea and Vomiting: The recommended IV dosage of ZOFRAN is a single 32-mg dose or three 0.15-mg/kg doses. A single 32-mg dose is infused over 15 minutes beginning 30 minutes before the start of emetogenic chemotherapy. The recommended infusion rate should not be exceeded (see OVERDOSAGE). With the three-dose (0.15-mg/kg) regimen, the first dose is infused over 15 minutes beginning 30 minutes before the start of emetogenic chemotherapy. Subsequent doses (0.15 mg/kg) are administered 4 and 8 hours after the first dose of ZOFRAN.

ZOFRAN Injection should not be mixed with solutions for which physical and chemical compatibility have not been established. In particular, this applies to alkaline solutions as a precipitate may form.

Vial: DILUTE BEFORE USE. ZOFRAN Injection should be diluted in 50 mL of 5% Dextrose Injection or 0.9% Sodium Chloride Injection before administration.

Flexible Plastic Container. ZOFRAN Injection Premixed, 32 mg in 5% dextrose, 50 mL, REQUIRES NO DILUTION.

Pediatric Use: On the basis of the limited available information (see CLINICAL TRIALS: Pediatric Studies and CLINICAL PHARMACOLOGY: Pharmacokinetics), the dosage in pediatric patients 4 to 18 years of age should be three 0.15-mg/kg doses (see above). Little information is available about dosage in pediatric patients 3 years of age or younger.

Use in the Elderly: The dosage recommendation is the same as for the general population.

Prevention of Postoperative Nausea and Vomiting: The recommended IV dosage of ZOFRAN for adults is 4 mg undiluted administered intravenously in not less than 30 seconds, preferably over 2 to 5 minutes, immediately before induction of anesthesia, or postoperatively if the patient experiences nausea and/or vomiting occurring shortly after surgery. Alternatively, 4 mg undiluted may be administered intramuscularly as a single injection for adults.

Vial: ZOFRAN Injection REQUIRES NO DILUTION FOR ADMINISTRATION FOR POSTOPERATIVE NAUSEA AND VOMITING.

Repeat dosing for patients who continue to experience nausea and/or vomiting postoperatively has not been studied. While recommended as a fixed dose for patients weighing more than 40 kg, few patients above 80 kg have been studied.

Pediatric Use: The recommended IV dosage of ZOFRAN for pediatric patients (2 to 12 years of age) is a single 0.1-mg/kg dose for pediatric patients weighing 40 kg or less, or a single 4-mg dose for pediatric patients weighing more than 40 kg. The rate of administration should not be less than 30 seconds, preferably over 2 to 5 minutes. Little information is available about dosage in pediatric patients younger than 2 years of age.

Use in the Elderly: The dosage recommendation is the same as for the general population.

Dosage Adjustment for Patients With Impaired Renal Function: No specific studies have been conducted in patients with renal insufficiency.

Dosage Adjustment for Patients With Impaired Hepatic Function: In patients with severe hepatic impairment according to Child-Pugh[1] criteria, a single maximal daily dose of 8 mg to be infused over 15 minutes beginning 30 minutes before the start of the emetogenic chemotherapy is recommended. There is no experience beyond first-day administration of ondansetron.

ZOFRAN Injection Premixed in Flexible Plastic Containers: Instructions for Use: *To Open:* Tear outer wrap at notch and remove solution container. Check for minute leaks by squeezing container firmly. If leaks are found, discard unit as sterility may be impaired.

Preparation for Administration: Use aseptic technique.

1. Close flow control clamp of administration set.
2. Remove cover from outlet port at bottom of container.
3. Insert piercing pin of administration set into port with a twisting motion until the pin is firmly seated. NOTE: See full directions on administration set carton.
4. Suspend container from hanger.
5. Squeeze and release drip chamber to establish proper fluid level in chamber during infusion of ZOFRAN Injection Premixed.
6. Open flow control clamp to expel air from set. Close clamp.
7. Attach set to venipuncture device. If device is not indwelling, prime and make venipuncture.
8. Perform venipuncture.
9. Regulate rate of administration with flow control clamp.

Caution: ZOFRAN Injection Premixed in flexible plastic containers is to be administered by IV drip infusion only. ZOFRAN Injection Premixed should not be mixed with solutions for which physical and chemical compatibility have not been established. In particular, this applies to alkaline solutions as a precipitate may form. If used with a primary IV fluid system, the primary solution should be discontinued during ZOFRAN Injection Premixed infusion.

Do not administer unless solution is clear and container is undamaged.

Warning: Do not use flexible plastic container in series connections.

Stability: ZOFRAN Injection is stable at room temperature under normal lighting conditions for 48 hours after dilution with the following IV fluids: 0.9% Sodium Chloride Injection, 5% Dextrose Injection, 5% Dextrose and 0.9% Sodium Chloride Injection, 5% Dextrose and 0.45% Sodium Chloride Injection, and 3% Sodium Chloride Injection.

Although ZOFRAN Injection is chemically and physically stable when diluted as recommended, sterile precautions should be observed because diluents generally do not contain preservative. After dilution, do not use beyond 24 hours.

Continued on next page

This product information is based on labeling in effect on June 1, 1998. For further information, contact via direct mail, phone, or web site Medical Information: Glaxo Wellcome Inc., PO Box 13398, Research Triangle Park, NC 27709. Healthcare Professionals (Medical Information): 800-334-0089 Patients (Customer Response Center): 888-TALK2GW (1-888-825-5249) Glaxo Wellcome Corporate Web Site: www.glaxowellcome.com

Zofran Injection—Cont.

Note: Parenteral drug products should be inspected visually for particulate matter and discoloration before administration whenever solution and container permit.

Precaution: Occasionally, ondansetron precipitates at the stopper/vial interface in vials stored upright. Potency and safety are not affected. If a precipitate is observed, resolubilize by shaking the vial vigorously.

HOW SUPPLIED

ZOFRAN Injection, 2 mg/mL, is supplied as follows:
NDC 0173-0442-02 2-mL single-dose vials (Carton of 5)
NDC 0173-0442-00 20-mL multidose vials (Singles)
Store between 2° and 30°C (36° and 86°F). Protect from light.

ZOFRAN Injection Premixed, 32 mg/50 mL, in 5% Dextrose, contains no preservatives and is supplied as a sterile, premixed solution for IV administration in single-dose, flexible plastic containers (NDC 0173-0461-00) (case of 6).
Store between 2° and 30°C (36° and 86°F). Protect from light. Avoid excessive heat. Protect from freezing.

REFERENCE

1. 1. Pugh RNH, Murray-Lyon IM, Dawson JL, Pietroni MC, Williams R. Transection of the oesophagus for bleeding oesophageal varices. *Brit J Surg.* 1973; 60:646-649.

© Copyright 1996 Glaxo Wellcome Inc. All rights reserved.
November 1997/RL-503

Shown in Product Identification Guide, page 315

ZOFRAN® ℞
[zō'-frăn]
(ondansetron hydrochloride)
Tablets

ZOFRAN® ℞
(ondansetron hydrochloride)
Oral Solution

DESCRIPTION

The active ingredient in ZOFRAN Tablets and ZOFRAN Oral Solution is ondansetron hydrochloride (HCl) as the dihydrate, the racemic form of ondansetron and a selective blocking agent of the serotonin 5-HT_3 receptor type. Chemically it is (±) 1, 2, 3, 9-tetrahydro-9-methyl-3-[(2-methyl-1H-imidazol-1-yl)methyl]-4H-carbazol-4-one, monohydrochloride, dihydrate.

The empirical formula is $C_{18}H_{19}N_3O{\cdot}HCl{\cdot}2H_2O$, representing a molecular weight of 365.9.

Ondansetron HCl dihydrate is a white to off-white powder that is soluble in water and normal saline.

Each 4-mg ZOFRAN Tablet for oral administration contains ondansetron HCl dihydrate equivalent to 4 mg of ondansetron. Each 8-mg ZOFRAN Tablet for oral administration contains ondansetron HCl dihydrate equivalent to 8 mg of ondansetron. Each tablet also contains the inactive ingredients lactose, microcrystalline cellulose, pregelatinized starch, hydroxypropyl methylcellulose, magnesium stearate, titanium dioxide, iron oxide yellow (8-mg tablet only), and sodium benzoate (4-mg tablet only).

Each 5 mL of ZOFRAN Oral Solution contains 5 mg of ondansetron HCl dihydrate equivalent to 4 mg of ondansetron. ZOFRAN Oral Solution contains the inactive ingredients citric acid anhydrous, purified water, sodium benzoate, sodium citrate, sorbitol, and strawberry flavor.

CLINICAL PHARMACOLOGY

Pharmacodynamics: Ondansetron is a selective 5-HT_3 receptor antagonist. While its mechanism of action has not been fully characterized, ondansetron is not a dopamine-receptor antagonist. Serotonin receptors of the 5-HT_3 type are present both peripherally on vagal nerve terminals and centrally in the chemoreceptor trigger zone of the area postrema. It is not certain whether ondansetron's antiemetic action is mediated centrally, peripherally, or in both sites. However, cytotoxic chemotherapy appears to be associated with release of serotonin from the enterochromaffin cells of the small intestine. In humans, urinary 5-HIAA (5-hydroxyindoleacetic acid) excretion increases after cisplatin administration in parallel with the onset of emesis. The released serotonin may stimulate the vagal afferents through the 5-HT_3 receptors and initiate the vomiting reflex.

In animals, the emetic response to cisplatin can be prevented by pretreatment with an inhibitor of serotonin synthesis, bilateral abdominal vagotomy and greater splanchnic nerve section, or pretreatment with a serotonin 5-HT_3 receptor antagonist.

In normal volunteers, single intravenous doses of 0.15 mg/kg of ondansetron had no effect on esophageal motility, gastric motility, lower esophageal sphincter pressure, or small intestinal transit time. Multiday administration of ondansetron has been shown to slow colonic transit in normal volunteers. Ondansetron has no effect on plasma prolactin concentrations.

Pharmacokinetics: Ondansetron is extensively metabolized in humans, with approximately 5% of a radiolabeled dose recovered from the urine as the parent compound. The primary metabolic pathway is hydroxylation on the indole ring followed by subsequent glucuronide or sulfate conjugation. Although some nonconjugated metabolites have pharmacologic activity, these are not found in plasma concentrations likely to significantly contribute to the biological activity of ondansetron.

Oral ondansetron is well absorbed and undergoes limited first-pass metabolism. Following the administration of a single 8-mg ondansetron tablet to healthy, young, male volunteers and from pooled studies, the time to peak plasma ondansetron concentration is approximately 1.7 hours, the terminal elimination half-life is approximately 3 hours, and bioavailability is approximately 56%. Gender differences were shown in the disposition of ondansetron given as a single dose. The extent and rate of ondansetron's absorption is greater in women than men. Slower clearance in women, a smaller apparent volume of distribution (adjusted for weight), and higher absolute bioavailability resulted in higher plasma ondansetron levels. These higher plasma levels may in part be explained by differences in body weight between men and women. It is not known whether these gender-related differences were clinically important. More detailed pharmacokinetic information is contained in the following table taken from one study.

[See table below]

Five milliliters (5 mL) of ZOFRAN Oral Solution (4 mg/5 mL) is bioequivalent to one 4-mg ZOFRAN Tablet and may be used interchangeably. Similarly, 10 mL of ZOFRAN Oral Solution (4 mg/5 mL) is bioequivalent to one 8-mg ZOFRAN Tablet or two 4-mg ZOFRAN Tablets.

Both AUC and C_{max} more than double on increasing the tablet dose from 8 to 16 mg (123% and 118%, respectively). This may result from saturation of first-pass metabolism leading to greater oral bioavailability at 16 mg than 8 mg.

The administration of oral ondansetron with food increases significantly (about 17%) the extent of absorption of ondansetron. The peak plasma concentration and time to peak plasma concentration are not significantly affected. This change in the extent of absorption is not believed to be of any clinical relevance.

There was no significant effect of antacid administration on the pharmacokinetics of orally administered ondansetron.

Because ondansetron undergoes extensive metabolism, the modest reduction in clearance in the over-75 age-group was not unexpected. However, since there was a difference in neither safety nor efficacy between patients over 65 years of age and those under 65 years of age, no adjustment in dosage is required in the elderly.

Plasma protein binding of ondansetron as measured in vitro was 70% to 76% over the concentration range of 10 to 500 ng/mL. Circulating drug also distributes into erythrocytes.

Pharmacokinetics in Normal Volunteers: Single 8-mg Tablet Dose

Age-group (years)		Mean Weight (kg)	n	Peak Plasma Concentration (ng/mL)	Time of Peak Plasma Concentration (h)	Mean Elimination Half-life (h)	Systemic Plasma Clearance L/h/kg	Absolute Bioavailability
18–40	M	69.0	6	26.2	2.0	3.1	0.403	0.483
	F	62.7	5	42.7	1.7	3.5	0.354	0.663
61–74	M	77.5	6	24.1	2.1	4.1	0.384	0.585
	F	60.2	6	52.4	1.9	4.9	0.255	0.643
≥75	M	78.0	5	37.0	2.2	4.5	0.277	0.619
	F	67.6	6	46.1	2.1	6.2	0.249	0.747

CLINICAL TRIALS

Chemotherapy-Induced Nausea and Vomiting: In one double-blind US study in 67 patients, ZOFRAN Tablets were significantly more effective than placebo in preventing vomiting induced by cyclophosphamide-based chemotherapy containing doxorubicin. Treatment response is based on the total number of emetic episodes over the 3-day study period. The results of this study are summarized below:

Emetic Episodes: Treatment Response

	Ondansetron 8-mg b.i.d. Tablets*	Placebo	*P* Value
Number of patients	33	34	
Treatment response			
0 Emetic episodes	20 (61%)	2 (6%)	<0.001
1–2 Emetic episodes	6 (18%)	8 (24%)	
More than 2 emetic episodes/withdrawn	7 (21%)	24 (71%)	<0.001
Median number of emetic episodes	0.0	Undefined†	
Median time to first emetic episode (h)	Undefined‡	6.5	

* The first dose was administered 30 minutes before the start of emetogenic chemotherapy, with a subsequent dose 8 hours after the first dose. An 8-mg tablet was administered twice a day for 2 days after completion of chemotherapy.
† Median undefined since at least 50% of the patients were withdrawn or had more than two emetic episodes.
‡ Median undefined since at least 50% of patients did not have any emetic episodes.

In one double-blind US study in 336 patients, ZOFRAN Tablets 8 mg administered twice a day were as effective as ZOFRAN Tablets 8 mg administered three times a day in preventing nausea and vomiting induced by cyclophosphamide-based chemotherapy containing either methotrexate or doxorubicin. Treatment response is based on the total number of emetic episodes over the 3-day study period. The results of this study are summarized below:

Emetic Episodes: Treatment Response

	Ondansetron 8-mg b.i.d. Tablets*	Ondansetron 8-mg t.i.d. Tablets†
Number of patients	165	171
Treatment response		
0 Emetic episodes	101 (61%)	99 (58%)
1–2 Emetic episodes	16 (10%)	17 (10%)
More than 2 emetic episodes/withdrawn	48 (29%)	55 (32%)
Median number of emetic episodes	0.0	0.0
Median time to first emetic episode (h)	Undefined‡	Undefined‡
Median nausea scores (0–100)§	6	6

* The first dose was administered 30 minutes before the start of emetogenic chemotherapy, with a subsequent dose 8 hours after the first dose. An 8-mg tablet was administered twice a day for 2 days after completion of chemotherapy.
† The first dose was administered 30 minutes before the start of emetogenic chemotherapy, with subsequent doses 4 and 8 hours after the first dose. An 8-mg tablet was administered three times a day for 2 days after completion of chemotherapy.
‡ Median undefined since at least 50% of patients did not have any emetic episodes.
§ Visual analog scale assessment: 0 = no nausea, 100 = nausea as bad as it can be.

Re-treatment: In uncontrolled trials, 148 patients receiving cyclophosphamide-based chemotherapy were re-treated with ZOFRAN Tablets 8 mg t.i.d. of oral ondansetron during subsequent chemotherapy for a total of 396 re-treatment courses. No emetic episodes occurred in 314 (79%) of the re-treatment courses, and only one to two emetic episodes occurred in 43 (11%) of the re-treatment courses.

Pediatric Studies: Three open-label, uncontrolled, foreign trials have been performed with 182 patients 4 to 18 years old with cancer who were given a variety of cisplatin or noncisplatin regimens. In these foreign trials, the initial dose of ZOFRAN® (ondansetron HCl) Injection ranged from 0.04 to 0.87 mg/kg for a total dose of 2.16 to 12 mg. This was followed by the administration of ZOFRAN Tablets ranging from 4 to 24 mg daily for 3 days. In these studies, 58% of the 170 evaluable patients had a complete response (no emetic episodes) on day 1. Two studies showed the response rates for patients less than 12 years of age who received ZOFRAN Tablets 4 mg three times a day to be similar to those in patients 12 to 18 years of age who received ZOFRAN Tablets 8 mg three times daily. Thus, prevention of emesis in these children was essentially the same as for patients older than 18 years of age. Overall, ZOFRAN Tablets were well tolerated in these pediatric patients.

Elderly Patients: One hundred thirty-seven (137) patients 65 years of age or older have received ZOFRAN Tablets.

Prevention of emesis was similar to that in patients younger than 65 years of age and adverse reactions were not seen in increased frequency.

Radiation-Induced Nausea and Vomiting: *Total Body Irradiation:* In a randomized, double-blind study in 20 patients, ZOFRAN Tablets (8 mg given 1.5 hours before each fraction of radiotherapy for 4 days) were significantly more effective than placebo in preventing vomiting induced by total body irradiation. Total body irradiation consisted of 11 fractions (120 cGy per fraction) over 4 days for a total of 1,320 cGy. Patients received three fractions for 3 days, then two fractions on day 4.

Single High-Dose Fraction Radiotherapy: Ondansetron was significantly more effective than metoclopramide with respect to complete control of emesis (0 emetic episodes) in a double-blind trial in 105 patients receiving single high-dose radiotherapy (800 to 1,000 cGy) over an anterior or posterior field size of ≥80 cm² to the abdomen. Patients received the first dose of ZOFRAN Tablets (8 mg) or metoclopramide (10 mg) 1 to 2 hours before radiotherapy. If radiotherapy was given in the morning, two additional doses of study treatment were given (one tablet late afternoon and one tablet before bedtime). If radiotherapy was given in the afternoon, patients took only one further tablet that day before bedtime. Patients continued the oral medication on a t.i.d. basis for 3 days.

Daily Fractionated Radiotherapy: Ondansetron was significantly more effective than prochlorperazine with respect to complete control of emesis (0 emetic episodes) in a double-blind trial in 135 patients receiving a 1- to 4-week course of fractionated radiotherapy (180 cGy doses) over a field size of ≥100 cm² to the abdomen. Patients received the first dose of ZOFRAN Tablets (8 mg) or prochlorperazine (10 mg) 1 to 2 hours before the patient received the first daily radiotherapy fraction, with two subsequent doses on a t.i.d. basis. Patients continued the oral medication on a t.i.d. basis on each day of radiotherapy.

Postoperative Nausea and Vomiting: Surgical patients who received ondansetron 1 hour before the induction of general balanced anesthesia (barbiturate: thiopental, methohexital, or thiamylal; opioid: alfentanil, sufentanil, morphine, or fentanyl; nitrous oxide; neuromuscular blockade: succinylcholine/curare or gallamine and/or vecuronium, pancuronium, or atracurium; and supplemental isoflurane or enflurane) were evaluated in two double-blind studies (one US study, one foreign) involving 865 patients. ZOFRAN Tablets (16 mg) were significantly more effective than placebo in preventing postoperative nausea and vomiting.

The study populations in all trials thus far consisted of women undergoing inpatient surgical procedures. No studies have been performed in males. No controlled clinical study comparing ZOFRAN Tablets to ZOFRAN Injection has been performed.

INDICATIONS AND USAGE

1. Prevention of nausea and vomiting associated with initial and repeat courses of moderately emetogenic cancer chemotherapy.
2. Prevention of nausea and vomiting associated with radiotherapy in patients receiving either total body irradiation, single high-dose fraction to the abdomen, or daily fractions to the abdomen.
3. Prevention of postoperative nausea and/or vomiting. As with other antiemetics, routine prophylaxis is not recommended for patients in whom there is little expectation that nausea and/or vomiting will occur postoperatively. In patients where nausea and/or vomiting must be avoided postoperatively, ZOFRAN Tablets and ZOFRAN Oral Solution are recommended even where the incidence of postoperative nausea and/or vomiting is low.

CONTRAINDICATIONS

ZOFRAN Tablets and ZOFRAN Oral Solution are contraindicated for patients known to have hypersensitivity to the drug.

WARNINGS

Hypersensitivity reactions have been reported in patients who have exhibited hypersensitivity to other selective 5-HT₃ receptor antagonists.

PRECAUTIONS

Ondansetron is not a drug that stimulates gastric or intestinal peristalsis. It should not be used instead of nasogastric suction. The use of ondansetron in patients following abdominal surgery or in patients with chemotherapy-induced nausea and vomiting may mask a progressive ileus and/or gastric distension.

Drug Interactions: Ondansetron does not itself appear to induce or inhibit the cytochrome P-450 drug-metabolizing enzyme system of the liver. Because ondansetron is metabolized by hepatic cytochrome P-450 drug-metabolizing enzymes, inducers or inhibitors of these enzymes may change the clearance and, hence, the half-life of ondansetron. On the basis of available data, no dosage adjustment is recommended for patients on these drugs. Tumor response to chemotherapy in the P 388 mouse leukemia model is not

affected by ondansetron. In humans, carmustine, etoposide, and cisplatin do not affect the pharmacokinetics of ondansetron.

Use in Surgical Patients: The coadministration of ondansetron had no effect on the pharmacokinetics and pharmacodynamics of temazepam.

Carcinogenesis, Mutagenesis, Impairment of Fertility: Carcinogenic effects were not seen in 2-year studies in rats and mice with oral ondansetron doses up to 10 and 30 mg/kg per day, respectively. Ondansetron was not mutagenic in standard tests for mutagenicity. Oral administration of ondansetron up to 15 mg/kg per day did not affect fertility or general reproductive performance of male and female rats.

Pregnancy: *Teratogenic Effects: Pregnancy Category B:* Reproduction studies have been performed in pregnant rats and rabbits at daily oral doses up to 15 and 30 mg/kg per day, respectively, and have revealed no evidence of impaired fertility or harm to the fetus due to ondansetron. There are, however, no adequate and well-controlled studies in pregnant women. Because animal reproduction studies are not always predictive of human response, this drug should be used during pregnancy only if clearly needed.

Nursing Mothers: Ondansetron is excreted in the breast milk of rats. It is not known whether ondansetron is excreted in human milk. Because many drugs are excreted in human milk, caution should be exercised when ondansetron is administered to a nursing woman.

Pediatric Use: Little information is available about dosage in children 4 years of age or younger (see CLINICAL PHARMACOLOGY and DOSAGE AND ADMINISTRATION sections for use in children 4 to 18 years of age).

Use in Elderly Patients: Dosage adjustment is not needed in patients over the age of 65 (see CLINICAL PHARMACOLOGY). Prevention of nausea and vomiting in elderly patients was no different than in younger age-groups.

ADVERSE REACTIONS

Chemotherapy-Induced Nausea and Vomiting: The following adverse events have been reported in adults receiving either 8 mg of ZOFRAN Tablets two or three times a day for 3 days or placebo in four trials. These patients were receiving concurrent chemotherapy, primarily cyclophosphamide-based regimens.

Principal Adverse Events in US Trials: 3 Days of Therapy With ZOFRAN Tablets

Event	Ondansetron 8 mg b.i.d. n = 242	Ondansetron 8 mg t.i.d. n = 415	Placebo n = 262
Headache	58 (24%)	113 (27%)	34 (13%)
Malaise/fatigue	32 (13%)	37 (9%)	6 (2%)
Constipation	22 (9%)	26 (6%)	1 (<1%)
Diarrhea	15 (6%)	16 (4%)	10 (4%)
Dizziness	13 (5%)	18 (4%)	12 (5%)
Abdominal pain	3 (1%)	13 (3%)	1 (<1%)
Xerostomia	5 (2%)	6 (1%)	1 (<1%)
Weakness	0 (0%)	7 (2%)	1 (<1%)

Central Nervous System: There have been rare reports consistent with, but not diagnostic of, extrapyramidal reactions in patients receiving ondansetron.

Hepatic: In 723 patients receiving cyclophosphamide-based chemotherapy in US clinical trials, AST and/or ALT values have been reported to exceed twice the upper limit of normal in approximately 1% to 2% of patients receiving ZOFRAN Tablets. The increases were transient and did not appear to be related to dose or duration of therapy. On repeat exposure, similar transient elevations in transaminase values occurred in some courses, but symptomatic hepatic disease did not occur. The role of cancer chemotherapy in these biochemical changes cannot be clearly determined. There have been reports of liver failure and death in patients with cancer receiving concurrent medications including potentially hepatotoxic cytotoxic chemotherapy and antibiotics. The etiology of the liver failure is unclear.

Integumentary: Rash has occurred in approximately 1% of patients receiving ondansetron.

Other: Rare cases of anaphylaxis, bronchospasm, tachycardia, angina (chest pain), hypokalemia, electrocardiographic alterations, vascular occlusive events, and grand mal seizures have been reported. Except for bronchospasm and anaphylaxis, the relationship to ZOFRAN was unclear.

Radiation-Induced Nausea and Vomiting: The adverse events reported in patients receiving ZOFRAN Tablets and concurrent radiotherapy were similar to those reported in patients receiving ZOFRAN Tablets and concurrent chemotherapy. The most frequently reported adverse events were headache, constipation, and diarrhea.

Postoperative Nausea and Vomiting: The following adverse events have been reported in ≥5% of patients receiving ZOFRAN Tablets at a dosage of 16 mg orally in clinical trials. With the exception of headache, rates of these events were not significantly different in the ondansetron and placebo groups. These patients were receiving multiple concomitant perioperative and postoperative medications.

Frequency of Adverse Events From Controlled Studies

Adverse Event	Ondansetron 16 mg (n = 550)	Placebo (n = 531)
Wound problem	152 (28%)	162 (31%)
Drowsiness/sedation	112 (20%)	122 (23%)
Headache	49 (9%)	27 (5%)
Hypoxia	49 (9%)	35 (7%)
Pyrexia	45 (8%)	34 (6%)
Dizziness	36 (7%)	34 (6%)
Gynecological disorder	36 (7%)	33 (6%)
Anxiety/agitation	33 (6%)	29 (5%)
Bradycardia	32 (6%)	30 (6%)
Shiver(s)	28 (5%)	30 (6%)
Urinary retention	28 (5%)	18 (3%)
Hypotension	27 (5%)	32 (6%)
Pruritus	27 (5%)	20 (4%)

DRUG ABUSE AND DEPENDENCE

Animal studies have shown that ondansetron is not discriminated as a benzodiazepine nor does it substitute for benzodiazepines in direct addiction studies.

OVERDOSAGE

There is no specific antidote for ondansetron overdose. Patients should be managed with appropriate supportive therapy. Individual intravenous doses as large as 145 mg and total daily intravenous doses as large as 252 mg have been inadvertently administered without significant adverse events. These doses are more than 10 times the recommended daily dose.

Hypotension (and faintness) occurred in a patient that took 48 mg of ZOFRAN Tablets. The events resolved completely.

DOSAGE AND ADMINISTRATION

Prevention of Nausea and Vomiting Associated With Moderately Emetogenic Cancer Chemotherapy: The recommended adult oral dosage of ZOFRAN is 8 mg or 10 mL (2 teaspoonfuls equivalent to 8 mg of ondansetron) given twice a day. The first dose should be administered 30 minutes before the start of emetogenic chemotherapy, with a subsequent dose 8 hours after the first dose. One 8-mg ZOFRAN Tablet or 10 mL (2 teaspoonfuls equivalent to 8 mg of ondansetron) of ZOFRAN Oral Solution should be administered twice a day (every 12 hours) for 1 to 2 days after completion of chemotherapy.

Pediatric Use: For patients 12 years of age and older, the dosage is the same as for adults. For patients 4 through 11 years of age, the dosage is one 4-mg tablet or 5 mL (1 teaspoonful equivalent to 4 mg of ondansetron) of oral solution given three times a day. The first dose should be administered 30 minutes before the start of emetogenic chemotherapy, with subsequent doses 4 and 8 hours after the first dose. One 4-mg ZOFRAN Tablet or 5 mL (1 teaspoonful equivalent to 4 mg of ondansetron) of ZOFRAN Oral Solution should be administered three times a day (every 8 hours) for 1 to 2 days after completion of chemotherapy.

Use in the Elderly: The dosage is the same as for the general population.

Prevention of Nausea and Vomiting Associated With Radiotherapy, Either Total Body Irradiation, or Single High-Dose Fraction or Daily Fractions to the Abdomen: The recommended oral dosage is one 8-mg tablet or 10 mL (2 teaspoonfuls equivalent to 8 mg of ondansetron) of oral solution given three times a day.

For total body irradiation, one 8-mg ZOFRAN Tablet or 10 mL (2 teaspoonfuls equivalent to 8 mg of ondansetron) of ZOFRAN Oral Solution should be administered 1 to 2 hours before each fraction of radiotherapy administered each day.

For single high-dose fraction radiotherapy to the abdomen, one 8-mg ZOFRAN Tablet or 10 mL (2 teaspoonfuls equivalent to 8 mg of ondansetron) of ZOFRAN Oral Solution should be administered 1 to 2 hours before radiotherapy, with subsequent doses every 8 hours after the first dose for 1 to 2 days after completion of radiotherapy.

For daily fractionated radiotherapy to the abdomen, one 8-mg ZOFRAN Tablet or 10 mL (2 teaspoonfuls equivalent to 8 mg of ondansetron) of ZOFRAN Oral Solution should be administered 1 to 2 hours before radiotherapy, with subsequent doses every 8 hours after the first dose for each day radiotherapy is given.

Continued on next page

This product information is based on labeling in effect on June 1, 1998. For further information, contact via direct mail, phone, or web site Medical Information: Glaxo Wellcome Inc., PO Box 13398, Research Triangle Park, NC 27709. Healthcare Professionals (Medical Information): 800-334-0089 Patients (Customer Response Center): 888-TALK2GW (1-888-825-5249) Glaxo Wellcome Corporate Web Site: www.glaxowellcome.com

Zofran Tablets—Cont.

Pediatric Use: There is no experience with the use of ZOFRAN Tablets or ZOFRAN Oral Solution in the prevention of radiation-induced nausea and vomiting in children.
Use in the Elderly: The dosage recommendation is the same as for the general population.
Postoperative Nausea and Vomiting: The recommended dosage is 16 mg given as two 8-mg ZOFRAN Tablets or 20 mL (4 teaspoonfuls equivalent to 16 mg of ondansetron) of ZOFRAN Oral Solution 1 hour before induction of anesthesia.
Pediatric Use: There is no experience with the use of ZOFRAN Tablets or ZOFRAN Oral Solution in the prevention of postoperative nausea and vomiting in children.
Use in the Elderly: The dosage is the same as for the general population.
Dosage Adjustment for Patients With Impaired Renal Function: No specific studies have been conducted in patients with renal insufficiency.
Dosage Adjustment for Patients With Impaired Hepatic Function: In patients with severe hepatic insufficiency, clearance is reduced, apparent volume of distribution is increased with a resultant increase in plasma half-life, and bioavailability approaches 100%. In such patients, a total daily dose of 8 mg should not be exceeded.

HOW SUPPLIED

ZOFRAN Tablets, 4 mg (ondansetron HCl dihydrate equivalent to 4 mg of ondansetron), are white, oval, film-coated tablets engraved with "Zofran" on one side and "4" on the other in daily unit dose packs of 3 tablets (NDC 0173-0446-04), bottles of 30 tablets (NDC 0173-0446-00), and unit dose packs of 100 tablets (NDC 0173-0446-02).
ZOFRAN Tablets, 8 mg (ondansetron HCl dihydrate equivalent to 8 mg of ondansetron), are yellow, oval, film-coated tablets engraved with "Zofran" on one side and "8" on the other in daily unit dose packs of 3 tablets (NDC 0173-0447-04), bottles of 30 tablets (NDC 0173-0447-00), and unit dose packs of 100 tablets (NDC 0173-0447-02).
Store between 2° and 30°C (36° and 86°F). Protect from light. Store blisters and bottles in cartons.
ZOFRAN Oral Solution, a clear, colorless to light yellow liquid with a characteristic strawberry odor, contains 5 mg of ondansetron HCl dihydrate equivalent to 4 mg of ondansetron per 5 mL in amber glass bottles of 50-mL with child-resistant closures (NDC 0173-0489-00).
Store upright between 15° and 30°C (59° and 86°F). Protect from light. Store bottles upright in cartons.
©Copyright 1996 Glaxo Wellcome Inc. All rights reserved.
October 1996/RL-371
Shown in Product Identification Guide, page 315

ZOVIRAX® Capsules ℞
ZOVIRAX® Tablets ℞
ZOVIRAX® Suspension ℞
[zō ″vī ′răx]
(acyclovir)

DESCRIPTION

ZOVIRAX is the brand name for acyclovir, an antiviral drug. ZOVIRAX Capsules, Tablets, and Suspension are formulations for oral administration. Each capsule of ZOVIRAX contains 200 mg of acyclovir and the inactive ingredients corn starch, lactose, magnesium stearate, and sodium lauryl sulfate. The capsule shell consists of gelatin, FD&C Blue No. 2, and titanium dioxide. May contain one or more parabens. Printed with edible black ink.
Each 800-mg tablet of ZOVIRAX contains 800 mg of acyclovir and the inactive ingredients FD&C Blue No. 2, magnesium stearate, microcrystalline cellulose, povidone, and sodium starch glycolate.
Each 400-mg tablet of ZOVIRAX contains 400 mg of acyclovir and the inactive ingredients magnesium stearate, microcrystalline cellulose, povidone, and sodium starch glycolate.
Each teaspoonful (5 mL) of ZOVIRAX Suspension contains 200 mg of acyclovir and the inactive ingredients methylparaben 0.1% and propylparaben 0.02% (added as preservatives), carboxymethylcellulose sodium, flavor, glycerin, microcrystalline cellulose, and sorbitol.
The chemical name of acyclovir is 2-amino-1,9-dihydro-9-[(2-hydroxyethoxy)methyl]-6*H*-purin-6-one.
Acyclovir is a white, crystalline powder with the molecular formula $C_8H_{11}N_5O_3$ and a molecular weight of 225. The maximum solubility in water at 37°C is 2.5 mg/mL. The pka's of acyclovir are 2.27 and 9.25.

VIROLOGY

Mechanism of Antiviral Action: Acyclovir is a synthetic purine nucleoside analogue with in vitro and in vivo inhibitory activity against herpes simplex virus types 1 (HSV-1), 2 (HSV-2), and varicella-zoster virus (VZV). In cell culture, acyclovir's highest antiviral activity is against HSV-1, followed in decreasing order of potency against HSV-2 and VZV.
The inhibitory activity of acyclovir is highly selective due to its affinity for the enzyme thymidine kinase (TK) encoded by HSV and VZV. This viral enzyme converts acyclovir into acyclovir monophosphate, a nucleotide analogue. The monophosphate is further converted into diphosphate by cellular guanylate kinase and into triphosphate by a number of cellular enzymes. In vitro, acyclovir triphosphate stops replication of herpes viral DNA. This is accomplished in three ways: 1) competitive inhibition of viral DNA polymerase, 2) incorporation into and termination of the growing viral DNA chain, and 3) inactivation of the viral DNA polymerase. The greater antiviral activity of acyclovir against HSV compared to VZV is due to its more efficient phosphorylation by the viral TK.
Antiviral Activities: The quantitative relationship between the in vitro susceptibility of herpes viruses to antivirals and the clinical response to therapy has not been established in humans, and virus sensitivity testing has not been standardized. Sensitivity testing results, expressed as the concentration of drug required to inhibit by 50% the growth of virus in cell culture (IC_{50}), vary greatly depending upon a number of factors. Using plaque-reduction assays, the IC_{50} against herpes simplex virus isolates ranges from 0.02 to 13.5 mcg/mL for HSV-1 and from 0.01 to 9.9 mcg/mL for HSV-2. The IC_{50} for acyclovir against most laboratory strains and clinical isolates of VZV ranges from 0.12 to 10.8 mcg/mL. Acyclovir also demonstrates activity against the Oka vaccine strain of VZV with a mean IC_{50} of 1.35 mcg/mL.
Drug Resistance: Resistance of VZV to antiviral nucleoside analogues can result from qualitative or quantitative changes in the viral TK or DNA polymerase. Clinical isolates of VZV with reduced susceptibility to acyclovir have been recovered from patients with AIDS. In these cases, TK-deficient mutants of VZV have been recovered.
Resistance of HSV to antiviral nucleoside analogues occurs by the same mechanisms as resistance to VZV. While most of the acyclovir-resistant mutants isolated thus far from immunocompromised patients have been found to be TK-deficient mutants, other mutants involving the viral TK gene (TK partial and TK altered) and DNA polymerase have also been isolated. TK-negative mutants may cause severe disease in immunocompromised patients. The possibility of viral resistance to acyclovir should be considered in patients who show poor clinical response during therapy.

CLINICAL PHARMACOLOGY

Pharmacokinetics: The pharmacokinetics of acyclovir after oral administration have been evaluated in healthy volunteers and in immunocompromised patients with herpes simplex or varicella-zoster virus infection. Acyclovir pharmacokinetic parameters are summarized in Table 1.

Table 1: Acyclovir Pharmacokinetic Characteristics (Range)

Parameter	Range
Plasma protein binding	9% to 33%
Plasma elimination half-life	2.5 to 3.3 hr
Average oral bioavailability	10% to 20%*

* Bioavailability decreases with increasing dose.

In one multiple-dose, cross-over study in healthy subjects (n = 23), it was shown that increases in plasma acyclovir concentrations were less than dose proportional with increasing dose, as shown in Table 2. The decrease in bioavailability is a function of the dose and not the dosage form.

Table 2: Acyclovir Peak and Trough Concentrations at Steady State

Parameter	200 mg	400 mg	800 mg
C^{SS}_{max}	0.83 mcg/mL	1.21 mcg/mL	1.61 mcg/mL
C^{SS}_{trough}	0.46 mcg/mL	0.63 mcg/mL	0.83 mcg/mL

There was no effect of food on the absorption of acyclovir (n = 6); therefore ZOVIRAX Capsules, Tablets, and Suspension may be adminstered with or without food.
The only known urinary metabolite is 9-[(carboxymethoxy)methyl]guanine.
Special Populations: *Adults with Impaired Renal Function:* The half-life and total body clearance of acyclovir are dependent on renal function. A dosage adustment is recommended for patients with reduced renal function (see DOSAGE AND ADMINSTRATION).
Pediatrics: In general, the pharmacokinetics of acyclovir in pediatric patients is similar to that of adults. Mean half-life after oral doses of 300 mg/m^2 and 600 mg/m^2 in pediatric patients ages 7 months to 7 years was 2.6 hours (range 1.59 to 3.74 hours).
Drug Interactions: Coadministration of probenecid with intravenous acyclovir has been shown to increase acyclovir half-life and systemic exposure. Urinary excretion and renal clearance were correspondingly reduced.
Clinical Trials: *Initial Genital Herpes:* Double-blind, placebo-controlled studies have demonstrated that orally administered ZOVIRAX significantly reduced the duration of acute infection and duration of lesion healing. The duration of pain and new lesion formation was decreased in some patient groups.
Recurrent Genital Herpes: Double-blind, placebo-controlled studies in patients with frequent recurrences (six or more episodes per year) have shown that orally administered ZOVIRAX given daily for 4 months to 10 years prevented or reduced the frequency and/or severity of recurrences in greater than 95% of patients.
In a study of patients who received ZOVIRAX 400 mg twice daily for 3 years, 45%, 52%, and 63% of patients remained free of recurrences in the first, second, and third years, respectively. Serial analyses of the 3-month recurrence rates for patients showed that 71% to 87% were recurrence-free in each quarter.
Herpes Zoster Infections: In a double-blind, placebo-controlled study of immunocompetent patients with localized cutaneous zoster infection, ZOVIRAX (800 mg five times daily for 10 day) shortened the times to lesion scabbing, healing, and complete cessation of pain, and reduced the duration of viral shedding and the duration of new lesion formation.
In a similar double-blind, placebo-controlled study, ZOVIRAX (800 mg five times daily for 7 days) shortened the times to complete lesion scabbing, healing, and cessation of pain, reduced the duration of new lesion formation, and reduced the prevalence of localized zoster-associated neurologic symptoms (paresthesia, dysesthesia, or hyperesthesia).
Treatment was begun within 72 hours of rash onset and was most effective if started within the first 48 hours.
Adults greater than 50 years of age showed greater benefit.
Chickenpox: Three randomized, double-blind, placebo controlled trials were conducted in 993 pediatric patients ages 2 to 18 years with chickenpox. All patients were treated within 24 hours after the onset of rash. In two trials, ZOVIRAX was administered at 20 mg/kg four times daily (up to 3200 mg per day) for 5 days. In the third trial, doses of 10, 15, or 20 mg/kg were administered four times daily for 5 to 7 days. Treatment with ZOVIRAX shortened the time to 50% healing, reduced the maximum number of lesions, reduced the median number of vesicles, decreased the median number of residual lesions on day 28, and decreased the proportion of patients with fever, anorexia, and lethargy by day 2. Treatment with ZOVIRAX did not affect varicella-zoster virus-specific humoral or cellular immune responses at 1 month or 1 year following treatment.

INDICATIONS AND USAGE

Herpes Zoster Infections: ZOVIRAX is indicated for the acute treatment of herpes zoster (shingles).
Genital Herpes: ZOVIRAX is indicated for the treatment of initial episodes and the managment of recurrent episodes of genital herpes.
Chickenpox: ZOVIRAX is indicated for the treatment of chickenpox (varicella).

CONTRAINDICATIONS

ZOVIRAX is contraindicated for patients who develop hypersensitivity or intolerance to the components of the formulations.

WARNINGS

ZOVIRAX Capsules, Tablets, and Suspension are intended for oral ingestion only.

PRECAUTIONS

Dosage adjustment is recommended when administering ZOVIRAX to patients with renal impairment (see DOSAGE AND ADMINISTRATION). Caution should also be exercised when administering ZOVIRAX to patients receiving potentially nephrotoxic agents since this may increase the risk of renal dysfunction and/or the risk of reversible central nervous system symptoms such as those that have been reported in patients treated with intravenous acyclovir.
Information for Patients: Patients are instructed to consult with their physician if they experience severe or troublesome adverse reactions, they become pregnant or intend to become pregnant, they intend to breastfeed while taking orally administered ZOVIRAX, or they have any other questions.
Herpes Zoster: There are no data on treatment initiated more than 72 hours after onset of the zoster rash. Patients should be advised to initiate treatment as soon as possible after a diagnosis of herpes zoster.
Genital Herpes Infections: Patients should be informed that ZOVIRAX is not a cure for genital herpes. There are no data evaluating whether ZOVIRAX will prevent transmission of infection to others. Because genital herpes is a sexually transitted disease, patients should avoid contact with le-

sions or intercourse when lesions and/or symptoms are present to avoid infecting partners. Genital herpes can also be transmitted in the absence of symptoms through asymptomatic viral shedding. If medical management of a genital herpes recurrence is indicated, patients should be advised to initiate therapy at the first sign or symptom of an episode.

Chickenpox: Chickenpox in otherwise healthy children is usually a self-limited disease of mild to moderate severity. Adolescents and adults tend to have more severe disease. Treatment was initiated within 24 hours of the typical chickenpox rash in the controlled studies, and there is no information regarding the effects of treatment begun later in the disease course.

Drug Interaction: See CLINICAL PHARMACOLOGY: Pharmacokinetics.

Carcinogenesis, Mutagenesis, Impairment of Fertility: The data presented below include references to peak steady-state plasma acyclovir concentrations observed in humans treated with 800 mg given orally six times a day (dosing appropriate for treatment of herpes zoster) or 200 mg given orally six times a day (dosing appropriate for treatment of genital herpes). Plasma drug concentrations in animal studies are expressed as multiples of human exposure to acyclovir at the higher and lower dosing schedules (see Pharmacokinetics).

Acyclovir was tested in lifetime bioassays in rats and mice at single daily doses of up to 450 mg/kg administered by gavage. There was no statistically significant difference in the incidence of tumors between treated and control animals, nor did acyclovir shorten the latency of tumors. Maximum plasma concentrations were three to six times human levels in the mouse bioassay and one to two times human levels in the rat bioassay.

Acyclovir was tested in 16 genetic toxicity assays. No evidence of mutagenicity was observed in four microbial assays. Acyclovir demonstrated mutagenic activity in two in vitro cytogenetic assays (one mouse lymphoma cell line and human lymphocytes). No mutagenic activity was observed in five in vitro cytogenetic assays (three Chinese hamster ovary cell lines and two mouse lymphoma cell lines).

A positive result was demonstrated in one of two in vitro cell transformation assays, and morphologically transformed cells obtained in this assay formed tumors when inoculated into immunosuppressed, syngeneic, weanling mice. No mutagenic activity was demonstrated in another, possibly less sensitive, in vitro cell transformation assay.

Acyclovir was clastogenic in Chinese hamsters at 380 to 760 times human dose levels. In rats, acyclovir produced a non-significant increase in chromosomal damage at 62 to 125 times human levels. No activity was observed in a dominant lethal study in mice at 36 to 73 times human levels.

Acyclovir did not impair fertility or reproduction in mice (450 mg/kg/day, PO) or in rats (25 mg/kg/day, SC). In the mouse study, plasma levels were 9 to 18 times human levels, while in the rat study, they were 8 to 15 times human levels. At higher doses (50 mg/kg per day, SC) in rats and rabbits (11 to 22 and 16 to 31 times human levels, respectively) implantation efficacy, but not litter size, was decreased. In a rat peri-and post-natal study at 50 mg/kg per day, SC, there was a statistically significant decrease in group mean number of corpora lutea, total implantation sites, and live fetuses.

No testicular abnormalities were seen in dogs given 50 mg/kg per day, IV for 1 month (21 to 41 times human levels) or in dogs given 60 mg/kg per day orally for 1 year (six to 12 times human levels). Testicular atrophy and aspermatogenesis were observed in rats and dogs at higher dose levels.

Pregnancy: *Teratogenic Effects:* Pregnancy Category B. Acyclovir was not teratogenic in the mouse (450 mg/kg per day, PO), rabbit (50 mg/kg per day, SC and IV), or rat (50 mg/kg per day, SC). These exposures resulted in plasma levels 9 and 18, 16 and 106, and 11 and 22 times, respectively, human levels. In a nonstandard test, rats were given three SC doses of 100 mg/kg acyclovir on gestation day 10, resulting in plasma levels 63 and 125 times human levels. In this test, there were fetal abnormalities, such as head and tail anomalies, and maternal toxicity.

There are no adequate and well-controlled studies in pregnant women. A prospective epidemiologic registry of acyclovir use during pregnancy has collected data since June, 1984. As of December 1997, outcomes of live births have been documented in 552 women exposed to systemic acyclovir during the first trimester of pregnancy. The occurrence rate of birth defects approximates that found in the general population. However, the small size of the registry is insufficient to evaulate the risk for specific defects or to permit definitive conclusions regarding the safety of acyclovir in pregnant women and their developing fetuses. Acyclovir should be used during pregnancy only if the potential benefit justifies the potential risk to the fetus.

Nursing Mothers: Acyclovir concentrations have been documented in breast milk in two women following oral administration of ZOVIRAX and ranged from 0.6 to 4.1 times corresponding plasma levels. These concentrations would potentially expose the nursing infant to a dose of acyclovir as high as 0.3 mg/kg per day. ZOVIRAX should be administered to a nursing mother with caution and only when indicated.

Table 3: Dosage Modification for Renal Impairment

Normal Dosage Regimen	Creatinine Clearance (mL/min/1.73 m^2)	Adjusted Dosage Regimen	
		Dose (mg)	Dosing Interval
200 mg every 4 hours	>10	200	every 4 hours, 5x daily
	0-10	200	every 12 hours
400 mg every 12 hours	>10	400	every 12 hours
	0–10	200	every 12 hours
800 mg every 4 hours	>25	800	every 4 hours, 5x daily
	10–25	800	every 8 hours
	0–10	800	every 12 hours

Geriatric Use: Clinical studies of ZOVIRAX did not include sufficient number of patients aged 65 and over to determine whether they respond differently than younger patients. Other reported clinical experience has not identified differences in responses between elderly and younger patients. In general, dose selection for an elderly patient should be cautious, usually starting at the low end of the dosing range, reflecting the greater frequency of decreased renal function, and of concomitant disease or other drug therapy.

Pediatric Use: Safety and effectiveness in pediatric patients less than 2 years of age have not been adequately studied.

ADVERSE REACTIONS

Herpes Simplex: *Short-Term Administration:* The most frequent adverse events reported during clinical trials of treatment of genital herpes with ZOVIRAX 200 mg administered orally five times daily every 4 hours for 10 days were nausea and/or vomiting in 8 of 298 patient treatments (2.7%). Nausea and/or vomiting occurred in 2 of 287 (0.7%) patients who received placebo.

Long-Term Administration: The most frequent adverse events reported in a clinical trial for the prevention of recurrences with continuous administration of 400 mg (two 200-mg capsules) two times daily for 1 year in 586 patients treated with ZOVIRAX were nausea (4.8%) and diarrhea (2.4%). The 589 control patients receiving intermittent treatment of recurrences with ZOVIRAX for 1 year reported diarrhea (2.7%), nausea (2.4%), and headache (2.2%).

Herpes Zoster: The most frequent adverse event reported during three clinical trials of treatment of herpes zoster (shingles) with 800 mg of oral ZOVIRAX five times daily for 7 to 10 days in 323 patients was malaise (11.5%). The 323 placebo recipients reported malaise (11.1%).

Chickenpox: The most frequent adverse event reported during three clinical trials of treatment of chickenpox with oral ZOVIRAX at doses of 10 to 20 mg/kg four times daily for 5 to 7 days or 800 mg four times daily for 5 days in 495 patients was diarrhea (3.2%). The 498 patients receiving placebo reported diarrhea (2.2%).

Observed During Clinical Practice: In addition to adverse events reported from clinical trials, the following events have been identified during post-approval use of acyclovir (ZOVIRAX). Because they are reported voluntarily from a population of unknown size, estimates of frequency cannot be made. These events have been chosen for inclusion due to a combination of their seriousness, frequency of reporting, or potential causal connection to ZOVIRAX.

General: Fever, headache, pain, peripheral edema, and rarely, anaphylaxis.

Nervous: Confusion, dizziness, hallucinations, paresthesia, seizure, somnolence (These symptoms may be marked, particularly in older adults.)

Digestive: Diarrhea, elevated liver function tests, gastrointestinal distress, nausea.

Hemic and Lymphatic: Leukopenia, lymphadenopathy.

Musculoskeletal: Myalgia.

Skin: Alopecia, erythema multiforme, pruritus, rash, Stevens-Johnson syndrome, toxic epidermal necrolysis, urticaria.

Special Senses: Visual abnormalities.

Urogenital: Elevated creatinine.

OVERDOSAGE

Patients have ingested intentional overdoses of up to 100 capsules (20 g) of ZOVIRAX, with no unexpected adverse effects. Precipitation of acyclovir in renal tubules may occur when the solubility (2.5 mg/mL) is exceeded in the intratubular fluid. In the event of acute renal failure and anuria, the patient may benefit from hemodialysis until renal function is restored (see DOSAGE AND ADMINISTRATION).

DOSAGE AND ADMINISTRATION

Acute Treatment of Herpes Zoster: 800 mg every 4 hours orally, five times daily for 7 to 10 days.

Genital Herpes: *Treatment of Initial Genital Herpes:* 200 mg every 4 hours, five times daily for 10 days.

Chronic Suppressive Therapy for Recurrent Disease: 400 mg two times daily for up to 12 months, followed by re-evaluation. Alternative regimens have included doses ranging from 200 mg three times daily to 200 mg five times daily. The frequency and severity of episodes of untreated genital herpes may change over time. After 1 year of therapy, the frequency and severity of the patient's genital herpes infection should be re-evaluated to assess the need for continuation of therapy with ZOVIRAX.

Intermittent Therapy: 200 mg every 4 hours, five times daily for 5 days. Therapy should be initiated at the earliest sign or symptom (prodrome) of recurrence.

Treatment of Chickenpox: *Children (2 years of age and older):* 20 mg/kg **per dose** orally four times daily (80 mg/kg per day) for 5 days. Children over 40 kg should receive the adult dose for chickenpox.

Adults and Children over 40 kg: 800 mg four times daily for 5 days.

Intravenous ZOVIRAX is indicated for the treatment of varicella-zoster infections in immunocompromised patients.

When therapy is indicated, it should be initiated at the earliest sign or symptom of chickenpox. There is no information about the efficacy of therapy initiated more than 24 hours after onset of signs and symptoms.

Patients With Acute or Chronic Renal Impairment: In patients with renal impairment, the dose of ZOVIRAX Capsules, Tablets, or Suspension should be modified as shown in Table 3:

[See table 3 above]

Hemodialysis: For patients who require hemodialysis, the mean plasma half-life of acyclovir during hemodialysis is approximately 5 hours. This results in a 60% decrease in plasma concentrations following a 6-hour dialysis period. Therefore, the patient's dosing schedule should be adjusted so that an additional dose is administered after each dialysis.

Peritoneal Dialysis: No supplemental dose appears to be necessary after adjustment of the dosing interval.

Bioequivalence of Dosage Forms: ZOVIRAX Suspension was shown to be bioequivalent to ZOVIRAX Capsules (n = 20) and one ZOVIRAX 800-mg tablet was shown to be bioequivalent to four ZOVIRAX 200-mg capsules (n = 24).

HOW SUPPLIED

ZOVIRAX Capsules (blue, opaque cap and body) containing 200 mg acyclovir and printed with "Wellcome ZOVIRAX 200"—Bottle of 100 (NDC 0173-0991-55) and unit dose pack of 100 (NDC 0173-0991-56).

Store at 15° to 25°C (59° to 77°F) and protect from moisture.

ZOVIRAX Tablets (light blue, oval) containing 800 mg acyclovir and engraved with "ZOVIRAX 800"—Bottle of 100 (NDC 0173-0945-55) and unit dose pack of 100 (NDC 0173-0945-56).

Store at 15° to 25°C (59° to 77°F) and protect from moisture.

ZOVIRAX Tablets (white, shield-shaped) containing 400 mg acyclovir and engraved with "ZOVIRAX" on one side and a triangle on the other side—Bottle of 100 (NDC 0173-0949-55).

Store at 15° to 25°C (59° to 77°F) and protect from moisture.

ZOVIRAX Suspension (off-white, banana-flavored) containing 200 mg acyclovir in each teaspoonful (5 mL)—Bottle of 1 pint (473 mL) (NDC 0173-0953-96).

Continued on next page

This product information is based on labeling in effect on June 1, 1998. For further information, contact via direct mail, phone, or web site Medical Information: Glaxo Wellcome Inc., PO Box 13398, Research Triangle Park, NC 27709. Healthcare Professionals (Medical Information): 800-334-0089 Patients (Customer Response Center): 888-TALK2GW (1-888-825-5249) Glaxo Wellcome Corporate Web Site: www.glaxowellcome.com

Zovirax—Cont.

Store at 15° to 25°C (59° to 77°F).
©Copyright 1996 Glaxo Wellcome Inc. All rights reserved.
May 1998/RL-577
Shown in Product Identification Guide, page 315

ZOVIRAX® Ointment 5% ℞
[*zō "vī 'răx*]
(acyclovir)

DESCRIPTION

ZOVIRAX is the brand name for acyclovir, an antiviral drug active against herpes viruses. ZOVIRAX Ointment 5% is a formulation for topical administration. Each gram of ZOVIRAX Ointment 5% contains 50 mg of acyclovir in a polyethylene glycol (PEG) base.
The chemical name of acyclovir is 2-amino-1,9-dihydro-9-[(2-hydroxyethoxy)methyl]-6*H*-purin-6-one.
Acyclovir is a white, crystalline powder with a molecular weight of 225 daltons, and a maximum solubility in water of 1.3 mg/mL.

CLINICAL PHARMACOLOGY

Acyclovir is a synthetic acyclic purine nucleoside analogue with in vitro inhibitory activity against Herpes simplex types 1 and 2 (HSV-1 and HSV-2), varicella-zoster, Epstein-Barr, and cytomegalovirus. In cell cultures, the inhibitory activity of acyclovir for Herpes simplex virus is highly selective. Cellular thymidine kinase does not effectively utilize acyclovir as a substrate. Herpes simplex virus-coded thymidine kinase, however, converts acyclovir into acyclovir monophosphate, a nucleotide. The monophosphate is further converted into diphosphate by cellular guanylate kinase and into triphosphate by a number of cellular enzymes.[1] Acyclovir triphosphate interferes with Herpes simplex virus DNA polymerase and inhibits viral DNA replication. Acyclovir triphosphate also inhibits cellular α-DNA polymerase but to a lesser degree. In vitro, acyclovir triphosphate can be incorporated into growing chains of DNA by viral DNA polymerase and to a much smaller extent by cellular α-DNA polymerase.[2] When incorporation occurs, the DNA chain is terminated.[3] Acyclovir is preferentially taken up and selectively converted to the active triphosphate form by herpes-virus-infected cells. Thus, acyclovir is much less toxic in vitro for normal uninfected cells because: 1) less is taken up; 2) less is converted to the active form; 3) cellular α-DNA polymerase is less sensitive to the effects of the active form.
The relationship between in vitro susceptibility of Herpes simplex virus to antiviral drugs and clinical response has not been established. The techniques and cell culture types used for determining in vitro susceptibility may influence the results obtained. Using a quantitative assay to determine the acyclovir concentration producing 50% inhibition of viral cytopathic effect (ID_{50}), 28 HSV-1 clinical isolates had a mean ID_{50} of 0.17 mcg/mL and 32 HSV-2 clinical isolates had a mean ID_{50} of 0.46 mcg/mL.* Results from other studies using different assays have yielded mean ID_{50} values for clinical HSV-1 isolates of 0.018, 0.03, and 0.043 mcg/mL and for clinical HSV-2 isolates of 0.027, 0.36, and 0.03 mcg/mL, respectively.[4,5,6]
Two clinical pharmacology studies were performed with ZOVIRAX Ointment 5% in adult immunocompromised patients at risk of developing mucocutaneous Herpes simplex virus infections or with localized varicella-zoster infections. These studies were designed to evaluate the dermal tolerance, systemic toxicity, and percutaneous absorption of acyclovir.
In one of these studies, which included 16 inpatients, the complete ointment or its vehicle were randomly administered in a dose of 1-cm strips (25 mg acyclovir) four times a day for 7 days to an intact skin surface area of 4.5 square inches. No local intolerance, systemic toxicity, or contact dermatitis were observed. In addition, no drug was detected in blood and urine by radioimmunoassay (sensitivity, 0.01 mcg/mL).
The other study included 11 patients with localized varicella-zoster. In this uncontrolled study, acyclovir was detected in the blood of nine patients and in the urine of all patients tested. Acyclovir levels in plasma ranged from <0.01 to 0.28 mcg/mL in eight patients with normal renal function, and from <0.01 to 0.78 mcg/mL in one patient with impaired renal function. Acyclovir excreted in the urine ranged from <0.02% to 9.4% of the daily dose. Therefore, systemic absorption of acyclovir after topical application is minimal.

INDICATIONS AND USAGE

ZOVIRAX (acyclovir) Ointment 5% is indicated in the management of initial herpes genitalis and in limited nonlife-threatening mucocutaneous Herpes simplex virus infections in immunocompromised patients. In clinical trials of initial herpes genitalis, ZOVIRAX Ointment 5% has shown a decrease in healing time and, in some cases, a decrease in duration of viral shedding and duration of pain. In studies in immunocompromised patients with mainly herpes labialis, there was a decrease in duration of viral shedding and a slight decrease in duration of pain.
By contrast, in studies of recurrent herpes genitalis and of herpes labialis in nonimmunocompromised patients, there was no evidence of clinical benefit; there was some decrease in duration of viral shedding.
Diagnosis: Whereas cutaneous lesions associated with Herpes simplex infections are often characteristic, the finding of multinucleated giant cells in smears prepared from lesion exudate or scrapings may assist in the diagnosis.[7] Positive cultures for Herpes simplex virus offer a reliable means for confirmation of the diagnosis. In genital herpes, appropriate examinations should be performed to rule out other sexually transmitted diseases.

CONTRAINDICATIONS

ZOVIRAX Ointment 5% is contraindicated for patients who develop hypersensitivity or chemical intolerance to the components of the formulation.

WARNINGS

ZOVIRAX Ointment 5% is intended for cutaneous use only and should not be used in the eye.

PRECAUTIONS

General: The recommended dosage, frequency of applications, and length of treatment should not be exceeded (see DOSAGE AND ADMINISTRATION). There exist no data which demonstrate that the use of ZOVIRAX Ointment 5% will either prevent transmission of infection to other persons or prevent recurrent infections when applied in the absence of signs and symptoms. ZOVIRAX Ointment 5% should not be used for the prevention of recurrent HSV infections. Although clinically significant viral resistance associated with the use of ZOVIRAX Ointment 5% has not been observed, this possibility exists.
Drug Interactions: Clinical experience has identified no interactions resulting from topical or systemic administration of other drugs concomitantly with ZOVIRAX Ointment 5%.
Carcinogenesis, Mutagenesis, Impairment of Fertility: Acyclovir was tested in lifetime bioassays in rats and mice at single daily doses of 50, 150, and 450 mg/kg/day given by gavage. These studies showed no statistically significant difference in the incidence of benign and malignant tumors produced in drug-treated as compared to control animals, nor did acyclovir induce the occurrence of tumors earlier in drug-treated animals as compared to controls. In two in vitro cell transformation assays, used to provide preliminary assessment of potential oncogenicity in advance of these more definitive lifetime bioassays in rodents, conflicting results were obtained. Acyclovir was positive at the highest dose used in one system and the resulting morphologically transformed cells formed tumors when inoculated into immunosuppressed, syngeneic, weanling mice. Acyclovir was negative in another transformation system.
No chromosome damage was observed at maximum tolerated parenteral doses of 100 mg/kg acyclovir in rats or Chinese hamsters; higher doses of 500 and 1000 mg/kg were clastogenic in Chinese hamsters. In addition, no activity was found in a dominant lethal study in mice. In nine of 11 microbial and mammalian cell assays, no evidence of mutagenicity was observed. In two mammalian cell assays (human lymphocytes and L5178Y mouse lymphoma cells in vitro), positive response for mutagenicity and chromosomal damage occurred, but only at concentrations at least 1000 times the plasma levels achieved in humans following topical application.
Acyclovir does not impair fertility or reproduction in mice at oral doses up to 450 mg/kg/day or in rats at subcutaneous doses up to 25 mg/kg/day. In rabbits given a high dose of acyclovir (50 mg/kg/day, SC), there was a statistically significant decrease in implantation efficiency.
Pregnancy: *Teratogenic Effects.* Pregnancy Category C. Acyclovir was not teratogenic in the mouse (450 mg/kg/day, PO), rabbit (50 mg/kg/day, SC and IV) or in standard tests in the rat (50 mg/kg/day, SC). In a non-standard test in rats, fetal abnormalities, such as head and tail anomalies, were observed following subcutaneous administration of acyclovir at very high doses associated with toxicity to the maternal rat. The clinical relevance of these findings is uncertain.[8] There are no adequate and well-controlled studies in pregnant women. Acyclovir should not be used during pregnancy unless the potential benefit justifies the potential risk to the fetus.
Nursing Mothers: It is not known whether topically applied acyclovir is excreted in breast milk. After oral administration of ZOVIRAX, acyclovir concentrations have been documented in breast milk in two women and ranged from 0.6 to 4.1 times the corresponding plasma levels.[9,10] Caution should be exercised when ZOVIRAX Ointment is administered to a nursing woman.
Pediatric Use: Safety and effectiveness in pediatric patients have not been established.

ADVERSE REACTIONS

Because ulcerated genital lesions are characteristically tender and sensitive to any contact or manipulation, patients may experience discomfort upon application of ointment. In the controlled clinical trials, mild pain (including transient burning and stinging) was reported by 103 (28.3%) of 364 patients treated with acyclovir and by 115 (31.1%) of 370 patients treated with placebo; treatment was discontinued in 2 of these patients. Other local reactions among acyclovir-treated patients included pruritus in 15 (4.1%), rash in 1 (0.3%), and vulvitis in 1 (0.3%). Among the placebo-treated patients, pruritus was reported by 17 (4.6%) and rash by 1 (0.3%).
In all studies, there was no significant difference between the drug and placebo group in the rate or type of reported adverse reactions nor were there any differences in abnormal clinical laboratory findings.
Observed During Clinical Practice: Based on clinical practice experience in patients treated with ZOVIRAX Ointment in the U.S., spontaneously reported adverse events are uncommon. Data are insufficient to support an estimate of their incidence or to establish causation. These events may also occur as part of the underlying disease process. Voluntary reports of adverse events which have been received since market introduction include:
General: edema and/or pain at the application site
Skin: pruritus, rash

OVERDOSAGE

Overdosage by topical application of ZOVIRAX Ointment 5% is unlikely because of limited transcutaneous absorption (see CLINICAL PHARMACOLOGY).

DOSAGE AND ADMINISTRATION

Apply sufficient quantity to adequately cover all lesions every 3 hours, 6 times per day for 7 days. The dose size per application will vary depending upon the total lesion area but should approximate a one-half inch ribbon of ointment per 4 square inches of surface area. A finger cot or rubber glove should be used when applying ZOVIRAX to prevent autoinoculation of other body sites and transmission of infection to other persons. **Therapy should be initiated as early as possible following onset of signs and symptoms.**

HOW SUPPLIED

ZOVIRAX Ointment 5% is supplied in 15-g tubes (NDC 0173-0993-94) and 3-g tubes (NDC 0173-0993-41). Each gram contains 50 mg acyclovir in a polyethylene glycol base.
Store at 15° to 25°C (59° to 77°F) in a dry place.

ANIMAL PHARMACOLOGY AND ANIMAL TOXICOLOGY

Topical treatment of guinea pigs with 10% acyclovir in polyethylene glycol ointment for 3 weeks did not result in cutaneous irritation or systemic toxicity. Also, a wide variety of animal tests by parenteral routes demonstrated that acyclovir has a low order of toxicity.
Acyclovir did not cause dermal sensitization in guinea pigs.

REFERENCES

1. Miller WH, Miller RL. Phosphorylation of acyclovir (acycloguanosine) monophosphate by GMP kinase. *J Biol Chem.* 1980;255:7204-7207.
2. Furman PA, St. Clair MH, Fyfe JA, et al. Inhibition of herpes simplex virus-induced DNA polymerase activity and viral DNA replication by 9-(2-hydroxyethoxymethyl)guanine and its triphosphate. *J Virol.* 1979; 32:72-77.
3. Derse D, Cheng YC, Furman PA, et al. Inhibition of purified human and herpes simplex virus-induced DNA polymerases by 9-(2-hydroxyethoxymethyl)guanine triphosphate: effects on primer-template function. *J Biol Chem.* 1981;256:11447-11451.
4. Collins P, Bauer DJ. The activity in vitro against herpes virus of 9-(2-hydroxyethoxymethyl)guanine (acycloguanosine), a new antiviral agent. *J Antimicrob Chemother.* 1979;5:431-436.
5. Crumpacker CS, Schnipper LE, Zaia JA, et al. Growth inhibition of acycloguanosine of herpesviruses isolated from human infections. *Antimicrob Agents Chemother.* 1979;15:642-645.
6. DeClercq E, Descamps J, Verhelst G, et al. Comparative efficacy of antiherpes drugs against different strains of herpes simplex virus. *J Infect Dis.* 1980;141:563-574.
7. Naib ZM, Nahmias AJ, Josey WE, et al. Relation of cytohistopathology of genital herpesvirus infection to cervical anaplasia. *Cancer Res.* 1973;33:1452-1463.
8. Stahlmann R, Klug S, Lewandowski C, et al. Teratogenicity of acyclovir in rats. *Infection.* 1987;15:261-262.
9. Lau RJ, Emery MG, Galinsky RE, et al. Unexpected accumulation of acyclovir in breast milk with estimate of infant exposure. *Obstet Gynecol.* 1987;69:468-471.
10. Meyer LJ, deMiranda P, Sheth N, et al. Acyclovir in human breast milk. *Am J Obstet Gynecol.* 1988;158: 586-588.

*Data on file at Glaxo Wellcome Inc.
U.S. Patent No. 4,199,574
©Copyright 1996 Glaxo Wellcome Inc. All rights reserved.
December 1997/RL-513
Shown in Product Identification Guide, page 315

ZOVIRAX® ℞

[zō "vī 'răx]

(acyclovir sodium)

Sterile Powder

FOR INTRAVENOUS INFUSION ONLY

DESCRIPTION

ZOVIRAX is the brand name for acyclovir, an antiviral drug active against herpesviruses. ZOVIRAX Sterile Powder is a formulation for intravenous administration. Each 5.49 mg of sterile lyophilized acyclovir sodium is equivalent to 5 mg acyclovir.

The chemical name of acyclovir sodium is 2-amino-1,9-dihydro-9-[(2-hydroxyethoxy)methyl]-6*H*-purin-6-one monosodium salt.

Acyclovir sodium is a white, crystalline powder with a molecular weight of 247 daltons, and a solubility in water exceeding 100 mg/mL. Each 500-mg or 1000-mg vial of ZOVIRAX Sterile Powder when reconstituted with 10 mL or 20 mL, respectively, sterile diluent yields 50 mg/mL acyclovir (pH approximately 11). Further dilution in any appropriate intravenous solution must be performed before infusion (see Method of Preparation). At physiologic pH, acyclovir exists as the un-ionized form with a molecular weight of 225 daltons and a maximum solubility of 2.5 mg/mL at 37°C.

CLINICAL PHARMACOLOGY

Mechanism of Antiviral Effects: Acyclovir is a synthetic purine nucleoside analogue with in vitro and in vivo inhibitory activity against human herpes viruses including herpes simplex types 1 (HSV-1) and 2 (HSV-2), varicella-zoster virus (VZV), Epstein-Barr virus (EBV), and cytomegalovirus (CMV). In cell culture, acyclovir has the highest antiviral activity against HSV-1, followed in decreasing order of potency against HSV-2, VZV, EBV, and CMV.[1]

The inhibitory activity of acyclovir for HSV-1, HSV-2 , VZV, and EBV is highly selective. The enzyme thymidine kinase (TK) of normal uninfected cells does not effectively use acyclovir as a substrate. However, TK encoded by HSV, VZV, and EBV[2] converts acyclovir into acyclovir monophosphate, a nucleotide analogue. The monophosphate is further converted into diphosphate by cellular guanylate kinase and into triphosphate by a number of cellular enzymes.[3] Acyclovir triphosphate interferes with Herpes simplex virus DNA polymerase and inhibits viral DNA replication. Acyclovir triphosphate also inhibits cellular α-DNA polymerase but to a lesser degree. In vitro, acyclovir triphosphate can be incorporated into growing chains of DNA by viral DNA polymerase and to a much smaller extent by cellular α-DNA polymerase.[4] When incorporation occurs, the DNA chain is terminated.[5,6] Acyclovir is preferentially taken up and selectively converted to the active triphosphate form by herpesvirus-infected cells. Thus, acyclovir is much less toxic in vitro for normal uninfected cells because: 1) less is taken up; 2) less is converted to the active form; 3) cellular α-DNA polymerase is less sensitive to the effects of the active form. The mode of acyclovir phosphorylation in cytomegalovirus-infected cells is not clearly established, but may involve virally induced cell kinases or an unidentified viral enzyme. Acyclovir is not efficiently activated in cytomegalovirus-infected cells, which may account for the reduced susceptibility of cytomegalovirus to acyclovir in vitro.

Microbiology: The quantitative relationship between the in vitro susceptibility of herpes simplex virus to acyclovir and the clinical response to therapy has not been established in humans, and virus sensitivity testing has not been standardized. Sensitivity testing results, expressed as the concentration of drug required to inhibit by 50% the growth of virus in cell culture (ID_{50}), vary greatly depending upon the particular assay used,[7] the cell type employed,[8] and the laboratory performing the test.[1] The ID_{50} of acyclovir against HSV-1 isolates may range from 0.02 mcg/mL (plaque reduction in Vero cells) to 5.9 to 13.5 mcg/mL (plaque reduction in green monkey kidney [GMK] cells).[1] The ID_{50} against HSV-2 ranges from 0.01 mcg/mL to 9.9 mcg/mL (plaque reduction in Vero and GMK cells, respectively).[1]

Using a dye-uptake method in Vero cells,[9] which gives ID_{50} values approximately 5- to 10-fold higher than plaque reduction assays, 1,417 isolates (553 HSV-1 and 864 HSV-2) from approximately 500 patients were examined over a 5-year period.[10] These assays found that 90% of HSV-1 isolates were sensitive to ≤ 0.9 mcg/mL acyclovir and 50% of all isolates were sensitive to ≤ 0.2 mcg/mL acyclovir. For HSV-2 isolates, 90% were sensitive to ≤ 2.2 mcg/mL and 50% of all isolates were sensitive to ≤ 0.7 mcg/mL of acyclovir. Isolates with significantly diminished sensitivity were found in 44 patients. It must be emphasized that neither the patients nor the isolates were randomly selected and, therefore, do not represent the general population.

Most of the less sensitive clinical isolates have been relatively deficient in the viral TK.[11-19] Strains with alterations in viral TK[20] or viral DNA polymerase[21] have also been reported. Prolonged exposure to low concentrations (0.1 mcg/mL) of acyclovir in cell culture has resulted in the emergence of a variety of acyclovir-resistant strains.[22]

The ID_{50} against VZV ranges from 0.17 to 1.53 mcg/mL (yield reduction, human foreskin fibroblasts) to 1.85 to 3.98 mcg/mL (foci reduction, human embryo fibroblasts [HEF]). Reproduction of EBV genome is suppressed by 50% in superinfected Raji cells or P3HR-1 lymphoblastoid cells by 1.5 mcg/mL acyclovir. CMV is relatively resistant to acyclovir with ID_{50} values ranging from 2.3 to 17.6 mcg/mL (plaque reduction, HEF cells) to 1.82 to 56.8 mcg/mL (DNA hybridization, HEF cells). The latent state of the genome of any of the human herpesviruses is not known to be sensitive to acyclovir.[1]

Pharmacokinetics: The pharmacokinetics of acyclovir has been evaluated in 95 patients (nine studies). Results were obtained in adult patients with normal renal function during Phase 1/2 studies after single doses ranging from 0.5 to 15 mg/kg and after multiple doses ranging from 2.5 to 15 mg/kg every 8 hours. Pharmacokinetics was also determined in pediatric patients with normal renal function ranging in age from 1 to 17 years at doses of 250 mg/m^2 or 500 mg/m^2 every 8 hours. In these studies, dose-independent pharmacokinetics is observed in the range of 0.5 to 15 mg/kg. Proportionality between dose and plasma levels is seen after single doses or at steady state after multiple dosing.[23] When ZOVIRAX was administered to adults at 5 mg/kg (approximately 250 mg/m^2) by 1-hour infusions every 8 hours, mean steady-state peak and trough concentrations of 9.8 mcg/mL (5.5 to 13.8 mcg/mL) and 0.7 mcg/mL (0.2 to 1.0 mcg/mL), respectively, were achieved. Similar concentrations are achieved in pediatric patients over 1 year of age when doses of 250 mg/m^2 are given by 1-hour infusions every 8 hours. At a dose of 10 mg/kg given by 1-hour infusion every 8 hours, mean steady-state peak and trough concentrations were 22.9 mcg/mL (14.1 to 44.1 mcg/mL) and 1.9 mcg/mL (0.5 to 2.9 mcg/mL). Similar concentrations were achieved in pediatric patients dosed at 500 mg/m^2 given by 1-hour infusion every 8 hours. Concentrations achieved in the cerebrospinal fluid are approximately 50% of plasma values. Plasma protein binding is relatively low (9% to 33%) and drug interactions involving binding site displacement are not anticipated.[23]

Renal excretion of unchanged drug by glomerular filtration and tubular secretion is the major route of acyclovir elimination accounting for 62% to 91% of the dose as determined by ^{14}C-labeled drug. The only major urinary metabolite detected is 9-carboxymethoxymethylguanine. This may account for up to 14.1% of the dose in patients with normal renal function. An insignificant amount of drug is recovered in feces and expired CO_2 and there is no evidence to suggest tissue retention.[23] However, postmortem examinations have shown that acyclovir is widely distributed in tissues and body fluids including brain, kidney, lung, liver, muscle, spleen, uterus, vaginal mucosa, vaginal secretions, cerebrospinal fluid, and herpetic vesicular fluid.

The half-life and total body clearance of acyclovir is dependent on renal function as shown below.[23]

Creatinine Clearance (mL/min/1.73m²)	Half-Life (hr)	Total Body Clearance (mL/min/1.73m²)
>80	2.5	327
50–80	3.0	248
15–50	3.5	190
0 (Anuric)	19.5	29

ZOVIRAX was administered at a dose of 2.5 mg/kg to six adult patients with severe renal failure. The peak and trough plasma levels during the 47 hours preceding hemodialysis were 8.5 mcg/mL and 0.7 mcg/mL, respectively.[24,25]

Consult DOSAGE AND ADMINISTRATION section for recommended adjustments in dosing based upon creatinine clearance. The half-life and total body clearance of acyclovir in pediatric patients over 1 year of age is similar to those in adults with normal renal function (see DOSAGE AND ADMINISTRATION).

INDICATIONS AND USAGE

ZOVIRAX Sterile Powder is indicated for the treatment of initial and recurrent mucosal and cutaneous Herpes simplex (HSV-1 and HSV-2) and varicella-zoster (shingles) infections in immunocompromised patients. It is also indicated for herpes simplex encephalitis in patients over 6 months of age and for severe initial clinical episodes of herpes genitalis in patients who are not immunocompromised.

Herpes Simplex Infections in Immunocompromised Patients: A multicenter trial of ZOVIRAX Sterile Powder at a dose of 250 mg/m^2 every 8 hours (750 mg/m^2/day) for 7 days was conducted in 98 immunocompromised patients (73 adults and 25 children) with oro-facial, esophageal, genital, and other localized infections (52 treated with ZOVIRAX and 46 with placebo). ZOVIRAX significantly decreased virus excretion, reduced pain, and promoted scabbing and rapid healing of lesions.[14,26,27,28]

Initial Episodes of Herpes Genitalis: In placebo-controlled trials, 58 patients with initial genital herpes were treated with intravenous ZOVIRAX 5 mg/kg or placebo (27 patients treated with ZOVIRAX and 31 treated with placebo) every 8 hours for 5 days. ZOVIRAX decreased the duration of viral excretion, new lesion formation, and duration of vesicles, and promoted healing of lesions.[28,29,30]

Herpes Simplex Encephalitis: Sixty-two patients ages 6 months to 79 years with brain biopsy-proven herpes simplex encephalitis were randomized to receive either ZOVIRAX (30 mg/kg/day) or adenine arabinoside (VIRA-A) (15 mg/kg/day) for 10 days (28 were treated with ZOVIRAX and 34 with VIRA-A).[31] Overall mortality at 6 months for patients treated with ZOVIRAX was 18% compared to 59% for patients treated with VIRA-A (P = 0.003). The proportion of patients treated with ZOVIRAX functioning normally or with only mild sequelae (e.g., decreased attention span) was 39% compared to 9% of patients treated with VIRA-A (P = 0.01). The remaining patients in both groups had moderate (e.g., hemiparesis, speech impediment, or seizure) or severe (continuous supportive care required) neurologic sequelae. After 12 months of follow-up, two additional patients treated with ZOVIRAX had died, resulting in an overall mortality of 25% compared to 59% for patients treated with VIRA-A (P = 0.02). Morbidity assessments at that time indicated that 32% of patients treated with ZOVIRAX were functioning normally, or with only mild sequelae compared to 12% of patients treated with VIRA-A (P = 0.06). Moderate to severe impairment was noted in all remaining patients in both groups who were available for evaluation. Patients less than 30 years of age and those who had the least severe neurologic involvement at time of entry into study had the best outcome with treatment with ZOVIRAX. An additional controlled study performed in Europe[32] demonstrated similar findings. The superiority of ZOVIRAX over VIRA-A for neonatal herpes encephalitis has not been demonstrated.

Varicella-Zoster Infections in Immunocompromised Patients: A multicenter trial of ZOVIRAX Sterile Powder at a dose of 500 mg/m^2 every 8 hours for 7 days was conducted in immunocompromised patients with zoster infections (shingles). Ninety-four (94) patients were evaluated (52 patients were treated with ZOVIRAX and 42 with placebo). ZOVIRAX halted progression of infection as determined by significant reductions in cutaneous dissemination, visceral dissemination, or the proportion of patients deemed treatment failures.[28,33]

A comparative trial of ZOVIRAX and vidarabine was conducted in 22 severely immunocompromised patients with zoster infections. ZOVIRAX was shown to be superior to vidarabine as demonstrated by significant differences in the time of new lesion formation, the time to pain reduction, the time to lesion crusting, the time to complete healing, the incidence of fever, and the duration of positive viral cultures. In addition, cutaneous dissemination occurred in none of the 10 patients treated with ZOVIRAX compared to 5 of the 10 vidarabine recipients who presented with localized dermatomal disease.[34]

Diagnosis: Diagnosis is confirmed by virus isolation. Accelerated viral culture assays or immunocytology allow more rapid diagnosis than standard viral culture. In initial episodes of genital herpes, appropriate examinations should be performed to rule out other sexually transmitted diseases. Whereas cutaneous lesions associated with Herpes simplex and varicella-zoster infections are often characteristic, the finding of multinucleated giant cells in smears prepared from lesion exudate or scrapings may assist in the diagnosis.[35]

The Tzanck smear does not distinguish varicella-zoster from herpes simplex infections. Culture of varicella-zoster is not widely available.

Herpes encephalitis should be confirmed by brain biopsy to obtain tissue for histologic examination and viral culture and to exclude other causes of neurologic disease. A presumptive diagnosis of herpes encephalitis may be made on the basis of focal changes in the temporal lobe visualized with various diagnostic methods including magnetic resonance imaging, computerized tomography, radionuclide scans, or electroencephalography. Culture of the cerebrospinal fluid for herpes simplex virus is unreliable.

CONTRAINDICATIONS

ZOVIRAX Sterile Powder is contraindicated for patients who develop hypersensitivity to the drug.

Continued on next page

This product information is based on labeling in effect on June 1, 1998. For further information, contact via direct mail, phone, or web site Medical Information: Glaxo Wellcome Inc., PO Box 13398, Research Triangle Park, NC 27709. Healthcare Professionals (Medical Information): 800-334-0089 Patients (Customer Response Center): 888-TALK2GW (1-888-825-5249) Glaxo Wellcome Corporate Web Site: www.glaxowellcome.com

Zovirax Powder—Cont.

WARNINGS

ZOVIRAX Sterile Powder is intended for intravenous infusion only, and should not be administered topically, intramuscularly, orally, subcutaneously, or in the eye. Intravenous infusions must be given over a period of at least 1 hour to reduce the risk of renal tubular damage (see PRECAUTIONS and DOSAGE AND ADMINISTRATION).

PRECAUTIONS

General: The recommended dosage, frequency, and length of treatment should not be exceeded (see DOSAGE AND ADMINISTRATION).

Although the aqueous solubility of acyclovir sodium (for infusion) is >100 mg/mL, precipitation of acyclovir crystals in renal tubules can occur if the maximum solubility of free acyclovir (2.5 mg/mL at 37°C in water) is exceeded or if the drug is administered by bolus injection. This complication causes a rise in serum creatinine and blood urea nitrogen (BUN), and a decrease in renal creatinine clearance. Ensuing renal tubular damage can produce acute renal failure.

Abnormal renal function (decreased creatinine clearance) can occur as a result of acyclovir administration and depends on the state of the patient's hydration, other treatments, and the rate of drug administration. Bolus administration of the drug leads to a 10% incidence of renal dysfunction, while in controlled studies, infusion of 5 mg/kg (250 mg/m^2) and 10 mg/kg (500 mg/m^2) over an hour was associated with a lower frequency—3.8%. Concomitant use of other nephrotoxic drugs, pre-existing renal disease, and dehydration make further renal impairment with acyclovir more likely. In most instances, alterations of renal function were transient and resolved spontaneously or with improvement of water and electrolyte balance, drug dosage adjustment, or discontinuation of drug administration. However, in some instances, these changes may progress to acute renal failure.

Administration of ZOVIRAX by intravenous infusion must be accompanied by adequate hydration. Since maximum urine concentration occurs within the first 2 hours following infusion, particular attention should be given to establishing sufficient urine flow during that period in order to prevent precipitation in renal tubules. Recommended urine output is ≥500 mL per gram of drug infused. In patients with encephalitis, the recommended hydration should be balanced by the risk of cerebral edema.

When dosage adjustments are required, they should be based on estimated creatinine clearance (see DOSAGE AND ADMINISTRATION).

Approximately 1% of patients receiving intravenous acyclovir have manifested encephalopathic changes characterized by either lethargy, obtundation, tremors, confusion, hallucinations, agitation, seizures, or coma. ZOVIRAX should be used with caution in those patients who have underlying neurologic abnormalities and those with serious renal, hepatic, or electrolyte abnormalities or significant hypoxia. It should also be used with caution in patients who have manifested prior neurologic reactions to cytotoxic drugs or those receiving concomitant intrathecal methotrexate or interferon.

Exposure of HSV isolates to acyclovir in vitro can lead to the emergence of less sensitive viruses. These viruses usually are deficient in thymidine kinase (required for acyclovir activation) and are less pathogenic in animals. Similar isolates have been observed in severely immunocompromised patients during the course of controlled and uncontrolled studies of intravenously administered ZOVIRAX. These occurred in patients with severe combined immunodeficiencies or following bone marrow transplantation. The presence of these viruses was not associated with a worsening of clinical illness and, in some instances, the virus disappeared spontaneously. The possibility of the appearance of less sensitive viruses must be recognized when treating such patients.[11-19] The relationship between the in vitro sensitivity of herpes simplex or varicella-zoster virus to acyclovir and clinical response to therapy has not been established.

Drug Interactions: Co-administration of probenecid with acyclovir has been shown to increase the mean half-life and the area under the concentration-time curve. Urinary excretion and renal clearance were correspondingly reduced.[36] The clinical effects of this combination have not been studied.

Carcinogenesis, Mutagenesis, Impairment of Fertility: The data presented below include references to peak steady-state plasma acyclovir concentrations observed in humans treated with 30 mg/kg/day (10 mg/kg/every 8 hours, dosing appropriate for treatment of herpes zoster or herpes encephalitis), or 15 mg/kg/day (5 mg/kg/every 8 hours, dosing appropriate for treatment of primary genital herpes or herpes simplex infections in immunocompromised patients). Plasma drug concentrations in animal studies are expressed as multiples of human exposure to acyclovir at the higher and lower dosing schedules (see CLINICAL PHARMACOLOGY: Pharmacokinetics).

Acyclovir was tested in lifetime bioassays in rats and mice at single daily doses of up to 450 mg/kg administered by gavage. There was no statistically significant difference in the incidence of tumors between treated and control animals, nor did acyclovir shorten the latency of tumors. At 450 mg/kg/day, plasma concentrations in both the mouse and rat bioassay were lower than concentrations in humans.

Acyclovir was tested in two in vitro cell transformation assays. Positive results were observed at the highest concentration tested (three to five times human levels) in one system and the resulting morphologically transformed cells formed tumors when inoculated into immunosuppressed, syngeneic, weanling mice. Acyclovir was negative (three to six times human levels) in the other, possibly less sensitive, transformation assay.

In acute cytogenetic studies, there was an increase, though not statistically significant, in the incidence of chromosomal damage at maximum tolerated parenteral doses of acyclovir (100 mg/kg) in rats (five to ten times human levels) but not in Chinese hamsters; higher doses of 500 and 1000 mg/kg were clastogenic in Chinese hamsters (31 to 61 times human levels). In addition, no activity was found after 5 days dosing in a dominant lethal study in mice (three to six times human levels). In all four microbial assays, no evidence of mutagenicity was observed. Positive results were obtained in two of seven genetic toxicity assays using mammalian cells in vitro. In human lymphocytes, a positive response for chromosomal damage was seen at concentrations 13 to 25 times the acyclovir plasma levels achieved in humans. At one locus in mouse lymphoma cells, mutagenicity was observed at concentrations 20 to 40 times human plasma levels. Results in the other five mammalian cell loci follow: at three loci in a Chinese hamster ovary cell line, the results were inconclusive at concentrations at least 150 times human levels; at two other loci in mouse lymphoma cells, no evidence of mutagenicity was observed at concentrations at least 120 times human levels.

Acyclovir has not been shown to impair fertility or reproduction in mice (450 mg/kg/day, PO) or in rats (25 mg/kg/day, SC). In the mouse study, plasma levels were the same as human levels. At 50 mg/kg/day, SC in the rat (one to two times human levels), there was a statistically significant increase in post-implantation loss, but no concomitant decrease in litter size. In female rabbits treated subcutaneously with acyclovir subsequent to mating, there was a statistically significant decrease in implantation efficiency but no concomitant decrease in litter size at a dose of 50 mg/kg/day (one to three times human levels). No effect upon implantation efficiency was observed when the same dose was administered intravenously (four to nine times human levels). In a rat peri- and postnatal study at 50 mg/kg/day, SC, (one to two times human levels), there was a statistically significant decrease in the group mean numbers of corpora lutea, total implantation sites, and live fetuses in the F_1 generation. Although not statistically significant, there was also a dose-related decrease in group mean numbers of live fetuses and implantation sites, at 12.5 mg/kg/day and 25 mg/kg/day, SC. The intravenous administration of 100 mg/kg/day, a dose known to cause obstructive nephropathy in rabbits, caused a significant increase in fetal resorptions and a corresponding decrease in litter size (plasma levels were not measured). However, at a maximum tolerated intravenous dose of 50 mg/kg/day in rabbits (four to nine times human levels), no drug-related reproductive effects were observed.

Intraperitoneal doses of 80 or 320 mg/kg/day acyclovir given to rats for 6 and 1 months, respectively, caused testicular atrophy. Plasma levels were not measured in the 1-month study and were two to four times human levels in the 6-month study. Testicular atrophy was persistent through the 4-week postdose recovery phase after 320 mg/kg/day; some evidence of recovery of sperm production was evident 30 days postdose. Intravenous doses of 100 and 200 mg/kg/day acyclovir given to dogs for 31 days caused aspermatogenesis. At 100 mg/kg/day, plasma levels were four to eight times human levels, while at 200 mg/kg/day, they were 13 to 25 times human levels. No testicular abnormalities were seen in dogs given 50 mg/kg/day IV for 1 month (two to three times human levels) and in dogs given 60 mg/kg/day orally for 1 year (the same as human levels).

Pregnancy: ***Teratogenic Effects:*** Pregnancy Category C. Acyclovir was not teratogenic in the mouse (450 mg/kg/day, PO), rabbit (50 mg/kg/day, SC and IV) or in standard tests in the rat (50 mg/kg/day, SC). These exposures resulted in plasma levels the same as, four and nine, and one and two times, respectively, human levels. In a non-standard test in rats, there were fetal abnormalities, such as head and tail anomalies, and maternal toxicity.[37] In this test, rats were given three SC doses of 100 mg/kg acyclovir on gestation day 10, resulting in plasma levels five and 10 times human levels. There are no adequate and well-controlled studies in pregnant women. Acyclovir should not be used during pregnancy unless the potential benefit justifies the potential risk to the fetus. Although acyclovir was not teratogenic in standard animal studies, the drug's potential for causing chromosome breaks at high concentration should be taken into consideration in making this determination.

Pregnancy Exposure Registry: To monitor maternal-fetal outcomes of pregnant women exposed to systemic acyclovir. Glaxo Wellcome Inc. maintains an Acyclovir in Pregnancy Registry. Physicians are encouraged to register patients by calling 1-888-825-5249, ext. 39441.

Nursing Mothers: Acyclovir concentrations have been documented in breast milk in two women following oral administration of ZOVIRAX and ranged from 0.6 to 4.1 times corresponding plasma levels.[38,39] These concentrations would potentially expose the nursing infant to a dose of acyclovir up to 0.3 mg/kg/day. Caution should be exercised when ZOVIRAX is administered to a nursing woman.

ADVERSE REACTIONS

The adverse reactions listed below have been observed in controlled and uncontrolled clinical trials in approximately 700 patients who received ZOVIRAX at ~5 mg/kg (250 mg/m^2) three times daily, and approximately 300 patients who received ~10 mg/kg (500 mg/m^2) three times daily.

The most frequent adverse reactions reported during administration of ZOVIRAX were inflammation or phlebitis at the injection site in approximately 9% of the patients, and transient elevations of serum creatinine or BUN in 5% to 10% (the higher incidence occurred usually following rapid [less than 10 minutes] intravenous infusion). Nausea and/or vomiting occurred in approximately 7% of the patients (the majority occurring in nonhospitalized patients who received 10 mg/kg). Itching, rash, or hives occurred in approximately 2% of patients. Elevation of transaminases occurred in 1% to 2% of patients.

Approximately 1% of patients receiving intravenous acyclovir have manifested encephalopathic changes characterized by either lethargy, obtundation, tremors, confusion, hallucinations, agitation, seizures, or coma (see PRECAUTIONS).

Adverse reactions which occurred at a frequency of less than 1% and which were probably or possibly related to intravenous administration of ZOVIRAX were: anemia, anuria, hematuria, hypotension, edema, anorexia, lightheadedness, thirst, headache, diaphoresis, fever, neutropenia, thrombocytopenia, abnormal urinalysis (characterized by an increase in formed elements in urine sediment), and pain on urination.

Other reactions have been reported with a frequency of less than 1% in patients receiving ZOVIRAX, but a causal relationship between ZOVIRAX and the reaction could not be determined. These include pulmonary edema with cardiac tamponade, abdominal pain, chest pain, thrombocytosis, leukocytosis, neutrophilia, ischemia of digits, hypokalemia, purpura fulminans, pressure on urination, hemoglobinemia, and rigors.

Observed During Clinical Practice: In addition to adverse events reported from clinical trials, the following events have been identified during post-approval use of ZOVIRAX for Injection in clinical practice. Because they are reported voluntarily from a population of unknown size, estimates of frequency cannot be made. These events have been chosen for inclusion due to either their seriousness, frequency of reporting, potential causal connection to ZOVIRAX, or a combination of these factors.

General: Fever, pain, and rarely, anaphylaxis.

Digestive: Elevated liver function tests, nausea.

Hemic and Lymphatic: Leukopenia.

Nervous: Agitation, coma, confusion, convulsions, delirium, hallucinations, obtundation, psychosis.

Skin: Alopecia, erythema multiforme, pruritus, rash, Stevens-Johnson syndrome, toxic epidermal necrolysis, urticaria.

Urogenital: Elevated blood urea nitrogen, elevated creatinine, renal failure.

OVERDOSAGE

Overdosage has been reported following administration of bolus injections, or inappropriately high doses, and in patients whose fluid and electrolyte balance was not properly monitored. This has resulted in elevations in BUN, serum creatinine, and subsequent renal failure. Lethargy, convulsions, and coma have been reported rarely.

Precipitation of acyclovir in renal tubules may occur when the solubility (2.5 mg/mL) in the intratubular fluid is exceeded (see PRECAUTIONS). Renal lesions related to obstruction of renal tubules by precipitated drug crystals occurred in the following species: rats treated with IV and IP doses of 20 mg/kg/day for 21 and 31 days, respectively, and at SC doses of 100 mg/kg/day for 10 days; rabbits at SC and IV doses of 50 mg/kg/day for 13 days; and dogs at IV doses of 100 mg/kg/day for 31 days. In the event of overdosage, sufficient urine flow must be maintained to prevent precipitation of drug in renal tubules. Recommended urine output is ≥500 mL per gram of drug infused. A 6-hour hemodialysis results in a 60% decrease in plasma acyclovir concentration. Data concerning peritoneal dialysis are incomplete but indicate that this method may be significantly less efficient in removing acyclovir from the blood. In the event of acute renal failure and anuria, the patient may benefit from hemodialysis until renal function is restored (see DOSAGE AND ADMINISTRATION).

DOSAGE AND ADMINISTRATION

CAUTION— RAPID OR BOLUS INTRAVENOUS AND INTRAMUSCULAR OR SUBCUTANEOUS INJECTION MUST BE AVOIDED. Therapy should be initiated as early as possible following onset of signs and symptoms. For diagnosis— see INDICATIONS.

Dosage: *Herpes Simplex Infections: Mucosal and Cutaneous Herpes Simplex (HSV-1 and HSV-2) Infections in Immunocompromised Patients:* 5 mg/kg infused at a constant rate over 1 hour, every 8 hours (15 mg/kg/day) for 7 days in adult patients with normal renal function. In pediatric patients under 12 years of age, more accurate dosing can be attained by infusing 250 mg/m^2 at a constant rate over 1 hour, every 8 hours (750 mg/m^2/day) for 7 days.

Severe Initial Clinical Episodes of Herpes Genitalis: The same dose given above—administered for 5 days.

Herpes Simplex Encephalitis: 10 mg/kg infused at a constant rate over at least 1 hour, every 8 hours for 10 days. In pediatric patients between 6 months and 12 years of age, more accurate dosing is achieved by infusing 500 mg/m^2, at a constant rate over at least 1 hour, every 8 hours for 10 days.

Varicella Zoster Infections: Zoster in Immunocompromised Patients: 10 mg/kg infused at a constant rate over 1 hour, every 8 hours for 7 days in adult patients with normal renal function. In pediatric patients under 12 years of age, equivalent plasma concentrations are attained by infusing 500 mg/m^2 at a constant rate over at least 1 hour, every 8 hours for 7 days. Obese patients should be dosed at 10 mg/kg (Ideal Body Weight). A maximum dose equivalent to 500 mg/m^2 every 8 hours should not be exceeded for any patient.

Patients with Acute or Chronic Renal Impairment: Refer to DOSAGE AND ADMINISTRATION section for recommended doses, and adjust the dosing interval as indicated in the table below.

Creatinine Clearance (mL/min/1.73 m^2)	Percent of Recommended Dose	Dosing Interval (hours)
>50	100%	8
25–50	100%	12
10–25	100%	24
0–10	50%	24

Hemodialysis: For patients who require dialysis, the mean plasma half-life of acyclovir during hemodialysis is approximately 5 hours. This results in a 60% decrease in plasma concentrations following a 6-hour dialysis period. Therefore, the patient's dosing schedule should be adjusted so that an additional dose is administered after each dialysis.[24,25]

Peritoneal Dialysis: No supplemental dose appears to be necessary after adjustment of the dosing interval.[40,41]

Method of Preparation: Each 10-mL vial contains acyclovir sodium equivalent to 500 mg of acyclovir. Each 20-mL vial contains acyclovir sodium equivalent to 1000 mg of acyclovir. The contents of the vial should be dissolved in Sterile Water for Injection as follows:

Contents of Vial	Amount of Diluent
500 mg	10 mL
1000 mg	20 mL

The resulting solution in each case contains 50 mg acyclovir per mL (pH approximately 11). Shake the vial well to assure complete dissolution before measuring and transferring each individual dose. DO NOT USE BACTERIOSTATIC WATER FOR INJECTION CONTAINING BENZYL ALCOHOL OR PARABENS.

Administration: The calculated dose should then be removed and added to any appropriate intravenous solution at a volume selected for administration during each 1-hour infusion. Infusion concentrations of approximately 7 mg/mL or lower are recommended. In clinical studies, the average 70-kg adult received between 60 and 150 mL of fluid per dose. Higher concentrations (e.g., 10 mg/mL) may produce phlebitis or inflammation at the injection site upon inadvertent extravasation. Standard, commercially available electrolyte and glucose solutions are suitable for intravenous administration; biologic or colloidal fluids (e.g., blood products, protein solutions, etc.) are not recommended.

Once in solution in the vial at a concentration of 50 mg/mL, the drug should be used within 12 hours. Once diluted for administration, each dose should be used within 24 hours. Refrigeration of reconstituted solutions may result in formation of a precipitate which will redissolve at room temperature.

HOW SUPPLIED

10-mL sterile vials, each containing acyclovir sodium equivalent to 500 mg of acyclovir, tray of 10 (NDC 0173-0995-01).

20-mL sterile vials, each containing acyclovir sodium equivalent to 1000 mg of acyclovir, tray of 10 (NDC 0173-0952-01).

Store at 15° to 25°C (59° to 77°F).

REFERENCES

1. O'Brien JJ, Campoli-Richards DM. Acyclovir—an updated review of its antiviral activity, pharmacokinetic properties and therapeutic efficacy. *Drugs.* 1989;37:233-309.
2. Littler E, Zeuthen J, McBride AA, et al. Identification of an Epstein-Barr virus-coded thymidine kinase. *EMBO J.* 1986;5:1959-1966.
3. Miller WH, Miller RL. Phosphorylation of acyclovir (acycloguanosine) monophosphate by GMP kinase. *J Biol Chem.* 1980;255:7204-7207.
4. Furman PA, St Clair MH, Fyfe JA, et al. Inhibition of herpes simplex virus-induced DNA polymerase activity and viral DNA replication by 9-(2-hydroxyethoxymethyl)guanine and its triphosphate. *J Virol.* 1979;32:72-77.
5. Derse D, Cheng YC, Furman PA, et al. Inhibition of purified human and herpes simplex virus-induced DNA polymerases by 9-(2-hydroxyethoxymethyl)guanine triphosphate: effects on primer-template function. *J Biol Chem.* 1981;256:11447-11451.
6. McGuirt PV, Shaw JE, Elion GB, et al. Identification of small DNA fragments synthesized in herpes simplex virus-infected cells in the presence of acyclovir. *Antimicrob Agents Chemother.* 1984;25:507-509.
7. Barry DW, Blum MR. Antiviral drugs: acyclovir. In: Turner P, Shand DG, eds. *Recent Advances in Clinical Pharmacology.* ed 3. New York: Churchill Livingstone, 1983: chap 4.
8. DeClercq E. Comparative efficacy of antiherpes drugs in different cell lines. *Antimicrob Agents Chemother.* 1982;21:661-663.
9. McLaren C, Ellis MN, Hunter GA. A colorimetric assay for the measurement of the sensitivity of herpes simplex viruses to antiviral agents. *Antiviral Res.* 1983;3:223-234.
10. Barry DW, Nusinoff-Lehrman S. Viral resistance in clinical practice: summary of five years experience with acyclovir. In: Kono R, Nakajima A, eds. *Herpes Viruses and Virus Chemotherapy (Ex Med Int Congr Ser 667).* New York: *Excerpta Medica,* 1985;269-270.
11. Dekker C, Ellis MN, McLaren C, et al. Virus resistance in clinical practice. *J Antimicrob Chemother.* 1983;12 (suppl B):137-152.
12. Sibrack CD, Gutman LT, Wilfert CM, et al. Pathogenicity of acyclovir-resistant herpes simplex virus type 1 from an immunodeficient child. *J Infect Dis.* 1982;146:673-682.
13. Crumpacker CS, Schnipper LE, Marlowe Sl, et al. Resistance to antiviral drugs of herpes simplex virus isolated from a patient treated with acyclovir. *N Engl J Med.* 1982;306:343-346.
14. Wade JC, Newton B, McLaren C, et al. Intravenous acyclovir to treat mucocutaneous herpes simplex virus infection after marrow transplantation: a double-blind trial. *Ann Intern Med.* 1982;96:265-269.
15. Burns WH, Saral R, Santos GW, et al. Isolation and characterization of resistant herpes simplex virus after acyclovir therapy. *Lancet.* 1982;1:421-423.
16. Straus SE, Takiff HE, Seidlin M, et al. Suppression of frequently recurring genital herpes: a placebo-controlled double-blind trial of oral acyclovir. *N Engl J Med.* 1984;310:1545-1550.
17. Collins P. Viral sensitivity following the introduction of acyclovir. *Am J Med.* 1988;85(suppl 2A):129-134.
18. Erlich KS, Mills J, Chatis P, et al. Acyclovir-resistant herpes simplex virus infections in patients with the acquired immunodeficiency syndrome. *N Engl J Med.* 1989;320:293-296.
19. Hill EL, Ellis MN, Barry DW. In: *28th Intersci Conf on Antimicrob Agents Chemother.* Los Angeles, 1988, Abst. No. 0840:260.
20. Ellis MN, Keller PM, Fyfe JA, et al. Clinical isolates of herpes simplex virus type 2 that induces a thymidine kinase with altered substrate specificity. *Antimicrob Agents Chemother.* 1987;31:1117-1125.
21. Collins P, Larder BA, Oliver NM, et al. Characterization of a DNA polymerase mutant of herpes simplex virus from a severely immunocompromised patient receiving acyclovir. *J Gen Virol.* 1989;70:375-382.
22. Field HJ, Darby G, Wildy P. Isolation and characterization of acyclovir-resistant mutants of herpes simplex virus. *J Gen Virol.* 1980;49:115-124.
23. Blum MR, Liao SH, deMiranda P. Overview of acyclovir pharmacokinetic disposition in adults and children. *Am J Med.* 1982;73:186-192.
24. Laskin OL, Longstreth JA, Whelton A, et al. Effect of renal failure on the pharmacokinetics of acyclovir. *Am J Med.* 1982;73:197-201.
25. Krasny HC, Liao SH, deMiranda P, et al. Influence of hemodialysis on acyclovir pharmacokinetics in patients with chronic renal failure. *Am J Med.* 1982;73:202-204.
26. Mitchell CD, Bean B, Gentry SR, et al. Acyclovir therapy for mucocutaneous herpes simplex infections in immunocompromised patients. *Lancet.* 1981;1:1389-1392.
27. Meyers JD, Wade JC, Mitchell CD, et al. Multicenter collaborative trial of intravenous acyclovir for treatment of mucocutaneous herpes simplex virus infection in the immunocompromised host. *Am J Med.* 1982;73: 229-235.
28. Data on file, Glaxo Wellcome Inc.
29. Corey L, Fife KH, Benedetti JK, et al. Intravenous acyclovir for the treatment of primary genital herpes. *Ann Intern Med.* 1983;98:914-921.
30. Mindel A, Adler MW, Sutherland S, et al. Intravenous acyclovir treatment for primary genital herpes. *Lancet.* 1982;1:697-700.
31. Whitley RJ, Alford CA, Hirsch MS, et al. Vidarabine versus acyclovir therapy in herpes simplex encephalitis. *N Engl J Med.* 1986;314:144-149.
32. Sköldenberg B, Forsgren M, Alestig K, et al. Acyclovir versus vidarabine in herpes simplex encephalitis: randomized multicenter study in consecutive Swedish patients. *Lancet.* 1984;2:707-711.
33. Balfour HH Jr, Bean B, Laskin OL, et al. Acyclovir halts progression of herpes zoster in immunocompromised patients. *N Engl J Med.* 1983;308:1448-1453.
34. Shepp DH, Danliker PS, Meyers JD. Treatment of varicella-zoster virus infection in severely immunocompromised patients. *N Engl J Med.* 1986;314:208-212.
35. Naib ZM, Nahmias AJ, Josey WE, et al. Relation of cytohistopathology of genital herpesvirus infection to cervical anaplasia. *Cancer Res.* 1973;33:1452-1463.
36. Laskin OL, deMiranda P, King DH, et al. Effects of probenecid on the pharmacokinetics and elimination of acyclovir in humans. *Antimicrob Agents Chemother.* 1982;21:804-807.
37. Stahlmann R, Klug S, Lewandowski C, et al. Teratogenicity of acyclovir in rats. *Infection.* 1987;15:261-262.
38. Lau RJ, Emery MG, Galinsky RE, et al. Unexpected accumulation of acyclovir in breast milk with estimate of infant exposure. *Obstet Gynecol.* 1987;69:468-471.
39. Meyer LJ, deMiranda P, Sheth N, et al. Acyclovir in human breast milk. *Am J Obstet Gynecol.* 1988;158:586-588.
40. Boelart J, Schurgers M, Daneels R, et al. Multiple dose pharmacokinetics of intravenous acyclovir in patients on continuous ambulatory peritoneal dialysis. *J Antimicrob Chemother.* 1987;20:69-76.
41. Shah GM, Winer RL, Krasny HC. Acyclovir pharmacokinetics in a patient on continuous ambulatory peritoneal dialysis. *Am J Kidney Dis.* 1986;7:507-510.

April 1998/RL-543

Shown in Product Identification Guide, page 315

ZYBAN™ ℞

[zī' ban]

**(bupropion hydrochloride)
Sustained-Release Tablets**

DESCRIPTION

ZYBAN (bupropion hydrochloride) Sustained-Release Tablets are a non-nicotine aid to smoking cessation. Initially developed and marketed as an antidepressant (WELLBUTRIN® [bupropion hydrochloride] Tablets and WELLBUTRIN® SR [bupropion hydrochloride] Sustained-Release Tablets), ZYBAN is chemically unrelated to tricyclic, tetracyclic, selective serotonin re-uptake inhibitor, or other known antidepressant agents. Its structure closely resembles that of diethylpropion; it is related to phenylethylamines. It is (±)-1-(3-chlorophenyl)-2-[(1,1-dimethylethyl)amino]-1-propanone hydrochloride. The molecular weight is 276.2. The molecular formula is $C_{13}H_{18}ClNO \cdot HCl$. Bupropion hydrochloride powder is white, crystalline, and highly soluble in water. It has a bitter taste and produces the sensation of local anesthesia on the oral mucosa.

ZYBAN is supplied for oral administration as 150-mg (purple), film-coated, sustained-release tablets. Each tablet contains the labeled amount of bupropion hydrochloride and the inactive ingredients carnauba wax, cysteine hydrochloride, hydroxypropyl methylcellulose, magnesium stearate, microcrystalline cellulose, polyethylene glycol, polysorbate

Continued on next page

This product information is based on labeling in effect on June 1, 1998. For further information, contact via direct mail, phone, or web site Medical Information: Glaxo Wellcome Inc., PO Box 13398, Research Triangle Park, NC 27709. Healthcare Professionals (Medical Information): 800-334-0089 Patients (Customer Response Center): 888-TALK2GW (1-888-825-5249) Glaxo Wellcome Corporate Web Site: www.glaxowellcome.com

Zyban—Cont.

80 and titanium dioxide and is printed with edible black ink. In addition, the 150-mg tablet contains FD&C Blue No. 2 Lake and FD&C Red No. 40 Lake.

CLINICAL PHARMACOLOGY

Pharmacodynamics: Bupropion is a relatively weak inhibitor of the neuronal uptake of norepinephrine, serotonin, and dopamine, and does not inhibit monoamine oxidase. The mechanism by which ZYBAN enhances the ability of patients to abstain from smoking is unknown. However, it is presumed that this action is mediated by noradrenergic and/or dopaminergic mechanisms.

Pharmacokinetics: Bupropion is a racemic mixture. The pharmacologic activity and pharmacokinetics of the individual enantiomers have not been studied. Bupropion follows biphasic pharmacokinetics best described by a two-compartment model. The terminal phase has a mean half-life (±% CV) of about 21 hours (±20%), while the distribution phase has a mean half-life of 3 to 4 hours.

Absorption: Bupropion has not been administered intravenously to humans; therefore, the absolute bioavailability of ZYBAN Sustained-Release Tablets in humans has not been determined. In rat and dog studies, the bioavailability of bupropion ranged from 5% to 20%.

Following oral administration of ZYBAN to healthy volunteers, peak plasma concentrations of bupropion are achieved within 3 hours. The mean peak concentration (C_{max}) values were 91 and 143 ng/mL from two single-dose (150-mg) studies. At steady state, the mean C_{max} following a 150-mg dose every 12 hours is 136 ng/mL.

In a single-dose study, food increased the C_{max} of bupropion by 11% and the extent of absorption as defined by area under the plasma concentration-time curve (AUC) by 17%. The mean time to peak concentration (t_{max}) was prolonged by 1 hour. This effect was of no clinical significance.

Distribution: In vitro tests show that bupropion is 84% bound to human plasma proteins at concentrations up to 200 mcg/mL. The extent of protein binding of the hydroxybupropion metabolite is similar to that for bupropion, whereas the extent of protein binding of the threohydrobupropion metabolite is about half that seen with bupropion. The volume of distribution (V_{ss}/F) estimated from a single 150-mg dose given to 17 subjects is 1,950 L (20% CV).

Metabolism: Bupropion is extensively metabolized in humans. There are three active metabolites: hydroxybupropion and the amino-alcohol isomers threohydrobupropion and erythrohydrobupropion, which are formed via hydroxylation of the *tert*-butyl group of bupropion and/or reduction of the carbonyl group. Oxidation of the bupropion side chain results in the formation of a glycine conjugate of meta-chlorobenzoic acid, which is then excreted as the major urinary metabolite. The potency and toxicity of the metabolites relative to bupropion have not been fully characterized; however, it has been demonstrated in mice that hydroxybupropion is comparable in potency to bupropion, while the other metabolites are one tenth to one half as potent. This may be of clinical importance because the plasma concentrations of the metabolites are higher than those of bupropion. In vitro findings suggest that cytochrome P450 2B6 (CYP2B6) is the principal isoenzyme involved in the formation of hydroxybupropion, while cytochrome P450 isoenzymes are not involved in the formation of threohydrobupropion.

Following a single dose in humans, peak plasma concentrations of hydroxybupropion occur approximately 6 hours after administration. Peak plasma concentrations of hydroxybupropion are approximately 10 times the peak level of the parent drug at steady state. The AUC at steady state is about 17 times that of bupropion. The times to peak concentrations for the erythrohydrobupropion and threohydrobupropion metabolites are similar to that of the hydroxybupropion metabolite, and steady-state AUCs are 1.5 and 7 times that of bupropion, respectively.

Elimination: The mean (±% CV) apparent clearance (Cl/F) estimated from two single-dose (150-mg) studies are 135 (±20%) and 209 L/hr (±21%). Following chronic dosing of 150 mg of ZYBAN every 12 hours for 14 days (n = 34), the mean Cl/F at steady state was 160 L/hr (±23%). The mean elimination half-life of bupropion estimated from a series of studies is approximately 21 hours. Estimates of the half-lives of the metabolites determined from a multiple-dose study were 20 hours (±25%) for hydroxybupropion, 37 hours (±35%) for threohydrobupropion, and 33 hours (±30%) for erythrohydrobupropion. Steady-state plasma concentrations of bupropion and metabolites are reached within 5 and 8 days, respectively.

Following oral administration of 200 mg of ^{14}C-bupropion in humans, 87% and 10% of the radioactive dose were recovered in the urine and feces, respectively. The fraction of the oral dose of bupropion excreted unchanged was only 0.5%.

The effects of cigarette smoking on the pharmacokinetics of bupropion were studied in 34 healthy male and female volunteers; 17 were chronic cigarette smokers and 17 were nonsmokers. Following oral administration of a single 150-mg dose of ZYBAN, there was no statistically significant difference in C_{max}, half-life, t_{max}, AUC, or clearance of bupropion or its major metabolites between smokers and nonsmokers.

Bupropion and its metabolites exhibit linear kinetics following chronic administration of 150 to 300 mg/day.

Population Subgroups: Factors or conditions altering metabolic capacity (e.g., liver disease, congestive heart failure, age, concomitant medications, etc.) or elimination may be expected to influence the degree and extent of accumulation of the active metabolites of bupropion. The elimination of the major metabolites of bupropion may be affected by reduced renal or hepatic function because they are moderately polar compounds and are likely to undergo further metabolism or conjugation in the liver prior to urinary excretion.

Hepatic: The disposition of bupropion following a single 200-mg oral dose was compared in eight healthy volunteers and eight weight- and age-matched volunteers with alcoholic liver disease. The half-life of hydroxybupropion was significantly prolonged in subjects with alcoholic liver disease (32 hours [±41%] versus 21 hours [±23%]). The differences in half-life for bupropion and the other metabolites in the two patient groups were minimal.

Renal: The effect of renal disease on the pharmacokinetics of bupropion has not been studied. The elimination of the major metabolites of bupropion may be affected by reduced renal function.

Left Ventricular Dysfunction: During a chronic dosing study with bupropion in 14 depressed patients with left ventricular dysfunction (history of congestive heart failure [CHF] or an enlarged heart on x-ray), no apparent effect on the pharmacokinetics of bupropion or its metabolites, compared to healthy normal volunteers, was revealed.

Age: The effects of age on the pharmacokinetics of bupropion and its metabolites have not been fully characterized, but an exploration of steady-state bupropion concentrations from several depression efficacy studies involving patients dosed in a range of 300 to 750 mg/day, on a three times a day schedule, revealed no relationship between age (18 to 83 years) and plasma concentration of bupropion. These data suggest there is no prominent effect of age on bupropion concentration (see PRECAUTIONS: Use in the Elderly).

Gender: A single-dose study involving 12 healthy male and 12 healthy female volunteers revealed no sex-related differences in the pharmacokinetic parameters of bupropion.

CLINICAL TRIALS

The efficacy of ZYBAN as an aid to smoking cessation was demonstrated in two placebo-controlled, double-blind trials in nondepressed chronic cigarette smokers (n = 1,508, ≥15 cigarettes per day). In these studies, ZYBAN was used in conjunction with individual smoking cessation counseling.

The first study was a dose-response trial conducted at three clinical centers. Patients in this study were treated for 7 weeks with one of three doses of ZYBAN (100, 150, or 300 mg/day) or placebo; quitting was defined as total abstinence during the last 4 weeks of treatment (weeks 4 through 7). Abstinence was determined by patient daily diaries and verified by carbon monoxide levels in expired air.

Results of this dose-response trial with ZYBAN demonstrated a dose-dependent increase in the percentage of patients able to achieve 4-week abstinence (weeks 4 through 7). Treatment with ZYBAN at both 150 and 300 mg/day was significantly more effective than placebo in this study.

Table 1 presents quit rates over time in the multicenter trial by treatment group. The quit rates are the proportions of all persons initially enrolled (i.e., intent to treat analysis) who abstained from week 4 of the study through the specified week. Treatment with ZYBAN (150 or 300 mg/day) was more effective than placebo in helping patients achieve 4-week abstinence. In addition, treatment with ZYBAN (7 weeks at 300 mg/day) was more effective than placebo in helping patients maintain continuous abstinence through week 26 (6 months) of the study.

[See table 1 below]

The second study was a comparative trial conducted at four clinical centers. Four treatments were evaluated: ZYBAN 300 mg/day, HABITROL® (nicotine transdermal system) (NTS) 21 mg/day, combination of ZYBAN 300 mg/day plus NTS 21 mg/day, and placebo. Patients were treated for 9 weeks. Treatment with ZYBAN was initiated at 150 mg/day while the patient was still smoking and was increased after 3 days to 300 mg/day given as 150 mg twice daily. NTS 21 mg/day was added to treatment with ZYBAN after approximately 1 week when the patient reached the target quit date. During weeks 8 and 9 of the study, NTS was tapered to 14 and 7 mg/day, respectively. Quitting, defined as total abstinence during weeks 4 through 7, was determined by patient daily diaries and verified by expired air carbon monoxide levels.

In this study, patients treated with either ZYBAN or NTS achieved greater 4-week abstinence rates than patients treated with placebo. In addition, patients treated with the combination of ZYBAN and NTS achieved higher abstinence rates than patients treated with either of the individual active treatments alone, although only the comparison with NTS achieved statistical significance.

Table 2 presents quit rates over time by treatment group for the comparative trial. Both ZYBAN and NTS were more effective than placebo in helping patients maintain abstinence through week 10 of the study. The treatment combination of ZYBAN and NTS displayed the highest rates of continuous abstinence throughout the study.

[See table 2 at top of next page]

Quit rates in clinical trials are influenced by the population selected. Quit rates in an unselected population may be lower than the above rates.

Treatment with ZYBAN reduced withdrawal symptoms compared to placebo. Reductions on the following withdrawal symptoms were most pronounced: irritability, frustration, or anger; anxiety; difficulty concentrating; restlessness; and depressed mood or negative affect. Depending on the study and the measure used, treatment with ZYBAN showed evidence of reduction in craving for cigarettes or urge to smoke compared to placebo.

INDICATIONS AND USAGE

ZYBAN is indicated as an aid to smoking cessation treatment.

CONTRAINDICATIONS

ZYBAN is contraindicated in patients with a seizure disorder.

ZYBAN is contraindicated in patients treated with WELLBUTRIN, WELLBUTRIN SR, or any other medications that contain bupropion because the incidence of seizure is dose dependent.

ZYBAN is contraindicated in patients with a current or prior diagnosis of bulimia or anorexia nervosa because of a higher incidence of seizures noted in patients treated for bulimia with the immediate-release formulation of bupropion.

The concurrent administration of ZYBAN and a monoamine oxidase (MAO) inhibitor is contraindicated. At least 14 days should elapse between discontinuation of an MAO inhibitor and initiation of treatment with ZYBAN.

ZYBAN is contraindicated in patients who have shown an allergic response to bupropion or the other ingredients that make up ZYBAN.

WARNINGS

Patients should be made aware that ZYBAN contains the same active ingredient found in WELLBUTRIN and WELLBUTRIN SR used to treat depression, and that ZYBAN should not be used in combination with WELLBUTRIN, WELLBUTRIN SR, or any other medications that contain bupropion.

Because the use of bupropion is associated with a dose-dependent risk of seizures, *clinicians should not prescribe doses over 300 mg/day for smoking cessation.* The risk of seizures is also related to patient factors, clinical situation, and concurrent medications, which must be considered in selection of patients for therapy with ZYBAN.

- **Dose:** ***For smoking cessation, doses above 300 mg/day***

Table 1: Dose-Response Trial: Quit Rates by Treatment Group

	Treatment Groups			
Abstinence From Week 4 Through Specified Week	Placebo (n = 151) % (95% Cl)	ZYBAN™ 100 mg/day (n = 153) % (95% Cl)	ZYBAN 150 mg/day (n = 153) % (95% Cl)	ZYBAN 300 mg/day (n = 156) % (95% Cl)
Week 7 (4-week quit)	17% (11-23)	22% (15-28)	27%* (20-35)	36%* (28-43)
Week 12	14% (8-19)	20% (13-26)	20% (14-27)	25%* (18-32)
Week 26	11% (6-16)	16% (11-22)	18% (12-24)	19%* (13-25)

* Significantly different from placebo ($P \leq 0.05$).

Table 2: Comparative Trial: Quit Rates by Treatment Group

	Treatment Groups			
Abstinence From Week 4 Through Specified Week	Placebo (n = 160) % (95% Cl)	Nicotine Transdermal System (NTS) 21 mg/day (n = 244) % (95% Cl)	ZYBAN™ 300 mg/day (n = 244) % (95% Cl)	ZYBAN 300 mg/day and NTS 21 mg/day (n = 245) % (95% Cl)
Week 7 (4-week quit)	23% (17-30)	36%* (30-42)	49%*† (43-56)	58%*†‡ (51-64)
Week 10	20% (14-26)	32%* (26-37)	46%*† (39-52)	51%*† (45-58)

* $P<0.01$ versus placebo.
† $P<0.01$ versus NTS.
‡ $P = 0.06$ versus ZYBAN.

***should not be used.* The seizure rate associated with doses of sustained-release bupropion up to 300 mg/day is approximately 0.1% (1/1,000). This incidence was prospectively determined during an 8-week treatment exposure in approximately 3,100 depressed patients. Data for the immediate-release formulation of bupropion revealed a seizure incidence of approximately 0.4% (4/1,000) in depressed patients treated at doses in a range of 300 to 450 mg/day. In addition, the estimated seizure incidence increases almost tenfold between 450 and 600 mg/day.**

- **Patient factors: Predisposing factors that may increase the risk of seizure with bupropion use include history of head trauma or prior seizure, central nervous system (CNS) tumor, and concomitant medications that lower seizure threshold.**
- **Clinical situations: Circumstances associated with an increased seizure risk include, among others, excessive use of alcohol; abrupt withdrawal from alcohol or other sedatives; addiction to opiates, cocaine, or stimulants; use of over-the-counter stimulants and anorectics; and diabetes treated with oral hypoglycemics or insulin.**
- **Concomitant medications: Many medications (e.g., antipsychotics, antidepressants, theophylline, systemic steroids) and treatment regimens (e.g., abrupt discontinuation of benzodiazepines) are known to lower seizure threshold.**

Recommendations for Reducing the Risk of Seizure: Retrospective analysis of clinical experience gained during the development of bupropion suggests that the risk of seizure may be minimized if

- **the total daily dose of ZYBAN does *not* exceed 300 mg (the maximum recommended dose for smoking cessation), and**
- **the recommended daily dose for most patients (300 mg/day) is administered in divided doses (150 mg twice daily).**
- **No single dose should exceed 150 mg to avoid high peak concentrations of bupropion and/or its metabolites.**
- **ZYBAN should be administered with extreme caution to patients with a history of seizure, cranial trauma, or other predisposition(s) toward seizure, or patients treated with other agents (e.g., antipsychotics, antidepressants, theophylline, systemic steroids, etc.) or treatment regimens (e.g., abrupt discontinuation of a benzodiazepine) that lower seizure threshold.**

Potential for Hepatotoxicity: In rats receiving large doses of bupropion chronically, there was an increase in incidence of hepatic hyperplastic nodules and hepatocellular hypertrophy. In dogs receiving large doses of bupropion chronically, various histologic changes were seen in the liver, and laboratory tests suggesting mild hepatocellular injury were noted.

PRECAUTIONS

General: *Allergic Reactions:* Anaphylactoid reactions characterized by symptoms such as pruritus, urticaria, angioedema, and dyspnea requiring medical treatment have been reported at a rate of about 1-3 per thousand in clinical trials of ZYBAN. In addition, there have been rare spontaneous postmarketing reports of erythema multiforme, Stevens-Johnson syndrome, and anaphylactic shock associated with bupropion.

Insomnia: In the dose-response smoking cessation trial, 29% of patients treated with 150 mg/day of ZYBAN and 35% of patients treated with 300 mg/day of ZYBAN experienced insomnia, compared to 21% of placebo-treated patients. Symptoms were sufficiently severe to require discontinuation of treatment in 0.6% of patients treated with ZYBAN and none of the patients treated with placebo.

In the comparative trial, 40% of the patients treated with 300 mg/day of ZYBAN, 28% of the patients treated with 21 mg/day of NTS, and 45% of the patients treated with the combination of ZYBAN and NTS experienced insomnia compared to 18% of placebo-treated patients. Symptoms were sufficiently severe to require discontinuation of treatment in 0.8% of patients treated with ZYBAN and none of the patients in the other three treatment groups.

Insomnia may be minimized by avoiding bedtime doses and, if necessary, reduction in dose.

Psychosis, Confusion, and Other Neuropsychiatric Phenomena: In clinical trials with ZYBAN conducted in nondepressed smokers, the incidence of neuropsychiatric side effects was generally comparable to placebo. Depressed patients treated with bupropion in depression trials have been reported to show a variety of neuropsychiatric signs and symptoms including delusions, hallucinations, psychosis, concentration disturbance, paranoia, and confusion. In some cases, these symptoms abated upon dose reduction and/or withdrawal of treatment.

Activation of Psychosis and/or Mania: Antidepressants can precipitate manic episodes in bipolar disorder patients during the depressed phase of their illness and may activate latent psychosis in other susceptible individuals. The sustained-release formulation of bupropion is expected to pose similar risks. There were no reports of activation of psychosis or mania in clinical trials with ZYBAN conducted in nondepressed smokers.

Use in Patients With Systemic Illness: There is no clinical experience establishing the safety of ZYBAN in patients with a recent history of myocardial infarction or unstable heart disease. Therefore, care should be exercised if it is used in these groups. Bupropion was well tolerated in depressed patients who had previously developed orthostatic hypotension while receiving tricyclic antidepressants, and was generally well tolerated in a group of 36 depressed inpatients with stable CHF. However, bupropion was associated with a rise in supine blood pressure in the study of patients with CHF, resulting in discontinuation of treatment in two patients for exacerbation of baseline hypertension.

In the comparative trial, 6.1% of patients treated with the combination of ZYBAN and NTS had treatment-emergent hypertension compared to 2.5%, 1.6%, and 3.1% of patients treated with ZYBAN, NTS, and placebo, respectively. The majority of these patients had evidence of preexisting hypertension. Three patients (1.2%) treated with the combination of ZYBAN and NTS and one patient (0.4%) treated with NTS had study medication discontinued due to hypertension compared to none of the patients treated with ZYBAN or placebo. Monitoring for treatment-emergent hypertension is recommended in patients receiving the combination of ZYBAN and NTS.

Because bupropion hydrochloride and its metabolites are almost completely excreted through the kidney and metabolites are likely to undergo conjugation in the liver prior to urinary excretion, treatment of patients with renal or hepatic impairment should be initiated at reduced dosage as bupropion and its metabolites may accumulate in such patients to a greater extent than usual. The patient should be closely monitored for possible toxic effects of elevated blood and tissue levels of drug and metabolites.

Information for Patients: See PATIENT INFORMATION at the end of this labeling for the text of the separate leaflet provided for patients. Physicians are advised to review the leaflet with their patients and to emphasize that ZYBAN contains the same active ingredient found in WELLBUTRIN and WELLBUTRIN SR used to treat depression and that ZYBAN should not be used in conjunction with WELLBUTRIN, WELLBUTRIN SR, or any other medications that contain bupropion hydrochloride.

Laboratory Tests: There are no specific laboratory tests recommended.

Drug Interactions: In vitro studies indicate that bupropion is primarily metabolized to hydroxybupropion by the CYP2B6 isoenzyme. Therefore, the potential exists for a drug interaction between ZYBAN and drugs that affect the CYP2B6 isoenzyme metabolism (e.g., orphenadrine and cyclophosphamide). The threohydrobupropion metabolite of bupropion does not appear to be produced by the cytochrome P450 isoenzymes. No systemic data have been collected on the metabolism of ZYBAN following concomitant administration with other drugs or, alternatively, the effect of concomitant administration of ZYBAN on the metabolism of other drugs.

Animal data indicated that bupropion may be an inducer of drug-metabolizing enzymes in humans. However, following chronic administration of bupropion, 100 mg t.i.d. to 8 healthy male volunteers for 14 days, there was no evidence of induction of its own metabolism. Because bupropion is extensively metabolized, the coadministration of other drugs may affect its clinical activity. In particular, certain drugs may induce the metabolism of bupropion (e.g., carbamazepine, phenobarbital, phenytoin), while other drugs may inhibit the metabolism of bupropion (e.g., cimetidine).

Studies in animals demonstrate that the acute toxicity of bupropion is enhanced by the MAO inhibitor phenelzine (see CONTRAINDICATIONS).

Limited clinical data suggest a higher incidence of adverse experiences in patients receiving concurrent administration of bupropion and levodopa. Administration of ZYBAN to patients receiving levodopa concurrently should be undertaken with caution, using small initial doses and gradual dose increases.

Concurrent administration of ZYBAN and agents (e.g., antipsychotics, antidepressants, theophylline, systemic steroids, etc.) or treatment regimens (e.g., abrupt discontinuation of benzodiazepines) that lower seizure threshold should be undertaken only with extreme caution (see WARNINGS).

Physiological changes resulting from smoking cessation itself, with or without treatment with ZYBAN, may alter the pharmacokinetics of some concomitant medications, which may require dosage adjustment.

Carcinogenesis, Mutagenesis, Impairment of Fertility: Lifetime carcinogenicity studies were performed in rats and mice at doses up to 300 and 150 mg/kg per day, respectively. These doses are approximately ten and two times the maximum recommended human dose (MRHD), respectively, on a mg/m^2 basis. In the rat study, there was an increase in nodular proliferative lesions of the liver at doses of 100 to 300 mg/kg per day (approximately three to ten times the MRHD on a mg/m^2 basis); lower doses were not tested. The question of whether or not such lesions may be precursors of neoplasms of the liver is currently unresolved. Similar liver lesions were not seen in the mouse study, and no increase in malignant tumors of the liver and other organs was seen in either study.

Bupropion produced a positive response (two to three times control mutation rate) in two of five strains in the Ames bacterial mutagenicity test and an increase in chromosomal aberrations in one of three in vivo rat bone marrow cytogenic studies.

A fertility study in rats at doses up to 300 mg/kg revealed no evidence of impaired fertility.

Pregnancy: *Teratogenic Effects: Pregnancy Category B:* Teratology studies have been performed at doses up to 450 mg/kg in rats (approximately 14 times the MRHD on a mg/m^2 basis), and at doses up to 150 mg/kg in rabbits (approximately 10 times the MRHD on a mg/m^2 basis). There is no evidence of impaired fertility or harm to the fetus due to bupropion. There are no adequate and well-controlled studies in pregnant women. Because animal reproduction studies are not always predictive of human response, this drug should be used during pregnancy only if clearly needed. Pregnant smokers should be encouraged to attempt cessation using educational and behavioral interventions before pharmacological approaches are used.

To monitor fetal outcomes of pregnant women exposed to ZYBAN, Glaxo Wellcome Inc. maintains a Bupropion Pregnancy Registry. Health care providers are encouraged to register patients by calling (800) 722-9292, ext. 39441.

Labor and Delivery: The effect of ZYBAN on labor and delivery in humans is unknown.

Nursing Mothers: Bupropion and its metabolites are secreted in human milk. Because of the potential for serious adverse reactions in nursing infants from ZYBAN, a decision should be made whether to discontinue nursing or to discontinue the drug, taking into account the importance of the drug to the mother.

Pediatric Use: Clinical trials with ZYBAN did not include individuals under the age of 18. Therefore, the safety and efficacy in a pediatric smoking population have not been established. The immediate-release formulation of bupropion

Continued on next page

This product information is based on labeling in effect on June 1, 1998. For further information, contact via direct mail, phone, or web site Medical Information: Glaxo Wellcome Inc., PO Box 13398, Research Triangle Park, NC 27709. Healthcare Professionals (Medical Information): 800-334-0089 Patients (Customer Response Center): 888-TALK2GW (1-888-825-5249) Glaxo Wellcome Corporate Web Site: www.glaxowellcome.com

Zyban—Cont.

was studied in 104 pediatric patients (age range, 6 to 16) in clinical trials of the drug for other indications. Although generally well tolerated, the limited exposure is insufficient to assess the safety of bupropion in pediatric patients.

Use in the Elderly: In general, older patients are known to metabolize drugs more slowly and to be more sensitive to the side effects of drugs. A single-dose pharmacokinetic study demonstrated that the disposition of bupropion and its metabolites in elderly subjects was similar to that of younger subjects (see CLINICAL PHARMACOLOGY). Of the approximately 5,600 patients who participated in clinical trials with bupropion sustained-release tablets (depression and smoking cessation studies), 303 were 60 to 69 years old and 88 were 70 years of age or older. The experience with patients 60 years of age or older was similar to that in younger patients.

ADVERSE REACTIONS

(see also WARNINGS and PRECAUTIONS)

The information included under ADVERSE REACTIONS is based primarily on data from the dose-response trial and the comparative trial that evaluated ZYBAN for smoking cessation (see CLINICAL TRIALS). Information on additional adverse events associated with the sustained-release formulation of bupropion in depression trials, as well as the immediate-release formulation of bupropion, is included in a separate section (see Other Events Observed During the Clinical Development and Postmarketing Experience of Bupropion).

Adverse Events Associated With the Discontinuation of Treatment: Adverse events were sufficiently troublesome to cause discontinuation of treatment in 8% of the 706 patients treated with ZYBAN and 5% of the 313 patients treated with placebo. The more common events leading to discontinuation of treatment with ZYBAN included nervous system disturbances (3.4%), primarily tremors, and skin disorders (2.4%), primarily rashes.

Incidence of Commonly Observed Adverse Events: The most commonly observed adverse events consistently associated with the use of ZYBAN were dry mouth and insomnia. The most commonly observed adverse events were defined as those that consistently occurred at a rate of five percentage points greater than that for placebo across clinical studies.

Dose Dependency of Adverse Events: The incidence of dry mouth and insomnia may be related to the dose of ZYBAN. The occurrence of these adverse events may be minimized by reducing the dose of ZYBAN. In addition, insomnia may be minimized by avoiding bedtime doses.

Adverse Events Occurring at an Incidence of 1% or More Among Patients Treated With ZYBAN: Table 3 enumerates selected treatment-emergent adverse events from the dose-response trial that occurred at an incidence of 1% or more and were more common in patients treated with ZYBAN compared to those treated with placebo. Table 4 enumerates selected treatment-emergent adverse events from the comparative trial that occurred at an incidence of 1% or more and were more common in patients treated with ZYBAN, NTS, or the combination of ZYBAN and NTS compared to those treated with placebo. Reported adverse events were classified using a COSTART-based dictionary.

Table 3: Treatment-Emergent Adverse Event Incidence in the Dose-Response Trial*

Body System/ Adverse Experience	ZYBAN™ 100 to 300 mg/day (n = 461) %	Placebo (n = 150) %
Body (General)		
Neck pain	2	<1
Allergic reaction	1	0
Cardiovascular		
Hot flashes	1	0
Hypertension	1	<1
Digestive		
Dry mouth	11	5
Increased appetite	2	<1
Anorexia	1	<1
Musculoskeletal		
Arthralgia	4	3
Myalgia	2	1
Nervous system		
Insomnia	31	21
Dizziness	8	7
Tremor	2	1
Somnolence	2	1
Thinking abnormality	1	0
Respiratory		
Bronchitis	2	0
Skin		
Pruritus	3	<1
Rash	3	<1
Dry skin	2	0
Urticaria	1	0
Special senses		
Taste perversion	2	<1

*Selected adverse events with an incidence of at least 1% of patients treated with ZYBAN and more frequent than in the placebo group.

[See table 4 at top of next page]

Other Events Observed During the Clinical Development and Postmarketing Experience of Bupropion: In addition to the adverse events noted above, the following events have been reported in clinical trials with the sustained-release formulation of bupropion in depressed patients and in nondepressed smokers, as well as in clinical trials and postmarketing clinical experience with the immediate-release formulation of bupropion.

Adverse events for which frequencies are provided below occurred in clinical trials with bupropion sustained-release. The frequencies represent the proportion of patients who experienced a treatment-emergent adverse event on at least one occasion in placebo-controlled studies for depression (n=987) or smoking cessation (n=1,013), or patients who experienced an adverse event requiring discontinuation of treatment in an open-label surveillance study with bupropion sustained-release tablets (n=3,100). All treatment-emergent adverse events are included except those listed in Tables 3 and 4, those events listed in other safety-related sections of the insert, those adverse events subsumed under COSTART terms that are either overly general or excessively specified so as to be uninformative, those events not reasonably associated with the use of the drug, and those events that were not serious and occurred in fewer than two patients.

Events are further categorized by body system and listed in order of decreasing frequency according to the following definitions of frequency: Frequent adverse events are defined as those occurring in at least 1/100 patients. Infrequent adverse events are those occurring in 1/100 to 1/1,000 patients, while rare events are those occurring in less than 1/1,000 patients.

Adverse events for which frequencies are not provided occurred in clinical trials or postmarketing experience with the immediate-release formulation of bupropion. Only those adverse events not previously listed for sustained-release bupropion are included. The extent to which these events may be associated with ZYBAN is unknown.

Body (General): Frequent were asthenia, fever, and headache. Infrequent were back pain, chills, inguinal hernia, musculoskeletal chest pain, pain, and photosensitivity. Rare was malaise.

Cardiovascular: Infrequent were flushing, migraine, postural hypotension, stroke, tachycardia, and vasodilation. Rare was syncope. Also observed were cardiovascular disorder, complete AV block, extrasystoles, hypotension, myocardial infarction, phlebitis, and pulmonary embolism.

Digestive: Frequent were dyspepsia, flatulence, and vomiting. Infrequent were abnormal liver function, bruxism, dysphagia, gastric reflux, gingivitis, glossitis, jaundice, and stomatitis. Rare was edema of tongue. Also observed were colitis, esophagitis, gastrointestinal hemorrhage, gum hemorrhage, hepatitis, increased salivation, intestinal perforation, liver damage, pancreatitis, stomach ulcer, and stool abnormality.

Endocrine: Also observed was syndrome of inappropriate antidiuretic hormone.

Hemic and Lymphatic: Infrequent was ecchymosis. Also observed were anemia, leukocytosis, leukopenia, lymphadenopathy, and pancytopenia.

Metabolic and Nutritional: Infrequent were edema, increased weight, and peripheral edema. Also observed was glycosuria.

Musculoskeletal: Infrequent were leg cramps and twitching. Also observed were arthritis and muscle rigidity/fever/rhabdomyolysis.

Nervous System: Frequent were agitation, depression, and irritability. Infrequent were abnormal coordination, CNS stimulation, confusion, decreased libido, decreased memory, depersonalization, emotional lability, hostility, hyperkinesia, hypertonia, hypesthesia, paresthesia, suicidal ideation, and vertigo. Rare were amnesia, ataxia, derealization, and hypomania. Also observed were abnormal electroencephalogram (EEG), akinesia, aphasia, coma, delirium, delusions, dysarthria, dyskinesia, dystonia, euphoria, extrapyramidal syndrome, hypokinesia, increased libido, manic reaction, neuralgia, neuropathy, paranoid reaction, and unmasking tardive dyskinesia.

Respiratory: Rare was bronchospasm. Also observed was pneumonia.

Skin: Frequent was sweating. Infrequent was acne and dry skin. Rare was maculopapular rash. Also observed were angioedema, exfoliative dermatitis, and hirsutism.

Special Senses: Frequent was amblyopia. Infrequent were accommodation abnormality and dry eye. Also observed were deafness, diplopia, and mydriasis.

Urogenital: Frequent was urinary frequency. Infrequent were impotence, polyuria, and urinary urgency. Also observed were abnormal ejaculation, cystitis, dyspareunia, dysuria, gynecomastia, menopause, painful erection, prostate disorder, salpingitis, urinary incontinence, urinary retention, urinary tract disorder, and vaginitis.

DRUG ABUSE AND DEPENDENCE

ZYBAN is likely to have a low abuse potential.

Humans: There have been few reported cases of drug dependence and withdrawal symptoms associated with the immediate-release formulation of bupropion. In human studies of abuse liability, individuals experienced with drugs of abuse reported that bupropion produced a feeling of euphoria and desirability. In these subjects, a single dose of 400 mg (1.33 times the recommended daily dose) of bupropion produced mild amphetamine-like effects compared to placebo on the Morphine-Benzedrine Subscale of the Addiction Research Center Inventories (ARCI), which is indicative of euphorigenic properties and a score intermediate between placebo and amphetamine on the Liking Scale of the ARCI.

Animals: Studies in rodents and primates have shown that bupropion exhibits some pharmacologic actions common to psychostimulants. In rodents, it has been shown to increase locomotor activity, elicit a mild stereotyped behavioral response, and increase rates of responding in several schedule-controlled behavior paradigms. In primate models to assess the positive reinforcing effects of psychoactive drugs, bupropion was self-administered intravenously. In rats, bupropion produced amphetamine- and cocaine-like discriminative stimulus effects in drug discrimination paradigms used to characterize the subjective effects of psychoactive drugs.

The possibility that bupropion may induce dependence should be kept in mind when evaluating the desirability of including the drug in smoking cessation programs of individual patients.

OVERDOSAGE

Human Overdose Experience: There has been very limited experience with overdosage of the sustained-release formulation of bupropion; three such cases were reported during clinical trials in depressed patients. One patient ingested 3,000 mg of bupropion sustained-release tablets and vomited quickly after the overdose; the patient experienced blurred vision and lightheadedness. A second patient ingested a "handful" of bupropion sustained-release tablets and experienced confusion, lethargy, nausea, jitteriness, and seizure. A third patient ingested 3,600 mg of bupropion sustained-release tablets and a bottle of wine; the patient experienced nausea, visual hallucinations, and "grogginess." None of the patients experienced further sequelae. There has been extensive experience with overdosages of the immediate-release formulation of bupropion. Thirteen overdoses occurred during clinical trials in depressed patients. Twelve patients ingested 850 to 4,200 mg and recovered without significant sequelae. Another patient who ingested 9,000 mg of the immediate-release formulation of bupropion and 300 mg of tranylcypromine experienced a grand mal seizure and recovered without further sequelae.

Since introduction, overdoses of up to 17,500 mg of the immediate-release formulation of bupropion have been reported. Seizure was reported in approximately one third of all cases. Other serious reactions reported with overdoses of the immediate-release formulation of bupropion alone included hallucinations, loss of consciousness, and sinus tachycardia. Fever, muscle rigidity, rhabdomyolysis, hypotension, stupor, coma, and respiratory failure have been reported when the immediate-release formulation of bupropion was part of multiple drug overdoses.

Although most patients recovered without sequelae, deaths associated with overdoses of the immediate-release formulation of bupropion alone have been reported rarely in patients ingesting massive doses of the drug. Multiple uncontrolled seizures, bradycardia, cardiac failure, and cardiac arrest prior to death were reported in these patients.

Management of Overdose: Following suspected overdose, hospitalization is advised. If the patient is conscious, vomiting should be induced by syrup of ipecac. Activated charcoal also may be administered every 6 hours during the first 12 hours after ingestion. Baseline laboratory values should be obtained. Electrocardiogram and EEG monitoring also are recommended for the next 48 hours. Adequate fluid intake should be provided.

If the patient is stuporous, comatose, or convulsing, airway intubation is recommended prior to undertaking gastric lavage. Although there is little clinical experience with lavage following an overdose of bupropion, it is likely to be of benefit within the first 12 hours after ingestion since absorption of the drug may not yet be complete.

Table 4: Treatment-Emergent Adverse Event Incidence in the Comparative Trial*

Adverse Experience (COSTART Term)	ZYBAN™ 300 mg/day (n = 243) %	Nicotine Transdermal System (NTS) 21 mg/day (n = 243) %	ZYBAN and NTS (n = 244) %	Placebo (n = 159) %
Body				
Abdominal pain	3	4	1	1
Accidental injury	2	2	1	1
Chest pain	<1	1	3	1
Neck pain	2	1	<1	0
Facial edema	<1	0	1	0
Cardiovascular				
Hypertension	1	<1	2	0
Palpitations	2	0	1	0
Digestive				
Nausea	9	7	11	4
Dry mouth	10	4	9	4
Constipation	8	4	9	3
Diarrhea	4	4	3	1
Anorexia	3	1	5	1
Mouth ulcer	2	1	1	1
Thirst	<1	<1	2	0
Musculoskeletal				
Myalgia	4	3	5	3
Arthralgia	5	3	4	2
Nervous system				
Insomnia	40	28	45	18
Dream abnormality	5	18	13	3
Anxiety	8	6	9	6
Disturbed concentration	9	3	9	4
Dizziness	10	2	8	6
Nervousness	4	<1	2	2
Tremor	1	<1	2	0
Dysphoria	<1	1	2	1
Respiratory				
Rhinitis	12	11	9	8
Increased cough	3	5	<1	1
Pharyngitis	3	2	3	0
Sinusitis	2	2	2	1
Dyspnea	1	0	2	1
Epistaxis	2	1	1	0
Skin				
Application site reaction†	11	17	15	7
Rash	4	3	3	2
Pruritus	3	1	5	1
Urticaria	2	0	2	0
Special Senses				
Taste perversion	3	1	3	2
Tinnitus	1	0	<1	0

* Selected adverse events with an incidence of at least 1% of patients treated with either ZYBAN, NTS, or the combination of ZYBAN and NTS and more frequent than in the placebo group.
† Patients randomized to ZYBAN or placebo received placebo patches.

While diuresis, dialysis, or hemoperfusion are sometimes used to treat drug overdosage, there is no experience with their use in the management of overdoses of bupropion. Because diffusion of bupropion and its metabolites from tissue to plasma may be slow, dialysis may be of minimal benefit. Based on studies in animals, it is recommended that seizures be treated with an intravenous benzodiazepine preparation and other supportive measures, as appropriate. Further information about the treatment of overdoses may be available from a poison control center.

DOSAGE AND ADMINISTRATION

ZYBAN: *Usual Dosage for Adults:* The recommended and maximum dose of ZYBAN is 300 mg/day, given as 150 mg twice daily. Dosing should begin at 150 mg/day given every day for the first 3 days, followed by a dose increase for most patients to the recommended usual dose of 300 mg/day. There should be an interval of at least 8 hours between successive doses. Doses above 300 mg/day should not be used (see WARNINGS). Treatment with ZYBAN should be initiated **while the patient is still smoking,** since approximately 1 week of treatment is required to achieve steady-state blood levels of bupropion. Patients should set a "target quit date" within the first 2 weeks of treatment with ZYBAN, generally in the second week. Treatment with ZYBAN should be continued for 7 to 12 weeks; duration of treatment should be based on the relative benefits and risks for individual patients. If a patient has not made significant progress towards abstinence by the seventh week of therapy with ZYBAN, it is unlikely that he or she will quit during that attempt, and treatment should probably be discontinued. Dose tapering of ZYBAN is not required when discontinuing treatment. It is important that patients continue to receive counseling and support throughout treatment with ZYBAN, and for a period of time thereafter.

Individualization of Therapy: Patients are more likely to quit smoking and remain abstinent if they are seen frequently and receive support from their physicians or other health care professionals. It is important to ensure that patients read the instructions provided to them and have their questions answered. Physicians should review the patient's overall smoking cessation program that includes treatment with ZYBAN. Patients should be advised of the importance of participating in the behavioral interventions, counseling, and/or support services to be used in conjunction with ZYBAN. See information for patients at the end of the package insert.

The goal of therapy with ZYBAN is complete abstinence. If a patient has not made significant progress towards abstinence by the seventh week of therapy with ZYBAN, it is unlikely that he or she will quit during that attempt, and treatment should be discontinued.

Patients who fail to quit smoking during an attempt may benefit from interventions to improve their chances for success on subsequent attempts. Patients who are unsuccessful should be evaluated to determine why they failed. A new quit attempt should be encouraged when factors that contributed to failure can be eliminated or reduced, and conditions are more favorable.

Maintenance: Although clinical data are not available regarding the long-term use (>12 weeks) of bupropion for smoking cessation, bupropion has been used for longer periods of time in the treatment of depression. Whether to continue treatment with ZYBAN for periods longer than 12 weeks for smoking cessation must be determined for individual patients.

Combination Treatment With ZYBAN and a Nicotine Transdermal System (NTS): Combination treatment with ZYBAN and NTS may be prescribed for smoking cessation. The prescriber should review the complete prescribing in-

formation for both ZYBAN and NTS before using combination treatment. See also CLINICAL TRIALS for methods and dosing used in the ZYBAN and NTS combination trial. Monitoring for treatment-emergent hypertension in patients treated with the combination of ZYBAN and NTS is recommended.

HOW SUPPLIED

ZYBAN Sustained-Release Tablets, 150 mg of bupropion hydrochloride, are purple, round, biconvex, film-coated tablets printed with "ZYBAN 150" in bottles of 60 (NDC 0173-0556-02) tablets and the ZYBAN Advantage Pack™ containing 1 bottle of 60 (NDC 0173-0556-01) tablets.

Store at controlled room temperature, 20° to 25°C (68° to 77°F) (see USP). Dispense in tight, light-resistant containers as defined in the USP.

PATIENT INFORMATION: The following wording is contained in a separate leaflet provided for patients.

Information for the Patient
ZYBAN™ (bupropion hydrochloride) Sustained-Release Tablets
Please read this information before you start taking ZYBAN. Also read this leaflet each time you renew your prescription, in case anything has changed. This information is not intended to take the place of discussions between you and your doctor. You and your doctor should discuss ZYBAN as part of your plan to stop smoking. Your doctor has prescribed ZYBAN for your use only. Do not let anyone else use your ZYBAN.

IMPORTANT WARNING:
There is a chance that approximately 1 out of every 1,000 people taking bupropion hydrochloride, the active ingredient in ZYBAN, will have a seizure. The chance of this happening increases if you:
• have a seizure disorder (for example, epilepsy);
• have or have had an eating disorder (for example, bulimia or anorexia nervosa);
• take more than the recommended amount of ZYBAN; or
• take other medicines with the same active ingredient that is in ZYBAN, such as WELLBUTRIN® (bupropion hydrochloride) Tablets and WELLBUTRIN® SR (bupropion hydrochloride) Sustained-Release Tablets. (Both of these medicines are used to treat depression.)
You can reduce the chance of experiencing a seizure by following your doctor's directions on how to take ZYBAN. You should also discuss with your doctor whether ZYBAN is right for you.

1. What is ZYBAN?
ZYBAN is a prescription medicine to help people quit smoking. Studies have shown that more than one third of people quit smoking for at least 1 month while taking ZYBAN and participating in a patient support program. For many patients, ZYBAN reduces withdrawal symptoms and the urge to smoke. ZYBAN should be used with a patient support program. It is important to participate in the behavioral program, counseling, or other support program your health care professional recommends.

2. Who should not take ZYBAN?
You should not take ZYBAN if you:
• have a seizure disorder (for example, epilepsy).
• are already taking WELLBUTRIN, WELLBUTRIN SR, or any other medicines that contain bupropion hydrochloride.
• have or have had an eating disorder (for example, bulimia or anorexia nervosa).
• are currently taking or have recently taken a monoamine oxidase inhibitor (MAOI).
• are allergic to bupropion.

3. Are there special concerns for women?
ZYBAN is not recommended for women who are pregnant or breast-feeding. Women should notify their doctor if they become pregnant or intend to become pregnant while taking ZYBAN.

4. How should I take ZYBAN?
• You should take ZYBAN as directed by your doctor. The usual recommended dosing is to take one 150-mg tablet in the morning for the first 3 days. On the fourth day, begin taking one 150-mg tablet in the morning and one 150-mg tablet in the early evening. Doses should be taken at least 8 hours apart.
• **Never take an "extra" dose of ZYBAN.** If you forget to take a dose, do not take an extra tablet to "catch up" for the dose you forgot. Wait and take your next tablet at the regular time. Do not take more tablets than your doctor prescribed. This is important so you do not increase your chance of having a seizure.
• It is important to swallow ZYBAN Tablets whole. Do not chew, divide, or crush tablets.

Continued on next page

This product information is based on labeling in effect on June 1, 1998. For further information, contact via direct mail, phone, or web site Medical Information: Glaxo Wellcome Inc., PO Box 13398, Research Triangle Park, NC 27709. Healthcare Professionals (Medical Information): 800-334-0089 Patients (Customer Response Center): 888-TALK2GW (1-888-825-5249) Glaxo Wellcome Corporate Web Site: www.glaxowellcome.com

Zyban—Cont.

5. How long should I take ZYBAN?
Most people should take ZYBAN for 7 to 12 weeks. Follow your doctor's instructions.

6. When should I stop smoking?
It takes about 1 week for ZYBAN to reach the right levels in your body to be effective. So, to maximize your chance of quitting, you should not stop smoking until you have been taking ZYBAN for 1 week. You should set a date to stop smoking during the second week you're taking ZYBAN.

7. Can I smoke while taking ZYBAN?
It is not physically dangerous to smoke and use ZYBAN at the same time. However, continuing to smoke after the date you set to stop smoking will seriously reduce your chance of breaking your smoking habit.

8. Can ZYBAN be used at the same time as nicotine patches?
Yes, ZYBAN and nicotine patches can be used at the same time but should only be used together under the supervision of your doctor. Using ZYBAN and nicotine patches together may raise your blood pressure. Your doctor will probably want to check your blood pressure regularly to make sure that it stays within acceptable levels.
DO NOT SMOKE AT ANY TIME if you are using a nicotine patch or any other nicotine product along with ZYBAN. It is possible to get too much nicotine and have serious side effects.

9. What are possible side effects of ZYBAN?
Like all medicines, ZYBAN may cause side effects.
- The most common side effects include dry mouth and difficulty sleeping. These side effects are generally mild and often disappear after a few weeks. If you have difficulty sleeping, avoid taking your medicine too close to bedtime.
- The most common side effects that caused people to stop taking ZYBAN during clinical studies were shakiness and skin rash.
- Contact your doctor or health care professional if you have a rash or other troublesome side effects.
- Use caution before driving a car or operating complex, hazardous machinery until you know if ZYBAN affects your ability to perform these tasks.

10. Can I drink alcohol while I am taking ZYBAN?
It is best to not drink alcohol at all or to drink very little while taking ZYBAN. If you drink a lot of alcohol and suddenly stop, you may increase your chance of having a seizure. Therefore, it is important to discuss your use of alcohol with your doctor before you begin taking ZYBAN.

11. Will ZYBAN affect other medicines I am taking?
ZYBAN may affect other medicines you're taking. It is important not to take medicines that may increase the chance for you to have a seizure. Therefore, you should make sure that your doctor knows about all medicines—prescription or over-the-counter—you are taking or plan to take.

12. Do ZYBAN Tablets have a characteristic odor?
ZYBAN Tablets may have a characteristic odor. If present, this odor is normal.

13. How should I store ZYBAN?
- Store ZYBAN at room temperature, out of direct sunlight.
- Keep ZYBAN in a tightly closed container.
- Keep ZYBAN out of the reach of children.
This summary provides important information about ZYBAN. This summary cannot replace the more detailed information that you need from your doctor. If you have any questions or concerns about either ZYBAN or smoking cessation, talk to your doctor or other health care professional.
HABITROL is a registered trademark of Ciba-Geigy Corporation.
U.S. Patent Nos. 5,427,798 and 5,358,970
©Copyright 1997 Glaxo Wellcome Inc. All rights reserved.
September 1997/RL-448
Shown in Product Identification Guide, page 315

ZYLOPRIM ®   ℞
[zī 'lō-prĭm]
(allopurinol)
**100 mg Scored Tablets and
300 mg Scored Tablets**

DESCRIPTION

ZYLOPRIM (allopurinol) is known chemically as 1,5-dihydro-4H-pyrazolo[3,4-d]pyrimidin-4-one. It is a xanthine oxidase inhibitor which is administered orally. Each scored white tablet contains 100 mg allopurinol and the inactive ingredients lactose, magnesium stearate, potato starch, and povidone. Each scored peach tablet contains 300 mg allopurinol and the inactive ingredients corn starch, FD&C Yellow No. 6 Lake, lactose, magnesium stearate, and povidone. Its solubility in water at 37°C is 80.0 mg/dL and is greater in an alkaline solution.

CLINICAL PHARMACOLOGY

ZYLOPRIM acts on purine catabolism, without disrupting the biosynthesis of purines. It reduces the production of uric acid by inhibiting the biochemical reactions immediately preceding its formation.
ZYLOPRIM is a structural analogue of the natural purine base, hypoxanthine. It is an inhibitor of xanthine oxidase, the enzyme responsible for the conversion of hypoxanthine to xanthine and of xanthine to uric acid, the end product of purine metabolism in man. ZYLOPRIM is metabolized to the corresponding xanthine analogue, oxipurinol (alloxanthine), which also is an inhibitor of xanthine oxidase.
It has been shown that reutilization of both hypoxanthine and xanthine for nucleotide and nucleic acid synthesis is markedly enhanced when their oxidations are inhibited by ZYLOPRIM and oxipurinol. This reutilization does not disrupt normal nucleic acid anabolism, however, because feedback inhibition is an integral part of purine biosynthesis. As a result of xanthine oxidase inhibition, the serum concentration of hypoxanthine plus xanthine in patients receiving ZYLOPRIM for treatment of hyperuricemia is usually in the range of 0.3 to 0.4 mg/dL compared to a normal level of approximately 0.15 mg/dL. A maximum of 0.9 mg/dL of these oxypurines has been reported when the serum urate was lowered to less than 2 mg/dL by high doses of ZYLOPRIM. These values are far below the saturation levels at which point their precipitation would be expected to occur (above 7 mg/dL).
The renal clearance of hypoxanthine and xanthine is at least 10 times greater than that of uric acid. The increased xanthine and hypoxanthine in the urine have not been accompanied by problems of nephrolithiasis. Xanthine crystalluria has been reported in only three patients. Two of the patients had Lesch-Nyhan syndrome, which is characterized by excessive uric acid production combined with a deficiency of the enzyme, hypoxanthineguanine phosphoribosyltransferase (HGPRTase). This enzyme is required for the conversion of hypoxanthine, xanthine, and guanine to their respective nucleotides. The third patient had lymphosarcoma and produced an extremely large amount of uric acid because of rapid cell lysis during chemotherapy.
ZYLOPRIM is approximately 90% absorbed from the gastrointestinal tract. Peak plasma levels generally occur at 1.5 hours and 4.5 hours for ZYLOPRIM and oxipurinol respectively, and after a single oral dose of 300 mg ZYLOPRIM, maximum plasma levels of about 3 mcg/mL of ZYLOPRIM and 6.5 mcg/mL of oxipurinol are produced.
Approximately 20% of the ingested ZYLOPRIM is excreted in the feces. Because of its rapid oxidation to oxipurinol and a renal clearance rate approximately that of glomerular filtration rate, ZYLOPRIM has a plasma half-life of about 1 to 2 hours. Oxipurinol, however, has a longer plasma half-life (approximately 15 hours) and therefore effective xanthine oxidase inhibition is maintained over a 24-hour period with single daily doses of ZYLOPRIM. Whereas ZYLOPRIM is cleared essentially by glomerular filtration, oxipurinol is reabsorbed in the kidney tubules in a manner similar to the reabsorption of uric acid.
The clearance of oxipurinol is increased by uricosuric drugs, and as a consequence, the addition of a uricosuric agent reduces to some degree the inhibition of xanthine oxidase by oxipurinol and increases to some degree the urinary excretion of uric acid. In practice, the net effect of such combined therapy may be useful in some patients in achieving minimum serum uric acid levels provided the total urinary uric acid load does not exceed the competence of the patient's renal function.
Hyperuricemia may be primary, as in gout, or secondary to diseases such as acute and chronic leukemia, polycythemia vera, multiple myeloma, and psoriasis. It may occur with the use of diuretic agents, during renal dialysis, in the presence of renal damage, during starvation or reducing diets, and in the treatment of neoplastic disease where rapid resolution of tissue masses may occur. Asymptomatic hyperuricemia is not an indication for treatment with ZYLOPRIM (see INDICATIONS AND USAGE).
Gout is a metabolic disorder which is characterized by hyperuricemia and resultant deposition of monosodium urate in the tissues, particularly the joints and kidneys. The etiology of this hyperuricemia is the overproduction of uric acid in relation to the patient's ability to excrete it. If progressive deposition of urates is to be arrested or reversed, it is necessary to reduce the serum uric acid level below the saturation point to suppress urate precipitation.
Administration of ZYLOPRIM generally results in a fall in both serum and urinary uric acid within 2 to 3 days. The degree of this decrease can be manipulated almost at will since it is dose-dependent. A week or more of treatment with ZYLOPRIM may be required before its full effects are manifested; likewise, uric acid may return to pretreatment levels slowly (usually after a period of 7 to 10 days following cessation of therapy). This reflects primarily the accumulation and slow clearance of oxipurinol. In some patients a dramatic fall in urinary uric acid excretion may not occur, particularly in those with severe tophaceous gout. It has been postulated that this may be due to the mobilization of urate from tissue deposits as the serum uric acid level begins to fall.
The action of ZYLOPRIM differs from that of uricosuric agents, which lower the serum uric acid level by increasing urinary excretion of uric acid. ZYLOPRIM reduces both the serum and urinary uric acid levels by inhibiting the formation of uric acid. The use of ZYLOPRIM to block the formation of urates avoids the hazard of increased renal excretion of uric acid posed by uricosuric drugs.
ZYLOPRIM can substantially reduce serum and urinary uric acid levels in previously refractory patients even in the presence of renal damage serious enough to render uricosuric drugs virtually ineffective. Salicylates may be given conjointly for their antirheumatic effect without compromising the action of ZYLOPRIM. This is in contrast to the nullifying effect of salicylates on uricosuric drugs.
ZYLOPRIM also inhibits the enzymatic oxidation of mercaptopurine, the sulfur-containing analogue of hypoxanthine, to 6-thiouric acid. This oxidation, which is catalyzed by xanthine oxidase, inactivates mercaptopurine. Hence, the inhibition of such oxidation by ZYLOPRIM may result in as much as a 75% reduction in the therapeutic dose requirement of mercaptopurine when the two compounds are given together.

INDICATIONS AND USAGE

THIS IS NOT AN INNOCUOUS DRUG. IT IS NOT RECOMMENDED FOR THE TREATMENT OF ASYMPTOMATIC HYPERURICEMIA.
ZYLOPRIM reduces serum and urinary uric acid concentrations. Its use should be individualized for each patient and requires an understanding of its mode of action and pharmacokinetics (see CLINICAL PHARMACOLOGY, CONTRAINDICATIONS, WARNINGS and PRECAUTIONS).
ZYLOPRIM is indicated in:
(1) the management of patients with signs and symptoms of primary or secondary gout (acute attacks, tophi, joint destruction, uric acid lithiasis and/or nephropathy).
(2) the management of patients with leukemia, lymphoma and malignancies who are receiving cancer therapy which causes elevations of serum and urinary uric acid levels. Treatment with ZYLOPRIM should be discontinued when the potential for overproduction of uric acid is no longer present.
(3) the management of patients with recurrent calcium oxalate calculi whose daily uric acid excretion exceeds 800 mg/day in male patients and 750 mg/day in female patients. Therapy in such patients should be carefully assessed initially and reassessed periodically to determine in each case that treatment is beneficial and that the benefits outweigh the risks.

CONTRAINDICATIONS

Patients who have developed a severe reaction to ZYLOPRIM should not be restarted on the drug.

WARNINGS

ZYLOPRIM SHOULD BE DISCONTINUED AT THE FIRST APPEARANCE OF SKIN RASH OR OTHER SIGNS WHICH MAY INDICATE AN ALLERGIC REACTION. In some instances a skin rash may be followed by more severe hypersensitivity reactions such as exfoliative, urticarial, and purpuric lesions as well as Stevens-Johnson syndrome (erythema multiforme exudativum), and/or generalized vasculitis, irreversible hepatotoxicity and on rare occasions death.
In patients receiving PURINETHOL® (mercaptopurine) or IMURAN® (azathioprine), the concomitant administration of 300 to 600 mg of ZYLOPRIM per day will require a reduction in dose to approximately one-third to one-fourth of the usual dose of mercaptopurine or azathioprine. Subsequent adjustment of doses of mercaptopurine or azathioprine should be made on the basis of therapeutic response and the appearance of toxic effects (see CLINICAL PHARMACOLOGY).
A few cases of reversible clinical hepatotoxicity have been noted in patients taking ZYLOPRIM, and in some patients, asymptomatic rises in serum alkaline phosphatase or serum transaminase have been observed. If anorexia, weight loss, or pruritus develop in patients on ZYLOPRIM, evaluation of liver function should be part of their diagnostic workup. In patients with pre-existing liver disease, periodic liver function tests are recommended during the early stages of therapy.
Due to the occasional occurrence of drowsiness, patients should be alerted to the need for due precaution when engaging in activities where alertness is mandatory.
The occurrence of hypersensitivity reactions to ZYLOPRIM may be increased in patients with decreased renal function receiving thiazides and ZYLOPRIM concurrently. For this reason, in this clinical setting, such combinations should be administered with caution and patients should be observed closely.

PRECAUTIONS

General: An increase in acute attacks of gout has been reported during the early stages of administration of

ZYLOPRIM, even when normal or subnormal serum uric acid levels have been attained. Accordingly, maintenance doses of colchicine generally should be given prophylactically when ZYLOPRIM is begun. In addition, it is recommended that the patient start with a low dose of ZYLOPRIM (100 mg daily) and increase at weekly intervals by 100 mg until a serum uric acid level of 6 mg/dL or less is attained but without exceeding the maximum recommended dose (800 mg per day). The use of colchicine or anti-inflammatory agents may be required to suppress gouty attacks in some cases. The attacks usually become shorter and less severe after several months of therapy. The mobilization of urates from tissue deposits which cause fluctuations in the serum uric acid levels may be a possible explanation for these episodes. Even with adequate therapy with ZYLOPRIM, it may require several months to deplete the uric acid pool sufficiently to achieve control of the acute attacks.

A fluid intake sufficient to yield a daily urinary output of at least two liters and the maintenance of a neutral or, preferably, slightly alkaline urine are desirable to (1) avoid the theoretical possibility of formation of xanthine calculi under the influence of therapy with ZYLOPRIM and (2) help prevent renal precipitation of urates in patients receiving concomitant uricosuric agents.

Some patients with pre-existing renal disease or poor urate clearance have shown a rise in BUN during administration of ZYLOPRIM. Although the mechanism responsible for this has not been established, patients with impaired renal function should be carefully observed during the early stages of administration of ZYLOPRIM and dosage decreased or the drug withdrawn if increased abnormalities in renal function appear and persist.

Renal failure in association with administration of ZYLOPRIM has been observed among patients with hyperuricemia secondary to neoplastic diseases. Concurrent conditions such as multiple myeloma and congestive myocardial disease were present among those patients whose renal dysfunction increased after ZYLOPRIM was begun. Renal failure is also frequently associated with gouty nephropathy and rarely with hypersensitivity reactions associated with ZYLOPRIM. Albuminuria has been observed among patients who developed clinical gout following chronic glomerulonephritis and chronic pyelonephritis.

Patients with decreased renal function require lower doses of ZYLOPRIM than those with normal renal function. Lower than recommended doses should be used to initiate therapy in any patients with decreased renal function and they should be observed closely during the early stages of administration of ZYLOPRIM. In patients with severely impaired renal function or decreased urate clearance, the half-life of oxipurinol in the plasma is greatly prolonged. Therefore, a dose of 100 mg per day or 300 mg twice a week, or perhaps less, may be sufficient to maintain adequate xanthine oxidase inhibition to reduce serum urate levels.

Bone marrow depression has been reported in patients receiving ZYLOPRIM, most of whom received concomitant drugs with the potential for causing this reaction. This has occurred as early as 6 weeks to as long as 6 years after the initiation of therapy of ZYLOPRIM. Rarely a patient may develop varying degrees of bone marrow depression, affecting one or more cell lines, while receiving ZYLOPRIM alone.

Information for Patients: Patients should be informed of the following:

(1) They should be cautioned to discontinue ZYLOPRIM and to consult their physician immediately at the first sign of a skin rash, painful urination, blood in the urine, irritation of the eyes, or swelling of the lips or mouth. (2) They should be reminded to continue drug therapy prescribed for gouty attacks since optimal benefit of ZYLOPRIM may be delayed for 2 to 6 weeks. (3) They should be encouraged to increase fluid intake during therapy to prevent renal stones. (4) If a single dose of ZYLOPRIM is occasionally forgotten, there is no need to double the dose at the next scheduled time. (5) There may be certain risks associated with the concomitant use of ZYLOPRIM and dicumarol, sulfinpyrazone, mercaptopurine, azathioprine, ampicillin, amoxicillin, and thiazide diuretics, and they should follow the instructions of their physician. (6) Due to the occasional occurrence of drowsiness, patients should take precautions when engaging in activities where alertness is mandatory. (7) Patients may wish to take ZYLOPRIM after meals to minimize gastric irritation.

Laboratory Tests: The correct dosage and schedule for maintaining the serum uric acid within the normal range is best determined by using the serum uric acid as an index.

In patients with pre-existing liver disease, periodic liver function tests are recommended during the early stages of therapy (see WARNINGS).

ZYLOPRIM and its primary active metabolite oxipurinol are eliminated by the kidneys; therefore, changes in renal function have a profound effect on dosage. In patients with decreased renal function or who have concurrent illnesses which can affect renal function such as hypertension and diabetes mellitus, periodic laboratory parameters of renal function, particularly BUN and serum creatinine or creatinine clearance, should be performed and the patient's dosage of ZYLOPRIM reassessed.

The prothrombin time should be reassessed periodically in the patients receiving dicumarol who are given ZYLOPRIM.

Drug Interactions: In patients receiving PURINETHOL (mercaptopurine) or IMURAN (azathioprine), the concomitant administration of 300 to 600 mg of ZYLOPRIM per day will require a reduction in dose to approximately one-third to one-fourth of the usual dose of mercaptopurine or azathioprine. Subsequent adjustment of doses of mercaptopurine or azathioprine should be made on the basis of therapeutic response and the appearance of toxic effects (see CLINICAL PHARMACOLOGY).

It has been reported that ZYLOPRIM prolongs the half-life of the anticoagulant, dicumarol. The clinical basis of this drug interaction has not been established but should be noted when ZYLOPRIM is given to patients already on dicumarol therapy.

Since the excretion of oxipurinol is similar to that of urate, uricosuric agents, which increase the excretion of urate, are also likely to increase the excretion of oxipurinol and thus lower the degree of inhibition of xanthine oxidase. The concomitant administration of uricosuric agents and ZYLOPRIM has been associated with a decrease in the excretion of oxypurines (hypoxanthine and xanthine) and an increase in urinary uric acid excretion compared with that observed with ZYLOPRIM alone. Although clinical evidence to date has not demonstrated renal precipitation of oxypurines in patients either on ZYLOPRIM alone or in combination with uricosuric agents, the possibility should be kept in mind.

The reports that the concomitant use of ZYLOPRIM and thiazide diuretics may contribute to the enhancement of allopurinol toxicity in some patients have been reviewed in an attempt to establish a cause-and-effect relationship and a mechanism of causation. Review of these case reports indicates that the patients were mainly receiving thiazide diuretics for hypertension and that tests to rule out decreased renal function secondary to hypertensive nephropathy were not often performed. In those patients in whom renal insufficiency was documented, however, the recommendation to lower the dose of ZYLOPRIM was not followed. Although a causal mechanism and a cause-and-effect relationship have not been established, current evidence suggests that renal function should be monitored in patients on thiazide diuretics and ZYLOPRIM even in the absence of renal failure, and dosage levels should be even more conservatively adjusted in those patients on such combined therapy if diminished renal function is detected.

An increase in the frequency of skin rash has been reported among patients receiving ampicillin or amoxicillin concurrently with ZYLOPRIM compared to patients who are not receiving both drugs. The cause of the reported association has not been established.

Enhanced bone marrow suppression by cyclophosphamide and other cytotoxic agents has been reported among patients with neoplastic disease, except leukemia, in the presence of ZYLOPRIM. However, in a well-controlled study of patients with lymphoma on combination therapy, ZYLOPRIM did not increase the marrow toxicity of patients treated with cyclophosphamide, doxorubicin, bleomycin, procarbazine, and/or mechlorethamine.

Tolbutamide's conversion to inactive metabolites has been shown to be catalyzed by xanthine oxidase from rat liver. The clinical significance, if any, of these observations is unknown.

Chlorpropamide's plasma half-life may be prolonged by ZYLOPRIM, since ZYLOPRIM and chlorpropamide may compete for excretion in the renal tubule. The risk of hypoglycemia secondary to this mechanism may be increased if ZYLOPRIM and chlorpropamide are given concomitantly in the presence of renal insufficiency.

Rare reports indicate that cyclosporine levels may be increased during concomitant treatment with ZYLOPRIM. Monitoring of cyclosporine levels and possible adjustment of cyclosporine dosage should be considered when these drugs are co-administered.

Drug/Laboratory Test Interactions: ZYLOPRIM is not known to alter the accuracy of laboratory tests.

Pregnancy: *Teratogenic Effects:* Pregnancy Category C. Reproductive studies have been performed in rats and rabbits at doses up to twenty times the usual human dose (5 mg/kg/day), and it was concluded that there was no impaired fertility or harm to the fetus due to allopurinol. There is a published report of a study in pregnant mice given 50 or 100 mg/kg allopurinol intraperitoneally on gestation days 10 or 13. There were increased numbers of dead fetuses in dams given 100 mg/kg allopurinol but not in those given 50 mg/kg. There were increased numbers of external malformations in fetuses at both doses of allopurinol on gestation day 10 and increased numbers of skeletal malformations in fetuses at both doses on gestation day 13. It cannot be determined whether this represented a fetal effect or an effect secondary to maternal toxicity. There are, however, no adequate or well-controlled studies in pregnant women. Because animal reproduction studies are not always predictive of human response, this drug should be used during pregnancy only if clearly needed.

Experience with ZYLOPRIM during human pregnancy has been limited partly because women of reproductive age rarely require treatment with ZYLOPRIM. There are two unpublished reports and one published paper of women giving birth to normal offspring after receiving ZYLOPRIM during pregnancy.

Nursing Mothers: Allopurinol and oxipurinol have been found in the milk of a mother who was receiving ZYLOPRIM. Since the effect of ZYLOPRIM on the nursing infant is unknown, caution should be exercised when ZYLOPRIM is administered to a nursing woman.

Pediatric Use: ZYLOPRIM is rarely indicated for use in children with the exception of those with hyperuricemia secondary to malignancy or to certain rare inborn errors of purine metabolism (see INDICATIONS AND USAGE and DOSAGE AND ADMINISTRATION).

ADVERSE REACTIONS

Data upon which the following estimates of incidence of adverse reactions are made are derived from experiences reported in the literature, unpublished clinical trials and voluntary reports since marketing of ZYLOPRIM (allopurinol) began. Past experience suggested that the most frequent event following the initiation of allopurinol treatment was an increase in acute attacks of gout (average 6% in early studies). An analysis of current usage suggests that the incidence of acute gouty attacks has diminished to less than 1%. The explanation for this decrease has not been determined but may be due in part to initiating therapy more gradually (see PRECAUTIONS and DOSAGE AND ADMINISTRATION).

The most frequent adverse reaction to ZYLOPRIM is skin rash. Skin reactions can be severe and sometimes fatal. Therefore, treatment with ZYLOPRIM should be discontinued immediately if a rash develops (see WARNINGS). Some patients with the most severe reaction also had fever, chills, arthralgias, cholestatic jaundice, eosinophilia and mild leukocytosis or leukopenia. Among 55 patients with gout treated with ZYLOPRIM for 3 to 34 months (average greater than 1 year) and followed prospectively, Rundles observed that 3% of patients developed a type of drug reaction which was predominantly a pruritic maculopapular skin eruption, sometimes scaly or exfoliative. However, with current usage, skin reactions have been observed less frequently than 1%. The explanation for this decrease is not obvious. The incidence of skin rash may be increased in the presence of renal insufficiency. The frequency of skin rash among patients receiving ampicillin or amoxicillin concurrently with ZYLOPRIM has been reported to be increased (see PRECAUTIONS).

Most Common Reactions* Probably Causally Related

Gastrointestinal: Diarrhea, nausea, alkaline phosphatase increase, SGOT/SGPT increase.

Metabolic and Nutritional: Acute attacks of gout.

Skin and Appendages: Rash, maculopapular rash.

*Early clinical studies and incidence rates from early clinical experience with ZYLOPRIM suggested that these adverse reactions were found to occur at a rate of greater than 1%. The most frequent event observed was acute attacks of gout following the initiation of therapy. Analyses of current usage suggest that the incidence of these adverse reactions is now less than 1%. The explanation for this decrease has not been determined, but it may be due to following recommended usage (see ADVERSE REACTIONS introduction, INDICATIONS AND USAGE, PRECAUTIONS and DOSAGE AND ADMINISTRATION).

Incidence Less Than 1% Probably Causally Related

Body as a whole: Ecchymosis, fever, headache.

Cardiovascular: Necrotizing angiitis, vasculitis.

Gastrointestinal: Hepatic necrosis, granulomatous hepatitis, hepatomegaly, hyperbilirubinemia, cholestatic jaundice, vomiting, intermittent abdominal pain, gastritis, dyspepsia.

Hemic and Lymphatic: Thrombocytopenia, eosinophilia, leukocytosis, leukopenia.

Musculoskeletal: Myopathy, arthralgias.

Nervous: Peripheral neuropathy, neuritis, paresthesia, somnolence.

Respiratory: Epistaxis.

Skin and Appendages: Erythema multiforme exudativum (Stevens-Johnson syndrome), toxic epidermal necrolysis (Lyell's syndrome), hypersensitivity vasculitis, purpura, ve-

Continued on next page

This product information is based on labeling in effect on June 1, 1998. For further information, contact via direct mail, phone, or web site Medical Information: Glaxo Wellcome Inc., PO Box 13398, Research Triangle Park, NC 27709. Healthcare Professionals (Medical Information): 800-334-0089 Patients (Customer Response Center): 888-TALK2GW (1-888-825-5249) Glaxo Wellcome Corporate Web Site: www.glaxowellcome.com

Zyloprim—Cont.

sicular bullous dermatitis, exfoliative dermatitis, eczematoid dermatitis, pruritus, urticaria, alopecia, onycholysis, lichen planus.

Special Senses: Taste loss/perversion.
Urogenital: Renal failure, uremia (see PRECAUTIONS).
Incidence Less Than 1% Causal Relationship Unknown
Body as a whole: Malaise.
Cardiovascular: Pericarditis, peripheral vascular disease, thrombophlebitis, bradycardia, vasodilation.
Endocrine: Infertility (male), hypercalcemia, gynecomastia (male).
Gastrointestinal: Hemorrhagic pancreatitis, gastrointestinal bleeding, stomatitis, salivary gland swelling, hyperlipidemia, tongue edema, anorexia.
Hemic and Lymphatic: Aplastic anemia, agranulocytosis, eosinophilic fibrohistiocytic lesion of bone marrow, pancytopenia, prothrombin decrease, anemia, hemolytic anemia, reticulocytosis, lymphadenopathy, lymphocytosis.
Musculoskeletal: Myalgia.
Nervous: Optic neuritis, confusion, dizziness, vertigo, foot drop, decrease in libido, depression, amnesia, tinnitus, asthenia, insomnia.
Respiratory: Bronchospasm, asthma, pharyngitis, rhinitis.
Skin and Appendages: Furunculosis, facial edema, sweating, skin edema.
Special Senses: Cataracts, macular retinitis, iritis, conjunctivitis, amblyopia.
Urogenital: Nephritis, impotence, primary hematuria, albuminuria.

OVERDOSAGE

Massive overdosing or acute poisoning by ZYLOPRIM has not been reported.

In mice the 50% lethal dose (LD_{50}) is 160 mg/kg given intraperitoneally (IP) with deaths delayed up to 5 days and 700 mg/kg orally (PO) (approximately 140 times the usual human dose) with deaths delayed up to 3 days. In rats the acute LD_{50} is 750 mg/kg IP and 6000 mg/kg PO (approximately 1200 times the human dose).

In the management of overdosage there is no specific antidote for ZYLOPRIM. There has been no clinical experience in the management of a patient who has taken massive amounts of ZYLOPRIM.

Both ZYLOPRIM and oxipurinol are dialyzable; however, the usefulness of hemodialysis or peritoneal dialysis in the management of an overdose of ZYLOPRIM is unknown.

DOSAGE AND ADMINISTRATION

The dosage of ZYLOPRIM to accomplish full control of gout and to lower serum uric acid to normal or near-normal levels varies with the severity of the disease. The average is 200 to 300 mg/day for patients with mild gout and 400 to 600 mg/day for those with moderately severe tophaceous gout. The appropriate dosage may be administered in divided doses or as a single equivalent dose with the 300-mg tablet. Dosage requirements in excess of 300 mg should be administered in divided doses. The minimal effective dosage is 100 to 200 mg daily and the maximal recommended dosage is 800 mg daily. To reduce the possibility of flare-up of acute gouty attacks, it is recommended that the patient start with a low dose of ZYLOPRIM (100 mg daily) and increase at weekly intervals by 100 mg until a serum uric acid level of 6 mg/dL or less is attained but without exceeding the maximal recommended dosage.

Normal serum urate levels are usually achieved in 1 to 3 weeks. The upper limit of normal is about 7 mg/dL for men and postmenopausal women and 6 mg/dL for premenopausal women. Too much reliance should not be placed on a single serum uric acid determination since, for technical reasons, estimation of uric acid may be difficult. By selecting the appropriate dosage and, in certain patients, using uricosuric agents concurrently, it is possible to reduce serum uric acid to normal or, if desired, to as low as 2 to 3 mg/dL and keep it there indefinitely.

While adjusting the dosage of ZYLOPRIM in patients who are being treated with colchicine and/or anti-inflammatory agents, it is wise to continue the latter therapy until serum uric acid has been normalized and there has been freedom from acute gouty attacks for several months.

In transferring a patient from a uricosuric agent to ZYLOPRIM, the dose of the uricosuric agent should be gradually reduced over a period of several weeks and the dose of ZYLOPRIM gradually increased to the required dose needed to maintain a normal serum uric acid level.

It should also be noted that ZYLOPRIM is generally better tolerated if taken following meals. A fluid intake sufficient to yield a daily urinary output of at least two liters and the maintenance of a neutral or, preferably, slightly alkaline urine are desirable.

Since ZYLOPRIM and its metabolites are primarily eliminated only by the kidney, accumulation of the drug can occur in renal failure, and the dose of ZYLOPRIM should consequently be reduced. With a creatinine clearance of 10 to 20 mL/min, a daily dosage of 200 mg of ZYLOPRIM is suit-

able. When the creatinine clearance is less than 10 mL/min the daily dosage should not exceed 100 mg. With extreme renal impairment (creatinine clearance less than 3 mL/min) the interval between doses may also need to be lengthened. The correct size and frequency of dosage for maintaining the serum uric acid just within the normal range is best determined by using the serum uric acid level as an index.

For the prevention of uric acid nephropathy during the vigorous therapy of neoplastic disease, treatment with 600 to 800 mg daily for 2 or 3 days is advisable together with a high fluid intake. Otherwise similar considerations to the above recommendations for treating patients with gout govern the regulation of dosage for maintenance purposes in secondary hyperuricemia.

The dose of ZYLOPRIM recommended for management of recurrent calcium oxalate stones in hyperuricosuric patients is 200 to 300 mg/day in divided doses or as the single equivalent. This dose may be adjusted up or down depending upon the resultant control of the hyperuricosuria based upon subsequent 24 hour urinary urate determinations. Clinical experience suggests that patients with recurrent calcium oxalate stones may also benefit from dietary changes such as the reduction of animal protein, sodium, refined sugars, oxalate-rich foods, and excessive calcium intake as well as an increase in oral fluids and dietary fiber. Children, 6 to 10 years of age, with secondary hyperuricemia associated with malignancies may be given 300 mg ZYLOPRIM daily while those under 6 years are generally given 150 mg daily. The response is evaluated after approximately 48 hours of therapy and a dosage adjustment is made if necessary.

HOW SUPPLIED

100 mg (white) scored, flat cylindrical tablets imprinted with "ZYLOPRIM 100" on a raised hexagon, bottles of 100 (NDC 0173-0996-55).
Store at 15° to 25°C (59° to 77°F) in a dry place.
300 mg (peach) scored, flat cylindrical tablets imprinted with "ZYLOPRIM 300" on a raised hexagon, bottles of 100 (NDC 0173-0998-55) and 500 (NDC 0173-0998-70).
Store at 15° to 25°C (59° to 77°F) in a dry place and protect from light.
© Copyright 1996 Glaxo Wellcome Inc. All rights reserved.
October 1997/RL-489
Shown in Product Identification Guide, page 315

Glenwood

82 N. SUMMIT STREET
TENAFLY, NJ 07670

Direct Inquiries to:
Professional Services Department
201-569-0050
(800) 542-0772

For Medical Information Contact:
In Emergencies:
Professional Services Department
201-569-0050
(800) 542-0772

BICHLORACETIC ACID® KAHLENBERG   ℞
Dichloroacetic Acid—Topical

DESCRIPTION

BICHLORACETIC ACID (dichloroacetic acid) Kahlenberg ($CHCl_2COOH$) is a clear, colorless liquid (sp. gr. 1.56) supplied full strength ready to use. It does not contain or require a solvent or diluent, is always uniform in potency. BICHLORACETIC ACID (dichloroacetic acid) remains colorless and retains its potency if kept in a tightly closed bottle and not contaminated with dissolved keratin or wooden applicators.

ACTIONS

BICHLORACETIC ACID (dichloroacetic acid) rapidly penetrates and cauterizes skin, keratin and other tissues. Its cauterizing effect is comparable to that obtained with such methods as electrocautery or freezing.

INDICATIONS

The lesions for which therapy with BICHLORACETIC ACID (dichloroacetic acid) is indicated are: calluses; hard and soft corns; xanthoma palpebrarum; seborrheic keratoses; ingrown nails; cysts and benign erosion of the cervix including endocervicitis and epistaxis.

CONTRAINDICATION

Topically applied chemical cauterant-keratolytics should not be used for the treatment of malignant or premalignant lesions.

WARNING

BICHLORACETIC ACID (dichloroacetic acid) is an extremely powerful keratolytic and cauterant. It should be restricted to those areas where these effects are desired.

ADMINISTRATION AND DOSAGE

The amount of BICHLORACETIC ACID (dichloroacetic acid) which should be applied varies with the nature of the lesion. Dense horny lesions such as corns and calluses require repeated extensive treatment. Lesions of light density such as xanthoma palpebrarum, soft corns, and seborrheic keratoses, should receive lighter applications.

Similarly, the number of treatments necessary will vary depending on the particular lesion being treated.

HOW SUPPLIED

Bichloracetic Acid® Kahlenberg
Complete Treatment Kit, NDC 0516-1004-11
Restocking Unit, NDC 0516-1006-77, 75 ml. bottle
Replenishment Unit, NDC 0516-1007-11, 10 ml. bottle

POTABA®   ℞
Systemic ANTIFIBROSIS THERAPY

PRODUCT OVERVIEW

KEY FACTS

Potaba® (Aminobenzoate Potassium) is considered a member of the vitamin B complex. It has been suggested that the antifibrotic action of Potaba® is due to its mediation of increased oxygen uptake at the tissue level.

MAJOR USES

Potaba® offers a means of treatment of serious and often chronic entities, such as scleroderma and Peyronie's Disease.

SAFETY INFORMATION

Contraindicated in patients taking sulfonamides. Anorexia, nausea, fever and rash have occurred infrequently and subside with omission of the drug. Often, desensitization can be accomplished and treatment resumed.

PRESCRIBING INFORMATION

POTABA®   ℞
Systemic ANTIFIBROSIS THERAPY

FORMULA

POTABA is chemically Aminobenzoate Potassium, U.S.P.

> **INDICATIONS**
> Based on a review of this drug by the National Academy of Sciences-National Research Council and/or other information, FDA has classified the indications as follows:
> "Possibly" effective: Potassium aminobenzoate is possibly effective in the treatment of scleroderma, dermatomyositis, morphea, linear scleroderma, pemphigus, and Peyronie's disease.
> Final classification of the less-than-effective indications requires further investigation.

ADVANTAGES

POTABA offers a means of treatment of serious and often chronic entities involving fibrosis and nonsuppurative inflammation.

PHARMACOLOGY

P-Aminobenzoate is considered a member of the vitamin B complex. Small amounts are found in cereal, eggs, milk and meats. Detectable amounts are normally present in human blood, spinal fluid, urine, and sweat. PABA is a component of several biologically important systems, and it participates in a number of fundamental biological processes. It has been suggested that the antifibrosis action of POTABA is due to its mediation of increased oxygen uptake at the tissue level. Fibrosis is believed to occur from either too much serotonin or too little monoamine oxidase activity over a period of time. Monoamine oxidase requires an adequate supply of oxygen to function properly. By increasing oxygen supply at the tissue level POTABA may enhance MAO activity and prevent or bring about regression of fibrosis.

CLINICAL USES

PEYRONIE'S DISEASE: 21 patients with Peyronie's disease were placed on POTABA therapy for periods ranging from 3 months to 2 years. Pain disappeared from 16 of 16 cases in which it had been present. There was objective improvement in penile deformity in 10 of 17 patients, and decrease in plaque size in 16 of 21. The authors suggest that this medication offers no hazard of further local injury as may result from other therapy. There were no significant untoward effects encountered on long term POTABA therapy.

SCLERODERMA: Of 135 patients with diffuse systemic sclerosis treated with POTABA every patient but one has

shown softening of the involved skin if treatment has been continued for 3 months or longer. The responses have been reported in a number of publications. The treatment program consists of systemic antifibrosis therapy with POTABA, physical therapy, including deep breathing exercises and dynamic traction splints where indicated, and bethanechol chloride for relief of dysphagia as well as small doses of reserpine for amelioration of Raynaud's phenomena.

DERMATOMYOSITIS: Five patients with scleroderma and 2 with dermatomyositis were treated with POTABA. There was striking clinical improvement in each patient. Doses of 15-20 grams per day were well tolerated, and patients were easily able to take these doses.

MORPHEA and LINEAR SCLERODERMA: All 14 patients with localized forms of scleroderma placed on long-term POTABA treatment showed softening of the sclerotic component of their disorder. Treatment is particularly indicated in patients where persistent compressive sclerosis may contribute even greater disfigurement or functional embarrassment from secondary pressure atrophy.

DOSAGE AND ADMINISTRATION

The average adult daily dose of POTABA is 12 grams, usually given in four to six divided doses. Tablets and capsules 0.5 gram are given at the rate of 4 tablets or capsules 6 times daily, or 6 given four times daily, usually with meals, and at bed-time with a snack. Tablets must be dissolved in an adequate amount of liquid to prevent gastrointestinal upset.

POTABA Envules contain 2 grams pure drug each, and 6 Envules are given for a total of 12 grams POTABA daily.

Children are given 1 gram POTABA daily in divided doses for each 10 lbs. of body weight.

SIDE EFFECTS

Anorexia, nausea, fever and rash have occurred infrequently and subside with omission of the drug. Often, desensitization can be accomplished and treatment resumed.

USAGE IN PREGNANCY

Safety for use in pregnancy or during lactation has not been established.

PRECAUTIONS

Should anorexia or nausea occur, therapy is interrupted until the patient is eating normally again. This permits prompt subsidence of symptoms and also avoids the possible development of hypoglycemia. Give cautiously to patients with renal disease. If a hypersensitivity reaction should occur, POTABA should be stopped.

CONTRAINDICATIONS

POTABA should not be administered to patients taking sulfonamides.

HOW SUPPLIED

POTABA Capsules—0.5 gm.
NDC 0516-0051-25 Bottle of 250
NDC 0516-0051-10 Bottle of 1000
POTABA Tablets—0.5 gm.
NDC 0516-0054-01 Bottle of 100
NDC 0516-0054-10 Bottle of 1000
POTABA Envules—2 gm.
NDC 0516-0052-50 Box of 50

Shown in Product Identification Guide, page 315

SCLEROMATE™ ℞

[skle "ro-māt]

MORRHUATE SODIUM INJECTION U.S.P.

DESCRIPTION

Morrhuate Sodium Injection, U.S.P. is a mixture of the sodium salts of the saturated and unsaturated fatty acids of Cod Liver Oil. SCLEROMATE Morrhuate Sodium Injection, U.S.P. is prepared by the saponification of selected Cod Liver Oils, it is overlaid with filtered Nitrogen to prevent discoloration that occurs on exposure to oxygen. Morrhuate Sodium occurs as a pale-yellowish, granular powder with a slight fishy odor and is soluble in water and in alcohol.

NOTE: Solid matter may develop a hazy appearance on standing and the injection should not be used if the solid matter does not dissolve completely on warming. The pH of the injection is adjusted to approximately 9.5.

CLINICAL PHARMACOLOGY

Morrhuate Sodium, when injected into the vein, causes inflammation of the intima and formation of a thrombus. This blood clot occludes the injected vein and fibrous tissue develops, resulting in the obliteration of the vein.

INDICATIONS AND USAGE

Morrhuate Sodium Injection is used for the obliteration of primary varicosed veins that consist of simple dilation with competent valves.

Sclerotherapy should not be used in patients with significant valvular or deep vein incompetence. (See Precautions.)

Although Morrhuate Sodium has been used as a sclerosing agent for the treatment of internal hemorrhoids, there is no substantial evidence that the drug is useful for this purpose. Most patients with symptomatic primary varicosed veins should be treated initially with compression stockings. If this treatment is inadequate, surgery may be required. Sclerosing agents may be useful as a supplement to venous ligation to obliterate residual varicosed veins or in patients who have conditions which increase the risk of surgery. However, many clinicians consider sclerotherapy if not effective may decrease the potential success of later surgery, should this be required.

CONTRAINDICATIONS

Morrhuate Sodium is contraindicated in patients who have shown a previous hypersensitivity reaction to the drug or to the fatty acids of cod liver oil. Continued administration of the drug is contraindicated when an unusual local reaction at the injection site or a systemic reaction occurs.

Thrombosis induced by Morrhuate Sodium may extend into the deep venous system in patients with significant valvular incompetence, therefore, valvular competency, deep vein patency, and deep vein competency should be determined by angiography and/or by tests such as the Trendelenberg and Perthes before injection of sclerosing agents. The drug is contraindicated for obliterations of superficial veins in patients with persistent occlusion of the deep veins. Morrhuate Sodium is also contraindicated in patients with acute superficial thrombophlebitis; underlying arterial disease; varicosities caused by abdominal and pelvic tumors, uncontrolled diabetes mellitus, thyrotoxicosis, tuberculosis, neoplasms, asthma, sepsis, blood dyscrasias, acute respiratory or skin disease; and in bedridden patients. Treatment with Morrhuate Sodium should be delayed in patients with acute local or systemic infections (including infected ulcers). Extensive therapy with the drug is inadvisable in patients who are severely debilitated or senile.

PRECAUTIONS

Burning or cramping sensations indicate local reactions. Urticaria may result. Sloughing and necrosis of tissue may occur with extravasation of the drug. Technique development is essential for optimal success in sclerotherapy, therefore the drug should be administered only by a physician familiar with proper injection technique. Drowsiness and headache may occur rarely. Pulmonary embolism has been reported.

Rarely, patients may have, or may develop hypersensitivity to Morrhuate Sodium, characterized by dizziness, weakness, vascular collapse, asthma, respiratory depression, gastrointestinal disturbances (i.e., nausea, vomiting), and urticaria. Anaphylactic reactions may occur within a few minutes after injection of the drug and are most likely to occur when therapy is reinstituted after an interval of several weeks. Morrhuate Sodium should only be administered when adequate facilities, drugs (i.e., epinephrine, antihistamines, corticosteroids), and personnel are available for the treatment of anaphylactic reactions.

PREGNANCY

Safety in use of Morrhuate Sodium during pregnancy has not been established.

DOSAGE

Morrhuate Sodium is administered only by INTRAVENOUS Injection. Care must be taken to avoid extravasation. (See Precautions.) Specialized references should be consulted for specific procedures and techniques of administration. When small veins are injected, or the injection solution is cold, or if solid matter has separated in the solution, the vial should be warmed by immersing in hot water. The solution should become clear on warming; only a clear solution should be used. Because the solution froths easily, a large bore needle should be used to fill the syringe, however, a small bore needle should be used for the injection.

To determine possible sensitivity to the drug, some clinicians recommend injection of 0.25–1 ml of 5% Morrhuate Sodium injection into a varicosity 24 hours before administration of a large dose.

Dosage of Morrhuate Sodium depends on the size and degree of varicosity. The usual adult dose for obliteration of small or medium veins is 50–100mg (1–2ml of the 5% injection). For large veins, 150–250 mg (3–5ml of the injection) is used. The drug may be given as multiple injections at one time or in single doses. Therapy may be repeated at 5–7 day intervals, according to the patient's response. Following injection of Morrhuate Sodium, the vein promptly becomes hard and swollen for 2–4 inches, depending on the size and response of the vein. After 24 hours, the vein is hard and slightly tender to the touch (with little or no periphlebitis). The skin around the injection becomes light-bronze; this color usually disappears shortly. An aching sensation and feeling of stiffness usually occur and last approximately 48 hours.

HOW SUPPLIED

MORRHUATE SODIUM INJECTION 5%

NDC 0516-0003-01 30ml multiple use vials

STORAGE

Store below 40 degrees C. (104 degrees F.) preferably in a refrigerator, or between 15–30 degrees C. (59–86 degrees F.).

Rev. July 1985

YOCON® ℞

[yō 'kon]

(brand of yohimbine hydrochloride)

DESCRIPTION

Yohimbine is a 3α-15α-20β-17α-hydroxy Yohimbine-16α-carboxylic acid methyl ester. The alkaloid is found in Rubaceae and related trees. Also in Rauwolfia Serpentina (L) Benth.

Yohimbine is an indolalkylamine alkaloid with chemical similarity to reserpine. It is a crystalline powder, odorless. Each compressed tablet contains (1/12 gr.) 5.4 mg of Yohimbine Hydrochloride.

ACTION

Yohimbine blocks presynaptic alpha-2 adrenergic receptors. Its action on peripheral blood vessels resembles that of reserpine, though it is weaker and of short duration. Yohimbine's peripheral autonomic nervous system effect is to increase parasympathetic (cholinergic) and decrease sympathetic (adrenergic) activity. It is to be noted that in male sexual performance, erection is linked to cholinergic activity and to alpha-2 adrenergic blockade which may theoretically result in increased penile inflow, decreased penile outflow or both.

Yohimbine exerts a stimulating action on the mood and may increase anxiety. Such actions have not been adequately studied or related to dosage although they appear to require high doses of the drug. Yohimbine has a mild anti-diuretic action, probably via stimulation of hypothalamic centers and release of posterior pituitary hormone.

Reportedly, Yohimbine exerts no significant influence on cardiac stimulation and other effects mediated by β-adrenergic receptors, its effect on blood pressure, if any, would be to lower it; however, no adequate studies are at hand to quantitate this effect in terms of Yohimbine dosage.

INDICATIONS

YOCON is indicated as a sympathicolytic and mydriatic. It may have activity as an aphrodisiac.

CONTRAINDICATIONS

Renal diseases, and patients sensitive to the drug. In view of the limited and inadequate information at hand, no precise tabulation can be offered of additional contraindications.

WARNING

Generally, this drug is not proposed for use in females and certainly must not be used during pregnancy. Neither is this drug proposed for use in pediatric, geriatric or cardio-renal patients with gastric or duodenal ulcer history. Nor should it be used in conjunction with mood-modifying drugs such as antidepressants, or in psychiatric patients in general.

ADVERSE REACTIONS

Yohimbine readily penetrates the (CNS) and produces a complex pattern of responses in lower doses than required to produce peripheral α-adrenergic blockade. These include anti-diuresis, a general picture of central excitation including elevation of blood pressure and heart rate, increased motor activity, irritability and tremor. Sweating, nausea and vomiting are common after parenteral administration of the drug.[1,2] Also dizziness, headache, skin flushing reported when used orally[1,3].

DOSAGE AND ADMINISTRATION

Experimental dosage reported in treatment of erectile impotence:[1,3,4] 1 tablet (5.4 mg) 3 times a day, to adult males taken orally. Occasional side effects reported with this dosage are nausea, dizziness or nervousness. In the event of side effects dosage is to be reduced to ½ tablet 3 times a day, followed by gradual increases to 1 tablet 3 times a day. Reported therapy not more than 10 weeks[3].

HOW SUPPLIED

Oral tablets of Yocon® 1/12 gr 5.4 mg in bottles of 100's **NDC** 0516-0001-01, 1000's **NDC** 0516-0001-10, and blister-paks of 30's **NDC** 0516-0001-30.

REFERENCES

1. A. Morales et al., New England Journal of Medicine: 1221. November 12, 1981.
2. Goodman, Gilman —The Pharmacological Basis of Therapeutics 6th ed., p. 176-188, McMillan
3. Weekly Urological Clinical letter, 27:2, July 4, 1983.
4. A. Morales et al., The Journal of Urology *128* : 45-47, 1982.

Rev. January 1985

YODOXIN® ℞
210 mg. & 650 mg. Tablets
(IODOQUINOL TABLETS U.S.P.)

PRODUCT OVERVIEW

KEY FACTS

Yodoxin (Iodoquinol) is amebicidal against the cyst and trophozoite forms of Entamoeba histolytica. Yodoxin® contains 64% organically bound iodine.

MAJOR USES

Yodoxin® is used in the treatment of intestinal amebiasis.

SAFETY INFORMATION

Contraindicated in patients with hepatic damage and in patients with known hypersensitivity to iodine and 8-hydroxyquinolines. Long term use of this drug should be avoided as optic neuritis, optic atrophy and peripheral neuropathy have been reported following prolonged high dosage with halogenated 8-hydroxyquinolines.

PRESCRIBING INFORMATION

YODOXIN® ℞
210 mg. & 650 mg. Tablets
(IODOQUINOL TABLETS U.S.P.)

DESCRIPTION

Iodoquinol is of a light yellowish to tan color, nearly odorless and stable in air. The compound is practically insoluble in water, and sparingly soluble in most other solvents. It contains 64 per cent organically bound iodine.

ACTION

Iodoquinol is amebicidal against Entamoeba histolytica and is considered effective against the trophozoite and cyst forms.

INDICATIONS

Iodoquinol is used in the treatment of intestinal amebiasis. Iodoquinol is not recommended for the treatment of nonspecific diarrhea.

CONTRAINDICATIONS

Known hypersensitivity to iodine and 8-hydroxyquinolines. Contraindicated in patients with hepatic damage.

WARNINGS

Optic neuritis, optic atrophy, and peripheral neuropathy have been reported following prolonged high dosage therapy with halogenated 8-hydroxyquinolines. Long term use of this drug should be avoided.

USE IN PREGNANCY

Safety for use in pregnancy or during lactation has not been established.

PRECAUTIONS

Iodoquinol should be used with caution in patients with thyroid disease.
Protein-bound serum iodine levels may be increased during treatment with iodoquinol and therefore interfere with certain thyroid function tests. These effects may persist for as long as six months after discontinuation of therapy. Discontinue the drug if hypersensitivity reactions occur.

ADVERSE REACTIONS

Skin: various forms of skin eruptions (acneiform papular and pustular; bullae; vegetating or tuberous iododerma), urticaria and pruritus. Gastrointestinal: nausea, vomiting, abdominal cramps, diarrhea, and pruritus ani.
Fever, chills, headache, vertigo and enlargement of thyroid have been reported. Optic neuritis, optic atrophy and peripheral neuropathy have been reported in association with prolonged high-dosage 8-hydroxyquinoline therapy.

DOSAGE AND ADMINISTRATION

Usual adult dose: (210 mg. each) 3 tablets three times daily, after meals for 20 days. Children 6 to 12 years: (210 mg. each) 2 tablets, t.i.d. Children under 6: (210 mg. each) one tablet per 15 pounds of body weight. Usual adult dose: (650 mg. each) one tablet three times a day for twenty days, to be taken after meals. Children (650 mg. each): For twenty days, 40 mg. per Kg. of body weight daily divided into 3 doses, not to exceed 1.95 grams in 24 hours, for 20 days.

HOW SUPPLIED

YODOXIN Tablets—210 mg.
NDC-0516-0092-01 Bottle of 100
YODOXIN Tablets—650 mg.
NDC-0516-0093-01 Bottle of 100

STORAGE

Store at Controlled Room Temperature 15–30°C. (59–86°F.)

CAUTION

Federal law prohibits dispensing without prescription.

A.C. Grace Co.
1100 QUITMAN ROAD
P.O. BOX 570
BIG SANDY, TX 75755

Direct Inquiries to:
Inquiries: (903) 636-4368
Orders Only: 800-833-4368

UNIQUE E™ OTC
NATURAL VITAMIN E COMPLEX
MIXED TOCOPHEROLS CONCENTRATE

DESCRIPTION

OUR SOLE PRODUCT! Established 1962! THE *VITAL* DIFFERENCE! NATURAL *UN*ESTERIFIED *HIGH ANTI-OXIDANT* MIXED TOCOPHEROLS CONCENTRATE. NOT ESTERIFIED TOCOPHER (YL) ACETATE, SUCCINATE, DL SYNTHETIC FORM, OR ANY ADULTERATED MIXTURE.

Each Bovine gelatin SOFTGEL capsule contains all natural *UN*ESTERIFIED form d-alpha, d-beta, d-GAMMA, d-delta tocopherols for high antioxidant protection against harmful free radical damage PLUS full biological activity and synergistic benefits of the complete natural Vitamin E Complex.

NO SOY or OTHER additive FILLER OILS in the capsule which can turn rancid even in sealed gelatin capsules and cause harmful free radical pathology. Contains NO ALLERGENS, PRESERVATIVES, COLOR OR FLAVORS.

Each UNIQUE E Softgel capsule is stabilized and Certified by Assay to provide not less than 700 mg of MIXED TOCOPHEROLS CONCENTRATE.

DOSAGE

Up to 6 capsules daily as directed by your physician according to individual weight or need, usually 1 capsule for each 40 lbs. of total body weight. Best results when entire daily dose is taken just before or with the morning meal.

HOW SUPPLIED

Bottles of 180 and 90 Softgel Capsules in safety-sealed, light protected plastic bottles.

Gray Pharmaceutical Co.
affiliate, The Purdue Frederick Company
100 CONNECTICUT AVENUE
NORWALK, CT 06850-3590

For Medical Information Contact:
Medical Department
(203) 853-0123

Senna
X-PREP® BOWEL EVACUANT LIQUID OTC
[ĕx 'prep]
(extract of senna concentrate)

INDICATIONS

An easy-to-administer, palatable, highly effective bowel evacuant for cleansing the colon prior to x-ray, endoscopic examination or surgery. Permits excellent visualization without residual oil droplets. X-PREP Liquid is fully prepared in a single dose container—all the patient has to do is drink the contents of one small bottle (2¹/₂ fl. oz.). Good patient cooperation is ensured because of highly pleasant taste. Predictable effectiveness helps reduce or eliminate the need for enemas prior to radiography.

DESCRIPTION

Each bottle contains 130 mg sennosides. Active Ingredient: Extract of Senna Concentrate. Inactive Ingredients: Alcohol 7%, by volume, Methyl paraben, Potassium sorbate, Propylparaben, Sodium lauryl sulfate, Sucrose, Water, Natural and Artificial Flavors and other ingredients.

CONTRAINDICATIONS

Acute surgical abdomen.

WARNINGS

Do not use this product unless directed by a physician. Do not use when abdominal pain, nausea or vomiting is present, unless directed by a physician. As with any drug, if you are pregnant or nursing a baby, seek the advice of a health professional before using this product. In case of accidental overdose, seek professional assistance or contact a Poison Control Center immediately. Keep out of children's reach.

CAUTION

In diabetic patients, the physician should be aware of the sugar content of X-PREP Liquid (50 grams per 2¹/₂ fl. oz. dose).

ADMINISTRATION AND DOSAGE

Recommended Dosage (or as directed by physician):
Adults and children 12 years of age and older: Take one bottle between 2 and 4 p.m. on day prior to x-ray or other diagnostic procedures. Drink entire contents. For children under 12 years of age, consult a doctor. A strong bowel action can be expected approximately 6 hours after drinking. After X-PREP Liquid is taken, diet should be confined to clear fluids.

HOW SUPPLIED

2¹/₂ fl. oz. bottles (alcohol 7% by volume), each providing a single, complete adult dose.
Also Available—Two X-PREP® Bowel Evacuant Kits.
Kit #1 contains: Two SENOKOT-S® Tablets (standardized senna concentrate and docusate sodium), one bottle of X-PREP Liquid 2¹/₂ fl. oz., and one RECTOLAX® Suppository (bisacodyl 10 mg), plus easy-to-follow patient instructions for hydration, clear liquid diet, and the correct time-sequence for administering the above laxatives.
Kit #2 contains: One dose CITRALAX® Granules 1.06 oz. (effervescent citrate/sulfate of magnesia), one bottle of X-PREP Liquid 2¹/₂ fl. oz., and one RECTOLAX® Suppository (bisacodyl 10 mg), plus easy-to-follow patient instructions.
Copyright © 1991, 1998, Gray Pharmaceutical Co., Norwalk, CT 06850-3590.

Guardian Laboratories
a division of United-Guardian, Inc.
P.O. Box 18050
HAUPPAUGE, N.Y. 11788

For Medical Information Contact:
Director of Medical Research
(516) 273-0900
(800) 645-5566

CLORPACTIN® WCS-90 OTC
[klor-pak 'tin]
(brand of sodium oxychlorosene)

COMPOSITION

Stabilized organic derivative of hypochlorous acid. A white, water soluble powder with a characteristic smell of hypochlorous acid. Active chlorine derived from calcium hypochlorite: 3–4%.

ACTION AND USES

For use as a topical antiseptic for treating localized infections, particularly when resistant organisms are present. Complete spectrum (bacteria, fungi, viruses, mold, yeast and spores); effective in cases of antibiotic resistance; nontoxic and non-allergenic in use concentrations.

ADMINISTRATION AND DOSAGE

Applied by irrigation, instillations, spray, soaks or wet compresses, preferably thoroughly cleansing with gravity flow irrigation or syringe to provide copious quantities of fresh solution to remove the organic wastes and debris from the site of the involvement. Also for preoperative skin preparation and postoperative protection. Generally applied as the 0.4% solution in water, or isotonic saline, but as the 0.1% to 0.2% in Urology and Ophthalmology.

CONTRAINDICATIONS

The use of this product is contraindicated where the site of the infection is not exposed to the direct contact with the solution. Not for systemic use.

HOW SUPPLIED

In boxes containing 5 x 2 gram bottles. NDC: 0327-0001-10
Store under refrigeration.

RENACIDIN® ℞
(Citric Acid, Glucono-delta-lactone, and Magnesium Carbonate)
Irrigation

DESCRIPTION

Renacidin® (Citric Acid, Glucono-delta-lactone, and Magnesium Carbonate) Irrigation is a sterile, non-pyrogenic irrigation for use within the urinary tract in the prevention and dissolution of calculi.
Each 100 ml. of Renacidin Irrigation contains:
Active ingredients:

Citric Acid (anhydrous), U.S.P.   6.602 grams
$C_6H_8O_7$

Glucono-delta-lactone   0.198 grams
$C_6H_{10}O_6$

Magnesium Carbonate, U.S.P.   3.177 grams
$(MgCO_3)_4 \cdot Mg(OH)_2 \cdot 3H_2O$

Citric Acid   **Glucono-delta-lactone**

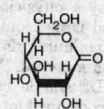

Magnesium Carbonate
$(MgCO_3)_4 \cdot Mg(OH)_2 \cdot 3H_2O$
Inert ingredients:
Benzoic Acid, U.S.P.   0.023 grams
Solution pH: 3.85 (3.50–4.20)

HOW SUPPLIED

Renacidin Irrigation is available as a sterile, non-pyrogenic solution in 500 ml containers, packaged in cartons of six. Exposure of Renacidin Irrigation to heat or cold should be minimized. Renacidin Irrigation should be stored at controlled room temperature, 59° to 86°F (15° to 30°C). Avoid excessive heat or cold (keep from freezing). Brief exposure to temperatures of up to 40°C or temperatures down to 5°C does not adversely affect the product.
NDC: 0327-0011-05
PRODUCT CODE: RN500

Healthpoint

**2600 AIRPORT FWY
FORT WORTH, TX 76111**

Direct Inquiries to:
800-441-8227

ACCUZYME™
PAPAIN-UREA DEBRIDING OINTMENT   ℞

DESCRIPTION

Each gram of Accuzyme enzymatic debriding ointment contains papain (1.1×10^6 USP units of activity) and 100mg urea in a hydrophilic ointment base composed of purified water, emulsifying wax, glycerin, isopropyl palmitate, potassium phosphate monobasic, fragrance, methylparaben and propylparaben.

CLINICAL PHARMACOLOGY

Papain, the proteolytic enzyme from the fruit of carica papaya, is a potent digestant of nonviable protein matter but is harmless to viable tissue. It is active over a pH range of 3 to 12. Papain is relatively ineffective when used alone as a debriding agent and requires the presence of activators to stimulate its digestive potency. In Accuzyme, papain is combined with urea, a denaturant of proteins, to bring about two supplemental chemical actions: (1) to expose by solvent action the activators of papain, and (2) to denature the nonviable protein matter in lesions and thereby render it more susceptible to enzymatic digestion. Pharmacologic studies have shown that the combination of papain and urea result in twice as much digestive activity as papain alone.

INDICATIONS AND USAGE

Accuzyme is indicated for debridement of necrotic tissue and liquefaction of slough in acute and chronic lesions such as pressure ulcers, varicose and diabetic ulcers, burns, post-operative wounds, pilonidal cyst wounds, carbuncles and miscellaneous traumatic or infected wounds.

CONTRAINDICATIONS

Accuzyme is contraindicated in patients who have shown sensitivity to papain or any other components of this preparation.

PRECAUTIONS

See Dosage and Administration. Not to be used in eyes.

ADVERSE REACTIONS

Accuzyme is generally well-tolerated and non-irritating. A transient "burning" sensation may be experienced by a small percentage of patients upon applying Accuzyme. Occasionally, the profuse exudate from enzymatic digestion may irritate the skin. In such cases, more frequent dressing changes will alleviate discomfort until exudate decreases.

DOSAGE AND ADMINISTRATION

Cleanse the wound with Allclenz™ Wound Cleanser or saline. Avoid cleansing with hydrogen peroxide solution as it may inactivate the papain. Apply Accuzyme directly to the wound, cover with appropriate dressing, secure into place. Daily or twice daily applications are preferred. Irrigate the wound at each redressing to remove any accumulation of liquefied necrotic material. NOTE: Papain may also be inactivated by the salts of heavy metals such as lead, silver and mercury. Contact with medications containing these metals should be avoided.

HOW SUPPLIED

30g tubes. Store in a cool place.
CAUTION: Federal law prohibits dispensing without prescription.
NDC–0064-1000-01
HEALTHPOINT®
Healthpoint, San Antonio, Texas 78215
1-800-441-8227
REORDER NO. 1000-01   126959-1195
Shown in Product Identification Guide, page 315

Heel, Inc.

**11600 COCHITI SE
ALBUQUERQUE, NM 87123**

Direct Inquiries to:
Medical Department
800–621–7644
(505) 293–3843
Fax: (505) 275–1672
http://www.heelbhi.com

TRAUMEEL® Tablets	**OTC**
Anti-inflammatory/Analgesic	
TRAUMEEL® Ointment	**OTC**
Anti-inflammatory/Analgesic	
TRAUMEEL® Oral Drops	**OTC**
Anti-inflammatory/Analgesic	
TRAUMEEL® Oral Liquid in Vials	**OTC**
Anti-inflammatory/Analgesic	

TRAUMEEL® Injection Solution   ℞

DESCRIPTION

TRAUMEEL® Injection Solution is an anti-inflammatory, analgesic, anti-edematous, anti-exudative combination formulation of 12 botanical substances and 1 mineral substance. TRAUMEEL® Injection Solution is officially classified as a homeopathic combination remedy (1).
1. Botanical ingredients:
Arnica montana, radix (mountain arnica)
Calendula officinalis (marigold)
Hamamelis virginiana (witch hazel)
Millefolium (milfoil)
Belladonna (deadly nightshade)
Aconitum napellus (monkshood)
Chamomilla (chamomile)
Symphytum officinale (comfrey)
Bellis perennis (daisy)
Echinacea angustifolia (narrow-leafed cone flower)
Echinacea purpurea (purple cone flower)
Hypericum perforatum (St. John's wort)
2. Mineral ingredients:
Hepar sulphuris calcareum (calcium sulfide)
Injection Solution: Each 2.0 ml ampule contains as active ingredients: Hepar sulphuris calcareum 8X 200.0 µl; Belladonna 3X 20.0 µl; Calendula officinalis 3X 20.0 µl; Chamomilla 4X 20.0 µl; Millefolium 4X 20.0 µl; Aconitum napellus 3X 12.0 µl; Bellis perennis 3X 10.0 µl; Hypericum perforatum 3X 6.0 µl; Echinacea angustifolia 3X 5.0 µl; Echinacea purpurea 3X 5.0 µl; Arnica montana, radix 2X 2.0 µl; Hamamelis virginiana 2X 2.0 µl; Symphytum officinale 6X 2.0 µl. Each 2.0 ml ampule contains as an inactive ingredient: Sterile isotonic sodium chloride solution.

CLINICAL PHARMACOLOGY

The exact mechanism of action of TRAUMEEL® Injection Solution is not fully understood. Various cellular and biochemical pathways appear to be modulated by the product ingredients. The mechanism of action of TRAUMEEL® Injection Solution does not appear to be the result of cyclooxygenase or lipoxygenase enzyme inhibition, as is the case with nonsteroidal anti-inflammatory drugs (NSAIDs). TRAUMEEL® Injection Solution does not inhibit the arachidonic acid pathway of prostaglandin synthesis. Instead, the mechanism of action of TRAUMEEL® Injection Solution appears to be the result of modulation of the release of oxygen radicals from activated neutrophils, and inhibition of the release of inflammatory mediators (possibly interleukin-1 from activated macrophages) and neuropeptides (2).

In vitro studies show that the ingredients in TRAUMEEL® Injection Solution are noncytotoxic to granulocytes, lymphocytes, platelets, and endothelia, which indicates that the defensive functions of these cells are preserved during treatment with TRAUMEEL® Injection Solution (3).
The anti-inflammatory, analgesic, anti-edematous, and anti-exudative effects of TRAUMEEL® Injection Solution have been demonstrated in clinical trials as well as in *in vivo* experimental models including the carrageenin-induced edema test and the adjuvant arthritis test (3).

INDICATIONS AND USAGE

TRAUMEEL® Injection Solution is indicated for the treatment of symptoms associated with inflammatory, exudative, and degenerative processes due to acute trauma (such as contusions, lacerations, fractures, sprains, post-operative wounds, etc.), repetitive or overuse injuries (such as tendonitis, bursitis, epicondylitis, etc.), and for minor aches and pains associated with such conditions. TRAUMEEL® Injection Solution is also indicated for the treatment of minor aches and pains associated with backache, muscular aches, and the minor pain from rheumatoid arthritis, osteoarthritis, gouty arthritis, and ankylosing spondylitis.

CONTRAINDICATIONS

TRAUMEEL® Injection Solution is contraindicated in patients with a known hypersensitivity to TRAUMEEL® Injection Solution or any of its ingredients (see **ADVERSE REACTIONS**).

WARNINGS

If pain persists or worsens, if new symptoms occur, or if redness or swelling is present, the patient should be carefully re-evaluated because these could be signs of a serious condition.

PRECAUTIONS

General:
Adverse effects with TRAUMEEL® Injection Solution are extremely rare. TRAUMEEL® Injection Solution exhibits no known adverse renal, hepatic, cardiovascular, gastrointestinal or central nervous system effects.
Information for Patients:
No harmful or potentially hazardous side effects such as central nervous system depression are known. TRAUMEEL® Injection Solution is generally well-tolerated. However, if symptoms persist or worsen, a physician should be consulted (see **WARNINGS**).
Drug Interactions:
TRAUMEEL® Injection Solution is not known to interact with other medications. Furthermore, the administration of TRAUMEEL® Injection Solution can be safely augmented by the application of a topical dosage form of TRAUMEEL®.
Drug/Laboratory Test Interactions:
TRAUMEEL® Injection Solution is not known to interact with any laboratory tests.
Carcinogenesis:
No studies have been performed to evaluate the carcinogenicity of TRAUMEEL® Injection Solution. In world-wide post-marketing surveillance studies no evidence of carcinogenicity has been found (2).
Pregnancy:
Pregnancy Category C. In general, medications such as TRAUMEEL® Injection Solution that are classified as homeopathic are not known to cause direct or indirect harm to the fetus. However, animal reproduction studies have not been performed and there are no well-controlled studies in pregnant women. In cases of pregnancy or suspected pregnancy, TRAUMEEL® Injection Solution should be used only if potential benefits justify potential risks to the fetus.
Nursing Mothers:
It is not known whether any of the ingredients in TRAUMEEL® Injection Solution are excreted in human milk. However, because many drugs are excreted in human milk, TRAUMEEL® Injection Solution should be administered with caution to nursing mothers.
Pediatric Use:
TRAUMEEL® Injection Solution can be safely administered to children as young as 2 years (see **DOSAGE AND ADMINISTRATION**).

ADVERSE REACTIONS

In rare cases, patients with hypersensitivity to botanicals of the Compositae family may experience an allergic reaction after the administration of TRAUMEEL® Injection Solution including anaphylactic reaction. TRAUMEEL® Injection Solution ingredients of the Compositae family are:
Arnica montana, radix (mountain arnica)
Calendula officinalis (marigold)
Millefolium (milfoil)
Chamomilla (chamomile)
Bellis perennis (daisy)
Echinacea angustifolia (narrow-leafed cone flower)
Echinacea purpurea (purple cone flower)

Continued on next page

Traumeel—Cont.

OVERDOSAGE

Due to the low concentration of active ingredients in homeopathic preparations such as TRAUMEEL® Injection Solution, adverse reactions following overdosage are extremely unlikely. However, care must be taken not to exceed the recommended dosage.

DOSAGE AND ADMINISTRATION

The dosage schedules listed below can be used as a general guide for the administration of TRAUMEEL® Injection Solution. TRAUMEEL® Injection Solution shows individual differences in clinical response. Therefore, the dosage for each patient should be individualized according to the patient's response to therapy. For best results, treatment with TRAUMEEL® Injection Solution should be initiated immediately following injury or at the first sign of symptoms. TRAUMEEL® Injection Solution may be administered until symptoms disappear.

TRAUMEEL® Injection Solution:

Adults: 1 ampule daily for acute disorders, or 1 to 2 ampules 1 to 3 times weekly.

Children (2 to 6 years): Half the adult dosage. Discard unused solution.

TRAUMEEL® Injection Solution may be administered intravenously, intramuscularly, subcutaneously or intradermally. TRAUMEEL® Injection Solution is indicated for peri-articular administration. However, TRAUMEEL® Injection Solution is not indicated for intra-articular use. If coadministration with a local anesthetic is desired, TRAUMEEL® Injection Solution may be mixed in a 1:1 ratio with 1% or 2% lidocaine hydrochloride. Similar local anesthetics may also be used. The required dose of TRAUMEEL® Injection Solution is first withdrawn from the ampule into the syringe. The local anesthetic is then withdrawn into the syringe, and the syringe is then shaken briefly. Normally, about 0.5 to 1.0 milliliters of each drug is withdrawn into the syringe.

TRAUMEEL® Injection Solution should be administered using a narrow gauge needle (e.g., 22 to 30 gauge). **Note:** Parenteral drug products like TRAUMEEL® Injection Solution should be inspected visually for particulate matter and discoloration prior to administration whenever solution and container permit. TRAUMEEL® Injection Solution is a clear, colorless solution. Discolored solutions should be discarded.

HOW SUPPLIED

TRAUMEEL® Injection Solution in 2.0 ml ampules: Packs of 10: NDC 50114-7000-1.

Avoid freezing and excessive heat. Store at controlled room temperature. Protect from light.

CAUTION: Rx only.

REFERENCES

(1) The Homeopathic Pharmacopoeia of the United States (HPUS), 8th edition, Falls Church, Virginia, 1979; and the Homeopathic Pharmacopoeia of the United States Revision Service (HPRS), 1988.

(2) Data on file, Heel GmbH, Baden-Baden, Germany.

(3) Conforti A, *et al.* Experimental Studies on the Anti-inflammatory Activity of a Homeopathic Preparation. *Biomedical Therapy XV* No.1:28-31, 1997.

This full prescribing information has been compiled in accordance with the Code of Federal Regulations (CFR), 21 sections 201.56 and 201.57.

VERTIGOHEEL® Tablets   ℞
VERTIGOHEEL® Oral Drops   ℞
VERTIGOHEEL® Oral Liquid in Vials   ℞

DESCRIPTION

VERTIGOHEEL® is a homeopathic combination formulation for the treatment of vertigo consisting of 2 botanical substances, 1 zoological substance, and 1 mineral substance (1, 2). VERTIGOHEEL® is officially classified as a homeopathic combination remedy.

1. Botanical ingredients:
   Conium maculatum (umbelliferae)
   Cocculus indicus (menispermaceae)
2. Zoological ingredient:
   Ambra grisea (ambergris)
3. Mineral ingredient:
   Petroleum (purified mineral oil)

Tablets: Each 300 mg tablet contains as active ingredients: Cocculus indicus 4X 210 mg; Conium maculatum 3X 30 mg; Ambra grisea 6X 30 mg; Petroleum 8X 30 mg; in a lactose base. Each 300 mg tablet contains as an inactive ingredient: Magnesium stearate.

Oral Drops: Each 100 ml of solution contains as active ingredients: Cocculus indicus 4X 70 ml; Conium maculatum 3X 10 ml; Ambra grisea 6X 10 ml; Petroleum 8X 10 ml. Contains ethyl alcohol 35% by volume.

Oral Liquid in Vials: Each 100 ml of solution contains as active ingredients: Cocculus indicus 3X 0.7 ml; Conium maculatum 2X 0.1 ml; Ambra grisea 5X 0.1 ml; Petroleum 7X 0.1 ml. Each 100 of solution contains as an inactive ingredient: Isotonic sodium chloride solution.

CLINICAL PHARMACOLOGY

The exact mechanism of action of VERTIGOHEEL® is not fully understood. Pharmacologic studies suggest that the effectiveness of VERTIGOHEEL® for the treatment of vertigo and nausea, and for improving vestibulo-ocular and proprioceptive symptoms, is due in part to central nervous system stimulation. Studies have confirmed that VERTIGOHEEL® activates the vestibular regulatory systems located in the brainstem area. Computer-processed brain mapping recordings indicate an increase in activity in the neuropathways, which connect the vestibulo-pathways with the corpora quadrigemina (3, 4).

INDICATIONS AND USAGE

VERTIGOHEEL® is indicated for the treatment of vertigo (3,4,5) and other related imbalance disorders, and related symptoms such as nausea. VERTIGOHEEL® is also indicated for the prevention and treatment of motion sickness (6).

CONTRAINDICATIONS

VERTIGOHEEL® is contraindicated in patients with a known hypersensitivity to VERTIGOHEEL® or any of its ingredients.

WARNINGS

VERTIGOHEEL® should not be administered for more than 10 days for adults or 5 days for children without follow-up assessment by a physician. If during the course of treatment symptoms persist or worsen, or if new symptoms occur, the patient should consult a physician because these could be signs of a serious condition requiring more aggressive therapy.

PRECAUTIONS

General:
Adverse effects with VERTIGOHEEL® are extremely rare. VERTIGOHEEL® exhibits no known adverse renal, hepatic, cardiovascular, gastrointestinal, or central nervous system effects.

Information for Patients:
No harmful or potentially hazardous side effects such as central nervous system depression are known. VERTIGOHEEL® is generally well-tolerated even during long term administration.

Drug Interactions:
VERTIGOHEEL® is not known to interact with other medications.

Drug/Laboratory Test Interactions:
VERTIGOHEEL® is not known to interact with any laboratory tests.

Carcinogenesis:
No studies have been performed to evaluate the carcinogenicity of VERTIGOHEEL®. In world-wide post-marketing surveillance no evidence of carcinogenicity has been found (5).

Pregnancy:
Pregnancy Category C. In general, medications such as VERTIGOHEEL® which are classified as homeopathic are not known to cause direct or indirect harm to the fetus. However, animal reproduction studies have not been performed and there are no well-controlled studies in pregnant women. In cases of pregnancy or suspected pregnancy, a physician should be consulted before administering VERTIGOHEEL®.

Nursing Mothers:
It is not known whether any of the ingredients in VERTIGOHEEL® are excreted in human milk. However, because many drugs are excreted in human milk, VERTIGOHEEL® should be administered with caution to nursing mothers.

Pediatric Use:
VERTIGOHEEL® Tablets and VERTIGOHEEL® Oral Liquid in Vials can be safely administered to children as young as 2 years (see DOSAGE AND ADMINISTRATION). However, due to its alcohol content (ethyl alcohol 35% by volume), VERTIGOHEEL® Oral Drops should be administered with caution to children below the age of 12 years.

ADVERSE REACTIONS

VERTIGOHEEL® exhibits no known adverse reactions.

OVERDOSAGE

Due to the low concentrations of active ingredients in homeopathic preparations such as VERTIGOHEEL®, adverse reactions following overdosage are extremely unlikely. However, care must be taken not to exceed the recommended dosage.

DOSAGE AND ADMINISTRATION

The dosage schedules listed below can be used as a general guide for the administration of VERTIGOHEEL®. The dosage for each patient should be individualized according to the patient's response to therapy. For the treatment or prevention of vertigo or motion sickness, the onset of action of VERTIGOHEEL® may not be immediate. Patients responding to VERTIGOHEEL® therapy will normally show benefit within one week (5,6). The frequency of administration of the 3 dosage forms may be increased to every 15 minutes over a 2-hour period for acute exacerbations of the symptoms of vertigo, in both children and adults, unless otherwise directed by a physician. VERTIGOHEEL® Tablets, Oral Drops, and Oral Liquid in Vials should be administered at least 30 minutes after meals and when the oral cavity is free of food material. For best results, treatment with VERTIGOHEEL® should be initiated at the first sign of symptoms and continued for a physician-specified period. If symptoms persist or worsen, the patient should contact a physician (see **WARNINGS**).

VERTIGOHEEL® Tablets:

Adults and Children above 6 years: 2 to 3 tablets sublingually or dissolved completely in the mouth 3 times daily.

Children 2 to 6 years: 1 to 2 tablets sublingually or dissolved completely in the mouth 3 times daily.

For best results, VERTIGOHEEL® Tablets should be dissolved under the tongue or in the mouth since the absorption is via the buccal lining. For small children tablets may be divided or crushed for easier administration.

VERTIGOHEEL® Oral Drops:

Adults and Children above 11 years: 15 to 20 drops taken sublingually 3 times daily.

Children 2 to 11 years: Half the adult dosage. Due to its alcohol content (ethyl alcohol 35% by volume), VERTIGOHEEL® Oral Drops should be administered with caution to children below the age of 12 years.

VERTIGOHEEL® Oral Drops may be added to clear, non-sparkling water prior to administration.

VERTIGOHEEL® Oral Liquid in Vials:

Adults and Children above 6 years: The contents of 1 vial taken orally 1 to 3 times daily.

Children 2 to 6 years: Half the contents of 1 vial taken orally 1 to 3 times daily.

VERTIGOHEEL® Oral Liquid in Vials may be added to clear, non-sparkling water prior to administration. **Note:** The unused portion of the open vials should be discarded. **NOT FOR INJECTION.**

HOW SUPPLIED

VERTIGOHEEL® Tablets (white, unscored with "Heel" impressed on one side) in bottles of 100: NDC 50114-1170-2. Avoid freezing and excessive heat. Store at room temperature. Keep container tightly closed. Protect from light and moisture.

VERTIGOHEEL® Oral Drops in 50 ml (1.6 fluid oz) bottles: NDC 50114-1170-4. Avoid freezing and excessive heat. Store at controlled room temperature. Keep container tightly closed. Protect from light.

VERTIGOHEEL® Oral Liquid in Vials, 1.1 ml packs of 10: NDC 50114-1122-4. Avoid freezing and excessive heat. Store at controlled room temperature. Protect from light.

CAUTION: Rx only.

REFERENCES

(1) The Homeopathic Pharmacopoeia of the United States (HPUS), 5th Edition, Falls Church, Virginia, 1979.

(2) The Homeopathic Pharmacopoeia of the United States Revision Service (HPRS), 1988.

(3) Claussen, CF. Treatment of the Syndrome of the Slowed Down Brainstem with Vertigoheel. *Biological Therapy,* Vol. V, No. 1, 1-24, 1987, and Vol. V, No. 2, 25-49, 1987.

(4) Claussen CF, Bergmann J, Bertora G, Claussen E. Clinico-experimental Study and Equilibrimetric Measurements Assessing the Therapeutic Efficacy of a Homeopathic Drug with the Ingredients Ambra, Cocculus, Conium, and Mineral Oil in Vertigo and Nausea Cases, *Arzneimittel-Forschung* (Drug Research) 34(ll), 12, 1791-1798, 1984.

(5) Data on file, Heel GmbH, Baden-Baden, Germany.

(6) Bruckner G. Vertigoheel in an Internal Medicine Practice, *Biomedical Therapy,* Vol. IV, No. 1, 2-5, 1986.

IDENTIFICATION PROBLEM?
Turn to the **Product Identification Guide,**
where you'll find more than
1600 products pictured in actual
size and full color.

High Chemical Co.
3901-A NEBRASKA ST.
LEVITTOWN, PA 19056

Direct Inquiries to:
800-447-8792

SARAPIN® ℞

DESCRIPTION
A sterile aqueous solution of soluble salts of the volatile bases from Sarraceniaceae (Pitcher Plant). Benzyl Alcohol 0.75%.

ACTIONS
The painful syndromes most commonly encountered in general practice which are relieved by SARAPIN® treatment are as follows:
Sciatic Pain
Intercostal Neuralgia
Alcoholic Neuritis
Occipital Neuritis
Brachial Plexus Neuralgia
Meralgia Paresthetica
Lumbar Neuralgia
Trigeminal Neuralgia

ADMINISTRATION
These and allied conditions may be treated with success in a majority of cases by nerve block or local infiltration:
Paravertebral—Careful localization of the zone of tenderness permits a determination of the corresponding trunk levels to be injected.
Perineural—In some instances, as in sciatica, the affected nerve can be injected at a site distant from its origin.
Local Infiltration—Multiple injections throughout an area of tenderness provide for diffusion into all the affected parts.

DOSAGE
Paravertebral Injections
Cervical .... 2–3 ml
Dorsal .... 5–10 ml
Lumbar .... 5–10 ml
Sacral .... 3–5 ml
Caudal Canal .... 10 ml
Sciatic Nerve .... 10 ml
Local Infiltration .... 5–10 ml

WARNINGS
Withdraw plunger of syringe to make sure the needle point is not in a blood vessel.

PRECAUTIONS
Procedure should be gentle and unhurried.
SARAPIN® is intended only for professional use. Its successful employment depends upon a thorough knowledge of the anatomy involved.

ADVERSE REACTIONS
Patients should be maintained in a recumbent position for 10 to 15 minutes following injection. A local sensation is to be expected, limited to the distribution of the nerve injected, and usually appearing as a temporary feeling of heaviness, although some cases will feel heat or a transitory aggravation of symptoms.

CONTRAINDICATIONS
SARAPIN® is non-toxic, has no side effects other than above and is contraindicated only in areas of local inflammation.

HOW SUPPLIED
50 ml Multiple Dose Vial.
NDC-10541-492-50
CAUTION: Federal law prohibits dispensing without prescription.

HIGH CHEMICAL COMPANY
3901-A Nebraska Street
Levittown, PA 19056-3333
800-447-8792

For information on over-the-counter drugs, consult **PDR For Nonprescription Drugs.**

Hill Dermaceuticals, Inc.
2650 SO. MELLONVILLE AVE.
SANFORD, FL 32773

Direct Inquiries to:
Rosario G. Ramirez
(407) 323-1887
FAX: (407) 649-9213/323-1871

DERMA-SMOOTHE/FS TOPICAL OIL ℞
Fluocinolone acetonide, 0.01%, Topical Oil

FS SHAMPOO, 0.01% ℞
Fluocinolone acetonide, 0.01%, Shampoo

HOECHST MARION ROUSSEL
10236 MARION PARK DRIVE
MAIL: P.O. BOX 9627
KANSAS CITY, MO 64134-0627

Direct Inquiries to:
Customer Information Center, Kl-M0928
P.O. Box 9627
Kansas City, MO 64134-0627
(800) 552-3656

For Medical Information Contact:
Generally:
Medical Informatics
P.O. Box 9627
Kansas City, MO 64134-0627
(800) 633-1610
After Hours and Weekend Emergencies:
(816) 966-5000

PRODUCT IDENTIFICATION
NUMERICAL SUMMARY
SOLID ORAL DOSAGE FORMS

Hoechst Marion Roussel
Kansas City, MO 64134
To provide quick and positive identification of Hoechst Marion Roussel prescription drug products, we have imprinted an identifying number and the name MARION on the following tablets or capsules.

1555 PAVABID® Capsules, 150 mg (papaverine hydrochloride)
1771 CARDIZEM® Tablets, 30 mg (diltiazem hydrochloride)
1772 CARDIZEM® Tablets, 60 mg (diltiazem hydrochloride)

ALLEGRA™ 60-mg capsules are imprinted in black ink, with "60 mg" on the cap and "1102" on the body, or "allegra" on the cap and "60 mg" on the body.
ALLEGRA-D™ extended-release tablets are engraved with "Allegra-D".
ALTACE® (ramipril) Capsules 1.25 mg are imprinted with "ALTACE 1.25 MG" on one end and "HOECHST" on the other.
ALTACE® (ramipril) Capsules 2.5 mg are imprinted with "ALTACE 2.5 MG" on one end and "HOECHST" on the other.
ALTACE® (ramipril) Capsules 5 mg are imprinted with "ALTACE 5 MG" on one end and "HOECHST" on the other.
ALTACE® (ramipril) Capsules 10 mg are imprinted with "ALTACE 10 MG" on one end and "HOECHST" on the other.
AMARYL® (glimepiride) Tablets 1 mg, 2 mg, and 4 mg are imprinted with "AMARYL" on one side and the Hoechst logo on both sides of the bisect on the other side.
ANZEMET® 50 mg tablets are imprinted with "ANZEMET 50" on one side.
ANZEMET® 100 mg tablets are imprinted with "100" on one side and "ANZEMET" on the other.
BENTYL® Capsules, 10 mg (dicyclomine hydrochloride USP) is imprinted BENTYL 10.
BENTYL® Tablets, 20 mg (dicyclomine hydrochloride USP) is debossed BENTYL 20.
BRICANYL® Tablets, 2.5 mg (terbutaline sulfate USP) is debossed BRICANYL 2½.
BRICANYL® Tablets, 5 mg (terbutaline sulfate USP) is debossed BRICANYL 5.

CANTIL® Tablets, 25 mg (mepenzolate bromide USP) is debossed MERRELL 37.
CARAFATE® Tablets, 1 g (sucralfate) is identified by the brand name CARAFATE embossed on one side and 1712 on the reverse side.
CARDIZEM® Tablets, 90 mg (diltiazem hydrochloride) is imprinted with the brand name CARDIZEM on one side and 90 mg on the reverse side.
CARDIZEM® Tablets, 120 mg (diltiazem hydrochloride) is imprinted with the brand name CARDIZEM on one side and 120 mg on the reverse side.
CARDIZEM® SR Capsules, 60 mg (diltiazem hydrochloride) is imprinted with the Cardizem logo on one end and Cardizem SR 60 mg on the other.
CARDIZEM® SR Capsules, 90 mg (diltiazem hydrochloride) is imprinted with the Cardizem logo on one end and Cardizem SR 90 mg on the other.
CARDIZEM® SR Capsules, 120 mg (diltiazem hydrochloride) is imprinted with the Cardizem logo on one end and Cardizem SR 120 mg on the other.
CARDIZEM® CD Capsules, 120 mg (diltiazem hydrochloride) is imprinted with Cardizem CD and 120 mg on one end.
CARDIZEM® CD Capsules, 180 mg (diltiazem hydrochloride) is imprinted with CARDIZEM CD and 180 mg on one end.
CARDIZEM® CD Capsules, 240 mg (diltiazem hydrochloride) is imprinted with CARDIZEM CD and 240 mg on one end.
CARDIZEM® CD Capsules, 300 mg (diltiazem hydrochloride) is imprinted with CARDIZEM CD and 300 mg on one end.
CLOMID® Tablets, 50 mg (clomiphene citrate) is debossed CLOMID 50.
DIAβETA® (glyburide) Tablets 1.25 mg, 2.5 mg, and 5 mg are imprinted with "Hoechst" on one side and "Diaβ" on the other side.
HIPREX® Tablets, 1 g (methenamine hippurate) is debossed MERRELL 277.
LASIX® (furosemide) Tablets 20 mg are imprinted with "Lasix® " on one side and "HOECHST" on the other.
LASIX® (furosemide) Tablets 40 mg are imprinted with "Lasix® 40" on one side and the Hoechst logo on the other.
LASIX® (furosemide) Tablets 80 mg are imprinted with "Lasix® 80" on one side and the Hoechst logo on the other.
NILANDRON® Tablets have a triangular logo on one face and an internal reference number (168) on the other.
NORPRAMIN® Tablets, 10 mg (desipramine hydrochloride USP) is imprinted 68-7.
NORPRAMIN® Tablets, 25 mg (desipramine hydrochloride USP) is imprinted NORPRAMIN 25.
NORPRAMIN® Tablets, 50 mg (desipramine hydrochloride USP) is imprinted NORPRAMIN 50.
NORPRAMIN® Tablets, 75 mg (desipramine hydrochloride USP) is imprinted NORPRAMIN 75.
NORPRAMIN® Tablets, 100 mg (desipramine hydrochloride USP) is imprinted NORPRAMIN 100.
NORPRAMIN® Tablets, 150 mg (desipramine hydrochloride USP) is imprinted NORPRAMIN 150.
NOVAFED® A Capsules, 120 mg pseudoephedrine hydrochloride and 8 mg chlorpheniramine maleate is imprinted NOVAFED A.
RIFADIN® Capsules, 150 mg (rifampin) is imprinted RIFADIN 150.
RIFADIN® Capsules, 300 mg (rifampin) is imprinted RIFADIN 300.
RIFAMATE® Capsules, 300 mg rifampin and 150 mg isoniazid is imprinted RIFAMATE.
RIFATER® Tablets, 120 mg rifampin, 50 mg isoniazid, and 300 mg pyrazinamide is imprinted RIFATER.
TECZEM extended-release tablets are coded "TECZEM 5/180".
TENUATE® Tablets, 25 mg (diethylpropion hydrochloride USP) is debossed TENUATE 25.
TENUATE® DOSPAN® Controlled-Release Tablets, 75 mg (diethylpropion hydrochloride USP) is debossed TENUATE 75.
TIAMATE 120 mg extended-release tablets are coded "TIAMATE 120".
TIAMATE 180 mg extended-release tablets are coded "TIAMATE 180".
TIAMATE 240 mg extended-release tablets are coded "TIAMATE 240".
TRENTAL® (pentoxifylline) Tablets are imprinted "TRENTAL".

ALLEGRA™ ℞
[ə-'lĕgra]
(fexofenadine hydrochloride) Capsules
60 mg

Prescribing Information as of December 1996

Continued on next page

Allegra—Cont.

DESCRIPTION

Fexofenadine hydrochloride, the active ingredient of ALLEGRA™, is a histamine H_1-receptor antagonist with the chemical name (±)-4-[1-hydroxy-4-[4-(hydroxydiphenylmethyl)-1-piperidinyl]-butyl]-α,α-dimethyl benzeneacetic acid hydrochloride. It has the following chemical structure:

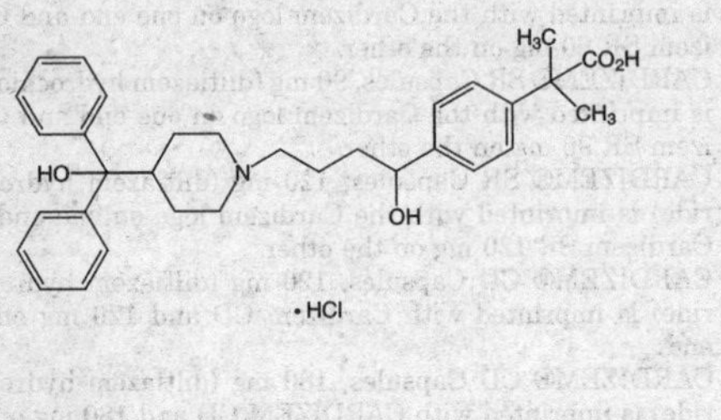

The molecular weight is 538.13 and the empirical formula is $C_{32}H_{39}NO_4$•HCl. Fexofenadine hydrochloride is a white to off-white crystalline powder. It is freely soluble in methanol and ethanol, slightly soluble in chloroform and water, and insoluble in hexane. Fexofenadine hydrochloride is a racemate and exists as a zwitterion in aqueous media at physiological pH. ALLEGRA™ is formulated as capsules for oral administration. Each capsule contains 60 mg fexofenadine hydrochloride and the following excipients: croscarmellose sodium, gelatin, lactose, microcrystalline cellulose, and pregelatinized starch. The printed capsule shell is made from gelatin, iron oxide, silicon dioxide, sodium lauryl sulfate, titanium dioxide, and other ingredients.

CLINICAL PHARMACOLOGY

Mechanism of Action

Fexofenadine, a metabolite of terfenadine, is an antihistamine with selective peripheral H_1-receptor antagonist activity. Fexofenadine inhibited antigen-induced bronchospasm in sensitized guinea pigs and histamine release from peritoneal mast cells in rats. In laboratory animals, no anticholinergic or alpha$_1$-adrenergic-receptor blocking effects were observed. Moreover, no sedative or other central nervous system effects were observed. Radiolabeled tissue distribution studies in rats indicated that fexofenadine does not cross the blood-brain barrier.

Pharmacokinetics

Fexofenadine hydrochloride was rapidly absorbed following oral administration of a single dose of two 60-mg capsules to healthy male volunteers with a mean time to maximum plasma concentration occurring at 2.6 hours postdose. After administration of a single 60-mg dose as an oral solution to healthy subjects, the mean plasma concentration was 209 ng/mL. Mean steady-state peak plasma concentrations of 286 ng/mL were observed when healthy volunteers were administered multiple doses of fexofenadine hydrochloride (60 mg oral solution every 12 hours for 10 doses). Fexofenadine pharmacokinetics were linear for oral doses up to 120 mg twice daily. Although the absolute bioavailability of fexofenadine hydrochloride capsules is unknown, the capsules are bioequivalent to an oral solution. The mean elimination half-life of fexofenadine was 14.4 hours following administration of 60 mg, twice daily, to steady-state in normal volunteers.

Human mass balance studies documented a recovery of approximately 80% and 11% of the [^{14}C] fexofenadine hydrochloride dose in the feces and urine, respectively. Approximately 5% of the total dose was metabolized. Because the absolute bioavailability of fexofenadine hydrochloride has not been established, it is unknown if the fecal component represents unabsorbed drug or the result of biliary excretion.

The pharmacokinetics of fexofenadine hydrochloride in seasonal allergic rhinitis patients were similar to those in healthy subjects. Peak fexofenadine plasma concentrations were similar between adolescent (12–16 years of age) and adult patients.

Fexofenadine is 60% to 70% bound to plasma proteins, primarily albumin and α_1-acid glycoprotein.

Special Populations

Special population pharmacokinetics (for age and renal and hepatic impairment), obtained after a single dose of 80 mg fexofenadine hydrochloride, were compared to those from normal subjects in a separate study of similar design. While subject weights were relatively uniform between studies, these special population patients were substantially older than the healthy, young volunteers. Thus, an age effect may be confounding the pharmacokinetic differences observed in some of the special populations.

Effect of Age. In older subjects (≥ 65 years old), peak plasma levels of fexofenadine were 99% greater than those observed in normal volunteers (< 65 years old). Mean elimination half-lives were similar to those observed in normal volunteers.

Renally Impaired. In patients with mild (creatinine clearance 41–80 mL/min) to severe (creatinine clearance 11–40 mL/min) renal impairment, peak plasma levels of fexofenadine were 87% and 111% greater, respectively, and mean elimination half-lives were 59% and 72% longer, respectively, than observed in normal volunteers. Peak plasma levels in patients on dialysis (creatinine clearance ≤ 10 mL/min) were 82% greater and half-life was 31% longer than observed in normal volunteers. Based on increases in bioavailability and half-life, a dose of 60 mg once daily is recommended as the starting dose in patients with decreased renal function. (See DOSAGE AND ADMINISTRATION.)

Hepatically Impaired. The pharmacokinetics of fexofenadine hydrochloride in patients with hepatic disease did not differ substantially from that observed in healthy subjects.

Effect of Gender. Across several trials, no clinically significant gender-related differences were observed in the pharmacokinetics of fexofenadine.

Pharmacodynamics

Wheal and Flare. Human histamine skin wheal and flare studies following single and twice daily doses of 20 mg and 40 mg fexofenadine hydrochloride demonstrated that the drug exhibits an antihistamine effect by 1 hour, achieves maximum effect at 2–3 hours, and an effect is still seen at 12 hours. There was no evidence of tolerance to these effects after 28 days of dosing.

Effects on QTc. In dogs, (10 mg/kg/day, orally for 5 days) and rabbits (10 mg/kg, intravenously over one hour) fexofenadine did not prolong QTc at plasma concentrations that were at least 28 and 63 times, respectively, the therapeutic plasma concentrations in man (based on a 60 mg twice daily fexofenadine hydrochloride dose). No effect was observed on calcium channel current, delayed K^+ channel current, or action potential duration in guinea pig myocytes, Na^+ current in rat neonatal myocytes, or on the delayed rectifier K^+ channel cloned from human heart at concentrations up to 1×10^{-5} M of fexofenadine. This concentration was at least 32 times the therapeutic plasma concentration in man (based on a 60-mg twice daily fexofenadine hydrochloride dose).

No statistically significant increase in mean QTc interval compared to placebo was observed in 714 seasonal allergic rhinitis patients given fexofenadine hydrochloride capsules in doses of 60 mg to 240 mg twice daily for two weeks or in 40 healthy volunteers given fexofenadine hydrochloride as an oral solution at doses up to 400 mg twice daily for 6 days.

Clinical Studies

In three, 2-week, multi-center, randomized, double-blind, placebo-controlled trials in patients 12–68 years of age with seasonal allergic rhinitis (n=1634), fexofenadine hydrochloride 60 mg twice daily significantly reduced total symptom scores (the sum of the individual scores for sneezing, rhinorrhea, itchy nose/palate/throat, itchy/watery/red eyes) compared to placebo. Statistically significant reductions in symptom scores were observed following the first 60-mg dose, with the effect maintained throughout the 12-hour interval. In general, there was no additional reduction in total symptom scores with higher doses of fexofenadine up to 240 mg twice daily. Although the number of subjects in some of the subgroups was small, there were no significant differences in the effect of fexofenadine hydrochloride across subgroups of patients defined by gender, age, and race. Onset of action for reduction in total symptom scores, excluding nasal congestion, was observed at 60 minutes compared to placebo following a single 60-mg fexofenadine hydrochloride dose administered to patients with seasonal allergic rhinitis who were exposed to ragweed pollen in an environmental exposure unit.

INDICATIONS AND USAGE

ALLEGRA™ is indicated for the relief of symptoms associated with seasonal allergic rhinitis in adults and children 12 years of age and older. Symptoms treated effectively include sneezing, rhinorrhea, itchy nose/palate/throat, itchy/watery/red eyes.

CONTRAINDICATIONS

ALLEGRA™ is contraindicated in patients with known hypersensitivity to any of its ingredients.

PRECAUTIONS

Drug Interactions

In two separate studies, fexofenadine hydrochloride 120 mg twice daily (twice the recommended dose) was co-administered with erythromycin 500 mg every 8 hours or ketoconazole 400 mg once daily under steady-state conditions to normal, healthy volunteers (n=24, each study). No differences in adverse events or QTc interval were observed when subjects were administered fexofenadine hydrochloride alone or in combination with erythromycin or ketoconazole. The findings of these studies are summarized in the following table:

Effects on Steady-State Fexofenadine Pharmacokinetics After 7 Days of Co-Administration with Fexofenadine Hydrochloride 120 mg Every 12 Hours (twice recommended dose) in Normal Volunteers (n=24)

Concomitant Drug	$C_{max,SS}$ *(Peak plasma concentration)*	$AUC_{SS}(0–12h)$ *(Extent of systemic exposure)*
Erythromycin (500 mg every 8 hrs)	+82%	+109%
Ketoconazole (400 mg once daily)	+135%	+164%

The mechanisms of these interactions are unknown, and the potential for interaction with other azole antifungal or macrolide agents has not been studied. These changes in plasma levels were within the range of plasma levels achieved in adequate and well-controlled clinical trials. Fexofenadine had no effect on the pharmacokinetics of erythromycin or ketoconazole.

Carcinogenesis, Mutagenesis, Impairment of Fertility

The carcinogenic potential and reproductive toxicity of fexofenadine hydrochloride were assessed using terfenadine studies with adequate fexofenadine exposure (based on plasma area-under-the-curve [AUC] values). No evidence of carcinogenicity was observed when mice and rats were given daily oral doses of 50 and 150 mg/kg of terfenadine for 18 and 24 months, respectively; these doses resulted in plasma AUC values of fexofenadine that were up to four times the human therapeutic value (based on a 60-mg twice-daily fexofenadine hydrochloride dose).

In in-vitro (Bacterial Reverse Mutation, CHO/HGPRT Forward Mutation, and Rat Lymphocyte Chromosomal Aberration assays) and in-vivo (Mouse Bone Marrow Micronucleus assay) tests, fexofenadine hydrochloride revealed no evidence of mutagenicity.

In rat fertility studies, dose-related reductions in implants and increases in postimplantation losses were observed at oral doses equal to or greater than 150 mg/kg of terfenadine; these doses produced plasma AUC values of fexofenadine that were equal to or greater than three times the human therapeutic value (based on a 60-mg twice-daily fexofenadine hydrochloride dose).

Pregnancy

Teratogenic Effects: Category C. There was no evidence of teratogenicity in rats or rabbits at oral terfenadine doses up to 300 mg/kg; these doses produced fexofenadine plasma AUC values that were up to 4 and 37 times the human therapeutic value (based on a 60-mg twice-daily fexofenadine hydrochloride dose), respectively.

There are no adequate and well-controlled studies in pregnant women. Fexofenadine hydrochloride should be used during pregnancy only if the potential benefit justifies the potential risk to the fetus.

Nonteratogenic Effects. Dose-related decreases in pup weight gain and survival were observed in rats exposed to oral doses equal to and greater than 150 mg/kg of terfenadine; at these doses the plasma AUC values of fexofenadine were equal to or greater than 3 times the human therapeutic values (based on a 60-mg twice-daily fexofenadine hydrochloride dose).

Nursing Mothers

There are no adequate and well-controlled studies in women during lactation. Because many drugs are excreted in human milk, caution should be exercised when fexofenadine hydrochloride is administered to a nursing woman.

Pediatric Use

Safety and effectiveness of ALLEGRA™ in pediatric patients under the age of 12 years have not been established. Across well-controlled clinical trials in patients with seasonal allergic rhinitis, a total of 205 patients between the ages of 12 to 16 years received doses ranging from 20 mg to 240 mg twice daily for up to two weeks. Adverse events were similar in this group compared to patients above the age of 16 years.

Geriatric Use

In placebo-controlled trials, 42 patients, age 60 to 68 years, received doses of 20 mg to 240 mg of fexofenadine twice daily for up to two weeks. Adverse events were similar in this group to patients under age 60 years.

ADVERSE REACTIONS

In placebo-controlled clinical trials, which included 2461 patients receiving fexofenadine hydrochloride at doses of 20 mg to 240 mg twice daily, adverse events were similar in fexofenadine hydrochloride and placebo-treated patients. The incidence of adverse events, including drowsiness, was not dose related and was similar across subgroups defined by age, gender, and race. The percent of patients who withdrew prematurely because of adverse events was 2.2% with fexofenadine hydrochloride vs 3.3% with placebo. All adverse events that were reported by greater than 1% of patients who received the recommended daily dose of fexofena-

dine hydrochloride (60 mg twice-daily), and that were more common with fexofenadine than placebo, are listed in the following table.

Adverse Experiences Reported in Placebo-Controlled Seasonal Allergic Rhinitis Clinical Trials at Rates of Greater Than 1%

Adverse Experience	*Fexofenadine 60 mg Twice Daily (n=679)*	*Placebo Twice Daily (n=671)*
Viral Infection (cold, flu)	2.5%	1.5%
Nausea	1.6%	1.5%
Dysmenorrhea	1.5%	0.3%
Drowsiness	1.3%	0.9%
Dyspepsia	1.3%	0.6%
Fatigue	1.3%	0.9%

Adverse events occurring in greater than 1% of fexofenadine hydrochloride-treated patients (60 mg twice daily), but that were more common in the placebo-treated group, include headache and throat irritation.
The frequency and magnitude of laboratory abnormalities were similar in fexofenadine hydrochloride and placebo-treated patients.

OVERDOSAGE

Information regarding acute overdosage is limited to experience from clinical trials conducted during the development of ALLEGRA™. Single doses of fexofenadine hydrochloride up to 800 mg (6 normal volunteers at this dose level), and doses up to 690 mg twice daily for one month (3 normal volunteers at this dose level), were administered without the development of clinically significant adverse events.
In the event of overdose, consider standard measures to remove any unabsorbed drug. Symptomatic and supportive treatment is recommended.
Hemodialysis did not effectively remove fexofenadine from blood (up to 1.7% removed) following terfenadine administration.
No deaths occurred at oral doses of fexofenadine hydrochloride up to 5000 mg/kg in mice (170 times the maximum recommended human daily oral dose based on mg/m^2) and up to 5000 mg/kg in rats (330 times the maximum recommended human daily oral dose based on mg/m^2). Additionally, no clinical signs of toxicity or gross pathological findings were observed. In dogs, no evidence of toxicity was observed at oral doses up to 2000 mg/kg (450 times the maximum recommended human daily oral dose based on mg/m^2).

DOSAGE AND ADMINISTRATION

The recommended dose of ALLEGRA™ is 60 mg twice daily for adults and children 12 years of age and older.
A dose of 60 mg once daily is recommended as the starting dose in patients with decreased renal function. (See CLINICAL PHARMACOLOGY.)

HOW SUPPLIED

ALLEGRA™ 60-mg capsules are available in: high-density polyethylene (HDPE) bottles of 60 (NDC 0088-1102-41); HDPE bottles of 100 (NDC 0088-1102-47); HDPE bottles of 500 (NDC 0088-1102-55); and aluminum-foil blister packs of 100 (NDC 0088-1102-49).
ALLEGRA™ capsules have a white opaque cap and a pink opaque body. The capsules are imprinted in black ink, with "60 mg" on the cap, and "1102" on the body or "allegra" on the cap and "60 mg" on the body.
Store ALLEGRA™ capsules at controlled room temperature 20–25°C (68–77°F). Foil-backed blister packs should be protected from excessive moisture.
Prescribing information as of December 1996
Hoechst Marion Roussel, Inc.
Kansas City, MO 64137 USA
US Patents 4,254,129; 5,375,693; 5,578,610.

Shown in Product Identification Guide, page 315

ALLEGRA-D™ ℞

[ə-'lĕgra-D]
(fexofenadine HCl 60 mg and pseudoephedrine HCl 120 mg) Extended-Release Tablets

Prescribing Information as of December 1997d

DESCRIPTION

ALLEGRA-D (fexofenadine hydrochloride and pseudoephedrine hydrochloride) Extended-Release Tablets for oral administration contain 60 mg fexofenadine hydrochloride for immediate-release and 120 mg pseudoephedrine hydrochloride for extended-release. Tablets also contain as excipients: microcrystalline cellulose, pregelatinized starch, croscarmellose sodium, magnesium stearate, carnauba wax, stearic acid, silicon dioxide, hydroxypropyl methylcellulose and polyethylene glycol.

Fexofenadine hydrochloride, one of the active ingredients of ALLEGRA-D, is a histamine H_1-receptor antagonist with the chemical name (±)-4-[1-hydroxy-4-[4-(hydroxydiphenylmethyl)-1-piperidinyl]-butyl]-α, α-dimethyl benzeneacetic acid hydrochloride and the following chemical structure:

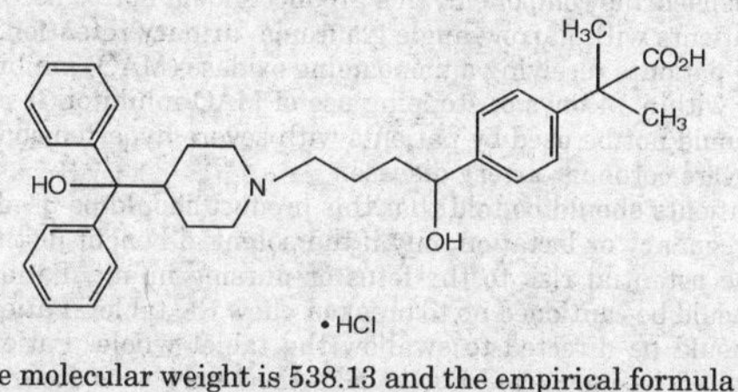

The molecular weight is 538.13 and the empirical formula is $C_{32}H_{39}NO_4$•HCl. Fexofenadine hydrochloride is a white to off-white crystalline powder. It is freely soluble in methanol and ethanol, slightly soluble in chloroform and water, and insoluble in hexane. Fexofenadine hydrochloride is a racemate and exists as a zwitterion in aqueous media at physiological pH.
Pseudoephedrine hydrochloride, the other active ingredient of ALLEGRA-D, is an adrenergic (vasoconstrictor) agent with the chemical name [S-(R*,R*)-α-[1-(methylamino) ethyl]-benzenemethanol hydrochloride and the following chemical structure:

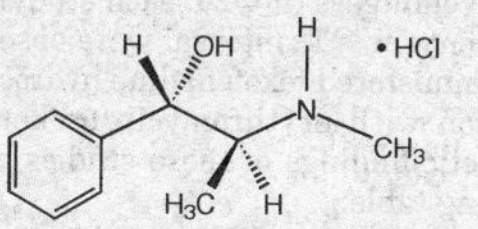

The molecular weight is 201.70. The molecular formula is $C_{10}H_{15}NO$•HCl. Pseudoephedrine hydrochloride occurs as fine, white to off-white crystals or powder, having a faint characteristic odor. It is very soluble in water, freely soluble in alcohol, and sparingly soluble in chloroform.

CLINICAL PHARMACOLOGY

Mechanism of Action

Fexofenadine hydrochloride, the major active metabolite of terfenadine, is an antihistamine with selective peripheral H_1-receptor antagonist activity. Fexofenadine hydrochloride inhibited antigen-induced bronchospasm in sensitized guinea pigs and histamine release from peritoneal mast cells in rats. In laboratory animals, no anticholinergic or alpha$_1$-adrenergic-receptor blocking effects were observed. Moreover, no sedative or other central nervous system effects were observed. Radiolabeled tissue distribution studies in rats indicated that fexofenadine does not cross the blood-brain barrier.
Pseudoephedrine hydrochloride is an orally active sympathomimetic amine and exerts a decongestant action on the nasal mucosa. Pseudoephedrine hydrochloride is recognized as an effective agent for the relief of nasal congestion due to allergic rhinitis. Pseudoephedrine produces peripheral effects similar to those of ephedrine and central effects similar to, but less intense than, amphetamines. It has the potential for excitatory side effects. At the recommended oral dose, it has little or no pressor effect in normotensive adults.

Pharmacokinetics

The pharmacokinetics of fexofenadine hydrochloride and pseudoephedrine hydrochloride when administered separately have been well characterized. Fexofenadine pharmacokinetics were linear for oral doses of fexofenadine hydrochloride up to 120 mg twice daily. The mean elimination half-life of fexofenadine was 14.4 hours following administration of 60 mg fexofenadine hydrochloride, twice daily, to steady-state in normal volunteers. Human mass balance studies documented a recovery of approximately 80% and 11% of the [^{14}C] fexofenadine hydrochloride dose in the feces and urine, respectively. Approximately 5% of the total dose was metabolized. Because the absolute bioavailability of fexofenadine hydrochloride has not been established, it is unknown if the fecal component is unabsorbed drug or the result of biliary excretion. The pharmacokinetics of fexofenadine hydrochloride in seasonal allergic rhinitis patients were similar to those in healthy subjects. Peak fexofenadine plasma concentrations were similar between adolescent (12–16 years of age) and adult patients.
Fexofenadine is 60% to 70% bound to plasma proteins, primarily albumin and α_1-acid glycoprotein.
Pseudoephedrine has been shown to have a mean elimination half-life of 4–6 hours which is dependent on urine pH. The elimination half-life is decreased at urine pH lower than 6 and may be increased at urine pH higher than 8.
The bioavailability of fexofenadine hydrochloride and pseudoephedrine hydrochloride from ALLEGRA-D Extended-Release Tablets is similar to that achieved with separate administration of the components. Coadministration of fexofenadine and pseudoephedrine does not significantly affect the bioavailability of either component.
Fexofenadine hydrochloride was rapidly absorbed following single-dose administration of the 60 mg fexofenadine hydrochloride/120 mg pseudoephedrine hydrochloride tablet with median time to mean maximum fexofenadine plasma concentration of 191 ng/mL occurring 2 hours postdose. Pseudoephedrine hydrochloride produced a mean single-dose pseudoephedrine peak plasma concentration of 206 ng/mL which occurred 6 hours postdose. Following multiple dosing to steady-state, a fexofenadine peak concentration of 255 ng/mL was observed 2 hours postdose. Following multiple dosing to steady-state, a pseudoephedrine peak concentration of 411 ng/mL was observed 5 hours postdose. Coadministration of ALLEGRA-D with a high-fat meal decreased fexofenadine plasma concentrations C_{max} (−46%) and AUC (−42%). Time to maximum concentration (T_{max}) was delayed by 50%. The rate or extent of pseudoephedrine absorption was not affected by food. It is recommended that the administration of ALLEGRA-D with food should be avoided. (See DOSAGE AND ADMINISTRATION).

Special Populations

Special population pharmacokinetics (for renal and hepatic impairment and age), obtained after a single dose of 80 mg fexofenadine hydrochloride, were compared to those from normal subjects in a separate study of similar design. While subject weights were relatively uniform between studies, these special population patients were substantially older than the healthy, young volunteers. Thus, an age effect may be confounding the pharmacokinetic differences observed in some of the special populations.
Effect of Age. In older subjects (≥65 years old), peak plasma levels of fexofenadine were 99% greater than those observed in younger subjects (<65 years old). Mean elimination half-lives were similar to those observed in younger subjects.
Renally Impaired. In patients with mild (creatinine clearance 41–80 mL/min) to severe (creatinine clearance 11–40 mL/min) renal impairment, peak plasma levels of fexofenadine were 87% and 111% greater, respectively, and mean elimination half-lives were 59% and 72% longer, respectively, than observed in normal volunteers. Peak plasma levels in patients on dialysis (creatinine clearance ≤10 mL / min) were 82% greater and half-life was 31% longer than observed in normal volunteers.
About 55–75% of an administered dose of pseudoephedrine hydrochloride is excreted unchanged in the urine; the remainder is apparently metabolized in the liver. Therefore, pseudoephedrine may accumulate in patients with renal insufficiency.
Based on increases in bioavailability and half-life of fexofenadine hydrochloride and pseudoephedrine hydrochloride, a dose of one tablet once daily is recommended as the starting dose in patients with decreased renal function (see DOSAGE AND ADMINISTRATION).
Hepatically Impaired. The pharmacokinetics of fexofenadine hydrochloride in patients with hepatic disease did not differ substantially from that observed in healthy subjects. The effect on pseudoephedrine pharmacokinetics is unknown.
Effect of Gender. Across several trials, no clinically significant gender-related differences were observed in the pharmacokinetics of fexofenadine hydrochloride.

Pharmacodynamics

Wheal and Flare. Human histamine skin wheal and flare studies following single and twice daily doses of 20 mg and 40 mg fexofenadine hydrochloride demonstrated that the drug exhibits an antihistamine effect by 1 hour, achieves maximum effect at 2–3 hours, and an effect is still seen at 12 hours. There was no evidence of tolerance to these effects after 28 days of dosing. The clinical significance of these observations is not known.
Effect on QT_c. In dogs, (10 mg/kg/day, orally for 5 days) and rabbits (10 mg/kg, intravenously over one hour) fexofenadine hydrochloride did not prolong QT_c at plasma concentrations that were at least 28 and 63 times, respectively, the therapeutic plasma concentrations in man (based on a 60 mg twice daily fexofenadine hydrochloride dose). No effect was observed on calcium channel current, delayed K^+ channel current, or action potential duration in guinea pig myocytes, Na^+ current in rat neonatal myocytes, or on the delayed rectifier K^+ channel cloned from human heart at concentrations up to 1×10^{-5} M of fexofenadine. This concentration was at least 32 times the therapeutic plasma concentration in man (based on a 60 mg twice daily fexofenadine hydrochloride dose).
No statistically significant increase in mean QT_c interval compared to placebo was observed in 714 seasonal allergic rhinitis patients given fexofenadine hydrochloride capsules in doses of 60 mg to 240 mg twice daily for two weeks or in 40 healthy volunteers given fexofenadine hydrochloride as an oral solution at doses up to 400 mg twice daily for 6 days.
A one year study designed to evaluate safety and tolerability of 240 mg of fexofenadine hydrochloride (n = 240) compared to placebo (n = 237) in healthy subjects, did not reveal a statistically significant increase in the mean QT_c interval for the fexofenadine hydrochloride treated group when evaluated pretreatment and after 1, 2, 3, 6, 9, and 12 months of treatment.

Continued on next page

Allegra-D—Cont.

Administration of the 60 mg fexofenadine hydrochloride/120 mg pseudoephedrine hydrochloride combination tablet for approximately 2 weeks to 213 patients with seasonal allergic rhinitis demonstrated no statistically significant increase in the mean QT$_c$ interval compared to fexofenadine hydrochloride administered alone (60 mg twice daily, n = 215), or compared to pseudoephedrine hydrochloride (120 mg twice daily, n = 215) administered alone.

Clinical Studies

In a 2-week, multicenter, randomized, double-blind, active-controlled trial in patients 12–65 years of age with seasonal allergic rhinitis due to ragweed allergy (n = 651), the 60 mg fexofenadine hydrochloride/120 mg pseudoephedrine hydrochloride combination tablet administered twice daily significantly reduced the intensity of sneezing, rhinorrhea, itchy nose/palate/throat, itchy/watery/red eyes, and nasal congestion.

In three, 2-week, multicenter, randomized, double-blind, placebo-controlled trials in patients 12–68 years of age with seasonal allergic rhinitis (n = 1634), fexofenadine hydrochloride 60 mg twice daily significantly reduced total symptom scores (the sum of the individual scores for sneezing, rhinorrhea, itchy nose/palate/throat, itchy/watery/red eyes) compared to placebo. Statistically significant reductions in symptom scores were observed following the first 60 mg dose, with the effect maintained throughout the 12-hour interval. In general, there was no additional reduction in total symptom scores with higher doses of fexofenadine hydrochloride up to 240 mg twice daily. Although the number of subjects in some of the subgroups was small, there were no significant differences in the effect of fexofenadine hydrochloride across subgroups of patients defined by gender, age, and race. Onset of action for reduction in total symptom scores, excluding nasal congestion, was observed at 60 minutes compared to placebo following a single 60 mg fexofenadine hydrochloride dose administered to patients with seasonal allergic rhinitis who were exposed to ragweed pollen in an environmental exposure unit.

INDICATIONS AND USAGE

ALLEGRA-D is indicated for the relief of symptoms associated with seasonal allergic rhinitis in adults and children 12 years of age and older. Symptoms treated effectively include sneezing, rhinorrhea, itchy nose/palate/ and/or throat, itchy/watery/red eyes, and nasal congestion. ALLEGRA-D should be administered when both the antihistaminic properties of fexofenadine hydrochloride and the nasal decongestant properties of pseudoephedrine hydrochloride are desired (see CLINICAL PHARMACOLOGY).

CONTRAINDICATIONS

ALLEGRA-D is contraindicated in patients with known hypersensitivity to any of its ingredients.

Due to its pseudoephedrine component, ALLEGRA-D is contraindicated in patients with narrow-angle glaucoma or urinary retention, and in patients receiving monoamine oxidase (MAO) inhibitor therapy or within fourteen (14) days of stopping such treatment (see Drug Interactions section). It is also contraindicated in patients with severe hypertension, or severe coronary artery disease, and in those who have shown hypersensitivity or idiosyncrasy to its components, to adrenergic agents, or to other drugs of similar chemical structures. Manifestations of patient idiosyncrasy to adrenergic agents include: insomnia, dizziness, weakness, tremor, or arrhythmias.

WARNINGS

Sympathomimetic amines should be used judiciously and sparingly in patients with hypertension, diabetes mellitus, ischemic heart disease, increased intraocular pressure, hyperthyroidism, renal impairment, or prostatic hypertrophy (see CONTRAINDICATIONS). Sympathomimetic amines may produce central nervous system stimulation with convulsions or cardiovascular collapse with accompanying hypotension.

PRECAUTIONS

General

Due to its pseudoephedrine component, ALLEGRA-D should be used with caution in patients with hypertension, diabetes mellitus, ischemic heart disease, increased intraocular pressure, hyperthyroidism, renal impairment, or prostatic hypertrophy (see WARNINGS and CONTRAINDICATIONS). Patients with decreased renal function should be given a lower initial dose (one tablet per day) because they have reduced elimination of fexofenadine and pseudoephedrine (See CLINICAL PHARMACOLOGY and DOSAGE AND ADMINISTRATION).

Information for Patients

Patients taking ALLEGRA-D tablets should receive the following information: ALLEGRA-D tablets are prescribed for the relief of symptoms of seasonal allergic rhinitis. Patients should be instructed to take ALLEGRA-D tablets only as prescribed. **Do not exceed the recommended dose.** If nervousness, dizziness, or sleeplessness occur, discontinue use

and consult the doctor. Patients should also be advised against the concurrent use of ALLEGRA-D tablets with over-the-counter antihistamines and decongestants.

The product should not be used by patients who are hypersensitive to it or to any of its ingredients. Due to its pseudoephedrine component, this product should not be used by patients with narrow-angle glaucoma, urinary retention, or by patients receiving a monoamine oxidase (MAO) inhibitor or within 14 days of stopping use of MAO inhibitor. It also should not be used by patients with severe hypertension or severe coronary artery disease.

Patients should be told that this product should be used in pregnancy or lactation only if the potential benefit justifies the potential risk to the fetus or nursing infant. Patients should be cautioned no to break or chew the tablet. Patients should be directed to swallow the tablet whole. Patients should be instructed not to take the tablet with food. Patients should also be instructed to store the medication in a tightly closed container in a cool, dry place, away from children.

Drug Interactions

Fexofenadine hydrochloride and pseudoephedrine hydrochloride do not influence the pharmacokinetics of each other when administered concomitantly.

In two separate studies, fexofenadine hydrochloride 120 mg twice daily (twice the recommended dose) was co-administered with erythromycin 500 mg every 8 hours or ketoconazole 400 mg once daily under steady-state conditions to normal, healthy volunteers (n = 24, each study). No differences in adverse events or QT$_c$ interval were observed when subjects were administered fexofenadine hydrochloride alone or in combination with erythromycin or ketoconazole. The pharmacokinetic findings of these studies are summarized in the following table:

Effects on Steady-State Fexofenadine Pharmacokinetics After 7 Days of Co-Administration with Fexofenadine Hydrochloride 120 mg Every 12 Hours (twice recommended dose) in Normal Volunteers (n=24)

Concomitant Drug	$C_{max}SS$ (Peak plasma concentration)	$AUC_{SS}(0–12h)$ (Extent of systemic exposure)
Erythromycin (500 mg every 8 hrs)	+82%	+109%
Ketoconazole (400 mg once daily)	+135%	+164%

The mechanisms of these interactions are unknown, and the potential for interaction with other azole antifungal or macrolide agents has not been studied. These changes in plasma levels were within the range of plasma levels achieved in adequate and well-controlled clinical trials. Fexofenadine had no effect on the pharmacokinetics of erythromycin or ketoconazole.

ALLEGRA-D tablets (pseudoephedrine component) are contraindicated in patients taking monoamine oxidase inhibitors and for 14 days after stopping use of an MAO inhibitor. Concomitant use with antihypertensive drugs which interfere with sympathetic activity (eg, methyldopa, mecamylamine, and reserpine) may reduce their antihypertensive effects. Increased ectopic pacemaker activity can occur when pseudoephedrine is used concomitantly with digitalis.

Care should be taken in the administration of ALLEGRA-D concomitantly with other sympathomimetic amines because combined effects on the cardiovascular system may be harmful to the patient (see WARNINGS).

Carcinogenesis, Mutagenesis, Impairment of Fertility

There are no animal or in vitro studies on the combination product fexofenadine hydrochloride and pseudoephedrine hydrochloride to evaluate carcinogenesis, mutagenesis, or impairment of fertility.

The carcinogenic potential and reproductive toxicity of fexofenadine hydrochloride were assessed using terfenadine studies with adequate fexofenadine exposure (area-under-the plasma concentration versus time curve [AUC]). No evidence of carcinogenicity was observed when mice and rats were given daily oral doses up to 150 mg/kg of terfenadine for 18 and 24 months, respectively. In both species, 150 mg/kg of terfenadine produced AUC values of fexofenadine that were approximately 3 times the human AUC at the maximum recommended daily oral dose in adults.

Two-year feeding studies in rats and mice conducted under the auspices of the National Toxicology Program (NTP) demonstrated no evidence of carcinogenic potential with ephedrine sulfate, a structurally related drug with pharmacological properties similar to pseudoephedrine, at doses up to 10 and 27 mg/kg, respectively (approximately 1/3 and 1/2, respectively, the maximum recommended daily oral dose of pseudoephedrine hydrochloride in adults on a mg/m² basis).

In in-vitro (Bacterial Reverse Mutation, CHO/HGPRT Forward Mutation, and Rat Lymphocyte Chromosomal Aberration assays) and in vivo (Mouse Bone Marrow Micronucleus assay) tests, fexofenadine hydrochloride revealed no evidence of mutagenicity.

Reproduction and fertility studies with terfenadine in rats produced no effect on male or female fertility at oral doses up to 300 mg/kg/day. However, reduced implants and post implantation losses were reported at 300 mg/kg. A reduction in implants was also observed at an oral dose of 150 mg/kg/day. Oral doses of 150 and 300 mg/kg of terfenadine produced AUC values of fexofenadine that were approximately 3 and 4 times, respectively, the human AUC at the maximum recommended daily oral dose in adults.

Pregnancy

Teratogenic Effects: Category C. Terfenadine alone was not teratogenic in rats and rabbits at oral doses up to 300 mg/kg; 300 mg/kg of terfenadine produced terfenadine AUC values that were approximately 4 and 30 times, respectively, the human AUC at the maximum recommended daily oral dose in adults.

The combination of terfenadine and pseudoephedrine hydrochloride in a ratio of 1:2 by weight was studied in rats and rabbits. In rats, an oral combination dose of 150/300

Adverse Experiences Reported in One Active-Controlled Seasonal Allergic Rhinitis Clinical Trial at Rates of Greater than 1%

Adverse Experience	60 mg Fexofenadine Hydrochloride/120 mg Pseudoephedrine Hydrochloride Combination Tablet Twice Daily (n=215)	Fexofenadine Hydrochloride 60 mg Twice Daily (n=218)	Pseudoephedrine Hydrochloride 120 mg Twice Daily (n=218)
Headache	13.0%	11.5%	17.4%
Insomnia	12.6%	3.2%	13.3%
Nausea	7.4%	0.5%	5.0%
Dry Mouth	2.8%	0.5%	5.5%
Dyspepsia	2.8%	0.5%	0.9%
Throat Irritation	2.3%	1.8%	0.5%
Dizziness	1.9%	0.0%	3.2%
Agitation	1.9%	0.0%	1.4%
Back Pain	1.9%	0.5%	0.5%
Palpitation	1.9%	0.0%	0.9%
Nervousness	1.4%	0.5%	1.8%
Anxiety	1.4%	0.0%	1.4%
Upper Respiratory Infection	1.4%	0.9%	0.9%
Abdominal Pain	1.4%	0.5%	0.5%

mg/kg produced reduced fetal weight and delayed ossification with a finding of wavy ribs. The dose of 150 mg/kg of terfenadine in rats produced an AUC value of fexofenadine that was approximately 3 times the human AUC at the maximum recommended daily oral dose in adults. The dose of 300 mg/kg of pseudoephedrine hydrochloride in rats was approximately 10 times the maximum recommended daily oral dose in adults on a mg/m^2 basis. In rabbits, an oral combination dose of 100/200 mg/kg produced decreased fetal weight. By extrapolation, the AUC of fexofenadine for 100 mg/kg orally of terfenadine was approximately 10 times the human AUC at the maximum recommended daily oral dose in adults. The dose of 200 mg/kg of pseudoephedrine hydrochloride was approximately 15 times the maximum recommended daily oral dose in adults on a mg/m^2 basis.

There are no adequate and well-controlled studies in pregnant women. ALLEGRA-D should be used during pregnancy only if the potential benefit justifies the potential risk to the fetus.

Nonteratogenic Effects. Dose-related decreases in pup weight gain and survival were observed in rats exposed to an oral dose of 150 mg/kg of terfenadine; this dose produced an AUC of fexofenadine that was approximately 3 times the human AUC at the maximum recommended daily oral dose in adults.

Nursing Mothers

It is not known if fexofenadine is excreted in human milk. Because many drugs are excreted in human milk, caution should be used when fexofenadine hydrochloride is administered to a nursing woman. Pseudoephedrine hydrochloride administered alone distributes into breast milk of lactating human females. Pseudoephedrine concentrations in milk are consistently higher than those in plasma. The total amount of drug in milk as judged by AUC is 2 to 3 times greater than the plasma AUC. The fraction of a pseudoephedrine dose excreted in milk is estimated to be 0.4% to 0.7%. A decision should be made whether to discontinue nursing or to discontinue the drug, taking into account the importance of the drug to the mother. Caution should be exercised when ALLEGRA-D is administered to nursing women.

Pediatric Use

Safety and effectiveness of ALLEGRA-D in pediatric patients under the age of 12 years have not been established.

Geriatric Use

Clinical studies of ALLEGRA-D did not include sufficient numbers of patients aged 65 and older to determine whether they respond differently from younger patients. Other reported clinical experience has not identified differences in responses between the elderly and younger patients, although the elderly are more likely to have adverse reactions to sympathomimetic amines. In general, dose selection for an elderly patient should be cautious, usually starting at the low end of the dosing range, reflecting the greater frequency of decreased hepatic, renal, or cardiac function, and of concomitant disease or other drug therapy. The pseudoephedrine component of ALLEGRA-D is known to be substantially excreted by the kidney, and the risk of toxic reactions to this drug may be greater in patients with impaired renal function. Because elderly patients are more likely to have decreased renal function, care should be taken in dose selection, and it may be useful to monitor renal function.

ADVERSE REACTIONS

ALLEGRA-D

In one clinical trial (n = 651) in which 215 patients with seasonal allergic rhinitis received the 60 mg fexofenadine hydrochloride/120 mg pseudoephedrine hydrochloride combination tablet twice daily for up to 2 weeks, adverse events were similar to those reported either in patients receiving fexofenadine hydrochloride 60 mg alone (n = 218 patients) or in patients receiving pseudoephedrine hydrochloride 120 mg alone (n = 218). A placebo group was not included in this study.

The percent of patients who withdrew prematurely because of adverse events was 3.7% for the fexofenadine hydrochloride/pseudoephedrine hydrochloride combination group, 0.5% for the fexofenadine hydrochloride group, and 4.1% for the pseudoephedrine hydrochloride group. All adverse events that were reported by greater than 1% of patients who received the recommended daily dose of the fexofenadine hydrochloride/pseudoephedrine hydrochloride combination are listed in the following table.

[See table at bottom of previous page]

Many of the adverse events occurring in the fexofenadine hydrochloride/pseudoephedrine hydrochloride combination group were adverse events also reported predominately in the pseudoephedrine hydrochloride group, such as insomnia, headache, nausea, dry mouth, dizziness, agitation, nervousness, anxiety, and palpitation.

Fexofenadine Hydrochloride

In placebo-controlled clinical trials, which included 2461 patients receiving fexofenadine hydrochloride at doses of 20 mg to 240 mg twice daily, adverse events were similar in fexofenadine hydrochloride and placebo-treated patients. The incidence of adverse events, including drowsiness, was not dose related and was similar across subgroups defined by age, gender, and race. The percent of patients who withdrew prematurely because of adverse events was 2.2% with fexofenadine hydrochloride vs 3.3% with placebo.

Pseudoephedrine Hydrochloride

Pseudoephedrine hydrochloride may cause mild CNS stimulation in hypersensitive patients. Nervousness, excitability, restlessness, dizziness, weakness, or insomnia may occur. Headache, drowsiness, tachycardia, palpitation, pressor activity, and cardiac arrhythmias have been reported. Sympathomimetic drugs have also been associated with other untoward effects such as fear, anxiety, tenseness, tremor, hallucinations, seizures, pallor, respiratory difficulty, dysuria, and cardiovascular collapse.

OVERDOSAGE

Information regarding acute overdosage is limited to experience from clinical trials conducted during the development of ALLEGRA and the marketing history of pseudoephedrine hydrochloride. Single doses of fexofenadine hydrochloride up to 800 mg (6 normal volunteers at this dose level), and doses up to 690 mg twice daily for one month (3 normal volunteers at this dose level), were administered without the development of clinically significant adverse events.

In large doses, sympathomimetics may give rise to giddiness, headache, nausea, vomiting, sweating, thirst, tachycardia, precordial pain, palpitations, difficulty in micturition, muscular weakness and tenseness, anxiety, restlessness, and insomnia. Many patients can present a toxic psychosis with delusions and hallucinations. Some may develop cardiac arrhythmias, circulatory collapse, convulsions, coma, and respiratory failure.

In the event of overdose, consider standard measures to remove any unabsorbed drug. Symptomatic and supportive treatment is recommended. Hemodialysis did not effectively remove fexofenadine from blood (up to 1.7% removed) following terfenadine administration.

The effect of hemodialysis on the removal of pseudoephedrine is unknown.

No deaths occurred in mature mice and rats at oral doses of fexofenadine hydrochloride up to 5000 mg/kg (approximately 170 and 340 times, respectively, the maximum recommended daily oral dose in adults on a mg/m^2 basis.) The median oral lethal dose in newborn rats was 438 mg/kg (approximately 30 times the maximum recommended daily oral dose in adults on a mg/m^2 basis). In dogs, no evidence of toxicity was observed at oral doses up to 2000 mg/kg (approximately 450 times the maximum recommended human daily oral dose in adults on a mg/m^2 basis). The oral median lethal dose of pseudoephedrine hydrochloride in rats was 1674 mg/kg (approximately 55 times the maximum recommended daily oral dose in adults on a mg/m^2 basis).

DOSAGE AND ADMINISTRATION

The recommended dose of ALLEGRA-D is one tablet twice daily for adults and children 12 years of age and older. It is recommended that the administration of ALLEGRA-D with food should be avoided. A dose of one tablet once daily is recommended as the starting dose in patients with decreased renal function. (See CLINICAL PHARMACOLOGY and PRECAUTIONS.)

HOW SUPPLIED

ALLEGRA-D (fexofenadine hydrochloride and pseudoephedrine hydrochloride) Extended-Release Tablets are available in: high-density polyethylene (HDPE) bottles of 60 (NDC 0088-1090-41) with a polypropylene child-resistant cap containing a pulp/wax liner with heat-sealed foil inner seal; HDPE bottles of 100 (NDC 0088-1090-47) with a polypropylene screw cap containing a pulp/wax liner with heat-sealed foil inner seal; HDPE bottles of 500 (NDC 0088-1090-55) with a polypropylene screw cap containing a pulp/wax liner with heat-sealed foil inner seal; and aluminum foil-backed clear blister packs of 100 (NDC 0088-1090-49).

ALLEGRA-D is a two-layer tablet, one white layer and one tan layer with a clear film coating on the tablet. The tablets are engraved with "Allegra-D" on the white layer.

Store ALLEGRA-D Extended-Release Tablets at 20–25°C (68–77°F).

(See USP Controlled Room Temperature.)

Prescribing Information as of December 1997d

Hoechst Marion Roussel, Inc.

Kansas City, MO 64137 USA

US Patents 4,254,129; 5,375,693; 5,578,610.

Shown in Product Identification Guide, page 315

ALTACE® ℞

[ŏl'tās]

(ramipril)*

Prescribing Information as of June 1996

USE IN PREGNANCY

When used in pregnancy during the second and third trimesters, ACE inhibitors can cause injury and even death to the developing fetus. When pregnancy is detected, ALTACE® should be discontinued as soon as possible. **See WARNINGS: Fetal/neonatal morbidity and mortality.**

DESCRIPTION

Ramipril is a 2-aza-bicyclo [3.3.0]-octane-3-carboxylic acid derivative. It is a white, crystalline substance soluble in polar organic solvents and buffered aqueous solutions. Ramipril melts between 105° C and 112° C.

The CAS Registry Number is 87333-19-5. Ramipril's chemical name is (2*S*,3a*S*,6a*S*)-1[(*S*)-*N*-[(*S*)-1-Carboxy-3-phenylpropyl]alanyl]octahydrocyclopenta[*b*]pyrrole-2-carboxylic acid, 1-ethyl ester; its structural formula is:

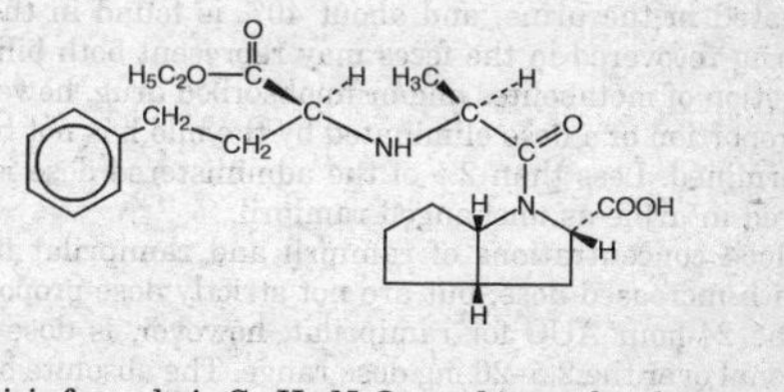

Its empiric formula is $C_{23}H_{32}N_2O_5$, and its molecular weight is 416.5.

Ramiprilat, the diacid metabolite of ramipril, is a non-sulfhydryl angiotensin converting enzyme inhibitor. Ramipril is converted to ramiprilat by hepatic cleavage of the ester group.

ALTACE® (ramipril) is supplied as hard shell capsules for oral administration containing 1.25 mg, 2.5 mg, 5 mg, and 10 mg of ramipril. The inactive ingredients present are pregelatinized starch NF, gelatin, and titanium dioxide. The 1.25 mg capsule shell contains yellow iron oxide, the 2.5 mg capsule shell contains D&C yellow #10 and FD&C red #40, the 5 mg capsule shell contains FD&C blue #1 and FD&C red #40, and the 10 mg capsule shell contains FD&C blue #1.

CLINICAL PHARMACOLOGY

Mechanism of Action

Ramipril and ramiprilat inhibit angiotensin-converting enzyme (ACE) in human subjects and animals. ACE is a peptidyl dipeptidase that catalyzes the conversion of anigotensin I to the vasoconstrictor substance, angiotensin II. Angiotensin II also stimulates aldosterone secretion by the adrenal cortex. Inhibition of ACE results in decreased plasma angiotensin II, which leads to decreased vasopressor activity and to decreased aldosterone secretion. The latter decrease may result in a small increase of serum potassium. In hypertensive patients with normal renal function treated with ALTACE® alone for up to 56 weeks, approximately 4% of patients during the trial had an abnormally high serum potassium and an increase from baseline greater than 0.75 mEq/L, and none of the patients had an abnormally low potassium and a decrease from baseline greater than 0.75 mEq/L. In the same study, approximately 2% of patients treated with ALTACE® and hydrochlorothiazide for up to 56 weeks had abnormally high potassium values and an increase from baseline of 0.75 mEq/L or greater, and approximately 2% had abnormally low values and decreases from baseline of 0.75 mEq/L or greater. (See PRECAUTIONS.)

Removal of angiotensin II negative feedback on renin secretion leads to increased plasma renin activity.

The effect of ramipril on hypertension appears to result at least in part from inhibition of both issue and circulating ACE activity, thereby reducing antiotensin II formation in tissue and plasma.

ACE is identical to kininase, an enzyme that degrades bradykinin. Whether increased levels of bradykinin, a potent vasodepressor peptide, play a role in the therapeutic effects of ALTACE® remains to be elucidated.

While the mechanism through which ALTACE® lowers blood pressure is believed to be primarily suppression of the renin-angiotensin-aldosterone system, ALTACE® has an antihypertensive effect even in patients with low-renin hypertension. Although ALTACE® was antihypertensive in all races studied, black hypertensive patients (usually a low-renin hypertensive population) had a smaller average response to monotherapy than non-black patients.

Pharmacokinetics and Metabolism

Following oral administration of ALTACE®, peak plasma concentrations of ramipril are reached within one hour. The extent of absorption is at least 50–60% and is not significantly influenced by the presence of food in the GI tract, although the rate of absorption is reduced.

In a trial in which subjects received ALTACE® capsules or the contents of identical capsules dissolved in water, dissolved in apple juice, or suspended in apple sauce, serum ramiprilat levels were essentially unrelated to the use or nonuse of the concomitant liquid or food.

Continued on next page

Altace—Cont.

Cleavage of the ester group (primarily in the liver) converts ramipril to its active diacid metabolite, ramiprilat. Peak plasma concentrations of ramiprilat are reached 2–4 hours after drug intake. The serum protein binding of ramipril is about 73% and that of ramiprilat about 56%; in vitro, these percentages are independent of concentration over the range of 0.01 to 10µg/mL.

Ramipril is almost completely metabolized to ramiprilat, which has about 6 times the ACE inhibitory activity of ramipril, and to the diketopiperazine ester, the diketopiperazine acid, and the glucuronides of ramipril and ramiprilat, all of which are inactive. After oral administration of ramipril, about 60% of the parent drug and its metabolites are eliminated in the urine, and about 40% is found in the feces. Drug recovered in the feces may represent both biliary excretion of metabolites and/or unabsorbed drug, however the proportion of a dose eliminated by the bile has not been determined. Less than 2% of the administered dose is recovered in urine as unchanged ramipril.

Blood concentrations of ramipril and ramiprilat increase with increased dose, but are not strictly dose-proportional. The 24-hour AUC for ramiprilat, however, is dose-proportional over the 2.5–20 mg dose range. The absolute bioavailabilities of ramipril and ramiprilat were 28% and 44%, respectively, when 5 mg of oral ramipril was compared with the same dose of ramipril given intravenously.

Plasma concentrations of ramiprilat decline in a triphasic manner (initial rapid decline, apparent elimination phase, terminal elimination phase). The initial rapid decline, which represents distribution of the drug into a large peripheral compartment and subsequent binding to both plasma and tissue ACE, has a half-life of 2–4 hours. Because of its potent binding to ACE and slow dissociation from the enzyme, ramiprilat shows two elimination phases. The apparent elimination phase corresponds to the clearance of free ramiprilat and has a half-life of 9–18 hours. The terminal elimination phase has a prolonged half-life (>50 hours) and probably represents the binding/dissociation kinetics of the ramiprilat/ACE complex. It does not contribute to the accumulation of the drug. After multiple daily doses of ramipril 5–10 mg, the half-life of ramiprilat concentrations within the therapeutic range was 13–17 hours.

After once-daily dosing, steady-state plasma concentrations of ramiprilat are reached by the fourth dose. Steady-state concentrations of ramiprilat are somewhat higher than those seen after the first dose of ALTACE®, especially at low doses (2.5 mg), but the difference is clinically insignificant. In patients with creatinine clearance less than 40 ml/min/1.73m², peak levels of ramiprilat are approximately doubled, and trough levels may be as much as quintupled. In multiple-dose regimens, the total exposure to ramiprilat (AUC) in these patients is 3–4 times as large as it is in patients with normal renal function who receive similar doses. The urinary excretion of ramipril, ramiprilat, and their metabolites is reduced in patients with impaired renal function. Compared to normal subjects, patients with creatinine clearance less than 40 ml/min/1.73m² had higher peak and trough ramiprilat levels and slightly longer times to peak concentrations. (See DOSAGE AND ADMINISTRATION.)

In patients with impaired liver function, the metabolism of ramipril to ramiprilat appears to be slowed, possibly because of diminished activity of hepatic esterases, and plasma ramipril levels in these patients are increased about 3-fold. Peak concentrations of ramiprilat in these patients, however, are not different from those seen in subjects with normal hepatic function, and the effect of a given dose of plasma ACE activity does not vary with hepatic function.

Pharmacodynamics

Single doses of ramipril of 2.5–20 mg produce approximately 60–80% inhibition of ACE activity 4 hours after dosing with approximately 40–60% inhibition after 24 hours. Multiple oral doses of ramipril of 2.0 mg or more cause plasma ACE activity to fall by more than 90% 4 hours after dosing, with over 80% inhibition of ACE activity remaining 24 hours after dosing. The more prolonged effect of even small multiple doses presumably reflects saturation of ACE binding sites by ramiprilat and relatively slow release from those sites.

Pharmacodynamics and Clinical Effects

Hypertension

Administration of ALTACE® to patients with mild to moderate hypertension results in a reduction of both supine and standing blood pressure to about the same extent with no compensatory tachycardia. Symptomatic postural hypotension is infrequent, although it can occur in patients who are salt- and/or volume-depleted. (See WARNINGS.) Use of ALTACE® in combination with thiazide diuretics gives a blood pressure lowering effect greater than that seen with either agent alone.

In single-dose studies, doses of 5–20 mg of ALTACE® lowered blood pressure within 1–2 hours, with peak reductions achieved 3–6 hours after dosing. The antihypertensive effect of a single dose persisted for 24 hours. In longer term (4–12

weeks) controlled studies, once-daily doses of 2.5–10 mg were similar in their effect, lowering supine or standing systolic and diastolic blood pressures 24 hours after dosing by about 6/4 mm Hg more than placebo. In comparisons of peak vs. trough effect, the trough effect represented about 50–60% of the peak response. In a titration study comparing divided (bid) vs. qd treatment, the divided regimen was superior, indicating that for some patients the antihypertensive effect with once-daily dosing is not adequately maintained. (See DOSAGE AND ADMINISTRATION).

In most trials, the antihypertensive effect of ALTACE® increased during the first several weeks of repeated measurements. The antihypertensive effect of ALTACE® has been shown to continue during long-term therapy for at least 2 years. Abrupt withdrawal of ALTACE® has not resulted in a rapid increase in blood pressure.

ALTACE® has been compared with other ACE inhibitors, beta-blockers, and thiazide diuretics. It was approximately as effective as other ACE inhibitors and as atenolol. In both caucasians and blacks, hydrochlorothiazide (25 or 50 mg) was significantly more effective than ramipril.

Except for thiazides, no formal interaction studies of ramipril with other antihypertensive agents have been carried out. Limited experience in controlled and uncontrolled trials combining ramipril with a calcium channel blocker, a loop diuretic, or triple therapy (beta-blocker, vasodilator, and a diuretic) indicate no unusual drug-drug interactions. Other ACE inhibitors have had less than additive effects with beta adrenergic blockers, presumably because both drugs lower blood pressure by inhibiting parts of the renin-angiotensin system.

ALTACE® was less effective in blacks than in caucasians. The effectiveness of ALTACE® was not influenced by age, sex, or weight.

In a baseline controlled study of 10 patients with mild essential hypertension, blood pressure reduction was accompanied by a 15% increase in renal blood flow. In healthy volunteers, glomerular filtration rate was unchanged.

Heart Failure post myocardial infarction

ALTACE® was studied in the Acute Infarction Ramipril Efficacy (AIRE) trial. This was a multinational (mainly European) 161-center, 2006-patient, double-blind, randomized, parallel-group study comparing ALTACE® to placebo in stable patients, 2-9 days after an acute myocardial infarction (MI), who had shown clinical signs of congestive heart failure (CHF) at any time after the MI. Patients in severe (NYHA class IV) heart failure, patients with unstable angina, patients with heart failure of congenital or valvular etiology, and patients with contraindications to ACE inhibitors were all excluded. The majority of patients had received thrombolytic therapy at the time of the index infarction, and the average time between infarction and initiation of treatment was 5 days.

Patients randomized to ramipril treatment were given an initial dose of 2.5 mg twice daily. If the initial regimen caused undue hypotension, the dose was reduced to 1.25 mg, but in either event doses were titrated upward (as tolerated) to a target regimen (achieved in 77% of patients randomized to ramipril) of 5 mg twice daily. Patients were then followed for an average of 15 months (range 6–46).

The use of ALTACE® was associated with a 27% reduction (p=0.002), in the risk of death from any cause; about 90% of the deaths that occurred were cardiovascular, mainly sudden death. The risks of progression to severe heart failure and of CHF-related hospitalization were also reduced, by 23% (p=0.017) and 26% (p=0.011), respectively. The benefits of ALTACE® therapy were seen in both genders, and they were not affected by the exact timing of the initiation of therapy, but older patients may have had a greater benefit than those under 65. The benefits were seen in patients on, and not on, various concomitant medications; at the time of randomization these included aspirin (about 80% of patients), diuretics (about 60%), organic nitrates (about 55%), beta-blockers (about 20%), calcium channel blockers (about 15%), and digoxin (about 12%).

INDICATIONS AND USAGE

Hypertension

ALTACE® is indicated for the treatment of hypertension. It may be used alone or in combination with thiazide diuretics. In using ALTACE®, consideration should be given to the fact that another angiotensin converting enzyme inhibitor, captopril, has caused agranulocytosis, particularly in patients with renal impairment or collagen-vascular disease. Available data are insufficient to show that ALTACE® does not have a similar risk. (See WARNINGS.)

In considering use of ALTACE®, it should be noted that in controlled trials ACE inhibitors have an effect on blood pressure that is less in black patients than in non-blacks. In addition, ACE inhibitors (for which adequate data are available) cause a higher rate of angioedema in black than in non-black patients. (See WARNINGS, Angioedema.)

Heart Failure post myocardial infarction

Ramipril is indicated in stable patients who have demonstrated clinical signs of congestive heart failure within the first few days after sustaining acute myocardial infarction.

Administration of ramipril to such patients has been shown to decrease the risk of death (principally cardiovascular death) and to decrease the risks of failure-related hospitalization and progression to severe/resistant heart failure. (See CLINICAL PHARMACOLOGY, Heart Failure post myocardial infarction for details and limitations of the survival trial.)

CONTRAINDICATIONS

ALTACE® is contraindicated in patients who are hypersensitive to this product and in patients with a history of angioedema related to previous treatment with an angiotensin converting enzyme inhibitor.

WARNINGS

Anaphylactoid and Possibly Related Reactions

Presumably because angiotensin-converting enzyme inhibitors affect the metabolism of eicosanoids and polypeptides, including endogenous bradykinin, patients receiving ACE inhibitors (including ALTACE®) may be subject to a variety of adverse reactions, some of them serious.

Angioedema

Patients with a history of angioedema unrelated to ACE inhibitor therapy may be at increased risk of angioedema while receiving an ACE inhibitor. (See also CONTRAINDICATIONS.)

Angioedema of the face, extremeties, lips, tongue, glottis, and larynx has been reported in patients treated with angiotensin converting enzyme inhibitors. Angioedema associated with laryngeal edema can be fatal. If laryngeal stridor or angioedema of the face, tongue, or glottis occurs, treatment with ALTACE® should be discontinued and appropriate therapy instituted immediately. **Where there is involvement of the tongue, glottis, or larynx, likely to cause airway obstruction, appropriate therapy, e.g., subcutaneous epinephrine solution 1:1,000 (0.3 ml to 0.5 ml) should be promptly administered. (See ADVERSE REACTIONS.)**

In a large U.S. postmarketing study, angioedema (defined as reports of angio, face, larynx, tongue, or throat edema) was reported in 3/1523 (0.20%) of black patients and in 8/8680 (0.09%) of white patients. These rates were not different statistically.

Anaphylactoid reactions during desensitization: Two patients undergoing desensitizing treatment with hymenoptera venom while receiving ACE inhibitors sustained life-threatening anaphylactoid reactions. In the same patients, these reactions were avoided when ACE inhibitors were temporarily withheld, but they reappeared upon inadvertent rechallenge.

Anaphylactoid reactions during membrane exposure: Anaphylactoid reactions have been reported in patients dialyzed with high-flux membranes and treated concomitantly with an ACE inhibitor. Anaphylactoid reactions have also been reported in patients undergoing low-density lipoprotein apheresis with dextran sulfate absorption.

Hypotension

ALTACE® can cause symptomatic hypotension, after either the initial dose or a later dose when the dosage has been increased. Like other ACE inhibitors, ramipril has been only rarely associated with hypotension in uncomplicated hypertensive patients. Symptomatic hypotension is most likely to occur in patients who have been volume- and/or salt-depleted as a result of prolonged diuretic therapy, dietary salt restriction, dialysis, diarrhea, or vomiting. Volume and/or salt depletion should be corrected before initiating therapy with ALTACE®.

In patients with congestive heart failure, with or without associated renal insufficiency, ACE inhibitor therapy may cause excessive hypotension, which may be associated with oliguria or azotemia and, rarely, with acute renal failure and death. In such patients, ALTACE® therapy should be started under close medical supervision; they should be followed closely for the first 2 weeks of treatment and whenever the dose of ramipril or diuretic is increased.

If hypotension occurs, the patient should be placed in a supine position and, if necessary, treated with intravenous infusion of physiological saline. ALTACE® treatment usually can be continued following restoration of blood pressure and volume.

Hepatic Failure

Rarely, ACE inhibitors have been associated with a syndrome that starts with cholestatic jaundice and progresses to fulminant hepatic necrosis and (sometimes) death. The mechanism of this syndrome is not understood. Patients receiving ACE inhibitors who develop jaundice or marked elevations of hepatic enzymes should discontinue the ACE inhibitor and receive appropriate medical follow-up.

Neutropenia/Agranulocytosis

Another angiotensin converting enzyme inhibitor, captopril, has been shown to cause agranulocytosis and bone marrow depression, rarely in uncomplicated patients, but more frequently in patients with renal impairment, especially if they also have a collagen-vascular disease such as systemic lupus erythematosus or scleroderma. Available data from clinical trials of ramipril are insufficient to show that ramipril does not cause agranulocytosis at similar rates. Moni-

toring of white blood cell counts should be considered in patients with collagen-vascular disease, especially if the disease is associated with impaired renal function.

Fetal/neonatal morbidity and mortality

ACE inhibitors can cause fetal and neonatal morbidity and death when administered to pregnant women. Several dozen cases have been reported in the world literature. When pregnancy is detected, ACE inhibitors should be discontinued as soon as possible.

The use of ACE inhibitors during the second and third trimesters of pregnancy has been associated with fetal and neonatal injury, including hypotension, neonatal skull hypoplasia, anuria, reversible or irreversible renal failure, and death. Oligohydramnios has also been reported, presumably resulting from decreased fetal renal function; oligohydramnios in this setting has been associated with fetal limb contractures, craniofacial deformation, and hypoplastic lung development. Prematurity, intrauterine growth retardation, and patent ductus arteriosus have also been reported, although it is not clear whether these occurrences were due to the ACE inhibitor exposure.

These adverse effects do not appear to have resulted from intrauterine ACE inhibitor exposure that has been limited to the first trimester. Mothers whose embryos and fetuses are exposed to ACE inhibitors only during the first trimester should be so informed. Nonetheless, when patients become pregnant, physicians should make every effort to discontinue the use of ALTACE® as soon as possible. Rarely (probably less often than once in every thousand pregnancies), no alternative to ACE inhibitors will be found. In these rare cases, the mothers should be apprised of the potential hazards to their fetuses, and serial ultrasound examinations should be performed to assess the intraamniotic environment.

If oligohydramnios is observed, ALTACE® should be discontinued unless it is considered life-saving for the mother. Contraction stress testing (CST), a nonstress test (NST), or biophysical profiling (BPP) may be appropriate, depending upon the week of pregnancy. Patients and physicians should be aware, however, that oligohydramnios may not appear until after the fetus has sustained irreversible injury.

Infants with histories of *in utero* exposure to ACE inhibitors should be closely observed for hypotension, oliguria, and hyperkalemia. If oliguria occurs, attention should be directed toward support of blood pressure and renal perfusion. Exchange transfusion or dialysis may be required as means of reversing hypotension and/or substituting for disordered renal function. ALTACE® which crosses the placenta can be removed from the neonatal circulation by these means, but limited experience has not shown that such removal is central to the treatment of these infants.

No teratogenic effects of ALTACE® were seen in studies of pregnant rats, rabbits, and cynomolgus monkeys. On a body surface area basis, the doses used were up to approximately 400 times (in rats and monkeys) and 2 times (in rabbits) the recommended human dose.

PRECAUTIONS

Impaired Renal Function: As a consequence of inhibiting the renin-angiotensin-aldosterone system, changes in renal function may be anticipated in susceptible individuals. In patients with severe congestive heart failure whose renal function may depend on the activity of the renin-angiotensin-aldosterone system, treatment with angiotensin converting enzyme inhibitors, including ALTACE®, may be associated with oliguria and/or progressive azotemia and (rarely) with acute renal failure and/or death.

In hypertensive patients with unilateral or bilateral renal artery stenosis, increases in blood urea nitrogen and serum creatinine may occur. Experience with another angiotensin converting enzyme inhibitor suggests that these increases are usually reversible upon discontinuation of ALTACE® and/or diuretic therapy. In such patients renal function should be monitored during the first few weeks of therapy.

Some hypertensive patients with no apparent pre-existing renal vascular disease have developed increases in blood urea nitrogen and serum creatinine, usually minor and transient, especially when ALTACE® has been given concomitantly with a diuretic. This is more likely to occur in patients with pre-existing renal impairment. Dosage reduction of ALTACE® and/or discontinuation of the diuretic may be required.

Evaluation of the hypertensive patient should always include assessment of renal function. (See DOSAGE AND ADMINISTRATION.)

Hyperkalemia: In clinical trials, hyperkalemia (serum potassium greater than 5.7 mEq/L) occurred in approximately 1% of hypertensive patients receiving ALTACE® (ramipril). In most cases, these were isolated values, which resolved despite continued therapy. None of these patients was discontinued from the trials because of hyperkalemia. Risk factors for the development of hyperkalemia include renal insufficiency, diabetes mellitus, and the concomitant use of potassium-sparing diuretics, potassium supplements, and/or potassium-containing salt substitutes which should be used cautiously, if at all, with ALTACE®. (See DRUG INTERACTIONS.)

Cough: Presumably due to the inhibition of the degradation of endogenous bradykinin, persistent nonproductive cough has been reported with all ACE inhibitors, always resolving after discontinuation of therapy. ACE inhibitor-induced cough should be considered in the differential diagnosis of cough.

Impaired Liver Function: Since ramipril is primarily metabolized by hepatic esterases to its active moiety, ramiprilat, patients with impaired liver function could develop markedly elevated plasma levels of ramipril. No formal pharmacokinetic studies have been carried out in hypertensive patients with impaired liver function.

Surgery/Anesthesia: In patients undergoing surgery or during anesthesia with agents that produce hypotension, ramipril may block angiotensin II formation that would otherwise occur secondary to compensatory renin release. Hypotension that occurs as a result of this mechanism can be corrected by volume expansion.

Information for Patients

Pregnancy: Female patients of childbearing age should be told about the consequences of second- and third-trimester exposure to ACE inhibitors, and they should also be told that these consequences do not appear to have resulted from intrauterine ACE inhibitor exposure that has been limited to the first trimester. These patients should be asked to report pregnancies to their physicians as soon as possible.

Angioedema: Angioedema, including laryngeal edema, can occur with treatment with ACE inhibitors, especially following the first dose. Patients should be so advised and told to report immediately any signs or symptoms suggesting angioedema (swelling of face, eyes, lips, or tongue, or difficulty in breathing) and to take no more drug until they have consulted with the prescribing physician.

Symptomatic Hypotension: Patients should be cautioned that lightheadedness can occur, especially during the first days of therapy, and it should be reported. Patients should be told that if syncope occurs, ALTACE® should be discontinued until the physician has been consulted.

All patients should be cautioned that inadequate fluid intake or excessive perspiration, diarrhea, or vomiting can lead to an excessive fall in blood pressure, with the same consequences of lightheadedness and possible syncope.

Hyperkalemia: Patients should be told not to use salt substitutes containing potassium without consulting their physician.

Neutropenia: Patients should be told to promply report any indication of infection (e.g., sore throat, fever), which could be a sign of neutropenia.

Drug Interactions

With diuretics: Patients on diuretics, especially those in whom diuretic therapy was recently instituted, may occasionally experience an excessive reduction of blood pressure after initiation of therapy with ALTACE®. The possibility of hypotensive effects with ALTACE® can be minimized by either discontinuing the diuretic or increasing the salt intake prior to initiation of treatment with ALTACE®. If this is not possible, the starting dose should be reduced. (See DOSAGE AND ADMINISTRATION.)

With potassium supplements and potassium-sparing diuretics: ALTACE® can attenuate potassium loss caused by thiazide diuretics. Potassium-sparing diuretics (spironolactone, amiloride, triamterene, and others) or potassium supplements can increase the risk of hyperkalemia. Therefore, if concomitant use of such agents is indicated, they should be given with caution, and the patient's serum potassium should be monitored frequently.

With lithium: Increased serum lithium levels and symptoms of lithium toxicity have been reported in patients receiving ACE inhibitors during therapy with lithium.These drugs should be coadministred with caution, and frequent monitoring of serum lithium levels is recommended. If a diuretic is also used, the risk of lithium toxicity may be increased.

Other: Neither ALTACE® nor its metabolites have been found to interact with food, digoxin, antacid, furosemide, cimetidine, indomethacin, and simvastatin. The combination of ALTACE® and propranolol showed no adverse effects on dynamic parameters (blood pressure and heart rate). The co-administration of ALTACE® and warfarin did not adversely affect the anticoagulant effects of the latter drug. Additionally, co-administration of ALTACE® with phenprocoumon did not affect minimum phenprocoumon levels or interfere with the subjects' state of anti-coagulation.

Carcinogenesis, Mutagenesis, Impairment of Fertility

No evidence of a tumorigenic effect was found when ramipril was given by gavage to rats for up to 24 months at doses of up to 500 mg/kg/day or to mice for up to 18 months at doses of up to 1000 mg/kg/day. (For either species, these doses are about 200 times the maximum recommended human dose when compared on the basis of body surface area.) No mutagenic activity was detected in the Ames test in bacteria, the micronucleus test in mice, unscheduled DNA synthesis in a human cell line, or a forward gene-mutation assay in a Chinese hamster ovary cell line. Several metabolites and degradation products of ramipril were also negative in the Ames test. A study in rats with dosages as great as 500 mg/kg/day did not produce adverse effects on fertility.

Pregnancy

Pregnancy Category C (first trimester) and D (second and third trimesters). See WARNINGS: Fetal/neonatal morbidity and mortality.

Nursing Mothers

Ingestion of single 10 mg oral dose of ALTACE® resulted in undetectable amounts of ramipril and its metabolites in breast milk. However, because multiple doses may produce low milk concentrations that are not predictable from single doses, women receiving ALTACE® should not breast feed.

Geriatric Use

Of the total number of patients who received ramipril in US clinical studies of ALTACE® 11.0% were 65 and over while 0.2% were 75 and over. No overall differences in effectiveness or safety were observed between these patients and younger patients, and other reported clinical experience has not identified differences in responses between the elderly and younger patients, but greater sensitivity of some older individuals cannot be ruled out.

One pharmacokinetic study conducted in hospitalized elderly patients indicated that peak ramiprilat levels and area under the plasma concentration time curve (AUC) for ramiprilat are higher in older patients.

Pediatric Use

Safety and effectiveness in pediatric patients have not been established.

ADVERSE REACTIONS

Hypertension

ALTACE® has been evaluated for safety in over 4,000 patients with hypertension; of these, 1,230 patients were studied in US controlled trials, and 1,107 were studied in foreign controlled trials. Almost 700 of these patients were treated for at least one year. The overall incidence of reported adverse events was similar in ALTACE® and placebo patients. The most frequent clinical side effects (possibly or probably related to study drug) reported by patients receiving ALTACE® in US placebo-controlled trials were: headache (5.4%), "dizziness" (2.2%) and fatigue or asthenia (2.0%), but only the last was more common in ALTACE® patients than in patients given placebo. Generally, the side effects were mild and transient, and there was no relation to total dosage within the range of 1.25 to 20 mg. Discontinuation of therapy because of a side effect was required in approximately 3% of US patients treated with ALTACE®. The most common reasons for discontinuation were: cough (1.0%), "dizziness" (0.5%), and impotence (0.4%).

The side effects considered possibly or probably related to study drug that occurred in US placebo-controlled trials in more than 1% of patients treated with ALTACE® are shown below.

PATIENTS IN US PLACEBO CONTROLLED STUDIES

	Altace® (N=651)		Placebo (N=286)	
	n	%	n	%
Headache	35	5.4	17	5.9
"Dizziness"	14	2.2	9	3.1
Asthenia (Fatigue)	13	2.0	2	0.7
Nausea/Vomiting	7	1.1	3	1.0

In placebo-controlled trials, there was also an excess of upper respiratory infection and flu syndrome in the ramipril group. As these studies were carried out before the relationship of cough to ACE inhibitors was recognized, some of these events may represent ramipril-induced cough. In a later 1-year study, increased cough was seen in almost 12% of ramipril patients, with about 4% of these patients requiring discontinuation of treatment.

Heart Failure post myocardial infarction

Adverse reactions (except laboratory abnormalities) considered possibly/probably related to study drug that occurred in more than one percent of patients with heart failure treated with ALTACE® are shown below. The incidences represent the experiences from the AIRE study. The follow-up time was between 6 and 46 months for this study.

Percentage of Patients with Adverse Events Possibly/Probably Related to Study Drug

Placebo-Controlled (AIRE) Mortality Study

Adverse Event	Ramipril (N=1004)	Placebo (N=982)
Hypotension	10.7	4.7
Cough Increased	7.6	3.7
Dizziness	4.1	3.2
Angina Pectoris	2.9	2.0
Nausea	2.2	1.4
Postural Hypotension	2.2	1.4
Syncope	2.1	1.4
Heart Failure Severe/Resistance	2.0	2.2

Continued on next page

Altace—Cont.

Heart Failure	2.0	3.0
Myocardial Infarct	1.7	1.7
Vomiting	1.6	0.5
Vertigo	1.5	0.7
Headache	1.2	0.8
Kidney Function	1.2	0.5
Abnormal Chest Pain	1.1	0.9
Diarrhea	1.1	0.4
Asthenia	0.3	0.8

Other adverse experiences reported in controlled clinical trials (in less than 1% of ramipril patients), or rarer events seen in postmarketing experience, include the following (in some, a causal relationship to drug use is uncertain):

Body As a Whole: Anaphylactoid reactions. (See WARNINGS.)

Cardiovascular: Symptomatic hypotension (reported in 0.5% of patients in US trials) (See WARNINGS and PRECAUTIONS), syncope (not reported in US trials), angina pectoris, arrhythmia, chest pain, palpitations, myocardial infarction, and cerebrovascular events.

Hematologic: Pancytopenia, hemolytic anemia and thrombocytopenia.

Renal: Some hypertensive patients with no apparent preexisting renal disease have developed minor, usually transient, increases in blood urea nitrogen and serum creatinine when taking ALTACE®, particularly when ALTACE® was given concomitantly with a diuretic. (See WARNINGS.)

Angioneurotic Edema: Angioneurotic edema has been reported in 0.3% of patients in US clinical trials. (See WARNINGS.)

Cough: A tickling, dry, persistent, nonproductive cough has been reported with the use of ACE inhibitors. Approximately 1% of patients treated with ALTACE® have required discontinuation because of cough. The cough disappears shortly after discontinuation of treatment. (See PRECAUTIONS, Cough subsection.)

Gastrointestinal Pancreatitis, abdominal pain (sometimes with enzyme changes suggesting pancreatitis), anorexia, constipation, diarrhea, dry mouth, dyspepsia, dysphagia, gastroenteritis, hepatitis, nausea, increased salivation, taste disturbance, and vomiting.

Dermatologic: Apparent hypersensitivity reactions (manifested by urticaria, pruritis, or rash, with or without fever), erythema multiforme, pemphigus, photosensitivity, and purpura.

Neurologic and Psychiatric: Anxiety, amnesia, convulsions, depression, hearing loss, insomnia, nervousness, neuralgia, neuropathy, paresthesia, somnolence, tinnitus, tremor, vertigo, and vision disturbances.

Miscellaneous: As with other ACE inhibitors, a symptom complex has been reported which may include a positive ANA, an elevated erythrocyte sedimentation rate, arthralgia/arthritis, myalgia, fever, vasculitis, eosinophilia, photosensitivity, rash and other dermatologic manifestations.

Fetal/neonatal morbidity and mortality. See **WARNINGS: Fetal/neonatal morbidity and mortality.**

Other: arthralgia, arthritis, dyspnea, edema, epistaxis, impotence, increased sweating, malaise, myalgia, and weight gain.

Clinical Laboratory Test Findings:

Creatinine and Blood Urea Nitrogen: Increases in creatinine levels occurred in 1.2% of patients receiving ALTACE® alone, and in 1.5% of patients receiving ALTACE® and a diuretic. Increases in blood urea nitrogen levels occurred in 0.5% of patients receiving ALTACE® alone and in 3% of patients receiving ALTACE® with a diuretic. None of these increases required discontinuation of treatment. Increases in these laboratory values are more likely to occur in patients with renal insufficiency or those pretreated with a diuretic and, based on experience with other ACE inhibitors, would be expected to be especially likely in patients with renal artery stenosis. (See WARNINGS and PRECAUTIONS.) Since ramipril decreases aldosterone secretion, elevation of serum potassium can occur. Potassium supplements and potassium-sparing diuretics should be given with caution, and the patient's serum potassium should be monitored frequently. (See WARNINGS and PRECAUTIONS.)

Hemoglobin and Hematocrit: Decreases in hemoglobin or hematocrit (a low value and a decrease of 5 g/dl or 5% respectively) were rare, occurring in 0.4% of patients receiving ALTACE® alone and in 1.5% of patients receiving ALTACE® plus a diuretic. No US patients discontinued treatment because of decreases in hemoglobin or hematocrit.

Other (causal relationships unknown): Clinically important changes in standard laboratory tests were rarely associated with ALTACE® administration. Elevations of liver enzymes, serum bilirubin, uric acid, and blood glucose have been reported, as have cases of hyponatremia and scattered incidents of leukopenia, eosinophilia, and proteinuria. In US trials, less than 0.2% of patients discontinued treatment for laboratory abnormalities: all of these were cases of proteinuria or abnormal liver-function tests.

OVERDOSAGE

Single oral doses in rats and mice of 10–11 g/kg resulted in significant lethality. In dogs, oral doses as high as 1 g/kg induced only mild gastrointestinal distress. Limited data on human overdosage are available. The most likely clinical manifestations would be symptoms attributable to hypotension.

Laboratory determinations of serum levels of ramipril and its metabolites are not widely available, and such determinations have, in any event, no established role in the management of ramipril overdose.

No data are available to suggest physiological maneuvers (e.g., maneuvers to change the pH of the urine) that might accelerate elimination of ramipril and its metabolites. Similarly, it is not known which, if any, of these substances can be usefully removed from the body by hemodialysis.

Angiotensin II could presumably serve as a specific antagonist-antidote in the setting of ramipril overdose, but angiotensin II is essentially unavailable outside of scattered research facilities. Because the hypotensive effect of ramipril is achieved through vasodilation and effective hypovolemia, it is reasonable to treat ramipril overdose by infusion of normal saline solution.

DOSAGE AND ADMINISTRATION

Hypertension

The recommended initial dose for patients not receiving a diuretic is 2.5 mg once a day. Dosage should be adjusted according to the blood pressure response. The usual maintenance dosage range is 2.5 to 20 mg per day administered as a single dose or in two equally divided doses. In some patients treated once daily, the antihypertensive effect may diminish toward the end of the dosing interval. In such patients, an increase in dosage or twice daily administration should be considered. If blood pressure is not controlled with ALTACE® alone, a diuretic can be added.

Heart Failure post myocardial infarction

For the treatment of post-infarction patients who have shown signs of congestive failure, the recommended starting dose of ALTACE® is 2.5 mg twice daily. A patient who becomes hypotensive at this dose may be switched to 1.25 mg twice daily, but all patients should then be titrated (as tolerated) toward a target dose of 5 mg twice daily.

After the initial dose of ALTACE®, the patient should be observed under medical supervision for at least two hours and until blood pressure has stabilized for at least an additional hour. (See WARNINGS and PRECAUTIONS, Drug Interactions.) If possible, the dose of any concomitant diuretic should be reduced which may diminish the likelihood of hypotension. The appearance of hypotension after the initial dose of ALTACE® does not preclude subsequent careful dose titration with the drug, following effective management of the hypotension.

The ALTACE® Capsule is usually swallowed whole. The ALTACE® Capsule can also be opened and the contents sprinkled on a small amount (about 4 oz.) of apple sauce or mixed in 4 oz. (120 ml) of water or apple juice. To be sure that ramipril is not lost when such a mixture is used, the mixture should be consumed in its entirety. The described mixtures can be pre-prepared and stored for up to 24 hours at room temperature or up to 48 hours under refrigeration.

Concomitant administration of ALTACE® with potassium supplements, potassium salt substitutes, or potassium-sparing diuretics can lead to increases of serum potassium (See PRECAUTIONS.)

In patients who are currently being treated with a diuretic, symptomatic hypotension occasionally can occur following the initial dose of ALTACE®. To reduce the likelihood of hypotension, the diuretic should, if possible, be discontinued two to three days prior to beginning therapy with ALTACE®. (See WARNINGS.) Then, if blood pressure is not controlled with ALTACE® alone, diuretic therapy should be resumed.

If the diuretic cannot be discontinued, an initial dose of 1.25 mg ALTACE® should be used to avoid excess hypotension.

Dosage Adjustment in Renal Impairment

In patients with creatinine clearance <40 ml/min/1.73m^2 (serum creatinine approximately >2.5 mg/dl) doses only 25% of those normally used should be expected to induce full therapeutic levels of ramiprilat. (See CLINICAL PHARMACOLOGY.)

Hypertension: For patients with hypertension and renal impairment, the recommended initial dose is 1.25 mg ALTACE® once daily. Dosage may be titrated upward until blood pressure is controlled or to a maximum total daily dose of 5 mg.

Heart Failure post myocardial infarction: For patients with heart failure and renal impairment, the recommended initial dose is 1.25 mg ALTACE® once daily. The dose may be increased to 1.25 mg b.i.d. and up to a maximum dose of 2.5 mg b.i.d. depending upon clinical response and tolerability.

HOW SUPPLIED

ALTACE® is available in potencies of 1.25 mg, 2.5 mg, 5 mg, and 10 mg in hard gelatin capsules, packaged in bottles of 100 capsules. ALTACE® is also supplied in blister packages (10 capsules/blister card).

ALTACE® 1.25 mg capsules are supplied as yellow, hard gelatin capsules in bottles of 100 (NDC 0039-0103-10), and Unit Dose packs of 100 (NDC 0039-0103-11).

ALTACE® 2.5 mg capsules are supplied as orange, hard gelatin capsules in bottles of 100 (NDC 0039-0104-10), and Unit Dose packs of 100 (NDC 0039-0104-11).

ALTACE® 5 mg capsules are supplied as red, hard gelatin capsules in bottles of 100 (NDC 0039-0105-10), and Unit Dose packs of 100 (NDC 0039-0105-11).

ALTACE® 10 mg capsules are supplied as Process Blue, hard gelatin capsules in bottles of 100 (NDC 0039-0106-10).

Dispense in well-closed container with safety closure.

Store at controlled room temperature (59 to 86° F).

Caution: Federal law prohibits dispensing without prescription.

*US Patent 4,587,258

ALTACE REG TM HOECHST AG Made in USA

Prescribing Information as of June 1996

Hoechst-Roussel Pharmaceuticals

Division of Hoechst Marion Roussel, Inc.

Kansas City, MO 64137

Shown in Product Identification Guide, page 316

AMARYL® ℞

(glimepiride* TABLETS 1, 2, and 4 mg)

Prescribing Information as of November 1996

DESCRIPTION

AMARYL® (glimepiride tablets) is an oral blood-glucose-lowering drug of the sulfonylurea class. Glimepiride is a white to yellowish-white, crystalline, odorless to practically odorless powder formulated into tablets of 1-mg, 2-mg, and 4-mg strengths for oral administration. AMARYL® tablets contain the active ingredient glimepiride and the following inactive ingredients: lactose (hydrous), sodium starch glycolate, povidone, microcrystalline cellulose, and magnesium stearate. In addition, AMARYL® 1-mg tablets contain Ferric Oxide Red, AMARYL® 2-mg tablets contain Ferric Oxide Yellow and FD&C Blue #2 Aluminum Lake, and AMARYL® 4-mg tablets contain FD&C Blue #2 Aluminum Lake.

Chemically, glimepiride is identified as 1-[[p-[2-(3-ethyl-4-methyl-2-oxo-3-pyrroline-1-carboxamido) ethyl]phenyl]-sulfonyl]-3-(trans-4-methylcyclohexyl)urea. The CAS Registry Number is 93479-97-1. The structural formula is:

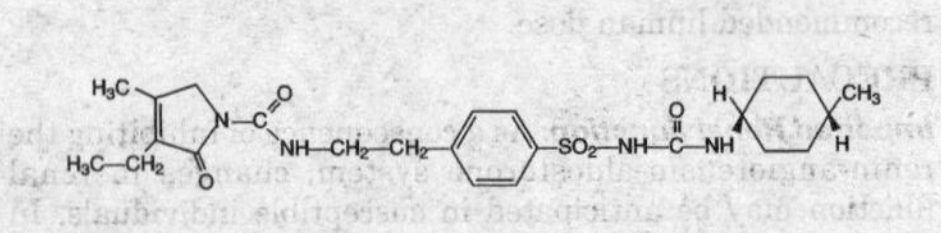

Molecular Formula: $C_{24}H_{34}N_4O_5S$

Molecular Weight: 490.62

Glimepiride is practically insoluble in water.

CLINICAL PHARMACOLOGY

Mechanism Of Action

The primary mechanism of action of glimepiride in lowering blood glucose appears to be dependent on stimulating the release of insulin from functioning pancreatic beta cells. In addition, extrapancreatic effects may also play a role in the activity of sulfonylureas such as glimepiride. This is supported by both preclinical and clinical studies demonstrating that glimepiride administration can lead to increased sensitivity of peripheral tissues to insulin. These findings are consistent with the results of a long-term, randomized, placebo-controlled trial in which AMARYL® therapy improved postprandial insulin/C-peptide responses and overall glycemic control without producing clinically meaningful increases in fasting insulin/C-peptide levels. However, as with other sulfonylureas, the mechanism by which glimepiride lowers blood glucose during long-term administration has not been clearly established.

Pharmacodynamics

A mild glucose-lowering effect first appeared following single oral doses as low as 0.5–0.6 mg in healthy subjects. The time required to reach the maximum effect (i.e., minimum blood glucose level [T_{min}]) was about 2 to 3 hours. In noninsulin-dependent (Type II) diabetes mellitus (NIDDM) patients, both fasting and 2-hour postprandial glucose levels were significantly lower with glimepiride (1, 2, 4, and 8 mg once daily) than with placebo after 14 days of oral dosing. The glucose-lowering effect in all active treatment groups was maintained over 24 hours.

In larger dose-ranging studies, blood glucose and HbA1c were found to respond in a dose-dependent manner over the range of 1 to 4 mg/day of AMARYL®. Some patients, particularly those with higher fasting plasma glucose (FPG) levels, may benefit from doses of AMARYL® up to 8 mg once daily. No difference in response was found when AMARYL® was administered once or twice daily.

In two 14-week, placebo-controlled studies in 720 subjects, the average net reduction in HbA1c for AMARYL® (glimepiride tablets) patients treated with 8 mg once daily was 2.0% in absolute units compared with placebo-treated patients. In a long-term, randomized, placebo-controlled study of NIDDM patients unresponsive to dietary management, AMARYL® therapy improved postprandial insulin/C-peptide responses, and 75% of patients achieved and maintained control of blood glucose and HbA1c. Efficacy results were not affected by age, gender, weight, or race.

In long-term extension trials with previously-treated patients, no meaningful deterioration in mean fasting blood glucose (FBG) or HbA1c levels was seen after $2^1/_2$ years of AMARYL® therapy.

Combination therapy with AMARYL® and insulin (70% NPH/30% regular) was compared to placebo/insulin in secondary failure patients whose body weight was >130% of their ideal body weight. Initially, 5–10 units of insulin were administered with the main evening meal and titrated upward weekly to achieve predefined FPG values. Both groups in this double-blind study achieved similar reductions in FPG levels but the AMARYL®/insulin therapy group used approximately 38% less insulin.

AMARYL® therapy is effective in controlling blood glucose without deleterious changes in the plasma lipoprotein profiles of patients treated for NIDDM.

Pharmacokinetics

Absorption. After oral administration, glimepiride is completely (100%) absorbed from the GI tract. Studies with single oral doses in normal subjects and with multiple oral doses in patients with NIDDM have shown significant absorption of glimepiride within 1 hour after administration and peak drug levels (C_{max}) at 2 to 3 hours. When glimepiride was given with meals, the mean T_{max} (time to reach C_{max}) was slightly increased (12%) and the mean C_{max} and AUC (area under the curve) were slightly decreased (8% and 9%, respectively).

Distribution. After intravenous (IV) dosing in normal subjects, the volume of distribution (Vd) was 8.8 L (113 mL/kg), and the total body clearance (CL) was 47.8 mL/min. Protein binding was greater than 99.5%.

Metabolism. Glimepiride is completely metabolized by oxidative biotransformation after either an IV or oral dose. The major metabolites are the cyclohexyl hydroxy methyl derivative (M1) and the carboxyl derivative (M2). Cytochrome P450 II C9 has been shown to be involved in the biotransformation of glimepiride to M1. M1 is further metabolized to M2 by one or several cytosolic enzymes. M1, but not M2, possesses about $^1/_3$ of the pharmacological activity as compared to its parent in an animal model; however, whether the glucose-lowering effect of M1 is clinically meaningful is not clear.

Excretion. When ^{14}C-glimepiride was given orally, approximately 60% of the total radioactivity was recovered in the urine in 7 days and M1 (predominant) and M2 accounted for 80–90% of that recovered in the urine. Approximately 40% of the total radioactivity was recovered in feces and M1 and M2 (predominant) accounted for about 70% of that recovered in feces. No parent drug was recovered from urine or feces. After IV dosing in patients, no significant biliary excretion of glimepiride or its M1 metabolite has been observed.

Pharmacokinetic Parameters. The pharmacokinetic parameters of glimepiride obtained from a single-dose, crossover, dose-proportionality (1, 2, 4, and 8 mg) study in normal subjects and from a single- and multiple-dose, parallel, dose-proportionality (4 and 8 mg) study in patients with NIDDM are summarized below.

[See table above]

	Volunteers			Patients with NIDDM					
	Single Dose Mean ± SD			Single Dose (Day 1) Mean ± SD			Multiple Dose (Day 10) Mean ± SD		
C_{max} (ng/mL)									
1 mg	103	±	34 (12)		___			___	
2 mg	177	±	44 (12)		___			___	
4 mg	308	±	69 (12)	352	±	222 (12)	309	±	134 (12)
8 mg	557	±	152 (12)	591	±	232 (14)	578	±	265 (11)
T_{max} (h)	2.4	±	0.8 (48)	2.5	±	1.2 (26)	2.8	±	2.2 (23)
CL/f (mL/min)	52.1	±	16.0 (48)	48.5	±	29.3 (26)	52.7	±	40.3 (23)
Vd/f (L)	21.8	±	13.9 (48)	19.8	±	12.7 (26)	37.1	±	18.2 (23)
$T^1/_2$ (h)	5.3	±	4.1 (48)	5.0	±	2.5 (26)	9.2	±	3.6 (23)

( ) = No. of subjects
CL/f = Total body clearance after oral dosing
Vd/f = Volume of distribution calculated after oral dosing

These data indicate that glimepiride did not accumulate in serum, and the pharmacokinetics of glimepiride were not different in healthy volunteers and in NIDDM patients. Oral clearance of glimepiride did not change over the 1–8-mg dose range, indicating linear pharmacokinetics.

Variability. In normal healthy volunteers, the intra-individual variabilities of C_{max}, AUC, and CL/f for glimepiride were 23%, 17%, and 15%, respectively, and the inter-individual variabilities were 25%, 29%, and 24%, respectively.

Special Populations

Geriatric. Comparison of glimepiride pharmacokinetics in NIDDM patients ≤ 65 years and those > 65 years was performed in a study using a dosing regimen of 6 mg daily. There were no significant differences in glimepiride pharmacokinetics between the two age groups. The mean AUC at steady state for the older patients was about 13% lower than that for the younger patients; the mean weight-adjusted clearance for the older patients was about 11% higher than that for the younger patients.

Pediatric. No studies were performed in pediatric patients.

Gender. There were no differences between males and females in the pharmacokinetics of glimepiride when adjustment was made for differences in body weight.

Race. No pharmacokinetic studies to assess the effects of race have been performed, but in placebo-controlled studies of AMARYL® (glimepiride tablets) in patients with NIDDM, the antihyperglycemic effect was comparable in whites (n=536), blacks (n=63), and Hispanics (n=63).

Renal Insufficiency. A single-dose, open-label study was conducted in 15 patients with renal impairment. AMARYL® (3 mg) was administered to 3 groups of patients with different levels of mean creatinine clearance (CLcr); (Group I, CLcr = 77.7 mL/min, n=5), (Group II, CLcr = 27.7 mL/min, n=3), and (Group III, CLcr = 9.4 mL/min, n=7). AMARYL® was found to be well tolerated in all 3 groups. The results showed that glimepiride serum levels decreased as renal function decreased. However, M1 and M2 serum levels (mean AUC values) increased 2.3 and 8.6 times from Group I to Group III. The apparent terminal half-life ($T_{1/2}$) for glimepiride did not change, while the half-lives for M1 and M2 increased as renal function decreased. Mean urinary excretion of M1 plus M2 as percent of dose, however, decreased (44.4%, 21.9%, and 9.3% for Groups I to III).

A multiple-dose titration study was also conducted in 16 NIDDM patients with renal impairment using doses ranging from 1–8 mg daily for 3 months. The results were consistent with those observed after single doses. All patients with a CLcr less than 22 mL/min had adequate control of their glucose levels with a dosage regimen of only 1 mg daily. The results from this study suggested that a starting dose of 1 mg AMARYL® may be given to NIDDM patients with kidney disease, and the dose may be titrated based on fasting blood glucose levels.

Hepatic Insufficiency. No studies were performed in patients with hepatic insufficiency.

Other Populations. There were no important differences in glimepiride metabolism in subjects identified as phenotypically different drug-metabolizers by their metabolism of sparteine.

The pharmacokinetics of glimepiride in morbidly obese patients were similar to those in the normal weight group, except for a lower C_{max} and AUC. However, since neither C_{max} nor AUC values were normalized for body surface area, the lower values of C_{max} and AUC for the obese patients were likely the result of their excess weight and not due to a difference in the kinetics of glimepiride.

Drug Interactions. The hypoglycemic action of sulfonylureas may be potentiated by certain drugs, including nonsteroidal anti-inflammatory drugs and other drugs that are highly protein bound, such as salicylates, sulfonamides, chloramphenicol, coumarins, probenecid, monoamine oxidase inhibitors, and beta adrenergic blocking agents. When these drugs are administered to a patient receiving AMARYL®, the patient should be observed closely for hypoglycemia. When these drugs are withdrawn from a patient receiving AMARYL®, the patient should be observed closely for loss of glycemic control.

Certain drugs tend to produce hyperglycemia and may lead to loss of control. These drugs include the thiazides and other diuretics, corticosteroids, phenothiazines, thyroid products, estrogens, oral contraceptives, phenytoin, nicotinic acid, sympathomimetics, and isoniazid. When these drugs are administered to a patient receiving AMARYL®, the patient should be closely observed for loss of control. When these drugs are withdrawn from a patient receiving AMARYL®, the patient should be observed closely for hypoglycemia.

Coadministration of aspirin (1 g tid) and AMARYL® led to a 34% decrease in the mean glimepiride AUC and, therefore, a 34% increase in the mean CL/f. The mean C_{max} had a decrease of 4%. Blood glucose and serum C-peptide concentrations were unaffected and no hypoglycemic symptoms were reported. Pooled data from clinical trials showed no evidence of clinically significant adverse interactions with uncontrolled concurrent administration of aspirin and other salicylates.

Coadministration of either cimetidine (800 mg once daily) or ranitidine (150 mg bid) with a single 4-mg oral dose of AMARYL® did not significantly alter the absorption and disposition of glimepiride, and no differences were seen in hypoglycemic symptomatology. Pooled data from clinical trials showed no evidence of clinicallly significant adverse interactions with uncontrolled concurrent administration of H2-receptor antagonists.

Concomitant administration of propranolol (40 mg tid) and AMARYL® significantly increased C_{max}, AUC, and $T_{1/2}$ of glimepiride by 23%, 22%, and 15%, respectively, and it decreased CL/f by 18%. The recovery of M1 and M2 from urine, however, did not change. The pharmacodynamic responses to glimepiride were nearly identical in normal subjects receiving propranolol and placebo. Pooled data from clinical trials in patients with NIDDM showed no evidence of clinically significant adverse interactions with uncontrolled concurrent administration of beta-blockers. However, if beta-blockers are used, caution should be exercised and patients should be warned about the potential for hypoglycemia.

Concomitant administration of AMARYL® (glimepiride tablets) (4 mg once daily) did not alter the pharmacokinetic characteristics of R- and S-warfarin enantiomers following administration of a single dose (25 mg) of racemic warfarin to healthy subjects. No changes were observed in warfarin plasma protein binding. AMARYL® treatment did result in a slight, but statistically significant, decrease in the pharmacodynamic response to warfarin. The reductions in mean area under the prothrombin time (PT) curve and maximum PT values during AMARYL® treatment were very small (3.3% and 9.9%, respectively) and are unlikely to be clinically important.

The responses of serum glucose, insulin, C-peptide, and plasma glucagon to 2 mg AMARYL® were unaffected by coadministration of ramipril (an ACE inhibitor) 5 mg once daily in normal subjects. No hypoglycemic symptoms were reported. Pooled data from clinical trials in patients with NIDDM showed no evidence of clinically significant adverse interactions with uncontrolled concurrent administration of ACE inhibitors.

A potential interaction between oral miconazole and oral hypoglycemic agents leading to severe hypoglycemia has been reported. Whether this interaction also occurs with the intravenous, topical, or vaginal preparations of miconazole is not known. Potential interactions of glimepiride with other drugs metabolized by cytochrome P450 II C9 also include phenytoin, diclofenac, ibuprofen, naproxen, and mefenamic acid.

Although no specific interaction studies were performed, pooled data from clinical trials showed no evidence of clinically significant adverse interactions with uncontrolled concurrent administration of calcium-channel blockers, estrogens, fibrates, NSAIDS, HMG CoA reductase inhibitors, sulfonamides, or thyroid hormone.

INDICATIONS AND USAGE

AMARYL® is indicated as an adjunct to diet and exercise to lower the blood glucose in patients with noninsulin-dependent (Type II) diabetes mellitus (NIDDM) whose hyperglycemia cannot be controlled by diet and exercise alone.

AMARYL® is also indicated for use in combination with insulin to lower blood glucose in patients whose hyperglycemia cannot be controlled by diet and exercise in conjunction with an oral hypoglycemic agent. Combined use of glimepiride and insulin may increase the potential for hypoglycemia.

In initiating treatment for noninsulin-dependent diabetes, diet and exercise should be emphasized as the primary form of treatment. Caloric restriction, weight loss, and exercise are essential in the obese diabetic patient. Proper dietary management and exercise alone may be effective in controlling the blood glucose and symptoms of hyperglycemia. In addition to regular physical activity, cardiovascular risk factors should be identified and corrective measures taken where possible.

Continued on next page

Amaryl—Cont.

If this treatment program fails to reduce symptoms and/or blood glucose, the use of an oral sulfonylurea or insulin should be considered. Use of AMARYL® must be viewed by both the physician and patient as a treatment in addition to diet and exercise and not as a substitute for diet and exercise or as a convenient mechanism for avoiding dietary restraint. Furthermore, loss of blood glucose control on diet and exercise alone may be transient, thus requiring only short-term administration of AMARYL®.

During maintenance programs, AMARYL® monotherapy should be discontinued if satisfactory lowering of blood glucose is no longer achieved. Judgments should be based on regular clinical and laboratory evaluations. Secondary failures to AMARYL® monotherapy can be treated with AMARYL®-insulin combination therapy.

In considering the use of AMARYL® in asymptomatic patients, it should be recognized that blood glucose control in NIDDM has not definitely been established to be effective in preventing the long-term cardiovascular and neural complications of diabetes. However, the Diabetes Control and Complications Trial (DCCT) demonstrated that control of HbA1c and glucose was associated with a decrease in retinopathy, neuropathy, and nephropathy for insulin-dependent diabetic (IDDM) patients.

CONTRAINDICATIONS

AMARYL® is contraindicated in patients with
1. Known hypersensitivity to the drug.
2. Diabetic ketoacidosis, with or without coma. This condition should be treated with insulin.

WARNINGS

SPECIAL WARNING ON INCREASED RISK OF CARDIOVASCULAR MORTALITY

The administration of oral hypoglycemic drugs has been reported to be associated with increased cardiovascular mortality as compared to treatment with diet alone or diet plus insulin. This warning is based on the study conducted by the University Group Diabetes Program (UGDP), a long-term, prospective clinical trial designed to evaluate the effectiveness of glucose-lowering drugs in preventing or delaying vascular complications in patients with non-insulin-dependent diabetes. The study involved 823 patients who were randomly assigned to one of four treatment groups (Diabetes, 19 supp. 2: 747–830, 1970).

UGDP reported that patients treated for 5 to 8 years with diet plus a fixed dose of tolbutamide (1.5 grams per day) had a rate of cardiovascular mortality approximately $2\frac{1}{2}$ times that of patients treated with diet alone. A significant increase in total mortality was not observed, but the use of tolbutamide was discontinued based on the increase in cardiovascular mortality, thus limiting the opportunity for the study to show an increase in overall mortality. Despite controversy regarding the interpretation of these results, the findings of the UGDP study provide an adequate basis for this warning. The patient should be informed of the potential risks and advantages of AMARYL® (glimepiride tablets) and of alternative modes of therapy.

Although only one drug in the sulfonylurea class (tolbutamide) was included in this study, it is prudent from a safety standpoint to consider that this warning may also apply to other oral hypoglycemic drugs in this class, in view of their close similarities in mode of action and chemical structure.

PRECAUTIONS

General

Hypoglycemia: All sulfonylurea drugs are capable of producing severe hypoglycemia. Proper patient selection, dosage, and instructions are important to avoid hypoglycemic episodes. Patients with impaired renal function may be more sensitive to the glucose-lowering effect of AMARYL®. A starting dose of 1 mg once daily followed by appropriate dose titration is recommended in those patients. Debilitated or malnourished patients, and those with adrenal, pituitary, or hepatic insufficiency are particularly susceptible to the hypoglycemic action of glucose-lowering drugs. Hypoglycemia may be difficult to recognize in the elderly and in people who are taking beta-adrenergic blocking drugs or other sympatholytic agents. Hypoglycemia is more likely to occur when caloric intake is deficient, after severe or prolonged exercise, when alcohol is ingested, or when more than one glucose-lowering drug is used.

Loss of control of blood glucose: When a patient stabilized on any diabetic regimen is exposed to stress such as fever, trauma, infection, or surgery, a loss of control may occur. At such times, it may be necessary to add insulin in combination with AMARYL® or even use insulin monotherapy. The effectiveness of any oral hypoglycemic drug, including AMARYL®, in lowering blood glucose to a desired level decreases in many patients over a period of time, which may be due to progression of the severity of the diabetes or to diminished responsiveness to the drug. This phenomenon is known as secondary failure, to distinguish it from primary failure in which the drug is ineffective in an individual patient when first given. Should secondary failure occur with

AMARYL® monotherapy, AMARYL®-insulin combination therapy may be instituted. Combined use of glimepiride and insulin may increase the potential for hypoglycemia.

Information for Patients

Patients should be informed of the potential risks and advantages of AMARYL® and of alternative modes of therapy. They should also be informed about the importance of adherence to dietary instructions, of a regular exercise program, and of regular testing of blood glucose.

The risks of hypoglycemia, its symptoms and treatment, and conditions that predispose to its development should be explained to patients and responsible family members. The potential for primary and secondary failure should also be explained.

Laboratory Tests

Fasting blood glucose should be monitored periodically to determine therapeutic response. Glycosylated hemoglobin should also be monitored, usually every 3 to 6 months, to more precisely assess long-term glycemic control.

Drug Interactions

(See CLINICAL PHARMACOLOGY, Drug Interactions.)

Carcinogenesis, Mutagenesis, and Impairment of Fertility

Studies in rats at doses of up to 5000 ppm in complete feed (approximately 340 times the maximum recommended human dose, based on surface area) for 30 months showed no evidence of carcinogenesis. In mice, administration of glimepiride for 24 months resulted in an increase in benign pancreatic adenoma formation which was dose related and is thought to be the result of chronic pancreatic stimulation. The no-effect dose for adenoma formation in mice in this study was 320 ppm in complete feed, or 46-54 mg/kg body weight/day. This is about 35 times the maximum human recommended dose of 8 mg once daily based on surface area. Glimepiride was non-mutagenic in a battery of *in vitro* and *in vivo* mutagenicity studies (Ames test, somatic cell mutation, chromosomal aberration, unscheduled DNA synthesis, mouse micronucleus test).

There was no effect of glimepiride on male mouse fertility in animals exposed up to 2500 mg/kg body weight (>1,700 times the maximum recommended human dose based on surface area). Glimepiride had no effect on the fertility of male and female rats administered up to 4000 mg/kg body weight (approximately 4,000 times the maximum recommended human dose based on surface area).

Pregnancy

Teratogenic Effects. Pregnancy Category C. Glimepiride did not produce teratogenic effects in rats exposed orally up to 4000 mg/kg body weight (approximately 4,000 times the maximum recommended human dose based on surface area) or in rabbits exposed up to 32 mg/kg body weight (approximately 60 times the maximum recommended human dose based on surface area). Glimepiride has been shown to be associated with intrauterine fetal death in rats when given in doses as low as 50 times the human dose based on surface area and in rabbits when given in doses as low as 0.1 times the human dose based on surface area. This fetotoxicity, observed only at doses inducing maternal hypoglycemia, has been similarly noted with other sulfonylureas, and is believed to be directly related to the pharmacologic (hypoglycemic) action of glimepiride.

There are no adequate and well-controlled studies in pregnant women. On the basis of results from animal studies, AMARYL® (glimepiride tablets) should not be used during pregnancy. Because recent information suggests that abnormal blood glucose levels during pregnancy are associated with a higher incidence of congenital abnormalities, many experts recommend that insulin be used during pregnancy to maintain glucose levels as close to normal as possible.

Nonteratogenic Effects. In some studies in rats, offspring of dams exposed to high levels of glimepiride during pregnancy and lactation developed skeletal deformities consisting of shortening, thickening, and bending of the humerus during the postnatal period. Significant concentrations of glimepiride were observed in the serum and breast milk of the dams as well as in the serum of the pups. These skeletal deformations were determined to be the result of nursing from mothers exposed to glimepiride.

Prolonged severe hypoglycemia (4 to 10 days) has been reported in neonates born to mothers who were receiving a sulfonylurea drug at the time of delivery. This has been reported more frequently with the use of agents with prolonged half-lives. Patients who are planning a pregnancy should consult their physician, and it is recommended that they change over to insulin for the entire course of pregnancy and lactation.

Nursing Mothers

In rat reproduction studies, significant concentrations of glimepiride were observed in the serum and breast milk of the dams, as well as in the serum of the pups. Although it is not known whether AMARYL® is excreted in human milk, other sulfonylureas are excreted in human milk. Because the potential for hypoglycemia in nursing infants may exist, and because of the effects on nursing animals, AMARYL® should be discontinued in nursing mothers. If AMARYL® is

discontinued, and if diet and exercise alone are inadequate for controlling blood glucose, insulin therapy should be considered. (See above **Pregnancy, Nonteratogenic Effects.**)

Pediatric Use

Safety and effectiveness in pediatric patients have not been established.

ADVERSE REACTIONS

The incidence of hypoglycemia with AMARYL®, as documented by blood glucose values <60 mg/dL, ranged from 0.9–1.7% in two large, well-controlled, 1-year studies. (See **WARNINGS** and **PRECAUTIONS**.)

AMARYL® has been evaluated for safety in 2,013 patients in US controlled trials, and in 1,551 patients in foreign controlled trials. More than 1,650 of these patients were treated for at least 1 year.

Adverse events, other than hypoglycemia, considered to be possibly or probably related to study drug that occurred in US placebo-controlled trials in more than 1% of patients treated with AMARYL® are shown below.

Adverse Events Occurring in ≥1% AMARYL® Patients

	AMARYL®		Placebo	
	No.	%	No.	%
Total Treated	746	100	294	100
Dizziness	13	1.7	1	0.3
Asthenia	12	1.6	3	1.0
Headache	11	1.5	4	1.4
Nausea	8	1.1	0	0.0

Gastrointestinal Reactions

Vomiting, gastrointestinal pain, and diarrhea have been reported, but the incidence in placebo-controlled trials was less than 1%. Isolated transaminase elevations have been reported. Cholestatic jaundice has been reported to occur rarely with sulfonylureas.

Dermatologic Reactions

Allergic skin reactions, e.g., pruritus, erythema, urticaria, and morbilliform or maculopapular eruptions, occur in less than 1% of treated patients. These may be transient and may disappear despite continued use of AMARYL®; if skin reactions persist, the drug should be discontinued. Porphyria cutanea tarda and photosensitivity reactions have been reported with sulfonylureas.

Hematologic Reactions

Leukopenia, agranulocytosis, thrombocytopenia, hemolytic anemia, aplastic anemia, and pancytopenia have been reported with sulfonylureas.

Metabolic Reactions

Hepatic porphyria reactions and disulfiram-like reactions have been reported with sulfonylureas; however, no cases have yet been reported with AMARYL® (glimepiride tablets). Cases of hyponatremia have been reported with glimepiride and all other sulfonylureas, most often in patients who are on other medications or have medical conditions known to cause hyponatremia or increase release of antidiuretic hormone. The syndrome of inappropriate antidiuretic hormone (SIADH) secretion has been reported with certain other sulfonylureas, and it has been suggested that these sulfonylureas may augment the peripheral (antidiuretic) action of ADH and/or increase release of ADH.

Other Reactions

Changes in accommodation and/or blurred vision may occur with the use of AMARYL®. This is thought to be due to changes in blood glucose, and may be more pronounced when treatment is initiated. This condition is also seen in untreated diabetic patients, and may actually be reduced by treatment. In placebo-controlled trials of AMARYL®, the incidence of blurred vision was placebo, 0.7%, and AMARYL®, 0.4%.

OVERDOSAGE

Overdosage of sulfonylureas, including AMARYL®, can produce hypoglycemia. Mild hypoglycemic symptoms without loss of consciousness or neurologic findings should be treated aggressively with oral glucose and adjustments in drug dosage and/or meal patterns. Close monitoring should continue until the physician is assured that the patient is out of danger. Severe hypoglycemic reactions with coma, seizure, or other neurological impairment occur infrequently, but constitute medical emergencies requiring immediate hospitalization. If hypoglycemic coma is diagnosed or suspected, the patient should be given a rapid intravenous injection of concentrated (50%) glucose solution. This should be followed by a continuous infusion of a more dilute (10%) glucose solution at a rate that will maintain the blood glucose at a level above 100 mg/dL. Patients should be closely monitored for a minimum of 24 to 48 hours, because hypoglycemia may recur after apparent clinical recovery.

DOSAGE AND ADMINISTRATION

There is no fixed dosage regimen for the management of diabetes mellitus with AMARYL® or any other hypoglycemic agent. The patient's fasting blood glucose and HbA1c must be measured periodically to determine the minimum effective dose for the patient; to detect primary failure, i.e., in-

adequate lowering of blood glucose at the maximum recommended dose of medication; and to detect secondary failure, i.e., loss of adequate blood glucose lowering response after an initial period of effectiveness. Glycosylated hemoglobin levels should be performed to monitor the patient's response to therapy.

Short-term administration of AMARYL® may be sufficient during periods of transient loss of control in patients usually controlled well on diet and exercise.

Usual Starting Dose

The usual starting dose of AMARYL® as initial therapy is 1–2 mg once daily, administered with breakfast or the first main meal. Those patients who may be more sensitive to hypoglycemic drugs should be started at 1 mg once daily, and should be titrated carefully. (See **PRECAUTIONS** Section for patients at increased risk.)

No exact dosage relationship exists between AMARYL® and the other oral hypoglycemic agents. The maximum starting dose of AMARYL® should be no more than 2 mg.

Failure to follow an appropriate dosage regimen may precipitate hypoglycemia. Patients who do not adhere to their prescribed dietary and drug regimen are more prone to exhibit unsatisfactory response to therapy.

Usual Maintenance Dose

The usual maintenance dose is 1 to 4 mg once daily. The maximum recommended dose is 8 mg once daily. After reaching a dose of 2 mg, dosage increases should be made in increments of no more than 2 mg at 1–2 week intervals based upon the patient's blood glucose response. Long-term efficacy should be monitored by measurement of HbA1c levels, for example, every 3 to 6 months.

AMARYL® -Insulin Combination Therapy

Combination therapy with AMARYL® and insulin may be used in secondary failure patients. The fasting glucose level for instituting combination therapy is in the range of >150 mg/dL in plasma or serum depending on the patient. The recommended AMARYL® dose is 8 mg once daily administered with the first main meal. After starting with low-dose insulin, upward adjustments of insulin can be done approximately weekly as guided by frequent measurements of fasting blood glucose. Once stable, combination-therapy patients should monitor their capillary blood glucose on an ongoing basis, preferably daily. Periodic adjustments of insulin may also be necessary during maintenance as guided by glucose and HbA1c levels.

Specific Patient Populations

AMARYL® (glimepiride tablets) is not recommended for use in pregnancy, nursing mothers, or children. In elderly, debilitated, or malnourished patients, or in patients with renal or hepatic insufficiency, the initial dosing, dose increments, and maintenance dosage should be conservative to avoid hypoglycemic reactions (See **CLINICAL PHARMACOLOGY, *Special Populations*** and **PRECAUTIONS, *General***).

Patients Receiving Other Oral Hypoglycemic Agents

As with other sulfonylurea hypoglycemic agents, no transition period is necessary when transferring patients to AMARYL®. Patients should be observed carefully (1–2 weeks) for hypoglycemia when being transferred from longer half-life sulfonylureas (e.g., chlorpropamide) to AMARYL® due to potential overlapping of drug effect.

HOW SUPPLIED

AMARYL® tablets are available in the following strengths and package sizes:

1 mg (pink, flat-faced, oblong with notched sides at double bisect, imprinted with "AMA RYL" on one side and the Hoechst logo on both sides of the bisect on the other side)
Bottles of 100 (NDC 0039-0221-10)

2 mg (green, flat-faced, oblong with notched sides at double bisect, imprinted with "AMA RYL" on one side and the Hoechst logo on both sides of the bisect on the other side)
Bottles of 100 (NDC 0039-0222-10)
Unit Dose Cartons (100) (NDC 0039-0222-11)

4 mg (blue, flat-faced, oblong with notched sides at double bisect, imprinted with "AMA RYL" on one side and the Hoechst logo on both sides of the bisect on the other side)
Bottles of 100 (NDC 0039-0223-10)
Unit Dose Cartons (100) (NDC 0039-0223-11)

Store between 59° and 86° F (15° to 30° C).
Dispense in well-closed containers with safety closures.
Caution: Federal law prohibits dispensing without a prescription.
AMARYL® REG TM HOECHST AG
*US Patent 4,379,785

ANIMAL TOXICOLOGY

Reduced serum glucose values and degranulation of the pancreatic beta cells were observed in beagle dogs exposed to 320 mg glimepiride/kg/day for 12 months (approximately 1,000 times the recommended human dose based on surface area). No evidence of tumor formation was observed in any organ. One female and one male dog developed bilateral subcapsular cataracts. Non-GLP studies indicated that glimepiride was unlikely to exacerbate cataract formation. Evaluation of the co-cataractogenic potential of glimepiride in several diabetic and cataract rat models was negative and there was no adverse effect of glimepiride on bovine ocular lens metabolism in organ culture.

HUMAN OPHTHALMOLOGY DATA

Ophthalmic examinations were carried out in over 500 subjects during long-term studies using the methodology of Taylor and West and Laties et al. No significant differences were seen between AMARYL® and glyburide in the number of subjects with clinically important changes in visual acuity, intra-ocular tension, or in any of the five lens-related variables examined.

Ophthalmic examinations were carried out during long-term studies using the method of Chylack et al. No significant or clinically meaningful differences were seen between AMARYL® and glipizide with respect to cataract progression by subjective LOCS II grading and objective image analysis systems, visual acuity, intraocular pressure, and general ophthalmic examination.

Prescribing Information as of November 1996

Hoechst-Roussel Pharmaceuticals
Division of Hoechst Marion Roussel, Inc.
Kansas City, MO 64137 USA

Shown in Product Identification Guide, page 315

ANZEMET® INJECTION ℞

[*an-zĕmĕt*]
(dolasetron mesylate injection)

Prescribing Information as of October 1997

DESCRIPTION

ANZEMET (dolasetron mesylate) is an antinauseant and antiemetic agent. Chemically, dolasetron mesylate is (2α,6α,8α,9aβ)-octahydro -3-oxo-2, 6-methano-2*H*-quinolizin-8-yl-1*H*-indole-3-carboxylate monomethanesulfonate, monohydrate. It is a highly specific and selective serotonin subtype 3 ($5\text{-}HT_3$) receptor antagonist both in vitro and in vivo. Dolasetron mesylate has the following structural formula:

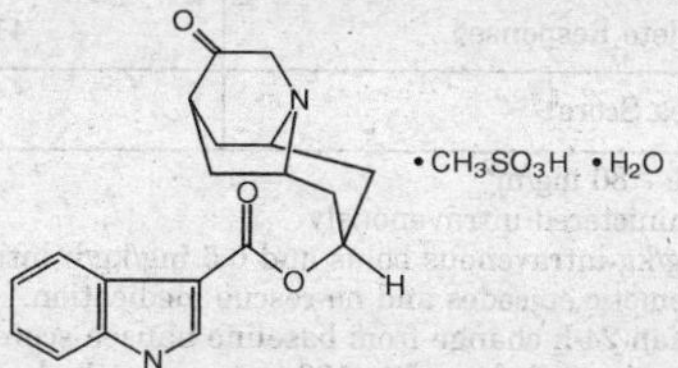

The empirical formula is $C_{19}H_{20}N_2O_3 \cdot CH_3SO_3H \cdot H_2O$, with a molecular weight of 438.50. Approximately 74% of dolasetron mesylate monohydrate is dolasetron base.

Dolasetron mesylate monohydrate is a white to off-white powder that is freely soluble in water and propylene glycol, slightly soluble in ethanol, and slightly soluble in normal saline.

ANZEMET Injection is a clear, colorless, nonpyrogenic, sterile solution for intravenous administration. Each milliliter of ANZEMET Injection contains 20 mg of dolasetron mesylate and 38.2 mg mannitol with an acetate buffer in water for injection. The pH of the resulting solution is 3.2 to 3.8.

CLINICAL PHARMACOLOGY

Dolasetron mesylate and its active metabolite, hydrodolasetron (MDL 74,156), are selective serotonin $5\text{-}HT_3$ receptor antagonists not shown to have activity at other known serotonin receptors and with low affinity for dopamine receptors. The serotonin $5\text{-}HT_3$ receptors are located on the nerve terminals of the vagus in the periphery and centrally in the chemoreceptor trigger zone of the area postrema. It is thought that chemotherapeutic agents produce nausea and vomiting by releasing serotonin from the enterochromaffin cells of the small intestine, and that the released serotonin then activates $5\text{-}HT_3$ receptors located on vagal efferents to initiate the vomiting reflex.

Acute, usually reversible, ECG changes (PR and QT_c prolongation; QRS widening), caused by dolasetron mesylate, have been observed in healthy volunteers and in controlled clinical trials. The active metabolites of dolasetron may block sodium channels, a property unrelated to its ability to block $5\text{-}HT_3$ receptors. QT_c prolongation is primarily due to QRS widening. Dolasetron appears to prolong both depolarization and, to a lesser extent, repolarization time. The magnitude and frequency of the ECG changes increased with dose (related to peak plasma concentrations of hydrodolasetron but not the parent compound). These ECG interval prolongations usually returned to baseline within 6 to 8 hours, but in some patients were present at 24 hour follow up. Dolasetron mesylate administration has little or no effect on blood pressure.

In healthy volunteers (N=64), dolasetron mesylate in single intravenous doses up to 5 mg/kg produced no effect on pupil size or meaningful changes in EEG tracings. Results from neuropsychiatric tests revealed that dolasetron mesylate did not alter mood or concentration. Multiple daily doses of dolasetron have had no effect on colonic transit in humans. Dolasetron mesylate has no effect on plasma prolactin concentrations.

Pharmacokinetics in Humans

Intravenous dolasetron mesylate is rapidly eliminated ($t_{1/2}$ <10 min) and completely metabolized to the most clinically relevant species, hydrodolasetron.

The reduction of dolasetron to hydrodolasetron is mediated by a ubiquitous enzyme, carbonyl reductase. Cytochrome P-450 (CYP)IID6 is primarily responsible for the subsequent hydroxylation of hydrodolasetron and both CYPIIIA and flavin monooxygenase are responsible for the N-oxidation of hydrodolasetron.

Hydrodolasetron is excreted in the urine unchanged (53.0% of administered intravenous dose). Other urinary metabolites include hydroxylated glucuronides and N-oxide.

Hydrodolasetron appeared rapidly in plasma, with a maximum concentration occurring approximately 0.6 hour after the end of intravenous treatment, and was eliminated with a mean half-life of 7.3 hours (%CV=24) and an apparent clearance of 9.4 mL/min/kg (%CV=28) in 24 adults. Hydrodolasetron is eliminated by multiple routes, including renal excretion and, after metabolism, mainly glucuronidation, and hydroxylation. Hydrodolasetron exhibits linear pharmacokinetics over the intravenous dose range of 50 to 200 mg and they are independent of infusion rate. Doses lower than 50 mg have not been studied. Two thirds of the administered dose is recovered in the urine and one third in the feces. Hydrodolasetron is widely distributed in the body with a mean apparent volume of distribution of 5.8 L/kg (%CV=25, N=24) in adults.

Sixty-nine to 77% of hydrodolasetron is bound to plasma protein. In a study with ^{14}C labeled dolasetron, the distribution of radioactivity to blood cells was not extensive. The binding of hydrodolasetron to α_1-acid glycoprotein is approximately 50%. The pharmacokinetics of hydrodolasetron are linear and similar in men and women.

Pediatric Patients

In a pharmacokinetic study in pediatric cancer patients (ages 3 to 11, N=25; ages 12 to 17, N=21) given a single 0.6, 1.2, 1.8, or 2.4 mg/kg dose of ANZEMET Injection intravenously, apparent clearance values were highest and half-lives were lowest in the youngest age group. For the 3 to 11 and the 12 to 17 year age groups, all receiving doses between 0.6 to 2.4 mg/kg, mean apparent clearances are 2 and 1.3 times greater, respectively, than for healthy adults receiving the same range of doses.

Thirty-two pediatric cancer patients ages 3 to 11 years (N=19) and 12 to 17 years (N=13), received 0.6, 1.2, or 1.8 mg ANZEMET Injection diluted with either apple or apple-grape juice and administered orally. In this study, the mean apparent clearances were 3 times greater in the younger pediatric group and 1.8 times greater in the older pediatric group than those observed in healthy adult volunteers. Across this spectrum of pediatric patients, maximum plasma concentrations were 0.6 to 0.7 times those observed in healthy adults receiving similar doses.

In a pharmacokinetic study in 18 pediatric patients (2 to 11 years of age) undergoing surgery with general anesthesia and administered a single 1.2 mg/kg intravenous dose of ANZEMET Injection, mean apparent clearance was greater (40%) and terminal half-life shorter (36%) for hydrodolasetron than in healthy adults receiving the same dose.

For 12 pediatric patients, ages 2 to 12 years receiving 1.2 mg/kg ANZEMET Injection diluted in apple or apple-grape juice and administered orally, the mean apparent clearance was 34% greater and half-life was 21% shorter than in healthy adults receiving the same dose. The pharmacokinetics of hydrodolasetron, in special and targeted patient populations following intravenous administration of ANZEMET Injection, are summarized in Table 1. The pharmacokinetics of hydrodolasetron are similar in adult healthy volunteers and in adult cancer patients receiving chemotherapeutic agents. The apparent clearance of hydrodolasetron in pediatric and adolescent patients is 1.4 times to twofold higher than in adults. The apparent clearance of hydrodolasetron is not affected by age in adult cancer patients. Following intravenous administration, the apparent clearance of hydrodolasetron remains unchanged with severe hepatic impairment and decreases 47% with severe renal impairment. No dose adjustment is necessary for elderly patients or for patients with hepatic or renal impairment.

[See table 1 at top of next page]

CLINICAL STUDIES

Prevention of Cancer Chemotherapy-Induced Nausea and Vomiting

ANZEMET Injection administered intravenously at a dose of 1.8 mg/kg gave similar results in preventing nausea and vomiting as the other selective serotonin $5\text{-}HT_3$ receptor antagonists studied as active comparators. It was more effec-

Continued on next page

Anzemet Injection—Cont.

tive than metoclopramide. Efficacy was based on complete response rates (0 emetic episodes and no rescue medication).

Cisplatin Based Chemotherapy
A randomized, double-blind trial compared single intravenous doses of ANZEMET Injection with metoclopramide in 226 (160 men and 66 women) adult cancer patients receiving $\geq$80 mg/m^2 cisplatin. ANZEMET Injection at a dose of 1.8 mg/kg was significantly more effective than metoclopramide in the prevention of chemotherapy-induced nausea and vomiting in this study (Table 2).
[See table 2 at right]
A second randomized, double-blind trial compared single intravenous doses of ANZEMET Injection with intravenous ondansetron in 609 (377 men and 232 women) adult cancer patients receiving $\geq$70 mg/m^2 cisplatin. A single intravenous 1.8 mg/kg dose of ANZEMET Injection was shown to be equivalent to a single intravenous 32 mg dose of ondansetron (Table 3).
[See table 3 at right]
Another randomized, double-blind trial compared single IV doses of ANZEMET with a single 3-mg IV dose of granisetron in 474 (315 men and 159 women) patients receiving $\geq$80 mg/m^2 cisplatin chemotherapy. A single intravenous 1.8-mg/kg dose of ANZEMET gave similar results as those from granisetron.

Cyclophosphamide Based Chemotherapy
In a study of ANZEMET Injection in 309 patients (96 men and 213 women) receiving moderately emetogenic chemotherapy such as cyclophosphamide based regimens, a single intravenous 1.8 mg/kg dose of ANZEMET Injection was equivalent to metoclopramide administered as a 2 mg/kg intravenous bolus followed by 3 mg/kg intravenously over 8 hours. Complete response rates were 63% and 52%, respectively, p=0.12.

Prevention of Postoperative Nausea and Vomiting
ANZEMET Injection administered intravenously at a dose of 12.5 mg approximately 15 minutes before the cessation of general balanced anesthesia (short-acting barbiturate, nitrous oxide, narcotic and analgesic, and skeletal muscle relaxant) was significantly more effective than placebo in preventing postoperative nausea and vomiting. No increased efficacy was seen with higher doses.
One trial compared single intravenous ANZEMET Injection doses of 12.5, 25, 50, and 100 mg with placebo in 635 women surgical patients undergoing laparoscopic procedures. ANZEMET Injection at a dose of 12.5 mg was statistically superior to placebo for complete response (no vomiting, no rescue medication) (p=.0003). Complete response rates were 50% and 31%, respectively.
Another trial compared single intravenous ANZEMET Injection doses of 12.5, 25, 50, and 100 mg with placebo in 1030 (722 women and 308 men) surgical patients. In women, the 12.5 mg dose was statistically superior to placebo for complete response. The complete response rates were 50% and 40% respectively. However, in men, there was no statistically significant difference in complete response between any ANZEMET dose and placebo.

Treatment of Postoperative Nausea and/or Vomiting
Two randomized, double-blinded trials compared single intravenous ANZEMET Injection doses of 12.5, 25, 50, and 100 mg with placebo in 124 male and 833 female patients who had undergone surgery with general balance anesthesia and presented with early postoperative nausea or vomiting requiring antiemetic treatment.
In both studies, the 12.5 mg intravenous dose of ANZEMET was statistically superior to placebo for complete response (no vomiting, no escape medication). No significant increased efficacy was seen with higher doses.

INDICATIONS AND USAGE
ANZEMET Injection is indicated for the following:
(1) **the prevention of nausea and vomiting associated with initial and repeat courses of emetogenic cancer chemotherapy, including high dose cisplatin;**
(2) **the prevention of postoperative nausea and vomiting.** As with other antiemetics, routine prophylaxis is not recommended for patients in whom there is little expectation that nausea and/or vomiting will occur postoperatively. In patients where nausea and/or vomiting must be avoided postoperatively, ANZEMET Injection is recommended even where the incidence of postoperative nausea and/or vomiting is low.
(3) **the treatment of postoperative nausea and/or vomiting.**

CONTRAINDICATIONS
ANZEMET Injection is contraindicated in patients known to have hypersensitivity to the drug.

WARNINGS
ANZEMET can cause ECG interval changes (PR, QT$_c$, JT prolongation and QRS widening). These changes are related in magnitude and frequency to blood levels of the active me-

Table 1. Pharmacokinetic Values for Plasma Hydrodolasetron Following Intravenous Administration of ANZEMET Injection*

	Age (years)	Dose	CL$_{app}$ (mL/min/kg)	t$_{1/2}$ (h)	C$_{max}$ (ng/mL)
Young Healthy Volunteers (N=24)	19-40	100 mg	9.4 (28%)	7.3 (24%)	320 (25%)
Elderly Healthy Volunteers (N=15)	65-75	2.4 mg/kg	8.3 (30%)	6.9 (22%)	620 (31%)
Cancer Patients					
Adults (N=273)	19-87	0.6-3.0 mg/kg	10.2 (34%)†	7.5 (43%)†	505 (26%)‡
Adolescents (N=21)	12-17	0.6-3.0 mg/kg	12.5 (37%)	5.5 (31%)	562 (45%)§
Children (N=25)	3-11	0.6-2.4 mg/kg	19.2 (30%)	4.4 (24%)	505 (100%)‖
Pediatric Surgery Patients (N=18)	2-11	1.2 mg/kg	13.1 (47%)	4.8 (23%)	255 (22%)
Patients with Severe Renal Impairment (N=12) (Creatinine clearance ≤10 mL/min)	28-74	200 mg	5.0 (33%)	10.9 (30%)	867 (31%)
Patients with Severe Hepatic Impairment (N=3)	42-52	150 mg	9.6 (19%)	11.7 (22%)	396 (45%)

CL$_{app}$: apparent clearance   t$_{1/2}$: terminal elimination half-life   ( ): coefficient of variation in %
* :   mean values
† :   results from population kinetic study
‡ :   results from adult cancer study (dose=1.8 mg/kg, N=8)
§ :   results from adolescents (dose=1.8 mg/kg, N=7)
‖ :   results from children (dose=1.8 mg/kg, N=5)

Table 2. Prevention of Chemotherapy-Induced Nausea and Emesis from Cisplatin Chemotherapy*

	ANZEMET Injection 1.8 mg/kg†	Metoclopramide‡	*P*-value
Number of Patients	72	69	
Response Over 24 Hours			
Complete Response§	41 (57%)	24 (35%)	0.0009
Nausea Score‖	4	30	0.0400

* :   Dose $\geq$80 mg/m^2
† :   Administered intravenously
‡ :   3 mg/kg intravenous bolus and 0.5 mg/kg/h intravenously over 8 h.
§ :   No emetic episodes and no rescue medication.
‖ :   Median 24-h change from baseline nausea score using visual analog scale (VAS): Score range 0="none" to 100="nausea as bad as it could be."

Table 3. Prevention of Chemotherapy-Induced Nausea and Emesis from Cisplatin Chemotherapy*

	ANZEMET Injection 1.8 mg/kg†	Ondansetron 32 mg‡	*P*-value
Number of Patients	198	206	
Response Over 24 Hours			
Complete Response§	88 (44%)	88 (43%)	NS
Nausea Score‖	10	16	NS

* :   Dose $\geq$70 mg/kg^2
† :   Administered intravenously
‡ :   Includes 12 patients who received 3 doses 0.15 mg/kg of ondansetron intravenously.
§ :   No emetic episodes and no rescue medication.
‖ :   Median 24-h change from baseline nausea score using visual analog scale (VAS): Score range 0="none" to 100="nausea as bad as it could be."

tabolite. These changes are self-limiting with declining blood levels. Some patients have interval prolongations for 24 hours or longer. Interval prolongation could lead to cardiovascular consequences, including heart block or cardiac arrhythmias. These have rarely been reported.
A cardiac conduction abnormality observed on an intraoperative cardiac rhythm monitor (interpreted as complete heart block) was reported in a 61 year old woman who received 200 mg ANZEMET for the prevention of postoperative nausea and vomiting. This patient was also taking verapamil. A similar event also interpreted as complete heart block was reported in one patient receiving placebo.
A 66-year-old man with Stage IV non-Hodgkins lymphoma died suddenly 6 hours after receiving 1.8 mg/kg (119 mg) intravenous ANZEMET Injection. This patient had other potential risk factors including substantial exposure to doxorubicin and concomitant cyclophosphamide.

PRECAUTIONS
General
Dolasetron should be administered with caution in patients who have or may develop prolongation of cardiac conduction intervals, particularly QT$_c$. These include patients with hypokalemia or hypomagnesemia, patients taking diuretics with potential for inducing electrolyte abnormalities, patients with congenital QT syndrome, patients taking anti-arrhythmic drugs or other drugs which lead to QT prolongation, and cumulative high dose anthracycline therapy.

Drug Interactions
The potential for clinically significant drug-drug interactions posed by dolasetron and hydrodolasetron appears to be low for drugs commonly used in chemotherapy or surgery, because hydrodolasetron is eliminated by multiple routes. See PRECAUTIONS, General for information about potential interaction with other drugs that prolong the QT$_c$ interval. Blood levels of hydrodolasetron increased 24% when dolasetron was coadministered with cimetidine (nonselective inhibitor of cytochrome P-450) for 7 days, and decreased 28% with coadministration of rifampin (potent inducer of cytochrome P-450) for 7 days.
ANZEMET Injection has been safely coadministered with drugs used in chemotherapy and surgery. As with other

Table 4. Adverse Events ≥ 2% from Chemotherapy-Induced Nausea and Vomiting Studies

Event	ANZEMET Injection 1.8 mg/kg (n=695)	Odansetron/ Granisetron* (n=356)
Headache	169 (24.3%)	73 (20.5%)
Diarrhea	86 (12.4%)	25 (7.0%)
Fever	30 (4.3%)	18 (5.1%)
Fatigue	25 (3.6%)	12 (3.4%)
Hepatic Function Abnormal †	25 (3.6%)	12 (3.4%)
Abdominal Pain	22 (3.2%)	7 (2.0%)
Hypertension	20 (2.9%)	9 (2.5%)
Pain	17 (2.4%)	7 (2.0%)
Dizziness	15 (2.2%)	7 (2.0 %)
Chills/Shivering	14 (2.0%)	6 (1.7%)

*: Ondansetron 32 mg intravenous, granisetron 3 mg intravenous.
†: Includes events coded as SGOT- and/or SGPT-increased (see also Liver and Biliary System below)

Table 5. Adverse Events ≥ 2% from Placebo-Controlled Postoperative Nausea and Vomiting Studies

Event	ANZEMET Injection 12.5 mg (n=615)	Placebo (n=739)
Headache	58 (9.4%)	51 (6.9%)
Dizziness	34 (5.5%)	23 (3.1%)
Drowsiness	15 (2.4%)	18 (2.4%)
Pain	15 (2.4%)	21 (2.8%)
Urinary Retention	12 (2.0%)	16 (2.2%)

ANZEMET® Injection
(dolasetron mesylate injection)
20 mg/mL

Strength	Description	NDC Number
12.5 mg	0.625-mL single use ampules (Box of 6)	0088-1208-65
100 mg/5 mL	5-mL single use vial	0088-1206-32

agents which prolong ECG intervals, caution should be exercised in patients taking drugs which prolong ECG intervals, particularly QT$_c$.
In patients taking furosemide, nifedipine, diltiazem, ACE inhibitors, verapamil, glyburide, propranolol, and various chemotherapy agents, no effect was shown on the clearance of hydrodolasetron. Clearance of hydrodolasetron decreased by about 27% when dolasetron mesylate was administered intravenously concomitantly with atenolol. ANZEMET does not influence anesthesia recovery time in patients. Dolasetron mesylate did not inhibit the antitumor activity of four chemotherapeutic agents (cisplatin, 5-fluorouracil, doxorubicin, cyclophosphamide) in four murine models.

Carcinogenesis, Mutagenesis, Impairment of Fertility
In a 24-month carcinogenicity study, there was a statistically significant (P <0.001) increase in the incidence of combined hepatocellular adenomas and carcinomas in male mice treated with 150 mg/kg/day and above. In this study, mice (CD-1) were treated orally with dolasetron mesylate 75, 150 or 300 mg/kg/day (225, 450 or 900 mg/m²/day). For a 50 kg person of average height (1.46 m² body surface area), these doses represent 3.4, 6.8 and 13.5 times the recommended clinical dose (66.6 mg/m², intravenous) on a body surface area basis. No increase in liver tumors was observed at a dose of 75 mg/kg/day in male mice and at doses up to 300 mg/kg/day in female mice.
In a 24-month rat (Sprague-Dawley) carcinogenicity study, oral dolasetron mesylate was not tumorigenic at doses up to 150 mg/kg/day (900 mg/m²/day, 13.5 times the recommended human dose based on body surface area) in male rats and 300 mg/kg/day (1800 mg/m²/day, 27 times the recommended human dose based on body surface area) in female rats.
Dolasetron mesylate was not genotoxic in the Ames test, the rat lymphocyte chromosomal aberration test, the Chinese hamster ovary (CHO) cell (HGPRT) forward mutation test, the rat hepatocyte unscheduled DNA synthesis (UDS) test or the mouse micronucleus test.

Dolasetron mesylate was found to have no effect on fertility and reproductive performance at oral doses up to 100 mg/kg/day (600 mg/m²/day, 9 times the recommended human dose based on body surface area) in female rats and up to 400 mg/kg/day (2400 mg/m²/day, 36 times the recommended human dose based on body surface area) in male rats.
Pregnancy: Teratogenic Effects, Pregnancy Category B.
Teratology studies have not revealed evidence of impaired fertility or harm to the fetus due to dolasetron mesylate. These studies have been performed in pregnant rats at intravenous doses up to 60 mg/kg/day (5.4 times the recommended human dose based on body surface area) and pregnant rabbits at intravenous doses up to 20 mg/kg/day (3.2 times the recommended human dose based on body surface area). There are, however, no adequate and well-controlled studies in pregnant women. Because animal reproduction studies are not always predictive of human response, this drug should be used during pregnancy only if clearly needed.
Nursing Mothers
It is not known whether dolasetron mesylate is excreted in human milk. Because many drugs are excreted in human milk, caution should be exercised when ANZEMET Injection is administered to a nursing woman.
Pediatric Use
Four open-label, noncomparative pharmacokinetic studies have been performed in a total of 108 pediatric patients receiving emetogenic chemotherapy or undergoing surgery with general anesthesia. These patients received ANZEMET Injection either intravenously or orally in juice. Pediatric patients from 2 to 17 years of age participated in these trials, which included intravenous ANZEMET Injection doses of 0.6, 1.2, 1.8 or 2.4 mg/kg, and oral doses of 0.6, 1.2, or 1.8 mg/kg. There is no experience in pediatric patients under 2 years of age. Overall, ANZEMET Injection was well tolerated in these pediatric patients. Efficacy information collected in pediatric patients receiving cancer chemotherapy are consistent with those obtained in adults. No efficacy information was collected in the pediatric postoperative nausea and vomiting studies.

Use in Elderly Patients
Dosage adjustment is not needed in patients over 65. Effectiveness in prevention of nausea and vomiting in elderly patients was no different than in younger age-groups.

ADVERSE REACTIONS
Chemotherapy Patients
In controlled clinical trials, 2265 adult patients received ANZEMET Injection. The overall adverse event rates were similar with 1.8 mg/kg ANZEMET Injection and ondansetron or granisetron. Patients were receiving concurrent chemotherapy, predominantly high-dose (≥50 mg/m²) cisplatin. Following is a combined listing of all adverse events reported in ≥2% of patients in these controlled trials (Table 4).
[See table 4 above]
Postoperative Patients
In controlled clinical trials with 2550 adult patients, headache and dizziness were reported more frequently with 12.5 mg ANZEMET Injection than with placebo. Rates of other adverse events were similar. Following is a listing of all adverse events reported in ≥2% of patients receiving either placebo or 12.5 mg ANZEMET Injection for the prevention or treatment of postoperative nausea and vomiting in controlled clinical trials (Table 5).
[See table 5 at left]
In clinical trials, the following infrequently reported adverse events, assessed by investigators as treatment-related or causality unknown, occurred following oral or intravenous administration of ANZEMET to adult patients receiving concomitant cancer chemotherapy or surgery:
Cardiovascular: Hypotension; rarely–edema, peripheral edema. The following events also occurred rarely and with a similar frequency as placebo and/or active comparator: Mobitz I AV block, chest pain, orthostatic hypotension, myocardial ischemia, syncope, severe bradycardia, and palpitations. See PRECAUTIONS section for information on potential effects on ECG.
In addition, the following asymptomatic treatment-emergent ECG changes were seen at rates less than or equal to those for active or placebo controls: bradycardia, tachycardia, T wave change, ST-T wave change, sinus arrhythmia, extrasystole (APCs or VPCs), poor R-wave progression, bundle branch block (left and right), nodal arrhythmia, U wave change, atrial flutter/fibrillation.
Dermatologic: Rash, increased sweating.
Gastrointestinal System: Constipation, dyspepsia, abdominal pain, anorexia; rarely–pancreatitis.
Hearing, Taste and Vision: Taste perversion, abnormal vision; rarely–tinnitus, photophobia.
Hematologic: Rarely–hematuria, epistaxis, prothrombin time prolonged, PTT increased, anemia, purpura/hematoma, thrombocytopenia.
Hypersensitivity: Rarely–anaphylactic reaction, facial edema, urticaria.
Liver and Biliary System: Transient increases in AST (SGOT) and/or ALT (SGPT) values have been reported as adverse events in less than 1% of adult patients receiving ANZEMET in clinical trials. The increases did not appear to be related to dose or duration of therapy and were not associated with symptomatic hepatic disease. Similar increases were seen with patients receiving active comparator. Rarely–hyperbilirubinemia, increased GGT.
Metabolic and Nutritional: Rarely–alkaline phosphatase increased.
Musculoskeletal: Rarely–myalgia, arthralgia.
Nervous System: Flushing, vertigo, paraesthesia, tremor; rarely–ataxia, twitching.
Psychiatric: Agitation, sleep disorder, depersonalization; rarely–confusion, anxiety, dreaming abnormal.
Respiratory System: Rarely–dyspnea, bronchospasm.
Urinary System: Rarely–dysuria, polyuria, acute renal failure.
Vascular (Extracardia): Rarely–peripheral ischemia, thrombophlebitis/phlebitis.

OVERDOSAGE

A 59-year old man with metastatic melanoma developed severe hypotension and dizziness 40 minutes after receiving a 15 minute intravenous infusion of 1000 mg (13 mg/kg) of dolasetron mesylate. Treatment for the overdose consisted of infusion of 500 mL of a plasma expander, dopamine, and atropine. The patient had normal sinus rhythm and prolongation of PR, QRS and QT$_c$ intervals on an ECG recorded 2 hours after the infusion. The patient's blood pressure was normal 3 hours after the event and the ECG intervals returned to baseline on follow-up. The patient was released from the hospital 6 hours after the event.
Following a suspected overdose of ANZEMET Injection, a patient found to have second-degree or higher AV conduction block should undergo cardiac telemetry monitoring.
There is no known specific antidote for dolasetron mesylate, and patients with suspected overdose should be managed

Continued on next page

Anzemet Injection—Cont.

with supportive therapy. Individual doses as large as 5 mg/kg intravenously or 400 mg orally have been safely given to healthy volunteers or cancer patients.
It is not known if dolasetron mesylate is removed by hemodialysis or peritoneal dialysis.
A 7-year-old boy received 6 mg/kg dolasetron mesylate orally before surgery. No symptoms occurred and no treatment was required.
Single intravenous doses of dolasetron mesylate at 160 mg/kg in male mice and 140 mg/kg in female mice and rats of both sexes (6.3 to 12.6 times the recommended human dose based on body surface area) were lethal. Symptoms of acute toxicity were tremors, depression and convulsions.

DOSAGE AND ADMINISTRATION

The recommended dose of ANZEMET Injection should not be exceeded.

Prevention of Cancer Chemotherapy-Induced Nausea and Vomiting

Adults: The recommended intravenous dosage of ANZEMET Injection from clinical trial results is 1.8 mg/kg given as a single dose approximately 30 minutes before chemotherapy (see Administration). Alternatively, for most patients, a fixed dose of 100 mg can be administered over 30 seconds.

Pediatric Patients: The recommended intravenous dosage in pediatric patients 2 to 16 years of age is 1.8 mg/kg given as a single dose approximately 30 minutes before chemotherapy, up to a maximum of 100 mg (see Administration). Safety and effectiveness in pediatric patients under 2 years of age have not been established.
ANZEMET Injection mixed in apple or apple-grape juice may be used for oral dosing of pediatric patients. When ANZEMET Injection is administered orally, the recommended dosage in pediatric patients 2 to 16 years of age is 1.8 mg/kg up to a maximum 100 mg dose given within 1 hour before chemotherapy.
The diluted product may be kept up to 2 hours at room temperature before use.

Use in the Elderly, in Renal Failure Patients, or in Hepatically Impaired Patients: No dosage adjustment is recommended.

Prevention or Treatment of Postoperative Nausea and/or Vomiting

Adults: The recommended intravenous dosage of ANZEMET Injection is 12.5 mg given as a single dose approximately 15 minutes before the cessation of anesthesia (prevention) or as soon as nausea or vomiting presents (treatment).

Pediatric Patients: The recommended intravenous dosage in pediatric patients 2 to 16 years of age is 0.35 mg/kg, with a maximum dose of 12.5 mg, given as a single dose approximately 15 minutes before the cessation of anesthesia or as soon as nausea or vomiting presents. Safety and effectiveness in pediatric patients under 2 years of age have not been established.
ANZEMET Injection mixed in apple or apple-grape juice may be used for oral dosing of pediatric patients. When ANZEMET Injection is administered orally, the recommended oral dosage in pediatric patients 2 to 16 years of age is 1.2 mg/kg up to a maximum 100-mg dose given within 2 hours before surgery. The diluted product may be kept up to 2 hours at room temperature before use.

Use in the Elderly, in Renal Failure Patients, or in Hepatically Impaired Patients: No dosage adjustment is recommended.

Administration

ANZEMET Injection can be safely infused intravenously as rapidly as 100 mg/30 seconds or diluted in a compatible intravenous solution (see below) to 50 mL and infused over a period of up to 15 minutes. ANZEMET Injection should not be mixed with other drugs. Flush the infusion line before and after administration of ANZEMET Injection.

Stability

After dilution, ANZEMET Injection is stable under normal lighting conditions at room temperature for 24 hours or under refrigeration for 48 hours with the following compatible intravenous fluids: 0.9% sodium chloride injection, 5% dextrose injection, 5% dextrose and 0.45% sodium chloride injection, 5% dextrose and Lactated Ringer's injection, Lactated Ringer's injection, and 10% mannitol injection. Although ANZEMET Injection is chemically and physically stable when diluted as recommended, sterile precautions should be observed because diluents generally do not contain preservative. After dilution, do not use beyond 24 hours, or 48 hours if refrigerated.
Parenteral drug products should be inspected visually for particulate matter and discoloration before administration whenever solution and container permit.

HOW SUPPLIED

ANZEMET Injection (dolasetron mesylate injection) is supplied in single-use ampuls and vials as a clear, colorless solution.

[See third table from top of previous page]
Store at controlled room temperature 20–25°C (68–77°F). Protect from light.

Prescribing information as of October 1997

Manufactured for Hoechst Marion Roussel, Inc.
Kansas City, MO 64137 USA

Manufactured by Ben Venue Laboratories, Inc.
Bedford, OH 44146 USA

Shown in Product Identification Guide, page 316

ANZEMET® Tablets ℞

[*an-zĕmĕt*]
(dolasetron mesylate)

Prescribing Information as of October 1997

DESCRIPTION

ANZEMET (dolasetron mesylate) is an antinauseant and antiemetic agent. Chemically, dolasetron mesylate is (2α,6α,8α,9aβ)-octahydro-3-oxo-2,6-methano-2*H*-quinolizin-8-yl-1*H*-indole-3-carboxylate monomethanesulfonate, monohydrate. It is a highly specific and selective serotonin subtype 3 ($5\text{-}HT_3$) receptor antagonist both in vitro and in vivo.
Dolasetron mesylate has the following structural formula:

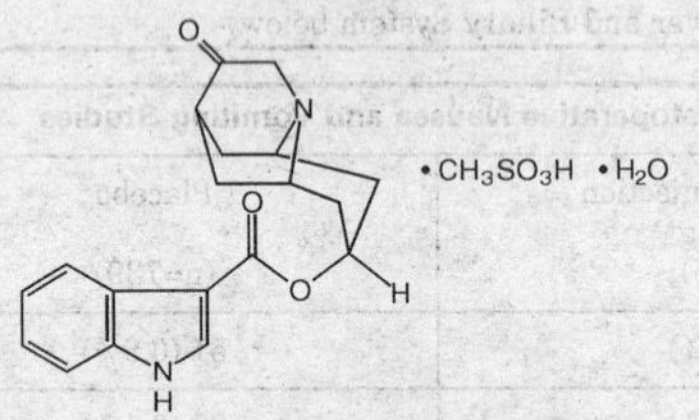

The empirical formula is $C_{19}H_{20}N_2O_3 \bullet CH_3SO_3H \bullet H_2O$, with a molecular weight of 438.50. Approximately 74% of dolasetron mesylate monohydrate is dolasetron base. Dolasetron mesylate monohydrate is a white to off-white powder that is freely soluble in water and propylene glycol, slightly soluble in ethanol, and slightly soluble in normal saline. Each ANZEMET Tablet for oral administration contains dolasetron mesylate (as the monohydrate) and also contains the inactive ingredients: carnauba wax, croscarmellose sodium, hydroxypropyl methylcellulose, lactose, magnesium stearate, polyethylene glycol, polysorbate 80, pregelatinized starch, synthetic red iron oxide, titanium dioxide, and white wax. The tablets are printed with black ink, which contains lecithin, pharmaceutical glaze, propylene glycol, and synthetic black iron oxide.

CLINICAL PHARMACOLOGY

Dolasetron mesylate and its active metabolite, hydrodolasetron (MDL 74,156), are selective serotonin $5\text{-}HT_3$ receptor antagonists not shown to have activity at other known serotonin receptors and with low affinity for dopamine receptors. The serotonin $5\text{-}HT_3$ receptors are located on the nerve terminals of the vagus in the periphery and centrally in the chemoreceptor trigger zone of the area postrema. It is thought that chemotherapeutic agents produce nausea and vomiting by releasing serotonin from the enterochromaffin cells of the small intestine, and that the released serotonin then activates $5\text{-}HT_3$ receptors located on vagal efferents to initiate the vomiting reflex.
Acute, usually reversible, ECG changes (PR and QT_c prolongation; QRS widening), caused by dolasetron mesylate, have been observed in healthy volunteers and in controlled clinical trials. The active metabolites of dolasetron may block sodium channels, a property unrelated to its ability to block $5\text{-}HT_3$ receptors. QT_c prolongation is primarily due to QRS widening. Dolasetron appears to prolong both depolarization and, to a lesser extent, repolarization time. The magnitude and frequency of the ECG changes increased with dose (related to peak plasma concentrations of hydrodolasetron but not the parent compound). These ECG interval prolongations usually returned to baseline within 6 to 8 hours, but in some patients were present at 24 hour follow up. Dolasetron mesylate administration has little or no effect on blood pressure.
In healthy volunteers (N=64), dolasetron mesylate in single intravenous doses up to 5 mg/kg produced no effect on pupil size or meaningful changes in EEG tracings. Results from neuropsychiatric tests revealed that dolasetron mesylate did not alter mood or concentration. Multiple daily doses of dolasetron have had no effect on colonic transit in humans. Dolasetron has no effect on plasma prolactin concentrations.

Pharmacokinetics in Humans

Oral dolasetron is well absorbed, although parent drug is rarely detected in plasma due to rapid and complete metabolism to the most clinically relevant species, hydrodolasetron.
The reduction of dolasetron to hydrodolasetron is mediated by a ubiquitous enzyme, carbonyl reductase. Cytochrome P-450 (CYP)IID6 is primarily responsible for the subsequent hydroxylation of hydrodolasetron and both CYPIIIA and flavin monooxygenase are responsible for the N-oxidation of hydrodolasetron.
Hydrodolasetron is excreted in the urine unchanged (61.0% of administered oral dose).
Other urinary metabolites include hydroxylated glucuronides and N-oxide.
Hydrodolasetron appears rapidly in plasma, with a maximum concentration occurring approximately 1 hour after dosing, and is eliminated with a mean half-life of 8.1 hours (%CV=18%) and an apparent clearance of 13.4 mL/min/kg (%CV=29%) in 30 adults. The apparent absolute bioavailability of oral dolasetron, determined by the major active metabolite hydrodolasetron, is approximately 75%. Orally administered dolasetron intravenous solution and tablets are bioequivalent. Food does not affect the bioavailability of dolasetron taken by mouth.
Hydrodolasetron is eliminated by multiple routes, including renal excretion and, after metabolism, mainly, glucuronidation and hydroxylation. Two thirds of the administered dose is recovered in the urine and one third in the feces. Hydrodolasetron is widely distributed in the body with a mean apparent volume of distribution of 5.8 L/kg (%CV=25%, N=24) in adults.
Sixty-nine to 77% of hydrodolasetron is bound to plasma protein. In a study with ^{14}C labeled dolasetron, the distribution of radioactivity to blood cells was not extensive. Approximately 50% of hydrodolasetron is bound to α_1-acid glycoprotein. The pharmacokinetics of hydrodolasetron are linear and similar in men and women.

Pediatric Patients

The pharmacokinetics of ANZEMET Tablets have not been studied in the pediatric population. However, the following pharmacokinetic data are available on intravenous ANZEMET Injection administered orally to children.
Thirty-two pediatric cancer patients ages 3 to 11 years (N=19) and 12 to 17 years (N=13), received 0.6, 1.2, or 1.8 mg ANZEMET Injection diluted with either apple or apple-grape juice and administered orally. In this study, the mean apparent clearances of hydrodolasetron were 3 times greater in the younger pediatric group and 1.8 times greater in the older pediatric group than those observed in healthy adult volunteers. Across this spectrum of pediatric patients, maximum plasma concentrations were 0.6 to 0.7 times those observed in healthy adults receiving similar doses.
For 12 pediatric patients, ages 2 to 12 years receiving 1.2 mg/kg ANZEMET Injection diluted in apple or apple-grape juice and administered orally, the mean apparent clearance was 34% greater and half-life was 21% shorter than in healthy adults receiving the same dose. The pharmacokinetics of hydrodolasetron, in special and targeted patient populations following oral administration of dolasetron, are summarized in Table 1. The pharmacokinetics of hydrodolasetron are similar in adult healthy volunteers and in adult cancer patients receiving chemotherapeutic agents.
The apparent clearance following oral administration of hydrodolasetron is approximately 1.6- to 3.4-fold higher in children and adolescents than in adults. The clearance following oral administration of hydrodolasetron is not affected by age in adult cancer patients. The apparent oral clearance of hydrodolasetron decreases 42% with severe hepatic impairment and 44% with severe renal impairment. No dose adjustment is necessary for elderly patients or for patients with hepatic or renal impairment.
[See table 1 at top of next page]

CLINICAL STUDIES

Prevention of Cancer Chemotherapy-Induced Nausea and Vomiting

Oral ANZEMET at a dose of 100 mg prevents nausea and vomiting associated with moderately emetogenic cancer therapy as shown by 24 hour efficacy data from two double-blind studies. Efficacy was based on complete response (ie, no vomiting, no rescue medication). The first randomized, double-blind trial compared single oral ANZEMET doses of 25, 50, 100 and 200 mg in 60 men and 259 women cancer patients receiving cyclophosphamide and/or doxorubicin. There was no statistically significant difference in complete response between the 100 mg and 200 mg dose. Results are summarized in Table 2.
[See table 2 at top of next page]
Another trial also compared single oral ANZEMET doses of 25, 50, 100 and 200 mg in 307 patients receiving moderately emetogenic chemotherapy. In this study, the 100 mg ANZEMET dose gave a 73% complete response rate.

Prevention of Postoperative Nausea and Vomiting

ANZEMET Tablets at a dose of 100 mg administered orally 1–2 hours before surgery and before general balanced anesthesia (short-acting barbiturate, nitrous oxide, narcotic analgesic, and skeletal muscle relaxant) was significantly more effective than placebo in preventing postoperative nausea and vomiting. Efficacy was based on complete response rates (0 emetic episodes and no rescue medication over 24 hours). No increased efficacy was seen with higher doses.

Table 1. Pharmacokinetic Values for Plasma Hydrodolasetron Following Oral Administration of ANZEMET*

	Age (years)	Dose	CL$_{app}$ (mL/min/kg)	t$_{1/2}$ (h)	C$_{max}$ (ng/mL)
Young Healthy Volunteers (N=30)	19–45	200 mg	13.4 (29%)	8.1 (18%)	556 (28%)
Elderly Healthy Volunteers (N=15)	65–75	2.4 mg/kg	9.5 (36%)	7.2 (32%)	662 (28%)
Cancer Patients Adults (N=61)†	24–84	25–200 mg	12.9 (49%)	7.9 (43%)	— ‡
Adolescents (N=13)	12–17	0.6–1.8 mg/kg	26.5 (67%)	6.4 (30%)	374 § (32%)
Children (N=19)	3–11	0.6–1.8 mg/kg	44.2 (49%)	5.5 (39%)	217 ‖ (67%)
Pediatric Surgery Patients (N=11)	2–12	1.2 mg/kg	20.8 (49%)	5.9 (24%)	159 (32%)
Patients with Severe Renal Impairment (N=12) (Creatinine clearance ≤10 mL/min)	28–74	200 mg	7.2 (48%)	10.7 (29%)	701 (21%)
Patients with Severe Hepatic Impairment (N=3)	42–52	150 mg	8.8 (57%)	11.0 (36%)	410 (12%)

CL$_{app}$: apparent clearance t$_{1/2}$: terminal elimination half-life ( ): coefficient of variation in %
*: mean values
†: analyzed by nonlinear mixed effect modeling with data pooled across dose strengths
‡: sampling times did not allow calculation
§: results from adolescents (dose=1.8 mg/kg, N=3)
‖: results from children (dose=1.8 mg/kg, N=7)

Table 2. Prevention of Chemotherapy-Induced Nausea and Vomiting from Moderately Emetogenic Chemotherapy

	ANZEMET Tablets				
Response Over 24 Hours	25 mg (N=78)	50 mg (N=83)	**100 mg† (N=80)**	200 mg (N=78)	P-value for Linear Trend
Complete Response‡	24 (31%)	34 (41%)	**49 (61%)**	46 (59%)	P<.0001
Nausea Score§	49	10	**11**	7	P=.0006

†: The recommended dose
‡: No emetic episodes and no rescue medication.
§: Median 24-h change from baseline nausea score using visual analog scale (VAS): Score range 0 = "none" to 100 = "nausea as bad as it can be."

Table 3. Prevention of Postoperative Nausea and Vomiting

	ANZEMET Tablets				
Response Over 24 Hours	25 mg (N=159)	50 mg (N=166)	**100 mg† (N=154)**	200 mg (N=154)	Placebo (N=156)
Complete Response‡	71 (45%)	95 (57%)*	**78 (51%)***	73 (47%)*	55 (35%)
Nausea Score§	5*	4*	**5***	6*	15

*: P<.05 vs placebo
†: The recommended dose
‡: No emetic episodes and no rescue medication.
§: Median 24-h change from baseline nausea score using visual analog scale (VAS): Score range 0 = "none" to 100 = "nausea as bad as it can be."

One trial compared single ANZEMET Tablet doses of 25, 50, 100 and 200 mg with placebo in 789 women undergoing gynecological surgery. In this study the 100 mg dose produced a complete response rate statistically superior to placebo. The study results are summarized in Table 3.
[See table 3 above]
Another trial also compared single oral ANZEMET doses of 25, 50, 100 and 200 mg with placebo in 373 women undergoing gynecological surgery. In this study, the 100 mg ANZEMET dose gave a 54% complete response rate as compared to the 29% rate of placebo.

INDICATIONS AND USAGE
ANZEMET Tablets are indicated for:
1) the prevention of nausea and vomiting associated with moderately-emetogenic cancer chemotherapy, including initial and repeat courses;
2) the prevention of postoperative nausea and vomiting.

CONTRAINDICATIONS
ANZEMET Tablets are contraindicated in patients known to have hypersensitivity to the drug.

WARNINGS
ANZEMET can cause ECG interval changes (PR, QT$_C$, JT prolongation and QRS widening). These changes are related in magnitude and frequency to blood levels of the active metabolite. These changes are self-limiting with declining blood levels. Some patients have interval prolongations for 24 hours or longer. Interval prolongation could lead to cardiovascular consequences, including heart block or cardiac arrhythmias. These have rarely been reported.
A cardiac conduction abnormality observed on an intraoperative cardiac rhythm monitor (interpreted as complete heart block) was reported in a 61 year old woman who received 200 mg ANZEMET for the prevention of postoperative nausea and vomiting. This patient was also taking verapamil. A similar event also interpreted as complete heart block was reported in one patient receiving placebo.
A 66-year-old man with Stage IV non-Hodgkins lymphoma died suddenly 6 hours after receiving 1.8 mg/kg (119 mg) intravenous ANZEMET Injection. This patient had other potential risk factors including substantial exposure to doxorubicin and concomitant cyclophosphamide.

PRECAUTIONS
General
Dolasetron should be administered with caution in patients who have or may develop prolongation of cardiac conduction intervals, particularly QT$_c$. These include patients with hypokalemia or hypomagnesemia, patients taking diuretics with potential for inducing electrolyte abnormalities, patients with congenital QT syndrome, patients taking anti-arrhythmic drugs or other drugs which lead to QT prolongation, and cumulative high dose anthracycline therapy.
Drug Interactions
The potential for clinically significant drug-drug interactions posed by dolasetron and hydrodolasetron appears to be low for drugs commonly used in chemotherapy or surgery, because hydrodolasetron is eliminated by multiple routes. See PRECAUTIONS, General for information about potential interaction with other drugs that prolong the QT$_c$ interval. Blood levels of hydrodolasetron increased 24% when dolasetron was coadministered with cimetidine (nonselective inhibitor of cytochrome P-450) for 7 days, and decreased 28% with coadministration of rifampin (potent inducer of cytochrome P-450) for 7 days.
ANZEMET has been safely coadministered with drugs used in chemotherapy and surgery. As with other agents which prolong ECG intervals, caution should be exercised in patients taking drugs which prolong ECG intervals, particularly QT$_c$.
In patients taking furosemide, nifedipine, diltiazem, ACE inhibitors, verapamil, glyburide, propranolol, and various chemotherapy agents, no effect was shown on the clearance of hydrodolasetron. Clearance of hydrodolasetron decreased by about 27% when dolasetron mesylate was administered intravenously concomitantly with atenolol. ANZEMET does not influence anesthesia recovery time in patients. Dolasetron mesylate did not inhibit the antitumor activity of four chemotherapeutic agents (cisplatin, 5-fluorouracil, doxorubicin, cyclophosphamide) in four murine models.

Carcinogenesis, Mutagenesis, Impairment of Fertility
In a 24-month carcinogenicity study, there was a statistically significant (P<0.001) increase in the incidence of combined hepatocellular adenomas and carcinomas in male mice treated with 150 mg/kg/day and above. In this study, mice (CD-1) were treated orally with dolasetron mesylate 75, 150 or 300 mg/kg/day (225, 450 or 900 mg/m^2/day). For a 50 kg person of average height (1.46 m^2 body surface area), these doses represent 3, 6, and 12 times the recommended clinical dose (74 mg/m^2) on a body surface area basis. No increase in liver tumors was observed at a dose of 75 mg/kg/day in male mice and at doses up to 300 mg/kg/day in female mice.
In a 24-month rat (Sprague-Dawley) carcinogenicity study, oral dolasetron mesylate was not tumorigenic at doses up to 150 mg/kg/day (900 mg/m^2/day, 12 times the recommended human dose based on body surface area) in male rats and 300 mg/kg/day (1800 mg/m^2/day, 24 times the recommended human dose based on body surface area) in female rats.
Dolasetron mesylate was not genotoxic in the Ames test, the rat lymphocyte chromosomal aberration test, the Chinese hamster ovary (CHO) cell (HGPRT) forward mutation test, the rat hepatocyte unscheduled DNA synthesis (UDS) test or the mouse micronucleus test.
Dolasetron mesylate was found to have no effect on fertility and reproductive performance at oral doses up to 100 mg/kg/day (600 mg/m^2/day, 8 times the recommended human dose based on body surface area) in female rats and up to 400 mg/kg/day (2400 mg/m^2/day, 32 times the recommended human dose based on body surface area) in male rats.
Pregnancy: Teratogenic Effects, Pregnancy Category B.
Teratology studies have not revealed evidence of impaired fertility or harm to the fetus due to dolasetron mesylate. These studies have been performed in pregnant rats at oral doses up to 100 mg/kg/day (8 times the recommended human dose based on body surface area) and pregnant rabbits at oral doses up to 100 mg/kg/day (16 times the recommended human dose based on body surface area). There are, however, no adequate and well-controlled studies in pregnant women. Because animal reproduction studies are not always predictive of human response, this drug should be used during pregnancy only if clearly needed.
Nursing Mothers
It is not known whether dolasetron mesylate is excreted in human milk. Because many drugs are excreted in human milk, caution should be exercised when ANZEMET Tablets are administered to a nursing woman.
Pediatric Use
ANZEMET Tablets are expected to be as safe and effective as when ANZEMET Injection is given orally to pediatric patients. ANZEMET Tablets are recommended for children old enough to swallow tablets (see CLINICAL PHARMACOLOGY, Pharmacokinetics in Humans).
Elderly
Dosage adjustment is not needed in patients over 65. Effectiveness in prevention of nausea and vomiting in elderly patients was no different than in younger age groups.

ADVERSE REACTIONS
Chemotherapy Patients
In controlled clinical trials, 943 adult cancer patients received ANZEMET Tablets. These patients were receiving concurrent chemotherapy, predominantly cyclophosphamide and doxorubicin regimens. The following adverse events were reported in ≥2% of patients receiving either ANZEMET 25 mg or ANZEMET 100 mg tablets for prevention of cancer chemotherapy induced nausea and vomiting in controlled clinical trials (Table 4).

Continued on next page

Anzemet Tablets—Cont.

Table 4. Adverse Events ≥2% from Chemotherapy-Induced Nausea and Vomiting Studies

Event	ANZEMET	
	25 mg (N=235)	100 mg (N=227)
Headache	42 (17.9%)	52 (22.9%)
Fatigue	6 (2.6%)	13 (5.7%)
Diarrhea	5 (2.1%)	12 (5.3%)
Bradycardia	12 (5.1%)	9 (4.0%)
Dizziness	3 (1.3%)	7 (3.1%)
Pain	0	7 (3.1%)
Tachycardia	7 (3.0%)	6 (2.6%)
Dyspepsia	7 (3.0%)	5 (2.2%)
Chills/Shivering	3 (1.3%)	5 (2.2%)

Postoperative Patients

In controlled clinical trials, 936 adult female patients have received oral ANZEMET for the prevention of postoperative nausea and vomiting. Following is a listing of all adverse events reported in ≥2% of patients receiving either placebo or ANZEMET for prevention of postoperative nausea and vomiting in controlled clinical trials (Table 5).

Table 5. Adverse Events ≥ 2% from Placebo-Controlled Postoperative Nausea and Vomiting Studies

Event	ANZEMET 100 mg (N=228)	Placebo (N=231)
Headache	16 (7.0%)	11 (4.8%)
Hypotension	12 (5.3%)	15 (6.5%)
Dizziness	10 (4.4%)	0 (0.0%)
Fever	8 (3.5%)	7 (3.0%)
Pruritus	7 (3.1%)	8 (3.5%)
Oliguria	6 (2.6%)	3 (1.3%)
Hypertension	5 (2.2%)	7 (3.0%)
Tachycardia	5 (2.2%)	2 (0.9%)

In clinical trials, the following infrequently reported adverse events, assessed by investigators as treatment-related or causality unknown, occurred following oral or intravenous administration of ANZEMET to adult patients receiving concomitant cancer chemotherapy or surgery:

Cardiovascular: Hypotension; rarely-edema, peripheral edema. The following events also occurred rarely and with a similar frequency as placebo and/or active comparator: Mobitz I AV block, chest pain, orthostatic hypotension, myocardial ischemia, syncope, severe bradycardia, and palpitations. See PRECAUTIONS section for information on potential effects on ECG.

In addition, the following asymptomatic treatment-emergent ECG changes were seen at rates less than or equal to those for active or placebo controls: bradycardia, T wave change, ST-T wave change, sinus arrhythmia, extrasystole (APCs or VPCs), poor R-wave progression, bundle branch block (left and right), nodal arrhythmia, U wave change, atrial flutter/fibrillation.

Dermatologic: Rash, increased sweating.

Gastrointestinal System: Constipation, dyspepsia, abdominal pain, anorexia; rarely—pancreatitis.

Hearing, Taste and Vision: Taste perversion, abnormal vision; rarely—tinnitus, photophobia.

Hematologic: Rarely—hematuria, epistaxis, prothrombin time prolonged, PTT increased, anemia, purpura/hematoma, thrombocytopenia.

Hypersensitivity: Rarely—anaphylactic reaction, facial edema, urticaria.

Liver and Biliary System: Transient increases in AST (SGOT) and/or ALT (SGPT) values have been reported as adverse events in less than 1% of adult patients receiving ANZEMET in clinical trials. The increases did not appear to be related to dose or duration of therapy and were not associated with symptomatic hepatic disease. Similar increases were seen with patients receiving active comparator. Rarely—hyperbilirubinemia, increased GGT.

Metabolic and Nutritional: Rarely—alkaline phosphatase increased.

Musculoskeletal: Rarely—myalgia, arthralgia.

Nervous System: Flushing, vertigo, paresthesia, tremor; rarely—ataxia, twitching.

Psychiatric: Agitation, sleep disorder, depersonalization; rarely—confusion, anxiety, dreaming abnormal.

Respiratory System: Rarely—dyspnea, bronchospasm.

Urinary System: Rarely—dysuria, polyuria, acute renal failure.

Vascular (Extracardiac): Rarely—peripheral ischemia, thrombophlebitis/phlebitis.

OVERDOSAGE

A 59-year-old man with metastatic melanoma developed severe hypotension and dizziness 40 minutes after receiving a 15 minute intravenous infusion of 1000 mg (13 mg/kg) of dolasetron mesylate. Treatment for the overdose consisted of infusion of 500 mL of a plasma expander, dopamine, and atropine. The patient had normal sinus rhythm and prolongation of PR, QRS and QT$_c$ intervals on an ECG recorded 2 hours after the infusion. The patient's blood pressure was normal 3 hours after the event and the ECG intervals returned to baseline on follow-up. The patient was released from the hospital 6 hours after the event. Following a suspected overdose of ANZEMET Injection, a patient found to have second-degree or higher AV conduction block should undergo cardiac telemetry monitoring.

There is no known specific antidote for dolasetron mesylate, and patients with suspected overdose should be managed with supportive therapy. Individual doses as large as 5 mg/kg intravenously or 400 mg orally have been safely given to healthy volunteers or cancer patients.

It is not known if dolasetron mesylate is removed by hemodialysis or peritoneal dialysis.

A 7-year-old boy received 6 mg/kg of dolasetron mesylate orally before surgery. No symptoms occurred and no treatment was required.

Single intravenous doses of dolasetron mesylate at 160 mg/kg in male mice and 140 mg/kg in female mice and rats of both sexes (6.3 to 12.6 times the recommended human dose based on body surface area) were lethal. Symptoms of acute toxicity were tremors, depression and convulsions.

DOSAGE AND ADMINISTRATION

The recommended doses of ANZEMET Tablets should not be exceeded.

Prevention of Cancer Chemotherapy-Induced Nausea and Vomiting

Adults: The recommended oral dosage of ANZEMET (dolasetron mesylate) is 100 mg given within one hour before chemotherapy.

Pediatric Patients: The recommended oral dosage in pediatric patients 2 to 16 years of age is 1.8 mg/kg given within one hour before chemotherapy, up to a maximum of 100 mg. Safety and effectiveness in pediatric patients under 2 years of age have not been established.

Use in the Elderly, Renal Failure Patients, or Hepatically Impaired Patients: No dosage adjustment is recommended. (See Pharmacokinetics in Humans.)

Prevention of Postoperative Nausea and Vomiting

Adults: The recommended oral dosage of ANZEMET (dolasetron mesylate) is 100 mg within two hours before surgery.

Pediatric Patients: The recommended oral dosage in pediatric patients 2 to 16 years of age is 1.2 mg/kg given within

two hours before surgery, up to a maximum of 100 mg. Safety and effectiveness in pediatric patients under 2 years of age have not been established.

Use in the Elderly, Renal Failure Patients, or Hepatically Impaired Patients:

No dosage adjustment is recommended. (See Pharmacokinetics in Humans.)

HOW SUPPLIED

[See table below]

Store at controlled room temperature 20–25°C (68–77°F). Protect from light.

Prescribing Information as of October 1997

Hoechst Marion Roussel, Inc.

Kansas City, MO 64137 USA

Shown in Product Identification Guide, page 316

A/T/S®

(erythromycin)

2% ACNE TOPICAL SOLUTION FOR DERMATOLOGIC USE ONLY. NOT FOR USE IN EYES.

℞

Prescribing Information as of August 1991

DESCRIPTION

A/T/S® (erythromycin) is an antibiotic produced from a strain of *Streptomyces erythraeus*. It is basic and readily forms salts with acids. Each mL of A/T/S® Topical Solution contains 20 mg of erythromycin base in a vehicle consisting of alcohol USP (66%), propylene glycol USP, and citric acid USP to adjust pH. The CAS Registry Number is 114-07-8.

ACTIONS

Although the mechanism of action by which A/T/S® Topical Solution acts in reducing inflammatory lesions of acne vulgaris is unknown, it is presumably due to its antibiotic action.

INDICATIONS

A/T/S® is indicated for the topical control of acne vulgaris.

CONTRAINDICATION

A/T/S® is contraindicated in persons who have shown hypersensitivity to any of its ingredients.

WARNING

The safe use of A/T/S® Topical Solution during pregnancy or lactation has not been established.

PRECAUTIONS

General: The use of antibiotic agents may be associated with the overgrowth of antibiotic-resistant organisms. If this occurs, administration of the drug should be discontinued and appropriate measures taken.

Information for Patients: A/T/S® (erythromycin) is for external use only and should be kept away from the eyes, nose, mouth, and other mucous membranes. Concomitant topical acne therapy should be used with caution because a cumulative irritant effect may occur, especially with the use of peeling, desquamating, or abrasive agents.

Carcinogenesis, Mutagenesis, Impairment of Fertility: Long-term animal studies to evaluate carcinogenic potential, mutagenicity, or the effect on fertility of erythromycin have not been performed.

Pregnancy: Pregnancy Category C. Animal reproduction studies have not been conducted with erythromycin. It is also not known whether erythromycin can cause fetal harm when administered to a pregnant woman or can affect reproduction capacity. Erythromycin should be given to a pregnant woman only if clearly needed.

Nursing Mothers: Erythromycin is excreted in breast milk. Caution should be exercised when erythromycin is administered to a nursing woman.

ADVERSE REACTIONS

Adverse conditions reported with the use of erythromycin topical solutions include dryness, tenderness, pruritus, desquamation, erythema, oiliness, and burning sensation. Irritation of the eyes has also been reported. A case of generalized urticarial reaction, possibly related to the drug, which required the use of systemic steroid therapy has been reported.

Of a total of 90 patients exposed to A/T/S® during clinical effectiveness studies, 17 experienced some type of adverse effect. These included dry skin, scaly skin, pruritis, irritation of the eye, and burning sensation.

DOSAGE AND ADMINISTRATION

A/T/S® Topical Solution should be applied to the affected area twice a day after the skin is thoroughly washed with warm water and soap and patted dry. Moisten the applicator or a pad with A/T/S®, then rub over the affected area. Acne lesions of the face, neck, shoulder, chest, and back may be treated in this manner.

ANZEMET®
(dolasetron mesylate)
Tablets

Strength	Quantity	NDC Number	Description
50 mg	5 ct Bottle 10 ct Unit Dose 5 ct Blister Pack	0088-1202-05 0088-1202-43 0088-1202-29	Light pink, film coated, round tablet imprinted with "ANZEMET 50" on one side.
100 mg	5 ct Bottle 10 ct Unit Dose 5 ct Blister Pack	0088-1203-05 0088-1203-43 0088-1203-29	Pink, film coated, elongated oval tablet imprinted with "100" on one side and "ANZEMET" on the other.

HOW SUPPLIED

A/T/S® 2% Acne Topical Solution—60 mL
Store at controlled room temperature (59–86°F).
Prescribing Information as of August 1991
Distributed by:
Hoechst-Roussel Pharmaceuticals
Division of Hoechst Marion Roussel, Inc.
Kansas City, MO 64137 USA
Shown in Product Identification Guide, page 315

A/T/S®   Rx
(Erythromycin Topical Gel USP) 2%
FOR DERMATOLOGIC USE ONLY
NOT FOR OPTHALMIC USE

DESCRIPTION

A/T/S® Topical Gel contains erythromycin. Erythromycin is a macrolide antibiotic obtained from cultures of *Streptomyces erythraeus.*

Structural Formula

Erythromycin
Empirical Formula: $C_{37}H_{67}NO_{13}$
Molecular Weight: 733.94
Contains: erythromycin, USP .... 2% (20 mg/g)
with: alcohol 92% and hydroxypropyl cellulose.

CLINICAL PHARMACOLOGY

The exact mechanism by which erythromycin reduces lesions of acne vulgaris is not fully known; however, the effect appears to be due in part to the antibacterial activity of the drug.

MICROBIOLOGY

Erythromycin appears to inhibit protein synthesis in susceptible organisms by reversibly binding to ribosomal subunits, thereby inhibiting translocation of aminoacyl transfer-RNA and inhibiting polypeptide synthesis. Antagonism has been demonstrated between erythromycin, lincomycin, chloramphenicol, and clindamycin.

INDICATIONS AND USAGE

A/T/S® is indicated for the topical treatment of acne vulgaris.

CONTRAINDICATIONS

A/T/S® is contraindicated in those individuals who have shown hypersensitivity to any of its components.

PRECAUTIONS

General: For topical use only; not for ophthalmic use. Concomitant topical acne therapy should be used with caution since a possible cumulative irritancy effect may occur, especially with the use of peeling, desquamating or abrasive agents.
Avoid contact with eyes and all mucous membranes. The use of antibiotic agents may be associated with the overgrowth of antibiotic-resistant organisms. If this occurs, discontinue use and take appropriate measures.
Carcinogenesis, mutagenesis, impairment of fertility: Animal studies to evaluate carcinogenic and mutagenic potential, or effects on fertility have not been performed with erythromycin.
Pregnancy Category B:
There was no evidence of teratogenicity or any other adverse effect on reproduction in female rats fed erythromycin base (up to 0.25% of diet) prior to and during mating, during gestation and through weaning of two successive litters. There are, however, no adequate and well-controlled studies in pregnant women. Because animal reproduction studies are not always predictive of human response, this drug should be used in pregnancy only if clearly needed. Erythromycin has been reported to cross the placental barrier in humans, but fetal plasma levels are generally low.
Nursing Mothers:
It is not known whether topically applied erythromycin is excreted in human milk. A decision should be made whether to discontinue nursing or to discontinue the drug, taking into account the importance of the drug to the mother.
Pediatric Use:
Safety and effectiveness in children have not been established.

ADVERSE REACTIONS

The most common adverse reaction reported with A/T/S® (Erythromycin Topical Gel USP) 2% was burning. The following have been reported occasionally: peeling, dryness, itching, erythema, and oiliness, irritation of the eyes and tenderness of the skin have also been reported with the topical use of erythromycin. A generalized urticarial reaction, possibly related to the use of erythromycin, which required systemic steroid therapy has been reported.

DOSAGE AND ADMINISTRATION

Apply sparingly as a thin film once or twice a day to the affected area(s) after the skin is thoroughly cleansed and patted dry. If there has been no improvement after 6 to 8 weeks, or if the condition becomes worse, treatment should be discontinued, and the physician should be consulted. Spread the medication lightly rather than rubbing it in. The hands should be washed after application. There are no data directly comparing the safety and efficacy of b.i.d. versus q.d. dosing.

HOW SUPPLIED

A/T/S® (Erythromycin Topical Gel USP) 2% - 30 gram plastic tubes (NDC 0039-0116-30).
Note: FLAMMABLE. Keep away from heat and flame. Keep tube tightly closed. Store between 15° and 25°C (59° and 77°F).
CAUTION: Federal law prohibits dispensing without prescription.
Manufactured by:
ALLERGAN Herbert
Skin Care Division of ALLERGAN, INC.
Irvine, CA 92715
Distributed by:
Hoechst-Roussel Pharmaceuticals
Division of Hoechst Marion Roussel, Inc.
Kansas City, MO 64137 USA

711600-12/93

Shown in Product Identification Guide, page 315

AVC™   Rx
(sulfanilamide)
Cream/Suppositories

Prescribing information as of March 1996

DESCRIPTION

AVC™ is a preparation for vaginal administration for the treatment of *Candida albicans* infections and available in the following forms:
AVC Cream
Each tube contains:
Sulfanilamide 15.0%
in a water-miscible, non-staining base made from lactose, propylene glycol, stearic acid, diglycol stearate, methylparaben, propylparaben, trolamine, and water; buffered with lactic acid to an acid pH of approximately 4.3.
AVC Suppositories
Each suppository contains:
Sulfanilamide .... 1.05 g
with lactose, in a base made from polyethylene glycol 400, polysorbate 80, polyethylene glycol 3350, and glycerin, buffered with lactic acid to an acid pH of approximately 4.5. AVC Suppositories have an inert, white, non-staining covering, which dissolves promptly in the vagina. The covering is composed of gelatin, glycerin, water, methylparaben, propylparaben, and coloring.
Sulfanilamide is an anti-infective agent. It is *p*-amino-benzenesulfonamide with the chemical structure:

Sulfanilamide occurs as a white odorless crystalline powder with a slightly bitter taste and sweet aftertaste. It is slightly soluble in water, alcohol, acetone, glycerin, propylene glycol, hydrochloric acid, and solutions of potassium and sodium hydroxide. It is practically insoluble in chloroform, ether, benzene, and petroleum ether.

CLINICAL PHARMACOLOGY

Sulfanilamide has been a useful ingredient of vaginal formulations for about four decades. It blocks certain metabolic processes essential for the growth of susceptible bacteria. In AVC, the sulfanilamide is in a specially compounded base buffered to the pH (about 4.3) of the normal vagina to encourage the presence of the normally occurring Döderlein's bacilli of the vagina.
The use of AVC for the treatment of vulvovaginitis caused by *Candida albicans* is supported by three clinical investigations. The three studies show AVC with sulfanilamide to be significantly more effective (p≤0.01) than placebo as follows:

In Study I, the ratio of effectiveness was 71% for the AVC with sulfanilamide versus 49% for placebo with 30 days of treatment;
In Study II, the percentages were 48% and 24%, respectively, with 15 days of treatment;
In Study III, the percentages were 66% versus 33%, respectively, with 30 days of treatment.

INDICATIONS AND USAGE

For the treatment of vulvovaginitis caused by *Candida albicans.* (See CLINICAL PHARMACOLOGY.)

CONTRAINDICATIONS

AVC should not be used in patients known to be sensitive to this product or to the sulfonamides.

PRECAUTIONS

General
Because sulfonamides are absorbed from the vaginal mucosa, the usual precautions for oral sulfonamides apply. Patients should be observed for skin rash or evidence of systemic toxicity, and if these develop, the medications should be discontinued.
Deaths associated with administration of oral sulfonamides have reportedly occurred from hypersensitivity reactions, agranulocytosis, aplastic anemia, and other blood dyscrasias.
Goiter production, diuresis, and hypoglycemia have reportedly occurred rarely in patients receiving oral sulfonamides. Cross-sensitivity may exist with these agents. Rats appear to be especially susceptible to the goitrogenic effects of sulfonamides, and long-term administration has reportedly produced thyroid malignancies in this species.
Vaginal applicators or inserters should be used with caution after the seventh month of pregnancy.
Information For Patients
The doctor should advise the patient that in the event unusual local itching and burning occur, or other unusual symptoms develop, medication should be discontinued and not restarted without further consultation.
Drug Interactions
Drug interactions have not been documented with AVC.
Carcinogenesis, Mutagenesis, Impairment of Fertility
No data are available on long-term potential of AVC for carcinogenicity, mutagenicity, or impairment of fertility in animals or humans.
Pregnancy
Teratogenic Effects. Pregnancy Category C: Animal reproductive studies have been conducted with sulfonamides, including sulfanilamide (see below). It is not known whether AVC can cause fetal harm when administered to a pregnant woman or can affect reproductive capacity. AVC should be given to a pregnant woman only if clearly needed.
Sulfonamides, including sulfanilamide, readily pass through the placenta and reach fetal circulation. The concentration in the fetus is from 50–90% of that in the maternal blood and if high enough, can cause toxic effects. The safe use of sulfonamides, including sulfanilamide, in pregnancy has not been established. The teratogenic potential of most sulfonamides has not been thoroughly investigated in either animals or humans. However, a significant increase in the incidence of cleft palate and other bony abnormalities of offspring has been observed with certain sulfonamides of the short-, intermediate-, and long-acting types (including sulfanilamide) when given to pregnant rats and mice at high oral doses (seven to 25 times the human therapeutic oral dose).
Nursing Mothers
Sulfanilamide should be avoided in nursing mothers because absorbed sulfonamides will appear in maternal milk, and have caused kernicterus in the newborn. Because of the potential for serious adverse reactions in nursing infants from sulfonamides, a decision should be made whether to discontinue nursing or to discontinue the drug.
Pediatric Use
Safety and effectiveness of AVC in pediatric patients have not been established.

ADVERSE REACTIONS

Local sensitivity reactions such as increased discomfort or a burning sensation have occasionally been reported following the use of topical sulfonamides. With the use of AVC Cream, sensitivity reactions (only local) were reported for 0.2% of the investigational patients.
Treatment should be discontinued if either local or systemic manifestations of sulfonamide toxicity or sensitivity occur.

DRUG ABUSE AND DEPENDENCE

Tolerance, abuse, or dependence with AVC have not been reported.

OVERDOSAGE

There have been no reports of accidental overdosage with AVC.
The acute oral LD_{50} of sulfanilamide is 3700–4200 mg/kg in mice.

Continued on next page

AVC—Cont.

The minimum human lethal dose of AVC has not been established.
It is not known if AVC is dialyzable.

DOSAGE AND ADMINISTRATION

One applicatorful (about 6 g) or one suppository intravaginally once or twice daily. Improvements in symptoms should occur within a few days, but treatment should be continued for a period of 30 days.
Douching with a suitable solution before insertion may be recommended for hygienic purposes.

HOW SUPPLIED

AVC Cream
NDC 0068-0099-04 4 oz tube with applicator
Store at room temperature, below 86°F. Protect from cold.
Product darkens with age. Potency is maintained throughout labeled shelf life when stored as directed.
AVC Suppositories
NDC 0068-0098-16 Box of 16 white gelatin suppositories with inserter
Store at room temperature, below 86°F. Protect from excessive cold and moisture.
Prescribing information as of March 1996
Suppositories Manufactured by
R.P. Scherer, North America
Saint Petersburg, Florida 33716
for
Merrell Pharmaceuticals Inc.
Subsidiary of Hoechst Marion Roussel, Inc.
Kansas City, MO 64137 USA

BRICANYL® ℞

[*brĭk 'ă-nĭl*]
(terbutaline sulfate USP)
Subcutaneous Injection

Prescribing Information as of February 1996

DESCRIPTION

BRICANYL (terbutaline sulfate USP) Subcutaneous Injection is a sterile, isotonic solution. Each mL of solution contains 1 mg terbutaline sulfate (equivalent to 0.82 mg free base) and 8.9 mg sodium chloride in water for injection. Hydrochloric acid is used to adjust pH to 3–5. Filled under nitrogen.
Terbutaline sulfate (5-[2-[(1,1-dimethylethyl)amino]-1-hydroxyethyl]-1,3-benzenediol sulfate) is a β-adrenergic agonist bronchodilator having the chemical structure:

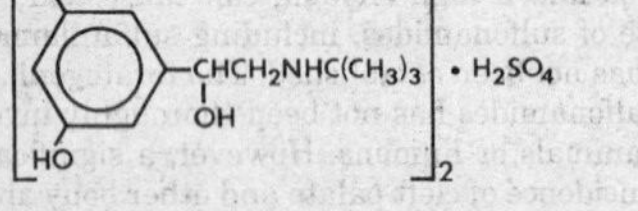
HO
CHCH2NHC(CH3)3
OH
HO
• H2SO4
2

CLINICAL PHARMACOLOGY

BRICANYL is a β-adrenergic receptor agonist which has been shown by in vitro and in vivo pharmacologic studies in animals to exert a preferential effect on β_2-adrenergic receptors, such as those located in bronchial smooth muscle. However, controlled clinical studies of patients who were administered the drug have not revealed a preferential β_2-adrenergic effect.
It has been postulated that β-adrenergic agonists produce many of their pharmacologic effects by activation of adenyl cyclase, the enzyme which catalyzes the conversion of adenosine triphosphate to cyclic adenosine monophosphate.
BRICANYL Injection has been shown in controlled clinical studies to relieve acute bronchospasm in acute and chronic obstructive pulmonary disease, resulting in a clinically significant increase in pulmonary flow rates, e.g., an increase of 15% or greater in FEV_1 in some patients. Following administration of 0.25 mg by subcutaneous injection, a measurable change in flow rate is usually observed within five minutes, and a clinically significant increase in FEV_1 occurs by 15 minutes following the injection. The maximum effect usually occurs within 30–60 minutes and clinically significant bronchodilator activity has been observed to persist for 90 minutes to four hours in most patients. The duration of clinically significant improvement is comparable to that found with equimilligram doses of epinephrine.
Subcutaneously administered BRICANYL shows peak plasma concentrations 15–30 minutes after injection (0.5 mg dose, mean peak plasma level 7.6 μg/L). Approximately one-third is metabolized (inactive), the majority of the dose being excreted in urine unchanged. A half-life of 3–4 hours has been reported.
Terbutaline crosses the placenta. After single dose IV administration of terbutaline to 22 women in late pregnancy who were delivered by elective Caesarean section due to clinical reasons, umbilical blood levels of terbutaline were found to range from 11 to 48% of the maternal blood levels.
Recent studies in laboratory animals (minipigs, rodents, and dogs) recorded the occurrence of cardiac arrhythmias and sudden death (with histologic evidence of myocardial necrosis) when β agonists and methylxanthines were administered concurrently. The significance of these findings when applied to humans is currently unknown.

INDICATIONS AND USAGE

BRICANYL is indicated as a bronchodilator for the relief of reversible bronchospasm in patients with obstructive airway diseases such as asthma, bronchitis, and emphysema.

CONTRAINDICATIONS

BRICANYL is contraindicated in patients with a history of hypersensitivity to any of its components or sympathomimetic amines.

WARNINGS

Usage in Labor and Delivery: BRICANYL is not indicated and should not be used for the management of preterm labor. Serious adverse reactions have been reported following administration of terbutaline sulfate to women in labor. These reports have included transient hypokalemia, pulmonary edema (sometimes after delivery), and hypoglycemia in the mother and/or the neonatal child. Maternal death has been reported with terbutaline sulfate and other drugs of this class.
There have been rare reports of seizures occurring in patients receiving terbutaline, which do not recur when the drug is discontinued and have not been explained on any other basis.

PRECAUTIONS

General
Terbutaline sulfate is a sympathomimetic amine and as such should be used with caution in patients with cardiovascular disorders (including arrhythmias, coronary insufficiency, and hypertension), in patients with hyperthyroidism or diabetes mellitus, history of seizures, or in patients who are unusually responsive to sympathomimetic amines.
Age-related differences in the hemodynamic response to β-adrenergic receptor stimulation have been reported.
Patients susceptible to hypokalemia should be monitored because transient early falls in serum potassium levels have been reported with β agonists.
Immediate hypersensitivity reactions and exacerbation of bronchospasm have been reported after terbutaline administration.
Preparation of Other Dosage Forms: Use of the subcutaneous injection for preparation of other dosage forms, e.g., IV infusion, is not appropriate. Sterility, stability, and accurate dosing cannot be assured if the ampuls are not used in accordance with information in DOSAGE AND ADMINISTRATION.
Large doses of intravenous terbutaline sulfate have been reported to aggravate preexisting diabetes and ketoacidosis.
Information for Patients
Patients should be advised regarding the potential adverse reactions associated with BRICANYL.
Drug Interactions
Other sympathomimetic bronchodilators or epinephrine should not be used concomitantly with terbutaline sulfate since their combined effect on the cardiovascular system may be deleterious to the patient.
Terbutaline sulfate should be administered with caution in patients being treated with monoamine oxidase (MAO) inhibitors or tricyclic antidepressants, since the action of terbutaline sulfate on the vascular system may be potentiated.
β-adrenergic receptor blocking agents not only block the pulmonary effect of terbutaline but may produce severe asthmatic attacks in asthmatic patients. Therefore, patients requiring treatment for both bronchospastic disease and hypertension should be treated with medication other than β-adrenergic blocking agents for hypertension.
Carcinogenesis, Mutagenesis, Impairment of Fertility
A 2 year, oral carcinogenesis bioassay of terbutaline sulfate (50, 500, 1000, and 2000 mg/kg, corresponding to 5,000, 50,000, 100,000, and 200,000 times the recommended daily adult subcutaneous dose, respectively) in the Sprague-Dawley rat revealed drug-related changes in the female genital system. Females showed dose-related increases in leiomyomas of the mesovarium: 3 (5%) at 50 mg/kg, 17 (28%) at 500 mg/kg, 21 (35%) at 1000 mg/kg, and 23 (38%) at 2000 mg/kg, which were significant at the three highest levels. None occurred in female controls. The incidence of ovarian cysts was significantly elevated at all dose levels except at 2000 mg/kg and hyperplasia of the mesovarium was increased significantly at 500 and 2000 mg/kg. A 21-month oral study of terbutaline sulfate (5, 50 and 200 mg/kg, corresponding to 500, 5,000 and 20,000 times the recommended daily adult subcutaneous dose, respectively) in the mouse revealed no evidence of carcinogenicity.
Studies of terbutaline sulfate have not been conducted to determine mutagenic potential.
An oral reproduction study of terbutaline sulfate up to 50 mg/kg (corresponding to 5,000 times the human subcutaneous dose) in the rat revealed no adverse effects on fertility.
Pregnancy
Teratogenic Effects. Pregnancy Category B: Reproduction studies in mice (up to 1.1 mg/kg subcutaneously, corresponding to 110 times the human subcutaneous dose) and in rats and rabbits (up to 50 mg/kg orally, corresponding to 5,000 times the human subcutaneous dose) have revealed no evidence of impaired fertility or harm to the fetus due to terbutaline. There are, however, no adequate and well-controlled studies in pregnant women. Because animal reproduction studies are not always predictive of human response, this drug should be used during pregnancy only if clearly needed.
Labor and Delivery
Usage in Labor and Delivery: The safe use of BRICANYL for the management of preterm labor or for other uses during labor and delivery has not been established and the drug should not be used. (See WARNINGS.)
Nursing Mothers
Terbutaline is excreted in breast milk. Caution should be exercised when BRICANYL is administered to a nursing woman.
Pediatric Use
Safety and effectiveness in pediatric patients below the age of 12 have not been established.

ADVERSE REACTIONS

The adverse reactions of terbutaline sulfate are similar to those of other sympathomimetic agents.
The most commonly observed side effects are tremor and nervousness. These occur more frequently at doses in excess of 0.25 mg. Other commonly reported reactions include increased heart rate, palpitations and dizziness. Other reported reactions include headache, drowsiness, vomiting, nausea, sweating, and muscle cramps. These reactions are generally transient and usually do not require treatment.
There have been rare reports of elevations in liver enzymes and of hypersensitivity vasculitis.

OVERDOSAGE

Overdosage information is limited. Excessive adrenergic-receptor stimulation may augment the signs and symptoms listed under ADVERSE REACTIONS and may be accompanied by other adrenergic effects.
Signs and symptoms of overdosage may include the following:
Cardiovascular: tachycardia of varying degrees, transient arrhythmias, and extrasystoles. A significant drop in blood pressure may occur due to peripheral vasodilation.
Neuromuscular: tremors of varying degrees, nervousness, drowsiness, muscle cramps, headache, and sweating.
Gastrointestinal: nausea and vomiting.
Endocrine: varying degrees of hyperglycemia and rise in insulin levels which could be followed by rebound hypoglycemia. Hypokalemia in the early stages may occur. The duration of these signs and symptoms will be dependent on the degree of overdosage.
In the case of terbutaline overdosage, the patient should be treated symptomatically for sympathomimetic overdosage with careful consideration to the appropriateness of any chosen therapy and possible effect on the patient's underlying disease state. (See also WARNINGS.)
Studies in mice, rats, rabbits, and dogs have established the LD_{50} of terbutaline to be 1–9 g/kg orally and 0.3–1.6 g/kg subcutaneously.
It is not known whether terbutaline is dialyzable.

DOSAGE AND ADMINISTRATION

Parenteral drug products should be inspected visually for particulate matter and discoloration prior to administration, whenever solution and container permit.
The usual subcutaneous dose of BRICANYL is 0.25 mg (0.25 mL, 1/4 ampul contents) injected into the lateral deltoid area. If significant clinical improvement does not occur by 15–30 minutes, a second dose of 0.25 mg may be administered. A total dose of 0.5 mg should not be exceeded within a four-hour period. If a patient fails to respond to a second 0.25 mg (0.25 mL) dose within 15–30 minutes, other therapeutic measures should be considered.

HOW SUPPLIED

Each 2 mL size ampul contains 1 mL of solution (1 mg terbutaline sulfate). Note: 0.25 mL of solution will provide the usual clinical dose of 0.25 mg.
NDC 0068-0702-20: package of 10 ampuls
Solutions of terbutaline sulfate are sensitive to excessive heat and light. Ampuls should, therefore, be stored at controlled room temperature 15–30°C (59–86°F) in their original carton to provide protection from light until dispensed.
Solutions should not be used if discolored.
Prescribing Information as of February 1996
Manufactured for
Merrell Pharmaceuticals Inc.
Subsidiary of Hoechst Marion Roussel, Inc.

Kansas City, MO 64137 USA
Shown in Product Identification Guide, page 316

BRICANYL® ℞
[*brĭk 'ă-nĭl*]
(terbutaline sulfate USP)
Tablets

Prescribing Information as of February 1996

DESCRIPTION

BRICANYL (terbutaline sulfate USP) Tablets for oral administration contain 2.5 or 5 mg of terbutaline sulfate (equivalent to 2.05 and 4.1 mg free base, respectively). Both the 2.5 and 5 mg tablets contain the following inactive ingredients: corn starch (or pregelatinized corn starch), lactose, magnesium stearate, microcrystalline cellulose, and povidone.
Terbutaline sulfate (5-[2-[(1,1-dimethylethyl)amino]-1-hydroxyethyl]-1,3-benzenediol sulfate) is a β-adrenergic agonist bronchodilator having the chemical structure:

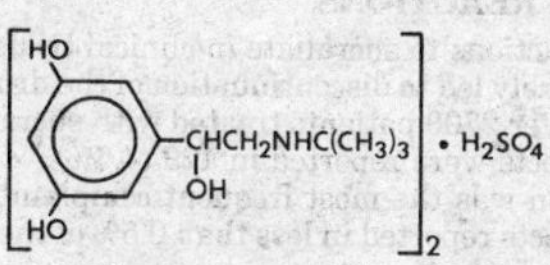

CLINICAL PHARMACOLOGY

BRICANYL is a β-adrenergic receptor agonist which has been shown by in vitro and in vivo pharmacologic studies in animals to exert a preferential effect on β_2-adrenergic receptors, such as those located in bronchial smooth muscle. However, controlled clinical studies on patients who were administered the drug have not revealed a preferential β_2-adrenergic effect.
It has been postulated that β-adrenergic agonists produce many of their pharmacologic effects by activation of adenyl cyclase, the enzyme which catalyzes the conversion of adenosine triphosphate to cyclic adenosine monophosphate.
BRICANYL Tablets have been shown in controlled clinical studies to relieve bronchospasm in chronic obstructive pulmonary disease, such as asthma, chronic bronchitis, and emphysema. This action was manifested by a clinically significant increase in pulmonary function as demonstrated by an increase of 15% or greater in FEV_1 in some patients. A measurable change in pulmonary function usually occurs within 30 minutes following oral administration. The maximum effect usually occurs within 120–180 minutes. There is a clinically significant decrease in airway and pulmonary resistance which persists for at least 4 hours or longer in most patients. Significant bronchodilator action, as measured by various pulmonary function determinations (airway resistance, MMEFR, PEFR) has been demonstrated in studies for periods up to 8 hours in many patients.
Clinical studies have evaluated the effectiveness of oral BRICANYL for periods up to 12 months and the drug continued to produce significant improvement of pulmonary function throughout the period of treatment.
Orally administered terbutaline sulfate is 30–70% absorbed in the GI tract (food reduces bioavailability by one-third). Sixty percent of the absorbed oral dose is metabolized via first pass conjugation in the gut wall and liver. There are no known active metabolites. After single oral doses, peak concentrations are found 30 minutes to 5 hours after administration. Each mg of orally administered terbutaline sulfate (in fasting adults) produces an average peak serum concentration of approximately 1 μg/L. Terbutaline has a half-life of 3–4 hours and is excreted in the urine.
Terbutaline crosses the placenta. After single dose IV administration of terbutaline to 22 women in late pregnancy who were delivered by elective Caesarean section due to clinical reasons, umbilical blood levels of terbutaline were found to range from 11 to 48% of the maternal blood levels.
Recent studies in laboratory animals (minipigs, rodents, and dogs) recorded the occurrence of cardiac arrhythmias and sudden death (with histologic evidence of myocardial necrosis) when β agonists and methylxanthines were administered concurrently. The significance of these findings when applied to humans is currently unknown.

INDICATIONS AND USAGE

BRICANYL is indicated as a bronchodilator for the relief of reversible bronchospasm in patients with obstructive airway diseases, such as asthma, bronchitis, and emphysema.

CONTRAINDICATIONS

BRICANYL is contraindicated in patients with a history of hypersensitivity to any of its components or sympathomimetic amines.

WARNINGS

Usage in Labor and Delivery. BRICANYL is not indicated and should not be used for the management of preterm labor. Serious adverse reactions have been reported following administration of terbutaline sulfate to women in labor. These reports have included transient hypokalemia, pulmonary edema (sometimes after delivery), and hypoglycemia in the mother and/or the neonatal pediatric patient. Maternal death has been reported with terbutaline sulfate and other drugs of this class.
There have been rare reports of seizures occurring in patients receiving terbutaline, which do not recur when the drug is discontinued and have not been explained on any other basis.

PRECAUTIONS

General

Terbutaline sulfate is a sympathomimetic amine and as such should be used with caution in patients with cardiovascular disorders (including arrhythmias, coronary insufficiency, and hypertension), in patients with hyperthyroidism or diabetes mellitus, history of seizures, or in patients who are unusually responsive to sympathomimetic amines.
Age-related differences in the hemodynamic response to β-adrenergic receptor stimulation have been reported.
Patients susceptible to hypokalemia should be monitored because transient early falls in serum potassium levels have been reported with β agonists.
Large doses of intravenous terbutaline sulfate have been reported to aggravate preexisting diabetes and ketoacidosis. The relevance of this observation to the use of BRICANYL Tablets is unknown.
Immediate hypersensitivity reactions and exacerbation of bronchospasm have been reported after terbutaline administration.

Information for Patients

The patient should be advised regarding the potential adverse reactions associated with BRICANYL and that: (1) the action of BRICANYL Tablets may last up to 8 hours and, therefore, should not be used more frequently than recommended, (2) the number or frequency of doses should not be increased without medical consultation, (3) medical consultation should be sought promptly if symptoms get worse, and (4) other medicines should not be used while taking BRICANYL without consulting the physician.

Drug Interactions

Other sympathomimetic bronchodilators or epinephrine should not be used concomitantly with terbutaline sulfate, since their combined effect on the cardiovascular system may be deleterious to the patient. This recommendation does not preclude the judicious use of an aerosol bronchodilator of the adrenergic stimulant type in patients receiving BRICANYL Tablets.
Such concomitant use, however, should be individualized and not given on a routine basis. If regular coadministration is required, alternative therapy should be considered. Terbutaline sulfate should be administered with caution in patients being treated with monoamine oxidase (MAO) inhibitors or tricyclic antidepressants, since the action of terbutaline sulfate on the vascular system may be potentiated.
β-Adrenergic receptor blocking agents not only block the pulmonary effect of terbutaline, but may produce severe asthmatic attacks in asthmatic patients. Therefore, patients requiring treatment for both bronchospastic disease and hypertension should be treated with medication other than β-adrenergic blocking agents for hypertension.

Carcinogenesis, Mutagenesis, Impairment of Fertility

A 2-year, oral carcinogenesis bioassay of terbutaline sulfate (50, 500, 1000 and 2000 mg/kg, corresponding to 167, 1667, 3333, and 6667 times the recommended daily adult oral dose, respectively) in the Sprague-Dawley rat revealed drug-related changes in the female genital system. Females showed dose-related increases in leiomyomas of the mesovarium: 3 (5%) at 50 mg/kg, 17 (28%) at 500 mg/kg, 21 (35%) at 1000 mg/kg, and 23 (38%) at 2000 mg/kg, which were significant at the three highest levels. None occurred in female controls. The incidence of ovarian cysts was significantly elevated at all dose levels except at 2000 mg/kg and hyperplasia of the mesovarium was increased significantly at 500 and 2000 mg/kg. A 21-month oral study of terbutaline sulfate (5, 50 and 200 mg/kg, corresponding to 17, 167 and 667 times the recommended daily adult oral dose, respectively) in the mouse revealed no evidence of carcinogenicity.
Studies of terbutaline sulfate have not been conducted to determine mutagenic potential.
An oral reproduction study of terbutaline sulfate up to 50 mg/kg (corresponding to 167 times the human oral dose) in the rat revealed no adverse effects on fertility.

Pregnancy

Teratogenic Effects. Pregnancy Category B: Reproduction studies in mice (up to 1.1 mg/kg subcutaneously, corresponding to four times the human oral dose) and in rats and rabbits (up to 50 mg/kg orally, corresponding to 167 times the human oral dose) have revealed no evidence of impaired fertility or harm to the fetus due to terbutaline. There are, however, no adequate and well-controlled studies in pregnant women. Because animal reproduction studies are not always predictive of human response, this drug should be used during pregnancy only if clearly needed.

Labor and Delivery

Usage in Labor and Delivery. The safe use of BRICANYL for the mangement of preterm labor or for other uses during labor and delivery has not been established and the drug should not be used. (See WARNINGS.)

Nursing Mothers

Terbutaline is excreted in breast milk. Caution should be exercised when BRICANYL is administered to a nursing woman.

Pediatric Use

Safety and effectiveness in pediatric patients below the age of 12 have not been established.

ADVERSE REACTIONS

The adverse reactions of terbutaline sulfate are similar to those of other sympathomimetic agents.
The most commonly observed side effects are tremor and nervousness. The frequency of these side effects appear to diminish with continued therapy. Other commonly reported reactions include increased heart rate, palpitations, and dizziness. Other reported reactions include headache, drowsiness, vomiting, nausea, sweating, and muscle cramps. These reactions are generally transient and usually do not require treatment.
There have been rare reports of elevations in liver enzymes and of hypersensitivity vasculitis.

OVERDOSAGE

Overdosage information is limited. Excessive adrenergic-receptor stimulation may augment the signs and symptoms listed under ADVERSE REACTIONS and may be accompanied by other adrenergic effects.
Signs and symptoms of overdosage may include the following:
Cardiovascular: tachycardia of varying degrees, transient arrhythmias, and extrasystoles. A significant drop in blood pressure may occur due to peripheral vasodilation.
Neuromuscular: tremors of varying degrees, nervousness, drowsiness, muscle cramps, headache, and sweating.
Gastrointestinal: nausea and vomiting.
Endocrine: varying degrees of hyperglycemia and rise in insulin levels which could be followed by rebound hypoglycemia. Hypokalemia in the early stages may occur. The duration of these sign and symptoms will be dependent on the degree of overdosage.
Treat the alert patient who has taken excessive oral medication by emptying the stomach by means of induced emesis, followed by gastric lavage. In the unconscious patient, secure the airway with a cuffed endotracheal tube before beginning lavage (do not induce emesis). Instillation of activated charcoal slurry may help reduce absorption of terbutaline sulfate. Maintain adequate respiratory exchange. Provide cardiac and respiratory support as needed. Continue observation until symptom-free.
Careful consideration should be given to the appropriateness of any chosen therapy and possible effect on the patient's underlying disease state. (See also WARNINGS.)
Studies in mice, rats, rabbits, and dogs have established the LD_{50} of terbutaline to be 1–9 g/kg orally and 0.3–1.6 g/kg subcutaneously.
It is not known whether terbutaline is dialyzable.

DOSAGE AND ADMINISTRATION

Adults. Usual dose is 5 mg three times daily. Dosing may be initiated at 2.5 mg three or four times daily and titrated upward depending on clinical response. A total dose of 15 mg in a 24-hour period should not be exceeded.
Pediatric patients. (12–15 yrs): 2.5 mg three times daily.
If a previously effective dosage regimen fails to provide the usual relief, medical advice should be sought immediately as this is often a sign of seriously worsening asthma which would require reassessment of therapy.

HOW SUPPLIED

2.5 mg tablets (round, white, debossed "BRICANYL $2^1/_2$"):
NDC 0068-0725-61: Bottle of 100
5.0 mg tablets (square, white, scored, debossed "BRICANYL 5"):
NDC 0068-0750-61: Bottle of 100
Store at controlled room temperature 15°–30°C (59°–86°F).
Prescribing Information as of February 1996
Merrell Pharmaceuticals Inc.
Subsidiary of Hoechst Marion Roussel, Inc.
Kansas City, MO 64137
Shown in Product Identification Guide, page 316

CARAFATE® Tablets ℞
[*kăr 'afăt*]
(sucralfate)
Prescribing Information as of May 1996

DESCRIPTION

CARAFATE Tablets contain sucralfate and sucralfate is an α-D-glucopyranoside, β-D-fructofuranosyl-, octakis-(hydrogen sulfate), aluminum complex.
[See chemical structure at top of next column]

Continued on next page

Carafate Tablets—Cont.

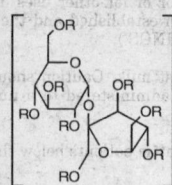

[Al(OH)₃] x [H₂O] γ
(χ = 8 to 10 and γ = 22 to 31)

R = SO₃Al(OH)₂

Tablets for oral administration contain 1 g of sucralfate. Also contain: D&C Red #30 Lake, FD&C Blue #1 Lake, magnesium stearate, microcrystalline cellulose, and starch. Therapeutic category: antiulcer.

CLINICAL PHARMACOLOGY

Sucralfate is only minimally absorbed from the gastrointestinal tract. The small amounts of the sulfated disaccharide that are absorbed are excreted primarily in the urine.

Although the mechanism of sucralfate's ability to accelerate healing of duodenal ulcers remains to be fully defined, it is known that it exerts its effect through a local, rather than systemic, action. The following observations also appear pertinent:

1. Studies in human subjects and with animal models of ulcer disease have shown that sucralfate forms an ulcer-adherent complex with proteinaceous exudate at the ulcer site.
2. In vitro, a sucralfate-albumin film provides a barrier to diffusion of hydrogen ions.
3. In human subjects, sucralfate given in doses recommended for ulcer therapy inhibits pepsin activity in gastric juice by 32%.
4. In vitro, sucralfate adsorbs bile salts.

These observations suggest that sucralfate's antiulcer activity is the result of formation of an ulcer-adherent complex that covers the ulcer site and protects it against further attack by acid, pepsin, and bile salts. There are approximately 14 to 16 mEq of acid-neutralizing capacity per 1-g dose of sucralfate.

CLINICAL TRIALS

Acute Duodenal Ulcer

Over 600 patients have participated in well-controlled clinical trials worldwide. Multicenter trials conducted in the United States, both of them placebo-controlled studies with endoscopic evaluation at 2 and 4 weeks, showed:

STUDY 1

Treatment Groups	Ulcer Healing/No. Patients	
	2 wk	4 wk (Overall)
Sucralfate	37/105 (35.2%)	82/109 (75.2%)
Placebo	26/106 (24.5%)	68/107 (63.6%)

STUDY 2

Treatment Groups	Ulcer Healing/No. Patients	
	2 wk	4 wk (Overall)
Sucralfate	8/24 (33%)	22/24 (92%)
Placebo	4/31 (13%)	18/31 (58%)

The sucralfate-placebo differences were statistically significant in both studies at 4 weeks but not at 2 weeks. The poorer result in the first study may have occurred because sucralfate was given 2 hours after meals and at bedtime rather than 1 hour before meals and at bedtime, the regimen used in international studies and in the second United States study. In addition, in the first study liquid antacid was utilized as needed, whereas in the second study antacid tablets were used.

Maintenance Therapy After Healing of Duodenal Ulcer

Two double-blind randomized placebo-controlled U.S. multicenter trials have demonstrated that sucralfate (1 g bid) is effective as maintenance therapy following healing of duodenal ulcers.

In one study, endoscopies were performed monthly for 4 months. Of the 254 patients who enrolled, 239 were analyzed in the intention-to-treat life table analysis presented below.

Duodenal Ulcer Recurrence Rate (%)

Drug	n	Months of Therapy			
		1	2	3	4
CARAFATE	122	20*	30*	38†	42†
Placebo	117	33	46	55	63

*P<0.05, †P<0.01

In this study, prn antacids were not permitted.

In the other study, scheduled endoscopies were performed at 6 and 12 months, but for-cause endoscopies were permitted as symptoms dictated. Median symptom scores between the sucralfate and placebo groups were not significantly different. A life table intention-to-treat analysis for the 94 patients enrolled in the trial had the following results:

Duodenal Ulcer Recurrence Rate (%)

Drug	n	6 months	12 months
CARAFATE	48	19*	27*
Placebo	46	54	65

*P<0.002

In this study, prn antacids were permitted.

Data from placebo-controlled studies longer than 1 year are not available.

INDICATIONS AND USAGE

CARAFATE® (sucralfate) is indicated in:
- Short-term treatment (up to 8 weeks) of active duodenal ulcer. While healing with sucralfate may occur during the first week or two, treatment should be continued for 4 to 8 weeks unless healing has been demonstrated by x-ray or endoscopic examination.
- Maintenance therapy for duodenal ulcer patients at reduced dosage after healing of acute ulcers.

CONTRAINDICATIONS

There are no known contraindications to the use of sucralfate.

PRECAUTIONS

Duodenal ulcer is a chronic, recurrent disease. While short-term treatment with sucralfate can result in complete healing of the ulcer, a successful course of treatment with sucralfate should not be expected to alter the posthealing frequency or severity of duodenal ulceration.

Special Populations: Chronic Renal Failure and Dialysis Patients

When sucralfate is administered orally, small amounts of aluminum are absorbed from the gastrointestinal tract. Concomitant use of sucralfate with other products that contain aluminum, such as aluminum-containing antacids, may increase the total body burden of aluminum. Patients with normal renal function receiving the recommended doses of sucralfate and aluminum-containing products adequately excrete aluminum in the urine. Patients with chronic renal failure or those receiving dialysis have impaired excretion of absorbed aluminum. In addition, aluminum does not cross dialysis membranes because it is bound to albumin and transferrin plasma proteins. Aluminum accumulation and toxicity (aluminum osteodystrophy, osteomalacia, encephalopathy) have been described in patients with renal impairment. Sucralfate should be used with caution in patients with chronic renal failure.

Drug Interactions

Some studies have shown that simultaneous sucralfate administration in healthy volunteers reduced the extent of absorption (bioavailability) of single doses of the following: cimetidine, digoxin, fluoroquinolone antibiotics, ketoconazole, l-thyroxine, phenytoin, quinidine, ranitidine, tetracycline, and theophylline. Subtherapeutic prothrombin times with concomitant warfarin and sucralfate therapy have been reported in spontaneous and published case reports. However, two clinical studies have demonstrated no change in either serum warfarin concentration or prothrombin time with the addition of sucralfate to chronic warfarin therapy.

The mechanism of these interactions appears to be nonsystemic in nature, presumably resulting from sucralfate binding to the concomitant agent in the gastrointestinal tract. In all cases studied to date (cimetidine, ciprofloxacin, digoxin, norfloxacin, ofloxacin, and ranitidine), dosing the concomitant medication 2 hours before sucralfate eliminated the interaction. Because of the potential of CARAFATE to alter the absorption of some drugs, CARAFATE should be administered separately from other drugs when alterations in bioavailability are felt to be critical. In these cases, patients should be monitored appropriately.

Carcinogenesis, Mutagenesis, Impairment of Fertility

Chronic oral toxicity studies of 24 months' duration were conducted in mice and rats at doses up to 1 g/kg (12 times the human dose). There was no evidence of drug-related tumorigenicity. A reproduction study in rats at doses up to 38 times the human dose did not reveal any indication of fertility impairment. Mutagenicity studies were not conducted.

Pregnancy

Teratogenic effects. Pregnancy Category B. Teratogenicity studies have been performed in mice, rats, and rabbits at doses up to 50 times the human dose and have revealed no evidence of harm to the fetus due to sucralfate. There are, however, no adequate and well-controlled studies in pregnant women. Because animal reproduction studies are not always predictive of human response, this drug should be used during pregnancy only if clearly needed.

Nursing Mothers

It is not known whether this drug is excreted in human milk. Because many drugs are excreted in human milk, caution should be exercised when sucralfate is administered to a nursing woman.

Pediatric Use

Safety and effectiveness in pediatric patients have not been established.

ADVERSE REACTIONS

Adverse reactions to sucralfate in clinical trials were minor and only rarely led to discontinuation of the drug. In studies involving over 2700 patients treated with sucralfate tablets, adverse effects were reported in 129 (4.7%).

Constipation was the most frequent complaint (2%). Other adverse effects reported in less than 0.5% of the patients are listed below by body system:

Gastrointestinal: diarrhea, nausea, vomiting, gastric discomfort, indigestion, flatulence, dry mouth
Dermatological: pruritus, rash
Nervous System: dizziness, insomnia, sleepiness, vertigo
Other: back pain, headache

Postmarketing reports of hypersensitivity reactions, including urticaria (hives), angioedema, respiratory difficulty, rhinitis laryngospasm, and facial swelling have been reported in patients receiving sucralfate tablets. Similar events were reported with sucralfate suspension. However, a causal relationship has not been established.

Bezoars have been reported in patients treated with sucralfate. The majority of patients had underlying medical conditions that may predispose to bezoar formation (such as delayed gastric emptying) or were receiving concomitant enteral tube feedings.

Inadvertent injection of insoluble sucralfate and its insoluble excipients has led to fatal complications, including pulmonary and cerebral emboli. Sucralfate is **not** intended for intravenous administration.

OVERDOSAGE

Due to limited experience in humans with overdosage of sucralfate, no specific treatment recommendations can be given. Acute oral toxicity studies in animals, however, using doses up to 12 g/kg body weight, could not find a lethal dose. Sucralfate is only minimally absorbed from the gastrointestinal tract. Risks associated with acute overdosage should, therefore, be minimal. In rare reports describing sucralfate overdose, most patients remained asymptomatic. Those few reports where adverse events were described included symptoms of dyspepsia, abdominal pain, nausea, and vomiting.

DOSAGE AND ADMINISTRATION

Active Duodenal Ulcer: The recommended adult oral dosage for duodenal ulcer is 1 g four times a day on an empty stomach.

Antacids may be prescribed as needed for relief of pain but should not be taken within one-half hour before or after sucralfate.

While healing with sucralfate may occur during the first week or two, treatment should be continued for 4 to 8 weeks unless healing has been demonstrated by x-ray or endoscopic examination.

Maintenance Therapy: The recommended adult oral dosage is 1 g twice a day.

HOW SUPPLIED

CARAFATE (sucralfate) 1-g tablets are supplied in bottles of 100 (NDC 0088-1712-47), 120 (NDC 0088-1712-53), and 500 (NDC 0088-1712-55) and in Unit Dose Identification Paks of 100 (NDC 0088-1712-49). Light pink, scored, oblong tablets are embossed with CARAFATE on one side and 1712 on the other.

Prescribing Information as of May 1996
Hoechst Marion Roussel, Inc.
Kansas City, MO 64137 USA

Shown in Product Identification Guide, page 316

CARAFATE®   ℞
[kăr 'afāt]
(sucralfate)
Suspension

Prescribing Information as of November 1997

DESCRIPTION

CARAFATE Suspension contains sucralfate and sucralfate is an α-D-glucopyranoside, β-D-fructofuranosyl-, octakis-(hydrogen sulfate), aluminum complex.

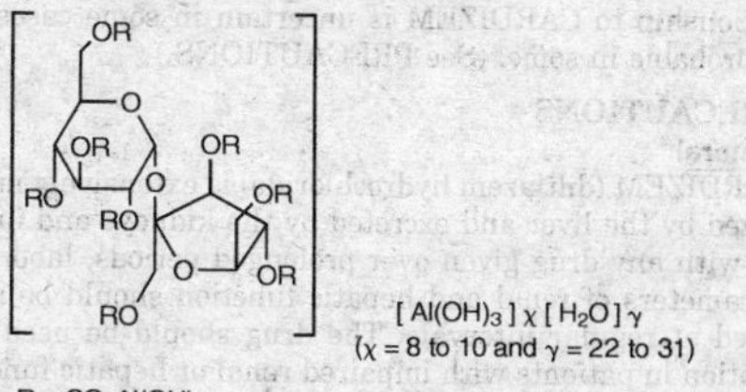
OR
O
OR
OR
RO
RO
OR
O
OR
RO
OR
[Al(OH)3]x[H2O]y
(x = 8 to 10 and y = 22 to 31)

$R = SO_3Al(OH)_2$

CARAFATE Suspension for oral administration contains 1 g of sucralfate per 10 mL.
CARAFATE Suspension also contains: colloidal silicon dioxide NF, FD&C Red #40, flavor, glycerin USP, methylcellulose USP, methylparaben NF, microcrystalline cellulose NF, purified water USP, simethicone USP, and sorbitol solution USP.
Therapeutic category: antiulcer.

CLINICAL PHARMACOLOGY

Sucralfate is only minimally absorbed from the gastrointestinal tract. The small amounts of the sulfated disaccharide that are absorbed are excreted primarily in the urine.
Although the mechanism of sucralfate's ability to accelerate healing of duodenal ulcers remains to be fully defined, it is known that it exerts its effect through a local, rather than systemic, action. The following observations also appear pertinent:

1. Studies in human subjects and with animal models of ulcer disease have shown that sucralfate forms an ulcer-adherent complex with proteinaceous exudate at the ulcer site.
2. In vitro, a sucralfate-albumin film provides a barrier to diffusion of hydrogen ions.
3. In human subjects, sucralfate given in doses recommended for ulcer therapy inhibits pepsin activity in gastric juice by 32%.
4. In vitro, sucralfate adsorbs bile salts.

These observations suggest that sucralfate's antiulcer activity is the result of formation of an ulcer-adherent complex that covers the ulcer site and protects it against further attack by acid, pepsin, and bile salts. There are approximately 14 to 16 mEq of acid-neutralizing capacity per 1-g dose of sucralfate.

CLINICAL TRIALS

In a multicenter, double-blind, placebo-controlled study of CARAFATE Suspension, a dosage regimen of 1 g (10 mL) four times daily was demonstrated to be superior to placebo in ulcer healing.

Results From Clinical Trials
Healing Rates for Acute Duodenal Ulcer

Treatment	n	Week 2 Healing Rates	Week 4 Healing Rates	Week 8 Healing Rates
CARAFATE Suspension	145	23(16%)*	66(46%)†	95(66%)‡
Placebo	147	10(7%)	39(27%)	58(39%)

* P=0.016 †P=0.001 ‡P=0.0001

Equivalence of sucralfate suspension to sucralfate tablets has not been demonstrated.

INDICATIONS AND USAGE

CARAFATE (sucralfate) Suspension is indicated in the short-term (up to 8 weeks) treatment of active duodenal ulcer.

CONTRAINDICATIONS

There are no known contraindications to the use of sucralfate.

PRECAUTIONS

Duodenal ulcer is a chronic, recurrent disease. While short-term treatment with sucralfate can result in complete healing of the ulcer, a successful course of treatment with sucralfate should not be expected to alter the posthealing frequency or severity of duodenal ulceration.

Special Populations: Chronic Renal Failure and Dialysis Patients
When sucralfate is administered orally, small amounts of aluminum are absorbed from the gastrointestinal tract. Concomitant use of sucralfate with other products that contain aluminum, such as aluminum-containing antacids, may increase the total body burden of aluminum. Patients with normal renal function receiving the recommended doses of sucralfate and aluminum-containing products adequately excrete aluminum in the urine. Patients with chronic renal failure or those receiving dialysis have impaired excretion of absorbed aluminum. In addition, aluminum does not cross dialysis membranes because it is bound to albumin and transferrin plasma proteins. Aluminum accumulation and toxicity (aluminum osteodystrophy, osteomalacia, encephalopathy) have been described in patients with renal impairment. Sucralfate should be used with caution in patients with chronic renal failure.

Drug Interactions
Some studies have shown that simultaneous sucralfate administration in healthy volunteers reduced the extent of absorption (bioavailability) of single doses of the following: cimetidine, digoxin, fluoroquinolone antibiotics, ketoconazole, l-thyroxine, phenytoin, quinidine, ranitidine, tetracycline, and theophylline. Subtherapeutic prothrombin times with concomitant warfarin and sucralfate therapy have been reported in spontaneous and published case reports. However, two clinical studies have demonstrated no change in either serum warfarin concentration or prothrombin time with the addition of sucralfate to chronic warfarin therapy.
The mechanism of these interactions appears to be nonsystemic in nature, presumably resulting from sucralfate binding to the concomitant agent in the gastrointestinal tract. In all cases studied to date (cimetidine, ciprofloxacin, digoxin, norfloxacin, ofloxacin, and ranitidine), dosing the concomitant medication 2 hours before sucralfate eliminated the interaction. Because of the potential of CARAFATE to alter the absorption of some drugs, CARAFATE should be administered separately from other drugs when alterations in bioavailability are felt to be critical. In these cases, patients should be monitored appropriately.

Carcinogenesis, Mutagenesis, Impairment of Fertility
Chronic oral toxicity studies of 24 months' duration were conducted in mice and rats at doses up to 1 g/kg (12 times the human dose). There was no evidence of drug-related tumorigenicity. A reproduction study in rats at doses up to 38 times the human dose did not reveal any indication of fertility impairment. Mutagenicity studies were not conducted.

Pregnancy
Teratogenic effects. Pregnancy Category B. Teratogenicity studies have been performed in mice, rats, and rabbits at doses up to 50 times the human dose and have revealed no evidence of harm to the fetus due to sulcralfate. There are, however, no adequate and well-controlled studies in pregnant women. Because animal reproduction studies are not always predictive of human response, this drug should be used during pregnancy only if clearly needed.

Nursing Mothers
It is not known whether this drug is excreted in human milk. Because many drugs are excreted in human milk, caution should be exercised when sucralfate is administered to a nursing woman.

Pediatric Use
Safety and effectiveness in pediatric patients have not been established.

ADVERSE REACTIONS

Adverse reactions to sucralfate tablets in clinical trials were minor and only rarely led to discontinuation of the drug. In studies involving over 2700 patients treated with sucralfate, adverse effects were reported in 129 (4.7%).
Constipation was the most frequent complaint (2%). Other adverse effects reported in less than 0.5% of the patients are listed below by body system:
Gastrointestinal: diarrhea, dry mouth, flatulence, gastric discomfort, indigestion, nausea, vomiting
Dermatological: pruritus, rash
Nervous System: dizziness, insomnia, sleepiness, vertigo
Other: back pain, headache
Postmarketing reports of hypersensitivity reactions, including urticaria (hives), angioedema, respiratory difficulty, rhinitis, laryngospasm, and facial swelling have been reported in patients receiving sucralfate tablets. Similar events were reported with sucralfate suspension. However, a causal relationship has not been established.
Bezoars have been reported in patients treated with sucralfate. The majority of patients had underlying medical conditions that may predispose to bezoar formation (such as delayed gastric emptying) or were receiving concomitant enteral tube feedings.
Inadvertent injection of insoluble sucralfate and its insoluble excipients has led to fatal complications, including pulmonary and cerebral emboli. Sucralfate is **not** intended for intravenous administration.

OVERDOSAGE

Due to limited experience in humans with overdosage of sucralfate, no specific treatment recommendations can be given. Acute oral studies in animals, however, using doses up to 12 g/kg body weight, could not find a lethal dose. Sucralfate is only minimally absorbed from the gastrointestinal tract. Risks associated with acute overdosage should, therefore, be minimal. In rare reports describing sucralfate overdose, most patients remained asymptomatic. Those few reports where adverse events were described included symptoms of dyspepsia, abdominal pain, nausea, and vomiting.

DOSAGE AND ADMINISTRATION

Active Duodenal Ulcer. The recommended adult oral dosage for duodenal ulcer is 1 g (10 mL/2 teaspoonfuls) four times per day. CARAFATE should be administered on an empty stomach.
Antacids may be prescribed as needed for relief of pain but should not be taken within one-half hour before or after sucralfate.
While healing with sucralfate may occur during the first week or two, treatment should be continued for 4 to 8 weeks unless healing has been demonstrated by x-ray or endoscopic examination.

HOW SUPPLIED

CARAFATE (sucralfate) Suspension 1 g/10 mL is a pink suspension supplied in bottles of 14 fl oz (NDC 0088-1700-15).
SHAKE WELL BEFORE USING
Store at controlled room temperature 20–25°C (68–77°F). [see USP]. Avoid freezing.
Prescribing Information as of November 1997
Hoechst Marion Roussel, Inc.
Kansas City, MO 64137

CARDIZEM® CD ℞

[kar' diz-em]
(diltiazem HCl)
Capsules

Prescribing Information as of December 1995A

DESCRIPTION

CARDIZEM® (diltiazem hydrochloride) is a calcium ion influx inhibitor (slow channel blocker or calcium antagonist). Chemically, diltiazem hydrochloride is 1,5-benzothiazepin-4(5H)one,3-(acetyloxy)-5-[2-(dimethylamino)ethyl]-2,3-dihydro-2-(4-methoxyphenyl)-, monohydrochloride,(+)-cis. The chemical structure is:

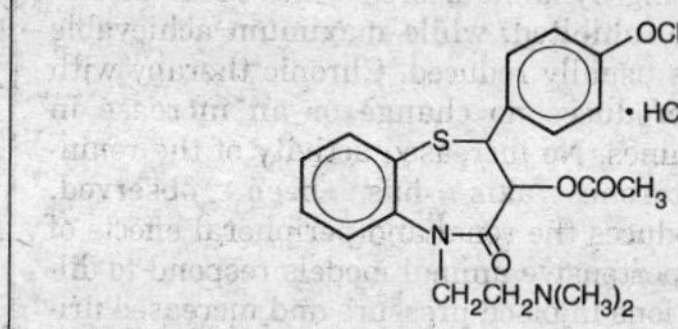
OCH3
• HCl
S
OCOCH3
N
O
CH2CH2N(CH3)2

Diltiazem hydrochloride is a white to off-white crystalline powder with a bitter taste. It is soluble in water, methanol, and chloroform. It has a molecular weight of 450.98. CARDIZEM CD is formulated as a once-a-day extended release capsule containing either 120 mg, 180 mg, 240 mg, or 300 mg diltiazem hydrochloride.
Also contains: black iron oxide, ethylcellulose, FD&C Blue #1, fumaric acid, gelatin-NF, sucrose, starch, talc, titanium dioxide, white wax, and other ingredients.
For oral administration.

CLINICAL PHARMACOLOGY

The therapeutic effects of CARDIZEM CD are believed to be related to its ability to inhibit the influx of calcium ions during membrane depolarization of cardiac and vascular smooth muscle.

Mechanisms of Action
Hypertension. CARDIZEM CD produces its antihypertensive effect primarily by relaxation of vascular smooth muscle and the resultant decrease in peripheral vascular resistance. The magnitude of blood pressure reduction is related to the degree of hypertension; thus hypertensive individuals experience an antihypertensive effect, whereas there is only a modest fall in blood pressure in normotensives.
Angina. CARDIZEM CD has been shown to produce increases in exercise tolerance, probably due to its ability to reduce myocardial oxygen demand. This is accomplished via reductions in heart rate and systemic blood pressure at submaximal and maximal work loads. Diltiazem has been shown to be a potent dilator of coronary arteries, both epicardial and subendocardial. Spontaneous and ergonovine-induced coronary artery spasm are inhibited by diltiazem.
In animal models, diltiazem interferes with the slow inward (depolarizing) current in excitable tissue. It causes excitation-contraction uncoupling in various myocardial tissues without changes in the configuration of the action potential.
Diltiazem produces relaxation of coronary vascular smooth muscle and dilation of both large and small coronary arteries at drug levels which cause little or no negative inotropic effect. The resultant increases in coronary blood flow (epicardial and subendocardial) occur in ischemic and nonis-

Continued on next page

Cardizem CD—Cont.

chemic models and are accompanied by dose-dependent decreases in systemic blood pressure and decreases in peripheral resistance.

Hemodynamic and Electrophysiologic Effects

Like other calcium channel antagonists, diltiazem decreases sinoatrial and atrioventricular conduction in isolated tissues and has a negative inotropic effect in isolated preparations. In the intact animal, prolongation of the AH interval can be seen at higher doses.

In man, diltiazem prevents spontaneous and ergonovine-provoked coronary artery spasm. It causes a decrease in peripheral vascular resistance and a modest fall in blood pressure in normotensive individuals and, in exercise tolerance studies in patients with ischemic heart disease, reduces the heart rate-blood pressure product for any given work load. Studies to date, primarily in patients with good ventricular function, have not revealed evidence of a negative inotropic effect; cardiac output, ejection fraction, and left ventricular end diastolic pressure have not been affected. Such data have no predictive value with respect to effects in patients with poor ventricular function, and increased heart failure has been reported in patients with preexisting impairment of ventricular function. There are as yet few data on the interaction of diltiazem and beta-blockers in patients with poor ventricular function. Resting heart rate is usually slightly reduced by diltiazem.

In hypertensive patients, CARDIZEM CD produces antihypertensive effects both in the supine and standing positions. In a double-blind, parallel, dose-response study utilizing doses ranging from 90 to 540 mg once daily, CARDIZEM CD lowered supine diastolic blood pressure in an apparent linear manner over the entire dose range studied. The changes in diastolic blood pressure, measured at trough, for placebo, 90 mg, 180 mg, 360 mg, and 540 mg were –2.9, –4.5, –6.1, –9.5, and –10.5 mm Hg, respectively. Postural hypotension is infrequently noted upon suddenly assuming an upright position. No reflex tachycardia is associated with the chronic antihypertensive effects. CARDIZEM CD decreases vascular resistance, increases cardiac output (by increasing stroke volume), and produces a slight decrease or no change in heart rate. During dynamic exercise, increases in diastolic pressure are inhibited, while maximum achievable systolic pressure is usually reduced. Chronic therapy with CARDIZEM CD produces no change or an increase in plasma catecholamines. No increased activity of the renin-angiotensin-aldosterone axis has been observed. CARDIZEM CD reduces the renal and peripheral effects of angiotensin II. Hypertensive animal models respond to diltiazem with reductions in blood pressure and increased urinary output and natriuresis without a change in urinary sodium/potassium ratio.

In a double-blind, parallel dose-response study of doses from 60 mg to 480 mg once daily, CARDIZEM CD increased time to termination of exercise in a linear manner over the entire dose range studied. The improvement in time to termination of exercise utilizing a Bruce exercise protocol, measured at trough, for placebo, 60 mg, 120 mg, 240 mg, 360 mg, and 480 mg was 29, 40, 56, 51, 69, and 68 seconds, respectively. As doses of CARDIZEM CD were increased, overall angina frequency was decreased. CARDIZEM CD, 180 mg once daily, or placebo was administered in a double-blind study to patients receiving concomitant treatment with long-acting nitrates and/or beta-blockers. A significant increase in time to termination of exercise and a significant decrease in overall angina frequency was observed. In this trial the overall frequency of adverse events in the CARDIZEM CD treatment group was the same as the placebo group.

Intravenous diltiazem in doses of 20 mg prolongs AH conduction time and AV node functional and effective refractory periods by approximately 20%. In a study involving single oral doses of 300 mg of CARDIZEM in six normal volunteers, the average maximum PR prolongation was 14% with no instances of greater than first-degree AV block. Diltiazem-associated prolongation of the AH interval is not more pronounced in patients with first-degree heart block. In patients with sick sinus syndrome, diltiazem significantly prolongs sinus cycle length (up to 50% in some cases). Chronic oral administration of CARDIZEM to patients in doses of up to 540 mg/day has resulted in small increases in PR interval, and on occasion produces abnormal prolongation. (See WARNINGS.)

Pharmacokinetics and Metabolism

Diltiazem is well absorbed from the gastrointestinal tract and is subject to an extensive first-pass effect, giving an absolute bioavailability (compared to intravenous administration) of about 40%. CARDIZEM undergoes extensive metabolism in which only 2% to 4% of the unchanged drug appears in the urine. Drugs which induce or inhibit hepatic microsomal enzymes may alter diltiazem disposition.

Total radioactivity measurement following short IV administration in healthy volunteers suggests the presence of other unidentified metabolites, which attain higher concentrations than those of diltiazem and are more slowly eliminated; half-life of total radioactivity is about 20 hours compared to 2 to 5 hours for diltiazem.

In vitro binding studies show CARDIZEM is 70% to 80% bound to plasma proteins. Competitive in vitro ligand binding studies have also shown CARDIZEM binding is not altered by therapeutic concentrations of digoxin, hydrochlorothiazide, phenylbutazone, propranolol, salicylic acid, or warfarin. The plasma elimination half-life following single or multiple drug administration is approximately 3.0 to 4.5 hours. Desacetyl diltiazem is also present in the plasma at levels of 10% to 20% of the parent drug and is 25% to 50% as potent as a coronary vasodilator as diltiazem. Minimum therapeutic plasma diltiazem concentrations appear to be in the range of 50 to 200 ng/mL. There is a departure from linearity when dose strengths are increased; the half-life is slightly increased with dose. A study that compared patients with normal hepatic function to patients with cirrhosis found an increase in half-life and a 69% increase in bioavailability in the hepatically impaired patients. A single study in nine patients with severely impaired renal function showed no difference in the pharmacokinetic profile of diltiazem compared to patients with normal renal function.

CARDIZEM CD Capsules. When compared to a regimen of CARDIZEM tablets at steady-state, more than 95% of drug is absorbed from the CARDIZEM CD formulation. A single 360-mg dose of the capsule results in detectable plasma levels within 2 hours and peak plasma levels between 10 and 14 hours; absorption occurs throughout the dosing interval. When CARDIZEM CD was coadministered with a high fat content breakfast, the extent of diltiazem absorption was not affected. Dose-dumping does not occur. The apparent elimination half-life after single or multiple dosing is 5 to 8 hours. A departure from linearity similar to that seen with CARDIZEM tablets and CARDIZEM SR capsules is observed. As the dose of CARDIZEM CD capsules is increased from a daily dose of 120 mg to 240 mg, there is an increase in the area-under-the-curve of 2.7 times. When the dose is increased from 240 mg to 360 mg there is an increase in the area-under-the-curve of 1.6 times.

INDICATIONS AND USAGE

CARDIZEM CD is indicated for the treatment of hypertension. It may be used alone or in combination with other antihypertensive medications.

CARDIZEM CD is indicated for the management of chronic stable angina and angina due to coronary artery spasm.

CONTRAINDICATIONS

CARDIZEM is contraindicated in (1) patients with sick sinus syndrome except in the presence of a functioning ventricular pacemaker, (2) patients with second- or third-degree AV block except in the presence of a functioning ventricular pacemaker, (3) patients with hypotension (less than 90 mm Hg systolic), (4) patients who have demonstrated hypersensitivity to the drug, and (5) patients with acute myocardial infarction and pulmonary congestion documented by x-ray on admission.

WARNINGS

1. **Cardiac Conduction.** CARDIZEM prolongs AV node refractory periods without significantly prolonging sinus node recovery time, except in patients with sick sinus syndrome. This effect may rarely result in abnormally slow heart rates (particularly in patients with sick sinus syndrome) or second- or third-degree AV block (13 of 3290 patients or 0.40%). Concomitant use of diltiazem with beta-blockers or digitalis may result in additive effects on cardiac conduction. A patient with Prinzmetal's angina developed periods of asystole (2 to 5 seconds) after a single dose of 60 mg of diltiazem. (See ADVERSE REACTIONS section.)
2. **Congestive Heart Failure.** Although diltiazem has a negative inotropic effect in isolated animal tissue preparations, hemodynamic studies in humans with normal ventricular function have not shown a reduction in cardiac index nor consistent negative effects on contractility (dp/dt). An acute study of oral diltiazem in patients with impaired ventricular function (ejection fraction 24% ± 6%) showed improvement in indices of ventricular function without significant decrease in contractile function (dp/dt). Worsening of congestive heart failure has been reported in patients with preexisting impairment of ventricular function. Experience with the use of CARDIZEM (diltiazem hydrochloride) in combination with beta-blockers in patients with impaired ventricular function is limited. Caution should be exercised when using this combination.
3. **Hypotension.** Decreases in blood pressure associated with CARDIZEM therapy may occasionally result in symptomatic hypotension.
4. **Acute Hepatic Injury.** Mild elevations of transaminases with and without concomitant elevation in alkaline phosphatase and bilirubin have been observed in clinical studies. Such elevations were usually transient and frequently resolved even with continued diltiazem treatment. In rare instances, significant elevations in enzymes such as alkaline phosphatase, LDH, SGOT, SGPT, and other phenomena consistent with acute hepatic injury have been noted. These reactions tended to occur early after therapy initiation (1 to 8 weeks) and have been reversible upon discontinuation of drug therapy. The relationship to CARDIZEM is uncertain in some cases, but probable in some. (See PRECAUTIONS.)

PRECAUTIONS

General

CARDIZEM (diltiazem hydrochloride) is extensively metabolized by the liver and excreted by the kidneys and in bile. As with any drug given over prolonged periods, laboratory parameters of renal and hepatic function should be monitored at regular intervals. The drug should be used with caution in patients with impaired renal or hepatic function. In subacute and chronic dog and rat studies designed to produce toxicity, high doses of diltiazem were associated with hepatic damage. In special subacute hepatic studies, oral doses of 125 mg/kg and higher in rats were associated with histological changes in the liver which were reversible when the drug was discontinued. In dogs, doses of 20 mg/kg were also associated with hepatic changes; however, these changes were reversible with continued dosing.

Dermatological events (see ADVERSE REACTIONS section) may be transient and may disappear despite continued use of CARDIZEM. However, skin eruptions progressing to erythema multiforme and/or exfoliative dermatitis have also been infrequently reported. Should a dermatologic reaction persist, the drug should be discontinued.

Drug Interactions

Due to the potential for additive effects, caution and careful titration are warranted in patients receiving CARDIZEM concomitantly with other agents known to affect cardiac contractility and/or conduction. (See WARNINGS.) Pharmacologic studies indicate that there may be additive effects in prolonging AV conduction when using beta-blockers or digitalis concomitantly with CARDIZEM. (See WARNINGS.)

As with all drugs, care should be exercised when treating patients with multiple medications. CARDIZEM undergoes biotransformation by cytochrome P-450 mixed function oxidase. Coadministration of CARDIZEM with other agents which follow the same route of biotransformation may result in the competitive inhibition of metabolism. Especially in patients with renal and/or hepatic impairment, dosages of similarly metabolized drugs, particularly those of low therapeutic ratio, may require adjustment when starting or stopping concomitantly administered diltiazem to maintain optimum therapeutic blood levels.

Beta-blockers. Controlled and uncontrolled domestic studies suggest that concomitant use of CARDIZEM and beta-blockers is usually well tolerated, but available data are not sufficient to predict the effects of concomitant treatment in patients with left ventricular dysfunction or cardiac conduction abnormalities.

Administration of CARDIZEM (diltiazem hydrochloride) concomitantly with propranolol in five normal volunteers resulted in increased propranolol levels in all subjects and bioavailability of propranolol was increased approximately 50%. In vitro, propranolol appears to be displaced from its binding sites by diltiazem. If combination therapy is initiated or withdrawn in conjunction with propranolol, an adjustment in the propranolol dose may be warranted. (See WARNINGS.)

Cimetidine. A study in six healthy volunteers has shown a significant increase in peak diltiazem plasma levels (58%) and area-under-the-curve (53%) after a 1-week course of cimetidine at 1200 mg per day and a single dose of diltiazem 60 mg. Ranitidine produced smaller, nonsignificant increases. The effect may be mediated by cimetidine's known inhibition of hepatic cytochrome P-450, the enzyme system responsible for the first-pass metabolism of diltiazem. Patients currently receiving diltiazem therapy should be carefully monitored for a change in pharmacological effect when initiating and discontinuing therapy with cimetidine. An adjustment in the diltiazem dose may be warranted.

Digitalis. Administration of CARDIZEM with digoxin in 24 healthy male subjects increased plasma digoxin concentrations approximately 20%. Another investigator found no increase in digoxin levels in 12 patients with coronary artery disease. Since there have been conflicting results regarding the effect of digoxin levels, it is recommended that digoxin levels be monitored when initiating, adjusting, and discontinuing CARDIZEM therapy to avoid possible over- or under-digitalization. (See WARNINGS.)

Anesthetics. The depression of cardiac contractility, conductivity, and automaticity as well as the vascular dilation associated with anesthetics may be potentiated by calcium channel blockers. When used concomitantly, anesthetics and calcium blockers should be titrated carefully.

Cyclosporine. A pharmacokinetic interaction between diltiazem and cyclosporine has been observed during studies involving renal and cardiac transplant patients. In renal and cardiac transplant recipients, a reduction of cyclosporine dose ranging from 15% to 48% was necessary to maintain cyclosporine through concentrations similar to those

seen prior to the addition of diltiazem. If these agents are to be administered concurrently, cyclosporine concentrations should be monitored, especially when diltiazem therapy is initiated, adjusted, or discontinued.

The effect of cyclosporine on diltiazem plasma concentrations has not been evaluated.

Carbamazepine. Concomitant administration of diltiazem with carbamazepine has been reported to result in elevated serum levels of carbamazepine (40% to 72% increase), resulting in toxicity in some cases. Patients receiving these drugs concurrently should be monitored for a potential drug interaction.

Carcinogenesis, Mutagenesis, Impairment of Fertility

A 24-month study in rats at oral dosage levels of up to 100 mg/kg/day and a 21-month study in mice at oral dosage levels of up to 30 mg/kg/day showed no evidence of carcinogenicity. There was also no mutagenic response in vitro or in vivo in mammalian cell assays or in vitro in bacteria. No evidence of impaired fertility was observed in a study performed in male and female rats at oral dosages of up to 100 mg/kg/day.

Pregnancy

Category C. Reproduction studies have been conducted in mice, rats and rabbits. Administration of doses ranging from five to ten times greater (on a mg/kg basis) than the daily recommended therapeutic dose has resulted in embryo and fetal lethality. These doses, in some studies, have been reported to cause skeletal abnormalities. In the perinatal/postnatal studies, there was an increased incidence of stillbirths at doses of 20 times the human dose or greater.

There are no well-controlled studies in pregnant women; therefore, use CARDIZEM in pregnant women only if the potential benefit justifies the potential risk to the fetus.

Nursing Mothers

Diltiazem is excreted in human milk. One report suggests that concentrations in breast milk may approximate serum levels. If use of CARDIZEM is deemed essential, an alternative method of infant feeding should be instituted.

Pediatric Use

Safety and effectiveness in pediatric patients have not been established.

ADVERSE REACTIONS

Serious adverse reactions have been rare in studies carried out to date, but it should be recognized that patients with impaired ventricular function and cardiac conduction abnormalities have usually been excluded from these studies. The following table presents the most common adverse reactions reported in placebo-controlled angina and hypertension trials in patients receiving CARDIZEM CD up to 360 mg with rates in placebo patients shown for comparison.

CARDIZEM CD Capsule Placebo-Controlled Angina and Hypertension Trials Combined

Adverse Reactions	Cardizem CD (n=607)	Placebo (n=301)
Headache	5.4%	5.0%
Dizziness	3.0%	3.0%
Bradycardia	3.3%	1.3%
AV Block First Degree	3.3%	0.0%
Edema	2.6%	1.3%
ECG Abnormality	1.6%	2.3%
Asthenia	1.8%	1.7%

In clinical trials of CARDIZEM CD capsules, CARDIZEM tablets, and CARDIZEM SR capsules involving over 3200 patients, the most common events (ie, greater than 1%) were edema (4.6%), headache (4.6%), dizziness (3.5%), asthenia (2.6%), first-degree AV block (2.4%), bradycardia (1.7%), flushing (1.4%), nausea (1.4%), and rash (1.2%).

In addition, the following events were reported infrequently (less than 1%) in angina or hypertension trials:

Cardiovascular: Angina, arrhythmia, AV block (second- or third-degree), bundle branch block, congestive heart failure, ECG abnormalities, hypotension, palpitations, syncope, tachycardia, ventricular extrasystoles

Nervous System: Abnormal dreams, amnesia, depression, gait abnormality, hallucinations, insomnia, nervousness, paresthesia, personality change, somnolence, tinnitus, tremor

Gastrointestinal: Anorexia, constipation, diarrhea, dry mouth, dysgeusia, dyspepsia, mild elevations of SGOT, SGPT, LDH, and alkaline phosphatase (see hepatic warnings), thirst, vomiting, weight increase

Dermatological: Petechiae, photosensitivity, pruritus, urticaria

Other: Amblyopia, CPK increase, dyspnea, epistaxis, eye irritation, hyperglycemia, hyperuricemia, impotence, muscle cramps, nasal congestion, nocturia, osteoarticular pain, polyuria, sexual difficulties

The following postmarketing events have been reported infrequently in patients receiving CARDIZEM: allergic reactions, alopecia, angioedema (including facial or periorbital

edema), asystole, erythema multiforme (including Stevens-Johnson syndrome, toxic epidermal necrolysis), exfoliative dermatitis, extrapyramidal symptoms, gingival hyperplasia, hemolytic anemia, increased bleeding time, leukopenia, purpura, retinopathy, and thrombocytopenia. In addition, events such as myocardial infarction have been observed which are not readily distinguishable from the natural history of the disease in these patients. A number of well-documented cases of generalized rash, some characterized as leukocytoclastic vasculitis, have been reported. However, a definitive cause and effect relationship between these events and CARDIZEM therapy is yet to be established.

OVERDOSAGE

The oral LD$_{50}$'s in mice and rats range from 415 to 740 mg/kg and from 560 to 810 mg/kg, respectively. The intravenous LD$_{50}$'s in these species were 60 and 38 mg/kg, respectively. The oral LD$_{50}$ in dogs is considered to be in excess of 50 mg/kg, while lethality was seen in monkeys at 360 mg/kg.

The toxic dose in man is not known. Due to extensive metabolism, blood levels after a standard dose of diltiazem can vary over tenfold, limiting the usefulness of blood levels in overdose cases. There have been 29 reports of diltiazem overdose in doses ranging from less than 1 g to 10.8 g. Sixteen of these reports involved multiple drug ingestions. Twenty-two reports indicated patients had recovered from diltiazem overdose ranging from less than 1 g to 10.8 g. There were seven reports with a fatal outcome; although the amount of diltiazem ingested was unknown, multiple drug ingestions were confirmed in six of the seven reports.

Events observed following diltiazem overdose included bradycardia, hypotension, heart block, and cardiac failure. Most reports of overdose described some supportive medical measure and/or drug treatment. Bradycardia frequently responded favorably to atropine as did heart block, although cardiac pacing was also frequently utilized to treat heart block. Fluids and vasopressors were used to maintain blood pressure, and in cases of cardiac failure, inotropic agents were administered. In addition, some patients received treatment with ventilatory support, gastric lavage, activated charcoal and/or intravenous calcium. Evidence of the effectiveness of intravenous calcium administration to reverse the pharmacological effects of diltiazem overdose was conflicting.

In the event of overdose or exaggerated response, appropriate supportive measures should be employed in addition to gastrointestinal decontamination. Diltiazem does not appear to be removed by peritoneal or hemodialysis. Limited data suggest that plasmapheresis or charcoal hemoperfusion may hasten diltiazem elimination following overdose. Based on the known pharmacological effects of diltiazem and/or reported clinical experiences, the following measures may be considered:

Bradycardia: Administer atropine (0.60 to 1.0 mg). If there is no response to vagal blockade, administer isoproterenol cautiously.

High-degree AV Block: Treat as for bradycardia above. Fixed high-degree AV block should be treated with cardiac pacing.

Cardiac Failure: Administer inotropic agents (isoproterenol, dopamine, or dobutamine) and diuretics.

Hypotension: Vasopressors (eg, dopamine or levarterenol bitartrate).

Actual treatment and dosage should depend on the severity of the clinical situation and the judgment and experience of the treating physician.

CARDIZEM® CD (diltiazem hydrochloride) Capsules

Strength	Quantity	NDC Number	Description
120 mg	30 btl 90 btl 100 UDIP®	0088-1795-30 0088-1795-42 0088-1795-49	Light turquoise blue/light turquoise blue capsule imprinted with CARDIZEM CD and 120 mg on one end.
180 mg	30 btl 90 btl 100 UDIP®	0088-1796-30 0088-1796-42 0088-1796-49	Light turquoise blue/blue capsule imprinted with CARDIZEM CD and 180 mg on one end.
240 mg	30 btl 90 btl 100 UDIP®	0088-1797-30 0088-1797-42 0088-1797-49	Blue/blue capsule imprinted with CARDIZEM CD and 240 mg on one end.
300 mg	30 btl 90 btl 100 UDIP®	0088-1798-30 0088-1798-42 0088-1798-49	Light gray/blue capsule imprinted with CARDIZEM CD and 300 mg on one end.

DOSAGE AND ADMINISTRATION

Patients controlled on diltiazem alone or in combination with other medications may be switched to CARDIZEM CD capsules at the nearest equivalent total daily dose. Higher doses of CARDIZEM CD may be needed in some patients. Patients should be closely monitored. Subsequent titration to higher or lower doses may be necessary and should be initiated as clinically warranted. There is limited general clinical experience with doses above 360 mg, but doses to 540 mg have been studied in clinical trials. The incidence of side effects increases as the dose increases with first-degree AV block, dizziness, and sinus bradycardia bearing the strongest relationship to dose.

Hypertension. Dosage needs to be adjusted by titration to individual patient needs. When used as monotherapy, reasonable starting doses are 180 to 240 mg once daily, although some patients may respond to lower doses. Maximum antihypertensive effect is usually observed by 14 days of chronic therapy; therefore, dosage adjustments should be scheduled accordingly. The usual dosage range studied in clinical trials was 240 to 360 mg once daily. Individual patients may respond to higher doses of up to 480 mg once daily.

Angina. Dosages for the treatment of angina should be adjusted to each patient's needs, starting with a dose of 120 or 180 mg once daily. Individual patients may respond to higher doses of up to 480 mg once daily. When necessary, titration may be carried out over a 7- to 14-day period.

Concomitant Use With Other Cardiovascular Agents.

1. **Sublingual NTG.** May be taken as required to abort acute anginal attacks during CARDIZEM CD (diltiazem hydrochloride) therapy.

2. **Prophylactic Nitrate Therapy.** CARDIZEM CD may be safely coadministered with short- and long-acting nitrates.

3. **Beta-blockers.** (See WARNINGS and PRECAUTIONS.)

4. **Antihypertensives.** CARDIZEM CD has an additive antihypertensive effect when used with other antihypertensive agents. Therefore, the dosage of CARDIZEM CD or the concomitant antihypertensives may need to be adjusted when adding one to the other.

HOW SUPPLIED

[See table above]

Storage Conditions: Store at controlled room temperature 59–86°F (15–30°C). Avoid excessive humidity.
Prescribing Information as of December 1995A
Hoechst Marion Roussel, Inc.
Kansas City, MO 64137 USA
Shown in Product Identification Guide, page 316

CARDIZEM® Injectable   ℞
[*kar'diz-em*]
(diltiazem HCl injection)
CARDIZEM® Lyo-Ject® Syringe
(diltiazem HCl)
CARDIZEM® Monovial®
(diltiazem HCl for injection)

Prescribing Information as of June 1997

DESCRIPTION

CARDIZEM® (diltiazem hydrochloride) is a calcium ion influx inhibitor (slow channel blocker or calcium channel an-

Continued on next page

Cardizem Injectable—Cont.

tagonist). Chemically, diltiazem hydrochloride is 1,5-benzothiazepin-4(5H)one,3-(acetyloxy)-5-[2-(dimethyl-amino) ethyl]-2, 3-dihydro-2-(4-methoxyphenyl)-, monohydrochloride,(+)-cis-. The chemical structure is:

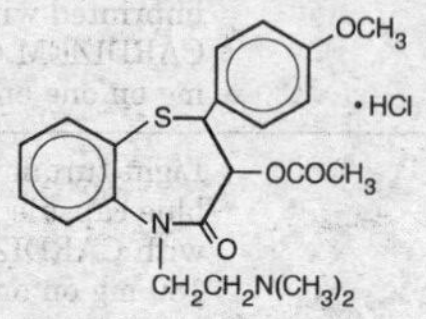

Diltiazem hydrochloride is a white to off-white crystalline powder with a bitter taste. It is soluble in water, methanol, and chloroform. It has a molecular weight of 450.98.

CARDIZEM Injectable (diltiazem hydrochloride injection) is a clear, colorless, sterile, nonpyrogenic solution. It has a pH range of 3.7 to 4.1.

CARDIZEM Injectable is for direct intravenous bolus injection and continuous intravenous infusion.

25-mg, 5-mL vial—each sterile vial contains 25 mg diltiazem hydrochloride, 3.75 mg citric acid USP, 3.25 mg sodium citrate dihydrate USP, 357 mg sorbitol solution USP, and water for injection USP up to 5 mL. Sodium hydroxide or hydrochloric acid is used for pH adjustment.

50-mg, 10-mL vial—each sterile vial contains 50 mg diltiazem hydrochloride, 7.5 mg citric acid USP, 6.5 mg sodium citrate dihydrate USP, 714 mg sorbitol solution USP, and water for injection USP up to 10 mL. Sodium hydroxide or hydrochloric acid is used for pH adjustment.

CARDIZEM Lyo-Ject Syringe (diltiazem hydrochloride) after reconstitution contains a clear, colorless, sterile, nonpyrogenic solution. It has a pH range of 4.0 to 7.0.

CARDIZEM Lyo-Ject Syringe after reconstitution is for direct intravenous bolus injection and continuous intravenous infusion.

CARDIZEM Lyo-Ject Syringe 25-mg syringe is available in a dual chamber, disposable syringe. Chamber 1 contains lyophilized powder comprised of diltiazem hydrochloride 25 mg and mannitol USP 37.5 mg. Chamber 2 contains sterile diluent composed of 5 mL water for injection with 0.5% benzyl alcohol NF, and 0.6% sodium chloride USP.

CARDIZEM Monovial (diltiazem hydrochloride for injection), after reconstitution in an infusion bag, produces a clear, colorless, sterile nonpyrogenic solution.

CARDIZEM Monovial for continuous intravenous infusion is available in a glass vial with transfer needle set. The vial contains lyophilized powder comprised of diltiazem hydrochloride 100 mg and mannitol USP 75 mg.

CLINICAL PHARMACOLOGY

Mechanism of Action

CARDIZEM inhibits the influx of calcium (Ca^{2+}) ions during membrane depolarization of cardiac and vascular smooth muscle. The therapeutic benefits of CARDIZEM in supraventricular tachycardias are related to its ability to slow AV nodal conduction time and prolong AV nodal refractoriness. CARDIZEM exhibits frequency (use) dependent effects on AV nodal conduction such that it may selectively reduce the heart rate during tachycardias involving the AV node with little or no effect on normal AV nodal conduction at normal heart rates.

CARDIZEM slows the ventricular rate in patients with a rapid ventricular response during atrial fibrillation or atrial flutter. CARDIZEM converts paroxysmal supraventricular tachycardia (PSVT) to normal sinus rhythm by interrupting the reentry circuit in AV nodal reentrant tachycardias and reciprocating tachycardias, eg, Wolff-Parkinson-White syndrome (WPW).

CARDIZEM prolongs the sinus cycle length. If has no effect on the sinus node recovery time or on the sinoatrial conduction time in patients without SA nodal dysfunction. CARDIZEM has no significant electrophysiologic effects on tissues in the heart that are fast sodium channel dependent, eg, His-Purkinje tissue, atrial and ventricular muscle, and extranodal accessory pathways.

Like other calcium channel antagonists, because of its effect on vascular smooth muscle, CARDIZEM decreases total peripheral resistance resulting in a decrease in both systolic and diastolic blood pressure.

Hemodynamics

In patients with cardiovascular disease, CARDIZEM Injectable (diltiazem hydrochloride injection) administered intravenously in single bolus doses, followed in some cases by a continuous infusion, reduced blood pressure, systemic vascular resistance, the rate-pressure product, and coronary vascular resistance and increased coronary blood flow. In a limited number of studies of patients with compromised myocardium (severe congestive heart failure, acute myocardial infarction, hypertrophic cardiomyopathy), administration of intravenous diltiazem produced no significant effect on contractility, left ventricular end diastolic pressure, or pulmonary capillary wedge pressure. The mean ejection fraction and cardiac output/index remained unchanged or increased. Maximal hemodynamic effects usually occurred within 2 to 5 minutes of an injection. However, in rare instances, worsening of congestive heart failure has been reported in patients with preexisting impaired ventricular function.

Pharmacodynamics

The prolongation of PR interval correlated significantly with plasma diltiazem concentration in normal volunteers using the Sigmoidal E_{max} model. Changes in heart rate, systolic blood pressure, and diastolic blood pressure did not correlate with diltiazem plasma concentrations in normal volunteers. Reduction in mean arterial pressure correlated linearly with diltiazem plasma concentration in a group of hypertensive patients.

In patients with atrial fibrillation and atrial flutter, a significant correlation was observed between the percent reduction in HR and plasma diltiazem concentration using the Sigmoidal E_{max} model. Based on this relationship, the mean plasma diltiazem concentration required to produce a 20% decrease in heart rate was determined to be 80 ng/mL. Mean plasma diltiazem concentrations of 130 ng/mL and 300 ng/mL were determined to produce reductions in heart rate of 30% and 40%.

Pharmacokinetics and Metabolism

Following a single intravenous injection in healthy male volunteers, CARDIZEM appears to obey linear pharmacokinetics over a dose range of 10.5 to 21.0 mg. The plasma elimination half-life is approximately 3.4 hours. The apparent volume of distribution of CARDIZEM is approximately 305 L. CARDIZEM is extensively metabolized in the liver with a systemic clearance of approximately 65 L/h.

After constant rate intravenous infusion to healthy male volunteers, diltiazem exhibits nonlinear pharmacokinetics over an infusion range of 4.8 to 13.2 mg/h for 24 hours. Over this infusion range, as the dose is increased, systemic clearance decreases from 64 to 48 L/h while the plasma elimination half-life increases from 4.1 to 4.9 hours. The apparent volume of distribution remains unchanged (360 to 391 L). In patients with atrial fibrillation or atrial flutter, diltiazem systemic clearance has been found to be decreased compared to healthy volunteers. In patients administered bolus doses ranging from 2.5 mg to 38.5 mg, systemic clearance averaged 36 L/h. In patients administered continuous infusions at 10 mg/h or 15 mg/h for 24 hours, diltiazem systemic clearance averaged 42 L/h and 31 L/h, respectively.

Based on the results of pharmacokinetic studies in healthy volunteers administered different ***oral*** CARDIZEM formulations, constant rate intravenous infusions of CARDIZEM at 3, 5, 7, and 11 mg/h are predicted to produce steady-state plasma diltiazem concentrations equivalent to 120-, 180-, 240-, and 360-mg total daily oral doses of CARDIZEM tablets or CARDIZEM SR capsules.

After oral administration, CARDIZEM undergoes extensive metabolism in man by deacetylation, N-demethylation, and O-demethylation via cytochrome P-450 (oxidative metabolism) in addition to conjugation. Metabolites N-monodesmethyldiltiazem, desacetyldiltiazem, desacetyl-N-monodesmethyldiltiazem, desacetyl-O-desmethyldiltiazem, and desacetyl-N, O-desmethyldiltiazem have been identified in human urine. Following oral administration, 2% to 4% of the unchanged CARDIZEM appears in the urine. Drugs which induce or inhibit hepatic microsomal enzymes may alter diltiazem disposition.

Following single intravenous injection of CARDIZEM, however, plasma concentrations of N-monodesmethyldiltiazem and desacetyldiltiazem, two principal metabolites found in plasma after oral administration, are typically not detected. These metabolites are observed, however, following 24 hour constant rate intravenous infusion. Total radioactivity measurement following short IV administration in healthy volunteers suggests the presence of other unidentified metabolites which attain higher concentrations than those of diltiazem and are more slowly eliminated; half-life of total radioactivity is about 20 hours compared to 2 to 5 hours for diltiazem.

CARDIZEM is 70% to 80% bound to plasma proteins. In vitro studies suggest alpha$_1$-acid glycoprotein binds approximately 40% of the drug at clinically significant concentrations. Albumin appears to bind approximately 30% of the drug, while other constituents bind the remaining bound fraction. Competitive in vitro ligand binding studies have shown that CARDIZEM binding is not altered by therapeutic concentrations of digoxin, phenytoin, hydrochlorothiazide, indomethacin, phenylbutazone, propranolol, salicylic acid, tolbutamide, or warfarin.

Renal insufficiency, or even end-stage renal disease, does not appear to influence diltiazem disposition following ***oral*** administration. Liver cirrhosis was shown to reduce diltiazem's apparent ***oral*** clearance and prolong its half-life.

INDICATIONS AND USAGE

CARDIZEM Injectable, CARDIZEM Lyo-Ject Syringe, or CARDIZEM Monovial (diltiazem hydrochloride for injection) are indicated for the following:

Atrial Fibrillation or Atrial Flutter. Temporary control of rapid ventricular rate in atrial fibrillation or atrial flutter. It should not be used in patients with atrial fibrillation or atrial flutter associated with an accessory bypass tract such as in Wolff-Parkinson-White (WPW) syndrome or short PR syndrome.

In addition, CARDIZEM Injectable or CARDIZEM Lyo-Ject Syringe are indicated for:

Paroxysmal Supraventricular Tachycardia. Rapid conversion of paroxysmal supraventricular tachycardias (PSVT) to sinus rhythm. This includes AV nodal reentrant tachycardias and reciprocating tachycardias associated with an extranodal accessory pathway such as the WPW syndrome or short PR syndrome. Unless otherwise contraindicated, appropriate vagal maneuvers should be attempted prior to administration of CARDIZEM Injectable or CARDIZEM Lyo-Ject Syringe.

The use of CARDIZEM Injectable, CARDIZEM Lyo-Ject Syringe, or CARDIZEM Monovial should be undertaken with caution when the patient is compromised hemodynamically or is taking other drugs that decrease any or all of the following: peripheral resistance, myocardial filling, myocardial contractility, or electrical impulse propagation in the myocardium.

For either indication and particularly when employing continuous intravenous infusion, the setting should include continuous monitoring of the ECG and frequent measurement of blood pressure. A defibrillator and emergency equipment should be readily available.

In domestic controlled trials in patients with atrial fibrillation or atrial flutter, bolus administration of CARDIZEM Injectable was effective in reducing heart rate by at least 20% in 95% of patients. CARDIZEM Injectable rarely converts atrial fibrillation or atrial flutter to normal sinus rhythm. Following administration of one or two intravenous bolus doses of CARDIZEM Injectable, response usually occurs within 3 minutes and maximal heart rate reduction generally occurs in 2 to 7 minutes. Heart rate reduction may last from 1 to 3 hours. If hypotension occurs, it is generally short-lived, but may last from 1 to 3 hours.

A 24-hour continuous infusion of CARDIZEM Injectable in the treatment of atrial fibrillation or atrial flutter maintained at least a 20% heart rate reduction during the infusion in 83% of patients. Upon discontinuation of infusion, heart rate reduction may last from 0.5 hours to more than 10 hours (median duration 7 hours). Hypotension, if it occurs, may be simply persistent.

In the controlled clinical trials, 3.2% of patients required some form of intervention (typically, use of intravenous fluids or the Trendelenburg position) for blood pressure support following CARDIZEM Injectable.

In domestic controlled trials, bolus administration of CARDIZEM Injectable was effective in converting PSVT to normal sinus rhythm in 88% of patients within 3 minutes of the first or second bolus dose.

Symptoms associated with the arrhythmia were improved in conjunction with decreased heart rate or conversion to normal sinus rhythm following administration of CARDIZEM Injectable.

CONTRAINDICATIONS

Injectable forms of diltiazem are contraindicated in:

1. Patients with sick sinus syndrome except in the presence of a functioning ventricular pacemaker.
2. Patients with second- or third-degree AV block except in the presence of a functioning ventricular pacemaker.
3. Patients with severe hypotension or cardiogenic shock.
4. Patients who have demonstrated hypersensitivity to the drug.
5. Intravenous diltiazem and intravenous beta-blockers should not be administered together or in close proximity (within a few hours).
6. Patients with atrial fibrillation or atrial flutter associated with an accessory bypass tract such as in WPW syndrome or short PR syndrome.
   As with other agents which slow AV nodal conduction and do not prolong the refractoriness of the accessory pathway (eg, verapamil, digoxin), in rare instances patients in atrial fibrillation or atrial flutter associated with an accessory bypass tract may experience a potentially life-threatening increase in heart rate accompanied by hypotension when treated with injectable forms of diltiazem. As such, the initial use of injectable forms of diltiazem should be, if possible, in a setting where monitoring and resuscitation capabilities, including DC cardioversion/defibrillation, are present (see OVERDOSAGE). Once familiarity of the patient's response is established, use in an office setting may be acceptable.
7. Patients with ventricular tachycardia. Administration of other calcium channel blockers to patients with wide complex tachycardia (QRS ≥0.12 seconds) has resulted in hemodynamic deterioration and ventricular fibrillation. It is important that an accurate pretreatment diagnosis distinguish wide complex QRS tachycardia of supraventricular origin from that of ventricular origin prior to administration of injectable forms of diltiazem.

8. In newborns, due to the presence of benzyl alcohol (CARDIZEM Lyo-Ject Syringe only).

WARNINGS

1. **Cardiac Conduction.** Diltiazem prolongs AV nodal conduction and refractoriness that may rarely result in second- or third-degree AV block in sinus rhythm. Concomitant use of diltiazem with agents known to affect cardiac conduction may result in additive effects (see Drug Interactions). If high-degree AV block occurs in sinus rhythm, intravenous diltiazem should be discontinued and appropriate supportive measures instituted (see OVERDOSAGE).

2. **Congestive Heart Failure.** Although diltiazem has a negative inotropic effect in isolated animal tissue preparations, hemodynamic studies in humans with normal ventricular function and in patients with a compromised myocardium, such as severe CHF, acute MI, and hypertrophic cardiomyopathy, have not shown a reduction in cardiac index nor consistent negative effects on contractility (dp/dt). Administration of oral diltiazem in patients with acute myocardial infarction and pulmonary congestion documented by x-ray on admission is contraindicated. Experience with the use of CARDIZEM Injectable in patients with impaired ventricular function is limited. Caution should be exercised when using the drug in such patients.

3. **Hypotension.** Decreases in blood pressure associated with CARDIZEM Injectable therapy may occasionally result in symptomatic hypotension (3.2%). The use of intravenous diltiazem for control of ventricular response in patients with supraventricular arrhythmias should be undertaken with caution when the patient is compromised hemodynamically. In addition, caution should be used in patients taking other drugs that decrease peripheral resistance, intravascular volume, myocardial contractility or conduction.

4. **Acute Hepatic Injury.** In rare instances, significant elevations in enzymes such as alkaline phosphatase, LDH, SGOT, SGPT, and other phenomena consistent with acute hepatic injury have been noted following oral diltiazem. Therefore, the potential for acute hepatic injury exists following administration of intravenous diltiazem.

5. **Ventricular Premature Beats (VPBs).** VPBs may be present on conversion of PSVT to sinus rhythm with CARDIZEM Injectable. These VPBs are transient, are typically considered to be benign, and appear to have no clinical significance. Similar ventricular complexes have been noted during cardioversion, other pharmacologic therapy, and during spontaneous conversion of PSVT to sinus rhythm.

PRECAUTIONS

General

CARDIZEM (diltiazem hydrochloride) is extensively metabolized by the liver and excreted by the kidneys and in bile. The drug should be used with caution in patients with impaired renal or hepatic function (see WARNINGS). High intravenous dosages (4.5 mg/kg tid) administered to dogs resulted in significant bradycardia and alterations in AV conduction. In subacute and chronic dog and rat studies designed to produce toxicity, high oral doses of diltiazem were associated with hepatic damage. In special subacute hepatic studies, oral doses of 125 mg/kg and higher in rats were associated with histological changes in the liver, which were reversible when the drug was discontinued. In dogs, oral doses of 20 mg/kg were also associated with hepatic changes; however, these changes were reversible with continued dosing.

Dermatologic events progressing to erythema multiforme and/or exfoliative dermatitis have been infrequently reported following oral diltiazem. Therefore, the potential for these dermatologic reactions exists following exposure to intravenous diltiazem. Should a dermatologic reaction persist, the drug should be discontinued.

Drug Interactions

Due to potential for additive effects, caution is warranted in patients receiving CARDIZEM Injectable, CARDIZEM Lyo-Ject Syringe, or CARDIZEM Monovial concomitantly with other agent(s) known to affect cardiac contractility and/or SA or AV node conduction (see WARNINGS).

As with all drugs, care should be exercised when treating patients with multiple medications. CARDIZEM undergoes extensive metabolism by the cytochrome P-450 mixed function oxidase system. Although specific pharmacokinetic drug-drug interaction studies have not been conducted with single intravenous injection or constant rate intravenous infusion, coadministration of injectable diltiazem with other agents which primarily undergo the same route of biotransformation may result in competitive inhibition of metabolism.

Digitalis. Intravenous diltiazem has been administered to patients receiving either intravenous or oral digitalis therapy. The combination of the two drugs was well tolerated without serious adverse effects. However, since both drugs affect AV nodal conduction, patients should be monitored for excessive slowing of the heart rate and/or AV block.

CARDIZEM Injectable or CARDIZEM Lyo-Ject Syringe

Diluent Volume	Quantity of CARDIZEM Injectable or CARDIZEM Lyo-Ject to Add	Final Concentration	Administration	
			Dose*	Infusion Rate
100 mL	125 mg (25 mL) Final Volume 125 mL	1 mg/mL	10 mg/h 15 mg/h	10 mL/h 15 mL/h
250 mL	250 mg (50 mL) Final Volume 300 mL	0.83 mg/mL	10 mg/h 15 mg/h	12 mL/h 18 mL/h
500 mL	250 mg (50 mL) Final Volume 550 mL	0.45 mg/mL	10 mg/h 15 mg/h	22 mL/h 33 mL/h

*5 mg/h may be appropriate for some patients

CARDIZEM Monovial

Diluent Volume	Quantity of CARDIZEM Monovial to Add	Final Concentration	Administration	
			Dose*	Infusion Rate
100 mL	100 mg (1 monovial)	1 mg/mL	10 mg/h 15 mg/h	10 mL/h 15 mL/h
250 mL	200 mg (2 monovials)	0.80 mg/mL	10 mg/h 15 mg/h	12.5 mL/h 18.8 mL/h
500 mL	200 mg (2 monovials)	0.40 mg/mL	10 mg/h 15 mg/h	25 mL/h 37.5 mL/h

*5 mg/h may be appropriate for some patients

Beta-blockers. Intravenous diltiazem has been administered to patients on chronic oral beta-blocker therapy. The combination of the two drugs was generally well tolerated without serious adverse effects. If intravenous diltiazem is administered to patients receiving chronic oral beta-blocker therapy, the possibility for bradycardia, AV block, and/or depression of contractility should be considered (see CONTRAINDICATIONS). *Oral* administration of diltiazem with propranolol in five normal volunteers resulted in increased propranolol levels in all subjects and bioavailability of propranolol was increased approximately 50%. In vitro, propranolol appears to be displaced from its binding sites by diltiazem.

Anesthetics. The depression of cardiac contractility, conductivity, and automaticity as well as the vascular dilation associated with anesthetics may be potentiated by calcium channel blockers. When used concomitantly, anesthetics and calcium blockers should be titrated carefully.

Cyclosporine. A pharmacokinetic interaction between diltiazem and cyclosporine has been observed during studies involving renal and cardiac transplant patients. In renal and cardiac transplant recipients, a reduction of cyclosporine dose ranging from 15% to 48% was necessary to maintain cyclosporine trough concentrations similar to those seen prior to the addition of diltiazem. If these agents are to be administered concurrently, cyclosporine concentrations should be monitored, especially when diltiazem therapy is initiated, adjusted or discontinued.

The effect of cyclosporine on diltiazem plasma concentrations has not been evaluated.

Carbamazepine. Concomitant administration of *oral* diltiazem with carbamazepine has been reported to result in elevated plasma levels of carbamazepine (by 40 to 72%), resulting in toxicity in some cases. Patients receiving these drugs concurrently should be monitored for a potential drug interaction.

Carcinogenesis, Mutagenesis, Impairment of Fertility

A 24-month study in rats at oral dosage levels of up to 100 mg/kg/day and a 21-month study in mice at oral dosage levels of up to 30 mg/kg/day showed no evidence of carcinogenicity. There was also no mutagenic response in vitro or in vivo in mammalian cell assays or in vitro in bacteria. No evidence of impaired fertility was observed in a study performed in male and female rats at oral dosages of up to 100 mg/kg/day.

Pregnancy

Category C. Reproduction studies have been conducted in mice, rats, and rabbits.

Administration of oral doses ranging from five to ten times greater (on a mg/kg basis) than the daily recommended oral antianginal therapeutic dose has resulted in embryo and fetal lethality. These doses, in some studies, have been reported to cause skeletal abnormalities. In the perinatal/postnatal studies there was some reduction in early individual pup weights and survival rates. There was an increased incidence of stillbirths at doses of 20 times the human oral antianginal dose or greater.

There are no well-controlled studies in pregnant women; therefore, use CARDIZEM in pregnant women only if the potential benefit justifies the potential risk to the fetus.

Nursing Mothers

Diltiazem is excreted in human milk. One report with oral diltiazem suggests that concentrations in breast milk may approximate serum levels. If use of CARDIZEM is deemed essential, an alternative method of infant feeding should be instituted.

Pediatric Use

Safety and effectiveness in pediatric patients have not been established.

ADVERSE REACTIONS

The following adverse reaction rates are based on the use of CARDIZEM Injectable in over 400 domestic clinical trial patients with atrial fibrillation/flutter or PSVT under double-blind or open-label conditions. Worldwide experience in over 1300 patients was similar.

Adverse events reported in controlled and uncontrolled clinical trials were generally mild and transient. Hypotension was the most commonly reported adverse event during clinical trials. Asymptomatic hypotension occurred in 4.3% of patients. Symptomatic hypotension occurred in 3.2% of patients. When treatment for hypotension was required, it generally consisted of administration of saline or placing the patient in the Trendelenburg position. Other events reported in at least 1% of the diltiazem-treated patients were injection site reactions (eg, itching, burning) 3.9%, vasodilation (flushing) 1.7%, and arrhythmia (junctional rhythm or isorhythmic dissociation) 1.0%.

In addition, the following events were reported infrequently (less than 1%):

Cardiovascular: Asystole, atrial flutter, AV block first degree, AV block second degree, bradycardia, chest pain, congestive heart failure, sinus pause, sinus node dysfunction, syncope, ventricular arrhythmia, ventricular fibrillation, ventricular tachycardia

Dermatologic: Pruritus, sweating

Gastrointestinal: Constipation, elevated SGOT or alkaline phosphatase, nausea, vomiting

Nervous System: Dizziness, paresthesia

Other: Amblyopia, asthenia, dry mouth, dyspnea, edema, headache, hyperuricemia

Although not observed in clinical trials with CARDIZEM Injectable, the following events associated with oral diltiazem may occur:

Cardiovascular: AV block (third degree), bundle branch block, ECG abnormality, palpitations, syncope, tachycardia, ventricular extrasystoles

Dermatologic: Alopecia, erythema multiforme (including Stevens-Johnson syndrome, toxic epidermal necrolysis), exfoliative dermatitis, leukocytoclastic vasculitis, petechiae, photosensitivity, purpura, rash, urticaria

Continued on next page

Cardizem Injectable—Cont.

Gastrointestinal: Anorexia, diarrhea, dysgeusia, dyspepsia, mild elevations of SGPT and LDH, thirst, weight increase
Nervous System: Abnormal dreams, amnesia, depression, extrapyramidal symptoms, gait abnormality, hallucinations, insomnia, nervousness, personality change, somnolence, tremor
Other: Allergic reactions, angioedema (including facial or periorbital edema), CPK elevation, epistaxis, eye irritation, gingival hyperplasia, hemolytic anemia, hyperglycemia, impotence, increased bleeding time, leukopenia, muscle cramps, nasal congestion, nocturia, osteoarticular pain, polyuria, retinopathy, sexual difficulties, thrombocytopenia, tinnitus
Events such as myocardial infarction have been observed which are not readily distinguishable from the natural history of the disease for the patient.

OVERDOSAGE

Overdosage experience is limited. In the event of overdosage or an exaggerated response, appropriate supportive measures should be employed. The following measures may be considered:
Bradycardia: Administer atropine (0.60 to 1.0 mg). If there is no response to vagal blockade administer isoproterenol cautiously.
High-degree AV Block: Treat as for bradycardia above. Fixed high-degree AV block should be treated with cardiac pacing.
Cardiac Failure: Administer inotropic agents (isoproterenol, dopamine, or dobutamine) and diuretics.
Hypotension: Vasopressors (eg, dopamine or levarterenol bitartrate).
Actual treatment and dosage should depend on the severity of the clinical situation and the judgment and experience of the treating physician.
Diltiazem does not appear to be removed by peritoneal or hemodialysis. Limited data suggest that plasmapheresis or charcoal hemoperfusion may hasten diltiazem elimination following overdose.
The intravenous LD_{50}'s in mice and rats were 60 and 38 mg/kg, respectively. The toxic dose in man is not known.

DOSAGE AND ADMINISTRATION

Direct Intravenous Single Injections (Bolus)
The initial dose of CARDIZEM Injectable or CARDIZEM Lyo-Ject Syringe (see instructions for reconstitution of Lyo-Ject Syringe in blister pack) should be 0.25 mg/kg actual body weight as a bolus administered over 2 minutes (20 mg is a reasonable dose for the average patient). If response is inadequate, a second dose may be administered after 15 minutes. The second bolus dose of CARDIZEM Injectable or CARDIZEM Lyo-Ject Syringe should be 0.35 mg/kg actual body weight administered over 2 minutes (25 mg is a reasonable dose for the average patient). Subsequent intravenous bolus doses should be individualized for each patient. Patients with low body weights should be dosed on a mg/kg basis. Some patients may respond to an initial dose of 0.15 mg/kg, although duration of action may be shorter. Experience with this dose is limited.
Continuous Intravenous Infusion
For continued reduction of the heart rate (up to 24 hours) in patients with atrial fibrillation or atrial flutter, an intravenous infusion of CARDIZEM Injectable, CARDIZEM Lyo-Ject Syringe, or CARDIZEM Monovial may be administered. (For reconstitution of CARDIZEM Lyo-Ject Syringe or CARDIZEM Monovial, see instructions contained within packaging.) Immediately following bolus administration of 20 mg (0.25 mg/kg) or 25 mg (0.35 mg/kg) CARDIZEM Injectable or CARDIZEM Lyo-Ject Syringe, and reduction of heart rate, begin an intravenous infusion of CARDIZEM Injectable, CARDIZEM Lyo-Ject Syringe, or CARDIZEM Monovial. The recommended initial infusion rate of CARDIZEM Injectable, CARDIZEM Lyo-Ject Syringe, or CARDIZEM Monovial is 10 mg/h. Some patients may maintain response to an initial rate of 5 mg/h. The infusion rate may be increased in 5 mg/h increments up to 15 mg/h as needed, if further reduction in heart rate is required. The infusion may be maintained for up to 24 hours.
Diltiazem shows dose-dependent, non-linear pharmacokinetics. Duration of infusion longer than 24 hours and infusion rates greater than 15 mg/h have not been studied. Therefore, infusion duration exceeding 24 hours and infusion rates exceeding 15 mg/h are not recommended.
Dilution: To prepare CARDIZEM Injectable, CARDIZEM Lyo-Ject Syringe, or CARDIZEM Monovial for continuous intravenous infusion, aseptically transfer the appropriate quantity (see charts) of CARDIZEM to the desired volume of either Normal Saline, D5W, or D5W/0.45% NaCl. Mix thoroughly. Keep diluted CARDIZEM Injectable refrigerated until use. Diluted CARDIZEM Lyo-Ject Syringe and CARDIZEM Monovial may be stored at room temperature 15–30°C (59–86°F). Use within 24 hours.
[See tables at top of previous page]

Compatibility: CARDIZEM Injectable, CARDIZEM Lyo-Ject Syringe, and CARDIZEM Monovial were tested for compatibility with three commonly used intravenous fluids at a maximal concentration of 1 mg diltiazem hydrochloride per milliliter. CARDIZEM Injectable, CARDIZEM Lyo-Ject Syringe, and CARDIZEM Monovial were found to be physically compatible and chemically stable in the following parenteral solutions for at least 24 hours when stored in glass (CARDIZEM Injectable/CARDIZEM Lyo-Ject Syringe only) or polyvinylchloride (PVC) bags at controlled room temperature 15–30°C (59–86°F) or under refrigeration 2–8°C (36–46°F).
- dextrose (5%) injection USP
- sodium chloride (0.9%) injection USP
- dextrose (5%) and sodium chloride (0.45%) injection USP.

Physical Incompatibilities:
Because of potential physical incompatibilities, it is recommended that CARDIZEM Injectable, CARDIZEM Lyo-Ject Syringe, or CARDIZEM Monovial not be mixed with any other drugs in the same container. If possible, it is recommended that CARDIZEM Injectable, CARDIZEM Lyo-Ject Syringe, or CARDIZEM Monovial not be co-infused in the same intravenous line. Parenteral drug products should be inspected visually for particulate matter and discoloration prior to administration whenever solution and container permit.
CARDIZEM Injectable/CARDIZEM Lyo-Ject Syringe. Physical incompatibilities (precipitate formation or cloudiness) were observed when CARDIZEM Injectable or CARDIZEM Lyo-Ject Syringe was infused in the same intravenous line with the following drugs: acetazolamide, acyclovir, aminophylline, ampicillin, ampicillin sodium/sulbactam sodium, cefamandole, cefoperazone, diazepam, furosemide, hydrocortisone sodium succinate, insulin, (regular: 100 units/mL), methylprednisolone sodium succinate, mezlocillin, nafcillin, phenytoin, rifampin, and sodium bicarbonate.
NOTE: CARDIZEM Lyo-Ject Syringe was found to be compatible with insulin (regular, 100 units/mL).
CARDIZEM Monovial. Physical incompatibilities (precipitate formation or cloudiness) were observed when CARDIZEM Monovial at a concentration of 1 mg/mL diluted in normal saline was infused in the same intravenous line with the following drugs: acetazolamide, acyclovir, cefoperazone sodium, diazepam, furosemide, phenytoin and rifampin.
NOTE: CARDIZEM Monovial at a concentration of 1 mg/mL diluted in normal saline was infused in the same intravenous line and was found to be compatible with the following drugs: aminophylline, ampicillin sodium, ampicillin sodium/sulbactam sodium, cefamandole, hydrocortisone sodium succinate, regular insulin (100 units/mL), methylprednisolone sodium succinate, mezlocillin sodium, nafcillin sodium and sodium bicarbonate.
Transition to Further Antiarrhythmic Therapy
Transition to other antiarrhythmic agents following administration of CARDIZEM Injectable is generally safe. However, reference should be made to the respective agent manufacturer's package insert for information relative to dosage and administration.
In controlled clinical trials, therapy with antiarrhythmic agents to maintain reduced heart rate in atrial fibrillation or atrial flutter or for prophylaxis of PSVT was generally started within 3 hours after bolus administration of CARDIZEM Injectable. These antiarrhythmic agents were intravenous or oral digoxin, Class 1 antiarrhythmics (eg, quinidine, procainamide), calcium channel blockers, and oral beta-blockers.
Experience in the use of antiarrhythmic agents following maintenance infusion of CARDIZEM Injectable is limited. Patients should be dosed on an individual basis and reference should be made to the respective manufacturer's package insert for information relative to dosage and administration.

HOW SUPPLIED

CARDIZEM® Injectable (diltiazem hydrochloride injection) is supplied in boxes of six 5-mL vials with each vial containing 25 mg of diltiazem hydrochloride (5 mg/mL) (NDC 0088-1790-32) and boxes of six 10-mL vials with each vial containing 50 mg diltiazem hydrochloride (5 mg/mL) (NDC 0088-1790-33). STORE PRODUCT UNDER REFRIGERATION 2–8°C (36–46°F). DO NOT FREEZE. MAY BE STORED AT ROOM TEMPERATURE FOR UP TO 1 MONTH. DESTROY AFTER 1 MONTH AT ROOM TEMPERATURE. SINGLE-USE CONTAINERS. DISCARD UNUSED PORTION.
CARDIZEM Lyo-Ject 25-mg syringe is supplied in a single molded nonsterile tray in cartons of 6 syringes (NDC 0088-1789-17—formerly NDC 0088-1790-17). PRODUCT IS TO BE STORED AT ROOM TEMPERATURE 15–30°C (59–86°F). DO NOT FREEZE. RECONSTITUTED MATERIAL IS STABLE FOR 24 HOURS AT CONTROLLED ROOM TEMPERATURE. SINGLE-USE CONTAINERS. DISCARD UNUSED PORTION.
CARDIZEM Monovial for continuous infusion (100 mg) is supplied in a glass vial with transfer needle set (NDC 0088-1788-16). PRODUCT IS TO BE STORED AT ROOM TEMPERATURE 15–30°C (59–86°F). DO NOT FREEZE. RECONSTITUTED MATERIAL IS STABLE FOR 24 HOURS AT CONTROLLED ROOM TEMPERATURE. SINGLE-USE VIAL.
Monovial® is a registered trademark of Becton Dickinson S.A.
Cardizem® is a registered trademark of Carderm Capital L.P.
Lyo-Ject® is a registered trademark of Arzneimittel GmbH Apotheker Vetter & Company.
Prescribing Information as of June 1997
Manufactured for:
Hoechst Marion Roussel, Inc.
Kansas City, MO 64137 USA
Shown in Product Identification Guide, page 316

CARDIZEM® SR ℞

[kar 'diz-em]
(diltiazem HCl)
Sustained Release Capsules

Prescribing Information as of April 1996

DESCRIPTION

CARDIZEM® (diltiazem hydrochloride) is a calcium ion influx inhibitor (slow channel blocker or calcium antagonist). Chemically, diltiazem hydrochloride is 1,5-Benzothiazepin-4(5H)one,3-(acetyloxy)-5-[2-(dimethylamino)ethyl]-2, 3-dihydro-2-(4-methoxyphenyl)-,monohydrochloride,(+)-cis-. The chemical structure is:

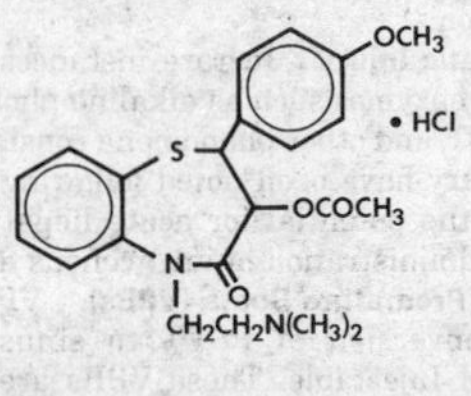

Diltiazem hydrochloride is a white to off-white crystalline powder with a bitter taste. It is soluble in water, methanol, and chloroform. It has a molecular weight of 450.98. Each CARDIZEM SR capsule contains either 60 mg, 90 mg, or 120 mg diltiazem hydrochloride. Also contains: D&C Yellow #10, FD&C Blue #1, FD&C Red #40, FD&C Yellow #6, fumaric acid, povidone, starch, sucrose, talc, titanium dioxide, and other ingredients.
For oral administration.

CLINICAL PHARMACOLOGY

The therapeutic effects of CARDIZEM are believed to be related to its ability to inhibit the influx of calcium ions during membrane depolarization of cardiac and vascular smooth muscle.
Mechanisms of Action
CARDIZEM SR produces its antihypertensive effect primarily by relaxation of vascular smooth muscle and the resultant decrease in perpheral vascular resistance. The magnitude of blood pressure reduction is related to the degree of hypertension; thus hypertensive individuals experience an antihypertensive effect, whereas there is only a modest fall in blood pressure in normotensives.
Hemodynamic and Electrophysiologic Effects
Like other calcium antagonists, diltiazem decreases sinoatrial and atrioventricular conduction in isolated tissues and has a negative inotropic effect in isolated preparations. In the intact animal, prolongation of the AH interval can be seen at higher doses.
In man, diltiazem prevents spontaneous and ergonovine-provoked coronary artery spasm. It causes a decrease in peripheral vascular resistance and a modest fall in blood pressure in normotensive individuals and, in exercise tolerance studies in patients with ischemic heart disease, reduces the heart rate-blood pressure product for any given work load. Studies to date, primarily in patients with good ventricular function, have not revealed evidence of a negative inotropic effect, cardiac output, ejection fraction, and left ventricular end diastolic pressure have not been affected. Increased heart failure has, however, been reported in occasional patients with preexisting impairment of ventricular function. There are as yet few data on the interaction of diltiazem and beta-blockers in patients with poor ventricular function. Resting heart rate is usually slightly reduced by diltiazem. CARDIZEM SR produces antihypertensive effects both in the supine and standing positions. Postural hypotension is infrequently noted upon suddenly assuming an upright position. No reflex tachycardia is associated with the chronic antihypertensive effects. CARDIZEM SR decreases vascular resistance, increases cardiac output (by increasing stroke volume), and produces a slight decrease or no change in

heart rate. During dynamic exercise, increases in diastolic pressure are inhibited while maximum achievable systolic pressure is usually reduced. Heart rate at maximum exercise does not change or is slightly reduced. Chronic therapy with CARDIZEM produces no change or an increase in plasma catecholamines. No increased activity of the renin-angiotensin-aldosterone axis has been observed. CARDIZEM SR antagonizes the renal and peripheral effects of angiotensin II. Hypertensive animal models respond to diltiazem with reductions in blood pressure and increased urinary output and natriuresis without a change in urinary sodium/potassium ratio.

Intravenous diltiazem in doses of 20 mg prolongs AH conduction time and AV node functional and effective refractory periods by approximately 20%. In a study involving single oral doses of 300 mg of CARDIZEM in six normal volunteers, the average maximum PR prolongation was 14% with no instances of greater than first-degree AV block. Diltiazem-associated prolongation of the AH interval is not more pronounced in patients with first-degree heart block. In patients with sick sinus syndrome, diltiazem significantly prolongs sinus cycle length (up to 50% in some cases). Chronic oral administration of CARDIZEM in doses of up to 360 mg/day has resulted in small increases in PR interval, and on occasion produces abnormal prolongation. (See WARNINGS.)

Pharmacokinetics and Metabolism

Diltiazem is well absorbed from the gastrointestinal tract and is subject to an extensive first-pass effect, giving an absolute bioavailability (compared to intravenous administration) of about 40%. CARDIZEM undergoes extensive metabolism in which 2% to 4% of the unchanged drug appears in the urine. In vitro binding studies show CARDIZEM is 70% to 80% bound to plasma proteins. Competitive in vitro ligand binding studies have also shown CARDIZEM binding is not altered by therapeutic concentrations of digoxin, hydrochlorothiazide, phenylbutazone, propranolol, salicylic acid, or warfarin. The plasma elimination half-life following single or multiple drug administration is approximately 3.0 to 4.5 hours. Desacetyl diltiazem is also present in the plasma at levels of 10% to 20% of the parent drug and is 25% to 50% as potent a coronary vasodilator as diltiazem. Minimum therapeutic plasma levels of CARDIZEM appear to be in the range of 50–200 ng/mL. There is a departure from linearity when dose strengths are increased; the half-life is slightly increased with dose. A study that compared patients with normal hepatic function to patients with cirrhosis found an increase in half-life and a 69% increase in bioavailability in the hepatically impaired patients. A single study in nine patients with severely impaired renal function showed no difference in the pharmacokinetic profile of diltiazem compared to patients with normal renal function.

CARDIZEM SR Capsules. Diltiazem is absorbed from the capsule formulation to about 92% of a reference solution at steady-state. A single 120-mg dose of the capsule results in detectable plasma levels within two to three hours and peak plasma levels at six to 11 hours. The apparent elimination half-life after single or multiple dosing is five to seven hours. A departure from linearity similar to that observed with the CARDIZEM tablet is observed. As the dose of CARDIZEM SR capsules is increased from a daily dose of 120 mg (60 mg bid) to 240 mg (120 mg bid) daily, there is an increase in area-under-the-curve of 2.6 times. When the dose is increased from 240 mg to 360 mg daily, there is an increase in area-under-the-curve of 1.8 times. The average plasma levels of the capsule dosed twice daily at steady-state are equivalent to the tablet dosed four times daily when the same total daily dose is administered.

INDICATIONS AND USAGE

CARDIZEM SR is indicated for the treatment of hypertension. It may be used alone or in combination with other antihypertensive medications, such as diuretics.

CONTRAINDICATIONS

CARDIZEM is contraindicated in (1) patients with sick sinus syndrome except in the presence of a functioning ventricular pacemaker, (2) patients with second- or third-degree AV block except in the presence of a functioning ventricular pacemarker, (3) patients with hypotension (less than 90 mm Hg systolic), (4) patients who have demonstrated hypersensitivity to the drug, and (5) patients with acute myocardial infarction and pulmonary congestion documented by x-ray on admission.

WARNINGS

1. **Cardiac Conduction.** CARDIZEM prolongs AV node refractory periods without significantly prolonging sinus node recovery time, except in patients with sick sinus syndrome. This effect may rarely result in abnormally slow heart rates (particularly in patients with sick sinus syndrome) or second- or third-degree AV block (nine of 2,111 patients or 0.43%). Concomitant use of diltiazem with beta-blockers or digitalis may result in additive effects on cardiac conduction. A patient with Prinzmetal's angina developed periods of asystole (2 to 5 seconds) after a single dose of 60 mg of diltiazem. (See ADVERSE REACTIONS section.)

CARDIZEM® SR
(diltiazem hydrochloride)
Sustained Release Capsules

Strength	Quantity	NDC Number	Description
60 mg	100 btl	0088-1777-47	Ivory/brown capsule imprinted with CARDIZEM logo on one end and CARDIZEM SR 60 mg on the other
90 mg	100 btl	0088-1778-47	Gold/brown capsule imprinted with CARDIZEM logo on one end and CARDIZEM SR 90 mg on the other
120 mg	100 btl	0088-1779-47	Caramel/brown capsule imprinted with CARDIZEM logo on one end and CARDIZEM SR 120 mg on the other

2. **Congestive Heart Failure.** Although diltiazem has a negative inotropic effect in isolated animal tissue preparations, hemodynamic studies in humans with normal ventricular function have not shown a reduction in cardiac index nor consistent negative effects on contractility (dp/dt). An acute study of oral diltiazem in patients with impaired ventricular function (ejection fraction 24% ± 6%) showed improvement in indices of ventricular function without significant decrease in contractile function (dp/dt). Experience with the use of CARDIZEM (diltiazem hydrochloride) in combination with beta-blockers in patients with impaired ventricular function is limited. Caution should be exercised when using this combination.

3. **Hypotension.** Decreases in blood pressure associated with CARDIZEM therapy may occasionally result in symptomatic hypotension.

4. **Acute Hepatic Injury.** Mild elevations of transaminases with and without concomitant elevation in alkaline phosphatase and bilirubin have been observed in clinical studies. Such elevations were usually transient and frequently resolved even with continued diltiazem treatment. In rare instances, significant elevations in enzymes such as alkaline phosphatase, LDH, SGOT, SGPT, and other phenomena consistent with acute hepatic injury have been noted. These reactions tended to occur early after therapy initiation (1 to 8 weeks) and have been reversible upon discontinuation of drug therapy. The relationship to CARDIZEM is uncertain in some cases, but probable in some. (See PRECAUTIONS.)

PRECAUTIONS
General

CARDIZEM (diltiazem hydrochloride) is extensively metabolized by the liver and excreted by the kidneys and in bile. As with any drug given over prolonged periods, laboratory parameters of renal and hepatic function should be monitored at regular intervals. The drug should be used with caution in patients with impaired renal or hepatic function. In subacute and chronic dog and rat studies designed to produce toxicity, high doses of diltiazem were associated with hepatic damage. In special subacute hepatic studies, oral doses of 125 mg/kg and higher in rats were associated with histological changes in the liver which were reversible when the drug was discontinued. In dogs, doses of 20 mg/kg were also associated with hepatic changes; however, these changes were reversible with continued dosing.

Dermatological events (see ADVERSE REACTIONS section) may be transient and may disappear despite continued use of CARDIZEM. However, skin eruptions progressing to erythema multiforme and/or exfoliative dermatitis have also been infrequently reported. Should a dermatologic reaction persist, the drug should be discontinued.

Drug Interactions

Due to the potential for additive effects, caution and careful titration are warranted in patients receiving CARDIZEM concomitantly with any agents known to affect cardiac contractility and/or conduction. (See WARNINGS.) Pharmacologic studies indicate that there may be additive effects in prolonging AV conduction when using beta-blockers or digitalis concomitantly with CARDIZEM. (See WARNINGS.)

As with all drugs, care should be exercised when treating patients with multiple medications. CARDIZEM undergoes biotransformation by cytochrome P-450 mixed function oxidase. Coadministration of CARDIZEM with other agents which follow the same route of biotransformation may result in the competitive inhibition of metabolism. Especially in patients with renal and/or hepatic impairment, dosages of similarly metabolized drugs, particularly those of low therapeutic ratio may require adjustment when starting or stopping concomitantly administered diltiazem to maintain optimum therapeutic blood levels.

Beta-blockers. Controlled and uncontrolled domestic studies suggest that concomitant use of CARDIZEM and beta-blockers is usually well tolerated, but available data are not sufficient to predict the effects of concomitant treatment in patients with left ventricular dysfunction or cardiac conduction abnormalities.

Administration of CARDIZEM (diltiazem hydrochloride) concomitantly with propranolol in five normal volunteers

resulted in increased propranolol levels in all subjects and bioavailability of propranolol was increased approximately 50%. In vitro, propranolol appears to be displaced from its binding sites by diltiazem. If combination therapy is initiated or withdrawn in conjunction with propranolol, an adjustment in the propranolol dose may be warranted. (See WARNINGS.)

Cimetidine. A study in six healthy volunteers has shown a significant increase in peak diltiazem plasma levels (58%) and area-under-the-curve (53%) after a 1-week course of cimetidine at 1,200 mg per day and a single dose of diltiazem 60 mg. Ranitidine produced smaller, nonsignificant increases. The effect may be mediated by cimetidine's known inhibition of hepatic cytochrome P-450, the enzyme system responsible for the first-pass metabolism of diltiazem. Patients currently receiving diltiazem therapy should be carefully monitored for a change in pharmacological effect when initiating and discontinuing therapy with cimetidine. An adjustment in the diltiazem dose may be warranted.

Digitalis. Administration of CARDIZEM with digoxin in 24 healthy male subjects increased plasma digoxin concentrations approximately 20%. Another investigator found no increase in digoxin levels in 12 patients with coronary artery disease. Since there have been conflicting results regarding the effect of digoxin levels, it is recommended that digoxin levels be monitored when initiating, adjusting, and discontinuing CARDIZEM therapy to avoid possible over- or under-digitalization. (See WARNINGS.)

Anesthetics. The depression of cardiac contractility, conductivity, and automaticity as well as the vascular dilation associated with anesthetics may be potentiated by calcium channel blockers. When used concomitantly, anesthetics and calcium blockers should be titrated carefully.

Cyclosporine. A pharmacokinetic interaction between diltiazem and cyclosporine has been observed during studies involving renal and cardiac transplant patients. In renal and cardiac transplant recipients, a reduction of cyclosporine dose ranging from 15% to 48% was necessary to maintain cyclosporine trough concentrations similar to those seen prior to the addition of diltiazem. If these agents are to be administered concurrently, cyclosporine concentrations should be monitored, especially when diltiazem therapy is initiated, adjusted or discontinued. The effect of cyclosporine on diltiazem plasma concentrations has not been evaluated.

Carbamazepine. Concomitant administration of diltiazem with carbamazepine has been reported to result in elevated serum levels of carbamazepine (40 to 72% increase), resulting in toxicity in some cases. Patients receiving these drugs concurrently should be monitored for a potential drug interaction.

Carcinogenesis, Mutagenesis, Impairment of Fertility

A 24-month study in rats and a 21-month study in mice showed no evidence of carcinogenicity. There was also no mutagenic response in in vitro bacterial tests. No intrinsic effect on fertility was observed in rats.

Pregnancy

Category C. Reproduction studies have been conducted in mice, rats, and rabbits. Administration of doses ranging from five to ten times greater (on a mg/kg basis) than the daily recommended therapeutic dose has resulted in embryo and fetal lethality. These doses, in some studies, have been reported to cause skeletal abnormalities. In the perinatal/postnatal studies, there was some reduction in early individual pup weights and survival rates. There was an increased incidence of stillbirths at doses of 20 times the human dose or greater.

There are no well-controlled studies in pregnant women; therefore, use CARDIZEM in pregnant women only if the potential benefit justifies the potential risk to the fetus.

Nursing Mothers

Diltiazem is excreted in human milk. One report suggests that concentrations in breast milk may approximate serum levels. If use of CARDIZEM is deemed essential, an alternative method of infant feeding should be instituted.

Continued on next page

Cardizem SR—Cont.

Pediatric Use
Safety and effectiveness in pediatric patients have not been established.

ADVERSE REACTIONS

Serious adverse reactions have been rare in studies carried out to date, but it should be recognized that patients with impaired ventricular function and cardiac conduction abnormalities have usually been excluded from these studies.
The adverse events described below represent events observed in clinical studies of hypertensive patients receiving either CARDIZEM Tablets or CARDIZEM SR Capsules as well as experiences observed in studies of angina and during marketing. The most common events in hypertension studies are shown in a table with rates in placebo patients shown for comparison. Less common events are listed by body system; these include any adverse reactions seen in angina studies that were not observed in hypertension studies. In all hypertensive patients studied (over 900), the most common adverse events were edema (9%), headache (8%), dizziness (6%), asthenia (5%), sinus bradycardia (3%), flushing (3%), and first-degree AV block (3%). Only edema and perhaps bradycardia and dizziness were dose related. The most common events observed in clinical studies (over 2,100 patients) of angina patients and hypertensive patients receiving CARDIZEM Tablets or CARDIZEM SR Capsules were (ie, greater than 1%) edema (5.4%), headache (4.5%), dizziness (3.4%), asthenia (2.8%), first-degree AV block (1.8%), flushing (1.7%), nausea (1.6%), bradycardia (1.5%), and rash (1.5%).

Double Blind Placebo Controlled Hypertension Trials

Adverse	Diltiazem n = 315 # pts (%)	Placebo n = 211 # pts (%)
headache	38 (12%)	17 (8%)
AV block first degree	24 (7.6%)	4 (1.9%)
dizziness	22 (7%)	6 (2.8%)
edema	19 (6%)	2 (0.9%)
bradycardia	19 (6%)	3 (1.4%)
ECG abnormality	13 (4.1%)	3 (1.4%)
asthenia	10 (3.2%)	1 (0.5%)
constipation	5 (1.6%)	2 (0.9%)
dyspepsia	4 (1.3%)	1 (0.5%)
nausea	4 (1.3%)	2 (0.9%)
palpitations	4 (1.3%)	2 (0.9%)
polyuria	4 (1.3%)	2 (0.9%)
somnolence	4 (1.3%)	—
alk phos increase	3 (1%)	1 (0.5%)
hypotension	3 (1%)	1 (0.5%)
insomnia	3 (1%)	1 (0.5%)
rash	3 (1%)	1 (0.5%)
AV block second degree	2 (0.6%)	—

In addition, the following events were reported infrequently (less than 1%) with CARDIZEM SR Capsules or CARDIZEM Tablets or have been observed in angina or hypertension trials.
Cardiovascular: Angina, arrhythmia, second- or third-degree AV block (see conduction warning), bundle branch block, congestive heart failure, syncope, tachycardia, ventricular extrasystoles.
Nervous System: Abnormal dreams, amnesia, depression, gait abnormality, hallucinations, nervousness, paresthesia, personality change, tremor.
Gastrointestinal: Anorexia, diarrhea, dry mouth, dysgeusia, mild elevations of SGOT, SGPT, and LDH (see hepatic warnings), thirst, vomiting, weight increase.
Dermatological: Petechiae, photosensitivity, pruritus, urticaria
Other: Amblyopia, CPK increase, dyspnea, epistaxis, eye irritation, hyperglycemia, hyperuricemia, impotence, muscle cramps, nasal congestion, nocturia, osteoarticular pain, sexual difficulties, tinnitus.
The following postmarketing events have been reported infrequently in patients receiving CARDIZEM: allergic reactions, alopecia, angioedema (including facial or periorbital edema), asystole, erythema multiforme (including Stevens-Johnson syndrome, toxic epidermal necrolysis), extrapyramidal symptoms, gingival hyperplasia, hemolytic anemia, increased bleeding time, leukopenia, purpura, retinopathy, and thrombocytopenia. There have been observed cases of a generalized rash, some characterized as leukocytoclastic vasculitis. In addition, events such as myocardial infarction have been observed which are not readily distinguishable from the natural history of the disease in these patients. A definitive cause and effect relationship between these events and CARDIZEM therapy cannot yet be established. Exfoliative dermatitis (proven by rechallenge) has also been reported.

OVERDOSAGE OR EXAGGERATED RESPONSE

The oral LD_{50} 's in mice and rats range from 415 to 740 mg/kg and from 560 to 810 mg/kg, respectively. The intravenous LD_{50} 's in these species were 60 and 38 mg/kg, respectively. The oral LD_{50} in dogs is considered to be in excess of 50 mg/kg, while lethality was seen in monkeys at 360 mg/kg.
The toxic dose in man is not known. Due to extensive metabolism, blood levels after a standard dose of diltiazem can vary over tenfold, limiting the usefulness of blood levels in overdose cases.
There have been 29 reports of diltiazem overdose in doses ranging from less than 1 g to 10.8 g. Sixteen of these reports involved multiple drug ingestions.
Twenty-two reports indicated patients had recovered from diltiazem overdose ranging from less than 1 g to 10.8 g. There were seven reports with a fatal outcome; although the amount of diltiazem ingested was unknown, multiple drug ingestions were confirmed in six of the seven reports.
Events observed following diltiazem overdose included bradycardia, hypotension, heart block, and cardiac failure. Most reports of overdose described some supportive medical measure and/or drug treatment. Bradycardia frequently responded favorably to atropine, as did heart block, although cardiac pacing was also frequently utilized to treat heart block. Fluids and vasopressors were used to maintain blood pressure and in cases of cardiac failure inotropic agents were administered. In addition, some patients received treatment with ventilatory support, gastric lavage, activated charcoal, and/or intravenous calcium. Evidence of the effectiveness of intravenous calcium administration to reverse the pharmacological effects of diltiazem overdose was conflicting.
In the event of overdose or exaggerated response, appropriate supportive measures should be employed in addition to gastrointestinal decontamination. Diltiazem does not appear to be removed by peritoneal or hemodialysis. Limited data suggest that plasmapheresis or charcoal hemoperfusion may hasten diltiazem elimination following overdose. Based on the known pharmacological effects of diltiazem and/or reported clinical experiences the following measures may be considered.
Bradycardia: Administer atropine (0.60 to 1.0 mg). If there is no response to vagal blockade, administer isoproterenol cautiously.
High-Degree AV Block: Treat as for bradycardia above. Fixed high-degree AV block should be treated with cardiac pacing.
Cardiac Failure: Administer inotropic agents (isoproterenol, dopamine, or dobutamine) and diuretics.
Hypotension: Vasopressors (eg, dopamine or levarterenol bitartrate).
Actual treatment and dosage should depend on the severity of the clinical situation and the judgment and experience of the treating physician.

DOSAGE AND ADMINISTRATION

Dosages must be adjusted to each patient's needs, starting with 60 to 120 mg twice daily. Maximum antihypertensive effect is usually observed by 14 days of chronic therapy; therefore, dosage adjustments should be scheduled accordingly. Although individual patients may respond to lower doses, the usual optimum dosage range in clinical trials was 240 to 360 mg/day.
CARDIZEM SR has an additive antihypertensive effect when used with other antihypertensive agents. Therefore, the dosage of CARDIZEM SR or the concomitant antihypertensives may need to be adjusted when adding one to the other. See WARNINGS and PRECAUTIONS regarding use with beta-blockers.

HOW SUPPLIED

[See table at top of previous page]
Storage Conditions: Store at controlled room temperature 59–86°F (15–30°C)
Prescribing Information as of April 1996
Hoechst Marion Roussel, Inc.
Kansas City, MO 64137 USA
Shown in Product Identification Guide, page 316

CARDIZEM® ℞
[kar 'diz-em]
(diltiazem hydrochloride)
Direct Compression Tablets

Prescribing Information as of May 1996

DESCRIPTION

CARDIZEM® (diltiazem hydrochloride) is a calcium ion influx inhibitor (slow channel blocker or calcium antagonist). Chemically, diltiazem hydrochloride is 1, 5-Benzothiazepin-4(5H) one,3-(acetyloxy)-5-[2-(dimethyl-amino)ethyl]-2,3-dihydro-2-(4-methoxyphenyl)-,monohydrochloride,(+)-cis-. The chemical structure is:
[See chemical structure at top of next column]

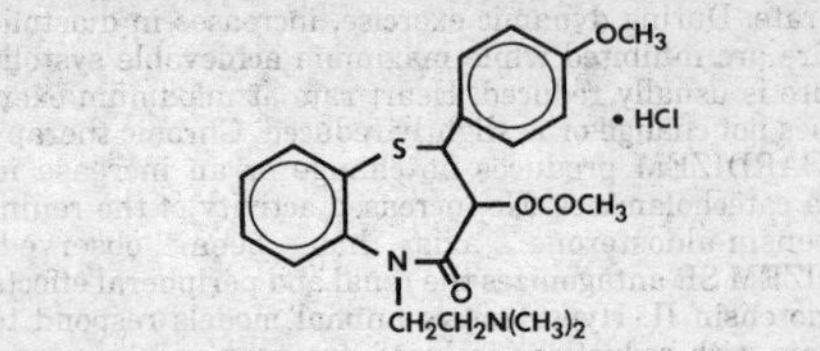

Diltiazem hydrochloride is a white to off-white crystalline powder with a bitter taste. It is soluble in water, methanol, and chloroform. It has a molecular weight of 450.98. Each tablet of CARDIZEM contains 30 mg, 60 mg, 90 mg, or 120 mg diltiazem hydrochloride. Also contains: D&C Yellow #10 Aluminum Lake, FD&C Yellow #6 Aluminum Lake (60 mg and 120 mg), FD&C Blue #1 Aluminum Lake (30 mg and 90 mg), hydroxypropyl methylcellulose, lactose, magnesium stearate, methylparaben, microcrystalline cellulose, silicon dioxide and other ingredients.
For oral administration.

CLINICAL PHARMACOLOGY

The therapeutic benefits achieved with CARDIZEM are believed to be related to its ability to inhibit the influx of calcium ions during membrane depolarization of cardiac and vascular smooth muscle.

Mechanisms of Action
Although precise mechanisms of its antianginal actions are still being delineated, CARDIZEM is believed to act in the following ways:
1. **Angina Due to Coronary Artery Spasm.** CARDIZEM has been shown to be a potent dilator of coronary arteries both epicardial and subendocardial. Spontaneous and ergonovine-induced coronary artery spasm are inhibited by CARDIZEM.
2. **Exertional Angina.** CARDIZEM has been shown to produce increases in exercise tolerance, probably due to its ability to reduce myocardial oxygen demand. This is accomplished via reductions in heart rate and systemic blood pressure at submaximal and maximal exercise workloads.

In animal models, diltiazem interferes with the slow inward (depolarizing) current in excitable tissue. It causes excitation-contraction uncoupling in various myocardial tissues without changes in the configuration of the action potential. Diltiazem produces relaxation of coronary vascular smooth muscle and dilation of both large and small coronary arteries at drug levels which cause little or no negative inotropic effect. The resultant increases in coronary blood flow (epicardial and subendocardial) occur in ischemic and nonischemic models and are accompanied by dose-dependent decreases in systemic blood pressure and decreases in peripheral resistance.

Hemodynamic and Electrophysiologic Effects
Like other calcium antagonists, diltiazem decreases sinoatrial and atrioventricular conduction in isolated tissues and has a negative inotropic effect in isolated preparations. In the intact animal, prolongation of the AH interval can be seen at higher doses.
In man, diltiazem prevents spontaneous and ergonovine-provoked coronary artery spasm. It causes a decrease in peripheral vascular resistance and a modest fall in blood pressure and, in exercise tolerance studies in patients with ischemic heart disease, reduces the heart rate-blood pressure product for any given workload. Studies to date, primarily in patients with good ventricular function, have not revealed evidence of a negative inotropic effect; cardiac output, ejection fraction, and left ventricular end-diastolic pressure have not been affected. There are as yet few data on the interaction of diltiazem and beta-blockers. Resting heart rate is usually unchanged or slightly reduced by diltiazem.
Intravenous diltiazem in doses of 20 mg prolongs AH conduction time and AV node functional and effective refractory periods approximately 20%. In a study involving single oral doses of 300 mg of CARDIZEM in six normal volunteers, the average maximum PR prolongation was 14% with no instances of greater than first-degree AV block. Diltiazem-associated prolongation of the AH interval is not more pronounced in patients with first-degree heart block. In patients with sick sinus syndrome, diltiazem significantly prolongs sinus cycle length (up to 50% in some cases).
Chronic oral administration of CARDIZEM in doses of up to 240 mg/day has resulted in small increases in PR interval, but has not usually produced abnormal prolongation.

Pharmacokinetics and Metabolism
Diltiazem is well absorbed from the gastrointestinal tract and is subject to an extensive first-pass effect, giving an absolute bioavailability (compared to intravenous dosing) of about 40%. CARDIZEM undergoes extensive metabolism in which 2% to 4% of the unchanged drug appears in the urine. In vitro binding studies show CARDIZEM is 70% to 80% bound to plasma proteins. Competitive in vitro ligand binding studies have also shown CARDIZEM binding is not altered by therapeutic concentrations of digoxin, hydrochlorothiazide, phenylbutazone, propranolol, salicylic acid, or warfarin. The plasma elimination half-life following single or multiple drug administration is approximately 3.0 to 4.5 hours. Desacetyl diltiazem is also present in the plasma at levels of 10% to 20% of the parent drug and is 25% to 50% as

potent as a coronary vasodilator as diltiazem. Minimum therapeutic plasma levels of CARDIZEM appear to be in the range of 50–200 ng/mL. There is a departure from linearity when dose strengths are increased. A study that compared patients with normal hepatic function to patients with cirrhosis found an increase in half-life and a 69% increase in AUC (area-under-the-plasma concentration vs time curve) in the hepatically impaired patients. A single study in nine patients with severely impaired renal functions showed no difference in the pharmacokinetic profile of diltiazem as compared to patients with normal renal function.

CARDIZEM Tablets. Diltiazem is absorbed from the tablet formulation to about 98% of a reference solution. Single oral doses of 30 to 120 mg of CARDIZEM tablets result in detectable plasma levels within 30 to 60 minutes and peak plasma levels 2 to 4 hours after drug administration. As the dose of CARDIZEM tablets is increased from a daily dose of 120 mg (30 mg qid) to 240 mg (60 mg qid) daily, there is an increase in area-under-the-curve of 2.3 times. When the dose is increased from 240 mg to 360 mg daily, there is an increase in area-under-the-curve of 1.8 times.

INDICATIONS AND USAGE

CARDIZEM is indicated for the management of chronic stable angina and angina due to coronary artery spasm.

CONTRAINDICATIONS

CARDIZEM is contraindicated in (1) patients with sick sinus syndrome except in the presence of a functioning ventricular pacemaker, (2) patients with second- or third-degree AV block except in the presence of a functioning ventricular pacemaker, (3) patients with hypotension (less than 90 mm Hg systolic), (4) patients who have demonstrated hypersensitivity to the drug, and (5) patients with acute myocardial infarction and pulmonary congestion documented by x-ray on admission.

WARNINGS

1. **Cardiac Conduction.** CARDIZEM prolongs AV node refractory periods without significantly prolonging sinus node recovery time, except in patients with sick sinus syndrome. This effect may rarely result in abnormally slow heart rates (particularly in patients with sick sinus syndrome) or second- or third-degree AV block (six of 1243 patients for 0.48%). Concomitant use of diltiazem with beta-blockers or digitalis may result in additive effects on cardiac conduction. A patient with Prinzmetal's angina developed periods of asystole (2 to 5 seconds) after a single dose of 60 mg of diltiazem. (See ADVERSE REACTIONS section.)

2. **Congestive Heart Failure.** Although diltiazem has a negative inotropic effect in isolated animal tissue preparations, hemodynamic studies in humans with normal ventricular function have not shown a reduction in cardiac index nor consistent negative effects on contractility (dp/dt). Experience with the use of CARDIZEM alone or in combination with beta-blockers in patients with impaired ventricular function is very limited. Caution should be exercised when using the drug in such patients.

3. **Hypotension.** Decreases in blood pressure associated with CARDIZEM therapy may occasionally result in symptomatic hypotension.

4. **Acute Hepatic Injury.** In rare instances, significant elevations in enzymes such as alkaline phosphatase, LDH, SGOT, SGPT, and other phenomena consistent with acute hepatic injury have been noted. These reactions have been reversible upon discontinuation of drug therapy. The relationship to CARDIZEM is uncertain in most cases, but probable in some. (See PRECAUTIONS.)

PRECAUTIONS

General
CARDIZEM (diltiazem hydrochloride) is extensively metabolized by the liver and excreted by the kidneys and in bile. As with any drug given over prolonged periods, laboratory parameters of renal and hepatic function should be monitored at regular intervals. The drug should be used with caution in patients with impaired renal or hepatic function. In subacute and chronic dog and rat studies designed to produce toxicity, high doses of diltiazem were associated with hepatic damage. In special subacute hepatic studies, oral doses of 125 mg/kg and higher in rats were associated with histological changes in the liver, which were reversible when the drug was discontinued. In dogs, doses of 20 mg/kg were also associated with hepatic changes; however, these changes were reversible with continued dosing.

Dermatological events (see ADVERSE REACTIONS section) may be transient and may disappear despite continued use of CARDIZEM. However, skin eruptions progressing to erythema multiforme and/or exfoliative dermatitis have also been infrequently reported. Should a dermatologic reaction persist, the drug should be discontinued.

Drug Interactions
Due to the potential for additive effects, caution and careful titration are warranted in patients receiving CARDIZEM concomitantly with any agents known to affect cardiac contractility and/or conduction. (See WARNINGS.)

Pharmacologic studies indicate that there may be additive effects in prolonging AV conduction when using beta-blockers or digitalis concomitantly with CARDIZEM. (See WARNINGS.)

As with all drugs, care should be exercised when treating patients with multiple medications. CARDIZEM undergoes biotransformation by cytochrome P-450 mixed function oxidase. Coadministration of CARDIZEM with other agents which follow the same route of biotransformation may result in the competitive inhibition of metabolism. Especially in patients with renal and/or hepatic impairment, dosages of similarly metabolized drugs, particularly those of low therapeutic ratio, may require adjustment when starting or stopping concomitantly administered diltiazem to maintain optimum therapeutic blood levels.

Beta-blockers. Controlled and uncontrolled domestic studies suggest that concomitant use of CARDIZEM and beta-blockers is usually well tolerated. Available data are not sufficient, however, to predict the effects of concomitant treatment, particularly in patients with left ventricular dysfunction of cardiac conduction abnormalities.

Administration of CARDIZEM (diltiazem hydrochloride) concomitantly with propranolol in five normal volunteers resulted in increased propranolol levels in all subjects, and bioavailability of propranolol was increased approximately 50%. In vitro, propranolol appears to be displaced from its binding sites by diltiazem. If combination therapy is initiated or withdrawn in conjunction with propranolol, an adjustment in the propranolol dose may be warranted. (See WARNINGS.)

Cimetidine. A study in six healthy volunteers has shown a significant increase in peak diltiazem plasma levels (58%) and area-under-the-curve (53%) after a 1-week course of cimetidine at 1200 mg per day and a single dose of diltiazem 60 mg. Ranitidine produced smaller, nonsignificant increases. The effect may be mediated by cimetidine's known inhibition of hepatic cytochrome P-450, the enzyme system responsible for the first-pass metabolism of diltiazem. Patients currently receiving diltiazem therapy should be carefully monitored for a change in pharmacological effect when initiating and discontinuing therapy with cimetidine. An adjustment in the diltiazem dose may be warranted.

Digitalis. Administration of CARDIZEM with digoxin in 24 healthy male subjects increased plasma digoxin concentrations approximately 20%. Another investigator found no increase in digoxin levels in 12 patients with coronary artery disease. Since there have been conflicting results regarding the effect of digoxin levels, it is recommended that digoxin levels be monitored when initiating, adjusting, and discontinuing CARDIZEM therapy to avoid possible over- or under-digitalization. (See WARNINGS.)

Anesthetics. The depression of cardiac contractility, conductivity, and automaticity, as well as the vascular dilation associated with anesthetics, may be potentiated by calcium channel blockers. When used concomitantly, anesthetics and calcium blockers should be titrated carefully.

Cyclosporine. A pharmacokinetic interaction between diltiazem and cyclosporine has been observed during studies involving renal and cardiac transplant patients. In renal and cardiac transplant recipients, a reduction of cyclosporine trough dose ranging from 15% to 48% was necessary to maintain concentrations similar to those seen prior to the addition of diltiazem. If these agents are to be administered concurrently, cyclosporine concentrations should be monitored, especially when diltiazem therapy is initiated, adjusted, or discontinued. The effect of cyclosporine on diltiazem plasma concentrations has not been evaluated.

Carbamazepine. Concomitant administration of diltiazem with carbamazepine has been reported to result in elevated serum levels of carbamazepine (40% to 72% increase) resulting in toxicity in some cases. Patients receiving these drugs concurrently should be monitored for a potential drug interaction.

Carcinogenesis, Mutagenesis, Impairment of Fertility
A 24-month study in rats and a 21-month study in mice showed no evidence of carcinogenicity. There was also no mutagenic response in in vitro bacterial tests. No intrinsic effect on fertility was observed in rats.

Pregnancy
Category C. Reproduction studies have been conducted in mice, rats, and rabbits. Administration of doses ranging from five to ten times greater (on a mg/kg basis) than the daily recommended therapeutic dose has resulted in embryo and fetal lethality. These doses, in some studies, have been reported to cause skeletal abnormalities. In the perinatal/postnatal studies, there was some reduction in early individual pup weights and survival rates. There was an increased incidence of stillbirths at doses of 20 times the human dose or greater.

There are no well-controlled studies in pregnant women; therefore, use CARDIZEM in pregnant women only if the potential benefit justifies the potential risk to the fetus.

Nursing Mothers
Diltiazem is excreted in human milk. One report suggests that concentrations in breast milk may approximate serum levels. If use of CARDIZEM is deemed essential, an alternative method of infant feeding should be instituted.

Pediatric Use
Safety and effectiveness in pediatric patients have not been established.

ADVERSE REACTIONS

Serious adverse reactions have been rare in studies carried out to date, but it should be recognized that patients with impaired ventricular function and cardiac conduction abnormalities usually have been excluded.

In domestic placebo-controlled angina trials, the incidence of adverse reactions reported during CARDIZEM therapy was not greater than that reported during placebo therapy. The following represent occurrences observed in clinical studies of angina patients. In many cases, the relationship to CARDIZEM has not been established. The most common occurrences from these studies, as well as their frequency of presentation, are edema (2.4%), headache (2.1%), nausea (1.9%), dizziness (1.5%), rash (1.3%), and asthenia (1.2%). In addition, the following events were reported infrequently (less than 1%):

Cardiovascular: Angina, arrhythmia, AV block (first degree), AV block (second or third degree—see conduction warning), bradycardia, bundle branch block, congestive heart failure, ECG abnormality, flushing, hypotension, palpitations, syncope, tachycardia, ventricular extrasystoles

Nervous System: Abnormal dreams, amnesia, depression, gait abnormality, hallucinations, insomnia, nervousness, paresthesia, personality change, somnolence, tremor

Gastrointestinal: Anorexia, constipation, diarrhea, dysgeusia, dyspepsia, mild elevations of alkaline phosphatase, SGOT, SGPT, and LDH (see hepatic warnings), thirst, vomiting, weight increase

Dermatological: Petechiae, photosensitivity, pruritus, urticaria

Other: Amblyopia, CPK elevation, dry mouth, dyspnea, epistaxis, eye irritation, hyperglycemia, hyperuricemia, impotence, muscle cramps, nasal congestion, nocturia, osteoarticular pain, polyuria, sexual difficulties, tinnitus

The following postmarketing events have been reported infrequently in patients receiving CARDIZEM: allergic reactions, alopecia, angioedema (including facial or periorbital edema), asystole, erythema multiforme (including Stevens-Johnson syndrome, toxic epidermal necrolysis), extrapyramidal symptoms, gingival hyperplasia, hemolytic anemia, increased bleeding time, leukopenia, purpura, retinopathy, and thrombocytopenia. There have been observed cases of a generalized rash, some characterized as leukocytoclastic vasculitis. In addition, events such as myocardial infarction have been observed, which are not readily distinguishable from the natural history of the disease in these patients. A definitive cause and effect relationship between these events and CARDIZEM therapy cannot yet be established. Exfoliative dermatitis (proven by rechallenge) has also been reported.

OVERDOSAGE OR EXAGGERATED RESPONSE

The oral LD_{50}s in mice and rats range from 415 to 740 mg/kg and from 560 to 810 mg/kg, respectively. The intravenous LD_{50}s in these species were 60 and 38 mg/kg, respectively. The oral LD_{50} in dogs is considered to be in excess of 50 mg/kg, while lethality was seen in monkeys at 360 mg/kg.

The toxic dose in man is not known. Due to extensive metabolism, blood levels after a standard dose of diltiazem can vary over tenfold, limiting the usefulness of blood levels in overdose cases.

There have been 29 reports of diltiazem overdose in doses ranging from less than 1 g to 10.8 g. Sixteen of these reports involved multiple drug ingestions.

Twenty-two reports indicated patients had recovered from diltiazem overdose ranging from less than 1 g to 10.8 g. There were seven reports with a fatal outcome; although the amount of diltiazem ingested was unknown, multiple drug ingestions were confirmed in six of the seven reports.

Events observed following diltiazem overdose included bradycardia, hypotension, heart block, and cardiac failure. Most reports of overdose described some supportive medical measure and/or drug treatment. Bradycardia frequently responded favorably to atropine, as did heart block, although cardiac pacing was also frequently utilized to treat heart block. Fluids and vasopressors were used to maintain blood pressure, and in cases of cardiac failure, inotropic agents were administered. In addition, some patients received treatment with ventilatory support, gastric lavage, activated charcoal, and/or intravenous calcium. Evidence of the effectiveness of intravenous calcium administration to reverse the pharmacological effects of diltiazem overdose was conflicting.

In the event of overdose or exaggerated response, appropriate supportive measures should be employed in addition to gastrointestinal decontamination. Diltiazem does not appear to be removed by peritoneal or hemodialysis. Limited data suggest that plasmapheresis or charcoal hemoperfusion may hasten diltiazem elimination following overdose.

Continued on next page

Cardizem Tablets—Cont.

Based on the known pharmacological effects of diltiazem and/or reported clinical experiences, the following measures may be considered:

Bradycardia: Administer atropine (0.60 to 1.0 mg). If there is no response to vagal blockade, administer isoproterenol cautiously.

High-Degree AV Block: Treat as for bradycardia above. Fixed high-degree AV block should be treated with cardiac pacing.

Cardiac Failure: Administer inotropic agents (isoproterenol, dopamine, or dobutamine) and diuretics.

Hypotension: Vasopressors (eg, dopamine or levarterenol bitartrate).

Actual treatment and dosage should depend on the severity of the clinical situation and the judgment and experience of the treating physician.

DOSAGE AND ADMINISTRATION

Exertional Angina Pectoris Due to Atherosclerotic Coronary Artery Disease or Angina Pectoris at Rest Due to Coronary Artery Spasm.

Dosage must be adjusted to each patient's needs. Starting with 30 mg four times daily, before meals, and at bedtime, dosage should be increased gradually (given in divided doses three or four times daily) at 1- to 2-day intervals until optimum response is obtained. Although individual patients may respond to any dosage level, the average optimum dosage range appears to be 180 to 360 mg/day. There are no available data concerning dosage requirements in patients with impaired renal or hepatic function. If the drug must be used in such patients, titration should be carried out with particular caution.

Concomitant Use With Other Cardiovascular Agents

1. **Sublingual NTG** may be taken as required to abort acute anginal attacks during CARDIZEM (diltiazem hydrochloride) therapy.
2. **Prophylactic Nitrate Therapy.** CARDIZEM may be safely coadministered with short- and long-acting nitrates, but there have been no controlled studies to evaluate the antianginal effectiveness of this combination.
3. **Beta-blockers.** (See WARNINGS and PRECAUTIONS.)

HOW SUPPLIED

CARDIZEM 30-mg tablets are supplied in bottles of 100 (NDC 0088-1771-47) and 500 (NDC 0088-1771-55) and in Unit Dose Identification Paks of 100 (NDC 0088-1771-49). Each green tablet is engraved with MARION on one side and 1771 on the other.

CARDIZEM 60-mg scored tablets are supplied in bottles of 100 (NDC 0088-1772-47) and 500 (NDC 0088-1772-55) and in Unit Dose Identification Paks of 100 (NDC 0088-1772-49). Each yellow tablet is engraved with MARION on one side and 1772 on the other.

CARDIZEM 90-mg scored tablets are supplied in bottles of 100 (NDC 0088-1791-47) and in Unit Dose Identification Paks of 100 (NDC 0088-1791-49). Each green oblong tablet is engraved with CARDIZEM on one side and 90 mg on the other.

CARDIZEM 120-mg scored tablets are supplied in bottles of 100 (NDC 0088-1792-47) and in Unit Dose Identification Paks of 100 (NDC 0088-1792-49). Each yellow oblong tablet is engraved with CARDIZEM on one side and 120 mg on the other.

Store at controlled room temperature 59–86°F (15–30°C).

Prescribing information as of May 1996

Hoechst Marion Roussel, Inc.
Kansas City, MO 64137 USA

Shown in Product Identification Guide, page 316

CLAFORAN® ℞

[*kla 'fər-an*]

Sterile (sterile cefotaxime sodium) and Injection (cefotaxime sodium injection)

Prescribing Information as of October 1996

DESCRIPTION

Sterile CLAFORAN® (cefotaxime sodium) is a semisynthetic, broad spectrum cephalosporin antibiotic for parenteral administration. It is the sodium salt of 7-[2-(2-amino-4-thiazolyl) glyoxylamido]-3-(hydroxymethyl)-8-oxo-5-thia-1-azabicyclo [4.2.0] oct-2-ene-2-carboxylate 7^2 (Z)-(o-methyloxime), acetate (ester). CLAFORAN® contains approximately 50.5 mg (2.2 mEq) of sodium per gram of cefotaxime activity. Solutions of CLAFORAN® range from very pale yellow to light amber depending on the concentration and the diluent used. The pH of the injectable solutions usually ranges from 5.0 to 7.5. The CAS Registry Number is 64485-93-4.

[See chemical structure at top of next column]

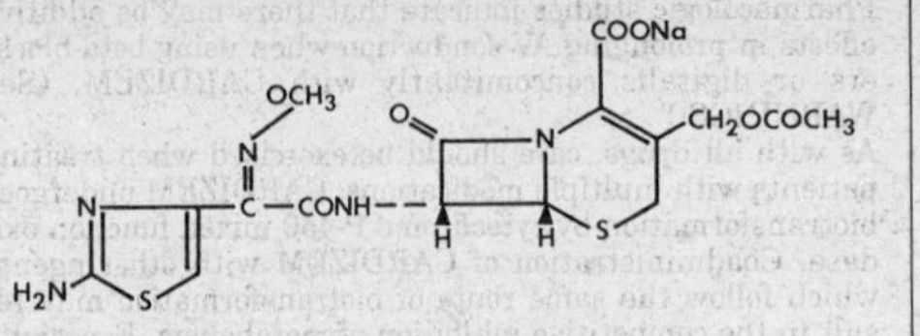

CLAFORAN® is supplied as a dry powder in conventional and ADD-Vantage® System compatible vials, infusion bottles, pharmacy bulk package bottles, and as a frozen, premixed, iso-osmotic injection in a buffered diluent solution in plastic containers. CLAFORAN®, equivalent to 1 gram and 2 grams cefotaxime, is supplied as frozen, premixed iso-osmotic injections in plastic containers. Solutions range from very pale yellow to light amber. Dextrose Hydrous, USP has been added to adjust osmolality (approximately 1.7 g and 700 mg to the 1 g and 2 g cefotaxime dosages, respectively). The injections are buffered with sodium citrate hydrous, USP. The pH is adjusted with hydrochloric acid and may be adjusted with sodium hydroxide.

The plastic container is fabricated from a specially designed multilayer plastic (PL 2040). Solutions are in contact with the polyethylene layer of this container and can leach out certain chemical components of the plastic in very small amounts within the expiration period. The suitability of the plastic has been confirmed in tests in animals according to the USP biological tests for plastic containers, as well as by tissue culture toxicity studies.

CLINICAL PHARMACOLOGY

Following IM administration of a single 500 mg or 1 g dose of CLAFORAN® to normal volunteers, mean peak serum concentrations of 11.7 and 20.5 µg/mL respectively were attained within 30 minutes and declined with an elimination half-life of approximately 1 hour. There was a dose-dependent increase in serum levels after the IV administration of 500 mg, 1 g, and 2 g of CLAFORAN® (38.9, 101.7, and 214.4 µg/mL respectively) without alteration in the elimination half-life. There is no evidence of accumulation following repetitive IV infusion of 1 g doses every 6 hours for 14 days as there are no alterations of serum or renal clearance. About 60% of the administered dose was recovered from urine during the first 6 hours following the start of the infusion.

Approximately 20–36% of an intravenously administered dose of ^{14}C-cefotaxime is excreted by the kidney as unchanged cefotaxime and 15–25% as the desacetyl derivative, the major metabolite. The desacetyl metabolite has been shown to contribute to the bactericidal activity. Two other urinary metabolites (M_2 and M_3) account for about 20–25%. They lack bactericidal activity.

A single 50 mg/kg dose of CLAFORAN® was administered as an intravenous infusion over a 10- to 15-minute period to 29 newborn infants grouped according to birth weight and age. The mean half-life of cefotaxime in infants with lower birth weights (≤1500 grams), regardless of age, was longer (4.6 hours) than the mean half-life (3.4 hours) in infants whose birth weight was greater than 1500 grams. Mean serum clearance was also smaller in the lower birth weight infants. Although the differences in mean half-life values are statistically significant for weight, they are not clinically important. Therefore, dosage should be based solely on age. (See DOSAGE AND ADMINISTRATION section.)

Additionally, no disulfiram-like reactions were reported in a study conducted in 22 healthy volunteers administered CLAFORAN® and ethanol.

Microbiology

The bactericidal activity of cefotaxime sodium results from inhibition of cell wall synthesis. Cefotaxime sodium has *in vitro* activity against a wide range of gram-positive and gram-negative organisms. CLAFORAN® has a high degree of stability in the presence of beta-lactamases, both penicillinases and cephalosporinases, of gram-negative and gram-positive bacteria. Cefotaxime sodium has been shown to be a potent inhibitor of β-lactamases produced by certain gram-negative bacteria. Cefotaxime sodium is usually active against the following microorganisms both *in vitro* and in clinical infections (see INDICATIONS AND USAGE).

Aerobes, Gram-positive: *Staphylococcus aureus,* including penicillinase and non-penicillinase producing strains, *Staphylococcus epidermidis, Enterococcus* species, *Streptococcus pyogenes* (Group A beta-hemolytic streptococci), *Streptococcus agalactiae* (Group B streptococci), *Streptococcus pneumoniae* (formerly *Diplococcus pneumoniae*).

Aerobes, Gram-negative: *Citrobacter* species, *Enterobacter* species, *Escherichia coli, Haemophilus influenzae* (including ampicillin-resistant *H. influenzae*), *Haemophilus parainfluenzae, Klebsiella* species (including *K. pneumoniae*), *Neisseria gonorrhoeae* (including penicillinase and nonpenicillinase producing strains), *Neisseria meningitidis, Proteus mirabilis, Proteus vulgaris, Proteus inconstans,* Group B, *Morganella morganii, Providencia rettgeri, Serratia* species, and *Acinetobacter* species.

NOTE: Many strains of the above organisms that are multiply resistant to other antibiotics, e.g., penicillins, cephalosporins, and aminoglycosides, are susceptible to cefotaxime sodium.

Cefotaxime sodium is active against some strains of *Pseudomonas aeruginosa.*

Anaerobes: *Bacteroides* species, including some strains of *B. fragilis, Clostridium* species (NOTE: Most strains of *C. difficile* are resistant.), *Peptococcus* species, *Peptostreptococcus* species, and *Fusobacterium* species (including *F. nucleatum*).

Cefotaxime sodium is highly stable *in vitro* to four of the five major classes of β-lactamases described by Richmond et al., including type IIIa (TEM) which is produced by many gram-negative bacteria. The drug is also stable to β-lactamase (penicillinase) produced by staphylococci. In addition, cefotaxime sodium shows high affinity for penicillin-binding proteins in the cell wall, including PBP, Ib and III.

Cefotaxime sodium also demonstrates *in vitro* activity against the following microorganisms although clinical significance is unknown: *Salmonella* species (including *S. typhi*), *Providencia* species, and *Shigella* species.

Cefotaxime sodium and aminoglycosides have been shown to be synergistic *in vitro* against some strains of *Pseudomonas aeruginosa.*

Susceptibility Tests

Quantitative methods that require measurement of zone diameters give the most precise estimate of antibiotic susceptibility. One such procedure[1] has been recommended for use with discs to test susceptibility to cefotaxime sodium. Interpretation involves correlation of the diameters obtained in the disc test with minimum inhibitory concentration (MIC) values for cefotaxime sodium.

Reports from the laboratory giving results of the standardized single-disc susceptibility test using a 30 µg cefotaxime sodium disc should be interpreted according to the following criteria:

Susceptible organisms produce zones of 20 mm or greater, indicating that the tested organism is likely to respond to therapy.

Organisms that produce zones of 15 to 19 mm are expected to be susceptible if high dosage is used or if the infection is confined to tissues and fluids (e.g., urine) in which high antibiotic levels are attained.

Resistant organisms produce zones of 14 mm or less, indicating that other therapy should be selected.

Organisms should be tested with the cefotaxime sodium disc, since cefotaxime sodium has been shown by *in vitro* tests to be active against certain strains found resistant when other beta lactam discs are used. The cefotaxime sodium disc should not be used for testing susceptibility to other cephalosporins. Organisms having zones of less than 18 mm around the cephalothin disc are not necessarily of intermediate susceptibility or resistant to cefotaxime sodium.

A bacterial isolate may be considered susceptible if the MIC value for cefotaxime sodium is not more than 16 µg/mL. Organisms are considered resistant to cefotaxime sodium if the MIC is equal to or greater than 64 µg/mL. Organisms having an MIC value of less than 64 µg/mL but greater than 16 µg/mL are expected to be susceptible if high dosage is used or if the infection is confined to tissues and fluids (e.g., urine) in which high antibiotic levels are attained.

INDICATIONS AND USAGE

Treatment

CLAFORAN® is indicated for the treatment of patients with serious infections caused by susceptible strains of the designated microorganisms in the diseases listed below.

(1) **Lower respiratory tract infections,** including pneumonia, caused by *Streptococcus pneumoniae* (formerly *Diplococcus pneumoniae*), *Streptococcus pyogenes** (Group A streptococci) and other streptococci (excluding enterococci, e.g., *Streptococcus faecalis*), *Staphylococcus aureus* (penicillinase and non-penicillinase producing), *Escherichia coli, Klebsiella* species, *Haemophilus influenzae* (including ampicillin resistant strains), *Haemophilus parainfluenzae, Proteus mirabilis, Serratia marcescens*, Enterobacter* species, indole positive *Proteus* and *Pseudomonas* species (including *P. aeruginosa*).

(2) **Genitourinary infections.** Urinary tract infections caused by *Enterococcus* species, *Staphylococcus epidermidis, Staphylococcus aureus*,* (penicillinase and non-penicillinase producing), *Citrobacter* species, *Enterobacter* species, *Escherichia coli, Klebsiella* species, *Proteus mirabilis, Proteus vulgaris*, Proteus inconstans* group B, *Morganella morganii*, Providencia rettgeri*, Serratia marcescens* and *Pseudomonas* species (including *P. aeruginosa*). Also, uncomplicated gonorrhea (cervical/urethral and rectal) caused by *Neisseria gonorrhoeae,* including penicillinase producing strains.

(3) **Gynecologic infections,** including pelvic inflammatory disease, endometritis and pelvic cellulitis caused by *Staphylococcus epidermidis, Streptococcus* species, *Enterococcus* species, *Enterobacter* species*, *Klebsiella* species*, *Escherichia coli, Proteus mirabilis, Bacteroides* species (including *Bacteroides fragilis**), *Clostridium* species, and anaerobic cocci (including *Peptostreptococcus* species and *Peptococcus* species) and *Fusobacterium* species (including *F. nucleatum**).

CLAFORAN®, like other cephalosporins, has no activity against *Chlamydia trachomatis.* Therefore, when cephalosporins are used in the treatment of patients with pelvic inflammatory disease and *C. trachomatis* is one of the suspected pathogens, appropriate antichlamydial coverage should be added.

(4) **Bacteremia/Septicemia** caused by *Escherichia coli, Klebsiella* species, *Serratia marcescens, Staphylococcus aureus,* and *Streptococcus* species (including *S. pneumoniae*).

(5) **Skin and skin structure infections** caused by *Staphylococcus aureus* (penicillinase and non-penicillinase producing), *Staphylococcus epidermidis, Streptococcus pyogenes* (Group A streptococci) and other streptococci, *Enterococcus* species, *Acinetobacter* species*, *Escherichia coli, Citrobacter* species (including *C. freundii**). *Enterobacter* species, *Klebsiella* species, *Proteus mirabilis, Proteus vulgaris**, *Morganella morganii, Providencia rettgeri**, *Pseudomonas* species, *Serratia marcescens, Bacteroides* species, and anaerobic cocci (including *Peptostreptococcus** species and *Peptococcus* species).

(6) **Intra-abdominal infections** including peritonitis caused by *Streptococcus* species*, *Escherichia coli, Klebsiella* species, *Bacteroides* species, and anaerobic cocci (including *Peptostreptococcus** species and *Peptococcus** species), *Proteus mirabilis**, and *Clostridium* species*.

(7) **Bone and/or joint infections** caused by *Staphylococcus aureus* (penicillinase and non-penicillinase producing strains), *Streptococcus* species (including *S. pyogenes**), *Pseudomonas* species (including *P. aeruginosa**), and *Proteus mirabilis**.

(8) **Central nervous system infections,** e.g., meningitis and ventriculitis, caused by *Neisseria meningitidis, Haemophilus influenzae, Streptococcus pneumoniae, Klebsiella pneumoniae** and *Escherichia coli**.

(*) Efficacy for this organism, in this organ system, has been studied in fewer than 10 infections.

Although many strains of enterococci (e.g., *S. faecalis*) and *Pseudomonas* species are resistant to cefotaxime sodium *in vitro,* CLAFORAN® has been used successfully in treating patients with infections caused by susceptible organisms.

Specimens for bacteriologic culture should be obtained prior to therapy in order to isolate and identify causative organisms and to determine their susceptibilities to CLAFORAN®. Therapy may be instituted before results of susceptibility studies are known; however, once these results become available, the antibiotic treatment should be adjusted accordingly.

In certain cases of confirmed or suspected gram-positive or gram-negative sepsis or in patients with other serious infections in which the causative organism has not been identified, CLAFORAN® may be used concomitantly with an aminoglycoside. The dosage recommended in the labeling of both antibiotics may be given and depends on the severity of the infection and the patient's condition. Renal function should be carefully monitored, especially if higher dosages of the aminoglycosides are to be administered or if therapy is prolonged, because of the potential nephrotoxicity and ototoxicity of aminoglycoside antibiotics. It is possible that nephrotoxicity may be potentiated if CLAFORAN® is used concomitantly with an aminoglycoside.

Prevention

The administration of CLAFORAN® preoperatively reduces the incidence of certain infections in patients undergoing surgical procedures (e.g., abdominal or vaginal hysterectomy, gastrointestinal and genitourinary tract surgery) that may be classified as contaminated or potentially contaminated.

In patients undergoing cesarean section, intraoperative (after clamping the umbilical cord) and postoperative use of CLAFORAN® may also reduce the incidence of certain postoperative infections. (See DOSAGE AND ADMINISTRATION section.)

Effective use for elective surgery depends on the time of administration. To achieve effective tissue levels, CLAFORAN® should be given $^1/_2$ to $1^1/_2$ hours before surgery. (See DOSAGE AND ADMINISTRATION section.)

For patients undergoing gastrointestinal surgery, preoperative bowel preparation by mechanical cleansing as well as with a non-absorbable antibiotic (e.g., neomycin) is recommended.

If there are signs of infection, specimens for culture should be obtained for identification of the causative organism so that appropriate therapy may be instituted.

CONTRAINDICATIONS

CLAFORAN® is contraindicated in patients who have shown hypersensitivity to cefotaxime sodium or the cephalosporin group of antibiotics.

WARNINGS

BEFORE THERAPY WITH CLAFORAN® IS INSTITUTED, CAREFUL INQUIRY SHOULD BE MADE TO DETERMINE WHETHER THE PATIENT HAS HAD PREVIOUS HYPERSENSITIVITY REACTIONS TO CEFOTAXIME SODIUM, CEPHALOSPORINS, PENICILLINS, OR OTHER DRUGS. THIS PRODUCT SHOULD BE GIVEN WITH CAUTION TO PATIENTS WITH TYPE I HYPERSENSITIVITY REACTIONS TO PENICILLIN. ANTIBIOTICS SHOULD BE ADMINISTERED WITH CAUTION TO ANY PATIENT WHO HAS DEMONSTRATED SOME FORM OF ALLERGY, PARTICULARLY TO DRUGS. IF AN ALLERGIC REACTION TO CLAFORAN® OCCURS, DISCONTINUE TREATMENT WITH THE DRUG. SERIOUS HYPERSENSITIVITY REACTIONS MAY REQUIRE EPINEPHRINE AND OTHER EMERGENCY MEASURES.

During post-marketing surveillance, a potentially life-threatening arrhythmia was reported in each of six patients who received a rapid (less than 60 seconds) bolus injection of cefotaxime through a central venous catheter. Therefore, cefotaxime should only be administered as instructed in the DOSAGE AND ADMINISTRATION section.

Pseudomembranous colitis has been reported with nearly all antibacterial agents, including cefotaxime, and may range from mild to life threatening. Therefore, it is important to consider its diagnosis in patients with diarrhea subsequent to the administration of antibacterial agents.

Treatment with antibacterial agents alters the normal flora of the colon and may permit overgrowth of Clostridia. Studies indicate that a toxin produced by *Clostridium difficile* is one primary cause of antibiotic-associated colitis.

After the diagnosis of pseudomembranous colitis has been established, appropriate therapeutic measures should be initiated. Mild cases of colitis may respond to drug discontinuance alone. In moderate to severe cases, consideration should be given to management with fluids and electrolytes, protein supplementation, and treatment with an antibacterial drug clinically effective against *Clostridium difficile* colitis.

When the colitis is not relieved by drug discontinuance or when it is severe, oral vancomycin is the treatment of choice for antibiotic-associated pseudomembranous colitis produced by *C. difficile.* Other causes of colitis should also be considered.

PRECAUTIONS

CLAFORAN® should be prescribed with caution in individuals with a history of gastrointestinal disease, particularly colitis.

Because high and prolonged serum antibiotic concentrations can occur from usual doses in patients with transient or persistent reduction of urinary output because of renal insufficiency, the total daily dosage should be reduced when CLAFORAN® is administered to such patients. Continued dosage should be determined by degree of renal impairment, severity of infection, and susceptibility of the causative organism.

Although there is no clinical evidence supporting the necessity of changing the dosage of cefotaxime sodium in patients with even profound renal dysfunction, it is suggested that, until further data are obtained, the dose of cefotaxime sodium be halved in patients with estimated creatinine clearances of less than 20 mL/min/1.73 m^2.

When only serum creatinine is available, the following formula[2] (based on sex, weight, and age of the patient) may be used to convert this value into creatinine clearance. The serum creatinine should represent a steady state of renal function.

Males: $\dfrac{\text{Weight (kg)} \times (140 - \text{age})}{72 \times \text{serum creatinine}}$

Females: $0.85 \times$ above value

As with other antibiotics, prolonged use of CLAFORAN® may result in overgrowth of nonsusceptible organisms. Repeated evaluation of the patient's condition is essential. If superinfection occurs during therapy, appropriate measures should be taken.

As with other beta-lactam antibiotics, granulocytopenia and, more rarely, agranulocytosis may develop during treatment with CLAFORAN®, particularly if given over long periods. For courses of treatment lasting longer than 10 days, blood counts should therefore be monitored.

CLAFORAN®, like other parenteral anti-infective drugs, may be locally irritating to tissues. In most cases, perivascular extravasation of CLAFORAN® responds to changing of the infusion site. In rare instances, extensive perivascular extravasation of CLAFORAN® may result in tissue damage and require surgical treatment. To minimize the potential for tissue inflammation, infusion sites should be monitored regularly and changed when appropriate.

Drug Interactions: Increased nephrotoxicity has been reported following concomitant administration of cephalosporins and aminoglycoside antibiotics.

Carcinogenesis, Mutagenesis: Long-term studies in animals have not been performed to evaluate carcinogenic potential. Mutagenic tests included a micronucleus and an Ames test. Both tests were negative for mutagenic effects.

Pregnancy (Category B): Reproduction studies have been performed in mice and rats at doses up to 30 times the usual human dose and have revealed no evidence of impaired fertility or harm to the fetus because of cefotaxime sodium. However, there are no well-controlled studies in pregnant women. Because animal reproductive studies are not always predictive of human response, this drug should be used during pregnancy only if clearly needed.

Nonteratogenic Effects: Use of the drug in women of childbearing potential requires that the anticipated benefit be weighed against the possible risks.

In perinatal and postnatal studies with rats, the pups in the group given 1200 mg/kg of CLAFORAN® were significantly lighter in weight at birth and remained smaller than pups in the control group during the 21 days of nursing.

Nursing Mothers: CLAFORAN® is excreted in human milk in low concentrations. Caution should be exercised when CLAFORAN® is administered to a nursing woman.

Pediatric Use: See Precautions above regarding perivascular extravasation. The potential for toxic effects in pediatric patients from chemicals that may leach from the plastic in single dose Galaxy® containers (premixed CLAFORAN® Injection) has not been determined.

ADVERSE REACTIONS

CLAFORAN® is generally well tolerated. The most common adverse reactions have been local reactions following IM or IV injection. Other adverse reactions have been encountered infrequently.

The most frequent adverse reactions (greater than 1%) are:

Local (4.3%)—Injection site inflammation with IV administration. Pain, induration, and tenderness after IM injection.

Hypersensitivity (2.4%)—Rash, pruritus, fever, and eosinophilia and less frequently urticaria and anaphylaxis.

Gastrointestinal (1.4%)—Colitis, diarrhea, nausea, and vomiting.

Symptoms of pseudomembranous colitis can appear during or after antibiotic treatment.

Nausea and vomiting have been reported rarely.

Less frequent adverse reactions (less than 1%) are:

Cardiovascular System—Potentially life-threatening arrhythmias following rapid (less than 60 seconds) bolus administration via central venous catheter have been observed.

Hematologic System—Neutropenia, transient leukopenia, eosinophilia, thrombocytopenia and agranulocytosis have been reported. Some individuals have developed positive direct Coombs Tests during treatment with CLAFORAN® (cefotaxime sodium injection) and other cephalosporin antibiotics. Rare cases of hemolytic anemia have been reported.

Genitourinary System—Moniliasis, vaginitis.

Central Nervous System—Headache.

Liver—Transient elevations in SGOT, SGPT, serum LDH, and serum alkaline phosphatase levels have been reported.

Kidney—As with some other cephalosporins, interstitial nephritis and transient elevations of BUN and creatinine have been occasionally observed with CLAFORAN®.

DOSAGE AND ADMINISTRATION

Adults

Dosage and route of administration should be determined by susceptibility of the causative organisms, severity of the infection, and the condition of the patient (see table for dosage guideline).

GUIDELINES FOR DOSAGE OF CLAFORAN®

Type of Infection	Daily Dose (grams)	Frequency and Route
Gonococcal urethritis/cervicitis in males and females	0.5	0.5 gram IM (single dose)
Rectal gonorrhea in females	0.5	0.5 gram IM (single dose)
Rectal gonorrhea in males	1	1 gram IM (single dose)
Uncomplicated Infections	2	1 gram every 12 hours IM or IV
Moderate to severe infections	3-6	1-2 grams every 8 hours IM or IV
Infections commonly needing antibiotics in higher dosage (e.g., septicemia)	6-8	2 grams every 6-8 hours IV
Life-threatening infections	up to 12	2 grams every 4 hours IV

Continued on next page

Claforan—Cont.

age guidelines). CLAFORAN® may be administered IM or IV after reconstitution. Premixed CLAFORAN® Injection is intended for IV administration after thawing. The maximum daily dosage should not exceed 12 grams.
[See table at top of previous page]

If *C. trachomatis* is a suspected pathogen, appropriate antichlamydial coverage should be added, because cefotaxime sodium has no activity against this organism.

To prevent postoperative infection in contaminated or potentially contaminated surgery, the recommended dose is a single 1 gram IM or IV administered 30 to 90 minutes prior to start of surgery.

Cesarean Section Patients

The first dose of 1 gram is administered intravenously as soon as the umbilical cord is clamped. The second and third doses should be given as 1 gram intravenously or intramuscularly at 6 and 12 hours after the first dose.

Neonates, Infants, and Children

The following dosage schedule is recommended:
Neonates (birth to 1 month):

0–1 week of age	50 mg/kg per dose every 12 hours IV
1–4 weeks of age	50 mg/kg per dose every 8 hours IV

It is not necessary to differentiate between premature and normal-gestational age infants.

Infants and Children (1 month to 12 years): For body weights less than 50 kg, the recommended daily dose is 50 to 180 mg/kg IM or IV body weight divided into four to six equal doses. The higher dosages should be used for more severe or serious infections, including meningitis. For body weights 50 kg or more, the usual adult dosage should be used; the maximum daily dosage should not exceed 12 grams.

Impaired Renal Function —see PRECAUTIONS section.

NOTE: As with antibiotic therapy in general, administration of CLAFORAN® should be continued for a minimum of 48 to 72 hours after the patient defervesces or after evidence of bacterial eradication has been obtained; a minimum of 10 days of treatment is recommended for infections caused by Group A beta-hemolytic streptococci in order to guard against the risk of rheumatic fever or glomerulonephritis; frequent bacteriologic and clinical appraisal is necessary during therapy of chronic urinary tract infection and may be required for several months after therapy has been completed; persistent infections may require treatment of several weeks and doses smaller than those indicated above should not be used.

PREPARATION OF CLAFORAN® STERILE

CLAFORAN® for IM or IV administration should be reconstituted as follows:

Strength	Diluent (mL)	Withdrawable Volume (mL)	Approximate Concentration (mg/mL)
500 mg via* (IM)	2	2.2	230
1g vial* (IM)	3	3.4	300
2g vial* (IM)	5	6.0	330
500 mg vial* (IV)	10	10.2	50
1g vial* (IV)	10	10.4	95
2g vial* (IV)	10	11.0	180
1g infusion	50–100	50–100	20–10
2g infusion	50–100	50–100	40–20
10g bottle	47	52.0	200
10g bottle	97	102.0	100

*In conventional vials

Shake to dissolve; inspect for particulate matter and discoloration prior to use. Solutions of CLAFORAN® range from very pale yellow to light amber, depending on concentration, diluent used, and length and condition of storage.

For intramuscular use: Reconstitute VIALS with Sterile Water for Injection or Bacteriostatic Water for Injection as described above.

For intravenous use: Reconstitute VIALS with at least 10 mL of Sterile Water for Injection. Reconstitute INFUSION BOTTLES with 50 or 100 mL of 0.9% Sodium Chloride Injection or 5% Dextrose Injection. For other diluents, see COMPATIBILITY AND STABILITY section.

Pharmacy Bulk Package: Reconstitute with 47 mL of diluent for an approximate concentration of 200 mg/mL or 97 mL of diluent for an approximate concentration of 100 mg/mL. Stock solutions may be further diluted for IV infusion with diluents as listed in COMPATIBILITY AND STABILITY section.

NOTE: Solutions of CLAFORAN® must not be admixed with aminoglycoside solutions. If CLAFORAN® and aminoglycosides are to be administered to the same patient, they must be administered separately and not as mixed injection.

A SOLUTION OF 1 G CLAFORAN® IN 14 ML OF STERILE WATER FOR INJECTION IS ISOTONIC.

IM Administration: As with all IM preparations, CLAFORAN® should be injected well within the body of a relatively large muscle such as the upper outer quadrant of the buttock (i.e., gluteus maximus); aspiration is necessary to avoid inadvertent injection into a blood vessel. Individual IM doses of 2 grams may be given if the dose is divided and is administered in different intramuscular sites.

IV Administration: The IV route is preferable for patients with bacteremia, bacterial septicemia, peritonitis, meningitis, or other severe or life-threatening infections, or for patients who may be poor risks because of lowered resistance resulting from such debilitating conditions as malnutrition, trauma, surgery, diabetes, heart failure, or malignancy, particularly if shock is present or impending.

For intermittent IV administration, a solution containing 1 gram or 2 grams in 10 mL of Sterile Water for Injection can be injected over a period of three to five minutes. Cefotaxime should not be administered over a period of less than three minutes. (See WARNINGS.) With an infusion system, it may also be given over a longer period of time through the tubing system by which the patient may be receiving other IV solutions. However, during infusion of the solution containing CLAFORAN®, it is advisable to discontinue temporarily the administration of other solutions at the same site. For the administration of higher doses by continuous IV infusion, a solution of CLAFORAN® may be added to IV bottles containing the solutions discussed below.

DIRECTIONS FOR USE OF CLAFORAN® (cefotaxime sodium injection) IN GALAXY CONTAINER (PL 2040 PLASTIC)

CLAFORAN® Injection in Galaxy containers (PL 2040 plastic) is for continuous or intermittent infusion using sterile equipment.

Storage

Store in a freezer capable of maintaining a temperature of −20°C/−4°F.

Thawing of Plastic Container

Thaw frozen container at room temperature or under refrigeration (at or below 5°C). [DO NOT FORCE THAW BY IMMERSION IN WATER BATHS OR BY MICROWAVE IRRADIATION.]

Check for minute leaks by squeezing container firmly. If leaks are detected, discard solution as sterility may be impaired.

DO NOT ADD SUPPLEMENTARY MEDICATION.

The container should be visually inspected. Components of the solution may precipitate in the frozen state and will dissolve upon reaching room temperature with little or no agitation. Potency is not affected. Agitate after solution has reached room temperature. If after visual inspection the solution remains cloudy or if an insoluble precipitate is noted or if any seals or outlet ports are not intact, the container should be discarded.

The thawed solution is stable for 10 days under refrigeration (at or below 5°C) or 24 hours at or below 22°C. Do not refreeze thawed antibiotics.

CAUTION: Do not use plastic containers in series connections. Such use could result in air embolism due to residual air being drawn from the primary container before administration of the fluid from the secondary container is complete.

Preparation for Intravenous Administration:

1. Suspend container from eyelet support.
2. Remove protector from outlet port at bottom of container.
3. Attach administration set. Refer to complete directions accompanying set.

PREPARATION OF CLAFORAN® STERILE IN ADD-VANTAGE® SYSTEM

CLAFORAN® Sterile 1 g or 2 g may be reconstituted in 50 mL or 100 mL of 5% Dextrose or 0.9% Sodium Chloride in the ADD-Vantage® diluent container. Refer to enclosed, separate INSTRUCTIONS FOR ADD-VANTAGE SYSTEM.

COMPATIBILITY AND STABILITY

Solutions of CLAFORAN® Sterile reconstituted as described above (Preparation of CLAFORAN® Sterile) remain chemically stable (potency remains above 90%) as follows when stored in original containers and disposable plastic syringes:
[See table below]

Reconstituted solutions stored in original containers and plastic syringes remain stable for 13 weeks frozen.

For the 10 g bottle withdraw reconstituted contents immediately. However, if it is not possible, aliquoting operations must be completed within four hours of reconstitution. Discard the reconstituted stock solution 4 hours after initial entry.

Reconstituted solutions may be further diluted up to 1000 mL with the following solutions and maintain satisfactory potency for 24 hours at or below 22°C, and at least 5 days under refrigeration (at or below 5°C): 0.9% Sodium Chloride Injection; 5 or 10% Dextrose Injection; 5% Dextrose and 0.9% Sodium Chloride Injection; 5% Dextrose and 0.45% Sodium Chloride Injection; 5% Dextrose and 0.2% Sodium Chloride Injection; Lactated Ringers Solution; Sodium Lactate Injection (M/6); 10% Invert Sugar Injection, 8.5% TRAVASOL® (Amino Acid) Injection without Electrolytes. Solutions of CLAFORAN® Sterile reconstituted in 0.9% Sodium Chloride Injection or 5% Dextrose Injection in Viaflex® plastic containers maintain satisfactory potency for 24 hours at or below 22°C, 5 days under refrigeration (at or below 5°C) and 13 weeks frozen. Solutions of CLAFORAN® Sterile reconstituted in 0.9% Sodium Chloride Injection or 5% Dextrose Injection in the ADD-Vantage® flexible containers maintain satisfactory potency for 24 hours at or below 22°C. DO NOT FREEZE.

NOTE: CLAFORAN® solutions exhibit maximum stability in the pH 5–7 range. Solutions of CLAFORAN® should not be prepared with diluents having a pH above 7.5, such as Sodium Bicarbonate Injection.

HOW SUPPLIED

Sterile CLAFORAN® is a dry off-white to pale yellow crystalline powder supplied in vials and bottles containing cefotaxime sodium as follows:

500 mg cefotaxime (free acid equivalent) in vials in packages of 10 (NDC 0039-0017-10).

1 g cefotaxime (free acid equivalent) in vials in packages of 10 (NDC 0039-0018-10), packages of 25 (NDC 0039-0018-25), packages of 50 (NDC 0039-0018-50); infusion bottles in packages of 10 (NDC 0039-0018-11).

2 g cefotaxime (free acid equivalent) in vials in packages of 10 (NDC 0039-0019-10), packages of 25 (NDC 0039-0019-25), packages of 50 (NDC 0039-0019-50); infusion bottles in packages of 10 (NDC 0039-0019-11).

10 g cefotaxime (free acid equivalent) in bottles (NDC 0039-0020-01).

1 g cefotaxime (free acid equivalent) in ADD-Vantage® System vials in packages of 25 (NDC 0039-0023-25) and 50 (NDC 0039-0023-50).

2 g cefotaxime (free acid equivalent) in ADD-Vantage® System vials in packages of 25 (NDC 0039-0024-25) and 50 (NDC 0039-0024-50).

ADD-Vantage® System diluents (5% Dextrose or 0.9% Sodium Chloride) are available from Abbott Laboratories.

NOTE: CLAFORAN® in the dry state should be stored below 30°C. The dry material as well as solutions tend to darken depending on storage conditions and should be protected from elevated temperatures and excessive light.

Premixed CLAFORAN® Injection is supplied as a frozen, iso-osmotic, sterile, nonpyrogenic solution in 50 mL single dose Galaxy® containers (PL 2040 plastic) as follows:

1 g cefotaxime (free acid equivalent) in packages of 12 (NDC 0039-0037-05) 2G3518.

2 g cefotaxime (free acid equivalent) in packages of 12 (NDC 0039-0038-05) 2G3519.

NOTE: Store Premixed CLAFORAN® Injection at or below −20°C/−4°F. [See DIRECTIONS FOR USE OF CLAFORAN® (cefotaxime sodium injection) IN GALAXY® CONTAINERS (PL 2040 PLASTIC)].

CLAFORAN® Injection supplied as a frozen, iso-osmotic, sterile, nonpyrogenic solution in Galaxy® containers (PL

Strength	Reconstituted Concentration mg/mL	Stability at or below 22°C	Stability under Refrigeration (at or below 5°C)	
			Original Containers	Plastic Syringes
500 mg vial IM	200	12 hours	7 days	5 days
1g vial IM	300	12 hours	7 days	5 days
2g vial IM	330	12 hours	7 days	5 days
500 mg vial IV	50	24 hours	7 days	5 days
1g vial IV	95	24 hours	7 days	5 days
2g vial IV	180	12 hours	7 days	5 days
1g infusion bottle	10–20	24 hours	10 days	
2g infusion bottle	20–40	24 hours	10 days	

2040 plastic) is manufactured for Hoechst-Roussel Pharmaceuticals, a Division of Hoechst Marion Roussel, Inc. by Baxter Healthcare Corporation.

REFERENCES

1) Bauer, A.W.; Kirby, W.M.M.; Sherris, J.C.; and Turck, M. Antibiotic Susceptibility Testing by a Standardized Single Disk Method, *Am J Clin Pathol.* 1966;45:493. Standardized Disc Susceptibility Test, Federal Register, 39: 19182-4, 1974. National Committee for Clinical Laboratory Standards, Approved Standard: ASM-2, Performance Standards for Antimicrobial Disc Susceptibility Tests, July, 1975.
2) Cockcroft, D.W. and Gault, M.H.: Prediction of Creatinine Clearance from Serum Creatinine. *Nephron.* 1976;16:31-41.

Sterile cefotaxime sodium US Patents 4,152,432; 4,224,371; 4,298,606; cefotaxime sodium injection US Patents 4,152,432; 4,298,606.
Claforan REG TM ROUSSEL-UCLAF.
Galaxy and PL 2040 REG TM Baxter International Inc.
ADD-Vantage REG TM Abbott Laboratories
US Patents ADD-Vantage System: 4,614,267; 4,614,515; 4,757,911; 4,703,864; 4,784,658; 4,784,259; 4,948,000; 4,936,445.
Prescribing Information as of October 1996.
Hoechst-Roussel Pharmaceuticals
Division of Hoechst Marion Roussel, Inc.
Kansas City, MO 64137

Shown in Product Identification Guide, page 316

CLOMID® ℞
(clomiphene citrate tablets USP)

Prescribing Information as of February 1996

DESCRIPTION

CLOMID (clomiphene citrate tablets USP) is an orally administered, nonsteroidal, ovulatory stimulant designated chemically as 2-[p-(2-chloro-1,2-diphenylvinyl)phenoxy] triethylamine citrate (1:1). It has the molecular formula of $C_{26}H_{28}ClNO \cdot C_6H_8O_7$ and a molecular weight of 598.09. It is represented structurally as:

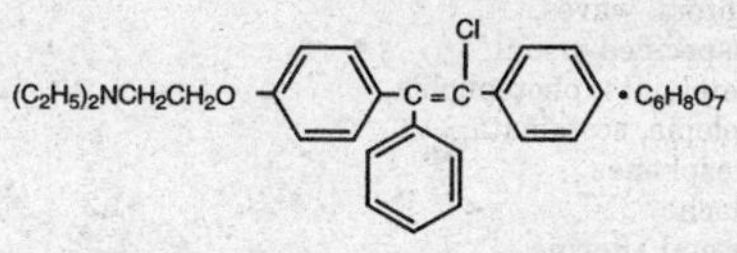

Clomiphene citrate is a white to pale yellow, essentially odorless, crystalline powder. It is freely soluble in methanol; soluble in ethanol; slightly soluble in acetone, water, and chloroform; and insoluble in ether.

CLOMID is a mixture of two geometric isomers [cis (zuclomiphene) and trans (enclomiphene)] containing between 30% and 50% of the cis-isomer.

Each white scored tablet contains 50 mg clomiphene citrate USP. The tablet also contains the following inactive ingredients: corn starch, lactose, magnesium stearate, pregelatinized corn starch, and sucrose.

CLINICAL PHARMACOLOGY

Action

CLOMID is a drug of considerable pharmacologic potency. With careful selection and proper management of the patient, CLOMID has been demonstrated to be a useful therapy for the anovulatory patient desiring pregnancy.

Clomiphene citrate is capable of interacting with estrogen-receptor-containing tissues, including the hypothalamus, pituitary, ovary, endometrium, vagina, and cervix. It may compete with estrogen for estrogen-receptor-binding sites and may delay replenishment of intracellular estrogen receptors. Clomiphene citrate initiates a series of endocrine events culminating in a preovulatory gonadotropin surge and subsequent follicular rupture. The first endocrine event in response to a course of clomiphene therapy is an increase in the release of pituitary gonadotropins. This initiates steroidogenesis and folliculogenesis, resulting in growth of the ovarian follicle and an increase in the circulating level of estradiol. Following ovulation, plasma progesterone and estradiol rise and fall as they would in a normal ovulatory cycle.

Available data suggest that both the estrogenic and antiestrogenic properties of clomiphene may participate in the initiation of ovulation. The two clomiphene isomers have been found to have mixed estrogenic and antiestrogenic effects, which may vary from one species to another. Some data suggest that zuclomiphene has greater estrogenic activity then enclomiphene.

Clomiphene citrate has no apparent progestational, androgenic, or antiandrogenic effects and does not appear to interfere with pituitary-adrenal or pituitary-thyroid function.

Although there is no evidence of a "carryover effect" of CLOMID, spontaneous ovulatory menses have been noted in some patients after CLOMID therapy.

Pharmacokinetics

Based on early studies with ^{14}C-labeled clomiphene citrate, the drug was shown to be readily absorbed orally in humans and excreted principally in the feces. Cumulative urinary and fecal excretion of the ^{14}C averaged about 50% of the oral dose and 37% of an intravenous dose after 5 days. Mean urinary excretion was approximately 8% with fecal excretion of about 42%.

Some ^{14}C label was still present in the feces 6 weeks after administration. Subsequent single-dose studies in normal volunteers showed that zuclomiphene (cis) has a longer half-life than enclomiphene (trans). Detectable levels of zuclomiphene persisted for longer than a month in these subjects. This may be suggestive of stereo-specific enterohepatic recycling or sequestering of the zuclomiphene. Thus, it is possible that some active drug may remain in the body during early pregnancy in women who conceive in the menstrual cycle during CLOMID therapy.

CLINICAL STUDIES

During clinical investigations, 7578 patients received CLOMID, some of whom had impediments to ovulation other than ovulatory dysfunction (see INDICATIONS AND USAGE). In those clinical trials, successful therapy characterized by pregnancy occurred in approximately 30% of these patients.

There were a total of 2635 pregnancies reported during the clinical trial period. Of those pregnancies, information on outcome was only available for 2369 of the cases. Table 1 summarizes the outcome of these cases.

Of the reported pregnancies, the incidence of multiple pregnancies was 7.98%: 6.9% twin, 0.5% triplet, 0.3% quadruplet, and 0.1% quintuplet. Of the 165 twin pregnancies for which sufficient information was available, the ratio of monozygotic to dizygotic twins was about 1:5. Table 1 reports the survival rate of the live multiple births.

A sextuplet birth was reported after completion of original clinical studies; none of the sextuplets survived (each weighed less than 400 g), although each appeared grossly normal.

Table 1. Outcome of Reported Pregnancies in Clinical Trials (n = 2369)

Outcome	Total Number of Pregnancies	Survival Rate
Pregnancy Wastage		
Spontaneous Abortions	483*	
Stillbirths	24	
Live Births		
Single Births	1697	98.16%†
Multiple Births	165	83.26%†

* Includes 28 ectopic pregnancies, 4 hydatiform moles, and 1 fetus papyraceous.
† Indicates percentage of surviving infants from these pregnancies.

The overall survival of infants from multiple pregnancies including spontaneous abortions, stillbirths, and neonatal deaths is 73%.

INDICATIONS AND USAGE

CLOMID is indicated for the treatment of ovulatory dysfunction in women desiring pregnancy. Impediments to achieving pregnancy must be excluded or adequately treated before beginning CLOMID therapy. Those patients most likely to achieve success with clomiphene therapy include patients with polycystic ovary syndrome (see WARNINGS: Ovarian Hyperstimulation Syndrome), amenorrhea-galactorrhea syndrome, psychogenic amenorrhea, post-oral-contraceptive amenorrhea, and certain cases of secondary amenorrhea of undetermined etiology.

Properly timed coitus in relationship to ovulation is important. A basal body temperature graph or other appropriate tests may help the patient and her physician determine if ovulation occurred. Once ovulation has been established, each course of CLOMID should be started on or about the 5th day of the cycle. Long-term cyclic therapy is not recommended beyond a total of about six cycles (including three ovulatory cycles). See DOSAGE AND ADMINISTRATION and PRECAUTIONS.)

CLOMID is indicated only in patients with demonstrated ovulatory dysfunction who meet the conditions described below (see CONTRAINDICATIONS):

1. Patients who are not pregnant.
2. Patients without ovarian cysts. CLOMID should not be used in patients with ovarian enlargement except those with polycystic ovary syndrome. Pelvic examination is necessary prior to the first and each subsequent course of CLOMID treatment.
3. Patients without abnormal vaginal bleeding. If abnormal vaginal bleeding is present, the patient should be carefully evaluated to ensure that neoplastic lesions are not present.
4. Patients with normal liver function.

In addition, patients selected for CLOMID therapy should be evaluated in regard to the following:

1. **Estrogen Levels.** Patients should have adequate levels of endogenous estrogen (as estimated from vaginal smears, endometrial biopsy, assay of urinary estrogen, or from bleeding in response to progesterone). Reduced estrogen levels, while less favorable, do not preclude successful therapy.
2. **Primary Pituitary or Ovarian Failure.** CLOMID therapy cannot be expected to substitute for specific treatment of other causes of ovulatory failure.
3. **Endometriosis and Endometrial Carcinoma.** The incidence of endometriosis and endometrial carcinoma increases with age as does the incidence of ovulatory disorders. Endometrial biopsy should always be performed prior to CLOMID therapy in this population.
4. **Other Impediments to Pregnancy.** Impediments to pregnancy can include thyroid disorders, adrenal disorders, hyperprolactinemia, and male factor infertility.
5. **Uterine Fibroids.** Caution should be exercised when using CLOMID in patients with uterine fibroids due to the potential for further enlargement of the fibroids.

There are no adequate or well-controlled studies that demonstrate the effectiveness of CLOMID in the treatment of male infertility. In addition, testicular tumors and gynecomastia have been reported in males using clomiphene. The cause and effect relationship between reports of testicular tumors and the administration of CLOMID is not known.

Although the medical literature suggests various methods, there is no universally accepted standard regimen for combined therapy (ie, CLOMID in conjunction with other ovulation-inducing drugs). Similarly, there is no standard CLOMID regimen for ovulation-induction in *in vitro* fertilization programs to produce ova for fertilization and reintroduction. Therefore, CLOMID is not recommended for these uses.

CONTRAINDICATIONS

Hypersensitivity

CLOMID is contraindicated in patients with a known hypersensitivity or allergy to clomiphene citrate or to any of its ingredients.

Pregnancy

CLOMID should not be administered during pregnancy. CLOMID may cause fetal harm in animals (see Animal Fetotoxicity). Although no causative evidence of a deleterious effect of CLOMID therapy on the human fetus has been established, there have been reports of birth anomalies which, during clinical studies, occurred at an incidence within the range reported for the general population (see Fetal/Neonatal Anomalies and Mortality; ADVERSE REACTIONS).

To avoid inadvertent CLOMID administration during early pregnancy, appropriate tests should be utilized during each treatment cycle to determine whether ovulation occurs. The patient should be evaluated carefully to exclude pregnancy, ovarian enlargement, or ovarian cyst formation between each treatment cycle. The next course of CLOMID therapy should be delayed until these conditions have been excluded.

Fetal/Neonatal Anomalies and Mortality. The following fetal abnormalities have been reported subsequent to pregnancies following ovulation induction therapy with CLOMID during clinical trials. Each of the following fetal abnormalities were reported at a rate of <1% (experiences are listed in order of decreasing frequency): Congenital heart lesions, Down syndrome, club foot, congenital gut lesions, hypospadias, microcephaly, harelip and cleft palate, congenital hip, hemangioma, undescended testicles, polydactyly, conjoined twins and teratomatous malformation, patent ductus arteriosus, amaurosis, arteriovenous fistula, inguinal hernia, umbilical hernia, syndactyly, pectus excavatum, myopathy, dermoid cyst of scalp, omphalocele, spina bifida occulta, ichthyosis, and persistent lingual frenulum. Neonatal death and fetal death/stillbirth in infants with birth defects have also been reported at a rate of <1%. The overall incidence of reported birth anomalies from pregnancies associated with maternal CLOMID ingestion during clinical studies was within the range of that reported for the general population.

In addition, reports of birth anomalies have been received during postmarketing surveillance of CLOMID (see ADVERSE REACTIONS).

Animal Fetotoxicity. Oral administration of clomiphene citrate to pregnant rats during organogenesis at doses of 1 to 2 mg/kg/day resulted in hydramnion and weak, edematous fetuses with wavy ribs and other temporary bone changes. Doses of 8 mg/kg/day or more also caused increased resorptions and dead fetuses, dystocia, and delayed parturition,

Continued on next page

Clomid—Cont.

and 40 mg/kg/day resulted in increased maternal mortality. Single doses of 50 mg/kg caused fetal cataracts, while 200 mg/kg caused cleft palate.
Following injection of clomiphene citrate 2 mg/kg to mice and rats during pregnancy, the offspring exhibited metaplastic changes of the reproduction tract. Newborn mice and rats injected during the first few days of life also developed metaplastic changes in uterine and vaginal mucosa, as well as premature vaginal opening and anovulatory ovaries. These findings are similar to the abnormal reproductive behavior and sterility described with other estrogens and antiestrogens.
In rabbits, some temporary bone alterations were seen in fetuses from dams given oral doses of 20 or 40 mg/kg/day during pregnancy, but not following 8 mg/kg/day. No permanent malformations were observed in those studies. Also, rhesus monkeys given oral doses of 1.5 to 4.5 mg/kg/day for various periods during pregnancy did not have any abnormal offspring.
Liver Disease. CLOMID therapy is contraindicated in patients with liver disease or a history of liver dysfunction (see also INDICATIONS AND USAGE and ADVERSE REACTIONS).
Abnormal Uterine Bleeding. CLOMID is contraindicated in patients with abnormal uterine bleeding of undetermined origin (see INDICATIONS AND USAGE).
Ovarian Cysts. CLOMID is contraindicated in patients with ovarian cysts or enlargement not due to polycystic ovarian syndrome (see INDICATIONS AND USAGE and WARNINGS).
Other. CLOMID is contraindicated in patients with uncontrolled thyroid or adrenal dysfunction or in the presence of an organic intracranial lesion such as pituitary tumor (see INDICATIONS AND USAGE).

WARNINGS

Visual Symptoms
Patients should be advised that blurring or other visual symptoms such as spots or flashes (scintillating scotomata) may occasionally occur during therapy with CLOMID. These visual symptoms increase in incidence with increasing total dose or therapy duration and generally disappear within a few days or weeks after CLOMID is discontinued. Patients should be warned that these visual symptoms may render such activities as driving a car or operating machinery more hazardous than usual, particularly under conditions of variable lighting.
These visual symptoms appear to be due to intensification and prolongation of afterimages. Symptoms often first appear or are accentuated with exposure to a brightly lit environment. While measured visual acuity usually has not been affected, a study patient taking 200 mg CLOMID daily developed visual blurring on the 7th day of treatment, which progressed to severe diminution of visual acuity by the 10th day. No other abnormaltiy was found, and the visual acuity returned to normal on the 3rd day after treatment was stopped.
Ophthalmologically definable scotomata and retinal cell function (electroretinographic) changes have also been reported. A patient treated during clinical studies developed phosphenes and scotomata during prolonged CLOMID administration, which disappeared by the 32nd day after stopping therapy.
Postmarketing surveillance of adverse events has also revealed other visual signs and symptoms during CLOMID therapy (see ADVERSE REACTIONS).
While the etiology of these visual symptoms is not yet understood, patients with any visual symptoms should discontinue treatment and have a complete ophthalmological evaluation carried out promptly.

Ovarian Hyperstimulation Syndrome
The ovarian hyperstimulation syndrome (OHSS) has been reported to occur in patients receiving clomiphene citrate therapy for ovulation induction. In some cases, OHSS occurred following cyclic use of clomiphene citrate therapy or when clomiphene citrate was used in combination with gonadotropins. Transient liver function test abnormalities suggestive of hepatic dysfunction, which may be accompanied by morphologic changes on liver biopsy, have been reported in association with ovarian hyperstimulation syndrome (OHSS).
OHSS is a medical event distinct from uncomplicated ovarian enlargement. The clinical signs of this syndrome in severe cases can include gross ovarian enlargement, gastrointestinal symptoms, ascites, dyspnea, oliguria, and pleural effusion. In addition, the following symptoms have been reported in association with this syndrome: pericardial effusion, anasarca, hydrothorax, acute abdomen, hypotension, renal failure, pulmonary edema, intraperitoneal and ovarian hemorrhage, deep venous thrombosis, torsion of the ovary, and acute respiratory distress. The early warning signs of OHSS are abdominal pain and distention, nausea, vomiting, diarrhea, and weight gain. Elevated urinary steroid levels, varying degrees of electrolyte imbalance, hypovolemia, hemoconcentration, and hypoproteinemia may occur. Death due to hypovolemic shock, hemoconcentration, or thromboembolism has occurred. Due to fragility of enlarged ovaries in severe cases, abdominal and pelvic examination should be performed very cautiously. If conception results, rapid progression to the severe form of the syndrome may occur.
To minimize the hazard associated with occasional abnormal ovarian enlargement associated with CLOMID therapy, the lowest dose consistent with expected clinical results should be used. Maximal enlargement of the ovary, whether physiologic or abnormal, may not occur until several days after discontinuation of the recommended dose of CLOMID. Some patients with polycystic ovary syndrome who are unusually sensitive to gonadotropin may have an exaggerated response to usual doses of CLOMID. Therefore, patients with polycystic ovary syndrome should be started on the lowest recommended dose and shortest treatment duration for the first course of therapy (see DOSAGE AND ADMINISTRATION).
If enlargement of the ovary occurs, additional CLOMID therapy should not be given until the ovaries have returned to pretreatment size, and the dosage or duration of the next course should be reduced. Ovarian enlargement and cyst formation associated with CLOMID therapy usually regress spontaneously within a few days or weeks after discontinuing treatment. The potential benefit of subsequent CLOMID therapy in these cases should exceed the risk. Unless surgical indication for laparotomy exists, such cystic enlargement should always be managed conservatively.
A causal relationship between ovarian hyperstimulation and ovarian cancer has not been determined. However, because a correlation between ovarian cancer and nulliparity, infertility, and age has been suggested, if ovarian cysts do not regress spontaneously, a thorough evaluation should be performed to rule out the presence of ovarian neoplasia.

PRECAUTIONS

General
Careful attention should be given to the selection of candidates for CLOMID therapy. Pelvic examination is necessary prior to CLOMID treatment and before each subsequent course (see CONTRAINDICATIONS and WARNINGS).

Information for Patients
The purpose and risks of CLOMID therapy should be presented to the patient before starting treatment. It should be emphasized that the goal of CLOMID therapy is ovulation for subsequent pregnancy. The physician should counsel the patient with special regard to the following potential risks:
Visual Symptoms: Advise that blurring or other visual symptoms occasionally may occur during or shortly after CLOMID therapy. Warn that visual symptoms may render such activities as driving a car or operating machinery more hazardous than usual, particularly under conditions of variable lighting (see WARNINGS).
The patient should be instructed to inform the physician whenever any unusual visual symptoms occur. If the patient has any visual symptoms, treatment should be discontinued and complete ophthalmologic evaluation performed.
Abdominal/Pelvic Pain or Distention: Ovarian enlargement may occur during or shortly after therapy with CLOMID. To minimize the risks associated with ovarian enlargement, the patient should be instructed to inform the physician of any abdominal or pelvic pain, weight gain, discomfort, or distention after taking CLOMID (see WARNINGS).
Multiple Pregnancy: Inform the patient that there is an increased chance of multiple pregnancy, including bilateral tubal pregnancy and coexisting tubal and intrauterine pregnancy, when conception occurs in relation to CLOMID therapy. The potential complications and hazards of multiple pregnancy should be explained.
Pregnancy Wastage and Birth Anomalies: The physician should explain the assumed risk of any pregnancy, whether ovulation is induced with the aid of CLOMID or occurs naturally. The patient should be informed of the greater risks associated with certain characteristics or conditions of any pregnant woman, eg, age of female and male partner, history of spontaneous abortions, Rh genotype, abnormal menstrual history, infertility history, organic heart disease, diabetes, exposure to infectious agents such as rubella, familial history of birth anomaly, that may be pertinent to the patient for whom CLOMID is being considered. Based upon the evaluation of the patient, genetic counseling may be indicated.
The overall incidence of reported birth anomalies from pregnancies associated with maternal CLOMID ingestion during the investigational studies was within the range of that reported in published references for the general population. (See CONTRAINDICATIONS: Pregnancy.)
During clinical investigation, the experience from patients with known pregnancy outcome (Table 1) shows a spontaneous abortion rate of 20.4% and stillbirth rate of 1.0%. (See CLINICAL PHARMACOLOGY.)

Drug Interactions
Drug interactions with CLOMID have not been documented.

Carcinogenesis, Mutagenesis, Impairment of Fertility
Long-term toxicity studies in animals have not been performed to evaluate the carcinogenic or mutagenic potential of clomiphene citrate.
Oral administration of CLOMID to male rats at doses of 0.3 or 1 mg/kg/day caused decreased fertility, while higher doses caused temporary infertility. Oral doses of 0.1 mg/kg/day in female rats temporarily interrupted the normal cyclic vaginal smear pattern and prevented conception. Doses of 0.3 mg/kg/day slightly reduced the number of ovulated ova and corpora lutea, while 3 mg/kg/day inhibited ovulation.

Pregnancy
Pregnancy Category X. (See CONTRAINDICATIONS).

Nursing Mothers
It is not known whether CLOMID is excreted in human milk. Because many drugs are excreted in human milk, caution should be exercised if CLOMID is administered to a nursing woman. In some patients, CLOMID may reduce lactation.

Ovarian Cancer
Prolonged use of clomiphene citrate tablets USP may increase the risk of a borderline or invasive ovarian tumor (see ADVERSE REACTIONS).

ADVERSE REACTIONS

Clinical Trial Adverse Events. CLOMID, at recommended dosages, is generally well tolerated. Adverse reactions usually have been mild and transient and most have disappeared promptly after treatment has been discontinued. Adverse experiences reported in patients treated with clomiphene citrate during clinical studies are shown in Table 2.

Table 2. Incidence of Adverse Events In Clinical Studies (Events Greater than 1%) (n = 8029*)

Adverse Event	%
Ovarian Enlargement	13.6
Vasomotor Flushes	10.4
Abdominal-Pelvic Discomfort/ Distention/Bloating	5.5
Nausea and Vomiting	2.2
Breast Discomfort	2.1
Visual Symptoms Blurred vision, lights, floaters, waves, unspecified visual complaints, photophobia, diplopia, scotomata, phosphenes	1.5
Headache	1.3
Abnormal Uterine Bleeding Intermenstrual spotting, menorrhagia	1.3

* Includes 498 patients whose reports may have been duplicated in the event totals and could not be distinguished as such. Also, excludes 47 patients who did not report symptom data.

The following adverse events have been reported in fewer than 1% of patients in clinical trials: Acute abdomen, appetite increase, constipation, dermatitis or rash, depression, diarrhea, dizziness, fatigue, hair loss/dry hair, increased urinary frequency/volume, insomnia, light-headedness, nervous tension, vaginal dryness, vertigo, weight gain/loss.
Patients on prolonged CLOMID therapy may show elevated serum levels of desmosterol. This is most likely due to a direct interference with cholesterol synthesis. However, the serum sterols in patients receiving the recommended dose of CLOMID are not significantly altered. Ovarian cancer has been infrequently reported in patients who have received fertility drugs. Infertility is a primary risk factor for ovarian cancer; however, epidemiology data suggest that prolonged use of clomiphene may increase the risk of a borderline or invasive ovarian tumor.

Postmarketing Adverse Events
The following adverse experiences were reported spontaneously with CLOMID: The cause and effect relationship of the listed events to the administration of CLOMID is not known.
Dermatologic: Acne, allergic reaction, erythema, erythema multiforme, erythema nodosum, hypertrichosis, pruritus
Central Nervous System: Migraine headache, paresthesia, seizure, stroke, syncope
Psychiatric: Anxiety, irritability, mood changes, psychosis
Visual Disorders: Abnormal accommodation, cataract, eye pain, macular edema, optic neuritis, photopsia, posterior vitreous detachment, retinal hemorrhage, retinal thrombosis, retinal vascular spasm, temporary loss of vision
Cardiovascular: Arrhythmia, chest pain, edema, hypertension, palpitation, phlebitis, pulmonary embolism, shortness of breath, tachycardia, thrombophlebitis
Musculoskeletal: Arthralgia, back pain, myalgia

Hepatic: Transaminases increased, hepatitis
Neoplasms: Liver (hepatic hemangiosarcoma, liver cell adenoma, hepatocellular carcinoma); breast (fibrocystic disease, breast carcinoma); endometrium (endometrial carcinoma); nervous system (astrocytoma, pituitary tumor, prolactinoma, neurofibromatosis, glioblastoma, multiforme, brain abcess); ovary (luteoma of pregnancy, dermoid cyst of the ovary, ovarian carcinoma); trophoblastic (hydatiform mole, choriocarcinoma); miscellaneous (melanoma, myeloma, perianal cysts, renal cell carcinoma, Hodgkin's lymphoma, tongue carcinoma, bladder carcinoma); and neoplasms of offspring (neuroectodermal tumor, thyroid tumor, hepatoblastoma, lymphocytic leukemia)
Genitourinary: Endometriosis, ovarian cyst (ovarian enlargement or cysts could, as such, be complicated by adnexal torsion), ovarian hemorrhage, tubal pregnancy, uterine hemorrhage
Body as a Whole: Fever, tinnitus, weakness
Other: Leukocytosis, thyroid disorder
Fetal/Neonatal anomalies. The following fetal abnormalities have also been reported during postmarketing surveillance: delayed development; abnormal bone development including skeletal malformations of the skull, face, nasal passages, jaw, hand, limb (ectromelia including amelia, hemimelia, and phocomelia); foot, and joints; tissue malformations including imperforate anus, tracheoesophageal fistula, diaphragmatic hernia, renal agenesis and dysgenesis, and malformations of the eye and lens (cataract), ear, lung, heart (ventricular septal defect and tetralogy of Fallot), and genitalia; as well as dwarfism, deafness, mental retardation, chromosomal disorders, and neural tube defects (including anencephaly).

DRUG ABUSE AND DEPENDENCE

Tolerance, abuse, or dependence with CLOMID has not been reported.

OVERDOSAGE

Signs and Symptoms

Toxic effects accompanying acute overdosage of CLOMID have not been reported. Signs and symptoms of overdosage as a result of the use of more than the recommended dose during CLOMID therapy include nausea, vomiting, vasomotor flushes, visual blurring, spots or flashes, scotomata, ovarian enlargement with pelvic or abdominal pain. (See CONTRAINDICATIONS: Ovarian Cyst.)

Oral LD_{50}. The acute oral LD_{50} of CLOMID is 1700 mg/kg in mice and 5750 mg/kg in rats. The toxic dose in humans is not known.

Dialysis: It is not known if CLOMID is dialyzable.

Treatment

In the event of overdose, appropriate supportive measures should be employed in addition to gastrointestinal decontamination.

DOSAGE AND ADMINISTRATION

General Considerations

The workup and treatment of candidates for CLOMID therapy should be supervised by physicians experienced in management of gynecologic or endocrine disorders. Patients should be chosen for therapy with CLOMID only after careful diagnostic evaluation (see INDICATIONS AND USAGE). The plan of therapy should be outlined in advance. Impediments to achieving the goal of therapy must be excluded or adequately treated before beginning CLOMID. The therapeutic objective should be balanced with potential risks and discussed with the patient and others involved in the achievement of a pregnancy.

Ovulation most often occurs from 5 to 10 days after a course of CLOMID. Coitus should be timed to coincide with the expected time of ovulation. Appropriate tests to determine ovulation may be useful during this time.

Recommended Dosage

Treatment of the selected patient should begin with a low dose, 50 mg daily (1 tablet) for 5 days. The dose should be increased only in those patients who do not ovulate in response to cyclic 50 mg CLOMID. A low dosage or duration of treatment course is particularly recommended if unusual sensitivity to pituitary gonadotropin is suspected, such as in patients with polycystic ovary syndrome (see WARNINGS: Ovarian Hyperstimulation Syndrome).

The patient should be evaluated carefully to exclude pregnancy, ovarian enlargement, or ovarian cyst formation between each treatment cycle.

If progestin-induced bleeding is planned, or if spontaneous uterine bleeding occurs prior to therapy, the regimen of 50 mg daily for 5 days should be started on or about the 5th day of the cycle. Therapy may be started at any time in the patient who has had no recent uterine bleeding. when ovulation occurs at this dosage, there is no advantage to increasing the dose in subsequent cycles of treatment. If ovulation does not appear to occur after the first course of therapy, a second course of 100 mg daily (two 50 mg tablets given as a single daily dose) for 5 days should be given. This course may be started as early as 30 days after the previous one after precautions are taken to exclude the presence of pregnancy. Increasing the dosage or duration of therapy beyond 100 mg/day for 5 days is not recommended.

The majority of patients who are going to ovulate will do so after the first course of therapy. If ovulation does not occur after three courses of therapy, further treatment with CLOMID is not recommended and the patient should be reevaluated. If three ovulatory responses occur, but pregnancy has not been achieved, further treatment is not recommended. If menses does not occur after an ovulatory response, the patient should be reevaluated. Long-term cyclic therapy is not recommended beyond a total of about six cycles (see PRECAUTIONS).

HOW SUPPLIED

NDC 0068-0226-30: 50 mg tablets in cartons of 30
Tablets are round, white, scored, and debossed CLOMID 50.
Store tablets at controlled room temperature 59–86°F (15–30°C).
Protect from heat, light, and excessive humidity, and store in closed containers.
Prescribing Information as of February 1996
Merrell Pharmaceuticals Inc.
Subsidiary of Hoechst Marion Roussel, Inc.
Kansas City, MO 64137 USA

Shown in Product Identification Guide, page 316

DIAβETA® ℞

[dī ″ə-bū ′ta]
(glyburide)
Tablets 1.25, 2.5 and 5 mg
Prescribing Information as of November 1996

DESCRIPTION

Diaβeta® (glyburide) is an oral blood-glucose-lowering drug of the sulfonylurea class. It is a white, crystalline compound, formulated as tablets of 1.25 mg, 2.5 mg, and 5 mg strengths for oral administration. Diaβeta® tablets contain the active ingredient glyburide and the following inactive ingredients: dibasic calcium phosphate USP, magnesium stearate NF, microcrystalline cellulose NF, sodium alginate NF, talc USP. Diaβeta® 1.25 mg tablets also contain D&C Yellow #10 Aluminum Lake and FD&C Red #40 Aluminum Lake. Diaβeta® 2.5 mg tablets also contain FD&C Red #40 Aluminum Lake. Diaβeta® 5 mg tablets also contain D&C Yellow #10 Aluminum Lake, and FD&C Blue #1. Chemically, Diaβeta® is identified as 1-[[p-[2-(5-Chloro-*o*-anisamido)ethyl]phenyl]sulfonyl]-3-cyclohexylurea.

The CAS Registry Number is 10238-21-8.

The structural formula is:

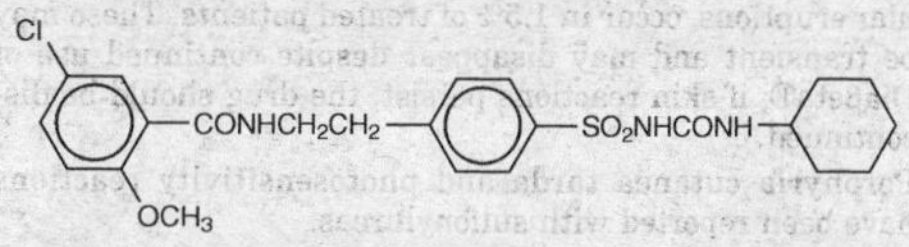

The molecular weight is 493.99. The aqueous solubility of Diaβeta® increases with pH as a result of salt formation.

CLINICAL PHARMACOLOGY

Diaβeta® appears to lower the blood glucose acutely by stimulating the release of insulin from the pancreas, an effect dependent upon functioning beta cells in the pancreatic islets. The mechanism by which Diaβeta® lowers blood glucose during long-term administration has not been clearly established.

With chronic administration in Type II diabetic patients, the blood glucose lowering effect persists despite a gradual decline in the insulin secretory response to the drug. Extrapancreatic effects may play a part in the mechanism of action of oral sulfonylurea hypoglycemic drugs.

In addition to its blood glucose lowering actions, Diaβeta® produces a mild diuresis by enhancement of renal free water clearance. Clinical experience to date indicates an extremely low incidence of disulfiram-like reactions in patients while taking Diaβeta®.

Pharmacokinetics

Single-dose studies with Diaβeta® in normal subjects demonstrate significant absorption within one hour, peak drug levels at about four hours, and low but detectable levels at twenty-four hours. Mean serum levels of glyburide, as reflected by areas under the serum concentration-time curve, increase in proportion to corresponding increases in dose. Multiple-dose studies with Diaβeta® in diabetic patients demonstrate drug level concentration-time curves similar to single-dose studies, indicating no build-up of drug in tissue depots. The decrease of glyburide in the serum of normal healthy individuals is biphasic, the terminal half-life being about 10 hours. In single-dose studies in fasting normal subjects, the degree and duration of blood glucose lowering is proportional to the dose administered and to the area under the drug level concentration-time curve. The blood glucose lowering effect persists for 24 hours following single morning doses in non-fasting diabetic patients. Under conditions of repeated administration in diabetic patients, however, there is no reliable correlation between blood drug levels and fasting blood glucose levels. A one-year study of diabetic patients treated with Diaβeta® showed no reliable correlation between administered dose and serum drug level.

The major metabolite of Diaβeta® is the 4-trans-hydroxy derivative. A second metabolite, the 3-cis-hydroxy derivative, also occurs. These metabolites contribute no significant hypoglycemic action since they are only weakly active (1/400th and 1/40th, respectively, as glyburide) in rabbits.

Diaβeta® is excreted as metabolites in the bile and urine, approximately 50% by each route. This dual excretory pathway is qualitatively different from that of other sulfonylureas, which are excreted primarily in the urine.

Sulfonylurea drugs are extensively bound to serum proteins. Displacement from protein binding sites by other drugs may lead to enhanced hypoglycemic action. *In vitro*, the protein binding exhibited by Diaβeta® is predominantly non-ionic, whereas that of other sulfonylureas (chlorpropamide, tolbutamide, tolazamide) is predominantly ionic. Acidic drugs such as phenylbutazone, warfarin, and salicylates displace the ionic-binding sulfonylureas from serum proteins to a far greater extent than the non-ionic binding Diaβeta®. It has not been shown that this difference in protein binding will result in fewer drug-drug interactions with Diaβeta® in clinical use.

INDICATIONS AND USAGE

Diaβeta® is indicated as an adjunct to diet to lower the blood glucose in patients with non-insulin-dependent diabetes mellitus (Type II) whose hyperglycemia cannot be controlled by diet alone.

In initiating treatment for non-insulin-dependent diabetes, diet should be emphasized as the primary form of treatment. Caloric restriction and weight loss are essential in the obese diabetic patient. Proper dietary management alone may be effective in controlling the blood glucose and symptoms of hyperglycemia. The importance of regular physical activity should also be stressed, and cardiovascular risk factors should be identified and corrective measures taken where possible.

If this treatment program fails to reduce symptoms and/or blood glucose, the use of an oral sulfonylurea or insulin should be considered. Use of Diaβeta® must be viewed by both the physician and patient as a treatment in addition to diet, and not as a substitute for diet or as a convenient mechanism for avoiding dietary restraint. Furthermore, loss of blood glucose control on diet alone may be transient, thus requiring only short-term administration of Diaβeta®.

During maintenance programs, Diaβeta® should be discontinued if satisfactory lowering of blood glucose is no longer achieved. Judgments should be based on regular clinical and laboratory evaluations.

In considering the use of Diaβeta® in asymptomatic patients, it should be recognized that controlling the blood glucose in non-insulin dependent diabetes has not been definitely established to be effective in preventing the long-term cardiovascular or neural complications of diabetes.

CONTRAINDICATIONS

Diaβeta® is contraindicated in patients with:

1. Known hypersensitivity to the drug.
2. Diabetic ketoacidosis, with or without coma.
   This condition should be treated with insulin.

WARNINGS

SPECIAL WARNING ON INCREASED RISK OF CARDIOVASCULAR MORTALITY

The administration of oral hypoglycemic drugs has been reported to be associated with increased cardiovascular mortality as compared to treatment with diet alone or diet plus insulin. This warning is based on the study conducted by the University Group Diabetes Program (UGDP), a long-term prospective clinical trial designed to evaluate the effectiveness of glucose-lowering drugs in preventing or delaying vascular complications in patients with non-insulin-dependent diabetes. The study involved 823 patients who were randomly assigned to one of four treatment groups (Diabetes 19 (supp. 2): 747-830, 1970).

UGDP reported that patients treated for 5 to 8 years with diet plus a fixed dose of tolbutamide (1.5 grams per day) had a rate of cardiovascular mortality approximately 2-½ times that of patients treated with diet alone. A significant increase in total mortality was not observed, but the use of tolbutamide was discontinued based on the increase in cardiovascular mortality, thus limiting the opportunity for the study to show an increase in overall mortality. Despite controversy regarding the interpretation of these results, the findings of the UGDP study provide an adequate basis for this warning. The patient should be informed of the potential risks and advantages of Diaβeta® and of alternative modes of therapy.

Although only one drug in the sulfonylurea class (tolbutamide) was included in this study, it is prudent from a safety standpoint to consider that this warning may also apply to

Continued on next page

DiaBeta—Cont.

other oral hypoglycemic drugs in this class, in view of their close similarities in mode of action and chemical structure.

PRECAUTIONS

General

Hypoglycemia: All sulfonylurea drugs are capable of producing severe hypoglycemia. Proper patient selection, dosage, and instructions are important to avoid hypoglycemic episodes. Renal or hepatic insufficiency may cause elevated blood levels of Diaβeta® and the latter may also diminish gluconeogenic capacity, both of which increase the risk of serious hypoglycemic reactions. Elderly, debilitated or malnourished patients, and those with adrenal or pituitary insufficiency are particularly susceptible to the hypoglycemic action of glucose-lowering drugs. Hypoglycemia may be difficult to recognize in the elderly, and in people who are taking beta-adrenergic blocking drugs or other sympatholytic agents. Hypoglycemia is more likely to occur when caloric intake is deficient, after severe or prolonged exercise, when alcohol is ingested, or when more than one glucose-lowering drug is used. Loss of control of blood glucose: When a patient stabilized on any diabetic regimen is exposed to stress such as fever, trauma, infection, or surgery, a loss of control may occur. At such times, it may be necessary to discontinue Diaβeta® and administer insulin.

The effectiveness of any oral hypoglycemic drug, including Diaβeta®, in lowering blood glucose to a desired level decreases in many patients over a period of time, which may be due to progression of the severity of the diabetes or to diminished responsiveness to the drug. This phenomenon is known as secondary failure, to distinguish it from primary failure in which the drug is ineffective in an individual patient when first given.

Information for Patients

Patients should be informed of the potential risks and advantages of Diaβeta® and of alternative modes of therapy. They should also be informed about the importance of adherence to dietary instructions, of a regular exercise program, and of regular testing of blood glucose.

The risks of hypoglycemia, its symptoms and treatment, and conditions that predispose to its development should be explained to patients and responsible family members. Primary and secondary failure should also be explained.

Laboratory Tests

Periodic fasting blood glucose measurements should be performed to monitor therapeutic response. A glycosylated hemoglobin determination should also be performed periodically.

Drug Interactions

The hypoglycemic action of sulfonylureas may be potentiated by certain drugs including nonsteroidal anti-inflammatory agents and other drugs that are highly protein bound, salicylates, sulfonamides, chloramphenicol, probenecid, monoamine oxidase inhibitors and beta adrenergic blocking agents. When such drugs are administered to a patient receiving Diaβeta®, the patient should be observed closely for hypoglycemia. When such drugs are withdrawn from a patient receiving Diaβeta®, the patient should be observed closely for loss of control.

A possible interaction between glyburide and fluoroquinolone antibiotics has been reported resulting in a potentiation of the hypoglycemic action of glyburide. The mechanism for this interaction is not known.

Possible interactions between glyburide and coumarin derivatives have been reported that may either potentiate or weaken the effects of coumarin derivatives. The mechanism of these interactions is not known.

Certain drugs tend to produce hyperglycemia and may lead to loss of control. These drugs include the thiazides and other diuretics, corticosteroids, phenothiazines, thyroid products, estrogens, oral contraceptives, phenytoin, nicotinic acid, sympathomimetics, calcium channel blocking drugs, and isoniazid. When such drugs are administered to a patient receiving Diaβeta®, the patient should be closely observed for loss of control. When such drugs are withdrawn from a patient receiving Diaβeta®, the patient should be observed closely for hypoglycemia. A potential interaction between oral miconazole and oral hypoglycemic agents leading to severe hypoglycemia has been reported. Whether this interaction also occurs with the intravenous, topical or vaginal preparations of miconazole is not known.

Carcinogenesis, Mutagenesis, and Impairment of Fertility

Diaβeta® is non-mutagenic when studied in the Salmonella microsome test (Ames test) and in the DNA damage/alkaline elution assay. Studies in rats at doses up to 300 mg/kg/day for 18 months showed no carcinogenic effects.

No drug related effects were noted in any of the criteria evaluated in the two year oncogenicity study of glyburide in mice.

Pregnancy

Teratogenic Effects: Pregnancy Category C

Diaβeta® has been shown to effect the maturation of the long bones (humerus and femur) in rat pups when given in doses 6250 times the maximum recommended human dose. These effects, which were seen during the period of lactation and not during organogenesis, are a shortening of the bones with effects to various structures of the long bones, especially in humerus and femur.

There are no adequate and well-controlled studies in pregnant women. Because animal reproduction studies are not always predictive of human response, Diaβeta® should be used during pregnancy only if the potential benefit justifies the risk to the fetus. Because recent information suggests that abnormal blood glucose levels during pregnancy are associated with a higher incidence of congenital abnormalities, many experts recommend that insulin be used during pregnancy to maintain blood glucose levels as close to normal as possible.

Nonteratogenic Effects: Prolonged severe hypoglycemia (4 to 10 days) has been reported in neonates born to mothers who were receiving a sulfonylurea drug at the time of delivery. This has been reported more frequently with the use of agents with prolonged half-lives. If Diaβeta® is used during pregnancy, it should be discontinued at least two weeks before the expected delivery date.

Nursing Mothers

Although it is not known whether Diaβeta® (glyburide) is excreted in human milk, some sulfonylureas are known to be excreted in human milk. Because of the potential for hypoglycemia in nursing infants may exist, a decision should be made whether to discontinue nursing or to discontinue administering the drug, taking into account the importance of the drug to the mother. If Diaβeta® is discontinued and if diet alone is inadequate for controlling blood glucose, insulin therapy should be considered.

PEDIATRIC USE

Safety and effectiveness in pediatric patients have not been established.

ADVERSE REACTIONS

Hypoglycemia: See PRECAUTIONS and OVERDOSAGE Sections.

Gastrointestinal Reactions: Cholestatic jaundice and hepatitis may occur rarely; Diaβeta® should be discontinued if this occurs. Liver function abnormalities, including isolated transaminase elevations, have been reported. Gastrointestinal disturbances, e.g., nausea, epigastric fullness, and heartburn, are the most common reactions and occur in 1.8% of treated patients. They tend to be dose-related and may disappear when dosage is reduced.

Dermatologic Reactions: Allergic skin reactions, e.g., pruritus, erythema, urticaria, and morbilliform or maculopapular eruptions, occur in 1.5% of treated patients. These may be transient and may disappear despite continued use of Diaβeta®; if skin reactions persist, the drug should be discontinued.

Porphyria cutanea tarda and photosensitivity reactions have been reported with sulfonylureas.

Hematologic Reactions: Leukopenia, agranulocytosis, thrombocytopenia, which occasionally may present as purpura, hemolytic anemia, aplastic anemia, and pancytopenia have been reported with sulfonylureas.

Metabolic Reactions: Hepatic porphyria reactions have been reported with sulfonylureas; however, these have not been reported with Diaβeta®. Disulfiram-like reactions have been reported very rarely with Diaβeta®. Cases of hyponatremia have been reported with glyburide and all other sulfonylureas, most often in patients who are on other medications or have medical conditions known to cause hyponatremia or increase release of antidiuretic hormone. The syndrome of inappropriate antidiuretic hormone (SIADH) secretion has been reported with certain other sulfonylureas, and it has been suggested that these sulfonylureas may augment the peripheral (antidiuretic) action of ADH and/or increase release of ADH.

Other Reactions: Changes in accommodation and/or blurred vision have been reported with glyburide and other sulfonylureas. These are thought to be related to fluctuation in glucose levels.

In addition to dermatologic reactions, allergic reactions such as angioedema, arthralgia, myalgia and vasculitis have been reported.

OVERDOSAGE

Overdosage of sulfonylureas, including Diaβeta®, can produce hypoglycemia. Mild hypoglycemic symptoms without loss of consciousness or neurologic findings should be treated aggressively with oral glucose and adjustments in drug dosage and/or meal patterns. Close monitoring should continue until the physician is assured that the patient is out of danger. Severe hypoglycemic reactions with coma, seizure, or other neurological impairment occur infrequently, but constitute medical emergencies requiring immediate hospitalization. If hypoglycemic coma is diagnosed or suspected, the patient should be given a rapid intravenous injection of concentrated (50%) glucose solution. This should be followed by a continuous infusion of a more dilute (10%) glucose solution at a rate that will maintain the blood glucose at a level above 100 mg/mL. Patients should be closely monitored for a minimum of 24 to 48 hours, since hypoglycemia may recur after apparent clinical recovery.

DOSAGE AND ADMINISTRATION

There is no fixed dosage regimen for the management of diabetes mellitus with Diaβeta® or any other hypoglycemic agent. The patient's fasting blood glucose must be measured periodically to determine the minimum effective dose for the patient; to detect primary failure, i.e., inadequate lowering of blood glucose at the maximum recommended dose of medication; and to detect secondary failure, i.e., loss of adequate blood glucose lowering response after an initial period of effectiveness. Periodic glycosylated hemoglobin determinations should be performed.

Short-term administration of Diaβeta® may be sufficient during periods of transient loss of control in patients usually controlled well on diet.

1. Usual Starting Dose

The usual starting dose of Diaβeta® as initial therapy is 2.5 to 5 mg daily, administered with breakfast or the first main meal. Those patients who may be more sensitive to hypoglycemic drugs should be started at 1.25 mg daily. (See PRECAUTIONS Section for patients at increased risk). Failure to follow an appropriate dosage regimen may precipitate hypoglycemia. Patients who do not adhere to their prescribed dietary and drug regimen are more prone to exhibit unsatisfactory response to therapy.

Transfer of patients from other oral antidiabetic regimens to Diaβeta® should be done conservatively and the initial daily dose should be 2.5 to 5 mg. When transferring patients from oral hypoglycemic agents other than chlorpropamide, to Diaβeta®, no transition period and no initial priming dose is necessary. When transferring patients from chlorpropamide, particular care should be exercised during the first two weeks because the prolonged retention of chlorpropamide in the body and subsequent overlapping drug effects may provoke hypoglycemia.

Bioavailability studies have demonstrated that Glynase® PresTab® Tablets 3 mg are not bioequivalent to Diaβeta® Tablets 5 mg. Therefore, these products are not substitutable and patients should be retitrated if transferred.

Some Type II diabetic patients being treated with insulin may respond satisfactorily to Diaβeta®. If the insulin dose is less than 20 units daily, substitution of Diaβeta® 2.5 to 5 mg as a single daily dose may be tried. If the insulin dose is between 20 and 40 units daily, the patient may be placed directly on Diaβeta® 5 mg daily as a single dose. If the insulin dose is more than 40 units daily, a transition period is required for conversion to Diaβeta®. In these patients, insulin dosage is decreased by 50% and Diaβeta® 5 mg daily is started. Please refer to Usual Maintenance Dose for further explanation.

2. Usual Maintenance Dose

The usual maintenance dose is in the range of 1.25 to 20 mg daily, which may be given as a single dose or in divided doses (See Dosage Interval Section). Dosage increases should be made in increments of no more than 2.5 mg at weekly intervals based upon the patient's blood glucose response.

No exact dosage relationship exists between Diaβeta® and the other oral hypoglycemic agents. Although patients may be transferred from the maximum dose of other sulfonylureas, the maximum starting dose of 5 mg of Diaβeta® should be observed. A maintenance dose of 5 mg Diaβeta® provides approximately the same degree of blood glucose control as 250 to 375 mg chlorpropamide, 250 to 375 mg tolazamide, 500 to 750 mg acetohexamide, or 1000 to 1500 mg tolbutamide.

When transferring patients receiving more than 40 units of insulin daily, they may be started on a daily dose of Diaβeta® 5 mg concomitantly with a 50% reduction in insulin dose. Progressive withdrawal of insulin and increase of Diaβeta® in increments of 1.25 to 2.5 mg every 2 to 10 days is then carried out. During this conversion period when both insulin and Diaβeta® are being used, hypoglycemia may rarely occur. During insulin withdrawal, patients should self-test their blood for glucose and their urine for acetone at least 3 times daily and report results to their physician. Self-testing of urinary glucose is a less desirable alternative. The appearance of persistent acetonuria with glycosuria indicates that the patient is a Type I diabetic who requires insulin therapy.

3. Maximum Dose

Daily doses of more than 20 mg are not recommended.

4. Dosage Interval

Once-a-day therapy is usually satisfactory, based upon usual meal patterns and a 10 hour half-life of Diaβeta®. Some patients, particularly those receiving more than 10 mg daily, may have a more satisfactory response with twice-a-day dosage.

In elderly patients, debilitated or malnourished patients, and patients with impaired renal or hepatic function, the initial and maintenance dosing should be conservative to avoid hypoglycemic reactions. (See PRECAUTIONS Section.)

HOW SUPPLIED

Diaβeta® (glyburide) tablets are available in the following strengths and package sizes:

1.25 mg (peach oblong, scored tablets with beveled edges, imprinted with "Hoechst" on one side and "Dia β" on the other side).

Bottles of 50	(NDC 0039-0053-05)

2.5 mg (pink oblong, scored tablets with beveled edges, imprinted with "Hoechst" on one side and "Dia β" on the other side).

Bottles of 100	(NDC 0039-0051-10)
Bottles of 500	(NDC 0039-0051-50)
Unit Dose Cartons of 100	(NDC 0039-0051-11)

5 mg (green oblong, scored tablets with beveled edges, imprinted with "Hoechst" on one side and "Dia β" on the other side).

Bottles of 100	(NDC 0039-0052-10)
Bottles of 500	(NDC 0039-0052-50)
Bottles of 1000	(NDC 0039-0052-70)
Unit Dose Cartons of 100	(NDC 0039-0052-11)

Store between 59 and 86° F (15° and 30° C).

Dispense in well-closed containers with safety closures.

Caution: Federal law prohibits dispensing without a prescription.

Prescribing Information as of November 1996.

Glynase and PresTab are registered trademarks of The Upjohn Company

Diaβeta REG TM HRPI

Made in USA

Hoechst-Roussel Pharmaceuticals

Division of Hoechst Marion Roussel, Inc.

Kansas City, MO 64137

Shown in Product Identification Guide, page 316

LASIX® ℞

[la ' siks]

(furosemide)

Tablets 20, 40, and 80 mg

Prescribing Information as of January 1996

WARNING

LASIX® (furosemide) is a potent diuretic which, if given in excessive amounts, can lead to a profound diuresis with water and electrolyte depletion. Therefore, careful medical supervision is required and dose and dose schedule must be adjusted to the individual patient's needs. (See "DOSAGE AND ADMINISTRATION".)

DESCRIPTION

LASIX® is a diuretic which is an anthranilic acid derivative. LASIX tablets for oral administration contain furosemide as the active ingredient and the following inactive ingredients: lactose USP, magnesium stearate NF, starch NF and talc USP. Chemically, it is 4-chloro-N-furfuryl-5-sulfamoylanthranilic acid. LASIX is available as white tablets for oral administration in dosage strengths of 20, 40, and 80 mg. Furosemide is a white to off-white odorless crystalline powder. It is practically insoluble in water, sparingly soluble in alcohol, freely soluble in dilute alkali solutions and insoluble in dilute acids.

The CAS Registry Number is 54-31-9.

The structural formula is as follows:

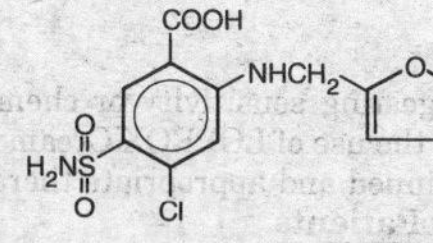

CLINICAL PHARMACOLOGY

Investigations into the mode of action of LASIX® have utilized micropuncture studies in rats, stop flow experiments in dogs and various clearance studies in both humans and experimental animals. It has been demonstrated that LASIX inhibits primarily the absorption of sodium and chloride not only in the proximal and distal tubules but also in the loop of Henle. The high degree of efficacy is largely due to the unique site of action. The action on the distal tubule is independent of any inhibitory effect on carbonic anhydrase and aldosterone.

Recent evidence suggests that furosemide glucuronide is the only or at least the major biotransformation product of furosemide in man. Furosemide is extensively bound to plasma proteins, mainly to albumin. Plasma concentrations ranging from 1 to 400 μg/mL are 91 to 99% bound in healthy individuals. The unbound fraction averages 2.3 to 4.1% at therapeutic concentrations.

The onset of diuresis following oral administration is within 1 hour. The peak effect occurs within the first or second hour. The duration of diuretic effect is 6 to 8 hours.

In fasted normal men, the mean bioavailability of furosemide from LASIX Tablets and LASIX Oral Solution is 64% and 60%, respectively, of that from an intravenous injection of the drug. Although furosemide is more rapidly absorbed from the oral solution (50 minutes) than from the tablet (87 minutes), peak plasma levels and area under the plasma concentration-time curves do not differ significantly. Peak plasma concentrations increase with increasing dose but times-to-peak do not differ among doses. The terminal half-life of furosemide is approximately 2 hours.

Significantly more furosemide is excreted in urine following the IV injection than after the tablet or oral solution. There are no significant differences between the two oral formulations in the amount of unchanged drug excreted in urine.

INDICATIONS AND USAGE

Edema

LASIX is indicated in adults, and pediatric patients for the treatment of edema associated with congestive heart failure, cirrhosis of the liver, and renal disease, including the nephrotic syndrome. LASIX is particularly useful when an agent with greater diuretic potential is desired.

Hypertension

Oral LASIX may be used in adults for the treatment of hypertension alone or in combination with other antihypertensive agents. Hypertensive patients who cannot be adequately controlled with thiazides will probably also not be adequately controlled with LASIX alone.

CONTRAINDICATIONS

LASIX® is contraindicated in patients with anuria and in patients with a history of hypersensitivity to furosemide.

WARNINGS

In patients with hepatic cirrhosis and ascites, LASIX therapy is best initiated in the hospital. In hepatic coma and in states of electrolyte depletion, therapy should not be instituted until the basic condition is improved. Sudden alterations of fluid and electrolyte balance in patients with cirrhosis may precipitate hepatic coma; therefore, strict observation is necessary during the period of diuresis. Supplemental potassium chloride and, if required, an aldosterone antagonist are helpful in preventing hypokalemia and metabolic alkalosis.

If increasing azotemia and oliguria occur during treatment of severe progressive renal disease, LASIX should be discontinued.

Cases of tinnitus and reversible or irreversible hearing impairment have been reported. Usually, reports indicate that LASIX ototoxicity is associated with rapid injection, severe renal impairment, doses exceeding several times the usual recommended dose, or concomitant therapy with aminoglycoside antibiotics, ethacrynic acid, or other ototoxic drugs. If the physician elects to use high dose parenteral therapy, controlled intravenous infusion is advisable (for adults, an infusion rate not exceeding 4 mg LASIX per minute has been used).

PRECAUTIONS

General

Excessive diuresis may cause dehydration and blood volume reduction with circulatory collapse and possibly vascular thrombosis and embolism, particularly in elderly patients. As with any effective diuretic, electrolyte depletion may occur during LASIX therapy, especially in patients receiving higher doses and a restricted salt intake. Hypokalemia may develop with LASIX, especially with brisk diuresis, inadequate oral eletrolyte intake, when cirrhosis is present, or during concomitant use of corticosteroids or ACTH. Digitalis therapy may exaggerate metabolic effects of hypokalemia, especially myocardial effects.

All patients receiving LASIX therapy should be observed for these signs or symptoms of fluid or electrolyte imbalance (hyponatremia, hypochloremic alkalosis, hypokalemia, hypomagnesemia or hypocalcemia): dryness of mouth, thirst, weakness, lethargy, drowsiness, restlessness, muscle pains or cramps, muscular fatigue, hypotension, oliguria, tachycardia, arrhythmia, or gastrointestinal disturbances such as nausea and vomiting. Increases in blood glucose and alterations in glucose tolerance tests (with abnormalities of the fasting and 2-hour postprandial sugar) have been observed, and rarely, precipitation of diabetes mellitus has been reported.

Asymptomatic hyperuricemia can occur and gout may rarely be precipitated. Patients allergic to sulfonamides may also be allergic to LASIX. The possibility exists of exacerbation or activation of systemic lupus erythematosus.

As with many other drugs, patients should be observed regularly for the possible occurrence of blood dyscrasias, liver or kidney damage, or other idiosyncratic reactions.

Information for Patients

Patients receiving LASIX should be advised that they may experience symptoms from excessive fluid and/or electrolyte losses. The postural hypotension that sometimes occurs can usually be managed by getting up slowly. Potassium supplements and/or dietary measures may be needed to control or avoid hypokalemia.

Patients with daibetes mellitus should be told that furosemide may increase blood glucose levels and thereby affect urine glucose tests. The skin of some patients may be more sensitive to the effects of sunlight while taking furosemide.

Hypertensive patients should avoid medications that may increase blood pressure, including over-the-counter products for appetite suppression and cold symptoms.

Laboratory Tests

Serum electrolytes (particularly potassium), CO_2, creatinine and BUN should be determined frequently during the first few months of LASIX therapy and periodically thereafter. Serum and urine electrolyte determinations are particularly important when the patient is vomiting profusely or receiving parenteral fluids. Abnormalities should be corrected or the drug temporarily withdrawn.

Other medications may also influence serum electrolytes.

Reversible elevations of BUN may occur and are associated with dehydration, which should be avoided, particularly in patients with renal insufficiency.

Urine and blood glucose should be checked periodically in diabetics receiving LASIX, even in those suspected of latent diabetes.

LASIX may lower serum levels of calcium (rarely cases of tetany have been reported) and magnesium. Accordingly, serum levels of these electrolytes should be determined periodically.

Drug Interactions

LASIX may increase the ototoxic potential of aminoglycoside antibiotics, especially in the presence of impaired renal function. Except in life-threatening situations, avoid this combination.

LASIX should not be used concomitantly with ethacrynic acid because of the possibility of ototoxicity. Patients receiving high doses of salicylates concomitantly with LASIX, as in rheumatic disease, may experience salicylate toxicity at lower doses because of competitive renal excretory sites.

LASIX has a tendency to antagonize the skeletal muscle relaxing effect of tubocurarine and may potentiate the action of succinylcholine.

Lithium generally should not be given with diuretics because they reduce lithium's renal clearance and add a high risk of lithium toxicity.

LASIX may add to or potentiate the therapeutic effect of other antihypertensive drugs. Potentiation occurs with ganglionic or peripheral adrenergic blocking drugs.

LASIX may decrease arterial responsiveness to norepinephrine However, norepinephrine may still be used effectively.

Simultaneous administration of sucralfate and LASIX tablets may reduce the natriuretic and antihypertensive effects of LASIX. Patients receiving both drugs should be observed closely to determine if the desired diuretic and/or antihypertensive effect of LASIX is achieved. The intake of LASIX and sucralfate should be separated by at least two hours.

One study in six subjects demonstrated that the combination of furosemide and acetylsalicylic acid temporarily reduced creatinine clearance in patients with chronic renal insufficiency. There are case reports of patients who developed increased BUN, serum creatinine and serum potassium levels, and weight gain when furosemide was used in conjunction with NSAIDs.

Literature reports indicate that coadministration of indomethacin may reduce the natriuretic and antihypertensive effects of LASIX (furosemide) in some patients by inhibiting prostaglandin synthesis. Indomethacin may also affect plasma renin levels, aldosterone excretion, and renin profile evaluation. Patients receiving both indomethacin and LASIX should be observed closely to determine if the desired diuretic and/or antihypertensive effect of LASIX is achieved.

Carcinogenesis, Mutagenesis, Impairment of Fertility

Furosemide was tested for carcinogenicity by oral administration in one strain of mice and one strain of rats. A small but significantly increased incidence of mammary gland carcinomas occurred in female mice at a dose 17.5 times the maximum human dose of 600 mg. There were marginal increases in uncommon tumors in male rats at a dose of 15 mg/kg (slightly greater than the maximum human dose) but not at 30 mg/kg.

Furosemide was devoid of mutagenic activity in various strains of *Salmonella typhimurium* when tested in the presence or absence of an *in vitro* metabolic activation system, and questionably positive for gene mutation in mouse lymphoma cells in the presence of rat liver S9 at the highest dose tested. Furosemide did not induce sister chromatid exchange in human cells *in vitro*, but other studies on chromosomal aberrations in human cells *in vitro* gave conflicting results. In Chinese hamster cells it induced chromosomal damage but was questionably positive for sister chromatic exchange. Studies on the induction by furosemide of chromosomal aberrations in mice were inconclusive. The urine of rats treated with this drug did not induce gene conversion in *Saccharomyces cerevisiae*.

LASIX produced no impairment of fertility in male or female rats, at 100 mg/kg/day (the maximum effective diuretic dose in the rate and 8 times the maximal human dose of 600 mg/day).

Continued on next page

Lasix—Cont.

Pregnancy

PREGNANCY CATEGORY C—Furosemide has been shown to cause unexplained maternal deaths and abortions in rabbits at 2, 4, and 8 times the maximal recommended human dose. There are no adequate and well-controlled studies in pregnant women. LASIX should be used during pregnancy only if the potential benefit justifies the potential risk to the fetus.

The effects of furosemide on embryonic and fetal development and on pregnant dams were studied in mice, rats and rabbits.

Furosemide caused unexplained maternal deaths and abortions in the rabbit at the lowest dose of 25 mg/kg (2 times the maximal recommended human dose of 600 mg/day). In another study, a dose of 50 mg/kg (4 times the maximal recommended human dose of 600 mg/day) also caused maternal deaths and abortions when administered to rabbits between Days 12 and 17 of gestation. In a third study, none of the pregnant rabbits survived a dose of 100 mg/kg. Data from the above studies indicate fetal lethality that can precede maternal deaths.

The results of the mouse study and one of the three rabbit studies also showed an increased incidence and severity of hydronephrosis (distention of the renal pelvis and, in some cases, of the ureters) in fetuses derived from the treated dams as compared with the incidence in fetuses from the control group.

Nursing Mothers

Because it appears in breast milk, caution should be exercised when LASIX is administered to a nursing mother.

ADVERSE REACTIONS

Adverse reactions are categorized below by organ system and listed by decreasing severity.

Gastrointestinal System Reactions

1. pancreatitis
2. jaundice (intrahepatic cholestatic jaundice)
3. anorexia
4. oral and gastric irritation
5. cramping
6. diarrhea
7. constipation
8. nausea
9. vomiting

Systemic Hypersensitivity Reactions

1. systemic vasculitis
2. interstitial nephritis
3. necrotizing angiitis

Central Nervous System Reactions

1. tinnitus and hearing loss
2. paresthesias
3. vertigo
4. dizziness
5. headache
6. blurred vision
7. xanthopsia

Hematologic Reactions

1. aplastic anemia (rare)
2. thrombocytopenia
3. agranulocytosis (rare)
4. hemolytic anemia
5. leukopenia
6. anemia

Dermatologic-Hypersensitivity Reactions

1. exfoliative dermatitis
2. erythema multiforme
3. purpura
4. photosensitivity
5. urticaria
6. rash
7. pruritus

Cardiovascular Reaction

Orthostatic hypotension may occur and be aggravated by alcohol, barbiturates or narcotics.

Other Reactions

1. hyperglycemia
2. glycosuria
3. hyperuricemia
4. muscle spasm
5. weakness
6. restlessness
7. urinary bladder spasm
8. thrombophlebitis
9. fever

Whenever adverse reactions are moderate or severe, LASIX dosage should be reduced or therapy withdrawn.

OVERDOSAGE

The principal signs and symptoms of overdose with LASIX are dehydration, blood volume reduction, hypotension, electrolyte imbalance, hypokalemia and hypochloremic alkalosis, and are extensions of its diuretic action.

The acute toxicity of LASIX has been determined in mice, rats and dogs. In all three, the oral LD_{50} exceeded 1000 mg/kg body weight, while the intravenous LD_{50} ranged from 300 to 680 mg/kg. The acute intragastric toxicity in neonatal rats is 7 to 10 times that of adult rats.

The concentration of LASIX in biological fluids associated with toxicity or death is not known.

Treatment of overdosage is supportive and consists of replacement of excessive fluid and electrolyte losses. Serum electrolytes, carbon dioxide level and blood pressure should be determined frequently. Adequate drainage must be assured in patients with urinary bladder outlet obstruction (such as prostatic hypertrophy).

Hemodialysis does not accelerate furosemide elimination.

DOSAGE AND ADMINISTRATION

Edema

Therapy should be individualized according to patient response to gain maximal therapeutic response and to determine the minimal dose needed to maintain that response.

Adults – The usual initial dose of LASIX® is 20 to 80 mg given as a single dose. Ordinarily a prompt diuresis ensues. If needed, the same dose can be administered 6 to 8 hours later or the dose may be increased. The dose may be raised by 20 or 40 mg and given not sooner than 6 to 8 hours after the previous dose until the desired diuretic effect has been obtained. The individually determined single dose should then be given once or twice daily (eg. at 8 am and 2 pm). The dose of LASIX may be carefully titrated up to 600 mg/day in patients with clinically severe edematous states.

Edema may be most efficiently and safely mobilized by giving LASIX on 2 to 4 consecutive days each week.

When doses exceeding 80 mg/day are given for prolonged periods, careful clinical observation and laboratory monitoring are particularly advisable. (See **PRECAUTIONS: Laboratory Tests.**)

Pediatric patients – The usual initial dose of oral LASIX® in pediatric patients is 2 mg/kg body weight, given as a single dose. If the diuretic response is not satisfactory after the initial dose, dosage may be increased by 1 or 2 mg/kg no sooner than 6 to 8 hours after the previous dose. Doses greater than 6 mg/kg body weight are not recommended. For maintenance therapy in pediatric patients, the dose should be adjusted to the minimum effective level.

Hypertension

Therapy should be individualized according to the patient's response to gain maximal therapeutic response and to determine the minimal dose needed to maintain the therapeutic response.

Adults – The usual initial dose of LASIX for hypertension is 80 mg, usually divided into 40 mg twice a day. Dosage should then be adjusted according to response. If response is not satisfactory, add other antihypertensive agents.

Changes in blood pressure must be carefully monitored when LASIX is used with other antihypertensive drugs, especially during initial therapy. To prevent excessive drop in blood pressure, the dosage of other agents should be reduced by at least 50 percent when LASIX is added to the regimen. As the blood pressure falls under the potentiating effect of LASIX, a further reduction in dosage or even discontinuation of other antihypertensive drugs may be necessary.

HOW SUPPLIED

LASIX (furosemide) Tablets 20 mg are supplied as white, oval, monogrammed tablets in Bottles of 100 (NDC 0039-0067-10), 500 (NDC 0039-0067-50), 1000 (NDC 0039-0067-70), and in Unit Dose Packs of 100 (NDC 0039-0067-11). The 20 mg tablets are imprinted with "Lasix®" on one side and "HOECHST" on the other.

LASIX Tablets 40 mg are supplied as white, round, monogrammed, scored tablets in Bottles of 100 (NDC 0039-0060-13), 500 (NDC 0039-0060-50), 1000 (NDC 0039-0060-70), and Unit Dose Packs of 100 (NDC 0039-0060-11). The 40 mg tablets are imprinted with "Lasix® 40"on one side and the Hoechst logo on the other.

LASIX Tablets 80 mg are supplied as white, round, monogrammed, facetted edge tablets in Bottles of 50 (NDC 0039-0066-05), 500 (NDC 0039-0066-50), and in Unit Dose Packs of 100 (NDC 0039-0066-11). The 80 mg tablets are imprinted with "Lasix® 80" on one side and the Hoechst logo on the other.

Note: Dispense in well-closed, light-resistant containers. Exposure to light might cause a slight discoloration. Discolored tablets should not be dispensed.

Tested by USP Dissolution Test 2

Prescribing Information as of January 1996

Hoechst-Roussel Pharmaceuticals
Division of Hoechst Marion Roussel, Inc.
Kansas City, MO 64137

Shown in Product Identification Guide, page 316

LOPROX® ℞

(ciclopirox olamine)
Cream 1%

Prescribing Information as of October 1996
FOR DERMATOLOGIC USE ONLY. NOT FOR USE IN EYES.

DESCRIPTION

LOPROX® (ciclopirox olamine) Cream 1% is for topical use. Each gram of LOPROX Cream 1% contains 10 mg ciclopirox olamine in a water miscible vanishing cream base consisting of purified water USP, octyldodecanol NF, mineral oil USP, stearyl alcohol NF, cetyl alcohol NF, cocamide DEA, polysorbate 60 NF, myristyl alcohol NF, sorbitan monostearate NF, lactic acid USP, and benzyl alcohol NF (1%) as preservative.

LOPROX Cream 1% contains a synthetic, broad-spectrum, antifungal agent ciclopirox olamine. The chemical name is 6-cyclohexyl-1-hydroxy-4-methyl-2(1*H*)-pyridone, 2-aminoethanol salt.

The CAS Registry Number is 41621-49-2.

The chemical structure is:

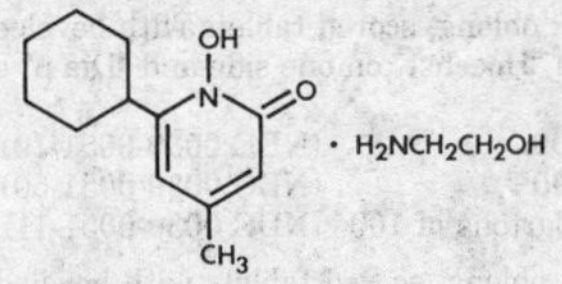

LOPROX Cream 1% has a pH of 7.

CLINICAL PHARMACOLOGY

Ciclopirox olamine is a broad-spectrum, antifungal agent that inhibits the growth of pathogenic dermatophytes, yeasts, and *Malassezia furfur*. Ciclopirox olamine exhibits fungicidal activity *in vitro* against isolates of *Trichophyton rubrum, Trichophyton mentagrophytes, Epidermophyton floccosum, Microsporum canis,* and *Candida albicans.*

Pharmacokinetic studies in men with tagged 1% ciclopirox olamine solution in polyethylene glycol 400 showed an average of 1.3% absorption of the dose when it was applied topically to 750 cm^2 on the back followed by occlusion for 6 hours. The biological half-life was 1.7 hours and excretion occurred via the kidney. Two days after application only 0.01% of the dose applied could be found in the urine. Fecal excretion was negligible.

Penetration studies in human cadaverous skin from the back, with LOPROX (ciclopirox olamine) Cream 1% with tagged ciclopirox olamine showed the presence of 0.8 to 1.6% of the dose in the stratum corneum 1.5 to 6 hours after application. The levels in the dermis were still 10 to 15 times above the minimum inhibitory concentrations.

Autoradiographic studies with human cadaverous skin showed that ciclopirox olamine penetrates into the hair and through the epidermis and hair follicles into the sebaceous glands and dermis, while a portion of the drug remains in the stratum corneum.

Draize Human Sensitization Assay, 21-Day Cumulative Irritancy study, Phototoxicity study, and Photo-Draize study conducted in a total of 142 healthy male subjects showed no contact sensitization of the delayed hypersensitivity type, no irritation, no phototoxicity, and no photo-contact sensitization due to LOPROX Cream 1%.

INDICATIONS AND USAGE

LOPROX Cream 1% is indicated for the topical treatment of the following dermal infections: tinea pedis, tinea cruris and tinea corporis due to *Trichophyton rubrum, Trichophyton mentagrophytes, Epidermophyton floccosum,* and *Microsporum canis; candidiasis* (moniliasis) due to *Candida albicans*; and tinea (pityriasis) versicolor due to *Malassezia furfur.*

CONTRAINDICATIONS

LOPROX Cream 1% is contraindicated in individuals who have shown hypersensitivity to any of its components.

WARNINGS

General

LOPROX (ciclopirox olamine) Cream 1% is not for ophthalmic use.

PRECAUTIONS

If a reaction suggesting sensitivity or chemical irritation should occur with the use of LOPROX Cream 1%, treatment should be discontinued and appropriate therapy instituted.

Information for Patients

The patient should be told to:

1. Use the medication for the full treatment time even though symptoms may have improved and notify the physician if there is no improvement after four weeks.
2. Inform the physician if the area of application shows signs of increased irritation (redness, itching, burning, blistering, swelling, oozing) indicative of possible sensitization.
3. Avoid the use of occlusive wrappings or dressings.

Carcinogenesis, Mutagenesis, Impairment of Fertility

A carcinogenicity study in female mice dosed cutaneously twice per week for 50 weeks followed by a 6-month drug-free observation period prior to necropsy revealed no evidence of tumors at the application site.

The following *in vitro* and *in vivo* genotoxicity tests have been conducted with ciclopirox olamine: studies to evaluate gene mutation in the Ames *Salmonella*/Mammalian Microsome Assay (negative) and Yeast Saccharomyces Cerevisiae Assay (negative) and studies to evaluate chromosome aberrations *in vivo* in the Mouse Dominant Lethal Assay and in the Mouse Micronucleus Assay at 500 mg/kg (negative).

The following battery of *in vitro* genotoxicity tests were conducted with *ciclopirox*: a chromosome aberration assay in V79 Chinese Hamster Cells, with and without metabolic

activation (positive); a gene mutation assay in the HGPRT-test with V79 Chinese Hamster Cells (negative); and a primary DNA damage assay (i.e., unscheduled DNA Synthesis Assay in A549 Human Cells (negative)). An *in vitro* Cell Transformation Assay in BALB/C3T3 Cells was negative for cell transformation. In an *in vivo* Chinese Hamster Bone Marrow Cytogenetic Assay, ciclopirox was negative for chromosome aberrations at 5000 mg/kg.

Pregnancy Category B

Reproduction studies have been performed in the mouse, rat, rabbit, and monkey, (via various routes of administration) at doses 10 times or more the topical human dose and have revealed no significant evidence of impaired fertility or harm to the fetus due to ciclopirox olamine. There are, however, no adequate or well-controlled studies in pregnant women. Because animal reproduction studies are not always predictive of human response this drug should be used during pregnancy only if clearly needed.

Nursing Mothers

It is not known whether this drug is excreted in human milk. Because many drugs are excreted in human milk, caution should be exercised when LOPROX (ciclopirox olamine) Cream 1% is administered to a nursing woman.

Pediatric Use

Safety and effectiveness in pediatric patients below the age of 10 years have not been established.

ADVERSE REACTIONS

In all controlled clinical studies with 514 patients using LOPROX Cream 1% and in 296 patients using the vehicle cream, the incidence of adverse reactions was low. This included pruritus at the site of application in one patient and worsening of the clinical signs and symptoms in another patient using ciclopirox olamine cream 1% and burning in one patient and worsening of the clinical signs and symptoms in another patient using the vehicle cream.

DOSAGE AND ADMINISTRATION

Gently massage LOPROX Cream 1% into the affected and surrounding skin areas twice daily, in the morning and evening. Clinical improvement with relief of pruritus and other symptoms usually occurs within the first week of treatment. If a patient shows no clinical improvement after four weeks of treatment with LOPROX Cream 1%, the diagnosis should be redetermined. Patients with tinea versicolor usually exhibit clinical and mycological clearing after two weeks of treatment.

HOW SUPPLIED

LOPROX (ciclopirox olamine) Cream 1% is supplied in 15 gram (NDC 0039-0009-15), 30 gram (NDC 0039-0009-30), and 90 gram (NDC 0039-0009-90) tubes.
Store between 59 and 86° F (15 and 30°C).
Caution: Federal law prohibits dispensing without prescription.
Prescribing Information as of October 1996
Loprox REG TM HOECHST AG
Hoechst-Roussel Pharmaceuticals
Division of Hoechst Marion Roussel, Inc.
Kansas City, MO 64137

Shown in Product Identification Guide, page 316

LOPROX®
[lō-proks]
(ciclopirox olamine)
Lotion 1%

℞

Prescribing Information as of March 1995

FOR DERMATOLOGIC USE ONLY.
NOT FOR USE IN EYES.

DESCRIPTION

Loprox® (ciclopirox olamine) Lotion 1% is for topical use. Each gram of Loprox® Lotion 1% contains 10 mg of ciclopirox olamine in a water miscible lotion base consisting of purified water USP, cocamide DEA, octyldodecanol NF, mineral oil USP, stearyl alcohol NF, cetyl alcohol NF, polysorbate 60 NF, myristyl alcohol NF, sorbitan monostearate NF, lactic acid USP, and benzyl alcohol NF (1%) as preservative. Loprox® Lotion contains a synthetic, broad-spectrum, antifungal agent ciclopirox olamine. The chemical name is 6-cyclohexyl-1-hydroxy-4-methyl-2(1*H*)-pyridone, 2-aminoethanol salt.
The CAS Registry Number is 41621-49-2.
The chemical structure is:

Loprox® Lotion 1% has a pH of 7.

CLINICAL PHARMACOLOGY

Ciclopirox olamine is a broad-spectrum, antifungal agent that inhibits the growth of pathogenic dermatophytes, yeasts, and *Malassezia furfur*. Ciclopirox olamine exhibits fungicidal activity *in vitro* against isolates of *Trichophyton rubrum*, *Trichophyton mentagrophytes*, *Epidermophyton floccosum*, *Microsporum canis*, and *Candida albicans*.
Pharmacokinetic studies in men with radiolabeled 1% ciclopirox olamine solution in polyethylene glycol 400 showed an average of 1.3% absorption of the dose when it was applied topically to 750 cm² on the back followed by occlusion for 6 hours. The biological half-life was 1.7 hours and excretion occurred via the kidney. Two days after application, only 0.01% of the dose applied could be found in the urine. Fecal excretion was negligible. Autoradiographic studies with human cadaver skin showed that ciclopirox olamine penetrates into the hair and through the epidermis and hair follicles into the sebaceous glands and dermis, while a portion of the drug remains in the stratum corneum.
In vitro penetration studies in frozen or fresh excised human cadaver and pig skin indicated that the penetration of Loprox® (ciclopirox olamine) Lotion 1% is equivalent to that of Loprox® Cream 1%. Therapeutic equivalence of cream and lotion formulations also was indicated by studies of experimentally induced guinea pig and human trichophytosis.

INDICATIONS AND USAGE

Loprox® (ciclopirox olamine) Lotion 1% is indicated for the topical treatment of the following dermal infections: tinea pedis, tinea cruris and tinea corporis due to *Trichophyton rubrum*, *Trichophyton mentagrophytes*, *Epidermophyton floccosum*, and *Microsporum canis*; cutaneous candidiasis (moniliasis) due to *Candida albicans*; and tinea (pityriasis) versicolor due to *Malassezia furfur*.

CONTRAINDICATIONS

Loprox® Lotion 1% is contraindicated in individuals who have shown hypersensitivity to any of its components.

WARNINGS

General: Loprox® Lotion 1% is not for ophthalmic use.

PRECAUTIONS

If a reaction suggesting sensitivity or chemical irritation should occur with the use of Loprox® Lotion 1%, treatment should be discontinued and appropriate therapy instituted.
Information for Patients
The patient should be told to:
1. Use the medication for the full treatment time even though signs/symptoms may have improved and notify the physician if there is no improvement after four weeks.
2. Inform the physician if the area of application shows signs of increased irritation (redness, itching, burning, blistering, swelling, oozing) indicative of possible sensitization.
3. Avoid the use of occlusive wrappings or dressings.

Carcinogenesis, Mutagenesis, Impairment of Fertility:
A carcinogenicity study in female mice dosed cutaneously twice per week for 50 weeks followed by a 6-month drug-free observation period prior to necropsy revealed no evidence of tumors at the application site. The following *in vitro* and *in vivo* genotoxicity tests have been conducted with ciclopirox olamine: studies to evaluate gene mutation in the Ames *Salmonella I* Mammalian Microsome Assay (negative) and Yeast Saccharomyces Cerevisiae Assay (negative) and studies to evaluate chromosome aberrations *in vivo* in the Mouse Dominant Lethal Assay and in the Mouse Micronucleus Assay at 500 mg/kg (negative). The following battery of *in vitro* genotoxicity tests were conducted with *ciclopirox*: a chromosome aberration assay in V79 Chinese Hamster Cells, with and without metabolic activation (positive); a gene mutation assay in the HGPRT - test with V79 Chinese Hamster Cells (negative); and a primary DNA damage assay (i.e., unscheduled DNA Synthesis Assay in A549 Human Cells (negative)). An *in vitro* Cell Transformation Assay in BALB/C3T3 Cells was negative for cell transformation. In an *in vivo* Chinese Hamster Bone Marrow Cytogenetic Assay, ciclopirox was negative for chromosome aberrations at 5000 mg/kg.

Pregnancy Category B:
Reproduction studies have been performed in the mouse, rat, rabbit, and monkey, via various routes of administration, at doses 10 times or more the topical human dose and have revealed no significant evidence of impaired fertility or harm to the fetus due to ciclopirox olamine. There are, however, no adequate or well-controlled studies in pregnant women. Because animal reproduction studies are not always predictive of human response, this drug should be used during pregnancy only if clearly needed.

Nursing Mothers:
It is not known whether this drug is excreted in human milk. Caution should be exercised when Loprox® (ciclopirox olamine) Lotion 1% is administered to a nursing woman.

Pediatric Use:

Safety and effectiveness in pediatric patients below the age of 10 years have not been established.

ADVERSE REACTIONS

In the controlled clinical trial with 89 patients using Loprox® Lotion 1% and 89 patients using the vehicle, the incidence of adverse reactions was low.
Those considered possibly related to treatment or occurring in more than one patient were pruritus, which occurred in two patients using ciclopirox olamine lotion 1% and one patient using the lotion vehicle, and burning, which occurred in one patient using ciclopirox olamine lotion 1%.

DOSAGE AND ADMINISTRATION

Gently massage Loprox® (ciclopirox olamine) Lotion 1% into the affected and surrounding skin areas twice daily, in the morning and evening. Clinical improvement with relief of pruritus and other symptoms usually occurs within the first week of treatment. If a patient shows no clinical improvement after four weeks of treatment with Loprox® Lotion 1% the diagnosis should be redetermined. Patients with tinea versicolor usually exhibit clinical and mycological clearing after two weeks of treatment.

HOW SUPPLIED

Loprox® Lotion 1% is supplied in 30 mL bottles (NDC 0039-0008-30) and 60 mL bottles (NDC 0039-0008-06).
Bottle space provided to allow for vigorous shaking before each use.
Store between 41 and 77°F (5 and 25°C).
Caution: Federal law prohibits dispensing without prescription.
Loprox REG TM HOECHST AG
HOECHST-ROUSSEL
Pharmaceuticals Incorporated
Somerville, NJ 08876-1258

708000-3/95

Shown in Product Identification Guide, page 316

NILANDRON™
(nilutamide)
Tablets

℞

Prescribing Information as of September 1996
DESCRIPTION
NILANDRON™ tablets contain nilutamide, a nonsteroidal, orally active antiandrogen having the chemical name 5,5-dimethyl 3-[4-nitro 3-(trifluoromethyl) phenyl] 2,4-imidazolidinedione with the following structural formula:

Nilutamide is a microcrystalline, white to practically white powder with a molecular weight of 317.25.
It is freely soluble in ethyl acetate, acetone, chloroform, ethyl alcohol, dichloromethane, and methanol. It is slightly soluble in water [< 0.1% W/V at 25°C (77°F)]. It melts between 153°C and 156°C (307.4°F and 312.8°F).
Each NILANDRON tablet contains 50 mg nilutamide. Other ingredients in NILANDRON tablets are corn starch, lactose, providone, docusate sodium, magnesium stearate, and talc.

CLINICAL PHARMACOLOGY
Mechanism of Action
Prostate cancer is known to be androgen sensitive and responds to androgen ablation. In animal studies, nilutamide has demonstrated antiandrogenic activity without other hormonal (estrogen, progesterone, mineralocorticoid, and glucocorticoid) effects. In vitro, nilutamide blocks the effects of testosterone at the androgen receptor level. In vivo, nilutamide interacts with the androgen receptor and prevents the normal androgenic response.
Pharmacokinetics
Absorption: Analysis of blood, urine, and feces samples following a single oral 150-mg dose of [¹⁴C]-nilutamide in patients with metastatic prostate cancer showed that the drug is rapidly and completely absorbed and that it yields high and persistent plasma concentrations.
Distribution: After absorption of the drug, there is a detectable distribution phase. There is moderate binding of the drug to plasma proteins and low binding to erythrocytes. The binding is nonsaturable except in the case of al-

Continued on next page

Nilandron—Cont.

pha-1-glycoprotein, which makes a minor contribution to the total concentration of proteins in the plasma. The results of binding studies do not indicate any effects that would cause nonlinear pharmacokinetics.

Metabolism: The results of a human metabolism study using ^{14}C-radiolabelled tablets show that nilutamide is extensively metabolized and less than 2% of the drug is excreted unchanged in urine after 5 days. Five metabolites have been isolated from human urine. Two metabolites display an asymmetric center, due to oxidation of a methyl group, resulting in the formation of D- and L-isomers. One of the metabolites was shown, in vitro, to possess 25 to 50% of the pharmacological activity of the parent drug, and the D-isomer of the active metabolite showed equal or greater potency compared to the L-isomer. However, the pharmacokinetics and the pharmacodynamics of the metabolites have not been fully investigated.

Elimination: The majority (62%) of orally administered [^{14}C]-nilutamide is eliminated in the urine during the first 120 hours after a single 150-mg dose. Fecal elimination is negligible, ranging from 1.4% to 7% of the dose after 4 to 5 days. Excretion of radioactivity in urine likely continues beyond 5 days. The mean elimination half-life of nilutamide determined in studies in which subjects received a single dose of 100–300 mg ranged from 38.0 to 59.1 hours with most values between 41 and 49 hours. The elimination of at least one metabolite is generally longer than that of unchanged nilutamide (59–126 hours). During multiple dosing of 3 × 50 mg twice a day, steady state was reached within 2 to 4 weeks for most patients, and mean steady state AUC_{0-12} was 110% higher than the $AUC_{0-\infty}$ obtained from the first dose of 3 × 50 mg. These data and in vitro metabolism data suggest that, upon multiple dosing, metabolic enzyme inhibition may occur for this drug.

Clinical Studies

Nilutamide through its antiandrogenic activity can complement surgical castration, which suppresses only testicular androgens. The effects of the combined therapy were studied in patients with previously untreated metastatic prostate cancer. In a double-blind, randomized, multicenter study that enrolled 457 patients (225 treated with orchiectomy and NILANDRON, 232 treated with orchiectomy and placebo), the NILANDRON group showed a statistically significant benefit in time to progression and time to death. The results are summarized below.

[See table below]

INDICATIONS AND USAGE

Metastatic Prostate Cancer

NILANDRON tablets are indicated for use in combination with surgical castration for the treatment of metastatic prostate cancer (Stage D_2).

For maximum benefit, NILANDRON treatment must begin on the same day as or on the day after surgical castration.

CONTRAINDICATIONS

NILANDRON tablets are contraindicated in patients:

- with severe hepatic impairment (baseline hepatic enzymes should be evaluated prior to treatment)
- with severe respiratory insufficiency
- with hypersensitivity to nilutamide or any component of this preparation.

WARNINGS

Interstitial pneumonitis

Interstitial pneumonitis has been reported in 2% of patients in controlled clinical trials in patients exposed to nilutamide. Patients typically presented with progressive exertional dyspnea, and possibly with cough, chest pain, and fever. X-rays showed interstitial or alveolo-interstitial changes. The suggestive signs of pneumonitis most often occurred within the first three months of NILANDRON treatment.

A routine chest X-ray should be performed before treatment, and patients should be told to report immediately any dyspnea or aggravation of pre-existing dyspnea. At the onset of dyspnea or worsening of pre-existing dyspnea at any time during treatment, NILANDRON should be interrupted until it can be determined if respiratory symptoms are drug related. A chest X-ray should be obtained, and if there are findings suggestive of interstitial pneumonitis, treatment with NILANDRON should be discontinued. The pneumonitis is almost always reversible when treatment is discontinued.

If the chest X-ray appears normal, pulmonary function tests including DL_{CO} (diffusing capacity of the lung for carbon monoxide) should be performed. If a significant decrease of DL_{CO} and/or a restrictive pattern is observed on pulmonary function testing, NILANDRON treatment should be terminated. In the absence of chest X-ray and pulmonary function test findings consistent with interstitial pneumonitis, treatment with NILANDRON can be restarted under close monitoring of pulmonary symptoms.

Because interstitial pneumonitis was reported in 8 of 47 patients (17%) in a small study performed in Japan, specific caution should be observed in the treatment of Asian patients.

Hepatitis

Hepatitis or marked increases in liver enzymes leading to drug discontinuation occurred in 1% of NILANDRON patients in controlled clinical trials:

Serum hepatic enzyme levels should be measured at baseline and at regular intervals (3 months); if transaminases increase over 2–3 times the upper limit of normal, treatment should be discontinued.

Appropriate laboratory testing should be done at the first symptom/sign of liver injury (e.g., jaundice, dark urine, fatigue, abdominal pain, or unexplained gastrointestinal symptoms) and NILANDRON treatment must be discontinued immediately if transaminases exceed 3 times the upper limit of normal.

There has been a report of elevated hepatic enzymes followed by death in a 65-year-old patient being treated with nilutamide.

Other

Foreign postmarketing surveillance has revealed isolated cases of aplastic anemia in which a causal relationship with NILANDRON could not be ascertained.

PRECAUTIONS

Information for Patients

Patients should be informed that NILANDRON tablets should be started on the day of, or on the day after, surgical castration. They should also be informed that they should not interrupt their dosing of NILANDRON or stop taking this medication without consulting their physician.

Because of the possibility of interstitial pneumonitis, patients should also be told to report immediately any dyspnea or aggravation of pre-existing dyspnea.

Because of the possibility of hepatitis, patients should be told to consult with their physician should nausea, vomiting, abdominal pain, or jaundice occur.

Because of the possibility of an intolerance to alcohol (facial flushes, malaise, hypotension) following ingestion of NILANDRON, it is recommended that intake of alcoholic beverages be avoided by patients who experience this reaction. This effect has been reported in about 5% of patients treated with NILANDRON.

In clinical trials, 13% to 57% of patients receiving NILANDRON reported a delay in adaptation to dark, ranging from seconds to a few minutes, when passing from a lighted area to a dark area. This effect sometimes does not abate as drug treatment is continued. Patients who experience this effect should be cautioned about driving at night or through tunnels. This effect can be alleviated by the wearing of tinted glasses.

Drug Interactions

In vitro, nilutamide has been shown to inhibit the activity of liver cytochrome P-450 isoenzymes and, therefore, may reduce the metabolism of compounds requiring these systems. Consequently, drugs with a low therapeutic margin, such as vitamin K antagonists, phenytoin, and theophylline, could have a delayed elimination and increases in their serum half-life leading to a toxic level. The dosage of these drugs or others with a similar metabolism may need to be modified if they are administered concomitantly with nilutamide. For example, when vitamin K antagonists are administered concomitantly with nilutamide, prothrombin time should be carefully monitored and, if necessary, the dosage of vitamin K antagonists should be reduced.

Carcinogenesis, Mutagenesis, Impairment of Fertility

Administration of nilutamide to rats for 18 months at doses of 0, 5, 15, or 45 mg/kg/day produced benign Leydig cell tumors in 35% of the high-dose male rats (AUC exposures in high-dose rats were approximately 1–2 times human AUC exposures with therapeutic doses). The increased incidence of Leydig cell tumors is secondary to elevated luteinizing hormone (LH) concentrations resulting from loss of feedback inhibition at the pituitary. Elevated LH and testosterone concentrations are not observed in castrated men receiving NILANDRON. Nilutamide had no effect on the incidence, size, or time of onset of any spontaneous tumor in rats.

Nilutamide displayed no mutagenic effects in a variety of in vitro and in vivo tests (Ames test, mouse micronucleus test, and two chromosomal aberration tests).

In reproduction studies in rats, nilutamide had no effect on the reproductive function of males and females, and no lethal, teratogenic, or growth-suppressive effects on fetuses were found. The maximal dose at which nilutamide did not affect reproductive function in either sex or have an effect on fetuses was estimated to be 45 mg/kg orally (AUC exposures in rats approximately 1–2 times human therapeutic AUC exposures).

Pregnancy

Pregnancy Category C; Animal reproduction studies have not been conducted with nilutamide. It is also not known whether nilutamide can cause fetal harm when administered to a pregnant woman or can affect reproductive capacity. Nilutamide should be given to a pregnant woman only if clearly needed.

Pediatric Use

Safety and effectiveness in pediatric patients have not been determined.

Animal Pharmacology and Toxicology

Administration of NILANDRON to beagle dogs resulted in drug-related deaths at dose levels that produce AUC exposures in dogs much lower than the AUC exposures of men receiving the therapeutic doses of 150 and 300 mg/day. Nilutamide-induced toxicity in dogs was cumulative with progressively lower doses producing death when given for longer durations. Nilutamide given to dogs at 60 mg/kg/day (1–2 times human AUC exposure) for 1 month produced 100% mortality. Administration of 20 and 30 mg/kg/day nilutamide ($^1/_2$–1 times human AUC exposure) for 6 months resulted in 20% and 70% mortality in treated dogs. Administration to dogs of 3, 6, and 12 mg/kg/day nilutamide ($^1/_{10}$–$^1/_2$) human AUC exposure) for 1 year resulted in 8%, 33%, and 50% mortality, respectively. **A "no-effect level" for nilutamide-induced mortality in dogs was not identified.** Pathology data from the one-year oral toxicity study suggest that the deaths in dogs were secondary to liver toxicity. Marked-to-massive hepatocellular swelling and vacuolization were observed in affected dogs. Liver toxicity in dogs was not consistently associated with elevations of liver enzymes.

Administration of nilutamide to rats at a dose level of 45 mg/kg/day (AUC exposure in rats 1–2 times human therapeutic AUC exposures) for 18 months increased the incidence of lung pathology (granulomatous inflammation and chronic alveolitis).

The hepatic and pulmonary adverse effects observed in nilutamide-treated animals and men are similar to effects observed with another nitroaromatic compound, nitrofurantoin. Nilutamide and nitrofurantoin are both metabolized in vitro to nitroanion free-radicals by microsomal NADPH-cytochrome P450 reductase in the lungs and liver of rats and humans.

ADVERSE REACTIONS

The following adverse experiences were reported during a multicenter clinical trial comparing NILANDRON + surgical castration versus placebo + surgical castration. The most frequently reported (greater than 5%) adverse experiences during treatment with NILANDRON tablets in combination with surgical castration are listed below. For comparison, adverse experiences seen with surgical castration and placebo are also listed.

[See first table at bottom of next page]

The overall incidence of adverse experiences was 86% (194/225) for the NILANDRON group and 81% (188/232) for the placebo group.

The following adverse experiences were reported during a multicenter clinical trial comparing NILANDRON + leuprolide versus placebo + leuprolide. The most frequently reported (greater than 5%) adverse experiences during treatment with NILANDRON tablets in combination with leuprolide are listed below.

For comparison, adverse experiences seen with leuprolide and placebo are also listed.

[See second table at bottom of next page]

The overall incidence of adverse experiences is 99.5% (208/209) for the NILANDRON group and 98.5% (199/202) for the placebo group.

Some frequently occurring adverse experiences, for example hot flushes, impotence, and decreased libido, are known to be associated with low serum androgen levels and known to occur with medical or surgical castration alone. Notable was the higher incidence of visual disturbances (variously described as impaired adaptation to darkness, abnormal vision, and colored vision), which led to treatment discontinuation in 1% to 2% of patients.

Interstitial pneumonitis occurred in one (<1%) patient receiving NILANDRON in combination with surgical castration and in seven patients (3%) receiving NILANDRON in combination with leuprolide and one patient receiving pla-

	NILANDRON	PLACEBO
Median Survival (months)	27.3	23.6
Progression-Free Survival (months)	21.1	14.9
Complete or Partial Regression	41%	24%
Improvement in Bone Pain	54%	37%

cebo in combination with leuprolide. Overall, it has been reported in 2% of patients receiving NILANDRON. This included a report of interstitial pneumonitis in 8 of 47 patients (17%) in a small study performed in Japan.

In addition, the following adverse experiences were reported in 2 to 5% of patients treated with NILANDRON in combination with leuprolide or orchiectomy.

Body as a Whole: Malaise (2%).
Cardiovascular System: Angina (2%), heart failure (3%), syncope (2%).
Digestive System: Diarrhea (2%), gastrointestinal disorder (2%), gastrointestinal hemorrhage (2%), melena (2%).
Metabolic and Nutritional System: Alcohol intolerance (5%), edema (2%), weight loss (2%).

Musculoskeletal System: Arthritis (2%).
Nervous System: Dry mouth (2%), nervousness (2%), paresthesia (3%).
Respiratory System: Cough increased (2%), interstitial lung disease (2%), lung disorder (4%), rhinitis (2%).
Skin and Appendages: Pruritus (2%).
Special Senses: Cataract (2%), photophobia (2%).
Laboratory Values: Haptoglobin increased (2%), leukopenia (3%), alkaline phosphatase increased (3%), BUN increased (2%), creatinine increased (2%), hyperglycemia (4%).

Adverse Experience	NILANDRON + surgical castration (N=225) % All	Placebo + surgical castration (N=232) % All
Cardiovascular System		
Hypertension	5.3	2.6
Digestive System		
Nausea	9.8	6.0
Constipation	7.1	3.9
Endocrine System		
Hot flushes	28.4	22.4
Metabolic and Nutritional System		
Increased AST	8.0	3.9
Increased ALT	7.6	4.3
Nervous System		
Dizziness	7.1	3.4
Respiratory System		
Dyspnea	6.2	7.3
Special Senses		
Impaired adaptation to dark	12.9	1.3
Abnormal vision	6.7	1.7
Urogenital System		
Urinary tract infection	8.0	9.1

Adverse Experience	NILANDRON + leuprolide (N=209) % All	Placebo + leuprolide (N=202) % All
Body as a Whole		
Pain	26.8	27.7
Headache	13.9	10.4
Asthenia	19.1	20.8
Back pain	11.5	16.8
Abdominal pain	10.0	5.4
Chest pain	7.2	4.5
Flu syndrome	7.2	3.0
Fever	5.3	6.4
Cardiovascular System		
Hypertension	9.1	9.9
Digestive System		
Nausea	23.9	8.4
Constipation	19.6	16.8
Anorexia	11.0	6.4
Dyspepsia	6.7	4.5
Vomiting	5.7	4.0
Endocrine System		
Hot flushes	66.5	59.4
Impotence	11.0	12.9
Libido decreased	11.0	4.5
Hemic and Lymphatic System		
Anemia	7.2	6.4
Metabolic and Nutritional System		
Increased AST	12.9	13.9
Peripheral edema	12.4	17.3
Increased ALT	9.1	8.9
Musculo Skeletal System		
Bone Pain	6.2	5.0
Nervous System		
Insomnia	16.3	15.8
Dizziness	10.0	11.4
Depression	8.6	7.4
Hypesthesia	5.3	2.0
Respiratory System		
Dyspnea	10.5	7.4
Upper respiratory infection	8.1	10.9
Pneumonia	5.3	3.5
Skin and Appendages		
Sweating	6.2	3.0
Body hair loss	5.7	0.5
Dry skin	5.3	2.5
Rash	5.3	4.0
Special Senses		
Impaired adaptation to dark	56.9	5.4
Chromatopsia	8.6	0.0
Impaired adaptation to light	7.7	1.0
Abnormal vision	6.2	4.5
Urogenital System		
Testicular atrophy	16.3	12.4
Gynecomastia	10.5	11.9
Urinary tract infection	8.6	21.3
Hematuria	8.1	7.9
Urinary tract disorder	7.2	10.4
Nocturia	6.7	6.4

OVERDOSAGE

One case of massive overdosage has been published. A 79-year-old man attempted suicide by ingesting 13 g of nilutamide (i.e., 43 times the maximum recommended dose). Despite immediate gastric lavage and oral administration of activated charcoal, plasma nilutamide levels peaked at 6 times the normal range 2 hours after ingestion. There were no clinical signs or symptoms or changes in parameters such as transaminases or chest X-ray. Maintenance treatment (150 mg/day) was resumed 30 days later.

In repeated-dose tolerance studies, doses of 600 mg/day and 900 mg/day were administered to 9 and 4 patients, respectively. The ingestion of these doses was associated with gastrointestinal disorders, including nausea and vomiting, malaise, headache, and dizziness. In addition, a transient elevation in hepatic enzyme levels was noted in one patient. Since nilutamide is protein bound, dialysis may not be useful as treatment for overdose. As in the management of overdosage with any drug, it should be borne in mind that multiple agents may have been taken. If vomiting does not occur spontaneously, it should be induced if the patient is alert. General supportive care, including frequent monitoring of the vital signs and close observation of the patient, is indicated.

DOSAGE AND ADMINISTRATION

The recommended dose is six tablets (50 mg each) once a day for a total daily dose of 300 mg for 30 days followed thereafter by three tablets (50 mg each) once a day for a total daily dosage of 150 mg. NILANDRON tablets can be taken with or without food.

HOW SUPPLIED

White, biconvex (with a triangular logo on one face and an internal reference number [168] on the other), cylindrical (about 7 mm in diameter) NILANDRON tablets containing 50 mg of nilutamide are available in "child-resistant" PVC blister pack with an aluminum foil backing in

Boxes of 90 tablets (6 blisters of 15 tablets each) NDC 0088-1110-35

Store at room temperature between 15°C and 30°C (59° and 86°F). Protect from light.

Prescribing Information as of September 1996
Manufactured by Usiphar, 60200 Compiegne, France for:
Hoechst Marion Roussel, Inc.
Kansas City, MO 64137 USA

Shown in Product Identification Guide, page 316

NITRO-BID® IV   ℞
[ni' tro-bid]
(nitroglycerin injection USP)

Prescribing Information as of January 1997
FOR INTRAVENOUS USE ONLY. NOT FOR DIRECT INTRAVENOUS INJECTION. NITRO-BID® MUST BE DILUTED IN DEXTROSE (5%) INJECTION USP OR SODIUM CHLORIDE (0.9%) INJECTION USP PRIOR TO ITS INFUSION (SEE DOSAGE AND ADMINISTRATION SECTION). THE ADMINISTRATION SET USED FOR INFUSION WILL AFFECT THE AMOUNT OF NITRO-BID IV DELIVERED TO THE PATIENT. (SEE WARNINGS AND DOSAGE AND ADMINISTRATION SECTIONS.)

CAUTION
SEVERAL PREPARATIONS OF NITROGLYCERIN FOR INJECTION ARE AVAILABLE. THEY DIFFER IN CONCENTRATION AND/OR VOLUME PER VIAL. WHEN SWITCHING FROM ONE PRODUCT TO ANOTHER, ATTENTION MUST BE PAID TO THE DILUTION AND DOSAGE AND ADMINISTRATION INSTRUCTIONS.

DESCRIPTION
Nitroglycerin is 1,2,3-propanetriol trinitrate, an organic nitrate whose structural formula is:

$$H_2CONO_2$$
$$HCONO_2$$
$$H_2CONO_2$$

Continued on next page

Nitro-Bid IV—Cont.

whose molecular formula is $C_3H_5N_3O_9$, and whose molecular weight is 227.09. The organic nitrates are vasodilators, active on both arteries and veins.
NITRO-BID IV (nitroglycerin injection USP) is a clear, practically colorless additive solution or intravenous infusion after dilution. Each milliliter contains 5 mg nitroglycerin and 45 mg propylene glycol dissolved in 70% ethanol.
The solution is sterile, nonpyrogenic, and nonexplosive.

CLINICAL PHARMACOLOGY

The principal pharmacological action of NITRO-BID IV (nitroglycerin) is relaxation of vascular smooth muscle and consequent dilatation of peripheral arteries and veins, especially the latter. Dilatation of the veins promotes peripheral pooling of blood and decreases venous return to the heart, thereby reducing left ventricular end diastolic pressure and pulmonary capillary wedge pressure (preload). Arteriolar relaxation reduces systemic vascular resistance, systolic arterial pressure, and mean arterial pressure (afterload). Dilatation of the coronary arteries also occurs. The relative importance of preload reduction, afterload reduction, and coronary dilatation remains undefined.
Dosing regimens for most chronically used drugs are designed to provide plasma concentrations that are continuously greater than a minimally effective concentration. This strategy is inappropriate for organic nitrates. Several well-controlled clinical trials have used exercise testing to assess the antianginal efficacy of continuously delivered nitrates. In the large majority of these trials, active agents were indistinguishable from placebo after 24 hours (or less) of continuous therapy. Attempts to overcome nitrate tolerance by dose escalation, even to doses far in excess of those used acutely, have consistently failed. Only after nitrates have been absent from the body for several hours has their antianginal efficacy been restored.

Pharmacokinetics

The volume of distribution of nitrolgycerin is about 3 L/kg, and nitroglycerin is cleared from this volume at extremely rapid rates, with a resulting serum half-life of about 3 minutes. The observed clearance rates (close to 1 L/kg/min) greatly exceed hepatic blood flow; known sites of extrahepatic metabolism include red blood cells and vascular walls. The first products in the metabolism of nitroglycerin are inorganic nitrate and the 1,2- and 1,3-dinitroglycerols. The dinitrates are less effective vasodilators than nitroglycerin, but they are longer lived in the serum, and their net contribution to the overall effect of chronic nitroglycerin regimens is not known. The dinitrates are further metabolized to (nonvasoactive) mononitrates and, ultimately, to glycerol and carbon dioxide.
To avoid development of tolerance to nitroglycerin, drug-free intervals of 10 to 12 hours are known to be sufficient; shorter intervals have not been well studied. In one well-controlled clinical trial, subjects receiving nitroglycerin appeared to exhibit a rebound or withdrawal effect, so that their exercise tolerance at the end of the daily drug-free interval was *less* than that exhibited by the parallel group receiving placebo.

Clinical Trials

Blinded, placebo-controlled trials of intravenous nitroclycerin have not been reported, but multiple investigators have reported open-label studies, and there are scattered reports of studies in which intravenous nitroglycerin was tested in blinded fashion against sodium nitroprusside.
In each of these studies, therapeutic doses of intravenous nitroglycerin were found to reduce systolic and diastolic arterial blood pressure. The heart rate was usually increased, presumably as a reflexive response to the fall in blood pressure. Coronary perfusion pressure was usually, but not always, maintained.
Intravenous nitroglycerin reduced central venous pressure (CVP), right atrial pressure (RAP), pulmonary arterial pressure (PAP), pulmonary capillary wedge pressure (PCWP), pulmonary vascular resistance (PVR), and systemic vascular resistance (SVR). When these parameters were elevated, reducing them toward normal usually caused a rise in cardiac output. Conversely, intravenous nitroglycerin usually *reduced* cardiac output when it was given to patients whose CVP, RAP, PAP, PCWP, PVR, and SVR were all normal.
Most clinical trials of intravenous nitroglycerin have been brief; they have typically followed hemodynamic parameters during a single surgical procedure. In one careful study, one of the few that lasted more than a few hours, continuous intravenous nitroglycerin had lost almost all of its hemodynamic effect after 48 hours. In the same study, patients who received nitroglycerin infusions for only 12 hours out of each 24 demonstrated no similar attenuation of effect. These results are consistent with those seen in multiple large, double-blind, placebo-controlled trials of other formulations of nitroglycerin and other nitrates.

INDICATIONS AND USAGE

NITRO-BID IV (nitroglycerin) is indicated for treatment of perioperative hypertension, for control of congestive heart failure in the setting of acute myocardial infarction, for treatment of angina pectoris in patients who have not responded to sublingual nitroglycerin and beta-blockers, and for induction of intraoperative hypotension.

CONTRAINDICATIONS

Allergic reactions to organic nitrates are extremely rare, but they do occur. NITRO-BID IV is contraindicated in patients who are allergic to it.
In patients with pericardial tamponade, restrictive cardiomyopathy, or constrictive pericarditis, cardiac output is dependent upon venous return. Intravenous nitroglycerin is contraindicated in patients with these conditions.

WARNINGS

Nitroglycerin readily migrates into many plastics, including the polyvinyl chloride (PVC) plastics commonly used for intravenous administration sets. Nitroglycerin absorption by PVC tubing is increased when the tubing is long, the flow rates are low, and the nitroglycerin concentration of the solution is high. The delivered fraction of the solution's original nitroglycerin content has been 20% to 60% in published studies using PVC tubing; the fraction varies with time during a single infusion, and no simple correction factor can be used. PVC tubing has been used in most published studies of intravenous nitroglycerin, but the reported doses have been calculated by simply multiplying the flow rate of the solution by the solution's original concentration of nitroglycerin. *The actual doses delivered have been less, sometimes much less, than those reported.* Some in-line intravenous filters also absorb nitroglycerin; these filters should be avoided.
Because of the absorption problem, the use of the least absorptive infusion tubing available (ie, non-PVC tubing) for infusions of NITRO-BID IV is recommended (see DOSAGE AND ADMINISTRATION).

DOSING INSTRUCTIONS MUST BE FOLLOWED WITH CARE. WHEN THE APPROPRIATE INFUSION SETS ARE USED, THE CALCULATED DOSE WILL BE DELIVERED TO THE PATIENT, BECAUSE THE LOSS OF NITRO-BID IV SEEN WITH STANDARD PVC TUBING WILL BE AVOIDED. THE DOSAGES REPORTED IN PUBLISHED STUDIES UTILIZED GENERAL-USE PVC ADMINISTRATION SETS, AND RECOMMENDED DOSES BASED ON THIS EXPERIENCE WILL BE TOO HIGH IF THE LOW-ABSORBING INFUSION SETS ARE USED.

PRECAUTIONS

General

Severe hypotension and shock may occur with even small doses of NITRO-BID IV (nitroglycerin). This drug should, therefore, be used with caution in patients who may be volume-depleted; who, for whatever reason, are already hypotensive; or who, because of inadequate circulation to the brain or to other vital organs, would be unusually compromised by undue hypotension. Hypotension induced by nitroglycerin may be accompanied by paradoxical bradycardia and increased angina pectoris.
Nitrate therapy may aggravate the angina caused by hypertrophic cardiomyopathy.
As tolerance to other forms of nitroglycerin develops, the effect of sublingual nitroglycerin on exercise tolerance, although still observable, is somewhat blunted.
In industrial workers who have had long-term exposure to unknown (presumably high) doses of organic nitrates, tolerance clearly occurs. Chest pain, acute myocardial infarction, and even sudden death have occurred during temporary withdrawal of nitrates from these workers, demonstrating the existence of true physical dependence.
Some clinical trials in angina patients have provided nitroglycerin for about 12 continuous hours of every 24-hour day. During the nitrate-free intervals in some of the trials, angina attacks have been more easily provoked than before treatment, and patients have demonstrated hemodynamic rebound and *decreased* exercise tolerance. The importance of these observations to the routine, clinical use of intravenous nitroglycerin is not known.
Lower concentrations of nitroglycerin increase the potential precision of dosing, but these concentrations increase the total fluid volume that must be delivered to the patient. Total fluid load may be a dominant consideration in patients with compromised function of the heart, liver, and/or kidneys.
Nitrolgycerin infusions should be administered only via a pump that can maintain a constant infusion rate.
Intracoronary injection of nitroglycerin infusions has not been studied.

Laboratory Tests

Because of the propylene glycol content of intravenous nitroglycerin, serum triglyceride assays that rely on glycerol oxidase may give falsely elevated results in patients receiving this medication.

Drug Interactions

The vasodilating effects of nitroglycerin may be additive with those of other vasodilators.
Administration of nitroglycerin infusions through the same infusion set as blood can result in pseudoagglutination and hemolysis. More generally, nitroglycerin in 5% dextrose or sodium chloride 0.9% should not be mixed with any other medication of any kind.
Intravenous nitroglycerin interferes, at least in some patients, with the anticoagulant effect of heparin. In patients receiving intravenous nitroglycerin, concomitant heparin therapy should be guided by frequent measurement of the activated partial thromboplastin time.

Carcinogenesis, Mutagenesis, Impairment of Fertility

Animal carcinogenesis studies with injectable nitroglycerin have not been performed.
Rats receiving up to 434 mg/kg/day of dietary nitroglycerin for 2 years developed dose-related fibrotic and neoplastic changes in liver, including carcinomas, and interstitial cell tumors in testes. At high dose, the incidences of hepatocellular carcinomas in both sexes were 52% vs 0% in controls, and incidences of testicular tumors were 52% vs 8% in controls. Lifetime dietary administration of up to 1058 mg/kg/day of nitroglycerin was not tumorigenic in mice.
Nitroglycerin was weakly mutagenic in Ames tests performed in two different laboratories. There was no evidence of mutagenicity in an in vivo dominant lethal assay with male rats treated with doses up to about 363 mg/kg/day, po, or in vitro cytogenetic tests in rat and dog tissues.
In a three-generation reproduction study, rats received dietary nitroglycerin at doses up to about 434 mg/kg/day for 6 months prior to mating of the F_0 generation with treatment continuing through successive F_1 and F_2 generations. The high dose was associated with decreased feed intake and body weight gain in both sexes at all matings. No specific effect on the fertility of the F_0 generation was seen. Infertility noted in subsequent generations, however, was attributed to increased interstitial cell tissue and aspermatogenesis in the high-dose males. In this three-generation study there was no clear evidence of teratogenicity.

Pregnancy

Pregnancy Category C. Animal teratology studies have not been conducted with nitroglycerin injection. Teratology studies in rats and rabbits, however, were conducted with topically applied nitroglycerin ointment at doses up to 80 mg/kg/day and 240 mg/kg/day, respectively. No toxic effects on dams or fetuses were seen at any dose tested. There are no adequate and well-controlled studies in pregnant women. Nitroglycerin should be given to a pregnant woman only if clearly needed.

Nursing Mothers

It is not known whether nitroglycerin is excreted in human milk. Because many drugs are excreted in human milk, caution should be exercised when NITRO-BID IV is administered to a nursing woman.

Pediatric Use

Safety and effectiveness in pediatric patients have not been established.

ADVERSE REACTIONS

Adverse reactions to NITRO-BID IV (nitroglycerin) are generally dose related, and almost all of these reactions are the result of nitroglycerin's activity as a vasodilator. Headache, which may be severe, is the most commonly reported side effect. Headache may be recurrent with each daily dose, especially at higher doses. Transient episodes of light-headedness, occasionally related to blood pressure changes, may also occur. Hypotension occurs infrequently, but in some patients, it may be severe enough to warrant discontinuation of therapy. Syncope, crescendo angina, and rebound hypertension have been reported but are uncommon.
Allergic reactions to nitroglycerin are also uncommon, and the great majority of those reported have been cases of contact dermatitis or fixed drug eruptions in patients receiving nitroglycerin in ointments or patches. There have been a few reports of genuine anaphylactoid reactions, and these reactions can probably occur in patients receiving nitroglycerin by any route.
Extremely rarely, ordinary doses of organic nitrates have caused methemoglobinemia in normal-seeming patients; for further discussion of its diagnosis and treatment, see OVERDOSAGE.
Data are not available to allow estimation of the frequency of adverse reactions during treatment with nitroglycerin injection.

OVERDOSAGE

Hemodynamic Effects

The ill effects of NITRO-BID IV (nitroglycerin) overdose are generally the result of nitroglycerin's capacity to induce vasodilatation, venous pooling, reduced cardiac output, and hypotension. These hemodynamic changes may have protean manifestations, including increased intracranial pressure, with any or all of the following: persistent throbbing headache, confusion, and moderate fever; vertigo; palpitation; visual disturbances; nausea and vomiting (possibly with colic and even bloody diarrhea); syncope (especially in the upright posture); air hunger and dyspnea, later followed by reduced ventilatory effort; diaphoresis, with the skin either flushed or cold and clammy; heart block and bradycardia; paralysis; coma; seizures; and death.

Laboratory determinations of serum levels of NITRO-BID IV and its metabolites are not widely available, and such determinations have, in any event, no established role in the management of NITRO-BID IV overdose.
No data are available to suggest physiological maneuvers (eg, maneuvers to change the pH of the urine) that might accelerate elimination of nitroglycerin and its active metabolites. Similarly, it is not known which, if any, of these substances can usefully be removed from the body by hemodialysis.
No specific antagonist to the vasodilator effects of NITRO-BID IV is known, and no intervention has been subject to controlled study as a therapy of nitroglycerin overdose. Because the hypotension associated with nitroglycerin overdose is the result of venodilatation and arterial hypovolemia, prudent therapy in this situation should be directed toward increase in central fluid volume. Passive elevation of the patient's legs may be sufficient, but intravenous infusion of normal saline or similar fluid may also be necessary.
The use of epinephrine or other arterial vasoconstrictors in this setting is likely to do more harm than good.
In patients with renal disease or congestive heart failure, therapy resulting in central volume expression is not without hazard.
Treatment of NITRO-BID IV overdose in these patiens may be subtle and difficult, and invasive monitoring may be required.

Methemoglobinemia

Nitrate ions liberated during metabolism of nitroglycerin can oxidize hemoglobin into methemoglobin. Even in patients totally without cytochrome b_5 reductase activity, however, and even assuming that the nitrate moieties of nitroglycerin are quantitatively applied to oxidation of hemoglobin, about 1 mg/kg of nitroglycerin should be required before any of these patients manifests clinically significant (≥10%) methemoglobinemia. In patients with normal reductase function, significant production of methemoglobin should require even larger doses of nitroglycerin. In one study in which 36 patients received 2 to 4 weeks of continuous nitroglycerin therapy at 3.1 to 4.4 mg/h, the average methemoglobin level measured was 0.2%; this was comparable to that observed in parallel patients who received placebo.
Notwithstanding these observations, there are case reports of significant methemoglobinemia in association with moderate overdoses of organic nitrates. None of the affected patients had been thought to be unusually susceptible.
Methemoglobin levels are available from most clinical laboratories. The diagnosis should be suspected in patients who exhibit signs of impaired oxygen delivery despite adequate cardiac output and adequate arterial pO_2. Classically, methemoglobinemic blood is described as chocolate brown, without color change on exposure to air.
When methemoglobinemia is diagnosed, the treatment of choice is methylene blue, 1 to 2 mg/kg intravenously.

DOSAGE AND ADMINISTRATION

NOT FOR DIRECT INTRAVENOUS INJECTION.

NITRO-BID IV (NITROGLYCERIN) IS A CONCENTRATED, POTENT DRUG, WHICH MUST BE DILUTED IN DEXTROSE (5%) INJECTION USP OR SODIUM CHLORIDE (0.9%) INJECTION USP PRIOR TO ITS INFUSION. NITRO-BID IV SHOULD NOT BE MIXED WITH OTHER DRUGS.

1. Initial Dilution:

Aseptically transfer the contents of one NITRO-BID IV vial (containing 25 or 50 mg of nitroglycerin) into a 500-mL *glass* bottle of either dextrose (5%) injection USP or sodium chloride (0.9%) injection USP. This yields a final concentration of 50 mcg/mL or 100 mcg/mL. Diluting 5 mg NITRO-BID IV into 100 mL will also yield a final concentration of 50 mcg/mL.

2. Maintenance Dilution:

It is important to consider the fluid requirements of the patient as well as the expected duration of infusion in selecting the appropriate dilution of NITRO-BID IV (nitroglycerin).
After the initial dosage titration, the concentration of the solution may be increased, if necessary, to limit fluids given to the patient. The NITRO-BID IV concentration should not exceed 400 mcg/mL (See tables).

Dilution Table

Diluent Volume	Quantity of NITRO-BID IV (5 mg/mL)	Approximate Final Concentration
100 mL	10 mg (2 mL)	100 mcg/mL
100 mL	20 mg (4 mL)	200 mcg/mL
100 mL	40 mg (8 mL)	400 mcg/mL
250 mL	25 mg (5 mL)	100 mcg/mL
250 mL	50 mg (10 mL)	200 mcg/mL
250 mL	100 mg (20 mL)	400 mcg/mL
500 mL	50 mg (10 mL)	100 mcg/mL
500 mL	100 mg (20 mL)	200 mcg/mL
500 mL	200 mg (40 mL)	400 mcg/mL

Administration Table
(60 microdrops = 1 milliliter)

Concentration (mcg/mL)	100	200	400
Dose (mcg/min)	Flow Rate (microdrops/min = mL/h)		
5	3	—	—
10	6	3	—
15	9	—	—
20	12	6	3
30	18	9	—
40	24	12	6
60	36	18	9
80	48	24	12
120	72	36	18
160	96	48	24
240	—	72	36
320	—	96	48
480	—	—	72
640	—	—	96

NOTE:
If the concentration is adjusted, it is imperative to flush or replace the infusion set before a new concentration is utilized. If the set is not flushed or replaced, it could take minutes to hours, depending upon the flow rate and the dead space of the set, for the new concentration to reach the patient.

Invert the glass parenteral bottle several times to assure uniform dilution of NITRO-BID IV.
Dosage is affected by the type of container and administration set used. (See WARNINGS.)
Although the usual starting adult dose range reported in clinical studies was 25 mcg/min or more, these studies used PVC administration sets. THE USE OF NONABSORBING TUBING WILL RESULT IN THE NEED FOR REDUCED DOSES.
If a peristaltic action infusion pump is used, an appropriate administration set should be selected with a drip chamber that delivers approximately 60 microdrops/mL. The NITRO-BID IV Dilution and Administration tables may be used to calculate NITRO-BID dilution and flow rate in microdrops/minute to achieve the desired NITRO-BID IV administration rate.
If a volumetric infusion pump is used, the NITRO-BID IV Dilution and Administration table may still be used; however, flow rate will be determined directly by the infusion pump, independent of the drop size of the drip chambers. Thus, the reference to "MICRODROPS/MIN" is not applicable, and the corresponding flow rate in mL/h should be used to determine pump settings.
When using a nonabsorbing infusion set, initial dosage should be 5 mcg/min delivered through an infusion pump capable of exact and constant delivery of the drug. Subsequent titration must be adjusted to the clinical situation, with dose increments becoming more cautious as partial response is seen. Initial titration should be in 5 mcg/min increments, with increases every 3 to 5 minutes until some response is noted. If no response is seen at 20 mcg/min, increments of 10 and later 20 mcg/min can be used. Once a partial blood pressure response is observed, the dose increase should be reduced and the interval between increases should be lengthened.
Some patients with normal or low left ventricular filling pressures or pulmonary capillary wedge pressure (eg, angina patients without other complications) may be hypersensitive to the effects of NITRO-BID IV and may respond fully to doses as small as 5 mcg/min. These patients require especially careful titrating and monitoring.
There is no fixed optimum dose of NITRO-BID IV. Due to variations in the responsiveness of individual patients to the drug, each patient must be titrated to the desired level of hemodynamic function.
Therefore, continuous monitoring of physiologic parameters (ie, blood pressure and heart rate in all patients and other measurements such as pulmonary capillary wedge pressure, as appropriate) MUST be performed to achieve the correct dose. Adequate systemic blood pressure and coronary perfusion pressure must be maintained.
As with all parenteral drug products, NITRO-BID IV should be inspected visually for particulate matter and discoloration prior to administration, whenever solution and container permit.

HOW SUPPLIED

NITRO-BID® IV is supplied in boxes of ten 1-mL vials (NDC 0088-1800-31), each vial containing 5 mg of nitroglycerin (5 mg/mL); ten 5-mL vials (NDC 0088-1800-32), each vial containing 25 mg nitroglycerin (5 mg/mL); and five 10-mL vials (NDC 0088-1800-33), each vial containing 50 mg nitroglycerin (5 mg/mL).
PROTECT FROM LIGHT BY RETAINING PRODUCT IN CARTON UNTIL READY TO USE.
NITRO-BID IV VIALS ARE INTENDED FOR SINGLE-DOSE USE ONLY. PROPERLY DISCARD ANY UNUSED PORTION.
Protect from freezing.
Store at controlled room temperature 20–25°C (68–77°F) [See USP].
Prescribing Information as of January 1997
Manufactured for:
Hoechst Marion Roussel, Inc.
Kansas City, MO 64137 USA

NITRO-BID® OINTMENT 2% ℞

[*ni' trō*-bid]
(nitroglycerin ointment USP)
Prescribing Information as of February 1996

DESCRIPTION

Nitroglycerin is 1,2,3,-propanetriol trinitrate, an organic nitrate whose structural formula is:

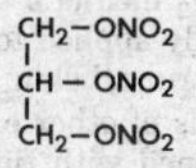

and whose molecular weight is 227.09. The organic nitrates are vasodilators, active on both arteries and veins.
NITRO-BID Ointment contains lactose and 2% nitroglycerin in a base of lanolin and white petrolatum. Each inch (2.5 cm), as squeezed from the tube, contains approximately 15 mg of nitroglycerin.

CLINICAL PHARMACOLOGY

The principal pharmacological action of nitroglycerin is relaxation of vascular smooth muscle and consequent dilatation of peripheral arteries and veins, especially the latter. Dilatation of the veins promotes peripheral pooling of blood and decreases venous return to the heart, thereby reducing left ventricular end-diastolic pressure and pulmonary capillary wedge pressure (preload). Arteriolar relaxation reduces systemic vascular resistance, systolic arterial pressure, and mean arterial pressure (afterload). Dilatation of the coronary arteries also occurs. The relative importance of preload reduction, afterload reduction, and coronary dilatation remains undefined.
Dosing regimens for most chronically used drugs are designed to provide plasma concentrations that are continuously greater than a minimally effective concentration. This strategy is inappropriate for organic nitrates. Several well-controlled clinical trials have used exercise testing to assess the antianginal efficacy of continuously delivered nitrates. In the large majority of these trials, active agents were indistinguishable from placebo after 24 hours (or less) of continuous therapy. Attempts to overcome nitrate tolerance by dose escalation, even to doses far in excess of those used acutely, have consistently failed. Only after nitrates had been absent from the body for several hours was their antianginal efficacy restored.

Pharmacokinetics

The volume of distribution of nitroglycerin is about 3 L/kg, and nitroglycerin is cleared from this volume at extremely rapid rates, with a resulting serum half-life of about 3 minutes. The observed clearance rates (close to 1 L/kg/min) greatly exceed hepatic blood flow; known sites of extrahepatic metabolism include red blood cells and vascular walls. The first products in the metabolism of nitroglycerin are inorganic nitrate and the 1,2- and 1,3-dinitroglycerols. The dinitrates are less effective vasodilators than nitroglycerin but they are longer-lived in the serum, and their net contribution to the overall effect of chronic nitroglycerin regimens is not known. The dinitrates are further metabolized to (nonvasoactive) mononitrates and, ultimately, to glycerol and carbon dioxide.
To avoid development of tolerance to nitrolglycerin, drug-free intervals of 10 to 12 hours are known to be sufficient; shorter intervals have not been well studied. In one well-controlled clinical trial, subjects receiving nitroglycerin appeared to exhibit a rebound or withdrawal effect, so that their exercise tolerance at the end of the daily drug-free interval was less than that exhibited by the parallel group receiving placebo.
Reliable assay techniques for plasma nitroglycerin levels have only recently become available, and studies using

Continued on next page

Nitro-Bid Ointment—Cont.

these techniques to define the pharmacokinetics of nitroglycerin ointment have not been reported. Published studies using older techniques provide results that often differ, in similar experimental settings, by an order of magnitude. The data are consistent, however, in suggesting that nitroglycerin levels rise to a steady state within an hour or so of application of ointment, and that after removal of nitroglycerin ointment, levels wane with a half-life of about half an hour.

The onset of action of transdermal nitroglycerin is not sufficiently rapid for this product to be useful in aborting an acute anginal episode.

The maximal achievable daily duration of antianginal activity provided by nitroglycerin ointment therapy has not been studied. Recent studies of other formulations of nitroglycerin suggest that the maximal achievable daily duration of anti-anginal effect from nitrogylcerin ointment will be about 12 hours.

It is reasonable to believe that the rate and extent of nitroglycerin absorption from ointment may vary with the site and square measure of the skin over which a given dose of ointment is spread, but these relationships have not been adequately studied.

Clinical Trials

Controlled trials have demonstrated that nitroglycerin ointment can effectively reduce exercise-related angina for up to 7 hours after a single application. Doses used in clinical trials have ranged from 1/2 inch (1.3 cm; 7.5 mg) to 2 inches (5.1 cm; 30 mg), typically applied to 36 square inches (232 square centimeters) of truncal skin.

In some controlled trials of other organic nitrate formulations, efficacy has declined with time. Because controlled, long-term trials of nitroglycerin ointment have not been reported, it is not known how the efficacy of NITRO-BID Ointment may vary during extended therapy.

INDICATIONS AND USAGE

Nitroglycerin ointment is indicated for the prevention of angina pectoris due to coronary artery disease. The onset of action of transdermal nitroglycerin is not sufficiently rapid for this product to be useful in aborting an acute anginal episode.

CONTRAINDICATIONS

Allergic reactions to organic nitrates are extremely rare, but they do occur. Nitroglycerin is contraindicated in patients who are allergic to it.

WARNINGS

The benefits of transdermal nitroglycerin in patients with acute myocardial infarction or congestive heart failure have not been established. If one elects to use nitroglycerin in these conditions, careful clinical or hemodynamic monitoring must be used to avoid the hazards of hypotension and tachycardia.

PRECAUTIONS

General

Severe hypotension, particularly with upright posture, may occur with even small doses of nitroglycerin. This drug should, therefore, be used with caution in patients who may be volume depleted or who, for whatever reason, are already hypotensive. Hypotension induced by nitroglycerin may be accompanied by paradoxical bradycardia and increased angina pectoris.

Nitrate therapy may aggravate the angina caused by hypertrophic cardiomyopathy.

As tolerance to other forms of nitroglycerin develops, the effect of sublingual nitroglycerin on exercise tolerance, although still observable, is somewhat blunted.

In industrial workers who have had long-term exposure to unknown (presumably high) doses of organic nitrates, tolerance clearly occurs.

Chest pain, acute myocardial infarction, and even sudden death have occurred during temporary withdrawal of nitrates from these workers, demonstrating the existence of true physical dependence.

Some clinical trials in angina patients have provided nitroglycerin for about 12 continuous hours of every 24-hour day. During the nitrate-free intervals in some of these trials, anginal attacks have been more easily provoked than before treatment, and patients have demonstrated hemodynamic rebound and *decreased* exercise tolerance. The importance of these observations to the routine clinical use of transdermal nitroglycerin is not known.

Information for Patients

Daily headaches sometimes accompany treatment with nitroglycerin. In patients who get these headaches, the headaches are a marker of the activity of the drug. Patients should resist the temptation to avoid headaches by altering the schedule of their treatment with nitroglycerin since loss of headache is likely to be associated with simultaneous loss of antianginal efficacy.

Treatment with nitroglycerin may be associated with lightheadedness on standing, especially just after rising from a recumbent or seated position.

This effect may be more frequent in patients who have also consumed alcohol.

Drug Interactions

The vasodilating effects of nitroglycerin may be additive with those of other vasodilators. Alcohol, in particular, has been found to exhibit additive effects of this variety.

Marked symptomatic orthostatic hypotension has been reported when calcium channel blockers and organic nitrates were used in combination. Dose adjustments of either class of agents may be necessary.

Carcinogenesis, Mutagenesis, and Impairment of Fertility

Studies to evaluate the carcinogenic or mutagenic potential of nitroglycerin have not been performed. Nitroglycerin's effect upon reproductive capacity is similarly unknown.

Pregnancy

Category C. Animal reproduction studies have not been conducted with nitroglycerin. It is also not known whether nitroglycerin can cause fetal harm when administered to a pregnant woman or whether it can affect reproductive capacity. Nitroglycerin should be given to a pregnant woman only if clearly needed.

Nursing Mothers

It is not known whether nitroglycerin is excreted in human milk. Because many drugs are excreted in human milk, caution should be exercised when nitroglycerin is administered to a nursing woman.

Pediatric Use

Safety and effectiveness in pediatric patients have not been established.

ADVERSE REACTIONS

Adverse reactions to nitroglycerin are generally dose-related, and almost all of these reactions are the result of nitroglycerin's activity as a vasodilator. Headache, which may be severe, is the most commonly reported side effect. Headache may be recurrent with each daily dose, especially at higher doses. Transient episodes of light-headedness, occasionally related to blood pressure changes, also may occur. Hypotension occurs infrequently, but in some patients it may be severe enough to warrant discontinuation of therapy. Syncope, crescendo angina, and rebound hypertension have been reported but are uncommon.

Allergic reactions to nitroglycerin are also uncommon, and the great majority of those reported have been cases of contact dermatitis or fixed drug eruptions in patients receiving nitroglycerin in ointments of patches. There have been a few reports of genuine anaphylactoid reactions, and these reactions can probably occur in patients receiving nitroglycerin by any route.

Extremely rarely, ordinary doses of organic nitrates have caused methemoglobinemia in normal-seeming patients; for further discussion of its diagnosis and treatment, see OVERDOSAGE.

Data are not available to allow estimation of the frequency of adverse reactions during treatment with NITRO-BID Ointment.

OVERDOSAGE

Hemodynamic Effects

The ill effects of nitroglycerin overdose are generally the result of nitroglycerin's capacity to induce vasodilation, venous pooling, reduced cardiac output, and hypotension. These hemodynamic changes may have protean manifestations, including increased intracranial pressure, with any or all of the following: persistent throbbing headache, confusion, and moderate fever; vertigo; palpitations; visual disturbances; nausea and vomiting (possibly with colic and even bloody diarrhea); syncope (especially in the upright posture); air hunger and dyspnea, later followed by reduced ventilatory effort: diaphoresis, with the skin either flushed or cold and clammy; heart block and bradycardia; paralysis; coma; seizures; and death.

Laboratory determinations of serum levels of nitroglycerin and its metabolites are not widely available, and such determinations, in any event, have no established role in the management of nitroglycerin overdose.

No data are available to suggest physiological maneuvers (eg, maneuvers to change the pH of the urine) that might accelerate elimination of nitroglycerin and its active metabolites. Similarly, it is not known which, if any, of these substances can usefully be removed from the body by hemodialysis.

No specific antagonist to the vasodilator effects of nitroglycerin is known, and no intervention has been subject to controlled study as a therapy for nitroglycerin overdose. Because the hypotension associated with nitroglycerin overdose is the result of venodilatation and arterial hypovolemia, prudent therapy in this situation should be directed toward increase in central fluid volume. Passive elevation of the patient's legs may be sufficient, but intravenous infusion of normal saline or similar fluid may also be necessary.

The use of epinephrine or other arterial vasoconstrictors in this setting is likely to do more harm than good.

In patients with renal disease or congestive heart failure, therapy resulting in central volume expansion is not without hazard. Treatment of nitroglycerin overdose in these patients may be subtle and difficult, and invasive monitoring may be required.

Methemoglobinemia

Nitrate ions liberated during metabolism of nitroglycerin can oxidize hemoglobin into methemoglobin. Even in patients totally without cytochrome b_5 reductase activity, however, and even assuming that the nitrate moieties of nitroglycerin are quantitatively applied to oxidation of hemoglobin, about 1 mg/kg of nitroglycerin should be required before any of these patients manifests clinically significant ($\geq$10%) methemoglobinemia. In patients with normal reductase function, significant production of methemoglobin should require even larger doses of nitroglycerin. In one study in which 36 patients received 2 to 4 weeks of continuous nitroglycerin therapy at 3.1 to 4.4 mg/hr, the average methemoglobin level measured was 0.2%; this was comparable to that observed in parallel patients who received placebo.

Notwithstanding these observations, there are case reports of significant methemoglobinemia in association with moderate overdoses of organic nitrates. None of the affected patients had been thought to be unusually susceptible.

Methemoglobin levels are available from most clinical laboratories. The diagnosis should be suspected in patients who exhibit signs of impaired oxygen delivery despite adequate cardiac output and adequate arterial pO_2. Classically, methemoglobinemic blood is described as chocolate brown without color change on exposure to air.

When methemoglobinemia is diagnosed, the treatment of choice is methylene blue, 1 to 2 mg/kg intravenously.

DOSAGE AND ADMINISTRATION

As noted above (CLINICAL PHARMACOLOGY), controlled trials have demonstrated that nitroglycerin ointment can effectively reduce exercise-related angina for up to 7 hours after a single application. Doses used in clinical trials have ranged from 1/2 inch (1.3 cm; 7.5 mg) to 2 inches (5.1 cm; 30 mg), typically applied to 36 square inches (232 square centimeters) of truncal skin.

It is reasonable to believe that the rate and extent of nitroglycerin absorption from ointment may vary with the site and square measure of the skin over which a given dose of ointment is spread, but these relationships have not been adequately studied.

Controlled trials with other formulations of nitroglycerin have demonstrated that, if plasma levels are maintained continuously, all antianginal efficacy is lost within 24 hours. This tolerance cannot be overcome by increasing the dose of nitroglycerin. As a result, any regimen of NITRO-BID Ointment administration should include a daily nitrate-free interval. The minimum necessary length of such an interval has not been defined, but studies with other nitroglycerin formulations have shown that 10 to 12 hours is sufficient.

Thus, one appropriate dosing schedule for NITRO-BID Ointment would begin with two daily 1/2-inch (7.5-mg) doses, one applied on rising in the morning and one applied 6 hours later. The dose could be doubled, and even doubled again, in patients tolerating this dose but failing to respond to it.

Each tube of ointment is supplied with a pad of ruled, impermeable paper applicators. These applicators allow ointment to be absorbed through a much smaller area of skin that used in any of the reported clinical trials, and the significance of this difference is not known. To apply the ointment using one of the applicators, place the applicator on a flat surface, printed side down. Squeeze the necessary amount of ointment from the tube onto the applicator, place the applicator (ointment side down) on the desired area of skin, and tape the applicator into place.

HOW SUPPLIED

NITRO-BID® Ointment 2% (nitroglycerin ointment USP) is available in 20-g (NDC 0088-1552-20) and 60-g (NDC 0088-1552-60) tubes and in Unit Dose Identification Paks of 100 1-g foil pouches (NDC 0088-1552-49).

Prescribing Information as of February 1996
Hoechst Marion Roussel, Inc.
Kansas City, MO 64137 USA

NORPRAMIN® ℞

[*nor-pram' in*]
(desipramine hydrochloride tablets USP)

Prescribing Information as of January 1996

DESCRIPTION

NORPRAMIN (desipramine hydrochloride USP) is an antidepressant drug of the tricyclic type, and is chemically: 5*H*-Dibenz[*bf*]azepine-5-propanamine, 10,11- dihydro-*N*-methyl-, monohydrochloride.

[See chemical structure at top of next column]

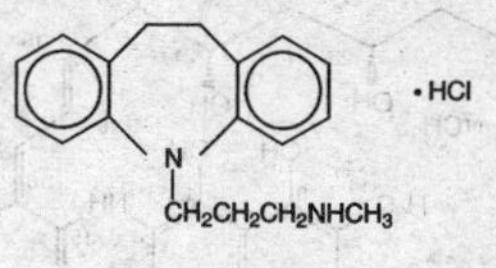

Inactive Ingredients
The following inactive ingredients are contained in all dosage strengths: acacia, calcium carbonate, corn starch, D&C Red No. 30 and D&C Yellow No. 10 (except 10 mg and 150 mg), FD&C Blue No. 1 (except 50 mg, 75 mg, and 100 mg), hydrogenated soy oil, iron oxide, light mineral oil, magnesium stearate, mannitol, polyethylene glycol 8000, pregelatinized corn starch, sodium benzoate (except 150 mg), sucrose, talc, titanium dioxide, and other ingredients.

CLINICAL PHARMACOLOGY

Mechanism of Action
Available evidence suggests that many depressions have a biochemical basis in the form of a relative deficiency of neurotransmitters such as norepinephrine and serotonin. Norepinephrine deficiency may be associated with relatively low urinary 3-methoxy-4-hydroxyphenyl glycol (MHPG) levels, while serotonin deficiencies may be associated with low spinal fluid levels of 5-hydroxyindoleacetic acid.
While the precise mechanism of action of the tricyclic antidepressants is unknown, a leading theory suggests that they restore normal levels of neurotransmitters by blocking the re-uptake of these substances from the synapse in the central nervous system. Evidence indicates that the secondary amine tricyclic antidepressants, including NORPRAMIN, may have greater activity in blocking the re-uptake of norepinephrine. Tertiary amine tricyclic antidepressants, such as amitriptyline, may have greater effect on serotonin re-uptake.
NORPRAMIN (desipramine hydrochloride) is not a monoamine oxidase (MAO) inhibitor and does not act primarily as a central nervous system stimulant. It has been found in some studies to have a more rapid onset of action than imipramine. Earliest therapeutic effects may occasionally be seen in 2 to 5 days, but full treatment benefit usually requires 2 to 3 weeks to obtain.

Metabolism
Tricyclic antidepressants, such as desipramine hydrochloride, are rapidly absorbed from the gastrointestinal tract. Tricyclic antidepressants or their metabolites are to some extent excreted through the gastric mucosa and reabsorbed from the gastrointestinal tract. Desipramine is metabolized in the liver, and approximately 70% is excreted in the urine.
The rate of metabolism of tricyclic antidepressants varies widely from individual to individual, chiefly on a genetically determined basis. Up to a 36-fold difference in plasma level may be noted among individuals taking the same oral dose of desipramine. In general, the elderly metabolize tricyclic antidepressants more slowly than do younger adults.
Certain drugs, particularly the psychostimulants and the phenothiazines, increase plasma levels of concomitantly administered tricyclic antidepressants through competition for the same metabolic enzyme systems. Concurrent administration of cimetidine and tricyclic antidepressants can produce clinically significant increases in the plasma concentrations of the tricyclic antidepressants. Conversely, decreases in plasma levels of the tricyclic antidepressants have been reported upon discontinuation of cimetidine, which may result in the loss of the therapeutic efficacy of the tricyclic antidepressant. Other substances, particularly barbiturates and alcohol, induce liver enzyme activity and thereby reduce tricyclic antidepressant plasma levels. Similar effects have been reported with tobacco smoke.
Research on the relationship of plasma level to therapeutic response with the tricyclic antidepressants has produced conflicting results. While some studies report no correlation, many studies cite therapeutic levels for most tricyclics in the range of 50 to 300 nanograms per milliliter. The therapeutic range is different for each tricyclic antidepressant. For desipramine, an optimal range of therapeutic plasma levels has not been established.

INDICATIONS AND USAGE

NORPRAMIN (desipramine hydrochloride) is indicated for the treatment of depression.

CONTRAINDICATIONS

Desipramine hydrochloride should not be given in conjunction with, or within 2 weeks of, treatment with an MAO inhibitor drug; hyperpyretic crises, severe convulsions, and death have occurred in patients taking MAO inhibitors and tricyclic antidepressants. When NORPRAMIN (desipramie hydrochloride) is substituted for an MAO inhibitor, at least 2 weeks should elapse between treatments. NORPRAMIN should then be started cautiously and should be increased gradually.
The drug is contraindicated in the acute recovery period following myocardial infarction. It should not be used in those who have shown prior hypersensitivity to the drug. Cross-sensitivity between this and other dibenzazepines is a possibility.

WARNINGS

Extreme caution should be used when this drug is given in the following situations:

a. In patients with cardiovascular disease, because of the possibility of conduction defects, arrhythmias, tachycardias, strokes, and acute myocardial infarction.
b. In patients with a history of urinary retention or glaucoma, because of the anticholinergic properties of the drug.
c. In patients with thyroid disease or those taking thyroid medication, because of the possibility of cardiovascular toxicity, including arrhythmias.
d. In patients with a history of seizure disorder, because this drug has been shown to lower the seizure threshold.

This drug is capable of blocking the antihypertensive effect of guanethidine and similarly acting compounds.
The patient should be cautioned that this drug may impair the mental and/or physical abilities required for the performance of potentially hazardous tasks such as driving a car or operating machinery.
In patients who may use alcohol excessively, it should be borne in mind that the potentiation may increase the danger inherent in any suicide attempt or overdosage.

Use in Pregnancy
Safe use of desipramine hydrochloride during pregnancy and lactation has not been established; therefore, if it is to be given to pregnant patients, nursing mothers, or women of childbearing potential, the possible benefits must be weighed against the possible hazards to mother and child. Animal reproductive studies have been inconclusive.

Use in Children
NORPRAMIN (desipramine hydrochloride) is not recommended for use in children since safety and effectiveness in the pediatric age group have not been established. (See ADVERSE REACTIONS, Cardiovascular.)

PRECAUTIONS

General
It is important that this drug be dispensed in the least possible quantities to depressed outpatients, since suicide has been accomplished with this class of drug. Ordinary prudence requires that children not have access to this drug or to potent drugs of any kind; if possible, this drug should be dispensed in containers with child-resistant safety closures. Storage of this drug in the home must be supervised responsibly.
If serious adverse effects occur, dosage should be reduced or treatment should be altered.
NORPRAMIN (desipramine hydrochloride) therapy in patients with manic-depressive illness may induce a hypomanic state after the depressive phase terminates.
The drug may cause exacerbation of psychosis in schizophrenic patients.
Both elevation and lowering of blood sugar levels have been reported.
Leukocyte and differential counts should be performed in any patient who develops fever and sore throat during therapy; the drug should be discontinued if there is evidence of pathologic neutrophil depression.
Clinical experience in the concurrent administration of ECT and antidepressant drugs is limited. Thus, if such treatment is essential, the possibility of increased risk relative to benefits should be considered.
This drug should be discontinued as soon as possible prior to elective surgery because of possible cardiovascular effects. Hypertensive episodes have been observed during surgery in patients taking desipramine hydrochloride.

Drug Interactions
Drugs Metabolized by P450 2D6. The biochemical activity of the drug metabolizing isozyme cytochrome P450 2D6 (debrisoquin hydroxylase) is reduced in a subset of the Caucasian population (about 7% to 10% of Caucasians are so called "poor metabolizers"); reliable estimates of the prevalence of reduced P450 2D5 isozyme activity among Asian, African and other populations are not yet available. Poor metabolizers have higher than expected plasma concentrations of tricyclic antidepressants (TCAs) when given usual doses. Depending on the fraction of drug metabolized by P450 2D6, the increase in plasma concentration may be small, or quite large (8 fold increase in plasma AUC of the TCA).
In addition, certain drugs inhibit the activity of this isozyme and make normal metabolizers resemble poor metabolizers. An individual who is stable on a given dose of TCA may become abruptly toxic when given one of these inhibiting drugs as concomitant therapy. The drugs that inhibit cytochrome P450 2D6 include some that are not metabolized by the enzyme (quinidine; cimetidine) and many that are substrates for P450 2D6 (many other antidepressants, phenothiazines, and the Type 1C antiarrhythmics propafenone and flecainide). While all the selective serotonin reuptake inhibitors (SSRIs), e.g., fluoxetine, sertraline, paroxetine, inhibit P450 2D6, they may vary in the extent of inhibition. The extent to which SSRI TCA interactions may pose clinical problems will depend on the degree of inhibition and the pharmacokinetics of the SSRI involved. Nevertheless, caution is indicated in the co-administration of TCAs with any of the SSRIs and also in switching from one class to the other. Of particular importance, sufficient time must elapse before initiating TCA treatment in a patient withdrawn from fluoxetine, given the long half-life of the parent and active metabolite (at least 5 weeks may be necessary).
Concomitant use of tricyclic antidepressants with drugs that can inhibit cytochrome P450 2D6 may require lower doses than usually prescribed for either the tricyclic antidepressant or the other drug. Furthermore, whenever one of these other drugs is withdrawn from co-therapy, an increased dose of tricyclic antidepressant may be required. It is desirable to monitor TCA plasma levels whenever a TCA is going to be co-administered with another drug known to be an inhibitor of P450 2D6.
Close supervision and careful adjustment of dosage are required when this drug is given concomitantly with anticholinergic or sympathomimetic drugs.
Patients should be warned that while taking this drug their response to alcoholic beverages may be exaggerated.
If NORPRAMIN (desipramine hydrochloride) is to be combined with other psychotropic agents such as tranquilizers or sedative/hypnotics, careful consideration should be given to the pharmacology of the agents employed since the sedative effects of NORPRAMIN and benzodiazepines (e.g., chlordiazepoxide or diazepam) are additive. Both the sedative and anticholinergic effects of the major tranquilizers are also additive to those of NORPRAMIN.

ADVERSE REACTIONS

Included in the following listing are a few adverse reactions that have not been reported with this specific drug. However, the pharmacologic similarities among the tricyclic antidepressant drugs require that each of the reactions be considered when NORPRAMIN (desipramine hydrochloride) is given.
Cardiovascular: hypotension, hypertension, palpitations, heart block, myocardial infarction, stroke, arrhythmias, premature ventricular contractions, tachycardia, ventricular tachycardia, ventricular fibrillation, sudden death
There has been a report of an "acute collapse" and "sudden death" in an 8-year-old (18 kg) male, treated for 2 years for hyperactivity.
There have been additional reports of sudden death in children. (See WARNINGS, Use in Children.)
Psychiatric: confusional states (especially in the elderly) with hallucinations, disorientation, delusions; anxiety, restlessness, agitation; insomnia and nightmares; hypomania; exacerbation of psychosis
Neurologic: numbness, tingling, paresthesias of extremities; incoordination, ataxia, tremors; peripheral neuropathy; extrapyramidal symptoms; seizures; alterations in EEG patterns; tinnitus
Symptoms attributed to Neuroleptic Malignant Syndrome have been reported during desipramine use with and without concomitant neuroleptic therapy.
Anticholinergic: dry mouth, and rarely associated sublingual adenitis; blurred vision, disturbance of accommodation, mydriasis, increased intraocular pressure; constipation, paralytic ileus; urinary retention, delayed micturition, dilation of urinary tract
Allergic: skin rash, petechiae, urticaria, itching, photosensitization (avoid excessive exposure to sunlight), edema (of face and tongue or general), drug fever, cross-sensitivity with other tricyclic drugs
Hematologic: bone marrow depressions including agranulocytosis, eosinophilia, purpura, thrombocytopenia
Gastrointestinal: anorexia, nausea and vomiting, epigastric distress, peculiar taste, abdominal cramps, diarrhea, stomatitis, black tongue, hepatitis, jaundice (simulating obstructive), altered liver function, elevated liver function tests, increased pancreatic enzymes
Endocrine: gynecomastia in the male, breast enlargement and galactorrhea in the female; increased or decreased libido, impotence, painful ejaculation, testicular swelling; elevation or depression of blood sugar levels; syndrome of inappropriate antidiuretic hormone secretion (SIADH)
Other: weight gain or loss; perspiration, flushing; urinary frequency, nocturia; parotid swelling; drowsiness, dizziness, weakness and fatigue, headache; fever; alopecia; elevated alkaline phosphatase
Withdrawal Symptoms: Though not indicative of addiction, abrupt cessation of treatment after prolonged therapy may produce nausea, headache, and malaise.

OVERDOSAGE*

Deaths may occur from overdosage with this class of drugs. Multiple drug ingestion (including alcohol) is common in deliberate tricyclic antidepressant overdose. As the manage-

Continued on next page

Norpramin—Cont.

ment is complex and changing, it is recommended that the physician contact a poison control center for current information on treatment. Signs and symptoms of toxicity develop rapidly after tricyclic antidepressant overdose; therefore, hospital monitoring is required as soon as possible. There is no specific antidote for desipramine overdosage.

* Poisindex®: Toxicologic Management
Topic: Antidepressants, Tricyclic
Micromedex Inc. Vol. 85

Oral LD_{50}

The oral LD_{50} of desipramine is 290 mg/kg in male mice and 320 mg/kg in female rats.

Manifestations of Overdosage

Critical manifestations of overdose include: cardiac dysrhythmias, severe hypotension, convulsions, and CNS depression, including coma. Changes in the electrocardiogram, particularly in QRS axis or width, are clinically significant indicators or tricyclic antidepressant toxicity.

Other signs of overdose may include: confusion, disturbed concentration, transient visual hallucinations, dilated pupils, agitation, hyperactive reflexes, stupor, drowsiness, muscle rigidity, vomiting, hypothermia, hyperpyrexia, or any of the symptoms listed under ADVERSE REACTIONS.

Management

Aggressive supportive care and serum alkalinization are the mainstays of therapy.

General. Obtain an ECG and immediately initiate cardiac monitoring. Protect the patient's airway, establish an intravenous line, and initiate gastric decontamination. A minimum of 6 hours of observation with cardiac monitoring and observation for signs of CNS or respirator depression, hypotension, cardiac dysrhythmias and/or conduction blocks, and seizures is necessary. If signs of toxicity occur at any time during this period, extended monitoring is required. Follow ECG, renal function, CPK, and arterial blood gasses as clinically indicated. There are case reports of patients succumbing to fatal dysrhythmias late after overdose; these patients had clinical evidence of significant poisoning prior to death, and most received inadequate gastrointestinal decontamination. Monitoring of plasma drug levels should not guide management of the patient.

Gastrointestinal Decontamination. All patients suspected of tricyclic antidepressant overdose should receive gastrointestinal decontamination. This should include large volume gastric lavage followed by activated charcoal. If consciousness is impaired, the airway should be secured prior to lavage. Emesis is contraindicated.

Cardiovascular. A maximal limb-lead QRS duration of ≥0.10 seconds may be the best indication of the severity of the overdose. Serum alkalinization, to a pH of 7.45 to 7.55, using intravenous sodium bicarbonate and hyperventilation (as needed) should be instituted for patients with dysrhythmias and/or QRS widening. A pH >7.60 or a pCO_2 <20mm Hg is undesirable. Dysrhythmias unresponsive to sodium bicarbonate therapy/hyperventilation may respond to lidocaine, bretylium or phenytoin. Type IA and IC antiarrhythmics are generally contraindicated (eg, quinidine, disopyramide, and procainamide).

In rare instances, hemoperfusion may be beneficial in acute refractory cardiovascular instability in patients with acute toxicity. However, hemodialysis, peritoneal dialysis, exchange transfusions, and forced diuresis generally have been reported as ineffective in tricyclic antidepressant poisoning.

CNS. In patients with CNS depression, early intubation is advised because of the potential for abrupt deterioration. Seizures should be controlled with benzodiazepines. If these are ineffective or seizures recur, other anticonvulsants (eg, phenobarbital, phenytoin) may be used. Physostigmine is not recommended except to treat life-threatening symptoms that have been unresponsive to other therapies, and then only in consultation with a poison control center.

Psychiatric Follow-up. Since overdosage is often deliberate, patients may attempt suicide by other means during the recovery phase. Psychiatric referral may be appropriate.

Pediatric Management. The principles of management of child and adult overdosages are similar. It is strongly recommended that the physician contact the local poison control center for specific pediatric treatment.

DOSAGE AND ADMINISTRATION

Not recommended for use in children (see WARNINGS).

Lower dosages are recommended for elderly patients and adolescents. Lower dosages are also recommended for outpatients compared to hospitalized patients, who are closely supervised. Dosage should be initiated at a low level and increased according to clinical response and any evidence of intolerance. Following remission, maintenance medication may be required for a period of time and should be at the lowest dose that will maintain remission.

Usual Adult Dose

The usual adult dose is 100 to 200 mg per day. In more severely ill patients, dosage may be further increased gradually to 300 mg/day if necessary. Dosages above 300 mg/day are not recommended.

Dosage should be initiated at a lower level and increased according to tolerance and clinical response.

Treatment of patients requiring as much as 300 mg should generally be initiated in hospitals, where regular visits by the physician, skilled nursing care, and frequent electrocardiograms (ECGs) are available.

The best available evidence of impending toxicity from very high doses of NORPRAMIN is prolongation of the QRS or QT intervals on the ECG. Prolongation of the PR interval is also significant, but less closely correlated with plasma levels. Clinical symptoms of intolerance, especially drowsiness, dizziness, and postural hypotension, should also alert the physician to the need for reduction in dosage. Plasma desipramine measurement would constitute the optimal guide to dosage monitoring.

Initial therapy may be administered in divided doses or a single daily dose.

Maintenance therapy may be given on a once-daily schedule for patient convenience and compliance.

Adolescent and Geriatric Dose

The usual adolescent and geriatric dose is 25 to 100 mg daily.

Dosage should be initiated at a lower level and increased according to tolerance and clinical response to a usual maximum of 100 mg daily. In more severely ill patients, dosage may be further increased to 150 mg/day. Doses above 150 mg/day are not recommended in these age groups.

Initial therapy may be administered in divided doses or a single daily dose.

Maintenance therapy may be given on a once-daily schedule for patient convenience and compliance.

HOW SUPPLIED

10 mg blue coated tablets imprinted 68-7
NDC 0068-0007-01: bottles of 100

25 mg yellow coated tablets imprinted NORPRAMIN 25
NDC 0068-0011-01: bottles of 100
NDC 0068-0011-61: unit dose dispenser of 100

50 mg green coated tablets imprinted NORPRAMIN 50
NDC 0068-0015-01: bottles of 100
NDC 0068-0015-61: unit dose dispenser of 100

75 mg orange coated tablets imprinted NORPRAMIN 75
NDC 0068-0019-01: bottles of 100

100 mg peach coated tablets imprinted NORPRAMIN 100
NDC 0068-0020-01: bottles of 100

150 mg white coated tablets imprinted NORPRAMIN 150
NDC 0068-0021-50: bottles of 50

NORPRAMIN tablets should be stored at room temperature, preferably below 86°F (30°C). Protect from excessive heat.

Prescribing Information as of January 1996
Merrell Pharmaceuticals Inc.
Subsidiary of Hoechst Marion Roussel, Inc.
Kansas City, MO 64137 USA

Shown in Product Identification Guide, page 316

PRIFTIN® ℞

[prĭf-tĭn]
(rifapentine)
150 mg Tablets

Prescribing Information as of June 1998

DESCRIPTION

PRIFTIN® (rifapentine) for oral administration contains 150 mg of the active ingredient rifapentine per tablet.

The 150 mg tablets also contain, as inactive ingredients: calcium stearate, disodium EDTA, FD&C Blue No. 2 aluminum lake, hydroxypropyl cellulose, hydroxypropyl methylcellulose, microcrystalline cellulose, polyethylene glycol, pregelatinized starch, propylene glycol, sodium ascorbate, sodium lauryl sulfate, sodium starch glycolate, synthetic red iron oxide, and titanium dioxide. Rifapentine is a rifamycin derivative antibiotic and has a similar profile of microbiological activity to rifampin (rifampicin). The molecular weight is 877.04.

The molecular formula is $C_{47}H_{64}N_4O_{12}$.

The chemical name for rifapentine is rifamycin, 3-[[(4-cyclopentyl-1-piperazinyl)imino]methyl]- or 3-[N-(4-Cyclopentyl-1-piperazinyl)formimidoyl] rifamycin or 5,6,9,17,19,21-hexahydroxy-23-methoxy-2,4,12,16,18,20,22-heptamethyl-8-[N-(4-cyclopentyl-l-piperazinyl)-formimidoyl]-2,7-(epoxypentadeca[1,11,13]trienimino)naphtho[2,1-b]furan-1,11(2H)-dione 21-acetate. It has the following structure:

[See chemical structure at top of next column]

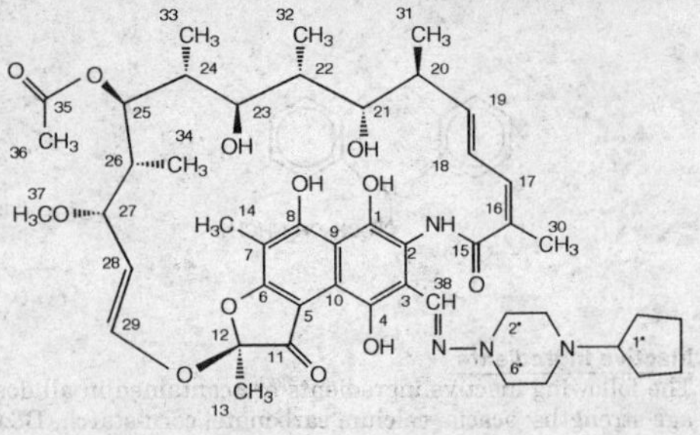

ACTIONS/CLINICAL PHARMACOLOGY

Pharmacokinetics

Absorption

The absolute bioavailability of rifapentine has not been determined. The relative bioavailability (with an oral solution as a reference) of rifapentine after a single 600 mg dose to healthy adult volunteers was 70%. The maximum concentrations were achieved from 5 to 6 hours after administration of the 600 mg rifapentine dose. Food (850 total calories: 33 g protein, 55 g fat and 58 g carbohydrate) increased AUC (0–∞) and C_{max} by 43% and 44%, respectively over that observed when administered under fasting conditions. When oral doses of rifapentine were administered once daily or once every 72 hours to healthy volunteers for 10 days, single dose AUC (0–∞) value of rifapentine was similar to its steady-state AUC_{ss} (0–24h) or AUC_{ss} (0–72h) values, suggesting no significant auto-induction effect on steady-state pharmacokinetics of rifapentine. Steady-state conditions were achieved by day 10 following daily administration of rifapentine 600 mg. The pharmacokinetic characteristics of rifapentine and 25-desacetyl rifapentine (active metabolite) on day 10 following oral administration of 600 mg rifapentine every 72 hours to healthy volunteers are contained in the following table.

[See table below]

Distribution

In a population pharmacokinetic analysis in 351 tuberculosis patients who received 600 mg rifapentine in combination with isoniazid, pyrazinamide and ethambutol, the estimated apparent volume of distribution was 70.2 ± 9.1 L. In healthy volunteers, rifapentine and 25-desacetyl rifapentine were 97.7% and 93.2% bound to plasma proteins, respectively. Rifapentine was mainly bound to albumin. Similar extent of protein binding was observed in healthy volunteers, asymptomatic HIV-infected subjects and hepatically impaired subjects.

Metabolism/Excretion

Following a single 600 mg oral dose of radiolabelled rifapentine to healthy volunteers (n=4), 87% of the total ^{14}C rifapentine was recovered in the urine (17%) and feces (70%). Greater than 80% of the total ^{14}C rifapentine dose was excreted from the body within 7 days. Rifapentine was hydrolyzed by an esterase enzyme to form a microbiologically active 25-desacetyl rifapentine. Rifapentine and 25-desacetyl rifapentine accounted for 99% of the total radioactivity in plasma. Plasma AUC(0-∞) and C_{max} values of the 25-desacetyl rifapentine metabolite were one-half and one-third those of the rifapentine, respectively. Based upon relative in vitro activities and AUC(0-∞) values, rifapentine and 25-desacetyl rifapentine potentially contributes 62% and 38% to the clinical activities against *M tuberculosis*, respectively.

Special Populations

Gender: In a population pharmacokinetics analysis of sparse blood samples obtained from 351 tuberculosis patients who received 600 mg rifapentine in combination with isoniazid, pyrazinamide and ethambutol, the estimated apparent oral clearance of rifapentine for males and females was 2.51 ± 0.14 L/h and 1.69 ± 0.41 L/h, respectively. The clinical significance of the difference in the estimated apparent oral clearance is not known.

Elderly: Following oral administration of a single 600 mg dose of rifapentine to elderly (≥65 years) male healthy volunteers (n=14), the pharmacokinetics of rifapentine and 25-desacetyl metabolite were similar to that observed for young (18 to 45 years) healthy male volunteers (n=20).

Pediatric (Adolescents): In a pharmacokinetics study of rifapentine in healthy adolescents (age 12 to 15), 600 mg rifapentine was administered to those weighing ≥45 kg

Parameter	Rifapentine	25-desacetyl Rifapentine
	Mean ± SD (n=12)	
C_{max} (μg/mL)	15.05 ± 4.62	6.26 ± 2.06
AUC (0–72) (μg*h/mL)	319.54 ± 91.52	215.88 ± 85.96
$T_{1/2}$ (h)	13.19 ± 1.38	13.35 ± 2.67
T_{max} (h)	4.83 ± 1.80	11.25 ± 2.73
Clpo (L/h)	2.03 ± 0.60	–

(n=10) and 450 mg was administered to those weighing <45 kg (n=2). The pharmacokinetics of rifapentine were similar to those observed in healthy adults.

Renal Impaired Patients: The pharmacokinetics of rifapentine have not been evaluated in renal impaired patients. Although only about 17% of an administered dose is excreted via the kidneys, the clinical significance of impaired renal function on the disposition of rifapentine and its 25-desacetyl metabolite is not known.

Hepatic Impaired Patients: Following oral administration of a single 600 mg dose of rifapentine to mild to severe hepatic impaired patients (n=15), the pharmacokinetics of rifapentine and 25-desacetyl metabolite were similar in patients with various degrees of hepatic impairment and to that observed in another study for healthy volunteers (n=12). Since the elimination of these agents are primarily via the liver, the clinical significance of impaired hepatic function on the disposition of rifapentine and its 25-desacetyl metabolite is not known.

Asymptomatic HIV-Infected Volunteers: Following oral administration of a single 600 mg dose of rifapentine to asymptomatic HIV-infected volunteers (n=15) under fasting conditions, mean C_{max} and AUC(0–∞) of rifapentine were lower (20–32%) than that observed in other studies in healthy volunteers (n=55). In a cross-study comparison, mean C_{max} and AUC values of the 25-desacetyl metabolite of rifapentine, when compared to healthy volunteers were higher (6–21%) in one study (n=20), but lower (15–16%) in a different study (n=40). The clinical significance of this observation is not known. Food (850 total calories: 33 g protein, 55 g fat, and 58 g carbohydrate) increases the mean AUC and C_{max} of rifapentine observed under fasting conditions in asymptomatic HIV-infected volunteers by about 51% and 53%, respectively.

Microbiology

Mechanism of Action

Rifapentine, a cyclopentyl rifamycin, inhibits DNA-dependent RNA polymerase in susceptible strains of *Mycobacterium tuberculosis* but not in mammalian cells. At therapeutic levels, rifapentine exhibits bactericidal activity against both intracellular and extracellular *M. tuberculosis* organisms. Both rifapentine and the 25-desacetyl metabolite accumulate in human monocyte-derived macrophages with intracellular/extracellular ratios of approximately 24:1 and 7:1, respectively.

Resistance Development

In the treatment of tuberculosis (see INDICATIONS AND USAGE), a small number of resistant cells present within large populations of susceptible cells can rapidly become predominant. Rifapentine resistance development in *M. tuberculosis* strains is principally due to one of several single point mutations that occur in the rpoB portion of the gene coding for the beta subunit of the DNA-dependent RNA polymerase. The incidence of rifapentine resistant mutants in an otherwise susceptible population of *M. tuberculosis* strains is approximately one in 10^7 to 10^8 bacilli. Due to the potential for resistance development to rifapentine, appropriate susceptibility tests should be performed in the event of persistently positive cultures.

M. tuberculosis organisms resistant to other rifamycins are likely to be resistant to rifapentine. A high level of cross resistance between rifampin and rifapentine has been demonstrated with *M. tuberculosis* strains. Cross resistance does not appear between rifapentine and non-rifamycin antimycobacterial agents such as isoniazid streptomycin.

In Vitro Activity of Rifapentine against *M. tuberculosis*

Rifapentine and its 25-desacetyl metabolite have demonstrated in vitro activity against rifamycin-susceptible strains of *Mycobacterium tuberculosis* including cidal activity against phagocytized *M. tuberculosis* organisms grown in activated human macrophages.

In vitro results indicate that rifapentine MIC values for *M. tuberculosis* organisms are influenced by study conditions. Rifapentine MIC values were substantially increased employing egg-based medium compared to liquid or agar-based solid media. The addition of Tween 80 in these assays has been shown to lower MIC values for rifamycin compounds. In mouse infection studies a therapeutic effect, in terms of enhanced survival time or reduction of organ bioburden, has been observed in *M. tuberculosis*-infected animals treated with various intermittent rifapentine-containing regimens. Animal studies have shown that the activity of rifapentine is influenced by dose and frequency of administration.

Susceptibility testing for *Mycobacterium tuberculosis*

Breakpoints to determine whether clinical isolates of *M. tuberculosis* are susceptible or resistant to rifapentine have not been established. The clinical relevance of rifapentine in vitro susceptibility test results for other mycobacterial species has not been determined.

CLINICAL TRIALS

A total of 722 patients were enrolled in Clinical Study 008, an open label, prospective, randomized, parallel group, active controlled trial, for the treatment of pulmonary tuberculosis. This population was mostly comprised of Black (>60%) or Multiracial (>31%) patients and the mean ± stan-

Table 2-1. Dose of Rifapentine, Rifampin, Isoniazid, Pyrazinamide, and Ethambutol

Rifapentine Combination Treatment

Intensive Phase	Rifapentine (mg)	Isoniazid (mg)	Pyrazinamide (mg)	Ethambutol* (mg)
	Twice Weekly	Daily	Daily	Daily
Patient Weight				
<50 kg	600	300	1500	800
≥50 kg	600	300	2000	1200
Continuation Phase	Rifapentine (mg)	Isoniazid (mg)		
	Once Weekly	Once Weekly		
Patient Weight				
<50 kg	600	600		
≥50 kg	600	900		

Rifampin Combination Treatment

Intensive Phase	Rifampin (mg)	Isoniazid (mg)	Pyrazinamide (mg)	Ethambutol (mg)
	Daily	Daily	Daily	Daily
Patient Weight				
<50 kg	450	300	1500	800
≥50 kg	600	300	2000	1200
Continuation Phase	Rifampin (mg)	Isoniazid (mg)		
	Twice Weekly	Twice Weekly		
Patient Weight				
<50 kg	450	600		
≥50 kg	600	900		

*Ethambutol was to be discontinued once baseline susceptibility test results were available

dard deviation age was 37 ± 11 years. Treatment groups were comparable with respect to age and race. The percentage of male patients was higher in the rifapentine combination group (80%) than in the rifampin combination group (73%). The study was divided into two phases on the basis of dosing frequency. For the first phase, designated as the Intensive Phase, 361 patients were randomized to receive rifapentine, isoniazid, pyrazinamide, and ethambutol for 60 days and 361 patients were randomized to receive rifampin, isoniazid, pyrazinamide, and ethambutol for 60 days. (Ethambutol was to be discontinued once baseline susceptibility test results were available.) Rifapentine and isoniazid were each administered at a fixed dose regardless of body weight. Rifampin, pyrazinamide, and ethambutol were administered based on body weight according to Table 2-1. **Note:** All drugs were administered *daily* in the Intensive Phase **except for rifapentine** which was administered twice weekly. During the second phase, designated as the Continuation Phase, 317 patients who had received rifapentine in the Intensive Phase continued to receive rifapentine and isoniazid once weekly for up to 120 days. Three hundred four patients who had received rifampin in the Intensive Phase continued to receive rifampin and isoniazid during the Continuation Phase twice weekly for up to 120 days. Rifampin and isoniazid were administered based on body weight according to Table 2-1.

Patients in either treatment group were scheduled to receive study drug over a 180-day period with a subsequent 24-month follow-up. Additionally, both treatment groups received pyridoxine (Vitamin B_6) over the 180-day treatment period.

The indication for treatment of pulmonary tuberculosis with PRIFTIN is based on the 6 month follow-up treatment outcome observed in Clinical Study 008 as a surrogate for the 2 year follow-up generally accepted as evidence of efficacy in the treatment of pulmonary tuberculosis.

[See table 2-1 above]

Table 2-2 presents clinical outcome in Study 008.

[See table 2-2 at top of next page]

Risk of relapse was higher in the rifapentine regimen. During the Intensive Phase of treatment the rate of noncompliance with companion medications was somewhat higher for the rifapentine regimen than for the rifampin regimen. Most of the relapses occurred among those with poor compliance with these companion medications and this group also had the largest risk of relapse for the rifapentine regimen relative to the rifampin regimen. This factor appears to explain most, but not all, of the higher relapse rate observed in the rifapentine arm. Failure to convert sputum after two months of treatment (ie, end of Intensive Phase) was associated with a greater risk of relapse for both treatment regi-

mens. Relapse rates were also higher for males in both regimens. Relapse in the rifapentine group was not associated with development of mono-resistance to rifampin.

In vitro susceptibility testing was conducted against initial and subsequent *M. tuberculosis* isolates recovered from 620 patients enrolled in the study. Rifapentine and rifampin MIC values were determined employing the radiometric susceptibility testing method utilizing 7H12 broth at pH 6.8 (NCCLS procedure M24-T). Six hundred and fourteen patients with rifampin susceptible (MIC ≤0.5 µg/ml) strains of *M. tuberculosis* had rifapentine MICs of ≤0.125 µg/ml. The remaining six patients with rifampin resistant (MIC > 8.0 µg/ml). *M. tuberculosis* isolates had rifapentine MICs of >8.0 µg/ml. Four of these represented baseline values for patients with multiresistant tuberculosis. One rifampin resistant isolate was from a rifapentine relapse patient while the remaining isolate was from a rifampin relapse patient. Restriction fragment length polymorphism (RFLP) studies showed the rifapentine relapse isolate to be genetically different from the baseline strain while RFLP data on the matched rifampin isolate is pending. This information is provided for comparative purposes only as rifapentine breakpoints have not been established.

INDICATIONS AND USAGE

PRIFTIN is indicated for the treatment of pulmonary tuberculosis. This indication is based on the 6 month follow-up treatment outcome observed in the controlled clinical trial as a surrogate for the 2 year follow-up generally accepted as evidence of efficacy in the treatment of pulmonary tuberculosis. PRIFTIN must always be used in conjunction with at least one other antituberculosis drug to which the isolate is susceptible. In the intensive phase of the short-course treatment of pulmonary tuberculosis, **PRIFTIN should be administered twice weekly for two months,** with an interval of no less than 3 days (72 hours) between doses, as part of an appropriate regimen which includes daily companion drugs (Table 2-1). It may also be necessary to add either streptomycin or ethambutol until the results of susceptibility testing are known. *Compliance with all drugs in the Intensive Phase (ie, PRIFTIN, isoniazid, pyrazinamide, ethambutol or streptomycin) is imperative to assure early sputum conversion and protection against relapse.* Following the intensive phase, Continuation Phase treatment should be continued with PRIFTIN for 4 months. **During this phase, PRIFTIN should be administered on a once-weekly basis** in combination with an appropriate antituberculous agent for susceptible organisms (Table 2-1) (see DOSAGE AND ADMINISTRATION section).

In the treatment of tuberculosis, the small number of resistant cells present within large populations of susceptible

Continued on next page

Priftin—Cont.

cells can rapidly become the predominant type. Consequently, clinical samples for mycobacterial culture and susceptibility testing should be obtained prior to the initiation of therapy, as well as during treatment to monitor therapeutic response. The susceptibility of *M. tuberculosis* organisms to isoniazid, rifampin, pyrazinamide, ethambutol, rifapentine and other appropriate agents should be measured. If test results show resistance to any of these drugs and the patient is not responding to therapy, the drug regimen should be modified.

Table 2-2. Clinical Outcome in Study 008*

	Rifapentine Combination	Rifampin Combination
Status at End of Treatment		
Converted	87% (249/286)	81% (229/284)
Not Converted	1% (4/286)	3% (8/284)
Lost to Follow-up	12% (33/286)	17% (47/284)
Status in Follow-up:		
Relapsed	10% (25/249)	5% (11/229)
Sputum negative, Still being followed	81% (201/249)	90% (205/229)
Lost to Follow-up	9% (23/249)	6% (13/229)

* All data through 8 July 1997 for patients with confirmed susceptible MTB (rifapentine combination, n=286; rifampin combination, n=284).

CONTRAINDICATIONS

This product is contraindicated in patients with a history of hypersensitivity to any of the rifamycins (eg, rifampin and rifabutin).

WARNINGS

Poor compliance with the dosage regimen, particularly the daily administered non-rifamycin drugs in the Intensive Phase, was associated with late sputum conversion and a high relapse rate in the rifapentine arm of Clinical Study 008. Therefore, compliance with the full course of therapy must be emphasized, and the importance of not missing any doses must be stressed. (See PRECAUTIONS and DOSAGE AND ADMINISTRATION.)

Since antituberculosis multidrug treatments, including the rifamycin class, are associated with serious hepatic events, patients with abnormal liver tests and/or liver disease should only be given rifapentine in cases of necessity and then with caution and under strict medical supervision. In these patients, careful monitoring of liver tests (especially serum transaminases) should be carried out prior to therapy and then every 2 to 4 weeks during therapy. If signs of liver disease occur or worsen, rifapentine should be discontinued.

Hyperbilirubinemia resulting from competition for excretory pathways between rifapentine and bilirubin cannot be excluded since competition between the related drug rifampin and bilirubin can occur. An isolated report showing a moderate rise in bilirubin and/or transaminase level is not in itself an indication for interrupting treatment; rather, the decision should be made after repeating the tests, noting trends in the levels and considering them in conjunction with the patient's clinical condition. Pseudomembranous colitis has been reported to occur with various antibiotics, including other rifamycins. Diarrhea, particularly if severe and/or persistent, occurring during treatment or in the initial weeks following treatment may be symptomatic of *Clostridium difficile*-associated disease, the most severe form of which is pseudomembranous colitis. If pseudomembranous colitis is suspected, rifapentine should be stopped immediately and the patient should be treated with supportive and specific treatment without delay (eg, oral vancomycin). Products inhibiting peristalsis are contraindicated in this clinical situation.

Experience in HIV-infected patients is limited. In an ongoing CDC TB trial, five out of 30 HIV-infected patients randomized to once weekly rifapentine (plus INH) in the Continuation Phase who completed treatment, relapsed. Four of these patients developed rifampin mono-resistant (RMR) TB. Each RMR patient had late-stage HIV infection, low CD4 counts and extrapulmonary disease, and documented co-administration of antifungal azoles. These findings are consistent with the literature in which an emergence of RMR TB in HIV-infected TB patients has been reported in recent years. Further study in this sub-population is warranted. As with other antituberculous treatments, when rifapentine is used in HIV-infected patients, a more aggressive regimen should be employed (eg, more frequent dosing). Based on results to date of the CDC trial (see above), once weekly dosing during the Continuation Phase of treatment is not recommended at this time.

Because rifapentine has been shown to increase indinavir metabolism (see DRUG INTERACTIONS), it should be used with extreme caution, if at all, in patients who are also taking protease inhibitors.

PRECAUTIONS

General

Rifapentine may produce a predominately red-orange discoloration of body tissues and/or fluids (eg, skin, teeth, tongue, urine, fecces, saliva, sputum, tears, sweat, and cerebrospinal fluid).

Contact lenses may become permanently stained.

Information for Patients

The patient should be told that PRIFTIN may produce a reddish coloration of the urine, sweat, sputum, and tears, and the patient should be forewarned that contact lenses may be permanently stained. The patient should be advised that the reliability of oral or other systemic hormonal contraceptives may be affected; consideration should be given to using alternative contraceptive measures. For those patients with a propensity to nausea, vomiting, or gastrointestinal upset, administration of PRIFTIN with food may be useful. Patients should be instructed to notify their physician promptly if they experience any of the following: fever, loss of appetite, malaise, nausea and vomiting, darkened urine, yellowish discoloration of the skin and eyes, and pain or swelling of the joints.

Compliance with the full course of therapy must be emphasized, and the importance of not missing any doses of the daily administered companion medications in the Intensive Phase must be stressed. (see DOSAGE AND ADMINISTRATION and WARNINGS).

Laboratory Tests

Adults treated for tuberculosis with rifapentine should have baseline measurements of hepatic enzymes, bilirubin, a complete blood count, and a platelet count (or estimate). Patients should be seen at least monthly during therapy and should be specifically questioned concerning symptoms associated with adverse reactions. All patients with abnormalities should have follow-up, including laboratory testing, if necessary. Routine laboratory monitoring for toxicity in people with normal baseline measurements is generally not necessary.

Therapeutic concentrations of rifampin have been shown to inhibit standard microbiological assays for serum folate and Vitamin B_{12}. Similar drug-laboratory interactions should be considered for rifapentine; thus, alternative assay methods should be considered.

Drug Interaction

Rifapentine-Indinavir Interaction: In a study in which 600 mg rifapentine was administered twice weekly for 14 days followed by rifapentine twice weekly plus 800 mg indinavir 3 times a day for an additional 14 days, indinavir C_{max} decreased by 55% while AUC reduced by 70%. Clearance of indinavir increased by 3-fold in the presence of rifapentine while half-life did not change. But when indinavir was administered for 14 days followed by coadministration with rifapentine for an additional 14 days, indinavir did not affect the pharmacokinetics of rifapentine. **Rifpentine should be used with extreme caution, it at all, in patients who are also taking protease inhibitors.** (See WARNINGS and DOSAGE AND ADMINISTRATION.) (See Reference 1.)

Rifapentine is an inducer of cytochromes P4503A4 and P4502C8/9. Therefore, rifapentine may increse the metabolism of other coadministered durgs that are metabolized by these enzymes. Induction of enzyme activities by rifapentine occurred within 4 days after the first dose. Enzyme activities returned to baseline levels 14 days after discontinuing rifapentine. In addition, the magnitude of enzyme induction by rifapentine was dose and dosing frequency dependent; less enzyme induction occurred when 600 mg oral doses of rifapentine were given once every 72 hours versus daily. In vitro and in vivo enzyme induction studies have suggested rifapentine induction potential may be less than rifampin but more potent than rifabutin. Rifampin has been reported to accelerate the metabolism and may reduce the activity of the following drugs; hence, rifapentine may also increase the metabolism and decrease the activity of these drugs. Dosage adjustments of the following drugs or of drugs metabolized by cytochrome P4503A4 or P4502C8/9 may be necesary if they are given concurrently with rifapentine. Patients using oral or other systemic hormonal contraceptives should be advised to change to nonhormonal methods of birth control.

Anticonvulsants: eg, phenytoin
Antiarrrhythmics: eg, disopyramide, mexiletine, quinidine, tocainide
Antibiotics: eg, chloramphenicol, clarithromycin, dapsone, doxycycline, fluoroquinolones (such as ciprofloxacin)
Oral antiacoagulants: eg, warfarin
Antifungals: eg, fluconazole, itraconazole, ketoconazole
Barbiturates
Benzodiazepines: eg, diazepam
Beta-blockers, calcium channel blockers: eg, diltiazem, nifedipine, verapamil
Corticosteroids
Cardiac glycoside preparations
Clofibrate
Oral or other systemic hormonal contraceptives
Haloperidol
HIV protease inhibitors: eg, indinavir, ritonavir, nelfinavir, saquinavir (see Rifapentine-Indinavir Interaction above)
Oral hypoglycemic agents: eg, sulfonylureas
Immunosuppressants: eg, cyclosporine, tacrolimus
Levothyroxine
Narcotic analgesics: eg, methadone
Progestins
Quinine
Reverse transcriptase inhibitors: eg, delavirdine, zidovudine
Sildenafil
Theophylline
Tricyclic antidepressants: eg, amitriptyline, nortriptyline

The conversion of rifapentine to 25-desacetyl rifapentine is mediated by an esterase enzyme. There is minimal potential for rifapentine metabolism to be inhibited or induced by another drug, or for rifapentine to inhibit the metabolism of another drug based upon the characteristics of the esterase enzymes. Rifapentine does not induce its own metabolism. Since rifapentine is highly bound to albumin, drug displacement interactions may also occur.

In Clinical Study 008 patients were advised to take rifapentine at least 1 hour before or 2 hours after ingestion of antacids.

Carcinogenesis, Mutagenesis, Impairment of Fertility

Carcinogenicity studies with rifapentine have not been completed. Rifapentine was negative in the following genotoxicity tests: in vitro gene mutation assay in bacteria (Ames test); in vitro point mutation test in *Aspergillus nidulans*; in vitro gene conversion assay in *Saccharomyces cerevisiae*; host-mediated (mouse) gene conversion assay with *Saccharomyces cerevisiae*; in vitro Chinese hamster ovary cell/hypoxanthine-guanine-phosphoribosyl transferase (CHO/HGPRT) forward mutation assay; in vitro chromosomal aberration assay utilizing rat lymphocytes; and in vivo mouse bone marrow micronucleus assay. Fertility and reproductive performance were not affected by oral administration of rifapentine to male and female rats at doses of up to one-third of the human dose (based on body surface area conversions).

Pregnancy Category C

Teratogenic Effects

Rifapentine has been shown to be teratogenic in rats and rabbits. In rats, when given in doses 0.6 times the human dose (based on body surface area comparisons) during the period of organogenesis, pups showed cleft palates, right aortic arch and increased incidence of delayed ossification and increased number of ribs. Rabbits treated with drug at doses between 0.3 and 1.3 times the human dose (based on body surface area comparison) displayed major malformations including ovarian agenesis, pes varus, arhinia, microphthalmia and irregularities of the ossified facial tissues (4 of 321 examined fetuses).

Nonteratogenic Effects

In rats, rifapentine administration was associated with increased resorption rate and post implantation loss, decreased mean fetus weight, increased number of stillborn pups and slightly increased mortality during lactation. Rabbits given 1.3 times the human dose (based on body surface area comparisons) showed higher post-implantation losses and an increased incidence of stillborn pups.

When rifapentine was administered at 0.3 times the human dose (based on body surface area comparisons) to mated female rats late in gestation (from day 15 of gestation to day 21 postpartum), pup weights and gestational survival (live pups born/pups born) were reduced compared to controls.

Pregnancy—Human Experience

There are no adequate and well-controlled studies in pregnant women. In Clinical Study 008, six patients randomized to rifapentine became pregnant; two had normal deliveries; two had first trimester spontaneous abortions, one had an elective abortion and one patient was lost to follow-up. Of the two patients who spontaneously aborted, co-morbid conditions of ethanol abuse in one and HIV infection in the other were noted.

When administered during the last few weeks of pregnancy, rifampin can cause postnatal hemorrhages in the mother and infant for which treatment with Vitamin K may be indicated. Thus, patients and infants who receive rifapentine during the last few weeks of pregnancy should have appropriate clotting parameters evaluated.

Rifapentine should be used during pregnancy only if the potential benefit justifies the potential risk to the fetus.

Nursing Mothers

It is not known whether rifapentine is excreted in human milk. Because many drugs are excreted in human milk and because of the potential for serious adverse reactions in

nursing infants, a decision should be made whether to discontinue nursing or discontinue the drug, taking into account the importance of the drug to the mother.

Pediatric Use

The safety and effectiveness of rifapentine in pediatric patients under the age of 12 have not been established. A pharmacokinetic study was conducted in 12- to 15-year-old healthy volunteers. (See ACTIONS/CLINICAL PHARMACOLOGY Special Populations for pharmacokinetic information).

ADVERSE REACTIONS

The investigators in the tuberculosis treatment clinical trial (Study 008) assessed the causality of adverse events as definitely, probably, possibly, unlikely or not related to one of the two drug regimens teted. The following table (Table 2-3) presents treatment-related adverse events deemed by the investigators to be at least possibly related to any of the four drugs in the regimens (rifapentine/rifampin, isoniazid, pyrazinamide, or ethambutol) which occurred in ≥1% of patients. Hyperuricemia was the most frequently reported event that was assessed as treatment related and was most likely related to the pyrazinamide since no cases were reported in the Continuation Phase when this drug was no longer included in the treatment regimen.

[See table 2-3 above]

Treatment-related adverse events of moderate or severe intensity in <1% of the rifapentine combination therapy patients in Study 008 are presented below by body system.

Hepatic & Biliary: bilirubinemia, hepatitis

Dermatologic: urticaria, skin discoloration

Hematologic: thrombocytopenia, neutrophilia, leukocytosis, purpura, hematoma

Metabolic & Nutritional: hyperkalemia, hypovolemia, alkaline phosphatase increased, LDH increased

Body as a Whole – General: peripheral edema, fatigue

Gastrointestinal: constipation, esophagitis, gastritis, pancreatitis

Musculoskeletal: gout, arthrosis

Psychiatric: aggressive reaction

Three patients (two rifampin combination therapy patients and one rifapentine combination therapy patient) were discontinued in the Intensive Phase as a result of hepatitis with increased liver function tests (ALT, AST, LDH, and bilirubin). Concomitant medications for all three patients included isoniazid, pyrazinamide, ethambutol, and pyridoxine. The two rifampin patients and one rifapentine patient recovered without sequelae.

Eighteen deaths occurred in Study 008 (nine in the rifampin combination therapy group and nine in the rifapentine combination therapy group). None of the deaths were attributed to study medication. In the study, 18/361 (5.0%) rifampin combination therapy patients discontinued the study due to an adverse event compared to 9/361 (2.5%) rifapentine combination therapy patients.

The overall occurrence rate of treatment-related adverse events was higher in males with the rifapentine combination regimen (50%) versus the rifampin combination regimen (43%), while in females the overall rate was greater in the rifampin combination group (68%) compared to the rifapentine combination group (59%). However, there were higher frequencies of treatment-related hematuria and ALT increases for female patients in both treatment groups compared to those for male patients.

Adverse events associated with rifampin may occur with rifapentine: effects of enzyme induction to increase metabolism resulting in decreased concentration of endogenous substrates, including adrenal hormones, thyroid hormones, and vitamin D.

OVERDOSAGE

There is no experience with the treatment of acute overdose with rifapentine at doses exceeding 1200 mg per dose.

In a pharmacokinetic study involving healthy volunteers (n=9), single oral doses up to 1200 mg have been administered without serious adverse events. The only adverse events reported with the 1200 mg dose were heartburn (3/8), headache (2/8) and increased urinary frequency (1/8). In clinical trials, tuberculosis patients ranging in age from 20 to 74 years accidentally received continuous daily doses of rifapentine 600 mg. Some patients received continuous daily dosing for up to 20 days without evidence of serious adverse effects. One patient experienced a transient elevation in SGPT and glucose (the latter attributed to pre-existing diabetes); a second patient experienced slight pruritus. While there is no experience with the treatment of acute overdose with rifapentine, clinical experience with rifamycins suggests that gastric lavage to evacuate gastric contents (within a few hours of overdose), followed by instillation of an activated charcoal slurry into the stomach, may help adsorb any remaining drug from the gastrointestinal tract.

Rifapentine and 25-desacetyl rifapentine are 97.7% and 93.2% plasma protein bound, respectively. Rifapentine and related compounds excreted in urine account for only 17% of the administered dose, therefore, neither hemodialysis nor forced diuresis is expected to enhance the systemic elimination of unchanged rifapentine from the body of a patient with PRIFTIN overdose.

DOSAGE AND ADMINISTRATION

PRIFTIN should not be used alone, in initial treatment or in retreatment of pulmonary tuberculosis. In the intensive phase of short-course therapy which is to continue for 2 months, 600 mg **(four 150 mg tablets)** of PRIFTIN should be given twice weekly with an interval of not less than 3 days (72 hours) between doses. For those patients with propensity to nausea, vomiting or gastrointestinal upset, administration of PRIFTIN with food may be useful. In the Intensive Phase, PRIFTIN must be administered in combination as part of an appropriate regimen which includes daily companion drugs. *Compliance with all drugs in the Intensive Phase (ie, PRIFTIN, isoniazid, pyrazinamide, ethambutol, or streptomycin), especially on days when rifapentine is not administered, is imperative to assure early sputum conversion and protection against relapse.* The Advisory Council for the Elimination of Tuberculosis, the American Thoracic Society and the Centers for Disease Control and Prevention also recommend that either streptomycin or ethambutol be added to the regimen unless the likelihood of isoniazid resistance is very low. The need for streptomycin or ethambutol should be reassessed when the results of susceptibility testing are known. An initial treatment regimen with less than four drugs may be considered if there is little possibility of drug resistance (that is, less than 4% primary resistance to isoniazid in the community, and the patient has had no previous treatment with antituberculosis medications, is not from a country with a high prevalence of drug resistance, and has no known exposure to a drug-resistant case) (see Reference 2).

Following the intensive phase, treatment should be continued with PRIFTIN once weekly for 4 months in combination with isoniazid or an appropriate agent for susceptible organisms. If the patient is still sputum smear or culture positive, if resistant organisms are present, or if the patient is HIV positive, follow the ATS/CDC treatment guidelines (see Reference 2).

Concomitant administration of pyridoxine (Vitamin B6) is recommended in the malnourished, in those predisposed to neuropathy (eg, alcoholics and diabetics), and in adolescents.

The above recommendations apply to patients with drug-susceptible organisms. Patients with drug-resistant organisms may require longer duration treatment with other drug regimens.

Table 2-3. Treatment-Related Adverse Events Occurring in ≥1% of the Patients in Study 008

Preferred Term	Intensive Phase[1] Rifapentine Combination (N=361) N (%)	Intensive Phase[1] Rifampin Combination (N=361) N (%)	Continuation Phase[2] Rifapentine Combination (N=321) N (%)	Continuation Phase[2] Rifampin Combination (N=306) N (%)	Total Rifapentine Combination (N=361) N (%)	Total Rifampin Combination (N=361) N (%)
Hyperuricemia	77 (21.3)	55 (15.2)	0	0	77 (21.3)	55 (15.2)
ALT increased	14 (3.9)	17 (4.7)	5 (1.6)	7 (2.3)	19 (5.3)	24 (6.6)
AST increased	12 (3.3)	16 (4.4)	5 (1.6)	7 (2.3)	16 (4.4)	23 (6.4)
Neutropenia	7 (1.9)	9 (2.5)	12 (3.7)	9 (2.9)	18 (5.0)	18 (5.0)
Pyuria	12 (3.3)	10 (2.8)	6 (1.9)	2 (0.7)	15 (4.2)	12 (3.3)
Proteinuria	15 (4.2)	10 (2.8)	2 (0.6)	1 (0.3)	17 (4.7)	11 (3.0)
Hematuria	10 (2.8)	11 (3.0)	4 (1.2)	3 (1.0)	13 (3.6)	14 (3.9)
Lymphopenia	14 (3.9)	13 (3.6)	3 (0.9)	1 (0.3)	16 (4.4)	14 (3.9)
Urinary casts	11 (3.0)	3 (0.8)	4 (1.2)	0	14 (3.9)	3 (0.8)
Rash	9 (2.5)	20 (5.5)	4 (1.2)	3 (1.0)	13 (3.6)	22 (6.1)
Pruritus	8 (2.2)	15 (4.2)	1 (0.3)	1 (0.3)	9 (2.5)	16 (4.4)
Acne	5 (1.4)	3 (0.8)	2 (0.6)	1 (0.3)	7 (1.9)	4 (1.1)
Anorexia	6 (1.7)	8 (2.2)	3 (0.9)	4 (1.3)	8 (2.2)	10 (2.8)
Anemia	7 (1.9)	9 (2.5)	2 (0.6)	1 (0.3)	9 (2.5)	10 (2.8)
Leukopenia	4 (1.1)	4 (1.1)	3 (0.9)	5 (1.6)	7 (1.9)	8 (2.2)
Arthralgia	9 (2.5)	7 (1.9)	0	0	9 (2.5)	7 (1.9)
Pain	7 (1.9)	5 (1.4)	0	1 (0.3)	7 (1.9)	6 (1.7)
Nausea	7 (1.9)	2 (0.6)	0	1 (0.3)	7 (1.9)	3 (0.8)
Vomiting	4 (1.1)	6 (1.7)	1 (0.3)	1 (0.3)	5 (1.4)	7 (1.9)
Headache	3 (0.8)	4 (1.1)	1 (0.3)	3 (1.0)	4 (1.1)	7 (1.9)
Dyspepsia	3 (0.8)	5 (1.4)	2 (0.6)	3 (1.0)	4 (1.1)	8 (2.2)
Hypertension	3 (0.8)	0 (0.0)	1 (0.3)	1 (0.3)	4 (1.1)	1 (0.3)
Dizziness	4 (1.1)	0	0	1 (0.3)	4 (1.1)	1 (0.3)
Thrombocytosis	4 (1.1)	2 (0.6)	0	0	4 (1.1)	2 (0.6)
Diarrhea	4 (1.1)	0	0	0	4 (1.1)	0
Rash maculopapular	4 (1.1)	3 (0.8)	0	0	4 (1.1)	3 (0.8)
Hemoptysis	2 (0.6)	0	2 (0.6)	0	4 (1.1)	0

Note: ≥1% refers to rifapentine in the TOTAL column.

Note: A patient may have experienced the same adverse event more than once during the course of the study, therefore, patient counts across the columns may not equal the patient counts in the TOTAL column.

[1] Intensive Phase consisted of therapy with either rifapentine or rifampin combined with isoniazid, pyrazinamide, and ethambutol administered daily (rifapentine twice weekly) for 60 days.

[2] Continuation Phase consisted of therapy with either rifapentine or rifampin combined with isoniazid for 120 days. Rifapentine patients were dosed once weekly; rifampin patients were dosed twice weekly. Events recorded in this phase includes those reported up to 3 months after Continuation Phase therapy was completed.

Continued on next page

Priftin—Cont.

HOW SUPPLIED

PRIFTIN (rifapentine) 150 mg pink film-coated tablets are packaged in aluminum foil blisters in cartons of 32 tablets (NDC 0088-2100-03).
Store at 25°C (77°F); excursions permitted 15–30°C (59–86°F) (see USP Controlled Room Temperature). Protect from excessive heat and humidity.
Prescribing Information as of June 1998
Manufactured by:
Gruppo Lepitit S.p.A.
20020 Lainate, Italy
Manufactured for:
Hoechst Marion Roussel, Inc.
Kansas City, MO 64137 USA
MADE IN ITALY

References:

1. Update on US Public Health Service (USPHS) Study 22: A trial of once weekly isoniazid (INH) & rifapentine (RPT) in the continuation phase of TB treatment. The USPHS Rifapentine Trial Group, A Vernon, et al. Am J Respir Crit Care Med. 157: (suppl) A467 (abstract). March 1998.
2. American Thoracic Society, CDC. Treatment of tuberculosis and tuberculosis infection in adults and children. Am J Respir Crit Care Med. 149: 1359–1374, 1994.

REFLUDAN™ ℞

[*rĕ flu'-dăn*]
[lepirudin (rDNA) for injection]

Prescribing Information as of March 1998

DESCRIPTION

REFLUDAN [lepirudin (rDNA) for injection] is a highly specific direct inhibitor of thrombin. Lepirudin (chemical designation: [Leu[1], Thr[2]]-63-desulfohirudin) is a recombinant hirudin derived from yeast cells. The polypeptide composed of 65 amino acids has a molecular weight of 6979.5 daltons. Natural hirudin is produced in trace amounts as a family of highly homologous isopolypeptides by the leech *Hirudo medicinalis*. The biosynthetic molecule (lepirudin) is identical to natural hirudin except for substitution of leucine for isoleucine at the N-terminal end of the molecule and the absence of a sulfate group on the tyrosine at position 63.
The activity of lepirudin is measured in a chromogenic assay. One antithrombin unit (ATU) is the amount of lepirudin that neutralizes one unit of World Health Organization preparation 89/588 of thrombin. The specific activity of lepirudin is approximately 16,000 ATU/mg. Its mode of action is independent of antithrombin III. Platelet factor 4 does not inhibit lepirudin. One molecule of lepirudin binds to one molecule of thrombin and thereby blocks the thrombogenic activity of thrombin. As a result, all thrombin-dependent coagulation assays are affected, eg, activated partial thromboplastin time (aPTT) values increase in a dose-dependent fashion (*Roethig 1991*).
REFLUDAN is supplied as a sterile, white, freeze-dried powder for injection or infusion and is freely soluble in Water for Injection USP or 0.9% Sodium Chloride Injection USP.
Each vial of REFLUDAN contains 50 mg lepirudin. Other ingredients are 40 mg mannitol and sodium hydroxide for adjustment of pH to approximately 7.

CLINICAL PHARMACOLOGY

Pharmacokinetic Properties

The pharmacokinetic properties of lepirudin following intravenous administration are well described by a two-compartment model. Distribution is essentially confined to extracellular fluids and is characterized by an initial half-life of approximately 10 minutes. Elimination follows a first-order process and is characterized by a terminal half-life of about 1.3 hours in young healthy volunteers. As the intravenous dose is increased over the range of 0.1 to 0.4 mg/kg, the maximum plasma concentration and the area-under-the-curve increase proportionally.
Lepirudin is thought to be metabolized by release of amino acids via catabolic hydrolysis of the parent drug. However, conclusive data are not available. About 48% of the administered dose is excreted in the urine which consists of unchanged drug (35%) and other fragments of the parent drug. The systemic clearance of lepirudin is proportional to the glomerular filtration rate or creatinine clearance. Dose adjustment based on creatinine clearance is recommended (see DOSAGE AND ADMINISTRATION: Monitoring and Adjusting Therapy; Use in Renal Impairment). In patients with marked renal insufficiency (creatinine clearance below 15 mL/min) and on hemodialysis, elimination half-lives are prolonged up to 2 days.
The systemic clearance of lepirudin in women is about 25% lower than in men. In elderly patients, the systemic clearance of lepirudin is 20% lower than in younger patients. This may be explained by the lower creatinine clearance in elderly patients compared to younger patients.
Table 1 summarizes systemic clearance (Cl) and volume of distribution at steady state (Vss) of lepirudin for various study populations.

Table 1: Systemic clearance (Cl) and volume of distribution at steady state (Vss) of lepirudin

	Cl (mL/min) Mean (% CV*)	Vss (L) Mean (% CV*)
Healthy young subjects (n = 18, age 18-60 years)	164 (19.3%)	12.2 (16.4%)
Healthy elderly subjects (n = 10, age 65-80 years)	139 (22.5%)	18.7 (20.6%)
Renally impaired patients (n = 16, creatinine clearance below 80 mL/min)	61 (89.4%)	18.0 (41.1%)
HIT† patients (n = 73)	114 (46.8%)	32.1 (98.9%)

* CV: Coefficient of variation
†HIT: Heparin-induced thrombocytopenia

Pharmacodynamic Properties

The pharmacodynamic effect of REFLUDAN on the proteolytic activity of thrombin was routinely assessed as an increase in aPTT. This was observed with increasing plasma concentrations of lepirudin, with no saturable effect up to the highest tested dose (0.5 mg/kg body weight intravenous bolus). Thrombin time (TT) frequently exceeded 200 seconds even at low plasma concentrations of lepirudin, which renders this test unsuitable for routine monitoring of REFLUDAN therapy.
The pharmacodynamic response defined by the aPTT ratio (aPTT at a time after REFLUDAN administration over an aPTT reference value, usually median of the laboratory normal range for aPTT) depends on plasma drug levels which in turn depend on the individual patient's renal function (see CLINICAL PHARMACOLOGY: Pharmacokinetic Properties). For patients undergoing additional thrombolysis, elevated aPTT ratios were already observed at low lepirudin plasma concentrations, and further response to increasing plasma concentrations was relatively flat. In other populations, the response was steeper. At plasma concentrations of 1500 ng/mL, aPTT ratios were nearly 3.0 for healthy volunteers, 2.3 for patients with heparin-induced thrombocytopenia, and 2.1 for patients with deep venous thrombosis.

CLINICAL TRIAL DATA

Heparin-induced thrombocytopenia (HIT) is described as an allergy-like adverse reaction to heparin. It can be found in about 1% to 2% of patients treated with heparin for more than 4 days. The clinical picture of HIT is characterized by thrombocytopenia alone or in combination with thromboembolic complications (TECs). These complications comprise the entire spectrum of venous and arterial thromboembolism including deep venous thrombosis, pulmonary embolism, myocardial infarction, ischemic stroke, and occlusion of limb arteries, which may ultimately result in necroses requiring amputation. Furthermore, there is evidence to suggest that warfarin-induced venous limb gangrene may be associated with HIT. Without further treatment, the mortality in HIT patients with new TECs is about 20% to 30% (*Fondu 1995; Greinacher 1995; Warkentin, Chong, et al., Warkentin, Elavathil, et al. 1997*).
The conclusion that REFLUDAN is an effective treatment for HIT is based upon the data of two prospective, historically controlled clinical trials ("HAT-1" study and "HAT-2" study). The trials were comparable with regard to study design, primary and secondary objectives, and dosing regimens, as well as general study outline and organization. They both used the same historical control group for comparison. This historical control was mainly compiled from a recent retrospective registry of HIT patients.
Overall, 198 (HAT-1: 82, HAT-2: 116) patients were treated with REFLUDAN and 182 historical control patients were treated with other therapies. All except 5 (HAT-1: 1, HAT-2: 4) prospective patients and all historical control patients were diagnosed with HIT using the heparin-induced platelet activation assay (HIPAA) or equivalent assays for testing. In total, 113 (HAT-1: 54, HAT-2: 59) prospective patients ("REFLUDAN") and 91 historical control patients ("historical control") presented with TECs at baseline (day of positive test result) and qualified for direct comparison of clinical endpoints.
The gender distribution was found to be similar in REFLUDAN patients and historical control patients. Overall, REFLUDAN patients tended to be younger than historical control patients. Table 2 summarizes the demographic baseline characteristics of patients presenting with TECs at baseline.

Table 2: Demographic baseline characteristics of patients presenting with TECs

	REFLUDAN		Historical Control
	HAT-1 (n = 54)	HAT-2 (n = 59)	(n = 91)
Males	27.8%	44.1%	35.2%
Females	72.2%	55.9%	64.8%
Age <65 years	63.0%	67.8%	44.0%
Age ≥65 years	37.0%	32.2%	56.0%
Mean age ± SD (years)	57 ± 17	58 ± 12	64 ± 14

The key criteria of efficacy from a laboratory standpoint (n = 115 evaluable patients) were platelet recovery (increase in platelet count by at least 30% of nadir to values >100,000) and effective anticoagulation (aPTT ratio >1.5 with a maximum total 40% increase in the initial infusion rate). The proportions of REFLUDAN patients presenting with TECs at baseline who showed platelet recovery, effective anticoagulation, or both (laboratory responders) are shown in Table 3. Comparable rates for the historical control group cannot be given, because (1) platelet counts were not monitored as closely as in the REFLUDAN group, and (2) most historical control patients did not receive therapies affecting aPTT.

Table 3: Proportions of laboratory responders among REFLUDAN patients presenting with TECs

	HAT-1	HAT-2
Number of evaluable patients	55	60
Platelet recovery	90.9%	95.0%
Effective anticoagulation	81.8%	75.0%
Both	72.7%	71.7%

Comparisons of clinical efficacy were made between REFLUDAN patients and historical control patients with regard to the combined and individual incidences of death, limb amputation, or new TEC.
The original main analyses included all events that occurred after laboratory confirmation of HIT. This approach was revealed to be substantially confounded by the relative contribution of the pretreatment period (time between laboratory confirmation of HIT and start of treatment). Although short in duration (mean length 1.5 days in HAT-1 and 2.0 days in HAT-2), the pretreatment period accounted for 45% and 26% of events observed in the main analyses of HAT-1 REFLUDAN patients and HAT-2 REFLUDAN patients, respectively. Therefore, initiation of treatment was set as the starting point for the analyses. For the historical control group, the first treatment selected within 2 days of laboratory confirmation of HIT was used for reference.
Seven days after start of treatment, the cumulative risk of death, limb amputation, or new TEC was 3.7% in the HAT-1 REFLUDAN patients and 16.9% in the HAT-2 REFLUDAN patients, as compared to 24.9% in the historical control group. At 35 days, when approximately 10% of patients were still at risk, the cumulative risk was 13.0% in the HAT-1 REFLUDAN patients and 28.9% in the HAT-2 REFLUDAN patients, as compared to 47.8% in the historical control group.
In an additional meta-analysis, the pooled REFLUDAN patients of the HAT-1 and HAT-2 studies who presented with TECs at baseline were compared to the respective historical control patients. Seven and 35 days after start of treatment, the cumulative risks of death were 4.4% and 8.9% in the REFLUDAN group, as compared to 1.4% and 17.6% in the historical control group. The cumulative risks of limb amputation were 2.7% and 6.5% in the REFLUDAN group, as compared to 2.6% and 10.4% in the historical control group. Most importantly, the cumulative risks of new TEC were 6.3% and 10.1% in the REFLUDAN group, as compared to 22.2% and 27.2% in the historical control group. As shown in Fig 1, the differences in the cumulative risk of death, limb amputation, or new TEC between the groups were statistically significant in favor of REFLUDAN in the analysis of time to event ($P = 0.004$ according to log-rank test).
[See graphic at top of next page]
The immediate impact of treatment on the combined risk of death, limb amputation, or new TEC is demonstrated by comparing pretreatment period and treatment period in regard to average combined event rates per patient day. In the pretreatment period, these rates were found to be 0.075 in the HAT-1 REFLUDAN patients, 0.052 in the HAT-2 REFLUDAN patients, and 0.040 in the historical control

Fig 1: Cumulative risk of death, limb amputation, or new thromboembolic complication after start of treatment

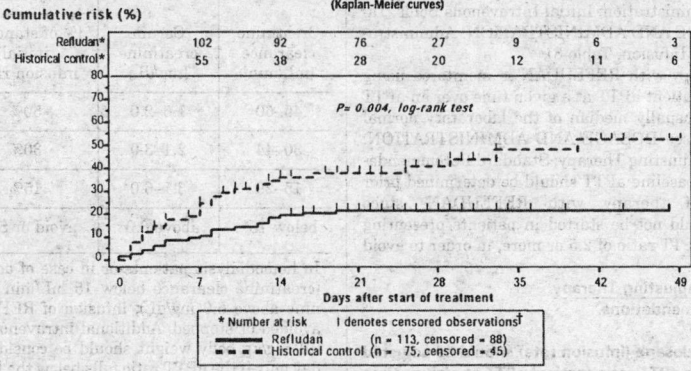

† Censored observations: Patients who did not reach a disease endpoint during their period of follow-up

group. In the treatment period, the rates showed a marked reduction in the REFLUDAN patients, where they dropped to 0.005 (HAT-1) and to 0.018 (HAT-2), while there was only a moderate decrease to 0.030 in the historical control group. In conclusion, REFLUDAN substantially reduced the risk of serious sequelae of HIT in comparison to a historical control group.

INDICATIONS AND USAGE

REFLUDAN is indicated for anticoagulation in patients with heparin-induced thrombocytopenia (HIT) and associated thromboembolic disease in order to prevent further thromboembolic complications.

CONTRAINDICATIONS

REFLUDAN is contraindicated in patients with known hypersensitivity to hirudins.

WARNINGS

Hemorrhagic Events

Intracranial bleeding following concomitant thrombolytic therapy with rt-PA or streptokinase may be life-threatening (see also ADVERSE REACTIONS: Adverse Events Reported in Other Populations; Intracranial Bleeding).

For patients with increased risk of bleeding, a careful assessment weighing the risk of REFLUDAN administration vs its anticipated benefit has to be made by the treating physician.

In particular, this includes the following conditions:

- **Recent puncture of large vessels or organ biopsy**
- **Anomaly of vessels or organs**
- **Recent cerebrovascular accident, stroke, intracerebral surgery, or other neuraxial procedures.**
- **Severe uncontrolled hypertension**
- **Bacterial endocarditis**
- **Advanced renal impairment (see also WARNINGS: Renal Impairment)**
- **Hemorrhagic diathesis**
- **Recent major surgery**
- **Recent major bleeding (eg, intracranial, gastrointestinal, intraocular, or pulmonary bleeding)**

Renal Impairment

With renal impairment, relative overdose might occur even with standard dosage regimen. Therefore, the bolus dose and the rate of infusion must be reduced in patients with known or suspected renal insufficiency (see CLINICAL PHARMACOLOGY: Pharmacokinetic Properties and DOSAGE AND ADMINISTRATION: Monitoring and Adjusting Therapy; Use in Renal Impairment).

PRECAUTIONS

General

Antibodies. Formation of antihirudin antibodies was observed in about 40% of HIT patients treated with REFLUDAN. This may increase the anticoagulant effect of REFLUDAN possibly due to delayed renal elimination of active lepirudin-antihirudin complexes (see also PRECAUTIONS: Animal Pharmacology and Toxicology). Therefore, strict monitoring of aPTT is necessary also during prolonged therapy (see also PRECAUTIONS: Laboratory Tests and DOSAGE AND ADMINISTRATION: Monitoring and Adjusting Therapy; Standard Recommendations). No evidence of neutralization of REFLUDAN or of allergic reactions associated with positive antibody test results was found.

Liver injury. Serious liver injury (eg, liver cirrhosis) may enhance the anticoagulant effect of REFLUDAN due to coagulation defects secondary to reduced generation of vitamin K-dependent coagulation factors.

Reexposure. Clinical trials have provided limited information to support any recommendations for reexposure to REFLUDAN. A total of 13 patients were reexposed in the HAT-1 and HAT-2 studies. One of these patients experienced a mild allergic skin reaction during the second treatment cycle. No further adverse experience was observed in relation to reexposure.

Laboratory Tests

In general, the dosage (infusion rate) should be adjusted according to the aPTT ratio (patient aPTT at a given time over an aPTT reference value, usually median of the laboratory normal range for aPTT); for full information, see DOSAGE AND ADMINISTRATION: Monitoring and Adjusting Therapy; Standard Recommendations. Other thrombin-dependent coagulation assays are changed by REFLUDAN (see also DESCRIPTION).

Drug Interactions

Concomitant treatment with thrombolytics (eg, rt-PA or streptokinase) may:

- increase the risk of bleeding complications
- considerably enhance the effect of REFLUDAN on aPTT prolongation

(See also WARNINGS: Hemorrhagic Events, ADVERSE REACTIONS: Adverse Events Reported in Other Populations; Intracranial Bleeding DOSAGE AND ADMINISTRATION: Monitoring and Adjusting Therapy; Concomitant Use With Thrombolytic Therapy)

Concomitant treatment with coumarin derivatives (vitamin K antagonists) and drugs that affect platelet may also increase the risk of bleeding (see also DOSAGE AND ADMINISTRATION: Monitoring and Adjusting Therapy; Use in Patients Scheduled for a Switch to Oral Anticoagulation).

Animal Pharmacology and Toxicology

General Toxicity. Lepirudin caused bleeding in animal toxicity studies. Antibodies against hirudin which appeared in several monkeys treated with lepirudin resulted in a prolongation of the terminal half-life and an increase of AUC plasma values of lepirudin.

Carcinogenesis, Mutagenesis, Impairment of Fertility. Long-term animal studies to evaluate the potential for carcinogenesis have not been performed with lepirudin. Lepirudin was not genotoxic in the Ames test, the Chinese hamster cell (V79/HGPRT) forward mutation test, the A549 human cell line unscheduled DNA synthesis (UDS) test, the Chinese hamster V79 cell chromosome aberration test, or the mouse micronucleus test. An effect on fertility and reproductive performance of male and female rats was not seen with lepirudin at intravenous doses up to 30 mg/kg/day (180 mg/m^2/day, 1.2 times the recommended maximum human total daily dose based on body surface area of 1.45m^2 for a 50 kg subject).

Pregnancy

Teratogenic Effects: Category B. Teratology studies with lepirudin performed in pregnant rats at intravenous doses up to 30 mg/kg/day (180 mg/m^2/day, 1.2 times the recommended maximum human total daily dose based on body surface area) and in pregnant rabbits at intravenous doses up to 30 mg/kg/day (360 mg/m^2/day, 2.4 times the recommended maximum human total daily dose based on body surface area) have revealed no evidence of harm to the fetus due to lepirudin. There are, however, no adequate and well-controlled studies in pregnant women. Because animal reproduction studies are not always predictive of human response, this drug should be used during pregnancy only if clearly needed.

Lepirudin (1 mg/kg) by intravenous administration crosses the placental barrier in pregnant rats. It is not known whether the drug crosses the placental barrier in humans. Following intravenous administration of lepirudin at 30 mg/kg/day (180 mg/m^2/day, 1.2 times the recommended maximum human total daily dose based on body surface area) during organogenesis and perinatal-postnatal periods, pregnant rats showed an increased maternal mortality due to undetermined causes.

Nursing Mothers

It is not known whether REFLUDAN is excreted in human milk. Because many drugs are excreted in human milk and because of the potential for serious adverse reactions in nursing infants from REFLUDAN, a decision should be made whether to discontinue nursing or to discontinue the drug, taking into account the importance of the drug to the mother.

Pediatric Use

Safety and effectiveness in pediatric patients have not been established. In the HAT-2 study, two children, an 11-year-old girl and a 12-year-old boy, were treated with REFLUDAN. Both children presented with TECs at baseline. REFLUDAN doses given ranged from 0.15 mg/kg/h to 0.22 mg/kg/h for the girl, and from 0.1 mg/kg/h (in conjunction with urokinase) to 0.7 mg/kg/h for the boy. Treatment with REFLUDAN was completed after 8 and 58 days, respectively, without serious adverse events (*Schiffmann 1997*).

ADVERSE REACTIONS

Adverse Events Reported in HIT Patients

The following safety information is based on all 198 patients treated with REFLUDAN in the HAT-1 and HAT-2 studies. The safety profile of 113 REFLUDAN patients from these studies who presented with TECs at baseline is compared to 91 such patients in the historical control.

Hemorrhagic Events. Bleeding was the most frequent adverse event observed in patients treated with REFLUDAN. Table 4 gives an overview of all hemorrhagic events which occurred in at least two patients.

Table 4: Hemorrhagic Events*

	HAT-1 HAT-2 (All patients) (n = 198)	Patients with TECs	
		REFLUDAN (n = 113)	Historical control (n = 91)
Bleeding from puncture sites and wounds	14.1%	10.6%	4.4%
Anemia or isolated drop in hemoglobin	13.1%	12.4%	1.1%
Other hematoma and unclassified bleeding	11.1%	10.6%	4.4%
Hematuria	6.6%	4.4%	0
Gastrointestinal and rectal bleeding	5.1%	5.3%	6.6%
Epistaxis	3.0%	4.4%	1.1%
Hemothorax	3.0%	0	1.1%
Vaginal bleeding	1.5%	1.8%	0
Intracranial bleeding	0	0	2.2%

*Patients may have suffered more than one event.

Other hemorrhagic events (hemoperitoneum, hemoptysis, liver bleeding, lung bleeding, mouth bleeding, retroperitoneal bleeding) each occurred in one individual among all 198 patients treated with REFLUDAN.

Nonhemorrhagic events. Table 5 gives an overview of the most frequently observed nonhemorrhagic events.

Table 5: Nonhemorrhagic adverse events*

	HAT-1 HAT-2 (All patients) (n = 198)	Patients with TECs	
		REFLUDAN (n = 113)	Historical control (n = 91)
Fever	6.1%	4.4%	8.8%
Abnormal liver function	6.1%	5.3%	0
Pneumonia	4.0%	4.4%	5.5%
Sepsis	4.0%	3.5%	5.5%
Allergic skin reactions	3.0%	3.5%	1.1%

Continued on next page

Refludan—Cont.

Heart failure	3.0%	1.8%	2.2%
Abnormal kidney function	2.5%	1.8%	4.4%
Unspecified infections	2.5%	1.8%	1.1%
Multiorgan failure	2.0%	3.5%	0
Pericardial effusion	1.0%	0	1.1%
Ventricular fibrillation	1.0%	0	0

*Patients may have suffered more than one event.

Adverse Events Reported in Other Populations

The following safety information is based on a total of 2302 individuals who were treated with REFLUDAN in clinical pharmacology studies (n = 323) or for clinical indications other than HIT (n = 1979).

Intracranial Bleeding. Intracranial bleeding was the most serious adverse reaction found in populations other than HIT patients. However, it only occurred in patients with acute myocardial infarction who were started on both REFLUDAN and thrombolytic therapy with rt-PA or streptokinase. The overall frequency of this potentially life-threatening complication among patients receiving both REFLUDAN and thrombolytic therapy was 0.6% (7 out of 1134 patients). No intracranial bleeding was observed in 1168 subjects or patients who did not receive concomitant thrombolysis.

Allergic Reactions. Allergic reactions or suspected allergic reactions in populations other than HIT patients include (in descending order of frequency*):

- Airway reactions (cough, bronchospasm, stridor, dyspnea): common
- Unspecified allergic reactions: uncommon
- Skin reactions (pruritus, urticaria, rash, flushes, chills): uncommon
- General reactions (anaphylactoid or anaphylactoid reactions): uncommon
- Edema (facial edema, tongue edema, larynx edema, angioedema): rare

* The CIOMS (Council for International Organization of Medical Sciences) III standard categories are used for classification of frequencies:

very common	10% or more
common (frequent)	1 to <10%
uncommon (infrequent)	0.1 to <1%
rare	0.01 to <0.1%
very rare	0.01% or less

About 53% (n = 46) of all allergic reactions or suspected allergic reactions occurred in patients who concomitantly received thrombolytic therapy (eg, streptokinase) for acute myocardial infarction and/or contrast media for coronary angiography.

OVERDOSAGE

In case of overdose (eg, suggested by excessively high aPTT values) the risk of bleeding is increased.

No specific antidote for REFLUDAN is available. If life-threatening bleeding occurs and excessive plasma levels of lepirudin are suspected, the following steps should be followed:

- Immediately STOP REFLUDAN administration
- Determine aPTT and other coagulation levels as appropriate
- Determine hemoglobin and prepare for blood transfusion
- Follow the current guidelines for treating patients with shock

Individual clinical case reports and in vitro data suggest that either hemofiltration or hemodialysis (using high-flux dialysis membranes with a cutoff point of 50,000 daltons, eg, AN/69) may be useful in this situation.

In studies in pigs, the application of von Willebrand Factor (vWF, 66 IU/kg body weight) markedly reduced the bleeding time. The clinical significance of this data is unknown.

DOSAGE AND ADMINISTRATION

Initial Dosage

Anticoagulation in adult patients with HIT and associated thromboembolic disease:

- 0.4 mg/kg body weight (up to 110 kg) slowly intravenously (eg, over 15 to 20 seconds) as a bolus dose,
- followed by 0.15 mg/kg body weight (up to 110 kg)/hour as a continuous intravenous infusion for 2 to 10 days or longer if clinically needed.

Normally the initial dosage depends on the patient's body weight. This is valid up to a body weight of 110 kg. In patients with a body weight exceeding 110 kg, the initial dosage should not be increased beyond the 110 kg body weight dose (maximal initial bolus dose of 44 mg, maximal initial infusion dose of 16.5 mg/h; see also DOSAGE AND ADMINISTRATION: Administration; Initial Intravenous Bolus, Table 7 and DOSAGE AND ADMINISTRATION: Administration; Intravenous Infusion, Table 8).

In general, therapy with REFLUDAN is monitored using the aPTT ratio (patient aPTT at a given time over an aPTT reference value, usually median of the laboratory normal range for aPTT, see DOSAGE AND ADMINISTRATION: Monitoring and Adjusting Therapy; Standard Recommendations). A patient baseline aPTT should be determined prior to initiation of therapy with REFLUDAN, since REFLUDAN should not be started in patients presenting with a baseline aPTT ratio of 2.5 or more, in order to avoid initial overdosing.

Monitoring and Adjusting Therapy

Standard Recommendations.

Monitoring.

- **In general, the dosage (infusion rate) should be adjusted according to the aPTT ratio (patient aPTT at a given time over an aPTT reference value, usually median of the laboratory normal range for aPTT).**
- **The target range for the aPTT ratio during treatment (therapeutic window) should be 1.5 to 2.5. Data from clinical trials in HIT patients suggest that with aPTT ratios higher than this target range, the risk of bleeding increases, while there is no incremental increase in clinical efficacy.**
- **As stated in DOSAGE AND ADMINISTRATION: Initial Dosage, REFLUDAN should not be started in patients presenting with a baseline aPTT ratio of 2.5 or more, in order to avoid initial overdosing.**
- **The first aPTT determination for monitoring treatment should be done 4 hours after start of the REFLUDAN infusion.**
- **Follow-up aPTT determinations are recommended at least once daily, as long as treatment with REFLUDAN is ongoing.**
- **More frequent aPTT monitoring is highly recommended in patients with renal impairment or serious liver injury (see DOSAGE AND ADMINISTRATION: Monitoring and Adjusting Therapy; Use in Renal Impairment) or with an increased risk of bleeding.**

Dose Modifications.

- **Any aPTT ratio out of the target range is to be confirmed at once before drawing conclusions with respect to dose modifications, unless there is a clinical need to react immediately.**
- **If the confirmed aPTT ratio is above the target range, the infusion should be stopped for two hours. At restart, the infusion rate should be decreased by 50% (no additional intravenous bolus should be administered). The aPTT ratio should be determined again 4 hours later.**
- **If the confirmed aPTT ratio is below the target range, the infusion rate should be increased in steps of 20%. The aPTT ratio should be determined again 4 hours later.**
- **In general, an infusion rate of 0.21 mg/kg/h should not be exceeded without checking for coagulation abnormalities which might be preventive of an appropriate aPTT response.**

Use in Renal Impairment

AS REFLUDAN is almost exclusively excreted in the kidneys (see also CLINICAL PHARMACOLOGY: Pharmacokinetic Properties), individual renal function should be considered prior to administration. In case of renal impairment, relative overdose might occur even with the standard dosage regimen. Therefore, the bolus dose and the infusion rate must be reduced in case of known or suspected renal insufficiency (creatinine clearance below 60 mL/min or serum creatinine above 1.5 mg/dL).

There is only limited information on the therapeutic use of REFLUDAN in HIT patients with significant renal impairment. The following dosage recommendations are mainly based on single-dose studies in a small number of patients with renal impairment. Therefore, these recommendations are only tentative.

Dose adjustments should be based on creatinine clearance values, whenever available, as obtained from a reliable method (24 h urine sampling). If creatinine clearance is not available, the dose adjusments should be based on the serum creatinine.

In all patients with renal insufficiency, the bolus dose is to be reduced to 0.2 mg/kg body weight.

The standard initial infusion rate given in DOSAGE AND ADMINISTRATION: Initial Dosage and DOSAGE AND ADMINISTRATION: Administration; Intravenous Infusion, Table 8 must be reduced according to the recommendations given in Table 6. Additional aPTT monitoring is highly recommended.

Table 6: Reduction of infusion rate in patients with renal impairment

Creatinine clearance [mL/min]	Serum creatinine [mg/dL]	Adjusted infusion rate [% of standard initial infusion rate]	Adjusted infusion rate [mg/kg/h]
45–60	1.6–2.0	50%	0.075
30–44	2.1–3.0	30%	0.045
15–29	3.1–6.0	15%	0.0225
below 15*	above 6.0*	avoid or STOP infusion!*	

*In hemodialysis patients or in case of acute renal failure (creatinine clearance below 15 mL/min or serum creatinine above 6.0 mg/dL), infusion of REFLUDAN is to be avoided or stopped. Additional intravenous bolus doses of 0.1 mg/kg body weight should be considered every other day only if the aPTT ratio falls below the lower therapeutic limit of 1.5 (see also DOSAGE AND ADMINISTRATION: Monitoring and Adjusting Therapy; Standard Recommendations).

Concomitant Use With Thrombolytic Therapy.

Clinical trials in HIT patients have provided only limited information on the combined use of REFLUDAN and thrombolytic agents. The following dosage regimen of REFLUDAN was used in a total of 9 HIT patients in the HAT-1 and HAT-2 studies who presented with TECs at baseline and were started on both REFLUDAN and thrombolytic therapy (rt-PA, urokinase or streptokinase):

- Initial intravenous bolus: 0.2 mg/kg body weight
- Continuous intravenous infusion: 0.1 mg/kg body weight/h

The number of patients receiving combined therapy was too small to identify differences in clinical outcome of patients who were started on REFLUDAN and thrombolytic therapy as compared to those who were started on REFLUDAN alone. The combined incidences of death, limb amputation, or new TEC were 22.2% and 20.7%, respectively. While there was a 47% relative increase in the overall bleeding rate in patients who were started on both REFLUDAN and thrombolytic therapy (55.6% vs 37.9%), there were no differences in the rates of serious bleeding events (fatal or life-threatening bleeds, bleeds that were permanently or significantly disabling, overt bleeds requiring transfusion of 2 or more units of packed red blood cells, bleeds necessitating surgical intervention, intracranial bleeds) between the groups (11.1% vs 11.2%). Although no intracranial bleeding has been observed in any of these patients, the risk of this potentially life-threatening complication may be increased in conjunction with thrombolytic agents (see ADVERSE REACTIONS: Adverse Events Reported in Other Populations; Intracranial Bleeding).

Special attention should be paid to the fact that thrombolytic agents per se may increase the aPTT ratio. Therefore, aPTT ratios with a given plasma level of lepirudin are usually higher in patients who receive concomitant thrombolysis than in those who do not (see also CLINICAL PHARMACOLOGY: Pharmacodynamic Properties).

Use in Patients Scheduled for a Switch to Oral Anticoagulation.

If a patient is scheduled to receive coumarin derivatives (vitamin K antagonists) for oral anticoagulation after REFLUDAN therapy, the dose of REFLUDAN should first be gradually reduced in order to reach an aPTT ratio just above 1.5 before initiating oral anticoagulation. As soon as an international normalized ratio (INR) of 2.0 is reached, REFLUDAN therapy should be stopped.

Administration

Directions on Preparation and Dilution.

REFLUDAN should not be mixed with other drugs except for Water for Injection USP, 0.9% Sodium Chloride Injection USP or 5% Dextrose Injection.

Use REFLUDAN before the expiration date given on the carton and container.

Reconstitution and further dilution are to be carried out under sterile conditions:

- For reconstitution, Water for Injection USP or 0.9% Sodium Chloride Injection USP are to be used.
- For further dilution, 0.9% Sodium Chloride Injection USP or 5% Dextrose Injection are suitable.
- For rapid, complete reconstitution, inject 1 mL of diluent into the vial and shake it gently. After reconstitution a clear, colorless solution is usually obtained in a few seconds, but definitely in less than 3 minutes.
- Parenteral drug products should be inspected visually for particulate matter and discoloration prior to administration whenever solution and container permit. Do not use solutions that are cloudy or contain particles.

- The reconstituted solution is to be used immediately. It remains stable for up to 24 hours at room temperature, (eg, during infusion).
- The preparation should be warmed to room temperature before administration.
- Discard any unused solution appropriately.

Initial Intravenous Bolus

For intravenous bolus injection, use a solution with a concentration of 5 mg/mL.
Preparation of a REFLUDAN solution with a concentration of 5 mg/mL:

- Reconstitute one vial (50 mg of lepirudin) with 1 mL of Water for Injection USP or 0.9% Sodium Chloride Injection USP.
- The final concentration of 5 mg/mL is obtained by transferring the contents of the vial into a sterile, single-use syringe (of at least 10 mL capacity) and diluting the solution to a total volume of 10 mL, using Water for Injection USP, 0.9% Sodium Chloride Injection USP or 5% Dextrose Injection.
- The final solution is to be administered according to body weight (see Table 7 below and DOSAGE AND ADMINISTRATION: Initial Dosage).

Intravenous injection of the bolus is to be carried out slowly (eg, over 15 to 20 seconds).

Table 7:   Standard bolus injection volumes according to body weight for a 5 mg/mL concentration

Body Weight [kg]	Injection volume	
	Dosage 0.4 mg/kg	Dosage 0.2 mg/kg*
50	4.0 mL	2.0 mL
60	4.8 mL	2.4 mL
70	5.6 mL	2.8 mL
80	6.4 mL	3.2 mL
90	7.2 mL	3.6 mL
100	8.0 mL	4.0 mL
≥110	8.8 mL	4.4 mL

*Dosage recommended for all patients with renal insufficiency (see DOSAGE AND ADMINISTRATION: Monitoring and Adjusting Therapy; Use in Renal Impairment)

Intravenous Infusion

For continuous intravenous infusion, solutions with concentration of 0.2 mg/mL or 0.4 mg/mL may be used.
Preparation of a REFLUDAN solution with a concentration of 0.2 or 0.4 mg/mL:

- Reconstitute two vials (each containing 50 mg of lepirudin) with 1 mL each using either Water for Injection USP or 0.9% Sodium Chloride Injection USP.
- The final concentrations of 0.2 mg/mL or 0.4 mg/mL are obtained by transferring the contents of both vials into an infusion bag containing 500 mL or 250 mL of 0.9% Sodium Chloride Injection USP or 5% Dextrose Injection.

The infusion rate [mL/h] is to be set according to body weight (see Table 8 below and DOSAGE AND ADMINISTRATION: Initial Dosage).

Table 8:   Standard infusion rates according to body weight

Body Weight [kg]	Infusion rate at 0.15 mg/kg/h	
	500-mL infusion bag 0.2 mg/mL	250-mL infusion bag 0.4 mg/mL
50	38 mL/h	19 mL/h
60	45 mL/h	23 mL/h
70	53 mL/h	26 mL/h
80	60 mL/h	30 mL/h
90	68 mL/h	34 mL/h
100	75 mL/h	38 mL/h
≥110	83 mL/h	41 mL/h

HOW SUPPLIED

REFLUDAN [lepirudin (rDNA) for injection] is supplied in boxes of 10 vials, each vial containing 50 mg lepirudin (NDC 0088-2150-57). STORE UNOPENED VIALS AT 2 to 25°C (36 to 77°F). USE REFLUDAN BEFORE THE EXPIRA-TION DATE GIVEN ON THE CARTON AND CONTAINER. ONCE RECONSTITUTED, USE REFLUDAN IMMEDIATELY.

REFERENCES

1. Fondu P, Heparin associated thrombocytopenia: an update. *Acta Clinica Belgica. 1995;50(6):343–357.*
2. Greinacher A. Antigen generation in heparin-associated thrombocytopenia: the nonimmunologic type and the immunologic type are closely linked in their pathogenesis. *Seminars Thromb Hemost. 1995;21:106–116.*
3. Roethig HJ, Maree JS, Meyer BH. Clinical pharmacology of hirudin (HBW 023). In: Reidenberg, MM ed. *The clinical pharmacology of biotechnology products.* Elsevier Publishers; 1991:227–236.
4. Schiffmann H, Unterhalt M, Harms K, Figula HR, Voelpel H, Greinacher A. Successful treatment of heparin-induced thrombocytopenia (HIT) type II in childhood with recombinant hirudin. *Monatsschr Kinderheilkd.* 1997; 145:606–612.
5. Warkentin TE, Chong BH, Greinacher A. Heparin-induced thrombocytopenia: towards consensus. *Thromb Haemostas.* 1998; 79:1–7.
6. Warkentin TE, Elavathil LJ, Hayward CPM, Johnston MA, Russett JI, Kelton JG. The pathogenesis of venous limb gangrene associated with heparin-induced thrombocytopenia. *Ann Intern Med. 1997; 127:804–812.*

Prescribing Information as of March 1998

Manufactured by:
Hoechst Marion Roussel
Deutschland GmbH
D-65926 Frankfurt am Main
Germany
Manufactured for:
Hoechst Marion Roussel, Inc.
Kansas City, MO 64137
www.hmri.com

RIFADIN®   ℞
[*rĭf ' uh-din*]
(rifampin capsules)
and
RIFADIN® IV
(rifampin for injection)

Prescribing Information as of July 1997

DESCRIPTION

RIFADIN (rifampin) capsules for oral administration contain 150 mg or 300 mg of rifampin per capsule. The 150 mg and 300 mg capsules also contain, as inactive ingredients: corn starch, D&C Red No. 28, FD&C Blue No. 1, FD&C Red No. 40, gelatin, magnesium stearate, and titanium dioxide. RIFADIN IV (rifampin for injection) contains rifampin 600 mg, sodium formaldehyde sulfoxylate 10 mg, and sodium hydroxide to adjust pH.

Rifampin is a semisynthetic antibiotic derivative of rifamycin SV. Rifampin is a red-brown crystalline powder very slightly soluble in water at neutral pH, freely soluble in chloroform, soluble in ethyl acetate and in methanol. Its molecular weight is 822.95 and its chemical formula is $C_{43}H_{58}N_4O_{12}$. The chemical name for rifampin is either:

3-[[(4-Methyl-1-piperazinyl)imino]methyl]rifamycin

or

5,6,9,17,19,21-hexahydroxy-23-methoxy-2,4,12,16,20,22-heptamethyl-8-[N-(4-methyl-1-piperazinyl)formimidoyl]-2,7-(epoxypentadeca [1,11,13]trienimino)naphtho[2,1-*b*]furan-1,11(2H)-dione 21-acetate.

Its structural formula is:

CLINICAL PHARMACOLOGY

Oral Administration

Rifampin is readily absorbed from the gastrointestinal tract. Peak serum concentrations in healthy adults and pediatric populations vary widely from individual to individual. Following a single 600 mg oral dose of rifampin in healthy adults, the peak serum concentration averages 7 µg/mL but may vary from 4 to 32 µg/mL. Absorption of rifampin is reduced by about 30% when the drug is ingested with food.

Rifampin is widely distributed throughout the body. It is present in effective concentrations in many organs and body fluids, including cerebrospinal fluid. Rifampin is about 80% protein bound. Most of the unbound fraction is not ionized and, therefore, diffuses freely into tissues.

In healthy adults, the mean biological half-life of rifampin in serum averages 3.35 ± 0.66 hours after a 600 mg oral dose, with increases up to 5.08 ± 2.45 hours reported after a 900 mg dose. With repeated administration, the half-life decreases and reaches average values of approximately 2 to 3 hours. The half-life does not differ in patients with renal failure at doses not exceeding 600 mg daily, and consequently, no dosage adjustment is required. Following a single 900 mg oral dose of rifampin in patients with varying degrees of renal insufficiency, the mean half-life increased from 3.6 hours in healthy adults to 5.0, 7.3, and 11.0 hours in patients with glomerular filtration rates of 30 to 50 mL/min, less than 30 mL/min, and in anuric patients, respectively. Refer to the WARNINGS section for information regarding patients with hepatic insufficiency.

Rifampin is rapidly eliminated in the bile, and an enterohepatic circulation ensues. During this process, rifampin undergoes progressive deacetylation so that nearly all the drug in the bile is in this form in about 6 hours. This metabolite is microbiologically active. Intestinal reabsorption is reduced by deacetylation, and elimination is facilitated. Up to 30% of a dose is excreted in the urine, with about half of this being unchanged drug.

Intravenous Administration

After intravenous administration of a 300 or 600 mg dose of rifampin infused over 30 minutes to healthy male volunteers (n=12), mean peak plasma concentrations were 9.0 ± 3.0 and 17.5 ± 5.0 µg/mL, respectively. Total body clearance after the 300 and 600 mg IV doses were 0.19 ± 0.06 and 0.14 ± 0.03 L/hr/kg, respectively. Volumes of distribution at steady state were 0.66 ± 0.14 and 0.64 ± 0.11 L/kg for the 300 and 600 mg IV doses, respectively. After intravenous administration of 300 or 600 mg doses, rifampin plasma concentrations in these volunteers remained detectable for 8 and 12 hours, respectively (see Table).

[See table at bottom of next page]

Plasma concentrations after the 600 mg dose, which were disproportionately higher (up to 30% greater than expected) than those found after the 300 mg dose, indicated that the elimination of larger doses was not as rapid.

After repeated once-a-day infusions (3 hr duration) of 600 mg in patients (n=5) for 7 days, concentrations of IV rifampin decreased from 5.81 ± 3.38 µg/mL 8 hours after the infusion on day 1 to 2.6 ± 1.88 µg/mL 8 hours after the infusion on day 7.

Rifampin is widely distributed throughout the body. It is present in effective concentrations in many organs and body fluids, including cerebrospinal fluid. Rifampin is about 80% protein bound. Most of the unbound fraction is not ionized and therefore diffuses freely into tissues.

Rifampin is rapidly eliminated in the bile and undergoes progressive enterohepatic circulation and deacetylation to the primary metabolite, 25-desacetyl-rifampin. This metabolite is microbiologically active. Less than 30% of the dose is excreted in the urine as rifampin or metabolites. Serum concentrations do not differ in patients with renal failure at a studied dose of 300 mg and consequently, no dosage adjustment is required.

Pediatrics

Oral Administration. In one study, pediatric patients 6 to 58 months old were given rifampin suspended in simple syrup or as dry powder mixed with applesauce at a dose of 10 mg/kg body weight. Peak serum concentrations of 10.7 ± 3.7 and 11.5 ± 5.1 µg/mL were obtained 1 hour after preprandial ingestion of the drug suspension and the applesauce mixture, respectively. After the administration of either preparation, the $t_{1/2}$ of rifampin averaged 2.9 hours. It should be noted that in other studies in pediatric populations, at doses of 10 mg/kg body weight, mean peak serum concentrations of 3.5 µg/mL to 15 µg/mL have been reported.

Intravenous Administration. In pediatric patients 0.25 to 12.8 years old (n=12), the mean peak serum concentration of rifampin at the end of a 30 minute infusion of approximately 300 mg/m^2 was 25.9 ± 1.3 µg/mL; individual peak concentrations 1 to 4 days after initiation of therapy ranged from 11.7 to 41.5 µg/mL; individual peak concentrations 5 to 14 days after initiation of therapy were 13.6 to 37.4 µg/mL. The individual serum half-life of rifampin changed from 1.04 to 3.81 hours early in therapy to 1.17 to 3.19 hours 5 to 14 days after therapy was initiated.

Microbiology

Rifampin inhibits DNA-dependent RNA polymerase activity in susceptible cells. Specifically, it interacts with bacterial RNA polymerase but does not inhibit mammalian enzyme. Rifampin at therapeutic levels has demonstrated bactericidal activity against both intracellular and extracellular *Mycobacterium tuberculosis* organisms.

Organisms resistant to rifampin are likely to be resistant to other rifamycins.

Rifampin has bactericidal activity against slow and intermittently growing *M tuberculosis* organisms. It also has significant activity against *Neisseria meningitidis* isolates (see INDICATIONS AND USAGE).

Continued on next page

Rifadin—Cont.

In the treatment of both tuberculosis and the meningococcal carrier state (see INDICATIONS AND USAGE), the small number of resistance cells present within large populations of susceptible cells can rapidly become predominant. In addition, resistance to rifampin has been determined to occur as single-step mutations of the DNA-dependent RNA polymerase. Since resistance can emerge rapidly, appropriate susceptibility tests should be performed in the event of persistent positive cultures.

Rifampin has been shown to be active against most strains of the following microorganisms, both in vitro and in clinical infections as described in the INDICATIONS AND USAGE section.

Aerobic Gram-Negative Microorganisms:
Neisseria meningitidis

"Other" Microorganisms:
Mycobacterium tuberculosis

The following in vitro data are available, but their clinical significance is unknown.

Rifampin exhibits in vitro activity against most strains of the following microorganisms; however, the safety and effectiveness of rifampin in treating clinical infections due to these microorganisms have not been established in adequate and well-controlled trials.

Aerobic Gram-Positive Microorganisms:
Staphylococcus aureus (including Methicillin-Resistant *S. aureus*/MRSA)
Staphylococcus epidermidis

Aerobic Gram-Negative Microorganisms:
Haemophilus influenzae

"Other" Microorganisms:
Mycobacterium leprae

β-lactamase production should have no effect on rifampin activity.

Susceptibility Tests

Prior to initiation of therapy, appropriate specimens should be collected for identification of the infecting organism and in vitro susceptibility tests.

In vitro testing for *Mycobacterium tuberculosis* isolates:

Two standardized in vitro susceptibility methods are available for testing rifampin against *M tuberculosis* organisms. The agar proportion method (CDC or NCCLS[1] M24-P) utilizes Middlebrook 7H10 medium impregnated with rifampin at a final concentration of 1.0 μg/mL to determine drug resistance. After three weeks of incubation MIC_{99} values are calculated by comparing the quantity of organisms growing in the medium containing drug to the control cultures. Mycobacterial growth in the presence of drug, of at least 1% of the growth in the control culture, indicates resistance.

The radiometric broth method employs the BACTEC 460 machine to compare the growth index from untreated control cultures to cultures grown in the presence of 2.0 μg/mL of rifampin. Strict adherence to the manufacturer's instructions for sample processing and data interpretation is required for this assay.

Susceptibility test results obtained by the two different methods can only be compared if the appropriate rifampin concentration is used for each test method as indicated above. Both procedures require the use of *M tuberculosis* H37Rv ATCC 27294 as a control organism.

The clinical relevance of in vitro susceptibility test results for mycobacterial species other than *M tuberculosis* using either the radiometric or the proportion method has not been determined.

In vitro testing for *Neisseria meningitidis* isolates:

Dilution Techniques: Quantitative methods that are used to determine minimum inhibitory concentrations provide reproducible estimates of the susceptibility of bacteria to antimicrobial compounds. One such standardized procedure uses a standardized dilution method[2,4] (broth, agar, or microdilution) or equivalent with rifampin powder. The MIC values obtained should be interpreted according to the following criteria for *Neisseria meningitidis*:

MIC (μg/mL)	Interpretation
≤1	(S) Susceptible
2	(I) Intermediate
≥4	(R) Resistant

A report of "susceptible" indicates that the pathogen is likely to be inhibited by usually achievable concentrations of the antimicrobial compound in the blood. A report of "intermediate" indicates that the result should be considered equivocal, and if the microorganism is not fully susceptible to alternative, clinically feasible drugs, the test should be repeated. This category implies possible clinical applicability in body sites where the drug is physiologically concentrated or in situations where the maximum acceptable dose of drug can be used. This category also provides a buffer zone that prevents small uncontrolled technical factors from causing major discrepancies in interpretation. A report of "resistant" indicates that usually achievable concentrations of the antimicrobial compound in the blood are unlikely to be inhibitory and that other therapy should be selected.

Measurement of MIC or minimum bactericidal concentrations (MBC) and achieved antimicrobial compound concentrations may be appropriate to guide therapy in some infections. (See CLINICAL PHARMACOLOGY section for further information on drug concentrations achieved in infected body sites and other pharmacokinetic properties of this antimicrobial drug product.)

Standardized susceptibility test procedures require the use of laboratory control microorganisms. The use of these microorganisms does not imply clinical efficacy (see INDICATIONS AND USAGE); they are used to control the technical aspects of the laboratory procedures. Standard rifampin powder should give the following MIC values:

Microorganism		MIC (μg/mL)
Staphylococcus aureus	ATCC 29213	0.008-0.06
Enterococcus faecalis	ATCC 29212	1-4
Escherichia coli	ATCC 25922	8-32
Pseudomonas aeruginosa	ATCC 27853	32-64
Haemophilus influenzae	ATCC 49247	0.25-1

Diffusion Techniques: Quantitative methods that require measurement of zone diameters provide reproducible estimates of the susceptibility of bacteria to antimicrobial compounds. One such standardized procedure[3,4] that has been recommended for use with disks to test the susceptibility of microorganisms to rifampin uses the 5 μg rifampin disk. Interpretation involves correlation of the diameter obtained in the disk test with the MIC for rifampin.

Reports from the laboratory providing results of the standard single-disk susceptibility test with a 5 μg rifampin disk should be interpreted according to the following criteria for *Neisseria meningitidis*:

Zone Diameter (mm)	Interpretation
≥20	(S) Susceptible
17-19	(I) Intermediate
≤16	(R) Resistant

Interpretation should be as stated above for results using dilution techniques.

As with standard dilution techniques, diffusion methods require the use of laboratory control microorganisms. The use of these microorganisms does not imply clinical efficacy (see INDICATIONS AND USAGE); they are used to control the technical aspects of the laboratory procedures. The 5 μg rifampin disk should provide the following zone diameters in these quality control strains:

Microorganism		Zone Diameter (mm)
S. aureus	ATCC 25923	26-34
E. coli	ATCC 25922	8-10
H. influenzae	ATCC 49247	22-30

INDICATIONS AND USAGE

In the treatment of both tuberculosis and the meningococcal carrier state, the small number of resistant cells present within large populations of susceptible cells can rapidly become the predominant type. Bacteriologic cultures should be obtained before the start of therapy to confirm the susceptibility of the organism to rifampin and they should be repeated throughout therapy to monitor the response to treatment. Since resistance can emerge rapidly, susceptibility tests should be performed in the event of persistent positive cultures during the course of treatment. If test results show resistance to rifampin and the patient is not responding to therapy, the drug regimen should be modified.

Tuberculosis

Rifampin is indicated in the treatment of all forms of tuberculosis.

A three-drug regimen consisting of rifampin, isoniazid, and pyrazinamide (eg, RIFATER®) is recommended in the initial phase of short-course therapy which is usually continued for 2 months. The Advisory Council for the Elimination of Tuberculosis, the American Thoracic Society, and Centers for Disease Control and Prevention recommend that either streptomycin or ethambutol be added as a fourth drug in a regimen containing isoniazid (INH), rifampin, and pyrazinamide for initial treatment of tuberculosis unless the likelihood of INH resistance is very low. The need for a fourth drug should be reassessed when the results of susceptibility testing are unknown. If community rates of INH resistance are currently less than 4%, an initial treatment regimen with less than four drugs may be considered.

Following the initial phase, treatment should be continued with rifampin and isoniazid (eg, RIFAMATE®) for at least 4 months. Treatment should be continued for longer if the patient is still sputum or culture positive, if resistant organisms are present, or if the patient is HIV positive.

RIFADIN IV is indicated for the initial treatment and retreatment of tuberculosis when the drug cannot be taken by mouth.

Meningococcal Carriers

Rifampin is indicated for the treatment of asymptomatic carriers of *Neisseria meningitidis* to eliminate meningococci from the nasopharynx. **Rifampin is not indicated for the treatment of meningococcal infection because of the possibility of the rapid emergence of resistant organisms.** (See WARNINGS.)

Rifampin should not be used indiscriminately, and therefore, diagnostic laboratory procedures, including serotyping and susceptibility testing, should be performed for establishment of the carrier state and the correct treatment. So that the usefulness of rifampin in the treatment of asymptomatic meningococcal carriers is preserved, the drug should be used only when the risk of meningococcal disease is high.

CONTRAINDICATIONS

Rifampin is contraindicated in patients with a history of hypersensitivity to any of the rifamycins. (See WARNINGS.)

WARNINGS

Rifampin has been shown to produce liver dysfunction. Fatalities associated with jaundice have occurred in patients with liver disease and in patients taking rifampin with other hepatotoxic agents. Patients with impaired liver function should be given rifampin only in cases of necessity and then with caution and under strict medical supervision. In these patients, careful monitoring of liver function, especially SGPT/ALT and SGOT/AST should be carried out prior to therapy and then every 2 to 4 weeks during therapy. If signs of hepatocellular damage occur, rifampin should be withdrawn.

In some cases, hyperbilirubinemia resulting from competition between rifampin and bilirubin for excretory pathways of the liver at the cell level can occur in the early days of treatment. An isolated report showing a moderate rise in bilirubin and/or transaminase level is not in itself an indication for interrupting treatment; rather, the decision should be made after repeating the tests, noting trends in the levels, and considering them in conjunction with the patient's clinical condition.

Rifampin has enzyme-inducing properties, including induction of delta amino levulinic acid synthetase. Isolated reports have associated porphyria exacerbation with rifampin administration.

The possibility of rapid emergence of resistant meningococci restricts the use of RIFADIN to short-term treatment of the asymptomatic carrier state. **RIFADIN is not to be used for the treatment of meningococcal disease.**

PRECAUTIONS

General

For the treatment of tuberculosis, rifampin is usually administered on a daily basis. Doses of rifampin greater than 600 mg given once or twice weekly have resulted in a higher incidence of adverse reactions, including the "flu syndrome" (fever, chills and malaise), hematopoietic reactions (leukopenia, thrombocytopenia, or acute hemolytic anemia), cutaneous, gastrointestinal, and hepatic reactions, shortness of breath, shock, anaphylaxis, and renal failure. Recent studies indicate that regimens using twice-weekly doses of rifampin 600 mg plus isoniazid 15 mg/kg are much better tolerated.

Intermittent therapy may be used if the patient cannot (or will not) self-administer drugs on a daily basis. Patients on intermittent therapy should be closely monitored for compliance and cautioned against intentional or accidental interruption of prescribed therapy, because of the increased risk of serious adverse reactions.

Rifampin has enzyme induction properties that can enhance the metabolism of endogenous substrates including adrenal hormones, thyroid hormones, and vitamin D. Rifampin and isoniazid have been reported to alter vitamin D metabolism. In some cases, reduced levels of circulating 25-hydroxy vitamin D and 1,25-dihydroxy vitamin D have been accompanied by reduced serum calcium and phosphate, and elevated parathyroid hormone.

Plasma Concentrations (mean ± standard deviation, μg/mL)

Rifampin Dosage IV	30 min	1 hr	2 hr	4 hr	8 hr	12 hr
300 mg	8.9±2.9	4.9±1.3	4.0±1.3	2.5±1.0	1.1±0.6	<0.4
600 mg	17.4±5.1	11.7±2.8	9.4±2.3	6.4±1.7	3.5±1.4	1.2±0.6

RIFADIN IV

For intravenous infusion only. Must not be administered by intramuscular or subcutaneous route. Avoid extravasation during injection: local irritation and inflammation due to extravascular infiltration of the infusion have been observed. If these occur, the infusion should be discontinued and restarted at another site.

Information for Patients

The patient should be told that rifampin may produce a reddish coloration of the urine, sweat, sputum, and tears, and the patient should be forewarned of this. Soft contact lenses may be permanently stained.

The patients should be advised that the reliability of oral or other systemic hormonal contraceptives may be affected; consideration should be given to using alternative contraceptive measures.

Patients should be instructed to take rifampin either 1 hour before or 2 hours after a meal with a full glass of water.

Patients should be instructed to notify their physicians promptly if they experience any of the following: fever, loss of appetite, malaise, nausea and vomiting, darkened urine, yellowish discoloration of the skin and eyes, and pain or swelling of the joints.

Compliance with the full course of therapy must be emphasized, and the importance of not missing any doses must be stressed.

Laboratory Tests

Adults treated for tuberculosis with rifampin should have baseline measurements of hepatic enzymes, bilirubin, serum creatinine, a complete blood count, and a platelet count (or estimate). Baseline tests are unnecessary in pediatric patients unless a complicating condition is known or clinically suspected.

Patients should be seen at least monthly during therapy and should be specifically questioned concerning symptoms associated with adverse reactions. All patients with abnormalities should have follow-up, including laboratory testing, if necessary. Routine laboratory monitoring for toxicity in people with normal baseline measurements is generally not necessary.

Drug Interactions

ENZYME INDUCTION: Rifampin is known to induce certain cytochrome P-450 enzymes. Administration of rifampin with drugs that undergo biotransformation through these metabolic pathways may accelerate elimination of coadministered drugs. To maintain optimum therapeutic blood levels, dosages of drugs metabolized by these enzymes may require adjustment when starting or stopping concomitantly administered rifampin.

Rifampin has been reported to accelerate the metabolism of the following drugs: anticonvulsants (eg, phenytoin), antiarrhythmics (eg, disopyramide, mexiletine, quinidine, tocainide), oral anticoagulants, antifungals (eg, fluconazole, itraconazole, ketoconazole), barbiturates, beta-blockers, calcium channel blockers (eg, diltiazem, nifedipine, verapamil), chloramphenicol, clarithromycin, corticosteroids, cyclosporine, cardiac glycoside preparations, clofibrate, oral or other systemic hormone contraceptives, dapsone, diazepam, doxycycline, fluoroquinolones (eg ciprofloxacin), haloperidol, oral hypoglycemic agents (sulfonylureas), levothyroxine, methadone, narcotic analgesics, nortriptyline, progestins, quinine, tacrolimus, theophylline tricyclic antidepressants (eg, amitriptyline, nortriptyline), and zidovudine. It may be necessary to adjust the dosages of these drugs if they are given concurrently with rifampin.

Patients using oral or other systemic hormonal contraceptives should be advised to change to nonhormonal methods of birth control during rifampin therapy.

Rifampin has been observed to increase the requirements for anticoagulant drugs of the coumarin type. In patients receiving anitcoagulants and rifampin concurrently, it is recommended that the prothrombin time be performed daily or as frequently as necessary to establish and maintain the required dose of anticoagulant.

Diabetes may become more difficult to control.

OTHER INTERACTIONS: When the two drugs were taken concomitantly, decreased concentrations of atovaquone and increased concentrations of rifampin were observed.

Concurrent use of ketoconazole and rifampin has resulted in decreased serum concentrations of both drugs. Concurrent use of rifampin and enalapril has resulted in decreased concentrations of enalaprilat, the active metabolite of enalapril. Dosage adjustments should be made if indicated by the patient's clinical condition. Concomitant antacid administration may reduce the absorption of rifampin. Daily doses of rifampin should be given at least 1 hour before the ingestion of antacids.

Probenecid and cotrimoxazole have been reported to increase the blood level of rifampin.

When rifampin is given concomitantly with either halothane or isoniazid, the potential for hepatotoxicity is increased. The concomitant use of rifampin and halothane should be avoided. Patients receiving both rifampin and isoniazid should be monitored close for hepatotoxicity.

Plasma concentrations of sulfapyridine may be reduced following the concomitant administration of sulfasalazine and rifampin. This finding may be the result of alteration in the colonic bacteria responsible for the reduction of sulfasalazine to sulfapyridine and mesalamine.

Drug/Laboratory Interactions

Cross-reactivity and false-positive urine screening tests for opiates have been reported in patients receiving rifampin when using the KIMS (Kinetic Interaction of Microparticles in Solution) method (eg, Abuscreen OnLine opiates assay; Roche Diagnostic Systems). Confirmatory tests, such as gas chromatography/mass spectrometry, will distinguish rifampin from opiates.

Therapeutic levels of rifampin have been shown to inhibit standard microbiological assays for serum folate and vitamin B_{12}. Thus, alternate assay methods should be considered. Transient abnormalities in liver function tests (eg, elevation in serum bilirubin, alkaline phosphatase, and serum transaminases) and reduced biliary excretion of contrast media used for visualization of the gallbladder have also been observed. Therefore, these tests should be performed before the morning dose of rifampin.

Carcinogenesis, Mutagenesis, Impairment of Fertility

There are no known human data on long-term potential for carinogenicity, mutagenicity, or impairment of fertility. A few cases of accelerated growth of lung carcinoma have been reported in man, but a causal relationship with the drug has not been established. An increase in the incidence of hepatomas in female mice (of a strain known to be particularly susceptible to the spontaneous development of hepatomas) was observed when rifampin was administered in doses 2 to 10 times the average daily human dose for 60 weeks, followed by an observation period of 46 weeks. No evidence of carcinogenicity was found in male mice of the same strain, mice of a different strain, or rats under similar experimental conditions.

Rifampin has been reported to possess immunosuppressive potential in rabbits, mice, rats, guinea pigs, human lymphocytes in vitro, and humans. Antitumor activity in vitro has also been shown with rifampin.

There was no evidence of mutagenicity in bacteria, *Drosophila melanogaster*, or mice. An increase in chromotid breaks was noted when whole blood cell cultures were treated with rifampin. Increased frequency of chromosomal aberrations was observed in vitro in lymphocytes obtained from patients treated with combinations of rifampin, isoniazid, and pyrazinamide and combinations of streptomycin, rifampin, isoniazid, and pyrazinamide.

Pregnancy—Teratogenic Effects

Category C. Rifampin has been shown to be teratogenic in rodents given oral doses of rifampin 15 to 25 times the human dose. Although rifampin has been reported to cross the placental barrier and appear in cord blood, the effect of RIFADIN, alone or in combination with other antituberculosis drugs, on the human fetus is not known . Neonates of rifampin-treated mothers should be carefully observed for any evidence of adverse effects. Isolated cases of fetal malformations have been reported; however, there are no adequate and well-controlled studies in pregnant women. Rifampin should be used during pregnancy only if the potential benefit justifies the potential risk to the fetus. Rifampin in oral doses of 150 to 250 mg/kg produced teratogenic effects in mice and rats. Malformations were primarily cleft palate in the mouse and spina bifida in the rat. The incidence of these anomalies was dose-dependent. When rifampin was given to pregnant rabbits in doses up to 20 times the usual daily human dose, imperfect osteogenesis and embryotoxicity were reported.

Pregnancy—Non-Teratogenic Effects

When administered during the last few weeks of pregnancy, rifampin can cause post-natal hemorrhages in the mother and infant for which treatment with vitamin K may be indicated.

Nursing Mothers

Because of the potential for tumorigenicity shown for rifampin in animal studies, a decision should be made whether to discontinue nursing or discontinue the drug, taking into account the importance of the drug to the mother.

Pediatric Use

See CLINICAL PHARMACOLOGY—Pediatrics; see also DOSAGE AND ADMINISTRATION.

ADVERSE REACTIONS

Gastrointestinal

Heartburn, epigastric distress, anorexia, nausea, vomiting, jaundice, flatulence, cramps, and diarrhea have been noted in some patients. Although *Clostridium difficile* has been shown in vitro to be sensitive to rifampin, pseudomembranous colitis has been reported with the use of rifampin (and other broad spectrum antibiotics). Therefore, it is important to consider this diagnosis in patients who develop diarrhea in association with antibiotic use. Rarely, hepatitis or a shock-like syndrome with hepatic involvement and abnormal liver function tests has been reported.

Hematologic

Thrombocytopenia has occurred primarily with high dose intermittent therapy, but has also been noted after resumption of interrupted treatment. It rarely occurs during well supervised daily therapy. This effect is reversible if the drug is discontinued as soon as purpura occurs. Cerebral hemorrhage and fatalities have been reported when rifampin administration has been continued or resumed after the appearance of purpura.

Rare reports of disseminated intravascular coagulation have been observed.

Transient leukopenia, hemolytic anemia, and decreased hemoglobin have been observed.

Central Nervous System

Headache, fever, drowsiness, fatigue, ataxia, dizziness, inability to concentrate, mental confusion, behavioral changes, pain in extremities, and generalized numbness have been observed.

Psychoses have been rarely reported.

Ocular

Visual disturbances have been observed.

Endocrine

Menstrual disturbances have been observed.

Rare reports of adrenal insufficiency in patients with compromised adrenal function have been observed.

Renal

Elevations in BUN and serum uric acid have been reported. Rarely, hemolysis, hemoglobinuria, hematuria, interstitial nephritis, acute tubular necrosis, renal insufficiency, and acute renal failure have been noted. These are generally considered to be hypersensitivity reactions. They usually occur during intermittent therapy or when treatment is resumed following intentional or accidental interruption of a daily dosage regimen, and are reversible when rifampin is discontinued and appropriate therapy instituted.

Dermatologic

Cutaneous reactions are mild and self-limiting and do not appear to be hypersensitivity reactions. Typically, they consist of flushing and itching with or without a rash. More serious cutaneous reactions which may be due to hypersensitivity occur but are uncommon.

Hypersensitivity Reactions

Occasionally, pruritus, urticaria, rash, pemphigoid reaction, erythema multiforme including Stevens-Johnson Syndrome, toxic epidermal necrolysis, vasculitis, eosinophilia, sore mouth, sore tongue, and conjunctivitis have been observed.

Anaphylaxis has been reported rarely.

Miscellaneous

Rare reports of myopathy and muscular weakness have also been observed. Edema of the face and extremities has been reported. Other reactions reported to have occurred with intermittent dosage regimens include "flu syndrome" (such as episodes of fever, chills, headache, dizziness, and bone pain), shortness of breath, wheezing, decrease in blood pressure and shock. The "flu syndrome" may also appear if rifampin is taken irregularly by the patient or if daily administration is resumed after a drug free interval.

OVERDOSAGE

Signs and Symptoms

Nausea, vomiting, abdominal pain, pruritus, headache, and increasing lethargy will probably occur within a short time after ingestion; unconsciousness may occur when there is severe hepatic disease. Transient increases in liver enzymes and/or bilirubin may occur. Brownish-red or orange discoloration of the skin, urine, sweat, saliva, tears, and feces will occur, and its intensity is proportional to the amount ingested.

Facial or periorbital edema has also been reported in pediatric patients. Hypotension, sinus tachycardia, ventricular arrhythmias, seizures and cardiac arrest were reported in some fatal cases.

Acute Toxicity

The LD_{50} of rifampin is approximately 885 mg/kg in the mouse, 1720 mg/kg in the rat, and 2120 mg/kg in the rabbit. The minimum acute lethal or toxic dose is not well established. However, nonfatal acute overdoses in adults have been reported with doses ranging from 9 to 12 gm rifampin. Fatal acute overdoses in adults have been reported with doses ranging from 14 to 60 gm. Alcohol or a history of alcohol abuse was involved in some of the fatal and nonfatal reports. Nonfatal overdoses in pediatric patients ages 1 to 4 years old of 100 mg/kg for one to two doses has been reported.

Treatment

Intensive support measures should be instituted and individual symptoms treated as they arise. Since nausea and vomiting are likely to be present, gastric lavage is probably preferable to induction of emesis. Following evacuation of the gastric contents, the instillation of activated charcoal slurry into the stomach may help absorb any remaining drug from the gastrointestinal tract. Antiemetic medication may be required to control severe nausea and vomiting. Active diuresis (with measured intake and output) will help promote excretion of the drug. Hemodialysis may be of value in some patients.

Continued on next page

Rifadin—Cont.

DOSAGE AND ADMINISTRATION

Rifampin can be administered by the oral route or by IV infusion (see INDICATIONS AND USAGE).

See CLINICAL PHARMACOLOGY for dosing information in patients with renal failure.

Tuberculosis

Adults: 10 mg/kg, in a single daily administration, not to exceed 600 mg/day, oral or IV

Pediatric Patients: 10–20 mg/kg, not to exceed 600 mg/day, oral or IV

It is recommended that oral rifampin be administered once daily, either 1 hour before or 2 hours after a meal with a full glass of water.

Rifampin is indicated in the treatment of all forms of tuberculosis. A three-drug regimen consisting of rifampin, isoniazid, and pyrazinamide (eg, RIFATER®) is recommended in the initial phase of short-course therapy which is usually continued for 2 months. The Advisory Council for the Elimination of Tuberculosis, the American Thoracic Society, and the Centers for Disease Control and Prevention recommend that either streptomycin or ethambutol be added as a fourth drug in a regimen containing isoniazid (INH), rifampin and pyrazinamide for initial treatment of tuberculosis unless the likelihood of INH resistance is very low. The need for a fourth drug should be reassessed when the results of susceptibility testing are known. If community rates of INH resistance are currently less than 4%, an initial treatment regimen with less than four drugs may be considered.

Following the initial phase, treatment should be continued with rifampin and isoniazid (eg, RIFAMATE®) for at least four months. Treatment should be continued for longer if the patient is still sputum or culture positive, if resistant organisms are present, or if the patient is HIV positive.

Preparation of Solution for IV Infusion: Reconstitute the lyophilized powder by transferring 10 mL of sterile water for injection to a vial containing 600 mg of rifampin for injection. Swirl vial gently to completely dissolve the antibiotic. The reconstituted solution contains 60 mg rifampin per mL and is stable at room temperature for 24 hours. Prior to administration, withdraw from the reconstituted solution a volume equivalent to the amount of rifampin calculated to be administered and add to 500 mL of infusion medium. Mix well and infuse at a rate allowing for complete infusion within 3 hours. Alternatively, the amount of rifampin calculated to be administered may be added to 100 mL of infusion medium and infused in 30 minutes.

Dilutions in dextrose 5% for injection (D5W) are stable at room temperature for up to 4 hours and should be prepared and used within this time. Precipitation of rifampin from the infusion solution may occur beyond this time. Dilutions in normal saline are stable at room temperature for up to 24 hours and should be prepared and used within this time. Other infusion solution are not recommended.

Incompatibilities: Physical incompatibility (precipitate) was observed with undiluted (5 mg/mL) and diluted (1 mg/mL in normal saline) diltiazem hydrochloride and rifampin (6 mg/mL in normal saline) during simulated Y-site administration.

Meningococcal Carriers

Adults: For adults, it is recommended that 600 mg rifampin be administered twice daily for two days.

Pediatric Patients: Pediatric patients 1 month of age or older: 10 mg/kg (not to exceed 600 mg per dose) every 12 hours for two days.

Pediatric patients under 1 month of age: 5 mg/kg every 12 hours for two days.

Preparation of Extemporaneous Oral Suspension

For pediatric and adult patients in whom capsule swallowing is difficult or where lower doses are needed, a liquid suspension may be prepared as follows:

RIFADIN 1% w/v suspension (10 mg/mL) can be compounded using one of four syrups—Simple Syrup (Syrup NF), Simple Syrup (Humco Laboratories), Syrpalta® Syrup (Emerson Laboratories), or Raspberry Syrup (Humco Laboratories).

1. Empty the contents of four RIFADIN 300 mg capsules or eight RIFADIN 150 mg capsules onto a piece of weighing paper.
2. If necessary, gently crush the capsule contents with a spatula to produce a fine powder.
3. Transfer the rifampin powder blend to a 4-ounce amber glass or plastic (high density polyethylene [HDPE], polypropylene, or procarbonate) prescription bottle.
4. Rinse the paper and spatula with 20 mL of one of the above-mentioned syrups, and add the rinse to the bottle. Shake vigorously.
5. Add 100 mL of syrup to the bottle and shake vigorously.

This compound procedure results in a 1% w/v suspension containing 10 mg rifampin/mL. Stability studies indicate that the suspension is stable when stored at room temperature (25 ± 3°C) or in a refrigerator (2–8°C) for four weeks. This extemporaneously prepared suspension must be shaken well prior to administration.

HOW SUPPLIED

150 maroon and scarlet capsules imprinted "RIFADIN 150".
Bottles of 30 (NDC 0068-0510-30)

300 maroon and scarlet capsules imprinted "RIFADIN 300".
Bottles of 30 (NDC 0068-0508-30)
Bottles of 60 (NDC 0068-0508-60)
Bottles of 100 (NDC 0068-0508-61)

Storage: Keep tightly closed. Store in a dry place. Avoid excessive heat.

RIFADIN IV (rifampin for injection) is available in glass vials containing 600 mg rifampin (NDC 0068-0597-01).

Storage: Avoid excessive heat (temperatures above 40°C or 104°F). Protect from light.

References:

1. National Committee for Clinical Laboratory Standards, Antimycobacterial Susceptibility Testing. Proposed Standard NCCLS Document M24-P, Vol. 10, No. 10, NNCLS, Villanova, PA, 1990.
2. National Committee for Clinical Laboratory Standards. Methods for Dilution Antimicrobial Susceptibility Tests for Bacteria that Grow Aerobically—Third Edition. Approved Standard NCCLS Document M7-A3, Vol. 13, No. 25, NCCLS, Villanova, PA, December 1993.
3. National Committee for Clinical Laboratory Standards. Performance Standards for Antimicrobial Disk Susceptibility Tests—Fifth Edition. Approved Standard NCCLS Document M2-A5, Vol. 13, No. 24, NCCLS, Villanova, PA, December 1993.
4. National Committee for Clinical Laboratory Standards. Performance Standards for Antimicrobial Susceptibility Testing; Fifth Informational Supplement, NCCLS Document M100-S5, Vol. 14, No. 16, NCCLS, Villanova, PA, December 1994.

Prescribing Information as of July 1997

Merrell Pharmaceuticals Inc.
Subsidiary of Hoechst Marion Roussel, Inc.
Kansas City, MO 64137 USA

Rifadin IV (rifampin for injection) is manufactured by:
GRUPPO LEPETIT S.p.A.
20020 Lainate, Italy

Shown in Product Identification Guide, page 316

RIFAMATE® ℞

[*rĭf 'uh-māt*]

(rifampin and isoniazid capsules)

Prescribing Information as of March 1996

WARNING

Severe and sometimes fatal hepatitis associated with isoniazid therapy may occur and may develop even after many months of treatment. The risk of developing hepatitis is age related. Approximate case rates by age are: 0 per 1,000 for persons under 20 years of age, 3 per 1,000 for persons in the 20–34 year age group, 12 per 1,000 for persons in the 35–49 year age group, 23 per 1,000 for persons in the 50–64 year age group, and 8 per 1,000 for persons over 65 years of age. The risk of hepatitis is increased with daily consumption of alcohol. Precise data to provide a fatality rate for isoniazid-related hepatitis is not available; however, in a U.S. Public Health Service Surveillance Study of 13,838 persons taking isoniazid, there were 8 deaths among 174 cases of hepatitis.

Therefore, patients given isoniazid should be carefully monitored and interviewed at monthly intervals. Serum transaminase concentration becomes elevated in about 10–20 percent of patients, usually during the first few months of therapy, but it can occur at any time. Usually enzyme levels return to normal despite continuance of drug, but in some cases progressive liver dysfunction occurs. Patients should be instructed to report immediately any of the prodromal symptoms of hepatitis, such as fatigue, weakness, malaise, anorexia, nausea, or vomiting. If these symptoms appear or if signs suggestive of hepatic damage are detected, isoniazid should be discontinued promptly, since continued use of the drug in these cases has been reported to cause a more severe form of liver damage.

Patients with tuberculosis should be given appropriate treatment with alternative drugs. If isoniazid must be reinstituted, it should be reinstituted only after symptoms and laboratory abnormalities have cleared. The drug should be restarted in very small and gradually increasing doses and should be withdrawn immediately if there is any indication of recurrent liver involvement.

Treatment should be deferred in persons with acute hepatic diseases.

DESCRIPTION

RIFAMATE is a combination capsule containing 300 mg rifampin and 150 mg isoniazid. The capsules also contain as inactive ingredients: colloidal silicon dioxide, FD&C Blue No. 1, FD&C Red No. 40, gelatin, magnesium stearate, sodium starch glycolate, and titanium dioxide.

Rifampin is a semisynthetic antibiotic derivative of rifamycin B. The chemical name for rifampin is 3-(4-methyl-1-piperazinyliminomethyl) rifamycin SV.

Isoniazid is the hydrazide of isonicotinic acid. It exists as colorless or white crystals or as a white, crystalline powder that is water soluble, odorless, and slowly affected by exposure to air and light.

ACTIONS

Rifampin

Rifampin inhibits DNA-dependent RNA polymerase activity in susceptible cells. Specifically, it interacts with bacterial RNA polymerase but does not inhibit the mammalian enzyme. This is the mechanism of action by which rifampin exerts its therapeutic effect. Rifampin cross resistance has only been shown with other rifamycins.

In a study of 14 normal human adult males, peak blood levels of rifampin occured 1 $^1/_2$ to 3 hours following oral administration of two RIFAMATE capsules. The peaks ranged from 6.9 to 14 mcg/ml with an average of 10 mcg/ml.

In normal subjects the $T^1/_2$ (biological half-life) of rifampin in blood is approximately 3 hours. Elimination occurs mainly through the bile and, to a much lesser extent, the urine.

Isoniazid

Isoniazid acts against actively growing tubercle bacilli.

After oral administration isoniazid produces peak blood levels within 1 to 2 hours which decline to 50% or less within 6 hours. It diffuses readily into all body fluids (cerebrospinal, pleural, and ascitic fluids), tissues, organs and excreta (saliva, sputum, and feces). The drug also passes through the placental barrier and into milk in concentrations comparable to those in the plasma. From 50 to 70% of a dose of isoniazid is excreted in the urine in 24 hours.

Isoniazid is metabolized primarily by acetylation and dehydrazination. The rate of acetylation is genetically determined. Approximately 50% of Blacks and Caucasians are "slow inactivators"; the majority of Eskimos and Orientals are "rapid inactivators."

The rate of acetylation does not significantly alter the effectiveness of isoniazid. However, slow acetylation may lead to higher blood levels of the drug, and thus an increase in toxic reactions.

Pyridoxine deficiency (B_6) is sometimes observed in adults with high doses of isoniazid and is considered probably due to its competition with pyridoxal phosphate for the enzyme apotryptophanase.

INDICATIONS

For pulmonary tuberculosis in which organisms are susceptible, and when the patient has been titrated on the individual components and it has therefore been established that this fixed dosage is therapeutically effective.

This fixed-dosage combination drug is not recommended for initial therapy of tuberculosis or for preventive therapy.

In the treatment of tuberculosis, small numbers of resistant cells, present within large populations of susceptible cells, can rapidly become the predominating type. Since rapid emergence of resistance can occur, culture and susceptibility tests should be performed in the event of persistent positive cultures.

This drug is not indicated for the treatment of meningococcal infections or asymptomatic carriers of *N. meningitidis* to eliminate meningococci from the nasopharynx.

CONTRAINDICATIONS

Previous isoniazid-associated hepatic injury; severe adverse reactions to isoniazid, such as drug fever, chills, and arthritis; acute liver disease of any etiology. A history of previous hypersensitivity reaction to any of the rifamycins or to isoniazid, including drug-induced hepatitis.

WARNINGS

RIFAMATE (rifampin-isoniazid) is a combination of two drugs, each of which has been associated with liver dysfunction. Liver function tests should be performed prior to therapy with RIFAMATE and periodically during treatment.

Rifampin

Rifampin has been shown to produce liver dysfunction. There have been fatalities associated with jaundice in patients with liver disease or receiving rifampin concomitantly with other hepatoxic agents. Since an increased risk may exist for individuals with liver disease, benefits must be weighed carefully against the risk of further liver damage.

Several studies of tumorigenicity potential have been done in rodents. In one strain of mice known to be particularly susceptible to the spontaneous development of hepatomas, rifampin given at a level 2–10 times the maximum dosage used clinically resulted in a significant increase in the occurrence of hepatomas in female mice of this strain after one year of administration.

There was no evidence of tumorigenicity in the males of this strain, in males or females of another mouse strain, or in rats.

Isoniazid

See the boxed warning.

PRECAUTIONS

Rifampin

Rifampin is not recommended for intermittent therapy; the patient should be cautioned against intentional or accidental interruption of the daily dosage regimen since rare renal hypersensitivity reactions have been reported when therapy was resumed in such cases.

Rifampin has been observed to increase the requirements for anticoagulant drugs of the coumarin type. The cause of the phenomenon is unknown. In patients receiving anticoagulants and rifampin concurrently, it is recommended that the prothrombin time be performed daily or as frequently as necessary to establish and maintain the required dose of anticoagulant.

Urine, feces, saliva, sputum, sweat and tears may be colored red-orange by rifampin and its metabolites. Soft contact lenses may be permanently stained. Individuals to be treated should be made aware of these possibilities.

It has been reported that the reliability of oral contraceptives may be affected in some patients being treated for tuberculosis with rifampin in combination with at least one other antituberculosis drug. In such cases, alternative contraceptive measures may need to be considered.

It has also been reported that rifampin given in combination with other antituberculosis drugs may decrease the pharmacologic activity of methadone, oral hypoglycemics, digitoxin, quinidine, disopyramide, dapsone, and corticosteroids. In these cases, dosage adjustment of the interacting drugs is recommended.

Therapeutic levels of rifampin have been shown to inhibit standard microbiological assays for serum folate and vitamin B_{12}. Alternative methods must be considered when determining folate and vitamin B_{12} concentrations in the presence of rifampin.

Since rifampin has been reported to cross the placental barrier and appear in cord blood and in maternal milk, neonates and newborns of rifampin-treated mothers should be carefully observed for any evidence of untoward effects.

Isoniazid

All drugs should be stopped and an evaluation of the patient should be made at the first sign of a hypersensitivity reaction.

Use of isoniazid should be carefully monitored in the following:

1. Patients who are receiving phenytoin (diphenylhydantoin) concurrently. Isoniazid may decrease the excretion of phenytoin or may enhance its effects. To avoid phenytoin intoxication, appropriate adjustment of the anticonvulsant dose should be made.
2. Daily users of alcohol. Daily ingestion of alcohol may be associated with a higher incidence of isoniazid hepatitis.
3. Patients with current chronic liver disease or severe renal dysfunction.

Periodic ophthalmoscopic examination during isoniazid therapy is recommended when visual symptoms occur.

Usage in Pregnancy and Lactation

Rifampin

Although rifampin has been reported to cross the placental barrier and appear in cord blood, the effect of rifampin, alone or in combination with other antituberculosis drugs, on the human fetus is not known. An increase in congenital malformations, primarily spina bifida and cleft palate, has been reported in the offspring of rodents given oral doses of 150–250 mg/kg/day of rifampin during pregnancy.

The possible teratogenic potential in women capable of bearing children should be carefully weighed against the benefits of therapy.

Isoniazid

It has been reported that in both rats and rabbits, isoniazid may exert an embryocidal effect when administered orally during pregnancy, although no isoniazid-related congenital anomalies have been found in reproduction studies in mammalian species (mice, rats, and rabbits). Isoniazid should be prescribed during pregnancy only when therapeutically necessary. The benefit of preventive therapy should be weighed against a possible risk to the fetus. Preventive treatment generally should be started after delivery because of the increased risk of tuberculosis for new mothers.

Since isoniazid is known to cross the placental barrier and to pass into maternal breast milk, neonates and breast-fed infants of isoniazid treated mothers should be carefully observed for any evidence of adverse effects.

Carcinogenesis: Isoniazid has been reported to induce pulmonary tumors in a number of strains of mice.

ADVERSE REACTIONS

Rifampin

Nervous system reactions: headache, drowsiness, fatigue, ataxia, dizziness, inability to concentrate, mental confusion, visual disturbances, muscular weakness, pain in extremities, and generalized numbness

Gastrointestinal disturbances: in some patients heartburn, epigastric distress, anorexia, nausea, vomiting, gas, cramps, and diarrhea

Hepatic reactions: transient abnormalities in liver function tests (e.g., elevations in serum bilirubin, BSP, alkaline phosphatase, serum transaminases) have been observed. Rarely, hepatitis or a shocklike syndrome with hepatic involvement and abnormal liver function tests

Renal reactions: elevations in BUN and serum uric acid have been reported. Rarely, hemolysis, hemoglobinuria, hematuria, interstitial nephritis, renal insufficiency, and acute renal failure have been noted. These are generally considered to be hypersensitivity reactions. They usually occur during intermittent therapy or when treatment is resumed following intentional or accidental interruption of a daily dosage regimen, and are reversible when rifampin is discontinued and appropriate therapy instituted.

Hematologic reactions: thrombocytopenia, transient leukopenia, hemolytic anemia, eosinophilia, and decreased hemoglobin have been observed. Thrombocytopenia has occurred when rifampin and ethambutol were administered concomitantly according to an intermittent dose schedule twice weekly and in high doses.

Allergic and immunological reactions: occasionally pruritus, urticaria, rash, pemphigoid reaction, eosinophilia, sore mouth, sore tongue, and exudative conjunctivitis. Rarely, hemolysis, hemoglobinuria, hematuria, renal insufficiency or acute renal failure have been reported which are generally considered to be hypersensitivity reactions. These have usually occurred during intermittent therapy or when treatment was resumed following intentional or accidental interruption of a daily dosage regimen and were reversible when rifampin was discontinued and appropriate therapy instituted.

Although rifampin has been reported to have an immunosuppressive effect in some animal experiments, available human data indicate that this has no clinical significance.

Metabolic reactions: elevations in BUN and serum uric acid have occurred.

Miscellaneous reactions: fever and menstrual disturbances have been noted.

Isoniazid

The most frequent reactions are those affecting the nervous system and the liver.

Nervous system reactions: peripheral neuropathy is the most common toxic effect. It is dose-related, occurs most often in the malnourished and in those predisposed to neuritis (e.g., alcoholics and diabetics), and is usually preceded by paresthesias of the feet and hands. The incidence is higher in "slow inactivators."

Other neurotoxic effects, which are uncommon with conventional doses, are convulsions, toxic encephalopathy, optic neuritis and atrophy, memory impairment, and toxic psychosis.

Gastrointestinal reactions: nausea, vomiting, and epigastric distress

Hepatic reactions: elevated serum transaminases (SGOT; SGPT), bilirubinemia, bilirubinuria, jaundice, and occasionally severe and sometimes fatal hepatitis. The common prodromal symptoms are anorexia, nausea, vomiting, fatigue, malaise, and weakness. Mild and transient elevations of serum transaminase levels occurs in 10 to 20 percent of persons taking isoniazid. The abnormality usually occurs in the first 4 to 6 months of treatment but can occur at any time during therapy. In most instances, enzyme levels return to normal with no necessity to discontinue medication. In occasional instances, progressive liver damage occurs, with accompanying symptoms. In these cases, the drug should be discontinued immediately. The frequency of progressive liver damage increases with age. It is rare in persons under 20, but occurs in up to 2.3 percent of those over 50 years of age.

Hematologic reactions: agranulocytosis, hemolytic sideroblastic or aplastic anemia, thrombocytopenia and eosinophilia

Hypersensitivity reactions: fever, skin eruptions (morbilliform, maculopapular, purpuric, or exfoliative), lymphadenopathy and vasculitis

Metabolic and endocrine reactions: pyridoxine deficiency, pellagra, hyperglycemia, metabolic acidosis, and gynecomastia

Miscellaneous reactions: rheumatic syndrome and systemic lupus erythematosus-like syndrome

OVERDOSAGE

Rifampin

Signs and Symptoms

Nausea, vomiting, and increasing lethargy will probably occur within a short time after ingestion; actual unconsciousness may occur with severe hepatic involvement. Brownish-red or orange discoloration of the skin, urine, sweat, saliva, tears, and feces is proportional to amount ingested.

Liver enlargement, possibly with tenderness, can develop within a few hours after severe overdosage, and jaundice may develop rapidly. Hepatic involvement may be more marked in patients with prior impairment of hepatic function. Other physical findings remain essentially normal.

Direct and total bilirubin levels may increase rapidly with severe overdosage; hepatic enzyme levels may be affected, especially with prior impairment of hepatic function. A direct effect upon hemopoietic system, electrolyte levels, or acid-base balance is unlikely.

Isoniazid

Signs and Symptoms

Isoniazid overdosage produces signs and symptoms within 30 minutes to 3 hours. Nausea, vomiting, dizziness, slurring of speech, blurring of vision, visual hallucinations (including bright colors and strange designs), are among the early manifestations. With marked overdosage, respiratory distress and CNS depression, progressing rapidly from stupor to profound coma, are to be expected, along with severe, intractable seizures. Severe metabolic acidosis, acetonuria, and hyperglycemia are typical laboratory findings.

RIFAMATE (rifampin and isoniazid capsules)

Treatment

The airway should be secured and adequate respiratory exchange established. Only then should gastric emptying (lavage-aspiration) be attempted; this may be difficult because of seizures. Since nausea and vomiting are likely to be present, gastric lavage is probably preferable to induction of emesis.

Activated charcoal slurry instilled into the stomach following evacuation of gastric contents can help absorb any remaining drug in the GI tract. Antiemetic medication may be required to control severe nausea and vomiting.

Blood samples should be obtained for immediate determination of gases, electrolytes, BUN, glucose, etc. Blood should be typed and crossmatched in preparation for possible hemodialysis.

Rapid control of metabolic acidosis is fundamental to management. Intravenous sodium bicarbonate should be given at once and repeated as needed, adjusting subsequent dosage on the basis of laboratory findings (i.e. serum sodium, pH, etc.). At the same time, anticonvulsants should be given intravenously (i.e., barbiturates, diphenylhydantoin, diazepam) as required, and large doses of intravenous pyridoxine.

Forced osmotic diuresis must be started early and should be continued for some hours after clinical improvement to hasten renal clearance of drug and help prevent relapse. Fluid intake and output should be monitored.

Bile drainage may be indicated in presence of serious impairment of hepatic function lasting more than 24–48 hours. Under these circumstances and for severe cases, extracorporeal hemodialysis may be required; if this is not available, peritoneal dialysis can be used along with forced diuresis.

Along with measures based on initial and repeated determination of blood gases and other laboratory tests as needed, meticulous respiratory and other intensive care should be utilized to protect against hypoxia, hypotension, aspiration, pneumonitis, etc.

In patients with previously adequate hepatic function, reversal of liver enlargement and impaired hepatic excretory function probably will be noted within 72 hours, with rapid return toward normal thereafter.

Untreated or inadequately treated cases of gross isoniazid overdosage can terminate fatally, but good response has been reported in most patients brought under adequate treatment within the first few hours after drug ingestion.

DOSAGE AND ADMINISTRATION

In general, therapy should be continued until bacterial conversion and maximal improvement have occurred.

Adults: Two RIFAMATE (rifampin-isoniazid) capsules (600 mg rifampin, 300 mg isoniazid) once daily, administered one hour before or two hours after a meal.

Concomitant administration of pyridoxine (B_6) is recommended in the malnourished, in those predisposed to neuropathy (e.g., diabetic), and in adolescents.

Susceptibility Testing

Rifampin

Rifampin susceptibility powders are available for both direct and indirect methods of determining the susceptibility of strains of mycobacteria. The MIC's of susceptible clinical isolates when determined in 7H10 or other non-egg-containing media have ranged from 0.1 to 2 mcg/ml.

Quantitative methods that require measurement of zone diameters give the most precise estimates of antibiotic susceptibility. One such procedure has been recommended for use with discs for testing susceptibility to rifampin. Interpretations correlate zone diameters from the disc test with MIC (minimal inhibitory concentration) values for rifampin.

HOW SUPPLIED

Capsules (opaque red), containing 300 mg rifampin and 150 mg isoniazid; bottles of 60 (NDC 0068-0509-60).

Continued on next page

Rifamate—Cont.

Prescribing Information as of March 1996
Merrell Pharmaceuticals Inc.
Subsidiary of Hoechst Marion Roussel, Inc.
Kansas City, MO 64137
Shown in Product Identification Guide, page 316

RIFATER®

[rif ' uh-ter]
(rifampin, isoniazid
and pyrazinamide)
Tablets

R_x

Prescribing Information as of December 1995

WARNING

Severe and sometimes fatal hepatitis associated with isoniazid therapy may occur and may develop even after many months of treatment. The risk of developing hepatitis is age related. Approximate case rates by age are: 0 per 1,000 for persons under 20 years of age, 3 per 1,000 for persons in the 20 to 34 year age group, 12 per 1,000 for persons in the 35 to 49 year age group, 23 per 1,000 for persons in the 50 to 64 year age group, and 8 per 1,000 for persons over 65 years of age. The risk of hepatitis is increased with daily consumption of alcohol. Precise data to provide a fatality rate for isoniazid-related hepatitis is not available; however, in a U.S. Public Health Service Surveillance Study of 13,838 persons taking isoniazid, there were 8 deaths amount 174 cases of hepatitis.

Therefore, patients given isoniazid should be carefully monitored and interviewed at monthly intervals. Serum transaminase concentration becomes elevated in about 10% to 20% of patients, usually during the first few months of therapy, but it can occur at any time. Usually enzyme levels return to normal despite continuance of drug, but in some cases progressive liver dysfunction occurs. Patients should be instructed to report immediately any of the prodromal symptoms of hepatitis, such as fatigue, weakness, malaise, anorexia, nausea, or vomiting. If these symptoms appear or if signs of suggestive of hepatic damage are detected, isoniazid should be discontinued promptly since continued use of the drug in these cases has been reported to cause a more severe form of liver damage.

Patients with tuberculosis should be given appropriate treatment with alternative drugs. If isoniazid must be reinstituted, it should be reinstituted only after symptoms and laboratory abnormalities have cleared. The drug should be restarted in very small and gradually increasing doses and should be withdrawn immediately if there is any indication of recurrent liver involvement. Treatment should be deferred in persons with acute hepatic diseases.

DESCRIPTION

RIFATER (rifampin/isoniazid/pyrazinamide) tablets are combination tablets containing 120 mg rifampin, 50 mg isoniazid, and 300 mg pyrazinamide for use in antibacterial therapy. The tablets also contain as inactive ingredients: povidone, carboxymethylcellulose sodium, calcium stearate, sodium lauryl sulfate, sucrose, talc, acacia, titanium dioxide, kaolin, magnesium carbonate, colloidal silicon dioxide, dried aluminum hydroxide gel, ferric oxide, black iron oxide, carnauba wax, white beeswax, colophony, hard paraffin, lecithin, shellac, and propylene glycol. The RIFATER triple therapy combinaion was developed for dosing convenience. Rifampin is a semisynthetic antibiotic derivative of rifamycin SV. Rifampin is a red-brown crystalline powder very slightly soluble in water at neutral pH, freely soluble in chloroform, soluble in ethyl acetate and methanol. Its molecular weight is 822.95 and its chemical formula is $C_{43}H_{58}N_4O_{12}$. The chemical name for rifampin is either: 3-[[(4-methyl-1-piperazinyl) imino]-methyl]-rifamycin; or 5, 6, 9, 17, 19, 21-hexahydroxy-23methoxy-2,4,12,16,18,20,22 heptamethyl-8-[N-(4-methyl-1-piperazinyl) formimidoyl]-2,7-(epoxypentadeca [1,11,13]trienimino)naphtho[2,1-b]furan-1, 11 (2H)-dione 21-acetate.

Its structural formula is:

Isoniazid is the hydroxide of isonicotinic acid. It is a colorless or white crystalline powder or white crystals. It is odorless and slowly affected by exposure to air and light. It is freely soluble in water, sparingly soluble in alcohol and slightly soluble in chloroform and in ether. Its molecular weight is 137.14 and its chemical formula is $C_6H_7N_3O$. The chemical name for isoniazid is 4-pyridinecarboxylic acid, hydrazide and its structural formula is:

Pyrazinamide, the pyrazine analogue of nicotinamide, is a white, crystalline powder, stable at room temperature, and sparingly soluble in water. The chemical name for pyrazinamide is pyrazinecarboxamide and its molecular weight is 123.11. Its chemical formula is $C_5H_5N_3O$ and its structural formula is:

CLINICAL PHARMACOLOGY

General

Rifampin. Rifampin is readily absorbed from the gastrointestinal tract. Peak serum levels in normal adults and pediatric populations vary widely from individual to individual. Following a single 600 mg oral dose of rifampin in healthy adults, the peak serum level averages 7µg/mL but may vary from 4 to 32 µg/mL. Absorption of rifampin is reduced when the drug is ingested with food.

In normal subjects, the biological half-life of rifampin in serum averages about 3 hours after a 600 mg oral dose, with increases up to 5.1 hours reported after a 900 mg dose. With repeated administration, the half-life decreases and reaches average values of approximately 2 to 3 hours. The half-life dos not differ in patients with renal failure at doses not exceeding 600 mg daily and, consequently no dosage adjustment is required. The half-life of rifampin at a dose of 720 mg daily has not been established in patients with renal failure. Following a single 900 mg oral dose of rifampin in patients with varying degrees of renal insufficiency, the half-life increased from 3.6 hours in normal subjects to 5.0, 7.3 and 11.0 hours in patients with glomerular filtration rates of 30–50 mL/min, less than 30 mL/min, and in anuric patients, respectively. Refer to the WARNINGS section for information regarding patients with hepatic insufficiency.

After absorption, rifampin is rapidly eliminated in the bile, and an enterohepatic circulation ensues. During this process, rifampin undergoes progressive deacetylation so that nearly all the drug in the bile is in this form in about 6 hours. This metabolite has antibacterial activity. Intestinal reabsorption is reduced by deacetylation, and elimination is facilitated. Up to 30% of a dose is excreted in the urine, with about half as unchanged drug.

Rifampin is widely distributed throughout the body. It is present in effective concentration in many organs and body fluids, including cerebrospinal fluid. Rifampin is about 80% protein bound. Most of the unbound fraction is not ionized and therefore is diffused freely in tissues.

Isoniazid. After oral administration, isoniazid is readily absorbed from the GI tract and produces peak blood levels within 1 to 2 hours. It diffuses readily into all body fluids (cerebrospinal, pleural, and ascitic fluids), tissues, organs, and excreta (saliva, sputum, and feces). Isoniazid is not substantially bound to plasma proteins. The drug also passes through the placental barrier and into milk in concentrations comparable to those in the plasma. the plasma half-life of isoniazid in patients with normal renal and hepatic function ranges from 1–4 hours, depending on the rate of metabolism. From 50% to 70% of a dose of isoniazid is excreted in the urine within 24 hours, mostly as metabolites. Isoniazid is metabolized in the liver mainly by acetylation and dehydrazination. The rate of acetylation is genetically determined. Approximately 50% of African Americans and Caucasians are "slow inactivators" and the rest are "rapid inactivators"; the majority of Eskimos and Asians are "rapid inactivators." The rate of acetylation does not significantly alter the effectiveness of isoniazid. However, slow acetylation may lead to higher blood levels of the drug, and thus, an increase in toxic reactions.

Pyridoxin (B_6) deficiency is sometimes observed in adults with high doses of isoniazid and is probably due to its competition with pyridoxal phosphate for the enzyme apotryphtophanase.

Pyrazinamide. Pyrazinamide is well absorbed from the gastrointestinal tract and attains peak plasma concentrations within 2 hours. Plasma concentrations generally range from 30 to 50 µg/mL with doses of 20 to 25 mg/kg. It is widely distributed in body tissues and fluids including the liver, lungs, and cerebrospinal fluid (CSF). The CSF concentration is approximately equal to concurrent steady-state plasma concentrations in patients with inflamed meninges. Pyrazinamide is approximately 10% bound to plasma proteins. The plasma half-life of pyrazinamide is 9 to 10 hours in patients with normal renal and hepatic function. The half-life of the drug may be prolonged in patients with impaired renal or hepatic function. Pyrazinamide is hydrolyzed in the liver to its major active metabolite, pyrazinoic acid. Pyrazinoic acid is hydroxylated to the main excretory product, 5-hydroxypyrazinoic acid.

Within 24 hours, approximately 70% of an oral dose of pyrazinamide is excreted in urine, mainly by glomerular filtration. About 4% to 14% of the dose is excreted as unchanged drug; the remainder is excreted as metabolites.

RIFATER

In a single-dose bioavailabilty study of five RIFATER tablets (Treatment A, n=23) versus RIFADIN 600 mg, isoniazid 250 mg, and pyrazinamide 1500 mg (Treatment B, n=24) administered concurrently in normal subjects, there was no difference in extent of absorption, as measured by the area under the plasma concentration versus time curve (AUC), of all three components. However, the mean peak plasma concentration of rifampin was approximately 18% lower following the single-dose administration of RIFATER tablets as compared to RIFADIN administered in combination with pyrazinamide and isoniazid. Mean (±SD) pharmacokinetic parameters are summarized in the following table.
[See table below]
The effect of food on the pharmacokinetics of RIFATER tablets was not studied.

Microbiology

Rifampin, isoniazid, and pyrazinamide at therapeutic levels have demonstrated bactericidal activity against both intracellular and extracellular *Mycobacterium tuberculosis* organisms.

Mechanism of Action

Rifampin. Rifampin inhibits DNA-dependent RNA polymerase activity in susceptible *Mycobacterium tuberculosis* organisms. Specifically, it interacts with bacterial RNA polymerase, but does not inhibit the mammalian enzyme. Organisms resistant to rifampin are likely to be resistant to other rifamycins.

Isoniazid. Isoniazid kills actively growing tubercle bacilli by inhibiting the biosynthesis of mycolic acids which are major components of the cell wall of *Mycobacterium tuberculosis*.

Pyrazinamide. The exact mechanism of action by which pyrazinamide inhibits the growth of *Mycobacterium tuberculosis* organisms is unknown. *In vitro* and *in vivo* studies have demonstrated that pyrazinamide is only active at a slightly acidic pH (pH 5.5).

Susceptibility Testing

Prior to initiation of therapy, appropriate specimens should be collected for identification of the infecting organism and *in vitro* susceptibility tests

Two standardized *in vitro* susceptibility methods are available for testing isoniazid, rifampin, and pyrazinamide against *Mycobacterium tuberculosis* organisms. The agar proportion method (CDC or NCCLS M24-P) utilizes Middlebrook 7H10 medium impregnated with isoniazid at 0.2 and 1.0 µg/mL for the final concentration of drug. The final con-

Parameter	C_{max} (µg/mL)		Half-life (hr)		Apparent Oral Clearance (L/hr)		Bioavailability (%)
Treatment	A	B	A	B	A	B	A
Isoniazid	3.09 ± 0.88	3.14 ± 0.92	2.80 ± 1.02	2.80 ± 1.11	24.02 ± 15.29	25.72 ± 18.38	100.6 ± 16.6
Rifampin	11.04 ± 3.08	13.61 ± 3.96	3.19 ± 0.63	3.41 ± 0.86	9.62 ± 3.00	8.30 ± 2.50	88.8 ± 16.5
Pyrazinamide	28.02 ± 4.52	29.21 ± 4.35	10.04 ± 1.54	10.08 ± 1.29	3.82 ± 0.65	3.70 ± 0.59	96.8 ± 7.6

centration for pyrazinamide is 25.0 μg/mL at pH 5.5. After 3 weeks of incubation MIC_{99} values are calculated by comparing the quantity of organisms growing in the medium containing drug to the control cultures. Mycobacterial growth in the presence of drug ≥1% of the control indicates resistance.

The radiometric broth method employs the BACTEC 460 machine to compare the growth index from untreated control cultures to cultures grown in the presence of 0.2 and 1.0 μg/mL of isoniazid and 2.0 μg/mL of rifampin. Strict adherence to the manufacturer's instructions for sample processing and data interpretation is required for this assay. The radiometric broth method has not been approved for the testing of pyrazinamide.

Susceptibility test results obtained by the two different methods can only be compared if the appropriate rifampin or isoniazid concentration are used for each test method as indicated above. Both test procedures require the use of *Mycobacterium tuberculosis* H37Rv, ATCC 27294, as a control organism.

The clinical relevance of *in vitro* susceptibility test results for mycobacterial species other than *Mycobacterium tuberculosis* using either the radiometric broth method or the proportion method has not been determined.

CLINICAL TRIALS

A total of 250 patients were enrolled in an open label, prospective, randomized, parallel group, active controlled trial, for the treatment of pulmonary tuberculosis. there were 241 patients evaluable for efficacy, 123 patients received isoniazid, rifampin and pyrazinamide at separate tablets and capsules for 56 days, and 118 patients received 4 to 6 RIFATER tablets based on body weight for 56 days. RIFATER tablets and the drugs dosed as separate tablets and capsules were administered based on body weight during the intensive phase of treatment according to the following table.

[See first table above]

Dose of Isoniazid, Rifampin and Pyrazinamide Administered as Separate Drugs

Patient Weight	Isoniazid (mg)	Rifampin (mg)	Pyrazinamide (mg)
<50 kg	300	450	1500
≥50 kg	300	600	2000

Dose of Isoniazid, Rifampin and Pyrazinamide Administered as RIFATER

Patient Weight	Number of Tablets	Isoniazid (mg)	Rifampin (mg)	Pyrazinamide (mg)
≤44 kg	4	200	480	1200
45 to 54 kg	5	250	600	1500
≥55 kg	6	300	720	1800

During the continuation phase, both treatment groups received 450 mg of rifampin and 300 mg of isoniazid per day for 4 months if the patient weighed <50 kg or 600 mg of rifampin and 300 mg of isoniazid per day for 4 months if the patient weighed ≥50 kg. Patients were followed for occurrence of relapses for up to 30 months after the end of therapy.

There were no significant differences in the negative bacteriological sputum results (available in a subset of patients) between the two treatments at 2 and 6 months during the trial and during the follow-up period. See table below.

[See second table above]

	Neative Sputums/No. of Patients (Percent Negative)		
Treatment	2 Months	6 Months	Follow-up Period*
RIFATER	91/96 (95%)	100/104 (96%)	99/101 (98%)
Separate†	99/108 (92%)	95/96 (99%)	105/106 (99%)

* The median follow-up time for all the RIFATER patients was 756 days with a range of 42 to 1325 days and 745 days with a range of 50 to 1427 days for the patients dosed with seperate tablets and capsules.

† Isoniazid, rifampin, and pyrazinamide dosed as separate tablets and capsules.

For adverse events, see ADVERSE REACTIONS section.

INDICATIONS AND USAGE

RIFATER is indicated in the initial phase of the short-course treatment of pulmonary tuberculosis. During this phase, which should last 2 months, RIFATER should be administered on a daily, continuous basis (see DOSAGE AND ADMINISTRATION section).

Following the initial phase and treatment with RIFATER, treatment should be continued with rifampin and isoniazid (eg, RIFAMATE) for at least 4 months. Treatment should be continued for a longer period of time if the patient is still sputum or culture positive, if resistant organisms are present, or if the patient is HIV positive.

In the treatment of tuberculosis, the small number of resistant cells present within large populations of susceptible cells can rapidly become the predominant type. since resistance can emerge rapidly, susceptibility tests should be performed in the event of persistent positive cultures during the course of treatment. Bacteriologic smears or cultures should be obtained before the start of therapy to confirm the susceptibility of the organism to rifampin, isoniazid, and pyrazinamide and they should be repeated throughout therapy to monitor response to the treatment. If test results show resistance to any of the components of RIFATER and the patient is not responding to therapy, the drug regimen should be modified.

CONTRAINDICATIONS

RIFATER is contraindicated in patients with a history of hypersensitivity to rifampin, isoniazid, pyrazinamide, or any of the components. Other contraindications include patients with severe hepatic damage; severe adverse reactions to isoniazid, such as drug fever, chills, and arthritis; patients with acute liver disease of any etiology; and patients with acute gout.

WARNINGS

RIFATER is a combination of the three drugs, rifampin, isoniazid, and pyrazinamide. Each of these individual drugs has been associated with liver dysfunction.

Rifampin. Rifampin has been shown to produce liver dysfunction. fatalities associated with jaundice have occurred in patients with liver disease and in patients taking rifampin with other hepatoxic agents. Because RIFATER contains both rifampin and isoniazid, it should only be given with caution and under strict medical supervision to patients with impaired liver function. In these patients, careful monitoring of liver function, especially serum glutamic pyruvic transaminase (SGPT) and serum glutamic oxaloacetic transaminase (SGOT) should be carried out prior to therapy and then every 2 to 4 weeks during therapy. If signs of hepatocellular damage occur, RIFATER should be withdrawn.

In some cases, hyperbilirubinemia resulting from competition between rifampin and bilirubin for excretory pathways of the liver at the cell level can occur in the early days of treatment. An isolated report showing a moderate rise in bilirubin and/or transminase level is not in itself an indication for interrupting treatment; rather, the decision should be made after repeating the tests, noting trends in the levels, and considering them in conjunction with the patient's clinical condition.

Rifampin has enzyme-inducing properties, including induction of delta amino levulinic acid synthetase. Isolated reports have associated porphyria exacerbation with rifampin administration.

Isoniazid. See the boxed WARNING.

Since RIFATER contains isoniazid, ophthalmologic examinations (including ophthalmoscopy) should be done before treatment is started and periodically thereafter, even without occurrence of visual symptoms.

Pyrazinamide. Since RIFATER contains pyrazinamide, patients started on RIFATER should have baseline serum uric acid and liver function determinations. Patients with preexisting liver disease or those patients at increased risk for drug related hepatitis (eg, alcohol abusers) should be followed closely.

Because it contains pyrazinamide, RIFATER should be discontinued and not be resumed if signs of hepatocellular damage or hyperuricemia accompanied by an acute gouty arthritis appear. If hyperuricemia accompanied by an acute gouty arthritis occurs without liver dysfunction, the patient should be transferred to a regimen not containing pyrazinamide.

PRECAUTIONS

General

RIFATER should be used with caution in patients with a history of diabetes mellitus, as diabetes management may be more difficult.

Rifampin. For treatment of tuberculosis, rifampin is usually administered on a daily basis. Doses of rifampin (>600 mg) given once or twice weekly have resulted in a higher incidence of adverse reactions, including the "flu syndrome" (fever, chills and malaise); hematopoietic reactions (leukopenia, thrombocytopenia, or acute hemolytic anemia); cutaneous gastrointestinal, and hepatic reactions; shortness of breath; shock and renal failure.

The patient should be advised that the reliability of oral contraceptives may be affected; consideration should be given to using alternative contraceptive measures.

Isoniazid. all drugs should be stopped and an evaluation of the patient should be made at the first sign of a hypersensitivity reaction. Use of RIFATER, because it contains isoniazid, should be carefully monitored in the following:

1. Patients who are receiving phenytoin (diphenylhydantoin) concurrently. Isoniazid may decrease the excretion of phenytoin or may enhance its effects. To avoid phenytoin intoxication, appropriate adjustment of the anticonvulsant dose should be made.
2. Daily users of alcohol. Daily ingestion of alcohol may be associated with a higher incidence of isoniazid hepatitis.
3. Patients with current chronic liver disease or severe renal dysfunction.

Pyrazinamide. Pyrazinamide inhibits renal excretion of urates, frequently resulting in hyperuricemia which is usually asymptomatic. If hyperuricemia is accompanied by acute gouty arthritis, RIFATER, because it contains pyrazinamide, should be discontinued.

Information for Patients

Food Interaction: Because isoniazid has some monoamine oxidase inhibiting activity, an interaction with tyramine-containing foods (cheese, red wine) may occur. Diamine oxidase may also be inhibited, causing exaggerated response (eg, headache, sweating, palpitations, flushing, hypotension) to foods containing histamine (eg, skipjack, tuna, other tropical fish). Tyramine- and histamine-containing foods should be avoided in patients receiving RIFATER.

RIFATER, because it contains rifampin, may produce a reddish coloration of the urine, sweat, sputum, and tears, and the patient should be forewarned of this. Soft contact lenses may be permanently stained.

Patients should be instructed to take RIFATER either 1 hour before or 2 hours after a meal.

Patients should be instructed to notify their physicians promptly if they experience any of the following: fever, loss of appetite, malaise, nausea and vomiting, darkened urine, yellowish discoloration of the skin and eyes, pain or swelling of the joints.

Compliance with the full course of therapy must be emphasized, and the importance of not missing any doses must be stressed.

Laboratory Tests

A complete blood count (CBC), liver function tests, and blood uric acid determinations should be obtained prior to instituting therapy and periodically throughout the course of therapy. Because of a possible transient rise in transaminase and bilirubin values, blood for baseline clinical chemistries should be obtained before RIFATER dosing.

Drug Interactions

Rifampin. Enzyme Induction: Rifampin is known to induce certain cytochrome P-450 enzymes. Coadministration of RIFATER, because it contains rifampin, with drugs that undergo biotransformation through these metabolic pathways may accelerate elimination. To maintain optimum therapeutic blood levels, dosages of drugs metabolized by these enzymes may require adjustment when starting or stopping concomitantly administered rifampin.

Rifampin has been reported to accelerate the metabolism of the following drugs: anticonvulsants (eg, phenytoin), antiarrhythmics (eg, disopyramide, mexiletine, quinidine, tocainide), anticoagulants, antifungals (eg, fluconazole, itraconazole, ketoconazole), barbiturates, beta-blockers, calcium channel blockers (eg, diltiazem, nifedipine, verapamil), chloramphenicol, ciprofloxacin, corticosteroids, cyclosporine, cardiac glycoside preparations, clofibrate, oral contraceptives, dapsone, diazepam, haloperidol, oral hypoglycemic agents (sulfonylureas), methadone, narcotic analgesics, nortriptyline, progestins, and theophylline. It may be necessary to adjust dosages of these drugs if they are given concurrently with RIFATER since it contains rifampin.

Rifampin has been observed to increase the requirements for anticoagulant drugs of the coumarin type. In patients receiving anticoagulants and RIFATER concurrently, it is

Continued on next page

Rifater—Cont.

recommended that the prothrombin time be performed daily or as frequently as necessary to establish and maintain the required dose of anticoagulant.

Concurrent use of ketoconazole and rifampin has resulted in decreased serum concentration of both drugs. Concurrent use of rifampin and enalapril has resulted in decreased concentrations of enalaprilat, the active metabolite of enalapril. Since RIFATER contains rifampin, dosage adjustments should be made if RIFATER is concurrently administered with ketoconazole or enalapril if indicated by the patient's clinical condition.

Other Interactions: Concomitant antacid administration may reduce the absorption of rifampin. Daily doses of RIFATER, because it contains rifampin, should be given at least 1 hour before the ingestion of antacids.

Probenecid and cotrimoxazole have been reported to increase the blood level of rifampin.

When rifampin is given concomitantly with either halothane or isoniazid the potential for hepatotoxicity is increased. The concomitant use of RIFATER, because it contains both rifampin and isoniazid, and halothane should be avoided. Patients receiving both rifampin and isoniazid as in RIFATER should be monitored closely for hepatotoxicity. See the boxed WARNING.

Plasma concentrations of sulfapyridine may be reduced following the concomitant administration of sulfasalazine and RIFATER, because it contains rifampin. This finding may be the result of alteration in the colonic bacteria responsible for the reduction of sulfasalazine to sulfapyridine and mesalamine.

Isoniazid. Enzyme Inhibition: Isoniazid is known to inhibit certain cytochrome P-450 enzymes. Coadministration of isoniazid with drugs that undergo biotransformation through these metabolic pathways may decrease elimination. Consequently, dosages of drugs metabolized by these enzymes may require adjustment when starting or stopping concomitantly administered RIFATER, because it contains isoniazid, to maintain optimum therapeutic blood levels.

Isoniazid has been reported to inhibit the metabolism of the following drugs: anticonvulsants (eg, carbamazepine, phenytoin, primidone, valproic acid), benzodiazepines (eg, diazepam), haloperidol, ketoconazole, theophylline, and warfarin. It may be necessary to adjust the dosages of these drugs if they are given concurrently with RIFATER because it contains isoniazid. The impact of the competing effects of rifampin and isoniazid on the metabolism of these drugs is unknown.

Other Interactions: Concomitant antacid administration may reduce the absorption of isoniazid. Ingestion with food may also reduce the absorption of isoniazid. Daily doses of RIFATER, because it contains isoniazid, should be given on an empty stomach at least 1 hour before the ingestion of antacids or food.

Corticosteroids (eg, prednisolone) may decrease the serum concentration of isoniazid by increasing acetylation rate and/or renal clearance. Para-aminosalicylic acid may increase the plasma concentration and elimination half-life of isoniazid by competition of acetylating enzymes.

Pharmacodynamic Interactions: Daily ingestion of alcohol may be associated with a higher incidence of isoniazid hepatitis. Isoniazid, when given concomitantly with rifampin, has been reported to increase with hepatotoxicity of both drugs. Patients receiving both rifampin and isoniazid as in RIFATER should be monitored closely for hepatotoxicity.

The CNS effects of meperidine (drowsiness), cycloserine (dizziness, drowsiness), and disulfiram (acute behavioral and coordination changes) may be exaggerated when concomitant RIFATER, because it contains isoniazid, is given.

Concurrent RIFATER, because it contains isoniazid, and levodopa administration may produce symptoms of excess catecholamine stimulation (agitation, flushing, palpitations) or lack of levodopa effect.

Isoniazid may produce hyperglycemia and lead to loss of glucose control in patients on oral hypoglycemics.

Fast acetylation of isoniazid may produce high concentrations of hydrazine which facilitate deflorination of enflurane. Renal function should be monitored in patients receiving both RIFATER and enflurane.

Food Interactions: Because isoniazid has some monoamine oxidase inhibiting activity, an interaction with tyramine-containing foods (cheese, red wine) may occur. Diamine oxidase may also be inhibited, causing exaggerated response (eg, headache, sweating, palpitations, flushing, hypotension) to foods containing histamine (eg, skipjack, tuna, other tropical fish). Tyramine- and histamine-containing foods should be avoided by patients receiving RIFATER.

Drug/Laboratory Tests Interaction

Rifampin. Therapeutic levels of rifampin have been shown to inhibit standard microbiological assays for serum folate and vitamin B_{12}. Therefore, alternative assay methods should be considered. Transient abnormalities in liver function tests (eg, elevation in serum bilirubin, abnormal bromsulphalein [BSP] excretion, alkaline phosphatase and serum transaminases), and reduced biliary excretion of contrast media used for visualization of the gallbladder have also been observed. Therefore, these tests should be performed before the morning dose of RIFATER.

Rifampin and isoniazid have been reported to alter vitamin D metabolism. In some cases, reduced levels of circulating 25-hydroxy vitamin D and 1,25-dihydroxy vitamin D have been accompanied by reduced serum calcium and phosphate, and elevated parathyroid hormone.

Pyrazinamide. Pyrazinamide has been reported to interfere with ACETEST® and KETOSTIX® urine tests to produce a pink-brown color.

Carcinogenesis, Mutagenesis, Impairment of Fertility

Increased frequency of chromosomal aberrations was observed *in vitro* in lymphocytes obtained from patients treated with combination of rifampin, isoniazid, and pyrazinamide and combinations of streptomycin, rifampin, isoniazid, and pyrazinamide.

Rifampin. There are no known human data on long-term potential for carcinogenicity, mutagenicity, or impairment of fertility. A few cases of accelerated growth of lung carcinoma have been reported in man, but a causal relationship with the drug has not been established. An increase in the incidence of hepatomas in female mice (of a strain known to be particularly susceptible to the spontaneous development of hepatomas) was observed when rifampicin was administered in doses two to ten times the average daily human dose for 60 weeks followed by an observation period of 46 weeks. No evidence of carcinogenicity was found in male mice of the same strain, mice of a different strain, or rats under similar experimental conditions.

Rifampin has been reported to possess immunosuppressive potential in rabbits, mice, rats, guinea pigs, human lymphocytes *in vitro*, and humans. Antitumor activity *in vitro* has also been shown with rifampin.

There was no evidence of mutagenicity in bacteria, *Drosophila melanogaster*, or mice. An increase in chromatid breaks was noted when whole blood cell cultures were treated with rifampin.

Isoniazid. Isoniazid has been reported to induce pulmonary tumors in a number of strains of mice.

Pyrazinamide. In lifetime bioassays in rats and mice, pyrazinamide was administered in the diet at concentrations of up to 10,000 ppm. This resulted in estimated daily doses of 2 g/kg for the mouse, or 40 times the maximum human dose, and 0.5 g/kg for the rat, or 10 times the maximum human dose. Pyrazinamide was not carcinogenic in rats or male mice and no conclusion was possible for female mice.

Pyrazinamide was not mutagenic in the Ames bacterial test, but induced chromosomal aberrations in human lymphocyte cell cultures.

Pregnancy—Teratogenic Effects

Category C. Animal reproduction studies have not been conducted with RIFATER. It is also not known whether RIFATER can cause fetal harm when administered to a pregnant woman. RIFATER should be given to a pregnant woman only if clearly needed.

Rifampin. Although rifampin has been reported to cross the placental barrier and appear in cord blood, the effect of rifampin, alone in combination with other antituberculosis drugs, on the human fetus is not known. An increase in congenital malformations, primarily spina bifida and cleft palate, has been reported in the offspring of rodents given oral doses of 150 to 250 mg/kg/day of rifampin during pregnancy. The possible teratogenic potential in women capable of bearing children should be carefully weighed against the benefits of RIFATER therapy.

Isoniazid. It has been reported that in both rats and rabbits, isoniazid may exert an embryocidal effect when administered orally during pregnancy, although no isoniazid-related congenital anomalies have been found in reproduction studies in mammalian species (mice, rats, and rabbits). RIFATER, because it contains isoniazid, should be prescribed during pregnancy only when therapeutically necessary. The benefit of preventive therapy should be weighed against a possible risk to the fetus. Preventive treatment generally should be started after delivery because of the increased risk of tuberculosis for new mothers.

Pyrazinamide. Animal reproduction studies have not been conducted with pyrazinamide. It is also not known whether pyrazinamide can cause fetal harm when administered to a pregnant woman. RIFATER, because it contains pyrazinamide, should be given to a pregnant women only if clearly needed.

Pregnancy—Non-Teratogenic Effects

It is not known whether RIFATER can affect reproduction capacity.

Rifampin. When administered during the last few weeks of pregnancy, rifampin can cause postnatal hemorrhages in the mother and infant. In this case, treatment with vitamin K may be indicated for postnatal hemorrhage.

Nursing Mothers

Since rifampin, isoniazid, and pyrazinamide are known to pass into maternal breast milk, a decision should be made whether to discontinue nursing or to discontinue RIFATER, taking into account the importance of the drug to the mother.

Pediatric Use

Safety and effectiveness in pediatric patients under the age of 15 have not been established.

ADVERSE REACTIONS

Adverse Experiences During the Clinical Trial

Adverse event data reported for the RIFATER and the separate drug treatment groups during the first 2 months of the trial are shown in the table below.

Adverse Events Reported During the Clinical Study

	Number of Patients With Adverse Events*	
Adverse Events by Body Systems During First 2 Months of Trial	RIFATER n = 122‡	Separate† n = 123‡
Cutaneous (rash, erythrodema, erythema, exfoliative dermatitis, Lyell syndrome, urticaria, localized skin rash, diffuse skin rash, pruritus, generalized hypersensitivity)	8 (7%)	21 (17%)
Gastrointestinal (nausea, vomiting, digestive pain, diarrhea)	8 (7%)	14 (11%)
Musculoskeletal (arthralgia, long bones pain, phlebitis localized joint pain, diffuse joint pain, edema of the legs)	5 (4%)	8 (7%)
Hearing and Vestibular(tinnitus, vertigo, vertigo with loss of equilibrium)	3 (2%)	6 (5%)
Liver and Biliary (hepatitis with conjunctival jaundice, hepatitis with deep jaundice)	0 (0%)	2 (2%)
Central and Peripheral Nervous System (sweating, headache, insomnia, diffuse paresthesia of the legs, anxiety, diabetic coma)	5 (4%)	4 (3%)
Total body (spiking fever, persistent fever)	2 (2%)	4 (3%)
Cardiorespiratory (tightness in chest, coughing, diffuse chest pain, hemoptysis, angina, palpitation, total pneumothorax)	8 (7%)	3 (2%)
Total number of patients with one or more adverse events	29	43

* A given patient may have experienced ≥1 adverse event.
† Isoniazid, rifampin and pyrazinamide dosed as separate tablets and capsules.
‡ A total of 250 patients (124 RIFATER; 126 separate) were originally enrolled in the study. Five patients (2 RIFATER; 3 separate) were excluded due to admission errors.

No serious adverse events were reported in the patients receiving RIFATER tablets. Three serious adverse events were reported in the patients given isoniazid, rifampin, and pyrazinamide as separate tablets and capsules. The three serious adverse events were two general hypersensitivity reactions and one jaundice reaction.

There were no significant differences between the two treatment groups in standard liver function, renal function and hematologic laboratory test values measured at baseline and after 8 weeks of treatment. As would be expected for these drugs, there were alterations in liver enzymes (SGOT, SGPT) and serum uric acid levels. the adverse reactions reported during therapy with RIFATER are consistent with those described below for the individual components.

Adverse Reactions Reported for Individual Components

Rifampin, Gastrointestinal: Heartburn, epigastric distress, anorexia, nausea, vomiting, jaundice, flatulence, cramps, and diarrhea have been noted in some patients. Although *Clostridium difficile* has been shown *in vitro* to be sensitive to rifampin, pseudomembranous colitis has been reported with the use of rifampin (and other broad spectrum antibiotics). Therefore, it is important to consider this diagnosis in patients who develop diarrhea in association with antibiotic use. Rarely, hepatitis or a shocklike syndrome with hepatic involvement and abnormal liver function tests has been reported.

Hematologic: Thrombocytopenia has occurred primarily with high dose intermittent therapy, but has also been noted after resumption of interrupted treatment. It rarely occurs during well-supervised daily therapy. This effect is

reversible if the drug is discontinued as soon as purpura occurs. Cerebral hemorrhage and fatalities have been reported when rifampin administration has been continued or resumed after the appearance of purpura.
Transient leukopenia, hemolytic anemia, and decreased hemoglobin have been observed.
Central Nervous System: Headache, fever, drowsiness, fatigue, ataxia, dizziness, inability to concentrate, mental confusion, behavioral changes, muscular weakness, pains in extremities, and generalized numbness have been observed.
Rare reports of myopathy have also been observed.
Ocular: Visual disturbances have been observed.
Endocrine: Menstrual disturbances have been observed.
Renal: Elevations in BUN and serum uric acid have been reported. Rarely, hemolysis, hemoglobinuria, hematuria, interstitial nephritis, renal insufficiency, and acute renal failure have been noted. These are generally considered to be hypersensitivity reactions. They usually occur during intermittent therapy or when treatment is resumed following intentional or accidental interruption of a daily dosage regimen, and are reversible when rifampin is discontinued and appropriate therapy instituted.
Dermatologic: Cutaneous reactions are mild and self-limiting and do not appear to be hypersensitivity reactions. Typically, they consist of flushing and itching with or without a rash. More serious cutaneous reactions which may be due to hypersensitivity occur but are uncommon.
Hypersensitivity Reactions: Occasionally pruritus, urticaria, rash, pemphigoid reaction, eosinophilia, sore mouth, sore tongue and conjunctivitis have been observed.
Miscellaneous: Edema of the face and extremities have been reported. Other reactions which have occurred with intermittent dosage regimens include "flu" syndrome (such as episodes of fever, chills, headache, dizziness, and bone pain), shortness of breath, wheezing, decrease in blood pressure and shock. The "flu" syndrome may also appear if rifampin is taken irregularly by the patient or if daily administration is resumed after a drug free interval.
Isoniazid. The most frequent reactions are those affecting the nervous system and the liver. See the boxed WARNING.
Nervous System: Peripheral neuropathy is the most common toxic effect. It is dose-related, occurs most often in the malnourished and in those predisposed to neuritis (eg, alcoholics and diabetics), and is usually preceded by paresthesias of the feet and hands. The incidence is higher in "slow inactivators."
Other neurotoxic effects, which are uncommon with conventional doses, are convulsions, toxic encephalopathy, optic neuritis and atrophy, memory impairment and toxic psychosis.
Gastrointestinal: Nausea, vomiting, and epigastric distress.
Hepatic: Elevated serum transaminases (SGOT, SGPT) bilirubinemia, bilirubinuria, jaundice, and occasionally severe and sometimes fatal hepatitis. The common prodromal symptoms are anorexia, nausea, vomiting, fatigue, malaise, and weakness. Mild and transient elevation of serum transaminase levels occurs in 10 to 20% of persons taking isoniazid. The abnormality usually occurs in the first 4 to 6 months of treatment but can occur at any time during therapy. In most instances, enzyme levels return to normal with no necessity to discontinue medication. In occasional instances, progressive liver damage occurs, with accompanying symptoms. In these cases, the drug should be discontinued immediately. The frequency of progressive liver damage increases with age. It is rare in persons under 20, but occurs in up to 2.3% of those over 50 years of age.
Hematologic: Agranulocytosis; hemolytic, sideroblastic, or aplastic anemia; thrombocytopenia; and eosinophilia.
Hypersensitivity Reactions: Fever, skin eruptions (morbilliform, maculopapular, purpuric, or exfoliative), lymphadenopathy, and vasculitis.
Metabolic and Endocrine: Pyridoxine deficiency, pellagra, hyperglycemia, metabolic acidosis, and gynecomastia.
Miscellaneous: Rheumatic syndrome and systemic lupus erythematosus-like syndrome.
Pyrazinamide. The principal adverse effect is a hepatic reaction (see WARNINGS). Hepatotoxicity appears to be dose related and may appear at any time during therapy. Pyrazinamide can cause hyeruricemia and gout (see PRECAUTIONS).
Gastrointestinal: GI disturbances including nausea, vomiting, and anorexia have also been reported.
Hematologic and Lymphatic: Thrombocytopenia and sideroblastic anemia with erythroid hyperplasia, vacuolation of erythrocytes and increased serum concentration have occurred rarely with this drug. Adverse effects on blood clotting mechanisms have also been rarely reported.
Other: Mild arthralgia and myalgia have been reported frequently. Hypersensitivity reactions including rashes, urticaria, and pruritus have been reported. Fever, acne, photosensitivity, porphyria, dysuria, and interstitial nephritis have been reported rarely.

OVERDOSAGE

RIFATER. There is no human experience with RIFATER overdosage.
Rifampin. Non-fatal overdoses with as high as 12 g of rifampin have been reported.
One case of fatal overdose is known: A 26-year old man died after self-administering 60 g of rifampin.
Isoniazid. Untreated or inadequately treated cases of gross isoniazid overdosage can be fatal, but good response has been reported in most patients treated within the first few hours after drug ingestion.
Ingested acutely, as little as 1.5 g isoniazid may cause toxicity in adults. Doses of 35 to 40 mg/kg have resulted in seizures. Ingestion of 80 to 150 mg/kg isoniazid has been associated with severe toxicity and, if untreated, significant mortality.
Pyrazinamide. Overdosage experience with pyrazinamide is limited.

Signs and Symptoms

The following signs and symptoms have been seen with each individual component in an overdosage situation.
Rifampin. Nausea, vomiting, and increasing lethargy will probably occur within a short time after rifampin overdosage; unconsciousness may occur when there is severe hepatic disease. Brownish red or orange discoloration of the skin, urine, sweat, saliva, tears, and feces will occur, and its intensity is proportional to the amount ingested.
Liver enlargement, possibly with tenderness, can develop within a few hours after severe overdosage; bilirubin levels may increase and jaundice may develop rapidly. Hepatic involvement may be more marked in patients with prior impairment of hepatic function. Other physical findings remain essentially normal. A direct effect upon the hematopoietic system, electrolyte levels, or acid-base balance is unlikely.
Isoniazid. Isoniazid overdosage produces signs and symptoms within 30 minutes to 3 hours. Nausea, vomiting, dizziness, slurring of speech, blurring of vision, and visual hallucinations (including bright colors and strange designs) are among the early manifestation. With marked overdosage, respiratory distress and CNS depression progressing rapidly from stupor to profound coma, are to be expected along with severe, intractable seizures. Severe metabolic acidosis, acetonuria, and hyperglycemia are typical laboratory findings.
Pyrazinamide. In one case of pyrazinamide overdosage, abnormal liver function tests developed. These spontaneously reverted to normal when the drug was stopped.

Treatment

The airway should be secured and adequate respiratory exchange should be established in cases of overdosage with RIFATER.
Obtain blood samples for immediate determination of gases, electrolytes, BUN, glucose, etc; type and cross-match blood in preparation for possible hemodialysis.
Gastric lavage within the first 2 to 3 hours after ingestion is advised, but it should not be attempted until convulsions are under control. To treat convulsions, administer IV diazepam or short-acting barbiturates, and IV pyridoxine (usually 1 mg/1 mg isoniazid ingested). Following evacuation of gastric contents, the instillation of activated charcoal slurry into the stomach may help absorb any remaining drug from the gastrointestinal tract. Antiemetic medication may be required to control severe nausea and vomiting.
RAPID CONTROL OF METABOLIC ACIDOSIS IS FUNDAMENTAL TO MANAGEMENT, Give IV sodium bicarbonate at once and repeat as needed, adjusting subsequent dosage on the basis of laboratory findings (ie, serum sodium, pH, etc).
Forced osmotic diuresis must be started early and should be continued for some hours after clinical improvement to hasten renal clearance of drug and help prevent relapse; monitor fluid intake and output.
Hemodialysis is advised for severe cases; if this is not available, peritoneal dialysis can be used along with forced diuresis.
Along with measures based on initial and repeated determination of blood gases and other laboratory tests as needed, utilize meticulous respiratory and other intensive care to protect against hypoxia, hypotension, aspiration pneumonitis, etc.

DOSAGE AND ADMINISTRATION

Adults: Patients should be given the following single daily dose of RIFATER either 1 hour before or 2 hours after a meal with a full glass of water.
Patients weighing ≤ 44 kg—4 tablets
Patients weighing between 45–54 kg—5 tablets
Patients weighing ≥55 kg—6 tablets
Pediatric Patients: The ratio of the drugs in RIFATER may not be appropriate in pediatric patients under the age of 15 (eg, higher mg/kg doses of isoniazid are usually given in pediatric patients than adults).
RIFATER is recommended in the initial phase of short-course therapy which is usually continued for 2 months. The Advisory Council for the Elimination of Tuberculosis, the American Thoracic Society, and the Centers for disease Control and Prevention recommend that either streptomycin or ethambutol be added as a fourth drug in a regimen containing isoniazid (INH), rifampin and pyrazinamide for initial treatment of tuberculosis unless the likelihood of INH or rifampin resistance is very low. The need for a fourth drug should be reassessed when the results of susceptibility testing are known. If community rates of INH resistance are currently less than 4%, an initial treatment regimen with less than four drugs may be considered.
Following the initial phase, treatment should be continued with rifampin and isoniazid (eg, RIFAMATE®) for at least 4 months. Treatment should be continued for longer if the patient is still sputum or culture positive, if resistant organisms are present, or if the patient is HIV positive.
Concomitant administration of pyridoxine (B_6) is recommended in the malnourished, in those predisposed to neuropathy (eg, alcoholics and diabetics), and in adolescents.
See CLINICAL PHARMACOLOGY: General for dosing information in patients with renal failure.

HOW SUPPLIED

RIFATER tablets are light beige, smooth, round, and shiny sugar-coated tablets imprinted with "RIFATER" in black ink and contain 120 mg rifampin, 50 mg isoniazid, and 300 mg pyrazinamide, and are supplied as:
Bottles of 60 tablets (NDC 0088-0576-41).
Storage Conditions: Store at controlled room temperature 59-86°F (15–30°C). Protect from excessive humidity.

Reference: 1. National Committee for Clinical Laboratory Standards. 1990. Antimycobacterial Susceptibility Testing (Proposed Standard). Document M24-P.

Prescribing information as of December 1995
Merrell Pharmaceuticals Inc.
Subsidiary of Hoechst Marion Roussel, Inc.
Kansas City, MO 64137 USA
Rifater Tablets are manufactured by:
GRUPPO LEPETIT S.p.A.
20020 Lainate, Italy
Shown in Product Identification Guide, page 316

TECZEM™ ℞

[tĕc zĕm]
(Enalapril Maleate/Diltiazem Malate Extended Release Tablets)

Prescribing Information as of July 1996

USE IN PREGNANCY
When used in pregnancy during the second and third trimesters, ACE inhibitors can cause injury and even death to the developing fetus. When pregnancy is detected, TECZEM should be discontinued as soon as possible. See WARNINGS, Pregnancy, Enalapril Maleate, Fetal Neonatal/Morbidity and Mortality.

DESCRIPTION

TECZEM™ (enalapril maleate/diltiazem malate extended release tablets) combines an angiotensin converting enzyme inhibitor, enalapril maleate, and a calcium ion influx inhibitor, diltiazem malate.
Enalapril maleate is the maleate salt of enalapril, the ethyl ester of a long-acting angiotensin converting enzyme inhibitor, enalaprilat.
Enalapril maleate is chemically described as (*S*)-1-[*N*-[1-(ethoxycarbonyl)-3-phenylpropyl]-L-alanyl]-L-proline, (*Z*)-2-butenedioate salt (1:1). Its empirical formula is $C_{20}H_{28}N_2O_5 \cdot C_4H_4O_4$, and its structural formula is:

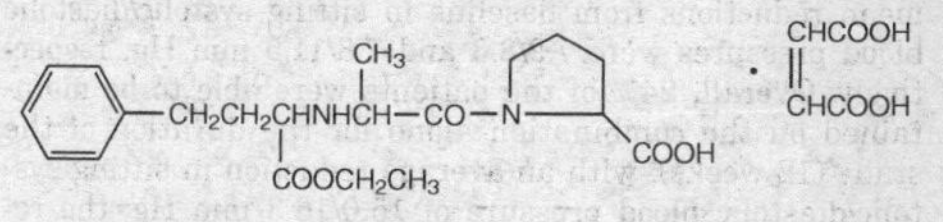

Enalapril maleate is a white to off-white crystalline powder with a molecular weight of 492.53. It is sparingly soluble in water, soluble in ethanol, and freely soluble in methanol.
Enalapril is a pro-drug; following oral administration, it is bioactivated by hydrolysis of the ethyl ester to enalaprilat, which is the active angiotensin converting enzyme inhibitor.
Diltiazem malate is a calcium ion influx inhibitor (slow channel blocker or calcium antagonist). Chemically, diltiazem malate is described as (+)-(2*S*,3*S*)-5-[2-(Dimethylamino)ethyl]-2,3-dihydro-3-hydroxy-2-(*p*-methoxyphenyl)-1,5-benzothiazepin- 4(*5H*)-one acetate (ester), (*S*)-malate (1:1). Its empirical formula is $C_{22}H_{26}N_2O_4S \cdot C_4H_6O_5$ and the chemical structure is:
[See chemical structure at top of next column]
Diltiazem malate is a white to off-white crystalline powder and has a molecular weight of 548.61. It is moderately soluble in isotonic saline, water, and methanol, and slightly soluble in acetonitrile and ethanol. TECZEM is formulated as a once-a-day extended release tablet containing 5 mg

Continued on next page

Teczem—Cont.

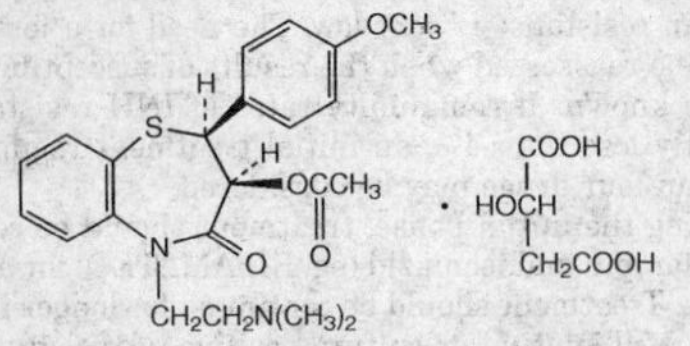

enalapril maleate and 219 mg diltiazem malate, which corresponds to a dose of 180 mg of diltiazem hydrochloride.
In addition to the active ingredients, each TECZEM tablet contains the following inactive ingredients: cellulose acetates, hydroxypropylcellulose, hydroxypropylmethylcellulose, iron oxide (0.65 mg/tablet as elemental iron), magnesium stearate, polyethylene glycol, povidone, sodium bicarbonate, sodium hydrogen tartrate, stearic acid, sucrose, and titanium dioxide.

CLINICAL PHARMACOLOGY

The therapeutic effects of diltiazem are believed to be related to its ability to inhibit the influx of calcium ions during membrane depolarization of cardiac and vascular smooth muscle. Administration of enalapril maleate blocks the renin-angiotensin-aldosterone axis.
The antihypertensive effects of TECZEM have been evaluated principally from the results of three double-blind, placebo-controlled trials which randomized 1458 patients with mild to moderate hypertension. Enalapril doses studied in these three trials varied from 5 to 20 mg, once-a-day and diltiazem malate extended release tablet doses (expressed as hydrochloride equivalents) varied from 60 to 360 mg, once-a-day. Blood pressure reduction was significantly greater for TECZEM than for either of the components used alone.
Compared to placebo, the combination of enalapril (as an immediate release tablet) and diltiazem malate extended release tablets produced increasing reductions of blood pressure as the doses of each component increased. When enalapril 5 mg was combined with diltiazem doses ranging from 60 to 240 mg, the placebo-adjusted reductions of trough sitting systolic/diastolic blood pressure ranged from 4.5/3.6 to 11.8/7.1 mm Hg. In contrast, when enalapril 20 mg was combined with diltiazem doses ranging from 60 to 360 mg, the placebo-adjusted reductions of trough sitting systolic/diastolic blood pressure ranged from 8.5/7.7 to 13.2/10.6 mm Hg. Placebo-adjusted peak effects, measured 4 to 6 hours after dosing, were greater than those at trough, ranging from 11.3/8.3 to 19.8/15.3 mm Hg for sitting systolic/diastolic blood pressure. Standing systolic and diastolic blood pressures were similarly affected by combinations of enalapril and extended release diltiazem. These antihypertensive effects were sustained for 24 hours in most patients. In spite of substantial decreases in blood pressure, changes in pulse rate were generally not of clinical significance. In long-term therapy lasting up to one year, the antihypertensive effects were generally well-maintained on combination treatment.
Of 109 patients with severe hypertension (sitting diastolic blood pressure ≥ 115 mm Hg at the time of randomization) who were randomized to one of two treatment arms (enalapril 5 mg/diltiazem 120 mg or enalapril 5 mg/diltiazem 180 mg), the initial reductions from baseline in sitting systolic/diastolic blood pressure were 3.9/3.7 and 2.8/6.3 mm Hg, respectively. Following a doubling of the dose (to enalapril 10 mg/diltiazem 240 mg or enalapril 10 mg/diltiazem 360 mg) for patients whose blood pressures were not controlled, mean reductions from baseline in sitting systolic/diastolic blood pressures were 7.9/8.3 and 7.8/11.5 mm Hg, respectively. Overall, 24% of the patients were able to be maintained on the combination alone for the duration of the study (12 weeks), with an average reduction in sitting systolic/diastolic blood pressure of 15.0/16.3 mm Hg; the remaining patients required the addition of one or more antihypertensive agents.

Enalapril Maleate

Mechanism of Action: Enalapril, after hydrolysis to enalaprilat, inhibits angiotensin converting enzyme (ACE) in human subjects and animals. ACE is a peptidyl dipeptidase that catalyzes the conversion of angiotensin I to the vasoconstrictor substance, angiotensin II. Angiotensin II also stimulates aldosterone secretion by the adrenal cortex. The beneficial effects of enalapril in hypertension appear to result primarily from suppression of the renin-angiotensin-aldosterone system. Inhibition of ACE results in decreased plasma angiotensin II, which leads to decreased vasopressor activity and to decreased aldosterone secretion. Although the latter decrease is small, it results in small increases of serum potassium. In hypertensive patients treated with enalapril maleate alone for up to 48 weeks, mean increase in serum potassium of approximately 0.2 mEq/L was observed. In patients treated with enalapril maleate plus a thiazide diuretic, there was essentially no change in serum potassium. (See PRECAUTIONS.) Removal of angiotensin II negative feedback on renin secretion leads to increased plasma renin activity.
ACE is identical to kininase, an enzyme that degrades bradykinin. Whether increased levels of bradykinin, a potent vasodepressor peptide, play a role in the therapeutic effects of enalapril remains to be elucidated.
While the mechanism through which enalapril lowers blood pressure is believed to be primarily suppression of the renin-angiotensin-aldosterone system, enalapril is antihypertensive even in patients with low-renin hypertension. Although enalapril was antihypertensive in all races studied, black hypertensive patients (usually a low-renin hypertensive population) had a smaller average response to enalapril maleate monotherapy than non-black patients.
Pharmacokinetics and Metabolism: The pharmacokinetics of enalapril are not changed by the concurrent use of diltiazem. Following oral administration of enalapril maleate, peak serum concentrations of enalapril occur within about one hour. Based on urinary recovery, the extent of absorption of enalapril is approximately 60 percent. Enalapril absorption is not influenced by the presence of food in the gastrointestinal tract. Following absorption, enalapril is hydrolyzed to enalaprilat, which is a more potent angiotensin converting enzyme inhibitor than enalapril; enalaprilat is poorly absorbed when administered orally. Peak serum concentrations of enalaprilat occur three to four hours after an oral dose of enalapril maleate. Excretion of enalaprilat and enalapril is primarily renal. Approximately 94 percent of the dose is recovered in the urine and feces as enalaprilat or enalapril. The principal components in urine are enalaprilat, accounting for about 40 percent of the dose, and intact enalapril. There is no evidence of metabolites of enalapril, other than enalaprilat.
The serum concentration profile of enalaprilat exhibits a prolonged terminal phase, apparently representing a small fraction of the administered dose that has been bound to ACE. The amount bound does not increase with dose, indicating a saturable site of binding. The effective half-life for accumulation of enalaprilat following multiple doses of enalapril maleate is 11 hours.
The disposition of enalapril and enalaprilat in patients with renal insufficiency is similar to that in patients with normal renal function until the glomerular filtration rate is 30 mL/min or less. With glomerular filtration rate ≤30 mL/min, peak and trough enalaprilat levels increase, time to peak concentration increases and time to steady state may be delayed. The effective half-life of enalaprilat following multiple doses of enalapril maleate is prolonged at this level of renal insufficiency. Enalaprilat is dialyzable at the rate of 62 mL/min.
Studies in dogs indicate that enalapril crosses the blood-brain barrier poorly, if at all; enalaprilat does not enter the brain. Multiple doses of enalapril maleate in rats do not result in accumulation in any tissues. Milk of lactating rats contains radioactivity following administration of ^{14}C-enalapril maleate. Radioactivity was found to cross the placenta following administration of labeled drug to pregnant hamsters. (See WARNINGS.)
Pharmacodynamics: Administration of enalapril maleate to patients with hypertension of severity ranging from mild to severe results in a reduction of both supine and standing blood pressure usually with no orthostatic component. Symptomatic postural hypotension is infrequent with enalapril alone but it can be anticipated in volume-depleted patients. (See WARNINGS.) In most patients studied, after oral administration of a single dose of enalapril maleate, onset of antihypertensive activity was seen at one hour with peak reduction of blood pressure achieved by four to six hours. At recommended doses, antihypertensive effects of enalapril maleate monotherapy have been maintained for at least 24 hours. In some patients the effects may diminish toward the end of the dosing interval.
Achievement of optimal blood pressure reduction may require several weeks of enalapril therapy in some patients.
The antihypertensive effects of enalapril have continued during long term therapy. Abrupt withdrawal of enalapril has not been associated with a rapid increase in blood pressure.
In hemodynamic studies in patients with essential hypertension, blood pressure reduction produced by enalapril was accompanied by a reduction in peripheral arterial resistance with an increase in cardiac output and little or no change in heart rate. Following administration of enalapril maleate, there is an increase in renal blood flow; glomerular filtration rate is usually unchanged. The effects appear to be similar in patients with renovascular hypertension.
In a clinical pharmacology study, indomethacin or sulindac was administered to hypertensive patients receiving enalapril maleate. In this study there was no evidence of a blunting of the antihypertensive action of enalapril maleate.

Diltiazem Malate

Mechanism of Action: Diltiazem produces its antihypertensive effect primarily by relaxation of vascular smooth muscle and the resultant decrease in peripheral vascular resistance. The magnitude of blood pressure reduction is related to the degree of hypertension; thus hypertensive individuals experience an antihypertensive effect, whereas there is only a modest fall in blood pressure in normotensives.
Hemodynamic and Electrophysiologic Effects: Like other calcium channel antagonists, diltiazem decreases sinoatrial and atrioventricular conduction in isolated tissues and has a negative inotropic effect in isolated preparations. In the intact animal, prolongation of the AH interval can be seen at higher doses.
In man, diltiazem prevents spontaneous and ergonovine-provoked coronary artery spasm. It causes a decrease in peripheral vascular resistance and a modest fall in blood pressure in normotensive individuals, and in exercise tolerance studies in patients with ischemic heart disease, reduces the heart rate-blood pressure product for any given work load. Studies to date, primarily in patients with good ventricular function, have not revealed evidence of a negative inotropic effect; cardiac output, ejection fraction, and left ventricular end diastolic pressure have not been affected. Such data have no predictive value with respect to effects in patients with poor ventricular function, and increased heart failure has been reported in patients with preexisting impairment of ventricular function. There are as yet few data on the interaction of diltiazem and beta-blockers in patients with poor ventricular function. Resting heart rate is usually slightly reduced by diltiazem. Three placebo-controlled studies establish that diltiazem malate extended release tablets produce an antihypertensive effect both in the sitting and standing positions. In one trial (a placebo-controlled, parallel group, dose-ranging trial) the mean, trough reduction of sitting diastolic blood pressure was 3.2, 4.2, 3.6, and 7.6 mm Hg greater than placebo for the 120, 180, 240, and 480 mg once-daily diltiazem malate extended release tablet arms, respectively, and was sustained for 24 hours in most patients. Reduction of sitting diastolic blood pressure measured 4 to 6 hours after dosing, approximately peak effect, was 6.0, 6.3, 8.9, and 14.2 mm Hg greater than placebo for the 120, 180, 240, and 480 mg once-daily arms, respectively. Postural hypotension was infrequently noted upon suddenly assuming an upright position. The antihypertensive effect of diltiazem malate extended release tablets was sustained during long term therapy.
The antihypertensive effect of diltiazem malate extended release tablets was not significantly influenced by patient age or race; however, the antihypertensive effect was somewhat greater in females.
Diltiazem decreases vascular resistance, increases cardiac output (by increasing stroke volume), and produces a slight decrease or no change in heart rate. During dynamic exercise, increases in diastolic pressure are inhibited while maximum achievable systolic pressure is usually reduced. Chronic therapy with diltiazem produces no change or an increase in plasma catecholamines. No increased activity of the renin-angiotensin-aldosterone axis has been observed. Diltiazem reduces the renal and peripheral effects of angiotensin II. Hypertensive animal models respond to diltiazem with reductions in blood pressure and increased urinary output and natriuresis without a change in urinary sodium/potassium ratio.
Following administration of single oral doses of 300 mg diltiazem hydrochloride in six normal volunteers, the average maximum PR prolongation was 14% with no instances of greater than first-degree AV block. Diltiazem-associated prolongation of the AH interval is not more pronounced in patients with first-degree heart block. In patients with sick sinus syndrome, diltiazem significantly prolongs sinus cycle length (up to 50% in some cases).
Chronic oral administration of diltiazem hydrochloride in patients in doses up to 540 mg/day has resulted in small increases in PR interval, and on occasion produces abnormal prolongation. (See WARNINGS.)
Pharmacokinetics and Metabolism: The pharmacokinetics of diltiazem are not changed by the concurrent use of enalapril. Diltiazem is well absorbed from the gastrointestinal tract and is subject to extensive first pass metabolism, giving a bioavailability, compared to intravenous administration of 40–50%. Following intravenous or oral administration of ^{14}C-diltiazem, approximately 71% of the radiolabel is excreted in urine and approximately 16% is excreted in feces.
Drugs that induce or inhibit hepatic microsomal enzymes may alter diltiazem disposition.
Diltiazem is extensively metabolized with major metabolic pathways including deacetylation, N-demethylation, O-demethylation, and aromatic oxidation followed by conversion to glucuronide and sulfate conjugates. The major metabolites are N-desmethyldiltiazem (DMD) and desacetyldiltiazem (DAD), both of which are pharmacologically less active than diltiazem. Following oral doses of diltiazem, plasma concentrations of DAD or DMD are approximately 30% and 10%, respectively, of those for diltiazem. These metabolites are eliminated via biliary and urinary excretion. Less than 4% of a dose is excreted in urine as unchanged drug, and even smaller amounts in bile. Total radioactivity measurement following short intravenous administration in healthy volunteers suggests the presence of other unidenti-

fied metabolites which attain higher concentrations than those of diltiazem and are more slowly eliminated; apparent half-life of total radioactivity is about 20 hours compared to 2 to 5 hours for diltiazem. Diltiazem is 70 to 80% bound to plasma protein (α_1-acid glycoprotein and albumin) over the therapeutic range of plasma concentrations. In vitro studies have shown that therapeutic concentrations of digoxin, hydrochlorothiazide, phenylbutazone, propranolol, salicylic acid, or warfarin do not affect the protein binding of diltiazem.

Following oral administration of the extended release formulation of diltiazem malate, peak plasma concentrations of diltiazem increase with dose and occur an average of 9 to 16 hours after drug administration. Compared to the intravenous administration of 20 mg of diltiazem, diltiazem malate extended release tablets are approximately 40% bioavailable. Dose-dumping was not noted in any of the pharmacokinetic studies with diltiazem malate extended release tablets even when it was administered immediately following a high-fat breakfast.

Diltiazem malate extended release tablets, as other diltiazem preparations, exhibited nonlinear pharmacokinetics. Steady state AUC, normalized for dose, showed increases of approximately 30% and 60% for the 240 and 360 mg, respectively, relative to the 120 mg dose. Additional non-linearity is anticipated at higher than 360 mg doses.

Mean AUC was slightly (approximately 16%) higher when diltiazem malate extended release tablets were given postprandially compared to fasting conditions. Release of diltiazem from diltiazem malate extended release tablets is dependent on gastrointestinal transit times. Release of 70% or more of diltiazem requires transit times of 10 hours or greater, shorter transit times result in proportionally less diltiazem released. A study in healthy elderly subjects (aged 65 to 77) showed an approximately 50% increase in mean AUC relative to young subjects following oral and intravenous administration due to slower elimination in the elderly. The bioavailability of diltiazem malate extended release tablets is unaffected by patient age.

INDICATIONS AND USAGE

TECZEM is indicated for the treatment of hypertension.

This fixed combination drug is not indicated for the initial therapy of hypertension. (See DOSAGE AND ADMINISTRATION.)

In using TECZEM, consideration should be given to the fact that an angiotensin converting enzyme inhibitor, captopril, has caused agranulocytosis, particularly in patients with renal impairment or collagen vascular disease, and that available data are insufficient to show that enalapril does not have a similar risk. (See WARNINGS, Neutropenia/Agranulocytosis.)

In considering use of TECZEM, it should be noted that in controlled clinical trials, the addition of enalapril to a regimen of diltiazem had an effect on blood pressure that was notably less in black patients than in non-blacks. In addition, it should be noted that black patients receiving ACE inhibitors have been reported to have a higher incidence of angioedema compared to non-blacks. (See WARNINGS, Angioedema.)

CONTRAINDICATIONS

TECZEM is contraindicated in patients who are hypersensitive to any component of this product. Due to the enalapril component, TECZEM is contraindicated in patients with a history of angioedema related to previous treatment with an angiotensin converting enzyme inhibitor. Due to the diltiazem component, TECZEM is also contraindicated in (1) patients with sick sinus syndrome except in the presence of a functioning ventricular pacemaker, (2) patients with second or third-degree AV block except in the presence of a functioning ventricular pacemaker, (3) patients with hypotension (less than 90 mm Hg systolic), and (4) patients with acute myocardial infarction and pulmonary congestion documented by x-ray on admission.

WARNINGS

General

Enalapril Maleate

Anaphylactoid and Possibly Related Reactions: Presumably because angiotensin-converting enzyme inhibitors affect the metabolism of eicosanoids and polypeptides, including endogenous bradykinin, patients receiving ACE inhibitors (including TECZEM) may be subject to a variety of adverse reactions, some of them serious.

Angioedema: Angioedema of the face, extremities, lips, tongue, glottis, and/or larynx has been reported in patients treated with angiotensin converting enzyme inhibitors, including enalapril. This may occur at any time during treatment. In such cases TECZEM should be promptly discontinued and appropriate therapy and monitoring should be provided until complete and sustained resolution of signs and symptoms has occurred. In instances where swelling has been confined to the face and lips, the condition has generally resolved without treatment, although antihistamines have been useful in relieving symptoms. Angioedema associated with laryngeal edema may be fatal. **Where there is involvement of the tongue, glottis or larynx, likely to cause airway obstruction, appropriate therapy, e.g., subcutaneous epinephrine solution 1:1000 (0.3 mL to 0.5 mL) and/or measures necessary to ensure a patent airway, should be promptly provided.** (See ADVERSE REACTIONS.)

Patients with a history of angioedema unrelated to ACE inhibitor therapy may be at increased risk of angioedema while receiving an ACE inhibitor. (See also INDICATIONS AND USAGE and CONTRAINDICATIONS.)

Anaphylactoid Reactions During Desensitization: Two patients undergoing desensitizing treatment with hymenoptera venom while receiving ACE inhibitors sustained life-threatening anaphylactoid reactions. In the same patients, these reactions were avoided when ACE inhibitors were temporarily withheld, but they reappeared upon inadvertent rechallenge.

Anaphylactoid Reactions During Membrane Exposure: Anaphylactoid reactions have been reported in patients dialyzed with high-flux membranes and treated concomitantly with an ACE inhibitor. Anaphylactoid reactions have also been reported in patients undergoing low-density lipoprotein apheresis with dextran sulfate absorption (a procedure dependent upon devices not approved in the United States).

Hypotension: Excessive hypotension is rare in uncomplicated hypertensive patients treated with enalapril maleate alone. Patients at risk for excessive hypotension, sometimes associated with oliguria and/or progressive azotemia, and rarely with acute renal failure and/or death, include those with the following conditions or characteristics: heart failure, hyponatremia, high dose diuretic therapy, recent intensive diuresis or increase in diuretic dose, renal dialysis, or severe volume and/or salt depletion of any etiology. It may be advisable to eliminate the diuretic (except in patients with heart failure), reduce the diuretic dose or increase salt intake cautiously before initiating therapy with enalapril maleate in patients at risk for excessive hypotension who are able to tolerate such adjustments. (See PRECAUTIONS, Drug Interactions and ADVERSE REACTIONS.) In patients at risk for excessive hypotension, therapy should be started under very close medical supervision. Such patients should be followed closely for the first two weeks of treatment and whenever the dose of enalapril and/or diuretic is increased. Similar considerations may apply to patients with ischemic heart or cerebrovascular disease, in whom an excessive fall in blood pressure could result in a myocardial infarction or cerebrovascular accident.

If excessive hypotension occurs, the patient should be placed in the supine position and, if necessary, receive an intravenous infusion of normal saline. A transient hypotensive response is not a contraindication to further doses of enalapril maleate, which usually can be given without difficulty once the blood pressure has stabilized. If symptomatic hypotension develops, a dose reduction or discontinuation of enalapril maleate or diuretic may be necessary.

Neutropenia/Agranulocytosis: Another angiotensin converting enzyme inhibitor, captopril, has been shown to cause agranulocytosis and bone marrow depression, rarely in uncomplicated patients but more frequently in patients with renal impairment especially if they also have a collagen vascular disease. Available data from clinical trials of enalapril are insufficient to show that enalapril does not cause agranulocytosis at similar rates. Marketing experience has revealed several cases of neutropenia or agranulocytosis in which a causal relationship to enalapril cannot be excluded. Periodic monitoring of white blood cell counts in patients with collagen vascular disease and renal disease should be considered.

Hepatic Failure: Rarely, ACE inhibitors have been associated with a syndrome that starts with cholestatic jaundice and progresses to fulminant hepatic necrosis and (sometimes) death. The mechanism of this syndrome is not understood. Patients receiving ACE inhibitors who develop jaundice or marked elevations of hepatic enzymes should discontinue the ACE inhibitor and receive appropriate medical follow-up.

Diltiazem Malate

Cardiac Conduction: Diltiazem prolongs AV node refractory periods without significantly prolonging sinus node recovery time, except in patients with sick sinus syndrome. This effect may rarely result in abnormally slow heart rates (particularly in patients with sick sinus syndrome) or second or third-degree AV block. Concomitant use of diltiazem with beta-blockers or digitalis may result in additive effects on cardiac conduction. A patient with Prinzmetal's angina developed periods of asystole (2 to 5 seconds) after a single dose of 60 mg of diltiazem.

Congestive Heart Failure: Although diltiazem has a negative inotropic effect in isolated animal tissue preparations, hemodynamic studies in humans with normal ventricular function have not shown a reduction in cardiac index nor consistent negative effects on contractility (dp/dt). Worsening of congestive heart failure has been reported in patients with pre-existing impairment of ventricular function. Experience with the use of diltiazem in combination with beta-blockers in patients with impaired ventricular function is limited. Caution should be exercised when using this combination.

Hypotension: Decreases in blood pressure associated with diltiazem therapy may occasionally result in symptomatic hypotension.

Acute Hepatic Injury: Mild elevations of transaminases with and without concomitant elevations in alkaline phosphatase and bilirubin have been observed in clinical studies with diltiazem. Such elevations were usually transient and frequently resolved even with continued treatment. In rare instances, significant elevations in enzymes such as alkaline phosphatase, LDH, SGOT, SGPT, and other phenomena consistent with acute hepatic injury have been noted after administration of diltiazem. These reactions tended to occur early after therapy initiation (1 to 8 weeks) and have been reversible upon discontinuation of drug therapy. The relationship to diltiazem is uncertain in some cases, but probable in some. (See PRECAUTIONS).

Pregnancy

Enalapril-Diltiazem

There was no developmental toxicity in mice given up to 0.5/6 mg/kg/day of enalapril/diltiazem (approximately 3/0.9 times the maximum daily human dose of enalapril/diltiazem in the combination based on body weight, 0.29/0.079 times the maximum daily human dose based on body surface area) or in rats given up to 5/60 mg/kg/day of enalapril/diltiazem (approximately 30/9 times the maximum daily human dose of enalapril/diltiazem in the combination based on body weight, 5.7/1.6 times the maximum daily human dose based on body surface area). In rats given a high dose of 12.5/150 mg/kg/day of enalapril/diltiazem (83/22 times the maximum human dose of the combination based on body weight, 14.3/4 times the maximum daily human dose based on body surface area) there was a decrease in fetal weight, an increase in incidence of fetuses with visceral anomalies (thin diaphragm with protruding liver and dilated renal pelvis/ureter), and a decrease in pup survival. In mice given a high dose of 2.5/30 mg/kg/day of enalapril/diltiazem (17/4.5 times the maximum daily human dose of the combination based on body weight, 1.4/0.4 times the maximum daily human dose based on body surface area), there was an increase in post-implantation loss and a decrease in fetal weight.

When used in pregnant women during the second and third trimesters, ACE inhibitors can cause injury and even death to the developing fetus. When pregnancy is detected, TECZEM should be discontinued as soon as possible. (See Enalapril Maleate, Fetal Neonatal/Morbidity and Mortality, below.)

Enalapril Maleate

Fetal Neonatal/Morbidity and Mortality: ACE inhibitors can cause fetal and neonatal morbidity and death when administered to pregnant women. Several dozen cases have been reported in the world literature.

When pregnancy is detected, ACE inhibitors should be discontinued as soon as possible.

The use of ACE inhibitors during the second and third trimesters of pregnancy has been associated with fetal and neonatal injury, including hypotension, neonatal skull hypoplasia, anuria, reversible or irreversible renal failure, and death. Oligohydramnios have also been reported, presumably resulting from decreased fetal renal function; oligohydramnios in this setting has been associated with fetal limb contractures, craniofacial deformation, and hypoplastic lung development. Prematurity, intrauterine growth retardation, and patent ductus arteriosus have also been reported, although it is not clear whether these occurrences were due to the ACE-inhibitor exposure.

These adverse effects do not appear to have resulted from intrauterine ACE-inhibitor exposure that has been limited to the first trimester. Mothers whose embryos and fetuses are exposed to ACE inhibitors only during the first trimester should be so informed. Nonetheless, when patients become pregnant, physicians should make every effort to discontinue the use of TECZEM as soon as possible.

Rarely (probably less often than once in every thousand pregnancies), no alternative to ACE inhibitors will be found. In these rare cases, the mothers should be apprised of the potential hazards to their fetuses, and serial ultrasound examinations should be performed to assess the intra-amniotic environment.

If oligohydramnios is observed, TECZEM should be discontinued unless it is considered lifesaving for the mother. Contraction stress testing (CST), a non-stress test (NST), or biophysical profiling (BPP) may be appropriate, depending upon the week of pregnancy. Patients and physicians should be aware, however, that oligohydramnios may not appear until after the fetus has sustained irreversible injury.

Infants with histories of in utero exposure to ACE inhibitors should be closely observed for hypotension, oliguria, and hyperkalemia. If oliguria occurs, attention should be directed toward support of blood pressure and renal perfusion. Exchange transfusion or dialysis may be required as means of reversing hypotension and/or substituting for disordered re-

Continued on next page

Teczem—Cont.

nal function. Enalapril, which crosses the placenta, has been removed from neonatal circulation by peritoneal dialysis with some clinical benefit, and theoretically may be removed by exchange transfusion, although there is no experience with the latter procedure.
No teratogenic effects of enalapril were seen in studies of pregnant rats, and rabbits. On a body surface area basis, the doses used were 57 times and 12 times, respectively, the maximum recommended human daily dose (MRHDD).

Diltiazem Malate
Reproduction studies have been conducted in mice, rats, and rabbits. Embryo and fetal lethality were observed in all three species, with doses of 200 or more mg diltiazem/kg/day in rats, 50 or more mg diltiazem/kg/day in mice, and 35 or more mg diltiazem/kg/day in rabbits. In rabbits and mice, these doses have also been associated with skeletal (primarily vertebral) malformations. On a mg/m^2 basis, these doses are similar to or lower than the maximum recommended human dose. Abnormalities of retina and tongue were associated with doses of 30 or more mg diltiazem/kg/day in a peri-post natal study in which only dead rat pups were examined for such anomalies. Prolonged gestation and dystocia leading to pup death/stillbirths occurred when rats were administered approximately 1.5 times (on a mg/m^2 basis) the daily recommended therapeutic dose immediately prior to, and throughout the period of parturition.

PRECAUTIONS

General
As with any other non-deformable material, caution should be used when administering TECZEM in patients with preexisting severe gastrointestinal narrowing (pathologic or iatrogenic). There have been reports of obstructive symptoms in patients with known strictures in association with the use of other non-deformable drug formulations.

Enalapril Maleate
Impaired Renal Function: As a consequence of inhibiting the renin-angiotensin-aldosterone system, changes in renal function may be anticipated in susceptible individuals. In patients with severe congestive heart failure whose renal function may depend on the activity of the renin-angiotensin-aldosterone system, treatment with angiotensin converting enzyme inhibitors, including enalapril, may be associated with oliguria and/or progressive azotemia and rarely with acute renal failure and/or death.
In clinical studies in hypertensive patients with unilateral or bilateral renal artery stenosis, increases in blood urea nitrogen and serum creatinine were observed in 20 percent of patients. These increases were almost always reversible upon discontinuation of enalapril and/or diuretic therapy. In such patients renal function should be monitored during the first few weeks of therapy.
Some patients with hypertension or heart failure with no apparent pre-existing renal vascular disease have developed increases in blood urea and serum creatinine, usually minor and transient, especially when enalapril has been given concomitantly with a diuretic. This is more likely to occur in patients with pre-existing renal impairment. Dosage reduction of enalapril and/or discontinuation of the diuretic may be required.
Evaluation of the hypertensive patient should always include assessment of renal function.
Hyperkalemia: Elevated serum potassium (greater than 5.7 mEq/L) was observed in approximately one percent of hypertensive patients in clinical trials treated with enalapril alone. In most cases there were isolated values which resolved despite continued therapy, although hyperkalemia was a cause of discontinuation of therapy in 0.28 percent of hypertensive patients. Risk factors for the development of hyperkalemia include renal insufficiency, diabetes mellitus, and the concomitant use of potassium-sparing diuretics, potassium supplements and/or potassium-containing salt substitutes, which should be used cautiously, if at all, with enalapril. (See Drug Interactions.)
Cough: Presumably due to the inhibition of the degradation of endogenous bradykinin, persistent nonproductive cough has been reported with the use of ACE inhibitors, always resolving after discontinuation of therapy. ACE inhibitor-induced cough should be considered as part of the differential diagnosis of cough.
Surgery/Anesthesia: In patients undergoing major surgery or during anesthesia with agents that produce hypotension, enalapril may block angiotensin II formation secondary to compensatory renin release. If hypotension occurs and is considered to be due to this mechanism, it can be corrected by volume expansion.

Diltiazem Malate
Diltiazem is extensively metabolized by the liver and excreted by the kidneys and in bile. As with any drug given over prolonged periods, laboratory parameters of renal and hepatic function should be monitored at regular intervals. The drug should be used with caution in patients with impaired renal or hepatic function. In subacute and chronic dog and rat studies designed to produce toxicity, high doses of diltiazem were associated with hepatic changes. In dogs, sporadic and occasionally transient elevations of transaminase values occurred in a one-year oral toxicity study at doses of 10 to 20 mg/kg/day.
Dermatological events (see ADVERSE REACTIONS section) may be transient and may disappear despite continued use of diltiazem. However, skin eruptions progressing to erythema multiforme and/or exfoliative dermatitis have also been infrequently reported with diltiazem. Should a dermatologic reaction persist, the drug should be discontinued.

Information for Patients
Patients should be instructed to take TECZEM tablets whole and not to break, crush, or chew the tablets. Patients should also be instructed not to be concerned if they notice something in their stool that looks like a tablet. In TECZEM, the diltiazem component is contained within a nonabsorbable shell that has been specially designed to slowly release drug for the patient's body to absorb. When this process is completed, the empty tablet is eliminated from the body.
Angioedema: Angioedema, including laryngeal edema, may occur at any time during treatment with angiotensin converting enzyme inhibitors, including enalapril. Patients should be so advised and told to report immediately any signs or symptoms suggesting angioedema (swelling of face, extremities, eyes, lips, tongue, difficulty in swallowing or breathing) and to take no more drug until they have consulted with the prescribing physician.
Hypotension: Patients should be cautioned to report lightheadedness especially during the first few days of therapy. If actual syncope occurs, the patients should be told to discontinue the drug until they have consulted with the prescribing physician.
All patients should be cautioned that excessive perspiration and dehydration may lead to an excessive fall in blood pressure because of reduction in fluid volume. Other causes of volume depletion such as vomiting or diarrhea may also lead to a fall in blood pressure; patients should be advised to consult with the physician.
Hyperkalemia: Patients should be told not to use salt substitutes containing potassium without consulting their physician.
Neutropenia: Patients should be told to report promptly any indication of infection (e.g., sore throat, fever) which may be a sign of neutropenia.
Pregnancy: Female patients of chilbearing age should be told about the consequences of second and third trimester exposure to ACE inhibitors, and they should also be told that these consequences do not appear to have resulted from intrauterine ACE-inhibitor exposure that has been limited to the first trimester. These patients should be asked to report pregnancies to their physicians as soon as possible.
NOTE: As with many other drugs, certain advice to patients being treated with TECZEM is warranted. This information is intended to aid in the safe and effective use of this medication. It is not a disclosure of all possible adverse or intended effects.

Drug Interactions
Enalapril Maleate
Hypotension—Patients on Diuretic Therapy: Patients on diuretics and especially those in whom diuretic therapy was recently instituted, may occasionally experience an excessive reduction of blood pressure after initiation of therapy with enalapril. The possibility of hypotensive effects with enalapril can be minimized by either discontinuing the diuretic or increasing the salt intake prior to initiation of treatment with enalapril. If it is necessary to continue the diuretic, provide medical supervision for at least two hours and until blood pressure has stabilized for at least an additional hour. (See WARNINGS, and DOSAGE AND ADMINISTRATION.)
Agents Causing Renin Release: The antihypertensive effect of enalapril is augmented by antihypertensive agents that cause renin release (e.g., diuretics).
Other Cardiovascular Agents: Enalapril has been used concomitantly with beta adrenergic-blocking agents, methyldopa, nitrates, calcium-blocking agents, hydralazine and prazosin without evidence of clinically significant adverse interactions.
Agents Increasing Serum Potassium: Enalapril attenuates diuretic-induced potassium loss. Potassium-sparing diuretics (e.g., spironolactone, triamterene, or amiloride), potassium supplements, or potassium-containing salt substitutes may lead to significant increases in serum potassium. Therefore, if concomitant use of these agents is indicated because of demonstrated hypokalemia they should be used with caution and with frequent monitoring of serum potassium.
Lithium: Lithium toxicity has been reported in patients receiving lithium concomitantly with drugs which cause elimination of sodium, including ACE inhibitors. A few cases of lithium toxicity have been reported in patients receiving concomitant enalapril and lithium and were reversible upon discontinuation of both drugs. It is recommended that serum lithium levels be monitored frequently if enalapril is administered concomitantly with lithium.

Diltiazem Malate
Due to the potential for additive effects, caution and careful titration are warranted in patients receiving diltiazem concomitantly with any agents known to affect cardiac contractility and/or conduction. (See WARNINGS.) Pharmacologic studies indicate that there may be additive effects in prolonging AV conduction when using beta-blockers or digitalis concomitantly with diltiazem. (See WARNINGS.)
As with all drugs, care should be exercised when treating patients with multiple medications. Diltiazem undergoes biotransformation by cytochrome P-450 mixed function oxidase. Coadministration of diltiazem with other agents which follow the same route of biotransformation may result in the competitive inhibition of metabolism. Especially in patients with renal and/or hepatic impairment, dosages of similarly metabolized drugs, particularly those of low therapeutic ratio, may require adjustment when starting or stopping concomitantly administered diltiazem to maintain optimum therapeutic blood levels.
The following interactions have been seen with diltiazem hydrochloride and can be anticipated to occur with the diltiazem malate salt.
Beta-blockers: Clinical trials with diltiazem suggest that concomitant use of diltiazem and beta-blockers is usually well-tolerated, but available data are not sufficient to predict the effects of concomitant treatment with beta-blockers in patients with left ventricular dysfunction or cardiac conduction abnormalities.
Administration of diltiazem hydrochloride concomitantly with propranolol in five normal volunteers resulted in increased propranolol levels in all subjects and bioavailability of propranolol was increased approximately 50%. In vitro, propranolol appears to be displaced from its binding sites by diltiazem. If combination therapy is initiated or withdrawn in conjuction with propranolol, an adjustment in the propranolol dose may be warranted. (See WARNINGS.)
Cimetidine: A study in six healthy volunteers has shown a significant increase in peak diltiazem plasma levels (58%) and area under the curve (53%) after a one-week course of cimetidine at 1,200 mg per day and a single dose of diltiazem 60 mg. Ranitidine produced smaller, nonsignificant increases. The effect may be mediated by cimetidine's known inhibition of hepatic cytochrome P-450, the enzyme system responsible for the first-pass metabolism of diltiazem. Patients currently receiving diltiazem therapy should be carefully monitored for a change in pharmacological effect when initiating and discontinuing therapy with cimetidine. An adjustment in the diltiazem dose may be warranted.
Digitalis: Administration of diltiazem with digoxin in 24 healthy male subjects increased plasma digoxin concentrations approximately 20%. Another investigator found no increase in digoxin levels in 12 patients with coronary artery disease. Since there have been conflicting results regarding the effect of digoxin levels, it is recommended that digoxin levels be monitored when initiating, adjusting, and discontinuing diltiazem therapy to avoid possible over- or under-digitalization. (See WARNINGS.)
Anesthetics: The depression of cardiac contractility, conductivity, and automaticity as well as the vascular dilation associated with anesthetics may be potentiated by calcium channel blockers. When used concomitantly, anesthetics and calcium blockers should be titrated carefully.
Cyclosporine: A pharmacokinetic interaction between diltiazem and cyclosporine has been observed during studies involving renal and cardiac transplant patients. In renal and cardiac transplant recipients, a reduction of cyclosporine dose ranging from 15% to 48% was necessary to maintain trough concentrations similar to those seen prior to the addition of diltiazem. If these agents are to be administered concurrently, cyclosporine concentrations should be monitored, especially when diltiazem therapy is initiated, adjusted, or discontinued. The effect of cyclosporine on diltiazem plasma concentrations has not been evaluated.
Carbamazepine: Concomitant administration of diltiazem with carbamazepine has been reported to result in elevated serum levels of carbamazepine (40% to 72% increase) resulting in toxicity in some cases. Patients receiving these agents concomitantly should be monitored for a potential drug interaction.

Carcinogenesis, Mutagenesis, Impairment of Fertility
Enalapril - Diltiazem
Carcinogenicity studies have not been conducted with enalapril in combination with diltiazem. Enalapril in combination with diltiazem was not mutagenic in the Ames microbial mutagen test with or without metabolic activation. Enalapril in combination with diltiazem did not produce DNA single strand breaks in an in vitro alkaline elution assay in rat hepatocytes or chromosomal aberrations in an in vivo mouse bone marrow assay. However, in an in vitro cytogenetics assay of enalapril in combination with diltiazem, increases in chromosomal aberrations were seen (including endoreduplication, a form of polyploidy), similar to increases seen when diltiazem malate was given alone. No evidence of impaired fertility was observed in studies in rats performed at oral dosages of 10/120 mg/kg/day of enalapril/

diltiazem in females and 8/96 mg/kg/day in males. On a body surface area basis, these doses were 12/3 times and 9/2.5 times, respectively, the maximum recommended human daily dose. However, in the female fertility study a slight decrease in litter size due to preimplantation loss at 10/120 mg/kg/day was considered of uncertain relationship to treatment.

Enalapril Maleate

There was no evidence of a tumorigenic effect when enalapril was administered for 106 weeks to male and female rats at doses up to 90 mg/kg/day or for 94 weeks to male and female mice at doses up to 90 and 180 mg/kg/day, respectively. These doses are 26 times (in rats and female mice) and 13 times (in male mice) the maximum recommended human daily dose (MRHDD) when compared on a body surface area basis. Neither enalapril maleate nor the active diacid was mutagenic in the Ames microbial mutagen test with or without metabolic activation. Enalapril was also negative in the following genotoxicity studies: rec-assay, reverse mutation assay with *E. coli* sister chromatid exchange with cultured mammalian cells, and the micronucleus test with mice, as well as in an in vivo cytogenic study using mouse bone marrow.

There were no adverse effects on reproductive performance in male and female rats treated with up to 90 mg/kg/day of enalapril (26 times the MRHDD when compared on a body surface area basis).

Diltiazem Malate

Oral administration of diltiazem hydrochloride to male and female rats for up to 104 weeks and to male mice for up to 92 weeks at doses up to 100 mg diltiazem/kg/day [approximately 2 and 1 times, respectively, the maximum recommended human dose (MRHD) of 480 mg/day on a mg/m² basis] revealed no evidence of a tumorigenic effect of diltiazem. In female mice receiving doses of 100 mg diltiazem/kg/day for 92 weeks, an increased incidence of benign ovarian granulosa cell tumor was observed. A similar effect was not apparent at doses as high as 200 mg diltiazem/kg/day administered for up to 78 weeks.

Diltiazem was negative in vitro for mutagenic effects in bacteria (Ames Test) and Chinese hamster lung cells and for induction of DNA strand breaks in rat hepatocytes (Alkaline Elution Assay). Diltiazem was also negative in vivo for chromosomal aberrations in mouse and Chinese hamster bone marrow, and for induction of micronuclei in Chinese hamster bone marrow. Diltiazem was, however, positive in vitro for induction of chromosomal aberrations in Chinese hamster ovary cells at concentrations approximately 500 times the human clinical plasma levels.

No evidence of impaired fertility or reproductive performance was observed in studies in rats at doses of up to 30 mg/kg/day. However, decreased reproductive performance (mating) was observed at 100 mg/kg/day in studies in which males were treated at this dosage level.

Pregnancy

Pregnancy Categories C (first trimester) and D (Second and third trimesters). (See WARNINGS, Pregnancy, Enalapril Maleate, Fetal Neonatal/Morbidity and Mortality.)

Nursing Mothers

Enalapril and enalaprilat are detected in human milk in trace amounts. Diltiazem is excreted in human milk. Concentrations of diltiazem in breast milk have been reported to approximate serum levels. If the use of TECZEM is deemed essential, an alternative method of infant feeding other than breast feeding should be instituted.

Pediatric Use

Safety and effectiveness in pediatric patients have not been established.

Geriatric Use

Of the total number of patients who received enalapril maleate/diltiazem malate extended release tablets in clinical studies, 18% were 65 or older. Overall differences in effectiveness or safety were not observed between these patients and younger patients, but greater sensitivity of some older individuals cannot be ruled out.

ADVERSE REACTIONS

Enalapril maleate/diltiazem malate combinations, including TECZEM, have been evaluated for safety in more than 1950 patients, including over 350 patients treated for one year or more. In clinical trials with enalapril maleate/diltiazem malate combinations, including TECZEM, no adverse experiences peculiar to this combination drug have been reported. Adverse experiences reported have been limited to those that have been previously reported with enalapril or diltiazem.

Generally, adverse experiences were mild and transient in nature. Discontinuation rates for adverse experiences reported in controlled trials were similar for enalapril maleate/diltiazem malate combinations, including TECZEM, and placebo-treated patients. All clinical adverse experiences, whether drug related or not, reported in greater than one percent of patients treated with enalapril maleate/diltiazem malate combinations, including TECZEM (in total

PERCENT OF PATIENTS IN CONTROLLED TRIALS

Body System Adverse Experience	All Adverse Experiences		Drug-Related Adverse Experiences*	
	Enalapril/Diltiazem Including TECZEM (N = 1283) Incidence %	Placebo (N = 260) Incidence %	Enalapril/Diltiazem Including TECZEM (N = 1283) Incidence %	Placebo (N = 260) Incidence %
Nervous				
Headache	7.2	13.5	2.7	4.6
Dizziness	3.2	3.5	1.9	1.2
Body as a Whole				
Edema/Swelling	3.4	4.6	2.3	2.3
Asthenia/Fatigue	3.0	2.3	2.0	0.4
Chest Pain	1.6	2.7	0.5	0.0
Abdominal Pain	1.2	1.2	0.5	0.4
Respiratory				
Upper Respiratory				
Infection	5.4	7.3	0.0	0.0
Cough	3.4	2.3	2.3	0.4
Sinusitis	1.2	3.1	0.0	0.4
Influenza	1.2	1.2	0.0	0.0
Skin				
Rash	2.0	1.5	1.3	0.4
Digestive				
Diarrhea	2.1	2.3	0.5	0.8
Nausea	1.5	2.3	0.6	0.0
Musculoskeletal				
Back Pain	1.1	3.5	0.1	0.0

*Considered possibly, probably, or definitely related to study drug by investigators.

TECZEM
(Enalapril Maleate/Diltiazem Malate Extended Release Tablets)

Strength	Quantity	NDC Number	Description
5 mg enalapril maleate/180 mg diltiazem malate*	100 unit of use bottle (with desiccant)	0088-1765-47	Gold-hued, film-coated, capsule-shaped, extended release tablets coded TECZEM 5/180.

*Expressed as the corresponding diltiazem hydrochloride doses. (See DESCRIPTION.)

daily doses up to 20 mg/360 mg, respectively), in controlled clinical trials, and the corresponding incidence of drug-related clinical adverse experiences, are shown below. [See first table above]

Clinical adverse experiences, regardless of drug relationship, reported in 0.5 to 1.0 percent of patients in controlled trials included:

Cardiovascular: First-degree AV block, palpitation
Digestive: Constipation, dental infection, dental pain
Musculoskeletal: Joint swelling
Nervous System/Psychiatric: Depression, insomnia, somnolence
Respiratory: Bronchitis, nasal congestion, pharyngitis, sinus disorder
Skin: Flushing
Urogenital: Impotence

Clinical Laboratory Test Findings

Creatinine, Blood Urea Nitrogen: In controlled clinical trials minor increases in blood urea nitrogen and serum creatinine, reversible upon discontinuation of therapy, were reported infrequently. More marked increases have been reported in other enalapril experience. Increases are more likely to occur in patients with renal artery stenosis. (See PRECAUTIONS.)

Hemoglobin and Hematocrit: Small decreases in hemoglobin and hematocrit occurred infrequently in hypertensive patients treated with enalapril maleate/diltiazem malate combinations but were rarely of clinical importance unless another cause of anemia coexisted. In clinical trials, less than 0.1 percent of patients discontinued therapy due to anemia.

Other: In controlled clinical trials minor increases in serum potassium, alanine transaminase, aspartate transaminase, alkaline phosphatase, and/or bilirubin, and minor decreases in serum sodium, generally reversible upon discontinuation, were reported. (See WARNINGS and PRECAUTIONS.)

Other adverse experiences, regardless of drug relationship, that have been reported in clinical trials or postmarketing experience with the individual components include the following and they should be considered as potential adverse reactions for TECZEM.

Enalapril Maleate

Body as a Whole: Anaphylactoid reaction (See WARNINGS), orthostatic effects, symptoms suggestive of facial edema or angioedema (see WARNINGS), syncope
Cardiovascular: Angina pectoris; atrial fibrillation; cardiac arrest; hypotension; myocardial infarction or cerebrovascular accident, possibly secondary to excessive hypotension in high-risk patients (see WARNINGS, Hypotension); ortho-

static hypotension; pulmonary edema; pulmonary embolism and infarction; rhythm disturbances including atrial tachycardia and bradycardia.
Digestive: Anorexia, dry mouth, dyspepsia, glossitis, hepatic failure, hepatitis (hepatocellular [proven on rechallenge] or cholestatic jaundice) (See WARNINGS, Hepatic Failure), ileus, melena, pancreatitis, stomatitis, vomiting
Hematologic: Hemolytic anemia, including cases of hemolysis in patients with G-6-PD deficiency, has been reported; a causal relationship to enalapril cannot be excluded. Rare cases of neutropenia, thrombocytopenia and bone marrow depression
Musculoskeletal: Muscle cramps
Nervous System/Psychiatric: Ataxia, confusion, nervousness, peripheral neuropathy (eg, paresthesia, dysesthesia), vertigo
Respiratory: Asthma, bronchospasm, dyspnea, pneumonia, pulmonary infiltrates, rhinorrhea, sore throat and hoarseness
Skin: Alopecia, diaphoresis, erythema multiforme, exfoliative dermatitis, herpes zoster, pemphigus, photosensitivity, pruritus, Stevens-Johnson syndrome, toxic epidermal necrolysis, urticaria
Special Senses: Anosmia, blurred vision, conjunctivitis, dry eyes, taste alteration, tearing, tinnitus
Urogenital: Flank pain, gynecomastia, oliguria, renal dysfunction (see PRECAUTIONS and DOSAGE AND ADMINISTRATION), renal failure, urinary tract infection
Angioedema: Angioedema has been reported in patients receiving enalapril, with an incidence higher in black than in non-black patients. Angioedema associated with laryngeal edema may be fatal. If angioedema of the face, extremities, lips, tongue, glottis and/or larynx occurs, treatment with TECZEM should be discontinued and appropriate therapy instituted immediately. (See WARNINGS.)
Miscellaneous: A symptom complex has been reported which may include a positive ANA, an elevated erythrocyte sedimentation rate, arthralgia/arthritis, myalgia/myositis, fever, serositis, vasculitis, leukocytosis, eosinophilia, photosensitivity, rash and other dermatologic manifestations.
Fetal/Neonatal Morbidity and Mortality: See WARNINGS, Pregnancy, Enalapril Maleate, Fetal/Neonatal Morbidity and Mortality.

Diltiazem Malate or Other Formulations of Diltiazem

Body as a Whole: Facial edema, fever, flu-like illness, orthostatic effects, pain, syncope, vasovagal reaction
Cardiovascular: Angina, arrhythmia, atrial fibrillation, AV block-second degree, AV block-third degree, bundle branch block, congestive heart failure, ECG abnormality, heart murmur, hypotension, myocardial infarction (not readily

Continued on next page

Teczem—Cont.

distinguishable from the natural history of the disease of the patients receiving diltiazem), myocardial ischemia, sinus bradycardia, tachycardia, ventricular extrasystoles

Digestive: Acid regurgitation, anorexia, dry mouth, dysgeusia, dyspepsia, flatulence, gingival hyperplasia, thirst, tongue edema, vomiting, weight gain

Hematologic: Hemolytic anemia, increased bleeding time, leukopenia, thrombocytopenia

Metabolic: Hyperglycemia, hyperuricemia, hypokalemia, increased creatine phosphokinase

Musculoskeletal: Arthralgia, foot pain, gout, knee pain, muscle cramp, osteoarticular pain, shoulder pain, stiffness, strain

Nervous System/Psychiatric: Abnormal dreams, amnesia, decreased libido, extrapyramidal symptoms, gait abnormalities, hallucinations, hypesthesia, migraine, muscle weakness, nervousness, paresthesia, personality changes, tremor

Respiratory: Allergic rhinitis, dyspnea, epistaxis, pharyngeal edema

Skin: Alopecia, erythema multiforme, exfoliative dermatitis, leukocytoclastic vasculitis, petechiae, photosensitivity, pruritus, purpura, urticaria

Special Senses: Amblyopia, eye infection, eye irritation, eyelid edema, otitis media, retinopathy, tinnitus

Urogenital: Flank pain, hematuria, nocturia, polyuria, proteinuria, pyuria, sexual difficulties, urinary frequency, urinary tract infection

OVERDOSAGE

No specific information is available on the treatment of overdosage with TECZEM. Treatment is symptomatic and supportive. Therapy with TECZEM should be discontinued and the patient observed closely. Suggested measures include induction of emesis and/or gastric lavage, and correction of hypotension, bradycardia, heart block, and heart failure by established procedures.

Enalapril Maleate

Limited data are available in regard to overdosage of enalapril maleate in humans. The oral LD_{50} of enalapril is 2000 mg/kg in mice and rats. The most likely manifestation of overdosage would be hypotension, for which the usual treatment would be intravenous infusion of normal saline solution. Enalaprilat may be removed from general circulation by hemodialysis and has been removed from neonatal circulation by peritoneal dialysis.

Diltiazem Malate

The oral LD_{50}'s of diltiazem malate in mice and rats range from 424 to 554 mg/kg and from 736 to 844 mg/kg, respectively. The intravenous LD_{50}'s in these species ranged from 40.6 to 44.1 and 39.9 to 40.2 mg/kg, respectively. The LD_{50}'s of the hydrochloride salt of diltiazem in mice and rats were comparable to that of the malate salt. The LD_{50} of the hydrochloride salt of diltiazem in dogs is considered to be in excess of 50 mg/kg, while lethality was seen in monkeys at 360 mg/kg.

The toxic dose in man is not known. Due to extensive metabolism, blood levels after a standard dose of diltiazem can vary over tenfold, limiting the usefulness of blood levels in overdose cases.

There have been several reports of diltiazem hydrochloride overdose in doses ranging up to 10.8g. In the majority of the cases, patients recovered from the reported overdose. In the few cases with a fatal outcome, multiple drug ingestions were usually involved. No specific information is available on overdose in humans with diltiazem malate.

Events observed following diltiazem overdose included bradycardia, hypotension, heart block, and cardiac failure. Most reports of overdose described some supportive medical measure and/or drug treatment. Bradycardia frequently responded favorably to atropine as did heart block, although cardiac pacing was also frequently utilized to treat heart block. Fluids and vasopressors were used to maintain blood pressure, and in cases of cardiac failure, inotropic agents were administered. In addition, some patients received treatment with ventilatory support, gastric lavage, activated charcoal, and/or intravenous calcium. Evidence of the effectiveness of intravenous calcium administration to reverse the pharmacological effects of calcium channel blockers overdose was conflicting.

In the event of overdose or exaggerated response, appropriate supportive measures should be employed in addition to gastrointestinal decontamination. Diltiazem does not appear to be removed by peritoneal or hemodialysis. Based on the known pharmacological effects of diltiazem and/or reported clinical experience, the following measures may be considered:

Bradycardia: Administer atropine (0.60 to 1.0 mg). If there is no response to vagal blockade, administer isoproterenol cautiously.

High-Degree AV Block: Treat as for bradycardia above. Fixed high-degree AV block should be treated with cardiac pacing.

Cardiac Failure: Administer inotropic agents (isoproterenol, dopamine, or dobutamine) and diuretics.

Hypotension: Vasopressors (eg, dopamine or levarterenol bitartrate).

Actual treatment and dosage should depend on the severity of the clinical situation and the judgment and experience of the treating physician.

DOSAGE AND ADMINISTRATION

The recommended initial dose of enalapril maleate for hypertension in patients not receiving diuretics is 5 mg once a day. The usual dosage range of enalapril maleate for hypertension is 10–40 mg per day administered in a single dose or two divided doses. In some patients treated once daily with enalapril, the antihypertensive effect may diminish toward the end of the dosing interval. In such patients, an increase in dosage or twice daily administration should be considered. The recommended usual dosage range of controlled-release formulations of diltiazem for hypertension is 120 to 540 mg, once-a-day.

In clinical trials of enalapril maleate/diltiazem malate controlled release formulation, administered once daily, the antihypertensive effect of the combination generally increased as the dose of each ingredient was increased. In the combination trials, the doses studied were 1.25 to 20 mg of enalapril maleate and 60 to 360 mg of diltiazem malate (dosage expressed as diltiazem hydrochloride).

The adverse events (see WARNINGS and ADVERSE REACTIONS) of enalapril are generally independent of dose; those of diltiazem are a mixture of dose-dependent phenomena (primarily dizziness, AV block, sinus bradycardia, and to a lesser extent peripheral edema) and dose-independent phenomena, the former much more common than the latter. Therapy with any combination of enalapril and diltiazem will thus be associated with both sets of dose-independent adverse events.

Rarely, the dose-independent adverse events associated with enalapril or diltiazem are serious. To minimize dose-independent adverse events, it is usually appropriate to begin therapy with TECZEM only after (a) a patient has failed to achieve the desired antihypertensive effect with one or the other monotherapy (see above) or (b) the dose of one or the other monotherapy cannot be increased further because of dose limiting side effects.

Replacement Therapy: For convenience, patients receiving enalapril and diltiazem as separate dosage forms may instead wish to receive tablets of TECZEM containing the same component doses.

Use in Renal Impairment: The usual regimens of therapy with TECZEM need not be adjusted as long as the patient's creatinine clearance is >30 mL/min/1.73m^2 (serum creatinine approximately ≤3 mg/dL or 265 µmol/L). In patients with more severe renal impairment, i.e., creatinine clearance ≤30 mL/min/1.73m^2 (serum creatinine >3 mg/dL or 265 µmol/L), titration of the individual components must be done prior to switching to TECZEM. (See PRECAUTIONS, Enalapril Maleate; Impaired Renal Function.)

HOW SUPPLIED

[See second table at top of previous page]

Storage: Store in a well-closed container at room temperature, 15–30°C (59–86°F). Protect from moisture.

Prescribing Information as of July 1996

Manufactured by:
Merck & Co., Inc.
West Point, PA 19486 USA
for
Hoechst Marion Roussel, Inc.
Kansas City, MO 64137 USA

Shown in Product Identification Guide, page 316

TOPICORT® (desoximetasone) ℞
Emollient Cream 0.25%
and
TOPICORT® LP (desoximetasone)
Emollient Cream 0.05%

Prescribing Information as of February 1996
FOR DERMATOLOGIC USE ONLY.
NOT FOR USE IN EYES.

DESCRIPTION

TOPICORT (desoximetasone) Emollient Cream 0.25% and TOPICORT LP (desoximetasone) Emollient Cream 0.05% contain the active synthetic corticosteroid desoximetasone. The topical corticosteroids constitute a class of primarily synthetic steroids used as anti-inflammatory and anti-pruritic agents.

Each gram of TOPICORT Emollient Cream 0.25% contains 2.5 mg of desoximetasone in an emollient cream consisting of white petrolatum USP, purified water USP, isopropyl myristate NF, lanolin alcohols NF, mineral oil USP, cetostearyl alcohol NF, aluminum stearate and magnesium stearate.

Each gram of TOPICORT LP Emollient Cream 0.05% contains 0.5 mg desoximetasone in an emollient cream consisting of white petrolatum USP, purified water USP, isopropyl myristate NF, lanolin alcohols NF, mineral oil USP, cetostearyl alcohol NF, aluminum stearate, edetate disodium USP, lactic acid USP and magnesium stearate.

The chemical name of desoximetasone is Pregna-1,4-diene-3, 20-dione, 9-fluoro-11, 21-dihydroxy-16-methyl-, (11β, 16α)-.

Desoximetasone has the empirical formula $C_{22}H_{29}FO_4$ and a molecular weight of 376.47.

The CAS Registry Number is 382-67-2. The chemical structure is:

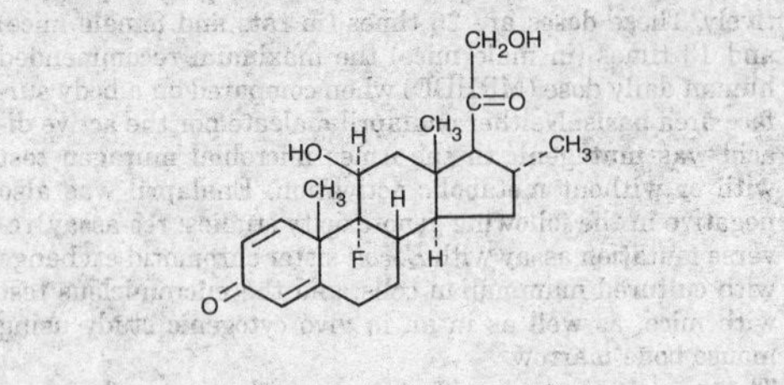

CLINICAL PHARMACOLOGY

Topical corticosteroids share anti-inflammatory, anti-pruritic and vasoconstrictive actions.

The mechanism of anti-inflammatory activity of the topical corticosteroids is unclear. Various laboratory methods, including vasoconstrictor assays, are used to compare and predict potencies and/or clinical efficacies of the topical corticosteroids. There is some evidence to suggest that a recognizable correlation exists between vasoconstrictor potency and therapeutic efficacy in man.

Pharmacokinetics

The extent of percutaneous absorption of topical corticosteroids is determined by many factors including the vehicle, the integrity of the epidermal barrier, and the use of occlusive dressings.

Topical corticosteroids can be absorbed from normal intact skin. Inflammation and/or other disease processes in the skin increase percutaneous absorption. Occlusive dressings substantially increase the percutaneous absorption of topical corticosteroids. Thus, occlusive dressings may be a valuable therapeutic adjunct for treatment of resistant dermatoses.

Once absorbed through the skin, topical corticosteroids are handled through pharmacokinetic pathways similar to systemically administered corticosteroids. Corticosteroids are bound to plasma proteins in varying degrees. Corticosteroids are metabolized primarily in the liver and are then excreted by the kidneys. Some of the topical corticosteroids and their metabolites are also excreted into the bile.

Pharmacokinetic studies in men with TOPICORT (desoximetasone) Emollient Cream 0.25% with tagged desoximetasone showed a total of 5.2% ± 2.9% excretion in urine (4.1% ± 2.3%) and feces (1.1% ± 0.6%) and no detectable level (limit of sensitivity: 0.005 µg/mL) in the blood when it was applied topically on the back followed by occlusion for 24 hours. Seven days after application, no further radioactivity was detected in urine or feces. The half-life of the material was 15 ± 2 hours (for urine) and 17 ± 2 hours (for feces) between the third and fifth trial day. Studies with other similarly structured steroids have shown that predominant metabolite reaction occurs through conjugation to form the glucuronide and sulfate ester.

INDICATIONS AND USAGE

TOPICORT Emollient Cream 0.25% and TOPICORT LP (desoximetasone) Emollient Cream 0.05% are indicated for the relief of the inflammatory and pruritic manifestations of corticosteroid-responsive dermatoses.

CONTRAINDICATIONS

Topical corticosteroids are contraindicated in those patients with a history of hypersensitivity to any of the components of the preparation.

PRECAUTIONS

General

Systemic absorption of topical corticosteroids has produced reversible hypothalamic-pituitary-adrenal (HPA) axis suppression, manifestations of Cushing's syndrome, hyperglycemia, and glucosuria in some patients.

Conditions which augment systemic absorption include the application of the more potent steroids, use over large surface areas, prolonged use, and the addition of occlusive dressings.

Therefore, patients receiving a large dose of a potent topical steroid applied to a large surface area or under an occlusive dressing should be evaluated periodically for evidence of HPA axis suppression by using the urinary free cortisol and ACTH stimulation tests. If HPA axis suppression is noted, an attempt should be made to withdraw the drug, to reduce the frequency of application, or to substitute a less potent steroid. Recovery of HPA axis function is generally prompt

and complete upon discontinuation of the drug. Infrequently, signs and symptoms of steroid withdrawal may occur, requiring supplemental systemic corticosteroids.

Pediatric patients may absorb proportionally larger amounts of topical corticosteroids and thus be more susceptible to systemic toxicity. (See PRECAUTIONS—Pediatric Use). If irritation develops, topical corticosteroids should be discontinued and appropriate therapy instituted.

In the presence of dermatological infections, the use of an appropriate antifungal or antibacterial agent should be instituted. If a favorable response does not occur promptly, the corticosteroid should be discontinued until the infection has been adequately controlled.

Information for the Patient

Patients using topical corticosteroids should receive the following information and instructions:

1. This medication is to be used as directed by the physician. It is for external use only. Avoid contact with the eyes.
2. Patients should be advised not to use this medication for any disorder other than for which it was prescribed.
3. The treated skin area should not be bandaged or otherwise covered or wrapped as to be occlusive unless directed by the physician.
4. Patients should report any signs of local adverse reactions especially under occlusive dressing.
5. Parents of pediatric patients should be advised not to use tight-fitting diapers or plastic pants on a child being treated in the diaper area, as these garments may constitute occlusive dressings.

Laboratory Tests

The following tests may be helpful in evaluating the HPA axis suppression: Urinary free cortisol test and ACTH stimulation test.

Carcinogenesis, Mutagenesis, and Impairment of Fertility

Long-term animal studies have not been performed to evaluate the carcinogenic potential or the effect on fertility of topical corticosteroids.

Studies to determine mutagenicity with prednisolone and hydrocortisone have revealed negative results. Desoximetasone did not show potential for mutagenic activity *in vitro* in the Ames microbial mutagent test with or without metabolic activation.

Pregnancy Category C

Corticosteroids are generally teratogenic in laboratory animals when administered systemically at relatively low dosage levels. The more potent corticosteroids have been shown to be teratogenic after dermal application in laboratory animals.

Desoximetasone has been shown to be teratogenic and embryotoxic in mice, rats, and rabbits when given by subcutaneous or dermal routes of administration in doses 3 to 30 times the human dose of TOPICORT (desoximetasone) Emollient Cream 0.25% or 15 to 150 times the human dose of TOPICORT LP (desoximetasone) Emollient Cream 0.05%.

There are no adequate and well-controlled studies in pregnant women on teratogenic effects from topically applied corticosteroids. Therefore, TOPICORT Emollient Cream 0.25% and TOPICORT LP Emollient Cream 0.05% should be used during pregnancy only if the potential benefit justifies the potential risk to the fetus. Drugs of this class should not be used extensively on pregnant patients, in large amounts, or for prolonged periods of time.

Nursing Mothers

It is not known whether topical administration of corticosteroids could result in sufficient systemic absorption to produce detectable quantities in breast milk. Systemically administered corticosteroids are secreted into breast milk in quantities not likely to have a deleterious effect on the infant. Nevertheless, caution should be exercised when topical corticosteroids are administered to a nursing woman.

Pediatric Use

Pediatric patients may demonstrate greater susceptibility to topical corticosteroid-induced HPA axis suppression and Cushing's syndrome than mature patients because of a larger skin surface area to body weight ratio.

Hypothalamic-pituitary-adrenal (HPA) axis suppression, Cushing's syndrome, and intracranial hypertension have been reported in pediatric patients receiving topical corticosteroids. Manifestations of adrenal suppression in pediatric patients include linear growth retardation, delayed weight gain, low plasma cortisol levels, and absence of response to ACTH stimulation. Manifestations of intracranial hypertension include bulging fontanelles, headaches, and bilateral papilledema.

Administration of topical corticosteroids to pediatric patients should be limited to the least amount compatible with an effective therapeutic regimen. Chronic corticosteroid therapy may interfere with the growth and development of pediatric patients.

ADVERSE REACTIONS

The following local adverse reactions are reported infrequently with topical corticosteroids, but may occur more frequently with the use of occlusive dressings. These reactions are listed in an approximate decreasing order of occurrence:

burning, itching, irritation, dryness, folliculitis, hypertrichosis, acneiform eruptions, hypopigmentation, perioral dermatitis, allergic contact dermatitis, maceration of the skin, secondary infection, skin atropy, striae, miliaria.

In controlled clinical studies the incidence of adverse reactions was low (0.8%) for TOPICORT (desoximetasone) Emollient Cream 0.25% and included burning, folliculitis and folliculo-pustular lesions. The incidence of adverse reactions was also 0.8% for TOPICORT LP (desoximetasone) Emollient Cream 0.05% and included pruritus, erythema, vesiculation and burning sensation.

OVERDOSAGE

Topically applied corticosteroids can be absorbed in sufficient amounts to produce systemic effects. (See PRECAUTIONS).

DOSAGE AND ADMINISTRATION

Apply a thin film of TOPICORT Emollient Cream 0.25% or TOPICORT LP Emollient Cream 0.05% to the affected skin areas twice daily. Rub in gently.

HOW SUPPLIED

TOPICORTt® (desoximetasone) Emollient Cream 0.25% is supplied in 15 gram (NDC 0039-0011-23), 60 gram (NDC 0039-0011-60), and 4 ounce (NDC 0039-0011-04) tubes.

TOPICORT® LP (desoximetasone) Emollient Cream 0.05% is supplied in 15 gram (NDC 0039-0012-23) and 60 gram (NDC 0039-0012-60) tubes.

Store at controlled room temperature (59 to 86° F).

CAUTION: FEDERAL LAW PROHIBITS DISPENSING WITHOUT PRESCRIPTION.

TOPICORT REG TM ROUSSEL UCLAF

Prescribing Information as of February 1996

Hoechst-Roussel Pharmaceuticals

Division of Hoechst Marion Roussel. Inc.

Kansas City, MO 64137

Shown in Product Identification Guide, page 316

TOPICORT® Gel ℞
(desoximetasone) 0.05%

Prescribing Information as of February 1996

FOR DERMATOLOGIC USE ONLY.
NOT FOR USE IN EYES.

DESCRIPTION

TOPICORT® GEL (desoximetasone) 0.05% contains the active synthetic corticosteroid desoximetasone. The topical corticosteroids constitute a class of primarily synthetic steroids used as anti-inflammatory and anti-pruritic agents.

Each gram of TOPICORT GEL 0.05% contains 0.5 mg desoximetasone in a gel consisting of purified water USP, SD alcohol 40 (20% w/w), isopropyl myristate NF, carbomer 940, trolamine NF, edetate disodium USP, and docusate sodium USP.

The chemical name of desoximetasone is Pregna-1, 4-diene-3, 20-dione, 9-fluoro-11, 21-dihydroxy-16-methyl-, (11β, 16α)-.

Desoximetasone has the empirical formula $C_{22}H_{29}FO_4$ and a molecular weight of 376.47.

The CAS Registry Number is 382-67-2.

The chemical structure is:

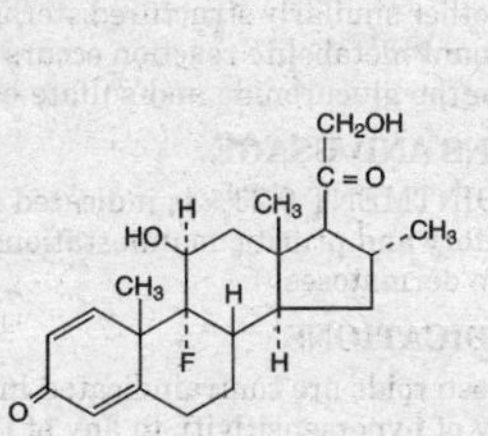

CLINICAL PHARMACOLOGY

Topical corticosteroids share anti-inflammatory, anti-pruritic and vasoconstrictive actions.

The mechanism of anti-inflammatory activity of the topical corticosteroids in unclear. Various laboratory methods, including vasoconstrictor assays, are used to compare and predict potencies and/or clinical efficacies of the topical corticosteroids. There is some evidence to suggest that a recognizable correlation exists between vasoconstrictor potency and therapeutic efficacy in man.

Pharmacokinetics

The extent of percutaneous absorption to topical corticosteroids is determined by many factors including the vehicle, the integrity of the epidermal barrier, and the use of occlusive dressings.

Topical corticosteroids can be absorbed from normal intact skin. Inflammation and/or other disease processes in the skin increase percutaneous absorption. Occlusive dressings substantially increase the percutaneous absorption of topical corticosteroids. Thus, occlusive dressings may be a valuable therapeutic adjunct for treatment of resistant dermatoses.

Once absorbed through the skin, topical corticosteroids are handled through pharmacokinetic pathways similar to systemically administered corticosteroids. Corticosteroids are bound to plasma proteins in varying degrees. Corticosteroids are metabolized primarily in the liver and are then excreted by the kidneys. Some of the topical corticosteroids and their metabolites are also excreted into the bile. Pharmacokinetics studies in men with TOPICORT® (desoximetasone) Emollient Cream 0.25% with tagged desoximetasone showed a total of 5.2% ± 2.9% excretion in urine (4.1% ± 2.3%) and feces (1.1% ± 0.6%) and no detectable level (limit of sensitivity: 0.005 μg/mL) in the blood when it was applied topically on the back followed by occlusion for 24 hours. Seven days after application, no further radioactivity was detected in urine or feces. The half-life of the material was 15 ± 2 hours (for urine) and 17 ± 2 hours (for feces) between the third and fifth trial day. Studies with other similarly structured steroids have shown that predominant metabolite reaction occurs through conjugation to form the glucuronide and sulfate ester.

INDICATIONS AND USAGE

TOPICORT GEL 0.05% is indicated for the relief of the inflammatory and pruritic manifestations of corticosteroid-responsive dermatoses.

CONTRAINDICATIONS

Topical corticosteroids are contraindicated in those patients with a history of hypersensitivity to any of the components of the preparation.

PRECAUTIONS

General

Systemic absorption of topical corticosteroids has produced reversible hypothalamic-pituitary-adrenal (HPA) axis suppression, manifestations of Cushing's syndrome, hyperglycemia, and glucosuria in some patients.

Conditions which augment systemic absorption include the application of the more potent steroids, use over large surface areas, prolonged use, and the addition of occlusive dressings.

Therefore, patients receiving a large dose of a potent topical steroid applied to a large surface area or under an occlusive dressing should be evaluated periodically for evidence of HPA axis suppression by using the urinary free cortisol and ACTH stimulation tests. If HPA axis suppression is noted, an attempt should be made to withdraw the drug, to reduce the frequency of application, or to substitute a less potent steroid. Recovery of HPA axis function is generally prompt and complete upon discontinuation of the drug. Infrequently, signs and symptoms of steroid withdrawal may occur, requiring supplemental systemic corticosteroids.

Pediatric patients may absorb proportionally larger amounts of topical corticosteroids and thus be more susceptible to systemic toxicity. (See PRECAUTIONS—Pediatric Use). If irritation develops, topical corticosteroids should be discontinued and appropriate therapy instituted.

In the presence of dermatological infections, the use of an appropriate antifungal or antibacterial agent should be instituted. If a favorable response does not occur promptly, the corticosteroid should be discontinued until the infection has been adequately controlled.

Information for the Patient

Patients using topical corticosteroids should receive the following information and instructions:

1. This medication is to be used as directed by the physician. It is for external use only. Avoid contact with the eyes.
2. Patients should be advised not to use this medication for any disorder other than for which it was prescribed.
3. The treated skin area should not be bandaged or otherwise covered or wrapped as to be occlusive unless directed by the physician.
4. Patients should report any signs of local adverse reactions especially under occlusive dressing.
5. Parents of pediatric patients should be advised not to use tight-fitting diapers or plastic pants on a child being treated in the diaper area, as these garments may constitute occlusive dressings.

Laboratory Tests

The following tests may be helpful in evaluating the HPA axis suppression:

Urinary free cortisol test
ACTH stimulation test

Carcinogenesis, Mutagenesis, and Impairment of Fertility

Long-term animal studies have not been performed to evaluate the carcinogenic potential or the effect on fertility of topical corticosteroids.

Studies to determine mutagenicity with prednisolone and hydrocortisone have revealed negative results. Desoximeta-

Continued on next page

Topicort Gel—Cont.

sone did not show potential for mutagenic activity *in vitro* in the Ames microbial mutagen test with or without metabolic activation.

Pregnancy Category C

Corticosteroids are generally teratogenic in laboratory animals when administered systemically at relatively low dosage levels. The more potent corticosteroids have been shown to be teratogenic after dermal application in laboratory animals.

Desoximetasone has been shown to be teratogenic and embryotoxic in mice, rats, and rabbits when given by subcutaneous or dermal routes of administration in doses 15 to 150 times the human dose of TOPICORT GEL (desoximetasone) 0.05%.

There are no adequate and well-controlled studies in pregnant women on teratogenic effects from topically applied corticosteroids. Therefore, TOPICORT GEL 0.05% should be used during pregnancy only if the potential benefit justifies the potential risk to the fetus. Drugs of this class should not be used extensively on pregnant patients, in large amounts, or for prolonged periods of time.

Nursing Mothers

It is not known whether topical administration of corticosteroids could result in sufficient systemic absorption to produce detectable quantities in breast milk. Systemically administered corticosteroids are secreted into breast milk in quantities not likely to have a deleterious effect on the infant. Nevertheless, caution should be exercised when topical corticosteroids are administered to a nursing woman.

Pediatric Use

Pediatric patients may demonstrate greater susceptibility to topical corticosteroid-induced HPA axis suppression and Cushing's syndrome than mature patients because of a larger skin surface area to body weight ratio.

Hypothalamic-pituitary-adrenal (HPA) axis suppression, Cushing's syndrome, and intracranial hypertension have been reported in pediatric patients receiving topical corticosteroids. Manifestations of adrenal suppression in pediatric patients include linear growth retardation, delayed weight gain, low plasma cortisol levels, and absence of response to ACTH stimulation. Manifestations of intracranial hypertension include bulging fontanelles, headaches, and bifateral papilledema.

Administration of topical corticosteroids to pediatric patients should be limited to the least amount compatible with an effective therapeutic regimen. Chronic corticosteroid therapy may interfere with the growth and development of pediatric patients.

ADVERSE REACTIONS

The following local adverse reactions are reported infrequently with topical corticosteroids, but may occur more frequently with the use of occlusive dressings. These reactions are listed in an approximate decreasing order of occurrence: burning, itching, irritation, dryness, folliculitis, perioral dermatitis, allergic contact dermatitis, hypertrichosis, acneiform eruptions, hypopigmentation, maceration of the skin, secondary infection, skin atrophy, striae, miliaria.

OVERDOSAGE

Topically applied corticosteroids can be absorbed in sufficient amounts to produce systermic effects. (See PRECAUTIONS.)

DOSAGE AND ADMINISTRATION

Apply a thin film of TOPICORT® GELl (desoxlmetasone) 0.05% to the affected skin areas twice daily. Rub in gently.

HOW SUPPLIED

TOPICORT GEL 0.05% is supplied in 15 gram (NDC 0039-0014-23) and 60 gram (NDC 0039-0014-60) tubes.

Store at controlled room temperature (59 to 86°F).

CAUTION: Federal Law Prohibits Dispensing Without Prescription.

TOPICORT REG TM ROUSSEL UCLAF

Prescribing Information as of February 1996

Hoechst-Roussel Pharmaceuticals
Division of Hoechst Marion Roussel, Inc.
Kansas City, MO 64137

Shown in Product Identification Guide, page 316

TOPICORT® OINTMENT ℞

[tä p' i-kôrt]

(desoximetasone) 0.25%

FOR DERMATOLOGIC USE ONLY.
NOT FOR USE IN EYES

Prescribing Information as of April 1996

DESCRIPTION

TOPICORT® OINTMENT (desoximetasone) 0.25% contains the active synthetic corticosteroid desoximetasone. The topical corticosteroids constitute a class of primarily synthetic steroids used as anti-inflammatory and anti-pruritic agents.

Each gram of TOPICORT OINTMENT 0.25% contains 2.5 mg of desoximetasone in a base consisting of white petrolatum USP, propylene glycol USP, sorbitan sesquioleate, beeswax, fatty alcohol citrate fatty acid pentaerythritol ester, aluminum stearate, citric acid, and butylated hydroxyanisole.

The chemical name of desoximetasone is Pregna-1, 4-diene-3, 20-dione, 9-fluoro-11, 21-dihydroxy-16-methyl-, (11β, 16α)-.

Desoximetasone has the empirical formula $C_{22}H_{29}FO_4$ and a molecular weight of 376.47.

The CAS Registry Number is 382-67-2. The chemical structure is:

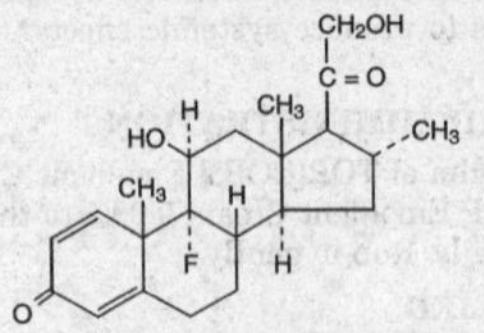

CLINICAL PHARMACOLOGY

Topical corticosteroids share anti-inflammatory, anti-pruritic and vasoconstrictive actions.

The mechanism of anti-inflammatory activity of the topical corticosteroids is unclear. Various laboratory methods, including vasoconstrictor assays, are used to compare and predict potencies and/or clinical efficacies of the topical corticosteroids. There is some evidence to suggest that a recognizable correlation exists between vasoconstrictor potency and therapeutic efficacy in man.

Pharmacokinetics

The extent of percutaneous absorption of topical corticosteroids is determined by many factors including the vehicle, the itegrity of the epidermal barrier, and the use of occlusive dressings.

Topical corticosteroids can be absorbed from normal intact skin. Inflammation and/or other disease processes in the skin increase percutaneous absorption. Occlusive dressings substantially increase the percutaneous absorption of topical corticosteroids. Thus, occlusive dressings may be a valuable therapeutic adjunct for treatment of resistant dermatoses.

Once absorbed through the skin, topical corticosteroids are handled through pharmacokinetic pathways similar to systemically administered corticosteroids. Corticosteroids are bound to plasma proteins in varying degrees. Corticosteroids are metabolized primarily in the liver and are then excreted by the kidneys. Some of the topical corticosteroids and their metabolites are also excreted into the bile.

Pharmacokinetic studies in men with TOPICORT OINTMENT (desoximetasone) 0.25% with tagged desoximetasone showed no detectable level (limit of sensitivity: 0.003 µg/mL) in 1 subject and 0.004 and 0.006 µg/mL in the remaining 2 subjects in the blood when it was applied topically on the back followed by occlusion for 24 hours. The extent of absorption for the ointment was 7% based on radioactivity recovered from urine and feces. Seven days after application. no further radioactivity was detected in urine or feces. Studies with other similarly structured steroids have shown that predominant metabolite reaction occurs through conjugation to form the glucuronide and sulfate ester.

INDICATIONS AND USAGE

TOPICORT OINTMENT 0.25% is indicated for the relief of the inflammatory and pruritic manifestations of corticosteroid-responsive dermatoses.

CONTRAINDICATIONS

Topical corticosteroids are contraindicated in those patients with a history of hypersensitivity to any of the components of the preparation.

PRECAUTIONS

General

Systemic absorption of topical corticosteroids has produced reversible hypothalamic-pituitary-adrenal (HPA) axis suppression, manifestations of Cushing's syndrome, hyperglycemia, and glucosuria in some patients.

Conditions which augment systemic absorption include the application of the more potent steroids, use over large surface areas, prolonged use, and the addition of occlusive dressings.

Therefore, patients receiving a large dose of a potent topical steroid applied to a large surface area or under an occlusive dressing should be evaluated periodically for evidence of HPA axis suppression by using the urinary free cortisol and ACTH stimulation tests. If HPA axis suppression is noted, an attempt should be made to withdraw the drug, to reduce the frequency of application, or to substitute a less potent steroid.

Recovery of HPA axis function is generally prompt and complete upon discontinuation of the drug. Infrequently, signs and symptoms of steroid withdrawal may occur, requiring supplemental systemic corticosteroids.

Pediatric patients may absorb proportionally larger amounts of topical corticosteroids and thus be more susceptible to systemic toxicity. (See PRECAUTIONS— Pediatric Use.)

If irritation develops, topical corticosteroids should be discontinued and appropriate therapy instituted.

In the presence of dermatological infections, the use of an appropriate antifungal or antibacterial agent should be instituted. If a favorable response does not occur promptly, the corticosteroid should be discontinued until the infection has been adequately controlled.

Information for the Patient

Patients using topical corticosteroids should receive the following information and instructions:

1. This medication is to be used as directed by the physician. It is for external use only. Avoid contact with the eyes.
2. Patients should be advised not to use this medication for any disorder other than for which it was prescribed.
3. The treated skin area should not be bandaged or otherwise covered or wrapped as to be occlusive unless directed by the physician.
4. Patients should report any signs of local adverse reactions especially under occlusive dressing.
5. Parents of pediatric patients should be advised not to use tight-fitting diapers or plastic pants on a child being treated in the diaper area, as these garments may constitute occlusive dressings.

Laboratory Tests

The following tests may be helpful in evaluating the HPA axis suppression:

Urinary free cortisol test
ACTH stimulation test

Carcinogenesis, Mutagenesis, and Impairment of Fertility

Long-term animal studies have not been performed to evaluate the carcinogenic potential or the effect on fertility of topical corticosteroids.

Studies to determine mutagenicity with prednisolone and hydrocortisone have revealed negative results. Desoximetasone did not show potential for mutagenic activity *in vitro* in the Ames microbial mutagen test with or without metabolic activation.

Pregnancy Category C

Corticosteroids are generally teratogenic in laboratory animals when administered systemically at relatively low dosage levels. The more potent corticosteroids have been shown to be teratogenic after dermal application in laboratory animals.

Desoximetasone has been shown to be teratogenic and embryotoxic in mice, rats, and rabbits when given by subcutaneous or dermal routes of administration in doses 3 to 30 times the human dose of TOPICORT OINTMENT (desoximetasone) 0.25%.

There are no adequate and well-controlled studies in pregnant women on teratogenic effects from topically applied corticosteroids. Therefore, TOPICORT OINTMENT 0.25% should be used during pregnancy only if the potential benefit justifies the potential risk to the fetus. Drugs of this class should not be used extensively on pregnant patients, in large amounts, or for prolonged periods of time.

Nursing Mothers

It is not known whether topical administration of corticosteroids could result in sufficient systemic absorption to produce detectable quantities in breast milk. Systemically administered corticosteroids are secreted into breast milk in quantities not likely to have a deleterious effect on the infant. Nevertheless, caution should be exercised when topical corticosteroids are administered to a nursing woman.

Pediatric Use

Pediatric patients may demonstrate greater susceptibility to topical corticosteroid-induced HPA axis suppression and Cushing's syndrome than mature patients because of a larger skin surface area to body weight ratio.

Hypothalamic-pituitary-adrenal (HPA) axis suppression. Cushing's syndrome, and intracranial hypertension have been reported in pediatric patients receiving topical corticosteroids. Manifestations of adrenal suppression in pediatric patients include linear growth retardation, delayed weight gain, low plasma cortisol levels, and absence of response to ACTH stimulation. Manifestations of intracranial hypertension include bulging fontanelles, headaches, and bilateral papilledema.

Administration of topical corticosteroids to pediatric patients should be limited to the least amount compatible with an effective therapeutic regimen.

Chronic corticosteroid therapy may interfere with the growth and development of pediatric patients. Safety and effectiveness of Topicort® Ointment (desoximetasone) 0.25% in pediatric patients below the age of 10 have not been established.

ADVERSE REACTIONS

The following local adverse reactions are reported infrequently with topical corticosteroids, but may occur more frequently with the use of occlusive dressings. These reactions are listed in an approximate decreasing order of occurrence: burning, itching, irritation, dryness, folliculitis, hypertrichosis, acneiform eruptions, hypopigmentation, perioral dermatitis, allergic contact dermatitis, maceration of the skin, secondary infection, skin atrophy, striae, miliaria.

In controlled clinical studies the incidence of adverse reactions was low (0.3%) for TOPICORT OINTMENT 0.25% and consisted of development of comedones at the site of application.

OVERDOSAGE

Topically applied corticosteroids can be absorbed in sufficient amounts to produce systemic effects. (See PRECAUTIONS.)

DOSAGE AND ADMINISTRATION

Apply a thin film of TOPICORT OINTMENT 0.25% to the affected skin areas twice daily. Rub in gently.

HOW SUPPLIED

TOPICORT® OINTMENT 0.25% is supplied in 15 gram (NDC 0039-0025-15) and 60 gram (NDC 0039-0025-60) tubes.

Store at controlled room temperature (59 to 86°F).

CAUTION: Federal law Prohibits Dispensing Without Prescription.

TOPICORT REG TM ROUSSEL UCLAF

Prescribing Information as of April 1996

Hoechst-Roussel Pharmaceuticals

Division of Hoechst Marion Roussel, Inc.

Kansas City, MO 64137

Shown in Product Identification Guide, page 316

TRENTAL®   ℞

[tren 'tal]

(pentoxifylline)*

Tablets, 400 mg

Prescribing Information as of April 1997

DESCRIPTION

TRENTAL® (pentoxifylline) tablets for oral administration contain 400 mg of the active drug and the following inactive ingredients: benzyl alcohol NF, D&C Red No. 27 Aluminum Lake or FD&C Red No. 3, hydroxypropyl methylcellulose USP, magnesium stearate NF, polyethylene glycol NF, povidone USP, talc USP, titanium dioxide USP, and other ingredients in a controlled-release formulation. Trental® is a trisubstituted xanthine derivative designated chemically as 1-(5-oxohexyl)-3, 7-dimethylxanthine that, unlike theophylline, is a hemorrheologic agent, i.e. and agent that affects blood viscosity. Pentoxifylline is soluble in water and ethanol, and sparingly soluble in toluene. The CAS Registry Number is 6493-05-6.

The chemical structure is:

$$CH_3CCH_2CH_2CH_2CH_2\text{—}N \quad N\text{—}CH_3$$

CLINICAL PHARMACOLOGY

Mode of Action

Pentoxifylline and its metabolites improve the flow properties of blood by decreasing its viscosity. In patients with chronic peripheral arterial disease, this increases blood flow to the affected microcirculation and enhances tissue oxygenation. The precise mode of action of pentoxifylline and the sequence of events leading to clinical improvement are still to be defined. Pentoxifylline administration has been shown to produce dose related hemorrheologic effects, lowering blood viscosity, and improving erythrocyte flexibility. Leukocyte properties of hemorrheologic importance have been modified in animal and in vitro human studies. Pentoxifylline has been shown to increase leukocyte deformability and to inhibit neutrophil adhesion and activation. Tissue oxygen levels have been shown to be significantly increased by therapeutic doses of pentoxifylline in patients with peripheral arterial disease.

Pharmacokinetics and Metabolism

After oral administration in aqueous solution pentoxifylline is almost completely absorbed. It undergoes a first-pass effect and the various metabolites appear in plasma very soon after dosing. Peak plasma levels of the parent compound and its metabolites are reached within 1 hour. The major metabolites are Metabolite I (1-[5-hydroxyhexyl]-3,7-dimethylxanthine) and Metabolite V (1-[3-carboxypropyl]-3,7-

INCIDENCE (%) OF SIDE EFFECTS

(Numbers of Patients at Risk)	Controlled-Release Tablets Commercially Available TRENTAL (321)	Placebo (128)	Immediate-Release Capsules Used only for Controlled Clinical Trials TRENTAL (177)	Placebo (138)
Discontinued for Side Effect	3.1	0	9.6	7.2
CARDIOVASCULAR SYSTEM				
Angina/Chest pain	0.3	—	1.1	2.2
Arrhythmia/Palpitation	—	—	1.7	0.7
Flushing	—	—	2.3	0.7
DIGESTIVE SYSTEM				
Abdominal Discomfort	—	—	4.0	1.4
Belching/Flatus/Bloating	0.6	—	9.0	3.6
Diarrhea	—	—	3.4	2.9
Dyspepsia	2.8	4.7	9.6	2.9
Nausea	2.2	0.8	28.8	8.7
Vomiting	1.2	—	4.5	0.7
NERVOUS SYSTEM				
Agitation/Nervousness	—	—	1.7	0.7
Dizziness	1.9	3.1	11.9	4.3
Drowsiness	—	—	1.1	5.8
Headache	1.2	1.6	6.2	5.8
Insomnia	—	—	2.3	2.2
Tremor	0.3	0.8	—	—
Blurred Vision	—	—	2.3	1.4

dimethylxanthine), and plasma levels of these metabolites are 5 and 8 times greater, respectively, than pentoxifylline. Following oral administration of aqueous solutions containing 100 to 400 mg of pentoxifylline, the pharmacokinetics of the parent compound and Metabolite I are dose-related and not proportional (non-linear), with half-life and area under the blood-level time curve (AUC) increasing with dose. The elimination kinetics of Metabolite V are not dose-dependent. The apparent plasma half-life of pentoxifylline varies from 0.4 to 0.8 hours and the apparent plasma half-lives of its metabolites vary from 1 to 1.6 hours. There is no evidence of accumulation or enzyme induction (Cytochrome P450) following multiple oral doses.

Excretion is almost totally urinary; the main biotransformation product is Metabolite V. Essentially no parent drug is found in the urine. Despite large variations in plasma levels of parent compound and its metabolites, the urinary recovery of Metabolite V is consistent and shows dose proportionality. Less than 4% of the administered dose is recovered in feces. Food intake shortly before dosing delays absorption of an immediate-release dosage form but does not affect total absorption. The pharmacokinetics and metabolism of TRENTAL have not been studied in patients with renal and/or hepatic dysfunction, but AUC was increased and elimination rate decreased in an older population (60–68 years) compared to younger individuals (22–30 years).

After administration of the 400 mg controlled-release TRENTAL tablet, plasma levels of the parent compound and its metabolites reach their maximum within 2 to 4 hours and remain constant over an extended period of time. The controlled release of pentoxifylline from the tablet eliminates peaks and troughs in plasma levels for improved gastrointestinal tolerance.

INDICATIONS AND USAGE

TRENTAL is indicated for the treatment of patients with intermittent claudication on the basis of chronic occlusive arterial disease of the limbs. TRENTAL can improve function and symptoms but is not intended to replace more definitive therapy, such as surgical bypass, or removal of arterial obstructions when treating peripheral vascular disease.

CONTRAINDICATIONS

Trental® should not be used in patients with recent cerebral and/or retinal hemorrhage or in patients who have previously exhibited intolerance to this product or methylxanthines such as caffeine, theophylline, and theobromine.

PRECAUTIONS

General: Patients with chronic occlusive arterial disease of the limbs frequently show other manifestations of arteriosclerotic disease. TRENTAL has been used safely for treatment of peripheral arterial disease in patients with concurrent coronary artery and cerebrovascular diseases, but there have been occasional reports of angina, hypotension, and arrhythmia. Controlled trials do not show that TRENTAL causes such adverse effects more often than placebo, but, as it is a methylxanthine derivative, it is possible some individuals will experience such responses. Patients on Warfarin should have more frequent monitoring of prothrombin times, while patients with other risk factors complicated by hemorrhage (e.g., recent surgery, peptic ulceration, cerebral and/or retinal bleeding) should have periodic examinations for bleeding including, hematocrit and/or hemoglobin.

Drug Interactions

Although a causal relationship has not been established, there have been reports of bleeding and/or prolonged pro-

thrombin time in patients treated with TRENTAL with and without anticoagulants or platelet aggregation inhibitors. Patients on Warfarin should have more frequent monitoring of prothrombin times, while patients with other risk factors complicated by hemorrhage (e.g., recent surgery, peptic ulceration) should have periodic examinations for bleeding including hematocrit and/or hemoglobin. Concomitant administration of TRENTAL and theophylline-containing drugs leads to increased theophylline levels and theophylline toxicity in some individuals. Such patients should be closely monitored for signs of toxicity and have their theophylline dosage adjusted as necessary. TRENTAL has been used concurrently with antihypertensive drugs, beta blockers, digitalis, diuretics, antidiabetic agents, and antiarrhythmics, without observed problems. Small decreases in blood pressure have been observed in some patients treated with TRENTAL; periodic systemic blood pressure monitoring is recommended for patients receiving concomitant antihypertensive therapy. If indicated, dosage of the antihypertensive agents should be reduced.

Carcinogenesis, Mutagenesis and Impairment of Fertility

Long-term studies of the carcinogenic potential of pentoxifylline were conducted in mice and rats by dietary administration of the drug at doses up to 450 mg/kg (approximately 19 times) the maximum recommended human daily dose (MRHD) in both species when based on body weight 1.5 times the MRHD in the mouse and 3.3 times the MRHD in the rat when based on body surface area). In mice, the drug was administered for 18 months, whereas in rats, the drug was administered for 18 months followed by an additional 6 months without drug exposure. In the rat study, there was a statistically significant increase in benign mammary fibroadenomas in females of the 450 mg/kg group. The relevance of this finding to human use is uncertain. Pentoxifylline was devoid of mutagenic activity in various strains of *Salmonella* (Ames test) and in cultured mammalian cells (unscheduled DNA synthesis test) when tested in the presence and absence of metabolic activation. It was also negative in the in vivo mouse micronucleus test.

Pregnancy

Category C. Teratogenic studies have been performed in rats and rabbits using oral doses up to 576 and 264 mg/kg, respectively. On a weight basis, these doses are 24 and 11 times the maximum recommended human daily dose (MRHD); on a body-surface-area basis, they are 4.2 and 3.5 times the MRHD. No evidence of fetal malformation was observed. Increased resorption was seen in rats of the 576 mg/kg group.

There are no adequate and well controlled studies in pregnant women. TRENTAL (pentoxifylline) should be used during pregnancy only if the potential benefit justifies the potential risk to the fetus.

Nursing Mothers

Pentoxifylline and its metabolites are excreted in human milk. Because of the potential for tumorigenicity shown for pentoxifylline in rats, a decision should be made whether to discontinue nursing or discontinue the drug, taking into account the importance of the drug to the mother.

Pediatric Use

Safety and effectiveness in pediatric patients have not been established.

ADVERSE REACTIONS

Clinical trials were conducted using either controlled-release TRENTAL tablets for up to 60 weeks or immediate-

Continued on next page

Trental—Cont.

release TRENTAL capsules for up to 24 weeks. Dosage ranges in the tablet studies were 400 mg bid to tid and in the capsule studies, 200–400 mg tid. The table summarizes the incidence (in percent) of adverse reactions considered drug related, as well as the numbers of patients who received controlled-release TRENTAL tablets, immediate-release TRENTAL capsules, or the corresponding placebos. The incidence of adverse reactions was higher in the capsule studies (where dose related increases were seen in digestive and nervous system side effects) than in the tablet studies. Studies with the capsule include domestic experience, whereas studies with the controlled-release tablets were conducted outside the U.S. The table indicates that in the tablet studies few patients discontinued because of adverse effects.

[See table at top of previous page]

TRENTAL been marketed in Europe and elsewhere since 1972. In addition to the above symptoms, the following have been reported spontaneously since marketing or occurred in other clinical trials with an incidence of less than 1%; the causal relationship was uncertain:

Cardiovascular—dyspnea, edema, hypotension.
Digestive—anorexia, cholecystitis, constipation, dry mouth/thirst.
Nervous—anxiety, confusion, depression, seizures.
Respiratory—epistaxis, flu-like symptoms, laryngitis, nasal congestion.
Skin and Appendages—brittle fingernails, pruritus, rash, urticaria, angiodema.
Special Senses—blurred vision, conjunctivitis, earache, scotoma.
Miscellaneous—bad taste, excessive salivation, leukopenia, malaise, sore throat/swollen neck glands, weight change.

A few rare events have been reported spontaneously worldwide since marketing in 1972. Although they occurred under circumstances in which a causal relationship with pentoxifylline could not be established, they are listed to serve as information for physicians: "Cardiovascular—angina, arrhythmia, tachycardia anaphylactoid reactions." Digestive—hepatitis, jaundice, increased liver enzymes; and Hemic and Lymphatic—decreased serum fibrinogen, pancytopenia, aplastic anemia, leukemia, purpura, thrombocytopenia.

OVERDOSAGE

Overdosage with TRENTAL been reported in pediatric patients and adults. Symptoms appear to be dose related. A report from a poison control center on 44 patients taking overdoses of enteric-coated pentoxifylline tablets noted that symptoms usually occurred 4–5 hours after ingestion and lasted about 12 hours. The highest amount ingested was 80 mg/kg; flushing, hypotension, convulsions, somnolence, loss of consciousness, fever, and agitation occurred. All patients recovered. In addition to symptomatic treatment and gastric lavage, special attention must be given to supporting respiration, maintaining systemic blood pressure, and controlling convulsions. Activated charcoal has been used to absorb pentoxifylline in patients who have overdosed.

DOSAGE AND ADMINISTRATION

The usual dosage of TRENTAL in controlled-release tablet form is one tablet (400 mg) three times a day with meals. While the effect of TRENTAL may be seen within 2 to 4 weeks, it is recommended that treatment be continued for at least 8 weeks. Efficacy has been demonstrated in double-blind clinical studies of 6 months duration.

Digestive and central nervous system side effects are dose related. If patients develop these side effects it is recommended that the dosage be lowered to one tablet twice a day (800 mg/day). If side effects persist at this lower dosage, the administration of TRENTAL should be discontinued.

HOW SUPPLIED

TRENTAL is available for oral administration as 400 mg pink film-coated oblong tablets imprinted Trental®; supplied in bottles of 100 (NDC 0039-0078-10), Bulk Pack 5000 (NDC 0039-0078-80, and Unit Dose Packs of 100 (NDC 0039-0078-11).

Store between 59 and 86°F (15 and 30°C).
Dispense in well-closed, light-resistant containers.
Protect blisters from light.
Prescribing Information as of April 1997.
*US Patents 3,737,433 & 4,189,469
US Patent 3,737,433 patent term has been extended.
Hoechst-Roussel Pharmaceuticals
Division of Hoechst Marion Roussel, Inc.
Kansas City, MO 64137 USA
Shown in Product Identification Guide, page 316

Horizon Pharmaceutical Corporation
1125 NORTHMEADOW PARKWAY
SUITE 130
ROSWELL, GA 30076

Direct Inquiries to:
Greg Hauck
(770) 442-9707
FAX: (770) 442-9594
Medical Emergency Contact:
800-849-9707
FAX: (770) 442-9594

DEFEN—L.A. Tablets   ℞
[dē-fĕn]

DESCRIPTION

Each dye-free, film-coated tablet imprinted DEFEN and scored contains:
Pseudoephedrine HCl .... 60 mg
Guaifenesin .... 600 mg

HOW SUPPLIED

Bottles of 100

MESCOLOR® TABLETS   ℞
[mĕs-cō-lŏr]

DESCRIPTION

Each dye-free, film-coated, tablet imprinted HP 15 and scored contains:
Chlorpheniramine Maleate .... 8.0 mg
Pseudoephedrine HCl .... 120.0 mg
Methscopolamine Nitrate .... 2.5 mg

HOW SUPPLIED

Bottles of 100

PROTUSS® LIQUID   Ⓒ ℞
[prō-təs]

DESCRIPTION

Each teaspoonful (5 mL) grape flavored liquid contains:
Hydrocodone Bitartrate .... 5 mg
    (Warning: May be habit forming)
Potassium Guaiacolsulfonate .... 400 mg

HOW SUPPLIED

Bottles of 4 oz and 16 oz.

PROTUSS®-D LIQUID   Ⓒ ℞
[prō-təs-D]

DESCRIPTION

Each teaspoonful (5 mL) contains:
Hydrocodone Bitartrate .... 5 mg
    (Warning: May be habit forming)
Potassium Guaiacolsulfonate .... 300 mg
Pseudoephedrine HCl .... 30 mg

HOW SUPPLIED

Bottles of 4 oz and 16 oz

PROTUSS®-DM TABLETS   ℞
[prō-təs-DM]

DESCRIPTION

Each dye-free, film-coated tablet imprinted PRO DM and scored contains:
Dextromethorphan HBr .... 30 mg
Pseudoephedrine HCl .... 60 mg
Guaifenesin .... 600 mg

HOW SUPPLIED

Bottles of 100

TANAFED® SUSPENSION   ℞
[tan-ă-fed]

DESCRIPTION

Each teaspoonful (5 mL) strawberry/banana flavored suspension contains:

Chlorpheniramine Tannate .... 4.5 mg
Pseudoephedrine Tannate .... 75.0 mg

HOW SUPPLIED

Bottles of 4 oz and 16 oz

ZOTO®-HC EAR DROPS   ℞
[zō-tō]

DESCRIPTION

Each 1 mL contains:
Chloroxylenol .... 1 mg
Pramoxine HCl .... 10 mg
Hydrocortisone .... 10 mg

HOW SUPPLIED

Plastic dropper vials of 10 mL.

ICN Pharmaceuticals, Inc.
ICN PLAZA
3300 HYLAND AVENUE
COSTA MESA, CA 92626

Direct Inquiries to:
Medical Emergency Contact
Boanerges Rubalcava, Ph.D., M.D.
(800) 548-5100, ext. 3531
FAX: (714) 641-7287

8-MOP® CAPSULES   ℞
(Methoxsalen Capsules, USP, 10 mg)

CAUTION: FEDERAL LAW PROHIBITS DISPENSING WITHOUT PRESCRIPTION.
CAUTION: METHOXSALEN IS A POTENT DRUG. READ ENTIRE BROCHURE PRIOR TO PRESCRIBING OR DISPENSING THIS MEDICATION.

> Methoxsalen with UV radiation should be used only by physicians who have special competence in the diagnosis and treatment of psoriasis and vitiligo and who have special training and experience in photochemotherapy. Psoralen and ultraviolet radiation therapy should be under constant supervision of such a physician. For the treatment of patients with psoriasis, photochemotherapy should be restricted to patients with severe, recalcitrant, disabling psoriasis which is not adequately responsive to other forms of therapy, and only when the diagnosis has been supported by biopsy. Because of the possibilities of ocular damage, aging of the skin, and skin cancer (including melanoma), the patient should be fully informed by the physician of the risks inherent in this therapy. When methoxsalen is used in combination with photopheresis, refer to the UVAR* System Operator's Manual for specific warnings, cautions, indications, and instructions related to photopheresis.

> CAUTION: 8-MOP® Capsules (Methoxsalen Hard Gelatin Capsules) may not be interchanged with Oxsoralen-Ultra® Capsules (Methoxsalen Soft Gelatin Capsules) without retitration of the patient.

I.   **DESCRIPTION**

8-MOP (Methoxsalen, 8-Methoxypsoralen) Capsules, 10mg. Methoxsalen is a naturally occurring photoactive substance found in the seeds of the **Ammi majus** (Umbelliferae) plant. It belongs to a group of compounds known as psoralens, or furocoumarins. The chemical name of methoxsalen is 9-methoxy-7 H-furo[3,2-g][1]-benzopyran-7-one; it has the following structure:
[See chemical structure at top of next column]

II.   **CLINICAL PHARMACOLOGY**

The combination treatment regimen of psoralen (P) and ultraviolet radiation of 320–400 nm wavelength commonly referred to as UVA is known by the acro-

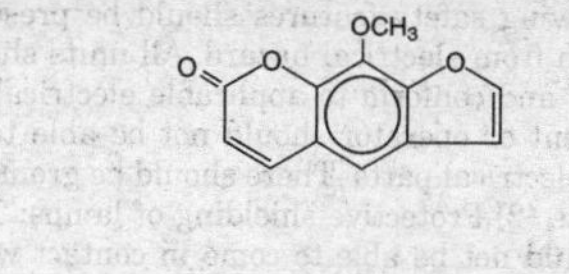

nym, PUVA. Skin reactivity to UVA (320–400 nm) radiation is markedly enhanced by the ingestion of methoxsalen. The drug reaches its maximum bioavailability $1\frac{1}{2}$–3 hours after oral administration and may last for up to 8 hours (Pathak et al., 1974)[1]. Methoxsalen is reversibly bound to serum albumin and is also preferentially taken up by epidermal cells (Artuc et al. 1979)[2]. At a dose which is six times larger than that used in humans, it induces mixed function oxidases in the liver of mice (Mandula et al. 1978)[3]. In both mice and man, methoxsalen is rapidly metabolized. Approximately 95% of the drug is excreted as a series of metabolites in the urine within 24 hours (Pathak et al. 1977)[4].

The exact mechanism of action of methoxsalen with the epidermal melanocyctes and keratinocytes is not known. The best known biochemical reaction of methoxsalen is with DNA. Methoxsalen, upon photoactiviation, conjugates and forms covalent bonds with DNA which leads to the formation of both monofunctional (addition to a single strand of DNA) and bifunctional adducts (crosslinking of psoralen to both strands of DNA) (Dall' Acqua et al., 1971[5]; Cole, 1970[6]; Musajo et al., 1974[7]; Dall' Acqua et al., 1979[8]). Reactions with proteins have also been described (Yoshikawa, et al., 1979[9]).

Methoxsalen acts as a photosensitizer. Administration of the drug and subsequent exposure to UVA can lead to cell injury. Orally administered methoxsalen reaches the skin via the blood and UVA penetrates well into the skin. If sufficient cell injury occurs in the skin, an inflammatory reaction occurs. The most obvious manifestation of this reaction is delayed erythema, which may not begin for several hours and peaks at 48–72 hours. The inflammation is followed, over several days to weeks, by repair which is manifested by increased melanization of the epidermis and thickening of the stratum corneum. The mechanisms of therapy are not known. In the treatment of vitiligo, it has been suggested that melanocytes in the hair follicle are stimulated to move up the follicle and to repopulate the epidermis (Ortonne et al, 1979[10]). In the treatment of psoriasis, the mechanism is most often assumed to be DNA photodamage and resulting decrease in cell proliferation but other vascular, leukocyte, or cell regulatory mechanisms may also be playing some role. Psoriasis is a hyperproliferative disorder and other agents known to be therapeutic for psoriasis are known to inhibit DNA synthesis.

III. INDICATIONS AND USAGE

A. Photochemotherapy (methoxsalen with long wave UVA radiation) is indicated for the symptomatic control of severe, recalcitrant, disabling psoriasis not adequately responsive to other forms of therapy and when the diagnosis has been supported by biopsy. Photochemotherapy is intended to be administered only in conjunction with a schedule of controlled doses of long wave ultraviolet radiation.

B. Photochemotherapy (methoxsalen with long wave ultraviolet radiation) is indicated for the repigmentation of idiopathic vitiligo.

C. Photopheresis (methoxsalen with long wave ultraviolet radiation of white blood cells) is indicated for use with the UVAR* System in the palliative treatment of the skin manifestations of cutaneous T-cell lymphoma (CTCL) in persons who have not been responsive to other forms of treatment. While this dosage form of methoxsalen has been approved for use in combination with photopheresis, Oxsoralen Ultra® Capsules have not been approved for that use.

IV. CONTRAINDICATIONS

A. Patients exhibiting idiosyncratic reactions to psoralen compounds.

B. Patients possessing a specific history of light sensitive disease states should not initiate methoxsalen therapy. Diseases associated with photosensitivity include lupus erythematosus, porphyria cutanea tarda, erythropoietic protoporphyria, variegate porphyria, xeroderma pigmentosum, and albinism.

C. Patients exhibiting melanoma or possessing a history of melanoma.

D. Patients exhibiting invasive squamous cell carcinomas.

E. Patients with aphakia, because of the significantly increased risk of retinal damage due to the absence of lenses.

V. WARNINGS—GENERAL

A. SKIN BURNING: Serious burns from either UVA or sunlight (even through window glass) can result if the recommended dosage of the drug and/or exposure schedules are not maintained.

B. CARCINOGENICITY:

1. ANIMAL STUDIES: Topical or intraperitoneal methoxsalen has been reported to be a potent photocarcinogen in albino mice and hairless mice. However, methoxsalen given by the oral route to albino mice or by any route in pigmented mice is considerably less phototoxic or carcinogenic (Hakim et al. 1960[11]; Pathak et al. 1959[12]).

2. HUMAN STUDIES: A prospective study of 1380 patients over 5 years revealed an approximately ninefold increase in risks of squamous cell carcinoma among PUVA treated patients (Stern et al. 1979[13] and Stern et al. 1980[14]). This increase in risk appears greatest among patients who are fair skinned or had pre-PUVA exposure to 1) prolonged tar and UVB treatment, 2) ionizing radiation, or 3) arsenic.

In addition, an approximately two-fold increase in the risk of basal cell carcinoma was noted in this study. Roenigk et al. 1980[15] studied 690 patients for up to 4 years and found no increase in the risk of non-melanoma skin cancer. However, patients in this cohort had significantly less exposure to PUVA than in the Stern et al study. After 5 years, two of 1380 patients in the Stern et al PUVA study have developed malignant melanoma. In addition, more than 1/5 of patients in this cohort have developed macular pigmented lesions on the buttocks. While there is no evidence that an increased risk of melanoma exists in PUVA treated patients, these observations indicate the need for continued evaluation of melanoma risk in PUVA treated patients.

In a study in Indian patients treated for 4 years for vitiligo, 12 percent developed keratoses, but not cancer, in the depigmented, vitiliginous areas (Mosher, 1980[16]). Clinically, the keratoses were keratotic papules, actinic keratosis-like macules, nonscaling dome-shaped papules, and lichenoid porokeratotic-like papules.

C. CATARACTOGENICITY:

1. ANIMAL STUDIES: Exposure to large doses of UVA causes cataracts in animals, and this effect is enhanced by the administration of methoxsalen (Cloud et al. 1960[17]; Cloud et al. 1961[18]; Freeman et al. 1969[19]).

2. HUMAN STUDIES: It has been found that the concentration of methoxsalen in the lens is proportional to the serum level. If the lens is exposed to UVA during the time methoxsalen is present in the lens, photochemical action may lead to irreversible binding of methoxsalen to proteins and the DNA components of the lens (Lerman et al. 1980[20]). However, if the lens is shielded from UVA, the methoxsalen will diffuse out of the lens in a 24 hour period[20]. Patients should be told emphatically to wear UVA-absorbing, wrap-around sunglasses for the twenty-four (24) hour period following ingestion of methoxsalen, whether exposed to direct or indirect sunlight in the open or through a window glass.

Among patients using proper eye protection, there is no evidence for a significantly increased risk of cataracts in association with PUVA therapy.[13] Thirty-five of 1380 patients have developed cataracts in the five years since their first PUVA treatment. This incidence is comparable to that expected in a population of this size and age distribution. No relationship between PUVA dose and cataract risk in this group has been noted.

D. ACTINIC DEGENERATION: Exposure to sunlight and/or ultraviolet radiation may result in "premature aging" of the skin.

E. BASAL CELL CARCINOMAS: Patients exhibiting multiple basal cell carcinomas or having a history of basal cell carcinomas should be diligently observed and treated.

F. RADIATION THERAPY: Patients having a history of previous x-ray therapy or grenz ray therapy should be diligently observed for signs of carcinoma.

G. ARSENIC THERAPY: Patients having a history of previous arsenic therapy should be diligently observed for signs of carcinoma.

H. HEPATIC DISEASES: Patients with hepatic insufficiency should be treated with caution since hepatic biotransformation is necessary for drug urinary excretion.

I. CARDIAC DISEASES: Patients with cardiac diseases or others who may be unable to tolerate prolonged standing or exposure to heat stress should not be treated in a vertical UVA chamber.

J. TOTAL DOSAGE: The total cumulative dose of UVA that can be given over long periods of time with safety has not as yet been established.

K. CONCOMITANT THERAPY: Special care should be exercised in treating patients who are receiving concomitant therapy (either topically or systemically) with known photosensitizing agents such as anthralin, coal tar or coal tar derivatives, griseofulvin, phenothiazines, nalidixic acid, halogenated salicylanilides (bacteriostatic soaps), sulfonamides, tetracyclines, thiazides, and certain organic staining dyes such as methylene blue, toluidine blue, rose bengal, and methyl orange.

VI. PRECAUTIONS

A. GENERAL—APPLICABLE TO BOTH VITILIGO AND PSORIASIS TREATMENT:

1. BEFORE METHOXSALEN INGESTION

Patients must not sunbathe during the 24 hours prior to methoxsalen ingestion and UV exposure. The presence of a sunburn may prevent an accurate evaluation of the patient's response to photochemotherapy.

2. AFTER METHOXSALEN INGESTION

a. UVA-absorbing wrap-around sunglasses should be worn during daylight for 24 hours after methoxsalen ingestion. The protective eyewear must be designed to prevent entry of stray radiation to the eyes, including that which may enter from the sides of the eyewear. The protective eyewear is used to prevent the irreversible binding of methoxsalen to the proteins and DNA components of the lens. Cataracts form when enough of the binding occurs. Visual discrimination should be permitted by the eyewear for patient well-being and comfort.

b. Patients must avoid sun exposure, even through window glass or cloud cover, for at least 8 hours after methoxsalen ingestion. If sun exposure cannot be avoided, the patient should wear protective devices such as a hat and gloves, and/or apply sunscreens which contain ingredients that filter out UVA radiation (e.g., sunscreens containing benzophenone and/or PABA esters which exhibit a sun protective factor equal to or greater than 15). These chemical sunscreens should be applied to all areas that might be exposed to the sun (including lips). Sunscreens should not be applied to areas affected by psoriasis until after the patient has been treated in the UVA chamber.

3. DURING PUVA THERAPY

a. Total UVA-absorbing/blocking goggles mechanically designed to give maximal ocular protection must be worn. Failure to do so may increase the risk of cataract formation. A reliable radiometer can be used to verify elimination of UVA transmission through the goggles.

b. Abdominal skin, breasts, genitalia, and other sensitive areas should be protected for approximately 1/3 of the initial exposure time until tanning occurs.

c. Unless affected by disease, male genitalia should be shielded.

4. AFTER COMBINED METHOXSALEN/UVA THERAPY

a. UVA-absorbing wrap-around sunglasses should be worn during the daylight for 24 hours after combined methoxsalen/UVA therapy.

b. Patients should not sunbathe for 48 hours after therapy. Erythema and/or burning due to photochemotherapy and sunburn due to sun exposure are additive.

5. VITILIGO THERAPY

a. The dosage of methoxsalen should not be increased above 0.6 mg/kg since overdosage may result in serious burning of the skin.

b. Eye and skin sun protection as described in the Precautions—General section should be observed.

B. INFORMATION FOR PATIENTS: See accompanying Patient Package Insert.

C. LABORATORY TESTS:

1. Patients should have an ophthalmologic examination prior to the start of therapy, and thence yearly.

2. Patients should have the following tests prior to the start of therapy and should be retested 6–12 months subsequently. Additional tests at more extended time periods should be conducted as clinically indicated.

a. Complete Blood Count (Hemoglobin or Hematocrit; White Blood Count—if abnormal, a differential count).

b. Anti-nuclear Antibodies.

c. Liver Function Tests.

d. Renal Function Tests (Creatinine or Blood Urea Nitrogen).

D. DRUG INTERACTIONS: See Warnings Section.

E. CARCINOGENESIS: See Warnings Section.

F. PREGNANCY:

Pregnancy Category C. Animal reproduction studies have not been conducted with methoxsalen. It is also not known whether methoxsalen can cause fetal harm when administered to a pregnant woman or can

Continued on next page

8-Mop—Cont.

affect reproduction capacity. Methoxsalen should be given to a woman only if clearly needed.

G. NURSING MOTHERS:

It is not known whether this drug is excreted in human milk. Because many drugs are excreted in human milk, caution should be exercised when methoxsalen is administered to a nursing woman.

H. PEDIATRIC USE:

Safety in children has not been established. Potential hazards of long-term therapy include the possibilities of carcinogenicity and cataractogenicity as described in the Warnings Section as well as the probability of actinic degeneration which is also described in the Warnings Section.

VII. ADVERSE REACTIONS

A. METHOXSALEN:

The most commonly reported side effect of methoxsalen alone is nausea, which occurs with approximately 10% of all patients. This effect may be minimized or avoided by instructing the patient to take methoxsalen with milk or food, or to divide the dose into two portions, taken approximately one-half hour apart. Other effects include nervousness, insomnia, and psychological depression.

B. COMBINED METHOXSALEN/UVA THERAPY:

1. PRURITUS: This adverse reaction occurs with approximately 10% of all patients. In most cases, pruritus can be alleviated with frequent application of bland emollients or other topical agents; severe pruritus may require systemic treatment. If pruritus is unresponsive to these measures, shield pruritic areas from further UVA exposure until the condition resolves. If intractable pruritus is generalized, UVA treatment should be discontinued until the pruritus disappears.

2. ERYTHEMA: Mild, transient erythema at 24–48 hours after PUVA therapy is an expected reaction and indicates that a therapeutic interaction between methoxsalen and UVA occurred. Any area showing moderate erythema (greater than Grade 2—See Table 1 for grades of erythema) should be shielded during subsequent UVA exposures until the erythema has resolved. Erythema greater than Grade 2 which appears within 24 hours after UVA treatment may signal a potentially severe burn. Erythema may become progressively worse over the next 24 hours, since the peak erythemal reaction characteristically occurs 48 hours or later after methoxsalen ingestion. The patient should be protected from further UVA exposures and sunlight, and should be monitored closely.

3. IMPORTANT DIFFERENCES BETWEEN PUVA ERYTHEMA AND SUNBURN: PUVA-induced inflammation differs from sunburn or UVB phototherapy in several ways. The **in situ** depth of photochemistry is deeper within the tissue because UVA is transmitted further into the skin. The DNA lesions induced by PUVA are very different from UV-induced thymine dimers and may lead to a DNA crosslink. This DNA lesion may be more problematic to the cell because crosslinks are more lethal and psoralen-DNA photoproducts may be "new" or unfamiliar substrates for DNA repair enzymes. DNA synthesis is also suppressed longer after PUVA. The time course of delayed erythema is different with PUVA and may not involve the usual mediators seen in sunburn. PUVA-induced redness may be just beginning at 24 hours, when UVB erythema has already passed its peak. The erythema dose-response curve is also steeper for PUVA. Compared to equally erythemogenic doses of UVB, the histologic alterations induced by PUVA show more dermal vessel damage and longer duration of epidermal and dermal abnormalities.

4. OTHER ADVERSE REACTIONS: Those reported include edema, dizziness, headache, malaise, depression, hypopigmentation, vesiculation and bullae for-

mation, non-specific rash, herpes simplex, miliaria, urticaria, folliculitis, gastrointestinal disturbances, cutaneous tenderness, leg cramps, hypotension, and extension of psoriasis.

VIII. OVERDOSAGE

In the event of methoxsalen overdosage, induce emesis and keep the patient in a darkened room for at least 24 hours. Emesis is beneficial only within the first 2 to 3 hours after ingestion of methoxsalen, since maximum blood levels are reached by this time.

IX. DRUG DOSAGE & ADMINISTRATION

A. VITILIGO THERAPY

1. DRUG DOSAGE: Two capsules (10 mg each) in one dose taken with milk or in food two to four hours before ultraviolet light exposure.

2. LIGHT EXPOSURE: The exposure time to sunlight should comply with the following guide:

	Basic Skin Color		
	Light	Medium	Dark
Initial Exposure	15 min.	20 min.	25 min.
Second Exposure	20 min.	25 min.	30 min.
Third Exposure	25 min.	30 min.	35 min.
Fourth Exposure	30 min.	35 min.	40 min.

Subsequent Exposure: Gradually increase exposure based on erythema and tenderness of the amelanotic skin.

Therapy should be on alternate days and never two consecutive days.

B. PSORIASIS THERAPY

1. DRUG DOSAGE—INITIAL THERAPY: The methoxsalen capsules should be taken 2 hours before UVA exposure with some food or milk according to the following table:

	Patient's Weight	Dose
(kg)	(lbs)	(mg)
<30	<65	10
30–50	66–110	20
51–65	111–145	30
66–80	146–175	40
81–90	176–200	50
91–115	201–250	60
>115	>250	70

Additional drug dosage directions are as follows:

a. Weight Change: In the event that the weight of a patient changes during treatment such that he/she falls into an adjacent weight range/dose category, no change in the dose of methoxsalen is usually required. If, in the physician's opinion, however, a weight change is sufficiently great to modify the drug dose, then an adjustment in the time of exposure to UVA should be made.

b. Dose/Week: The number of doses per week of methoxsalen capsules will be determined by the patient's schedule of UVA exposures. In no case should treatments be given more often than once every other day because the full extent of phototoxic reactions may not be evident until 48 hours after each exposure.

c. Dosage Increase: Dosage may be increased by 10 mg. after the fifteenth treatment under the conditions outlined in section XI.B.4.b.

X. UFA RADIATION SOURCE SPECIFICATIONS & INFORMATION

A. IRRADIANCE UNIFORMITY: (For photopheresis, refer to the UVAR* System Operator's Manual.)

The following specifications should be met with the window of the detector held in a vertical plane:

1. Vertical variation: For readings taken at any point along the vertical center axis of the chamber (to within 15 cm from the top and bottom), the lowest reading should not be less than 70 percent of the highest reading.

2. Horizontal variation: Throughout any specific horizontal plane, the lowest reading must be at least 80 percent of the highest reading, excluding the peripheral 3 cm of the patient treatment space:

B. PATIENT SAFETY FEATURES:

The following safety features should be present: (1) Protection from electrical hazard: All units should be grounded and conform to applicable electrical codes. The patient or operator should not be able to touch any live electrical parts. There should be ground fault protection. (2) Protective shielding of lamps: The patient should not be able to come in contact with the bare lamps. In the event of lamp breakage, the patient should not be exposed to broken lamp components. (3) Hand rails and hand holds: Appropriate supports should be available to the patient. (4) Patient viewing window: A window which blocks UV should be provided for viewing the patient during treatment. (5) Door and latches: Patients should be able to open the door from the inside with only slight pressure to the door. (6) Non-skid floor: The floor should be of a non-skid nature. (7) Thermoregulation: Sufficient air flow should be provided for patient safety and comfort, limiting temperature within the UVA radiator cabinet to approximately less than 100° F. (8) Timer: The irradiator should be equipped with an automatic timer which terminates the exposure at the conclusion of a pre-set time interval. (9) Patient alarm device: An alarm device within the UVA irradiator chamber should be accessible to the patient for emergency activation. (10) Danger label: The unit should have a label prominently displayed which reads as follows:
DANGER—Ultraviolet Radiation—Follow your physician's instructions—Failure to use protective eyewear may result in eye injury.

C. UVA EXPOSURE DOSIMETRY MEASUREMENTS:

The maximum radiant exposure or irradiance (within ± 15 percent) of UVA (320–400 nm) delivered to the patient should be determined by using an appropriate radiometer calibrated to be read in Joules/cm^2 or mW/cm^2. In the absence of a standard measuring technique approved by the National Bureau of Standards, the system should use a detector corrected to a cosine spatial response. The use and recalibration frequency of such a radiometer for a specific UVA irradiator chamber should be specified by the manufacturer because the UVA dose (exposure) is determined by the design of the irradiator, the number of lamps, and the age of the lamps. If irradiance is measured, the radiometer reading in mW/cm^2 is used to calculate the exposure time in minutes to deliver the required UVA dose in Joules/cm^2 to a patient in the UVA irradiator cabinet. The equation is:

$$\text{Exposure Time in minutes} = \frac{\text{Desired UVA Dose (J/cm}^2)}{0.06 \times \text{Irradiance (mW/cm}^2)}$$

Overexposure due to human error should be minimized by using an accurate automatic timing device, which is set by the operator and controlled by energizing and de-energizing the UVA irradiator lamp. The timing device calibration interval should be specified by the manufacturer. Safety systems should be included to minimize the possibility of delivering a UVA exposure which exceeds the prescribed dose, in the event the timer or radiometer should malfunction.

D. UVA SPECTRAL OUTPUT DISTRIBUTION:

The spectral distributions of the lamps should meet the following specifications:

Wavelength Band (Nanometers)	Output [1]
<310	<1
310 to 320	1 to 3
320 to 330	4 to 8
330 to 340	11 to 17
340 to 350	18 to 25
350 to 360	19 to 28
360 to 370	15 to 23
370 to 380	8 to 12
380 to 390	3 to 7
390 to 400	1 to 3

[1]As a percentage of total irradiance between 320 and 400 nanometers.

XI. PUVA TREATMENT PROTOCOL

A. INITIAL EXPOSURE: The initial UVA exposure should be conducted according to the guidelines presented previously under IX.B.1 and 2, Psoriasis therapy, Drug dosage-initial Therapy and Exposure.
[See table at left]

B. CLEARING PHASE: Specific recommendations for patient treatment are as follows:

1. SKIN TYPES I, II & III. Patients with skin types I, II and III may be treated 2 or 3 times per week. UVA exposure may be held constant or increased by up to 1.0 Joule/cm^2 at each treatment, according to the patient's response. If erythema occurs, however, do not increase exposure time until erythema resolves. The

Skin Type	History	Recommended Joules/cm^2
I	Always burn, never tan (Patients with Erythrodermic psoriasis are to be classed as Type I for determination of UVA dosage.)	0.5 J/cm^2
II	Always burn, but sometimes tan	1.0 J/cm^2
III	Sometimes burn, but always tan	1.5 J/cm^2
IV	Never burn, always tan	2.0 J/cm^2
	Physician Examination	
V*	Moderately pigmented	2.5 J/cm^2
VI*	Blacks	3.0 J/cm^2

[*Patients with natural pigmentation of these types should be classified into a lower skin type category if the sunburning history so indicates.]

severity and extent of the patient's erythema may be used to determine whether the next exposure should be shortened, omitted, or maintained at the previous dosage. See Adverse Reactions section for additional information.

2. SKIN TYPES IV, V & VI. Patients with skin types IV, V and VI may be treated 2 or 3 times per week. UVA exposure may be held constant or increased by up to 1.5 Joules/cm^2 at each treatment unless erythema occurs. If erythema occurs, follow instructions outlined above in the procedures for patients with skin types I, II and III.

3. ERYTHRODERMIC PSORIASIS. Patients with erythrodermic psoriasis should be treated with special attention because pre-existing erythema may obscure observations of possible treatment-related phototoxic erythema. These patients may be treated 2 or 3 times per week, as a Type I patient.

4. MISCELLANEOUS SITUATIONS:

a. If there is no response after a total of 10 treatments, the exposure of UVA energy may be increased by an additional 0.5–1.0 Joules/cm^2 above the prior incremental increases for each treatment. (Example: a patient whose exposure dosage is being increased by 1.0 Joule/cm^2 may now have all subsequent doses increased by 1.5–2.0 Joules/cm^2.)

b. If there is no response, or only minimal response, after 15 treatments, the dosage of methoxsalen may be increased by 10 mg. (a one-time increase in dosage). This increased dosage may be continued for the remainder of the course of treatment but should not be exceeded.

c. If a patient misses a treatment, the UVA exposure time of the next treatment should not be increased. If more than one treatment is missed, reduce the exposure by 0.5 Joules/cm^2 for each treatment missed.

d. If the lower extremities are not responding as well as the rest of the body and do not show erythema, cover all other body area and give 25 percent of the present exposure dose as an additional exposure to the lower extremities. This additional exposure to the lower extremities should be terminated if erythema develops on these areas.

e. Non-responsive psoriasis: If a patient's generalized psoriasis is not responding, or if the condition appears to be worsening during treatment, the possibility of a generalized phototoxic reaction should be considered. This may be confirmed by the improvement of the condition following temporary discontinuance of this therapy for two weeks. If no improvement occurs during the interruption of treatment, this patient may be considered a treatment failure.

C. ALTERNATIVE EXPOSURE SCHEDULE:

As an alternative to increasing the UVA exposure at each treatment, the following schedule may be followed; this schedule may reduce the total number of Joules/cm^2 received by the patient over the entire course of therapy.

1. Incremental increases in UVA exposure for all patients may range from 0.5 to 1.5 Joules/cm^2, according to the patient's response to therapy.

2. Once Grade 2 clearing (see Table 2) has been reached and the patient is progressing adequately, UVA dosage is held constant. This dosage is maintained until Grade 4 clearing is reached.

3. If the rate of clearing significantly decreases, exposure dosage may be increased at each treatment (0.1–1.5 Joules/cm^2) until Grade 3 clearing and a satisfactory progress rate is attained. The UVA exposure will be held constant again until Grade 4 clearing is attained. These increases may be used also if the rate of clearing significantly decreases between Grade 3 and Grade 4 response. However, the possibility of a phototoxic reaction should be considered; see Non-responsive Psoriasis, above.

4. In summary, this schedule raises slightly the increments (Joules/cm^2) of UVA dosage, but limits these increases to those periods when the patient is not responding adequately. Otherwise, the UVA exposure is held at the lowest effective dose.

D. MAINTENANCE PHASE:

The goal of maintenance treatment is to keep the patient as symptom-free as possible with the least amount of UVA exposure.

1. SCHEDULE OF EXPOSURES: When patients have achieved 95 percent clearing, or Grade 4 response (Table 2), they may be placed on the following maintenance schedules (M_1–M_4), in sequence. It is recommended that each maintenance schedule be adhered to for at least 2 treatments (unless erythema or psoriatic flare occurs, in which case see (2a) and (2b) below).

Maintenance Schedules

M_1–once/week

M_2–once/2 week

M_3–once/3 weeks

M_4–p.r.n. (i.e., for flares)

Table 2. Response to Therapy

Grade	Criteria	Percent Improvement (compared to original extent of disease
−1	Psoriasis worse	0
0	No change	0
1	Minimal improvement—slightly less scale and/or erythema	5–20
2	Definite improvement—partial flattening of all plaques—less scaling and less erythema	20–50
3	Considerable improvement—nearly complete flattening of all plaques but borders of plaques still palpable	50–95
4	Clearing; complete flattening of plaques including borders; plaques may be outlined by pigmentation	95

2. LENGTH OF EXPOSURE: The UVA exposure for the first maintenance treatment of any schedule (except M_4 as noted below) is the same as that of the patient's last treatment under the previous schedule. For skin types I-IV, however, it is recommended that the maximum UVA dosage during maintenance treatments not exceed the following:

Skin Types	Joules/cm^2/treatment
I	12
II	14
III	18
IV	22

If the patient develops erythema or new lesions of psoriasis, proceed as follows:

a. Erythema: During maintenance therapy, the patient's tan and threshold dose for erythema may gradually decrease. If maintenance treatments produce significant erythema, the exposure to UVA should be decreased by 25 percent until further treatments no longer produce erythema.

b. Psoriasis: If the patient develops new areas of psoriasis during maintenance therapy (but still is classified as having a Grade 4 response), the exposure to UVA may be increased by 0.5–1.5 Joules/cm^2 at each treatment; this is appropriate for all types of patients. These increases are continued until the psoriasis is brought under control and the patient is again clear. The exposure being administered when this clearing is reached should be used for further maintenance treatment.

3. FLARES DURING MAINTENANCE: If the patient flares during maintenance treatment (i.e., develops psoriasis on more than 5 percent of the originally involved areas of the body) his maintenance treatment schedule may be changed to the preceding maintenance or clearing schedule. The patient may be kept on his schedule until again 95 percent clear. If the original maintenance treatment schedule is unable to control the psoriasis, the schedule may be changed to a more frequent regimen. If a flare occurs less than 6 weeks after the last treatment, 25 percent of the maximum exposure received during the clearing phase, may be used and then proceed with the clearing schedule previously followed for this patient. (At 95 percent clearing follow regular maintenance until the optimum maintenance schedule is determined for the patient.) If more than 6 weeks have elapsed since the last treatment was given, treat patients as if they were beginning therapy insofar as exposure dosages are concerned, since their threshold for erythema may have decreased.

Table 1. Grades of Erythema

Grade	Erythema Level
0	No erythema
1	Minimally perceptible erythema—faint pink
2	Marked erythema but with no edema
3	Fiery erythema with edema
4	Fiery erythema with edema and blistering

[See table 2 above]

XII. HOW SUPPLIED

8-MOP Capsules, each containing 10 mg. of methoxsalen (8-methoxypsoralen) packaged in amber glass bottles of 50 (NDC 0187-0651-42).

BIBLIOGRAPHY

1. Pathak, M.A., Kramer, D.M., Fitzpatrick, T.B.: Photobiology and Photochemistry of Furocoumarins (Psoralens), SUNLIGHT AND MAN: Normal and Abnormal Photobiologic Responses. Edited by M.A. Pathak, L.C. Harber, M. Seiji et al. University of Tokyo Press. 1974, pp. 335–368.
2. Artuc, M., Stuettgen, G., Schalla, W., Schaefer, H., and Gazith, J.: Reversible binding of 5- and 8-methoxypsoralen to human serum proteins (albumin) and to epidermis in vitro: Brit. J. Dermat. 101, pp. 669–677 (1979).
3. Mandula, B.B., Pathak, M.A., Nakayama, Y., and Davidson, S.J.: Induction of mixed-function oxidases in mouse liver by psoralens., Ibid, 99, pp. 687–692 (1978).
4. Pathak, M.A., Fitzpatrick, T.B., Parrish, J.A.: PSORIASIS, Proceedings of the Second International Symposium. Edited by E.M. Farber, A.J. Cox, Yorke Medical Books, pp. 262–265 (1977).
5. Dall'Acqua, F., Marciani, S., Ciavatta, L, Rodighiero, G.: Formation of interstrand cross-linkings in the photoreactions between furocoumarins and DNA; Z Naturforsch (B), 26, pp. 561–569 (1971).
6. Cole, R.S.: Light-induced cross-linkings of DNA in the presence of a furocoumarin (psoralen), Biochem. Biophys. Acta, 217, pp. 30–39 (1970).
7. Musajo, L., Rodighiero, G., Caporale, G., Dall'Acqua, F., Marciani, S., Bordin, F., Baccichetti, F., Bevilacqua, R.: Photoreactions between Skin-Photosensitizing Furocoumarins and Nucleic Acids, SUNLIGHT AND MAN; Normal and Abnormal Photobiologic Responses. Edited by M.A. Pathak, L.C. Harber, M. Seiji et al. University of Tokyo Press, pp. 369–387 (1974).
8. Dall'Acqua, F., Vedaldi, D., Bordin, F., and Rodighiero, G.: New studies in the interaction between 8-methoxypsoralen and DNA in vitro; J. Investigative Dermat., 73, pp. 191–197 (1979).
9. Yoshikawa, K., Mori, N., Sakakibara, S., Mizuno, N., Song, P.: Photo-Conjugation of 8-methoxypsoralen with Proteins; Photochem. & Photobiol. 29, pp. 1127–1133 (1979).
10. Ortonne, J. P., MacDonald, D.M., Micoud, A., Thivolet, J.: PUVA-induced repigmentation of vitiligo: a histochemical (split-DOPA) and ultra-structural study: Brit. J. of Dermat., 101, pp. 1–12 (1979).
11. Hakim, R.E., Griffin, A.C., Knox, J.M.: Erythema and tumor formation in methoxsalen treated mice exposed to fluorescent light; Arch. Dermatol. 82, 572–577 (1960).
12. Pathak, M.A., Daniels, F., Hopkins, C.E., Fitzpatrick, T.B.: Ultraviolet carcinogenesis in albino and pigmented mice receiving furocoumarins: psoralens and 8-methoxypsoralen, Nature 183, pp. 728–730 (1959).
13. Stern, R.S., Thibodeau, L.A., Kleinerman, R.A., Parrish, J.A., Fitzpatrick, T.B., and 22 Participating Investigators: Risk of Cutaneous Carcinoma in Patients Treated with Oral Methoxsalen Photochemotherapy for Psoriasis: NEJM, 300. No. 15, pp. 809–813 (1979).
14. Stern, R.S., Parrish, J.A., Zierler, S.: Skin Carcinoma in Patients with Psoriasis Treated with Topical Tar and Artificial Ultraviolet Radiation. Lancet, 1, pp. 732–735 (1980).
15. Roenigk, Jr., H.H., and 12 Cooperating Investigators: Skin Cancer in the PUVA-48 Cooperative Study of Psoriasis. Program for Forty-First Annual Meeting for The Society of Investigative Dermatology, Inc., Sheraton Washington Hotel, Washington, D.C., May 12, 13, and 14, 1980. Abstracts JID, 74, No. 4, p. 250 (April, 1980).
16. Mosher, D.B., Pathak, M.A., Harris, T.J., Fitzpatrick, T.B.: Development of Cutaneous Lesions in Vitiligo During Long-Term PUVA Therapy. Program for Forty-First Annual Meeting for The Society for Investigative Dermatology, Inc., Sheraton Washington Hotel, Washington, D.C., May 12, 13, and 14, 1980. Abstracts JID, 74, No. 4, p. 259 (April, 1980).
17. Cloud, T.M., Hakim, R., Griffin, A.C.: Photosensitization of the eye with methoxsalen. I. Acute effects; Arch. Ophthalmol. 64, pp. 346–352 (1960).
18. Cloud, T.M., Hakim, R., Griffen, A.C.: Photosensitization of the eye with methoxsalen. II. Chronic effects, Ibid, 66, pp. 689–694 (1961).
19. Freeman, R.G., Troll, D.: Photosensitization of the eye by 8-methoxypsoralen, JID, 53, pp. 449–453 (1969).
20. Lerman, S., Megaw, J., Willis, I.: Potential ocular complications from PUVA therapy and their prevention; J. Invest. Dermat., 74, pp. 197–199 (1980).

2579-01 EL ICN Pharmaceuticals, Inc. Rev. 9-97
3300 Hyland Ave.
Costa Mesa, CA 92626

Shown in Product Identification Guide, page 317

Continued on next page

ANCOBON® ℞

[*an 'co-bon*]
brand of flucytosine
CAPSULES

> **WARNING**
> **Use with extreme caution in patients with impaired renal function. Close monitoring of hematologic, renal and hepatic status of all patients is essential. These instructions should be thoroughly reviewed before administration of Ancobon.**

DESCRIPTION

Ancobon (flucytosine), an antifungal agent, is available as 250-mg and 500-mg capsules for oral administration. Each capsule also contains corn starch, lactose and talc. Gelatin capsule shells contain parabens (butyl, methyl, propyl) and sodium propionate, with the following dye systems: 250-mg capsules—black iron oxide, FD&C Blue No. 1, FD&C Yellow No. 6, D&C Yellow No. 10 and titanium dioxide; 500-mg capsules—black iron oxide and titanium dioxide. Chemically, flucytosine is 5-fluorocytosine, a fluorinated pyrimidine which is related to fluorouracil and floxuridine. It is a white to off-white crystalline powder with a molecular weight of 129.09.

CLINICAL PHARMACOLOGY

Flucytosine is rapidly and virtually completely absorbed following oral administration. Bioavailability estimated by comparing the area under the curve of serum concentrations after oral and intravenous administration showed 78% to 89% absorption of the oral dose. Peak blood concentrations of 30 to 40 mcg/mL were reached within 2 hours of administration of a 2-gm oral dose to normal subjects. The mean blood concentrations were approximately 70 to 80 mcg/mL 1 to 2 hours after a dose in patients with normal renal function who received a 6-week regimen of flucytosine (150 mg/kg/day given in divided doses every 6 hours) in combination with amphotericin B. The half-life in the majority of normal subjects ranged between 2.4 and 4.8 hours. Flucytosine is excreted via the kidneys by means of glomerular filtration without significant tubular reabsorption. More than 90% of the total radioactivity after oral administration was recovered in the urine as intact drug. Approximately 1% of the dose is present in the urine as the α-fluoro-β-ureido-propionic acid metabolite. A small portion of the dose is excreted in the feces.

The half-life of flucytosine is prolonged in patients with renal insufficiency; the average half-life in nephrectomized or anuric patients was 85 hours (range: 29.9 to 250 hours). A linear correlation was found between the elimination rate constant of flucytosine and creatinine clearance.

In vitro studies have shown that 2.9% to 4% of flucytosine is protein-bound over the range of therapeutic concentrations found in the blood. Flucytosine readily penetrates the blood-brain barrier, achieving clinically significant concentrations in cerebrospinal fluid. Studies in pregnant rats have shown that flucytosine injected intraperitoneally crosses the placental barrier (see PRECAUTIONS).

Microbiology

Flucytosine has in vitro and in vivo activity against Candida and Cryptococcus. Although the exact mode of action is unknown, it has been proposed that flucytosine acts directly on fungal organisms by competitive inhibition of purine and pyrimidine uptake and indirectly by intracellular metabolism to 5-fluorouracil. Flucytosine enters the fungal cell via cytosine permease; thus, flucytosine is metabolized to 5-fluorouracil within fungal organisms. The 5-fluorouracil is extensively incorporated into fungal RNA and inhibits synthesis of both DNA and RNA. The result is unbalanced growth and death of the fungal organism. Antifungal synergism between Ancobon and polyene antibiotics, particularly amphotericin B, has been reported.

Actions

Flucytosine has in vitro and in vivo activity against Candida and Cryptococcus. The exact mode of action against these fungi is not known. Ancobon is not metabolized significantly when given orally to man.

Susceptibility

Cryptococcus: Most strains initially isolated from clinical material have shown flucytosine minimal inhibitory concentrations (MIC's) ranging from .46 to 7.8 mcg/mL. Any isolate with an MIC greater than 12.5 mcg/mL is considered resistant. In vitro resistance has developed in originally susceptible strains during therapy. It is recommended that clinical cultures for susceptibility testing be taken initially and at weekly intervals during therapy. The initial culture should be reserved as a reference in susceptibility testing of subsequent isolates.

Candida: As high as 40% to 50% of the pretreatment clinical isolates of Candida have been reported to be resistant to flucytosine. It is recommended that susceptibility studies be performed as early as possible and be repeated during therapy. An MIC value greater than 100 mcg/mL is considered resistant.

Interference with in vitro activity of flucytosine occurs in complex or semisynthetic media. In order to rely upon the recommended in vitro interpretations of susceptibility, it is essential that the broth medium and the testing procedure used be that described by Shadomy.[1]

INDICATIONS AND USAGE

Ancobon is indicated only in the treatment of serious infections caused by susceptible strains of Candida and/or Cryptococcus. *Candida:* Septicemia, endocarditis and urinary system infections have been effectively treated with flucytosine. Limited trials in pulmonary infections justify the use of flucytosine. *Cryptococcus:* Meningitis and pulmonary infections have been treated effectively. Studies in septicemias and urinary tract infections are limited, but good responses have been reported.

CONTRAINDICATIONS

Ancobon should not be used in patients with a known hypersensitivity to the drug.

WARNINGS

Ancobon must be given with extreme caution to patients with impaired renal function. Since Ancobon is excreted primarily by the kidneys, renal impairment may lead to accumulation of the drug. Ancobon blood concentrations should be monitored to determine the adequacy of renal excretion in such patients.[1] Dosage adjustments should be made in patients with renal insufficiency to prevent progressive accumulation of active drug.

Ancobon must be given with extreme caution to patients with bone marrow depression. Patients may be more prone to depression of bone marrow function if they: 1) have a hematologic disease, 2) are being treated with radiation or drugs which depress bone marrow, or 3) have a history of treatment with such drugs or radiation. Bone marrow toxicity can be irreversible and may lead to death in immunosuppressed patients. Frequent monitoring of hepatic function and of the hematopoietic system is indicated during therapy.

PRECAUTIONS

General: Before therapy with Ancobon is instituted, electrolytes (because of hypokalemia) and the hematologic and renal status of the patient should be determined (see WARNINGS). Close monitoring of the patient during therapy is essential.

Laboratory Tests: Since renal impairment can cause progressive accumulation of the drug, blood concentrations and kidney function should be monitored during therapy. Hematologic status (leucocyte and thrombocyte count) and liver function (alkaline phosphatase, SGOT and SGPT) should be determined at frequent intervals during treatment as indicated.

Drug Interactions: Cytosine arabinoside, a cytostatic agent, has been reported to inactivate the antifungal activity of Ancobon by competitive inhibition. Drugs which impair glomerular filtration may prolong the biological half-life of flucytosine. Antifungal synergism between Ancobon and polyene antibiotics, particularly amphotericin B, has been reported.

Drug/Laboratory Test Interactions: Measurement of serum creatinine levels should be determined by the Jaffe method, since Ancobon does not interfere with the determination of creatinine values by this method, as it does when the dry-slide enzymatic method with the Kodak Ektachem analyzer is used.

Carcinogenesis, Mutagenesis, Impairment of Fertility: Flucytosine has not undergone adequate animal testing to evaluate carcinogenic potential. The mutagenic potential of flucytosine was evaluated in Ames-type studies with five different mutants of *S. typhimurium* and no mutagenicity was detected in the presence or absence of activating enzymes. Flucytosine was nonmutagenic in three different repair assay systems.

There have been no adequate trials in animals on the effects of flucytosine on fertility or reproductive performance. The fertility and reproductive performance of the offspring (F_1 generation) of mice treated with 100, 200 or 400 mg/kg/day of flucytosine on days 7 to 13 of gestation was studied; the *in utero* treatment had no adverse effect on the fertility or reproductive performance of the offspring.

Pregnancy: Teratogenic Effects. Pregnancy Category C. Although standard segment II studies have not been done, flucytosine was shown to be teratogenic (vertebral fusions) in the rat at doses of 40 mg/kg/day (0.27 times the maximum human dose, based on nominal dose). At higher doses (700 mg/kg/day, 4.7 times the maximum human dose, based on nominal dose), cleft lip and palate and micrognathia were reported. Flucytosine was not teratogenic in rabbits up to a dose of 100 mg/kg/day (0.68 times the maximum human dose, based on nominal dose). In mice, 400 mg/kg/day of flucytosine (2.7 times the maximum human dose, based on nominal dose) was associated with a low incidence of cleft palate that was not statistically significant. There are no adequate and well-controlled studies in pregnant women. Ancobon should be used during pregnancy only if the potential benefits justifies the potential risk to the fetus.

Nursing Mothers: It is not known whether this drug is excreted in human milk. Because many drugs are excreted in human milk and because of the potential for serious adverse reactions in nursing infants from Ancobon, a decision should be made whether to discontinue nursing or to discontinue the drug, taking into account the importance of the drug to the mother.

Pediatric Use: Safety and effectiveness in children have not been established.

ADVERSE REACTIONS

The adverse reactions which have occurred during treatment with Ancobon are grouped according to organ system affected.

Cardiovascular: Cardiac arrest, myocardial toxicity, ventricular dysfunction.

Respiratory: Respiratory arrest, chest pain, dyspnea.

Dermatologic: Rash, pruritus, urticaria, photosensitivity.

Gastrointestinal: Nausea, emesis, abdominal pain, diarrhea, anorexia, dry mouth, duodenal ulcer, gastrointestinal hemorrhage, acute hepatic injury with possible fatal outcome in debilitated patients, hepatic dysfunction, jaundice, ulcerative colitis, bilirubin elevation.

Genitourinary: Azotemia, creatinine and BUN elevation, crystalluria, renal failure.

Hematologic: Anemia, agranulocytosis, aplastic anemia, eosinophilia, leukopenia, pancytopenia, thrombocytopenia.

Neurologic: Ataxia, hearing loss, headache, paresthesia, parkinsonism, peripheral neuropathy, pyrexia, vertigo, sedation, convulsions.

Psychiatric: Confusion, hallucinations, psychosis.

Miscellaneous: Fatigue, hypoglycemia, hypokalemia, weakness, allergic reactions, Lyell's syndrome.

OVERDOSAGE

There is no experience with intentional overdosage. It is reasonable to expect that overdosage may produce pronounced manifestations of the known clinical adverse reactions. Prolonged serum concentrations in excess of 100 mcg/mL may be associated with an increased incidence of toxicity, especially gastrointestinal (diarrhea, nausea, vomiting), hematologic (leukopenia, thrombocytopenia) and hepatic (hepatitis).

In the management of overdosage, prompt gastric lavage or the use of an emetic is recommended. Adequate fluid intake should be maintained, by the intravenous route if necessary, since Ancobon is excreted unchanged via the renal tract. The hematologic parameters should be monitored frequently; liver and kidney function should be carefully monitored. Should any abnormalities appear in any of these parameters, appropriate therapeutic measures should be instituted. Since hemodialysis has been shown to rapidly reduce serum concentrations in anuric patients, this method may be considered in the management of overdosage.

DOSAGE AND ADMINISTRATION

The usual dosage of Ancobon is 50 to 150 mg/kg/day administered in divided doses at 6-hour intervals. Nausea or vomiting may be reduced or avoided if the capsules are given a few at a time over a 15-minute period. If the BUN or the serum creatinine is elevated, or if there are other signs of renal impairment, the initial dose should be at the lower level (see WARNINGS).

HOW SUPPLIED

Capsules, 250 mg (gray and green), imprinted ANCOBON® 250 ROCHE; bottles of 100 (NDC 0004-0077-01). *Capsules,* 500 mg (gray and white), imprinted ANCOBON® 500 ROCHE, bottles of 100 (NDC 0004-0079-01).

REFERENCE

1. Shadomy S: *Appl Microbiol.* June 1969, 17: 871–877.

Revised: December 1996

Shown in Product Identification Guide, page 316

ANDROID® Ⓒ III

Brand of
Methyltestosterone
Capsules USP, 10 mg

DESCRIPTION

The androgens are steroids that develop and maintain primary and secondary male sex characteristics.

Androgens are derivatives of cyclopentanoperhydrophenanthrene. Endogenous androgens are C-19 steroids with a side chain at C-17, and with two angular methyl groups. Testosterone is the primary endogenous androgen. In their active form, all drugs in the class have a 17-beta hydroxy group. 17-alpha alkylation (methyltestosterone) increases the pharmacologic activity per unit weight compared to testosterone when given orally.

Methyltestosterone, a synthetic derivative of testosterone, is an androgenic preparation given by the oral route in a

capsule form. Each capsule contains 10 mg of Methyltestosterone USP. It has the following structural formula:

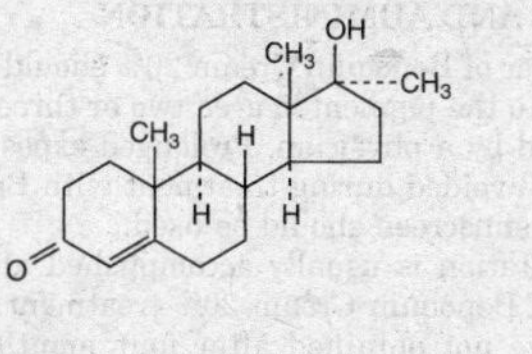

$C_{20}H_{30}O_2$ M.W. 302.46
17-β-hydroxy-17-methylandrost-4-en-3-one

Methyltestosterone occurs as white or creamy white crystals or powder, which is soluble in various organic solvents but is practically insoluble in water.

Each capsule, for oral administration, contains 10 mg of Methyltestosterone. In addition, each capsule contains the following inactive ingredients: Corn starch NF, Gelatin NF, FD&C Blue #1, FD&C Red #40.

CLINICAL PHARMACOLOGY

Endogenous androgens are responsible for the normal growth and development of the male sex organs and for maintenance of secondary sex characteristics. These effects include the growth and maturation of prostate, seminal vesicles, penis, and scrotum. The development of male hair distribution, such as beard, pubic, chest, and axillary hair; laryngeal enlargement, vocal chord thickening, alterations in body musculature, and fat distribution. Drugs in this class also cause retention of nitrogen, sodium, potassium, phosphorus, and decreased urinary excretion of calcium. Androgens have been reported to increase protein anabolism and decrease protein catabolism. Nitrogen balance is improved only when there is sufficient intake of calories and protein.

Androgens are responsible for the growth spurt of adolescence and for the eventual termination of linear growth which is brought about by fusion of the epiphyseal growth centers. In children, exogenous androgens accelerate linear growth rates, but may cause a disproportionate advancement in bone maturation. Use over long periods may result in fusion of the epiphyseal growth centers and termination of growth process. Androgens have been reported to stimulate the production of red blood cells by enhancing the production of erythropoietic stimulating factor.

During exogenous administration of androgens, endogenous testosterone release is inhibited through feedback inhibition of pituitary luteinizing hormone (LH). At large doses of exogenous androgens, spermatogenesis may also be suppressed through feedback inhibition of pituitary follicle stimulating hormone (FSH).

There is a lack of substantial evidence that androgens are effective in fractures, surgery, convalescence and functional uterine bleeding.

Pharmacokinetics

Testosterone given orally is metabolized by the gut and 44 percent is cleared by the liver of the first pass. Oral doses as high as 400 mg per day are needed to achieve clinically effective blood levels for full replacement therapy. The synthetic androgen, methyltestosterone, is less extensively metabolized by the liver and has a longer half-life. It is more suitable than testosterone for oral administration.

Testosterone in plasma is 98 percent bound to a specific testosterone-estradiol binding globulin, and about 2 percent is free. Generally, the amount of this sex-hormone binding globulin in the plasma will determine the distribution of testosterone between free and bound forms, and the free testosterone concentration will determine its half-life.

About 90 percent of a dose of testosterone is excreted in the urine as glucuronic and sulfuric acid conjugates of testosterone and its metabolites: and 6 percent of a dose is excreted in the feces, mostly in the unconjugated form. Inactivation of testosterone occurs primarily in the liver. Testosterone is metabolized to various 17-keto steroids through two different pathways. There are considerable variations of the half-life of testosterone as reported in the literature, ranging from 10 to 100 minutes.

In many tissues the activity of testosterone appears to depend on reduction to dihydrotestosterone, which binds to cytosol receptor proteins. The steroid-receptor complex is transported to the nucleus where it initiates transcription events and cellular changes related to androgen action.

INDICATIONS AND USAGE

1. Males

Androgens are indicated for replacement therapy in conditions associated with a deficiency or absence of endogenous testosterone.

a. Primary hipogonadism (congenital or acquired) — (testicular failure due to cryptorchidism, bilateral torsions, orchitis, vanishing testis syndrome; or orchidectomy.
b. Hypogonadotropic hypogonadism (congenital or acquired) — idiopathic gonadotropin or LHRH deficiency, or pituitary hypothalamic injury from tumors, trauma, or radiation. If the above conditions occur prior to puberty, androgen replacement therapy will be needed during the adolescent years for development of secondary sexual characteristics. Prolonged androgen treatment will be required to maintain sexual characteristics in these and other males who develop testosterone deficiency after puberty.
c. Androgens may be used to stimulate puberty in carefully selected males with clearly delayed puberty. These patients usually have a familial pattern of delayed puberty that is not secondary to a pathological disorder; puberty is expected to occur spontaneously at a relatively late date. Brief treatment with conservative doses may occasionally be justified in these patients if they do not respond to psychological support. The potential adverse effect on bone maturation should be discussed with the patient and parents prior to androgen administration. An X-ray of the hand and wrist to determine bone age should be obtained every 6 months to assess the effect of treatment on the epiphyseal centers (see WARNINGS).

2. Females

Androgens may be used secondarily in women with advancing inoperable metastatic (skeletal) mammary cancer who are 1 to 5 years postmenopausal. Primary goals of therapy in these women include ablation of the ovaries. Other methods of counteracting estrogen activity are adrenalectomy, hypophysectomy, and/or antiestrogen therapy. This treatment has also been used in premenopausal women with breast cancer who have benefited from oophorectomy and are considered to have a hormone-responsive tumor. Judgment concerning androgen therapy should be made by an oncologist with expertise in this field.

CONTRAINDICATIONS

Androgens are contraindicated in men with carcinomas of the breast or with known or suspected carcinomas of the prostate, and in women who are or may become pregnant. When administered to pregnant woman, androgens cause virilization of the external genitalia of the female fetus. This virilization includes clitoromegaly, abnormal vaginal development, and fusion of genital folds to form a scrotal-like structure. The degree of masculinization is related to the amount of drug given and the age of the fetus, and is most likely to occur in the female fetus when the drugs are given in the first trimester. If the patients becomes pregnant while taking these drugs, she should be apprised of the potential hazard to the fetus.

WARNINGS

In patients with breast cancer, androgen therapy may cause hypercalcemia by stimulating osteolysis. In this case, the drug should be discontinued.

Prolonged use of high doses of adrogens has been associated with the development of peliosis hepatis and hepatic neoplasms including hepatocellular carcinoma. (See PRECAUTIONS—Carcinogenesis). Peliosis hepatis can be a life-threatening or fatal complication.

Cholestatic hepatitis and jaundice occur with 17-alpha-alkylandrogens at a relatively low dose. If cholestatic hepatitis with jaundice appears or if liver function tests become abnormal, the androgen should be discontinued and the etiology should be determined. Drug-induced jaundice is reversible when the medication is discontinued.

Geriatric patients treated with androgens may be at an increased risk for the development of prostatic hypertrophy and prostatic carcinoma.

Edema with or without congestive heart failure may be a serious complication in patients with preexisting cardiac, renal, or hepatic disease. In addition to discontinuation of the drug, diuretic therapy may be required.

Gynecomastia frequently develops and occasionally persists in patients being treated for hypogonadism.

Androgen therapy should be used cautiously in healthy males with delayed puberty. The effect on bone maturation should be monitored by assessing bone age of the wrist and hand every 6 months. In children, androgen treatment may accelerate bone maturation without producing compensatory gain in linear growth. This adverse effect may result in compromised adult stature. The younger the child the greater the risk of compromising final mature height.

This drug has not been shown to be safe and effective for the enhancement of athletic performance. Because of the potential risk of serious adverse health effects, this drug should not be used for such purpose.

PRECAUTIONS

General

Women should be observed for signs of virilization (deepening of the voice, hirsutism, acne, clitoromegaly and menstrual irregularities). Discontinuation of drug therapy at the time of evidence of mild virilism is necessary to prevent irreversible virilization. Such virilization is usual following androgen use at high doses. A decision may be made by the patient and the physician that some virilization will be tolerated during treatment for breast carcinoma.

Information for the Patient

The physician should instruct patients to report any of the following side effects of androgens:

Adult or Adolescent Males:	Too frequent or persistent erections of the penis. Any male adolescent patient receiving androgens for delayed puberty should have bone development checked every six months.
Women:	Hoarseness, acne, changes in menstrual periods or more hair on the face.
All Patients:	Any nausea, vomiting, changes in skin color or ankle swelling.

Laboratory Tests

1. Women with disseminated breast carcinoma should have frequent determination of urine and serum calcium levels during the course of androgen therapy (See WARNINGS).
2. Because of the hepatotoxicity associated with the use of 17-alpha-alkylated androgens, liver function tests should be obtained periodically.
3. Periodic (every 6 months) X-ray examinations of bone age should be made during treatment of prepubertal males to determine the rate of bone maturation and the effects of androgen therapy on the epiphyseal centers.
4. Hemoglobin and hematocrit should be checked periodically for polycythemia in patients who are receiving high doses of androgens.

Drug Interactions

1. Anticoagulants: C-17 substituted derivatives of testosterone, such as methandrostenolone, have been reported to decrease the anticoagulant requirements of patients receiving oral anticoagulants. Patients receiving oral anticoagulant therapy require close monitoring, especially when androgens are started or stopped.

2. Oxyphenbutazone: Concurrent administration of oxyphenbutazone and androgens may result in elevated serum levels of oxyphenbutazone.

3. Insulin: In diabetic patients the metabolic effects of androgens may decrease blood glucose and insulin requirements.

Drug/Laboratory Test Interferences

Androgens may decrease levels of thyroxine-binding globulin, resulting in decreased total T4 serum levels and increased resin uptake of T3 and T4. Free thyroid hormone levels remain unchanged, however, and there is no clinical evidence of thyroid dysfunction.

Carcinogenesis

Animal Data

Testosterone has been tested by subcutaneous injection and implantation in mice and rats. The implant induced cervical-uterine tumors in mice, which metastasized in some cases. There is suggestive evidence that injection of testosterone into some strains of female mice increases their susceptibility to hepatoma. Testosterone is also known to increase the number of tumors and decrease the degree of differentiation of chemically induced carcinomas of the liver in rats.

Human Data

There are rare reports of hepatocellular carcinoma in patients receiving long-term therapy with androgens in high doses. Withdrawal of the drugs did not lead to regression of the tumors in all cases.

Geriatric patients treated with androgens may be at an increased risk for the development of prostatic hypertrophy and prostatic carcinoma.

Pregnancy

Teratogenic effects. Pregnacy Category X (See CONTRAINDICATIONS).

Nursing Mothers

It is not known whether androgens are excreted in human milk. Because many drugs are excreted in human milk and because of the potential for serious adverse reactions in nursing infants from androgens, a decision should be made whether to discontinue nursing or to discontinue the drug, taking into account the importance of the drug to the mother.

Pediatric Use

Androgen therapy should be used very cautiously in children and only by specialists who are aware of the adverse effects on bone maturation. Skeletal maturation must be monitored every six months by an X-ray of hand and wrist (See INDICATIONS AND USAGE and WARNINGS).

ADVERSE REACTIONS

Endocrine and Urogenital

Female: The most common side effects of androgen therapy are amenorrhea and other menstrual irregularities, inhibition of gonadotropin secretion and virilization, including deepening of the voice and clitoral enlargement. The latter usually is not reversible after androgens are discontinued. When administered to a pregnant woman androgens cause virilization of external genitalia of the female fetus.

Continued on next page

Android—Cont.

Male: Gynecomastia, and excesssive frequency and duration of penile erections. Oligosperma may occur at high dosages (see CLINICAL PHARMACOLOGY).

Skin and appendages: Hirsutism, male pattern of baldness, and acne.

Fluid and Electrolyte Disturbances: Retention of sodium, chloride, water, potassium, calcium and inorganic phosphates.

Gastrointestinal: Nausea, cholestatic jaundice, alterations in liver function tests, rarely hepatocellular neoplasms and peliosis hepatitis (see WARNINGS).

Hematologic: Suppression of clotting factors II, V, VII, and X, bleeding in patients on concomitant anticoagulant therapy and polycythemia.

Nervous System: Increased or decreased libido, headache, anxiety, depression, and generalized paresthesia.

Metabolic: Increased serum cholesterol.

Miscellaneous: Rarely anaphylactoid reactions.

DRUG ABUSE AND DEPENDENCE

Methyltestosterone Capsules are classified as a schedule III Controlled Substance under the Anabolic Steroids Act of 1990.

OVERDOSAGE

There have been no reports of acute overdosage with the androgens.

DOSAGE AND ADMINISTRATION

Methyltestosterone capsules are administered orally. The suggested dosage for androgens varies depending on the age, sex, and diagnosis of the individual patient. Dosage is adjusted according to the patient's response and the appearance of adverse reactions.

Replacement therapy in androgen-deficient males is 10 to 50 mg of methyltestosterone daily. Various dosage regimens have been used to induce pubertal changes in hypogonadal males, some experts have advocated lower dosages initially, gradually increasing the dose as puberty progresses with or without a decrease to maintenance levels. Other experts emphasize that higher dosages are needed to induce pubertal changes and lower dosages can be used for maintenance after puberty. The chronological and skeletal ages must be taken into consideration both in determining the initial dose and in adjusting the dose.

Doses used in delayed puberty generally are in the lower range of that given above, and for a limited duration, for example 4 to 6 months.

Women with metastatic breast carcinoma must be followed closely because androgen therapy occasionally appears to accelerate the disease. Thus, many experts prefer to use the shorter acting androgen preparations rather than those with prolonged activity for treating breast carcinoma, particularly during the early stages of androgen therapy. The dosage of methyltestosterone for androgen therapy in breast carcinoma in females is from 50–200 mg daily.

HOW SUPPLIED

Methyltestosterone capsules USP 10 mg are red capsules imprinted "ICN 0901" on both sections. They are available in bottles of 100.

CAUTION: Federal (USA) law prohibits dispensing without prescription.

ICN Pharmaceuticals, Inc.
ICN Plaza
3300 Hyland Avenue
Costa Mesa, CA 92626
(714)545-0100

Rev. 7/94

BENOQUIN® CREAM 20% ℞
(Monobenzone, Cream)

FEDERAL (U.S.A.) LAW PROHIBITS DISPENSING WITHOUT PRESCRIPTION.

FOR EXTERNAL USE ONLY

DESCRIPTION

Monobenzone is the monobenzyl ether of hydroquinone. Monobenzone occurs as a white, almost tasteless crystalline powder, soluble in alcohol and practically insoluble in water. Chemically, monobenzone is designated as p-(benzyloxy)phenol; the empirical formula is $C_{13}H_{12}O_2$; molecular weight 200.24. The structural formula is:

$C_{13}H_{12}O_2$ 200.24

Each gram of Benoquin Cream contains 200 mg of monobenzone USP, in a water-washable base consisting of purified water USP, cetyl alcohol NF, propylene glycol USP, sodium lauryl sulfate NF and white wax NF.

CLINICAL PHARMACOLOGY

Benoquin Cream 20% is a depigmenting agent whose mechanism of action is not fully understood.

The topical application of monobenzone in animals, increases the excretion of melanin from the melanocytes. The same action is thought to be responsible for the depigmenting effect of the drug in humans. Monobenzone may cause destruction of melanocytes and permanent depigmentation. This effect is erratic and may take one to four months to occur while existing melanin is lost with normal sloughing of the stratum corneum. Hyperpigmented skin appears to fade more rapidly than does normal skin, and exposure to sunlight reduces the depigmenting effect of the drug. The histology of the skin after depigmentation with topical monobenzone is the same as that seen in vitiligo; the epidermis is normal except for the absence of identifiable melanocytes.

INDICATIONS AND USAGE

Benoquin Cream 20% is indicated for final depigmentation in extensive Vitiligo.

Benoquin Cream 20% is applied topically to permanently depigment normal skin surrounding vitiliginous lesions in patients with disseminated (greater than 50 percent of body surface area) idiopathic vitiligo.

Benoquin Cream 20% is not recommended in freckling; hyperpigmentation caused by photosensitization following the use of certain perfumes (berlock dermatitis); melasma (chloasma) of pregnancy; or hyperpigmentation resulting from inflammation of the skin. Benoquin Cream 20% is not effective for the treatment of cafe-au-lait spots, pigmented nevi, malignant melanoma or pigmentation resulting from pigments other than melanin (e.g.: bile, silver, or artificial pigments).

CONTRAINDICATIONS

Benoquin Cream 20% contains a potent depigmenting agent and is not a cosmetic skin bleach. Use of Benoquin Cream 20% is contraindicated in any conditions other than disseminated vitiligo. Benoquin Cream 20% frequently produces irreversible depigmentation, and it must not be used as a substitute for hydroquinone.

Benoquin Cream 20% is also contraindicated in individuals with a history of sensitivity or allergic reactions to this product, or any of its ingredients.

WARNINGS

Benoquin Cream 20% is a potent depigmenting agent, not a mild cosmetic bleach. Do not use except for final depigmentation in extensive vitiligo.

Keep this, and all medications out of the reach of children. In case of accidental ingestion, call a physician or a Poison Control Center immediately.

PRECAUTIONS (See Warnings)

General. Benoquin Cream 20% is for External Use Only. Following therapy with Benoquin Cream 20%, the skin will be sensitive for the rest of the patient's life. He/she must use sunscreens during exposure to the sun.

Information for the Patient. Benoquin Cream 20% contains a potent depigmenting agent and is not a cosmetic skin bleach. Use of Benoquin Cream 20% is contraindicated in any conditions other than disseminated vitiligo. Use only for final depigmentation in extensive vitiligo. Areas of normal skin distant to the site of Benoquin Cream 20% application may become depigmented, and irregular, excessive, unsightly, and frequently permanent depigmentation may occur.

Carcinogenesis, mutagenesis, impairment of fertility. No long term studies have been performed to evaluate carcinogenic potential.

Pregnancy: Category C. Animal reproduction studies have not been conducted with Benoquin Cream 20%. It is also not known whether Benoquin Cream 20% can cause fetal harm when administered to a pregnant woman, or can affect reproduction capacity. Benoquin Cream 20% should be given to a pregnant woman only if clearly needed.

Nursing Mothers. It is not known whether this drug is excreted in human milk. Because many drugs are excreted in human milk, caution should be exercised when Benoquin Cream 20% is administered to a nursing woman.

Pediatric Use. The safety and effectiveness of Benoquin Cream 20% in pediatric patients below the age of 12 years have not been established.

ADVERSE REACTIONS

Mild, transient skin irritation and sensitization, including erythematous and eczematous reactions have occurred following topical application of Benoquin Cream 20%. Although those reactions are usually transient, treatment with Benoquin Cream 20% should be discontinued if irritation, a burning sensation, or dermatitis occur. Areas of normal skin distant to the site of Benoquin Cream 20% appli-

cation frequently have become depigmented, and irregular, excessive, unsightly, and frequently permanent depigmentation has occurred.

DOSAGE AND ADMINISTRATION

A thin layer of Benoquin Cream 20% should be applied and rubbed into the pigmented area two or three times daily, or as directed by a physician. Prolonged exposure to sunlight should be avoided during treatment with Benoquin Cream 20%, or a sunscreen should be used.

Depigmentation is usually accomplished after one to four months of Benoquin Cream 20% treatment. If satisfactory results are not obtained after four months of Benoquin Cream 20% treatment, the drug should be discontinued. When the desired degree of depigmentation is obtained, Benoquin Cream 20% should be applied only as often as needed to maintain depigmentation (usually only two times weekly).

HOW SUPPLIED

Benoquin Cream 20% in $1^1/_4$ oz. tubes (35.4 g) (NDC 0187-0380-34).

Benoquin Cream 20% should be stored at room temperature (15–30°C) (59–86°F)

ICN Pharmaceuticals, Inc.
3300 Hyland Ave.
Costa Mesa, CA 92626
(714) 545–0100
Rev. 4-96
2393-03EL

EFUDEX ® ℞
[*ef 'u-dex*]
brand of fluorouracil
TOPICAL SOLUTIONS AND CREAM

**For Topical Dermatological Use Only —
Not for Ophthalmic Use**

DESCRIPTION

Efudex Solutions and Cream are topical preparations containing the fluorinated pyrimidine 5-fluorouracil, an antineoplastic antimetabolite.

Efudex Solution consists of 2% or 5% fluorouracil on a weight/weight basis, compounded with propylene glycol, tris(hydroxymethyl)aminomethane, hydroxypropylcellulose, parabens (methyl and propyl) and disodium edetate.

Efudex Cream contains 5% fluorouracil in a vanishing cream base consisting of white petrolatum, stearyl alcohol, propylene glycol, polysorbate 60 and parabens (methyl and propyl).

Chemically, fluorouracil is 5-fluoro-2,4(1H,3H)-pyrimidinedione. It is a white to practically white, crystalline powder which is sparingly soluble in water and slightly soluble in alcohol. One gram of fluorouracil is soluble in 100 mL of propylene glycol. The molecular weight of 5-fluorouracil is 130.08 and the structural formula is:

CLINICAL PHARMACOLOGY

There is evidence that the metabolism of fluorouracil in the anabolic pathway blocks the methylation reaction of deoxyuridylic acid to thymidylic acid. In this manner fluorouracil interferes with the synthesis of deoxyribonucleic acid (DNA) and to a lesser extent inhibits the formation of ribonucleic acid (RNA). Since DNA and RNA are essential for cell division and growth, the effect of fluorouracil may be to create a thymine deficiency which provokes unbalanced growth and death of the cell. The effects of DNA and RNA deprivation are most marked on those cells which grow more rapidly and take up fluorouracil at a more rapid rate. The catabolic metabolism of fluorouracil results in degradation products (eg, CO_2, urea, α-fluoro-β-alanine) which are inactive.

Systemic absorption studies of topically applied fluorouracil have been performed on patients with actinic keratoses using tracer amounts of ^{14}C-labeled fluorouracil added to a 5% preparation. All patients had been receiving nonlabeled fluorouracil until the peak of the inflammatory reaction occurred (2 to 3 weeks), ensuring that the time of maximum absorption was used for measurement. One gram of labeled preparation was applied to the entire face and neck and left in place for 12 hours. Urine samples were collected. At the end of 3 days, the total recovery ranged between 0.48% and 0.94% with an average of 0.76%, indicating that approximately 5.98% of the topical dose was absorbed systematically. If applied twice daily, this would indicate systemic absorption of topical fluorouracil to be in the range of 5 to 6 mg per daily dose of 100 mg. In an additional study, negligible

amounts of labeled material were found in plasma, urine and expired CO_2 after 3 days of treatment with topically applied ^{14}C-labeled fluorouracil.

INDICATIONS AND USAGE

Efudex is recommended for the topical treatment of actinic or solar keratoses. In the 5% strength it is also useful in the treatment of superficial basal cell carcinomas when conventional methods are impractical, such as with multiple lesions or difficult treatment sites. Safety and efficacy in other indications have not been established.

The diagnosis should be established prior to treatment, since this method has not been proven effective in other types of basal cell carcinomas. With isolated, easily accessible basal cell carcinomas, surgery is preferred since success with such lesions is almost 100%. The success rate with Efudex Cream and Solution is approximately 93%, based on 113 lesions in 54 patients.Twenty-five lesions treated with the solution produced 1 failure and 88 lesions treated with the cream produced 7 failures.

CONTRAINDICATIONS

Efudex may cause fetal harm when administered to a pregnant woman.

There are no adequate and well-controlled studies in pregnant women with either the topical or parenteral forms of fluorouracil. One birth defect (cleft lip and palate) has been reported in the newborn of a patient using Efudex as recommended. One birth defect (ventricular septal defect) and cases of miscarriage have been reported when Efudex was applied to mucous membrane areas. Multiple birth defects have been reported in a fetus of a patient treated with intravenous fluorouracil.

Animal reproduction studies have not been conducted with Efudex. Fluorouracil administered parenterally has been shown to be teratogenic in mice, rats, and hamsters when given at doses equivalent to the usual human intravenous dose; however, the amount of fluorouracil absorbed systemically after topical administration to actinic keratoses is minimal (see CLINICAL PHARMACOLOGY). Fluorouracil exhibited maximum teratogenicity when given to mice as single intraperitoneal injections of 10 to 40 mg/kg on Day 10 or 12 of gestation. Similarly, intraperitoneal doses of 12 to 37 mg/kg given to rats between Days 9 and 12 of gestation and intramuscular doses of 3 to 9 mg/kg given to hamsters between Days 8 and 11 of gestation were teratogenic and/or embryotoxic (ie, resulted in increased resorptions or embryolethality). In monkeys, divided doses of 40 mg/kg given between Days 20 and 24 of gestation were not teratogenic. Doses higher than 40 mg/kg resulted in abortion.

Efudex is contraindicated in women who are or may become pregnant during therapy. If this drug is used during pregnancy, or if the patient becomes pregnant while using this drug, the patient should be apprised of the potential hazard to the fetus.

Efudex is also contraindicated in patients with known hypersensitivity to any of its components.

WARNINGS: Application to mucous membranes should be avoided due to the possibility of local inflammation and ulceration. Additionally, cases of miscarriage and a birth defect (ventricular septal defect) have been reported when Efudex was applied to mucous membrane areas during pregnancy.

Occlusion of the skin with resultant hydration has been shown to increase precutaneous penetration of several topical preparations. If any occlusive dressing is used in treatment of basal cell carcinoma, there may be an increase in the severity of inflammatory reactions in the adjacent normal skin. A porous gauze dressing may be applied for cosmetic reasons without increase in reaction.

Exposure to ultraviolet rays should be minimized during and immediately following treatment with Efudex because the intensity of the reaction may be increased.

PRECAUTIONS: *General:* There is a possibility of increased absorption through ulcerated or inflamed skin.

Information for Patients: Patients should be forewarned that the reaction in the treated areas may be unsightly during therapy and, usually, for several weeks following cessation of therapy. Patients should be instructed to avoid exposure to ultraviolet rays during and immediately following treatment with Efudex because the intensity of the reaction may be increased. If Efudex is applied with the fingers, the hands should be washed immediately afterward. Efudex should not be applied on the eyelids or directly into the eyes, nose or mouth because irritation may occur.

Laboratory Tests: Solar keratoses which do not respond should be biopsied to confirm the diagnosis. Follow-up biopsies should be performed as indicated in the management of superficial basal cell carcinoma.

Carcinogenesis, Mutagenesis, Impairment of Fertility: Adequate long-term studies in animals to evaluate carcinogenic potential have not been conducted with fluorouracil. Studies with the active ingredient of Efudex, 5-fluorouracil, have shown positive effects in in vitro tests for mutagenicity and on impairment of fertility.

5-Fluorouracil was positive in three in vitro cell neoplastic transformation assays. In the C3H/10T½ clone 8 mouse embryo cell system, the resulting morphologically transformed cells formed tumors when inoculated into immunosuppressed syngeneic mice.

While no evidence for mutagenic activity was observed in the Ames test (3 studies), fluorouracil has been shown to be mutagenic in the survival count rec-assay with *Bacillus subtilis* and in the Drosophilia wing-hair spot test. Fluorouracil produced petite mutations in *Saccharomyces cerevisiae* and was positive in the mironucleus test (bone marrow cells of male mice).

Fluorouracil was clastogenic in vitro (ie, chromatid gaps, breaks and exchanges) in Chinese hamster fibroblasts at concentrations of 1.0 and 2.0 µg/mL and has been shown to increase sister chromatid exchange in vitro in human lymphocytes. In addition, 5-fluorouracil has been reported to produce an increase in numerical and structural chromosome aberrations in peripheral lymphocytes of patients with this product.

Doses of 125 to 250 mg/kg, administered intraperitoneally, have been shown to induce chromosomal aberrations and changes in chromosome organization of spermatogonia in rats. Spermatogonial differentiation was also inhibited by fluorouracil, resulting in transient infertility. However, in studies with a strain of mouse which is sensitive to the induction of sperm head abnormalities after exposure to a range of chemical mutagens and carcinogens, fluorouracil was inactive at oral doses of 5 to 80 mg/kg/day. In female rats, fluorouracil administered intraperitoneally at doses of 25 and 50 mg/kg during the preovulatory phase of oogenesis significantly reduced the incidence of fertile matings, delayed the development of preimplantation and postimplantation embryos, increased the incidence of preimplantation lethality and induced chromosomal anomalies in these embryos. Single dose intravenous and intraperitoneal injections of 5-fluorouracil have been reported to kill differentiated spermatogonia and spermatocytes (at 500 mg/kg) and to produce abnormalities in spermatids (at 50 mg/kg) in mice.

Pregnancy: Pregnancy: **Teratogenic Effects: Pregnancy Category X:** See CONTRAINDICATIONS section.

Nursing Mothers: It is not known whether Efudex is excreted in human milk. Because there is some systemic absorption of fluorouracil after topical administration (see CLINICAL PHARMACOLOGY), because many drugs are excreted in human milk, and because of the potential for serious adverse reactions in nursing infants, a decision should be made whether to discontinue nursing or to discontinue use of the drug, taking into account the importance of the drug to the mother.

Pediatric Use: Safety and effectiveness in children have not been established.

ADVERSE REACTIONS

The most frequent adverse reactions to Efudex occur locally and are often related to an extension of the pharmacological activity of the drug. These include burning, crusting, allergic contact dermatitis, erosions, erythema, hyperpigmentation, irritation, pain, photosensitivity, pruritus, scarring, rash, soreness and ulceration. Ulcerations, other local reactions, cases of miscarriage and a birth defect (ventricular septal defect) have been reported when Efudex was applied to mucous membrane areas. Leukocytosis is the most frequent hematological side effect.

Although a causal relationship is remote, other adverse reactions which have been reported infrequently are:

Central Nervous System: Emotional upset, insomnia, irritability.

Gastrointestinal: Medicinal taste, stomatitis.

Hematological: Eosinophilia, thrombocytopenia, toxic granulation.

Integumentary: Alopecia, blistering, bullous pemphigoid, discomfort, ichthyosis, scaling, suppuration, swelling, telangiectasia, tenderness, urticaria, skin rash.

Special Senses: Conjunctival reaction, corneal reaction, lacrimation, nasal irritaiton.

Miscellaneous: Herpes simplex.

OVERDOSAGE

There have been no reports of overdosage with Efudex. The oral LD_{50} for the 5% topical cream was 234 mg/kg in rats and 39 mg/kg in dogs. These doses represented 11.7 and 1.95 mg/kg of fluorouracil, respectively. Studies with a 5% topical solution yielded an oral LD_{50} of 214 mg/kg in rats and 28.5 in dogs, corresponding to 10.7 and 14.3 mg/kg of fluorouracil, respectively. The topical application of the 5% cream to rats yielded an LD_{50} of greater than 500 mg/kg.

DOSAGE AND ADMINISTRATION

When Efudex is applied to a lesion, a response occurs with the following sequence; erythema, usually followed by vesiculation, desquamation, erosion and reepithelialization.

Efudex should be applied preferably with a nonmetal applicator or suitable glove. If Efudex is applied with the fingers, the hands should be washed immediately afterward.

Actinic or Solar Keratosis: Apply cream or solution twice daily in an amount sufficient to cover the lesions. Medication should be continued until the inflammatory response reaches the erosion state, at which time use of the drug should be terminated. The usual duraton of therapy is from 2 to 4 weeks. Complete healing of the lesions may not be evident for 1 to 2 months following cessation of Efudex therapy.

Superficial Basal Cell Carcinomas: **Only the 5% strength is recommended.** Apply cream or solution twice daily in an amount sufficient to cover the lesions. Treatment should be continued for at least 3 to 6 weeks. Therapy may be required for as long as 10 to 12 weeks before the lesions are obliterated. As in any neoplastic condition, the patient should be followed for a reasonable period of time to determine if a cure has been obtained.

HOW SUPPLIED

Efudex Solution is available in 10-mL drop dispensers containing either 2% (NDC 0187-3202-10) or 5% (NDC 0187-3203-10 fluorouracil on a weight/weight basis compounded with propylene glycol, tris(hydroxymethyl)aminomethane, hyroxypropyl cellulose, parabens (methyl and propyl) and disodium edetate.

Efudex Cream is available in 25-gm tubes containing 5% fluorouracil (NDC 0187-3204-26) in a vanishing cream base consisting of white petrolatum, stearyl alcohol, propylene glycol, polysorbate 60 and parabens (methyl and propyl).

Store at 25°C (77°F); excursion permitted to 15°C–30°C (59°F–86°F).

Manufactured for ICN Pharmaceuticals Inc.
Costa Mesa, CA 92626
by Hoffman-La Roche Inc.
Nutley, N.J. 07110
ICN Pharmaceuticals, Inc.
ICN Plaza
3300 Hyland Avenue
Costa Mesa, California 92626
714-545-0100

Revised: February 1998

ELDOQUIN FORTE® 4% Cream ℞
(Hydroquinone USP, 4%)
(Skin Bleaching Cream)
ELDOPAQUE FORTE® 4% Cream
(Hydroquinone USP, 4%)
(Skin Bleaching Cream with Sunblock)
SOLAQUIN FORTE® 4% Cream
(Hydroquinone USP, 4%)
(Skin Bleaching Cream with Sunscreens, SPF 17)
SOLAQUIN FORTE® 4% Gel
(Hydroquinone USP, 4%)
(Skin Bleaching Gel with Sunscreens)

FOR EXTERNAL USE ONLY

DESCRIPTION

Hydroquinone is 1,4-benzenediol. Hydroquinone is structurally related to monobenzone. Hydroquinone occurs as fine, white needles. The drug is freely soluble in water and in alcohol and has a pK_a of 9.96. Chemically, hydroquinone is designated as p-dihydroxybenzene; the empirical formula is $C_6H_6O_2$; molecular weight 110.0.

The structural formula is:

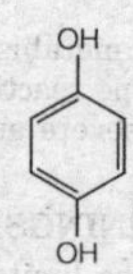

$C_6H_6O_2$

Each gram of Eldoquin Forte 4% Cream contains 40 mg of Hydroquinone USP in a vanishing cream base of purified water USP, stearic acid NF, propylene glycol USP, polyoxyl 40 stearate NF, polyoxyethylene (25) propylene glycol stearate, glycerol monostearate, light mineral oil NF, squalane NF, propylparaben NF and sodium metabisulfite NF.

Each gram of Eldopaque Forte 4% Cream contains 40 mg of Hydroquinone USP in a tinted sunblocking cream base of purified water USP, stearic acid NF, talc USP, polyoxyl 40 stearate NF, polyoxyethylene (25) propylene glycol stearate, propylene glycol USP, glycerol monostearate, iron oxides, light mineral oil NF, squalane NF, edetate disodium USP, sodium metabisulfite NF and potassium sorbate NF.

Each gram of Solaquin Forte 4% Cream contains 40 mg of Hydroquinone USP, 80 mg Padimate O USP, 30 mg Dioxybenzone USP and 20 mg Oxybenzone USP in a vanishing cream base of purified water USP, glycerol monostearate and polyoxyethylene stearate, ootyldodecyl stearoyl stearate, glyceryl dilaurate, quaternium-26, cetearyl alcohol and ceteareth-20, stearyl alcohol NF, propylene glycol USP, diethylaminoethyl stearate, polydimethylsiloxane, polysor-

Continued on next page

Eldoquin/Eldopaque/Solaquin—Cont.

bate 80 NF, lactic acid USP, ascorbic acid USP, hydroxyethyl cellulose, quaternium-14 and myristalkonium chloride, edetate disodium USP and sodium metabisulfite NF.
Each gram of Solaquin Forte 4% Gel contains 40 mg of Hydroquinone USP, 50 mg of Padimate O USP and 30 mg Dioxybenzone USP, in a hydro-alcoholic base of alcohol USP, purified water USP, propylene glycol USP, entprol, carbomer 940, edetate disodium USP and sodium metabisulfite NF.

CLINICAL PHARMACOLOGY

Topical application of hydroquinone produces a reversible depigmentation of the skin by inhibition of the enzymatic oxidation of tyrosine to 3,4-dihydroxyphenylalanine (dopa) (Denton, C. et al., 1952)[1] and suppression of other melanocyte metabolic processes (Jimbow, K. et al., 1974).[2] Exposure to sunlight or ultraviolet light will cause repigmentation of bleached areas which may be prevented by the sunblocking agents contained in Eldopaque Forte 4% Cream and by the broad spectrum sunscreen agents contained in Solaquin Forte 4% Cream and Solaquin Forte 4% Gel (Parrish, J.A. et al., 1978).[3]

INDICATIONS AND USAGE

For the gradual bleaching of hyperpigmented skin conditions such as chloasma, melasma, freckles, senile lentigines and other unwanted areas of melanin hyperpigmentation.

CONTRAINDICATIONS

Prior history of sensitivity or allergic reaction to these products or any of the ingredients. The safety of topical hydroquinone use during pregnancy or in children (12 years and under) has not been established.

WARNINGS

Caution: Hydroquinone is a skin bleaching agent which may produce unwanted cosmetic effects if not used as directed. The physician should be familiar with the contents of the package insert before prescribing or dispensing these medications.
Test for skin sensitivity before using by applying a small amount to an unbroken patch of skin and check in 24 hours. Minor redness is not a contraindication, but where there is itching or vesicle formation or excessive inflammatory response, further treatment is not advised. Close patient supervision is recommended. Contact with the eyes should be avoided. If no bleaching or lightening effect is noted after 2 months of treatment use, the medication should be discontinued. Eldoquin Forte 4% Cream, Eldopaque Forte 4% Cream, Solaquin Forte 4% Cream and Solaquin Forte 4% Gel are formulated for use as skin bleaching agents and should not be used for the prevention of sunburn.
Sunscreen use is an essential aspect of hydroquinone therapy because even minimal sunlight sustains melanocytic activity. The sunblock in Eldopaque Forte 4% Cream and the sunscreens in Solaquin Forte 4% Cream, and Solaquin Forte 4% Gel provide the necessary sun protection during skin bleaching therapy.
After clearing and during maintenance therapy, sun exposure should be avoided on bleached skin by application of a sunscreen or sunblock agent or protective clothing to prevent repigmentation
Keep this and all medication out of the reach of children. In case of accidental ingestion, call a physician or a poison control center immediately.
Warning: Contains sodium metabisulfite, a sulfite that may cause serious allergic type reactions (e.g., hives, itching, wheezing, anaphylaxis, severe asthma attack) in certain susceptible persons.

PRECAUTIONS (SEE WARNINGS)

General. Treatment should be limited to relatively small areas of the body at one time since some patients experience a transient skin reddening and a mild burning sensation which does not preclude treatment.
Pregnancy Category C. Animal reproduction studies have not been conducted with topical hydroquinone. It is also not known whether hydroquinone can cause fetal harm when used topically on a pregnant woman or affect reproductive capacity. It is not known to what degree, if any, topical hydroquinone is absorbed systemically. Topical hydroquinone should be used in pregnant women only when clearly indicated.
Nursing mothers. It is not known whether topical hydroquinone is absorbed or excreted in human milk. Caution is advised when topical hydroquinone is used by a nursing mother.
Pediatric usage. Safety and effectiveness in pediatric patients below the age of 12 years have not been established.

ADVERSE REACTIONS

No systemic adverse reactions have been reported. Occasional hypersensitivity (localized contact dermatitis) may occur, in which case the medication should be discontinued and the physician notified immediately.

DOSAGE AND ADMINISTRATION

Solaquin Forte 4% Cream and Solaquin Forte 4% Gel should be applied to the affected area and rubbed in well twice daily or as directed by a physician.
Eldopaque Forte 4% Cream should be applied to the affected area twice daily or as directed by a physician. Do not rub in.
Eldoquin Forte 4% Cream should be applied to the affected area and rubbed in well twice daily or as directed by a physician. During the day, an effective broad spectrum sunscreen should be used and unnecessary solar exposure avoided, or protective clothing should be worn to cover bleached skin in order to prevent repigmentation from occurring.

HOW SUPPLIED

ELDOQUIN FORTE 4% CREAM is available as follows:

SIZE	NDC NUMBER
1.0 ounce tube (28.4 grams)	0187-0394-31

ELDOPAQUE FORTE 4% CREAM is available as follows:

SIZE	NDC NUMBER
1.0 ounce tube (28.4 grams)	0187-0395-31

SOLAQUIN FORTE 4% CREAM is available as follows:

SIZE	NDC NUMBER
1.0 ounce tube (28.4 grams)	0187-0396-31

SOLAQUIN FORTE 4% GEL is available as follows:

SIZE	NDC NUMBER
1.0 ounce tube (28.4 grams)	0187-0523-31

Store at 25°C (77°F); excursion permitted to 15°C–30°C (59°–86°F)
Rx only

REFERENCES

1. Denton, C., A.B. Lerner and T.B. Fitzpatrick, "Inhibition of Melanin Formation by Chemical Agents," *Journal of Investigative Dermatology*, 18:119–135, 1952.
2. Jimbow, K., H. Obata, M. Pathak and T.B. Fitzpatrick, "Mechanism of Depigmentation by Hydroquinone," *Journal of Investigative Dermatology*, 62:436–449, 1974.
3. Parrish, J.A., R.R. Anderson, F. Urbach, D. Pitts, "UVA, Biological Effects of Ultraviolet Radiation with Emphasis on Human Responses to Longwave Ultraviolet," *Plenum Press*, New York and London, 1978, p. 151.

2614-00 EL Orig. 8/97
ICN PHARMACEUTICALS, INC.
3300 Hyland Avenue
Costa Mesa, CA 92626, U.S.A.
(714) 545-0100

FOTOTAR® CREAM OTC
PSORIASIS AND SEBORRHEIC DERMATITIS CREAM

DESCRIPTION

FOTOTAR® Cream contains coal tar extract (equivalent to 2% Coal Tar, USP) in an emollient, moisturizing cream base.

INDICATIONS

For the relief of itching, irritation, and skin flaking associated with psoriasis and seborrheic dermatitis.

CONTRAINDICATIONS

FOTOTAR® Cream is contraindicated in patients with a history of sensitivity to this product or to other coal tar products. FOTOTAR® Cream should not be used on patients who have a disease characterized by photosensitivity, such as lupus erythematosus or allergy to sunlight.

DIRECTIONS FOR USE

Apply to affected areas one to four times daily or as directed by a physician.

WARNINGS

FOR EXTERNAL USE ONLY.
Avoid contact with eyes. If contact occurs, rinse eyes thoroughly with water. If condition worsens or does not improve after regular use of this product as directed, consult a physician. Use caution in exposing skin to sunlight after applying this product. It may increase your tendency to sunburn for up to 24 hours after application. Do not use this product in or around the rectum or in the genital area or groin except on the advice of a physician. Do not use for prolonged periods without consulting a physician. Do not use this product with other forms of psoriasis therapy, such as ultraviolet radiation or prescription drugs, unless directed by a physician. If condition covers a large area of the body, consult your physician before using this product.
Keep out of reach of children. In case of accidental ingestion, seek professional assistance or contact a Poison Control Center immediately.

PRECAUTIONS

Staining of clothing may occur which is normally removed by standard laundry methods. Use on the scalp may cause temporary staining of light colored hair.

HOW SUPPLIED

FOTOTAR® Cream is available as follows:

SIZE	NDC NUMBER
3.0 oz. (85.05g) Tube	0187-0526-03
1 lb. (453g) Jar	0187-0526-05

STORAGE
FOTOTAR® Cream should be stored at controlled room temperature (15°– 30°C) 59°– 86°F.
Manufactured by
ICN PHARMACEUTICALS, INC.
3300 Hyland Ave.
Costa Mesa, CA 92626
U.S.A.
239–03EL Rev. 3/96

LEVO-DROMORAN® Ⓒ℞
[lee "vo dro 'mo-ran]
brand of
levorphanol tartrate
AMPULS, VIALS, TABLETS

WARNING: May be habit forming

DESCRIPTION

Levo-Dromoran (levorphanol tartrate) is a potent opioid analgesic with empirical formula $C_{17}H_{23}NO{\cdot}C_4H_6O_6{\cdot}2H_2O$ and molecular weight 443.5. Each mg of levorphanol tartrate is equivalent to 0.58 mg levorphanol base. Chemically levorphanol is levo-3-hydroxy-N-methylmorphinan. The USP nomenclature is 17-methylmorphinan 3-ol tartrate (1:1)(Salt) dihydrate. The material has 3 asymmetric carbon atoms.
Levorphanol tartrate is a white crystalline powder, soluble in water and ether but insoluble in chloroform.
Each 1-mL ampul contains 2 mg levorphanol tartrate, 1.8 mg methyl paraben preservative, 0.2 mg propyl paraben preservative, sodium hydroxide to adjust pH to approximately 4.3 and Water for Injection.
Each milliliter in the 10 mL vials contains 2 mg levorphanol tartrate, 4.5 mg phenol preservative, sodium hydroxide to adjust pH to approximately 4.3 and Water for Injection.
Each tablet contains 2 mg levorphanol tartrate, lactose, corn starch, stearic acid and talc.

CLINICAL PHARMACOLOGY

Pharmacodynamics: Levo-Dromoran is a potent synthetic opioid similar to morphine in its actions. Like other mu-agonist opioids it is believed to act at receptors in the periventricular and periaqueductal gray matter in both the brain and spinal cord to alter the transmission and perception of pain. Onset of analgesia and peak analgesic effect following administration of levorphanol are similar to morphine when administered at equianalgesic doses.
Levorphanol produces a degree of respiratory depression similar to that produced by morphine at equianalgesic doses, and like many mu-opioid drugs, levorphanol produces euphoria or has a positive effect on mood in many individuals. Two mg of intramuscular levorphanol tartrate depresses respiration to a degree approximately equivalent to that produced by 10 to 15 mg of intramuscular morphine in man. The hemodynamic changes after intravenous administration of levorphanol have not been studied in man but are expected to clinically resemble those seen after morphine.
As with other opioids, the blood levels required for analgesia are determined by the opioid tolerance of the patient and are likely to rise with chronic use. The rate of development of tolerance is highly variable and is determined by the dose, dosing interval, age, use of concomitant drugs and physical status of the patient. While blood levels of opioid drugs may be helpful in assessing individual cases, dosage is usually adjusted by careful clinical observation of the patient.
Pharmacokinetics: The pharmacokinetics of levorphanol have been studied in a limited number of cancer patients following intravenous (IV), intramuscular (IM) and oral (PO) administration. Following IV administration, plasma concentrations of levorphanol decline in a triexponential manner with a terminal half-life of approximately 11 to 16 hours and a clearance of 0.78 to 1.1 L/kg/hr. Based on terminal half-life, steady-state plasma concentrations should be achieved by the third day of dosing. Levorphanol is rapidly distributed (<1 hr) and redistributed (1 to 2 hours) following IV administration and has a steady-state volume of distribution of 10 to 13 L/kg. In vitro studies of protein binding indicate that levorphanol is only 40% bound to plasma proteins.
No pharmacokinetic studies of the absorption of IM levorphanol are available, but clinical data suggests that absorption is rapid with onset of effects within 15 to 30 minutes of administration.
Levorphanol is well absorbed after PO administration with peak plasma concentrations occurring approximately 1 hour after dosing. The bioavailability of levorphanol tablets compared to IM or IV administration is not known.

Plasma concentrations of levorphanol following chronic administration in patients with cancer increased with the dose, but the analgesic effect was dependent on the degree of opioid tolerance of the patient. Expected steady-state plasma concentrations for a 6-hour dosing interval can reach 2 to 5 times those following a single dose, depending on the patient's individual clearance of the drug. Very high plasma concentrations of levorphanol can be reached in patients on chronic therapy due to the long half-life of the drug. One study in 11 patients using the drug for control of cancer pain reported plasma concentrations from 5 to 10 ng/mL after a single 2-mg dose up to 50 to 100 ng/mL after repeated oral doses of 20 to 50 mg/day.

Animal studies suggest that levorphanol is extensively metabolized in the liver and is eliminated as the glucuronide metabolite. This renally excreted inactive glucuronide metabolite accumulates with chronic dosing in plasma at concentrations that reach fivefold that of the parent compound.

The effects of age, gender, hepatic and renal disease on the pharmacokinetics of levorphanol are not known. As with all drugs of this class, patients at the extremes of age are expected to be more susceptible to adverse effects because of a greater pharmacodynamic sensitivity and probable increased variability in pharmacokinetics due to age or disease.

CLINICAL TRIALS

Clinical trials have been reported in the medical literature that investigated the use of Levo-Dromoran as a preoperative medication, as a postoperative analgesic and in the management of chronic pain due primarily to malignancy. In each of these clinical settings Levo-Dromoran has been shown to be an effective analgesic of the mu-opioid type and similar to morphine, meperidine or fentanyl.

A single 2 mg intramuscular dose of Levo-Dromoran was studied as a routine preoperative medication in 100 patients as part of a blinded 1500 patient trial of a number of synthetic opioids and was found to provide sedation similar to that observed with 100 mg meperidine or 10 mg of methadone.

Levo-Dromoran has been studied in chronic cancer patients. Dosages were individualized to each patient's level of opioid tolerance. In one study, starting doses of 2 mg twice a day often had to be advanced by 50% or more within a few weeks of starting therapy. A study of levorphanol indicates that the relative potency is approximately 4 to 8 times that of morphine, depending on the specific circumstances of use. In postoperative patients, intramuscular levorphanol was determined to be about 8 times as potent as intramuscular morphine, whereas in cancer patients with chronic pain, it was found to be only about 4 times as potent.

INDIVIDUALIZATION OF DOSAGE

Accepted medical practice dictates that the dose of any opioid analgesic be appropriate to the degree of pain to be relieved, the clinical setting, the physical condition of the patient, and the kind and dose of concurrent medication. This is especially important during recovery from anesthesia because of the residual CNS-depressant effects of anesthetic agents and the adverse effects of surgery on respiratory reserve. In consequence, the dose of Levo-Dromoran should be reduced under circumstances likely to increase the patient's sensitivity to the adverse effects of opioids. As there is substantial redistribution involved in the kinetics of levorphanol, the duration of effect of a single dose may vary and physicians must judge the need for a repeat dose based on the clinical response of the patient. Clinicians are advised to remember that while the long terminal half-life of levorphanol may reduce the need for postoperative analgesics, the administration of an excessive dose preoperatively may cause a delay in the return of spontaneous respirations or prolonged hypoventilation in the postoperative period. In addition, accumulation of the drug following excessive dosage postoperatively may prolong or result in hypoventilation.

Levo-Dromoran has a long half-life similar to methadone or other slowly excreted opioids, rather than quickly excreted agents such as morphine or meperidine. Slowly excreted drugs may have some advantages in the management of chronic pain. Unfortunately, the duration of pain relief after a single dose of a slowly excreted opioid cannot always be predicted from pharmacokinetic principles, and the interdose interval may have to be adjusted to suit the patient's individual pharmacodynamic response.

Levo-Dromoran is 4 to 8 times as potent as morphine and has a longer half-life. Because there is incomplete cross-tolerance among opioids, when converting a patient from morphine to Levo-Dromoran, the total *daily* dose of oral Levo-Dromoran should begin at approximately $1/15$ to $1/12$ of the total *daily* dose of oral morphine that such patients had previously required and then the dose should be adjusted to the patient's clinical response. If a patient is to be placed on fixed-schedule dosing (round-the-clock) with this drug, care should be taken to allow adequate time after each dose change (approximately 72 hours) for the patient to reach a new steady-state before a subsequent dose adjustment to avoid excessive sedation due to drug accumulation.

INDICATIONS

Levo-Dromoran is indicated for the management of moderate to severe pain or as a preoperative medication where an opioid analgesic is appropriate.

CONTRAINDICATIONS

Levo-Dromoran is contraindicated in patients hypersensitive to levorphanol tartrate.

WARNINGS

Respiratory Depression: Levo-Dromoran, like morphine, may be expected to produce serious or potentially fatal respiratory depression if given in an excessive dose, too frequently, or if given in full dosage to compromised or vulnerable patients. This is because the doses required to produce analgesia in the general clinical population may cause serious respiratory depression in vulnerable patients. Safe usage of this potent opioid requires that the dose and dosage interval be individualized to each patient based on the severity of the pain, weight, age, diagnosis and physical status of the patient, and the kind and dose of concurrently administered medication.

The initial dose of Levo-Dromoran should be reduced by 50% or more when the drug is given to patients with any condition affecting respiratory reserve or in conjunction with other drugs affecting the respiratory center. Subsequent doses should then be individually titrated according to the patient's response. Respiratory depression produced by levorphanol tartrate can be reversed by naloxone, a specific antagonist (see OVERDOSAGE).

Preexisting Pulmonary Disease: Because Levo-Dromoran causes respiratory depression, it should be administered with caution to patients with impaired respiratory reserve or respiratory depression from some other cause (eg, from other medication, uremia, severe infection, obstructive respiratory conditions, restrictive respiratory diseases, intrapulmonary shunting or chronic bronchial asthma). As with other strong opioids, use of Levo-Dromoran in acute or severe bronchial asthma is not recommended (see *Respiratory Depression*).

Head Injury and Increased Intracranial Pressure: The respiratory depressant effects of Levo-Dromoran with carbon dioxide retention and secondary elevation of cerebral spinal fluid pressure may be markedly exaggerated in the presence of head injury, other intracranial lesions or pre-existing increase in intracranial pressure. Opioids, including Levo-Dromoran, produce effects that may obscure neurological signs of further increase in pressure in patients with head injuries. In addition, Levo-Dromoran may affect level of consciousness that may complicate neurological evaluation.

Cardiovascular Effects: The use of Levo-Dromoran in acute myocardial infarction or in cardiac patients with myocardial dysfunction or coronary insufficiency should be limited because the effects of levorphanol on the work of the heart are unknown.

Hypotensive Effect: The administration of Levo-Dromoran may result in severe hypotension in the postoperative patient or in any individual whose ability to maintain blood pressure has been compromised by a depleted blood volume or by administration of drugs, such as phenothiazines or general anesthetics. Opioids may produce orthostatic hypotension in ambulatory patients.

Use in Liver Disease: Levo-Dromoran should be administered with caution to patients with extensive liver disease who may be vulnerable to excessive sedation due to increased pharmacodynamic sensitivity or impaired metabolism of the drug.

Biliary Surgery: Levo-Dromoran has been shown to cause moderate to marked rises in pressure in the common bile duct when given in analgesic doses. It is not recommended for use in biliary surgery.

Use in Alcoholism or Drug Dependence: Levo-Dromoran has an abuse potential as great as morphine, and the prescription of this drug must always balance the prospective benefits against the risk of abuse and dependence. The use of levorphanol in patients with a history of alcohol or other drug dependence, either active or in remission, has not been specifically studied (see DRUG ABUSE AND DEPENDENCE).

PRECAUTIONS

General: As with other opioids, the administration of Levo-Dromoran may obscure the diagnosis or clinical course in patients with acute abdominal conditions. Levo-Dromoran should be administered with caution and the initial dose should be reduced in patients who are elderly or debilitated and in those patients with severe impairment of hepatic or renal function, hypothyroidism, Addison's disease, toxic psychosis, prostatic hypertrophy or urethral stricture, acute alcoholism, or delirium tremens.

Information for Patients: If Levo-Dromoran is administered to ambulatory patients, they should be cautioned against engaging in hazardous occupations requiring complete mental alertness such as operating machinery or driving a motor vehicle. They should also be warned that concurrent use of Levo-Dromoran with central nervous system depressants (eg, alcohol, sedatives, hypnotics, other opioids, barbiturates, tricyclic antidepressants, phenothiazines, tranquilizers, skeletal muscle relaxants and antihistamines) may result in additive central nervous system depressant effects. Patients should be made aware of the risk of orthostatic hypotension, dizziness and syncope in ambulatory patients taking Levo-Dromoran.

Drug Interactions: *Interactions with Other CNS Agents:* Concurrent use of Levo-Dromoran with all central nervous system depressants (eg, alcohol, sedatives, hypnotics, other opioids, general anesthetics, barbiturates, tricyclic antidepressants, phenothiazines, tranquilizers, skeletal muscle relaxants and antihistamines) may result in additive central nervous system depressant effects. Respiratory depression, hypotension, and profound sedation or coma may occur. When such combined therapy is contemplated, the dose of one or both agents should be reduced. Although no interaction between MAO inhibitors and Levo-Dromoran has been observed, it is not recommended for use with MAO inhibitors.

Most cases of serious or fatal adverse events involving Levo-Dromoran reported to the manufacturer or the FDA have involved either the administration of large initial doses or too frequent doses of the drug to nonopioid tolerant patients, or the simultaneous administration of levorphanol with other drugs affecting respiration (see INDIVIDUALIZATION OF DOSAGE and WARNINGS). The initial dose of levorphanol should be reduced by approximately 50% or more when it is given to patients along with another drug affecting respiration.

Interactions with Mixed Agonist/Antagonist Opioid Analgesics: Agonist/antagonist analgesics (eg, pentazocine, nalbuphine, butorphanol, dezocine and buprenorphine) should NOT be administered to a patient who has received or is receiving a course of therapy with a pure agonist opioid analgesic such as Levo-Dromoran. In opioid-dependent patients, mixed agonist/antagonist analgesics may precipitate withdrawal symptoms.

Use in Ambulatory Patients: Levo-Dromoran has been used in both inpatient and outpatient settings, but both physicians and patients must be aware of the risk of orthostatic hypotension, dizziness and syncope in ambulatory patients.

As with other opioids, the use of Levo-Dromoran may impair mental and/or physical abilities required for the performance of potentially hazardous tasks or for the exercise of normal good judgement and patients and staff should be advised accordingly.

Concurrent use of Levo-Dromoran with central nervous system depressants (eg, alcohol, sedatives, hypnotics, other opioids, barbiturates, tricyclic antidepressants, phenothiazines, tranquilizers, skeletal muscle relaxants and antihistamines) may result in additive central nervous system depressant effects.

Carcinogenesis, Mutagenesis, Impairment of Fertility: No information about the effects of Levo-Dromoran on carcinogenesis, mutagenesis, or fertility is available.

Pregnancy: Teratogenic Effects: Pregnancy Category C. Levo-Dromoran has been shown to be teratogenic in mice when given at a single oral dose of 25 mg/kg. The tested dose caused a near 50% mortality of the mouse embryos. There are no adequate and well-controlled studies in pregnant women. Levo-Dromoran should be used in pregnancy only if the potential benefit justifies the potential risk to the fetus.

Nonteratogenic Effects: Babies born to mothers who have been taking opioids regularly prior to delivery may be physically dependent.

A study in rabbits has demonstrated that at doses of 1.5 to 20 mg/kg, Levo-Dromoran administered intravenously crosses the placental barrier and depresses fetal respiration.

Labor and Delivery: The use of Levo-Dromoran in labor and delivery in humans has not been studied. However, as with other opioids, administration of Levo-Dromoran to the mother during labor and delivery may result in respiratory depression in the newborn. Therefore, its use during labor and delivery is not recommended.

Nursing Mothers: Studies of levorphanol concentrations in breast milk have not been performed. However, morphine, which is structurally similar to levorphanol, is excreted in human milk. Because of the potential for serious adverse reactions from Levo-Dromoran in nursing infants, a decision should be made whether to discontinue nursing or to discontinue the drug, taking into account the importance of the drug to the mother.

Pediatric Use: Levo-Dromoran is not recommended in children under the age of 18 years as the safety and efficacy of the drug in this population has not been established.

Geriatric Use: The initial dose of Levo-Dromoran should be reduced by 50% or more in the infirm elderly patient, even though there have been no reports of unexpected adverse events in older populations. All drugs of this class may

Continued on next page

Levo-Dromoran—Cont.

be associated with a profound or prolonged effect in elderly patients for both pharmacokinetic and pharmacodynamic reasons and caution is indicated.

ADVERSE REACTIONS

In approximately 1400 patients treated with Levo-Dromoran in controlled clinical trials, the type and incidence of side effects were those expected of an opioid analgesic, and no unforeseen or unusual toxicity was reported.

Drugs of this type are expected to produce a cluster of typical opioid effects in addition to analgesia, consisting of nausea, vomiting, altered mood and mentation, pruritus, flushing, difficulties in urination, constipation and biliary spasm. The frequency and intensity of these effects appears to be dose related. Although listed as adverse events these are expected pharmacologic actions of these drugs and should be interpreted as such by the clinician.

The following adverse events have been reported with the use of Levo-Dromoran:

Body as a Whole: abdominal pain, dry mouth, sweating

Cardiovascular System: cardiac arrest, shock, hypotension, arrhythmias including bradycardia and tachycardia, palpitations, extra-systoles

Digestive System: nausea, vomiting, dyspepsia, biliary tract spasm

Nervous System: coma, suicide attempt, convulsions, depression, dizziness, confusion, lethargy, abnormal dreams, abnormal thinking, nervousness, drug withdrawal, hypokinesia, dyskinesia, hyperkinesia, CNS stimulation, personality disorder, amnesia, insomnia

Respiratory System: apnea, cyanosis, hypoventilation

Skin & Appendages: pruritus, urticaria, rash, injection site reaction

Special Senses: abnormal vision, pupillary disorder, diplopia

Urogenital System: kidney failure, urinary retention, difficulty urinating

DRUG ABUSE AND DEPENDENCE

Warning: May be Habit Forming

Levo-Dromoran is a Schedule II Controlled Substance. All drugs of this class (mu-opioids of the morphine type) are habit forming and should be stored, prescribed, used and disposed of accordingly. Psychological/physical dependence and tolerance may develop upon repeated administration of Levo-Dromoran.

Discontinuation of Levo-Dromoran after chronic use has been reported to result in withdrawal syndromes, and some reports of overuse and self-reported addiction have been received. Neither withdrawal nor withdrawal symptoms are usually expected in postoperative patients who used the drug for less than a week or in patients who are gradually tapered off the drug after longer use.

OVERDOSAGE

Most reports of overdosage known to the manufacturer and to the FDA involve three clinical situations. These are: 1. the use of larger than recommended doses or too frequent doses, 2. administration of the drug to children or small adults without any reduction in dosage, and 3. the use of the drug in ordinary dosage in patients compromised by concurrent illness.

As with all opioids, overdose can occur due to accidental or intentional misuse of this product, especially in infants and children who may gain access to the drug in the home. Based on its pharmacology, levorphanol overdosage would be expected to produce signs of respiratory depression, cardiovascular failure (especially in predisposed patients) and/or central nervous system depression. Serious overdosage with Levo-Dromoran is characterized by respiratory depression (a decrease in respiratory rate and/or tidal volume, periodic breathing, cyanosis), extreme somnolence progressing to stupor or coma, skeletal muscle flaccidity, cold and clammy skin, constricted pupils, and sometimes bradycardia and hypotension. In severe overdosage, apnea, circulatory collapse, cardiac arrest and death may occur.

Treatment: The specific treatment of suspected levorphanol tartrate overdosage is immediate establishment of an adequate airway and ventilation, followed (if necessary) by intravenous naloxone. The respiratory and cardiac status of the patient should be continuously monitored and appropriate supportive measures instituted, such as oxygen, intravenous fluids and/or vasopressors, if required. Physicians are reminded that the duration of levorphanol action far exceeds the duration of action of naloxone, and repeated dosing with naloxone may be required. Naloxone should be administered cautiously to persons known or suspected to be physically dependent on Levo-Dromoran. In such cases an abrupt and complete reversal of opioid effects may precipitate an acute abstinence syndrome. If necessary to administer naloxone to the physically dependent patient, the antagonist should be administered with extreme care and by titration with smaller than usual doses of the antagonist.

DOSAGE AND ADMINISTRATION

Intravenous: The usual recommended starting dose for IV administration is up to 1 mg, given in divided doses, by slow injection. This may be repeated in 3 to 6 hours as needed, provided the patient is assessed for signs of hypoventilation or excessive sedation. Dosage should be adjusted according to the severity of the pain; age, weight and physical status of the patient; the patient's underlying diseases; use of concomitant medications; and other factors (see INDIVIDUALIZATION OF DOSAGE, WARNINGS and PRECAUTIONS). Total *daily* doses or more than 4 to 8 mg IV in 24 hours are generally not recommended as starting doses in nonopioid tolerant patients; lower total *daily* doses may be appropriate.

Intramuscular or Subcutaneous: The usual recommended starting dose for IM or SC administration is 1 to 2 mg. This may be repeated in 6 to 8 hours as needed, provided the patient is assessed for signs of hypoventilation or excessive sedation. Dosage should be adjusted according to the severity of the pain; age, weight and physical status of the patient; the patient's underlying diseases; use of concomitant medications; and other factors (see INDIVIDUALIZATION OF DOSAGE, WARNINGS and PRECAUTIONS). Total *daily* doses of more than 3 to 8 mg IM in 24 hours are generally not recommended as starting doses in nonopioid tolerant patients; lower total *daily* doses may be appropriate.

Oral: The usual recommended starting dose for oral administration is 2 mg. This may be repeated in 6 to 8 hours as needed, provided the patient is assessed for signs of hypoventilation and excessive sedation. If necessary, the dose may be increased to up to 3 mg every 6 to 8 hours, after adequate evaluation of the patient's response. Higher doses may be appropriate in opioid tolerant patients. Dosage should be adjusted according to the severity of the pain; age, weight and physical status of the patient; the patient's underlying diseases; use of concomitant medications; and other factors (see INDIVIDUALIZATION OF DOSAGE, WARNINGS and PRECAUTIONS). Total oral *daily* doses of more than 6 to 12 mg in 24 hours are generally not recommended as starting doses in nonopioid tolerant patients; lower total *daily* doses may be appropriate.

Use in Chronic Pain: The dosage of Levo-Dromoran in patients with cancer or with other conditions for which chronic opioid therapy is indicated must be individualized (see INDIVIDUALIZATION OF DOSAGE). Levo-Dromoran is 4 to 8 times as potent as morphine and has a longer half-life. Because there is incomplete cross-tolerance among opioids, when converting a patient from morphine to Levo-Dromoran, the total *daily* dose of oral Levo-Dromoran should begin at approximately $^1/_{15}$ to $^1/_{12}$ of the total *daily* dose of oral morphine that such patients had previously required and then the dose should be adjusted to the patient's clinical response. If a patient is to be placed on fixed-schedule dosing (round-the-clock) with this drug, care should be taken to allow adequate time after each dose change (approximately 72 hours) for the patient to reach a new steady-state before a subsequent dose adjustment to avoid excessive sedation due to drug accumulation.

Use in The Perioperative Period: Levo-Dromoran has been used for analgesic action during premedication and the postoperative period. Factors to be considered in determining the dosage include age, body weight, physical status, underlying pathological condition, use of other drugs, type of anesthesia used, the surgical procedure involved and the severity of pain (see INDIVIDUALIZATION OF DOSAGE, WARNINGS and PRECAUTIONS).

Premedication: The preoperative medication dose of Levo-Dromoran should be individualized (see INDIVIDUALIZATION OF DOSAGE, WARNINGS and PRECAUTIONS). The usual dose for healthy young adults is 1 to 2 mg intramuscularly or subcutaneously, administered 60 to 90 minutes before surgery. Older or debilitated patients usually require less drug. Two mg of Levo-Dromoran is approximately equivalent to 10 to 15 mg of morphine or 100 mg of meperidine.

NOTE: Parenteral drug products should be inspected visually for particulate matter and discoloration prior to administration, whenever solution and container permit.

Pharmaceutical Incompatibilities of Levo-Dromoran: Levorphanol tartrate injection has been reported to be physically incompatible with solutions containing aminophylline, ammonium chloride, amobarbital sodium, chlorothiazide sodium, heparin sodium, methicillin sodium, nitrofurantoin sodium, novobiocin sodium, pentobarbital sodium, perphenazine, phenobarbital sodium, phenytoin sodium, secobarbital sodium, sodium bicarbonate, sodium iodide, sulfadiazine sodium, sulfisoxazole diethanolamine and thiopental sodium.

Safety and Handling: Levo-Dromoran is packaged in sealed systems that have a low risk of accidental exposure to health care workers. Ordinary care should be taken to avoid aerosol generation while preparing a syringe for use. Significant absorption from accidental dermal exposure is unlikely, and spilled Levo-Dromoran should be washed from the skin by rinsing with cool water. As with all controlled substances, abuse by health care personnel is possible and the drug should be handled accordingly.

HOW SUPPLIED

Ampuls: 1 mL, 2 mg/mL levorphanol tartrate—boxes of 10 (NDC 0004-1910-06).

Multiple-Dose Vials: 10 mL, 2 mg/mL levorphanol tartrate—boxes of 1 (NDC 0004-1911-06).

Scored Oral Tablets: 2 mg levorphanol tartrate—bottles of 100 (NDC 0004-0044-01).

Storage: Tablets should be stored at 59° to 86°F (15° to 30°C).

Dispense in tight containers as defined in USP/NF.

Parenteral dosage forms should be stored at 59° to 86° F (15° to 30°C).

WARNING: May be habit forming.

DEA Order Form Required.

Revised: January 1995

Shown in Product Identification Guide, page 316

LIBRIUM® ℂ IV

[*lib 'ree-um*]

brand of chlordiazepoxide HCl

CAPSULES

DESCRIPTION

Librium, the original chlordiazepoxide HCl and prototype for the benzodiazepine compounds, was synthesized and developed at Hoffmann-La Roche Inc. It is a versatile therapeutic agent of proven value for the relief of anxiety. Librium is among the safer of the effective psychopharmacologic compounds available, as demonstrated by extensive clinical evidence.

Librium is available as capsules containing 5 mg, 10 mg or 25 mg chlordiazepoxide HCl. Each capsule also contains corn starch, lactose and talc. Gelatin capsule shells may contain methyl and propyl parabens and potassium sorbate, with the following dye systems: 5-mg capsules—FD&C Yellow No. 6 plus D&C Yellow No. 10 and either FD&C Blue No. 1 or FD&C Green No. 3. 10-mg capsules—FD&C Yellow No. 6 plus D&C Yellow No. 10 and either FD&C Blue No. 1 plus FD&C Red No. 3 or FD&C Green No. 3 plus FD&C Red No. 40. 25-mg capsules—D&C Yellow No. 10 and either FD&C Green No. 3 or FD&C Blue No. 1.

Chlordiazepoxide hydrochloride is 7-chloro-2-(methylamino)-5-phenyl-3H-1,4-benzodiazepine 4-oxide hydrochloride. A white to practically white crystalline substance, it is soluble in water. It is unstable in solution and the powder must be protected from light. The molecular weight is 336.22.

ACTIONS

Librium (chlordiazepoxide HCl) has antianxiety, sedative, appetite-stimulating and weak analgesic actions. The precise mechanism of action is not known. The drug blocks EEG arousal from stimulation of the brain stem reticular formation. It takes several hours for peak blood levels to be reached and the half-life of the drug is between 24 and 48 hours. After the drug is discontinued plasma levels decline slowly over a period of several days. Chlordiazepoxide is excreted in the urine, with 1% to 2% unchanged and 3% to 6% as a conjugate.

Animal Pharmacology: The drug has been studied extensively in many species of animals and these studies are suggestive of action on the limbic system of the brain, which recent evidence indicates is involved in emotional responses.

Hostile monkeys were made tame by oral drug doses which did not cause sedation. Chlordiazepoxide HCl revealed a "taming" action with the elimination of fear and aggression. The taming effect of chlordiazepoxide HCl was further demonstrated in rats made vicious by lesions in the septal area of the brain. The drug dosage which effectively blocked the vicious reaction was well below the dose which caused sedation in these animals.

The LD_{50} of parenterally administered chlordiazepoxide HCl was determined in mice (72 hours) and rats (5 days), and calculated according to the method of Miller and Tainter, with the following results: mice, IV, 123 ±12 mg/kg; mice, IM, 366 ±7 mg/kg; rats, IV, 120 ±7 mg/kg; rats, IM, >160 mg/kg.

Effects on Reproduction: Reproduction studies in rats fed 10, 20 and 80 mg/kg daily and bred through one or two matings showed no congenital anomalies, nor were there adverse effects on lactation of the dams or growth of the newborn. However, in another study at 100 mg/kg daily there was noted a significant decrease in the fertilization rate and a marked decrease in the viability and body weight of offspring which may be attributable to sedative activity, thus resulting in lack of interest in mating and lessened maternal nursing and care of the young. One neonate in each of the first and second matings in the rat reproduction study at the 100 mg/kg dose exhibited major skeletal defects. Further studies are in progress to determine the significance of these findings.

INDICATIONS

Librium is indicated for the management of anxiety disorders or for the short-term relief of symptoms of anxiety, withdrawal symptoms of acute alcoholism, and preoperative apprehension and anxiety. Anxiety or tension associated with the stress of everyday life usually does not require treatment with an anxiolytic.

The effectiveness of Librium in long-term use, that is, more than 4 months, has not been assessed by systematic clinical studies. The physician should periodically reassess the usefulness of the drug for the individual patient.

CONTRAINDICATIONS

Librium is contraindicated in patients with known hypersensitivity to the drug.

WARNINGS

Chlordiazepoxide HCl may impair the mental and/or physical abilities required for the performance of potentially hazardous tasks such as driving a vehicle or operating machinery. Similarly, it may impair mental alertness in children. The concomitant use of alcohol or other central nervous system depressants may have an additive effect. PATIENTS SHOULD BE WARNED ACCORDINGLY.

Usage in Pregnancy: An increased risk of congenital malformations associated with the use of minor tranquilizers (chlordiazepoxide, diazepam and meprobamate) during the first trimester of pregnancy has been suggested in several studies. Because use of these drugs is rarely a matter of urgency, their use during this period should almost always be avoided. The possibility that a woman of childbearing potential may be pregnant at the time of institution of therapy should be considered. Patients should be advised that if they become pregnant during therapy or intend to become pregnant they should communicate with their physicians about the desirability of discontinuing the drug.

Withdrawal symptoms of the barbiturate type have occurred after the discontinuation of benzodiazepines. (See DRUG ABUSE AND DEPENDENCE section.)

PRECAUTIONS

In elderly and debilitated patients, it is recommended that the dosage be limited to the smallest effective amount to preclude the development of ataxia or oversedation (10 mg or less per day initially, to be increased gradually as needed and tolerated). In general, the concomitant administration of Librium and other psychotropic agents is not recommended. If such combination therapy seems indicated, careful consideration should be given to the pharmacology of the agents to be employed — particularly when the known potentiating compounds such as the MAO inhibitors and phenothiazines are to be used. The usual precautions in treating patients with impaired renal or hepatic function should be observed.

Paradoxical reactions, eg, excitement, stimulation and acute rage, have been reported in psychiatric patients and in hyperactive aggressive pediatric patients, and should be watched for during Librium therapy. The usual precautions are indicated when Librium is used in the treatment of anxiety states where there is any evidence of impending depression; it should be borne in mind that suicidal tendencies may be present and protective measures may be necessary.

Although clinical studies have not established a cause and effect relationship, physicians should be aware that variable effects on blood coagulation have been reported very rarely in patients receiving oral anticoagulants and Librium. In view of isolated reports associating chlordiazepoxide with exacerbation of porphyria, caution should be exercised in prescribing chlordiazepoxide to patients suffering from this disease.

Pediatric Use: Because of the varied response of pediatric patients to CNS-acting drugs, therapy should be initiated with the lowest dose and increased as required (see DOSAGE AND ADMINISTRATION). Since clinical experience with Librium in pediatric patients under 6 years of age is limited, use in this age group is not recommended. Hyperactive aggressive pediatric patients should be monitored for paradoxical reactions to Librium (see PRECAUTIONS).

Information for Patients: To assure the safe and effective use of benzodiazepines, patients should be informed that, since benzodiazepines may produce psychological and physical dependence it is advisable that they consult with their physician before either increasing the dose or abruptly discontinuing this drug.

ADVERSE REACTIONS

The necessity of discontinuing therapy because of undesirable effects has been rare. Drowsiness, ataxia and confusion have been reported in some patients — particularly the elderly and debilitated. While these effects can be avoided in almost all instances by proper dosage adjustment, they have occasionally been observed at the lower dosage ranges. In a few instances syncope has been reported.

Other adverse reactions reported during therapy include isolated instances of skin eruptions, edema, minor menstrual irregularities, nausea and constipation, extrapyramidal symptoms, as well as increased and decreased libido. Such side effects have been infrequent and are generally controlled with reduction of dosage. Changes in EEG patterns (low-voltage fast activity) have been observed in patients during and after Librium treatment.

Blood dyscrasias (including agranulocytosis), jaundice and hepatic dysfunction have occasionally been reported during therapy. When Librium treatment is protracted, periodic blood counts and liver function tests are advisable.

DRUG ABUSE AND DEPENDENCE

Chlordiazepoxide hydrochloride capsules are classified by the Drug Enforcement Administration as a Schedule IV controlled substance.

Withdrawal symptoms, similar in character to those noted with barbiturates and alcohol (convulsions, tremor, abdominal and muscle cramps, vomiting and sweating), have occurred following abrupt discontinuance of chlordiazepoxide. The more severe withdrawal symptoms have usually been limited to those patients who had received excessive doses over an extended period of time. Generally milder withdrawal symptoms (eg, dysphoria and insomnia) have been reported following abrupt discontinuance of benzodiazepines taken continuously at therapeutic levels for several months. Consequently, after extended therapy, abrupt discontinuation should generally be avoided and a gradual dosage tapering schedule followed. Addiction-prone individuals (such as drug addicts or alcoholics) should be under careful surveillance when receiving chlordiazepoxide or other psychotropic agents because of the predisposition of such patients to habituation and dependence.

OVERDOSAGE

Manifestations of Librium overdosage include somnolence, confusion, coma and diminished reflexes. Respiration, pulse and blood pressure should be monitored, as in all cases of drug overdosage, although, in general, these effects have been minimal following Librium overdosage. General supportive measures should be employed, along with immediate gastric lavage. Intravenous fluids should be administered and an adequate airway maintained. Hypotension may be combated by the use of Levophed® (norepinephrine) or Aramine (metaraminol). Dialysis is of limited value. There have been occasional reports of excitation in patients following chlordiazepoxide HCl overdosage; if this occurs barbiturates should not be used. As with the management of intentional overdosage with any drug, it should be borne in mind that multiple agents may have been ingested.

Flumazenil, a specific benzodiazepine-receptor antagonist, is indicated for the complete or partial reversal of the sedative effects of benzodiazepines and may be used in situations when an overdose with a benzodiazepine is known or suspected. Prior to the administration of flumazenil, necessary measures should be instituted to secure airway, ventilation and intravenous access. Flumazenil is intended as an adjunct to, not as a substitute for, proper management of benzodiazepine overdose. Patients treated with flumazenil should be monitored for resedation, respiratory depression and other residual benzodiazepine effects for an appropriate period after treatment. **The prescriber should be aware of a risk of seizure in association with flumazenil treatment, particularly in long-term benzodiazepine users and in cyclic antidepressant overdose.** The complete flumazenil package insert, including CONTRAINDICATIONS, WARNINGS and PRECAUTIONS, should be consulted prior to use.

DOSAGE AND ADMINISTRATION

Because of the wide range of clinical indications for Librium, the optimum dosage varies with the diagnosis and response of the individual patient. The dosage, therefore, should be individualized for maximum beneficial effects.

ADULTS	*USUAL DAILY DOSE*
Relief of Mild and Moderate Anxiety Disorders and Symptoms of Anxiety	5 mg or 10 mg, 3 or 4 times daily
Relief of Severe Anxiety Disorders and Symptoms of Anxiety	20 mg or 25 mg, 3 or 4 times daily
Geriatric Patients, or in the presence of debilitating disease	5 mg, 2 to 4 times daily

Preoperative Apprehension and Anxiety:

On days preceding surgery, 5 to 10 mg orally, 3 or 4 times daily. If used as preoperative medication, 50 to 100 mg IM* 1 hour prior to surgery.

PEDIATRIC PATIENTS	*USUAL DAILY DOSE*
Because of the varied response of pediatric patients to CNS-acting drugs, therapy should be initiated with the lowest dose and increased as required. Since clinical experience in pediatric patients under 6 years of age is limited, the use of the drug in this age group is not recommended.	5 mg, 2 to 4 times daily (may be increased in some pediatric patients to 10 mg, 2 to 3 times daily)

For the relief of withdrawal symptoms of acute alcoholism, the parenteral form* is usually used initially. If the drug is administered orally, the suggested initial dose is 50 to 100 mg, to be followed by repeated doses as needed until agitation is controlled — up to 300 mg per day. Dosage should then be reduced to maintenance levels.

* See package insert for Injectable Librium (chlordiazepoxide HCl).

HOW SUPPLIED

Librium (chlordiazepoxide HCl) capsules — 5 mg, green and yellow — bottles of 100 (NDC 0140-0001-01) and 500 (NDC 0140-0001-14); 10 mg, green and black — bottles of 100 (NDC 0140-0002-01) and 500 (NDC 0140-0002-14); 25 mg, green and white — bottles of 100 (NDC 0140–0003–01) and 500 (NDC 0140–0003–14).

Revised: December 1996

Shown in Product Identification Guide, page 316

LIBRIUM® FOR INJECTION Ⓒ

[*lib 'ree-um*]

brand of chlordiazepoxide HCl

DESCRIPTION

Librium is a versatile therapeutic agent of proven value for the relief of anxiety and tension.

Librium is the first of a new class, unrelated chemically and pharmacologically to other types of tranquilizers. Librium promptly relieves anxiety and is among the safer of the effective psychopharmacologic compounds available.

Chlordiazepoxide HCl is 7-chloro-2-methylamino-5-phenyl-3H-1,4-benzodiazepine 4-oxide hydrochloride. A colorless, crystalline substance, it is soluble in water. It is unstable in solution and the powder must be protected from light. The molecular weight is 336.22.

ANIMAL PHARMACOLOGY

The drug has been studied extensively in many species of animals and these studies are suggestive of action on the limbic system of the brain, which recent evidence indicates is involved in emotional responses.

Hostile monkeys were made tame by oral drug doses which did not cause sedation. Librium revealed a "taming" action with the elimination of fear and aggression. The taming effect of Librium was further demonstrated in rats made vicious by lesions in the septal area of the brain. The drug dosage which effectively blocked the vicious reaction was well below the dose which caused sedation in these animals.

The LD_{50} of parenterally administered chlordiazepoxide HCl was determined in mice (72 hours) and rats (5 days), and calculated according to the method of Miller and Tainter, with the following results: mice, IV, 123 ± 12 mg/kg; mice, IM, 366 ± 7 mg/kg; rats, IV, 120 ± 7 mg/kg; rats, IM, >160 mg/kg.

Effects on Reproduction: Reproduction studies in rats fed 10, 20 and 80 mg/kg daily and bred through one or two matings showed no congenital anomalies, nor were there adverse effects on lactation of the dams or growth of the newborn. However, in another study at 100 mg/kg daily there was noted a significant decrease in the fertilization rate and a marked decrease in the viability and body weight of offspring which may be attributable to sedative activity, thus resulting in lack of interest in mating and lessened maternal nursing and care of the young. One neonate in each of the first and second matings in the rat reproduction study at the 100 mg/kg dose exhibited major skeletal defects. Further studies are in progress to determine the significance of these findings.

INDICATIONS

Injectable Librium is indicated for the management of anxiety disorders or for the short-term relief of symptoms of anxiety, withdrawal symptoms of acute alcoholism, and preoperative apprehension and anxiety. Anxiety or tension associated with the stress of everyday life usually does not require treatment with an anxiolytic.

CONTRAINDICATIONS

Librium is contraindicated in patients with known hypersensitivity to the drug.

WARNINGS

As in the case of other CNS-acting drugs, patients receiving Librium should be cautioned about possible combined effects with alcohol and other CNS depressants.

Continued on next page

Librium Injectable—Cont.

As is true of all preparations containing CNS-acting drugs, patients receiving Librium should be cautioned against hazardous occupations requiring complete mental alertness such as operating machinery or driving a motor vehicle.

Usage in Pregnancy: **An increased risk of congenital malformations associated with the use of minor tranquilizers (chlordiazepoxide, diazepam and meprobamate) during the first trimester of pregnancy has been suggested in several studies. Because use of these drugs is rarely a matter of urgency, their use during this period should almost always be avoided. The possibility that a woman of childbearing potential may be pregnant at the time of institution of therapy should be considered. Patients should be advised that if they become pregnant during therapy or intend to become pregnant they should communicate with their physicians about the desirability of discontinuing the drug.**

Management of Overdosage: Manifestations of Librium overdosage include somnolence, confusion, coma and diminished reflexes. Respiration, pulse and blood pressure should be monitored, as in all cases of drug overdosage, although, in general, these effects have been minimal following Librium overdosage. General supportive measures should be employed, along with immediate gastric lavage.

Intravenous fluids should be administered and an adequate airway maintained. Hypotension may be combated by the use of Levophed® (levarterenol) or Aramine (metaraminol). Dialysis is of limited value. There have been occasional reports of excitation in patients following Librium overdosage; if this occurs barbiturates should not be used. As with the management of intentional overdosage with any drug, it should be borne in mind that multiple agents may have been ingested.

Flumazenil, a specific benzodiazepine-receptor antagonist, is indicated for the complete or partial reversal of the sedative effects of benzodiazepines and may be used in situations when an overdose with a benzodiazepine is known or suspected. Prior to the administration of flumazenil, necessary measures should be instituted to secure airway, ventilation and intravenous access. Flumazenil is intended as an adjunct to, not as a substitute for, proper management of benzodiazepine overdose. Patients treated with flumazenil should be monitored for resedation, respiratory depression and other residual benzodiazepine effects for an appropriate period after treatment. **The prescriber should be aware of a risk of seizure in association with flumazenil treatment, particularly in long-term benzodiazepine users and in cyclic antidepressant overdose.** The complete flumazenil package insert, including CONTRAINDICATIONS, WARNINGS and PRECAUTIONS, should be consulted prior to use.

Withdrawal symptoms of the barbiturate type have occurred after the discontinuation of benzodiazepines. (See DRUG ABUSE AND DEPENDENCE section.)

PRECAUTIONS

Injectable Librium (intramuscular or intravenous) is indicated primarily in acute states, and patients receiving this form of therapy should be kept under observation, preferably in bed, for a period of up to 3 hours. Ambulatory patients should not be permitted to operate a vehicle following an injection. Injectable Librium should not be given to patients in shock or comatose states. Reduced dosage (usually 25 to 50 mg) should be used for elderly or debilitated patients. In general, the concomitant administration of Librium and other psychotropic agents is not recommended. If such combination therapy seems indicated, careful consideration should be given to the pharmacology of the agents to be employed—particularly when the known potentiating compounds such as the MAO inhibitors and phenothiazines are to be used. The usual precautions in treating patients with impaired renal or hepatic function should be observed.

Paradoxical reactions, eg, excitement, stimulation and acute rage, have been reported in psychiatric patients and in hyperactive aggressive pediatric patients, and should be watched for during Librium therapy. The usual precautions are indicated when Librium is used in the treatment of anxiety states where there is any evidence of impending depression; it should be borne in mind that suicidal tendencies may be present and protective measures may be necessary.

Although clinical studies have not established a cause and effect relationship, physicians should be aware that variable effects on blood coagulation have been reported very rarely in patients receiving oral anticoagulants and Librium. In view of isolated reports associating chlordiazepoxide with exacerbation of porphyria, caution should be exercised in prescribing chlordiazepoxide to patients suffering from this disease.

Pediatric Use: Reduced dosage (usually 25 to 50 mg) should be used for pediatric patients age 12 years and older (see DOSAGE AND ADMINISTRATION). Since clinical experience in pediatric patients under 12 years of age is limited, the use of the drug in this age group is not recommended. Hyperactive aggressive pediatric patients should be monitored for paradoxical reactions to Librium (see PRECAUTIONS).

ADVERSE REACTIONS

The necessity of discontinuing therapy because of undesirable effects has been rare. Drowsiness, ataxia and confusion are more commonly seen in the elderly and debilitated.

Other adverse reactions reported during therapy include isolated instances of syncope, hypotension, tachycardia, skin eruptions, edema, minor menstrual irregularities, nausea and constipation, extrapyramidal symptoms, blurred vision, as well as increased and decreased libido. Such side effects have been infrequent and are generally controlled with reduction of dosage. Similarly, hypotension associated with spinal anesthesia has occurred. Pain following intramuscular injection has been reported. Changes in EEG patterns (low-voltage fast activity) have been observed in patients during and after Librium treatment.

Blood dyscrasias (including agranulocytosis), jaundice and hepatic dysfunction, have occasionally been reported during therapy. When Librium treatment is protracted, periodic blood counts and liver function tests are advisable.

DRUG ABUSE AND DEPENDENCE

Withdrawal symptoms, similar in character to those noted with barbiturates and alcohol (convulsions, tremor, abdominal and muscle cramps, vomiting and sweating), have occurred following abrupt discontinuance of chlordiazepoxide. The more severe withdrawal symptoms have usually been limited to those patients who had received excessive doses over an extended period of time. Generally milder withdrawal symptoms (eg, dysphoria and insomnia) have been reported following abrupt discontinuance of benzodiazepines taken continuously at therapeutic levels for several months. Consequently, after extended therapy, abrupt discontinuation should generally be avoided and a gradual dosage tapering schedule followed. Addiction-prone individuals (such as drug addicts or alcoholics) should be under careful surveillance when receiving chlordiazepoxide or other psychotropic agents because of the predisposition of such patients to habituation and dependence.

PREPARATION AND ADMINISTRATION OF SOLUTIONS

Solutions of Librium for intramuscular or intravenous use should be prepared aseptically. Sterilization by heating should not be attempted.

Intramuscular: Add 2 mL of *Special Intramuscular Diluent* to contents of 5-mL dry-filled amber ampul of Librium Sterile Powder (100 mg). Avoid excessive pressure in injecting this special diluent into the ampul containing the powder since bubbles will form on the surface of the solution. Agitate gently until completely dissolved. Solution should be prepared immediately before administration. Any unused solution should be discarded. Deep intramuscular injection should be given *slowly* into the upper outer quadrant of the gluteus muscle.

Caution: Librium solution made with the Special Intramuscular Diluent should not be given intravenously because of the air bubbles which form when the intramuscular diluent is added to the Librium powder. Do not use diluent solution if it is opalescent or hazy.

Intravenous: In most cases, intramuscular injection is the preferred route of administration of Injectable Librium since beneficial effects are usually seen within 15 to 30 minutes. When, in the judgment of the physician, even more rapid action is mandatory, Injectable Librium may be administered intravenously. A suitable solution for intravenous administration may be prepared as follows: Add 5 mL of *sterile physiological saline* or *sterile water for injection* to contents of 5-mL dry-filled amber ampul of Librium Sterile Powder (100 mg). Agitate gently until thoroughly dissolved. Solution should be prepared immediately before administration. Any unused portion should be discarded. *Intravenous injection should be given slowly over a 1-minute period.*

Caution: Librium solution made with physiological saline or sterile water for injection should not be given intramuscularly because of pain on injection.

DOSAGE

Dosage should be individualized according to the diagnosis and the response of the patient. While 300 mg may be given during a 6-hour period, this dose should not be exceeded in any 24-hour period.

INDICATION	*ADULT DOSAGE**
Withdrawal Symptoms of Acute Alcoholism	50 to 100 mg IM or IV initially; repeat in 2 to 4 hours, if necessary
Acute or Severe Anxiety Disorders or Symptoms of Anxiety	50 to 100 mg IM or IV initially; then 25 to 50 mg 3 or 4 times daily, if necessary
Preoperative Apprehension and Anxiety	50 to 100 mg IM 1 hour prior to surgery

* Lower doses (usually 25 to 50 mg) should be used for elderly or debilitated patients, and for pediatric patients age 12 years and older. Because of limited clinical experience in pediatric patients under 12 years of age, the use of the drug in this age group is not recommended.

In most cases, acute symptoms may be rapidly controlled by parenteral administration so that subsequent treatment, if necessary, may be given orally. (See package insert for Oral Librium.)

HOW SUPPLIED

For Parenteral Administration: Ampuls—Duplex package consisting of a 5-mL dry-filled ampul containing 100 mg chlordiazepoxide HCl in dry crystalline form, and a 2-mL ampul of Special Intramuscular Diluent (for intramuscular administration) compounded with 1.5% benzyl alcohol, 4% polysorbate 80, 20% propylene glycol, 1.6% maleic acid and sodium hydroxide to adjust pH to approximately 3. Boxes of 10 (NDC 0140-1912-06).

CAUTION

Before preparing solution for intramuscular or intravenous administration, please read instructions for PREPARATION AND ADMINISTRATION OF SOLUTIONS.

Manufactured by Hoffmann-La Roche Inc., Nutley, NJ 07110

Revised: December 1996

LIMBITROL® Ⓒ

[lim 'bit-roll]

(chlordiazepoxide and amitriptyline HCl)
DS (double strength) TABLETS
TABLETS
Tranquilizer—Antidepressant

DESCRIPTION

Limbitrol combines for oral administration, chlordiazepoxide, an agent for the relief of anxiety and tension, and amitriptyline, an antidepressant. It is available in DS (double strength) white, film-coated tablets, each containing 10 mg chlordiazepoxide and 25 mg amitriptyline (as the hydrochloride salt); and in blue, film-coated tablets, each containing 5 mg chlordiazepoxide and 12.5 mg amitriptyline (as the hydrochloride salt). Each tablet also contains corn starch, hydroxypropyl cellulose, hydroxypropyl methylcellulose, lactose, magnesium stearate, polyethylene glycol, povidone and propylene glycol; Limbitrol tablets contain the following colorant system—FD&C Blue No. 1 aluminum lake and titanium dioxide; Limbitrol DS tablets contain titanium dioxide.

Chlordiazepoxide is a benzodiazepine with the formula 7-chloro-2-(methylamino)-5-phenyl-3*H*-1,4-benzodiazepine 4-oxide. It is a slightly yellow crystalline material and is insoluble in water. The molecular weight is 299.76.

Amitriptyline is a dibenzocycloheptadiene derivative. The formula is 10,11-dihydro-*N,N*-dimethyl-5H-dibenzo [a,d] cycloheptene-$\Delta^{5,\gamma}$-propylamine hydrochloride. It is a white or practically white crystalline compound that is freely soluble in water. The molecular weight is 313.87.

ACTIONS

Both components of Limbitrol exert their action in the central nervous system. Extensive studies with chlordiazepoxide in many animal species suggest action in the limbic system. Recent evidence indicates that the limbic system is involved in emotional response. Taming action was observed in some species. The mechanism of action of amitriptyline in man is not known, but the drug appears to interfere with the reuptake of norepinephrine into adrenergic nerve endings. This action may prolong the sympathetic activity of biogenic amines.

INDICATIONS

Limbitrol is indicated for the treatment of patients with moderate to severe depression associated with moderate to severe anxiety.

The therapeutic response to Limbitrol occurs earlier and with fewer treatment failures than when either amitriptyline or chlordiazepoxide is used alone.

Symptoms likely to respond in the first week of treatment include: insomnia, feelings of guilt or worthlessness, agitation, psychic and somatic anxiety, suicidal ideation and anorexia.

CONTRAINDICATIONS

Limbitrol is contraindicated in patients with hypersensitivity to either benzodiazepines or tricyclic antidepressants. It should not be given concomitantly with a monoamine oxidase inhibitor. Hyperpyretic crises, severe convulsions and deaths have occurred in patients receiving a tricyclic antidepressant and a monoamine oxidase inhibitor simultaneously. When it is desired to replace a monoamine oxidase

inhibitor with Limbitrol, a minimum of 14 days should be allowed to elapse after the former is discontinued. Limbitrol should then be initiated cautiously with gradual increase in dosage until optimum response is achieved.

This drug is contraindicated during the acute recovery phase following myocardial infarction.

WARNINGS

Because of the atropine-like action of the amitriptyline component, great care should be used in treating patients with a history of urinary retention or angle-closure glaucoma. In patients with glaucoma, even average doses may precipitate an attack. Severe constipation may occur in patients taking tricyclic antidepressants in combination with anticholinergic-type drugs.

Patients with cardiovascular disorders should be watched closely. Tricyclic antidepressant drugs, particularly when given in high doses, have been reported to produce arrhythmias, sinus tachycardia and prolongation of conduction time. Myocardial infarction and stroke have been reported in patients receiving drugs of this class.

Because of the sedative effects of Limbitrol, patients should be cautioned about combined effects with alcohol or other CNS depressants. The additive effects may produce a harmful level of sedation and CNS depression.

Patients receiving Limbitrol should be cautioned against engaging in hazardous occupations requiring complete mental alertness, such as operating machinery or driving a motor vehicle.

Usage in Pregnancy: Safe use of Limbitrol during pregnancy and lactation has not been established. Because of the chlordiazepoxide component, please note the following:

An increased risk of congenital malformations associated with the use of minor tranquilizers (chlordiazepoxide, diazepam and meprobamate) during the first trimester of pregnancy has been suggested in several studies. Because use of these drugs is rarely a matter of urgency, their use during this period should almost always be avoided. The possibility that a woman of childbearing potential may be pregnant at the time of institution of therapy should be considered. Patients should be advised that if they become pregnant during therapy or intend to become pregnant they should communicate with their physicians about the desirability of discontinuing the drug.

Withdrawal symptoms of the barbiturate type have occurred after the discontinuation of benzodiazepines. (See DRUG ABUSE AND DEPENDENCE section.)

PRECAUTIONS

General: Use with caution in patients with a history of seizures.

Close supervision is required when Limbitrol is given to hyperthyroid patients or those on thyroid medication.

The usual precautions should be observed when treating patients with impaired renal or hepatic function.

Patients with suicidal ideation should not have easy access to large quantities of the drug. The possibility of suicide in depressed patients remains until significant remission occurs.

Essential Laboratory Tests: Patients on prolonged treatment should have periodic liver function tests and blood counts.

Drug and Treatment Interactions: Because of its amitriptyline component, Limbitrol may block the antihypertensive action of guanethidine or compounds with a similar mechanism of action.

Drugs Metabolized by P450 2D6: The biochemical activity of the drug metabolizing isozyme cytochrome P450 2D6 (debrisoquin hydroxylase) is reduced in a subset of the caucasian population (about 7% to 10% of caucasians are so called "poor metabolizers"); reliable estimates of the prevalence of reduced P450 2D6 isozyme activity among Asian, African and other populations are not yet available. Poor metabolizers have higher than expected plasma concentrations of tricyclic antidepressants (TCAs) when given usual doses. Depending on the fraction of drug metabolized by P450 2D6, the increase in plasma concentration may be small or quite large (8-fold increase in plasma AUC of the TCA).

In addition, certain drugs inhibit the activity of this isozyme and make normal metabolizers resemble poor metabolizers. An individual who is stable on a given dose of TCA may become abruptly toxic when given one of these inhibiting drugs as concomitant therapy. The drugs that inhibit cytochrome P450 2D6 include some that are not metabolized by the enzyme (quinidine; cimetidine) and many that are substrates for P450 2D6 (many other antidepressants, phenothiazines, and the type 1c antiarrhythmics propafenone and flecainide). While all the selective serotonin reuptake inhibitors (SSRIs), eg, fluoxetine, sertraline and paroxetine, inhibit P450 2D6, they may vary in the extent of inhibition. The extent to which SSRI TCA interactions may pose clinical problems will depend on the degree of inhibition and the pharmacokinetics of the SSRI involved. Nevertheless, caution is indicated in the coadministration of TCAs with any of the SSRIs and also in switching from one class to the other. Of particular importance, sufficient time must elapse before initiating TCA treatment in a patient being withdrawn from fluoxetine, given the long half-life of the parent and active metabolite (at least 5 weeks may be necessary).

Concomitant use of tricyclic antidepressants with drugs that can inhibit cytochrome P450 2D6 may require lower doses than usually prescribed for either the tricyclic antidepressant or the other drug. Furthermore, whenever one of these other drugs is withdrawn from cotherapy, an increased dose of tricyclic antidepressant may be required. It is desirable to monitor TCA plasma levels whenever a TCA is going to be coadministered with another drug known to be an inhibitor of P450 2D6.

The effects of concomitant administration of Limbitrol and other psychotropic drugs have not been evaluated. Sedative effects may be additive.

Cimetidine is reported to reduce hepatic metabolism of certain tricyclic antidepressants and benzodiazepines, thereby delaying elimination and increasing steady-state concentrations of these drugs. Clinically significant effects have been reported with the tricyclic antidepressants when used concomitantly with cimetidine (Tagamet).

The drug should be discontinued several days before elective surgery.

Concurrent administration of ECT and Limbitrol should be limited to those patients for whom it is essential.

Pregnancy: See WARNINGS section.

Nursing Mothers: It is not known whether this drug is excreted in human milk. As a general rule, nursing should not be undertaken while a patient is on a drug, since many drugs are excreted in human milk.

Pediatric Use: Safety and effectiveness in children below the age of 12 years have not been established.

Elderly Patients: In elderly and debilitated patients it is recommended that dosage be limited to the smallest effective amount to preclude the development of ataxia, oversedation, confusion or anticholinergic effects.

Information for Patients: To assure the safe and effective use of benzodiazepines, patients should be informed that, since benzodiazepines may produce psychological and physical dependence, it is advisable that they consult with their physician before either increasing the dose or abruptly discontinuing this drug.

ADVERSE REACTIONS

Adverse reactions to Limbitrol are those associated with the use of either component alone. Most frequently reported were drowsiness, dry mouth, constipation, blurred vision, dizziness and bloating. Other side effects occurring less commonly included vivid dreams, impotence, tremor, confusion and nasal congestion. Many symptoms common to the depressive state, such as anorexia, fatigue, weakness, restlessness and lethargy, have been reported as side effects of treatment with both Limbitrol and amitriptyline.

Granulocytopenia, jaundice and hepatic dysfunction of uncertain etiology have also been observed rarely with Limbitrol. When treatment with Limbitrol is prolonged, periodic blood counts and liver function tests are advisable.

Note: Included in the listing which follows are adverse reactions which have not been reported with Limbitrol. However, they are included because they have been reported during therapy with one or both of the components or closely related drugs.

Cardiovascular: Hypotension, hypertension, tachycardia, palpitations, myocardial infarction, arrhythmias, heart block, stroke.

Psychiatric: Euphoria, apprehension, poor concentration, delusions, hallucinations, hypomania and increased or decreased libido.

Neurologic: Incoordination, ataxia, numbness, tingling and paresthesias of the extremities, extrapyramidal symptoms, syncope, changes in EEG patterns.

Anticholinergic: Disturbance of accommodation, paralytic ileus, urinary retention, dilatation of urinary tract.

Allergic: Skin rash, urticaria, photosensitization, edema of face and tongue, pruritus.

Hematologic: Bone marrow depression including agranulocytosis, eosinophilia, purpura, thrombocytopenia.

Gastrointestinal: Nausea, epigastric distress, vomiting, anorexia, stomatitis, peculiar taste, diarrhea, black tongue.

Endocrine: Testicular swelling and gynecomastia in the male, breast enlargement, galactorrhea and minor menstrual irregularities in the female, elevation and lowering of blood sugar levels, and syndrome of inappropriate ADH (antidiuretic hormone) secretion.

Other: Headache, weight gain or loss, increased perspiration, urinary frequency, mydriasis, jaundice, alopecia, parotid swelling.

DRUG ABUSE AND DEPENDENCE

Withdrawal symptoms, similar in character to those noted with barbiturates and alcohol (convulsions, tremor, abdominal and muscle cramps, vomiting and sweating), have occurred following abrupt discontinuance of chlordiazepoxide. The more severe withdrawal symptoms have usually been limited to those patients who had received excessive doses over an extended period of time. Generally milder withdrawal symptoms (eg, dysphoria and insomnia) have been reported following abrupt discontinuance of benzodiazepines taken continuously at therapeutic levels for several months. Withdrawal symptoms (eg, nausea, headache and malaise) have also been reported in association with abrupt amitriptyline discontinuation. Consequently, after extended therapy, abrupt discontinuation should generally be avoided and a gradual dosage tapering schedule followed. Addiction-prone individuals (such as drug addicts or alcoholics) should be under careful surveillance when receiving chlordiazepoxide or other psychotropic agents because of the predisposition of such patients to habituation and dependence.

OVERDOSAGE*

Deaths may occur from overdosage with this class of drugs. Multiple drug ingestion (including alcohol) is common in deliberate tricyclic antidepressant overdose. As the management is complex and changing, it is recommended that the physician contact a poison control center for current information on treatment. Signs and symptoms of toxicity develop rapidly after tricyclic antidepressant overdose; therefore, hospital monitoring is required as soon as possible.

Manifestations: Critical manifestations of overdose include: cardiac dysrhythmias, severe hypotension, convulsions and CNS depression, including coma. Changes in the electrocardiogram, particularly in QRS axis or width, are clinically significant indicators of tricyclic antidepressant toxicity.

Other signs of overdose may include: confusion, disturbed concentration, transient visual hallucinations, dilated pupils, agitation, hyperactive reflexes, stupor, drowsiness, muscle rigidity, vomiting, hypothermia, hyperpyrexia or any of the symptoms listed under ADVERSE REACTIONS.

Management: *General:* Obtain an ECG and immediately initiate cardiac monitoring. Protect the patient's airway, establish an intravenous line and initiate gastric decontamination. A minimum of 6 hours of observation with cardiac monitoring and observation for signs of CNS or respiratory depression, hypotension, cardiac dysrhythmias and/or conduction blocks, and seizures is necessary. If signs of toxicity occur at any time during this period, extended monitoring is required. *There are case reports of patients succumbing to fatal dysrhythmias late after overdose; these patients had clinical evidence of significant poisoning prior to death and most received inadequate gastrointestinal decontamination.* Monitoring of plasma drug levels should not guide management of the patient.

Gastrointestinal Decontamination: All patients suspected of tricyclic antidepressant overdose should receive gastrointestinal decontamination. This should include large volume gastric lavage followed by activated charcoal. If consciousness is impaired, the airway should be secured prior to lavage. Emesis is contraindicated.

Cardiovascular: A maximal limb-lead QRS duration of $\geq$ 0.10 seconds may be the best indication of the severity of the overdose. Serum alkalinization, to a pH of 7.45 to 7.56, using intravenous sodium bicarbonate and hyperventilation (as needed) should be instituted for patients with dysrhythmias and/or QRS widening. A pH $>$ 7.60 or a $pCO_2 < 20$ mm Hg is undesirable. Dysrhythmias unresponsive to sodium bicarbonate therapy/hyperventilation may respond to lidocaine, bretylium or phenytoin. Type *1A and 1C* antiarrhythmics are generally contraindicated (eg, quinidine, disopyramide and procainamide).

In rare instances, hemoperfusion may be beneficial in acute refractory cardiovascular instability in patients with acute toxicity. However, hemodialysis, peritoneal dialysis, exchange transfusions and forced diuresis generally have been reported as ineffective in tricyclic antidepressant poisoning.

CNS: In patients with CNS depression, early intubation is advised because of the potential for abrupt deterioration. Seizures should be controlled with benzodiazepines, or if these are ineffective, other anticonvulsants (eg, phenobarbital, phenytoin). *Physostigmine is not recommended except to treat life-threatening symptoms that have been unresponsive to other therapies,* and then only in consultation with a poison control center.

Psychiatric Follow-up: Since overdosage is often deliberate, patients may attempt suicide by other means during the recovery phase. Psychiatric referral may be appropriate.

Pediatric Management: The principles of management of child and adult overdosages are similar. It is strongly recommended that the physician contact the local poison control center for specific pediatric treatment.

*Poisindex® Toxicologic Management. Topic: Antidepressants, Tricyclic. *Micromedex Inc.* Vol. 85.

Chlordiazepoxide Overdosage: Manifestations of benzodiazepine overdosage include somnolence, confusion, coma and diminished reflexes. Dialysis is of limited value. There have been occasional reports of excitation in patients following benzodiazepine overdosage; if this occurs, barbiturates should not be used. Withdrawal symptoms of the barbiturate type have occurred after the discontinuation of benzodiazepines (see DRUG ABUSE AND DEPENDENCE sec-

Continued on next page

Limbitrol—Cont.

tion). Since Limbitrol contains amitriptyline, it is important to note that use of the benzodiazepine antagonist flumazenil is contraindicated in patients who are showing signs of serious cyclic antidepressant overdose.

DOSAGE AND ADMINISTRATION

Optimum dosage varies with the severity of the symptoms and the response of the individual patient. When a satisfactory response is obtained, dosage should be reduced to the smallest amount needed to maintain the remission. The larger portion of the total daily dose may be taken at bedtime. In some patients, a single dose at bedtime may be sufficient. In general, lower dosages are recommended for elderly patients.

Limbitrol DS (double strength) Tablets are recommended in an initial dosage of 3 or 4 tablets daily in divided doses; this may be increased to 6 tablets daily as required. Some patients respond to smaller doses and can be maintained on 2 tablets daily.

Limbitrol Tablets in an initial dosage of 3 or 4 tablets daily in divided doses may be satisfactory in patients who do not tolerate higher doses.

HOW SUPPLIED

DS (double strength) Tablets, containing 10 mg chlordiazepoxide and 25 mg amitriptyline (as the hydrochloride salt)—bottles of 100 and 500.

Tablets, containing 5 mg chlordiazepoxide and 12.5 mg amitriptyline (as the hydrochloride salt)—bottles of 100 and 500.

Revised: June 1996

Shown in Product Identification Guide, pages 316 and 317

MESTINON® INJECTABLE ℞

[*mes 'tin-on*]

(pyridostigmine bromide)

DESCRIPTION

Mestinon (pyridostigmine bromide) Injectable is an active cholinesterase inhibitor. Chemically, pyridostigmine bromide is 3-hydroxy-1-methylpyridinium bromide dimethylcarbamate. Its structural formula is:

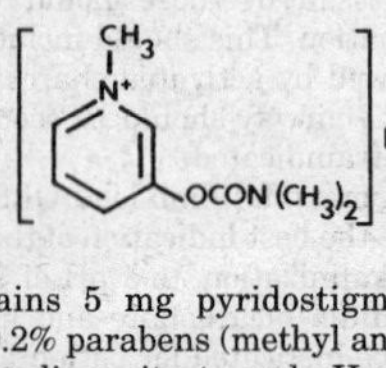

Each ml contains 5 mg pyridostigmine bromide compounded with 0.2% parabens (methyl and propyl) as preservatives, 0.02% sodium citrate and pH adjusted to approximately 5.0 with citric acid and, if necessary, sodium hydroxide.

ACTIONS

Mestinon facilitates the transmission of impulses across the myoneural junction by inhibiting the destruction of acetylcholine by cholinesterase. Pyridostigmine is an analog of neostigmine (Prostigmin®) but differs from it clinically by having fewer side effects. Currently available data indicate that pyridostigmine may have a significantly lower degree and incidence of bradycardia, salivation and gastrointestinal stimulation. Animal studies using the injectable form of pyridostigmine and human studies using the oral preparation have indicated that pyridostigmine has a longer duration of action than does neostigmine measured under similar circumstances.

INDICATIONS

Mestinon Injectable is useful in the treatment of myasthenia gravis and as a reversal agent or antagonist to nondepolarizing muscle relaxants such as curariform drugs and gallamine triethiodide.

CONTRAINDICATIONS

Known hypersensitivity to anticholinesterase agents; intestinal and urinary obstructions of mechanical type.

WARNINGS

Mestinon Injectable should be used with particular caution in patients with bronchial asthma or cardiac dysrhythmias. Transient bradycardia may occur and be relieved by atropine sulfate. Atropine should also be used with caution in patients with cardiac dysrhythmias. When large doses of Mestinon are administered, as during reversal of muscle relaxants, the prior or simultaneous injection of atropine sulfate is advisable. Because of the possibility of hypersensitivity in an occasional patient, atropine and antishock medication should always be readily available.

As is true of all cholinergic drugs, overdosage of Mestinon may result in cholinergic crisis, a state characterized by increasing muscle weakness which, through involvement of the muscles of respiration, may lead to death. Myasthenic crisis due to an increase in the severity of the disease is also accompanied by extreme muscle weakness and thus may be difficult to distinguish from cholinergic crisis on a symptomatic basis. Such differentiation is extremely important, since increases in doses of Mestinon or other drugs in this class in the presence of cholinergic crisis or of a refractory or "insensitive" state could have grave consequences. Osserman and Genkins[1] indicate that the two types of crisis may be differentiated by the use of Tensilon® (edrophonium chloride) as well as by clinical judgment. The treatment of the two conditions obviously differs radically. Whereas the presence of *myasthenic crisis* requires more intensive anticholinesterase therapy, *cholinergic crisis,* according to Osserman and Genkins,[1] calls for the prompt withdrawal of all drugs of this type. The immediate use of atropine in cholinergic crisis is also recommended. A syringe containing 1 mg of atropine sulfate should be immediately available to be given in aliquots intravenously to counteract severe cholinergic reactions.

Atropine may also be used to abolish or obtund gastrointestinal side effects or other muscarinic reactions; but such use, by masking signs of overdosage, can lead to inadvertent induction of cholinergic crisis.

For detailed information on the management of patients with myasthenia gravis, the physician is referred to one of the excellent reviews such as those by Osserman and Genkins,[2] Grob[3] or Schwab.[4,5]

When used as an antagonist to nondepolarizing muscle relaxants, adequate recovery of voluntary respiration and neuromuscular transmission must be obtained prior to discontinuation of respiratory assistance and there should be continuous patient observation. Satisfactory recovery may be defined by a combination of clinical judgment, respiratory measurements and observation of the effects of peripheral nerve stimulation. If there is any doubt concerning the adequacy of recovery from the effects of the nondepolarizing muscle relaxant, artificial ventilation should be continued until all doubt has been removed.

Usage in Pregnancy: The safety of Mestinon during pregnancy or lactation in humans has not been established. Therefore, use of Mestinon in women who may become pregnant requires weighing the drug's potential benefits against its possible hazards to mother and child.

ADVERSE REACTIONS

The side effects of Mestinon are most commonly related to overdosage and generally are of two varieties, muscarinic and nicotinic. Among those in the former group are nausea, vomiting, diarrhea, abdominal cramps, increased peristalsis, increased salivation, increased bronchial secretions, miosis and diaphoresis. Nicotinic side effects are comprised chiefly of muscle cramps, fasciculation and weakness. Muscarinic side effects can usually be counteracted by atropine, but for reasons shown in the preceding section the expedient is not without danger. As with any compound containing the bromide radical, a skin rash may be seen in an occasional patient. Such reactions usually subside promptly upon discontinuance of the medication. Thrombophlebitis has been reported subsequent to intravenous administration.

DOSAGE AND ADMINISTRATION

For Myasthenia Gravis —To supplement oral dosage, pre- and postoperatively, during labor and postpartum, during myasthenic crisis, or whenever oral therapy is impractical, approximately 1/30th of the oral dose of Mestinon may be given parenterally, either by intramuscular or *very slow* intravenous injection. *The patient must be closely observed for cholinergic reactions, particularly if the intravenous route is used.*

For details regarding the management of myasthenic patients who are to undergo major surgical procedures, see the article by Foldes.[6]

Neonates of myasthenic mothers may have transient difficulty in swallowing, sucking and breathing. Injectable Mestinon may be indicated—by symptomatology and use of the Tensilon® (edrophonium chloride) test—until Mestinon Syrup can be taken. To date the world literature consists of less than 100 neonate patients.[7] Of these only 5 were treated with injectable pyridostigmine, with the vast majority of the remaining neonates receiving neostigmine. Dosage requirements of Mestinon Injectable are minute, ranging from 0.05 mg to 0.15 mg/kg of body weight given intramuscularly. It is important to differentiate between cholinergic and myasthenic crises in neonates. (See **WARNINGS.**)

Mestinon given parenterally one hour before completion of second stage labor enables patients to have adequate strength during labor and provides protection to infants in the immediate postnatal state. For further information on the use of Mestinon Injectable in neonates of myasthenic mothers, see the article by Namba.[7]

NOTE: For information on a diagnostic test for myasthenia gravis, and on the evaluation and stabilization of therapy, please see product information on Tensilon® (edrophonium chloride).

For Reversal of Nondepolarizing Muscle Relaxants: When Mestinon Injectable is given intravenously to reverse the action of muscle relaxant drugs, it is recommended that atropine sulfate (0.6 to 1.2 mg) also be given intravenously immediately prior to the Mestinon. Side effects, notably excessive secretions and bradycardia, are thereby minimized. Usually 10 or 20 mg of Mestinon will be sufficient for antagonism of the effects of the nondepolarizing muscle relaxants. Although full recovery may occur within 15 minutes in most patients, others may require a half hour or more. Satisfactory reversal can be evident by adequate voluntary respiration, respiratory measurements and use of a peripheral nerve stimulator device. It is recommended that the patient be well ventilated and a patent airway maintained until complete recovery of normal respiration is assured. Once satisfactory reversal has been attained, recurarization has not been reported. For additional information on the use of Mestinon for antagonism of nondepolarizing muscle relaxants see the article by Katz[8] and McNall.[9]

Failure of Mestinon Injectable to provide prompt (within 30 minutes) reversal may occur, *e.g.,* in the presence of extreme debilitation, carcinomatosis, or with concomitant use of certain broad spectrum antibiotics or anesthetic agents, notably ether. Under these circumstances ventilation must be supported by artificial means until the patient has resumed control of his respiration.

HOW SUPPLIED

Mestinon is available in 2-ml ampuls (boxes of 10) (NDC 0187-3011-10).

REFERENCES

1. Osserman, KE, Genkins G, Studies in myasthenia gravis: Reduction in mortality rate after crisis. *JAMA. Jan 1963; 183; 97-101.*
2. Osserman, KE, Genkins G, Studies in myasthenia gravis. *NY State J Med.* June 1961; 61:2076-2085.
3. Grob D. Myasthenia gravis. A review of pathogenesis and treatment. *Arch Intern Med.* Oct 1961; 108:615-638.
4. Schwab RS. Management of myasthenia gravis. *New Eng J Med.* Mar 1963; 268:596-597.
5. Schwab RS. Management of myasthenia gravis. *New Eng J Med.* Mar 1963; 268:717-719.
6. Cronnelly R, Stanski DR, Miller RD, Sheiner LB. Pyridostigmine kinetics with and without renal function. *Clin Pharmacol Ther.* 1980; 28:No. 1, 78-81.
7. Miller RD. Pharmacodynamics and pharmacokinetics of anticholinesterase. In: Ruegheimer E, Zindler M, ed. *Anaesthesiology.* (Hamburg, Germany: Congress; Sep 14–21, 1980; 222-223.) (Int Congr. No. 538), Amsterdam, Netherlands: Excerpta Medica; 1981.
8. Breyer-Pfaff U, Maier U, Brinkmann AM, Schumm F. Pyridostigmine kinetics in healthy subjects and pathients with myasthenia gravis. *Clin Pharmacol Ther.* 1985; 5:495-501.
9. Foides FF, McNall PG. Myasthenia gravis: A guide for anesthesiologists. *Anesthesiology.* 23:837-872 Nov-Dec 1962.
10. Namba T. Brown SB, Grob D. Neonatal myasthenia gravis: Report of two cases and review of the literature. *Pediatrics.* 45(3):Mar 1970; 455-504.
11. Katz RL. Pyridostigmine (mestinon) as an antagonist of d-turbocurarine. *Anesthesiology.* 28(3):May-June 1967; 528-534.
12. McNail PG, Wolfson B, Tuazon JG, Siker ES. *Anesth Analg.* 48(6): Nov-Dec 1969;1026-1032.

Manufactured for ICN Pharmaceuticals, Inc.
Costa Mesa, CA 92626
by Hoffmann-La Roche Inc.
Nutley, N.J. 07110
Rev. 9-95

MESTINON® ℞

[*mes 'tin-on*]

(pyridostigmine bromide)
TABLETS, SYRUP and
TIMESPAN® TABLETS

DESCRIPTION

Mestinon (pyridostigmine bromide) is an orally active cholinesterase inhibitor. Chemically, pyridostigmine bromide is 3-hydroxy-1-methylpyridinium bromide dimethylcarbamate. Its structural formula is:

[See chemical structure at top of next column]

Mestinon is available in the following forms: Syrup containing 60 mg pyridostigmine bromide per teaspoonful in a vehicle containing 5% alcohol, glycerin, lactic acid, sodium benzoate, sorbitol, sucrose, FD&C Red No. 40, FD&C Blue No. 1, flavors and water. *Tablets* containing 60 mg pyridostigmine bromide; each tablet also contains lactose, silicon dioxide and stearic acid. *Timespan Tablets* containing 180 mg pyridostigmine bromide; each tablet also contains carnauba wax, corn-derived proteins, magnesium stearate, silica gel and tribasic calcium phosphate.

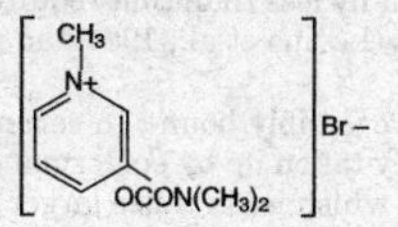

ACTIONS

Mestinon inhibits the destruction of acetylcholine by cholinesterase and thereby permits freer transmission of nerve impulses across the neuromuscular junction. Pyridostigmine is an analog of neostigmine (Prostigmin®), but differs from it in certain clinically significant respects; for example, pyridostigmine is characterized by a longer duration of action and fewer gastrointestinal side effects.

INDICATION

Mestinon is useful in the treatment of myasthenia gravis.

CONTRAINDICATIONS

Mestinon is contraindicated in mechanical intestinal or urinary obstruction, and particular caution should be used in its administration to patients with bronchial asthma. Care should be observed in the use of atropine for counteracting side effects, as discussed below.

WARNINGS

Although failure of patients to show clinical improvement may reflect underdosage, it can also be indicative of overdosage. As is true of all cholinergic drugs, overdosage of Mestinon may result in cholinergic crisis, a state characterized by increasing muscle weakness which, through involvement of the muscles of respiration, may lead to death. Myasthenic crisis due to an increase in the severity of the disease is also accompanied by extreme muscle weakness, and thus may be difficult to distinguish from cholinergic crisis on a symptomatic basis. Such differentiation is extremely important, since increases in doses of Mestinon or other drugs of this class in the presence of cholinergic crisis or of a refractory or "insensitive" state could have grave consequences. Osserman and Genkins[1] indicate that the differential diagnosis of the two types of crisis may require the use of Tensilon® (edrophonium chloride) as well as clinical judgment. The treatment of the two conditions obviously differs radically. Whereas the presence of myasthenic crisis suggests the need for more intensive anticholinesterase therapy, the diagnosis of cholinergic crisis, according to Osserman and Genkins,[1] calls for the prompt *withdrawal* of all drugs of this type. The immediate use of atropine in cholinergic crisis is also recommended.

Atropine may also be used to abolish or obtund gastrointestinal side effects or other muscarinic reactions; but such use, by masking signs of overdosage, can lead to inadvertent induction of cholinergic crisis.

For detailed information on the management of patients with myasthenia gravis, the physician is referred to one of the excellent reviews such as those by Osserman and Genkins,[2] Grob[3] or Schwab.[4,5]

Usage in Pregnancy: The safety of Mestinon during pregnancy or lactation in humans has not been established. Therefore, use of Mestinon in women who may become pregnant requires weighing the drug's potential benefits against its possible hazards to mother and child.

Pediatric Use: Safety and effectiveness in pediatric patients have not been established.

PRECAUTION

Pyridostigmine is mainly excreted unchanged by the kidney.[6,7,8] Therefore, lower doses may be required in patients with renal disease, and treatment should be based on titration of drug dosage to effect.[6,7]

ADVERSE REACTIONS

The side effects of Mestinon are most commonly related to overdosage and generally are of two varieties, muscarinic and nicotinic. Among those in the former group are nausea, vomiting, diarrhea, abdominal cramps, increased peristalsis, increased salivation, increased bronchial secretions, miosis and diaphoresis. Nicotinic side effects are comprised chiefly of muscle cramps, fasciculation and weakness. Muscarinic side effects can usually be counteracted by atropine, but for reasons shown in the preceding section the expedient is not without danger. As with any compound containing the bromide radical, a skin rash may be seen in an occasional patient. Such reactions usually subside promptly upon discontinuance of the medication.

DOSAGE AND ADMINISTRATION

Mestinon is available in three dosage forms:

Syrup —raspberry-flavored, containing 60 mg pyridostigmine bromide per teaspoonful (5 ml). This form permits accurate dosage adjustment for children and "brittle" myasthenic patients who require fractions of 60-mg doses. It is more easily swallowed, especially in the morning, by patients with bulbar involvement.

Conventional tablets —each containing 60 mg pyridostigmine bromide.

Timespan tablets —each containing 180 mg pyridostigmine bromide. This form provides uniformly slow release, hence prolonged duration of drug action; it facilitates control of myasthenic symptoms with fewer individual doses daily. The immediate effect of a 180-mg Timespan tablet is about equal to that of a 60-mg conventional tablet; however, its duration of effectiveness, although varying in individual patients, averages 2½ times that of a 60-mg dose.

Dosage: The size and frequency of the dosage must be adjusted to the needs of the individual patient.

Syrup and conventional tablets —The average dose is ten 60-mg tablets or ten 5-ml teaspoonfuls daily, spaced to provide maximum relief when maximum strength is needed. In severe cases as many as 25 tablets or teaspoonfuls a day may be required, while in mild cases one to six tablets or teaspoonfuls a day may suffice.

Timespan tablets —One to three 180-mg tablets, once or twice daily, will usually be sufficient to control symptoms; however, the needs of certain individuals may vary markedly from this average. The interval between doses should be at least six hours. For optimum control, it may be necessary to use the more rapidly acting regular tablets or syrup in conjunction with Timespan therapy.

Note: For information on a diagnostic test for myasthenia gravis, and for the evaluation and stabilization of therapy, please see product literature on Tensilon® (edrophonium chloride).

HOW SUPPLIED

Syrup, 60 mg pyridostigmine bromide per teaspoonful (5 ml) and 5% alcohol—bottles of 16 fluid ounces (1 pint) (NDC 0187-3012-20).

Tablets, scored, 60 mg pyridostigmine bromide each—bottles of 100 (NDC 0187-3010-30) and 500 (NDC 0187-3010-40).

Timespan tablets, scored, 180 mg pyridostigmine bromide each—bottles of 30 (NDC 0187-3013-30).

Note: Because of the hygroscopic nature of the Timespan tablets, mottling may occur. This does not affect their efficacy.

REFERENCES

1. Osserman KE, Genkins G. Studies in myasthenia gravis: Reduction in mortality rate after crisis. *JAMA.* Jan 1963; 183:97–101.
2. Osserman KE, Genkins G. Studies in myasthenia gravis. *NY State J. Med.* June 1961; 61:2076–2085.
3. Grob D. Myasthenia gravis. A review of pathogenesis and treatment. *Arch Intern Med.* Oct 1961; 108:615–638.
4. Schwab RS. Management of myasthenia gravis. *New Eng J Med.* Mar 1963; 268:596–597.
5. Schwab RS.Management of myasthenia gravis. *New Eng J Med.* Mar 1963; 268:717–719.
6. Cronnelly R, Stanski DR, Miller RD, Sheiner LB. Pyridostigmine kinetics with and without renal function. *Clin Pharmacol Ther.* 1980; 28:No. 1, 78–81.
7. Miller RD. Pharmacodynamics and pharmacokinetics of anticholinesterase. In: Ruegheimer E, Zindler M, ed. *Anaesthesiology.* (Hamburg, Germany: Congress; Sep 14–21, 1980; 222–223.) (Int Congr. No. 538), Amsterdam, Netherlands: Excerpta Medica; 1981.
8. Breyer-Pfaff U, Maier U, Brinkmann AM, Schumm F. Pyridostigmine kinetics in healthy subjects and patients with myasthenia gravis. *Clin Pharmacol Ther.* 1985;5: 495–501.

Manufactured for ICN Pharmaceuticals, Inc.
Costa Mesa, CA 92626
by Hoffmann-La Roche Inc.
Nutley, N.J. 07110
Rev. 1/97

Shown in Product Identification Guide, page 317

OXSORALEN® LOTION 1% ℞

[*ox 'sore "a-len*]
(methoxsalen USP, 1%)

CAUTION: FEDERAL (U.S.A.) LAW PROHIBITS DISPENSING WITHOUT A PRESCRIPTION.

CAUTION: METHOXSALEN LOTION IS A POTENT TOPICAL DRUG. READ ENTIRE BROCHURE BEFORE PRESCRIBING OR USING THIS MEDICATION.

WARNING: METHOXSALEN LOTION IS A POTENT DRUG CAPABLE OF PRODUCING SEVERE BURNS IF IMPROPERLY USED. IT SHOULD BE APPLIED ONLY BY A PHYSICIAN UNDER CONTROLLED CONDITIONS FOR LIGHT EXPOSURE AND SUBSEQUENT LIGHT SHIELDING.

THIS PREPARATION SHOULD NEVER BE DISPENSED TO A PATIENT.

I. DESCRIPTION

Each ml. of Oxsoralen Lotion contains 10 mg methoxsalen in an inert vehicle containing alcohol (71% v/v), propylene glycol, acetone, and purified water.

Methoxsalen is a naturally occurring substance found in the seeds of the **Ammi majus** (Umbelliferae) plant; it belongs to a group of compounds known as psoralens or furocoumarins. The chemical name of methoxsalen is 9-methoxy-7H-furo(3, 2g) (1)-benzopyran-7-one. It has the following structure:

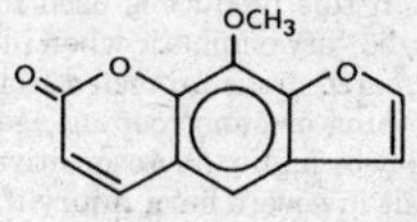

II. CLINICAL PHARMACOLOGY

The exact mechanism of action of methoxsalen with the epidermal melanocytes and keratinocytes is not known. Psoralens given orally are preferentially taken up by epidermal cells (Artuc et al, 1979).[1] The best known biochemical reaction of methoxsalen is with DNA. Methoxsalen, upon photoactivation, conjugates and forms covalent bonds with DNA which leads to the formation of both monofunctional (addition to a single strand of DNA) and bifunctional adducts (crosslinking of psoralen to both strands of DNA) (Dall'Acqua et al, 1971).[2] Reactions with proteins have also been described (Yoshikawa et al, 1979).[3]

Methoxsalen acts as a photosensitizer. Topical application of this drug and subsequent exposure to UVA, whether artificial or sunlight, can cause cell injury. If sufficient cell injury occurs in the skin an inflammatory reaction will result. The most obvious manifestation of this reaction is delayed erythema which may not begin for several hours and may not peak for 2 to 3 days or longer. It is crucial to realize that the length of time the skin remains sensitized or when the maximum erythema will occur is quite variable from person to person. The erythematous reaction is followed over several days or weeks by repair which is manifested by increased melanization of the epidermis and thickening of the stratum corneum. The exact mechanics are unknown but it has been suggested melanocytes in the hair follicles are stimulated to move up the follicle and to repopulate the epidermis. (Ortonne, et al, 1979).[4]

III. INDICATIONS AND USAGE

As a topical repigmenting agent in vitiligo in conjunction with controlled doses of ultraviolet A (320–400 nm) or sunlight.

IV. CONTRAINDICATIONS

A. Patients exhibiting idiosyncratic reactions to psoralen compounds or a history of sensitivity reactions to them.
B. Patients exhibiting melanoma or with a history of melanoma.
C. Patients exhibiting invasive skin carcinoma generally.
D. Patients with photosensitivity diseases such as porphyria, acute lupus erythematosus, xeroderma pigmentosum, etc.
E. Children under 12 since clinical studies to determine the efficacy and safety of treatment in this age group have not been done.

V. WARNINGS

A. Skin Burns

Serious skin burns from either UVA or sunlight (even through window glass) can result if recommended exposure schedule is exceeded and/or protective covering or sunscreens are not used. The blistering of the skin sometimes encountered after UVA exposure generally heals without complication or scarring. (Farrington Daniels, Jr, M.D., personal communication). Suitable covering of the area of application or a topical sunblock should follow the therapeutic UVA exposure.

B. Carcinogenicity

1. Animal Studies. Topical methoxsalen has been reported to be a potent photocarcinogen in certain strains of mice. (Pathak et al 1959).[5]

2. Human Studies. None of our clinical investigators reported skin cancer as a complication of topical treatment for vitiligo. However, it is recommended that caution be exercised when the patient is fair-skinned or has a history of prior coal tar UVA treatment, or has had ionizing radiation or taken arsenical compounds. Such patients who subsequently have oral psoralen—UVA treatment (PUVA) are at increased risk for developing skin cancer.

C. Concomitant Therapy

Special care should be exercised in treating patients who are receiving concomitant therapy (either topically or systemically) with known photosensitizing agents such as an-

Continued on next page

Oxsoralen Lotion—Cont.

thralin, coal tar or coal tar derivatives, griseofulvin, phenothiazines, nalidixic acid, halogenated salicylanilides (bacteriostatic soaps), sulfonamides, tetracyclines, thiazides, and certain organic staining dyes such as methylene blue, toluidine blue, rose bengal, and methyl orange.

VI. PRECAUTIONS

A. This product should be applied only in small well defined lesions and preferably on lesions which can be protected by clothing or a sunscreen from subsequent exposure to radiant UVA. If this product is used to treat vitiligo of face or hands, be very emphatic when instructing patient to keep the treated areas protected from light by use of protective clothing or sunscreening agents. The area of application may be highly photosensitive for several days and may result in severe burn injury if exposed to additional UVA or sunlight.

B. CARCINOGENESIS: See Warning Section

C. Pregnancy Category C. Animal reproduction studies have not been conducted with topical methoxsalen. It is also not known whether methoxsalen can cause fetal harm when used topically on a pregnant woman or affect reproductive capacity. It is not known to what degree, if any, topical methoxsalen is absorbed systemically. Topical methoxsalen should be used in pregnant women only when clearly indicated.

D. Nursing Mothers. It is not known whether topical methoxsalen is absorbed or excreted in human milk. Caution is advised when topical methoxsalen is used in a nursing mother.

E. Pediatric Usage. Safety and effectiveness in children below the age of 12 years have not been established.

VII. ADVERSE REACTIONS

Systemic adverse reactions have not been reported. The most common adverse reaction is severe burns of the treated area from overexposure to UVA, including sunlight. TREATMENT MUST BE INDIVIDUALIZED. Minor blistering of the skin is not a contraindication to further treatment and generally heals without incident. Treatment would be the standard for burn therapy. Since 1953, many studies have demonstrated the safety and effectiveness of topical methoxsalen and UVA for the treatment of vitiligo when used as directed. (Lerner, A.B., et al, 1953)[6] (Fitzpatrick, T.B., et al, 1966)[7] (Fulton, James F. et al, 1969)[8].

VIII. OVERDOSAGE

This does not apply to topical usage. In the unlikely event that the lotion is ingested, standard procedures for poisoning should be followed, including gastric lavage. Protection from UVA or daylight for hours or days would also be necessary. The patient should be kept in a darkened room.

IX. ADMINISTRATION

OXSORALEN® Lotion is applied to a well-defined area of vitiligo by the physician and the area is then exposed to a suitable source of UVA. Initial exposure time should be conservative and not exceed that which is predicted to be one-half the minimal erythema dose. Treatment intervals should be regulated by the erythema response; generally once a week is recommended or less often depending on the results. The hands and fingers of the person applying the medication should be protected by gloves or finger cots to avoid photosensitization and possible burns.

Pigmentation may begin after a few weeks but significant repigmentation may require up to 6 to 9 months of treatment. Periodic re-treatment may be necessary to retain all of the new pigment. Idiopathic vitiligo is reversible but not equally reversible in every patient. Treatment must be individualized. Repigmentation will vary in completeness, time of onset, and duration. Repigmentation occurs more rapidly in fleshy areas such as face, abdomen, and buttocks and less rapidly over less fleshy areas such as the dorsum of the hands or feet.

X. HOW SUPPLIED

Oxsoralen Lotion containing 1% methoxsalen (8-methoxypsoralen) packaged in 1 ounce (29.57 ml) amber glass bottles (NDC 0187-0402-31).

Store at controlled room temperature (15–30°C) (59–86°F).

REFERENCES

1. Artuc, M.; Stuettgen, G.; Schalla, W.; Schaefer, H.; Gazith, J.: Reversible binding of 5- and 8-methoxypsoralen to human serum proteins (albumin) and to epidermis **in vitro; Brit. J. Dermat., 101**, pp. 669–677 (1979).
2. Dall'Acqua, F.; Marciani, S.; Ciavatta, L.; Rodighiero, G.: formation of interstrand cross-linkings in the photoreactions between furocoumarins and DNA.; **Z Naturforsch** (B), **26**, pp. 561–569 (1971).
3. Yoshikawa, K; Mori, N.; Sakakibara, S.; Mizuno, N.; Song, P.: Photo-Conjugation of 8-methoxypsoralen with Proteins; **Photochem & Photobiol, 29**, pp. 1127–1133 (1979).
4. Ortonne, J.P.; MacDonald, D.M.; Micoud, A.; Thivolet, J.: PUVA-induced repigmentation of vitiligo: a histochemical (split-DOPA) and ultra-structural study; **Brit. J. Dermat., 101**, pp. 1–12 (1979).
5. Pathak, M.A.; Daniels, F.; Hopkins, C.E.; Fitzpatrick, T.B.: Ultraviolet carcinogenesis in albino and pigmented mice receiving furocoumarins: psoralens and 8-methoxypsoralen, **Nature, 183**, pp. 728–730 (1959).
6. Lerner, A.B.; Denton, C.R.; Fitzpatrick, T.B.: Clinical and experimental studies with 8-methoxypsoralen in vitiligo; **J. Invest. Derm., 20**, pp. 299–314 (April, 1953).
7. Fitzpatrick, T.B.; Arndt, K.A.; El Mofty, A.M.: Hydroquinone and psoralens in the therapy of hypermelanosis and vitiligo; **Arch Derm., 93**, pp. 589–599 (May, 1966).
8. Fulton, James F.; Leyden, James; Papa, Christopher: Treatment of vitiligo with topical methoxsalen and blacklite; **Arch. Derm., 101**, pp. 224–229 (1969).

Rev. 4–96
2398-02 EL

OXSORALEN–ULTRA® CAPSULES ℞

[ox '-sore "a-len]
(Methoxsalen, 10 mg)

CAUTION: FEDERAL LAW PROHIBITS DISPENSING WITHOUT PRESCRIPTION.
CAUTION: METHOXSALEN IS A POTENT DRUG, READ ENTIRE BROCHURE PRIOR TO PRESCRIBING OR DISPENSING THIS MEDICATION.

Methoxsalen with UV radiation should be used only by physicians who have special competence in the diagnosis and treatment of psoriasis and who have special training and experience in photochemotherapy. The use of Psoralen and ultraviolet radiation therapy should be under constant supervision of such a physician. For the treatment of patients with psoriasis, photochemotherapy should be restricted to patients with severe, recalcitrant, disabling psoriasis which is not adequately responsive to other forms of therapy, and only when the diagnosis has been supported by biopsy. Because of the possibilities of ocular damage, aging of the skin, and skin cancer (including melanoma), the patient should be fully informed by the physician of the risks inherent in this therapy.

CAUTION: Oxsoralen-Ultra® should not be used interchangeably with regular Oxsoralen®. This new dosage form of methoxsalen exhibits significantly greater bioavailability and earlier photosensitization onset time than previous methoxsalen dosage forms. Patients should be treated in accordance with the dosimetry specifically recommended for this product. The minimum phototoxic dose (MPD) and phototoxic peak time after drug administration prior to onset of photochemotherapy with this dosage form should be determined.

I. DESCRIPTION

Oxsoralen-Ultra (methoxsalen, 8-methoxypsoralen) Capsules, 10 mg. Methoxsalen is a naturally occurring photoactive substance found in the seeds of the **Ammi majus** (Umbelliferae) plant. It belongs to a group of compounds known as psoralens, or furocoumarins. The chemical name of methoxsalen is 9-methoxy-7H-furo [3,2-g] [1]benzopyran-7-one; it has the following structure:

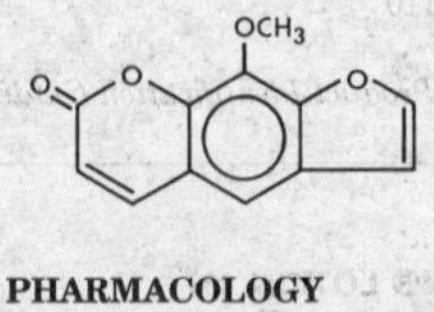

II. CLINICAL PHARMACOLOGY

The combination treatment regimen of psoralen (P) and ultraviolet radiation of 320–400 nm wavelength commonly referred to as UVA is known by the acronym, PUVA. Skin reactivity to UVA (320–400nm) radiation is markedly enhanced by the ingestion of methoxsalen. In a well controlled bioavailability study, Oxsoralen-Ultra Capsules reached peak drug levels in the blood of test subjects between 0.5 and 4 hours (Mean = 1.8 hours) as compared to between 1.5 and 6 hours (Mean = 3.0 hours) for regular Oxsoralen when administered with 8 ounces of milk. Peak drug levels were 2 to 3 fold greater when the overall extent of drug absorption was approximately two fold greater for Oxsoralen-Ultra Capsules as compared to regular Oxsoralen Capsules. Detectable methoxsalen levels were observed up to 12 hours post dose. The drug half-life is approximately 2 hours. Photosensitivity studies demonstrate a shorter time of peak photosensitivity of 1.5 to 2.1 hours vs. 3.9 to 4.25 hours for regular Oxsoralen capsules. In addition, the mean minimal erythema dose (MED), J/cm^2, for the Oxsoralen-Ultra Capsules is substantially less than that required for regular Oxsoralen Capsules (Levins et al., 1984 and private communication[1]).

Methoxsalen is reversibly bound to serum albumin and is also preferentially taken up by epidermal cells (Artuc et al., 1979[2]). At a dose which is six times larger than that used in humans, it induces mixed function oxidases in the liver of mice (Mandula et al., 1978[3]). In both mice and man, methoxsalen is rapidly metabolized. Approximately 95% of the drug is excreted as a series of metabolites in the urine within 24 hours (Pathak et al., 1977[4]). The exact mechanism of action of methoxsalen with the epidermal melanocytes and keratinocytes is not known. The best known biochemical reaction of methoxsalen is with DNA. Methoxsalen, upon photoactivation, conjugates and forms covalent bonds with DNA which leads to the formation of both monofunctional (addition to a single strand of DNA) and bifunctional (crosslinking of psoralen to both strands of DNA) adducts (Dall' Acqua et al., 1971[5]; Cole, 1970[6]; Musajo et al., 1974[7]; Dall' Acqua et al., 1979[8]). Reactions with proteins have also been described (Yoshikawa, et al., 1979[9]).

Methoxsalen acts as a photosensitizer. Administration of the drug and subsequent exposure to UVA can lead to cell injury. Orally administered methoxsalen reaches the skin via the blood and UVA penetrates well into the skin. If sufficient cell injury occurs in the skin, an inflammatory reaction occurs. The most obvious manifestation of this reaction is delayed erythema, which may not begin for several hours and peaks at 48–72 hours. The inflammation is followed, over several days to weeks, by repair which is manifested by increased melanization of the epidermis and thickening of the stratum corneum. The mechanisms of therapy are not known. In the treatment of psoriasis, the mechanism is most often assumed to be DNA photodamage and resulting decrease in cell proliferation but other vascular, leukocyte, or cell regulatory mechanisms may also be playing some role. Psoriasis is a hyper-proliferative disorder and other agents known to be therapeutic for psoriasis are known to inhibit DNA synthesis.

III. INDICATIONS AND USAGE

Photochemotherapy (Methoxsalen with long wave UVA radiation) is indicated for the symptomatic control of severe, recalcitrant, disabling psoriasis not adequately responsive to other forms of therapy and when the diagnosis has been supported by biopsy. Methoxsalen is intended to be administered only in conjunction with a schedule of controlled doses of long wave ultraviolet radiation.

IV. CONTRAINDICATIONS

A. Patients exhibiting idiosyncratic reactions to psoralen compounds.

B. Patients possessing a specific history of light sensitive disease states should not initiate methoxsalen therapy except under special circumstances. Diseases associated with photosensitivity include lupus erythematosus, porphyria cutanea tarda, erythropoietic protoporphyria, variegate porphyria, xeroderma pigmentosum, and albinism.

C. Patients with melanoma or with a history of melanoma.

D. Patients with invasive squamous cell carcinomas.

E. Patients with aphakia, because of the significantly increased risk of retinal damage due to the absence of lenses.

V. WARNINGS—GENERAL

A. SKIN BURNING: Serious burns from either UVA or sunlight (even through window glass) can result if the recommended dosage of the drug and/or exposure schedules are exceeded.

B. CARCINOGENICITY:

1. ANIMAL STUDIES: Topical or intraperitoneal methoxsalen has been reported to be a potent photocarcinogen in albino mice and hairless mice (Hakim et al., 1960[10]). However, methoxsalen given by the oral route to Swiss albino mice suggests this agent exerts a protective effect against ultraviolet carcinogenesis; mice given 8-methoxypsoralen in their diet showed 38% ear tumors 180 days after the start of ultraviolet therapy compared to 62% for controls (O'Neal et al., 1957[11]).

2. HUMAN STUDIES: A 5.7 year prospective study of 1380 psoriasis patients treated with oral methoxsalen and ultraviolet A photochemotherapy (PUVA) demonstrated that the risk of cutaneous squamous-cell carcinoma developing at least 22 months following the first PUVA exposure was approximately 12.8 times higher in the high dose patients than in the low dose patients (Stern et al., 1979[12], Stern et al., 1980[13], and Stern et al., 1984[14]). The substantial dose-dependent increase was observed in patients with neither a prior history of skin cancer nor significant exposure to cutaneous carcinogens. Reduction in PUVA dosage significantly reduces the risk. No substantial dose related increase was noted for basal cell carcinoma according to Stern et al., 1984[14]. Increases

appear greatest in patients who have pre-PUVA exposure to 1) prolonged tar and UVB treatment, 2) ionizing radiation, or 3) arsenic.

Roenigk et al., 1980[15], studied 690 patients for up to 4 years and found no increase in the risk of non-melanoma skin cancer, although patients in this cohort had significantly less exposure to PUVA than in the Stern et al. study. After 5 years, two of 1380 patients in the Stern et al. PUVA study have developed malignant melanoma. In addition, more than $^1/_5$ of the patients in this cohort have developed macular pigmented lesions on the buttocks. While there is no evidence that an increased risk of melanoma exists in PUVA treated patients, these observations indicate the need for continued evaluation of melanoma risk of PUVA treated patients.

In a study in Indian patients treated for 4 years for vitiligo, 12 percent developed keratoses, but not cancer, in the depigmented, vitiliginous areas (Mosher, 1980[16]). Clinically, the keratoses were keratotic papules, actinic keratosis-like macules, nonscaling dome-shaped papules, and lichenoid porokeratotic-like papules.

C. CATARACTOGENICITY:

1. ANIMAL STUDIES: Exposure to large doses of UVA causes cataracts in animals, and this effect is enhanced by the administration of methoxsalen (Cloud et al, 1960[17]; Cloud et al, 1961[18]; Freeman et al, 1969[19]).

2. HUMAN STUDIES: It has been found that the concentration of methoxsalen in the lens is proportional to the serum level. If the lens is exposed to UVA during the time methoxsalen is present in the lens, photochemical action may lead to irreversible binding of methoxsalen to proteins and the DNA components of the lens (Lerman et al, 1980[20]). However, if the lens is shielded from UVA, the methoxsalen will diffuse out of the lens in a 24 hour period (Lerman et al., 1980[20]). Patients should be told emphatically to wear UVA-absorbing, wrap-around sunglasses for the twenty-four (24) hour period following ingestion of methoxsalen, whether exposed to direct or indirect sunlight in the open or through a window glass. Among patients using proper eye protection, there is no evidence for a significantly increased risk of cataracts in association with PUVA therapy. (Stern et al., 1979[12]). Thirty-five of 1380 patients have developed cataracts in the five years since their first PUVA treatment. This incidence is comparable to that expected in a population of this size and age distribution. No relationship between PUVA dose and cataract risk in this group has been noted.

D. ACTINIC DEGENERATION: Exposure to sunlight and/or ultraviolet radiation may result in "premature aging" of the skin.

E. BASAL CELL CARCINOMAS: Patients exhibiting multiple basal cell carcinomas or having a history of basal cell carcinomas should be diligently observed and treated.

F. RADIATION THERAPY: Patients having a history of previous x-ray therapy or grenz ray therapy should be diligently observed for signs of carcinoma.

G. ARSENIC THERAPY: Patients having a history of previous arsenic therapy should be diligently observed for signs of carcinoma.

H. HEPATIC DISEASES: Patients with hepatic insufficiency should be treated with caution since hepatic biotransformation is necessary for drug urinary excretion.

I. CARDIAC DISEASES: Patients with cardiac diseases or others who may be unable to tolerate prolonged standing or exposure to heat stress should not be treated in a vertical UVA chamber.

J. TOTAL DOSAGE: The total cumulative dose of UVA that can be given over long periods of time with safety has not as yet been established.

K. CONCOMITANT THERAPY: Special care should be exercised in treating patients who are receiving concomitant therapy (either topically or systemically) with known photosensitizing agents such as anthralin, coal tar or coal tar derivatives, griseofulvin, phenothiazines, nalidixic acid, halogenated salicylanilides (bacteriostatic soaps), sulfonamides, tetracyclines, thiazides and certain organic staining dyes such as methylene blue, toluidine blue, rose bengal, and methyl orange.

VI. PRECAUTIONS

A. GENERAL—APPLICABLE TO PSORIASIS TREATMENT

1. BEFORE METHOXSALEN INGESTION
Patients must not sunbathe during the 24 hours prior to methoxsalen ingestion and UV exposure. The presence of a sunburn may prevent an accurate evaluation of the patient's response to photochemotherapy.

2. AFTER METHOXSALEN INGESTION
a. UVA-absorbing wrap-around sunglasses should be worn during daylight for 24 hours after methoxsalen ingestion. The protective eyewear must be designed to prevent entry of stray radiation to the eyes, including that which may enter from the sides of the eyewear. The protective eyewear is used to prevent the irreversible binding of methoxsalen to the proteins and DNA components of the lens. Cataracts form when enough of the binding occurs. Visual discrimination should be permitted by the eyewear for patient well-being and comfort.
b. Patients must avoid sun exposure, even through window glass or cloud cover, for at least 8 hours after methoxsalen ingestion. If sun exposure cannot be avoided, the patient should wear protective devices such as a hat and gloves, and/or apply sunscreens which contain ingredients that filter out UVA radiation (e.g. sunscreens containing benzophenone and/or PABA esters which exhibit a sun protective factor equal to or greater than 15). These chemical sunscreens should be applied to all areas that might be exposed to the sun (including lips). Sunscreens should not be applied to areas affected by psoriasis until after the patient has been treated in the UVA chamber.

3. DURING PUVA THERAPY
a. Total UVA-absorbing/blocking goggles mechanically designed to give maximal ocular protection must be worn. Failure to do so may increase the risk of cataract formation. A reliable radiometer can be used to verify elimination of UVA transmission through the goggles.
b. Abdominal skin, breasts, genitalia, and other sensitive areas should be protected for approximately $^1/_3$ of the initial exposure time until tanning occurs.
c. Unless affected by disease, male genitalia should be shielded.

4. AFTER COMBINED METHOXSALEN/UVA THERAPY
a. UVA-absorbing wrap-around sunglasses should be worn during daylight for 24 hours after combined methoxsalen/UVA therapy.
b. Patients should not sunbathe for 48 hours after therapy. Erythema and/or burning due to photochemotherapy and sunburn due to sun exposure are additive.

B. INFORMATION FOR PATIENTS: See accompanying Patient Package Insert.

C. LABORATORY TESTS:

1. Patients should have an ophthalmologic examination prior to start of therapy, and thence yearly.
2. Patients should have routine laboratory tests prior to the start of therapy and at regular periods thereafter if patients are on extended treatments.

D. DRUG INTERACTIONS: See Warnings Section.

E. CARCINOGENESIS: See Warnings Section.

F. PREGNANCY:
Pregnancy Category C. Animal reproduction studies have not been conducted with methoxsalen. It is also not known whether methoxsalen can cause fetal harm when administered to a pregnant woman or can affect reproduction capacity. Methoxsalen should be given to a woman with reproductive capacity only if clearly needed.

G. NURSING MOTHERS:
It is not known whether this drug is excreted in human milk. Because many drugs are excreted in human milk, either methoxsalen ingestion or nursing should be discontinued.

H. PEDIATRIC USE:
Safety in children has not been established. Potential hazards of long-term therapy include the possibilities of carcinogenicity and cataractogenicity as described in the Warnings Section as well as the probability of actinic degeneration which is also described in the Warnings Section.

VII. ADVERSE REACTIONS

A. METHOXSALEN:
The most commonly reported side effect of methoxsalen alone is nausea, which occurs with approximately 10% of all patients. This effect may be minimized or avoided by instructing the patient to take methoxsalen in milk or food, or to divide the dose into two portions, taken approximately one-half hour apart. Other effects include nervousness, insomnia, and depression.

B. COMBINED METHOXSALEN/UVA THERAPY:

1. PRURITUS: This adverse reaction occurs with approximately 10% of all patients. In most cases, pruritus can be alleviated with frequent application of bland emollients or other topical agents; severe pruritus may require systemic treatment. If pruritus is unresponsive to these measures, shield pruritic areas from further UVA exposure until the condition resolves. If intractable pruritus is generalized, UVA treatment should be discontinued until the pruritus disappears.

2. ERYTHEMA: Mild, transient erythema at 24–48 hours after PUVA therapy is an expected reaction and indicates that a therapeutic interaction between methoxsalen and UVA occurred. Any area showing moderate erythema (greater than Grade 2—See Table 1 for grades of erythema) should be shielded during subsequent UVA exposures until the erythema has resolved. Erythema greater than Grade 2 which appears within 24 hours after UVA treatment may signal a potentially severe burn. Erythema may become progressively worse over the next 24 hours, since the peak erythemal reaction characteristically occurs 48 hours or later after methoxsalen ingestion. The patient should be protected from further UVA exposures and sunlight, and should be monitored closely.

3. IMPORTANT DIFFERENCES BETWEEN PUVA ERYTHEMA AND SUNBURN: PUVA-induced inflammation differs from sunburn or UVB phototherapy in several ways. The percent transmission of UVB varies between 0% to 34% through skin whereas UVA varies between 1% to 80% transmission; thus, UVA is transmitted to a larger percent through the skin. (Diffey, 1982[21]). The DNA lesions induced by PUVA are very different from UV-induced thymine dimers and may lead to a DNA crosslink. This DNA lesion may be more problematic to the cell because crosslinks are more lethal and psoralen-DNA photoproducts may be "new" or unfamiliar substrates for DNA repair enzymes. DNA synthesis is also suppressed longer after PUVA. The time course of delayed erythema is different with PUVA and may not involve the usual mediators seen in sunburn. PUVA-induced redness may be just beginning at 24 hours, when UVB erythema has already passed its peak. The erythema dose-response curve is also steeper for PUVA. Compared to equally erythemogenic doses of UVB, the histologic alterations induced by PUVA show more dermal vessel damage and longer duration of epidermal and dermal abnormalities.

4. OTHER ADVERSE REACTIONS: Those reported include edema, dizziness, headache, malaise, depression, hypopigmentation, vesiculation and bullae formation, non-specific rash, herpes simplex, miliaria, urticaria, folliculitis, gastrointestinal disturbances, cutaneous tenderness, leg cramps, hypotension, and extension of psoriasis.

VIII. OVERDOSAGE

In the event of methoxsalen overdosage, induce emesis and keep the patient in a darkened room for at least 24 hours. Emesis is most beneficial within the first 2 to 3 hours after ingestion of methoxsalen, since maximum blood levels are reached by this time.

IX. DRUG DOSAGE AND ADMINISTRATION

CAUTION: Oxsoralen-Ultra represents a new dose form of methoxsalen. This new dosage form of methoxsalen exhibits significantly greater bioavailability and earlier photosensitization onset time than previous methoxsalen dosage forms. Each patient should be evaluated by determining the minimum phototoxic dose (MPD) and phototoxic peak time after drug administration prior to onset of photochemotherapy with this dosage form. Human bioavailability studies have indicated the following drug dosage and administration directions are to be used as a guideline only.

PSORIASIS THERAPY

1. DRUG DOSAGE-INITIAL THERAPY: The methoxsalen capsules should be taken $1^1/_2$ to 2 hours before UVA exposure with some low fat food or milk according to the following table:

Patient's Weight (kg)	(lbs)	Dose (mg)
<30	<65	10
30–50	65–100	20
51–65	101–145	30
66–80	146–175	40
81–90	176–200	50
91–115	201–250	60
>115	>250	70

2. INITIAL EXPOSURE: The initial UVA exposure energy level and corresponding time of exposure is determined by the patient's skin characteristics for sunburning and tanning as follows:

Skin Type	History	Recommended Joules/cm²
I	Always burn, never tan (patients with erythrodermic psoriasis are to be classed as Type I for determination of UVA dosage.)	0.5 J/cm²
II	Always burn, but sometimes tan	1.0 J/cm²
III	Sometimes burn, but always tan	1.5 J/cm²
IV	Never burn, always tan	2.0 J/cm²
Skin Type	**Physician Examination**	**Joules/cm²**
V*	Moderately pigmented	2.5 J/cm²
VI*	Blacks	3.0 J/cm²

Continued on next page

Oxsoralen–Ultra—Cont.

(*Patients with natural pigmentation of these types should be classified into a lower skin type category if the sunburning history so indicates.)

If the MPD is done, start at 1/2 MPD.
Additional drug dosage directions are as follows:
a. Weight Change: In the event that the weight of a patient changes during treatment such that he/she falls into an adjacent weight range/dose category, no change in the dose of methoxsalen is usually required. If, in the physician's opinion, however, a weight change is sufficiently great to modify the drug dose, then an adjustment in the time of exposure to UVA should be made.
b. Dose/Week: The number of doses per week of methoxsalen capsules will be determined by the patient's schedule of UVA exposures. In no case should treatments be given more often than once every other day because the full extent of phototoxic reactions may not be evident until 48 hours after each exposure.
c. Dosage Increase: Dosage may be increased by 10 mg after the fifteenth treatment under the conditions outlined in section XI. B. 4b.

X. UVA RADIATION SOURCE SPECIFICATIONS & INFORMATION

A. IRRADIANCE UNIFORMITY

The following specifications should be met with the window of the detector held in a vertical plane:
1. Vertical variation: For readings taken at any point along the vertical center axis of the chamber (to within 15 cm from the top and bottom), the lowest reading should not be less than 70 percent of the highest reading.
2. Horizontal variation: Throughout any specific horizontal plane, the lowest reading must be at least 80 percent of the highest reading, excluding the peripheral 3 cm of the patient treatment space.

B. PATIENT SAFETY FEATURES:

The following safety features should be present: (1) Protection from electrical hazard: All units should be grounded and conform to applicable electrical codes. The patient or operator should not be able to touch any live electrical parts. There should be ground fault protection. (2) Protective shielding of lamps: The patient should not be able to come in contact with the bare lamps. In the event of lamp breakage, the patient should not be exposed to broken lamp components. (3) Hand rails and hand holds: Appropriate supports should be available to the patient. (4) Patient viewing window: A window which blocks UV should be provided for viewing the patient during treatment. (5) Door and latches: Patients should be able to open the door from the inside with only slight pressure to the door. (6) Non-skid floor: The floor should be of a non-skid nature. (7) Thermoregulation: Sufficient air flow should be provided for patient safety and comfort, limiting temperature within the UVA radiator cabinet to approximately less than 100°F. (8) Timer: The irradiator should be equipped with an automatic timer which terminates the exposure at the conclusion of a preset time interval. (9) Patient alarm device: An alarm device within the UVA irradiator chamber should be accessible to the patient for emergency activation. (10) Danger label: The unit should have a label prominently displayed which reads as follows:
DANGER—Ultraviolet Radiation—Follow your physician's instructions—Failure to use protective eyewear may result in eye injury.

C. UVA EXPOSURE DOSIMETRY MEASUREMENTS:

The maximum radiant exposure or irradiance (within ± 15 percent) of UVA (320–400 nm) delivered to the patient should be determined by using an appropriate radiometer calibrated to be read in Joules/cm² or mW/cm². In the absence of a standard measuring technique approved by the National Bureau of Standards, the system should use a detector corrected to a cosine spatial response. The use and recalibration frequency of such a radiometer for a specific UVA irradiator chamber should be specified by the manufacturer because the UVA dose (exposure) is determined by the design of the irradiator, the number of lamps, and the age of the lamp. If irradiance is measured, the radiometer reading in mW/cm² is used to calculate the exposure time in minutes to deliver the required UVA in Joules/cm² to a patient in the UVA irradiator cabinet. The equation is:

$$\text{Exposure Time (minutes)} = \frac{\text{Desired UVA Dose (J/cm}^2\text{)}}{0.06 \times \text{Irradiance (mW/cm}^2\text{)}}.$$

Overexposure due to human error should be minimized by using an accurate automatic timing device, which is set by the operator and controlled by energizing and deenergizing the UVA irradiator lamp. The timing device calibration interval should be specified by the manufacturer. Safety systems should be included to minimize the possibility of delivering a UVA exposure which exceeds the prescribed dose, in the event the timer or radiometer should malfunction.

D. UVA SPECTRAL OUTPUT DISTRIBUTION:

The spectral distributions of the lamps should meet the following specifications:

Wavelength band (nanometers)	Output[1]
<310	<1
310 to 320	1 to 3
320 to 330	4 to 8
330 to 340	11 to 17
340 to 350	18 to 25
350 to 360	19 to 28
360 to 370	15 to 23
370 to 380	8 to 12
380 to 390	3 to 7
390 to 400	1 to 3

[1] As a percentage of total irradiance between 320 and 400 nanometers.

XI. PUVA TREATMENT PROTOCOL

INTRODUCTION:

The Oxsoralen-Ultra® Capsules reach their maximum bioavailability in 1 1/2 to 2 hours after ingestion.
On average, the serum level achieved with Oxsoralen-Ultra is twice that obtained with 8-MOP (formerly Oxsoralen) and reach their peak concentration in less than 1/2 the time of the 8-MOP capsules.
As a result the mean MED J/cm² for the Oxsoralen-Ultra Capsules is substantially less than that required for 8-MOP (Levins et al., 1984 and private communication[1]).
Photosensitivity studies demonstrate a shorter time of peak photosensitivity of 1.5 to 2.1 hours vs. 3.9 to 4.25 hours for regular methoxsalen capsules.

A. INITIAL EXPOSURE: The initial UVA exposures should be conducted according to the guidelines presented previously under IX.B.1 and 2, Psoriasis Therapy, Drug Dosage-initial Therapy and Exposure.

B. CLEARING PHASE: Specific recommendations for patient treatment are as follows:
1. SKIN TYPES I, II, & III. Patients with skin types I, II, and III may be treated 2 or 3 times per week. UVA exposure may be held constant or increased by up to 1.0 Joule/cm² at each treatment, according to the patient's response. If erythema occurs, however, do not increase exposure time until erythema resolves. The severity and extent of the patient's erythema may be used to determine whether the next exposure should be shortened, omitted, or maintained at the previous dosage. See Adverse Reactions section for additional information.
2. SKIN TYPES IV, V, & VI. Patients with skin types IV, V, and VI may be treated 2 or 3 times per week. UVA exposure may be held constant or increased by up to 1.5 Joules/cm² at each treatment unless erythema occurs. If erythema occurs, follow instructions outlined above in the procedures for patients with skin types I, II, and III.
3. ERYTHRODERMIC PSORIASIS. Patients with erythrodermic psoriasis should be treated with special attention because pre-existing erythema may obscure observations of possible treatment-related phototoxic erythema. These patients may be treated 2 or 3 times per week, as a Type I patient.
4. MISCELLANEOUS SITUATIONS:
a. If there is no response after a total of 10 treatments, the exposure of UVA energy may be increased by an additional 0.5-1.0 Joules/cm² above the prior incremental increases for each treatment. (Example: a patient whose exposure dose is being increased by 1.0 Joule/cm² may now have all subsequent doses increased by 1.5-2.0 Joules/cm².)
b. If there is no response, or only minimal response, after 15 treatments, the dosage of methoxsalen may be increased by 10 mg (a one-time increase in dosage). This increased dosage may be continued for the remainder of the course of treatment but should not be exceeded.
c. If a patient misses a treatment, the UVA exposure time of the next treatment should not be increased. If more than one treatment is missed, reduce the exposure by 0.5 Joules/cm² for each treatment missed.
d. If the lower extremities are not responding as well as the rest of the body and do not show erythema, cover all other body areas and give 25 percent of the present exposure dose as an additional exposure to the lower extremities. This additional exposure to the lower extremities should be terminated if erythema develops on these areas.
e. Non-responsive psoriasis: If a patient's generalized psoriasis is not responding, or if the condition appears to be worsening during treatment, the possibility of a generalized phototoxic reaction should be considered. This may be confirmed by the improvement of the condition following temporary discontinuance of this therapy for two weeks. If no improvement occurs during the interruption of treatment, this patient may be considered a treatment failure.

C. ALTERNATIVE EXPOSURE SCHEDULE:

As an alternative to increasing the UVA exposure at each treatment, the following schedule may be followed; this schedule may reduce the total number of Joules/cm² received by the patient over the entire course of therapy.
1. Incremental increases in UVA exposure for all patients may range from 0.5 to 1.5 Joules/cm², according to the patient's response to therapy.
2. Once Grade 2 clearing (see Table 2) has been reached and the patient is progressing adequately, UVA dosage is held constant. The dosage is maintained until Grade 4 clearing is reached.
3. If the rate of clearing significantly decreases, exposure dosage may be increased at each treatment (0.1–1.5 Joules/cm²) until Grade 3 clearing and a satisfactory progress rate is attained. The UVA exposure will be held constant again until Grade 4 clearing is attained. These increases may be used also if the rate of clearing significantly decreases between Grade 3 and Grade 4 response. However, the possibility of a phototoxic reaction should be considered; see Non-responsive Psoriasis, above.
4. In summary, this schedule raises slightly the increments (Joules/cm²) of UVA dosage, but limits these increases to those periods when the patient is not responding adequately. Otherwise, the UVA exposure is held at the lowest effective dose.

D. MAINTENANCE PHASE:

The goal of maintenance treatment is to keep the patient as symptom-free as possible with the least amount of UVA exposure.
1. SCHEDULE OF EXPOSURES: When patients have achieved 95 percent clearing, or Grade 4 response (Table 2), they may be placed on the following maintenance schedules (M_1–M_4), in sequence. It is recommended that each maintenance schedule be adhered to for at least 2 treatments (unless erythema or psoriatic flare occurs, in which case see (2a) and (2b) below).

Maintenance Schedules
M_1—once/week
M_2—once/2 weeks
M_3—once/3 weeks
M_4—p.r.n. (i.e. for flares)

2. LENGTH OF EXPOSURE: The UVA exposure for the first maintenance treatment of any schedule (except M_4 as noted below) is the same as that of the patient's last treatment under the previous schedule. For skin types I–IV, however, it is recommended that the maximum UVA dosage during maintenance treatments not exceed the following:

Skin Types	Joules/cm²/treatment
I	12
II	14
III	18
IV	22

If the patient develops erythema or new lesions of psoriasis, proceed as follows:
a. Erythema: During maintenance therapy, the patient's tan and threshold dose for erythema may gradually decrease. If maintenance treatments produce significant erythema, the exposure to UVA should be decreased by 25 percent until further treatments no longer produce erythema.
b. Psoriasis: If the patient develops new areas of psoriasis during maintenance therapy (but still is classified as having a Grade 4 response), the exposure to UVA may be increased by 0.5–1.5 Joules/cm² at each treatment; this is appropriate for all types of patients. These increases are continued until the psoriasis is brought under control and the patient is again clear. The exposure being administered when this clearing is reached should be used for further maintenance treatment.
3. FLARES DURING MAINTENANCE: If the patient flares during maintenance treatment (i.e., develops psoriasis on more than 5 percent of the originally involved areas of the body) his maintenance treatment schedule may be changed to the preceding maintenance or clearing schedule. The patient may be kept on his schedule until again 95 percent clear. If the original maintenance treatment schedule is unable to control the psoriasis, the schedule may be changed to a more frequent regimen. If a flare occurs less than 6 weeks after the last treatment, 25 percent of the maximum exposure received during the clearing phase, with the clearing schedule received during the clearing phase, may be used and then proceed with the clearing schedule previously followed for this patient. (At 95 percent clearing, follow regular maintenance until the optimum maintenance schedule is determined for the patient.) If more than 6 weeks have elapsed since the last treatment was given, treat patients as if they were beginning therapy insofar as exposure dosages are concerned, since their threshold for erythema may have decreased.

Table 1. Grades of Erythema

Grades	Erythema
0	No erythema
1	Minimally perceptible erythema—faint pink
2	Marked erythema but with no edema
3	Fiery erythema with edema
4	Fiery erythema with edema and blistering

Table 2. Response to Therapy

Grade	Criteria	Percent Improvement (compared to original extent of disease)
−1	Psoriasis worse	0
0	No change	0
1	Minimal improvement— slightly less scale and/or erythema	5–20
2	Definite improvement— partial flattening of all plaques— less scaling and less erythema	20–50
3	Considerable improvement— nearly complete flattening of all plaques but borders of plaques still palpable	50–95
4	Clearing; complete flattening of plaques including borders; plaques may be outlined by pigmentation	95

XII. HOW SUPPLIED

Oxsoralen-Ultra Capsules, each containing 10 mg of methoxsalen (8-methoxypsoralen) in a soft gelatin capsule packaged in amber glass bottles are available as follows:

Unit Count	NDC Number
50	0187-0650-42

ICN Pharmaceuticals, Inc. Rev. 9-96
Costa Mesa, Ca 92626 2400–01 EL

BIBLIOGRAPHY

1. Levins, P.C., Gange, R.W., Momtaz-T.K., Parrish, J.A., and Fitzpatrick, T.B.: A New Liquid Formulation of 8-Methoxypsoralen: Bioactivity and Effect of Diet: JID, *82,* No. 2, pp. 185–187 (1984) and private communication.
2. Artuc, M., Stuettgen, G. Schalla, W., Schaefer, H., and Gazith, J.: Reversible binding of 5- and 8-methoxypsoralen to human serum proteins (albumin) and to epidermis in vitro: Brit. J. Dermat. *101,* pp. 669–677 (1979).
3. Mandula, B.B., Pathak, M.A., Nakayama, T., and Davidson, S.J.: Induction of mixed-function oxidases in mouse liver by psoralens., Ibid, *99,* pp. 687–692 (1978).
4. Pathak, M.A., Fitzpatrick, T.B., Parrish, J.A.: PSORIASIS, Proceedings of the Second International Symposium. Edited by E.M. Farber, A.J. Cox, Yorke Medical Books, pp. 262–265 (1977).
5. Dall'Acqua, F., Marciani, S., Ciavatta, L., Rodighiero, G.: Formation of interstrand cross-linkings in the photoreactions between furocoumarins and DNA; Z Naturforsch (B), *26,* pp. 561–569 (1971).
6. Cole, R.S.: Light-induced cross-linkings of DNA in the presence of a furocoumarin (psoralen), Biochem. Biophys. Acta, *217,* pp. 30–39 (1970).
7. Musajo, L, Rodighiero, G., Caporale, G., Dall'Acqua, F, Marciani, S., Bordin, F., Baccichetti, F., Bevilacqua, R.: Photoreactions between Skin-Photosensitizing Furocoumarins and Nucleic Acids, *Sunlight and Man;* Normal and Abnormal Photobiologic Responses. Edited by M.A. Pathak, LC. Harber, M. Seiji et al. University of Tokyo Press, pp. 369–387 (1974).
8. Dall'Acqua, F., Vedaldi, D., Bordin, F., and Rodighiero, G.: New studies in the interaction between 8-methoxypsoralen and DNA *in vitro:* JID, *73,* pp. 191–197 (1979).
9. Yoshikawa, K., Mori, N., Sakakibara, S., Mizuno, N. Song, P.: Photo Conjugation of 8-methoxypsoralen with Proteins; Photochem. & Photobiol. *29,* pp. 1127–1133 (1979).
10. Hakim, R.E., Griffin, A.C.: Knox, J.M.: Erythema and tumor formation in methoxsalen treated mice exposed to fluorescent light; Arch. Dermatol. *82,* pp. 572–577 (1960).
11. O'Neal, M.A., Griffin, A.C.: The Effect of Oxypsoralen upon Ultraviolet Carcinogenesis in Albino Mice, Cancer Res., *17,* pp. 911–916 (1957).
12. Stern, R.S., Unpublished personal communication.
13. Stern, R.S., Parrish, J.A., Zierler, S.: Skin Carcinoma in Patients with Psoriasis Treated with Topical Tar and Artificial Ultraviolet Radiation. Lancet, *1,* pp. 732–735 (1980).
14. Stern, R.S., Laird, N., Melski, J. Parrish, J.A., Fitzpatrick, T.B., Bleich, H.L.: Cutaneous Squamous-Cell Carcinoma in Patients Treated with PUVA: NEJM, *310,* No. 18, pp. 1156–1161 (1984).
15. Roenigk, Jr., H.H., and 12 Cooperating Investigators: Skin Cancer in the PUVA-48 Cooperative Study of Psoriasis. Program for Forty-First Annual Meeting for The Society of Investigative Dermatology, Inc., Sheraton Washington Hotel, Washington, D.C., May 12, 13, and 14, 1980). Abstracts JID, *74,* No. 4, p. 250 (April, 1980).
16. Mosher, D.B., Pathak, M.A., Harris, T.J., Fitzpatrick, T.B.: Development of Cutaneous Lesions in Vitiligo During Long-Term PUVA Therapy. Program for Forty-First Annual Meeting for the Society for Investigative Dermatology, Inc., Sheraton Washington Hotel, Washington, D.C., May 12, 13, and 14, 1980. Abstracts JID, *74,* No. 4, p 259 (April, 1980).
17. Cloud, T.M. Hakim, R., Griffin, A.C.: Photosensitization of the eye with methoxsalen. I. Acute effects; Arch. Ophthalmol. *64,* pp. 346–352 (1960).
18. Cloud, T.M. Hakim, R., Griffin, A.C.: Photosensitization of the eye with methoxsalen. II. Chronic effects, Ibid, *66,* pp. 689–694 (1961).
19. Freeman, R.G., Troll, D.: Photosensitization of the eye by 8-methoxypsoralen, JID, *53,* pp. 449–453 (1969).
20. Lerman, S., Megaw, J., Willis, I.:Potential ocular complications from PUVA therapy and their prevention; JID, *74,* pp. 197–199 (1980).
21. Diffey, B.L., Medical Physics Handbook 11, Ultraviolet Radiation in Medicine, Adam Hilger, Ltd., Bristol, p. 86 (1982).

Shown in Product Identification Guide, page 317

PROSTIGMIN® ℞

[*pro-stig 'min*]
(neostigmine methylsulfate)
INJECTABLE

DESCRIPTION

Prostigmin (neostigmine methylsulfate) Injectable, an anticholinesterase agent, is a sterile aqueous solution intended for intramuscular, intravenous or subcutaneous administration.

Prostigmin Injectable is available in the following concentrations:

Prostigmin 1:2000 Ampuls — each ml contains 0.5 mg neostigmine methylsulfate compounded with 0.2% parabens (methyl and propyl) as preservatives and sodium hydroxide to adjust pH to approximately 5.9.

Prostigmin 1:1000 Multiple Dose Vials — each ml contains 1 mg neostigmine methylsulfate compounded with 0.45% phenol as preservative, 0.2 mg sodium acetate, and acetic acid and sodium hydroxide to adjust pH to approximately 5.9.

Prostigmin 1:2000 Multiple Dose Vials — each ml contains 0.5 mg neostigmine methylsulfate compounded with 0.45% phenol as preservative, 0.2 mg sodium acetate, and acetic acid and sodium hydroxide to adjust pH to approximately 5.9.

Chemically, neostigmine methylsulfate is (*m*-hydroxyphenyl)trimethylammonium methylsulfate dimethylcarbamate. It has a molecular weight of 334.39 and the following structural formula:

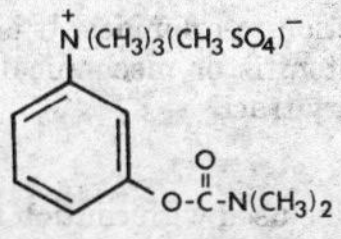

N (CH3)3(CH3 SO4)−
O
O-C-N(CH3)2

CLINICAL PHARMACOLOGY

Neostigmine inhibits the hydrolysis of acetylcholine by competing with acetylcholine for attachment to acetylcholinesterase at sites of cholinergic transmission. It enhances cholinergic action by facilitating the transmission of impulses across neuromuscular junctions. It also has a direct cholinomimetic effect on skeletal muscle and possibly on autonomic ganglion cells and neurons of the central nervous system. Neostigmine undergoes hydrolysis by cholinesterase and is also metabolized by microsomal enzymes in the liver. Protein binding to human serum albumin ranges from 15 to 25 percent.

Following intramuscular administration, neostigmine is rapidly absorbed and eliminated. In a study of five patients with myasthenia gravis, peak plasma levels were observed at 30 minutes, and the half-life ranged from 51 to 90 minutes. Approximately 80 percent of the drug was eliminated in urine within 24 hours; approximately 50% as the unchanged drug, and 30 percent as metabolites. Following intravenous administration, plasma half-life ranges from 47 to 60 minutes have been reported with a mean half-life of 53 minutes.

The clinical effects of neostigmine usually begin within 20 to 30 minutes after intramuscular injection and last from 2.5 to 4 hours.

INDICATIONS AND USAGE

Prostigmin is indicated for:

— the symptomatic control of myasthenia gravis when oral therapy is impractical.
— the prevention and treatment of postoperative distention and urinary retention after mechanical obstruction has been excluded.
— reversal of effects of nondepolarizing neuromuscular blocking agents (*e.g.,* tubocurarine, metocurine, gallamine, or pancuronium) after surgery.

CONTRAINDICATIONS

Prostigmin is contraindicated in patients with known hypersensitivity to the drug. It is also contraindicated in patients with peritonitis or mechanical obstruction of the intestinal or urinary tract.

WARNINGS

Prostigmin should be used with caution in patients with epilepsy, bronchial asthma, bradycardia, recent coronary occlusion, vagotonia, hyperthyroidism, cardiac arrhythmias or peptic ulcer. When large doses of Prostigmin are administered, the prior or simultaneous injection of atropine sulfate may be advisable. Separate syringes should be used for the Prostigmin and atropine. Because of the possibility of hypersensitivity in an occasional patient, atropine and antishock medication should always be readily available.

PRECAUTIONS

General: It is important to differentiate between myasthenic crisis and cholinergic crisis caused by overdosage of Prostigmin. Both conditions result in extreme muscle weakness but require radically different treatment. (See OVERDOSAGE section.)

Drug Interactions: Prostigmin does not antagonize, and may in fact prolong, the Phase I block of *depolarizing* muscle relaxants such as succinylcholine or decamethonium. Certain antibiotics, especially neomycin, streptomycin and kanamycin, have a mild but definite nondepolarizing blocking action which may accentuate neuromuscular block. These antibiotics should be used in the myasthenic patient only where definitely indicated, and then careful adjustment should be made of the anticholinesterase dosage. Local and some general anesthetics, antiarrhythmic agents and other drugs that interfere with neuromuscular transmission should be used cautiously, if at all, in patients with myasthenia gravis; the dose of Prostigmin may have to be increased accordingly.

Carcinogenesis, Mutagenesis and Impairment of Fertility: There have been no studies with Prostigmin which would permit an evaluation of its carcinogenic or mutagenic potential. Studies on the effect of Prostigmin on fertility and reproduction have not been performed.

Pregnancy:

Teratogenic Effects: Pregnancy Category C. There are no adequate or well-controlled studies of Prostigmin in either laboratory animals or in pregnant women. It is not known whether Prostigmin can cause fetal harm when administered to a pregnant woman or can affect reproductive capacity. Prostigmin should be given to a pregnant woman only if clearly needed.

Nonteratogenic Effects: Anticholinesterase drugs may cause uterine irritability and induce premature labor when given intravenously to pregnant women near term.

Nursing Mothers: It is not known whether Prostigmin is excreted in human milk. Because many drugs are excreted in human milk and because of the potential for serious adverse reactions from Prostigmin in nursing infants, a decision should be made whether to discontinue nursing or to discontinue the drug, taking into account the importance of the drug to the mother.

Pediatric Use: Safety and effectiveness in children have not been established.

ADVERSE REACTIONS

Side effects are generally due to an exaggeration of pharmacological effects of which salivation and fasciculation are the most common. Bowel cramps and diarrhea may also occur. The following additional adverse reactions have been reported following the use of either neostigmine bromide or neostigmine methylsulfate:

Allergic: Allergic reactions and anaphylaxis.

Neurologic: Dizziness, convulsions, loss of consciousness, drowsiness, headache, dysarthria, miosis and visual changes.

Cardiovascular: Cardiac arrhythmias (including bradycardia, tachycardia, A-V block and nodal rhythm) and nonspecific EKG changes have been reported, as well as cardiac arrest, syncope and hypotension. These have been predominantly noted following the use of the injectable form of Prostigmin.

Respiratory: Increased oral, pharyngeal and bronchial secretions, dyspnea, respiratory depression, respiratory arrest and bronchospasm.

Dermatologic: Rash and urticaria.

Gastrointestinal: Nausea, emesis, flatulence and increased peristalsis.

Continued on next page

Prostigmin Injectable—Cont.

Genitourinary: Urinary frequency.
Musculoskeletal: Muscle cramps and spasms, arthralgia.
Miscellaneous: Diaphoresis, flushing and weakness.

OVERDOSAGE

Overdosage of Prostigmin can cause cholinergic crisis, which is characterized by increasing muscle weakness, and through involvement of the muscles of respiration, may result in death. Myasthenic crisis, due to an increase in the severity of the disease, is also accompanied by extreme muscle weakness and may be difficult to distinguish from cholinergic crisis on a symptomatic basis. However, such differentiation is extremely important because increases in the dose of Prostigmin or other drugs in this class, in the presence of cholinergic crisis or of a refractory or "insensitive" state, could have grave consequences. The two types of crises may be differentiated by the use of Tensilon® (edrophonium chloride) as well as by clinical judgment.

Treatment of the two conditions differs radically. Whereas the presence of *myasthenic crisis* requires more intensive anticholinesterase therapy, *cholinergic crisis* calls for the prompt withdrawal of all drugs of this type. The immediate use of atropine in cholinergic crisis is also recommended.

Atropine may also be used to abolish or minimize gastrointestinal side effects or other muscarinic reactions; but such use, by masking signs of overdosage, can lead to inadvertent induction of cholinergic crisis.

The LD_{50} of neostigmine methylsulfate in mice is 0.3 ± 0.02 mg/kg intravenously, 0.54 ± 0.03 mg/kg subcutaneously, and 0.395 ± 0.025 mg/kg intramuscularly; in rats the LD_{50} is 0.315 ± 0.019 mg/kg intravenously, 0.445 ± 0.032 mg/kg subcutaneously, and 0.423 ± 0.032 mg/kg intramuscularly.

DOSAGE AND ADMINISTRATION

Symptomatic control of myasthenia gravis: One ml of the 1:2000 solution (0.5 mg) subcutaneously or intramuscularly. Subsequent doses should be based on the individual patient's response. In most patients, however, oral treatment with Prostigmin (neostigmine bromide) tablets, 15 mg each, is adequate for control of symptoms.

Prevention of postoperative distention and urinary retention: One ml of the 1:4000 solution (0.25 mg) subcutaneously or intramuscularly as soon as possible after operation; repeat every 4 to 6 hours for two or three days.

Treatment of postoperative distention: One ml of the 1:2000 solution (0.5 mg) subcutaneously or intramuscularly, as required.

Treatment of urinary retention: One ml of the 1:2000 solution (0.5 mg) subcutaneously or intramuscularly. If urination does not occur within an hour, the patient should be catheterized. After the patient has voided, or the bladder has been emptied, continue the 0.5 mg injections every three hours for at least 5 injections.

Reversal of Effects of Nondepolarizing Neuromuscular Blocking Agents: When Prostigmin is administered intravenously, it is recommended that atropine sulfate (0.6 to 1.2 mg) also be given intravenously using separate syringes. Some authorities have recommended that the atropine be injected several minutes before the Prostigmin rather than concomitantly. The usual dose is 0.5 to 2 mg Prostigmin given by *slow* intravenous injection, repeated as required. Only in exceptional cases should the total dose of Prostigmin exceed 5 mg. It is recommended that the patient be well ventilated and a patent airway maintained until complete recovery of normal respiration is assured. The optimum time for administration of the drug is during hyperventilation when the carbon dioxide level of the blood is low. It should never be administered in the presence of high concentrations of halothane or cyclopropane. In cardiac cases and severely ill patients, it is advisable to titrate the exact dose of Prostigmin required, using a peripheral nerve stimulator device. In the presence of bradycardia, the pulse rate should be increased to about 80/minute with atropine before administering Prostigmin.

Parenteral drug products should be inspected visually for particulate matter and discoloration prior to administration, whenever solution and container permit.

HOW SUPPLIED

Prostigmin 1:2000 (0.5 mg neostigmine methylsulfate/ml), 1-ml ampuls — boxes of 10 (NDC 0187-3101-30).
Prostigmin 1:4000 (0.25 mg neostigmine methylsulfate/mL), 1-mL ampuls — boxes of 10 (NDC 0187-3102-40).
Prostigmin 1:1000 (1 mg neostigmine methylsulfate/ml), 10-ml multiple dose vials — boxes of 10 (NDC 0187-3103-50).
Prostigmin 1:2000 (0.5 mg neostigmine methylsulfate/ml), 10-ml multiple dose vials — boxes of 10 (NDC 0187-3104-60).

Manufactured for ICN Pharmaceuticals, Inc.
Costa Mesa, CA 92626
by Hoffmann-La Roche Inc.
Nutley, N.J. 07110
Rev. 7/90

PROSTIGMIN® ℞

[*pro-stig 'min*]
(neostigmine bromide)
TABLETS

DESCRIPTION

Prostigmin (neostigmine bromide), an anticholinesterase agent, is available for oral administration in 15-mg tablets. Each tablet also contains gelatin, lactose, corn starch, stearic acid, sugar and talc.

Chemically, neostigmine bromide is (*m* -hydroxyphenyl)trimethylammonium bromide dimethylcarbamate. It is a white, crystalline, bitter powder, soluble 1:1 in water, with a molecular weight of 303.20 and the following structural formula:

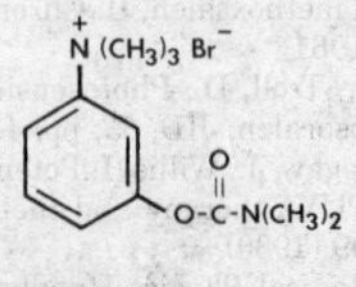

CLINICAL PHARMACOLOGY

Neostigmine inhibits the hydrolysis of acetylcholine by competing with acetylcholine for attachment to acetylcholinesterase at sites of cholinergic transmission. It enhances cholinergic action by facilitating the transmission of impulses across neuromuscular junctions. It also has a direct cholinomimetic effect on skeletal muscle and possibly on autonomic ganglion cells and neurons of the central nervous system. Neostigmine undergoes hydrolysis by cholinesterase and is also metabolized by microsomal enzymes in the liver. Protein binding to human serum albumin ranges from 15 to 25 percent.

Neostigmine bromide is poorly absorbed from the gastrointestinal tract following oral administration. As a rule, 15 mg of neostigmine bromide orally is equivalent to 0.5 mg of neostigmine methylsulfate parenterally, due to poor absorption of the tablet from the intestinal tract. In a study in fasting myasthenic patients, the extent of absorption was estimated to be 1 to 2 percent of the ingested 30-mg single oral dose. Peak concentrations in plasma occurred 1 to 2 hours following drug ingestion, with considerable individual variations. The half-life ranged from 42 to 60 minutes with a mean half-life of 52 minutes.

INDICATIONS AND USAGE

Prostigmin is indicated for the symptomatic treatment of myasthenia gravis. Its greatest usefulness is in prolonged therapy where no difficulty in swallowing is present. In acute myasthenic crisis where difficulty in breathing and swallowing is present, the parenteral form (neostigmine methylsulfate) should be used. The patient can be transferred to the oral form as soon as it can be tolerated.

CONTRAINDICATIONS

Prostigmin is contraindicated in patients with known hypersensitivity to the drug. Because of the presence of the bromide ion, it should not be used in patients with a previous history of reaction to bromides. It is contraindicated in patients with peritonitis or mechanical obstruction of the intestinal or urinary tract.

WARNINGS

Prostigmin should be used with caution in patients with epilepsy, bronchial asthma, bradycardia, recent coronary occlusion, vagotonia, hyperthyroidism, cardiac arrhythmias or peptic ulcer. As a rule, 15 mg of neostigmine bromide orally is equivalent to 0.5 mg of neostigmine methylsulfate parenterally, due to poor absorption of the tablet from the intestinal tract. Large doses should be avoided in situations where there might be an increased absorption rate from the intestinal tract. It should be used with caution when coadministered with anticholinergic drugs, in order to avoid reduction of intestinal motility.

PRECAUTIONS

General: It is important to differentiate between myasthenic crisis and cholinergic crisis caused by overdosage of Prostigmin. Both conditions result in extreme muscle weakness but require radically different treatment. (See OVERDOSAGE section.)

Drug Interactions: Certain antibiotics, especially neomycin, streptomycin and kanamycin, have a mild but definite nondepolarizing blocking action which may accentuate neuromuscular block. These antibiotics should be used in the myasthenic patient only where definitely indicated, and then careful adjustment should be made of adjunctive anticholinesterase dosage.

Local and some general anesthetics, antiarrhythmic agents and other drugs that interfere with neuromuscular transmission should be used cautiously, if at all, in patients with myasthenia gravis; the dose of Prostigmin may have to be increased accordingly.

Carcinogenesis, Mutagenesis and Impairment of Fertility: There have been no studies with Prostigmin which would permit an evaluation of its carcinogenic or mutagenic potential. Studies on the effect of Prostigmin on fertility and reproduction have not been performed.

Pregnancy:
Teratogenic Effects: Pregnancy Category C. There are no adequate or well-controlled studies of Prostigmin in either laboratory animals or in pregnant women. It is not known whether Prostigmin can cause fetal harm when administered to a pregnant woman or can affect reproductive capacity. Prostigmin should be given to a pregnant woman only if clearly needed.

Nonteratogenic Effects: Anticholinesterase drugs may cause uterine irritability and induce premature labor when given intravenously to pregnant women near term.

Nursing Mothers: It is not known whether Prostigmin is excreted in human milk. Because many drugs are excreted in human milk and because of the potential for serious adverse reactions from Prostigmin in nursing infants, a decision should be made whether to discontinue nursing or to discontinue the drug, taking into account the importance of the drug to the mother.

Pediatric Use: Safety and effectiveness in children have not been established.

ADVERSE REACTIONS

Side effects are generally due to an exaggeration of pharmacological effects of which salivation and fasciculation are the most common. Bowel cramps and diarrhea may also occur. The following additional adverse reactions have been reported following the use of either neostigmine bromide or neostigmine methylsulfate:

Allergic: Allergic reactions and anaphylaxis.
Neurologic: Dizziness, convulsions, loss of consciousness, drowsiness, headache, dysarthria, miosis and visual changes.
Cardiovascular: Cardiac arrhythmias (including bradycardia, tachycardia, A-V block and nodal rhythm) and nonspecific EKG changes have been reported, as well as cardiac arrest, syncope and hypotension. These have been predominantly noted following the use of the injectable form of Prostigmin.
Respiratory: Increased oral, pharyngeal and bronchial secretions, and dyspnea. Respiratory depression, respiratory arrest and bronchospasm have been reported following the use of the injectable form of Prostigmin.
Dermatologic: Rash and urticaria.
Gastrointestinal: Nausea, emesis, flatulence and increased peristalsis.
Genitourinary: Urinary frequency.
Musculoskeletal: Muscle cramps and spasms, arthralgia.
Miscellaneous: Diaphoresis, flushing and weakness.

OVERDOSAGE

Overdosage of Prostigmin can cause cholinergic crisis, which is characterized by increasing muscle weakness, and through involvement of the muscles of respiration, may result in death. Myasthenic crisis, due to an increase in the severity of the disease, is also accompanied by extreme muscle weakness and may be difficult to distinguish from cholinergic crisis on a symptomatic basis. However, such differentiation is extremely important because increases in the dose of Prostigmin or other drugs in this class, in the presence of cholinergic crisis or of a refractory or "insensitive" state, could have grave consequences. The two types of crises may be differentiated by the use of Tensilon® (edrophonium chloride) as well as by clinical judgment.

Treatment of the two conditions differs radically. Whereas the presence of *myasthenic crisis* requires more intensive anticholinesterase therapy, *cholinergic crisis* calls for the prompt withdrawal of all drugs of this type. The immediate use of atropine in cholinergic crisis is also recommended.

Atropine may also be used to abolish or minimize gastrointestinal side effects or other muscarinic reactions; but such use, by masking signs of overdosage, can lead to inadvertent induction of cholinergic crisis.

The LD_{50} of neostigmine methylsulfate in mice is 0.3 ± 0.02 mg/kg intravenously, 0.54 ± 0.03 mg/kg subcutaneously, and 0.395 ± 0.025 mg/kg intramuscularly; in rats the LD_{50} is 0.315 ± 0.019 mg/kg intravenously, 0.445 ± 0.032 mg/kg subcutaneously, and 0.423 ± 0.032 mg/kg intramuscularly.

DOSAGE AND ADMINISTRATION

The onset of action of Prostigmin given orally is slower than when given parenterally, but the duration of action is longer and the intensity of action more uniform. Dosage requirements for optimal results vary from 15 mg to 375 mg per day. In some instances it may be necessary to exceed these dosages, but the possibility of cholinergic crisis must be recognized. The average dose is 10 tablets (150 mg) administered over a 24-hour period. The interval between doses is of paramount importance. The dosage schedule should be adjusted for each patient and changed as the need arises. Frequently, therapy is required day and night. Larger portions of the total daily dose may be given at times when the patient is more prone to fatigue (afternoon, mealtimes, etc.).

The patient should be encouraged to keep a daily record of his or her condition to assist the physician in determining an optimal therapeutic regimen.

HOW SUPPLIED

Scored, white tablets containing 15 mg neostigmine bromide — bottles of 100 (NDC 0187-3100-10). Imprint on tablets: (front) PROSTIGMIN 15: (back) ICN.
Manufactured for ICN Pharmaceuticals, Inc.
Costa Mesa, CA 92626
by Hoffmann-La Roche Inc.
Nutley, N.J. 07110
Rev. 9/97

Shown in Product Identification Guide, page 317

TENSILON®   ℞

[ten 'sil-on]
(edrophonium chloride)
Injectable Solution
ampuls • vials

DESCRIPTION

Tensilon is a short and rapid-acting cholinergic drug. Chemically, edrophonium chloride is ethyl (*m*- hydroxyphenyl)dimethylammonium chloride.
10-ml vials: Each ml contains, in a sterile solution, 10 mg edrophonium chloride compounded with 0.45% phenol and 0.2% sodium sulfite as preservatives, buffered with sodium citrate and citric acid, and pH adjusted to approximately 5.4.
1-ml ampuls: Each ml contains, in a sterile solution, 10 mg edrophonium chloride compounded with 0.2% sodium sulfite, buffered with sodium citrate and citric acid, and pH adjusted to approximately 5.4.

ACTIONS

Tensilon is an anticholinesterase drug. Its pharmacological action is due primarily to the inhibition of acetylcholinesterase at sites of cholinergic transmission. Its effect is manifest within 30 to 60 seconds after injection and lasts an average of 10 minutes.

INDICATIONS

Tensilon is recommended for the differential diagnosis of myasthenia gravis and as an adjunct in the evaluation of treatment requirements in this disease. It may also be used for evaluating emergency treatment in myasthenic crises. Because of its brief duration of action, it is not recommended for maintenance therapy in myasthenia gravis.
Tensilon is also useful whenever a curare antagonist is needed to reverse the neuromuscular block produced by curare, tubocurarine, gallamine triethiodide or dimethyl-tubocurarine. It is *not* effective against decamethonium bromide and succinylcholine chloride. It may be used adjunctively in the treatment of respiratory depression caused by curare overdosage.

CONTRAINDICATIONS

Known hypersensitivity to anticholinesterase agents; intestinal and urinary obstructions of mechanical type.

WARNINGS

Whenever anticholinesterase drugs are used for testing, a syringe containing 1 mg of atropine sulfate should be immediately available to be given in aliquots intravenously to counteract severe cholinergic reactions which may occur in the hypersensitive individual, whether he is normal or myasthenic. Tensilon should be used with caution in patients with bronchial asthma or cardiac dysrhythmias. The transient bradycardia which sometimes occurs can be relieved by atropine sulfate. Isolated instances of cardiac and respiratory arrest following administration of Tensilon have been reported. It is postulated that these are vagotonic effects.
Tensilon solution contains sodium sulfite, a sulfite that may cause allergic-type reactions, including anaphylactic symptoms and life-threatening or less severe asthmatic episodes in certain susceptible people. The overall prevalence of sulfite sensitivity in the general population is unknown and probably low. Sulfite sensitivity is seen more frequently in asthmatic than in nonasthmatic people.
Usage in Pregnancy: The safety of Tensilon during pregnancy or lactation in humans has not been established. Therefore, use of Tensilon in women who may become pregnant requires weighing the drug's potential benefits against its possible hazards to mother and child.

PRECAUTIONS

Patients may develop "anticholinesterase insensitivity" for brief or prolonged periods. During these periods the patients should be carefully monitored and may need respiratory assistance. Dosages of anticholinesterase drugs should be reduced or withheld until patients again become sensitive to them.

	Myasthenic*	Adequate†	Cholinergic‡
Muscle Strength (ptosis, diplopia, dysphonia, dysphagia, dysarthria, respiration, limb strength)	Increased	No change	Decreased
Fasciculations (orbicularis oculi, facial muscles, limb muscles)	Absent	Present or absent	Present or absent
Side reactions (lacrimation, diaphoresis, salivation, abdominal cramps, nausea, vomiting, diarrhea)	Absent	Minimal	Severe

---

* Myasthenic Response—occurs in untreated myasthenics and may serve to establish diagnosis; in patients under treatment, indicates that therapy is inadequate.
† Adequate Response—observed in treated patients when therapy is stabilized; a typical response in normal individuals. In addition to this response in nonmyasthenics, the phenomenon of forced lid closure is often observed in psychoneurotics.[1]
‡ Cholinergic Response—seen in myasthenics who have been overtreated with anticholinesterase drugs.

ADVERSE REACTIONS

Careful observation should be made for severe cholinergic reactions in the hyperreactive individual. The myasthenic patient in crisis who is being tested with Tensilon should be observed for bradycardia or cardiac standstill and cholinergic reactions if an overdose is given. The following reactions common to anticholinesterase agents may occur, although not all of these reactions have been reported with the administration of Tensilon, probably because of its short duration of action and limited indications: **Eye:** Increased lacrimation, pupillary constriction, spasm of accommodation, diplopia, conjunctival hyperemia. **CNS:** Convulsions, dysarthria, dysphonia, dysphagia. **Respiratory:** Increased tracheobronchial secretions, laryngospasm, bronchiolar constriction, paralysis of muscles of respiration, central respiratory paralysis. **Cardiac:** Arrhythmias (especially bradycardia), fall in cardiac output leading to hypotension. **G.I.:** Increased salivary, gastric and intestinal secretion, nausea, vomiting, increased peristalsis, diarrhea, abdominal cramps. **Skeletal Muscle:** Weakness, fasciculations. **Miscellaneous:** Increased urinary frequency and incontinence, diaphoresis.

DOSAGE AND ADMINISTRATION

Tensilon Test in the Differential Diagnosis of Myasthenia Gravis:[1–8]
Intravenous Dosage (Adults): A tuberculin syringe containing 1 ml (10 mg) of Tensilon is prepared with an intravenous needle, and 0.2 ml (2 mg) is injected intravenously within 15 to 30 seconds. The needle is left *in situ. Only* if no reaction occurs after 45 seconds is the remaining 0.8 ml (8 mg) injected. If a cholinergic reaction (muscarinic side effects, skeletal muscle fasciculations and increased muscle weakness) occurs after injection of 0.2 ml (2 mg), the test is discontinued and atropine sulfate 0.4 mg to 0.5 mg is administered intravenously. After one-half hour the test may be repeated.
Intramuscular Dosage (Adults): In adults with inaccessible veins, dosage for intramuscular injection is 1 ml (10 mg) of Tensilon. Subjects who demonstrate hyperreactivity to this injection (cholinergic reaction), should be retested after one-half hour with 0.2 ml (2 mg) of Tensilon intramuscularly to rule out false-negative reactions.
Dosage (Children): The intravenous testing dose of Tensilon in children weighing up to 75 lbs is 0.1 ml (1 mg); above this weight, the dose is 0.2 ml (2 mg). If there is no response after 45 seconds, it may be titrated up to 0.5 ml (5 mg) in children under 75 lbs, given in increments of 0.1 ml (1 mg) every 30 to 45 seconds and up to 1 ml (10 mg) in heavier children. In infants, the recommended dose is 0.05 ml (0.5 mg). Because of technical difficulty with intravenous injection in children, the intramuscular route may be used. In children weighing up to 75 lbs, 0.2 ml (2 mg) is injected intramuscularly. In children weighing more than 75 lbs, 0.5 ml (5 mg) is injected intramuscularly. All signs which would appear with the intravenous test appear with the intramuscular test except that there is a delay of two to ten minutes before a reaction is noted.
Tensilon Test for Evaluation of Treatment Requirements in Myasthenia Gravis: The recommended dose is 0.1 ml to 0.2 ml (1 mg to 2 mg) of Tensilon, administered intravenously one hour after oral intake of the drug being used in treatment.[1–5] Response will be myasthenic in the undertreated patient, adequate in the controlled patient, and cholinergic in the overtreated patient. Responses to Tensilon in myasthenic and nonmyasthenic individuals are summarized in the following chart:[2]
[See table above]
Tensilon Test in Crisis: The term *crisis* is applied to the myasthenic whenever severe respiratory distress with objective ventilatory inadequacy occurs and the response to medication is not predictable. This state may be secondary to a sudden increase in severity of myasthenia gravis (myasthenic crisis), or to overtreatment with anticholinesterase drugs (cholinergic crisis).
When a patient is apneic, controlled ventilation must be secured immediately in order to avoid cardiac arrest and irreversible central nervous system damage. No attempt is made to test with Tensilon until respiratory exchange is adequate. *Dosage used at this time is most important:* If the patient is cholinergic, Tensilon will cause increased oropharyngeal secretions and further weakness in the muscles of respiration. If the crisis is myasthenic, the test clearly improves respiration and the patient can be treated with longer-acting intravenous anticholinesterase medication. When the test is performed, there should not be more than 0.2 ml (2 mg) Tensilon in the syringe. An intravenous dose of 0.1 ml (1 mg) is given initially. The patient's heart action is carefully observed. If, after an interval of one minute, this dose does not further impair the patient, the remaining 0.1 ml (1 mg) can be injected. If no clear improvement of respiration occurs after 0.2 ml (2 mg) dose, it is usually wisest to discontinue all anticholinesterase drug therapy and secure controlled ventilation by tracheostomy with assisted respiration.[5]
For Use as a Curare Antagonist: Tensilon should be administered by intravenous injection in 1 ml (10 mg) doses given slowly over a period of 30 to 45 seconds so that the onset of cholinergic reaction can be detected. This dosage may be repeated whenever necessary. The maximal dose for any one patient should be 4 ml (40 mg). Because of its brief effect, Tensilon should not be given prior to the administration of curare, tubocurarine, gallamine triethiodide or dimethyl-tubocurarine; it should be used at the time when its effect is needed. When given to counteract curare overdosage, the effect of each dose on the respiration should be carefully observed before it is repeated, and assisted ventilation should always be employed.

DRUG INTERACTIONS

Care should be given when administering this drug to patients with symptoms of myasthenic weakness who are also on anticholinesterase drugs. Since symptoms of anticholinesterase overdose (cholinergic crisis) may mimic underdosage (myasthenic weakness), their condition may be worsened by the use of this drug. (See OVERDOSAGE section for treatment.)

OVERDOSAGE

With drugs of this type, muscarine-like symptoms (nausea, vomiting, diarrhea, sweating, increased bronchial and salivary secretions and bradycardia) often appear with overdosage (cholinergic crisis). An important complication that can arise is obstruction of the airway by bronchial secretions. These may be managed with suction (especially if tracheostomy has been performed) and by the use of atropine. Many experts have advocated a wide range of dosages of atropine *(for Tensilon, see atropine dosage below),* but if there are copious secretions, up to 1.2 mg intravenously may be given initially and repeated every 20 minutes until secretions are controlled. Signs of atropine overdosage such as dry mouth, flush and tachycardia should be avoided as tenacious secretions and bronchial plugs may form. A total dose of atropine of 5 to 10 mg or even more may be required. The following steps should be taken in the management of overdosage of Tensilon:

1. Adequate respiratory exchange should be maintained by assuring an open airway, and the use of assisted respiration augmented by oxygen.
2. Cardiac function should be monitored until complete stabilization has been achieved.
3. Atropine sulfate in doses of 0.4 to 0.5 mg should be administered intravenously. This may be repeated every 3 to 10 minutes. Because of the short duration of action of Tensilon the total dose required will seldom exceed 2 mg.
4. If convulsions or shock is present, appropriate measures should be instituted.

HOW SUPPLIED

Multiple Dose Vials, 10 ml, boxes of 10 (NDC 0187-3200-20).
Ampuls, 1 ml, boxes of 10 (NDC 0187-3200-10).

REFERENCES

1. Osserman, K.E. and Kaplan, L.I., *J.A.M.A.,* 150: 265, 1952.

Continued on next page

Tensilon—Cont.

2. Osserman, K.E., Kaplan, L.I. and Besson, G., *J. Mt. Sinai Hosp., 20:* 165, 1953.
3. Osserman, K.E. and Kaplan, L.I., *Arch. Neurol. & Psychiat., 70:* 385, 1953.
4. Osserman, K.E. and Teng, P., *J.A.M.A., 160:* 153, 1956.
5. Osserman, K.E. and Genkins, G., *Ann. N.Y. Acad. Sci., 135:* 312, 1966.
6. Tether, J.E., Second International Symposium Proceedings, Myasthenia Gravis, 1961, p. 444.
7. Tether, J.E., in H.F. Conn: *Current Therapy 1960,* Philadelphia, W. B. Saunders Company, p. 551.
8. Tether, J.E., in H.F. Conn: *Current Therapy 1965,* Philadelphia, W. B. Saunders Company, p. 556.
9. Grob, D. and Johns, R.J., *J.A.M.A., 166:* 1855, 1958.

Manufactured for ICN Pharmaceuticals, Inc.
Costa Mesa, CA 92626
by Hoffmann-La Roche Inc.
Nutley, NJ 07110
Rev. 11/93

TESTRED® Ⓒ℞

Brand of
Methyltestosterone Capsules, USP 10 mg

DESCRIPTION

The androgens are steroids that develop and maintain primary and secondary male sex characteristics. Androgens are derivatives of cyclopentanoperhydrophenanthrene. Endogenous androgens are C-19 steroids with a side chain at C-17, and with two angular methyl groups. Testosterone is the primary endogenous androgen. In their active form, all drugs in the class have a 17-beta-hydroxy group. 17-alpha alkylation (methyltestosterone) increases the pharmacologic activity per unit weight compared to testosterone when given orally. Methyltestosterone, a synthetic derivative of testosterone, is an androgenic preparation given by the oral route in a capsule form. Each capsule contains 10 mg of methyltestosterone USP. It has the following structural formula:

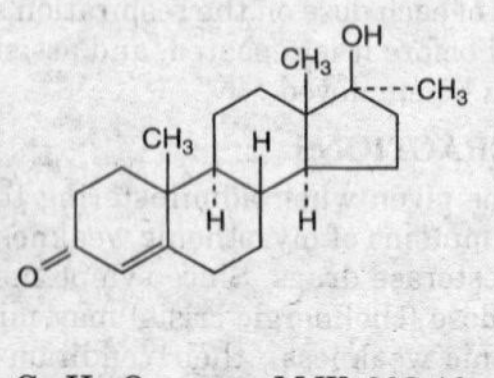

$C_{20}H_{30}O_2$ M.W. 302.46
17β-hydroxy-17-methylandrost-4-en-3-one

Methyltestosterone occurs as white or creamy white crystals or powder, which is soluble in various organic solvents but is practically insoluble in water.

Each capsule, for oral administration, contains 10 mg of methyltestosterone. In addition, each capsule contains the following inactive ingredients: Corn starch NF, Gelatin NF, FD&C Blue #1, FD&C Red #40.

CLINICAL PHARMACOLOGY

Endogenous androgens are responsible for the normal growth and development of the male sex organs and for maintenance of secondary sex characteristics. These effects include the growth and maturation of prostate, seminal vesicles, penis, and scrotum. The development of male hair distribution, such as beard, pubic, chest, and axillary hair; laryngeal enlargement, vocal chord thickening, alterations in body musculature and fat distribution. Drugs in this class also cause retention of nitrogen, sodium, potassium, phosphorus, and decreased urinary excretion of calcium. Androgens have been reported to increase protein anabolism and decrease protein catabolism. Nitrogen balance is improved only when there is sufficient intake of calories and protein.

Androgens are responsible for the growth spurt of adolescence and for the eventual termination of linear growth which is brought about by fusion of the epiphyseal growth centers. In children, exogenous androgens accelerate linear growth rates, but may cause a disproportionate advancement in bone maturation. Use over long periods may result in fusion of the epiphyseal growth centers and termination of growth process. Androgens have been reported to stimulate the production of red blood cells by enhancing the production of erythropoietic stimulating factor.

During exogenous administration of androgens, endogenous testosterone release is inhibited through feedback inhibition of pituitary luteinizing hormone (LH). At large doses of exogenous androgens, spermatogenesis may also be suppressed through feedback inhibition of pituitary follicle stimulating hormone (FSH).

There is a lack of substantial evidence that androgens are effective in fractures, surgery, convalescence and functional uterine bleeding.

Pharmacokinetics

Testosterone given orally is metabolized by the gut and 44 percent is cleared by the liver of the first pass. Oral doses as high as 400 mg per day are needed to achieve clinically effective blood levels for full replacement therapy. The synthetic androgen, methyltestosterone, is less extensively metabolized by the liver and has a longer half-life. It is more suitable than testosterone for oral administration.

Testosterone in plasma is 98 percent bound to a specific testosterone-estradiol binding globulin, and about 2 percent is free. Generally, the amount of this sex-hormone binding globulin in the plasma will determine the distribution of testosterone between free and bound forms, and the free testosterone concentration will determine its half-life.

About 90 percent of a dose of testosterone is excreted in the urine as glucuronic and sulfuric acid conjugates of testosterone and its metabolites; about 6 percent of a dose is excreted in the feces, mostly in the unconjugated form. Inactivation of testosterone occurs primarily in the liver. Testosterone is metabolized to various 17-keto steroids through two different pathways. There are considerable variations of the half-life of testosterone as reported in the literature, ranging from 10 to 100 minutes.

In many tissues the activity of testosterone appears to depend on reduction to dihydrotestosterone, which binds to cytosol receptor proteins. The steroid-receptor complex is transported to the nucleus where it initiates transcription events and cellular changes related to androgen action.

INDICATIONS AND USAGE

1. Males

Androgens are indicated for replacement therapy in conditions associated with a deficiency or absence of endogenous testosterone;

a. Primary hypogonadism (congenital or acquired)—testicular failure due to cryptorchidism, bilateral torsions, orchitis, vanishing testis syndrome; or orchidectomy.

b. Hypogonadotropic hypogonadism (congenital or acquired)—idiopathic gonadotropin or LHRH deficiency, or pituitary-hypothalamic injury from tumors, trauma or radiation.

   If the above conditions occur prior to puberty, androgen replacement therapy will be needed during the adolescent years for development of secondary sexual characteristics. Prolonged androgen treatment will be required to maintain sexual characteristics in these and other males who develop testosterone deficiency after puberty.

c. Androgens may be used to stimulate puberty in carefully selected males with clearly delayed puberty. These patients usually have a familial pattern of delayed puberty that is not secondary to a pathological disorder; puberty is expected to occur spontaneously at a relatively late date. Brief treatment with conservative doses may occasionally be justified in these patients if they do not respond to psychological support. The potential adverse effect on bone maturation should be discussed with the patient and parents prior to androgen adminstration. An X-ray of the hand and wrist to determine bone age should be obtained every 6 months to assess the effect of treatment on the epiphyseal centers (see WARNINGS).

2. Females

Androgens may be used secondarily in women with advancing inoperable metastatic (skeletal) mammary cancer who are 1 to 5 years postmenopausal. Primary goals of therapy in these women include ablation of the ovaries. Other methods of counteracting estrogen activity are adrenalectomy, hypophysectomy, and/or antiestrogen therapy. This treatment has also been used in premenopausal women with breast cancer who have benefited from oophorectomy and are considered to have a hormone-responsive tumor. Judgment concerning androgen therapy should be made by an oncologist with expertise in this field.

CONTRAINDICATIONS

Androgens are contraindicated in men with carcinomas of the breast or with known or suspected carcinomas of the prostate, and in women who are or may become pregnant. When administered to pregnant women, androgens cause virilization of the external genitalia of the female fetus. This virilization includes clitoromegaly, abnormal vaginal development, and fusion of genital folds to form a scrotal-like structure. The degree of masculinization is related to the amount of drug given and the age of the fetus, and is most likely to occur in the female fetus when the drugs are given in the first trimester. If the patient becomes pregnant while taking these drugs, she should be apprised of the potential hazard to the fetus.

WARNINGS

In patients with breast cancer, androgen therapy may cause hypercalcemia by stimulating osteolysis. In this case, the drug should be discontinued.

Prolonged use of high doses of androgens has been associated with the development of peliosis hepatis and hepatic neoplasms including hepatocellular carcinoma. (See PRECAUTIONS-Carcinogenesis). Peliosis hepatis can be a life-threatening or fatal complication.

Cholestatic hepatitis and jaundice occur with 17-alpha-alkylandrogens at a relatively low dose. If cholestatic hepatitis with jaundice appears or if liver function tests become abnormal, the androgen should be discontinued and the etiology should be determined. Drug-induced jaundice is reversible when the medication is discontinued.

Geriatric patients treated with androgens may be at an increased risk for the development of prostatic hypertrophy and prostatic carcinoma.

Edema with or without congestive heart failure may be a serious complication in patients with preexisting cardiac, renal, or hepatic disease. In addition to discontinuation of the drug, diuretic therapy may be required.

Gynecomastia frequently develops and occasionally persists in patients being treated for hypogonadism. Androgen therapy should be used cautiously in healthy males with delayed puberty. The effect on bone maturation should be monitored by assessing bone age of the wrist and hand every 6 months. In children, androgen treatment may accelerate bone maturation without producing compensatory gain in linear growth. This adverse effect may result in compromised adult stature. The younger the child the greater the risk of compromising final mature height.

This drug has not been shown to be safe and effective for the enhancement of athletic performance. Because of the potential risk of serious adverse health effects, this drug should not be used for such purpose.

PRECAUTIONS

General

Women should be observed for signs of virilization (deepening of the voice, hirsutism, acne, clitoromegaly and menstrual irregularities). Discontinuation of drug therapy at the time of evidence of mild virilism is necessary to prevent irreversible virilization. Such virilization is usual following androgen use at high doses. A decision may be made by the patient and the physician that some virilization will be tolerated during treatment for breast carcinoma.

Information for the Patient

The physician should instruct patients to report any of the following side effects of androgens:

Adult or Adolescent Males:	Too frequent or persistent erections of the penis. Any male adolescent patient receiving androgens for delayed puberty should have bone development checked every six months.
Women:	Hoarseness, acne, changes in menstrual periods, or more hair on the face.
All Patients:	Any nausea, vomiting, changes in skin color or ankle swelling.

Laboratory Tests

1. Women with disseminated breast carcinoma should have frequent determination of urine and serum calcium levels during the course of androgen therapy. (See WARNINGS).
2. Because of the hepatotoxicity associated with the use of 17-alpha-alkylated androgens, liver function tests should be obtained periodically.
3. Periodic (every 6 months) x-ray examinations of bone age should be made during treatment of prepubertal males to determine the rate of bone maturation and the effects of androgen therapy on the epiphyseal centers.
4. Hemoglobin and hematocrit should be checked periodically for polycythemia in patients who are receiving high doses of androgens.

Drug Interactions

1. **Anticoagulants:** C-17 substituted derivatives of testosterone, such as methandrostenolone, have been reported to decrease the anticoagulant requirements of patients receiving oral anticoagulants. Patients receiving oral anticoagulant therapy require close monitoring, especially when androgens are started or stopped.
2. **Oxyphenbutazone:** Concurrent administration of oxyphenbutazone and androgens may result in elevated serum levels of oxyphenbutazone.
3. **Insulin:** In diabetic patients the metabolic effects of androgens may decrease blood glucose and insulin requirements.

Drug/Laboratory Test Interferences

Androgens may decrease levels of thyroxine-binding globulin, resulting in decreased total T4 serum levels and increased resin uptake of T3 and T4. Free thyroid hormone levels remain unchanged, however, and there is no clinical evidence of thyroid dysfunction.

Carcinogenesis
Animal Data
Testosterone has been tested by subcutaneous injection and implantation in mice and rats. The implant induced cervical-uterine tumors in mice, which metastasized in some cases. There is suggestive evidence that injection of testosterone into some strains of female mice increases their susceptibility to hepatoma. Testosterone is also known to increase the number of tumors and decrease the degree of differentiation of chemically induced carcinomas of the liver in rats.
Human Data
There are rare reports of hepatocellular carcinoma in patients receiving long-term therapy with androgens in high doses. Withdrawal of the drugs did not lead to regression of the tumors in all cases.
Geriatric patients treated with androgens may be at an increased risk for the development of prostatic hypertrophy and prostatic carcinoma.
Pregnancy
Teratogenic effects. Pregnancy Category X (See CONTRAINDICATIONS).
Nursing Mothers
It is not known whether androgens are excreted in human milk. Because many drugs are excreted in human milk and because of the potential for serious adverse reactions in nursing infants from androgens, a decision should be made whether to discontinue nursing or to discontinue the drug, taking into account the importance of the drug to the mother.
Pediatric Use
Androgen therapy should be used very cautiously in children and only by specialists who are aware of the adverse effects on bone maturation. Skeletal maturation must be monitored every six months by an x-ray of hand and wrist (See INDICATIONS AND USAGE and WARNINGS).

ADVERSE REACTIONS

Endocrine and Urogenital
Female: The most common side effects of androgen therapy are amenorrhea and other menstrual irregularities, inhibition of gonadotropin secretion, and virilization, including deepening of the voice and clitoral enlargement. The latter usually is not reversible after androgens are discontinued. When administered to a pregnant woman androgens cause virilization of external genitalia of the female fetus.
Male: Gynecomastia, and excessive frequency and duration of penile erections. Oligospermia may occur at high dosages (see CLINICAL PHARMACOLOGY).
Skin and appendages: Hirsutism, male pattern of baldness, and acne.
Fluid and Electrolyte Disturbances: Retention of sodium, chloride, water, potassium, calcium, and inorganic phosphates.
Gastrointestinal: Nausea, cholestatic jaundice, alterations in liver function tests, rarely hepatocellular neoplasms and peliosis hepatis (see WARNINGS).
Hematologic: Suppression of clotting factors II, V, VII, and X, bleeding in patients on concomitant anticoagulant therapy, and polycythemia.
Nervous System: Increased or decreased libido, headache, anxiety, depression, and generalized paresthesia.
Metabolic: Increased serum cholesterol.
Miscellaneous: Rarely anaphylactoid reactions.

DRUG ABUSE AND DEPENDENCE

Testred Capsules are classified as a schedule III Controlled Substance under the Anabolic Steroids Act of 1990.

OVERDOSAGE

There have been no reports of acute overdosage with the androgens.

DOSAGE AND ADMINISTRATION

Methyltestosterone capsules are administered orally. The suggested dosage for androgens varies depending on the age, sex, and diagnosis of the individual patient. Dosage is adjusted according to the patient's response and the appearance of adverse reactions.
Replacement therapy in androgen-deficient males is 10 to 50 mg of methyltestosterone daily. Various dosage regimens have been used to induce pubertal changes in hypogonadal males; some experts have advocated lower dosages initially, gradually increasing the dose as puberty progresses, with or without a decrease to maintenance levels. Other experts emphasize that higher dosages are needed to induce pubertal changes and lower dosages can be used for maintenance after puberty. The chronological and skeletal ages must be taken into consideration, both in determining the initial dose and in adjusting the dose.
Doses used in delayed puberty generally are in the range of that given above, and for a limited duration, for example, 4 to 6 months.
Women with metastatic breast carcinoma must be followed closely because androgen therapy occasionally appears to accelerate the disease. Thus, many experts prefer to use the shorter acting androgen preparations rather than those with prolonged activity for treating breast carcinoma, particularly during the early stages of androgen therapy. The dosage of methyltestosterone for androgen therapy in breast carcinoma in females is from 50–200 mg daily.

HOW SUPPLIED

Methyltestosterone capsules USP 10 mg are red capsules imprinted "ICN 0901" on both sections. They are available in bottles of 100.
CAUTION: Federal (U.S.A.) law prohibits dispensing without prescription.

Revision July 1994

ICN Pharmaceuticals, Inc.
ICN Plaza
3300 Hyland Avenue
Costa Mesa, CA 92626
(714) 545-0100

Shown in Product Identification Guide, page 317

TRISORALEN® * ℞

[*trī* 'sore "a-len]
(Trioxsalen USP, 5 mg)

To facilitate repigmentation in vitiligo, increase tolerance to solar exposure and enhance pigmentation.
CAUTION: THIS IS A POTENT DRUG.
CAUTION: Federal (U.S.A.) law prohibits dispensing without prescription.

DESCRIPTION

Trisoralen Tablets 5 mg.
TRISORALEN (TRIOXSALEN) is the first synthetic psoralen compound made available to the medical profession. It possesses greater activity than Methoxsalen (1) (2) (3) (4), yet the LD 50 of (TRIOXSALEN) is six times that of Methoxsalen.

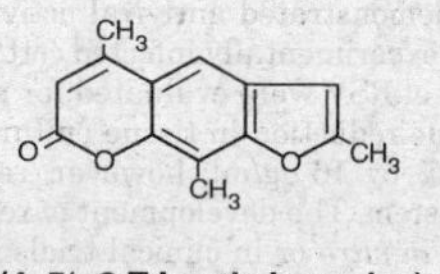

(4, 5', 8-Trimethylpsoralen)

ACTIONS

Pigment formation with TRISORALEN (TRIOXSALEN)
The normal pigmentation of the skin is due to melanin which is produced in the cytoplasm of the melanocytes located in the basal layers of the epidermis at its junction with the dermis. Melanin is formed by the oxidation of tyrosine to DOPA (Dihydroxyphenylalanine) with tyrosinase as catalyst. This enzymatic reaction, however, must be activated by radiant energy in the form of ultraviolet light, preferably between 2900 and 3800 angstroms (black light) (10).
The exact mechanism of the action of psoralens in the process of melanogenesis is not known. One group of investigators feel that the psoralens have a specific effect on the epidermis or, more specifically, on the melanocytes. Another group feels that the primary response to the psoralens is an inflammatory one and that the process of melanogenesis is secondary.

INDICATIONS

TRISORALEN (TRIOXSALEN), taken approximately two hours before measured periods of exposure to ultraviolet facilitates:

1. **Repigmentation of idiopathic vitiligo.** (12) (13) (14) Repigmentation, not equally reversible in every patient, will vary in completeness, time of onset, and duration. The rate of completeness of pigmentation with respect to locations of lesions, occurs more rapidly on fleshy regions, such as the face, abdomen, and buttocks, and less rapidly over bony areas such as the dorsum of the hands and feet. Repigmentation may begin after a few weeks; however, significant results may take as long as six to nine months, and repigmentation, at the optimum level, may, in some cases, require maintenance dosage to retain the new pigment. If follicular repigmentation is not apparent after three months of daily treatment, treatment should be discontinued as a failure.
2. **Increasing tolerance to sunlight.** (14) In blond persons and those with fair complexions who suffer painful reactions when exposed to sunlight, TRISORALEN (TRIOXSALEN) aids in increasing resistance to solar damage. Certain persons who are allergic to sunlight or exhibit sun sensitivity may be benefited by the protective action of TRISORALEN (TRIOXSALEN) (5). In albinism, TRISORALEN (TRIOXSALEN) will increase the tolerance of the skin to sunlight, although no pigment is formed (6) (7) (8). This protective action seems to be related to the thickening of the horny layer and retention of melanin which produced a thickened, melanized stratum corneum and formation of a stratum lucidum (9) (10).
3. **Enhancing pigmentation** (3) (4). The use of TRISORALEN (TRIOXSALEN) accelerates pigmentation only when the administration of the drug is followed by exposure of the skin to sunlight or ultraviolet irradiation. The increase in pigmentation is not immediate but occurs gradually within a few days of repeated exposure and may become equivalent in a degree to that achieved by a full summer of sun exposure. Since sufficient pigmentation will have been formed within two weeks of continuous therapy, the use of TRISORALEN (TRIOXSALEN) should not be continued beyond this period. Pigmentation can be maintained by periodic exposure to sunlight.

CONTRAINDICATIONS

In those diseases associated with photosensitivity, such as porphyria, acute lupus erythematosus, or leukoderma of infectious origin. To date, the safety of this drug in young persons (12 and under), has not been established and is, therefore contraindicated. No preparation with any photosensitizing capacity, internal or external should be used concomitantly with TRISORALEN (TRIOXSALEN) therapy.

WARNINGS

TRISORALEN IS A POTENT DRUG.
Read entire brochure before prescribing or dispensing this medication. The dosage of this medication should not be increased. The dosage of TRISORALEN (TRIOXSALEN) and exposure time should not be increased. Overdosage and/or overexposure may result in serious burning and blistering. When used to increase tolerance to sunlight or accelerate tanning, TRISORALEN (TRIOXSALEN) total dosage should not exceed 28 tablets, taken in daily single doses of two tablets on a continuous or interrupted regimen. To prevent harmful effects, the physician should carefully instruct the patient to adhere to the prescribed dosage schedule and procedure.
*U.S. Patent 3,201,421

PRECAUTIONS

ACCIDENTAL OVERDOSAGE:
If an overdose of TRISORALEN (TRIOXSALEN) or ultraviolet light has been taken, emesis should be encouraged. The individual should be kept in a darkened room for eight hours or until cutaneous reactions subside. The treatment for severe reactions resulting from overdosage or over-exposure should follow accepted procedures for treatment of severe burns. There have not been any clinical reports or tests to verify that more severe reactions may result from the concomitant ingestion of furocoumarin-containing food while on TRISORALEN (TRIOXSALEN) therapy; but the physician should warn the patient that taking limes, figs, parsley, parsnips, mustard, carrots and celery, might be dangerous.

ADVERSE REACTIONS AND SIDE EFFECTS

Severe burns can result from excessive sunlight or sun lamp ultraviolet exposure. Occasionally, there may occur gastric discomfort; to minimize this gastric effect, the tablets may be taken with milk or after a meal. Some patients who are unable to tolerate 10 mg. will tolerate 5 mg. This dosage produces the same therapeutic effect but more slowly.

DOSAGE

(Adults and children over 12 years of age)
VITILIGO: Two tablets daily, taken two to four hours before measured periods of ultraviolet exposure or fluorescent black light (10). (See suggested sun exposure guide.)
To increase tolerance to sunlight and/or enhance pigmentation: Two tablets daily, taken two hours before measured periods of exposure to sun or ultraviolet irradiation. Not to be continued for longer than 14 days. The dosage should **NOT** be increased, as severe burning may occur. (See suggested sun exposure guide.)

SUGGESTED SUN EXPOSURE GUIDE
The exposure time to sunlight should be limited according to the following plan:

	Basic Skin Color	
	Light	**Medium**
Initial Exposure	15 min.	20 min.
Second Exposure	20 min.	25 min.
Third Exposure	25 min.	30 min.
Fourth Exposure	30 min.	35 min.

Subsequent Exposure: Gradually increase exposure based on erythema and tenderness.

Sunglasses should be worn during exposure and the lips protected with a light-screening lipstick (10).

SUN-LAMP EXPOSURE: Should be initiated according to directions of the sun-lamp manufacturer.

HOW SUPPLIED

TRISORALEN Tablets 5 mg.

UNIT COUNT	NDC NO.
28	0187-0303-28
100	0187-0303-01
1000	0187-0303-10

Store at controlled room temperature (15°–30°C) 59°–86°F.

Continued on next page

Trisoralen—Cont.

REFERENCES

1. Pathak, M.A., and Fitzpatrick, T.B.: Bioassay of Natural and Synthetic Furocoumarins (Psoralens). J. Invest. Dermat. 32, 509–518, 1959.
2. Pathak, M.A.; Fellman, J.H.; and Kaufman, K.D.,: The Effect of Structural Alterations on the Erytheral Activity of Furocoumarins: Psoralens. J. Invest. Dermat. 35, 165–183, 1960.
3. Lerner, R.M., and Lerner, A.B.,: Dermatologic Medications, Second Edition. Year book Publishers, Pages 98–99.
4. Pathak, M.A., and Fitzpatrick, T.B.,: Relationship of Molecular Configuration to the Activity of Furocoumarins Which Increase the Cutaneous Responses Following Long Wave Ultraviolet Radiation. J. Invest. Dermat. 32, No. 2, 255–262, 1959.
5. Becker, S.W., Jr.,: Prevention of Sunburn and Light Allergy with Methoxsalen. G.P. 19, 115–117, 1959.
6. Hu, F.; Fosnaugh, R.P.; and Lesney, P.F.,: Studies on Albinism, Arch. Dermat. 83, 723–729, 1961.
7. Lerner, A.B.,; Denton, C.R.; and Fitzpatrick, T.B.,: Clinical and Experimental Studies on 8-Methoxypsoralen in Vitiligo. J. Invest. Dermat. 20, 878, 1958.
8. Sulzberger, M.B., and Lerner, A.B.,: Suntanning-Potentiation with Oral Medication. J.A.M.A., 167, 2077–2079, 1958.
9. Becker, S.W., Jr.,: Effects of 8-Methoxypsoralen and Ultraviolet Light on Human Skin. Science, 127, 878, 1958.
10. Stegmaier, O.C.,: The Use of Methoxsalen in Suntanning. J. Invest. Dermat. 32, No. 2, 345–349, 1959.
11. Fitzpatrick, T.B.,: Current Therapy, W.B. Saunders Co., Page 515, 1958.
12. Fitzpatrick, T.B.; Arndt, K.A.; El Mofty, A.M. and Pathak, M.A.: Hydroquinone and Psoralens in Therapy of Hypermelanosis and Vitiligo, ARCH. DERM. 93, 589–600, 1966.
13. Becker, S.W., Jr.,: Psoralen Phototherapeutic Agents, J.A.M.A., 202, 422–424, 1967.
14. El Mofty, A.M.; Vitiligo and Psoralens, PERGAMON PRESS INC., Long Island City, New York, 1st Edition, 1968.

ICN PHARMACEUTICALS, INC.
3300 Hyland Ave.
Costa Mesa, CA 92626 USA

Revised 2-96
2399-03

Shown in Product Identification Guide, page 317

VIRAZOLE® ℞

[*vira 'zahl'*]
(Ribavirin for Inhalation Solution)

WARNINGS:
USE OF AEROSOLIZED VIRAZOLE IN PATIENTS REQUIRING MECHANICAL VENTILATOR ASSISTANCE SHOULD BE UNDERTAKEN ONLY BY PHYSICIANS AND SUPPORT STAFF FAMILIAR WITH THE SPECIFIC VENTILATOR BEING USED AND THIS MODE OF ADMINISTRATION OF THE DRUG. STRICT ATTENTION MUST BE PAID TO PROCEDURES THAT HAVE BEEN SHOWN TO MINIMIZE THE ACCUMULATION OF DRUG PRECIPITATE, WHICH CAN RESULT IN MECHANICAL VENTILATOR DYSFUNCTION AND ASSOCIATED INCREASED PULMONARY PRESSURES (SEE WARNINGS).
SUDDEN DETERIORATION OF RESPIRATORY FUNCTION HAS BEEN ASSOCIATED WITH INITIATION OF AEROSOLIZED VIRAZOLE USE IN INFANTS. RESPIRATORY FUNCTION SHOULD BE CAREFULLY MONITORED DURING TREATMENT. IF INITIATION OF AEROSOLIZED VIRAZOLE TREATMENT APPEARS TO PRODUCE SUDDEN DETERIORATION OF RESPIRATORY FUNCTION, TREATMENT SHOULD BE STOPPED AND REINSTITUTED ONLY WITH EXTREME CAUTION, CONTINUOUS MONITORING AND CONSIDERATION OF CONCOMITANT ADMINISTRATION OF BRONCHODILATORS (SEE WARNINGS).
VIRAZOLE IS NOT INDICATED FOR USE IN ADULTS. PHYSICIANS AND PATIENTS SHOULD BE AWARE THAT RIBAVIRIN HAS BEEN SHOWN TO PRODUCE TESTICULAR LESIONS IN RODENTS AND TO BE TERATOGENIC IN ALL ANIMAL SPECIES IN WHICH ADEQUATE STUDIES HAVE BEEN CONDUCTED (RODENTS AND RABBITS); (SEE CONTRAINDICATIONS).

DESCRIPTION

Virazole® is a brand name for ribavirin, a synthetic nucleoside with antiviral activity. VIRAZOLE for inhalation solution is a sterile, lyophilized powder to be reconstituted for aerosol administration. Each 100 ml glass vial contains 6 grams of ribavirin, and when reconstituted to the recommended volume of 300 ml with sterile water for injection or sterile water for inhalation (no preservatives added), will contain 20 mg of ribavirin per ml, pH approximately 5.5. Aerosolization is to be carried out in a Small Particle Aerosol Generator (SPAG-2) nebulizer only.
Ribavirin is 1-beta-D-ribofuranosyl-1H-1,2,4-triazole-3-carboxamide, with the following structural formula:

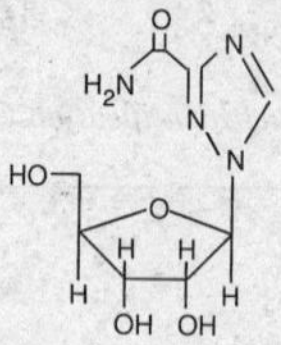

Ribavirin is a stable, white, crystalline compound with a maximum solubility in water of 142 mg/ml at 25°C and with only a slight solubility in ethanol. The empirical formula is $C_8H_{12}N_4O_5$ and the molecular weight is 244.21.

CLINICAL PHARMACOLOGY

Mechanism of Action
In cell cultures the inhibitory activity of ribavirin for respiratory syncytial virus (RSV) is selective. The mechanism of action is unknown. Reversal of the *in vitro* antiviral activity by guanosine or xanthosine suggests ribavirin may act as an analogue of these cellular metabolites.

Microbiology
Ribavirin has demonstrated antiviral activity against RSV *in vitro*[1] and in experimentally infected cotton rats.[2] Several clinical isolates of RSV were evaluated for ribavirin susceptibility by plaque reduction in tissue culture. Plaques were reduced 85–98% by 16 µg/ml; however, results may vary with the test system. The development of resistance has not been evaluated *in vitro* or in clinical trials.
In addition to the above, ribavirin has been shown to have *in vitro* activity against influenza A and B viruses and herpes simplex virus, but the clinical significance of these data is unknown.

Immunologic Effects
Neutralizing antibody responses to RSV were decreased in aerosolized VIRAZOLE treated infants compared to placebo treated infants.[3] One study also showed that RSV-specific IgE antibody in bronchial secretions was decreased in patients treated with aerosolized VIRAZOLE. In rats, ribavirin administration resulted in lymphoid atrophy of the thymus, spleen, and lymph nodes. Humoral immunity was reduced in guinea pigs and ferrets. Cellular immunity was also mildly depressed in animal studies. The clinical significance of these observations is unknown.

Pharmacokinetics
Assay for VIRAZOLE in human materials is by a radioimmunoassay which detects ribavirin and at least one metabolite.
VIRAZOLE brand of ribavirin, when administered by aerosol, is absorbed systemically. Four pediatric patients inhaling VIRAZOLE aerosol administered by face mask for 2.5 hours each day for 3 days had plasma concentrations ranging from 0.44 to 1.55 µM, with a mean concentration of 0.76 µM. The plasma half-life was reported to be 9.5 hours. Three pediatric patients inhaling aerosolized VIRAZOLE administered by face mask or mist tent for 20 hours each day for 5 days had plasma concentrations ranging from 1.5 to 14.3 µM, with a mean concentration of 6.8 µM.
The bioavailability of aerosolized VIRAZOLE is unknown and may depend on the mode of aerosol delivery. After aerosol treatment, peak plasma concentrations of ribavirin are 85% to 98% less than the concentration that reduced RSV plaque formation in tissue culture. After aerosol treatment, respiratory tract secretions are likely to contain ribavirin in concentrations many fold higher than those required to reduce plaque formation. However, RSV is an intracellular virus and it is unknown whether plasma concentrations or respiratory secretion concentrations of the drug better reflect intracellular concentrations in the respiratory tract.
In man, rats, and rhesus monkeys, accumulation of ribavirin and/or metabolites in the red blood cells has been noted, plateauing in red cells in man in about 4 days and gradually declining with an apparent half-life of 40 days (the half-life of erythrocytes). The extent of accumulation of ribavirin following inhalation therapy is not well defined.

Animal Toxicology
Ribavirin, when administered orally or as an aerosol, produced cardiac lesions in mice, rats, and monkeys, when given at doses of 30, 36 and 120 mg/kg or greater for 4 weeks or more (estimated human equivalent doses of 4.8, 12.3 and 111.4 mg/kg for a 5 kg child, or 2.5, 5.1 and 40 mg/kg for a 60 kg adult, based on body surface area adjustment). Aerosolized ribavirin administered to developing ferrets at 60 mg/kg for 10 or 30 days resulted in inflammatory and possibly emphysematous changes in the lungs. Proliferative changes were seen in the lungs following exposure at 131 mg/kg for 30 days. The significance of these findings to human administration is unknown.

INDICATIONS AND USAGE

VIRAZOLE is indicated for the treatment of hospitalized infants and young children with severe lower respiratory tract infections due to respiratory syncytial virus. Treatment early in the course of severe lower respiratory tract infection may be necessary to achieve efficacy.
Only severe RSV lower respiratory tract infection should be treated with VIRAZOLE. The vast majority of infants and children with RSV infection have disease that is mild, self-limited, and does not require hospitalization or antiviral treatment. Many children with mild lower respiratory tract involvement will require shorter hospitalization than would be required for a full course of VIRAZOLE aerosol (3 to 7 days) and should not be treated with the drug. Thus the decision to treat with VIRAZOLE should be based on the severity of the RSV infection.
The presence of an underlying condition such as prematurity, immunosuppression or cardiopulmonary disease may increase the severity of clinical manifestations and complications of RSV infection.
Use of aerosolized VIRAZOLE in patients requiring mechanical ventilator assistance should be undertaken only by physicians and support staff familiar with this mode of administration and the specific ventilator being used (see Warnings, and Dosage and Administration).

Diagnosis
RSV infection should be documented by a rapid diagnostic method such as demonstration of viral antigen in respiratory tract secretions by immunofluorescence[3,4] or ELISA[5] before or during the first 24 hours of treatment. Treatment may be initiated while awaiting rapid diagnostic test results. However, treatment should not be continued without documentation of RSV infection.
Non-culture antigen detection techniques may have false positive or false negative results. Assessment of the clinical situation, the time of year and other parameters may warrant reevaluation of the laboratory diagnosis.

Description of Studies
Non-Mechanically-Ventilated Infants: In two placebo controlled trials in infants hospitalized with RSV lower respiratory tract infection, aerosolized VIRAZOLE treatment had a therapeutic effect, as judged by the reduction in severity of clinical manifestations of disease by treatment day 3.[3,4] Treatment was most effective when instituted within the first 3 days of clinical illness. Virus titers in respiratory secretions were also significantly reduced with VIRAZOLE in one of these original studies.[4] Additional controlled studies conducted since these initial trials of aerosolized VIRAZOLE in the treatment of RSV infection have supported these data.
Mechanically-Ventilated Infants: A randomized, double-blind, placebo controlled evaluation of aerosolized VIRAZOLE at the recommended dose was conducted in 28 infants requiring mechanical ventilation for respiratory failure caused by documented RSV infection.[6] Mean age was 1.4 months (SD, 1.7 months). Seven patients had underlying diseases predisposing them to severe infection and 21 were previously normal. Aerosolized VIRAZOLE treatment significantly decreased the duration of mechanical ventilation required (4.9 vs. 9.9 days, p=0.01) and duration of required supplemental oxygen (8.7 vs 13.5 days, p=0.01). Intensive patient management and monitoring techniques were employed in this study. These included endotracheal tube suctioning every 1 to 2 hours; recording of proximal airway pressure, ventilatory rate, and F_1O_2 every hour; and arterial blood gas monitoring every 2 to 6 hours. To reduce the risk of VIRAZOLE precipitation and ventilator malfunction, heated wire tubing, two bacterial filters connected in series in the expiratory limb of the ventilator (with filter changes every 4 hours), and water column pressure release valves to monitor internal ventilator pressures were used in connecting ventilator circuits to the SPAG-2.
Employing these techniques, no technical difficulties with VIRAZOLE administration were encountered during the study. Adverse events consisted of bacterial pneumonia in one case, staphyloccus bacteremia in one case and two cases of post-extubation stridor. None were felt to be related to VIRAZOLE administration.

CONTRAINDICATIONS

VIRAZOLE is contraindicated in individuals who have shown hypersensitivity to the drug or its components, and in women who are or may become pregnant during exposure

to the drug. Ribavirin has demonstrated significant teratogenic and/or embryocidal potential in all animal species in which adequate studies have been conducted (rodents and rabbits). Therefore, although clinical studies have not been performed, it should be assumed that VIRAZOLE may cause fetal harm in humans. Studies in which the drug has been administered systemically demonstrate that ribavirin is concentrated in the red blood cells and persists for the life of the erythrocyte.

WARNINGS

SUDDEN DETERIORATION OF RESPIRATORY FUNCTION HAS BEEN ASSOCIATED WITH INITIATION OF AEROSOLIZED VIRAZOLE USE IN INFANTS. Respiratory function should be carefully monitored during treatment. If initiation of aerosolized VIRAZOLE treatment appears to produce sudden deterioration of respiratory function, treatment should be stopped and reinstituted only with extreme caution, continuous monitoring, and consideration of concomitant administration of bronchodilators.

Use with Mechanical Ventilators

USE OF AEROSOLIZED VIRAZOLE IN PATIENTS REQUIRING MECHANICAL VENTILATOR ASSISTANCE SHOULD BE UNDERTAKEN ONLY BY PHYSICIANS AND SUPPORT STAFF FAMILIAR WITH THIS MODE OF ADMINISTRATION AND THE SPECIFIC VENTILATOR BEING USED. Strict attention must be paid to procedures that have been shown to minimize the accumulation of drug precipitate, which can result in mechanical ventilator dysfunction and associated increased pulmonary pressures. These procedures include the use of bacteria filters in series in the expiratory limb of the ventilator circuit with frequent changes (every 4 hours), water column pressure release valves to indicate elevated ventilator pressures, frequent monitoring of these devices and verification that ribavirin crystals have not accumulated within the ventilator circuitry, and frequent suctioning and monitoring of the patient (see Clinical Studies).

Those administering aersolized VIRAZOLE in conjunction with mechanical ventilator use should be thoroughly familiar with detailed descriptions of these procedures as outlined in the SPAG-2 manual.

PRECAUTIONS

General: Patients with severe lower respiratory tract infection due to respiratory syncytial virus require optimum monitoring and attention to respiratory and fluid status (see SPAG-2 manual).

Drug Interactions

Clinical studies of interactions of VIRAZOLE with other drugs commonly used to treat infants with RSV infections, such as digoxin, bronchodilators, other antiviral agents, antibiotics, or anti-metabolites have not been conducted. Interference by VIRAZOLE with laboratory tests has not been evaluated.

Carcinogenesis and Mutagenesis

Ribavirin increased the incidence of cell transformations and mutations in mouse Balb/c 3T3 (fibroblasts) and L5178Y (lymphoma) cells at concentrations of 0.015 and 0.03–5.0 mg/ml, respectively (without metabolic activation.) Modest increases in mutation rates (3–4x) were observed at concentrations between 3.75–10.0 mg/ml in L5178Y cells *in vitro* with the addition of a metabolic activation fraction. In the mouse micronucleus assay, ribavirin was clastogenic at intravenous doses of 20–200 mg/kg, (estimated human equivalent of 1.67–16.7 mg/kg, based on body surface area adjustment for a 60 kg adult). Ribavirin was not mutagenic in a dominant lethal assay in rats at intraperitoneal doses between 50–200 mg/kg when administered for 5 days (estimated human equivalent of 7.14–28.6 mg/kg, based on body surface area adjustment; see Pharmacokinetics).

In vivo carcinogenicity studies with ribavirin are incomplete. However, results of a chronic feeding study with ribavirin in rats, at doses of 16–100 mg/kg/day (estimated human equivalent of 2.3–14.3 mg/kg/day, based on body surface area adjustment for the adult), suggest that ribavirin may induce benign mammary, pancreatic, pituitary and adrenal tumors. Preliminary results of 2 oral gavage oncogenicity studies in the mouse and rat (18–24 months; doses of 20–75 and 10–40 mg/kg/day, respectively [estimated human equivalent of 1.67–6.25 and 1.43–5.71 mg/kg/day, respectively, based on body surface area adjustment for the adult]) are inconclusive as to the carcinogenic potential of ribavirin (see Pharmacokinetics). However, these studies have demonstrated a relationship between chronic ribavirin exposure and increased incidences of vascular lesions (microscopic hemorrhages in mice) and retinal degeneration (in rats).

Impairment of Fertility

The fertility of ribavirin-treated animals (male or female) has not been fully investigated. However, in the mouse, administration of ribavirin at doses between 35–150 mg/kg/day (estimated human equivalent of 2.92–12.5 mg/kg/day, based on body surface area adjustment for the adult) resulted in significant seminiferous tubule atrophy, decreased sperm concentrations, and increased numbers of sperm with abnormal morphology. Partial recovery of sperm production was apparent 3–6 months following dose cessation. In several additional toxicology studies, ribavirin has been shown to cause testicular lesions (tubular atrophy), in adult rats at oral dose levels as low as 16 mg/kg/day (estimated human equivalent of 2.29 mg/kg/day, based on body surface area adjustment; see Pharmacokinetics). Lower doses were not tested. The reproductive capacity of treated male animals has not been studied.

Pregnancy: Category X

Ribavirin has demonstrated significant teratogenic and/or embryocidal potential in all animal species in which adequate studies have been conducted. Teratogenic effects were evident after single oral doses of 2.5 mg/kg or greater in the hamster, and after daily oral doses of 0.3 and 1.0 mg/kg in the rabbit and rat, respectively (estimated human equivalent doses of 0.12 and 0.14 mg/kg, based on body surface area adjustment for the adult). Malformations of the skull, palate, eye, jaw, limbs, skeleton, and gastrointestinal tract were noted. The incidence and severity of teratogenic effects increased with escalation of the drug dose. Survival of fetuses and offspring was reduced. Ribavirin caused embryolethality in the rabbit at daily oral dose levels as low as 1 mg/kg. No teratogenic effects were evident in the rabbit and rat administered daily oral doses of 0.1 and 0.3 mg/kg, respectively with estimated human equivalent doses of 0.01 and 0.04 mg/kg, based on body surface area adjustment (see Pharmacokinetics). These doses are considered to define the "No Observable Teratogenic Effects Level" (NOTEL) for ribavirin in the rabbit and rat.

Following oral administration of ribavirin in the pregnant rat (1.0 mg/kg) and rabbit (0.3 mg/kg), mean plasma levels of drug ranged from 0.10–0.20 μM [0.024–0.049 μg/ml] at 1 hour after dosing, to undetectable levels at 24 hours. At 1 hour following the administration of 0.3 or 0.1 mg/kg in the rat and rabbit (NOTEL), respectively, mean plasma levels of drug in both species were near or below the limit of detection (0.05 μM; see Pharmacokinetics),

Although clinical studies have not been performed, VIRAZOLE may cause fetal harm in humans. As noted previously, ribavirin is concentrated in red blood cells and persists for the life of the cell. Thus the terminal half-life for the systemic elimination of ribavirin is essentially that of the half-life of circulating erythrocytes. The minimum interval following exposure to VIRAZOLE before pregnancy may be safely initiated is unknown (see Contraindications, Warnings, and Information for Health Care Personnel).

Nursing Mothers

VIRAZOLE has been shown to be toxic to lactating animals and their offspring. It is not known if VIRAZOLE is excreted in human milk.

Information for Health Care Personnel

Health care workers directly providing care to patients receiving aerosolized VIRAZOLE should be aware that ribavirin has been shown to be teratogenic in all animal species in which adequate studies have been conducted (rodents and rabbits). Although no reports of teratogenesis in offspring of mothers who were exposed to aerosolized VIRAZOLE during pregnancy have been confirmed, no controlled studies have been conducted in pregnant women. Studies of environmental exposure in treatment settings have shown that the drug can disperse into the immediate bedside area during routine patient care activities with highest ambient levels closest to the patient and extremely low levels outside of the immediate bedside area. Adverse reactions resulting from actual occupational exposure in adults are described below (see Adverse Events in Health Care Workers). Some studies have documented ambient drug concentrations at the bedside that could potentially lead to systemic exposures above those considered safe for exposure during pregnancy (1/1000 of the NOTEL dose in the most sensitive animal species).[7,8,9]

A 1992 study conducted by the National Institute of Occupational Safety and Health (NIOSH) demonstrated measurable urine levels of ribavirin in health care workers exposed to aerosol in the course of direct patient care.[7] Levels were lowest in workers caring for infants receiving aerosolized VIRAZOLE with mechanical ventilation and highest in those caring for patients being administered the drug via an oxygen tent or hood. This study employed a more sensitive assay to evaluate ribavirin levels in urine than was available for several previous studies of environmental exposure that failed to detect measurable ribavirin levels in exposed workers. Creatinine adjusted urine levels in the NIOSH study ranged from less than 0.001 to 0.140 μM of ribavirin per gram of creatinine in exposed workers. However, the relationship between urinary ribavirin levels in exposed workers, plasma levels in animal studies, and the specific risk of teratogenesis in exposed pregnant women is unknown.

It is good practice to avoid unnecessary occupational exposure to chemicals wherever possible. Hospitals are encouraged to conduct training programs to minimize potential occupational exposure to VIRAZOLE. Health care workers who are pregnant should consider avoiding direct care of patients receiving aerosolized VIRAZOLE. If close patient contact cannot be avoided, precautions to limit exposure should be taken. These include administration of VIRAZOLE in negative pressure rooms; adequate room ventilation (at least six air exchanges per hour); the use of VIRAZOLE aerosol scavenging devices; turning off the SPAG-2 device for 5 to 10 minutes prior to prolonged patient contact, and wearing appropriately fitted respirator masks. Surgical masks do not provide adequate filtration of VIRAZOLE particles. Further information is available from NIOSH's Hazard Evaluation and Technical Assistance Branch and additional recommendations have been published in an Aerosol Consensus Statement by the American Respiratory Care Foundation and the American Association for Respiratory Care.[10]

ADVERSE REACTIONS

The description of adverse reactions is based on events from clinical studies (approximately 200 patients) conducted prior to 1986, and the controlled trial of aerosolized VIRAZOLE conducted in 1989–1990. Additional data from spontaneous post-marketing reports of adverse events in individual patients have been available since 1986.

Deaths

Deaths during or shortly after treatment with aerosolized VIRAZOLE have been reported in 20 cases of patients treated with VIRAZOLE (12 of these patients were being treated for RSV infections). Several cases have been characterized as "possibly related" to VIRAZOLE by the treating physician; these were in infants who experienced worsening respiratory status related to bronchospasm while being treated with the drug. Several other cases have been attributed to mechanical ventilator malfunction in which VIRAZOLE precipitation within the ventilator apparatus led to excessively high pulmonary pressures and diminished oxygenation. In these cases the monitoring procedures described in the current package insert were not employed (see Description of Studies, Warnings, and Dosage and Administration).

Pulmonary and Cardiovascular

Pulmonary function significantly deteriorated during aerosolized VIRAZOLE treatment in six of six adults with chronic obstructive lung disease and in four of six asthmatic adults. Dyspnea and chest soreness were also reported in the latter group. Minor abnormalities in pulmonary function were also seen in healthy adult volunteers.

In the original study population of approximately 200 infants who received aerosolized VIRAZOLE, several serious adverse events occurred in severely ill infants with life-threatening underlying diseases, many of whom required assisted ventilation. The role of VIRAZOLE in these events is indeterminate. Since the drug's approval in 1986, additional reports of similar serious, though non-fatal, events have been filed infrequently. Events associated with aerosolized VIRAZOLE use have included the following:

Pulmonary: Worsening of respiratory status, bronchospasm, pulmonary edema, hypoventilation, cyanosis, dyspnea, bacterial pneumonia, pneumothorax, apnea, atelectasis and ventilator dependence.

Cardiovascular: Cardiac arrest, hypotension, bradycardia and digitalis toxicity. Bigeminy, bradycardia and tachycardia have been described in patients with underlying congenital heart disease.

Some subjects requiring assisted ventilation experienced serious difficulties, due to inadequate ventilation and gas exchange. Precipitation of drug within the ventilatory apparatus, including the endotracheal tube, has resulted in increased positive end expiratory pressure and increased positive inspiratory pressure. Accumulation of fluid in tubing ("rain out") has also been noted. Measures to avoid these complications should be followed carefully (see Dosage and Administration).

Hematologic

Although anemia was not reported with use of aerosolized VIRAZOLE in controlled clinical trials, most infants treated with the aerosol have not been evaluated 1 to 2 weeks post-treatment when anemia is likely to occur. Anemia has been shown to occur frequently with experimental oral and intravenous VIRAZOLE in humans. Also, cases of anemia (type unspecified), reticulocytosis and hemolytic anemia associated with aerosolized VIRAZOLE use have been reported through post-marketing reporting systems. All have been reversible with discontinuation of the drug.

Other

Rash and conjunctivitis have been associated with the use of aerosolized VIRAZOLE. These usually resolve within hours of discontinuing therapy. Seizures and asthenia associated with experimental intravenous VIRAZOLE therapy have also been reported.

Adverse Events in Health Care Workers

Studies of environmental exposure to aerosolized VIRAZOLE in health care workers administering care to patients receiving the drug have not detected adverse signs or symptoms related to exposure. However, 152 health care workers have reported experiencing adverse events through post-marketing surveillance. Nearly all were in individuals providing direct care to infants receiving aerosolized VIRA-

Continued on next page

Virazole—Cont.

ZOLE. Of 358 events from these 152 individual health care worker reports, the most common signs and symptoms were headache (51% of reports), conjunctivitis (32%), and rhinitis, nausea, rash, dizziness, pharyngitis, or lacrimation (10–20% each). Several cases of bronchospasm and/or chest pain were also reported, usually in individuals with known underlying reactive airway disease. Several case reports of damage to contact lenses after prolonged close exposure to aerosolized VIRAZOLE have also been reported. Most signs and symptoms reported as having occurred in exposed health care workers resolved within minutes to hours of discontinuing close exposure to aerosolized VIRAZOLE (also see Information for Health Care Personnel).

The symptoms of RSV in adults can include headache, conjunctivitis, sore throat and/or cough, fever, hoarseness, nasal congestion and wheezing, although RSV infections in adults are typically mild and transient. Such infections represent a potential hazard to uninfected hospital patients. It is unknown whether certain symptoms cited in reports from health care workers were due to exposure to the drug or infection with RSV. Hospitals should implement appropriate infection control procedures.

Overdosage

No overdosage with VIRAZOLE by aerosol administration has been reported in humans. The LD_{50} in mice is 2 gm orally and is associated with hypoactivity and gastrointestinal symptoms (estimated human equivalent dose of 0.17gm/kg, based on body surface area conversion). The mean plasma half-life after administration of aerosolized VIRAZOLE for pediatric patients is 9.5 hours. VIRAZOLE is concentrated and persists in red blood cells for the life of the erythrocyte (see Pharmacokinetics).

DOSAGE AND ADMINISTRATION

BEFORE USE, READ THOROUGHLY THE ICN SMALL PARTICLE AEROSOL GENERATOR MODEL SPAG-2 OPERATOR'S MANUAL FOR SMALL PARTICLE AEROSOL GENERATOR OPERATING INSTRUCTIONS. AEROSOLIZED VIRAZOLE SHOULD NOT BE ADMINISTERED WITH ANY OTHER AEROSOL GENERATING DEVICE.

The recommended treatment regimen is 20 mg/ml VIRAZOLE as the starting solution in the drug reservoir of the SPAG-2 unit, with continuous aerosol administration for 12–18 hours per day for 3 to 7 days. Using the recommended drug concentration of 20 mg/ml the average aerosol concentration for a 12 hour delivery period would be 190 micrograms/liter of air. Aerosolized VIRAZOLE should not be administered in a mixture for combined aerosolization or simultaneously with other aerosolized medications.

Non-mechanically ventilated infants

VIRAZOLE should be delivered to an infant oxygen hood from the SPAG-2 aerosol generator. Administration by face mask or oxygen tent may be necessary if a hood cannot be employed (see SPAG-2 manual). However, the volume and condensation area are larger in a tent and this may alter delivery dynamics of the drug.

Mechanically ventilated infants

The recommended dose and administration schedule for infants who require mechanical ventilation is the same as for those who do not. Either a pressure or volume cycle ventilator may be used in conjunction with the SPAG-2. In either case, patients should have their endotracheal tubes suctioned every 1–2 hours, and their pulmonary pressures monitored frequently (every 2–4 hours). For both pressure and volume ventilators, heated wire connective tubing and bacteria filters in series in the expiratory limb of the system (which must be changed frequently, i.e., every 4 hours) must be used to minimize the risk of VIRAZOLE precipitation in the system and the subsequent risk of ventilator dysfunction. Water column pressure release valves should be used in the ventilator circuit for pressure cycled ventilators, and may be utilized with volume cycled ventilators (SEE SPAG-2 MANUAL FOR DETAILED INSTRUCTIONS).

Method of Preparation

VIRAZOLE brand of ribavirin is supplied as 6 grams of lyophilized powder per 100 ml vial for aerosol administration only. By sterile technique, reconstitute drug with a minimum of 75 ml of **sterile USP water for injection or inhalation** in the original 100 ml glass vial. Shake well. Transfer to the clean, sterilized 500 ml SPAG-2 reservoir and further dilute to a final volume of 300 ml with Sterile Water for Injection, USP, or Inhalation. The final concentration should be 20 mg/ml. **Important:** This water should NOT have had any antimicrobial agent or other substance added. The solution should be inspected visually for particulate matter and discoloration prior to administration. Solutions that have been placed in the SPAG-2 unit should be discarded at least every 24 hours and when the liquid level is low before adding newly reconstituted solution.

HOW SUPPLIED

VIRAZOLE (ribavirin for inhalation solution) is supplied in 100 ml glass vials with 6 grams of sterile, lyophilized drug which is to be reconstituted with 300 ml Sterile Water for Injection or Sterile Water for Inhalation (no preservatives added) and administered only by a small particle aerosol generator (SPAG-2). Vials containing the lyophilized drug powder should be stored in a dry place at 15–25°C (59–78°F). Reconstituted solutions may be stored, under sterile conditions, at room temperature (20–30°C, 68–86°F) for 24 hours. Solutions which have been placed in the SPAG-2 unit should be discarded at least every 24 hours.

REFERENCES

1. Hruska JF, Bernstein JM, Douglas Jr., RG, and Hall CB. Effects of Virazole on respiratory syncytial virus in vitro. Antimicrob Agents Chemother 17:770–775, 1 1980.
2. Hruska JF, Morrow PE, Suffin SC, and Douglas Jr., RG. In vivo inhibition of respiratory syncytial virus by Virazole. Antimicrob Agents Chemother 21:125–130, 1982.
3. Taber LH, Knight V, Gilbert BE, McClung HW et al. Virazole aerosol treatment of bronchiolitis associated with respiratory tract infection in infants. Pediatrics 72:613–618, 1983.
4. Hall CB, McBride JT, Walsh EE, Bell DM et al. Aerosolized Virazole treatment of infants with respiratory syncytial viral infection. N Engl J Med 308:1443–7, 1983.
5. Hendry RM, McIntosh K, Fahnestock ML, and Pierik LT. Enzyme-linked immunosorbent assay for detection of respiratory syncytial virus infection. J Clin Microbiol 16:329–33, 1982.
6. Smith, David W., Frankel, Lorry R., Mather, Larry H., Tang, Allen T.S., Ariagno, Ronald L., Prober, Charles G. A Controlled Trial of Aerosolized Ribavirin in Infants Receiving Mechanical Ventilation for Severe Respiratory Syncytial Virus Infection. The New England Journal of Medicine 1991; 325:24–29.
7. Decker, John, Shultz, Ruth A., Health Hazard Evaluation Report: Florida Hospital, Orlando, Florida, Cincinnati OH: U.S. Department of Health and Human Services, Public Health Service, Centers for NIOSH Report No. HETA 91-104-2229.*
8. Barnes, D.J. and Doursew, M. Reference dose: Description and use in health risk assessments. Regul Tox. and Pharm. Vol. 8; p. 471–486, 1988.
9. Federal Register Vol. 53 No. 126 Thurs. June 30, 1988 p. 24834–24847.
10. American Association for Respirtory Care [1991]. Aerosol Consensus Statement-1991. Respiratory Care 36(9): 916–921.

*Copies of the Report may be purchased from National Technical Information Service, 5285 Port Royal Road, Springfield, VA 22161; Ask for Publication PB 93119-345.

1957-06 EL
Rev. 5-96

ICN PHARMACEUTICALS, INC.
ICN Plaza
3300 Hyland Avenue
Costa Mesa, California 92626
714-545-0100

IDEC Pharmaceuticals Corporation

11011 TORREYANA RD.
SAN DIEGO, CA 92121

Direct Inquiries to:
(619) 550-8500

RITUXAN™ ℞

[rī-tǝks-ǎn]
Rituximab

DESCRIPTION

The RITUXAN (Rituximab) antibody is a genetically engineered chimeric murine/human monoclonal antibody directed against the CD20 antigen found on the surface of normal and malignant B lymphocytes. The antibody is an IgG_1 kappa immunoglobulin containing murine light- and heavy-chain variable region sequences and human constant region sequences. Rituximab is composed of two heavy chains of 451 amino acids and two light chains of 213 amino acids (based on cDNA analysis) and has an approximate molecular weight of 145 kD. Rituximab has a binding affinity for the CD20 antigen of approximately 8.0 nM.

The chimeric anti-CD20 antibody is produced by mammalian cell (Chinese Hamster ovary) suspension culture in a nutrient medium containing the antibiotic gentamicin. Gentamicin is not detectable in the final product. The anti-CD20 antibody is purified by affinity and ion exchange chromatography. The purification process includes specific viral inactivation and removal procedures. Rituximab drug product is manufactured from either bulk drug substance manufactured by Genentech, Inc. (US License No. 1048), or utilizing formulated bulk Rituximab supplied by IDEC Pharmaceuticals Corporation (US License No. 1235) under a shared manufacturing arrangement.

RITUXAN is a sterile, clear, colorless, preservative-free liquid concentrate for intravenous (IV) administration. RITUXAN is supplied at a concentration of 10 mg/mL in either 100 mg (10 mL) or 500 mg (50 mL) single-use vials. The product is formulated for intravenous administration in 9.0 mg/mL sodium chloride, 7.35 mg/mL sodium citrate dihydrate, 0.7 mg/mL polysorbate 80, and Sterile Water for Injection. The pH is adjusted to 6.5.

CLINICAL PHARMACOLOGY

General

Rituximab binds specifically to the antigen CD20 (human B-lymphocyte-restricted differentiation antigen, Bp35), a hydrophobic transmembrane protein with a molecular weight of approximately 35 kD located on pre-B and mature B lymphocytes.[1,2] The antigen is also expressed on >90% of B-cell non-Hodgkin's lymphomas (NHL)[3] but is not found on hematopoietic stem cells, pro-B cells, normal plasma cells or other normal tissues.[4] CD20 regulates an early step(s) in the activation process for cell cycle initiation and differentiation,[4] and possibly functions as a calcium ion channel.[5] CD20 is not shed from the cell surface and does not internalize upon antibody binding.[6] Free CD20 antigen is not found in the circulation.[2]

Pre-clinical Pharmacology and Toxicology

Mechanism of Action: The Fab domain of Rituximab binds to the CD20 antigen on B-lymphocytes and the Fc domain recruits immune effector functions to mediate B-cell lysis *in vitro*. Possible mechanisms of cell lysis include complement-dependent cytotoxicity (CDC)[7] and antibody-dependent cell mediated cytotoxicity (ADCC). The antibody has been shown to induce apoptosis in the DHL-4 human B-cell lymphoma line.[8]

Normal Tissue Cross-reactivity: Rituximab binding was observed on lymphoid cells in the thymus, the white pulp of the spleen, and a majority of B-lymphocytes in peripheral blood and lymph nodes. Little or no binding was observed in non-lymphoid tissues examined.

Human Pharmacokinetics/Pharmacodynamics

In patients given single doses at 10, 50, 100, 250 or 500 mg/m^2 as an IV infusion, serum levels and the half-life of Rituximab were proportional to dose. In 9 patients given 375 mg/m^2 as an IV infusion for four doses, the mean serum half-life was 59.8 hours (range 11.1 to 104.6 hours) after the first infusion and 174 hours (range 26 to 442 hours) after the fourth infusion. The wide range of half-lives may reflect the variable tumor burden among patients and the changes in CD20 positive (normal and malignant) B-cell populations upon repeated administrations.

Rituximab at a dose of 375 mg/m^2 was administered as an IV infusion at weekly intervals for four doses to 166 patients. The peak and trough serum levels of Rituximab were inversely correlated with baseline values for the number of circulating CD20 positive B cells and measures of disease burden. Median steady-state serum levels were higher for responders compared to nonresponders; however, no difference was found in the rate of elimination as measured by serum half-life. Serum levels were higher in patients with International Working Formulation (IWF) subtypes B, C, and D as compared to those with subtype A. Rituximab was detectable in the serum of patients three to six months after completion of treatment.

The pharmacokinetic profile of Rituximab when administered as six infusions of 375 mg/m^2 in combination with six cycles of CHOP chemotherapy was similar to that seen with Rituximab alone.

Administration of RITUXAN resulted in a rapid and sustained depletion of circulating and tissue-based B cells. Lymph node biopsies performed 14 days after therapy showed a decrease in the percentage of B-cells in seven of eight patients who had received single doses of Rituximab ≥100 mg/m^2.[9] Among the 166 patients in the pivotal study, circulating B-cells (measured as CD19 positive cells) were depleted within the first three doses with sustained depletion for up to 6 to 9 months post-treatment in 83% of patients. One of the responding patients (1%), failed to show significant depletion of CD19 positive cells after the third infusion of Rituximab as compared to 19% of the nonresponding patients. B-cell recovery began at approximately six months following completion of treatment. Median B-cell levels returned to normal by twelve months following completion of treatment.

There were sustained and statistically significant reductions in both IgM and IgG serum levels observed from 5 through 11 months following Rituximab administration. However, only 14% of patients had reductions in IgG and/or IgM serum levels, resulting in values below the normal range.

CLINICAL STUDIES

A multicenter, open-label, single-arm study was conducted in 166 patients with relapsed or refractory low-grade or fol-

licular B-cell NHL who received 375 mg/m^2 of RITUXAN given as an IV infusion weekly for four doses. Patients with tumor masses >10 cm or with >5,000 lymphocytes/μL in the peripheral blood were excluded from the study. The overall response rate (ORR) was 48% (80/166) with a 6% (10/166) complete response (CR) and a 42% (70/166) partial response (PR) rate. Disease-related signs and symptoms (including B-symptoms) were present in 23% (39/166) of patients at study entry and resolved in 64% (25/39) of those patients. The median time to onset of response was 50 days and the median duration of response is projected to be 10 to 12 months.

In a multivariate analysis, the ORR was higher in patients with IWF B, C, and D histologic subtypes as compared to IWF A subtype (58% vs. 12%), higher in patients whose largest lesion was <5 cm vs. >7 cm in greatest diameter (53% vs. 38%), and higher in patients with chemosensitive relapse as compared to chemoresistant (defined as duration of response <3 months) relapse (53% vs. 36%). ORR in patients previously treated with autologous bone marrow transplant was 78% (18/23). The following factors were not associated with a lower response rate: age ≥60 years, extranodal disease, prior anthracycline therapy, and bone marrow involvement.

In a second multicenter, multiple-dose study, 37 patients with relapsed or refractory B-cell NHL received 375 mg/m^2 of RITUXAN as an IV infusion once weekly for four doses.[10,11] The ORR was 46% with a median duration of response of 8.6 months (range 2.6 to 26.2+). Single doses of up to 500 mg/m^2 were well-tolerated.[9]

Twenty patients have received two courses and one patient has received three courses of RITUXAN as 4 weekly infusions of 375 mg/m^2 per infusion. The percentage of patients reporting adverse events upon retreatment was similar to that reported following the first course, although the incidence of specific adverse events differed (see ADVERSE EVENTS). All patients had obtained an objective clinical response (CR or PR) to the first course of RITUXAN; upon retreatment, 6 of 12 patients evaluable for response obtained a complete or partial remission.

Twenty-nine patients with relapsed or refractory, bulky (single lesion of >10 cm in diameter), low grade NHL received 375 mg/m^2 of RITUXAN as four weekly infusions. The overall incidence of adverse events and the incidence of Grade 3 and 4 adverse events was higher in patients with bulky disease than in patients with non-bulky disease (see ADVERSE EVENTS). Ten of 21 patients evaluable for response have obtained a complete or partial remission.

INDICATIONS AND USAGE

RITUXAN is indicated for the treatment of patients with relapsed or refractory low-grade or follicular, CD20 positive, B-cell non-Hodgkin's lymphoma.

CONTRAINDICATIONS

RITUXAN is contraindicated in patients with known Type I hypersensitivity or anaphylactic reactions to murine proteins or to any component of this product. (See WARNINGS.)

WARNINGS

RITUXAN rapidly decreases CD20 positive cells that are both benign and malignant. Tumor lysis syndrome has been reported to occur within 12 to 24 hours after the first RITUXAN infusion in patients with high numbers of circulating malignant lymphocytes. Other patients with high tumor burden may also be at risk. Consideration should be given to prophylactic treatment of tumor lysis syndrome in patients who are considered to be at high risk.

RITUXAN is associated with hypersensitivity reactions which may respond to adjustments in the infusion rate. Hypotension, bronchospasm, and angioedema have occurred in association with RITUXAN infusion as part of an infusion-related symptom complex. RITUXAN infusion should be interrupted for severe reactions and can be resumed at a 50% reduction in rate (e.g., from 100 mg/hr to 50 mg/hr) when symptoms have completely resolved. Treatment of these symptoms with diphenhydramine and acetaminophen is recommended; additional treatment with bronchodilators or IV saline may be indicated. In most cases, patients who have experienced non-life-threatening reactions have been able to complete the full course of therapy. (See DOSAGE and ADMINISTRATION.) Medications for the treatment of hypersensitivity reactions, e.g., epinephrine, antihistamines and corticosteroids should be available for immediate use in the event of a reaction during administration.

Infusions should be discontinued in the event of serious or life-threatening cardiac arrhythmias. Patients who develop clinically significant arrhythmias should undergo cardiac monitoring during and after subsequent infusions of RITUXAN. Patients with preexisting cardiac conditions including arrhythmias and angina have had recurrences of these events during RITUXAN therapy and should be monitored throughout the infusion and immediate post-infusion period.

PRECAUTIONS

Laboratory Monitoring: Complete blood counts (CBC) and platelet counts should be obtained at regular intervals during RITUXAN therapy and more frequently in patients who develop cytopenias (see ADVERSE EVENTS). In patients who appear to be at risk for developing tumor lysis syndrome, appropriate laboratory studies should be monitored and prophylactic treatment used (see WARNINGS).

Drug/Laboratory Interactions: There have been no formal drug interaction studies performed with RITUXAN.

HAMA/HACA Formation: Human anti-murine antibody (HAMA) was not detected in 67 patients evaluated. Less than 1.0% (3/355) of patients evaluated for human anti-chimeric antibody (HACA) were positive. Patients who develop HAMA/HACA titers may have allergic or hypersensitivity reactions when treated with this or other murine or chimeric monoclonal antibodies.

Immunization: The safety of immunization with any vaccine, particularly live viral vaccines, following RITUXAN therapy has not been studied. The ability to generate a primary or anamnestic humoral response to any vaccine has also not been studied.

Carcinogenesis, Mutagenesis, Impairment of Fertility: No long-term animal studies have been performed to establish the carcinogenic or mutagenic potential of RITUXAN, or to determine its effects on fertility in males or females. Individuals of childbearing potential should use effective contraceptive methods during treatment and for up to 12 months following RITUXAN therapy.

Pregnancy Category C: Animal reproduction studies have not been conducted with RITUXAN. It is not known whether RITUXAN can cause fetal harm when administered to a pregnant woman or whether it can affect reproductive capacity. Human IgG is known to pass the placental barrier, and thus may potentially cause fetal B-cell depletion; therefore, RITUXAN should be given to a pregnant woman only if clearly needed.

Nursing Mothers: It is not known whether RITUXAN is excreted in human milk. Because human IgG is excreted in human milk and the potential for absorption and immunosuppression in the infant is unknown, women should be advised to discontinue nursing until circulating drug levels are no longer detectable. (See CLINICAL PHARMACOLOGY.)

Pediatric Use: The safety and effectiveness of RITUXAN in children have not been established.

ADVERSE REACTIONS

Safety data are based on 315 patients treated in five single-agent studies of RITUXAN. This includes patients with bulky disease (lesions >10 cm), those who have received more than one course of RITUXAN, and patients receiving 375 mg/m^2 for eight doses.

Infusion-Related Events: An infusion-related symptom complex consisting of fever and chills/rigors occurred in the majority of patients during the first RITUXAN infusion. Other frequent infusion-related symptoms included nausea, urticaria, fatigue, headache, pruritus, bronchospasm, dyspnea, sensation of tongue or throat swelling (angioedema), rhinitis, vomiting, hypotension, flushing, and pain at disease sites. These reactions generally occurred within 30 minutes to 2 hours of beginning the first infusion, and resolved with slowing or interruption of the RITUXAN infusion and with supportive care (IV saline, diphenhydramine, and acetaminophen). The incidence of infusion-related events decreased from 80% (7% Grade 3/4) during the first infusion to approximately 40% (5% to 10% Grade 3/4) with subsequent infusions. Mild to moderate hypotension requiring interruption of RITUXAN infusion with or without the administration of IV saline occurred in 32 (10%) patients. Isolated occurrences of severe reactions requiring epinephrine have been reported in patients receiving RITUXAN for other indications. Angioedema was reported in 41 (13%) patients and was serious in one patient. Bronchospasm occurred in 24 (8%) patients; one-quarter of these patients were treated with bronchodilators. A single report of bronchiolitis obliterans was noted.

Immunologic Events: RITUXAN induced B-cell depletion in 70 to 80% of patients and was associated with decreased

Table 1. Adverse Events ≥5% of Patients (N=315)

	Incidence All Grades	
	N	%
Any Adverse Event	275	87
Body As A Whole		
Fever	154	49
Chills	102	32
Asthenia	49	16
Headache	43	14
Throat Irritation	19	6
Abdominal Pain	18	6
Cardiovascular System		
Hypotension	32	10
Digestive System		
Nausea	55	18
Vomiting	23	7
Hemic and Lymphatic System		
Leukopenia	33	11
Thrombocytopenia	25	8
Neutropenia	21	7
Metabolic and Nutritional System		
Angioedema	41	13
Musculo-Skeletal System		
Myalgia	21	7
Nervous System		
Dizziness	23	7
Respiratory System		
Rhinitis	25	8
Bronchospasm	24	8
Skin and Appendages		
Pruritus	32	10
Rash	31	10
Urticaria	24	8

Continued on next page

Rituxan—Cont.

serum immunoglobulins in a minority of patients. The incidence of infection did not appear to be increased. During the treatment period, 50 patients in the pivotal trial developed 68 infectious events; 6 (9%) were Grade 3 in severity and none were Grade 4 events. Of the 6 serious infectious events, none were associated with neutropenia. The serious bacterial events included sepsis due to Listeria (n=1), Staphylococcal bacteremia (n=1) and polymicrobial sepsis (n=1). In the post-treatment period (30 days to 11 months following the last dose), bacterial infections included sepsis (n=1); significant viral infections included herpes simplex infections (n=2) and herpes zoster (n=3).

Retreatment Events: Twenty-one patients have received more than one course of RITUXAN. The percentage of patients reporting any adverse event upon retreatment was similar to the percentage of patients reporting adverse events upon initial exposure. The following adverse events were reported more frequently in retreated subjects: asthenia, throat irritation, flushing, tachycardia, anorexia, leukopenia, thrombocytopenia, anemia, peripheral edema, dizziness, depression, respiratory symptoms, night sweats, and pruritus.

Hematologic Events: During the treatment period (up to 30 days following last dose) severe thrombocytopenia occurred in 1.3% of patients, severe neutropenia occurred in 1.9% of patients, and severe anemia occurred in 1.0% of patients. A single occurrence of transient aplastic anemia (pure red cell aplasia) and two occurrences of hemolytic anemia following RITUXAN therapy were reported.

Cardiac Events: Four patients developed arrhythmias during RITUXAN infusion. One of the four discontinued treatment because of ventricular tachycardia and supraventricular tachycardias. The other three patients experienced trigeminy (1) and irregular pulse (2) and did not require discontinuation of therapy. Angina was reported during infusion and myocardial infarction occurred 4 days post-infusion in one subject with a prior history of myocardial infarction.

[See table at top of previous page]

Severe and life-threatening (Grade 3 and 4) events were reported in 10% (32/315) of patients. The following Grade 3 and 4 adverse events were reported: neutropenia (1.9%), chills (1.6%), leukopenia and thrombocytopenia (1.3% for each), hypotension, anemia, bronchospasm, and urticaria (1.0% for each), headache, abdominal pain, arrhythmia (0.6% for each), and asthenia, hypertension, nausea, vomiting, coagulation disorder, angioedema, arthralgia, pain, rhinitis, increased cough, dyspnea, bronchiolitis obliterans, hypoxia, asthma, pruritus, and rash (one patient each, 0.3%).

The following adverse events occurred in ≥1.0% but <5.0% of patients, in order of decreasing incidence: flushing, arthralgia, diarrhea, anemia, cough increase, hypertension, lacrimation disorder, pain, hyperglycemia, back pain, peripheral edema, paresthesia, dyspepsia, chest pain, anorexia, anxiety, malaise, tachycardia, agitation, insomnia, sinusitis, conjunctivitis, abdominal enlargement, postural hypotension, LDH increase, hypocalcemia, hypesthesia, respiratory disorder, tumor pain, pain at injection site, bradycardia, hypertonia, nervousness, bronchitis, and taste perversion.

The proportion of patients reporting any adverse event was similar in patients with bulky disease and those with lesions <10 cm in diameter. However, the incidence of dizziness, neutropenia, thrombocytopenia, myalgia, anemia and chest pain was higher in patients with lesions >10 cm. The incidence of any Grade 3 and 4 event was higher (31% vs. 13%) and the incidence of Grade 3 or 4 neutropenia, anemia, hypotension, and dyspnea was also higher in patients with bulky disease compared with patients with lesions <10 cm.

OVERDOSAGE

There has been no experience with overdosage in human clinical trials. Single doses higher than 500 mg/m² have not been tested.

DOSAGE AND ADMINISTRATION

Usual Dose:

The recommended dosage of RITUXAN is 375 mg/m² given as an IV infusion once weekly for four doses (days 1, 8, 15, and 22). RITUXAN may be administered in an outpatient setting. **DO NOT ADMINISTER AS AN INTRAVENOUS PUSH OR BOLUS. (See Administration.)**

Instructions for Administration

Preparation for Administration: Use appropriate aseptic technique. Withdraw the necessary amount of RITUXAN and dilute to a final concentration of 1 to 4 mg/mL into an infusion bag containing either 0.9% Sodium Chloride USP or 5% Dextrose in Water USP. Gently invert the bag to mix the solution. Discard any unused portion left in the vial. Parenteral drug products should be inspected visually for particulate matter and discoloration prior to administra-

RITUXAN solutions for infusion are stable at 2° to 8° C (36° to 46° F) for 24 hours and at room temperature for an additional 12 hours. No incompatibilities between RITUXAN and polyvinylchloride or polyethylene bags have been observed.

Administration: **DO NOT ADMINISTER AS AN INTRAVENOUS PUSH OR BOLUS.** Hypersensitivity reactions may occur (see WARNINGS). Premedication, consisting of acetaminophen and diphenhydramine, should be considered before each infusion of RITUXAN. Premedication may attenuate infusion-related events. Since transient hypotension may occur during RITUXAN infusion, consideration should be given to withholding anti-hypertensive medications 12 hours prior to RITUXAN infusion.

First Infusion: The RITUXAN solution for infusion should be administered intravenously at an initial rate of 50 mg/hr. RITUXAN should not be mixed or diluted with other drugs. If hypersensitivity or infusion-related events do not occur, escalate the infusion rate in 50 mg/hr increments every 30 minutes, to a maximum of 400 mg/hr. If hypersensitivity or an infusion-related event develops, the infusion should be temporarily slowed or interrupted (see WARNINGS). The infusion can continue at one-half the previous rate upon improvement of patient symptoms.

Subsequent Infusions: Subsequent RITUXAN infusions can be administered at an initial rate of 100 mg/hr, and increased by 100 mg/hr increments at 30-minute intervals, to a maximum of 400 mg/hr as tolerated.

Stability and Storage: RITUXAN vials are stable at 2° to 8° C (36° to 46° F). Do not use beyond expiration date stamped on carton. RITUXAN vials should be protected from direct sunlight.

HOW SUPPLIED

RITUXAN is supplied as 100 mg and 500 mg of sterile, preservative-free, single-use vials.

Single unit 100 mg carton: Contains one 10 mL vial of RITUXAN (10 mg/mL). NDC 50242-051-21

Single unit 500 mg carton: Contains one 50 mL vial of RITUXAN (10 mg/mL). NDC 50242-053-06

REFERENCES

1. Valentine MA, Meier KE, Rossie S, et al. Phosphorylation of the CD20 phosphoprotein in resting B lymphocytes. J. Biol. Chem. 1989 264(19): 11282–11287.
2. Einfeld DA, Brown JP, Valentine MA, et al. Molecular cloning of the human B cell CD20 receptor predicts a hydrophobic protein with multiple transmembrane domains. EMBO J. 1988 7(3):711–717.
3. Anderson KC, Bates MP, Slaughenhoupt BL, et al. Expression of human B cell-associated antigens on leukemias and lymphomas: A model of human B cell differentiation. Blood 1984 63(6):1424–1433.
4. Tedder TF, Boyd AW, Freedman AS, et al. The B cell surface molecule B1 is functionally linked with B cell activation and differentiation. J. Immunol. 1985 135(2): 973–979.
5. Tedder TF, Zhou LJ, Bell PD, et al. The CD20 surface molecule of B lymphocytes functions as a calcium channel. J. Cell. Biochem. 1990 14D:195.
6. Press OW, Applebaum F, Ledbetter JA, Martin PJ, Zarling J, Kidd P, et al. Monoclonal antibody 1F5 (anti-CD20) serotherapy of human B-cell lymphomas. Blood 1987 69(2):584–591.
7. Reff ME, Carner C, Chambers KS, Chinn PC, Leonard JE, Raab R, et al. Depletion of B cells in vivo by a chimeric mouse human monoclonal antibody to CD20. Blood 1994 83(2):435–445.
8. Demidem A, Lam T, Alas S, Hariharan K, Hanna N, and Bonavida B. Chimeric anti-CD20 (IDEC-C2B8) monoclonal antibody sensitizes a B cell lymphoma cell line to cell killing by cytotoxic drugs. Cancer Chemotherapy & Radiopharmaceuticals 1997 12(3):177–186.
9. Maloney DG, Liles TM, Czerwinski C, Waldichuk J, Rosenberg J, Grillo-López A, et al. Phase I clinical trial using escalating single-dose infusion of chimeric anti-CD20 monoclonal antibody (IDEC-C2B8) in patients with recurrent B-cell lymphoma. Blood 1994 84(8):2457–2466.
10. Maloney DG, Grillo-López AJ, Bodkin D, White CA, Liles T-M, Royston I, et al. IDEC-C2B8: Results of a phase I multiple-dose trial in patients with relapsed non-Hodgkin's lymphoma. J. Clin. Oncol. 1997 15(10): 3266–3274.
11. Maloney DG, Grillo-López AJ, White CA, Bodkin D, Schilder RJ, Neidhart JA, et al. IDEC-C2B8 (Rituximab) anti-CD20 monoclonal antibody therapy in patients with relapsed low-grade non-Hodgkin's lymphoma. Blood 1997 90(6):2188–2195.

Jointly Marketed by:
IDEC Pharmaceuticals Corporation
11011 Torreyana Road
San Diego, CA 92121

Genentech, Inc.
1 DNA Way
South San Francisco, CA 94080-4990
© 1998 IDEC Pharmaceuticals Corporation and Genentech, Inc.   4809702
Revised July, 1998
Shown in Product Identification Guide, page 317

Immunex Corporation
51 UNIVERSITY STREET
SEATTLE, WA 98101

For Medical Information Contact:
Generally:
Professional Services
(800) 466-8639
FAX: (800) 221-6820
FAX: (206) 223-5525
In Emergencies:
Professional Services
(800) 466-8639
FAX: (800) 221-6820
FAX: (206) 223-5525

AMICAR®   ℞
(Aminocaproic Acid)
Syrup, Tablets and Injection

DESCRIPTION

AMICAR (aminocaproic acid) is 6-aminohexanoic acid, which acts as an inhibitor of fibrinolysis. Its chemical structure is:

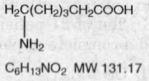

$$H_2C(CH_2)_3CH_2COOH$$
$$|$$
$$NH_2$$
$$C_6H_{13}NO_2 \quad MW \ 131.17$$

AMICAR is soluble in water, acid and alkaline solutions; it is sparingly soluble in methanol and practically insoluble in chloroform.

AMICAR (aminocaproic acid) Injection, for intravenous administration, is a sterile pyrogen-free solution containing 250 mg/mL of aminocaproic acid with benzyl alcohol 0.9% as preservative and Water for Injection. Hydrochloric acid may be added to adjust pH to approximately 6.8 during manufacture.

AMICAR (aminocaproic acid) Syrup, 25%, for oral administration, contains 250 mg/mL of aminocaproic acid with potassium sorbate 0.2% and sodium benzoate 0.1% as preservatives and the following inactive ingredients: citric acid, flavorings, sodium saccharin, and sorbitol solution.

Each AMICAR (aminocaproic acid) Tablet, for oral administration, contains 500 mg of aminocaproic acid and the following inactive ingredients: magnesium stearate, stearic acid and povidone.

CLINICAL PHARMACOLOGY

The fibrinolysis-inhibitory effects of AMICAR appear to be exerted principally via inhibition of plasminogen activators and to a lesser degree through antiplasmin activity.

In adults, oral absorption appears to be a zero-order process with an absorption rate of 5.2 g/hr. The mean lag time in absorption is 10 minutes. After a single oral dose of 5 g, absorption was complete (F=1). Mean ± SD peak plasma concentrations (164 ± 28 mcg/mL) were reached within 1.2 ± 0.45 hours.

After oral administration, the apparent volume of distribution was estimated to be 23.1 ± 6.6 L (mean ± SD). Correspondingly, the volume of distribution after intravenous administration has been reported to be 30.0 ± 8.2 L. After prolonged administration, AMICAR has been found to distribute throughout extravascular and intravascular compartments of the body, penetrating human red blood cells as well as other tissue cells.

Renal excretion is the primary route of elimination, whether AMICAR is administered orally or intravenously. Sixty-five percent of the dose is recovered in the urine as unchanged drug and 11% of the dose appears as the metabolite adipic acid. Renal clearance (116 mL/min) approximates endogenous creatinine clearance. The total body clearance is 169 mL/min. The terminal elimination half-life for AMICAR is approximately 2 hours.

INDICATIONS AND USAGE

AMICAR is useful in enhancing hemostasis when fibrinolysis contributes to bleeding. In life-threatening situations, fresh whole blood transfusions, fibrinogen infusions, and other emergency measures may be required.

Fibrinolytic bleeding may frequently be associated with surgical complications following heart surgery (with or without cardiac bypass procedures) and portacaval shunt; hematological disorders such as aplastic anemia; abruptio placentae; hepatic cirrhosis; neoplastic disease such as carcinoma of the prostate, lung, stomach, and cervix.

Urinary fibrinolysis, usually a normal physiological phenomenon, may frequently be associated with life-threatening complications following severe trauma, anoxia, and shock. Symptomatic of such complications is surgical hematuria (following prostatectomy and nephrectomy) or nonsurgical hematuria (accompanying polycystic or neoplastic diseases of the genitourinary system). (See **WARNINGS**.)

CONTRAINDICATIONS

AMICAR should not be used when there is evidence of an active intravascular clotting process.

When there is uncertainty as to whether the cause of bleeding is primary fibrinolysis or disseminated intravascular coagulation (DIC), this distinction must be made before administering AMICAR.

The following tests can be applied to differentiate the two conditions:

- Platelet count is usually decreased in DIC but normal in primary fibrinolysis.
- Protamine paracoagulation test is positive in DIC; a precipitate forms when protamine sulfate is dropped into citrated plasma. The test is negative in the presence of primary fibrinolysis.
- The euglobulin clot lysis test is abnormal in primary fibrinolysis but normal in DIC.

AMICAR must not be used in the presence of DIC without concomitant heparin.

WARNINGS

In patients with upper urinary tract bleeding, AMICAR administration has been known to cause intrarenal obstruction in the form of glomerular capillary thrombosis or clots in the renal pelvis and ureters. For this reason, AMICAR should not be used in hematuria of upper urinary tract origin, unless the possible benefits outweigh the risk.

Subendocardial hemorrhages have been observed in dogs given intravenous infusions of 0.2 times the maximum human therapeutic dose of AMICAR and in monkeys given 8 times the maximum human therapeutic dose of AMICAR.

Fatty degeneration of the myocardium has been reported in dogs given intravenous doses of AMICAR at 0.8 to 3.3 times the maximum human therapeutic dose and in monkeys given intravenous doses of AMICAR at 6 times the maximum human therapeutic dose.

Rarely, skeletal muscle weakness with necrosis of muscle fibers has been reported following prolonged administration. Clinical presentation may range from mild myalgias with weakness and fatigue to a severe proximal myopathy with rhabdomyolysis, myoglobinuria, and acute renal failure. Muscle enzymes, especially creatine phosphokinase (CPK) are elevated. CPK levels should be monitored in patients on long-term therapy. AMICAR administration should be stopped if a rise in CPK is noted. Resolution follows discontinuation of AMICAR; however, the syndrome may recur if AMICAR is restarted.

The possibility of cardiac muscle damage should also be considered when skeletal myopathy occurs. One case of cardiac and hepatic lesions observed in man has been reported. The patient received 2 g of aminocaproic acid every 6 hours for a total dose of 26 g. Death was due to continued cerebrovascular hemorrhage. Necrotic changes in the heart and liver were noted at autopsy.

PRECAUTIONS
General

AMICAR Injection contains benzyl alcohol as a preservative and is not recommended for use in newborns.

AMICAR inhibits both the action of plasminogen activators and to a lesser degree, plasmin activity. The drug should NOT be administered without a definite diagnosis and/or laboratory finding indicative of hyperfibrinolysis (hyperplasminemia).[1]

Rapid intravenous administration of the drug should be avoided since this may induce hypotension, bradycardia, and/or arrhythmia.

Inhibition of fibrinolysis by aminocaproic acid may theoretically result in clotting or thrombosis. However, there is no definite evidence that administration of aminocaproic acid has been responsible for the few reported cases of intravascular clotting which followed this treatment. Rather, it appears that such intravascular clotting was most likely due to the patient's preexisting clinical condition, e.g., the presence of DIC. It has been postulated that extravascular clots formed *in vivo* may not undergo spontaneous lysis as do normal clots.

Reports have appeared in the literature of an increased incidence of certain neurological deficits such as hydrocephalus, cerebral ischemia, or cerebral vasospasm associated with the use of antifibrinolytic agents in the treatment of subarachnoid hemorrhage (SAH). All of these events have also been described as part of the natural course of SAH, or as a consequence of diagnostic procedures such as angiography. Drug relatedness remains unclear.

Thrombophlebitis, a possibility with all intravenous therapy, should be guarded against by strict attention to the proper insertion of the needle and the fixing of its position. Thrombosis with severe sequelae (acute myocardial infarction, gangrene) has been rarely reported in patients with hemophilia receiving combined treatment with Factor IX concentrate and AMICAR. AMICAR should not be administered concomitantly with prothrombin complex concentrates or with activated prothrombin concentrates unless the increased risk of thrombosis is outweighed by the anticipated clinical benefit.

Laboratory Tests

The use of AMICAR should be accompanied by tests designed to determine the amount of fibrinolysis present. There are presently available: (a) general tests such as those for the determination of the lysis of a clot of blood or plasma; and (b) more specific tests for the study of various phases of fibrinolytic mechanisms. These latter tests include both semiquantitative and quantitative techniques for the determination of profibrinolysin, fibrinolysin, and antifibrinolysin.

Drug Laboratory Test Interactions

Prolongation of the template bleeding time has been reported during continuous intravenous infusion of AMICAR at dosages exceeding 24 g/day. Platelet function studies in these patients have not demonstrated any significant platelet dysfunction. However, *in vitro* studies have shown that at high concentrations (7.4 mMol/L or 0.97 mg/mL and greater) EACA inhibits ADP and collagen-induced platelet aggregation, the release of ATP and serotonin, and the binding of fibrinogen to the platelets in a concentration-response manner. Following a 10 g bolus of AMICAR, transient peak plasma concentrations of 4.6 mMol/L or 0.60 mg/mL have been obtained. The concentration of AMICAR necessary to maintain inhibition of fibrinolysis is 0.99 mMol/L or 0.13 mg/mL. Administration of a 5 g bolus followed by 1 to 1.25 g/hr should achieve and sustain plasma levels of 0.13 mg/mL. Thus, concentrations which have been obtained *in vivo* clinically in patients with normal renal function are considerably lower than the *in vitro* concentrations found to induce abnormalities in platelet function tests. However, higher plasma concentrations of AMICAR may occur in patients with severe renal failure.

Carcinogenesis, Mutagenesis, Impairment of Fertility

Long-term studies in animals to evaluate the carcinogenic potential of AMICAR and studies to evaluate its mutagenic potential have not been conducted. Dietary administration of an equivalent of the maximum human therapeutic dose of AMICAR to rats of both sexes impaired fertility as evidenced by decreased implantations, litter sizes and number of pups born.

Pregnancy

Pregnancy Category C. Animal teratological studies have not been conducted with AMICAR. It is also not known whether AMICAR can cause fetal harm when administered to a pregnant woman or can affect reproduction capacity. AMICAR should be given to a pregnant woman only if clearly needed.

Nursing Mothers

It is not known whether this drug is excreted in human milk. Because many drugs are excreted in human milk, caution should be exercised when AMICAR is administered to a nursing woman.

Pediatric Use

Safety and effectiveness in pediatric patients have not been established.

ADVERSE REACTIONS

AMICAR is generally well tolerated. The following adverse experiences have been reported:

General: Edema, fever, headache, hemorrhage, malaise.
Hypersensitivity Reactions: Allergic and anaphylactoid reactions, anaphylaxis.
Local Reactions: Injection site reactions, pain and necrosis.
Cardiovascular: Bradycardia, hypotension, ischemia, thrombosis.
Gastrointestinal: Abdominal pain, diarrhea, nausea, vomiting.
Hematologic: Agranulocytosis, coagulation disorder, leukopenia, thrombocytopenia.
Musculoskeletal: CPK increased, muscle weakness, myalgia, myopathy (see **WARNINGS**), myositis, rhabdomyolysis.
Neurologic: Confusion, convulsions, delirium, dizziness, hallucinations, intracranial hypertension, stroke, syncope.
Respiratory: Dyspnea, nasal congestion, pulmonary embolism.
Skin: Pruritus, rash.

Special Senses: Deafness, glaucoma, tinnitus, vision decreased, watery eyes.
Urogenital: BUN increased, ejaculatory disorder, renal failure.

OVERDOSAGE

A few cases of acute overdosage with AMICAR administered intravenously have been reported. The effects have ranged from no reaction to transient hypotension to severe acute renal failure leading to death. One patient with a history of brain tumor and seizures experienced seizures after receiving an 8 gram bolus injection of AMICAR. The single dose of AMICAR causing symptoms of overdosage or considered to be life-threatening is unknown. Patients have tolerated doses as high as 100 grams while acute renal failure has been reported following a dose of 12 grams.

The intravenous and oral LD_{50} of AMICAR were 3.0 and 12.0 g/kg, respectively, in the mouse and 3.2 and 16.4 g/kg, respectively, in the rat. An intravenous infusion dose of 2.3 g/kg was lethal in the dog. On intravenous administration, tonic-clonic convulsions were observed in dogs and mice.

No treatment for overdosage is known, although evidence exists that AMICAR is removed by hemodialysis and may be removed by peritoneal dialysis. Pharmacokinetic studies have shown that total body clearance of AMICAR is markedly decreased in patients with severe renal failure.

DOSAGE AND ADMINISTRATION
Intravenous

AMICAR (aminocaproic acid) Injection is administered by infusion, utilizing the usual compatible intravenous vehicles (e.g., Sterile Water for Injection, Sodium Chloride for Injection, 5% Dextrose or Ringer's Injection). Although Sterile Water for Injection is compatible for intravenous injection the resultant solution is hypo-osmolar. RAPID INJECTION OF AMICAR INJECTION UNDILUTED INTO A VEIN IS NOT RECOMMENDED.

For the treatment of acute bleeding syndromes due to elevated fibrinolytic activity, it is suggested that 16 to 20 mL (4 to 5 g) of AMICAR Injection in 250 mL of diluent be administered by infusion during the first hour of treatment, followed by a continuing infusion at the rate of 4 mL (1 g) per hour in 50 mL of diluent. This method of treatment would ordinarily be continued for about 8 hours or until the bleeding situation has been controlled.

Parenteral drug products should be inspected visually for particulate matter and discoloration prior to administration, whenever solution and container permit.

Oral Therapy

If the patient is able to take medication by mouth, an identical dosage regimen may be followed by administering AMICAR Tablets or AMICAR Syrup, 25% as follows: For the treatment of acute bleeding syndromes due to elevated fibrinolytic activity, it is suggested that 10 tablets (5 g) or 4 teaspoonfuls of syrup (5 g) of AMICAR be administered during the first hour of treatment, followed by a continuing rate of 2 tablets (1 g) or 1 teaspoonful of syrup (1.25 g) per hour. This method of treatment would ordinarily be continued for about 8 hours or until the bleeding situation has been controlled.

HOW SUPPLIED

AMICAR® (aminocaproic acid) Injection, supplied as follows:

Each 20 mL vial contains 5 g of aminocaproic acid (250 mg/mL) as an aqueous solution with benzyl alcohol 0.9% as preservative.

20 mL vial - NDC 58406-610-12

Each 96 mL single-use infusion vial contains 24 g of aminocaproic acid (250 mg/mL) as an aqueous solution with benzyl alcohol 0.9% as preservative.

96 mL vial - NDC 58406-610-13

STORE BETWEEN 15°–30°C (59°–86°F).
DO NOT FREEZE.
Manufactured for IMMUNEX CORPORATION, Seattle, WA 98101
by LEDERLE PARENTERALS, INC., Carolina, Puerto Rico 00987

AMICAR® (aminocaproic acid) Syrup, 25%, supplied as follows:

Each mL of raspberry-flavored syrup contains 250 mg of aminocaproic acid.

16 Fl. Oz. (473 mL) Bottle - NDC 58406-611-90

STORE BETWEEN 15°–30°C (59°–86°F).
Dispense in tight containers.
DO NOT FREEZE.

AMICAR® (aminocaproic acid) Tablets, supplied as follows:
Each round, white tablet, engraved with LL on one side and scored on the other with A to the left of the score and 10 on the right, contains 500 mg of aminocaproic acid.

Bottle of 100 - NDC 58406-612-61

STORE BETWEEN 15°–30°C (59°–86°F).
Dispense in tight containers.

Continued on next page

Amicar—Cont.

Manufactured for
IMMUNEX CORPORATION
Seattle, WA 98101
by
LEDERLE LABORATORIES DIVISION
American Cyanamid Company
Pearl River, NY 10965

REFERENCES

1. Stefanini M, Dameshek W: The Hemorrhagic Disorders, Ed. 2, New York, Grune and Stratton. 1962; pp. 510-514.

Rev 0162-02
CI 4545-1
Issued 5/96
©1996 Immunex Corporation

AMICAR® ℞
(Aminocaproic Acid)
Syrup, Tablets and Injection

DESCRIPTION

AMICAR (aminocaproic acid) is 6-aminohexanoic acid, which acts as an inhibitor of fibrinolysis.
Its chemical structure is:

$$H_2C(CH_2)_3CH_2COOH$$
$$|$$
$$NH_2$$

$C_6H_{13}NO_2$ MW 131.17

AMICAR is soluble in water, acid and alkaline solutions; it is sparingly soluble in methanol and practically insoluble in chloroform.

AMICAR (aminocaproic acid) Injection, for intravenous administration, is a sterile pyrogen-free solution containing 250 mg/mL of aminocaproic acid with benzyl alcohol 0.9% as preservative and Water for Injection. Hydrochloric acid may be added to adjust pH to approximately 6.8 during manufacture.

AMICAR (aminocaproic acid) Syrup, 25%, for oral administration, contains 250 mg/mL of aminocaproic acid with potassium sorbate 0.2% and sodium benzoate 0.1% as preservatives and the following inactive ingredients: citric acid, flavorings, sodium saccharin, and sorbitol solution.

Each AMICAR (aminocaproic acid) Tablet, for oral administration, contains 500 mg of aminocaproic acid and the following inactive ingredients: magnesium stearate, stearic acid and povidone.

CLINICAL PHARMACOLOGY

The fibrinolysis-inhibitory effects of AMICAR appear to be exerted principally via inhibition of plasminogen activators and to a lesser degree through antiplasmin activity.

In adults, oral absorption appears to be a zero-order process with an absorption rate of 5.2 g/hr. The mean lag time in absorption is 10 minutes. After a single oral dose of 5 g, absorption was complete (F=1). Mean ± SD peak plasma concentrations (164 ± 28 mcg/mL) were reached within 1.2 ± 0.45 hours.

After oral administration, the apparent volume of distribution was estimated to be 23.1 ± 6.6 L (mean ± SD). Correspondingly, the volume of distribution after intravenous administration has been reported to be 30.0 ± 8.2 L. After prolonged administration, AMICAR has been found to distribute throughout extravascular and intravascular compartments of the body, penetrating human red blood cells as well as other tissue cells.

Renal excretion is the primary route of elimination, whether AMICAR is administered orally or intravenously. Sixty-five percent of the dose is recovered in the urine as unchanged drug and 11% of the dose appears as the metabolite adipic acid. Renal clearance (116 mL/min) approximates endogenous creatinine clearance. The total body clearance is 169 mL/min. The terminal elimination half-life for AMICAR is approximately 2 hours.

INDICATIONS AND USAGE

AMICAR is useful in enhancing hemostasis when fibrinolysis contributes to bleeding. In life-threatening situations, fresh whole blood transfusions, fibrinogen infusions, and other emergency measures may be required.

Fibrinolytic bleeding may frequently be associated with surgical complications following heart surgery (with or without cardiac bypass procedures) and portacaval shunt; hematological disorders such as aplastic anemia; abruptio placentae; hepatic cirrhosis; neoplastic disease such as carcinoma of the prostate, lung, stomach, and cervix.

Urinary fibrinolysis, usually a normal physiological phenomenon, may frequently be associated with life-threatening complications following severe trauma, anoxia, and shock. Symptomatic of such complications is surgical hematuria (following prostatectomy and nephrectomy) or nonsurgical hematuria (accompanying polycystic or neoplastic diseases of the genitourinary system). (See **Warnings**.)

CONTRAINDICATIONS

AMICAR should not be used when there is evidence of an active intravascular clotting process.

When there is uncertainty as to whether the cause of bleeding is primary fibrinolysis or disseminated intravascular coagulation (DIC), this distinction must be made before administering AMICAR.

The following tests can be applied to differentiate the two conditions:

- Platelet count is usually decreased in DIC but normal in primary fibrinolysis.
- Protamine paracoagulation test is positive in DIC; a precipitate forms when protamine sulfate is dropped into citrated plasma. The test is negative in the presence of primary fibrinolysis.
- The euglobulin clot lysis test is abnormal in primary fibrinolysis but normal in DIC.

AMICAR must not be used in the presence of DIC without concomitant heparin.

WARNINGS

In patients with upper urinary tract bleeding, AMICAR administration has been known to cause intrarenal obstruction in the form of glomerular capillary thrombosis or clots in the renal pelvis and ureters. For this reason, AMICAR should not be used in hematuria of upper urinary tract origin, unless the possible benefits outweigh the risk.

Subendocardial hemorrhages have been observed in dogs given intravenous infusions of 0.2 times the maximum human therapeutic dose of AMICAR and in monkeys given 8 times the maximum human therapeutic dose of AMICAR. Fatty degeneration of the myocardium has been reported in dogs given intravenous doses of AMICAR at 0.8 to 3.3 times the maximum human therapeutic dose and in monkeys given intravenous doses of AMICAR at 6 times the maximum human therapeutic dose.

Rarely, skeletal muscle weakness with necrosis of muscle fibers has been reported following prolonged administration. Clinical presentation may range from mild myalgias with weakness and fatigue to a severe proximal myopathy with rhabdomyolysis, myoglobinuria, and acute renal failure. Muscle enzymes, especially creatine phosphokinase (CPK) are elevated. CPK levels should be monitored in patients on long-term therapy. AMICAR administration should be stopped if a rise in CPK is noted. Resolution follows discontinuation of AMICAR; however, the syndrome may recur if AMICAR is restarted.

The possibility of cardiac muscle damage should also be considered when skeletal myopathy occurs. One case of cardiac and hepatic lesions observed in man has been reported. The patient received 2 g of aminocaproic acid every 6 hours for a total dose of 26 g. Death was due to continued cerebrovascular hemorrhage. Necrotic changes in the heart and liver were noted at autopsy.

PRECAUTIONS

GENERAL

AMICAR Injection contains benzyl alcohol as a preservative and is not recommended for use in newborns.

AMICAR inhibits both the action of plasminogen activators and to a lesser degree, plasmin activity. The drug should NOT be administered without a definite diagnosis and/or laboratory finding indicative of hyperfibrinolysis (hyperplasminemia).[1]

Rapid intravenous administration of the drug should be avoided since this may induce hypotension, bradycardia, and/or arrhythmia.

Inhibition of fibrinolysis by aminocaproic acid may theoretically result in clotting or thrombosis. However, there is no definite evidence that administration of aminocaproic acid has been responsible for the few reported cases of intravascular clotting which followed this treatment. Rather, it appears that such intravascular clotting was most likely due to the patient's preexisting clinical condition, e.g., the presence of DIC. It has been postulated that extravascular clots formed in vivo may not undergo spontaneous lysis as do normal clots.

Reports have appeared in the literature of an increased incidence of certain neurological deficits such as hydrocephalus, cerebral ischemia, or cerebral vasospasm associated with the use of antifibrinolytic agents in the treatment of subarachnoid hemorrhage (SAH). All of these events have also been described as part of the natural course of SAH, or as a consequence of diagnostic procedures such as angiography. Drug relatedness remains unclear.

Thrombophlebitis, a possibility with all intravenous therapy, should be guarded against by strict attention to the proper insertion of the needle and the fixing of its position. Thrombosis with severe sequelae (acute myocardial infarction, gangrene) has been rarely reported in patients with hemophilia receiving combined treatment with Factor IX concentrate and AMICAR. AMICAR should not be administered concomitantly with prothrombin complex concentrates or with activated prothrombin concentrates unless the increased risk of thrombosis is outweighed by the anticipated clinical benefit.

LABORATORY TESTS

The use of AMICAR should be accompanied by tests designed to determine the amount of fibrinolysis present. There are presently available: (a) general tests such as those for the determination of the lysis of a clot of blood or plasma; and (b) more specific tests for the study of various phases of fibrinolytic mechanisms. These latter tests include both semiquantitative and quantitative techniques for the determination of profibrinolysin, fibrinolysin, and antifibrinolysin.

DRUG LABORATORY TEST INTERACTIONS

Prolongation of the template bleeding time has been reported during continuous intravenous infusion of AMICAR at dosages exceeding 24 g/day. Platelet function studies in these patients have not demonstrated any significant platelet dysfunction. However, in vitro studies have shown that at high concentrations (7.4 mMol/L or 0.97 mg/mL and greater) EACA inhibits ADP and collagen-induced platelet aggregation, the release of ATP and serotonin, and the binding of fibrinogen to the platelets in a concentration-response manner. Following a 10 g bolus of AMICAR, transient peak plasma concentrations of 4.6 mMol/L or 0.60 mg/mL have been obtained. The concentration of AMICAR necessary to maintain inhibition of fibrinolysis is 0.99 mMol/L or 0.13 mg/mL. Administration of a 5 g bolus followed by 1 to 1.25 g/hr should achieve and sustain plasma levels of 0.13 mg/mL. Thus, concentrations which have been obtained in vivo clinically in patients with normal renal function are considerably lower than the in vitro concentrations found to induce abnormalities in platelet function tests. However, higher plasma concentrations of AMICAR may occur in patients with severe renal failure.

CARCINOGENESIS, MUTAGENESIS, IMPAIRMENT OF FERTILITY

Long-term studies in animals to evaluate the carcinogenic potential of AMICAR and studies to evaluate its mutagenic potential have not been conducted. Dietary administration of an equivalent of the maximum human therapeutic dose of AMICAR to rats of both sexes impaired fertility as evidenced by decreased implantations, litter sizes and number of pups born.

PREGNANCY

Pregnancy Category C. Animal teratological studies have not been conducted with AMICAR. It is also not known whether AMICAR can cause fetal harm when administered to a pregnant woman or can affect reproduction capacity. AMICAR should be given to a pregnant woman only if clearly needed.

NURSING MOTHERS

It is not known whether this drug is excreted in human milk. Because many drugs are excreted in human milk, caution should be exercised when AMICAR is administered to a nursing woman.

PEDIATRIC USE

Safety and effectiveness in pediatric patients have not been established.

ADVERSE REACTIONS

AMICAR is generally well tolerated. The following adverse experiences have been reported:

General: Edema, fever, headache, hemorrhage, malaise.

Hypersensitivity Reactions: Allergic and anaphylactoid reactions, anaphylaxis.

Local Reactions: Injection site reactions, pain and necrosis.

Cardiovascular: Bradycardia, hypotension, ischemia, thrombosis.

Gastrointestinal: Abdominal pain, diarrhea, nausea, vomiting.

Hematologic: Agranulocytosis, coagulation disorder, leukopenia, thrombocytopenia.

Musculoskeletal: CPK increased, muscle weakness, myalgia, myopathy (see **Warnings**), myositis, rhabdomyolysis.

Neurologic: Confusion, convulsions, delirium, dizziness, hallucinations, intracranial hypertension, stroke, syncope.

Respiratory: Dyspnea, nasal congestion, pulmonary embolism.

Skin: Pruritus, rash.

Special Senses: Deafness, glaucoma, tinnitus, vision decreased, watery eyes.

Urogenital: BUN increased, ejaculatory disorder, renal failure.

OVERDOSAGE

A few cases of acute overdosage with AMICAR administered intravenously have been reported. The effects have ranged from no reaction to transient hypotension to severe acute renal failure leading to death. One patient with a history of brain tumor and seizures experienced seizures after receiving an 8 gram bolus injection of AMICAR. The single dose of AMICAR causing symptoms of overdose or considered to be life-threatening is unknown. Patients have tolerated doses as high as 100 grams while acute renal failure has been reported following a dose of 12 grams.

The intravenous and oral LD$_{50}$ of AMICAR were 3.0 and 12.0 g/kg, respectively, in the mouse and 3.2 and 16.4 g/kg, respectively, in the rat. An intravenous infusion dose of 2.3 g/kg was lethal in the dog. On intravenous administration, tonic-clonic convulsions were observed in dogs and mice. No treatment for overdosage is known, although evidence exists that AMICAR is removed by hemodialysis and may be

removed by peritoneal dialysis. Pharmacokinetic studies have shown that total body clearance of AMICAR is markedly decreased in patients with severe renal failure.

DOSAGE AND ADMINISTRATION

INTRAVENOUS

AMICAR (aminocaproic acid) Injection is administered by infusion, utilizing the usual compatible intravenous vehicles (e.g., Sterile Water for Injection, Sodium Chloride for Injection, 5% Dextrose or Ringer's Injection). Although Sterile Water for Injection is compatible for intravenous injection the resultant solution is hypo-osmolar. RAPID INJECTION OF AMICAR INJECTION UNDILUTED INTO A VEIN IS NOT RECOMMENDED.

For the treatment of acute bleeding syndromes due to elevated fibrinolytic activity, it is suggested that 16 to 20 mL (4 to 5 g) of AMICAR Injection in 250 mL of diluent be administered by infusion during the first hour of treatment, followed by a continuing infusion at the rate of 4 mL (1 g) per hour in 50 mL of diluent. This method of treatment would ordinarily be continued for about 8 hours or until the bleeding situation has been controlled.

Parenteral drug products should be inspected visually for particulate matter and discoloration prior to administration, whenever solution and container permit.

ORAL THERAPY

If the patient is able to take medication by mouth, an identical dosage regimen may be followed by administering AMICAR Tablets or AMICAR Syrup, 25% as follows: For the treatment of acute bleeding syndromes due to elevated fibrinolytic activity, it is suggested that 10 tablets (5 g) or 4 teaspoonfuls of syrup (5 g) of AMICAR be administered during the first hour of treatment, followed by a continuing rate of 2 tablets (1 g) or 1 teaspoonful of syrup (1.25 g) per hour. This method of treatment would ordinarily be continued for about 8 hours or until the bleeding situation has been controlled.

HOW SUPPLIED

AMICAR® (aminocaproic acid) Injection, supplied as follows:

Each 20 mL vial contains 5 g of aminocaproic acid (250 mg/mL) as an aqueous solution with benzyl alcohol 0.9% as preservative.

20 mL vial - NDC 58406-610-12

Each 96 mL single-use infusion vial contains 24 g of aminocaproic acid (250 mg/mL) as an aqueous solution with benzyl alcohol 0.9% as preservative.

96 mL vial - NDC 58406-610-13

STORE BETWEEN 15°-30°C (59°-86°F).

DO NOT FREEZE.

Manufactured for IMMUNEX CORPORATION, Seattle, WA 98101

by LEDERLE PARENTERALS, INC., Carolina, Puerto Rico 00987

AMICAR® (aminocaproic acid) Syrup, 25%, supplied as follows:

Each mL of raspberry-flavored syrup contains 250 mg of aminocaproic acid.

16 Fl. Oz. (473 mL) Bottle - NDC 58406-611-90

STORE BETWEEN 15°-30°C (59°-86°F).

Dispense in tight containers.

DO NOT FREEZE.

AMICAR® (aminocaproic acid) Tablets, supplied as follows: Each round, white tablet, engraved with LL on one side and scored on the other with A to the left of the score and 10 on the right, contains 500 mg of aminocaproic acid.

Bottle of 100 - NDC 58406-612-61

STORE BETWEEN 15°-30°C (59°-86°F).

Dispense in tight containers.

Manufactured for

IMMUNEX CORPORATION

Seattle, WA 98101

by LEDERLE LABORATORIES DIVISION

American Cyanamid Company, Pearl River, NY 10965

REFERENCES

1. Stefanini M, Dameshek W: The Hemorrhagic Disorders, Ed. 2, New York, Grune and Stratton. 1962; pp. 510-514.

REV 0197-02

CI 4565-2 Revised June 12, 1996 Printed in USA

LEUCOVORIN CALCIUM FOR INJECTION ℞

DESCRIPTION

Leucovorin is one of several active, chemically reduced derivatives of folic acid. It is useful as an antidote to drugs which act as folic acid antagonists.

Also known as folinic acid, Citrovorum factor, or 5-formyl-5,6,7,8 tetrahydrofolic acid, this compound has the chemical designation of L-Glutamic acid, N-[4-[[(2-amino-5-formyl-1,4,5,6,7,8-hexahydro-4-oxo-6 pteridinyl)methyl]amino]benzoyl]-,calcium salt (1:1). The formula weight is 511.51 and the structural formula of leucovorin calcium is:

[See chemical structure at top of next column]

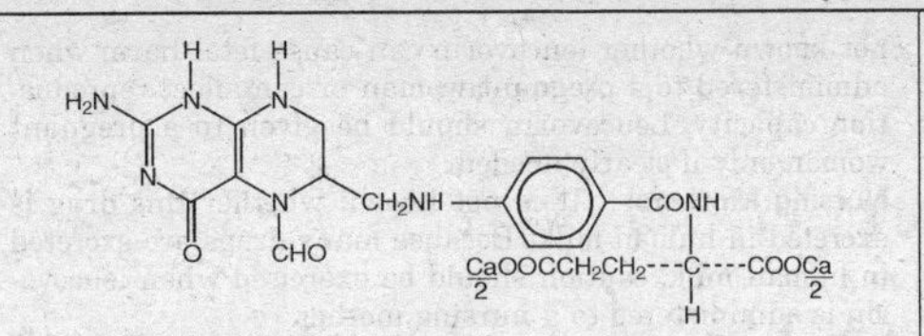

Leucovorin Calcium for Injection

Leucovorin Calcium for Injection is indicated for intravenous or intramuscular administration and is supplied as a sterile lyophilized powder. The 350 mg vial is preservative free. The inactive ingredient is sodium chloride 140 mg/vial for the 350 mg vial. Sodium hydroxide and/or hydrochloric acid are used to adjust the pH to approximately 8.1 during manufacture. One milligram of leucovorin calcium contains 0.002 mmol of leucovorin and 0.002 mmol of calcium.

CLINICAL PHARMACOLOGY

Leucovorin is a mixture of the diastereoisomers of the 5-formyl derivative of tetrahydrofolic acid (THF). The biologically active compound of the mixture is the (-)-*l*-isomer, known as Citrovorum factor or (-) folinic acid. Leucovorin does not require reduction by the enzyme dihydrofolate reductase in order to participate in reactions utilizing folates as a source of "one-carbon" moieties. *l*-Leucovorin (*l*-5 formyltetrahydrofolate) is rapidly metabolized (via 5,10 methenyltetrahydrofolate then 5,10-methylenetetrahydrofolate) to *l*-5 methyltetrahydrofolate. *l*-5-Methyltetrahydrofolate can in turn be metabolized via other pathways back to 5,10-methylenetetrahydrofolate, which is converted to 5-methyltetrahydrofolate by an irreversible, enzyme catalyzed reduction using the cofactors FADH2 and NADPH.

Administration of leucovorin can counteract the therapeutic and toxic effects of folic acid antagonists such as methotrexate, which act by inhibiting dihydrofolate reductase.

In contrast, leucovorin can enhance the therapeutic and toxic effects of fluoropyrimidines used in cancer therapy, such as 5-fluorouracil. Concurrent administration of leucovorin does not appear to alter the plasma pharmacokinetics of 5-fluorouracil. 5-Fluorouracil is metabolized to fluorodeoxyuridylic acid, which binds to and inhibits the enzyme thymidylate synthase (an enzyme important in DNA repair and replication).

Leucovorin is readily converted to another reduced folate, 5,10 methylenetetrahydrofolate, which acts to stabilize the binding of fluorodeoxyuridylic acid to thymidylate synthase and thereby enhances the inhibition of this enzyme.

The pharmacokinetics after intravenous, intramuscular, and oral administration of a 25 mg dose of leucovorin were studied in male volunteers. After intravenous administration, serum total reduced folates (as measured by *Lactobacillus casei* assay) reached a mean peak of 1259 ng/mL (range 897-1625). The mean time to peak was 10 minutes. This initial rise in total reduced folates was primarily due to the parent compound 5-formyl-THF (measured by *Streptococcus faecalis* assay) which rose to 1206 ng/mL at 10 minutes. A sharp drop in parent compound followed and coincided with the appearance of the active metabolite 5 methyl-THF which became the predominant circulating form of the drug.

The mean peak of 5-methyl-THF was 258 ng/mL and occurred at 1.3 hours. The terminal half-life for total reduced folates was 6.2 hours. The area under the concentration versus time curves (AUCs) for *l*-leucovorin, *d*-leucovorin and 5-methyltetrahydrofolate were 28.4 ± 3.5, 956 ± 97 and 129 ± 12 (mg.min/L ± S.E.). When a higher dose of *d,l*-leucovorin (200 mg/m^2) was used, similar results were obtained. The *d*-isomer persisted in plasma at concentrations greatly exceeding those of the *l*-isomer.

After intramuscular injection, the mean peak of serum total reduced folates was 436 ng/mL (range 240-725) and occurred at 52 minutes. Similar to IV administration, the initial sharp rise was due to the parent compound. The mean peak of 5-formyl-THF was 360 ng/mL and occurred at 28 minutes. The level of the metabolite 5-methyl-THF increased subsequently over time until at 1.5 hours it represented 50% of the circulating total folates. The mean peak of 5-methyl-THF was 226 ng/mL at 2.8 hours. The terminal half-life of total reduced folates was 6.2 hours. There was no difference of statistical significance between IM and IV administration in the AUC for total reduced folates, 5-formyl-THF, or 5 methyl-THF.

After oral administration of leucovorin reconstituted with aromatic elixir, the mean peak concentration of serum total reduced folates was 393 ng/mL (range 160-550). The mean time to peak was 2.3 hours and the terminal half-life was 5.7 hours. The major component was the metabolite 5-methyltetrahydrofolate to which leucovorin is primarily converted in the intestinal mucosa. The mean peak of 5-methyl-THF was 367 ng/mL at 2.4 hours. The peak level of the parent compound was 51 ng/mL at 1.2 hours. The AUC of total reduced folates after oral administration of the 25 mg dose was 92% of the AUC after intravenous administration.

Following oral administration, leucovorin is rapidly absorbed and expands the serum pool of reduced folates. At a dose of 25 mg, almost 100% of the *l*-isomer but only 20% of the *d*-isomer is absorbed. Oral absorption of leucovorin is saturable at doses above 25 mg. The apparent bioavailability of leucovorin was 97% for 25 mg, 75% for 50 mg, and 37% for 100 mg.

In a randomized clinical study conducted by the Mayo Clinic and the North Central Cancer Treatment Group (Mayo/NCCTG) in patients with advanced metastatic colorectal cancer three treatment regimens were compared: Leucovorin (LV) 200 mg/m^2 and 5-fluorouracil (5-FU) 370 mg/m2 versus LV 20 mg/m^2 and 5-FU 425 mg/m^2 versus 5-FU 500 mg/m^2. All drugs were administered by slow intravenous infusion daily for 5 days repeated every 28-35 days. Response rates were 26% (p = 0.04 versus 5-FU alone), 43% (p = 0.001 versus 5-FU alone) and 10% for the high dose leucovorin, low dose leucovorin and 5-FU alone groups respectively. Respective median survival times were 12.2 months (p = 0.037), 12 months (p = 0.050), and 7.7 months. The low dose LV regimen gave a statistically significant improvement in weight gain of more than 5%, relief of symptoms, and improvement in performance status. The high dose LV regimen gave a statistically significant improvement in performance status and trended toward improvement in weight gain and in relief of symptoms but these were not statistically significant.

In a second Mayo/NCCTG randomized clinical study the 5-FU alone arm was replaced by a regimen of sequentially administered methotrexate (MTX), 5-FU, and LV. Response rates with LV 200 mg/m^2 and 5-FU 370 mg/m2 versus LV 20 mg/m^2 and 5-FU 425 mg/m^2 versus sequential MTX and 5-FU and LV were respectively 31% (p = <.01), 42% (p = <.01), and 14%. Respective median survival times were 12.7 months (p = <.04), 12.7 months (p = <.01), and 8.4 months. No statistically significant difference in weight gain of more than 5% or in improvement in performance status was seen between the treatment arms.

INDICATIONS AND USAGE

Leucovorin calcium rescue is indicated after high-dose methotrexate therapy in osteosarcoma. Leucovorin calcium is also indicated to diminish the toxicity and counteract the effects of impaired methotrexate elimination and of inadvertent overdosages of folic acid antagonists.

Leucovorin calcium is indicated in the treatment of megaloblastic anemias due to folic acid deficiency when oral therapy is not feasible.

Leucovorin is also indicated for use in combination with 5-fluorouracil to prolong survival in the palliative treatment of patients with advanced colorectal cancer. Leucovorin should not be mixed in the same infusion as 5-fluorouracil because a precipitate may form.

CONTRAINDICATIONS

Leucovorin is improper therapy for pernicious anemia and other megaloblastic anemias secondary to the lack of vitamin B_{12}. A hematologic remission may occur while neurologic manifestations continue to progress.

WARNINGS

In the treatment of accidental overdosages of folic acid antagonists, intravenous leucovorin should be administered as promptly as possible. As the time interval between antifolate administration [eg, methotrexate (MTX)] and leucovorin rescue increases, leucovorin's effectiveness in counteracting toxicity decreases. In the treatment of accidental overdosages of intrathecally administered folic acid antagonists, do not administer leucovorin intrathecally. LEUCOVORIN MAY BE HARMFUL OR FATAL IF GIVEN INTRATHECALLY.

Monitoring of the serum MTX concentration is essential in determining the optimal dose and duration of treatment with leucovorin.

Delayed MTX excretion may be caused by a third space fluid accumulation (ie, ascites, pleural effusion), renal insufficiency, or inadequate hydration. Under such circumstances, higher doses of leucovorin or prolonged administration may be indicated. Doses higher than those recommended for oral use must be given intravenously.

Because of the benzyl alcohol contained in certain diluents used for Leucovorin Calcium for Injection, when doses greater than 10 mg/m2 are administered, Leucovorin Calcium for Injection should be reconstituted with Sterile Water for Injection, USP, and used immediately. (See DOSAGE AND ADMINISTRATION.)

Because of the calcium content of the leucovorin solution, no more than 160 mg of leucovorin should be injected intravenously per minute (16 mL of a 10 mg/mL, or 8 mL of a 20 mg/mL solution per minute).

Leucovorin enhances the toxicity of 5-fluorouracil. When these drugs are administered concurrently in the palliative therapy of advanced colorectal cancer, the dosage of 5-fluorouracil must be lower than usually administered. Although the toxicities observed in patients treated with the combination of leucovorin plus 5-fluorouracil are qualitatively similar to those observed in patients treated with 5-fluoro-

Continued on next page

Leucovorin Calcium for Inj.—Cont.

uracil alone, gastrointestinal toxicities (particularly stomatitis and diarrhea) are observed more commonly and may be more severe and of prolonged duration in patients treated with the combination.

In the first Mayo/NCCTG controlled trial, toxicity, primarily gastrointestinal, resulted in 7% of patients requiring hospitalization when treated with 5-fluorouracil alone or 5-fluorouracil in combination with 200 mg/m^2 of leucovorin and 20% when treated with 5-fluorouracil in combination with 20 mg/m^2 of leucovorin. In the second Mayo/NCCTG trial, hospitalizations related to treatment toxicity also appeared to occur more often in patients treated with the low dose leucovorin/5-fluorouracil combination than in patients treated with the high dose combination — 11% versus 3%. Therapy with leucovorin/5-fluorouracil must not be initiated or continued in patients who have symptoms of gastrointestinal toxicity of any severity, until those symptoms have completely resolved. Patients with diarrhea must be monitored with particular care until the diarrhea has resolved, as rapid clinical deterioration leading to death can occur. In an additional study utilizing higher weekly doses of 5-FU and leucovorin, elderly and/or debilitated patients were found to be at greater risk for severe gastrointestinal toxicity.

Seizures and/or syncope have been reported rarely in cancer patients receiving leucovorin, usually in association with fluoropyrimidine administration, and most commonly in those with CNS metastases or other predisposing factors, however, a causal relationship has not been established.

The concomitant use of leucovorin with trimethoprim-sulfamethoxazole for the acute treatment of Pneumocystis carinii pneumonia in patients with HIV infection was associated with increased rates of treatment failure and morbidity in a placebo-controlled study.

PRECAUTIONS
General
Parenteral administration is preferable to oral dosing if there is a possibility that the patient may vomit or not absorb the leucovorin. Leucovorin has no effect on non-hematologic toxicities of MTX such as the nephrotoxicity resulting from drug and/or metabolite precipitation in the kidney. **Since leucovorin enhances the toxicity of fluorouracil, leucovorin/5 fluorouracil combination therapy for advanced colorectal cancer should be administered under the supervision of a physician experienced in the use of antimetabolite cancer chemotherapy. Particular care should be taken in the treatment of elderly or debilitated colorectal cancer patients, as these patients may be at increased risk of severe toxicity.**

Laboratory Tests
Patients being treated with the leucovorin/5-fluorouracil combination should have a CBC with differential and platelets prior to each treatment. During the first two courses a CBC with differential and platelets has to be repeated weekly and thereafter once each cycle at the time of anticipated WBC nadir. Electrolytes and liver function tests should be performed prior to each treatment for the first three cycles then prior to every other cycle. Dosage modifications of fluorouracil should be instituted as follows, based on the most severe toxicities:

Diarrhea and/or Stomatitis	WBC/mm^3 Nadir	Platelets/mm^3 Nadir	5-FU Dose
Moderate	1,000-1,900	25-75,000	decrease 20%
Severe	<1,000	<25,000	decrease 30%

If no toxicity occurs, the 5-fluorouracil dose may increase 10%. Treatment should be deferred until WBCs are 4,000/mm^3 and platelets 130,000/mm^3. If blood counts do not reach these levels within two weeks, treatment should be discontinued. Patients should be followed up with physical examination prior to each treatment course and appropriate radiological examination as needed. Treatment should be discontinued when there is clear evidence of tumor progression.

Drug Interactions
Folic acid in large amounts may counteract the antiepileptic effect of phenobarbital, phenytoin and primidone, and increase the frequency of seizures in susceptible pediatric patients.

Preliminary animal and human studies have shown that small quantities of systemically administered leucovorin enter the CSF primarily as 5 methyltetrahydrofolate and, in humans, remain 1–3 orders of magnitude lower than the usual methotrexate concentrations following intrathecal administration. However, high doses of leucovorin may reduce the efficacy of intrathecally administered methotrexate.
Leucovorin may enhance the toxicity of 5-fluorouracil. (See WARNINGS.)

Pregnancy: Teratogenic Effects:
"Pregnancy Category C." Adequate animal reproduction studies have not been conducted with leucovorin. It is also not known whether leucovorin can cause fetal harm when administered to a pregnant woman or can affect reproduction capacity. Leucovorin should be given to a pregnant woman only if clearly needed.

Nursing Mothers: It is not known whether this drug is excreted in human milk. Because many drugs are excreted in human milk, caution should be exercised when leucovorin is administered to a nursing mother.

Pediatric Use: See Drug Interactions.

ADVERSE REACTIONS
Allergic sensitization, including anaphylactoid reactions and urticaria, has been reported following administration of both oral and parenteral leucovorin. No other adverse reactions have been attributed to the use of leucovorin per se. The following table summarizes significant adverse events occurring in 316 patients treated with the leucovorin-5-fluorouracil combinations compared against 70 patients treated with 5-fluorouracil alone for advanced colorectal carcinoma. These data are taken from the Mayo/NCCTG large multicenter prospective trial evaluating the efficacy and safety of the combination regimen.
[See first table below]

OVERDOSAGE
Excessive amounts of leucovorin may nullify the chemotherapeutic effect of folic acid antagonists.

DOSAGE AND ADMINISTRATION
Advanced Colorectal Cancer: Either of the following two regimens is recommended:
1. Leucovorin is administered at 200 mg/m^2 by slow intravenous injection over a minimum of 3 minutes, followed by 5-fluorouracil at 370 mg/m^2 by intravenous injection.
2. Leucovorin is administered at 20 mg/m^2 by intravenous injection followed by 5-fluorouracil at 425 mg/m^2 by intravenous injection.

5-Flurouracil and leucovorin should be administered separately to avoid the formation of a precipitate.
Treatment is repeated daily for five days. This five-day treatment course may be repeated at 4 week (28-day) intervals, for 2 courses and then repeated at 4–5 week (28–35 day) intervals provided that the patient has completely recovered from the toxic effects of the prior treatment course. In subsequent treatment courses, the dosage of 5-fluorouracil should be adjusted based on patient tolerance of the prior treatment course. The daily dosage of 5-fluorouracil should be reduced by 20% for patients who experienced moderate hematologic or gastrointestinal toxicity in the prior treatment course, and by 30% for patients who experienced severe toxicity (see PRECAUTIONS: Laboratory Tests). For patients who experienced no toxicity in the prior treatment course, 5-fluorouracil dosage may be increased by 10%. Leucovorin dosages are not adjusted for toxicity.

Several other doses and schedules of leucovorin/5-fluorouracil therapy have also been evaluated in patients with advanced colorectal cancer; some of these alternative regimens may also have efficacy in the treatment of this disease. However, further clinical research will be required to confirm the safety and effectiveness of these alternative leucovorin/5-fluorouracil treatment regimens.

Leucovorin Rescue After High-Dose Methotrexate Therapy. The recommendations for leucovorin rescue are based on a methotrexate dose of 12–15 grams/m^2 administered by intravenous infusion over 4 hours (see methotrexate package insert for full prescribing information).

Leucovorin rescue at a dose of 15 mg (approximately 10 mg/m^2) every 6 hours for 10 doses starts 24 hours after the beginning of the methotrexate infusion. In the presence of gastrointestinal toxicity, nausea or vomiting, leucovorin should be administered parenterally. Do not administer leucovorin intrathecally.

Serum creatinine and methotrexate levels should be determined at least once daily. Leucovorin administration, hydration, and urinary alkalinization (pH of 7.0 or greater) should be continued until the methotrexate level is below 5 x 10-8 M (0.05 micromolar). The leucovorin dose should be adjusted or leucovorin rescue extended based on the above guidelines.
[See second table below]
Patients who experience delayed early methotrexate elimination are likely to develop reversible renal failure. In addition to appropriate leucovorin therapy, these patients require continuing hydration and urinary alkalinization, and close monitoring of fluid and electrolyte status, until the serum methotrexate level has fallen to below 0.05 micromolar and the renal failure has resolved.

Some patients will have abnormalities in methotrexate elimination or renal function following methotrexate administration, which are significant but less severe than the abnormalities described in the table above. These abnormalities may or may not be associated with significant clinical toxicity. If significant clinical toxicity is observed, leucovorin rescue should be extended for an additional 24 hours (total of 14 doses over 84 hours) in subsequent courses of

---

**PERCENTAGE OF PATIENTS TREATED WITH LEUCOVORIN/FLUOROURACIL
FOR ADVANCED COLORECTAL CARCINOMA
REPORTING ADVERSE EXPERIENCES OR HOSPITALIZED FOR TOXICITY**

	(High LV)/5-FU (N=155)		(Low LV)/5-FU (N=161)		5-FU Alone (N=70)	
	Any (%)	Grade 3+ (%)	Any (%)	Grade 3+ (%)	Any (%)	Grade 3+ (%)
Leukopenia	69	14	83	23	93	48
Thrombocytopenia	8	2	8	1	18	3
Infection	8	1	3	1	7	2
Nausea	74	10	80	9	60	6
Vomiting	46	8	44	9	40	7
Diarrhea	66	18	67	14	43	11
Stomatitis	75	27	84	29	59	16
Constipation	3	0	4	0	1	–
Lethargy/Malaise/Fatigue	13	3	12	2	6	3
Alopecia	42	5	43	6	37	7
Dermatitis	21	2	25	1	13	–
Anorexia	14	1	22	4	14	–
Hospitalization for Toxicity	5%		15%		7%	

High LV = Leucovorin 200 mg/m^2, Low LV = Leucovorin 20 mg/m^2
Any = percentage of patients reporting toxicity of any severity
Grade 3+ = percentage of patients reporting toxicity of Grade 3 or higher

---

**GUIDELINES FOR LEUCOVORIN DOSAGE AND ADMINISTRATION
DO NOT ADMINISTER LEUCOVORIN INTRATHECALLY**

Clinical Situation	Laboratory Findings	Leucovorin Dosage and Duration
Normal Methotrexate Elimination	Serum methotrexate level approximately 10 micromolar at 24 hours after administration, 1 micromolar at 48 hours, and less than 0.2 micromolar at 72 hours.	15 mg PO, IM, or IV q 6 hours for 60 hours (10 doses starting at 24 hours after start of methotrexate infusion)
Delayed Late Methotrexate Elimination	Serum methotrexate level remaining above 0.2 micromolar at 72 hours, and more than 0.05 micromolar at 96 hours after administration.	Continue 15 mg PO, IM, or IV q 6 hours, until methotrexate level is less than 0.05 micromolar.
Delayed Early Methotrexate Elimination and/or Evidence of Acute Renal Injury	Serum methotrexate level of 50 micromolar or more at 24 hours, or 5 micromolar or more at 48 hours after administration, OR; a 100% or greater increase in serum creatinine level at 24 hours after methotrexate administration (eg, an increase from 0.5 mg/dL to a level of 1 mg/dL or more)	150 mg IV q 3 hours, until methotrexate level is less than 1 micromolar; then 15 mg IV q 3 hours until methotrexate level is less than 0.05 micromolar.

therapy. The possibility that the patient is taking other medications which interact with methotrexate (eg, medications which may interfere with methotrexate elimination or binding to serum albumin) should always be reconsidered when laboratory abnormalities or clinical toxicities are observed.

Impaired Methotrexate Elimination or Inadvertent Overdosage: Leucovorin rescue should begin as soon as possible after an inadvertent overdosage and within 24 hours of methotrexate administration when there is delayed excretion (see WARNINGS). Leucovorin 10 mg/m^2 should be administered IV, IM, or PO every 6 hours until the serum methotrexate level is less than 10^{-8} M. In the presence of gastrointestinal toxicity, nausea, or vomiting, leucovorin should be administered parenterally. Do not administer leucovorin intrathecally.

Serum creatinine and methotrexate levels should be determined at 24 hour intervals. If the 24 hour serum creatinine has increased 50% over baseline or if the 24 hour methotrexate level is greater than 5 × 10^{-6} M or the 48 hour level is greater than 9 × 10^{-7} M, the dose of leucovorin should be increased to 100 mg/m^2 IV every 3 hours until the methotrexate level is less than 10^{-8} M.

Hydration (3 L/d) and urinary alkalinization with sodium bicarbonate solution should be employed concomitantly. The bicarbonate dose should be adjusted to maintain the urine pH at 7.0 or greater.

Megaloblastic Anemia Due to Folic Acid Deficiency: Up to 1 mg daily. There is no evidence that doses greater than 1 mg/day have greater efficacy than those of 1 mg; additionally, loss of folate in urine becomes roughly logarithmic as the amount administered exceeds 1 mg.

Each 350 mg vial of Leucovorin Calcium for Injection when reconstituted with 17 mL of sterile diluent yields a leucovorin concentration of 20 mg leucovorin per mL. Leucovorin Calcium for Injection contains no preservative. Reconstitute with Bacteriostatic Water for Injection, USP, which contains benzyl alcohol, or with Sterile Water for Injection, USP. When reconstituted with Bacteriostatic Water for Injection, USP, the resulting solution must be used within 7 days. If the product is reconstituted with Sterile Water for Injection, USP, it must be used immediately.

Because of the benzyl alcohol contained in Bacteriostatic Water for Injection, USP, when doses greater than 10 mg/m^2 are administered Leucovorin Calcium for Injection should be reconstituted with Sterile Water for Injection, USP, and used immediately. (See WARNINGS.) Because of the calcium content of the leucovorin solution, no more than 160 mg of leucovorin should be injected intravenously per minute (16 mL of a 10 mg/mL, or 8 mL of a 20 mg/mL solution per minute).

Parenteral drug products should be inspected visually for particulate matter and discoloration prior to administration, whenever solution and container permit. Leucovorin should not be mixed in the same infusion as 5-fluorouracil, since this may lead to the formation of a precipitate.

HOW SUPPLIED

Leucovorin Calcium for Injection is supplied in sterile, single-use vials

NDC 58406-623-07 - 350 mg Vial
STORE AT 25°C (77°F); EXCURSIONS PERMITTED TO 15–30°C (59°–86°F).
PROTECT FROM LIGHT.
Manufactured for
IMMUNEX CORPORATION,
Seattle, WA 98101
by LEDERLE PARENTERALS, INC.,
Carolina, Puerto Rico 00987
©1997 Immunex Corporation
CI 4820-4
Rev 0163-04   Issued 12/97

LEUCOVORIN CALCIUM TABLETS   ℞
[lu-cō-vor-in căl-sēē-um]

DESCRIPTION

Leucovorin is one of several active, chemically reduced derivatives of folic acid. It is useful as an antidote to drugs which act as folic acid antagonists. Also known as folinic acid, Citrovorum factor, or 5-formyl-5,6,7,8-tetrahydrofolic acid, this compound has the chemical designation of L-Glutamic acid, N-[4-[[(2-amino-5-formyl-1,4,5,6,7,8-hexa hydro-4-oxo-6-pteridinyl)methyl]amino]benzoyl]-,calcium salt (1:1). The formula weight is 511.51 and the structural formula of leucovorin calcium is:
[See chemical structure at top of next column]
Leucovorin Calcium Tablets, 5 mg, contain 5 mg of leucovorin (equivalent to 5.40 mg of anhydrous leucovorin calcium) and the following inactive ingredients: Corn Starch, Dibasic Calcium Phosphate, Magnesium Stearate, and Pregelatinized Starch.
Leucovorin Calcium Tablets, 15 mg, contain 15 mg of leucovorin (equivalent to 16.20 mg of anhydrous leucovorin cal-

cium) and the following inactive ingredients: Lactose, Magnesium Stearate, Microcrystalline Cellulose, Pregelatinized Starch, and Sodium Starch Glycolate.
Leucovorin Calcium Tablets are indicated for oral administration only.

CLINICAL PHARMACOLOGY

Leucovorin is a mixture of the diastereoisomers of the 5-formyl derivative of tetrahydrofolic acid. The biologically active component of the mixture is the (-)-L-isomer, known as Citrovorum factor, or (-)-folinic acid. Leucovorin does not require reduction by the enzyme dihydrofolate reductase in order to participate in reactions utilizing folates as a source of "one-carbon" moieties. Following oral administration, leucovorin is rapidly absorbed and enters the general body pool of reduced folates.

The increase in plasma and serum reduced folate activity (determined microbiologically with *Lactobacillus casei*) seen after oral administration of leucovorin is predominantly due to 5-methyltetrahydrofolate.

Following a 20 mg dose of leucovorin calcium, the mean maximum serum total reduced folate concentrations were:

Tablet	364 ± 12.1 ng/mL at 2.0	± 0.07 hours
Oral Solution	375 ± 12.8 ng/mL at 2.1	± 0.11 hours
Parenteral	355 ± 17.2 ng/mL at 0.96	± 0.10 hours

The half-life of plasma 5-formyltetrahydrofolate was 1.5 ± 0.08 hours and that of the 5-methyltetrahydrofolate was 3.0 ± 0.09 hours.

Oral tablets produced equivalent bioavailability (8% difference) when compared to the parenteral administration. The parenteral solution also provided equal bioavailability to the tablets when administered orally (2% difference). Oral absorption of leucovorin is saturable at doses above 25 mg. The apparent bioavailability of leucovorin was 97% for 25 mg, 75% for 50 mg and 37% for 100 mg.

INDICATIONS

Leucovorin calcium rescue is indicated after high-dose methotrexate therapy in osteosarcoma. Leucovorin is also indicated to diminish the toxicity and counteract the effects of impaired methotrexate elimination and of inadvertent overdosages of folic acid antagonists.

CONTRAINDICATIONS

Leucovorin is improper therapy for pernicious anemia and other megaloblastic anemias secondary to the lack of vitamin B$_{12}$. A hematologic remission may occur while neurologic manifestations remain progressive.

WARNINGS

In the treatment of accidental overdosages of folic acid antagonists, leucovorin should be administered as promptly as possible. As the time interval between antifolate administration [eg, methotrexate (MTX)] and leucovorin rescue increases, leucovorin's effectiveness in counteracting toxicity diminishes.

Monitoring of serum MTX concentration is essential in determining the optimal dose and duration of treatment with leucovorin.

Delayed MTX excretion may be caused by a third space fluid accumulation (ie, ascites, pleural effusion), renal insufficiency, or inadequate hydration. Under such circumstances, higher doses of leucovorin or prolonged administration may be indicated. Doses higher than those recommended for oral use must be given intravenously.

Leucovorin may enhance the toxicity of fluorouracil. Deaths from severe enterocolitis, diarrhea, and dehydration have been reported in elderly patients receiving weekly leucovorin and fluorouracil.[1] Concomitant granulocytopenia and fever were present in some but not all of the patients.

Seizures and/or syncope have been reported rarely in cancer patients receiving leucovorin, usually in association with fluoropyrimidine administration, and most commonly in those with CNS metastases or other predisposing factors, however, a causal relationship has not been established.[2]

PRECAUTIONS

General
Parenteral administration is preferable to oral dosing if there is a possibility that the patient may vomit or not absorb the leucovorin. Leucovorin has no effect on other established toxicities of MTX such as the nephrotoxicity resulting from drug and/or metabolite precipitation in the kidney.

Drug Interactions
Folic acid in large amounts may counteract the antiepileptic effect of phenobarbital, phenytoin and primidone, and increase the frequency of seizures in susceptible children. Preliminary animal and human studies have shown that small quantities of systemically administered leucovorin enter the CSF primarily as 5-methyltetrahydrofolate and, in humans, remain 1–3 orders of magnitude lower than the usual methotrexate concentrations following intrathecal administration. However, high doses of leucovorin may reduce the efficacy of intrathecally administered methotrexate.
Leucovorin may enhance the toxicity of fluorouracil (see WARNINGS).

Pregnancy: Teratogenic Effects
"Pregnancy Category C." Animal reproduction studies have not been conducted with leucovorin. It is also not known whether leucovorin can cause fetal harm when administered to a pregnant woman or can affect reproduction capacity. Leucovorin should be given to a pregnant woman only if clearly needed.

Nursing Mothers: It is not known whether this drug is excreted in human milk. Because many drugs are excreted in human milk, caution should be exercised when leucovorin is administered to a nursing mother.

Pediatric Use: see **Drug Interactions**.

ADVERSE REACTIONS

Allergic sensitization, including anaphylactoid reactions and urticaria, has been reported following the administration of both oral and parenteral leucovorin.

OVERDOSAGE

Excessive amounts of leucovorin may nullify the chemotherapeutic effect of folic acid antagonists.

DOSAGE AND ADMINISTRATION

Leucovorin Calcium Tablets are intended for oral administration. Because absorption is saturable, oral administration of doses greater than 25 mg is not recommended.

Leucovorin Rescue after High-Dose Methotrexate Therapy: The recommendations for leucovorin rescue are based on a methotrexate dose of 12–15 grams/m^2 administered by intravenous infusion over 4 hours (see methotrexate package insert for full prescribing information).[3] Leuco-

Continued on next page

GUIDELINES FOR LEUCOVORIN DOSAGE AND ADMINISTRATION
DO NOT ADMINISTER LEUCOVORIN INTRATHECALLY

Clinical Situation	Laboratory Findings	Leucovorin Dosage and Duration
Normal Methotrexate Elimination	Serum methotrexate level approximately 10 micromolar at 24 hours after administration, 1 micromolar at 48 hours, and less than 0.2 micromolar at 72 hours.	15 mg PO, IM, or IV q 6 hours for 60 hours (10 doses starting at 24 hours after start of methotrexate infusion).
Delayed Late Methotrexate Elimination	Serum methotrexate level remaining above 0.2 micromolar at 72 hours, and more than 0.05 micromolar at 96 hours after administration.	Continue 15 mg PO, IM, or IV q 6 hours, until methotrexate level is less than 0.05 micromolar.
Delayed Early Methotrexate Elimination and/or Evidence of Acute Renal Injury	Serum methotrexate level of 50 micromolar or more at 24 hours, or 5 micromolar or more at 48 hours after administration, OR; a 100% or greater increase in serum creatinine level at 24 hours after methotrexate administration (eg, an increase from 0.5 mg/dL to a level of 1 mg/dL or more).	150 mg IV q 3 hours, until methotrexate level is less than 1 micromolar; then 15 mg IV q 3 hours until methotrexate level is less than 0.05 micromolar.

Leucovorin Calcium Tablets—Cont.

vorin rescue at a dose of 15 mg (approximately 10 mg/m²) every 6 hours for 10 doses starts 24 hours after the beginning of the methotrexate infusion. In the presence of gastrointestinal toxicity, nausea or vomiting, leucovorin should be administered parenterally.

Serum creatinine and methotrexate levels should be determined at least once daily. Leucovorin administration, hydration, and urinary alkalinization (pH of 7.0 or greater) should be continued until the methotrexate level is below 5 × 10⁻⁸ M (0.05 micromolar). The leucovorin dose should be adjusted or leucovorin rescue extended based on the following guidelines:

[See table at bottom of previous page]

Patients who experience delayed early methotrexate elimination are likely to develop reversible renal failure. In addition to appropriate leucovorin therapy, these patients require continuing hydration and urinary alkalinization, and close monitoring of fluid and electrolyte status, until the serum methotrexate level has fallen to below 0.05 micromolar and the renal failure has resolved.

Some patients will have abnormalities in methotrexate elimination or renal function following methotrexate administration, which are significant but less severe than the abnormalities described in the table above. These abnormalities may or may not be associated with significant clinical toxicity. If significant clinical toxicity is observed, leucovorin rescue should be extended for an additional 24 hours (total of 14 doses over 84 hours) in subsequent courses of therapy. The possibility that the patient is taking other medications which interact with methotrexate (eg, medications which may interfere with methotrexate elimination or binding to serum [albumin]) should always be reconsidered when laboratory abnormalities or clinical toxicities are observed.

Impaired Methotrexate Elimination or Inadvertent Overdosage: The same dosage and administration guidelines may be used. However, leucovorin administration should begin as soon as possible after an inadvertent overdosage is recognized.

HOW SUPPLIED

Leucovorin Calcium Tablets, 5 mg are round, convex, yellowish-white, engraved LL above 5 on one side, scored in half on the other side and engraved C above the score and 33 below, each containing 5 mg of leucovorin as the calcium salt, supplied as follows:

NDC 58406-624-62 - Bottle of 30 with CRC
NDC 58406-624-67 - Bottle of 100

Leucovorin Calcium Tablets, 15 mg are oval, convex, yellowish-white, engraved LL on left and 15 on right on one side, scored in half on the other side and engraved C to the left of the score and 35 to the right, each containing 15 mg of leucovorin as the calcium salt, supplied as follows:

NDC 58406-626-68 - Bottle of 12 with CRC
NDC 58406-626-74 - Bottle of 24 with CRC

STORE BETWEEN 15°-30°C (59°-86°F). PROTECT FROM LIGHT.

REFERENCES

Grem JL, Shoemaker DD, Petrelli NJ, Douglas HO, "Severe and Fatal Toxic Effects Observed in Treatment with High- and Low-Dose Leucovorin Plus 5-Fluorouracil for Colorectal Carcinoma," *Cancer Treat Rep* 1987; 71:1122.
Meropol NJ, Creaven PJ, White RM, et al, "Seizures Associated With Leucovorin Administration in Cancer Patients." *J NCI* 1995; 87(1):56-58.
Link MP, Goorin AM, Miser AW, et al, "The Effect of Adjuvant Chemotherapy on Relapse-Free Survival in Patients with Osteosarcoma of the Extremity." *N Engl J Med* 1986; 314:1600-1606.

IMMUNEX®
Manufactured for
IMMUNEX CORPORATION
Seattle, WA 98101
by
LEDERLE LABORATORIES DIVISION
Pearl River, NY 10965
©1996 Immunex Corporation   Rev 0164-01 Issued 3/96
CI 4819-1

LEUKINE®   ℞
SARGRAMOSTIM

Caution: Federal law prohibits dispensing without prescription.

DESCRIPTION

LEUKINE® (sargramostim) is a recombinant human granulocyte-macrophage colony stimulating factor (rhu GM-CSF) produced by recombinant DNA technology in a yeast (*S. cerevisiae*) expression system. GM-CSF is a hematopoietic growth factor which stimulates proliferation and differentiation of hematopoietic progenitor cells. LEUKINE is a glycoprotein of 127 amino acids characterized by 3 primary molecular species having molecular masses of 19,500, 16,800 and 15,500 daltons. The amino acid sequence of LEUKINE differs from the natural human GM-CSF by a substitution of leucine at position 23, and the carbohydrate moiety may be different form the native protein. Sargramostim has been selected as the proper name for yeast-derived rhu GM-CSF.

The LEUKINE Liquid presentation is formulated as a sterile, preserved (1.1% benzyl alcohol), injectable solution (500 mcg/mL) in a vial. Lyophilized LEUKINE is a sterile, white, preservative-free powder (250 mcg) that requires reconstitution with 1 mL Sterile Water for Injection, USP or 1 mL Bacteriostatic Water for Injection, USP.

LEUKINE Liquid and reconstituted lyophilized LEUKINE are clear, colorless liquids suitable for subcutaneous injection or intravenous infusion. LEUKINE Liquid contains 500 mcg (2.8 × 10⁶ IU/mL) sargramostim and 1.1% benzyl alcohol in a 1 mL solution. The vial of lyophilized LEUKINE contains 250 mcg (1.4 × 10⁶ IU/vial) sargramostim. The LEUKINE Liquid vial and reconstituted lyophilized LEUKINE vial also contain 40 mg/mL mannitol, USP; 10 mg/mL sucrose, NF; and 1.2 mg/mL tromethamine, USP, as excipients. Biological potency is expressed in International Units (IU) as tested against the WHO First International Reference Standard. The specific activity of LEUKINE is approximately 5.6 × 10⁶ IU/mg.

CLINICAL PHARMACOLOGY

General GM-CSF belongs to a group of growth factors termed colony stimulating factors which support survival, clonal expansion, and differentiation of hematopoietic progenitor cells. GM-CSF induces partially committed progenitor cells to divide and differentiate in the granulocyte-macrophage pathways.

GM-CSF is also capable of activating mature granulocytes and macrophages. GM-CSF is a multilineage factor and, in addition to dose-dependent effects on the myelomonocytic lineage, can promote the proliferation of megakaryocytic and erythroid progenitors.[1] However, other factors are required to induce complete maturation in these two lineages. The various cellular responses (i.e., division, maturation, activation) are induced through GM-CSF binding to specific receptors expressed on the cell surface of target cells.[2]

In vitro **Studies of LEUKINE in Human Cells** The biological activity of GM-CSF is species-specific. Consequently, *in vitro* studies have been performed on human cells to characterize the pharmacological activity of LEUKINE. *In vitro* exposure of human bone marrow cells to LEUKINE at concentrations ranging from 1–100 ng/mL results in the proliferation of hematopoietic progenitors and in the formation of pure granulocyte, pure macrophage and mixed granulocyte-macrophage colonies.[3] Chemotactic, anti-fungal and anti-parasitic[4] activities of granulocytes and monocytes are increased by exposure to LEUKINE *in vitro*. LEUKINE increases the cytotoxicity of monocytes toward certain neoplastic cell lines[3] and activates polymorphonuclear neutrophils to inhibit the growth of tumor cells.

In vivo **Primate Studies of LEUKINE** Pharmacology/toxicology studies of LEUKINE were performed in cynomolgus monkeys. An acute toxicity study revealed an absence of treatment-related toxicity following a single IV bolus injection at a dose of 300 mcg/kg. Two subacute studies were performed using IV injection (maximum dose 200 mcg/kg/day × 14 days) and subcutaneous injection (maximum dose 200 mcg/kg/day × 28 days). No major visceral organ toxicity was documented. Notable histopathology findings included increased cellularity in hematologic organs and heart and lung tissues. A dose-dependent increase in leukocyte count, which consisted primarily of segmented neutrophils, occurred during the dosing period; increases in monocytes, basophils, eosinophils and lymphocytes were also noted. Leukocyte counts decreased to pretreatment values over a 1–2 week recovery period.

Pharmacokinetics Pharmacokinetic profiles have been analyzed in controlled studies of 24 normal male volunteers. Liquid and lyophilized LEUKINE, at the recommended dose of 250 mcg/m², have been determined to be bioequivalent based on the statistical evaluation of AUC.[5]

When LEUKINE (either liquid or lyophilized) was administered IV over 2 hours to normal volunteers, the mean beta half-life was approximately 60 minutes. Peak concentrations of GM-CSF were observed in blood samples obtained during or immediately after completion of LEUKINE infusion. For LEUKINE Liquid, the mean maximum concentration (Cmax) was 5.0 ng/mL, the mean clearance rate was approximately 420 mL/min/m² and the mean AUC (0–inf) was 640 ng·L. Corresponding results for lyophilized LEUKINE in the same subjects were mean Cmax of 5.4 ng/mL, mean clearance rates of 431 mL/min/m², and mean AUC (0–inf) of 677 ng/mL·min. GM-CSF was last detected in the blood samples obtained at 3 to 6 hours.

When LEUKINE (either liquid or lyophilized) was administered SC to normal volunteers, GM-CSF was detected in the serum at 15 minutes, the first sample point. The mean beta half-life was approximately 162 minutes. Peak level occurred at 1 to 3 hours post injection, and LEUKINE remained undetectable for up to 6 hours after injection. The mean Cmax was 1.5 ng/mL. For LEUKINE Liquid, the mean clearance was 549 mL/min/m² and the mean AUC (0–inf) was 549 ng/mL·min. For lyophilized LEUKINE, the mean clearance was 529 mL/min/m² and the mean AUC (0–inf) was 501 ng/mL·min.

Antibody Formation Serum samples collected before and after LEUKINE treatment from 214 patients with a variety of underlying diseases have been examined for the presence of antibodies. Neutralizing antibodies were detected in 5 of 214 patients (2.3%) after receiving LEUKINE by continuous IV infusion (3 patients) or subcutaneous injection (2 patients) for 28 to 84 days in multiple courses. All 5 patients had impaired hematopoiesis before the administration of LEUKINE and consequently the effect of the development of anti-GM-CSF antibodies on normal hematopoiesis could not be assessed. Drug-induced neutropenia, neutralization of endogenous GM-CSF activity and diminution of the therapeutic effect of LEUKINE secondary to formation of neutralizing antibody remain a theoretical possibility.

INDICATIONS AND USAGE

Use Following Induction Chemotherapy in Acute Myocardial Leukemia LEUKINE is indicated for use following induction chemotherapy in older adult patients with acute myelogenous leukemia (AML) to shorten time to neutrophil recovery and to reduce the incidence of severe and life-threatening infections and infections resulting in death. The safety and efficacy of LEUKINE have not been assessed in patients with AML under 55 years of age.

The term acute myelogenous leukemia, also referred to as acute non-lymphocytic leukemia (ANLL), encompasses a heterogeneous group of leukemias arising from various nonlymphoid cell lines which have been defined morphologically by the French-American-British (FAB) system of classification.

Use in Mobilization and Following Transplantation of Autologous Peripheral Blood Progenitor Cells LEUKINE is indicated for the mobilization of hematopoietic progenitor cells into peripheral blood for collection by leukapheresis. Mobilization allows for the collection of increased numbers of progenitor cells capable of engraftment as compared with collection without mobilization. After myeloablative chemotherapy, the transplantation of an increased number of progenitor cells can lead to more rapid engraftment, which may result in a decreased need for supportive care. Myeloid reconstitution is further accelerated by administration of LEUKINE following peripheral blood progenitor cell transplantation.

Use in Myeloid Reconstitution After Autologous Bone Marrow Transplantation LEUKINE is indicated for acceleration of myeloid recovery in patients with non-Hodgkin's lymphoma (NHL), acute lymphoblastic leukemia (ALL) and Hodgkin's disease undergoing autologous bone marrow transplantation (BMT). After autologous BMT in patients with NHL, ALL, or Hodgkin's disease, LEUKINE has been found to be safe and effective in accelerating myeloid engraftment, decreasing median duration of antibiotic administration, reducing the median duration of infectious episodes and shortening the median duration of hospitalization. Hematologic response to LEUKINE can be detected by complete blood count (CBC) with differential performed twice per week.

Use in Myeloid Reconstitution After Allogeneic Bone Marrow Transplantation LEUKINE is indicated for acceleration of myeloid recovery in patients undergoing allogeneic BMT from HLA-matched related doners LEUKINE has been found to be safe and effective in accelerating myeloid engraftment, reducing the incidence of bacteremia and other culture positive infections, and shortening the median duration of hospitalization.

Use in Bone Marrow Transplantation Failure or Engraftment Delay LEUKINE is indicated in patients who have undergone allogeneic or autologous bone marrow transplantation (BMT) in whom engraftment is delayed or has failed. LEUKINE has been found to be safe and effective in prolonging survival of patients who are experiencing graft failure or enlargement delay, in the presence of absence of infection, following autologous or allogeneic BMT. Survival benefit may be relatively greater in those patients who demonstrate one or more of the following characteristics: autologous BMT failure or engraftment delay, no previous total body irradiation, malignancy other than leukemia or a multiple organ failure (MOF) score ≤ 2 (see CLINICAL EXPERIENCE). Hematologic response to LEUKINE can be detected by complete blood count (CBC) with differential performed twice per week.

CLINICAL EXPERIENCE

Acute Myelogenous Leukemia The safety and efficacy of sargramostim in patients with AML who are younger than

Hematological Recovery (in Days): Induction

Dataset	sargramostim n=52* Median (25%, 75%)	Placebo n=47 Median (25%, 75%)	p-value**
ANC>500/mm[3a]	13 (11, 16)	17 (13, 25)	0.009
ANC>1000/mm[3b]	14 (12, 18)	21 (13, 34)	0.003
PLT>20,000/mm[3c]	11 (7, 14)	12 (9, ≥42)	0.10
RBC[§]	12 (9, 24)	14 (9. 42)	0.53

** Patients with missing data censored.*
[a] 2 patients on sargramostim and 4 patients on placebo had missing values.
[b] 2 patients on sargramostim and 3 patients on placebo had missing values.
[c] 4 patients on placebo had missing values.
§ 3 patients on sargramostim and 4 patients on placebo had missing values.
*** p=Generalized Wilcoxon*

ANC and Platelet Recovery after PBPC Transplant

	Route for Mobilization	Post-transplant LEUKINE	ENGRAFTMENT (median value in days)	
			ANC>500/mm^3	Last platelet transfusion
No Mobilization	-	no	29	28
LEUKINE	IV	no	21	24
250 mcg/m^2	IV	yes	12	19
	SC	yes	12	17

55 years of age have not been determined. Based on Phase II data suggesting the best therapeutic effects could be achieved in patients at highest risk for severe infections and mortality while neutropenic, the Phase III clinical trial was conducted in older patients. The safety and efficacy of LEUKINE in the treatment of AML were evaluated in a multicenter, randomized, double-blind placebo-controlled trial of 99 newly diagnosed adult patients, 55–70 years of age, receiving induction with or without consolidation.[5] A combination of standard doses of daunorubicin (days 1–3) and ara-C (days 1–7) was administered during induction and high dose ara-C was administered days 1–6 as a single course of consolidation, if given. Bone marrow evaluation was performed on day 10 following induction chemotherapy. If hypoplasia with <5% blasts was not achieved, patients immediately received a second cycle of induction chemotherapy. If the bone marrow was hypoplastic with <5% blasts on day 10 or 4 days following the second cycle of induction chemotherapy, LEUKINE (250 mcg/m^2/day) or placebo was given IV over 4 hours each day, starting 4 days after the completion of chemotherapy. Study drug was continued until an ANC ≥1500/mm^3 for three consecutive days was attained or a maximum of 42 days. LEUKINE or placebo was also administered after the single course of consolidation chemotherapy if delivered (ara-C 3–6 weeks after induction following neutrophil recovery). Study drug was discontinued immediately if leukemic regrowth occurred.

[See first table above]

LEUKINE (sargramostim) significantly shortened the median duration of ANC <500/mm^3 by 7 days following induction (see table at right), 75% of patients receiving LEUKINE achieved ANC >500/mm^3 by day 16, compared to day 25 for patients receiving placebo. The proportion of patients receiving 1 cycle (70%) for 2 cycles (30%) of induction was similar in both treatment groups; LEUKINE significantly shortened the median times to neutrophil recovery whether one cycle (12 versus 15 days) or two cycles (14 versus 23 days) of induction chemotherapy was administered. Median times to platelet (>20,000/mm^3) and RBC transfusion independence were not significantly different between treatment groups.

During the consolidation phase of treatment, LEUKINE did not shorten the median time to recovery of ANC to 500/mm^3 (13 days) or 1000/mm^3 (14.5 days) compared to placebo. There were no significant differences in time to platelet and RBC transfusion independence.

The incidence of severe infections and deaths associated with infections was significantly reduced in patients who received LEUKINE. During induction or consolidation, 27 of 52 patients receiving LEUKINE and 35 of 47 patients receiving placebo had at least one grade 3, 4 or 5 infection (p=0.02). Twenty-five patients receiving LEUKINE and 30 patients receiving placebo experienced severe and fatal infections during induction only. There were significantly fewer deaths from infectious causes in the sargramostim arm (3 versus 11, p=0.02). The majority of deaths due in the placebo group were associated with fungal infections with pneumonia as the primary infection.

Disease outcomes were not adversely affected by the use of LEUKINE. The proportion of patients achieving complete remission (CR) was higher in the LEUKINE group (69% as compared to 55% for the placebo group), but the difference was not significant (p=0.21). There was no significant difference in relapse rates; 12 of 36 patients who received LEUKINE and 5 of 26 patients who received placebo relapsed within 180 days of documented CR (p=0.26). The overall median survival was 378 days for patients receiving LEUKINE and 268 days for those on placebo (p=0.17). The study was not sized to assess the impact of LEUKINE treatment on response or survival.

Mobilization and Engraftment of PBPC A retrospective review was conducted on data from patients with cancer undergoing collection of peripheral blood progenitor cells (PBPC) at a single transplant center. Mobilization of PBPC and myeloid reconstitution post-transplant were compared between four groups of patients (n=196) receiving LEUKINE for mobilization and a historical control group who did not receive any mobilization treatment [progenitor cells collected by leukapheresis without mobilization (n=100)]. Sequential cohorts received LEUKINE. The cohorts differed by dose (125 or 250 mcg/m^2/day), route (IV over 24 hours or SC) and use of LEUKINE post-transplant. Leukaphereses were initiated for all mobilization groups after the WBC reached 10,000/mm^3. Leukaphereses continued until both a minimum number of mononucleated cells (MNC) were collected (6.5 or 8.0 × 10^8/kg body weight) and a minimum number of phereses (5–8) were performed. Both minimum requirements varied by treatment cohort and planned conditioning regimen. If subjects failed to reach a WBC of 10,000 cells/mm^3 by day 5, another cytokine was substituted for LEUKINE; these subjects were all successfully leukapheresed and transplanted. The most marked mobilization and post-transplant effects were seen in patients administered the higher dose of LEUKINE (250 mcg/m^2) either IV (n=63) or SC (n=41).

PBPCs from patients treated at the 250 mcg/m^2/day dose had significantly higher number of granulocyte-macrophage colony-forming units (CFU-GM) than those collected without mobilization. The mean value after thawing was 11.41 × 10^4 CFU-GM/kg for all LEUKINE-mobilized patients, compared to 0.96 × 10^4/kg for the non-mobilized group. A similar difference was observed in the mean number of erythrocyte burst-forming units (BFU-E) collected (23.96 × 10^4/kg for patients mobilized with 250 mcg/m^2 doses of LEUKINE administered SC vs. 1.63 × 10^4/kg for non-mobilized patients).

[See second table above]

After transplantation, mobilized subjects had shorter times to myeloid engraftment and fewer days between transplantation and the last platelet transfusion compared to non-mobilized subjects. Neutrophil recovery (ANC >500/mm^3) was more rapid in patients administered LEUKINE following PBPC transplantation with LEUKINE-mobilized cells (see table at right). Mobilized patients also had fewer days to the last platelet transfusion and last RBC transfusion, and a shorter duration of hospitalization than did non-mobilized subjects.

A second retrospective review of data from patients undergoing PBPC at another single transplant center was also conducted. LEUKINE was given SC at 250 mcg/m^{2}day once a day (n=10) or twice a day (n=21) until completion of the pheresis. Phereses were begun on day 5 of LEUKINE administration and continued until the targeted MNC count of 9 × 10^8/kg or CD34+ cell count of 1 × 10^5/kg was reached. There was no difference in CD34+ cell count in patients receiving LEUKINE once or twice a day. The median time to ANC>500/mm^3 was 12 days and to platelet recovery (>25,000/mm^3) was 23 days.

Survival studies comparing mobilized study patients to the non-mobilized patients and to an autologous historical bone marrow transplant group showed no differences in median survival time.

Autologous Bone Marrow Transplantation[7] Following a dose-ranging Phase I/II trial in patients undergoing autologous BMT for lymphoid malignancies,[8, 9] three single center, randomized, placebo-controlled and double-blind studies were conducted to evaluate the safety and efficacy of LEUKINE for promoting hematopoietic reconstitution following autologous BMT. A total of 128 patients (65 LEUKINE, 63 placebo) were enrolled in these 3 studies. The majority of the patients had lymphoid malignancy (87 NHL, 17 ALL), 23 patients had Hodgkin's disease, and 1 patient had acute myeloblastic leukemia (AML). In 72 patients with NHL or ALL, the bone marrow harvest was purged prior to storage with one of several monoclonal antibodies. No chemical agent was used for *in vitro* treatment of the bone marrow. Preparative regimens in the 3 studies included cyclophosphamide (total dose 120–150 mg/kg) and total body irradiation (total dose 1,200–1,575 rads). Other regimens used in patients with Hodgkin's disease and NHL without radiotherapy consisted of 3 or more of the following in combination (expressed as total dose): cytosine arabinoside (400 mg/m^2) and carmustine (300 mg/m^2), cyclophosphamide (140–150 mg/kg), hydroxyurea (4.5 grams/m^2) and etoposide (375–450 mg/m^2).

Compared to placebo, administration of LEUKINE in 2 studies (n=44 and 47) significantly improved the following hematologic and clinical endpoints: time to neutrophil engraftment, duration of hospitalization and infection experience or antibacterial usage. In the third study (n=37) there was a positive trend toward earlier myeloid engraftment in favor of LEUKINE. This latter study differed from the other 2 in having enrolled a large number of patients with Hodgkin's disease who had also received extensive radiation and chemotherapy prior to harvest of autologous bone marrow. A subgroup analysis of the data from all 3 studies revealed that the median time to engraftment for patients with Hodgkin's disease, regardless of treatment, was 6 days longer when compared to patients with NHL and ALL, but that the overall beneficial LEUKINE treatment was the same. In the following combined analysis of the 3 studies, these 2 subgroups (NHL and ALL vs Hodgkin's disease) are presented separately.

Patients with Lymphoid Malignancy (Non-Hodgkin's Lymphoma and Acute Lymphoblastic Leukemia): Myeloid engraftment (absolute neutrophil count [ANC] ≥ 500 cells/mm^3) in 54 patients receiving LEUKINE was observed 6 days earlier than in 50 patients treated with placebo (see table at right).

[See table at top of next page]

Accelerated myeloid engraftment was associated with significant clinical benefits. The median duration of hospitalization was 6 days shorter with the LEUKINE group than for the placebo group. Median duration of infectious episodes (defined as fever and neutropenia; or 2 positive cultures of the same organism; or fever >38°C and 1 positive blood culture; or clinical evidence of infection) was 3 days less in the group treated with LEUKINE. The median duration of antibacterial administration in the post-transplantation period was 4 days shorter for the patients treated with LEUKINE than for the placebo-treated patients. The study was unable to detect a significant difference between the treatment groups in rate of disease relapse 24 months post-transplantation. As a group, leukemic subjects received LEUKINE derived less benefit than NHL subjects. However, both the leukemic and NHL groups receiving LEUKINE engrafted earlier than controls.

Patients with Hodgkin's Disease: If patients with Hodgkin's disease are analysed separately, a trend toward earlier myeloid engraftment is noted. LEUKINE-treated patients engrafted earlier (by 5 days) than the placebo-treated patients (p=0.189, Wilcoxon) but the number of patients was small (n=22). Studies are in progress to confirm statistically the trend toward earlier engraftment with LEUKINE in patients with Hodgkin's disease.

Allogeneic Bone Marrow Transplantation: A multi-center, randomized, placebo-controlled, and double-blinded study was conducted to evaluate the safety and efficacy of LEUKINE for promoting hematopoietic reconstitution following allogeneic BMT. A total of 109 patients (53 LEUKINE, 56 placebo) were enrolled in the study. Twenty-three patients (11 LEUKINE, 12 placebo) were 18 years old or younger. Sixty-seven patients had myeloid malignancies (33 AML, 34 CML), 17 had lymphoid malignancies (12 ALL, 5 NHL), 3 patients had Hodgkin's disease, 6 had multiple myeloma, 9 had myelodysplastic disease, and 7 patients had aplastic anemia. In 22 patients at one of the seven study sites, bone marrow harvests were depleted of T cells. Preparative regi-

Continued on next page

Leukine—Cont.

mens included cyclophosphamide, busulfan, cytosine arabinoside, etoposide, methotrexate, corticosteroids, and asparaginase. Some patients also received total body, splenic, or testicular irradiation. Primary graft-versus-host disease (GVHD) prophylaxis was cyclosporine A and a corticosteroid.

Accelerated myeloid engraftment was associated with significant laboratory and clinical benefits. Compared to placebo, administration of LEUKINE significantly improved following: time to neutrophil engraftment, duration of hospitalization, number of patients with bacteremia and overall incidence of infection (see table at right).

[See second table at right]

Median time to myeloid engraftment (ANC ≥500 cells/mm³) in 53 patients receiving LEUKINE (sargramostim) was 4 days less than in 56 patients treated with placebo (see table at right). The number of patients with bacteremia and infection was significantly lower in the LEUKINE group compared to the placebo group (9/53 versus 19/56 and 30/53 versus 42/56, respectively). There were a number of secondary laboratory and clinical endpoints. Of these, only the incidence of severe (grade 3/4) mucositis was significantly improved in the LEUKINE group (4/53) compared to the placebo group (16/56) at p<0.05. LEUKINE-treated patients also had a shorter median duration of post-transplant IV antibiotic infusions, and shorter median number of days to last platelet and RBC transfusions compared to placebo patients, but none of these differences reached statistical significance.

Bone Marrow Transplantation Failure or Engraftment Delay A historically controlled study was conducted in patients experiencing graft failure following allogeneic or autologous BMT to determine whether LEUKINE improved survival after BMT failure.

Three categories of patients were eligible for this study:

1) patients displaying a delay in engraftment (ANC ≤ 100 cells/mm³ by day 28 post-transplantation);

2) patients displaying a delay in engraftment (ANC ≤ 100 cells/mm³ by day 21 post-transplantation) and who had evidence of an active infection, and

3) patients who lost their marrow graft after a transient engraftment (manifested by an average of ANC ≥ 500 cells/mm³ for at least one week followed by loss of engraftment with ANC <500 cells/mm³ for at least one week beyond day 21 post-transplantation).

A total of 140 eligible patients from 35 institutions were treated with LEUKINE and evaluated in comparison to 103 historical control patients from a single institution. One hundred sixty-three patients had lymphoid or myeloid leukemia, 24 patients had non-Hodgkin's lymphoma, 19 patients had Hodgkin's disease and 37 patients had other diseases, such as aplastic anemia, myelodysplasia or non-hematologic malignancy. The majority of patients (223 out of 243) had received prior chemotherapy with or without radiotherapy and/or immunotherapy prior to preparation for transplantation.

One hundred day survival was improved in favor of the patients treated with LEUKINE after graft failure following either autologous or allogeneic BMT. In addition, the median survival was improved by greater than 2-fold. The median survival of patients treated with LEUKINE after autologus failure was 474 days versus 161 days for the historical patients. Similarly, after allogeneic failure, the median survival was 97 days with LEUKINE treatment and 35 days for the historical controls. Improvement in survival was better in patients with fewer impaired organs.

The MOF score is a simple clinical laboratory assessment of 7 major organ systems: cardiovascular, respiratory, gastrointestinal, hematologic, renal, hepatic and neurologic.[10] Assessment of the MOF score is recommended as an additional method of determining the need to initiate treatment with LEUKINE in patients with graft failure or delay in engraftment following autologous or allogeneic BMT.

[See third table above]

Factors that Contribute to Survival: The probability of survival was relatively greater for patients with any one of the following characteristics: autologous BMT failure or delay in engraftment, exclusion of total body irradiation from the preparative regimen, a non-leukemic malignancy or MOF score ≤ 2 (0, 1 or 2 dysfunctional organ systems). Leukemic subjects derived less benefit than other subjects.

CONTRAINDICATIONS

LEUKINE is contraindicated:

1) in patients with excessive leukemic myeloid blasts in the bone marrow or peripheral blood (≥ 10%).

2) in patients with known hypersensitivity to GM-CSF yeast-derived products or any component of the product.

3) for concomitant use with chemotherapy or radiotherapy. Due to the potential sensitivity of rapidly dividing hematopoietic progenitor cells, LEUKINE should not be administered simultaneously with cytotoxic chemotherapy or radiotherapy or within 24 hours preceding or following chemotherapy or radiotherapy. In one controlled study,

Autologous BMT: Combined Analysis from Placebo-Controlled Clinical Trials of Responses in Patients with NHL and ALL
Median Value (days)

	ANC ≥500/mm³	ANC ≥1000/mm³	Duration of Hospitalization	Duration of Infection	Duration of Antibacterial Therapy
LEUKINE (n=54)	18*#	24*#	25*	1*	21*
Placebo (n=50)	24	32	31	4	25

* p<0.05 Wilcoxon or CMH ridit chi-squared
\# p<0.05 Log rank
Note: The single AML patient was not included.

Allogeneic BMT: Analysis of Data from Placebo-Controlled Clinical Trial
Median Values (days or number of patients)

	ANC ≥ 500/mm³	ANC ≥ 1000/mm³	Number of Patients with Infections	Number of Patients with Bacteremia	Days of Hospitalization
LEUKINE (n=53)	13*	14*	30*	9**	25*
Placebo (n=56)	17	19	42	19	26

* p<0.05 generalized Wilcoxon test
** p<0.05 simple chi-square test

Median Survival by Multiple Organ failure (MOF) Category
Median Survival (days)

	MOF ≤ 2 Organs	MOF ≤ 2 Organs	MOF (Composite of Both Groups)
Autologous BMT			
LEUKINE	474 (n=58)	78.5 (n=10)	474 (n=68)
Historical	165 (n=14)	39 (n=3)	161 (n=17)
Allogeneic BMT			
LEUKINE	174 (n =50)	27 (n=22)	97 (n=72)
Historical	52.5 (n=60)	15.5 (n=26)	35 (n=86)

patients with small cell lung cancer received LEUKINE and concurrent thoracic radiotherapy and chemotherapy or the identical radiotherapy and chemotherapy without LEUKINE. The patients randomized to LEUKINE had significantly higher incidence of adverse events, including higher mortality and a higher incidence of grade 3 and 4 infections and grade 3 and 4 thrombocytopenia.[11]

WARNINGS

Pediatric Use Benzyl alcohol is a constituent of LEUKINE Liquid and Bacteriostatic Water for Injection diluent. Benzyl alcohol has been reported to be associated with a fatal "Gasping Syndrome" in premature infants **Liquid solutions containing benzyl alcohol (including LEUKINE Liquid) or lyophilized LEUKINE reconstituted with Bacteriostatic Water for Injection, USP (0.9% benzyl alcohol) should not be administered to neonates** (see PRECAUTIONS and DOSAGE AND ADMINISTRATION).

Fluid Retention Edema, capillary leak syndrome, pleural and/or pericardial effusion have been reported in patients after LEUKINE administration. In 156 patients enrolled in placebo-controlled studies using LEUKINE at a dose of 250 mcg/m²/day by 2-hour IV infusion, the reported incidences of fluid retention (LEUKINE vs. placebo) were as follows: peripheral edema, 11% vs. 7%; pleural effusion, 1% vs. 0%; and pericardial effusion, 4% vs. 1%. Capillary leak syndrome was not observed in this limited number of studies; based on other uncontrolled studies and reports from users of marketed LEUKINE, the incidence is estimated to be less than 1%. In patients with preexisting pleural and pericardial effusions, administration of LEUKINE may aggravate fluid retention; however, fluid retention associated with or worsened by LEUKINE has been reversible after interruption or dose reduction of LEUKINE with or without diuretic therapy. LEUKINE should be used with caution in patients with preexisting fluid retention, pulmonary infiltrates or congestive heart failure.

Respiratory Symptoms Sequestration of granulocytes in the pulmonary circulation has been documented following LEUKINE infusion,[12] and dyspnea has been reported occasionally in patients treated with LEUKINE. Special attention should be given to respiratory symptoms during or immediately following LEUKINE infusion, especially in patients with preexisting lung disease. In patients displaying dyspnea during LEUKINE administration, the rate of infusion should be reduced by half. If respiratory symptoms worsen despite infusion rate reduction, the infusion should be discontinued. Subsequent IV infusions may be administered following the standard dose schedule with careful monitoring. LEUKINE should be administered with caution in patients with hypoxia.

Cardiovascular Symptoms Occasional transient supraventricular arrhythmias has been reported in uncontrolled studies during LEUKINE administration, particularly in patients with a previous history of cardiac arrhythmia. However, these arrhythmias have been reversible after discontinuation of LEUKINE. LEUKINE should be used with caution in patients with preexisting cardiac disease.

Renal and Hepatic Dysfunction In some patients with preexisting renal or hepatic dysfunction enrolled in uncontrolled clinical trials, administration of LEUKINE has induced elevation of serum creatinine or bilirubin and hepatic enzymes. Dose reduction or interruption of LEUKINE administration has resulted in a decrease to pretreatment values. However, in controlled clinical trials the incidences of renal and hepatic dysfunction were comparable between LEUKINE (250 mcg/m²/day by 2-hour IV infusion) and placebo-treated patients. Monitoring of renal and hepatic function in patients displaying renal or hepatic dysfunction prior to initiation of treatment is recommended at least every other week during LEUKINE administration.

PRECAUTIONS

General Parenteral administration of recombinant proteins should be attended by appropriate precautions in case an allergic or untoward reaction occurs. Serious allergic or anaphylactic reactions have been reported. If any serious allergic or anaphylactic reaction occurs, LEUKINE therapy should immediately be discontinued and appropriate therapy initiated.

A syndrome characterized by respiratory distress, hypoxia, flushing, hypotension, syncope, and/or tachycardia has been reported following the first administration of LEUKINE (sargramostim) in a particular cycle. These signs have resolved with symptomatic treatment and usually do not recur with subsequent doses in the same cycle of treatment. Stimulation of marrow precursors with LEUKINE may result in a rapid rise in white blood cell (WBC) count. If the ANC exceeds 20,000 cells/mm³ or if the platelet count exceeds 500,000/mm³, LEUKINE administration should be interrupted or the dose reduced by half. The decision to reduce the dose or interrupt treatment should be based on the clinical condition of the patient. Excessive blood counts have returned to normal or baseline levels within 3 to 7 days following cessation of LEUKINE therapy. Twice weekly monitoring of CBC with differential (including examination for the presence of blast cells) should be performed to preclude development of excessive counts.

Growth Factor Potential LEUKINE is a growth factor that primarily stimulates normal myeloid precursors. However, the possibility that LEUKINE can act as a growth factor for any tumor type, particularly myeloid malignancies, cannot

be excluded. Because of the possibility of tumor growth potentiation, precaution should be exercised when using this drug in any malignancy with myeloid characteristics.

Should disease progression be detected during LEUKINE treatment, LEUKINE therapy should be discontinued.

LEUKINE has been administered to patients with myelodysplastic syndromes (MDS) in uncontrolled studies without evidence of increased relapse rates.[13, 14, 15] Controlled studies have not been performed in patients with MDS.

Use in Patients Receiving Purged Bone Marrow LEUKINE is effective in accelerating myeloid recovery in patients receiving bone marrow purged by anti-B lymphocyte monoclonal antibodies. Data obtained from uncontrolled studies suggest that if *in vitro* marrow purging with chemical agents causes a significant decrease in the number of responsive hematopoietic progenitors, the patient may not respond to LEUKINE. When the bone marrow purging process preserves a sufficient number of progenitors (>1.2 × 10^4/kg), a beneficial effect of LEUKINE on myeloid engraftment has been reported.[16]

Use in Patients Previously Exposed to Intensive Chemotherapy/Radiotherapy In patients who before autologous BMT, have received extensive radiotherapy to hematopoietic sites for the treatment of primary disease in the abdomen or chest, or have been exposed to multiple myelotoxic agents (alkylating agents, anthracycline antibiotics and antimetabolites), the effect of LEUKINE on myeloid reconstitution may be limited.

Use in Patients with Malignancy Undergoing LEUKINE-Mobilized PBPC Collection When using LEUKINE to mobilize PBPC, the limited *in vitro* data suggest that tumor cells may be released and reinfused into the patient in the leukapheresis product. The effect of reinfusion of tumor cells has not been well studied and the data are inconclusive.

Patient Monitoring LEUKINE can induce variable increases in WBC and/or platelet counts. In order to avoid potential complications of excessive leukocytosis (WBC >50,000 cells/mm^3; ANC >20,000 cells/mm^3), a CBC is recommended twice per week during LEUKINE therapy. Monitoring of renal and hepatic function in patients displaying renal or hepatic dysfunction prior to initiation of treatment is recommended at least biweekly during LEUKINE administration. Body weight and hydration status should be carefully monitored during LEUKINE administration.

Drug Interaction Interactions between LEUKINE and other drugs have not been fully evaluated. Drugs which may potentiate the myeloproliferative effects of LEUKINE, such as lithium and corticosteroids, should be used with caution.

Carcinogenesis, Mutagenesis, Impairment of Fertility Animal studies have not been conducted with LEUKINE to evaluate the carcinogenic potential or the effect on fertility.

Pregnancy (Category C) Animal reproduction studies have not been conducted with LEUKINE. It is not known whether LEUKINE can cause fetal harm when administered to a pregnant woman or can affect reproductive capability. LEUKINE should be given to a pregnant woman only if clearly needed.

Nursing Mothers It is not known whether LEUKINE is excreted in human milk. Because many drugs are excreted in human milk, LEUKINE should be administered to a nursing women only if clearly needed.

Pediatric Use Safety and effectiveness in pediatric patients have not been established; however, available safety data indicate that LEUKINE does not exhibit any greater toxicity in pediatric patients than in adults. A total of 124 pediatric subjects between the ages of 4 months and 18 years have been treated with LEUKINE in clinical trials at doses ranging from 60–1,000 mcg/m^2/day intravenously and 4–1,500 mcg/m^2/day subcutaneously. In 53 pediatric patients enrolled in controlled studies at a dose of 250 mcg/m^2/day by 2-hour IV infusion, the type and frequency of adverse events were comparable to those reported for the adult population. **Liquid solutions containing benzyl alcohol (including LEUKINE Liquid) or lyophilized LEUKINE reconstituted with Bacteriostatic Water for Injection, USP (0.9% benzyl alcohol) should not be administered to neonates (see WARNINGS).**

ADVERSE REACTIONS

Autologous and Allogeneic Bone Marrow Transplantation LEUKINE is generally well tolerated. In 3 placebo-controlled studies enrolling a total of 156 patients after autologous BMT or peripheral blood progenitor cell transplantation, events reported in at least 10% of patients who received IV LEUKINE or placebo were as reported at right:

[See table above]

Percent of AuBMT Patients Reporting Events

Events by Body System	LEUKINE (n=79)	Placebo (n=77)	Events by Body System	LEUKINE (n=79)	Placebo (n=77)
Body, General			**Metabolic/Nutritional Disorder**		
Fever	95	96	Edema	34	35
Mucous membrane disorder	75	78	Peripheral edema	11	7
Asthenia	66	51	**Respiratory System**		
Malaise	57	51	Dyspnea	28	31
Sepsis	11	14	Lung disorder	20	23
Digestive System			**Hemic and Lymphatic System**		
Nausea	90	96	Blood dyscrasia	25	27
Diarrhea	89	82	**Cardiovascular System**		
Vomiting	85	90	Hemorrhage	23	30
Anorexia	54	58	**Urogenital System**		
GI disorder	37	47	Urinary tract disorder	14	13
GI hemorrhage	27	33	Kidney function abnormal	8	10
Stomatitis	24	29	**Nervous System**		
Liver damage	13	14	CNS disorder	11	16
Skin and Appendages					
Alopecia	73	74			
Rash	44	38			

No significant differences were observed between LEUKINE and placebo-treated patients in the type or frequency of laboratory abnormalities, including renal and hepatic parameters. In some patients with preexisting renal or hepatic dysfunction enrolled in uncontrolled clinical trials, administration of LEUKINE has induced elevation of serum creatinine or bilirubin and hepatic enzymes (see WARNINGS). In addition, there was no significant difference in relapse rate and 24 month survival between the LEUKINE and placebo-treated patients.

In the placebo-controlled trial of 109 patients after allogeneic BMT, events reported in at least 10% of patients who received IV LEUKINE or placebo were as reported at right:

[See table at top of next page]

There were no significant differences in the incidence or severity of GVHD, relapse rates and survival between the LEUKINE and placebo-treated patients.

Adverse events observed for the patients treated with LEUKINE (sargramostim) in the historically controlled BMT failure study were similar to those reported in the placebo-controlled studies. In addition, headache (26%), pericardial effusion (25%), arthralgia (21%) and myalgia (18%) were also reported in patients treated with LEUKINE in the graft failure study.

In uncontrolled Phase I/II studies with LEUKINE in 215 patients, the most frequent adverse events were fever, asthenia, headache, bone pain, chills and myalgia. These systemic events were generally mild to moderate and were usually prevented or reversed by the administration of analgesics and antipyretics such as acetaminophen. In these uncontrolled trials, other infrequent events reported were dyspnea, peripheral edema, and rash.

Reports of events occurring marketed LEUKINE include arrhythmia, fainting, eosinophilia, dizziness, hypotension, injection site reactions, pain (including abdominal, back, chest, and joint pain), tachycardia, thrombosis, and transient liver function abnormalities.

In patients with preexisting edema, capillary leak syndrome, pleural and/or pericardial effusion, administration of LEUKINE may aggravate fluid retention (see WARNINGS). Body weight and hydration status should be carefully monitored during LEUKINE administration.

Adverse events observed in pediatric patients in controlled studies were comparable to those observed in adult patients.

Acute Myelogenous Leukemia Adverse events reported in at least 10% of patients who received LEUKINE or placebo were as reported at right:

[See second table at top of next page]

Nearly all patients reported leukopenia, thrombocytopenia and anemia. The frequency and type of adverse events observed following induction were similar between LEUKINE and placebo groups. The only significant difference in the rates of these adverse events was an increase in skin associated events in the LEUKINE group (p=0.002). No significant differences were observed in laboratory results, renal or hepatic toxicity. No significant differences were observed between the LEUKINE- and placebo-treated patients for adverse events following consolidation. There was no significant difference in response rate or relapse rate.

In a historically controlled study of 86 patients with acute myelogenous leukemia (AML), the LEUKINE treated group exhibited an increased incidence of weight gain (p=0.007), low serum proteins and prolonged prothrombin time (p=0.02) when compared to the control group. Two LEUKINE treated patients had progressive increase in circulating monocytes and promonocytes and blasts in the marrow which reversed when LEUKINE was discontinued. The historical control group exhibited an increased incidence of cardiac events (p=0.018), liver function abnormalities (p=0.008), and neurocortical hemorrhagic events (p=0.025).[15]

Overdosage The maximum amount of LEUKINE that can be safely administered in single or multiple doses has not been determined. Doses up to 100 mcg/kg/day (4,000 mcg/m^2/day or 16 times the recommended dose) were administered to 4 patients in a Phase I uncontrolled clinical study by continuous IV infusion for 7 to 18 days. Increases in WBC up to 200,000 cells/mm^3 were observed. Adverse events reported were dyspnea, malaise, nausea, fever, rash, sinus tachycardia, headache and chills. All these events were reversible after discontinuation of LEUKINE.

In case of overdosage, LEUKINE therapy should be discontinued and the patient carefully monitored for WBC increase and respiratory symptoms.

DOSAGE AND ADMINISTRATION

Neutrophil Recovery Following Chemotherapy in Acute Myelogenous Leukemia The recommended dose is 250 mcg/m^2/day administered intravenously over a 4 hour period starting approximately on day 11 or 4 days following the completion of induction chemotherapy, if the day 10 bone marrow is hypoplastic with <5% blasts. If a second cycle of induction chemotherapy is necessary, LEUKINE should be administered approximately 4 days after the completion of chemotherapy if the bone marrow is hypoplastic with <5% blasts. LEUKINE should be continued until an ANC >1500 cells/mm^3 for 3 consecutive days or a maximum of 42 days. LEUKINE should be discontinued immediately if leukemic regrowth occurs. If a severe adverse reaction occurs, the dose can be reduced by 50% or temporarily discontinued until the reaction abates.

In order to avoid potential complications of excessive leukocytosis (WBC >50,000 cells/mm^3 or ANC >20,000 cells/mm^3) a CBC with differential is recommended twice per week during LEUKINE therapy. LEUKINE treatment should be interrupted or the dose reduced by half if the ANC exceeds 20,000 cells/mm^3.

Mobilization of Peripheral Blood Progenitor Cells The recommended dose is 250 mcg/m^2/day administered IV over 24 hours or SC once daily. Dosing should continue at the same dose through the period of PBPC collection. The optimal schedule for PBPC collection has not been established. In clinical studies, collection of PBPC was usually begun by day 5 and performed daily until protocol specified targets were achieved (see CLINICAL EXPERIENCE, Mobilization and Engraftment of PBPC). If WBC >50,000 cells/mm^3, the LEUKINE dose should be reduced by 50%. If adequate numbers of progenitor cells are not collected, other mobilization therapy should be considered.

Post Peripheral Blood Progenitor Cell Transplantation The recommended dose is 250 mcg/m^2/day administered IV over 24 hours or SC once daily beginning immediately following infusion of progenitor cells and continuing until an ANC>1500 cells/mm^3 for 3 consecutive days is attained.

Myeloid Reconstitution After Autologous or Allogeneic Bone Marrow Transplantation The recommended dose is 250 mcg/m^2/day administered IV over a 2-hour period beginning 2 to 4 hours after bone marrow infusion, and not less than 24 hours after the last dose of chemotherapy or radiotherapy. Patients should not receive LEUKINE until the post marrow infusion ANC is less than 500 cells/mm^3. LEUKINE should be continued until an ANC >1500 cells/mm^3 for 3 consecutive days is attained. If a severe adverse reaction occurs, the dose can be reduced by 50% of temporarily discontinued until the reaction abates. LEUKINE should be discontinued immediately if blast cells appear or disease progression occurs.

In order to avoid potential complications of excessive leukocytosis (WBC >50,000 cells/mm^3 ANC >20,000 cells/mm^3) a CBC with differential is recommended twice per week during LEUKINE therapy. LEUKINE treatment should be interrupted or the dose reduced by 50% if the ANC exceeds 20,000 cells/mm^3.

Bone Marrow Transplantation Failure or Engraftment Delay The recommended dose is 250 mcg/m^2/day for 14 days as a 2-hour IV infusion. The dose can be repeated after 7 days off therapy if engraftment has not occurred. If engraftment still has not occurred, a third course of 500 mcg/m^2/

Continued on next page

Leukine—Cont.

day for 14 days may be tried after another 7 days off therapy. If there is still no improvement, it is unlikely that further dose escalation will be beneficial. If a severe adverse reaction occurs, the dose can be reduced by 50% or temporarily discontinued until the reaction abates. LEUKINE should be discontinued immediately if blast cells appear or disease progression occurs.

In order to avoid potential complications of excessive leukocytosis (WBC >50,000 cells/mm^3 and ANC >20,000 cells/mm^3) a CBC with differential is recommended twice per week during LEUKINE therapy. LEUKINE treatment should be interrupted or the dose reduced by half if the ANC exceeds 20,000 cells/mm^3.

Preparation of LEUKINE

1. LEUKINE Liquid is formulated as a sterile, preserved (1.1% benzyl alcohol), injectable solution (500 mcg/mL) in a vial. Lyophilized LEUKINE is a sterile, white, preservative-free powder (250 mcg) that requires reconstitution with 1 mL Sterile Water for Injection, USP, or 1 mL Bacteriostatic Water for Injection, USP.
2. LEUKINE Liquid may be stored for up to 20 days at 2–8°C once the vial has been entered. Discard any remaining solution after 20 days.
3. Lyophilized LEUKINE (250 mcg) should be reconstituted aseptically with 1.0 mL of diluent (see below). The contents of vials reconstituted with different diluents should not be mixed together.

Sterile Water for Injection, USP (without preservative): Lyophilized LEUKINE vials contain no antibacterial preservative, and therefore solutions prepared with Sterile Water for Injection, USP should be administered as soon as possible, and within 6 hours following reconstitution and/or dilution for IV infusion. The vial should not be reentered or reused. Do not save any unused portion for administration more than 6 hours following reconstitution. *Bacteriostatic Water for Injection, USP (0.9% benzyl alcohol):* Reconstituted solutions prepared with Bacteriostatic Water for Injection, USP (0.9% benzyl alcohol) may be stored for up to 20 days at 2–8°C prior to use. Discard reconstituted solution after 20 days. Previously reconstituted solutions mixed with freshly reconstituted solutions must be administered within 6 hours following mixing. **Preparations containing benzyl alcohol (including LEUKINE Liquid and lyophilized LEUKINE reconstituted with Bacteriostatic Water for Injection) should not be used in neonates (see WARNINGS).**

4. During reconstitution of lyophilized LEUKINE the diluent should be directed at the side of the vial and the contents gently swirled to avoid foaming during dissolution. Avoid excessive or vigorous agitation; do not shake.
5. LEUKINE should be used for SC injection without further dilution. Dilution for IV infusion should be performed in 0.9% Sodium Chloride Injection, USP. If the final concentration of LEUKINE is below 10 mcg/mL, Albumin (Human) at a final concentration of 0.1% should be added to the saline prior to addition of LEUKINE to prevent adsorption to the components of the drug delivery system. To obtain a final concentration of 0.1% Albumin (Human), add 1 mg Albumin (Human) per 1 mL 0.9% Sodium Chloride Injection, USP (e.g., use 1 mL 5% Albumin [Human] in 50 mL 0.9% Sodium Chloride Injection, USP).
6. An in-line membrane filter should NOT be used for intravenous infusion of LEUKINE.
7. Store LEUKINE Liquid and reconstituted lyophilized LEUKINE solutions under refrigeration at 2–8°C (36–46°F); DO NOT FREEZE.
8. In the absence of compatibility and stability information, no other medication should be added to infusion solutions containing LEUKINE. Use only 0.9% Sodium Chloride Injection, USP to prepare IV infusion solutions.
9. Aseptic technique should be employed in the preparation of all LEUKINE solutions. To assure correct concentration following reconstitution, care should be exercised to eliminate any air bubbles from the needle hub of the syringe used to prepare the diluent. Parenteral drug products should be inspected visually for particulate matter and discoloration prior to administration whenever solution and container permit.

HOW SUPPLIED

LEUKINE Liquid is available in vials containing 500 mcg/mL (2.8 × 10^6 IU/mL) sargramostim. Lyophilized LEUKINE is available in vials containing 250 mcg (1.4 × 10^6 IU/vial) sargramostim.

Each dosage form is supplied as follows:
Carton of 5 vials of lyophilized LEUKINE 250 mcg (NDC 58406-002-33).
Carton of 5 multiple-dose vials; each vial contains 1 mL of preserved 500 mcg/mL LEUKINE Liquid (NDC 58406-050-30).

STORAGE

LEUKINE should be refrigerated at 2–8°C (36–46°F). Do not freeze or shake. Do not use beyond the expiration date printed on the vial.

Percent of Allogeneic BMT Patients Reporting Events

Events by Body System	LEUKINE (n=53)	Placebo (n=56)
Body, General		
Fever	77	80
Abdominal pain	38	23
Headache	36	36
Chills	25	20
Pain	17	36
Asthenia	17	20
Chest pain	15	9
Back pain	9	18
Digestive System		
Diarrhea	81	66
Nausea	70	66
Vomiting	70	57
Stomatitis	62	63
Anorexia	51	57
Dyspepsia	17	20
Hematemesis	13	7
Dysphagia	11	7
GI hemorrhage	11	5
Constipation	8	11
Skin and Appendages		
Rash	70	73
Alopecia	45	45
Pruritis	23	13
Musculo-skeletal System		
Bone pain	21	5
Arthralgia	11	4
Special Senses		
Eye hemorrhage	11	0
Cardiovascular System		
Hypertension	34	32
Tachycardia	11	9

Events by Body System	LEUKINE (n=53)	Placebo (n=56)
Metabolic/Nutritional Disorders		
Bilirubinemia	30	27
Hyperglycemia	25	23
Peripheral edema	15	21
Increased creatinine	15	14
Hypomagnesemia	15	9
Increased SGPT	13	16
Edema	13	11
Increased alk. phosphatase	8	14
Respiratory System		
Pharyngitis	23	13
Epistaxis	17	16
Dyspnea	15	14
Rhinitis	11	14
Hemic and Lymphatic System		
Thrombocytopenia	19	34
Leukopenia	17	29
Petechia	6	11
Agranulocytosis	6	11
Urogenital System		
Hematuria	9	21
Nervous System		
Paresthesia	11	13
Insomnia	11	9
Anxiety	11	2
Laboratory Abnormalities*		
High glucose	41	49
Low albumin	27	36
High BUN	23	17
Low calcium	2	7
High cholesterol	17	8

* *Grade 3 and 4 laboratory abnormalities only. Denominators may vary due to missing laboratory measurements.*

Percent of AML Patients Reporting Events

Events by Body System	LEUKINE (n=52)	Placebo (n=47)
Body General		
Fever (no injection)	81	74
Infection	65	68
Weight loss	37	28
Weight gain	8	21
Chills	19	26
Allergy	12	15
Sweats	6	13
Digestive System		
Nausea	58	55
Liver	77	83
Diarrhea	52	53
Vomiting	46	34
Stomatitis	42	43
Anorexia	13	11
Abdominal distention	4	13
Skin and Appendages		
Skin	77	45
Alopecia	37	51

Events by Body System	LEUKINE (n=52)	Placebo (n=47)
Metabolic/Nutritional Disorder		
Metabolic	58	49
Edema	25	23
Respiratory System		
Pulmonary	48	64
Hemic and Lymphatic System		
Coagulation	19	21
Cardiovascular System		
Hemorrhage	29	43
Hypertension	25	32
Cardiac	23	32
Hypotension	13	26
Urogenital System		
GU	50	57
Nervous System		
Neuro-clinical	42	53
Neuro-motor	25	26
Neuro-psych	15	26
Neuro-sensory	6	11

REFERENCES

1. Metcalf D. The molecular biology and functions of the granulocyte-macrophage colony-stimulating factors. Blood 1986; 67(2):257–267.
2. Park LS, Friend D, Gillis S, Urdal DL. Characterization of the cell surface receptor for human granulocyte/macrophage colony stimulating factor. J Exp Med 1986; 164: 251–262.
3. Grabstein KH, Urdal DL, Tushinski RJ, et al. Induction of macrophage tumoricidal activity by granulocyte-macrophage colony-stimulating factors. Science 1986; 232: 506–508.
4. Reed SG, Nathan CF, Pihl DL, et al. Recombinant granulocyte/macrophage colony-stimulating factor activates macrophages to inhibit Trypanosoma cruzi and release hydrogen peroxide. J Exp Med 1987; 166:1734–1746.
5. Data on file Immunex Corporation; Seattle, WA.
6. Rowe JM, Andersen JW, Mazza JJ, et al. A randomized placebo-controlled phase III study of granulocyte-macrophage colony-stimulating factor in adult patients (>55 to 70 years of age) with acute myelogenous leukemia: a study of the Eastern Cooperative Oncology Group (E1490). Blood 1995; 86(2):457–462.
7. Nemunaitis J, Rabinowe SN, Singer JW, et al. Recombinant human granulocyte-macrophage colony-stimulating factor after autologous bone marrow transplantation for lymphoid malignancy: Pooled results of a randomized, double-blind, placebo controlled trial. NEJM 1991; 324(25):1773–1778.
8. Nemunaitis J, Singer JW, Buckner CD, et al. Use of recombinant human granulocyte-macrophages colony-stimulating factor in autologous bone marrow transplantation for lymphoid malignancies. Blood 1988; 72(2):834–836.
9. Nemunaitis J, Singer JW, Buckner CD, et al. Long-term follow-up of patients who received recombinant human granulocyte-macrophage colony-stimulating factor after autologous bone marrow transplantation for lymphoid malignancy. BMT 1991; 7:49–52.
10. Goris RJA, Boekhorst TPA, Nuytinck JKS, et al. Multiple organ failure: Generalized auto-destructive inflammation? Arch Surg 1985; 120:1109–1115.
11. Bunn P, Crowley J, Kelly J, et al. Chemoradiotherapy with or without granulocyte-macrophage colony-stimulating factor in the treatment of limited-state small-cell lung cancer: a prospective phase III randomized study of the southwest oncology group JCO 1995; 13(7):1632–1641.
12. Hermann F, Schultz G, Lindemann A, et al. Yeast-expressed granulocyte-macrophage colony-stimulating factor in cancer patients: A phase lb clinical study. In Behring Institute Research Communications. Colony Stimulating Factors-CSF. International Symposium, Garmisch-Partenkirchen, West Germany, 1988; 83:107–118.
13. Estey EH, Dixon D, Kantarjian H, et al. Treatment of poor-prognosis, newly diagnosed acute myeloid leukemia with Ara-C and recombinant human granulocyte-macrophage colony-stimulating factor. Blood 1990; 75(9):1766–1769.
14. Vadhan-Raj S, Keating M, LeMaistre A, et al. Effects of recombinant human granulocyte-macrophage colony-stimulating factor in patients with myelodysplastic syndromes. NEJM 1987; 317:1545–1552.

15. Buchner BR, Hiddemann W, Koenigsmann M, *et al*. Recombinant human granylocyte-macrophage colony stimulating factor after chemotherapy in patients with acute myeloid leukemia at higher age or after relapse. Bloodd 1991; 78(5):1190–1197.

16. Blazar BR, Kersey JH, McGlave, *et al. In vivo* administration of recombinant human granylocyte/macrophage colony-stimulating factor in acute lymphoblastic patients receiving purged autographs. Blood 1989; 73(3): 849–857.

IMMUNEX®

LEUKINE® is a registered trademark of Immunex Corporation, Seattle WA 98101

© 1998 Immunex Corporation. All rights reserved. Immunex U.S. Patent Nos. 5,391,485; 5,393,870; and 5,229,496. Licensed under Research Corporation Technologies U.S. Patent No. 5,602,007.

Rev 0230-02
Issued 02/98

METHOTREXATE SODIUM TABLETS ℞
METHOTREXATE SODIUM FOR INJECTION ℞
METHOTREXATE LPF® SODIUM ℞
(METHOTREXATE Sodium Injection) and
METHOTREXATE SODIUM INJECTION ℞

WARNINGS

METHOTREXATE SHOULD BE USED ONLY BY PHYSICIANS WHOSE KNOWLEDGE AND EXPERIENCE INCLUDE THE USE OF ANTIMETABOLITE THERAPY.

BECAUSE OF THE POSSIBILITY OF SERIOUS TOXIC REACTIONS (WHICH CAN BE FATAL):

METHOTREXATE SHOULD BE USED ONLY IN LIFE THREATENING NEOPLASTIC DISEASES, OR IN PATIENTS WITH PSORIASIS OR RHEUMATOID ARTHRITIS WITH SEVERE, RECALCITRANT, DISABLING DISEASE WHICH IS NOT ADEQUATELY RESPONSIVE TO OTHER FORMS OF THERAPY.

DEATHS HAVE BEEN REPORTED WITH THE USE OF METHOTREXATE IN THE TREATMENT OF MALIGNANCY, PSORIASIS, AND RHEUMATOID ARTHRITIS.

PATIENTS SHOULD BE CLOSELY MONITORED FOR BONE MARROW, LIVER, LUNG AND KIDNEY TOXICITIES. (See **PRECAUTIONS**.)

PATIENTS SHOULD BE INFORMED BY THEIR PHYSICIAN OF THE RISKS INVOLVED AND BE UNDER A PHYSICIAN'S CARE THROUGHOUT THERAPY.

THE USE OF METHOTREXATE HIGH DOSE REGIMENS RECOMMENDED FOR OSTEOSARCOMA REQUIRES METICULOUS CARE. (See **DOSAGE AND ADMINISTRATION**.) HIGH DOSE REGIMENS FOR OTHER NEOPLASTIC DISEASES ARE INVESTIGATIONAL AND A THERAPEUTIC ADVANTAGE HAS NOT BEEN ESTABLISHED.

METHOTREXATE FORMULATIONS AND DILUENTS CONTAINING PRESERVATIVES MUST NOT BE USED FOR INTRATHECAL OR HIGH DOSE METHOTREXATE THERAPY.

1. Methotrexate has been reported to cause fetal death and/or congenital anomalies. Therefore, it is not recommended for women of childbearing potential unless there is clear medical evidence that the benefits can be expected to outweigh the considered risks. Pregnant women with psoriasis or rheumatoid arthritis should not receive methotrexate. (See **CONTRAINDICATIONS**.)
2. Methotrexate elimination is reduced in patients with impaired renal function, ascites, or pleural effusions. Such patients require especially careful monitoring for toxicity, and require dose reduction or, in some cases, discontinuation of methotrexate administration.
3. Unexpectedly severe (sometimes fatal) bone marrow suppression and gastrointestinal toxicity have been reported with concomitant administration of methotrexate (usually in high dosage) along with some nonsteroidal anti-inflammatory drugs (NSAIDs). (See **PRECAUTIONS, Drug Interactions.**)
4. Methotrexate causes hepatotoxicity, fibrosis and cirrhosis, but generally only after prolonged use. Acutely, liver enzyme elevations are frequently seen. These are usually transient and asymptomatic, and also do not appear predictive of subsequent hepatic disease. Liver biopsy after sustained use often shows histologic changes, and fibrosis and cirrhosis have been reported; these latter lesions may not be preceded by symptoms or abnormal liver function tests in the psoriasis population. For this reason, periodic liver biopsies are usually recommended for psoriatic patients who are under long-term treatment. Persistent abnormalities in liver function tests may precede appearance of fibrosis or cirrhosis in the rheumatoid arthritis population. (See **PRECAUTIONS, Organ System Toxicity,** *Hepatic*.)
5. Methotrexate-induced lung disease is a potentially dangerous lesion, which may occur acutely at any time during therapy and which has been reported at doses as low as 7.5 mg/week. It is not always fully reversible. Pulmonary symptoms (especially a dry, nonproductive cough) may require interruption of treatment and careful investigation.
6. Diarrhea and ulcerative stomatitis require interruption of therapy; otherwise, hemorrhagic enteritis and death from intestinal perforation may occur.
7. Malignant lymphomas, which may regress following withdrawal of methotrexate, may occur in patients receiving low-dose methotrexate and, thus, may not require cytotoxic treatment. Discontinue methotrexate first and, if the lymphoma does not regress, appropriate treatment should be instituted.
8. Like other cytotoxic drugs, methotrexate may induce "tumor lysis syndrome" in patients with rapidly growing tumors. Appropriate supportive and pharmacologic measures may prevent or alleviate this complication.
9. Severe, occasionally fatal, skin reactions have been reported following single or multiple doses of methotrexate. Reactions have occurred within days of oral, intramuscular, intravenous, or intrathecal methotrexate administration. Recovery has been reported with discontinuation of therapy. (See **PRECAUTIONS, Organ System Toxicity,** *Skin*)
10. Potentially fatal opportunistic infections, especially *Pneumocystis carinii* pneumonia, may occur with methotrexate therapy.

DESCRIPTION

Methotrexate (formerly Amethopterine) is an antimetabolite used in the treatment of certain neoplastic diseases, sever psoriasis, and adult rheumatoid arthritis.

Chemically methotrexate is *N*-[4[[(2,4-diamino-6-pteridinyl) methyl]methylamino]benzoyl]-L-glutamic acid The structural formula is:

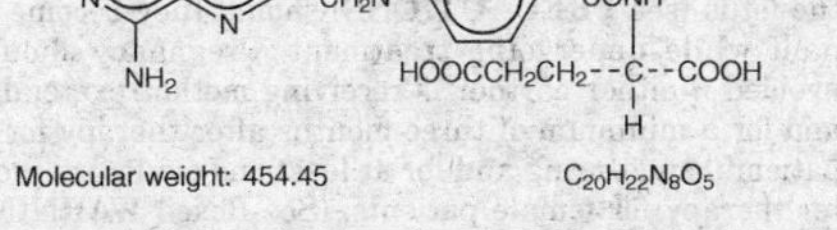

Molecular weight: 454.45 $C_{20}H_{22}N_8O_5$

Methotrexate Sodium Tablets for oral administration are available in bottles of 100 and in a packaging system designated as the RHEUMATREX® Methotrexate Sodium Dose Pack for therapy with a weekly dosing schedule of 5 mg, 7.5 mg, 10 mg, 12.5 mg and 15 mg. Methotrexate Sodium Tablets contain an amount of methotrexate sodium equivalent to 2.5 mg of methotrexate and the following inactive ingredients: Lactose, Magnesium Stearate and Pregelatinized Starch. May also contain Corn Starch.

Methotrexate Sodium Injection and for injection products are sterile and non-pyrogenic and may be given by the intramuscular, intravenous, intra-arterial or intrathecal route. (See **DOSAGE AND ADMINISTRATION.**) However, the preservative formulation contains Benzyl Alcohol and must not be used for intrathecal or high dose therapy.

Methotrexate Sodium Injection, Isotonic Liquid, Contains Preservative is available in 25 mg/mL, 2 mL (50 mg) and 10 mL (250 mg) vials.

Each 25 mg/mL, 2 mL and 10 mL vial contains methotrexate sodium equivalent to 50 mg and 250 mg methotrexate respectively, 0.90% w/v of Benzyl Alcohol as a preservative, and the following inactive ingredients: Sodium Chloride 0.260% w/v and Water for Injection qs ad 100% v. Sodium Hydroxide and, if necessary, Hydrochloric Acid are added to adjust the pH to approximately 8.5.

Methotrexate LPF® Sodium (methotrexate sodium injection), Isotonic Liquid, Preservative Free, for single use only, is available in 25 mg/mL, 2 mL (50 mg), 4 mL (100 mg), 8 mL (200 mg) and 10 mL (250 mg) vials.

Each 25 mg/mL, 2 mL, 4 mL, 8 mL and 10 mL vial contains methotrexate sodium equivalent to 50 mg, 100 mg, 200 mg and 250 mg methotrexate respectively, and the following inactive ingredients: Sodium Chloride 0.490% w/v and Water for Injection qs ad 100% v. Sodium Hydroxide and, if necessary, Hydrochloric Acid are added to adjust the pH to approximately 8.5. The 2 mL, 4 mL, 8 mL and 10 mL solutions contain approximately 0.43 mEq, 0.86 mEq, 1.72 mEq and 2.15 mEq of Sodium per vial, respectively, and are isotonic solutions.

Methotrexate Sodium for Injection, Lyophilized, Preservative Free, for single use only, is available in 20 mg and 1 gram vials.

Each 20 mg and 1 g vial of lyophilized powder contains methotrexate sodium equivalent to 20 mg and 1 g methotrexate respectively. Contains no preservative. Sodium Hydroxide and, if necessary, Hydrochloric Acid are added during manufacture to adjust the pH. The 20 mg vial contains approximately 0.14 mEq of Sodium and the 1 g vial contains approximately 7 mEq Sodium.

CLINICAL PHARMACOLOGY

Methotrexate inhibits dihydrofolic acid reductase. Dihydrololates must be reduced to tetrahydrofolates by this enzyme before they can be utilized as carriers of one-carbon groups in the synthesis of purine nucleotides and thymidylate. Therefore, methotrexate interferes with DNA synthesis, repair, and cellular replication. Actively proliferating tissues such as malignant cells, bone marrow, fetal cells, buccal and intestinal mucosa, and cells of the urinary bladder are in general more sensitive to this effect of methotrexate. When cellular proliferation in malignant tissues is greater than in most normal tissues, methotrexate may impair malignant growth without irreversible damage to normal tissues.

The mechanism of action in rheumatoid arthritis is unknown, it may affect immune function. Two reports describe *in vitro* methotrexate inhibition of DNA precursor uptake by stimulated mononuclear cells, and another describes in animal polyarthritis partial correction by methotrexate of spleen cell hyporesponsiveness and suppressed IL 2 production. Other laboratories, however, have been unable to demonstrate similar effects. Clarification of methotrexate's effect on immune activity and its relation to rheumatoid immunopathogenesis await further studies.

In patients with rheumatoid arthritis, effects of methotrexate on articular swelling and tenderness can be seen as early as 3 to 6 weeks. Although methotrexate clearly ameliorates symptoms of inflammation (pain, swelling, stiffness), there is no evidence that it induces remission of rheumatoid arthritis nor has a beneficial effect been demonstrated on bone erosions and other radiologic changes which result in impaired joint use, functional disability, and deformity.

Most studies of methotrexate in patients with rheumatoid arthritis are relatively short term (3 to 6 months). Limited data from long-term studies indicate that an initial clinical improvement is maintained for at least two years with continued therapy.

In psoriasis, the rate of production of epithelial cells in the skin is greatly increased over normal skin. This differential in proliferation rates is the basis for the use of methotrexate to control the psoriatic process.

Methotrexate in high doses, followed by leucovorin rescue, is used as a part of the treatment of patients with non-metastatic osteosarcoma. The original rationale for high dose methotrexate therapy was based on the concept of selective rescue of normal tissues by leucovorin. More recent evidence suggests that high dose methotrexate may also overcome methotrexate resistance caused by impaired active transport, decreased affinity of dihydrofolic acid reductase for methotrexate, increased levels of dihydrofolic acid reductase resulting from gene amplification, or decreased polyglutamation of methotrexate. The actual mechanism of action is unknown.

Two Pediatric Oncology Group studies (one randomized and one non-randomized) demonstrated a significant improvement in relapse-free survival in patients with non-metastatic osteosarcoma when high dose methotrexate with leucovorin rescue was used in combination with other chemotherapeutic agents following surgical resection of the primary tumor. These studies were not designed to demonstrate the specific contribution of high dose methotrexate/leucovorin rescue therapy to the efficacy of the combination. However, a contribution can be inferred from the reports of objective responses to this therapy in patients with metastatic osteosarcoma, and from reports to extensive tumor necrosis following preoperative administration of this therapy to patients with non-metastatic osteosarcoma.

Pharmacokinetics

Absorption — In adults, oral absorption appears to be dose dependent. Peak serum levels are reached within one to two hours. At doses of 30 mg/m^2 or less, methotrexate is generally well absorbed with a mean bioavailability of about 60%. The absorption of doses greater than 80 mg/m^2 is significantly less, possibly due to a saturation effect.

In leukemic pediatric patients, oral absorption has been reported to vary widely (23% to 95%). A twenty fold difference between highest and lowest peak levels (C_{max}: 0.11 to 2.3 micromolar after a 20 mg/m^2 dose) has been reported. Significant interindividual variability has also been noted in time to peak concentration (T_{max}: 0.67 to 4 hrs after a 15 mg/m^2 dose) and fraction of dose absorbed. Food has been shown to delay absorption and reduce peak concentration.

Continued on next page

Methotrexate Sodium—Cont.

Methotrexate is generally completely absorbed from parenteral routes of injection. After intramuscular injection, peak serum concentrations occur in 30 to 60 minutes.

Distribution — After intravenous administration, the initial volume of distribution is approximately 0.18 L/kg (18% of body weight) and steady-state volume of distribution is approximately 0.4 to 0.8 L/kg (40% to 80% of body weight). Methotrexate competes with reduced folates for active transport across cell membranes by means of a single carrier-mediated active transport process. At serum concentrations greater than 100 micromolar, passive diffusion becomes a major pathway by which effective intracellular concentrations can be achieved. Methotrexate in serum is approximately 50% protein bound. Laboratory studies demonstrate that it may be displaced from plasma albumin by various compounds including sulfonamides, salicylates, tetracyclines, chloramphenicol, and phenytoin.

Methotrexate does not penetrate the blood-cerebrospinal fluid barrier in therapeutic amounts when given orally or parenterally. High CSF concentrations of the drug may be attained by intrathecal administration.

In dogs, synovial fluid concentrations after oral dosing were higher in inflamed than uninflamed joints. Although salicylates did not interfere with this penetration, prior prednisone treatment reduced penetration into inflamed joints to the level of normal joints.

Metabolism — After absorption, methotrexate undergoes hepatic and intracellular metabolism to polyglutamated forms which can be converted back to methotrexate by hydrolase enzymes. These polyglutamates act as inhibitors of dihydrolase reductase and thymidylate synthetase. Small amounts of methotrexate polyglutamates may remain in tissues for extended periods. The retention and prolonged drug action of these active metabolites vary among different cells, tissues and tumors. A small amount of metabolism to 7-hydroxymethotrexate may occur at doses commonly prescribed. Accumulation of this metabolite may become significant at the high doses used in osteogenic sarcoma. The aqueous solubility of 7-hydroxymethotrexate is 3 to 5 fold lower than the parent compound. Methotrexate is partially metabolized by intestinal flora after oral administration.

Half Life — The terminal half life reported for methotrexate is approximately three to ten hours for patients receiving treatment for psoriasis, or rheumatoid arthritis or low dose antineoplastic therapy (less than 30 mg/m^2). For patients receiving high doses of methotrexate, the terminal half-life is eight to 15 hours.

Excretion — Renal excretion is the primary route of elimination and is dependent upon dosage and route of administration. With IV administration, 80% to 90% of the administered dose is excreted unchanged in the urine within 24 hours. There is limited biliary excretion amounting to 10% or less of the administered dose. Enterohepatic recirculation of methotrexate has been proposed.

Renal excretion occurs by glomerular filtration and active tubular secretion. Nonlinear elimination due to saturation of renal tubular reabsorption has been observed in psoriatic patients at doses between 7.5 and 30 mg. Impaired renal function, as well as concurrent use of drugs such as weak organic acids that also undergo tubular secretion, can markedly increase methotrexate serum levels. Excellent correlation has been reported between methotrexate clearance and endogenous clearance.

Methotrexate clearance rates vary widely and are generally decreased at higher doses. Delayed drug clearance has been identified as one of the major factors responsible for methotrexate toxicity. It has been postulated that the toxicity of methotrexate for normal tissues is more dependent upon the duration of exposure to the drug rather than the peak level achieved. When a patient has delayed drug elimination due to compromised renal function, a third space effusion, or other causes, methotrexate serum concentrations may remain elevated for prolonged periods.

The potential for toxicity from high dose regimens or delayed excretion is reduced by the administration of leucovorin calcium during the final phase of methotrexate plasma elimination. Pharmacokinetic monitoring of methotrexate serum concentrations may help identify those patients at high risk for methotrexate toxicity and aid in proper adjustment of leucovorin dosing. Guidelines for monitoring serum methotrexate levels, and for adjustment of leucovorin dosing to reduce the risk of methotrexate toxicity, are provided below in **DOSAGE AND ADMINISTRATION**.

Methotrexate has been detected in human breast milk. The highest breast milk to plasma concentration ratio reached 0.08:1.

INDICATIONS AND USAGE

Neoplastic Diseases

Methotrexate is indicated in the treatment of gestational choriocarcinoma, chorioadenoma destruens and hydatidiform mole.

In acute lymphocytic leukemia, methotrexate is indicated in the prophylaxis of meningeal leukemia and is used in maintenance therapy in combination with other chemotherapeutic agents. Methotrexate is also indicated in the treatment of meningeal leukemia.

Methotrexate is used alone or in combination with other anticancer agents in the treatment of breast cancer, epidermoid cancers of the head and neck, advanced mycosis fungoides, and lung cancer, particularly squamous cell and small cell types. Methotrexate is also used in combination with other chemotherapeutic agents in the treatment of advanced stage non-Hodgkin's lymphomas.

Methotrexate in high doses followed by leucovorin rescue in combination with other chemotherapeutic agents is effective in prolonging relapse-free survival in patients with non-metastatic osteosarcoma who have undergone surgical resection or amputation for the primary tumor.

Psoriasis

Methotrexate is indicated in the symptomatic control of severe, recalcitrant, disabling psoriasis that is not adequately responsive to other forms of therapy, *but only when the diagnosis has been established, as by biopsy and/or after dermatologic consultation.* It is important to ensure that a psoriasis "flare" is not due to an undiagnosed concomitant disease affecting immune responses.

Rheumatoid Arthritis

Methotrexate is indicated in the management of selected adults with severe, active, classical or definite rheumatoid arthritis (ARA criteria) who have had an insufficient therapeutic response to, or are intolerant of, an adequate trial of first-line therapy including full dose NSAIDs and usually a trial of at least one or more disease-modifying antirheumatic drugs.

Aspirin, nonsteroidal anti-inflammatory agents, and/or low dose steroids may be continued, although the possibility of increased toxicity with concomitant use of NSAIDs including salicylates has not been fully explored. (See **PRECAUTIONS, Drug Interactions.**) Steroids may be reduced gradually in patients who respond to methotrexate. Combined use of methothrexate with gold, penicillamine, hydroxychloroquine, sulfasalazine, or cytotoxic agents, has not been studied and may increase the incidence of adverse effects. Rest and physiotherapy as indicated should be continued.

CONTRAINDICATIONS

Methotrexate can cause fetal death or teratogenic effects when administered to a pregnant woman. Methotrexate is contraindicated in pregnant women with psoriasis or rheumatoid arthritis and should be used in the treatment of neoplastic diseases only when the potential benefit outweighs the risk to the fetus. Women of childbearing potential should not be started on methotrexate until pregnancy is excluded and should be fully counseled on the serious risk to the fetus (see **PRECAUTIONS**) should they become pregnant while undergoing treatment. Pregnancy should be avoided if either partner is receiving methotrexate; during and for a minimum of three months after therapy for male patients, and during and for at least one ovulatory cycle after therapy for female patients. (See Boxed **WARNINGS.**)

Because of the potential for serious adverse reactions from methotrexate in breast fed infants, it is contraindicated in nursing mothers.

Patients with psoriasis or rheumatoid arthritis with alcoholism, alcoholic liver disease or other chronic liver disease should not receive methotrexate.

Patients with psoriasis or rheumatoid arthritis who have overt or laboratory evidence of immunodeficiency syndromes should not receive methotrexate.

Patients with psoriasis or rheumatoid arthritis who have preexisting blood dyscrasias, such as bone marrow hypoplasia, leukopenia, thrombocytopenia or significant anemia, should not receive methotrexate.

Patients with a known hypersensitivity to methotrexate should not receive the drug.

WARNINGS—SEE BOXED WARNINGS.

PRECAUTIONS

General

Methotrexate has the potential for serious toxicity. (See Boxed **WARNINGS.**) Toxic effects may be related in frequency and severity to dose or frequency of administration but have been seen at all doses. Because they can occur at any time during therapy, it is necessary to follow patients on methotrexate closely. Most adverse reactions are reversible if detected early. When such reactions do occur, the drug should be reduced in dosage or discontinued and appropriate corrective measures should be taken. If necessary, this could include the use of leucovorin calcium. (See **OVERDOSAGE.**) If methotrexate therapy is reinstituted, it should be carried out with caution, with adequate consideration of further need for the drug and with increased alertness as to possible recurrence of toxicity.

The clinical pharmacology of methotrexate has not been well studied in older individuals. Due to adminished hepatic and renal function as well as decreased folate stores in this population, relatively low doses should be considered, and these patients should be closely monitored for early signs of toxicity.

Information for Patients

Patients should be informed of the early signs and symptoms of toxicity, of the need to see their physician promptly if they occur, and the need for close follow-up, including periodic laboratory tests to monitor toxicity.

Both the physician and pharmacist should emphasize to the patient that the recommended dose is taken weekly in rheumatoid arthritis and psoriasis, and that mistaken daily use of the recommended dose has led to fatal toxicity. Patients should be encouraged to read the Patients Instructions sheet within the Dose Pack. Prescriptions should not be written or refilled on a PRN basis.

Patients should be informed of the potential benefit and risk in the use of methotrexate. The risk of effects on reproduction should be discussed with both male and female patients taking methotrexate.

Laboratory Tests

Patients undergoing methotrexate therapy should be closely monitored so that toxic effects are detected promptly. Baseline assessment should include a complete blood count with differential and platelet counts, hepatic enzymes, renal function tests, and a chest X-ray. During therapy of rheumatoid arthritis and psoriasis, monitoring of these parameters is recommended: hematology at least monthly, renal function and liver function every 1 to 2 months. More frequent monitoring is usually indicated during antineoplastic therapy. *During initial or changing doses*, or during periods of increased risk of elevated methotrexate blood levels (eg. dehydration), more frequent monitoring may also be indicated.

Transient liver function test abnormalities are observed frequently after methotrexate administration and are usually not cause for modification of methotrexate therapy. Persistent liver function test abnormalities, and/or depression of serum albumin may be indicators of serious liver toxicity and require evaluation. (See **PRECAUTIONS, Organ System Toxicity,** *Hepatic*

A relationship between abnormal liver function tests and fibrosis or cirrhosis of the liver has not been established for patients with psoriasis. Persistent abnormalities in liver function tests may precede appearance of fibrosis or cirrhosis in the rheumatoid arthritis population.

Pulmonary function tests may be useful if methotrexate induced lung disease is suspected, especially if baseline measurements are available.

Drug Interactions

Nonsteroidal anti-inflammatory drugs should not be administered prior to or concomitantly with the high doses of methotrexate used in the treatment of osteosarcoma. Concomitant administration of some NSAIDs with high dose methotrexate therapy has been reported to elevate and prolong serum methotrexate levels, resulting in deaths from severe hematologic and gastrointestinal toxicity.

Caution should be used when NSAIDs and salicylates are administered concomitantly with lower doses of methotrexate. These drugs have been reported to reduce the tubular secretion of methotrexate in an animal model and may enhance its toxicity.

Despite the potential interactions, studies of methotrexate in patients with rheumatoid arthritis have usually included concurrent use of constant dosage regimens of NSAIDs, without apparent problems. It should be appreciated, however, that the doses used in rheumatoid arthritis (7.5 to 15 mg/week) are somewhat lower than those used in psoriasis and that larger doses could lead to unexpected toxicity.

Methotrexate is partially bound to serum albumin, and toxicity may be increased because of displacement by certain drugs, such as salicylates, phenylbutazone, phenytoin, and sulfonamides. Renal tubular transport is also diminished by probenecid; use of methotrexate with this drug should be carefully monitored.

In the treatment of patients with osteosarcoma, caution must be exercised if high-dose methotrexate is administered in combination with a potentially nephrotoxic chemotherapeutic agent (eg, cisplatin).

Oral antibiotics such as tetracycline, chloramphenicol, and nonabsorbable broad spectrum antibiotics, may decrease intestinal absorption of methotrexate or interfere with the enterohepatic circulation by inhibiting bowel flora and suppressing metabolism of the drug by bacteria.

Penicillins may reduce the renal clearance of methotrexate, increased serum concentrations of methotrexate with concomitant hematologic and gastrointestinal toxicity have been observed with high and low dose methotrexate. Use of methotrexate with penicillins should be carefully monitored.

Patients receiving concomitant therapy with methotrexate and etretinate or other retinoids should be monitored closely for possible increased risk of hepatotoxicity.

Methotrexate may decrease the clearance of theophylline; theophylline levels should be monitored when used concurrently with methotrexate.

Vitamin preparations containing folic acid or its derivatives may decrease responses to systemically administered methotrexate. Preliminary animal and human studies have shown that small quantities of intravenously administered

leucovorin enter the CSF primarily as 5-methyltetrahydrofolate and, in humans, remain 1–3 orders of magnitude lower than the usual methotrexate concentrations following intrathecal administration. However, high doses of leucovorin may reduce the efficacy of intrathecally administered methotrexate.

Folate deficiency states may increase methotrexate toxicity. Trimethoprim/sulfamethoxazole has been reported rarely to increase bone marrow suppression in patients receiving methotrexate, probably by an additive antifolate effect.

Carcinogenesis, Mutagenesis, and Impairment of Fertility

No controlled human data exist regarding the risk of neoplasia with methotrexate. Methotrexate has been evaluated in a number of animal studies for carcinogenic potential with inconclusive results. Although there is evidence that methotrexate causes chromosomal damage to animal somatic cells and human bone marrow cells, the clinical significance remains uncertain. Non-Hodgkin's lymphoma and other tumors have been reported in patients receiving low-dose oral methotrexate. However, there have been instances of malignant lymphoma arising during treatment with low dose oral methotrexate, which have regressed completely following withdrawal of methotrexate, without requiring active anti-lymphoma treatment. Benefits should be weighed against the potential risks before using methotrexate alone or in combination with other drugs, especially in pediatric patients or young adults. Methotrexate causes embryotoxicity, abortion, and fetal defects in humans. It has also been reported to cause impairment of fertility, oligospermia and menstrual dysfunction in humans, during and for a short period after cessation of therapy.

Pregnancy

Psoriasis and rheumatoid arthritis: Methotrexate is in Pregnancy Category X. See **CONTRAINDICATIONS**.

Nursing Mothers

See **CONTRAINDICATIONS**

Pediatric Use

Safety and effectiveness in pediatric patients have not been established, other than in cancer chemotherapy.

Organ System Toxicity

Gastrointestinal If vomiting, diarrhea, or stomatitis occur, which may result in dehydration, methotrexate should be discontinued until recovery occurs. Methotrexate should be used with extreme caution in the presence of peptic ulcer disease or ulcerative colitis.

Hematologic: Methotrexate can suppress hematopoiesis and cause anemia, leukopenia, and/or thrombocytopenia. In patients with malignancy and preexisting hematopoietic impairment, the drug should be used with caution, if at all. In controlled clinical trials in rheumatoid arthritis (n=128), leukopenia (WBC <3000/mm^3) was seen in 2 patients, thrombocytopenia (platelets <100,000/mm^3) in 6 patients, and pancytopenia in 2 patients.

In psoriasis and rheumatoid arthritis, methotrexate should be stopped immediately if there is a significant drop in blood counts. In the treatment of neoplastic diseases, methotrexate should be continued only if the potential benefit warrants the risk of severe myelosuppression. Patients with profound granulocytopenia and fever should be evaluated immediately and usually require parenteral broad-spectrum antibiotic therapy.

Hepatic: Methotrexate has the potential for acute (elevated transaminases) and chronic (fibrosis and cirrhosis) hepatotoxicity. Chronic toxicity is potentially fatal, it generally has occurred after prolonged use (generally two years or more) and after a total dose of at least 1.5 grams. In studies in psoriatic patients, hepatotoxicity appeared to be a function of total cumulative dose and appeared to be enhanced by alcoholism, obesity, diabetes and advanced age. An accurate incidence rate has not been determined; the rate of progression and reversibility of lesions is not known. Special caution is indicated in the presence of preexisting liver damage or impaired hepatic function.

In psoriasis, liver function tests, including serum albumin, should be performed periodically prior to dosing but are often normal in the face of developing fibrosis or cirrhosis. These lesions may be detectable only by biopsy. The usual recommendation is to obtain a liver biopsy at 1) pretherapy or shortly after initiation of therapy (2–4 months), 2) a total cumulative dose of 1.5 grams, and 3) after each additional 1.0 to 1.5 grams.[1] Moderate fibrosis or any cirrhosis normally leads to discontinuation of the drug; mild fibrosis normally suggests a repeat biopsy in 6 months. Milder histologic findings such as fatty change and low grade portal inflammation are relatively common pretherapy. Although these mild changes are usually not a reason to avoid or discontinue methotrexate therapy, the drug should be used with caution.

In rheumatoid arthritis, age at first use of methotrexate and duration of therapy have been reported as risk factors for hepatotoxicity; other risk factors, similar to those observed in psoriasis, may be present in rheumatoid arthritis but have not been confirmed to date. Persistent abnormalities in liver function tests may precede appearance of fibrosis or cirrhosis in this population. There is a combined reported experience in 217 rheumatoid arthritis patients with liver biopsies both before and during treatment (after a cumulative dose of at least 1.5 g) and in 714 patients with a biopsy only during treatment. There are 64 (7%) cases of fibrosis and 1 (0.1%) case of cirrhosis. Of the 64 cases of fibrosis, 60 were deemed mild. The reticulin stain is more sensitive for early fibrosis and its use may increase these figures. It is unknown whether even longer use will increase these risks.

Liver function tests should be performed at baseline and at 4–8 week intervals in patients receiving methotrexate for rheumatoid arthritis. Pretreatment liver biopsy should be performed for patients with a history of excessive alcohol consumption, persistently abnormal baseline liver function test values or chronic hepatitis B or C infection. During therapy, liver biopsy should be performed if there are persistent liver function test abnormalities or there is a decrease in serum albumin below the normal range (in the setting of well controlled rheumatoid arthritis).

If the results of a liver biopsy show mild changes (Roenigk grades I, II, IIIa), methotrexate may be continued and the patient monitored as per recommendations listed above. Methotrexate should be discontinued in any patient who displays persistently abnormal liver function tests and refuses liver biopsy or in any patient whose liver biopsy shows moderate to severe changes (Roenigk grade IIIb or IV).[2]

Infection or Immunologic States: Methotrexate should be used with extreme caution in the presence of active infection, and is usually contraindicated in patients with overt or laboratory evidence of immunodeficiency syndromes. Immunization may be ineffective when given during methotrexate therapy. Immunization with live virus vaccines is generally not recommended. There have been reports of disseminated vaccinia infections after smallpox immunization in patients receiving methotrexate therapy. Hypogammaglobulinemia has been reported rarely.

Potentially fatal opportunistic infections, especially *Pneumocystis carinii* pneumonia, may occur with methotrexate therapy. When a patient presents with pulmonary symptoms, the possibility of *Pneumocystis carinii* pneumonia should be considered.

Neurologic: There have been reports of leukoencephalopathy following intravenous administration of methotrexate to patients who have had craniospinal irradiation. Serious neurotoxicity, frequently manifested as generalized or local seizures, has been reported with unexpectedly increased frequency among pediatric patients with acute lymphoblastic leukemia who were treated wtih intermediate-dose intravenous methotrexate (1 gm/m^2). Symptomatic patients were commonly noted to have leukoencephalopathy and/or microangiopathic calcifications on diagnostic imaging studies. Chronic leukoencephalopathy has also been reported in patients who received repeated doses of high-dose methotrexate with leucovorin rescue even without cranial irradiation. Discontinuation of methotrexate does not always result in complete recovery.

A transient acute neurologic syndrome has been observed in patients treated with high dosage regimens. Manifestations of this stroke-like encephalopathy may include confusion, hemiparesis, seizures and coma. The exact cause is unknown.

After the intrathecal use of methotrexate, the central nervous system toxicity which may occur can be classified as follows: acute chemical arachnoiditis manifested by such symptoms as headache, back pain, nuchal rigidity, and fever; sub-acute myelopathy characterized by paraparesis/paraplegia associated with involvement with one or more spinal nerve roots; chronic leukoencephalopathy manifested by confusion, irritability, somnolence, ataxia, dementia, seizures and coma. This condition can be progressive and even fatal.

Pulmonary: Pulmonary symptoms (especially a dry nonproductive cough) or a nonspecific pneumonitis occurring during methotrexate therapy may be indicative of a potentially dangerous lesion and require interruption of treatment and careful investigation. Although clinically variable, the typical patient with methotrexate induced lung disease presents with fever, cough, dyspnea, hypoxemia, and an infiltrate on chest X-ray; infection needs to be excluded. This lesion can occur at all dosages.

Renal: High doses of methotrexate used in the treatment of osteosarcoma may cause renal damage leading to acute renal failure. Nephrotoxicity is due primarily to the precipitation of methotrexate and 7-hydroxymethotrexate in the renal tubules. Close attention to renal function including adequate hydration, urine alkalinization and measurement of serum methotrexate and creatinine levels are essential for safe administration.

Skin: Severe, occasionally fatal, dermatologic reactions, including toxic epidermal necrolysis. Stevens-Johnson syndrome, exfoliative dermatitis, skin necrosis, and erythema multiforme, have been reported in children and adults, within days of oral, intramuscular, intravenous, or intrathecal methotrexate administration. Reactions were noted after single or multiple, low, intermediate or high doses of methotrexate in patients with neoplastic and non-neoplastic diseases.

Other Precautions: Methotrexate should be used with extreme caution in the presence of debility.

Methotrexate exists slowly from third space compartments (eg, pleural effusions or ascites). This results in a prolonged terminal plasma half-life and unexpected toxicity. In patients with significant third space accumulations, it is advisable to evacuate the fluid before treatment and to monitor plasma methotrexate levels.

Lesions of psoriasis may be aggravated by concomitant exposure to ultraviolet radiation. Radiation dermatitis and sunburn may be "recalled" by the use of methotrexate.

ADVERSE REACTIONS

IN GENERAL, THE INCIDENCE AND SEVERITY OF ACUTE SIDE EFFECTS ARE RELATED TO DOSE AND FREQUENCY OF ADMINISTRATION. THE MOST SERIOUS REACTIONS ARE DISCUSSED ABOVE UNDER ORGAN SYSTEM TOXICITY IN THE PRECAUTION SECTION. THAT SECTION SHOULD ALSO BE CONSULTED WHEN LOOKING FOR INFORMATION ABOUT ADVERSE REACTIONS WITH METHOTREXATE.

The most frequently reported adverse reactions include ulcerative stomatitis, leukopenia, nausea, and abdominal distress. Other frequently reported adverse effects are malaise, undue fatigue, chills and fever, dizziness and decreased resistance to infection.

Other adverse reactions that have been reported with methotrexate are listed below by organ system. In the oncology setting, concomitant treatment and the underlying disease make specific attribution of a reaction to methotrexate difficult.

Alimentary System: gingivitis, pharyngitis, stomatitis, anorexia, nausea, vomiting, diarrhea, hematemesis, melena, gastrointestinal ulceration and bleeding, enteritis, pancreatitis.

Cardiovascular: pericarditis, pericardial effusion, hypotension, and thromboembolic events (including arterial thrombosis, cerebral thrombosis, deep vein thrombosis, retinal vein thrombosis, thrombophlebitis, and pulmonary embolus).

Central Nervous System: headaches, drowsiness, blurred vision. Aphasia, hemiparesis, paresis and convulsions have also occurred following administration of methotrexate. Following low doses, there have been occasional reports of transient subtle cognitive dysfunction, mood alteration, unusual cranial sensation, leukoencephalopathy, or encephalopathy.

Infection: There have been case reports of sometimes fatal opportunistic infections in patients receiving methotrexate therapy for neoplastic and non-neoplastic diseases. *Pneumocystis carinii* pneumonia was the most common infection. Other reported infections included nocardiosis; histoplasmosis, cryptococcosis, *Herpes zoster, H. simplex* hepatitis, and disseminated *H. simplex*.

Ophthalmic: conjunctivitis, serious visual changes of unknown etiology.

Pulmonary System: intestinal pneumonitis deaths have been reported, and chronic interstitial obstructive pulmonary disease has occasionally occurred.

Skin: erythematous rashes, pruritus, urticaria, photosensitivity, pigmentary changes, alopecia, ecchymosis, telangiectasia, acne furunculosis, erythema multiforme, toxic epidermal necrolysis, Stevens-Johnson syndrome, skin necrosis, and exfoliative dermatitis.

Urogenital System: severe nephropathy or renal failure, azotemia, cystitis, hematuria; defective oogenesis or spermatogenesis, transient oligospermia, menstrual dysfunction, vaginal discharge, and gynecomastia; infertility, abortion, fetal defects.

Other rarer reactions related to or attributed to the use of methotrexate such as nodulosis, vasculitis, arthralgia/myalgia, loss of libido/impotence, diabetes, osteoporosis, sudden death, reversible lymphomas, and tumor lysis syndrome. Anaphylactoid reactions have been reported.

Adverse Reactions in Double-Blind Rheumatoid Arthritis Studies

The approximate incidences of methotrexate-attributed (ie, placebo rate subtracted) adverse reactions in 12 to 18 week double-blind studies of patients (n=128) with rheumatoid arthritis treated with low-dose oral (7.5 to 15 mg/week) pulse methotrexate are listed below. Virtually all of these patients were on concomitant nonsteroidal anti-inflammatory drugs and some were also taking low dosages of corticosteroids.

Incidence greater than 10%: Elevated liver function tests 15%, nausea/vomiting 10%.3.

Incidence 3% to 10%. Stomatitis, thrombocylopenia (platelet count less than 100,000/mm^3).

Incidence 1% to 3%: Rash/pruritus/dermatitis, diarrhea, alopecia, leukopenia (WBC less than 3000/mm^3), pancytopenia, dizziness.

No pulmonary toxicity was seen in these two trials. Thus, the incidence is probably less than 2.5% (95% C.L.). Hepatic histology was not examined in these short-term studies. (See **PRECAUTIONS**.)

Continued on next page

Methotrexate Sodium—Cont.

Other less common reactions included decreased hematocrit, headache, upper respiratory infection, anorexia, arthralgias, chest pain, coughing, dysuria, eye discomfort, epistaxis, fever, infection, sweating, tinnitus, and vaginal discharge.

Adverse Reactions in Psoriasis

There are no recent placebo-controlled trials in patients with psoriasis. There are two literature reports (Roenigk, 1969 and Nylors, 1978) describing large series (n=204, 248) of psoriasis patients treated with methotrexate. Dosages ranged up to 25 mg per week and treatment was administered for up to four years. With the exception of alopecia, photosensitivity, and "burning of skin lesions" (each 3% to 10%), the adverse reaction rates in these reports were very similar to those in the rheumatoid arthritis studies.

OVERDOSAGE

Leucovorin is indicated to diminish the toxicity and counteract the effect of inadvertently administered overdosages of methotrexate. Leucovorin administration should begin as promptly as possible. As the time interval between methotrexate administration and leucovorin initiation increases, the effectiveness of leucovorin in counteracting toxicity decreases. Monitoring of the serum methotrexate concentration is essential in determining the optimal dose and duration of treatment with leucovorin.

In cases of massive overdosage, hydration and urinary alkalinization may be necessary to prevent the precipitation of methotrexate and/or its metabolites in the renal tubules. Neither hemodialysis nor peritoneal dialysis have been shown to improve methotrexate elimination.

Accidental intrathecal overdosage may require intensive systemic support, high-dose systemic leucovorin, alkaline diuretics and rapid CSF drainage and ventriculolumbar perfusion.

DOSAGE AND ADMINISTRATION

Neoplastic Diseases

Oral administration in tablet form is often preferred when low doses are being administered since absorption is rapid and effective serum levels are obtained. Methotrexate sodium injection and for injection may be given by the intramuscular, intravenous, intra-arterial or intrathecal route. However, the preserved formulation contains Benzyl Alcohol and must not be used for intrathecal or high dose therapy. Parenteral drug products should be inspected visually for particulate matter and discoloration prior to administration, whenever solution and container permit.

Choriocarcinoma and similar trophoblastic diseases: Methotrexate is administered orally or intramuscularly in doses of 15 to 30 mg daily for a five-day course. Such courses are usually repeated for 3 to 5 times as required, with rest periods of one or more weeks interposed between courses, until any manifesting toxic symptoms subside. The effectiveness of therapy is ordinarily evaluated by 24 hour quantitative analysis of urinary chorionic gonadotropin (hCG), which should return to normal or less than 50 IU/24 hr usually after the third or fourth course and usually be followed by a complete resolution of measurable lesions in 4 to 6 weeks. One to two courses of methotrexate after normalization of hCG is usually recommended. Before each course of the drug careful clinical assessment is essential. Cyclic cmbination therapy of methotrexate with other antitumor drugs has been reported as being useful.

Since hydatidiforme mole may precede choriocarcinoma, prophylactic chemotherapy with methotrexate has been recommended.

Chorioadenoma destruens is considered to be an invasive form of hydatidiform mole. Methotrexate is administered in these disease states in doses similar to those recommended for choriocarcinoma.

Leukemia: Acute lymphoblastic leukemia in pediatric patients and young adolescents is the most responsive to present day chemotherapy. In young adults and older patients, clinical remission is more difficult to obtain and early relapse is more common.

Methotrexate alone or in combination with steroids was used initially for induction of remission in acute lymphoblastic leukemias. More recently corticosteroid therapy, in combination with other antileukemic drugs or in cyclic combinations with methotrexate included, has appeared to produce rapid and effective remissions. When used for induction, methotrexate in doses of 3.3 mg/m^2 in combination with 60 mg/m^2 of prednisone, given daily, produced remissions in 50% of patients treated, usually within a period of 4 to 6 weeks. Methotrexate in combination with other agents appears to be the drug of choice for securing maintenance of drug-induced remissions. When remission is achieved and supportive care has produced general clinical improvement, maintenance therapy is initiated, as follows: Methotrexate is administered 2 times weekly either by mouth or intramuscularly in total weekly doses of 30 mg/m^2 It has also been given in doses of 2.5 mg/kg intravenously every 14 days. If and when relapse does occur, reinduction of remission can again usually be obtained by repeating the initial induction regimen.

A variety of combination chemotherapy regimens have been used for both induction and maintenance therapy in acute lymphoblastic leukemia. The physician should be familiar with the new advances in antileukemic therapy.

Meningeal Leukemia: In the treatment of prophylaxis of meningeal leukemia, methotrexate must be administered intrathecally. Preservative free methotrexate is diluted to a concentration of 1 mg/mL in an appropriate sterile, preservative free medium such as 0.9% Sodium Chloride Injection, USP.

The cerebrospinal fluid volume is dependent on age and not on body surface area. The CSF is at 40% of the adult volume at birth and reaches the adult volume in several years.

Intrathecal methotrexate administration at a dose of 12 mg/m^2 (maximum 15 mg) has been reported to result in low CSF methotrexate concentrations and reduced efficacy in pediatric patients and high concentrations and neurotoxicity in adults. The following dosage regimen is based on age instead of body surface area:

Age (years)	Dose (mg)
<1	6
1	8
2	10
3 or older	12

In one study in patients under the age of 40, this dosage regimen appeared to result in more consistent CSF methotrexate concentrations and less neurotoxicity. Another study in pediatric patients with acute lymphocytic leukemia compared this regimen to a dose of 12 mg/m^2 (maximum 15 mg), a significant reduction in the rate of CNS relapse was observed in the group whose dose was based on age.

Because the CSF volume and turnover may decrease with age, a dose reduction may be indicated in elderly patients. For the treatment of meningeal leukemia, intrathecal methotrexate may be given at intervals of 2 to 5 days. However, administration at intervals of less than 1 week may result in increased subacute toxicity. Methotrexate is administered until the cell count of the cerebrospinal fluid returns to normal. At this point one additional dose is advisable. For prophylaxis against meningeal leukemia, the dosage is the same as for treatment except for the intervals of administration. On this subject, it is advisable for the physician to consult the medical literature.

Untoward side effects may occur with any given intrathecal injection and are commonly neurological in character. Large doses may cause convulsions. Methotrexate given by the intrathecal route appears significantly in the systemic circulation and may cause systemic methotrexate toxicity. Therefore, systemic antileukemic therapy with the drug should be appropriately adjusted reduced, or discontinued. Focal leukemic involvement of the central nervous system may not respond to intrathecal chemotherapy and is best treated with radiotherapy.

Lymphomas: In Burkitt's tumor, Stages I–II, methotrexate has produced prolonged remissions in some cases. Recommended dosage is 10 to 25 mg/day orally for 4 to 8 days. In Stage III, methotrexate is commonly given concomitantly with other antitumor agents. Treatment in all stages usually consists of several courses of the drug interposed with 7 to 10 day rest periods. Lymphosarcomas in Stage III may respond to combined drug therapy with methotrexate given in doses of 0.625 to 2.5 mg/kg daily.

Mycosis Fungoides: Therapy with methotrexate appears to produce clinical remissions in one half of the cases treated. Dosage is usually 2.5 to 10 mg daily by mouth for weeks or months. Dose levels of drug and adjustment of dose regimen by reduction or cessation of drug are guided by patient response and hematologic monitoring. Methotrexate has also been given intramuscularly in doses of 50 mg once weekly or 25 mg 2 times weekly.

Osteosarcoma: An effective adjuvant chemotherapy regimen requires the administration of several cytotoxic chemotherapeutic agents. In addition to high-dose methotrexate with leucovorin rescue, these agents may include doxorubicin, cisplatin, and the combination of bleomycin, cyclophosphamide and dactinomycin (BCD) in the doses and schedule shown in the table below. The starting dose for high dose methotrexate treatment is 12 grams/m^2. If this dose is not sufficient to produce a peak serum methotrexate concentration of 1,000 micromolar (10^{-3} mol/L) at the end of the methotrexate infusion, the dose may be escalated to 15 grams/m^2 in subsequent treatments. If the patient is vomiting or is unable to tolerate oral medication, leucovorin is given IV or IM at the same dose and schedule.

Drug*	Dose*	Treatment Week After Surgery
Methotrexate	12 g/m^2 IV as 4 hour infusion (starting dose)	4,5,6,7,11,12,15, 16,29,30,44,45
Leucovorin	15 mg orally every six hours for 10 doses starting at 24 hours after start of methotrexate infusion.	
Doxorubicin† as a single drug	30 mg/m^2/day IV × 3 days	8,17
Doxorubicin†	50 mg/m^2 IV	20,23,33,36
Cisplatin†	100 mg/m^2 IV	20,23,33,36
Bleomycin†	15 units/m^2 IV × 2 days	2,13,26,39,42
Cyclophosphamide†	600 mg/m^2 IV × 2 days	2,13,26,39,42
Dactinomycin†	0.6 mg/m^2 IV × 2 days	2,13,26,39,42

* Link MP, Goorin AM, Miser AW, et al: The effect of adjuvant chemotherapy on relapse-free survival in patients with osteosarcoma of the extremity. *N Engl J of Med* 1986; 314(No.25):1600–1606.

† See each respective package insert for full prescribing information. Dosage modifications may be necessary because of drug-induced toxicity.

When these higher doses of methotrexate are to be administered, the following safety guidelines should be closely observed.

GUIDELINES FOR METHOTREXATE THERAPY WITH LEUCOVORIN RESCUE

1. Administration of methotrexate should be delayed until recovery if
   - the WBC count is less than 1500/microliter
   - the neutrophil count is less than 200/microliter
   - the platelet count is less than 75,000/microliter
   - the serum bilirubin level is greater than 1.2 mg/dL
   - the SGPT level is greater than 450 U
   - mucositis is present, until there is evidence of healing
   - persistent pleural effusion is present; this should be drained dry prior to infusion.
2. Adequate renal function must be documented.
   a. Serum creatinine must be normal, and creatinine clearance must be greater than 60 mL/min, before initiation of therapy.
   b. Serum creatinine must be measured prior to each subsequent course of therapy. If serum creatinine has increased by 50% or more compared to a prior value, the creatinine clearance must be measured and documented to be greater than 60 mL/min (even if the serum creatinine is still within the normal range).
3. Patients must be well hydrated, and must be treated with sodium bicarbonate for urinary alkalinization.
   a. Administer 1,000 mL/m^2 of intravenous fluid over 6 hours prior to initiation of the methotrexate infusion. Continue hydration at 125 mL/m^2/hr (3 liters/m^2/day) during the methotrexate infusion, and for 2 days after the infusion has been completed.
   b. Alkalinize urine to maintain pH above 7.0 during methotrexate infusion and leucovorin calcium therapy. This can be accomplished by the administration of sodium bicarbonate orally or by incorporation into a separate intravenous solution.
4. Repeat serum creatinine and serum methotrexate 24 hours after starting methotrexate and at least once daily until the methotrexate level is below (0.05 micromolar).
5. The table below provides guidelines for leucovorin calcium dosage based upon serum methotrexate levels. (See table below.‡)
   Patients who experience delayed early methotrexate elimination are likely to develop nonreversible oliguric renal failure. In addition to appropriate leucovorin therapy, these patients require continuing hydration and urinary alkalinization, and close monitoring of fluid and electrolyte status, until the serum methotrexate level has fallen to below 0.05 micromolar and the renal failure has resolved.
6. Some patients will have abnormalities in methotrexate elimination, or abnormalities in renal function following methotrexate administration, which are significant but less severe than the abnormalities described in the table below. These abnormalities may or may not be associated with significant clinical toxicity. If significant clinical toxicity is observed, leucovorin rescue should be extended for an additional 24 hours (total 14 doses over 84 hours) in subsequent courses of therapy. The possibility that the

patient is taking other medications which interact with methotrexate (eg, medications which may interfere with methotrexate binding to serum albumin, or elimination) should always be reconsidered when laboratory abnormalities or clinical toxicities are observed.

CAUTION: DO NOT ADMINISTER LEUCOVORIN INTRATHECALLY.

Psoriasis and Rheumatoid Arthritis

The patient should be fully informed of the risks involved and should be under constant supervision of the physician. (See **Information for Patients** Under **PRECAUTIONS**.) Assessment of hematologic, hepatic, renal, and pulmonary function should be made by history, physical examination, and laboratory tests before beginning, periodically during, and before reinstituting methotrexate therapy. (See **PRECAUTIONS**.) Appropriate steps should be taken to avoid conception during methotrexate therapy. (See **PRECAUTIONS** and **CONTRAINDICATIONS**.)

Weekly therapy may be instituted with the RHEUMATREX® Methotrexate Sodium 2.5 mg Tablet Dose Packs which are designed to provide doses over a range of 5 mg to 15 mg administered as a single weekly dose. The dose packs are not recommended for administration of methotrexate in weekly doses greater than 15 mg. All schedules should be continually tailored to the individual patient. An initial test dose may be given prior to the regular dosing schedule to detect any extreme sensitivity to adverse effects. (See **ADVERSE REACTIONS**.) Maximal myelosuppression usually occurs in seven to ten days.

Psoriasis: Recommended Starting Dose Schedules

1. Weekly single oral, IM or IV dose schedule: 10 to 25 mg per week until adequate response is achieved.
2. Divide oral dose schedule: 2.5 mg at 12-hour intervals for three doses.

Dosages in each schedule may be gradually adjusted to achieve optimal clinical response; 30 mg/week should not ordinarily be exceeded.

Once optimal clinical response has been achieved, each dosage schedule should be reduced to the lowest possible amount of drug and to the longest possible rest period. The use of methotrexate may permit the return to conventional topical therapy, which should be encouraged.

Rheumatoid Arthritis: Recommended Starting Dosage Schedules

1. Single oral doses of 7.5 mg once weekly.
2. Divide oral dosages of 2.5 mg at 12 hour intervals for 3 doses given as a course once weekly.

Dosages in each schedule may be adjusted gradually to achieve an optimal response, but not ordinarily to exceed a total weekly dose of 20 mg. Limited experience shows a significant increase in the incidence and severity of serious toxic reactions, especially bone marrow suppression, at doses greater than 20 mg/wk.

Once response has been achieved, each schedule should be reduced, if possible, to the lowest possible effective dose. Therapeutic response usually begins within 3 to 6 weeks and the patient may continue to improve for another 12 weeks or more.

The optimal duration of therapy is unknown. Limited data available from long-term studies indicate that the initial clinical improvement is maintained for at least two years with continued therapy. When methotrexate is discontinued, the arthritis usually worsens within 3 to 6 weeks.

HANDLING AND DISPOSAL

Procedures for proper handling and disposal of anticancer drugs should be considered. Several guidelines on this subject have been published.[3-8] There is no general agreement that all of the procedures recommended in the guidelines are necessary or appropriate.

RECONSTITUTION OF LYOPHILIZED POWDERS

Reconstitute immediately prior to use.

Methotrexate Sodium for Injection should be reconstituted with an appropriate sterile, preservative free medium such as 5% Dextrose Solution, USP, or Sodium Chloride Injection, USP. Reconstitute the 20 mg vial to a concentration no greater than 25 mg/mL. **The 1 gram vial should be reconstituted with 19.4 mL to a concentration of 50 mg/mL.** When high doses of methotrexate are administered by IV infusion, the total dose is diluted in 5% Dextrose Solution. For intrathecal injection, reconstitute to a concentration of 1 mg/mL with an appropriate sterile, preservative free medium such as Sodium Chloride Injection, USP.

DILUTION INSTRUCTIONS FOR LIQUID METHOTREXATE SODIUM INJECTION PRODUCTS

Methotrexate Sodium Injection, Isotonic Liquid, Contains Preservatives

If desired, the solution may be further diluted with a compatible medium such as Sodium Chloride Injection, USP. Storage for 24 hours at a temperature of 21 to 25°C results in a product which is within 90% of label potency.

Methotrexate LPF® Sodium (methotrexate sodium injection), Isotonic Liquid, Preservative Free, for Single Use Only

If desired, the solution may be further diluted immediately prior to use with an appropriate sterile, preservative free medium such as 5% Dextrose Solution, USP or Sodium Chloride Injection, USP.

LEUCOVORIN RESCUE SCHEDULES FOLLOWING TREATMENT WITH HIGHER DOSES OF METHOTREXATE

Clinical Situation	Laboratory Findings	Leucovorin Dosage and Duration
Normal Methotrexate Elimination	Serum methotrexate level approximately 10 micromolar at 24 hours after administration, 1 micromolar at 48 hours, and less than 0.2 micromolar at 72 hours.	15 mg PO, IM or IV q 6 hours for 60 hours (10 doses starting at 24 hours after start of methotrexate infusion).
Delayed Late Methotrexate Elimination	Serum methotrexate level remaining above 0.2 micromolar at 72 hours, and more than 0.05 micromolar at 96 hours after administration.	Continue 15 mg PO, IM or IV q six hours, until methotrexate level is less than 0.05 micromolar.
Delayed Early Methotrexate Elimination and/or Evidence of Acute Renal Injury	Serum methotrexate level of 50 micromolar or more at 24 hours, or 5 micromolar or more at 48 hours after administration, OR; a 100% or greater increase in serum creatinine level at 24 hours after methotrexate administration (eg, an increase from 0.5 mg/dL to a level of 1 mg/dL or more).	150 mg IV q three hours, until methotrexate level is less than 1 micromolar; then 15 mg IV q three hours, until methotrexate level is less than 0.05 micromolar.

HOW SUPPLIED

Parenteral:

Methotrexate Sodium for Injection, Lyophilized, Preservative Free, for Single Use Only. Each 20 mg and 1 g vial of lyophilized powder contains methotrexate sodium equivalent to 20 mg and 1 g methotrexate respectively.

20 mg Vial — NDC 58406-673-01 (Dark Blue Cap)

1 g Vial — NDC 58406-671-05 (Red Cap)

Methotrexate LPF® Sodium (methotrexate sodium injection), Isotonic Liquid, Preservative Free, for Single Use Only. Each 25 mg/mL, 2 mL, 4 mL, 8 mL and 10 mL vial contains methotrexate sodium equivalent to 50 mg, 100 mg, 200 mg and 250 mg methotrexate respectively.

50 mg — 2 mL Vial— NDC 58406-683-15 (Brown Cap)

100 mg — 4 mL Vial— NDC 58406-683-18 (Light Blue Cap)

200 mg — 8 mL Vial— NDC 58406-683-12 (Orange Cap)

250 mg —10 mL Vial— NDC 58406-683-16 (Violet Cap)

Methotrexate Sodium Injection, Isotonic Liquid, Contains Preservative. Each 25 mg/mL, 2 mL and 10 mL vial contains methotrexate sodium equivalent to 50 mg and 250 mg methotrexate respectively.

50 mg — 2 mL Vial — NDC 58406-681-14 (Red Cap)

250 mg — 10 mL Vial — NDC 58406-681-17 (Brown Cap)

Store at 25°C (77°F); excursions permitted to 15°–30°C (59°–86°F) [see USP Controlled Room Temperature]. Protect from light.

IMMUNEX®

Manufactured for

IMMUNEX CORPORATION, Seattle, WA 98101

by

LEDERLE PARENTERALS, INC., Carolina, Puerto Rico 00987

Oral:

Description

Methotrexate Sodium Tablets contain an amount of methotrexate sodium equivalent to 2.5 mg of methotrexate and are round, convex, yellow tablets, engraved with LL on one side, scored in half on the other side, and engraved with M above the score, and 1 below.

NDC 0005-4507-23 — Bottle of 100

RHEUMATREX® Methotrexate Sodium Tablet 2.5 mg Dose Packs — (each tablet equivalent to 2.5 mg of methotrexate)

NDC 0005-4507-04—RHEUMATREX® Methotrexate Sodium Tablets Dose Pack—4 cards each containing two 2.5 mg tablets, ie, 5 mg per week.

NDC 0005-4507-05—RHEUMATREX® Methotrexate Sodium Tablets Dose Pack—4 cards each containing three 2.5 mg tablets, ie, 7.5 mg per week.

NDC 0005-4507-07—RHEUMATREX® Methotrexate Sodium Tablets Dose Pack—4 cards each containing four 2.5 mg tablets, ie, 10 mg per week.

NDC 0005-4507-09—RHEUMATREX® Methotrexate Sodium Tablets Dose Pack—4 cards each containing five 2.5 mg tablets, ie, 12.5 mg per week.

NDC 0005-4507-91—RHEUMATREX® Methotrexate Sodium Tablets Dose Pack—4 cards each containing six 2.5 mg tablets, ie, 15 mg per week.

Store at 25°C (77°F); excursions permitted to 15°–30°C (59°–86°F) [see USP Controlled Room Temperature]. Protect from light.

LEDERLE PHARMACEUTICAL DIVISION
of American Cyanamid Company
Pearl River, NY 10965
CI 4814-3   Revised 11/97
REV 0168-04
©1997

REFERENCES

1. Roenigk HH, Auerbach R, Maibach HI, et al. Methotrexate in Psoriasis: Revised Guidelines. *J Am Acad Dermatol* 1988; 19:145–156.
2. Kremer JM, et al. Methotrexate for Rheumatoid Arthritis: Suggested Guidelines for Monitoring Liver Toxicity. *Arth Rheum* 1994; 37:316–328.
3. Recommendations for the Safe Handling of Parenteral Antineoplastic Drugs. NIH Publication No. 83-2621. For sale by the Superintendent of Documents, US Government Printing Office, Washington, DC 20402.
4. AMA Council Report. Guidelines for Handling Parenteral Antineoplastics. *JAMA,* March 15, 1985.
5. National Study Commission on Cytotoxic Exposure - Recommendations for Handling Cytotoxic Agents. Available from Louis P. Jeffrey, ScD, Chairman, National Study Commission on Cytotoxic Exposure, Massachusetts College of Pharmacy and Allied Health Sciences, 179 Longwood Avenue, Boston, Massachusetts 02115.
6. Clinical Oncological Society of Australia: Guidelines and Recommendations for Safe Handling of Antineoplastic Agents. *Med J Australia* 1983; 1:426–428.
7. Jones RB, et al. Safe Handling of Chemotherapeutic Agents: A Report from the Mount Sinai Medical Center. Ca - *A Cancer Journal for Clinicians* Sept/Oct 1983; 258-263.
8. American Society of Hospital Pharmacists Technical Assistance Bulletin on Handling Cytotoxic and Hazardous Drugs. *Am J Hosp Pharm* 1990; 47:1033–1049.

[See table above]

NOVANTRONE®   ℞
mitoxantrone for injection concentrate

> **WARNING**
>
> NOVANTRONE® (mitoxantrone for injection concentrate) should be administered under the supervision of a physician experienced in the use of cancer chemotherapeutic agents.
>
> Except for the treatment of acute nonlymphocytic leukemia, NOVANTRONE® therapy generally should not be given to patients with baseline neutrophil counts of less than 1,500 cells/mm³. In order to monitor the occurrence of bone marrow suppression, primarily neutropenia, which may be severe and result in infection, it is recommended that frequent peripheral blood cell counts be performed on all patients receiving NOVANTRONE®.

DESCRIPTION

NOVANTRONE® (mitoxantrone hydrochloride) is a synthetic antineoplastic anthracenedione for intravenous use. The molecular formula is $C_{22}H_{28}N_4O_6 \cdot 2HCl$ and the molecular weight is 517.41. It is supplied as a concentrate which MUST BE DILUTED PRIOR TO INJECTION. The concentrate is a sterile, nonpyrogenic, dark blue aqueous solution containing mitoxantrone hydrochloride equivalent to 2 mg/mL mitoxantrone free base, with sodium chloride (0.80% w/v), sodium acetate (0.005% w/v), and acetic acid (0.046% w/v) as inactive ingredients. The solution has a pH of 3.0 to 4.5 and contains 0.14 mEq of sodium per mL. The product does not contain preservatives. The chemical name is 1,4-

Continued on next page

Novantrone—Cont.

dihydroxy-5,8-bis[[2-[(2-hydroxyethyl) amino]ethyl]amino]-9,10-anthracenedione dihydrochloride and the structural formula is:

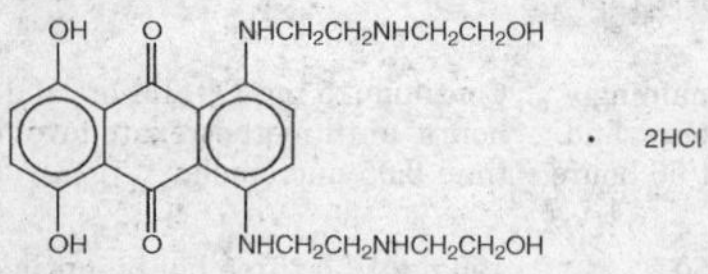

CLINICAL PHARMACOLOGY

Mechanism of Action

Although its mechanism of action is not fully elucidated, mitoxantrone is a DNA-reactive agent. It has a cytocidal effect on both proliferating and nonproliferating cultured human cells, suggesting lack of cell cycle phase specificity.

Pharmacokinetics

Pharmacokinetics of mitoxantrone in patients following a single intravenous administration can be characterized by a three-compartment model. The mean alpha half-life of mitoxantrone is 6 to 12 minutes, the mean beta half-life is 0.1 to 3.1 hours and the mean gamma (terminal or elimination) half-life is 23 to 215 hours (median approximately 75 hours). Pharmacokinetic studies have not been performed in humans receiving multiple daily dosing. Distribution to tissues is extensive: steady-state volume of distribution exceeds 1,000 L/m^2 . Tissue concentrations of mitoxantrone appear to exceed those in the blood during the terminal elimination phase. In the monkey, distribution to brain, spinal cord, eye, and spinal fluid is low.

In patients administered 15-90 mg/m^2 of mitoxantrone intravenously, there is a linear relationship between dose and the area under the concentration-time curve.

Mitoxantrone is 78% bound to plasma proteins in the observed concentration range of 26-455 ng/mL. This binding is independent of concentration and is not affected by the presence of phenytoin, doxorubicin, methotrexate, prednisone, prednisolone, heparin, or aspirin.

Metabolism and Elimination: Metabolism and elimination of mitoxantrone are not well characterized. Eleven percent of the dose is recovered in the urine, and 25% or less is recovered in the feces, within five days after drug administration. Of the material recovered in the urine, 65% is unchanged drug. The remaining 35% is comprised primarily of a mono- and a dicarboxylic acid derivative and their glucurocide conjugates. These carboxylic acid metabolites are not DNA-reactive/cytocidal, and their route of formation is unknown.

Special Populations:

Gender: The effect of gender on mitoxantrone pharmacokinetics is unknown.

Geriatric: Mitoxantrone pharmacokinetics in the elderly are unknown.

Pediatric: Mitoxantrone pharmacokinetics in the pediatric population are unknown.

Race: The effect of race on mitoxantrone pharmacokinetics is unknown.

Renal Impairment: Mitoxantrone pharmacokinetics in patients with renal impairment are unknown.

Hepatic Impairment: Mitoxantrone clearance is reduced by hepatic impairment. Patients with severe hepatic dysfunction (bilirubin greater than 3.4 mg/dL) have an AUC more than 3-fold that of patients with normal hepatic function receiving the same dose. For patients with hepatic impairment, there is at present no laboratory measurement that allows for dose adjustment recommendations.

Drug Interactions: Pharmacokinetic studies of the interaction of mitoxantrone with concomitantly administered medications have not been performed. The interaction of mitoxantrone with the human P450 system has not been investigated.

Clinical Trials

Advanced Hormone-Refractory Prostate Cancer

A multicenter phase 2 trial of NOVANTRONE and low-dose prednisone (N + P) was conducted in 27 symptomatic patients with hormone-refractory prostate cancer. Using NPCP (National Prostate Cancer Project) criteria for disease response, there was one partial responder and 12 patients with stable disease. However, nine patients or 33% achieved a palliative response defined on the basis of reduction in analgesic use or pain intensity.

These findings lead to the initiation of a randomized multicenter trial (CCI-NOV22) comparing the effectiveness of (N + P) to low-dose prednisone alone (P). Eligible patients were required to have metastatic or locally advanced disease that had progressed on standard hormonal therapy, a castrate serum testosterone level, and at least mild pain at study entry. NOVANTRONE was administered at a dose of 12 mg/m^2 by short IV infusion every three weeks. Prednisone was administered orally at a dose of 5 mg twice a day. Patients randomized to the prednisone arm were crossed over to the N + P arm if they progressed or if they were not improved after a minimum of six weeks of therapy with prednisone alone.

A total of 161 patients were randomized, 80 to the N + P arm and 81 to the P arm. The median NOVANTRONE dose administered was 12 mg/m^2 per cycle. The median cumulative NOVANTRONE dose administered was 73 mg/m^2 (range of 12 to 212 mg/m^2).

A primary palliative response (defined as a 2-point decrease in pain intensity in a 6-point pain scale, associated with stable analgesic use, and lasting a minimum of 6 weeks) was achieved in 29% of patients randomized to N + P compared to 12% of patients randomized to P alone (p = 0.011). Two responders left the study after meeting primary response criterion for two consecutive cycles. For the purposes of analysis of duration of response, these two patients are assigned a value of zero. A secondary palliative response was defined as a 50% or greater decrease in analgesic use, associated with stable pain intensity, and lasting a minimum of 6 weeks. An overall palliative response (defined as primary plus secondary responses) was achieved in 38% of patients randomized to N + P compared to 21% of patients randomized to P (p = 0.025).

The median duration of primary palliative response for patients randomized to N + P was 7.6 months compared to 2.1 months for patients randomized to P alone (p = 0.0009). The median duration of overall palliative response for patients randomized to N + P was 5.6 months compared to 1.9 months for patients randomized to P alone (p = 0.0004).

Time to progression was defined as a 1-point increase in pain intensity, or a >25% increase in analgesic use, or evidence of disease progression on radiographic studies, or requirement for radiotherapy. The median time to progression for all patients randomized to N + P was 4.4 months compared to 2.3 months for all patients randomized to P alone (p = 0.0001). Median time to death was 11.3 months for all patients on the N + P arm compared to 10.8 months for all patients on P alone (p = 0.2324).

Forty-eight patients on the P arm crossed over to receive N + P. Of these, thirty patients had progressed on P, while 18 had stable disease on P. The median cycle of crossover was 5 cycles (range of 2 to 16 cycles). Time trends for pain intensity prior to crossover were significantly worse for patients who crossed over than for those who remained on P alone (p = 0.012). Nine patients (19%) demonstrated a palliative response on N + P after crossover. The median time to death for patients who crossed over to N + P was 12.7 months.

The clinical significance of a fall in prostate specific antigen (PSA) concentrations after chemotherapy is unclear. On the CCI-NOV22 trial, a PSA fall of 50% or greater for two consecutive follow-up assessments after baseline was reported in 33% of all patients randomized to the N+P arm and 9% of all patients randomized to the P arm. These findings should be interpreted with caution since PSA responses were not defined prospectively. A number of patients were inevaluable for response, and there was an imbalance between treatment arms in the numbers of evaluable patients. In addition, PSA reduction did not correlate precisely with palliative response, the primary efficacy endpoint of this study. For example, among the 26 evaluable patients randomized to the N+P arm who had a ≥50% reduction in PSA, only 13 had a primary palliative response. Also, among 42 evaluable patients on this arm who did not have this reduction in PSA, 8 nonetheless had a primary palliative response.

Investigators at Cancer and Leukemia Group B (CALGB) conducted a phase III comparative trial of NOVANTRONE plus hydrocortisone (N + H) versus hydrocortisone alone (H) in patients with hormone-refractory prostate cancer (CALGB 9182). Eligible patients were required to have metastatic disease that had progressed despite at least one hormonal therapy. Progression at study entry was defined on the basis of progressive symptoms, increases in measurable or osseous disease, or rising PSA levels. NOVANTRONE was administered intravenously at a dose of 14 mg/m^2 every 21 days and hydrocortisone was administered orally at a daily dose of 40 mg. A total of 242 subjects were randomized, 119 to the N + H arm and 123 to the H arm. There were no differences in survival between the two arms, with a median of 11.1 months in the N + H arm, and 12 months in the H arm (p = 0.3298).

Using NPCP criteria for response, partial responses were achieved in 10 patients (8.4%) randomized to the N + H arm compared with 2 patients (1.6%) randomized to the H arm (p = 0.018). The median time to progression, defined by NPCP criteria, for patients randomized to the N + H arm was 7.3 months compared to 4.1 months for patients randomized to H alone (p = 0.0654).

Approximately 60% of patients on each arm required analgesics at baseline. Analgesic use was measured in this study using a 5-point scale. The best percent change from baseline in mean analgesic use was -17% for 61 patients with available data on the N + H arm, compared with +17% for 61 patients on H alone (p = 0.014). A time trend analysis for analgesic use in individual patients also showed a trend favoring the N + H arm over H alone but was not statistically significant.

Pain intensity was measured using the Symptom Distress Scale (SDS) Pain Item 2 (a 5-point scale). The best percent change from baseline in mean pain intensity was -14% for 37 patients with available data on the N + H arm, compared with +8% for 38 patients on H alone (p = 0.057). A time trend analysis for pain intensity in individual patients showed no difference between treatment arms.

Acute Nonlymphocytic Leukemia

In two large randomized multicenter trials, remission induction therapy for acute nonlymphocytic leukemia (ANLL) with NOVANTRONE 12 mg/m^2 daily for 3 days as a 10-minute intravenous infusion and cytarabine 100 mg/m^2 for 7 days given as a continuous 24-hour infusion was compared with daunorubicin 45 mg/m^2 daily by intravenous infusion for 3 days plus the same dose and schedule of cytarabine used with NOVANTRONE. Patients who had an incomplete antileukemic response received a second induction course in which NOVANTRONE or daunorubicin was administered for 2 days and cytarabine for 5 days using the same daily dosage schedule. Response rates and median survival information for both the U.S. and international multicenter trials are given in the following table:

[See table below]

In these studies, two consolidation courses were administered to complete responders on each arm. Consolidation therapy consisted of the same drug and daily dosage used for remission induction, but only 5 days of cytarabine and 2 days of NOVANTRONE or daunorubicin were given. The first consolidation course was administered 6 weeks after the start of the final induction course if the patient achieved a complete remission. The second consolidation course was generally administered 4 weeks later. Full hematologic recovery was necessary for patients to receive consolidation therapy. For the U.S. trial, median granulocyte nadirs for patients receiving NOVANTRONE + cytarabine for consolidation courses 1 and 2 were 10/mm^3 for both courses, and for those patients receiving daunorubicin + cytarabine nadirs were 170/mm^3 and 260/mm^3, respectively. Median platelet nadirs for patients who received NOVANTRONE + cytarabine for consolidation courses 1 and 2 were 17,000/mm^3 and 14,000/mm^3, respectively, and were 33,000/mm^3 and 22,000/mm^3 in courses 1 and 2 for those patients who received daunorubicin + cytarabine. The benefit of consolidation therapy in ANLL patients who achieve a complete remission remains controversial. However, in the only well-controlled prospective, randomized multicenter trials with NOVANTRONE in ANLL, consolidation therapy was given to all patients who achieved a complete remission. During consolidation in the U.S. study, two myelosuppression-related deaths occurred on the NOVANTRONE arm and one on the daunorubicin arm. However, in the international study there were eight deaths on the NOVANTRONE arm during consolidation which were related to the myelosuppression and none on the daunorubicin arm where less myelosuppression occurred.

INDICATIONS AND USAGE

NOVANTRONE in combination with corticosteroids is indicated as initial chemotherapy for the treatment of patients with pain related to advanced hormone-refractory prostate cancer.

NOVANTRONE in combination with other approved drug(s) is indicated in the initial therapy of acute nonlymphocytic leukemia (ANLL) in adults. This category includes myelogenous, promyelocytic, monocytic, and erythroid acute leukemias.

CONTRAINDICATIONS

NOVANTRONE is contraindicated in patients who have demonstrated prior hypersensitivity to it.

WARNINGS

WHEN NOVANTRONE IS USED IN DOSES INDICATED FOR THE TREATMENT OF LEUKEMIA, SEVERE MYELOSUPPRESSION WILL OCCUR. THEREFORE, IT IS RECOMMENDED THAT NOVANTRONE BE ADMINISTERED ONLY BY PHYSICIANS EXPERIENCED IN THE

Trial	% Complete Response (CR)		Median Time to CR (days)		Median Survival (days)	
	NOV	DAUN	NOV	DAUN	NOV	DAUN
U.S.	63 (62/98)	53 (54/102)	35	42	312	237
International	50 (56/112)	51 (62/123)	36	42	192	230

NOV = NOVANTRONE® + cytarabine
DAUN = daunorubicin + cytarabine

CHEMOTHERAPY OF THIS DISEASE. LABORATORY AND SUPPORTIVE SERVICES MUST BE AVAILABLE FOR HEMATOLOGIC AND CHEMISTRY MONITORING AND ADJUNCTIVE THERAPIES, INCLUDING ANTIBIOTICS. BLOOD AND BLOOD PRODUCTS MUST BE AVAILABLE TO SUPPORT PATIENTS DURING THE EXPECTED PERIOD OF MEDULLARY HYPOPLASIA AND SEVERE MYELOSUPPRESSION. PARTICULAR CARE SHOULD BE GIVEN TO ASSURING FULL HEMATOLOGIC RECOVERY BEFORE UNDERTAKING CONSOLIDATION THERAPY (IF THIS TREATMENT IS USED) AND PATIENTS SHOULD BE MONITORED CLOSELY DURING THIS PHASE.

Patients with preexisting myelosuppression as the result of prior drug therapy should not receive NOVANTRONE unless it is felt that the possible benefit from such treatment warrants the risk of further medullary suppression.

The safety of NOVANTRONE in patients with hepatic insufficiency is not established. (See **CLINICAL PHARMACOLOGY** section.)

Safety for use by routes other than intravenous administration has not been established.

Pregnancy - NOVANTRONE may cause fetal harm when administered to a pregnant woman. In treated rats, at doses of ≥0.1 mg/kg (0.05 fold the recommended human dose on a mg/m^2 basis) low fetal birth weight and retarded development of the fetal kidney were seen in greater frequency. In treated rabbits, an increased incidence of premature delivery was observed at doses ≥0.01 mg/kg (0.01 fold the recommended human dose on a mg/m^2 basis). NOVANTRONE was not teratogenic in rabbits. There are no adequate and well-controlled studies in pregnant women. If this drug is used during pregnancy, or if the patient becomes pregnant while taking this drug, the patient should be apprised of the potential hazard to the fetus. Women of childbearing potential should be advised to avoid becoming pregnant.

Topoisomerase II inhibitors, including NOVANTRONE, in combination with other antineoplastic agents, have been associated with the development of acute leukemia.

Cardiac Effects

Because of the possible danger of cardiac effects in patients previously treated with daunorubicin or doxorubicin, the benefit-to-risk ratio of NOVANTRONE therapy in such patients should be determined before starting therapy.

General - Functional cardiac changes including decreases in left ventricular ejection fraction (LVEF) and irreversible congestive heart failure can occur with NOVANTRONE. Cardiac toxicity may be more common in patients with prior treatment with anthracyclines, prior mediastinal radiotherapy, or with preexisting cardiovascular disease. Such patients should have regular cardiac monitoring of LVEF from the initiation of therapy. In investigational trials of intermittent single doses in other tumor types, patients who received up to the cumulative dose of 140 mg/m^2 had a cumulative 2.6% probability of clinical congestive heart failure. The overall cumulative probability rate of moderate or serious decreases in LVEF at this dose was 13% in comparative trials.

Leukemia - Acute congestive heart failure may occasionally occur in patients treated with NOVANTRONE for ANLL. In first-line comparative trials of NOVANTRONE + cytarabine *vs* daunorubicin + cytarabine in adult patients with previously untreated ANLL, therapy was associated with congestive heart failure in 6.5% of patients on each arm. A causal relationship between drug therapy and cardiac effects is difficult to establish in this setting since myocardial function is frequently depressed by the anemia, fever and infection, and hemorrhage which often accompany the underlying disease.

Hormone-Refractory Prostate Cancer - Functional cardiac changes such as decreases in LVEF and congestive heart failure may occur in patients with hormone-refractory prostate cancer treated with NOVANTRONE. In a randomized comparative trial of NOVANTRONE plus low-dose prednisone vs low-dose prednisone, 7 of 128 patients (5.5%) treated with NOVANTRONE had a cardiac event defined as any decrease in LVEF below the normal range, congestive heart failure (n = 3), or myocardial ischemia. Two patients had a prior history of cardiac disease. The total NOVANTRONE dose administered to patients with cardiac effects ranged from >48 to 212 mg/m^2.

Among 112 patients evaluable for safety on the NOVANTRONE + hydrocortisone arm of the CALGB trial, 18 patients (19%) had a reduction in cardiac function, 5 patients (5%) had cardiac ischemia, and 2 patients (2%) experienced pulmonary edema. The range of total NOVANTRONE doses administered to these patients is not available.

PRECAUTIONS

General: Therapy with NOVANTRONE should be accompanied by close and frequent monitoring of hematologic and chemical laboratory parameters, as well as frequent patient observation.

Systemic infections should be treated concomitantly with or just prior to commencing therapy with NOVANTRONE.

	ALL INDUCTION [percentage of pts entering induction]		ALL CONSOLIDATION [percentage of pts entering consolidation]	
	NOV N=102	DAUN N=102	NOV N=55	DAUN N=49
Cardiovascular	26	28	11	24
CHF	5	6	0	0
Arrhythmias	3	3	4	4
Bleeding	37	41	20	6
GI	16	12	2	2
Petechiae/Ecchymoses	7	9	11	2
Gastrointestinal	88	85	58	51
Nausea/Vomiting	72	67	31	31
Diarrhea	47	47	18	8
Abdominal Pain	15	9	9	4
Mucositis/Stomatitis	29	33	18	8
Hepatic	10	11	14	2
Jaundice	3	8	7	0
Infections	66	73	60	43
UTI	7	2	7	2
Pneumonia	9	7	9	0
Sepsis	34	36	31	18
Fungal Infections	15	13	9	6
Renal Failure	8	6	0	2
Fever	78	71	24	18
Alopecia	37	40	22	16
Pulmonary	43	43	24	14
Cough	13	9	9	2
Dyspnea	18	20	6	0
CNS	30	30	34	35
Seizures	4	4	2	8
Headache	10	9	13	8
Eye	7	6	2	4
Conjunctivitis	5	1	0	0

Information for Patients: NOVANTRONE may impart a blue-green color to the urine for 24 hours after administration, and patients should be advised to expect this during therapy. Bluish discoloration of the sclera may also occur. Patients should be advised of the signs and symptoms of myelosuppression.

Laboratory Tests: Serial complete blood counts and liver function tests are necessary for appropriate dose adjustments. (See **DOSAGE AND ADMINISTRATION** section.) In leukemia treatment, hyperuricemia may occur as a result of rapid lysis of tumor cells by NOVANTRONE. Serum uric acid levels should be monitored and hypouricemic therapy instituted prior to the initiation of antileukemic therapy.

Carcinogenesis, Mutagenesis, Impairment of Fertility

Carcinogenesis: Intravenous treatment of rats and mice, once every 21 days for 24 months, with NOVANTRONE resulted in an increased incidence of fibroma and external auditory canal tumors in rats at a dose of 0.03 mg/kg (0.02 fold the recommended human dose, on a mg/m^2 basis), and hepatocellular adenoma in male mice at a dose of 0.1 mg/kg (0.03 fold the recommended human dose, on a mg/m^2 basis). Mutagenesis: NOVANTRONE produced a clastogenic effect *in vivo* (rat bone marrow metaphase analysis) and *in vitro* (induced DNA damage in primary rat hepatocytes and SCE in CHO cells), and is mutagenic in bacterial (Ames/Salmonella and *E.Coli*) and mammalian (L5178Y TK+/-mouse lymphoma) test systems.

Impairment of Fertility: Daily treatment of male rats (71 days prior to, and during the mating period, and until confirmation of pregnancy in females) and female rats (15 days prior to, and during the mating period) with NOVANTRONE i.v. doses up to 0.03 mg/kg (0.02 fold the recommended human dose, on a mg/m^2 basis) had no effects on fertility.

Drug Interactions: There is no evidence for drug-drug interactions when NOVANTRONE is administered with corticosteroids.

Pregnancy: Pregnancy Category D: (See **WARNINGS** section.)

Nursing Mothers: It is not known whether NOVANTRONE is excreted in human milk. Because of the potential for serious adverse reactions in infants from NOVANTRONE, breast feeding should be discontinued before starting treatment.

Pediatric Use: Safety and effectiveness in pediatric patients have not been established.

ADVERSE REACTIONS

Leukemia - NOVANTRONE® (mitoxantrone for injection concentrate) has been studied in approximately 600 patients with ANLL. The table below represents the adverse reaction experience in the large U.S. comparative study of mitoxantrone + cytarabine vs daunorubicin + cytarabine. Experience in the large international study was similar. A much wider experience in a variety of other tumor types revealed no additional important reactions other than cardiomyopathy. (See WARNINGS section.) It should be appreciated that the listed adverse reaction categories include overlapping clinical symptoms related to the same condition,

e.g., dyspnea, cough and pneumonia. In addition, the listed adverse reactions cannot all necessarily be attributed to chemotherapy as it is often impossible to distinguish effects of the drug and effects of the underlying disease. It is clear, however, that the combination of NOVANTRONE + cytarabine was responsible for nausea and vomiting, alopecia, mucositis/stomatitis, and myelosuppression.

The following table summarizes adverse reactions occurring in patients treated with NOVANTRONE + cytarabine in comparison with those who received daunorubicin + cytarabine for therapy of ANLL in a large multicenter randomized prospective U.S. trial. Adverse reactions are presented as major categories and selected examples of clinically significant subcategories.

[See table above]

Hormone-Refractory Prostate Cancer - Detailed safety information is available for a total of 353 patients with hormone-refractory prostate cancer treated with NOVANTRONE, including 274 patients who received NOVANTRONE in combination with corticosteroids.

The following table summarizes adverse reactions of all grades occurring in ≥5% of patients in Trial CCI-NOV22.

Adverse Events of Any Intensity Occurring in ≥5% of Patients Trial CCI-NOV22

Event	N+P (n = 80) %	P (n = 81) %
Nausea	61	35
Fatigue	39	14
Alopecia	29	0
Anorexia	25	6
Constipation	16	14
Dyspnea	11	5
Nail bed changes	11	0
Edema	10	4
Systemic Infection	10	7
Mucositis	10	4
UTI	9	4
Emesis	9	5
Pain	8	9
Fever	6	5
Hemorrhage/bruise	6	1
Anemia	5	3
Cough	5	0
Decreased LVEF	5	0
Anxiety/depression	5	3
Dyspepsia	5	6
Skin infection	5	3
Blurred vision	3	5

No non-hematologic adverse events of Grade 3/4 were seen in >5% of patients.

The next table summarizes adverse events of all grades occurring in ≥5% of patients in Trial CALGB 9182.

Continued on next page

Novantrone—Cont.

Adverse Events of Any Intensity Occurring in ≥5% of Patients Trial CALGB 9182

Event	M+H (n = 112) n	M+H (n = 112) %	H (n = 113) n	H (n = 113) %
Decreased WBC	96	87	4	4
Granulocytes/bands	88	79	3	3
Decreased hemoglobin	83	75	42	39
Lymphocytes	78	72	27	25
Pain	45	41	44	39
Platelets	43	39	8	7
Alkaline Phosphatase	41	37	42	38
Malaise/fatigue	37	34	16	14
Hyperglycemia	33	31	32	30
Edema	31	30	15	14
Nausea	28	26	9	8
Anorexia	24	22	16	14
BUN	24	22	22	20
Transaminase	22	20	16	14
Alopecia	20	20	1	1
Cardiac function	19	18	0	0
Infection	18	17	4	4
Weight loss	18	17	13	12
Dyspnea	16	15	9	8
Diarrhea	16	14	4	4
Fever in absence of infection	5	14	7	6
Weight gain	15	14	16	15
Creatinine	14	13	11	10
Other gastrointestinal	13	14	11	11
Vomiting	12	11	6	5
Other neurologic	11	11	5	5
Hypocalcemia	10	10	5	5
Hematuria	9	11	5	6
Hyponatremia	9	9	3	3
Sweats	9	9	2	2
Other liver	8	8	8	8
Stomatitis	8	8	1	1
Cardiac dysrrhythmia	7	7	3	3
Hypokalemia	7	7	4	4
Neuro/constipation	7	7	2	2
Neuro/motor	7	7	3	3
Neuro/mood	6	6	2	2
Skin	6	6	4	4
Cardiac ischemia	5	5	1	1
Chills	5	5	0	0
Hemorrhage	5	5	3	3
Myalgias/arthralgias	5	5	3	3
Other kidney/bladder	5	5	3	3
Other endocrine	5	6	3	4
Other pulmonary	5	5	3	3
Hypertension	4	4	5	5
Impotence/libido	4	7	2	3
Proteinuria	4	6	2	3
Sterility	3	5	2	3

General

Allergic Reaction: Hypotension, urticaria, dyspnea, and rashes have been reported occasionally.

Cutaneous: Injection site reactions including phlebitis have been reported infrequently at the site of infusion. There have been rare reports of tissue necrosis following extravasation. Skin discoloration has also been reported.

Hematologic: Topoisomerase II inhibitors, including NOVANTRONE in combination with other antineoplastic agents, have been associated with the development of acute leukemia.

Leukemia - Myelosuppression is rapid in onset and is consistent with the requirement to produce significant marrow hypoplasia in order to achieve a response in acute leukemia. The incidences of infection and bleeding seen in the U.S. trial are consistent with those reported for other standard induction regimens.

Hormone-Refractory Prostate Cancer - In a randomized study where dose escalation was required for neutrophil counts greater than 1000/mm^3, Grade 4 neutropenia (ANC < 500 /mm^3) was observed in 54% of patients treated with NOVANTRONE + low-dose prednisone. In a separate randomized trial where patients were treated with 14 mg/m^2, Grade 4 neutropenia in 23% of patients treated with NOVANTRONE + hydrocortisone was observed. Neutropenic fever/infection occurred in 11% and 10% of patients receiving NOVANTRONE + corticosteroids, respectively, on the two trials. Platelets < 50,000/mm^3 were noted in 4% and 3% of patients receiving NOVANTRONE + corticosteroids on these trials, and there was one patient death on NOVANTRONE + hydrocortisone due to intracranial hemorrhage after a fall.

Gastrointestinal: Nausea and vomiting occurred acutely in most patients and may have contributed to reports of dehydration, but were generally mild to moderate and could be controlled through the use of antiemetics. Stomatitis/mucositis occurred within 1 week of therapy.

Cardiovascular: Congestive heart failure, tachycardia, EKG changes including arrhythmias, chest pain, and asymptomatic decreases in left ventricular ejection fraction have occurred. (See **WARNINGS** section.)

OVERDOSAGE

There is no known specific antidote for NOVANTRONE. Accidental overdoses have been reported. Four patients receiving 140 - 180 mg/m^2 as a single bolus injection died as a result of severe leukopenia with infection. Hematologic support and antimicrobial therapy may be required during prolonged periods of medullary hypoplasia.

Although patients with severe renal failure have not been studied, NOVANTRONE is extensively tissue bound and it is unlikely that the therapeutic effect or toxicity would be mitigated by peritoneal or hemodialysis.

DOSAGE AND ADMINISTRATION (See WARNINGS section.)

Hormone-Refractory Prostate Cancer: Based on data from two Phase III comparative trials of NOVANTRONE plus corticosteroids versus corticosteroids alone, the recommended dosage of NOVANTRONE is 12 to 14 mg/m^2 given as a short intravenous infusion every 21 days.

Combination Initial Therapy for ANLL in Adults: For induction, the recommended dosage is 12 mg/m^2 of NOVANTRONE daily on days 1-3 given as an intravenous infusion, and 100 mg/m^2 of cytarabine for 7 days given as a continuous 24-hour infusion on days 1-7.

Most complete remissions will occur following the initial course of induction therapy. In the event of an incomplete antileukemic response, a second induction course may be given. NOVANTRONE should be given for 2 days and cytarabine for 5 days using the same daily dosage levels.

If severe or life-threatening nonhematologic toxicity is observed during the first induction course, the second induction course should be withheld until toxicity clears.

Consolidation therapy which was used in 2 large randomized multicenter trials consisted of NOVANTRONE, 12 mg/m^2 given by intravenous infusion daily on days 1 and 2 and cytarabine, 100 mg/m^2 for 5 days given as a continuous 24-hour infusion on days 1-5. The first course was given approximately 6 weeks after the final induction course, the second was generally administered 4 weeks after the first. Severe myelosuppression occurred. (See **CLINICAL PHARMACOLOGY** section.)

Hepatic Impairment: For patients with hepatic impairment, there is at present no laboratory measurement that allows for dose adjustment recommendations. (See **CLINICAL PHARMACOLOGY**, Special Populations: *Hepatic Impairment*)

Preparation and Administration Precautions: NOVANTRONE CONCENTRATE MUST BE DILUTED PRIOR TO USE.

Parenteral drug products should be inspected visually for particulate matter and discoloration prior to administration whenever solution and container permit.

The dose of NOVANTRONE should be diluted to at least 50 mL with either 0.9% Sodium Chloride Injection (USP) or 5% Dextrose Injection (USP). NOVANTRONE may be further diluted into Dextrose 5% in Water, Normal Saline or Dextrose 5% with Normal Saline and used immediately. DO NOT FREEZE.

NOVANTRONE should not be mixed in the same infusion as heparin since a precipitate may form. Because specific compatibility data are not available, it is recommended that NOVANTRONE not be mixed in the same infusion with other drugs. The diluted solution should be introduced slowly into the tubing as a freely running intravenous infusion of 0.9% Sodium Chloride Injection (USP) or 5% Dextrose Injection (USP) over a period of not less than 3 minutes. Unused infusion solutions should be discarded immediately in an appropriate fashion. In the case of multidose use, after penetration of the stopper, the remaining portion of the undiluted NOVANTRONE concentrate should be stored not longer than 7 days between 15°-25° C (59°-77° F) or 14 days under refrigeration. DO NOT FREEZE. CONTAINS NO PRESERVATIVE.

If extravasation occurs, the administration should be stopped immediately and restarted in another vein. The nonvesicant properties of NOVANTRONE minimize the possibility of severe local reactions following extravasation. However, care should be taken to avoid extravasation at the infusion site and to avoid contact of NOVANTRONE with the skin, mucous membranes or eyes.

Skin accidentally exposed to NOVANTRONE should be rinsed copiously with warm water and if the eyes are involved, standard irrigation techniques should be used immediately. The use of goggles, gloves, and protective gowns is recommended during preparation and administration of the drug. Spills on equipment and environmental surfaces may be cleaned using an aqueous solution of calcium hypochlorite (5.5 parts calcium hypochlorite in 13 parts by weight of water for each 1 part of NOVANTRONE). Absorb the solution with guaze or towels and dispose of these in a safe manner. Appropriate safety equipment such as goggles and gloves should be worn while working with calcium hypochlorite.

Procedures for proper handling and disposal of anticancer drugs should be considered. Several guidelines on this subject have been published.[2-8] There is no general agreement that all of the procedures recommended in the guidelines are necessary or appropriate.

REFERENCES

1. Recommendations for the Safe Handling of Parenteral Antineoplastic Drugs. NIH Publication No. 83-2621. For sale by the Superintendent of Documents, US Government Printing Office, Washington, DC 20402.
2. AMA Council Report. Guidelines for Handling Parenteral Antineoplastics. *JAMA*. 1985; 253 (11) :1590-1592.
3. National Study Commission on Cytotoxic Exposure - Recommendations for Handling Cytotoxic Agents. Available from Louis P. Jeffrey, Sc D, Chairman, National Study Commission on Cytotoxic Exposure, Massachusetts College of Pharmacy and Allied Health Sciences, 179 Longwood Avenue, Boston, Massachusetts 02115.
4. Clinical Oncological Society of Australia: Guidelines and recommendations for safe handling of antineoplastic agents. *Med J Australia.*1983; 1:426-428.
5. Jones RB, et al. Safe handling of chemotherapeutic agents: A report from the Mount Sinai Medical Center. Ca - *A Cancer Journal for Clinicians*. Sept/Oct 1983; 258-263.
6. American Society of Hospital Pharmacists technical assistance bulletin on handling cytotoxic and hazardous drugs. *Am J Hosp Pharm.* 1990; 47:1033-1049.
7. OSHA Work-Practice guidelines for personnel dealing with cytotoxic (antineoplastic) drugs. *Am J Hosp Pharm* 1986; 43:1193-1204.

HOW SUPPLIED

NOVANTRONE® (mitoxantrone for injection concentrate) is a sterile aqueous solution containing mitoxantrone hydrochloride at a concentration equivalent to 2 mg mitoxantrone free base per mL supplied in vials for multidose use as follows:

NDC 58406-640-03 - 10 mL/multidose vial (20 mg)
NDC 58406-640-05 - 12.5 mL/multidose vial (25 mg)
NDC 58406-640-07 - 15 mL/multidose vial (30 mg)

NOVANTRONE® (mitoxantrone for injection concentrate) should be stored between 15°-25°C (59°-77°F). DO NOT FREEZE.

Manufactured for IMMUNEX CORPORATION, Seattle, WA 98101
by LEDERLE PARENTERALS, INC., Carolina, Puerto Rico 00987

Rev 0166-04 CI 4606-2
Revised 06/97

THIOPLEX® ℞

(Thiotepa For Injection)
15 mg/Vial

DESCRIPTION

THIOPLEX® (thiotepa for injection) is an ethylenimine-type compound. It is supplied as a non-pyrogenic, sterile lyophilized powder for intravenous, intracavitary or intravesical administration, containing 15 mg of thiotepa. THIOPLEX is a synthetic product with antitumor activity. The chemical name for thiotepa is Aziridine, 1,1′,1″-phosphinothioylidynetris-, or Tris (1-aziridinyl) phosphine sulfide.

Thiotepa has the following structural formula:

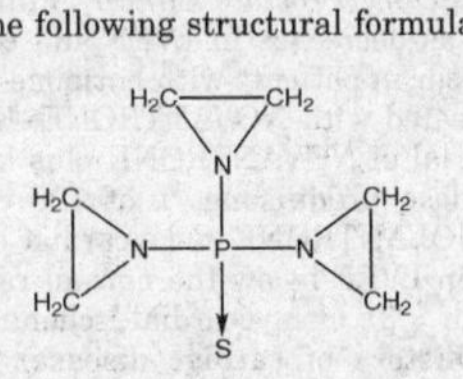

Thiotepa has the empirical formula $C_6H_{12}N_3PS$ and a molecular weight of 189.22. When reconstituted with Sterile Water for Injection, the resulting solution has a pH of approximately 5.5 - 7.5. Thiotepa is stable in alkaline medium and unstable in acid medium.

CLINICAL PHARMACOLOGY

Thiotepa is a cytotoxic agent of the polyfunctional type, related chemically and pharmacologically to nitrogen mustard. The radiomimetic action of thiotepa is believed to occur through the release of ethylenimine radicals which, like irradiation, disrupt the bonds of DNA. One of the principal bond disruptions is initiated by alkylation of guanine at the N-7 position, which severs the linkage between the purine base and the sugar and liberates alkylated guanines.

The pharmacokinetics of thiotepa and TEPA in thirteen female patients (45 - 84 years) with advanced stage ovarian

Pharmacokinetic Parameters	Mean ± SEM			
	Thiotepa		TEPA	
(units)	60 mg	80 mg	60 mg	80 mg
Peak Serum concentration (ng/mL)	1331 ± 119	1828 ± 135	273 ± 46	353 ± 46
Elimination half-life (h)	2.4 ± 0.3	2.3 ± 0.3	17.6 ± 3.6	15.7 ± 2.7
Area under the curve (ng/h/mL)	2832 ± 412	4127 ± 668	4789 ± 1022	7452 ± 1667
Total body clearance (mL/min)	446 ± 63	419 ± 56		

Label Claim (mg/vial)	Actual Content (mg/vial)	Amount of Diluent to be Added (mL)	Approximate Withdrawable Volume (mL)	Approximate Withdrawable Amount (mg/vial)	Approximate Reconstituted Concentration (mg/mL)
15.0	15.6	1.5	1.4	14.7	10.4

cancer receiving 60 mg and 80 mg thiotepa by intravenous infusion on subsequent courses given at 4-week intervals are presented in the following table:
[See first table above]
TEPA, which possesses cytotoxic activity, appears to be the major metabolite of thiotepa found in human serum and urine. Urinary excretion of ^{14}C-labeled thiotepa and metabolites in a 34-year old patient with metastatic carcinoma of the cecum who received a dose of 0.3 mg/kg intravenously was 63%. Thiotepa and TEPA in urine each accounts for less than 2% of the administered dose.
The pharmacokinetics of thiotepa in renal and hepatic dysfunction patients have not been evaluated. Possible pharmacokinetic interactions of thiotepa with any concomitantly administered medications have not been formally investigated.

INDICATIONS AND USAGE

Thiotepa has been tried with varying results in the palliation of a wide variety of neoplastic diseases. However, the most consistent results have been seen in the following tumors:

1. Adenocarcinoma of the breast.
2. Adenocarcinoma of the ovary.
3. For controlling intracavitary effusions secondary to diffuse or localized neoplastic diseases of various serosal cavities.
4. For the treatment of superficial papillary carcinoma of the urinary bladder.

While now largely superseded by other treatments, thiotepa has been effective against other lymphomas, such as lymphosarcoma and Hodgkin's disease.

CONTRAINDICATIONS

THIOPLEX is contraindicated in patients with a known hypersensitivity (allergy) to this preparation.
Therapy is probably contraindicated in cases of existing hepatic, renal, or bone-marrow damage. However, if the need outweighs the risk in such patients, thiotepa may be used in low dosage, and accompanied by hepatic, renal and hemopoietic function tests.

WARNINGS

Death has occurred after intravesical administration, caused by bone-marrow depression from systematically absorbed drug.
Death from septicemia and hemorrhage has occurred as a direct result of hematopoietic depression by thiotepa.
Thiotepa is highly toxic to the hematopoietic system. A rapidly falling white blood cell or platelet count indicates the necessity for discontinuing or reducing the dosage of thiotepa. Weekly blood and platelet counts are recommended during therapy and for at least 3 weeks after therapy has been discontinued.
Thiotepa can cause fetal harm when administered to a pregnant woman. Thiotepa given by the intraperitoneal (IP) route was teratogenic in mice at doses ≥1 mg/kg (3.2 mg/m^2), approximately 8-fold less than the maximum recommended human therapeutic dose (0.8 mg/kg, 27 mg/m^2), based on body-surface area. Thiotepa given by the IP route was teratogenic in rats at doses ≥3 mg/kg (21 mg/m^2), approximately equal to the maximum recommended human therapeutic dose, based on body-surface area. Thiotepa was lethal to rabbit fetuses at a dose of 3 mg/kg (41 mg/m^2), approximately two times the maximum recommended human therapeutic dose based on body-surface area.
Effective contraception should be used during thiotepa therapy if either the patient or partner is of childbearing potential. There are no adequate and well-controlled studies in pregnant women. If thiotepa is used during pregnancy, or if pregnancy occurs during thiotepa therapy, the patient and partner should be apprised of the potential hazard to the fetus.
Thiotepa is a polyfunctional alkylating agent, capable of cross-linking the DNA within a cell and changing its nature. The replication of the cell is, therefore, altered, and thiotepa may be described as mutagenic. An *in vitro* study has shown that it causes chromosomal aberrations of the chromatid type and that the frequency of induced aberrations increases with the age of the subject.
Like many alkylating agents, thiotepa has been reported to be carcinogenic when administered to laboratory animals. Carcinogenicity is shown most clearly in studies using mice, but there is some evidence of carcinogenicity in man. In patients treated with thiotepa, cases of myelodysplastic syndromes and acute non-lymphocytic leukemia have been reported.

PRECAUTIONS

General
The serious complication of excessive thiotepa therapy, or sensitivity to the effects of thiotepa, is bone-marrow depression. If proper precautions are not observed thiotepa may cause leukopenia, thrombocytopenia, and anemia.

Information for Patients
The patient should notify the physician in the case of any sign of bleeding (epistaxis, easy bruising, change in color of urine, black stool) or infection (fever, chills) or for possible pregnancy to patient or partner.
Effective contraception should be used during thiotepa therapy if either the patient or the partner is of childbearing potential.

Laboratory Tests
The most reliable guide to thiotepa toxicity is the white blood cell count. If this falls to 3000 or less, the dose should be discontinued. Another good index of thiotepa toxicity is the platelet count; if this falls to 150,000, therapy should be discontinued. Red blood cell count is a less accurate indicator of thiotepa toxicity. If the drug is used in patients with hepatic or renal damage (see **CONTRAINDICATIONS** section), regular assessment of hepatic and renal function tests are indicated.

Drug Interactions
It is not advisable to combine, simultaneously or sequentially, cancer chemotherapeutic agents or a cancer chemotherapeutic agent and a therapeutic modality having the same mechanism of action. Therefore, thiotepa combined with other alkylating agents such as nitrogen mustard or cyclophosphamide or thiotepa combined with irradiation would serve to intensify toxicity rather than to enhance therapeutic response. If these agents must follow each other, it is important that recovery from the first agent, as indicated by white blood cell count, be complete before therapy with the second agent is instituted.
Other drugs which are known to produce bone-marrow depression should be avoided.

Carcinogenesis, Mutagenesis and Impairment of Fertility
Also see **WARNINGS** section.

Carcinogenesis
In mice, repeated IP administration of thiotepa (1.15 or 2.3 mg/kg three times per week for 52 or 43 weeks, respectively) produced a significant increase in the combined incidence of squamous-cell carcinomas of the skin, preputial gland, and ear canal, and combined incidence of lymphoma and lymphocytic leukemia. In other studies in mice, repeated IP administration of thiotepa (4 or 8 mg/kg three times per week for 4 weeks followed by a 20-week observation period or 1.8 mg/kg three times per week for 4 weeks followed by a 35-week observation period) resulted in an increased incidence of lung tumors. In rats, repeated IP administration of thiotepa (0.7 or 1.4 mg/kg three times per week for 52 or 34 weeks, respectively) produced significant increases in the incidence of squamous-cell carcinomas of the skin or ear canal, combined hematopoietic neoplasms, and uterine adenocarcinomas. Thiotepa given intravenously (IV) to rats (1 mg/kg once per week for 52 weeks) produced an increased incidence of malignant tumors (abdominal cavity sarcoma, lymphosarcoma, myelosis, seminoma, fibrosarcoma, salivary gland hemangioendothelioma, mammary sarcoma, pheochromocytoma) and benign tumors.
The lowest reported carcinogenic dose in mice (1.15 mg/kg, 3.68 mg/m^2) is approximately 7-fold less than the maximum recommended human therapeutic dose based on body-surface area. The lowest reported carcinogenic dose in rats (0.7 mg/kg, 4.9 mg/m^2) is approximately 6-fold less than the maximum recommended human therapeutic dose based on body-surface area.

Mutagenesis
Thiotepa was mutagenic in *in vitro* assays in *Salmonella typhimurium*, *E. coli*, Chinese hamster lung and human lymphocytes. Chromosomal aberrations and sister chromatid exchanges were observed *in vitro* with thiotepa in bean root tips, human lymphocytes, Chinese hamster lung, and monkey lymphocytes. Mutations were observed with oral thiotepa in mouse at doses >2.5 mg/kg (8 mg/m^2). The mouse micronucleus test was positive with IP administration of >1 mg/kg (3.2 mg/m^2). Other positive *in vivo* chromosomal aberration or mutation assays included *Drosophila melanogaster*, Chinese hamster marrow, murine marrow, monkey lymphocyte, and murine germ cell.

Impairment of Fertility
Thiotepa impaired fertility in male mice at PO or IP doses ≥0.7 mg/kg (2.24 mg/m^2), approximately 12-fold less than the maximum recommended human therapeutic dose based on body-surface area. Thiotepa (0.5 mg) inhibited implantation in female rats when instilled into the uterine cavity. Thiotepa interfered with spermatogenesis in mice at IP doses ≥0.5 mg/kg (1.6 mg/m^2), approximately 17-fold less than the maximum recommended human therapeutic dose based on body-surface area. Thiotepa interfered with spermatogenesis in hamsters at an IP dose of 1 mg/kg (4.1 mg/m^2), approximately 7-fold less than the maximum recommended human therapeutic dose based on body-surface area.

Pregnancy
Category D: See **WARNINGS** section.
Thiotepa can cause fetal harm when administered to a pregnant woman. Thiotepa given by the IP route was teratogenic in mice at doses ≥1 mg/kg (3.2 mg/m^2), approximately 8-fold less than the maximum recommended human therapeutic dose based on body-surface area. Thiotepa given by the IP route was teratogenic in rats at doses ≥3 mg/kg (21 mg/m^2), approximately equal to the maximum recommended human therapeutic dose based on body-surface area. Thiotepa was lethal to rabbit fetuses at a dose of 3 mg/kg (41 mg/m^2), approximately 2 times the maximum recommended human therapeutic dose based on body-surface area. Patients of childbearing potential should be advised to avoid pregnancy. There are no adequate and well-controlled studies in pregnant women. If thiotepa is used during pregnancy, or if pregnancy occurs during thiotepa therapy, the patient and partner should be apprised of the potential hazard to the fetus.

Nursing Mothers
It is not known whether thiotepa is excreted in human milk. Because many drugs are excreted in human milk and because of the potential for tumorigenicity shown for thiotepa in animal studies, a decision should be made whether to discontinue nursing or to discontinue the drug, taking into account the importance of the drug to the mother.

Pediatric Use
Safety and effectiveness in pediatric patients have not been established.

ADVERSE REACTIONS

In addition to its effect on the blood-forming elements (see **WARNINGS** and **PRECAUTIONS** sections), thiotepa may cause other adverse reactions.
General: Fatigue, weakness. Febrile reaction and discharge from a subcutaneous lesion may occur as the result of breakdown of tumor tissue.
Hypersensitivity Reactions: Allergic reactions - rash, urticaria, laryngeal edema, asthma, anaphylactic shock, wheezing.
Local Reactions: Contact dermatitis, pain at the injection site.
Gastrointestinal: Nausea, vomiting, abdominal pain, anorexia.
Renal: Dysuria, urinary retention. There have been rare reports of chemical cystitis or hemorrhagic cystitis following intravesical, but not parenteral administration of thiotepa.
Respiratory: Prolonged apnea has been reported when succinylcholine was administered prior to surgery, following combined use of thiotepa and other anticancer agents. It was theorized that this was caused by decrease of pseudocholinesterase activity caused by the anticancer drugs.
Neurologic: Dizziness, headache, blurred vision.
Skin: Dermatitis, alopecia. Skin depigmentation has been reported following topical use.
Special Senses: Conjunctivitis.
Reproductive: Amenorrhea, interference with spermatogenesis.

OVERDOSAGE

Hematopoietic toxicity can occur following overdose, manifested by a decrease in the white cell count and/or platelets. Red blood cell count is a less accurate indicator of thiotepa

Continued on next page

Thioplex—Cont.

toxicity. Bleeding manifestations may develop. The patient may become more vulnerable to infection, and less able to combat such infection.
Dosages within and minimally above the recommended therapeutic doses have been associated with potentially life-threatening hematopoietic toxicity. Thiotepa has a toxic effect on the hematopoietic system that is dose related.
Thiotepa is dialyzable.
There is no known antidote for overdosage with thiotepa. Transfusions of whole blood or platelets have proven beneficial to the patient in combating hematopoietic toxicity.

DOSAGE AND ADMINISTRATION

Since absorption from the gastrointestinal tract is variable, thiotepa should not be administered orally.
Dosage must be carefully individualized. A slow response to thiotepa does not necessarily indicate a lack of effect. Therefore, increasing the frequency of dosing may only increase toxicity. After maximum benefit is obtained by initial therapy, it is necessary to continue the patient on maintenance therapy (1 to 4 week intervals). In order to continue optimal effect, maintenance doses should not be administered more frequently than weekly in order to preserve correlation between dose and blood counts.
Preparation and Administration Precautions: Thiotepa is a cytotoxic anticancer drug and as with other potentially toxic compounds, caution should be exercised in handling and preparation of thiotepa. Skin reactions associated with accidental exposure to thiotepa may occur. The use of gloves is recommended. If thiotepa solution contacts the skin, immediately wash the skin thoroughly with soap and water. If thiotepa contacts mucous membranes, the membranes should be flushed thoroughly with water.
Preparation of Solution: THIOPLEX (thiotepa for injection) should be reconstituted with **1.5 mL** of Sterile Water for Injection resulting in a drug concentration of approximately **10 mg/mL**. The actual withdrawable quantities and concentration achieved are illustrated in the following table:
[See second table at top of previous page]
The reconstituted solution is hypotonic and should be further diluted with Sodium Chloride Injection (0.9% sodium chloride) before use.
When reconstituted with Sterile Water for Injection, solutions of THIOPLEX should be stored in a refrigerator and used within 8 hours. Reconstituted solutions further diluted with Sodium Chloride Injection should be used immediately.
In order to eliminate haze, filter solutions through a 0.22 micron filter* prior to administration. Filtering does not alter solution potency. Reconstituted solutions should be clear. Solutions that remain opaque or precipitate after filtration should not be used.
* Polysulfone membrane (Gelman's Sterile Acrodisc®, Single Use) or triton-free mixed ester of cellulose/PVC (Millipore's MILLEX®-GS Filter Unit).
Parenteral drug products should be inspected visually for particulate matter and discoloration prior to administration, whenever solution and container permit.
Initial and Maintenance Doses: Initially the higher dose in the given range is commonly administered. The maintenance dose should be adjusted weekly on the basis of pretreatment control blood counts and subsequent blood counts.
Intravenous Administration: Thiotepa may be given by rapid intravenous administration in doses of 0.3 to 0.4 mg/kg. Doses should be given at 1 to 4 week intervals.
Intracavitary Administration: The dosage recommended is 0.6 - 0.8 mg/kg. Administration is usually effected through the same tubing which is used to remove the fluid from the cavity involved.
Intravesical Administration: Patients with papillary carcinoma of the bladder are dehydrated for 8 to 12 hours prior to treatment. Then 60 mg of thiotepa in 30 - 60 mL of Sodium Chloride Injection is instilled into the bladder by catheter. For maximum effect, the solution should be retained for 2 hours. If the patient finds it impossible to retain 60 mL for 2 hours, the dose may be given in a volume of 30 mL. If desired, the patient may be positioned every 15 minutes for maximum area contact. The usual course of treatment is once a week for 4 weeks. The course may be repeated if necessary, but second and third courses must be given with caution since bone-marrow depression may be increased. Deaths have occurred after intravesical administration, caused by bone-marrow depression from systemically absorbed drug.
Handling and Disposal: Follow safe cytotoxic agent handling procedures. Several guidelines on this subject have been published.[1–6] There is no general agreement that all of the procedures recommended in the guidelines are necessary or appropriate.

HOW SUPPLIED

THIOPLEX® (thiotepa for injection), for single use only, is available in vials containing 15 mg of non-pyrogenic, sterile lyophilized powder, supplied as follows:
NDC 58406-661-31 - 6 x 15 mg/vial

STORAGE

Store in refrigerator between 2-8°C (36-46°F). PROTECT FROM LIGHT AT ALL TIMES.

REFERENCES

1. Recommendations for the Safe Handling of Parenteral Antineoplastic Drugs. NIH Publication No. 83-2621. For sale by the Superintendent of Documents, US Government Printing Office, Washington, DC 20402.
2. AMA Council Report. Guidelines for Handling Parenteral Antineoplastics. *JAMA*. 1985; 253(11):1590-1592.
3. National Study Commission on Cytotoxic Exposure - Recommendations for Handling Cytotoxic Agents. Available from Louis P. Jeffrey, Sc D, Chairman, National Study Commission on Cytotoxic Exposure, Massachusetts College of Pharmacy and Allied Health Sciences, 179 Longwood Avenue, Boston, Massachusetts 02115.
4. Clinical Oncological Society of Australia: Guidelines and recommendations for safe handling of antineoplastic agents. *Med J Australia*. 1983; 1:426-428.
5. Jones RB, et al. Safe handling of chemotherapeutic agents: A report from the Mount Sinai Medical Center. Ca - *A Cancer Journal for Clinicians*. Sept/Oct 1983; 258-263.
6. American Society of Hospital Pharmacists technical assistance bulletin on handling cytotoxic and hazardous drugs. *Am J Hosp Pharm*. 1990; 47:1033-1049.

Manufactured for IMMUNEX CORPORATION, Seattle, WA 98101
by LEDERLE PARENTERALS, INC., Carolina, Puerto Rico 00987
 Rev 0167-01 Issued 4/97
CI 4506-1

Immuno
1200 PARKDALE ROAD
ROCHESTER, MI 48307 USA

Direct Inquiries to:
(800) 423-2090

ALBUMIN (HUMAN) ℞
5% SOLUTION

DESCRIPTION

Albumin (Human) 5% is a sterile aqueous solution for intravenous use containing the albumin component of human plasma. The solution is approximately isotonic and isooncotic with human plasma. The effective oncotic pressure of the solution depends largely on its albumin content. Sodium bicarbonate is used to adjust the pH to 6.9 ± 0.5. The sodium content of the solution ranges between 130 and 160 meq/L. 0.08 millimole sodium caprylate/g albumin and 0.08 millimole sodium N- acetyltryptophanate/g albumin are added as stabilizers to prevent denaturation during heating. The solution has been heat-treated at 60°C for 10 hours for inactivation of hepatitis viruses.

CLINICAL PHARMACOLOGY

Albumin is a very soluble, globular protein (MW 66,500) accounting for 70–80% of the colloid osmotic pressure of plasma. Albumin (Human) 5% is an effective and long acting agent for plasma volume expansion. The rationale for this is the Starling concept of the capillary balance of hydrostatic and oncotic pressure gradients across the capillary walls as the determinant of the fluid-i.e., volume-distribution between the intravascular and interstitial compartments (10). Albumin is distributed throughout the extracellular water; more than 60% of the body albumin pool is located in the extravascular fluid compartment. The total body albumin in a 70 kg man is approximately 320 g. Albumin has a half life of 15–20 days in the circulation (2,7) with a turnover of approximately 15 g per day.
When injected intravenously, Albumin (Human) 5% will increase the circulating plasma volume by an amount approximately equal to the amount infused. The additional fluid will reduce the hemoconcentration and decrease blood viscosity. The degree and duration of volume expansion depend upon the initial blood volume. In patients with diminished blood volume, the effect of infused Albumin (human) may persist many hours. The hemodilution lasts for a much shorter time when albumin is administered to individuals with normal blood volume.
Albumin is a transport protein which binds naturally occurring therapeutic and toxic materials in the circulation. The binding properties of albumin may, in special circumstances, provide an indication for its clinical use. For such purposes, however, Albumin (Human) 25% should be used.

INDICATIONS AND USAGE

Conditions For Which Albumin (Human) 5% Is Recommended:
Shock
The definitive treatment of major hemorrhage is the transfusion of red blood cells for restoring the normal oxygen transport capacity of the blood. Since, however, the life-threatening event in major hemorrhage is the loss of blood volume and not the erythrocyte deficit, the blood volume should, as an emergency measure, be supported by Albumin (Human) 5% or another rapidly acting plasma substitute if blood is not immediately available. This will restore cardiac output and abolish circulatory failure with tissue anoxia. In the presence of dehydration, electrolyte solutions such as Ringer's lactate should be administered in conjunction with Albumin (Human).
Burns
Apart from damage to the respiratory tract, the development of burn shock is the most life-threatening event in the immediate care of the burned patient. An optimum regimen for the use of Albumin (Human), electrolytes, and fluid in the treatment of burns has not been established. Therapy during the first 24 hours after a severe burn is usually directed at the administration of large volumes of crystalloid solutions and lesser amounts of Albumin (Human) to maintain an adequate plasma volume. For continuation of therapy beyond 24 hours, larger amounts of Albumin (Human) and lesser amounts of crystalloid are generally used (12).
Conditions For Which Albumin (Human) 5% May Be Useful:
Pancreatitis and Peritonitis
Albumin (Human) 5% may be useful in the early therapy of shock associated with acute hemorrhagic pancreatitis and peritonitis. It has been found that the correction of the blood volume deficit and adequate fluid therapy are mandatory in the acute stage of pancreatitis and peritonitis when there is loss of fluid into the peritoneal cavity or the retroperitoneal space (1).
Conditions For Which Albumin (Human) 5% Is Usually Not Recommended:
Postoperative albumin loss
It is now recognized that intraoperative damage to capillary walls, e.g., by blunt handling and sharp dissection of tissue, leads to substantial postoperative losses of circulating albumin, over and above those due to bleeding. However, this internal redistribution rarely causes clinically significant hypovolemia or adversely affects wound healing, and treatment of this condition with Albumin (Human) 5% is usually not indicated.
Hypoproteinemia with an oncotic deficit
In subacute or chronic hypoproteinemia, efforts should always be made to determine the underlying cause and to improve circulating protein levels by dietary means. Most commonly, such states are due to protein-calorie malnutrition, defective absorption in gastrointestinal disorders, faulty albumin synthesis in chronic hepatic failure, increased protein catabolism after operation or in sepsis, and abnormal renal losses of albumin in chronic kidney disease. In all these situations, the circulating plasma volume is usually maintained by the renal retention of sodium and water, but this is associated with tissue edema due to the hypoalbuminemia and with an oncotic deficit. Though relief of the basic pathology is the definitive therapy for restoration of the plasma protein level, Albumin (Human) is effective in the rapid correction of an oncotic deficit occurring in the aforementioned acute complications of chronic hypoproteinemia. For this purpose, however, Albumin (Human) 25% is the preferable therapeutic agent, possibly in conjunction with a diuretic. It is emphasized that whereas Albumin (Human) may be needed to treat the acute complications of chronic hypoproteinemia, it is NOT indicated for treatment of the chronic disease itself.

CONTRAINDICATIONS

The use of Albumin (Human) is contraindicated in patients with a history of an incompatibility reaction to such preparations (see Adverse Reactions). In addition, the Albumin (Human) may be contraindicated in patients with cardiac failure, pulmonary edema or severe anemia because of the risk of acute circulatory overload. Also, Albumin (Human) has been reported to contain trace amounts of aluminum (4,5). Accumulations of aluminum in patients with chronic renal insufficiencies has led to toxic manifestations such as hypercalcemia, vitamin D-refractory osteodystrophy, anemia, and severe progressive encephalopathy (5,6,13). Therefore, when large volumes of Albumin (Human) are contemplated for administration to such patients, serious consideration of these potential risks relative to the anticipated benefits should be given.

WARNINGS

ALBUMIN (HUMAN) 5% MUST NOT BE USED IF THE SOLUTION IS TURBID.
ALBUMIN (HUMAN) 5% MUST BE INFUSED IMMEDIATELY AND WITHOUT INTERRUPTION AFTER PERFORATION OF THE R/C BOTTLE. DO NOT BEGIN ADMINISTRATION MORE THAN 4 HOURS AFTER THE CONTAINER HAS BEEN ENTERED. PARTIALLY USED BOTTLES MUST BE DISCARDED.
ALBUMIN (HUMAN) 5% MUST NOT BE GIVEN THROUGH INFUSION SETS WHICH HAVE ALREADY BEEN USED OR ARE INTENDED FOR SIMULTANEOUS INFUSION OF PROTEIN HYDROLYSATE OR SOLUTIONS CONTAINING ALCOHOL.

PRECAUTIONS

Adequate precautions should be taken against circulatory overload; this can be done, for example, by measurement of the pulmonary wedge pressure. Special caution is indicated in patients with stabilized chronic anemia or renal insufficiency.

The rapid rise in blood pressure following infusion necessitates careful observation of injured or postoperative patients to detect and treat severed blood vessels that may not have bled at the lower blood pressure.

Certain components used in the packaging of this product contain natural rubber latex.

PREGNANCY CATEGORY C. Albumin (Human) 5% - Animal reproduction studies have not been conducted with Albumin (Human) 5%. It is also not known whether Albumin (Human) 5% can cause fetal harm when administered to a pregnant woman or can affect reproduction capacity. Albumin (Human) 5% should be given to a pregnant woman only if clearly needed.

ADVERSE REACTIONS

Though very rare, adverse reactions such as chills, fever, tachycardia, hypotension, urticaria, skin rash and nausea may occur (3,8,9,11). These symptoms may disappear if the infusion is slowed or stopped for a short period of time. If necessary, the intravenous administration of 50 to 200 mg of prednisolone may be useful (9).

DOSAGE AND ADMINISTRATION

Upon administration of Albumin (Human) 5% there is a rapid increase of the plasma volume about equal to the volume infused. The initial dose for adults is 250 to 500 mL. The quantity given may be increased to a total of 0.5 g albumin per pound of body weight (i.e., 10 mL/pound), but administration should be monitored by careful observation of the patient. The rate of infusion and the total volume administered are determined by the condition and the response of the patient. A rate of 1–2 mL per minute is usually suitable in the absence of overt shock, whereas the capacity of the administration set is the only limit in the exsanguinated patient. During resuscitation, constant monitoring of the patient provides the guidelines for treatment. For children, a dose of 10 to 15 mL per pound of body weight is usually adequate and close surveillance of the small patient is essential. In severely injured or septic patients, administration of Albumin (Human) 5% should always be guided by an appropriate hemodynamic monitoring of the patient.

Parenteral drug products should be inspected visually for particulate matter and discoloration prior to administration, whenever solution and container permit.

To prepare Albumin (Human) 5% for administration, remove outer seal to expose central portion of rubber stopper, cleanse stopper with germicidal solution and follow directions for use of intravenous injection set.

Albumin (Human) 5% must be administered INTRAVENOUSLY. The venipuncture site should not be infected or traumatized, and should be prepared with standard aseptic technique. The solution is compatible with whole blood or packed red cells as well as the usual electrolyte and carbohydrate solutions intended for intravenous use. By contrast, it should not be mixed with protein hydrolysates, amino acid mixtures, or solutions containing alcohol. It is ready for use as contained in the bottle and may be given without regard to the blood group of the recipient.

Only clear solutions of a light yellowish color should be administered.

HOW SUPPLIED

Puncture vial containing 50 mL of Albumin (Human) 5%.
Puncture vial containing 250 mL of Albumin (Human) 5%.
Puncture vial containing 500 mL of Albumin (Human) 5%.
The package may be supplied with an intravenous injection set.

STORAGE

Albumin (Human) 5% can be stored for 3 years at a temperature not exceeding 30°C (86°F).
Protect from freezing.

REFERENCES
1. CLOWES, G.H.A., Jr., VUCINIC, M., and WEIDNER, M.G.: Ann. Surg. 163, 866 (1966).
2. JANEWAY, C.A. In: Sgouris, J.T. and Rene A. (eds.): Proceedings of the Workshop of Albumin, DHEW Publication No. (NIH) 76-925, U.S. Government Printing Office, Washington, D.C., p. 3–21 (1976).
3. LOWENSTEIN, E. In: Sgouris, J.T. and Rene A. (eds.): Proceedings of the Workshop on Albumin, DHEW Publication No. (NIH) 76-925, U.S. Government Printing Office, Washington, D.C., p. 302 (1976).
4. MAHARAJ, D., FELL, G.S., BOYCE, B.F., NG, J.P., SMITHE, G.D., BOULTON-JONES, J.M., CUMMING, R.L., and DAVIDSON, J.F.: Brit. Med. J. 295, 693–696 (1987).
5. MILLINER, D.S., SHINABERGER, J.H., SHUMAN, P., and COBURN, J.W.: N. Engl. J. Med. 312, 165–167 (1985).
6. OTT, S.M., MALONEY, N.A., KLEIN, G.L., ALFREY, A.C., AMENT, M.E., COBURN, J.W., and SHERRAND, D.J.: Ann. of Inter. Med. 98, 910–914 (1983).
7. PETERS, T., Jr., In: Putnam, F.W. (ed.): Plasma Proteins, 2nd Edition, Vol. 1, Academic Press, New York, p. 133–181 (1975).
8. RING, J. and MESSMER, K.: Lancet 1, 466 (1977).
9. RING, J., SEIFERT, J., LOB, G., COULIN, K., and BRENDEL, W.: W. Klin, Wschr. 52, 595 (1974).
10. STARLING, E.H.: J Physiol. (London) 19, 312 (1896).
11. TULLIS, J.L.: J.A.M.A. 237, 355 (1977).
12. TULLIS, J.L.: J.A.M.A. 237, 460 (1977).
13. WILLIS, M.R., and SAVORY, J.A.: Lancet 2, 29–34 (1983).

IMMUNO-U.S., INC.
1200 Parkdale Road
Rochester, MI 48307 USA
Distributed in Canada by:
IMMUNO (Canada) LTD.
U.S. License No. 850
Canadian License No. 227
Rev. July, 1997

ALBUMIN (HUMAN) 25% SOLUTION ℞

DESCRIPTION

Albumin (Human) 25% is a sterile aqueous solution for intravenous use, mainly containing the albumin component of human plasma. The effective oncotic pressure of the 25% solution largely depends on its albumin content and is approximately five times that of human plasma. Sodium bicarbonate is used to adjust the pH to 6.9 ± 0.5. The sodium content of the solution ranges between 130 and 160 meq/L, 0.08 millimole sodium caprylate and 0.08 millimole sodium N-acetyltryptophanate per gram albumin are added as stabilizers to prevent denaturation during heating. The solution is heat-treated at 60°C for 10 hours for inactivation of hepatitis viruses.

CLINICAL PHARMACOLOGY

Albumin is a very soluble, globular protein (MW66,500) accounting for 70–80% of the colloid osmotic pressure of plasma which is the predominant reason for its clinical use. The rationale for this is the Starling concept of the capillary balance of hydrostatic and oncotic pressure gradients across the capillary walls as the determinant of the fluid-i.e., volume-distribution between the intravascular and the interstitial compartments (12). Albumin is distributed throughout the extracellular water; more than 60% of the body albumin pool is located in the extravascular fluid compartment. The total body albumin in a 70 kg man is approximately 320 g. Albumin has a half life of 15–20 days in the circulation (2,8), with a turnover of approximately 15 g per day.

When injected intravenously, Albumin (Human) 25% will draw approximately 3.5 times its volume of additional fluid into the circulation within 15 minutes, if the recipient is adequately hydrated. The additional fluid will reduce the hemoconcentration and decrease blood viscosity. The degree and duration of volume expansion depends upon the initial blood volume. In patients with diminished blood volume, the effect of infused Albumin (Human) may persist many hours. The hemodilution lasts for a much shorter time when Albumin (Human) is administered to individuals with normal blood volume. The minimum plasma albumin level necessary to prevent or reverse peripheral edema is unknown. Although it varies from patient to patient, there is some evidence that it is approximately 2.5 g/dL. This concentration provides a plasma oncotic pressure of 20 mm Hg (the equivalent of a total protein concentration of 5.2 g/dL).

Albumin is a transport protein which binds naturally occurring therapeutic and toxic materials in the circulation. The binding properties of albumin may provide an indication for its use in severe hemolytic disease of the newborn, where it may lower the plasma concentration of free bilirubin pending or in conjunction with an exchange transfusion (14). This effect may also be relevant in certain cases of acute liver failure with rapidly increasing levels of serum billirubin, particularly in the presence of severe hypoproteinemia. Albumin (Human) 25% offers minimal risk of hemorrhagic diathesis or blockage of the reticuloendothelial system. It does not impair coagulation or platelet function. Antibodies, including isoagglutinins, have been removed, thus enabling the product to be used without regard to the patient's blood group or blood factors.

INDICATIONS AND USAGE

General Principles

The two main indications for the use of Albumin (Human) 25% - are a plasma or blood volume deficit and the oncotic deficit resulting from hypoproteinemia.

Volume Deficit

Since the oncotic pressure of Albumin (Human) 25% solution is about five times that of normal human serum, it will expand the plasma volume if interstitial water is available for an inflow through the capillary walls. However, many patients suffering from an acute volume deficit also have some degree of interstitial dehydration. In the absence of overhydration, the treatment of an acute volume deficit with Albumin (Human) 25% should, therefore, include isotonic electrolyte solutions with an albumin: electrolyte ratio of 1:3 or 1:4. By contrast, chronic volume deficits have usually been at least partially compensated for by the renal retention of sodium and water with some degree of tissue edema, and in these circumstances a trial with Albumin (Human) 25% only is indicated.

Oncotic Deficit

The common causes of hypoproteinemia are protein-calorie malnutrition, defective absorption in gastrointestinal disorders, faulty albumin synthesis (e.g., in chronic hepatic failure), increased protein catabolism after operation or in sepsis, and abnormal renal losses of albumin in chronic kidney disease. In these situations, the circulating plasma volume is usually maintained by the renal retention of sodium and water, but this is associated with tissue edema and an oncotic deficit. Though relief of the underlying pathology is the definitive therapy for the restoration of the plasma protein level, this process takes time to become effective and the rapid correction of an oncotic deficit by the administration of Albumin (Human) 25%, possibly in conjunction with a diuretic, may be indicated.

It is emphasized that whereas Albumin (Human) may be necessary to prevent or treat the aforementioned acute complication of hypoproteinemia, it is NOT indicated for treatment of the chronic condition itself.

SPECIFIC INDICATIONS

Acute Circumstances In Which
Albumin (Human) 25%
Use Is Usually Appropriate:

Shock

The definitive treatment of major hemorrhage is the transfusion of red blood cells restoring a normal oxygen transport capacity of the blood. However, the life-threatening event in major hemorrhage is the loss of blood volume and not the erythrocyte deficit. Therefore, the blood volume should, as an emergency measure, be supported by Albumin (Human) 5% or another rapidly acting plasma substitute if blood is not immediately available. This will restore cardiac output and abolish circulatory failure with tissue anoxia. If Albumin (Human) 5% is not available, Albumin (Human) 5% can be prepared by diluting Albumin (Human) 25% with 4 volumes of an appropriate electrolyte solution, such as Ringer's lactate. Alternatively, the two solutions may be administered concurrently. If the patients is severely dehydrated, additional electrolyte solutions may be required.

Burns

An optimal regimen for the use of Albumin (Human), electrolytes, and water in the treatment of burns has not been established. Therapy during the first 24 hours after a severe burn is usually directed at the administration of crystalloid solutions in order to maintain an adequate plasma volume. For continuation of therapy beyond 24 hours, larger amounts of Albumin (Human) and lesser amounts of crystalloid are generally used (14).

Adult Respiratory Distress Syndrome

Several factors are usually involved in the development of the state now commonly called the adult respiratory distress syndrome, one of these being a hypoproteinemic fluid overload. In its initial phase, this may be corrected by the use of Albumin (Human) 25% and a diuretic (11,14) along with careful hemodynamic and respiratory monitoring of the patient. It must be recognized, however, that the beneficial effects of Albumin (Human) in this condition depend on the integrity of the pulmonary microvasculature. Increased permeability to albumin can negate these beneficial effects, and in such circumstances Albumin (Human) could actually contribute to the respiratory distress.

Cardiopulmonary Bypass

An adequate blood volume during cardiopulmonary bypass can be maintained with crystalloids or colloids (albumin). A commonly employed program is an Albumin (Human) and crystalloid pump prime adjusted so as to achieve a hematocrit of 20% and a plasma albumin level of 2.5 g/100 mL in the patient, but the level to which either may be lowered safely has not yet been defined (14).

Hemolytic Disease of the Newborn

Albumin (Human) 25% may be indicated in order to bind and thus detoxify free serum bilirubin in severely hemolytic infants pending an exchange transfusion (14). Caution is recommended in hypervolemic infants.

Acute nephrosis

Patients with acute nephrosis may prove refractory to cyclophosphamide or steroid therapy and their edema may even be aggravated initially by steroids. In such cases, a response may be elicited by combining Albumin (Human) 25% with an appropriate diuretic, after which the patient may react satisfactorily to drug therapy (14).

Continued on next page

Albumin (Human) 25%—Cont.

Circumstances In which albumin (Human) 25% Is Usually Not Justified:

Postoperative Hypoproteinemia
Intraoperative damage of capillary walls, e.g., by blunt dissection, leads to substantial losses of circulating albumin over and above those due to bleeding. However, this redistribution of albumin in the body rarely causes clinically significant hypovolemia, and treatment of the resultant plasma oncotic defect with Albumin (Human) 25% is not usually indicated.

Red Cell Resuspension Media
As a rule, the use of Albumin (Human) for resuspending red cells can be dispensed with. However, in exceptional circumstances such as certain types of exchange transfusions and the use of very large volumes of erythrocyte concentrates and frozen or washed red cells, the addition of Albumin (Human) to the resuspension medium may be indicated in order to provide sufficient volume and/or avoid excessive hypoproteinemia during the subsequent transfusion. If necessary, 20–25 g or more of albumin per liter of red cells should be added as a concentrated solution to the isotonic electrolyte suspension of erythrocytes immediately before transfusion.

Renal Dialysis
Patients undergoing long-term hemodialysis may need Albumin (Human) for the treatment of a volume or an oncotic deficit. The patients should be carefully observed for signs of a circulatory overload to which they are particularly sensitive.

Acute Liver Failure
In acute liver failure, Albumin (Human) may serve the triple purpose of stabilizing the circulation, correcting an oncotic deficit and binding excessive serum bilirubin. The therapeutic approach is guided by the individual circumstances (14).

Ascites
The use of Albumin (Human) for blood volume support may be indicated if circulatory instability follows the withdrawal of large amounts (>1500 mL) of ascitic fluid.

Third Space Problems of Infectious Origin
The sequestration of protein-rich fluid during acute peritonitis, pancreatitis, mediastinitis or extensive cellulitis will very rarely be of sufficient magnitude to require the treatment of a volume or an oncotic deficit with Albumin (Human)(1).

There is no valid reason for the use of Albumin (Human) as an intravenous nutrient.

CONTRAINDICATIONS
The use of albumin (Human) is contraindicated in patients with a history of an incompatibility reaction to such preparations (see Adverse Reactions). In addition, the Albumin (Human) may be contraindicated in patients with cardiac failure, pulmonary edema or severe anemia because of the risk of acute circulatory overload. Also, Albumin (Human) has been reported to contain trace amounts of aluminum (5,6). Accumulations of aluminum in patients with chronic renal insufficiencies has led to toxic manifestations such as hypercalcemia, vitamin D-refractory osteodystrophy, anemia, and severe progressive encephalopathy (6,7,15). Therefore, when large volumes of Albumin (Human) are contemplated for administration to such patients, serious consideration of these potential risks relative to the anticipated benefits should be given.

WARNINGS
ALBUMIN (HUMAN) 25% MUST NOT BE USED IF THE SOLUTIONS TURBID.
ALBUMIN (HUMAN) 25% MUST BE INFUSED IMMEDIATELY AND WITHOUT INTERRUPTION AFTER PERFORATION OF THE R/C BOTTLE. DO NOT BEGIN ADMINISTRATION MORE THAN 4 HOURS AFTER THE CONTAINER HAS BEEN ENTERED. PARTIALLY USED BOTTLES MUST BE DISCARDED.
ALBUMIN (HUMAN) 25% MUST NOT BE GIVEN THROUGH INFUSION SETS WHICH HAVE ALREADY BEEN USED OR ARE INTENDED FOR SIMULTANEOUS INFUSION OF PROTEIN HYDROLYSATE OR SOLUTIONS CONTAINING ALCOHOL.

PRECAUTIONS
Adequate precautions should be taken against circulatory overload; this can be done, for example, by the measurement of the pulmonary wedge pressure. Special caution is indicated in patients with stabilized chronic anemia or renal insufficiency. A rapid rise in blood pressure following infusion necessitates careful observation of injured or postoperative patients to detect and treat severed blood vessels that may not have bled at a lower blood pressure.
Certain components used in the packaging of this product contain natural rubber latex.
PREGNANCY CATEGORY C. Albumin (Human) 25% - Animal reproduction studies have not been conducted with Albumin (Human) 25%. It is also not known whether Albumin (Human) 25% can cause fetal harm when administered

to a pregnant woman or can affect reproduction capacity. Albumin (Human) 25% should be given to a pregnant woman only if clearly needed.

ADVERSE REACTIONS
Though very rare, adverse reactions such as chills, fever, tachycardia, hypotension, urticaria, skin rash and nausea may occur (4,9,10,13).
The symptoms may disappear if the infusion is slowed or stopped for a short period of time. If necessary, the intravenous administration of 50 to 200 mg of prednisolone may be useful (10).

DOSAGE AND ADMINISTRATION
The dosage of Albumin (Human) 25% is based on the principles outlined in the section on Indications and Usage but should always be adapted to the individual situation. The quantities required may be underestimated because of hidden extravascular deficits, and the effect of Albumin (Human) infusion on the serum protein level should therefore, be checked by laboratory analysis.
The appropriate Albumin (Human) 25% dose for the treatment of a volume deficit should be estimated from the recipient's hemodynamic response (3) and precautions taken to safeguard against circulatory overload. In the absence of active hemorrhage, the total dose should not exceed the normal circulating albumin mass, i.e., 2 g per kg body weight. Patients with acute nephrosis may respond to a combination of 100 mL of Albumin (Human) 25% and an appropriate diuretic, repeated daily for about one week. For hemolytic disease of the newborn, the dosage is 4 mL of albumin (Human) 25% /kg body mass, to be given about one hour prior to ordering exchange transfusion. If Albumin (Human) is considered necessary for a renal dialysis patient, the initial dose should not exceed 100 mL of the 25% solution.
Parenteral drug products should be inspected visually for particulate matter and discoloration prior to administration, whenever solution and container permit.
To prepare Albumin (Human) 25% for administration, remove outer seal to expose central portion of rubber stopper and cleanse stopper with germicidal solution before use in syringes. Follow directions for use if the solution is administered by an intravenous injection set.
Albumin (Human) 25% must be administered INTRAVENOUSLY. The venipuncture site should not be infected or traumatized, and should be prepared with standard aseptic technique. The solution is compatible with whole blood or packed red cells as well as the usual electrolyte and carbohydrate solutions intended for intravenous use. By contrast, it should not be mixed with protein hydrolysates, amino acid mixtures, or solutions containing alcohol. It is ready for use as contained in the bottle and may be given without regard to the blood group of the recipient.
Only clear solutions of a light yellowish or amber color should be administered.

HOW SUPPLIED
Puncture vial containing 20 mL of Albumin (Human) 25%.
Puncture vial containing 50 mL of Albumin (Human) 25%.
Puncture vial containing 100 mL of Albumin (Human) 25%.
The package may be supplied with an intravenous injection set.

STORAGE
Albumin (Human) 25% can be stored for 3 years at a temperature not exceeding 30°C (86°F).
Protect from freezing.

REFERENCES
1. CLOWES, G.H.A., Jr., VUCINIC, M., and WEIDNER, M.G.: Ann Surg. 163, 866 (1966).
2. JANEWAY, C.A.: In: Sgouris, J.T. and Rene A. (eds,): Proceedings of the Workshop on Albumin, DHEW Publication No. (NIH) 76-925, U.S.Government Printing Office, Washington, D.C., p. 3-21 (1976).
3. KINNEY, J.M., EGDAHL, R.H. and ZUIDEMA, G.D.: manual of Preoperative and Postoperative Care, American College of Surgeons, W.B. Saunders Co., Philadelphia (1971).
4. LOWENSTEIN, E. In: Sgouris, J.T. and Rene A. (eds.): Proceedings of the Workshop on Albumin, DHEW Publication No. (NIH) 76-925, U.S. Government Printing Office, Washington, D.C., p. 302 (1976).
5. MAHARAJ, D., FELL, G.S., BOYCE, B.F., NG, J.P., SMITHE, G.D., BOULTON-JONES, J.M., CUMMING, R.L., and DAVIDSON, J.F.: Brit. Med. J. 295, 693–696 (1987).
6. MILLINER, D.S., SHINABERGER, J.H., SHUMAN, P., and COBURN, J.W.: N. Engl. J. Med. 312, 165–167 (1985).
7. OTT, S.M., MALONEY, N.A., KLEIN, G.L., ALFREY, A.C., AMENT, M.E., COBURN, J.W., and SHERAND, D.J.: Ann. of Inter, Med. 98, 910–914 (1983).
8. PETERS, T., Jr., In: Putnam, F.W. (ed.): Plasma Proteins, 2nd Edition, Vol. 1, Academic Press, New York, p. 133–181 (1975).
9. RING, J. and MESSMER, K.: Lancet 1, 466 (1977).
10. RING, J., SEIFERT, J., LOB, G., COULIN, K., and BRENDEL, W.: W. Klin, Wschr. 52, 595 (1974).
11. SKILLMAN, J.J., PARIKH, B.M., and TANENBAUM, B.J.: Amer. J. Surg. 119, 440 (1970).
12. STARLING, E.H.: J. Physiol. (London) 19, 312 (1896).
13. TULLIS, J.L.: J.A.M.A. 237, 355 (1977).
14. TULLIS, J.L.: J.A.M.A. 237, 460 (1977).
15. WILLIS, MR.R., and SAVORY, J.A.: Lancet 2, 29–34 (1983).

IMMUNO-U.S., INC.
1200 Parkdale Road
Rochester, MI 48307 USA
Distributed in Canada By:
IMMUNO (Canada) LTD.
U.S. License No. 850
Canadian License No. 227
Rev. July, 1997

BEBULIN® VH IMMUNO ℞
FACTOR IX COMPLEX, VAPOR HEATED

DESCRIPTION
FACTOR IX COMPLEX, VAPOR HEATED, BEBULIN VH IMMUNO is a purified, sterile, stable, freeze-dried concentrate of the coagulation Factors IX (Christmas Factor) as well as II (Prothrombin) and X (Stuart Prower Factor) and low amounts of Factor VII. In addition, the product contains small amounts of heparin (≤0.15 I.U. heparin per I.U. Factor IX).
FACTOR IX COMPLEX, VAPOR HEATED, BEBULIN VH IMMUNO is standardized in terms of Factor IX content and each vial is labeled for the Factor IX content indicated in International Units (I.U.). One International Unit of Factor IX (according to the current International Standard for Human Blood Coagulation Factors II, IX, and X in Concentrates, Code 84/681) corresponds to the activity of Factor IX in 1 mL of fresh normal human plasma.

CLINICAL PHARMACOLOGY
FACTOR IX COMPLEX, VAPOR HEATED, BEBULIN VH IMMUNO is a combination of vitamin K-dependent clotting factors found in normal plasma. The administration of FACTOR IX COMPLEX, VAPOR HEATED, BEBULIN VH IMMUNO provides an increase in plasma levels of Factor IX and can temporarily correct the coagulation defect of patients with Factor IX deficiency. Plasma levels of Factors II and X will also be increased. However, no clinical studies have been conducted to show benefit from this product for treating deficiencies other than Factor IX deficiency.
In vivo recovery of FACTOR IX COMPLEX, VAPOR HEATED, BEBULIN VH IMMUNO was determined by investigators in Germany, Japan, and the United States using the former International Standard, WHO 72/32 and found to be 53.3% ±9.6%, 57.5% ±21.8%, and 53.24% ±16.95%, respectively. In the same studies, using different methodologies, half-lives were determined to be 19.4 hrs ±3.8 hrs, 24.6 hrs ±3.2 hrs, and 19.97 hrs ±8.24 hrs, respectively (1,2, 3).
The product has been subjected to virus inactivation by vapor heating where vapor is first applied for 10 hours at 60°C ±0.5°C and an excess pressure of 190 ±25 mbar followed by 1 hour at 80°C ±0.5°C and an excess pressure of 375 ±35 mbar (4). The effectiveness of vapor heating was evaluated in vitro using Human Immunodeficiency Virus (HIV-1) and Sindbis Virus. Lyophilization followed by vapor heat treatment at 60°C inactivated >5.8 logs of HIV-1 and 4.0 logs of Sindbis Virus within 3 hours. Lyophilization with vapor heating at 60°C for 10 hours resulted in no detectable Sindbis Virus (>4.5 log reduction). Vapor heating at 80°C inactivated >3.5 logs of HIV-1 and >4.4 logs of Sindbis Virus within one hour.
In the context of two prospective clinical studies (5, 6) and a retrospective survey (7) FACTOR IX COMPLEX, VAPOR HEATED, BEBULIN VH IMMUNO was followed up for the risk of transfusion-transmitted viral infections. All patients received blood products for the first time. Using criteria established by the ICTH, 16 patients could be followed up for nonA, nonB hepatitis, 9 for HCV seroconversion, 3 for hepatitis B, and 24 for HIV seroconversion. None tested positive for any of these infections. An additional 3 patients with 2 or more consecutive test samples missing tested negative for nonA, nonB hepatitis for all samples available. Three studies using ICTH criteria for testing (5, 6, 8), a retrospective survey (7), and a case report (9) on other vapor heated factors of the prothrombin complex that were subjected to the same inactivation process as BEBULIN VH gave the following results: 27 patients tested negative for nonA, nonB hepatitis, 15 for HCV seroconversion, 25 for hepatitis B, and 75 for HIV seroconversion.

INDICATIONS AND USAGE
FACTOR IX COMPLEX, VAPOR HEATED, BEBULIN VH IMMUNO is indicated for the prevention and control of hemorrhagic episodes in hemophilia B patients.

FACTOR IX COMPLEX, VAPOR HEATED, BEBULIN VH IMMUNO is not indicated for use in the treatment of Factor VII deficiency. No clinical studies have been conducted to show benefit from this product for treating deficiencies other than Factor IX deficiency.

CONTRAINDICATIONS

None known.

WARNINGS

This product is prepared from pooled human plasma which may contain the causative agents of hepatitis and other viral diseases. Prescribed manufacturing procedures utilized at the plasma collection centers, plasma testing laboratories, and the fractionation facilities are designed to reduce the risk of transmitting viral infection. However, the risk of viral infectivity from this product cannot be totally eliminated.

Individuals who receive infusions of blood or plasma products may develop signs and/or symptoms of some viral infections, particularly nonA, nonB hepatitis. Hepatitis B vaccination is essential for patients with hemophilia and it is recommended that this be done at birth or diagnosis.

The risk of thromboembolic complications including DIC and hyperfibrinolysis is present with the administration of Factor IX Complex, particularly in the postoperative period and in patients with risk factors predisposing to thrombosis.

PRECAUTIONS

In patients with risk factors predisposing to thrombosis the Factor IX level should not be raised to more than approximately 60% of normal (10). In addition, it is recommended that such patients as well as patients who require high doses of Factor IX because of major surgical interventions be monitored for the possible development of DIC and/or thrombosis. In case changes occur in blood pressure or pulse rate or symptoms such as respiratory distress, chest pain or cough, treatment should be stopped immediately.

Information for Patients

Patients should be informed of the early signs of hypersensitivity reactions such as fever, urticaria, rashes, nausea or retching and should be advised to discontinue use of the product and contact their physician if these symptoms occur.

Pregnancy Category C.

Animal reproduction studies have not been conducted with FACTOR IX COMPLEX, VAPOR HEATED, BEBULIN VH IMMUNO. It is also not known whether FACTOR IX COMPLEX, VAPOR HEATED, BEBULIN VH IMMUNO can cause fetal harm when administered to a pregnant woman or can affect reproduction capacity. FACTOR IX COMPLEX, VAPOR HEATED, BEBULIN VH IMMUNO should be given to a pregnant woman only if clearly needed.

ADVERSE REACTIONS

As with any other infused plasma derivatives, anaphylactoid or anaphylactic reactions may occur in rare cases. The occurrence of these reactions (e.g. fever, urticarial rashes, nausea, retching, dyspnea, anaphylactic shock) necessitates the interruption of replacement therapy. Mild reactions can be managed with antihistamines; severe hypotensive reactions require immediate intervention using current principles of shock therapy.

DOSAGE AND ADMINISTRATION

General

FACTOR IX COMPLEX, VAPOR HEATED, BEBULIN VH IMMUNO is intended for intravenous administration only. As a general rule, 1 International Unit of Factor IX activity/kg will increase the plasma level of Factor IX by 0.8%. Accordingly, the following formula is provided for dosage calculations:

$$\text{Number of Factor IX I.U. required} = \text{bodyweight (kg)} \times \text{desired Factor IX increase (\% of normal)} \times 1.2$$

It must, however, be emphasized that the response to treatment will vary from patient to patient and that occasionally larger doses than those derived from the above formula will be required, particularly if treatment is delayed. Exact dosage determination should be based on localization and extent of hemorrhage, and the level of Factor IX to be achieved.

It must be emphasized that particularly with severe hemorrhage and major surgery close laboratory monitoring of the Factor IX level is required to determine proper dosage.

Management of Specific Types of Bleeding (10, 11, 12, 13, 14)

Approximate Factor IX levels, typical initial doses, and the average duration of treatment are suggested in the table below. For minor bleeding a single dose will usually be sufficient, otherwise a second dose may be given after 24 hours. More severe hemorrhage will require the administration of several doses at approximately 24 hour intervals. For maintenance therapy usually two thirds of the initial dose is infused.

Type of Bleeding	Approximate Factor IX Level (% Normal)	Typical Initial Dose (I.U./kg)	Average Duration of Treatment Days
Minor early hemarthrosis, minor epistaxis, and gingival bleeding, mild hematuria	20	25–35	1
Moderate severe joint bleeding, early hematoma, major open bleeding, minor trauma, minor hemoptysis hematemesis, and melena, major hematuria	40	40–55	2 or until adequate wound healing
Major severe hematoma, major trauma, severe hemoptysis, hematemesis, and melena	≥60*	60–70	2–3 or until adequate wound healing

* For patients predisposing to thrombosis see "PRECAUTIONS" section.

Management of Surgical Procedures (10, 11, 12, 13, 14)

Dosage guidelines for surgical procedures are suggested below. The preoperative loading dose should be administered one hour prior to surgery. Depending on the type of surgery replacement therapy has to be continued over one to several weeks until adequate wound healing is achieved. The average treatment interval will initially be 12 hours, while in the later postoperative period 24 hours are generally adequate.

[See table below]

For tooth extraction the same initial dose as for minor surgery is recommended. Generally, one infusion will be sufficient. In case of extraction of several teeth, replacement therapy for up to one week may be necessary using the same doses as for minor surgery (12, 13, 14).

Long-Term Prophylactic Treatment

Prophylactic doses of 20–30 I.U./kg administered once, or preferably up to twice a week have been shown to significantly reduce the frequency of spontaneous hemorrhage (12, 15). It is, however, recommended that prophylactic dosage regimens be tailored to individual needs.

Reconstitution

FACTOR IX COMPLEX, VAPOR HEATED, BEBULIN VH IMMUNO should be reconstituted immediately before application. The solution does not contain a preservative and must be used within 3 hours of reconstitution.

For reconstitution proceed as follows:

1. Warm both diluent and concentrate in unopened vials to room temperature (not above 37°C, 98°F).
2. Remove caps from both vials to expose central portions of the rubber stoppers.
3. Cleanse exposed surface of the rubber stoppers with germicidal solution and allow to dry.
4. Using aseptic technique, remove protective covering from one end of the double-ended needle, and insert the exposed end through the diluent vial stopper.

5. Remove protective covering from the other end of the double-ended needle, taking care not to touch the exposed end. Invert diluent vial over the concentrate vial, then insert free end of the needle through the concentrate vial stopper. Diluent will be drawn into the concentrate vial by vacuum.
6. Disconnect the two vials by removing needle from the concentrate vial stopper. Gently agitate or rotate the concentrate vial until all material is dissolved.

Do not refrigerate after reconstitution!

Administration

Parenteral drug products should be inspected for particulate matter and discoloration prior to administration, whenever solution and container permit.

Intravenous Injection:

1. After reconstituting the concentrate as described above attach the enclosed filter needle to a sterile disposable syringe using aseptic technique. Insert filter needle through the concentrate vial stopper.
2. Inject air and withdraw solution into the syringe.
3. Remove and discard filter needle. Attach a suitable intravenous needle or infusion set with winged adapter.
4. Administer the solution intravenously at a rate comfortable to the patient (maximum rate 2 ml per minute).

HOW SUPPLIED

FACTOR IX COMPLEX, IMMUNO, VAPOR HEATED, BEBULIN VH is supplied in single dose vials with Sterile Water for Injection, U.S.P. (This Product Contains Dry Natural Rubber.), double-ended needle, and filter needle for reconstitution and withdrawal.

FACTOR IX activity in International Units is stated on the label of each vial.

Rx only

STORAGE

When stored at refrigerator temperature (2°C–8°C, 35°F–46°F), FACTOR IX COMPLEX, VAPOR HEATED, BEBULIN VH IMMUNO is stable for the period indicated by the expiration date on its label.

Avoid freezing, which may damage the diluent vial.

REFERENCES

1. H.H. Brackmann: A Study to Investigate the In Vivo Recovery and Half-Life Time of Factor IX Concentrate S-TIM 4. Unpublished Report, 1985.
2. T. Abe et al.: Clinical Study with BENOBIL TIM 4, Steam-Treated Factor IX Complex, Single Administration. Jap. Pharm. & Ther., 14, 1986, 1, pp. 19–31.
3. C. Kasper, A. Andes, L.M. Aledort: Clinical Study of Recovery and Half-Life of Factor IX Complex (Human) IMMUNO, Vapor Heated, Bebulin VH. Unpublished Report, 1990.
4. F. Elsinger, G. Wöber, F. Dorner, J. Eibl, Y. Linnau, A. Philapitsch, O. Schwarz: Steam Treatment of Freeze-Dried Plasma Fractions. In: N.L. Ciavarella, Z.M. Ruggeri, Th.S. Zimmermann (Eds.): Factor VII/von Willebrand Factor–Biological and Clinical Advances. Milano: Wichtig Editore srl, 1986, pp. 297–302.
5. Kl. Schimpf: Klinische Studien zur Infektiosität von konventionellen und virusinaktivierten Gerinnungsfaktorenkonzentraten. In: G. Landbeck, Kl. Schimpf (Eds.): 3. Rundtischgespräch über aktuelle Probleme der Substitutionstherapie Hämophiler. Berlin: Springer Verlag, 1986, pp. 69–79.
6. A Study to Determine the Safety of Virus Inactivated Factor Concentrates in Hemophiliacs Naive to Blood Product Administration. Data on file.
7. Kl. Schimpf: Substitutionstherapie bei angeborenen Gerinnungsstörungen. In: O. H. Just, C. Krier (Eds.): Haemostasis in Anaesthesia and Intensive Medicine. Berlin: Springer Verlag, 1988, pp. 17–31.
8. D. U. Preiss, B. Eberspächer, D. Abdullah, I. Rosner: Safety of Vapour Heated Prothrombin Complex Concentrate (PCC) Prothromplex S-TIM 4. Thrombosis Research, 63, 1991, pp. 651–659.
9. M. Köhler, P. Hellstern, G. Pindur, E. Wenzel, G. v. Blohn: Factor VII Half-Life after Transfusion of a Steam-Treated Prothrombin Complex Concentrate in a Patient with Homozygous Factor VII Deficiency. Vox Sang., 56, 1989, pp. 200–201.
10. P.H. Levine: Clinical Manifestations and Therapy of Hemophilias A and B. In: R.W. Colman, J. Hirsh, V.J. Marder, E.W. Salzman (Eds.): Hemostasis and Thrombosis. Philadelphia: J.B. Lippincott Company, 1987, pp. 97–111.
11. C. R. Rizza, P. Jones: Management of patients with inherited blood coagulation defects. In: A.L. Bloom, D.P. Thomas (Eds.): Hemostasis and Thrombosis. Edinburgh: Churchill Livingstone, 1987, pp. 465–493.
12. T. Abe, M. Kazama: An International Survey on the Appropriate Dosage of Hemophilias and Related Congeni-

Type of Surgery	Day of Operation		Init. Postop. Period (1st to 2nd Week)		Late Postop. Period (from 3rd Week Onwards)	
	Approx. Level F IX (% Normal)	Dose (I.U./kg)	Approx. Level F IX (% Normal)	Dose (I.U./kg)	Approx. Level F IX (% Normal)	Dose (I.U./kg)
Major	≥60*	70–95	60→20	70→35	20	35→25
Minor	40–60	50–60	40→20	55→25		

* For patients predisposing to thrombosis see "PRECAUTIONS" section.

Continued on next page

Bebulin VH—Cont.

tal Coagulopathies. In: Proceedings of the 3rd International Symposion on Haemostasis and Thrombosis, 1982, pp. 273–304.
13. I.M. Nilsson Å. Ahlberg, G. Björlin: Clinical Experience with a Swedish Factor IX Concentrate. Acta Med. Scand., 190, 1971, pp. 257–266.
14. J.N. George, R. T. Breckenridge: The Use of Factor VIII and Factor IX Concentrates During Surgery. JAMA, 214, 1970, 9, pp. 1673–1676.
15. E. Ludwig, K. Lechner. Prophylaktische Behandlung bei schwerer Hämophilie B mit einem Faktor-IX-Konzentrat. Dtsch. Med. Wschr., 99 1974 25 pp. 1355–1361.

Manufactured by
ÖSTERREICHISCHES INSTITUT FÜR HAEMODERIVATE GES.M.B.H.
Subsidiary of **IMMUNO AG**
A-1220 Vienna, Austria
U.S. Establishment Licence 258
U.S. Pat. Nos. 4,640,834 and 4,388,232
Distributed by
IMMUNO U.S., Inc.
1200 Parkdale Road
Rochester, Michigan 48307

Issued April 1998
6205212EH03

FEIBA® VH IMMUNO ℞
ANTI-INHIBITOR, COAGULANT COMPLEX, VAPOR HEATED

DESCRIPTION

Anti-Inhibitor Coagulant Complex, Vapor Heated, FEIBA® VH IMMUNO, is a freeze-dried sterile human plasma fraction with Factor VIII inhibitor bypassing activity. In vitro, FEIBA® VH IMMUNO shortens the activated partial thromboplastin time (APTT) of plasma containing Factor VIII inhibitor. Factor VIII inhibitor bypassing activity is expressed in arbitrary units. One IMMUNO Unit of activity is defined as that amount of Anti-Inhibitor Coagulant Complex, Vapor Heated, FEIBA® VH IMMUNO which shortens the APTT of a high titer Factor VIII inhibitor reference plasma to 50% of the blank value. The product is intended for intravenous administration.

Anti-Inhibitor Coagulant Complex, Vapor Heated, FEIBA® VH IMMUNO contains Factors II, IX, and X, mainly non-activated, and Factor VII[1–3] mainly in the activated form. The product contains approximately equal unitages of Factor VIII inhibitor bypassing activity and Prothrombin Complex Factors. In addition, 1–6 units of Factor VIII coagulant antigen (F VIII C: Ag) per mL are present. The preparation contains only traces of factors of the kinin generating system. It contains no heparin.

Reconstituted Anti-Inhibitor Coagulant Complex, Vapor Heated, FEIBA® VH IMMUNO contains 4 mg of trisodium citrate and 8 mg of sodium chloride per mL.

Anti-Inhibitor Coagulant Complex, Vapor Heated, FEIBA® VH IMMUNO has been prepared from Source Plasma and/or Plasma.

The produce has been subjected to in-process virus inactivation where vapor is first applied for 10 hours at 60° ± 0.5°C and an excess pressure of 190 ± 20 mbar followed by 1 hour at 80° ± 0.5°C and an excess pressure of 370 ± 30 mbar. (Refer to Clinical Pharmacology and Warnings sections.)

CLINICAL PHARMACOLOGY

In a preclinical study to determine the virus inactivating efficacy of vapor heating, samples of bulk Anti-Inhibitor Coagulant Complex, FEIBA® IMMUNO were spiked with 2×10^6/mL infectious units of HIV and subjected to vapor heat treatment. The residual virus titer was found to be less than 1 infectious unit/0.5 mL. A clinical study[4] testing Antihemophilic Factor treated by a similar vapor heating procedure has shown none of 4 lots used in the study to produce nonA, nonB hepatitis in intensively followed patients naive to blood product administration

The safety and efficacy of Anti-Inhibitor Coagulant Complex, FEIBA® IMMUNO has been demonstrated by two prospective clinical trials[5–7]. The first, conducted by Sixma and collaborators during 1979 and early 1980, was a randomized double-blind study comparing the effect of Anti-Inhibitor Coagulant Complex, FEIBA® IMMUNO, and PROTHROMPLEX IMMUNO (a non-activated prothrombin complex concentrate) in 15 patients with hemophilia A and inhibitors to Factor VIII. A total of 150 bleeding episodes (primarily joint and musculoskeletal plus a few mucocutaneous) were treated. A single dose of 88 IMMUNO Units per kg of body weight was used uniformly for treatments with Anti-Inhibitor Coagulant Complex, FEIBA® IMMUNO. The study showed that, based on subjective patient evaluation, FEIBA® IMMUNO was fully effective in 41.0% and partly effective in 24.6% of episodes (i.e. combined effectiveness of 65.6%), while PROTHROMPLEX IMMUNO was rated fully effective in 25.0% and partly effective in 21.4% of episodes (i.e. combined effectiveness of 46.4%).

The second study with FEIBA® IMMUNO was a multiclinic study conducted by Hilgartner et al. It was designed to evaluate the efficacy of FEIBA® IMMUNO in the treatment of joint, mucous membrane, musculocutaneous and emergency bleeding episodes such as central nervous system hemorrhages and surgical bleedings. In 49 patients with inhibitor titers of greater than 5 Bethesda Units (from nine cooperating hemophilia centers), 489 single doses were given for the treatment of 165 bleeding episodes. The usual dosage was 50 IMMUNO Units per kg of body weight, repeated at 12-hour intervals (6-hour intervals in mucous membrane bleedings), if necessary. Bleeding was controlled in 153 episodes (93%). In 130 (78%) of the episodes hemostasis was achieved with one or more infusions within 36 hours. Of these 36% were controlled with one infusion within 12 hours. An additional 14% of episodes responded after more than 36 hours.

Of the 489 single doses only 18 (3.7%) caused minor transient reactions in recipients. 10 out of 49 patients (20%) showed a rise in their inhibitor titers. In 5 of these patients (10%) the rise was tenfold or more. However, of these 10 patients 3 had received Factor VIII or Factor IX concentrates within 2 weeks prior to treatment with FEIBA® IMMUNO. These anamnestic rises have not been observed to interfere with the efficacy of Anti-Inhibitor Coagulant Complex, FEIBA® IMMUNO.

INDICATIONS AND USAGE

Anti-Inhibitor Coagulant Complex, Vapor Heated, FEIBA® VH IMMUNO is indicated for the control of spontaneous bleeding episodes or to cover surgical interventions in hemophilia A and B patients with inhibitors.

In addition, the use of Anti-Inhibitor Coagulant Complex, FEIBA® IMMUNO has been described in a few non-hemophiliacs with acquired inhibitors to Factors VIII, XI, and XII[8–12]. One case has been reported where Anti-Inhibitor Coagulant Complex, FEIBA® IMMUNO was effective in a patient with von Willebrand's disease with an inhibitor[16].

Clinical experience suggests that patients with a Factor VIII inhibitor titer of less than 5 B.U. may be successfully treated with Antihemophilic Factor. Patients with titers ranging between 5 and 10 B.U. may either be treated with Antihemophilic Factor or Anti-Inhibitor Coagulant Complex, Vapor Heated, FEIBA® VH IMMUNO. Cases with Factor VIII inhibitor titers greater than 10 B.U. have generally been refractory to treatment with Antihemophilic Factor.

Guidelines to First and Second Choice Treatment:

AICC = Anti-Inhibitor Coagulant Complex, Vapor Heated, FEIBA® VH IMMUNO
AHF = Antihemophilic Factor

Patient's Inhibitor Titer	Clinical Situation: Minor Bleeding	Major Bleeding	Surgery (Emergency)
less than 5 B.U.	AHF	AHF	AHF
5 to 10 B.U.	AHR	AHF	AHF
	AICC	AICC	AICC
more than 10 B.U.	AICC	AICC	AICC

Inadequate response to treatment may result from an abnormal platelet count or impaired platelet function[13–15] which were present before treatment with Anti-Inhibitor Coagulant Complex, Vapor Heated, FEIBA® VH IMMUNO.

CONTRAINDICATIONS

The use of Anti-Inhibitor Coagulant Complex, Vapor Heated, FEIBA® VH IMMUNO is contraindicated in patients who are known to have a normal coagulation mechanism.

WARNINGS

Anti-Inhibitor Coagulant Complex, Vapor Heated, FEIBA® VH IMMUNO must be used only in patients with circulating inhibitors to one or more coagulation factors and should not be used for the treatment of bleeding episodes resulting from coagulation factor deficiencies. It should not be given to patients with significant signs of disseminated intravascular coagulation (DIC) or fibrinolysis.

In the course of treatment with preparations containing the prothrombin complex thromboembolic events may occur, particularly following the administration of high doses and/or in patients with thrombotic risk factors.

Single doses of 100 units per kg of body weight of FEIBA® VH IMMUNO and daily doses of 200 units per kg of body weight of FEIBA® VH IMMUNO should not be exceeded. Patients receiving more than 100 units per kg of body weight of Anti-Inhibitor Coagulant Complex, Vapor Heated, FEIBA® VH IMMUNO must be monitored for the development of DIC and/or symptoms of acute coronary ischemia (see Adverse Reactions section).

High doses of FEIBA® VH IMMUNO should be given only as long as absolutely necessary to stop bleeding.

It has been reported that Anti-Inhibitor Coagulant Complex, Vapor Heated, FEIBA® VH IMMUNO and antifibrinolytics have been given simultaneously without complications. It is, however, recommended not to use antifibrinolytics until 12 hours after the administration of Anti-Inhibitor Coagulant Complex, Vapor Heated, FEIBA® VH IMMUNO.

Anamnestic responses with rise in Factor VIII inhibitor titer have been observed in 20% of the cases (see Clinical Pharmacology section).

This product is prepared from pooled human plasma which may contain the causative agents of hepatitis and other viral diseases. Prescribed manufacturing procedures utilized at the plasma collection centers, plasma testing laboratories, and the fractionation facilities are designed to reduce the risk of transmitting viral infection. However, the risk of viral infectivity from this product cannot be totally eliminated.

Individuals who receive infusions of blood or plasma products may develop signs and/or symptoms of some viral infections, particularly nonA, nonB hepatitis.

PRECAUTIONS

Monitoring of Therapy

If clinical signs of intravascular coagulation occur, which include changes in blood pressure, pulse rate, respiratory distress, chest pain and cough, the infusion should be stopped promptly and appropriate diagnostic and therapeutic measures are to be initiated.

Laboratory indications of DIC are decreased fibrinogen, decreased platelet count, and/or presence of fibrin-fibrinogen degradation products (FDP). Other indications of DIC include significantly prolonged thrombin time, prothrombin time, or partial thromboplastin time.

Non Hemophilic Patients

Non hemophilic patients with acquired inhibitors against Factors VIII, IX or XII may have both a bleeding tendency and an increased risk of thrombosis at the same time.

Laboratory Tests and Clinical Efficacy

Tests used to control efficacy such as APTT, WBCT, and TEG do not correlate with clinical improvement. For this reason, attempts at normalizing these values by increasing the dose of Anti-Inhibitor Coagulant Complex, Vapor Heated, FEIBA® VH IMMUNO may not be successful and are strongly discouraged because of the potential hazard of producing DIC by overdosage.

Pregnancy Category C. Animal reproduction studies have not been conducted with Anti-Inhibitor Coagulant Complex, Vapor Heated, FEIBA® VH IMMUNO. It is also not known whether Anti-Inhibitor Coagulant Complex, Vapor Heated, FEIBA® VH IMMUNO can cause fetal harm when administered to a pregnant woman or can affect reproduction capacity.

Anti-Inhibitor Coagulant Complex, Vapor Heated, FEIBA® VH IMMUNO should be given to a pregnant woman only if clearly needed.

Pediatric Use

No data are available regarding the use of Anti-Inhibitor Coagulant Complex, Vapor Heated, FEIBA® VH IMMUNO in newborns.

ADVERSE REACTIONS

In the course of treatment with preparations containing the prothrombin complex thromboembolic events may occur, particularly after high doses and/or in patients with thrombotic risk factors.

After application of high doses (single infusion of beyond 100 units per kg of body weight, and daily doses of 200 units per kg of body weight) of Anti-Inhibitor Coagulant Complex, Vapor Heated, FEIBA® VH IMMUNO laboratory and/or clinical signs of DIC have occasionally been observed.

In individual instances myocardial infarction was found to occur after high doses and/or prolonged administration and/or in the presence of risk factors predisposing to myocardial infarction.

As will all human plasma products, any kind of allergic reaction may be seen, ranging from mild, short-term urticarial rashes to severe anaphylactoid reactions.

Administration of Anti-Inhibitor Coagulant Complex, Vapor Heated, FEIBA® VH IMMUNO should be discontinued immediately, if such signs appear. Allergic reactions should be treated with antihistamines and glucocorticoids. Shock should be treated in the usual way.

DOSAGE AND ADMINISTRATION

Parenteral drug products should be inspected visually for particulate matter and discoloration prior to administration, whenever solution and container permit.

Clinical trials[5–7] have demonstrated that the response to treatment with Anti-Inhibitor Coagulant Complex, FEIBA® IMMUNO, may differ from patient to patient with no correlation to the patient's inhibitor titer. Response may also vary between different types of hemorrhage (e.g. joint hemorrhage vs. CNS hemorrhage).

As a general guideline a dosage range of 50 to 100 IMMUNO Units of Anti-Inhibitor Coagulant Complex, Vapor

Heated, FEIBA® VH IMMUNO per kg of body weight is recommended. However, care should be taken to distinguish between the following four indications, all of which have undergone careful clinical evaluation:

Joint Hemorrhage

In joint hemorrhage, a dose of 50 units per kg of body weight is recommended at 12-hour intervals, which may be increased to doses of 100 units per kg of body weight at 12-hour intervals.

Treatment should be continued until clear signs of clinical improvement appear, such as relief of pain, reduction of swelling or mobilization of the joint.

Mucous Membrane Bleeding

A dose of 50 units per kg of body weight is recommended to be given at 6-hour intervals under careful monitoring (visible bleeding site, repeated measurements of the patient's hematocrit). Again, if hemorrhage does not stop, the dose may be increased to 100 units per kg of body weight at 6-hour intervals. However, 2 such administrations or 200 units per kg of body weight a day should not be exceeded.

Soft Tissue Hemorrhage

For serious soft tissue bleeding, such as retroperitoneal bleeding, doses of 100 units per kg of body weight at 12-hour intervals are recommended. A daily dosage of 200 units per kg of body weight should not be exceeded.

Other Severe Hemorrhages

Severe hemorrhages, such as CNS bleedings have been effectively treated with doses of 100 units per kg of body weight at 12-hour intervals. Sometimes, Anti-Inhibitor Coagulant Complex, Vapor Heated, FEIBA® VH IMMUNO may be indicated at 6-hour intervals until clear clinical improvement is achieved.

Reconstitution

1. Warm the unopened bottle containing Sterile Water for Injection (diluent) to room temperature (not above 37°C, 98°F).
2. Remove caps from the concentrate and diluent bottles to expose central portions of the rubber stoppers.
3. Cleanse exposed surface of the rubber stoppers with germicidal solution and allow to dry.
4. Using aseptic technique, remove protective covering from one end of the double-ended needle, and completely insert the exposed end through the diluent bottle stopper.
5. Remove protective covering from the other end of the double-ended needle, taking care not to touch the exposed end. Invert diluent bottle over the concentrate bottle, then rapidly insert free end of the needle to its full length through the concentrate bottle stopper. Diluent will be drawn into the concentrate bottle by vacuum.
6. Disconnect the two bottles by removing needle from the concentrate bottle stopper. Gently agitate or rotate the concentrate bottle until all material is dissolved.

Do not refrigerate after reconstitution!

After complete reconstitution of Anti-Inhibitor Coagulant Complex, Vapor Heated, FEIBA® VH IMMUNO, its injection or infusion should be commenced as promptly as practicable, but must be completed within three hours following reconstitution.

The solution must be given by intravenous injection or intravenous drip infusion and the **maximum injection or infusion rate must not exceed 2 units per kg per body weight per minute.** In a patient with a body weight of 75 kg, this corresponds to an infusion rate of 2.5–7.5 mL per minute depending on the number of units per vial (see label on vial).

For Intravenous Injection:

1. After reconstituting the concentrate as described under **Reconstitution,** attach the enclosed filter needle to a sterile disposable syringe. Insert filter needle through the concentrate bottle stopper.
2. Inject air and withdraw solution into the syringe.
3. Remove and discard the filter needle. Attach a suitable intravenous needle or infusion set with winged adapter, and inject solution intravenously.

For Intravenous Infusion:

Prepare a solution of Anti-Inhibitor Coagulant Complex, Vapor Heated, FEIBA® VH IMMUNO as described under **Reconstitution.**

Follow manufacturer's instructions for the administration set used. Make sure that the set contains an adequate filter.

HOW SUPPLIED

Anti-Inhibitor Coagulant Complex, Vapor Heated, FEIBA® VH IMMUNO is supplied as freeze-dried powder, accompanied by a suitable volume of Sterile Water for Injection, U.S.P. (This Product Contains Dry Natural Rubber.), a sterile double-ended needle, and a sterile filter needle.

The number of IMMUNO Units of Factor VIII inhibitor bypassing activity is stated on the label of each bottle.

STORAGE

Store at refrigerator temperature (2° to 8°C, 35° to 46°F).
Avoid freezing, which may damage the diluent bottle.

REFERENCES

1. ELSINGER F.: Aktivierter Faktor VII in Prothrombinkomplex-Konzentraten, 23rd Annual Meeting of "Deutsche Arbeitsgemeinschaft für Blutgerinnungsforschung" (DAB), Heidelberg, 1979. F. K. Schattauer Verlag, Stuttgart-New York, 367, 1980.
2. SELIGSOHN U., ØSTERUD B., RAPAPORT S.I.: Coupled Amidolytic Assay for Factor VII: Its Use With a Clotting Assay to Determine the Activity State of Factor VII. Blood 52: 978, 1978.
3. SELIGSOHN U., KASPER C. K., ØSTERUD B., RAPAPORT S.I.: Activated Factor VII: Presence in Factor IX Concentrates and Persistence in the Circulation After Infusion. Blood 53: 828, 1979.
4. MANNUCCI P. M.: Personal communication.
5. SJAMSOEDIN L. J. M., HEIJNEN L., MAUSER-BUNSCHOTEN E. P., van GEIJLSWIJK J. L., van HOUWELINGEN H., van ASTEN P., SIXMA J. J.: The Effect of Activated Prothrombin-Complex Concentrate (FEIBA) on Joint and Muscle Bleeding in Patients with Hemophilia A and Antibodies to Factor VIII. The New England. J. of Med. 305: 717, 1981.
6. ROBERTS H. R.: Hemophiliacs with inhibitors. Therapeutic Options. The New Engl. J. of Med. 305: 757, 1981.
7. HILGARTNER M. W., KNATTERUD G. AND THE FEIBA-STUDY GROUP: The Use of Factor-Eight-Inhibitor-By-Passing-Activity (FEIBA Immuno) Product for Treatment of Bleeding Episodes in Hemophiliacs with Inhibitors. Blood 61: 36, 1983.
8. THOMAS T., WILLIAMS H., WILLIAMS Y., HUNT J.: FEIBA in Haemophiliacs with Factor VIII Inhibitor. Brit. Med. J. 1: 52, 1977.
9. ROLOVIC Z., ELEZOVIC I., OBRENOVIC B.: Life-Threatening Bleeding Due to an Acquired Inhibitor to Factor XII–XI Successfully Treated with FEIBA. Proceedings of Joint Meeting of the 18th Congress of the International Society of Hematology and 16th Congress of the International Society of Blood Transfusion, Montreal. Abstract 703, 1980.
10. DORMANDY K.: Unpublished data.
11. VINAZZER H.: Personal communication.
12. PRESTON F. E.: A Review of Cases Treated with FEIBA in 1977/78. Presentation at the Second Workshop on Factor VIII Inhibitor Patients, Vienna, 1979.
13. VERMYLEN J., SCHETZ J., SEMERARO N., MERTENS F., VERSTRAETE M.: Evidence that 'Activated' Prothrombin Concentrates Enhance Platelet Coagulant Activity. Brit. J. Haematol. 38: 235, 1978.
14. SEMERARO N., VERMYLEN J.: Evidence that Washed Human Platelets Possess Factor-X Activator Activity. Brit. J. Haematol 36: 107, 1977.
15. WENSLEY R. T.: General Summary of the Use of FEIBA in Haemophiliacs with Inhibitors to F VIII. Presentation at the Second Workshop on Factor VIII Inhibitor Patients, Vienna, 1979.
16. HILGARTNER M. W.: Personal communication.

Issued April 1998
(C) 1993 IMMUNO AG,
All Rights Reserved

Manufactured by
ÖSTERREICHISCHES INSTITUT FÜR HAEMODERIVATE GES.M.B.H.
Subsidiary of **IMMUNO AG**
A-1220 Vienna, Austria
U.S. Establishment Licence 258
U.S. Pat. Nos. 4,364,861, 4,391,746, 4,395,396, and 4,640,834
Distributed by
IMMUNO-U.S., Inc.
1200 Parkdale Road
Rochester, Michigan 48307

6205820EH15

IVEEGAM®   ℞
IMMUNE GLOBULIN INTRAVENOUS (HUMAN)

DESCRIPTION

Immune Globulin Intravenous (Human), IVEEGAM®, is a sterile freeze-dried concentrate of immunoglobulin G (IgG). Reconstitution of the freeze-dried powder with the accompanying quantity of Sterile Water for Injection, U.S.P. gives a 5% protein solution suitable for intravenous administration. This final solution contains, per mL, 50 ± 5 mg of IgG, 50 mg of glucose as a stabilizer, and 3 mg of sodium chloride. Trace amounts of IgM and IgA are also present. The reconstituted solution is clear, colorless, and free of detectable aggregates. It contains no preservative.

IVEEGAM® is prepared from large pools of human plasma. The pooled plasma is fractionated by a modified cold ethanol process. Cohn Fraction II is subjected to treatment with immobilized trypsin and purified by sequential precipitation steps with polyethylene glycol. Polyethylene glycol may be present in the final product at levels below 0.5 g/dL.

CLINICAL PHARMACOLOGY

Patients with primary humoral immunodeficiency are at high risk for the development of acute and chronic bacterial infections because of their low levels of circulation IgG (1, 2). Immune Globulin Intravenous (Human), IVEEGAM® provides a broad spectrum of IgG antibodies (3). The opsonizing, neutralizing, and complement binding activities of these antibodies help prevent or attenuate a multiplicity of infectious diseases.

When administered intravenously, 100% of the IgG antibodies are available in the circulation immediately. The distribution of the intravenously administered preparation between intra- and extravascular compartments requires several days to reach an equilibrium. The serum IgG level therefore drops to approximately 40–50% of the peak level during the first week postinfusion (4, 5).

IVEEGAM® has a half-life of approximately three to four weeks, which is in agreement with that reported for intramuscular immunoglobulin (4, 6). In six agammaglobulinemic patients, the half-life was determined by measuring the activity of tetanus antibody during a four week period after infusion of 150 mg/kg body mass. The half-life ranged from 23 to 29 days (6). Variation in half-life has been observed among patients and is important in determining the dosage regimen for each patient.

IgG serum levels were measured in 21 patients with primary immunodeficiencies treated with IVEEGAM® with an average monthly dose of 225 mg/kg body mass for approximately 16 months. Serum levels increased from an average preinfusion level of 406 mg IgG/dL to an average of 762 mg IgG/dL postinfusion. The average increase in individual patients calculated per 100 mg IgG/kg body mass varied from 44 to 309 mg IgG/dL.

Infections were evaluated in 12 primary immunodeficient children receiving one of two dose levels of IVEEGAM®: 150 mg/kg (low dose) or 500 mg/kg (high dose). Eight children had been previously treated with fresh plasma for up to two years. The number of days with infections was reduced when comparing low dose IVEEGAM® to plasma and when comparing high dose to low dose IVEEGAM®. The geometric means and ranges (mg/dL) of serum IgG levels for eight patients were: plasma: 169 (62–435), low dose IVEEGAM®: 212 (68–425), and high dose IVEEGAM®: 557 (315–810) (7). Studies were performed to monitor for the presence of antibody to Human Immunodeficiency Virus (HIV) and markers for viral hepatitis. No evidence of viral transmission has been observed in more than 30 patients on various dosage regimens followed for periods of 4 to 12 months and tested at intervals ranging from 3 to 6 weeks.

Reports of reactions from clinical trials and clinical experience in Europe and Canada have been infrequent and no serious adverse reactions have been observed (7, 8). See Adverse Reaction Section.

In order to evaluate the efficacy and safety of IVEEGAM® in the treatment of Kawasaki syndrome (KS), two controlled, multi-center, randomized studies were performed. The first study compared the efficacy and safety of IVEEGAM® plus aspirin with that of aspirin alone in reducing the frequency of coronary artery abnormalities in children with acute KS (9). Children randomly assigned to the immune globulin group received IVEEGAM®, 400 mg/kg of body mass per day, for four consecutive days. Both treatment groups received aspirin, 100 mg/kg of body mass each day through the fourteenth day of illness, and 3 to 5 mg/kg each day thereafter for approximately five weeks. Two weeks after enrollment, coronary artery abnormalities were present in 18 of 78 children (23%) in the aspirin only group as compared to 6 of 75 (8%) in the IVEEGAM® group (p<0.01). Seven weeks after enrollment, abnormalities were present in 14 of 79 patients (18%) in the aspirin only group and 3 of 79 (4%) of the IVEEGAM® group (p<0.005). It was concluded that high-dose IVEEGAM® is safe and effective in reducing the prevalence of coronary artery abnormalities when administered early in the course of KS.

The second clinical trial was a multi-center, randomized trial involving 549 children with acute KS (10). Children were randomly assigned to receive IVEEGAM® either in a single infusion of 2 g/kg over 10 hours or in daily infusions of 400 mg/kg for four consecutive days. Both treatment groups received aspirin, 100 mg/kg each day through the fourteenth day of illness, then 3 to 5 mg/kg each day thereafter. Results showed that at two weeks after enrollment coronary artery abnormalities were present in 24 of 263 children (9.1%) in the four-day group as compared to 12 of 260 (4.6%) in the single-infusion group (p<0.05). Seven weeks after enrollment abnormalities were present in 7.2% of the four-day group and in 3.9% in the single-infusion group (p<0.1). The two groups had a similar incidence of adverse effects, occurring in approximately 3% of children overall.

The second study thus supports the efficacy of IVEEGAM® in treating acute KS, and further demonstrates that a single dose of 2 g/kg of IVEEGAM® infused over 10 hours is at least as effective as four smaller daily doses of 400 mg/kg.

INDICATIONS AND USAGE
Immunodeficiency Syndromes

Immune Globulin Intravenous (Human), IVEEGAM® is indicated for replacement therapy in patients with primary

Continued on next page

Iveegam—Cont.

immunodeficiency syndromes such as congenital agammaglobulinemia, common variable immunodeficiency, x-linked agammaglobulinemia (with or without hyper IgM) and Wiskott-Aldrich syndrome (2).
Patients with severe combined immunodeficiency have, in addition to a T-cell defect, an impairment of antibody production. They may benefit from replacement therapy with IVEEGAM® even though this therapy will not correct the cellular immune defect.
IVEEGAM® is especially useful when high levels or rapid elevation of circulating antibodies are desired or when intramuscular injections are contraindicated.

Kawasaki Syndrome
IVEEGAM® is indicated in the treatment of Kawasaki syndrome. When administered in conjunction with aspirin, within ten days of onset of disease, treatment with either a single dose of 2000 mg/kg body mass given over a ten hour period, or 400 mg/kg body mass on four consecutive days resulted in a 65% to 78% decrease in the incidence of coronary artery abnormalities compared to treatment with aspirin alone (9, 10).

CONTRAINDICATIONS
IVEEGAM® is contraindicated in individuals who are known to have had an anaphylactic or severe systemic response to Immune Globulin (Human).
Individuals with selective IgA deficiency should not receive IVEEGAM® since these patients may experience severe reactions to the IgA which may be present.

WARNINGS
IVEEGAM® should be administered only intravenously as the intramuscular and subcutaneous routes have not been evaluated.
Although not observed in the clinical studies with this product, severe anaphylactic reactions have been observed following administration of other immunoglobulin preparations (11, 12, 13, 14). These reactions have been attributed to the presence of immunoglobulin A in certain preparations, and in certain instances, to antigen-antibody interactions, if patients had antigenemia and the respective antibodies were present in the product (12).
IF ANAPHYLACTIC OR SEVERE ANAPHYLACTOID REACTIONS OCCUR, THE INFUSION IS TO BE DISCONTINUED IMMEDIATELY. Whenever IVEEGAM® is administered, appropriate therapy should be available to treat a severe anaphylactic reaction, e.g. epinephrine.

PRECAUTIONS
General
Any vial which has been reconstituted should be used promptly. Partially used vials should be discarded.
Patients with severe antibody deficiency syndromes are more likely to react adversely to the initial infusions of homologous immunoglobulin. Modified dosage regimens have been used to prevent such reactions. See Dosage and Administration Section.

Drug Interactions
Reconstituted Immune Globulin Intravenous (Human), IVEEGAM® may be diluted with 5% dextrose or saline. If administered with other preparations, always use separate infusion lines.
Interactions or incompatibilities with other drugs have not been evaluated.
It is reported that antibodies in immune globulin preparations may interfere with the responses by pediatric patients to live viral vaccines such as measles, mumps, and rubella. Immunizing physicians should be informed of recent therapy with Immune Globulin Intravenous (Human), so that appropriate precautions may be taken.

Pregnancy Category C
Animal reproduction studies have not been carried out with Immune Globulin Intravenous (Human), IVEEGAM®. It is also not known whether IVEEGAM® can cause fetal harm when administered to a pregnant woman or can affect reproduction capacity. IVEEGAM® should be given to a pregnant woman only if clearly needed.

ADVERSE REACTIONS
Reported reactions to IVEEGAM® in patients with primary humoral immunodeficiency have been mild and transient in nature, and have included flushing, rise in blood pressure, malaise, headache, nausea, vomiting, low-grade fever, and rash. In clinical trials involving more than 1300 infusions, reaction rates have ranged from 0.3% to 0.8% (4, 6, 7, 8).
Although not observed in clinical trials with IVEEGAM®, severe anaphylactic reactions have been reported with other immunoglobulin preparations.
In the first clinical trial of IVEEGAM® in the treatment of Kawasaki syndrome, mild congestive heart failure developed with comparable frequency in the aspirin only group (5%) and in the aspirin plus IVEEGAM® group (4%). In each of the latter cases, the child tolerated subsequent infusions without difficulty. After the first infusion, one child had shaking chills and itching, which resolved after treatment with diphenhydramine. These symptoms did not recur with subsequent infusions. One child had sepsis secondary to an intravenous line. One child treated with IVEEGAM® had neutropenia and splenomegaly for several months after treatment; one child in the aspirin group also had neutropenia.
In the second clinical trial, 3.3% of children overall had possible complications attributable to IVEEGAM®. Two children (0.36%) had hypotension, two (0.36%) had pruritus, nine (1.6%) had mild worsening of congestive heart failure, and five (0.91%) had other events, including infiltrates at the site of the i.v. line and skin slough (1), generalized edema without congestive heart failure (2), acute onset of nasal congestion and cough without urticaria, pruritus, or hypotension, responding to Benadryl without interruption of infusion (1), and probably autoimmune hemolytic anemia (1). There were no life-threatening complications in either study.
No long-term hematological or biochemical changes attributable to IVEEGAM® therapy were detected during the course of either study. No evidence for the transmission of non-A/non-B hepatitis or human immunodeficiency virus was associated with the use of IVEEGAM®.

DOSAGE AND ADMINISTRATION
Immune Globulin Intravenous (Human), IVEEGAM® must be administered intravenously after reconstitution. The usual rate of administration is 1 mL per minute up to a maximum of 2 mL per minute for the 5% solution.
Parenteral drug products should be inspected visually for particulate matter and discoloration prior to administration whenever solution and container permit. Reconstituted vials found to contain particles or to be discolored should not be used.

Immunodeficiency Syndromes
A dosage of 200 mg/kg per month is recommended for treatment of primary humoral immunodeficiency syndromes.
If the desired clinical results are not obtained, the dosage may be increased up to 4-fold or intervals shortened. Doses of Immune Globulin Intravenous (Human), IVEEGAM® up to 800 mg/kg body mass per month were tolerated by immunodeficient patients (6).
If adequate doses are given at regular intervals, pre-infusion IgG levels may be expected to rise steadily over a period of 6–12 months until a plateau is reached. The minimum serum concentration of IgG necessary for protection has not been established.
Dosage regimens have been modified in an attempt to prevent adverse reactions in previously untreated, severe, immunodeficient patients. In a limited number of such patients, treatment has been initiated with lower doses of IVEEGAM® diluted with saline or 5% dextrose. With gradually increasing dosage levels and protein concentrations (up to 5% protein) adverse reactions were not observed (6).

Kawasaki Syndrome
Treatment with IVEEGAM® should be initiated within ten days of onset of the disease. Either a dosage of 400 mg/kg body mass daily for four consecutive days or a single dose of 2000 mg/kg given over a ten hour period may be used. Because all studies of this product to date have involved concurrent administration of aspirin, the treatment regimen should include aspirin, 100 mg/kg each day through the fourteenth day of illness, then 3 to 5 mg/kg each day thereafter for a period of five weeks.

Reconstitution
Reconstitution with the Sterile Water for Injection, U.S.P. provided in each package results in a 5% solution.

1. Remove protective caps from the concentrate and solvent bottles (Fig. 1) and disinfect rubber stoppers of both bottles.
2. Remove protective covering from one end of the accompanying double-ended spike and insert the exposed spike through the diluent bottle stopper (Fig. 2).
3. Remove protective cap from the other end of the double-ended spike. Do not touch exposed spike end!
4. Turn diluent bottle upside down and insert free end of the spike into the concentrate bottle stopper to its full length, then invert the connected bottles (Fig. 3). Diluent will be drawn into the concentrate bottle by vacuum.
5. Disconnect the two bottles leaving the spike on the solvent bottle (Fig. 4). Accelerate reconstitution by agitating or rotating the concentrate bottle. DO NOT SHAKE VIGOROUSLY!
6. Either draw up the clear solution into a syringe using the accompanying filter needle (Fig. 5, 500 mg and 1000 mg sizes) or administer the solution directly using the accompanying infusion set with filter (2500 mg and 5000 mg sizes).

[See figures 1-5 at top of next column]

HOW SUPPLIED
Immune Globulin Intravenous (Human), IVEEGAM® 500 mg:
1 vial containing 500 mg of freeze-dried Immune Globulin Intravenous (Human), IVEEGAM®
1 vial containing 10 ml of Sterile Water for Injection, U.S.P., (This Product Contains Dry Natural Rubber.)

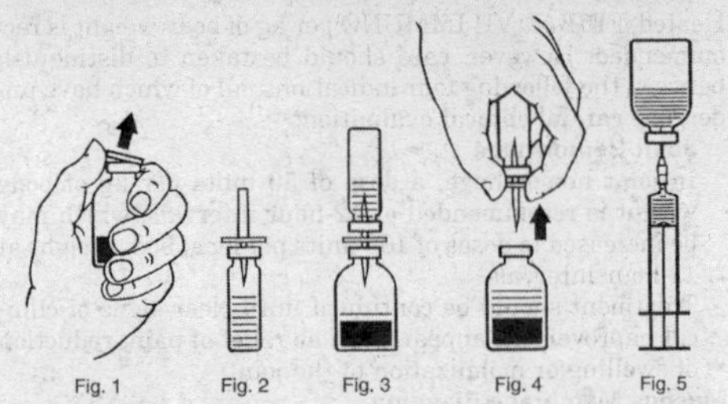

Fig. 1 Fig. 2 Fig. 3 Fig. 4 Fig. 5

1 double-ended spike,
1 filter needle.
Immune Globulin Intravenous (Human), IVEEGAM® 1000 mg:
1 vial containing 1000 mg of freeze-dried Immune globulin Intravenous (Human), IVEEGAM®
1 vial containing 20 ml of Sterile Water for Injection, U.S.P., (This Product Contains Dry Natural Rubber.)
1 double-ended spike,
1 filter needle.
Immune Globulin Intravenous (Human), IVEEGAM® 2500 mg:
1 infusion bottle containing 2500 mg of freeze-dried Immune Globulin Intravenous (Human), IVEEGAM®
1 vial containing 50 ml of Sterile Water for Injection, U.S.P., (This Product Contains Dry Natural Rubber.)
1 double-ended spike.
1 infusion set with filter.
Immune globulin Intravenous (Human), IVEEGAM® 5000 mg:
1 infusion bottle containing 5000 mg of freeze-dried Immune Globulin Intravenous (Human), IVEEGAM®
1 vial containing 100 ml of Sterile Water for Injection, U.S.P.,
(This Product Contains Dry Natural Rubber.)
1 double-ended spike,
1 infusion set with filter.
Rx only

STORAGE
Store at +2°C to +8°C (+35°F to +46°F).
Avoid freezing, which may damage the diluent bottle.
Do not use after expiration date.

REFERENCES

1. JANEWAY C. A., ROSEN F. S.: The Gamma Globulins: IV. Therapeutic Uses of Gamma Globulin, N. Engl. J. Med. 275, 1966, pp. 826–831
2. ROSEN F. S., WEDGWOOD R. J., EIBL M.: Primary Immunodeficiency Diseases. Report of a WHO Scientific Group. Clin. Immunol. Immunopathol. 40, 1986, pp. 166–196
3. EIBL M.: Treatment of Defect of Humoral Immunity. In: Primary Immunodeficiency Diseases; Birth Defects: Original Article Series. Edited by R. J. WEDGWOOD and F. S. ROSEN. Alan R. Liss, Inc. New York, Vol. 19, No. 3, 1983, pp. 193–200
4. EIBL M.: Intravenous Immunoglobulins: Clinical and Experimental Studies. In: Immunoglobulins: Characteristics and Uses of Intravenous Preparations. Edited by B. M. ALVING and J. S. FINLAYSON. U.S. Department of Health and Human Services, Public Health Service, FDA, DHHS Publication No. (FDA)-80-9005, 1979, pp. 23–30
5. WALDMANN T. A., et al.: Metabolism of Immunoglobulins. In: Progress in Allergy. Edited by P. KALLOS and B. H. WAKSMAN, Karger, Basel, Vol. 13, 1969, pp. 1–110
6. Data on File, IMMUNO AG, Vienna.
7. BERNATOWSKA E., et al: Results of a Prospective Controlled Two-Dose Crossover Study with Intravenous Immunoglobulin and Comparison (Retrospective) with Plasma Treatment. Clin. Immunol. Immunopathol. 43, 1987, pp. 153–162
8. EIBL M., et al.: Safety and Efficacy of a Monomeric, Functionally Intact Intravenous IgG Preparation in Patients with Primary Immunodeficiency Syndromes. Clin. Immunol. Immunopathol. 31, 1984, pp. 151–160
9. NEWBURGER J. W., et al.: The Treatment of Kawasaki Syndrome with Intravenous Gamma Globulin. N. Engl. J. Med., 315, 1986, pp. 341–347
10. NEWBURGER J. W., et al.: A Single Intravenous Infusion of Gamma Globulin as Compared with Four Infusions in the Treatment of Acute Kawasaki Syndrome. N. Engl. J. Med., 324, 1991, pp. 1633–1639
11. BURKS A.W., et al.: Anaphylactic Reactions after Gammaglobulin Administration in Patients with Hypogammaglobulinemia. Detection of IgG Antibodies to IgA. N. Engl. J. Med. 314, 1986, pp. 560–564
12. CUNNINGHAM-RUNDLES C., et al.: Reactions to Intravenous Gammaglobulin Infusions and Immune Complex Formation. In: Immuno Hemotherapy. A Guide to Immunoglobulin Prophylaxis and Therapy. Edited by U.E. NYDEGGER. Academic Press, London, 1982, pp. 447–450

13. LEIKOLA J., et al.: IgA-Induced Anaphylactic Transfusion Reactions: A Report of Four Cases. Blood 42, 1973, pp. 111–119
14. THOMPSON R. A., REES-JONES A.: The Antibody Deficiency Syndrome: A Report on Current Management. J. Infect. 1, 1979, pp. 49–60

BIBLIOGRAPHY

ALVING B. M., FINLAYSON J. S. (Eds.): Immunoglobulins: Characteristics and Uses of Intravenous Preparations. U.S. Department of Health and Human Services, Public Health Service, DHHS Publication No. (FDA)-80-9005, 1979

AMMANN A. J., ASHMAN R. F., BUCKLEY R. H., HARDIE W. R., KRANTMANN H. J., NELSON J., OCHS H., STIEHM R., TILLER T., WARA D. W., WEDGWOOD R.: Use of Intravenous γ-Globulin in Antibody Immunodeficiency: Results of a Multicenter Controlled Trial. Clin. Immunol. Immunopathol. 22, 1982, pp. 60–67

BARANDUN S., SKVARIL F., MORELL A.: Prophylaxe und Therapie mit γ-Globulin. Allgemeine Charakterisierung und klinische Anwendung von γ-Globulin-Präparaten. Schweiz. med. Wschr. 106, 1976, pp. 533–542

BARANDUN S., MORELL A., SKVARIL F.: Clinical Use of Intravenous Gamma-Globulin. Biblthca haemat. 46, 1980, pp. 170–174

BUCKLEY R. H.: Long Term Use of Intravenous Immune Globulin in Patients with Primary Immunodeficiency Diseases: Inadequacy of Current Dosage Practices and Approaches to the Problem. J. Clin. Immunol. 2 (Suppl.) 1982, pp. 15S–21S

EIBL, M.: Treatment of Defects of Humoral Immunity. In: Primary Immunodeficiency Diseases: Birth Defects.: Original Articles Series, Edited by R. J. WEDGWOOD and F. S. ROSEN, Alan R. Liss, Inc. New York, Vol. 19, No. 3, 1983, pp. 193–200

KISHIMOTO S.: The Application of Immunoglobulin Preparations. Proc. Symp. Immunoglob., 1979, pp. 24–29

KOBAYASHI M.: Replacement Therapy for Immunodeficiency Syndrome. Proc. Symp. on Immunoglobulin Therapy (Ed.: K. Mashimo) Tokyo, 1979, pp. 94–100

LITMAN G. W., GOOD R. A. (Eds.): Immunoglobulins. Comprehensive Immunology 5. (Series editors: R. A. Good, S. B. Day). Plenum Medical Book Company, New York and London, 1978

MAGILAVY D. B., CASSIDY J. T., TUBERGEN D. G., PETTY R. E., CHISHOLM R. McCALL K.: Intravenous Gamma Globulin in the Management of Patients with Hypogammaglobulinemia. J. Allergy Clin. Immunol. 61, 1978, pp. 378–383

MAZZUCCONI M. G., MELONI G., BOTTINI F., ROMOLI D.: Sperimentazione Clinica e Tollerablità di un Nuovo Preparato di Immunoglobuline per Uso Endovenoso. Quaderni di Medicina e Chirurgia, 43; Suppl. a Malattie del Torace e Cardiovascolari, Vol. VII, 1975

MORELL A., SCHÜRCH B., RYSER D., HOFER F., SKVARIL F., BARANDUN S.: In vivo Behaviour of Gamma Globulin Preparations. Vox Sang. 38, 1980, pp. 272–283

MORELL A., BARANDUN S.: Substitution mit Immunglobulinen bei primärem Antikörpermangel-syndrom. Beitr. Infusionstherapie klin. Ernähr. 9, 1982, pp. 16–24

NOLTE M. T., PIROFSKY B., GERRITZ G. A., GOLDING B.: Intravenous Immunoglobulin Theray for Antibody Deficiency. Clin. Exp. Immunol. 36, 1979, pp. 237–243

RÖMER J., MORGENTHALER J.-J., SCHERZ R., SKVARIL F.: Characterization of Various Immunoglobulin Preparations for Intravenous Application. I. Protein Composition and Antibody Content. Vox. Sang. 42, 1982, pp. 62–73

RÖMER J., SPÄTH P. J., SKVARIL F., NYDEGGER U.E.: Characterization of Various Immunoglobulin Preparations for Intravenous Application. II. Complement Activation and Binding to Staphylococcus Protein A. Vox. Sang. 42, 1982, pp. 74–80

ROSEN F. S.: The Immunodeficiency Syndromes. In: Immunological Diseases. (Ed.: M. Samter). Third Edition, Vol. 1. Little, Brown and Comp., Boston, 1978, pp. 472–498

ROSEN F. S. in: Panel Discussion on Indications and Limitations of Immunoglobulin Prophylaxis and Therapy. In: Immuno Hemotherapy. A Guide to Immunoglobulin Prophylaxis and Therapy, 1981, pp. 451–460

SKVARIL F., PROBST M., AUDRAN R., STEINBUCH M.: Distribution of IgG Subclasses in Commercial and Some Experimental γ-Globulin Preparations. Vox Sang. 32, 1977, pp. 335–338

Issued April 1998
© 1992 IMMUNO AG
All Rights Reserved

Manufactured by
ÖSTERREICHISCHES INSTITUT FÜR HAEMODERIVATE GES.M.B.H.
Subsidiary of IMMUNO AG, A-1220 Vienna, Austria
U.S. Establishment License No. 258
U.S. Pat. Nos. 4,276,283 and 4,886,758

Distributed by
IMMUNO U.S., Inc.
1200 Parkdale Road
Rochester, Michigan 48307

6224000EH08

Interferon Sciences, Inc.
783 JERSEY AVENUE
NEW BRUNSWICK, NJ 08901-3660

Direct Inquiries to:
J.R. Knill, M.D.
(732) 249-3250, ext. 565
FAX: (732) 249-0623
For Medical Information Contact:
In Emergencies:
J.R. Knill, M.D.
(732) 249-3250, ext. 565
(800) 591-4483 after business hours

Prescribing information for the product Alferon N Injection® is listed under Interferon Sciences, Inc.

ALFERON N INJECTION® ℞
Interferon alfa-n3
(human leukocyte derived)

DESCRIPTION

Alferon N Injection® [Interferon alfa-n3 (human leukocyte derived)] is a sterile aqueous formulation of purified, natural, human interferon alpha proteins for use by injection. Alferon N Injection® consists of interferon alpha proteins comprising approximately 166 amino acids ranging in molecular weights from 16,000 to 27,000 daltons. The specific activity of Interferon alfa-n3 is approximately equal to, or greater than, 2×10^8 IU/mg of protein.

Alferon N Injection® is manufactured from pooled units of human leukocytes which have been induced by incomplete infection with a murine virus (Sendai virus) to produce Interferon alfa-n3. The manufacturing process includes immunoaffinity chromatography with a murine monoclonal antibody, acidification (pH 2) for 5 days at 4°C, and gel filtration chromatography.

Since Alferon N Injection® is manufactured using source leukocytes, human donor screening is performed to minimize the risk that the leukocytes could contain infectious agents. In addition, the manufacturing process contains steps which have been shown to inactivate viruses. There has been no evidence of infection transmission to recipients in clinical trials. The laboratory and clinical data obtained support the conclusion that Alferon N Injection® is equivalent to other products derived from human blood or plasma which are free of risk of transmission of infectious agents, such as immunoglobulin and albumin.

The Alferon N Injection® manufacturing process was evaluated for quantitative removal or inactivation of model pathogenic viruses. The viruses were deliberately added to the leukocytes in amounts far exceeding those present in contaminated blood, i.e., $\geq 10^9$ infectious units per milliliter. The manufacturing process yielded a cumulative reduction of $\geq 10^{14}$ of infectious HIV-1, i.e., $\geq 10^{6.5}$ removal by acid inactivation and $\geq 10^{7.9}$ removal by the purification process. In the validation studies, there was 10^8 reduction in the titer of hepatitis B virus as determined by HBsAg assay, and a 10^9 reduction in the infectious titer of herpes simplex virus-1 (HSV-1). Cultivation of Alferon N Injection® [Interferon alfa-n3 (human leukocyte derived)] Purified Drug Concentrate with human indicator cells, i.e., MRC-5 cells, peripheral blood leukocytes in the presence of Cyclosporin A, and fetal cord blood cells, did not detect the presence of infectious viruses.

As part of a validation study, Alferon N Injection® was examined for the presence of the following viruses; Sendai virus (SV), HIV-1, HTLV-l, HBV, HSV-1, CMV, and EBV. Alferon N Injection® contained no detectable quantities of these viruses. In addition, other studies, i.e., Polymerase Chain Reaction (PCR) and Dot Blot Hybridization (DBH), have shown no detectable genetic material from these viruses in Alferon N Injection®. The sensitivity of the PCR was 10 copies for HIV-1 (env gene probe) and 10 copies for HBV (S/P gene probe). The sensitivity of the DBH was 1 pg for EBV, < 10 pg for CMV, < 10 pg for HSV-1, and < 2 pg for SV. Furthermore, sera from 105 patients treated with Alferon N Injection® (95 with condylomata acuminata and 10 with cancer) were tested for antibody to HIV-1 and HIV p24 antigen. There was no evidence to suggest transmission of HIV-1 by Alferon N Injection®. Sera from 135 patients with condylomata acuminata treated with Alferon N Injection®

were tested to determine abnormal SGOT laboratory values. There was no evidence to suggest transmission of hepatitis by Alferon N Injection® based on both SGOT results and patient data collected during clinical trials.

Alferon N Injection® has been extensively purified using immunoaffinity chromatography with a murine monoclonal antibody, acidification (pH 2) for 5 days at 4°C, and gel filtration chromatography. Alferon N Injection® has been subjected to the acid treatment for five days during its manufacture in order to reduce the risk of viral transmission. Subsequent analyses of the Alferon N Injection® [Interferon alfa-n3 (human leukocyte derived)] Purified Drug Concentrate confirm the absence of detectable infectious or non-infectious viral particles.

The leukocyte nutrient medium contains the antibiotic neomycin sulfate at a concentration of 35 mg/L; however, neomycin sulfate is not detectable in the final product, i.e., < 0.64 μg/ml.

Murine immunoglobulin (IgG) is detected in the Alferon N Injection® Purified Drug Concentrate at levels below 0.15% of the Interferon alfa-n3 protein. This equates to levels less than 8 ng of murine IgG per million of IU Interferon alfa-n3 (range of 0.9 to 5.6 ng typically found).

Alferon N Injection® is available in an injectable solution containing 5 million IU Interferon alfa-n3 per vial for intralesional injection. The solution is clear and colorless. Each milliliter (ml) contains five million IU of Interferon alfa-n3 in phosphate-buffered saline (8.0 mg sodium chloride, 1.74 mg sodium phosphate dibasic, 0.20 mg potassium phosphate monobasic, and 0.20 mg potassium chloride) containing 3.3 mg phenol as a preservative and 1 mg Albumin (Human) as a stabilizer.

CLINICAL PHARMACOLOGY

General Interferons are naturally occurring proteins with antiviral, antiproliferative, and immunoregulatory properties. They are produced and secreted in response to viral infections and to a variety of other synthetic and biological inducers. Four major families of interferons have been identified: alpha, beta, gamma, and omega. The interferon alpha family contains 13 different non-allelic molecular species. Their molecular weights range from 16,000 to 27,000 daltons.

Interferons bind to specific membrane receptors on cell surfaces. Interferon alfa-n3 has been shown to bind to the same receptors as Interferon alfa-2b. The receptors have a high degree of selectivity for the binding of human but not mouse interferon. This correlates with the high species specificity found in laboratory studies.

Binding of interferon to membrane receptors initiates a series of events including induction of protein synthesis. These actions are followed by a variety of cellular responses, including inhibition of virus replication and suppression of cell proliferation. Immunomodulation, including enhancement of phagocytosis by macrophages, augmentation of the cytotoxicity of lymphocytes and enhancement of human leukocyte antigen expression occurs in response to exposure to interferons. One or more of these activities may contribute to the therapeutic effect of interferon.

Pharmacokinetics In a study of intralesional use of Alferon N Injection® [Interferon alfa-n3 (human leukocyte derived)] for the treatment of condylomata acuminata, plasma concentrations of interferon were below the detection limit of the assay, i.e., ≤ 3 IU/ml. Minor systemic effects (e.g., myalgias, fever, and headaches) were noted, indicating that some of the injected interferon entered the systemic circulation (See ADVERSE REACTIONS).

Condylomata Acuminata Condylomata acuminata (venereal or genital warts) are associated with infections of human papilloma virus (HPV), especially HPV type-6 and possibly type-11. Given the antiviral and antiproliferative activities of interferons and the viral etiology of condylomata, a placebo-controlled clinical trial was conducted to evaluate the safety and efficacy of intralesional injection of Alferon N Injection® in the treatment of condylomata acuminata.

In a multicenter, randomized, double-blind, placebo-controlled, clinical trial, intralesional administration of Alferon N Injection® was an effective treatment for condylomata acuminata.[1-4] One hundred fifty-six (156) patients were evaluable for efficacy (81 Alferon N Injection® patients and 75 placebo patients). Patients had a mean of five warts (range was 2-14) and all warts were treated. Patients were injected intralesionally with a mean of 225,000 IU of Alferon N Injection® per wart 2 times a week for up to 8 weeks.

Overall, 80% ($^{65}/_{81}$) of patients treated with Alferon N Injection® had a complete or partial resolution of warts compared with 44% ($^{33}/_{75}$) of placebo-treated patients (p < 0.001). Alferon N Injection® was significantly more effective than placebo in producing a complete resolution of warts (p < 0.001), as shown by the following table:

[See table 1 at top of next page]

Of the patients who had a complete resolution of warts, approximately half ($^{21}/_{44}$) the patients had complete resolution of warts by the end of treatment, and half ($^{23}/_{44}$) had com-

Continued on next page

Alferon N—Cont.

plete resolution of warts during the three months after the cessation of treatment. Patients with complete resolution of warts were followed for a median of 48 weeks. Overall, 76% ($^{31}/_{41}$) of Alferon N Injection® [Interferon alfa-n3 (human leukocyte derived)]-treated patients who achieved complete resolution of warts remained clear of all treated lesions during follow-up, while 79% ($^{11}/_{14}$) of the placebo-treated patients remained clear of all treated lesions during follow-up. A total of 762 evaluable warts were injected in this trial. Of the 407 Alferon N Injection®-treated warts, 73% ($^{297}/_{407}$) completely resolved, as compared to 35% ($^{125}/_{355}$) of the placebo-treated warts ($p < 0.0001$). Alferon N Injection® was effective in treating lesions of all sizes, and there was no difference in resolution for perianal, penile, or vulvar lesions.

There was no difference in resolution for patients who had received prior treatment of their warts and for those who had not. Among patients with recalcitrant warts (i.e., warts that were refractory to previous treatment or recurring), 82% ($^{58}/_{71}$) of the evaluable patients had complete or partial resolution of warts due to intralesional administration of Alferon N Injection® as compared to 43% ($^{29}/_{67}$) of placebo patients ($p < 0.001$). Fifty-four percent ($^{38}/_{71}$) of the evaluable Alferon N Injection® patients had complete resolution of warts as compared to 18% ($^{12}/_{67}$) of placebo patients ($p < 0.001$). Patients with primary occurrence of genital warts (i.e., no prior treatment of warts) had a similar resolution rate compared to the patients with recalcitrant warts: 70% ($^{7}/_{10}$) had complete or partial resolution of warts due to Alferon N Injection® [Interferon alfa-n3 (human leukocyte derived)] treatment and 60% ($^{6}/_{10}$) had complete resolution of warts, as compared to 50% ($^{4}/_{8}$) of placebo recipients who had complete or partial resolution of warts and 38% ($^{3}/_{8}$) who had complete resolution. Overall, 83% ($^{5}/_{6}$) of Alferon N Injection®-treated patients with primary occurrence, who achieved complete resolution of warts, remained clear of all treated lesions during a median follow-up of 52 weeks. Because the number of patients with primary occurrence of warts was small (10 Alferon N Injection® recipients and 8 placebo recipients), the difference between Alferon N Injection® and placebo treatment was not statistically significant. However, when the resolution of primary warts was examined, 75% ($^{33}/_{44}$) of the Alferon N Injection®-treated primary warts resolved completely as compared to 39% ($^{11}/_{28}$) of the placebo-treated primary warts ($p = 0.003$).

In an open clinical trial using a once-a-week treatment schedule for up to 16 weeks, 28 patients were evaluable for efficacy. Eighty-nine percent ($^{25}/_{28}$) of patients had a complete or partial resolution of warts following treatment with Alferon N Injection®. The condylomata acuminata resolved completely in 46% ($^{13}/_{28}$) of the patients. Of the 154 warts treated, 77% ($^{118}/_{154}$) resolved completely.

After injections of Alferon N Injection®, side effects were minor and transient. After 4 weeks of treatment, the frequency of adverse reactions was similar in Alferon N Injection® and placebo treatment groups. The most frequent side effects were myalgias, fever, and headache (See ADVERSE REACTIONS).

Antigenicity

1. Alferon N Injection®
   One hundred five (105) patients treated with Alferon N Injection® [Interferon alfa-n3 (human leukocyte derived)] during clinical trials were tested for the presence of anti-interferon antibodies using three different antibody assays: Immunoradiometric Assay (IRMA), Enzyme Linked Immunosorbent Assay (ELISA), and neutralization by the Cytopathic Effect Assay (CPE). To date, no antibodies to Interferon alfa-n3 have been detected in any of the patients.
2. Mouse Proteins
   No hypersensitivity reactions to the components in Alferon N Injection® have been observed. Alferon N Injection® uses a murine monoclonal antibody in one of the purification procedures. A possibility exists that patients treated with Alferon N Injection® may develop hypersensitivity to the mouse proteins. However, none of the patients receiving Alferon N Injection® during clinical trials developed antibodies or hypersensitivity to mouse proteins (See CONTRAINDICATIONS).
3. Egg Protein
   The initial stage in the manufacture of Alferon N Injection® uses Sendai virus which was grown in chicken-embryonated eggs as the specific Interferon alfa-n3 inducer. Although no egg protein (ovalbumin) has been detected in the initial stage of interferon manufacture using an ELISA (sensitivity of 16 ng/ml), a possibility exists that patients treated with Alferon N Injection® may develop hypersensitivity to egg protein (See CONTRAINDICATIONS).

INDICATIONS AND USAGE

Alferon N Injection® is indicated for the intralesional treatment of refractory or recurring external condylomata acuminata in patients 18 years of age or older (See DOSAGE AND ADMINISTRATION).

Table 1

Degree of Resolution as Measured By Total Wart Volume per Patient

	Percent of Patients with: Complete Resolution	Partial Resolution (≥50% resolution)	Minor Resolution (<50% resolution)	Progression/ No change
Alferon (n = 81)	54%	26%	15%	5%
Placebo (n = 75)	20%	24%	13%	43%

The physician should select patients for treatment with Alferon N Injection® after consideration of a number of factors: the locations and sizes of the lesions, past treatment and response thereto, and the patient's ability to comply with the treatment regimen. Alferon N Injection® is particularly useful for patients who have not responded satisfactorily to other treatment modalities, e.g., podophyllin resin, surgery, laser or cryotherapy.

There have been no studies with this product in adolescents. This product is not recommended for use in patients less than 18 years of age.

CONTRAINDICATIONS

Alferon N Injection® [Interferon alfa-n3 (human leukocyte derived)] is contraindicated in patients with known hypersensitivity to human interferon alpha proteins or any component of the product. The product is also contraindicated in patients who have anaphylactic sensitivity to mouse immunoglobulin (IgG), egg protein or neomycin.

WARNINGS

Because of the fever and other "flu-like" symptoms associated with Alferon N Injection® (See ADVERSE REACTIONS), it should be used cautiously in patients with debilitating medical conditions such as cardiovascular disease (e.g., unstable angina and uncontrolled congestive heart failure), severe pulmonary disease (e.g., chronic obstructive pulmonary disease), or diabetes mellitus with ketoacidosis. Alferon N Injection® should be used cautiously in patients with coagulation disorders (e.g., thrombophlebitis, pulmonary embolism and hemophilia), severe myelosuppression, or seizure disorders. Acute, serious hypersensitivity reactions (e.g., urticaria, angioedema, bronchoconstriction, and anaphylaxis) have not been observed in patients receiving Alferon N Injection®. However, if such reactions develop, drug administration should be discontinued immediately and appropriate medical therapy should be instituted.

PRECAUTIONS

General Patients being treated with Alferon N Injection® should be informed of the benefits and risks associated with the treatment. Because the manufacturing process, strength, and type of interferon (e.g., natural, human leukocyte interferon versus single-species recombinant interferon) may vary for different interferon formulations, changing brands may require a change in dosage. Therefore, physicians are cautioned not to change from one interferon product to another without considering these factors.

Information for Patients Patients should be informed of the early signs of hypersensitivity reactions including hives, generalized urticaria, tightness of the chest, wheezing, hypotension, and anaphylaxis, and should be advised to contact their physician if these symptoms occur.

Patients being treated with Alferon N Injection® [Interferon alfa-n3 (human leukocyte derived)] should be informed of benefits and risks associated with treatment.

Patients should be cautioned not to change brands of interferon without medical consultation, as a change in dosage may occur.

Carcinogenesis, Mutagenesis, Impairment of Fertility Studies with Alferon N Injection® have not been performed to determine carcinogenicity, mutagenicity, or the effect on fertility. In studies with adult females, interferon alpha has been shown to affect the menstrual cycle and decrease serum estradiol and progesterone levels[5].

Alferon N Injection® should be used with caution in fertile men. Fertile women should be cautioned to use effective contraception while being treated with Alferon N Injection®.

Changes in the menstrual cycle and abortions have been reported to occur in non-human primates given extremely high doses of recombinant interferon alpha[6]. In these studies, Macaca mulatta (rhesus monkeys) were given interferon daily by intramuscular injection. When given at daily intramuscular doses 326 times the average intralesional dose of Alferon N Injection® (120 times the maximum recommended dose), this recombinant interferon formulation produced menstrual cycle changes in the monkeys.

In human clinical trials with Alferon N Injection®, menstrual cycle data were reported by 51 patients (36 Alferon N Injection® and 15 placebo). There was no significant difference between Alferon N Injection® and placebo treatment groups with regard to menstrual cycle changes.

PREGNANCY Pregnancy Category C Animal reproduction studies have not been conducted with Alferon N Injection®. It is also not known whether Alferon N Injection® [Interferon alfa-n3 (human leukocyte derived)] can cause fetal harm when administered to a pregnant woman or can affect reproductive capacity. Alferon N Injection® should be given to a pregnant woman only if clearly needed.

Changes in the menstrual cycle and abortions have been reported to occur in non-human primates given extremely high doses of recombinant interferon alpha. In these studies, Macaca mulatta (rhesus monkeys) were given interferon daily by intramuscular injection. Abortifacient effects were noted when the recombinant interferon alpha was given daily during early to mid-gestation at intramuscular doses of 978 times the average intralesional dose of Alferon N Injection® (360 times the maximum recommended dose).

Nursing Mothers It is not known whether Alferon N Injection® is excreted in human milk. Studies in mice have shown that mouse interferons are excreted in milk[7]. Because many drugs are excreted in human milk and because of the potential for serious adverse reactions in nursing infants, a decision should be made whether to discontinue nursing or to not initiate drug treatment, taking into account the importance of the drug to the mother and the potential risk to the infant.

Pediatric Use Safety and effectiveness have not been established in patients below the age of 18 years.

ADVERSE REACTIONS

Adverse reactions were evaluated in 202 patients with condylomata acuminata receiving Alferon N Injection® by intralesional administration and in 31 patients with cancer receiving Alferon N Injection® by systemic administration.

In the double-blind efficacy trial for the treatment of condylomata acuminata, 104 patients were treated with doses of Alferon N Injection® of 0.05 million to 2.5 million IU per treatment session (average dose = 0.92 million IU per treatment session) by intralesional injection. In open trials, an additional 98 patients received a dose range of 0.05 to 4.6 million IU of Alferon N Injection® per treatment session (average dose = 1.12 million IU per treatment session). Patients with cancer were given doses of Alferon N Injection® [Interferon alfa-n3 (human leukocyte derived)] of 3 million, 9 million, or 15 million IU per day for ten days by intramuscular injection.

Adverse Reactions in Patients with Condylomata Acuminata

A total of 104 patients with condylomata acuminata was treated with Alferon N Injection® during the double-blind clinical trial. Adverse reactions were reported to be likely, unlikely, or not known to be related to Alferon N Injection®. Adverse reactions consisted primarily of "flu-like" symptoms (myalgias, fever, and/or headache) which were in most cases mild or moderate, and transient, and did not interfere with treatment.

The "flu-like" adverse reactions, consisting of fever, myalgias, and/or headache, occurred primarily after the first treatment session and were reported by 30% of the patients. The frequency of "flu-like" adverse reactions abated with repeated dosing of Alferon N Injection® so that the incidences due to Alferon N Injection® and placebo were similar after three to four weeks of treatment (after six to eight treatment sessions). "Flu-like" symptoms were relieved by administration of acetaminophen.

Adverse reactions were reported at least once during the course of treatment in the following percentages of patients in each treatment group:

Table 2

Percent of Patients with Adverse Reactions

Adverse Reactions:	Alferon (n = 104)	Placebo (n = 85)
Autonomic Nervous System		
Sweating	2%	1%
Vasovagal Reaction	2%	0%

Body as a Whole

Fever	40%	19%
Chills	14%	2%
Fatigue	14%	6%
Malaise	9%	9%

Skin

Generalized Pruritis	2%	0%

Central & Peripheral Nervous System

Dizziness	9%	4%
Insomnia	2%	1%

Gastrointestinal System

Nausea	4%	7%
Vomiting	3%	0%
Dyspepsia/Heartburn	3%	1%
Diarrhea	2%	2%

Musculoskeletal System

Arthralgia	5%	1%
Back Pain	4%	1%
Myalgias	45%	15%
Headache	31%	15%

Psychiatric Disorders

Depression	2%	1%

Noasopharyngeal

Nose/sinus drainage	2%	2%

Most of the systemic adverse reactions were mild or moderate. Severe systemic adverse reactions were reported by 18% of Alferon N Injection® [Interferon alfa-n3 (human leukocyte derived)]-treated patients and 13% of placebo-treated patients (not a statistically significant difference). Most of the severe systemic adverse reactions reported were "flu-like". Other severe systemic adverse reactions included back pain, insomnia, and sensitivity to allergens. Those adverse reactions which were reported by 1% of patients treated with Alferon N Injection® in the double-blind trial include: left groin lymph node swelling, tongue hyperaesthesia, thirst, tingling of legs/feet, hot sensation on bottom of feet, strange taste in mouth, increased salivation, heat intolerance, visual disturbances, pharyngitis, sensitivity to allergens, muscle cramps, nosebleed, throat tightness, and papular rash on neck. Additional adverse reactions which were reported by 1% of patients treated with placebo include: pharyngitis, oral pain, penile discharge, cold, knuckle stiffness, herpes outbreak, cough, disorientation, and weight/appetite loss.

Additional adverse reactions which occurred only in open clinical trials of intralesional use of Alferon N Injection® [Interferon alfa-n3 (human leukocyte derived)] for treatment of condylomata acuminata were herpes labialis, hot flashes, nervousness, decrease in concentration, dysuria, photosensitivity, and swollen lymph nodes. These reactions occurred in 1% of the patients. One patient with a history of epilepsy, who was not taking anticonvulsant medication, had a grand mal seizure while being treated with Alferon N Injection®; this seizure was judged to be unrelated to Alferon N Injection® administration.

Application Site Disorders The frequency of application site disorders (such as itching and pain) for patients treated with Alferon N Injection® was significantly less than that reported with placebo (12% versus 26%). No severe application site disorders were reported by patients treated with Alferon N Injection®, while 7% of placebo-treated patients reported severe disorders.

Labortory Test Values Abnormalities were seen with statistically equivalent frequencies in both the Alferon N Injection® and placebo groups. None of the laboratory abnormalities were considered clinically significant. The abnormalities in the Alferon N Injection®-treated patients consisted primarily of decreased WBC (11%). Decreases also occurred in 4% of the placebo patients (not a statistically significant difference). The abnormalities in Alferon N Injection®-treated patients involved increases of only one WHO grade.

Adverse Reactions in Patients with Cancer Thirty-one (31) patients with cancer were treated with a maximum of ten intramuscular injections of Alferon N Injection® in doses of 3 million IU, 9 million IU, or 15 million IU per treatment session. The occurrence of adverse reactions was judged to be unrelated to the dose of Alferon N Injection®. The following adverse reactions were reported at least once (the per-centage of patients experiencing the reaction is indicated in parentheses): chills (87%), fever (81%), anorexia (68%), malaise (65%), nausea (48%), vomiting (29%), myalgias (16%), arthralgia (10%), chest pains (10%), soreness at injection site (10%), sleepiness (10%), headache (10%), diarrhea (6%), fatigue (6%), low blood pressure (6%), sore mouth/stomatitis (6%), and blurred vision (6%). Those adverse reactions which were each reported by only one patient treated with Alferon N Injection® [Interferon alfa-n3 (human leukocyte derived)] include: stiff shoulders, flushed face, edema, dry mouth, mucositis, coughing, numbness, numbness in hands, numbness in fingers, pain on ocular rotation, shakes/shivers, ringing in ears, cramps, constipation, muscle soreness, confusion, light-headedness, depression, upset stomach, and sweating. The following adverse reactions were reported as severe by at least one patient (the percentage of patients experiencing the reaction is indicated in parentheses): fever (55%), malaise (54%), anorexia (45%), chills (45%), nausea (16%), myalgias (13%), vomiting (10%), fatigue (6%), low blood pressure (6%), chest pains (6%), sore mouth/stomatitis (6%), headache (3%), diarrhea (3%), sleepiness (3%), arthralgia (3%), blurred vision (3%), stiff shoulders (3%), numbness (3%), pain on ocular rotation (3%), muscle soreness (3%), confusion (3%), light-headedness (3%), depression (3%), and sweating (3%).

The number and percentage of patients with cancer who experienced a significant abnormal laboratory test value (values that changed from WHO Grades 0, 1, or 2 at baseline to WHO Grades 3 or 4 during or after treatment) at least once during the trials are shown in the following table:

Table 3

Abnormal Laboratory Test Values

	Cancer (n = 31)
Hemoglobin Level	2 (7%)
White Blood Cell Count	1 (3%)
Platelet Count	1 (3%)
GGT	1 (6%)
SGOT	1 (3%)
Alkaline Phosphatase	2 (8%)
Total Bilirubin	1 (4%)

DOSAGE AND ADMINISTRATION

The recommended dose of Alferon N Injection® for the treatment of condylomata acuminata is 0.05 ml (250,000 IU) per wart. Alferon N Injection® should be administered twice weekly for up to 8 weeks. The maximum recommended dose per treatment session is 0.5 ml (2.5 million IU). Alferon N Injection® [Interferon alfa-n3 (human leukocyte derived)] should be injected into the base of each wart, preferably using a 30 gauge needle. For large warts, Alferon N Injection® may be injected at several points around the periphery of the wart, using a total dose of 0.05 ml per wart. The minimum effective dose of Alferon N Injection® for the treatment of condylomata acuminata has not been established. Moderate to severe adverse experiences may require modification of the dosage regimen or, in some cases, termination of therapy with Alferon N Injection®.

Genital warts usually begin to disappear after several weeks of treatment with Alferon N Injection®. Treatment should continue for a maximum of 8 weeks. In clinical trials with Alferon N Injection®, many patients who had partial resolution of warts during treatment experienced further resolution of their warts after cessation of treatment. Of the patients who had complete resolution of warts due to treatment, half the patients had complete resolution of warts by the end of the treatment and half had complete resolution of warts during the 3 months after cessation of treatment. Thus, it is recommended that no further therapy (Alferon N Injection® or conventional therapy) be administered for 3 months after the initial 8-week course of treatment unless the warts enlarge or new warts appear. Studies to determine the safety and efficacy of a second course of treatment with Alferon N Injection® have not been conducted.

Parenteral drug products should be inspected visually for particulate matter and discoloration prior to administration, whenever solution and container permit.

HOW SUPPLIED

Injectable Solution: Each vial contains 1 ml of Alferon N Injection®. Each ml of Alferon N Injection® contains 5 million IU of Interferon alfa-n3, 3.3 mg of phenol, and 1 mg of Albumin (Human) in a pH 7.4 phosphate-buffered saline solution (8.0 mg/ml sodium chloride, 1.74 mg/ml sodium phosphate dibasic, 0.20 mg/ml potassium phosphate monobasic, and 0.20 mg/ml potassium chloride). One vial per box. (NDC 54746-001-01).

STORAGE

Alferon N Injection® [Interferon alfa-n3 (human leukocyte derived)] should be stored at 2° to 8°C (36° to 46°F). Do not freeze. Do not shake.

CAUTION: FEDERAL (U.S.A.) LAW PROHIBITS DISPENSING WITHOUT PRESCRIPTION.

REFERENCES

1. Friedman-Kien, AE; Eron, LJ; Conant, M; et al., *JAMA* 1988; *259:* 533–538.
2. Kirby, P; (editorial comment), *JAMA* 1988; *259:* 570–572.
3. Friedman-Kien, AE; Plasse, TF; et al., *Papilloma Viruses: Molecular and Clinical Aspects* [Howley, PM, Broker, TR (eds)], New York, Alan R. Liss, Inc.; 1986; 217–233.
4. Geffen, JR; Klein, RJ; Friedman-Kien, AE; *J. Infect. Dis.* 1984; *150:* 612–615.
5. Kauppila; A; et al., *Int. J. Cancer* 1982; *29:* 291–294.
6. Trown, PW; et al., *Cancer* 1986; *57 (Suppl):* 1648–1656.
7. Schafer, TW; et al., *Science* 1972; *176:* 1326–1327.

Manufactured and Distributed by:
Interferon Sciences, Inc.
783 Jersey Avenue
New Brunswick, NJ 08901-3660
U.S. Lic. No. 930
Copyright © 1989, 1990, 1997 Interferon Sciences, Inc.
New Brunswick, NJ 08901-3660.
All rights reserved.
7/97

Shown in Product Identification Guide, page 317

Jacobus Pharmaceutical Co., Inc.

37 CLEVELAND LANE
P.O. BOX 5290
PRINCETON, NJ 08540

Direct Inquiries to:
Professional Services
(609) 921-7447
FAX: (609) 799-1176

For Medical Information Contact:
In Emergencies:
Medical Department
(609) 921-7447
FAX: (609) 799-1176

DAPSONE TABLETS USP ℞
[dap 'sōne]
25 mg. & 100 mg.

PRODUCT OVERVIEW

KEY FACTS

Dapsone is a sulfone for the primary treatment of Dermatitis herpetiformis and an antibacterial drug for susceptible cases of leprosy.

MAJOR USES

Dapsone is used to control the dermatologic symptoms of Dermatitis herpetiformis. Dapsone is used alone or in combination with other anti-leprosy drugs for leprosy.

SAFETY INFORMATION

Dapsone is contraindicated in patients with Dapsone hypersensitivity. Complete blood counts and laboratory monitoring should be done frequently. See labeling.

PRODUCT INFORMATION

DAPSONE TABLETS USP ℞
[dap 'sōne]
25 mg. & 100 mg.

DESCRIPTION

Dapsone-USP, 4,4'-diaminodiphenylsulfone (DDS) is a primary treatment for Dermatitis herpetiformis. It is an antibacterial drug for susceptible cases of leprosy. It is a white, odorless crystalline powder, practically insoluble in water and insoluble in fixed and vegetable oils.

Dapsone is issued on prescription in tablets of 25 and 100 mg. for oral use.

$$NH_2 - - SO_2 - - NH_2$$

Inactive Ingredients: Colloidal silicone dioxide, magnesium stearate, microcrystalline cellulose, and corn starch.

CLINICAL PHARMACOLOGY

Actions: The mechanism of action in Dermatitis herpetiformis has not been established. By the kinetic method in mice, Dapsone is bactericidal as well as bacteriostatic against *Mycobacterium leprae.*

Continued on next page

Dapsone—Cont.

Absorption and Excretion: Dapsone, when given orally, is rapidly and almost completely absorbed. About 85 percent of the daily intake is recoverable from the urine mainly in the form of water-soluble metabolites. Excretion of the drug is slow and a constant blood level can be maintained with the usual dosage.

Blood Levels: Detected a few minutes after ingestion, the drug reaches peak concentration in 4–8 hours. Daily administration for at least eight days is necessary to achieve a plateau level. With doses of 200 mg. daily, this level averaged 2.3 µg/ml with a range of 0.1–7.0 µg/ml. The half-life in the plasma in different individuals varies from ten hours to fifty hours and averages twenty-eight hours. Repeat tests in the same individual are constant. Daily administration (50–100 mg.) in leprosy patients will provide blood levels in excess of the usual minimum inhibitory concentration even for patients with a short Dapsone half-life.

INDICATIONS AND USAGE
Dermatitis herpetiformis: (D.H.)
Leprosy: All forms of leprosy except for cases of proven Dapsone resistance.

CONTRAINDICATION
Hypersensitivity to Dapsone and/or its derivatives.

WARNINGS
The patient should be warned to respond to the presence of clinical signs such as sore throat, fever, pallor, purpura or jaundice. Deaths associated with the administration of Dapsone have been reported from agranulocytosis, aplastic anemia and other blood dyscrasias. Complete blood counts should be done frequently in patients receiving Dapsone. The FDA Dermatology Advisory Committee recommended that, when feasible counts should be done weekly for the first month, monthly for six months and semi-annually thereafter. If a significant reduction in leucocytes, platelets or hemopoiesis is noted, Dapsone should be discontinued and the patient followed intensively. Folic acid antagonists have similar effects and may increase the incidence of hematologic reactions; if co-administered with Dapsone the patient should be monitored more frequently. Patients on weekly Pyrimethamine and Dapsone have developed agranulocytosis during the second and third month of therapy. Severe anemia should be treated prior to initiation of therapy and hemoglobin monitored. Hemolysis and methemoglobin may be poorly tolerated by patients with severe cardio-pulmonary disease.

Cutaneous reactions, especially bullous, include exfoliative dermatitis and are probably one of the most serious, though rare, complications of sulfone therapy. They are directly due to drug sensitization. Such reactions include toxic erythema, erythema multiforme, toxic epidermal necrolysis, morbilliform and scarlatiniform reactions, urticaria and erythema nodosum. If new or toxic dermatologic reactions occur, sulfone therapy must be promptly discontinued and appropriate therapy instituted.

Leprosy reactional states, including cutaneous, are not hypersensitivity reactions to Dapsone and do not require discontinuation. See special section.

PRECAUTIONS
General: Hemolysis and Heinz body formation may be exaggerated in individuals with a glucose-6-phosphate dehydrogenase (G6PD) deficiency, or methemoglobin reductase deficiency, or hemoglobin M. This reaction is frequently dose-related. Dapsone should be given with caution to these patients or if the patient is exposed to other agents or conditions such as infection or diabetic ketosis capable of producing hemolysis. Drugs or chemicals which have produced significant hemolysis in G6PD or methemoglobin reductase deficient patients include Dapsone, sulfanilamide, nitrite, aniline, phenylhydrazine, napthalene, niridazole, nitrofurantoin and 8-amino-antimalarials such as primaquine.

Toxic hepatitis and cholestatic jaundice have been reported early in therapy. Hyperbilirubinemia may occur more often in G6PD deficient patients. When feasible, baseline and subsequent monitoring of liver function is recommended. If abnormal, Dapsone should be discontinued until the source of the abnormality is established.

Drug Interactions: Rifampin lowers Dapsone levels 7 to 10-fold by accelerating plasma clearance; in leprosy this reduction has not required a change in dosage.
Folic acid antagonists such as pyrimethamine may increase the likelihood of hematologic reactions.
A modest interaction has been reported for patients receiving 100 mg Dapsone od in combination with trimethoprim 5 mg/kg q6h. On Day 7, the serum Dapsone levels averaged 2.1 ± 1.0 µg/mL in comparison to 1.5 ± 0.5 µg/mL for Dapsone alone. On Day 7, trimethoprim levels averaged 18.4 ± 5.2 µg/mL in comparison to 12.4 ± 4.5 µg/mL for patients not receiving Dapsone. Thus, there is a mutual interaction between Dapsone and trimethoprim in which each raises the level of the other about 1.5 times.

Carcinogenesis, mutagenesis: Dapsone has been found carcinogenic (sarcomagenic) for male rats and female mice causing mesenchymal tumors in the spleen and peritoneum, and thyroid carcinoma in female rats. Dapsone is not mutagenic with or without microsomal activation in *S. typhimurium* tester strains 1535, 1537, 1538, 98, or 100.

Pregnancy Category C: Animal reproduction studies have not been conducted with Dapsone. Extensive, but uncontrolled experience and two published surveys on the use of Dapsone in pregnant women have not shown that Dapsone increases the risk of fetal abnormalities if administered during all trimesters of pregnancy or can affect reproduction capacity. Because of the lack of animal studies or controlled human experience, Dapsone should be given to a pregnant woman only if clearly needed. In general, for leprosy, USPHS at Carville recommends maintenance of Dapsone. Dapsone has been important for the management of some pregnant D.H. patients.

Nursing Mothers: Dapsone is excreted in breast milk in substantial amounts. Hemolytic reactions can occur in neonates. See section on hemolysis. Because of the potential for tumorgenicity shown for Dapsone in animal studies a decision should be made whether to discontinue nursing or discontinue the drug taking into account the importance of the drug to the mother.

Pediatric Use: Children are treated on the same schedule as adults but with correspondingly smaller doses. Dapsone is generally not considered to have an effect on the later growth, development and functional development of the child.

ADVERSE REACTIONS
In addition to the warnings listed above, the following syndromes and serious reactions have been reported in patients on Dapsone.

Hematologic Effects: Dose-related hemolysis is the most common adverse effect and is seen in patients with or without G6PD deficiency. Almost all patients demonstrate the interrelated changes of a loss of 1–2g of HB, an increase in the reticulocytes (2–12%), a shortened red cell life span and a rise in methemoglobin. G6PD deficient patients have greater responses.

Nervous System Effects: Peripheral neuropathy is a definite but unusual complication of Dapsone therapy in nonleprosy patients. Motor loss is predominent. If muscle weakness appears, Dapsone should be withdrawn. Recovery on withdrawal is usually substantially complete. The mechanism of recovery is reportedly by axonal regeneration. Some recovered patients have tolerated retreatment at reduced dosage. In leprosy this complication may be difficult to distinguish from a leprosy reactional state.

Body As A Whole: In addition to the warnings and adverse effects reported above, additional adverse reactions include: nausea, vomiting, abdominal pains, pancreatitis, vertigo, blurred vision, tinnitus, insomnia, fever, headache, psychosis, phototoxicity, pulmonary eosinophilia, tachycardia, albuminuria, the nephrotic syndrome, hypoalbuminemia without proteinuria, renal papillary necrosis, male infertility, drug-induced Lupus erythematosus and an infectious mononucleosis-like syndrome. In general, with the exception of the complications of severe anoxia from overdosage (retinal and optic nerve damage, etc.) these adverse reactions have regressed off drug.

OVERDOSAGE
Nausea, vomiting, hyperexcitability can appear a few minutes up to 24 hours after ingestion of an overdose. Methemoglobin induced depression, convulsions and severe cyanosis requires prompt treatment. In normal and methemoglobin reductase deficient patients, methylene blue, 1–2 mg/kg of body weight, given slowly intravenously is the treatment of choice. The effect is complete in 30 minutes, but may have to be repeated if methemoglobin reaccumulates. For nonemergencies, if treatment is needed, methylene blue may be given orally in doses of 3–5 mg/kg every 4–6 hours.
Methylene blue reduction depends on G6PD and should not be given to fully expressed G6PD deficient patients.

DOSAGE AND ADMINISTRATION
Dermatitis herpetiformis: The dosage should be individually titrated starting in adults with 50 mg. daily and correspondingly smaller doses in children. If full control is not achieved within the range of 50–300 mg. daily, higher doses may be tried. Dosage should be reduced to a minimum maintenance level as soon as possible. In responsive patients there is a prompt reduction in pruritus followed by clearance of skin lesions. There is no effect on the gastrointestinal component of the disease.
Dapsone levels are influenced by acetylation rates. Patients with high acetylation rates, or who are receiving treatment affecting acetylation may require an adjustment in dosage.
A strict gluten free diet is an option for the patient to elect, permitting many to reduce or eliminate the need for Dapsone; the average time for dosage reduction is 8 months with a range of 4 months to 2½ years and for dosage elimination 29 months with a range of 6 months to 9 years.

Leprosy: In order to reduce secondary Dapsone resistance, the WHO Expert Committee on Leprosy and the USPHS at Carville, LA, recommend that Dapsone should be commenced in combination with one or more anti-leprosy drugs. In the multi-drug program Dapsone should be maintained at the full dosage of 100 mg. daily without interruption (with correspondingly smaller doses for children) and provided to all patients who have sensitive organisms with new or recrudescent disease or who have not yet completed a two year course of Dapsone monotherapy. For advice and other drugs, the USPHS at Carville, LA, (1 800-642-2477) should be contacted. Before using other drugs consult appropriate product labeling.
In bacteriologically negative tuberculoid and indeterminate disease, the recommendation is the coadministration of Dapsone 100 mg. daily with six months of Rifampin 600 mg. daily. Under WHO, daily Rifampin may be replaced by 600 mg. Rifampin monthly, if supervised. The Dapsone is continued until all signs of clinical activity are controlled—usually after an additional six months. Then Dapsone should be continued for an additional three years for tuberculoid and indeterminate patients and for five years for borderline tuberculoid patients.
In lepromatous and borderline lepromatous patients, the recommendation is the coadministration of Dapsone 100 mg. daily with two years of Rifampin 600 mg. daily. Under WHO, daily Rifampin may be replaced by 600 mg. Rifampin monthly, if supervised. One may elect the concurrent administration of a third anti-leprosy drug, usually either Clofazamine 50–100mg. daily or Ethionamide 250–500 mg. daily. Dapsone 100 mg. daily is continued 3–10 years until all signs of clinical activity are controlled with skin scrapings and biopsies negative for one year. Dapsone should then be continued for an additional 10 years for borderline patients and for life for lepromatous patients.
Secondary Dapsone resistance should be suspected whenever a lepromatous or borderline lepromatous patient receiving Dapsone treatment relapses clinically and bacteriologically, solid staining bacilli being found in the smears taken from the new active lesions. If such cases show no response to regular and supervised Dapsone therapy within three to six months or good compliance for the past 3–6 months can be assured, Dapsone resistance should be considered confirmed clinically. Determination of drug sensitivity using the mouse footpad method is recommended and, after prior arrangement, is available without charge from the USPHS, Carville, LA. Patients with proven Dapsone resistance should be treated with other drugs.

LEPROSY REACTIONAL STATES
Abrupt changes in clinical activity occur in leprosy with any effective treatment and are known as reactional states. The majority can be classified into two groups.
The "Reversal" reaction (Type 1) may occur in borderline or tuberculoid leprosy patients often soon after chemotherapy is started. The mechanism is presumed to result from a reduction in the antigenic load: the patient is able to mount an enhanced delayed hypersensitivity response to residual infection leading to swelling ("Reversal") of existing skin and nerve lesions. If severe, or if neuritis is present, large doses of steroids should always be used. If severe, the patient should be hospitalized. In general anti-leprosy treatment is continued and therapy to suppress the reaction is indicated such as analgesics, steroids, or surgical decompression of swollen nerve trunks. USPHS at Carville, LA should be contacted for advice in management.
Erythema nodosum leprosum (ENL) (lepromatous reaction) (Type 2 reaction) occurs mainly in lepromatous patients and small numbers of borderline patients. Approximately 50% of treated patients show this reaction in the first year. The principal clinical features are fever and tender erythematous skin nodules sometimes associated with malaise, neuritis, orchitis, albuminuria, joint swelling, iritis, epistaxis or depression. Skin lesions can become pustular and/or ulcerate. Histologically there is a vasculitis with an intense polymorphonuclear infiltrate. Elevated circulating immune complexes are considered to be the mechanism of reaction. If severe, patients should be hospitalized. In general, anti-leprosy treatment is continued. Analgesics, steroids, and other agents available from USPHS, Carville, LA, are used to suppress the reaction.

HOW SUPPLIED
Rx: Dapsone 25 mg, round white scored tablet, debossed "25" above and "102" below the score and on the obverse "Jacobus" in light and child-resistant bottles, of 100, NDC 49938-102-01.
Dapsone 100 mg, round white scored tablet, debossed "100" above and "101" below the score and on the obverse "Jacobus" in light and child-resistant bottles of 100, NDC 49938-101-01.
Store at controlled room temperature, 20°–25°C (68°–77°F). Protect from light.
CAUTION: Federal law prohibits dispensing without prescription.
Dispense this product in a well-closed child-resistant container.

JACOBUS PHARMACEUTICAL CO., INC.
P.O. Box 5290
Princeton, NJ 08540

9J JUNE, 1997

PASER® GRANULES ℞
(aminosalicylic acid granules)

DESCRIPTION

PASER granules are a delayed release granule preparation of aminosalicylic acid (p-aminosalicylic acid: 4–aminosalicylic acid) for use with other anti-tuberculosis drugs for the treatment of all forms of active tuberculosis due to susceptible strains of tubercle bacilli. The granules are designed for gradual release to avoid high peak levels not useful (and perhaps toxic) with bacteriostatic drugs. Aminosalicylic acid is rapidly degraded in acid media; the protective acid-resistant outer coating is rapidly dissolved in neutral media so a mildly acidic food such as orange, apple or tomato juice, yogurt or apple sauce should be used.

Aminosalicylic acid (p-aminosalicylic acid) is 4–Amino-2-hydroxybenzoic acid. PASER granules are the free base of aminosalicylic acid and do NOT contain sodium or a sugar. The molecular formula is $C_7H_7NO_3$ with a molecular weight of 153.14. With heat p-aminosalicylic acid is decarboxylated to produce CO_2 and m-aminophenol. If the airtight packets are swollen, storage has been improper. DO NOT USE if packets are swollen or the granules have lost their tan color and are dark brown or purple.

The structural formula is:

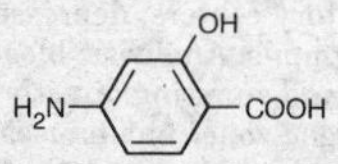

PASAR granules are supplied as off-white tan colored granules with an average diameter of 1.5 mm and an average content of 60% aminosalicylic acid by weight. The acid resistant outer coating will be completely removed by a few minutes at a neutral pH. The inert ingredients are:

colloidal silicon dioxide
dibutyl sebacate
hydroxypropyl methyl cellulose
methacrylic acid copolymer
microcystalline cellulose
talc

The packets contain 4 grams of aminosalicylic acid for oral administration three times a day by sprinkling an apple sauce or yogurt to be eaten without chewing. Suspension in an acidic fruit drink such as orange juice or tomato juice will protect the coating for at least 2 hours. Swirling the juice in the glass will help resuspend the granules if they sink.

CLINICAL PHARMACOLOGY

Mechanism of Action: Aminosalicylic acid is bacteriostatic against Mycobacterium tuberculosis. It inhibits the onset of bacterial resistance to streptomycin and isoniazid. The mechanism of action has been postulated to be inhibition of folic acid synthesis (but without potentiation with antifolic compounds) and/or inhibition of synthesis of the cell wall component, mycobactin, thus reducing iron uptake by M. tuberculosis.

Characteristics: The two major considerations in the clinical pharmacology of aminosalicylic acid are the prompt production of a toxic inactive metabolite under acid conditions and the short serum half life of one hour for the free drug. Both are discussed below.

After two hours in simulated gastric fluid, 10% of unprotected aminosalicylic acid is decarboxylated to form meta-aminophenol, a known hepatotoxin. The acid-resistant coating of the PASER granules protects against degradation in the stomach. The small granules are designed to escape the usual restriction on gastric emptying of large particles. Under neutral conditions such as are found in the small intestine or in neutral foods, the acid-resistant coating is dissolved within one minute. Care must be taken in the administration of these granules to protect the acid-resistant coating by maintaining the granules in an acidic food during dosage administration. Patients who have neutralized gastric acid with antacids will not need to protect the acid resistant coating with an acidic food since no acid is present to spoil the drug. Antacids may influence the absorption of other medications and are not necessary for PASER consumed with an acidic food.

Because PASER granules are protected by an enteric coating absorption does not commence until they leave the stomach; the soft skeletons of the granules remain and may be seen in the stool.

Absorption and excretion: In a single 4 gram pharmacokinetic study with food in normal volunteers the initial time to a 2 µg/mL serum level of aminosalicylic acid was 2 hours with a range of 45 minutes to 24 hours; the median time to peak was 6 hours with a range of 1.5 to 24 hours; the mean peak level was 20 µg/mL with a range of 9 to 35 µg/mL; a level of 2 µg/mL was maintained for an average of 7.9 hours with a range of 5 to 9; a level of 1 µg/mL was maintained for an average of 8.8 hours with a range of 6 to 11.5 hours. The recommended schedule is 4 grams every 8 hours.

80% of aminosalicylic acid is excreted in the urine, with 50% or more of the dosage excreted in acetylated form. The acetylation process is not genetically determined as is the case for isoniazid. Aminosalicylic acid is excreted by glomerular filtration; although previously reported otherwise, probenecid, a tubular blocking agent, does not enhance plasma concentration. In a 1954 study thyroxine synthesis but not iodide uptake was reported reduced about 40% when the sodium salt (not PASER granules) of aminosalicylic acid was administered one hour before radio-iodine; the sodium salt typically produces a serum level over 120 µg/mL at one hour lasting one hour. Occasional goiter development can be prevented by the administration of thyroxine but not iodide. Penetration into the cerebrospinal fluid occurs only if the meninges are inflamed.

Approximately 50–60% of aminosalicylic acid is protein bound; binding is reported to be reduced 50% in kwashiorkor.

Microbiology: The aminosalicylic acid MIC for M. tuberculosis in 7H11 agar was less than 1.0 µg/mL for nine strains including three multidrug resistant strains, but 4 and 8 µg/mL for two other multidrug resistant strains. The 90% inhibition in 7H12 broth (Bactec) showed little dose response but was interpreted as being less than or equal to 0.12–0.25 µg/mL for eight strains of which three were multiresistant, 0.50 µg/mL for one resistant strain, questionable for four nonresistant strains and greater than 1 µg/mL for one non-resistant and three resistant strains. Aminosalicylic acid is not active in vitro against M. avium.

INDICATIONS AND USAGE

PASER is indicated for the treatment of tuberculosis in combination with other active agents. It is most commonly used in patients with Multi-drug Resistant TB (MDR-TB) or in situations when therapy with isoniazid and rifampin is not possible due to a combination of resistance and/or intolerance. When PASER is added to the treatment regimen in patients with proven or suspected drug resistance, it should be accompanied by at least one and preferably two other new agents to which the patient's organism is known or expected to be susceptible.

CONTRAINDICATIONS

Hypersensitivity to any component of this medication.
Severe renal disease.

Patients with severe renal disease will accumulate aminosalicylic acid and its acetyl metabolite but will continue to acetylate, thus leading exclusively to the inactive acetylated form; deacetylation, if any, is not significant.

The half life of free aminosalicylic acid in renal disease is 30.8 minutes in comparison to 26.4 minutes in normal volunteers, but the half life of the inactive metabolite is 309 minutes in uremic patients in comparison to 51 minutes in normal volunteers. Although aminosalicylic acid passes dialysis membranes, the frequency of dialysis usually is not comparable to the half-life of 50 minutes for the free acid. Patients with end stage renal disease should not receive aminosalicylic acid.

WARNINGS

Liver Function

In one retrospective study of 7492 patients on rapidly absorbed aminosalicylic acid preparations, drug-induced hepatitis occurred in 38 patients (0.5%); in these 38 the first symptom usually appeared within three months of the start of therapy with a rash as the most common event followed by fever and much less frequently by GI disturbances of anorexia, nausea or diarrhea. Only one patient was diagnosed on routine biochemistry.

Premonitory symptoms in 90% of these 38 patients preceded jaundice by a few days to several weeks with the mean time of onset 33 days with a range of 7–90 days. Half of the adverse reactions occurred during the third, fourth or fifth weeks. When aminosalicylic acid-induced hepatitis was diagnosed, hepatomegaly was invariably present with lymphadenopathy in 46%, leucocytosis in 79%, and eosinophilia in 55%. Prompt recognition with discontinuation led to the recovery of all 38 patients. If recognized in the premonitory stage, the reaction is reported to "settle" in 24 hours and no jaundice ensues. From other reported studies failure to recognize the reaction can result in a mortality of up to 21%. The patient must be monitored carefully during the first three months of therapy and treatment must be discontinued immediately at the first sign of a rash, fever or other premonitory signs of intolerance.

PRECAUTIONS

(1) General:

All drugs should be stopped at the first sign suggesting a hypersensitivity reaction. They may be restarted one at a time in very small but gradually increasing doses to determine whether the manifestations are drug-induced and, if so, which drug is responsible.

Desensitization has been accomplished successfully in 15 of 17 patients starting with 10 mg aminosalicylic acid given as a single dose. The dosage is doubled every 2 days until reaching a total of 1 gram after which the dosage is divided to follow the regular schedule of administration. If a mild temperature rise or skin reaction develops, the increment is to be dropped back one level or the progression held for one cycle. Reactions are rare after a total dosage of 1.5 grams.

Patients with hepatic disease may not tolerate aminosalicylic acid as well as normal patients, even though the metabolism in patients with hepatic disease has been reported to be comparable to that in normal volunteers.

(2) Information for Patients:

The patient should be advised that the first signs of hypersensitivity include a rash, often followed by fever, and much less frequently, GI disturbances of anorexia, nausea or diarrhea. If such symptoms develop, the patient should immediately cease taking the medication and arrange for a prompt clinical visit.

Patients should be advised that poor compliance in taking anti-TB medication often leads to treatment failure, and, not infrequently, to the development of resistance of the organisms in the individual patient.

Patients should be advised that the skeleton of the granules may be seen in the stool.

The coating to protect the PASER granules dissolves promptly under neutral conditions; the granules therefore should be administered by sprinkling on acidic foods such as apple sauce or yogurt or by suspension in a fruit drink which will protect the coating, but the granules sink and will have to be swirled. The coating will last at least 2 hours in either system. All juices tested to date have been satisfactory; tested are: tomato, orange, grapefruit, grape, cranberry, apple, "fruit punch".

Patients should be advised to store PASER in a refrigerator or freezer. PASER packets may be stored at room temperature for short periods of time.

Patients should be advised NOT to use if the packets are swollen or the granules have lost their tan color and are dark brown or purple. The patient should inform the pharmacist or physician immediately and return the medication.

(3) Laboratory Tests:

Aminosalicylic acid has been reported to interfere technically with the serum determinations of albumin by dye-binding. SGOT by the azoene dye method and with qualitative urine tests for ketones, bilirubin, urobilinogen or porphobilinogen.

(4) Drug Interactions:

Aminosalicytic acid at a dosage of 12 grams in a rapidly available form has been reported to produce a 20 percent reduction in the acetylation of isoniazid, especially in patients who are rapid acetylators; INH serum levels, half lives and excretions in fast acetylators still remain half of the levels seen in slow acetylators with or without p-aminosalicylic acid. The effect is dose related and, while it has not been studied with the current delayed release preparation, the lower serum levels with this preparation will result in a reduced effect on the acetylation of INH.

Aminosalicylic acid has previously been reported to block the absorption of rifampin. A subsequent report has shown that this blockade was due to an excipient not included in PASER granules. Oral administration of a solution containing both aminosalicylic acid and rifampin showed full absorption of each product.

As a result of competition, Vitamin B_{12} absorption has been reduced 55% by 5 grams of aminosalicylic acid with clinically significant erythrocyte abnormalities developing after depletion; patients on therapy of more than one month should be considered for maintenance B_{12}.

A malabsorption syndrome can develop in patients on aminosalicylic acid but is usually not complete. The complete syndrome includes steatorrhea, an abnormal small bowel pattern on x-ray, villus atrophy, depressed cholesterol, reduced D-xylose and iron absorption. Triglyceride absorption always is normal.

In one literature report 8 hours after the last dosage of aminosalicylic acid at 2 gm qid serum digoxin levels were reduced 40% in two of ten patients but not changed in the remaining eight.

(5) Carcinogenesis, mutagenesis, impairment of fertility: Sodium aminosalicylate produced an occipital bone defect, probably with a dose response, when administered to ten pregnant Wistar rats at five doses from 3.85 to 385 mg/kg from days 6 to 14. There were no significant changes from controls in any group in corpora lutea, early resorptions, total resorptions, fetal death, litter size, or hematomas. For all except the 77 mg/kg group, fetal weights were significantly greater than controls. Chinchilla rabbits on 5 mg/kg

Continued on next page

Paser—Cont.

from days 7 to 14 did not show any significant differences as compared to controls for the same parameters studied. Sodium aminosalicylic acid was not mutagenic in Ames tester strain TA 100. In human lymphocyte cultures in-vitro clastogenic effects of achromatic, chromatid, isochromatic breaks or chromatid translocations were not seen at 153 or 600 µg/mL. At 1500 and 3000 µg/mL there was a dose related increase in chromatid aberrations.

Patients on isoniazid and aminosalicylic acid have been reported to have an increased number of chromosomal aberrations as compared to controls.

(6) Pregnancy: Pregnancy Category C:

Aminosalicylic acid has been reported to produce occipital malformations in rats when given at doses within the human dose range. Although there probably is a dose response, the frequency of abnormalities was comparable to controls at the highest level tested (two times the human dosage). When administered to rabbits at 5 mg/kg, throughout all three trimesters, no teratologic embryocidal effects were seen. Literature reports on aminosalicylic acid in pregnant women always report coadministration of other medications. Because there are no adequate and well controlled studies of aminosalicylic acid in humans, PASER granules should be given to a pregnant woman only if clearly needed.

(8) Nursing mothers:

After administration of a different preparation of aminosalicylic acid to one patient, the maximum concentration in the milk was 1 µg/mL at 3 hours with a half-life of 2.5 hours; the maximum maternal plasma concentration was 70 µg/mL at two hours.

ADVERSE EFFECTS

The most common side effect is gastrointestinal intolerance manifested by nausea, vomiting, diarrhea, and abdominal pain.

Hypersensitivity reactions: Fever, skin eruptions of various types, including exfoliative dermatitis, infectious mononucleosis-like, or lymphoma-like syndrome, leucopenia, agranulocytosis, thrombocytopenia, Coombs' positive hemolytic anemia, jaundice, hepatitis, pericarditis, hypoglycemia, optic neuritis, encephalopathy, Loeffler's syndrome, and vasculitis and a reduction in prothrombin.

Crystalluria may be prevented by the maintenance of urine at a neutral or an alkaline pH.

OVERDOSAGE

Overdosage has not been reported.

DOSAGE AND ADMINISTRATION

PASER granules should be administered with other drugs to which the organism is known or expected to be susceptible. It is most commonly administered to patients with Multi-drug Resistant TB (MDR-TB) or in other situations in which therapy with isoniazid or rifampin is not possible due to a combination of resistance and/or tolerance. The adult dosage of four grams (one packet) three times per day or correspondingly smaller doses in children should be given by sprinkling on apple sauce or yogurt or by swirling in the glass to suspend the granules in an acidic drink such as tomato or orange juice.

DO NOT USE if the packet is swollen or the granules have lost their tan color, turning dark brown or purple.

HOW SUPPLIED

Carton of 30 PASER packets (NDC 49938-107-04). Each packet contains four grams aminosalicylic acid. PASER granules are supplied in packets containing 4 grams of aminosalicylic acid for administration three times a day by suspension in an acidic drink or food with a pH less than 5. Examples include apple sauce, yogurt, tomato or orange juice.

Distributors and Pharmacists: Store below 59°F (15°C) (in a refrigerator or freezer).

Patients are urged to store PASER in a refrigerator or freezer. PASER packets may be stored at room temperature for short periods of time.

AVOID EXCESSIVE HEAT. DO NOT USE if packet is swollen or the granules have lost their tan color, turning dark brown or purple.

Caution: Federal, law prohibits dispensing without prescription.

JACOBUS PHARMACEUTICAL CO., INC.
P.O. Box 5290
Princeton, NJ 08540

2A JULY, 1996

Janssen Pharmaceutica Inc.
1125 TRENTON-HARBOURTON ROAD
P.O. BOX 200
TITUSVILLE, NJ 08560-0200

For Medical Information Monday through Friday 8 am-8 pm EST Contact:
Generally:
(800) JANSSEN
FAX: (609) 730-2461
After Hours and Weekends:
(800) JANSSEN

DURAGESIC® Ⓒ Ɽ
[dūr-a-jē 'sik]
(fentanyl transdermal system)

Full Prescribing Information

> BECAUSE SERIOUS OR LIFE-THREATENING HYPOVENTILATION COULD OCCUR, DURAGESIC® IS CONTRAINDICATED:
> - In the management of acute or post-operative pain, including use in out-patient surgeries
> - In the management of mild or intermittent pain responsive to PRN or non--opioid therapy
> - In doses exceeding 25 µg/hour at the initiation of opioid therapy
> (See CONTRAINDICATIONS for further information.)
> DURAGESIC® SHOULD NOT BE ADMINISTERED TO CHILDREN UNDER 12 YEARS OF AGE OR PATIENTS UNDER 18 YEARS OF AGE WHO WEIGH LESS THAN 50 KG (110 LBS) EXCEPT IN AN AUTHORIZED INVESTIGATIONAL RESEARCH SETTING. (See PRECAUTIONS - Pediatric Use.)
> DURAGESIC® is indicated for treatment of chronic pain (such as that of malignancy) that:
> - cannot be managed by lesser means such as acetaminophen-opioid combinations, non-steroidal analgesics, or PRN dosing with short-acting opioids and
> - requires continuous opioid administration.
> The 50, 75, and 100 mcg/hour dosages should ONLY be used in patients who are already on and are tolerant to opioid therapy.

WARNING: May be habit forming.

DESCRIPTION

DURAGESIC® is a transdermal system providing continuous systemic delivery of fentanyl, a potent opioid analgesic, for 72 hours. The chemical name is N-Phenyl-N-(1-2-phenylethyl-4-piperidyl) propanamide. The structural formula is

$$CH_3CH_2CON \quad N-CH_2 CH_2$$

The molecular weight of fentanyl base is 336.5, and the empirical formula is $C_{22}H_{28}N_2O$. The n-octanol:water partition coefficient is 860:1. The pKa is 8.4.

System Components and Structure

The amount of fentanyl released from each system per hour is proportional to the surface area (25 µg/h per 10 cm²). The composition per unit area of all system sizes is identical. Each system also contains 0.1 mL of alcohol USP per 10 cm².

Dose* (µg/h)	Size (cm²)	Fentanyl Content (mg)
25	10	2.5
50 **	20	5
75 **	30	7.5
100 **	40	10

* Nominal delivery rate per hour
** FOR USE ONLY IN OPIOID TOLERANT PATIENTS

DURAGESIC® is a rectangular transparent unit comprising a protective liner and four functional layers. Proceeding from the outer surface toward the surface adhering to skin, these layers are:

1) a backing layer of polyester film; 2) a drug reservoir of fentanyl and alcohol USP gelled with hydroxyethyl cellulose;3) an ethylene-vinyl acetate copolymer membrane that controls the rate of fentanyl delivery to the skin surface; and4) a fentanyl containing silicone adhesive. Before use, a protective liner covering the adhesive layer is removed and discarded.

[See figure at top of next column]

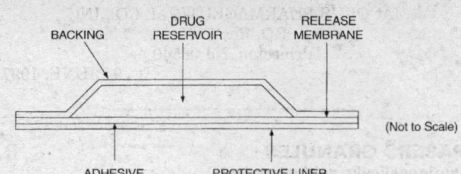

BACKING · DRUG RESERVOIR · RELEASE MEMBRANE · ADHESIVE · PROTECTIVE LINER · (Not to Scale)

The active component of the system is fentanyl. The remaining components are pharmacologically inactive. Less than 0.2 mL of alcohol is also released from the system during use.

Do not cut or damage DURAGESIC®. If the DURAGESIC® system is cut or damaged, controlled drug delivery will not be possible.

CLINICAL PHARMACOLOGY

Pharmacology

Fentanyl is an opioid analgesic. Fentanyl interacts predominately with the opioid µ-receptor. These µ-binding sites are discretely distributed in the human brain, spinal cord, and other tissues.

In clinical settings, fentanyl exerts its principal pharmacologic effects on the central nervous system. Its primary actions of therapeutic value are analgesia and sedation. Fentanyl may increase the patient's tolerance for pain and decrease the perception of suffering, although the presence of the pain itself may still be recognized.

In addition to analgesia, alterations in mood, euphoria and dysphoria, and drowsiness commonly occur. Fentanyl depresses the respiratory centers, depresses the cough reflex, and constricts the pupils. Analgesic blood levels of fentanyl may cause nausea and vomiting directly by stimulating the chemoreceptor trigger zone, but nausea and vomiting are significantly more common in ambulatory than in recumbent patients, as is postural syncope.

Opioids increase the tone and decrease the propulsive contractions of the smooth muscle of the gastrointestinal tract. The resultant prolongation in gastrointestinal transit time may be responsible for the constipating effect of fentanyl. Because opioids may increase biliary tract pressure, some patients with biliary colic may experience worsening rather than relief of pain.

While opioids generally increase the tone of urinary tract smooth muscle, the net effect tends to be variable, in some cases producing urinary urgency, in others, difficulty in urination.

At therapeutic dosages, fentanyl usually does not exert major effects on the cardiovascular system. However, some patients may exhibit orthostatic hypotension and fainting.

Histamine assays and skin wheal testing in man indicate that clinically significant histamine release rarely occurs with fentanyl administration. Assays in man show no clinically significant histamine release in dosages up to 50 µg/kg.

Pharmacokinetics (see graph and tables)

DURAGESIC® releases fentanyl from the reservoir at a nearly constant amount per unit time. The concentration gradient existing between the saturated solution of drug in the reservoir and the lower concentration in the skin drives drug release. Fentanyl moves in the direction of the lower concentration at a rate determined by the copolymer release membrane and the diffusion of fentanyl through the skin layers. While the actual rate of fentanyl delivery to the skin varies over the 72 hour application period, each system is labeled with a nominal flux which represents the average amount of drug delivered to the systemic circulation per hour across average skin.

While there is variation in dose delivered among patients, the nominal flux of the systems (25, 50, 75, and 100 µg of fentanyl per hour) are sufficiently accurate as to allow individual titration of dosage for a given patient. The small amount of alcohol which has been incorporated into the system enhances the rate of drug flux through the rate-limiting copolymer membrane and increases the permeability of the skin to fentanyl.

Following DURAGESIC® application, the skin under the system absorbs fentanyl, and a depot of fentanyl concentrates in the upper skin layers. Fentanyl then becomes available to the systemic circulation. Serum fentanyl concentrations increase gradually following initial DURAGESIC® application, generally leveling off between 12 and 24 hours and remaining relatively constant, with some fluctuation, for the remainder of the 72 hour application period. Peak serum levels of fentanyl generally occurred between 24 and 72 hours after initial application (see Table A). Serum fentanyl concentrations achieved are proportional to the DURAGESIC® delivery rate. With continuous use, serum fentanyl concentrations continue to rise for the first few system applications. After several sequential 72-hour applications, patients reach and maintain a steady state

serum concentration that is determined by individual variation in skin permeability and body clearance of fentanyl (see graph and Table B).

After system removal, serum fentanyl concentrations decline gradually, falling about 50% in approximately 17 (range 13–22) hours. Continued absorption of fentanyl from the skin accounts for a slower disappearance of the drug from the serum than is seen after an IV infusion, where the apparent half-life is approximately 7 (range 3–12) hours. [See graphic at right]

[See table A at top of next page]

[See table B at top of next page]

Fentanyl plasma protein binding capacity decreases with increasing ionization of the drug. Alterations in pH may affect its distribution between plasma and the central nervous system. Fentanyl accumulates in the skeletal muscle and fat and is released slowly into the blood.

The average volume of distribution for fentanyl is 6 L/kg (range 3–8, N=8). The average clearance in patients undergoing various surgical procedures is 46 L/h (range 27–75, N=8). The kinetics of fentanyl in geriatric patients has not been well studied, but in geriatric patients the clearance of IV fentanyl may be reduced and the terminal half-life greatly prolonged (see PRECAUTIONS).

Fentanyl is metabolized primarily in the liver. In humans the drug appears to be metabolized primarily by N-dealkylation to norfentanyl and other inactive metabolites that do not contribute materially to the observed activity of the drug. Within 72 hours of IV fentanyl administration, approximately 75% of the is excreted in urine, mostly as metabolites with less than 10% representing unchanged drug. Approximately 9% of the dose is recovered in the feces, primarily as metabolites. Mean values for unbound fractions of fentanyl in plasma are estimated to be between 13 and 21%.

Skin does not appear to metabolize fentanyl delivered transdermally. This was determined in a human keratinocyte cell assay and in clinical studies in which 92% of the dose delivered from the system was accounted for as unchanged fentanyl that appeared in the systemic circulation.

Pharmacodynamics

Analgesia

DURAGESIC® is a strong opioid analgesic. In controlled clinical trials in non-opioid tolerant patients, 60 mg/day IM morphine was considered to provide analgesia approximately equivalent to DURAGESIC® 100 µg/h in an acute pain model.

Minimum effective analgesic serum concentrations of fentanyl in opioid naive patients range from 0.2 to 1.2 ng/mL; side effects increase in frequency at serum levels above 2 ng/mL. Both the minimum effective concentration and the concentration at which toxicity occurs rise with increasing tolerance. The rate of development of tolerance varies widely among individuals.

Ventilatory Effects

At equivalent analgesic serum concentrations, fentanyl and morphine produce a similar degree of hypoventilation. A small number of patients have experienced clinically significant hypoventilation with DURAGESIC®. Hypoventilation was manifest by respiratory rates of less than 8 breaths/minute or a pCO_2 greater than 55 mm Hg. In clinical trials of 357 postoperative (acute pain) patients treated with DURAGESIC®, 13 patients experienced hypoventilation. In these studies the incidence of hypoventilation was higher in nontolerant women (10) than in men (3) and in patients weighing less than 63 kg (9 of 13). Although patients with impaired respiration were not common in the trials, they had higher rates of hypoventilation. In addition, post-marketing reports have been received of opioid-naive post-operative patients who have experienced clinically significant hypoventilation with DURAGESIC®. DURAGESIC® is contraindicated in the treatment of postoperative and acute pain.

While most patients using DURAGESIC® chronically develop tolerance to fentanyl induced hypoventilation, episodes of slowed respirations may occur at any time during therapy; medical intervention generally was not required in these instances.

Hypoventilation can occur throughout the therapeutic range of fentanyl serum concentrations. However, in non-opioid-tolerant patients the risk of hypoventilation increases at serum fentanyl concentrations greater than 2 ng/mL, especially for patients who have an underlying pulmonary condition or who receive usual doses of opioids or other CNS drugs associated with hypoventilation in addition to DURAGESIC®. The use of DURAGESIC® should be monitored by clinical evaluation. As with other drug level measurements, serum fentanyl concentrations may be useful clinically, although they do not reflect patient sensitivity to fentanyl and should not be used by physicians as a sole indicator of effectiveness or toxicity.

See BOX WARNING, CONTRAINDICATIONS, WARNINGS, PRECAUTIONS, ADVERSE REACTIONS, and OVERDOSAGE for additional information on hypoventilation.

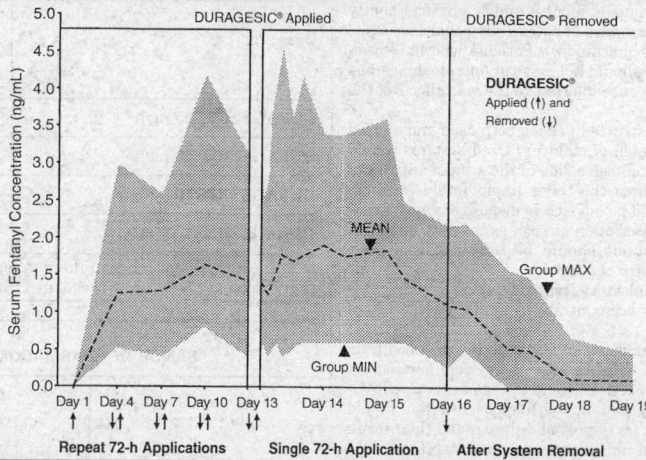

Serum Fentanyl Concentrations Following Multiple Applications of DURAGESIC® 100 µg/h (n=10)

Cardiovascular Effects

Intravenous fentanyl may infrequently produce bradycardia. The incidence of bradycardia in clinical trials with DURAGESIC® was less than 1%.

CNS Effects

In opioid naive patients, central nervous system effects increase when serum fentanyl concentrations are greater than 3 ng/mL.

CLINICAL TRIALS

DURAGESIC® (fentanyl transdermal system) was studied in patients with acute and chronic pain (postoperative and cancer pain models); however, DURAGESIC® is contraindicated for postoperative analgesia.

The analgesic efficacy of DURAGESIC® was demonstrated in an acute pain model with surgical procedures expected to produce various intensities of pain (eg hysterectomy, major orthopedic surgery). Clinical use and safety was evaluated in patients experiencing chronic pain due to malignancy. Based on the results of these trials, DURAGESIC® was determined to be effective in both populations, but safe only for use in patients with chronic pain. Because of the risk of hypoventilation (4% incidence) in postoperative patients with actue pain, DURAGESIC® is contraindicated for postoperative analgesia. (See BOX WARNING and CONTRAINDICATIONS.)

DURAGESIC® as therapy for pain due to cancer has been studied in 153 patients. In this patient population, DURAGESIC® has been administered in doses of 25 µg/h to 600 µg/h. Individual patients have used DURAGESIC® continuously for up to 866 days. At one month after initiation of DURAGESIC® therapy, patients generally reported lower pain intensity scores as compared to a prestudy analgesic regimen of oral morphine (see graph).

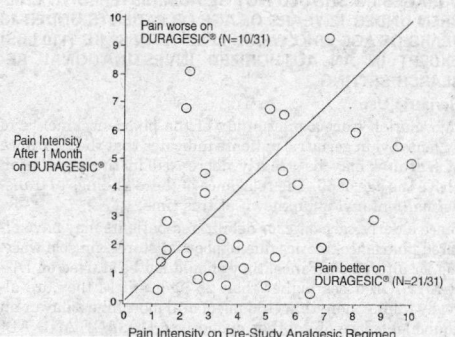

Visual Analogue Score of Pain Intensity Ratings at Entry in the Study and After One Month of DURAGESIC® Use

INDICATIONS AND USAGE

DURAGESIC® (fentanyl transdermal system) is indicated in the management of chronic pain in patients who require continuous opioid analgesia for pain that cannot be managed by lesser means such as acetaminophen-opioid combinations, non-steroidal analgesics, or PRN dosing with short-acting opioids.

DURAGESIC® should not be used in the management of acute or postoperative pain because serious or life-threatening hypoventilation could result. (See BOX WARNING and CONTRAINDICATIONS.)

In patients with chronic pain, it is possible to individually titrate the dose of the transdermal system to minimize the risk of adverse effects while providing analgesia. In properly selected patients, DURAGESIC® is a safe and effective alternative to other opioid regimens. (See DOSAGE AND ADMINISTRATION.)

CONTRAINDICATIONS

BECAUSE SERIOUS OR LIFE-THREATENING HYPOVENTILATION COULD OCCUR, DURAGESIC® IS CONTRAINDICATED:

- **in the management of acute or post-operative pain, including use in out-patient surgeries because there is no opportunity for proper dose titration (See CLINICAL PHARMACOLOGY and DOSAGE AND ADMINISTRATION),**
- **in the management of mild or intermittent pain that can otherwise be managed by lesser means such as acetaminophen-opioid combinations, non-steriodal analgesics, or PRN dosing with short-acting opioids, and**
- **in doses exceeding 25 µg/hour at the initiation of opioid therapy because of the need to individualize dosing by titrating to the desired analgesic effect.**

DURAGESIC® is also contraindicated in patients with known hypersensitivity to fentanyl or adhesives.

WARNINGS

DURAGESIC® (FENTANYL TRANSDERMAL SYSTEM) SHOULD NOT BE ADMINISTERED TO CHILDREN UNDER 12 YEARS OF AGE OR PATIENTS UNDER 18 YEARS OF AGE WHO WEIGH LESS THAN 50 KG (110 LBS) EXCEPT IN AN AUTHORIZED INVESTIGATIONAL RESEARCH SETTING. (See PRECAUTIONS-Pediatric Use.)

PATIENTS WHO HAVE EXPERIENCED ADVERSE EVENTS SHOULD BE MONITORED FOR AT LEAST 12 HOURS AFTER DURAGESIC® REMOVAL SINCE SERUM FENTANYL CONCENTRATIONS DECLINE GRADUALLY AND REACH AN APPROXIMATE 50% REDUCTION IN SERUM CONCENTRATIONS 17 HOURS AFTER SYSTEM REMOVAL.

DURAGESIC® SHOULD BE PRESCRIBED ONLY BY PERSONS KNOWLEDGEABLE IN THE CONTINUOUS ADMINISTRATION OF POTENT OPIOIDS, IN THE MANAGEMENT OF PATIENTS RECEIVING POTENT OPIOIDS FOR TREATMENT OF PAIN, AND IN THE DETECTION AND MANAGEMENT OF HYPOVENTILATION INCLUDING THE USE OF OPIOID ANTAGONISTS.

THE CONCOMITANT USE OF OTHER CENTRAL NERVOUS SYSTEM DEPRESSANTS, INCLUDING OTHER OPIOIDS, SEDATIVES OR HYPNOTICS, GENERAL ANESTHETICS, PHENOTHIAZINES, TRANQUILIZERS, SKELETAL MUSCLE RELAXANTS, SEDATING ANTIHISTAMINES, AND ALCOHOLIC BEVERAGES MAY PRODUCE ADDITIVE DEPRESSANT EFFECTS. HYPOVENTILATION, HYPOTENSION AND PROFOUND SEDATION OR COMA MAY OCCUR. WHEN SUCH COMBINED THERAPY IS CONTEMPLATED, THE DOSE OF ONE OR BOTH AGENTS SHOULD BE REDUCED BY AT LEAST 50%.

ALL PATIENTS SHOULD BE ADVISED TO AVOID EXPOSING THE DURAGESIC® APPLICATION SITE TO DIRECT EXTERNAL HEAT SOURCES, SUCH AS HEATING PADS OR ELECTRIC BLANKETS, HEAT LAMPS, SUANAS, HOT TUBS, AND HEATED WATER BEDS, ETC. WHILE WEARING THE SYSTEM. THERE IS A POTENTIAL FOR TEMPERATURE-DEPENDENT INCREASES IN FENTANYL RELEASE FROM THE SYSTEM. (See PRECAUTIONS, Patients with Fever/External Heat.)

PRECAUTIONS

General

DURAGESIC® doses greater than 25 µg/h are too high for initiation of therapy in non opioid-tolerant patients and should not be used to begin DURAGESIC® therapy in these patients. (See BOX WARNING.)

Continued on next page

Duragesic—Cont.

DURAGESIC® may impair mental and/or physical ability required for the performance of potentially hazardous tasks (eg driving, operating machinery). Patients who have been given DURAGESIC® should not drive or operate dangerous machinery unless they are tolerant to the side effects of the drug.

Patients should be instructed to keep both used and unused systems out of the reach of children. Used systems should be folded so that the adhesive side of the system adheres to itself and flushed down the toilet immediately upon removal. Patients should be advised to dispose of any systems remaining from a prescription as soon as they are no longer needed. Unused systems should be removed from their pouch and flushed down the toilet.

Hypoventilation (Respiratory Depression)
Hypoventilation may occur at any time during the use of DURAGESIC®.

Because significant amounts of fentanyl are absorbed from the skin for 17 hours or more after the system is removed, hypoventilation may persist beyond the removal of DURAGESIC®. Consequently, patients with hypoventilation should be carefully observed for degree of sedation and their respiratory rate monitored until respiration has stabilized.

The use of concomitant CNS active drugs requires special patient care and observation. See WARNINGS.

Chronic Pulmonary Disease
Because potent opioids can cause hypoventilation, DURAGESIC® (fentanyl transdermal system) should be administered with caution to patients with preexisting medical conditions predisposing them to hypoventilation. In such patients, normal analgesic doses of opioids may further decrease respiratory drive to the point of respiratory failure.

Head Injuries and Increased Intracranial Pressure
DURAGESIC® should not be used in patients who may be particularly susceptible to the intracranial effects of CO_2 retention such as those with evidence of increased intracranial pressure, impaired consciousness, or coma. Opioids may obscure the clinical course of patients with head injury. DURAGESIC® should be used with caution in patients with brain tumors.

Cardiac Disease
Intravenous fentanyl may produce bradycardia. Fentanyl should be administered with caution to patients with bradyarrhythmias.

Hepatic or Renal Disease
At the present time insufficient information exists to make recommendations regarding the use of DURAGESIC® in patients with impaired renal or hepatic function. If the drug is used in these patients, it should be used with caution because of the hepatic metabolism and renal excretion of fentanyl.

Patients with Fever/External Heat
Based on a pharmacokinetic model, serum fentanyl concentrations could theoretically increase by approximately one third for patients with a body temperature of 40°C (104°F) due to temperature-dependent increases in fentanyl release from the system and increased skin permeability. Therefore, patients wearing DURAGESIC® systems who develop fever should be monitored for opioid side effects and the DURAGESIC® dose should be adjusted if necessary.

ALL PATIENTS SHOULD BE ADVISED TO AVOID EXPOSING THE DURAGESIC® APPLICATION SITE TO DIRECT EXTERNAL HEAT SOURCES, SUCH AS HEATING PADS OR ELECTRIC BLANKETS, HEAT LAMPS, SAUNAS, HOT TUBS, AND HEATED WATER BEDS, ETC. WHILE WEARING THE SYSTEM. THERE IS A POTENTIAL FOR TEMPERATURE-DEPENDENT INCREASES IN FENTANYL RELEASE FROM THE SYSTEM.

Central Nervous System Depressants
When patients are receiving DURAGESIC®, the dose of additional opioids or other CNS depressant drugs (including benzodiazepines) should be reduced by at least 50%. With the concomitant use of CNS depressants, hypotension may occur.

Drug or Alcohol Dependence
Use of DURAGESIC® in combination with alcoholic beverages and/or other CNS depressants can result in increased risk to the patient. DURAGESIC® should be used with caution in individuals who have a history of drug or alcohol abuse, especially if they are outside a medically controlled environment.

Ambulatory Patients
Strong opioid analgesics impair the mental or physical abilities required for the performance of potentially dangerous tasks such as driving a car or operating machinery. Patients who have been given DURAGESIC® should not drive or operate dangerous machinery unless they are tolerant to the effects of the drug.

Carcinogenesis, Mutagenesis, and Impairment of Fertility
Because long-term animal studies have not been conducted, the potential carcinogenic effects of DURAGESIC® are unknown. There was no evidence of mutagenicity in the Ames *Salmonella typhimurium* mutagenicity assay, the primary

TABLE A
FENTANYL PHARMACOKINETIC PARAMETERS FOLLOWING FIRST 72-HOUR APPLICATION OF DURAGESIC®

Dose	Mean (SD) Time to Maximal Concentration T_{max} (h)	Mean (SD) Maximal Concentration C_{max} (ng/mL)
DURAGESIC® 25 µg/h	38.1 (18.0)	0.6 (0.3)
DURAGESIC® 50 µg/h	34.8 (15.4)	1.4 (0.5)
DURAGESIC® 75 µg/h	33.5 (14.5)	1.7 (0.7)
DURAGESIC® 100 µg/h	36.8 (15.7)	2.5 (1.2)

NOTE: After system removal there is continued systemic absorption from residual fentanyl in the skin so that serum concentrations fall 50%, on average, in 17 hours.

TABLE B
RANGE OF PHARMACOKINETIC PARAMETERS OF INTRAVENOUS FENTANYL IN PATIENTS

	Clearance (L/h) Range [70 kg]	Volume of Distribution V_{ss} (L/kg) Range	Half-Life $t\frac{1}{2}$ (h) Range
Surgical Patients	27–75	3–8	3–12
Hepatically Impaired Patients	3–80+	0.8–8+	4–12+
Renally Impaired Patients	30–78	—	—

+Estimated
NOTE: Information on volume of distribution and half-life not available for renally impaired patients.

rat hepatocyte unscheduled DNA synthesis assay, the BALB/c-3T3 transformation test, the mouse lymphoma assay, the human lymphocyte and CHO chromosomal aberration in-vitro assays or the in-vivo micronucleus test.

Pregnancy—Pregnancy Category C
Fentanyl has been shown to impair fertility and to have an embryocidal effect in rats when given in intravenous doses 0.3 times the human dose for a period of 12 days. No evidence of teratogenic effects has been observed after administration of fentanyl to rats. There are no adequate and well-controlled studies in pregnant women. DURAGESIC® should be used during pregnancy only if the potential benefit justifies the potential risk to the fetus.

Labor and Delivery
DURAGESIC® is not recommended for analgesia during labor and delivery.

Nursing Mothers
Fentanyl is excreted in human milk; therefore DURAGESIC® is not recommended for use in nursing women because of the possibility of effects in their infants.

Pediatric Use
The safety and efficacy of DURAGESIC® in children has not been established. (See BOX WARNING and CONTRAINDICATIONS.)

DURAGESIC® SHOULD NOT BE ADMINISTERED TO CHILDREN UNDER 12 YEARS OF AGE OR PATIENTS UNDER 18 YEARS OF AGE WHO WEIGH LESS THAN 50 KG (110 LBS) EXCEPT IN AN AUTHORIZED INVESTIGATIONAL RESEARCH SETTING.

Geriatric Use
Information from a pilot study of the pharmacokinetics of IV fentanyl in geriatric patients indicates that the clearance of fentanyl may be greatly decreased in the population above the age of 60. The relevance of these findings to transdermal fentanyl is unknown at this time.

Since elderly, cachectic, or debilitated patients may have altered pharmacokinetics due to poor fat stores, muscle wasting, or altered clearance, they should not be started on DURAGESIC® doses higher than 25 µg/h unless they are already taking more than 135 mg of oral morphine a day or an equivalent dose of another opioid (see DOSAGE AND ADMINISTRATION).

Information for Patients
A patient instruction sheet is included in the package of DURAGESIC® systems dispensed to the patient.

Disposal of DURAGESIC®
DURAGESIC® should be kept out of the reach of children. DURAGESIC® systems should be folded so that the adhesive side of the system adheres to itself, then the system should be flushed down the toilet immediately upon removal. Patients should dispose of any systems remaining from a prescription as soon as they are no longer needed. Unused systems should be removed from their pouch and flushed down the toilet.

If the gel from the drug reservoir accidentally contacts the skin, the area should be washed with clear water.

ADVERSE REACTIONS

In post-marketing experience, deaths from hypoventilation due to inappropriate use of DURAGESIC® have been reported. (See BOX WARNING and CONTRAINDICATIONS.)

Pre-marketing Clinical Trial Experience:
The safety of DURAGESIC® has been evaluated in 357 postoperative patients and 153 cancer patients for a total of 510 patients. Patients with acute pain used DURAGESIC® for 1 to 3 days. The duration of DURAGESIC® use varied in cancer patients; 56% of patients used DURAGESIC® for over 30 days, 28% continued treatment for more than 4 months, and 10% used DURAGESIC® for more than 1 year.

Hypoventilation was the most serious adverse reaction observed in 13 (4%) postoperative patients and in 3 (2%) of the cancer patients. Hypotension and hypertension were observed in 11 (3%) and 4 (1%) of the opioid-naive patients. Various adverse events were reported; a causal relationship to DURAGESIC® was not always determined. The frequencies presented here reflect the actual frequency of each adverse effect in patients who received DURAGESIC®. There has been no attempt to correct for a placebo effect, concomitant use of other opioids, or to subtract the frequencies reported by placebo-treated patients in controlled trials.

The following adverse reactions were reported in 153 cancer patients at a frequency of 1% or greater; similar reactions were seen in the 357 postoperative patients studied.
Body as a Whole: abdominal pain*, headache*
Cardiovascular: arrhythmia, chest pain
Digestive: nausea**, vomiting**, constipation**, dry mouth**, anorexia*, diarrhea*, dyspepsia*, flatulence
Nervous: somnolence**, confusion**, asthenia**, dizziness*, nervousness*, hallucinations*, anxiety*, depression*, euphoria*, tremor, abnormal coordination, speech disorder, abnormal thinking, abnormal gait, abnormal dreams, agitation, paresthesia, amnesia, syncope, paranoid reaction
Respiratory: dyspnea*, hypoventilation*, apnea*, hemoptysis, pharyngitis, hiccups
Skin and Appendages: sweating**, pruritus*, rash, application site reaction - erythema, papules, itching, edema
Urogenital: urinary retention*
*Reactions occurring in 3%–10% of DURAGESIC® patients
**Reactions occurring in 10% or more of DURAGESIC® patients

The following adverse effects have been reported in less than 1% of the 510 postoperative and cancer patients studied; the association between these events and DURAGESIC® administration is unknown. This information is listed to serve as alerting information for the physician.
Digestive: abdominal distention
Nervous: aphasia, hypertonia, vertigo, stupor, hypotonia, depersonalization, hostility
Respiratory: stertorous breathing, asthma, respiratory disorder
Skin and Appendages, General: exfoliative dermatitis, pustules

Special Senses: amblyopia
Urogenital: bladder pain, oliguria, urinary frequency

DRUG ABUSE AND DEPENDENCE

Fentanyl is a Schedule II controlled substance and can produce drug dependence similar to that produced by morphine. DURAGESIC® (fentanyl transdermal system) therefore has the potential for abuse. Tolerance, physical and psychological dependence may develop upon repeated administration of opioids. Iatrogenic addiction following opioid administration is relatively rare. Physicians should not let concerns of physical dependence deter them from using adequate amounts of opioids in the management of severe pain when such use is indicated.

OVERDOSAGE

Clinical Presentation

The manifestations of fentanyl overdosage are an extension of its pharmacologic actions with the most serious significant effect being hypoventilation.

Treatment

For the management of hypoventilation immediate countermeasures include removing the DURAGESIC® (fentanyl transdermal system) system and physically or verbally stimulating the patient. These actions can be followed by administration of a specific narcotic antagonist such as naloxone. The duration of hypoventilation following an overdose may be longer than the effects of the narcotic antagonist's action (the half-life of naloxone ranges from 30 to 81 minutes). The interval between IV antagonist doses should be carefully chosen because of the possibility of re-narcotization after system removal; repeated administration of naloxone may be necessary. Reversal of the narcotic effect may result in acute onset of pain and the release of catecholamines.

If the clinical situation warrants, ensure a patent airway is established and maintained, administer oxygen and assist or control respiration as indicated and use an oropharyngeal airway or endotracheal tube if necessary. Adequate body temperature and fluid intake should be maintained.

If severe or persistent hypotension occurs, the possibility of hypovolemia should be considered and managed with appropriate parenteral fluid therapy.

DOSAGE AND ADMINISTRATION

With all opioids, the safety of patients using the products is dependent on health care practitioners prescribing them in strict conformity with their approved labeling with respect to patient selection, dosing, and proper conditions for use.

As with all opioids, dosage should be individualized. The most important factor to be considered in determining the appropriate dose is the extent of preexisting opioid tolerance. (See BOX WARNING and CONTRAINDICATIONS.) Initial doses should be reduced in elderly or debilitated patients (see PRECAUTIONS).

DURAGESIC® (fentanyl transdermal system) should be applied to non-irritated and non-irradiated skin on a flat surface such as chest, back, flank or upper arm. Hair at the application site should be clipped (not shaved) prior to system application. If the site of DURAGESIC® application must be cleansed prior to application of the system, do so with clear water. Do not use soaps, oils, lotions, alcohol, or any other agents that might irritate the skin or alter its characteristics. Allow the skin to dry completely prior to system application.

DURAGESIC® should be applied immediately upon removal from the sealed package. Do not alter the system, e.g., cut, in any way prior to application.

The transdermal system should be pressed firmly in place with the palm of the hand for 30 seconds, making sure the contact is complete, especially around the edges.

Each DURAGESIC® may be worn continuously for 72 hours. If analgesia for more than 72 hours is required, a new system should be applied to a different skin site after removal of the previous transdermal system.

DURAGESIC® should be kept out of the reach of children. Used systems should be folded so that the adhesive side of the system adheres to itself, then the system should be flushed down the toilet immediately upon removal. Patients should dispose of any systems remaining from a prescription as soon as they are no longer needed. Unused systems should be removed from their pouch and flushed down the toilet.

Dose Selection

DOSES MUST BE INDIVIDUALIZED BASED UPON THE STATUS OF EACH PATIENT AND SHOULD BE ASSESSED AT REGULAR INTERVALS AFTER DURAGESIC® APPLICATION. REDUCED DOSES OF DURAGESIC® ARE SUGGESTED FOR THE ELDERLY AND OTHER GROUPS DISCUSSED IN PRECAUTIONS.

DURAGESIC® DOSES GREATER THAN 25 µG/H SHOULD NOT BE USED FOR INITIATION OF DURAGESIC® THERAPY IN NON-OPIOID TOLERANT PATIENTS.

In selecting an initial DURAGESIC® dose, attention should be given to 1) the daily dose, potency, and characteristics of the opioid the patient has been taking previously (eg

whether it is a pure agonist or mixed agonist-antagonist), 2) the reliability of the relative potency estimates used to calculate the DURAGESIC® dose needed (potency estimates may vary with the route of administration), 3) the degree of opioid tolerance, if any, and 4) the general condition and medical status of the patient. Each patient should be maintained at the lowest dose providing acceptable pain control.

Initial DURAGESIC® Dose Selection

There has been no systematic evaluation of DURAGESIC® as an initial opioid analgesic in the management of chronic pain, since most patients in the clinical trials were converted to DURAGESIC® from other narcotics. Therefore, unless the patient has pre-existing opioid tolerance, the lowest DURAGESIC® dose, 25 µg/h, should be used as the initial dose.

To convert patients from oral or parenteral opioids to DURAGESIC® use the following methodology:

1. Calculate the previous 24-hour analgesic requirement.
2. Convert this amount to the equianalgesic oral morphine dose using Table C.
3. Table D displays the range of 24-hour oral morphine doses that are recommended for conversion to each DURAGESIC® dose. Use this table to find the calculated 24-hour morphine dose and the corresponding DURAGESIC® dose. Initiate DURAGESIC® treatment using the recommended dose and titrate patients upwards (no more frequently than every 3 days after the initial dose or than every 6 days thereafter) until analgesic efficacy is attained. The recommended starting dose when converting from other opioids to DURAGESIC® is likely too low for 50% of patients. This starting dose is recommended to minimize the potential for overdosing patients with the first dose. For delivery rates in excess of 100 µg/h, multiple systems may be used.

TABLE Cᵃ
EQUIANALGESIC POTENCY CONVERSION

Name	Equianalgesic Dose (mg)	
	IMᵇᶜ	PO
morphine	10	60 (30)ᵈ
hydromorphone (Dilaudid®)	1.5	7.5
methadone (Dolophine®)	10	20
oxycodone (Percocet®)	15	30
levorphanol (Levo-Dromoran®)	2	4
oxymorphone (Numorphan®)	1	10 (PR)
heroin	5	60
meperidine (Demerol®)	75	—
codeine	130	200

ᵃ All IM and PO doses in this chart are considered equivalent to 10 mg of IM morphine in analgesic effect. IM denotes intramuscular, PO oral, and PR rectal.
ᵇ Based on single-dose studies in which an intramuscular dose of each drug listed was compared with morphine to establish the relative potency. Oral doses are those recommended when changing from parenteral to an oral route.
ᶜ Although controlled studies are not available, in clinical practice it is customary to consider the doses of opioid given IM, IV or subcutaneously to be equivalent. There may be some differences in pharmacokinetic parameters such as C_{max} and T_{max}.
ᵈ The conversion ratio of 10 mg parenteral morphine = 30 mg oral morphine is based on clinical experience in patients with chronic pain. The conversion ratio of 10 mg parenteral morphine = 60 mg oral morphine is based on a potency study in acute pain. Reference: Foley, K.M. (1985) The treatment of cancer pain. NEJM 313(2):84-95. Reference: Ashburn and Lipman (1993) Management of pain in the cancer patient. Anesth Analg 76: 402–416.

TABLE D
RECOMMENDED DURAGESIC® DOSE BASED UPON DAILY ORAL MORPHINE DOSE

Oral 24-hour Morphine (mg/day)	DURAGESIC® Dose (µg/hr)
45–134	25
135–224	50
225–314	75
315–404	100
405–494	125
495–584	150
585–674	175
675–764	200
765–854	225
855–944	250
945–1034	275
1035–1124	300

NOTE: In clinical trials these ranges of daily oral morphine doses were used as a basis for conversion to DURAGESIC®.

¹THIS TABLE SHOULD NOT BE USED TO CONVERT FROM DURAGESIC® TO OTHER THERAPIES, BECAUSE THIS CONVERSION TO DURAGESIC® IS CONSERVATIVE. USE OF TABLE D FOR CONVERSION TO OTHER ANALGESIC THERAPIES CAN OVERESTIMATE THE DOSE OF THE NEW AGENT. OVERDOSAGE OF THE NEW ANALGESIC AGENT IS POSSIBLE. (See DOSAGE AND ADMINISTRATION—Discontinuation of DURAGESIC®.)

The majority of patients are adequately maintained with DURAGESIC® administered every 72 hours. A small number of patients may not achieve adequate analgesia using this dosing interval and may require systems to be applied every 48 hours rather than every 72 hours. An increase in the DURAGESIC® dose should be evaluated before changing dosing intervals in order to maintain patients on a 72-hour regimen.

Because of the increase in serum fentanyl concentration over the first 24 hours following initial system application, the initial evaluation of the maximum analgesic effect of DURAGESIC® cannot be made before 24 hours of wearing. The initial DURAGESIC® dosage may be increased after 3 days (see Dose Titration).

During the initial application of DURAGESIC®, patients should use short-acting analgesics for the first 24 hours as needed until analgesic efficacy with DURAGESIC® is attained. Thereafter, some patients still may require periodic supplemental doses of other short-acting analgesics for 'breakthrough' pain.

Dose Titration

The recommended initial DURAGESIC® dose based upon the daily oral morphine is conservative, and 50% of patients are likely to require a dose increase after initial application of DURAGESIC®. The initial DURAGESIC® dosage may be increased after 3 days, based on the daily dose of supplemental analgesics required by the patient in the second or third day of the initial application.

Physicians are advised that it may take up to 6 days after increasing the dose of DURAGESIC® for the patient to reach equilibrium on the new dose (see graph in CLINICAL PHARMACOLOGY). Therefore, patients should wear a higher dose through two applications before any further increase in dosage is made on the basis of the average daily use of a supplemental analgesic.

Appropriate dosage increments should be based on the daily dose of supplementary opioids, using the ratio of 90 mg/24 hours of oral morphine to a 25 µg/h increase in DURAGESIC® dose.

Discontinuation of DURAGESIC®

To convert patients to another opioid, remove DURAGESIC® and titrate the dose of the new analgesic based upon the patient's report of pain until adequate analgesia has been attained. Upon system removal, 17 hours or more are required for a 50% decrease in serum fentanyl concentrations. For patients requiring discontinuation of opioids, a gradual downward titration is recommended since it is not known what dose level the opioid may be discontinued without producing the signs and symptoms of abrupt withdrawal.

TABLE D SHOULD NOT BE USED TO CONVERT FROM DURAGESIC® TO OTHER THERAPIES. BECAUSE THE CONVERSION TO DURAGESIC® IS CONSERVATIVE, USE OF TABLE D FOR CONVERSION TO OTHER ANALGESIC THERAPIES CAN OVERESTIMATE THE DOSE OF THE NEW AGENT. OVERDOSAGE OF THE NEW ANALGESIC AGENT IS POSSIBLE.

HOW SUPPLIED

DURAGESIC® is supplied in cartons containing 5 individually packaged systems. See chart for information regarding individual systems.

DURAGESIC® Dose (µg/h)	System Size (cm²)	Fentanyl Content (mg)	NDC Number
DURAGESIC®-25	10	2.5	50458-033-05
DURAGESIC®-50*	20	5	50458-034-05
DURAGESIC®-75*	30	7.5	50458-035-05
DURAGESIC®-100*	40	10	50458-036-05

* FOR USE ONLY IN OPIOID TOLERANT PATIENTS.

Safety and Handling

DURAGESIC® is supplied in sealed transdermal systems which pose little risk of exposure to health care workers. If the gel from the drug reservoir accidentally contacts the

Continued on next page

Duragesic—Cont.

skin, the area should be washed with copious amounts of water. Do not use soap, alcohol, or other solvents to remove the gel because they may enhance the drug's ability to penetrate the skin. Do not cut or damage DURAGESIC®. If the DURAGESIC® system is cut or damaged, controlled drug delivery will not be possible.
Do not store above 77°F (25°C). Apply immediately after removal from individual sealed package. Do not use if the seal is broken. **For transdermal use only.**
CAUTION: Federal law prohibits dispensing without prescription
DEA order form required. A schedule CII narcotic.
Manufactured by:
ALZA Corporation
Palo Alto, CA 94304
Distributed by:
JANSSEN PHARMACEUTICA
Titusville, NJ 08560
June 1994, June 1997 7500310
Shown in Product Identification Guide, page 317

ERGAMISOL® ℞

[*ər-gam 'ə-, sōl*]
(levamisole hydrochloride)
Tablets

DESCRIPTION

ERGAMISOL® (levamisole hydrochloride) is an immunomodulator available in tablets for oral administration containing the equivalent of 50 mg as levamisole base. Fifty-nine (59) mg of levamisole HCl is equivalent to 50 mg of levamisole base. Inactive ingredients are colloidal silicon dioxide, hydrogenated vegetable oil, hydroxypropyl methylcellulose, lactose, microcystalline cellulose, polyethylene glycol 6000, polysorbate 80, and talc.
Levamisole hydrochloride is (-)-(S)-2,3,5,6-tetrahydro-6-phenylimidazo [2,1-b] thiazole monohydrochloride.
Levamisole hydrochloride is a white to almost white crystalline powder which is almost odorless and is freely soluble in water. It is quite stable in acid aqueous media but hydrolyzes in alkaline or neutral solutions. It has a molecular weight of 240.75.

CLINICAL PHARMACOLOGY

Two clinical trials having essentially the same design have demonstrated an increase in survival and a reduction in recurrence rate in the subset of patients with resected Dukes' C colon cancer treated with a regimen of ERGAMISOL® (levamisole hydrochloride) plus fluorouracil[1,2]. After surgery, patients were randomized to no further therapy, ERGAMISOL® alone, or ERGAMISOL® plus fluorouracil.
In one clinical trial in which 408 Dukes' B and C colorectal cancer patients were studied, 262 Dukes' C patients were evaluated for a minimum follow-up of five years[1]. A subset analysis of these Dukes' C patients showed the estimated reduction in death rate was 27% for ERGAMISOL® plus fluorouracil (p = 0.11) and 28% for ERGAMISOL® alone (p = 0.11)[3]. The estimated reduction in recurrence rate was 36% for ERGAMISOL® plus fluorouracil (p = 0.025) and 28% for ERGAMISOL® alone (p = 0.11)[3]. In another clinical trial designed to confirm the above results, 929 Dukes' C colon cancer patients were evaluated for a minimum follow-up of 2 years[2]. The estimated reduction in death rate was 33% for ERGAMISOL® plus fluorouracil (p = 0.006). The estimated reduction in recurrence rate was 41% for ERGAMISOL® plus fluorouracil (p<0.0001). The ERGAMISOL® alone group did not show advantage over no treatment on improving recurrence or survival rates. There are presently insufficient data to evaluate the effect of the combination of ERGAMISOL® plus fluorouracil in Dukes' B patients.
There are also insufficient data to evaluate the effect of ERGAMISOL® plus fluorouracil in patients with rectal cancer because only 12 patients with rectal cancer were treated with the combination in the first study and none in the second study.
The mechanism of action of ERGAMISOL® in combination with fluorouracil is unknown. The effects of levamisole on the immune system are complex. The drug appears to restore depressed immune function rather than to stimulate response to above-normal levels. Levamisole can stimulate formation of antibodies to various antigens, enhance T-cell responses by stimulating T-cell activation and proliferation, potentiate monocyte and macrophage functions including phagocytosis and chemotaxis, and increase neutrophil mobility, adherence, and chemotaxis. Other drugs have similar short-term effects and the clinical relevance is unclear.
Besides its immunomodulatory function, levamisole has other mammalian pharmacologic activities, including inhibition of alkaline phosphatase, and cholinergic activity.
The pharmacokinetics of ERGAMISOL® have not been studied in the dosage regimen recommended with fluorouracil. After administration of a single oral dose of 50 mg of a research formulation of ERGAMISOL®, it appears that levamisole is rapidly absorbed from the gastrointestinal tract. Mean peak plasma concentrations of 0.13 mcg/ml are attained within 1.5 to 2 hours. The plasma elimination half-life of levamisole is between 3-4 hours. Following a 150-mg radio-labelled dose, levamisole is extensively metabolized by the liver in humans and the metabolities excreted mainly by the kidneys (70% over 3 days). The elimination half-life of metabolite excretion is 16 hours. Approximately 5% is excreted in the feces. Less than 5% is excreted unchanged in the urine and less than 0.2% in the feces. Approximately 12% is recovered in the urine as the glucuronide of p-hydroxy-levamisole. The clinical significance of these data are unknown since a 150-mg dose may not be proportional to a 50-mg dose. In the presence of cirrhosis the C_{max} of ERGAMISOL® is not clearly increased but the AUC increases four-fold.

INDICATIONS AND USAGE

ERGAMISOL® (levamisole hydrochloride) is only indicated as adjuvant treatment in combination with fluorouracil after surgical resection in patients with Dukes' stage C colon cancer.

CONTRAINDICATIONS

ERGAMISOL® (levamisole hydrochloride) is contraindicated in patients with a known hypersensitivity to the drug or its components.

WARNINGS

Cases of an encephalopathy-like syndrome associated with demyelination have been reported in patients treated with ERGAMISOL® (levamisole hydrochloride). Worldwide post-marketing experience with the combination therapy of ERGAMISOL® and fluorouracil has also included reports of peripheral neuropathy and multifocal inflammatory leukoencephalopathy. The onset of symptoms and the clinical presentation in these cases are quite varied. Symptoms may include coma, confusion, lethargy, memory loss, muscle weakness, paresthesia, seizures, and speech disturbances. This condition has been associated with MRI and CT scan findings of demyelinating lesions in the white matter. If an acute neurological syndrome occurs, ERGAMISOL® and fluorouracil should be discontinued immediately. Patients have generally recovered/improved with drug discontinuation, but in some cases patients have not recovered/improved and deaths have been reported. Patients are generally treated with corticosteroids, but the efficacy of corticosteroids has not been proven.
ERGAMISOL® has been associated with agranulocytosis, sometimes fatal. The onset of agranulocytosis is frequently accompanied by a flu-like syndrome (fever, chills, etc.); however, in a small number of patients it is asymptomatic. A flu-like syndrome may also occur in the absence of agranulocytosis. It is essential that appropriate hematological monitoring be done routinely during therapy with ERGAMISOL® and fluorouracil. Neutropenia is usually reversible following discontinuation of therapy. Patients should be instructed to report immediately any flu-like symptoms.
Higher than recommended doses of ERGAMISOL® may be associated with an increased incidence of agranulocytosis, so the recommended dose should not be exceeded.
In the presence of cirrhosis the C_{max} of ERGAMISOL® is not clearly increased but the AUC increases four-fold. Dose modification or discontinuation of ERGAMISOL® may be necessary if adverse experiences are observed. The combination of ERGAMISOL® and fluorouracil has been associated with frequent neutropenia, anemia and thrombocytopenia.

PRECAUTIONS

Before beginning this combination adjuvant treatment, the physician should become familiar with the labeling for fluorouracil.
Information for Patients: The patient should be informed that if flu-like symptoms or malaise occurs, the physician should be notified immediately.
Drug Interactions: ERGAMISOL® (levamisole hydrochloride) has been reported to produce "ANTABUSE®"-like side effects when given concomitantly with alcohol. Concomitant administration of phenytoin and ERGAMISOL® plus fluorouracil has led to increased plasma levels of phenytoin. The physician is advised to monitor plasma levels of phenytoin and to decrease the dose if necessary.
Because of reports of prolongation of the prothrombin time beyond the therapeutic range in patients taking concurrent levamisole and warfarin sodium, it is suggested that the prothrombin time be monitored carefully, and the dose of warfarin sodium or other coumarin-like drugs should be adjusted accordingly, in patients taking both drugs.
Laboratory Tests: On the first day of therapy with ERGAMISOL®/fluorouracil, patients should have a CBC with differential and platelets, electrolytes and liver function tests performed. Thereafter, a CBC with differential and platelets should be performed weekly prior to each treatment with fluorouracil with electrolytes and liver function tests peformed every 3 months for a total of one year. Dosage modifications should be instituted as follows: If WBC is 2500-3500/mm^3 defer the fluorouracil dose until WBC is >3500/mm^3. If WBC is < 2500/mm^3, defer the fluorouracil dose until WBC is > 3500/mm^3; then resume the fluorouracil dose reduced by 20%. If WBC remains < 2500/mm^3 for over 10 days despite deferring fluorouracil, discontinue administration of ERGAMISOL®. Both drugs should be deferred unless enough platelets are present (≥ 100,000/mm^3).
Carcinogenesis, Mutagenesis, Impairment of Fertility: Adequate animal carcinogenicity studies have not been conducted with levamisole. Studies of levamisole administered in drinking water at 5, 20, and 80 mg/kg/day to mice for up to 18 months or admnistered to rats in the diet at 5, 20, and 80 mg/kg/day for 24 months showed no evidence of neoplastic effects. These studies were not conducted at the maximum tolerated dose, therefore the animals may not have been exposed to a reasonable drug challenge. No mutagenic effects were demonstrated in dominant lethal studies in male and female mice, in an Ames test, and in a study to detect chromosomal aberrations in cultured peripheral human lymphocytes.
Adverse effects were not observed on male or female fertility when levamisole was administered to rats in the diet at doses of 2.5, 10, 40, and 160 mg/kg. In a rat gavage study at doses of 20, 60, and 180 mg/kg, the copulation period was increased, the duration of pregnancy was slightly increased, and fertility, pup viability and weight, lactation index, and number of fetuses were decreased at 60 mg/kg. No negative reproductive effects were present when the offspring were allowed to mate and litter.
Pregnancy: Pregnancy Category C: Teratogenicity studies have been performed in rats and rabbits at oral doses up to 180 mg/kg. Fetal malformations were not observed. In rats, embryotoxicity was present at 160 mg/kg and in rabbits, significant embryotoxicity was observed at 180 mg/kg. There are no adequate and well-controlled studies in pregnant women and ERGAMISOL® should not be administered unless the potential benefits outweigh the risks. Women taking the combination of ERGAMISOL® and fluorouracil should be advised not to become pregnant.
Nursing Mothers: It is not known whether ERGAMISOL® is excreted in human milk; it is excreted in cows' milk. Because of the potential for serious adverse reactions in nursing infants from ERGAMISOL®, a decision should be made whether to discontinue nursing or to discontinue the drug, taking into account the importance of the drug to the mother.
Pediatric Use: Safety and effectiveness of ERGAMISOL® in children have not been established.

ADVERSE REACTIONS

Almost all patients receiving ERGAMISOL® (levamisole hydrochloride) and fluorouracil reported adverse experiences. Tabulated below is the incidence of adverse experiences that occurred in at least 1% of patients enrolled in two clinical trials who were adjuvantly treated with either ERGAMISOL® or ERGAMISOL® plus fluorouracil following colon surgery. In the larger clinical trial, 66 of 463 patients (14%) discontinued the combination of ERGAMISOL® plus fluorouracil because of adverse reactions. Forty-three of these patients (9%) developed isolated or a combination of gastrointestinal toxicities. (e.g., nausea, vomiting, diarrhea, stomatitis and anorexia). Ten patients developed rash and/or pruritus. Five patients discontinued therapy because of flu-like symptoms or fever with chills; ten patients developed central nervous system symptoms such as dizziness, ataxia, depression, confusion, memory loss, weakness, inability to concentrate, and headache; two patients developed reversible neutropenia and sepsis; one patient because of thrombocytopenia; one patient because of hyperbilirubinemia. One patient in the ERGAMISOL® plus fluorouracil group developed agranulocytosis and sepsis and died.
In the ERGAMISOL® alone arm of the trial, 15 of 310 patients (4.8%) discontinued therapy because of adverse experiences. Six of these (2%) discontinued because of rash, six because of arthralgia/myalgia, and one each for fever and neutropenia, urinary infection, and cough.
[See table at bottom of next page]
In worldwide experience with ERGAMISOL®, less frequent adverse experiences included exfoliative dermatitis, fixed drug eruptions, periorbital edema, vaginal bleeding, anaphylaxis, confusion, convulsions, hallucinations, impaired concentration, renal failure, pancreatitis, elevated serum creatinine, and increased alkaline phosphatase.
Reports of hyperlipidemia have been observed in patients receiving combination therapy of ERGAMISOL® and fluorouracil; elevations in triglyceride levels have been greater than increases in cholesterol levels. In worldwide postmarketing experience with the combination therapy, there have been rare cases of elevated hepatic enzymes and hepatosteatosis in patients.
The following additional adverse experiences have been reported for fluorouracil alone: esophagopharyngitis, pancytopenia, myocardial ischemia, angina, gastrointestinal ulcer-

ation and bleeding, anaphylaxis and generalized allergic reactions, acute cerebellar syndrome, nystagmus, dry skin, fissuring, photosensitivity, lacrimal duct stenosis, photophobia, euphoria, thrombophlebitis, and nail changes.

OVERDOSAGE

Fatalities have been reported in a three-year-old child who ingested 15 mg/kg and in an adult who ingested 32 mg/kg. No further clinical information is available. In cases of overdosage, gastric lavage is recommended together with symptomatic and supportive measures.

DOSAGE AND ADMINISTRATION

The adjuvant use of ERGAMISOL® (levamisole hydrochloride) and fluorouracil is limited to the following dosage schedule:

Initial Therapy:
ERGAMISOL®: 50 mg p.o.   (starting 7–30 days
q8h for 3 days   post-surgery)
fluorouracil: 450 mg/m^2/day (starting 21–34 days
IV for 5 days   post-surgery)
concomitant with a 3-day course
of ERGAMISOL®

Maintenance:
ERGAMISOL®: 50 mg p.o. q8h for 3 days every 2 weeks.
fluorouracil: 450 mg/m^2/day IV once a week beginning 28 days after the initiation of the 5-day course.

Treatment: ERGAMISOL®, administered orally, should be initiated no earlier than 7 and no later than 30 days post surgery at a dose of 50 mg q8h × 3 days repeated every 14 days for 1 year. Fluorouracil therapy should be initiated no earlier than 21 days and no later than 35 days after surgery providing the patient is out of the hospital, ambulatory, maintaining normal oral nutrition, has well-healed wounds, and is fully recovered from any postoperative complications. If ERGAMISOL® has been initiated from 7 to 20 days after surgery, initiation of fluorouracil therapy should be coincident with the second course of ERGAMISOL®, i.e., at 21 to 34 days. If ERGAMISOL® is initiated from 21 to 30 days after surgery, fluorouracil should be initiated simultaneously with the first course of ERGAMISOL®. Since the AUC of ERGAMISOL® is markedly increased in cirrhotic patients, such patients should be observed closely for adverse effects. Dose reduction or discontinuation of ERGAMISOL® may be warranted if adverse experiences are noted. Fluorouracil should be administered by rapid IV push at a dosage of 450 mg/m^2/day for 5 consecutive days. Dosage calculation is based on actual weight (estimated dry weight if there is evidence of fluid retention). *This course should be discontinued before the full 5 doses are administered if the patient develops any stomatitis or diarrhea (5 or more loose stools).* Twenty-eight days after initiation of this course, weekly fluorouracil should be instituted at a dosage of 450 mg/m^2/week and continued for a total treatment time of 1 year. If stomatitis or diarrhea develop during weekly ther-

apy, the next dose of fluorouracil should be deferred until these side effects have subsided. If these side effects are moderate to severe, the fluorouracil dose should be reduced 20% when it is resumed.
Dosage modifications should be instituted as follows: If WBC is 2500-3500/mm^3 defer the fluorouracil dose until WBC is >3500/mm^3. If WBC is <2500/mm^3, defer the fluorouracil dose until WBC is >3500/mm^3; then resume the fluorouracil dose reduced by 20%. If WBC remains <2500/mm^3 for over 10 days despite deferring fluorouracil, discontinue administration of ERGAMISOL®. Both drugs should be deferred unless platelets are adequate (≥100,000/mm^3).
ERGAMISOL® should not be used at doses exceeding the recommended dose or frequency. Clinical studies suggest a relationship between ERGAMISOL® adverse experiences and increasing dose, and since some of these, e.g. agranulocytosis, may be life-threatening, the recommended dosage regimen should not be exceeded (see **"WARNINGS"**).
Before beginning this combination adjuvant treatment, the physician should become familiar with the labeling for fluorouracil.

HOW SUPPLIED

ERGAMISOL® (levamisole hydrochloride) is available in white, coated tablets containing the equivalent of 50 mg of levamisole base, debossed "JANSSEN" and "L"/"50".
They are supplied in blister packages of 36 tablets (NDC 50458-270-36).
Store at room temperature, 15°–30°C (59°–86°F).
Protect from moisture.

REFERENCES

1. Laurie JA, Moertel CG, Fleming TR, et al. Surgical adjuvant therapy of large-bowel carcinoma: An evaluation of levamisole and the combination of levamisole and fluorouracil. *J Clin Oncol.* 1989; 7:1447–1456.
2. Moertel CG, Fleming TR, Macdonald JS, et al. Levamisole and fluorouracil for adjuvant therapy of resected colon carcinoma. *New Engl J Med.* 1990; 322:352–358.
3. Data on file, Janssen Pharmaceutica Inc.
Manufactured by:
Janssen Pharmaceutica, nv
Beerse, Belgium
Distributed by:
Janssen Pharmaceutica Inc.
Titusville, NJ 08560
Edition July 1996, September 1997
U.S. Patent Number 4,584,305
Shown in Product Identification Guide, page 317

Adverse experience	ERGAMISOL® N = 440 %	ERGAMISOL® plus fluorouracil N = 599 %
Gastrointestinal		
Nausea	22	65
Diarrhea	13	52
Stomatitis	3	39
Vomiting	6	20
Anorexia	2	6
Abdominal pain	2	5
Constipation	2	3
Flatulence	<1	2
Dyspepsia	<1	1
Hematological		
Leukopenia		
<2000/mm^3	<1	1
≥2000 to <4000/mm^3	4	19
≥4000/mm^3	2	33
unscored category	0	<1
Thrombocytopenia		
<50,000/mm^3	0	0
≥50,000 to <130,000/mm^3	1	8
≥130,000/mm^3	1	10
Anemia	0	6
Granulocytopenia	<1	2
Epistaxis	0	1
Skin and Appendages		
Dermatitis	8	23
Alopecia	3	22
Pruritus	1	2
Skin discoloration	0	2
Urticaria	<1	0
Body as a Whole		
Fatigue	6	11
Fever	3	5
Rigors	3	5
Chest pain	<1	1
Edema	1	1
Resistance Mechanisms		
Infection	5	12
Special Senses		
Taste Perversion	8	8
Altered sense of smell	1	1
Musculoskeletal System		
Arthralgia	5	4
Myalgia	3	2
Central and peripheral nervous system		
Dizziness	3	4
Headache	3	4
Paresthesia	2	3
Ataxia	0	2
Psychiatric		
Somnolence	3	2
Depression	1	2
Nervousness	1	2
Insomnia	1	1
Anxiety	1	1
Forgetfulness	0	1
Vision		
Abnormal tearing	0	4
Blurred vision	1	2
Conjunctivitis	<1	2
Liver and biliary system		
Hyperbilirubinemia	<1	1

HISMANAL® ℞
[*his 'ma-nal*]
(astemizole) Tablets

WARNING BOX
QT PROLONGATION/VENTRICULAR ARRHYTHMIAS
RARE CASES OF SERIOUS CARDIOVASCULAR ADVERSE EVENTS INCLUDING DEATH, CARDIAC ARREST, QT PROLONGATION, TORSADES DE POINTES, AND OTHER VENTRICULAR ARRHYTHMIAS HAVE BEEN OBSERVED IN PATIENTS EXCEEDING RECOMMENDED DOSES OF ASTEMIZOLE. WHILE THE MAJORITY OF SUCH EVENTS HAVE OCCURRED FOLLOWING SUBSTANTIAL OVERDOSES OF ASTEMIZOLE, TORSADES DE POINTES (ARRHYTHMIAS) HAVE VERY RARELY OCCURRED AT REPORTED DOSES AS LOW AS 20–30 MG DAILY (2–3 TIMES THE RECOMMENDED DAILY DOSE). DATA SUGGEST THAT THESE EVENTS ARE ASSOCIATED WITH ELEVATION OF ASTEMIZOLE AND/OR ASTEMIZOLE METABOLITE LEVELS, RESULTING IN ELECTROCARDIOGRAPHIC QT PROLONGATION.
THESE EVENTS HAVE ALSO OCCURRED AT 10 MG DAILY IN A FEW PATIENTS WITH POSSIBLE AUGMENTING CIRCUMSTANCES (SEE CONTRAINDICATIONS AND WARNINGS). IN VIEW OF THE POTENTIAL FOR CARDIAC ARRHYTHMIAS, ADHERENCE TO THE RECOMMENDED DOSE SHOULD BE EMPHASIZED.
DO NOT EXCEED THE RECOMMENDED DOSE OF 10 MG (ONE TABLET) DAILY.
SOME PATIENTS APPEAR TO INCREASE THE DOSE OF HISMANAL® (ASTEMIZOLE) TABLETS IN AN ATTEMPT TO ACCELERATE THE ONSET OF ACTION. PATIENTS SHOULD BE ADVISED NOT TO DO THIS AND NOT TO USE HISMANAL® ON AN AS-NEEDED BASIS (I.E., P R N) FOR IMMEDIATE RELIEF OF SYMPTOMS.
CONCOMITANT ADMINISTRATION OF ASTEMIZOLE WITH SYSTEMIC KETOCONAZOLE, ITRACONAZOLE, ERYTHROMYCIN, CLARITHROMYCIN, TROLEANDOMYCIN, MIBEFRADIL OR QUININE IS CONTRAINDICATED (SEE CONTRAINDICATIONS AND PRECAUTIONS: DRUG INTERACTIONS).

Continued on next page

Hismanal—Cont.

> SINCE ASTEMIZOLE IS EXTENSIVELY METABOLIZED BY THE LIVER, THE USE OF ASTEMIZOLE IN PATIENTS WITH SIGNIFICANT HEPATIC DYSFUNCTION IS CONTRAINDICATED.
> IN SOME CASES, SEVERE ARRHYTHMIAS HAVE BEEN PRECEDED BY EPISODES OF SYNCOPE. SYNCOPE IN PATIENTS RECEIVING ASTEMIZOLE SHOULD LEAD TO IMMEDIATE DISCONTINUATION OF TREATMENT AND APPROPRIATE CLINICAL EVALUATION, INCLUDING ELECTRO-CARDIOGRAPHIC TESTING (LOOKING FOR QT PROLONGATION AND VENTRICULAR ARRHYTHMIA).
> (SEE CLINICAL PHARMACOLOGY, CONTRAINDICATIONS, WARNINGS, PRECAUTIONS, OVERDOSAGE, AND DOSAGE AND ADMINISTRATION.)

DESCRIPTION

HISMANAL® (astemizole) is a histamine H_1-receptor antagonist available in scored white tablets for oral use. Each tablet contains 10 mg of astemizole, and, as inactive ingredients: lactose, cornstarch, microcrystalline cellulose, pregelatinized starch, povidone K90, magnesium stearate, colloidal silicon dioxide, and sodium lauryl sulfate. Astemizole is chemically designated as 1-[(4-fluorophenyl)-methyl]-N-[1-[2-(4-methoxyphenyl)ethyl]-4-piperidinyl]-1H-benzimidazol-2-amine, with a molecular weight of 458.58. The empirical formula is $C_{28}H_{31}FN_4O$.

Astemizole is a white to slightly off-white powder; it is insoluble in water, slightly soluble in ethanol and soluble in chloroform and methanol.

CLINICAL PHARMACOLOGY

Mechanism of Action

Astemizole is a long-acting, selective histamine H_1-receptor antagonist. Receptor binding studies in animals demonstrated that at pharmacological doses, astemizole occupies peripheral H_1-receptors but does not reach H_1-receptors in the brain. Whole body autoradiographic studies in rats, radiolabel tissue distribution studies in dogs and radioligand binding studies of guinea pig brain H_1-receptors have shown that astemizole does not readily cross the blood-brain barrier. Screening studies in rats at effective antihistaminic doses showed no anticholinergic effects. Studies in humans using the recommended dosage regimens have not been performed to determine whether astemizole is associated with a different frequency of anticholinergic effects than therapeutic doses of other antihistamines.

Pharmacokinetics

The absorption of astemizole is reduced by 60% when taken with meals. In single oral dose studies, astemizole was rapidly absorbed from the gastrointestinal tract; peak plasma concentrations of unchanged astemizole were reached within one hour. Due to extensive first pass metabolism and significant tissue distribution, plasma concentrations of unchanged drug were low. Elimination of unchanged astemizole occurred with a half-life of approximately one day. Elimination of astemizole plus hydroxylated metabolites, considered together to represent the pharmacologically active fraction in plasma, was biphasic with half-lives of 20 hours for the distribution phase and 7–11 days for the elimination phase. The pharmacokinetics of astemizole plus hydroxylated metabolites are dose proportional following single doses of 10 to 30 mg.

Following chronic administration, steady state plasma concentrations of astemizole plus hydroxylated metabolites (mainly desmethylastemizole) were reached within four to eight weeks; concentrations of the metabolites are substantially higher than those of unchanged astemizole. Astemizole plus hydroxylated metabolites decayed biphasically with an initial half-life of 7–9 days, with plasma concentrations being reduced by 75% within this phase, and with a terminal half-life of about 19 days. The initial phase ($t_{1/2}$=7–9 days) appears to determine the time to reach steady state plasma concentrations of astemizole plus hydroxylated metabolites. Steady state plasma concentrations of unchanged astemizole were reached by 6 days (with a range of 6–9 days); unchanged astemizole was eliminated from plasma with a half-life of approximately 2 days (with a range of 1–2.5 days).

The in-vitro plasma protein binding of unchanged astemizole (100 ng/mL) as 96.7% with 2.3% being found as free drug in the plasma water. In human blood with an astemizole concentration of 100 ng/mL, 61.5% of astemizole was bound to the plasma proteins, with 36.2% being distributed to the blood cell fraction. The concentration of astemizole found in the blood was the same as that found in the plasma fraction of the blood. Binding studies for the astemizole metabolite(s) which achieve much higher concentrations than astemizole under chronic dosing conditions have not been conducted.

Metabolism

Excretion and metabolism studies with ^{14}C-labeled astemizole in volunteers demonstrated that the drug is almost completely metabolized and primarily excreted in the feces.

In-vitro metabolism studies with human liver microsomes indicate that astemizole is metabolized to its principle circulating metabolite, desmethylastemizole, predominantly by a specific cytochrome P-450 isozyme, CYP 3A4. These in-vitro studies also indicate that the P-450 isozymes CYP 1A2 and CYP 2D6 are involved in the minor metabolic pathways of astemizole. The relative contributions of the CYP 3A4 isozymes in the liver and gastrointestinal mucosa to the presystemic clearance of astemizole are unknown. Concurrent administration of astemizole with the CYP 3A4 inhibitors ketoconazole or erythromycin to healthy volunteers was associated with significantly increased plasma concentrations of astemizole. (See WARNING BOX; CONTRAINDICATIONS; WARNINGS; PRECAUTIONS, Drug Interactions; ADVERSE REACTIONS; and DOSAGE AND ADMINISTRATION.)

Special Populations

Elevated levels of unmetabolized astemizole, whether due to significant hepatic dysfunction, concomitant use of interacting medications, or overdose, have been associated with QTC interval prolongation and serious cardiac events. (See WARNING BOX; CONTRAINDICATIONS; WARNINGS; PRECAUTIONS, Drug Interactions; ADVERSE REACTIONS; and DOSAGE AND ADMINISTRATION.)

Interpatient variability in pharmacokinetic parameters may be greater in patients with liver disease as compared to normal subjects. Systematic evaluation of the pharmacokinetics in patients with hepatic or renal dysfunction has not been performed.

Effects on Cardiac Repolarization

In controlled clinical trials, small mean increases from baseline in corrected QT interval (QTC) of approximately 7 milliseconds were observed at daily doses of 10 mg.

Clinical Trials

Seasonal Allergic Rhinitis

Clinical trials supporting the approval of HISMANAL® (astemizole) Tablets for seasonal allergic rhinitis involved 425 patients aged 12 and over who received either HISMANAL® once daily or another antihistamine and/or placebo in double-blind randomized controlled studies. HISMANAL® was superior to placebo in effects on nasal and non-nasal symptoms of seasonal allergic rhinitis. In these and other clinical studies, the efficacy of HISMANAL® versus placebo was not demonstrated until several days after beginning dosing.

Idiopathic Chronic Urticaria

Clinical trials supporting the approval of HISMANAL® for idiopathic chronic urticaria involved 142 patients aged 12 and over who received either HISMANAL® once daily or another antihistamine and/or placebo in double-blind randomized controlled studies. HISMANAL® was superior to placebo in the management of idiopathic chronic urticaria as demonstrated by reduction in associated itching, erythema, and hives. The onset of efficacy of HISMANAL® versus placebo in this condition has not been adequately studied.

INDICATIONS AND USAGE

HISMANAL® (astemizole) Tablets are indicated for the relief of symptoms associated with seasonal allergic rhinitis and chronic idiopathic urticaria. HISMANAL® should not be used on an as-needed (i.e., p r n) basis for immediate relief of symptoms. Patients should be advised not to increase the dose in an attempt to accelerate the onset of action. Clinical studies have not been conducted to evaluate the effectiveness of HISMANAL® in the common cold.

CONTRAINDICATIONS

CONCOMITANT ADMINISTRATION OF ASTEMIZOLE WITH SYSTEMIC KETOCONAZOLE, ITRACONAZOLE, ERYTHROMYCIN, CLARITHROMYCIN, TROLEANDOMYCIN, MIBEFRADIL DIHYDROCHLORIDE OR QUININE IS CONTRAINDICATED. ASTEMIZOLE IS ALSO CONTRAINDICATED IN PATIENTS WITH SEVERE HEPATIC IMPAIRMENT OR WHO ARE TAKING OTHER CONCOMITANT MEDICATIONS KNOWN TO IMPAIR ITS METABOLISM. QT PROLONGATION HAS BEEN DEMONSTRATED IN PATIENTS TAKING ASTEMIZOLE IN THESE SETTINGS AND CASES OF SERIOUS CARDIOVASCULAR EVENTS, INCLUDING DEATH. CARDIAC ARREST, AND TORSADES DE POINTES, HAVE BEEN REPORTED IN THESE PATIENT POPULATIONS. (See WARNING BOX; WARNINGS; PRECAUTIONS, Special Populations; PRECAUTIONS, Drug Interactions; ADVERSE REACTIONS; and DOSAGE AND ADMINISTRATION.)

HISMANAL® is contraindicated in patients with known hypersensitivity to astemizole or any of the inactive ingredients.

WARNINGS

Astemizole undergoes extensive presystemic metabolism to its major active metabolite predominantly by the cytochrome P-450 3A4 isozyme. Cytochromes P-450 1A2 and 2D6 contribute to the overall metabolism of astemizole to a lesser extent. These metabolic pathways may be impaired in patients with hepatic dysfunction (e.g., alcoholic cirrhosis, hepatitis) or who are taking drugs systemically such as ketoconazole, itraconazole, erythromycin, clarithromycin, troleandomycin, mibefradil dihydrochloride, other potent inhibitors of this isozyme or quinine. Interference with this metabolism can lead to elevated astemizole and/or desmethylastemizole plasma levels associated with QT prolongation and increased risk of ventricular tachyarrhythmias (such as torsades de pointes, ventricular tachycardia, and ventricular fibrillation) at the recommended dose. HISMANAL® (astemizole) Tablets are contraindicated for use by patients with these conditions. (See WARNING BOX; CONTRAINDICATIONS; PRECAUTIONS, Special Populations; PRECAUTIONS, Drug Interactions; and DOSAGE AND ADMINISTRATION.)

Patients known to have conditions leading to QT prolongation may experience QT prolongation and/or ventricular arrhythmia with astemizole at recommended doses. The effect of astemizole in patients who are receiving other agents which alter the QT interval is unknown. However, in view of astemizole's known potential for QT prolongation, it is advisable to avoid its use in 1) patients with congenital QT prolongation syndrome, 2) those taking medications which are reported to prolong QT intervals (including certain antiarrhythmics, bepridil, certain psychotropics, cisapride, sparfloxacin or terfenadine [this list may not be all inclusive]), 3) patients with electrolyte abnormalities such as hypokalemia or hypomagnesemia, or 4) those taking diuretics with the potential for inducing electrolyte abnormalities.

The relationship of underlying cardiac disease to the development of ventricular tachyarrhythmias while on HISMANAL® therapy is unclear; nonetheless, HISMANAL® should also be used with caution in these patients.

PRECAUTIONS

General

Elevated concentrations of astemizole and/or its principal metabolite, desmethylastemizole, whether due to overdose, significant hepatic dysfunction, or concomitant medications, have been associated with altered cardiac repolarization and/or serious cardiac arrhythmias. Patients with impaired hepatic function or those receiving treatment with significant inhibitors of CYP 3A4 or quinine may experience QT prolongation and/or ventricular arrhythmias, including torsades de pointes, at the recommended dose. Patients having conditions leading to QT prolongation may also be at risk for these cardiovascular events. (See WARNING BOX; CLINICAL PHARMACOLOGY; CONTRAINDICATIONS; WARNINGS; PRECAUTIONS, Special Populations; PRECAUTIONS, Drug Interactions; ADVERSE REACTIONS; and DOSAGE AND ADMINISTRATION.)

Rare cases of anaphylaxis, including anaphylactic shock, have been reported.

Caution should also be used when treating patients with renal impairment.

Information for Patients

Patients taking HISMANAL® (astemizole) Tablets should receive the following information and instructions. Antihistamines are prescribed to reduce allergic symptoms. Patients taking HISMANAL® should be advised 1) to adhere to the recommended dose, and 2) that the use of excessive doses may lead to serious cardiovascular events. Some patients appear to increase the dose of HISMANAL® in an attempt to accelerate the onset of action. PATIENTS SHOULD BE ADVISED NOT TO DO THIS and not to use HISMANAL® on an as-needed (i.e., p r n) basis for immediate relief of symptoms. Patients should be questioned about the use of any other prescriptions or over-the-counter medication, and should be cautioned regarding the potential for life-threatening arrhythmias with concurrent use of ketoconazole, itraconazole, erythromycin, clarithromycin, troleandomycin, mibefradil dihydrochloride, or quinine. Limited human data indicate that although beverages containing quinine (up to 80 mg/day or about 32 ounces of tonic water) may elevate plasma levels of astemizole and desmethylastemizole, this effect is small and is not accompanied by significant prolongation of the QT interval. Patients should be advised to consult their physician before concurrent use of other medications with astemizole. Patients should also be advised that HISMANAL® should not be taken with grapefruit juice. Patients should be questioned about pregnancy or lactation before starting HISMANAL® therapy, since the drug should be used in pregnancy or lactation only if the potential benefit justifies the potential risk to fetus or baby (see Pregnancy subsection). In addition, patients should be instructed to take HISMANAL® on an empty stomach, e.g., at least 2 hours after a meal. No additional food should be taken for at least 1 hour after dosing. Patients should also be instructed to store this medication in a tightly closed container in a cool, dry place, away from heat or direct sunlight, and away from children.

Drug Interactions

Before prescribing or adding a newly available drug to the regimen of a patient receiving astemizole, the package insert of the new drug and/or the medical literature should be consulted to determine if an interaction between the new drug and astemizole has been reported.

Astemizole is predominantly metabolized by the cytochrome P-450 3A4 (CYP 3A4) isozyme with some metabolism by the 1A2 and 2D6 isozymes. Inhibition of CYP 3A4 in patients taking HISMANAL® can result in markedly elevated plasma concentrations of astemizole and/or its principal metabolite, desmethylastemizole. This could increase or prolong both the therapeutic effect and adverse events. Presence of elevated astemizole/desmethylastemizole concentrations is associated with significant prolongation of the QT and QTC intervals. (See BOX WARNING; CONTRAINDICATIONS; WARNINGS; PRECAUTIONS, Drug Interactions; ADVERSE REACTIONS; and DOSAGE AND ADMINISTRATION.)

Concomitant administration of the drugs in Table A with astemizole is contraindicated.

Table A
Drugs Contraindicated for Use with Astemizole

> Azole antifungals: ketoconazole, itraconazole
> Macrolide antibiotics: clarithromycin, erythromycin, troleandomycin
> Other: mibefradil, quinine

The drugs noted below have been demonstrated to be inhibitors of CYP 3A4 in-vitro and have been shown to have clinically significant pharmacokinetic interactions with other substrates of this isozyme. Because of the potential for these drugs to influence the metabolism of astemizole and until the clinical significance of these findings is fully established, concomitant use of astemizole with the drugs in Table B is not recommended.

Table B
Drugs Not Recommended for Use with Astemizole

> Other antifungals: fluconazole, metronidazole, miconazole i.v.
> Serotonin Reuptake Inhibitors (SRI): fluoxetine, fluvoxamine, nefazodone, paroxetine, sertraline
> HIV Protease Inhibitors: ritonavir, indinavir, saquinavir, nelfinavir
> Other: grapefruit juice, zileuton, other potent CYP 3A4 inhibitors

Ketoconazole/Itraconazole
Concomitant administration of ketoconazole or itraconazole with astemizole results in markedly elevated concentrations of astemizole and its principal metabolite, desmethylastemizole. Therefore, concomitant administration of HISMANAL® with ketoconazole or itraconazole is contraindicated.

Other Antifungals
Due to the chemical similarity of fluconazole, metronidazole, and miconazole i.v. to ketoconazole, concomitant use of these products with astemizole is not recommended.

Macrolide Antibiotics
Concomitant administration of erythromycin with astemizole results in markedly elevated concentrations of astemizole and its principal metabolite, desmethylastemizole. Because of the chemical similarity of clarithromycin and troleandomycin to erythromycin and the known relative inhibitory potencies of these macrolides, concomitant administration of erythromycin, clarithromycin or troleandomycin with astemizole is also contraindicated.

Mibefradil dihydrochloride
Mibefradil is an inhibitor of the P-450 isozyme primarily responsible for the metabolism of astemizole (CYP 3A4). Coadministration of mibefradil with terfenadine (also metabolized by CYP 3A4) in healthy subjects results in inhibition of terfenadine metabolism and accumulation of unmetabolized terfenadine with resulting clinically significant repolarization abnormalities. Because of the potential for mibefradil to influence the metabolism of astemizole, concomitant use of astemizole with mibefradil dihydrochloride is contraindicated.

Quinine
Although quinine is not known to be an inhibitor of CYP 3A4, concomitant administration of quinine with astemizole results in markedly elevated concentrations of astemizole and its principal metabolite, desmethylastemizole. The mechanism of this interaction is not known. Concomitant administration of astemizole with quinine is therefore contraindicated.

Other 3A4 Inhibitors
Astemizole is metabolized by the cytochrome P-450 3A4 isozyme (CYP 3A4). Inhibition of this enzyme in patients taking HISMANAL® results in increased plasma concentrations of astemizole and/or its principal metabolite, desmethylastemizole. Presence of elevated astemizole/desmethylastemizole concentrations is associated with significant prolongation of the QT and QTC intervals. The drugs noted below have been demonstrated to be inhibitors of CYP 3A4 in-vitro and have been shown to have clinically significant pharmacokinetic interactions with other substrates of this isozyme. Because of the potential for these drugs to influence the metabolism of astemizole and until the clinical significance is fully established, concomitant use of astemizole and the drugs below is not recommended.

> Serotonin Reuptake Inhibitors: fluoxetine, fluvoxamine, nefazodone, paroxetine, sertraline
> HIV Protease Inhibitors: ritonavir, indinavir, saquinavir, nelfinavir
> Grapefruit juice
> Zileuton
> Other potent CYP 3A4 inhibitors

Carcinogenesis, Mutagenesis, Impairment of Fertility
Astemizole did not reveal any carcinogenic potential at oral doses up to 80 mg/kg/day for 24 months in rats and 18 months in mice (approximately 65 and 30 times, respectively, the maximum recommended daily oral dose in adults on a mg/m^2 basis). Micronucleus, dominant lethal, sister chromatid exchange and Ames tests of astemizole have not revealed mutagenic activity. No impairment of fertility was observed in rats at oral doses up to 40 mg/kg/day (approximately 30 times the maximum recommended daily oral dose in adults on a mg/m^2 basis).

Pregnancy: Pregnancy Category C
Teratogenic effects were not observed in rats at oral doses up to 160 mg/kg/day (approximately 130 times the maximum recommended daily oral dose in adults on a mg/m^2 basis) and in rabbits at oral doses up to 40 mg/kg/day (approximately 65 times the maximum recommended daily oral dose in adults on a mg/m^2 basis). Maternal mortality was seen in rabbits at oral doses of 10 mg/kg/day and above (approximately 16 times the maximum recommended daily oral dose in adults on a mg/m^2 basis). Embryocidal effects accompanied by maternal effects were observed in rats at oral doses of 40 mg/kg/day and above (approximately 30 times the maximum recommended daily oral dose in adults on a mg/m^2 basis). Embryotoxicity was not observed in rats at an oral dose of 10 mg/kg/day (approximately 8 times the maximum recommended daily oral dose in adults on a mg/m^2 basis) and maternal toxicity was not reported in rabbits at an oral dose of 2.5 mg/kg/day (approximately 4 times the maximum recommended daily oral dose in adults on a mg/m^2 basis). There are no adequate and well-controlled studies in pregnant women. HISMANAL® should be used during pregnancy only if the potential benefit justifies the potential risk to the fetus. Metabolites may remain in the body for as long as 4 months after the end of dosing, calculated on the basis of 6 times the terminal half-life (see CLINICAL PHARMACOLOGY section).

Nursing Mothers
Astemizole is excreted in the milk of dogs. It is not known whether astemizole is excreted in human milk. Because certain drugs are known to be excreted in human milk, caution should be exercised when HISMANAL® is administered to a nursing woman.

Pediatric Use
Safety and efficacy in children under 12 years of age have not been demonstrated.

ADVERSE REACTIONS
Cardiovascular Adverse Events
Rare reports of serious cardiovascular effects have been received which include ventricular tachyarrhythmias (torsades de pointes, ventricular tachycardia, ventricular fibrillation, and cardiac arrest), hypotension, syncope, and dizziness. Rare reports of deaths resulting from ventricular tachyarrhythmias have been received. In most instances, astemizole overdoses, QT-prolonging conditions, drug interactions leading to impaired astemizole metabolism or other factors which could have contributed to the events, were observed. (See WARNING BOX; CONTRAINDICATIONS; WARNINGS; PRECAUTIONS, Drug Interactions; and DOSAGE AND ADMINISTRATION.) Hypotension, palpitations, syncope, and dizziness could reflect undetected ventricular arrhythmia. IN SOME PATIENTS, DEATH, CARDIAC ARREST, OR TORSADES DE POINTES HAVE BEEN PRECEDED BY EPISODES OF SYNCOPE (see WARNINGS). Rare reports of serious cardiovascular adverse events have been received, some involving QT prolongation and torsades de pointes, in apparently normal individuals without identifiable risk factors and at recommended doses. There is not conclusive evidence of a causal relationship of these events with astemizole.

Reports of serious cardiovascular effects associated with patients intentionally taking more than the recommended daily dose of astemizole in an attempt to accelerate the onset of action have been received. Patients should be cautioned not to exceed the recommended daily dose (see PRECAUTIONS, Information for Patients).

General Adverse Events
The reported incidences of adverse reactions listed in the following table are derived from controlled clinical studies in adults. In these studies the usual maintenance dose of HISMANAL® (astemizole) Tablets was 10 mg once daily. [See table above]

Adverse reaction information has been obtained from more than 7500 patients in all clinical trials. Weight gain has been reported in 3.6% of astemizole treated patients involved in controlled studies, with an average treatment duration of 53 days. In 46 of the 59 patients for whom actual weight gain data was available, the average weight gain was 3.2 kg.

Less frequently occurring adverse experiences reported in clinical trials or spontaneously from marketing experience with HISMANAL® include: angioedema, asymptomatic liver enzyme elevations, bronchospasm, depression, edema, epistaxis, hepatitis, myalgia, palpitation, paresthesia, photosensitivity, pruritus, and rash.

Rare cases of anaphylaxis, including anaphylactic shock, have been reported.

Marketing experiences include isolated cases of convulsions. A causal relationship with HISMANAL® has not been established.

OVERDOSAGE

In the event of overdosage, supportive measures including gastric lavage and emesis should be employed. Substantial overdoses of HISMANAL® (astemizole) Tablets can cause death, cardiac arrest, QT prolongation, torsades de pointes, and other ventricular arrhythmias. These events can also occur, although rarely, at doses (20–30 mg) close to the recommended dose (10 mg/daily). Patients should be advised not to take more than the daily recommended dose of HISMANAL® in attempts to accelerate the onset of action. (See WARNING BOX; CONTRAINDICATIONS; WARNINGS; PRECAUTIONS, Information for Patients; PRECAUTIONS, Drug Interactions; ADVERSE REACTIONS; and DOSAGE AND ADMINISTRATION.)

Seizures and syncope have also been reported with overdose and may be associated with a cardiac event.

ADVERSE EVENT	Percent of Patients Reporting Controlled Studies*		
	HISMANAL® (N=1630) %	PLACEBO (N=1109) %	ACTIVE CONTROLS** (N=304) %
Central Nervous System			
Drowsiness	7.1	6.4	22.0
Headache	6.7	9.2	3.3
Fatigue	4.2	1.6	11.8
Appetite increase	3.9	1.4	0.0
Weight increase	3.6	0.7	1.0
Nervousness	2.1	1.2	0.3
Dizziness	2.0	1.8	1.0
Gastrointestinal System			
Nausea	2.5	2.9	1.3
Diarrhea	1.8	2.0	0.7
Abdominal pain	1.4	1.2	0.7
Eye, Ear, Nose, and Throat			
Mouth dry	5.2	3.8	7.9
Pharyngitis	1.7	2.3	0.3
Conjunctivitis	1.2	1.2	0.7
Other			
Arthralgia	1.2	1.6	0.0

*Duration of treatment in controlled studies ranged from 7 to 182 days
**Active Controls: Clemastine (N=137); Chlorpheniramine (N=100); Pheniramine Maleate (N=47); d-Chlorpheniramine (N=20)

Continued on next page

Hismanal—Cont.

Overdose patients should be carefully monitored as long as the QT interval is prolonged or arrhythmias are present. In some cases, this has been up to six days. In overdose cases in which ventricular arrhythmias are associated with significant QT prolongation, treatment with antiarrhythmics known to prolong QT intervals is not recommended. HISMANAL® does not appear to be dialyzable.

Oral median lethal doses for astemizole were 2052 mg/kg in mice (approximately 830 times the maximum recommended daily oral dose in adults on a mg/m² basis) and 3154 mg/kg in rats (approximately 2600 times the maximum recommended daily dose in adults on a mg/m² basis). In neonatal rats, the oral median lethal dose was 1070 mg/kg (approximately 870 times the maximum recommended daily oral dose in adults on a mg/m² basis).

DOSAGE AND ADMINISTRATION

The recommended dosage for adults and children 12 years of age and older is 10 mg (1 tablet) once daily.

DO NOT EXCEED THE RECOMMENDED DOSE. Patients should be advised not to increase the dose of HISMANAL® (astemizole) Tablets in an attempt to accelerate the onset of action. USE OF HISMANAL® IN PATIENTS WITH SIGNIFICANT HEPATIC DYSFUNCTION OR IN PATIENTS TAKING KETOCONAZOLE, ITRACONAZOLE, ERYTHROMYCIN, CLARITHROMYCIN, TROLEANDOMYCIN, MIBEFRADIL DIHYDROCHLORIDE, OR QUININE IS CONTRAINDICATED. (See WARNING BOX; CONTRAINDICATIONS; WARNINGS; PRECAUTIONS, Information for Patients; PRECAUTIONS, Drug Interactions; ADVERSE REACTIONS; OVERDOSAGE; and DOSAGE AND ADMINISTRATION.)

Studies evaluating the need for dosage adjustments for patients with hepatic or renal dysfunction have not been performed. Since astemizole is extensively metabolized by the liver, use of HISMANAL® in patients with significant hepatic dysfunction is contraindicated.

HISMANAL® should be taken on an empty stomach, e.g., at least two hours after a meal. There should be no additional food intake for at least one hour post-dosing.

HOW SUPPLIED

HISMANAL® (astemizole) Tablets are available as white, scored tablets containing 10 mg of astemizole debossed "JANSSEN" and on the reverse side debossed "Ast/10."

NDC 50458-510-10 (HDPE bottles of 100 tablets)

NDC 50458-510-13 (HDPE bottles of 30 tablets with a child resistant closure)

Store at controlled room temperature 59°–77°F (15°–25°C). Protect from moisture.

7500212

U.S. Patent 4,219,559

Revised January 1997, February 1998

© Janssen Pharmaceutica Inc. 1998

JANSSEN
PHARMACEUTICA
Titusville, NJ 08560

PATIENT INFORMATION

HISMANAL®

Generic name: astemizole
10 mg tablets

This leaflet is a summary of important information about HISMANAL®. Be sure to ask your doctor if you have any questions or want to known more.

What is HISMANAL® and What Is It Used For?

HISMANAL® is an antihistamine (astemizole). It is used to relieve symptoms of seasonal allergies or hay fever. These symptoms may include runny nose, sneezing, itching of the nose or throat, and itchy, watery eyes. HISMANAL® may also be prescribed by your doctor to treat the symptoms and skin manifestations of hives (urticaria). These symptoms include generalized itching and redness of the skin.

HISMANAL® has not been demonstrated to be effective in relieving the symptoms of the common cold.

How Do I Take HISMANAL®?

— The recommended dose of HISMANAL® is ONE tablet taken ONCE A DAY. DO NOT TAKE MORE OFTEN THAN ONE TABLET ONCE A DAY.

— HISMANAL® does not work immediately and therefore should not be used for immediate relief. Because taking more than the recommended dose can increase your risk of having a serious side effect, you should not take more than one tablet once a day to try to get it to work faster.

— If you miss your daily dose of HISMANAL®, do not take extra HISMANAL® tablets to make up for it.

— HISMANAL® should be taken on an empty stomach (at least 2 hours after having a meal). Also, don't eat any food for at least 1 hour after taking your HISMANAL®.

What Are Important Warnings About Using HISMANAL®?

— **WARNING: DO NOT TAKE HISMANAL® IF YOUR ARE USING KETOCONAZOLE (NIZORAL®), ITRACONAZOLE (SPORANOX®), ERYHTROMYCIN, CLARITHROMYCIN (BIAXIN®), TROLEANDOMYCIN (TAO®), QUININE, OR MIBEFRADIL (POSICOR®). IF YOU HAVE ANY LIVER OR HEART PROBLEMS, TALK TO YOUR DOCTOR BEFORE YOU USE HISMANAL®.**

— Do not use HISMANAL® with any other prescription or nonprescription medicines without first talking to your doctor and pharmacist.

— Do not take HISMANAL® with grapefruit juice.

— If you faint, become dizzy, have unusual heartbeats, or any other unusual symptoms while using HISMANAL®, contact your doctor.

— If you become pregnant or are nursing a baby, talk to your doctor about whether you should take HISMANAL®. Your doctor will decide whether you should take HISMANAL® based on the benefits and risks.

What Are the Risks of Using HISMANAL®?

The side effects which occur most often are drowsiness, fatigue, and dry mouth. Increased appetite and weight gain have also been reported by patients taking HISMANAL®.

In rare cases, HISMANAL® has caused IRREGULAR HEARTBEATS which may cause serious problems such as fainting, dizziness, cardiac arrest, or death.

In these rare cases, this occurred most often when HISMANAL® was taken:

— in more than the recommended dose (Remember, do not take more than one tablet once a day);

— with antifungal drugs such as ketoconazole (Nizoral) or itraconazole (Sporanox);

— with the antibiotic drugs erythromycin, clarithromycin (Biaxin), or troleandomycin (TAO);

— with oral quinine preparations;

— by patients with severe liver disease.

How Do I Store HISMANAL®?

HISMANAL® should be stored in a tightly closed container, at room temperature out of direct sunlight. It should be kept away from children.

Shown in Product Identification Guide, page 317

IMODIUM®
(loperamide HCl) Capsules

℞

DESCRIPTION

IMODIUM® (loperamide hydrochloride), 4-(p-chlorophenyl)-4-hydroxy-N, N-dimethyl-α,α-dipheny-1-piperidinebutyramide monohydrochloride, is a synthetic antidiarrheal for oral use.

IMODIUM® is available in 2 mg capsules.

The inactive ingredients are: Lactose, cornstarch, talc, and magnesium stearate. IMODIUM® capsules contain FD&C Yellow No. 6.

CLINICAL PHARMACOLOGY

In vitro and animal studies show that IMODIUM® (loperamide hydrochloride) acts by slowing intestinal motility and by affecting water and electrolyte movement through the bowel. IMODIUM® inhibits peristaltic activity by a direct effect on the circular and longitudinal muscles of the intestinal wall.

In man, IMODIUM® prolongs the transit time of the intestinal contents. It reduces the daily fecal volume, increases the viscosity and bulk density, and diminishes the loss of fluid and electrolytes. Tolerance to the antidiarrheal effect has not been observed.

Clinical studies have indicated that the apparent elimination half-life of loperamide in man is 10.8 hours with a range of 9.1–14.4 hours. Plasma levels of unchanged drug remain below 2 nanograms per ml after the intake of a 2 mg capsule of IMODIUM®. Plasma levels are highest approximately five hours after administration of the capsule and 2.5 hours after the liquid. The peak plasma levels of loperamide were similar for both formulations. Of the total excreted in urine and feces, most of the administered drug was excreted in feces.

In those patients in whom biochemical and hematological parameters were monitored during clinical trials, no trends toward abnormality during IMODIUM® therapy were noted. Similarly, urinalyses, EKG and clinical ophthalmological examinations did not show trends toward abnormality.

INDICATIONS AND USAGE

IMODIUM® (loperamide hydrochloride) is indicated for the control and symptomatic relief of acute nonspecific diarrhea and of chronic diarrhea associated with inflammatory bowel disease. IMODIUM® is also indicated for reducing the volume of discharge from ileostomies.

CONTRAINDICATIONS

IMODIUM® (loperamide hydrochloride) is contraindicated in patients with known hypersensitivity to the drug and in those in whom constipation must be avoided.

WARNINGS

IMODIUM® (loperamide hydrochloride) should not be used in the case of acute dysentery, which is characterized by blood in stools and high fever.

Fluid and electrolyte depletion often occur in patients who have diarrhea. In such cases, administration of appropriate fluid and electrolytes is very important. The use of IMODIUM® does not preclude the need for appropriate fluid and electrolyte therapy.

In some patients with acute ulcerative colitis, and in pseudomembranous colitis associated with broad-spectrum antibiotics, agents which inhibit intestinal motility or delay intestinal transit time have been reported to induce toxic megacolon.

IMODIUM® therapy should be discontinued promptly if abdominal distention, constipation, or ileus occurs.

IMODIUM® should be used with special caution in young children because of the greater variability of response in this age group. Dehydration, particularly in younger children, may further influence the variability of response to IMODIUM®.

PRECAUTIONS

General

Extremely rare allergic reactions including anaphylaxis and anaphylactic shock have been reported.

In acute diarrhea, if clinical improvement is not observed in 48 hours, the administration of IMODIUM® (loperamide hydrochloride) should be discontinued. Patients with hepatic dysfunction should be monitored closely for signs of CNS toxicity because of the apparent large first pass biotransformation.

Information for Patients

Patients should be advised to check with their physician if their diarrhea does not improve after a couple of days or if they note blood in their stools or develop a fever.

Drug Interactions

There was no evidence in clinical trials of drug interactions with concurrent medications.

Carcinogenesis, mutagenesis, impairment of fertility

In an 18-month rat study with doses up to 133 times the maximum human dose (on a mg/kg basis), there was no evidence of carcinogenesis. Mutagenicity studies were not conducted. Reproduction studies in rats indicated that high doses (150–200 times the human dose) could cause marked female infertility and reduced male fertility.

Pregnancy

Teratogenic Effects

Pregnancy Category B

Reproduction studies in rats and rabbits have revealed no evidence of impaired fertility or harm to the fetus at doses up to 30 times the human dose. Higher doses impaired the survival of mothers and nursing young. The studies offered no evidence of teratogenic activity. There are, however, no adequate and well controlled studies in pregnant women. Because animal reproduction studies are no always predictive of human response, this drug should be used during pregnancy only if clearly needed.

Nursing Mothers

It is not known whether this drug is excreted in human milk. Because many drugs are excreted in human milk, caution should be exercised when IMODIUM® is administered to a nursing woman.

Pediatric Use

See the "Warnings" Section for information on the greater variability of response in this age group.

In case of accidental overdosage of IMODIUM® by children, see "Overdosage" Section for suggested treatment.

ADVERSE REACTIONS

The adverse effects reported during clinical investigations of IMODIUM® (loperamide hydrochloride) are difficult to distinguish from symptoms associated with the diarrheal syndrome. Adverse experiences recorded during clinical studies with IMODIUM® were generally of a minor and self-limiting nature. They were more commonly observed during the treatment of chronic diarrhea.

The following adverse events have been reported: hypersensitivity reactions such as skin rash and urticaria, and extremely rare cases of anaphylactic shock and bullous eruption including Toxic Epidermal Necrolysis. In the majority of these cases, the patients were on other medications which may have caused or contributed to the reactions.

The following patient complaints have also been reported: abdominal pain, distention or discomfort, nausea, vomiting, constipation, tiredness, drowsiness or dizziness and dry mouth.

There have been rare reports of paralytic ileus associated with abdominal distention. Most of these reports occurred in the setting of acute dysentery, overdose, and with very young children of less than two years of age.

DRUG ABUSE AND DEPENDENCE

Abuse

A specific clinical study designed to assess the abuse potential of loperamide at high doses resulted in a finding of extremely low abuse potential.

Dependence

Studies in morphine-dependent monkeys demonstrated that loperamide hydrochloride at doses above those recommended for humans prevented signs of morphine withdrawal. However, in humans, the naloxone challenge pupil test, which when positive indicates opiate-like effects, performed after a single high dose, or after more than two years of therapeutic use of IMODIUM® (loperamide hydrochloride), was negative. Orally administered IMODIUM® (loperamide formulated with magnesium stearate) is both highly insoluble and penetrates the CNS poorly.

OVERDOSAGE

In cases of overdosage, paralytic ileus and CNS depression may occur. Children may be more sensitive to CNS effects than adults. Clinical trials have demonstrated that a slurry of activated charcoal administered promptly after ingestion of loperamide hydrochloride can reduce the amount of drug which is absorbed into the systemic circulation by as much as ninefold. If vomiting occurs spontaneously upon ingestion, a slurry of 100 gms of activated charcoal should be administered orally as soon as fluids can be retained.

If vomiting has not occurred, gastric lavage should be performed followed by administration of 100 gms of the activated charcoal slurry through the gastric tube. In the event of overdosage, patients should be monitored for signs of CNS depression for at least 24 hours. Children may be more sensitive to central nervous system effects than adults. If CNS depression is observed, naloxone may be administered. If responsive to naloxone, vital signs must be monitored carefully for recurrence of symptoms of drug overdose for at least 24 hours after the last dose of naloxone.

In view of the prolonged action of loperamide and the short duration (one to three hours) of naloxone, the patient must be monitored closely and treated repeatedly with naloxone as indicated. Since relatively little drug is excreted in the urine, forced diuresis is not expected to be effective for IMODIUM® (loperamide hydrochloride) overdosage.

In clinical trials an adult who took three 20 mg doses within a 24 hour period was nauseated after the second dose and vomited after the third dose. In studies designed to examine the potential for side effects, intentional ingestion of up to 60 mg of loperamide hydrochloride in a single dose to healthy subjects resulted in no significant adverse effects.

DOSAGE AND ADMINISTRATION

(1 capsule = 2 mg)

Patients should receive appropriate fluid and electrolyte replacement as needed.

Acute Diarrhea

Adults: The recommended initial dose is 4 mg (two capsules) followed by 2 mg (one capsule) after each unformed stool. Daily dosage should not exceed 16 mg (eight capsules). Clinical improvement is usually observed within 48 hours.

Children: IMODIUM® (loperamide hydrochloride) use is not recommended for children under 2 years of age. In children 2 to 5 years of age (20 kg or less), the non-prescription liquid formulation (IMODIUM A-D 1 mg/5 ml) should be used; for ages 6 to 12, either IMODIUM® Capsules of IMODIUM® A-D liquid may be used. For children 2 to 12 years of age, the following schedule for capsules or liquid will usually fulfill initial dosage requirements:

Recommended First Day Dosage Schedule

Two to five years: 1 mg t.i.d. (3 mg daily dose) (13 to 20 kg)
Six to eight years: 2 mg b.i.d. (4 mg daily dose) (20 to 30 kg)
Eight to twelve years: 2 mg t.i.d. (6 mg daily dose) (greater than 30 kg)

Recommended Subsequent Daily Dosage

Following the first treatment day, it is recommended that subsequent IMODIUM® doses (1 mg/10 kg body weight) be administered only after a loose stool. Total daily dosage should not exceed recommended dosages for the first day.

Chronic Diarrhea

Children: Although IMODIUM® has been studied in a limited number of children with chronic diarrhea, the therapeutic dose for the treatment of chronic diarrhea in a pediatric population has not been established.

Adults: The recommended initial dose is 4 mg (two capsules) followed by 2 mg (one capsule) after each unformed stool until diarrhea is controlled, after which the dosage of IMODIUM® should be reduced to meet individual requirements. When the optimal daily dosage has been established, this amount may then be administered as a single dose or in divided doses.

The average daily maintenance dosage in clinical trials was 4 to 8 mg (two to four capsules). A dosage of 16 mg (eight capsules) was rarely exceeded. If clinical improvement is not observed after treatment with 16 mg per day for at least 10 days, symptoms are unlikely to be controlled by further administration. IMODIUM® administration may be continued if diarrhea cannot be adequately controlled with diet or specific treatment.

HOW SUPPLIED

Capsules—each capsule contains 2 mg of loperamide hydrochloride. The capsules have a light green body and a dark green cap with "JANSSEN" imprinted on one segment and "IMODIUM" on the other segment. IMODIUM® capsules are supplied in bottles of 100.

NDC 50458-400-10
(100 capsules)
Store at 15°–25°C (59°–77°F).
Revised September 1996, July 1998
©Janssen Pharmaceutica Inc. 1998
CAUTION: FEDERAL LAW PROHIBITS DISPENSING WITHOUT A PRESCRIPTION
U.S. Patent 3,714,159 7502205
JANSSEN PHARMACEUTICA
Titusville, New Jersey 08560
Shown in Product Identification Guide, page 317

NIZORAL® ℞
[nī 'zōr-ăl]
(ketoconazole) 2% Cream

DESCRIPTION

NIZORAL® (ketoconazole) 2% Cream contains the broad-spectrum synthetic antifungal agent, ketoconazole 2%, formulated in an aqueous cream vehicle consisting of propylene glycol, stearyl and cetyl alcohols, sorbitan monostearate, polysorbate 60, isopropyl myristate, sodium sulfite anhydrous, polysorbate 80 and purified water.

Ketoconazole is cis -1-acetyl-4-[4-[[2-(2,4-dichlorophenyl)-2-(1H -imidazol -1- ylmethyl) -1, 3- dioxolan -4- yl] methoxy]phenyl]piperazine.

CLINICAL PHARMACOLOGY

When NIZORAL® (ketoconazole) 2% Cream was applied dermally to intact or abraded skin of Beagle dogs for 28 consecutive days at a dose of 80 mg, there were no detectable plasma levels using an assay method having a lower detection limit of 2 ng/ml.

After a single topical application to the chest, back and arms of normal volunteers, systemic absorption of ketoconazole was not detected at the 5 ng/ml level in blood over a 72-hour period.

Two dermal irritancy studies, a human sensitization test, a phototoxicity study and a photoallergy study conducted in 38 male and 62 female volunteers showed no contact sensitization of the delayed hypersensitivity type, no irritation, no phototoxicity and no photoallergenic potential due to NIZORAL® (ketoconazole) 2% Cream.

Microbiology: Ketoconazole is a broad spectrum synthetic antifungal agent which inhibits the in vitro growth of the following common dermatophytes and yeasts by altering the permeability of the cell membrane: dermatophytes: Trichophyton rubrum, T. mentagrophytes, T. tonsurans, Microsporum canis, M. audouini, M. gypseum and Epidermophyton floccosum; yeasts: Candida albicans, Malassezia ovale (Pityrosporum ovale) and C. tropicalis; and the organism responsible for tinea versicolor, Malassezia furfur (Pityrosporum orbiculare). Only those organisms listed in the INDICATIONS AND USAGE Section have been proven to be clinically affected. Development of resistance to ketoconazole has not been reported.

Mode of Action: In vitro studies suggest that ketoconazole impairs the synthesis of ergosterol, which is a vital component of fungal cell membranes. It is postulated that the therapeutic effect of ketoconazole in seborrheic dermatitis is due to the reduction of M. ovale, but this has not been proven.

INDICATIONS AND USAGE

NIZORAL® (ketoconazole) 2% Cream is indicated for the topical treatment of tinea corporis, tinea cruris and tinea pedis caused by Trichophyton rubrum, T. mentagrophytes and Epidermophyton floccosum; in the treatment of tinea (pityriasis) versicolor caused by Malassezia furfur (Pityrosporum orbiculare); in the treatment of cutaneous candidiasis caused by Candida spp. and in the treatment of seborrheic dermatitis.

CONTRAINDICATIONS

NIZORAL® (ketoconazole) 2% Cream is contraindicated in persons who have shown hypersensitivity to the active or excipient ingredients of this formulation.

WARNINGS

NIZORAL® (ketoconazole) 2% Cream is not for ophthalmic use.

NIZORAL® (ketoconazole) 2% Cream contains sodium sulfite anhydrous, a sulfite that may cause allergic-type reactions including anaphylactic symptoms and life-threatening or less severe asthmatic episodes in certain susceptible people. The overall prevalence of sulfite sensitivity in the general population is unknown and probably low. Sulfite sensitivity is seen more frequently in asthmatic than in nonasthmatic people.

PRECAUTIONS

General: If a reaction suggesting sensitivity or chemical irritation should occur, use of the medication should be discontinued. Hepatitis (1:10,000 reported incidence) and, at high doses, lowered testosterone and ACTH induced corticosteroid serum levels have been seen with orally administered ketoconazole; these effects have not been seen with topical ketoconazole.

Carcinogenesis, Mutagenesis, Impairment of Fertility: A long-term feeding study in Swiss Albino mice and in Wistar rats showed no evidence of oncogenic activity. The dominant lethal mutation test in male and female mice revealed that single oral doses of ketoconazole as high as 80 mg/kg produced no mutation in any stage of germ cell development. The Ames' Salmonella microsomal activator assay was also negative.

Pregnancy: Teratogenic effects: Pregnancy Category C: Ketoconazole has been shown to be teratogenic (syndactylia and oligodactylia) in the rat when given orally in the diet at 80 mg/kg/day, (10 times the maximum recommended human oral dose). However, these effects may be related to maternal toxicity, which was seen at this and higher dose levels.

There are no adequate and well-controlled studies in pregnant women. Ketoconazole should be used during pregnancy only if the potential benefit justifies the potential risk to the fetus.

Nursing Mothers: It is not known whether NIZORAL® (ketoconazole) 2% Cream administered topically could result in sufficient systemic absorption to produce detectable quantities in breast milk. Nevertheless, a decision should be made whether to discontinue nursing or discontinue the drug, taking into account the importance of the drug to the mother.

Pediatric Use: Safety and effectiveness in children have not been established.

ADVERSE REACTIONS

During clinical trials 45 (5.0%) of 905 patients treated with NIZORAL® (ketoconazole) 2% Cream and 5 (2.4%) of 208 patients treated with placebo reported side effects consisting mainly of severe irritation, pruritus and stinging. One of the patients treated with NIZORAL® Cream developed a painful allergic reaction.

In worldwide postmarketing experience, rare reports of contact dermatitis have been associated with NIZORAL Cream or one of its excipients, namely sodium sulfite or propylene glycol.

DOSAGE AND ADMINISTRATION

Cutaneous candidiasis, tinea corporis, tinea cruris, tinea pedis, and tinea (pityriasis) versicolor: It is recommended that NIZORAL® (ketoconazole) 2% Cream be applied once daily to cover the affected and immediate surrounding area. Clinical improvement may be seen fairly soon after treatment is begun; however, candidal infections and tinea cruris and corporis should be treated for two weeks in order to reduce the possibility of recurrence. Patients with tinea versicolor usually require two weeks of treatment. Patients with tinea pedis require six weeks of treatment.

Seborrheic dermatitis: NIZORAL® (ketoconazole) 2% Cream should be applied to the affected area twice daily for four weeks or until clinical clearing.

If a patient shows no clinical improvement after the treatment period, the diagnosis should be redetermined.

HOW SUPPLIED

NIZORAL® (ketoconazole) 2% Cream is supplied in 15 (NDC 50458-221-15), 30 (NDC 50458-221-30) and 60 (NDC 50458-221-60) gm tubes.
Store below 77°F (25°C)
Revised July 1994, April 1995
U.S. Patent No. 4,335,125
JANSSEN PHARMACEUTICA
Titusville, NJ 08560
Shown in Product Identification Guide, page 317

NIZORAL® ℞
[nī 'zōr-ăl]
(ketoconazole) 2% Shampoo

DESCRIPTION

NIZORAL® (ketoconazole) 2% Shampoo is a red-orange liquid for topical application, containing the broad-spectrum synthetic antifungal agent ketoconazole in a concentration of 2% in an aqueous suspension. It also contains: coconut fatty acid diethanolamide, disodium monolauryl ether sulfosuccinate, F.D. & C. Red No. 40, hydrochloric acid, imidurea, laurdimonium hydrolyzed animal collagen, macrogol 120 methyl-glucose dioleate, perfume bouquet, sodium chloride, sodium hydroxide, sodium lauryl ether sulfate, and purified water.

Continued on next page

Nizoral Shampoo—Cont.

Ketoconazole is cis-1-acetyl-4-[4-[[2-(2,4-di-chlorophenyl)-2-(1H-imidazol-1-ylmethyl)-1,3-dioxolan-4-yl]methoxy]phenyl]piperazine.

CLINICAL PHARMACOLOGY

Tinea (pityriasis) versicolor is a non-contagious infection of the skin caused by *Pityrosporum orbiculare (Malassezia furfur)*. This commensal organism is part of the normal skin flora. In susceptible individuals the condition is often recurrent and may give rise to hyperpigmented or hypopigmented patches on the trunk which may extend to the neck, arms and upper thighs. Treatment of the infection may not immediately result in restoration of pigment to the affected sites. Normalization of pigment following successful therapy is variable and may take months, depending on individual skin type and incidental skin exposure. The rate of recurrence of infection is variable.

When ketoconazole 2% shampoo was applied dermally to intact or abraded skin of rabbits for 28 days at doses up to 50 mg/kg and allowed to remain one hour before being washed away, there were no detectable plasma ketoconazole levels using an assay method having a lower detection limit of 5 ng/mL. NIZORAL® (ketoconazole) was not detected in plasma in 39 patients who shampooed 4–10 times per week for 6 months or in 33 patients who shampooed 2–3 times per week for 3–26 months (mean: 16 months).

An exaggerated use washing test on the sensitive antecubital skin of 10 subjects twice daily for five consecutive days showed that the irritancy potential of ketoconazole 2% shampoo was significantly less than that of 2.5% selenium sulfide shampoo.

A human sensitization test, a phototoxicity study, and a photoallergy study conducted in 38 male and 22 female volunteers showed no contact sensitization of the delayed hypersensitivity type, no phototoxicity and no photoallergenic potential due to NIZORAL® (ketoconazole) 2% Shampoo.

Mode of Action: Interpretations of *in vivo* studies suggest that ketoconazole impairs the synthesis of ergosterol, which is a vital component of fungal cell membranes. It is postulated, but not proven, that the therapeutic effect of ketoconazole in tinea (pityriasis) versicolor is due to the reduction of *Pityrosporum orbiculare (Malassezia furfur)* and that the therapeutic effect in dandruff is due to the reduction of *Pityrosporum ovale*. Support for the therapeutic effect in tinea versicolor comes from a three-arm, parallel, double-blind, placebo-controlled study in patients who had moderately severe tinea (pityriasis) versicolor. Successful response rates in the primary efficacy population for each of both three-day and single-day regimens of ketoconazole 2% shampoo were statistically significantly greater (73% and 69%, respectively) than a placebo regimen (5%). There had been mycological confirmation of fungal disease in all cases at baseline. Mycological clearing rates were 84% and 78%, respectively, for the three-day and one-day regimens of the 2% shampoo and 11% in the placebo regimen. While the differences in the rates of successful response between either of the two active treatments and placebo were statistically significant, the difference between the two active regimens was not.

Microbiology: NIZORAL® (ketoconazole) is a broad-spectrum synthetic antifungal agent which inhibits the growth of the following common dermatophytes and yeasts by altering the permeability of the cell membrane: dermatophytes: *Trichophyton rubrum, T. mentagrophytes, T. tonsurans, Microsporum canis, M. audouini, M. gypseum* and *Epidermophyton floccosum;* yeasts: *Candida albicans, C. tropicalis, Pityrosporum ovale (Malassezia ovale)* and *Pityrosporum orbiculare (M. furfur)*. Development of resistance by these microorganisms to ketoconazole has not been reported.

INDICATIONS AND USAGE

NIZORAL® (ketoconazole) 2% Shampoo is indicated for the treatment of tinea (pityriasis) versicolor caused by or presumed to be caused by *Pityrosporum orbiculare* (also known as *Malassezia furfur* or *M. orbiculare*).

Note: Tinea (pityriasis) versicolor may give rise to hyperpigmented or hypopigmented patches on the trunk which may extend to the neck, arms and upper thighs. Treatment of the infection may not immediately result in normalization of pigment to the affected sites. Normalization of pigment following successful therapy is variable and may take months, depending on individual skin type and incidental sun exposure. Although tinea versicolor is not contagious, it may recur because the organism that causes the disease is part of the normal skin flora.

CONTRAINDICATIONS

NIZORAL® (ketoconazole) 2% Shampoo is contraindicated in persons who have shown hypersensitivity to the active ingredient or excipients of this formulation.

PRECAUTIONS

General: If a reaction suggesting sensitivity or chemical irritation should occur, use of the medication should be discontinued.

Information for Patients: May be irritating to mucous membranes of the eyes and contact with this area should be avoided.

There have been reports that use of the shampoo resulted in removal of the curl from permanently waved hair.

Carcinogenesis, Mutagenesis, Impairment of Fertility: The dominant lethal mutation test in male and female mice revealed that single oral doses of ketoconazole as high as 80 mg/kg produced no mutation in any stage of germ cell development. The Ames Salmonella microsomal activator assay was also negative. A long-term feeding study of ketoconazole in Swiss Albino mice and in Wistar rats showed no evidence of oncogenic activity.

Pregnancy: Teratogenic effects: Pregnancy Category C: Ketoconazole is not detected in plasma after chronic shampooing. Ketoconazole has been shown to be teratogenic (syndactylia and oligodactylia) in the rat when given orally in the diet at 80 mg/kg/day (10 times the maximum recommended human oral dose). However, these effects may be related to maternal toxicity, which was seen at this and higher dose levels.

There are no adequate and well-controlled studies in pregnant women. Ketoconazole should be used during pregnancy only if the potential benefit justifies the potential risk to the fetus.

Nursing mothers: Ketoconazole is not detected in plasma after chronic shampooing. Nevertheless, caution should be exercised when NIZORAL® (ketoconazole) 2% Shampoo is administered to a nursing woman.

Pediatric Use: Safety and effectiveness in children have not been established.

ADVERSE REACTIONS

In 11 double-blind trials in 264 patients using ketoconazole 2% shampoo for the treatment of dandruff or seborrheic dermatitis, an increase in normal hair loss and irritation occurred in less than 1% of patients. In three open-label safety trials in which 41 patients shampooed 4–10 times weekly for six months, the following adverse experiences each occurred once: abnormal hair texture, scalp pustules, mild dryness of the skin, and itching. As with other shampoos, oiliness and dryness of hair and scalp have been reported.

In a double-blind, placebo-controlled trial in which patients with tinea versicolor were treated with either a single application of NIZORAL® (ketoconazole) 2% Shampoo (n=106), a daily application for three consecutive days (n=107), or placebo (n=105), drug-related adverse events occurred in 5 (5%), 7 (7%) and 4 (4%) of patients, respectively. The only events that occurred in more than one patient in any one of the three treatment groups were pruritus, application site reaction, and dry skin; none of these events occurred in more than 3% of the patients in any one of the three groups.

OVERDOSAGE

NIZORAL® (ketoconazole) 2% Shampoo is intended for external use only. In the event of accidental ingestion, supportive measures should be employed. Induced emesis and gastric lavage should usually be avoided.

DOSAGE AND ADMINISTRATION

Apply the shampoo to the damp skin of the affected area and a wide margin surrounding this area. Lather, leave in place for 5 minutes, and then rinse off with water.

One application of the shampoo should be sufficient.

HOW SUPPLIED

NIZORAL® (ketoconazole) 2% Shampoo is a red-orange liquid supplied in a 4-fluid ounce nonbreakable plastic bottle (NDC 50458-223-04).

Storage conditions: Store at a temperature not above 25°C (77°F). Protect from light.

Manufactured by:
Janssen Cilag SPA
Latina, Italy
Distributed by:
Janssen Pharmaceutica Inc.
Titusville, NJ 08560
Revised June 1996, August 1997
U.S. Patent No. 4,335,125

Shown in Product Identification Guide, page 317

NIZORAL® ℞

[*nī 'zōr-ăl*]
(ketoconazole)
Tablets

WARNING: When used orally, ketoconazole has been associated with hepatic toxicity, including some fatalities. Patients receiving this drug should be informed by the physician of the risk and should be closely monitored. See WARNINGS and PRECAUTIONS sections.

Coadministration of terfenadine with ketoconazole tablets is contraindicated. Rare cases of serious cardiovascular adverse events, including death, ventricular tachycardia and torsades de pointes have been observed in patients taking ketoconazole tablets concomitantly with terfenadine, due to increased terfenadine concentrations induced by ketoconazole tablets. See CONTRAINDICATIONS, WARNINGS, and PRECAUTIONS sections.

Pharmacokinetic data indicate that oral ketoconazole inhibits the metabolism of astemizole, resulting in elevated plasma levels of astemizole and its active metabolite desmethylastemizole which may prolong QT intervals. Coadministration of astemizole with ketoconazole tablets is therefore contraindicated. See CONTRAINDICATIONS, WARNINGS, and PRECAUTIONS sections.

Coadministration of cisapride with ketoconazole is contraindicated. Serious cardiovascular adverse events including ventricular tachycardia, ventricular fibrillation and torsades de pointes have occurred in patients taking ketoconazole concomitantly with cisapride. See CONTRAINDICATIONS, WARNINGS, and PRECAUTIONS sections.

DESCRIPTION

NIZORAL® (ketoconazole) is a synthetic broad-spectrum antifungal agent available in scored white tablets, each containing 200 mg ketoconazole base for oral administration. Inactive ingredients are colloidal silicon dioxide, corn starch, lactose, magnesium stearate, microcrystalline cellulose, and povidone. Ketoconazole is cis-1-acetyl-4-[4-[[2-(2,4-dichlorophenyl) -2- (1H-imidazol-1-ylmethyl)-1,3-dioxolan-4-yl] methoxyl]phenyl] piperazine.

Ketoconazole is a white to slightly beige, odorless powder, soluble in acids, with a molecular weight of 531.44.

CLINICAL PHARMACOLOGY

Mean peak plasma levels of approximately 3.5 µg/mL are reached within 1 to 2 hours, following oral administration of a single 200 mg dose taken with a meal. Subsequent plasma elimination is biphasic with a half-life of 2 hours during the first 10 hours and 8 hours thereafter. Following absorption from the gastrointestinal tract, NIZORAL® (ketoconazole) is converted into several inactive metabolites. The major identified metabolic pathways are oxidation and degradation of the imidazole and piperazine rings, oxidative O-dealkylation and aromatic hydroxylation. About 13% of the dose is excreted in the urine, of which 2 to 4% is unchanged drug. The major route of excretion is through the bile into the intestinal tract. *In vitro,* the plasma protein binding is about 99% mainly to the albumin fraction. Only a negligible proportion of ketoconazole reaches the cerebral-spinal fluid. Ketoconazole is a weak dibasic agent and thus requires acidity for dissolution and absorption.

NIZORAL® Tablets are active against clinical infections with *Blastomyces dermatitidis, Candida spp., Coccidioides immitis, Histoplasma capsulatum, Paracoccidioides brasiliensis,* and *Phialophora spp.* NIZORAL® Tablets are also active against *Trichophyton spp., Epidermophyton spp.,* and *Microsporum spp.* Ketoconazole is also active *in vitro* against a variety of fungi and yeast. In animal models, activity has been demonstrated against *Candida spp., Blastomyces dermatitidis, Histoplasma capsulatum, Malassezia furfur, Coccidioides immitis,* and *Cryptococcus neoformans.*

Mode of Action: In vitro studies suggest that ketoconazole impairs the synthesis of ergosterol, which is a vital component of fungal cell membranes.

INDICATIONS AND USAGE

NIZORAL® (ketoconazole) Tablets are indicated for the treatment of the following systemic fungal infections: candidiasis, chronic mucocutaneous candidiasis, oral thrush, candiduria, blastomycosis, coccidioidomycosis, histoplasmosis, chromomycosis, and paracoccidioidomycosis. NIZORAL® Tablets should not be used for fungal meningitis because it penetrates poorly into the cerebral-spinal fluid.

NIZORAL® Tablets are also indicated for the treatment of patients with severe recalcitrant cutaneous dermatophyte infections who have not responded to topical therapy or oral griseofulvin, or who are unable to take griseofulvin.

CONTRAINDICATIONS

Coadministration of terfenadine or astemizole with ketoconazole tablets is contraindicated. (See BOX WARNING, WARNINGS, and PRECAUTIONS sections.)

Concomitant administration of NIZORAL® Tablets with cisapride is contraindicated. (See BOX WARNING, WARNINGS, and PRECAUTIONS sections.)

Concomitant administration of NIZORAL® Tablets with oral triazolam is contraindicated. (See PRECAUTIONS section.)

NIZORAL® is contraindicated in patients who have shown hypersensitivity to the drug.

WARNINGS

Hepatotoxicity, primarily of the hepatocellular type, has been associated with the use of NIZORAL® (ketoconazole) Tablets, including rare fatalities. The reported incidence of hepatotoxicity has been about 1:10,000 exposed patients, but this probably represents some degree of under-reporting, as is the case for most reported adverse reactions to drugs. The median duration of NIZORAL® Tablet therapy in patients who developed symptomatic hepatotoxicity was about 28 days, although the range extended to as low as 3 days. The hepatic injury has usually, but not always, been reversible upon discontinuation of NIZORAL® Tablet treatment. Several cases of hepatitis have been reported in children.

Prompt recognition of liver injury is essential. Liver function tests (such as SGGT, alkaline phosphatase, SGPT, SGOT and bilirubin) should be measured before starting treatment and at frequent intervals during treatment. Patients receiving NIZORAL® Tablets concurrently with other potentially hepatotoxic drugs should be carefully monitored, particularly those patients requiring prolonged therapy or those who have had a history of liver disease.

Most of the reported cases of hepatic toxicity have to date been in patients treated for onychomycosis. Of 180 patients worldwide developing idiosyncratic liver dysfunction during NIZORAL® Tablet therapy, 61.3% had onychomycosis and 16.8% had chronic recalcitrant dermatophytoses.

Transient minor elevations in liver enzymes have occurred during treatment with NIZORAL® Tablets. The drug should be discontinued if these persist, if the abnormalities worsen, or if the abnormalities become accompanied by symptoms of possible liver injury.

In rare cases anaphylaxis has been reported after the first dose. Several cases of hypersensitivity reactions including urticaria have also been reported.

Coadministration of ketoconazole tablets and terfenadine has led to elevated plasma concentrations of terfenadine which may prolong QT intervals, sometimes resulting in life-threatening cardiac dysrhythmias. Cases of torsades de pointes and other serious ventricular dysrhythmias, in rare cases leading to fatality, have been reported among patients taking terfenadine concurrently with ketoconazole tablets. Coadministration of ketoconazole tablets and terfenadine is contraindicated.

Coadministration of astemizole with ketoconazole tablets is contraindicated. (See BOX WARNING, CONTRAINDICATIONS, and PRECAUTIONS sections.)

Concomitant administration of NIZORAL® Tablets with cisapride is contraindicated because it has resulted in markedly elevated cisapride plasma concentrations and prolonged QT interval, and has rarely been associated with ventricular arrhythmias and torsades de pointes. (See BOX WARNINGS, CONTRAINDICATIONS and PRECAUTIONS sections.)

In European clinical trials involving 350 patients with metastatic prostatic cancer, eleven deaths were reported within two weeks of starting treatment with high doses of ketoconazole tablets (1200 mg/day). It is not possible to ascertain from the information available whether death was related to ketoconazole therapy in these patients with serious underlying disease. However, high doses of ketoconazole tablets are known to suppress adrenal corticosteroid secretion.

In female rats treated three to six months with ketoconazole at dose levels of 80 mg/kg and higher, increased fragility of long bones, in some cases leading to fracture, was seen. The maximum "no-effect" dose level in these studies was 20 mg/kg (2.5 times the maximum recommended human dose). The mechanism responsible for this phenomenon is obscure. Limited studies in dogs failed to demonstrate such an effect on the metacarpals and ribs.

PRECAUTIONS

General: NIZORAL® (ketoconazole) Tablets have been demonstrated to lower serum testosterone. Once therapy with NIZORAL® Tablets has been discontinued, serum testosterone levels return to baseline values. Testosterone levels are impaired with doses of 800 mg per day and abolished by 1600 mg per day. NIZORAL® Tablets also decrease ACTH induced corticosteroid serum levels at similar high doses. The recommended dose of 200 mg–400 mg daily should be followed closely.

In four subjects with drug-induced achlorhydria, a marked reduction in ketoconazole absorption was observed. NIZORAL® Tablets require acidity for dissolution. If concomitant antacids, anticholinergics, and H_2-blockers are needed, they should be given at least two hours after administration of NIZORAL® Tablets. In cases of achlorhydria, the patients should be instructed to dissolve each tablet in 4 mL aqueous solution of 0.2 N HCl. For ingesting the resulting mixture, they should use a drinking straw so as to avoid contact with the teeth. This administration should be followed with a cup of tap water.

Information for Patients: Patients should be instructed to report any signs and symptoms which may suggest liver dysfunction so that appropriate biochemical testing can be done. Such signs and symptoms may include unusual fatigue, anorexia, nausea and/or vomiting, jaundice, dark urine or pale stools (see WARNINGS section).

Drug Interactions: Ketoconazole is a potent inhibitor of the cytochrome P450 3A4 enzyme system. Coadministration of NIZORAL® Tablets and drugs primarily metabolized by the cytochrome P450 3A4 enzyme system may result in increased plasma concentrations of the drugs that could increase or prolong both therapeutic and adverse effects. Therefore, unless otherwise specified, appropriate dosage adjustments may be necessary. The following drug interactions have been identified involving NIZORAL® Tablets and other drugs metabolized by the cytochrome P450 3A4 enzyme system.

Ketoconazole tablets inhibit the metabolism of terfenadine, resulting in an increased plasma concentration of terfenadine and a delay in the elimination of its acid metabolite. The increased plasma concentration of terfenadine or its metabolite may result in prolonged QT intervals. (See BOX WARNING, CONTRAINDICATIONS, and WARNINGS sections.)

Pharmacokinetic data indicate that oral ketoconazole inhibits the metabolism of astemizole, resulting in elevated plasma levels of astemizole and its active metabolite desmethylastemizole which may prolong QT intervals. Coadministration of astemizole with ketoconazole tablets is therefore contraindicated. (See BOX WARNING, CONTRAINDICATIONS, and WARNINGS sections.)

Human pharmacokinetics data indicate that oral ketoconazole potently inhibits the metabolism of cisapride resulting in a mean eight-fold increase in AUC of cisapride. Data suggest that coadministration of oral ketoconazole and cisapride can result in prolongation of the QT interval on the ECG. Therefore concomitant administration of ketoconazole tablets with cisapride is contraindicated. (See BOX WARNING, CONTRAINDICATIONS, and WARNINGS sections.)

Ketoconazole tablets may alter the metabolism of cyclosporine, tacrolimus, and methylprednisolone, resulting in elevated plasma concentrations of the latter drugs. Dosage adjustment may be required if cyclosporine, tacrolimus, or methylprednisolone are given concomitantly with NIZORAL® Tablets.

Coadministration of NIZORAL® Tablets with midazolam or triazolam has resulted in elevated plasma concentrations of the latter two drugs. This may potentiate and prolong hypnotic and sedative effects, especially with repeated dosing or chronic administration of these agents. These agents should not be used in patients treated with NIZORAL® Tablets. If midazolam is administered parenterally, special precaution is required since the sedative effect may be prolonged.

Rare cases of elevated plasma concentrations of digoxin have been reported. It is not clear whether this was due to the combination of therapy. It is, therefore, advisable to monitor digoxin concentrations in patients receiving ketoconazole.

When taken orally, imidazole compounds like ketoconazole may enhance the anticoagulant effect of coumarin-like drugs. In simultaneous treatment with imidazole drugs and coumarin drugs, the anticoagulant effect should be carefully titrated and monitored.

Because severe hypoglycemia has been reported in patients concomitantly receiving oral miconazole (an imidazole) and oral hypoglycemic agents, such a potential interaction involving the latter agents when used concomitantly with ketoconazole tablets (an imidazole) can not be ruled out.

Concomitant administration of ketoconazole tablets with phenytoin may alter the metabolism of one or both of the drugs. It is suggested to monitor both ketoconazole and phenytoin.

Concomitant administration of rifampin with ketoconazole tablets reduces the blood levels of the latter. INH (Isoniazid) is also reported to affect ketoconazole concentrations adversely. These drugs should not be given concomitantly.

After the coadministration of 200 mg oral ketoconazole twice daily and one 20 mg dose of loratadine to 11 subjects, the AUC and C_{max} of loratadine averaged 302% (± 142 S.D.) and 251% (± 68 S.D.), respectively, of those obtained after co-treatment with placebo. The AUC and C_{max} of descarboethoxyloratadine, an active metabolite, averaged 155% (± 27 S.D.) and 141% (± 35 S.D.), respectively. However, no related changes were noted in the QT_c on ECG taken at 2, 6, and 24 hours after the coadministration. Also, there were no clinically significant differences in adverse events when loratadine was administered with or without ketoconazole.

Rare cases of disulfiram-like reaction to alcohol have been reported. These experiences have been characterized by flushing, rash, peripheral edema, nausea, and headache. Symptoms resolved within a few hours.

Carcinogenesis, Mutagenesis, Impairment of Fertility: The dominant lethal mutation test in male and female mice revealed that single oral doses of ketoconazole as high as 80 mg/kg produced no mutation in any stage of germ cell development. The *Ames Salmonella* microsomal activator assay was also negative. A long term feeding study in Swiss Albino mice and in Wistar rats showed no evidence of oncogenic activity.

Pregnancy: Teratogenic effects: *Pregnancy Category C:* Ketoconazole has been shown to be teratogenic (syndactylia and oligodactylia) in the rat when given in the diet at 80 mg/kg/day (10 times the maximum recommended human dose). However, these effects may be related to maternal toxicity, evidence of which also was seen at this and higher dose levels.

There are no adequate and well controlled studies in pregnant women. NIZORAL® Tablets should be used during pregnancy only if the potential benefit justifies the potential risk to the fetus.

Nonteratogenic Effects: Ketoconazole has also been found to be embryotoxic in the rat when given in the diet at doses higher than 80 mg/kg during the first trimester of gestation. In addition, dystocia (difficult labor) was noted in rats administered oral ketoconazole during the third trimester of gestation. This occurred when ketoconazole was administered at doses higher than 10 mg/kg (higher than 1.25 times the maximum human dose).

It is likely that both the malformations and the embryotoxicity resulting from the administration of oral ketoconazole during gestation are a reflection of the particular sensitivity of the female rat to this drug. For example, the oral LD_{50} of ketoconazole given by gavage to the female rat is 166 mg/kg whereas in the male rat the oral LD_{50} is 287 mg/kg.

Nursing Mothers: Since ketoconazole is probably excreted in the milk, mothers who are under treatment should not breast feed.

Pediatric Use: NIZORAL® (ketoconazole) Tablets have not been systematically studied in children of any age, and essentially no information is available on children under 2 years. NIZORAL® Tablets should not be used in pediatric patients unless the potential benefit outweighs the risks.

ADVERSE REACTIONS

In rare cases, anaphylaxis has been reported after the first dose. Several cases of hypersensitivity reactions including urticaria have also been reported. However, the most frequent adverse reactions were nausea and/or vomiting in approximately 3%, abdominal pain in 1.2%, pruritus in 1.5%, and the following in less than 1% of the patients: headache, dizziness, somnolence, fever and chills, photophobia, diarrhea, gynecomastia, impotence, thrombocytopenia, leukopenia, hemolytic anemia, and bulging fontanelles. Oligospermia has been reported in investigational studies with the drug at dosages above those currently approved. Oligospermia has not been reported at dosages up to 400 mg daily, however sperm counts have been obtained infrequently in patients treated with these dosages. Most of these reactions were mild and transient and rarely required discontinuation of NIZORAL® (ketoconazole) Tablets. In contrast, the rare occurrences of hepatic dysfunction require special attention (see WARNINGS section).

In worldwide postmarketing experience with NIZORAL® Tablets there have been rare reports of alopecia, paresthesia, and signs of increased intracranial pressure including bulging fontanelles and papilledema. Hypertriglyceridemia has also been reported but a causal association with NIZORAL® Tablets is uncertain.

Neuropsychiatric disturbances, including suicidal tendencies and severe depression, have occurred rarely in patients using NIZORAL® Tablets.

Ventricular dysrhythmias (prolonged QT intervals) have occurred with the concomitant use of terfenadine with ketoconazole tablets. (See BOX WARNING, CONTRAINDICATIONS, and WARNINGS sections.) Data suggest that coadministration of ketoconazole tablets and cisapride can result in prolongation of the QT interval and has rarely been associated with ventricular arrhythmias. (See CONTRAINDICATIONS, WARNINGS, and PRECAUTIONS sections.)

OVERDOSAGE

In the event of accidental overdosage, supportive measures, including gastric lavage with sodium bicarbonate, should be employed.

DOSAGE AND ADMINISTRATION

Adults: The recommended starting dose of NIZORAL® (ketoconazole) Tablets is a single daily administration of 200 mg (one tablet). In very serious infections or if clinical responsiveness is insufficient within the expected time, the dose of NIZORAL® Tablets may be increased to 400 mg (two tablets) once daily.

Children: In small numbers of children over 2 years of age, a single daily dose of 3.3 to 6.6 mg/kg has been used. NIZORAL® Tablets have not been studied in children under 2 years of age.

There should be laboratory as well as clinical documentation of infection prior to starting ketoconazole therapy. Treatment should be continued until tests indicate that active fungal infection has subsided. Inadequate periods of treatment may yield poor response and lead to early recurrence of clinical symptoms. Minimum treatment for candidiasis is one or two weeks. Patients with chronic mucocutaneous candidiasis usually require maintenance therapy. Minimum treatment for the other indicated systemic mycoses is six months.

Continued on next page

Nizoral Tablets—Cont.

Minimum treatment for recalcitrant dermatophyte infections is four weeks in cases involving glabrous skin. Palmar and plantar infections may respond more slowly. Apparent cures may subsequently recur after discontinuation of therapy in some cases.

HOW SUPPLIED

NIZORAL® (ketoconazole) is available as white, scored tablets containing 200 mg of ketoconazole debossed "JANSSEN" and on the reverse side debossed "NIZORAL". They are supplied in bottles of 100 tablets (NDC 50458-220-10) and in blister packs of 10 × 10 tablets (NDC 50458-220-01).
Store at controlled room temperature
15°–25°C(59°–77°C). Protect from moisture
U.S. Patent 4,335,125
Rev. June 1996, March 1997
JANSSEN PHARMACEUTICA
Titusville, NJ 08560-0200
Shown in Product Identification Guide, page 317

PROPULSID® ℞

[*prō-pəl 'sid*]
(cisapride)
TABLETS/SUSPENSION

Warning: Serious cardiac arrhythmias including ventricular tachycardia, ventricular fibrillation, torsades de pointes, and QT prolongation have been reported in patients taking PROPULSID®. Many of these patients also took drugs expected to increase cisapride blood levels by inhibiting the cytochrome P450 3A4 enzymes that metabolize cisapride. These drugs include clarithromycin, erythromycin, troleandomycin, nefazodone, fluconazole, itraconazole, ketoconazole, indinavir and ritonavir. Some of these events have been fatal. PROPULSID® is contraindicated in patients taking any of these drugs. (See CONTRAINDICATIONS, WARNINGS, PRECAUTIONS and DRUG INTERACTIONS).
QT prolongation, torsades de pointes (sometimes with syncope), cardiac arrest and sudden death have been reported in patients taking PROPULSID® without the above-mentioned contraindicated drugs. Most patients had disorders that may have predisposed them to arrhythmias with cisapride. PROPULSID® is contraindicated for those patients with: history of prolonged electrocardiographic QT intervals; renal failure; history of ventricular arrhythmias, ischemic heart disease, and congestive heart failure; uncorrected electrolyte disorders (hypokalemia, hypomagnesemia); respiratory failure; and concomitant medications known to prolong the QT interval and increase the risk of arrhythmia, such as certain antiarrhythmics, including those of Class 1A (such as quinidine and procainamide) and Class III (such as sotalol); tricyclic antidepressants (such as amitriptyline); certain tetracyclic antidepressants (such as maprotiline); certain antipsychotic medications (such as certain phenothiazines and sertindole); astemizole, bepridil, sparfloxacin and terodiline. **(The preceding lists of drugs are not comprehensive.)**
Recommended doses of PROPULSID® should not be exceeded.

DESCRIPTION

PROPULSID® (cisapride) Tablets and Suspension contain cisapride as the monohydrate, which is an oral gastrointestinal agent chemically designated as (±)-cis-4-amino-5-chloro-N-[1-[3-(4-fluorophenoxy)propyl]-3-methoxy-4-piperidinyl]-2-methoxybenzamide monohydrate. Its empirical formula is $C_{23}H_{29}ClFN_3O_4 \bullet H_2O$. The molecular weight is 483.97 and the structural formula is:

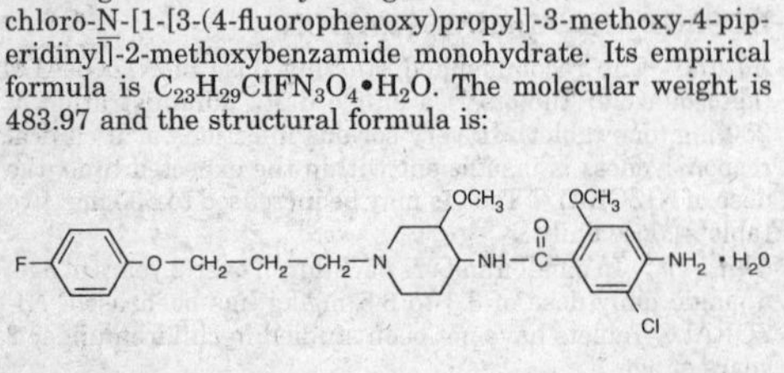

Cisapride as the monohydrate is a white to slightly beige odorless powder. It is practically insoluble in water, sparingly soluble in methanol, and soluble in acetone. Each 1.04 mg of cisapride as the monohydrate is equivalent to one mg of cisapride.
PROPULSID® is available for oral use in tablets containing cisapride as the monohydrate equivalent to 10 mg or 20 mg of cisapride and as a suspension containing the equivalent of 1 mg/mL of cisapride. The inactive ingredients in the tablets are colloidal silicon dioxide, lactose monohydrate, magnesium stearate, microcrystalline cellulose, polysorbate 20, povidone, and starch (corn). The 20 mg tablets also contain FD&C Blue No. 2 aluminum lake. The inactive ingredients in the suspension are hydroxypropyl methylcellulose, methylparaben, microcrystalline cellulose and carboxymethylcellulose sodium, polysorbate 20, propylparaben, sodium chloride, sorbitol, and water. The 1 mg/mL suspension also contains artificial cherry cream flavor and FD&C Red No. 40.

CLINICAL PHARMACOLOGY

Pharmacokinetics
Cisapride is metabolized mainly via the cytochrome P450 3A4 enzyme. PROPULSID® (cisapride) is extensively metabolized; unchanged drug accounts for less than 10% of urinary and fecal recovery following oral administration. Norcisapride, formed by N-dealkylation, is the principal metabolite in plasma, feces and urine. PROPULSID® is rapidly absorbed after oral administration; peak plasma concentrations are reached 1 to 1.5 hours after dosing. The absolute bioavailability of PROPULSID® is 35–40%. When gastric acidity was reduced by high dose histamine H_2 receptor blocker and sodium bicarbonate in fasting subjects, there was a decrease in the rate, and to a lesser degree the extent, of PROPULSID® tablet absorption. (This has not been established for the suspension.) PROPULSID® binds to an extent of 97.5–98% to plasma proteins, mainly to albumin. The volume of distribution of PROPULSID® is about 180 L, indicating extensive tissue distribution.
The plasma clearance of PROPULSID® is about 100 mL/min. The mean terminal half-life reported for PROPULSID® ranges from 6 to 12 hours; longer half-lives, up to 20 hours, have been reported following intravenous (IV) administration.
There was no unusual drug accumulation due to time-dependent or non-linear changes in pharmacokinetics. After cessation of the repeated dosing, the elimination half-lives (8 to 10 hr) were in the same order as after single dosing. The degree of accumulation of PROPULSID® and/or its metabolites may be somewhat higher in patients with hepatic or renal impairment and in elderly patients compared to young healthy volunteers, but the differences are not consistent. Dose adjustments are recommended in patients with hepatic impairment. (See DOSAGE AND ADMINISTRATION.)
The pharmacokinetics of cisapride in pediatric patients are not well characterized. Therefore, it is unknown if the dose-response relationship in the adult population can be extrapolated to the pediatric population.
Pharmacodynamics
The onset of pharmacological action of cisapride is approximately 30 to 60 minutes after oral administration. Cisapride promotes gastric motility. The mechanism of action of cisapride is thought to be primarily enhancement of release of acetylcholine at the myenteric plexus. Cisapride does not induce muscarinic or nicotinic receptor stimulation, nor does it inhibit acetylcholinesterase activity. It is less potent than metoclopramide in dopamine receptor-blocking effects in rats. It does not increase or decrease basal or pentagastrin-induced gastric acid secretion.
In vitro studies have shown that cisapride is a serotonin-4 ($5\text{-}HT_4$) receptor agonist.
Electrophysiological studies *in vivo* anesthetized guinea pig and rabbit models and *in vitro* isolated rabbit Purkinje fibers and ventricular papillary muscle and isolated rabbit ventricular myocyte models, have shown that cisapride prolonged cardiac repolarization without slowing conduction by selectively blocking the rapid component of the delayed rectifying K^+ current (I_{kr}) which lead to a lengthening of the action potential (QT Syndrome).
Esophagus: Twenty milligrams oral cisapride given once to healthy volunteers increased LESP, starting 45 minutes after dosing, with a peak response at 75 minutes. The full duration of the effect was not monitored, and doses smaller than 20 mg were ineffective. Ten milligrams oral cisapride, administered 3 times daily for several days to patients with GERD, resulted in a significant increase in LESP, and an increased esophageal acid clearance.
Stomach: Cisapride (single 10 mg doses or 10 mg given orally 3 times daily up to six weeks) significantly accelerated gastric emptying of both liquids and solids. Acceleration of gastric emptying, measured over a four hour period following a radio-labeled test meal given at lunch time, was greatest when 10 mg cisapride was given both in the morning and again before the test meal, intermediate when 20 mg was given as a single administration in the morning and least when only 10 mg was given on the morning of the test meal. The increases in gastric emptying were proportional to the plasma levels of cisapride measured in these subjects over the same 4 hours that the gastric emptying test was conducted.
Clinical Trials
Clinical trials have shown that cisapride can reduce the severity of symptoms of nocturnal heartburn associated with gastroesophageal reflux disease. Two placebo-controlled studies, one using a dose of 10 mg q.i.d., the other both 10 and 20 mg q.i.d., showed effects on nighttime heartburn, although the 10 mg dose in the second study was only marginally effective. There were no consistent effects on daytime heartburn, symptoms of regurgitation, or histopathology of the esophagus. Use of antacids was only infrequently affected and slightly decreased. In a third controlled trial of similar design to the others, neither 10 mg nor 20 mg taken 4 times daily was superior to placebo. In these clinical trials cisapride did not show a significant effect on LESP.
In a clinical trial comparing 10 mg cisapride to placebo, pH probe evaluation, in a relatively small number of patients, did not reveal a significant difference in pH.

INDICATIONS AND USAGE

PROPULSID® (cisapride) is indicated for the symptomatic treatment of adult patients with nocturnal heartburn due to gastroesophageal reflux disease. Because of the risk of serious, and sometimes fatal, ventricular arrhythmias (see Boxed Warning), PROPULSID® should generally be reserved for patients who do not respond adequately to lifestyle modifications (See PRECAUTIONS: Information for Patients), antacids and gastric acid reducing agents.

CONTRAINDICATIONS

Serious cardiac arrhythmias including ventricular tachycardia, ventricular fibrillation, torsades de pointes, and QT prolongation have been reported in patients taking PROPULSID® (cisapride) with other drugs that inhibit cytochrome P450 3A4. Some of these events have been fatal. Concomitant oral or intravenous administration of the following drugs with cisapride may lead to elevated cisapride blood levels and is contraindicated (See WARNINGS, PRECAUTIONS and DRUG INTERACTIONS):
Antibiotics: Oral or i.v. erythromycin, clarithromycin (BIAXIN®), troleandomycin (TAO®)
Antidepressants: Nefazodone (SERZONE®)
Antifungals: Oral or i.v. fluconazole (DIFLUCAN®), itraconazole (SPORANOX®), oral ketoconazole (NIZORAL®)
Protease inhibitors: Indinavir (CRIXIVAN®), ritonavir (NORVIR®)
PROPULSID® is also contraindicated for patients with: history of prolonged electrocardiographic QT intervals; renal failure; history of ventricular arrhythmias, ischemic heart disease, and congestive heart failure; uncorrected electrolyte disorders (hypokalemia, hypomagnesemia); respiratory failure; and concomitant medications known to prolong the QT interval and increase the risk of arrhythmia, such as certain antiarrhythmics, certain antipsychotics, certain antidepressants, astemizole, bepridil, sparfloxacin and terodiline. The preceding lists of drugs are not comprehensive.
PROPULSID® should not be used in patients with uncorrected hypokalemia or hypomagnesemia or who might experience rapid reduction of plasma potassium such as those administered potassium-wasting diuretics and/or insulin in acute settings.
PROPULSID® should not be used in patients in whom an increase in gastrointestinal motility could be harmful, e.g., in the presence of gastrointestinal hemorrhage, mechanical obstruction, or perforation. PROPULSID® is contraindicated in patients with known sensitivity or intolerance to the drug.

WARNINGS

PROPULSID® (cisapride) undergoes metabolism mainly by the hepatic cytochrome P450 3A4 isoenzyme. Drugs which inhibit this enzyme such as clarithromycin (BIAXIN®), erythromycin, troleandomycin (TAO®), nefazodone (SERZONE®), fluconazole (DIFLUCAN®), itraconazole (SPORANOX®), ketoconazole (NIZORAL®), indinavir (CRIXIVAN®) and ritonavir (NORVIR®) can lead to elevated cisapride blood levels.
Numerous cases of serious cardiac arrhythmias, including ventricular arrhythmias and torsades de pointes associated with QT prolongation, have been reported in patients taking cisapride with clarithromycin (BIAXIN®), erythromycin, troleandomycin (TAO®), nefazodone (SERZONE®), fluconazole (DIFLUCAN®), itraconazole (SPORANOX®), ketoconazole (NIZORAL®), indinavir (CRIXIVAN®) or ritonavir (NORVIR®). Some of these patients did not have cardiac disease; however, most had been receiving multiple other medications and had pre-existing cardiac disease or risk factors for arrhythmias. Some of these cases have been fatal.
QT prolongation, torsades de pointes (sometimes with syncope), cardiac arrest and sudden death have been reported in patients taking PROPULSID® without the above-mentioned contraindicated drugs. Most patients had disorders that may have predisposed them to arrhythmias with cisapride.
ECG should be considered prior to initiation of cisapride. Cisapride should not be used in patients with a prolonged QT interval at baseline, those with a history of torsades de pointes, or those with long QT syndrome. Cisapride should also be avoided in patients with sinus node dysfunction, and in those with second or third degree atrioventricular block. Cisapride should not be used concomitantly with other drugs known to prolong the QT interval: certain antiarrhythmics, including those of Class IA (such as quinidine and procainamide) and Class III (such as sotalol); tricyclic

antidepressants (such as amitriptyline); certain tetracyclic antidepressants (such as maprotiline); certain antipsychotic medications (such as certain phenothiazines and sertindole); astemizole, bepridil, sparfloxacin and terodiline. (See CONTRAINDICATIONS, PRECAUTIONS and DRUG INTERACTIONS.) The preceding lists of drugs are not comprehensive.

PRECAUTIONS

General: Potential benefits should be weighed against risks prior to administration of cisapride to patients who have or may develop prolongation of cardiac conduction intervals, particularly QT_c. These include patients with conditions that could predispose them to the development of serious arrhythmias, such as multiple organ failure, COPD, apnea and advanced cancer. (See CONTRAINDICATIONS.) PROPULSID® (cisapride) should not be used in patients with uncorrected hypokalemia or hypomagnesemia, such as those with severe dehydration, vomiting or malnutrition, or those taking potassium-wasting diuretics. PROPULSID® should not be used in patients who might experience rapid reduction of plasma potassium, such as those administered potassium-wasting diuretics and/or insulin in acute settings.

Information for Patients: Patients should be warned against concomitant use of clarithromycin (BIAXIN®), erythromcyin, troleandomycin (TAO®), nefazodone (SERZONE®), fluconazole (DIFLUCAN®), itraconazole (SPORANOX®), ketoconazole (NIZORAL®), indinavir (CRIXIVAN®) or ritonavir (NORVIR®).

Recommended doses should not be exceeded.

Patients should be advised to seek medical attention if they faint or become faint, dizzy, experience an irregular heartbeat or pulse, or any other unusual symptoms while using cisapride.

Patients should inform their physician of any concomitant medication use.

Although PROPULSID® does not affect psychomotor function nor does it induce sedation or drowsiness when used alone, patients should be advised that the sedative effects of benzodiazepines and of alcohol may be enhanced by PROPULSID®.

Patients should be advised that generally the following lifestyle changes should be tried before using any drug for nighttime heartburn, including PROPULSID®: avoiding alcohol, quitting/decreasing cigarette smoking, elevating the head of the bed, avoiding large meals/meals just before bedtime, losing weight, avoiding fatty foods, chocolate, caffeine, or citrus.

Drug Interactions: Cisapride is metabolized mainly via the cytochrome P450 3A4 enzyme. In some cases where serious ventricular arrhythmias, QT prolongation, and torsades de pointes have occurred when cisapride was taken in conjunction with one of the cytochrome P450 3A4 inhibitors, elevated blood cisapride levels were noted at the time of the QT prolongation.

Antibiotics: *In vitro* and/or *in vivo* data show that **clarithromycin, erythromycin** and **troleandomycin** markedly inhibit the metabolism of PROPULSID®, which can result in an increase in plasma cisapride levels and prolongation of the QT interval on the ECG.

Anticholinergics: Concurrent administration of certain anticholinergic compounds, such as belladonna alkaloids and dicyclomine, would be expected to compromise the beneficial effects of PROPULSID®.

Anticoagulants (oral): In patients receiving oral anticoagulants, the coagulation times were increased in some cases. It is advisable to check coagulation time within the first few days after the start and discontinuation of PROPULSID® therapy, with an appropriate adjustment of the anticoagulant dose, if necessary.

Antidepressants: *In vitro* data indicate that **nefazodone** inhibits the metabolism of PROPULSID®, which can result in an increase in plasma cisapride levels and prolongation of the QT interval in the ECG.

Antifungals: *In vitro* and/or *in vivo* data indicate that **fluconazole, itraconazole** and **oral ketoconazole** markedly inhibit the metabolism of PROPULSID®, which can result in an increase in plasma cisapride levels and prolongation of the QT interval on the ECG. Human pharmacokinetic data indicate that oral ketoconazole markedly inhibits the metabolism of cisapride, resulting in a mean eight-fold increase in AUC of cisapride. A study in 14 normal male and female volunteers suggests that coadministration of PROPULSID® and ketoconazole can result in prolongation of the QT interval on the ECG.

H_2 receptor antagonists: **Cimetidine** coadministration leads to an increased peak plasma concentration and AUC of PROPULSID®; there is no effect on PROPULSID® absorption when it is coadministered with **ranitidine**. The gastrointestinal absorption of cimetidine and ranitidine is accelerated when they are coadministered with PROPULSID®.

Protease inhibitors: *In vitro* data that indicate that **indinavir** and **ritonavir** markedly inhibit the metabolism of PROPULSID® which can result in an increase in plasma cisapride levels and prolongation of the QT interval on the ECG.

Cisapride should not be used concomitantly with other drugs known to prolong the QT interval: certain antiarrhythmics, including those of Class IA (such as quinidine and procainamide) and Class III (such as sotalol); tricyclic antidepressants (such as amitriptyline); certain tetracyclic antidepressants (such as maprotiline); certain antipsychotic medications (such as sertindole); astemizole, bepridil, sparfloxacin and terodiline. The preceding lists of drugs are not comprehensive.

The acceleration of gastric emptying by PROPULSID® could affect the rate of absorption of other drugs. Patients receiving narrow therapeutic ratio drugs or other drugs that require careful titration should be followed closely; if plasma levels are being monitored, they should be reassessed.

Carcinogenesis, mutagenesis, impairment of fertility: In a twenty-five month oral carcinogenicity study in rats, cisapride at daily doses up to 80 mg/kg was not tumorigenic. For a 50 kg person of average height (1.46 m^2 body surface area), this dose represents 50 times the maximum recommended human dose (1.6 mg/kg/day) on a mg/kg basis and 7 times the maximum recommended human dose (54.4 mg/m^2) on a body surface area basis. In a nineteen month oral carcinogenicity study in mice, cisapride at daily doses up to 80 mg/kg was not tumorigenic. This dose represents 50 times the maximum recommended human dose on a mg/kg basis and about 4 time the maximum recommended human dose on a body surface area basis.

Cisapride was not mutagenic in the *in vitro* Ames test, human lymphocyte chromosomal aberration test, mouse lymphoma cell forward mutation test, and rat hepatocyte UDS test and *in vivo* rat micronucleus test, male and female mouse dominant lethal mutations tests, and sex linked recessive lethal test in male *Drosophila melanogaster.*

Fertility and reproductive performance studies were conducted in male and female rats. Cisapride was found to have no effect on fertility and reproductive performance of male rats at oral doses up to 160 mg/kg/day (100 times the maximum recommended human dose on a mg/kg basis and 14 times the maximum recommended human dose on a mg/m^2 basis). In the female rats, cisapride at oral doses of 40 mg/kg/day and higher prolonged the breeding interval required for impregnation. Similar effects were also observed at maturity in the female offspring (F_1) of the female rats (F_0) treated with oral doses of cisapride at 10 mg/kg/day or higher. Cisapride at an oral dose of 160 mg/kg/day also exerted contragestational/pregnancy disrupting effects in female rats (F_0).

Pregnancy: Teratogenic effects: Pregnancy category C: Oral teratology studies have been conducted in rats (doses up to 160 mg/kg/day) and rabbits (doses up to 40 mg/kg/day). There was no evidence of a teratogenic potential of cisapride in rats or rabbits. Cisapride was embryotoxic and fetotoxic in rats at a dose of 160 mg/kg/day (100 times the maximum recommended human dose on a mg/kg basis and 14 times the maximum recommended human dose on a mg/m^2 basis) and in rabbits at a dose of 20 mg/kg/day (approximately 12 times the maximum recommended human dose on a mg/kg basis) or higher. It also produced reduced birth weights of pups in rats at 40 and 160 mg/kg/day and adversely affected the pup survival. There are no adequate and well-controlled studies in pregnant women. Cisapride should be used during pregnancy only if the potential benefit to the mother justifies the potential risk to the mother and the fetus.

Nursing Mothers: Cisapride is excreted in human milk at concentrations approximately one twentieth of those observed in plasma. Caution should be exercised when PROPULSID® is administered to a nursing woman, and particular care must be taken if the nursing infant or the mother is taking a drug that might alter PROPULSID®'s metabolism in the infant. (See CONTRAINDICATIONS, WARNINGS, PRECAUTIONS and DRUG INTERACTIONS.)

Pediatric Use: Safety and effectiveness in pediatric patients have not been established. Although causality has not been established, serious adverse events, including death, have been reported in infants and children treated with cisapride. Several pediatric deaths were due to cardiovascular events (third degree heart block and ventricular tachycardia). Pediatric deaths have been associated with seizures and there has been at least one case of "sudden unexplained death" in a 3-month-old infant. Other unlabeled potentially serious events which have been reported in pediatric patients include: antinuclear antibody (ANA) positive, anemia, hemolytic anemia, methemoglobinemia, hyperglycemia, hypoglycemia with acidosis, unexplained apneic episodes, confusion, impaired concentration, depression, apathy, visual changes accompanied by amnesia, and severe photosensitivity reaction.

A one-month-old male infant received 2 mg/kg cisapride four times per day for 5 days. The patient developed third degree heart block and subsequently died of right ventricular perforation caused by pacemaker wire insertion.

Geriatric Use: Steady-state plasma levels are generally higher in older than in younger patients, due to a moderate prolongation of the elimination half-life. Therapeutic doses, however, are similar to those used in younger adults.

The rate of common adverse experiences in patients greater than 65 years of age in clinical trials was similar to that in younger adults.

ADVERSE REACTIONS

In the U.S. clinical trial population of 1728 patients (comprising 506 with gastroesophageal reflux disorders, and the remainder with other disorders) the following adverse experiences were reported in more than 1% of patients treated with PROPULSID® (cisapride) and at least as often on PROPULSID® as on placebo.

System/Adverse Event	PROPULSID® N=1042	Placebo N=686
Central & Peripheral Nervous Systems		
Headache	19.3%	17.1%
Gastrointestinal		
Diarrhea	14.2	10.3
Abdominal pain	10.2	7.7
Nausea	7.6	7.6
Constipation	6.7	3.4
Flatulence	3.5	3.1
Dyspepsia	2.7	1.0
Respiratory System		
Rhinitis	7.3	5.7
Sinusitis	3.6	3.5
Coughing	1.5	1.2
Resistance Mechanism		
Viral infection	3.6	3.2
Upper respiratory tract infection	3.1	2.8
Body as a Whole		
Pain	3.4	2.3
Fever	2.2	1.5
Urinary System		
Urinary tract infection	2.4	1.9
Micturition frequency	1.2	0.6
Psychiatric		
Insomnia	1.9	1.3
Anxiety	1.4	1.0
Nervousness	1.4	0.7
Skin & Appendages		
Rash	1.6	1.6
Pruritus	1.2	1.0
Musculoskeletal System		
Arthralgia	1.4	1.2
Vision		
Abnormal vision	1.4	0.3
Reproductive, Female		
Vaginitis	1.2	0.9

The following adverse events also reported in more than 1% of PROPULSID® patients were more frequently reported on placebo: dizziness, vomiting, pharyngitis, chest pain, fatigue, back pain, depression, dehydration, and myalgia.

Diarrhea, abdominal pain, constipation, flatulence and rhinitis all occurred more frequently in patients using 20 mg of PROPULSID® than in patients using 10 mg.

Additional adverse experiences reported to occur in 1% or less of patients in the U.S. clinical studies are: dry mouth, somnolence, palpitation, migraine, tremor and edema.

In other U.S. and international trials and in postmarketing experience, there have been rare reports of seizures and extrapyramidal effects. Also reported have been tachycardia, elevated liver enzymes, hepatitis, thrombocytopenia, leukopenia, aplastic anemia, pancytopenia, and granulocytopenia. The relationship of PROPULSID® to the event was not clear in these cases.

Cardiac arrhythmias, including ventricular tachycardia, ventricular fibrillation, torsades de pointes, and QT prolongation, in some cases resulting in death, have been reported. (See CONTRAINDICATIONS, WARNINGS, PRECAUTIONS and DRUG INTERACTIONS.)

Postmarketing Reports: In addition to the cardiovascular adverse events, the following events have been identified during post-approval use of cisapride in clinical practice. Because they are reported voluntarily from a population of unknown size, estimates of frequency cannot be made. These events have been chosen for inclusion in this insert due to a combination of their seriousness, frequency of re-

Continued on next page

Propulsid—Cont.

porting, or potential causal connection to cisapride: allergic reactions, including bronchospasm, urticaria, and angioedema; possible exacerbation of asthma; psychiatric events, including confusion, depression, suicide attempt, and hallucinations; gynecomastia, female breast enlargement, urinary incontinence, hyperprolactinemia and galactorrhea.

The following events were specifically reported in the pediatric population: antinuclear antibody (ANA) positive, anemia, hemolytic anemia, methemoglobinemia, hyperglycemia, hypoglycemia with acidosis, unexplained apneic episodes, confusion, impaired concentration, depression, apathy, visual changes accompanied by amnesia, and severe photosensitivity reaction.

There have been rare cases of sinus tachycardia reported. Rechallenge precipitated the tachycardia again in some of those patients.

OVERDOSAGE

With overdose, rare cases of QT prolongation and ventricular arrhythmia have been reported.

A one-month-old infant received 2 mg/kg of cisapride four times per day for 5 days. The patient developed third degree heart block and subsequently died of right ventricular perforation caused by pacemaker wire insertion.

In instances of overdose, patients should be evaluated for possible QT prolongation and ventricular arrhythmias, including torsades de pointes. Treatment should include gastric lavage and/or activated charcoal, close observation and general supportive measures.

Reports of overdosage with PROPULSID® (cisapride) also include an adult who took 540 mg and for 2 hours experienced retching, borborygmi, flatulence, stool frequency and urinary frequency.

Single oral doses of cisapride at 4000 mg/kg, 160 mg/kg, 1280 mg/kg and 640 mg/kg were lethal in adult rats, neonatal rats, mice, and dogs, respectively. Symptoms of acute toxicity were ptosis, tremors, convulsions, dyspnea, loss of righting reflex, catalepsy, catatonia, hypotonia and diarrhea.

DOSAGE AND ADMINISTRATION

5 mL (1 teaspoon) suspension = 5 mg.

Adults: Initiate therapy with one 10 mg tablet of PROPULSID® (cisapride) or 10 mL of the suspension 4 times daily at least 15 minutes before meals and at bedtime. In some patients the dosage will need to be increased to 20 mg, given as above, to obtain a satisfactory result.

PROPULSID® should be discontinued if relief of nocturnal heartburn does not occur. The minimum effective dose should be used. Recommended doses of PROPULSID® should not be exceeded.

It is recommended that the daily dose be halved in patients with hepatic insufficiency.

In elderly patients, steady-state plasma levels are generally higher due to a moderate prolongation of the elimination half-life. Therapeutic doses, however, are similar to those used in younger adults.

HOW SUPPLIED

PROPULSID® (cisapride) Tablets are provided as scored white tablets debossed "Janssen" and P/10 containing the equivalent of 10 mg of cisapride in blister packages of 100 (NDC 50458-430-01) and in bottles of 100 (NDC 50458-430-10) and 500 (NDC 50458-430-50). PROPULSID® is also provided as blue tablets, debossed "Janssen" and P/20, containing the equivalent of 20 mg cisapride in blister packages of 100 (NDC 50458-440-01) and in bottles of 100 (NDC 50458-440-10) and bottles of 250 (NDC 50458-440-25).

PROPULSID® Suspension is provided as a bright pink homogeneous suspension containing the equivalent of 1 mg/mL of cisapride in 16 oz. bottles containing 450 mL (NDC 50458-440-45).

Store at 15°–25°C (59°–77°F). Protect the tablets from moisture. The 20 mg tablets should also be protected from light.

JANSSEN PHARMACEUTICA Titusville, NJ 08560

7502614

U.S. Patent No. 4,962,115

Revised September 1997, June 1998

©Janssen Pharmaceutica Inc. 1998

Shown in Product Identification Guide, page 317

RISPERDAL®   ℞

[ris 'pər dăl]

(risperidone) Tablets/Oral Solution

DESCRIPTION

RISPERDAL® (risperidone) is an antipsychotic agent belonging to a new chemical class, the benzisoxazole derivatives. The chemical designation is 3-[2-[4-(6-fluoro-1,2-benzisoxazol-3-yl)-1-piperidinyl]ethyl]-6,7,8,9-tetrahydro-2-methyl-4H-pyrido[1,2-a]pyrimidin-4-one. Its molecular formula is $C_{23}H_{27}FN_4O_2$ and its molecular weight is 410.49.

Risperidone is a white to slightly beige powder. It is practically insoluble in water, freely soluble in methylene chloride, and soluble in methanol and 0.1 N HCl.

RISPERDAL® tablets are available in tablets of 1 mg (white, scored), 2 mg (orange), 3 mg (yellow), and 4 mg (green) strengths. Inactive ingredients are colloidal silicon dioxide, hydroxypropyl methylcellulose, lactose, magnesium stearate, microcrystalline cellulose, propylene glycol, sodium lauryl sulfate, and starch (corn). Tablets of 2, 3, and 4 mg also contain talc and titanium dioxide. The 2 mg tablets contain FD&C Yellow No. 6 Aluminum Lake; the 3 mg and 4 mg tablets contain D&C Yellow No. 10; the 4 mg tablets contain FD&C Blue No. 2 Aluminum Lake.

RISPERDAL® is also available as a 1 mg/mL oral solution. The inactive ingredients for this solution are; tartaric acid, benzoic acid, sodium hydroxide and purified water (formulation F68).

CLINICAL PHARMACOLOGY

Pharmacodynamics

The mechanism of action of RISPERDAL® (risperidone), as with other antipsychotic drugs, is unknown. However, it has been proposed that this drug's antipsychotic activity is mediated through a combination of dopamine type 2 (D_2) and serotonin type 2 ($5HT_2$) antagonism. Antagonism at receptors other than D_2 and $5HT_2$ may explain some of the other effects of RISPERDAL®.

RISPERDAL® is a selective monoaminergic antagonist with high affinity (Ki of 0.12 to 7.3 nM) for the serotonin type 2 ($5HT_2$), dopamine type 2 (D_2), α_1 and α_2 adrenergic, and H_1 histaminergic receptors. RISPERDAL® antagonizes other receptors, but with lower potency. RISPERDAL® has low to moderate affinity (Ki of 47 to 253 nM) for the serotonin $5HT_{1C}$, $5HT_{1D}$, and $5HT_{1A}$ receptors, weak affinity (Ki of 620 to 800 nM) for the dopamine D_1 and haloperidol-sensitive sigma site, and no affinity (when tested at concentrations $>10^{-5}$ M) for cholinergic muscarinic or β_1 and β_2 adrenergic receptors.

Pharmacokinetics

Risperidone is well absorbed, as illustrated by a mass balance study involving a single 1 mg oral dose of ^{14}C-risperidone as a solution in three healthy male volunteers. Total recovery of radioactivity at one week was 85%, including 70% in the urine and 15% in the feces.

Risperidone is extensively metabolized in the liver by cytochrome $P_{450}IID_6$ to a major active metabolite, 9-hydroxyrisperidone, which is the predominant circulating specie, and appears approximately equi-effective with risperidone with respect to receptor binding activity and some effects in animals. (A second minor pathway is N-dealkylation). Consequently, the clinical effect of the drug likely results from the combined concentrations of risperidone plus 9-hydroxyrisperidone. Plasma concentrations of risperidone, 9-hydroxyrisperidone, and risperidone plus 9-hydroxyrisperidone are dose proportional over the dosing range of 1 to 16 mg daily (0.5 to 8 mg BID). The relative oral bioavailability of risperidone from a tablet was 94% (CV=10%) when compared to a solution. Food does not affect either the rate or extent of absorption of risperidone. Thus, risperidone can be given with or without meals. The absolute oral bioavailability of risperidone was 70% (CV=25%).

The enzyme catalyzing hydroxylation of risperidone to 9-hydroxyrisperidone is cytochrome $P_{450}IID_6$, also called debrisoquin hydroxylase, the enzyme responsible for metabolism of many neuroleptics, antidepressants, antiarrhythmics, and other drugs. Cytochrome $P_{450}IID_6$ is subject to genetic polymorphism (about 6-8% of Caucasians, and a very low percent of Asians have little or no activity and are "poor metabolizers") and to inhibition by a variety of substrates and some non-substrates, notably quinidine. Extensive metabolizers convert risperidone rapidly into 9-hydroxyrisperidone, while poor metabolizers convert it much more slowly. Extensive metabolizers, therefore, have lower risperidone and higher 9-hydroxyrisperidone concentrations than poor metabolizers. Following oral administration of solution or tablet, mean peak plasma concentrations occurred at about 1 hour. Peak 9-hydroxyrisperidone occurred at about 3 hours in extensive metabolizers, and 17 hours in poor metabolizers. The apparent half-life of risperidone was three hours (CV=30%) in extensive metabolizers and 20 hours (CV=40%) in poor metabolizers. The apparent half-life of 9-hydroxyrisperidone was about 21 hours (CV=20%) in extensive metabolizers and 30 hours (CV=25%) in poor metabolizers. Steady-state concentrations of risperidone are reached in 1 day in extensive metabolizers and would be expected to reach steady state in about 5 days in poor metabolizers. Steady-state concentrations of 9-hydroxyrisperidone are reached in 5-6 days (measured in extensive metabolizers).

Because risperidone and 9-hydroxyrisperidone are approximately equi-effective, the sum of their concentrations is pertinent. The pharmacokinetics of the sum of risperidone and 9-hydroxyrisperidone, after single and multiple doses, were similar in extensive and poor metabolizers, with an overall mean elimination half-life of about 20 hours. In analyses comparing adverse reaction rates in extensive and poor metabolizers in controlled and open studies, no important differences were seen.

Risperidone could be subject to two kinds of drug-drug interactions. First, inhibitors of cytochrome $P_{450}IID_6$ could interfere with conversion of risperidone to 9-hydroxyrisperidone. This in fact occurs with quinidine, giving essentially all recipients a risperidone pharmacokinetic profile typical of poor metabolizers. The favorable and adverse effects of risperidone in patients receiving quinidine have not been evaluated, but observations in a modest number (n is approximately equal to 70) of poor metabolizers given risperidone do not suggest important differences between poor and extensive metabolizers. It would also be possible for risperidone to interfere with metabolism of other drugs metabolized by cytochrome $P_{450}IID_6$. Relatively weak binding of risperidone to the enzyme suggests this is unlikely (See PRECAUTIONS and DRUG INTERACTIONS).

The plasma protein binding of risperidone was about 90% over the in vitro concentration range of 0.5 to 200 ng/mL and increased with increasing concentrations of α_1-acid glycoprotein. The plasma binding of 9-hydroxyrisperidone was 77%. Neither the parent nor the metabolite displaced each other from the plasma binding sites. High therapeutic concentrations of sulfamethazine (100 μg/mL), warfarin (10 μg/mL) and carbamazepine (10 μg/mL) caused only a slight increase in the free fraction of risperidone at 10 ng/mL and 9-hydroxyrisperidone at 50 ng/mL, changes of unknown clinical significance.

Special Populations

Renal Impairment: In patients with moderate to severe renal disease, clearance of the sum of risperidone and its active metabolite decreased by 60% compared to young healthy subjects. RISPERDAL® doses should be reduced in patients with renal disease (See PRECAUTIONS and DOSAGE AND ADMINISTRATION).

Hepatic Impairment: While the pharmacokinetics of risperidone in subjects with liver disease were comparable to those in young healthy subjects, the mean free fraction of risperidone in plasma was increased by about 35% because of the diminished concentration of both albumin and α_1-acid glycoprotein. RISPERDAL® doses should be reduced in patients with liver disease (See PRECAUTIONS and DOSAGE AND ADMINISTRATION).

Elderly: In healthy elderly subjects renal clearance of both risperidone and 9-hydroxyrisperidone was decreased, and elimination half-lives were prolonged compared to young healthy subjects. Dosing should be modified accordingly in the elderly patients (See DOSAGE AND ADMINISTRATION).

Race and Gender Effects: No specific pharmacokinetic study was conducted to investigate race and gender effects, but a population pharmacokinetic analysis did not identify important differences in the disposition of risperidone due to gender (whether corrected for body weight or not) or race.

Clinical Trials

The efficacy of RISPERDAL® in the management of the manifestations of psychotic disorders was established in four short-term (4- to 8-week) controlled trials of psychotic inpatients who met DSM-III-R criteria for schizophrenia.

Several instruments were used for assessing psychiatric signs and symptoms in these studies, among them the Brief Psychiatric Rating Scale (BPRS), a multi-item inventory of general psychopathology traditionally used to evaluate the effects of drug treatment in psychosis. The BPRS psychosis cluster (conceptual disorganization, hallucinatory behavior, suspiciousness, and unusual thought content) is considered a particularly useful subset for assessing actively psychotic schizophrenic patients. A second traditional assessment, the Clinical Global Impression (CGI), reflects the impression of a skilled observer, fully familiar with the manifestations of schizophrenia, about the overall clinical state of the patient. In addition, two more recently developed, but less well evaluated scales, were employed; these included the Positive and Negative Syndrome Scale (PANSS) and the Scale for Assessing Negative Symptoms (SANS).

The results of the trials follow:

(1) In a 6-week, placebo-controlled trial (n=160) involving titration of RISPERDAL® in doses up to 10 mg/day (BID schedule), RISPERDAL® was generally superior to placebo on the BPRS total score, on the BPRS psychosis cluster, and marginally superior to placebo on the SANS.

(2) In an 8-week, placebo-controlled trial (n=513) involving 4 fixed doses of RISPERDAL® (2, 6, 10, and 16 mg/day, on a BID schedule), all 4 RISPERDAL® groups were generally superior to placebo on the BPRS total score, BPRS psychosis cluster, and CGI severity score; the 3 highest RISPERDAL® dose groups were generally superior to placebo on the PANSS negative subscale. The most consistently positive responses on all measures were seen for the 6 mg dose group, and there was no suggestion of increased benefit from larger doses.

(3) In an 8-week, dose comparison trial (n=1356) involving 5 fixed doses of RISPERDAL® (1, 4, 8, 12, and 16 mg/day, on a BID schedule), the four highest RISPERDAL® dose groups were generally superior to the 1 mg RISPERDAL® dose group on BPRS total score, BPRS psychosis cluster, and CGI severity score. None of the dose groups were supe-

rior to the 1 mg group on the PANSS negative subscale. The most consistently positive responses were seen for the 4 mg dose group.

(4) In a 4-week, placebo-controlled dose comparison trial (n=246) involving 2 fixed doses of RISPERDAL® (4 and 8 mg/day on a QD schedule), both RISPERDAL® dose groups were generally superior to placebo on several PANSS measures, including a response measure (> 20% reduction in PANSS total score), PANSS total score, and the BPRS psychosis cluster (derived from PANSS). The results were generally stronger for the 8 mg than for the 4 mg dose group.

INDICATIONS AND USAGE

RISPERDAL® (risperidone) is indicated for the management of the manifestations of psychotic disorders.

The antipsychotic efficacy of RISPERDAL® was established in short-term (6 to 8-weeks) controlled trials of schizophrenic inpatients (See CLINICAL PHARMACOLOGY).

The effectiveness of RISPERDAL® in long-term use, that is, more than 6 to 8-weeks, has not been systematically evaluated in controlled trials. Therefore, the physician who elects to use RISPERDAL® for extended periods should periodically re-evaluate the long-term usefulness of the drug for the individual patient. (See DOSAGE AND ADMINISTRATION).

CONTRAINDICATIONS

RISPERDAL® (risperidone) is contraindicated in patients with a known hypersensitivity to the product.

WARNINGS

Neuroleptic Malignant Syndrome (NMS)

A potentially fatal symptom complex sometimes referred to as Neuroleptic Malignant Syndrome (NMS) has been reported in association with antipsychotic drugs. Clinical manifestations of NMS are hyperpyrexia, muscle rigidity, altered mental status and evidence of autonomic instability (irregular pulse or blood pressure, tachycardia, diaphoresis and cardiac dysrhythmia). Additional signs may include elevated creatine phosphokinase, myoglobinuria (rhabdomyolysis), and acute renal failure.

The diagnostic evaluation of patients with this syndrome is complicated. In arriving at a diagnosis, it is important to identify cases where the clinical presentation includes both serious medical illness (e.g., pneumonia, systemic infection, etc.) and untreated or inadequately treated extrapyramidal signs and symptoms (EPS). Other important considerations in the differential diagnosis include central anticholinergic toxicity, heat stroke, drug fever, and primary central nervous system pathology.

The management of NMS should include: 1) immediate discontinuation of antipsychotic drugs and other drugs not essential to concurrent therapy; 2) intensive symptomatic treatment and medical monitoring; and 3) treatment of any concomitant serious medical problems for which specific treatments are available. There is no general agreement about specific pharmacological treatment regimens for uncomplicated NMS.

If a patient requires antipsychotic drug treatment after recovery from NMS, the potential reintroduction of drug therapy should be carefully considered. The patient should be carefully monitored, since recurrences of NMS have been reported.

Tardive Dyskinesia

A syndrome of potentially irreversible, involuntary, dyskinetic movements may develop in patients treated with antipsychotic drugs. Although the prevalence of the syndrome appears to be highest among the elderly, especially elderly women, it is impossible to rely upon prevalence estimates to predict, at the inception of antipsychotic treatment, which patients are likely to develop the syndrome. Whether antipsychotic drug products differ in their potential to cause tardive dyskinesia is unknown.

The risk of developing tardive dyskinesia and the likelihood that it will become irreversible are believed to increase as the duration of treatment and the total cumulative dose of antipsychotic drugs administered to the patient increase. However, the syndrome can develop, although much less commonly, after relatively brief treatment periods at low doses.

There is no known treatment for established cases of tardive dyskinesia, although the syndrome may remit, partially or completely, if antipsychotic treatment is withdrawn. Antipsychotic treatment, itself, however, may suppress (or partially suppress) the signs and symptoms of the syndrome and thereby may possibly mask the underlying process. The effect that symptomatic suppression has upon the long-term course of the syndrome is unknown.

Given these considerations, RISPERDAL® (risperidone) should be prescribed in a manner that is most likely to minimize the occurrence of tardive dyskinesia. Chronic antipsychotic treatment should generally be reserved for patients who suffer from a chronic illness that (1) is known to respond to antipsychotic drugs, and (2) for whom alternative, equally effective, but potentially less harmful treatments are not available or appropriate. In patients who do require chronic treatment, the smallest dose and the shortest dura-

tion of treatment producing a satisfactory clinical response should be sought. The need for continued treatment should be reassessed periodically.

If signs and symptoms of tardive dyskinesia appear in a patient on RISPERDAL®, drug discontinuation should be considered. However, some patients may require treatment with RISPERDAL® despite the presence of the syndrome.

Potential for Proarrhythmic Effects: Risperidone and/or 9-hydroxyrisperidone appears to lengthen the QT interval in some patients, although there is no average increase in treated patients, even at 12–16 mg/day, well above the recommended dose. Other drugs that prolong the QT interval have been associated with the occurrence of torsades de pointes, a life-threatening arrhythmia. Bradycardia, electrolyte imbalance, concomitant use with other drugs that prolong QT, or the presence of congenital prolongation in QT can increase the risk for occurrence of this arrhythmia.

PRECAUTIONS

General

Orthostatic Hypotension: RISPERDAL® (risperidone) may induce orthostatic hypotension associated with dizziness, tachycardia, and in some patients, syncope, especially during the initial dose-titration period, probably reflecting its alpha-adrenergic antagonistic properties. Syncope was reported in 0.2% (6/2607) of RISPERDAL® treated patients in phase 2–3 studies. The risk of orthostatic hypotension and syncope may be minimized by limiting the initial dose to 2 mg total (either QD or 1 mg BID) in normal adults and 0.5 mg BID in the elderly and patients with renal or hepatic impairment (See DOSAGE AND ADMINISTRATION). A dose reduction should be considered if hypotension occurs. RISPERDAL® should be used with particular caution in patients with known cardiovascular disease (history of myocardial infarction or ischemia, heart failure, or conduction abnormalities), cerebrovascular disease, and conditions which would predispose patients to hypotension e.g., dehydration and hypovolemia. Clinically significant hypotension has been observed with concomitant use of RISPERDAL® and antihypertensive medication.

Seizures: During premarketing testing, seizures occurred in 0.3% (9/2607) of RISPERDAL® treated patients, two in association with hyponatremia. RISPERDAL® should be used cautiously in patients with a history of seizures.

Hyperprolactinemia: As with other drugs that antagonize dopamine D_2 receptors, risperidone elevates prolactin levels and the elevation persists during chronic administration. Tissue culture experiments indicate that approximately one-third of human breast cancers are prolactin dependent in vitro, a factor of potential importance if the prescription of these drugs is contemplated in a patient with previously detected breast cancer. Although disturbances such as galactorrhea, amenorrhea, gynecomastia, and impotence have been reported with prolactin-elevating compounds, the clinical significance of elevated serum prolactin levels is unknown for most patients. As is common with compounds which increase prolactin release, an increase in pituitary gland, mammary gland, and pancreatic islet cell hyperplasia and/or neoplasia was observed in the risperidone carcinogenicity studies conducted in mice and rats (See CARCINOGENESIS). However, neither clinical studies nor epidemiologic studies conducted to date have shown an association between chronic administration of this class of drugs and tumorigenesis in humans; the available evidence is considered too limited to be conclusive at this time.

Potential for Cognitive and Motor Impairment: Somnolence was a commonly reported adverse event associated with RISPERDAL® treatment, especially when ascertained by direct questioning of patients. This adverse event is dose related, and in a study utilizing a checklist to detect adverse events, 41% of the high dose patients (RISPERDAL® 16 mg/day) reported somnolence compared to 16% of placebo patients. Direct questioning is more sensitive for detecting adverse events than spontaneous reporting, by which 8% of RISPERDAL® 16 mg/day patients and 1% of placebo patients reported somnolence as an adverse event. Since RISPERDAL® has the potential to impair judgment, thinking, or motor skills, patients should be cautioned about operating hazardous machinery, including automobiles, until they are reasonably certain that RISPERDAL® therapy does not affect them adversely.

Priapism: Rare cases of priapism have been reported. While the relationship of the events to RISPERDAL® use has not been established, other drugs with alpha-adrenergic blocking effects have been reported to induce priapism, and it is possible that RISPERDAL® may share this capacity. Severe priapism may require surgical intervention.

Thrombotic Thrombocytopenic Purpura (TTP): A single case of TTP was reported in a 28 year-old female patient receiving RISPERDAL® in a large, open premarketing experience (approximately 1300 patients). She experienced jaundice, fever, and bruising, but eventually recovered after receiving plasmapheresis. The relationship to RISPERDAL® therapy is unknown.

Antiemetic effect: Risperidone has an antiemetic effect in animals; this effect may also occur in humans, and may

mask signs and symptoms of overdosage with certain drugs or of conditions such as intestinal obstruction, Reye's syndrome, and brain tumor.

Body Temperature Regulation: Disruption of body temperature regulation has been attributed to antipsychotic agents. Both hyperthermia and hypothermia have been reported in association with RISPERDAL® use. Caution is advised when prescribing for patients who will be exposed to temperature extremes.

Suicide: The possibility of a suicide attempt is inherent in schizophrenia, and close supervision of high risk patients should accompany drug therapy. Prescriptions for RISPERDAL® should be written for the smallest quantity of tablets consistent with good patient management, in order to reduce the risk of overdose.

Use in Patients with Concomitant Illness: Clinical experience with RISPERDAL® in patients with certain concomitant systemic illnesses is limited. Caution is advisable in using RISPERDAL® in patients with diseases or conditions that could affect metabolism or hemodynamic responses. RISPERDAL® has not been evaluated or used to any appreciable extent in patients with a recent history of myocardial infarction or unstable heart disease. Patients with these diagnoses were excluded from clinical studies during the product's premarket testing. The electrocardiograms of approximately 380 patients who received RISPERDAL® and 120 patients who received placebo in two double-blind, placebo-controlled trials were evaluated and the data revealed one finding of potential concern, i.e., 8 patients taking RISPERDAL® whose baseline QTc interval was less than 450 msec were observed to have QTc intervals greater than 450 msec during treatment; no such prolongations were seen in the smaller placebo group. There were 3 such episodes in the approximately 125 patients who received haloperidol. Because of the risks of orthostatic hypotension and QT prolongation, caution should be observed in cardiac patients (See WARNINGS AND PRECAUTIONS).

Increased plasma concentrations of risperidone and 9-hydroxyrisperidone occur in patients with severe renal impairment (creatinine clearance <30 mL/min/1.73 m^2), and an increase in the free fraction of the risperidone is seen in patients with severe hepatic impairment. A lower starting dose should be used in such patients (See DOSAGE AND ADMINISTRATION).

Information for Patients

Physicians are advised to discuss the following issues with patients for whom they prescribe RISPERDAL®:

Orthostatic Hypotension: Patients should be advised of the risk of orthostatic hypotension, especially during the period of initial dose titration.

Interference With Cognitive and Motor Performance: Since RISPERDAL® has the potential to impair judgment, thinking, or motor skills, patients should be cautioned about operating hazardous machinery, including automobiles, until they are reasonably certain that RISPERDAL® therapy does not affect them adversely.

Pregnancy: Patients should be advised to notify their physician if they become pregnant or intend to become pregnant during therapy.

Nursing: Patients should be advised not to breast feed an infant if they are taking RISPERDAL®.

Concomitant Medication: Patients should be advised to inform their physicians if they are taking, or plan to take, any prescription or over-the-counter drugs, since there is a potential for interactions.

Alcohol: Patients should be advised to avoid alcohol while taking RISPERDAL®.

Laboratory Tests

No specific laboratory tests are recommended.

Drug Interactions

The interactions of RISPERDAL® and other drugs have not been systematically evaluated. Given the primary CNS effects of risperidone, caution should be used when RISPERDAL® is taken in combination with other centrally acting drugs and alcohol.

Because of its potential for inducing hypotension, RISPERDAL® may enhance the hypotensive effects of other therapeutic agents with this potential.

RISPERDAL® may antagonize the effects of levodopa and dopamine agonists.

Chronic administration of carbamazepine with risperidone may increase the clearance of risperidone.

Chronic administration of clozapine with risperidone may decrease the clearance of risperidone.

Drugs that Inhibit Cytochrome $P_{450}IID_6$ and Other P_{450} Isozymes: Risperidone is metabolized to 9-hydroxyrisperidone by cytochrome $P_{450}IID_6$, an enzyme that is polymorphic in the population and that can be inhibited by a variety of psychotropic and other drugs (See CLINICAL PHARMACOLOGY). Drug interactions that reduce the metabolism of risperidone to 9-hydroxyrisperidone would increase the plasma concentrations of risperidone and lower the concentrations of 9-hydroxyrisperidone. Analysis of clinical studies involving a modest number of poor metabolizers (n is ap-

Continued on next page

Risperdal—Cont.

proximately equal to 70) does not suggest that poor and extensive metabolizers have different rates of adverse effects. No comparison of effectiveness in the two groups has been made.

In vitro studies showed that drugs metabolized by other P_{450} isozymes, including 1A1, 1A2, IIC9, MP, and IIIA4, are only weak inhibitors of risperidone metabolism.

Drugs Metabolized by Cytochrome $P_{450}IID_6$: In vitro studies indicate that risperidone is a relatively weak inhibitor of cytochrome $P_{450}IID_6$. Therefore, RISPERDAL® is not expected to substantially inhibit the clearance of drugs that are metabolized by this enzymatic pathway. However, clinical data to confirm this expectation are not available.

Carcinogenesis, Mutagenesis, Impairment of Fertility

Carcinogenesis: Carcinogenicity studies were conducted in Swiss albino mice and Wistar rats. Risperidone was administered in the diet at doses of 0.63, 2.5, and 10 mg/kg for 18 months to mice and for 25 months to rats. These doses are equivalent to 2.4, 9.4 and 37.5 times the maximum human dose (16 mg/day) on a mg/kg basis or 0.2, 0.75 and 3 times the maximum human dose (mice) or 0.4, 1.5, and 6 times the maximum human dose (rats) on a mg/m² basis. A maximum tolerated dose was not achieved in male mice. There were statistically significant increases in pituitary gland adenomas, endocrine pancreas adenomas and mammary gland adenocarcinomas. The following table summarizes the multiples of the human dose on a mg/m² (mg/kg) basis at which these tumors occurred.

TUMOR TYPE	SPECIES	SEX	MULTIPLE OF MAXIMUM HUMAN DOSE in mg/m² (mg/kg): LOWEST EFFECT LEVEL	HIGHEST NO EFFECT LEVEL
Pituitary adenomas	mouse	female	0.75 (*9.4*)	0.2 (*2.4*)
Endocrine pancreas adenomas	rat	male	1.5 (*9.4*)	0.4 (*2.4*)
Mammary gland adeno-carcinomas	mouse	female	0.2 (*2.4*)	none
	rat	female	0.4 (*2.4*)	none
	rat	male	6 (*37.5*)	1.5 (*9.4*)
Mammary gland neoplasms, Total	rat	male	1.5 (*9.4*)	0.4 (*2.4*)

Antipsychotic drugs have been shown to chronically elevate prolactin levels in rodents. Serum prolactin levels were not measured during the risperidone carcinogenicity studies; however, measurements during subchronic toxicity studies showed that risperidone elevated serum prolactin levels 5 to 6 fold in mice and rats at the same doses used in the carcinogenicity studies. An increase in mammary, pituitary, and endocrine pancreas neoplasms has been found in rodents after chronic administration of other antipsychotic drugs and is considered to be prolactin mediated. The relevance for human risk of the findings of prolactin-mediated endocrine tumors in rodents is unknown (See Hyperprolactinemia under PRECAUTIONS, GENERAL).

Mutagenesis: No evidence of mutagenic potential for risperidone was found in the Ames reverse mutation test, mouse lymphoma assay, in vitro rat hepatocyte DNA-repair assay, in vivo micronucleus test in mice, the sex-linked recessive lethal test in Drosophila, or the chromosomal aberration test in human lymphocytes or Chinese hamster cells.

Impairment of Fertility: Risperidone (0.16 to 5 mg/kg) was shown to impair mating, but not fertility, in Wistar rats in three reproductive studies (two Segment I and a multigenerational study) at doses 0.1 to 3 times the maximum recommended human dose on a mg/m² basis. The effect appeared to be in females since impaired mating behavior was not noted in the Segment I study in which males only were treated. In a subchronic study in Beagle dogs in which risperidone was administered at doses of 0.31 to 5 mg/kg, sperm motility and concentration were decreased at doses 0.6 to 10 times the human dose on a mg/m² basis. Dose-related decreases were also noted in serum testosterone at the same doses. Serum testosterone and sperm parameters partially recovered but remained decreased after treatment was discontinued. No no-effect doses were noted in either rat or dog.

Pregnancy

Pregnancy Category C: The teratogenic potential of risperidone was studied in three Segment II studies in Sprague-Dawley and Wistar rats and in one Segment II study in New Zealand rabbits. The incidence of malformations was not increased compared to control in offspring of rats or rabbits given 0.4 to 6 times the human dose on a mg/m² basis. In three reproductive studies in rats (two Segment III and a multigenerational study), there was an increase in pup deaths during the first 4 days of lactation at doses 0.1 to 3 times the human dose on a mg/m² basis. It is not known whether these deaths were due to a direct effect on the fetuses or pups or to effects on the dams. There was no no-effect dose for increased rat pup mortality. In one Segment III study, there was an increase in stillborn rat pups at a dose 1.5 times higher than the human dose on a mg/m² basis.

Placental transfer of risperidone occurs in rat pups. There are no adequate and well-controlled studies in pregnant women. However, there was one report of a case of agenesis of the corpus callosum in an infant exposed to risperidone in utero. The causal relationship to RISPERDAL® therapy is unknown.

RISPERDAL® should be used during pregnancy only if the potential benefit justifies the potential risk to the fetus.

Labor and Delivery

The effect of RISPERDAL® on labor and delivery in humans is unknown.

Nursing Mothers

It is not known whether or not risperidone is excreted in human milk. In animal studies, risperidone and 9-hydroxyrisperidone were excreted in breast milk. Therefore, women receiving RISPERDAL® should not breast feed.

Pediatric Use

Safety and effectiveness in children have not been established.

Geriatric Use

Clinical studies of RISPERDAL® did not include sufficient numbers of patients aged 65 and over to determine whether they respond differently from younger patients. In general, a lower starting dose is recommended for an elderly patient, reflecting a decreased pharmacokinetic clearance in the elderly, as well as a greater frequency of decreased hepatic, renal, or cardiac function, and a greater tendency to postural hypotension (See CLINICAL PHARMACOLOGY and DOSAGE AND ADMINISTRATION).

ADVERSE REACTIONS

Associated with Discontinuation of Treatment

Approximately 9% percent (244/2607) of RISPERDAL® (risperidone)-treated patients in phase 2–3 studies discontinued treatment due to an adverse event, compared with about 7% on placebo and 10% on active control drugs. The more common events (≥0.3%) associated with discontinuation and considered to be possibly or probably drug-related included:

Adverse Event	RISPERDAL®	Placebo
Extrapyramidal symptoms	2.1%	0%
Dizziness	0.7%	0%
Hyperkinesia	0.6%	0%
Somnolence	0.5%	0%
Nausea	0.3%	0%

Suicide attempt was associated with discontinuation in 1.2% of RISPERDAL® treated patients compared to 0.6% of placebo patients, but, given the almost 40-fold greater exposure time in RISPERDAL® compared to placebo patients, it is unlikely that suicide attempt is a RISPERDAL® related adverse event (See PRECAUTIONS). Discontinuation for extrapyramidal symptoms was 0% in placebo patients but 3.8% in active-control patients in the phase 2–3 trials.

Incidence in Controlled Trials

Commonly Observed Adverse Events in Controlled Clinical Trials: In two 6- to 8-week placebo-controlled trials, spontaneously-reported, treatment-emergent adverse events with an incidence of 5% or greater in at least one of the RISPERDAL® groups and at least twice that of placebo were: anxiety, somnolence, extrapyramidal symptoms, dizziness, constipation, nausea, dyspepsia, rhinitis, rash, and tachycardia.

Adverse events were also elicited in one of these two trials (i.e., in the fixed-dose trial comparing RISPERDAL® at doses of 2, 6, 10, and 16 mg/day with placebo) utilizing a checklist for detecting adverse events, a method that is more sensitive than spontaneous reporting. By this method, the following additional common and drug-related adverse events were present at least 5% and twice the rate of placebo: increased dream activity, increased duration of sleep, accommodation disturbances, reduced salivation, micturition disturbances, diarrhea, weight gain, menorrhagia, diminished sexual desire, erectile dysfunction, ejaculatory dysfunction, and orgastic dysfunction.

Adverse Events Occurring at an Incidence of 1% or More Among RISPERDAL®-Treated Patients: The table that follows enumerates adverse events that occurred at an incidence of 1% or more, and were at least as frequent among RISPERDAL® treated patients treated at doses of ≤10 mg/day than among placebo-treated patients in the pooled results of two 6- to 8-week controlled trials. Patients received RISPERDAL® doses of 2, 6, 10, or 16 mg/day in the dose comparison trial, or up to a maximum dose of 10 mg/day in the titration study. This table shows the percentage of patients in each dose group (≤10 mg/day or 16 mg/day) who spontaneously reported at least one episode of an event at some time during their treatment. Patients given doses of 2, 6, or 10 mg did not differ materially in these rates. Reported adverse events were classified using the World Health Organization preferred terms.

The prescriber should be aware that these figures cannot be used to predict the incidence of side effects in the course of usual medical practice where patient characteristics and other factors differ from those which prevailed in this clinical trial. Similarly, the cited frequencies cannot be compared with figures obtained from other clinical investigations involving different treatments, uses and investigators. The cited figures, however, do provide the prescribing physician with some basis for estimating the relative contribution of drug and nondrug factors to the side effect incidence rate in the population studied.

Table 1: Treatment-Emergent Adverse Experience Incidence in 6- to 8-Week Controlled Clinical Trials[1]

Body System/ Preferred Term	RISPERDAL® ≤10 mg/day (N=324)	RISPERDAL® 16 mg/day (N=77)	Placebo (N=142)
Psychiatric Disorders			
Insomnia	26%	23%	19%
Agitation	22%	26%	20%
Anxiety	12%	20%	9%
Somnolence	3%	8%	1%
Aggressive reaction	1%	3%	1%
Nervous System			
Extrapyramidal symptoms[2]	17%	34%	16%
Headache	14%	12%	12%
Dizziness	4%	7%	1%
Gastrointestinal System			
Constipation	7%	13%	3%
Nausea	6%	4%	3%
Dyspepsia	5%	10%	4%
Vomiting	5%	7%	4%
Abdominal pain	4%	1%	0%
Saliva increased	2%	0%	1%
Toothache	2%	0%	0%
Respiratory System			
Rhinitis	10%	8%	4%
Coughing	3%	3%	1%
Sinusitis	2%	1%	1%
Pharyngitis	2%	3%	0%
Dyspnea	1%	0%	0%
Body as a Whole			
Back pain	2%	0%	1%
Chest pain	2%	3%	1%
Fever	2%	3%	0%
Dermatological			
Rash	2%	5%	1%
Dry skin	2%	4%	0%
Seborrhea	1%	0%	0%
Infections			
Upper respiratory	3%	3%	1%
Visual			
Abnormal vision	2%	1%	1%
Musculo-Skeletal			
Arthralgia	2%	3%	0%
Cardiovascular			
Tachycardia	3%	5%	0%

[1] Events reported by at least 1% of patients treated with RISPERDAL® ≤10 mg/day are included, and are rounded to the nearest %. Comparative rates for RISPERDAL® 16 mg/day and placebo are provided as well. Events for which the RISPERDAL® incidence (in both dose groups) was equal to or less than placebo are not listed in the table, but included the following: nervousness, injury, and fungal infection.

[2] Includes tremor, dystonia, hypokinesia, hypertonia, hyperkinesia, oculogyric crisis, ataxia, abnormal gait, involuntary muscle contractions, hyporeflexia, akathisia and extrapyramidal disorders. Although the incidence of 'extrapyramidal symptoms' does not appear to differ for the '≤10 mg/day' group and placebo, the data for individual dose groups in fixed dose trials do suggest a dose/response relationship (See DOSE DEPENDENCY OF ADVERSE EVENTS).

Dose Dependency of Adverse Events:

Extrapyramidal symptoms: Data from two fixed dose trials provided evidence of dose-relatedness for extrapyramidal symptoms associated with risperidone treatment.

Two methods were used to measure extrapyramidal symptoms (EPS) in an 8-week trial comparing four fixed doses of risperidone (2, 6, 10, and 16 mg/day), including (1) a parkinsonism score (mean change from baseline) from the Extrapyramidal Symptom Rating Scale and (2) incidence of spontaneous complaints of EPS:

Dose Groups	Placebo	Ris 2	Ris 6	Ris 10	Ris 16
Parkinsonism	1.2	0.9	1.8	2.4	2.6
EPS Incidence	13%	13%	16%	20%	31%

Similar methods were used to measure extrapyramidal symptoms (EPS) in an 8-week trial comparing five fixed doses of risperidone (1, 4, 8, 12, and 16 mg/day):

Dose Groups	Ris 1	Ris 4	Ris 8	Ris 12	Ris 16
Parkinsonism	0.6	1.7	2.4	2.9	4.1
EPS Incidence	7%	12%	18%	18%	21%

Other Adverse Events: Adverse event data elicited by a checklist for side effects from a large study comparing 5 fixed doses of RISPERDAL® (1, 4, 8, 12, and 16 mg/day) were explored for dose-relatedness of adverse events. A Cochran-Armitage Test for trend in these data revealed a positive trend ($p<0.05$) for the following adverse events: sleepiness, increased duration of sleep, accommodation disturbances, orthostatic dizziness, palpitations, weight gain, erectile dysfunction, ejaculatory dysfunction, orgastic dysfunction, asthenia/lassitude/increased fatiguability, and increased pigmentation.

Vital Sign Changes: RISPERDAL® is associated with orthostatic hypotension and tachycardia (See PRECAUTIONS).

Weight changes: The proportions of RISPERDAL® and placebo-treated patients meeting a weight gain criterion of ≥ 7% of body weight were compared in a pool of 6- to 8-week placebo-controlled trials, revealing a statistically significantly greater incidence of weight gain for RISPERDAL® (18%) compared to placebo (9%).

Laboratory Changes: A between group comparison for 6- to 8-week placebo-controlled trials revealed no statistically significant RISPERDAL®/placebo differences in the proportions of patients experiencing potentially important changes in routine serum chemistry, hematology, or urinalysis parameters. Similarly, there were no RISPERDAL®/placebo differences in the incidence of discontinuations for changes in serum chemistry, hematology, or urinalysis. However, RISPERDAL® administration was associated with increases in serum prolactin (See PRECAUTIONS).

ECG Changes: The electrocardiograms of approximately 380 patients who received RISPERDAL® and 120 patients who received placebo in two double-blind, placebo-controlled trials were evaluated and revealed one finding of potential concern; i.e., 8 patients taking RISPERDAL® whose baseline QTc interval was less than 450 msec were observed to have QTc intervals greater than 450 msec during treatment (See WARNINGS). Changes of this type were not seen among about 120 placebo patients, but were seen in patients receiving haloperidol (3/126).

Other Events Observed During the Pre-Marketing Evaluation of RISPERDAL®

During its premarketing assessment, multiple doses of RISPERDAL® (risperidone) were administered to 2607 patients in phase 2 and 3 studies. The conditions and duration of exposure to RISPERDAL® varied greatly, and included (in overlapping categories) open and double-blind studies, uncontrolled and controlled studies, inpatient and outpatient studies, fixed-dose and titration studies, and short-term or longer-term exposure. In most studies, untoward events associated with this exposure were obtained by spontaneous report and recorded by clinical investigators using terminology of their own choosing. Consequently, it is not possible to provide a meaningful estimate of the proportion of individuals experiencing adverse events without first grouping similar types of untoward events into a smaller number of standardized event categories. In two large studies, adverse events were also elicited utilizing the UKU (direct questioning) side effect rating scale, and these events were not further categorized using standard terminology (Note: These events are marked with an asterisk in the listings that follow).

In the listings that follow, spontaneously reported adverse events were classified using World Health Organization (WHO) preferred terms. The frequencies presented, therefore, represent the proportion of the 2607 patients exposed to multiple doses of RISPERDAL® who experienced an event of the type cited on at least one occasion while receiving RISPERDAL®. All reported events are included except those already listed in Table 1, those events for which a drug cause was remote, and those event terms which were so general as to be uninformative. It is important to emphasize that, although the events reported occurred during treatment with RISPERDAL®, they were not necessarily caused by it.

Events are further categorized by body system and listed in order of decreasing frequency according to the following definitions: frequent adverse events are those occurring in at least 1/100 patients (only those not already listed in the tabulated results from placebo controlled trials appear in this listing); infrequent adverse events are those occurring in 1/100 to 1/1000 patients; rare events are those occurring in fewer than 1/1000 patients.

Psychiatric Disorders: *Frequent:* increased dream activity*, diminished sexual desire*, nervousness. *Infrequent:* impaired concentration, depression, apathy, catatonic reaction, euphoria, increased libido, amnesia. *Rare:* emotional lability, nightmares, delirium, withdrawal syndrome, yawning.

Central and Peripheral Nervous System Disorders: *Frequent:* increased sleep duration*. *Infrequent:* dysarthria, vertigo, stupor, paraesthesia, confusion. *Rare:* aphasia, cholinergic syndrome, hypoesthesia, tongue paralysis, leg cramps, torticollis, hypotonia, coma, migraine, hyperreflexia, choreoathetosis.

Gastro-intestinal Disorders: *Frequent:* anorexia, reduced salivation*. *Infrequent:* flatulence, diarrhea, increased appetite, stomatitis, melena, dysphagia, hemorrhoids, gastritis. *Rare:* fecal incontinence, eructation, gastroesophageal reflux, gastroenteritis, esophagitis, tongue discoloration, cholelithiasis, tongue edema, diverticulitis, gingivitis, discolored feces, GI hemorrhage, hematemesis.

Body as a Whole/General Disorders: *Frequent:* fatigue. *Infrequent:* edema, rigors, malaise, influenza-like symptoms. *Rare:* pallor, enlarged abdomen, allergic reaction, ascites, sarcoidosis, flushing.

Respiratory System Disorders: *Infrequent:* hyperventilation, bronchospasm, pneumonia, stridor. *Rare:* asthma, increased sputum, aspiration.

Skin and Appendage Disorders: *Frequent:* increased pigmentation*, photosensitivity*. *Infrequent:* increased sweating, acne, decreased sweating, alopecia, hyperkeratosis, pruritus, skin exfoliation. *Rare:* bullous eruption, skin ulceration, aggravated psoriasis, furunculosis, verruca, dermatitis lichenoid, hypertrichosis, genital pruritus, urticaria.

Cardiovascular Disorders: *Infrequent:* palpitation, hypertension, hypotension, AV block, myocardial infarction. *Rare:* ventricular tachycardia, angina pectoris, premature atrial contractions, T wave inversions, ventricular extrasystoles, ST depression, myocarditis.

Vision Disorders: *Infrequent:* abnormal accommodation, xerophthalmia. *Rare:* diplopia, eye pain, blepharitis, photopsia, photophobia, abnormal lacrimation.

Metabolic and Nutritional Disorders: *Infrequent:* hyponatremia, weight increase, creatine phosphokinase increase, thirst, weight decrease, diabetes mellitus. *Rare:* decreased serum iron, cachexia, dehydration, hypokalemia, hypoproteinemia, hyperphosphatemia, hypertriglyceridemia, hyperuricemia, hypoglycemia.

Urinary System Disorders: *Frequent:* polyuria/polydipsia*. *Infrequent:* urinary incontinence, hematuria, dysuria. *Rare:* urinary retention, cystitis, renal insufficiency.

Musculo-skeletal System Disorders: *Infrequent:* myalgia. *Rare:* arthrosis, synostosis, bursitis, arthritis, skeletal pain.

Reproductive Disorders, Female: *Frequent:* menorrhagia*, orgastic dysfunction*, dry vagina*. *Infrequent:* nonpuerperal lactation, amenorrhea, female breast pain, leukorrhea, mastitis, dysmenorrhea, female perineal pain, intermenstrual bleeding, vaginal hemorrhage.

Liver and Biliary System Disorders: *Infrequent:* increased SGOT, increased SGPT. *Rare:* hepatic failure, cholestatic hepatitis, cholecystitis, cholelithiasis, hepatitis, hepatocellular damage.

Platelet, Bleeding and Clotting Disorders: *Infrequent:* epistaxis, purpura. *Rare:* hemorrhage, superficial phlebitis, thrombophlebitis, thrombocytopenia.

Hearing and Vestibular Disorders: *Rare:* tinnitus, hyperacusis, decreased hearing.

Red Blood Cell Disorders: *Infrequent:* anemia, hypochromic anemia. *Rare:* normocytic anemia.

Reproductive Disorders, Male: *Frequent:* erectile dysfunction*. *Infrequent:* ejaculation failure.

White Cell and Resistance Disorders: *Rare:* leukocytosis, lymphadenopathy, leucopenia, Pelger-Huet anomaly.

Endocrine Disorders: *Rare:* gynecomastia, male breast pain, antidiuretic hormone disorder.

Special Senses: *Rare:* bitter taste.

* Incidence based on elicited reports.

Post introduction Reports: Adverse events reported since market introduction which were temporally (but not necessarily causally) related to RISPERDAL® therapy, include the following: anaphylactic reaction, angioedema, apnea, atrial fibrillation, cerebrovascular disorder, diabetes mellitus aggravated, including diabetic ketoacidosis intestinal obstruction, jaundice, mania, pancreatitis, Parkinson's disease aggravated, pulmonary embolism. There have been rare reports of sudden death and/or cardiopulmonary arrest in patients receiving RISPERDAL®. A causal relationship with RISPERDAL® has not been established. It is important to note that sudden and unexpected death may occur in psychotic patients whether they remain untreated or whether they are treated with other antipsychotic drugs.

DRUG ABUSE AND DEPENDENCE

Controlled Substance Class: RISPERDAL® (risperidone) is not a controlled substance.

Physical and Psychologic Dependence: RISPERDAL® has not been systematically studied in animals or humans for its potential for abuse, tolerance or physical dependence. While the clinical trials did not reveal any tendency for any drug-seeking behavior, these observations were not systematic and it is not possible to predict on the basis of this limited experience the extent to which a CNS-active drug will be misused, diverted and/or abused once marketed. Consequently, patients should be evaluated carefully for a history of drug abuse, and such patients should be observed closely for signs of RISPERDAL® misuse or abuse (e.g., development of tolerance, increases in dose, drug-seeking behavior).

OVERDOSAGE

Human Experience: Premarketing experience included eight reports of acute RISPERDAL® overdosage with estimated doses ranging from 20 to 300 mg and no fatalities. In general, reported signs and symptoms were those resulting from an exaggeration of the drug's known pharmacological effects, i.e., drowsiness and sedation, tachycardia and hypotension, and extrapyramidal symptoms. One case, involving an estimated overdose of 240 mg, was associated with hyponatremia, hypokalemia, prolonged QT, and widened QRS. Another case, involving an estimated overdose of 36 mg, was associated with a seizure. Postmarketing experience includes reports of acute RISPERDAL® overdosage, with estimated doses of up to 360 mg. In general, the most frequently reported signs and symptoms are those resulting from an exaggeration of the drug's known pharmacological effects, i.e., drowsiness, sedation, tachycardia and hypotension. Other adverse events reported since market introduction which were temporally, (but not necessarily causally) related to RISPERDAL® overdose, include prolonged QT interval, convulsions, cardiopulmonary arrest, and rare fatality associated with multiple drug overdose.

Management of Overdosage: In case of acute overdosage, establish and maintain an airway and ensure adequate oxygenation and ventilation. Gastric lavage (after intubation, if patient is unconscious) and administration of activated charcoal together with a laxative should be considered. The possibility of obtundation, seizures or dystonic reaction of the head and neck following overdose may create a risk of aspiration with induced emesis. Cardiovascular monitoring should commence immediately and should include continuous electrocardiographic monitoring to detect possible arrhythmias. If antiarrhythmic therapy is administered, disopyramide, procainamide and quinidine carry a theoretical hazard of QT-prolonging effects that might be additive to those of risperidone. Similarly, it is reasonable to expect that the alpha-blocking properties of bretylium might be additive to those of risperidone, resulting in problematic hypotension.

There is no specific antidote to RISPERDAL®. Therefore appropriate supportive measures should be instituted. The possibility of multiple drug involvement should be considered. Hypotension and circulatory collapse should be treated with appropriate measures such as intravenous fluids and/or sympathomimetic agents (epinephrine and dopamine should not be used, since beta stimulation may worsen hypotension in the setting of risperidone-induced alpha blockade). In cases of severe extrapyramidal symptoms, anticholinergic medication should be administered. Close medical supervision and monitoring should continue until the patient recovers.

DOSAGE AND ADMINISTRATION

Usual Initial Dose: RISPERDAL® (risperidone) can be administered on either a BID or a QD schedule. In early clinical trials, RIPSERDAL® was generally administered at 1 mg BID initially, with increases in increments of 1 mg BID on the second and third day, as tolerated, to a target dose of 3 mg BID by the third day. Subsequent controlled trials have indicated that total daily risperidone doses of up to 8 mg on a QD regimen are also safe and effective. However, regardless of which regimen is employed, in some patients a slower titration may be medically appropriate. Further dosage adjustments, if indicated, should generally occur at intervals of not less than 1 week, since steady state for the active metabolite would not be achieved for approximately 1 week in the typical patient. When dosage adjustments are necessary, small increments/decrements of 1–2 mg are recommended.

Continued on next page

Risperdal—Cont.

Antipsychotic efficacy was demonstrated in a dose range of 4 to 16 mg/day in the clinical trials supporting effectiveness of RISPERDAL®, however, maximal effect was generally seen in a range of 4 to 8 mg/day. Doses above 6 mg/day for BID dosing were not demonstrated to be more efficacious than lower doses, were associated with more extrapyramidal symptoms and other adverse effects, and are not generally recommended. In a single study supporting QD dosing, the efficacy results were generally stronger for 8 mg than for 4 mg. The safety of doses above 16 mg/day has not been evaluated in clinical trials.

Pediatric Use: Safety and effectiveness in pediatric patients have not been established.

Dosage in Special Populations: The recommended initial dose is 0.5 mg BID in patients who are elderly or debilitated, patients with severe renal or hepatic impairment, and patients either predisposed to hypotension or for whom hypotension would pose a risk. Dosage increases in these patients should be in increments of no more than 0.5 mg BID. Increases to dosages above 1.5 mg BID should generally occur at intervals of at least 1 week. In some patients, slower titration may be medically appropriate.

Elderly or debilitated patients, and patients with renal impairment, may have less ability to eliminate RISPERDAL® than normal adults. Patients with impaired hepatic function may have increases in the free fraction of the risperidone, possibly resulting in an enhanced effect (See CLINICAL PHARMACOLOGY). Patients with a predisposition to hypotensive reactions or for whom such reactions would pose a particular risk likewise need to be titrated cautiously and carefully monitored (See PRECAUTIONS).

If a once-a-day dosing regimen in the elderly or debilitated patient is being considered, it is recommended that the patient be titrated on a twice-a-day regimen for 2–3 days at the target dose. Subsequent switches to a once-a-day dosing regimen can be done thereafter.

Maintenance Therapy: While there is no body of evidence available to answer the question of how long the patient treated with RISPERDAL® should remain on it, the effectiveness of maintenance treatment is well established for many other antipsychotic drugs. It is recommended that responding patients be continued on RISPERDAL®, but at the lowest dose needed to maintain remission. Patients should be periodically reassessed to determine the need for maintenance treatment.

Reinitiation of Treatment in Patients Previously Discontinued: Although there are no data to specifically address reinitiation of treatment, it is recommended that when restarting patients who have had an interval off RISPERDAL®, the initial titration schedule should be followed.

Switching from Other Antipsychotics: There are no systematically collected data to specifically address switching from other antipsychotics to RISPERDAL®, or concerning concomitant administration with other antipsychotics. While immediate discontinuation of the previous antipsychotic treatment may be acceptable for some patients, more gradual discontinuation may be most appropriate for other patients. In all cases, the period of overlapping antipsychotic administration should be minimized. When switching patients from depot antipsychotics, if medically appropriate, initiate RISPERDAL® therapy in place of the next scheduled injection. The need for continuing existing EPS medication should be reevaluated periodically.

HOW SUPPLIED

RISPERDAL® (risperidone) tablets are imprinted "JANSSEN", and "R" and the strength "1", "2", "3", or "4".

1 mg white, scored, tablet: bottles of 60 NDC 50458-300-06, blister pack of 100 NDC 50458-300-01, bottles of 500 NDC 50458-300-50

2 mg orange tablet: bottles of 60 NDC 50458-320-06, blister pack of 100 NDC 50458-320-01, bottles of 500 NDC 50458-320-50

3 mg yellow tablet: bottles of 60 NDC 50458-330-06, blister pack of 100 NDC 50458-330-01, bottles of 500 NDC 50458-330-50

4 mg green tablet: bottles of 60 NDC 50458-350-06, blister pack of 100 NDC 50458-350-01.

RISPERDAL® (risperidone) 1 mg/mL oral solution (NDC 50458-305-03) is supplied in 30mL bottles with a calibrated (in milligrams and milliliters) pipette. The minimum calibrated volume is 0.25 mL, while the maximum calibrated volume is 3 mL.

Patient Instructions (including illustrations) for using the RISPERDAL® (risperidone) calibrated dispensing-pipette are provided. Tests indicate that RISPERDAL® (risperidone) oral solution is compatible in the following beverages: water, coffee, orange juice and low-fat milk; it is NOT compatible with either cola or tea, however.

STORAGE AND HANDLING - RISPERDAL® tablets should be stored at controlled room temperature (59°–77°F/15°–25°C) away from children, and should be protected from light and moisture.

RISPERDAL® 1 mg/mL oral solution should be stored at controlled room temperature (59°–77°F/15°–25°C) away from children, and should be protected from light and freezing.

US Patent 4,804,663

Revised June 1998

JANSSEN PHARMACEUTICA

Titusville, NJ 08560

Shown in Product Identification Guide, page 317

SPORANOX ℞

[*spər 'ah-näks"*]

(Itraconazole)

100 mg capsules

> **WARNING:** Coadministration of terfenadine, astemizole, and cisapride with SPORANOX® (itraconazole) Capsules or Oral Solution is contraindicated. SPORANOX® is a potent inhibitor of the cytochrome P450 3A enzyme system and may raise plasma concentrations of drugs metabolized by this pathway. Serious cardiovascular events, including death, ventricular tachycardia, and torsades de pointes have occurred in patients taking itraconazole concomitantly with terfenadine or cisapride, which are metabolized by the cytochrome P450 3A system. See CONTRAINDICATIONS, WARNINGS, and PRECAUTIONS: DRUG INTERACTIONS for more information.

DESCRIPTION

SPORANOX® is the brand name for itraconazole, a synthetic triazole antifungal agent. Itraconazole is a 1:1:1:1 racemic mixture of four diastereomers (two enantiomeric pairs), each possessing three chiral centers. It may be represented by the following nomenclature:

(±)-1-[(R*)-sec-butyl]-4-[p-[4-[p-[[(2R*,4S*)-2- (2,4-dichlorophenyl)-2-(1H-1,2,4-triazol-1-ylmethyl)- 1,3-dioxolan-4-yl]methoxy]phenyl]-1-piperazinyl]phenyl] -Δ^{2}-1,2,4-triazolin-5-one mixture with (±)-1 -[(R*)-sec-butyl]-4-[p-[4- [p-[[(2S*,4R*)-2-(2,4-dichlorophenyl)-2-(1H-1,2,4-triazol-1-ylmethyl)-1,3-dioxolan-4-yl]methoxy]phenyl]-1- piperazinyl]-phenyl]-Δ^{2}-1,2,4-triazolin-5-one

or

(±)-1-[(RS)-sec-butyl]-4-[p-[4-[p-[[(2R,4S)-2-(2,4-dichlorophenyl)-2-(1H-1,2,4-triazol-1-ylmethyl)-1,3-dioxolan-4-yl-]methoxy]phenyl]-1-piperazinyl]phenyl]-Δ^{2}-1,2,4-triazolin-5-one

Itraconazole has a molecular formula of $C_{35}H_{38}Cl_2N_8O_4$ and a molecular weight of 705.64. It is a white to slightly yellowish powder. It is insoluble in water, very slightly soluble in alcohols, and freely soluble in dichloromethane. It has a pKa of 3.70 (based on extrapolation of values obtained from methanolic solutions) and a log (n-octanol/water) partition coefficient of 5.66 at pH 8.1.

SPORANOX® Capsules contains 100 mg of itraconazole coated on sugar spheres. Inactive ingredients are gelatin, hydroxypropyl methylcellulose, polyethylene glycol (PEG) 20,000, starch, sucrose, titanium dioxide, FD&C Blue No. 1, FD&C Blue No. 2, D&C Red No. 22 and D&C Red No. 28.

MICROBIOLOGY

Mechanism of Action: *In vitro* studies have demonstrated that itraconazole inhibits the cytochrome P-450-dependent synthesis of ergosterol, which is a vital component of fungal cell membranes.

Activity in vitro and in vivo: Itraconazole exhibits *in vitro* activity against *Blastomyces dermatitidis, Histoplasma capsulatum, Histoplasma duboisii, Aspergillus flavus, Aspergillus fumigatus, Candida albicans* and *Cryptococcus neoformans.* Itraconazole also exhibits varying *in vitro* activity against *Sporothrix schenckii,* Trichophyton spp., *Candida krusei* and other Candida spp. The bioactive metabolite, hydroxyitraconazole, has not been evaluated against *Histoplasma capsulatum* and *Blastomyces dermatitidis.* Correlation between *in vitro* minimum inhibitory concentration (MIC) results and clinical outcome has yet to be established for azole antifungal agents.

Itraconazole administered orally was active in a variety of animal models of fungal infection using standard laboratory strains of fungi. Fungistatic activity has been demonstrated against disseminated fungal infections caused by *Blastomyces dermatitidis, Histoplasma duboisii, Aspergillus fumigatus, Coccidioides immitis, Cryptococcus neoformans, Paracoccidioides brasiliensis, Sporothrix schenckii, Trichophyton rubrum* and *Trichophyton mentagrophytes.*

Itraconazole administered at 2.5 mg/kg and 5.0 mg/kg via the oral and parenteral routes increased survival rates and sterilized organ systems in normal and immunosuppressed guinea pigs with disseminated *Aspergillus fumigatus* infections. Oral itraconazole administered daily at 40 mg/kg and 80 mg/kg increased survival rates in normal rabbits with disseminated disease and immunosuppressed rats with pulmonary *Aspergillus fumigatus* infection, respectively. Itraconazole has demonstrated antifungal activity in a variety of animal models infected with *Candida albicans* and other Candida species.

In vivo studies suggest that the activity of amphotericin B may be suppressed by azole antifungal therapy. As with other azoles, itraconazole inhibits the ^{14}C-demethylation step in the synthesis of ergosterol, a cell wall component of fungi. Ergosterol is the active site for amphotericin B. In one study the antifungal activity of amphotericin B against *Aspergillus fumigatus* infections in mice was inhibited by ketoconazole therapy. The clinical significance of test results obtained in this study is unknown.

Several *in vitro* studies have reported that some fungal clinical isolates, including Candida species, with reduced susceptibility to one azole antifungal agent may also be less susceptible to other azole derivatives. The finding of cross-resistance is dependent upon a number of factors, including the species evaluated, its clinical history, the particular azole compounds compared and the type of susceptibility test that is performed. The relevance of these *in vitro* susceptibility data to clinical outcome remains to be elucidated.

CLINICAL PHARMACOLOGY

Pharmacokinetics and Metabolism: NOTE: The plasma concentrations reported below were measured by high performance liquid chromatography (HPLC) specific for itraconazole. When itraconazole in plasma is measured by a bioassay, values reported are approximately 3.3 times higher than those obtained by HPLC due to the presence of the bioactive metabolite, hydroxyitraconazole. (See MICROBIOLOGY.)

The pharmacokinetics of itraconazole after intravenous administration and its absolute oral bioavailability from an oral solution were studied in a randomized crossover study using six healthy male volunteers. The observed absolute oral bioavailability of itraconazole was 55%.

The oral bioavailability of itraconazole is maximal when SPORANOX® (itraconazole) Capsules are taken with a full meal. The pharmacokinetics of itraconazole were studied using six healthy male volunteers who received, in a crossover design, single 100 mg doses of itraconazole as a polyethylene glycol capsule, with or without a full meal. The same six volunteers also received 50 mg or 200 mg with a full meal in a crossover design. In this study, only itraconazole plasma concentrations were measured. Presented in the table below are the respective pharmacokinetic parameters for itraconazole:

	50 mg (fed)	100 mg (fed)	100 mg (fasted)	200 mg (fed)
C_{max} (ng/mL)	45 ± 16*	132 ± 67	38 ± 20	289 ± 100
T_{max} (hours)	3.2 ± 1.3	4.0 ± 1.1	3.3 ± 1.0	4.7 ± 1.4
$AUC_{0-\infty}$ (ng·h/mL)	567 ± 264	1899 ± 838	722 ± 289	5211 ± 2116

*mean ± standard deviation

Doubling the SPORANOX® dose results in approximately a three-fold increase in the itraconazole plasma concentrations.

Values given in the table below represent data from a crossover pharmacokinetics study in which 27 healthy male volunteers each took a single 200 mg dose of SPORANOX® Capsules with or without a full meal:

	Itraconazole		Hydroxyitraconazole	
	Fed	Fasted	Fed	Fasted
C_{max} (ng/mL)	239 ± 85*	140 ± 65	397 ± 103	286 ± 101
T_{max} (hours)	4.5 ± 1.1	3.9 ± 1.0	5.1 ± 1.6	4.5 ± 1.1
$AUC_{0-\infty}$ (ng·h/mL)	3423 ± 1154	2094 ± 905	7978 ± 2648	5191 ± 2489
$t_{1/2}$ (hours)	21 ± 5	21 ± 7	12 ± 3	12 ± 3

*mean ± standard deviation

Absorption of itraconazole under fasted conditions in individuals with relative or absolute achlorhydria, such as patients with AIDS or volunteers taking gastric acid secretion suppressors (e.g., H_2inhibitors), was increased when SPORANOX® Capsules were administered with a cola beverage. Eighteen males with AIDS received single 200 mg doses of SPORANOX® Capsules under fasted conditions with 8 ounces of water or 8 ounces of a cola beverage in a crossover design. The absorption of itraconazole was increased when SPORANOX® Capsules were coadministered with a cola beverage with AUC_{0-24} and C_{max} increasing 75 ± 121% and 95 ± 128%, respectively. Thirty healthy males received sin-

gle 200 mg doses of SPORANOX® Capsules under fasted conditions either 1) with water; 2) with water, after ranitidine 150 mg b.i.d. for 3 days; or 3) with cola, after ranitidine 150 mg b.i.d. for 3 days. When SPORANOX® Capsules were administered after ranitidine pretreatment, itraconazole was absorbed to a lesser extent than when SPORANOX® Capsules were administered alone, with decreases in AUC_{0-24} and C_{max} of 39 ± 37% and 42 ± 39%, respectively. When SPORANOX® Capsules were administered with cola after ranitidine pretreatment, itraconazole absorption was comparable to that observed when SPORANOX® Capsules were administered alone.

Steady-state concentrations were reached within 15 days following oral doses of 50–400 mg daily. Values given in the table below are data at steady-state from a pharmacokinetics study in which 27 healthy male volunteers took 200 mg SPORANOX® Capsules b.i.d. (with a full meal) for 15 days:

	Itraconazole	Hydroxyitraconazole
C_{max} (ng/mL)	2282 ± 514*	3488 ± 742
C_{min} (ng/mL)	1855 ± 535	3349 ± 761
T_{max} (hours)	4.6 ± 1.8	3.4 ± 3.4
AUC_{0-12h} (ng·h/mL)	22569 ± 5375	38572 ± 8450
$t_{1/2}$ (hours)	64 ± 32	56 ± 24

*mean ± standard deviation

Results of the pharmacokinetics study suggest that itraconazole may undergo saturation metabolism with multiple dosing.

The plasma protein binding of itraconazole is 99.8% and that of hydroxyitraconazole is 99.5%. Following intravenous administration, the volume of distribution of itraconazole averaged 796 ± 185 L.

Itraconazole is extensively metabolized resulting in the formation of several metabolites including hydroxyitraconazole, the major metabolite. Results of a pharmacokinetics study suggest that itraconzole may undergo saturable metabolism with multiple dosing. Fecal excretion of the parent drug varies between 3–18% of the dose. Renal excretion of the parent drug is less than 0.03% of the dose. About 40% of the dose is excreted as inactive metabolites in the urine. No single excreted metabolite represents more than 5% of a dose. Itraconazole total plasma clearance averaged 381 ± 95 mL/min following intravenous administration.

Special populations:

Renal Insufficiency: Plasma concentrations of itraconazole in patients with mild to severe renal insufficiency, including patients receiving hemodialysis, were comparable to those obtained in healthy subjects.

Hepatic Insufficiency: The effect of hepatic impairment on plasma concentrations of itraconazole is unknown. It is recommended that patients with hepatic impairment be carefully monitored when taking itraconazole.

INDICATIONS AND USAGE

SPORANOX® (itraconazole) Capsules are indicated for the treatment of the following fungal infections in immunocompromised and non-immunocompromised patients:

1. Blastomycosis, pulmonary and extrapulmonary;
2. Histoplasmosis, including chronic cavitary pulmonary disease and disseminated, non-meningeal histoplasmosis; and
3. Aspergillosis, pulmonary and extrapulmonary, in patients who are intolerant of or who are refractory to amphotericin B therapy.

SPORANOX® Capsules are also indicated for the treatment of the following fungal infections in non-immunocompromised patients:

1. Onychomycosis of the toenail with or without fingernail involvement due to dermatophytes (tinea unguium);
2. Onychomycosis of the fingernail due to dermatophytes (tinea unguium).

Specimens for fungal cultures and other relevant laboratory studies (wet mount, histopathology, serology) should be obtained prior to therapy to isolate and identify causative organisms. Therapy may be instituted before the results of the cultures and other laboratory studies are known; however, once these results become available, anti-infective therapy should be adjusted accordingly.

Description of Clinical Studies:

Blastomycosis: Analyses were conducted on data from two open-label, non-concurrently controlled studies (n=73 combined) in patients with normal or abnormal immune status. The median dose was 200 mg/day. A response for most signs and symptoms was observed within the first two weeks, and all cleared between 3 and 6 months. Results of these two studies demonstrated substantial evidence of the effectiveness of itraconazole, for the treatment of blastomycosis, compared to the natural history of untreated cases.

Histoplasmosis: Analyses were conducted on data from two open-label, non-concurrently controlled studies (n=34 combined) in patients with normal or abnormal immune status (not including HIV-infected patients). The median dose was 200 mg/day. A response for most signs and symptoms was observed within the first 2 weeks, and all cleared between 3 and 12 months. Results of these two studies demonstrated substantial evidence of the effectiveness of itraconazole, for the treatment of histoplasmosis, compared to the natural history of untreated cases.

Histoplasmosis in HIV-infected patients: Data from a small number of HIV-infected patients suggested that the response rate of histoplasmosis in HIV-infected patients is similar to non-HIV-infected patients. The clinical course of histoplasmosis in HIV-infected patients is more severe and usually requires maintenance therapy to prevent relapse.

Aspergillosis: Analyses were conducted on data from an open-label, "single-patient-use" protocol designed to make itraconazole available in the U.S. for patients who either failed or were intolerant to amphotericin B therapy (n=190). The findings were corroborated by two smaller open-label studies (n=31 combined) in the same patient population. Most adult patients were treated with a daily dose of 200 to 400 mg with a median duration of 3 months. Results of these studies demonstrated substantial evidence of effectiveness of itraconazole, as a second-line therapy for the treatment of aspergillosis, compared to the natural history of the disease in patients who either failed or were intolerant to amphotericin B therapy.

Onychomycosis of the toenail: Analyses were conducted on data from three double-blind, placebo-controlled studies (n=214 total; 110 given SPORANOX® Capsules) in which patients with onychomycosis of the toenails received 200 mg of SPORANOX® Capsules q.d. for 12 consecutive weeks. Results of these studies demonstrated mycological cure, defined as simultaneous occurrence of negative KOH plus negative culture, in 54% of patients. Thirty-five percent (35%) of patients were considered an overall success (mycological cure plus clear or minimal nail involvement with significantly decreased signs) and 14% of patients demonstrated mycological cure plus clinical cure (clearance of all signs, with or without residual nail deformity). The mean time to overall success was approximately 10 months. Twenty-one (21) percent of the overall success group had a relapse (worsening of the global score or conversion of KOH or culture from negative to positive).

Onychomycosis of the fingernail: Analyses were conducted on data from a double-blind, placebo-controlled study (n=73 total; 37 given SPORANOX® Capsules) in which patients with onychomycosis of the fingernails received two pulses of 200 mg of SPORANOX® Capsules b.i.d. for one week separated by a 3-week period without SPORANOX®. Results demonstrated mycological cure in 61% of patients. Fifty-six percent (56%) of patients were considered an overall success and 47% of patients demonstrated mycological cure plus clinical cure. The mean time to overall success was approximately 5 months. None of the patients who achieved overall success relapsed.

CONTRAINDICATIONS

Coadministration of SPORANOX® (itraconazole) Capsules or Oral Solution with certain drugs metabolized by the P450 3A enzyme system may result in increased plasma concentrations of those drugs leading to potentially serious and/or life-threatening adverse events. Terfenadine, astemizole, oral triazolam, oral midazolam and cisapride are specifically contraindicated with SPORANOX®. HMG-CoA reductase inhibitors metabolized by this system (e.g., lovastatin and simvastatin) should also be discontinued during SPORANOX® therapy. (See PRECAUTIONS: DRUG INTERACTIONS.)

SPORANOX® should not be administered for the treatment of onychomycosis to pregnant patients or to women contemplating pregnancy.

SPORANOX® is contraindicated in patients who have shown hypersensitivity to the drug or its excipients. There is no information regarding cross hypersensitivity between itraconazole and other azole antifungal agents. Caution should be used in prescribing SPORANOX® to patients with hypersensitivity to other azoles.

WARNINGS

SPORANOX® (itraconazole) Capsules and SPORANOX® Oral Solution should not be used interchangeably. This is because drug exposure is greater with the Oral Solution than with the Capsules when the same dose of drug is given. Additionally, the topical effects of mucosal exposure may be different between the two formulations. Only the Oral Solution has been demonstrated effective for oral and/or esophageal candidiasis.

Hepatitis: There have been rare cases of reversible idiosyncratic hepatitis reported among patients taking SPORANOX® (itraconazole) Capsules. SPORANOX® has been associated with rare cases of serious hepatotoxicity, including fatalities, primarily in patients with serious underlying medical conditions taking multiple medications. The causal association with SPORANOX® is uncertain. If clinical signs and symptoms develop that are consistent with liver disease and may be attributable to itraconazole, SPORANOX® should be discontinued.

Cardiac Dysrhythmias: There have been rare cases of life-threatening cardiac dysrhythmia and death reported in patients receiving terfenadine and itraconazole. Coadministration of terfenadine, astemizole and cisapride with SPORANOX® is contraindicated. (See BOX WARNING, CONTRAINDICATIONS, and PRECAUTIONS: DRUG INTERACTIONS.)

PRECAUTIONS

General: Hepatic enzyme test values should be monitored in patients with preexisting hepatic function abnormalities. Hepatic enzyme test values should be monitored periodically in all patients receiving continuous treatment for more than one month or at any time a patient develops signs or symptoms suggestive of liver dysfunction.

SPORANOX® (itraconazole) Capsules should be administered after a full meal. (See CLINICAL PHARMACOLOGY: PHARMACOKINETICS and METABOLISM.)

Under fasted conditions, itraconazole absorption was decreased in the presence of decreased gastric acidity. The absorption of itraconazole may be decreased with the concomitant administration of antacids or gastric acid secretion suppressors. Studies conducted under fasted conditions demonstrated that administration with 8 ounces of a cola beverage resulted in increased absorption of itraconazole in AIDS patients with relative or absolute achlorhydria. This increase relative to the effects of a full meal is unknown. (See CLINICAL PHARMACOLOGY: PHARMACOKINETICS and METABOLISM.)

Information for patients: Patients should be aware that SPORANOX® (itraconazole) Capsules is a different preparation than SPORANOX® Oral Solution, and these should not be used interchangeably. This is because drug exposure is greater with the Oral Solution than with the Capsules when the same dose of drug is given. Additionally, the topical effects of mucosal exposure may be different between the two formulations. Only the Oral Solution has been demonstrated effective for oral and/or esophageal candidiasis.

Patients should be instructed to take SPORANOX® Capsules with a full meal.

Patients should be instructed to report any signs and symptoms that may suggest liver dysfunction so that the appropriate laboratory testing can be done. Such signs and symptoms may include unusual fatigue, anorexia, nausea and/or vomiting, jaundice, dark urine or pale stool.

Patients should be instructed to contact their physician before taking any concomitant medications with itraconazole to insure there are no potential drug interactions.

Drug interactions: Both itraconazole and its major metabolite, hydroxyitraconazole, are inhibitors of the cytochrome P450 3A enzyme system. Coadministration of SPORANOX® and drugs primarily metabolized by the cytochrome P450 3A enzyme system may result in increased plasma concentrations of the other drug that could increase or prolong both its therapeutic and adverse effects. Therefore, unless otherwise specified, concomitant medications metabolized by the P450 3A enzyme system should be discontinued as medically indicated.

Table of Selected Drugs That Are Predicted to Have Plasma Concentrations Increased by Itraconazole+

Anticoagulants: warfarin
Antihistamines: terfenadine*, astemizole*
Anti-HIV protease inhibitors: ritonavir, indinavir
Antineoplastic agents: vinca alkaloids
Benzodiazepines: midazolam*†, triazolam*, diazepam
Calcium channel blockers: dihydropyridines
Cholesterol-lowering agents: lovastatin*, simvastatin*
GI motility agents: cisapride*
Immunosuppressive agents: cyclosporine, tacrolimus
Steroids: methylprednisolone
Other: digoxin, quinidine

\+ This table is not all inclusive.

* Specifically contraindicated with SPORANOX® based on clinical and/or pharmacokinetics studies (see WARNINGS and below).

† See paragraph below on *Benzodiazepines* for information on parenteral administration.

Table of Selected Drugs That Are Predicted to Decrease Itraconazole Plasma Concentrations+‡

Anticonvulsants: phenytoin, phenobarbital, carbamazepine
Antimycobacterial agents: isoniazid, rifampin, rifabutin

\+ This table is not all inclusive.

‡ SPORANOX® may not be effective due to decreased itraconazole plasma concentrations in patients using these agents concomitantly.

Anticoagulants: It has been reported that SPORANOX® enhances the anticoagulant effect of coumarin-like drugs. Therefore, prothrombin time should be carefully monitored in patients receiving SPORANOX® and coumarin-like drugs simultaneously.

Continued on next page

Sporanox Capsules—Cont.

Anticonvulsants: Reduced plasma concentrations of itraconazole were reported when SPORANOX® was coadministered with phenytoin. The physician is advised to monitor the plasma concentrations of itraconazole when phenytoin is taken concurrently, and to increase the dose of SPORANOX® if necessary.

Antihistamines: Coadministration of terfenadine with SPORANOX® has led to elevated plasma concentrations of terfenadine, resulting in rare instances of life-threatening cardiac dysrhythmia and death. Coadministration of astemizole with SPORANOX® has led to elevated plasma concentrations of astemizole and desmethylastemizole which may prolong the QT intervals. Therefore, concomitant administration of SPORANOX® with astemizole is contraindicated. (See BOX WARNING, CONTRAINDICATIONS, and WARNINGS.)

Anti-HIV protease inhibitors: Coadministration of SPORANOX® with protease inhibitors primarily metabolized by the cytochrome P450 3A enzyme system, such as ritonavir or indinavir, may result in changes in plasma concentrations of both drugs. Caution is advised when these drugs are used concomitantly.

Anti-HIV reverse transcriptase inhibitors: The results from a study in which eight HIV-infected individuals were treated with zidovudine, 8 ± 0.4 mg/kg/day, showed that the pharmacokinetics of zidovudine were not affected during concomitant administration of SPORANOX® Capsules, 100 mg b.i.d. Other agents have not been studied.

Antimycobacterial agents: Plasma concentrations of azole antifungal agents are reduced when given concurrently with isoniazid or rifampin. Alternative antifungal therapy should be considered if isoniazid or rifampin therapy is necessary. A similar effect may be expected with rifabutin.

Antineoplastic agents: The metabolism of vinca alkaloids may be inhibited by itraconazole. Therefore, patients receiving SPORANOX® concomitantly with vinca alkaloids should be monitored for an increase and/or prolongation of the effects of the latter drug product, including adverse effects such as peripheral neuropathy and ileus, and the dose of the vinca alkaloid should be adjusted appropriately.

Benzodiazepines: Coadministration of SPORANOX® with oral midazolam or triazolam has resulted in elevated plasma concentrations of the latter two drugs. This may potentiate and prolong hypnotic and sedative effects. These agents should not be used in patients treated with SPORANOX®. If midazolam is administered parenterally, special precaution and patient monitoring is required since the sedative effect may be prolonged. (See CONTRAINDICATIONS.)

Calcium channel blockers: Edema has been reported in patients concomitantly receiving SPORANOX® and dihydropyridine calcium channel blockers. Appropriate dosage adjustments may be necessary.

Cholesterol-lowering agents: Human pharmacokinetic data indicate that SPORANOX® inhibits the metabolism of lovastatin resulting in significantly elevated plasma concentrations of lovastatin or lovastatin acid, which have been associated with rhabdomyolysis. Use of HMG-CoA reductase inhibitors metabolized by the P450 3A enzyme system, such as lovastatin or simvastatin, should be temporarily discontinued during SPORANOX® therapy. (See CONTRAINDICATIONS.)

Digoxin: Coadministration of SPORANOX® and digoxin has led to increased plasma concentrations of digoxin. Digoxin concentrations should be monitored at the initiation of SPORANOX® therapy and frequently thereafter, and the dose of digoxin should be adjusted appropriately.

GI motility agents: Human pharmacokinetic data indicate that oral ketoconazole potently inhibits the metabolism of cisapride resulting in significantly elevated plasma concentrations of cisapride. Data suggest that coadministration of oral ketoconazole and cisapride can result in prolongation of the QT interval on the ECG. *In vitro* data suggest that itraconazole also markedly inhibits the biotransformation system mainly responsible for the metabolism of cisapride; therefore, concomitant administration of SPORANOX® with cisapride is contraindicated. (See BOX WARNING, CONTRAINDICATIONS, and WARNINGS.)

H_2 antagonists: Reduced plasma concentrations of itraconazole were reported when SPORANOX® Capsules were coadministered with H_2 antagonists.

Immunosuppressive agents: Coadministration of SPORANOX® and cyclosporine or tacrolimus has led to increased plasma concentrations of the latter two agents. Cyclosporine and tacrolimus concentrations should be monitored at the initiation of SPORANOX® therapy and frequently thereafter, and the dose of cyclosporine or tacrolimus should be adjusted appropriately.

Oral hypoglycemic agents: Severe hypoglycemia has been reported in patients concomitantly receiving azole antifungal agents and oral hypoglycemic agents. Blood glucose concentrations should be carefully monitored when SPORANOX® and oral hypoglycemic agents are coadministered.

Quinidine: Tinnitus and decreased hearing have been reported in patients concomitantly receiving SPORANOX® and quinidine.

Steroids: The metabolism of methylprednisolone may be inhibited by itraconazole. Therefore, patients receiving SPORANOX® concomitantly with methylprednisolone should be monitored for an increase and/or prolongation of the effects of the latter drug product, including adverse effects, and the dose of methylprednisolone should be adjusted appropriately.

Carcinogenesis, Mutagenesis and Impairment of Fertility: Itraconazole showed no evidence of carcinogenicity potential in mice treated orally for 23 months at dosage levels up to 80 mg/kg/day [approximately 10× the maximum recommended human dose (MRHD)]. Male rats treated with 25 mg/kg/day (3.1× MRHD) had a slightly increased incidence of soft tissue sarcoma. These sarcomas may have been a consequence of hypercholesterolemia, which is a response of rats, but not dogs or humans, to chronic itraconazole administration. Female rats treated with 50 mg/kg/day (6.25× MRHD) had an increased incidence of squamous cell carcinoma of the lung (2/50) as compared to the untreated group. Although the occurrence of squamous cell carcinoma in the lung is extremely uncommon in untreated rats, the increase in this study was not statistically significant.

Itraconazole produced no mutagenic effects when assayed in a DNA repair test (unscheduled DNA synthesis) in primary rat hepatocytes, in Ames tests with Salmonella typhimurium (six strains) and Escherichia coli, in the mouse lymphoma gene mutation tests, in a sex-linked recessive lethal mutation (Drosophila melanogaster) test, in chromosome aberration tests in human lymphocytes, in a cell transformation test with C3H/10T$^1/_2$ C18 mouse embryo fibroblasts cells, in a dominant lethal mutation test in male and female mice, and in micronucleus tests in mice and rats.

Itraconazole did not affect the fertility of male or female rats treated orally with dosage levels of up to 40 mg/kg/day (5x MRHD) even though parental toxicity was present at this dosage level. More severe signs of parental toxicity, including death, were present in the next higher dosage level, 160 mg/kg/day (20x MRHD).

Pregnancy: Teratogenic Effects. Pregnancy Category C: Itraconazole was found to cause a dose-related increase in maternal toxicity, embryotoxicity and teratogenicity in rats at dosage levels of approximately 40–160 mg/kg/day (5–20×MRHD) and in mice at dosage levels of approximately 80 mg/kg/day (10× MRHD). In rats, the teratogenicity consisted of major skeletal defects; in mice it consisted of encephaloceles and/or macroglossia.

There are no studies in pregnant women. SPORANOX® should be used for the treatment of systemic fungal infections in pregnancy only if the benefit outweighs the potential risk. SPORANOX® should not be administered for the treatment of onychomycosis to pregnant patients or to women contemplating pregnancy. SPORANOX® should not be administered to women of child-bearing potential for the treatment of onychomycosis unless they are taking effective measures to prevent pregnancy and the patient begins therapy on the second or third day following the onset of menses. Effective contraception should be continued throughout SPORANOX® therapy and for 2 months following the end of treatment.

Nursing Mothers: Itraconazole is excreted in human milk; therefore, the expected benefits of SPORANOX® therapy for the mother should be weighed against the potential risk from exposure of itraconazole to the infant. The U.S. Public Health Service Centers for Disease Control and Prevention advises HIV-infected women not to breast-feed to avoid potential transmission of HIV to uninfected infants.

Pediatric Use: The efficacy and safety of SPORANOX® have not been established in pediatric patients. No pharmacokinetic data on capsules are available in children. A small number of patients age 3 to 16 years have been treated with 100 mg/day of itraconazole capsules for systemic fungal infections and no serious unexpected adverse effects have been reported. SPORANOX® Oral Solution (5 mg/kg/day) has been administered to pediatric patients (n=26, age 0.5–12 years) for two weeks and no serious unexpected adverse events were reported.

In three toxicology studies using rats, itraconazole induced bone defects at dosage levels as low as 20 mg/kg/day (2.5×MRHD). The induced defects included reduced bone plate activity, thinning of the zona compacta of the large bones and increased bone fragility. At a dosage level of 80 mg/kg/day (10× MRHD) over one year or 160 mg/kg/day (20× MRHD) for six months, itraconazole induced small tooth pulp with hypocellular appearance in some rats. While no such bone toxicity has been reported in adult patients, the long term effect of itraconazole in pediatric patients is unknown.

HIV-infected Patients: Because hypochlorhydria has been reported in HIV-infected individuals, the absorption of itraconazole in these patients may be decreased.

ADVERSE REACTIONS

There have been rare cases of reversible idiosyncratic hepatitis reported among patients taking SPORANOX® (itraconazole) Capsules. SPORANOX® has been associated with rare cases of serious hepatotoxicity, including fatalities, primarily in patients with serious underlying medical conditions taking multiple medications. The causal association with SPORANOX® is uncertain. If clinical signs and symptoms develop that are consistent with liver disease and may be attributable to itraconazole, SPORANOX® should be discontinued. (See WARNINGS.)

ONYCHOMYCOSIS OF THE TOENAIL **(Continuous dosing regimen of 200 mg q.d. for 12 consecutive weeks):** Adverse events in the following table led to either temporary or permanent discontinuation of treatment:

Body System/Adverse Event	Incidence (%) (n=112)
Elevated Liver Enzymes (>2× normal range)	4%
Gastrointestinal Disorders	4%
Rash	3%
Hypertension	2%
Orthostatic Hypotension	1%
Headache	1%
Malaise	1%
Myalgia	1%
Vasculitis	1%
Vertigo	1%

Adverse events reported with an incidence of >1% in patients given SPORANOX® (200 mg q.d. for 12 consecutive weeks; n=112) in clinical trials of toenail onychomycosis were: headache (11; 10%), rhinitis (10; 9%), upper respiratory tract infection (9; 8%), sinusitis (8; 7%), injury (8; 7%), diarrhea (5; 4%), dyspepsia (5; 4%), flatulence (5; 4%), abdominal pain (4; 4%), dizziness (4; 4%), rash (4; 4%), nausea (3; 3%), cystitis (3; 3%), urinary tract infection (3; 3%), liver function abnormality (3; 3%), myalgia (3; 3%), appetite increased (2; 2%), constipation (2; 2%), gastritis (2; 2%), gastroenteritis (2; 2%), pharyngitis (2; 2%), asthenia (2; 2%), fever (2; 2%), pain (2; 2%), tremor (2; 2%), herpes zoster (2; 2%) and abnormal dreaming (2; 2%).

ONYCHOMYCOSIS OF THE FINGERNAIL **(Pulse regimen consisting of two one-week treatment periods with 200 mg b.i.d. separated by a 3-week period without SPORANOX®):**

Adverse events in the following table led to either temporary or permanent discontinuation of treatment:

Body System/Adverse Event	Incidence (%) (n=37)
Rash/pruritus	3%
Hypertriglyceridemia	3%

Adverse events reported with an incidence of >1% in patients given SPORANOX® (two one-week treatment periods with 200 mg b.i.d., separated by a 3-week period without SPORANOX®; n=37) in the clinical trial of fingernail onychomycosis were: headache (3; 8%), pruritus (2; 5%), nausea (2; 5%), rhinitis (2; 5%), rash (1; 3%), bursitis (1; 3%), anxiety (1; 3%), depression (1; 3%), constipation (1; 3%), abdominal pain (1; 3%), dyspepsia (1; 3%), ulcerative stomatitis (1; 3%), gingivitis (1; 3%), hypertriglyceridemia (1; 3%), sinusitis (1; 3%), fatigue (1; 3%), malaise (1; 3%), pain (1; 3%) and injury (1; 3%).

SYSTEMIC FUNGAL INFECTIONS:

Adverse experience data in the following table are derived from 602 patients treated for systemic fungal disease in U.S. clinical trials, who were immunocompromised or receiving multiple concomitant medications. Of these patients, treatment was discontinued in 10.5% of patients due to adverse events. The median duration before discontinuation of therapy was 81 days, with a range of 2–776 days. The table lists adverse events reported by at least 1% of patients.

Body System/Adverse Event (Incidence ≥ 1%)	Incidence (%)
Gastrointestinal disorders	
Nausea	10.6
Vomiting	5.1
Diarrhea	3.3
Abdominal pain	1.5
Anorexia	1.2
Body as a whole	
Edema	3.5
Fatigue	2.8
Fever	2.5
Malaise	1.2
Skin and appendages disorders	
Rash	8.6*
Pruritus	2.5

Central/peripheral Nervous system	
Headache	3.8
Dizziness	1.7
Psychiatric disorders	
Libido decreased	1.2
Somnolence	1.2
Cardiovascular disorders	
Hypertension	3.2
Metabolic and nutritional Disorders	
Hypokalemia	2.0
Urinary system disorders	
Albuminuria	1.2
Liver and biliary system Disorders	
Hepatic function abnormal	2.7
Reproductive disorders, male	
Impotence	1.2

* Rash tends to occur more frequently in immunocompromised patients receiving immunosuppressive medications.

Adverse events infrequently reported in all studies included: constipation, gastritis, depression, insomnia, tinnitus, menstrual disorder, adrenal insufficiency, gynecomastia and male breast pain.

In worldwide postmarketing experience with SPORANOX® Capsules, allergic reactions including rash, pruritus, urticaria, angioedema and in rare instances, anaphylaxis and Stevens-Johnson syndrome, have been reported. Marketing experiences have also included reports of elevated liver enzymes and rare hepatitis. Although the causal association with SPORANOX® is uncertain, rare alopecia, hypertriglyceridemia, neutropenia and isolated cases of neuropathy have also been reported.

OVERDOSAGE

Itraconazole is not removed by dialysis. In the event of accidental overdosage, supportive measures, including gastric lavage with sodium bicarbonate, should be employed.

There are limited data on the outcomes of patients ingesting high doses of itraconazole. In patients taking either 1000 mg of SPORANOX® (itraconazole) Oral Solution or up to 3000 mg of SPORANOX® Capsules, the adverse event profile was similar to that observed at recommended doses.

DOSAGE AND ADMINISTRATION

SPORANOX® (itraconazole) Capsules should be taken with a full meal to ensure maximal absorption.

Treatment of blastomycosis and histoplasmosis: The recommended dose is 200 mg once daily (2 capsules). If there is no obvious improvement or there is evidence of progressive fungal disease, the dose should be increased in 100 mg increments to a maximum of 400 mg daily. Doses above 200 mg per day should be given in two divided doses.

Treatment of aspergillosis: A daily dose of 200 to 400 mg is recommended.

In life-threatening situations: Although these studies did not provide for a loading dose, it is recommended, based on pharmacokinetic data, that a loading dose of 200 mg (2 capsules) t.i.d. (600 mg/day) be given for the first three days.

Treatment should be continued for a minimum of three months and until clinical parameters and laboratory tests indicate that the active fungal infection has subsided. An inadequate period of treatment may lead to recurrence of active infection. The above recommendations for the treatment of blastomycosis and histoplasmosis are based on the results of two open-label studies of patients with blastomycosis (n=73) and histoplasmosis (n=34) where results were compared to the expected outcome for untreated patients from historical controls. The recommendation for the treatment of aspergillosis is based primarily on the results of an open-label, single-patient use protocol designed to make itraconazole available in the U.S. for patients who either failed or were intolerant to amphotericin B therapy (n=190), and is supported by two smaller open-label studies (n=31 combined) in the same patient population.

Onychomycosis: Toenails with or without fingernail involvement: The recommended dose is 200 mg (2 capsules) q.d. for 12 consecutive weeks. Fingernails only: The recommended dosing regimen is two treatment pulses, each consisting of 200 mg (2 capsules) b.i.d. (400 mg/day) for one week. The pulses are separated by a 3-week period without SPORANOX®.

SPORANOX® Capsules and SPORANOX® Oral Solution should not be used interchangeably. Only the Oral Solution has been demonstrated effective for oral and/or esophageal candidiasis.

HOW SUPPLIED

SPORANOX® (itraconazole) Capsules are available containing 100 mg of itraconazole, with a blue opaque cap and pink transparent body, imprinted with "JANSSEN" and "SPORANOX 100." The capsules are supplied in unit-dose blister packs of 3 × 10 capsules (NDC 50458-290-01), bottles of 30 capsules (NDC 50458–290-04) and in the PulsePak™ containing 7 blister packs × 4 capsules each (NDC 50458-290-28).

Store at controlled room temperature (59°–77°F/15°–25°C).
Protect from light and moisture.
U.S. Patent No. 4,267,179
Rev. February 1997, August 1997

Distributed by:
JANSSEN PHARMACEUTICA INC.
Titusville, NJ 08560

Capsule contents manufactured by:
JANSSEN PHARMACEUTICA N.V.
Beerse, Belgium

Shown in Product Identification Guide, page 317

SPORANOX® ℞
(ITRACONAZOLE) ORAL SOLUTION
[spər 'ah-n äks"]

> **WARNING**: Coadministration of terfenadine, astemizole, and cisapride with SPORANOX® (itraconazole) Capsules or Oral Solution is contraindicated. SPORANOX® is a potent inhibitor of the cytochrome P450 3A enzyme system and may raise plasma concentrations of drugs metabolized by this pathway. Serious cardiovascular events, including death, ventricular tachycardia, and torsades de pointes have occurred in patients taking itraconazole concomitantly with terfenadine or cisapride, which are metabolized by the cytochrome P450 3A system. See CONTRAINDICATIONS, WARNINGS, and PRECAUTIONS: DRUG INTERACTIONS for more information.

DESCRIPTION

SPORANOX® is the brand name for itraconazole, a synthetic triazole antifungal agent. Itraconazole is a 1:1:1:1 racemic mixture of four diastereomers (two enantiomeric pairs), each possessing three chiral centers. It may be represented by the following structural formula and nomenclature:

(±)-1-[(R*)-sec-butyl]-4-[p-[4-[p-[[(2R*,4S*)-2-(2,4-dichlorophenyl)-2-(1H-1,2,4-triazol-1-ylmethyl)-1,3-dioxolan-4-yl]methoxy]phenyl]-1-piperazinyl]phenyl]-Δ^2-1,2,4-triazolin-5-one mixture with (±)-1-[(R*)-sec-butyl]-4-[p-[4-[p-[[(2S*,4R*)-2-(2,4-dichlorophenyl)-2-(1H-1,2,4-triazol-1-ylmethyl)-1,3-dioxolan-4-yl]methoxy]phenyl]-1-piperazinyl]-phenyl]-Δ^2-1,2,4-triazolin-5-one

or

(±)-1-[(RS)-sec-butyl]-4-[p-[4-[p-[[(2R,4S)-2-(2,4-dichlorophenyl)-2-(1H-1,2,4-triazol-1-ylmethyl)-1,3-dioxolan-4-yl]methoxy]phenyl]-1-piperazinyl]phenyl]-Δ^2-1,2,4-triazolin-5-one.

Itraconazole has a molecular formula of $C_{35}H_{38}Cl_2N_8O_4$ and a molecular weight of 705.64. It is a white to slightly yellowish powder. It is insoluble in water, very slightly soluble in alcohols, and freely soluble in dichloromethane. It has a pKa of 3.70 (based on extrapolation of values obtained from methanolic solutions) and a log (n-octanol/water) partition coefficient of 5.66 at pH 8.1.

SPORANOX® (itraconazole) Oral Solution contains 10 mg of itraconazole per mL, solubilized by hydroxypropyl-β-cyclodextrin (400 mg/mL) as a molecular inclusion complex. SPORANOX® Oral Solution is clear and yellowish in color with a target pH of 2. Other ingredients are hydrochloric acid, propylene glycol, purified water, sodium hydroxide, sodium saccharin, sorbitol, cherry flavor 1, cherry flavor 2 and caramel flavor.

MICROBIOLOGY

Mechanism of Action: In vitro studies have demonstrated that itraconazole inhibits the cytochrome P-450-dependent synthesis of ergosterol, which is a vital component of fungal cell membranes.

Activity in vitro and in vivo: Itraconazole exhibits *in vitro* activity against *Blastomyces dermatitidis, Histoplasma capsulatum, Histoplasma duboisii, Aspergillus flavus, Aspergillus fumigatus, Candida albicans* and *Cryptococcus neoformans.* Itraconazole also exhibits varying *in vitro* activity against *Sporothrix schenckii,* Trichophyton spp., *Candida krusei* and other Candida spp. The bioactive metabolite, hydroxyitraconazole, has not been evaluated against *Histoplasma capsulatum* and *Blastomyces dermatitidis.* Correlation between *in vitro* minimum inhibitory concentration (MIC) results and clinical outcome has yet to be established for azole antifungal agents.

Itraconazole administered orally was active in a variety of animal models of fungal infection using standard laboratory strains of fungi. Fungistatic activity has been demonstrated against disseminated fungal infections caused by *Blastomyces dermatitidis, Histoplasma duboisii, Aspergillus fumigatus, Coccidioides immitis, Cryptococcus neoformans, Paracoccidioides brasiliensis, Sporothrix schenckii, Trichophyton rubrum* and *Trichophyton mentagrophytes.*

Itraconazole administered at 2.5 mg/kg and 5.0 mg/kg via the oral and parenteral routes increased survival rates and sterilized organ systems in normal and immunosuppressed guinea pigs with disseminated *Aspergillus fumigatus* infections. Oral itraconazole administered daily at 40 mg/kg and 80 mg/kg increased survival rates in normal rabbits with disseminated disease and immunosuppressed rats with pulmonary *Aspergillus fumigatus* infection, respectively. Itraconazole has demonstrated antifungal activity in a variety of animal models infected with *Candida albicans* and other Candida species.

In vivo studies suggest that the activity of amphotericin B may be suppressed by azole antifungal therapy. As with other azoles, itraconazole inhibits the ^{14}C-demethylation step in the synthesis of ergosterol, a cell wall component of fungi. Ergosterol is the active site for amphotericin B. In one study the antifungal activity of amphotericin B against *Aspergillus fumigatus* infections in mice was inhibited by ketoconazole therapy. The clinical significance of test results obtained in this study is unknown.

Several *in vitro* studies have reported that some fungal clinical isolates, including Candida species, with reduced susceptibility to one azole antifungal agent may also be less susceptible to other azole derivatives. The finding of cross-resistance is dependent upon a number of factors, including the species evaluated, its clinical history, the particular azole compounds compared and the type of susceptibility test that is performed. The relevance of these *in vitro* susceptibility data to clinical outcome remains to be elucidated.

CLINICAL PHARMACOLOGY

Pharmacokinetics and Metabolism: NOTE: The plasma concentrations reported below were measured by high performance liquid chromatography (HPLC) specific for itraconazole. When itraconazole in plasma is measured by a bioassay, values reported are approximately 3.3 times higher than those obtained by HPLC due to the presence of the bioactive metabolite, hydroxyitraconazole. (See MICROBIOLOGY.)

The absolute bioavailability of itraconazole administered as a non-marketed solution formulation under fed conditions as 55% in six healthy male volunteers. However, the bioavailability of SPORANOX® (itraconazole) Oral Solution is increased under fasted conditions reaching higher maximum plasma concentrations (C_{max}) in a shorter period of time. In 27 healthy male volunteers, the steady state area under the plasma concentration versus time curve (AUC_{0-24h}) of itraconazole (SPORANOX® Oral Solution, 200 mg daily for 15 days) under fasted conditions was 131 ± 30% of that obtained under fed conditions. Therefore, unlike SPORANOX® Capsules, it is recommeded that SPORANOX® Oral Solution be administered without food. Presented in the table below are the steady-state (Day 15) pharmacokinetic parameters for itraconazole and hydroxyitraconazole (SPORANOX® Oral Solution) under fasted and fed conditions:

[See table below]

The bioavailability of SPORANOX® Oral Solution relative to SPORANOX® Capsules was studied in 30 healthy male volunteers who received 200 mg of itraconazole as the oral solution and capsules under fed conditions. The $AUC_{0-\infty}$ from SPORANOX® Oral Solution was 149 ± 68% of that obtained from SPORANOX® Capsules; a similar increase was observed for hydroxyitraconazole. In addition, a cross study comparison of itraconazole and hydroxyitraconazole pharmacokinetics following the administration of single 200 mg doses of SPORANOX® Oral Solution (under fasted conditions) or SPORANOX® Capsules (under fed conditions) indicates that when these two formulations are administered under conditions which optimize their systemic absorption, the bioavailability of the solution relative to cap-

Continued on next page

	Itraconazole		Hydroxyitraconazole	
	Fasted	Fed	Fasted	Fed
C_{max} (ng/mL)	1963 ± 601*	1435 ± 477	2055 ± 487	1781 ± 397
T_{max} (hours)	2.5 ± 0.8	4.4 ± 0.7	5.3 ± 4.3	4.3 ± 1.2
AUC_{0-24h} (ng·h/mL)	29271 ± 10285	22815 ± 7098	45184 ± 10981	38823 ± 8907
$t_{1/2}$ (hours)	39.7 ± 13	37.4 ± 13	27.3 ± 13	26.1 ± 10

*mean ± standard deviation

Sporanox Oral Solution—Cont.

sules is expected to be increased further. Therefore, it is recommended that SPORANOX® Oral Solution and SPORANOX® Capsules not be used interchangeably. The following table contains pharmacokinetic parameters for itraconazole and hydroxyitraconazole following single 200 mg doses of SPORANOX® Oral Solution (n=27) or SPORANOX® Capsules (n=30) administered to healthy male volunteers under fasted and fed conditions, respectively:
[See table at bottom of page]
The plasma protein binding of itraconazole is 99.8% and that of hydroxyitraconazole is 99.5%. Following intravenous administration, the volume of distribution of itraconazole averaged 796 ± 185 L.

Itraconazole is extensively metabolized resulting in the formation of several metabolites including hydroxitraconazole, the major metabolite. Results of a pharmacokinetics study suggest that itraconazole may undergo saturable metabolism with multiple dosing. Fecal excretion of the parent drug varies between 3–18% of the dose. Renal excretion of the parent drug is less than 0.03% of the dose. About 40% of the dose is excreted as inactive metabolites in the urine. No single excreted metabolite represents more than 5% of a dose. Itraconazole total plasma clearance averaged 381 ± 95 mL/min following intravenous administration.

Special Populations:
Pediatrics: The pharmacokinetics of SPORANOX® Oral Solution were studied in 26 pediatric patients requiring systemic antifungal therapy. Patients were stratified by age: 6 months to 2 years (n=8), 2 to 5 years (n=7) and 5 to 12 years (n=11), and received itraconazole oral solution 5 mg/kg once daily for 14 days. Pharmacokinetic parameters at steady state (Day 14) were not significantly different among the age strata and are summarized in the table below for all 26 patients:

	Itraconazole	Hydroxyitraconazole
C_{max} (ng/mL)	582.5 ± 382.4*	692.4 ± 355.0
C_{min} (ng/mL)	187.5 ± 161.4	403.8 ± 336.1
AUC_{0-24h} (ng·h/mL)	7706.7 ± 5245.2	13356.4 ± 8942.4
$t_{1/2}$ (hours)	35.8 ± 35.6	17.7 ± 13.0

* mean ± standard deviation

Renal Insufficiency: Plasma concentrations of itraconazole in patients with mild to severe renal insufficiency, including patients receiving hemodialysis, were comparable to those obtained in healthy subjects.
Hepatic Insufficiency: The effect of hepatic impairment on plasma concentrations of itraconazole is unknown. It is recommended that patients with hepatic impairment be carefully monitored when taking itraconazole.

INDICATIONS AND USAGE

SPORANOX® (itraconazole) Oral Solution is indicated for the treatment of oropharyngeal and esophageal candidiasis.
Description of Clinical Studies:
Oropharyngeal candidiasis: Two randomized, controlled studies for the treatment of oropharyngeal candidiasis have been conducted (total n=344). In one trial, clinical response to either 7 or 14 days of itraconazole oral solution, 200 mg/day, was similar to fluconazole tablets and averaged 84% across all arms. Clinical response in this study was defined as cured or improved (only minimal signs and symptoms with no visible lesions). Approximately 5% of subjects were lost to follow-up before any evaluations could be performed. Response to 14 days therapy of itraconazole oral solution was associated with a lower relapse rate than 7 days of itraconazole therapy. In another trial, the clinical response rate (defined as cured or improved) for itraconazole oral solution was similar to clotrimazole troches and averaged approximately 71% across both arms, with approximately 3% of subjects lost to follow-up before any evaluations could be performed. Ninety-two percent of the patients in these studies were HIV seropositive.
In an uncontrolled, open-label study of selected patients clinically unresponsive to fluconazole tablets (n=74, all patients HIV seropositive), patients were treated with itraconazole oral solution 100 mg b.i.d. (Clinically unresponsive to fluconazole in this study was defined as having received a dose of fluconazole tablets at least 200 mg/day for a minimum of 14 days.) Treatment duration was 14–28 days based

on response. Approximately 55% of patients had complete resolution of oral lesions. Of patients who responded and then entered a follow-up phase (n=22), all relapsed within 1 month (median 14 days) when treatment was discontinued. Although baseline endoscopies had not been performed, several patients in this study developed symptoms of esophageal candidiasis while receiving therapy with itraconazole oral solution. Itraconazole oral solution has not been directly compared to other agents in a controlled trial of similar patients.
Esophageal candidiasis: A double-blind randomized study (n=119, 111 of whom were HIV seropositive) compared itraconazole oral solution (100 mg/day) to fluconazole tablets (100 mg/day). The dose of each was increased to 200 mg/day for patients not responding initially. Treatment continued for 2 weeks following resolution of symptoms, for a total duration of treatment of 3–8 weeks. Clinical response (a global assessment of cured or improved) was not significantly different between the two study arms, and averaged approximately 86% with 8% lost to follow-up. Six of 53 (11%) itraconazole-treated patients and 12/57 (21%) fluconazole-treated patients were escalated to the 200 mg dose in this trial. Of the subgroup of patients who responded and entered a follow-up phase (n=88), approximately 23% relapsed across both arms within 4 weeks.

CONTRAINDICATIONS

Coadministration of SPORANOX® (itraconazole) Capsules or Oral Solution with certain drugs metabolized by the P450 3A enzyme system may result in increased plasma concentrations of those drugs leading to potentially serious and/or life-threatening adverse events. Terfenadine, astemizole, oral triazolam, oral midazolam and cisapride are specifically contraindicated with SPORANOX®. HMG-CoA reductase inhibitors metabolized by this system (e.g., lovastatin and simvastatin) should also be discontinued during SPORANOX® therapy. (See PRECAUTIONS: DRUG INTERACTIONS.)
SPORANOX® is contraindicated in patients who have shown hypersensitivity to the drug or its excipients. There is no information regarding cross hypersensitivity between itraconazole and other azole antifungal agents; however, caution should be used in prescribing SPORANOX® to patients with hypersensitivity to other azoles.

WARNINGS

SPORANOX® (itraconazole) Oral Solution and SPORANOX® Capsules should not be used interchangeably. Only SPORANOX® Oral Solution has been demonstrated effective for oral and/or esophageal candidiasis. SPORANOX® Oral Solution contains the excipient hydroxypropyl-β-cyclodextrin which produced pancreatic adenocarcinomas in a rat carcinogenicity study. These findings were not observed in a similar mouse carcinogenicity study. The clinical relevance of these findings is unknown. (See CARCINOGENESIS, MUTAGENESIS, AND IMPAIRMENT OF FERTILITY.)
Hepatitis: There have been rare cases of reversible idiosyncratic hepatitis reported among patients taking SPORANOX® Capsules. SPORANOX® has been associated with rare cases of serious hepatotoxicity, including fatalities, primarily in patients with serious underlying medical conditions taking multiple medications. The causal association with SPORANOX® is uncertain. If clinical signs and symptoms develop that are consistent with liver disease and may be attributable to itraconazole, SPORANOX® should be discontinued.
Cardiac Dysrhythmias: There have been rare cases of life-threatening cardiac dysrhythmia and death reported in patients receiving terfenadine and itraconazole. Coadministration of terfenadine, astemizole and cisapride with SPORANOX® is contraindicated. (See BOX WARNING, CONTRAINDICATIONS and PRECAUTIONS: DRUG INTERACTIONS.)

PRECAUTIONS

General: Hepatic enzyme test values should be monitored in patients with preexisting hepatic function abnormalities. Hepatic enzyme test values should be monitored periodically in all patients receiving continuous treatment for more than one month or at any time a patient develops signs or symptoms suggestive of liver dysfunction.
Information for patients: Patients should be aware that SPORANOX® (itraconazole) Oral Solution is a different preparation than SPORANOX® Capsules, and these should not be used interchangeably. Only SPORANOX® Oral Solu-

tion has been demonstrated effective for oral and/or esophageal candidiasis. SPORANOX® Oral Solution contains the excipient hydroxypropyl-β-cyclodextrin which produced pancreatic adenocarcinomas in a rat carcinogenicity study. These findings were not observed in a similar mouse carcinogenicity study. The clinical relevance of these findings is unknown. (See CARCINOGENESIS, MUTAGENESIS, AND IMPAIRMENT OF FERTILITY.)
Taking SPORANOX® Oral Solution under fasted conditions improves the systemic availability of itraconazole. Therefore, patients should be instructed to take SPORANOX® Oral Solution without food, if possible.
Patients should be instructed to report any signs and symptoms that may suggest liver dysfunction so that the appropriate laboratory testing can be done. Such signs and symptoms may include unusual fatigue, anorexia, nausea and/or vomiting, jaundice, dark urine or pale stool.
Patients should be instructed to contact their physician before taking any concomitant medications with itraconazole to insure there are no potential drug interactions.
Drug Interactions: Both itraconazole and its major metabolite, hydroxyitraconazole, are inhibitors of the cytochrome P450 3A enzyme system. Coadministration of SPORANOX® and drugs primarily metabolized by the cytochrome P450 3A enzyme system may result in increased plasma concentrations of the other drug that could increase or prolong both its therapeutic and adverse effects. Therefore, unless otherwise specified, concomitant medications metabolized by the P450 3A enzyme system should be discontinued as medically indicated.

Table of Selected Drugs That Are Predicted to Have Plasma Concentrations Increased by Itraconazole+

> *Anticoagulants:* warfarin
> *Antihistamines:* terfenadine*, astemizole*
> *Anti-HIV protease inhibitors:* ritonavir, indinavir
> *Antineoplastic agents:* vinca alkaloids
> *Benzodiazepines:* midazolam*†, triazolam*, diazepam
> *Calcium channel blockers:* dihydropyridines
> *Cholesterol-lowering agents:* lovastatin*, simvastatin*
> *GI motility agents:* cisapride*
> *Immunosuppressive agents:* cyclosporine, tacrolimus
> *Steroids:* methylprednisolone
> *Other:* digoxin, quinidine

+This table is not all inclusive.
*Specifically contraindicated with SPORANOX® based on clinical and/or pharmacokinetics studies (see WARNINGS and below).
†See paragraph below on *Benzodiazepines* for information on parenteral administration.

Table of Selected Drugs That Are Predicted to Decrease Itraconazole Plasma Concentrations+‡

> *Anticonvulsants:* phenytoin, phenobarbital, carbamazepine
> *Antimycobacterial agents:* isoniazid, rifampin, rifabutin

+This table is not all inclusive.
‡SPORANOX® may not be effective due to decreased itraconazole plasma concentrations in patients using these agents concomitantly.

Anticoagulants: It has been reported that SPORANOX® enhances the anticoagulant effect of coumarin-like drugs. Therefore, prothrombin time should be carefully monitored in patients receiving SPORANOX® and coumarin-like drugs simultaneously.
Anticonvulsants: Reduced plasma concentrations of itraconazole were reported when SPORANOX® was coadministered with phenytoin. The physician is advised to monitor the plasma concentrations of itraconazole when phenytoin is taken concurrently, and to increase the dose of SPORANOX® if necessary.
Antihistamines: Coadministration of terfenadine with SPORANOX® has led to elevated plasma concentrations of terfenadine, resulting in rare instances of life-threatening cardiac dysrhythmia and death. Coadministration of astemizole with SPORANOX® has led to elevated plasma concentrations of astemizole and desmethylastemizole which may prolong the QT intervals. Therefore, concomitant administration of SPORANOX® with astemizole is contraindicated. (See BOX WARNING, CONTRAINDICATIONS, and WARNINGS.)
Anti-HIV protease inhibitors: Coadministration of SPORANOX® with protease inhibitors primarily metabolized by the cytochrome P450 3A enzyme system, such as ritonavir or indinavir, may result in changes in plasma concentrations of both drugs. Caution is advised when these drugs are used concomitantly.
Anti-HIV reverse transcriptase inhibitors: The results from a study in which eight HIV-infected individuals were treated with zidovudine, 8 ± 0.4 mg/kg/day, showed that the pharmacokinetics of zidovudine were not affected during concomitant administration of SPORANOX® Capsules, 100 mg b.i.d. Other agents have not been studied.

	Itraconazole		Hydroxyitraconazole	
	Oral Solution fasted	Capsules fed	Oral Solution fasted	Capsules fed
C_{max} (ng/mL)	544 ± 213*	302 ± 119	622 ± 116	504 ± 132
T_{max} (hours)	2.2 ± 0.8	5 ± 0.8	3.5 ± 1.2	5 ± 1
AUC_{0-24h} (ng·h/mL)	4505 ± 1670	2682 ± 1084	9552 ± 1835	7293 ± 2144

* mean ± standard deviation

Antinycobacterial agents: Plasma concentrations of azole antifungal agents are reduced when given concurrently with isoniazid or rifampin. Alternative antifungal therapy should be considered if rifampin or isoniazid therapy is necessary. A similar effect may be expected with rifabutin.

Antineoplastic agents: The metabolism of vinca alkaloids may be inhibited by itraconazole. Therefore, patients receiving SPORANOX® concomitantly with vinca alkaloids should be monitored for an increase and/or prolongation of the effects of the latter drug product, including adverse effects such as peripheral neuropathy and ileus, and the dose of the vinca alkaloid should be adjusted appropriately.

Benzodiazepines: Coadministration of SPORANOX® with oral midazolam or triazolam has resulted in elevated plasma concentrations of the latter two drugs. This may potentiate and prolong hypnotic and sedative effects. These agents should not be used in patients treated with SPORANOX®. If midazolam is administered parenterally, special precaution and patient monitoring is required since the sedative effect may be prolonged. (See CONTRAINDICATIONS.)

Calcium channel blockers: Edema has been reported in patients concomitantly receiving SPORANOX® and dihydropyridine calcium channel blockers. Appropriate dosage adjustments may be necessary.

Cholesterol-lowering agents: Human pharmacokinetic data indicate that SPORANOX® inhibits the metabolism of lovastatin resulting in significantly elevated plasma concentrations of lovastatin or lovastatin acid, which have been associated with rhabdomyolysis. Use of HMG-CoA reductase inhibitors metabolized by the P450 3A enzyme system, such as lovastatin or simvastatin, should be temporarily discontinued during SPORANOX® therapy. (See CONTRAINDICATIONS.)

Digoxin: Coadministration of SPORANOX® and digoxin has led to increased plasma concentrations of digoxin. Digoxin concentrations should be monitored at the initiation of SPORANOX® therapy and frequently thereafter, and the dose of digoxin should be adjusted appropriately.

GI motility agents: Human pharmacokinetic data indicate that oral ketoconazole potently inhibits the metabolism of cisapride resulting in significantly elevated plasma concentrations of cisapride. Data suggest that coadministration of oral ketoconazole and cisapride can result in prolongation of the QT interval on the ECG. *In vitro* data suggest that itraconazole also markedly inhibits the biotransformation system mainly responsible for the metabolism of cisapride; therefore, concomitant administration of SPORANOX® with cisapride is contraindicated. (See BOX WARNING, CONTRAINDICATIONS and WARNINGS.)

H_2 antagonists: Reduced plasma concentrations of itraconazole were reported when SPORANOX® Capsules were coadministered with H_2 antagonists. However, as itraconazole is already dissolved in SPORANOX® Oral Solution, the effect of H_2 antagonists is expected to be substantially less than with the capsules. Nevertheless, caution is advised when the two drugs are coadministered.

Immunosuppressive agents: Coadministration of SPORANOX® and cyclosporine or tacrolimus has led to increased plasma concentrations of the latter two agents. Cyclosporine and tacrolimus concentrations should be monitored at the initiation of SPORANOX® therapy and frequently thereafter, and the dose of cyclosporine or tacrolimus should be adjusted appropriately.

Oral hypoglycemic agents: Severe hypoglycemia has been reported in patients concomitantly receiving azole antifungal agents and oral hypoglycemic agents. Blood glucose concentrations should be carefully monitored when SPORANOX® and oral hypoglycemic agents are coadministered.

Quinidine: Tinnitus and decreased hearing have been reported in patients concomitantly receiving SPORANOX® and quinidine.

Steroids: The metabolism of methylprednisolone may be inhibited by itraconazole. Therefore, patients receiving SPORANOX® concomitantly with methylprednisolone should be monitored for an increase and/or prolongation of the effects of the latter drug product, including adverse effects, and the dose of methylprednisolone should be adjusted appropriately.

Carcinogenesis, Mutagenesis and Impairment of Fertility: Itraconazole showed no evidence of carcinogenicity potential in mice treated orally for 23 months at dosage levels up to 80 mg/kg/day [approximately 10x the maximum recommended human dose (MRHD)]. Male rats treated with 25 mg/kg/day (3.1x MRHD) had a slightly increased incidence of soft tissue sarcoma. These sarcomas may have been a consequence of hypercholesterolemia, which is a response of rats, but not dogs or humans, to chronic itraconazole administration. Female rats treated with 50 mg/kg/day (6.25x MRHD) had an increased incidence of squamous cell carcinoma of the lung (2/50) as compared to the untreated group. Although the occurrence of squamous cell carcinoma in the lung is extremely uncommon in untreated rats, the increase in this study was not statistically significant.

Hydroxypropyl-β-cyclodextrin (HP-β-CD), the solubilizing excipient used in SPORANOX® Oral Solution, was found to produce pancreatic exocrine hyperplasia and neoplasia when administered orally to rats at doses of 500, 2000 or 5000 mg/kg/day for 25 months. Adenocarcinomas of the exocrine pancreas produced in the treated animals were not seen in the untreated group and are not reported in the historical controls. Development of these tumors may be related to a mitogenic action of cholecystokinin. This finding was not observed in the mouse carcinogenicity study at doses of 500, 2000 or 5000 mg/kg/day for 22–23 months; however, the clinical relevance of these findings is unknown. Based on body surface area comparisons, the exposure to humans of HP-β-CD at the recommended clinical dose of SPORANOX® Oral Solution, is approximately equivalent to 1.7 times the exposure at the lowest dose in the rat study.

Body System/Adverse Event	Itraconazole Total n=350*	Itraconazole All controlled Studies n=272	Fluconazole n=125**	Clotrimazole n=81***
Gastrointestinal disorders				
Nausea	11.1%	10.3%	11.2%	4.9%
Diarrhea	10.9%	10.3%	10.4%	3.7%
Vomiting	7.1%	5.5%	8.0%	1.2%
Abdominal Pain	5.7%	4.0%	7.2%	7.4%
Constipation	2.0%	2.2%	0.8%	0%
Body as a whole				
Fever	6.6%	6.3%	8.0%	4.9%
Chest pain	2.6%	2.9%	2.4%	0%
Pain	2.3%	1.8%	4.0%	0%
Fatigue	2.0%	1.1%	1.6%	0%
Respiratory disorders				
Coughing	4.0%	4.4%	9.6%	0%
Dyspnea	2.3%	2.6%	4.8%	1.2%
Pneumonia	2.0%	1.5%	0%	0%
Sinusitis	2.0%	1.8%	4.0%	0%
Sputum increased	2.0%	2.6%	3.2%	1.2%
Skin and appendages disorders				
Rash	4.0%	4.8%	4.0%	6.2%
Increased sweating	3.4%	3.7%	6.4%	1.2%
Skin disorder, unspecified	2.3%	2.2%	2.4%	1.2%
Central/peripheral nervous system				
Headache	4.3%	4.4%	5.6%	6.2%
Dizziness	2.0%	1.5%	4.0%	1.2%
Resistance mechanism disorders				
Pneumocystis carinii infection	2.3%	1.5%	1.6%	0%
Psychiatric disorders				
Depression	2.0%	1.1%	0%	1.2%

* Of the 350 patients, 209 were treated for oropharyngeal candidiasis in controlled studies, 63 were treated for esophageal candidiasis in controlled studies and 78 were treated for oropharyngeal candidiasis in an open study.
** Of the 125 patients, 62 were treated for oropharyngeal candidiasis and 63 were treated for esophageal candidiasis.
*** All 81 patients were treated for oropharyngeal candidiasis.

Itraconazole produced no mutagenic effects when assayed in a DNA repair test (unscheduled DNA synthesis) in primary rat hepatocytes, in Ames test with Salmonella typhimurium (six strains) and Escherichia coli, in the mouse lymphoma gene mutation test, in a sex-linked recessive lethal mutation (Drosophila melanogaster) test, in chromosome aberration tests in human lymphocytes, in a cell transformation test with C3H/10T$^1/_2$ C18 mouse embryo fibroblasts cells, in a dominant lethal mutation test in male and female mice, and in micronucleus tests in mice and rats.

Itraconazole did not affect the fertility of male or female rats treated orally with dosage levels of up to 40 mg/kg/day (5x MRHD) even though parental toxicity was present at this dosage level. More severe signs of parental toxicity, including death, were present in the next higher dosage level, 160 mg/kg/day (20x MRHD).

Pregnancy: Teratogenic Effects. Pregnancy Category C: Itraconazole was found to cause a dose-related increase in maternal toxicity, embryotoxicity and teratogenicity in rats at dosage levels of approximately 40–160 mg/kg/day (5–20x MRHD) and in mice at dosage levels of approximately 80 mg/kg/day (10x MRHD). In rats, the teratogenicity consisted of major skeletal defects; in mice it consisted of encephaloceles and/or macroglossia.

There are no studies in pregnant women. SPORANOX® should be used in pregnancy only if the benefit outweighs the potential risk

Nursing Mothers: Itranconazole is excreted in human milk; therefore, the expected benefits of SPORANOX® therapy for the mother should be weighed against the potential risk from exposure of itraconazole to the infant. The U.S. Public Health Service Centers for Disease Control and Prevention advises HIV-infected women not to breast-feed to avoid potential transmission of HIV to uninfected infants.

Pediatric Use: The efficacy and safety of SPORANOX® have not been established in pediatric patients. A pharmacokinetic study was conducted with SPORANOX® Oral Solution in 26 pediatric patients, aged 6 months to 12 years, requiring systemic antifungal treatment. Itraconazole was dosed at 5 mg/kg once daily for two weeks and no serious unexpected adverse events were reported. (See CLINICAL PHARMACOLOGY.)

In three toxicology studies using rats, itraconazole induced bone defects at dosage levels as low as 20 mg/kg/day (2.5x MRHD). The induced defects included reduced bone plate activity, thinning of the zona compacta of the large bones and increased bone fragility. At a dosage level of 80 mg/kg/day (10x MRHD) over one year or 160 mg/kg/day (20x MRHD) for six months, intraconazole induced small tooth pulp with hypocellular appearance in some rats. While no such bone toxicity has been reported in adult patients, the long term effect of itraconazole in pediatric patients is unknown.

ADVERSE REACTIONS

There have been rare cases of reversible idiosyncratic hepatitis reported among patients taking SPORANOX® (itraconazole) Capsules. SPORANOX® has been associated with rare cases of serious hepatotoxicity, including fatalities, primarily in patients with serious underlying medical conditions taking multiple medications. The causal association with SPORANOX® is uncertain. If clinical signs and symptoms develop that are consistent with liver disease and may be attributable to itraconazole, SPORANOX® should be discontinued. (See WARNINGS.)

U.S. adverse experience data are derived from 350 immunocompromised patients (332 HIV seropositive/AIDS) treated for oropharyngeal or esophageal candidiasis. The table below lists adverse events reported by at least 2% of patients treated with SPORANOX® Oral Solution in U.S. clinical trials. Data on patients receiving comparator agents in these trials are included for comparison.

[See table above]

Adverse events reported by less than 2% of patients in U.S. clinical trials with SPORANOX® included: adrenal insufficiency, asthenia, back pain, dehydration, dyspepsia, dysphagia, flatulence, gynecomastia, hematuria, hemorrhoids, hot flushes, implantation complication, infection unspecified, injury, insomnia, male breast pain, myalgia, pharyngitis, pruritus, rhinitis, rigors, stomatitis ulcerative, taste perversion, tinnitus, upper respiratory tract infection, vi-

Continued on next page

Sporanox Oral Solution—Cont.

sion abnormal, and weight decrease. Edema, hypokalemia and menstrual disorders have been reported in clinical trials with itraconazole capsules.

In worldwide postmarketing experience with SPORANOX® Capsules, allergic reactions including rash, pruritus, urticaria, angioedema and in rare instances, anaphylaxis and Stevens-Johnson syndrome, have been reported. Marketing experiences have also included reports of elevated liver enzymes and rare hepatitis. Although the causal association with SPORANOX® is uncertain, rare alopecia, hypertriglyceridemia, neutropenia and isolated cases of neuropathy have also been reported.

OVERDOSAGE

Itraconazole is not removed by dialysis. In the event of accidental overdosage, supportive measures, including gastric lavage with sodium bicarbonate, should be employed.

There are limited data on the outcomes of patients ingesting high doses of itraconazole. In patients taking either 1000 mg of SPORANOX® (itraconazole) Oral Solution or up to 3000 mg of SPORANOX® Capsules, the adverse event profile was similar to that observed at recommended doses.

DOSAGE AND ADMINISTRATION

The solution should be vigorously swished in the mouth (10 mL at a time) for several seconds and swallowed.

The recommended dosage of SPORANOX® (itraconazole) Oral Solution for oropharyngeal candidiasis is 200 mg (20 mL) daily for 1 to 2 weeks. Clinical signs and symptoms of oropharyngeal candidiasis generally resolve within several days.

For patients with oropharyngeal candidiasis unresponsive/refractory to treatment with fluconazole tablets, the recommended dose is 100 mg (10 mL) b.i.d. For patients responding to therapy, clinical response will be seen in 2 to 4 weeks. Patients may be expected to relapse shortly after discontinuing therapy. Limited data on the safety of long-term use (>6 months) of SPORANOX® Oral Solution are available at this time.

The recommended dosage of SPORANOX® Oral Solution for esophageal candidiasis is 100 mg (10 mL) daily for a minimum treatment of three weeks. Treatment should continue for 2 weeks following resolution of symptoms. Doses up to 200 mg (20 mL) per day may be used based on medical judgement of the patient's response to therapy.

SPORANOX® Oral Solution and SPORANOX® Capsules should not be used interchangeably. Patients should be instructed to take SPORANOX® Oral Solution without food, if possible. Only SPORANOX® Oral Solution has been demonstrated effective for oral and/or esophageal candidiasis.

HOW SUPPLIED

SPORANOX® (itraconazole) Oral Solution is available in 150 mL amber glass bottles (NDC 50458-295-15) containing 10 mg of itraconazole per mL.

Store at or below 25°C (77°F). Do not freeze.

U.S. Patent 4,267,179

January 1997, February 1997

©JANSSEN PHARMACEUTICA, INC. 1997

Manufactured by:

Janssen Pharmaceutica N.V.

Beerse, Belgium

Distributed by:

Janssen Pharmaceutica Inc.

Titusville, NJ 08560

Shown in Product Identification Guide, page 317

VERMOX®

R

[*vĕr ´mŏx*]

(mebendazole)

Chewable Tablets

DESCRIPTION

VERMOX® (mebendazole) is a (synthetic) broad-spectrum anthelmintic available as chewable tablets, each containing 100 mg of mebendazole. Inactive ingredients are: colloidal silicon dioxide, corn starch, hydrogenated vegetable oil, magnesium stearate, microcrystalline cellulose, sodium lauryl sulfate, sodium saccharin, sodium starch glycolate, talc, tetrarome orange, and FD&C yellow No. 6.

Mebendazole is methyl 5-benzoylbenzimidazole-2-carbamate.

Mebendazole is a white to slightly yellow powder with a molecular weight of 295.29. It is less than 0.05% soluble in water, dilute mineral acid solutions, alcohol, ether and chloroform, but is soluble in formic acid.

CLINICAL PHARMACOLOGY

Following administration of 100 mg twice daily for three consecutive days, plasma levels of VERMOX® (mebendazole) and its primary metabolite, the 2-amine, do not exceed 0.03 µg/ml and 0.09 µg/ml, respectively. All metabolites are devoid of anthelmintic activity. In man, approximately 2% of administered VERMOX® is excreted in urine and the remainder in the feces as unchanged drug or a primary metabolite.

Mode of Action: VERMOX® inhibits the formation of the worms' microtubules and causes the worms' glucose depletion.

INDICATIONS AND USAGE

VERMOX® (mebendazole) is indicated for the treatment of *Enterobius vermicularis* (pinworm), *Trichuris trichiura* (whipworm), *Ascaris lumbricoides* (common roundworm), *Ancylostoma duodenale* (common hookworm), *Necator americanus* (American hookworm) in single or mixed infections.

Efficacy varies as a function of such factors as pre-existing diarrhea and gastrointestinal transit time, degree of infection, and helminth strains. Efficacy rates derived from various studies are shown in the table below:

[See first table above]

CONTRAINDICATIONS

VERMOX® (mebendazole) is contraindicated in persons who have shown hypersensitivity to the drug.

WARNINGS

There is no evidence that VERMOX® (mebendazole), even at high doses, is effective for hydatid disease. There have been rare reports of neutropenia and agranulocytosis, when VERMOX® was taken for prolonged periods and at dosages substantially above those recommended.

PRECAUTIONS

General: Periodic assessment of organ system functions, including hematopoietic and hepatic, is advisable during prolonged therapy.

Information for Patients: Patients should be informed of the potential risk to the fetus in women taking VERMOX® (mebendazole) during pregnancy, especially during the first trimester (see Use in Pregnancy).

Patients should also be informed that cleanliness is important to prevent reinfection and transmission of the infection.

Drug Interactions: Preliminary evidence suggests that cimetidine inhibits mebendazole metabolism and may result in an increase in plasma concentrations of mebendazole.

Carcinogenesis, Mutagenesis, Impairment of Fertility: In carcinogenicity tests of mebendazole in mice and rats, no carcinogenic effects were seen at doses as high as 40 mg/kg (one to two times the human dose, based on mg/m²) given daily over two years. Dominant lethal mutation tests in mice showed no mutagenicity at single doses as high as 640 mg/kg (18 times the human dose, based on mg/m²). Neither the spermatocyte test, the F_1 translocation test, nor the Ames test indicated mutagenic properties. Doses up to 40 mg/kg in mice (equal to the human dose, based on mg/m²), given to males for 60 days and to females for 14 days prior to gestation, had no effect upon fetuses and offspring, though there was slight maternal toxicity.

Pregnancy: Teratogenic effects. Pregnancy Category C. Mebendazole has shown embryotoxic and teratogenic activity in pregnant rats at single oral doses as low as 10 mg/kg (approximately equal to the human dose, based on mg/m²). In view of these findings the use of VERMOX® is not recommended in pregnant women. Although there are no adequate and well-controlled studies in pregnant women, a post-marketing survey has been done of a limited number of women who inadvertently had consumed VERMOX® during the first trimester of pregnancy. The incidence of spontaneous abortion and malformation did not exceed that in the general population. In 170 deliveries on term, no teratogenic risk of VERMOX® was identified.

Nursing Mothers: It is not known whether VERMOX® is excreted in human milk. Because many drugs are excreted in human milk, caution should be exercised when VERMOX® is administered to a nursing woman.

Pediatric Use: The drug has not been extensively studied in children under two years; therefore, in the treatment of children under two years the relative benefit/risk should be considered.

ADVERSE REACTIONS

Gastrointestinal: Transient symptoms of abdominal pain and diarrhea in cases of massive infection and expulsion of worms.

Hypersensitivity: Rash, urticaria and angioedema have been observed on rare occasions.

Central Nervous System: Very rare cases of convulsions have been reported.

Liver: There have been liver function test elevations [AST (SGOT), ALT (SGPT), AND GGT] and rare reports of hepatitis when VERMOX® was taken for prolonged periods and at dosages substantially above those recommended.

Hematologic: Neutropenia and agranulocytosis. (See WARNINGS).

OVERDOSAGE

In the event of accidental overdosage gastrointestinal complaints lasting up to a few hours may occur. Vomiting and purging should be induced.

DOSAGE AND ADMINISTRATION

The same dosage schedule applies to children and adults. The tablet may be chewed, swallowed, or crushed and mixed with food.

[See second table above]

If the patient is not cured three weeks after treatment, a second course of treatment is advised. No special procedures, such as fasting or purging, are required.

HOW SUPPLIED

VERMOX® (mebendazole) is available as chewable tablets, each containing 100 mg of mebendazole, and is supplied in boxes of twelve tablets.

Store at controlled room temperature (59°–77°F/15°–25°C).

JANSSEN PHARMACEUTICA INC.

Titusville, NJ 08560-0200

Rev. February 1998, February 1998

NDC 50458-110-01 (blister package of 12)

U.S. Patent 3,657,267

Shown in Product Identification Guide, page 317

Vermox®	Pinworm (enterobiasis)	Whipworm (trichuriasis)	Common Roundworm (ascariasis)	Hookworm
Cure rates mean	95%	68%	98%	96%
Egg reduction mean	—	93%	99%	99%

Vermox®	Pinworm (enterobiasis)	Whipworm (trichuriasis)	Common Roundworm (ascariasis)	Hookworm
Dose	1 tablet, once	1 tablet morning and evening for 3 consecutive days.	1 tablet morning and evening for 3 consecutive days.	1 tablet morning and evening for 3 consecutive days.

IDENTIFICATION PROBLEM?

Turn to the **Product Identification Guide,**

where you'll find more than

1600 products pictured in actual

size and full color.

Johnson & Johnson • MERCK
Consumer Pharmaceuticals Co.
CAMP HILL ROAD
FORT WASHINGTON, PA 19034

Direct Inquiries to:
Consumer Affairs Department
Fort Washington, PA 19034
(215) 233-7000
For Medical Information Contact:
In Emergencies:
(215) 233-7000

CHILDREN'S MYLANTA®
UPSET STOMACH RELIEF   OTC
CALCIUM CARBONATE/ANTACID
LIQUID AND TABLETS

DESCRIPTION
Children's Mylanta is a specially formulated antacid to quickly and effectively relieve the upset stomach kids sometime experience.

ACTIVE INGREDIENTS
Each tablet or 5 ml teaspoonful contains 400 mg of calcium carbonate.

INACTIVE INGREDIENTS
Tablets: Citric acid, confectioner's sugar, D&C Red #27, flavors, magnesium stearate, sorbitol, starch.
Liquid: Butylparaben, cellulose, flavor propylparaben, purified water, D&C Red #22, D&C Red #28, simethicone, sodium saccharin, sorbitol, xanthan gum, may contain tartaric acid.
Acid Neutralizing Capacity:

Tablet	Liquid
8 mEq	8 mEq

INDICATIONS
For the relief of acid indigestion, sour stomach, or heartburn and upset stomach associated with these conditions, or overindulgence in food and drink.

DIRECTIONS
Find the right dose on the chart below. If possible use weight as your dosing guide; otherwise use age. Repeat dosing as needed. DO NOT USE MORE THAN THREE TIMES PER DAY.

WEIGHT (LB)	AGE (YR)	TABLET	LIQUID (TSP)
Under 24	Under 2	Consult Physician	
24–47	2–5	1	1
48–95	6–11	2	2

WARNINGS
Keep this and all drugs out of the reach of children. Do not take more than 3 tablets or 3 teaspoonfuls (2–5 years) or 6 tablets or 6 teaspoonfuls (6–11 years) in a 24-hour period, or use the maximum dosage of this product for more than two weeks, except under the advice and supervision of a physician.

DRUG INTERACTION PRECAUTION
Antacids may interact with certain prescription drugs. If your child is presently taking a prescription drug, do not give this product without checking with your physician or other health professional.

HOW SUPPLIED
Children's Mylanta Upset Stomach Relief is supplied as a liquid and chewable tablets in bubble gum flavor.
NDC 16837-810   Bubble Gum tablets
NDC 16837-820   Bubble Gum liquid
Shown in Product Identification Guide, page 318

INFANTS' MYLICON® Drops   OTC
[my 'li-con]
Antiflatulent

INGREDIENTS
Each 0.6 mL of drops contains: Active: simethicone, 40 mg. Inactive: carbomer 934P, citric acid, flavors, hydroxypropyl methylcellulose, purified water, Red 3, saccharin calcium, sodium benzoate, sodium citrate.

INDICATIONS
For relief of the symptoms of excess gas in the digestive tract. Such gas is frequently caused by excessive swallowing of air or by eating foods that disagree. The defoaming action of INFANTS' MYLICON® Drops relieves flatulence by dispersing and preventing the formation of mucus-surrounded gas pockets in the gastrointestinal tract. INFANTS' MYLICON® Drops act in the stomach and intestines to change the surface tension of gas bubbles enabling them to coalesce, thereby freeing and eliminating the gas more easily by belching or passing flatus.

DIRECTIONS
Infants (under 2 years): 0.3 ml four times daily after meals and at bedtime, or as directed by a physician. The dosage can also be mixed with 1 oz of cool water, infant formula or other suitable liquids to ease administration.
Adults and children: 0.6 ml four times daily, after meals and at bedtime, or as directed by a physician.

WARNINGS
Do not exceed 12 doses per day except under the advice and supervision of a physician. Keep this and all drugs out of the reach of children.

HOW SUPPLIED
INFANTS' MYLICON® Drops are available in bottles of 15 ml (0.5 fl oz) and 30 ml (1.0 fl oz) pink, pleasant tasting liquid. NDC 16837-630.
Shown in Product Identification Guide, page 318

MYLANTA AR ACID REDUCER™   OTC

DESCRIPTION
ACTIVE INGREDIENT: Famotidine 10 mg per tablet.
INACTIVE INGREDIENTS: Hydroxypropyl cellulose, hydroxypropyl methylcellulose, magnesium stearate, microcrystalline cellulose, starch, talc, titanium dioxide.

PRODUCT BENEFITS
- **1 tablet** relieves heartburn and acid indigestion.
- Mylanta AR Acid Reducer prevents heartburn and acid indigestion brought on by consuming food and beverages.
- It contains famotidine, a prescription-proven medicine.
The ingredient in Mylanta AR Acid Reducer, famotidine, has been prescribed by doctors for years to treat millions of patients safely and effectively. The active ingredient in Mylanta AR Acid Reducer has been taken safely with many frequently prescribed medications.
Action: It is normal for the stomach to produce acid, especially after consuming food and beverages. However, acid in the wrong place (the esophagus), or too much acid, can cause burning pain and discomfort that interfere with everyday activities.
- **Heartburn—Caused by acid in the esophagus**

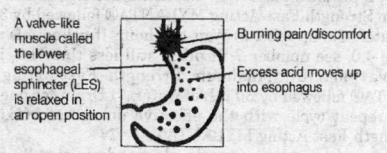

- **In clinical studies, Mylanta AR Acid Reducer was significantly better than placebo pills in relieving and preventing heartburn.**

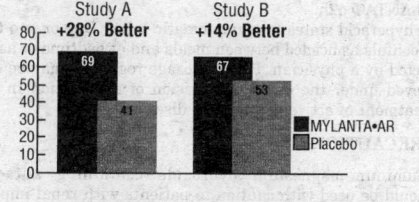

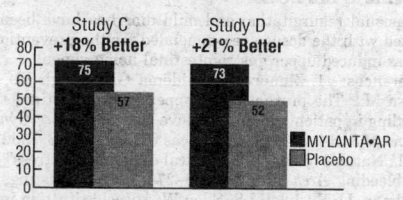

USES
- **For Relief** of heartburn, acid indigestion, and sour stomach;
- **For Prevention** of these symptoms brought on by consuming food and beverages.
How to help avoid symptoms
- Do not lie down soon after eating.
- If your are overweight, lose weight.
- If you smoke, stop or cut down.
- Avoid or limit foods such as caffeine, chocolate, fatty foods and alcohol.
- Do not eat just before bedtime.

WARNINGS
- Do not take the maximum daily dosage (2 tablets) for more than 2 weeks continuously except under the advice and supervision of a doctor.
- Do not use with other acid reducers.
- As with any drug, if you are pregnant or nursing a baby, seek the advice of a health professional before using this product.
- If you have trouble swallowing, or persistent abdominal pain, see your doctor promptly. You may have a serious condition that may need different treatment.
- Keep this and all drugs out of the reach of children.
- In case of accidental overdose, seek professional assistance or contact a poison control center immediately.

CAUTION
Heartburn and acid indigestion are common, but you should see your doctor promptly if:
- You have trouble swallowing or persistent abdominal pain. You may have a serious condition that may need different treatment.
- You have used the maximum dosage every day for two weeks continously.
Important: As with any drug, if you are pregnant or nursing a baby, seek the advice of a health professional before using this product. This product should not be given to children under 12 years old, unless directed by a doctor. Keep this and all drugs out of the reach of children. In case of accidental overdose, seek professional assistance or contact a poison control center immediately.

DIRECTIONS
- For **Relief** of symptoms **swallow 1 tablet with water.**
- For **Prevention** of symptoms brought on by consuming food and beverages **swallow 1 tablet with water 1 hour before eating a meal you expect to cause symptoms.**
- Can be used up to twice daily (up to 2 tablets in 24 hours).
- This product should not be given to children under 12 years old unless directed by a doctor.

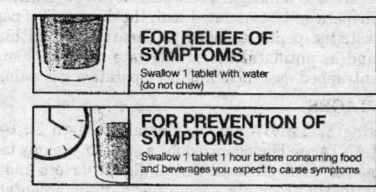

HOW SUPPLIED
Mylanta AR Acid Reducer is available as a white colored tablet identified as "MYL 10."
Mylanta AR is available in blister packs in boxes of 8, 16 and 30 tablets. NDC 16837-877.
- Read the directions and warnings before use.
- Keep the carton. It contains important information.
Store at temperatures up to 30°C (86°F).
Protect from moisture.
DO NOT USE IF THE INDIVIDUAL BLISTER UNIT IS OPEN OR BROKEN.

FAST-ACTING MYLANTA® AND   OTC
MAXIMUM-STRENGTH FAST-ACTING
MYLANTA®
[my-lan'ta]
Aluminum, Magnesium and Simethicone
Liquid
Antacid/Anti-Gas

DESCRIPTION
Fast-acting MYLANTA® and Maximum Strength Fast-Acting MYLANTA® are well-balanced, pleasant-tasting, antacid/anti-gas medications that provide consistent, effective relief of symptoms associated with gastric hyperacidity and excess gas. Non-constipating and very low sodium Fast-Acting MYLANTA® and Maximum Strength Fast-Acting MYLANTA® contain two proven antacids, aluminum hydroxide and magnesium hydroxide, plus simethicone for gas relief.

ACTIVE INGREDIENTS
Each 5 mL teaspoon contains:

Continued on next page

Fast-Acting Mylanta Liq.—Cont.

	MYLANTA®	MYLANTA® Double Strength
Aluminum Hydroxide	200 mg	400 mg
Magnesium Hydroxide	200 mg	400 mg
Simethicone	20 mg	40 mg

INACTIVE INGREDIENTS

LIQUIDS:
Butylparaben, carboxymethylcellulose sodium, flavors, hydroxypropyl methylcellulose, microcrystalline cellulose, propylparaben, purified water, saccharin sodium, and sorbitol.

SODIUM CONTENT

Each 5 mL teaspoon contains the following amount of sodium:

	MYLANTA®	MYLANTA® Double Strength
Liquid	0.68 mg	1.14 mg
	(0.03 mEq)	(0.05 mEq)

ACID NEUTRALIZING CAPACITY

Two teaspoonfuls have the following acid neutralizing capacity:

	Fast Acting MYLANTA®	Maximum Strength Fast Acting MYLANTA®
Liquid	25.4 mEq	50.8 mEq

INDICATIONS

Fast-Acting MYLANTA® and Maximum Strength Fast-Acting MYLANTA® are indicated for the relief of acid indigestion, heartburn, sour stomach, and symptoms of gas and upset stomach associated with those conditions. Fast-Acting MYLANTA® and Maximum Strength Fast-Acting MYLANTA® are also indicated as antacids for the symptomatic relief of hyperacidity associated with the diagnosis of peptic ulcer, gastritis, peptic esophagitis, heartburn and hiatal hernia and as antiflatulents to alleviate the symptoms of mucus-entrapped gas, including postoperative gas pain.

ADVANTAGES

Fast-Acting MYLANTA and Maximum Strength Fast-Acting MYLANTA are homogenized for a smooth, creamy taste. The choice of three pleasant-tasting liquid flavors and the non-constipating formula encourage patient acceptance, thereby minimizing the skipping of prescribed doses. Fast-Acting MYLANTA and Maximum Strength Fast-Acting MYLANTA are also available in tablets, and both the liquid and tablet forms are very low in sodium. Fast-Acting MYLANTA and Maximum Strength Fast-Acting MYLANTA provide consistent relief in patients suffering from distress associated with hyperacidity, mucus-entrapped gas, or swallowed air.

DIRECTIONS

Liquid:
Shake well. 2-4 teaspoonfuls between meals and at bedtime, or as directed by a physician.

WARNINGS

Keep this and all drugs out of the reach of children. Do not take more than 24 tsps of Fast-Acting MYLANTA® or 12 tsps of Maximum Strength Fast-Acting MYLANTA® in a 24-hour period or use the maximum dose of this product for more than two weeks, except under the advice and supervison of a physician. Do not use this product if you have kidney disease.

Prolonged use of aluminum-containing antacids in patients with renal failure may result in or worsen dialysis osteomalacia. Elevated tissue aluminum levels contribute to the development of the dialysis encephalopathy and osteomalacia syndromes. Small amounts of aluminum are absorbed from the gastrointestinal tract and renal excretion of aluminum is impaired in renal failure. Aluminum is not well removed by dialysis because it is bound to albumin and transferrin, which do not cross dialysis membranes. As a result, aluminum is deposited in bone, and dialysis osteomalacia may develop when large amounts of aluminum are ingested orally by patients with impaired renal function.

Aluminum forms insoluble complexes with phosphate in the gastrointestinal tract, thus decreasing phosphate absorption. Prolonged use of aluminum-containing antacids by normophosphatemic patients may result in hypophosphatemia if phosphate intake is not adequate. In its more severe forms, hypophosphatemia can lead to anorexia, malaise, muscle weakness, and osteomalacia.

DRUG INTERACTION PRECAUTION

Antacids may interact with certain prescription drugs. If you are presently taking a prescription drug, do not take this product without checking with your physician or other health professional.

HOW SUPPLIED

Fast-Acting MYLANTA® and Maximum Strength Fast-Acting MYLANTA® are available as white liquid suspensions in pleasant-tasting flavors, Original, Cherry Creme and Cool Mint Creme. Liquids are supplied in bottles of 5 oz, 12 oz, and 24 oz. Also available for hospital use in liquid unit dose bottles of 1 oz and bottles of 5 oz.

MYLANTA®
NDC 16837-610 ORIGINAL LIQUID
NDC 16837-629 COOL MINT CREME LIQUID
NDC 16837-621 CHERRY CREME LIQUID
NDC 16837-817 Lemon Twist Liquid
MYLANTA® Maximum Strength
NDC 16837-652 ORIGINAL LIQUID
NDC 16837-624 COOL MINT CREME LIQUID
NDC 16837-622 CHERRY CREME LIQUID
NDC 16837-818 Lemon Twist Liquid

Professional Labeling

INDICATIONS

Stress-induced upper gastrointestinal hemorrhage: Maximum Strength Fast-Acting MYLANTA® is indicated for the prevention of stress-induced upper gastrointestinal hemorrhage. Hyperacidic conditions: As an antacid, for the symptomatic relief of hyperacidity associated with the diagnosis of peptic ulcer and other gastrointestinal conditions where a high degree of acid neutralization is desired.

DIRECTIONS

Prevention of stress-induced upper gastrointestinal hemorrhage: 1) Aspirate stomach via nasogastric tube* and record pH. 2) Instill 10 mL of Maximum Strength Fast-Acting MYLANTA® followed by 30 mL of water via nasogastric tube. Clamp tube. 3) Wait one hour. Aspirate stomach and record pH. 4a) If pH equals or exceeds 4.0, apply drainage or intermittent suction for one hour, then repeat the cycle. 4b) If pH is less than 4.0, instill double (20 mL) Maximum Strength Fast-Acting MYLANTA® followed by 30 mL of water. Clamp tube. 5) Wait one hour. If pH equals or exceeds 4.0, see number 7, if pH is still less than 4.0, instill double (40 mL) Maximum Strength Fast-Acting MYLANTA® followed by 30 mL of water. Clamp tube. 6) Wait one hour. If pH equals or exceeds 4.0, see number 7. If pH is still less than 4.0, instill double (80 mL)† Maximum Strength Fast-Acting MYLANTA® followed by 30 mL of water. 7) Drain for one hour and repeat cycle with the effective dosage of Maximum Strength Fast-Acting MYLANTA®.

*If nasogastric tube is not in place, administer 20 mL of Maximum Strength Fast-Acting MYLANTA® orally q2h.
† In a recent clinical study[1] 20 mL of Maximum Strength Fast-Acting MYLANTA®, q2h, was sufficient in more than 85 percent of the patients. No patient studied required more than 80 mL of Maximum Strength Fast-Acting MYLANTA® q2h.

In hyperacid states for symptomatic relief: One or two teaspoonfuls as needed between meals and at bedtime or as directed by a physician. Higher dosage regimens may be employed under the direct supervision of a physician in the treatment of active peptic ulcer disease.

PRECAUTIONS

Aluminum-magnesium hydroxide containing antacids should be used with caution in patients with renal impairment.

ADVERSE EFFECTS

Occasional regurgitation and mild diarrhea have been reported with the dosage recommended for the prevention of stress-induced upper gastrointestinal hemorrhage.
References: 1. Zinner MJ, Zuidema GD, Smigh PL, Mignosa M: The prevention of upper gastrointestinal tract bleeding in patients in an intensive care unit. *Surg Gynecol Obster* 153:214–220, 1981. 2. Lucas CE, Sugawa C, Riddle J, et al.: Natural history and surgical dilemma of "stress" gastric bleeding. *Arch Surg* 102:266–273, 1971. 3. Hastings PR, Skillman JJ, Bushnell LS, Silen W: Antacid titration in the prevention of acute gastrointestinal bleeding: a controlled, randomized trial in 100 critically ill patients. *N Engl J Med* 298:1042–1045, 1978. 4. Day SB, MacMillan BG, Altemeier WA: *Curling's Ulcer, An Experience of Nature.* Springfield, IL, Charles C Thomas Co., 1972, p. 205. 5. Skillman JJ, Bushnell LS, Goldman H, Silen W: Respiratory failure, hypotension, sepsis, and jaundice. A clinical syndrome associated with lethal hemorrhage from acute stress ulceration of the stomach. *Am J Surg* 117:523–530, 1969. 6. Priebe HJ,

Skillman J, Bushnell LS, et al. Antacid versus cimetidine in preventing acute gastrointestinal bleeding. *N Engl J Med* 302:426–430, 1980. 7. Silen W: The prevention and management of stress ulcers. *Hosp Pract* 15:93–97, 1980. 8. Herrmann V, Kaminski DL: Evaluation of intragastric pH in acutely ill patients. *Arch Surg* 114:511–514, 1979. 9. Martin LF, Staloch DK, Simonowitz DA, et al.: Failure of cimetidine prophylaxis in the critically ill. *Arch Surg* 114:492–496, 1979. 10. Zinner MJ, Turtinen L, Gurll NJ, Reynolds DG: The effect of metiamide on gastric mucosal injury in rat restraint. *Clin Res* 23:484A, 1975. 11. Zinner M, Turtinen BA, Gurll NJ: The role of acid and ischemia in production of stress ulcers during canine hemorrhagic shock. *Surgery* 77:807–816, 1975. 12. Winans CS: Prevention and treatment of stress ulcer bleeding: Antacids or cimetidine? *Drug Ther Bull* (hospital) 12:37–45, 1981.
Shown in Product Identification Guide, page 317

FAST-ACTING MYLANTA AND MAXIMUM STRENGTH FAST ACTING MYLANTA   OTC
[mylan 'ta]
Calcium Carbonate and Magnesium Hydroxide Tablets Antacid

DESCRIPTION

Fast-Acting MYLANTA and Maximum Strength Fast-Acting MYLANTA are well balanced, pleasant tasting antacid medications that provide consistent, effective relief of symptoms associated with gastric hyperacidity. Non-constipating and very low in sodium, Fast-Acting MYLANTA and Maximum Strength Fast-Acting MYLANTA contain two proven antacids, calcium carbonate and magnesium hydroxide.
Active Ingredients
Each tablet contains:

	Fast-Acting MYLANTA	Maximum Strength Fast-Acting MYLANTA
Calcium Carbonate	350mg	700mg
Magnesium Hydroxide	150mg	300mg

Inactive Ingredients
Citric acid, confectioner's sugar, flavors, magnesium stearate, sorbitol, FD&C Blue 1 or D&C Yellow 10 or D&C Red 27

Sodium Content
Each chewable tablet contains the following amount of sodium:

Fast-Acting MYLANTA	Maximum Strength Fast-Acting MYLANTA
0.3mg	0.6mg

Acid Neutralizing Capacity
Two chewable tablets have the following acid neutralizing capacity:

Fast-Acting MYLANTA	Maximum Strength Fast-Acting MYLANTA
24.0mEq	48.0mEq

INDICATIONS

Fast-Acting MYLANTA and Maximum Strength Fast-Acting MYLANTA are indicated for the relief of heartburn, acid indigestion, sour stomach and upset stomach associated with these conditions. Fast-Acting MYLANTA and Maximum Strength Fast-Acting MYLANTA are also indicated as antacids for the symptomatic relief of hyperacidity associated with the diagnosis of peptic ulcer, gastritis, peptic esophagitis, heartburn and hiatal hernia.

DIRECTIONS

Thoroughly chew 2–4 tablets between meals, at bedtime or as directed by a physician.

WARNINGS

Keep this and all drugs out of the reach of children. Do not take more than 20 tablets of Fast-Acting MYLANTA or 10 tablets of MYLANTA Maximum Strength Fast-Acting in a 24-hour period, or use the maximum dosage for more than two weeks. Do not use this product if you have kidney disease, except under the advise and supervision of a physician.

DRUG INTERACTION PRECAUTION

Antacids may interact with certain prescription drugs. If you are presently taking a prescription drug, do not take this product without checking with your physician or other health professional.

HOW SUPPLIED

Fast-Acting MYLANTA is available as a green Cool Mint Creme chewable tablet. Maximum Strength Fast-Acting MYLANTA is available as a green Cool Mint Creme Chewable tablet and pink Cherry Creme chewable tablet.

Fast-Acting Mylanta
NDC 16837-848 Cool Mint Creme
Maximum Strength Fast-Acting MYLANTA
NDC 16837-869 Cherry Creme
NDC 16837-849 Cool Mint Creme
Shown in Product Identification Guide, page 317

MYLANTA® GAS Relief Tablets   OTC
Maximum Strength MYLANTA® GAS
Relief Tablets
MYLANTA® Gas Relief Gelcaps
[*My-lan '-ta*]
Antiflatulent

ACTIVE INGREDIENTS

Each chewable tablet contains:

	Simethicone
MYLANTA® GAS Relief	80 mg
Maximum Strength-	
MYLANTA® GAS Relief	125 mg
MYLANTA® GAS Relief Gelcaps	62.5 mg

INACTIVE INGREDIENTS

TABLETS: Dextrates, flavor, sorbitol, stearic acid, tricalcium phosphate. Cherry: Red 7.
GELCAPS: Benzyl alcohol, butylparaben, castor oil, croscarmellose sodium, D&C Red 28, D&C Yellow 10, dextrose, dibasic calcium phosphate dihydrate, edetate calcium disodium, FD&C Blue 1, FD&C Red 28, gelatin, hydroxypropyl methylcellulose, maltodextrin, methylparaben, microcrystalline cellulose, propylene glycol, propylparaben, silicon dioxide, sodium lauryl sulfate, sodium propionate, sorbitol, stearic acid, titanium dioxide, tribasic calcium phosphate.

INDICATIONS

For relief of the symptoms of excess gas in the digestive tract. Such gas is frequently caused by excessive swallowing of air or by eating foods that disagree. MYLANTA® GAS Relief Gelcaps, MYLANTA® GAS Relief, and Maximum Strength MYLANTA® GAS Relief Tablets are high capacity antiflatulents for adjunctive treatment of many conditions in which the retention of gas may be a problem, such as the following: air swallowing, postoperative gaseous distention, peptic ulcer, spastic or irritable colon, diverticulosis. If condition persists, consult your physician.
MYLANTA® GAS Relief Gelcap, MYLANTA® GAS Relief, and Maximum Strength MYLANTA® GAS Relief Tablets have a defoaming action that relieves flatulence by dispersing and preventing the formation of mucus-surrounded gas pockets in the gastrointestinal tract. MYLANTA® GAS Relief Gelcaps, MYLANTA® GAS Relief, and Maximum Strength MYLANTA® GAS Relief Tablets act in the stomach and intestines to change the surface tension of gas bubbles enabling them to coalesce, thereby freeing and eliminating the gas more easily by belching or passing flatus.

DIRECTIONS

MYLANTA® GAS Relief Tablets
One tablet four times daily after meals and at bedtime. May also be taken as needed up to six tablets daily or as directed by a physician.
Maximum Strength MYLANTA® GAS Relief Tablets
One tablet four times daily after meals and at bedtime or as directed by a physician.
TABLETS SHOULD BE CHEWED THOROUGHLY
MYLANTA® GAS Relief Gelcaps
Swallow 2-4 gelcaps as needed after meals and at bedtime. Do not exceed 8 gelcaps per day unless directed by a physician.

WARNINGS

Keep this and all drugs out of the reach of children.

HOW SUPPLIED

MYLANTA® GAS Relief Tablets are available as white (mint) or pink (cherry) scored, chewable tablets identified "MYL GAS 80." Mint flavor is available in bottles of 60 and 100 tablets and individually wrapped 12 and 30 tablet packages. Cherry flavor is available in packages of 12 individually wrapped tablets. Mint NDC 16837-858. Cherry NDC 16837-859.
Maximum Strength MYLANTA® GAS Relief Tablets are available as white, scored, chewable tablets identified "MYL GAS 125" in individually wrapped 12 and 24 tablet packages and economical 48 tablet bottles. NDC 16837-455.
MYLANTA® Gas Relief Gelcaps are available as blue and yellow gelcaps identified as 'MYLANTA GAS' in individually wrapped 24 tablet packages. NDC 16837-626.
Shown in Product Identification Guide, pages 317 and 318

PEPCID AC® ACID CONTROLLER™   OTC

DESCRIPTION

ACTIVE INGREDIENT: Famotidine 10 mg per tablet.
INACTIVE INGREDIENTS: Hydroxypropyl cellulose, hydroxypropyl methylcellulose, red iron oxide, magnesium stearate, microcrystalline cellulose, starch, talc, titanium dioxide.

Product Benefits:

- 1 tablet relieves heartburn and acid indigestion.
- Pepcid AC Acid Controller prevents heartburn and acid indigestion brought on by consuming food and beverages. It contains famotidine, a prescription-proven medicine.

The ingredient in PEPCID AC Acid Controller, famotidine, has been prescribed by doctors for years to treat millions of patients safely and effectively. The active ingredient in PEPCID AC Acid Controller has been taken safely with many frequently prescribed medications.
Action: It is normal for the stomach to produce acid, especially after consuming food and beverages. However, acid in the wrong place (the esophagus), or too much acid, can cause burning pain and discomfort that interfere with everyday activities.

- **Heartburn—Caused by acid in the esophagus**

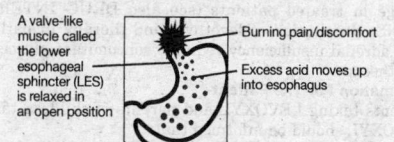

A valve-like muscle called the lower esophageal sphincter (LES) is relaxed in an open position
Burning pain/discomfort
Excess acid moves up into esophagus

In clinical studies, PEPCID AC Acid Controller was significantly better than placebo pills in relieving and preventing heartburn.

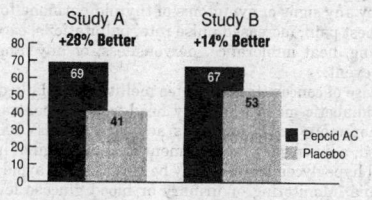

Study A +28% Better: Pepcid AC 69, Placebo 41
Study B +14% Better: Pepcid AC 67, Placebo 53

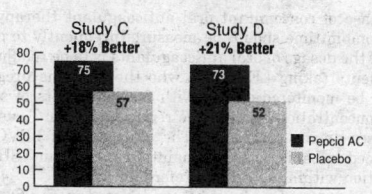

Study C +18% Better: Pepcid AC 75, Placebo 57
Study D +21% Better: Pepcid AC 73, Placebo 52

Uses:

- **For Relief** of heartburn, acid indigestion, and sour stomach;
- **For Prevention** of these symptoms brought on by consuming food and beverages.

How to help avoid symptoms

- Do not lie down soon after eating.
- If your are overweight, lose weight.
- If you smoke, stop or cut down.
- Avoid or limit foods such as caffeine, chocolate, fatty foods and alcohol.
- Do not eat just before bedtime.

WARNINGS

- Do not take the maximum daily dosage for more than 2 weeks continuously except under the advice and supervision of a doctor.
- Do not use with other acid reducers.
- As with any drug, if you are pregnant or nursing a baby, seek the advice of a health professional before using this product.
- If you have trouble swallowing, or persistent abdominal pain, see your doctor promptly. You may have a serious condition that may need different treatment.
- Keep this and all drugs out of the reach of children.
- In case of accidental overdose, seek professional assistance or contact a poison control center immediately.

Caution:
Heartburn and acid indigestion are common, but you should see your doctor promptly if:

- You have trouble swallowing or persistent abdominal pain. You may have a serious condition that may need different treatment.
- You have used the maximum dosage every day for two weeks continously.

Important: As with any drug, if you are pregnant or nursing a baby, seek the advice of a health professional before

using this product. This product should not be given to children under 12 years old, unless directed by a doctor. Keep this and all drugs out of the reach of children. In case of accidental overdose, seek professional assistance or contact a poison control center immediately.

DIRECTIONS

- **For Relief** of symptoms **swallow 1 tablet with water.**
- **For Prevention** of symptoms brought on by consuming food and beverages **swallow 1 tablet with water 1 hour before eating a meal you expect to cause symptoms.**
- Can be used up to twice daily (up to 2 tablets in 24 hours).
- This product should not be given to children under 12 years old unless directed by a doctor.

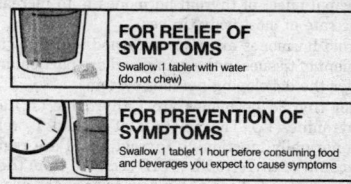

FOR RELIEF OF SYMPTOMS
Swallow 1 tablet with water (do not chew)

FOR PREVENTION OF SYMPTOMS
Swallow 1 tablet 1 hour before consuming food and beverages you expect to cause symptoms

HOW SUPPLIED

Pepcid AC Acid Controller is available as a rose-colored tablet identified as 'PEPCID AC'.
Pepcid AC is available in blister packs in boxes of 6, 12, 18, 30, 50, and 80 tablets. NDC 16837-872

- Read the directions and warnings before use.
- Keep the carton. It contains important information.

Store at temperatures up to 30°C (86°F).
Protect from moisture.
DO NOT USE IF THE INDIVIDUAL BLISTER UNIT IS OPEN OR BROKEN.
Shown in Product Identification Guide, page 318

Jones Medical Industries, Inc.

1945 CRAIG ROAD
PO BOX 46903
ST LOUIS, MO 63146

Direct Inquiries to:
Customer Service:
314-576-6100
Fax:
314-469-5749

BREVITAL® SODIUM   ℂ ℞
METHOHEXITAL SODIUM
FOR INJECTION, USP
For Intravenous Use

CYTOMEL®   ℞
[*sigh "toe 'mel*]
brand of liothyronine sodium
tablets

LEVOXYL®   ℞
(Levothyroxine Sodium Tablets, USP)
FOR ORAL ADMINISTRATION

DESCRIPTION

Each LEVOXYL (Levothyroxine Sodium, USP) tablet contains synthetic crystalline levothyroxine sodium (L-thyroxine). L-thyroxine is the principle hormone secreted by the normal thyroid gland. Chemically, L-thyroxine is designated as L-tyrosine, 0-(4-hydroxy-3,5-diiodophenyl) - 3,5-diiodo-, monosodium salt, hydrate. The molecular formula is $C_{15}H_{10}I_4N$ NaO_4 and the structural formula is:

$$HO \text{—} \bigcirc \text{—} O \text{—} \bigcirc \text{—} CH_2 \text{—} \underset{H}{\overset{NH_2}{C}} \text{—} COONa \cdot xH_2O$$

INACTIVE INGREDIENTS: lactose, microcrystalline cellulose, pre-gelatinized starch, magnesium stearate. The following are the color additives per tablet strength:

Strength (mcg)		Strength (mcg)	
Color Additive(s)		(Color Additive(s)	
25	FD&C Yellow No. 6	125	FD&C Red No. 40
50	none		D&C Yellow No. 10
75	FD&C Blue No. 1	137	FD&C Blue No. 1
	D&C Red No. 30	150	FD&C Blue No. 1

Continued on next page

Levoxyl—Cont.

88	FD&C Yellow No. 6 FD&CBlue No. 1 D&C Yellow No. 10		D&C Red No. 30
		175	D&C Blue No. 1 D&C Yellow No. 10
100	FD&C Yellow No. 6 D&C Yellow No. 10	200	D&C Red No. 30 D&C Yellow No. 10
112	FD&C Yellow No. 6 FD&C Red No. 40 D&C Red No. 30	300	FD&C Yellow No. 6 FD&C Blue No. 1 D&C Yellow No. 10

CLINICAL PHARMACOLOGY

The principal effect of thyroid hormones is to increase the metabolic rate of most body tissues.

The thyroid hormones are also concerned with growth and development of tissues in the young and are particularly important for the developing nervous system.

The major thyroid hormones are L-thyroxine (T_4) and L-triiodothyronine (T_3). The amounts of T_4 and T_3 released from the normally functioning thyroid gland are regulated by the amount of thyrotropin (TSH) secreted from the anterior pituitary gland. T_4 is the major component of normal thyroid gland secretions and is therefore the primary determinant of normal thyroid functions. T_4 acts as a substrate for physiologic deiodination to T_3 in the peripheral tissues. The physiologic effects of thyroid hormones are largely mediated at the cellular level primarily by T_3. LEVOXYL (L-thyroxine) tablets taken orally provide T_4 which upon absorption cannot be distinguished from T_4 secreted endogenously. Oral T_4 is absorbed in the small intestine, mainly in the jejunum and ileum; about two-thirds to three-quarters of the oral dose is actually absorbed. Absorption may be less than expected in patients with malabsorptive bowel disease, such as sprue, or with short bowel syndromes. Absorption is also affected by food and is slightly higher in the fasting state compared to when an oral dose is taken with food; the difference, however, is usually not of much clinical consequence. Certain other medications taken concomitantly by mouth can diminish absorption of T_4 from intestinal lumen; these include aluminum hydroxide, sucralfate, ferrous sulfate, soybean-based foods (often taken for medical reasons), and binding resins used to lower cholesterol.

Once in the blood stream, T_4 is bound to plasma proteins, mainly to thyroxine-binding globulin (TBG); nevertheless, T_4 gains access to the tissues where it acts because the small fraction of T_4 that is not bound to plasma proteins ("free T_4") does cross all membranes. A small fraction of circulating T_4 is also converted to circulating triiodothyronine (T_3), mainly in the liver; T_3 is also largely bound to circulating plasma proteins but not as tightly as is T_4. Once inside responsive cells, T_4 is converted to T_3 which is the major thyroid hormone acting intracellularly; circulating T_3 also gains access to the intracellular space and contributes to the action of thyroid hormone.

Circulating T_4 is gradually eliminated from the body with a plasma half-life of about seven days. Thus, an oral dose given once daily, once the dose is stabilized, results in a fairly stable level of serum T_4 over the course of the next 24 hours except for a slight rise of 10% to 15% in the few hours after the oral dose. The circulating T_3 formed from circulating T_4, on the other hand, is cleared from the blood much more rapidly with a plasma half-life of about 1 to 1 1/2 days. Thus, the oral dosing of T_4 results in a steady, stable serum level of T_4 which in turn provides an equally stable level of serum T_3. Oral T_3 given alone, on the other hand, results in a fairly rapid rise and fall in the serum T_3 level after each and fails to mimic the normal pattern of serum T_3.

INDICATIONS AND USAGE

LEVOXYL (L-thyroxine) tablets are indicated as:

1. Replacement therapy for any form of diminished or absent thyroid function, e.g., as in cretinism, myxedema, or hypopituitarism, and including hypothyroidism seen in children, in pregnancy and in the elderly. The hypothyroidism may result from functional deficiency, primary atrophy, or partial or complete absence of the thyroid gland; from the effects of surgery, radiation or antithyroid agents on the thyroid gland; or from pituitary or hypothalamic disease. LEVOXYL therapy must usually be maintained continuously to control the hypothyroidism. When hypothyroidism is due to subacute or postpartum thyroiditis, it may be temporary and treatment need not be permanent.
2. A means of suppressing pituitary secretion of TSH in euthyroid patients in order to treat or prevent the recurrence of various types of goiter, including thyroid nodules, lymphocytic thyroiditis(Hashimoto's), multinodular goiter, and as part of the management of thyroid cancer. An exception is a patient with euthyroid autonomous function wherein the goiter is not under the control of pituitary TSH; T_4 therapy is not indicated in such patients (see below under CONTRAINDICATIONS).
3. A diagnostic agent in suppression tests to aid in the diagnosis of suspected mild hyperthyroidism or thyroid gland autonomy; this should be done rarely, only when clinically indicated and only when other tests such as stimulation with thyrotropin-releasing hormone (TRH) have not resolved the problem.

CONTRAINDICATIONS

L-thyroxine therapy is contraindicated in untreated thyrotoxicosis, in other states of thyroid autonomy, acute myocardial infarction and uncorrected adrenal insufficiency.

WARNINGS

Drugs with thyroid hormone activity, alone or together with other therapeutic agents, have been used for the treatment of obesity. In euthyroid patients, doses within the range of daily hormonal requirements are ineffective for weight reduction. Larger doses may produce serious or even life-threatening manifestations of toxicity, particularly when given in association with sympathomimetic amines such as those used for their anorectic effects.

PRECAUTIONS

General—Caution must be exercised in the administration of this drug to patients with cardiovascular disease. Development of chest pain or other aggravation of the cardiovascular disease may preclude its use or require a reduction of dosage in treated patients (see also DRUG INTERACTIONS). Institution of levothyroxine therapy in patients with adrenal insufficiency requires concomitant glucocorticoid therapy.

Information For The Patient-

Patients taking LEVOXYL and parents of children taking LEVOXYL should be informed that:

1. Replacement therapy is to be taken essentially for life, with the exception of cases of transient hypothyroidism, usually associated with thyroiditis, and in those patients receiving a therapeutic tiral of the drug.
2. They should immediately report during the course of therapy any signs or symptoms of thyroid hormone toxicity, e.g., chest pain, increased pulse rate, palpitations, excessive sweating, heat intolerance, nervousness, or any other unusual event.
3. In case of concomitant diabetes mellitus, the daily dosage of antidiabetic medication may need readjustment as thyroid horomone replacement is achieved. If LEVOXYL is stopped, a downward readjustment of the dosage of insulin or oral hypoglycemic agent may be necessary to avoid hypoglycemia. Monitoring or urinary or blood glucose levels is mandatory in such patients during changes in thyroid medication.
4. In case of concomitant oral anticoagulant therapy, the prothrombin time should be measured frequently to determine if the dosage of oral anticoagulants is to be readjusted.
5. Patients taking LEVOXYL who then become pregnant should be monitored closely with measurements of serum TSH concentration because the requirement for T_4 usually increases during pregnancy. The daily dose of LEVOXYL may need to be increased to maintain the serum TSH concentration within the normal reference range.
6. Partial loss of hair may be experienced in the first few months of thyroid therapy, but this is usually a transient phenomenon and later recovery is the rule.

Laboratory Tests—The patient's response to thyroid replacement can be followed by laboratory tests such as serum levels of thyroxine (T_4, serum triiodothyronine (T_3), free thyroxine index and thyroid stimulating hormone (TSH). The principal test used to monitor treatment in primary hypothyroidism is the serum TSH level. In hypopituitarism, the serum TSH level is not usually useful and monitoring should be done with measurement of serum total or free T_4. In euthyroid goiter patients or those with thyroid cancer, the serum TSH should be suppressed below the reference range; how far below the reference range depends on the clinical goal.

Drug Interactions—In patients with diabetes mellitus, addition of oral T_4 therapy may cause an increase in the required dosage of insulin or oral hypoglycemic agents. Therefore, patients with diabetes mellitus should be observed closely for possible changes in antidiabetic drug dosage requirements.

Patients stabilized on oral anticoagulants who are found to require thyroid replacement therapy should be watched very closely when therapy is started; successful treatment with LEVOXYL in a patient who is initially hypothyroid may result in a need for a lower dose of oral anticoagulant. No special precautions appear to be necessary when oral anticoagulant therapy is begun in a patient already stabilized on maintenance LEVOXYL therapy. Cholestyramine and colestipol binding T_4 in the intestine, thus impairing its absorption. In vitro studies indicate that the binding is not easily reversed. Therefore, four to five hours should elapse between administration of cholestyramine and oral T_4. Other medications that interfere with absorption of oral T_4 from the gut include sucralfate, ferrous sulfate, aluminum hydroxide and soy-containing dietary supplements.

Estrogens tend to increase serum thyronine-binding globulin (TBG). In a patient with a non-functioning thyroid gland who is receiving thyroid replacement therapy, free thyroxine may be decreased when etrogens are started thus increasing LEVOXYL requirements. Therefore, patients without a functioning thyrid gland who are on thyroid replacement therapy may need to increase their dosage of LEVOXYL if estrogens or estrogen-containing oral contraceptives are given. This need can be assessed by measurement of the serum TSH level. Similarly, androgen therapy in hypogonadal men, or women with breast cancer, can decrease TBG; the result may be a decreased need for oral T_4 and so the dosage of LEVOXYL may need to be decreased. Again, measurement of the serum TSH level is a good method of assessing this possibility.

Drug/Laboratory Test Interactions—The following drugs or moieties are known to interfere with laboratory tests performed on patients taking thyroid hormone: androgens, corticosteroids, estrogens, oral contraceptives containing estrogens, iodine-containing preparations, and salicylates. In some instances, e.g., the use of androgens, estrogens, or oral contraceptives, patients' thyroid status may be affected and monitoring with serum TSH measurement may be indicated.

1. Pregnancy, estorgens, and estrogen-containing oral contraceptives increase TBG concentrations. TBG may also be increased during infectious hepatitis. Decreases in TBG concentrations can occur in nephrosis, acromegaly, or during androgen or corticosteroid therapy. Familial hyper- or hypo-thyroxne-binding-globulinemias have been described. The binding of thyroxine by thyroid-binding pre-albumin (TBPA) is inhibited by salicylates. In all these cases of changes in L-T_4 binding to serum proteins, the serum T_4 level may change. Measurement of the serum TSH level will determine the clinical significance of any change in serum T_4.
2. A high iodine intake interferes with radio-iodine uptake (RAIU) in normal persons but the RAIU would be low in those taking thyroxine in any case; this test has little use in patients treated with oral T_4 and the interference of a high iodine intake is of little clinical relevance.
3. Continued evidence of hypothyroidism in spite of apparently adequate dosage replacement indicated poor patient compliance, poor absorption, excessive fecal loss, interference by conocomitantly ingested food, or inactivity of the preparation. Poor compliance is the most common cause but each possible cause should be considered.

Carcinogenesis, Mutagenesis, and Impairment of Fertility—A reportedly apparent association between prolonged thyroid therapy and breast cancer has not been confirmed and patients taking LEVOXYL for established indications should not discontinue therapy. There are no data suggesting that L-T_4 is mutagenic or impairs fertility; such studies in animals over the long term have not been performed.

Pregnancy—Category A—Thyroid hormones do not readily cross the placental barrier. Clinical experience to date does not indicate any adverse effect on fetuses when thyroid hormones are administered to pregnant women. On the basis of current knowledge, LEVOXYL replacement therapy to hypothyroid women should not be discontinued during pregnancy. During pregnancy, LEVOXYL requirements may increase; dosage should be guided pby periodic measurements of serum TSH concentration.

Nursing Mothers—Some thyroid hormone is excreted in human milk but this is usually insufficient for hypothyroid nursing neonates. L-T_4 taken by nursing mothers is not associated with serious adverse reactions and does not have a known tumorigenic potential; properly indicated LEVOXYL therapy should be continued.

Pediatric Use—Congenital hypothyroidism is uncommon (1: 4,000) and is not prevented by the small amounts of hormone that cross the placenta. Determination of serum T_4 and/or TSH is needed to make the diagnosis in neonates and must be done within a few days of birth to prevent the serious effects of hypothyroidism on growth and development, particularly of the brain and nervous system. Treatment should be initiated immediately upon diagnosis, and maintained for life, unless transient hypothyroidism is suspected in which case therapy may be interrupted for 2 to 8 weeks after the age of 3 years to reassess the condition. Cessation of therapy is justified in patients who have maintained a normal TSH during those 2 to 8 weeks.

ADVERSE REACTIONS

Adverse reactions are due to overdosage and are those of induced hyperthyroidism.

OVERDOSAGE

Excessive dosage of thyroid medication may result in symptoms of hyperthyroidism. Since, however, the effects do not appear at once, the symptoms may not appear for one to three weeks after an excessive dose is begun. The most common signs and symptoms of overdosage are weight loss, palpitation, nervousness, diarrhea or abdominal cramps, sweating, tachycardia, cardiac arrhythmias, angina pectoris, tremors, headache, insomnia, and intolerance to heat. If symptoms of overdosage appear, discontinue the medication for several days and reinstitute treatment at a lower dosage level.

Laboratory tests such as serum T_4, serum T_3 and the free thyroxine index will be elevated during the period of overdosage and the hallmark is a clearly suppressed serum TSH level. Complications as a result of the induced hypermetabolic state may include cardiac failure and death due to arrhythmia or failure.

TREATMENT OF OVERDOSAGE—Dosage should be reduced or therapy temporarily discontinued if signs and symptoms of overdosage appear. Treatment may be reinstituted at a lower dosage.

Treatment of acute massive thyroid hormone overdosage is aimed at reduing gastrointestinal absorption of the drugs and counteracting central and peripheral effects, mainly those of increased sympathetic activity. Vomiting may be induced initially if further gastrointestinal absorption can reasonably be prevented provided there are no contraindications such as coma, convulsions, or loss of the gag reflex. Treatment is mainly symptomatic and supportive. Oxygen may be administered and ventilation maintained. Cardiac glycosides may be indicated if congestive heart failure develops. Measures to control fever, hypoglycemia, or fluid loss should be instituted if needed. Antiadrenergic agents, particularly propranolol, have been used advantageously in the treatment of increased sympathetic activity. Propranolol may be administered intravenously at a dosage of 1 to 3 mg over a 10 minute period or orally, 80 to 160 mg/day, especially when no contraindications exist for its use.

DOSAGE AND ADMINISTRATION

Primary Hypothyroidism—The goal of therapy in primary hypothyroidism should be the restoration of euthyroidism as judged by clinical response and confirmed by appropriate laboratory tests such as serum thyroxine (T_4), serum triiodothyronine (T_3), free thyroxine index and serum TSH; the principal measure in primary hypothyroidism is the serum TSH level. The age and general condition of the patient, the severity and duration of hypothyroid symptoms, and whether or not the serum TSH level remains high or has become normal determine the starting dose of LEVOXYL and the rate of incremental dosage increase leading to a final maintenance dosage.

In otherwise healthy adults with primary hypothyroidism, the recommended initial dosage of LEVOXYL is 25 to 100 mcg (0.025 to 0.1 mg) daily, while the predicted full maintenance dose of 100 to 200 mcg (0.1 to 0.2 mg) daily may be achieved in several months.

In the elderly patient with primary hypothyroidism, particularly in those with long-standing or severe primary hypothyroidism or with evidence of cardiovascular dysfunction, the initial dose of LEVOXYL may be as little as 12.5 mcg (0.0125 mg) per day; incremental increases of 25 mcg (0.025 mg) per day at 4 to 6 week intervals may be instituted depending on patient response. It is the physician's judgement of the severity of the disease and close observation of patient response and of the serum TSH level which determine the rate and extent of dosage increase.

Once the serum TSH level in those with primary hypothyroidism has fallen to the normal reference range during LEVOXYL treatment and the serum TSH concentration has been stable at this level for 4 to 8 weeks, the daily dose being taken is then the maintenance dose. To monitor the adequacy of this dose and patient compliance, periodic assessment of the serum TSh level should be done. The aim is the maintenance of the serum TSH level in the normal reference range. There are no data showing the optimum frequency of measurement of serum TSH concentration in this circumstance but common practice is 1 to 3 times per year; if there is reason to suspect poor compliance with therapy or other potential problems, the serum TSH measurement should be done more often, even when the dose of oral T_4 is unchanged.

Severe Hypothyroidism—Sometimes referred to as "myxedema coma", far-advanced hypothyroidism is an uncommon but dangerous and potentially lethal state. Often precipitated by another event, such as infection or injury, in an already hypothyroid patient and often characterized by hypothermia and somnolence or actual coma, severe hypothyroidism is a medical emergency. Other characteristics are slow pulse, electrolyte abnormalities such as hyponatremia, respiratory failure with CO_2 retention, and hypotension. The principal treatment initially is aimed at supportive therapy, treatment of infection if present, gentle warming if indicated, and correction of non-thyroid abnormalities such as abnormal electrolyte values or cardiac arrhythmias. Glucocorticoid therapy is often given, although there are no data showing clear benefit. In addition, replacement therapy with levothyroxine is essential. While oral T_4 appears to be well absorbed in such patients, there are no data showing in a controlled trial whether it is better to give the L-T_4 by mouth, by nasogastric tube, or parenterally. Nevertheless, many prefer to give the LT-$_4$ parenterally. Similarly, there is no clear consensus on the dose of L-T_4 to be used; some prefer to give enough to replace the entire deficiency of circulating T_4 (often 400 to 600 mcg, usually parenterally, as a single dose or given over a few hours) while other physicians prefer to begin with smaller doses, e.g., 75 to 150 mcg, (0.075-0.15 mg) given by mouth, if possible, or parenterally, if not. Further dosing of L-T_4 depends on patient response which in turn requires intensive monitoring for at least a few days. The total daily dose of L-T_4 given after the initial dose should in general not exceed the daily dose required previously by the patient or the average daily dose taken by similar patients. Clinical judgement is a major determinant of the details of treatment because laboratory results will usually not be available initially.

Secondary Hypothyroidism—Hypothyroidism due to pituitary or hypothalamic disease, or secondary hypothyroidism, is uncommon; the vast majority of hypothyroid patients have primary hypothyroidism. Secondary hypothyroidism is suspected whenever there is known hypothalamic or pituitary disease, such as pituitary tumor or diabetes insipidus; it is characterized by a low serum concentration of total T_4 or free T_4 without a clearly raised serum TSH concentration; the serum TSH level may be slightly raised, in the reference range, or low. The serum TSH level cannot be used to monitor the dosage of LEVOXYL as it is in primary hypothyroidism. The initial dose of LEVOXYL should be chosen as it is in the primary hypothyroidism, observing the same guidelines and precautions (see **Primary Hypothyroidism**). Further dose increases, if any, are based on the clinical response using clinical judgement and measurement of serum total or free T_4.

Suppression of Pituitary Secretion of TSH—In selected patients with goiter, thyroid nodules, or papillary or follicular thyroid cancer, LEVOXYL can be used in an attempt to inhibit growth or prevent re-growth of the abnormal thyroid tissue; the overall management may include other therapies such as surgery or radioactive iodine. The suppressive action of LEVOXYL is based on the known ability of oral T_4 to suppress pituitary secretion of TSH even when patients are initially euthyroid (a hypothyroid person with any of the above conditions should be treated with LEVOXYL in any case for the hypothyroidism). Because most persons with these conditions are euthyroid and so have a normal serum TSH concentration, the goal of LEVOXYL therapy is to suppress the serum TSH level to below the reference range. In so doing, some patients with these conditions may have an inhibition of further growth of the abnormal thyroid tissue. Because various clinical trials have reached different conclusions on the efficacy of oral T_4 in the treatment of thyroid nodules or goiter and there are no controlled trials on its use in papillary or follicular thyroid cancer or on the degree to which the serum TSH level needs to be suppressed, the use of LEVOXYL in these conditions needs to be individualized; continued use depends on the clincial response balanced against the possibility of induced hyperthyroidism. In general, the suppression of serum TSH concentration should be to the level of 0.1 to 0.2 mU/L although some prefer to suppress the serum TSH concentration to less than 0.1 mu/L in patients with differentiated thyroid carcinoma.

Pediatric Hypothyroidism—In infants and children there is a great urgency to achieve full thyroid replacement because of the critical importance of thyroid hormone is sustaining growth and maturation as well as development of the brain and intellectual function. Despite the smaller body size, the dosage needed to sustain a full rate of growth, development and general thriving is higher in the child than in the adult. The recommended daily replaceent dosage of L-thyroxine in childhood is: 0–6 months: 8–10 mcg/kg; 6–12 months: 6–8 mcg/kg; 1–5 years: 5–6 mg/kg; 6–12 years: 4–5 mcg/kg of body weight daily.

HOW SUPPLIED

LEVOXYL (L-thyroxine) tablets are supplied as oval, color-coded, potency marked tablets in 12 strengths:

25 mcg-Orange:
Bottles of 100, NDC 0689-1117-01
Bottles of 1000, NDC 0689-1117-10
Unit dose cartons of 100, NDC 0689-1117-05

50 mcg-White:
Bottles of 100, NDC 0689-1118-01
Bottles of 1000, NDC 0689-1118-10
Unit dose cartons of 100, NDC 0689-1118-05

75 mcg-Purple:
Bottles of 100, NDC 0689-1119-01
Bottles of 100, NDC 0689-1119-10
Unit dose cartons of 100, NDC 0689-1119-05

88 mcg-Olive;
Bottles of 100, NDC 0689-1132-01
Bottles of 1000, NDC 0689-1132-10

100 mcg-Yellow:
Bottles of 100, NDC 0689-1110-01
Bottles of 1000, NDC 0689-1110-10
Unit dose cartons of 100, NDC 0689-1110-05

112 mcg-Rose:
Bottles of 100, NDC 0689-1130-01
Bottles of 1000, NDC 0689-1130-10

125 mcg-Brown:
Bottles of 100, NDC 0689-1120-01
Bottles of 1000, NDC 0689-1120-10
Unit dose cartons of 100, NDC 0689-1120-05

137 mcg-Dark Blue:
Bottles of 100, NDC 0689-1135-01
Bottles of 1000, NDC 0689-1135-10

150 mcg-Blue:
Bottles of 100, NDC 0689-1111-01
Bottles of 1000, NDC 0689-1111-10
Unit dose cartons of 100, NDC 0689-1111-05

175 mcg-Turquoise:
Bottles of 100, NDC 0689-1122-01
Bottles of 1000, NDC 0689-1122-10

200 mcg-Pink:
Bottles of 100, NDC 0689-1112-01
Bottles of 1000, NDC 0689-1112-10
Unit dose cartons of 100, NDC 0689-1112-05

300 mcg-Green:
Bottles of 100, NDC 0689-1121-01
Bottles of 1000, NDC 0689-1121-10

Store at controlled room temperature 15°–30°C (59°–86°F)
Caution: Federal (USA) law prohibits dispensing without a prescription.

JONES MEDICAL INDUSTRIES, INC.
1945 Craig Road
ST. LOUIS, MO 63146
(NASDAQ: JMED)
800-525-8466 Revised May 1996

Shown in Product Identification Guide, page 318

TABLETS
TAPAZOLE® ℞
METHIMAZOLE TABLETS, USP

DESCRIPTION

Tapazole® (Methimazole Tablets, USP) (1–methylimidazole-2-thiol) is a white, crystalline substance that is freely soluble in water. It differs chemically from the drugs of the thiouracil series primarily because it has a 5-instead of a 6–membered ring.

Each tablet contains 5 or 10 mg (43.8 or 87.6 µmol) methimazole, an orally administered antithyroid drug.

Each tablet also contains lactose, magnesium stearate, starch, and talc.

The molecular weight is 114.16, and the empirical formula is $C_4H_6N_2S$. The structural formula is as follows:

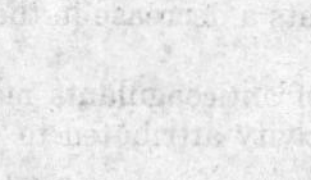

CLINICAL PHARMACOLOGY

Methimazole inhibits the synthesis of thyroid hormones and thus is effective in the treatment of hyperthyroidism. The drug does not inactivate existing thyroxine and triiodothyronine that are stored in the thyroid or circulating in the blood nor does it interfere with the effectiveness of thyroid hormones given by mouth or by injection.

The actions and use of methimazole are similar to those of propylthiouracil. On a weight basis, the drug is at least 10 times as potent as propylthiouracil, but methimazole, may be less consistent in action.

Methimazole is readily absorbed from the gastrointestinal tract. It is metabolized rapidly and requires frequent administration. Methimazole is excreted in the urine.

In laboratory animals, various regimens that continuously suppress thyroid function and thereby increase TSH secretion result in thyroid tissue hypertrophy. Under such conditions, the appearance of thyroid and pituitary neoplasms has also been reported. Regimens that have been studied in this regard include antithyroid agents, as well as dietary iodine deficiency, subtotal thyroidectomy, implantation of autonomous thyrotropic hormone-secreting pituitary tumors, and administration of chemical goitrogens.

INDICATIONS AND USAGE

Tapazole is indicated in the medical treatment of hyperthyroidism. Long-term therapy may lead to remission of the disease. Tapazole may be used to ameliorate hyperthyroidism in preparation for subtotal thyroidectomy or radioactive iodine therapy. Tapazole is also used when thyroidectomy is contraindicated or not advisable.

CONTRAINDICATIONS

Tapazole is contraindicated in the presence of hypersensitivity to the drug and in nursing mothers because the drug is excreted in milk.

WARNINGS

Agranulocytosis is potentially a serious side effect. Patients should be instructed to report to their physicians any symptoms of agranulocytosis, such as fever or sore throat. Leukopenia, thrombocytopenia, and aplastic anemia (pancytopenia) may also occur. The drug should be discontinued in

Continued on next page

Tapazole—Cont.

the presence of agranulocytosis, aplastic anemia (pancytopenia), hepatitis, or exfoliative dermatitis. The patient's bone marrow function should be monitored.

Due to the similar hepatic toxicity profiles of Tapazole and propylthiouracil, attention is drawn to the severe hepatic reactions which have occurred with both drugs. There have been rare reports of fulminant hepatitis, hepatic necrosis, encephalopathy, and death. Symptoms suggestive of hepatic dysfunction (anorexia, pruritus, right upper quadrant pain, etc) should prompt evaluation of liver function. Drug treatment should be discontinued promptly in the event of clinically significant evidence of liver abnormality including hepatic transaminase values exceeding 3 times the upper limit of normal.

Tapazole can cause fetal harm when administered to a pregnant woman. Tapazole readily crosses the placental membranes and can induce goiter and even cretinism in the developing fetus. In addition, rare instances of aplasia cutis, as manifested by scalp defects, have occurred in infants born to mothers who received Tapazole during pregnancy. If Tapazole is used during pregnancy or if the patient becomes pregnant while taking this drug, the patient should be warned of the potential hazard to the fetus.

Since scalp defects have not been reported in offspring of patients treated with propylthiouracil, that agent may be preferable to Tapazole in pregnant women requiring treatment with antithyroid drugs.

Postpartum patients receiving Tapazole should not nurse their babies.

PRECAUTIONS

General—Patients who receive Tapzole should be under close surveillance and should be cautioned to report immediately any evidence of illness, particularly sore throat, skin eruptions, fever, headache, or general malaise. In such cases, white-blood-cell and differential counts should be made to determine whether agranulocytosis has developed. Particular care should be exercised with patients who are receiving additional drugs known to cause agranulocytosis.

Laboratory Tests—Because Tapazole may cause hypoprothrombinemia and bleeding, prothrombin time should be monitored during therapy with the drug, especially before surgical procedures (*see* General *under* Precautions).

Periodic monitoring thyroid function is warranted, and the finding of an elevated TSH warrants a decrease in the dosage of Tapazole.

Drug Interactions—The activity of anticoagulants may be potentiated by anti-vitamin-K activity attributed to Tapazole.

Carcinogenesis, Mutagenesis, Impairment of Fertility—In a 2 year study, rats were given methimazole at doses of 0.5, 3, and 18 mg/kg/day. These doses were 0.3, 2, and 12 times the 15 mg/day maximum human maintenance dose (when calculated on the basis of surface area). Thyroid hyperplasia, adenoma, and carcinoma developed in rats at the two higher doses. The clinical significance of these findings is unclear.

Pregnancy Category D—See Warnings—Tapazole used judiciously is an effective drug in hyperthyroidism complicated by pregnancy. In many pregnant women, the thyroid dysfunction diminishes as the pregnancy proceeds; consequently, a reduction in dosage may be possible. In some instances, use of Tapazole can be discontinued 2 or 3 weeks before delivery.

Nursing Mothers—The drug appears in human breast milk and its use is contraindicated in nursing mothers (*see* Warnings).

Usage in Children—See Dosage and Administration.

ADVERSE REACTIONS

Major adverse reactions (which occur with much less frequency than the minor adverse reactions) include inhibition of myelopoiesis (agranulocytosis, granulocytopenia, and thrombocytopenia), aplastic anemia, drug fever, a lupuslike syndrome, insulin autoimmune syndrome (which can result in hypoglycemia coma), hepatitis (jaundice may persist for several weeks after discontinuation of the drug), periarteritis, and hypoprothrombinemia. Nephritis occurs very rarely. Minor adverse reactions include skin rash, urticaria, nausea, vomiting, epigastric distress, arthralgia, paresthesia, loss of taste, abnormal loss of hair, myalgia, headache, pruritus, drowsiness, neuritis, edema, vertigo, skin pigmentation, jaundice, sialadenopathy, and lymphadenopathy.

It should be noted that about 10% of patients with untreated hyperthyroidism have leukopenia (white-blood-cell count of less than 4,000/mm^3), often with relative granulopenia.

OVERDOSAGE

Signs and Symptoms—Symptoms may include nausea, vomiting, epigastric distress, headache, fever, joint pain, pruritus, and edema. Aplastic anemia (pancytopenia) or agranulocytosis may be mainfested in hours to days. Less frequent events are hepatitis, nephrotic syndrome, exfolia-

tive dermatitis, neuropathies, and CNS stimulation or depression. Although not well studied, methimazole-induced agranulocytosis is generally associated with doses of 40 mg or more in patients older than 40 years of age.

No information is available on the median lethal dose of the drug or the concentration of methimazole in biologic fluids associated with toxicity and/or death.

Treatment—To obtain up-to-date information about the treatment of overdose, a good resource is your certified Regional Poison Control Center. Telephone numbers of certified poison control centers are listed in the *Physicians' Desk Reference (PDR)*. In managing overdosage, consider the possibility of multiple drug overdoses, interaction among drugs, and unusual drug kinetics in your patient.

Protect the patient's airway and support ventilation and perfusion. Meticulously monitor and maintain, within acceptable limits, the patient's vital signs, blood gases, serum electrolytes, etc. The patient's bone marrow function should be monitored. Absorption of drugs from the gastrointestinal tract may be decreased by giving activated charcoal, which, in many cases, is more effective than emesis or lavage; consider charcoal instead of or in addition to gastric emptying. Repeated doses of charcoal over time may hasten elimination of some drugs that have been absorbed. Safeguard the patient's airway when employing gastric emptying or charcoal.

Forced diuresis, peritoneal dialysis, hemodialysis, or charcoal hemoperfusion have not been established as beneficial for an overdose of methimazole.

DOSAGE AND ADMINSTRATION

Tapazole is administered orally. It is usually given in 3 equal doses at approximately 8-hour intervals.

Adult—The initial daily dosage is 15 mg for mild hyperthyroidism, 30 to 40 mg for moderately severe hyperthyroidism, and 60 mg for severe hyperthyroidism, divided into 3 doses at 8-hour intervals. The maintenance dosage is 5 to 15 mg daily.

Pediatric—Initially, the daily dosage is 0.4 mg/kg of body weight divided into 3 doses and given at 8-hour intervals. The maintenance dosage is approximately $\frac{1}{2}$ of the initial dose.

HOW SUPPLIED

Tapazole® Tablets, are available in:

The 5-mg tablets (UC5385) are white in color, round, beveled, scored, and debossed with "J94".

They are available as follows:

   Bottles of 100   NDC 52604-1094-1
    (No. 1765)

The 10-mg tablets (UC5386) are white in color, round, beveled, scored, and debossed with "J95".

They are available as follows:

   Bottles of 100   NDC 52604-1095-1
    (No. 1770)

Store at controlled room temperature, 59° to 86°F (15° to 30°C).

CAUTION—Federal (USA) law prohibits dispensing without prescription.

Literature issued May 1, 1996

Distributed Exclusively by
Jones Medical Industries, Inc.
St. Louis, MO 63146
Mfd. by Eli Lilly and Company
Indianapolis, IN 46285
PV 0370 UCP

THROMBIN, TOPICAL U.S.P.
(BOVINE ORIGIN)

THROMBIN-JMI™   R

TRIOSTAT™   R
[*try 'o-stat*]
brand of
liothyronine sodium
injection
(T₃)

For information on over-the-counter drugs, consult **PDR For Nonprescription Drugs**.

Key Pharmaceuticals, Inc.
GALLOPING HILL ROAD
KENILWORTH, NJ 07033

For Medical Information Contact:
Generally:
Drug Information Services
(800) 526-4099
(9:00 AM to 5:00 PM EST)

After Hours and Weekends:
(908) 298-4000

Product Identification Codes

To provide quick and positive identification of Key Products, we have imprinted the product identification number of the National Drug Code on most tablets and capsules. In some cases, identification letters also appear.

Additionally: the following telephone numbers are provided for inquiries:

Drug Information Services
9:00 AM to 5:00 PM EST
1-800-526-4099
After regular hours and on weekends (908) 298-4000

IMDUR®   R
(isosorbide mononitrate)
Extended Release Tablets

DESCRIPTION

Isosorbide mononitrate (ISMN), an organic nitrate and the major biologically active metabolite of isosorbide dinitrate (ISDN), is a vasodilator with effects on both arteries and veins.

IMDUR Tablets contain 30 mg, 60 mg, or 120 mg of isosorbide mononitrate in an extended-release formulation. The inactive ingredients are aluminum silicate, colloidal silicon dioxide, hydroxypropyl cellulose, hydroxypropyl methylcellulose, iron oxide, magnesium stearate, paraffin wax, polyethylene glycol, titanium dioxide, and trace amounts of ethanol.

The chemical name for ISMN is 1,4:3,6-dianhydro-, D-glucitol 5-nitrate; the compound has the following structural formula:

ISMN is a white, crystalline, odorless compound which is stable in air and in solution, has a melting point of about 90°C, and an optical rotation of +144° (2% in water, 20°C). Isosorbide mononitrate is freely soluble in water, ethanol, methanol, chloroform, ethyl acetate, and dichloromethane.

CLINICAL PHARMACOLOGY

Mechanism of Action The IMDUR® product is an oral extended-release formulation of ISMN, the major active metabolite of isosorbide dinitrate; most of the clinical activity of the dinitrate is attributable to the mononitrate.

The principal pharmacological action of ISMN and all organic nitrates in general is relaxation of vascular smooth muscle, producing dilatation of peripheral arteries and veins, especially the latter. Dilatation of the veins promotes peripheral pooling of blood, decreases venous return to the heart, thereby reducing left ventricular end-diastolic pressure and pulmonary capillary wedge pressure (preload). Arteriolar relaxation reduces systemic vascular resistance, and systolic arterial pressure and mean arterial pressure (afterload). Dilatation of the coronary arteries also occurs. The relative importance of preload reduction, afterload reduction, and coronary dilatation remains undefined.

Pharmacodynamics Dosing regimens for most chronically used drugs are designed to provide plasma concentrations that are continuously greater than a minimally effective concentration. This strategy is inappropriate for organic nitrates. Several well-controlled clinical trials have used exercise testing to assess the antianginal efficacy of continuously delivered nitrates. In the large majority of these trials, active agents were indistinguishable from placebo after 24 hours (or less) of continuous therapy. Attempts to overcome tolerance by dose escalation, even to doses far in excess of those used acutely, have consistently failed. Only after nitrates have been absent from the body for several hours has their antianginal efficacy been restored. IMDUR Tablets during long-term use over 42 days dosed at 120 mg once daily continued to improve exercise performance at 4 hours and at 12 hours after dosing but its effects (although

better than placebo) are less than or at best equal to the effects of the first dose of 60 mg.

Pharmacokinetics and Metabolism After oral administration of ISMN as a solution or immediate-release tablets, maximum plasma concentrations of ISMN are achieved in 30 to 60 minutes, with an absolute bioavailability of approximately 100%. After intravenous administration, ISMN is distributed into total body water in about 9 minutes with a volume of distribution of approximately 0.6-0.7 L/kg. Isosorbide mononitrate is approximately 5% bound to human plasma proteins and is distributed into blood cells and saliva. Isosorbide mononitrate is primarily metabolized by the liver, but unlike oral isosorbide dinitrate, it is not subject to first-pass metabolism. Isosorbide mononitrate is cleared by denitration to isosorbide and glucuronidation as the mononitrate, with 96% of the administered dose excreted in the urine within 5 days and only about 1% eliminated in the feces. At least six different compounds have been detected in urine, with about 2% of the dose excreted as the unchanged drug and at least five metabolites. The metabolites are not pharmacologically active. Renal clearance accounts for only about 4% of total body clearance. The mean plasma elimination half-life of ISMN is approximately 5 hours.

The disposition of ISMN in patients with various degrees of renal insufficiency, liver cirrhosis, or cardiac dysfunction was evaluated and found to be similar to that observed in healthy subjects. The elimination half-life of ISMN was not prolonged, and there was no drug accumulation in patients with chronic renal failure after multiple oral dosing.

The pharmacokinetics and/or bioavailability of IMDUR Tablets have been studied in both normal volunteers and patients following single- and multiple-dose administration. Data from these studies suggest that the pharmacokinetics of ISMN administered as IMDUR Tablets are similar between normal healthy volunteers and patients with angina pectoris. In single- and multiple-dose studies, the pharmacokinetics of ISMN were dose proportional between 30 mg and 240 mg.

In a multiple-dose study, the effect of age on the pharmacokinetic profile of IMDUR 60 mg and 120 mg (2 x 60 mg) Tablets was evaluated in subjects ≥45 years. The results of that study indicate that there are no significant differences in any of the pharmacokinetic variables of ISMN between elderly (≥65 years) and younger individuals (45-64 years) for the IMDUR Tablets 120 mg (2 x 60 mg tablets every 24 hours for 7 days) produced a dose-proportional increase in C_{max} and AUC, without changes in T_{max} or the terminal half-life. The older group (65-74 years) showed 30% lower apparent oral clearance (Cl/F) following the higher dose, ie, 120 mg, compared to the younger group (45-64 years); Cl/F was not different between the two groups following the 60 mg regimen. While Cl/F was independent of dose in the younger group, the older group showed slightly lower Cl/F following the 120 mg regimen compared to the 60 mg regimen. Differences between the two age groups, however, were not statistically significant. In the same study, females showed a slight (15%) reduction in clearance when the dose was increased. Females showed higher AUCs and C_{max} compared to males, but these differences were accounted for by differences in body weight between the two groups. When the data were analyzed using age as a variable, the results indicated that there were no significant differences in any of the pharmacokinetic variables of ISMN between older (≥65 years) and younger individuals (45-64 years). The results of this study, however, should be viewed with caution due to the small numbers of subjects in each age subgroup and consequently the lack of sufficient statistical power.

The following table summarizes key pharmacokinetic parameters of ISMN after single- and multiple-dose administration of ISMN as an oral solution of IMDUR Tablets:

[See table above]

	SINGLE-DOSE STUDIES		MULTIPLE-DOSE STUDIES	
PARAMETER	ISMN 60 mg	IMDUR 60 mg	IMDUR 60 mg	IMDUR 120 mg
C_{max} (ng/mL)	1242-1534	424-541	557-572	1151-1180
T_{max} (hr)	0.6-0.7	3.1-4.5	2.9-4.2	3.1-3.2
AUC (ng•hr/mL)	8189-8313	5990-7452	6625-7555	14241-16800
$t_{1/2}$ (hr)	4.8-5.1	6.3-6.6	6.2-6.3	6.2-6.4
Cl/F (mL/min)	120-122	151-187	132-151	119-140

Food Effects The influence of food on the bioavailability of ISMN after single-dose administration of IMDUR Tablets 60 mg was evaluated in three different studies involving either a "light" breakfast or a high-calorie, high-fat breakfast. Results of these studies indicate that concomitant food intake may decrease the rate (increase in T_{max}) but not the extent (AUC) of absorption of ISMN.

CLINICAL TRIALS

Controlled trials with IMDUR Tablets have demonstrated antianginal activity following acute and chronic dosing. Administration of IMDUR Tablets once daily, taken early in the morning on arising, provided at least 12 hours of antianginal activity.

In a placebo-control parallel study 30, 60, 120, and 240 mg of IMDUR Tablets were administered once daily for up to 6 weeks. Prior to randomization, all patients completed a 1- to 3-week single-blind placebo phase to demonstrate nitrate responsiveness and total exercise treadmill time reproducibility. Exercise tolerance tests using the Bruce Protocol were conducted prior to and at 4 and 12 hours after the morning dose on days 1, 7, 14, 28, and 42 of the double-blind period. IMDUR Tablets 30 and 60 mg (only doses evaluated acutely) demonstrated a significant increase from baseline in total treadmill time relative to placebo at 4 and 12 hours after the administration of the first dose. At day 42, the 120 and 240 mg dose of IMDUR Tablets demonstrated a significant increase in total treadmill time at 4 and 12 hours postdosing, but by day 42 the 30 and 60 mg doses no longer were differentiable from placebo. Throughout chronic dosing rebound was not observed in any IMDUR treatment group.

Pooled data from two other trials, comparing IMDUR Tablets 60 mg once daily, ISDN 30 mg QID, and placebo QID in patients with chronic stable angina using a randomized, double-blind, three-way crossover design found statistically significant increases in exercise tolerance times for IMDUR Tablets compared to placebo at hours 4, 8, and 12 and to ISDN at hour 4. The increases in exercise tolerance on day 14, although statistically significant compared to placebo, were about half of that seen on day 1 of the trial.

INDICATIONS AND USAGE

IMDUR Tablets are indicated for the prevention of angina pectoris due to coronary artery disease. The onset of action of oral isosorbide mononitrate is not sufficiently rapid for this product to be useful in aborting an acute anginal episode.

CONTRAINDICATIONS

IMDUR Tablets are contraindicated to patients who have shown hypersensitivity or idiosyncratic reactions to other nitrates or nitrites.

WARNINGS

The benefits of ISMN in patients with acute myocardial infarction or congestive heart failure have not been established; because the effects of isosorbide mononitrate are difficult to terminate rapidly, this drug is not recommended in these settings.

If isosorbide mononitrate is used in these conditions, careful clinical or hemodynamic monitoring must be used to avoid the hazards of hypotension and tachycardia.

PRECAUTIONS

General Severe hypotension, particularly with upright posture, may occur with even small doses of isosorbide mononitrate. This drug should therefore be used with caution in patients who may be volume depleted or who, for whatever reason, are already hypotensive. Hypotension induced by isosorbide mononitrate may be accompanied by paradoxical bradycardia and increased angina pectoris.

Nitrate therapy may aggravate the angina caused by hypertrophic cardiomyopathy.

In industrial workers who have had long-term exposure to unknown (presumably high) doses of organic nitrates, tolerance clearly occurs. Chest pain, acute myocardial infarction, and even sudden death have occurred during temporary withdrawal of nitrates from these workers, demonstrating the existence of true physical dependence. The importance of these observations to the routine, clinical use of oral isosorbide mononitrate is not known.

Information for Patients Patients should be told that the antianginal efficacy of IMDUR Tablets can be maintained by carefully following the prescribed schedule of dosing. For most patients, this can be accomplished by taking the dose on arising.

As with other nitrates, daily headaches sometimes accompany treatment with isosorbide mononitrate. In patients who get these headaches, the headaches are a marker of the activity of the drug. Patients should resist the temptation to avoid headaches by altering the schedule of their treatment with isosorbide mononitrate, since loss of headache may be associated with simultaneous loss of antianginal efficacy. Aspirin or acetaminophen often successfully relieves isosorbide mononitrate-induced headaches with no deleterious effect on isosorbide mononitrate's antianginal efficacy.

Treatment with isosorbide mononitrate may be associated with light-headedness on standing, especially just after rising from a recumbent or seated position. This effect may be more frequent in patients who have also consumed alcohol.

Drug Interactions The vasodilating effects of isosorbide mononitrate may be additive with those of other vasodilators. Alcohol, in particular, has been found to exhibit additive effects of this variety.

Marked symptomatic orthostatic hypotension has been reported when calcium channel blockers and organic nitrates were used in combination. Dose adjustments of either class of agents may be necessary.

Drug/Laboratory Test Interactions Nitrates and nitrites may interfere with the Zlatkis-Zak color reaction, causing falsely low readings in serum cholesterol determinations.

Carcinogenesis, Mutagenesis, Impairment of Fertility No evidence of carcinogenicity was observed in rats exposed to isosorbide mononitrate in their diets at doses of up to 900 mg/kg/day for the first 6 months and 500 mg/kg/day for the remaining duration of a study in which males were dosed for up to 121 weeks and females were dosed for up to 137 weeks.

Isosorbide mononitrate did not produce gene mutations (Ames test, mouse lymphoma test) or chromosome aberrations (human lymphocyte and mouse micronucleus tests) at biologically relevant concentrations.

No effects on fertility were observed in a study in which male and female rats were administered doses of up to 750 mg/kg/day beginning, in males, 9 weeks prior to mating, and in females, 2 weeks prior to mating.

PREGNANCY

Teratogenic Effects *Pregnancy Category B.* In studies designed to detect effects of isosorbide mononitrate on embryofetal development, doses of up to 240 or 248 mg/kg/day, administered to pregnant rats and rabbits, were unassociated with evidence of such effects. These animal doses are about 100 times the maximum recommended human dose (120 mg in a 50 kg woman) when comparison is based on body weight; when comparison is based on body surface area, the rat dose is about 17 times the human dose and the rabbit dose is about 38 times the human dose. There are, however, no adequate and well-controlled studies in pregnant women. Because animal reproduction studies are not always predictive of human response, IMDUR Tablets should be used during pregnancy only if clearly needed.

Nonteratogenic Effects Neonatal survival and development and incidence of stillbirths were adversely affected when pregnant rats were administered oral doses of 750 (but not 300) mg isosorbide mononitrate/kg/day during late gestation and lactation. This dose (about 312 times the human dose when comparison is based on body weight and 54 times the human dose when comparison is based on body surface area) was associated with decreases in maternal weight gain and motor activity and evidence of impaired lactation.

Nursing Mothers It is not known whether this drug is excreted in human milk. Because many drugs are excreted in human milk, caution should be exercised when ISMN is administered to a nursing mother.

Pediatric Use The safety and effectiveness of ISMN in children have not been established.

ADVERSE REACTIONS

The table below shows the frequencies of the adverse events that occurred in >5% of the subjects in three placebo-controlled North American studies, in which patients in the active treatment arm received 30 mg, 60 mg, 120 mg, or 240 mg of isosorbide mononitrate as IMDUR Tablets once daily. In parentheses, the same table shows the frequencies with which these adverse events were associated with the discontinuation of treatment. Overall, 8% of the patients who received 30 mg, 60 mg, 120 mg or 240 mg of isosorbide mononitrate in the three placebo-controlled North American studies discontinued treatment because of adverse events. Most of these discontinued because of headache. Dizziness was rarely associated with withdrawal from these studies. Since headache appears to be a dose-related adverse effect and tends to disappear with continued treatment, it is recommended that IMDUR treatment be initiated at low doses for several days before being increased to desired levels.

[See table at top of next page]

In addition, the three North American trials were pooled with 11 controlled trials conducted in Europe. Among the 14 controlled trials, a total of 711 patients were randomized to IMDUR Tablets. When the pooled data were reviewed, headache and dizziness were the only adverse events that were reported by >5% of patients. Other adverse events, each reported by ≤5% of exposed patients, and in many cases of uncertain relation to drug treatment, were:

Autonomic Nervous System Disorders: Dry mouth, hot flushes.

Continued on next page

Imdur—Cont.

Body as a Whole: Asthenia, back pain, chest pain, edema, fatigue, fever, flu-like symptoms, malaise, rigors.
Cardiovascular Disorder, General: Cardiac Failure, hypertension, hypotension.
Central and Peripheral Nervous System Disorders: Dizziness, headache, hypoesthesia, migraine, neuritis, paresis, paresthesia, ptosis, tremor, vertigo.
Gastrointestinal System Disorders: Abdominal pain, constipation, diarrhea, dyspepsia, flatulence, gastric ulcer, gastritis, glossitis, hemorrhagic gastric ulcer, hemorrhoids, loose stools, melena, nausea, vomiting.
Hearing and Vestibular Disorders: Earache, tinnitus, tympanic membrane perforation.
Heart Rate and Rhythm Disorders: Arrhythmia, arrhythmia atrial, atrial fibrillation, bradycardia, bundle branch block, extrasystole, palpitation, tachycardia, ventricular tachycardia.
Liver and Biliary System Disorders: SGOT increase, SGPT increase.
Metabolic and Nutritional Disorders: Hyperuricemia, hypokalemia.
Musculoskeletal System Disorders: Arthralgia, frozen shoulder, muscle weakness, musculoskeletal pain, myalgia, myositis, tendon disorder, torticollis.
Myo-, Endo-, Pericardial, and Valve Disorders: Angina pectoris aggravated, heart murmur, heart sound abnormal, myocardial infarction, Q wave abnormality.
Platelet, Bleeding, and Clotting Disorders: Purpura, thrombocytopenia.
Psychiatric Disorders: Anxiety, concentration impaired, confusion, decreased libido, depression, impotence, insomnia, nervousness, paroniria, somnolence.
Red Blood Cell Disorder: Hypochromic anemia.
Reproductive Disorders, Female: Atrophic vaginitis, breast pain.
Resistance Mechanism Disorders: Bacterial infection, moniliasis, viral infection.
Respiratory System Disorders: Bronchitis, bronchospasm, coughing, dyspnea, increased sputum, nasal congestion, pharyngitis, pneumonia, pulmonary infiltration, rales, rhinitis, sinusitis.
Skin and Appendages Disorders: Acne, hair texture abnormal, increased sweating, pruritus, rash, skin nodule.
Urinary System Disorders: Polyuria, renal calculus, urinary tract infection.
Vascular (Extracardiac) Disorders: Flushing, intermittent claudication, leg ulcer, varicose vein.
Vision Disorders: Conjunctivitis, photophobia, vision abnormal.
In addition, the following spontaneous adverse event has been reported during the marketing of isosorbide mononitrate: syncope.

OVERDOSAGE

Hemodynamic Effects The ill effects of isosorbide mononitrate overdose are generally the results of isosorbide mononitrate's capacity to induce vasodilatation, venous pooling, reduced cardiac output, and hypotension. These hemodynamic changes may have protean manifestations, including increased intracranial pressure, with any or all of persistent throbbing headache, confusion, and moderate fever; vertigo; palpitations; visual disturbances; nausea and vomiting (possibly with colic and even bloody diarrhea); syncope (especially in the upright posture); air hunger and dyspnea, later followed by reduced ventilatory effort; diaphoresis, with the skin either flushed or cold and clammy; heart block and bradycardia; paralysis; coma; seizures; and death.
Laboratory determinations of serum levels of isosorbide mononitrate and its metabolites are not widely available, and such determinations have in any event, no established role in the management of isosorbide mononitrate overdose. There are no data suggesting what dose of isosorbide mononitrate is likely to be life threatening in humans. In rats and mice, there is significant lethality at doses of 2000 mg/kg and 3000 mg/kg, respectively.
No data are available to suggest physiological maneuvers (eg. maneuvers to change the pH of the urine) that might accelerate elimination of isosorbide mononitrate. In particular, dialysis is known to be ineffective in removing isosorbide mononitrate from the body.
No specific antagonist to the vasodilator effects of isosorbide mononitrate is known, and no intervention has been subject to controlled study as a therapy of isosorbide mononitrate overdose. Because the hypotension associated with isosorbide mononitrate overdose is the result of venodilatation and arterial hypovolemia, prudent therapy in this situation should be directed toward an increase in central fluid volume. Passive elevation of the patient's legs may be sufficient, but intravenous infusion of normal saline or similar fluid may also be necessary.
The use of epinephrine or other arterial vasoconstrictors in this setting is likely to do more harm than good.
In patients with renal disease or congestive heart failure, therapy resulting in central volume expansion is not with-

FREQUENCY AND ADVERSE EVENTS (DISCONTINUED)*

Three Controlled North American Studies

Dose	Placebo	30 mg	60 mg	120 mg**	240 mg**
Patients	96	60	102	65	65
Headache	15% (0%)	38% (5%)	51% (8%)	42% (5%)	57% (8%)
Dizziness	4% (0%)	8% (0%)	11% (1%)	9% (2%)	9% (2%)

* Some individuals discontinued for multiple reasons.
** Patients were started on 60 mg and titrated to their final dose.

out hazard. Treatment of isosorbide mononitrate overdose in these patients may be subtle and difficult, and invasive monitoring may be required.
Methemoglobinemia Methemoglobinemia has been reported in patients receiving other organic nitrates, and it probably could also occur as a side effect of isosorbide mononitrate. Certainly nitrate ions liberated during metabolism of isosorbide mononitrate can oxidize hemoglobin into methemoglobin. Even in patients totally without cytochrome b_5 reductase activity, however, and even assuming that the nitrate moiety of isosorbide mononitrate is quantitatively applied to oxidation of hemoglobin about 2 mg/kg of isosorbide mononitrate should be required before any of these patients manifest clinically significant ($\geq$10%) methemoglobinemia. In patients with normal reductase function, significant production of methemoglobin should require even larger doses of isosorbide mononitrate. In one study in which 36 patients received 2-4 weeks of continuous nitroglycerin therapy at 3.1 to 4.4 mg/hr (equivalent, in total administered dose of nitrate ions, to 7.8-11.1 mg of isosorbide mononitrate per hour), the average methemoglobin level measured was 0.2%; this was comparable to that observed in parallel patients who received placebo.
Notwithstanding these observations, there are case reports of significant methemoglobinemia in association with moderate overdoses of organic nitrates. None of the affected patients had been thought to be unusually susceptible.
Methemoglobin levels are available from most clinical laboratories. The diagnosis should be suspected in patients who exhibit signs of impaired oxygen delivery despite adequate cardiac output and adequate arterial pO_2. Classically, methemoglobinemic blood is described as chocolate brown, without color change on exposure to air.
When methemoglobinemia is diagnosed, the treatment of choice is methylene blue, 1-2 mg/kg intravenously.

DOSAGE AND ADMINISTRATION

The recommended starting dose of IMDUR Tablets is 30 mg (given as a single 30 mg tablet or as ½ of a 60 mg tablet) or 60 mg (given as a single tablet) once daily. After several days the dosage may be increased to 120 mg (given as a single 120 mg tablet or as two 60 mg tablets) once daily. Rarely, 240 mg may be required. The daily dose of IMDUR Tablets should be taken in the morning on arising IMDUR Extended Release Tablets should not be chewed or crushed and should be swallowed together with a half-glassful of fluid.

HOW SUPPLIED

IMDUR Extended Release Tablets
30 mg: rose-colored tablets, scored on both sides and branded with the tradename ("IMDUR") on one side and the strength on the other.
Bottles of 30 .... NDC 0085-3306-02
Bottles of 100 .... NDC 0085-3306-03
Unit Dose 100 (10 x 10 blister strips) NDC 0085-3306-01
Unit Dose 90 (9 x 10 blister strips)
　Institutional Pack for
　Inpatient Use Only .... NDC 0085-3306-04
60 mg: yellow-colored tablets, scored on both sides and branded with the tradename ("IMDUR") on one side and the strength on the other.
Bottles of 100 .... NDC 0085-4110-03
Unit Dose 100 (10 x 10 blister strips) NDC 0085-4110-01
Unit Dose 90 (9 x 10 blister strips)
　Institutional Pack for
　Inpatient Use Only .... NDC 0085-4110-05
120 mg: white-colored tablets, branded with the tradename ("IMDUR") on one side and the strength on the other.
Bottles of 100 .... NDC 0085-1153-03
Unit Dose 100 (10 x 10 blister strips) NDC 0085-1153-04
Unit Dose 90 (9 x 10 blister strips)
　Institutional Pack for
　Inpatient Use Only .... NDC 0085-1153-07
Store at controlled room temperature 20°-25°C (68°-77°F) [see USP].
Protect unit dose from excessive moisture.

IMDUR®
(isosorbide mononitrate)
Extended Release Tablets

Manufactured for Key Pharmaceuticals, Inc.,
Kenilworth, NJ 07033 by A.B. ASTRA, Sweden.

Shown in Product Identification Guide, page 318

INTEGRILIN™　　　　　　　　　　　　　　　　　　℞
[ĭn-tĕg-rĭl-in]
(eptifibatide)
Injection

For Intravenous Administration

DESCRIPTION

Eptifibatide is a cyclic heptapeptide containing six amino acids and one mercaptopropionyl (des-amino cysteinyl) residue. An interchain disulfide bridge is formed between the cysteine amide and the mercaptopropionyl moieties. Chemically it is N^6-(aminoiminomethyl)-N^2-(3-mercapto-1-oxopropyl-L-lysylglycyl-L-α-aspartyl-L-tryptophyl-L-prolyl-L-cysteinamide, cyclic (1→6)-disulfide. Eptifibatide binds to the platelet receptor glycoprotein (GP) IIb/IIIa of human platelets and inhibits platelet aggregation.
The eptifibatide peptide is produced by solution-phase peptide synthesis, and is purified by preparative reverse-phase liquid chromatography and lyophilized. The structural formula is:

$C_{35}H_{49}N_{11}O_9S_2$　　　　　　　　Mol. Wt. 831.96

INTEGRILIN (eptifibatide) Injection is a clear, colorless, sterile, non-pyrogenic solution for intravenous (IV) use. Each 10-mL vial contains 2 mg/mL of eptifibatide and each 100-mL vial contains 0.75 mg/mL of eptifibatide. Each vial of either size also contains 5.25 mg/mL citric acid and sodium hydroxide to adjust the pH to 5.25.

CLINICAL PHARMACOLOGY

Mechanism of Action. Eptifibatide reversibly inhibits platelet aggregation by preventing the binding of fibrinogen, von Willebrand factor, and other adhesive ligands to GP IIb/IIIa. When administered intravenously, eptifibatide inhibits *ex vivo* platelet aggregation in a dose- and concentration-dependent manner. Platelet aggregation inhibition is reversible following cessation of the eptifibatide infusion; this is thought to result from dissociation of eptifibatide from the platelet.
Pharmacodynamics. Infusion of eptifibatide into baboons caused a dose-dependent inhibition of *ex vivo* platelet aggregation, with complete inhibition of aggregation achieved at infusion rates greater than 5 µg/kg/min. In a baboon model that is refractory to aspirin and heparin, doses of eptifibatide that inhibit aggregation prevented acute thrombosis with only a modest prolongation (2- to 3-fold) of the bleeding time. Platelet aggregation in dogs was also inhibited by infusions of eptifibatide, with complete inhibition at 2 µg/kg/min. This infusion dose completely inhibited canine coronary thrombosis induced by coronary artery injury (Folts model).
Human pharmacodynamic data were obtained in healthy subjects and in patients presenting with unstable angina (UA) or non-Q-wave myocardial infarction (NQMI) and/or

undergoing percutaneous coronary interventions. Studies in healthy subjects enrolled only males; patient studies enrolled approximately one third women. In these studies, eptifibatide inhibited *ex vivo* platelet aggregation induced by adenosine diphosphate (ADP) and other agonists in a dose- and concentration-dependent manner. The effect of eptifibatide was observed immediately after administration of a 180 μg/kg intravenous bolus. Table 1 shows the effects on platelet function and bleeding time of the doses of eptifibatide used in the two principal clinical studies.

Table 1
Platelet Inhibition and Bleeding Time

	IMPACT II 135/0.5	PURSUIT 180/2.0
Inhibition of platelet aggregation 15 min. after bolus	69%	84%
Inhibition of platelet aggregation at steady state	40–50%	>90%
Bleeding-time prolongation at steady state	<5×	<5×
Inhibition of platelet aggregation 4h after infusion discontinuation	<30%	<50%
Bleeding-time prolongation 6h after infusion discontinuation	1×	1.4×

When administered alone, eptifibatide has no measurable effect on prothrombin time (PT) or activated partial thromboplastin time (aPTT). (See also PRECAUTIONS: Drug Interactions.)

There were no important differences between men and women or between age groups in the pharmacodynamics properties of eptifibatide. Differences among ethnic groups have not been assessed.

Pharmacokinetics. The pharmacokinetics of eptifibatide are linear and dose-proportional for bolus doses ranging from 90 to 250 μg/kg and infusion rates from 0.5 to 3 μg/kg/min. Plasma elimination half-life is approximately 2.5 hours. The recommended regimens of a bolus followed by an infusion produce an early peak level, followed by a small decline with attainment of steady state within 4–6 hours. The extent of eptifibatide binding to human plasma protein is about 25%.

Excretion and Metabolism. Clearance in patients with coronary artery disease is 55–58 mL/kg/h. In healthy subjects, renal clearance accounts for approximately 50% of total body clearance, with the majority of the drug excreted in the urine as eptifibatide, deamidated eptifibatide, and other, more polar metabolites. No major metabolites have been detected in human plasma. Clinical studies have included 2418 patients with serum creatinine between 1 and 2 mg/dL (for the 180 μg/kg bolus and the 2 μg/kg/min infusion) and 7 patients with serum creatinine between 2 and 4 mg/dL (for the 135 μg/kg bolus and the 0.5 μg/kg/min infusion), without dose adjustment. No data are available in patients with more severe degrees of renal impairment, but plasma eptifibatide levels are expected to be higher in such patients (see CONTRAINDICATIONS).

Special Populations. Patients in clinical studies were older than the subjects in clinical pharmacology studies, and they had lower total body eptifibatide clearance and higher eptifibatide plasma levels. Clinical studies were conducted in patients aged 20 to 94 years with coronary artery disease without dose adjustment for age. Because patients over 75 years of age were enrolled into the PURSUIT clinical study only if their body weight exceeded 50 kg, minimal data are available on lighter-weight patients over 75 years of age. Men and women showed no important differences in the pharmacokinetics of eptifibatide.

CLINICAL STUDIES

Eptifibatide was studied in two placebo-controlled, randomized studies, one (PURSUIT) in patients with acute coronary syndrome (unstable angina (UA) or non-Q-wave myocardial infarction (NQMI)), the other (IMPACT II) in patients about to undergo a percutaneous cardiovascular intervention (PCI; balloon angioplasty in most cases, but sometimes directional atherectomy, transluminal extraction catheter atherectomy, rotational ablation atherectomy, or excimer-laser angioplasty).

Acute coronary syndrome is defined as prolonged (≥10 minutes) symptoms of cardiac ischemia within the previous 24 hours associated with either ST-segment changes (elevation between 0.6 mm and 1 mm or depression >0.5 mm), T-wave inversion (>1 mm), or positive CK-MB. This definition includes "unstable angina" and "non-Q-wave myocardial infarction" but excludes myocardial infarction that is associated with Q waves or greater degrees of ST-segment elevation.

PURSUIT was a 726-center, 27-country, double-blind, randomized, placebo-controlled study in 10,948 patients presenting with UA or NQMI. Patients could be enrolled only if they had experienced cardiac ischemia at rest (≥10 minutes) within the previous 24 hours and had either ST-segment changes (elevations between 0.6 mm and 1 mm or depression >0.5 mm), T-wave inversion (>1 mm), or increased CK-MB. Important exclusion criteria included a history of bleeding diathesis, evidence of abnormal bleeding within the previous 30 days, uncontrolled hypertension, major surgery within the previous 6 weeks, stroke within the previous 30 days, any history of hemorrhagic stroke, serum creatinine >2 mg/dL, dependency on renal dialysis, or platelet count <100,000/mm^3.

Table 2
Clinical Events in The PURSUIT Study

Death or MI	Placebo (n = 4739) n (%)	Eptifibatide (180/2.0) (n = 4722) n (%)	p-value
3 days	359 (7.6%)	279 (5.9%)	0.001
7 days	552 (11.6%)	477 (10.1%)	0.016
30 days			
Death or MI (Primary Endpoint)	745 (15.7%)	672 (14.2%)	0.042
Death	177 (3.7%)	165 (3.5%)	
Nonfatal MI	568 (12.0%)	507 (10.7%)	

Patients were randomized to either placebo, eptifibatide 180 μg/kg bolus followed by a 2 μg/kg/min infusion (180/2.0), or eptifibatide 180 μg/kg bolus followed by a 1.3 μg/kg/min infusion (180/1.3). The infusion was continued for 72 hours, until hospital discharge, or until the time of coronary artery bypass grafting (CABG), whichever occurred first, except that if PCI was performed, the eptifibatide infusion was continued for 24 hours after the procedure, allowing for a duration of infusion up to 96 hours.

The lower-infusion-rate arm was stopped after the first interim analysis when the two active-treatment arms appeared to have the same incidence of bleeding.

Patient age ranged from 20 to 94 (mean 63) years, and 65% were male. The patients were 89% Caucasian, 6% Hispanic, and 5% Black, recruited in the United States and Canada (40%), Western Europe (39%), Eastern Europe (16%), and Latin America (5%).

This was a "real world" study; each patient was managed according to the usual standards of the investigational site; frequencies of angiography, PCI, and CABG therefore differed widely from site to site and from country to country. Of the patients in PURSUIT, 13% were managed with PCI during drug infusion, of whom 50% received intracoronary stents; 87% were managed medically (without PCI during drug infusion).

The majority of patients received aspirin (75–325 mg once daily). Heparin was administered intravenously or subcutaneously, at the physician's discretion, most commonly as an intravenous bolus of 5000 U followed by a continuous infusion of 1000 U/h. For patients weighing less than 70 kg, the recommended heparin bolus dose was 60 U/kg followed by a continuous infusion of 12 U/kg/h. A target aPTT of 50–70 seconds was recommended. A total of 1250 patients underwent PCI within 72 hours after randomization, in which case they received intravenous heparin to maintain an activated clotting time (ACT) of 300–350 seconds.

The primary endpoint of the study was the occurrence of death from any cause or new myocardial infarction (MI) (evaluated by a blinded Clinical Endpoints Committee) within 30 days of randomization.

Compared to placebo, eptifibatide administered as a 180 μg/kg bolus followed by a 2 μg/kg/min infusion significantly (p=0.042) reduced the incidence of endpoint events (see Table 2). The reduction in the incidence of endpoint events in patients receiving eptifibatide was evident early during treatment, and this reduction was maintained through at least 30 days (see Figure 1). Table 2 also shows the incidence of the components of the primary endpoint, death (whether or not preceded by an MI) and new MI in surviving patients at 30 days.

[See table 2 above]

Figure 1
Kaplan-Meier Plot of Time to Death or Myocardial Infarction Within 30 Days of Randomization

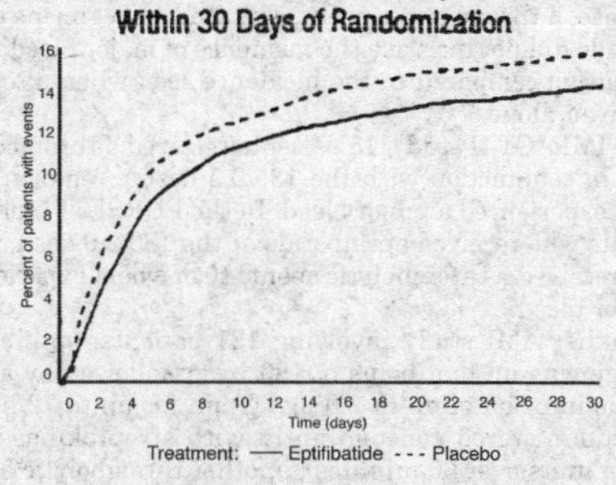

The effect of eptifibatide in PURSUIT did not appear to vary with patients' age. There were too few non-Caucasian patients to reach any conclusion as to possible differences related to race. Analysis of the PURSUIT results reveals a complex interaction of treatment, gender, and region. Throughout the world, eptifibatide was significantly less beneficial in women than in men, and in the overall study eptifibatide in women was nonsignificantly worse than placebo. These results were, however, strikingly heterogeneous across the several regions; eptifibatide appeared much worse than placebo in women in Latin America, while effects in men and women were scarcely distinguishable (relative risk reductions of 23% and 18%, respectively) in the U.S. and Canada. These results may reflect (a) genuine biological interactions between eptifibatide and gender, (b) interactions between eptifibatide and unknown international differences in concomitant therapy delivered to men and women, and (c) the play of chance, but the relative contributions of these possible factors are unknown. Treatment with eptifibatide reduced clinical events in patients undergoing PCI during drug administration and in those receiving medical management alone. Table 3 shows the incidence of death or MI within 72 hours of randomization.

Table 3
Clinical Events (Death or MI) in the PURSUIT Study Within 72 Hours of Randomization

	Placebo	Eptifibatide 180/2.0
Overall Patient Population	n=4739	n=4722
–At 72 hours	7.6%	5.9%
Patients undergoing early PCI	n=631	n=619
–Pre-procedure (nonfatal MI only)	5.5%	1.8%
–At 72 hours	14.4%	9.0%
Patients not undergoing early PCI	n=4108	n=4103
–At 72 hours	6.5%	5.4%

All of the effect of eptifibatide was established within 72 hours (during the period of drug infusion), regardless of management strategy. Moreover, for patients undergoing early PCI, a reduction in events was evident prior to the procedure.

IMPACT II was a multi-center, double-blind, randomized, placebo-controlled study conducted in the United States in 4010 patients undergoing PCI. Major exclusion criteria included a history of bleeding diathesis, major surgery within 6 weeks of treatment, gastrointestinal bleeding within 30 days, any stroke or structural CNS abnormality, uncontrolled hypertension, PT >1.2 times control, hematocrit <30%, platelet count <100,000/mm^3, and pregnancy.

Patient age ranged from 24 to 89 (mean 60) years, and 75% were male. The patients were 92% Caucasian, 5% Black, and 3% Hispanic. Patients were randomly assigned to one of three treatment regimens, each incorporating a bolus dose initiated immediately prior to PCI followed by a continuous infusion lasting 20–24 hours: 1) 135 μg/kg bolus followed by a continuous infusion of 0.5 μg/kg/min of eptifibatide (135/0.5); 2) 135 μg/kg bolus followed by a continuous infusion of 0.75 μg/kg/min of eptifibatide (135/0.75); or 3) a matching placebo bolus followed by a matching placebo continuous infusion. Each patient received aspirin and an intravenous heparin bolus of 100 U/kg, with additional bolus infusions of up to 2000 additional units of heparin every 15 minutes to maintain an activated clotting time (ACT) of 300–350 seconds.

The primary endpoint was the composite of death, MI, or urgent revascularization, analyzed at 30 days after randomization in all patients who received at least one dose of study drug.

As shown in Table 4, each eptifibatide regimen reduced the rate of death, MI, or urgent intervention, although at 30 days, this finding was statistically significant only in the

Continued on next page

Integrilin—Cont.

lower-dose eptifibatide group. As in the PURSUIT study, the effects of eptifibatide were seen early and persisted throughout the 30-day period.

[See table 4 at right]

At the time of randomization, approximately 25% of the IMPACT II patients suffered from only chronic stable angina, or had had no angina at all since a remote (more than 14 days prior) myocardial infarction. At the other extreme, approximately 40% of the IMPACT II patients had ongoing acute coronary syndromes, including patients with rest angina, others with refractory recurrent angina, others with early post-infarction angina, and others about to receive percutaneous interventions during or immediately following acute myocardial infarction. The remaining patients had various histories of recent and remote acute coronary syndromes; data are not available to describe what fraction of these underwent PCI within only a day or two of an acute episode. The IMPACT II study was not powered to obtain stable estimates of efficacy in subpopulations defined by degree of acuity, but (as shown in Table 5) the data suggest that the benefit of eptifibatide was not limited to patients with ongoing acute coronary syndromes.

[See table 5 at right]

INDICATIONS AND USAGE

INTEGRILIN is indicated:

• For the treatment of patients with acute coronary syndrome (UA/NQMI), including patients who are to be managed medically and those undergoing percutaneous coronary intervention (PCI). In this setting, INTEGRILIN has been shown to decrease the rate of a combined endpoint of death or new myocardial infarction.

• For the treatment of patients undergoing PCI. In this setting, INTEGRILIN has been shown to decrease the rate of a combined endpoint of death, new myocardial infarction, or need for urgent intervention.

In the clinical studies of eptifibatide, most patients received heparin and aspirin, as described in CLINICAL TRIALS.

CONTRAINDICATIONS

Treatment with eptifibatide is contraindicated in patients with:

• A history of bleeding diathesis, or evidence of active abnormal bleeding within the previous 30 days.

• Severe hypertension (systolic blood pressure >200 mm Hg or diastolic blood pressure >110 mm Hg) not adequately controlled on antihypertensive therapy.

• Major surgery within the preceding 6 weeks.

• History of stroke within 30 days or any history of hemorrhagic stroke.

• Current or planned administration of another parenteral GP IIb/IIIa inhibitor.

• Platelet count <100,000/mm³.

• Serum creatinine ≥2.0 mg/dL (for the 180 µg/kg bolus and the 2 µg/kg/min infusion) or ≥4.0 mg/dL (for the 135 µg/kg bolus and the 0.5 µg/kg/min infusion).

• Dependency on renal dialysis.

• Known hypersensitivity to any component of the product.

WARNINGS

Bleeding. Bleeding is the most common complication encountered during eptifibatide therapy. Administration of eptifibatide is associated with an increase in major and minor bleeding, as classified by the criteria of the Thrombolysis in Myocardial Infarction Study group (TIMI), (see ADVERSE REACTIONS). Most major bleeding associated with eptifibatide has been at the arterial access site for cardiac catheterization or from the gastrointestinal or genitourinary tract.

In patients undergoing percutaneous coronary interventions, patients receiving eptifibatide experience an increased incidence of major bleeding compared to those receiving placebo. Special care should be employed to minimize the risk of bleeding among these patients (see PRECAUTIONS).

If bleeding cannot be controlled with pressure, infusion of eptifibatide and concomitant heparin should be stopped immediately.

PRECAUTIONS

Bleeding Precautions

Care of the Femoral Artery Access Site in Patients Undergoing Percutaneous Coronary Intervention (PCI). In patients undergoing PCI, treatment with eptifibatide is associated with an increase in major and minor bleeding at the site of arterial sheath placement. After PCI, eptifibatide infusion should be continued for 20–24 hours. The femoral artery sheath may be removed during treatment with eptifibatide, but only after heparin has been discontinued and its effects largely reversed. In the IMPACT II study, heparin use was discouraged after the PCI procedure if the coronary lesion appeared angiographically stable. Early sheath removal was encouraged in both the IMPACT II and the PURSUIT studies while study drug was being infused. Prior to

removing the sheath, it was recommended that heparin be discontinued for 3–4 hours and that an aPTT of <45 seconds be documented. In any case, both heparin and eptifibatide should be discontinued and sheath hemostasis should be achieved by standard compressive techniques at least 4 hours before hospital discharge.

Use of Thrombolytics, Anticoagulants, and Other Antiplatelet Agents. In the IMPACT II and PURSUIT studies, eptifibatide was used concomitantly with heparin and aspirin (see CLINICAL STUDIES). Because eptifibatide inhibits platelet aggregation, caution should be employed when it is used with other drugs that affect hemostasis, including **thrombolytics, oral anticoagulants, non-steroidal anti-inflammatory drugs, dipyridamole, ticlopidine, and clopidogrel.** To avoid potentially additive pharmacologic effects, concomitant treatment with **other inhibitors of platelet receptor GP IIb/IIIa** should be avoided.

There is only a small experience with concomitant use of eptifibatide and **thrombolytics.** In a study of 180 patients with acute myocardial infarction (AMI), eptifibatide (in regimens up to a bolus of 180 µg/kg followed by a continuous infusion of 0.75 µg/kg/min for 24 hours) was administered concomitantly with the approved "accelerated" regimen of alteplase, a thrombolytic agent. The studied regimens of eptifibatide did not increase the incidence of major bleeding or transfusion compared to the incidence seen when alteplase was given alone.

In the IMPACT II study, 15 patients received a thrombolytic agent in conjunction with the 135/0.5 dosing regimen, 2 of whom experienced a major bleed. In the PURSUIT study, 40 patients who received eptifibatide at the 180/2.0 dosing regimen received a thrombolytic agent, 10 of whom experienced a major bleed.

In another AMI study involving 181 patients, eptifibatide (in regimens up to a bolus of 180 µg/kg followed by a continuous infusion of up to 2.0 µg/kg/min for up to 72 hours) was administered concomitantly with streptokinase (1.5 million units over 60 minutes), another thrombolytic agent. At the highest studied infusion rates (1.3 µg/kg/min and 2.0

µg/kg/min), eptifibatide was associated with an increase in the incidence of bleeding and transfusions compared to the incidence seen when streptokinase was given alone.

These limited data on the use of eptifibatide in patients receiving thrombolytic agents do not allow an estimate of the bleeding risk associated with concomitant use of thrombolytics. Systemic thrombolytic therapy should be used with caution in patients who have received eptifibatide.

Minimization of Vascular and Other Trauma. Arterial and venous punctures, intramuscular injections, and the use of urinary catheters, nasotracheal intubation, and nasogastric tubes should be minimized. When obtaining intravenous access, noncompressible sites (e.g., subclavian or jugular veins) should be avoided.

Laboratory Tests. Before infusion of eptifibatide, the following laboratory tests should be performed to identify pre-existing hemostatic abnormalities: hematocrit or hemoglobin, platelet count, serum creatinine, and PT/aPTT. In patients undergoing PCI, the activated clotting time (ACT) should also be measured.

Maintaining Target aPTT and ACT. The aPTT should be maintained between 50 and 70 seconds unless PCI is to be performed. During PCI, the ACT should be maintained between 300 and 350 seconds.

The aPTT should be checked prior to arterial sheath removal. The sheath should not be removed unless the aPTT is <45 seconds. In patients treated with heparin, bleeding can be minimized by close monitoring of the aPTT. Table 6 displays the risk of major bleeding according to the maximum aPTT attained within 72 hours in the PURSUIT study.

[See table 6 above]

Thrombocytopenia. If the patient experiences a confirmed platelet decrease to <100,000/mm³, INTEGRILIN and heparin should be discontinued and the condition appropriately monitored and treated.

Renal Insufficiency. Based on results of clinical studies with eptifibatide (which did not adjust dose for renal func-

Table 4
Clinical Events in the IMPACT II Study

	Placebo n (%)	Eptifibatide (135/0.5) n (%)	Eptifibatide (135/0.75) n (%)
Patients	1285	1300	1286
Abrupt Closure	65 (5.1%)	36 (2.8%)	43 (3.3%)
p-value vs. placebo		0.003	0.030
Death, MI, or Urgent Intervention			
24 hours	123 (9.6%)	86 (6.6%)	89 (6.9%)
p-value vs. placebo		0.006	0.014
48 hours	131 (10.2%)	99 (7.6%)	102 (7.9%)
p-value vs. placebo		0.021	0.045
30 days (primary endpoint)	149 (11.6%)	118 (9.1%)	128 (10.0%)
p-value vs. placebo		0.035	0.179
Death or MI			
30 days	110 (8.6%)	89 (6.8%)	95 (7.4%)
p-value vs. placebo		0.102	0.272
6 months	151 (11.9%)*	136 (10.6%)*	130 (10.3%)*
p-value vs. placebo		0.297	0.182

*Kaplan-Meier estimate of event rate

Table 5
Clinical Events at 30 Days in the IMPACT II Study, Stratified by Acuity at Time of Randomization

Classification of Patients (%)	Placebo n (%)	Eptifibatide 135/0.5 n (%)	Eptifibatide 135/0.75 n (%)
Ongoing ACS, MI ongoing or within past 24h(41.3%)	538 (11.5%)	532 (10.0%)	527 (10.6%)
Others (58.7%)	747 (11.6%)	768 (8.5%)	759 (9.5%)

Table 6
Major Bleeding by Maximal aPTT Within 72 Hours in the PURSUIT Study

	Placebo n (%)	Eptifibatide 180/1.3* n (%)	Eptifibatide 180/2.0 n (%)
Maximum aPTT (seconds)			
<50	44/721(6.1%)	21/244(8.6%)	44/743(5.9%)
50–70 (recommended)	92/908(10.1%)	28/259(10.8%)	99/883(11.2%)
>70	281/2786(10.1%)	99/891(11.1%)	345/2811(12.3%)

*Administered only until the first interim analysis

tion) and the fact that the drug is cleared equally by renal and nonrenal mechanisms, dose adjustment is unnecessary for patients with mild to moderate renal impairment (serum creatinine <2 mg/dL for the 180 µg/kg bolus and the 2.0 µg/kg/min infusion and <4 mg/dL for the 135 µg/kg bolus and the 0.5 µg/kg/min infusion). Plasma eptifibatide levels are expected to be higher in patients with more severe renal impairment, but no data are available for such patients or for patients on renal dialysis. *In vitro* studies have indicated that eptifibatide may be cleared from plasma by dialysis.

Geriatric Use. The PURSUIT and IMPACT II clinical studies enrolled patients up to the age of 94 years (45% were age 65 and over; 12% were age 75 and older). There was no apparent difference in efficacy between older and younger patients treated with eptifibatide. The incidence of bleeding complications was higher in the elderly in both placebo and eptifibatide groups, and the incremental risk of eptifibatide-associated bleeding was greater in the older patients. No dose adjustment was made for elderly patients, but patients over 75 years of age had to weigh at least 50 kg to be enrolled in the PURSUIT study because of concern about an increased risk of bleeding in this subgroup (see also ADVERSE REACTIONS).

Carcinogenesis, Mutagenesis, Impairment of Fertility. No long-term studies in animals have been performed to evaluate the carcinogenic potential of eptifibatide. Eptifibatide was not genotoxic in the Ames test, the mouse lymphoma cell (L 5178Y, TK$^{+/-}$) forward mutation test, the human lymphocyte chromosome aberration test, or the mouse micronucleus test. Administered by continuous intravenous infusion at total daily doses up to 72 mg/kg/day (about 4 times the recommended maximum daily human dose on a body surface area basis), eptifibatide had no effect on fertility and reproductive performance of male and female rats.

Pregnancy. Pregnancy Category B. Teratology studies have been performed by continuous intravenous infusion of eptifibatide in pregnant rats at total daily doses of up to 72 mg/kg/day (about 4 times the recommended maximum daily human dose on a body surface area basis) and in pregnant rabbits at total daily doses of up to 36 mg/kg/day (also about 4 times the recommended maximum daily human dose on a body surface area basis). These studies revealed no evidence of harm to the fetus due to eptifibatide. There are, however, no adequate and well-controlled studies in pregnant women with eptifibatide. Because animal reproduction studies are not always predictive of human response, eptifibatide should be used during pregnancy only if clearly needed.

Pediatric Use. Safety and effectiveness of eptifibatide in pediatric patients have not been studied.

Nursing Mothers. It is not known whether eptifibatide is excreted in human milk. Because many drugs are excreted in human milk, caution should be exercised when eptifibatide is administered to a nursing mother.

ADVERSE REACTIONS

A total of 14,718 patients were treated in the two Phase III clinical trials (PURSUIT and IMPACT II). Of these, 8737 received eptifibatide: 1300 at 135/0.5 for up to 24 hours, 1286 at 135/0.75 for up to 24 hours, 1472 at 180/1.3 for up to 72 hours, and 4679 at 180/2.0 for up to 72 hours. The other 5981 patients received placebo. These 14,718 patients had a mean age of 62 years (range 20 to 94 years). Eighty-nine percent of the patients were Caucasian, with the remainder being predominantly Black (5%) and Hispanic (5%). Sixty-seven percent were men.

Because of the different regimens used in PURSUIT and IMPACT II, data from the two studies were not pooled.

Bleeding. The incidences of bleeding events and transfusions in the PURSUIT and IMPACT II studies are shown in Table 7. Bleeding was classified as major or minor by the criteria of the TIMI study group. Major bleeding events consisted of intracranial hemorrhage and other bleeding that led to decreases in hemoglobin greater than 5 g/dL. Minor bleeding events included spontaneous gross hematuria, spontaneous hematemesis, other observed blood loss with a hemoglobin decrease of more than 3 g/dL, and other hemoglobin decreases that were greater than 4 g/dL but less than 5 g/dL. In patients who received transfusions, the corresponding loss in hemoglobin was estimated through an adaptation period of the method of Landefeld *et al.*

[See table 7 above]

As shown in Tables 8 and 9, the overall incidence of major bleeding in these studies was strongly related to the incidence of coronary artery bypass graft (CABG) surgery; the excess bleeding seen with eptifibatide, however, was seen only among the patients who did not undergo CABG.

In the PURSUIT study, the greatest increase in major bleeding in eptifibatide-treated patients compared to placebo was associated with bleeding at the femoral artery access site (2.8% versus 1.3%). Oropharyngeal (primarily gingival), genitourinary, gastrointestinal, and retroperitoneal bleeding were also seen more commonly in eptifibatide-treated patients compared to placebo. Among patients experiencing a major bleed in the IMPACT II study, an increase in bleeding on eptifibatide versus placebo was observed only for the femoral artery access site (3.2% versus 2.8%).

Table 7
Bleeding Events and Transfusions in the PURSUIT and IMPACT II Studies

	PURSUIT		
	Placebo n (%)	Eptifibatide 180/1.3* n (%)	Eptifibatide 180/2.0 n (%)
Patients	4696	1472	4679
Major bleeding[a]	425 (9.3%)	152 (10.5%)	498 (10.8%)
Minor bleeding[a]	347 (7.6%)	152 (10.5%)	604 (13.1%)
Requiring Transfusions[b]	490 (10.4%)	188 (12.8%)	601 (12.8%)

	IMPACT II		
	Placebo n (%)	Eptifibatide 135/0.5 n (%)	Eptifibatide 135/0.75 n (%)
Patients	1285	1300	1286
Major bleeding[a]	55 (4.5%)	55 (4.4%)	58 (4.7%)
Minor bleeding[a]	115 (9.3%)	146 (11.7%)	177 (14.2%)
Requiring Transfusions[b]	66 (5.1%)	71 (5.5%)	74 (5.8%)

Note: denominator is based on patients for whom data are available
* Administered only until the first interim analysis
[a] For major and minor bleeding, patients are counted only once according to the most severe classification.
[b] Includes transfusions of whole blood, packed red blood cells, fresh frozen plasma, cryoprecipitate, platelets, and autotransfusion during the initial hospitalization.

Table 8
Major Bleeding by Procedures in the PURSUIT Study

	Placebo n (%)	Eptifibatide 180/1.3* n (%)	Eptifibatide 180/2.0 n (%)
Patients	4577	1451	4604
Overall Incidence of Major Bleeding	425 (9.3%)	152 (10.5%)	498 (10.8%)
Breakdown by Procedure:			
CABG	375 (8.2%)	123 (8.5%)	377 (8.2%)
Angioplasty without CABG	27 (0.6%)	16 (1.1%)	64 (1.4%)
Angiography without angioplasty or CABG	11 (0.2%)	7 (0.5%)	29 (0.6%)
Medical Therapy Only	12 (0.3%)	6 (0.4%)	28 (0.6%)

Denominators are based on the total number of patients whose TIMI classification was resolved.
* Administered only until the first interim analysis

Table 9
Major Bleeding by Procedures in the IMPACT II Study

	Placebo n (%)	Eptifibatide 135/0.5 n (%)	Eptifibatide 135/0.75 n (%)
Patients	1230	1249	1245
Overall Incidence of Major Bleeding	55 (4.5%)	55 (4.4%)	58 (4.7%)
Breakdown of Bleeding by Procedure:			
CABG	35 (2.8%)	23 (1.8%)	26 (2.1%)
Angioplasty without CABG	20 (1.6%)	32 (2.6%)	32 (2.7%)

Denominators are based on the total number of patients whose TIMI classification was resolved.

Tables 8 and 9 display the incidence of TIMI major bleeding according to the cardiac procedures carried out in the PURSUIT and IMPACT II studies, respectively. The most common bleeding complications were related to cardiac revascularization (CABG-related or femoral artery access site bleeding).
[See table 8 above]
[See table 9 above]
In the PURSUIT study, the risk of major bleeding with eptifibatide increased inversely with patient weight. This relationship was most apparent for patients weighing less than 70 kg. These trends were not apparent in the IMPACT II study.
Bleeding adverse events resulting in discontinuation of study drug were more frequent among patients receiving eptifibatide than placebo (8% versus 1% in PURSUIT, 3.5% versus 1.9% in IMPACT II).

Intracranial Hemorrhage and Stroke. Intracranial hemorrhage was rare in the PURSUIT clinical study, with only 3 patients in the placebo group, 1 patient in the group treated with eptifibatide 180/1.3 and 5 patients in the group treated with eptifibatide 180/2.0 experiencing a hemorrhagic stroke. The overall incidence of stroke was 0.5% in patients receiving eptifibatide 180/1.3, 0.7% in patients receiving eptifibatide 180/2.0, and 0.8% in placebo patients.

In the IMPACT II study, intracranial hemorrhage was experienced by 1 patient treated with eptifibatide 135/0.5, 2 patients treated with eptifibatide 135/0.75 and 2 patients in the placebo group. The overall incidence of stroke was 0.5% in patients receiving 135/0.5 eptifibatide, 0.7% in patients receiving eptifibatide 135/0.75 and 0.7% in the placebo group.

Thrombocytopenia. In the PURSUIT and IMPACT II studies, the incidence of thrombocytopenia (<100,000/mm^3 or ≥50% reduction from baseline) and the incidence of platelet transfusions were similar between patients treated with eptifibatide and placebo.

Allergic Reactions. In the IMPACT II study, anaphylaxis was reported in 1 patient (0.08%) on placebo and in no patients on eptifibatide. In the PURSUIT study, anaphylaxis was reported in 7 patients receiving placebo (0.15%) and 7 patients receiving eptifibatide 180/2.0 (0.16%). In the IM-

Continued on next page

Integrilin—Cont.

PACT II study, 2 patients (1 patient (0.04%) receiving eptifibatide and 1 patient (0.08%) receiving placebo) discontinued study drug because of allergic reactions. In the PURSUIT study, anaphylaxis was given as a reason for drug discontinuation in 3 patients (0.05%) who received eptifibatide and in none of the patients who received placebo.

Other Adverse Reactions. Serious non-bleeding events occurred in 19% of the eptifibatide and 19% of the placebo patients in the PURSUIT study. The only serious non-bleeding adverse event that occurred at a rate of at least 1% and was more common with eptifibatide than placebo (7% versus 6%) was hypotension. Most of the serious non-bleeding events consisted of cardiovascular events typical of an unstable angina population. In the IMPACT II study, serious non-bleeding events that occurred in greater than 1% of patients were uncommon and similar in incidence between placebo- and eptifibatide-treated patients.

Discontinuation of study drug due to adverse events other than bleeding was uncommon in both the PURSUIT and IMPACT II studies, with no single event occurring in >0.5% of the study population. In the PURSUIT study, non-bleeding adverse events leading to discontinuation occurred in the eptifibatide and placebo groups in the following body systems with an incidence of ≥0.1%: cardiovascular system (0.3% and 0.3%), digestive system (0.1% and 0.1%), hemic/lymphatic system (0.1% and 0.1%), nervous system (0.3% and 0.4%), urogenital system (0.1% and 0.1%), and whole body system (0.2% and 0.2%). In the IMPACT II study, non-bleeding adverse events leading to discontinuation occurred in the 135/0.5 eptifibatide and placebo groups in the following body systems with an incidence of ≥0.1%: whole body (0.3% and 0.1%), cardiovascular system (1.4% and 1.4%), digestive system (0.2% and 0%), hemic/lymphatic system (0.2% and 0%), nervous system (0.3% and 0.2%), and respiratory system (0.1% and 0.1%).

OVERDOSAGE

There has been only limited experience with overdosage of eptifibatide. There were 8 patients in the IMPACT II study and 9 patients in the PURSUIT study who received bolus doses and/or infusion doses more than double those called for in the protocols, or who were identified by the investigator as having received an overdose. None of these patients experienced an intracranial bleed or other major bleeding. Eptifibatide was not lethal to rats, rabbits, or monkeys when administered by continuous intravenous infusion for 90 minutes at a total dose of 45 mg/kg (about 2 to 5 times the recommended maximum daily human dose on a body surface area basis). Symptoms of acute toxicity were loss of righting reflex, dyspnea, ptosis, and decreased muscle tone in rabbits and petechial hemorrhages in the femoral and abdominal areas of monkeys.

DOSAGE AND ADMINISTRATION

The safety and efficacy of eptifibatide has been established in clinical studies that employed concomitant use of heparin and aspirin. Different dose regimens of eptifibatide were used in the major clinical studies. (See CLINICAL STUDIES.)

Acute Coronary Syndrome. The recommended adult dosage of eptifibatide in patients with acute coronary syndrome is an intravenous bolus of 180 μg/kg as soon as possible following diagnosis, followed by a continuous infusion of 2 μg/kg/min until hospital discharge or initiation of CABG surgery, up to 72 hours. If a patient is to undergo a percutaneous coronary intervention (PCI) while receiving eptifibatide, consideration can be given to decreasing the infusion rate to 0.5 μg/kg/min (the infusion rate in IMPACT II) at the time of the procedure. Infusion should be continued for an additional 20–24 hours after the procedure, allowing for up to 96 hours of therapy. In the PURSUIT study, patients weighing more than 121 kg received a maximum bolus of 22.6 mg (11.3 mL of the 2 mg/mL injection) followed by a maximum infusion of 15 mg (20 mL of the 0.75 mg/mL injection) per hour.

Percutaneous Coronary Intervention (PCI) in patients not presenting with an acute coronary syndrome. The recommended adult dosage of eptifibatide in patients undergoing PCI and not presenting with an acute coronary syndrome is an intravenous bolus of 135 μg/kg administered immediately before the initiation of PCI followed by a continuous infusion of 0.5 μg/kg/min for 20–24 hours. In the IMPACT II study, there was little experience in patients weighing more than 143 kg.

In patients who undergo coronary artery bypass graft surgery, eptifibatide infusion should be discontinued prior to surgery.

In the clinical trials that showed eptifibatide to be effective, most patients received concomitant aspirin and heparin. The aspirin doses used in the clinical studies were as follows:

1. INTEGRILIN Dosing Chart by Weight for Patients With Acute Coronary Syndrome (180 μg/kg Bolus and 2μg/kg/min Infusion)

Patient Weight (kg)	Bolus Volume (2 mg/mL)	Infusion Rate (0.75 mg/mL)
37–41	3.4 mL	6 mL/h
42–46	4	7
47–53	4.5	8
54–59	5	9
60–65	5.6	10
66–71	6.2	11
72–78	6.8	12
79–84	7.3	13
85–90	7.9	14
91–96	8.5	15
97–103	9	16
104–109	9.5	17
110–115	10.2	18
116–121	10.7	19
>121	11.3	20

2. INTEGRILIN Dosing Chart by Weight for Patients Without Acute Coronary Syndromes Undergoing PCI (135 μg/kg Bolus and 0.5 μg/kg/min Infusion)

Patient Weight (kg)	Bolus Volume (2 mg/mL)	Infusion Rate (0.75 mg/mL)
40–55	3.4 mL	2 mL/h
56–68	4.2	2.5
69–80	5.1	3
81–93	5.9	3.5
94–105	6.8	4
106–118	7.6	4.5
119–131	8.4	5
132–143	9.2	5.5

Acute Coronary Syndrome (PURSUIT Study)	Angioplasty (IMPACT II Study)
160 mg initially, then 75–325 mg daily	75–325 mg 1–24 hours prior to intervention

The initial target aPTT in the PURSUIT study was 50–70 seconds, and the recommended heparin dosing was:
- if weight ≥70 kg, 5000 U bolus followed by infusion of 1000 U/h
- if weight <70 kg, 60 U/kg bolus followed by infusion of 12 U/kg/h

When these patients were to undergo PCI, the target ACT was 300–350 seconds, and the recommended heparin doses were:

Initial Heparin Bolus

ACT (seconds)	Heparin Bolus
<150	100 U/kg (10,000 U maximum)
151–225	75 U/kg
226–299	50 U/kg
≥300	none

Repeat Heparin Bolus*

ACT (seconds)	Heparin Bolus
<275	50 U/kg
275–299	25 U/kg
≥300	none

*based on hourly ACT determinations

In the IMPACT II study, the target ACT was 300–350 seconds before the procedure and ≤ 350 seconds thereafter. The recommended heparin doses were:
- prior to intervention: 100 U/kg bolus
- during intervention: up to 2000 U bolus q15min
- after intervention: infusion at physician's discretion

Patients requiring thrombolytic therapy had eptifibatide infusions stopped and were discontinued from the studies.

Instructions for Administration

1. Like other parenteral drug products, INTEGRILIN solutions should be inspected visually for particulate matter and discoloration prior to administration, whenever solution and container permit.
2. INTEGRILIN may be administered in the same intravenous line as alteplase, atropine, dobutamine, heparin, lidocaine, meperidine, metoprolol, midazolam, morphine, nitroglycerin, or verapamil. INTEGRILIN should not be administered through the same intravenous line as furosemide.
3. INTEGRILIN may be administered in the same IV line with 0.9% NaCl or 0.9% NaCl/5% dextrose. With either vehicle, the infusion may also contain up to 60 mEq/L of potassium chloride. No incompatibilities have been observed with intravenous administration sets. No compatibility studies have been performed with PVC bags.

4. The bolus dose of INTEGRILIN should be withdrawn from the 10-mL vial into a syringe. The bolus dose should be administered by IV push over 1–2 minutes.
5. Immediately following the bolus dose administration, a continuous infusion of INTEGRILIN should be initiated. When using an intravenous infusion pump, INTEGRILIN should be administered undiluted directly from the 100-mL vial. The 100-mL vial should be spiked with a vented infusion set. Care should be taken to center the spike within the circle on the stopper top.

INTEGRILIN is to be administered by volume according to patient weight. Patients should receive study drug according to the following table:

[See tables 1 & 2 above]

HOW SUPPLIED

INTEGRILIN (eptifibatide) Injection is supplied as a sterile solution in 10-mL vials containing 20 mg of eptifibatide (NDC 0085-1177-01) and 100-mL vials containing 75 mg of eptifibatide (NDC 0085-1136-01).

Vials should be stored refrigerated at 2–8°C (36–46°F). Protect from light until administration. Do not use beyond the expiration date. Discard any unused portion left in the vial.

Rx only

Marketed By:
COR Therapeutics, Inc.
South San Francisco, CA 94080
and
Key Pharmaceuticals, Inc.
Kenilworth, NJ 07033

Distributed By:
Key Pharmaceuticals, Inc.
Kenilworth, NJ 07033

Issued May 1998
Rev 0

K–DUR®
Microburst Release System®
(Potassium Chloride) USP
Extended Release Tablets

℞

DESCRIPTION

K-DUR® 20 is an immediately dispersing extended release oral dosage form of potassium chloride containing 1500 mg of microencapsulated potassium chloride USP equivalent to 20 mEq of potassium in a tablet.

K-DUR® 10 is an immediately dispersing extended release oral dosage form of potassium chloride containing 750 mg of microencapsulated potassium chloride USP equivalent to 10 mEq of potassium in a tablet.

These formulations are intended to slow the release of potassium so that the likelihood of a high localized concentration of potassium chloride within the gastrointestinal tract is reduced.

K-DUR is an electrolyte replenisher. The chemical name of the active ingredient is potassium chloride, and the structural formula is KCl. Potassium chloride USP occurs as a white, granular powder or as colorless crystals. It is odorless and has a saline taste. Its solutions are neutral to litmus. It is freely soluble in water and insoluble in alcohol.

K-DUR is a tablet formulation (not enteric coated or wax matrix) containing individually microencapsulated potassium chloride crystals which disperse upon tablet disintegration. In simulated gastric fluid at 37°C and in the absence of outside agitation, K-DUR begins disintegrating into microencapsulated crystals within seconds and completely disintegrates within one minute. The microencapsulated crystals are formulated to provide an extended release of potassium chloride.

Inactive Ingredients: Crospovidone, Ethylcellulose, Hydroxypropyl Cellulose, Magnesium Stearate, and Microcrystalline Cellulose.

CLINICAL PHARMACOLOGY

The potassium ion is the principal intracellular cation of most body tissues. Potassium ions participate in a number of essential physiological processes including the maintenance of intracellular tonicity, the transmission of nerve impulses, the contraction of cardiac, skeletal and smooth muscle and the maintenance of normal renal function.

The intracellular concentration of potassium is approximately 150 to 160 mEq per liter. The normal adult plasma concentration is 3.5 to 5 mEq per liter. An active ion transport system maintains this gradient across the plasma membrane.

Potassium is a normal dietary constituent and under steady state conditions the amount of potassium absorbed from the gastrointestinal tract is equal to the amount excreted in the urine. The usual dietary intake of potassium is 50 to 100 mEq per day.

Potassium depletion will occur whenever the rate of potassium loss through renal excretion and/or loss from the gastrointestinal tract exceeds the rate of potassium intake. Such depletion usually develops as a consequence of therapy with diuretics, primary or secondary hyperaldosteronism, diabetic ketoacidosis, or inadequate replacement of potassium in patients on prolonged parenteral nutrition. Depletion can develop rapidly with severe diarrhea, especially if associated with vomiting. Potassium depletion due to these causes is usually accompanied by a concomitant loss of chloride and is manifested by hypokalemia and metabolic alkalosis. Potassium depletion may produce weakness, fatigue, disturbances of cardiac rhythm (primarily ectopic beats), prominent U-waves in the electrocardiogram, and in advanced cases, flaccid paralysis and/or impaired ability to concentrate urine.

If potassium depletion associated with metabolic alkalosis cannot be managed by correcting the fundamental cause of the deficiency, e.g., where the patient requires long term diuretic therapy, supplemental potassium in the form of high potassium food or potassium chloride may be able to restore normal potassium levels.

In rare circumstances (e.g., patients with renal tubular acidosis) potassium depletion may be associated with metabolic acidosis and hyperchloremia. In such patients potassium replacement should be accomplished with potassium salts other than the chloride, such as potassium bicarbonate, potassium citrate, potassium acetate, or potassium gluconate.

INDICATIONS AND USAGE

BECAUSE OF REPORTS OF INTESTINAL AND GASTRIC ULCERATION AND BLEEDING WITH CONTROLLED RELEASE POTASSIUM CHLORIDE PREPARATIONS, THESE DRUGS SHOULD BE RESERVED FOR THOSE PATIENTS WHO CANNOT TOLERATE OR REFUSE TO TAKE LIQUID OR EFFERVESCENT POTASSIUM PREPARATIONS OR FOR PATIENTS IN WHOM THERE IS A PROBLEM OF COMPLIANCE WITH THESE PREPARATIONS.

1. For the treatment of patients with hypokalemia with or without metabolic alkalosis, in digitalis intoxication and in patients with hypokalemic familial periodic paralysis. If hypokalemia is the result of diuretic therapy, consideration should be given to the use of a lower dose of diuretic, which may be sufficient without leading to hypokalemia.
2. For the prevention of hypokalemia in patients who would be at particular risk if hypokalemia were to develop, e.g., digitalized patients or patients with significant cardiac arrhythmias.

The use of potassium salts in patients receiving diuretics for uncomplicated essential hypertension is often unnecessary when such patients have a normal dietary pattern and when low doses of the diuretic are used. Serum potassium should be checked periodically, however, and if hypokalemia occurs, dietary supplementation with potassium-containing foods may be adequate to control milder cases. In more severe cases, and if dose adjustment of the diuretic is ineffective or unwarranted, supplementation with potassium salts may be indicated.

CONTRAINDICATIONS

Potassium supplements are contraindicated in patients with hyperkalemia since a further increase in serum potassium concentration in such patients can produce cardiac arrest. Hyperkalemia may complicate any of the following conditions: chronic renal failure, systemic acidosis such as diabetic acidosis, acute dehydration, extensive tissue breakdown as in severe burns, adrenal insufficiency, or the administration of a potassium-sparing diuretic (e.g., spironolactone, triamterene, amiloride) (see **OVERDOSAGE**).

Controlled release formulations of potassium chloride have produced esophageal ulceration in certain cardiac patients with esophageal compression due to enlarged left atrium. Potassium supplementation, when indicated in such patients, should be given as a liquid preparation or as an aqueous (water) suspension of K-DUR (see **PRECAUTIONS; Information for Patients,** and **DOSAGE AND ADMINISTRATION** sections).

All solid oral dosage forms of potassium chloride are contraindicated in any patient in whom there is structural, pathological (e.g., diabetic gastroparesis) or pharmacologic (use of anticholinergic agents or other agents with anticholinergic properties at sufficient doses to exert anticholinergic effects) cause for arrest or delay in tablet passage through the gastrointestinal tract.

WARNINGS

Hyperkalemia (see **OVERDOSAGE**)—In patients with impaired mechanisms for excreting potassium, the administration of potassium salts can produce hyperkalemia and cardiac arrest. This occurs most commonly in patients given potassium by the intravenous route but may also occur in patients given potassium orally. Potentially fatal hyperkalemia can develop rapidly and be asymptomatic. The use of potassium salts in patients with chronic renal disease, or any other condition which impairs potassium excretion, requires particularly careful monitoring of the serum potassium concentration and appropriate dosage adjustment.

Interaction with Potassium Sparing Diuretics—Hypokalemia should not be treated by the concomitant administration of potassium salts and a potassium-sparing diuretic (e.g., spironolactone, triamterene or amiloride) since the simultaneous administration of these agents can produce severe hyperkalemia.

Interaction with Angiotensin Converting Enzyme Inhibitors—Angiotensin converting enzyme (ACE) inhibitors (e.g., captopril, enalapril) will produce some potassium retention by inhibiting aldosterone production. Potassium supplements should be given to patients receiving ACE inhibitors only with close monitoring.

Gastrointestinal Lesions—Solid oral dosage forms of potassium chloride can produce ulcerative and/or stenotic lesions of the gastrointestinal tract. Based on spontaneous adverse reaction reports, enteric coated preparations of potassium chloride are associated with an increased frequency of small bowel lesions (40–50 per 100,000 patient years) compared to sustained release wax matrix formulations (less than one per 100,000 patient years). Because of the lack of extensive marketing experience with microencapsulated products, a comparison between such products and wax matrix or enteric coated products is not available. K-DUR is a tablet formulated to provide a controlled rate of release of microencapsulated potassium chloride and thus to minimize the possibility of a high local concentration of potassium near the gastrointestinal wall.

Prospective trials have been conducted in normal human volunteers in which the upper gastrointestinal tract was evaluated by endoscopic inspection before and after one week of solid oral potassium chloride therapy. The ability of this model to predict events occurring in usual clinical practice is unknown. Trials which approximated usual clinical practice did not reveal any clear differences between the wax matrix and microencapsulated dosage forms. In contrast, there was a higher incidence of gastric and duodenal lesions in subjects receiving a high dose of a wax matrix controlled release formulation under conditions which did not resemble usual or recommended clinical practice (i.e., 96 mEq per day in divided doses of potassium chloride administered to fasted patients, in the presence of an anticholinergic drug to delay gastric emptying). The upper gastrointestinal lesions observed by endoscopy were asymptomatic and were not accompanied by evidence of bleeding (Hemoccult testing). The relevance of these findings to the usual conditions (i.e., non-fasting, no anticholinergic agent, smaller doses) under which controlled release potassium chloride products are used is uncertain; epidemiologic studies have not identified an elevated risk, compared to microencapsulated products, for upper gastrointestinal lesions in patients receiving wax matrix formulations. K-DUR should be discontinued immediately and the possibility of ulceration, obstruction or perforation considered if severe vomiting, abdominal pain, distention, or gastrointestinal bleeding occurs.

Metabolic Acidosis—Hypokalemia in patients with metabolic acidosis should be treated with an alkalinizing potassium salt such as potassium bicarbonate, potassium citrate, potassium acetate, or potassium gluconate.

PRECAUTIONS

General: The diagnosis of potassium depletion is ordinarily made by demonstrating hypokalemia in a patient with a clinical history suggesting some cause for potassium depletion. In interpreting the serum potassium level, the physician should bear in mind that acute alkalosis per se can produce hypokalemia in the absence of a deficit in total body potassium while acute acidosis per se can increase the serum potassium concentration into the normal range even in the presence of a reduced total body potassium. The treatment of potassium depletion, particularly in the presence of cardiac disease, renal disease, or acidosis requires careful attention to acid-base balance and appropriate monitoring of serum electrolytes, the electrocardiogram, and the clinical status of the patient.

Information for Patients: Physicians should consider reminding the patient of the following:

To take each dose with meals and with a full glass of water or other liquid.

To take each dose without crushing, chewing, or sucking the tablets. If those patients are having difficulty swallowing whole tablets, they may try one of the following alternate methods of administration:

a. Break the tablet in half, and take each half separately with a glass of water.

b. Prepare an aqueous (water) suspension as follows:
1. Place the whole tablet(s) in approximately one-half glass of water (4 fluid ounces).
2. Allow approximately 2 minutes for the tablet(s) to disintegrate.
3. Stir for about half a minute after the tablet(s) has disintegrated.
4. Swirl the suspension and consume the entire contents of the glass immediately by drinking or by the use of a straw.
5. Add another one fluid ounce of water, swirl, and consume immediately.
6. Then, add an additional one fluid ounce of water, swirl, and consume immediately.

Aqueous suspension of K-DUR tablets that is not taken immediately should be discarded. The use of other liquids for suspending K-DUR tablets is not recommended.

To take this medicine following the frequency and amount prescribed by the physician. This is especially important if the patient is also taking diuretics and/or digitalis preparations.

To check with the physician at once if tarry stools or other evidence of gastrointestinal bleeding is noticed.

Laboratory Tests: When blood is drawn for analysis of plasma potassium it is important to recognize that artifactual elevations can occur after improper venipuncture technique or as a result of in-vitro hemolysis of the sample.

Drug Interactions: Potassium-sparing diuretics, angiotensin converting enzyme inhibitors (see **WARNINGS**).

Carcinogenesis, Mutagenesis, Impairment of Fertility: Carcinogenicity, mutagenicity and fertility studies in animals have not been performed. Potassium is a normal dietary constituent.

Pregnancy Category C: Animal reproduction studies have not been conducted with K-DUR. It is unlikely that potassium supplementation that does not lead to hyperkalemia would have an adverse effect on the fetus or would affect reproductive capacity.

Nursing Mothers: The normal potassium ion content of human milk is about 13 mEq per liter. Since oral potassium becomes part of the body potassium pool, so long as body potassium is not excessive, the contribution of potassium chloride supplementation should have little or no effect on the level in human milk.

Pediatric Use: Safety and effectiveness in children have not been established.

ADVERSE REACTIONS

One of the most severe adverse effects is hyperkalemia (see **CONTRAINDICATIONS, WARNINGS,** and **OVERDOSAGE**). There have also been reports of upper and lower gastrointestinal conditions including obstruction, bleeding, ulceration, and perforation (see **CONTRAINDICATIONS** and **WARNINGS**).

The most common adverse reactions to oral potassium salts are nausea, vomiting, flatulence, abdominal pain/discomfort, and diarrhea. These symptoms are due to irritation of the gastrointestinal tract and are best managed by diluting the preparation further, taking the dose with meals or reducing the amount taken at one time.

OVERDOSAGE

The administration of oral potassium salts to persons with normal excretory mechanisms for potassium rarely causes serious hyperkalemia. However, if excretory mechanisms are impaired or if potassium is administered too rapidly intravenously, potentially fatal hyperkalemia can result (see **CONTRAINDICATIONS** and **WARNINGS**). It is important to recognize that hyperkalemia is usually

Continued on next page

K-Dur—Cont.

asymptomatic and may be manifested only by an increased serum potassium concentration (6.5–8.0 mEq/L) and characteristic electrocardiographic changes (peaking of T-waves, loss of P-waves, depression of S-T segment, and prolongation of the QT-interval). Late manifestations include muscle-paralysis and cardiovascular collapse from cardiac arrest. (9–12 mEq/L).

Treatment measures for hyperkalemia include the following:

1. Elimination of foods and medications containing potassium and of any agents with potassium-sparing properties.
2. Intravenous administration of 300 to 500 mL/hr of 10% dextrose solution containing 10–20 units of crystalline insulin per 1,000 mL.
3. Correction of acidosis, if present, with intravenous sodium bicarbonate.
4. Use of exchange resins, hemodialysis, or peritoneal dialysis.

In treating hyperkalemia, it should be recalled that in patients who have been stabilized on digitalis, too rapid a lowering of the serum potassium concentration can produce digitalis toxicity.

DOSAGE AND ADMINISTRATION

The usual dietary intake of potassium by the average adult is 50 to 100 mEq per day. Potassium depletion sufficient to cause hypokalemia usually requires the loss of 200 or more mEq of potassium from the total body store.

Dosage must be adjusted to the individual needs of each patient. The dose for the prevention of hypokalemia is typically in the range of 20 mEq per day. Doses of 40–100 mEq per day or more are used for the treatment of potassium depletion. Dosage should be divided if more than 20 mEq per day is given such that no more than 20 mEq is given in a single dose.

Each K-DUR 20 tablet provides 20 mEq of potassium chloride.

Each K-DUR 10 tablet provides 10 mEq of potassium chloride.

K-DUR tablets should be taken with meals and with a glass of water or other liquid. This product should not be taken on an empty stomach because of its potential for gastric irritation (see **WARNINGS**).

Patients having difficulty swallowing whole tablets may try one of the following alternate methods of administration:

a. Break the tablet in half, and take each half separately with a glass of water.
b. Prepare an aqueous (water) suspension as follows:
   1. Place the whole tablet(s) in approximately one-half glass of water (4 fluid ounces).
   2. Allow approximately 2 minutes for the tablet(s) to disintegrate.
   3. Stir for about half a minute after the tablet(s) has disintegrated.
   4. Swirl the suspension and consume the entire contents of the glass immediately by drinking or by the use of a straw.
   5. Add another one fluid ounce of water, swirl, and consume immediately.
   6. Then, add an additional one fluid ounce of water, swirl, and consume immediately.

Aqueous suspension of K-DUR tablets that is not taken immediately should be discarded. The use of other liquids for suspending K-DUR tablets is not recommended.

HOW SUPPLIED

K-DUR 20 mEq Extended Release Tablets are available in bottles of 100 (NDC 0085-0787-01); bottles of 500 (NDC 0085-0787-06); bottles of 1000 (NDC 0085-0787-10) and boxes of 100 for unit dose dispensing (NDC 0085-0787-81). K-DUR 20 mEq tablets are white, oblong, imprinted K-DUR 20 and scored for flexibility of dosing.

K-DUR 10 mEq Extended Release Tablets are available in bottles of 100 (NDC 0085-0263-01) and boxes of 100 for unit dose dispensing (NDC 0085-0263-81). K-DUR 10 mEq tablets are white, oblong, imprinted K-DUR 10.

STORAGE CONDITIONS

Keep tightly closed. Store at controlled room temperature 15–30°C (59–86°F).

CAUTION

Federal law prohibits dispensing without prescription.

Rev. 4/90 14274766

Copyright © 1986, 1989, 1990, Key Pharmaceuticals, Inc. All rights reserved.

Shown in Product Identification Guide, page 318

NITRO-DUR® ℞
(nitroglycerin)
Transdermal Infusion System

DESCRIPTION

Nitroglycerin is 1,2,3-propanetriol trinitrate, an organic nitrate whose structural formula is:

[See chemical structure at top of next column]

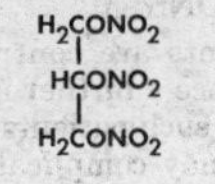

and whose molecular weight is 227.09. The organic nitrates are vasodilators, active on both arteries and veins.

The NITRO-DUR (nitroglycerin) Transdermal Infusion System is a flat unit designed to provide continuous controlled release of nitroglycerin through intact skin. The rate of release of nitroglycerin is linearly dependent upon the area of the applied system; each cm^2 of applied system delivers approximately 0.02 mg of nitroglycerin per hour. Thus, the 5-, 10-, 15-, 20-, 30-, and 40-cm^2 systems deliver approximately 0.1, 0.2, 0.3, 0.4, 0.6, and 0.8 mg of nitroglycerin per hour, respectively.

The remainder of the nitroglycerin in each system serves as a reservoir and is not delivered in normal use. After 12 hours, for example, each system has delivered approximately 6% of its original content of nitroglycerin.

The NITRO-DUR transdermal system contains nitroglycerin in acrylic-based polymer adhesives with a resinous cross-linking agent to provide a continuous source of active ingredient. Each unit is sealed in a paper polyethylene-foil pouch.

Cross section of the system.

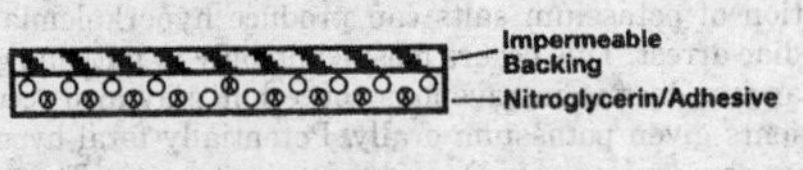

CLINICAL PHARMACOLOGY

The principal pharmacological action of nitroglycerin is relaxation of vascular smooth muscle and consequent dilatation of peripheral arteries and veins, especially the latter. Dilatation of the veins promotes peripheral pooling of blood and decreases venous return to the heart, thereby reducing left ventricular end-diastolic pressure and pulmonary capillary wedge pressure (preload). Arteriolar relaxation reduces systemic vascular resistance, systolic arterial pressure, and mean arterial pressure (afterload). Dilatation of the coronary arteries also occurs. The relative importance of preload reduction, afterload reduction, and coronary dilatation remains undefined.

Dosing regimens for most chronically used drugs are designed to provide plasma concentrations that are continuously greater than a minimally effective concentration. This strategy is inappropriate for organic nitrates. Several well-controlled clinical trials have used exercise testing to assess the antianginal efficacy of continuously delivered nitrates. In the large majority of these trials, active agents were indistinguishable from placebo after 24 hours (or less) of continuous therapy. Attempts to overcome nitrate tolerance by dose escalation, even to doses far in excess of those used acutely, have consistently failed. Only after nitrates have been absent from the body for several hours has their antianginal efficacy been restored.

Pharmacokinetics: The volume of distribution of nitroglycerin is about 3 L/kg, and nitroglycerin is cleared from this volume at extremely rapid rates, with a resulting serum half-life of about 3 minutes. The observed clearance rates (close to 1 L/kg/min) greatly exceed hepatic blood flow; known sites of extrahepatic metabolism include red blood cells and vascular walls.

The first products in the metabolism of nitroglycerin are inorganic nitrate and the 1,2- and 1,3-dinitroglycerols. The dinitrates are less effective vasodilators than nitroglycerin, but they are longer-lived in the serum, and their net contribution to the overall effect of chronic nitroglycerin regimens is not known. The dinitrates are further metabolized to (nonvasoactive) mononitrates and, ultimately, to glycerol and carbon dioxide.

To avoid development of tolerance to nitroglycerin, drug-free intervals of 10–12 hours are known to be sufficient; shorter intervals have not been well studied. In one well-controlled clinical trial, subjects receiving nitroglycerin appeared to exhibit a rebound or withdrawal effect, so that their exercise tolerance at the end of the daily drug-free interval was *less* than that exhibited by the parallel group receiving placebo.

In healthy volunteers, steady-state plasma concentrations of nitroglycerin are reached by about 2 hours after application of a patch and are maintained for the duration of wearing the system (observations have been limited to 24 hours). Upon removal of the patch, the plasma concentration declines with a half-life of about an hour.

Clinical Trials: Regimens in which nitroglycerin patches were worn for 12 hours daily have been studied in well-controlled trials up to 4 weeks in duration. Starting about 2 hours after application and continuing until 10–12 hours after application, patches that deliver at least 0.4 mg of nitroglycerin per hour have consistently demonstrated greater antianginal activity than placebo. Lower-dose patches have not been as well studied, but in one large, well-controlled trial in which higher-dose patches were also studied, patches delivering 0.2 mg/hr had significantly *less* antianginal activity than placebo.

It is reasonable to believe that the rate of nitroglycerin absorption from patches may vary with the site of application, but this relationship has not been adequately studied.

INDICATIONS AND USAGE

Transdermal nitroglycerin is indicated for the prevention of angina pectoris due to coronary artery disease. The onset of action of transdermal nitroglycerin is not sufficiently rapid for this product to be useful in aborting an acute attack.

CONTRAINDICATIONS

Allergic reactions to organic nitrates are extremely rare, but they do occur. Nitroglycerin is contraindicated in patients who are allergic to it. Allergy to the adhesives used in nitroglycerin patches has also been reported, and it similarly constitutes a contraindication to the use of this product.

WARNINGS

The benefits of transdermal nitroglycerin in patients with acute myocardial infarction or congestive heart failure have not been established. If one elects to use nitroglycerin in these conditions, careful clinical or hemodynamic monitoring must be used to avoid the hazards of hypotension and tachycardia.

A cardioverter/defibrillator should not be discharged through a paddle electrode that overlies a NITRO-DUR patch. The arcing that may be seen in this situation is harmless in itself, but it may be associated with local current concentration that can cause damage to the paddles and burns to the patient.

PRECAUTIONS

General: Severe hypotension, particularly with upright posture, may occur with even small doses of nitroglycerin. This drug should therefore be used with caution in patients who may be volume depleted or who, for whatever reason, are already hypotensive. Hypotension induced by nitroglycerin may be accompanied by paradoxical bradycardia and increased angina pectoris.

Nitrate therapy may aggravate the angina caused by hypertrophic cardiomyopathy.

As tolerance to other forms of nitroglycerin develops, the effects of sublingual nitroglycerin on exercise tolerance, although still observable, is somewhat blunted.

In industrial workers who have had long-term exposure to unknown (presumably high) doses of organic nitrates, tolerance clearly occurs. Chest pain, acute myocardial infarction, and even sudden death have occurred during temporary withdrawal of nitrates from these workers, demonstrating the existence of true physical dependence.

Several clinical trials in patients with angina pectoris have evaluated nitroglycerin regimens which incorporated a 10- to 12-hour, nitrate-free interval. In some of these trials, an increase in the frequency of anginal attacks during the nitrate-free interval was observed in a small number of patients. In one trial, patients had decreased exercise tolerance at the end of the nitrate-free interval. Hemodynamic rebound has been observed only rarely; on the other hand, few studies were so designed that rebound, if it had occurred, would have been detected. The importance of these observations to the routine, clinical use of transdermal nitroglycerin is unknown.

Information for Patients: Daily headaches sometimes accompany treatment with nitroglycerin. In patients who get these headaches, the headaches may be a marker of the activity of the drug. Patients should resist the temptation to avoid headaches by altering the schedule of their treatment with nitroglycerin, since loss of headache may be associated with simultaneous loss of antianginal efficacy.

Treatment with nitroglycerin may be associated with lightheadedness on standing, especially just after rising from a recumbent or seated position. This effect may be more frequent in patients who have also consumed alcohol.

After normal use, there is enough residual nitroglycerin in discarded patches that they are a potential hazard to children and pets.

A patient leaflet is supplied with the systems.

Drug Interactions: The vasodilating effects of nitroglycerin may be additive with those of other vasodilators. Alcohol, in particular, has been found to exhibit additive effects of this variety.

Carcinogenesis, Mutagenesis, Impairment of Fertility: Animal carcinogenesis studies with topically applied nitroglycerin have not been performed.

Rats receiving up to 434 mg/kg/day of dietary nitroglycerin for 2 years developed dose-related fibrotic and neoplastic changes in liver, including carcinomas, and interstitial cell tumors in testes. At high dose, the incidences of hepatocellular carcinomas in both sexes were 52% vs. 0% in controls, and incidences of testicular tumors were 52% vs. 8% in controls. Lifetime dietary administration of up to 1058 mg/kg/day of nitroglycerin was not tumorigenic in mice.

Nitroglycerin was weakly mutagenic in Ames tests performed in two different laboratories. Nevertheless, there

was no evidence of mutagenicity in an *in vivo* dominant lethal assay with male rats treated with doses up to about 363 mg/kg/day, p.o., or in *in vitro* cytogenetic tests in rat and dog tissues.

In a three-generation reproduction study, rats received dietary nitroglycerin at doses up to about 434 mg/kg/day for 6 months prior to mating of the F_0 generation with treatment continuing through successive F_1 and F_2 generations. The high dose was associated with decreased feed intake and body weight gain in both sexes at all matings. No specific effect on the fertility of the F_0 generation was seen. Infertility noted in subsequent generations, however, was attributed to increased interstitial cell tissue and aspermatogenesis in the high-dose males. In this three-generation study there was no clear evidence of teratogenicity.

Pregnancy: Pregnancy Category C:
Animal teratology studies have not been conducted with nitroglycerin transdermal systems. Teratology studies in rats and rabbits, however, were conducted with topically applied nitroglycerin ointment at doses up to 80 mg/kg/day and 240 mg/kg/day, respectively. No toxic effects on dams or fetuses were seen at any dose tested. There are no adequate and well-controlled studies in pregnant women. Nitroglycerin should be given to a pregnant woman only if clearly needed.

Nursing Mothers: It is not known whether nitroglycerin is excreted in human milk. Because many drugs are excreted in human milk, caution should be exercised when nitroglycerin is administered to a nursing woman.

Pediatric Use: Safety and effectiveness in children have not been established.

ADVERSE REACTIONS

Adverse reactions to nitroglycerin are generally dose related, and almost all of these reactions are the result of nitroglycerin's activity as a vasodilator. Headache, which may be severe, is the most commonly reported side effect. Headache may be recurrent with each daily dose, especially at higher doses. Transient episodes of lightheadedness, occasionally related to blood pressure changes, may also occur. Hypotension occurs infrequently, but in some patients it may be severe enough to warrant discontinuation of therapy. Syncope, crescendo angina, and rebound hypertension have been reported but are uncommon.

Allergic reactions to nitroglycerin are also uncommon, and the great majority of those reported have been cases of contact dermatitis or fixed drug eruptions in patients receiving nitroglycerin in ointments or patches. There have been few reports of genuine anaphylactoid reactions, and these reactions can probably occur in patients receiving nitroglycerin by any route.

Extremely rarely, ordinary doses of organic nitrates have caused methemoglobinemia in normal-seeming patients. Methemoglobinemia is so infrequent at these doses that further discussion of its diagnosis and treatment is deferred (see **OVERDOSAGE**).

Application-site irritation may occur but is rarely severe.

In two placebo-controlled trials of intermittent therapy with nitroglycerin patches at 0.2 to 0.8 mg/hr, the most frequent adverse reactions among 307 subjects were as follows:

	Placebo	Patch
Headache	18%	63%
Lightheadedness	4%	6%
Hypotension, and/or Syncope	0%	4%
Increased Angina	2%	2%

OVERDOSAGE

Hemodynamic Effects: The ill effects of nitroglycerin overdose are generally the results of nitroglycerin's capacity to induce vasodilatation, venous pooling, reduced cardiac output, and hypotension. These hemodynamic changes may have protean manifestations, including increased intracranial pressure, with any or all of persistent throbbing headache, confusion, and moderate fever; vertigo; palpitations; visual disturbances; nausea and vomiting (possibly with colic and even bloody diarrhea); syncope (especially in the upright posture); air hunger and dyspnea, later followed by reduced ventilatory effort; diaphoresis, with the skin either flushed or cold and clammy; heart block and bradycardia; paralysis; coma; seizures; and death.

Laboratory determinations of serum levels of nitroglycerin and its metabolites are not widely available, and such determinations have, in any event, no established role in the management of nitroglycerin overdose.

No data are available to suggest physiological maneuvers (eg, maneuvers to change the pH of the urine) that might accelerate elimination of nitroglycerin and its active metabolites. Similarly, it is not known which—if any—of these substances can usefully be removed from the body by hemodialysis.

No specific antagonist to the vasodilator effects of nitroglycerin is known, and no intervention has been subject to controlled study as a therapy of nitroglycerin overdose. Because the hypotension associated with nitroglycerin overdose is the result of venodilatation and arterial hypovolemia, prudent therapy in this situation should be directed toward increase in central fluid volume. Passive ele-

vation of the patient's legs may be sufficient, but intravenous infusion of normal saline or similar fluid may also be necessary.

The use of epinephrine or other arterial vasoconstrictors in this setting is likely to do more harm than good.

In patients with renal disease or congestive heart failure, therapy resulting in central volume expansion is not without hazard. Treatment of nitroglycerin overdose in these patients may be subtle and difficult, and invasive monitoring may be required.

Methemoglobinemia: Nitrate ions liberated during metabolism of nitroglycerin can oxidize hemoglobin into methemoglobin. Even in patients totally without cytochrome b_5 reductase activity, however, and even assuming that the nitrate moieties of nitroglycerin are quantitatively applied to oxidation of hemoglobin, about 1 mg/kg of nitroglycerin should be required before any of these patients manifests clinically significant ($\geq 10\%$) methemoglobinemia. In patients with normal reductase function, significant production of methemoglobin should require even larger doses of nitroglycerin. In one study in which 36 patients received 2–4 weeks of continuous nitroglycerin therapy at 3.1 to 4.4 mg/hr, the average methemoglobin level measured was 0.2%; this was comparable to that observed in parallel patients who received placebo.

Notwithstanding these observations, there are case reports of significant methemoglobinemia in association with moderate overdoses of organic nitrates. None of the affected patients had been thought to be unusually susceptible.

Methemoglobin levels are available from most clinical laboratories. The diagnosis should be suspected in patients who exhibit signs of impaired oxygen delivery despite adequate cardiac output and adequate arterial PO_2. Classically, methemoglobinemic blood is described as chocolate brown, without color change on exposure to air.

When methemoglobinemia is diagnosed, the treatment of choice is methylene blue, 1–2 mg/kg intravenously.

DOSAGE AND ADMINISTRATION

The suggested starting dose is between 0.2 mg/hr* and 0.4 mg/hr*. Doses between 0.4 mg/hr* and 0.8 mg/hr* have shown continued effectiveness for 10–12 hours daily for at least 1 month (the longest period studied) of intermittent administration. Although the minimum nitrate-free interval has not been defined, data show that a nitrate-free interval of 10–12 hours is sufficient (see **CLINICAL PHARMACOLOGY**). Thus, an appropriate dosing schedule for nitroglycerin patches would include a daily patch-on period of 12–14 hours and a daily patch-off period of 10–12 hours.

*Release rates were formerly described in terms of drug delivered per 24 hours. In these terms, the supplied NITRO-DUR systems would be rated at 2.5 mg/24 hours (0.1 mg/hour), 5 mg/24 hours (0.2 mg/hour), 7.5 mg/24 hours (0.3 mg/hour), 10 mg/24 hours (0.4 mg/hour), and 15 mg/24 hours (0.6 mg/hour).

NITRO-DUR System Rated Release *In Vivo**	Total Nitroglycerin Content	System Size	Package Size
0.1 mg/hr	20 mg	5 cm^2	Unit Dose 30 (NDC 0085-3305-30) Hospital Unit Dose 100 (NDC 0085-3305-01) Institutional Package 30 (NDC 0085-3305-35)
0.2 mg/hr	40 mg	10 cm^2	Unit Dose 30 (NDC 0085-3310-30) Hospital Unit Dose 100 (NDC 0085-3310-01) Institutional Package 30 (NDC 0085-3310-35)
0.3 mg/hr	60 mg	15 cm^2	Unit Dose 30 (NDC 0085-3315-30) Hospital Unit Dose 100 (NDC 0085-3315-01) Institutional Package 30 (NDC 0085-3315-35)
0.4 mg/hr	80 mg	20 cm^2	Unit Dose 30 (NDC 0085-3320-30) Hospital Unit Dose 100 (NDC 0085-3320-01) Institutional Package 30 (NDC 0085-3320-35)
0.6 mg/hr	120 mg	30 cm^2	Unit Dose 30 (NDC 0085-3330-30) Hospital Unit Dose 100 (NDC 0085-3330-01) Institutional Package 30 (NDC 0085-3330-35)
0.8 mg/hr	160 mg	40 cm^2	Unit Dose 30 (NDC 0085-0819-30) Hospital Unit Dose 100 (NDC 0085-0819-01) Institutional Package 30 (NDC 0085-0819-35)

* Release rates were formerly described in terms of drug delivered per 24 hours. In these terms, the supplied NITRO-DUR systems would be rated at 2.5 mg/24 hours (0.1 mg/hour), 5 mg/24 hours (0.2 mg/hour), 7.5 mg/24 hours (0.3 mg/hour), 10 mg/24 hours (0.4 mg/hour), and 15 mg/24 hours (0.6 mg/hour).

Although some well-controlled clinical trials using exercise tolerance testing have shown maintenance of effectiveness when patches are worn continuously, the large majority of such controlled trials have shown the development of tolerance (ie, complete loss of effect) within the first 24 hours after therapy was initiated. Dose adjustment, even to levels much higher than generally used, did not restore efficacy.

HOW SUPPLIED

[See table above]

Store between 15° and 30°C (59° and 86°F). Do not refrigerate.

CAUTION: Federal law prohibits dispensing without prescription.

Key Pharmaceuticals, Inc.
Kenilworth, NJ 07033 USA
Rev. 7/95
18143615
I030167

U. S. Patent No. 5,186,938
Shown in Product Identification Guide, page 318

THEO-DUR® ℞
(theophylline)
Extended-Release Tablets

Some of the information contained in this insert (eg, information regarding pediatric patients under the age of 12) was derived from FDA's Class Labeling Guidance for Immediate-Release Theophylline Products and is intended for informational purposes only.

DESCRIPTION

THEO-DUR® Extended-Release Tablets contain anhydrous theophylline in an extended-release formulation for oral administration which allows a 12-hour dosing interval for a majority of patients and a 24-hour dosing interval for selected patients (see **DOSAGE AND ADMINISTRATION** for a description of appropriate patient populations).

Theophylline:
Theophylline is a bronchodilator, structurally classified as a methylxanthine. It occurs as a white, odorless, crystalline powder with a bitter taste. Anhydrous theophylline has the chemical name 1H-Purine-2,6-dione,3,7-dihydro-1,3-dimethyl-, and is represented by the following structural formula:

[See chemical structure at top of next page]

The molecular formula of anhydrous theophylline is $C_7H_8N_4O_2$ with a molecular weight of 180.17.

Continued on next page

Theo-Dur—Cont.

THEO-DUR Extended-Release Tablets contain no color additives and are available in four strengths: 100 mg, 200 mg, 300 mg, and 450 mg.

The inactive ingredients for THEO-DUR 100 mg Extended-Release Tablets include: acacia, NF; acetone; alcohol, NF; cellulose acetate phthalate, NF; cetyl alcohol, NF; chloroform; confectioner's sugar 6X, NF; corn starch, NF; diethyl phthalate, NF; ethyl acetate, NF; glyceryl monostearate; isopropyl alcohol, USP; hydrous spray dried lactose, NF; magnesium stearate, NF; myristyl alcohol, NF; nonpareil seeds 18–20 mesh, NF; purified water, USP; sodium lauryl sulfate, NF; talc, USP; and white wax, NF.

The inactive ingredients for THEO-DUR 200 mg, 300 mg, and 450 mg Extended-Release Tablets include: acetone; cellulose acetate phthalate, NF; cetyl alcohol, NF; diethyl phthalate; glyceryl monostearate; hydroxypropyl methylcellulose 2910, USP; isopropyl alcohol, NF; anhydrous lactose, NF; magnesium stearate, NF; myristyl alcohol; nonpareil seeds 18–20 mesh, NF; purified water, USP; and white wax, NF.

CLINICAL PHARMACOLOGY
Mechanism of Action:
Theophylline has two distinct actions in the airways of patients with reversible obstruction; smooth muscle relaxation (ie, bronchodilation) and suppression of the response of the airways to stimuli (ie, nonbronchodilator prophylactic effects). While the mechanisms of action of theophylline are not known with certainty, studies in animals suggest that bronchodilation is mediated by the inhibition of two isozymes of phosphodiesterase (PDE III and, to a lesser extent, PDE IV) while nonbronchodilator prophylactic actions are probably mediated through one or more different molecular mechanisms that do not involve inhibition of PDE III

or antagonism of adenosine receptors. Some of the adverse effects associated with theophylline appear to be mediated by inhibition of PDE III (eg, hypotension, tachycardia, headache, and emesis) and adenosine receptor antagonism (eg, alterations in cerebral blood flow).

Theophylline increases the force of contraction of diaphragmatic muscles. This action appears to be due to enhancement of calcium uptake through an adenosine-mediated channel.

Serum Concentration-Effect Relationship:
Bronchodilation occurs over the serum theophylline concentration range of 5–20 mcg/mL. Clinically important improvement in symptom control has been found in most studies to require peak serum theophylline concentrations >10 mcg/mL, but patients with mild disease may benefit from lower concentrations. At serum theophylline concentrations >20 mcg/mL, both the frequency and severity of adverse reactions increase. In general, maintaining peak serum theophylline concentrations between 10 and 15 mcg/mL will achieve most of the drug's potential therapeutic benefit while minimizing the risk of serious adverse events.

Pharmacokinetics:
Overview Theophylline is rapidly and completely absorbed after oral administration in solution or immediate-release solid oral dosage form. Theophylline does not undergo any appreciable presystemic elimination, distributes freely into fat-free tissues, and is extensively metabolized in the liver. The pharmacokinetics of theophylline vary widely among similar patients and cannot be predicted by age, sex, body weight, or other demographic characteristics. In addition, certain concurrent illnesses and alterations in normal physiology (See **Table I**) and coadministration of other drugs (see **Table II**) can significantly alter the pharmacokinetic characteristics of theophylline. Within-subject variability in metabolism has also been reported in some studies, especially in acutely ill patients. It is, therefore, recommended that serum theophylline concentrations be measured frequently in acutely ill patients (eg, at 24-hour intervals) and periodically in patients receiving long-term therapy (eg, at 6- to 12-month intervals). More frequent measurements should be made in the presence of any condition that may significantly alter theophylline clearance (see **PRECAUTIONS, Monitoring Serum Theophylline Concentrations**, and **DOSAGE AND ADMINISTRATION**).

[See table I below]

Note: In addition to the factors listed above, theophylline clearance is increased and half-life decreased by low-carbohydrate/ high-protein diets, parenteral nutrition, and daily consumption of charcoal-broiled beef. A high-carbohydrate/ low-protein diet can decrease the clearance and prolong the half-life of theophylline.

Absorption Theophylline is rapidly and completely absorbed after oral administration in solution or immediate-release solid oral dosage form. After a single immediate-release theophylline dose of 5 mg/kg in adults, a mean peak serum concentration of about 10 mcg/mL (range 5–15 mcg/mL) can be expected 1–2 hours after the dose. Coadministration of theophylline with food or antacids does not cause clinically significant changes in the absorption of theophylline from immediate-release dosage forms.

THEO-DUR Product Pharmacokinetics
THEO-DUR (100, 200, 300, and 450 mg) Extended-Release Tablets:
In single-dose studies with 18 normal fasting subjects, the THEO-DUR product at 8 mg/kg body weight (300–700 mg/dose) produced mean peak theophylline plasma levels of 7.5 ± 1.9 mcg/mL at 9.2 ± 1.9 hours following administration. In multiple-dose, steady-state 3- and 5-day studies with 12 normal subjects, THEO-DUR administered at 8 mg/kg (300–600 mg/dose) twice daily, achieved an average peak-trough difference of 4 mcg/mL. The C_{max} and C_{min} were 13.9 ± 6.9 and 9.9 ± 6.0, respectively. The mean % fluctuation ± S.D. of the plasma concentration at steady state [% fluctuation = 100 $(C_{max}-C_{min})/C_{min}$] was 54.2 ± 45.7%. These pharmacokinetic parameters were measured under fasting conditions.

THEO-DUR (200, 300, and 450 mg) Extended-Release Tablets:
In a multiple-dose (300–500 mg BID) steady-state, 5-day study involving 14 normal, nonfasting subjects with theophylline half-lives between 5.8 and 12.3 hours (mean 8.0 ± 1.8 hours), THEO-DUR dosed twice daily, produced mean C_{max} and C_{min} levels of 12.2 ± 2.0 and 10.2 ± 1.6 mcg/mL, respectively, over the AM dosing interval and C_{max} and C_{min} of 11.6 ± 1.6 and 8.7 ± 1.8 mcg/mL, respectively, over the PM dosing interval. The mean % fluctuation ± S.D. over the AM dosing interval was 30.4 ± 12.9% and 33.7 ± 13.1% over the PM dosing interval. In the same subjects, the THEO-DUR product given once daily, in the morning, in doses ranging from 600–1000 mg (same daily dose as for BID above) produced a mean C_{max} and C_{min} of 14.4 ± 2.2 and 5.5 ± 2.0, respectively, and a mean % fluctuation ± S.D. of 195.8 ± 106.0%. Average peak-trough differences over 24 hours were 8.9 ± 1.3 and 3.7 ± 1.2 mcg/mL when THEO-DUR was given once or twice daily, respectively. In both the twice-daily and once-daily dosing regimens, THEO-DUR exhibited complete bioavailability when compared to an immediate-release product.

THEO-DUR (200, 300, and 450 mg) Extended-Release Tablets:
In a single-dose bioavailability study in eleven subjects, 1000 mg of the THEO-DUR product was administered under fasting conditions and immediately following a high-fat content (62 g) breakfast of approximately 1100 kcal. The rate and extent of absorption of theophylline from THEO-DUR administered in fasting and fed conditions were similar.

Distribution Once theophylline enters the systemic circulation, about 40% is bound to plasma protein, primarily albumin. Unbound theophylline distributes throughout body water, but distributes poorly into body fat. The apparent volume of distribution of theophylline is approximately 0.45 L/kg (range 0.3–0.7 L/kg) based on ideal body weight. Theophylline passes freely across the placenta, into breast milk, and into the cerebrospinal fluid (CSF). Saliva theophylline concentrations approximate unbound serum concentrations, but are not reliable for routine or therapeutic monitoring unless special techniques are used. An increase in the volume of distribution of theophylline, primarily due to reduction in plasma protein binding, occurs in premature neonates, patients with hepatic cirrhosis, uncorrected acidemia, the elderly, and in women during the third trimester of pregnancy. In such cases, the patient may show signs of toxicity at total (bound + unbound) serum concentrations of theophylline in the therapeutic range (10–20 mcg/mL) due to elevated concentrations of the pharmacologically active unbound drug. Similarly, a patient with decreased theophylline binding may have a subtherapeutic total drug concentration while the pharmacologically active unbound concentration is in the therapeutic range. If only total serum theophylline concentration is measured, this may lead to an unnecessary and potentially dangerous dose increase. In patients with reduced protein binding, measurement of unbound serum theophylline concentration provides a more reliable means of dosage adjustment than measurement of total serum theophylline concentration. Generally, concentrations of unbound theophylline should be maintained in the range of 6–12 mcg/mL.

Metabolism Following oral dosing, theophylline does not undergo any measurable first-pass elimination. In adults

Table I. Mean and range of total body clearance and half-life of theophylline related to age and altered physiological states.¶

Population characteristics	Total body clearance* mean (range)†† (mL/kg/min)	Half-life mean (range)†† (hr)
Age		
Premature neonates		
postnatal age 3–15 days	0.29 (0.09–0.49)	30 (17–43)
postnatal age 25–57 days	0.64 (0.04–1.2)	20 (9.4–30.6)
Term infants		
postnatal age 1–2 days	NR†	25.7 (25–26.5)
postnatal age 3–30 weeks	NR†	11 (6–29)
Children		
1–4 years	1.7 (0.5–2.9)	3.4 (1.2–5.6)
4–12 years	1.6 (0.8–2.4)	NR†
13–15 years	0.9 (0.48–1.3)	NR†
6–17 years	1.4 (0.2–2.6)	3.7 (1.5–5.9)
Adults (16–60 years)		
otherwise healthy nonsmoking asthmatics	0.65 (0.27–1.03)	8.7 (6.1–12.8)
Elderly (>60 years)		
nonsmokers with normal cardiac, liver, and renal function	0.41 (0.21–0.61)	9.8 (1.6–18)
Concurrent illness or altered physiological state		
Acute pulmonary edema	0.33** (0.07–2.45)	19** (3.1–82)
COPD >60 years, stable nonsmoker >1 year	0.54 (0.44–0.64)	11 (9.4–12.6)
COPD with cor pulmonale	0.48 (0.08–0.88)	NR†
Cystic fibrosis (14–28 years)	1.25 (0.31–2.2)	6.0 (1.8–10.2)
Fever associated with acute viral respiratory illness (children 9–15 years)	NR†	7.0 (1.0–13)
Liver disease - cirrhosis	0.31** (0.1–0.7)	32** (10–56)
acute hepatitis	0.35 (0.25–0.45)	19.2 (16.6–21.8)
cholestasis	0.65 (0.25–1.45)	14.4 (5.7–31.8)
Pregnancy - 1st trimester	NR†	8.5 (3.1–13.9)
2nd trimester	NR†	8.8 (3.8–13.8)
3rd trimester	NR†	13.0 (8.4–17.6)
Sepsis with multi-organ failure	0.47 (0.19–1.9)	18.8 (6.3–24.1)
Thyroid disease - hypothyroid	0.38 (0.13–0.57)	11.6 (8.2–25)
hyperthyroid	0.8 (0.68–0.97)	4.5 (3.7–5.6)

¶ For various North American patient populations from literature reports. Different rates of elimination and consequent dosage requirements have been observed among other peoples.

* Clearance represents the volume of blood completely cleared of theophylline by the liver in 1 minute. Values listed were generally determined at serum theophylline concentrations <20 mcg/mL; clearance may decrease and half-life may increase at higher serum concentrations due to nonlinear pharmacokinetics.

†† Reported range or estimated range (mean ± 2 S.D.) where actual range not reported.

† NR = not reported or not reported in a comparable format.

** Median

and children beyond 1 year of age, approximately 90% of the dose is metabolized in the liver. Biotransformation takes place through demethylation to 1-methylxanthine and 3-methylxanthine and hydroxylation to 1,3-dimethyluric acid. 1-methylxanthine is further hydroxylated, by xanthine oxidase, to 1-methyluric acid. About 6% of a theophylline dose is N-methylated to caffeine. Theophylline demethylation to 3methylxanthine is catalyzed by cytochrome P450 1A2, while cytochromes P450 2E1 and P450 3A3 catalyze the hydroxylation to 1,3-dimethyluric acid. Demethylation to 1--methylxanthine appears to be catalyzed either by cytochrome P450 1A2 or a closely related cytochrome. In neonates, the N-demethylation pathway is absent while the function of the hydroxylation pathway is markedly deficient. The activity of these pathways slowly increases to maximal levels by 1 year of age.

Caffeine and 3-methylxanthine are the only theophylline metabolites with pharmacologic activity. 3-methylxanthine has approximately one tenth the pharmacologic activity of theophylline and serum concentrations in adults with normal renal function are <1 mcg/mL. In patients with end-stage renal disease, 3-methylxanthine may accumulate to concentrations that approximate the unmetabolized theophylline concentration. Caffeine concentrations are usually undetectable in adults regardless of renal function. In neonates, caffeine may accumulate to concentrations that approximate the unmetabolized theophylline concentration and thus, exert a pharmacologic effect.

Both the N-demethylation and hydroxylation pathways of theophylline biotransformation are capacity-limited. Due to the wide intersubject variability of the rate of theophylline metabolism, nonlinearity of elimination may begin in some patients at serum theophylline concentrations <10 mcg/mL. Since this nonlinearity results in more than proportional changes in serum theophylline concentrations with changes in dose, it is advisable to make increases or decreases in dose in small increments in order to achieve desired changes in serum theophylline concentrations (see **DOSAGE AND ADMINISTRATION, Table V**). Accurate prediction of dose dependency of theophylline metabolism in patients *a priori* is not possible, but patients with very high initial clearance rates (ie, low steady-state serum theophylline concentrations at above average doses) have the greatest likelihood of experiencing large changes in serum theophylline concentration in response to dosage changes.

Excretion In neonates, approximately 50% of the theophylline dose is excreted unchanged in the urine. Beyond the first 3 months of life, approximately 10% of the theophylline dose is excreted unchanged in the urine. The remainder is excreted in the urine mainly as 1,3-dimethyluric acid (35%–40%), 1-methyluric acid (20%–25%), and 3-methylxanthine (15%–20%). Since little theophylline is excreted unchanged in the urine and since active metabolites of theophylline (ie, caffeine, 3-methylxanthine) do not accumulate to clinically significant levels even in the face of end-stage renal disease, no dosage adjustment for renal insufficiency is necessary in adults and children >3 months of age. In contrast, the large fraction of the theophylline dose excreted in the urine as unchanged theophylline and caffeine in neonates requires careful attention to dose reduction and frequent monitoring of serum theophylline concentrations in neonates with reduced renal function (see **WARNINGS**).

Serum Concentrations at Steady State After multiple doses of immediate-release theophylline, steady state is reached in 30–65 hours (average 40 hours) in adults. At steady state, on a dosage regimen with 6-hour intervals, the expected mean trough concentration is approximately 60% of the mean peak concentration, assuming a mean theophylline half-life of 8 hours. The difference between peak and trough concentrations is larger in patients with more rapid theophylline clearance. In patients with high theophylline clearance and half-lives of about 4–5 hours, such as children age 1 to 9 years, the trough serum theophylline concentration may be only 30% of peak with a 6-hour dosing interval. In these patients a slow-release formulation would allow a longer dosing interval (8–12 hours) with a smaller peak/trough difference.

Special Populations (see Table I for mean clearance and half-life values)

Geriatric: The clearance of theophylline is decreased by an average of 30% in healthy elderly adults (>60 yrs) compared to healthy young adults. Careful attention to dose reduction and frequent monitoring of serum theophylline concentrations are required in elderly patients (see **WARNINGS**).

Pediatrics: The clearance of theophylline is very low in neonates (see **WARNINGS**). Theophylline clearance reaches maximal values by 1 year of age, remains relatively constant until about 9 years of age and then slowly decreases by approximately 50% to adult values at about age 16. Renal excretion of unchanged theophylline in neonates amounts to about 50% of the dose, compared to about 10% in children older than 3 months and in adults. Careful attention to dosage selection and monitoring of serum theophylline concentrations are required in pediatric patients (see **WARNINGS** and **DOSAGE AND ADMINISTRATION**).

Gender: Gender differences in theophylline clearance are relatively small and unlikely to be of clinical significance. Significant reduction in theophylline clearance, however, has been reported in women on the 20th day of the menstrual cycle and during the third trimester of pregnancy.

Race: Pharmacokinetic differences in theophylline clearance due to race have not been studied.

Renal Insufficiency: Only a small fraction, eg, about 10%, of the administered theophylline dose is excreted unchanged in the urine of children greater than 3 months of age and adults. Since little theophylline is excreted unchanged in the urine and since active metabolites of theophylline (ie, caffeine, 3-methylxanthine) do not accumulate to clinically significant levels even in the face of end-stage renal disease, no dosage adjustment for renal insufficiency is necessary in adults and children >3 months of age. In contrast, approximately 50% of the administered theophylline dose is excreted unchanged in the urine in neonates. Careful attention to dose reduction and frequent monitoring of serum theophylline concentrations are required in neonates with decreased renal function (see **WARNINGS**).

Hepatic Insufficiency: Theophylline clearance is decreased by 50% or more in patients with hepatic insufficiency (eg, cirrhosis, acute hepatitis, cholestasis). Careful attention to dose reduction and frequent monitoring of serum theophylline concentrations are required in patients with reduced hepatic function (see **WARNINGS**).

Congestive Heart Failure (CHF): Theophylline clearance is decreased by 50% or more in patients with CHF. The extent of reduction in theophylline clearance in patients with CHF appears to be directly correlated to the severity of the cardiac disease. Since theophylline clearance is independent of liver blood flow, the reduction in clearance appears to be due to impaired hepatocyte function rather than reduced perfusion. Careful attention to dose reduction and frequent monitoring of serum theophylline concentrations are required in patients with CHF (see **WARNINGS**).

Smokers: Tobacco and marijuana smoking appear to increase the clearance of theophylline by induction of metabolic pathways. Theophylline clearance has been shown to increase by approximately 50% in young adult tobacco smokers and by approximately 80% in elderly tobacco smokers compared to nonsmoking subjects. Passive smoke exposure has also been shown to increase theophylline clearance by up to 50%. Abstinence from tobacco smoking for 1 week causes a reduction of approximately 40% in theophylline clearance. Careful attention to dose reduction and frequent monitoring of serum theophylline concentrations are required in patients who stop smoking (see **WARNINGS**). Use of nicotine gum has been shown to have no effect on theophylline clearance.

Fever: Fever, regardless of its underlying cause, can decrease the clearance of theophylline. The magnitude and duration of the fever appear to be directly correlated to the degree of decrease of theophylline clearance. Precise data are lacking, but a temperature of 39°C (102°F) for at least 24 hours or lesser temperature elevations for longer periods, are probably required to produce a clinically significant increase in serum theophylline concentrations. Children with rapid rates of theophylline clearance (ie, those who require a dose that is substantially larger than average [eg, >22 mg/kg/day] to achieve a therapeutic peak serum theophylline concentration when afebrile) may be at greater risk of toxic effects from decreased clearance during sustained fever. Careful attention to dose reduction and frequent monitoring of serum theophylline concentrations are required in patients with sustained fever (see **WARNINGS**).

Miscellaneous: Other factors associated with decreased theophylline clearance include the third trimester of pregnancy, sepsis with multiple organ failure, and hypothyroidism. Careful attention to dose reduction and frequent monitoring of serum theophylline concentrations are required in patients with any of these conditions (see **WARNINGS**). Other factors associated with increased theophylline clearance include hyperthyroidism and cystic fibrosis.

Clinical Studies:

In patients with chronic asthma, including patients with severe asthma requiring inhaled corticosteroids or alternate-day oral corticosteroids, many clinical studies have shown that theophylline decreases the frequency and severity of symptoms, including nocturnal exacerbations, and decreases the "as needed" use of inhaled $beta_2$-agonists. Theophylline has also been shown to reduce the need for short courses of daily oral prednisone to relieve exacerbations of airway obstruction that are unresponsive to bronchodilators in asthmatics.

In patients with chronic obstructive pulmonary disease (COPD), clinical studies have shown that theophylline decreases dyspnea, air trapping, the work of breathing, and improves contractility of diaphragmatic muscles with little or no improvement in pulmonary function measurements.

INDICATIONS AND USAGE

THEO-DUR Extended-Release Tablets are indicated for the treatment of the symptoms and reversible airflow obstruction associated with chronic asthma and other chronic lung diseases, eg, emphysema and chronic bronchitis.

CONTRAINDICATIONS

THEO-DUR Extended-Release Tablets are contraindicated in patients with a history of hypersensitivity to theophylline or other components in the product.

WARNINGS

Serious side effects such as ventricular arrhythmias, convulsions, or even death may appear as the first sign of toxicity without any recognized prior warning. Less serious signs of theophylline toxicity (eg, nausea and restlessness) may occur frequently when initiating therapy but are usually transient. When such signs are persistent during maintenance therapy, they are often associated with serum concentrations above 20 mcg/mL. Stated differently, serious toxicity is not reliably preceded by less severe side effects.

Concurrent Illness:

Theophylline should be used with extreme caution in patients with the following clinical conditions due to the increased risk of exacerbation of the concurrent condition:

Active peptic ulcer disease (peptic ulcer disease should be controlled with appropriate therapy since theophylline is known to increase peptic acid secretion)

Seizure disorders

Cardiac arrhythmias (not including bradyarrhythmias)

Conditions That Reduce Theophylline Clearance:

There are several readily identifiable causes of reduced theophylline clearance. ***If the total daily dose is not appropriately reduced so as to lower serum theophylline levels to within the therapeutic range in the presence of these risk factors, severe and potentially fatal theophylline toxicity can occur.*** Careful consideration must be given to the benefits and risks of theophylline use and the need for more intensive monitoring of serum theophylline concentrations in patients with the following risk factors:

Age:

Neonates (term and premature)
Children <1 year
Elderly (>60 years)

Concurrent Diseases:

Acute pulmonary edema
Congestive heart failure
Cor pulmonale
Fever; ≥102°F for 24 hours or more; or lesser temperature elevations for longer periods
Hypothyroidism
Liver disease; cirrhosis, acute hepatitis
Reduced renal function in infants <3 months of age
Sepsis with multi-organ failure
Shock

Cessation of Smoking

Drug Interactions:

Adding a drug that inhibits theophylline metabolism (eg, cimetidine, erythromycin, tacrine) or stopping a concurrently administered drug that enhances theophylline metabolism (eg, carbamazepine, rifampin). (See **PRECAUTIONS, Drug Interactions, Table II.**)

When Signs or Symptoms of Theophylline Toxicity Are Present:

Whenever a patient receiving theophylline develops nausea or vomiting, particularly repetitive vomiting, or other signs or symptoms consistent with theophylline toxicity (even if another cause may be suspected), additional doses of theophylline should be withheld and a serum theophylline concentration should be measured immediately. Patients should be instructed not to continue any dosage that causes adverse effects and to withhold subsequent doses until the symptoms have resolved, at which time the clinician may instruct the patient to resume the drug at a lower dosage (see **DOSAGE AND ADMINISTRATION, Dosage Guidelines, Table V**).

Dosage Increases:

Increases in the dose of theophylline should not be made in response to an acute exacerbation of symptoms of chronic lung disease since theophylline provides little added benefit to inhaled $beta_2$-selective agonists and systematically administered corticosteroids in this circumstance and increases the risk of adverse effects. A *peak* steady-state serum theophylline concentration should be measured before increasing the dose in response to persistent chronic symptoms to ascertain whether an increase in dose is safe. Before increasing the theophylline dose on the basis of a low serum concentration, the clinician should consider whether the blood sample was obtained at an appropriate time in relationship to the dose and whether the patient has adhered to the prescribed regimen (see **PRECAUTIONS, Monitoring Serum Theophylline Concentrations**).

As the rate of theophylline clearance may be dose dependent (ie, steady-state serum concentrations may increase disproportionately to the increase in dose), an increase in dose based upon a subtherapeutic serum concentration measurement should be conservative. In general, limiting dose increases to about 25% of the previous total daily dose

Continued on next page

Theo-Dur—Cont.

will reduce the risk of unintended excessive increases in serum theophylline concentration (see **DOSAGE AND ADMINISTRATION, Table V**).

PRECAUTIONS

THEO-DUR TABLETS SHOULD *NOT* BE CHEWED OR CRUSHED AND SHOULD *BE BROKEN ONLY AT THE SCORE.*

General:

Careful consideration of the various interacting drugs (including recently discontinued medications), physiologic conditions, and other factors such as smoking that can alter theophylline clearance and require dosage adjustment should occur prior to initiation of theophylline therapy, prior to increases in theophylline dose, and during follow up (see **WARNINGS**). The dose of theophylline selected for initiation of therapy should be low and, *if tolerated*, increased slowly over a period of a week or longer with the final dose guided by monitoring serum theophylline concentrations and the patient's clinical response (see **DOSAGE AND ADMINISTRATION, Table IV**).

Monitoring Serum Theophylline Concentrations:

Serum theophylline concentration measurements are readily available and should be used to determine whether the dosage is appropriate. Specifically, the serum theophylline concentration should be measured as follows:

1. When initiating therapy to guide final dosage adjustment after titration.
2. Before making a dose increase to determine whether the serum concentration is subtherapeutic in a patient who continues to be symptomatic.
3. Whenever signs or symptoms of theophylline toxicity are present.
4. Whenever there is a new illness, worsening of a chronic illness, or a change in the patient's treatment regimen that may alter theophylline clearance [eg, fever (see **CLINICAL PHARMACOLOGY,** *Fever*), hepatitis, or drugs listed in **Table II** are added or discontinued].

To guide a dose increase, the blood sample should be obtained at the time of the expected peak serum theophylline concentration; 4 to 8 hours when medication is taken every 12 hours or 8 hours when taken once daily. It is important that the patient has not missed or taken additional doses during the previous 48 hours and that the dosing intervals were reasonably equally spaced. A trough concentration (ie, at the end of the dosing interval) provides no additional useful information and may lead to an inappropriate dose increase since the peak serum theophylline concentration can be two or more times greater than the trough concentration with an immediate-release formulation. If the serum sample is drawn more than 8 hours after the dose, the results must be interpreted with caution since the concentration may not be reflective of the peak concentration. In contrast, when signs or symptoms of theophylline toxicity are present, the serum sample should be obtained as soon as possible, analyzed immediately, and the result reported to the clinician without delay. In patients in whom decreased serum protein binding is suspected (eg, cirrhosis, women during the third trimester of pregnancy), the concentration of unbound theophylline should be measured and the dosage adjusted to achieve an unbound concentration of 6–12 mcg/mL.

Saliva concentrations of theophylline cannot be used reliably to adjust dosage without special techniques.

Effects on Laboratory Tests:

As a result of its pharmacological effects, theophylline at serum concentrations within the 10–20 mcg/mL range modestly increases plasma glucose (from a mean of 88 mg% to 98 mg%), uric acid (from a mean of 4 mg/dL to 6 mg/dL), free fatty acids (from a mean of 451 μeq/L to 800 μeq/L), total cholesterol (from a mean of 140 vs 160 mg/dL), HDL (from a mean of 36 to 50 mg/dL), HDL/LDL ratio (from a mean of 0.5 to 0.7), and urinary free cortisol excretion (from a mean of 44 to 63 mcg/24 hr). Theophylline at serum concentrations within the 10–20 mcg/mL range may also transiently decrease serum concentrations of triiodothyronine (144 before, 131 after 1 week and 142 ng/dL after 4 weeks of theophylline). The clinical importance of these changes should be weighed against the potential therapeutic benefit of theophylline in individual patients.

Information for Patients:

This information is intended to aid in the safe and effective use of this medication. It is not a disclosure of all adverse or intended effects.

The patient (or parent/caregiver) should be instructed to seek medical advice whenever nausea, vomiting, persistent headache, insomnia, restlessness, or rapid heartbeat occurs during treatment with theophylline, even if another cause is suspected. The patient should be instructed to contact their clinician if they develop a new illness, especially if accompanied by a persistent fever, if they experience worsening of a chronic illness, if they start or stop smoking cigarettes or marijuana, or if another clinician adds a new medication or discontinues a previously prescribed medication. Patients

should be informed that theophylline interacts with a wide variety of drugs (see **Table II**). They should be instructed to inform all clinicians involved in their care that they are taking theophylline, especially when a medication is being added or deleted from their treatment. Patients should be instructed to not alter the dose, timing of the dose, or frequency of administration without first consulting their clinician. If a dose is missed, the patient should be instructed to take the next dose at the usually scheduled time and to not attempt to make up for the missed dose.

THEO-DUR Tablets *should not be chewed or crushed*. When dosing THEO-DUR Extended-Release Tablets on a once-daily (q24h) basis, tablets should be taken whole and not split.

Drug Interactions

Drug/Drug Interactions:

Theophylline interacts with a wide variety of drugs. The interaction may be pharmacodynamic, ie, alterations in the therapeutic response to theophylline or another drug or occurrence of adverse effects without a change in serum theophylline concentration. More frequently, however, the interaction is pharmacokinetic, ie, the rate of theophylline clearance is altered by another drug resulting in increased or decreased serum theophylline concentrations. Theophylline only rarely alters the pharmacokinetics of other drugs. The drugs listed in **Table II** have the potential to produce clinically significant pharmacodynamic or pharmacokinetic interactions with theophylline. The information in the **"Effect"** column of **Table II** assumes that the interacting drug is being added to a steady-state theophylline regimen. If theophylline is being initiated in a patient who is already taking a drug that inhibits theophylline clearance (eg, cimetidine, erythromycin), the dose of theophylline required to achieve a therapeutic serum theophylline concentration will be smaller. Conversely, if theophylline is being initiated in a patient who is already taking a drug that enhances theophylline clearance (eg, rifampin), the dose of theophylline required to achieve a therapeutic serum theophylline concentration will be larger. Discontinuation of a concomitant drug that increases theophylline clearance will result in accumulation of theophylline to potentially toxic levels, unless the theophylline dose is appropriately reduced. Discontinuation of a concomitant drug that inhibits theophylline clearance will result in decreased serum theophylline concentrations, unless the theophylline dose is appropriately increased.

The listing of drugs in **Table II** is current as of February 9, 1995. New interactions are continuously being reported for theophylline, especially with new chemical entities. **The clinician should not assume that a drug does not interact with theophylline if it is not listed in Table II.** Before addition of a newly available drug in a patient receiving theophylline, the package insert of the new drug and/or the medical literature should be consulted to determine if an interaction between the new drug and theophylline has been reported.

[See table II at top of next page]

Drug/Food Interactions:

THEO-DUR 100 mg Extended-Release Tablets have not been adequately studied to determine whether their bioavailability is altered when given with food. Available data suggest that drug administration at the time of food ingestion may influence the absorption characteristics of theophylline controlled-release products resulting in serum values different from those found after administration in the fasting state.

A drug-food effect, if any, would likely have its greatest clinical significance when high theophylline serum levels are being maintained and/or when large single doses (> 13 mg/kg or 900 mg) of a controlled-release theophylline product are given.

THEO-DUR (200, 300, and 450 mg) Extended-Release Tablets: The rate and extent of absorption of theophylline from THEO-DUR 200 mg, 300 mg, and 450 mg tablets are similar when administered fasting or immediately after a high-fat content breakfast such as 8 oz. whole milk, egg/cheese/bacon on muffin, 1 blueberry muffin with margarine, and 1 serving of hash brown potatoes (about 1100 kcal, including approximately 62 g of fat) (see **CLINICAL PHARMACOLOGY, Pharmacokinetics**).

The Effect of Other Drugs on Theophylline Serum Concentration Measurements:

Most serum theophylline assays in clinical use are immunoassays which are specific for theophylline. Other xanthines such as caffeine, dyphylline, and pentoxifylline are not detected by these assays. Some drugs (eg, cefazolin, cephalothin), however, may interfere with certain HPLC techniques. Caffeine and xanthine metabolites in neonates or patients with renal dysfunction may cause the reading from some dry reagent office methods to be higher than the actual serum theophylline concentration.

Carcinogenesis, Mutagenesis, and Impairment of Fertility:

Long-term carcinogenicity studies have been carried out in mice (oral doses 30–150 mg/kg) and rats (oral doses 5–75 mg/kg). Results are pending.

Theophylline has been studied in Ames salmonella, *in vivo* and *in vitro* cytogenetics, micronucleus, and Chinese hamster ovary test systems and has not been shown to be genotoxic.

In a 14-week continuous breeding study, theophylline, administered to mating pairs of B6C3F$_1$ mice at oral doses of 120, 270, and 500 mg/kg (approximately 1.0–3.0 times the human dose on a mg/m^2 basis) impaired fertility, as evidenced by decreases in the number of live pups per litter, decreases in the mean number of litters per fertile pair, and increases in the gestation period at the high dose as well as decreases in the proportion of pups born alive at the mid and high dose. In 13-week toxicity studies, theophylline was administered to F344 rats and B6C3F$_1$ mice at oral doses of 40–300 mg/kg (approximately 2.0 times the human dose on a mg/m^2 basis). At the high dose, systemic toxicity was observed in both species including decreases in testicular weight.

Pregnancy:

Category C There are no adequate and well-controlled studies in pregnant women. Additionally, there are no teratogenicity studies in nonrodents (eg, rabbits). Theophylline was not shown to be teratogenic in CD-1 mice at oral doses up to 400 mg/kg, approximately 2.0 times the recommended human dose on a mg/m^2 basis or CD-1 rats at oral doses up to 260 mg/kg, approximately 3.0 times the recommended human dose on a mg/m^2 basis. At a dose of 220 mg/kg, embryotoxicity was observed in rats in the absence of maternal toxicity.

Nursing Mothers:

Theophylline is excreted into breast milk and may cause irritability or other signs of mild toxicity in nursing human infants. The concentration of theophylline in breast milk is about equivalent to the maternal serum concentration. An infant ingesting a liter of breast milk containing 10–20 mcg/mL of theophylline a day is likely to receive 10–20 mg of theophylline per day. Serious adverse effects in the infant are unlikely unless the mother has toxic serum theophylline concentrations.

Pediatric Use:

Safety and effectiveness of THEO-DUR Extended-Release Tablets administered:

1. Every 24 hours in pediatric patients under 12 years of age have not been established.
2. Every 12 hours in pediatric patients under 6 years of age have not been established.

Other theophylline formulations, however, are safe and effective for the approved indications in pediatric patients under the ages listed above. The maintenance dose of theophylline must be selected with caution in pediatric patients since the rate of theophylline clearance is highly variable across the age range of neonates to adolescents (see **CLINICAL PHARMACOLOGY, Table I, WARNINGS,** and **DOSAGE AND ADMINISTRATION, Table IV**).

Geriatric Use:

Elderly patients are at significantly greater risk of experiencing serious toxicity from theophylline than younger patients due to pharmacokinetic and pharmacodynamic changes associated with aging. Theophylline clearance is reduced in patients greater than 60 years of age, resulting in increased serum theophylline concentrations in response to a given theophylline dose. Protein binding may be decreased in the elderly resulting in a large proportion of the total serum theophylline concentration in the pharmacologically active unbound form. Elderly patients also appear to be more sensitive to the toxic effects of theophylline after chronic overdosage than younger patients. For these reasons, the maximum daily dose of theophylline in patients greater than 60 years of age ordinarily should not exceed 400 mg/day unless the patient continues to be symptomatic and the peak steady-state serum theophylline concentration is <10 mcg/mL (see **DOSAGE AND ADMINISTRATION**). Theophylline doses greater than 400 mg/day should be prescribed with caution in elderly patients.

ADVERSE REACTIONS

Adverse reactions associated with theophylline are generally mild when peak serum theophylline concentrations are <20 mcg/mL and mainly consist of transient caffeine-like adverse effects such as nausea, vomiting, headache, and insomnia. When peak serum theophylline concentrations exceed 20 mcg/mL, however, theophylline produces a wide range of adverse reactions including persistent vomiting, cardiac arrhythmias, and intractable seizures which can be lethal (see **OVERDOSAGE**). The transient caffeine-like adverse reactions occur in about 50% of patients when theophylline therapy is initiated at doses higher than recommended initial doses (eg, >300 mg/day in adults and >12 mg/kg/day in children beyond >1 year of age). During the initiation of theophylline therapy, caffeine-like adverse effects may transiently alter patient behavior, especially in school-age children, but this response rarely persists. Initiation of theophylline therapy at a low dose with subsequent slow titration to a predetermined age-related maximum dose will significantly reduce the frequency of these transient adverse effects (see **DOSAGE AND ADMINISTRA-**

Table II. Drug	Clinically significant drug interactions with theophylline.* Type of Interaction	Effect**
Adenosine	Theophylline blocks adenosine receptors.	Higher doses of adenosine may be required to achieve desired effect.
Alcohol	A single large dose of alcohol (eg, 3 mL/kg of whiskey) decreases theophylline clearance for up to 24 hours.	30% increase
Allopurinol	Decreases theophylline clearance at allopurinol doses ≥600 mg/day.	25% increase
Aminoglutethimide	Increases theophylline clearance by induction of microsomal enzyme activity.	25% decrease
Carbamazepine	Similar to aminoglutethimide.	30% decrease
Cimetidine	Decreases theophylline clearance by inhibiting cytochrome P45 1A2.	70% increase
Ciprofloxacin	Similar to cimetidine.	40% increase
Clarithromycin	Similar to erythromycin.	25% increase
Diazepam	Benzodiazepines increase CNS concentrations of adenosine, a potent CNS depressant, while theophylline blocks adnosine receptors.	Larger diazepam doses may be required to produce desired level of sedation. Discontinuation of theophylline without reduction of diazepam dose may result in respiratory depression.
Disulfiram	Decreases theophylline clearance by inhibiting hydroxylation and demethylation.	50% increase
Enoxacin	Similar to cimetidine.	300% increase
Ephedrine	Synergistic CNS effects.	Increased frequency of nausea, nervousness, and insomnia.
Erythromycin	Erythromycin metabolite decreases theophylline clearance by inhibiting cytochrome P450 3A3.	35% increase. Erythromycin steady-state serum concentrations decrease by a similar amount.
Estrogen	Estrogen-containing oral contraceptives decrease theophylline clearance in a dose-dependent fashion. The effect of progesterone on theophylline clearance is unknown.	30% increase
Flurazepam	Similar to diazepam.	Similar to diazepam.
Fluvoxamine	Similar to cimetidine.	Similar to cimetidine.
Halothane	Halothane sensitizes the myocardium to catecholamines; theophylline increases release of endogenous catecholamines.	Increased risk of ventricular arrhythmias.
Interferon, human recombinant alpha-A	Decreases theophylline clearance.	100% increase
Isoproterenol (IV)	Increases theophylline clearance.	20% decrease
Ketamine	Pharmacologic.	May lower theophylline seizure threshold.
Lithium	Theophylline increases renal lithium clearance.	Lithium dose required to achieve a therapeutic serum concentration increased an average of 60%.
Lorazepam	Similar to diazepam.	Similar to diazepam.
Methotrexate (MTX)	Decreases theophylline clearance.	20% increase after low dose MTX; higher dose MTX may have a greater effect.
Mexiletine	Similar to disulfiram.	80% increase
Midazolam	Similar to diazepam.	Similar to diazepam.
Moricizine	Increases theophylline clearance.	25% decrease
Norfloxacin	Increases serum theophylline levels.	
Ofloxacin	Increases serum theophylline levels.	
Pancuronium	Theophylline may antagonize nondepolarizing neuromuscular blocking effects; possibly due to phosphodiesterase inhibition.	Larger dose of pancuronium may be required to achieve neuromuscular blockade.
Pentoxifylline	Decreases theophylline clearance.	30% increase
Phenobarbital (PB)	Similar to aminoglutethimide.	25% decrease after 2 weeks of concurrent PB.
Phenytoin	Phenytoin increases theophylline clearance by increasing microsomal enzyme activity. Theophylline decreases phenytoin absorption.	Serum theophylline and phenytoin concentrations decrease about 40%.
Propafenone	Decreases theophylline clearance and pharmacologic interaction.	40% increase. Beta₂-blocking effect may decrease efficacy of theophylline.
Propranolol	Similar to cimetidine and pharmacologic interaction.	100% increase. Beta₂-blocking effect may decrease efficacy of theophylline.
Rifampin	Increases theophylline clearance by increasing cytochrome P450 1A2 and 3A3 activity.	20%–40% decrease
Ritonavir	Increases theophylline clearance (mechanism unknown).	43% decrease in AUC.
Sucralfate	Reduced absorption of theophylline.	
Sulfinpyrazone	Increases theophylline clearance by increasing demethylation and hydroxylation. Decreases renal clearance of theophylline.	20% decrease
Tacrine	Similar to cimetidine, also increases renal clearance of theophylline.	90% increase
Thiabendazole	Decreases theophylline clearance.	190% increase
Ticlopidine	Decreases theophylline clearance.	60% increase
Troleandomycin	Similar to erythromycin.	33%–100% increase depending on troleandomycin dose.
Verapamil	Similar to disulfiram.	

* Refer to **PRECAUTIONS, Drug Interactions** for further information regarding table.

** Average effect on steady-state theophylline concentration or other clinical effect for pharmacologic interactions. Individual patients may experience larger changes in serum theophylline concentration than the value listed.

TION, Table IV). In a small percentage of patients (<3% of children and <10% of adults), the caffeine-like adverse effects persist during maintenance therapy, even at peak serum theophylline concentrations within the therapeutic range (ie, 10–20 mcg/mL). Dosage reduction may alleviate the caffeine-like adverse effects in these patients, however, persistent adverse effects should result in a reevaluation of the need for continued theophylline therapy and the potential therapeutic benefit of alternative treatment.

Other adverse reactions that have been reported to occur at serum theophylline concentrations less than 20 mcg/mL include diarrhea, irritability, restlessness, fine skeletal muscle tremors, alopecia, muscle twitching/spasms, palpitations, rash, reflex hyperexcitability, transient diuresis, and ventricular arrhythmia. Whether or not theophylline caused these reported events is not known. In patients with hypoxia secondary to COPD, multifocal atrial tachycardia and flutter have been reported at serum theophylline concentrations ≥ 15 mcg/mL. There have been a few isolated reports of seizures at serum theophylline concentrations <20 mcg/mL in patients with an underlying neurological disease or in elderly patients. The occurrence of seizures in elderly patients with serum theophylline concentrations <20 mcg/mL may be secondary to decreased protein binding resulting in a larger proportion of the total serum theophylline concentration in the pharmacologically active unbound form. The clinical characteristics of the seizures reported in patients with serum theophylline concentration <20 mcg/mL have generally been milder than seizures associated with excessive serum theophylline concentrations resulting from an overdose (ie, they have generally been transient, often stopped without anticonvulsant therapy, and did not result in neurological residua).

[See table III at top of next page]

OVERDOSAGE
General:

The chronicity and pattern of theophylline overdosage significantly influences clinical manifestations of toxicity, management, and outcome. There are two common presentations: (1) *acute overdose*, ie, ingestion of a single large excessive dose (>10 mg/kg) as occurs in the context of an attempted suicide or isolated medication error, and (2) *chronic overdosage*, ie, ingestion of repeated doses that are excessive for the patient's rate of theophylline clearance. The most common causes of chronic theophylline overdosage include patient or caregiver error in dosing, clinician prescribing of an excessive dose or a normal dose in the presence of factors known to decrease the rate of theophylline clearance, and increasing the dose in response to an exacerbation of symptoms without first measuring the serum theophylline concentration to determine whether a dose increase is safe.

Severe toxicity from theophylline overdose is a relatively rare event. In one health maintenance organization, the frequency of hospital admissions for chronic overdosage of theophylline was about 1 per 1000 person-years exposure. In another study, among 6000 blood samples obtained for measurement of serum theophylline concentration, for any reason, from patients treated in an emergency department, 7% were in the 20–30 mcg/mL range and 3% were >30 mcg/mL. Approximately two thirds of the patients with serum theophylline concentrations in the 20–30 mcg/mL range had one or more manifestations of toxicity while >90% of patients with serum theophylline concentrations >30 mcg/mL were clinically intoxicated. Similarly, in other reports, serious toxicity from theophylline is seen principally at serum concentrations >30 mcg/mL.

Several studies have described the clinical manifestations of theophylline overdose and attempted to determine the factors that predict life-threatening toxicity. In general, patients who exeperience an acute overdose are less likely to experience seizures than patients who have experienced a chronic overdosage, unless the peak serum theophylline concentration is >100 mcg/mL. After a chronic overdosage, generalized seizures, life-threatening cardiac arrhythmias, and death may occur at serum theophylline concentrations >30 mcg/mL. The severity of toxicity after chronic overdosage is more strongly correlated with the patient's age than the peak serum theophylline concentration; patients >60 years are at the greatest risk for severe toxicity and mortality after a chronic overdosage. Pre-existing or concurrent disease may also significantly increase the susceptibility of a patient to a particular toxic manifestation, eg, patients with neurologic disorders have an increased risk of seizures and patients with cardiac disease have an increased risk of cardiac arrhythmias for a given serum theophylline concentration compared to patients without the underlying disease.

The frequency of various reported manifestations of theophylline overdose according to the mode of overdose are listed in **Table III.**

Other manifestations of theophylline toxicity include increases in serum calcium, creatine kinase, myoglobin, and

Continued on next page

Theo-Dur—Cont.

leukocyte count; decreases in serum phosphate and magnesium, acute myocardial infarction, and urinary retention in men with obstructive uropathy.

Seizures associated with serum theophylline concentrations >30 mcg/mL are often resistant to anticonvulsant therapy and may result in irreversible brain injury if not rapidly controlled. Death from theophylline toxicity is most often secondary to cardiorespiratory arrest and/or hypoxic encephalopathy following prolonged generalized seizures or intractable cardiac arrhythmias causing hemodynamic compromise.

Overdose Management:

General Recommendations for Patients with Symptoms of Theophylline Overdose or Serum Theophylline Concentrations >30 mcg/mL. (Note: Serum theophylline concentrations may continue to increase after presentation of the patient for medical care.)

1. While simultaneously instituting treatment, contact a regional poison center to obtain updated information and advice on individualizing the recommendations that follow.
2. Institute supportive care, including establishment of intravenous access, maintenance of the airway, and electrocardiographic monitoring.
3. *Treatment of seizures:* Because of the high morbidity and mortality associated with theophylline-induced seizures, treatment should be rapid and aggressive. Anticonvulsant therapy should be initiated with an intravenous benzodiazepine, eg, diazepam, in increments of 0.1–0.2 mg/kg every 1–3 minutes until seizures are terminated. Repetitive seizures should be treated with a loading dose of phenobarbital (20 mg/kg infused over 30–60 minutes). Animal studies and case reports of theophylline overdose in humans suggest that phenytoin is ineffective in terminating theophylline-induced seizures. The doses of benzodiazepines and phenobarbital required to terminate theophylline-induced seizures are close to the doses that may cause severe respiratory depression or respiratory arrest; the clinician should therefore be prepared to provide assisted ventilation. Elderly patients and patients with COPD may be more susceptible to the respiratory depressant effects of anticonvulsants. Barbiturate-induced coma or administration of general anesthesia may be required to terminate repetitive seizures or status epilepticus. General anesthesia should be used with caution in patients with theophylline overdose because fluorinated volatile anesthetics may sensitize the myocardium to endogenous catecholamines released by theophylline. Enflurane appears less likely to be associated with this effect than halothane and may, therefore, be safer. Neuromuscular blocking agents alone should not be used to terminate seizures since they abolish the musculoskeletal manifestations without terminating seizure activity in the brain.
4. *Anticipate need for anticonvulsants:* In patients with theophylline overdose who are at high risk for theophylline-induced seizures, eg, patients with acute overdoses and serum theophylline concentrations >100 mcg/mL or chronic overdosage in patients >60 years of age with serum theophylline concentrations >30 mcg/mL, the need for anticonvulsant therapy should be anticipated. A benzodiazepine such as diazepam should be drawn into a syringe and kept at the patient's bedside and medical personnel qualified to treat seizures should be immediately available. In selected patients at high risk for theophylline-induced seizures, consideration should be given to the administration of prophylactic anticonvulsant therapy. Situations where prophylactic anticonvulsant therapy should be considered in high-risk patients include anticipated delays in instituting methods for extracorporeal removal of theophylline (eg, transfer of a high-risk patient from one healthcare facility to another for extracorporeal removal) and clinical circumstances that significantly interfere with efforts to enhance theophylline clearance (eg, a neonate where dialysis may not be technically feasible or a patient with vomiting unresponsive to antiemetics who is unable to tolerate multiple-dose oral activated charcoal). In animal studies, prophylactic administration of phenobarbital, *but not phenytoin,* has been shown to delay the onset of theophylline-induced generalized seizures and to increase the dose of theophylline required to induce seizures (ie, markedly increases the LD_{50}). Although there are no controlled studies in humans, a loading dose of intravenous phenobarbital (20 mg/kg infused over 60 minutes) may delay or prevent life-threatening seizures in high-risk patients while efforts to enhance theophylline clearance are continued. Phenobarbital may cause respiratory depression, particularly in elderly patients and patients with COPD.
5. *Treatment of cardiac arrhythmias:* Sinus tachycardia and simple ventricular premature beats are not harbingers of life-threatening arrhythmias, they do not require treatment in the absence of hemodynamic compromise, and they resolve with declining serum theophylline concentrations. Other arrhythmias, especially those associated with hemodynamic compromise, should be treated with antiarrhythmic therapy appropriate for the type of arrhythmia.
6. *Gastrointestinal decontamination:* Oral activated charcoal (0.5 g/kg up to 20 g and repeat at least once 1–2 hours after the first dose) is extremely effective in blocking the absorption of theophylline throughout the gastrointestinal tract, even when administered several hours after ingestion. If the patient is vomiting, the charcoal should be administered through a nasogastric tube or after administration of an antiemetic. Phenothiazine antiemetics such as prochlorperazine or perphenazine should be avoided since they can lower the seizure threshold and frequently cause dystonic reactions. A single dose of sorbitol may be used to promote stooling to facilitate removal of theophylline bound to charcoal from the gastrointestinal tract. Sorbitol, however, should be dosed with caution since it is a potent purgative which can cause profound fluid and electrolyte abnormalities, particularly after multiple doses. Commercially available fixed combinations of liquid charcoal and sorbitol should be avoided in young children and after the first dose in adolescents and adults since they do not allow for individualization of charcoal and sorbitol dosing. Ipecac syrup should be avoided in theophylline overdoses. Although ipecac induces emesis, it does not reduce the absorption of theophylline unless administered within 5 minutes of ingestion and even then is less effective than oral activated charcoal. Moreover, ipecac-induced emesis may persist for several hours after a single dose and significantly decrease the retention and the effectiveness of oral activated charcoal.
7. *Serum theophylline concentration monitoring:* The serum theophylline concentration should be measured immediately upon presentation, 2–4 hours later, and then at sufficient intervals, eg, every 4 hours, to guide treatment decisions and to assess the effectiveness of therapy. Serum theophylline concentrations may continue to increase after presentation of the patient for medical care as a result of continued absorption of theophylline from the gastrointestinal tract. Serial monitoring of serum theophylline serum concentrations should be continued until it is clear that the concentration is no longer rising and has returned to nontoxic levels.
8. *General monitoring procedures:* Electrocardiographic monitoring should be initiated on presentation and continued until the serum theophylline level has returned to a nontoxic level. Serum electrolytes and glucose should be measured on presentation and at appropriate intervals indicated by clinical circumstances. Fluid and electrolyte abnormalities should be promptly corrected. **Monitoring and treatment should be continued until the serum concentration decreases below 20 mcg/mL.**
9. *Enhance clearance of theophylline:* Multiple-dose oral activated charcoal (eg, 0.5 mg/kg up to 20 g, every 2 hours) increases the clearance of theophylline at least twofold by absorption of theophylline secreted into gastrointestinal fluids. Charcoal must be retained in, and pass through, the gastrointestinal tract to be effective; emesis should therefore be controlled by administration of appropriate antiemetics. Alternatively, the charcoal can be administered continuously through a nasogastric tube in conjunction with appropriate antiemetics. A single dose of sorbitol may be administered with the activated charcoal to promote stooling to facilitate clearance of the adsorbed theophylline from the gastrointestinal tract. Sorbitol alone does not enhance clearance of theophylline and should be dosed with caution to prevent excessive stooling which can result in severe fluid and electrolyte imbalances. Commercially available fixed combinations of liquid charcoal and sorbitol should be avoided in young children and after the first dose in adolescents and adults since they do not allow for individualization of charcoal and sorbitol dosing. In patients with intractable vomiting, extracorporeal methods of theophylline removal should be instituted (see **OVERDOSAGE, Extracorporeal Removal**).

Specific Recommendations:

Acute Overdose

A. Serum Concentration >20 <30 mcg/mL
   1. Administer a single dose of oral activated charcoal.
   2. Monitor the patient and obtain a serum theophylline concentration in 2–4 hours to ensure that the concentration is not increasing.

B. Serum Concentration >30 <100 mcg/mL
   1. Administer multiple-dose oral activated charcoal and measures to control emesis.
   2. Monitor the patient and obtain serial theophylline concentrations every 2–4 hours to gauge the effectiveness of therapy and to guide further treatment decisions.
   3. Institute extracorporeal removal if emesis, seizures, or cardiac arrhythmias cannot be adequately controlled (see **OVERDOSAGE, Extracorporeal Removal**).

C. Serum Concentration >100 mcg/mL
   1. Consider prophylactic anticonvulsant therapy.
   2. Administer multiple-dose oral activated charcoal and measures to control emesis.

Table III. Manifestations of theophylline toxicity.*

Sign/Symptom	Percentage of patients reported with sign or symptom: Acute Overdose (Large Single Ingestion) Study 1 (n=157)	Acute Overdose Study 2 (n=14)	Chronic Overdosage (Multiple Excessive Doses) Study 1 (n=92)	Chronic Overdosage Study 2 (n=102)
Asymptomatic	NR**	0	NR**	6
Gastrointestinal				
Vomiting	73	93	30	61
Abdominal pain	NR**	21	NR**	12
Diarrhea	NR**	0	NR**	14
Hematemesis	NR**	0	NR**	2
Metabolic/Other				
Hypokalemia	85	79	44	43
Hyperglycemia	98	NR**	18	NR**
Acid/base disturbance	34	21	9	5
Rhabdomyolysis	NR**	7	NR**	0
Cardiovascular				
Sinus tachycardia	100	86	100	62
Other supraventricular tachycardias	2	21	12	14
Ventricular premature beats	3	21	10	19
Atrial fibrillation or flutter	1	NR**	12	NR**
Multifocal atrial tachycardia	0	NR**	2	NR**
Ventricular arrhythmias with hemodynamic instability	7	14	40	0
Hypotension/shock	NR**	21	NR**	8
Neurologic				
Nervousness	NR**	64	NR**	21
Tremors	38	29	16	14
Disorientation	NR**	7	NR**	11
Seizures	5	14	14	5
Death	3	21	10	4

* These data are derived from two studies in patients with serum theophylline concentrations >30 mcg/mL. In the first study (Study #1-Shanon, *Ann Intern Med.* 1993;119:1161-67), data were prospectively collected from 249 consecutive cases of theophylline toxicity referred to a regional poison center for consultation. In the second study (Study #2-Sessler, *Am J Med.* 1990;88:567-76), data were retrospectively collected from 116 cases with serum theophylline concentrations >30 mcg/mL among 6000 blood samples obtained for measurement of serum theophylline concentrations in three emergency departments. Differences in the incidence of manifestations of theophylline toxicity between the two studies may reflect sample selection as a result of study design (eg, in Study #1, 48% of the patients had acute intoxications versus only 10% in Study #2) and different methods of reporting results.

** NR = Not reported in a comparable manner.

3. Consider extracorporeal removal, even if the patient has not experienced a seizure (see **OVERDOSAGE, Extracorporeal Removal**).
4. Monitor the patient and obtain serial theophylline concentrations every 2–4 hours to gauge the effectiveness of therapy and to guide further treatment decisions.

Chronic Overdosage

A. Serum Concentration >20 <30 mcg/mL (with manifestations of theophylline toxicity)
1. Administer a single dose of oral activated charcoal.
2. Monitor the patient and obtain a serum theophylline concentration in 2–4 hours to ensure that the concentration is not increasing.

B. Serum Concentration >30 mcg/mL in patients <60 years of age
1. Administer multiple-dose oral activated charcoal and measures to control emesis.
2. Monitor the patient and obtain serial theophylline concentrations every 2–4 hours to gauge the effectiveness of therapy and to guide further treatment decisions.
3. Institute extracorporeal removal if emesis, seizures, or cardiac arrhythmias cannot be adequately controlled (see **OVERDOSAGE, Extracorporeal Removal**).

C. Serum Concentration >30 mcg/mL in patients ≥60 years of age
1. Consider prophylactic anticonvulsant therapy.
2. Administer multiple-dose oral activated charcoal and measures to control emesis.
3. Consider extracorporeal removal even if the patient has not experienced a seizure (see **OVERDOSAGE, Extracorporeal Removal**).
4. Monitor the patient and obtain serial theophylline concentrations every 2–4 hours to gauge the effectiveness of therapy and to guide further treatment decisions.

Extracorporeal Removal:

Increasing the rate of theophylline clearance by extracorporeal methods may rapidly decrease serum concentrations, but the risks of the procedure must be weighed against the potential benefit. Charcoal hemoperfusion is the most effective method of extracorporeal removal, increasing theophylline clearance up to sixfold, but serious complications, including hypotension, hypocalcemia, platelet consumption, and bleeding diatheses may occur. Hemodialysis is about as efficient as multiple-dose oral activated charcoal and has a lower risk of serious complications than charcoal hemoperfusion. Hemodialysis should be considered as an alternative when charcoal hemoperfusion is not feasible and multiple-dose oral charcoal is ineffective because of intractable emesis. Serum theophylline concentrations may rebound 5–10 mcg/mL after discontinuation of charcoal hemoperfusion or hemodialysis due to redistribution of theophylline from the tissue compartment. Peritoneal dialysis is ineffective for theophylline removal; exchange transfusions in neonates have been minimally effective.

DOSAGE AND ADMINISTRATION

THEO-DUR Extended-Release Tablets should not be chewed or crushed. When dosing THEO-DUR Extended-Release Tablets on a once-daily (q24h) basis, tablets should be taken whole and not split.

THEO-DUR (200, 300, and 450 mg) Extended-Release Tablets: The rate and extent of absorption of theophylline from THEO-DUR 200, 300, and 450 mg tablets when administered fasting or immediately after a high-fat content breakfast are similar (see **CLINICAL PHARMACOLOGY, Pharmacokinetics**).

THEO-DUR 100 mg Extended-Release Tablets have not been adequately studied for their bioavailability when administered with food (see **PRECAUTIONS, Drug/Food Interactions**).

General Considerations:

The steady-state peak serum theophylline concentration is a function of the dose, the dosing interval, and the rate of theophylline absorption and clearance in the individual patient. Because of marked individual differences in the rate of theophylline clearance, the dose required to achieve a peak serum theophylline concentration in the 10–20 mcg/mL range varies fourfold among otherwise similar patients in the absence of factors known to alter theophylline clearance (eg, 400–1600 mg/day in adults <60 years old and 10–36 mg/kg/day in children 1–9 years old). For a given population there is no single theophylline dose that will provide both safe and effective serum concentrations for all patients. Administration of the median theophylline dose required to achieve a therapeutic serum theophylline concentration in a given population may result in either subtherapeutic or potentially toxic serum theophylline concentrations in individual patients. For example, at a dose of 900 mg/day in adults <60 years or 22 mg/kg/day in children 1–9 years, the steady-state peak serum theophylline concentration will be <10 mcg/mL in about 30% of patients, 10–20 mcg/mL in about 50%, and 20–30 mcg/mL in about 20% of patients. **The dose of theophylline must be individualized on the basis of peak serum theophylline concentration measurements in order to achieve a dose that will provide maximum potential benefit with minimal risk of adverse effects.**

Table IV. Dosing initiation and titration (as anhydrous theophylline).*

A. Children (6–15 years) and adults (16–60 years) without risk factors for impaired clearance.

Titration Step	*Children <45 kg*	*Children >45 kg and adults*
1. Starting dosage:	12–14 mg/kg/day up to a maximum of 300 mg/day divided Q12 hrs*	300 mg/day divided Q12 hrs*
2. After 3 days, *if tolerated*, increase dose to:	16 mg/kg/day up to a maximum of 400 mg/day divided Q12 hrs*	400 mg/day divided Q12 hrs*
3. After 3 more days, *if tolerated*, increase dose to:	20 mg/kg/day up to a maximum of 600 mg/day divided Q12 hrs*	600 mg/day divided Q12 hrs*

B. **Patients With Risk Factors For Impaired Clearance, The Elderly (>60 Years), And Those In Whom It Is Not Feasible To Monitor Serum Theophylline Concentrations:**

In children 6–15 years of age, the final theophylline dose should not exceed 16 mg/kg/day up to a maximum of 400 mg/day in the presence of risk factors for reduced theophylline clearance (see **WARNINGS**) or if it is not feasible to monitor serum theophylline concentrations.

In adolescents ≥16 years and adults, including the elderly, the final theophylline dose should not exceed 400 mg/day in the presence of risk factors for reduced theophylline clearance (see **WARNINGS**) or if it is not feasible to monitor serum theophylline concentrations.

* Patients with more rapid metabolism, clinically identified by higher than average dose requirements, should receive a smaller dose more frequently (every 8 hours) to prevent breakthrough symptoms resulting from low trough concentrations before the next dose.

Table V. Dosage adjustment guided by serum theophylline concentration.

Peak Serum Concentration	**Dosage Adjustment**
<9.9 mcg/mL	If symptoms are not controlled and current dosage is tolerated, increase dose about 25%. Recheck serum concentration after 3 days for further dosage adjustment.
10 to 14.9 mcg/mL	If symptoms are controlled and current dosage is tolerated, maintain dose and recheck serum concentration at 6- to 12-month intervals.¶ If symptoms are not controlled and current dosage is tolerated, consider adding additional medication(s) to treatment regimen.
15–19.9 mcg/mL	Consider 10% decrease in dose to provide greater margin of safety even if current dosage is tolerated.¶
20–24.9 mcg/mL	Decrease dose by 25% even if no adverse effects are present. Recheck serum concentration after 3 days to guide further dosage adjustment.
25–30 mcg/mL	Skip next dose and decrease subsequent doses at least 25% even if no adverse effects are present. Recheck serum concentration after 3 days to guide further dosage adjustment. If symptomatic, consider whether overdose treatment is indicated (see recommendations for chronic overdosage).
>30 mcg/mL	Treat overdose as indicated (see recommendations for chronic overdosage). If theophylline is subsequently resumed, decrease dose by at least 50% and recheck serum concentration after 3 days to guide further dosage adjustment.

¶ Dose reduction and/or serum theophylline concentration measurement is indicated whenever adverse effects are present, physiologic abnormalities that can reduce theophylline clearance occur (eg, sustained fever), or a drug that interacts with theophylline is added or discontinued (see **WARNINGS**).

Transient caffeine-like adverse effects and excessive serum concentrations in slow metabolizers can be avoided in most patients by starting with a sufficiently low dose and slowly increasing the dose, *if judged to be clinically indicated,* in small increments (see **Table IV**). Dose increases should only be made if the previous dosage is well tolerated and at intervals of not less than 3 days to allow serum theophylline concentrations to reach the new steady state. Dosage adjustment should be guided by serum theophylline concentration measurement (see **PRECAUTIONS, Monitoring Serum Theophylline Concentrations**, and **DOSAGE AND ADMINISTRATION, Table V**). Healthcare providers should instruct patients and caregivers to discontinue any dosage that causes adverse effects, to withhold the medication until these symptoms are gone, and to then resume therapy at a lower, previously tolerated dosage (see **WARNINGS**).

In the patient's symptoms are well controlled, there are no apparent adverse effects, and no intervening factors that might alter dosage requirements (see **WARNINGS** and **PRECAUTIONS**), serum theophylline concentrations should be monitored at 6-month intervals for rapidly growing children and at yearly intervals for all others. In acutely ill patients, serum theophylline concentrations should be monitored at frequent intervals, eg, every 24 hours.

Theophylline distributes poorly into body fat, therefore, mg/kg dose should be calculated on the basis of ideal body weight.

Table IV contains theophylline dosing titration schema recommended for patients in various age groups and clinical circumstances.

Table V contains recommendations for theophylline dosage adjustment based upon serum theophylline concentrations.

Application of these general dosing recommendations to individual patients must take into account the unique clinical characteristics of each patient. In general, these recommendations should serve as the upper limit for dosage adjustments in order to decrease the risk of potentially serious adverse events associated with unexpected large increases in serum theophylline concentration.

[See table IV above]

[See table V above]

Once-Daily Dose:

The slow absorption rate of this preparation may allow once-daily administration in adult nonsmokers with appropriately total body clearance and other patients with low dosage requirements. Once-daily dosing should be considered only after the patient has been gradually and satisfactorily titrated to therapeutic levels with q12h dosing. Once-daily dosing (twice the q12h dose) should be based on the dosing guidelines in **Table IV** and **Table V** and should be initiated at the end of the last q12h dosing interval. The trough concentration (C_{min}) obtained following conversion to once-daily dosing may be lower (especially in high-clearance patients) and the peak concentration (C_{max}) may be higher (especially in low-clearance patients) than that obtained with q12h dosing. If symptoms recur, or signs of toxicity appear during the once-daily dosing interval, dosing on the q12h basis should be reinstituted.

It is essential that serum theophylline concentrations be monitored before and after transfer to once-daily dosing.

Food and posture, along with changes associated with circadian rhythm, may influence the rate of absorption and/or clearance rates of theophylline from controlled-release dosage forms administered at night. The exact relationship of these and other factors to nighttime serum concentrations and the clinical significance of such findings require additional study. Therefore, it is not recommended that THEO-DUR, when used as a once-a-day product, be administered at night. THEO-DUR, when used as a once-a-day product, must be taken whole and not broken.

HOW SUPPLIED

THEO-DUR 100 mg, 200 mg, and 300 mg Extended-Release Tablets are available in bottles of 100, 500, 1000, and 5000, and in unit-dose packages of 100. THEO-DUR 450 mg Extended-Release Tablets are available in bottles of 100, and unit-dose packages of 100.

100 mg tablet; NDC 0085-0487; round, white to off-white, debossed THEO-DUR 100 on one side and scored on the other side.

200 mg tablet; NDC 0085-0933; oval, white to off-white, debossed THEO-DUR 200 on one side and scored on the other side.

Continued on next page

Theo-Dur—Cont.

300 mg tablet; NDC 0085-0584; capsule shaped, white to off-white, debossed THEO-DUR 300 on one side and scored on the other side.
450 mg tablet; NDC 0085-0806; capsule shaped, white to off-white, scored debossed THEO-DUR 450 on one side.

STORAGE CONDITIONS
Keep tightly closed. Store at controlled room temperature 15°–30°C (59°–86°F).
CAUTION: Federal law prohibits dispensing without prescription.
Key Pharmaceuticals Inc,
Kenilworth, NJ 07033 USA
Copyright ©1995, 1996, 1997,
Key Pharmaceuticals, Inc. All rights reserved.
Rev. 3/97 B-19767710
Shown in Product Identification Guide, page 318

TRINALIN® ℞

brand of azatadine maleate, USP and pseudoephedrine sulfate, USP
Long-Acting Antihistamine/Decongestant
REPETABS® Tablets

DESCRIPTION

TRINALIN Long-Acting Antihistamine/Decongestant REPETABS (brand of repeat-action tablets) Tablets contain 1 mg azatadine maleate, USP in the tablet coating and 120 mg pseudoephedrine sulfate, USP, equally distributed between the tablet coating and the barrier-coated core. Following ingestion, the two active components in the coating are quickly liberated; release of the decongestant in the core is delayed for several hours.
Azatadine maleate is an antihistamine having the empirical formula, $C_{20}H_{22}N_2 \cdot 2C_4H_4O_4$, the chemical name, 6,11-Dihydro-11-(-methyl-4-piperidylidene)-5*H* -benzo [5,6] cyclohepta [1,2-*b*]pyridine maleate (1:2), and the chemical structure:

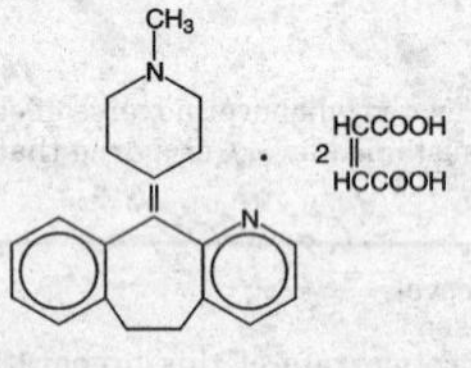

The molecular weight of azatadine maleate is 522.54. Azatadine maleate is a white to off-white powder and is very soluble in water and soluble in alcohol.
Pseudoephedrine sulfate, a sympathomimetic amine, is a salt of pseudoephedrine, one of the naturally occurring alkaloids obtained from various species of the plant *Ephedra.* The empirical formula for pseudoephedrine sulfate is $(C_{10}H_{15}NO)_2 \cdot H_2SO_4$; the chemical name is Benzenemethanol, α-[1-(methylamino)ethyl]-, [*S*-(*R**, *R**)]-, sulfate (2:1) (salt), and the chemical structure is:

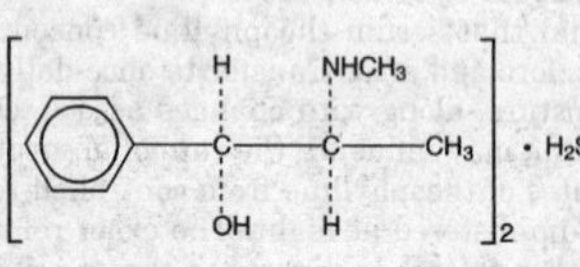

The molecular weight of pseudoephedrine sulfate is 428.56. It is a white to off-white crystal or powder, very soluble in water, freely soluble in alcohol, and sparingly soluble in chloroform.
The inactive ingredients for TRINALIN REPETABS Tablets are: acacia, butylparaben, calcium sulfate, carnauba wax, corn starch, D&C Red No. 30 Al Lake, FD&C Yellow No. 6 Al Lake, gelatin, lactose, magnesium stearate, neutral soap, oleic acid, povidone, rosin, sugar, talc, white wax, and zein.

CLINICAL PHARMACOLOGY

Azatadine maleate is an antihistamine, related to cyproheptadine, with antiserotonin, anticholinergic (drying), and sedative effects. Antihistamines appear to compete with histamine for histamine H_1-receptor sites on effector cells. The antihistamines antagonize those pharmacological effects of histamine which are mediated through activation of H_1-receptor sites and thereby reduce the intensity of allergic reactions and tissue injury response involving histamine release. Antihistamines antagonize the vasodilator effect of endogenously released histamine, especially in small vessels, and mitigate the effect of histamine which results in increased capillary permeability and edema formation. As consequences of these actions, antihistamines antagonize the physiological manifestations of histamine release in the nose following antigen-antibody interaction, such as congestion related to vascular engorgement, mucosal edema, and profuse, watery secretion, and irritation and sneezing resulting from histamine action on afferent nerve terminals.
Pseudoephedrine sulfate (d-isoephedrine sulfate) is an orally effective nasal decongestant which appears to exert its sympathomimetic effect indirectly, predominantly through release of adrenergic mediators from post-ganglionic nerve terminals. In effective recommended oral dosage, pseudoephedrine sulfate produces minimal other sympathomimetic effects, such as pressor activity and CNS stimulation. Use of an orally administered vasoconstrictor for shrinkage of congested nasal mucosa has several advantages: a) it produces a gradual but sustained decongestant effect, causing little, if any "rebound" congestion; b) it facilitates shrinkage of swollen mucosa in upper respiratory areas that are relatively inaccessible to topically applied sprays or drops; c) it relieves nasal obstruction without the additional irritation that may result from local medication.
Pseudoephedrine passes through the blood-brain and placental barriers. While the antihistamines have not been studied systematically for passage through these barriers, the occurrence of pharmacologic effects in the central nervous system and in newborns indicate presence of the drug.
Following administration of the two drugs to normal volunteers in either a single TRINALIN REPETABS Tablet or similar doses in two conventional pseudoephedrine sulfate tablets and a conventional tablet of azatadine maleate, the blood levels of pseudoephedrine and the urinary excretion of azatadine showed that the TRINALIN REPETABS Tablets are bioequivalent to the conventional dosage forms. The apparent elimination half-life of pseudoephedrine in TRINALIN REPETABS Tablets was approximately $6^1/_2$ hours. The apparent elimination of half-life of azatadine maleate (available from the outer layer of the TRINALIN REPETABS Tablets or from the conventional azatadine maleate tablet) was approximately 12 hours.

INDICATIONS AND USAGE

TRINALIN Long-Acting Antihistamine/Decongestant REPETABS Tablets are indicated for the relief of the symptoms of upper respiratory mucosal congestion in perennial and allergic rhinitis, and for the relief of nasal congestion and eustachian tube congestion. Analgesics, antibiotics, or both may be administered concurrently, when indicated.

CONTRAINDICATIONS

Antihistamines should not be used to treat lower respiratory tract symptoms, including asthma.
This product is contraindicated in patients with narrow-angle glaucoma or urinary retention, and in patients receiving monoamine oxidase (MAO) inhibitor therapy or within ten days of stopping such treatment. (See **Drug Interactions** section.) It is also contraindicated in patients with severe hypertension, severe coronary artery disease, hyperthyroidism, and in those who have shown hypersensitivity or idiosyncrasy to its components, to adrenergic agents, or to other drugs of similar chemical structures. Manifestations of patient idiosyncrasy to adrenergic agents include: insomnia, dizziness, weakness, tremor, or arrhythmias.

WARNINGS

TRINALIN REPETABS Tablets should be used with considerable caution in patients with: stenosing peptic ulcer, pyloroduodenal obstruction, urinary bladder obstruction due to symptomatic prostatic hypertrophy, or narrowing of the bladder neck. It should also be administered with caution to patients with: cardiovascular disease, including hypertension or ischemic heart disease; increased intraocular pressure (see **CONTRAINDICATIONS**); diabetes mellitus, or in patients receiving digitalis or oral anticoagulants.
Central nervous system stimulation and convulsions or cardiovascular collapse with accompanying hypotension may be produced by sympathomimetics.
Do not exceed recommended dosage.
Use in Activities Requiring Mental Alertness: Patients should be warned about engaging in activities requiring mental alertness, such as driving a car or operating appliances, machinery, etc.
Use in Patients Approximately 60 Years and Older: Antihistamines are more likely to cause dizziness, sedation, and hypotension in patients over 60 years of age. In these patients, sympathomimetics are also more likely to cause adverse reactions, such as confusion, hallucinations, convulsions, CNS depression, and death. For this reason, before considering the use of a repeat-action formulation, the safe use of a short-acting sympathomimetic in that particular patient should be demonstrated.

PRECAUTIONS

General: Because of the atropine-like action of antihistamines, this product should be used with caution in patients with a history of bronchial asthma.

Information for Patients:

1. Products containing antihistamines may cause drowsiness.
2. Patients should not engage in activities requiring mental alertness, such as driving or operating machinery or appliances.
3. Alcohol or other sedative drugs may enhance the drowsiness caused by antihistamines.
4. Patients should not take TRINALIN REPETABS Tablets if they are receiving a monoamine oxidase inhibitor or within 2 weeks of stopping such treatment, or if they are receiving oral anticoagulants.
5. This medication should not be given to children less than 12 years of age.

Drug Interactions: MAO inhibitors prolong and intensify the effects of antihistamines. Concomitant use of antihistamines with alcohol, tricyclic antidepressants, barbiturates, or other central nervous system depressants may have an additive effect.
When sympathomimetic drugs are given to patients receiving monoamine oxidase inhibitors, hypertensive reactions, including hypertensive crises, may occur. The antihypertensive effects of methyldopa, mecamylamine, reserpine, and veratrum alkaloids may be reduced by sympathomimetics. Beta-adrenergic blocking agents may also interact with sympathomimetics. Increased ectopic pacemaker activity can occur when pseudoephedrine is used concomitantly with digitalis. Antacids increase the rate of absorption of pseudoephedrine, while kaolin decreases it.
Drug/Laboratory Test Interactions: The *in vitro* addition of pseudoephedrine to sera containing the cardiac isoenzyme MB of serum creatine phosphokinase progressively inhibits the activity of the enzyme. The inhibition becomes complete over 6 hours.
Carcinogenesis, Mutagenesis, and Impairment of Fertility: There is no animal or laboratory study of the mixture of azatadine maleate and pseudoephedrine sulfate to evaluate carcinogenesis or mutagenesis. Reproduction studies of this mixture in rats showed no evidence of impaired fertility.
Pregnancy Category C: Retarded fetal development and the presence of angulated hyoid wings were seen in the offspring of pregnant rabbits administered TRINALIN REPETABS Tablets at about 12.5 times and 5 times the recommended human dosage, respectively; increased resorption was noted at about 25 times the human dosage. A decreased survival rate at day 21 was seen in rat pups born of mothers given TRINALIN REPETABS Tablets during pregnancy at a dose about 12.5 times the human dosage. There are no adequate and well-controlled studies in pregnant women. TRINALIN REPETABS Tablets should be used during pregnancy only if the potential benefits to the mother justify the potential risks to the infant. (See **Nonteratogenic Effects.**)
Nonteratogenic Effects: Antihistamines should not be used in the third trimester of pregnancy because newborns and premature infants may have severe reactions to them, such as convulsions.
Nursing Mothers: It is not known whether these drugs are excreted in human milk. However, certain antihistamines and sympathomimetics are known to be excreted in human milk. Because of the higher risks of antihistamines for infants generally and for newborns and prematures in particular, a decision should be made whether to discontinue nursing or to discontinue the drug, taking into account the importance of the drug to the mother.
There is a report of irritability, excessive crying, and disturbed sleeping patterns in a nursing infant whose mother had taken a product containing an antihistamine and pseudoephedrine.
Pediatric Use: Safety and effectiveness in children below the age of 12 years have not been established.

ADVERSE REACTIONS

The following adverse reactions are associated with antihistamine and sympathomimetic drugs. (Those adverse reactions which occur most frequently with the antihistamines are underlined.)
General: Urticaria, drug rash, anaphylactic shock, photosensitivity, excessive perspiration, chills, dryness of mouth, nose, and throat.
Cardiovascular: Hypertension (see **CONTRAINDICATIONS** and **WARNINGS**), hypotension, arrhythmias and cardiovascular collapse, headache, palpitations, extrasystoles, tachycardia, angina.
Hematologic: Hemolytic anemia, hypoplastic anemia, thrombocytopenia, agranulocytosis.
Central Nervous System: Sedation, sleepiness, dizziness, vertigo, tinnitus, acute labyrinthitis, disturbed coordination, fatigue, mydriasis, confusion, restlessness, excitation, nervousness, tension, tremor, irritability, insomnia, euphoria, paresthesias, blurred vision, hysteria, neuritis, convulsions, fear, anxiety, hallucinations, CNS depression, weakness, pallor.

Gastrointestinal: Epigastric distress, anorexia, nausea, vomiting, diarrhea, constipation, abdominal cramps.
Genitourinary: Urinary frequency, urinary retention, dysuria, early menses.
Respiratory: Thickening of bronchial secretions, tightness of chest and wheezing, nasal stuffiness, respiratory difficulty.

DRUG ABUSE AND DEPENDENCE

There is no information to indicate that abuse or dependency occurs with azatadine maleate.
Pseudoephedrine, like other central nervous system stimulants, has been abused. At high doses, subjects commonly experience an elevation of mood, a sense of increased energy and alertness, and decreased appetite. Some individuals become anxious, irritable, and loquacious. In addition to the marked euphoria, the user experiences a sense of markedly enhanced physical strength and mental capacity. With continued use, tolerance develops, the user increases the dose, and toxic signs and symptoms appear. Depression may follow rapid withdrawal.

OVERDOSAGE

In the event of overdosage, emergency treatment should be started immediately.
Manifestations of overdosage may vary from central nervous system depression (sedation, apnea, diminished mental alertness, cyanosis, coma, cardiovascular collapse) to stimulation (insomnia, hallucinations, tremors, or convulsions) to death. Other signs and symptoms may be euphoria, excitement, tachycardia, palpitations, thirst, perspiration, nausea, dizziness, tinnitus, ataxia, blurred vision, and hypertension or hypotension. Stimulation is particularly likely in children, as are atropine-like signs and symptoms (dry mouth; fixed, dilated pupils; flushing; hyperthermia; and gastrointestinal symptoms).
In large doses sympathomimetics may give rise to giddiness, headache, nausea, vomiting, sweating, thirst, tachycardia, precordial pain, palpitations, difficulty in micturition, muscular weakness and tenseness, anxiety, restlessness, and insomnia. Many patients can present a toxic psychosis with delusions and hallucinations. Some may develop cardiac arrhythmias, circulatory collapse, convulsions, coma, and respiratory failure.
The oral LD_{50} of the mixture of the two drugs in mature rats and mice was greater than 1700 mg/kg and 600 mg/kg, respectively.
Treatment —The patient should be induced to vomit, even if emesis has occurred spontaneously. Pharmacologically induced vomiting by the administration of ipecac syrup is a preferred method. However, vomiting should not be induced in patients with impaired consciousness. The action of ipecac is facilitated by physical activity and by the administration of eight to twelve fluid ounces of water. If emesis does not occur within 15 minutes, the dose of ipecac should be repeated. Precautions against aspiration must be taken, especially in infants and children. Following emesis, any drug remaining in the stomach may be adsorbed by activated charcoal administered as a slurry with water. If vomiting is unsuccessful or contraindicated, gastric lavage should be performed. Isotonic and one-half isotonic saline are the lavage solutions of choice. Saline cathartics, such as milk of magnesia, draw water into the bowel by osmosis and therefore may be valuable for their action in rapid dilution of bowel content. Dialysis is of little value in antihistamine poisoning. After emergency treatment the patient should continue to be medically monitored.
Treatment of the signs and symptoms of overdosage is symptomatic and supportive. Stimulants (analeptic agents) should not be used. Vasopressors may be used to treat hypotension. Short-acting barbiturates, diazepam, or paraldehyde, may be administered to control seizures. Hyperpyrexia, especially in children, may require treatment with tepid water sponge baths or a hypothermic blanket. Apnea is treated with ventilatory support.

DOSAGE AND ADMINISTRATION

TRINALIN REPETABS Tablets ARE NOT INTENDED FOR USE IN CHILDREN UNDER 12 YEARS OF AGE. The usual adult dosage is one tablet twice a day.

HOW SUPPLIED

TRINALIN REPETABS Tablets contain 1 mg azatadine maleate and 120 mg pseudoephedrine sulfate. TRINALIN REPETABS Tablets are coral-colored, sugar-coated tablets branded in black with the product name (TRINALIN) and product identification numbers, 703; bottle of 100 (NDC 0085-0703-04).
Store between 2° and 30°C (36° and 86°F).
TRINALIN®
brand of azatadine maleate, USP and
pseudoephedrine sulfate, USP
Long-Acting Antihistamine/
Decongestant REPETABS® Tablets
Key Pharmaceuticals, Inc.
Kenilworth, NJ 07033 USA
Rev. 10/96 17070916

Shown in Product Identification Guide, page 318

UNI-DUR® ℞
(theophylline)
Extended-release Tablets

Some of the information contained in this insert (eg, information regarding pediatric patients under the age of 12) was derived from FDA's Class Labeling Guidance for Immediate-Release Theophylline Products and is intended for informational purposes only.

DESCRIPTION

UNI-DUR® Extended-release Tablets for oral administration contain 400 or 600 mg anhydrous theophylline in an extended-release system which allows a 24-hour dosing interval for appropriate patients.
Theophylline is a bronchodilator, structurally classified as a methylxanthine. It occurs as a white, odorless, crystalline powder with a bitter taste. Anhydrous theophylline has the chemical name 1*H*-Purine-2,6-dione,3,7-dihydro-1,3-dimethyl-, and is represented by the following structural formula:

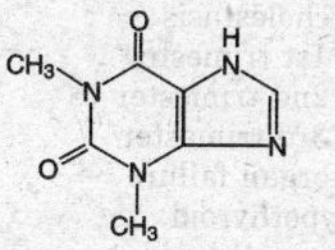

The molecular formula of anhydrous theophylline is $C_7H_8N_4O_2$ with a molecular weight of 180.17.
The inactive ingredients for UNI-DUR 400 and 600 mg Extended-release Tablets include: acacia, NF; acetone; cellulose acetate phthalate, NF; cetyl alcohol, NF; confectioner's sugar, NF; corn starch, NF; diethyl phthalate, NF; glyceryl monostearate; lactose monohydrate, NF; magnesium stearate, NF; myristyl alcohol, NF; nonpareil seeds (sugar spheres), NF; and white wax, NF.

CLINICAL PHARMACOLOGY

Mechanism of Action:
Theophylline has two distinct actions in the airways of patients with reversible obstruction; smooth muscle relaxation (ie, bronchodilation) and suppression of the response of the airways to stimuli (ie, non-bronchodilator prophylactic effects). While the mechanisms of action of theophylline are not known with certainty, studies in animals suggest that bronchodilation is mediated by the inhibition of two isozymes of phosphodiesterase (PDE III and, to a lesser extent, PDE IV) while non-bronchodilator prophylactic actions are probably mediated through one or more different molecular mechanisms that do not involve inhibition of PDE III or antagonism of adenosine receptors. Some of the adverse effects associated with theophylline appear to be mediated by inhibition of PDE III (eg, hypotension, tachycardia, headache, and emesis) and adenosine receptor antagonism (eg, alterations in cerebral blood flow).
Theophylline increases the force of contraction of diaphragmatic muscles. This action appears to be due to enhancement of calcium uptake through an adenosine-mediated channel.
Serum Concentration-Effect Relationship:
Bronchodilation occurs over the serum theophylline concentration range of 5–20 mcg/mL. Clinically important improvement in symptom control has been found in most studies to require peak serum theophylline concentration >10 mcg/mL, but patients with mild disease may benefit from lower concentrations. At serum theophylline concentrations >20 mcg/mL, both the frequency and severity of adverse reactions increase. In general, maintaining peak serum theophylline concentrations between 10 and 15 mcg/mL will achieve most of the drug's potential therapeutic benefit while minimizing the risk of serious adverse events.
Pharmacokinetics:
Overview Theophylline is rapidly and completely absorbed after oral administration in solution or immediate-release solid oral dosage form. Theophylline does not undergo any appreciable pre-systemic elimination, distributes freely into fat-free tissues, and is extensively metabolized in the liver.
The pharmacokinetics of theophylline vary widely among similar patients and cannot be predicted by age, sex, body weight, or other demographic characteristics. In addition, certain concurrent illnesses and alterations in normal physiology (see **Table I**) and coadministration of other drugs (see **Table II**) can significantly alter the pharmacokinetic characteristics of theophylline. Within-subject variability in metabolism has also been reported in some studies, especially in acutely ill patients. It is, therefore, recommended that serum theophylline concentrations be measured frequently in acutely ill patients (eg, at 24-hour intervals) and periodically in patients receiving long-term therapy (eg, at 6- to 12-month intervals). More frequent measurements should be made in the presence of any condition that may significantly alter theophylline clearance (see **PRECAUTIONS, Monitoring Serum Theophylline Concentrations** and **DOSAGE AND ADMINISTRATION**).
[See table I at top of next page]
Note: In addition to the factors listed above, theophylline clearance is increased and half-life decreased by low-carbohydrate/high-protein diets, parenteral nutrition, and daily consumption of charcoal-broiled beef. A high-carbohydrate/low-protein diet can decrease the clearance and prolong the half-life of theophylline.
Absorption Theophylline is rapidly and completely absorbed after oral administration in solution or immediate-release solid oral dosage form. After a single immediate-release theophylline dose of 5 mg/kg in adults, a mean peak serum concentration of about 10 mcg/mL (range 5–15 mcg/mL) can be expected 1–2 hours after the dose. Coadministration of theophylline with food or antacids does not cause clinically significant changes in the absorption of theophylline from immediate-release dosage forms.
UNI-DUR Pharmacokinetics
Following the single-dose crossover administration of a 600 mg UNI-DUR Tablet to 20 healthy male subjects after an overnight fast, a peak serum theophylline concentration of 5.3 ± 1.3 mcg/mL was obtained at 13.6 ± 3.7 hours and the mean area under the curve extrapolated to infinity (AUC_{inf}) was 132.7 ± 45.1 mcg hr/mL. When taken immediately after a high-fat breakfast, the mean AUC_{inf} was 136.0 ± 36.7 mcg hr/mL with a mean peak theophylline serum level of 5.2 ± 1.5 mcg/mL at 17.1 ± 6.3 hours. While food did not affect the extent of absorption as evidenced by the similar AUC_{inf} values, food did prolong the time to peak concentration. The absorption from half tablets of the 600 mg product was also evaluated and found to be bioequivalent to that of the whole tablets. The relative extent of absorption of theophylline from the 600 mg UNI-DUR Tablet, fasting, when compared to an immediate-release theophylline tablet, was 84.3%; and the nonfasting treatment was 88.7%.
In a separate multiple-dose study, two 400 mg UNI-DUR Tablets were compared to one 600 mg UNI-DUR Tablet. This study was a two-way, randomized, crossover multiple-dose study in 17 nonsmoking healthy males. Both products were dosed once a day in the morning after an overnight fast and 1 hour prior to a meal for 5 days. There was no significant difference in any of the pharmacokinetic parameters when corrected for dose.
The mean dose AUC_{ss} (corrected to the 600 mg dose) for the two 400 mg UNI-DUR Tablets was 179.7 ± 62.9 mcg hr/mL and for the 600 mg UNI-DUR Tablet was 170.9 ± 75.2 mcg hr/mL. The two 400 mg UNI-DUR Tablets reached dose corrected maximum serum concentration of 9.8 ± 2.6 mcg/mL and the 600 mg UNI-DUR Tablet reached a maximum of 9.7 ± 3.5 mcg/mL. The minimum concentrations were 4.9 ± 2.6 mcg/mL and 4.4 ± 2.6 mcg/mL for the two 400 mg and 600 mg UNI-DUR Tablets, respectively.
Steady-state pharmacokinetics were determined in a multiple-dose, crossover study with 24 healthy nonsmoking male subjects having an average theophylline clearance of 5.70 ± 2.36 (S.D.) liters per hour. Following an overnight fast, a UNI-DUR 600 mg Extended-release Tablet was administered once daily in the morning for 5 consecutive days. The UNI-DUR Tablet exhibited better extended-release characteristics compared with a reference extended-release q12h product (2 × 300 mg) administered once daily in the morning following an overnight fast for 5 consecutive days. The results are noted as follows (mean values ± S.D.):
[See second table at top of next page]
The mean percent fluctuation [$(C_{max}-C_{min}/C_{min}) \times 100$] was 130% for the once-daily UNI-DUR regimen and 389% for the reference q12h product administered once daily. The extent of theophylline absorption from UNI-DUR Tablets relative to the reference q12h product was 74.9% (95% C.I. = 67–84).
In a randomized, multiple-dose crossover study with 18 healthy male subjects, a 600 mg UNI-DUR Extended-release Tablet was administered once daily either in the morning or evening for 5 consecutive days. The theophylline AUC_{ss} for the 24-hour period following the dose given on day 5 was equivalent for morning (177 ± 89 mcg hr/mL) and evening (175 ± 76 mcg hr/mL) administration. The peak theophylline concentrations (C_{max}) at steady state were also equivalent for morning (10.6 ± 4.9 mcg/mL) and evening (10.3 ± 4.0 mcg/mL) administration.
Steady-state pharmacokinetics comparing UNI-DUR Tablets once-daily administration with twice-daily administration were determined in a multiple-dose, crossover study with 24 healthy, nonsmoking male subjects having an aver-

Continued on next page

Uni-Dur—Cont.

age theophylline clearance of 4.53 ± 1.21 (S.D.) liters per hour. Using UNI-DUR 400 mg Extended-release Tablets, a total daily theophylline dose of 800 mg was administered for 5 consecutive days either once daily as two tablets in the morning (8 AM) with a standardized breakfast or twice daily as one tablet in the morning (8 AM) with a standardized breakfast or twice daily as one tablet in the morning (8 AM) with a standardized breakfast and one tablet in the evening (8 PM). The once-daily UNI-DUR regimen was bioequivalent to the twice-daily UNI-DUR regimen. The results are noted as follows (mean values ± S.D.):

[See table at bottom of page]

The mean percent fluctuation [$(C_{max}-C_{min}/C_{min}) \times 100$] was 78% for the once-daily UNI-DUR regimen and 17% for the twice-daily UNI-DUR regimen. The extent of theophylline absorption from the once-daily UNI-DUR regimen relative to the twice-daily UNI-DUR regimen was 100% (95% C.I. = 95–105).

Distribution Once theophylline enters the systemic circulation, about 40% is bound to plasma protein, primarily albumin. Unbound theophylline distributes throughout body water, but distributes poorly into body fat. The apparent volume of distribution of theophylline is approximately 0.45 L/kg (range 0.3–0.7 L/kg) based on ideal body weight. Theophylline passes freely across the placenta, into breast milk, and into the cerebrospinal fluid (CSF). Saliva theophylline concentrations approximate unbound serum concentrations, but are not reliable for routine or therapeutic monitoring unless special techniques are used. An increase in the volume of distribution of theophylline, primarily due to reduction in plasma protein binding, occurs in premature neonates, patients with hepatic cirrhosis, uncorrected acidemia, the elderly, and in women during the third trimester of pregnancy. In such cases, the patient may show signs of toxicity at total (bound + unbound) serum concentration of theophylline in the therapeutic range (10–20 mcg/mL) due to elevated concentrations of the pharmacologically active unbound drug. Similarly, a patient with decreased theophylline binding may have a subtherapeutic total drug concentration while the pharmacologically active unbound concentration is in the therapeutic range. If only total serum theophylline concentration is measured, this may lead to an unnecessary and potentially dangerous dose increase. In patients with reduced protein binding, measurement of unbound serum theophylline concentration provides a more reliable means of dosage adjustment than measurement of total serum theophylline concentration. Generally, concentrations of unbound theophylline should be maintained in the range of 6–12 mcg/mL.

Metabolism Following oral dosing, theophylline does not undergo any measurable first-pass elimination. In adults and children beyond 1 year of age, approximately 90% of the dose is metabolized in the liver. Biotransformation takes place through demethylation to 1-methylxanthine and 3-methylxanthine and hydroxylation to 1,3-dimethyluric acid. 1-methylxanthine is further hydroxylated by xanthine oxidase, to 1-methyluric acid. About 6% of a theophylline dose is N-methylated to caffeine. Theophylline demethylation 3-methylxanthine is catalyzed by cytochrome P450 1A2, while cytochromes P450 2E1 and P450 3A3 catalyze the hydroxylation to 1,3-dimethyluric acid. Demethylation to 1-methylxanthine appears to be catalyzed either by cytochrome P450 1A2 or a closely related cytochrome. In neonates, the N-demethylation pathway is absent while the function of the hydroxylation pathway is markedly deficient. The activity of these pathways slowly increases to maximal levels by 1 year of age.

Caffeine and 3 methylxanthine are the only theophylline metabolites with pharmacologic activity. 3-methylxanthine has approximately one tenth the pharmacologic activity of theophylline and serum concentration in adults with normal renal function are <1 mcg/mL. In patients with end-stage renal disease, 3-methylxanthine may accumulate to concentrations that approximate the unmetabolized theophylline concentration. Caffeine concentrations are usually undetectable in adults regardless of renal function. In neonates, caffeine may accumulate to concentrations that approximate the unmetabolized theophylline concentration and thus, exert a pharmacologic effect.

Both the N-demethylation and hydroxylation pathways of theophylline biotransformation are capacity-limited. Due to the wide intersubject variability of the rate of theophylline metabolism, nonlinearity of elimination may begin in some patients at serum theophylline concentrations <10 mcg/mL. Since this nonlinearity results in more than proportional changes in serum theophylline concentrations with changes in dose, it is advisable to make increases or decreases in dose in small increments in order to achieve desired changes in serum theophylline concentrations (see **DOSAGE AND ADMINISTRATION**, Table V). Accurate prediction of dose-dependency of theophylline metabolism in patients *a priori* is not possible, but patients with very high initial clearance rates (ie, low steady-state serum theophylline concentrations at above average doses) have the greatest likelihood of experiencing large changes in serum theophylline concentration in response to dosage changes.

Excretion In neonates, approximately 50% of the theophylline dose is excreted unchanged in the urine. Beyond the first 3 months of life, approximately 10% of the theophylline dose is excreted unchanged in the urine. The remainder is excreted in the urine mainly as 1,3-dimethyluric acid (35%–40%), 1-methyluric acid (20%–25%), and 3-methylxanthine (15%–20%). Since little theophylline is excreted unchanged in the urine and since active metabolites of theophylline (ie, caffeine, 3-methylxanthine) do not accumulate to clinically significant levels even in the face of end-stage renal disease, no dosage adjustment for renal insufficiency is necessary in adults and children >3 months of age. In contrast, the large fraction of the theophylline dose excreted in the urine as unchanged theophylline and caffeine in neonates requires careful attention to dose reduction and frequent monitoring of serum theophylline concentrations in neonates with reduced renal function (see **WARNINGS**).

Serum Concentration at Steady State After multiple doses of immediate-release theophylline, steady state is reached in 30–65 hours (average 40 hours) in adults. At steady state, on a dosage regimen with 6-hour intervals, the expected mean trough concentration is approximately 60% of the mean peak concentration, assuming a mean theophylline half-life of 8 hours. The difference between peak and trough concentrations is larger in patients with more rapid theophylline clearance. In patients with high theophylline clearance and half-lives of about 4–5 hours, such as children aged 1 to 9 years, the trough serum theophylline concentration may be only 30% of peak with a 6-hour dosing interval. In these patients a slow-release formulation would allow a longer dosing interval (8–12 hours) with a smaller peak/trough difference.

Special Populations (See Table I for mean clearance and half-life values.)

Geriatric: The clearance of theophylline is decreased by an average of 30% in healthy elderly adults (>60 yrs) compared to healthy young adults. Careful attention to dose reduction and frequent monitoring of serum theophylline concentrations are required in elderly patients (see **WARNINGS**).

Pediatrics: The clearance of theophylline is very low in neonates (see **WARNINGS**). Theophylline clearance reaches maximal values by 1 year of age, remains relatively constant until about 9 years of age, and then slowly decreases by approximately 50% to adult values at about age 16. Renal excretion of unchanged theophylline in neonates amounts to about 50% of the dose, compared to about 10% in children older than 3 months and in adults. Careful attention to dosage selection and monitoring or serum theophylline concentrations are required in pediatric patients (see **WARNINGS** and **DOSAGE AND ADMINISTRATION**).

Gender: Gender differences in theophylline clearance are relatively small and unlikely to be of clinical significance. Significant reduction in theophylline clearance, however, has been reported in women on the 20th day of the menstrual cycle and during the third trimester of pregnancy.

Race: Pharmacokinetic differences in theophylline clearance due to race have not been studied.

Renal Insufficiency: Only a small fraction, eg, about 10% of the administered theophylline dose is excreted unchanged in the urine of children greater than 3 months of age and adults. Since little theophylline is excreted unchanged in the urine and since active metabolites of theophylline (ie, caffeine, 3-methylxanthine) do not accumulate to clinically significant levels even in the face of end-stage renal disease, no dosage adjustment for renal insufficiency is necessary in adults and children >3 months of age. In contrast, approximately 50% of the administered theophylline dose is excreted unchanged in the urine in neonates. Careful attention to dose reduction and frequent monitoring of serum theophylline concentrations are required in neonates with decreased renal function (see **WARNINGS**).

Table I. Mean and range of total body clearance and half-life of theophylline related to age and altered physiological states.¶

Population characteristics	Total body clearance* mean (range)†† (mL/kg/min)		Half-life mean (range)†† (hr)	
Age				
Premature neonates				
postnatal age 3–15 days	0.29	(0.09–0.49)	30	(17–43)
postnatal age 25–57 days	0.64	(0.04–1.2)	20	(9.4–30.6)
Term infants				
postnatal age 1–2 days	NR†		25.7	(25–26.5)
postnatal age 3–30 weeks	NR†		11	(6–29)
Children				
1–4 years	1.7	(0.5–2.9)	3.4	(1.2–5.6)
4–12 years	1.6	(0.8–2.4)	NR†	
13–15 years	0.9	(0.48–1.3)	NR†	
6–17 years	1.4	(0.2–2.6)	3.7	(1.5–5.9)
Adults (16–60 years)				
otherwise healthy nonsmoking asthmatics	0.65	(0.27–1.03)	8.7	(6.1–12.8)
Elderly (>60 years) nonsmokers with normal cardiac, liver, and renal function	0.41	(0.21–0.61)	9.8	(1.6–18)
Concurrent illness or altered physiological state				
Acute pulmonary edema	0.33**	(0.07–2.45)	19**	(3.1–82)
COPD->60 years, stable nonsmoker >1 year	0.54	(0.44–0.64)	11	(9.4–12.6)
COPD with cor pulmonale	0.48	(0.08–0.88)	NR†	
Cystic fibrosis (14–28 years)	1.25	(0.31–2.2)	6.0	(1.8–10.2)
Fever associated with acute viral respiratory illness (children 9–15 years)	NR†		7.0	(1.0–13)
Liver disease- cirrhosis	0.31**	(0.1–0.7)	32**	(10–56)
acute hepatitis	0.35	(0.25–0.45)	19.2	(16.6–21.8)
cholestasis	0.65	(0.25–1.45)	14.4	(5.7–31.8)
Pregnancy- 1st trimester	NR†		8.5	(3.1–13.9)
2nd trimester	NR†		8.8	(3.8–13.8)
3rd trimester	NR†		13.0	(8.4–17.6)
Sepsis with multi-organ failure	0.47	(0.19–1.9)	18.8	(6.3–24.1)
Thyroid disease-hypothyroid	0.38	(0.13–0.57)	11.6	(8.2–25)
hyperthyroid	0.8	(0.68–0.97)	4.5	(3.7–5.6)

¶ For various North American patient populations from literature reports. Different rates of elimination and consequent dosage requirements have been observed among other peoples.

* Clearance represents the volume of blood completely cleared of theophylline by the liver in 1 minute. Values listed were generally determined at serum theophylline concentrations <20 mcg/mL; clearance may decrease and half-life may increase at higher serum concentrations due to nonlinear pharmacokinetics.

†† Reported range or estimated range (mean ± 2 S.D.) where actual range not reported.

† NR = not reported or not reported in a comparable format.

** Median

	AUC_{ss} (mcg hr/mL)	C_{max} (mcg/mL)	C_{min} (mcg/mL)	T_{max} (hr)
UNI-DUR	119 ± 36	6.9 ± 2.4	3.7 ± 1.3	11.5 ± 5.7
Reference	154 ± 37	10.5 ±2.3	2.5 ± 1.1	7.6 ± 1.7

	AUC_{ss} (mcg hr/mL)	C_{max} (mcg/mL)	C_{min} (mcg/mL)	T_{max} (hr)
QD Regimen	187 ± 45	10.4 ± 2.9	6.0 ± 1.3	12.0 ± 3.7
q12h Regimen	187 ± 43	9.4 ± 2.2	8.4 ± 2.6	14.5 ± 6.6

Hepatic Insufficiency: Theophylline clearance is decreased by 50% or more in patients with hepatic insufficiency (eg, cirrhosis, acute hepatitis, cholestasis). Careful attention to dose reduction and frequent monitoring of serum theophylline concentrations are required in patients with reduced hepatic function (see **WARNINGS**).

Congestive Heart Failure (CHF): Theophylline clearance is decreased by 50% or more in patients with CHF. The extent of reduction in theophylline clearance in patients with CHF appears to be directly correlated to the severity of the cardiac disease. Since theophylline clearance is independent of liver blood flow, the reduction in clearance appears to be due to impaired hepatocyte function rather than reduced perfusion. Careful attention to dose reduction and frequent monitoring of serum theophylline concentrations are required in patients with CHF (see **WARNINGS**).

Smokers: Tobacco and marijuana smoking appear to increase the clearance of theophylline by induction of metabolic pathways. Theophylline clearance has been shown to increase by approximately 50% in young adult tobacco smokers and by approximately 80% in elderly tobacco smokers compared to nonsmoking subjects. Passive smoke exposure has also been shown to increase theophylline clearance by up to 50%. Abstinence from tobacco smoking for 1 week causes a reduction of approximately 40% in theophylline clearance. Careful attention to dose reduction and frequent monitoring of serum theophylline concentrations are required in patients who stop smoking (see **WARNINGS**). Use of nicotine gum has been shown to have no effect on theophylline clearance.

Fever: Fever, regardless of its underlying cause, can decrease the clearance of theophylline. The magnitude and duration of the fever appear to be directly correlated to the degree of decrease of theophylline clearance. Precise data are lacking, but a temperature of 39°C (102°F) for at least 24 hours or lesser temperature elevations for longer periods, are probably required to produce a clinically significant increase in serum theophylline concentrations. Children with rapid rates of theophylline clearance (ie, those who require a dose that is substantially larger than average [eg, >22 mg/kg/day] to achieve a therapeutic peak serum theophylline concentration when afebrile) may be at greater risk of toxic effects from decreased clearance during sustained fever. Careful attention to dose reduction and frequent monitoring of serum theophylline concentrations are required in patients with sustained fever (see **WARNINGS**).

Miscellaneous: Other factors associated with decreased theophylline clearance include the third trimester of pregnancy, sepsis with multiple organ failure, and hypothyroidism. Careful attention to dose reduction and frequent monitoring of serum theophylline concentrations are required in patients with any of these conditions (see **WARNINGS**). Other factors associated with increased theophylline clearance include hyperthyroidism and cystic fibrosis.

Clinical Studies:
In patients with chronic asthma, including patients with severe asthma requiring inhaled corticosteroids or alternate-day oral corticosteroids, many clinical studies have shown that theophylline decreases the frequency and severity of symptoms, including nocturnal exacerbations, and decreases the "as needed" use of inhaled beta₂-agonists. Theophylline has also been shown to reduce the need for short courses of daily oral prednisone to relieve exacerbations of airway obstruction that are unresponsive to bronchodilators in asthmatics.

In patients with chronic obstructive pulmonary disease (COPD), clinical studies have shown that theophylline decreases dyspnea, air trapping, the work of breathing, and improves contractility of diaphragmatic muscles with little or no improvement in pulmonary function measurements.

INDICATIONS AND USAGE

UNI-DUR Extended-release Tablets are indicated for the treatment of the symptoms and reversible airflow obstruction associated with chronic asthma and other chronic lung diseases, eg, emphysema and chronic bronchitis.

CONTRAINDICATIONS

UNI-DUR Extended-release Tablets are contraindicated in patients with a history of hypersensitivity to theophylline or other components in the product.

WARNINGS

Serious side effects such as ventricular arrhythmias, convulsions, or even death may appear as the first sign of toxicity without any recognized prior warnings. Less serious signs of theophylline toxicity (eg, nausea and restlessness) may occur frequently when initiating therapy but are usually transient. When such signs are persistent during maintenance therapy, they are often associated with serum concentrations above 20 mcg/mL. Stated differently, serious toxicity is not reliably preceded by less severe side effects.

Concurrent Illness:
Theophylline should be used with extreme caution in patients with the following clinical conditions due to the increased risk of exacerbation of the concurrent condition:

Active peptic ulcer disease (peptic ulcer disease should be controlled with appropriate therapy since theophylline is known to increase peptic-acid secretion)
Seizure disorders
Cardiac arrhythmias (not including bradyarrhythmias)

Conditions That Reduce Theophylline Clearance:
There are several readily identifiable causes of reduced theophylline clearance. *If the total daily dose is not appropriately reduced so as to lower serum theophylline levels to within the therapeutic range in the presence of these risk factors, severe and potentially fatal theophylline toxicity can occur.* Careful consideration must be given to the benefits and risks of theophylline use and the need for more intensive monitoring of serum theophylline concentrations in patients with the following risk factors:

Age:
Neonates (term and premature)
Children <1 year
Elderly (>60 years)
Concurrent Diseases:
Acute pulmonary edema
Congestive heart failure
Cor pulmonale
Fever; ≥102°F for 24 hours or more; or lesser temperature elevations for longer periods
Hypothyroidism
Liver disease; cirrhosis, acute hepatitis
Reduced renal function in infants <3 months of age
Sepsis with multi-organ failure
Shock
Cessation of Smoking
Drug Interactions:
Adding a drug that inhibits theophylline metabolism (eg, cimetidine, erythromycin, tacrine) or stopping a concurrently administered drug that enhances theophylline metabolism (eg, carbamazepine, rifampin). (See **PRECAUTIONS, Drug Interactions, Table II**.)

When Signs or Symptoms of Theophylline Toxicity Are Present:
Whenever a patient receiving theophylline develops nausea or vomiting, particularly repetitive vomiting, or other signs or symptoms consistent with theophylline toxicity (even if another cause may be suspected), additional doses of theophylline should be withheld and a serum theophylline concentration should be measured immediately. Patients should be instructed not to continue any dosage that causes adverse effects and to withhold subsequent doses until the symptoms have resolved, at which time the clinician may instruct the patient to resume the drug at a lower dosage (see **DOSAGE AND ADMINISTRATION, Dosage Guidelines, Table V**).

Dosage Increases:
Increases in the dose of theophylline should not be made in response to an acute exacerbation of symptoms of chronic lung disease since theophylline provides little added benefit to inhaled beta₂-selective agonists and systemically administered corticosteroids in this circumstance and increases the risk of adverse effects. A *peak* steady-state serum theophylline concentration should be measured before increasing the dose in response to persistent chronic symptoms to ascertain whether an increase in dose is safe. Before increasing the theophylline dose on the basis of a low serum concentration, the clinician should consider whether the blood sample was obtained at an appropriate time in relationship to the dose and whether the patient has adhered to the prescribed regimen (see **PRECAUTIONS, Monitoring Serum Theophylline Concentrations**).

As the rate of theophylline clearance may be dose-dependent (ie, steady-state serum concentrations may increase disproportionately to the increase in dose), an increase in dose based upon a subtherapeutic serum concentration measurement should be conservative. In general, limiting dose increases to about 25% of the previous total daily dose will reduce the risk of unintended excessive increases in serum theophylline concentration (see **DOSAGE AND ADMINISTRATION, Table V**).

PRECAUTIONS

UNI-DUR TABLETS SHOULD *NOT* BE CHEWED OR CRUSHED AND SHOULD *BE BROKEN ONLY AT THE SCORE.*
General:
Careful consideration of the various interacting drugs (including recently discontinued medications), physiologic conditions, and other factors such as smoking that can alter theophylline clearance and require dosage adjustment should occur prior to initiation of theophylline therapy, prior to increases in theophylline dose, and during follow up (see **WARNINGS**). The dose of theophylline selected for initiation of therapy should be low and, *if tolerated*, increased slowly over a period of a week or longer with the final dose guided by monitoring serum theophylline concentrations and the patient's clinical response (see **DOSAGE AND ADMINISTRATION, Table IV**).

Monitoring Serum Theophylline Concentrations:
Serum theophylline concentration measurements are readily available and should be used to determine whether the dosage is appropriate. Specifically, the serum theophylline concentration should be measured as follows:

1. When initiating therapy to guide final dosage adjustment after titration.
2. Before making a dose increase to determine whether the serum concentration is subtherapeutic in a patient who continues to be symptomatic.
3. Whenever signs or symptoms of theophylline toxicity are present.
4. Whenever there is a new illness, worsening of a chronic illness, or a change in the patient's treatment regimen that may alter theophylline clearance [eg, fever (see **CLINICAL PHARMACOLOGY**, *Fever*), hepatitis, or drugs listed in **Table II** are added or discontinued].

To guide a dose increase, the blood sample should be obtained at the time of the expected peak serum theophylline concentration; 8 to 12 hours after a UNI-DUR dose at steady state. For most patients, steady state will be reached after 4 days of dosing with UNI-DUR Tablets when no doses have been missed, no extra doses have been added, and none of the doses have been taken at unequal intervals. A trough concentration (ie, at the end of the dosing interval) provides no additional useful information and may lead to an inappropriate dose increase since the peak serum theophylline concentration can be two or more times greater than the trough concentration with an immediate-release formulation. If the serum sample is drawn more than 12 hours after the dose, the results may be interpreted with caution since the concentration may not be reflective of the peak concentration. In contrast, when signs or symptoms of theophylline toxicity are present, the serum sample should be obtained as soon as possible, analyzed immediately, and the result reported to the clinician without delay. In patients in whom decreased serum protein binding is suspected (eg, cirrhosis, women during the third trimester of pregnancy), the concentration of unbound theophylline should be measured and the dosage adjusted to achieve an unbound concentration of 6–12 mcg/mL.

Saliva concentrations of theophylline cannot be used reliably to adjust dosage without special techniques.

Effects on Laboratory Tests:
As a result of its pharmacological effects, theophylline at serum concentrations within the 10–20 mcg/mL range modestly increases plasma glucose (from a mean of 88 mg% to 98 mg%), uric acid (from a mean of 4 mg/dL to 6 mg/dL), free fatty acids (from a mean of 451 μeq/L to 800 μeq/L), total cholesterol (from a mean of 140 vs 160 mg/dL), HDL (from a mean of 36 to 50 mg/dL), HDL/LDL ratio (from a mean of 0.5 to 0.7), and urinary free cortisol excretion (from a mean of 44 to 63 mcg/24 hr). Theophylline at serum concentrations within the 10–20 mcg/mL range may also transiently decrease serum concentrations of triiodothyronine (144 before, 131 after 1 week and 142 ng/dL after 4 weeks of theophylline). The clinical importance of these changes should be weighed against the potential therapeutic benefit of theophylline in individual patients.

Information for Patients:
This information is intended to aid in the safe and effective use of this medication. It is not a disclosure of all adverse or intended effects.

The patient (or parent/caregiver) should be instructed to seek medical advice whenever nausea, vomiting, persistent headache, insomnia, restlessness, or rapid heartbeat occurs during treatment with theophylline, even if another cause is suspected. The patient should be instructed to contact their clinician if they develop a new illness, especially if accompanied by a persistent fever, if they experience worsening of a chronic illness, if they start or stop smoking cigarettes or marijuana, or if another clinician adds a new medication or discontinues a previously prescribed medication. Patients should be informed that theophylline interacts with a wide variety of drugs (see **Table II**). They should be instructed to inform all clinicians involved in their care that they are taking theophylline, especially when a medication is being added or deleted from their treatment. Patients should be instructed to not alter the dose, timing of the dose, or frequency of administration without first consulting their clinician. If a dose is missed, the patient should be instructed to take the next dose at the usually scheduled time and to not attempt to make up for the missed dose. UNI-DUR Tablets *should not be chewed or crushed.* Information relating to taking UNI-DUR Tablets in relation to meals or fasting should be provided.

Drug Interactions
Drug/Drug Interactions:
Theophylline interacts with a wide variety of drugs. The interaction may be pharmacodynamic, ie, alterations in the therapeutic response to theophylline or another drug or occurrence of adverse effects without a change in serum theophylline concentration. More frequently, however, the interaction is pharmacokinetic, ie, the rate of theophylline

Continued on next page

Uni-Dur—Cont.

clearance is altered by another drug resulting in increased or decreased serum theophylline concentrations. Theophylline only rarely alters the pharmacokinetics of other drugs. The drugs listed in **Table II** have the potential to produce clinically significant pharmacodynamic or pharmacokinetic interactions with theophylline. The information in the **"Effect"** column of **Table II** assumes that the interacting drug is being added to a steady-state theophylline regimen. If theophylline is being initiated in a patient who is already taking a drug that inhibits theophylline clearance (eg, cimetidine, erythromycin), the dose of theophylline required to achieve a therapeutic serum theophylline concentration will be smaller. Conversely, if theophylline is being initiated in a patient who is already taking a drug that enhances theophylline clearance (eg, rifampin), the dose of theophylline required to achieve therapeutic serum theophylline concentration will be larger. Discontinuation of a concomitant drug that increases theophylline clearance will result in accumulation of theophylline to potentially toxic levels, unless the theophylline dose is appropriately reduced. Discontinuation of a concomitant drug that inhibits theophylline clearance will result in decreased serum theophylline concentrations, unless the theophylline dose is appropriately increased.

The listing of drugs in **Table II** is current as of February 9, 1995. New interactions are continuously being reported for theophylline, especially with new chemical entities. **The clinician should not assume that a drug does not interact with theophylline if it is not listed in Table II.** Before addition of a newly available drug in a patient receiving theophylline, the package insert of the new drug and/or the medical literature should be consulted to determine if an interaction between the new drug and theophylline has been reported.

[See table II above]

Drug/Food Interactions:
The extent of theophylline absorption from UNI-DUR® Extended-release Tablets is similar when administered fasting or immediately after a high-fat content breakfast. However, the time to peak concentration was delayed following the high-fat content breakfast (see **CLINICAL PHARMACOLOGY, Pharmacokinetics**). This breakfast contained 729 total kilocalories of which 55% were derived from 45 g of fat; and it consisted of two scrambled eggs, two strips of bacon, one slice of toast with 1 pat of butter, 3 oz. of hash brown potatoes, and 180 mL of whole milk. The influence of the type and amount of other foods, as well as the time interval between drug and food has not been studied.

The Effect of Other Drugs on Theophylline Serum Concentration Measurements:
Most serum theophylline assays in clinical use are immunoassays which are specific for theophylline. Other xanthines such as caffeine, dyphylline, and pentoxifylline are not detected by these assays. Some drugs (eg, cefazolin, cephalothin), however, may interfere with certain HPLC techniques. Caffeine and xanthine metabolites in patients with renal dysfunction may cause the reading from some dry reagent office methods to be higher than the actual serum theophylline concentration.

Carcinogenesis, Mutagenesis, and Impairment of Fertility:
Long-term carcinogenicity studies have been carried out in mice (oral doses 30–150 mg/kg) and rats (oral doses 5–75 mg/kg). Results are pending.
Theophylline has been studied in Ames salmonella, *in vivo* and *in vitro* cytogenetics, micronucleus, and Chinese hamster ovary test systems and has not been shown to be genotoxic.
In a 14-week continuous breeding study, theophylline, administered to mating pairs of B6C3F$_1$ mice at oral doses of 120, 270, and 500 mg/kg (approximately 1.0–3.0 times the human dose on a mg/m^2 basis) impaired fertility, as evidenced by decreases in the number of live pups per litter, decreases in the mean number of litters per fertile pair, and increases in the gestation period at the high dose as well as decreases in the proportion of pups born alive at the mid and high dose. In 13-week toxicity studies, theophylline was administered to F344 rats and B6C3F$_1$ mice at oral doses of 40–300 mg/kg (approximately 2.0 times the human dose on a mg/m^2 basis). At the high dose, systemic toxicity was observed in both species including decreases in testicular weight.

Pregnancy:
Category C There are no adequate and well-controlled studies in pregnant women. Additionally, there are no teratogenicity studies in nonrodents (eg, rabbits). Theophylline was not shown to be teratogenic in CD-1 mice at oral doses up to 400 mg/kg, approximately 2.0 times the recommended human dose on a mg/m^2 basis or CD-1 rats at oral doses up to 260 mg/kg, approximately 3.0 times the recommended human dose on a mg/m^2 basis. At a dose of 220 mg/kg, embryotoxicity was observed in rats in the absence of maternal toxicity.

Nursing Mothers:
Theophylline is excreted into breast milk and may cause irritability or other signs of mild toxicity in nursing human

Table II.

Drug	Type of Interaction	Effect**
Adenosine	Theophylline blocks adenosine receptors.	Higher doses of adenosine may be required to achieve desired effect.
Alcohol	A single large dose of alcohol (eg, 3 mL/kg of whiskey) decreases theophylline clearance for up to 24 hours.	30% increase
Allopurinol	Decreases theophylline clearance at allopurinol doses ≥600 mg/day.	25% increase
Aminoglutethimide	Increases theophylline clearance by induction of microsomal enzyme activity.	25% decrease
Carbamazepine	Similar to aminoglutethimide.	30% decrease
Cimetidine	Decreases theophylline clearance by inhibiting cytochrome P450 1A2.	70% increase
Ciprofloxacin	Similar to cimetidine.	40% increase
Clarithromycin	Similar to erythromycin.	25% increase
Diazepam	Benzodiazepines increase CNS concentrations of adenosine, a potent CNS depressant, while theophylline blocks adenosine receptors.	Larger diazepam doses may be required to produce desired level of sedation. Discontinuation of theophylline without reduction of diazepam dose may result in respiratory depression.
Disulfiram	Decreases theophylline clearance by inhibiting hydroxylation and demethylation.	50% increase
Enoxacin	Similar to cimetidine.	300% increase
Ephedrine	Synergistic CNS effects.	Increased frequency of nausea, nervousness, and insomnia.
Erythromycin	Erythromycin metabolite decreases theophylline clearance by inhibiting cytochrome P450 3A3.	35% increase. Erythromycin steady-state serum concentrations decrease by a similar amount.
Estrogen	Estrogen-containing oral contraceptives decrease theophylline clearance in a dose-dependent fashion. The effect of progesterone on theophylline clearance is unknown.	30% increase
Flurazepam	Similar to diazepam.	Similar to diazepam.
Fluvoxamine	Similar to cimetidine.	Similar to cimetidine.
Halothane	Halothane sensitizes the myocardium to catecholamines; theophylline increases release of endogenous catecholamines.	Increased risk of ventricular arrhythmias.
Interferon, human recombinant alpha-A	Decreases theophylline clearance.	100% increase
Isoproterenol (IV)	Increases theophylline clearance.	20% decrease
Ketamine	Pharmacologic.	May lower theophylline seizure threshold.
Lithium	Theophylline increases renal lithium clearance.	Lithium dose required to achieve a therapeutic serum concentration increased an average of 60%.
Lorazepam	Similar to diazepam.	Similar to diazepam.
Methotrexate (MTX)	Decreases theophylline clearance.	20% increase after low dose MTX; higher dose MTX may have a greater effect.
Mexiletine	Similar to disulfiram.	80% increase
Midazolam	Similar to diazepam.	Similar to diazepam.
Moricizine	Increases theophylline clearance.	25% decrease
Norfloxacin	Increases serum theophylline levels.	
Ofloxacin	Increases serum theophyllline levels.	
Pancuronium	Theophylline may antagonize nondepolarizing neuromuscular blocking effects; possibly due to phosphodiesterase inhibition.	Larger dose of pancuronium may be required to achieve neuromuscular blockade.
Pentoxifylline	Decreases theophylline clearance.	30% increase
Phenobarbital (PB)	Similar to aminoglutethimide.	25% decrease after 2 weeks of concurrent PB.
Phenytoin	Phenytoin increases theophylline clearance by increasing microsomal enzyme activity. Theophylline decreases phenytoin absorption.	Serum theophylline *and* phenytoin concentrations decrease about 40%.
Propafenone	Decreases theophylline clearance and pharmacologic interaction.	40% increase. Beta$_2$-blocking effect may decrease efficacy of theophylline.
Propranolol	Similar to cimetidine and pharmacologic interaction.	100% increase. Beta$_2$-blocking effect may decrease efficacy of theophylline.
Rifampin	Increases theophylline clearance by increasing cytochrome P450 1A2 and 3A3 activity.	20%–40% decrease
Ritonavir	Increases theophylline clearance (mechanism unknown)	43% decrease in AUC
Sucralfate	Reduced absorption of theophylline.	
Sulfinpyrazone	Increases theophylline clearance by increasing demethylation and hydroxylation. Decreases renal clearance of theophylline.	20% decrease
Tacrine	Similar to cimetidine, also increases renal clearance of theophylline.	90% increase
Thiabendazole	Decreases theophylline clearance.	190% increase
Ticlopidine	Decreases theophylline clearance.	60% increase
Troleandomycin	Similar to erythromycin.	33%–100% increase depending on troleandomycin dose.
Verapamil	Similar to disulfiram.	20% increase

Clinically significant drug interactions with theophylline.*

* Refer to **PRECAUTIONS, Drug Interactions** for further information regarding table.
** Average effect on steady-state theophylline concentration or other clinical effect for pharmacologic interactions. Individual patients may experience larger changes in serum theophylline concentration than the value listed.

infants. The concentration of theophylline in breast milk is about equivalent to the maternal serum concentration. An infant ingesting a liter of breast milk containing 10–20 mcg/mL of theophylline a day is likely to receive 10–20 mg of theophylline per day. Serious adverse effects in the infant are unlikely unless the mother has toxic serum theophylline concentrations.

Pediatric Use:
Safety and effectiveness of UNI-DUR Extended-release Tablets in pediatric patients under 12 years of age have not been established. Other theophylline formulations, however, are safe and effective for the approved indications in pediatric patients under the age of 12. The maintenance dose of theophylline must be selected with caution in pediatric patients under the age of 12. The maintenance dose of theophylline must be selected with caution in pediatric patients since the rate of theophylline clearance is highly variable across the age range of neonates to adolescents (see **CLINICAL PHARMACOLOGY, Table I, WARNINGS,** and **DOSAGE AND ADMINISTRATION, Table IV**).

Geriatric Use:
Elderly patients are at significantly greater risk of experiencing serious toxicity from theophylline than younger patients due to pharmacokinetic and pharmacodynamic changes associated with aging. Theophylline clearance is reduced in patients greater than 60 years of age, resulting in increased serum theophylline concentrations in response to a given theophylline dose. Protein binding may be decreased in the elderly resulting in a larger proportion of the total serum theophylline concentration in the pharmacologically active unbound form. Elderly patients also appear to be more sensitive to the toxic effects of theophylline after chronic overdosage than younger patients. For these reasons, the maximum daily dose of theophylline in patients greater than 60 years of age ordinarily should not exceed 400 mg/day unless the patient continues to be symptomatic and the peak steady-state serum theophylline concentration is <10 mcg/mL (see **DOSAGE AND ADMINISTRATION**). Theophylline doses greater than 400 mg/day should be prescribed with caution in elderly patients.

ADVERSE REACTIONS

Adverse reactions associated with theophylline are generally mild when peak serum theophylline concentrations are <20 mcg/mL and mainly consist of transient caffeine-like adverse effects such as nausea, vomiting, headache, and insomnia. When peak serum theophylline concentrations exceed 20 mcg/mL, however, theophylline produces a wide range of adverse reactions including persistent vomiting, cardiac arrhythmias, and intractable seizures, which can be lethal (see **OVERDOSAGE**). The transient caffeine-like adverse reactions occur in about 50% of patients when theophylline therapy is initiated at doses higher than recommended initial doses (eg, >300 mg/day in adults and >12 mg/kg/day in children beyond >1 year of age). During the initiation of theophylline therapy, caffeine-like adverse effects may transiently alter patient behavior, especially in school-age children, but this response rarely persists. Initiation of theophylline therapy at a low dose with subsequent slow titration to a predetermined age-related maximum dose will significantly reduce the frequency of these transient adverse effects (see **DOSAGE AND ADMINISTRATION, Table IV**). In a small percentage of patients (<3% of children and <10% of adults), the caffeine-like adverse effects persist during maintenance therapy, even at peak serum theophylline concentrations within the therapeutic range (ie, 10–20 mcg/mL). Dosage reduction may alleviate the caffeine-like adverse effects in these patients; however, persistent adverse effects should result in a re-evaluation of the need for continued theophylline therapy and the potential therapeutic benefit of alternative treatment.

Other adverse reactions that have been reported to occur at serum theophylline concentrations less than 20 mcg/mL include diarrhea, irritability, restlessness, fine skeletal muscle tremors, alopecia, muscle twitching/spasms, palpitations, rash, reflex hyperexcitability, transient diuresis, and ventricular arrhythmias. Whether or not theophylline caused these reported events is not known. In patients with hypoxia secondary to COPD, multifocal atrial tachycardia and flutter have been reported at serum theophylline concentrations ≥ 15 mcg/mL. There have been a few isolated reports of seizures at serum theophylline concentrations <20 mcg/mL in patients with an underlying neurological disease or in elderly patients. The occurrence of seizures in elderly patients with serum theophylline concentrations <20 mcg/mL may be secondary to decreased protein binding resulting in a larger proportion of the total serum theophylline concentration in the pharmacologically active unbound form. The clinical characteristics of the seizures reported in patients with serum theophylline concentrations <20 mcg/mL have generally been milder than seizures associated with excessive serum theophylline concentrations resulting from an overdose (ie, they have generally been transient, often stopped without anticonvulsant therapy, and did not result in neurological residua).

[See table III above]

Table III. Manifestations of theophylline toxicity.*

Sign/Symptom	Percentage of patients reported with sign or symptom: Acute Overdose (Large Single Ingestion) Study 1 (n=157)	Acute Overdose Study 2 (n=14)	Chronic Overdosage (Multiple Excessive Doses) Study 1 (n=92)	Chronic Overdosage Study 2 (n=102)
Asymptomatic	NR**	0	NR**	6
Gastrointestinal				
Vomiting	73	93	30	61
Abdominal pain	NR**	21	NR**	12
Diarrhea	NR**	0	NR**	14
Hematemesis	NR**	0	NR**	2
Metabolic/Other				
Hypokalemia	85	79	44	43
Hyperglycemia	98	NR**	18	NR**
Acid/base disturbance	34	21	9	5
Rhabdomyolysis	NR**	7	NR**	0
Cardiovascular				
Sinus tachycardia	100	86	100	62
Other supraventricular tachycardias	2	21	12	14
Ventricular premature beats	3	21	10	19
Atrial fibrillation or flutter	1	NR**	12	NR**
Multifocal atrial tachycardia	0	NR**	2	NR**
Ventricular arrhythmias with hemodynamic instability	7	14	40	0
Hypotension/shock	NR**	21	NR**	8
Neurologic				
Nervousness	NR**	64	NR**	21
Tremors	38	29	16	14
Disorientation	NR**	7	NR**	11
Seizures	5	14	14	5
Death	3	21	10	4

* These data are derived from two studies in patients with serum theophylline concentrations >30 mcg/mL. In the first study (Study #1-Shanon, *Ann Intern Med.* 1993;119:1161-67), data were prospectively collected from 249 consecutive cases of theophylline toxicity referred to a regional poison center for consultation. In the second study (Study #2-Sessler, *Am J Med.* 1990;88:567-76), data were retrospectively collected from 116 cases with serum theophylline concentrations >30 mcg/mL among 6000 blood samples obtained for measurement of serum theophylline concentrations in three emergency departments. Differences in the incidence of manifestations of theophylline toxicity between the two studies may reflect sample selection as a result of study design (eg, in Study #1, 48% of the patients had acute intoxications versus only 10% in Study #2) and different methods of reporting results.

** NR = Not reported in a comparable manner.

OVERDOSAGE

General:
The chronicity and pattern of theophylline overdosage significantly influences clinical manifestations of toxicity, management, and outcome. There are two common presentations: (1) *acute overdose*, ie, ingestion of a single large excessive dose (>10 mg/kg) as occurs in the context of an attempted suicide or isolated medication error, and (2) *chronic overdosage*, ie, ingestion of repeated doses that are excessive for the patient's rate of theophylline clearance. The most common causes of chronic theophylline overdosage include patient or caregiver error in dosing, clinician prescribing of an excessive dose or a normal dose in the presence of factors known to decrease the rate of theophylline clearance, and increasing the dose in response to an exacerbation of symptoms without first measuring the serum theophylline concentration to determine whether a dose increase is safe.

Severe toxicity from theophylline overdose is a relatively rare event. In one health maintenance organization, the frequency of hospital admissions for chronic overdosage of theophylline was about 1 per 1000 person-years exposure. In another study, among 6000 blood samples obtained for measurement of serum theophylline concentration, for any reason, from patients treated in an emergency department, 7% were in the 20–30 mcg/mL range and 3% were >30 mcg/mL. Approximately two thirds of the patients with serum theophylline concentrations in the 20–30 mcg/mL range had one or more manifestations of toxicity while >90% of patients with serum theophylline concentrations >30 mcg/mL were clinically intoxicated. Similarly, in other reports, serious toxicity from theophylline is seen principally at serum concentrations >30 mcg/mL.

Several studies have described the clinical manifestations of theophylline overdose and attempted to determine the factors that predict life-threatening toxicity. In general, patients who experience an acute overdose are less likely to experience seizures than patients who have experienced a chronic overdosage, unless the peak serum theophylline concentration is >100 mcg/mL. After a chronic overdosage, generalized seizures, life-threatening cardiac arrhythmias, and death may occur at serum theophylline concentrations >30 mcg/mL. The severity of toxicity after chronic overdosage is more strongly correlated with the patient's age than the peak serum theophylline concentration; patients >60 years are at the greatest risk for severe toxicity and mortality after a chronic overdosage. Pre-existing or concurrent disease may also significantly increase the susceptibility of a patient to a particular toxic manifestation, eg, patients with neurologic disorders have an increased risk of seizures and patients with cardiac disease have an increased risk of cardiac arrhythmias for a given serum theophylline concentration compared to patients without the underlying disease.

The frequency of various reported manifestations of theophylline overdose according to the mode of overdose are listed in **Table III.**

Other manifestations of theophylline toxicity include increases in serum calcium, creatine kinase, myoglobin, and leukocyte count, decreases in serum phosphate and magnesium, acute myocardial infarction, and urinary retention in men with obstructive uropathy.

Seizures associated with serum theophylline concentrations >30 mcg/mL are often resistant to anticonvulsant therapy and may result in irreversible brain injury if not rapidly controlled. Death from theophylline toxicity is most often secondary to cardiorespiratory arrest and/or hypoxic encephalopathy following prolonged generalized seizures or intractable cardiac arrhythmias causing hemodynamic compromise.

Overdose Management:

General Recommendations for Patients With Symptoms of Theophylline Overdose or Serum Theophylline Concentrations >30 mcg/mL. (Note: Serum theophylline concentrations may continue to increase after presentation of the patient for medical care.)

1. While simultaneously instituting treatment, contact a regional poison center to obtain updated information and advice on individualizing the recommendations that follow.
2. Institute supportive care, including establishment of intravenous access, maintenance of the airway, and electrocardiographic monitoring.
3. *Treatment of seizures:* Because of the high morbidity and mortality associated with theophylline-induced seizures, treatment should be rapid and aggressive. Anticonvulsant therapy should be initiated with an intravenous benzodiazepine, eg, diazepam, in increments of 0.1–0.2 mg/kg every 1–3 minutes until seizures are terminated. Repetitive seizures should be treated with a loading dose of phenobarbital (20 mg/kg infused over 30–60 minutes). Animal studies and case reports of theophylline overdose in humans suggest that phenytoin is ineffective in terminating theophylline-induced seizures. The doses of benzodiazepines and phenobarbital required to terminate theophylline-induced seizures are close to the doses that may cause severe respiratory depression or respiratory arrest; the clinician should therefore be prepared to provide assisted ventilation. Elderly patients and patients with COPD may be more susceptible to the respiratory depressant effects of anticonvulsants. Barbi-

Continued on next page

Uni-Dur—Cont.

turate-induced coma or administration of general anesthesia may be required to terminate repetitive seizures or status epilepticus. General anesthesia should be used with caution in patients with theophylline overdose because fluorinated volatile anesthetics may sensitize the myocardium to endogenous catecholamines released by theophylline. Enflurane appears less likely to be associated with this effect than halothane and may, therefore, be safer. Neuromuscular blocking agents alone should not be used to terminate seizures since they abolish the musculoskeletal manifestations without terminating seizure activity in the brain.

4. *Anticipate need for anticonvulsants:* In patients with theophylline overdose who are at high risk for theophylline-induced seizures, eg, patients with acute overdoses and serum theophylline concentrations >100 mcg/mL or chronic overdosage in patients >60 years of age with serum theophylline concentrations >30 mcg/mL, the need for anticonvulsant therapy should be anticipated. A benzodiazepine such as diazepam should be drawn into a syringe and kept at the patient's bedside and medical personnel qualified to treat seizures should be immediately available. In selected patients at high risk for theophylline-induced seizures, consideration should be given to the administration of prophylactic anticonvulsant therapy. Situations where prophylactic anticonvulsant therapy should be considered in high-risk patient include anticipated delays in instituting methods for extracorporeal removal of theophylline (eg, transfer of a high-risk patient from one healthcare facility to another for extracorporeal removal) and clinical circumstances that significantly interfere with efforts to enhance theophylline clearance (eg, a neonate where dialysis may not be technically feasible or patient with vomiting unresponsive to antiemetics who is unable to tolerate multiple-dose oral activated charcoal). In animal studies, prophylactic administration of phenobarbital, *but not phenytoin,* has been shown to delay the onset of theophylline-induced generalized seizures and to increase the dose of theophylline required to induce seizures (ie, markedly increases the LD_{50}). Although there are no controlled studies in humans, a loading dose of intravenous phenobarbital (20 mg/kg infused over 60 minutes) may delay or prevent life-threatening seizures in high-risk patients while efforts to enhance theophylline clearance are continued. Phenobarbital may cause respiratory depression, particularly in elderly patients and patients with COPD.

5. *Treatment of cardiac arrhythmias:* Sinus tachycardia and simple ventricular premature beats are not harbingers of life-threatening arrhythmias, they do not require treatment in the absence of hemodynamic compromise, and they resolve with declining serum theophylline concentrations. Other arrhythmias, especially those associated with hemodynamic compromise, should be treated with antiarrhythmic therapy appropriate for the type of arrhythmia.

6. *Gastrointestinal decontamination:* Oral activated charcoal (0.5 g/kg up to 20 g and repeat at least once 1–2 hours after the first dose) is extremely effective in blocking the absorption of theophylline throughout the gastrointestinal tract, even when administered several hours after ingestion. If the patient is vomiting, the charcoal should be administered through a nasogastric tube or after administration of an antiemetic. Phenothiazine antiemetics such as prochlorperazine or perphenazine should be avoided since they can lower the seizure threshold and frequently cause dystonic reactions. A single dose of sorbitol may be used to promote stooling to facilitate removal of theophylline bound to charcoal from the gastrointestinal tract. Sorbitol, however, should be dosed with caution since it is a potent purgative which can cause profound fluid and electrolyte abnormalities, particularly after multiple doses. Commercially available fixed combinations of liquid charcoal and sorbitol should be avoided in young children and after the first dose in adolescents and adults since they do not allow for individualization of charcoal and sorbitol dosing. Ipecac syrup should be avoided in theophylline overdoses. Although ipecac induces emesis, it does not reduce the absoprtion of theophylline unless administered within 5 minutes of ingestion and even then is less effective than oral activated charcoal. Moreover, ipecac-induced emesis may persist for several hours after a single dose and significantly decrease the retention and the effectiveness of oral activated charcoal.

7. *Serum theophylline concentration monitoring:* The serum theophylline concentration should be measured immediately upon presentation, 2–4 hours later, and then at sufficient intervals, eg, every 4 hours, to guide treatment decisions and to assess the effectiveness of therapy. Serum theophylline concentrations may continue to increase after presentation of the patient for medical care as a result of continued absorption of theo-

phylline from the gastrointestinal tract. Serial monitoring of serum theophylline serum concentrations should be continued until it is clear that the concentration is no longer rising and has returned to nontoxic levels.

8. *General monitoring procedures:* Electrocardiographic monitoring should be initiated on presentation and continued until the serum theophylline level has returned to a nontoxic level. Serum electrolytes and glucose should be measured on presentation and at appropriate intervals indicated by clinical circumstances. Fluid and electrolyte abnormalities should be promptly corrected. **Monitoring and treatment should be continued until the serum concentration decreases below 20 mcg/mL.**

9. *Enhance clearance of theophylline:* Multiple-dose oral activated charcoal (eg, 0.5 mg/kg up to 20 g, every 2 hours) increases the clearance of theophylline at least twofold by absorption of theophylline secreted into gastrointestinal fluids. Charcoal must be retained in, and pass through, the gastrointestinal tract to be effective; emesis should therefore be controlled by administration of appropriate antiemetics. Alternatively, the charcoal can be administered continuously through a nasogastric tube in conjunction with appropriate antiemetics. A single dose of sorbitol may be administered with the activated charcoal to promote stooling to facilitate clearance of the adsorbed theophylline from the gastrointestinal tract. Sorbitol alone does not enhance clearance of theophylline and should be dosed with caution to prevent excessive stooling which can result in severe fluid and electrolyte imbalances. Commercially available fixed combinations of liquid charcoal and sorbitol should be avoided in young children and after the first dose in adolescents and adults since they do not allow for individualization of charcoal and sorbitol dosing. In patients with intractable vomiting, extracorporeal methods of theophylline removal should be instituted (see **OVERDOSAGE, Extracorporeal Removal**).

Specific Recommendations:

Acute Overdose

A. Serum Concentration >20 <30 mcg/mL
  1. Administer a single dose of oral activated charcoal.
  2. Monitor the patient and obtain a serum theophylline concentrations in 2–4 hours to ensure that the concentration is not increasing.

B. Serum Concentration >30 <100 mcg/mL
  1. Administer multiple-dose oral activated charcoal and measures to control emesis.
  2. Monitor the patient and obtain serial theophylline concentrations every 2–4 hours to gauge the effectiveness of therapy and to guide further treatment decisions.
  3. Institute extracorporeal removal if emesis, seizures, or cardiac arrhythmias cannot be adequately controlled (see **OVERDOSAGE, Extracorporeal Removal**).

C. Serum Concentration >100 mcg/mL
  1. Consider prophylactic anticonvulsant therapy.
  2. Administer multiple-dose oral activated charcoal and measures to control emesis.
  3. Consider extracorporeal removal, even if the patient has not experienced a seizure (see **OVERDOSAGE, Extracorporeal Removal**).
  4. Monitor the patient and obtain serial theophylline concentrations every 2–4 hours to gauge the effectiveness of therapy and to guide further treatment decisions.

Chronic Overdosage

A. Serum Concentration >20 <30 mcg/mL (with manifestations of theophylline toxicity)
  1. Administer a single dose of oral activated charcoal.
  2. Monitor the patient and obtain a serum theophylline concentration in 2–4 hours to ensure that the concentration is not increasing.

B. Serum Concentration >30 mcg/mL in patients <60 years of age
  1. Administer multiple-dose oral activated charcoal and measures to control emesis.
  2. Monitor the patient and obtain serial theophylline concentrations every 2–4 hours to gauge the effectiveness of therapy and to guide further treatment deci- sions.

Table IV. Dosing initiation and titration (as anhydrous theophylline).*

A. Children (12–15 years) and adults (16–60 years) without risk factors for impaired clearance.

Titration Step	Children <45 kg	Children >45 kg and adults
1. Starting dosage:	12–14 mg/kg/day up to a maximum of 300 mg/day administered QD*	300–400 mg/day[1] administered QD*
2. After 3 days, *if tolerated*, increase dose to:	16 mg/kg/day up to a maximum of 400 mg/day administered QD*	400–600 mg/day[1] administered QD*
3. After 3 more days, *if tolerated*, increase dose to:	20 mg/kg/day upto a maximum of 600 mg/day administered QD*	As with all theophylline products, doses greater than 600 mg should be titrated according to blood level (see **Table V**).

B. **Patients With Risk Factors For Impaired Clearance, The Elderly (>60 Years), And Those In Whom It Is Not Feasible To Monitor Serum Theophylline Concentrations:**

In children 12–15 years of age, the final theophylline dose should not exceed 16 mg/kg/day up to a maximum of 400 mg/day in the presence of risk factors for reduced theophylline clearance (see **WARNINGS**) or if it is not feasible to monitor serum theophylline concentrations.

In adolescents ≥16 years and adults, including the elderly, the final theophylline dose should not exceed 400 mg/day in the presence of risk factors for reduced theophylline clearance (see **WARNINGS**) or if it is not feasible to monitor serum theophylline concentrations.

---

* Patients with more rapid metabolism, clinically identified by higher than average dose requirements, should receive a smaller dose more frequently (every 12 hours) to prevent breakthrough symptoms resulting from low trough concentrations before the next dose.

[1] If caffeine-like adverse effects occur, then consideration should be given to a lower dose and titrating the dose more slowly (see **ADVERSE REACTIONS**).

Table V. Dosage adjustment guided by serum theophylline concentration.

Peak Serum Concentration	Dosage Adjustment
<9.9 mcg/mL	If symptoms are not controlled and current dosage is tolerated, increase dose about 25%. Recheck serum concentration after 3 days for further dosage adjustment.
10 to 14.9 mcg/mL	If symptoms are controlled and current dosage is tolerated, maintain dose and recheck serum concentration at 6- to 12-month intervals.¶ If symptoms are not controlled and current dosage is tolerated, consider adding additional medication(s) to treatment regimen.
15–19.9 mcg/mL	Consider 10% decrease in dose to provide greater margin of safety even if current dosage is tolerated.¶
20–24.9 mcg/mL	Decrease dose by 25% even if no adverse effects are present. Recheck serum concentration after 3 days to guide further dosage adjustment.
25–30 mcg/mL	Skip next dose and decrease subsequent doses at least 25% even if no adverse effects are present. Recheck serum concentration after 3 days to guide further dosage adjustment. If symptomatic, consider whether overdose treatment is indicated (see recommendations for chronic overdosage).
>30 mcg/mL	Treat overdose as indicated (see recommendations for chronic overdosage). If theophylline is subsequently resumed, decrease dose by at least 50% and recheck serum concentration after 3 days to guide further dosage adjustment.

¶ Dose reduction and/or serum theophylline concentration measurement is indicated whenever adverse effects are present, physiologic abnormalities that can reduce theophylline clearance occur (eg, sustained fever), or a drug that interacts with theophylline is added or discontinued (see **WARNINGS**).

3. Institute extracorporeal removal if emesis, seizures, or cardiac arrhythmias cannot be adequately controlled (see **OVERDOSAGE, Extracorporeal Removal**).

C. Serum Concentration >30 mcg/mL in patients ≥60 years of age
1. Consider prophylactic anticonvulsant therapy.
2. Administer multiple-dose oral activated charcoal and measures to control emesis.
3. Consider extracorporeal removal even if the patient has not experienced a seizure (see **OVERDOSAGE, Extracorporeal Removal**).
4. Monitor the patient and obtain serial theophylline concentrations every 2–4 hours to gauge the effectiveness of therapy and to guide further treatment decisions.

Extracorporeal Removal:
Increasing the rate of theophylline by extracorporeal methods may rapidly decrease serum concentrations, but the risks of the procedure must be weighed against the potential benefit. Charcoal hemoperfusion is the most effective method of extracorporeal removal, increasing theophylline clearance up to sixfold, but serious complications, including hypotension, hypocalcemia, platelet consumption, and bleeding diatheses may occur. Hemodialysis is about as efficient as multiple-dose oral activated charcoal and has a lower risk of serious complications than charcoal hemoperfusion. Hemodialysis should be considered as an alternative when charcoal hemoperfusion is not feasible and multiple-dose oral charcoal is ineffective because of intractable emesis. Serum theophylline concentrations may rebound 5–10 mcg/mL after discontinuation of charcoal hemoperfusion or hemodialysis due to redistribution of theophylline from the tissue compartment. Peritoneal dialysis is ineffective for theophylline removal; exchange transfusions in neonates have been minimally effective.

DOSAGE AND ADMINISTRATION

The extent of absorption of theophylline from UNI-DUR Tablets when administered fasting or immediately after a high-fat content breakfast is similar. However, the time to peak concentration is delayed (see **PRECAUTIONS, Drug/Food Interactions**).
Effective use of theophylline (ie, the concentration of drug in the serum associated with optimal benefit and minimal risk of toxicity) is considered to occur when the theophylline concentration is maintained from 10 to 15 mcg/mL.
Patients who clear theophylline normally or relatively slowly, eg, nonsmokers, may be reasonable candidates for taking UNI-DUR Tablets once daily. However, certain patients, such as the young, smokers, and some nonsmoking adults are likely to metabolize theophylline more rapidly and may require dosing at 12-hour intervals. Such patients may experience symptoms of bronchospasm toward the end of a once-daily dosing interval and/or require a higher daily dose (higher than those recommended in labeling) and are more likely to experience relatively wide peak to trough differences in serum theophylline concentrations.
UNI-DUR Tablets may be administered either in the morning or in the evening.
UNI-DUR Tablets *should not be chewed or crushed.*

General Considerations:
The steady-state peak serum theophylline concentration is a function of the dose, the dosing interval, and the rate of theophylline absorption and clearance in the individual patient. Because of marked individual differences in the rate of theophylline clearance, the dose required to achieve a peak serum theophylline concentration in the 10–20 mcg/mL range varies fourfold among otherwise similar patients in the absence of factors known to alter theophylline clearance (eg, 400–1600 mg/day in adults <60 years old and 10–36 mg/kg/day in children 1–9 years old). For a given population there is no single theophylline dose that will provide both safe and effective serum concentrations for all patients. Administration of the median theophylline dose required to achieve a therapeutic serum theophylline concentration in a given population may result in either subtherapeutic or potentially toxic serum theophylline concentrations in individual patients. For example, at a dose of 900 mg/day in adults <60 years or 22 mg/kg/day in children 1–9 years, the steady-state peak serum theophylline concentration will be <10 mcg/mL in about 30% of patients, 10–20 mcg/mL in about 50%, and 20–30 mcg/mL in about 20% of patients. **The dose of theophylline must be individualized on the basis of peak serum theophylline concentration measurements in order to achieve a dose that will provide maximum potential benefit with minimal risk of adverse effects.**
Transient caffeine-like adverse effects and excessive serum concentrations in slow metabolizers can be avoided in most patients by starting with a sufficiently low dose and slowly increasing the dose, *if judged to be clinically indicated*, in small increments (see **Table IV**). Dose increases should only be made if the previous dosage is well tolerated and at intervals of no less than 3 days to allow serum theophylline concentrations to reach the new steady state. Dosage adjustment should be guided by serum theophylline concentration measurement (see **PRECAUTIONS, Monitoring Serum Theophylline Concentrations,** and **DOSAGE AND ADMINISTRATION, Table V**). Healthcare providers should instruct patients and caregivers to discontinue any dosage that causes adverse effects, to withhold the medication until these symptoms are gone, and to then resume therapy at lower, previously tolerated dosage (see **WARNINGS**).
If the patient's symptoms are well controlled, there are no apparent adverse effects, and no intervening factors that might alter dosage requirements (see **WARNINGS** and **PRECAUTIONS**), serum theophylline concentrations should be monitored at 6-month intervals for rapidly growing children and at yearly intervals for all others. In acutely ill patients, serum theophylline concentrations should be monitored at frequent intervals, eg, every 24 hours.
Theophylline distributes poorly into body fat, therefore, mg/kg dose should be calculated on the basis of ideal body weight.
Table IV contains theophylline dosing titration schema recommended for patients in various age groups and clinical circumstances. **Table V** contains recommendations for theophylline dosage adjustment based upon serum theophylline concentrations. **Application of these general dosing recommendations to individual patients must take into account the unique clinical characteristics of each patient. In general, these recommendations should serve as the upper limit for dose adjustments in order to decrease the risk of potentially serious adverse events associated with unexpected large increases in serum theophylline concentration.**

[See table IV at top of previous page]
[See table V at top of previous page]

HOW SUPPLIED

UNI-DUR Extended-release Tablets are supplied as controlled-release tablets containing either 400 mg or 600 mg of theophylline anhydrous. They are mottled white, capsule-shaped tablets; scored on one side and debossed with the product name and strength on the other.
UNI-DUR Extended-release Tablets 400 mg are available in bottles of 100's (NDC 0085-0694-01).
UNI-DUR Extended-release Tablets 600 mg are available in bottles of 100's (NDC 0085-0814-01).

STORAGE CONDITIONS
Keep bottles tightly closed. Store between 15° and 25°C (59° and 77°F).
CAUTION: Federal law prohibits dispensing without prescription.

Key Pharmaceuticals, Inc.
Kenilworth, NJ 07033 USA

Rev. 3/97 B-19767914

Shown in Product Identification Guide, page 318

Knoll Laboratories

**A Division of
Knoll Pharmaceutical Company
3000 CONTINENTAL DRIVE NORTH
MOUNT OLIVE, NJ 07828**

Direct Inquiries to:
Knoll Pharmaceutical Company
(973) 426-2600
Customer Operations Department:
(800) 526-0710

For Medical Information Contact:
(800) 526-0221

AKINETON® TABLETS AND AMPULES ℞
[*ā-kĭn 'ĕ-ton*]
biperiden hydrochloride and biperiden lactate

DESCRIPTION

Each AKINETON Tablet for oral administration contains 2 mg biperiden hydrochloride. Other ingredients may include corn syrup, lactose, magnesium stearate, potato starch and talc. Each 1 mL AKINETON Ampule for intramuscular or intravenous administration contains 5 mg biperiden lactate in an aqueous 1.4 percent sodium lactate solution. No added preservative. AKINETON is an anticholinergic agent. Biperiden is α-5-Norbornen-2-yl-α-phenyl-1-piperidine propanol. It is a white, crystalline, odorless powder, slightly soluble in water and alcohol. It is stable in air at normal temperatures. Biperiden may be represented by the following structural formula:

[See chemical structure at top of next column]

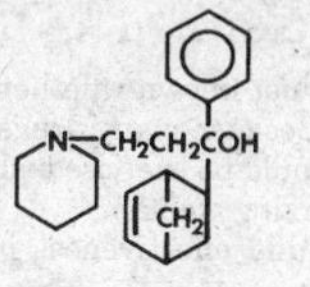

CLINICAL PHARMACOLOGY

AKINETON is a weak peripheral anticholinergic agent. It has, therefore, some antisecretory, antispasmodic and mydriatic effects. In addition, AKINETON possesses nicotinolytic activity. Parkinsonism is thought to result from an imbalance between the excitatory (cholinergic) and inhibitory (dopaminergic) systems in the corpus striatum. The mechanism of action of centrally active anticholinergic drugs such as AKINETON is considered to relate to competitive antagonism of acetylcholine at cholinergic receptors in the corpus striatum, which then restores the balance.
The parenteral form of AKINETON is an effective and reliable agent for the treatment of acute episodes of extrapyramidal disturbances sometimes seen during treatment with neuroleptic agents. Akathisia, akinesia, dyskinetic tremors, rigor, oculogyric crisis, spasmodic torticollis, and profuse sweating are markedly reduced or eliminated. With parenteral AKINETON, these drug-induced disturbances are rapidly brought under control. Subsequently, this can usually be maintained with oral doses which may be given with tranquilizer therapy in psychotic and other conditions requiring an uninterrupted therapeutic program.
Pharmacokinetics and Metabolism: Only limited pharmacokinetic studies of biperiden in humans are available The serum concentration at 1 to 1.5 hours following a single, 4 mg oral dose was 4–5 ng/mL. Plasma levels (0.1–0.2 ng/mL) could be determined up to 48 hours after dosing. Six hours after an oral dose of 250 mg/kg in rats, 87% of the drug had been absorbed. The metabolism of AKINETON is also incompletely understood, but does involve hydroxylation. In normal volunteers a single 10 mg intravenous dose of biperiden seemed to cause a transient rise in plasma cortisol and prolactin. No change in GH, LH, FSH, or TSH levels were seen. Biperiden lactate (10 mg/mL) was not irritating to the tissue of rabbits when injected intramuscularly (1.0 mL) into the sacrospinalis muscles and intradermally (0.25 mL) and subcutaneously (0.5 mL) into the shaved abdominal skin.

INDICATIONS AND USAGE

- As an adjunct in the therapy of all forms of parkinsonism (idiopathic, postencephalitic, arteriosclerotic)
- Control of extrapyramidal disorders secondary to neuroleptic drug therapy (e.g., phenothiazines)

CONTRAINDICATIONS

1) Hypersensitivity to biperiden 2) Narrow angle glaucoma 3) Bowel obstruction 4) Megacolon

WARNINGS

Isolated instances of mental confusion, euphoria, agitation and disturbed behavior have been reported in susceptible patients. Also, the central anticholinergic syndrome can occur as an adverse reaction to properly prescribed anticholinergic medication, although it is more frequently due to overdosage. It may also result from concomitant administration of an anticholinergic agent and a drug that has secondary anticholinergic actions (see Drug Interactions and Overdosage sections). Caution should be observed in patients with manifest glaucoma, though no prohibitive rise in intraocular pressure has been noted following either oral or parenteral administration. Patients with prostatism, epilepsy or cardiac arrhythmia should be given this drug with caution.
Occasionally, drowsiness may occur, and patients who drive a car or operate any other potentially dangerous machinery should be warned of this possibility. As with other drugs acting on the central nervous system, the consumption of alcohol should be avoided during AKINETON therapy.

PRECAUTIONS

Drug Interactions: The central anticholinergic syndrome can occur when anticholinergic agents such as AKINETON are administered concomitantly with drugs that have secondary anticholinergic actions, e.g., certain narcotic analgesics such as meperidine, the phenothiazines and other antipsychotics, tricyclic antidepressants, certain antiarrhythmics such as the quinidine salts, and antihistamines. See Overdosage section for signs and symptoms of the central anticholinergic syndrome, and for treatment.
Pregnancy: Pregnancy Category C. Animal reproduction studies have not been conducted with AKINETON. It is also not known whether AKINETON can cause fetal harm when administered to a pregnant woman or can affect reproduction capacity. AKINETON should be given to a pregnant woman only if clearly needed.

Continued on next page

Akineton—Cont.

Nursing Mothers: It is not known whether this drug is excreted in human milk. Because many drugs are excreted in human milk, caution should be exercised when AKINETON is administered to a nursing woman.
Pediatric Use: Safety and effectiveness in children have not been established.

ADVERSE REACTIONS

Atropine-like side effects such as dry mouth; blurred vision; drowsiness; euphoria or disorientation; urinary retention; postural hypotension; constipation; agitation; disturbed behavior may be seen. There usually are no significant changes in blood pressure or heart rate in patients who have been given the parenteral form of AKINETON. Mild transient postural hypotension and bradycardia may occur. These side effects can be minimized or avoided by slow intravenous administration. No local tissue reactions have been reported following intramuscular injection. If gastric irritation occurs following oral administration, it can be avoided by administering the drug during or after meals.
The central anticholinergic syndrome can occur as an adverse reaction to properly prescribed anticholinergic medication. See Overdosage section for signs and symptoms of the central anticholinergic syndrome, and for treatment.

OVERDOSAGE

Signs and Symptoms: Overdosage with AKINETON produces typical central symptoms of atropine intoxication (the central anticholinergic syndrome). Correct diagnosis depends upon recognition of the peripheral signs of parasympathetic blockade including dilated and sluggish pupils; warm, dry skin; facial flushing; decreased secretions of the mouth, pharynx, nose, and bronchi; foul-smelling breath; elevated temperature, tachycardia, cardiac arrhythmias, decreased bowel sounds, and urinary retention. Neuropsychiatric signs such as delirium, disorientation, anxiety, hallucinations, illusions, confusion, incoherence, agitation, hyperactivity, ataxia, loss of memory, paranoia, combativeness, and seizures may be present. The condition can progress to stupor, coma, paralysis, and cardiac and respiratory arrest and death.
Treatment: Treatment of acute overdose revolves around symptomatic and supportive therapy. If AKINETON was administered orally, gastric lavage or other measures to limit absorption should be instituted. A small dose of diazepam or a short acting barbiturate may be administered if CNS excitation is observed. Phenothiazines are contraindicated because the toxicity may be intensified due to their antimuscarinic action, causing coma. Respiratory support, artificial respiration or vasopressor agents may be necessary. Hyperpyrexia must be reversed, fluid volume replaced and acid-base balance maintained. Urinary catheterization may be necessary.
Routine use of physostigmine for overdose is controversial. Delirium, hallucinations, coma, and supraventricular tachycardia (not ventricular tachycardias or conduction defects) seem to respond. If indicated, 1 mg (half this amount for children or elderly) may be given intramuscularly or by slow intravenous infusion. If there is no response within 20 minutes, an additional 1 mg dose may be given; this may be repeated until a total of 4 mg has been administered, a reversal of the toxic effects occur or excessive cholinergic signs are seen. Frequent monitoring of clinical signs should be done. Since physostigmine is rapidly destroyed, additional injections may be required every one or two hours to maintain control. The relapse intervals tend to lengthen as the toxic anticholinergic agent is metabolized, so the patient should be carefully observed for 8 to 12 hours following the last relapse.
Toxicity in Animals: The LD_{50} of biperiden in the white mouse is 545 mg/kg orally, 195 mg/kg subcutaneously, and 56 mg/kg intravenously. The acute oral toxicity (LD_{50}) in rats is 750 mg/kg. The intraperitoneal toxicity (LD_{50}) of biperiden lactate in rats was 270 mg/kg and the intravenous toxicity (LD_{50}) in dogs is 222 mg/kg. In dogs under general anesthesia, respiratory arrest occurred at 33 mg/kg (intravenous) and circulatory standstill at 45 mg/kg (intravenous). The oral LD_{50} in dogs was 340 mg/kg. Chronic toxicity studies in both rat and dog have been reported.

DOSAGE AND ADMINISTRATION

Drug-Induced Extrapyramidal Symptoms:
Parenteral: The average adult dose is 2 mg intramuscularly or intravenously. May be repeated every half-hour until there is resolution of symptoms, but not more than four consecutive doses should be given in a 24-hour period.
Note: Parenteral drug products should be inspected visually for particulate matter and discoloration prior to administration, whenever solution and container permit.
Oral: One tablet one to three times daily.
Parkinson's Disease: Oral: The usual beginning dose is one tablet three or four times daily. The dosage should be individualized with the dose titrated upward to a maximum of 8 tablets (16 mg) per 24 hours.

HOW SUPPLIED

AKINETON Tablets, 2 mg each, white, embossed on one face with a triangle, bisected on the reverse and imprinted with the number "11."
Bottles of 100—NDC #0044-0120-02.
Bottles of 1000—NDC #0044-0120-04.
Storage: All dosage forms of AKINETON should be stored at 15°–30°C (59°–86°F). Dispense in tight, light-resistant container as defined in USP.
©1996 Knoll Pharmaceutical Company
AKINETON is a registered trademark of Knoll AG
Revised: July 1996
Knoll Laboratories
A Division of
Knoll Pharmaceutical Company
Mount Olive, New Jersey 07828
BASF Pharma 0900002-2
Shown in Product Identification Guide, page 318

COLLAGENASE SANTYL® Ointment ℞
[săn 'tĭl]

DESCRIPTION

Collagenase Santyl® Ointment is a sterile enzymatic debriding ointment which contains 250 collagenase units per gram of white petrolatum USP. The enzyme collagenase is derived from the fermentation by *Clostridium histolyticum.* It possesses the unique ability to digest collagen in necrotic tissue.

CLINICAL PHARMACOLOGY

Since collagen accounts for 75% of the dry weight of skin tissue, the ability of collagenase to digest collagen in the physiological pH and temperature range makes it particularly effective in the removal of detritus.[1] Collagenase thus contributes towards the formation of granulation tissue and subsequent epithelization of dermal ulcers and severely burned areas.[2, 3, 4, 5, 6] Collagen in healthy tissue or in newly formed granulation tissue is not attacked.[2, 3, 4, 5, 6, 7, 8] There is no information available on collagenase absorption through skin or its concentration in body fluids associated with therapeutic and/or toxic effects, degree of binding to plasma proteins, degree of uptake by a particular organ or in the fetus, and passage across the blood brain barrier.

INDICATIONS

Collagenase Santyl® Ointment is indicated for debriding chronic dermal ulcers[2, 3, 4, 5, 6, 8, 9, 10, 11, 12, 13, 14, 15, 16, 17, 18] and severely burned areas.[3, 4, 5, 7, 16, 19, 20, 21]

CONTRAINDICATIONS

Collagenase Santyl® Ointment is contraindicated in patients who have shown local or systemic hypersensitivity to collagenase.

PRECAUTIONS

The optimal pH range of collagenase is 6 to 8. Higher or lower pH conditions will decrease the enzyme's activity and appropriate precautions should be taken. The enzymatic activity is also adversely affected by detergents, and heavy metal ions such as mercury and silver which are used in some antiseptics. When it is suspected such materials have been used, the site should be carefully cleansed by repeated washings with normal saline before Collagenase Santyl® Ointment is applied. Soaks containing metal ions or acidic solutions should be avoided because of the metal ion and low pH. Cleansing materials such as hydrogen peroxide, Dakin's solution, and normal saline are compatible with Collagenase Santyl® Ointment.
Debilitated patients should be closely monitored for systemic bacterial infections because of the theoretical possibility that debriding enzymes may increase the risk of bacteremia.
A slight transient erythema has been noted occasionally in the surrounding tissue, particularly when Collagenase Santyl® Ointment was not confined to the wound. Therefore, the ointment should be applied carefully within the area of the wound. Safety and effectiveness in pediatric patients have not been established.

ADVERSE REACTIONS

No allergic sensitivity or toxic reactions have been noted in clinical use when used as directed. However, one case of systemic manifestations of hypersensitivity to collagenase in a patient treated for more than one year with a combination of collagenase and cortisone has been reported.

OVERDOSAGE

Action of the enzyme may be stopped, should this be desired, by the application of Burow's solution USP (pH 3.6–4.4) to the lesion.

DOSAGE AND ADMINISTRATION

Santyll Ointment should be applied once daily (or more frequently if the dressing becomes soiled, as from incontinence) in the following manner:

(1) Prior to application the lesion should be cleansed of debris and digested material by gently rubbing with a gauze pad saturated with hydrogen peroxide or Dakin's solution followed by sterile normal saline.
(2) Whenever infection is present it is desirable to use an appropriate topical antibiotic powder. The antibiotic should be applied to the lesion prior to the application of Santyll Ointment. Should the infection not respond, therapy with Santyll Ointment should be discontinued until remission of the infection.
(3) Santyll Ointment should be applied directly to deep lesions with a wooden tongue depressor or spatula. For shallow lesions, Santyll Ointment may be applied to a sterile gauze pad which is then applied to the wound and properly secured.
(4) Crosshatching thick eschar with a #10 blade allows collagenase more surface contact with necrotic debris. It is also desirable to remove, with forceps and scissors, as much loosened detritus as can be done readily.
(5) All excess ointment should be removed each time dressing is changed.
(6) Use of Santyll Ointment should be terminated when debridement of necrotic tissue is complete and granulation tissue is well established.

HOW SUPPLIED

Santyll Ointment contains 250 units of collagenase enzyme per gram of white petrolatum USP. The potency assay of collagenase is based on the digestion of undenatured collagen (from bovine Achilles tendon) at pH 7.2 and 37°C for 24 hours. The number of peptide bonds cleaved are measured by reaction with ninhydrin. Amino groups released by a trypsin digestion control are subtracted. One net collagenase unit will solubilize ninhydrin reactive material equivalent to 4 micromoles of leucine.
Collagenase Santyll Ointment 15g
NDC# 0044-5270-02
Collagenase Santyll Ointment 30g
NDC# 0044-5270-03

REFERENCES

1—Mandl, I., Adv. Enzymol. 23:163, 1961.
2—Boxer, A.M., Gottesman, N., Bernstein, H., Mandl, I., Geriatrics 24:75, 1969.
3—Mazurek, I., Med. Welt 22:150, 1971.
4—Zimmerman, W.E., in "Collagenase," I., Mandl, ed., Gordon & Breach, Science Publishers, New York, 1971, p. 131, p. 185.
5—Vetra, H., & Whittaker, D., Geriatrics 30:53, 1975.
6—Rao, D.B., Sane, P.G., & Georgiev, E.L., J. Am. Geriatrics Soc. 23:22, 1975.
7—Vrabec, R., Moserova, J., Konickova, Z., Behounkova, E., & Blaha, J., J. Hyg. Epidemiol. Microbiol. Immunol. 18:496, 1974.
8—Lippmann, H.I., Arch. Phys. Med. Rehabil. 54:588, 1973.
9—German, F.M., in "Collagenase," I., Mandl, ed., Gordon & Breach, Science Publishers, New York, 1971, p. 165.
10—Haimovici, H. & Strauch, B., in "Collagenase," I. Mandl, ed., Gordon & Breach, Science Publishers, New York, 1971, p. 177.
11—Lee, L.K., & Ambrus, J.L., Geriatrics 30:91, 1975.
12—Locke, R.K., & Heifitz, N.M., J. Am. Pod. Assoc. 65:242, 1975.
13—Varma, A.O., Bugatch, E., & German, F.M., Surg. Gynecol. Obstet. 136:281, 1973.
14—Barrett, D., Jr., & Klibanski, A., Am. J. Nurs. 73:849, 1973.
15—Bardfeld, L.A., J. Pod. Ed. 1:41, 1970.
16—Blum, G., Schweiz. Rundschau Med. Praxis 62:820, 1973. Abstr. in Dermatology Digest, Feb. 1974, p. 36.
17—Zaruba, F., Lettl, A., Brozkova, L., Skrdlantova, H., & Krs, V., J. Hyg. Epidemiol. Microbiol. Immunol. 18:499, 1974.
18—Altman, M.I., Goldstein, L., Horwitz, S., J. Am. Pod. Assoc. 68:11, 1978.
19—Rehn, V.J., Med. Klin. 58:799, 1963.
20—Krauss, H., Koslowski, L., & Zimmermann, W.E., Langenbecks Arch. Klin. Chir. 303:23, 1963.
21—Gruenagel, H.H., Med. Klin. 58:442, 1963.

Manufactured by
ADVANCE BIOFACTURES CORPORATION
A Subsidiary of
BIOSPECIFICS TECHNOLOGIES CORP.
35 Wilbur Street
Lynbrook, New York 11563
Distributed by
KNOLL LABORATORIES
A Division of
Knoll Pharmaceutical Company
3000 Continental Drive - North
Mount Olive, NJ 07828
©1997 Knoll Pharmaceutical Company
SANTYL is a registered trademark of Knoll Pharmaceutical Company
Revised: July 1997 0900020-3
Shown in Product Identification Guide, page 318

DILAUDID® Ⓒ℞

[*dī "law 'dĭd*]

hydromorphone hydrochloride

DESCRIPTION

DILAUDID (hydromorphone hydrochloride) (**WARNING**: May be habit forming), a hydrogenated ketone of morphine, is a narcotic analgesic. It is available in:

Ampules (for parenteral administration) containing:

1 mg, 2 mg, and 4 mg hydromorphone hydrochloride per mL with 0.2% sodium citrate, 0.2% citric acid solution. DILAUDID ampules are sterile.

Multiple Dose Vials (for parenteral administration) containing:

20 mL of solution. Each mL contains 2 mg hydromorphone hydrochloride and 0.5 mg edetate disodium with 1.8 mg methylparaben and 0.2 mg propylparaben as preservatives. Sodium hydroxide or hydrochloric acid is used for pH adjustment. DILAUDID multiple dose vials are sterile.

Color Coded Tablets (for oral administration) containing:

2 mg hydromorphone hydrochloride (orange tablet) and D&C red #30 Lake dye, D&C yellow #10 Lake dye, lactose, and magnesium stearate.

4 mg hydromorphone hydrochloride (yellow tablet) and D&C yellow #10 Lake dye, lactose, and magnesium stearate.

Suppositories (for rectal administration) containing:

3 mg hydromorphone hydrochloride in a cocoa butter base with silicon dioxide.

Non-Sterile Powder (for prescription compounding) containing hydromorphone hydrochloride. The structural formula of DILAUDID (hydromorphone hydrochloride) is:

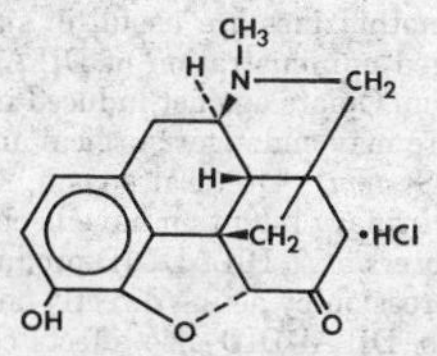

M.W. 321.8

CLINICAL PHARMACOLOGY

DILAUDID is a narcotic analgesic; its principal therapeutic effect is relief of pain. The precise mechanism of action of DILAUDID and other opiates is not known, although it is believed to relate to the existence of opiate receptors in the central nervous system. There is no intrinsic limit to the analgesic effect of DILAUDID; like morphine, adequate doses will relieve even the most severe pain. Clinically, however, dosage limitations are imposed by the adverse effects, primarily respiratory depression, nausea, and vomiting, which can result from high doses.

DILAUDID has diverse additional actions. It may produce drowsiness, changes in mood and mental clouding, depress the respiratory center and the cough center, stimulate the vomiting center, produce pinpoint constriction of the pupil, enhance parasympathetic activity, elevate cerebrospinal fluid pressure, increase biliary pressure, produce transient hyperglycemia.

Generally, the analgesic action of parenterally administered DILAUDID is apparent within 15 minutes and usually remains in effect for more than five hours. The onset of action of oral DILAUDID is somewhat slower, with measurable analgesia occurring within 30 minutes.

In human plasma the half-life of a DILAUDID 4 mg tablet is 2.6 hours. In a random crossover study in six subjects, 4 mg of oral DILAUDID produced a mean concentration/time curve similar to that of 2 mg DILAUDID I.V., after the first hour.

INDICATIONS AND USAGE

DILAUDID is indicatd for the relief of moderate to severe pain such as that due to:

- Surgery
- Cancer
- Trauma (soft tissue & bone)
- Biliary Colic
- Myocardial Infarction
- Burns
- Renal Colic

CONTRAINDICATIONS

DILAUDID is contraindicated in patients with a known hypersensitivity to hydromorphone; in the presence of an intracranial lesion associated with increased intracranial pressure; and whenever ventilatory function is depressed (chronic obstructive pulmonary disease, cor pulmonale, emphysema, kyphoscoliosis, status asthmaticus).

WARNINGS

Respiratory Depression: DILAUDID produces dose-related respiratory depression by acting directly on brain stem respiratory centers. DILAUDID also affects centers that control respiratory rhythm, and may produce irregular and periodic breathing.

Head Injury and Increased Intracranial Pressure: The respiratory depressant effects of narcotics and their capacity to elevate cerebrospinal fluid pressure may be markedly exaggerated in the presence of head injury, other intracranial lesions or a preexisting increase in intracranial pressure. Furthermore, narcotics produce effects which may obscure the clinical course of patients with head injuries.

Acute Abdominal Conditions: The administration of narcotics may obscure the diagnosis or clinical course of patients with acute abdominal conditions.

PRECAUTIONS

Special Risk Patients: DILAUDID should be used with caution in elderly or debilitated patients and those with impaired renal or hepatic function, hypothyroidism, Addison's disease, prostatic hypertrophy or urethral stricture. As with any narcotic analgesic agent, the usual precautions should be observed and the possibility of respiratory depression should be kept in mind.

Cough Reflex: DILAUDID suppresses the cough reflex; as with all narcotics, caution should be exercised when DILAUDID is used postoperatively and in patients with pulmonary disease.

Usage in Ambulatory Patients: Narcotics may impair the mental and/or physical abilities required for the performance of potentially hazardous tasks such as driving a car or operating machinery; patients should be cautioned accordingly

Drug Interactions: Patients receiving other narcotic analgesics, general anesthetics, phenothiazines, tranquilizers, sedative hypnotics, tricyclic antidepressants or other CNS depressants (including alcohol) concomitantly with DILAUDID may exhibit an additive CNS depression. When such combined therapy is contemplated, the dose of one or both agents should be reduced.

Parenteral Administration: The parenteral form of DILAUDID may be given intravenously, but the injection should be given very slowly. Rapid intravenous injection of narcotic analgesics increases the possibility of side effects such as hypotension and respiratory depression.

Pregnancy: Pregnancy Category C. DILAUDID has been shown to be teratogenic in hamsters when given in doses 600 times the human dose. There are no adequate and well-controlled studies in pregnant women. DILAUDID should be used during pregnancy only if the potential benefit justifies the potential risk to the fetus.

Nonteratogenic effects: Babies born to mothers who have been taking opioids regularly prior to delivery will be physically dependent. The withdrawal signs include irritability and excessive crying, tremors, hyperactive reflexes, increased respiratory rate, increased stools, sneezing, yawning, vomiting, and fever. The intensity of the syndrome does not always correlate with the duration of maternal opioid use or dose. There is no consensus on the best method of managing withdrawal. Chlorpromazine 0.7 to 1.0 mg/kg q6h, phenobarbital 2 mg/kg q6h, and paregoric 2 to 4 drops/kg q4h, have been used to treat withdrawal symptoms in infants. The duration of therapy is 4 to 28 days, with the dosages decreased as tolerated.

Labor and Delivery: As with all narcotics, administration of DILAUDID to the mother shortly before delivery may result in some degree of respiratory depression in the newborn, especially if higher doses are used.

Nursing Mothers: It is not known whether this drug is excreted in human milk. Because many drugs are excreted in human milk and because of the potential for serious adverse reactions in nursing infants from DILAUDID, a decision should be made whether to discontinue nursing or to discontinue the drug, taking into account the importance of the drug to the mother.

Pediatric Use: Safety and effectiveness in children have not been established.

ADVERSE REACTIONS

Central Nervous System: Sedation, drowsiness, mental clouding, lethargy, impairment of mental and physical performance, anxiety, fear, dysphoria, dizziness, psychic dependence, mood changes.

Gastrointestinal System: Nausea and vomiting occur infrequently; they are more frequent in ambulatory than in recumbent patients. The antiemetic phenothiazines are useful in suppressing these effects; however, some phenothiazine derivatives seem to be antianalgesic and to increase the amount of narcotic required to produce pain relief, while other phenothiazines reduce the amount of narcotic required to produce a given level of analgesia. Prolonged administration of DILAUDID may produce constipation. Opiate agonist-induced increase in intraluminal pressure may endanger surgical anastomosis.

Cardiovascular System: Circulatory depression, peripheral circulatory collapse and cardiac arrest have occurred after rapid intravenous injection Orthostatic hypotension and fainting may occur if a patient stands up suddenly after receiving an injection of DILAUDID.

Genitourinary System: Ureteral spasm, spasm of vesical sphincters and urinary retention have been reported.

Respiratory Depression: DILAUDID produces dose-related respiratory depression by acting directly on brain stem respiratory centers. DILAUDID also affects centers that control respiratory rhythm, and may produce irregular and periodic breathing. If significant respiratory depression occurs, it may be antagonized by the use of naloxone hydrochloride. The usual adult dose of 0.4 to 0.8 mg given *intramuscularly or intravenously*, promptly reverses the effects of morphine-like opioid agonists such as DILAUDID. In patients who are physically dependent, small doses of naloxone may be sufficient not only to antagonize respiratory depression, but also to precipitate withdrawal phenomena. The dose of naloxone should therefore be adjusted accordingly in such patients. Since the duration of action of DILAUDID may exceed that of the antagonist, the patient should be kept under continued surveillance, repeated doses of the antagonist may be required to maintain adequate respiration. Apply other supportive measures when indicated.

DRUG ABUSE AND DEPENDENCE

DILAUDID is a Schedule II narcotic. Psychic dependence, physical dependence, and tolerance may develop upon repeated administration of narcotics; therefore DILAUDID should be prescribed and administered with caution. However, psychic dependence is unlikely to develop when DILAUDID is used for a short time for the treatment of pain. Physical dependence, the condition in which continued administration of the drug is required to prevent the appearance of a withdrawal syndrome, usually assumes clinically significant proportions only after several weeks of continued narcotic use, although some mild degree of physical dependence may develop after a few days of narcotic therapy. Tolerance, in which increasingly large doses are required in order to produce the same degree of analgesia, is manifested initially by a shortened duration of analgesic effect, and subsequently by decreases in the intensity of analgesia. The rate of development of tolerance varies among patients.

OVERDOSAGE

Signs and Symptoms: Serious overdosage with DILAUDID is characterized by respiratory depression (a decrease in respiratory rate and/or tidal volume. Cheyne-Stokes respiration, cyanosis), extreme somnolence progressing to stupor or coma, skeletal muscle flaccidity, cold and clammy skin, and sometimes bradycardia and hypotension. In severe overdosage, particularly by the intravenous route, apnea, circulatory collapse, cardiac arrest, and death may occur.

Treatment: Primary attention should be given to the reestablishment of adequate respiratory exchange through provision of a patient airway and institution of assisted or controlled ventilation. The narcotic antagonist naloxone hydrochloride is a specific antidote against respiratory depression which may result from overdosage or unusual sensitivity to narcotics, including DILAUDID. Therefore, naloxone hydrochloride should be administered as described under *Adverse Reactions* (see *Respiratory Depression)* in conjunction with ventilatory assistance.

Since the duration of action of DILAUDID may exceed that of the antagonist, the patient should be kept under continued surveillance; repeated doses of the antagonist may be required to maintain adequate respiration. An antagonist should not be administered in the absence of clinically significant respiratory or cardiovascular depression. Oxygen, intravenous fluids vasopressors, and other supportive measures should be employed as indicated.

In cases of overdosage with oral DILAUDID, gastric lavage or induced emesis may be useful in removing unabsorbed drug from conscious patients.

DOSAGE AND ADMINISTRATION

Parenteral: The usual starting dose is 1–2 mg *subcutaneously* or *intramuscularly* every 4 to 6 hours as necessary for pain control. The dose should be adjusted according to the severity of pain, as well as the patient's underlying disease, age, and size. Patients with terminal cancer may be tolerant to narcotic analgesics and may, therefore, require higher doses for adequate pain relief. Intravenous or subcutaneous administration is usually not painful. Should intravenous administration be necessary, the injection should be given ***slowly***, over at least 2 to 3 minutes, depending on the dose. A gradual increase in dose may be required if analgesia is inadequate, tolerance occurs, or if pain severity increases. The first sign of tolerance is usually a reduced duration of effect.

NOTE: Parenteral drug products should be inspected visually for particulate matter and discoloration prior to administration, whenever solution and container permit. A slight yellowish discoloration may develop in DILAUDID ampules and multiple dose vials. No loss of potency has been demonstrated.

Oral: The usual oral dose is 2 mg every 4 to 6 hours as necessary. The dose must be individually adjusted according

Continued on next page

Dilaudid—Cont.

to severity of pain, patient response and patient size. More severe pain may require 4 mg or more every 4 to 6 hours. If the pain increases in severity, analgesia is not adequate or tolerance occurs, a gradual increase in dosage may be required. If pain is exceedingly severe, or if prompt response is desired, parenteral DILAUDID should be used initially in adequate amounts to control the pain.

Rectal: DILAUDID suppositories (3 mg) may provide longer duration of relief which could obviate additional medication during the sleeping hours. The usual adult dose is one (1) suppository inserted rectally every 6 to 8 hours or as directed by physician.

HOW SUPPLIED

Ampules: (One mL sterile solution for parenteral administration)

1 mg/mL ampules–Boxes of 10–
NDC #0044-1011-01.

2 mg/mL ampules–Boxes of 10–
NDC #0044-1012-01.
Boxes of 25-NDC #0044-1012-09.

4 mg/mL ampules–Boxes of 10–
NDC #0044-1014-01.

Multiple Dose Vials: (20 mL sterile solution for parenteral administration)

2 mg/mL–20 mL multiple dose vials-
NDC #0044-1062-05.

Oral Color Coded Tablets: (NOT FOR INJECTION)

2 mg tablet (orange)–Bottles of 100–
NDC #0044-1022-02.
Unit Dose of 100 (4×25)–
NDC #0044-1022-45.
Bottles of 500–NDC #0044-1022-03.

4 mg tablet (yellow)–Bottles of 100–
NDC #0044-1024-02.
Unit Dose of 100 (4×25)-
NDC #0044-1024-45.
Bottles of 500–NDC #0044-1024-03.

Rectal Suppositories: 3 mg suppositories-Boxes of 6–
NDC #0044-1053-01.

Non-Sterile Powder: For prescription compounding.
15 grain vial-NDC #0044-1040-01.

Storage: Parenteral and oral dosages of DILAUDID should be stored at 15°–30°C (59°–86°F). Protect from light. DILAUDID suppositories should be stored in a refrigerator. A Schedule Ⓒ Narcotic. DEA order form required.

© 1996 Knoll Pharmaceutical Company.
DILAUDID is a registered trademark of Knoll Pharmaceutical Company.

Revised: August 1996

Parenteral Products Manufactured for
Knoll Laboratories
A Division of Knoll Pharmaceutical Company
By Sanofi Winthrop, Inc.
McPherson, KS 67460

BASF Pharma

0900003A–2
Shown in Product Identification Guide, page 318

DILAUDID® COUGH SYRUP   Ⓒ ℞
[dĭ "law 'dĭd]
hydromorphone hydrochloride

DESCRIPTION

Each 5 mL (1 teaspoonful) contains 1 mg DILAUDID (hydromorphone hydrochloride) (WARNING: May be habit forming), and 100 mg guaifenesin in a peach-flavored syrup containing 5% alcohol. DILAUDID is a hydrogenated ketone of morphine; it is a narcotic analgesic and antitussive. The structural formula of DILAUDID (hydromorphone hydrochloride) is:

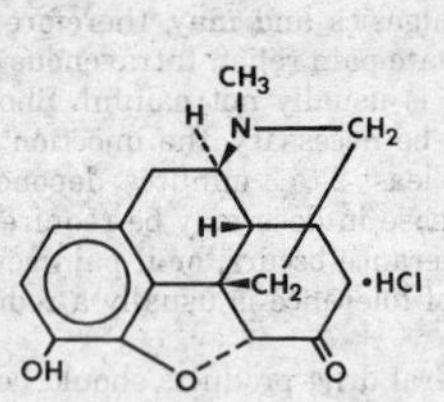

M.W. 321.8

CLINICAL PHARMACOLOGY

DILAUDID (hydromorphone hydrochloride) is a centrally acting narcotic antitussive which acts directly on the cough reflex center.

DILAUDID is also a narcotic analgesic; its principal therapeutic effect is relief of pain. The precise mechanism of action of DILAUDID and other opiates is not known, although it is believed to relate to the existence of opiate receptors in the central nervous system. There is no intrinsic limit to the analgesic effect of DILAUDID; like morphine, adequate doses will relieve even the most severe pain. Clinically, however, dosage limitations are imposed by the adverse effects, primarily respiratory depression, nausea, and vomiting, which can result from high doses.

DILAUDID has diverse additional actions. It produces drowsiness, changes in mood and mental clouding, depresses the respiratory center and the cough center, stimulates the vomiting center, produces pinpoint constriction of the pupil, enhances parasympathetic activity, elevates cerebrospinal fluid pressure, increases biliary pressure, produces transient hyperglycemia.

Generally, the analgesic action of parenterally administered DILAUDID is apparent within 15 minutes and usually remains in effect for more than five hours. The onset of action of oral DILAUDID is somewhat slower, with measurable analgesia occurring within 30 minutes.

Radioimmunoassay techniques have recently been developed for the analysis of DILAUDID in human plasma. In humans the half-life of a DILAUDID 4 mg tablet is 2.6 hours. In a random crossover study in six subjects, 4 mg of oral DILAUDID produced a mean concentration/time curve similar to that of 2 mg DILAUDID I.V., after the first hour. Guaifenesin (glyceryl guaiacolate) reduces the viscosity of secretions, thereby increasing the efficiency of the cough reflex and of ciliary action in removing accumulated secretions from the trachea and bronchi. Unlike many other expectorants, guaifenesin rarely causes gastric irritation.

INDICATIONS AND USAGE

DILAUDID Cough Syrup is indicated for the control of persistent, exhausting cough or dry, non-productive cough.

CONTRAINDICATIONS

DILAUDID Cough Syrup is contraindicated in patients known to have a hypersensitivity to hydromorphone; in the presence of an intracranial lesion associated with increased intracranial pressure; and whenever ventilatory function is depressed (chronic obstructive pulmonary disease, cor pulmonale, emphysema, kyphoscoliosis, status asthmaticus).

WARNINGS

Respiratory Depression: DILAUDID produces dose-related respiratory depression by acting directly on brain stem respiratory centers. DILAUDID also affects centers that control respiratory rhythm, and may produce irregular and periodic breathing.

Head Injury and Increased Intracranial Pressure: The respiratory depressant effects of narcotics and their capacity to elevate cerebrospinal fluid pressure may be markedly exaggerated in the presence of head injury, other intracranial lesions or a preexisting increase in intracranial pressure. Furthermore, narcotics produce adverse effects which may obscure the clinical course of patients with head injuries.

Acute Abdominal Conditions: The administration of narcotics may obscure the diagnosis or clinical course of patients with acute abdominal conditions.

PRECAUTIONS

Special Risk Patients: DILAUDID Cough Syrup should be used with caution in elderly or debilitated patients and those with impaired renal or hepatic function, hypothyroidism, Addison's disease, prostatic hypertrophy or urethral stricture. As with any narcotic analgesic agent, the usual precautions should be observed and the possibility of respiratory depression should be kept in mind.

Cough Reflex: DILAUDID Cough Syrup suppresses the cough reflex; as with all narcotics, caution should be exercised when DILAUDID Cough Syrup is used postoperatively and in patients with pulmonary disease.

Usage in Ambulatory Patients: Narcotics may impair the mental and/or physical abilities required for the performance of potentially hazardous tasks such as driving a car or operating machinery; patients should be cautioned accordingly.

Drug Interactions: Patients receiving other narcotic analgesics, general anesthetics, phenothiazines, tranquilizers, sedative-hypnotics, tricyclic antidepressants or other CNS depressants (including alcohol) concomitantly with DILAUDID Cough Syrup may exhibit an additive CNS depression. When such combined therapy is contemplated, the dose of one or both agents should be reduced.

Usage in Pregnancy: Pregnancy Category C. DILAUDID has been shown to be teratogenic in hamsters when given in doses 600 times the human dose. There are no adequate and well-controlled studies in pregnant women. DILAUDID Cough Syrup should be used during pregnancy only if the potential benefit justifies the potential risk to the fetus.

Nonteratogenic effects: Babies born to mothers who have been taking opioids regularly prior to delivery will be physically dependent. The withdrawal signs include irritability and excessive crying, tremors, hyperactive reflexes, increased respiratory rate, increased stools, sneezing, yawning, vomiting, and fever. The intensity of the syndrome does not always correlate with the duration of maternal opioid use or dose. There is no consensus on the best method of managing withdrawal. Chlorpromazine 0.7 to 1.0 mg/kg q6h, phenobarbital 2 mg/kg q6h, and paregoric 2 to 4 drops/kg q4h, have been used to treat withdrawal symptoms in infants. The duration of therapy is 4 to 28 days, with the dosage decreased as tolerated.

Labor and Delivery: As with all narcotics, administration of DILAUDID Cough Syrup to the mother shortly before delivery may result in some degree of respiratory depression in the newborn, especially if higher doses are used.

Nursing Mothers: It is not known whether this drug is excreted in human milk. Because many drugs are excreted in human milk and because of the potential for serious adverse reactions in nursing infants from DILAUDID Cough Syrup, a decision should be made whether to discontinue nursing or to discontinue the drug, taking into account the importance of the drug to the mother.

Pediatric Use: Safety and effectiveness in children have not been established.

FD&C Yellow No. 5: DILAUDID Cough Syrup contains FD&C Yellow No. 5 (tartrazine) dye which may cause allergic-type reactions (including bronchial asthma) in certain susceptible individuals. Although the overall incidence of FD&C Yellow No. 5 (tartrazine) dye sensitivity in the general population is low, it is frequently seen in patients who also have aspirin hypersensitivity.

ADVERSE REACTIONS

Central Nervous System: Sedation, drowsiness, mental clouding, lethargy, impairment of mental and physical performance, anxiety, fear, dysphoria, dizziness, psychic dependence, mood changes.

Gastrointestinal System: Nausea and vomiting occur more frequently in ambulatory than in recumbent patients. The antiemetic phenothiazines are useful in suppressing these effects. Prolonged administration of DILAUDID may produce constipation. Opiate agonist-induced increase in intraluminal pressure may endanger surgical anastomosis.

Genitourinary System: Ureteral spasm, spasm of vesical sphincters and urinary retention have been reported.

Respiratory Depression: DILAUDID produces dose-related respiratory depression by acting directly on brain stem respiratory centers. DILAUDID also affects centers that control respiratory rhythm, and may produce irregular and periodic breathing. If significant respiratory depression occurs, it may be antagonized by the use of naloxone hydrochloride. The usual adult dose of 0.4 to 0.8 mg given intramuscularly or intravenously, promptly reverses the effects of morphine-like opioid agonists such as DILAUDID. In patients who are physically dependent, small doses of naloxone may be sufficient not only to antagonize respiratory depression, but also to precipitate withdrawal phenomena. The dose of naloxone should therefore be adjusted accordingly in such patients. Since the duration of action of DILAUDID may exceed that of the antagonist, the patient should be kept under continued surveillance; repeated doses of the antagonist may be required to maintain adequate respiration. Apply other supportive measures when indicated.

DRUG ABUSE AND DEPENDENCE

DILAUDID is a Schedule Ⓒ narcotic. Psychic dependence, physical dependence, and tolerance may develop upon repeated administration of narcotics; therefore, DILAUDID should be prescribed and administered with caution. However, psychic dependence is unlikely to develop when DILAUDID Cough Syrup is used for a short time as indicated. Physical dependence, the condition in which continued administration of the drug is required to prevent the appearance of a withdrawal syndrome, usually assumes clinically significant proportions only after several weeks of continued narcotic use, although some mild degree of physical dependence may develop after few days of narcotic therapy.

OVERDOSAGE

Signs and Symptoms: Serious overdosage with DILAUDID is characterized by respiratory depression (a decrease in respiratory rate and/or tidal volume, Cheyne-Stokes respiration, cyanosis), extreme somnolence progressing to stupor or coma, skeletal muscle flaccidity, cold and clammy skin, and sometimes bradycardia and hypotension. In severe overdosage, particularly by the intravenous route, apnea, circulatory collapse, cardiac arrest, and death may occur.

Treatment: Primary attention should be given to the reestablishment of adequate respiratory exchange through provision of a patent airway and institution of assisted or controlled ventilation. The narcotic antagonist naloxone hydrochloride is a specific antidote against respiratory depression which may result from overdosage or unusual sensitivity to narcotics, including DILAUDID. Therefore, naloxone hydrochloride should be administered as described under ADVERSE REACTIONS (see Respiratory Depression) in conjunction with ventilatory assistance.

Since the duration of action of DILAUDID may exceed that of the antagonist, the patient should be kept under continued surveillance; repeated doses of the antagonist may be

required to maintain adequate respiration. An antagonist should not be administered in the absence of clinically significant respiratory or cardiovascular depression. Oxygen, intravenous fluids, vasopressors, and other supportive measures should be employed as indicated.

In cases of overdosage with oral DILAUDID, gastric lavage or induced emesis may be useful in removing unabsorbed drug from conscious patients.

DOSAGE AND ADMINISTRATION

The usual adult dose of DILAUDID Cough Syrup is one teaspoonful (5 mL) every 3 to 4 hours.

HOW SUPPLIED

Bottles of 1 pint (473 mL)—NDC #0044-1080-01.
Storage: Store at 15°–30°C (59°–86°F).
DEA order form required
A Schedule ⓒII Narcotic.
Knoll Laboratories
A Division of
Knoll Pharmaceutical Company
Mt. Olive, NJ 07828
BASF Pharma 0900013-1

DILAUDID–HP® INJECTION ⓒII

[*dī "law 'dĭd*]
10mg/mL
hydromorphone hydrochloride

WARNING: DILAUDID-HP® (HIGH POTENCY) IS A HIGHLY CONCENTRATED SOLUTION OF HYDROMORPHONE INTENDED FOR USE IN NARCOTIC-TOLERANT PATIENTS. DO NOT CONFUSE DILAUDID-HP WITH STANDARD PARENTERAL FORMULATIONS OF DILAUDID OR OTHER NARCOTICS. OVERDOSE AND DEATH COULD RESULT.

DESCRIPTION

DILAUDID (hydromorphone hydrochloride) (WARNING: May be habit forming), a hydrogenated ketone of morphine, is a narcotic analgesic. HIGH POTENCY DILAUDID is available in AMBER ampules or single dose vials for intravenous (IV), subcutaneous (SC), or intramuscular (IM) administration. Each 1 mL of sterile solution contains 10 mg hydromorphone hydrochloride with 0.2% sodium citrate, and 0.2% citric acid solution.

It is also available as lyophilized Dilaudid for intravenous (IV), subcutaneous (SC), or intramuscular (IM) administration. Each single dose vial contains 250mg sterile, lyophilized hydromorphone HCl to be reconstituted with 25mL of Sterile Water for Injection USP to provide a solution containing 10mg/mL.

The structural formula of DILAUDID (hydromorphone hydrochloride) is:

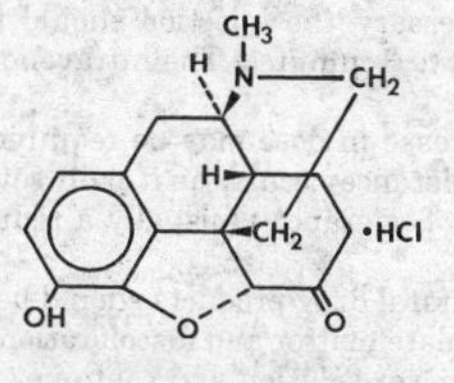

MW 321.8

CLINICAL PHARMACOLOGY

Many of the effects described below are common to the class of narcotic analgesics. In some instances, data may not exist to demonstrate that DILAUDID-HP possesses similar or different effects than those observed with other narcotic analgesics. However, in the absence of data to the contrary, it is assumed that DILAUDID-HP would possess these effects.

Central Nervous System: Narcotic analgesics have multiple actions but exert their primary effects on the central nervous system and organs containing smooth muscle. The principal actions of therapeutic value are analgesia and sedation. A significant feature of the analgesia is that it occurs without loss of consciousness. Narcotic analgesics also suppress the cough reflex and cause respiratory depression, mood changes, mental clouding, euphoria, dysphoria, nausea, vomiting and electroencephalographic changes. The precise mode of analgesic action of narcotic analgesics is unknown. However, specific CNS opiate receptors have been identified. Narcotics are believed to express their pharmacological effects by combining with these receptors.

Narcotics depress the cough reflex by direct effect on the cough center in the medulla.

Narcotics produce respiratory depression by direct effect on brain stem respiratory centers. The mechanism of respiratory depression also involves a reduction in the responsiveness of the brain stem respiratory centers to increases in carbon dioxide tension.

Narcotics cause miosis. Pinpoint pupils are a common sign of narcotic overdose but are not pathognomonic (e.g., pontine lesions of hemorrhagic or ischemic origin may produce similar findings) and marked mydriasis occurs when asphyxia intervenes.

Gastrointestinal Tract and Other Smooth Muscle: Gastric, biliary and pancreatic secretions are decreased by narcotics. Narcotics cause a reduction in motility associated with an increase in tone in the antrum portion of the stomach and duodenum. Digestion of food in the small intestine is delayed and propulsive contractions are decreased. Propulsive peristaltic waves in the colon are decreased, and tone may be increased to the point of spasm. The end result is constipation. Narcotics can cause a marked increase in biliary tract pressure as a result of spasm of the sphincter of Oddi.

Cardiovascular System: Certain narcotics produce peripheral vasodilation which may result in orthostatic hypotension. Release of histamine may occur with narcotics and may contribute to narcotic-induced hypotension. Other manifestations of histamine release and/or peripheral vasodilation may include pruritis, flushing, and red eyes.

Effects on the myocardium after i.v. administration of narcotics are not significant in normal persons, vary with different narcotic analgesic agents and vary with the hemodynamic state of the patient, state of hydration and sympathetic drive.

Pharmacokinetics: In normal human volunteers hydromorphone is metabolized primarily in the liver. It is excreted primarily as the glucuronidated conjugate, with small amounts of parent drug and minor amounts of 6-hydroxy reduction metabolites.

Following intravenous administration of DILAUDID to normal volunteers, the mean half-life of elimination was 2.64 ± 0.88 hours. The mean volume of distribution was 91.5 liters, suggesting extensive tissue uptake. DILAUDID is rapidly removed from the blood stream and distributed to skeletal muscle, kidneys, liver, intestinal tract, lungs, spleen and brain. DILAUDID also crosses the placental membranes.

In terms of area under the analgesic time-effect curve, hydromorphone is approximately 8 times more potent than morphine (i.e., 1.3 mg of hydromorphone produces analgesia equal to that produced by 10 mg of morphine). After intramuscular administration, hydromorphone has a slightly more rapid onset and slightly shorter duration of action than morphine. The duration of DILAUDID analgesia in the non-tolerant patient with usual doses may be up to 4–5 hours. However, in tolerant subjects, duration will vary substantially depending on tolerance and dose. Dose should be adjusted so that 3–4 hours of pain relief may be achieved.

INDICATIONS AND USAGE

DILAUDID-HP is indicated for the relief of moderate-to-severe pain in narcotic-tolerant patients who require larger than usual doses of narcotics to provide adequate pain relief. Because DILAUDID-HP contains 10 mg of hydromorphone per mL, a smaller injection volume can be used than with other parenteral narcotic formulations. Discomfort associated with the intramuscular or subcutaneous injection of an unusually large volume of solution can therefore be avoided.

CONTRAINDICATIONS

DILAUDID-HP is contraindicated in: patients who are not already receiving large amounts of parenteral narcotics, patients with known hypersensitivity to the drug, patients with respiratory depression in the absence of resuscitative equipment, and in patients with status asthmaticus. DILAUDID-HP is also contraindicated for use in obstetrical analgesia.

WARNINGS—DRUG DEPENDENCE

DILAUDID-HP can produce drug dependence of the morphine type and therefore has the potential for being abused. Psychic dependence, physical dependence and tolerance may develop upon repeated administration of DILAUDID-HP, and it should be prescribed and administered with the same degree of caution appropriate for the use of morphine. Since DILAUDID-HP is indicated for use in patients who are already tolerant to and hence physically dependent on narcotics, abrupt discontinuance in the administration of DILAUDID-HP is likely to result in a withdrawal syndrome. (See **Drug Abuse and Dependence**).

Infants born to mothers physically dependent on DILAUDID-HP will also be physically dependent and may exhibit respiratory difficulties and withdrawal symptoms (See **Drug Abuse and Dependence**).

Impaired Respiration: Respiratory depression is the chief hazard of DILAUDID-HP. Respiratory depression occurs most frequently in the elderly, in the debilitated, and in those suffering from conditions accompanied by hypoxia or hypercapnia when even moderate therapeutic doses may dangerously decrease pulmonary ventilation.

DILAUDID-HP should be used with extreme caution in patients with chronic obstructive pulmonary disease or cor pulmonale, patients having a substantially decreased respiratory reserve, hypoxia, hypercapnia, or preexisting respiratory depression. In such patients even usual therapeutic doses of narcotic analgesics may decrease respiratory drive while simultaneously increasing airway resistance to the point of apnea.

Head Injury and Increased Intracranial Pressure: The respiratory depressant effects of DILAUDID-HP with carbon dioxide retention and secondary elevation of cerebrospinal fluid pressure may be markedly exaggerated in the presence of head injury, other intracranial lesions, or preexisting increase in intracranial pressure. Narcotic analgesics including DILAUDID-HP may produce effects which can obscure the clinical course and neurologic signs of further increase in pressure in patients with head injuries.

Hypotensive Effect: Narcotic analgesics, including DILAUDID-HP, may cause severe hypotension in an individual whose ability to maintain his blood pressure has already been compromised by a depleted blood volume, or a concurrent administration of drugs such as phenothiazines or general anesthetics (see also **Precautions —Drug Interactions**). DILAUDID-HP may produce orthostatic hypotension in ambulatory patients.

DILAUDID-HP should be administered with caution to patients in circulatory shock, since vasodilation produced by the drug may further reduce cardiac output and blood pressure.

PRECAUTIONS

General: Because of its high concentration, the delivery of precise doses of DILAUDID-HP may be difficult if low doses of hydromorphone are required. Therefore, DILAUDID-HP should be used only if the amount of hydromorphone required can be delivered accurately with this formulation.

In general, narcotics should be given with caution and the initial dose should be reduced in the elderly or debilitated and those with severe impairment of hepatic, pulmonary or renal function; myxedema or hypothyroidism; adrenocortical insufficiency (e.g., Addison's Disease); CNS depression or coma; toxic psychoses; prostatic hypertrophy or urethral stricture; gall bladder disease; acute alcoholism; delirium tremens; or kyphoscoliosis.

In the case of DILAUDID-HP, however, the patient is presumed to be receiving a narcotic to which he or she exhibits tolerance and the initial dose of DILAUDID-HP selected should be estimated based on the relative potency of hydromorphone and the narcotic previously used by the patient. See **(Dosage and Administration)** section.

The administration of narcotic analgesics including DILAUDID-HP may obscure the diagnosis or clinical course in patients with acute abdominal conditions and may aggravate preexisting convulsions in patients with convulsive disorders.

Narcotic analgesics including DILAUDID-HP should also be used with caution in patients about to undergo surgery of the biliary tract since it may cause spasm of the sphincter of Oddi.

Drug Interactions: The concomitant use of other central nervous system depressants including sedatives or hypnotics, general anesthetics, phenothiazines, tranquilizers and alcohol may produce additive depressant effects. Respiratory depression, hypotension and profound sedation or coma may occur. When such combined therapy is contemplated, the dose of one or both agents should be reduced. Narcotic analgesics, including DILAUDID-HP may enhance the action of neuromuscular blocking agents and produce an increased degree of respiratory depression.

PREGNANCY—CATEGORY C:

Human: Adequate animal studies on reproduction have not been performed to determine whether hydromorphone affects fertility in males or females. There are no well-controlled studies in women. Reports based on marketing experience do not identify any specific teratogenic risks following routine (short-term) clinical use. Although there is no clearly defined risk, such reports do not exclude the possibility of infrequent or subtle damage to the human fetus. DILAUDID-HP should be used in pregnant women only when clearly needed (see ***Labor and Delivery*** and ***Drug Abuse and Dependence***).

Animal: Literature reports of hydromorphone hydrochloride administration to pregnant Syrian hamsters show that DILAUDID is teratogenic at a dose of 20 mg/kg which is 600 times the human dose. A maximal teratogenic effect (50% of fetuses affected) in the Syrian hamster was observed at a dose of 125 mg/kg.

Labor and Delivery: DILAUDID-HP is contraindicated in Labor and Delivery (see **Contraindications** section).

Nursing Mothers: Low levels of narcotic analgesics have been detected in human milk. As a general rule, nursing should not be undertaken while a patient is receiving DILAUDID-HP since it, and other drugs in this class, may be excreted in the milk.

Pediatric Use: Safety and effectiveness in children have not been established.

ADVERSE REACTIONS

The adverse effects of DILAUDID-HP are similar to those of other narcotic analgesics, and represent established phar-

Continued on next page

Dilaudid-HP—Cont.

macological effects of the drug class. The major hazards include respiratory depression and apnea. To a lesser degree, circulatory depression, respiratory arrest, shock and cardiac arrest have occurred.

The most frequently observed adverse effects are lightheadedness, dizziness, sedation, nausea, vomiting, and sweating. These effects seem to be more prominent in ambulatory patients and in those not experiencing severe pain. Some adverse reactions in ambulatory patients may be alleviated if the patient lies down.

Less Frequently Observed with Narcotic Analgesics:

General and CNS: Dysphoria, euphoria, weakness, headache, agitation, tremor, uncoordinated muscle movements, alterations of mood (nervousness, apprehension, depression, floating feelings, dreams), muscle rigidity, paresthesia, muscle tremor, blurred vision, nystagmus, diplopia and miosis, transient hallucinations* and disorientation, visual disturbances, insomnia and increased intracranial pressure may occur.

*Hallucinations, although unusual with pure agonist narcotics, have been observed in one patient following both a 6 mg and a 4 mg DILAUDID-HP dose. However, the patient was receiving several concomitant medications during the second episode and a causal relationship cannot be established.

Cardiovascular: Flushing of the face, chills, tachycardia, bradycardia, palpitation, faintness, syncope, hypotension and hypertension have been reported.

Respiratory: Bronchospasm and laryngospasm have been known to occur.

Gastrointestinal: Dry mouth, constipation, biliary tract spasm, anorexia, diarrhea, cramps and taste alterations have been reported.

Genitourinary: Urinary retention or hesitancy, and antidiuretic effects have been reported.

Dermatologic: Pruritis, urticaria, other skin rashes, wheal and flare over the vein with intravenous injection, and diaphoresis have been reported with narcotic analgesics.

Other: In clinical trials, neither local tissue irritation nor induration was observed at the site of subcutaneous injection of DILAUDID-HP; pain at the injection site was rarely observed. However, local irritation and induration have been seen following parenteral injection of other narcotic drug products.

DRUG ABUSE AND DEPENDENCE

Narcotic analgesics may cause psychological and physical dependence (see ***Warnings***). Physical dependence results in withdrawal symptoms in patients who abruptly discontinue the drug. Withdrawal symptoms also may be precipitated in the patient with physical dependence by the administration of a drug with narcotic antagonist activity, e.g., naloxone (see also ***Overdosage***). Physical dependence usually does not occur to a clinically significant degree until after several weeks of continued narcotic usage. Tolerance, in which increasingly large doses are required in order to produce the same degree of analgesia, is initially manifested by a shortened duration of analgesic effect, and subsequently, by decreases in the intensity of analgesia. In chronic pain patients, and in narcotic-tolerant cancer patients, the dose of DILAUDID-HP should be guided by the degree of tolerance manifested.

In chronic pain patients in whom narcotic analgesics including DILAUDID-HP are abruptly discontinued, a severe abstinence syndrome should be anticipated. This may be similar to the abstinence syndrome noted in patients who withdraw from heroin. The latter abstinence syndrome may be characterized by restlessness, lacrimation, rhinorrhea, yawning, perspiration, gooseflesh, restless sleep or "yen" and mydriasis during the first 24 hours. These symptoms may increase in severity and over the next 72 hours may be accompanied by increasing irritability, anxiety, weakness, twitching and spasms of muscles, kicking movements, severe backache, abdominal and leg pains, abdominal and muscle cramps, hot and cold flashes, insomnia, nausea, anorexia, vomiting, intestinal spasm, diarrhea, coryza and repetitive sneezing, increase in body temperature, blood pressure, respiratory rate and heart rate.

Because of excessive loss of fluids through sweating, or vomiting and diarrhea, there is usually marked weight loss, dehydration, ketosis, and disturbances in acid-base balance. Cardiovascular collapse can occur. Without treatment most observable symptoms disappear in 5–14 days; however, there appears to be a phase of secondary or chronic abstinence which may last for 2–6 months characterized by insomnia, irritability, muscular aches, and autonomic instability.

In the treatment of physical dependence on DILAUDID-HP, the patient may be detoxified by gradual reduction of the dosage, although this is unlikely to be necessary in the terminal cancer patient. If abstinence symptoms become severe, the patient may be given methadone. Temporary administration of tranquilizers and sedatives may aid in reducing patient anxiety. Gastrointestinal disturbances or dehydration should be treated accordingly.

OVERDOSAGE

Serious overdosage with DILAUDID-HP is characterized by respiratory depression, somnolence progressing to stupor or coma, skeletal muscle flaccidity, cold and clammy skin, constricted pupils, and sometimes bradycardia and hypotension. In serious overdosage, particularly following intravenous injection, apnea, circulatory collapse, cardiac arrest and death may occur.

In the treatment of overdosage primary attention should be given to the reestablishment of adequate respiratory exchange through provision of a patent airway and institution of assisted or controlled ventilation.

NARCOTIC-TOLERANT PATIENT: Since tolerance to the respiratory and CNS depressant effects of narcotics develops concomitantly with tolerance to their analgesic effects, serious respiratory depression due to an acute overdose is unlikely to be seen in narcotic-tolerant patients receiving DILAUDID-HP for chronic pain.

NOTE: In such an individual who is physically dependent on narcotics, administration of the usual dose of the antagonist will precipitate an acute withdrawal syndrome. The severity will depend on the degree of physical dependence and the dose of the antagonist administered. Use of a narcotic antagonist in such a person should be avoided. If necessary to treat serious respiratory depression in the physically dependent patient, the antagonist should be administered with extreme care and by titration with smaller than usual doses of the antagonist.

NON-TOLERANT PATIENT: The narcotic antagonist, naloxone, is a specific antidote against respiratory depression which may result from overdosage, or unusual sensitivity to DILAUDID-HP. A dose of naloxone (usually 0.4 to 2.0 mg) should be administered intravenously, if possible, simultaneously with respiratory resuscitation. The dose can be repeated in 3 minutes. Naloxone should not be administered in the absence of clinically significant respiratory or circulatory depression. Naloxone should be administered cautiously to persons who are known, or suspected to be physically dependent on DILAUDID-HP. In such cases, an abrupt or complete reversal of narcotic effects may precipitate an acute abstinence syndrome.

Since the duration of action of DILAUDID-HP may exceed that of the antagonist, the patient should be kept under continued surveillance; repeated doses of the antagonist may be required to maintain adequate respiration. Apply other supportive measures when indicated.

Supportive measures (including oxygen, vasopressors) should be employed in the management of circulatory shock and pulmonary edema accompanying overdose as indicated. Cardiac arrest or arrhythmias may require cardiac massage or defibrillation.

DOSAGE AND ADMINISTRATION

Parenteral: DILAUDID-HP SHOULD BE GIVEN ONLY TO PATIENTS WHO ARE ALREADY RECEIVING LARGE DOSES OF NARCOTICS. DILAUDID-HP is indicated for relief of moderate-to-severe pain in narcotic-tolerant patients. Thus, these patients will already have been treated with other narcotic analgesics. If the patient is being changed from regular DILAUDID to DILAUDID-HP, similar doses should be used, depending on the patient's clinical response to the drug. If DILAUDID-HP is substituted for a different narcotic analgesic, the following equivalency table should be used as a guide to determine the appropriate dose of DILAUDID-HP (hydromorphone hydrochloride).

[See table below]

In open clinical trials with DILAUDID-HP in patients with terminal cancer, doses ranged from 1–14 mg subcutaneously or intramuscularly; one patient received 30 mg subcutaneously on two occasions. In these trials, both subcutaneous and intramuscular injections of DILAUDID-HP were well-tolerated, with minimal pain and/or burning at the injection site. Mild erythema was rarely noted after intramuscular injection. There was no induration after either intramuscular or subcutaneous administration of DILAUDID-HP. Subcutaneous injections of DILAUDID-HP were particularly well accepted when administered with a short, 30 gauge needle.

Experience with administration of DILAUDID-HP by the intravenous route is limited. Should intravenous administration be necessary, the injection should be given slowly, over at least 2 to 3 minutes. The intravenous route is usually painless.

A gradual increase in dose may be required if analgesia is inadequate, tolerance occurs, or if pain severity increases. The first sign of tolerance is usually a reduced duration of effect.

NOTE: Parenteral drug products should be inspected visually for particulate matter and discoloration prior to administration, whenever solution and container permit. A slight yellowish discoloration may develop in DILAUDID-HP ampules. No loss of potency has been demonstrated. Dilaudid injection is physically compatible and chemically stable for at least 24 hours at 25°C protected from light in most common large volume parenteral solutions.

500mg/50mL Vial: To use this single dose presentation, do not penetrate the stopper with a syringe. Instead, remove both the aluminum flipseal and rubber stopper in a suitable work area such as under a laminar flow hood (or equivalent clean air compounding area). The contents may then be withdrawn for preparation of a single, large volume parenteral solution. Any unused portion should be discarded in an appropriate manner.

Reconstitution of sterile lyophilized Dilaudid HP 250mg: Reconstitution immediately prior to use with 25mL of Sterile Water for Injection USP to provide a sterile solution containing 10mg/mL.

HOW SUPPLIED

DILAUDID-HP *amber* ampules and single dose vials contain 10 mg hydromorphone hydrochloride per mL with 0.2% sodium citrate and 0.2% citric acid solution. No added preservative.

NOTE: DILAUDID-HP ampules are *amber* in color.

The lyophilized Dilaudid HP Single Dose Vial contains 250mg of sterile, lyophilized hydromorphone HCl.

HIGH POTENCY:
10 mg/1 mL
Box of 10 ampules
NDC 0044-1017-10
50 mg/5mL

STRONG ANALGESICS AND STRUCTURALLY RELATED DRUGS USED IN THE TREATMENT OF CANCER PAIN*

Nonproprietary (Trade) Names	IM OR SC ADMINISTRATION: Dose, mg Equianalgesic to 10 mg of IM Morphine†	IM OR SC ADMINISTRATION: Duration Compared With Morphine
Morphine sulfate	10	Same
Papaveretum (Pantopon)	20	Same
Hydromorphone (DILAUDID) hydrochloride	1.3	Slightly Shorter
Oxymorphone (Numorphan) hydrochloride	1.1	Slightly Shorter
Nalbuphine (Nubain) hydrochloride	12	Same
Heroin, diamorphine hydrochloride (NA in U.S.)	4–5	Slightly Shorter
Levorphanol (Levo-Dromoran) tartrate	2.3	Same
Butorphanol (Stadol) tartrate	1.5–2.5	Same
Pentazocine (Talwin) lactate or hydrochloride	60	Shorter
Meperidine, pethidine (Demerol) hydrochloride	80	Shorter
Methadone (Dolophine) hydrochloride	10	Same

* From Beaver WT.
Management of cancer pain with parenteral medication. J. Am. Med. Assoc. 244:2653–2657 (1980).
† (In terms of the area under the analgesic time-effect curve.)

Box of 10 ampules
NDC 0044-1017-25
*500 mg/50 mL
Single dose vial
NDC 0044-1017-06
*lyophilized 250mg
Single Dose Vial
NDC 0044-1911-01
*FOR USE IN THE PREPARATION OF LARGE VOLUME PARENTERAL SOLUTIONS
STORAGE: Parenteral forms of DILAUDID-HP should be stored at 15°–30°C (59°–86°F). Protect from light.
A Schedule Ⓒ Narcotic   DEA Order Form Required.
© 1997 Knoll Pharmaceutical Company.
DILAUDID HP is a registered trademark of Knoll Pharmaceutical Company.
Revised: September 1997

Parenteral Products

Manufactured for
Knoll Laboratories
A Division of Knoll Pharmaceutical Company
Mount Olive, New Jersey 07828
By Abbott Laboratories
North Chicago, IL 60064, USA
BASF Pharma   0900012A-3
Shown in Product Identification Guide, page 318

DILAUDID® ORAL LIQUID and
DILAUDID® 8 mg Tablets   Ⓒ ℞
(hydromorphone hydrochloride)
WARNING: May be habit forming

DESCRIPTION

DILAUDID (hydromorphone hydrochloride), a hydrogenated ketone of morphine, is a narcotic analgesic.
The structural formula of hydromorphone hydrochloride is:

M.W. 321.8

Each 5 mL (1 teaspoon) of DILAUDID ORAL LIQUID contains 5 mg of hydromorphone hydrochloride. In addition, other ingredients include purified water, methylparaben, propylparaben, sucrose, and glycerin. DILAUDID ORAL LIQUID may contain traces of sodium bisulfite.
Each DILAUDID 8 mg TABLET contains 8 mg hydromorphone hydrochloride. In addition, the tablets include lactose anhydrous, and magnesium stearate. DILAUDID 8 mg TABLET may contain traces of sodium bisulfite.

CLINICAL PHARMACOLOGY

Many of the effects described below are common to this class of mu-opioid agonist analgesics. In some instances, data may not exist to distinguish the effects of DILAUDID ORAL LIQUID and DILAUDID 8 mg TABLETS from those observed with other opioid analgesics. However, in the absence of data to the contrary, it is assumed that DILAUDID ORAL LIQUID and DILAUDID 8 mg TABLETS would possess all the actions of mu-agonist opioids.
Opioid analgesics exert their primary effects on the central nervous system and organs containing smooth muscle. The principal actions of therapeutic value are analgesia and sedation. A significant feature of the analgesia is that it can occur without loss of consciousness. Opioid analgesics also suppress the cough reflex and may cause respiratory depression, mood changes, mental clouding, euphoria, dysphoria, nausea, vomiting and electroencephalographic changes. The precise mode of analgesic action of opioid analgesics is unknown. However, specific CNS opiate receptors have been identified. Opioids are believed to express their pharmacological effects by combining with these receptors.
Opioids depress the cough reflex by direct effect on the cough center in the medulla.
Opioids depress the respiratory reflex by a direct effect on brain stem respiratory centers. The mechanism of respiratory depression also involves a reduction in the responsiveness of the brain stem respiratory centers to increases in carbon dioxide tension.
Opioids cause miosis. Pinpoint pupils are a common sign of opioid overdose but are not pathognomonic (e.g., pontine lesions of hemorrhagic or ischemic origin may produce similar findings) and marked mydriasis occurs with asphyxia.
Gastric, biliary and pancreatic secretions are decreased by opioids. Opioids cause a reduction in motility associated with an increase in tone in the gastric antrum and duodenum. Digestion of food in the small intestine is delayed and propulsive contractions are decreased. Propulsive peristaltic waves in the colon are decreased, and tone may be increased to the point of spasm. The end result is constipation. Opioids can cause a marked increase in biliary tract pressure as a result of spasm of the sphincter of Oddi.
Certain opioids produce peripheral vasodilation which may result in orthostatic hypotension. Release of histamine may occur with opioids and may contribute to drug-induced hypotension. Other manifestations of histamine release may include pruritus, flushing, and red eyes.
The dosage of opioid analgesics like hydromorphone should be individualized for any given patient, since adverse events can occur at doses that may not provide complete freedom from pain (see INDIVIDUALIZATION OF DOSAGE).

PHARMACOKINETICS

In a single-dose crossover study in 27 normal subjects the pharmacokinetics of DILAUDID 8 mg TABLETS was compared to that of 8 mL of DILAUDID ORAL LIQUID (1 mg/mL). Plasma hydromorphone concentration was determined using a sensitive and specific assay. The pharmacokinetic parameters from this study are outlined below.

Parameter Mean & (CV)	8 mg Tablet	8 mg Oral Liquid (1 mg/mL)
C_{max} (ng/mL)	5.5 (33%)	5.7 (31%)
T_{max} (hr)	0.74 (34%)	0.73 (71%)
$AUC_{0-\infty}$ (ng*hr/mL)	23.7 (28%)	24.6 (29%)
$T_{1/2}$ (hr)	2.6 (18%)	2.8 (20%)

Dose proportionality between the DILAUDID 8 mg TABLETS and other strengths of Dilaudid tablets has not been established.
In normal human volunteers hydromorphone is metabolized primarily in the liver. It is excreted in the urine primarily as the glucuronidated conjugate, with small amounts of parent drug and minor amounts of 6-hydroxy reduction metabolites. The effects of renal disease on the clearance of hydromorphone are unknown, but caution should be taken to guard against unanticipated accumulation if renal and/or hepatic functions are seriously impaired. Hydromorphone has been shown to cross placental membranes.

CLINICAL TRIALS

Analgesic effects of single doses of DILAUDID ORAL LIQUID administered to patients with post-surgical pain have been studied in double-blind controlled trials. In one study with 61 patients, both 5 mg and 10 mg of DILAUDID ORAL LIQUID provided significantly more analgesia than placebo. In another trial with 80 patients, 5 mg and 10 mg of DILAUDID ORAL LIQUID were compared to 30 mg and 60 mg of morphine sulfate oral liquid. The pain relief provided by 5 mg and 10 mg DILAUDID ORAL LIQUID was comparable to 30 mg and 60 mg oral morphine sulfate, respectively.

INDIVIDUALIZATION OF DOSAGE

Safe and effective administration of opioid analgesics to patients with acute or chronic pain depends upon a comprehensive assessment of the patient. The nature of the pain (severity, frequency, etiology, and pathophysiology) as well as the concurrent medical status of the patient will affect selection of the starting dosage.
In non-opioid-tolerant patients, therapy with hydromorphone is typically initiated at an oral dose of 2–4 mg every four hours, but elderly patients may require lower doses (see PRECAUTIONS—Geriatric Use).
In patients receiving opioids, both the dose and duration of analgesia will vary substantially depending on the patient's opioid tolerance. The dose should be selected and adjusted so that at least 3–4 hours of pain relief may be achieved. In patients taking opioid analgesics, the starting dose of DILAUDID should be based on the prior opioid usage. This should be done by converting the total daily usage of the previous opioid to an equivalent total daily dosage of oral DILAUDID using an equianalgesic table (see below). For opioids not in the table, first estimate the equivalent total daily usage of oral morphine, then use the table to find the equivalent total daily dosage of Dilaudid.
Once the total daily dosage of DILAUDID has been estimated, it should be divided into the desired number of doses. Since there is individual variation in response to different opioid drugs, only $1/2$ to $2/3$ of the estimated dose of DILAUDID calculated from equivalence tables should be given for the first few doses, then increased as needed according to the patient's response.
In chronic pain, doses should be administered around-the-clock. A supplemental dose of 5–15% of the total daily usage may be administered every two hours on an "as-needed" basis.
Periodic reassessment after the initial dosing is always required. If pain management is not satisfactory and in the absence of significant opioid-induced adverse events, the hydromorphone dose may be increased gradually. If excessive opioid side effects are observed early in the dosing interval, the hydromorphone dose should be reduced. If this results in breakthrough pain at the end of the dosing interval, the dosing interval may need to be shortened. Dose titration should be guided more by the need for analgesia than the absolute dose of opioid employed.
[See table above]
* Dosages, and ranges of dosages represented, are a compilation of estimated equipotent dosages from published references comparing opioid analgesics in cancer and severe pain.

INDICATIONS AND USAGE

DILAUDID ORAL LIQUID and DILAUDID 8 mg TABLETS are indicated for the management of pain in patients where an opioid analgesic is appropriate.

CONTRAINDICATIONS

DILAUDID ORAL LIQUID and DILAUDID 8 mg TABLETS are contraindicated in: patients with known hypersensitivity to hydromorphone, patients with respiratory depression in the absence of resuscitative equipment, and in patients with status asthmaticus. DILAUDID ORAL LIQUID and DILAUDID 8 mg TABLETS are also contraindicated for use in obstetrical analgesia.

WARNINGS

Impaired Respiration: Respiratory depression is the chief hazard of DILAUDID ORAL LIQUID and DILAUDID 8 mg TABLETS. Respiratory depression occurs most frequently in overdose situations, in the elderly, in the debilitated, and in those suffering from conditions accompanied by hypoxia or hypercapnia when even moderate therapeutic doses may dangerously decrease pulmonary ventilation.
DILAUDID ORAL LIQUID and DILAUDID 8 mg TABLETS should be used with extreme caution in patients with chronic obstructive pulmonary disease or cor pulmonale, patients having a substantially decreased respiratory depression, hypoxia, hypercapnia, or in patients with preexisting respiratory depression. In such patients even usual therapeutic doses of opioid analgesics may decrease respiratory drive while simultaneously increasing airway resistance to the point of apnea.
Drug Dependence: DILAUDID is a Schedule II narcotic. DILAUDID ORAL LIQUID and DILAUDID 8 mg TABLETS can produce drug dependence of the morphine type and therefore have the potential for being abused. Psychic dependence, physical dependence and tolerance may develop upon repeated administration of DILAUDID, which should be prescribed and administered with the degree of caution appropriate to the use of morphine. Abrupt discontinuance in the administration of DILAUDID ORAL LIQUID and DILAUDID 8 mg TABLETS in patients who are physically dependent on opioids is likely to result in a withdrawal syndrome (see DRUG ABUSE AND DEPENDENCE).
Sulfites: Contains sodium bisulfite, a sulfite that may cause allergic-type reactions including anaphylactic symptoms and life-threatening or less severe asthmatic episodes

OPIOID ANALGESIC EQUIVALENTS WITH APPROXIMATELY EQUIANALGESIC POTENCY*

Nonproprietary (Trade) Name	IM or SC Dose	ORAL dose
Morphine Sulfate	10 mg	40–60 mg
Hydromorphone HCl (DILAUDID)	1.3–2 mg	6.5–7.5 mg
Oxymorphone HCl (Numorphan)	1–1.1 mg	6.6 mg
Levorphanol tartrate (Levo-Dromoran)	2–2.3 mg	4 mg
Meperidine HCl (Demerol)	75–100 mg	300–400 mg
Methadone HCl (Dolophine)	10 mg	10–20 mg

Continued on next page

Dilaudid—Cont.

in certain susceptible people. The overall prevalence of sulfite sensitivity in the general population is unknown and probably low. Sulfite sensitivity is seen more frequently in asthmatic than in nonasthmatic people.

PRECAUTIONS

Special Risk Patients: In general, opioids should be given with caution and the initial dose should be reduced in the elderly or debilitated and those with severe impairment of hepatic, pulmonary or renal functions; myxedema or hypothyroidism; adrenocortical insufficiency (e.g., Addison's Disease); CNS depression or coma; toxic psychoses; prostatic hypertrophy or urethral stricture; gall bladder disease; acute alcoholism; delirium tremens; kyphoscoliosis or following gastrointestinal surgery.

The administration of opioid analgesics including DILAUDID ORAL LIQUID and DILAUDID 8 mg TABLETS may obscure the diagnoses or clinical course in patients with acute abdominal conditions and may aggravate preexisting convulsions in patients with convulsive disorders.

Head Injury and Increased Intracranial Pressure: The respiratory depressant effects of DILAUDID ORAL LIQUID and DILAUDID 8 mg TABLETS with carbon dioxide retention and secondary elevation of cerebrospinal fluid pressure may be markedly exaggerated in the presence of head injury, other intracranial lesions, or preexisting increase in intracranial pressure. Opioid analgesics including DILAUDID ORAL LIQUID and DILAUDID 8 mg TABLETS may produce effects which can obscure the clinical course and neurologic signs of further increase in intracranial pressure in patients with head injuries.

Hypotensive Effect: Opioid analgesics, including DILAUDID ORAL LIQUID and DILAUDID 8 mg TABLETS, may cause severe hypotension in an individual whose ability to maintain blood pressure has already been compromised by a depleted blood volume, or a concurrent administration of drugs such as phenothiazines or general anesthetics (see also PRECAUTIONS—Drug Interactions). Therefore, DILAUDID ORAL LIQUID and DILAUDID 8 mg TABLETS should be administered with caution to patients in circulatory shock, since vasodilation produced by the drug may further reduce cardiac output and blood pressure.

Use in Ambulatory Patients: DILAUDID ORAL LIQUID and DILAUDID 8 mg TABLETS may impair mental and/or physical ability required for the performance of potentially hazardous tasks (e.g. driving, operating machinery). Patients should be cautioned accordingly. DILAUDID may produce orthostatic hypotension in ambulatory patients. The addition of other CNS depressants to DILAUDID therapy may produce additive depressant effects, and DILAUDID should not be taken with alcohol.

Use in Biliary Surgery: Opioid analgesics including DILAUDID ORAL LIQUID and DILAUDID 8 mg TABLETS should also be used with caution in patients about to undergo surgery of the biliary tract since it may cause spasm of the sphincter of Oddi.

Use in Drug and Alcohol Dependent Patients: DILAUDID should be used with caution in patients with alcoholism and other drug dependencies due to the increased frequency of narcotic tolerance, dependence, and the risk of addiction observed in these patient populations. Abuse of DILAUDID in combination with other CNS depressant drugs can result in serious risk to the patient.

Drug Interactions: The concomitant use of other central nervous system depressants including sedatives or hypnotics, general anesthetics, phenothiazines, tranquilizers and alcohol may produce additive depressant effects. Respiratory depression, hypotension and profound sedation or coma may occur. When such combined therapy is contemplated, the dose of one or both agents should be reduced. Opioid analgesics, including DILAUDID ORAL LIQUID and DILAUDID 8 mg TABLETS, may enhance the action of neuromuscular blocking agents and produce an excessive degree of respiratory depression.

Carcinogenesis, Mutagenesis, Impairment of Fertility: Studies in animals to evaluate the drug's carcinogenic and mutagenic potential or the effect on fertility, have not been conducted.

Pregnancy—Pregnancy Category C: Literature reports of hydromorphone hydrochloride administration to pregnant Syrian hamsters show that DILAUDID is teratogenic at a dose of 20 mg/kg which is 600 times the human dose. A maximal teratogenic effect (50% of fetuses affected) in the Syrian hamster was observed at a dose of 125 mg/kg (738 mg/m^2). There are no well-controlled studies in women. Hydromorphone is known to cross placental membranes. DILAUDID ORAL LIQUID and DILAUDID 8 mg TABLETS should be used in pregnant women only if the potential benefit justifies the potential risk to the fetus (see *Labor and Delivery* and DRUG ABUSE AND DEPENDENCE).

Labor and Delivery: DILAUDID ORAL LIQUID and DILAUDID 8 mg TABLETS are contraindicated in Labor and Delivery (see CONTRAINDICATIONS).

Nursing Mothers: Low levels of opioid analgesics have been detected in human milk. As a general rule, nursing should not be undertaken while a patient is receiving DILAUDID ORAL LIQUID and DILAUDID 8 mg TABLETS since it, and other drugs in this class, may be excreted in the milk.

Pediatric Use: Safety and effectiveness in children have not been established.

Geriatric Use: DILAUDID has not been studied in geriatric patients. Elderly subjects have been shown to have at least twice the sensitivity (as measured by EEG changes) of young adults to some opioids. When administering DILAUDID to the elderly, the initial dose should be reduced (see INDIVIDUALIZATION OF DOSAGE and PRECAUTIONS).

ADVERSE REACTIONS

The adverse effects of DILAUDID ORAL LIQUID and DILAUDID 8 mg TABLETS are similar to those of other agonist analgesics, and represent established pharmacological effects of the drug class. The major hazards include respiratory depression and apnea. To a lesser degree, circulatory depression, respiratory arrest, shock and cardiac arrest have occurred.

The most frequently observed adverse effects are lightheadedness, dizziness, sedation, nausea, vomiting, sweating, dysphoria, euphoria, dry mouth, and pruritus. These effects seem to be more prominent in ambulatory patients and in those not experiencing severe pain. Syncopal reactions and related symptoms in ambulatory patients may be alleviated if the patient lies down.

Less Frequently Observed with Opioid Analgesics:

General and CNS: Weakness, headache, agitation, tremor, uncoordinated muscle movements, alterations of mood (nervousness, apprehension, depression, floating feelings, dreams), muscle rigidity, paresthesia, muscle tremor, blurred vision, nystagmus, diplopia and miosis, transient hallucinations and disorientation, visual disturbances, insomnia and increased intracranial pressure may occur.

Cardiovascular: Chills, tachycardia, bradycardia, palpitation, faintness, syncope, hypotension and hypertension have been reported.

Respiratory: Bronchospasm and laryngospasm have been known to occur.

Gastrointestinal: Constipation biliary tract spasm, ileus, anorexia, diarrhea, cramps and taste alteration have been reported.

Genitourinary: Urinary retention or hesitancy, and antidiuretic effects have been reported.

Dermatologic: Urticaria, other skin rashes, and diaphoresis.

DRUG ABUSE AND DEPENDENCE

DILAUDID is a Schedule II narcotic, similar to morphine. Opioid analgesics may cause psychological and physical dependence (see WARNINGS). Physical dependence results in withdrawal symptoms in patients who abruptly discontinue the drug. Withdrawal symptoms also may be precipitated in the patient with physical dependence by the administration of a drug with opioid antagonist activity, e.g., naloxone (see also OVERDOSAGE).

Physical dependence usually does not occur to a clinically significant degree until after several weeks of continued opioid usage, but it may become clinically detectable after as little as a week. Tolerance, in which increasingly large doses are required in order to produce the same degree of analgesia, is initially manifested by a shortened duration of analgesic effect, and subsequently, by decreases in the intensity of analgesia. In chronic pain patients, and in opioid-tolerant cancer patients, the dose of DILAUDID ORAL LIQUID and DILAUDID 8 mg TABLETS should be guided by the degree of tolerance manifested.

In chronic pain patients in whom opioid analgesics including DILAUDID ORAL LIQUID and DILAUDID 8 mg TABLETS are abruptly discontinued, a severe abstinence syndrome should be anticipated. This may be similar to the abstinence syndrome noted in patients who withdraw from heroin. Because of excessive loss of fluids through sweating, or vomiting and diarrhea, patients experiencing the syndrome usually exhibit marked weight loss, dehydration, ketosis, and disturbances in acid-base balance. Cardiovascular collapse can occur. Without treatment most observable symptoms disappear in 5–14 days; however, there appears to be a phase of secondary or chornic abstinence which may last for 2–6 months characterized by insomnia, irritability, muscular aches, and autonomic instability.

In the treatment of physical dependence on DILAUDID ORAL LIQUID and DILAUDID 8 mg TABLETS, the patient may be detoxified by gradual reduction of the dosage, although this is unlikely to be necessary in the terminal cancer patient. If abstinence symptoms become severe, the patient may be detoxified with methadone. Temporary administration of tranquilizers and sedatives may aid in reducing patient anxiety. Gastrointestinal disturbances or dehydration should be treated accordingly.

OVERDOSAGE

Serious overdosage with DILAUDID ORAL LIQUID and DILAUDID 8 mg TABLETS is characterized by respiratory depression, somnolence progressing to stupor or coma, skeletal muscle flaccidity, cold and clammy skin, constricted pupils, and sometimes bradycardia and hypotension. In serious overdosage, particularly following intravenous injection, apnea, circulatory collapse, cardiac arrest and death may occur.

In the treatment of overdosage, primary attention should be given to the reestablishment of adequate respiratory exchange through provision of a patent airway and institution of assisted or controlled ventilation. A potentially serious oral ingestion, if recent, should be managed with gut decontamination. In unconscious patients with a secure airway, instill activated charcoal (30–100 g in adults, 1–2 g/kg in infants) via a nasogastric tube. A saline cathartic or sorbitol may be added to the first dose of activated charcoal.

Opioid-tolerant patient: Since tolerance to the respiratory and CNS depressant effects of opioids develops concomitantly with tolerance to their analgesic effects, serious respiratory depression due to an acute overdose is unlikely to be seen in opioid-tolerant patients receiving the usual therapeutic dosage of DILAUDID ORAL LIQUID and DILAUDID 8 mg TABLETS for chronic pain.

Note: In an individual who is physically dependent on opioids, administration of the usual dose of an opioid antagonist will precipitate an acute withdrawal syndrome. The severity will depend on the degree of physical dependence and the dose of the antagonist administered. If necessary to treat serious respiratory depression in the physically-dependent patient, the opioid antagonist should be administered with care and by titration, using fractional (one fifth to one tenth) doses of the antagonist.

Non-tolerant patient: The opioid antagonist, naloxone, is a specific antidote against respiratory depression which may result from overdosage, or unusual sensitivity to DILAUDID ORAL LIQUID and DILAUDID 8 mg TABLETS. A dose of naloxone (usually given as a test dose of 0.4 mg, followed by up to 2.0 mg if needed) should be administered intravenously, if possible, simultaneously with respiratory resuscitation. The dose can be repeated in 3 minutes. Naloxone should not be administered in the absence of clinically significant respiratory or circulatory depression. Naloxone should be administered cautiously to persons who are known, or suspected to be physically dependent on DILAUDID ORAL LIQUID and DILAUDID 8 mg TABLETS (see Opioid tolerant patient).

Since the duration of action of DILAUDID ORAL LIQUID and DILAUDID 8 mg TABLETS may exceed that of the antagonist, the patient should be kept under continued surveillance; repeated doses of the antagonist may be required to maintain adequate respiration. Apply other supportive measures when indicated.

Supportive measures (including oxygen, vasopressors) should be employed in the management of circulatory shock and pulmonary edema accompanying overdose as indicated. Cardiac arrest or arrhythmias may require cardiac massage or defibrillation.

DOSAGE AND ADMINISTRATION

DILAUDID ORAL LIQUID: The usual adult oral dosage of DILAUDID ORAL LIQUID is one-half (2.5 mL) to two teaspoonfuls (10 mL) (2.5 mg–10 mg) every 3 to 6 hours as directed by the clinical situation. Oral dosages higher than the usual dosages may be required in some patients.

DILAUDID 8 mg TABLET: The usual starting dose for DILAUDID tablets is 2 mg to 4 mg, orally, every 4 to 6 hours. Appropriate use of the DILAUDID 8 mg TABLET must be decided by careful evaluation of each clinical situation.

A gradual increase in dose may be required if analgesia is inadequate, as tolerance develops, or if pain severity increases. The first sign of tolerance is usually a reduced duration of effect.

SAFETY AND HANDLING INSTRUCTIONS

DILAUDID ORAL LIQUID and DILAUDID 8 mg TABLETS pose little risk of direct exposure to health care personnel and should be handled and disposed of prudently in accordance with hospital or institutional policy. Significant absorption from dermal exposure is unlikely; accidental dermal exposure to DILAUDID ORAL LIQUID should be treated by removal of any contaminated clothing and rinsing the affected area with water. Patients and their families should be instructed to flush any DILAUDID ORAL LIQUID and DILAUDID 8 mg TABLETS that are no longer needed.

Access to abuseable drugs such as DILAUDID ORAL LIQUID and DILAUDID 8 mg TABLETS presents an occupational hazard for addiction in the health care industry. Routine procedures for handling controlled substances developed to protect the public may not be adequate to protect health care workers. Implementation of more effective accounting procedures and measures to restrict access to drugs of this class (appropriate to the practice setting) may minimize the risk of self-administration by health care providers.

HOW SUPPLIED

DILAUDID ORAL LIQUID is a clear, sweet, slightly viscous liquid. It is available in:
Bottles of 1 pint (473 mL)—NDC# 0044-1085-01
DILAUDID 8 mg TABLETS are white and triangular shaped, embossed with the number 8 on one side and bisected and embossed with a double "Knoll" triangle on the other side. They are available in:
Bottles of 100—NDC# 0044-1028-02
Storage: DILAUDID ORAL LIQUID and DILAUDID 8 mg TABLETS should be stored at 15–25°C (59–77°F). Protect from light.
A schedule II Narcotic DEA Order Form is Required.
© 1996 Knoll Pharmaceutical Company
DILAUDID is a registered trademark of Knoll Pharmaceutical Company
Revised: August 1996
Knoll Laboratories
A Division of
Knoll Pharmaceutical Company
Mount Olive, New Jersey 07828
BASF Pharma   0900016-2
Shown in Product Identification Guide, page 318

ISOPTIN® SR   ℞
(verapamil HCl)
Sustained Release Oral Tablets

DESCRIPTION

ISOPTIN SR® (verapamil hydrochloride) is a calcium ion influx inhibitor (slow channel blocker or calcium ion antagonist). ISOPTIN SR is available for oral administration as light green, capsule shaped, scored, film-coated tablets containing 240 mg verapamil hydrochloride, as light pink, oval shaped, scored, film-coated tablets containing 180 mg verapamil hydrochloride, and as light violet, oval shaped, film-coated tablets containing 120 mg verapamil hydrochloride. The tablets are designed for sustained release of the drug in the gastrointestinal tract, sustained release characters are not altered when the tablet is divided in half.
The structural formula of verapamil HCl is given below:

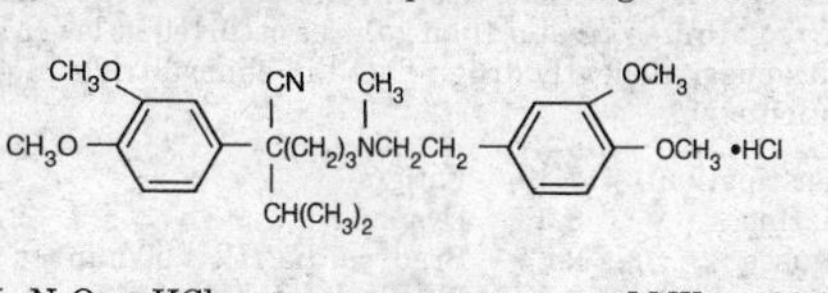

$$CH_3O-\text{—}-C(CH_2)_3N\text{—}CH_2CH_2-\text{—}-OCH_3 \cdot HCl$$

(with substituents CN, CH₃, CH(CH₃)₂, CH₃O, OCH₃)

$$C_{27}H_{38}N_2O_4 \cdot HCl \qquad M.W. = 491.08$$

Benzeneacetonitrile,
α-[[3-[[2-(3,4-dimethoxyphenyl) ethyl]
methylamino]
propyl]-3,4-dimethoxy-α-(1-methylethyl) hydrochloride

Verapamil HCl is an almost white, crystalline powder, practically free of odor, with a bitter taste. It is soluble in water, chloroform and methanol. Verapamil HCl is not chemically related to other cardioactive drugs.
In addition to verapamil HCl, the ISOPTIN SR tablet contains the following ingredients: alginate, hydroxypropyl methylcellulose, magnesium stearate, microcrystalline cellulose, polyethylene glycol, polyvinyl pyrrolidone, talc, and titanium dioxide. The following are the color additives per tablet strength:

Strength (mg)	Color Additive(s)
120	Iron Oxide
180	Iron Oxide
240	D&C yellow #10 Lake dye, and FD&C blue #2 Lake dye

CLINICAL PHARMACOLOGY

ISOPTIN is a calcium ion influx inhibitor (slow channel blocker or calcium ion antagonist) which exerts its pharmacologic effects by modulating the influx of ionic calcium across the cell membrane of the arterial smooth muscle as well as in conductile and contractile myocardial cells.
Mechanism of Action
Essential Hypertension
ISOPTIN exerts antihypertensive effects by decreasing systemic vascular resistance, usually without orthostatic decreases in blood pressure or reflex tachycardia; bradycardia (rate less than 50 beats/min) is uncommon (1.4%). During isometric or dynamic exercise ISOPTIN does not alter systolic cardiac function in patients with normal ventricular function. ISOPTIN does not alter total serum calcium levels. However, one report suggested that calcium levels above the normal range may alter the therapeutic effect of ISOPTIN.
Other Pharmacologic Actions of ISOPTIN Include the Following
ISOPTIN (verapamil HCl) dilates the main coronary arteries and coronary arterioles, both in normal and ischemic regions, and is a potent inhibitor of coronary artery spasm,

whether spontaneous or ergonovine-induced. This property increases myocardial oxygen delivery in patients with coronary artery spasm, and is responsible for the effectiveness of ISOPTIN in vasospastic (Prinzmetal's or variant) as well as unstable angina at rest. Whether this effect plays any role in classical effort angina is not clear, but studies of exercise tolerance have not shown an increase in the maximum exercise rate-pressure product, a widely accepted measure of oxygen utilization. This suggests that, in general, relief of spasm or dilation of coronary arteries is not an important factor in classical angina.
ISOPTIN regularly reduces the total systemic resistance (afterload) against which the heart works both at rest and at a given level of exercise by dilating peripheral arterioles. Electrical activity through the AV node depends, to a significant degree, upon calcium influx through the slow channel. By decreasing the influx of calcium, ISOPTIN prolongs the effective refractory period within the AV node and slows AV conduction in a rate-related manner.
Normal sinus rhythm is usually not affected, but in patients with sick sinus syndrome, ISOPTIN may interfere with sinus node impulse generation and may induce sinus arrest or sinoatrial block. Atrioventricular block can occur in patients without preexisting conduction defects (see WARNINGS).
ISOPTIN does not alter the normal atrial action potential or intraventricular conduction time, but depresses amplitude, velocity of depolarization and conduction in depressed atrial fibers. ISOPTIN may shorten the antegrade effective refractory period of accessory bypass tracts. Acceleration of ventricular rate and/or ventricular fibrillation has been reported in patients with atrial flutter or atrial fibrillation and a coexisting accessory AV pathway following administration of verapamil (see WARNINGS).
ISOPTIN has a local anesthetic action that is 1.6 times that of procaine on an equimolar basis. It is not known whether this action is important at the doses used in man.
Pharmacokinetics and Metabolism: With the immediate release formulation, more than 90% of the orally administered dose of ISOPTIN is absorbed. Because of rapid biotransformation of verapamil during its first pass through the portal circulation, bioavailability ranges from 20% to 35%. Peak plasma concentrations are reached between 1 and 2 hours after oral administration. Chronic oral administration of 120 mg of ISOPTIN every 6 hours resulted in plasma levels of verapamil ranging from 125 to 400 ng/mL with higher values reported occasionally. A nonlinear correlation between the verapamil dose administered and verapamil plasma levels does exist. No relationship has been established between the plasma concentration of verapamil and a reduction in blood pressure.
In early dose titration with verapamil a relationship exists between verapamil plasma concentrations and the prolongation of the PR interval. However, during chronic administration this relationship may disappear. The mean elimination half-life in single dose studies ranged from 2.8 to 7.4 hours. In these same studies, with repetitive dosing, the half-life increased to a range from 4.5 to 12.0 hours (after less than 10 consecutive doses given 6 hours apart). Half-life of verapamil may increase during titration.
Aging may affect the pharmacokinetics of verapamil. Elimination half-life may be prolonged in the elderly.
In multiple dose studies under fasting conditions the bioavailability measured by AUC of ISOPTIN SR was similar to ISOPTIN immediate release; rates of absorption were, of course, different. In a randomized, single-dose, crossover study using healthy volunteers, administration of 240 mg ISOPTIN SR with food produced peak plasma verapamil concentrations of 79 ng/mL, time to peak plasma verapamil concentrations of 7.71 hours, and AUC (0–24 hr) of 841 ng-hr/mL. When ISOPTIN SR was administered to fasting subjects, peak plasma verapamil concentration was 164 ng/mL; time to peak plasma verapamil concentration was 5.21 hours; and AUC (0–24 hr) was 1,478 ng-hr/mL. Similar results were demonstrated for plasma norverapamil. Food thus produces decreased bioavailability (AUC) but a narrower peak to trough ratio. Good correlation of dose and response is not available, but controlled studies of ISOPTIN SR have shown effectiveness of doses similar to the effective doses of ISOPTIN (immediate release).
In healthy man, orally administered ISOPTIN undergoes extensive metabolism in the liver. Twelve metabolites have been identified in plasma; all except norverapamil are present in trace amounts only. Norverapamil can reach steady-state plasma concentrations approximately equal to those of verapamil itself. The cardiovascular activity of norverapamil appears to be approximately 20% that of verapamil. Approximately 70% of an administered dose is excreted as metabolites in the urine and 16% or more in the feces within 5 days. About 3% to 4% is excreted in the urine as unchanged drug. Approximately 90% is bound to plasma proteins. In patients with hepatic insufficiency, metabolism of immediate release verapamil is delayed and elimination half-life prolonged up to 14 to 16 hours (see PRECAUTIONS); the volume of distribution is increased and plasma clearance reduced to about 30% of normal. Verapamil clear-

ance values suggest that patients with liver dysfunction may attain therapeutic verapamil plasma concentrations with one-third of the oral daily dose required for patients with normal liver function.
After four weeks of oral dosing (120 mg q.i.d.), verapamil and norverapamil levels were noted in the cerebrospinal fluid with estimated partition coefficient of 0.06 for verapamil and 0.04 for norverapamil.
Hemodynamics and Myocardial Metabolism:
ISOPTIN reduces afterload and myocardial contractility. Improved left ventricular diastolic function in patients with IHSS and those with coronary heart disease has also been observed with ISOPTIN therapy. In most patients, including those with organic cardiac disease, the negative inotropic action of ISOPTIN is countered by reduction of afterload and cardiac index is usually not reduced. In patients with severe left ventricular dysfunction however, (e.g., pulmonary wedge pressure above 20 mmHg or ejection fraction lower than 30%), or in patients on beta-adrenergic blocking agents or other cardiodepressant drugs, deterioration of ventricular function may occur (see DRUG INTERACTIONS).
Pulmonary Function: ISOPTIN does not induce bronchoconstriction and hence, does not impair ventilatory function.

INDICATIONS AND USAGE

ISOPTIN SR (verapamil HCl) is indicated for the management of essential hypertension.

CONTRAINDICATIONS

Verapamil HCl is contraindicated in:
1. Severe left ventricular dysfunction (see WARNINGS)
2. Hypotension (less than 90 mmHg systolic pressure) or cardiogenic shock
3. Sick sinus syndrome (except in patients with a functioning artificial ventricular pacemaker)
4. Second- or third-degree AV block (except patients with a functioning artificial ventricular pacemaker).
5. Patients with atrial flutter or atrial fibrillation and an accessory bypass tract (e.g., Wolff-Parkinson-White, Lown-Ganong-Levine syndromes). (see WARNINGS).
6. Patients with known hypersensitivity to verapamil hydrochloride.

WARNINGS

Heart Failure: Verapamil has a negative inotropic effect which, in most patients, is compensated by its afterload reduction (decreased systemic vascular resistance) properties without a net impairment of ventricular performance. In clinical experience with 4,954 patients, 87 (1.8%) developed congestive heart failure or pulmonary edema. Verapamil should be avoided in patients with severe left ventricular dysfunction (e.g., ejection fraction less than 30%, pulmonary wedge pressure above 20mm Hg, or severe symptoms of cardiac failure) and in patients with any degree of ventricular dysfunction if they are receiving a beta adrenergic blocker (see DRUG INTERACTIONS). Patients with milder ventricular dysfunction should, if possible, be controlled with optimum doses of digitalis and/or diuretics before verapamil treatment (Note interactions with digoxin under: PRECAUTIONS).
Hypotension: Occasionally, the pharmacologic action of verapamil may produce a decrease in blood pressure below normal levels which may result in dizziness or symptomatic hypotension. The incidence of hypotension observed in 4,954 patients enrolled in clinical trials was 2.5%. In hypertensive patients, decreases in blood pressure below normal are unusual. Tilt table testing (60 degrees) was not able to induce orthostatic hypotension.
Elevated Liver Enzymes: Elevations of transaminases with and without concomitant elevations in alkaline phosphatase and bilirubin have been reported. Such elevations has sometimes been transient and may disappear even in the face of continued verapamil treatment. Several cases of hepatocellular injury related to verapamil have been proven by rechallenge; half of these had clinical symptoms (malaise, fever, and/or right upper quadrant pain) in addition to elevations of SGOT, SGPT and alkaline phosphatase. Periodic monitoring of liver function in patients receiving verapamil is therefore prudent.
Accessory Bypass Tract (Wolff-Parkinson-White or Lown-Ganong-Levine): Some patients with paroxysmal and/or chronic atrial fibrillation or atrial flutter and a coexisting accessory AV pathway have developed increased antegrade conduction across the accessory pathway bypassing the AV node, producing a very rapid ventricular response or ventricular fibrillation after receiving intravenous verapamil (or digitalis). Although a risk of this occurring with oral verapamil has not been established, such patients receiving oral verapamil may be at risk and its use in these patients is contraindicated (see CONTRAINDICATIONS).
Treatment is usually DC-cardioversion. Cardioversion has been used safely and effectively after oral ISOPTIN.
Atrioventricular Block: The effect of verapamil on AV conduction and the SA node may lead to asympomtic first-

Continued on next page

Isoptin SR—Cont.

degree AV block and transient bradycardia, sometimes accompanied by nodal escape rhythms. PR interval prolongation is correlated with verapamil plasma concentrations, especially during the early titration phases of therapy. Higher degrees of AV block, however, were infrequently (0.8%) observed. Marked first-degree block or progressive development to second- or third-degree AV block requires a reduction in dosage or, in rare instances, discontinuation of verapamil HCl and institution of appropriate therapy depending upon the clinical situation.

Patients with Hypertrophic Cardiomyopathy (IHSS): In 120 patients with hypertrophic cardiomyopathy (most of them refractory or intolerant to propranolol) who received therapy with verapamil at doses up to 720 mg/day, a variety of serious adverse effects were seen. Three patients died in pulmonary edema; all had severe left ventricular outflow obstruction and a past history of left ventricular dysfunction. Eight other patients had pulmonary edema and/or severe hypotension; abnormally high (over 20 mmHg) capillary wedge pressure and a marked left ventricular outflow obstruction were present in most of these patients. Concomitant administration of quinidine (see DRUG INTERACTIONS) preceded the severe hypotension in 3 of the 8 patients (2 of whom developed pulmonary edema). Sinus bradycardia occurred in 11% of the patients, second-degree AV block in 4% and sinus arrest in 2%. It must be appreciated that this group of patients had a serious disease with a high mortality rate. Most adverse effects responded well to dose reduction and only rarely did verapamil have to be discontinued.

PRECAUTIONS
General
Use in Patients with Impaired Hepatic Functions: Since verapamil is highly metabolized by the liver, it should be administered cautiously to patients with impaired hepatic function. Severe liver dysfunction prolongs the elimination half-life of immediate release verapamil to about 14 to 16 hours; hence, approximately 30% of the dose given to patients with normal liver function should be administered to these patients. Careful monitoring for abnormal prolongation of the PR interval or other signs of excessive pharmacologic effects (see OVERDOSAGE) should be carried out.

Use in Patients with Attenuated (Decreased) Neuromuscular Transmission: It has been reported that verapamil decreases neuromuscular transmission in patients with Duchenne's muscular dystrophy, and that verapamil prolongs recovery from the neuromuscular blocking agent vecuronium. It may be necessary to decrease the dosage of verapamil when it is administered to patients with attenuated neuromuscular transmission.

Use in Patients with Impaired Renal Function: About 70% of an administered dose of verapamil is excreted as metabolites in the urine. Verapamil is not removed by hemodialysis. Until further data are available, verapamil should be administered cautiously to patients with impaired renal function. These patients should be carefully monitored for abnormal prolongation of the PR interval or other signs of overdosage (see OVERDOSAGE).

Drug Interactions
Beta Blockers: Concomitant therapy with beta-adrenergic blockers and verapamil may result in additive negative effects on heart rate, atrioventricular conduction, and/or cardiac contractility. The combination of sustained-release verapamil and beta-adrenergic blocking agents has not been studied. However, there have been reports of excessive bradycardia and AV block, including complete heart block, when the combination has been used for the treatment of hypertension. For hypertensive patients, the risks of combined therapy may outweigh the potential benefits. The combination should be used only with caution and close monitoring.

Asymptomatic bradycardia (36 beats/min) with a wandering atrial pacemaker has been observed in a patient receiving concomitant timolol (a beta-adrenergic blocker) eyedrops and oral verapamil.

A decrease in metoprolol and propranolol clearance has been observed when either drug is administered concomitantly with verapamil. A variable effect has been seen when verapamil and atenolol were given together.

Digitalis: Clinical use of verapamil in digitalized patients has shown the combination to be well tolerated if digoxin doses are properly adjusted. Chronic verapamil treatment can increase serum digoxin levels by 50 to 75% during the first week of therapy, and this can result in digitalis toxicity. In patients with hepatic cirrhosis the influence of verapamil on digoxin kinetics is magnified. Verapamil may reduce total body clearance and extrarenal clearance of digitoxin by 27% and 29%, respectively. Maintenance digitalis doses should be reduced when verapamil is administered, and the patient should be carefully monitored to avoid over- or underdigitalization. Whenever overdigitalization is suspected, the daily dose of digitalis should be reduced or temporarily

discontinued. Upon discontinuation of ISOPTIN (verapamil HCl), the patient should be reassessed to avoid underdigitalization.

Antihypertensive Agents: Verapamil administered concomitantly with oral antihypertensive agents (e.g., vasodilators, angiotensin-converting enzyme inhibitors, diuretics, beta blockers) will usually have an additive effect on lowering blood pressure. Patients receiving these combinations should be appropriately monitored. Concomitant use of agents that attenuate alpha-adrenergic function with verapamil may result in a reduction in blood pressure that is excessive in some patients. Such an effect was observed in one study following the concomitant administration of verapamil and prazosin.

Antiarrhythmic Agents
Disopyramide: Until data on possible interactions between verapamil and disopyramide phosphate are obtained, disopyramide should not be administered within 48 hours before or 24 hours after verapamil administration.

Flecainide: A study of healthy volunteers showed that the concomitant administration of flecainide and verapamil may have additive effects on myocardial contractility, AV conduction, and repolarization. Concomitant therapy with flecainide and verapamil may result in additive negative inotropic effect and prolongation of atrioventricular conduction.

Quinidine: In a small number of patients with hypertrophic cardiomyopathy (IHSS), concomitant use of verapamil and quinidine resulted in significant hypotension. Until further data are obtained, combined therapy of verapamil and quinidine in patients with hypertrophic cardiomyopathy should probably be avoided.

The electrophysiological effects of quinidine and verapamil on AV conduction were studied in 8 patients. Verapamil significantly counteracted the effects of quinidine on AV conduction. There has been a report of increased quinidine levels during verapamil therapy.

Nitrates: Verapamil has been given concomitantly with short- and long-acting nitrates without any undesirable drug interactions. The pharmacologic profile of both drugs and the clinical experience suggest beneficial interactions.

Other
Cimetidine: The interaction between cimetidine and chronically administered verapamil has not been studied. Variable results on clearance have been obtained in acute studies of healthy volunteers; clearance of verapamil was either reduced or unchanged.

Lithium: Increases sensitivity to the effects of lithium (neurotoxicity) has been reported during concomitant verapamil-lithium therapy; lithium levels have been observed sometimes to increase, sometimes to decrease, and sometimes to be unchanged. Patients receiving both drugs must be monitored carefully.

Carbamazepine: Verapamil therapy may increase carbamazepine concentrations during combined therapy. This may produce carbamazepine side effects such as diplopia, headache, ataxia, or dizziness.

Rifampin: Therapy with rifampin may markedly reduce oral verapamil bioavailability.

Phenobarbital: Phenobarbital therapy may increase verapamil clearance.

Cyclosporine: Verapamil therapy may increase serum levels of cyclosporine.

Theophylline: Verapamil may inhibit the clearance and increase the plasma levels of theophylline.

Inhalation Anesthetics: Animal experiments have shown that inhalation anesthetics depress cardiovascular activity by decreasing the inward movement of calcium ions. When used concomitantly, inhalation anesthetics and calcium antagonists, such as verapamil, should be titrated carefully to avoid excessive cardiovascular depression.

Neuromuscular Blocking Agents: Clinical data and animal studies suggest that verapamil may potentiate the activity of neuromuscular blocking agents (curare-like and depolarizing). It may be necessary to decrease the dose of verapamil and/or the dose of the neuromuscular blocking agent when the drugs are used concomitantly.

Carcinogenesis, Mutagenesis, Impairment of Fertility: An 18–month toxicity study in rats, at a low multiple (6 fold) of the maximum recommended human dose, and not the maximum tolerated dose, did not suggest a tumorigenic potential. There was no evidence of a carcinogenic potential of verapamil administered in the diet of rats for two years at doses of 10, 35, and 120 mg/kg per day or approximately 1×, 3.5×, and 12×, respectively, the maximum recommended human daily dose (480 mg per day or 9.6 mg/kg/day). Verapamil was not mutagenic in the Ames test in 5 test strains at 3 mg per plate, with or without metabolic activation.

Studies in female rats at daily dietary doses up to 5.5 times (55 mg/kg/day) the maximum recommended human dose did not show impaired fertility. Effects on male fertility have not been determined.

Pregnancy: Pregnancy Category C. Reproduction studies have been performed in rabbits and rats at oral doses up to 1.5 (15 mg/kg/day) and 6 (60 mg/kg/day) times the human

oral daily dose, respectively, and have revealed no evidence of teratogenicity. In the rat, however, this multiple of the human dose was embryocidal and retarded fetal growth and development, probably because of adverse maternal effects reflected in the reduced weight gains of the dams. This oral dose has also been shown to cause hypotension in rats. There are no adequate and well-controlled studies in pregnant women. Because animal reproduction studies are not always predictive of human response, this drug should be used during pregnancy only if clearly needed. ISOPTIN (verapamil HCl) crosses the placental barrier and can be detected in umbilical vein blood at delivery.

Labor and Delivery: It is not known whether the use of verapamil during labor or delivery has immediate or delayed adverse effects on the fetus, or whether it prolongs the duration of labor or increases the need for forceps delivery or other obstetric intervention. Such adverse experiences have not been reported in the literature, despite a long history of use of ISOPTIN in Europe in the treatment of cardiac side effects of beta-adrenergic agonist agents used to treat premature labor.

Nursing Mothers: ISOPTIN is excreted in human milk. Because of the potential for adverse reactions in nursing infants for verapamil, nursing should be discontinued while verapamil is administered.

Pediatric Use: Safety and efficacy of ISOPTIN in children below the age of 18 years have not been established.

Animal Pharmacology and/or Animal Toxicology: In chronic animal toxicology studies verapamil caused lenticular and/or suture line changes at 30 mg/kg/day or greater and frank cataracts at 62.5 mg/kg/day or greater in the beagle dog but not the rat. Development of cataracts due to verapamil has not been reported in man.

ADVERSE REACTIONS
Serious adverse reactions are uncommon when ISOPTIN (verapamil HCl) therapy is initiated with upward dose titration within the recommended single and total daily dose. See WARNINGS for discussion of heart failure, hypotension, elevated liver enzymes, AV block, and rapid ventricular response. Reversible (upon discontinuation of verapamil) non-obstructive, paralytic, ileus has been infrequently reported in association with the use of verapamil. The following reactions to orally administered ISOPTIN occurred at rates greater than 1.0% or occurred at lower rates but appeared clearly drug-related in clinical trials in 4,954 patients.

Constipation	7.3%	Fatigue	1.7%
Dizziness	3.3%	Dyspnea	1.4%
Nausea	2.7%	Bradycardia(HR <50/min)	1.4%
Hypotension	2.5%	AV Block-total (1°, 2°, 3°)	1.2%
Headache	2.2%	2° and 3°	0.8%
Edema	1.9%	Rash	1.2%
CHF/		Flushing	0.6%
Pulmonary			
Edema	1.8%		

Elevated Liver Enzymes (see WARNING)

In clinical trials related to the control of ventricular response in digitalized patients who had atrial fibrillation or atrial flutter, ventricular rates below 50/min at rest occurred in 15% of patients and asymptomatic hypotension occurred in 5% of patients.

The following reactions, reported in 1.0% or less of patients, occurred under conditions (open trials, marketing experience) where a causal relationship is uncertain; they are listed to alert the physician to a possible relationship.

Cardiovascular: angina pectoris, atrioventricular dissociation, chest pain, claudication, myocardial infarction, palpitations, purpura (vasculitis), syncope.

Digestive System: diarrhea, dry mouth, gastrointestinal distress, gingival hyperplasia.

Hemic and Lymphatic: ecchymosis or bruising.

Nervous System: cerebrovascular accident, confusion, equilibrium disorders, insomnia, muscle cramps, parathesia, psychotic symptoms, shakiness, somnolence.

Skin: arthralgia and rash, exanthema, hair loss, hyperkeratosis, maculae, sweating, urticaria, Stevens-Johnson syndrome, erythema multiforme.

Special Senses: blurred vision.

Urogenital: gynecomastia, impotence, galactorrhea/hyperprolactinemia, increased urination, spotty menstruation.

Treatment of Acute Cardiovascular Adverse Reactions: The frequency of cardiovascular adverse reactions which require therapy is rare, hence, experience with their treatment is limited. Whenever severe hypotension or complete AV block occur following oral administration of verapamil, the appropriate emergency measures should be applied immediately, e.g., intravenously administered isoproterenol HCl, levarterenol bitartrate, atropine (all in the usual doses), or calcium gluconate (10% solution). In patients with hypertrophic cardiomyopathy (IHSS), alphaadrenergic agents (phenylephrine, metaraminol bitartrate or methoxamine) should be used to maintain blood pressure, and isoproterenol and levarterenol should be avoided. If further support is necessary,

inotropic agents (dopamine or dobutamine) may be administered. Actual treatment and dosage should depend on the severity and the clinical situation and the judgment and experience of the treating physician.

OVERDOSAGE

Treat all verapamil overdoses as serious and maintain observation for at least 48 hours (especially Isoptin SR), preferably under continuous hospital care. Delayed pharmacodynamic consequences may occur with the sustained released formulation. Verapamil is known to decrease gastrointestinal transit time.

Treatment of overdosage should be supportive. Beta adrenergic stimulation or parenteral administration of calcium solutions may increase calcium ion flux across the slow channel, and have been used effectively in treatment of deliberate overdosage with verapamil. Verapamil cannot be removed by hemodialysis. Clinically significant hypotensive reactions or high degree AV block should be treated with vasopressor agents or cardiac pacing, respectively. Asystole should be handled by the usual measures including cardiopulmonary resuscitation.

DOSAGE AND ADMINISTRATION
Essential Hypertension

The dose of ISOPTIN SR should be individualized by titration and the drug should be administered with food. Initiate therapy with 180 mg of sustained-release verapamil HCl, ISOPTIN SR, given in the morning. Lower, initial doses of 120 mg a day may be warranted in patients who may have an increased response to verapamil (e.g., the elderly or small people etc.). Upward titration should be based on therapeutic efficacy and safety evaluated weekly and approximately 24 hours after the previous dose. The antihypertensive effects of ISOPTIN SR are evident within the first week of therapy.

If adequate response is not obtained with 180 mg of ISOPTIN SR, the dose may be titrated upward in the following manner:

a) 240 mg each morning,
b) 180 mg each morning plus 180 mg each evening, or 240 mg each morning plus 120 mg each evening
c) 240 mg every twelve hours.

When switching from immediate release ISOPTIN to ISOPTIN SR, the total daily dose in milligrams may remain the same.

HOW SUPPLIED

ISOPTIN® SR 240 mg tablets are supplied as light green, capsule shaped, scored, film-coated tablets containing 240 mg of verapamil hydrochloride. The tablet is embossed with a double Knoll triangle on one side and "ISOPTIN SR" on the other side. ISOPTIN® SR 180 mg tablets are supplied as light pink, oval shaped, scored, film-coated tablets containing 180 mg of verapamil hydrochloride. The tablet is embossed with "ISOPTIN SR" on one side, and "180 mg" on the other side. The ISOPTIN® SR 120 mg tablets are supplied as light violet, oval shaped, film-coated tablets containing 120 mg of verapamil hydrochloride. The tablet is embossed with "KNOLL" on one side and "120 SR" on the other side.

240 mg (light green)- Bottle of 30-
NDC #0044-1826-93
Bottle of 100-
NDC #0044-1826-02
Bottle of 500-
NDC #0044-1826-03
Hospital Unit Dose (100 Tablets-
10 Strips of 10)-NDC #0044-1826-10
180 mg (light pink)- Bottle of 100-
NDC #0044-1825-02
Bottle of 500-
NDC #0044-1825-03
Hospital Unit Dose (100 Tablets-
10 Strips of 10)-NDC #0044-1825-12
120 mg (light violet)- Bottle of 100-
NDC #0044-1827-02
Bottle of 500-
NDC #0044-1827-03
Hospital Unit Dose (100 Tablets-
10 Strips of 10) - NDC #0044-1827-12

Storage: 15° to 25°C (59° to 77°F)
Protect from light and moisture.
Dispense in a light, light-resistant container as defined in the USP.
© 1996 Knoll Pharmaceutical Company.
ISOPTIN is a registered trademark of Knoll AG.
Revised: June 1996
Knoll Laboratories
A Division of
Knoll Pharmaceutical Company
Mount Olive, New Jersey 07828   **BASF** Pharma
0900023-3

Shown in Product Identification Guide, page 318

RYTHMOL® TABLETS   ℞
(propafenone hydrochloride)

DESCRIPTION

RYTHMOL (propafenone hydrochloride) is an antiarrhythmic drug supplied in scored, film-coated tablets of 150, 225 and 300 mg for oral administration. Propafenone has some structural similarities to beta-blocking agents.
The structural formula of propafenone hydrochloride is given below:

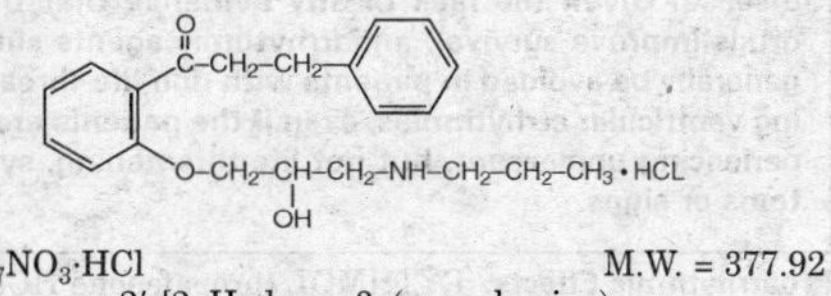

$C_{21}H_{27}NO_3 \cdot HCl$ M.W. = 377.92
2'-[2—Hydroxy-3—(propylamino)
-propoxy]-3-phenylpropiophenone
hydrochloride

Propafenone hydrochloride occurs as colorless crystals or white crystalline powder with a very bitter taste. It is slightly soluble in water (20°C), chloroform and ethanol. The following inactive ingredients are contained in the tablet: corn starch, hydroxypropyl methylcellulose, magnesium stearate, polyethylene glycol, polysorbate, povidone, propylene glycol, sodium starch glycolate and titanium dioxide.

CLINICAL PHARMACOLOGY

Mechanism of Action: RYTHMOL (propafenone HCl) is a Class 1C antiarrhythmic drug with local anesthetic effects, and a direct stablizing action on myocardial membranes. The electrophysiological effect of RYTHMOL manifests itself in a reduction of upstroke velocity (Phase 0) of the monophasic action potential. In Purkinje fibers, and to a lesser extent myocardial fibers, RYTHMOL reduces the fast inward current carried by sodium ions. Diastolic excitability threshold is increased and effective refractory period prolonged. Propafenone reduces spontaneous automaticity and depresses triggered activity.

Studies in anesthetized dogs and isolated organ preparations show that RYTHMOL has beta-sympatholytic activity at about 1/50 the potency of propranolol. Clinical studies employing isoproternol challenge and exercise testing after single doses of propafenone indicate a beta-adrenergic blocking potency (per mg) about 1/40 that of propranolol in man. In clinical trials, resting heart rate decreases of about 8% were noted at the higher end of the therapeutic plasma concentration range. At very high concentrations in vitro, propafenone can inhibit the slow inward current carried by calcium but this calcium antagonist effect probably does not contribute to antiarrhythmic efficacy. Propafenone has local anesthetic activity approximately equal to procaine.

Electrophysiology: Electrophysiology studies in patients with ventricular tachycardia have shown that RYTHMOL prolongs atrioventricular conduction which having little or no effect on sinus node function. Both AV nodal conduction time (AH interval) and His-Purkinje conduction time (HV interval) are prolonged. Propafenone has little or no effect on the atrial functional refractory period, but AV nodal functional and effective refractory periods are prolonged. In patients with WPW, RYTHMOL reduces conduction and increses the effective refractory period of the accessory pathway in both directions. Propafenone slows conduction and consequently produces dose related changes in the PR interval and QRS duration. QTc interval does not change.

Mean Changes in ECG Intervals*
Total Daily Dose (mg)

Interval	337.5 mg		450 mg		675 mg		900 mg	
	msec	%	msec	%	msec	%	msec	%
RR	−14.5	−1.8	30.6	3.8	31.5	3.9	41.7	5.1
PR	3.6	2.1	19.1	11.6	28.9	17.8	35.6	21.9
QRS	5.6	6.4	5.5	6.1	7.7	8.4	15.6	17.3
QTc	2.7	0.7	−7.5	−1.8	5.0	1.2	14.7	3.7

* Change and percent change based on mean baseline values for each treatment group.

In any individual patient, the above ECG changes cannot be readily used to predict either efficacy or plasma concentration.
RYTHMOL causes a dose-related and concentration-related decrease in the rate of single and multiple PVCs and can suppress recurrence of ventricular tachycardia. Based on the percent of patients attaining substantial (80–90%) suppression of ventricular ectopic activity, it appears that trough plasma levels of 0.2 to 1.5 µg/mL can provide good suppression, with higher concentrations giving a greater rate of good response.

When 600 mg/day propafenone was administered to patients with paroxysmal atrial tachyarrhythmias, mean heart rate during arrhythmia decreased 14 beats/min and 37 beats/min for PAF patients and PSVT patients, respectively.
Hemodynamics: Sympathetic stimulation may be a vital component supporting circulatory function in patients with congestive heart failure, and its inhibition by the beta blockade produced by RYTHMOL may in itself aggravate congestive heart failure.
Additionally, like other Class 1C antiarrhythmic drugs, studies in humans have shown that RYTHMOL exerts a negative inotropic effect on the myocardium. Cardiac catheterization studies in patients with moderately impaired ventricular function (mean C.I.=2.61 L/min/m^2) utilizing intravenous propafenone infusions (2 mg/kg over 10 min+2 mg/min for 30 min) that gave mean plasma concentrations of 3.0 µg/mL (well above the therapeutic range of 0.2–1.5 µg/mL) showed significant increases in pulmonary capillary wedge pressure, systemic and pulmonary vascular resistances and depression of cardiac output and cardiac index.
Pharmacokinetics and Metabolism: RYTHMOL is nearly completely absorbed after oral administration with peak plasma levels occurring approximately 3.5 hours after administration in most individuals. Propafenone exhibits extensive saturable presystemic biotransformation (first pass effect) resulting in a dose dependent and dosage form dependent absolute bioavailability; e.g., a 150 mg tablet had absolute bioavailability of 3.4%, while a 300 mg tablet had absolute bioavailability of 10.6%. A 300 mg solution which was rapidly aboosrbed, had absolute bioavailability of 21.4%. At still larger doses, above those recommended, bioavailability increases still further. Decreased liver function also increases bioavailability, bioavailability inversely related to indocyanine green clearance reaching 60–70% at clearances of 7 mL/min and below. The clearance of propafenone is reduced and the elimination half-life increased in patients with significant heptic dysunction (see PRECAUTIONS).
RYTHMOL follows a nonlinear pharmacokinetic disposition presumably due to saturation of first pass hepatic metabolism as the liver is exposed to higher concentrations of propafenone and shows a very high degree of interindividual variability. For example, for a three-fold increase in daily dose from 300 to 900 mg/day there is a tenfold increase in steady-slate plasma concentration.The top 25% of patients given 375 mg/day, however, had a mean concentration of propafenone larger than the bottom 25%, and about equal to the second 25%, of patients given a dose of 900 mg. Although food increased peak blood level and bioavailability in a single dose study, during multiple dose administration of propafenone to healthy volunteers food did not change bioavailability significantly.
There are two genetically determined patterns of propafenone metabolism. In over 90% of patients, the drug is rapidly and extensively metabolized with an elimination half life from 2–10 hours. These patients metabolize propafenone into two active metabolites: 5-hydroxy-propafenone and N-depropylpropafenone. In vitro preparations have shown these two metabolites to have antiarrhythmic activity comparable to propafenone but in man they both are usually present in concentrations less than 20% of propafenone. Nine additional metabolites have been identified, most in only trace amounts. It is the saturable hydroxylation pathway that is responsible for the nonlinear pharmacokinetic disposition.
In less than 10% of patients (and in any patient also receiving quindine, see PRECAUTIONS), metabolism of propafenone is slower because the 5-hydroxy metabolite is not formed or is minimally formed. The estimated propafenone elimination half-life ranges from 10–32 hours. Decreased ability to form the 5-hydroxy metabolite of propafernone is associated with a diminished ability to metabolize debrisoquine and a variety of other drugs (encainide, metoprolol, dextromethorphan). In these patients, the N-deproplpropafenone occurs in quantities comparable to the levels occurring in extensive metabolizers. In slow metabolizers propafenone pharmacokinetics are linear.
There are significant differences in plasma concentrations of propafenone in slow and extensive metabolizers, the former achieving concentrations 1.5 to 2.0 times those of the extensive metabolizers at daily doses of 675–900 mg/day. At low doses the differences are greater, with slow metabolizers attaining concentrations more than five times that of extensive metabolizers. Because the difference decreases at high doses and is mitigated by the lack of the active 5-hydroxy metabolite in the slow metabolizers, and because steady-slate conditions are achieved after 4–5 days of dosing in all patients, the recommended dosing regimen is the same for all patients. The greater variability in blood levels require that the drug be titrated carefully in patients with close attention paid to clinical and ECG evidence of toxicity (See DOSAGE AND ADMINISTRATION).
Clinical Trials: In two randomized, crossover, placebo-controlled, double-blind trials of 60–90 days duration in pa-

Continued on next page

Rythmol—Cont.

tients with paroxysmal supraventricular arrhythmias [paroxysmal atrial fibrillation/flutter (PAF), or paroxysmal supraventricular tachycardia (PSVT)], propafenone reduced the rate of both arrhythmias, as shown in the following table:

	Study 1		Study 2	
	Pro-pafenone	Placebo	Pro-pafenone	Placebo
PAF	n=30	n=30	n=9	n=9
Percent attack free	53%	13%	67%	22%
Median time to first recurrene	>98 days	8 days	62 days	5 days
PSVT	n=45	n=45	n=15	n=15
Percent attack free	47%	16%	38%	7%
Median time to first recurrence	>98 days	12 days	31 days	8 days

The patient population in the above trials was 50% male with a mean age of 57.3 years. Fifty percent of the patients had a diagnosis of PAF and 50% had PSVT. Eighty percent of the patients received 60 mg/day propafenone. No patient died in the above 2 studies.

In the U.S. long-term safety trials, 474 patients (mean age: 57.4 ± 14.5 years) with supraventricular arrhythmias [195 with PAF, 274 with PSVT and 5 with both PAF and PSVT] were treated up to 5 years (mean: 14.4 months) with propafenone. Fourteen of the patients died. When this mortality rate was compared to the rate in a similar patient population (n=194 patients; mean age: 43.0 ± 16.8 years) studied in an arrhythmia clinic, there was no age-adjusted difference in mortality. This comparison was not, however, a randomized trial and the 95% confidence interval around the comparison was large, such that neither a significant adverse or favorable effect could be ruled out.

INDICATIONS AND USAGE

In patients without structural heart disease, RYTHMOL (propafenone HCl) is indicated to prolong the time to recurrence of

— paroxysmal atrial fibrillation/flutter (PAF) associated with disabling symptoms.
— paroxysmal supraventricular tachycardia (PSVT) associated with disabling symptoms.

As with other agents, some patients with atrial flutter treated with propafenone have developed 1:1 conduction, producing an increase in ventricular rate. Concomitant treatment with drugs that increase the functional AV refractory period is recommended.

The use of Rythmol in patients with chronic atrial fibrillation has not been evaluated. Rythmol should not be used to control ventricular rate during atrial fibrillation.

RYTHMOL is also indicated for the treatment of
— documented ventricular arrhythmias, such as sustained ventricular tachycardia, that, in the judgement of the physician, are life-threatening. Because the proarrhythmic effects of RYTHMOL, its use with lesser ventricular arrhythmias is not recommended, even if patients are symptomatic, and any use of the drug should be reserved for patients in whom, in the opinion of the physician, the potential benefits outweigh the risks.

Initiation of RYTHMOL treatment, as with other anti-arrthythmics used to treat life-threatening ventricular arrhythmias, should be carried out in the hospital.

RYTHMOL, like other antiarrhythmic drugs, has not been shown to enhance survival in patients with ventricular or atrial arrhythmias.

CONTRAINDICATIONS

RYTHMOL (propafenone HCl) is contraindicated in the presence of uncontrolled congestive heart failure, cardiogenic shock, sinoatrial, atrioventricular and intraventricular disorders of impulse generation and/or conduction (e.g., sick sinus node syndrome, atrioventricular block) in the absence of an artificial pacemaker, bradycardia, marked hypotension, bronchospastic disorders, manifest electrolyte imbalance, and known hypersensitivity to the drug.

WARNINGS

Mortality: In the National Heart, Lung and Blood Institute's Cardiac Arrhythmia Suppression Trial (CAST), a long-term, multi-center, randomized, double-blind study in patients with asymptomatic non-life-threatening ventricular arrhythmias who had a myocardial infarction more than six days but less than two years previously, an increased rate of death or reversed cardiac

arrest (7.7%; 56/730) was seen in patients treated with encainide or flecainide (class 1C antiarrhythmics) compared with that seen in patients assigned to placebo (3.0%; 22/725). The average duration of treatment with encainide or flecainide in this study was ten months. The applicability of the CAST results to other populations (e.g., those without recent myocardial infarction) or other antiarrhythmic drugs is uncertain, but at present it is prudent to consider any 1C antiarrhythmic to have a significant risk in patients with structural heart disease. Given the lack of any evidence that these drugs improve survival, antiarrhythmic agents should generally be avoided in patients with non-life-threatening ventricular arrhythmias, even if the patients are experiencing unpleasant, but not life-threatening, symptoms or signs.

Proarrhythmic Effects: RYTHMOL (propafenone HCl), like other antiarrhythmic agents, may cause new or worsened arrhythmias. Such proarrhythmic effects range from an increase in frequency of PVCs to the development of more severe ventricular tachycardia, ventricular fibrillation or tosade de pointes; i.e., tachycardia that is more sustained or more rapid may lead to fatal consequences. It is therefore essential that each patient given RYTHMOL be evaluated electrocardiographically and clinically prior to, and during therapy to determine whether the response to RYTHMOL supports continued treatment.

Overall in clinical trials with propafenone. 4.7% of all patients had new or worsened ventricular arrhythmia possible representing a pro-arrthythmic event (0.7% was an increase in PVCs; 4.0% a worsening, or new appearance, of VT or VF). Of the patients who had worsening of VT (4%), 92% had a history of VT and/or VT/VF, 71% had coronary artery disease, and 68% had a prior myocardial infarction. The incidence of proarrhythmia in patients with less serious or benign arrhythmias, which include patients with an increase in frequency of PVCs, was 1.6%. Although most proarrhythmic events occurred during the first week of therapy, late events also were seen and the CAST study (see above) suggests that an increased risk is present throughout treatment.

In the 474 patient U.S. multicenter trial in patients with symptomatic SVT, 1.9% (9/474) of these patients experienced ventricular tachycardia (VT) or ventricular fibrillation (VF) during the study. However, in 4 of the 9 patients, the ventricular tachycardia was of atrial origin. Six of the nine patients that developed ventricular arrhythmias did so within 14 days of onset of therapy. About 2.3% (11/474) of all patients had a recurrence of SVT during the study which could have been a change in the patients' arrhythmia behavior or could represent a proarrhythmic event. Case reports in patients treated with RYTHMOL for atrial fibrillation/flutter have included increased PVCs, VT, VF, and death.

Nonallergic Bronchospasm (e.g., chronic bronchitis, emphysema): PATIENTS WITH BRONCHOPASTIC DISEASE SHOULD, IN GENERAL, NOT RECEIVE PROPAFENONE or other agents with beta-adrenergic-blocking activity.

Congestive Heart Failure: During treatment with oral propafenone in patients with depressed baseline function (mean EF=33.5%), no significant decreases in ejection fraction were seen. In clinical trial experience, new or worsened CHF has been reported in 3.7% of patients with ventricular arrhythmia, of those 0.9% were considered probably or definitely related to RYTHMOL. Of the patients with congestive heart failure probably related to propafenone, 80% had preexisting heart failure and 85% had coronary artery disease. CHF attributable to RYTHMOL developed rarely (<0.2%) in ventricular arrhythmia patients who had no previous history of CHF. CHF occurred in 1.9% of patients studied with PAF or PSVT.

As RYTHMOL exerts both beta blockade and a (dose-related) negative inotropic effect on cardiac muscle, patients with congestive heart failure should be fully compensated before receiving RYTHMOL. If congestive heart failure worsens, RYTHMOL should be discontinued (unless congestive heart failure is due to the cardiac arrhythmia) and, if indicated, restarted at a lower dosage only after adequate cardiac compensation has been established.

Conduction Disturbances: RYTHMOL slows atrioventricular conduction and also causes first degree AV block. Average PR interval prolongation and increases in QRS duration are closely correlated with dosage increases and concomitant increases in propafenone plasma concentrations. The incidence of first degree, second degree, and third degree AV block observed in 2,127 patients was 2.5%, 0.6%, and 0.2%, respectively. Development of second or third degree AV block requires a reduction in dosage or discontinuation of RYTHMOL. Bundle branch block (1.2%) and intraventricular conduction delay (1.1%) have been reported in patients receiving propafenone. Bradycardia has also been reported (1.5%). Experience in patients with sick sinus node syndrome is limited and these patients should not be treated with propafenone.

Effects on Pacemaker Threshold: RYTHMOL may alter both pacing and sensing thresholds of artificial pacemakers. Pacemakers should be monitored and programmed accordingly during therapy.

Hematologic Disturbances: Agranulocytosis (fever, chills, weakness, and neutropenia) has been reported in patients receiving propafenone. Generally, the agranulocytosis occurred within the first two months of propafenone therapy and upon discontinuation of therapy, the white count usually normalized by 14 days. Unexplained fever and/or decrease in white cell count, particularly during the initial three months of therapy, warrant consideration of possible agranulocytosis/granulocytopenia. Patients should be instructed to promptly report the development of any signs of infection such as fever, sore throat, or chills.

PRECAUTIONS

Hepatic Dysfunction: Propafenone is highly metabolized by the liver and should, therefore, be administered cautiously to patients with impaired hepatic function. Severe liver dysfunction increases the bioavailability of propafenone to approximately 70% compared to 3–40% for patients with normal liver function. In eight patients with moderate to severe liver disease, the mean half-life was approximately 9 hours. As a result, the dose of propafenone given to patients with impaired hepatic function should be approximately 20–30% of the dose given to patients with normal hepatic function (see DOSAGE AND ADMINISTRATION). Careful monitoring for excessive pharmacological effects (see OVERDOSE) should be carried out.

Renal Dysfunction: A considerable percentage of propafenone metabolites (18.5%-38% of the dose/48 hours) are excreted in the urine.

Until further data are available, RYTHMOL (propafenone HCl) should be administered cautiously to patients with impaired renal function. These patients should be carefully monitored for signs of overdosage (see OVERDOSAGE).

Elevated ANA Titers: Positive ANA titers have been reported in patients receiving propafenone. They have been reversible upon cessation of treatment and may disappear even in the face of continued propafenone therapy. These laboratory findings were usually not associated with clinical symptoms, but there is one published case of drug-induced lupus erythematosis (positive rechallenge); if resolved completely upon discontinuation of therapy. Patients who develop an abnormal ANA test should be carefully evaluated and, if persistent or worsening elevation of ANA titers is defected, consideration should be given to discontinuing therapy.

Impaired Spermatogenesis: Reversible disorders of spermatogenesis have been demonstrated in monkeys, dogs and rabbits after high dose intravenous administration. Evaluation of the effects of short-term propafenone administration on spermatogenesis in 11 normal subjects suggests that propafenone produced a reversible, short-term drop (within normal range) in sperm count. Subsequent evaluations in 11 patients receiving propafenone chronically have suggested no effect of propafenone on sperm count.

Neuromuscular Dysfunction: Exacerbation of myasthenia gravis has been reported during propafenone therapy.

Drug interactions:

Quinidine: Small doses of quinidine completely inhibit the hydroxylation metabolic pathway, making all patients, in effect, slow metabolizers (see CLINCAL PHARMACOLOGY). There is, as yet, too little information to recommend concomitant use of propafenone and quinidine.

Local Anesthetics: Concomitant use of local anesthetics (i.e., during pacemaker implantations, surgery, or dental use) may increase the risks of central nervous system side effects.

Digitalis: RYTHMOL (propafenone hydrochloride) produces dose-related increases in serum digoxin levels ranging from about 35% at 450 mg/day to 85% at 900 mg/day of propafenone without affecting digoxin renal clearance. These elevations of digoxin levels were maintained for up to 16 months during concomitant administration. Plasma digoxin levels were maintained for up to 16 months during concomitant administration. Plasma digoxin levels of patients on concomitant therapy should be measured, and digoxin dosage should ordinarily be reduced when propafenone is started, especially if a relatively large digoxin dose is used or if plasma concentrations are relatively high.

Beta-Antagonists: In a study involving healthy subjects, concomitant administration of propafenone and propranolol has resulted in substantial increases in propranolol plasma concentration and elimination half-life with no change in propafenone plasma levels from control values. Similar observations have been reported with metoprolol. Propafenone appears to inhibit the hydroxylation pathway for the two beta-antagonists (just as quinidine inhibits propafenone metabolism). Increased plasma concentrations of metoprolol could overcome its relative cardioselectivity. In propafenone clinical trials, patients who were receiving beta-blockers concurrently did not experience an increased incidence of side effects. While the therapeutic range for beta-blockers is

Adverse Reactions Reported for ≥1% of Ventricular Arrhythmia Patients
N=2127

	Incidence by Total Daily Dose			Total Incidence	% of Pts. Who Discont.
	450 mg	600 mg	≥900 mg		
	(N = 1430)	(N = 1337)	(N = 1333)	(N = 2127)	
Dizziness	4%	7%	11%	13%	2.4%
Nausea and/or Vomiting	2%	6%	9%	11%	3.4%
Unusual Taste	3%	5%	6%	9%	0.7%
Constipation	2%	4%	5%	7%	0.5%
Fatigue	2%	3%	4%	6%	1.0%
Dyspnea	2%	2%	4%	5%	1.6%
Proarrhythmia	2%	2%	3%	5%	4.7%
Angina	2%	2%	3%	5%	0.5%
Headache(s)	2%	3%	3%	5%	1.0%
Blurred Vision	1%	2%	3%	4%	0.8%
CHF	1%	2%	3%	4%	1.4%
Ventricular Tachycardia	1%	2%	3%	3%	1.2%
Dyspepsia	1%	2%	3%	3%	0.9%
Palpitations	1%	2%	3%	3%	0.5%
Rash	1%	1%	2%	3%	0.8%
AV Block First Degree	1%	1%	2%	3%	0.3%
Diarrhea	1%	2%	2%	3%	0.6%
Weakness	1%	2%	2%	2%	0.7%
Dry Mouth	1%	1%	1%	2%	0.2%
Syncope/Near Syncope	1%	1%	1%	2%	0.7%
QRS Duration, Increased	1%	1%	2%	2%	0.5%
Chest Pain	1%	1%	1%	2%	0.2%
Anorexia	1%	1%	2%	2%	0.4%
Abdominal Pain, Cramps	1%	1%	1%	2%	0.4%
Ataxia	0%	1%	2%	2%	0.2%
Insomnia	0%	1%	1%	2%	0.3%
Premature Ventricular Contraction(s)	1%	1%	1%	2%	0.1%
Bradycardia	1%	1%	1%	2%	0.5%
Anxiety	1%	1%	1%	2%	0.6%
Edema	1%	0%	1%	1%	0.2%
Tremor(s)	0%	1%	1%	1%	0.3%
Diaphoresis	1%	0%	1%	1%	0.3%
Bundle Branch Block	0%	1%	1%	1%	0.5%
Drowsiness	1%	1%	1%	1%	0.2%
Atrial Fibrillation	1%	1%	1%	1%	0.4%
Flatulence	0%	1%	1%	1%	0.1%
Hypotension	0%	1%	1%	1%	0.4%
Intraventricular Conduction Delay	0%	1%	1%	1%	0.1%
Pain, Joints	0%	0%	1%	1%	0.1%

wide, a reduction in dosage may be necessary during concomitant administration with propafenone.

Warfarin: In a study of eight healthy subjects receiving propafenone and warfarin concomitantly, mean steady-state warfarin plasma concentrations increased 39% with a corresponding increase in prothrombin times of approximately 25%. It is therefore recommended that prothrombin times be routinely monitored and the dose of warfarin be adjusted if necessary.

Cimetidine: Concomitant administration of propafenone and cimetidine in 12 healthy subjects resulted in a 20% increase in steady-state plasma concentrations of propafenone with no detectable changes in electrocardiographic parameters beyond that measured on propafenone alone.

Desipramine: Concomitant administration of propafenone and desipramine may result in elevated serum desipramine levels. Both desipramine, a tricyclic antidepressant, and propafenone are cleared by oxidative pathways of demethy-

lation and hydroxylation carried out by the hepatic P-450 cytochrome.

Cyclosporin: Propafenone therapy may increase levels of cyclosporin.

Theophylline: Propafenone may increase theophylline concentration during concomitant therapy with the development of theophylline toxicity.

Rifampin: Rifampin may accelerate the metabolism and decrease the plasma levels and antiarrhythmic efficacy of propafenone.

Other: Limited experience with propafenone combined with calcium antagonists and diuretics has been reported without evidence of clinically significant adverse reactions.

Carcinogenesis, Mutagenesis, impairment of Fertility: Lifetime maximally tolerated oral dose studies in mice (up to 360 mg/kg/day) and rats (up to 270 mg/kg/day) provided no evidence of a carcinogenic potential for propafenone. RYTHMOL was not mutagenic when assayed for genotoxicity in 1) mouse Dominant Lethal test. 2) rat bone marrow Chromosome Analysis, 3) Chinese hamster bone marrow and spermatogonia chromosome analysis, 4) Chinese hamster micronucleus test, and 5) Ames bacterial test. Propafenone administered intravenously to rabbits, dogs, and monkeys has been shown to decrease spermatogenesis. These effects were reversible, were not found following oral dosing of propafenone, were seen only at lethal or sublethal dose levels and were not seen in rats treated either orally or intravenously (see PRECAUTIONS, Impaired Spermatogenesis). Propafenone did not affect fertility rates when administered orally to male and female rats at doses up to 270 mg/kg/day or when administered orally or intravenously to male rabbits at doses of 120 mg/kg/day or 3.5 mg/kg/day, respectively. On a body weight basis, the above noted oral doses in rat and rabbit are 18 times and 8 times, respectively, the maximum recommended daily human dose of 900 mg (based on 60 kg human body weight).

Pregnancy-Teratogenic Effects:
Pregnancy Category C:
Propafenone has been shown to be embyotoxic in rabbits and rats when given in doses 10 and 40 times, respectively, the maximum recommended human dose. No teratogenic potential was apparent in either species. There are no adequate and well-controlled studies in pregnant women. Propafenone should be used during pregnancy only if the potential benefit justifies the potential risk to the fetus.

Pregnancy-Nonteratogenic Effects: In a perinatal and postnatal study in rats, propafenone, at dose levels of 6 or more times the maximum recommended human dose, produced dose dependent increses in maternal and neonatal mortality, decreased maternal and pup body weight gain and reduced neonatal physiological development.

Labor and Delivery: It is not know whether the use of propafenone during labor or delivery has immediate or delayed adverse effects on the fetus, or whether it prolongs the duration of labor or increases the need for forceps delivery or other obstetrical intervention.

Nursing Mothers: It is not known whether this drug is excreted in human milk. Because many drugs are excreted in human milk and because of the potential for serious adverse reactions in nursing infants from RYTHMOL, a decision should be made whether to discontinue nursing or to discontinue the drug, taking into account the importance of the drug to the mother.

Pediatric Use: The safety and effectiveness of RYTHMOL in pediatric patients have not been established.

Geriatric Use: There do not appear to be any age-related differences in adverse reaction rates in the most commonly reported adverse reactions. Because of the possible increased risk of impaired hepatic or renal function in this age group, RYTHMOL should be used with caution. The effective dose may be lower in these patients.

Animal Toxicology: Renal changes have been observed in the rat following 6 months of oral administration of propafenone at doses of 180 and 360 mg/kg/day (12–24 times the maximum recommended human dose) but not 90 mg/kg/day. Both inflammatory and non-inflammatory changes in the renal tubules with accompanying interstitial nephritis were observed. These lesions were reversible in that they were not found in rats treated at these dosage levels and allowed to recover for 6 weeks. Fatty degenerative changes of the liver were found in rats following chronic administration of propafenone at dose levels 19 times the maximum recommended human dose.

ADVERSE REACTIONS

Adverse reactions associated with RYTHMOL occur most frequently in the gastrointestinal, cardiovascular, and central nervous systems. About 20% of patients treated with RYTHMOL have discontinued treatment because of adverse reactions.

Adverse reactions reported for > 1.5% of 474 SVT patients who received propafenone in U.S. clinical trials are presented in the following table by incidence and percent discontinuation, reported to the nearest percent.

Continued on next page

Rythmol—Cont.

Adverse Reactions Reported for > 1.5% of SVT Patients

	Incidence (N=480)	% of Pts. who Discontinued
Unusual taste	14%	1.3%
Nausea and/or Vomiting	11%	2.9%
Dizziness	9%	1.7%
Constipation	8%	0.2%
Headache	6%	0.8%
Fatigue	6%	1.5%
Blurred Vision	3%	0.6%
Weakness	3%	1.3%
Dyspnea	2%	1.0%
Wide Complex Tachycardia	2%	1.9%
CHF	2%	0.6%
Bradycardia	2%	0.2%
Palpitations	2%	0.2%
Tremor	2%	0.4%
Anorexia	2%	0.2%
Diarrhea	2%	0.4%
Ataxia	2%	0.0%

Results of controlled trials in ventricular arrhythmia patients comparing adverse reaction rates on propafenone and placebo, and on propafenone and quinidine are shown in the following table. Adverse reactions reported in ≥ 1% of the patients receiving propafenone are shown, unless they were more frequent on placebo than propafenone. The most common events were unusual taste, dizziness, first degree AV block, intraventricular conduction delay, nausea and/or vomiting, and constipation. Headache was relatively common also, but was not increased compared to placebo.

Adverse Reactions Reported for ≥1% of Ventricular Arrhythmia Patients

	Prop./Placebo Trials		Prop./Quinidine Trial	
	Prop.	Placebo	Prop.	Quinidine
	(N=247)	(N=111)	(N=53)	(N=52)
Unusual Taste	7%	1%	23%	0%
Dizziness	7%	5%	15%	10%
First Degree AV Block	5%	1%	2%	0%
Headache(s)	5%	5%	2%	8%
Constipation	4%	0%	6%	6%
Intraventricular Conduction Delay	4%	0%	-	-
Nausea and/or Vomiting	3%	1%	6%	15%
Fatigue	-	-	4%	2%
Palpitations	2%	1%	-	-
Blurred Vision	2%	1%	6%	2%
Dry Mouth	2%	1%	6%	6%
Dyspnea	2%	3%	4%	0%
Abdominal Pain/Cramps	-	-	2%	8%
Dyspepsia	-	-	2%	8%

CHF	-	-	2%	0%
Fever	-	-	2%	10%
Tinnitus	-	-	2%	2%
Vision, Abnormal	-	-	2%	2%
Esophagitis	-	-	2%	0%
Gastroenteritis	-	-	2%	0%
Anxiety	2%	2%	-	-
Anorexia	2%	1%	-	2%
Proarrhythmia	1%	0%	2%	0%
Flatulence	1%	0%	2%	0%
Angina	1%	0%	2%	4%
Second Degree AV Block	1%	0%	-	-
Bundle Branch Block	1%	0%	2%	2%
Loss of Balance	1%	0%	-	-
Diarrhea	1%	1%	6%	39%

Adverse reactions reported for ≥ 1% of 2,127 ventricular arrhythmia patients who received propafenone in U.S. clinical trials are presented in the following table by propafenone daily dose. The most common adverse reactions in controlled clinical trials appeared dose related (but note that most patients spent more time at the larger doses), especially dizziness, nausea and/or vomiting, unusual taste, constipation, and blurred vision. Some less common reactions may also have been dose related such as first degree AV block, congestive heart failure, dyspepsia, and weakness. The principal causes of discontinuation were the most common events and are shown in the table.
[See table at top of previous page]
In addition, the following adverse reactions were reported less frequently than 1% either in clinical trials or in marketing experience (adverse events for marketing experience are given in italics). Causality and relationship to propafenone therapy cannot necessarily be judged from these events.

Cardiovascular System: Atrial flutter, AV dissociation, cardiac arrest, flushing, hot flashes, sick sinus syndrome, sinus pause or arrest, supraventricular tachycardia.
Nervous System: Abnormal dreams, abnormal speech, abnormal vision, apnea, coma, confusion, depression, memory loss, numbness paresthesias, psychosis/mania, seizures (0.3%), tinnitus, unusual smell sensation, vertigo.
Gastrointestinal: A number of patients with liver abnormalities associated with propafenone therapy have been reported in foreign post-marketing experience. Some appeared due to hepatocellular injury, some were cholestatic and some showed a mixed picture. Some of these reports were simply discovered through clinical chemistries, others because of clinical symptoms including fulminant hepatitis and death. One case was rechallenged with a positive outcome. Cholestasis (0.1%), elevated liver enzymes (alkaline phophatase, serum transaminases) (0.2%), gastroenteritis, hepatitis (0.03%).
Hematologic: Agranulocytosis, anemia, bruising, granulocytopenia, increased bleeding time, leukopenia, purpura, thrombocytopenia.
Other: Alopecia, eye irritation, hyponatremia/inappropriate ADH secretion, impotence, increased glucose, kidney failure, positive ANA (0.7%), lupus erythematosis, muscle cramps, muscle weakness, nephrotic syndrome, pain, pruritus.

OVERDOSAGE

The symptoms of overdosage, which are usually most severe within 3 hours of ingestion, may include hypotension, somnolence, bradycardia, intra-atrial and intraventricular conduction disturbances, and rarely convulsions and high grade ventricular arrhythmias. Defibrillation as well as infusion of dopamine and isproterenol have been effective in controlling rhythm and blood pressure. Convulsions have been alleviated with intravenous diazepam. General supportive measures such as mechanical respiratory assistance and external cardiac massage may be necessary.

DOSAGE AND ADMINISTRATION

The dose of RYTHMOL (propafenone HCl) must be individually titrated on the basis of response and tolerance. It is recommended that therapy be initiated with 150 mg propafenone given every eight hours (450 mg/day). Dosage may be increased at a minimum of 3 to 4 day intervals to 225 mg

every 8 hours (675 mg/day) and, if necessary, to 300 mg every 8 hours (900 mg/day). The usefulness and safety of dosages exceeding 900 mg per day have not been established. In those patients in whom significant widening of the QRS complex or second or third degree AV block occurs, dose reduction should be considered.
As with other antiarrhythmic agents, in the elderly or in patients with marked previous myocardial damage, the dose of RYTHMOL should be increased more gradually during the initial phase of treatment.

HOW SUPPLIED

RYTHMOL (propafenone HCl) tablets are supplied as scored, round, film-coated tablets containing either 150 mg, 225 mg or 300 mg of propafenone hydrochloride and embossed with 150, 225 or 300 and an arched triangle on the same side.
150 mg (white)– Bottle of 100–NDC#0044-5022-02
    Hospital Unit Dose (100 tablets-strips of 10)-NDC#0044-5022-10
225 mg (white)– Bottle of 100-NDC # 0044-5024-02
    Hospital Unit Dose (100 tablets- strips of 10)-NDC #0044-5024-10
300 mg (white)– Bottle of 100-NDC # 0044-5023-02
    Hospital Unit Dose (100 tablets-strips of 10)-NDC#0044-5023-10

Storage: Store at controlled room temperature 15°–30°C (59°–86°F). Dispense in a tight, light-resistant container as defined in the U.S.P.

©1998 Knoll Pharmaceutical Company
RYTHMOL is a registered trademark of Fieldmark, Inc. used under license by Knoll Pharmaceutical Company

Revised: January 1998

Knoll Laboratories
A Division of
Knoll Pharmaceutical Company
3000 Continental Drive- North
Mount Olive, NJ 07828-1234
BASF Pharma   0909001-5
Shown in Product Identification Guide, page 318

VICODIN HP™   Ⅽ Ŗ
[vĭkō-dĭn]
(hydrocodone bitartrate* and acetaminophen tablets, USP)
10 mg/660 mg
*Warning: May be habit forming.

DESCRIPTION

Hydrocodone bitartrate and acetaminophen is supplied in tablet form for oral administration.
Hydrocodone bitartrate is an opioid analgesic and antitussive and occurs as fine, white crystals or as a crystalline powder. It is affected by light. The chemical name is 4,5α-epoxy-3-methoxy-17-methylmorphinan-6-one tartrate (1:1) hydrate (2:5). It has the following structural formula:

$C_{18}H_{21}NO_3 \cdot C_4H_6O_6 \cdot 2^1/_2H_2O)$ M.W.=494.50

Acetaminophen, 4'-hydroxyacetanilide, a slightly bitter, white, odorless, crystalline powder, is a non-opiate, non-salicylate analgesic and antipyretic. It has the following structural formula:

$C_8H_9NO_2$ M.W.=151.17

Each VICODIN HP™ tablet contains:
Hydrocodone Bitartrate   10 mg
(**WARNING:** May be habit forming.)
Acetaminophen   660 mg

In addition each tablet contains the following inactive ingredients: colloidal silicon dioxide, croscarmellose sodium, magnesium stearate, microcrystalline cellulose, povidone, pregelatinized starch, and stearic acid.

CLINICAL PHARMACOLOGY

Hydrocodone is a semisynthetic narcotic analgesic and antitussive with multiple actions qualitatively similar to those of codeine. Most of these involve the central nervous system and smooth muscle. The precise mechanism of action of hydrocodone and other opiates is not known, although it is believed to relate to the existance of opiate receptors in the central nervous system. In addition to analgesia, narcotics may produce drowsiness, changes in mood and mental clouding.

The analgesic action of acetaminophen involves peripheral influences, but the specific mechanism is as yet undetermined. Antipyretic activity is mediated through hypothalamic heat regulating centers. Acetaminophen inhibits prostaglandin synthetase. Therapeutic doses of acetaminophen have negligible effects on the cardiovascular or respiratory systems; however, toxic doses may cause circulatory failure and rapid, shallow breathing.

Pharmacokinetics: The behavior of the individual components is described below.

Hydrocodone: Following a 10mg oral dose of hydrocodone administered to five adult male subjects, the mean peak concentration was 23.6 ± 5.2ng/mL. Maximum serum levels were achieved at 1.3 ± 0.3 hours and the half-life was determined to be 3.8 ± 0.3 hours. Hydrocodone exhibits a complex pattern of metabolism including O-demethylation, N-demethylation and 6-keto reduction to the corresponding 6-α- and 6-β- hydroxy-metabolites. See OVERDOSAGE for toxicity information.

Acetaminophen: Acetaminophen is rapidly absorbed from the gastrointestinal tract and is distributed throughout most body tissues. The plasma half-life is 1.25 to 3 hours, but may be increased by liver damage and following overdosage. Elimination of acetaminophen is principally by liver metabolism (conjugation) and subsequent renal excretion of metabolites. Approximately 85% of an oral dose appears in the urine within 24 hours of adminstration, most as the glucuronide conjugate, with small amounts of other conjugates and unchanged drug. See OVERDOSAGE for toxicity information.

INDICATIONS AND USAGE

VICODIN HP™ tablets are indicated for the relief of moderate to moderately severe pain.

CONTRAINDICATIONS

This product should not be administered to patients who have previously exhibited hypersensitivity to hydrocodone or acetaminophen.

WARNINGS

Respiratory Depression: At high doses or in sensitive patients, hydrocodone may produce dose-related respiratory depression by acting directly on the brain stem respiratory center. Hydrocodone also affects the center that controls respiratory rhythm, and may produce irregular and periodic breathing.

Head Injury and Increased Intracranial Pressure: The respiratory depressant effects of narcotics and their capacity to elevate cerebrospinal fluid pressure may be markedly exaggerated in the presence of head injury, other intracranial lesions or a preexisting increase in intracranial pressure. Furthermore, narcotics produce adverse reactions which may obscure the clinical course of patients with head injuries.

Acute Abdominal Conditions: The administration of narcotics may obscure the diagnosis or clinical course of patients with acute abdominal conditions.

PRECAUTIONS

General:

Special Risk Patients: As with any narcotic analgesic agent, VICODIN HP™ Tablets should be used with caution in elderly or debilitated patients, and those with severe impairment of hepatic or renal function, hypothyroidism, Addison's disease, prostatic hypertrophy or urethral stricture. The usual precautions should be observed and the possibility of respiratory depression should be kept in mind.

Cough Reflex: Hydrocodone suppresses the cough reflex; as with all narcotics, caution should be exercised when VICODIN HP™ Tablets are used postoperatively and in patients with pulmonary disease.

Information for Patients: Hydrocodone, like all narcotics, may impair the mental and/or physical abilities required for the performance of potentially hazardous tasks such as driving a car or operating machinery; patients should be cautioned accordingly.

Alcohol and other CNS depressants may produce an additive CNS depression, when taken with this combination product, and should be avoided.

Hydrocodone may be habit forming. Patients should take the drug only for as long as it is prescribed, in the amounts prescribed, and no more frequently than prescribed.

Laboratory Tests: In patients with severe hepatic or renal disease, effects of therapy should be monitored with serial liver and/or renal function tests.

Drug Interactions: Patients receiving narcotics, antihistamines, antipsychotics, antianxiety agents, or other CNS depressants (including alcohol) concomitantly with VICODIN HP™ Tablets may exhibit an additive CNS depression. When combined therapy is contemplated, the dose of one or both agents should be reduced.

The use of MAO inhibitors or tricyclic antidepressants with hydrocodone preparations may increase the effect of either the antidepressant or hydrocodone.

Drug/Laboratory Test Interactions: Acetaminophen may produce false-positive test results for urinary 5-hydroxyindoleacetic acid.

Carcinogenesis, Mutagenesis, Impairment of Fertility: No adequate studies have been conducted in animals to determine whether hydrocodone or acetaminophen have a potential for carcinogenesis, mutagenesis, or impairment of fertility.

Pregnancy:

Teratogenic Effects: Pregnancy Category C. There are no adequate and well-controlled studies in pregnant women. VICODIN HP™ Tablets should be used during pregnancy only if the potential benefit justifies the potential risk to the fetus.

Nonteratogenic Effects: Babies born to mothers who have been taking opioids regularly prior to delivery will be physically dependent. The withdrawal signs include irritability and excessive crying, tremors, hyperactive reflexes, increased respiratory rate, increased stools, sneezing, yawning, vomiting, and fever. The intensity of the syndrome does not always correlate with the duration of maternal opioid use or dose. There is no consensus on the best method of managing withdrawal.

Labor and Delivery: As with all narcotics, administration of VICODIN HP™ Tablets to the mother shortly before delivery may result in some degree of respiratory depression in the newborn, especially if higher doses are used.

Nursing Mothers: Acetaminophen is excreted in breast milk in small amounts, but the significance of its effects on nursing infants is not known. It is not known whether hydrocodone is excreted in human milk. Because many drugs are excreted in human milk and because of the potential for serious adverse reactions in nursing infants from hydrocodone and acetaminophen, a decision should be made whether to discontinue nursing or to discontinue the drug, taking into account the importance of the drug to the mother.

Pediatric Use: Safety and effectiveness in the pediatric population have not been established.

ADVERSE REACTIONS

The most frequently reported adverse reactions are lightheadedness, dizziness, sedation, nausea and vomiting. These effects seem to be more prominent in ambulatory than in nonambulatory patients, and some of these adverse reactions may be alleviated if the patient lies down.

Other adverse reactions include:

Central Nervous System: Drowsiness, mental clouding, lethargy, impairment of mental and physical performance, anxiety, fear, dysphoria, psychic dependence, mood changes.

Gastrointestinal System: Prolonged administration of VICODIN HP™ Tablets may produce constipation.

Genitourinary System: Ureteral spasm, spasm of vesical sphincters and urinary retention have been reported with opiates.

Respiratory Depression: Hydrocodone bitartrate may produce dose-related respiratory depression by acting directly on the brain stem respiratory centers (see OVERDOSAGE).

Dermatological: Skin rash, pruritus.

The following adverse drug events may be borne in mind as potential effects of acetaminophen: allergic reactions, rash, thrombocytompenia, agranulocytosis.

Potential effects of high dosage are listed in the OVERDOSAGE section.

DRUG ABUSE AND DEPENDENCE

Controlled Substance: VICODIN HP™ Tablets are classified as a Schedule C-III controlled substance.

Abuse and Dependence: Psychic dependence, physical dependence, and tolerance may develop upon repeated administration of narcotics; therefore, VICODIN HP™ Tablets should be prescribed and administered with caution. However, psychic dependence is unlikely to develop when VICODIN HP™ Tablets are used for a short time for the treatment of pain.

Physical dependence, the condition in which continued administration of the drug is required to prevent the appearance of a withdrawal syndrome, assumes clinically significant proportions only after several weeks of continued narcotic use, although some mild degree of physical dependence may develop after a few days of narcotic therapy. Tolerance, in which increasingly large doses are required in order to produce the same degree of analgesia, is manifested initially by a shortened duration of analgesic effect, and subsequently by decreases in the intensity of analgesia. The rate of development of tolerance varies among patients.

OVERDOSAGE

Following an acute overdosage, toxicity may result from hydrocodone or acetaminophen.

Signs and Symptoms:

Hydrocodone: Serious overdose with hydrocodone is characterized by respiratory depression (a decrease in respiratory rate and/or tidal volume, Cheyne-Stokes respiration, cyanosis), extreme somnolence progressing to stupor or coma, skeletal muscle flaccidity, cold and clammy skin, and sometimes bradycardia and hypotension. In severe overdosage, apnea, circulatory collapse, cardiac arrest and death may occur.

Acetaminophen: In acetaminophen overdosage: dose-dependent, potentially fatal hepatic necrosis is the most serious adverse effect. Renal tubular necrosis, hypoglycemic coma, and thrombocytopenia may also occur.

Early symptoms following a potentially hepatotoxic overdose may include: nausea, vomiting, diaphoresis and general malaise. Clinical and laboratory evidence of hepatic toxicity may not be apparent until 48 to 72 hours post-ingestion.

In adults, hepatic toxicity has rarely been reported with acute overdoses of less than 10 grams, or fatalities with less than 15 grams.

Treatment: A single or multiple overdose with hydrocodone and acetaminophen is a potentially lethal polydrug overdose, and consultation with a regional poison control center is recommended.

Immediate treatment includes support of cardiorespiratory function and measures to reduce drug absorption. Vomiting should be induced mechanically, or with syrup of ipecac, if the patient is alert (adequate pharyngeal and laryngeal reflexes). Oral activated charcoal (1 g/kg) should follow gastric emptying. The first dose should be accompanied by an appropriate cathartic. If repeated doses are used, the cathartic might be included with alternate doses as required. Hypotension is usually hypovolemic and should respond to fluids. Vasopressors and other supportive measures should be employed as indicated. A cuffed endo-tracheal tube should be inserted before gastric lavage of the unconscious patient and, when necessary, to provide assisted respiration.

Meticulous attention should be given to maintaining adequate pulmonary ventilation. In severe cases of intoxication, peritoneal dialysis, or preferably hemodialysis may be considered. If hypoprothombinemia occurs due to acetaminophen overdose, vitamin K should be administered intravenously.

Naoloxone, a narcotic antagonist, can reverse respiratory depression and coma associated with opioid overdose. Naloxone hydrochloride 0.4 mg to 2 mg is given parenterally. Since the duration of action of hydrocodone may exceed that of the naloxone, the patient should be kept under continuous surveillance and repeated doses of the antagonist should be administered as needed to maintain adequate respiration. A narcotic antagonist should not be administered in the absence of clinically significant respiratory or cardiovascular depression.

If the dose of acetaminophen may have exceeded 140 mg/kg, acetylcysteine should be administered as early as possible. Serum acetaminophen levels should be obtained, since levels four or more hours following ingestion help predict acetaminophen toxicity. Do not await acetaminophen assay results before initiating treatment. Hepatic enzymes should be obtained initially, and repeated at 24-hour intervals.

Methemoglobinemia over 30% should be treated with methylene blue by slow intravenous administration.

The toxic dose for adults for acetaminophen is 10 g.

DOSAGE AND ADMINISTRATION

Dosage should be adjusted according to severity of pain and the response of the patient. However, it should be kept in mind that tolerance to hydrocodone can develop with continued use and that the incidence of untoward effects is dose related.

The usual adult dosage is one tablet every four to six hours as needed for pain. The total daily dosage should not exceed 6 tablets.

HOW SUPPLIED

VICODIN HP™ (hydrocodone bitartrate and acetaminophen, 10 mg/660 mg) is supplied as a white, oval-shaped, tablet bisected on one side and debossed with "VICODIN HP" on the other side.

Bottles of 100-NDC #0044-0725-02

Bottles of 500-NDC #0044-0725-03

Storage: Store at controlled room temperature 15°–30°C (59°–86°F).

Dispense in a tight, light-resistant container as defined in the USP.

Caution: Federal law prohibits dispensing without prescription.

A Schedule C-III Narcotic.

Revised: May 1996

Knoll Laboratories

A Division of **BASF** Pharma

Knoll Pharmaceutical Company

Continued on next page

Vicodin HP—Cont.

Mount Olive, New Jersey 07828 0900005-3
Shown in Product Identification Guide, page 318

VICODIN® Ⓒ℞
(hydrocodone bitartrate* and acetaminophen tablets, USP)
5 mg/500 mg
*** Warning:** May be habit forming

DESCRIPTION
Hydrocodone bitartrate and acetaminophen is supplied in tablet form for oral administration.
Hydrocodone bitartrate is an opioid analgesic and antitussive and occurs as fine, white crystals or as a crystalline powder. It is affected by light. The chemical name is: 4,5α-epoxy-3-methoxy-17-methylmorphinan-6-one tartrate (1:1) hydrate (2:5). It has the following structural formula:

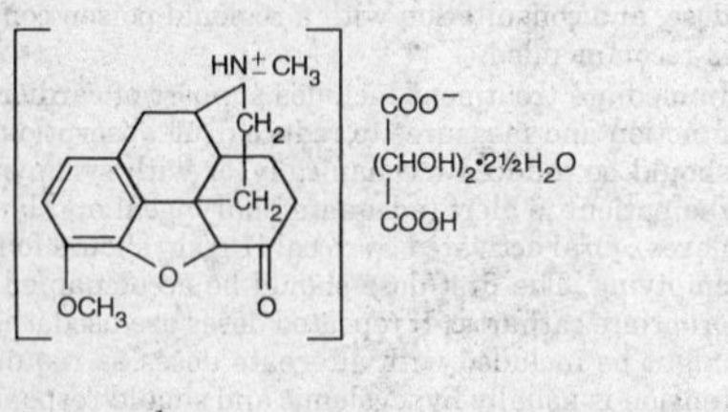

$C_{18}H_{21}NO_3C_4H_6O_6{\cdot}2^1/_2H_2O$ M.W. 494.50

Acetaminophen, 4′-hydroxyacetanilide, a slightly bitter, white, odorless, crystalline powder, is a non-opiate, non-salicylate analgesic and antipyretic. It has the following structural formula:

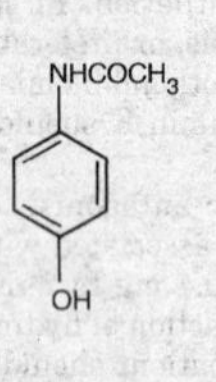

$C_8H_9NO_2$ M.W. 151.16

Each VICODIN® tablet contains:

Hydrocodone Bitartrate 5 mg
(**WARNING:** May be habit forming)
Acetaminophen 500 mg

In addition each tablet contains the following inactive ingredients: colloidal silicon dioxide, starch, croscarmellose sodium, dibasic calcium phosphate, magnesium stearate, microcrystalline cellulose, povidone, and stearic acid.

CLINICAL PHARMACOLOGY
Hydrocodone is a semisynthetic narcotic analgesic and antitussive with multiple actions qualitatively similar to those of codeine. Most of these involve the central nervous system and smooth muscle. The precise mechamism of action of hydrocodone and other opiates is not known, although it is believed to relate to the existence of opiate receptors in the central nervous system. In addition to analgesia, narcotics may produce drowsiness, changes in mood and mental clouding.
The analgesic action of acetaminophen involves peripheral influences, but the specific mechanism is as yet undetermined. Antipyretic activity is mediated through hypothalmic heat regulating centers. Acetaminophen inhibits prostaglandin synthetase. Therapeutic doses of acetaminophen have negligible effects on the cardiovascular or respiratory systems; however, toxic doses may cause circulatory failure and rapid, shallow breathing.
Pharmacokinetics: The behavior of the individual components is described below.
Hydrocodone: Following a 10mg oral dose of hydrocodone administered to five adult male subjects, the mean peak concentration was 23.6 ± 5.2ng/mL. Maximum serum levels were achieved at 1.3 ± 0.3 hours and the half-life was determined to be 3.8 ± 0.3 hours. Hydrocodone exhibits a complex pattern of metabolism including O-demethylation, N-demethylation and 6-keto reduction to the corresponding 6-α- and 6-β-hydroxymetabolites. See OVERDOSAGE for toxicity information.
Acetaminophen: Acetaminophen is rapidly absorbed from the gastrointestinal tract and is distributed throughout most body tissues. The plasma half-life is 1.25 to 3 hours, but may be increased by liver damage and following overdosage. Elimination of acetaminophen is principally by liver metabolism (conjugation) and subsequent renal excretion of metabolites. Approximately 85% of an oral dose appears in the urine within 24 hours of administration, most as the glucuronide conjugate, with small amounts of other conjugates and unchanged drug. See OVERDOSAGE for toxicity information.

INDICATIONS AND USAGE
VICODIN Tablets are indicated for the relief of moderate to moderately severe pain.

CONTRAINDICATIONS
This product should not be administered to patients who have previously exhibited hypersensitivity to hydrocodone or acetaminophen.

WARNINGS
Respiratory Depression: At high doses or in sensitive patients, hydrocodone may produce dose-related respiratory depression by acting directly on the brain stem respiratory center. Hydrocodone also affects the center that controls respiratory rhythm, and may produce irregular and periodic breathing.
Head Injury and Increased Intracranial Pressure: The respiratory depressant effects of narcotics and their capacity to elevate cerebrospinal fluid pressure may be markedly exaggerated in the presence of head injury, other intracranial lesions or a preexisting increase in intracranial pressure. Furthermore, narcotics produce adverse reactions which may obscure the clinical course of patients with head injuries.
Acute Abdominal Conditions: The administration of narcotics may obscure the diagnosis or clinical course of patients with acute abdominal conditions.

PRECAUTIONS
General:
Special Risk Patients: As with any narcotic analgesic agent, VICODIN Tablets should be used with caution in elderly or debilitated patients and those with severe impairment of hepatic or renal function, hypothyroidism, Addison's disease, prostatic hypertrophy or urethral stricture. The usual precautions should be observed and the possibility of respiratory depression should be kept in mind.
Cough Reflex: Hydrocodone suppresses the cough reflex; as with all narcotics, caution should be exercised when VICODIN Tablets are used postoperatively and in patients with pulmonary disease.
Information for Patients: Hydrocodone, like all narcotics, may impair the mental and/or physical abilities required for the performance of potentially hazardous tasks such as driving a car or operating machinery; patients should be cautioned accordingly.
Alcohol and other CNS depressants may produce an additive CNS depression, when taken with this combination product, and should be avoided.
Hydrocodone may be habit forming. Patients should take the drug only for as long as it is prescribed, in the amounts prescribed, and no more frequently than prescribed.
Laboratory Tests: In patients with severe hepatic or renal disease, effects of therapy should be monitored with serial liver and/or renal function tests.
Drug Interactions: Patients receiving other narcotic analgesics, antihistamines, antipsychotics, antianxiety agents, or other CNS depressants (including alcohol) concomitantly with VICODIN Tablets may exhibit an additive CNS depression. When combined therapy is contemplated, the dose of one or both agents should be reduced.
The use of MAO inhibitors or tricyclic antidepressants with hydrocodone preparations may increase the effect of either the antidepressant or hydrocodone.
Drug/Laboratory Test Interactions: Acetaminophen may produce false-positive test results for urinary 5-hydroxyindoleacetic acid.
Carcinogenesis, Mutagenesis, Impairment of Fertility: No adequate studies have been conducted in animals to determine whether hydrocodone or acetaminophen have a potential for carcinogenesis, mutagenesis, or impairment of fertility.
Pregnancy:
Teratogenic Effects: Pregnancy Category C. There are no adequate and well-controlled studies in pregnant women. VICODIN Tablets should be used during pregnancy only if the potential benefit justifies the potential risk to the fetus.
Nonteratogenic Effects: Babies born to mothers who have been taking opioids regularly prior to delivery will be physically dependent. The withdrawal signs include irritability and excessive crying, tremors, hyperactive reflexes, increased respiratory rate, increased stools, sneezing, yawning, vomiting, and fever. The intensity of the syndrome does not always correlate with the duration of maternal opioid use or dose. There is not consensus on the best method of managing withdrawal.
Labor and Delivery: As with all narcotics, administration of VICODIN Tablets to the mother shortly before delivery may result in some degree of respiratory depression in the newborn, especially if higher doses are used.
Nursing Mothers: Acetaminophen is excreted in breast milk in small amounts, but the significance of its effects on nursing infants is not known. It is not known whether hydrocodone is excreted in human milk. Because many drugs are excreted in human milk and because of the potential for serious adverse reactions in nursing infants from hydrocodone and acetaminophen, a decision should be made whether to discontinue nursing or to discontinue the drug, taking into account the importance of the drug to the mother.
Pediatric Use: Safety and effectiveness in the pediatric population have not been established.

ADVERSE REACTIONS
The most frequently reported adverse reactions include lightheadedness, dizziness, sedation, nausea and vomiting. These effects seem to be more prominent in ambulatory than in nonambulatory patients and some of these adverse reactions may be alleviated if the patient lies down.
Other adverse reactions include:
Central Nervous System: Drowsiness, mental clouding, lethargy, impairment of mental and physical performance, anxiety, fear, dysphoria, psychic dependence, mood changes.
Gastrointestinal System: Prolonged administration of VICODIN Tablets may produce constipation.
Genitourinary System: Ureteral spasm, spasm of vesical sphincters and urinary retention have been reported with opiates.
Respiratory Depression: Hydrocodone bitartrate may produce dose-related respiratory depression by acting directly on the brain stem respiratory center. (see OVERDOSAGE).
Dermatological: Skin rash, pruritus.
The following adverse drug events may be borne in mind as potential effects of acetaminophen: allergic reactions, rash, thrombocytopenia, agranulocytosis
Potential effects of high dosage are listed in the OVERDOSAGE section.

DRUG ABUSE AND DEPENDENCE
Controlled Substance: VICODIN Tablets are classified as a Schedule Ⓒ **controlled substance.**
Abuse Dependence: Psychic dependence, physical dependence, and tolerance may develop upon repeated administration of narcotics; therefore, VICODIN Tablets should be prescribed and administered with caution. However, psychic dependence is unlikely to develop when VICODIN Tablets are used for a short time for the treatment of pain.
Physical dependence, the condition in which continued administration of the drug is required to prevent the appearance of a withdrawal syndrome, assumes clinically significant proportions only after several weeks of continued narcotic use, although some mild degree of physical dependence may develop after a few days of narcotic therapy. Tolerance, in which increasingly large doses are required in order to produce the same degree of analgesia, is manifested initially by a shortened duration of analgesic effect, and subsequently by decreases in the intensity of analgesia. The rate of development of tolerance varies among patients.

OVERDOSAGE
Following an acute overdosage, toxicity may result from hydrocodone or acetaminophen.
Signs and Symptoms:
Hydrocodone: Serious overdose with hydrocodone is characterized by respiratory depression (a decrease in respiratory rate and/or tidal volume, Cheyne-Stokes respiration, cyanosis), extreme somnolence progressing to stupor or coma, skeletal muscle flaccidity, cold and clammy skin, and sometimes bradycardia and hypotension. In severe overdosage, apnea, circulatory collapse, cardiac arrest and death may occur.
Acetaminophen: In acetaminophen overdosage, dose-dependent, potentially fatal hepatic necrosis is the most serious adverse effect. Renal tubular necrosis, hypoglycemic coma, and thrombocytopenia may also occur.
Early symptoms following a potentially hepatotoxic overdose may include: nausea, vomiting, diaphoresis and general malaise. Clinical and laboratory evidence of hepatic toxicity may not be apparent until 48 to 72 hours post-ingestion.
In adults, hepatic toxicity has rarely been reported with acute overdoses of less than 15 grams.
Treatment:
A single or multiple overdose with hydrocodone and acetaminophen is a potentially lethal polydrug overdose, and consultation with a regional poison control center is recommended.
Immediate treatment includes support of cardiorespiratory function and measures to reduce drug absorption. Vomiting should be induced mechanically, or with syrup of ipecac, if the patient is alert (adequate pharyngeal and laryngeal reflexes). Oral activated charcoal (1 g/kg) should follow gastric emptying. The first dose should be accompanied by an appropriate cathartic. If repeated doses are used, the cathartic might be included with alternate doses as required. Hypotension is usually hypovolemic and should respond to fluids. Vasopressors and other supportive measures should be employed as indicated. A cuffed endo-tracheal tube should be inserted before gastric lavage of the unconscious patient and, when necessary to provide assisted respiration.
Meticulous attention should be given to maintaining adequate pulmonary ventilation. In severe cases of intoxica-

tion, peritoneal dialysis, or preferably hemodialysis may be considered. If hypoprothrombinemia occurs due to acetaminophen overdose, vitamin K should be administered intravenously.

Naloxone, a narcotic antagonist, can reverse respiratory depression and coma associated with opioid overdose. Naloxone hydrochloride 0.4 mg to 2 mg is given parenterally. Since the duration of action of hydrocodone may exceed that of the naloxone, the patient should be kept under continuous surveillance and repeated doses of the antagonist should be administered as needed to maintain adequate respiration. A narcotic antagonist should not be administered in the absence of clinically significant respiratory or cardiovascular depression.

If the dose of acetaminophen may have exceeded 140 mg/kg, acetylcysteine should be administered as early as possible. Serum acetaminophen levels should be obtained, since levels four or more hours following ingestion help predict acetaminophen toxicity. Do not await acetaminophen assay results before initiating treatment. Hepatic enzymes should be obtained initially, and repeated at 24-hour intervals. Methemoglobinemia over 30% should be treated with methylene blue by slow intravenous administration.

The toxic dose for adults for acetaminophen is 10 g.

DOSAGE AND ADMINISTRATION

Dosage should be adjusted according to the severity of the pain and the response of the patient. However, it should be kept in mind that tolerance to hydrocodone can develop with continued use and that the incidence of untoward effects is dose related.

The usual adult dosage is one or two tablets every four to six hours as needed for pain. The total daily dosage should not exceed 8 tablets.

HOW SUPPLIED

VICODIN is supplied as white, capsule-shaped tablets containing 5 mg hydrocodone bitartrate and 500 mg acetaminophen, bisected on one side and debossed with "VICODIN" on the other.

Bottles of 100—NDC #0044-0727-02.
Bottles of 500—NDC #0044-0727-03.
Hospital Unit Dose Package–100 tablets (4×25 tablets)—NDC#0044-0727-41.

Storage: Store at controlled room temperature 15°–30°C (59°–86°F).

Dispense in a tight, light-resistant container as defined in the USP.

A Schedule � Narcotic.

Revised: April, 1996

Knoll Laboratories
A Division of   **BASF** Pharma
Knoll Pharmaceutical Company
Mount Olive, New Jersey 07828

0900010-2

Shown in Product Identification Guide, page 318

VICODIN ES® TABLETS   ⑪ ℞
(hydrocodone bitartrate and
acetaminophen tablets, USP)
7.5 mg/750 mg

DESCRIPTION

Hydrocodone bitartrate and acetaminophen is supplied in tablet form for oral administration.

Hydrocodone bitartrate is an opioid analgesic and antitussive and occurs as fine, white crystals or as a crystalline powder. It is affected by light. The chemical name is: 4,5α-epoxy-3-methoxy-17-methylmorphinan-6-one tartrate (1:1) hydrate (2:5). It has the following structural formula:

$C_{18}H_{21}NO_3 \cdot C_4H_6O_6 \cdot 2\frac{1}{2} H_2O$ M.W. 494.50

Acetaminophen, 4'-hydroxyacetanilide, is a slightly bitter, white, odorless, crystalline powder, is a non-opiate, nonsalicylate analgesic and antipyretic. It has the following structural formula:

[See chemical structure at top of next column]

Each VICODIN ES® tablet contains:
    Hydrocodone Bitartrate 7.5 mg
    Acetaminophen   750 mg

In addition each tablet contains the following inactive ingredients: colloidal silicon dioxide, pregelatinized starch, magnesium stearate, microcrystalline cellulose, povidone, and stearic acid.

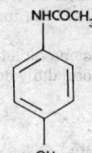

$C_8H_9NO_2$ M.W.151.16

CLINICAL PHARMACOLOGY

Hydrocodone is a semisynthetic narcotic analgesic and antitussive with multiple actions qualitatively similar to those of codeine. Most of these involve the central nervous system and smooth muscle. The precise mechanism of action of hydrocodone and other opiates is not known, although it is believed to relate to the existence of opiate receptors in the central nervous system. In addition to analgesia, narcotics may produce drowsiness, changes in mood and mental clouding.

The analgesic action of acetaminophen involves peripheral influences, but the specific mechanism is as yet undetermined. Antipyretic activity is mediated through hypothalmic heat regulating centers. Acetaminophen inhibits prostaglandin synthetase. Therapeutic doses of acetaminophen have negligible effects on the cardiovascular or respiratory systems; however, toxic doses may cause circulatory failure and rapid, shallow breathing.

Pharmacokinetics: The behavior of the individual components is described below.

Hydrocodone: Following a 10mg oral dose of hydrocodone administered to five adult male subjects, the mean peak concentration was 23.6 ± 5.2 ng/mL. Maximum serum levels were achieved at 1.3 ± 0.3 hours and the half-life was determined to be 3.8 ± 0.3 hours. Hydrocodone exhibits a complex pattern of metabolism including O-demethylation, N-demethylation and 6-keto reduction to the corresponding 6-α- and 6-β- hydroxymetabolites. See OVERDOSAGE for toxicity information.

Acetaminophen: Acetaminophen is rapidly absorbed from the gastrointestinal tract and is distributed throughout most body tissues. The plasma half-life is 1.25 to 3 hours, but may be increased by liver damage and following overdosage. Elimination of acetaminophen is principally by liver metabolism (conjugation) and subsequent renal excretion of metabolites. Approximately 85% of an oral dose appears in the urine within 24 hours of administration, most as the glucuronide conjugate, with small amounts of other conjugates and unchanged drug. See OVERDOSAGE for toxicity information.

INDICATIONS AND USAGE

VICODIN ES tablets are indicated for the relief of moderate to moderately severe pain.

CONTRAINDICATIONS

This product should not be administered to patients who have previously exhibited hypersensitivity to hydrocodone or acetaminophen.

WARNINGS

Respiratory Depression: At high doses or in sensitive patients, hydrocodone may produce dose-related respiratory depression by acting directly on the brain stem respiratory center. Hydrocodone also affects the center that controls respiratory rhythm, and may produce irregular and periodic breathing.

Head Injury and Increased Intracranial Pressure: The respiratory depressant effects of narcotics and their capacity to elevate cerebrospinal fluid pressure may be markedly exaggerated in the presence of head injury, other intracranial lesions or a preexisting increase in intracranial pressure. Furthermore, narcotics produce adverse reactions which may obscure the clinical course of patients with head injuries.

Acute Abdominal Conditions: The administration of narcotics may obscure the diagnosis or clinical course of patients with acute abdominal conditions.

PRECAUTIONS
General:

Special Risk Patients: As with any narcotic analgesic agent, VICODIN ES tablets should be used with caution in elderly or debilitated patients and those with severe impairment of hepatic or renal function, hypothyroidism, Addison's disease, prostatic hypertrophy or urethral stricture. The usual precautions should be observed and the possibility of respiratory depression should be kept in mind.

Cough Reflex: Hydrocodone suppresses the cough reflex; as with all narcotics, caution should be exercised when VICODIN ES Tablets are used postoperatively and in patients with pulmonary disease.

Information for Patients: Hydrocodone, like all narcotics, may impair the mental and/or physical abilities required for the performance of potentially hazardous tasks such as driving a car or operating machinery; patients should be cautioned accordingly.

Alcohol and other CNS depressants may produce an additive CNS depression, when taken with this combination product, and should be avoided.

Hydrocodone may be habit forming. Patients should take the drug only for as long as it is prescribed. In the amounts prescribed, and no more frequently than prescribed.

Laboratory Tests: In patients with severe hepatic or renal disease, effects of therapy should be monitored with serial liver and/or renal function tests.

Drug Interactions: Patients receiving other narcotic analgesics, antihistamines, antipsychotics, antianxiety agents, or other CNS depressants (including alcohol) concomitantly with VICODIN ES tablets may exhibit an additive CNS depression. When combined therapy is contemplated, the dose of one or both agents should be reduced.

The use of MAO inhibitors or tricyclic antidepressants with hydrocodone preparations may increase the effect of either the antidepressant or hydrocodone.

Drug/Laboratory Test Interaction: Acetaminophen may produce false-positive test results for urinary 5-hydroxyindoleacetic acid.

Carcinogenesis, Mutagenesis, Impairment of Fertility: No adequate studies have been conducted in animals to determine whether hydrocodone or acetaminophen have a potential for carcinogenesis, mutagenesis, or impairment of fertility.

Pregnancy:

Teratogenic Effects: Pregnancy Category C. There are no adequate and well-controlled studies in pregnant women. VICODIN ES tablets should be used during pregnancy only if the potential benefit justifies the potential risk to the fetus.

Nonteratogenic Effects: Babies born to mothers who have been taking opioids regularly prior to delivery will be physically dependent. The withdrawal signs include irritability and excessive crying, tremors, hyperactive reflexes, increased respiratory rate, increased stools, sneezing, yawning, vomiting, and fever. The intensity of the syndrome does not always correlate with the duration of maternal opioid use or dose. There is no consensus on the best method of managing withdrawal.

Labor and Delivery: As with all narcotics, administration of VICODIN ES tablets to the mother shortly before delivery may result in some degree of respiratory depression in the newborn, especially if higher doses are used.

Nursing Mothers: Acetaminophen is excreted in breast milk in small amounts, but the significance of its effects on nursing infants is not known. It is not known whether hydrocodone is excreted in human milk. Because many drugs are excreted in human milk and because of the potential for serious adverse reactions in nursing infants from hydrocodone and acetaminophen, a decision should be made whether to discontinue nursing or to discontinue the drug, taking into account the importance of the drug to the mother.

Pediatric Use: Safety and effectiveness in the pediatric population have not been established.

Geriatric Use: Clinical studies of VICODIN ES® (hydrocodone bitartrate 7.5 mg and acetaminophen 750 mg) did not include sufficient numbers of subjects aged 65 and over to determine whether they respond differently from younger subjects. Other reported clinical experience has not identified differences in responses between the elderly and younger patients. In general, dose selection for an elderly patient should be cautious, usually starting at the low end of the dosing range, reflecting the greater frequency of decreased hepatic, renal, or cardiac function, and of concomitant disease or other drug therapy.

ADVERSE REACTIONS

The most frequently reported adverse reactions include: lightheadedness, dizziness, sedation, nausea and vomiting. These effects seem to be more prominent in ambulatory than in nonambulatory patients and some of these adverse reactions may be alleviated if the patient lies down.

Other adverse reactions include:

Central Nervous System: Drowsiness, mental clouding, lethargy, impairment of mental and physical performance, anxiety, fear, dysphoria, psychic dependence, mood changes.

Gastrointestinal System: Prolonged administration of VICODIN ES tablets may produce constipation.

Genitourinary System: Ureteral spasm, spasm of vesical sphincters and urinary retention have been reported with opiates.

Respiratory Depression: Hydrocodone bitartrate may produce dose-related respiratory depression by acting directly on the brain stem respiratory center. (see OVERDOSAGE).

Dermatological: Skin rash, pruritus.

The following adverse drug events may be borne in mind as potential effects of acetaminophen: allergic reactions, rash, thrombocytopenia, agranulocytosis.

Potential effects of high dosage are listed in the OVERDOSAGE section.

Continued on next page

Vicodin ES—Cont.

DRUG ABUSE AND DEPENDENCE

Controlled Substance: VICODIN ES tablets are classified as a Schedule ⑩ controlled substance.

Abuse and Dependence: Psychic dependence, physical dependence, and tolerance may develop upon repeated administration of narcotics; therefore, VICODIN ES tablets should be prescribed and administered with caution. However, psychic dependence is unlikely to develop when VICODIN ES tablets are used for a short time for the treatment of pain.

Physical dependence, the condition in which continued administration of the drug is required to prevent the appearance of a withdrawal syndrome, assumes clinically significant proportions only after several weeks of continued narcotic use, although some mild degree of physical dependence may develop after a few days of narcotic therapy. Tolerance, in which increasingly large doses are required in order to produce the same degree of analgesia, is manifested initially by a shortened duration of analgesic effect, and subsequently by decreases in the intensity f analgesia. The rate of development of tolerance varies among patients.

OVERDOSAGE

Following an acute overdosage, toxicity may result from hydrocodone or acetaminophen.

Signs and Symptoms:

Hydrocodone: Serious overdose with hydrocodone is characterized by respiratory depression (a decrease in respiratory rate and/or tidal volume. Cheyne-Stokes respiration, cyanosis), extreme somnolence progressing to stupor or coma, skeletal muscle flaccidity, cold and clammy skin, and sometimes bradycardia and hypotension. In severe overdosage, apnea, circulatory collapse, cardiac arrest and death may occur.

Acetaminophen: In acetaminophen overdosage: dose-dependent, potentially fatal hepatic necrosis is the most serious adverse effect. Renal tubular necrosis, hypoglycemic coma, and thrombocytopenia may also occur.

Early symptoms following a potentially hepatotoxic overdose may include: nausea, vomiting, diaphoresis and general malaise. Clinical and laboratory evidence of hepatic toxicity may not be apparent until 48 to 72 hours post-ingestion.

In adults, hepatic toxicity has rarely been reported with acute overdoses of less than 10 grams and fatalities with less than 15 grams.

Treatment:

A single or multiple overdose with hydrocodone and acetaminophen is a potentially lethal polydrug overdose, and consultation with a regional poison control center is recommended.

Immediate treatment includes support of cardiorespiratory function and measures to reduce drug absorption. Vomiting should be induced mechanically, or with syrup of ipecac, if the patient is alert (adequate pharyngeal and laryngeal reflexes). Oral activated charcoal (1 g/kg) should follow gastric emptying. The first dose should be accompanied by an appropriate cathartic. If repeated doses are used, the cathartic might be included with alternate doses as required. Hypotension is usually hypovolemic and should respond to fluids. Vasopressors and other supportive measures should be employed as indicated. A cuffed endo-tracheal tube should be inserted before gastric lavage of the unconscious patient and, when necessary, to provide assisted respiration.

Meticulous attention should be given to maintaining adequate pulmonary ventilation. In severe cases of intoxication, peritoneal dialysis, or preferably hemodialysis may be considered. If hypoprothrombinemia occurs due to acetaminophen overdose, vitamin K should be administered intravenously.

Naloxone, a narcotic antagonist, can reverse respiratory depression and coma associated with opioid overdose. Naloxone hydrochloride 0.4 mg to 2 mg is given parenterally. Since the duration of action of hydrocodone may exceed that of the naloxone, the patient should be kept under continuous surveillance and repeated doses of the antagonist should be administered as needed to maintain adequate respiration. A narcotic antagonist should not be administered in the absence of clinically significant respiratory or cardiovascular depression.

If the dose of acetaminophen may have exceeded 140 mg/kg, acetylcysteine should be administered as early as possible. Serum acetaminophen levels should be obtained, since levels four or more hours following ingestion help predict acetaminophen toxicity. Do not await acetaminophen assay results before initiating treatment. Hepatic enzymes should be obtained initially, and repeated at 24-hour intervals. Methemoglobinemia over 30% should be treated with methylene blue by slow intravenous administration.

The toxic dose for adults for acetaminophen is 10 g.

DOSAGE AND ADMINISTRATION

Dosage should be adjusted according to the severity of the pain and the response of the patient. However, it should be

kept in mind that tolerance to hydrocodone can develop with continued use and that the incidence of untoward effects is dose related.

The usual adult dosage is one tablet every four to six hours as needed for pain. The total daily dosage should not exceed 5 tablets.

HOW SUPPLIED

White, oval-shaped, faceted edged tablet bisected on one side and imprinted with "VICODIN ES" on the other side.
Bottles of 100-NDC #0044-0728-02
Bottles of 500-NDC #0044-0728-03
Hospital Unit Dosage Package—100 tablets (4×25 tablets)—NDC #0044-0728-41.
Storage: Store at 25°C (77°F); excursions permitted to 15°–30°C (59°–86°F). [See USP Controlled Room Temperature]. Dispense in a tight, light-resistant container as defined in the USP.
A Schedule ⑩ Narcotic.

Rx only

VICODIN ES is a registered trademark of Knoll Pharmaceutical Company.

© 1998 Knoll Pharmaceutical Company
All rights reserved.

Revised: July, 1998

Knoll Laboratories
A Division of
Knoll Pharmaceutical Company
Mount Olive, New Jersey 07828

0900011-4

Shown in Product Identification Guide, page 318

VICODIN TUSS™
Expectorant
(hydrocodone bitartrate and guaifenesin)

⑩

DESCRIPTION

VICODIN TUSS™ Expectorant Syrup contains hydrocodone (dihydrocodeinone) bitartrate, semi-synthetic centrally-acting narcotic antitussive and guaifenesin, an expectorant for oral administration.
Each teaspoonful (5 mL) contains:
Hydrocodone bitartrate USP .... 5 mg
WARNING: May be habit forming
Guaifenesin USP .... 100 mg
VICODIN TUSS™ Expectorant Syrup also contains: glycerin, L-menthol, methylparaben, propylparaben, propylene glycol, sodium saccharin, sorbitol solution, artificial flavoring, and purified water.

CLINICAL PHARMACOLOGY

Clinical trials have proven hydrocodone bitartrate to be an effective antitussive agent which is pharmacologically 2 to 8 times as potent as codeine. At equi-effective doses, its sedative action is greater than codeine. The precise mechanism of action of hydrocodone and other opiates is not known, however, hydrocodone is believed to act by directly depressing the cough center. In excessive doses hydrocodone, like other opium derivatives, can depress respiration. The effects of hydrocodone in therapeutic doses on the cardiovascular system is insignificant. The constipation effects of hydrocodone are much weaker than that of morphine and no stronger than that of codeine. Hydrocodone can produce miosis, euphoria, physical and psychological dependence. At therapeutic antitussive doses, it does exert analgesic effects. Following a 10 mg oral dose of hydrocodone administered to five male human subjects the mean peak concentration was 23.6 ± 5.2 ng/mL. Maximum serum levels were achieved at 1.3 ± 0.3 hours and half-life was determined to be 3.8 ± 0.3 hours. Hydrocodone exhibits a complex pattern of metabolism including O-demethylation, N-demethylation and 6-ketoreduction to the corresponding 6-α- and 6-β-hydroxymetabolites.

The exact mechanism of action is not established but guaifenesin is believed to act by stimulating receptors in the gastric mucosa that initates a reflex secretion of respiratory tract fluid, thereby increasing the volume and decreasing the viscosity of bronchial secretions. Studies with guaifenesin indicate that it is rapidly absorbed from the gastrointestinal tract and has a half-life of one hour.

INDICATIONS AND USAGE

VICODIN TUSS™ Expectorant is indicated for the symptomatic relief of irritating non-productive cough associated with upper and lower respiratory tract congestion.

CONTRAINDICATIONS

VICODIN TUSS™ Expectorant is contraindicated in patients hypersensitive to hydrocodone or guaifenesin. Patients known to be hypersensitive to other opioids may exhibit cross sensitivity to VICODIN TUSS™ Expectorant. Hydrocodone is contraindicated in the presence of an intracranial lesion associated with increased intracranial pressure; and whenever ventilatory function is depressed.

WARNINGS

May be habit forming. Hydrocodone can produce drug dependence of the morphine type and therefore has the potential for being abused. Psychic dependence, physical dependence and tolerance may develop upon repeated administration of VICODIN TUSS™ Expectorant and it should be prescribed and administered with the same degree of caution appropriate to the use of other narcotic drugs (see DRUG ABUSE AND DEPENDENCE).

Respiratory Depression: VICODIN TUSS™ Expectorant produces dose-related respiratory depression by directly acting on the brain stem respiratory centers. If respiratory depression occurs, it may be antagonized by the use of naloxone hydrochloride and other supportive measures when indicated.

Head Injury and Increased Intracranial Pressure: The respiratory depressant properties of narcotics and their capacity to elevate cerebrospinal fluid pressure may be markedly exaggerated in the presence of head injury, other intracranial lesions or a pre-existing increase in intracranial pressure. Furthermore, narcotics produce adverse reactions which may obscure the clinical course of patients with head injuries.

Acute Abdominal Conditions: The administration of VICODIN TUSS™ Expectorant or other opioids may obscure the diagnosis or clinical course of patients with acute abdominal conditions.

PRECAUTIONS

Before prescribing medication to suppress or modify cough, it is important to ascertain that the underlying cause of cough is identified, that modification of cough does not increase the risk of clinical or physiologic complications, and that appropriate therapy for the primary disease is provided.

Usage in Ambulatory Patients: Hydrocodone, like all narcotics, may impair the mental and/or physical abilities required for the performance of potentially hazardous tasks such as driving a car or operating machinery, and patients should be warned accordingly.

Drug Interactions: Patients receiving other narcotic analgesics, general anesthetics, phenothiazines, other tranquilizers, sedative hypnotics or other CNS depressants (including alcohol) concomitantly with hydrocodone may exhibit an additive CNS depression. When such combined therapy is contemplated, the dose of one or both agents should be reduced (see WARNINGS).

Laboratory Interactions: The metabolite of guaifenesin has been found to produce an apparent increase in urinary 5-hydroxyindoleacetic acid, and guaifenesin therefore may interfere with the interpretation of this test for the diagnosis of carcinoid syndrome. Guaifenesin administration should be discontinued 24 hours prior to the collection of urine specimens for the determination of 5-hydroxyindoleacetic acid.

Carcinogenesis, mutagenesis, impairment of fertility: Carcinogenicity, mutagenicity and reproduction studies have not been conducted with VICODIN TUSS™ Expectorant.

Usage in Pregnancy: Pregnancy Category C. Animal reproduction studies have not been conducted with VICODIN TUSS™ Expectorant. It is also not known whether VICODIN TUSS™ Expectorant can cause fetal harm when administered to a pregnant woman or can affect reproductive capacity.

VICODIN TUSS™ Expectorant should be given to a pregnant woman only if clearly needed.

Nonteratogenic effects: Babies born to mothers who have been taking opioids regularly prior to delivery will be physically dependent. The withdrawal signs include irritability and excessive crying, tremors, hyperactive reflexes, increased respiratory rate, increased stools, sneezing, yawning, vomiting and fever. The intensity of the syndrome does not always correlate with the duration of maternal opioid use or dose. There is no consensus on the best method of managing withdrawal. Chlorpromazine 0.7–1.0 mg/kg q 6 h, phenobarbital 2 mg/kg q 6 h, and paregoric 2–4 drops/kg q 4 h, have been used to treat withdrawal symptoms in infants. The duration of therapy is 4 to 28 days, with the dosages decreased as tolerated.

Nursing mothers: It is not known whether this drug is excreted in human milk. Because many drugs are excreted in human milk and because of the potential for serious adverse reactions in nursing infants from VICODIN TUSS™ Expectorant, a decision should be made whether to discontinue nursing or discontinue the drug, taking into account the importance of the drug to the mother.

ADVERSE REACTIONS

Respiratory System: Hydrocodone produces dose-related respiratory depression by acting directly on brain stem respiratory centers.

Cardiovascular System: Hypertension, postural hypotension and palpitations.

Genitourinary System: Ureteral spasm, spasm of vesical sphincters and urinary retention have been reported with opiates.

Central Nervous System: Sedation, drowsiness, mental clouding, lethargy, impairment of mental and physical performance, anxiety, fear, dysphoria, dizziness, psychic dependence, mood changes and blurred vision.

Gastrointestinal System: Nausea and vomiting occur more frequently in ambulatory than in recumbent patients.

DRUG ABUSE DEPENDENCE

Special care should be exercised in prescribing hydrocodone for emotionally unstable patients and for those with a history of drug misuse. Such patients should be closely supervised when long-term therapy is contemplated.

VICODIN TUSS™ Expectorant is a Schedule III narcotic. Psychic dependence, physical dependence and tolerance may develop upon repeated administration of narcotics; therefore, VICODIN TUSS™ Expectorant should always be prescribed and administered with caution. Physical dependence is the condition in which continued administration of the drug is required to prevent the appearance of a withdrawal syndrome.

Patients physically dependent on opioids will develop an abstinence syndrome upon abrupt discontinuation of the opioid or following the administration of a narcotic antagonist. The character and severity of the withdrawal symptoms are related to the degree of physical dependence. Manifestations of opioid withdrawal are similar to but milder than that of morphine and include lacrimation, rhinorrhea, yawning, sweating, restlessness, dilated pupils, anorexia, goose-flesh, irritability and tremor. In more severe forms, nausea, vomiting, intestinal spasm and diarrhea, increased heart rate and blood pressure, chills, and pains in bones and muscles of the back and extremities may occur. Peak effects will usually be apparent at 48 to 72 hours.

Treatment of withdrawal is usually managed by providing sufficient quantities of an opioid to suppress **severe** withdrawal symptoms and then gradually reducing the dose of opioid over a period of several days.

OVERDOSAGE

Signs and Symptoms: Serious overdosage with VICODIN TUSS™ Expectorant is characterized by respiratory depression (a decrease in respiratory rate and/or tidal volume, Cheyne-Stokes respiration, cyanosis), extreme somnolence progressing to stupor or coma, skeletal muscle flaccidity, cold and clammy skin, and sometimes bradycardia and hypotension. In severe overdosage apnea, circulatory collapse, cardiac arrest, and death may occur.

Treatment: Primary attention should be given to the reestablishment of adequate respiratory exchange through provision of a patent airway and the institution of assisted or controlled ventilation. The narcotic antagonist naloxone hydrochloride is a specific antidote for respiratory depression which may result from overdosage or unusual sensitivity to narcotics including hydrocodone. Therefore, an appropriate dose of naloxone hydrochloride should be administered, preferably by the intravenous route, simultaneously with efforts at respiratory resuscitation. For further information, see full prescribing information for naloxone hydrochloride. An antagonist should not be administered in the absence of clinically significant respiratory depression. Oxygen, intravenous fluids, vasopressors and other supportive measures should be employed as indicated. Gastric emptying may be useful in removing unabsorbed drug. Activated charcoal may be of benefit.

DOSAGE AND ADMINISTRATION

Usual Adult Dose: One teaspoonful (5 mL) after meals and at bedtime, not less than 4 hours apart (not to exceed 6 teaspoonsful in a 24 hour period). Treatment should be initiated with one teaspoonful and subsequent doses, up to a maximum single dose of 3 teaspoonsful, adjusted if required.

Usual Children's Dose:

Over 12 years: Initial dose 1 teaspoonful; maximum single dose, 2 teaspoonsful.

6 to 12 years: Initial dose $^1/_2$ teaspoonful; maximum single dose, 1 teaspoonful.

HOW SUPPLIED

VICODIN TUSS™ Expectorant is available in bottles as a colorless, cherry-flavored syrup which contains no sugar, alcohol or dye.

One pint: NDC 0044-0730-16.

Store in a tight, light resistant container as defined in the USP. Keep tightly closed.

Store at controlled room temperature 15°–30°C (59°–86°F).

A Schedule Ⓒⅲ Narcotic. Oral prescription where permitted by State Law.

Revised: April, 1996

Knoll Laboratories
A Division of
Knoll Pharmaceutical Company
Mt. Olive, NJ 07828
BASF Pharma 0900007-2

Shown in Product Identification Guide, page 318

VICOPROFEN® Ⓒⅲ ℞

[*vī-cō-prōfen*]

(hydrocodone bitartrate* and ibuprofen tablets)
7.5 mg/200 mg
***Warning:** May be habit forming

DESCRIPTION

Each VICOPROFEN® tablet contains:

Hydrocodone Bitartrate*, USP 7.5 mg
(***WARNING:** May be habit forming.)
Ibuprofen, USP 200 mg

VICOPROFEN is supplied in a fixed combination tablet form for oral administration. VICOPROFEN combines the opioid analgesic agent, hydrocodone bitartrate, with the nonsteroidal anti-inflammatory (NSAID) agent, ibuprofen. Hydrocodone bitartrate is a semisynthetic and centrally acting opioid analgesic. Its chemical name is: 4,5 α-epoxy-3-methoxy-17-methylmorphinan-6-one tartrate (1:1) hydrate (2:5). Its chemical formula is: $C_{18}H_{21}NO_3 \bullet C_4H_6O_6 \bullet 2^1/_2H_2O$, and the molecular weight is 494.50. Its structural formula is:

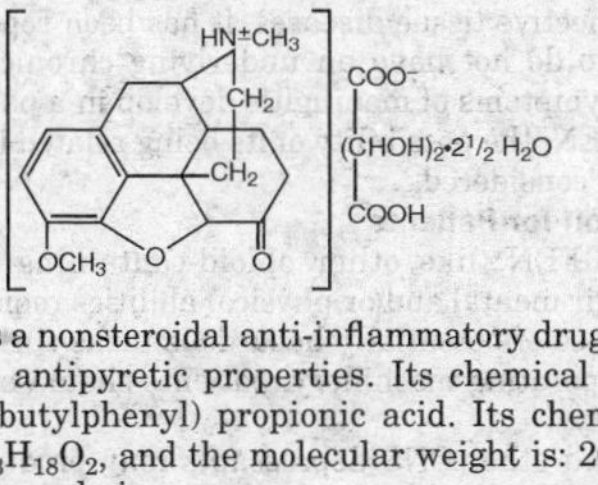

Ibuprofen is a nonsteroidal anti-inflammatory drug with analgesic and antipyretic properties. Its chemical name is: (±)-2-(*p*-isobutylphenyl) propionic acid. Its chemical formula is: $C_{13}H_{18}O_2$, and the molecular weight is: 206.29. Its structural formula is:

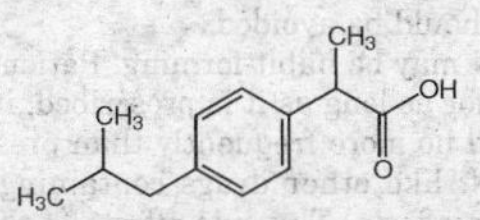

Inactive ingredients in VICOPROFEN tablets include: colloidal silicon dioxide, corn starch, croscarmellose sodium, hydroxypropyl methylcellulose, magnesium stearate, microcrystalline cellulose, polyethylene glycol, polysorbate 80, and titanium dioxide.

CLINICAL PHARMACOLOGY

Hydrocodone component: Hydrocodone is a semisynthetic opioid analgesic and antitussive with multiple actions qualitatively similar to those of codeine. Most of these involve the central nervous system and smooth muscle. The precise mechanism of action of hydrocodone and other opioids is not known, although it is believed to relate to the existence of opiate receptors in the central nervous system. In addition to analgesia, opioids may produce drowsiness, changes in mood, and mental clouding.

Ibuprofen component: Ibuprofen is a nonsteroidal anti-inflammatory agent that possesses analgesic and antipyretic activities. Its mode action, like that of other NSAIDs, is not completely understood, but may be related to inhibition of cyclooxygenase activity and prostaglandin synthesis. Ibuprofen is a peripherally acting analgesic. Ibuprofen does not have any known effects on opiate receptors.

Pharmacokinetics:

Absorption: After oral dosing with the VICOPROFEN tablet, a peak hydrocodone plasma level of 27 ng/mL is achieved at 1.7 hours, and a peak ibuprofen plasma level of 30 mcg/mL is achieved at 1.8 hours. The effect of food on the absorption of either component from the VICOPROFEN tablet has not been established.

Distribution: Ibuprofen is highly protein-bound (99%) like most other non-steroidal anti-inflammatory agents. Although the extent of protein binding of hydrocodone in human plasma has not been definitely determined, structural similarities to related opioid analgesics suggest that hydrocodone is not extensively protein bound. As most agents in the 5-ring morphinan group of semi-synthetic opioids bind plasma protein to a similar degree (range 19% [hydromorphone] to 45% [oxycodone]), hydrocodone is expected to fall within this range.

Metabolism: Hydrocodone exhibits a complex pattern of metabolism, including *O*-demethylation, *N*-demethylation, and 6-keto reduction to the corresponding 6-α-and 6-β-hydroxy metabolites. Hydromorphone, a potent opioid, is formed from the *O*-demethylation of hydrocodone and contributes to the total analgesic effect of hydrocodone. The *O*- and *N*-demethylation processes are mediated by separate P-450 isoenzymes: CYP2D6 and CYP3A4, respectively.

Ibuprofen is present in this product as a racemate, and following absorption it undergoes interconversion in the plasma from the R-isomer to the S-isomer. Both the R- and S- isomers are metabolized to two primary metabolites: (+)-2-4′-(2hydroxy-2-methyl-propyl) phenyl propionic acid and (+)-2-4′-(2carboxypropyl) phenyl propionic acid, both of which circulate in the plasma at low levels relative to the parent.

Elimination: Hydrocodone and its metabolites are eliminated primarily in the kidneys, with a mean plasma half-life of 4.5 hours. Ibuprofen is excreted in the urine, 50% to 60% as metabolites and approximately 15% as unchanged drug and conjugate. The plasma half-life is 2.2 hours.

Special Populations: No significant pharmacokinetic differences based on age or gender have been demonstrated. The pharmacokinetics of hydrocodone and ibuprofen from VICOPROFEN has not been evaluated in children.

Renal Impairment: The effect of renal insufficiency on the pharmacokinetics of the VICOPROFEN dosage form has not been determined.

CLINICAL STUDIES

In single-dose studies of post surgical pain (abdominal, gynecological, orthopedic), 940 patients were studied at doses of one or two tablets. VICOPROFEN produced greater efficacy than placebo and each of its individual components given at the same dose. No advantage was demonstrated for the two-tablet dose.

INDICATIONS AND USAGE

VICOPROFEN tablets are indicated for the short-term (generally less than 10 days) management of acute pain. VICOPROFEN is not indicated for the treatment of such conditions as osteoarthritis or rheumatoid arthritis.

CONTRAINDICATIONS

VICOPROFEN should not be administered to patients who previously have exhibited hypersensitivity to hydrocodone or ibuprofen. VICOPROFEN should not be given to patients who have experienced asthma, urticaria, or allergic-type reactions after taking aspirin or other NSAIDs. Severe, rarely fatal, anaphylactic-like reactions to NSAIDs have been reported in such patients (see WARNINGS - Anaphylactoid Reactions, and PRECAUTIONS - Pre-existing Asthma).

Patients known to be hypersensitive to other opioids may exhibit cross-sensitivity to hydrocodone.

WARNINGS

Abuse and Dependence: Hydrocodone can produce drug dependence of the morphine type and therefore has the potential for being abused. Psychic and physical dependence as well as tolerance may develop upon repeated administration of this drug and it should be prescribed and administered with the same degree of caution as other narcotic drugs (see DRUG ABUSE AND DEPENDENCE).

Respiratory Depression: At high doses or in opioid-sensitive patients, hydrocodone may produce dose-related respiratory depression by acting directly on the brain stem respiratory centers. Hydrocodone also affects the center that controls respiratory rhythm, and may produce irregular and periodic breathing.

Head Injury and Increased Intracranial Pressure: The respiratory depressant effects of opioids and their capacity to elevate cerebrospinal fluid pressure may be markedly exaggerated in the presence of head injury, intracranial lesions or a pre-existing increase in intracranial pressure. Furthermore, opioids produce adverse reactions which may obscure the clinical course of patients with head injuries.

Acute Abdominal Conditions: The administration of opioids may obscure the diagnosis or clinical course of patients with acute abdominal conditions.

Gastrointestinal (GI) Effects - Risk of GI Ulceration, Bleeding and Perforation: Serious gastrointestinal toxicity, such as inflammation, bleeding, ulceration, and perforation of the stomach, small intestine or large intestine, can occur at any time, with or without warning symptoms, in patients treated with nonsteroidal anti-inflammatory drugs (NSAIDs). Minor upper GI problems, such as dyspepsia, are common and may also occur at any time during NSAID therapy. Therefore, physicians and patients should remain alert for ulceration and bleeding even in the absence of previous GI tract symptoms. Patients should be informed about the signs and/or symptoms of serious GI toxicity and what steps to take if they occur. The utility of periodic laboratory monitoring has not been demonstrated, nor has it been adequately assessed. Only one in five patients, who develop a serious upper GI adverse event of NSAID therapy, is symptomatic. Even short term therapy is not without risk.

NSAIDs should be prescribed with extreme caution in those with a prior history of ulcer disease or gastrointestinal bleeding. Most spontaneous reports of fatal GI events are in elderly or debilitated patients and therefore special care should be taken in treating this population. To minimize the potential risk for an adverse GI event, the lowest effective dose should be used for the shortest possible duration. For high risk patients, alternate therapies that do not involve NSAIDs should be considered.

Studies have shown that patients with a prior history of peptic ulcer disease and/or gastrointestinal bleeding and who use NSAIDs, have a greater than 10-fold risk for developing a GI bleed than patients with neither of these risk factors. In addition to a past history of ulcer disease, pharmaco-epidemiological studies have identified several other co-therapies or co-morbid conditions that may increase the

Continued on next page

Vicoprofen—Cont.

risk for GI bleeding such as: treatment with oral corticosteroids, treatment with anticoagulants, longer duration of NSAID therapy, smoking, alcoholism, older age, and poor general health status.

Anaphylactoid Reactions: Anaphylactoid reactions may occur in patients without known prior exposure to VICOPROFEN. VICOPROFEN should not be given to patients with the aspirin triad. The triad typically occurs in asthmatic patients who experience rhinitis with or without nasal polyps, or who exhibit severe, potentially fatal bronchospasm after taking aspirin or other NSAIDs. Fatal reactions to NSAIDs have been reported in such patients (see CONTRAINDICATIONS and PRECAUTIONS - Pre-existing Asthma). Emergency help should be sought when anaphylactoid reaction occurs.

Advanced Renal Disease: In cases with advanced kidney disease, treatment with VICOPROFEN is not recommended. If NSAID therapy, however, must be initiated, close monitoring of the patient's kidney function is advisable (see PRECAUTIONS - Renal Effects).

Pregnancy: As with other NSAID-containing products, VICOPROFEN should be avoided in late pregnancy because it may cause premature closure of the ductus arteriosus.

PRECAUTIONS
General Precautions
Special Risk Patients: As with any opioid analgesic agent, VICOPROFEN tablets should be used with caution in elderly or debilitated patients, and those with severe impairment of hepatic or renal function, hypothyroidism, Addison's disease, prostatic hypertrophy or urethral stricture. The usual precautions should be observed and the possibility of respiratory depression should be kept in mind.

Cough Reflex: Hydrocodone suppresses the cough reflex; as with opioids, caution should be exercised when VICOPROFEN is used postoperatively and in patients with pulmonary disease.

Effect on Diagnostic Signs: The antipyretic and anti-inflammatory activity of ibuprofen may reduce fever and inflammation, thus diminishing their utility as diagnostic signs in detecting complications of presumed noninfectious, noninflammatory painful conditions.

Hepatic Effects: As with other NSAIDs, ibuprofen has been reported to cause borderline elevations of one or more liver enzymes; this may occur in up to 15% of patients. These abnormalities may progress, may remain essentially unchanged, or may be transient with continued therapy. Notable (3 times the upper limit of normal) elevations of SGPT (ALT) or SGOT (AST) occurred in controlled clinical trials in less than 1% of patients. A patient with symptoms and/or signs suggesting liver dysfunction, or in whom an abnormal liver test has occurred, should be evaluated for evidence of the development of more severe hepatic reactions while on therapy with VICOPROFEN. Severe hepatic reactions, including jaundice and cases of fatal hepatitis, have been reported with ibuprofen as with other NSAIDs. Although such reactions are rare, if abnormal liver tests persist or worsen, if clinical signs and symptoms consistent with liver disease develop, or if systemic manifestations occur (e.g. eosinophilia, rash, etc.), VICOPROFEN should be discontinued.

Renal Effects: Caution should be used when initiating treatment with VICOPROFEN in patients with considerable dehydration. It is advisable to rehydrate patients first and then start therapy with VICOPROFEN. Caution is also recommended in patients with pre-existing kidney disease (see WARNINGS - Advanced Renal Disease).

As with other NSAIDs, long-term administration of ibuprofen has resulted in renal papillary necrosis and other renal pathologic changes. Renal toxicity has also been seen in patients in which renal prostaglandins have a compensatory role in the maintenance of renal perfusion. In these patients, administration of a nonsteroidal anti-inflammatory drug may cause a dose-dependent reduction in prostaglandin formation and, secondarily, in renal blood flow, which may precipitate overt renal decompensation. Patients at greatest risk of this reaction are those with impaired renal function, heart failure, liver dysfunction, those taking diuretics and ACE inhibitors, and the elderly. Discontinuation of nonsteroidal anti-inflammatory drug therapy is usually followed by recovery to the pretreatment state.

Ibuprofen metabolites are eliminated primarily by the kidneys. The extent to which the metabolites may accumulate in patients with renal failure has not been studied. Patients with significantly impaired renal function should be more closely monitored.

Hematological Effects: Ibuprofen, like other NSAIDs, can inhibit platelet aggregation but the effect is quantitatively less and of shorter duration than that seen with aspirin. Ibuprofen has been shown to prolong bleeding time in normal subjects. Because this prolonged bleeding effect may be exaggerated in patients with underlying hemostatic defects, VICOPROFEN should be used with caution in persons with intrinsic coagulation defects and those on anticoagulant therapy.

Anemia is sometimes seen in patients receiving NSAIDs, including ibuprofen. This may be due to fluid retention, GI loss, or an incompletely described effect upon erythropoiesis.

Fluid Retention and Edema: Fluid retention and edema have been reported in association with ibuprofen, therefore, the drug should be used with caution in patients with a history of cardiac decompensation, hypertension or heart failure.

Pre-existing Asthma: Patients with asthma may have aspirin-sensitive asthma. The use of aspirin in patients with aspirin-sensitive asthma has been associated with severe bronchospasm, which may be fatal. Since cross-reactivity between aspirin and other NSAIDs has been reported in such aspirin-sensitive patients, VICOPROFEN should not be administered to patients with this form of aspirin sensitivity and should be used with caution in patients with pre-existing asthma.

Aseptic Meningitis: Aseptic meningitis with fever and coma has been observed on rare occasions in patients on ibuprofen therapy. Although it is probably more likely to occur in patients with systemic lupus erythematosus and related connective tissue diseases, it has been reported in patients who do not have an underlying chronic disease. If signs or symptoms of meningitis develop in a patient on VICOPROFEN, the possibility of its being related to ibuprofen should be considered.

Information for Patients
VICOPROFEN, like other opioid-containing analgesics, may impair mental and/or physical abilities required for the performance of potentially hazardous tasks such as driving a car or operating machinery; patients should be cautioned accordingly.

Alcohol and other CNS depressants may produce an additive CNS depression, when taken with this combination product, and should be avoided.

VICOPROFEN may be habit-forming. Patients should take the drug only for as long as it is prescribed, in the amounts prescribed, and no more frequently than prescribed.

VICOPROFEN, like other drugs containing ibuprofen, is not free of side effects. The side effects of these drugs can cause discomfort and, rarely, there are more serious side effects, such as gastrointestinal bleeding, which may result in hospitalization and even fatal outcomes. Patients should be instructed to report any signs and symptoms of gastrointestinal bleeding, blurred vision or other eye symptoms, skin rash, weight gain, or edema.

Laboratory Tests
A decrease in hemoglobin may occur during VICOPROFEN® (hydrocodone bitartrate 7.5 mg and ibuprofen 200 mg) therapy, and elevations of liver enzymes may be seen in a small percentage of patients during VICOPROFEN therapy (see PRECAUTIONS - Hematological Effects and PRECAUTIONS - Hepatic Effects).

In patients with severe hepatic or renal disease, effects of therapy should be monitored with liver and/or renal function tests.

Drug Interactions
ACE-Inhibitors: Reports suggest that NSAIDs may diminish the antihypertensive effect of ACE-inhibitors. This interaction should be given consideration in patients taking VICOPROFEN concomitantly with ACE-inhibitors.

Anticholinergics: The concurrent use of anticholinergics with hydrocodone preparations may produce paralytic ileus.

Antidepressants: The use of MAO inhibitors or tricyclic antidepressants with VICOPROFEN may increase the effect of either the antidepressant or hydrocodone.

Aspirin: As with other products containing NSAIDs, concomitant administration of VICOPROFEN and aspirin is not generally recommended because of the potential of increased adverse effects.

CNS Depressants: Patients receiving other opioids, antihistamines, antipsychotics, antianxiety agents, or other CNS depressants (including alcohol) concomitantly with VICOPROFEN may exhibit an additive CNS depression. When combined therapy is contemplated, the dose of one or both agents should be reduced.

Furosemide: Ibuprofen has been shown to reduce the natriuretic effect of furosemide and thiazides in some patients. This response has been attributed to inhibition of renal prostaglandin synthesis. During concomitant therapy with VICOPROFEN the patient should be observed closely for signs of renal failure (see PRECAUTIONS- Renal Effects), as well as diuretic efficacy.

Lithium: Ibuprofen has been shown to elevate plasma lithium concentration and reduce renal lithium clearance. This effect has been attributed to inhibition of renal prostaglandin synthesis by ibuprofen. Thus, when VICOPROFEN and lithium are administered concurrently, patients should be observed for signs of lithium toxicity.

Methotrexate: Ibuprofen, as well as other NSAIDs, has been reported to competitively inhibit methotrexate accumulation in rabbit kidney slices. This may indicate that ibuprofen could enhance the toxicity of methotrexate. Caution should be used when VICOPROFEN is administered concomitantly with methotrexate.

Warfarin: The effects of warfarin and NSAIDs on GI bleeding are synergistic, such that users of both drugs together have a risk of serious GI bleeding higher than users of either drug alone.

Carcinogenicity, Mutagenicity, and Impairment of Fertility
The carcinogenic and mutagenic potential of VICOPROFEN has not been investigated. The ability of VICOPROFEN to impair fertility has not been assessed.

Pregnancy: Pregnancy Category C.

Teratogenic Effects: VICOPROFEN, administered to rabbits of 95 mg/kg (5.72 and 1.9 times the maximum clinical dose based on body weight and surface area, respectively), a maternally toxic dose, resulted in an increase in the percentage of litters and fetuses with any major abnormality and an increase in the number of litters and fetuses with one or more nonossified metacarpals (a minor abnormality). VICOPROFEN, administered to rats at 166 mg/kg (10.0 and 1.66 times the maximum clinical dose based on body weight and surface area, respectively), a maternally toxic dose, did not result in any reproductive toxicity. There are no adequate and well-controlled studies in pregnant women. VICOPROFEN should be used during pregnancy only if the potential benefit justifies the potential risk to the fetus.

Nonteratogenic Effects: Because of the known effects of nonsteroidal anti-inflammatory drugs on the fetal cardiovascular system (closure of the ductus arteriosus), use during pregnancy (particularly late pregnancy) should be avoided. Babies born to mothers who have been taking opioids regularly prior to delivery will be physically dependent. The withdrawal signs include irritability and excessive crying, tremors, hyperactive reflexes, increased respiratory rate, increased stools, sneezing, yawning, vomiting, and fever. The intensity of the syndrome does not always correlate with the duration of maternal opioid use or dose. There is no consensus on the best method of managing withdrawal.

Labor and Delivery
As with other drugs known to inhibit prostaglandin synthesis, an increased incidence of dystocia and delayed parturition occurred in rats. Administration of VICOPROFEN is not recommended during labor and delivery.

Nursing Mothers
It is not known whether hydrocodone is excreted in human milk. In limited studies, an assay capable of detecting 1 mcg/mL did not demonstrate ibuprofen in the milk of lactating mothers. However, because of the limited nature of the studies, and the possible adverse effects of protaglandin-inhibiting drugs on neonates, VICOPROFEN is not recommended for use in nursing mothers.

Pediatric Use
The safety and effectiveness of VICOPROFEN in pediatric patients below the age of 16 have not been established.

Geriatric Use
In controlled clinical trials there was no difference in tolerability between patients <65 years of age and those ≥65, apart from an increased tendency of the elderly to develop constipation. However, because the elderly may be more sensitive to the renal and gastrointestinal effects of nonsteroidal anti-inflammatory agents as well as possible increased risk of respiratory depression with opioids, extra caution and reduced dosages should be used when treating the elderly with VICOPROFEN.

ADVERSE REACTIONS
VICOPROFEN was administered to approximately 300 pain patients in a safety study that employed dosages and a duration of treatment sufficient to encompass the recommended usage (see DOSAGE AND ADMINISTRATION). Adverse event rates generally increased with increasing daily dose. The event rates reported below are from approximately 150 patients who were in a group that received one tablet of VICOPROFEN an average of three to four times daily. The overall incidence rates of adverse experiences in the trials were fairly similar for this patient group and those who received the comparison treatment, acetaminophen 600 mg with codeine 60 mg.

The following lists adverse events that occurred with an incidence of 1% or greater in clinical trials of VICOPROFEN, without regard to the causal relationship of the events to the drug. To distinguish different rates of occurrence in clinical studies, the adverse events are listed as follows:

name of adverse event = less than 3%
adverse events marked with an asterisk * = 3% to 9%
adverse event rates over 9% are in parentheses.

Body as a Whole: Abdominal pain*; Asthenia*; Fever; Flu syndrome; Headache (27%); Infection*; Pain.

Cardiovascular: Palpitations; Vasodilation.

Central Nervous System: Anxiety*; Confusion; Dizziness (14%); Hypertonia; Insomnia*; Nervousness*; Paresthesia; Somnolence (22%); Thinking abnormalities.

Digestive: Anorexia; Constipation (22%); Diarrhea*; Dry mouth*; Dyspepsia (12%); Flatulence*; Gastritis; Melena; Mouth ulcers; Nausea (21%); Thirst; Vomiting*.

Metabolic and Nutritional Disorders: Edema*.

Respiratory: Dyspnea; Hiccups; Pharyngitis; Rhinitis.
Skin and Appendages: Pruritus*; Sweating*.
Special Senses: Tinnitus.
Urogenital: Urinary frequency.
Incidence less than 1%
Body as a Whole: Allergic reaction.
Cardiovascular: Arrhythmia; Hypotension; Tachycardia.
Central Nervous System: Agitation; Abnormal dreams; Decreased libido; Depression; Euphoria; Mood changes; Neuralgia; Slurred speech; Tremor, Vertigo.
Digestive: Chalky stool; "Clenching teeth"; Dysphagia; Esophageal spasm; Esophagitis; Gastroenteritis; Glossitis; Liver enzyme elevation.
Metabolic and Nutritional: Weight decrease.
Musculoskeletal: Arthralgia; Myalgia.
Respiratory: Asthma; Bronchitis; Hoarseness; Increased cough; Pulmonary congestion; Pneumonia; Shallow breathing; Sinusitis.
Skin and Appendages: Rash; Urticaria.
Special Senses: Altered vision; Bad taste; Dry eyes.
Urogenital: Cystitis; Glycosuria; Impotence; Urinary incontinence; Urinary retention.

DRUG ABUSE AND DEPENDENCE

Controlled Substance: VICOPROFEN Tablets are a Schedule III controlled substance.
Abuse: Psychic dependence, physical dependence, and tolerance may develop upon repeated administration of opioids; therefore, VICOPROFEN Tablets should be prescribed and administered with the same degree of caution appropriate to use of other oral narcotic medications.
Dependence: Physical dependence, the condition in which continued administration of the drug is required to prevent the appearance of a withdrawal syndrome, assumes clinically significant proportions only after several weeks of continued opioid use, although a mild degree of physical dependence may develop after a few days of opioid therapy. Tolerance, in which increasingly large doses are required in order to produce the same degree of analgesia, is manifested initially by a shortened duration of analgesic effect, and subsequently by decreases in the intensity of analgesia. The rate of development of tolerance varies among patients. However, psychic dependence is unlikely to develop when VICOPROFEN Tablets are used for a short time for the treatment of acute pain.

OVERDOSAGE

Following an acute overdosage, toxicity may result from hydrocodone and/or ibuprofen.
Signs and Symptoms:
Hydrocodone component: Serious overdose with hydrocodone is characterized by respiratory depression (a decrease in respiratory rate and/or tidal volume, Cheyne-Stokes respiration, cyanosis) extreme somnolence progressing to stupor or coma, skeletal muscle flaccidity, cold and clammy skin, and sometimes bradycardia and hypotension. In severe overdosage, apnea, circulatory collapse, cardiac arrest and death may occur.
Ibuprofen component: Symptoms include gastrointestinal irritation with erosion and hemorrhage or perforation, kidney damage, liver damage, heart damage, hemolytic anemia, agranulocytosis, thrombocytopenia, aplastic anemia, and meningitis. Other symptoms may include headache, dizziness, tinnitus, confusion, blurred vision, mental disturbances, skin rash, stomatitis, edema, reduced retinal sensitivity, corneal deposits, and hyperkalemia.
Treatment:
Primary attention should be given to the re-establishment of adequate respiratory exchange through provision of a patent airway and the institution of assisted or controlled ventilation. Naloxone, a narcotic antagonist, can reverse respiratory depression and coma associated with opioid overdose or unusual sensitivity to opioids, including hydrocodone. Therefore, an appropriate dose of naloxone hydrochloride should be administered intravenously with simultaneous efforts at respiratory resuscitation. Since the duration of action of hydrocodone may exceed that of the naloxone, the patient should be kept under continuous surveillance and repeated doses of the antagonist should be administered as needed to maintain adequate respiration. Supportive measures should be employed as indicated. Gastric emptying may be useful in removing unabsorbed drug. In cases where consciousness is impaired it may be inadvisable to perform gastric lavage. If gastric lavage is performed, little drug will likely be recovered if more than an hour has elapsed since ingestion. Ibuprofen is acidic and is excreted in the urine; therefore, it may be beneficial to administer alkali and induce diuresis. In addition to supportive measures the use of oral activated charcoal may help to reduce the absorption and reabsorption of ibuprofen. Dialysis is not likely to be effective for removal of ibuprofen because it is very highly bound to plasma proteins.

DOSAGE AND ADMINISTRATION

For the short-term (generally less than 10 days) management of acute pain, the recommended dose of VICOPROFEN is one tablet every 4 to 6 hours, as necessary. Dosage should not exceed 5 tablets in a 24-hour period. It should be kept in mind that tolerance to hydrocodone can develop with continued use and that the incidence of untoward effects is dose related.
The lowest effective dose or the longest dosing interval should be sought for each patient, especially in the elderly. After observing the initial response to therapy with VICOPROFEN, the dose and frequency of dosing should be adjusted to suit the individual patient's need, without exceeding the total daily dose recommended.

HOW SUPPLIED

VICOPROFEN tablets are available as:
White film-coated round convex tablets, engraved with "VP" over the Knoll triangle on one side and plain on the other side.
Bottles of 100-NDC #0044-0723-02
Bottles of 500-NDC #0044-0723-03
Hospital Unit Dosage Package-100 tablets
(4×25 tablets)-NDC #0044-0723-41
Storage: Store at 25° C (77° F); excursions permitted to 15° to 30° C (59°–86° F). [See USP Controlled Room Temperature].
Dispense in a tight, light-resistant container.
Caution: Federal law prohibits dispensing without prescription.
A Schedule Ⓒ Narcotic.
©1997 Knoll Pharmaceutical Company
VICOPROFEN is a registered trademark of Knoll Pharmaceutical Company
Revised: September 1997
Knoll Laboratories
A Division of
Knoll Pharmaceutical Company
3000 Continental Drive - North
Mount Olive, New Jersey 07828-1234   **BASF** Pharma
                                        0900001-3
Shown in Product Identification Guide, page 319

EDUCATIONAL MATERIAL

Continuing Education Booklets
"Controlling Severe Pain in the 1990s: An Update for Pharmacy Practitioners" (3 credits) Home Study Module—Pharmacists

---

Knoll Pharmaceutical Company
**3000 CONTINENTAL DRIVE NORTH
MOUNT OLIVE, NJ 07828**

BASF Group

Direct Inquiries to:
Knoll Pharmaceutical Company
(973) 426-2600
Customer Operations Department:
(800) 526-0710

For Medical Information Contact:
(800)526-0221

MAVIK®   ℞
[mă 'vick]
(Trandolapril) Tablets
PRESCRIBING INFORMATION

USE IN PREGNANCY
When used in pregnancy during the second and third trimesters, ACE inhibitors can cause injury and even death to the developing fetus. When pregnancy is detected, MAVIK® should be discontinued as soon as possible. See WARNINGS, Fetal/Neonatal Morbidity and Mortality.

DESCRIPTION

Trandolapril is the ethyl ester prodrug of a non-sulfhydryl angiotensin converting enzyme (ACE) inhibitor, trandolaprilat. Trandolapril is chemically described as (2S, 3aR, 7aS)-1-[(S)-N-[(S)-1-Carboxy-3-phenylpropyl]alanyl] hexahydro-2-indolinecarboxylic acid, 1-ethyl ester. Its empirical formula is $C_{24}H_{34}N_2O_5$ and its structural formula is [See chemical structure at top of next column]

R:- C_2H_5: Trandolapril
-H: Trandolaprilat (diacid)

M.W.=430.54
Melting Point=125°C

Trandolapril is a colorless, crystalline substance that is soluble (>100 mg/mL) in chloroform, dichloromethane, and methanol. MAVIK® tablets contain 1 mg, 2 mg, or 4 mg of trandolapril for oral administration. Each tablet also contains corn starch, croscarmellose sodium, hydroxypropyl methyl-cellulose, iron oxide, lactose, povidone, sodium stearyl fumarate.

CLINICAL PHARMACOLOGY
Mechanism of Action:
Trandolapril is deesterified to the diacid metabolite, trandolaprilat, which is approximately eight times more active as an inhibitor of ACE activity. ACE is a peptidyl dipeptidase that catalyzes the conversion of angiotensin 1 to the vasoconstrictor, angiotensin II. Angiotensin II is a potent peripheral vasoconstrictor that also stimulates secretion of aldosterone by the adrenal cortex and provides negative feedback for renin secretion. The effect of tradolapril in hypertension appears to result primarily from the inhibition of circulating and tissue ACE activity thereby reducing angiotensin II formation, decreasing vasoconstriction, decreasing aldosterone secretion, and increasing plasma renin. Decreased aldosterone secretion leads to diuresis, natriuresis, and a small increase of serum potassium. In controlled clinical trials, treatment with MAVIK® alone resulted in mean increases in potassium of 0.1 mEq/L. (See **PRECAUTIONS**).
ACE is identical to kininase II, an enzyme that degrades bradykinin, a potent peptide vasodilator; whether increased levels of bradykinin play a role in the therapeutic effect of trandolapril remains to be elucidated.
While the principal mechanism of antihypertensive effect is thought to be through the renin-angiotensin-aldosterone system, trandolapril exerts antihypertensive actions even in patients with low-renin hypertension. MAVIK® was an effective antihypertensive in all races studied. Both black patients (usually a predominantly low-renin group) and non-black patients responded to 2 to 4 mg of MAVIK®.
Pharmacokinetics and Metabolism:
Pharmacokinetics Trandolapril's ACE-inhibiting activity is primarily due to its diacid metabolite, trandolaprilat. Cleavage of the ester group of trandolapril, primarily in the liver, is responsible for conversion. Absolute bioavailability after oral administration of trandolapril is about 10% as trandolapril and 70% as trandolaprilat. After oral trandolapril under fasting conditions, peak trandolapril levels occur at about one hour and peak trandolaprilat levels occur between 4 and 10 hours. The elimination half lives of trandolapril and transolaprilat are about 6 and 10 hours, respectively, but, like all ACE inhibitors, trandolaprilat also has a prolonged terminal elimination phase, involving a small fraction of administered drug, probably representing binding to plasma and tissue ACE. During multiple dosing of trandolapril, there is no significant accumulation of trandolaprilat. Food slows absorption of trandolapril, but does not affect AUC or Cmax of trandolaprilat or Cmax of trandolapril.
Metabolism and Excretion After oral administration of trandolapril, about 33% of parent drug and metabolites are recovered in urine, mostly as trandolaprilat, with about 66% in feces. The extent of the absorbed dose which is biliary excreted has not been determined. Plasma concentrations (Cmax and AUC of trandolapril and Cmax of trandolaprilat) are dose proportional over the 1–4 mg range, but the AUC of trandolaprilat is somewhat less than dose proportional. In addition to trandolaprilat, at least 7 other metabolites have been found, principally glucuronides or deesterification products.
Serum protein binding of trandolapril is about 80%, and is independent of concentration. Binding of trandolaprilat is concentration-dependent, varying from 65% at 1000 ng/mL to 94% at 0.1 ng/mL, indicating saturation of binding with increasing concentration.
The volume of distribution of trandolapril is about 18 liters. Total plasma clearances of trandolapril and trandolaprilat after approximately 2 mg IV doses are about 52 liters/hour and 7 liters/hour respectively. Renal clearance of trandolaprilat varies from 1–4 liters/hour, depending on dose.

Continued on next page

Mavik—Cont.

Special populations:
Pediatric Trandolapril pharmacokinetics have not been evaluated in patients <18 years of age.

Geriatric and Gender Trandolapril pharmacokinetics have been investigated in the elderly (>65 years) and in both genders. The plasma concentration of trandolapril is increased in elderly hypertensive patients, but the plasma concentration of trandolaprilat and inhibition of ACE activity are similar in elderly and young hypertensive patients. The pharmacokinetics of trandolapril and trandolaprilat and inhibition of ACE activity are similar in male and female elderly hypertensive patients.

Race Pharmacokinetic differences have not been evaluated in different races.

Renal Insufficiency Compared to normal subjects, the plasma concentrations of trandolapril and trandolaprilat are approximately 2-fold greater and renal clearance is reduced by about 85% in patients with creatinine clearance below 30 ml/min and in patients on hemodialysis. Dosage adjustment is recommended in renally impaired patients. (See **DOSAGE** and **ADMINISTRATION**.)

Hepatic Insufficiency Following oral administration in patients with mild to moderate alcoholic cirrhosis, plasma concentrations of trandolapril and prandolaprilat were, respectively, 9-fold and 2-fold greater than in normal subjects, but inhibition of ACE activity was not affected. Lower doses should be considered in patients with hepatic insufficiency. (See **DOSAGE** and **ADMINISTRATION**.)

Drug Interactions Trandolapril did not affect the plasma concentration (pre-dose and 2 hours post-dose) of oral digoxin (0.25 mg). Coadministration of trandolapril and cimetidine led to an increase of about 44% in Cmax for trandolapril, but no difference in the pharmacokinetics of trandolaprilat or in ACE inhibition. Coadministration of trandolapril and furosemide led to an increase of about 25% in the renal clearance of trandolaprilat, but no effect was seen on the pharmacokinetics of furosemide or trandolaprilat or on ACE inhibition.

Pharmacodynamics and Clinical Effects:

A single 2–mg dose of MAVIK® produces 70 to 85% inhibition of plasma ACE activity at 4 hours with about 10% decline at 24 hours and about half the effect manifest at 8 days. Maximum ACE inhibition is achieved with a plasma trandolaprilat concentration of 2 ng/mL. ACE inhibition is a function of trandolaprilat concentration, not trandolapril concentration. The effect of trandolapril on exogenous angiotensin I was not measured.

Hypertension

Four placebo-controlled dose response studies were conducted using once-daily oral dosing of MAVIK® in doses from 0.25 to 16 mg per day in 827 black and non-black patients with mild to moderate hypertension. The minimal effective once-daily dose was 1 mg in non-black patients and 2 mg in black patients. Further decreases in trough supine diastolic blood pressure were obtained in non-black patients with higher doses, and no further response was seen with doses above 4 mg (up to 16 mg). The antihypertensive effect diminished somewhat at the end of the dosing interval, but trough/peak ratios are well above 50% for all effective doses. There was a slightly greater effect on the diastolic pressure, but no difference on systolic pressure with b.i.d. dosing. During chronic therapy, the maximum reduction in blood pressure with any dose is achieved within one week. Following 6 weeks of monotherapy in placebo-controlled trials in patients with mild to moderate hypertension, once-daily doses of 2 to 4 mg lowered supine or standing systolic/diastolic blood pressure 24 hours after dosing by an average of 7–10/4–5 mmHg below placebo responses in non-black patients. Once-daily doses of 2 to 4 mg lowered blood pressure 4–6/3–4 mmHg in black patients. Trough to peak ratios for effective doses ranged from 0.5 to 0.9. There were no differences in response between men and women, but responses were somewhat greater in patients under 60 than in patients over 60 years old. Abrupt withdrawal of MAVIK® has not been associated with a rapid increase in blood pressure. Administration of MAVIK® to patients with mild to moderate hypertension results in a reduction of supine, sitting and standing blood pressure to about the same extent without compensatory tachycardia.

Symptomatic hypotension is infrequent, although it can occur in patients who are salt- and/or volume-depleted. (See **WARNINGS**.) Use of MAVIK® in combination with thiazide diuretics gives a blood pressure lowering effect greater than that seen with either agent alone, and the additional effect of trandolapril is similar to the effect of monotherapy.

Heart Failure Post Myocardial Infarction or Left Ventricular Dysfunction Post Myocardial Infarction:

The Trandolapril Cardiac Evaluation (TRACE) Trial was a Danish, 27-center, double-blind, placebo controlled, parallel-group study of the effect of trandolapril on all-cause mortality in stable patients with echocardiographic evidence of left ventricular dysfunction 3 to 7 days after a myocardial infarction. Subjects with residual ischemia or overt heart fail-

ure were included. Patients tolerant of a test dose of 1 mg trandolapril were randomized to placebo (n=873) or trandolapril (n=876) and followed for 24 months. Among patients randomized to trandolapril, who began treatment on 1 mg, 62% were successfully titrated to a target dose of 4 mg once daily over a period of weeks. The use of trandolapril was associated with a 16% reduction in the risk of all-cause mortality (p=0.042), largely cardiovascular mortality. Trandolapril was also associated with a 20% reduction in the risk of progression of heart failure (p=0.047), defined by a time-to-first-event analysis of death attributed to heart failure, hospitalization for heart failure, or requirement for open-label ACE inhibitor for the treatment of heart failure. There was no significant effect of treatment on other endpoints: subsequent hospitalization, incidence of recurrent myocardial infarction, exercise tolerance, ventricular function, ventricular dimensions, or NYHA class.

The population in TRACE was entirely Caucasian and had less usage than would be typical in a U.S. population of other post-infarction interventions: 42% thrombolysis, 16% beta-adrenergic blockade, and 6.7% PTCA or CABG during the entire period of follow-up. Blood pressure control, especially in the placebo group, was poor: 47 to 53% of patients randomized to placebo and 32 to 40% of patients randomized to trandolapril had blood pressures >140/95 at 90-day follow-up visits.

INDICATIONS AND USAGE
Hypertension

MAVIK® is indicated for the treatment of hypertension. It may be used alone or in combination with other antihypertensive medication such as hydrochlorothiazide.

In considering the use of MAVIK®, it should be noted that in controlled trials ACE inhibitors (for which adequate data are available) cause a higher rate of angioedema in black than in non-black patients. (See **Warnings: Angioedema**.) When using MAVIK®, consideration should be given to the fact that another angiotensin converting enzyme inhibitor, captopril, has caused agranulocytosis, particularly in patients with renal impairment or collagen-vascular disease. Available data are insufficient to show that MAVIK® does not have a similar risk. (See **WARNINGS**.)

Heart Failure Post Myocardial Infarction or Left-Ventricular Dysfunction Post Myocardial Infarction:

MAVIK® is indicated in stable patients who have evidence of left-ventricular systolic dysfunction (identified by wall motion abnormalities) or who are symptomatic from congestive heart failure within the first few days after sustaining acute myocardial infarction. Administration of trandolapril to Caucasian patients has been shown to decrease the risk of death (principally cardiovascular death) and to decrease the risk of heart failure-related hospitalization (See **CLINICAL PHARMACOLOGY, Heart Failure or Left-Ventricular Dysfunction Post Myocardial Infarction** for details of the survival trial).

CONTRAINDICATIONS

MAVIK® is contraindicated in patients who are hypersensitive to this product and in patients with a history of angioedema related to previous treatment with an ACE inhibitor.

WARNINGS
Anaphylactoid and Possibly Related Reactions:

Presumably because angiotensin converting enzyme inhibitors affect the metabolism of eicosanoids and polypeptides, including endogenous bradykinin, patients receiving ACE inhibitors, including MAVIK®, may be subject to a variety of adverse reactions, some of them serious.

Angioedema:

Angioedema of the face, extremities, lips, tongue, glottis, and larynx has been reported in patients treated with ACE inhibitors including MAVIK®. Symptoms suggestive of angioedema or facial edema occurred in 0.13% of MAVIK®-treated patients. Two of the four cases were life-threatening and resolved without treatment or with medication (corticosteroids). Angioedema associated with laryngeal edema can be fatal. If laryngeal stridor or angioedema of the face, tongue or glottis occurs, treatment with MAVIK® should be discontinued immediately, the patient treated in accordance with accepted medical care and carefully observed until the swelling disappears. In instances where swelling is confined to the face and lips, the condition generally resolves without treatment; antihistamines may be useful in relieving symptoms. **Where there is involvement of the tongue, glottis, or larynx, likely to cause airway obstruction, emergency therapy, including but not limited to subcutaneous epinephrine solution 1:1,000 (0.3 to 0.5 mL) should be promptly administered.** (See **PRECAUTIONS**: Information for Patients and **ADVERSE REACTIONS**.)

Anaphylactoid Reactions During Densitization Two patients undergoing desentizing treatment with hymenoptera venom while receiving ACE inhibitors sustained life-threatening anaphylactoid reactions. In the same patients, these reactions did not occur when ACE inhibitors were temporarily withheld, but they reappeared when the ACE inhibitors were inadvertently readministered.

Anaphylactoid Reactions During Membrane Exposure Anaphylactoid reactions have been reported in patients

dialyzed with high-flux membranes and treated concomitantly with an ACE inhibitor. Anaphylactoid reactions have also been reported in patients undergoing low-density lipoprotein apheresis with dextran sulfate absorption.

Hypotension:

MAVIK® can cause symptomatic hypotension. Like other ACE inhibitors, MAVIK® has only rarely been associated with symptomatic hypotension in uncomplicated hypertensive patients. Symptomatic hypotension is most likely to occur in patients who have been sale- or volume-depleted as a result of prolonged treatment with diuretics, dietary sale restriction, dialysis, diarrhea, or vomiting. Volume and/or sale depletion should be corrected before initiating treatment with MAVIK®. (See **PRECAUTIONS**, Drug Interactions, and **ADVERSE REACTIONS**.) In controlled and uncontrolled studies, hypotension was reported as an adverse event in 0.6 percent of patients and led to discontinuations in 0.1% of patients.

In patients with concomitant congestive heart failure, with or without associated renal insufficiency, ACE inhibitor therapy may cause excessive hypotension, which may be associated with oliguria or azotemia, and rarely, with acute renal failure and death. In such patients, MAVIK® therapy should be started at the recommended dose under close medical supervision. These patients should be followed closely during the first 2 weeks of treatment and, thereafter, whenever the dosage of MAVIK® or diuretic is increased. (See **DOSAGE** and **ADMINISTRATION**.) Care in avoiding hypotension should also be taken in patients with ischemic heart disease, aortic stenosis, or cerebrovascular disease.

If symptomatic hypotension occurs, the patient should be placed in the supine position and, if necessary, normal saline may be administered intravenously. A transient hypotensive response is not a contraindication to further doses; however, lower doses of MAVIK® or reduced concomitant diuretic therapy should be considered.

Neutropenia/Agranulocytosis:

Another ACE inhibitor, captopril, has been shown to cause agranulocytosis and bone marrow depression rarely in patients with uncomplicated hypertension, but more frequently in patients with renal impairment, especially if they also have a collagen-vascular disease such as systemic lupus erythematosus or scleroderma. Available data from clinical trials of trandolapril are insufficient to show that trandolapril does not cause agranulocytosis at similar rates. As with other ACE inhibitors, periodic monitoring of white blood cell counts in patients with collagen-vascular disease and/or renal disease should be considered.

Hepatic Failure:

ACE inhibitors rarely have been associated with a syndrome of cholestatic jaundice, fulminant hepatic necrosis, and death. The mechanism of this syndrome is not understood. Patients receiving ACE inhibitors who develop jaundice should discontinue the ACE inhibitor and receive appropriate medical follow-up.

Fetal/Neonatal Morbidity and Mortality:

ACE inhibitors can cause fetal and neonatal morbidity and death when administered to pregnant women. Several dozen cases have been reported in the world literature. When pregnancy is detected, ACE inhibitors should be discontinued as soon as possible.

The use of ACE inhibitors during the second and third trimesters of pregnancy has been associated with fetal and neonatal injury, including hypotension, neonatal skull hypoplasia anuria, reversible or irreversible renal failure, and death. Oligohydramnios has also been reported, presumably resulting from decreased fetal renal function; oligohydramnios in this setting has been associated with fetal limb contractures, craniofacial deformation, and hypoplastic lung development. Prematurity, intrauterine growth retardation, and patent ductus arteriosus have also been reported, although it is not clear whether these occurrences were due to the ACE inhibitor exposure.

These adverse effects do not appear to have resulted from intrauterine ACE-inhibitor exposure that has been limited to the first trimester. Mothers whose embryos and fetuses are exposed to ACE inhibitors only during the first trimester should be so informed. Nonetheless, when patients become pregnant, physicians should make every effort to discontinue the use of trandolapril as soon as possible.

Rarely (probably less often than once in every thousand pregnancies), no alternative to ACE inhibitors will be found. In these rare cases, the mothers should be apprised of the potential hazards to their fetuses, and serial ultrasound examinations should be performed to assess the intra-amniotic environment.

If oligohydramnios is observed, trandolapril should be discontinued unless it is considered life-saving for the mother. Contraction stress testing (CST), a non-stress test (NST), or biophysical profiling (BPP) may be appropriate, depending upon the week of pregnancy.

Patients and physicians should be aware, however, that oligohydramnios may not appear until after the fetus has sustained irreversible injury.

Infants with histories of *in utero* exposure to ACE inhibitors should be closely observed for hypotension, oliguria, and hyperkalemia. If oliguria occurs, attention should be directed toward support of blood pressure and renal perfusion. Exchange transfusions or dialysis may be required as a means of reversing hypotension and/or substituting for disordered renal function.

Doses of 0.8 mg/kg/day (9.4 mg/m²/day) in rabbits, 1000 mg/kg/day (7000 mg/m²/day) in rats, and 25 mg/kg/day (295 mg/m²/day) in cynomoglus monkeys did not produce teratogenic effects. These doses represent 10 and 3 times (rabbits), 1250 and 2564 times (rats), and 312 and 108 times (monkeys) the maximum projected human dose of 4 mg based on body-weight and body-surface-area, respectively assuming a 50 kg woman.

PRECAUTIONS

General

Impaired Renal Function:

As a consequence of inhibiting the renin-angiotensin-aldosterone system, changes in renal function may be anticipated in susceptible individuals. In patients with severe heart failure whose renal function may depend on the activity of the renin-angiotensin-aldosterone system, treatment with ACE inhibitors, including MAVIK®, may be associated with oliguria and/or progressive azotemia and rarely with acute renal failure and/or death.

In hypertensive patients with unilateral or bilateral renal artery stenosis, increases in blood urea nitrogen and serum creatinine have been observed in some patients following ACE inhibitor therapy. These increases were almost always reversible upon discontinuation of the ACE inhibitor and/or diuretic therapy. In such patients, renal function should be monitored during the first few weeks of therapy.

Some hypertensive patients with no apparent preexisting renal vascular disease have developed increases in blood urea and serum creatinine, usually minor and transient, especially when ACE inhibitors have been given concomitantly with a diuretic. This is more likely to occur in patients with preexisting renal impairment. Dosage reduction and/or discontinuation of any diuretic and/or the ACE inhibitor may be required.

Evaluation of hypertensive patients should always include assessment of renal function. (See DOSAGE and ADMINISTRATION.)

Hyperkalemia and potassium-sparing diuretics:

In clinical trials, hyperkalemia (serum potassium > 6.00 mEq/L) occurred in approximately 0.4 percent of hypertensive patients receiving MAVIK®. In most cases, elevated serum potassium levels were isolated values, which resolved despite continued therapy. None of these patients were discontinued from the trials because of hyperkalemia. Risk factors for the development of hyperkalemia include renal insufficiency, diabetes mellitus, and the concomitant use of potassium-sparing diuretics, potassium supplements, and/or potassium-containing salt substitutes, which should be used cautiously, if at all, with MAVIK®. (See PRECAUTIONS: Drug Interactions.)

Cough:

Presumably due to the inhibition of the degradation of endogenous bradykinin, persistent nonproductive cough has been reported with all ACE inhibitors, always resolving after discontinuation of therapy. ACE inhibitor-induced cough should be considered in the differential diagnosis of cough. In controlled trials of trandolapril, cough was present in 2% of trandolapril patients and 0% of patients given placebo. There was no evidence of a relationship to dose.

Surgery/anesthesia:

In patients undergoing major surgery or during anesthesia with agnets that produce hypotension, MAVIK® will block angiotensin II formation secondary to compensatory renin release. If hypotension occurs and is considered to be due to this mechanism, it can be corrected by volume expansion.

Information for Patients

Angioedema:

Angioedema, including laryngeal edema, may occur at any time during treatment with ACE inhibitors, including MAVIK®. Patients should be so advised and told to report immediately any signs or symptoms suggesting angioedema (swelling of face, extremities, eyes, lips, tongue, difficulty in swallowing or breathing) and to stop taking the drug until they have consulted with their physician. (See WARNINGS and ADVERSE REACTIONS.)

Symptomatic Hypotension:

Patients should be cautioned that light-headedness can occur, especially during the first days of MAVIK® therapy, and should be reported to a physician. If actual syncope occurs, patients should be told to stop taking the drug until they have consulted with their physician (See WARNINGS.)

All patients should be cautioned that inadequate fluid intake, excessive perspiration, diarrhea, or vomiting, resulting in reduced fluid volume, may precipitate an excessive fall in blood pressure with the same consequences of light-headedness and possible syncope.

Patients planning to undergo any surgery and/or anesthesia should be told to inform their physician that they are taking an ACE inhibitor that has a long duration of action.

Hyperkalemia:

Patients should be told not to use potassium supplements or salt substitutes containing potassium without consulting their physician. (See PRECAUTIONS.)

Neutropenia:

Patients should be told to report promptly any indication of infection (e.g., sore throat, fever) which could be a sign of neutropenia.

Pregnancy:

Female patients of childbearing age should be told about the consequences of second- and third-trimester exposure to ACE inhibitors, and they should also be told that these consequences do not appear to have resulted from intrauterine ACE-inhibitor exposure that has been limited to the first trimester. These patients should be asked to report prepregnancies to their physicians as soon as possible.

NOTE: As with many other drugs, certain advice to patients being treated with MAVIK® is warranted. This information is intended to aid in the safe and effective use of this medication. It is not a disclosure of all possible adverse or intended effects.

Drug Interactions

Concomitant diuretic therapy:

As with other ACE inhibitors, patients on diuretics, especially those on recently instituted diuretic therapy, may experience an excessive reduction of blood pressure after initiation of therapy with MAVIK®. The possibility of exacerbation of hypotensive effects with MAVIK® may be minimized by either discontinuing the diuretic or cautiously increasing salt intake prior to initiation of treatment with MAVIK®. If it is not possible to discontinue the diuretic, the starting dose of trandolapril should be reduced (See DOSAGE and ADMINISTRATION.)

Agents increasing serum potassium:

Trandolapril can attenuate potassium loss caused by thiazide diuretics and increase serum potassium when used alone. Use of potassium-sparing diuretics (spironolactone, triamterene, or amiloride), potassium supplements, or potassium-containing salt substitutes concomitantly with ACE inhibitors can increase the risk of hyperkalemia. If concomitant use of such agents is indicated, they should be used with caution and with appropriate monitoring of serum potassium. (See PRECAUTIONS.)

Lithium:

Increased serum lithium levels and symptoms of lithium toxicity have been reported in patients receiving concomitant lithium and ACE inhibitor therapy. These drugs should be coadministered with caution, and frequent monitoring of serum lithium levels is recommended. If a diuretic is also used, the risk of lithium toxicity may be increased.

Other:

No clinically significant interaction has been found between trandolaprilat and food, cimetidine, digoxin, or furosemide. The anticoagulant effect of warfarin was not significantly changed by trandolapril.

Carcinogenesis, Mutagenesis, Impariment of Fertility

Long-term studies were conducted with oral trandolapril administered by gavage to mice (78 weeks) and rats (104 and 106 weeks). No evidence of carcinogenic potential was seen in mice dosed up to 25 mg/kg/day (85 mg/m²/day) or rats dosed up to 8 mg/kg/day (60 mg/m²/day). These doses are 313 and 32 times (mice), and 100 and 23 times (rats) the maximum recommended human daily dose (MRHDD) of 4 mg based on body-weight and body-surface-area, respectively assuming a 50 kg individual. The genotoxic potential of trandolapril was evaluated in the microbial mutagenicity (Ames) test, the point mutation and chromosome aberration assays in Chinese hamster V79 cells, and the micronucleus test in mice. There was no evidence of mutgenic or clastogenic potential in these in vitro and in vivo assays.

Reproduction studies in rats did not show any impairment of fertility at doses up to 100 mg/kg/day (710 mg/m²/day) of trandolapril, or 1250 and 260 times the MRHDD on the basis of body-weight and body-surface-area, respectively

Pregnancy

Pregnancy Categories C (first trimester) and D (second and third trimesters): See WARNINGS, Fetal/Neonatal Morbidity and mortality.

Nursing Mothers

Radiolabeled trandolapril or its metabolites are secreted in rat milk. MAVIK® (trandolapril) should not be administered to nursing mothers.

Geriatric Use

In placebo-controlled studies of MAVIK®, 31.1% of patients were 60 years and older, 20.1% were 65 years and older, and 2.3% were 75 years and older. No overall differences in effectiveness or safety were observed between these patients and younger patients. (Greater sensitivity of some older individual patients cannot be ruled out.)

Pediatric use

The safety and effectiveness of MAVIK® in pediatric patients have not been established.

ADVERSE REACTIONS

The safety experience in U.S. placebo-controlled trials included 1067 hypertensive patients, of whom 831 received MAVIK®. Nearly 200 hypertensive patients received MAVIK® for over one year in open-label trials. In controlled trials, withdrawals for adverse events were 2.1% on placebo and 1.4% on MAVIK®. Adverse events considered at least

possibly related to treatment occurring in 1% of MAVIK®-treated patients and more common on MAVIK® than placeob, pooled for all doses, are shown below, together with the frequency of discontinuation of treatment because of these events.

ADVERSE EVENTS IN PLACEBO-CONTROLLED HYPERTENSION TRIALS
Occurring at 1% or greater

	MAVIK (N=832) % Incidence (% Discontinuance)	PLACEBO (N=237) % Incidence (% Discontinuance)
Cough	1.9 (0.1)	0.4 (0.4)
Dizziness	1.3 (0.2)	0.4 (0.4)
Diarrhea	1.0 (0.0)	0.4 (0.0)

Headache and fatigue were all seen in more than 1% of MAVIK®-treated patients but were more frequently seen on placebo. Adverse events were not usually persistent or difficult to manage.

Left Ventricular Dysfunction Post Myocardial Infarction:
Adverse reactions related to Mavik®, occurring at a rate greater than that observed in placebo-treated patients with left ventricular dysfunction, are shown below. The incidences represent the experiences from the TRACE study. The follow-up time was between 24 and 50 months for this study.

Percentage of Patients with Adverse Events Greater Than Placebo

Adverse Event	Placebo-Controlled (TRACE) Mortality Study	
	Trandolapril N=876	Placebo N=873
Cough	35	22
Dizziness	23	17
Hypotension	11	6.8
Elevated Serum uric acid	15	13
Elevated BUN	9.0	7.6
PICA or CABG	7.3	6.1
Dyspepsia	6.4	6.0
Syncope	5.9	3.3
Hyperkalemia	5.3	2.8
Bradycardia	4.7	4.4
Hypocalcemia	4.7	3.9
Myalgia	4.7	3.1
Elevated Creatinine	4.7	2.4
Gastritis	4.2	3.6
Cardiogenic shock	3.8	<2
Intermittent claudication	3.8	<2
Stroke	3.3	3.2
Asthenia	3.3	2.6

Clinical adverse experiences possibly or probably related or of uncertain relationship to therapy occurring in 0.3% to 1.0% (except as noted) of the patients treated with MAVIK® (with or without concomitant calcium ion antagonist or diuretic) in controlled or uncontrolled trials (N=1134) and less frequent, clinically significant events seen in clinical trials or post-marketing experience (the rarer events are in italics) include (listed by body system):

General Body Function: chest pain.

Cardiovascular: AV first degree block, bradycardia, edema, flushing, hypotension, palpitations.

Central Nervous System: drowsiness, insomnia, paresthesia, vertigo.

Dermatologic: pruritus, rash, pemphigus.

Eye, Ear, Nose, Throat: epistaxis, throat inflammation, upper respiratory tract infection.

Emotional, Mental, Sexual States: anxiety, impotence, decreased libido.

Gastrointestinal: abdominal distention, abdominal pain/cramps, constipation, dyspepsia, diarrhea, vomiting, *pancreatitis*.

Hemopoietic: *decreased leukocytes, decreased neutrophils.*

Metabolism and Endocrine: *increased creatinine, increased potassium*, increased SGPT (ALT).

Musculoskeletal System: extremity pain, muscle cramps, gout.

Pulmonary: dyspnea.

Angioedema: Angioedema has been reported in 4 (0.13%) patients receiving MAVIK® in U.S. and foreign studies. Angioedema associated with laryngeal edema may be fatal. If angioedema of the face, extremities, lips, tongue, glottis, and/or larynx occurs, treatment with MAVIK® should be discontinued and appropriate therapy instituted immediately. (See WARNINGS.)

Hypotension: In hypertensive patients, symptomatic hypotension occurred in 0.6 percent and near syncope occurred in 0.2 percent. Hypotension or syncope was a cause for discontinuation of therapy in 0.1 percent of hypertensive patients.

Fetal/Neonatal Morbidity and Mortality: See WARNINGS, Fetal Neonatal Morbidity and Mortality.

Continued on next page

Mavik—Cont.

Cough: See **PRECAUTIONS,** Cough.
Clinical Laboratory Test Findings
Hematology: (See **WARNINGS.**) Low white blood cells, low neutrophils, low lymphocytes, thrombocytopenia.
Serum Electrolytes: Hyperkalemia (See **PRECAUTIONS,**) hyponatremia.
Creatinine and Blood Urea Nitrogen: Increases in creatinine levels occurred in 1.1 percent of patients receiving MAVIK® alone and 7.3 percent of patients treated with MAVIK®, a calcium ion antagonist and a diuretic. Increases in blood urea nitrogen levels occurred in 0.6 percent of patients receiving MAVIK® alone and 1.4 percent of patients receiving MAVIK®, a calcium ion antagonist, and a diuretic. None of these increases required discontinuation of treatment. Increases in these laboratory values are more likely to occur in patients with renal insufficiency or those pretreated with a diuretic and, based on experience with other ACE inhibitors, would be expected to be especially likely in patients with renal artery stenosis. (See **PRECAUTIONS** and **WARNINGS.**)
Liver function tests: Occasional elevation of transaminases at the rate of 3X upper normals occurred in 0.8% of patients and persistent increase in bilirubin occurred in 0.2% of patients. Discontinuation for elevated liver enzymes occurred in 0.2 percent of patients.

OVERDOSAGE

No data are available with respect to overdosage in humans. The oral LD_{50} of trandolapril in mice was 4875 mg/Kg in males and 3990 mg/Kg in females. In rats, an oral dose of 5000 mg/Kg caused low mortality (1 male out of 5; 0 females). In dogs, an oral dose of 1000 mg/Kg did not cause mortality and abnormal clinical signs were not observed. In humans the most likely clinical manifestation would be symptoms attributable to severe hypotension.

Laboratory determinations of serum levels of trandolapril and its metabolites are not widely available, and such determinations have, in any event, no established role in the management of trandolapril overdose. No data are available to suggest that physiological maneuvers (e.g., maneuvers to change the pH of the urine) might accelerate elimination of trandolapril and its metabolites. Trandolaprilat is removed by hemodialysis. Angiotension II could presumably serve as a specific antagonist antidote in the settling of trandolapril overdose, but angiotension II is essentially unavailable outside of scattered research facilities. Because the hypotensive effect of trandolapril is achieved through vasodilation and effective hypovolemia, it is reasonable to treat trandolapril overdose by infusion of normal saline solution.

DOSAGE AND ADMINISTRATION

The recommended initial dosage of MAVIK® for patients not receiving a diuretic is 1 mg once daily in non-black patients and 2 mg in black patients. Dosage should be adjusted according to the blood pressure response. Generally, dosage adjustments should be made at intervals of at least 1 week. Most patients have required dosages of 2 to 4 mg once daily. There is little clinical experience with doses above 8 mg.

Patients inadequately treated with once-daily dosing at 4 mg may be treated with twice-daily dosing. If blood pressure is not adequately controlled with MAVIK® monotherapy, a diuretic may be added.

In patients who are currently being treated with a diuretic, symptomatic hypotension occasionally can occur following the initial dose of MAVIK®. To reduce the likelihood of hypotension, the diuretic should, if possible, be discontinued two to three days prior to beginning therapy with MAVIK®. (See **WARNINGS.**) Then, if blood pressure is not controlled with MAVIK® alone, diuretic therapy should be resumed. If the diuretic cannot be discontinued, an initial dose of 0.5 mg MAVIK® should be used with careful medical supervision for several hours until blood pressure has stabilized. The dosage should subsequently be titrated (as described above) to the optimal response. (See **WARNINGS, PRECAUTIONS,** and **Drug Interactions.**)

Concomitant administration of MAVIK® with potassium supplements, potassium salt substitutes, or potassium-sparing diuretics can lead to increases of serum potassium. (See **PRECAUTIONS.**)

Dosage Adjustment in Renal Impairment or Hepatic Cirrhosis:

For patients with a creatinine clearance <30 mL/min. or with hepatic cirrhosis, the recommended starting dose, based on clinical and pharmacokinetic data, is 0.5 mg daily. Patients should subsequently have their dosage titrated (as described above) to the optimal response.

HOW SUPPLIED

MAVIK® tablets are supplied as follows:
1 mg tablet— salmon colored, round shaped, scored, compressed tablets, with code KNOLL 1 on one side.
   NDC (0048-5805-01-bottles of 100)
   NDC (0048-5805-41-unit dose packs of 100)

2 mg tablet— yellow colored, round shaped, compressed tablets with code KNOLL 2 on one side.
   NDC (0048-5806-01-bottles of 100)
   NDC (0048-5806-41-unit dose packs of 100)
4 mg tablet— rose colored, round shaped, compressed tablets, with code KNOLL 4 on one side.
   NDC (0048-5807-01-bottles of 100)
   NDC (0048-5807-41-unit dose packs of 100)
   Dispense in well-closed container with safety closure.
Storage: Store at controlled room temperature 20–25°C (68–77°F) see USP.
Caution: Federal law prohibits dispensing without prescription.
Revised: June 1997

Knoll Pharmaceutical Company
3000 Continental Drive-North
Mount Olive, New Jersey 07828-1234
BASF Pharma

0983000-3

Shown in Product Identification Guide, page 319

MERIDIA®   Ⓒⓥ ℞
[*mĕr-ĭdĭa*]
(sibutramine hydrochloride monohydrate) Capsules

DESCRIPTION

MERIDIA® (sibutramine hydrochloride monohydrate) is an orally administered agent for the treatment of obesity. Chemically, the active ingredient is a racemic mixture of the (+) and (−) enantiomers of cyclobutanemethanamine, 1-(4-chlorophenyl)-*N*, *N*-dimethyl-α-(2-methylpropyl)-, hydrochloride, monohydrate, and has an empirical formula of $C_{17}H_{29}Cl_2NO$. Its molecular weight is 334.33.
The structural formula is shown below:

Sibutramine hydrochloride monohydrate is a white to cream crystalline powder with a solubility of 2.9 mg/mL in pH 5.2 water. Its octanol:water partition coefficient is 30.9 at pH 5.0.
Each MERIDIA capsule contains 5 mg, 10 mg, 15 mg of sibutramine hydrochloride monohydrate. It also contains as inactive ingredients: lactose monohydrate, NF; microcrystalline cellulose, NF; colloidal silicon dioxide, NF; and magnesium stearate, NF in a hard-gelatin capsule [which contains titanium dioxide, USP; gelatin; FD&C Blue No. 2 (5- and 10-mg capsules only); D&C Yellow No. 10 (5- and 15-mg capsules only), and other inactive ingredients].

CLINICAL PHARMACOLOGY
Mode of Action
Sibutramine produces its therapeutic effects by norepinephrine, serotonin and dopamine reuptake inhibition. Sibutramine and its major pharmacologically active metabolites (M_1 and M_2) do not act via release of monoamines.
Pharmacodynamics
Sibutramine exerts its pharmacological actions predominantly via its secondary (M_1) and primary (M_2) amine metabolites. The parent compound, sibutramine, is a potent inhibitor of serotonin (5-hydroxytryptamine, 5-HT) and norepinephrine reuptake *in vivo*, but not *in vitro*. However, metabolites M_1 and M_2 inhibit the reuptake of these neurotransmitters both *in vitro* and *in vivo*.

In human brain tissue, M_1 and M_2 also inhibit dopamine reuptake *in vitro*, but with ~3-fold lower potency than for the reuptake inhibition of serotonin or norepinephrine.

Potencies of Sibutramine, M_1 and M_2 as *In Vitro* Inhibitors of Monoamine Reuptake in Human Brain

Potency to Inhibit Monoamine Reuptake (K_i; nM)

	Serotonin	Norepinephrine	Dopamine
Sibutramine	298	5451	943
M_1	15	20	49
M_2	20	15	45

A study using plasma samples taken from sibutramine-treated volunteers showed monoamine reuptake inhibition of norepinephrine > serotonin > dopamine; maximum inhibitions were norepinephrine = 73%, serotonin = 54% and dopamine = 16%.

Sibutramine and its metabolites (M_1 and M_2) are not serotonin, norepinephrine or dopamine releasing agents. Following chronic administration of sibutramine to rats, no depletion of brain monoamines has been observed.

Sibutramine, M_1 and M_2 exhibit no evidence of anticholinergic or antihistaminergic actions. In addition, receptor binding profiles show that sibutramine, M_1 and M_2 have low affinity for serotonin (5-HT$_1$, 5-HT$_{1A}$, 5-HT$_{1B}$, 5-HT$_{2A}$, 5-HT$_{2C}$), norepinephrine (β, β$_1$, β$_3$, α$_1$ and α$_2$), dopamine (D$_1$ and D$_2$), benzodiazepine, and glutamate (NMDA) receptors. These compounds also lack monoamine oxidase inhibitory activity *in vitro* and *in vivo*.
Pharmacokinetics
Absorption
Sibutramine is rapidly absorbed from the GI tract (T_{max} of 1.2 hours) following oral administration and undergoes extensive first-pass metabolism in the liver (oral clearance of 1750 L/h and half-life of 1.1 h) to form the pharmacologically active mono- and di- desmethyl metabolites M_1 and M_2. Peak plasma concentrations of M_1 and M_2 are reached within 3 to 4 hours. On the basis of mass balance studies, on average, at least 77% of a single oral dose of sibutramine is absorbed. The absolute bioavailability of sibutramine has not been determined.
Distribution
Radiolabeled studies in animals indicated rapid and extensive distribution into tissues: highest concentrations of radiolabeled material were found in the eliminating organs, liver and kidney. Tissue distribution was unaffected by pregnancy, with relatively low transfer to the fetus. *In vitro*, sibutramine, M_1 and M_2 are extensively bound (97%, 94% and 94%, respectively) to human plasma proteins at plasma concentrations seen following therapeutic doses.
Metabolism
Sibutramine is metabolized in the liver principally by the cytochrome P450(3A$_4$) isoenzyme, to desmethyl metabolites, M_1 and M_2. These active metabolites are further metabolized by hydroxylation and conjugation to pharmacologically inactive metabolites, M_5 and M_6. Following oral administration of radiolabeled sibutramine, essentially all of the peak radiolabeled material in plasma was accounted for by unchanged sibutramine (3%), M_1 (6%), M_2 (12%), M_5 (52%), and M_6 (27%).
M_1 and M_2 plasma concentrations reached steady-state within four days of dosing and were approximately two-fold higher than following a single dose. The elimination half-lives of M_1 and M_2, 14 and 16 hours, respectively, were unchanged following repeated dosing.
Excretion
Approximately 85% (range 68-95%) of a single orally administered radiolabeled dose was excreted in urine and feces

Summary of Pharmacokinetic Parameters

Mean (% CV) and 95% Confidence Intervals of Pharmacokinetic Parameters
(Dose = 15 mg)

Study Population	C_{max} (ng/mL)	T_{max} (h)	AUC† (ng*h/mL)	T½ (h)
Metabolite M_1				
Target Population:				
Obese Subjects	4.0 (42)	3.6 (28)	25.5 (63)	- -
(n=18)	3.2 – 4.8	3.1 – 4.1	18.1 – 32.9	
Special Population:				
Moderate Hepatic	2.2 (36)	3.3 (33)	18.7 (65)	
Impairment (n=12)	1.8 – 2.7	2.7 – 3.9	11.9 – 25.5	
Metabolite M_2				
Target Population:				
Obese Subjects	6.4 (28)	3.5 (17)	92.1 (26)	17.2 (58)
(n=18)	5.6 – 7.2	3.2 – 3.8	81.2 – 103	12.5 – 21.8
Special Population:				
Moderate Hepatic	4.3 (37)	3.8 (34)	90.5 (27)	22.7 (30)
Impairment (n=12)	3.4 – 5.2	3.1 – 4.5	76.9 – 104	18.9 – 26.5

† Calculated only up to 24 hr for M_1

over a 15-day collection period with the majority of the dose (77%) excreted in the urine. Major metabolites in urine were M_5 and M_6; unchanged sibutramine, M_1, and M_2 were not detected. The primary route of excretion for M_1 and M_2 is hepatic metabolism and for M_5 and M_6 is renal excretion.
[See table at bottom of previous page]

Effect of Food

Administration of a single 20 mg dose of sibutramine with a standard breakfast resulted in reduced peak M_1 and M_2 concentrations (by 27% and 32%, respectively) and delayed the time to peak by approximately three hours. However, the AUCs of M_1 and M_2 were not significantly altered.

Special Populations

Geriatric: Plasma concentrations of M_1 and M_2 were similar between elderly (ages 61 to 77 yr) and young (ages 19 to 30 yr) subjects following a single 15-mg oral sibutramine dose. Plasma concentrations of the inactive metabolites M_5 and M_6 were higher in the elderly; these differences are not likely to be of clinical significance. In general, dose selection for an elderly patient should be cautious, reflecting the greater frequency of decreased hepatic, renal, or cardiac function, and of concomitant disease or other drug therapy.

Pediatric: The safety and effectiveness of MERIDIA in pediatric patients under 16 years old have not been established.

Gender: Pooled pharmacokinetic parameters from 54 young, healthy volunteers (37 males and 17 females) receiving a 15-mg oral dose of sibutramine showed the mean C_{max} and AUC of M_1 and M_2 to be slightly (≤19% and ≤36%, respectively) higher in females than males. Somewhat higher steady-state trough plasma levels were observed in female obese patients from a large clinical efficacy trial. However, these differences are not likely to be of clinical significance. Dosage adjustment based upon the gender of a patient is not necessary (see "**DOSAGE AND ADMINISTRATION**").

Race: The relationship between race and steady-state trough M_1 and M_2 plasma concentrations was examined in a clinical trial in obese patients. A trend towards higher concentrations in Black patients over Caucasian was noted for M_1 and M_2. However, these differences are not considered to be of clinical significance.

Renal Insufficiency: The effect of renal disease has not been studied. However, since sibutramine and its active metabolites M_1 and M_2 are eliminated by hepatic metabolism, renal disease is unlikely to have a significant effect on their disposition. Elimination of the inactive metabolites M_5 and M_6, which are renally excreted, may be affected in this population. MERIDIA, should not be used in patients with severe renal impairment.

Hepatic Insufficiency: In 12 patients with moderate hepatic impairment receiving a single 15-mg oral dose of sibutramine, the combined AUCs of M_1 and M_2 were increased by 24% compared to healthy subjects while M_5 and M_6 plasma concentrations were unchanged. The observed differences in M_1 and M_2 concentrations do not warrant dosage adjustment in patients with mild to moderate hepatic impairment. MERIDIA should not be used in patients with severe hepatic dysfunction.

CLINICAL STUDIES

Observational epidemiologic studies have established a relationship between obesity and the risks for cardiovascular disease, non-insulin dependent diabetes mellitus (NIDDM), certain forms of cancer, gallstones, certain respiratory disorders, and an increase in overall mortality. These studies suggest that weight loss, if maintained, may produce health benefits for some patients with chronic obesity who may also be at risk for other diseases.

The long-term effects of MERIDIA on the morbidity and mortality associated with obesity have not been established. Weight loss was examined in 11 double-blind, placebo-controlled obesity trials with study durations of 12 to 52 weeks and doses ranging from 1 to 30 mg once daily. Weight was significantly reduced in a dose-related manner in sibutramine-treated patients compared to placebo over the dose range of 5 to 20 mg once daily. In two 12-month studies, maximal weight loss was achieved by 6 months and statistically significant weight loss was maintained over 12 months. The amount of placebo-subtracted weight loss achieved on MERIDIA was consistent across studies.

Analysis of the data in three long-term (≥6 months) obesity trials indicates that patients who lose at least 4 pounds in the first 4 weeks of therapy with a given dose of MERIDIA are most likely to achieve significant long-term weight loss on that dose of MERIDIA. Approximately 60% of such patients went on to achieve a placebo-subtracted weight loss of ≥5% of their initial body weight by month 6. Conversely, of those patients on a given dose of MERIDIA who did not lose at least 4 pounds in the first 4 weeks of therapy, approximately 80% did not go on to achieve a placebo-subtracted weight loss of ≥5% of their initial body weight on that dose by month 6.

Significant dose-related reductions in waist circumference, an indicator of intra-abdominal fat, have also been observed over 6 and 12 months in placebo-controlled clinical trials. In a 12-week placebo-controlled study of non-insulin dependent diabetes mellitus patients randomized to placebo or 15 mg per day of MERIDIA, Dual Energy X-Ray Absorptiometry (DEXA) assessment of changes in body composition showed that total body fat mass decreased by 1.8 kg in the MERIDIA group versus 0.2 kg in the placebo group (p<0.001). Similarly, truncal (android) fat mass decreased by 0.6 kg in the MERIDIA group versus 0.1 kg in the placebo group (p<0.01). The changes in lean mass, fasting blood sugar, and HbA_1 were not statistically different between the two groups.

Mean Weight Loss (lbs) in the Six-Month and One-Year Trials

Study/Patient Group	Placebo (n)	MERIDIA (mg) 5 (n)	10 (n)	15 (n)	20 (n)
Study 1					
All patients*	2.0	6.6	9.7	12.1	13.6
	(142)	(148)	(148)	(150)	(145)
Completers**	2.9	8.1	12.1	15.4	18.0
	(84)	(103)	(95)	(94)	(89)
Early responders***	8.5	13.0	16.0	18.2	20.1
	(17)	(60)	(64)	(73)	(76)
Study 2					
All patients*	3.5		9.8	14.0	
	(157)		(154)	(152)	
Completers**	4.8		13.6	15.2	
	(76)		(80)	(93)	
Early responders***	10.7		18.2	18.8	
	(24)		(57)	(76)	
Study 3****					
All patients*	15.2		28.4		
	(78)		(81)		
Completers**	16.7		29.7		
	(48)		(60)		
Early responders***	21.5		33.0		
	(22)		(46)		

* Data for all patients who received study drug and who had any post-baseline measurement (last observation carried forward analysis).

** Data for all patients who completed the entire 6-month (Study 1) or one-year period of dosing and have data recorded for the month 6 (Study 1) or month 12 visit.

*** Data for patients who lost at least 4 lbs in the first 4 weeks of treatment and completed the study.

**** Weight loss data shown describe changes in weight from the pre-VLCD; mean weight loss during the 4-week VLCD was 16.9 lbs for sibutramine and 16.3 lbs for placebo.

Eleven double-blind, placebo-controlled obesity trials with study durations of 12 to 52 weeks have provided evidence that MERIDIA does not adversely affect glycemia, serum lipid profiles, or serum uric acid in obese patients. Treatment with MERIDIA (5 to 20 mg once daily) is associated with mean increases in blood pressure of 1 to 3 mm Hg and with mean increases in pulse rate of 4 to 5 beats per minute relative to placebo. These findings are similar in normotensives and in patients with hypertension controlled with medication. Those patients who lose significant (≥ 5% weight loss) amounts of weight on MERIDIA tend to have smaller increases in blood pressure and pulse rate (see "**WARNINGS**").

In Study 1, a 6-month, double-blind, placebo-controlled study in obese patients, Study 2, a 1-year, double-blind, placebo-controlled study in obese patients, and Study 3, a 1-year, double-blind, placebo-controlled study in obese patients who lost at least 6 kg on a 4-week very low calorie diet (VLCD), MERIDIA produced significant reductions in weight, as shown above. In two 1-year studies, maximal weight loss was achieved by 6 months and statistically significant weight loss was maintained over 12 months.
[See table above]

MERIDIA induced weight loss has been accompanied by beneficial changes in serum lipids that are similar to those seen with nonpharmacologically-mediated weight loss. A combined, weighted analysis of the changes in serum lipids in 11 placebo-controlled obesity studies ranging in length from 12 to 52 weeks is shown at the bottom of the next page for the last observation carried forward (LOCF) analysis.
[See table at top of next page]

MERIDIA induced weight loss has been accompanied by reductions in serum uric acid. In one study, serum uric acid has been identified as an independent risk factor for death from coronary artery disease.

Certain centrally-acting weight loss agents that cause release of serotonin from nerve terminals have been associated with cardiac valve dysfunction. The possible occurrence of cardiac valve disease was specifically investigated in two studies. In one study 2-D and color Doppler echocardiography were performed on 210 patients (mean age, 54 years) receiving MERIDIA 15 mg or placebo daily for periods of 2 weeks to 16 months (mean duration of treatment, 7.6 months). In patients without a prior history of valvular heart disease, the incidence of valvular heart disease was 3/132 (2.3%) in the sibutramine treatment group (all three cases were mild aortic insufficiency) and 2/77 (2.6%) in the placebo treatment group (one case of mild aortic insufficiency and one case of severe aortic insufficiency). In another study, 25 patients underwent 2-D and color Doppler echocardiography before treatment with MERIDIA and again after treatment with MERIDIA 5 to 30 mg daily for three months; there were no cases of valvular heart disease.

INDICATIONS AND USAGE

MERIDIA is indicated for the management of obesity, including weight loss and maintenance of weight loss, and should be used in conjunction with a reduced calorie diet. MERIDIA is recommended for obese patients with an initial body mass index ≥ 30 kg/m², or ≥ 27 kg/m² in the presence of other risk factors (e.g., hypertension, diabetes, dyslipidemia).

Below is a chart of Body Mass Index (BMI) based on various heights and weights.

BMI is calculated by taking the patient's weight, in kg, and dividing by the patient's height, in meters, squared. Metric conversions are as follows: pounds ÷ 2.2 = kg; inches × 0.0254 = meters.

	BMI	25	26	27	28	29	30	31	32	33	34	35	40
		WEIGHT (lbs)											
	4'10"	119	124	129	134	138	143	149	153	158	163	167	191
	4'11"	124	128	133	138	143	148	154	158	164	169	173	198
	5'	128	133	138	143	148	153	159	164	169	175	179	204
	5'1"	132	137	143	148	153	158	165	169	175	180	185	211
	5'2"	136	142	147	153	158	164	170	175	181	186	191	218
H	5'3"	141	146	152	158	163	169	175	181	187	192	197	225
	5'4"	145	151	157	163	169	174	181	187	193	199	204	232
E	5'5"	150	156	162	168	174	180	187	193	199	205	210	240
	5'6"	155	161	167	173	179	186	192	199	205	211	216	247
I	5'7"	159	166	172	178	185	191	198	205	211	218	223	255
	5'8"	164	171	177	184	190	197	204	211	218	224	230	262
G	5'9"	169	176	182	189	196	203	210	217	224	231	236	270
	5'10"	174	181	188	195	202	207	216	223	230	237	243	278
H	5'11"	179	186	193	200	208	215	222	230	237	244	250	286
	6'	184	191	199	206	213	221	228	236	244	251	258	294
T	6'1"	189	197	204	212	219	227	236	243	251	258	265	302
	6'2"	194	202	210	218	225	233	241	250	258	265	272	311
	6'3"	200	208	216	224	232	240	248	256	264	272	279	319

CONTRAINDICATIONS

MERIDIA is contraindicated in patients receiving monoamine oxidase inhibitors (MAOIs) (see "**WARNINGS**").

MERIDIA is contraindicated in patients with hypersensitivity to sibutramine or any of the inactive ingredients of MERIDIA.

MERIDIA is contraindicated in patients who have anorexia nervosa.

MERIDIA is contraindicated in patients taking other centrally acting appetite suppressant drugs.

WARNINGS

Blood Pressure and Pulse

MERIDIA SUBSTANTIALLY INCREASES BLOOD PRESSURE IN SOME PATIENTS. REGULAR MONITORING OF BLOOD PRESSURE IS REQUIRED WHEN PRESCRIBING MERIDIA.

In placebo-controlled obesity studies, MERIDIA 5 to 20 mg once daily was associated with mean increases in systolic

Continued on next page

Meridia—Cont.

and diastolic blood pressure of approximately 1 to 3 mm Hg relative to placebo, and with mean increases in pulse rate relative to placebo of approximately 4 to 5 beats per minute. Larger increases were seen in some patients, particularly when therapy with MERIDIA was initiated at the higher doses (see table below). In pre-marketing placebo-controlled obesity studies, 0.4% of patients treated with MERIDIA were discontinued for hypertension (SBP ≥ 160 mm Hg or DBP ≥ 95 mm Hg), compared with 0.4% in the placebo group, and 0.4% of patients with MERIDIA were discontinued for tachycardia (pulse rate ≥ 100 bpm), compared with 0.1% in the placebo group. Blood pressure and pulse should be measured prior to starting therapy with MERIDIA and should be monitored at regular intervals thereafter. For patients who experience a sustained increase in blood pressure or pulse rate while receiving MERIDIA, either dose reduction or discontinuation should be considered. MERIDIA should be given with caution to those patients with a history of hypertension (see "**DOSAGE AND ADMINISTRATION**"), and should not be given to patients with uncontrolled or poorly controlled hypertension.

Percent Outliers in Studies 1 and 2

	%Outliers*		
Dose (mg)	SBP	DBP	Pulse
Placebo	9	7	12
5	6	20	16
10	12	15	28
15	13	17	24
20	14	22	37

*Outlier defined as increase from baseline of ≥ 15 mm Hg for three consecutive visits (SBP), ≥ 10 mm Hg for three consecutive visits (DBP), or pulse ≥ 10 bpm for three consecutive visits.

Potential Interaction With Monoamine Oxidase Inhibitors
MERIDIA is a norepinephrine, serotonin and dopamine reuptake inhibitor and should not be used concomitantly with MAOIs (see "**PRECAUTIONS**", Drug Interactions subsection). There should be at least a 2-week interval after stopping MAOIs before commencing treatment with MERIDIA. Similarly, there should be at least a 2-week interval after stopping MERIDIA before starting treatment with MAOIs.

Concomitant Cardiovascular Disease
Treatment with MERIDIA has been associated with increases in heart rate and/or blood pressure. Therefore, MERIDIA should not be used in patients with a history of coronary artery disease, congestive heart failure, arrhythmias, or stroke.

Glaucoma
Because MERIDIA can cause mydriasis, it should be used with caution in patients with narrow angle glaucoma.

Miscellaneous
Organic causes of obesity (e.g., untreated hypothyroidism) should be excluded before prescribing MERIDIA.

PRECAUTIONS

Pulmonary Hypertension
Certain centrally-acting weight loss agents that cause release of serotonin from nerve terminals have been associated with pulmonary hypertension (PPH), a rare but lethal disease. In pre-marketing clinical studies, no cases of PPH have been reported with MERIDIA. Because of the low incidence of this disease in the underlying population, however, it is not known whether or not MERIDIA may cause this disease.

Seizures
During premarketing testing, seizures were reported in < 0.1% of MERIDIA treated patients. MERIDIA should be used cautiously in patients with a history of seizures. It should be discontinued in any patient who develops seizures.

Gallstones
Weight loss can precipitate or exacerbate gallstone formation.

Renal/Hepatic Dysfunction
Patients with severe renal impairment or severe hepatic dysfunction have not been systematically studied; MERIDIA should therefore not be used in such patients.

Interference With Cognitive and Motor Performance
Although sibutramine did not affect psychomotor or cognitive performance in healthy volunteers, any CNS active drug has the potential to impair judgment, thinking or motor skills.

Information For Patients
Physicians should instruct their patients to read the patient package insert before starting therapy with MERIDIA and to reread it each time the prescription is renewed.

Combined Analysis (11 Studies) of Percentage Change in Serum Lipids (N) - LOCF

Category	TG	CHOL	LDL-C	HDL-C
All Placebo	0.53 (475)	-1.53 (475)	-0.09 (233)	-0.56 (248)
<5% Weight Loss	4.52 (382)	-0.42 (382)	-070 (205)	-0.71 (217)
≥5% Weight Loss	-15.30 (92)	-6.23 (92)	-6.19 (27)	0.94 (30)
All Sibutramine	-8.75 (1164)	-2.21 (1165)	-1.85 (642)	4.13 (664)
<5% Weight Loss	-0.54 (547)	0.17 (548)	-0.37 (320)	3.19 (331)
≥5% Weight Loss	-16.59 (612)	-4.87 (612)	-4.56 (317)	4.68 (328)

Baseline mean values:
Placebo: TG 187 mg/dL; CHOL 221 mg/dL; LDL-C 140 mg/dL; HDL-C 47 mg/dL
Sibutramine: TG 172 mg/dL; CHOL 215 mg/dL; LDL-C 140 mg/dL; HDL-C 47 mg/dL

Physicians should also discuss with their patients any part of the package insert that is relevant to them. In particular, the importance of keeping appointments for follow-up visits should be emphasized.
Patients should be advised to notify their physician if they develop a rash, hives, or other allergic reactions.
Patients should be advised to inform their physicians if they are taking, or plan to take, any prescription or over-the-counter drugs, especially weight-reducing agents, decongestants, antidepressants, cough suppressants, lithium, dihydroergotamine, sumatriptan (Imitrex®), or tryptophan, since there is a potential for interactions.
Patients should be reminded of the importance of having their blood pressure and pulse monitored at regular intervals.

Drug Interactions
CNS Active Drugs: The use of MERIDIA in combination with other CNS-active drugs, particularly serotonergic agents, has not been systematically evaluated. Consequently, caution is advised if the concomitant administration of MERIDIA with other centrally-acting drugs is indicated (see "**CONTRAINDICATIONS**" and "**WARNINGS**").
In patients receiving monoamine oxidase inhibitors (MAOIs) (e.g. phenelzine, selegiline) in combination with serotonergic agents (e.g. fluoxetine, fluvoxamine, paroxetine, sertraline, venlafaxine), there have been reports of serious, sometimes fatal, reactions ("serotonin syndrome;" see below). Because MERIDIA inhibits serotonin reuptake, MERIDIA should not be used concomitantly with MAOI (see "**CONTRAINDICATIONS**"). At least 2 weeks should elapse between discontinuation of a MAOI and initiation of treatment with MERIDIA. Similarly, at least 2 weeks should elapse between discontinuation of MERIDIA and initiation of treatment with MAOI.
The rare, but serious, constellation of symptoms termed "serotonin syndrome" has also been reported with the concomitant use of selective serotonin reuptake inhibitors and agents for migraine therapy, such as Imitrex® (sumatriptan succinate) and dihydroergotamine, certain opioids, such as dextramethorphan, meperidine, pentazocine and fentanyl, lithium, or tryptophan. Serotonin syndrome has also been reported with the concomitant use of two serotonin reuptake inhibitors. The syndrome requires immediate medical attention and may include one or more of the following symptoms: excitement, hypomania, restlessness, loss of consciousness, confusion, disorientation, anxiety, agitation, motor weakness, myoclonus, tremor, hemiballismus, hyperreflexia, ataxia, dysarthria, incoordination, hyperthermia, shivering, pupillary dilation, diaphoresis, emesis, and tachycardia.
Because MERIDIA inhibits serotonin reuptake, it should not be administered with other serotonergic agents such as those listed above.

Drugs That May Raise Blood Pressure and/or Heart Rate: Concomitant use of MERIDIA and other agents that may raise blood pressure or heart rate have not been evaluated. These include certain decongestants, cough, cold, and allergy medications that contain agents such as phenylpropanolamine, ephedrine, or pseudoephedrine. Caution should be used when prescribing MERIDIA to patients who use these medications.

Drugs That Inhibit Cytochrome P450(3A$_4$) Metabolism: *In vitro* studies indicated that the cytochrome P450(3A$_4$)-mediated metabolism of sibutramine was inhibited by ketoconazole and to a lesser extent by erythromycin. Clinical interaction trials were conducted on these substrates. The data indicate that there is a potential for such interactions, but the magnitude appears to be small.
Ketoconazole: Concomitant administration of 200 mg doses of ketoconazole twice daily and 20 mg sibutramine once daily for 7 days in 12 uncomplicated obese subjects resulted in moderate increases in AUC and $C_{max}$of 58% and 36% for M_1 and of 20% and 19% for M_2, respectively.
Erythromycin: The steady-state pharmacokinetics of sibutramine and metabolites M_1 and M_2 were evaluated in 12 uncomplicated obese subjects following concomitant administration of 500 mg of erythromycin three times daily and 20 mg of sibutramine once daily for 7 days. Concomitant erythromycin resulted in small increases in the AUC (less than 14%) for M_1 and M_2. A small reduction in C_{max} for M_1 (11%) and a slight increase in C_{max} for M_2 (10%) were observed.
Cimetidine: Concomitant administration of cimetidine 400 mg twice daily and sibutramine 15 mg once daily for 7 days in 12 volunteers resulted in small increases in combined (M_1 and M_2) plasma C_{max} (3.4%) and AUC (7.3%); these differences are unlikely to be of clinical significance.
Alcohol: In a double-blind, placebo controlled, crossover study in 19 volunteers, administration of a single dose of ethanol (0.5 mL/kg) together with 20 mg of sibutramine resulted in no psychomotor interactions of clinical significance between alcohol and sibutramine. However, the concomitant use of MERIDIA and excess alcohol is not recommended.
Oral Contraceptives: The suppression of ovulation by oral contraceptives was not inhibited by MERIDIA. In a crossover study, 12 healthy female volunteers on oral steroid contraceptives received placebo in one period and 15 mg sibutramine in another period over the course of 8 weeks. No clinically significant systemic interaction was observed; therefore, no requirement for alternative contraceptive precautions are needed when patients taking oral contraceptives are concurrently prescribed sibutramine.
Drugs Highly Bound to Plasma Proteins: Although sibutramine and its active metabolites M_1 and M_2 are extensively bound to plasma proteins (≥94%), the low therapeutic concentrations and basic characteristics of these compounds make them unlikely to result in clinically significant protein binding interactions with other highly protein bound drugs such as warfarin and phenytoin. *In vitro* protein binding interaction studies have not been conducted.

Carcinogenesis, Mutagenesis, Impairment of Fertility
Carcinogenicity
Sibutramine was administered in the diet to mice (1.25, 5 or 20 mg/kg/day) and rats (1, 3, or 9 mg/kg/day) for two years generating combined maximum plasma AUC's of the two major active metabolites equivalent to 0.5 and 21 times, respectively, those following the maximum daily human dose (20 mg). There was no evidence of carcinogenicity in mice or in female rats. In male rats there was a higher incidence of benign tumors of the testicular interstitial cells; such tumors are commonly seen in rats and are hormonally mediated. The relevance of these tumors to humans is not known.
Mutagenicity
Sibutramine was not mutagenic in the Ames test, *in vitro* Chinese hamster V79 cell mutation assay, *in vitro* clastogenicity assay in human lymphocytes or micronucleus assay in mice. Its two major active metabolites were found to have equivocal bacterial mutagenic activity in the Ames test. However, both metabolites gave consistently negative results in the *in vitro* Chinese hamster V79 cell mutation assay, *in vitro* clastogenicity assay in human lymphocytes, *in vitro* DNA-repair assay in HeLa cells, micronucleus assay in mice and *in vivo* unscheduled DNA-synthesis assay in rat hepatocytes.
Impairment of Fertility
In rats, there were no effects on fertility at doses generating combined plasma AUC's of the two major active metabolites up to 43 times those following the maximum human dose (20 mg). At 13 times the human combined AUC, there was maternal toxicity, and the dam's nest-building behavior was impaired, leading to a higher incidence of perinatal mortality; there was no effect at approximately 4 times the human combined AUC.

Pregnancy
Teratogenic Effects-Pregnancy Category C
In rats, there was no evidence of teratogenicity at doses of 1, 3, or 10 mg/kg/day generating combined plasma AUC's of the two major active metabolites up to approximately 43 times those following the maximum human dose (20 mg). In rabbits dosed at 3, 15, or 75 mg/kg/day, plasma AUC's greater than approximately 5 times those following the maximum human dose caused maternal toxicity. At markedly toxic doses, Dutch Belted rabbits had a slightly higher than control incidence of pups with a broad short snout, short rounded pinnae, short tail and, in some, shorter thickened long bones in the limbs; at comparably high doses in

New Zealand White rabbits, one study showed a slightly higher than control incidence of pups with cardiovascular anomalies while a second study showed a lower incidence than in the control group.

No adequate and well controlled studies with MERIDIA have been conducted in pregnant women. The use of MERIDIA during pregnancy is not recommended. Women of child-bearing potential should employ adequate contraception while taking MERIDIA. Patients should be advised to notify their physician if they become pregnant or intend to become pregnant during therapy.

Nursing Mothers

It is not known whether sibutramine or its metabolites are excreted in human milk. MERIDIA is not recommended for use in nursing mothers. Patients should be advised to notify their physician if they are breast-feeding.

Pediatric Use

The safety and effectiveness of MERIDIA in pediatric patients under 16 years of age have not been established.

Geriatric Use

Clinical studies of MERIDIA did not include sufficient numbers of patients aged 65 and over to determine whether they respond differently from younger patients. In general, dose selection for an elderly patient should be cautious, reflecting the greater frequency of decreased hepatic, renal, or cardiac function, and of concomitant disease or other drug therapy. Pharmacokinetics in elderly patients are discussed in "**CLINICAL PHARMACOLOGY.**"

ADVERSE REACTIONS

In placebo-controlled studies, 9% of patients treated with MERIDIA (n=2068) and 7% of patients treated with placebo (n=884) withdrew for adverse events.

In placebo-controlled obesity studies, the most common events were dry mouth, anorexia, insomnia, and constipation. Adverse events in these studies occurring in ≥ 1% of MERIDIA treated patients and more frequently than in the placebo group are shown in the following table.

[See table above]

The following additional adverse events were reported in ≥ 1% of all patients who received MERIDIA in controlled and uncontrolled pre-marketing studies.

Body as a Whole: fever.

Digestive System: diarrhea, flatulence, gastroenteritis, tooth disorder.

Metabolic and Nutritional: peripheral edema.

Musculoskeletal System: arthritis.

Nervous System: agitation, leg cramps, hypertonia, thinking abnormal.

Respiratory System: bronchitis, dyspnea.

Skin and Appendages: pruritus.

Special Senses: amblyopia.

Urogenital System: menstrual disorder.

Other Notable Adverse Events

Seizures: Convulsions were reported as an adverse event in three of 2068 (0.1%) MERIDIA treated patients and in none of 884 placebo-treated patients in placebo-controlled premarketing obesity studies. Two of the three patients with seizures had potentially predisposing factors (one had a prior history of epilepsy; one had a subsequent diagnosis of brain tumor). The incidence in all subjects who received MERIDIA (three of 4,588 subjects) was less than 0.1%.

Ecchymosis/Bleeding Disorders: Ecchymosis (bruising) was observed in 0.7% of MERIDIA treated patients and in 0.2% of placebo-treated patients in pre-marketing placebo-controlled obesity studies. One patient had prolonged bleeding of a small amount which occurred during minor facial surgery. MERIDIA may have an effect on platelet function due to its effect on serotonin uptake.

Interstitial Nephritis: Acute interstitial nephritis (confirmed by biopsy) was reported in one obese patient receiving MERIDIA during pre-marketing studies. After discontinuation of the medication, dialysis and oral corticosteroids were administered; renal function normalized. The patient made a full recovery.

Altered Laboratory Findings: Abnormal liver function tests, including increases in AST, ALT, GGT, LDH, alkaline phosphate and bilirubin, were reported as adverse events in 1.6% of MERIDIA-treated obese patients in placebo-controlled trials compared with 0.8% of placebo patients. In these studies, potentially clinically significant values (total bilirubin ≥ 2mg/dL; ALT, AST, GGT, LDH, or alkaline phosphatase ≥ 3× upper limit of normal) occurred in 0% (alkaline phosphatase) to 0.6% (ALT) of the MERIDIA treated patients and in none of the placebo-treated patients. Abnormal values tended to be sporadic, often diminished with continued treatment, and did not show a clear dose-response relationship.

DRUG ABUSE AND DEPENDENCE

Controlled Substance

MERIDIA is a controlled substance in Schedule IV of the Controlled Substances Act (CSA).

Abuse and Physical and Psychological Dependence

Physicians should carefully evaluate patients for history of drug abuse and follow such patients closely, observing them

BODY SYSTEM	Obese Patients in Placebo-Controlled Studies	
	MERIDIA® (n = 2068)	Placebo (n = 884)
Adverse Event	% incidence	% incidence
BODY AS A WHOLE		
Headache	30.3	18.6
Back pain	8.2	5.5
Flu syndrome	8.2	5.8
Injury accident	5.9	4.1
Asthenia	5.9	5.3
Abdominal pain	4.5	3.6
Chest pain	1.8	1.2
Neck pain	1.6	1.1
Allergic reaction	1.5	0.8
CARDIOVASCULAR SYSTEM		
Tachycardia	2.6	0.6
Vasodilation	2.4	0.9
Migraine	2.4	2.0
Hypertension/increased blood pressure	2.1	0.9
Palpitation	2.0	0.8
DIGESTIVE SYSTEM		
Anorexia	13.0	3.5
Constipation	11.5	6.0
Increased appetite	8.7	2.7
Nausea	5.9	2.8
Dyspepsia	5.0	2.6
Gastritis	1.7	1.2
Vomiting	1.5	1.4
Rectal disorder	1.2	0.5
METABOLIC & NUTRITIONAL		
Thirst	1.7	0.9
Generalized edema	1.2	0.8
MUSCULOSKELETAL SYSTEM		
Arthralgia	5.9	5.0
Myalgia	1.9	1.1
Tenosynovitis	1.2	0.5
Joint disorder	1.1	0.6
NERVOUS SYSTEM		
Dry mouth	17.2	4.2
Insomnia	10.7	4.5
Dizziness	7.0	3.4
Nervousness	5.2	2.9
Anxiety	4.5	3.4
Depression	4.3	2.5
Paresthesia	2.0	0.5
Somnolence	1.7	0.9
CNS stimulation	1.5	0.5
Emotional lability	1.3	0.6
RESPIRATORY SYSTEM		
Rhinitis	10.2	7.1
Pharyngitis	10.0	8.4
Sinusitis	5.0	2.6
Cough increase	3.8	3.3
Laryngitis	1.3	0.9
SKIN & APPENDAGES		
Rash	3.8	2.5
Sweating	2.5	0.9
Herpes simplex	1.3	1.0
Acne	1.0	0.8
SPECIAL SENSES		
Taste perversion	2.2	0.8
Ear disorder	1.7	0.9
Ear pain	1.1	0.7
UROGENITAL SYSTEM		
Dysmenorrhea	3.5	1.4
Urinary tract infection	2.3	2.0
Vaginal monilia	1.2	0.5
Metrorrhagia	1.0	0.8

for signs of misuse or abuse (e.g., drug development of tolerance, incrementation of doses, drug seeking behavior).

OVERDOSAGE

Human Experience

There is very limited experience of overdose with MERIDIA. Three cases of overdose have been reported with MERIDIA. The first was in a 2-year-old child of one patient who ingested up to eight 10 mg capsules. No complications were observed during the overnight hospitalization, and the child was discharged the following day with no sequela. The second report was in a 30-year-old male in a depression study who ingested approximately 100 mg of sibutramine in an attempt to commit suicide. The patient suffered no adverse effects or ECG abnormalities post-ingestion. The third report was in the 45-year-old husband of a patient in an obese dyslipidemic study. He ingested 400 mg of his wife's drug supply and was hospitalized for observation; a heart rate of 120 bpm was noted. He was discharged the next day with no apparent sequela.

Overdose Management

There is no specific antidote to MERIDIA. Treatment should consist of general measures employed in the management of overdosage: an airway should be established; cardiac and vi-

tal sign monitoring is recommended; general symptomatic and supportive measures should be instituted. Cautious use of β-blockers may be indicated to control elevated blood pressure or tachycardia. The benefits of forced diuresis and hemodialysis are unknown.

DOSAGE AND ADMINISTRATION

The recommended starting dose of MERIDIA is 10 mg administered once daily with or without food. If there is inadequate weight loss, the dose may be titrated after four weeks to a total of 15 mg once daily. The 5 mg dose should be reserved for patients who do not tolerate the 10 mg dose. Blood pressure and heart rate changes should be taken into account when making decisions regarding dose titration (see "**PRECAUTIONS**").

Doses above 15 mg daily are not recommended. In most clinical trials, MERIDIA was given in the morning.

Analysis of numerous variables has indicated that approximately 60% of patients who lose at least 4 pounds in the first 4 weeks of treatment with a given dose of MERIDIA in combination with a reduced-calorie diet lose at least 5% (placebo-subtracted) of their initial body weight by the end

Continued on next page

Meridia—Cont.

of 6 months to 1 year of treatment on that dose of ME-RIDIA. Conversely, approximately, 80% of patients who do not lose at least 4 pounds in the first 4 weeks of treatment with a given dose of MERIDIA do not lose at least 5% (placebo-subtracted) of their initial body weight by the end of 6 months to 1 year of treatment on that dose. If a patient has not lost at least 4 pounds in the first 4 weeks of treatment, the physician should consider reevaluation of therapy which may include increasing the dose or discontinuation of MERIDIA.

The safety and effectiveness of MERIDIA, as demonstrated in double-blind, placebo-controlled trials, have not been determined beyond 1 year at this time.

HOW SUPPLIED

MERIDIA (sibutramine hydrochloride monohydrate) Capsules contain 5 mg, 10 mg, or 15 mg sibutramine hydrochloride monohydrate and are supplied as follows:

5 mg, NDC 0048-0605-01, blue/yellow capsules imprinted with "MERIDIA" on the cap and "-5-" on the body, in bottles of 100 capsules.

10 mg, NDC 0048-0610-01, blue/white capsules imprinted with "MERIDIA" on the cap and "-10-" on the body, in bottles of 100 capsules.

15 mg, NDC 0048-0615-01, yellow/white capsules imprinted with "MERIDIA" on the cap and "-15-" on the body, in bottles of 100 capsules.

Storage: Store at 25°C (77°F); excursions permitted to 15-30°C (59-86°F) [see USP controlled room temperature]. Protect from heat and moisture. Dispense in a tight, light-resistant container as defined in USP.

Caution: Federal law prohibits dispensing without prescription.

MERIDIA is a registered trademark of Knoll Pharmaceutical Company.

IMITREX® is a registered trademark of Glaxo Group Limited.

Sibutramine is covered by US Patent Nos. 4,746,680; 4,929,629; and 5,436,272.

©1998 Knoll Pharmaceutical Company
All rights reserved
Revised: January 1998
0995010-2
Knoll Pharmaceutical Company
3000 Continental Drive - North
Mount Olive, New Jersey 07828-1234
BASF Pharma

Shown in Product Identification Guide, page 319

SYNTHROID®　　　　　　　　　　　　　　　　℞
[sĭn 'throid]
(levothyroxine sodium, USP)
SYNTHROID Tablets—for oral administration
SYNTHROID Injection—for parenteral administration

DESCRIPTION

SYNTHROID (levothyroxine sodium, USP) Tablets and Injection contain synthetic crystalline L-3,3′,5,5′,-tetraiodothyronine sodium salt [levothyroxine (T_4) sodium]. Synthetic T_4 is identical to that produced in the human thyroid gland.

Levothyroxine (T_4) Sodium has an empirical formula of $C_{15}H_{10}L_4NNaO_4xH_2O$, molecular weight of 798.86 (anhydrous), and structural formula as shown:

$$HO-\text{\textcircled{}}-O-\text{\textcircled{}}-CH_2-\overset{NH_2}{\underset{H}{C}}-COONa\cdot XH_2O$$

LEVOTHYROXINE SODIUM

Inactive Ingredients (SYNTHROID Tablets): acacia, confectioner's sugar (contains corn starch), lactose, magnesium stearate, providone, talc. The following are the color additives by tablet strength:

Strength (mcg)	Color Additive(s)
25	FD&C Yellow No. 6
50	None
75	FD&C Red No. 40, FD&C Blue No. 2
88	FD&C Blue No. 1, FD&C Yellow No. 6, D&C Yellow No. 10
100	D&C Yellow No. 10, FD&C Yellow No. 6
112	D&C Red No. 27 & 30
125	FD&C Yellow No. 6, FD&C Red No. 40, FD&C Blue No. 1
150	FD&C Blue No. 2
175	FD&C Blue No. 1, D&C Red No. 27 & 30
200	FD&C Red No. 40
300	D&C Yellow No. 10, FD&C Yellow No. 6, FD&C Blue No. 1

Inactive Ingredients (SYNTHROID Injection): 10 mg mannitol USP, 0.7 mg tribasic sodium phosphate, anhydrous (200 mcg/vial), 1.75 mg tribasic sodium phosphate, anhydrous (500 mcg/vial), sodium hydroxide, Q.S. for pH adjustment. Levothyroxine sodium powder for reconstitution for injection is a sterile preparation.

CLINICAL PHARMACOLOGY

The synthesis and secretion of the major thyroid hormones, L-thyroxine (T_4) and L-triiodothyronine (T_3), from the normally functioning thyroid gland are regulated by complex feedback mechanisms of the hypothalamic-pituitary-thyroid axis. The thyroid gland is stimulated to secrete thyroid hormones by the action of thyrotropin (thyroid stimulating hormone, TSH), which is produced in the anterior pituitary gland. TSH secretion is in turn controlled by thyrotropin-releasing hormone (TRH) produced in the hypothalamus, circulating thyroid hormones, and possibly other mechanisms. Thyroid hormones circulating in the blood act as feedback inhibitors of both TSH and TRH secretion. Thus, when serum concentrations of T_3 and T_4 are increased, secretion of TSH and TRH decreases. Conversely, when serum thyroid hormone concentrations are decreased, secretion of TSH and TRH is increased. Administration of exogenous thyroid hormones to euthyroid individuals results in suppression of endogenous thyroid hormone secretion.

The mechanisms by which thyroid hormones exert their physiologic actions have not been completely elucidated. T_4 and T_3 are transported into cells by passive and active mechanisms. T_3 in cell cytoplasm and T_3 generated from T_4 within the cell diffuse into the nucleus and bind to thyroid receptor proteins, which appear to be primarily attached to DNA. Receptor binding leads to activation or repression of DNA transcription, thereby altering the amounts of mRNA and resultant proteins. Changes in protein concentrations are responsible for the metabolic changes observed in organs and tissues.

Thyroid hormones enhance oxygen consumption of most body tissues and increase the basal metabolic rate and metabolism of carbohydrates, lipids, and proteins. Thus, they exert a profound influence on every organ system and are of particular importance in the development of the central nervous system. Thyroid hormones also appear to have direct effects on tissues, such as increased myocardial contractility and decreased systemic resistance.

The physiologic effects of thyroid hormones are produced primarily by T_3, a large portion of which is derived from the deiodination of T_4 in peripheral tissues. About 70 to 90 percent of peripheral T_3 is produced by monodeiodination of T_4 at the 5 position (inner ring) results in the formation of reverse triiodothyronine (rT_3), which is calorigenically inactive.

PHARMACOKINETICS: Few clinical studies have evaluated the kinetics of orally administered thyroid hormone. In animals, the most active sites of absorption appear to be the proximal and mid-jejunum. T_4 is not absorbed from the stomach and little, if any, drug is absorbed from the duodenum. There seems to be no absorption of T_4 from the distal colon in animals. A number of human studies have confirmed the importance of an intact jejunum and ileum for T_4 absorption and have shown some absorption from the duodenum. Studies involving radioiodinated T_4 fecal excretion methods, equilibration, and AUC methods have shown that absorption varies from 48 to 80 percent of the administered dose. The extent of absorption is increased in the fasting state and decreased in malabsorption syndromes, such as sprue. Absorption may also decrease with age. The degree of T_4 absorption is dependent on the product formulation as well as on the character of the intestinal contents, including plasma protein and soluble dietary factors, which bind thyroid hormone making if unavailable for diffusion. Decreased absorption may result from administration of infant soybean formula, ferrous sulfate, sodium polystyrene sulfonate, aluminum hydroxide, sucralfate or bile acid sequestrants. T_4 absorption following intramuscular administration is variable.

Distribution of thyroid hormones in human body tissues and fluids has not been fully elucidated. More than 99 percent of circulating hormones is bound to serum proteins, including thyroxine-binding globulin (TBG), thyroxine-binding prealbumin (TBPA), and albumin (TBA). T_4 is more extensively and firmly bound to serum proteins than is T_3. Only unbound thyroid hormone is metabolically active. The higher affinity of TBG and TBPA for T_4 partly explains the higher serum levels, slower metabolic clearance, and longer serum elimination half-life of this hormone.

Certain drugs and physiologic conditions can alter the binding of thyroid hormones to serum proteins and/or the concentrations of the serum proteins available for thyroid hormone binding. These effects must be considered when interpreting the results of thyroid function tests. (See **Drug Interactions** and **Laboratory Test Interactions.**)

T_4 is eliminated slowly from the body, with a half-life of 6 to 7 day. T_3 has a half-life of 1 to 2 days. The liver is the major site of degradation for both hormones. T_4 and T_3 are conjugated with glucuronic and sulfuric acids and excreted in the bile. There is an enterohepatic circulation of thyroid hormones, as they are liberated by hydrolysis in the intestine and reabsorbed. A portion of the conjugated material reaches the colon unchanged, is hydrolyzed there, and is eliminated as free compounds in the feces. In man, approximately 20 to 40 percent of T_4 is eliminated in the stool. About 70 percent of the T_4 secreted daily is deiodinated to yield equal amounts of T_3 and rT_3. Subsequent deiodination of T_3 and rT_4 yields multiple forms of diiodothyronine. A number of the minor T_4 metabolites have also been identified. Although some of these metabolites have biologic activity, their overall contribution to the therapeutic effect of T_4 is minimal.

INDICATIONS AND USAGE

SYNTHROID is indicated:

1. As replacement or supplemental therapy in patients of any age or state (including pregnancy) with hypothyroidism of any etiology except transient hypothyroidism during the recovery phase of subacute thyroiditis: primary hypothyroidism resulting from thyroid dysfunction, primary atrophy, or partial or total absence of the thyroid gland, or from the effects of surgery, radiation or drugs, with or without the presence of goiter, including subclinical hypothyroidism; secondary (pituitary hypothyroidism; and tertiary (hypothalamic) hypothyroidism (see **CONTRAINDICATIONS** and **PRECAUTIONS**). SYNTHROID Injection can be used intravenously when rapid repletion is required, and either intravenously or intramuscularly when the oral route is precluded.

2. As a pituitary TSH suppressant in the treatment or prevention of various types of euthyroid goiters, including thyroid modules, subacute or chronic lymphocytic thyroiditis (Hashimoto's), multinodular goiter, and in conjunction with surgery and radioactive iodine therapy in the management of thyrotropin-dependent well-differentiated papillary or follicular carcinoma of the thyroid.

CONTRAINDICATIONS

SYNTHROID is contraindicated in patients with untreated thyrotoxicosis of any etiology or an apparent hypersensitivity to thyroid hormones or any of the inactive product constituents. (The 50 mcg tablet is formulated without color additives for patients who are sensitive to dyes.) There is no well-documented evidence of true allergic or idiosyncratic reactions to thyroid hormone. SYNTHROID is also contraindicated in the patients with uncorrected adrenal insufficiency, as thyroid hormones increase tissue demands for adrenocortical hormones and may thereby precipitate acute adrenal crisis (**see PRECAUTIONS**).

> **WARNINGS:** Thyroid hormones, either alone or together with other therapeutic agents, should not be used for the treatment of obesity. In euthyroid patients, doses within the range of daily hormonal requirements are ineffective for weight reduction. Larger doses may produce serious or even life threatening manifestations of toxicity, particularly when given in association with sympathomimetic amines such as those used for their anorectic effects.

The use of SYNTHROID in the treatment of obesity, either alone or in combination with other drugs, is unjustified. The use of SYNTHROID is also unjustified in the treatment of male or female infertility unless this condition is associated with hypothyroidism.

PRECAUTIONS

General: SYNTHROID should be used with caution in patients with cardiovascular disorders, including angina, coronary artery disease, and hypertension, and in the elderly who have a greater likelihood of occult cardiac disease. Concomitant administration of thyroid hormone and sympathomimetic agents to patients with coronary artery disease may increase the risk of coronary insufficiency.

Use of SYNTHROID in patients with concomitant diabetes mellitus, diabetes insipidus or adrenal cortical insufficiency may aggravate the intensity of their symptoms. Appropriate adjustments of the various therapeutic measures directed at these concomitant endocrine diseases may therefore be required. Treatment of myxedema coma may require simultaneous administration of glucocorticoids (see **DOSAGE AND ADMINISTRATION**).

T_4 enhances the response to anticoagulant therapy. Prothrombin time should be closely monitored in patients taking both SYNTHROID and oral anticoagulants, and the dosage of anticoagulant adjusted accordingly.

Seizures have been reported rarely in association with the initiation of levothyroxine sodium therapy, and may be related to the effect of thyroid hormone on seizure threshold. Lithium blocks the TSH-mediated release of T_4 and T_3. Thyroid function should therefore be carefully monitored during

lithium initiation, stabilization, and maintenance. If hypothyroidism occurs during lithium treatment, a higher than usual SYNTHROID dose may be required.

Information for the Patient:

1. SYNTHROID is intended to replace a hormone that is normally produced by your thyroid gland. It is generally taken for life, except in cases of temporary hypothyroidism associated with an inflammation of the thyroid gland.

2. Before or at any time while using SYNTHROID you should tell your doctor if you are allergic to any foods or medicines, are pregnant or intend to become pregnant, are breastfeeding, are taking or start taking any other prescription or nonprescription (OTC) medications, or have any other medical problems (especially hardening of the arteries, heart disease, high blood pressure, or history of thyroid, adrenal or pituitary gland problems).

3. Use SYNTHROID only as prescribed by your doctor. Do not discontinue SYNTHROID or change the amount you take or how often you take it, except as directed by your doctor.

4. SYNTHROID, like all medicines obtained from your doctor, must be used only by you and for the condition determined appropriate by your doctor.

5. It may take a few weeks for SYNTHROID to begin working. Until it begins working, you may not notice any change in your symptoms.

6. You should notify your doctor if you experience any of the following symptoms, or if you experience any other unusual medical event: chest pain, shortness of breath, hives or skin rash, rapid or irregular heartbeat, headache, irritability, nervousness, sleeplessness, diarrhea, excessive sweating, heat intolerance, changes in appetite, vomiting, weight gain or loss, changes in menstrual periods, fever, hand tremors, leg cramps.

7. You should inform your doctor or dentist that you are taking SYNTHROID before having any kind of surgery.

8. You should notify your doctor if you become pregnant while taking SYNTHROID. Your dose of this medicine will likely have to be increased while you are pregnant.

9. If you have diabetes, your dose insulin or oral antidiabetic agent may need to be changed after starting SYNTHROID. You should monitor your blood or urinary glucose levels as directed by your doctor and report any changes to your doctor immediately.

10. If you are taking an oral anticoagulant drug such as warfarin, your dose may need to be changed after starting SYNTHROID. Your coagulation status should be checked often to determine if a change in dose is required.

11. Partial hair loss may occur rarely during the first few months of SYNTHROID therapy, but it is usually temporary.

12. SYNTHROID is the trade name for tablets, containing the thyroid hormone levothyroxine, manufactured by Knoll Pharmaceutical Company. Other manufacturers also makes tablets containing levothyroxine. You should not change to another manufacturer's product without discussing that change with your doctor first. Repeat blood tests and a change in the amount of levothyroxine you take may be required.

13. Keep SYNTHROID out of the reach of children. Store SYNTHROID away from heat and moisture.

Laboratory Tests: Treatment of patients with SYNTHROID requires periodic assessment of adequacy of titration by appropriate laboratory tests and clinical evaluation. Selection of appropriate tests for the diagnosis and management of thyroid disorders depends on patient variables such as presenting signs and symptoms, pregnancy, and concomitant medications. A combination of sensitive TSH assay and free T_4 estimate (free T_4, free T_4 index) are recommended to confirm a diagnosis of thyroid disease. Normal ranges for theses parameters are age-specific in newborns and younger children.

TSH alone or initially may be useful for thyroid disease screening and for monitoring therapy for primary hypothyroidism as a linear inverse correlation exists between serum TSH and free T_4. Measurement of total serum T_4 and T_3, resin T_3 uptake, and free T_3 concentrations may also be useful. Antithyroid microsomal antibodies are an indicator of autoimmune thyroid disease. The presence of positive microsomal antibodies in an euthyroid patient is a major risk factor for the future development of hypothyroidism. As elevated serum TSH in the presence of normal T_4 may indicate subclinical hypothyroidism. Intracellular resistance to thyroid hormone is quite rare, and is suggested by clinical signs and symptoms of hypothyroidism in the presence of high serum T_4 levels. Adequacy of SYNTHROID therapy for hypothyroidism of pituitary or hypothalamic origin should be assessed by measuring free T_4, which should be maintained in the upper half of the normal range. Measurement of TSH is not a reliable indicator of response to therapy for this condition. Adequacy of SYNTHROID therapy for congenital and acquired pediatric hypothyroidism should be assessed by measuring serum total T_4 or free T_4, which should be maintained in the upper half of the normal range. In congenital hypothyroidism, normalization of serum TSH levels may lag behind normalization of serum T_4 levels by 2 or 3

months or longer. In rare patients serum TSH remains relatively elevated despite clinical euthyroidism and age-specific normal levels of T_4 or free T_4.

Drug Interactions: The magnitude and relative clinical importance of the effects noted below are likely to be patient-specific and may vary by such factors as age, gender, race, intercurrent illnesses, dose of either agent, additional concomitant medications, and timing of drug administration. Any agent that alters thyroid hormone synthesis, secretion, distribution, effect on target tissues, metabolism, or elimination may alter the optimal therapeutic dose of SYNTHROID.

Levothyroxine sodium absorption—The following agents may bind and decrease absorption of levothyroxine sodium from the gastrointestinal tract: aluminum hydroxide, cholestyramine resin, colestipol hydrochloride, ferrous sulfate, sodium polystyrene sulfonate, soybean flour (e.g., infant formula), sucralfate.

Binding to serum proteins—The following agents may either inhibit levothyroxine sodium binding to serum proteins or alter the concentrations of serum binding proteins: androgens and related anabolic hormones, asparaginase, clofibrate, estrogens and estrogen-containing compounds, 5-fluorouracil, furosemide, glucocorticoids, meclofenamic acid, mefenamic acid, methadone, perphenazine, phenylbutazone, phenytoin, salicylates, tamoxifen.

Thyroid physiology—The following agents may alter thyroid hormone or TSH levels, generally by effects on thyroid hormone synthesis, secretion, distribution, metabolism, hormone action, or elimination, or altered TSH secretion: aminoglutethimide, p-aminosalicyclic acid, amiodarone, androgens and related anabolic hormones, complex anions (thiocyanate, perchlorate, pertechnetate), antithyroid drugs, β-adrenergic blocking agents, carbamazepine, chloral hydrate, diazepam, dopamine and dopamine agonists, ethionamide, glucocorticoids, heparin, hepatic enzyme inducers, insulin, iodinated cholestographic agents, iodine-containing compounds, levodopa, lovastatin, lithium, 6-mercaptopurine, metoclopramide, mitotane, nitroprusside, phenobarbital, phenytoin, resorcinol, rifampin, somatostatin analogs, sulfonamides, sulfonylureas, thiazide diuretics.

Adrenocorticoids—Metabolic clearance of adrenocorticoids is decreased in hypothyroid patients and increased in hyperthyroid patients, and may therefore change with changing thyroid status.

Amiodarone—Amiodarone therapy alone can cause hypothyroidism or hyperthyroidism.

Anticoagulants (oral)—The hypoprothrombinemic effect of anticoagulants may be potentiated, apparently by increased catabolism of vitamin K-dependent clotting factors.

Antidiabetic agents (insulin, sulfonylureas)—Requirements for insulin or oral antidiabetic agents may be reduced in hypothyroid patients with diabetes mellitus, and may subsequently increase with the initiation of thyroid hormone replacement therapy.

β-adrenergic blocking agents—Actions of some beta-blocking agents may be impaired when hypothyroid patients become euthyroid.

Cytokines (interferon, interleukin)—Cytokines have been reported to induce both hyperthyroidism and hypothyroidism.

Digitalis glycosides—Therapeutic effects of digitalis glycosides may be reduced. Serum digitalis levels may be decreased in hyperthyroidism or when a hypothyroid patient becomes euthyroid.

Ketamine—Marked hypertension and tachycardia have been reported in association with concomitant administration of levothyroxine sodium and ketamine.

Maprotiline—Risk of cardiac arrhythmias may increase.

Sodium iodide (^{123}I and ^{131}I), sodium pertechnetate Tc99m—Uptake of radiolabeled ions may be decreased.

Somatrem/somatropin—Excessive concurrent use of thyroid hormone may accelerate epiphyseal closure. Untreated hypothyroidism may interfere with the growth response to somatrem or somatropin.

Theophylline—Theophylline clearance may decrease in hypothyroid patients and return toward normal when a euthyroid state is achieved.

Tricyclic antidepressants—Concurrent use may increase the therapeutic and toxic effects of both drugs, possibly due to increased catecholamine sensitivity. Onset of action of tricyclics may be accelerated.

Sympathomimetic agents—Possible increased risk of coronary insufficiency in patients with coronary artery disease.

Laboratory Test Interactions: A number of drugs or moieties are known to alter serum levels of TSH, T_4 and T_3 and may thereby influence the interpretation of laboratory tests of thyroid function (see **Drug Interactions**).

1. Changes in TBG concentration should be taken into consideration when interpreting T_4 and T_3 values. Drugs such as estrogens and estrogen-containing oral contraceptives increase TBG concentrations. TBG concentrations may also be increased during pregnancy and in infectious hepatitis. Decreases in TBG concentrations are observed in nephrosis, acromegaly, and after androgen or corticosteroid therapy. Familial hyper- or hypo-thyroxine-binding-globulinemias have been described. The incidence of TBG deficiency is ap-

proximately 1 in 9000. Certain drugs such as salicylates inhibit the protein-binding of T_4. In such cases, the unbound (free) hormone should be measured. Alternatively, an indirect measure of free thyroxine, such as the FT_4I may be used.

2. Medicinal or dietary iodine interferes with *in vivo* tests of radioiodine uptake, producing low uptakes which may not indicate a true decrease in hormone synthesis.

3. Persistent clinical and laboratory evidence of hypothyroidism despite an adequate replacement dose suggests either poor patient compliance, impaired absorption, drug interactions, or decreased potency of the preparation due to improper storage.

Carcinogenesis, Mutagenesis, and Impairment of Fertility: Although animal studies to determine the mutagenic or carcinogenic potential of thyroid hormones have not been performed, synthetic T_4 is identical to that produced by the human thyroid gland. A reported association between prolonged thyroid hormone therapy and breast cancer has not been confirmed and patients receiving levothyroxine sodium for established indications should not discontinue therapy.

Pregnancy: Pregnancy Category A. Studies in pregnant women have not shown that levothyroxine sodium increases the risk of fetal abnormalities if administered during pregnancy. If levothyroxine sodium is used during pregnancy, the possibility of fetal harm appears remote. Because studies cannot rule out the possibility of harm, levothyroxine sodium should be used during pregnancy only if clearly needed.

Thyroid hormones cross the placental barrier to some extent. T_4 levels in the cord blood of athyroid fetuses have been shown to be about one-third of maternal levels. Nevertheless, maternal-fetal transfer of T_4 may not prevent *in utero* hypothyroidism.

Hypothyroidism during pregnancy is associated with a higher rate of complications, including spontaneous abortion and preeclampsia, and has been reported to have an adverse effect on fetal and childhood development. On the basis of current knowledge, SYNTHROID® (levothyroxine sodium, USP) should therefore not be discontinued during pregnancy, and hypothyroidism diagnosed during pregnancy should be treated. Studies have shown that during pregnancy T_4 concentrations may decrease and TSH concentrations may increase to values outside normal ranges. Postpartum values are similar to preconception values. Elevations in TSH may occur as early as 4 weeks gestation.

Pregnant women who are maintained on SYNTHROID should have their TSH measured periodically. An elevated TSH should be corrected by an increase in SYNTHROID dose. After pregnancy, the dose can be decreased to the optimal preconception dose.

Nursing Mothers: Minimal amounts of thyroid hormones are excreted in human milk. Thyroid hormones are not associated with serious adverse reactions and do not have known tumorigenic potential. While caution should be exercised when SYNTHROID is administered to a nursing woman, adequate replacement doses of levothyroxine sodium are generally needed to maintain normal lactation.

Pediatric Use: Congenital hypothyroidism: Rapid restoration of normal serum T_4 concentrations is essential for preventing the deleterious effects of neonatal thyroid hormone deficiency on intelligence, as well as on overall growth and development. SYNTHROID should be initiated immediately upon diagnosis, and is generally continued for life. The goal of therapy is to maintain the serum total T_4 or FT_4 in the upper half of the normal range and serum TSH in the normal range.

An initial starting dose of 10 to 15 mcg/kg/day (ages 0–3 months) will generally increase serum T_4 concentrations to the upper half of the normal range in less than 3 weeks. Clinical assessment of growth and development and thyroid status should be monitored frequently. In most cases, the dose of SYNTHROID per body weight will decrease gradually as the patient grows through infancy and childhood (see Table). Prolonged use of large doses in infants may be associated with later behavior problems.

Thyroid function tests (serum total T_4 or FT_4, and TSH) should be monitored closely and used to determine the adequacy of SYNTHROID therapy. Normalization of serum T_4 levels is usually followed by a rapid decline of TSH levels. Nevertheless, normalization of TSH may lag behind normalization of T_4 levels by 2 to 3 months or longer. The relative elevation of serum TSH is more marked during the early months of therapy, but can persist to some degree throughout life. In rare patients TSH remains relatively elevated despite clinical euthyroidism and age-specific normal levels of total T_4 or FT_4. Increasing the SYNTHROID dosage to suppress TSH into the normal range may result in overtreatment, with an elevated serum T_4 level and clinical features of hyperthyroidism, including irritability, increased appetite with diarrhea, and sleeplessness. Another risk of prolonged overtreatment in infants is premature cranial synostosis.

Continued on next page

Synthroid—Cont.

Assessment of permanence of hypothyroidism may be done when transient hypothyroidism is suspected. Levothyroxine therapy may be interrupted for 30 days after 3 years of age and serum measurement of T_4 and TSH levels obtained. If T_4 is low and the TSH level is elevated, permanent hypothyroidism is confirmed and therapy should be re-instituted. If T_4 and TSH remain in the normal range, a presumptive diagnosis of transient hypothyroidism can be made. In this instance, continued clinical monitoring and periodic reevaluation of thyroid function may be warranted.

Acquired hypothyroidism. The initial dose of SYNTHROID varies with age and body weight, and should be adjusted to maintain serum total T_4 or free T_4 levels in the upper half of the normal range. In general, in the absence of overriding clinical concerns, children should be started on a full replacement dose. Children with underlying heart disease should be started at lower doses, with careful upward titration. Children with severe, long-standing hypothyroidism may also be started on a lower initial dose with upward titration in an attempt to avoid premature closure of epiphyses. The recommended dose per body weight decreases with age (see Table).

Treated children may resume growth at a rate greater than normal (period of transient catch-up growth). In some cases catch-up growth may be adequate to normalize growth; however, in children with severe and prolonged hypothyroidism, adult height may be reduced. Excessive thyroxine replacement may initiate accelerated bone maturation resulting in disproportionate advancement in skeletal age and shortened adult stature.

Assessment of permanence of hypothyroidism may be done when transient hypothyroidism is suspected. Levothyroxine therapy may be interrupted for 30 days and serum measurement of T_4 and TSH levels obtained. If T_4 is low and the TSH level is elevated, permanent hypothyroidism is confirmed and therapy should be re-instituted. If T_4 and TSH remain in the normal range, a presumptive diagnosis of transient hypothyroidism can be made. In this instance, continued clinical monitoring and periodic reevaluation of thyroid function may be warranted.

ADVERSE REACTIONS

Adverse reactions other than those indicative of thyrotoxicosis as a result of therapeutic overdosage, either initially or during the maintenance periods, are rare (see **OVERDOSAGE**). Craniosynostosis has been associated with iatrogenic hyperthyroidism in infants receiving thyroid hormone replacement therapy. Inadequate doses of SYNTHROID may produce or fail to resolve symptoms of hypothyroidism. Hypersensitivity reactions to the product excipients, such as rash and urticaria, may occur. Partial hair loss may occur during the initial months of therapy, but is generally transient. The incidence of continued hair loss is unknown. Pseudotumor cerebri has been reported in pediatric patients receiving thyroid hormone replacement therapy.

OVERDOSAGE

Signs and Symptoms: Excessive doses of SYNTHROID result in a hypermetabolic state indistinguishable from thyrotoxicosis of endogenous origin. Signs and symptoms of thyrotoxicosis include weight loss, increased appetite, palpitations, nervousness, diarrhea, abdominal cramps, sweating, tachycardia, increased pulse and blood pressure, cardiac arrhythmias, tremors, insomnia, heat intolerance, fever, and menstrual irregularities. Symptoms are not always evident or may not appear until several days after ingestion.

Treatment of Overdosage: SYNTHROID should be reduced in dose or temporarily discontinued if signs and symptoms of overdosage appear.

In the treatment of acute massive SYNTHROID overdosage, symptomatic and supportive therapy should be instituted immediately. Treatment is aimed at reducing gastrointestinal absorption and counteracting central and peripheral effects, mainly those of increased sympathetic activity. The stomach should be emptied immediately by emesis or gastric lavage if not otherwise contraindicated (e.g., by coma, convulsions or loss of gag reflex). Cholestyramine and activated charcoal have also been used to decrease levothyroxine sodium absorption. Oxygen should be administered and ventilation maintained as necessary, β-receptor antagonists, particularly propranolol, are useful in counteracting many of the effects of increased sympathetic activity. Propranolol may be administered intravenously at a dosage of 1 to 3 mg over a 10 minute period or orally, 80 to 160 mg/day, especially when no contraindications exist for its use. Cardiac glycosides may be administered if congestive heart failure develops. Measures to control fever, hypoglycemia, or fluid loss should be initiated as necessary. Glucocorticoids may be administered to inhibit the conversion of T_4 to T_3. Since T_4 is extensively protein bound, very little drug will be removed by dialysis.

DOSAGE AND ADMINISTRATION

The dosage and rate of administration of SYNTHROID is determined by the indication, and must in every case be individualized according to patient response and laboratory findings.

Hypothyroidism: The goal of therapy for primary hypothyroidism is to achieve and maintain a clinical and biochemical euthyroid state with consequent resolution of hypothyroid signs and symptoms. The starting dose of SYNTHROID, the frequency of dose titration, and the optimal full replacement dose must be individualized for every patient, and will be influenced by such factors as age, weight, cardiovascular status, presence of other illness, and the severity and duration of hypothyroid symptoms.

The usual full replacement dose of SYNTHROID for younger, healthy adults is approximately 1.6 mcg/kg/day administered once daily. In the elderly, the full replacement dose may be altered by decreases in T_4 metabolism and levothyroxine sodium absorption. Older patients may require less than 1 mcg/kg/day. Children generally require higher doses (see **Pediatric Dosage**). Women who are maintained on SYNTHROID during pregnancy may require increased doses (see **Pregnancy**).

Therapy is usually initiated in younger, healthy adults at the anticipated full replacement dose. Clinical and laboratory evaluations should be performed at 6 to 8 week intervals (2 to 3 weeks in severely hypothyroid patients), and the dosage adjusted by 12.5 to 25 mcg increments until the serum TSH concentration is normalized and signs and symptoms resolve. In older patients or in younger patients with a history of cardiovascular disease, the starting dose should be 12.5 to 50 mcg once daily with adjustments of 12.5 to 25 mcg every 3 to 6 weeks until TSH is normalized. If cardiac symptoms develop or worsen, the cardiac disease should be evaluated and the dose of SYNTHROID reduced. Rarely, worsening angina or other signs of cardiac ischemia may prevent achieving a TSH in the normal range.

Treatment of subclinical hypothyroidism, when indicated, may require lower than usual replacement doses, e.g. 1.0 mcg/kg/day. Patients for whom treatment is not initiated should be monitored yearly for changes in clinical status, TSH, and thyroid antibodies.

In patients with hypothyroidism resulting from pituitary or hypothalamic disease, the possibility of secondary adrenal insufficiency should be considered, and if present, treated with glucocorticoids prior to initiation of SYNTHROID. The adequacy of SYNTHROID therapy should be assessed in these patients by measuring FT_4I, which should be maintained in the upper half of the normal range, in addition to clinical assessment. Measurement of TSH is not a reliable indicator of response to therapy for this condition.

Few patients require doses greater than 200 mcg/day. An inadequate response to daily doses of 300 to 400 mcg/day is rare, and may suggest malabsorption, poor patient compliance, and/or drug interactions.

Once optimal replacement is achieved, clinical and laboratory evaluations should be conducted at least annually or whenever warranted by a change in patient status. Levothyroxine sodium products from different manufacturers should not be used interchangeably unless retesting of the patient and retitration of the dosage, as necessary, accompanies the product switch.

SYNTHROID Injection by the intravenous of intramuscular route can be substituted for the oral dosage form when the oral administration is precluded. The initial parenteral dosage should be approximately one-half the previously established oral dosage of SYNTHROID Tablets. Close observation of the patient is recommended, with adjustment of the dosage as needed. Administration of SYNTHROID Injection by the subcutaneous route is not recommended as studies have shown that the influx of T_4 from the subcutaneous site is very slow, and depends on many factors such as volume of injectate, the anatomic site of injection, ambient temperature, and presence of venospasm.

Myxedema Coma: Myxedema coma represents the extreme expression of severe hypothyroidism and is considered a medical emergency. It is characterized by hypothermia, hypotension, hypoventilation, hyponatremia, and bradycardia. In addition to restoration of normal thyroid hormone levels, therapy should be directed at the correction of electrolyte disturbances and possible infection. Because the mortality rate of patients with untreated myxedema coma is high, treatment must be started immediately, and should include appropriate supportive therapy and corticosteroids to prevent adrenal insufficiency. Possible precipitating factors should also be identified and treated. SYNTHROID may be given via nasogastric tube, but the preferred route of administration is intravenous. A bolus dose of SYNTHROID is given immediately to replete the peripheral pool of T_4, usually 300 to 500 mcg. Although such a dose is usually well-tolerated even in the elderly, the rapid intravenous administration of large doses of levothyroxine sodium to patients with cardiovascular disease is clearly not without risks. Under such circumstances, intravenous therapy should not be undertaken without weighing the alternate risks of myxedema coma and the cardiovascular disease. Clinical judgement in this situation may dictate smaller intravenous doses of SYNTHROID. The initial dose is followed by daily intravenous doses of 75 to 100 mcg until the patient is stable and oral administration is feasible. Normal T_4 levels are usually achieved in 24 hours, followed by progressive increases in T_3. Improvement in cardiac output, blood pressure, temperature, and mental status generally occur within 24 hours, with improvement in many manifestations of hypothyroidism in 4 to 7 days.

TSH Suppression in Thyroid Cancer and Thyroid Nodules: The rationale for TSH suppression therapy is that a reduction in TSH secretion may decrease the growth and function of abnormal thyroid tissue. Exogenous thyroid hormone may inhibit recurrence of tumor growth and may produce regression of metastases from well-differentiated (follicular and papillary) carcinoma of the thyroid. It is used as ancillary therapy of these conditions following surgery or radioactive iodine therapy. Medullary and anaplastic carcinoma of the thyroid is unresponsive to TSH suppression therapy. TSH suppression is also used in treating nontoxic solitary nodules and multinodular goiters.

No controlled studies have compared the various degrees of TSH suppression in the treatment of either benign or malignant thyroid nodular disease. Further, the effectiveness of TSH suppression for benign nodular disease is controversial. The dose of SYNTHROID used for TSH suppression should therefore be individualized by the nature of the disease, the patient being treated, and the desired clinical response, weighing the potential benefits of therapy against the risks of iatrogenic thyrotoxicosis. In general, SYNTHROID should be given in the smallest dose that will achieve the desired clinical response.

For well-differentiated thyroid cancer, TSH is generally suppressed to less than 0.1 mU/L. Doses of SYNTHROID greater than 2 mcg/kg/day are usually required. The efficacy of TSH suppression in reducing the size of benign thyroid nodules and in preventing nodule regrowth after surgery are controversial. Nevertheless, when treatment with levothyroxine sodium is considered warranted, TSH is generally suppressed to a higher target range (e.g., 0.1 to 0.3 mU/L) than that employed for the treatment of thyroid cancer. SYNTHROID therapy may also be considered for patients with nontoxic multinodular goiter who have a TSH in the normal range, to moderately suppress TSH (e.g., 0.1 to 0.3 mU/L).

SYNTHROID should be administered with caution to patients in whom there is a suspicion of thyroid gland autonomy, in view of the fact that the effects of exogenous hormone administration will be additive to endogenous thyroid hormone production.

Pediatric Dosage: Congenital or acquired hypothyroidism: The dosage of SYNTHROID for pediatric hypothyroidism varies with age and body weight. SYNTHROID should be given at a dose that maintains the serum total T_4 or free T_4 concentrations in the upper half of the normal range and serum TSH in the normal range (see **Pediatric Use**).

SYNTHROID therapy is usually initiated at the full replacement dose (see Table). Infants and neonates with very low or undetectable serum T_4 levels (<5 mcg/dL) should start at the higher end of the dosage range (e.g., 50 mcg daily). A lower starting dosage (e.g., 25 mcg daily) should be considered for neonates at risk of cardiac failure, increasing every few days until a full maintenance dose is reached. In children with severe, long-standing hypothyroidism, SYNTHROID should be initiated gradually, with an initial dose of 25 mcg for two weeks, and then increasing the dose by 25 mcg every 2 to 4 weeks until the desired dose based on serum T_4 and TSH levels is achieved. (see **Pediatric Use**).

Serum T_4 and TSH measurements should be evaluated at the following intervals, with subsequent dosage adjustments to normalize serum total T_4 or FT_4, and TSH:

2 and 4 weeks after the initiation of SYNTHROID treatment;

every 1 to 2 months during the first year of life;

every 2 to 3 months between 1 and 3 years of age;

every 3 to 12 months thereafter until growth is completed.

Evaluation at more frequent intervals is advisable when compliance is questioned or abnormal values are obtained. Patient evaluation is also advisable approximately 6 to 8 weeks after any change in SYNTHROID dose.

SYNTHROID tablets may be given to infants and children who cannot swallow intact tablets by crushing the tablet and suspending the freshly crushed tablet in a small amount of water (5 to 10 mL), breast milk or non-soybean formula. The suspension can be given by spoon or dropper. **DO NOT STORE THE SUSPENSION FOR ANY PERIOD OF TIME.** The crushed tablet may also be sprinkled over a small amount of food, such as apple sauce. Foods or formula containing large amounts of soybean, fiber, or iron should not be used for administering SYNTHROID.

Dosing Guidelines for Pediatric Hypothyroidism

Age	Daily dose per kg body weight*
0-3 mos	10-15 mcg
3-6 mos	8-10 mcg
6-12 mos	6-8 mcg
1-5 yrs	5-6 mcg

6-12 yrs	4-5 mcg
>12 years	2-3 mcg
Growth & puberty complete	1.6 mcg

* To be adjusted on the basis of clinical response and laboratory tests (see Laboratory Tests).

HOW SUPPLIED

SYNTHROID® (levothyroxine sodium, USP) **Tablets:** round, color coded, scored tablet debossed with "FLINT" and potency.

25 mcg, orange
Bottles of 100, Code 3P1023   NDC 0048-1020-03
Bottles of 1000, Code 3P1025   NDC 0048-1020-05

50 mcg, white
Bottles of 100, Code 3P1043   NDC 0048-1040-03
Bottles of 1000, Code 3P1045   NDC 0048-1040-05
Unit Dose Cartons of 100,   NDC 0048-1040-13
  Code 3P1033

75 mcg, violet
Bottles of 100, Code 3P1053   NDC 0048-1050-03
Bottles of 1000, Code 3P1055   NDC 0048-1050-05
Unit Dose Cartons of 100,   NDC 0048-1050-13
  Code 3P1003

88 mcg, olive
Bottles of 100, Code 3P0883   NDC 0048-1060-03

100 mcg, yellow
Bottles of 100, Code 3P1073   NDC 0048-1070-03
Bottles of 1000, Code 3P1075   NDC 0048-1070-05
Unit Dose Cartons of 100,   NDC 0048-1070-13
  Code 3P1063

112 mcg, rose
Bottles of 100, Code 3P1183   NDC 0048-1080-03
Bottles of 1000, Code 3P1185   NDC 0048-1080-05

125 mcg, brown
Bottles of 100, Code 3P1103   NDC 0048-1130-03
Bottles of 1000, Code 3P1105   NDC 0048-1130-05
Unit Dose Cartons of 100,   NDC 0048-1130-13
  Code 3P1113

150 mcg, blue
Bottles of 100, Code 3P1093   NDC 0048-1090-03
Bottles of 1000, Code 3P1095   NDC 0048-1090-05
Unit Dose Cartons of 100,   NDC 0048-1090-13
  Code 3P1083

175 mg, lilac
Bottles of 100, Code 3P1153   NDC 0048-1100-03

200 mcg, pink
Bottles of 100, Code 3P1143   NDC 0048-1140-03
Bottles of 1000, Code 3P1145   NDC 0048-1140-05
Unit Dose Cartons of 100,   NDC 0048-1140-13
  Code 3P1133

300 mcg, green
Bottles of 100, Code 3P1173   NDC 0048-1170-03
Bottles of 1000, Code 3P1175   NDC 0048-1170-05

Store at controlled room temperature 15°-30°C (59°-86°F). SYNTHROID Tablets should be protected from light and moisture.
SYNTHROID® (levothyroxine sodium, USP) **Injection** is a lyophilized powder. It is supplied in color coded vials as follows:

200 mcg, gray
10 mL Single Dose Vial,   NDC 0048-1014-99
  Code 3P1312
500 mcg, yellow
10 mL Single Dose Vial,   NDC 0048-1012-99
  Code 3P1302

Store at controlled room temperature 15°- 30C (59 - 86°F).

DIRECTIONS FOR RECONSTITUTION: Reconstitute the lyophilized levothyroxine sodium by aseptically adding 5 mL of 0.9% Sodium Chloride Injection, USP (final volume approximately 5mL). Shake vial to insure complete mixing. Do not add to other intravenous fluids. Use immediately after reconstitution. Discard any unused portion.
CAUTION: Federal (USA) law prohibits dispensing without a prescription.

Tablets Manufactured by
BASF Pharmaceuticals
A Unit of BASF
Jayuya, Puerto Rico 00664
Injection Manufactured by
Ben Venue Laboratories, Inc.
Bedford, Ohio 44146 USA
For
Knoll Pharmaceutical Company
3000 Continental Drive-North
Mount Olive, NJ 07828–1234
BASF Pharma

Shown in Product Identification Guide, page 319

TARKA®   ℞
(Trandolapril/Verapamil
Hydrochloride ER Tablets)

> ### USE IN PREGNANCY
> **When used in pregnancy during the second and third trimesters, ACE inhibitors can cause injury and even death to the developing fetus.** When pregnancy is detected, TARKA® should be discontinued as soon as possible. See **WARNINGS**, Fetal/Neonatal Morbidity and Mortality.

DESCRIPTION

TARKA® (trandolapril/verapamil hydrochloride ER) combines a slow release formulation of a calcium channel blocker, verapamil hydrochloride, and an immediate release formulation of an angiotensin converting enzyme inhibitor, trandolapril.

Verapamil Component—Verapamil hydrochloride is chemically described as benzeneacetonitrile, α[3-[[2-(3,4-dimethoxyphenyl) ethyl] methylamino] propyl]-3,4-dimethoxy-α-(1-methylethyl) hydrochloride. Its empirical formula is $C_{27}H_{38}N_2O_4$ HCl and its structural formula is:

Verapamil hydrochloride is an almost white crystalline powder, with a molecular weight of 491.08. It is soluble in water, chloroform, and methanol. It is practically free of odor, with a bitter taste.

Trandolapril Component—Trandolapril is the ethyl ester prodrug of a nonsulfhydryl angiotensin converting enzyme (ACE) inhibitor, trandolaprilat. It is chemically described as (2S,3aR,7aS)-1-[(S)-N-[(S)-Carboxy-3-phenylpropyl]alanyl] hexahydro-2-indolinecarboxylic acid, 1-ethyl ester. Its empirical formula is $C_{24}H_{34}N_2O_5$ and its structural formula is:

Trandolapril is a colorless, crystalline substance with a molecular weight of 430.54. It is soluble (>100 mg/mL) in chloroform, dichloromethane, and methanol.
TARKA tablets are formulated for oral administration, containing verapamil hydrochloride as a controlled release formulation and trandolapril as an immediate release formulation. The tablet strengths are trandolapril 2 mg/verapamil hydrochloride ER 180 mg, trandolapril 1 mg/verapamil hydrochloride ER 240 mg, trandolapril 2 mg/verapamil hydrochloride ER 240 mg, and trandolapril 4 mg/verapamil hydrochloride ER 240 mg. The tablets also contain the following ingredients: corn starch, dioctyl sodium sulfosuccinate, ethanol, hydroxypropyl cellulose, hydroxypropyl methylcellulose, lactose, magnesium stearate, microcrystalline cellulose, polyethylene glycol, povidone, purified water, silicon dioxide, sodium alginate, sodium stearyl fumarate, synthetic iron oxides, talc, and titanium dioxide.

CLINICAL PHARMACOLOGY

Verapamil hydrochloride and trandolapril have been used individually and in combination for the treatment of hypertension. For the four dosing strengths, the antihypertensive effect of the combination is approximately additive to the individual components.
Verapamil Component—Verapamil is a calcium channel blocker that exerts its pharmacologic effects by modulating the influx of ionic calcium across the cell membrane of the arterial smooth muscle as well as in conductile and contractile myocardial cells. Verapamil exerts antihypertensive effects by decreasing systemic vascular resistance, usually without orthostatic decreases in blood pressure or reflex

tachycardia. During isometric or dynamic exercise, verapamil does not alter systolic cardiac function in patients with normal ventricular function. Verapamil does not alter total serum calcium levels.
Trandolapril Component—Trandolapril is de-esterified to its diacid metabolite, trandolaprilat. Both inhibit angiotensin-converting enzyme (ACE) in human subjects and in animals. Trandolaprilat is about 8 times more potent than trandolapril. ACE is a peptidyl dipeptidase that catalyzes the conversion of angiotensin I to the vasoconstrictor, angiotensin II. Angiotensin II also stimulates aldosterone secretion by the adrenal cortex.
Inhibition of ACE results in decreased plasma angiotensin II, which leads to decreased vasopressor activity and to decreased aldosterone secretion. The latter decrease may result in a small increase of serum potassium. In controlled clinical trials, treatment with TARKA resulted in mean increases in potassium of 0.1 mEq/L (see **PRECAUTIONS**). Removal of angiotensin II negative feedback on renin secretion leads to increased plasma renin activity (PRA).
ACE is identical to kininase II, an enzyme that degrades bradykinin. Whether increased levels of bradykinin, a potent vasodepressor peptide, play a role in the therapeutic effect of TARKA remains to be elucidated.
While the mechanism through which trandolapril lowers blood pressure is believed to be primarily suppression of the renin-angiotensin-aldosterone system, trandolapril has an antihypertensive effect even in patients with low renin hypertension. Trandolapril is an effective antihypertensive in all races studied. Both black patients (usually a predominantly low renin group) and non-black patients respond to 2 to 4 mg of trandolapril.

Pharmacokinetics and Metabolism: *TARKA*—Following a single oral dose of TARKA in healthy subjects, peak plasma concentrations are reached within 0.5–2 hours for trandolapril and within 4–15 hours for verapamil. Peak plasma concentrations of the active desmethyl metabolite of verapamil, norverapamil, are reached within 5–15 hours. Cleavage of the ester group converts trandolapril to its active diacid metabolite, trandolaprilat, which reaches peak plasma concentrations within 2–12 hours. The pharmacokinetics of trandolapril and trandolaprilat are not altered when trandolapril is administered in combination with verapamil, compared to monotherapy. The AUC and Cmax for both verapamil and norverapamil are increased when 240 mg of controlled release verapamil is administered concomitantly with 4 mg trandolapril. The increase in Cmax is 54 and 30% and the AUC is increased by 65 and 32% for verapamil and norverapamil, respectively. Administration of TARKA 4/240 (4 mg trandolapril and 240 mg verapamil hydrochloride ER) with a high-fat meal does not alter the bioavailability of trandolapril whereas verapamil peak concentrations and area under the curve (AUC) decrease 37% and 28%, respectively. Food thus decreases verapamil bioavailability and the time to peak plasma concentration for both verapamil and norverapamil are delayed by approximately 7 hours. Both optical isomers of verapamil are similarly affected.
Trandolaprilat has an effective elimination half-life of approximately 10 hours but like all ACE inhibitors, it has a prolonged terminal elimination half-life. The terminal half-life of verapamil is 6–11 hours. Steady-state plasma concentrations of the two components are achieved after about a week of once-daily dosing of TARKA. At steady-state, plasma concentrations of verapamil and trandolaprilat are up to two-fold higher than those observed after a single oral TARKA dose.
The pharmacokinetics of verapamil and trandolaprilat are significantly different in the elderly (≥65 years) than in younger subjects. The bioavailability of verapamil and norverapamil are increased by 87% and 77%, respectively, and that of trandolapril by approximately 35% in the elderly. AUCs are approximately 80% and 35% higher, respectively.
Verapamil Component—With the immediate release formulation, more than 90% of the orally administered dose is absorbed with peak plasma concentrations of verapamil observed 1 to 2 hours after dosing. A delayed rate but similar extent of absorption is observed for the sustained release formulation when compared to the immediate release formulation. Because of the rapid biotransformation of verapamil during its first pass through the portal circulation, absolute bioavailability ranges from 20% to 35%. A nonlinear correlation exists between verapamil dose and plasma concentrations.
In early dose titration with verapamil, a relationship exists between plasma concentrations of verapamil and prolongation of the PR interval. However, during chronic administration, this relationship may disappear. No relationship has been established between the plasma concentration of verapamil and reduction in blood pressure.
In healthy subjects, orally administered verapamil undergoes extensive metabolism in the liver. Twelve metabolites have been identified in plasma; all except norverapamil are

Continued on next page

Tarka—Cont.

present in trace amounts only. Approximately 70% of an administered dose is excreted as metabolites in the urine and 16% or more in the feces within 5 days. Urinary excretion of unchanged drug is about 3% to 4% of the dose. Verapamil is approximately 90% bound to plasma proteins.

In patients with hepatic insufficiency, verapamil clearance is decreased about 30% and the elimination half-life is prolonged up to 14 to 16 hours (see **PRECAUTIONS**). In patients with liver dysfunction, a dosage adjustment may be required. In the elderly (≥65 years), verapamil clearance is reduced resulting in increases in elimination half-life.

Trandolapril Component—Following oral administration of trandolapril, the absolute bioavailability of trandolapril is approximately 10% as trandolapril and 10% as trandolaprilat. Plasma concentrations of trandolaprilat but not trandolapril increase in proportion with dose. Plasma concentrations of trandolaprilat decline in a triphasic manner. The more prolonged terminal elimination phase probably represents a small fraction of dose saturably bound to ACE.

After an oral radiolabeled dose of trandolapril, excretion of trandolapril and metabolites account for 33% of the dose in the urine and about 66% in the feces. Less than 1% of the dose is excreted in the urine as unchanged drug. Serum protein binding of trandolapril is about 80%, and is independent of concentration. Binding of trandolaprilat is concentration-dependent, varying from 65% at 1000 ng/ml to 94% at 0.1 ng/ml, indicating saturation of binding with increasing concentration.

Compared to normal subjects, the plasma concentrations of trandolapril and trandolaprilat are approximately 2-fold greater and renal clearance is reduced by about 85% in patients with creatinine clearance below 30 ml/min and in patients on hemodialysis. Dosage adjustment is recommended in renally impaired patients. (See **DOSAGE AND ADMINISTRATION**).

Following oral administration in patients with mild to moderate alcoholic cirrhosis, plasma concentrations of trandolapril and trandolaprilat were, respectively, 9-fold and 2-fold greater than in normal subjects, but inhibition of ACE activity was not affected. Lower dosages should be considered in patients with hepatic insufficiency, (see **DOSAGE AND ADMINISTRATION**).

Pharmacodynamics: *TARKA*—Verapamil does not interfere with ACE inhibition by trandolapril. Trandolapril does not alter the effect of verapamil on intra-cardiac conduction.

Verapamil Component—Verapamil dilates the main coronary arteries, both in normal and ischemic regions, and is a potent inhibitor of coronary artery spasm. This property increases myocardial oxygen delivery in patients with coronary artery spasm, and is responsible for the effectiveness of verapamil in vasospastic (Prinzmetal's or variant) as well as unstable angina at rest.

Verapamil regularly reduces the total systemic resistance (afterload) by dilating peripheral arterioles. By decreasing the influx of calcium, verapamil prolongs the effective refractory period within the AV node and slows AV conduction in a rate-related manner.

Normal sinus rhythm is usually not affected, but in patients with sick sinus syndrome, verapamil may interfere with sinus node impulse generation and may induce sinus arrest or sinoatrial block. Atrioventricular block can occur in patients without preexisting conduction defects (see **WARNINGS**).

Verapamil does not alter the normal atrial action potential or intraventricular conduction time, but depresses amplitude, velocity of depolarization and conduction in depressed atrial fibers. Verapamil may shorten the antegrade effective refractory period of accessory bypass tracts. Acceleration of ventricular rate and/or ventricular fibrillation has been reported in patients with atrial flutter or atrial fibrillation and a coexisting accessory AV pathway following administration of verapamil (see **WARNINGS**).

Hemodynamics and Myocardial Metabolism: Verapamil reduces afterload and myocardial contractility. Improved left ventricular diastolic function in patients with idiopathic hypertrophic subaortic stenosis (IHSS) and those with coronary heart disease has also been observed with verapamil therapy. In most patients, including those with organic cardiac disease, the negative inotropic action of verapamil is countered by a reduction of afterload and cardiac index is usually not reduced. However, in patients with severe left ventricular dysfunction (e.g., pulmonary wedge pressure about 20 mmHg or ejection fraction less than 30%), or in patients taking beta-adrenergic blocking agents or other cardio-depressant drugs, deterioration of ventricular function may occur (see **DRUG INTERACTIONS**).

Pulmonary Function: Verapamil does not induce bronchoconstriction and hence, does not impair ventilatory function.

Trandolapril Component—After a single 2 mg dose of trandolapril, inhibition of ACE activity reaches a maximum (70-85%) at 4 hours with about 1% decline at 24 hours. Eight days after dosing, ACE inhibition is still 40%.

Four placebo-controlled dose response studies were conducted using once daily oral dosing of trandolapril in doses from 0.25 to 16 mg per day in 827 black and non-black patients with mild to moderate hypertension. The minimal effective once daily dose was 1.0 mg in non-black patients and 2.0 mg in black patients. Further decreases in trough supine diastolic blood pressure were obtained in non-black patients with higher doses, and no further response was seen in doses above 4 mg (up to 16 mg). The antihypertensive effect diminished somewhat at the end of the dosing interval.

During chronic therapy, the maximum reduction in blood pressure with any dose is achieved within one week. Following 6 weeks of monotherapy in placebo-controlled trials in patients with mild to moderate hypertension, once daily doses of 2 to 4 mg lowered supine or standing systolic/diastolic blood pressure 24 hours after dosing by an average 7-10/4-5 mmHg below placebo responses in non-black patients. Once daily doses of 2 to 4 mg lowered blood pressures 4-6/3-4 mmHg below placebo responses in black patients.

CLINICAL STUDIES

In controlled clinical trials, once daily doses of TARKA, trandolapril 4 mg/verapamil HCl ER 240 mg or trandolapril 2 mg/verapamil HCl ER 180 mg, decreased placebo-corrected seated pressure (systolic/diastolic) 24 hours after dosing by about 7-12/6-8 mmHg. Each of the components of TARKA added to the antihypertensive effect. Treatment effects were consistent across age groups (<65, ≥65 years), and gender (male, female).

Blood pressure reductions were significantly greater for the TARKA 4/240 combination than for either of the components used alone.

The antihypertensive effects of TARKA have continued during therapy for at least 1 year.

INDICATIONS AND USAGE

TARKA is indicated for treatment of hypertension.

This fixed combination drug is not indicated for the initial therapy of hypertension (see DOSAGE and ADMINISTRATION).

In using TARKA, consideration should be given to the fact that an angiotension converting enzyme inhibitor, captopril, has caused agranulocytosis, particularly in patients with renal impairment or collagen vascular disease, and that available data are insufficient to show that trandolapril does not have similar risk (see **WARNINGS: Neutropenia/Agranulocytosis**).

CONTRAINDICATIONS

TARKA is contraindicated in patients who are hypersensitive to any ACE inhibitor or verapamil.

Because of the verapamil component, TARKA is contraindicated in:

1. Severe left ventricular dysfunction (see **WARNINGS**).
2. Hypotension (systolic pressure less than 90 mmHg) or cardiogenic shock.
3. Sick sinus syndrome (except in patients with a functioning artificial ventricular pacemaker).
4. Second- or third-degree AV block (except in patients with a functioning artificial ventricular pacemaker).
5. Patients with atrial flutter or atrial fibrillation and an accessory bypass tract (e.g. Wolff-Parkinson-White, Lown-Ganong-Levine syndromes) (see **WARNINGS**).

Because of the trandolapril component, TARKA is contraindicated in patients with a history of angioedema related to previous treatment with angiotension converting enzyme (ACE) inhibitor.

WARNINGS

Heart Failure: *Verapamil Component*—Verapamil has a negative inotropic effect which, in most patients, is compensated by its afterload reduction (decreased systemic vascular resistance) properties without a net impairment of ventricular performance. In clinical experience with 4,954 patients, 87 (1.8%) developed congestive heart failure of pulmonary edema. Verapamil should be avoided in patients with severe left ventricular dysfunction (e.g., ejection fraction less than 30%, pulmonary wedge pressure above 20 mmHg, or severe symptoms of cardiac failure) and in patients with any degree of ventricular dysfunction if they are receiving a beta adrenergic blocker (see **DRUG INTERACTIONS**). Patients with milder ventricular dysfunction should, if possible, be controlled with optimum doses of digitalis and/or diuretics before verapamil treatment (Note interactions with digoxin under: **PRECAUTIONS**).

Trandolapril Component—Trandolapril, as an ACE inhibitor, may cause excessive hypotension in patients with congestive heart failure (see **WARNINGS, Hypotension**).

Hypotension: *Verapamil Component*—Occasionally, the pharmacologic action of verapamil may produce a decrease in blood pressure below normal levels which may result in dizziness or symptomatic hypotension.

Trandolapril Component—Trandolapril can cause symptomatic hypotension. Like other ACE inhibitors, trandolapril has only rarely been associated with symptomatic hypotension in uncomplicated hypertensive patients. Symptomatic hypotension is most likely to occur in patients who

are salt- or volume-depleted as a result of prolonged treatment with diuretics, dietary salt restriction, dialysis, diarrhea, or vomiting. Volume and/or salt depletion should be corrected before initiating treatment with trandolapril (see **PRECAUTIONS, Drug Interactions**, and **ADVERSE REACTIONS**).

In controlled studies, hypotension was observed in 0.6% of patients receiving any combination of trandolapril and verapamil HCl ER.

In patients with concomitant congestive heart failure, with or without associated renal insufficiency, ACE inhibitor therapy may cause excessive hypotension, which may be associated with oliguria or azotemia, and, rarely, with acute renal failure and death (see **DOSAGE AND ADMINISTRATION**).

If symptomatic hypotension occurs, the patients should be placed in the supine position and, if necessary, normal saline may be administered intravenously. A transient hypotensive response is not a contraindication to further doses; however, lower doses of verapamil HCl ER and/or trandolapril or reduced concomitant diuretic therapy should be considered.

Elevated Liver Enzymes/Hepatic Failure:

Verapamil Component—Elevations of transaminases with and without concomitant elevations in alkaline phosphatase and bilirubin have been reported. Such elevations have sometimes been transient and may disappear even in the face of continued verapamil treatment. Several cases of hepatocellular injury related to verapamil have been proven by rechallenge; half of these had clinical symptoms (malaise, fever, and/or right upper quadrant pain) in addition to elevations of SGOT, SGPT, and alkaline phosphatase.

Trandolapril Component—ACE inhibitors rarely have been associated with a syndrome of cholestatic jaundice, fulminant hepatic necrosis, and death. The mechanism of this syndrome is not understood. Patients receiving ACE inhibitors who develop jaundice should discontinue the ACE inhibitor and receive appropriate medical follow-up.

Liver abnormalities were noted in 3.2% of patients taking any of several combinations of trandolapril/verapamil doses. Periodic monitoring of liver function in patients taking TARKA is therefore prudent.

Accessory Bypass Tract (Wolff-Parkinson-White or Lown-Ganong-Levine Syndromes):

Verapamil Component—Some patients with paroxysmal and/or chronic atrial fibrillation or atrial flutter and a coexisting accessory AV pathway have developed increased antegrade conduction across the accessory pathway bypassing the AV node, producing a very rapid ventricular response or ventricular fibrillation after receiving intravenous verapamil (or digitalis). Although a risk of this occurring with oral verapamil has not been established, such patients receiving oral verapamil may be at risk and its use in these patients is contraindicated (see **CONTRAINDICATIONS**). Treatment is usually DC-cardioversion. Cardioversion has been used safely and effectively after oral verapamil.

Atrioventricular Block:

Verapamil Component—The effect of verapamil on AV conduction and the SA node may lead to asymptomatic first-degree AV block and transient bradycardia, sometimes accompanied by nodal escape rhythms. PR interval prolongation is correlated with verapamil plasma concentrations, especially during the early titration phases of therapy. Higher degrees of AV block, however, are infrequently (0.8%) observed. Marked first-degree block or progressive development to second- or third-degree AV block requires a reduction in dosage or, in rare instances, discontinuation of verapamil HCl and institution of appropriate therapy depending upon the clinical situation.

Patients with Hypertrophic Cardiomyopathy (IHSS):

Verapamil Component—In 120 patients with hypertrophic cardiomyopathy (most of them refractory or intolerant to propranolol) who received therapy with verapamil at doses up to 720 mg/day, a variety of serious adverse effects were seen. Three patients died in pulmonary edema; all had severe left ventricular outflow obstruction and a past history of left ventricular dysfunction. Eight other patients had pulmonary edema and/or severe hypotension; abnormally high (over 20 mmHg) capillary wedge pressure and a marked left ventricular outflow obstruction were present in most of these patients. Sinus bradycardia occurred in 11% of the patients, second-degree AV block in 4% and sinus arrest in 2%. It must be appreciated that this group of patients had a serious disease with a high mortality rate. Most adverse effects responded well to dose reduction and only rarely did verapamil have to be discontinued.

Anaphylactoid and Possibly Related Reactions:

Presumably because angiotensin-converting enzyme inhibitors affect the metabolism of eicosanoids and polypeptides, including endogenous bradykinin, patients receiving ACE inhibitors, including trandolapril may be subject to a variety of adverse reactions, some of them serious.

Angioedema:

Angioedema of the face, extremities, lips, tongue, glottis, and larynx has been reported in patients treated with ACE inhibitors including trandolapril. Symptoms suggestive of

angioedema or facial edema occurred in 0.13% of trandolapril-treated patients. Two of the four cases were life-threatening and resolved without treatment or with medication (corticosteroids). Angioedema associated with laryngeal edema can be fatal. If laryngeal stridor or angioedema of the face, tongue or glottis occurs, treatment with TARKA should be discontinued immediately, the patient treated in accordance with accepted medical care and carefully observed until the swelling disappears. In instances where swelling is confined to the face and lips, the condition generally resolves without treatment; antihistamines may be useful in relieving symptoms **Where there is involvement of the tongue, glottis, or larynx, likely to cause airway obstruction, emergency therapy, including but not limited to subcutaneous epinephrine solution 1:1,000 (0.3 to 0.5 mL) should be promptly administered.** (see **PRECAUTIONS: Information for Patients** and **ADVERSE REACTIONS**).

Anaphylactoid Reactions During Desensitization: Two patients undergoing desensitizing treatment with hymenoptera venom while receiving ACE inhibitors sustained life-threatening anaphylactoid reactions. In the same patients, these reactions did not occur when ACE inhibitors were temporarily withheld, but they reappeared when the ACE inhibitors were inadvertently readministered.

Anaphylactoid Reactions During Membrane Exposure: Anaphylactoid reactions have been reported in patients dialyzed with high-flux membranes and treated concomitantly with an ACE inhibitor. Anaphylactoid reactions have also been reported in patients undergoing low-density lipoprotein apheresis with dextran sulfate absorption.

Neutropenia/Agranulocytosis:

Trandolapril Component—Another ACE inhibitor, captopril, has been shown to cause agranulocytosis and bone marrow depression rarely in patients with uncomplicated hypertension, but more frequently in patients with renal impairment, especially if they also have a collagen-vascular disease such as systemic lupus erythematosus or scleroderma. Available data from clinical trials of trandolapril or TARKA are insufficient to show that trandolapril does not cause agranulocytosis at similar rates. As with other ACE inhibitors, periodic monitoring of white blood cell counts in patients with collagen-vascular disease and/or renal disease should be considered.

Fetal/Neonatal Morbidity and Mortality:

Trandolapril Component—ACE inhibitors can cause fetal and neonatal morbidity and death when administered to pregnant women. Several dozen cases have been reported in the world literature. When pregnancy is detected, ACE inhibitors should be discontinued as soon as possible.

The use of ACE inhibitors during the second and third trimesters of pregnancy has been associated with fetal and neonatal injury, including hypotension, neonatal skull hypoplasia, anuria, reversible or irreversible renal failure, and death. Oligohydramnios has also been reported, presumably resulting from decreased fetal renal function; oligohydramnios in this setting has been associated with fetal limb contractures, craniofacial deformation, and hypoplastic lung development. Prematurity, intrauterine growth retardation, and patent ductus arteriosus have also been reported, although it is not clear whether these occurrences were due to the ACE-inhibitor exposure.

These adverse effects do not appear to have resulted from intrauterine ACE-inhibitor exposure that has been limited to the first trimester. Mothers whose embryos and fetuses are exposed to ACE inhibitors only during the first trimester should be so informed. Nonetheless, when patients become pregnant, physicians should make every effort to discontinue the use of TARKA as soon as possible.

Rarely (probably less often than once in every thousand pregnancies), no alternative to ACE inhibitors will be found. In these rare cases, the mothers should be apprised of the potential hazards to their fetuses, and serial ultrasound examinations should be performed to assess the intra-amniotic environment.

If oligohydramnios is observed, TARKA should be discontinued unless it is considered life-saving for the mother. Contraction stress testing (CST), a non-stress test (NST), or biophysical profiling (BPP) may be appropriate, depending upon the week of pregnancy. Patients and physicians should be aware, however, that oligohydramnios may not appear until after the fetus has sustained irreversible injury.

Infants with histories of in utero exposure to ACE inhibitors should be closely observed for hypotension, oliguria, and hyperkalemia. If oliguria occurs, attention should be directed toward support of blood pressure and renal perfusion. Exchange transfusion or dialysis may be required as a means of reversing hypotension and/or substituting for disordered renal function.

Trandolapril in doses of 0.8 mg/kg/day in rabbits, 100.0 mg/kg/day in rats, and 25 mg/kg/day in cynomolgus monkeys (10, 1,250, and 312 times the maximum projected human dose, respectively, assuming a 50 kg woman) did not produce teratogenic effects.

PRECAUTIONS

Use in Patients with Impaired Hepatic Function:

TARKA has not been evaluated in subjects with impaired hepatic function.

Verapamil Component—Since verapamil is highly metabolized by the liver, it should be administered cautiously to patients with impaired hepatic function. Severe liver dysfunction prolongs the elimination half-life of immediate release verapamil to about 14 to 16 hours; hence, approximately 30% of the dose given to patients with normal liver function should be administered to these patients.

Careful monitoring for abnormal polongation of the PR interval or other signs of excessive pharmacologic effects (see **OVERDOSAGE**) should be carried out.

Trandolapril Component—Trandolapril and trandolaprilat concentrations increase in patients with impaired liver function.

Use in Patients with Impaired Renal Function:

TARKA has not been evaluated in patients with impaired renal function.

Verapamil Component—About 70% of an administered dose of verapamil is excreted as metabolites in the urine. Verapamil is not removed by hemodialysis. Until further data are available, verapamil should be administered cautiously to patients with impaired renal function. These patients should be carefully monitored for abnormal prolongation of the PR interval or other signs of overdosage (see **OVERDOSAGE**).

Trandolapril Component—As a consequence of inhibiting the renin-angiotensin-aldosterone system, changes in renal function may be anticipated in susceptible individuals. In patients with severe heart failure whose renal function may depend on the activity of the renin-angiotensin-aldosterone system, treatment with ACE inhibitors, including trandolapril, may be associated with oliguria and/or progressive azotemia and rarely with acute renal failure and/or death.

In hypertensive patients with unilateral or bilateral renal artery stenosis, increases in blood urea nitrogen and serum creatinine have been observed in some patients following ACE inhibitor therapy. These increases were almost always reversible upon discontinuation of the ACE inhibitor and/or diuretic therapy. In such patients, renal function should be monitored during the first few weeks of therapy.

Some hypertensive patients with no apparent preexisting renal vascular disease have developed increases in blood urea and serum creatinine, usually minor and transient, especially when ACE inhibitors have been given concomitantly with a diuretic. This is more likely to occur in patients with preexisting renal impairment. Dosage reduction and/or discontinuation of any diuretic and/or the ACE inhibitor may be required.

Evaluation of hypertensive patients should always include assessment of renal function (see **DOSAGE AND ADMINISTRATION**).

Use in Patients with Attenuated (Decreased) Neuromuscular Transmission:

Verapamil Component—It has been reported that verapamil decreases neuromuscular transmission in patients with Duchenne's muscular dystrophy, and that verapamil prolongs recovery from the neuromuscular blocking agent vecuronium. It may be necessary to decrease the dosage of verapamil when it is administered to patients with attenuated neuromuscular transmission. (See **PRECAUTIONS—Surgery/Anesthesia**)

Hyperkalemia and potassium-sparing diuretics:

Trandolapril Component—In clinical trials, hyperkalemia (serum potassium > 6.00 mEq/L) occurred in approximately 0.4 percent of hypertensive patients receiving trandolapril and in 0.8% of patients receiving a dose of trandolapril (0.5–8 mg) in combination with a dose of verapamil SR (120–240 mg). In most cases, elevated serum potassium levels were isolated values, which resolved despite continued therapy. None of these patients were discontinued from the trials because of hyperkalemia. Risk factors for the development of hyperkalemia include renal insufficiency, diabetes mellitus, and the concomitant use of potassium-sparing diuretics, potassium supplements, and/or potassium-containing salt substitutes, which should be used cautiously, if at all, with trandolapril (see **PRECAUTIONS, Drug Interactions**).

Cough:

Presumably due to the inhibition of the degradation of endogenous bradykinin, persistent nonproductive cough has been reported with all ACE inhibitors, always resolving after discontinuation of therapy. ACE inhibitor-induced cough should be considered in the differential diagnosis of cough. In controlled trials of trandolapril, cough was present in 2% of trandolapril patients and 0% of patients given placebo. There was no evidence of a relationship to dose.

Surgery/anesthesia:

Trandolapril Component—In patients undergoing major surgery or during anesthesia with agents that produce hypotension, trandolapril will block angiotensin II formation secondary to compensatory renin release. If hypotension occurs and is considered to be due to this mechanism, it can be corrected by volume expansion. (See **PRECAUTIONS—Use in Patients with Attenuated (Decreased) Neuromuscular Transmission**)

Drug Interactions:

Digitalis: Clinical use of verapamil in digitalized patients has shown the combination to be well tolerated if digoxin doses are properly adjusted. Chronic verapamil treatment can increase serum digoxin levels by 50 to 75% during the first week of therapy, and this can result in digoxin toxicity. In patients with hepatic cirrhosis, the influence of verapamil on digoxin kinetics is magnified. Verapamil may reduce total body clearance and extrarenal clearance of digitoxin by 27% and 29%, respectively. Maintenance digoxin doses should be reduced when verapamil is administered, and the patient should be carefully monitored to avoid over- or under-digitalization. Whenever overdigitalization is suspected, the daily dose of digoxin should be reduced or temporarily discontinued. Upon discontinuation of any verapamil-containing regime including TARKA, the patient should be reassessed to avoid underdigitalization. Neither trandolapril nor its metabolites have been found to interact with digoxin.

Lithium: Increased sensitivity to the effects of lithium (neurotoxicity) has been reported during concomitant verapamil-lithium therapy with either no change or an increase in serum lithium levels. Increased serum lithium levels and symptoms of lithium toxicity have been reported in patients receiving concomitant lithium and ACE inhibitor therapy. TARKA and lithium should be coadministered with caution, and frequent monitoring of serum lithium levels is recommended. If a diuretic is also used, the risk of lithium toxicity may be increased.

Cimetidine: The interaction between cimetidine and chronically administered verapamil has not been studied. Variable results on clearance have been obtained in acute studies of healthy volunteers; clearance of verapamil was either reduced or unchanged. Neither trandolapril nor its metabolites have been found to interact with cimetidine.

Beta Blockers: *Verapamil Component*—Concomitant therapy with beta-adrenergic blockers and verapamil may result in additive negative effects on heart rate, atrioventricular conduction, and/or cardiac contractility. The use of verapamil in combination with a beta-blocker should be used only with caution, and close monitoring.

Asymptomatic bradycardia (36 beats/min) with a wandering atrial pacemaker has been observed in a patient receiving concomitant timolol (a beta-adrenergic blocker) eyedrops and oral verapamil.

Antiarrhythmic Agents:

Verapamil Component—Disopyramide—Data on possible interactions between verapamil and disopyramide phosphate are not available. Therefore, disopyramide should not be administered within 48 hours before or 24 hours after verapamil administration.

Flecainide—A study of healthy volunteers showed that the concomitant administration of flecainide and verapamil may have additive effects on myocardial contractility, AV conduction, and repolarization. Concomitant therapy with flecainide and verapamil may result in additive negative inotropic effect and prolongation of atrioventricular conduction.

Quinidine—In a small number of patients with hypertrophic cardiomyopathy (IHSS), concomitant use of verapamil and quinidine resulted in significant hypotension. Until further data are obtained, combined therapy of verapamil and quinidine in patients with hypertrophic cardiomyopathy should probably be avoided.

The electrophysiological effects of quinidine and verapamil on AV conduction were studied in 8 patients. Verapamil significantly counteracted the effects of quinidine on AV conduction. There has been a report of increased quinidine levels during verapamil therapy.

Nitrates — Verapamil has been given concomitantly with short- and long-acting nitrates without any undesirable drug interactions. The pharmacologic profile of both drugs and the clinical experience suggest beneficial interactions.

Other: *Verapamil Component* — Carbamazepine — Verapamil may increase carbamazepine concentrations during combined therapy. This may produce carbamazepine side effects such as diplopia, headache, ataxia, or dizziness.

Rifampin — Therapy with rifampin may markedly reduce oral verapamil bioavailability.

Phenobarbital — Phenobarbital therapy may increase verapamil clearance.

Cyclosporin — Verapamil therapy may increase serum levels of cyclosporin.

Theophylline — Verapamil therapy may inhibit the clearance and increase the plasma levels of theophylline.

Inhalation Anesthetics — Animal experiments have shown that inhalation anesthetics depress cardiovascular activity by decreasing the inward movement of calcium ions. When used concomitantly, inhalation anesthetics and calcium antagonists, such as verapamil, should be titrated carefully to avoid excessive cardiovascular depression.

Neuromuscular Blocking Agents — Clinical data and animal studies suggest that verapamil may potentiate the activity of neuromuscular blocking agents (curare-like and de-

Continued on next page

Tarka—Cont.

polarizing). It may be necessary to decrease the dose of verapamil and/or the dose of the neuromuscular blocking agent when the drugs are used concomitantly.

Concomitant diuretic therapy:

Trandolapril Component — As with other ACE inhibitors, patients on diuretics, especially those on recently instituted diuretic therapy, may occasionally experience an excessive reduction of blood pressure after initiation of therapy with TARKA. The possibility of exacerbation of hypotensive effects with TARKA may be minimized by either discontinuing the diuretic or cautiously increasing salt intake prior to initiation of treatment with TARKA. If it is not possible to discontinue the diuretic, the starting dose of TARKA should be reduced (see **DOSAGE AND ADMINISTRATION**).

Agents increasing serum potassium:

Trandolapril can attenuate potassium loss caused by thiazide diuretics and increase serum potassium when used alone. Use of potassium-sparing diuretics (spironolactone, triamterene, or amiloride), potassium supplements, or potassium-containing salt substitutes concomitantly with ACE inhibitors can increase the risk of hyperkalemia. If concomitant use of such agents is indicated, they should be used with caution and with appropriate monitoring of serum potassium. (See **PRECAUTIONS.**)

Other: *Trandolapril Component* — Neither trandolapril nor its metabolites have been found to interact with furosemide or nifledipine. The anticoagulant effect of warfarin was not significantly changed by trandolapril.

Carcinogenesis, Mutagenesis, Impairment of Fertility:

Verapamil Component — An 18–month toxicity study in rats, at a low multiple (6 fold) of the maximum recommended human dose, and not the maximum tolerated dose, did not suggest a tumorigenic potential. There was no evidence of a carcinogenic potential of verapamil administered in the diet of rats for two years at doses of 10, 35, and 120 mg/kg per day or approximately 1x, 3.5x and 12x, respectively, the maximum recommended human daily dose (480 mg per day or 9.6 mg/kg/day).

Verapamil was not mutagenic in the Ames test in 5 test strains at 3 mg per plate, with or without metabolic activation.

Studies in female rats at daily doses up to 5.5 times (55 mg/kg/day) the maximum recommended human dose did not show impaired fertility. Effects on male fertility have not been determined.

Long-term studies were conducted with oral trandolapril administered by gavage to mice (78 weeks) and rats (104 and 106 weeks). No evidence of carcinogenic potential was seen in mice dosed up to 25 mg/kg/day (85 mg/m^2/day) or rats dosed up to 8 mg/kg/day (60 mg/m^2/day). These doses are 313 and 32 times (mice), and 100 and 23 times (rats) the maximum recommended human daily dose (MRHDD) of 4 mg based on body-weight and body-surface-area, respectively assuming a 50 kg individual. The genotoxic potential of trandolapril was evaluated in the microbial mutagenicity (Ames) test, the point mutation and chromosome aberration assays in Chinese hamster V79 cells, and the micronucleus test in mice. There was no evidence of mutagenic or clastogenic potential in these in vitro and in vivo assays.

Reproduction studies in rats did not show any impairment of fertility at doses up to 100 mg/kg/day (710 mg/m^2/day) of trandolapril, or 1250 and 260 times the MRHDD on the basis of body-weight and body-surface-area, respectively.

Pregnancy; Pregnancy Categories C (first trimester) and D (second and third trimesters). See WARNINGS, Fetal/Neonatal Morbidity and Mortality.

Nursing Mothers: Verapamil is excreted in human milk. Radiolabeled trandolapril or its metabolites are secreted in rat milk. TARKA should not be administered to nursing mothers.

Geriatric Use: In placebo-controlled studies, where 23% of patients receiving TARKA were 65 years and older, and 2.4% were 75 years and older, no overall differences in effectiveness or safety were observed between these patients and younger patients. However, greater sensitivity of some older individual patients cannot be ruled out.

Pediatric Use: The safety and effectiveness of TARKA in children below the age of 18 have not been established.

Animal Pharmacology and/or Animal Toxicology: In chronic animal toxicology studies, verapamil caused lenticular and/or suture line changes at 30 mg/kg/day or greater and frank cataracts at 62.5 mg/kg/day or greater in the beagle dog but not the rat. Development of cataracts due to verapamil has not been reported in man.

ADVERSE REACTIONS

TARKA has been evaluated in over 1,957 subjects and patients. Of these, 541 patients, including 23% elderly patients, participated in U.S. controlled clinical trials, and 251 were studied in foreign controlled clinical trials. In clinical trials with TARKA, no adverse experiences peculiar to this combination drug have been observed. Adverse experiences that have occurred have been limited to those that have been previously reported with verapamil or trandolapril. TARKA has been evaluated for long-term safety in 272 patients treated for 1 year or more. Adverse experiences were usually mild and transient.

Discontinuation of therapy because of adverse events in U.S. placebo-controlled hypertension studies was required in 2.6% and 1.9% of patients treated with TARKA and placebo, respectively.

Adverse experiences occurring in 1% or more of the 541 patients in placebo-controlled hypertension trials who were treated with a range of trandolapril (0.5–8 mg) and verapamil (120–240 mg) combinations are shown below.

[See table below]

Other clinical adverse experiences possibly, probably, or definitely related to drug treatment occurring in 0.3% or more of patients treated with trandolapril/verapamil combinations with or without concomitant diuretic in controlled or uncontrolled trials (N=990) and less frequent, clinically significant events (in italics) include the following.

Cardiovascular: angina, *AV block second degree, bundle branch block*, edema, flushing, hypotension, *myocardial infarction*, palpitations, premature ventricular contractions, nonspecific ST-T changes, near syncope, tachycardia.

Central Nervous System: drowsiness, *hypesthesia, insomnia, loss of balance, paresthesia, vertigo.*

Dermatologic: pruritus, rash.

Emotional, Mental, Sexual States: anxiety, impotence, *abnormal mentation.*

Eye, Ear, Nose, Throat: epistaxis, tinnitus, upper respiratory tract infection, *blurred vision.*

Gastrointestinal: diarrhea, dyspepsia, dry mouth, nausea.

General Body Function: chest pain, malaise, weakness.

Genitourinary: endometriosis, hematuria, nocturia, polyuria, proteinuria.

Hemopoietic: decreased leukocytes, *decreased neutrophils.*

Musculoskeletal System: arthralgias/myalgias, *gout (increased uric acid).*

Pulmonary: dyspnea.

Angioedema: Angioedema has been reported in 3 (0.15%) patients receiving TARKA in the U.S. and foreign studies (N=1,957). Angioedema associated with laryngeal edema may be fatal. If angioedema of the face, extremities, lips, tongue, glottis, and/or larynx occurs, treatment with TARKA should be discontinued and appropriate therapy instituted immediately (see **WARNINGS**).

Hypotension: (See **WARNINGS**). In hypertensive patients, hypotension occurred in 0.6% and near syncope occurred in 0.1%. Hypotension or syncope was a cause for discontinuation of therapy in 0.4% of hypertensive patients.

Treatment of Acute Cardiovascular Adverse Reactions: The frequency of cardiovascular adverse reactions which require therapy is rare, hence, experience with their treatment is limited. Whenever severe hypotension or complete AV block occur following oral administration of TARKA (verapamil component), the appropriate emergency measures should be applied immediately, e.g., intravenously administered isoproterenol HCl, levarterenol bitartrate, atropine (all in the usual doses), or calcium gluconate (10% solution). In patients with hypertrophic cardiomyopathy (IHSS), alpha-adrenergic agents (phenylephrine, metaraminol bitartrate or methoxamine) should be used to maintain blood pressure, and isoproterenol and levarterenol should be avoided. If further support is necessary, inotropic agents (dopamine or dobutamine) may be administered. Actual treatment and dosage should depend on the severity and the clinical situation and the judgment and experience of the treating physician.

Fetal/Neonatal Morbidity and Mortality: See **WARNINGS, Fetal Neonatal Morbidity and Mortality.**

Other adverse experiences (in addition to those in table and listed above) that have been reported with the individual components are listed below.

Verapamil Component:

Cardiovascular: (See **WARNINGS.**) CHF/pulmonary edema, AV block 3°, atrioventricular dissociation, claudication, purpura (vasculitis), syncope.

Digestive System: gingival hyperplasia. Reversible, (upon discontinuation of verapamil) nonobstructive, paralytic ileus has been infrequently reported in association with the use of verapamil.

Hemic and Lymphatic: ecchymosis or bruising.

Nervous System: cerebrovascular accident, confusion, psychotic symptoms, shakiness, somnolence.

Skin: exanthema, hair loss, hyperkeratosis, maculae, sweating, urticaria, Stevens-Johnson syndrome, erythema multiform.

Urogenital: gynecomastia, galactorrhea/hyperprolactinemia, increased urination, spotty menstruation.

Trandolapril Component:

Emotional, Mental, Sexual States: decreased libido.

Gastrointestinal: pancreatitis.

Clinical Laboratory Test Findings

Hematology: (See **WARNINGS.**) Low white blood cells, low neutrophils, low lymphocytes, low platelets.

Serum Electrolytes: Hyperkalemia (See **PRECAUTIONS**), hyponatremia

Renal Function Tests: Increases in creatinine and blood urea nitrogen levels occurred in 1.1 percent and 0.3 percent, respectively, of patients receiving TARKA with or without hydrochlorothiazide therapy. None of these increases required discontinuation of treatment. Increases in these laboratory values are more likely to occur in patients with renal insufficiency or those pretreated with a diuretic and, based on experience with other ACE inhibitors, would be expected to be especially likely in patients with renal artery stenosis. (See **PRECAUTIONS** and **WARNINGS.**)

Liver function tests: Elevations of liver enzymes (SGOT, SGPT, LDH, and alkaline phosphatase) and/or serum bilirubin occurred. Discontinuation for elevated liver enzymes occurred in 0.9 percent of patients. (see **WARNINGS.**)

OVERDOSAGE

No specific information is available on the treatment of overdosage with TARKA.

Verapamil Component—Overdose with verapamil may lead to pronounced hypotension, bradycardia, and conduction system abnormalities (e.g., junctional rhythm with AV dissociation and high degree AV block, including asystole). Other symptoms secondary to hypoperfusion (e.g., metabolic acidosis, hyperglycemia, hyperkalemia, renal dysfunction, and convulsions) may be evident.

Treat all verapamil overdoses as serious and maintain observation for at least 48 hours, preferably under continuous hospital care. Delayed pharmacodynamic consequences may

ADVERSE EVENTS OCCURRING IN ≥ 1% OF TARKA® PATIENTS IN U.S. PLACEBO-CONTROLLED TRIALS

	TARKA (N=541) % Incidence (% Discontinuance)	PLACEBO (N=206) % Incidence (% Discontinuance)
AV Block First Degree	3.9 (0.2)	0.5 (0.0)
Bradycardia	1.8 (0.0)	0.0 (0.0)
Bronchitis	1.5 (0.0)	0.5 (0.0)
Chest Pain	2.2 (0.0)	1.0 (0.0)
Constipation	3.3 (0.0)	1.0 (0.0)
Cough	4.6 (0.0)	2.4 (0.0)
Diarrhea	1.5 (0.2)	1.0 (0.0)
Dizziness	3.1 (0.0)	1.9 (0.5)
Dyspnea	1.3 (0.4)	0.0 (0.0)
Edema	1.3 (0.0)	2.4 (0.0)
Fatigue	2.8 (0.4)	2.4 (0.0)
Headache(s)+	8.9 (0.0)	9.7 (0.5)
Increased Liver Enzymes*	2.8 (0.2)	1.0 (0.0)
Nausea	1.5 (0.2)	0.5 (0.0)
Pain Extremity(ies)	1.1 (0.2)	0.5 (0.0)
Pain Back+	2.2 (0.0)	2.4 (0.0)
Pain Joint(s)	1.7 (0.0)	1.0 (0.0)
Upper Respiratory Tract infection(s)+	5.4 (0.0)	7.8 (0.0)
Upper Respiratory Tract Congestion+	2.4 (0.0)	3.4 (0.0)

* Also includes increase in SGPT, SGOT, Alkaline Phosphatase

+ Incidence of adverse events is higher in Placebo group than TARKA patients

occur with the sustained release formulation. Verapamil is known to decrease gastrointestinal transit time. In cases of overdose, tablets of ISOPTIN SR have occasionally been reported to form concretions within the stomach or intestines. These concretions have not been visible on plain radiographs of the abdomen, and no medical means of gastrointestinal emptying is of proven efficacy in removing them. Endoscopy might reasonably be considered in cases of overdose when symptoms are unusually prolonged. Verapamil cannot be removed by hemodialysis.

Treatment of overdosage should be supportive. Beta adrenergic stimulation or parenteral administration of calcium solutions may increase calcium ion flux across the slow channel, and have been used effectively in treatment of deliberate overdosage with verapamil. The following measures may be considered:

Bradycardia and conduction system abnormalities: Atropine, isoproterenol, and cardiac pacing.

Hypotension: Intravenous fluids, vasopressors (e.g., dopamine, dobutamine), calcium solutions (e.g., 10% calcium chloride solution)

Cardiac failures: Inotropic agents (e.g., isoproterenol, dopamine, dobutamine), diuretics. Asystole should be handled by the usual measures including cardiopulmonary resuscitation.

Trandolapril Component—The oral LD$_{50}$ of trandolapril in mice was 4875 mg/kg in males and 3990 mg/kg in females. In rats, an oral dose of 5000 mg/kg caused low mortality (1 male out of 5; 0 females). In dogs, an oral dose of 1000 mg/kg did not cause mortality and abnormal clinical signs were not observed.

In humans, the most likely clinical manifestation would be symptoms attributable to severe hypotension. Laboratory determinations of serum levels of trandolapril and its metabolites are not widely available, and such determinations have, in any event, no established role in the management of trandolapril overdose. No data are available to suggest that physiological maneuvers (e.g., maneuvers to change pH of the urine) might accelerate elimination of trandolapril and its metabolites. It is not known if trandolapril or trandolaprilat can be usefully removed from the body by hemodialysis.

Angiotensin II could presumably serve as a specific antagonist antidote in the setting of trandolapril overdose, but angiotensin II is essentially unavailable outside of scattered research facilities. Because the hypotensive effect of trandolapril is achieved through vasodilation and effective hypovolemia, it is reasonable to treat trandolapril overdose by infusion of normal saline solution.

DOSAGE AND ADMINISTRATION

The recommended usual dosage range of trandolapril for hypertension is 1 to 4 mg per day administered in a single dose or two divided doses. The recommended usual dosage range of Isoptin-SR for hypertension is 120 to 480 mg per day administered in a single dose or two divided doses.

The hazards (see **WARNINGS**) of trandolapril are generally independent of dose; those of verapamil are a mixture of dose-dependent phenomena (primarily dizziness, AV block, constipation) and dose-independent phenomena, the former much more common than the latter. Therapy with any combination of trandolapril and verapamil will thus be associated with both sets of dose-independent hazards. The dose-dependent side effects of verapamil have not been shown to be decreased by the addition of trandolapril nor visa versa.

Rarely, the dose-independent hazards of trandolapril are serious. To minimize dose-independent hazards, it is usually appropriate to begin therapy with TARKA only after a patient has either (a) failed to achieve the desired antihypertensive effect with one or the other monotherapy at its respective maximally recommended dose and shortest dosing interval, or (b) the dose of one or the other monotherapy cannot be increased further because of the dose-limiting side effects.

Clinical trials with TARKA have explored only once-a-day doses. The antihypertensive effect and or adverse effects of adding 4 mg of trandolapril once-a-day to a dose of 240 mg Isoptin-SR administered twice-a-day has not been studied, nor have the effects of adding as little of 180 mg of Isoptin-SR to 2 mg trandolapril administered twice-a-day been evaluated. Over the dose range of Isoptin-SR 120 to 240 mg once-a-day and trandolapril 0.5 to 8 mg once-a-day, the effects of the combination increase with increasing doses of either component.

Replacement therapy: For convenience, patients receiving trandolapril (up to 8 mg) and verapamil (up to 240 mg) in separate tablets, administered once-a-day, may instead wish to receive tablets of TARKA containing the same component doses. TARKA should be administered with food.

HOW SUPPLIED

TARKA 2/180 mg tablets are supplied as pink, oval, film-coated tablets containing 2 mg trandolapril in an immediate release form and 180 mg verapamil hydrochloride in a sustained release form. The tablet is embossed with the Knoll triangle and 182 on one side and TARKA on the other side.

NDC 0048-5921-80—bottles of 100

TARKA 1/240 mg tablets are supplied as white, oval, film-coated tablets containing 1 mg trandolapril in an immediate release form and 240 mg verapamil hydrochloride in a sustained release form. The tablet is embossed with the Knoll triangle and 241 on one side and TARKA on the other side.

NDC 0048-5912-40—bottles of 100

TARKA 2/240 mg tablets are supplied as gold, oval, film-coated tablets containing 2 mg trandolapril in an immediate release form and 240 mg verapamil hydrochloride in a sustained release form. The tablet is embossed with Knoll triangle and 242 on one side and TARKA on the other side.

NDC 0048-5922-40—bottles of 100

TARKA 4/240 mg tablets are supplied as reddish-brown, oval, film-coated tablets containing 4 mg trandolapril in an immediate release form and 240 mg verapamil hydrochloride in a sustained release form. The tablet is embossed with the Knoll triangle and 244 on one side and TARKA on the other side.

NDC 0048-5942-40—bottles of 100

Dispense in well-closed container with safety closure.

Storage: Store at 15°–25°C (59°–77°F) see USP.

Caution: Federal law prohibits dispensing without prescription.

©1997 Knoll Pharmaceutical Company.

TARKA is a registered trademark of Knoll AG.

Revised: February 1997

Knoll Pharmaceutical Company

3000 Continental Drive – North

Mount Olive, New Jersey 07828-1234

BASF Pharma   0900055-3

Shown in Product Identification Guide, page 319

EDUCATIONAL MATERIAL

"Compliance Counseling In Thyroid Disease Therapy" (2 credits) Home Study Module Pharmacists.

"The Orange Book-Drug Product Equivalence and Pharmacist Liability" (3 credits) Home Study Module Pharmacists.

KOS Pharmaceuticals, Inc.

1001 BRICKELL BAY DRIVE
25TH FLOOR
MIAMI, FL 33131

Direct inquiries to:
For medical information contact:

Drug Information Services
1-888-4-LIPIDS
1-888-454-7437

NIASPAN®   ℞

[nī*ă-span*]

(niacin extended-release tablets)

DESCRIPTION

Niaspan® (niacin extended-release tablets), contain niacin, a B-complex vitamin and antihyperlipidemic agent. Niacin (nicotinic acid, or 3-pyridinecarboxylic acid) is a white, crystalline powder, very soluble in water, with the following structural formula:

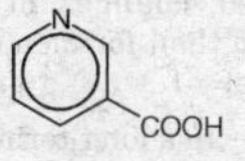

$C_6H_5NO_2$ M.W. = 123.11

Niaspan® is an unscored, off-white tablet for oral administration that contains no color additives and is available in four tablet strengths containing 375, 500, 750, and 1000mg niacin. Niaspan® tablets also contain the inactive ingredients methylcellulose, povidone, and stearic acid.

CLINICAL PHARMACOLOGY

Niacin functions in the body after conversion to nicotinamide adenine dinucleotide (NAD) in the NAD coenzyme system. Niacin (but not nicotinamide) in gram doses reduces total cholesterol (TC), low-density lipoprotein cholesterol (LDL-C) and triglycerides (TG), and increases high-density lipoprotein cholesterol (HDL-C). The magnitude of individual lipid and lipoprotein responses may be influenced by the severity and type of underlying lipid abnormality. The increase in total HDL-C is associated with a shift in the distribution of HDL subfractions (as defined by ultra-centrifugation) with an increase in the HDL$_2$:HDL$_3$ ratio; and an increase in apolipoprotein A1 (Apo A1) content. Niacin

treatment also decreases serum levels of apolipoprotein B-100 (Apo B), the major protein component of the very low-density lipoprotein (VLDL) and LDL fractions, and of lipoprotein a [Lp(a)], a variant form of LDL independently associated with coronary risk.[1] In addition, preliminary reports suggest that niacin causes favorable LDL particle size transformations, although the clinical relevance of this effect requires further investigation. The effect of niacin-induced changes in lipids/lipoproteins on cardiovascular morbidity or mortality in individuals without pre-existing coronary disease has not been established.

Mechanism of Action

The mechanism by which niacin alters lipid profiles has not been well defined. It may involve several actions including partial inhibition of release of free fatty acids from adipose tissue, and increased lipoprotein lipase activity, which may increase the rate of chylomicron triglyceride removal from plasma. Niacin decreases the rate of hepatic synthesis of VLDL and LDL, and does not appear to affect fecal excretion of fats, sterols, or bile acids.

Pharmacokinetics/Metabolism

Absorption

Niacin is rapidly and extensively absorbed (at least 60–76% of dose) when administered orally. To maximize bioavailability and reduce the risk of gastrointestinal (GI) upset, administration of Niaspan® with a low-fat meal or snack is recommended.

Single-dose bioavailability studies have demonstrated that Niaspan® tablet strengths are not interchangeable.

Distribution

Studies using radiolabeled niacin in mice show that niacin and its metabolites concentrate in the liver, kidney and adipose tissue.

Metabolism

The pharmacokinetic profile of niacin is complicated due to rapid and extensive first-pass metabolism, which is species and dose-rate specific. In humans, one pathway is through a simple conjugation step with glycine to form nicotinuric acid (NUA). NUA is then excreted in the urine, although there may be a small amount of reversible metabolism back to niacin. The other pathway results in the formation of nicotinamide adenine dinucleotide (NAD). It is unclear whether nicotinamide is formed as a precursor to, or following the synthesis of, NAD. Nicotinamide is further metabolized to at least N-methylnicotinamide (MNA) and nicotinamide-N-oxide (NNO). MNA is further metabolized to two other compounds, N-methyl-2-pyridone-5-carboxamide (2PY) and N-methyl-4-pyridone-5-carboxamide (4PY). The formation of 2PY appears to predominate over 4PY in humans. At the doses used to treat hyperlipidemia, these metabolic pathways are saturable, which explains the nonlinear relationship between niacin dose and plasma concentrations following multiple-dose Niaspan® administration (Table 1).

Nicotinamide does not have hypolipidemic activity; the activity of the other metabolites is unknown.

Table 1. Mean Steady-State Pharmacokinetic Parameters for Plasma Niacin

Niaspan® dose/day	given as	Niacin Peak Concentration (μg/mL)	Time to Peak (hrs)
1000mg	2x500mg	0.6	5
1500mg	2x750mg	4.9	4
2000mg	2x1000mg	15.5	5

Elimination

Niacin and its metabolites are rapidly eliminated in the urine. Following single and multiple doses, approximately 60–76% of the niacin dose administered as Niaspan® was recovered in urine as niacin and metabolites; up to 12% was recovered as unchanged niacin after multiple dosing. The ratio of metabolites recovered in the urine was dependent on the dose administered.

Special Populations

Hepatic

No studies have been performed. Niaspan® should be used with caution in patients with a past history of liver disease, who consume substantial quantities of alcohol, or have unexplained transaminase elevations. Niaspan® is contraindicated in patients with active liver disease (see WARNINGS).

Renal

There are no data in this population. Niaspan® should be used with caution in patients with renal disease (see PRECAUTIONS).

Gender

Steady-state plasma concentrations of niacin and metabolites after administration of Niaspan® are generally higher in women than in men, with the magnitude of the difference varying with dose and metabolite. Recovery of niacin and metabolites in urine, however, is generally similar for men

Continued on next page

Niaspan—Cont.

and women, indicating that absorption is similar for both genders. The gender differences observed in plasma levels of niacin and its metabolites may be due to gender-specific differences in metabolic rate or volume of distribution. Data from the clinical trials suggest that women have a greater hypolipidemic response than men at equivalent doses of Niaspan®.

Niacin Clinical Studies

The role of LDL-C in atherogenesis is supported by pathological observations, clinical studies, and many animal experiments. Observational epidemiological studies have clearly established that high total or LDL cholesterol and low HDL-C are risk factors for coronary heart disease (CHD). Additionally, elevated levels of Lp(a) have been shown to be independently associated with CHD risk.[1] The efficacy of niacin in improving lipoprotein lipid profiles, either alone or in combination with other lipid-altering drugs, as an adjunct to diet therapy in the treatment of hyperlipoproteinemia has been well documented.

Niacin's ability to reduce mortality and the risk of definite, nonfatal myocardial infarction (MI) has also been assessed in long-term studies. The Coronary Drug Project,[2] completed in 1975, was designed to assess the safety and efficacy of niacin and other lipid-altering drugs in men 30 to 64 years old with a history of myocardial infarction. Over an observation period of 5 years, niacin treatment was associated with a statistically significant reduction in nonfatal, recurrent myocardial infarctions. The incidence of definite, nonfatal MI was 8.9% for the 1,119 patients randomized to nicotinic acid versus 12.2% for the 2,789 patients who received placebo ($p<0.004$). Total mortality was similar in the two groups at 5 years (24.4% with nicotinic acid versus 25.4% with placebo; p=N.S.). At the time of a 15 year follow-up, there were 11% (69) fewer deaths in the niacin group compared to the placebo cohort (52.0% versus 58.2%; $p<0.0004$).[3] However, mortality at 15 years was not an original endpoint of the Coronary Drug Project. In addition, patients had not received niacin for approximately nine years, and confounding variables such as concomitant medication use and medical or surgical treatments were not controlled.

The Cholesterol-Lowering Atherosclerosis Study (CLAS) was a randomized, placebo-controlled, angiographic trial testing combined colestipol and niacin therapy in 162 non-smoking males with previous coronary bypass surgery.[4] The primary, per-subject cardiac endpoint was global coronary artery change score. After 2 years, 61% of patients in the placebo cohort showed disease progression by global change score (n=82), compared with only 38.8% of drug-treated subjects (n=80), when both native arteries and grafts were considered ($p<0.005$); disease regression also occurred more frequently in the drug-treated group (16.2% versus 2.4%; $p<0.002$). In a follow-up to this trial in a subgroup of 103 patients treated for 4 years, again, significantly fewer patients in the drug-treated group demonstrated progression than in the placebo cohort (48% versus 85%, respectively; $p<0.0001$).[5]

The Familial Atherosclerosis Treatment Study (FATS) in 146 men ages 62 and younger with apolipoprotein B levels ≥125 mg/dL, established coronary artery disease, and family histories of vascular disease, assessed change in severity of disease in the proximal coronary arteries by quantitative arteriography.[6] Patients were given dietary counseling and randomized to treatment with either conventional therapy with double placebo (or placebo plus colestipol if the LDL-C was elevated); lovastatin plus colestipol; or niacin plus colestipol. In the conventional therapy group, 46% of patients had disease progression (and no regression) in at least one of nine proximal coronary segments; regression was the only change in 11%. In contrast, progression (as the only change) was seen in only 25% in the niacin plus colestipol group, while regression was observed in 39%. Though not an original endpoint of the trial, clinical events (death, myocardial infarction, or revascularization for worsening angina) occurred in 10 of 52 patients who received conventional therapy, compared with 2 of 48 who received niacin plus colestipol.

The Harvard Atherosclerosis Reversibility Project (HARP) was a randomized placebo-controlled, 2.5 year study of the effect of a stepped-care antihyperlipidemic drug regimen on 91 patients (80 men and 11 women) with coronary heart disease and average baseline TC levels less than 250mg/dL and ratios of TC to HDL-C greater than 4.0.[7] Drug treatment consisted of an HMG-CoA reductase inhibitor administered alone as initial therapy followed by addition of varying dosages of either a slow-release nicotinic acid, cholestyramine, or gemfibrozil. Addition of nicotinic acid to the HMG-CoA reductase inhibitor resulted in further statistically significant mean reductions in total cholesterol, LDL-C, and triglycerides, as well as a further increase in HDL-C in a majority of patients (40 of 44 patients). The ratios of total cholesterol to HDL-C and LDL-C to HDL-C were also significantly reduced by this combination drug regimen (see WARNINGS, *Skeletal Muscle*).

Table 2. Lipid Response to Niaspan® Therapy

		Mean Percent Change from Baseline to Week 16*							
	n	TC	LDL-C	HDL-C	TC/HDL-C	TG	Lp(a)	Apo B	Apo A1
Niaspan® 1000mg q hs	41	-3	-5	+18	-17	-21	-13	-6	+9
Niaspan® 2000mg q hs	41	-10	-14	+22	-25	-28	-27	-16	+8
Placebo	40	0	-1	+4	-3	0	0	+1	+3
Niaspan® 1500mg q hs	76	-8	-12	+20	-20	-13	-15	-12	+8
Placebo	73	+2	+1	+2	+1	+12	+2	+1	+2

n = number of patients at baseline;
* Mean percent change from baseline for all Niaspan® doses was significantly different ($p<0.05$) from placebo for all lipid parameters shown except Apo A1 at 2000mg.

Table 3. Lipid Response in Dose-Escalation Study

		Mean Percent Change from Baseline*							
	(n)	TC	LDL-C	HDL-C	TC/HDL-C	TG	Lp(a)	Apo B	Apo A1
Placebo‡ q hs	(44)	-2	-1	+5	-7	-6	-5	-2	+4
Niaspan®	(87)								
500mg q hs		-2	-3	+10	-10	-5	-3	-2	+5
1000mg q hs		-5	-9	+15	-17	-11	-12	-7	+8
1500mg q hs		-11	-14	+22	-26	-28	-20	-15	+10
2000mg q hs		-12	-17	+26	-29	-35	-24	-16	+12

n = number of patients enrolled;
‡ Placebo data shown are after 24 weeks of placebo treatment.
* For all Niaspan® doses except 500mg, mean percent change from baseline was significantly different ($p<0.05$) from placebo for all lipid parameters shown except Lp(a) and Apo A1 which were significantly different from placebo starting with 1500mg and 2000mg, respectively.

Table 4. Effect of Gender on Niaspan® Dose Response

Niaspan®		Mean Percent Change from Baseline							
Dose	n (M/F)	LDL-C M	LDL-C F	HDL-C M	HDL-C F	TG M	TG F	Apo B M	Apo B F
500mg q hs	50/37	-2	-5	+11	+8	-3	-9	-1	-5
1000mg q hs	76/52	-6*	-11*	+14	+20	-10	-20	-5*	-10*
1500mg q hs	104/59	-12	-16	+19	+24	-17	-28	-13	-15
2000mg q hs	75/53	-15	-18	+23	+26	-30	-36	-16	-16

n = Number of male/female patients enrolled.
* Percent change significantly different between genders ($p<0.05$).

Niaspan® Clinical Studies

In two randomized, double-blind, parallel, multi-center, placebo-controlled trials, Niaspan® dosed at 1000, 1500 or 2000mg daily at bedtime with a low-fat snack for 16 weeks (including 4 weeks of dose escalation) favorably altered lipid profiles compared to placebo (Table 2). Women appeared to have a greater response than men at each Niaspan® dose level (see *Gender Effect*, below).

[See table 2 above]

In a double-blind, multi-center, forced dose-escalation study, monthly 500mg increases in Niaspan® dose resulted in incremental reductions of approximately 5% in LDL-C and Apo B levels in the daily dose range of 500mg through 2000mg (Table 3). Women again tended to have a greater response to Niaspan® than men (see *Gender Effect*, below).

[See table 3 above]

Gender Effect: Combined data from the three placebo-controlled Niaspan® studies suggest that, at each Niaspan® dose level studied, changes in lipid concentrations are greater for women than for men (Table 4).

[See table 4 above]

Long-term Study. In a long-term open-label study, patients received Niaspan® in doses titrated to individual response and tolerance. An HMG-CoA reductase inhibitor or a bile acid sequestrant (BAS) was added to Niaspan® therapy for patients whose response to Niaspan® alone (usually at 2000mg q hs) was insufficient, or who would not tolerate higher niacin doses. Preliminary data from 48 and 96 weeks of treatment (Table 5) suggest combination therapy enhanced total cholesterol and LDL-C response (see WARNINGS, *Skeletal Muscle*).

[See table 5 at top of next page]

INDICATIONS AND USAGE

Therapy with lipid-altering agents should be only one component of multiple risk factor intervention in individuals at significantly increased risk for atherosclerotic vascular disease due to hypercholesterolemia. Niacin therapy is indicated as an adjunct to diet when the response to a diet restricted in saturated fat and cholesterol and other nonpharmacologic measures alone has been inadequate (see also the NCEP treatment guidelines[8]). Prior to initiating therapy with niacin, secondary causes for hypercholesterolemia (e.g., poorly controlled diabetes mellitus, hypothyroidism, nephrotic syndrome, dysproteinemias, obstructive liver disease, other drug therapy, alcoholism) should be excluded, and a lipid profile obtained to measure total cholesterol, HDL-C, and triglycerides.

1. Niaspan® is indicated as an adjunct to diet for reduction of elevated total cholesterol, LDL cholesterol, Apo B and triglyceride levels in adult patients with primary hypercholesterolemia and mixed dyslipidemia (Types IIa and IIb; Table 6), when the response to an appropriate diet has been inadequate. The independent effect of niacin-induced lowering of triglyceride levels on the risk for coronary artery disease morbidity and mortality has not been determined.
2. Niaspan® in combination with a bile-acid binding resin is indicated as an adjunct to diet for reduction of elevated total and LDL cholesterol levels in adult patients with primary hypercholesterolemia (Type IIa; Table 6), when the response to an appropriate diet, or diet plus monotherapy, has been inadequate.
3. Niacin is also indicated as adjunctive therapy for treatment of adult patients with very high serum triglyceride levels (Types IV and V hyperlipidemia; Table 6) who present a risk of pancreatitis and who do not respond adequately to a determined dietary effort to control them. Such patients typically have serum triglyceride levels over 2000 mg/dL and have elevations of VLDL cholesterol as well as fasting chylomicrons (Type V hyperlipidemia; Table 6). Patients who consistently have total serum or plasma triglycerides below 1000 mg/dL are unlikely to develop pancreatitis. Therapy with niacin may be considered for those patients with triglyceride elevations between 1000 and 2000 mg/dL who have a history of pancreatitis or of recurrent abdominal pain typical of pancreatitis. Some Type IV patients with triglycerides under 1000 mg/dL may, through dietary or alcohol indiscretion, convert to a Type V pattern with massive triglyceride elevations accompanying fasting chylomicronemia, but the influence of niacin therapy on risk of pancreatitis in such situations has not been adequately studied. Drug therapy is not indicated for patients with Type I hyperlipoproteinemia, who have elevations of chylomicrons and plasma triglycerides, but who have normal levels of VLDL cholesterol. Inspection of plasma refrigerated for 14 hours is helpful in distinguishing Type I, IV, and V hyperlipoproteinemia.[9]

Table 5. Niaspan® Efficacy with Combination Therapy

Treatment	Duration	n	TC	LDL-C	HDL-C	TC/HDL-C	TG	Lp(a)*	Apo B*
					Mean Percent Change from Baseline				
Niaspan® Alone	Baseline	185	—	—	—	—	—	—	—
	48 weeks	101	-11	-18	+29	-29	-24	-36	-15
	96 weeks	74	-10	-18	+32	-30	-27	na	na
Niaspan® & HMG-CoA	Baseline	53	—	—	—	—	—	—	—
	48 weeks	45	-23	-32	+26	-38	-30	-19	-26
	96 weeks	37	-24	-32	+25	-38	-32	na	na
Niaspan® & BAS	Baseline	16	—	—	—	—	—	—	—
	48 weeks	15	-11	-20	+36	-33	-13	-24	-19
	96 weeks	7	-15	-28	+31	-34	+5	na	na

Note: Median Niaspan® dose was 2000mg q hs in each dose group. Mean duration of HMG-CoA combination therapy was approximately 47 weeks. Mean duration of BAS combination therapy was approximately 40 weeks.
* number of patients (n) are up to 33% lower at baseline and at 48 weeks; na = data are not available

Table 7. Treatment-Emergent Adverse Events by Dose Level in ≥5% of Patients,
Events Considered At Least Remotely Related to Study Medication

	Placebo-Controlled Studies Niaspan® Treatment†						
		Recommended Daily Maintenance Doses				Greater Than Recommended Daily Doses	
	Placebo (n=157) %	500mg‡ (n=87) %	1000mg (n=110) %	1500mg (n=136) %	2000mg (n=95) %	2500mg‡ (n=49) %	3000 mg‡ (n=46) %
Headache	15	5*	9	11	8	4*	4
Pain	3	1	2	5	3	0	2
Pain, Abdominal	3	3	2	3	5	0	0
Diarrhea	8	6	7	6	8	10	11
Dyspepsia	8	2	4	5	5	6	0
Nausea	4	2	5	3	8	10	4
Vomiting	2	2	2	3	8*	8	2
Rhinitis	7	2	5	4	3	0	0
Pruritus	1	6	<1	3	1	0	0
Rash	<1	5	5	4	0	0	0

Note: Percentages are calculated from the total number of patients in each column. AEs are reported at the lowest dose where they occurred.
† Pooled results from placebo-controlled studies; for Niaspan®, n=245 and mean treatment duration = 17 weeks. Number of Niaspan® patients (n) are not additive across doses.
‡ The 500mg, 2500mg and 3000mg/day doses are outside the recommended daily maintenance dosing range; see DOSAGE AND ADMINISTRATION.
* Significantly different from placebo at $p \leq 0.05$; Chi-square test (cell sizes>5), Fishers's Exact test (cell sizes≤5). In general, the incidence of adverse events was higher in women compared to men.

4. In patients with a history of myocardial infarction and hypercholesterolemia, niacin is indicated to reduce the risk of recurrent nonfatal myocardial infarction.
5. In patients with a history of coronary artery disease (CAD) and hypercholesterolemia, niacin, in combination with a bile acid binding resin, is indicated to slow progression or promote regression of atherosclerotic disease.

Table 6. Classification of Hyperlipoproteinemias

Type	Lipoproteins Elevated	Lipid Elevations	
		Major	Minor
I (rare)	chylomicrons	TG	$\uparrow \rightarrow$TC
IIa	LDL	TC	—
IIb	LDL, VLDL	TC	TG
III (rare)	IDL	TC/TG	—
IV	VLDL	TG	$\uparrow \rightarrow$TC
V (rare)	chylomicrons, VLDL	TG	$\uparrow \rightarrow$TC

TC = total cholesterol; TG = triglycerides; LDL = low-density lipoprotein;
VLDL = very low-density lipoprotein; IDL = intermediate-density lipoprotein
$\uparrow \rightarrow$ = increased or no change

CONTRAINDICATIONS

Niaspan® is contraindicated in patients with a known hypersensitivity to niacin or any component of this medication, significant or unexplained hepatic dysfunction, active peptic ulcer disease, or arterial bleeding.

WARNINGS

Niaspan® preparations should not be substituted for equivalent doses of immediate-release (crystalline) niacin. For patients switching from immediate-release niacin to Niaspan®, therapy with Niaspan® should be initiated with low doses (i.e., 375 mg q hs) and the Niaspan® dose should then be titrated to the desired therapeutic response (see DOSAGE AND ADMINISTRATION).

Liver Dysfunction

Cases of severe hepatic toxicity, including fulminant hepatic necrosis, have occurred in patients who have substituted sustained-release (modified-release, timed-release) niacin products for immediate-release (crystalline) niacin at equivalent doses.

Niaspan® should be used with caution in patients who consume substantial quantities of alcohol and/or have a past history of liver disease. Active liver diseases or unexplained transaminase elevations are contraindications to the use of Niaspan®.

Niacin preparations, like some other lipid-lowering therapies, have been associated with abnormal liver tests. In three placebo-controlled clinical trials involving titration to final daily Niaspan® doses ranging from 500–3000mg, 245 patients received Niaspan® for a mean duration of 17 weeks. No patient with normal serum transaminase levels (AST, ALT) at baseline experienced elevations to more than 3 times the upper limit of normal (ULN) during treatment with Niaspan®. In these studies, fewer than 1% (2/245) of Niaspan® patients discontinued due to transaminase elevations greater than two times the ULN.

An ongoing, long-term extension study involving more than 700 patients (617 who have been treated for a mean duration of 50 weeks) showed that less than 1% (4/717) of Niaspan®-treated patients with normal serum transaminase levels at baseline experienced elevations greater than 3× ULN (one of the four was receiving concomitant HMG-CoA reductase inhibitor therapy).

In the placebo-controlled clinical trials and the long-term extension study, elevations in transaminases did not appear to be related to treatment duration; elevations in AST levels did appear to be dose related. Transaminase elevations were reversible upon discontinuation of Niaspan®.

Liver tests should be performed on all patients during therapy with Niaspan®. Serum transaminase levels, including AST and ALT (SGOT and SGPT), should be monitored before treatment begins, every six weeks to twelve weeks for the first year, and periodically thereafter (e.g., at approximately 6-month intervals). Special attention should be paid to patients who develop elevated serum transaminase levels, and in these patients, measurements should be repeated promptly and then performed more frequently. If the transaminase levels show evidence of progression, particularly if they rise to three times the upper limit of normal and are persistent, or if they are associated with symptoms of nausea, fever, and/or malaise, the drug should be discontinued.

Skeletal Muscle

Rare cases of rhabdomyolysis have been associated with concomitant administration of lipid-altering doses (≥1 g/day) of niacin and HMG-CoA reductase inhibitors. Physicians contemplating combined therapy with HMG-CoA reductase inhibitors and Niaspan® should carefully weigh the potential benefits and risks and should carefully monitor patients for any signs and symptoms of muscle pain, tenderness, or weakness, particularly during the initial months of therapy and during any periods of upward dosage titration of either drug. Periodic serum creatinine phosphokinase (CPK) and potassium determinations should be considered in such situations, but there is no assurance that such monitoring will prevent the occurrence of severe myopathy.

PRECAUTIONS

General

Before instituting therapy with Niaspan®, an attempt should be made to control hyperlipidemia with appropriate diet, exercise, and weight reduction in obese patients, and to treat other underlying medical problems (see INDICATIONS AND USAGE).

Patients with a past history of jaundice, hepatobiliary disease, or peptic ulcer should be observed closely during Niaspan® therapy. Frequent monitoring of liver function tests and blood glucose should be performed to ascertain that the drug is producing no adverse effects on these organ systems. Diabetic patients may experience a dose-related rise in glucose intolerance, the clinical significance of which is unclear. Diabetic or potentially diabetic patients should be observed closely. Adjustment of diet and/or hypoglycemic therapy may be necessary.

Caution should also be used when Niaspan® is used in patients with unstable angina or in the acute phase of myocardial infarction, particularly when such patients are also receiving vasoactive drugs such as nitrates, calcium channel blockers, or adrenergic blocking agents.

Elevated uric acid levels have occurred with Niaspan® therapy, therefore Niaspan® should be used with caution in patients predisposed to gout.

Niaspan® has been associated with small but statistically significant dose-related reductions in platelet count (mean of -11% with 2000mg). In addition, Niaspan® has been associated with small but statistically significant increases in prothrombin time (mean of approximately +4%); accordingly, patients undergoing surgery should be carefully evaluated. Caution should be observed when Niaspan® is administered concomitantly with anticoagulants; prothrombin time and platelet counts should be monitored closely in such patients.

In placebo-controlled trials, Niaspan® has been associated with small but statistically significant, dose-related reductions in phosphorus levels (mean of -13% with 2000mg). Although these reductions were transient, phosphorus levels should be monitored periodically in patients at risk for hypophosphatemia.

Niacin is rapidly metabolized by the liver, and excreted through the kidneys. Niaspan® is contraindicated in patients with significant or unexplained hepatic dysfunction (see CONTRAINDICATIONS and WARNINGS) and should be used with caution in patients with renal dysfunction.

Information for Patients

Patients should be advised:
— to take Niaspan® at bedtime, after a low-fat snack. Administration on an empty stomach is not recommended;
— to carefully follow the prescribed dosing regimen, including the recommended titration schedule, in order to minimize side effects (see DOSAGE AND ADMINISTRATION);
— that flushing is a common side effect of niacin therapy that usually subsides after several weeks of consistent niacin use. Flushing may last for several hours after dosing and will, by taking Niaspan® at bedtime, most likely occur during sleep;
— that taking aspirin (approximately 30 minutes before taking Niaspan®) or a non-steroidal anti-inflammatory drug (e.g., ibuprofen) may minimize flushing;
— to avoid ingestion of alcohol or hot drinks around the time of Niaspan® administration, to minimize flushing;
— that if Niaspan® therapy is discontinued for an extended length of time, their physician should be contacted prior to re-starting therapy; re-titration is recommended (see DOSAGE AND ADMINISTRATION; Table 8);

Continued on next page

Niaspan—Cont.

— to notify their physician if they are taking vitamins or other nutritional supplements containing niacin or related compounds such as nicotinamide (see Drug Interactions);
— that Niaspan® tablets should not be broken, crushed or chewed, but should be swallowed whole.

Drug Interactions

HMG-CoA Reductase Inhibitors: see WARNINGS, *Skeletal Muscle.*

Antihypertensive Therapy: Niacin may potentiate the effects of ganglionic blocking agents and vasoactive drugs resulting in postural hypotension.

Aspirin: Concomitant aspirin may decrease the metabolic clearance of nicotinic acid. The clinical relevance of this finding is unclear.

Bile-Acid Sequestrants: An *in vitro* study was carried out investigating the niacin-binding capacity of colestipol and cholestyramine. About 98% of available niacin was bound to colestipol, with 10 to 30% binding to cholestyramine. These results suggest that 4–6 hours, or as great an interval as possible, should elapse between the ingestion of bile acid-binding resins and the administration of Niaspan®.

Other: Concomitant alcohol or hot drinks may increase the side effects of flushing and pruritus and should be avoided around the time of Niaspan® ingestion. Vitamins or other nutritional supplements containing large doses of niacin or related compounds such as nicotinamide may potentiate the adverse effects of Niaspan®.

Drug/Laboratory Test Interactions

Niacin may produce false elevations in some fluorometric determinations of plasma or urinary catecholamines. Niacin may also give false-positive reactions with cupric sulfate solution (Benedict's reagent) in urine glucose tests.

Carcinogenesis, Mutagenesis, Impairment of Fertility

Niacin administered to mice for a lifetime as a 1% solution in drinking water was not carcinogenic. The mice in this study received approximately 6 to 8 times a human dose of 3000 mg/day as determined on a mg/m^2 basis. Niacin was negative for mutagenicity in the Ames test. No studies on impairment of fertility have been performed. No studies have been conducted with Niaspan® regarding carcinogenesis, mutagenesis, or impairment of fertility.

Pregnancy

Pregnancy Category C.
Animal reproduction studies have not been conducted with niacin or with Niaspan®. It is also not known whether niacin at doses typically used for lipid disorders can cause fetal harm when administered to pregnant women or whether it can affect reproductive capacity. If a women receiving niacin for primary hypercholesterolemia (Types IIa or IIb) becomes pregnant, the drug should be discontinued. If a women being treated with niacin for hypertriglyceridemia (Types IV or V) conceives, the benefits and risks of continued therapy should be assessed on an individual basis.

Nursing Mothers

Niacin has been reported to be excreted in human milk. Because of the potential for serious adverse reactions in nursing infants from lipid-altering doses of nicotinic acid, a decision should be made whether to discontinue nursing or to discontinue the drug, taking into account the importance of the drug to the mother. No studies have been conducted with Niaspan® in nursing mothers.

Pediatric Use

Safety and effectiveness of niacin therapy in pediatric patients (≤16 years) have not been established. No studies in patients under 21 years of age have been conducted with Niaspan®.

ADVERSE REACTIONS

Niaspan® is generally well tolerated; adverse reactions have been mild and transient. In the placebo-controlled clinical trials, flushing episodes (i.e., warmth, redness, itching, and/or tingling) were the most common treatment-emergent adverse events (reported by as many as 88% of patients) for Niaspan®. In these studies, fewer than 6% (14/245) of Niaspan® patients discontinued due to flushing. In comparisons of immediate-release (IR) niacin and Niaspan®, although the proportion of patients who flushed was similar, fewer flushing episodes were reported by patients who received Niaspan®. Following 4 weeks of maintenance therapy at daily doses of 1500mg, the incidence of flushing over the 4-week period averaged 8.56 events per patient for IR niacin versus 1.88 following Niaspan®.

Other adverse events occurring in 5% or greater of patients treated with Niaspan®, at least remotely related to Niaspan®, are shown in Table 7 below.
[See table 7 on previous page]
The following adverse events have also been reported during treatment with niacin products.
Cardiovascular: atrial fibrillation and other cardiac arrhythmias; orthostasis; hypotension
Gastrointestinal: activation of peptic ulcers and peptic ulceration; jaundice
Skin: hyper-pigmentation; acanthosis nigricans; dry skin
Metabolic: decreased glucose tolerance; gout
Eye: toxic amblyopia, cystoid macular edema
Other: migraine
Clinical Laboratory Abnormalities

Chemistry: Elevations in serum transaminases (see WARNINGS—*Liver Dysfunction*), LDH, fasting glucose, uric acid, total bilirubin, and amylase; reductions in phosphorus

Hematology: Slight reductions in platelet counts and prolongation in prothrombin time (see WARNINGS)

DRUG ABUSE AND DEPENDENCE

Niacin is a non-narcotic drug. It has no known addiction potential in humans.

OVERDOSAGE

Supportive measures should be undertaken in the event of an overdosage.

DOSAGE AND ADMINISTRATION

Niaspan® should be taken at bedtime, after a low-fat snack, and doses should be individualized according to patient response. Therapy with Niaspan® must be initiated with the titration starter pack in order to reduce the incidence and severity of side effects which may occur during early therapy. The recommended dose escalation is shown in Table 8 below.
[See table 8 below]
Maintenance Dose:
The daily dosage of Niaspan® should not be increased by more than 500mg in any 4-week period. The recommended maintenance dose is 1000mg (two 500mg tablets) to 2000mg (two 1000mg tablets) once daily at bedtime. Doses greater than 2000mg daily are not recommended. Women may respond at lower Niaspan® doses than men (see CLINICAL PHARMACOLOGY, *Gender Effect*).

If lipid response to Niaspan® alone is insufficient, or if higher doses of Niaspan® are not well tolerated, some patients may benefit from combination therapy with a bile-acid binding resin or an HMG-CoA reductase inhibitor. (see WARNINGS, PRECAUTIONS, Drug Interactions, Concomitant Therapy below, and CLINICAL PHARMACOLOGY, Niaspan® Clinical Studies)

Flushing of the skin (see ADVERSE REACTIONS) may be reduced in frequency or severity by pretreatment with aspirin (taken 30 minutes prior to Niaspan® dose) or non-steroidal anti-inflammatory drugs. Tolerance to this flushing develops rapidly over the course of several weeks. Flushing, pruritus, and gastrointestinal distress are also greatly reduced by slowly increasing the dose of niacin and avoiding administration on an empty stomach.

Equivalent doses of Niaspan® should **not** be substituted for sustained-release (modified-release, timed-release) niacin preparations or immediate-release (crystalline) niacin (see WARNINGS). Patients previously receiving other niacin products should be started with the recommended Niaspan® titration schedule (see Table 8), and the dose should subsequently be individualized based on patient response. Single-dose bioavailability studies have demonstrated that Niaspan® tablet strengths are not interchangeable.

If Niaspan® therapy is discontinued for an extended period, reinstitution of therapy should include a titration phase (see Table 8).

Niaspan® tablets should be taken whole and should not be broken, crushed or chewed before swallowing.

Concomitant Therapy

Preliminary evidence suggests that the lipid-lowering effects of Niaspan® on total and LDL-C are enhanced with an HMG-CoA reductase inhibitor, e.g., lovastatin, pravastatin, simvastatin, and fluvastatin. Additive effects on LDL-C are also seen when niacin is combined with bile-acid binding resins. (see WARNINGS and PRECAUTIONS, Drug Interactions)

Dosage in Patients with Renal or Hepatic Insufficiency

Use of Niaspan® in patients with renal or hepatic insufficiency has not been studied. Niaspan® is contraindicated in patients with significant or unexplained hepatic dysfunction. Niaspan® should be used with caution in patients with renal insufficiency (see WARNINGS, PRECAUTIONS).

HOW SUPPLIED

Niaspan® is an unscored, off-white capsule-shaped tablet containing either 375, 500, 750, or 1000mg of niacin in an extended-release formulation. Tablets are debossed KOS on one side and the tablet strength (375, 500, 750 or 1000) on the other side. Tablets are supplied in a 21-day starter pack, and in bottles of 100 as shown below.

500mg tablets: bottles of 100—NDC# 60598-001-01
750mg tablets: bottles of 100—NDC# 60598-002-01
1000mg tablets: bottles of 100—NDC# 60598-003-01
Titration Starter pack: contains seven 375mg Niaspan® tablets for Days 1–7, seven 500mg Niaspan® tablets for Days 8–14, and seven 750mg Niaspan® tablets for Days 15–21—NDC# 60598-004-21 for commercial use; NDC# 60598-004-05 for professional sample pack
Store at room temperature, (20–25°C or 68–77°F).
CAUTION: Federal law prohibits dispensing without prescription.

REFERENCES

1. Boston AG et al. *JAMA.* 1996;276:544-548.
2. The Coronary Drug Project Research Group. *JAMA.* 1975;231:360-381.
3. Canner PL et al. *J Am Coll Cardiol.* 1986;8(6):1245-1255.
4. Blankenhorn DH et al. *JAMA.* 1987;257(23):3233-3240.
5. Cashin-Hemphill L et al. *JAMA.* 1990;264(23):3013-3017.
6. Brown G et al. *NEJM.* 1990;323:1289-1298.
7. Pastemak RC et al. *Annals Int Med.* 1996;125:529-540.
8. Summary of the Second Report of the National Cholesterol Education Program (NCEP) Expert Panel on Detection, Evaluation, and Treatment of High Blood Cholesterol in Adults (Adult Treatment Panel II), *JAMA.* 1993;269:3015-3023.
9. Nikkila EA. In: *The Metabolic Basis of Inherited Disease.* 5th ed. 1983;chap 30:622-642.

Manufactured by:
Kos Pharmaceuticals, Inc.
Miami, FL 33131

0897 ©1997 Kos Pharmaceuticals, Inc., Miami, FL 33131, USA

Shown in Product Identification Guide, page 319

Table 8. Recommended Dosing

	Week(s)	Niaspan® Dosage		Daily Niacin Dose	
INITIAL TITRATION SCHEDULE	1	Niaspan® 375mg	1 tablet at bedtime	375mg	TITRATION STARTER PACK
	2	Niaspan® 500mg	1 tablet at bedtime	500mg	
	3	Niaspan® 750mg	1 tablet at bedtime	750mg	
	4 - 7	Niaspan® 500mg	2 tablets at bedtime	1000mg	
	*	Niaspan® 750mg	2 tablets at bedtime	1500mg	
	*	Niaspan® 1000mg	2 tablets at bedtime	2000mg	

* After Week 7, titrate to patient response and tolerance. If response to 1000mg daily is inadequate, increase dose to 1500mg daily; may subsequently increase dose to 2000mg daily. Daily dose should not be increased more than 500mg in a 4-week period, and doses above 2000mg daily are not recommended. Women may respond at lower doses than men.

For information on over-the-counter drugs, consult **PDR For Nonprescription Drugs.**

Kramer Laboratories, Inc.
8778 S.W. 8TH STREET
MIAMI, FL 33174

Direct Inquiries to:
8778 S.W. 8th Street
Miami, FL 33174
(800) 824-4894

For Medical Information Contact:
In Emergencies:
Professional Director
(800) 824-4894

CHARCOAL PLUS DS® ENTERIC COATED OTC
250 mg Activated Charcoal Tablets

After every meal

RECOMMENDED CONSUMPTION
Two enteric coated tablets after eating as needed but do not exceed 20 tablets per day. Swallow the tablets whole. Do not chew.

CAUTION
If taking medication allow an interval of 1 hour between ingestion of this product and ingestion of any medication.

HOW SUPPLIED
Bottles of 120 tablets and 36 tablets.

WARNING
Activated Charcoal may cause darkening of the stool.

HALFPRIN®   OTC
162 mg. Enteric Coated Aspirin
Aspirin For Suspected Acute MI

DESCRIPTION
Halfprin® is the only 162 mg. enteric coated aspirin available for the indicated use to reduce the risk of vascular mortality in people with a suspected acute myocardial infarction (MI). The Halfprin® 162 mg. aspirin has been determined to be the indicated dose to reduce the risk of fatal and nonfatal cardiovascular and cerebrovascular events in subjects with a suspected acute MI.

INDICATIONS
Suspected Acute MI
The use of aspirin in patients with a suspected acute MI is supported by the results of a large, multicenter 2×2 factorial study of 17,187 subjects with suspected acute MI.(1). Subjects were randomized within 24 hours of the onset of symptoms so that 8,587 subjects received oral aspirin (162.5 milligrams, enteric-coated) daily for 1 month (the first dose crushed, sucked, or chewed) and 8,600 received oral placebo. Of the subjects 8,592 were also randomized to receive a single dose of streptokinase (1.5 million units) infused intravenously for about 1 hour, and 8,595 received a placebo infusion. Thus, 4,295 subject received aspirin plus placebo, 4,300 received streptokinase plus placebo, 4,292 received aspirin plus streptokinase, and 4,300 received double placebo.
Vascular mortality (attributed to cardiac, cerebral, hemorrhagic, other vascular, or unknown causes) occurred in 9.4 percent of subjects in the aspirin group and in 11.8 percent of subjects in the oral placebo group in the 35-day follow up. This represents an absolute reduction of 2.4 percent in the mean 35-day vascular mortality attributable to aspirin and a 23 percent reduction in odds of vascular death.
Significant absolute reductions in mortality and corresponding reductions in specific clinical events favoring aspirin were found for reinfarction (1.5 percent absolute reduction, 45 percent odds reduction, 2p<0.00001), cardiac arrest (1.2 percent absolute reduction, 14.2 percent odds reduction, 2p <0.01), and total stroke (0.4 percent absolute reduction, 41.5 percent odds reduction, 2p<0.01). The effect of aspirin over and above its effect on mortality was evidenced by small, but significant, reductions in vascular morbidity in those subjects who were discharged.
The beneficial effects of aspirin on mortality were present with or without streptokinase infusion. Aspirin reduced vascular mortality from 10.4 to 8.0 percent for days 0 to 35 in subjects given streptokinase and reduced vascular mortality from 13.2 to 10.7 percent in the effects of aspirin and thrombolytic therapy with streptokinase in this study were approximately additive. Subjects who received the combination of streptokinase infusion and daily aspirin had significantly lower vascular mortality at 35 days than those who received either active treatment alone (combination 8.0 percent, aspirin 10.7 percent, streptokinase 10.4 percent, and no treatment 13.2 percent. While this study demonstrated that aspirin has an additive benefit in patients given streptokinase, there is no reason to restrict its use to that specific thrombolytic.

ADVERSE REACTIONS
Gastrointestinal Reactions
Doses of 1,000 milligrams per day of aspirin caused gastrointestinal symptoms and bleeding that in some cases were clinically significant. In the Aspirin Myocardial Infarction Study (AMIS) (4) with 4,500 post infarction subjects, the percentage incidences of gastrointestinal symptoms for the aspirin (1,000 milligrams of a standard, solid—tablet formulation) and placebo-treated subjects, respectively, were: Stomach pain (14.5 percent, 4.4 percent); heartburn (11.9 percent, 4.8 percent); nausea and/or vomiting (7.6 percent, 2.1 percent); hospitalization for gastrointestinal disorder (4.8 percent, 3.5 percent). Symptoms and signs of gastrointestinal irritation were not significantly increased in subjects treated for instable angina with 325 milligrams buffered aspirin in solution.

Bleeding
In the AMIS and other trails, aspirin treated subjects had increased rates of gross gastrointestinal bleeding. In the ISIS—2 study (1), there was no significant difference in the incidence of major bleeding (bleeds requiring transfusion) between 8,587 subjects taking 162.5 milligrams aspirin daily and 8,600 subjects taking placebo (31 versus 33 subjects). There were five confirmed cerebral hemorrhage in the aspirin group compared with two in the placebo group, but the incidence of stroke of all causes was significantly reduced from 81 to 47 for the placebo versus aspirin group (0.4 percent absolute change). There was a small and statistically significant excess (0.6 percent) of minor bleeding in people taking aspirin (2.5 percent for aspirin, 1.9 percent for placebo). No other significant adverse effects were reported.

Cardiovascular and Biochemical
In the AMIS trail(4), the dosage of 1,000 milligrams per day of aspirin was associated with small increases in systolic blood pressure (BP) (average 1.5 to 2.1 millimeters Hg) and diastolic BP (0.5 to 0.6 millimeters Hg), depending upon whether maximal or last available readings were used. Blood urea nitrogen and uric acid levels were also increased, but by less than 1.0 milligram percent.
Subjects with marked hypertension or renal insufficiency had been excluded from the trail so that clinical importance of these observations for such subjects or for any subjects treated over more prolonged periods is not known. It is recommended that patients placed on long-term aspirin treatment, even at doses of 160 milligrams per day, be seen at regular intervals to assess changes in these measurements.

DOSAGE AND ADMINISTRATION
The recommended dose of aspirin to treat suspected acute MI is 160 to 162.5 milligrams taken as soon as the first infarct is suspected and then daily for at least 30 days. (One-half of a conventional 325-milligram aspirin tablet or two 80–81 milligram aspirin tablets may be taken.) This use of aspirin applies to both solid, oral dosage forms (buffered, plain, and enteric-coated aspirin) and buffered aspirin in solution. If using a solid dosage form, the first dose should be crushed, sucked, or chewed. After the 30-day treatment, physicians should consider further therapy based on the labeling for dosage and administration of aspirin for prevention of recurrent MI (reinfarction).

REFERENCES
(1) ISIS-2 (Second International Study of Infarct Survival) Collaborative Group. "Randomized Trail of Intravenous Streptokinase, Oral Aspirin, Both, or Neither Among 17,187 Cases of Suspected Acute Myocardial Infarction: ISIS-2," lancet, 2:349–360, August 13, 1988.

HOW SUPPLIED
Halfprin Tablets
162 mg. in bottle of 60* and 200
81 mg. in bottle of 90
*Easy to open bottle/ Not child-resistant caps.

Comments questions or sample request call toll free 1-800-824-4894

SAFE TUSSIN 30   OTC
EXPECTORANT/COUGH SUPPRESSANT

DESCRIPTION
Each 10 cc contains 200 mg Guaifenesin, U.S.P. and 30 mg Dextromethorphan Hydrobromide U.S.P.

INDICATIONS
For temporary relief of cough due to minor throat and bronchial irritation associated with the common cold or inhaled irritants. Helps loosen phlegm (mucus) and thin bronchial secretions to rid the bronchial passageways of bothersome mucus.

DIRECTIONS
Adults and children 12 years of age and over: 2 teaspoonfuls every 6 hours, not to exceed 8 teaspoonfuls in 24 hours. Children 6 to under 12 years of age: 1 teaspoonful every 6 hours not to exceed 4 teaspoonfuls in 24 hours. Children 2 to under 6 years of age: $\frac{1}{2}$ teaspoonful every 6 hours not to exceed 2 teaspoonfuls in 24 hours. Children under 2 years of age consult a physician.

INACTIVE INGREDIENTS
Citric Acid, Benzoic Acid U.S.P., Glycerin U.S.P., Sorbitol, Flavor (Peppermint, Menthol), Water.
Safe Tussin 30 does not contain antihistamines, sugar, alcohol, sodium, dyes, codeine; all of which may pose risks for certain patients. Each dose of Safe Tussin 30 contains .066g sorbitol, a non-nutritive caloric sweetener.

CONTRAINDICATIONS
Do not take if hypersensitive to Guaifenesin, Dextromethorphan or any of the ingredients listed above.

HOW SUPPLIED
Clear liquid in 4 oz bottles.

Laser, Inc.
2200 W. 97TH PLACE, P.O. BOX 905
CROWN POINT, IN 46307

Direct Inquiries to:
Joseph N. Allegretti, R.Ph.
(219) 663-1165

DALLERGY® CAPLETS, SYRUP, TABLETS   ℞

Each Extended-Release Caplet* (Capsule-shaped tablet) contains: Chlorpheniramine Maleate 8 mg, Phenylephrine Hydrochloride 20 mg, Methscopolamine Nitrate 2.5 mg. Each 5 mL of grape-flavored Syrup contains: Chlorpheniramine Maleate 2 mg, Phenylephrine Hydrochloride 10 mg, Methscopolamine Nitrate 0.625 mg. Each Tablet contains: Chlorpheniramine Maleate 4 mg, Phenylephrine Hydrochloride 10 mg, Methscopolamine Nitrate 1.25 mg.

*In a specially prepared base to provide a prolonged therapeutic effect.

DALLERGY® –JR. CAPSULES   ℞

Each Extended-Release Capsule* contains: Brompheniramine Maleate 6 mg, Pseudoephedrine Hydrochloride 60 mg.

*In a specially prepared base to provide prolonged action.

DONATUSSIN DC SYRUP   Ⓒ ℞

Each 5 mL contains: Hydrocodone* Bitartrate 2.5 mg *(WARNING: May be habit forming), Phenylephrine Hydrochloride 7.5 mg, Guaifenesin 50 mg. Red Syrup.

DONATUSSIN DROPS   ℞

Each mL contains: Chlorpheniramine Maleate 1 mg, Phenylephrine Hydrochloride 2 mg, Guaifenesin 20 mg. Peach-flavored, orange color.

DONATUSSIN SYRUP   ℞

Each 5 mL contains: Dextromethorphan HBr 7.5 mg, Chlorpheniramine Maleate 2 mg, Phenylephrine HCl 10 mg, Guaifenesin 100 mg. Red Syrup.

FUMATINIC® CAPSULES   ℞

Each Extended-Release FUMATINIC Capsule contains: Ferrous Fumarate* 200 mg (equivalent to 66 mg of elemental iron), Vitamin C* (Ascorbic Acid) 60 mg, Vitamin B-12 (Cyanocobalamin) 5 mcg with Intrinsic Factor.
*In a specially prepared base to provide prolonged action.

KIE® SYRUP   ℞

Each 5 mL contains: Potassium Iodide 150 mg, Ephedrine Hydrochloride 8 mg. Green Syrup.

LACTOCAL–F TABLETS   ℞

Multivitamin, Multimineral supplement for pregnant or lactating women. White coated dye free tablet.

Continued on next page

RESPAIRE®–SR CAPSULES 60 & 120 ℞

Each Extended-Release RESPAIRE-60 SR Capsule contains: Pseudoephedrine Hydrochloride* 60 mg and Guaifenesin† 200 mg. Each Extended-Release RESPAIRE-120 SR Capsule contains: Pseudoephedrine Hydrochloride* 120 mg and Guaifenesin† 250 mg.

* In a specially prepared base to provide prolonged action.
† Designed for immediate release to provide rapid action.

Lederle Piperacillin, Inc.
CAROLINA, PUERTO RICO 00630

Lederle Parenterals, Inc.
CAROLINA, PUERTO RICO 00630

LEDERLE LABORATORIES
Division American Cyanamid Company
Pearl River, NY 10965
US Gov't. License No. 17

For Medical Information Contact:
MARKETED ONCOLOGY PRODUCTS:
Immunex Corporation
Professional Services Department
51 University Street
Seattle, WA 98101
(800) IMMUNEX

OTHER MARKETED DRUG PRODUCTS:
Lederle Laboratories/Wyeth-Ayerst Laboratories
Medical Affairs Department
P.O. Box 8299
Philadelphia, PA 19101
Day: (800) 934-5556
8:30 AM to 4:30 PM
(Eastern Standard Time),
Weekdays only
Night: (610) 688-4400 (Emergencies only; non-emergencies should wait until the next day)

MARKETED VACCINES AND TINE TESTS:
Lederle Laboratories/Wyeth-Ayerst Laboratories
Medical Affairs Department
P.O. Box 8299
Philadelphia, PA 19101
Day: (800) 934-5556
8:30 AM to 4:30 PM
(Eastern Standard Time),
Weekdays only
Night: (610) 688-4400 (Emergencies only; non-emergencies should wait until the next day)

LEDERLE PRODUCTS

The following list of Lederle products includes the alphanumeric LEDERMARK® codes which provide quick and positive identification of Lederle capsules and tablets:

Product Identity Code No.	Product
	ACEL-IMUNE® Diphtheria and Tetanus Toxoids and Acellular Pertussis Vaccine Adsorbed
A11	ARTANE® Tabs., 2mg
A12	ARTANE® Tabs., 5mg
—	ARTANE® Elixir, 2mg/5mL
A13	ASENDIN® Tabs., 25mg
A15	ASENDIN® Tabs., 50mg
A17	ASENDIN® Tabs., 100mg
A18	ASENDIN® Tabs., 150mg
B1	ZEBETA® Tablets, 5mg
B3	ZEBETA® Tablets, 10mg
B12	ZIAC® Tablets, 2.5/6.25mg
B13	ZIAC® Tablets, 5/6.25mg
B14	ZIAC® Tablets, 10/6.25mg
D1	DIAMOX® Tablets, 125mg
D2	DIAMOX® Tablets, 250mg
D3	DIAMOX® SEQUELS® Capsules, 500mg
D11	DECLOMYCIN® Tabs., 150mg
D12	DECLOMYCIN® Tabs., 300mg
—	Diphtheria & Tetanus Toxoids Adsorbed PUROGENATED® for Pediatric Use
—	HibTITER® Haemophilus b Conjugate Vaccine
M1	RHEUMATREX® Tabs., 2.5mg
M6	MYAMBUTOL® Tabs., 100mg
M7	MYAMBUTOL® Tabs., 400mg
M45	MINOCIN® Pellet-Filled Caps., 50mg
M46	MINOCIN® Pellet-Filled Caps., 100mg
—	MINOCIN® IV, 100mg/vial
—	MINOCIN® Oral Suspension, 50mg/5mL
M55	MATERNA® Tabs.
—	ORIMUNE® Poliovirus Vaccine Live Oral Trivalent
—	PIPRACIL® 2g
—	PIPRACIL® 3g
—	PIPRACIL® 4g
—	PIPRACIL® 40g
—	PNU-IMUNE® 23 Pneumococcal Vaccine Polyvalent
—	PROSTEP® nicotine transdermal system, 11mg
—	PROSTEP® nicotine transdermal system, 22mg
S200	SUPRAX® Tablets, 200mg
S400	SUPRAX® Tablets, 400mg
—	SUPRAX® Powder for Oral Suspension
—	Tetanus Toxoid Adsorbed PUROGENATED®
—	Tetanus and Diphtheria Toxoids Adsorbed PUROGENATED® for Adult Use
—	TETRAMUNE® Diphtheria and Tetanus Toxoids and Pertussis Vaccine Adsorbed and Haemophilus b Conjugate Vaccine (Diphtheria CRM₁₉₇ Protein Conjugate)
—	TRI-IMMUNOL® Diphtheria and Tetanus Toxoids and Pertussis Vaccine Adsorbed
—	Tuberculin, Old, TINE TEST®
—	Tuberculin, Purified Protein Derivative PPD TINE TEST®
T1	TriHEMIC® 600 Tabs.
V7	VERELAN® Caps., 180mg
V8	VERELAN® Caps., 120mg
V9	VERELAN® Caps., 240mg
—	ZOSYN® 2.25g vial
—	ZOSYN® 3.375g vial
—	ZOSYN® 4.5g vial
—	ZOSYN® 40.5g pharmacy bulk vial

DIPHTHERIA and TETANUS TOXOIDS and ACELLULAR PERTUSSIS VACCINE ADSORBED
ACEL-IMUNE®
FOR ALL FIVE DOSES ℞

DESCRIPTION

Diphtheria and Tetanus Toxoids and Acellular Pertussis Vaccine Adsorbed (DTaP), ACEL-IMUNE, is a sterile combination of PUROGENATED® Diphtheria Toxoid, PUROGENATED® Tetanus Toxoid, and Acellular Pertussis Vaccine which is adsorbed to an aluminum adjuvant. The acellular pertussis vaccine component is produced by Takeda Chemical Industries, Ltd., Osaka, Japan and is combined with diphtheria and tetanus toxoids manufactured by Lederle Laboratories. The bulk vaccine is prepared by Lederle Laboratories. ACEL-IMUNE is filled, labeled, packaged, and released by Lederle Laboratories. ACEL-IMUNE is for intramuscular use only. After shaking, the vaccine is a homogeneous white suspension.

The diphtheria and tetanus toxoids are derived from *Corynebacterium diphtheriae* and *Clostridium tetani*, respectively, which are grown in media according to the method of Mueller and Miller.[1,2] *C. diphtheriae* is grown in a defined medium containing casamino acids and *C. tetani* in a medium containing beef heart infusion. They are detoxified by use of formaldehyde. The toxoids are refined by the Pillemer alcohol fractionation method[3] and are diluted with a solution containing sodium phosphate monobasic, sodium phosphate dibasic, glycine, and thimerosal (mercury derivative) as a preservative. The acellular pertussis vaccine component is prepared by growing Phase I *Bordetella pertussis* in Stainer-Scholte defined medium and harvesting the culture fluid. Purification of the acellular pertussis vaccine component is accomplished by ammonium sulfate fractionation steps and a final sucrose density gradient centrifugation. The acellular pertussis vaccine component is detoxified with formaldehyde and thimerosal (mercury derivative) is added as a preservative.

The diphtheria toxoid, tetanus toxoid, and acellular pertussis vaccine are combined, diluted in phosphate buffered saline (PBS), and adsorbed to aluminum adjuvant. The aluminum adjuvant is formulated to contain 0.23 mg aluminum per 0.5 mL dose as aluminum hydroxide and aluminum phosphate. The residual free formaldehyde content by assay is ≤0.02%. Thimerosal (mercury derivative) is present in a final concentration of 1:10,000. The final product may also contain gelatin and polysorbate 80 which are used in early stages of the manufacture of the pertussis component.

Each single dose of 0.5 mL of ACEL-IMUNE is formulated to contain 9 Lf of diphtheria toxoid and 5 Lf of tetanus toxoid (both toxoids induce not less than 2 units of antitoxin per mL in the guinea pig potency test) and 300 hemagglutinating (HA) units of acellular pertussis vaccine. A hemagglutination unit is that amount of material which completely agglutinates chicken red blood cells as measured by the HA assay.[4] The acellular pertussis vaccine component contains approximately 40 μg (but not more than 60 μg) of pertussis antigen protein per 0.5 mL dose with approximately 86% filamentous hemagglutinin (FHA), approximately 8% inactivated pertussis toxin (PT, also known as lymphocytosis promoting factor), approximately 4% per dose of 69-kilodalton outer membrane protein (pertactin), and approximately 2% type 2 fimbriae (pertussis-specific agglutinogen).

The potency of the pertussis component is evaluated by measurement of antibodies to FHA, PT, pertactin, and fimbriae in immunized mice by ELISA.

CLINICAL PHARMACOLOGY

Simultaneous immunization against diphtheria, tetanus, and pertussis (whooping cough) during infancy and childhood has been a routine practice in the United States since the late 1940s. It has played a major role in markedly reducing the incidence of cases and deaths from each of these diseases.

Diphtheria is primarily a localized and generalized intoxication caused by diphtheria toxin, an extracellular protein metabolite of toxinogenic strains of *C. diphtheriae*. While the incidence of diphtheria in the US has decreased from over 200,000 cases reported in 1921, before the general use of diphtheria toxoid, to only 15 cases reported from 1990 to 1994,[5] the case fatality rate has remained constant at about 5% to 10%. The highest case fatality rates are in the very young and in the elderly. Diphtheria remains a serious disease in some areas of the world as demonstrated by the recent epidemic in the former Soviet Union.[6]

Following adequate immunization with diphtheria toxoid it is thought that protection lasts for at least 10 years.[7] Antitoxin levels of at least 0.01 antitoxin units/mL are generally regarded as protective.[8] This significantly reduces both the risk of developing diphtheria and the severity of clinical illness. It does not, however, eliminate carriage of *C. diphtheriae* in the pharynx or on the skin.[7]

Tetanus is an intoxication manifested primarily by neuromuscular dysfunction caused by a potent exotoxin elaborated by *C. tetani*. The incidence of tetanus in the US has dropped dramatically with the routine use of tetanus toxoid, with an average of 57 cases reported annually from 1985–1994.[5] Spores of *C. tetani* are ubiquitous and there is essentially no natural immunity to tetanus toxin.

Thus, universal primary immunization with tetanus toxoid with subsequent maintenance of adequate antitoxin levels, by means of timed boosters, is recommended to protect all age groups.[7] Tetanus toxoid is a highly effective antigen and a completed primary series generally induces serum antitoxin levels of at least 0.01 antitoxin units, a level which has been reported to be protective.[9] It is thought that protection persists for at least 10 years.[7]

The toxoids of tetanus and diphtheria induce neutralizing antibodies to the toxins produced by the infecting organisms. In two clinical studies with ACEL-IMUNE, serum antitoxin levels to diphtheria and tetanus toxins were shown to be greater than 0.01 antitoxin units/mL in 100% of 140 infants following three doses.[10] These levels are generally regarded to be protective.[9,11]

Pertussis (whooping cough) is a highly communicable disease of the respiratory tract. Attack rates of over 90% have been reported in unimmunized household contacts.[9,12] Since immunization against pertussis (whooping cough) became widespread, the number of reported cases and associated mortality in the US has declined from about 120,000 cases and 1100 deaths in 1950,[13] to a historical low of 1010 cases in 1976. However, since the early 1980's, reported pertussis incidence has increased with peaks occurring in 1983, 1986, 1990, and 1993. Following the peak in reported cases in 1993, the numbers declined during 1994 and the first 2 quarters of 1995 — a pattern consistent with the previously observed 3–4 year periodicity in pertussis incidence.[14] An average of 4515 cases were reported annually from 1990–1994.[5] Precise data do not exist, since bacteriological confirmation of pertussis can be obtained in less than half of the suspected cases. In the US, most reported illness from *B. pertussis* occurs in infants and young children; approximately 80% of reported deaths occur in children less than 1 year old.[7] Older children and adults, in whom classic signs are often absent, may go undiagnosed and serve as reservoirs of disease.[7,15]

Pertussis disease (whooping cough) is caused by a gram-negative coccobacillus, *B. pertussis*. Several antigens that

are thought to play a role in protective immunity have been isolated from cultures of *B. pertussis*. These include FHA, PT, pertactin, and fimbriae.[16–18] Another biologically active component, endotoxin, may contribute to reactogenicity of pertussis vaccines.[19] The Takeda acellular pertussis vaccine component used in ACEL-IMUNE contains inactivated FHA, PT, pertactin, and type 2 fimbriae, with minimal endotoxin compared to that in whole-cell pertussis vaccine. The pertussis component induces immunity against pertussis disease in humans.

Efficacy of ACEL-IMUNE was assessed in infants in a prospective study conducted in Germany at 227 investigator sites. A total of 8532 infants were randomized to receive ACEL-IMUNE (n=4273) or Lederle whole-cell DTP (n=4259) at mean ages of 3, 5 and 7 months followed by a fourth dose of ACEL-IMUNE (n=3991) or DTP (n=3925) at a mean age of 17 months. By parental choice, 1739 additional infants received German-manufactured Diphtheria and Tetanus Toxoids (DT) at mean ages of 3 and 5 months followed by a third dose at a mean age of 17 months. In order to adjust for potential confounding, several variables were examined to determine which ones differed between the randomized and non-randomized groups and affected the risk of developing pertussis. Telephone calls were performed every 14 days by investigator personnel to ensure close surveillance of pertussis disease among study subjects and household members. Evaluation of a 7-day cough which was not improving included a nasopharyngeal specimen for culture and blood sample for acute serology. Subjects with greater than 14 days of cough were evaluated by central investigators and convalescent serology was scheduled for 6–8 weeks after cough onset. Completeness of surveillance to ascertain the presence and duration of cough illness was not directly assessed; however, study sites were monitored for compliance with the protocol.

A total of 154 cases were identified using a case definition of 21 days or more of cough with paroxysms, whoop or post-tussive vomiting plus confirmation by positive culture for *B. pertussis*, or household contact with a person with positive culture for *B. pertussis*, or by serologic confirmation (significant rise in PT IgG between acute and convalescent samples or PT IgA value significantly elevated above the normal limits). Case rates per 100 person-years of follow-up for each vaccine were: DTaP, 0.48; DTP, 0.22; and DT, 2.98. Adjusting for single adult households and households in which all siblings were unimmunized, the vaccine efficacy after 3 doses and before receipt of the fourth dose of ACEL-IMUNE or until 19 months of age was 73% (95% Cl 51 to 86) and after 4 doses 85% (95% Cl 76 to 90). DTP efficacy after 3 doses was 83% (95% Cl 65 to 92) and after 4 doses was 94% (95% Cl 89 to 97). For ACEL-IMUNE, there is no significant difference in efficacy between 3 and 4 doses (p=0.16). Considering all observation time, i.e., including from after the third dose until the fourth dose (approximately 40% of follow-up time) and from after the fourth dose until the end of the study (approximately 60% of follow-up time), the adjusted efficacy estimated for ACEL-IMUNE was 81% (95% Cl 73 to 87) compared to 91% for DTP (95% Cl 85 to 95). The relative risk for pertussis in the ACEL-IMUNE group compared to the DTP group was 1.5 (95% Cl 0.7 to 3.4) after 3 doses and 2.8 (95% Cl 1.3 to 5.9) after 4 doses.

Some subjects with 21 days or more of cough with paroxysms, whoop or post-tussive vomiting did not have complete laboratory tests. Of those subjects whose available tests were negative (DT, 113 subjects; DTaP, 241 subjects; and DTP, 239 subjects), 68% in the DT group, 69% in the ACEL-IMUNE group, and 68% in the Lederle whole-cell DTP group had at least one missing laboratory test. In the efficacy analysis these subjects were classified as non-cases. The effect of this classification was evaluated by applying missing value imputation procedures in which it was assumed that the probability of being a pertussis case was the same among subjects with and without all laboratory results; missing values were found to have minimal effect on vaccine efficacy.[10] It is possible, however, that the misclassification of such subjects due to missing laboratory values may have resulted in overestimates of ACEL-IMUNE and whole-cell DTP efficacy.

Vaccine efficacy was also estimated in a household contact analysis within the prospective German study. A primary case of pertussis was defined as cough for 21 or more days with paroxysms, whoop, or post-tussive vomiting plus laboratory confirmation. A total of 167 households had a member other than a study infant who met this definition. A secondary case of pertussis was defined as cough for 21 or more days with paroxysms, whoop, or post-tussive vomiting plus laboratory confirmation, with an onset within 7–28 days after onset of pertussis in a primary case in the household. Thirteen secondary cases were identified among study infants, resulting in secondary attack rates of 9.5% (ACEL-IMUNE), 2.0% (DTP), and 32% (DT). Based on this analysis, the vaccine efficacy for ACEL-IMUNE was 70% (95% Cl 11 to 90). Analysis of potentially confounding variables revealed none that were associated with both vaccine group and pertussis case status.[10]

Following primary immunization, US children (n=126) had antibody titers to pertussis antigens which were similar to those achieved in German children who participated in a pilot study (n=52) and a subset of children in the efficacy trial (n=52) where vaccine efficacy was demonstrated.[10]

In a clinical study conducted in the US, 77 infants received ACEL-IMUNE, HibTITER and Hepatitis B vaccine simultaneously at 2, 4 and 6 months of age. Ninety-four percent of the children demonstrated anti-PRP antibodies ≥1 μg/mL. All of the 74 infants evaluated for HBs responses had anti-HBs titers of >10 mIU/mL.[10]

Sera from 30 infants who received OPV simultaneously with ACEL-IMUNE at 2 and 4 months showed that at 6 months, 90 to 100% had protective neutralizing antibody to all three poliovirus types (comparable to results seen with simultaneous DTP administration with OPV).[10]

Ninety-two to 100% of 15–18 month old children (n=48) who received MMR simultaneously with ACEL-IMUNE had protective titers to measles, mumps, and rubella; similar results were seen for children who received DTP and MMR simultaneously.[20]

INDICATIONS AND USAGE

Diphtheria and Tetanus Toxoids and Acellular Pertussis Vaccine Adsorbed, ACEL-IMUNE, is indicated for active immunization of children from 6 weeks of age up to age 7 years (prior to seventh birthday) for protection against diphtheria, tetanus, and pertussis.

This product is not recommended for immunizing persons on or after their seventh birthday (see **DOSAGE AND ADMINISTRATION**).

Children who have recovered from culture-confirmed pertussis need not receive further doses of a pertussis-containing vaccine[7], but should complete the recommended series with Dipththeria and Tetanus Toxoids, Adsorbed for pediatric use (DT).

ACEL-IMUNE is intended for active immunization against diphtheria, tetanus, and pertussis, and is not to be used for treatment of actual infection.

If a contraindicating event to the pertussis vaccine component occurs, Diphtheria and Tetanus Toxoids Adsorbed for pediatric use (DT) should be substituted for each of the remaining doses. The Advisory Committee on Immunization Practices (ACIP) recommends that if an immediate anaphylactic reaction occurs, no further vaccination with any of the three antigens in DTP should be carried out.[7]

As with any vaccine, ACEL-IMUNE may not protect 100% of individuals receiving the vaccine.

If passive immunization is required, Tetanus Immune Globulin (TIG) or Diphtheria Antitoxin are recommended.

CONTRAINDICATIONS

HYPERSENSITIVITY TO ANY COMPONENT OF THE VACCINE, INCLUDING THIMEROSAL, A MERCURY DERIVATIVE, IS A CONTRAINDICATION.

THE DECISION TO ADMINISTER OR DELAY DTP VACCINATION BECAUSE OF A CURRENT OR RECENT FEBRILE ILLNESS DEPENDS LARGELY ON THE SEVERITY OF THE SYMPTOMS AND THEIR ETIOLOGY. ALTHOUGH A MODERATE OR SEVERE FEBRILE ILLNESS IS SUFFICIENT REASON TO POSTPONE VACCINATION, MINOR ILLNESSES SUCH AS A MILD UPPER RESPIRATORY INFECTION WITH OR WITHOUT LOW GRADE FEVER ARE NOT CONTRAINDICATIONS.[7,21,22]

ROUTINE IMMUNIZATION SHOULD BE DEFERRED DURING AN OUTBREAK OF POLIOMYELITIS PROVIDING THE PATIENT HAS NOT SUSTAINED AN INJURY THAT INCREASES THE RISK OF TETANUS AND PROVIDING AN OUTBREAK OF DIPHTHERIA OR PERTUSSIS DOES NOT OCCUR SIMULTANEOUSLY.[23]

DATA ON THE USE OF ACEL-IMUNE IN CHILDREN FOR WHOM WHOLE-CELL PERTUSSIS VACCINE IS CONTRAINDICATED ARE NOT AVAILABLE. UNTIL SUCH DATA ARE AVAILABLE, IT WOULD BE PRUDENT TO CONSIDER THE ACIP AND AMERICAN ACADEMY OF PEDIATRICS (AAP) CONTRAINDICATIONS TO WHOLE-CELL PERTUSSIS VACCINE AS CONTRAINDICATIONS TO ACEL-IMUNE.

IMMUNIZATION WITH ACEL-IMUNE IS CONTRAINDICATED IF THE CHILD HAS EXPERIENCED ANY EVENT FOLLOWING PREVIOUS IMMUNIZATION WITH ANY VACCINE CONTAINING A PERTUSSIS COMPONENT, WHICH IS CONSIDERED BY THE AAP OR ACIP TO BE A CONTRAINDICATION TO FURTHER DOSES OF PERTUSSIS VACCINE. THESE EVENTS ARE:

AN IMMEDIATE ANAPHYLACTIC REACTION. BECAUSE OF THE UNCERTAINTY AS TO WHICH COMPONENT OF THE VACCINE MIGHT BE RESPONSIBLE, NO FURTHER VACCINATION WITH ANY OF THE ANTIGENS IN DTP SHOULD BE CARRIED OUT. ALTERNATIVELY, BECAUSE OF THE IMPORTANCE OF TETANUS VACCINATION, SUCH INDIVIDUALS MAY BE REFERRED FOR EVALUATION BY AN ALLERGIST.[7,21,22]

ENCEPHALOPATHY (NOT DUE TO ANOTHER IDENTIFIABLE CAUSE) OCCURRING WITHIN 7 DAYS FOLLOWING VACCINATION. THIS IS DEFINED AS AN ACUTE, SEVERE CENTRAL NERVOUS SYSTEM DISORDER OCCURRING WITHIN 7 DAYS FOLLOWING VACCINATION, AND GENERALLY CONSISTING OF MAJOR ALTERATIONS IN CONSCIOUSNESS, UNRESPONSIVENESS, GENERALIZED OR FOCAL SEIZURES THAT PERSIST MORE THAN A FEW HOURS, WITH FAILURE TO RECOVER WITHIN 24 HOURS. EVEN THOUGH CAUSATION BY DTP CANNOT BE ESTABLISHED, NO SUBSEQUENT DOSES OF PERTUSSIS VACCINE SHOULD BE GIVEN.[7,21,22]

THE CLINICAL JUDGMENT OF THE ATTENDING PHYSICIAN SHOULD PREVAIL AT ALL TIMES.

WARNINGS

THE ACIP AND THE AAP STATE THAT IF ANY OF THE FOLLOWING EVENTS OCCUR IN TEMPORAL RELATION TO RECEIPT OF DTP OR DTaP, THE DECISION TO GIVE SUBSEQUENT DOSES OF VACCINE CONTAINING THE PERTUSSIS COMPONENT SHOULD BE CAREFULLY CONSIDERED. ALTHOUGH THESE EVENTS WERE ONCE CONSIDERED CONTRAINDICATIONS TO WHOLE-CELL DTP, THERE MAY BE CIRCUMSTANCES, SUCH AS A HIGH INCIDENCE OF PERTUSSIS, IN WHICH THE POTENTIAL BENEFITS OUTWEIGH THE POSSIBLE RISKS, PARTICULARLY BECAUSE THESE EVENTS HAVE NOT BEEN SHOWN TO CAUSE PERMANENT SEQUELAE.[7,21,22]

1. TEMPERATURE OF ≥40.5°C (105°F) WITHIN 48 HOURS NOT DUE TO IDENTIFIABLE CAUSE.
2. COLLAPSE OR SHOCK-LIKE STATE (HYPOTONIC-HYPORESPONSIVE EPISODE) WITHIN 48 HOURS.
3. PERSISTENT, INCONSOLABLE CRYING LASTING ≥3 HOURS, OCCURRING WITHIN 48 HOURS.
4. CONVULSIONS WITH OR WITHOUT FEVER OCCURRING WITHIN 3 DAYS.[7,21,22,24]

Data on the use of ACEL-IMUNE in children with a personal history of convulsion or an evolving or changing disorder of the central nervous system are not available. In the opinion of the manufacturer, the presence of a personal history of convulsion or an evolving disorder affecting the central nervous system is considered a warning against further immunization with this vaccine.

The ACIP and the AAP recommend considering deferral of immunization against pertussis in children with progressive neurologic disorders, personal history of convulsion, and known or suspected neurologic conditions which predispose to seizures or neurologic deterioration until the child's status has been fully assessed, a treatment regimen established, and the condition stabilized.[7,21,22,25]

Children with a personal or family history of convulsion may have an increased risk for seizures following DTP vaccination compared with children without such histories.[26,27] However, the ACIP states that children with stable central nervous system disorders, including well-controlled seizures or satisfactorily explained single seizures may receive pertussis vaccination. The ACIP and AAP do not consider a family history of seizures to be a contraindication to pertussis vaccination.[7,21,22] Data on the use of ACEL-IMUNE in such persons are not available.

Although there are no data on whether the prophylactic use of antipyretics can decrease the risk of febrile convulsions, data suggest that acetaminophen will reduce the incidence of postvaccination fever.[28] The ACIP and AAP recommend administering acetaminophen at age-appropriate doses at the time of vaccination and every 4 hours for 24 hours to children at higher risk for seizures than the general population.[7,22,29] The decision to administer a pertussis-containing vaccine to such children must be made by the physician on an individual basis, with consideration of all relevant factors, and assessment of potential risks and benefits for that individual. The physician should review the full text of ACIP and AAP guidelines prior to considering vaccination for such children.[7,22,29] The parent or guardian should be advised of the potential increased risk.

A detailed follow-up of the National Childhood Encephalopathy Study (NCES) indicated that children who had had a serious acute neurologic illness were significantly more likely than children in a control group without acute neurologic illness to have chronic nervous system dysfunction 10 years later.[30] These children with chronic nervous system dysfunction were more likely than children in the control group to have received DTP within 7 days of onset of the original serious acute neurologic illness (i.e., 12 [3.3%] of 367 children vs. six [0.8%] of 723 children).[21,30] After reviewing the follow-up data, a committee of the Institute of Medicine (IOM) concluded that the NCES provided evidence of an association between DTP and chronic nervous system dysfunction in children who had had a serious acute neurologic illness after vaccination with DTP.[31] However, IOM also concluded that the results were insufficient to determine whether DTP increases the overall risk for chronic nervous system dysfunction in children.[31] The ACIP indicated that the results of the NCES were insufficient to de-

Continued on next page

Acel-Imune—Cont.

termine whether DTP administration before the acute neurological event influenced the potential for neurologic dysfunction 10 years later.[21] Acute encephalopathy or permanent neurological injury have not been reported in clinical trials after administration of ACEL-IMUNE, but the experience with this vaccine is insufficient to rule this out (see **ADVERSE REACTIONS**).

ACEL-IMUNE should not be given to infants or children with thrombocytopenia or any coagulation disorder that would contraindicate intramuscular injection unless the potential benefit clearly outweighs the risk of administration. If the decision is made to administer ACEL-IMUNE to children with coagulation disorders, it should be given with caution (see **DRUG INTERACTIONS**).

PRECAUTIONS
General
CARE IS TO BE TAKEN BY THE HEALTH PROVIDER FOR SAFE AND EFFECTIVE USE OF THIS PRODUCT.
1. PRIOR TO ADMINISTRATION OF ANY DOSE OF ACEL-IMUNE, THE PARENT OR GUARDIAN SHOULD BE ASKED ABOUT THE PERSONAL HISTORY, FAMILY HISTORY, AND RECENT HEALTH STATUS OF THE VACCINE RECIPIENT. THE PHYSICIAN SHOULD ASCERTAIN PREVIOUS IMMUNIZATION HISTORY, CURRENT HEALTH STATUS, AND OCCURRENCE OF ANY SYMPTOMS AND/OR SIGNS OF AN ADVERSE EVENT AFTER PREVIOUS IMMUNIZATIONS IN THE CHILD TO BE IMMUNIZED, IN ORDER TO DETERMINE THE EXISTENCE OF ANY CONTRAINDICATION TO IMMUNIZATION WITH ACEL-IMUNE AND TO ALLOW AN ASSESSMENT OF BENEFITS AND RISKS.
2. BEFORE THE INJECTION OF ANY BIOLOGICAL, THE PHYSICIAN SHOULD TAKE ALL PRECAUTIONS KNOWN FOR THE PREVENTION OF ALLERGIC OR ANY OTHER SIDE REACTIONS. This should include a review of the patient's history regarding possible sensitivity; the ready availability of epinephrine 1:1000 and other appropriate agents used for control of immediate allergic reactions; and a knowledge of the recent literature pertaining to use of the biological concerned, including the nature of side effects and adverse reactions that may follow its use.
3. Children with impaired immune responsiveness, whether due to the use of immunosuppressive therapy (including irradiation, corticosteroids, antimetabolites, alkylating agents, and cytotoxic agents), a genetic defect, human immunodeficiency virus (HIV) infection, or other causes, may have reduced antibody response to active immunization procedures.[7,22,32,33] Deferral of administration of vaccine may be considered in individuals receiving immunosuppressive therapy.[7] Other groups should receive this vaccine according to the usual recommended schedule.[7,22,33,34] (see **DRUG INTERACTIONS**).
4. This product is not contraindicated for use in individuals with human immunodeficiency virus (HIV) infection.[35]
5. *Since this product is a suspension containing an adjuvant, shake vigorously to obtain a uniform suspension prior to withdrawing each dose from the multiple dose vial.*
6. A separate sterile syringe and needle or a sterile disposable unit should be used for each individual patient to prevent transmission of hepatitis or other infectious agents from one person to another. Needles should be disposed of properly and should not be recapped.
7. Special care should be taken to prevent injection into a blood vessel.

Information for Patient
PRIOR TO ADMINISTRATION OF ACEL-IMUNE, HEALTH CARE PERSONNEL SHOULD INFORM THE PARENT, GUARDIAN, OR OTHER RESPONSIBLE ADULT OF THE RECOMMENDED IMMUNIZATION SCHEDULE FOR PROTECTION AGAINST DIPHTHERIA, TETANUS, AND PERTUSSIS AND THE BENEFITS AND RISKS TO THE CHILD RECEIVING THIS VACCINE CONTAINING AN ACELLULAR PERTUSSIS COMPONENT. GUIDANCE SHOULD BE PROVIDED ON MEASURES TO BE TAKEN SHOULD ADVERSE EVENTS OCCUR, SUCH AS ANTIPYRETIC MEASURES FOR ELEVATED TEMPERATURES AND THE NEED TO REPORT ADVERSE EVENTS TO THE HEALTH CARE PROVIDER. PARENTS SHOULD BE PROVIDED WITH VACCINE INFORMATION MATERIALS AT THE TIME OF EACH VACCINATION, AS STATED IN THE NATIONAL CHILDHOOD VACCINE INJURY ACT.[36]
THE HEALTH CARE PROVIDER SHOULD INFORM THE PATIENT, PARENT, OR GUARDIAN OF THE IMPORTANCE OF COMPLETING THE IMMUNIZATION SERIES UNLESS CONTRAINDICATED.
PATIENTS, PARENTS, OR GUARDIANS SHOULD BE INSTRUCTED TO REPORT ANY SERIOUS ADVERSE REACTIONS TO THEIR HEALTH CARE PROVIDER

Drug Interactions
Children receiving immunosuppressive therapy may have a reduced response to active immunization procedures.[7,22,32,33] Although no specific studies with pertussis vaccine are available, if immunosuppressive therapy will be discontinued shortly, it would be reasonable to defer immunization until the patient has been off therapy for one month; otherwise, the patient should be vaccinated while still on therapy.[32]
As with other intramuscular injections, ACEL-IMUNE should be given with caution to children on anticoagulant therapy.
Tetanus Immune Globulin or Diphtheria Antitoxin, if used, should be given in a separate site with a separate needle and syringe if used at the same time as ACEL-IMUNE.
Please see **DOSAGE AND ADMINISTRATION** for information regarding simultaneous administration with other vaccines.

Carcinogenesis, Mutagenesis, Impairment of Fertility
ACEL-IMUNE has not been evaluated for its carcinogenic, mutagenic potential or impairment of fertility.

Pregnancy
Pregnancy Category C
Animal reproduction studies have not been conducted with ACEL-IMUNE. It is not known whether ACEL-IMUNE vaccine can cause fetal harm when administered to a pregnant woman or can affect reproductive capacity. ACEL-IMUNE vaccine is NOT recommended for use in a pregnant woman. THIS PRODUCT IS NOT RECOMMENDED FOR USE IN INDIVIDUALS 7 YEARS OF AGE OR OLDER.

Pediatric Use
The safety and effectiveness of ACEL-IMUNE in children below the age of 6 weeks have not been established (see **DOSAGE AND ADMINISTRATION**).
For immunization of children 7 years of age and older, Tetanus and Diphtheria Toxoids Adsorbed for Adults Use (Td) is recommended.[7,22]
Protection against the indicated diseases (tetanus, diphtheria, pertussis) is based on a full course of immunization.

ADVERSE REACTIONS
Adverse reactions associated with ACEL-IMUNE have been evaluated in a total of 6941 US and German infants administered a total of 20,390 doses for the first three doses in the series. A total of 5152 of these infants received ACEL-IMUNE for the fourth dose in a 4-dose DTaP series as toddlers and a total of 357 of these toddlers also received ACEL-IMUNE for the fifth dose in a 5-dose DTaP series at 4 to 6 years of age. Adverse event data were actively collected using parent diary cards, phone call follow-up, and/or by questioning the parents at clinic visits.
[See table 1 below]
In the German efficacy study where 8532 infants were randomized to receive DTaP or DTP, a total of 16,642 doses of ACEL-IMUNE were given. When compared to Lederle whole-cell pertussis DTP vaccine, ACEL-IMUNE produced significantly fewer local reactions and systemic events (see Table 1 below).
In other clinical studies of ACEL-IMUNE conducted in the US, 2593 children received 8601 doses for doses 1 through 4. In general, rates of local reactions and systemic events were comparable to those reported in the German efficacy study and lower than for whole-cell DTP. Rates of local reactions increased over the first 4 doses of ACEL-IMUNE: erythema >20mm from 1% (dose 1) to 8% (dose 4), induration >20mm from 1% (dose 1) to 6% (dose 4), and tenderness from 4% (dose 2) to 16% (dose 4). Rates of temperature $\geq$38.0°C increased over the 4-dose series from 2% (dose 1) to 18% (dose 4). With the exception of drowsiness which decreased over the 4-dose series from 20% (dose 1) to 5% (dose 4), similar rates for doses 1 through 4 were reported for other systemic events: fretfulness from 18% (dose 4) to 23% (doses 1 and 2), and loss of appetite from 9% (dose 1) to 12% (dose 4).[10]
In four clinical studies conducted in Germany and the US, a total of 357 children received a fifth dose of ACEL-IMUNE in a 5-dose DTaP series at 4 to 6 years of age. Two hundred seventy-eight subjects received vaccine formulated to contain 0.15 mg aluminum per dose and 79 subjects received vaccine formulated to contain 0.23 mg aluminum per dose. While there were no comparative DTP groups in these study segments, the reactogenicity of ACEL-IMUNE was no greater than that described for historical controls who received a fifth dose of whole-cell DTP after 4 previous doses of whole-cell DTP.[10,37,38]

Table 2
Percent of Adverse Events Occurring within 72 Hours Following the Fifth Dose of ACEL-IMUNE in Children Who Received Four Previous Consecutive Doses of ACEL-IMUNE

Symptom	DTaP[1] N = 357
Erythema	
Any	35
Significant[2]	20
Induration	
Any	30
Significant[2]	14
Tenderness	38
Fever $\geq$38.0°C	9
>39.0°C	3
Fretfulness	9
Drowsiness	10
Decreased appetite	8
Vomiting	3

[1] For some adverse events, information was not available for a small number of subjects
[2] Significant varied by protocol from >20mm–>24 mm

In the large German efficacy trial, 4273 subjects received 16,642 doses of ACEL-IMUNE and 4259 subjects received 16,420 doses of DTP. Adverse events (rates per 1000 doses) meeting AAP and ACIP criteria as absolute contraindications or precautions to further pertussis immunization and occurring within 72 hours following the immunizations were: persistent or unusual cry (1.14 for DTaP, 4.75 for DTP), fever $\geq$40.5°C (0.06 for DTaP, 0.18 for DTP), seizures, all of which were febrile (0.06 for DTaP, 0.18 for DTP) and hypotonic-hyporesponsive episode (0 for DTaP and 0.06 for DTP). When the total clinical trial experience with ACEL-IMUNE is considered (25,899 immunizations), rates per 1000 doses of ACEL-IMUNE were: persistent or unusual cry (1.27), fever $\geq$40.5°C (0.08), seizure (0.04), possible seizure (0.04), and hypotonic-hyporesponsive episode (0.04).[10]
Adverse reactions associated with ACEL-IMUNE have been evaluated in clinical trials in 911 children receiving this vaccine as the fourth or fifth dose in the DTP series when they had previously received 3 or 4 doses of whole-cell DTP. The percent of children experiencing common symptoms at any time within 72 hours following immunization is summarized in Table 3.

Table 1
Adverse Events Occurring Within 72 Hours Following DTaP and DTP
% OF CHILDREN

EVENT	ACEL-IMUNE				Lederle-Whole Cell DTP			
	Dose 1	Dose 2	Dose 3	Dose 4	Dose 1	Dose 2	Dose 3	Dose 4
Number of Children[a]	4273	4223	4155	3991	4259	4149	4087	3925
Local								
Erythema >23 mm[b]	2	3	5	10	15	11	11	13
Induration >23 mm[b]	2	4	6	9	17	13	11	13
Systemic								
Fever[c] $\geq$38.0°C[b]	7	12	16	26	44	35	40	50
Fever[c] >39.0°C[b]	0.3	1	1	2	1	2	3	4
Fretfulness[b]	18	18	16	15	47	33	28	31
Drowsiness[b]	23	16	12	11	40	25	19	21
Decreased Appetite[b]	10	9	7	9	21	14	12	17

[a] For each adverse event, information was not available for a small number of subjects; $^{2}/_{3}$ of all subjects received vaccinations in the thigh, $^{1}/_{3}$ in the buttocks
[b] p <0.001—when compared to whole-cell DTP for all doses
[c] Rectal temperature

Table 3
Percent of Children with Symptoms Following a
Fourth or Fifth Dose of ACEL-IMUNE
After 3 or 4 Doses of Whole-Cell DTP

Symptom	% of Children[1] Reporting Symptoms within 72 Hours of Immunization n = 911
Tenderness	26
Erythema (>2 cm)	10
Induration (>2 cm)	7
Increased injection site temperature	17
Fever[2] ≥38°C (100.4°F)	19
>39°C (102.2°F)	1.5
Drowsiness	6
Fretfulness	17
Vomiting	2

[1] Children 17 to 24 months of age (fourth dose) and 4 to 6 years of age (fifth dose)
[2] Rectal temperature for 17–24 month olds
Oral temperature for 4–6 year olds

In a large, post-marketing surveillance study, 28,095 doses of ACEL-IMUNE were administered to children as a fourth or fifth dose following previous doses with whole-cell DTP. The rates of local and systemic events reported in a subset of approximately 4400 subjects who were evaluated by telephone interview within 48 to 72 hours postimmunization were: tenderness, 31%; erythema ≥ 1 inch, 4%; induration ≥ 1 inch, 3.5%; perceived fever, 15%; irritability, 25%; and vomiting, 2%.[10]

As with other aluminum-containing vaccines, a nodule may occasionally be palpable at the injection site for several weeks. Sterile abscess formation or subcutaneous atrophy at the injection site may occur rarely.[39]

Urticaria, erythema multiforme or other rash, arthralgias,[40] and, more rarely, a severe anaphylactic reaction[7] (e.g., urticaria with swelling of the mouth, difficulty breathing, hypotension, or shock) have been reported following administration of preparations containing diphtheria, tetanus, and/or pertussis antigens.

Arthus-type hypersensitivity reactions, characterized by severe local reactions (generally starting 2 to 8 hours after an injection) may follow receipt of tetanus toxoid.

Whole-cell pertussis DTP has been associated with acute encephalopathy.[31] A detailed follow-up of the National Childhood Encephalopathy Study (NCES) indicated that children who had had a serious acute neurologic illness were significantly more likely than children in a control group without acute neurologic illness to have chronic nervous system dysfunction 10 years later.[30] These children with chronic nervous system dysfunction were more likely than children in the control group to have received DTP within 7 days of onset of the original serious acute neurologic illness (i.e., 12 [3.3%] of 367 children vs. six [0.8%] of 723 children).[21,30] After reviewing the follow-up data, a committee of the Institute of Medicine (IOM) concluded that the NCES provided evidence of an association between DTP and chronic nervous system dysfunction in children who had a serious acute neurologic illness after vaccination with DTP.[31] However, IOM also concluded that the results were insufficient to determine whether DTP increases the overall risk for chronic nervous system dysfunction in children.[31] The ACIP indicated that the results of the NCES were insufficient to determine whether DTP administration before the acute neurological event influenced the potential for neurologic dysfunction 10 years later.[21]

Onset of infantile spasms has occurred in infants who have recently received DTP and DT. Analysis of data from the NCES on children with infantile spasms showed that receipt of DT or DTP was not causally related to infantile spasms.[31,41] The incidence of onset of infantile spasms increases at 3 to 9 months of age, the time period in which the second and third doses of DTP are generally given. Therefore, some cases of infantile spasms can be expected to be related by chance alone to recent receipt of DTP.[7,31]

A bulging fontanelle associated with increased intracranial pressure which occurred within 24 hours following DTP immunization has been reported, although a causal relationship has not been established.[31,42-44]

The above findings regarding possible association of unusual neurologic events related only to DTP vaccine containing whole-cell pertussis. At this time there are insufficient data to determine their relevance to ACEL-IMUNE. Sudden Infant Death Syndrome (SIDS) has occurred in infants following administration of whole-cell pertussis DTP and DTaP. Large case-control studies of SIDS in the US have shown that receipt of whole-cell DTP was not causally related to SIDS.[45-47] A review by a committee of the IOM concluded that available evidence did not indicate a causal relation between DTP vaccine and SIDS.[31] The rate of SIDS in the German efficacy trial was 0.2 per thousand infants

and in US safety studies was 0.8 per thousand infants vaccinated with ACEL-IMUNE.[10] The reported rate of SIDS in the US from 1985 through 1991 was 1.5 per thousand live births.[48] Since SIDS occurs most commonly at the age when DTP primary immunizations are recommended, by chance alone, some cases of SIDS can be expected to follow receipt of whole-cell pertussis DTP and DTaP.

Neurological complications,[49] such as convulsions,[40] encephalopathy[40,50] and various mono- and polyneuropathies,[50-56] including Guillain-Barré syndrome,[57,58] have been reported following administration of preparations containing diphtheria, tetanus, and/or pertussis antigens. A review by the IOM found a causal relation between tetanus toxoid and brachial neuritis and Guillain-Barré syndrome.[59] Permanent neurological disability and death have been reported rarely in temporal relation to immunization with vaccines containing pertussis antigens; however, a causal relationship has not been established.

As with any vaccine, there is the possibility that broad use of ACEL-IMUNE could reveal adverse reactions not observed in clinical trials.

In clinical trials involving 25,899 immunizations with ACEL-IMUNE, there were no occurrences of anaphylaxis or encephalopathy. Six deaths were reported to study investigators. Causes of death included three SIDS and three accidental deaths. None of these events was determined to be vaccine-related and all occurred more than 4 weeks postimmunization. No deaths from invasive bacterial infections were reported in studies with ACEL-IMUNE.

Adverse Event Reporting

Any adverse reactions following immunization should be reported by the health care provider to the US Department of Health and Human Services (DHHS). The **National Childhood Vaccine Injury Act** requires that the manufacturer and lot number of the vaccine administered be recorded by the health care provider in the vaccine recipient's permanent medical record (or in a permanent office log or file), along with the date of administration of the vaccine and the name, address, and title of the person administering the vaccine. The Act further requires the health care provider to report to the Secretary of the Department of Health and Human Services, the occurrence following immunization of any event set forth in the Vaccine Injury Table, including anaphylaxis or anaphylactic shock within 4 hours; encephalopathy or encephalitis within 72 hours; or any sequela (including death) of an illness, disability, injury, or condition referred to above which illness, disability, injury, or condition arose within the time period prescribed or any event that would contraindicate further doses of vaccine, according to this ACEL-IMUNE package insert.[36,60]

The US Department of Health and Human Services has established Vaccine Adverse Event Reporting System (VAERS) to accept all reports of suspected adverse events after the administration of any vaccine including, but not limited to, the reporting of events required by the National Childhood Vaccine Injury Act of 1986.[36] The VAERS toll-free number for VAERS forms and information is 800-822-7967.

DOSAGE AND ADMINISTRATION

For intramuscular use only
The dose is 0.5 mL to be given intramuscularly.

Primary Immunization
For infants, the primary immunization series of ACEL-IMUNE consists of three doses of 0.5 mL each. The customary age for the first dose is 2 months of age but can be given as young as 6 weeks of age. The recommended dosing interval is 4 to 8 weeks. It is also recommended that ACEL-IMUNE be given for all three doses since no interchangeability data on DTaP vaccines exist for the primary series.
ACEL-IMUNE may be used to complete the primary series in infants who have received one or two doses of whole-cell pertussis DTP. However, the safety and efficacy of ACEL-IMUNE in such infants has not been evaluated.

Booster Immunization
When ACEL-IMUNE or DTP is given for the primary series, a fourth dose of ACEL-IMUNE is recommended at 15 to 20 months of age. The interval between the third and fourth dose should be at least 6 months. A fifth dose of 0.5 mL is recommended at 4 to 6 years of age, preferably prior to entrance into kindergarten or elementary school. If the fourth dose was administered on or after the fourth birthday, a fifth dose prior to school entry is not considered necessary.[7]
Preterm infants should be vaccinated according to their chronological age, calculated from date of birth.[7]
Interruption of the recommended schedules with a delay between doses does not interfere with the final immunity achieved; nor does it necessitate starting the series over again, regardless of the length of time elapsed between doses.[7]
In the case of anaphylaxis, no further vaccination with any of the three antigens in DTaP should be carried out. Alternatively, because of the importance of tetanus vaccination, such individuals may be referred for evaluation by an allergist.[7] If a contraindication to the pertussis vaccine compo-

nent occurs, Diphtheria and Tetanus Toxoids, Adsorbed, for pediatric use (DT), should be substituted for each of the remaining doses.
The use of reduced volume (fractional doses) is not recommended. The effect of such practices on the frequency of serious adverse events and on protection against disease has not been determined.
Shake vigorously to obtain a uniform suspension prior to withdrawing each dose from the multiple dose vial. The vaccine should not be used if it cannot be resuspended.
Parenteral drug products should be inspected visually for particulate matter and discoloration prior to administration (see **DESCRIPTION**).
The vaccine should be injected intramuscularly. The preferred sites are the anterolateral aspect of the thigh or the deltoid muscle of the upper arm. The vaccine should not be injected in the gluteal area or areas where there may be a major nerve trunk. Before injection, the skin at the injection site should be cleansed and prepared with a suitable germicide.
After insertion of the needle, aspirate to help avoid inadvertent injection into a blood vessel.
For booster immunization against tetanus and diphtheria of individuals 7 years of age or older, the use of Tetanus and Diphtheria Toxoids Adsorbed for Adult Use (Td) is recommended.
Routine simultaneous administration of DTaP, OPV (or IPV), Hib vaccine, MMR and Hepatitis B vaccine may be given to children who are the recommended age to receive these vaccines and for whom no specific contraindications exist at the time of the visit.[24]

HOW SUPPLIED
NDC 0005-1800-31 5.0 mL Vial
STORAGE
DO NOT FREEZE. STORE REFRIGERATED, AWAY FROM FREEZER COMPARTMENT, AT 2°C TO 8°C (36°F TO 46°F).

REFERENCES
1. Mueller JH, Miller PA. Production of diphtheria toxin of high potency (100 Lf) on a reproducible medium. *J Immunol.* 1941;40:21-32.
2. Mueller JH, Miller PA. Factors influencing the production of tetanus toxin. *J Immunol.* 1947;56:143-147.
3. Pillemer L, Grossberg DB, Wittler RG. The immunochemistry of toxins and toxoids. II. The preparation of immunologic evaluation of purified tetanal toxoid. *J Immunol.* 1946;54:213-224.
4. Arai H, Sato Y. Separation and characterization of two distinct hemagglutinins contained in purified leukocytosis promoter factor from *Bordetella pertussis. Biochimica et Biophysica Acta.* 1976;444:765-782.
5. CDC. Summary of Notifiable Diseases, United States, 1994. *MMWR.* 1995; 43(53):70-71.
6. Diphtheria Epidemic-New Independent States of the Former Soviet Union. 1990-1994. *MMWR.* 1995;44(10):177-181.
7. Diphtheria, tetanus and pertussis: Recommendations for vaccine use and other preventive measures—recommendations of the Immunization Practices Advisory Committee (ACIP). *MMWR.* 1991;40 (RR-10).
8. Ipsen J. Immunization of adults against diphtheria and tetanus. *NEJM.* 1954;251:459-466.
9. *Federal Register Notice,* Friday, December 13, 1985, Vol. 50, No. 240.
10. Unpublished data available from Lederle Laboratories.
11. Pappenheimer AM Jr. Diphtheria. In: Germanier R, ed. *Bacterial Vaccines.* New York, NY: Academic Press Inc; 1984:1-36.
12. Kendrick PL. Secondary familial attack rates from pertussis in vaccinated and unvaccinated children. *Am J. Hygiene.* 1940;32:89-91.
13. Reported incidence of notifiable diseases in the United States. *MMWR.* 1970;19(53):44.
14. Pertussis surveillance-United States, January 1992-June 1995. *MMWR.* 1995;44(28):525-529.
15. Mortimer JD Jr. Pertussis and its prevention: a family affair. *J Infect Dis.* 1990;161:473-479.
16. Cowell JL, Oda M, Burstyn DG, et al. Prospective protective antigens and animal models for pertussis. In: Leive L, Schlessinger D, eds, *Microbiology - 1984.* Washington, DC: American Society for Microbiology; 1984:172-175.
17. Shahin RD, Brennan MJ, Li ZM, et al. Characterization of the protective capacity and immunogenicity of the 69-kd outer membrane protein of *Bordetella pertussis. J Exper Med.* 1990;171(1):63-73.
18. Novotny P, Kobisch M, Cownley K, et al. Evaluation of *Bordetella bronchiseptica* vaccines in specific-pathogen-free piglets with bacterial cell surface antigens in enzyme linked immunosorbent assay. *Infect Immun.* 1985;50:190-198.
19. Manclark CR, Cowell JL. Pertussis vaccine. In: Germanier R, ed. *Bacterial Vaccines.* New York, NY: Academic Press, Inc; 1984;69-106.
20. Rothstein EP, Bernstein HH, Glode MP, et al. Simultaneous administration of a diphtheria and tetanus toxoids

Continued on next page

Acel-Imune—Cont.

and acellular pertussis vaccine with measles-mumps-rubella and oral poliovirus vaccines. *AJDC.* 1993;(147):854-857.

21. Update: Vaccine side effects, adverse reactions, contraindications, and precautions. *MMWR.* 1996;45 (RR-12):22-31.

22. American Academy of Pediatrics. *Report of the Committee on Infectious Diseases.* 23rd ed. Elk Grove Village, III: American Academy of Pediatrics; 1994.

23. Sutter RW, Patriarca PA, Suleiman, AJM, et al. Attributable risk of DTP (Diphtheria and Tetanus Toxoids and Pertussis Vaccines) injection in provoking paralytic poliomyelitis during a large outbreak in Oman. *J Infect Dis.* 1992;165:444-449.

24. Pertussis vaccination: acellular pertussis vaccine for reinforcing and booster use-supplementary ACIP statement. *MMWR* 1992;41(RR-1):1-10.

25. Livingstone S. Comprehensive management of epilepsy in infancy. Springfield, IL: Charles C. Thomas; 1972;159-66.

26. Livengood JR, Mullen JR, White JW, et al. Family history of convulsions and use of pertussis vaccine. *J Pediatr.* 1989;115:527-531.

27. Stetler HC, Orenstein WA, Bart KJ, et al. History of convulsion and use of pertussis vaccine. *J Pediatr.* 1985;107;175-9.

28. Ipp MM, Gold R, Greenberg S, et al. Acetaminophen prophylaxis of adverse reactions following vaccination of infants with diphtheria-pertussis-tetanus toxoids-polio vaccine. *Pediatr Infect Dis J.* 1987;6:721-725.

29. Pertussis immunization: family history of convulsions and use of antipyretics - supplementary ACIP statement. *MMWR.* 1987;36(18);281-282.

30. Miller D, Madge N, Diamond J, et al. Pertussis immunization and serious acute neurological illnesses in children. *BMJ.* 1993;307:1171-6.

31. Howson CP, Howe CJ, Fineberg HV. Adverse effects of pertussis and rubella vaccines, pertussis vaccines and CNS disorders. Institute of Medicine (IOM). Washington, DC: National Academy Press; 1991.

32. Recommendtions of the Advisory Committee on Immunization Practices (ACIP): Use of Vaccines and Immuno Globulins in Persons with Altered Immunocompetence. *MMWR.* 1993;42(RR-4).

33. Immunization of children infected with human immunodeficiency virus - supplementary ACIP statement. *MMWR.* 1988;37(12):181-183.

34. Recommendation of the ACIP: immunization of children infected with human T-lymphotropic virus type III/lymphadenopathy-associated virus. *MMWR.* 1986;35(38):595-606.

35. General Recommendations on Immunization—Recommendations of the Immunization Practices Advisory Committee (ACIP). *MMWR.* 1989;38(13):221.

36. CDC. Vaccine Adverse Event Reporting System—United States. *MMWR.* 1990;39:730-733.

37. Morgan CM, Blumberg DA, Cherry JD, et al. Comparison of acellular and whole-cell pertussis-component DTP vaccines. *AJDC.* 1990;144:41-45.

38. Cody CL, Baraff LJ, Cherry JP, et al. Nature and rates of adverse reactions associated with DTP and DT immunizations in infants and children. *Pediatrics.* 1981;68:(5):650-660.

39. Fawcett HA, Smith NP. Injection-site granuloma due to aluminum. *Arch Dermatol.* 1984;120:1318-1322.

40. Adverse events following immunization. *MMWR.* 1985;34(3):43-47.

41. Bellman MH, Ross EM, Miller DL. Infantile spasms and pertussis immunization. *Lancet*, 1983; 1:1031-1034.

42. Jacob J, Mannino F. Increased intracranial pressure after diphtheria, tetanus and pertussis immunization. *AJDC.* 1979;(133):217-218.

43. Mathur R, Kumari S. Bulging fontanel following triple vaccine. *Indian Pediatr.* 1981;18(6):417-418.

44. Shendurnikar N, Gandhi DJ, Patel J, et al. Bulging fontanel following DTP vaccine. *Indian Pediatr.* 1986;23(11):960.

45. Griffin MR, Ray Wa, Livengood JR, et al. Risk of sudden infant death syndrome after immunization with diphtheria-tetanus-pertussis vaccine. *NEJM* 1988;319(10):618-623.

46. Hoffman HJ, Hunter JC, Damus K, et al. Diphtheria-tetanus-pertussis immunization and sudden infant death: results of the National Institute of Child Health and Human Development Cooperative Epidemiological study of sudden infant death syndrome risk factors. *Pediatrics.* 1987:79:598-611.

47. Walker AM, Jick H, Perera DR, et al. Diphtheria-tetanus-pertussis immunization and sudden infant death syndrome. *Am J Pub Health.* 1987;77:945-951.

48. Willinger M, Hoffman HJ, Hartford RB. Infant sleep position and risk for sudden infant death syndrome: report of meeting held January 13 and 14, 1994, National Institutes of Health, Bethesda, MD. *Pediatrics.* 1994; 93(5):814-819.

49. Rutledge SL, Snead OC. Neurological complications of immunizations. *J Pediatr.* 1986;109:917-924.

50. Schlenska GK. Unusual neurological complications following tetanus toxoid administration. *J Neurol.* 1977;215: 299-302.

51. Blumstein GI, Kreithen H. Peripheral neuropathy following tetanus toxoid administration. *JAMA.* 1966;198: 1030-1031.

52. Reinstein L, Pargament JM, Goodman JS. Peripheral neuropathy after multiple tetanus toxoid injections. *Arch Phys Med Rehabil.* 1982;63:332-334.

53. Tsairis P, Dyck PJ, Mulder DW. Natural history of brachial plexus neuropathy. *Arch Neurol.* 1972;27:109-117.

54. Quast U, Hennessen W, Widmark RM. Mono- and polyneuritis after tetanus vaccination. *Dev Biol Stand.* 1979;43: 25-32.

55. Holliday PL, Bauer RB. Polyradiculoneuritis secondary to immunization with tetanus and diphtheria toxoids. *Arch Neurol.* 1983;40:56-57.

56. Fenichel GM. Neurological complications of tetanus toxoid. *Arch Neurol.* 1983;40:390.

57. Pollard JD, Selby G. Relapsing neuropathy due to tetanus toxoid. *J Neurol Sci.* 1978;37:113-125.

58. Newton N, Janati A. Guillain-Barré syndrome after vaccination with purified tetanus toxoid. *S Med J.* 1987;80: 1053-1054.

59. Stratton KR, Howe CJ, Johnston RB. Adverse events associated with childhood vaccines. Evidence bearing on causality. Institute of Medicine. Washington, DC: National Academy Press; 1994.

60. *Federal Register Final Rule,* Wednesday, February 8, 1995, Vo. 60, No. 26:7694.

Manufactured by:
LEDERLE LABORATORIES
Division American Cyanamid Company
Pearl River, NY 10965
US Gov't. License No. 17

Marketed by:
WYETH-LEDERLE VACCINES
Wyeth-Ayerst Laboratories
Philadelphia, PA 19101

Shown in Product Identification Guide, page 319

ACHROMYCIN® V ℞

[a-krō-mī-cin]
tetracycline HCl
for ORAL USE

DESCRIPTION

ACHROMYCIN V tetracycline hydrochloride is an antibiotic isolated from *Streptomyces aureofaciens.* Chemically it is the monohydrochloride of [4S -(4α,4aα,5aα,6β,12aα,)] -4-(Dimethylamino)-1,4,4a,5,5a,6,11,12a-octahydro-3, 6, 10, 12, 12a-pentahydroxy-6-methyl-1, 11-dioxo-2-naphthacenecarboxamide.

ACHROMYCIN V oral dosage forms contain the following inactive ingredients:

Capsules: Blue 1, FD&C Yellow No. 6, Gelatin, Lactose, Magnesium Stearate, Red 28, Titanium Dioxide, Yellow 10 and other ingredients.

CLINICAL PHARMACOLOGY

The tetracyclines are primarily bacteriostatic and are thought to exert their antimicrobial effect by the inhibition of protein synthesis. Tetracyclines are active against a wide range of gram-negative and gram-positive organisms.

The drugs in the tetracycline class have closely similar antimicrobial spectra, and cross-resistance among them is common.

Microorganisms may be considered susceptible if the MIC (minimum inhibitory concentration) is not more than 4 mcg/mL and intermediate if the MIC is 4 to 12.5 mcg/mL.

Susceptibility plate testing: A tetracycline disc may be used to determine microbial susceptibility to drugs in the tetracycline class. If the Kirby-Bauer method of disc susceptibility testing is used, a 30 mcg tetracycline HCl disc should give a zone of at least 19 mm when tested against a tetracycline-susceptible bacterial strain.

Tetracyclines are readily absorbed and are bound to plasma proteins in varying degrees. They are concentrated by the liver in the bile and excreted in the urine and feces at high concentrations and in a biologically active form.

INDICATIONS

ACHROMYCIN V is indicated in infections caused by the following microorganisms.

Rickettsiae: (Rocky Mountain spotted fever, typhus fever and the typhus group, Q fever, rickettsialpox, tick fevers).

Mycoplasma pneumoniae (PPLO, Eaton agent).

Agents of psittacosis and ornithosis.

Agents of lymphogranuloma venereum and granuloma inguinale.

The spirochetal agent of relapsing fever (*Borrelia recurrentis*).

The following gram-negative microorganisms:

Haemophilus ducreyi (chancroid),
Yersinia pestis and *Francisella tularensis,* formerly *Pasteurella pestis* and *Pasteurella tularensis,*
Bartonella bacilliformis,
Bacteroides species,
Vibrio comma and *Vibrio fetus,*
Brucella species (in conjunction with streptomycin).

Because many strains of the following groups of microorganisms have been shown to be resistant to tetracyclines, culture and susceptibility testing are recommended.

ACHROMYCIN is indicated for treatment of infections caused by the following gram-negative microorganisms, when bacteriologic testing indicates appropriate susceptibility to the drug:

Escherichia coli,
Enterobacter aerogenes (formerly *Aerobacter aerogenes*),
Shigella species,
Mima species and *Herellea* species,
Haemophilus influenzae (respiratory infections),
Klebsiella species (respiratory and urinary infections).

ACHROMYCIN is indicated for treatment of infections caused by the following gram-positive microorganisms, when bacteriologic testing indicates appropriate susceptibility to the drug:

Streptococcus species:

Up to 44% of strains of *Streptococcus pyogenes* and 74% of *Streptococcus faecalis* have been found to be resistant to tetracycline drugs. Therefore, tetracyclines should not be used for streptococcal disease unless the organism has been demonstrated to be sensitive.

For upper respiratory infections due to Group A beta-hemolytic streptococci, penicillin is the usual drug of choice, including prophylaxis of rheumatic fever.

Streptococcus pneumoniae,
Staphylococcus aureus, skin and soft tissue infections.

Tetracyclines are not the drug of choice in the treatment of any type of staphylococcal infection.

When penicillin is contraindicated, tetracyclines are alternative drugs in the treatment of infections due to:

Neisseria gonorrhoeae,
Treponema pallidum and *Treponema pertenue* (syphilis and yaws),
Listeria monocytogenes,
Clostridium species,
Bacillus anthracis,
Fusobacterium fusiforme (Vincent's infection),
Actinomyces species.

In acute intestinal amebiasis, the tetracyclines may be a useful adjunct to amebicides.

In severe acne, the tetracyclines may be useful adjunctive therapy.

ACHROMYCIN V is indicated in the treatment of trachoma, although the infectious agent is not always eliminated, as judged by immunofluorescence.

Inclusion conjunctivitis may be treated with oral tetracyclines or with a combination of oral and topical agents.

ACHROMYCIN is indicated for the treatment of uncomplicated urethral, endocervical or rectal infections in adults caused by *Chlamydia trachomatis.*[1]

CONTRAINDICATIONS

This drug is contraindicated in persons who have shown hypersensitivity to any of the tetracyclines.

WARNINGS

THE USE OF DRUGS OF THE TETRACYCLINE CLASS DURING TOOTH DEVELOPMENT (LAST HALF OF PREGNANCY, INFANCY AND CHILDHOOD TO THE AGE OF 8 YEARS) MAY CAUSE PERMANENT DISCOLORATION OF THE TEETH (YELLOW-GRAY-BROWN). This adverse reaction is more common during long-term use of the drugs but has been observed following repeated short-term courses. Enamel hypoplasia has also been reported. TETRACYCLINE DRUGS, THEREFORE, SHOULD NOT BE USED IN THIS AGE GROUP UNLESS OTHER DRUGS ARE NOT LIKELY TO BE EFFECTIVE OR ARE CONTRAINDICATED.

If renal impairment exists, even usual oral or parenteral doses may lead to excessive systemic accumulation of the drug and possible liver toxicity. Under such conditions, lower than usual total doses are indicated and, if therapy is prolonged, serum level determinations of the drug may be advisable.

Photosensitivity manifested by an exaggerated sunburn reaction has been observed in some individuals taking tetracyclines. Patients apt to be exposed to direct sunlight or ultraviolet light should be advised that this reaction can occur with tetracycline drugs, and treatment should be discontinued at the first evidence of skin erythema.

The anti-anabolic action of the tetracyclines may cause an increase in BUN. While this is not a problem in those with normal renal function, in patients with significantly impaired function, higher serum levels of tetracycline may lead to azotemia, hyperphosphatemia, and acidosis.

Usage in Pregnancy (See above **WARNINGS** about use during tooth development.) Results of animal studies indicate

that tetracyclines cross the placenta, are found in fetal tissues and can have toxic effects on the developing fetus (often related to retardation of skeletal development). Evidence of embryotoxicity has also been noted in animals treated early in pregnancy.

Usage in Newborns, Infants, and Children (See above **WARNINGS** about use during tooth development.)

All tetracyclines form a stable calcium complex in any bone forming tissue. A decrease in the fibula growth rate has been observed in prematures given oral tetracycline in doses of 25 mg/kg every six hours. This reaction was shown to be reversible when the drug was discontinued.

Tetracyclines are present in the milk of lactating women who are taking a drug in this class.

PRECAUTIONS

General

Pseudotumor cerebri (benign intracranial hypertension) in adults has been associated with the use of tetracyclines. The usual clinical manifestations are headache and blurred vision. Bulging fontanels have been associated with the use of tetracyclines in infants. While both of these conditions and related symptoms usually resolve soon after discontinuation of the tetracycline, the possibility for permanent sequelae exists.

As with other antibiotics preparations, use of this drug may result in overgrowth of nonsusceptible organisms, including fungi. If superinfection occurs, the antibiotic should be discontinued and appropriate therapy should be instituted.

In venereal diseases when coexistent syphilis is suspected, darkfield examination should be done before treatment is started and the blood serology repeated monthly for at least 4 months.

In long-term therapy, periodic laboratory evaluation of organ systems, including hematopoietic, renal and hepatic studies should be performed.

All infections due to Group A beta-hemolytic streptococci should be treated for at least ten days.

Drug Interactions

Because tetracyclines have been shown to depress plasma prothrombin activity, patients who are on anticoagulant therapy may require downward adjustment of their anticoagulant dosage.

Since bacteriostatic drugs, such as the tetracycline class of antibiotics, may interfere with the bactericidal action of penicillins, it is not advisable to administer these drugs concomitantly.

Concurrent use of tetracyclines with oral contraceptives may render oral contraceptives less effective. Breakthrough bleeding has been reported.

ADVERSE REACTIONS

Gastrointestinal: Anorexia, nausea, vomiting, diarrhea, glossitis, dysphagia, enterocolitis, pancreatitis, and inflammatory lesions (with monilial overgrowth) in the anogenital region, increases in liver enzymes, and hepatic toxicity have been reported rarely. Rare instances of esophagitis and esophageal ulcerations have been reported in patients taking the tetracycline-class antibiotics in capsule and tablet form. Most of these patients took the medication immediately before going to bed (see **DOSAGE AND ADMINISTRATION**).

Skin: Maculopapular and erythematous rashes. Exfoliative dermatitis has been reported but is uncommon. Fixed drug eruptions, including balanitis, have been rarely reported. Photosensitivity is discussed above. (See **WARNINGS.**)

Renal toxicity: Rise in BUN has been reported and is apparently dose related. (See **WARNINGS.**)

Hypersensitivity reactions: Urticaria, angioneurotic edema, anaphylaxis, anaphylactoid purpura, pericarditis and exacerbation of systemic lupus erythematosus.

Blood: Hemolytic anemia, thrombocytopenia, neutropenia and eosinophilia have been reported.

CNS: Pseudotumor cerebri (benign intracranial hypertension) in adults and bulging fontanels in infants. (See **PRECAUTIONS—General.**) Dizziness, tinnitus, and visual disturbances have been reported. Myasthenic syndrome has been reported rarely.

Other: When given over prolonged periods, tetracyclines have been reported to produce brown-black microscopic discoloration of thyroid glands. No abnormalities of thyroid function studies are known to occur.

DOSAGE AND ADMINISTRATION

Therapy should be continued for at least 24 to 48 hours after symptoms and fever have subsided.

Concomitant therapy: Antacids containing aluminum, calcium, or magnesium impair absorption and should not be given to patients taking oral tetracycline.

Foods and some dairy products also interfere with absorption. Oral forms of tetracycline should be given 1 hour before or 2 hours after meals.

In patients with renal impairment: (See **WARNINGS**). Total dosage should be decreased by reduction of recommended individual doses and/or by extending time intervals between doses.

In the treatment of streptococcal infections, a therapeutic dose of tetracycline should be administered for at least ten days.

Adults: Usual daily dose, 1–2 grams divided in two or four equal doses, depending on the severity of the infection.

For children above eight years of age: Usual daily dose, 10–20 mg (25–50 mg/kg) per pound of body weight divided in two or four equal doses.

For treatment of brucellosis, 500 mg tetracycline four times daily for 3 weeks should be accompanied by streptomycin, 1 gram intramuscularly twice daily the first week and once daily the second week.

For treatment of syphilis, a total of 30–40 grams in equally divided doses over a period of 10–15 days should be given. Close follow up, including laboratory tests, is recommended.

Gonorrhea patients sensitive to pencillin may be treated with tetracycline, administered as an initial oral dose of 1.5 grams followed by 0.5 gram every 6 hours for four days to a total dosage of 9 grams.

Uncomplicated urethral, endocervical, or rectal infection in adults caused by *Chlamydia trachomatis:* 500 mg, by mouth, 4 times a day for at least 7 days.[1]

HOW SUPPLIED

ACHROMYCIN® V tetracycline HCl oral dosage forms are available as follows:

CAPSULES

500 mg - Two-piece, hard shell, elongated, opaque capsules with a blue cap and a yellow body, printed with Lederle over A5 on one half and Lederle over 500 mg on the other in gray ink, supplied as follows:

NDC 0005-4875-23—Bottle of 100
NDC 0005-4875-34—Bottle of 1,000

250 mg - Two-piece, hard shell, opaque capsules with a blue cap and a yellow body, printed with Lederle over A3 on one half and Lederle over 250 mg on the other in gray ink, supplied as follows:

NDC 0005-4880-23—Bottle of 100
NDC 0005-4880-34—Bottle of 1,000

Store at Controlled Room Temperature 15°–30°C (59°–86°F).

Reference: 1. CDC Sexually Transmitted Diseases Treatment Guidelines 1982.

Manufactured by:

LEDERLE PHARMACEUTICAL DIVISION
American Cyanamid Company
Pearl River, NY 10965

ARTANE® ℞

[*ar-tāne*]
(trihexyphenidyl HCl)
For Oral Use

DESCRIPTION

ARTANE (trihexyphenidyl HCl) is a synthetic antispasmodic drug available in the following forms:

TABLETS: Containing 2 mg and 5 mg ARTANE (trihexyphenidyl HCl), each strength also containing as inactive ingredients: Corn Starch, Dibasic Calcium Phosphate, Magnesium Stearate and Pregelatinized Starch.

ELIXIR: Containing 2 mg/5 mL ARTANE (trihexyphenidyl HCl) in a clear, colorless, lime-mint flavored preparation, also containing as inactive ingredients: Alcohol 5%, Citric Acid, Flavorings, Methylparaben, Propylparaben, Sodium Chloride and Sorbitol Solution.

ACTIONS

ARTANE (trihexyphenidyl HCl) is the substituted piperidine salt, 3-(1-piperidyl)-1-phenyl-cyclohexyl-1-propanol hydrochloride, which exerts a direct inhibitory effect upon the parasympathetic nervous system. It also has a relaxing effect on smooth musculature; exerted both directly upon the muscle tissue itself and indirectly through an inhibitory effect upon the parasympathetic nervous system. Its therapeutic properties are similar to those of atropine although undesirable side effects are ordinarily less frequent and severe than with the latter.

INDICATIONS

This drug is indicated as an adjunct in the treatment of all forms of parkinsonism (postencephalitic, arteriosclerotic, and idiopathic). It is often useful as adjuvant therapy when treating these forms of parkinsonism with levodopa. Additionally, it is indicated for the control of extrapyramidal disorders caused by central nervous system drugs such as the dibenzoxazepines, phenothiazines, thioxanthenes, and butyrophenones.

WARNING

Patients to be treated with ARTANE should have a gonioscope evaluation and close monitoring of intraocular pressures at regular periodic intervals.

PRECAUTIONS

Although trihexyphenidyl HCl is not contraindicated for patients with cardiac, liver, or kidney disorders, or with hypertension, such patients should be maintained under close observation.

Since the use of trihexyphenidyl HCl may in some cases continue indefinitely and since it has atropine-like properties, patients should be subjected to constant and careful long-term observation to avoid allergic and other untoward reactions. Inasmuch as trihexyphenidyl HCl possesses some parasympatholytic activity, it should be used with caution in patients with glaucoma, obstructive disease of the gastrointestinal or genitourinary tracts, and in elderly males with possible prostatic hypertrophy. Geriatric patients, particularly over the age of 60, frequently develop increased sensitivity to the actions of drugs of this type, and hence, require strict dosage regulation. Incipient glaucoma may be precipitated by parasympatholytic drugs such as trihexyphenidyl HCl.

Tardive dyskinesia may appear in some patients on long-term therapy with antipsychotic drugs or may occur after therapy with these drugs has been discontinued. Antiparkinsonism agents do not alleviate the symptoms of tardive dyskinesia, and in some instances may aggravate them. However, parkinsonism and tardive dyskinesia often coexist in patients receiving chronic neuroleptic treatment, and anticholinergic therapy with ARTANE may relieve some of these parkinsonism symptoms.

ADVERSE REACTIONS

Minor side effects, such as dryness of the mouth, blurring of vision, dizziness; mild nausea or nervousness, will be experienced by 30 to 50 percent of all patients. These sensations, however, are much less troublesome with ARTANE (trihexyphenidyl HCl) than with belladonna alkaloids and are usually less disturbing than unalleviated parkinsonism. Such reactions tend to become less pronounced, and even to disappear, as treatment continues. Even before these reactions have remitted spontaneously, they may often be controlled by careful adjustment of dosage form, amount of drug, or interval between doses.

Isolated instances of suppurative parotitis secondary to excessive dryness of the mouth, skin rashes, dilatation of the colon, paralytic ileus, and certain psychiatric manifestations such as delusions and hallucinations, plus one doubtful case of paranoia all of which may occur with any of the atropine-like drugs, have been reported rarely with ARTANE.

Patients with arteriosclerosis or with a history of idiosyncrasy to other drugs may exhibit reactions of mental confusion, agitation, disturbed behavior, or nausea and vomiting. Such patients should be allowed to develop a tolerance through the initial administration of a small dose and gradual increase in dose until an effective level is reached. If a severe reaction should occur, administration of the drug should be discontinued for a few days and then resumed at a lower dosage. Psychiatric disturbances can result from indiscriminate use (leading to overdosage) to sustain continued euphoria.

Potential side effects associated with the use of any atropine-like drugs include constipation, drowsiness, urinary hesitancy or retention, tachycardia, dilation of the pupil, increased intraocular tension, weakness, vomiting, and headache.

The occurrence of angle-closure glaucoma due to long-term treatment with trihexyphenidyl hydrochloride has been reported.

DOSAGE AND ADMINISTRATION

Dosage should be individualized. The initial dose should be low and then increased gradually, especially in patients over 60 years of age. Whether ARTANE (trihexyphenidyl HCl) may best be given before or after meals should be determined by the way the patient reacts. Postencephalitic patients, who are usually more prone to excessive salivation, may prefer to take it after meals and may, in addition, require small amounts of atropine which, under such circumstances, is sometimes an effective adjuvant. If ARTANE® tends to dry the mouth excessively, it may be better to take it before meals, unless it causes nausea. If taken after meals, the thirst sometimes induced can be allayed by mint candies, chewing gum or water.

ARTANE (trihexyphenidyl HCl) in Idiopathic Parkinsonism

As initial therapy for parkinsonism, 1 mg of ARTANE® in tablet or elixir form may be administered the first day. The dose may then be increased by 2 mg increments at intervals of three to five days, until a total of 6 to 10 mg is given daily. The total daily dose will depend upon what is found to be the optimal level. Many patients derive maximum benefit from this daily total of 6 to 10 mg, but some patients, chiefly those in the postencephalitic group, may require a total daily dose of 12 to 15 mg.

Continued on next page

Artane—Cont.

ARTANE (trihexyphenidyl HCl) in Drug-Induced Parkinsonism

The size and frequency of dose of ARTANE needed to control extrapyramidal reactions to commonly employed tranquilizers, notably the phenothiazines, thioxanthenes, and butyrophenones, must be determined empirically. The total daily dosage usually ranges between 5 and 15 mg although, in some cases, these reactions have been satisfactorily controlled on as little as 1 mg daily. It may be advisable to commence therapy with a single 1 mg dose. If the extrapyramidal manifestations are not controlled in a few hours, the subsequent doses may be progressively increased until satisfactory control is achieved. Satisfactory control may sometimes be more rapidly achieved by temporarily reducing the dosage of the tranquilizer on instituting ARTANE (trihexyphenidyl HCl) therapy and then adjusting dosage of both drugs until the desired ataractic effect is retained without onset of extrapyramidal reactions.

It is sometimes possible to maintain the patient on a reduced ARTANE dosage after the reactions have remained under control for several days. Instances have been reported in which these reactions have remained in remission for long periods after ARTANE therapy was discontinued.

Concomitant Use of ARTANE (trihexyphenidyl HCl) with Levodopa

When ARTANE is used concomitantly with levodopa, the usual dose of each may need to be reduced. Careful adjustment is necessary, depending on side effects and degree of symptom control. ARTANE dosage of 3 to 6 mg daily, in divided doses, is usually adequate.

Concomitant Use of ARTANE (trihexyphenidyl HCl) with Other Parasympathetic Inhibitors

ARTANE (trihexyphenidyl HCl) may be substituted, in whole or in part, for other parasympathetic inhibitors. The usual technique is partial substitution initially, with progressive reduction in the other medication as the dose of trihexyphenidyl HCl is increased.

ARTANE TABLETS and ELIXIR—The total daily intake of ARTANE tablets or elixir is tolerated best if divided into 3 doses and taken at mealtimes. High doses (>10 mg daily) may be divided into 4 parts, with 3 doses administered at mealtimes and the fourth at bedtime.

HOW SUPPLIED

ARTANE® (trihexyphenidyl HCl) Elixir is available as follows:

2 mg/5mL – NDC 0005-4440-65 – Bottles of 16 fl oz.
Store at controlled room temperature 20°-25°C (68°-77°F). DO NOT FREEZE.
ALSO AVAILABLE IN TABLETS:
2 mg—round, flat, scored, white tablets; engraved ARTANE above 2 on one side and LL above A11 below the score on the other side, supplied as follows:

NDC 0005-4434-23—Bottle of 100
NDC 0005-4434-34—Bottle of 1000

5 mg—round, flat, scored, white tablets; engraved ARTANE above 5 on one side and LL above A12 below the score on the other side, supplied as follows:

NDC 0005-4436-23—Bottle of 100
NDC 0005-4436-34—Bottle of 1000

Store at controlled room temperature 20°-25°C (68°-77°F).
Manufactured by:
LEDERLE PHARMACEUTICAL DIVISION
American Cyanamid Company
Pearl River, NY 10965

Shown in Product Identification Guide, page 319

ASENDIN® ℞

[a-sen-din]
amoxapine tablets

DESCRIPTION

ASENDIN amoxapine is an antidepressant of the dibenzoxazepine class, chemically distinct from the dibenzazepines, dibenzocycloheptenes, and dibenzoxepines.

It is designated chemically as 2-chloro-11-(1-piperazinyl)dibenz-[b,f][1,4]oxazepine. The molecular weight is 313.8. The empirical formula is $C_{17}H_{16}ClN_3O$.

ASENDIN is supplied for oral administration as 25 mg, 50 mg, 100 mg, and 150 mg tablets.

Inactive Ingredients: All tablets contain Corn Starch, Dibasic Calcium Phosphate, Magnesium Stearate, Pregelatinized Starch, and Stearic Acid. Additionally, the 50 and 150 mg tablets contain FD&C Yellow No. 6 and the 100 mg tablet contains Blue 2.

CLINICAL PHARMACOLOGY

ASENDIN is an antidepressant with a mild sedative component to its action. The mechanism of its clinical action in man is not well understood. In animals, amoxapine reduced the uptake of norepinephrine and serotonin and blocked the response of dopamine receptors to dopamine. Amoxapine is not a monoamine oxidase inhibitor.

ASENDIN is absorbed rapidly and reaches peak blood levels approximately 90 minutes after ingestion. It is almost completely metabolized. The main route of excretion is the kidney. *In vitro* tests show that amoxapine binding to human serum is approximately 90%.

In man, amoxapine serum concentration declines with a half-life of eight hours. However, the major metabolite, 8-hydroxyamoxapine, has a biologic half-life of 30 hours. Metabolites are excreted in the urine in conjugated form as glucuronides.

Clinical studies have demonstrated that ASENDIN has a more rapid onset of action than either amitriptyline or imipramine. The initial clinical effect may occur within four to seven days and occurs within two weeks in over 80% of responders.

INDICATIONS AND USAGE

ASENDIN is indicated for the relief of symptoms of depression in patients with neurotic or reactive depressive disorders as well as endogenous and psychotic depressions. It is indicated for depression accompanied by anxiety or agitation.

CONTRAINDICATIONS

ASENDIN is contraindicated in patients who have shown prior hypersensitivity to dibenzoxazepine compounds. It should not be given concomitantly with monoamine oxidase inhibitors. Hyperpyretic crises, severe convulsions, and deaths have occurred in patients receiving tricyclic antidepressants and monoamine oxidase inhibitors simultaneously. When it is desired to replace a monoamine oxidase inhibitor with ASENDIN, a minimum of 14 days should be allowed to elapse after the former is discontinued. ASENDIN should then be initiated cautiously with gradual increase in dosage until optimum response is achieved. The drug is not recommended for use during the acute recovery phase following myocardial infarction.

WARNINGS

Tardive Dyskinesia

Tardive dyskinesia, a syndrome consisting of potentially irreversible, involuntary, dyskinetic movements may develop in patients treated with neuroleptic (ie, antipsychotics) drugs. (Amoxapine is not an antipsychotic, but it has substantive neuroleptic activity.) Although the prevalence of the syndrome appears to be highest among the elderly, especially elderly women, it is impossible to rely upon prevalence estimates to predict, at the inception of neuroleptic treatment, which patients are likely to develop the syndrome. Whether neuroleptic drug products differ in their potential to cause tardive dyskinesia is unknown.

Both the risk of developing the syndrome and the likelihood that it will become irreversible are believed to increase as the duration of treatment and the total cumulative dose of neuroleptic drugs administered to the patient increase. However, the syndrome can develop, although much less commonly, after relatively brief treatment periods at low doses.

There is no known treatment for established cases of tardive dyskinesia, although the syndrome may remit, partially or completely, if neuroleptic treatment is withdrawn. Neuroleptic treatment itself, however, may suppress (or partially suppress) the signs and symptoms of the syndrome and thereby may possibly mask the underlying disease process. The effect that symptomatic suppression has upon the long-term course of the syndrome is unknown.

Given these considerations, neuroleptics should be prescribed in a manner that is most likely to minimize the occurrence of tardive dyskinesia. Chronic neuroleptic treatment should generally be reserved for patients who suffer from a chronic illness that 1) is known to respond to neuroleptic drugs, and 2) for whom alternative, equally effective, but potentially less harmful treatments are not available or appropriate. In patients who do require chronic treatment, the smallest dose and the shortest duration of treatment producing a satisfactory clinical response should be sought. The need for continued treatment should be reassessed periodically.

If signs and symptoms of tardive dyskinesia appear in a patient on neuroleptics, drug discontinuation should be considered. However, some patients may require treatment despite the presence of the syndrome.

(For further information about the description of tardive dyskinesia and its clinical detection, please refer to **Information for the Patient** and **ADVERSE REACTIONS.**)

Neuroleptic Malignant Syndrome (NMS)

A potentially fatal symptom complex sometimes referred to as Neuroleptic Malignant Syndrome (NMS) has been reported in association with antipsychotic drugs and with amoxapine. Clinical manifestations of NMS are hyperpyrexia, muscle rigidity, altered mental status and evidence of autonomic instability (irregular pulse or blood pressure, tachycardia, diaphoresis, and cardiac dysrhythmias).

The diagnostic evaluation of patients with this syndrome is complicated. In arriving at a diagnosis, it is important to identify cases where the clinical presentation includes both serious medical illness (e.g., pneumonia, systemic infection, etc) and untreated or inadequately treated extrapyramidal signs and symptoms (EPS). Other important considerations in the differential diagnosis include central anticholinergic toxicity, heat stroke, drug fever, and primary central nervous system (CNS) pathology.

The management of NMS should include 1) immediate discontinuation of antipsychotic drugs and other drugs not essential to concurrent therapy, 2) intensive symptomatic treatment and medical monitoring, and 3) treatment of any concomitant serious medical problems for which specific treatments are available. There is no general agreement about specific pharmacological treatment regimens for uncomplicated NMS.

If a patient requires antipsychotic drug treatment after recovery from NMS, the potential reintroduction of drug therapy should be carefully considered. The patient should be carefully monitored since recurrences of NMS have been reported.

ASENDIN amoxapine should be used with caution in patients with a history of urinary retention, angle-closure glaucoma, or increased intraocular pressure. Patients with cardiovascular disorders should be watched closely. Tricyclic antidepressant drugs, particularly when given in high doses, can induce sinus tachycardia, changes in conduction time, and arrhythmias. Myocardial infarction and stroke have been reported with drugs of this class.

Extreme caution should be used in treating patients with a history of convulsive disorder or those with overt or latent seizure disorders.

PRECAUTIONS

General:
In prescribing the drug it should be borne in mind that the possibility of suicide is inherent in any severe depression, and persists until a significant remission occurs; the drug should be dispensed in the smallest suitable amount. Manic depressive patients may experience a shift to the manic phase. Schizophrenic patients may develop increased symptoms of psychosis; patients with paranoid symptomatology may have an exaggeration of such symptoms. This may require reduction of dosage or the addition of a major tranquilizer to the therapeutic regimen. Antidepressant drugs can cause skin rashes and/or "drug fever" in susceptible individuals. These allergic reactions may, in rare cases, be severe. They are more likely to occur during the first few days of treatment, but may also occur later. ASENDIN should be discontinued if rash and/or fever develop. Amoxapine possesses a degree of dopamine-blocking activity which may cause extrapyramidal symptoms in <1% of patients. Rarely, symptoms indicative of tardive dyskinesia have been reported.

Information for the Patient:
Given the likelihood that some patients exposed chronically to neuroleptics will develop tardive dyskinesia, it is advised that all patients in whom chronic use is contemplated be given, if possible, full information about this risk. The decision to inform patients and/or their guardians must obviously take into account the clinical circumstances and the competency of the patient to understand the information provided.

Patients should be warned of the possibility of drowsiness that may impair performance of potentially hazardous tasks such as driving an automobile or operating machinery.

Drug Interactions:
See **CONTRAINDICATIONS** about concurrent usage of tricyclic antidepressants and monoamine oxidase inhibitors. Paralytic ileus may occur in patients taking tricyclic antidepressants in combination with anticholinergic drugs. ASENDIN may enhance the response to alcohol and the effects of barbiturates and other CNS depressants. Serum levels of several tricyclic antidepressants have been reported to be significantly increased when cimetidine is administered concurrently. Although such an interaction has not been reported to date with ASENDIN, specific interaction studies have not been done, and the possibility should be considered.

Drugs Metabolized by P450 2D6: The biochemical activity of the drug metabolizing isozyme cytochrome P450 2D6 (debrisoquin hydroxylase) is reduced in a subset of the caucasian population (about 7–10% of caucasians are so-called "poor metabolizers"); reliable estimates of the prevalence of reduced P450 2D6 isozyme activity among Asian, African and other populations are not yet available. Poor metabolizers have higher than expected plasma concentrations of tricyclic antidepressants (TCAs) when given usual doses. Depending on the fraction of drug metabolized by P450 2D6, the increase in plasma concentration may be small, or quite large (8-fold increase in plasma AUC of the TCA).

In addition, certain drugs inhibit the activity of this isozyme and make normal metabolizers resemble poor metabolizers. An individual who is stable on a given dose of TCA may become abruptly toxic when given one of these inhibiting drugs as concomitant therapy. The drugs that inhibit cytochrome P450 2D6 include some that are not metabolized by the enzyme (quinidine; cimetidine) and many that are substrates for P450 2D6 (many other antidepressants, pheno-

thiazines, and the Type 1C antiarrhythmics propafenone and flecainide). While all the selective serotonin reuptake inhibitors (SSRIs), e.g., fluoxetine, sertraline, and paroxetine, inhibit P450 2D6, they may vary in the extent of inhibition. The extent to which SSRI TCA interactions may pose clinical problems will depend on the degree of inhibition and the pharmacokinetics of the SSRI involved. Nevertheless, caution is indicated in the co-administration of TCAs with any of the SSRIs and also in switching from one class to the other. Of particular importance, sufficient time must elapse before initiating TCA treatment in a patient being withdrawn from fluoxetine, given the long half-life of the parent and active metabolite (at least 5 weeks may be necessary). Concomitant use of tricyclic antidepressants with drugs that can inhibit cytochrome P450 2D6 may require lower doses than usually prescribed for either the tricyclic antidepressant or the other drug. Furthermore, whenever one of these other drugs is withdrawn from co-therapy, an increased dose of tricyclic antidepressant may be required. It is desirable to monitor TCA plasma levels whenever a TCA is going to be co-administered with another drug known to be an inhibitor of P450 2D6.

Therapeutic Interactions:
Concurrent administration with electroshock therapy may increase the hazards associated with such therapy.

Carcinogenesis, Impairment of Fertility:
In a 21-month toxicity study at three dose levels in rats, pancreatic islet cell hyperplasia occurred with slightly increased incidence at doses 5 to 10 times the human dose. Pancreatic adenocarcinoma was detected in low incidence in the mid-dose group only, and may possibly have resulted from endocrine-mediated organ hyperfunction. The significance of these findings to man is not known.
Treatment of male rats with 5–10 times the human dose resulted in a slight decrease in the number of fertile matings. Female rats receiving oral doses within the therapeutic range displayed a reversible increase in estrous cycle length.

Pregnancy: Pregnancy Category C:
Studies performed in mice, rats, and rabbits have demonstrated no evidence of teratogenic effect due to ASENDIN. Embryotoxicity was seen in rats and rabbits given oral doses approximating the human dose. Fetotoxic effects (intrauterine death, stillbirth, decreased birth weight) were seen in animals studied at oral doses 3–10 times the human dose. Decreased postnatal survival (between days 0–4) was demonstrated in the offspring of rats at 5–10 times the human dose. There are no adequate and well-controlled studies in pregnant women. ASENDIN should be used during pregnancy only if the potential benefit justifies the potential risk to the fetus.

Nursing Mothers:
ASENDIN, like many other systemic drugs, is excreted in human milk. Because effects of the drug on infants are unknown, caution should be exercised when ASENDIN is administered to nursing women.

Pediatric Use:
Safety and effectiveness in children below the age of 16 have not been established.

ADVERSE REACTIONS

Adverse reactions reported in controlled studies in the United States are categorized with respect to incidence below. Following this is a listing of reactions known to occur with other antidepressant drugs of this class but not reported to date with ASENDIN.

INCIDENCE GREATER THAN 1%
The most frequent types of adverse reactions occurring with ASENDIN in controlled clinical trials were sedative and anticholinergic: these included drowsiness (14%), dry mouth (14%), constipation (12%), and blurred vision (7%).
Less frequently reported reactions are:
CNS and Neuromuscular–anxiety, insomnia, restlessness, nervousness, palpitations, tremors, confusion, excitement, nightmares, ataxia, alterations in EEG patterns.
Allergic–edema, skin rash.
Endocrine–elevation of prolactin levels.
Gastrointestinal–nausea.
Other–dizziness, headache, fatigue, weakness, excessive appetite, increased perspiration.
INCIDENCE LESS THAN 1%
Anticholinergic–disturbances of accommodation, mydriasis, delayed micturition, urinary retention, nasal stuffiness.
Cardiovascular–hypotension, hypertension, syncope, tachycardia.
Allergic–drug fever, urticaria, photosensitization, pruritus, rarely vasculitis, hepatitis.
CNS and Neuromuscular–tingling, paresthesias of the extremities, tinnitus, disorientation, seizures, hypomania, numbness, incoordination, disturbed concentration, hyperthermia, extrapyramidal symptoms, including, rarely, tardive dyskinesia. Neuroleptic malignant syndrome has been reported. (See **WARNINGS**.)
Hematologic–leukopenia, agranulocytosis.
Gastrointestinal–epigastric distress, vomiting, flatulence, abdominal pain, peculiar taste, diarrhea.

Endocrine–increased or decreased libido, impotence, menstrual irregularity, breast enlargement and galactorrhea in the female, syndrome of inappropriate antidiuretic hormone secretion.
Other–lacrimation, weight gain or loss, altered liver function, painful ejaculation.

DRUG RELATIONSHIP UNKNOWN
The following reactions have been reported very rarely, and occurred under uncontrolled circumstances where a drug relationship was difficult to assess. These observations are listed to serve as alerting information to physicians.
Anticholinergic–paralytic ileus.
Cardiovascular–atrial arrhythmias (including atrial fibrillation), myocardial infarction, stroke, heart block.
CNS and Neuromuscular–hallucinations.
Hematologic–thrombocytopenia, eosinophilia, purpura, petechiae.
Gastrointestinal–parotid swelling.
Endocrine–change in blood glucose levels.
Other–pancreatitis, hepatitis, jaundice, urinary frequency, testicular swelling, anorexia, alopecia.

ADDITIONAL ADVERSE REACTIONS
The following reactions have been reported with other antidepressant drugs, but not with ASENDIN.
Anticholinergic–sublingual adenitis, dilation of the urinary tract.
CNS and Neuromuscular–delusions.
Gastrointestinal–stomatitis, black tongue.
Endocrine–gynecomastia.

OVERDOSAGE

Signs and Symptoms:
Toxic manifestations of ASENDIN overdosage differ significantly from those of other tricyclic antidepressants. Serious cardiovascular effects are seldom if ever observed. However, CNS effects—particularly grand mal convulsions—occur frequently, and treatment should be directed primarily toward prevention or control of seizures. Status epilepticus may develop and constitutes a neurologic emergency. Coma and acidosis are other serious complications of substantial ASENDIN overdosage in some cases.
Renal failure may develop two to five days after toxic overdosage in patients who may appear otherwise recovered. Acute tubular necrosis with rhabdomyolysis and myoglobinuria is the most common renal complication in such cases. This reaction probably occurs in less than 5% of overdose cases, and typically in those who have experienced multiple seizures.

Treatment:
Treatment of ASENDIN overdosage should be symptomatic and supportive, but with special attention to prevention or control of seizures. If the patient is conscious, induced emesis followed by gastric lavage with appropriate precautions to prevent pulmonary aspiration should be accomplished as soon as possible. Following lavage, activated charcoal may be administered to reduce absorption, and repeated administrations may facilitate drug elimination. An adequate airway should be established in comatose patients and assisted ventilation instituted if necessary. Seizures may respond to standard anticonvulsant therapy such as intravenous diazepam and/or phenytoin. The value of physostigmine appears less certain. Status epilepticus, should it develop, requires vigorous treatment such as that described by Delgado-Escueta et al (*N Engl J Med* 1982; 306:1337-1340).
Convulsions, when they occur, typically begin within 12 hours after ingestion. Because seizures may occur precipitously in some overdosage patients who appear otherwise relatively asymptomatic, the treating physician may wish to consider prophylactic administration of anticonvulsant medication during this period.
Treatment of renal impairment, should it occur, is the same as that for nondrug-induced renal dysfunction.
Serious cardiovascular effects are remarkably rare following ASENDIN overdosage, and the ECG typically remains within normal limits except for sinus tachycardia. Hence, prolongation of the QRS interval beyond 100 milliseconds within the first 24 hours is *not* a useful guide to the severity of overdosage with this drug.
Fatalities and, rarely, neurologic sequelae have resulted from prolonged status epilepticus in ASENDIN amoxapine overdosage patients. While the lethal dose appears higher than that of other tricyclic antidepressants (80% of lethal ASENDIN overdosages have involved ingestion of 3 grams or more), many factors other than amount ingested are important in assessing probability of survival. These include age and physical condition of the patient, concomitant ingestion of other drugs, and especially the interval between drug ingestion and initiation of emergency treatment.

DOSAGE AND ADMINISTRATION

Effective dosage of ASENDIN may vary from one patient to another. Usual effective dosage is 200 to 300 mg daily. Three weeks constitutes an adequate period of trial providing dosage has reached 300 mg daily (or lower level of tolerance) for at least two weeks. If no response is seen at 300 mg, dosage may be increased, depending upon tolerance, up to 400 mg daily. Hospitalized patients who have been refractory to an-

tidepressant therapy and who have no history of convulsive seizures may have dosage raised cautiously up to 600 mg daily in divided doses.
ASENDIN may be given in a single daily dose, not to exceed 300 mg, preferably at bedtime. If the total daily dosage exceeds 300 mg, it should be given in divided doses.

Initial Dosage for Adults:
Usual starting dosage is 50 mg two or three times daily. Depending upon tolerance, dosage may be increased to 100 mg two or three times daily by the end of the first week. (Initial dosage of 300 mg daily may be given, but notable sedation may occur in some patients during the first few days of therapy at this level.) Increases above 300 mg daily should be made only if 300 mg daily has been ineffective during a trial period of at least 2 weeks. When effective dosage is established, the drug may be given in a single dose (not to exceed 300 mg) at bedtime.

Elderly Patients:
In general, lower dosages are recommended for these patients. Recommended starting dosage of ASENDIN is 25 mg two or three times daily. If no intolerance is observed, dosage may be increased by the end of the first week to 50 mg two or three times daily. Although 100 to 150 mg daily may be adequate for many elderly patients, some may require higher dosage. Careful increases up to 300 mg daily are indicated in such cases.
Once an effective dosage is established, ASENDIN may conveniently be given in a single bedtime dose, not to exceed 300 mg.

Maintenance
Recommended maintenance dosage of ASENDIN amoxapine is the lowest dose that will maintain remission. If symptoms reappear, dosage should be increased to the earlier level until they are controlled.
For maintenance therapy at dosages of 300 mg or less, a single dose at bedtime is recommended.

HOW SUPPLIED

ASENDIN® amoxapine Tablets are supplied as follows:
25 mg—White, heptagon-shaped tablets, engraved on one side with LL above 25 and with A13 on the other scored side.
　NDC 0005-5389-23—Bottle of 100
50 mg—Orange, heptagon-shaped tablets, engraved on one side with LL above 50 and with A15 on the other scored side.
　NDC 0005-5390-23—Bottle of 100
　NDC 0005-5390-31—Bottle of 500
　NDC 0005-5390-60—10 (2 × 5) Strips
100 mg—Blue, heptagon-shaped tablets, engraved on one side with LL above 100 and with A17 on the other scored side.
　NDC 0005-5391-23—Bottle of 100
　NDC 0005-5391-60—10 (2 × 5) Strips
150 mg—Peach, heptagon-shaped tablets, engraved on one side with LL above 150 and with A18 on the other scored side.
　NDC 0005-5392-38—Bottle of 30 with CRC
Store at Controlled Room Temperature 15°–30° C (59°–86° F).
Manufactured by:
LEDERLE PHARMACEUTICAL DIVISION
American Cyanamid Company
Pearl River, NY 10965
　Shown in Product Identification Guide, page 319

DECLOMYCIN®　　　　　　　　　　　　　　　　　　　　℞
[děk-lō-mĭ-sĭn]
Demeclocycline Hydrochloride
For Oral Use

DESCRIPTION

DECLOMYCIN demeclocycline hydrochloride is an antibiotic isolated from a mutant strain of *Streptomyces aureofaciens*. Chemically it is 7-Chloro-4-(dimethylamino)-1,4,4a,5,5a,6,11,12a-octahydro - 3,6,10,12, 12a- pentahydroxy - 1,11-dioxo -2- naphthacenecarboxamide monohydrochloride.
DECLOMYCIN contains the following inactive ingredients: Tablets: Alginic Acid, Corn Starch, Ethylcellulose, Hydroxypropyl Methylcellulose, Magnesium Stearate, Red 7, Sorbitol, Titanium Dioxide, Yellow 10 and other ingredients. May also contain Sodium Lauryl Sulfate.

CLINICAL PHARMACOLOGY

The tetracyclines are primarily bacteriostatic and are thought to exert their antimicrobial effect by the inhibition of protein synthesis. Tetracyclines are active against a wide range of gram-negative and gram-positive organisms.
The drugs in the tetracycline class have closely similar antimicrobial spectra, and cross-resistance among them is common. Microorganisms may be considered susceptible if

Continued on next page

Declomycin—Cont.

the MIC (minimum inhibitory concentration) is not more than 4 mcg/mL and intermediate if the MIC is 4 to 12.5 mcg/mL.

Susceptibility plate testing: A tetracycline disc may be used to determine microbial susceptibility to drugs in the tetracycline class. If the Kirby-Bauer method of disc susceptibility testing is used, a 30 mcg tetracycline disc should give a zone of at least 19 mm when tested against a tetracycline-susceptible bacterial strain.

Tetracyclines are readily absorbed and are bound to plasma proteins in varying degrees. They are concentrated by the liver in the bile and excreted in the urine and feces at high concentrations and in a biologically active form.

INDICATIONS AND USAGE

DECLOMYCIN demeclocycline hydrochloride is indicated in infections caused by the following microorganisms:
Rickettsiae: (Rocky Mountain spotted fever, typhus fever and the typhus group, Q fever, rickettsialpox, tick fevers).
Mycoplasma pneumoniae (PPLO, Eaton agent).
Agents of psittacosis and ornithosis.
Agents of lymphogranuloma venereum and granuloma inguinale.
The spirochetal agent of relapsing fever (*Borrelia recurrentis*).
The following gram-negative microorganisms:
Haemophilus ducreyi (chancroid),
Yersinia pestis and *Francisella tularensis,* formerly *Pasteurella pestis* and *Pasteurella tularensis,*
Bartonella bacilliformis,
Bacteroides species,
Vibrio comma and *Vibrio fetus.*
Brucella species (in conjunction with streptomycin).
Because many strains of the following groups of microorganisms have been shown to be resistant to tetracyclines, culture and susceptibility testing are recommended.
Demeclocycline is indicated for treatment of infections caused by the following gram-negative microorganisms, when bacteriologic testing indicates appropriate susceptibility to the drug:
Escherichia coli,
Enterobacter aerogenes (formerly *Aerobacter aerogenes*),
Shigella species,
Mima species and *Herellea* species,
Haemophilus influenzae (respiratory infections),
Klebsiella species (respiratory and urinary infections).
DECLOMYCIN is indicated for treatment of infections caused by the following gram-positive microorganisms when bacteriologic testing indicates appropriate susceptibility to the drug:
Streptococcus species:
Up to 44% of strains of *Streptococcus pyogenes* and 74% of *Streptococcus faecalis* have been found to be resistant to tetracycline drugs. Therefore, tetracyclines should not be used for streptococcal disease unless the organism has been demonstrated to be sensitive.
For upper respiratory infections due to Group A beta-hemolytic streptococci, penicillin is the usual drug of choice, including prophylaxis of rheumatic fever.
Streptococcus pneumoniae,
Staphylococcus aureus, skin and soft tissue infections.
Tetracyclines are not the drugs of choice in the treatment of any type of staphylococcal infection.
When penicillin is contraindicated, tetracyclines are alternative drugs in the treatment of infections due to:
Neisseria gonorrhoeae,
Treponema pallidum and *Treponema pertenue* (syphilis and yaws),
Listeria monocytogenes,
Clostridium species,
Bacillus anthracis,
Fusobacterium fusiforme (Vincent's infection),
Actinomyces species.
In acute intestinal amebiasis, the tetracyclines may be a useful adjunct to amebicides.
DECLOMYCIN demeclocycline hydrochloride is indicated in the treatment of trachoma, although the infectious agent is not always eliminated, as judged by immunofluorescence. Inclusion conjunctivitis may be treated with oral tetracyclines or with a combination of oral and topical agents.

CONTRAINDICATIONS

This drug is contraindicated in persons who have shown hypersensitivity to any of the tetracyclines.

WARNINGS

THE USE OF DRUGS OF THE TETRACYCLINE CLASS DURING TOOTH DEVELOPMENT (LAST HALF OF PREGNANCY, INFANCY, AND CHILDHOOD TO THE AGE OF 8 YEARS) MAY CAUSE PERMANENT DISCOLORATION OF THE TEETH (YELLOW-GRAY-BROWN).

This adverse reaction is more common during long-term use of the drugs but has been observed following repeated short-term courses. Enamel hypoplasia has also been reported.

TETRACYCLINE DRUGS, THEREFORE, SHOULD NOT BE USED IN THIS AGE GROUP UNLESS OTHER DRUGS ARE NOT LIKELY TO BE EFFECTIVE OR ARE CONTRAINDICATED.

If renal impairment exists, even usual oral or parenteral doses may lead to excessive systemic accumulation of the drug and possible liver toxicity. Under such conditions, lower than usual total doses are indicated and, if therapy is prolonged, serum level determinations of the drug may be advisable.

Phototoxic reactions can occur in individuals taking demeclocycline, and are characterized by severe burns of exposed surfaces resulting from direct exposure of patients to sunlight during therapy with moderate or large doses of demeclocycline. Patients apt to be exposed to direct sunlight or ultraviolet light should be advised that this reaction can occur, and treatment should be discontinued at the first evidence of skin erythema.

The anti-anabolic action of the tetracyclines may cause an increase in BUN. While this is not a problem in those with normal renal function, in patients with significantly impaired function, higher serum levels of tetracycline may lead to azotemia, hyperphosphatemia, and acidosis.

Administration of DECLOMYCIN® has resulted in appearance of the diabetes insipidus syndrome (polyuria, polydipsia and weakness) in some patients on long-term therapy. The syndrome has been shown to be nephrogenic, dose-dependent and reversible on discontinuance of therapy.

Usage in pregnancy: (See above **WARNINGS** about use during tooth development.) Results of animal studies indicate that tetracyclines cross the placenta, are found in fetal tissues and can have toxic effects on the developing fetus (often related to retardation of skeletal development). Evidence of embryotoxicity has also been noted in animals treated early in pregnancy.

Usage in newborns, infants, and children: (See above **WARNINGS** about use during tooth development.)

All tetracyclines form a stable calcium complex in any bone forming tissue. A decrease in the fibula growth rate has been observed in prematures given oral tetracycline in doses of 25 mg/kg every six hours. This reaction was shown to be reversible when the drug was discontinued.

Tetracyclines are present in the milk of lactating women who are taking a drug in this class.

PRECAUTIONS

General

Pseudotumor cerebri (benign intracranial hypertension) in adults has been associated with the use of tetracyclines. The usual clinical manifestations are headache and blurred vision. Bulging fontanels have been associated with the use of tetracyclines in infants. While both of these conditions and related symptoms usually resolve soon after discontinuation of the tetracycline, the possibility for permanent sequelae exists.

As with other antibiotic preparations, use of this drug may result in overgrowth of nonsusceptible organisms, including fungi. If superinfection occurs, the antibiotic should be discontinued and appropriate therapy should be instituted.

In venereal diseases when coexistent syphilis is suspected, darkfield examination should be done before treatment is started and the blood serology repeated monthly for at least 4 months.

In long-term therapy, periodic laboratory evaluation of organ systems, including hematopoietic, renal and hepatic studies should be performed.

All infections due to Group A beta-hemolytic streptococci should be treated for at least ten days.

Interpretation of Bacteriologic Studies: Following a course of therapy, persistence for several days in both urine and blood of bacterio-suppressive levels of demeclocycline may interfere with culture studies. These levels should not be considered therapeutic.

Drug Interactions

Because the tetracyclines have been shown to depress plasma prothrombin activity, patients who are on anticoagulant therapy may require downward adjustment of their anticoagulant dosage.

Since bacteriostatic drugs, such as the tetracycline class of antibiotics, may interfere with the bactericidal action of penicillins, it is not advisable to administer these drugs concomitantly.

Concurrent use of tetracyclines with oral contraceptives may render oral contraceptives less effective. Breakthrough bleeding has been reported.

ADVERSE REACTIONS

Gastrointestinal: Anorexia, nausea, vomiting, diarrhea, glossitis, dysphagia, enterocolitis, pancreatitis, and inflammatory lesions (with monilial overgrowth) in the anogenital region, increases in liver enzymes, and hepatic toxicity has been reported rarely. Rare instances of esophagitis and esophageal ulcerations have been reported in patients taking the tetracycline-class antibiotics in capsule and tablet form. Most of these patients took the medication immediately before going to bed (see **DOSAGE AND ADMINISTRATION**).

Skin: Maculopapular and erythematous rashes. Exfoliative dermatitis has been reported but is uncommon. Fixed drug eruptions, including balanitis, have been rarely reported. Photosensitivity is discussed above. (See **WARNINGS**.)

Renal Toxicity: Rise in BUN has been reported and is apparently dose related. Nephrogenic diabetes insipidus. (See **WARNINGS**.)

Hypersensitivity Reactions: Urticaria, angioneurotic edema, anaphylaxis, anaphylactoid purpura, pericarditis and exacerbation of systemic lupus erythematosus.

Blood: Hemolytic anemia, thrombocytopenia, neutropenia and eosinophilia have been reported.

CNS: Pseudotumor cerebri (benign intracranial hypertension) in adults and bulging fontanels in infants (see **PRECAUTIONS—General**). Dizziness, tinnitus, and visual disturbances have been reported. Myasthenic syndrome has been reported rarely.

Other: When given over prolonged periods, tetracyclines have been reported to produce brown-black microscopic discoloration of thyroid glands. No abnormalities of thyroid function studies are known to occur.

DOSAGE AND ADMINISTRATION

Therapy should be continued for at least 24 to 48 hours after symptoms and fever have subsided.

Concomitant therapy: Antacids containing aluminum, calcium, or magnesium impair absorption and should not be given to patients taking oral tetracycline.

Foods and some dairy products also interfere with absorption. Oral forms of tetracycline should be given one hour before or two hours after meals.

In patients with renal impairment: (See **WARNINGS**.) Total dosage should be decreased by reduction of recommended individual doses and/or by extending time intervals between doses.

In the treatment of streptococcal infections, a therapeutic dose of demeclocycline should be administered for at least ten days.

Adults: Usual daily dose—Four divided doses of 150 mg each or two divided doses of 300 mg each.

For children above eight years of age: Usual daily dose, 3–6 mg per pound body weight per day, depending upon the severity of the disease, divided into two to four doses.

Gonorrhea patients sensitive to penicillin may be treated with demeclocycline administered as an initial oral dose of 600 mg followed by 300 mg every 12 hours for four days to a total of 3 grams.

HOW SUPPLIED

DECLOMYCIN® demeclocycline hydrochloride Tablets, 150 mg are round, convex, red, film coated tablets, engraved with LL on one side and D11 on the other, supplied as follows:

NDC 0005-9218-23—Bottle of 100

DECLOMYCIN® demeclocycline hydrochloride Tablets, 300 mg are round, convex, red, film coated tablets, engraved with LL on one side and D12 on the other, supplied as follows:

NDC 0005-9270-29—Bottle of 48

Store at controlled room temperature 20°–25°C (68–77°F).

Manufactured by:
LEDERLE PHARMACEUTICAL DIVISION
American Cyanamid Company
Pearl River, NY 10965

Shown in Product Identification Guide, page 319

DIAMOX®
Acetazolamide Tablets USP
and
DIAMOX®
Sterile Acetazolamide Sodium USP
Intravenous

℞

(For full prescribing information, please refer to the 1999 PDR for Ophthalmology.)

DIAMOX®
Acetazolamide
SEQUELS®
Sustained Release Capsules

℞

(For full prescribing information, please refer to the 1999 PDR for Ophthalmology.)

DIPHTHERIA AND TETANUS TOXOIDS ADSORBED
Aluminum Phosphate-Adsorbed
PUROGENATED®
For Pediatric Use

℞

DESCRIPTION

Diphtheria and Tetanus Toxoids Adsorbed, aluminum phosphate-adsorbed PUROGENATED is a sterile combination of

refined diphtheria and tetanus toxoids for intramuscular use only. After shaking, the vaccine is a homogeneous white suspension.

The diphtheria and tetanus toxins are produced according to the method of Mueller and Miller[1,2] and are detoxified by use of formaldehyde. The toxoids are refined by the Pillemer alcohol fractionation method[3] and are diluted with a solution containing sodium phosphate monobasic, sodium phosphate dibasic, aluminum phosphate, glycine and thimerosal (mercury derivative) as a preservative. The final concentration of thimerosal in the combined vaccine is 1:10,000. The aluminum content of the final product does not exceed 0.80 mg per 0.5 mL dose.

Each 0.5 mL dose is formulated to contain 12.5 Lf units of diphtheria toxoid, and 5 Lf units of tetanus toxoid.

CLINICAL PHARMACOLOGY

Diphtheria is primarily a localized and generalized intoxication caused by diphtheria toxin, an extracellular protein metabolite of toxinogenic strains of *Corynebacterium diphtheriae*. While the incidence of diphtheria in the U.S. has decreased from over 200,000 cases reported in 1921 before the general use of diphtheria toxoid, to only 15 cases reported from 1980 through 1983, the ratio of fatalities to attack rate has remained constant at about 5% to 10%.[4] The highest case fatality rates are in the very young and the elderly.

Following adequate immunization with diphtheria toxoid, which induces antitoxin, it is thought that protection lasts for at least 10 years.[4] This significantly reduces both the risk of developing diphtheria and the severity of clinical illness. It does not, however, eliminate carriage of *C diphtheriae* in the pharynx or on the skin.[4]

Tetanus is an intoxication manifested primarily by neuromuscular dysfunction, caused by a potent exotoxin elaborated by *Clostridium tetani*. The incidence of tetanus in the U.S. has dropped dramatically with the routine use of tetanus toxoid, remaining relatively constant over the last decade at about 90 cases reported annually.[4] Spores of *C tetani* are ubiquitous, and there is essentially no natural immunity to tetanus toxin. Thus, universal primary immunization with tetanus toxoid, and subsequent maintenance of adequate antitoxin levels by means of timed boosters, is necessary to protect all age groups.[4,6] Tetanus toxoid is a highly effective antigen, and a completed primary series generally induces protective levels of serum antitoxin that persist for at least 10 years.[4]

INDICATIONS AND USAGE

Diphtheria and Tetanus Toxoids Adsorbed is indicated for active immunization of infants and children from 2 months of age up to their seventh birthday both for routine protection and as a preventive measure against diphtheria and tetanus, in circumstances in which the use of a combined triple vaccine containing pertussis antigen is contraindicated.[4,5]

Tetanus or diphtheria infection may not confer immunity; therefore, initiation or completion of active immunization is indicated at the time of recovery from these infections.[4]

CONTRAINDICATIONS

HYPERSENSITIVITY TO ANY COMPONENT OF THE VACCINE, INCLUDING THIMEROSAL, A MERCURY DERIVATIVE, IS A CONTRAINDICATION.

THE OCCURRENCE OF ANY NEUROLOGICAL SYMPTOMS OR SIGNS FOLLOWING ADMINISTRATION OF THIS PRODUCT IS A CONTRAINDICATION TO FURTHER USE.

IMMUNIZATION SHOULD BE DEFERRED DURING THE COURSE OF ANY FEBRILE ILLNESS OR ACUTE INFECTION. A MINOR AFEBRILE ILLNESS SUCH AS A MILD UPPER RESPIRATORY INFECTION IS NOT USUALLY REASON TO DEFER IMMUNIZATION.[4,5]

The clinical judgment of the attending physician should prevail at all times.

Routine immunization should be deferred during an outbreak of poliomyelitis, providing the patient has not sustained an injury that increases the risk of tetanus and providing an outbreak of diphtheria does not occur simultaneously.

WARNINGS

THIS PRODUCT IS NOT RECOMMENDED FOR IMMUNIZING PERSONS ON OR AFTER THEIR SEVENTH BIRTHDAY.

For individuals 7 years of age or older, Tetanus and Diphtheria Toxoids Adsorbed For Adult Use (Td) should be used instead of Diphtheria and Tetanus Toxoids Adsorbed For Pediatric Use (DT). The concentration of diphtheria toxoid in preparations intended for use in persons 7 years of age or older is lower than that of the pediatric formulation; a lower dosage of diphtheria toxoid is recommended for persons 7 years of age or older because adverse reactions to the diphtheria component are thought to be related to both dose and age.[4]

THE OCCURRENCE OF A NEUROLOGICAL OR SEVERE HYPERSENSITIVITY REACTION FOLLOWING A PREVIOUS DOSE IS A CONTRAINDICATION TO FURTHER USE OF THIS PRODUCT.[4]

DT should not be given to infants or children with thrombocytopenia or any coagulation disorder that would contraindicate intramuscular injection unless the potential benefits clearly outweigh the risk of administration.

Patients with impaired immune responsiveness, whether due to the use of immunosuppressive therapy (including irradiation, corticosteroids, antimetabolites, alkylating agents, and cytotoxic agents), a genetic defect, human immunodeficiency virus (HIV) infection, or other causes, may have a reduced antibody response to active immunization procedures.[4,5,6] Deferral of administration of DT may be considered in individuals receiving immunosuppressive therapy.[4,5] Other groups should generally receive this vaccine according to the usual recommended schedule.[4-7]

Special care should be taken to prevent injection into a blood vessel.

PRECAUTIONS

General

1. THIS PRODUCT SHOULD BE USED FOR THE AGE GROUP BETWEEN 2 MONTHS AND THE SEVENTH BIRTHDAY.

2. PRIOR TO ADMINISTRATION OF ANY DOSE OF DT, THE PARENT OR GUARDIAN SHOULD BE ASKED ABOUT THE RECENT HEALTH STATUS OF THE INFANT OR CHILD TO BE IMMUNIZED IN ORDER TO DETERMINE THE EXISTENCE OF ANY CONTRAINDICATION TO IMMUNIZATION WITH DT (SEE **CONTRAINDICATIONS, WARNINGS**).

3. WHEN AN INFANT OR CHILD RETURNS FOR THE NEXT DOSE IN A SERIES, THE PARENT OR GUARDIAN SHOULD BE QUESTIONED CONCERNING OCCURRENCE OF ANY SYMPTOM AND/OR SIGN OF AN ADVERSE REACTION AFTER THE PREVIOUS DOSE (SEE **CONTRAINDICATIONS, ADVERSE REACTIONS**).

4. BEFORE THE INJECTION OF ANY BIOLOGICAL, THE PHYSICIAN SHOULD TAKE ALL PRECAUTIONS KNOWN FOR PREVENTION OF ALLERGIC OR ANY OTHER SIDE REACTIONS. This should include: a review of the patient's history regarding possible sensitivity; the ready availability of epinephrine 1:1,000 and other appropriate agents used for control of immediate allergic reactions; and a knowledge of the recent literature pertaining to use of the biological concerned, including the nature of side effects and adverse reactions that may follow its use.

5. A separate sterile syringe and needle or a sterile disposable unit should be used for each individual patient to prevent transmission of hepatitis or other infectious agents from one person to another.

6. *Shake vigorously before withdrawing each dose to resuspend the contents of the vial.*

7. NATIONAL CHILDHOOD VACCINE INJURY ACT OF 1986 (AS AMENDED IN 1987)

   This Act requires that the manufacturer and lot number of the vaccine administered be recorded by the health care provider in the vaccine recipient's permanent medical record, along with the date of administration of the vaccine and the name, address and title of the person administering the vaccine.

   The Act further requires the health care provider to report to a health department or to the FDA the occurrence following immunization of any event set forth in the Vaccine Injury Table including: anaphylaxis or anaphylactic shock within 24 hours, encephalopathy or encephalitis within 7 days, residual seizure disorder, any acute complication or sequelae (including death) of above events, or any event that would contraindicate further doses of vaccine, according to this package insert.[8]

Information for the Patient

PRIOR TO THE ADMINISTRATION OF THIS VACCINE, HEALTH CARE PERSONNEL SHOULD INFORM THE PARENT, GUARDIAN, OR OTHER RESPONSIBLE ADULT OF THE BENEFITS AND RISKS TO THE CHILD OF VACCINATION AGAINST DIPHTHERIA AND TETANUS.

Use in Pregnancy

This product is not recommended for administration to females of child-bearing age.

ADVERSE REACTIONS

Local reactions, manifested by varying degrees of erythema, induration, and tenderness, may occur after administration of DT.[9,10] Such local reactions are usually self-limited and require no therapy. Nodule,[11] sterile abscess formation, or subcutaneous atrophy may occur at the site of injection.

Systemic symptoms, including drowsiness, fretfulness, vomiting, anorexia, and persistent crying have been described following DT immunization.[9,10]

In one study, fever ≥38°C (100.4°F) was reported in 9.3% of DT recipients, and fever ≥39°C (102.2°F) was reported in 0.7% of recipients.[9]

Pallor, coldness, and hyporesponsiveness have been reported in a child receiving a DT vaccine.[10]

NEUROLOGICAL COMPLICATIONS,[12] SUCH AS CONVULSIONS,[13] ENCEPHALOPATHY,[13,14] AND VARIOUS MONO- AND POLYNEUROPATHIES,[14-20] INCLUDING GUILLAIN-BARRE SYNDROME,[21,22] HAVE BEEN REPORTED FOLLOWING ADMINISTRATION OF PREPARATIONS CONTAINING DIPHTHERIA AND/OR TETANUS ANTIGENS.

URTICARIA, ERYTHEMA MULTIFORME OR OTHER RASH, ARTHRALGIAS[13] AND, MORE RARELY, A SEVERE ANAPHYLACTIC REACTION (I.E., URTICARIA WITH SWELLING OF THE MOUTH, DIFFICULTY BREATHING, HYPOTENSION, OR SHOCK) HAVE BEEN REPORTED FOLLOWING ADMINISTRATION OF PREPARATIONS CONTAINING DIPHTHERIA, AND/OR TETANUS ANTIGENS.

DOSAGE AND ADMINISTRATION

For Intramuscular Use Only

Shake vigorously before withdrawing each dose to resuspend the contents of the vial.

Parenteral drug products should be inspected visually for particulate matter and discoloration prior to administration. (See **DESCRIPTION**.)

The vaccine should be injected intramuscularly, preferably into the midlateral muscles of the thigh or deltoid, with care to avoid major peripheral nerve trunks.

Before injection, the skin at the injection site should be cleansed and prepared with a suitable germicide.

After insertion of the needle, aspirate to help avoid inadvertent injection into a blood vessel.

This combined preparation against both diphtheria and tetanus is designed particularly to meet the need of children less than 7 years of age for whom the use of a combined triple vaccine containing pertussis antigen is contraindicated.

It is recommended that active immunization against diphtheria and tetanus be started at 2 months of age.

Unimmunized infants and children less than 1 year of age for whom vaccine containing pertussis antigen is contraindicated should receive three doses of 0.5 mL each of DT at 4 to 8 week intervals, followed by a fourth (reinforcing) dose of 0.5 mL, 6 to 12 months after the third dose, for the primary series.

Unimmunized children 1 year of age or older for whom vaccine containing pertussis antigen is contraindicated should receive two doses of 0.5 mL each of DT, 4 to 8 weeks apart, followed by a third (reinforcing) dose 6 to 12 months later, for the primary series.

If after beginning a DTP series, further doses of vaccine containing pertussis antigen become contraindicated, DT should be substituted for each of the remaining doses.[4,5]

The reinforcing dose is an integral part of the primary immunizing series.

Interruption of the recommended schedule with a delay between doses does not interfere with the final immunity achieved, nor does it necessitate starting the series over again, regardless of the length of time elapsed between doses.[4,5]

A booster dose of 0.5 mL is indicated at age 4 to 6 years, preferably prior to entrance into kindergarten or elementary school. However, if the last dose of the primary immunizing series was administered after the fourth birthday, a booster prior to school entry is not considered necessary.[4,5]

For either primary or booster immunization against tetanus and diphtheria of individuals 7 years of age and older, the use of Tetanus and Diphtheria Toxoids Adsorbed For Adult Use is recommended.[4,5]

Diphtheria Prophylaxis for Case Contacts

All case contacts, household and others, who have previously received fewer than three doses of diphtheria toxoid should receive an immediate dose of an appropriate diphtheria toxoid-containing preparation and should complete the series according to schedule. Case contacts who previously received three or more doses, but who have not received a dose of a preparation containing diphtheria toxoid within the previous 5 years, should receive a dose of a diphtheria toxoid-containing preparation appropriate for their age. This combined preparation against both diphtheria and tetanus is designed particularly to meet the need of children less than 7 years of age for whom the use of a combined triple vaccine containing pertussis antigen is contraindicated.

Tetanus Prophylaxis in Wound Management

For routine wound management of children under 7 years of age who are not completely immunized, DT should be used instead of single-antigen tetanus toxoid (if pertussis antigen is contraindicated or individual circumstances are such that potential febrile reactions following DTP might confound the management of the patient).[4] Completion of primary vaccination thereafter should be ensured.

For tetanus-prone wounds in children who have had fewer than three, or an unknown number of immunizations with a tetanus-toxoid containing product, passive immunization with human Tetanus-Immune Globulin (TIG) is also recommended.[4] A separate syringe and site of injection should be used.

Continued on next page

Diphtheria & Tetanus Toxoids —Cont

HOW SUPPLIED

NDC 0005-1858-31   5.0 mL vial

STORAGE

DO NOT FREEZE. STORE REFRIGERATED, AWAY FROM FREEZER COMPARTMENT, AT 2°C to 8°C (36°F to 46°F).

REFERENCES

1. Mueller JH, Miller PA: Production of diphtheria toxin of high potency (100Lf) on a reproducible medium. *J Immunol* 1941;40:21–32.
2. Mueller JH, Miller PA: Factors influencing the production of tetanal toxin. *J Immunol* 1947;56:143–147.
3. Pillemer L, Grossberg DB, Wittler RG: The immunochemistry of toxins and toxoids. II. The preparation and immunological evaluation of purified tetanal toxoid. *J Immunol* 1946;54:213–224.
4. Recommendation of the Immunization Practices Advisory Committee (ACIP): Diphtheria, tetanus and pertussis: Guidelines for vaccine prophylaxis and other preventive measures. *MMWR* 1985;34:405–426.
5. American Academy of Pediatrics: Report of the Committee on Infectious Diseases, ed 20. Elk Grove Village, IL, American Academy of Pediatrics, 1986.
6. Recommendation of the ACIP: Immunization of children infected with Human T-Lymphotrophic Virus Type III/Lymphadenopathy associated virus. *MMWR* 1986;35(38):595–606.
7. Immunization of children infected with Human Immunodeficiency Virus—Supplementary ACIP statement. *MMWR* 1988;37(12):181–183.
8. National Childhood Vaccine Injury Act: Requirements for permanent vaccination records and for reporting of selected events after vaccination. *MMWR* 1988;37(13):197–200.
9. Cody C, et al: Nature and rates of adverse reactions associated with DTP and DT immunizations in infants and children. *Pediatrics* 1981;68:650–660.
10. Feery BJ: Incidence and type of reactions to triple antigen (DTP) and DT (CDT) vaccines. *Med Jour of Australia* 1982;2:511–515.
11. Fawcett HA, Smith NP: Injection-site granuloma due to aluminum. *Arch Dermatol* 1984;120:1318–1322.
12. Rutledge SL, Snead OC: Neurological complications of immunizations. *J Pediatr* 1986;109:917–924.
13. Adverse Events Following Immunization. *MMWR* 1985;34(3):43–47.
14. Schlenska GK: Unusual neurological complications following tetanus toxoid administration. *J Neurol* 1977;215:299–302.
15. Blumstein GI, Kreithen H: Peripheral neuropathy following tetanus toxoid administration. *JAMA* 1966;198:1030–1031.
16. Reinstein L, Pargament JM, Goodman JS: Peripheral neuropathy after multiple tetanus toxoid injections. *Arch Phys Med Rehabil* 1982;63:332–334.
17. Tsairis P, Duck PJ, Mulder DW: Natural history of brachial plexus neuropathy. *Arch Neurol* 1972;27:109–117.
18. Quast U, Hennessen W, Widmark RM: Mono- and polyneuritis after tetanus vaccination. *Devel Bio Stand* 1979;43:25–32.
19. Holliday PL, Bauer RB: Polyradiculoneuritis secondary to immunization with tetanus and diphtheria toxoids. *Arch Neurol* 1983;40:56–57.
20. Fenichel GM: Neurological complications of tetanus toxoid. *Arch Neurol* 1983;40:390.
21. Pollard JD, Selby G: Relapsing neuropathy due to tetanus toxoid. *J Neurol Sci* 1978;37:113–125.
22. Newton N, Janati A: Guillain-Barre syndrome after vaccination with purified tetanus toxoid. *S Med J* 1987;80:1053–1054.

Manufactured by:
LEDERLE LABORATORIES
Division American Cyanamid Company
Pearl River, NY 10965
US Gov't. License No. 17
Marketed by:
WYETH-LEDERLE VACCINES
Wyeth-Ayerst Laboratories
Philadelphia, PA 19101

HAEMOPHILUS b CONJUGATE VACCINE   ℞
(Diphtheria CRM₁₉₇ Protein Conjugate)
HibTITER®

DESCRIPTION

Haemophilus b Conjugate Vaccine (Diphtheria CRM$_{197}$ Protein Conjugate) HibTITER is a sterile solution of a conjugate of oligosaccharides of the capsular antigen of *Haemophilus influenzae* type b (Haemophilus b) and diphtheria CRM$_{197}$ protein (CRM$_{197}$) dissolved in 0.9% sodium chloride.

The oligosaccharides are derived from highly purified capsular polysaccharide, polyribosylribitol phosphate, isolated from Haemophilus b strain Eagan grown in a chemically defined medium (a mixture of mineral salts, amino acids, and cofactors). The oligosaccharides are purified and sized by diafiltrations through a series of ultrafiltration membranes, and coupled by reductive amination directly to highly purified CRM$_{197}$.[1,2] CRM$_{197}$ is a nontoxic variant of diphtheria toxin isolated from cultures of *Corynebacterium diphtheriae* C7 (β197) grown in a casamino acids and yeast extract-based medium that is ultrafiltered before use. CRM$_{197}$ is purified through ultrafiltration, ammonium sulfate precipitation, and ion-exchange chromatography to high purity. The conjugate is purified to remove unreacted protein, oligosaccharides, and reagents; sterilized by filtration; and filled into vials. HibTITER is intended for intramuscular use.

The vaccine is a clear, colorless solution. Each single dose of 0.5 mL is formulated to contain 10 µg of purified Haemophilus b saccharide and approximately 25 µg of CRM$_{197}$ protein. Multidose vials contain thimerosal (mercurial derivative) 1:10,000 as a preservative. The potency of HibTITER is determined by chemical assay for polyribosylribitol.

CLINICAL PHARMACOLOGY

For several decades, *Haemophilus influenzae* type b (Haemophilus b) was the most common cause of invasive bacterial disease, including meningitis, in young children in the United States. Although nonencapsulated *H. influenzae* are common and six capsular polysaccharide types are known, strains with the type b capsule caused most of the invasive Haemophilus diseases.[3]

Haemophilus b diseases occurred primarily in children under 5 years of age prior to immunization with *Haemophilus influenzae* type b vaccines. In the US, the cumulative risk of developing invasive Haemophilus b disease during the first 5 years of life was estimated to be about 1 in 200. Approximately 60% of cases were meningitis. Cellulitis, epiglottitis, pericarditis, pneumonia, sepsis, or septic arthritis made up the remaining 40%. An estimated 12,000 cases of Haemophilus b meningitis occurred annually prior to the routine use of conjugate vaccines in toddlers.[3,4] The mortality rate can be 5%, and neurologic sequelae have been observed in up to 38% of survivors.[5]

The incidence of invasive Haemophilus b disease peaks between 6 months and 1 year of age, and approximately 55% of disease occurs between 6 and 18 months of age.[3] Interpersonal transmission of Haemophilus b occurs and risk of invasive disease is increased in children younger than 4 years of age who are exposed in the household to a primary case of disease. Clusters of cases in children in day care have been reported and recent studies suggest that the rate of secondary cases may also be increased among children exposed to a primary case in the day-care setting.[3,6]

The incidence of invasive Haemophilus b disease is increased in certain children, such as those who are native Americans, black, or from lower socioeconomic status, and those with medical conditions such as asplenia, sickle cell disease, malignancies associated with immunosuppression, and antibody deficiency syndromes.[3,4,6]

The protective activity of antibody to Haemophilus b polysaccharide was demonstrated by passive antibody studies in animals and in children with agammaglobulinemia or with Haemophilus b disease[7] and confirmed with the efficacy study of Haemophilus b polysaccharide (HbPs) vaccine.[8] Data from passive antibody studies indicate that a preexisting titer of antibody to HbPs of 0.15 µg/mL correlates with protection.[9] Data from a Finnish field trial in children 18 to 71 months of age indicate that a titer of >1.0 µg/mL 3 weeks after vaccination is associated with long-term protection.[10,11]

Linkage of Haemophilus b saccharides to a protein such as CRM$_{197}$ converts the saccharide (HbO) to a T-dependent (HbOC)-antigen, and results in an enhanced antibody response to the saccharide in young infants that primes for an anamnestic response and is predominantly of the IgG class.[12] Laboratory evidence indicates that the native state of the CRM$_{197}$ protein and the use of oligosaccharides in the formulation of HibTITER enhances its immunogenicity.[13–15] Haemophilus b conjugate vaccines with other carrier proteins will be recognized differently by the immune system.

Prior to licensure, the immunogenicity of HibTITER was evaluated in US infants and children.[15] Infants 1 to 6 months of age at first immunization received three doses at approximately 2-month intervals.[16] Children 7 to 11 and 12 to 14 months of age received 2 doses at the same interval.[15] Children 15 to 23 months of age received a single dose.[17] HibTITER was highly immunogenic in all age groups studied, with 97% to 100% of 1,232 infants attaining titers of ≥1 µg/mL and 92% to 100% for bactericidal activity.[15–17]

Long-term persistence of the antibody response was observed. More than 80% of the 235 infants who received three doses of vaccine had an anti-HbPs antibody level ≥1 µg/mL at 2 years of age.[18]

The vaccine generated an immune response characteristic of a protein antigen. IgG anti-HbPs antibodies of IgG$_1$ subclass predominated and the immune system was primed for

a booster response to HibTITER. There is some evidence suggesting natural increases in antibody levels over time after vaccination, most probably the result of contact with Haemophilus type b organisms or cross-reactive antigens.[18] These studies were carried out at a time when significant levels of Haemophilus b disease were still present in the community.

Antibody generated by HibTITER has been found to have high avidity, a measure of the functional affinity of antibody to bind to antigen. High-avidity antibody is more potent than low-avidity antibody in serum bactericidal assays.[19] The contribution to clinical protection is unknown.

Immunogenicity of HibTITER was evaluated in 26 children 22 months to 5 years of age who had not responded to earlier vaccination with Haemophilus b polysaccharide vaccine. One dose of HibTITER was immunogenic in all 26 children and generated titers of ≥1 µg/mL in 25 of the 26 infants.[20] HibTITER has been found to be immunogenic in children with sickle cell disease, a condition that may cause increased susceptibility to Haemophilus b disease.[21] HibTITER has also been shown to be immunogenic in native American infants, such as the group of 50 studied in Alaska who received three doses at 2, 4, and 6 months of age.[20] Antibody levels achieved were comparable to those seen in healthy US infants who received their first dose at 1 to 2 months of age and subsequent doses at 4 to 6 months of age.[15,16,20]

Postlicensure surveillance of immunogenicity was conducted during the distribution of the first 30 million doses of HibTITER and during the time period over which Haemophilus b disease in children has been decreasing significantly in areas of extensive vaccine usage.[20,22–29] After three doses, titers ranged from 2.37 to 8.45 µg/mL, with 67% to 94% attaining ≥1 µg/mL.[20,24,25]

Persistence of antibody was examined in several cohorts of subjects that received either a selected commercial lot or that were part of the initial efficacy trial in northern California. Geometric mean titers for these cohorts were between 0.51 and 1.96 just prior to boosting at 15 to 18 months. These lots not only induced persistent antibody but also provided effective priming for a booster dose with commercial lots, with postboosting titers greater than 1.0 µg/mL in 80% to 97% of subjects.[20]

HibTITER (HbOC) was shown to be effective in a large-scale controlled clinical trial in a multiethnic population in northern California carried out between February 1988 and June 1990.[30,31] There were no (0) vaccine failures in infants who received three doses of HibTITER and 12 cases of Haemophilus b disease (6 cases of meningitis) in the control group. The estimate of efficacy is 100% (*P* = .0002) with 95% confidence intervals of 68% to 100%. Through the end of 1991, with an additional 49,000 person-years of follow-up, there were still no cases of Haemophilus b disease in fully vaccinated infants less than 2 years of age.[22,23] One case of disease has been reported in a 3^1/$_2$-year-old child who did not receive a booster dose as recommended.

A comparative clinical trial was performed in Finland where approximately 53,000 infants received HibTITER at 4 and 6 months of age and a booster dose at 14 months in a trial conducted from January 1988 through December 1990. Only two children developed Haemophilus b disease after receiving the two-dose primary immunization schedule. One child became ill at 15 months of age and the other at 18 months of age; neither child received the scheduled booster at 14 months of age. No vaccine failure has been reported in children who received the two-dose primary series and the booster dose at 14 months of age. Based on more than 32,000 person-years of follow-up time, the estimate of efficacy is about 95% when compared to historical control groups followed between 1985 and 1988.[20] Historical controls were used since all infants received one of two Haemophilus b conjugate vaccines during the period of the trial.

Evidence of efficacy postlicensure includes significant reductions in Haemophilus b disease that are closely associated with increases in the net doses of Haemophilus b Conjugate Vaccine distributed in the US.[20,22–29] In the northern California Kaiser Permanente there has been a 94% decrease in Haemophilus disease incidence in 1991 for children younger than 18 months of age, compared to 1984–1988, when HibTITER was not available for this age group.[22,23] Furthermore, active surveillance by the Centers for Disease Control and Prevention (CDC) has shown a 71% decrease in Haemophilus b disease in children less than 15 months old, between 1989 and 1991, which corresponds temporally and geographically with increases in net doses of Haemophilus b conjugate vaccine distributed in the US.[26] As with all vaccines, this conjugate vaccine cannot be expected to be 100% effective. There have been rare reports to the Vaccine Adverse Event Reporting System (VAERS) of Haemophilus b disease following full primary immunization.

INDICATIONS AND USAGE

Haemophilus b Conjugate Vaccine (Diphtheria CRM$_{197}$ Protein Conjugate) HibTITER is indicated for the immunization of children 2 months to 71 months of age against invasive diseases caused by *H. influenzae* type b.

As with any vaccine, HibTITER may not protect 100% of individuals receiving the vaccine.

HibTITER may be administered simultaneously but at different sites from other routine pediatric vaccines, eg, Diphtheria and Tetanus Toxoids and Pertussis Vaccine Adsorbed (DTP), Oral Poliovirus Vaccine (OPV), and Measles-Mumps-Rubella Vaccine (MMR).[32,33]

CONTRAINDICATIONS

Hypersensitivity to any component of the vaccine, including diphtheria toxoid, or thimerosal in the multidose presentation, is a contraindication to use of HibTITER.

WARNINGS

HibTITER WILL NOT PROTECT AGAINST *H. INFLUENZAE* OTHER THAN TYPE b STRAINS, NOR WILL HibTITER PROTECT AGAINST OTHER MICROORGANISMS THAT CAUSE MENINGITIS OR SEPTIC DISEASE.

AS WITH ANY INTRAMUSCULAR INJECTION, HibTITER SHOULD BE GIVEN WITH CAUTION TO INFANTS OR CHILDREN WITH THROMBOCYTOPENIA OR ANY COAGULATION DISORDER THAT WOULD CONTRAINDICATE INTRAMUSCULAR INJECTION (SEE **DRUG INTERACTIONS**).

ANTIGENURIA HAS BEEN DETECTED FOLLOWING RECEIPT OF HAEMOPHILUS b CONJUGATE VACCINE[34] AND THEREFORE ANTIGEN DETECTION IN URINE MAY NOT HAVE DIAGNOSTIC VALUE IN SUSPECTED HAEMOPHILUS b DISEASE WITHIN 2 WEEKS OF IMMUNIZATION.

PRECAUTIONS

GENERAL

1. CARE IS TO BE TAKEN BY THE HEALTH CARE PROVIDER FOR SAFE AND EFFECTIVE USE OF THIS PRODUCT.
2. PRIOR TO ADMINISTRATION OF ANY DOSE OF HibTITER, THE PARENT OR GUARDIAN SHOULD BE ASKED ABOUT THE PERSONAL HISTORY, FAMILY HISTORY, AND RECENT HEALTH STATUS OF THE VACCINE RECIPIENT. THE HEALTH CARE PROVIDER SHOULD ASCERTAIN PREVIOUS IMMUNIZATION HISTORY, CURRENT HEALTH STATUS, AND OCCURRENCE OF ANY SYMPTOMS AND/OR SIGNS OF AN ADVERSE EVENT AFTER PREVIOUS IMMUNIZATION IN THE CHILD TO BE IMMUNIZED, IN ORDER TO DETERMINE THE EXISTENCE OF ANY CONTRAINDICATION TO IMMUNIZATION WITH HibTITER AND TO ALLOW AN ASSESSMENT OF BENEFITS AND RISKS.
3. BEFORE THE INJECTION OF ANY BIOLOGICAL, THE HEALTH CARE PROVIDER SHOULD TAKE ALL PRECAUTIONS KNOWN FOR THE PREVENTION OF ALLERGIC OR ANY OTHER SIDE REACTIONS. This should include: a review of the patient's history regarding possible sensitivity; the ready availability of epinephrine 1:1,000 and other appropriate agents used for control of immediate allergic reactions; and a knowledge of the recent literature pertaining to use of the biological concerned, including the nature of side effects and adverse reactions that may follow its use.
4. Children with impaired immune responsiveness, whether due to the use of immunosuppressive therapy (including irradiation, corticosteroids, antimetabolites, alkylating agents, and cytotoxic agents), a genetic defect, human immunodeficiency virus (HIV) infection, or other causes, may have reduced antibody response to active immunization procedures.[35,36] Deferral of administration of vaccine may be considered in individuals receiving immunosuppressive therapy.[35] Other groups should receive this vaccine according to the usual recommended schedule.[35-37] (See **DRUG INTERACTIONS**.)
5. This product is not contraindicated based on the presence of human immunodeficiency virus infection.[38]
6. Any acute infection or febrile illness is reason for delaying use of HibTITER except when in the opinion of the physician, withholding the vaccine entails a greater risk. A minor afebrile illness, such as a mild upper respiratory infection, is not usually reason to defer immunization.
7. As reported with Haemophilus b polysaccharide vaccine, cases of Haemophilus b disease may occur prior to the onset of the protective effects of the vaccine.[3,39]
8. The vaccine should not be injected intradermally since the safety and immunogenicity of this route have not been evaluated. The vaccine should be given intramuscularly.
9. A separate sterile syringe and needle or a sterile disposable unit should be used for each individual patient to prevent transmission of infectious agents from one person to another. Needles should be disposed of properly and should not be recapped.
10. Special care should be taken to prevent injection into a blood vessel.

The US Department of Health and Human Services has established a new Vaccine Adverse Event Reporting System

(VAERS) to accept all reports of suspected adverse events after the administration of any vaccine, including but not limited to the reporting of events required by the National Childhood Vaccine Injury Act of 1986.[40] The VAERS toll-free number for VAERS forms and information is 800-822-7967.

ALTHOUGH SOME ANTIBODY RESPONSE TO DIPHTHERIA TOXIN OCCURS, IMMUNIZATION WITH HibTITER DOES NOT SUBSTITUTE FOR ROUTINE DIPHTHERIA IMMUNIZATION.

INFORMATION FOR PATIENT

PRIOR TO ADMINISTRATION OF HibTITER, HEALTH CARE PERSONNEL SHOULD INFORM THE PARENT, GUARDIAN, OR OTHER RESPONSIBLE ADULT, OF THE RECOMMENDED IMMUNIZATION SCHEDULE FOR PROTECTION AGAINST HAEMOPHILUS b DISEASE AND THE BENEFITS AND RISKS TO THE CHILD RECEIVING THIS VACCINE. GUIDANCE SHOULD BE PROVIDED ON MEASURES TO BE TAKEN SHOULD ADVERSE EVENTS OCCUR, SUCH AS, ANTIPYRETIC MEASURES FOR ELEVATED TEMPERATURES AND THE NEED TO REPORT ADVERSE EVENTS TO THE HEALTH CARE PROVIDER. Parents should be provided with vaccine information pamphlets at the time of each vaccination, as stated in the National Childhood Vaccine Injury Act.[40]

PATIENTS, PARENTS, OR GUARDIANS SHOULD BE INSTRUCTED TO REPORT ANY SERIOUS ADVERSE REACTIONS TO THEIR HEALTH CARE PROVIDER.

DRUG INTERACTIONS

No impairment of the antibody response to the individual antigens was demonstrated when HibTITER was given at the same time but at separate sites as DTP plus OPV to children 2 to 20 months of age or MMR to children 15 ± 1 month of age.[20,41]

As with other intramuscular injections, HibTITER should be given with caution to children on anticoagulant therapy.

CARCINOGENESIS, MUTAGENESIS, IMPAIRMENT OF FERTILITY

HibTITER has not been evaluated for its carcinogenic, mutagenic potential, or impairment of fertility.

PREGNANCY

REPRODUCTIVE STUDIES—PREGNANCY CATEGORY C

Animal reproduction studies have not been conducted with HibTITER. It is also not known whether HibTITER can cause fetal harm when administered to a pregnant woman or can affect reproduction capability. HibTITER is NOT recommended for use in a pregnant woman.

PEDIATRIC USE

The safety and effectiveness of HibTITER in children below the age of 6 weeks have not been established.

ADVERSE REACTIONS

Adverse reactions associated with HibTITER have been evaluated in 401 infants who were vaccinated initially at 1 to 6 months of age and were given 1,118 doses independent of DTP vaccine. Observations were made during the day of vaccination and days 1 and 2 postvaccination. A temperature >38.3°C was recorded at least once during the observation period following 2% of the vaccinations. Local erythema, warmth, or swelling (≥2 cm) was observed following 3.3% of vaccinations. The incidence of temperature >38.3°C was greater during the first postvaccination day than during the day of vaccination or the second postvaccination day. The incidence of local erythema, warmth, or swelling was similar during the day of vaccination and the first postvaccination day; it was lower during the second postvaccination day. All side effects have been infrequent, mild, and transient with no serious sequelae (Table 1). No difference in the rates of these complaints was reported after dose 1, 2, or 3.
[See table 1 above]

The following complaints were also observed after 1,118 vaccinations with HibTITER: irritability (133), sleepiness (91), prolonged crying [≥ 4 hours] (38), appetite loss (23), vomiting (9), diarrhea (2), and rash (1).

Additional safety data with HibTITER are available from the efficacy studies conducted in young infants.[30] There were 79,483 doses given to 30,844 infants at approximately 2, 4, and 6 months of age in California, usually at the same time as DTP (but at a separate injection site) and OPV; approximately 100,000 doses have been given to 53,000 infants at 4 and 6 months in Finland at the same time as a combined DTP and inactivated polio (IPV) vaccine (but at a separate injection site). The rate and type of reactions associated with the vaccinations were no different from those seen when DTP or DTP-IPV was administered alone. These included fever, local reactions, rash, and one hyporesponsive episode with a single seizure. The safety of HibTITER was also evaluated in the California study by direct phone questioning of the parents or guardians of 6,887 vaccine recipients. The incidence and type of side effects reported within 24 hours of vaccination were similar to those cited in Table 1. In addition, analysis of emergency room (ER) visits within 30 days and hospitalization within 60 days after receipt of 23,800 doses of HibTITER showed no increase in the rates of any type of ER visit or hospitalization.

Table 2 details the side effects associated with a single vaccination of HibTITER given (without DTP) to infants of 15 to 23 months of age.

Similar results have been observed in the analysis of 2,285 subjects of 18 to 60 months of age, vaccinated as part of a postmarketing safety study of HibTITER.[20] These data were collected by telephone survey 24 to 48 hours postvaccination. Additional observations included irritability, restless sleep, and GI symptoms (diarrhea, vomiting, and loss of appetite) in the group that received HibTITER alone. A cause and effect relationship between these observations and the vaccinations has not been established.

TABLE 1
Number of Subjects (Percent) Manifesting
Side Effects Associated with HibTITER
Administered Independently from DTP*
(Infants Vaccinated Initially at 1–6 Months of Age)

Symptoms	Dose 1 n=401 Same Day As Vacc.	+1 Day	+2 Days	Dose 2 n=383 Same Day As Vacc.	+1 Day	+2 Days	Dose 3 n=334 Same Day As Vacc.	+1 Day	+2 Days
Temp >38.3°C	0	2	2	2	3	2	2	6	5
	—	<1%	<1%	<1%	<1%	<1%	<1%	1.8%	1.5%
Redness ≥2cm	1	0	0	1	6	0	5	4	0
	<1%	—	—	<1%	1.6%	—	1.5%	1.2%	—
Warmth ≥2cm	1	1	0	2	1	0	1	6	0
	<1%	<1%	—	<1%	<1%	—	<1%	1.8%	—
Swelling ≥2cm	5	1	0	2	2	0	1	0	0
	1.2%	<1%	—	<1%	<1%	—	<1%	—	—

*DTP and HibTITER given 2 weeks apart with DTP having been given first.

TABLE 2
Selected Adverse Reactions* in
Children of 15–23 Months of Age
Following Vaccination with HibTITER

Adverse Reaction	No. of Subjects	Reaction Within 24 h	% Postvaccination At 48 h
Fever >38.3°C	354	1.4	0.6
Erythema	354	2.0	—
Swelling	354	1.7	—
Tenderness	354	3.7	0.3

* The following complaints were reported after vaccination of these 354 children in the indicated number of children: diarrhea (9), vomiting (5), prolonged crying [>4 hours] (4), and rashes (2).

Rash, hives (urticaria), erythema multiforme, convulsions,[42] vomiting/diarrhea,[42] and Guillain-Barré syndrome[43] have been observed following the administration of Haemophilus b polysaccharide and Haemophilus b conjugate vaccines. However, a cause and effect relationship among any of these events and the vaccination has not been established.

DOSAGE AND ADMINISTRATION

HibTITER is for intramuscular use only.

Any parenteral drug product should be inspected visually for extraneous particulate matter and/or discoloration prior to administration whenever solution and container permit. If these conditions exist, HibTITER should not be administered.

Continued on next page

HibTITER—Cont.

Before injection, the skin over the site to be injected should be cleansed with a suitable germicide. After insertion of the needle, aspirate to help avoid inadvertent injection into a blood vessel.

The vaccine should be injected intramuscularly, preferably into the midlateral muscles of the thigh or deltoid, with care to avoid major peripheral nerve trunks.

HibTITER is indicated for children 2 months to 71 months of age for the prevention of invasive Haemophilus b disease. For infants 2 to 6 months of age, the immunizing dose is three separate injections of 0.5 mL given at approximately 2-month intervals. Previously unvaccinated infants from 7 through 11 months of age should receive two separate injections approximately 2 months apart. Children from 12 through 14 months of age who have not been vaccinated previously receive one injection. All vaccinated children receive a single booster dose at 15 months of age or older, but not less than 2 months after the previous dose. Previously unvaccinated children 15 to 71 months of age receive a single injection of HibTITER.[32,33] Preterm infants should be vaccinated with HibTITER according to their chronological age, from birth.[32]

Recommended Immunization Schedule

Age at First Immunization (Mo)	No. of Doses	Booster
2–6	3	Yes
7–11	2	Yes
12 –14	1	Yes
15 and over	1	No

Interruption of the recommended schedules with a delay between doses does not interfere with the final immunity achieved nor does it necessitate starting the series over again, regardless of the length of time elapsed between doses.[32,33]

NO DATA ARE AVAILABLE TO SUPPORT THE INTERCHANGEABILITY OF HibTITER OR OTHER HAEMOPHILUS b CONJUGATE VACCINES WITH ONE ANOTHER FOR THE PRIMARY IMMUNIZATION SERIES. THEREFORE, IT IS RECOMMENDED THAT THE SAME CONJUGATE VACCINE BE USED THROUGHOUT EACH IMMUNIZATION SCHEDULE, CONSISTENT WITH THE DATA SUPPORTING APPROVAL AND LICENSURE OF THE VACCINE.

Each dose of 0.5 mL is formulated to contain 10 µg of purified Haemophilus b saccharide and approximately 25 µg of CRM_{197} protein.

STORAGE

Stability studies indicate that HibTITER can be shipped at ambient temperatures and stored at 2°–8°C (36°–46°F). DO NOT FREEZE.

HOW SUPPLIED

Vial, 1 Dose (4 per package) —Product No. 0005-0104-41

Vial, 10 Dose —Product No. 0005-0201-10

REFERENCES

1. United States Patent Number 4,902,506 by Anderson PW, Eby RJ filed May 5, 1986 issued February 20, 1990.
2. Seid RC Jr, Boykins RA, Liu DF, et al. Chemical evidence for covalent linkage of a semi-synthetic glycoconjugate vaccine for Haemophilus influenzae type b disease. Glycoconjugate J. 1989;6:489–498.
3. Wenger JD, Ward JL, Broome CV. Prevention of Haemophilus influenzae type b disease: vaccines and passive prophylaxis. In: Remington JS, Swartz MS, eds. Current Clinical Topics in Infectious Diseases. New York, NY: McGraw-Hill Inc; 1989;10:306–339.
4. Recommendation of the Immunization Practices Advisory Committee (ACIP)–polysaccharide vaccine for prevention of Haemophilus influenzae type b disease. MMWR. 1985;34:201–205.
5. Sell SH. Long term sequelae of bacterial meningitis in children. Pediatr Infect Dis J. 1983;2:90–93.
6. Broome CV. Epidemiology of Haemophilus influenzae type b infections in the United States. Pediatr Infect Dis J. 1987;6:779–782.
7. Alexander HE. The productive or curative element in type b Haemophilus influenzae rabbit serum. Yale J Biol Med. 1944;16:425–434.
8. Peltola H, Kayhty H, Sivonen A. Haemophilus influenzae type b capsular polysaccharide vaccine in children: a double-blind field study of 100,000 vaccinees 3 months to 5 years of age in Finland. Pediatrics. 1977;60:730–737.
9. Robbins JB, Parke JC Jr, Schneerson R. Quantitative measurement of "natural" and immunization-induced Haemophilus influenzae type b capsular polysaccharide antibodies. Pediatr Res. 1973;7:103-110.
10. Kayhty H, Peltola H, Karanko V, et al. The protective level of serum antibodies to the capsular polysaccharide of Haemophilus influenzae type b. J Infect Dis. 1983;147:1100.
11. Kayhty H, Karanko, V, Peltola H, et al. Serum antibodies after vaccination with Haemophilus influenzae type b capsular polysaccharide and responses to reimmunization: no evidence of immunologic tolerance or memory. Pediatrics. 1984;74:857–865.
12. Weinberg GA, Granoff DM. Polysaccharide-protein conjugate vaccines for the prevention of Haemophilus influenzae type b disease. J Pediatr. 1988;113:621–631.
13. Makela O, Péterfy F, Outshoorn IG, et al. Immunogenic properties of a (1–6) dextran, its protein conjugates, and conjugates of its breakdown products in mice. Scand J Immunol. 1984;19:541–550.
14. Anderson P, Pichichero ME, Insel RA. Immunogens consisting of oligosaccharides from Haemophilus influenzae type b coupled to diphtheria toxoid or the toxin protein CRM_{197}. J Clin Invest. 1985;76:52–59.
15. Madore DV, Phipps DC, Eby R, et al. Immune response of young children vaccinated with Haemophilus influenzae type b conjugate vaccines. In: Cruse JM, Lewis RE, eds. Contributions to Microbiology and Immunology: Conjugate Vaccines. New York, NY: Karger Medical and Scientific Publishers; 1989;10:125–150.
16. Madore DV, Phipps DC, Eby R, et al. Safety and immunologic response to Haemophilus influenzae type b oligosaccharide-CRM_{197} conjugate vaccine in 1- to 6-month-old infants. Pediatrics. 1990;85:331–337.
17. Madore DV, Johnson CL, Phipps DC, et al. Safety and immunogenicity of Haemophilus influenzae type b oligosaccharide-CRM_{197} conjugate vaccine in infants aged 15–23 months. Pediatrics. 1990;86:527–534.
18. Rothstein EP, Madore DV, Long S. Antibody persistence four years after primary immunization of infants and toddlers with Haemophilus influenzae type b CRM_{197} conjugate vaccine. J Pediatrics. 1991;119:655–657.
19. Schlesinger Y, Granoff DM. Avidity and bactericidal activity of antibodies elicited by different Haemophilus influenzae type b conjugate vaccines. JAMA. 1992; 267:1489–1494.
20. Unpublished data available from Lederle Laboratories.
21. Gigliotti F, Feldman S, Wang WC, et al. Immunization of young infants with sickle cell disease with a Haemophilus influenzae type b saccharide-diphtheria CRM_{197} protein conjugate vaccine. J Pediatr. 1989;114:1006-1010.
22. Black SB, Shinefield HR, The Kaiser Permanente Pediatric Vaccine Study Group. Immunization with oligosaccharide conjugate Haemophilus influenzae type b (HbOC) vaccine on a large health maintenance organization population: extended follow-up and impact on Haemophilus influenzae disease epidemiology. Pediatr Infect Dis J. 1992;11:610–613.
23. Black SB, Shinefield HR, Fireman B, et al. Safety, immunogenicity, and efficacy in infancy of oligosaccharide conjugate Haemophilus influenzae type b vaccine in a United States Population: possible implications for optimal use. J Infect Dis. 1992;165 (suppl 1):S139–143.
24. Granoff DM, Anderson EL, Osterholm MT, et al. Differences in the immunogenicity of three Haemophilus influenzae type b conjugate vaccines in infants. J Pediatr. 1992;121:187–194.
25. Decker MD, Edwards KM, Bradley R, et al. Comparative trial in infants of four conjugate Haemophilus influenzae type b vaccines. J Pediatr. 1992;120:184–189.
26. Adams WG, Deaver KA, Cochi SL, et al. Decline of childhood Haemophilus influenzae type b (Hib) disease in the Hib vaccine era. JAMA. 1993;269:221–226.
27. Murphy TV, White KE, Pastor P, et al. Declining incidence of Haemophilus influenzae type b disease since introduction of vaccination. JAMA. 1993;269:246–248.
28. Broadhurst LE, Erickson RL, Kelley PW. Decreases in invasive Haemophilus influenzae diseases in US Army children, 1984 through 1991. JAMA. 1993;269:227–231.
29. Shapiro ED. Infections caused by Haemophilus influenzae type b: the beginning of the end? JAMA. 1993;269:264–266.
30. Black SB, Shinefield HR, Lampert D, et al. Safety and immunogenicity of oligosaccharide conjugate Haemophilus influenzae type b (HbOC) vaccine in infancy. Pediatr Infect Dis J. 1991;10:92–96.
31. Black SB, Shinefield HR, Fireman B, et al. Efficacy in infancy of oligosaccharide conjugate Haemophilus influenzae type b (HbOC) vaccine in a United States population of 61,080 children. Pediatr Infect Dis J. 1991;10:97–104.
32. Recommendations of the AAP: Haemophilus influenzae type b conjugate vaccines: recommendations for immunization of infants and children 2 months of age and older: update. Pediatrics. 1991;88:169–172.
33. Recommendation of the ACIP: Haemophilus b conjugate vaccines for prevention of Haemophilus influenzae type b disease among infants and children two months of age and older. MMWR. 1991;40:1–7.
34. Jones RG, Bass JW, Weisse ME, et al. Antigenuria after immunization with Haemophilus influenzae oligosaccharide CRM_{197} conjugate (HbOC) vaccine. Pediatr Infect Dis J. 1991;10:557–559.
35. American Academy of Pediatrics: Report of the Committee on Infectious Diseases. 22nd ed. Elk Grove Village, Ill: American Academy of Pediatrics; 1991.
36. Recommendation of the ACIP—immunization of children infected with human T-lymphotrophic virus type III/lymphadenopathy-associated virus. MMWR. 1986;35(38):595–606.
37. Immunization of children infected with human immunodeficiency virus—supplementary ACIP statement. MMWR. 1988;37(12):181–183.
38. General Recommendations on Immunization—recommendations of the Immunization Practices Advisory Committee (ACIP). MMWR. 1989;38(13):221.
39. Spinola SM, Sheaffer CI, Philbrick KB, et al. Antigenuria after Haemophilus influenzae type b polysaccharide immunization: a prospective study. J Pediatr. 1986;109:835–837.
40. CDC. Vaccine Adverse Event Reporting System—United States. MMWR. 1990;39:730–733.
41. Paradiso PR. Combined childhood immunizations. JAMA. 1992;268:1685.
42. Milstein JB, Gross TP, Kuritsky JN. Adverse reactions reported following receipt of Haemophilus influenzae type b vaccine: an analysis after one year of marketing. Pediatrics. 1987;80:270–274.
43. D'Cruz DF, Shapiro ED, Spiegelman KN, et al. Acute inflammatory demyelinating polyradiculoneuropathy (Guillain-Barré syndrome) after immunization with Haemophilus influenzae type b conjugate vaccine. J Pediatr. 1989;115:743–746.

Manufactured by:
LEDERLE LABORATORIES
Division American Cyanamid Company
Pearl River, NY 10965 USA
US Gov't. License No. 17
Marketed by:
WYETH-LEDERLE VACCINES
Wyeth-Ayerst Laboratories
Philadelphia, PA 19101
Shown in Product Identification Guide, page 319

MATERNA® ℞

[mă-tĕr-nă]
Prenatal Vitamin and Mineral Tablets
For Use Before, During & After Pregnancy

DESCRIPTION

One tablet daily provides:

VITAMINS	
A*	5,000 IU
(50% as Beta Carotene)	
D	400 IU
E (dl-alpha tocopheryl acetate)	30 IU
C (ascorbic acid)	120 mg
Folic Acid	1 mg
B_1 (thiamine mononitrate)	3 mg
B_2 (riboflavin)	3.4 mg
B_6 (pyridoxine hydrochloride)	10 mg
Niacinamide	20 mg
B_{12} (cyanocobalamin)	12 mcg
Biotin	30 mcg
Pantothenic Acid (calcium pantothenate)	10 mg
MINERALS	
Calcium (calcium carbonate)	200 mg
Iodine (potassium iodide)	150 mcg
Iron (ferrous fumarate)	27 mg
Magnesium (magnesium oxide)	25 mg
Copper (cupric oxide)	2 mg
Zinc (zinc oxide)	25 mg
Chromium (chromium chloride)	25 mcg
Molybdenum (sodium molybdate)	25 mcg
Manganese (manganese sulfate)	5 mg
Selenium (sodium selenate)	20 mcg

*Input as vitamin A acetate and beta carotene
MATERNA contains no artificial dyes, flavors or added sweeteners.

INDICATIONS

To provide vitamin and mineral supplementation prior to conception, throughout pregnancy desk during the postnatal period for both the lactating and nonlactating mother.

DOSAGE

Before, during and after pregnancy, one tablet daily, or as directed by a physician.

WARNING: Accidental overdose of iron-containing products is a leading cause of fatal poisoning in children under six. Keep this product out of the reach of children. In case of accidental overdose, call a doctor or poison control center immediately.

CAUTION
Rx only

PRECAUTIONS
Folic acid may partially correct the hematological damage due to vitamin B_{12} deficiency of pernicious anemia, while the associated neurological damage progresses. In rare instances, allergic hypersensitivity has been reported following administration of folic acid.

NOTICE: Contact with moisture may produce surface discoloration or erosion of the tablet.

HOW SUPPLIED
MATERNA is available as oblong-shaped, scored, sand-colored, film-coated tablets, engraved with "M" to the left of the score and "55" to the right of the score on one side of each tablet and "MATERNA" on the other side, in bottles of 100, NDC 0005-5586-11.

Store at room temperature, approximately 25°C; avoid excess heat. Dispense in well-closed, light-resistant container.

A child-resistant safety cap is standard as a safeguard against accidental ingestion by children.

Questions or Comments: 1-800-999-9384

Manufactured by:
LEDERLE PHARMACEUTICAL DIVISION
American Cyanamid Company
Pearl River, NY 10965

Shown in Product Identification Guide, page 319

MINOCIN® ℞

[mī-nō-sĭn]

Sterile
Minocycline Hydrochloride
Intravenous
100 mg/Vial

DESCRIPTION

MINOCIN minocycline hydrochloride, a semisynthetic derivative of tetracycline, is named [4S-(4α,4aα,5aα,12aα)]-4,7-bis(dimethylamino)-1,4,4a,5,5a,6,11,12a-octahydro-3,10,-12,12a-tetrahydroxy-1, 11-dioxo-2-naphthacenecarboxamide monohydrochloride.

Each vial, dried by cryodesiccation, contains sterile minocycline HCl equivalent to 100 mg minocycline. When reconstituted with 5 mL of Sterile Water for Injection USP, the pH ranges from 2.0 to 2.8.

ACTIONS

Microbiology

The tetracyclines are primarily bacteriostatic and are thought to exert their antimicrobial effect by the inhibition of protein synthesis. Minocycline HCl is a tetracycline with antibacterial activity comparable to other tetracyclines with activity against a wide range of gram-negative and gram-positive organisms.

Tube dilution testing: Microorganisms may be considered susceptible (likely to respond to minocycline therapy) if the minimum inhibitory concentration (MIC) is not more than 4 mcg/mL. Microorganisms may be considered intermediate (harboring partial resistance) if the MIC is 4 to 12.5 mcg/mL and resistant (not likely to respond to minocycline therapy) if the MIC is greater than 12.5 mcg/mL.

Susceptibility plate testing: If the Kirby-Bauer method of susceptibility testing (using a 30 mcg tetracycline disc) gives a zone of 18 mm or greater, the bacterial strain is considered to be susceptible to any tetracycline. Minocycline shows moderate *in vitro* activity against certain strains of staphylococci which have been found resistant to other tetracyclines. For such strains, minocycline susceptibility powder may be used for additional susceptibility testing.

Human Pharmacology

Following a single dose of 200 mg administered intravenously to 10 healthy male volunteers, serum levels ranged from 2.52 to 6.63 mcg/mL (average 4.18), after 12 hours they ranged from 0.82 to 2.64 mcg/mL (average 1.38). In a group of five healthy male volunteers, serum levels of 1.4 to 1.8 mcg/mL were maintained at 12 and 24 hours with doses of 100 mg every 12 hours for three days. When given 200 mg once daily for three days, the serum levels had fallen to approximately 1 mcg/mL at 24 hours. The serum half-life following I.V. doses of 100 mg every 12 hours or 200 mg once daily did not differ significantly and ranged from 15 to 23 hours. The serum half-life following a single 200 mg oral dose in 12 essentially normal volunteers ranged from 11 to 17 hours, in 7 patients with hepatic dysfunction ranged from 11 to 16 hours, and in 5 patients with renal dysfunction from 18 to 69 hours.

Intravenously administered minocycline appears similar to oral doses in excretion. The urinary and fecal recovery of oral minocycline when administered to 12 normal volunteers is one-half to one-third that of other tetracyclines.

INDICATIONS

MINOCIN is indicated in infections caused by the following microorganisms:

Rickettsiae: (Rocky Mountain spotted fever, typhus fever and the typhus group, Q fever, rickettsialpox, tick fevers).
Mycoplasma pneumoniae (PPLO, Eaton agent).
Agents of psittacosis and ornithosis.
Agents of lymphogranuloma venereum and granuloma inguinale.
The spirochetal agent of relapsing fever (*Borrelia recurrentis*).

The following gram-negative microorganisms:
Haemophilus ducreyi (chancroid),
Yersinia pestis and *Francisella tularensis,* formerly *Pasteurella pestis* and *Pasteurella tularensis,*
Bartonella bacilliformis,
Bacteroides species,
Vibrio comma and *Vibrio fetus,*
Brucella species (in conjunction with streptomycin).

Because many strains of the following groups of microorganisms have been shown to be resistant to tetracyclines, culture and susceptibility testing are recommended.

MINOCIN is indicated for treatment of infections caused by the following gram-negative microorganisms when bacteriologic testing indicates appropriate susceptibility to the drug:
Escherichia coli,
Enterobacter aerogenes (formerly *Aerobacter aerogenes*),
Shigella species,
Mima species and *Herellea* species,
Haemophilus influenzae (respiratory infections),
Klebsiella species (respiratory and urinary infections).

MINOCIN is indicated for treatment of infections caused by the following gram-positive microorganisms when bacteriologic testing indicates appropriate susceptibility to the drug:
Streptococcus species:
Up to 44% of strains of *Streptococcus pyogenes* and 74% of *Streptococcus faecalis* have been found to be resistant to tetracycline drugs. Therefore, tetracyclines should not be used for streptococcal disease unless the organism has been demonstrated to be sensitive.

For upper respiratory infections due to Group A beta-hemolytic streptococci, penicillin is the usual drug of choice, including prophylaxis of rheumatic fever.
Streptococcus pneumoniae,
Staphylococcus aureus, skin and soft tissue infections.

Tetracyclines are not the drugs of choice in the treatment of any type of staphylococcal infection.

When penicillin is contraindicated, tetracyclines are alternative drugs in the treatment of infections due to:
Neisseria gonorrhoeae, and *Neisseria meningitidis,*
Treponema pallidum and *Treponema pertenue* (syphilis and yaws),
Listeria monocytogenes,
Clostridium species,
Bacillus anthracis,
Fusobacterium fusiforme (Vincent's infection),
Actinomyces species.

In acute intestinal amebiasis, the tetracyclines may be a useful adjunct to amebicides.

MINOCIN minocycline HCl is indicated in the treatment of trachoma, although the infectious agent is not always eliminated, as judged by immunofluorescence.

Inclusion conjunctivitis may be treated with oral tetracyclines or with a combination of oral and topical agents.

CONTRAINDICATIONS

This drug is contraindicated in persons who have shown hypersensitivity to any of the tetracyclines.

WARNINGS

In the presence of renal dysfunction, particularly in pregnancy, intravenous tetracycline therapy in daily doses exceeding 2 g has been associated with deaths through liver failure.

When the need for intensive treatment outweighs its potential dangers (mostly during pregnancy or in individuals with known or suspected renal or liver impairment), it is advisable to perform renal and liver function tests before and during therapy. Also, tetracycline serum concentrations should be followed.

If renal impairment exists, even usual oral or parenteral doses may lead to excessive systemic accumulation of the drug and possible liver toxicity. Under such conditions, lower than usual total doses are indicated, and if therapy is prolonged, serum level determinations of the drug may be advisable. This hazard is of particular importance in the parenteral administration of tetracyclines to pregnant or postpartum patients with pyelonephritis. When used under these circumstances, the blood level should not exceed 15 mcg/mL and liver function tests should be made at frequent intervals. Other potentially hepatotoxic drugs should not be prescribed concomitantly.

THE USE OF TETRACYCLINES DURING TOOTH DEVELOPMENT (LAST HALF OF PREGNANCY, INFANCY, AND CHILDHOOD TO THE AGE OF 8 YEARS) MAY CAUSE PERMANENT DISCOLORATION OF THE TEETH (YELLOW-GRAY-BROWN). This adverse reaction is more common during long-term use of the drugs but has been observed following repeated short-term courses. Enamel hypoplasia has also been reported. TETRACYCLINES, THEREFORE, SHOULD NOT BE USED IN THIS AGE GROUP UNLESS OTHER DRUGS ARE NOT LIKELY TO BE EFFECTIVE OR ARE CONTRAINDICATED.

Photosensitivity manifested by an exaggerated sunburn reaction has been observed in some individuals taking tetracyclines. Patients apt to be exposed to direct sunlight or ultraviolet light should be advised that this reaction can occur with tetracycline drugs, and treatment should be discontinued at the first evidence of skin erythema. Studies to date indicate that photosensitivity is rarely reported with MINOCIN minocycline HCl.

The anti-anabolic action of the tetracyclines may cause an increase in BUN. While this is not a problem in those with normal renal function, in patients with significantly impaired function, higher serum levels of tetracycline may lead to azotemia, hyperphosphatemia, and acidosis.

CNS side effects including light-headedness, dizziness or vertigo have been reported. Patients who experience these symptoms should be cautioned about driving vehicles or using hazardous machinery while on minocycline therapy. These symptoms may disappear during therapy and usually disappear rapidly when the drug is discontinued.

Usage in Pregnancy

(See above **WARNINGS** about use during tooth development.)

Results of animal studies indicate that tetracyclines cross the placenta, are found in fetal tissues and can have toxic effects on the developing fetus (often related to retardation of skeletal development). Evidence of embryotoxicity has also been noted in animals treated early in pregnancy.

The safety of MINOCIN for use during pregnancy has not been established.

Usage in Newborns, Infants, and Children

(See above **WARNINGS** about use during tooth development.)

All tetracyclines form a stable calcium complex in any bone-forming tissue. A decrease in the fibula growth rate has been observed in prematures given oral tetracycline in doses of 25 mg/kg every 6 hours. This reaction was shown to be reversible when the drug was discontinued.

Tetracyclines are present in the milk of lactating women who are taking a drug in this class.

PRECAUTIONS

General

Pseudotumor cerebri (benign intracranial hypertension) in adults has been associated with the use of tetracyclines. The usual clinical manifestations are headache and blurred vision. Bulging fontanels have been associated with the use of tetracyclines in infants. While both of these conditions and related symptoms usually resolve soon after discontinuation of the tetracycline, the possibility for permanent sequelae exists.

As with other antibiotic preparations, use of this drug may result in overgrowth of nonsusceptible organisms, including fungi. If superinfection occurs, the antibiotic should be discontinued and appropriate therapy should be instituted.

In venereal diseases when coexistent syphilis is suspected, darkfield examination should be done before treatment is started and the blood serology repeated monthly for at least 4 months.

In long-term therapy, periodic laboratory evaluation of organ systems, including hematopoietic, renal, and hepatic studies should be performed.

All infections due to Group A beta-hemolytic streptococci should be treated for at least ten days.

Drug Interactions

Because tetracyclines have been shown to depress plasma prothrombin activity, patients who are on anticoagulant therapy may require downward adjustment of their anticoagulant dosage.

Since bacteriostatic drugs may interfere with the bactericidal action of penicillin, it is advisable to avoid giving tetracycline in conjunction with penicillin.

Concurrent use of tetracyclines with oral contraceptives may render oral contraceptives less effective.

ADVERSE REACTIONS

Gastrointestinal: Anorexia, nausea, vomiting, diarrhea, glossitis, dysphagia, enterocolitis, pancreatitis, inflammatory lesions (with monilial overgrowth) in the anogenital region, and increases in liver enzymes. Rarely, hepatitis and liver failure have been reported.

These reactions have been caused by both the oral and parenteral administration of tetracyclines.

Skin: Maculopapular and erythematous rashes. Exfoliative dermatitis has been reported but is uncommon. Fixed drug eruptions, including balanitis, have been rarely re-

Continued on next page

Minocin Intravenous—Cont.

ported. Erythema multiforme and rarely Stevens-Johnson syndrome have been reported. Photosensitivity is discussed above. (See **WARNINGS.**)

Pigmentation of the skin and mucous membranes has been reported.

Tooth discoloration has been reported, rarely, in adults.

Renal Toxicity: Rise in BUN has been reported and is apparently dose related. (See **WARNINGS.**) Reversible acute renal failure has been rarely reported.

Hypersensitivity Reactions: Urticaria, angioneurotic edema, polyarthralgia, anaphylaxis, anaphylactoid purpura, pericarditis, exacerbation of systemic lupus erythematosus, and rarely, pulmonary infiltrates with eosinophilia have been reported. A transient lupus-like syndrome has also been reported.

Blood: Hemolytic anemia, thrombocytopenia, neutropenia, and eosinophilia have been reported.

CNS: (See **WARNINGS.**) Pseudotumor cerebri (benign intracranial hypertension) in adults and bulging fontanels in infants. (See **PRECAUTIONS—General.**) Headache has also been reported.

Other: When given over prolonged periods, tetracyclines have been reported to produce brown-black microscopic discoloration of the thyroid glands. Very rare cases of abnormal thyroid function have been reported.

Decreased hearing has been rarely reported in patients on MINOCIN.

DOSAGE AND ADMINISTRATION

Note: Rapid administration is to be avoided. Parenteral therapy is indicated only when oral therapy is not adequate or tolerated. Oral therapy should be instituted as soon as possible. If intravenous therapy is given over prolonged periods of time, thrombophlebitis may result.

ADULTS: Usual adult dose: 200 mg followed by 100 mg every 12 hours and should not exceed 400 mg in 24 hours.

The cryodesiccated powder should be reconstituted with 5 mL Sterile Water for Injection USP and immediately further diluted to 500 mL to 1,000 mL with Sodium Chloride Injection USP, Dextrose Injection USP, Dextrose and Sodium Chloride Injection USP, Ringer's Injection USP, or Lactated Ringer's Injection USP, but not other solutions containing calcium because a precipitate may form. When further diluted in 500 mL to 1,000 mL compatible solutions (except Lactated Ringers), the pH usually ranges from 2.5 to 4.0. The pH of MINOCIN IV 100 mg in Lactated Ringers 500 mL to 1,000 mL usually ranges from 4.5 to 6.0.

Final dilutions (500 mL to 1,000 mL) should be administered immediately but product and diluents are compatible at room temperature for 24 hours without a significant loss of potency. Any unused portions must be discarded after that period.

For children above eight years of age: Usual pediatric dose: 4 mg/kg followed by 2 mg/kg every 12 hours.

In patients with renal impairment: (See **WARNINGS.**)

Total dosage should be decreased by reduction of recommended individual doses and/or by extending time intervals between doses.

Parenteral drug products should be inspected visually for particulate matter and discoloration prior to administration, whenever solution and container permit.

HOW SUPPLIED

MINOCIN® minocycline HCl Intravenous is supplied as 100 mg vials of sterile cryodesiccated powder.

Product No. NDC 0205-5305-94

Store at Controlled Room Temperature 15–30°C (59–86°F).

Manufactured by:

LEDERLE PARENTERALS, INC.

Carolina, Puerto Rico 00987

Shown in Product Identification Guide, page 319

MINOCIN® ℞
Minocycline Hydrochloride
Pellet-Filled Capsules

DESCRIPTION

MINOCIN minocycline hydrochloride, a semisynthetic derivative of tetracycline, is [4*S* -(4α,4aα,5aα,12aα)]-4,7-bis(dimethylamino)-1,4,4α,5,5α,6,11,12α-octahydro-3,10,12,12a-tetrahydroxy-1,11-dioxo-2-naphthacenecarboxamide monohydrochloride.

MINOCIN minocycline hydrochloride pellet-filled capsules for oral administration contain pellets of minocycline HCl equivalent to 50 mg or 100 mg of minocycline in microcrystalline cellulose.

The capsule shells contain the following inactive ingredients: Blue 1, Gelatin, Titanium Dioxide and Yellow 10. The 50 mg capsule shells also contain Black and Yellow Iron Oxides.

CLINICAL PHARMACOLOGY

MINOCIN minocycline hydrochloride pellet-filled capsules are rapidly absorbed from the gastrointestinal tract following oral administration. Following a single dose of two 100 mg pellet-filled capsules of MINOCIN minocycline HCl administered to 18 normal fasting adult volunteers, maximum serum concentrations were attained in 1 to 4 hours (average 2.1 hours) and ranged from 2.1 to 5.1 mcg/mL (average 3.5 mcg/mL). The serum half-life in the normal volunteers ranged from 11.1 to 22.1 hours (average 15.5 hours).

When MINOCIN minocycline hydrochloride pellet-filled capsules were given concomitantly with a meal which included dairy products, the extent of absorption of MINOCIN minocycline hydrochloride pellet-filled capsules was not noticeably influenced. The peak plasma concentrations were slightly decreased (11.2%) and delayed by one hour when administered with food, compared to dosing under fasting conditions.

In previous studies with other minocycline dosage forms, the minocycline serum half-life ranged from 11 to 16 hours in 7 patients with hepatic dysfunction, and from 18 to 69 hours in 5 patients with renal dysfunction. The urinary and fecal recovery of minocycline when administered to 12 normal volunteers is one-half to one-third that of other tetracyclines.

Microbiology

The tetracyclines are primarily bacteriostatic and are thought to exert their antimicrobial effect by the inhibition of protein synthesis. The tetracyclines, including minocycline, have similar antimicrobial spectra of activity against a wide range of gram-positive and gram-negative organisms. Cross-resistance of these organisms to tetracyclines is common.

While *in vitro* studies have demonstrated the susceptibility of most strains of the following microorganisms, clinical efficacy for infections other than those included in the **INDICATIONS AND USAGE** section has not been documented.

GRAM-NEGATIVE BACTERIA:

Bartonella bacilliformis
Brucella species
Calymmatobacterium granulomatis
Campylobacter fetus
Francisella tularensis
Haemophilus ducreyi
Haemophilus influenzae
Listeria monocytogenes
Neisseria gonorrhoeae
Vibrio cholerae
Yersinia pestis

Because many strains of the following groups of gram-negative microorganisms have been shown to be resistant to tetracyclines, culture and susceptibility tests are especially recommended:

Acinetobacter species
Bacteroides species
Enterobacter aerogenes
Escherichia coli
Klebsiella species
Shigella species

GRAM-POSITIVE BACTERIA:

Because many strains of the following groups of gram-positive microorganisms have been shown to be resistant to tetracyclines, culture and susceptibility testing are especially recommended. Up to 44 percent of *Streptococcus pyogenes* strains have been found to be resistant to tetracycline drugs. Therefore, tetracycline should not be used for streptococcal disease unless the organism has been demonstrated to be susceptible.

Enterococcus group [*Enterococcus faecalis* (formerly *Streptococcus faecalis*) and *Enterococcus faecium* (formerly *Streptococcus faecium*)]
Streptococcus pneumoniae
Streptococcus pyogenes
Viridans group streptococci

OTHER MICROORGANISMS:

Actinomyces species
Bacillus anthracis
Balantidium coli
Borrelia recurrentis
Chlamydia psittaci
Chlamydia trachomatis
Clostridium species
Entamoeba species
Fusobacterium fusiforme
Mycoplasma pneumoniae
Propionibacterium acnes
Rickettsiae
Treponema pallidum
Treponema pertenue
Ureaplasma urealyticum

Susceptibility Tests

Diffusion Techniques

The use of antibiotic disk susceptibility test methods which measure zone diameter gives an accurate estimation of susceptibility of microorganisms to MINOCIN. One such standard procedure[1] has been recommended for use with disks for testing antimicrobials. Either the 30 mcg tetracycline-class disk or the 30 mcg minocycline disk should be used for the determination of the susceptibility of microorganisms to minocycline.

With this type of procedure a report of "susceptible" from the laboratory indicates that the infecting organism is likely to respond to therapy. A report of "intermediate susceptibility" suggests that the organism would be susceptible if a high dosage is used or if the infection is confined to tissues and fluids (e.g., urine) in which high antibiotic levels are attained. A report of "resistant" indicates that the infecting organism is not likely to respond to therapy. With either the tetracycline-class disk or the minocycline disk, zone sizes of 19 mm or greater indicate susceptibility, zone sizes of 14 mm or less indicate resistance, and zone sizes of 15 to 18 mm indicate intermediate susceptibility.

Standardized procedures require the use of laboratory control organisms. The 30 mcg tetracycline disk should give zone diameters between 19 and 28 mm for *Staphylococcus aureus* ATCC 25923 and between 18 and 25 mm for *Escherichia coli* ATCC 25922. The 30 mcg minocycline disk should give zone diameters between 25 and 30 mm for *S. aureus* ATCC 25923 and between 19 and 25 mm for *E. coli* ATCC 25922.

Dilution Techniques

When using the NCCLS agar dilution or broth dilution (including microdilution) method[2] or equivalent, a bacterial isolate may be considered susceptible if the MIC (minimal inhibitory concentration) of minocycline is 4 mcg/mL or less. Organisms are considered resistant if the MIC is 16 mcg/mL or greater. Organisms with an MIC value of less than 16 mcg/mL but greater than 4 mcg/mL are expected to be susceptible if a high dosage is used or if the infection is confined to tissues and fluids (e.g., urine) in which high antibiotic levels are attained.

As with standard diffusion methods, dilution procedures require the use of laboratory control organisms. Standard tetracycline or minocycline powder should give MIC values of 0.25 mcg/mL to 1.0 mcg/mL for *S. aureus* ATCC 25923, and 1.0 mcg/mL to 4.0 mcg/mL for *E. coli* ATCC 25922.

INDICATIONS AND USAGE

MINOCIN minocycline hydrochloride pellet-filled capsules are indicated in the treatment of the following infections due to susceptible strains of the designated microorganisms:

Rocky Mountain spotted fever, typhus fever and the typhus group, Q fever, rickettsialpox and tick fevers caused by *Rickettsiae.*

Respiratory tract infections caused by *Mycoplasma pneumoniae.*

Lymphogranuloma venereum caused by *Chlamydia trachomatis.*

Psittacosis (Ornithosis) due to *Chlamydia psittaci.*

Trachoma caused by *Chlamydia trachomatis,* although the infectious agent is not always eliminated, as judged by immunofluorescence.

Inclusion conjunctivitis caused by *Chlamydia trachomatis.*

Nongonococcal urethritis in adults caused by *Ureaplasma urealyticum* or *Chlamydia trachomatis.*

Relapsing fever due to *Borrelia recurrentis.*

Chancroid caused by *Haemophilus ducreyi.*

Plague due to *Yersinia pestis.*

Tularemia due to *Francisella tularensis.*

Cholera caused by *Vibrio cholerae.*

Campylobacter fetus infections caused by *Campylobacter fetus.*

Brucellosis due to *Brucella* species (in conjunction with streptomycin).

Bartonellosis due to *Bartonella bacilliformis.*

Granuloma inguinale caused by *Calymmatobacterium granulomatis.*

Minocycline is indicated for treatment of infections caused by the following gram-negative microorganisms, when bacteriologic testing indicates appropriate susceptibility to the drug:

Escherichia coli.
Enterobacter aerogenes.
Shigella species.
Acinetobacter species.

Respiratory tract infections caused by *Haemophilus influenzae.*

Respiratory tract and urinary tract infections caused by *Klebsiella* species.

MINOCIN minocycline hydrochloride pellet-filled capsules are indicated for the treatment of infections caused by the following gram-positive microorganisms when bacteriologic testing indicates appropriate susceptibility to the drug:

Upper respiratory tract infections caused by *Streptococcus pneumoniae.*

Skin and skin structure infections caused by *Staphylococcus aureus.* (Note: Minocycline is not the drug of choice in the treatment of any type of staphylococcal infection.)

Uncomplicated urethritis in men due to *Neisseria gonorrhoeae* and for the treatment of other gonococcal infections when penicillin is contraindicated.

When penicillin is contraindicated, minocycline is an alternative drug in the treatment of the following infections:

Infections in women caused by *Neisseria gonorrhoeae*.

Syphilis caused by *Treponema pallidum*.

Yaws caused by *Treponema pertenue*.

Listeriosis due to *Listeria monocytogenes*.

Anthrax due to *Bacillus anthracis*.

Vincent's infection caused by *Fusobacterium fusiforme*.

Actinomycosis caused by *Actinomyces israelii*.

Infections caused by *Clostridium* species.

In *acute intestinal amebiasis,* minocycline may be a useful adjunct to amebicides.

In severe *acne,* minocycline may be useful adjunctive therapy.

Oral minocycline is indicated in the treatment of asymptomatic carriers of *Neisseria meningitidis* to eliminate meningococci from the nasopharynx. In order to preserve the usefulness of minocycline in the treatment of asymptomatic meningococcal carrier, diagnostic laboratory procedures, including serotyping and susceptibility testing, should be performed to establish the carrier state and the correct treatment. It is recommended that the prophylactic use of minocycline be reserved for situations in which the risk of meningococcal meningitis is high.

Oral minocycline is not indicated for the treatment of meningococcal infection.

Although no controlled clinical efficacy studies have been conducted, limited clinical data show that oral minocycline hydrochloride has been used successfully in the treatment of infections caused by *Mycobacterium marinum.*

CONTRAINDICATIONS

This drug is contraindicated in persons who have shown hypersensitivity to any of the tetracyclines.

WARNINGS

MINOCIN PELLET-FILLED CAPSULES, LIKE OTHER TETRACYCLINE-CLASS ANTIBIOTICS, CAN CAUSE FETAL HARM WHEN ADMINISTERED TO A PREGNANT WOMAN. IF ANY TETRACYCLINE IS USED DURING PREGNANCY OR IF THE PATIENT BECOMES PREGNANT WHILE TAKING THESE DRUGS, THE PATIENT SHOULD BE APPRISED OF THE POTENTIAL HAZARD TO THE FETUS. THE USE OF DRUGS OF THE TETRACYCLINE CLASS DURING TOOTH DEVELOPMENT (LAST HALF OF PREGNANCY, INFANCY, AND CHILDHOOD TO THE AGE OF 8 YEARS) MAY CAUSE PERMANENT DISCOLORATION OF THE TEETH (YELLOW-GRAY-BROWN).

This adverse reaction is more common during long-term use of the drug but has been observed following repeated short-term courses. Enamel hypoplasia has also been reported. TETRACYCLINE DRUGS, THEREFORE, SHOULD NOT BE USED DURING TOOTH DEVELOPMENT UNLESS OTHER DRUGS ARE NOT LIKELY TO BE EFFECTIVE OR ARE CONTRAINDICATED.

All tetracyclines form a stable calcium complex in any bone-forming tissue. A decrease in fibula growth rate has been observed in premature human infants given oral tetracycline in doses of 25 mg/kg every six hours. This reaction was shown to be reversible when the drug was discontinued.

Results of animal studies indicate that tetracyclines cross the placenta, are found in fetal tissues, and can have toxic effects on the developing fetus (often related to retardation of skeletal development). Evidence of embryotoxicity has been noted in animals treated early in pregnancy.

The anti-anabolic action of the tetracyclines may cause an increase in BUN. While this is not a problem in those with normal renal function, in patients with significantly impaired function, higher serum levels of tetracycline may lead to azotemia, hyperphosphatemia, and acidosis. If renal impairment exists, even usual oral or parenteral doses may lead to excessive systemic accumulations of the drug and possible liver toxicity. Under such conditions, lower than usual total doses are indicated, and if therapy is prolonged, serum level determinations of the drug may be advisable.

Photosensitivity manifested by an exaggerated sunburn reaction has been observed in some individuals taking tetracyclines. This has been reported rarely with minocycline.

Central nervous system side effects including lightheadedness, dizziness, or vertigo have been reported with minocycline therapy. Patients who experience these symptoms should be cautioned about driving vehicles or using hazardous machinery while on minocycline therapy. These symptoms may disappear during therapy and usually disappear rapidly when the drug is discontinued.

PRECAUTIONS

General

As with other antibiotic preparations, use of this drug may result in overgrowth of non-susceptible organisms, including fungi. If superinfection occurs, the antibiotic should be discontinued and appropriate therapy instituted.

Pseudotumor cerebri (benign intracranial hypertension) in adults has been associated with the use of tetracyclines. The usual clinical manifestations are headache and blurred vision. Bulging fontanels have been associated with the use of tetracyclines in infants. While both of these conditions and related symptoms usually resolve after discontinuation of the tetracycline, the possibility for permanent sequelae exists.

Incision and drainage or other surgical procedures should be performed in conjunction with antibiotic therapy when indicated.

Information For Patients

Photosensitivity manifested by an exaggerated sunburn reaction has been observed in some individuals taking tetracyclines. Patients apt to be exposed to direct sunlight or ultraviolet light should be advised that this reaction can occur with tetracycline drugs, and treatment should be discontinued at the first evidence of skin erythema. This reaction has been reported rarely with use of minocycline.

Patients who experience central nervous system symptoms (see **WARNINGS**) should be cautioned about driving vehicles or using hazardous machinery while on minocycline therapy.

Concurrent use of tetracycline may render oral contraceptives less effective (see **Drug Interactions**).

Laboratory Tests

In venereal disease when coexistent syphilis is suspected, a dark-field examination should be done before treatment is started and the blood serology repeated monthly for at least four months.

In long-term therapy, periodic laboratory evaluations of organ systems, including hematopoietic, renal, and hepatic studies, should be performed.

Drug Interactions

Because tetracyclines have been shown to depress plasma prothrombin activity, patients who are on anticoagulant therapy may require downward adjustment of their anticoagulant dosage.

Since bacteriostatic drugs may interfere with the bactericidal action of penicillin, it is advisable to avoid giving tetracycline-class drugs in conjunction with penicillin.

Absorption of tetracyclines is impaired by antacids containing aluminum, calcium or magnesium, and iron-containing preparations.

The concurrent use of tetracycline and methoxyflurane has been reported to result in fatal renal toxicity.

Concurrent use of tetracyclines with oral contraceptives may render oral contraceptives less effective.

Drug/Laboratory Test Interactions

False elevations of urinary catecholamine levels may occur due to interference with the fluorescence test.

Carcinogenesis, Mutagenesis, Impairment of Fertility

Dietary administration of minocycline in long term tumorigenicity studies in rats resulted in evidence of thyroid tumor production. Minocycline has also been found to produce thyroid hyperplasia in rats and dogs. In addition, there has been evidence of oncogenic activity in rats in studies with a related antibiotic, oxytetracycline (i.e., adrenal and pituitary tumors). Likewise, although mutagenicity studies of minocycline have not been conducted, positive results in *in vitro* mammalian cell assays (i.e., mouse lymphoma and Chinese hamster lung cells) have been reported for related antibiotics (tetracycline hydrochloride and oxytetracycline). Segment I (fertility and general reproduction) studies have provided evidence that minocycline impairs fertility in male rats.

Teratogenic Effects: Pregnancy: *Pregnancy Category D:* (See **WARNINGS**.) *Nonteratogenic Effects:* (See **WARNINGS**.)

Labor and Delivery

The effect of tetracyclines on labor and delivery is unknown.

Nursing Mothers

Tetracyclines are excreted in human milk. Because of the potential for serious adverse reactions in nursing infants from the tetracyclines, a decision should be made whether to discontinue nursing or discontinue the drug, taking into account the importance of the drug to the mother (see **WARNINGS**).

Pediatric Use: See **WARNINGS.**

ADVERSE REACTIONS

Due to oral minocycline's virtually complete absorption, side effects to the lower bowel, particularly diarrhea, have been infrequent. The following adverse reactions have been observed in patients receiving tetracyclines.

Gastrointestinal: Anorexia, nausea, vomiting, diarrhea, glossitis, dysphagia, enterocolitis, pancreatitis, inflammatory lesions (with monilial overgrowth) in the anogenital region, and increases in liver enzymes. Rarely, hepatitis and liver failure have been reported. Rare instances of esophagitis and esophageal ulcerations have been reported in patients taking the tetracycline-class antibiotics in capsule and tablet form. Most of these patients took the medication immediately before going to bed (see **DOSAGE AND ADMINISTRATION**).

Skin: Maculopapular and erythematous rashes. Exfoliative dermatitis has been reported but is uncommon. Fixed drug eruptions have been rarely reported. Lesions occurring on the glans penis have caused balanitis. Erythema multiforme and rarely Stevens-Johnson syndrome have been reported. Photosensitivity is discussed above (see **WARNINGS**). Pigmentation of the skin and mucous membranes has been reported.

Renal toxicity: Elevations in BUN have been reported and are apparently dose related (see **WARNINGS**). Reversible acute renal failure has been rarely reported.

Hypersensitivity reactions: Urticaria, angioneurotic edema, polyarthralgia, anaphylaxis, anaphylactoid purpura, pericarditis, exacerbation of systemic lupus erythematosus and rarely pulmonary infiltrates with eosinophilia have been reported. A transient lupus-like syndrome has also been reported.

Blood: Hemolytic anemia, thrombocytopenia, neutropenia, and eosinophilia have been reported.

Central nervous system: Bulging fontanels in infants and benign intracranial hypertension (Pseudotumor cerebri) in adults (see **PRECAUTIONS—General**) have been reported. Headache has also been reported.

Other: When given over prolonged periods, tetracyclines have been reported to produce brown-black microscopic discoloration of the thyroid glands. Very rare cases of abnormal thyroid function have been reported.

Decreased hearing has been rarely reported in patients on MINOCIN.

Tooth discoloration in children less than 8 years of age (see **WARNINGS**) and also, rarely, in adults has been reported.

OVERDOSAGE

Minocycline is not removed in significant quantities by hemodialysis or peritoneal dialysis. In one study, four patients received 200 mg oral doses 3 hours prior to hemodialysis, following flow rates of 100 to 200 mL/min there was no consistent difference between venous and arterial minocycline concentrations and no detectable minocycline was found in the dialysate. In another study, four patients were administered IP minocycline over 72 to 96 hours and achieved blood concentrations of 1.5 to 2 mcg/mL, over the following 12 hours drug free dialysate was used. No detectable minocycline was found to transfer from the blood to the dialysate. In case of overdosage, discontinue medication, treat symptomatically, and institute supportive measures.

DOSAGE AND ADMINISTRATION

THE USUAL DOSAGE AND FREQUENCY OF ADMINISTRATION OF MINOCYCLINE DIFFERS FROM THAT OF THE OTHER TETRACYCLINES. EXCEEDING THE RECOMMENDED DOSAGE MAY RESULT IN AN INCREASED INCIDENCE OF SIDE EFFECTS.

MINOCIN minocycline hydrochloride pellet-filled capsules may be taken with or without food (see **CLINICAL PHARMACOLOGY**).

ADULTS

The usual dosage of MINOCIN minocycline hydrochloride pellet-filled capsules is 200 mg initially followed by 100 mg every 12 hours. Alternatively, if more frequent doses are preferred, two or four 50 mg pellet-filled capsules may be given initially followed by one 50 mg capsule four times daily.

For children above 8 years of age

The usual dosage of MINOCIN minocycline hydrochloride pellet-filled capsules is 4 mg/kg initially followed by 2 mg/kg every 12 hours.

Uncomplicated gonococcal infections other than urethritis and anorectal infections in men: 200 mg initially, followed by 100 mg every 12 hours for a minimum of four days, with post therapy cultures within 2 to 3 days.

In the treatment of uncomplicated gonococcal urethritis in men, 100 mg every 12 hours for five days is recommended. For the treatment of syphilis, the usual dosage of MINOCIN minocycline hydrochloride pellet-filled capsules should be administered over a period of 10 to 15 days. Close follow-up, including laboratory tests, is recommended.

In the treatment of meningococcal carrier state, the recommended dosage is 100 mg every 12 hours for five days.

Mycobacterium marinum infections: Although optimal doses have not been established, 100 mg every 12 hours for 6 to 8 weeks have been used successfully in a limited number of cases.

Uncomplicated nongonococcal urethral infection in adults caused by *Chlamydia trachomatis* or *Ureaplasma urealyticum:* 100 mg orally, every 12 hours for at least seven days. Ingestion of adequate amounts of fluids along with capsule and tablet forms of drugs in the tetracycline-class is recommended to reduce the risk of esophageal irritation and ulceration.

In patients with renal impairment (see **WARNINGS**), the total dosage should be decreased by either reducing the recommended individual doses and/or by extending the time intervals between doses.

Continued on next page

Minocin Capsules—Cont.

HOW SUPPLIED

MINOCIN® minocycline hydrochloride pellet-filled capsules are supplied as capsules containing minocycline hydrochloride equivalent to 100 mg and 50 mg minocycline.

100 mg, two-piece, hard-shell capsule with an opaque light green cap and a transparent green body, printed in white ink with Lederle over M46 on one half and Lederle over 100 mg on the other half. Each capsule contains pellets of minocycline HCl equivalent to 100 mg of minocycline, supplied as follows:

NDC 0005-5344-18—Bottle of 50
NDC 0005-5344-27—Bottle of 250

50 mg, two-piece, hard-shell capsule with an opaque yellow cap and a transparent green body, printed in black ink with Lederle over M45 on one half and Lederle over 50 mg on the other half. Each capsule contains pellets of minocycline HCl equivalent to 50 mg of minocycline, supplied as follows:

NDC 0005-5343-23—Bottle of 100
NDC 0005-5343-27—Bottle of 250

Store at Controlled Room Temperature 15°–30°C (59°–86°F).

Protect from light, moisture and excessive heat.

ANIMAL PHARMACOLOGY AND TOXICOLOGY

MINOCIN minocycline HCl has been observed to cause a dark discoloration of the thyroid in experimental animals (rats, minipigs, dogs, and monkeys). In the rat, chronic treatment with MINOCIN has resulted in goiter accompanied by elevated radioactive iodine uptake and evidence of thyroid tumor production. MINOCIN has also been found to produce thyroid hyperplasia in rats and dogs.

REFERENCES

1. National Committee for Clinical Laboratory Standards, Approved Standard: *Performance Standards for Antimicrobial Disk Susceptibility Tests*, 3rd Edition, Vol. 4(16): M2-A3, Villanova, PA, December 1984.
2. National Committee for Clinical Laboratory Standards, Approved Standard: *Methods for Dilution Antimicrobial Susceptibility Tests for Bacteria that Grow Aerobically*, 2nd Edition, Vol. 5(22):M7-A, Villanova, PA, December 1985.

Manufactured by:
LEDERLE PHARMACEUTICAL DIVISION
American Cyanamid Company
Pearl River, NY 10965

Shown in Product Identification Guide, page 319

MINOCIN® ℞

[*mī-nō-sĭn*]

Minocycline Hydrochloride Oral Suspension

DESCRIPTION

MINOCIN minocycline hydrochloride, a semisynthetic derivative of tetracycline, is named [4*S*-(4α, 4aα, 5aα, 12aα)]-4,7-bis (dimethylamino)-1,4,4a,5,5a,6,11,12a-octahydro-3,10,12,12a-tetrahydroxy-1,11-dioxo-2-naphthacenecarboxamide monohydrochloride.

Its structural formula is:

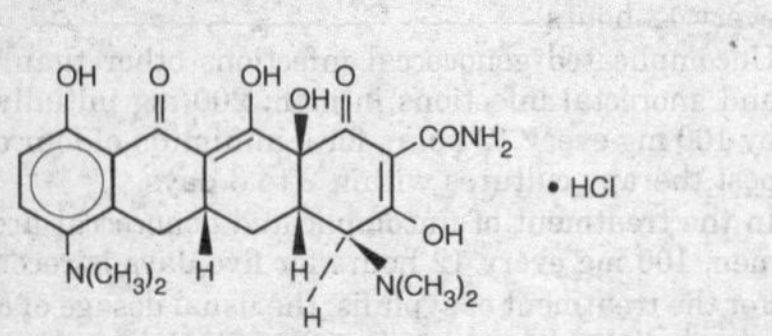

$C_{23}H_{27}N_3O_7 \cdot HCl$ M.W. 493.94

MINOCIN Oral Suspension contains minocycline HCl equivalent to 50 mg of minocycline per 5 mL (10 mg/mL) and the following inactive ingredients: Alcohol, Butylparaben, Calcium Hydroxide, Cellulose, Decaglyceryl Tetraoleate, Edetate Calcium Disodium, Glycol, Guar Gum, Polysorbate 80, Propylparaben, Propylene Glycol, Sodium Saccharin, Sodium Sulfite (see WARNINGS) and Sorbitol.

ACTIONS

Microbiology

The tetracyclines are primarily bacteriostatic and are thought to exert their antimicrobial effect by the inhibition of protein synthesis. Minocycline HCl is a tetracycline with antibacterial activity comparable to other tetracyclines with activity against a wide range of gram-negative and gram-positive organisms.

Tube dilution testing: Microorganisms may be considered susceptible (likely to respond to minocycline therapy) if the minimum inhibitory concentration (MIC) is not more than 4 mcg/mL. Microorganisms may be considered intermediate (harboring partial resistance) if the MIC is 4 to 12.5 mcg/mL and resistant (not likely to respond to minocycline therapy) if the MIC is greater than 12.5 mcg/mL.

Susceptibility plate testing: If the Kirby-Bauer method of susceptibility testing (using a 30 mcg tetracycline disc) gives a zone of 18 mm or greater, the bacterial strain is considered to be susceptible to any tetracycline. Minocycline shows moderate *in vitro* activity against certain strains of staphylococci which have been found resistant to other tetracyclines. For such strains minocycline susceptibility powder may be used for additional susceptibility testing.

Human Pharmacology

Following a single dose of two 100 mg minocycline HCl capsules administered to ten normal adult volunteers, serum levels ranged from 0.74 to 4.45 mcg/mL in one hour (average 2.24), after 12 hours, they ranged from 0.34 to 2.36 mcg/mL (average 1.25). The serum half-life following a single 200 mg dose in 12 essentially normal volunteers ranged from 11 to 17 hours. In seven patients with hepatic dysfunction it ranged from 11 to 16 hours, and in 5 patients with renal dysfunction from 18 to 69 hours. The urinary and fecal recovery of minocycline when administered to 12 normal volunteers is one half to one third that of other tetracyclines.

INDICATIONS

MINOCIN is indicated in infections caused by the following microorganisms:

Rickettsiae: (Rocky Mountain spotted fever, typhus fever and the typhus group, Q fever, rickettsialpox, tick fevers).

Mycoplasma pneumoniae (PPLO, Eaton agent).

Agents of psittacosis and ornithosis.

Agents of lymphogranuloma venereum and granuloma inguinale.

The spirochetal agent of relapsing fever (*Borrelia recurrentis*).

The following gram-negative microorganisms:

Haemophilus ducreyi (chancroid),

Yersinia pestis and *Francisella tularensis* (formerly *Pasteurella pestis* and *Pasteurella tularensis*),

Bartonella bacilliformis,

Bacteroides species,

Vibrio comma and *Vibrio fetus,*

Brucella species (in conjunction with streptomycin).

Because many strains of the following groups of microorganisms have been shown to be resistant to tetracyclines, culture and susceptibility testing are recommended.

MINOCIN is indicated for treatment of infections caused by the following gram-negative microorganisms when bacteriologic testing indicates appropriate susceptibility to the drug:

Escherichia coli,

Enterobacter aerogenes (formerly *Aerobacter aerogenes*),

Shigella species,

Acinetobacter calcoaceticus (formerly *Herellea, Mima*),

Haemophilus influenzae (respiratory infections),

Klebsiella species (respiratory and urinary infections).

MINOCIN is indicated for treatment of infections caused by the following gram-positive microorganisms when bacteriologic testing indicates appropriate susceptibility to the drug:

Streptococcus species:

Up to 44% of strains of *Streptococcus pyogenes* and 74% of *Streptococcus faecalis* have been found to be resistant to tetracycline drugs. Therefore, tetracyclines should not be used for streptococcal disease unless the organism has been demonstrated to be sensitive.

For upper respiratory infections due to Group A beta-hemolytic streptococci, penicillin is the usual drug of choice, including prophylaxis of rheumatic fever.

Streptococcus pneumoniae (formerly Diplococcus pneumoniae),

Staphylococcus aureus, skin and soft tissue infections.

Tetracyclines are not the drugs of choice in the treatment of any type of staphylococcal infection.

MINOCIN is indicated for the treatment of uncomplicated gonococcal urethritis in men due to *Neisseria gonorrhoeae.*

When penicillin is contraindicated, tetracyclines are alternative drugs in the treatment of infections due to:

Neisseria gonorrhoeae (in women),

Treponema pallidum and *Treponema pertenue* (syphilis and yaws),

Listeria monocytogenes,

Clostridium species,

Bacillus anthracis,

Fusobacterium fusiforme (Vincent's infection),

Actinomyces species.

In acute intestinal amebiasis, the tetracyclines may be a useful adjunct to amebicides.

In severe acne, the tetracyclines may be useful adjunctive therapy.

MINOCIN minocycline HCl is indicated in the treatment of trachoma, although the infectious agent is not always eliminated, as judged by immunofluorescence.

MINOCIN is indicated for the treatment of uncomplicated urethral, endocervical or rectal infections in adults caused by *Chlamydia trachomatis* or *Ureaplasma urealyticum.*[1]

Inclusion conjunctivitis may be treated with oral tetracyclines or with a combination of oral and topical agents.

MINOCIN is indicated in the treatment of asymptomatic carriers of *Neisseria meningitidis* to eliminate meningococci from the nasopharynx.

In order to preserve the usefulness of MINOCIN in the treatment of asymptomatic meningococcal carriers, diagnostic laboratory procedures, including serotyping and susceptibility testing, should be performed to establish the carrier state and the correct treatment. It is recommended that the drug be reserved for situations in which the risk of meningococcal meningitis is high.

MINOCIN by oral administration is not indicated for the treatment of meningococcal infection.

Although no controlled clinical efficacy studies have been conducted, limited clinical data show that oral MINOCIN has been used successfully in the treatment of infections caused by Mycobacterium marinum.

CONTRAINDICATIONS

This drug is contraindicated in persons who have shown hypersensitivity to any of the tetracyclines.

WARNINGS

THE USE OF DRUGS OF THE TETRACYCLINE CLASS DURING TOOTH DEVELOPMENT (LAST HALF OF PREGNANCY, INFANCY, AND CHILDHOOD TO THE AGE OF 8 YEARS) MAY CAUSE PERMANENT DISCOLORATION OF THE TEETH (YELLOW-GRAY-BROWN). This adverse reaction is more common during long-term use of the drugs but has been observed following repeated short-term courses. Enamel hypoplasia has also been reported. TETRACYCLINE DRUGS, THEREFORE, SHOULD NOT BE USED IN THIS AGE GROUP UNLESS OTHER DRUGS ARE NOT LIKELY TO BE EFFECTIVE OR ARE CONTRAINDICATED.

If renal impairment exists, even usual oral or parenteral doses may lead to excessive systemic accumulations of the drug and possible liver toxicity. Under such conditions, lower than usual total doses are indicated, and if therapy is prolonged, serum level determinations of the drug may be advisable.

Photosensitivity manifested by an exaggerated sunburn reaction has been observed in some individuals taking tetracyclines. Patients apt to be exposed to direct sunlight or ultraviolet light should be advised that this reaction can occur with tetracycline drugs, and treatment should be discontinued at the first evidence of skin erythema. Studies to date indicate that photosensitivity is rarely reported with MINOCIN minocycline HCl.

The anti-anabolic action of the tetracyclines may cause an increase in BUN. While this is not a problem in those with normal renal function, in patients with significantly impaired function, higher serum levels of tetracycline may lead to azotemia, hyperphosphatemia, and acidosis.

CNS side effects including light-headedness, dizziness, or vertigo have been reported. Patients who experience these symptoms should be cautioned about driving vehicles or using hazardous machinery while on minocycline therapy. These symptoms may disappear during therapy and usually disappear rapidly when the drug is discontinued.

MINOCIN Oral Suspension contains sodium sulfite, a sulfite that may cause allergic-type reactions including anaphylactic symptoms and life-threatening or less severe asthmatic episodes in certain susceptible people. The overall prevalence of sulfite sensitivity in the general population is unknown and probably low. Sulfite sensitivity is seen more frequently in asthmatic than in nonasthmatic people.

Usage in Pregnancy (See above **WARNINGS** about use during tooth development.) Results of animal studies indicate that tetracyclines cross the placenta, are found in fetal tissues and can have toxic effects on the developing fetus (often related to retardation of skeletal development). Evidence of embryotoxicity has also been noted in animals treated early in pregnancy.

The safety of MINOCIN for use during pregnancy has not been established.

Usage in Newborns, Infants, and Children (See above **WARNINGS** about use during tooth development.)

All tetracyclines form a stable calcium complex in any bone forming tissue. A decrease in the fibula growth rate has been observed in prematures given oral tetracycline in doses of 25 mg/kg every six hours. This reaction was shown to be reversible when the drug was discontinued.

Tetracyclines are present in the milk of lactating women who are taking a drug in this class.

PRECAUTIONS

General

Pseudotumor cerebri (benign intracranial hypertension) in adults has been associated with the use of tetracyclines. The usual clinical manifestations are headache and blurred vision. Bulging fontanels have been associated with the use of tetracyclines in infants. While both of these conditions and related symptoms usually resolve soon after discontinuation of the tetracycline, the possibility for permanent sequelae exists.

As with other antibiotic preparations, use of this drug may result in overgrowth of non-susceptible organisms, including fungi. If superinfection occurs, the antibiotic should be discontinued and appropriate therapy should be instituted.
In venereal diseases when coexistent syphilis is suspected, darkfield examination should be done before treatment is started and the blood serology repeated monthly for at least 4 months.
In long-term therapy, periodic laboratory evaluation of organ systems, including hematopoietic, renal and hepatic studies should be performed.
All infections due to Group A beta-hemolytic streptococci should be treated for at least ten days.

Drug Interactions

Because tetracyclines have been shown to depress plasma prothrombin activity, patients who are on anticoagulant therapy may require downward adjustment of their anticoagulant dosage.
Since bacteriostatic drugs may interfere with the bactericidal action of penicillin, it is advisable to avoid giving tetracycline in conjunction with penicillin.
Concurrent use of tetracyclines with oral contraceptives may render oral contraceptives less effective.

ADVERSE REACTIONS

Gastrointestinal: Anorexia, nausea, vomiting, diarrhea, glossitis, dysphagia, enterocolitis, pancreatitis, inflammatory lesions (with monilial overgrowth) in the anogenital region and increases in liver enzymes. Rarely, hepatitis and liver failure have been reported.
These reactions have been caused by both the oral and parenteral administration of tetracyclines.
Skin: Maculopapular and erythematous rashes. Exfoliative dermatitis has been reported but is uncommon. Fixed drug eruptions, including balanitis, have been rarely reported. Erythema multiforme and rarely Stevens-Johnson syndrome have been reported. Photosensitivity is discussed above. (See **WARNINGS.**)
Pigmentation of the skin and mucous membranes has been reported.
Tooth discoloration has been reported rarely in adults.
Renal toxicity: Rise in BUN has been reported and is apparently dose related. (See **WARNINGS.**) Reversible acute renal failure has been rarely reported.
Hypersensitivity reactions: Urticaria, angioneurotic edema, polyarthralgia, anaphylaxis, anaphylactoid purpura, pericarditis, exacerbation of systemic lupus erythematosus and rarely pulmonary infiltrates with eosinophilia have been reported. A transient lupus-like syndrome has also been reported.
Blood: Hemolytic anemia, thrombocytopenia, neutropenia and eosinophilia have been reported.
CNS: (See **WARNINGS.**) Pseudotumor cerebri (benign intracranial hypertension) in adults and bulging fontanels in infants. (See **PRECAUTIONS—General.**) Headache has also been reported.
Other: When given over prolonged periods, tetracyclines have been reported to produce brown-black microscopic discoloration of the thyroid glands. Very rare cases of abnormal thyroid function have been reported.
Decreased hearing has been rarely reported in patients on MINOCIN.

DOSAGE AND ADMINISTRATION

Therapy should be continued for at least 24 to 48 hours after symptoms and fever have subsided.
Concomitant therapy: Antacids containing aluminum, calcium, or magnesium impair absorption and should not be given to patients taking oral tetracycline.
Studies to date have indicated that the absorption of MINOCIN is not notably influenced by foods and dairy products.
In patients with renal impairment: (See **WARNINGS.**) Total dosage should be decreased by reduction of recommended individual doses and/or extending time intervals between doses.
In the treatment of streptococcal infections, a therapeutic dose of tetracycline should be administered for at least ten days.
ADULTS: The usual dosage of MINOCIN is 200 mg initially followed by 100 mg every 12 hours.
For children above eight years of age: The usual dosage of MINOCIN minocycline HCl is 4 mg/kg initially followed by 2 mg/kg every 12 hours.
For treatment of syphilis, the usual dosage of MINOCIN should be administered over a period of 10 to 15 days. Close follow up, including laboratory tests, is recommended.
Gonorrhea patients sensitive to penicillin may be treated with MINOCIN, administered as 200 mg initially followed by 100 mg every twelve hours for a minimum of four days, with post-therapy cultures within 2 to 3 days.
In the treatment of meningococcal carrier state, recommended dosage is 100 mg every 12 hours for five days.
Mycobacterium marinum infections: Although optimal doses have not been established, 100 mg twice a day for 6 to 8 weeks have been used successfully in a limited number of cases.
Uncomplicated urethral, endocervical, or rectal infection in adults caused by *Chlamydia trachomatis* or *Ureaplasma urealyticum:* 100 mg, by mouth, 2 times a day for at least seven days.[1]
In the treatment of uncomplicated gonococcal urethritis in men, 100 mg twice a day orally for five days is recommended.

HOW SUPPLIED

MINOCIN® minocycline hydrochloride Oral Suspension contains minocycline hydrochloride equivalent to 50 mg minocycline per teaspoonful (5 mL). Preserved with propylparaben 0.10% and butylparaben 0.06% with Alcohol USP 5% v/v, Custard-flavored.
NDC 0005-5313-56 Bottle 2 fl. oz. (60 mL)
Store at Controlled Room Temperature 15–30°C (59–86°F).
DO NOT FREEZE.

ANIMAL PHARMACOLOGY AND TOXICOLOGY

MINOCIN has been found to produce high blood concentrations following oral dosage to various animal species and to be extensively distributed to all tissues examined in ^{14}C-labeled drug studies in dogs. MINOCIN has been found experimentally to produce discoloration of the thyroid glands. This finding has been observed in rats and dogs. Changes in thyroid function have also been found in these animal species. However, no change in thyroid function has been observed in humans.

Reference: 1. CDC Sexually Transmitted Diseases Treatment Guidelines 1982.

Manufactured by:
LEDERLE PHARMACEUTICAL DIVISION
American Cyanamid Company
Pearl River, NY 10965

Shown in Product Identification Guide, page 319

MYAMBUTOL® ℞
[*mī-am-bū-tōl*]
Ethambutol Hydrochloride
Tablets
100 mg and 400 mg

DESCRIPTION

MYAMBUTOL ethambutol hydrochloride is an oral chemotherapeutic agent which is specifically effective against actively growing microorganisms of the genus *Mycobacterium,* including *M. tuberculosis.*
MYAMBUTOL 100 mg and 400 mg tablets contain the following inactive ingredients: Gelatin, Hydroxypropyl Methylcellulose, Magnesium Stearate, Sodium Lauryl Sulfate, Sorbitol, Stearic Acid, Sucrose, Titanium Dioxide, and other ingredients.

ACTION

MYAMBUTOL following a single oral dose of 25 mg/kg of body weight, attains a peak of 2 to 5 micrograms/mL in serum 2 to 4 hours after administration. When the drug is administered daily for longer periods of time at this dose, serum levels are similar. The serum level of MYAMBUTOL falls to undetectable levels by 24 hours after the last dose except in some patients with abnormal renal function. The intracellular concentrations of erythrocytes reach peak values approximately twice those of plasma and maintain this ratio throughout the 24 hours.
During the 24-hour period following oral administration of MYAMBUTOL approximately 50% of the initial dose is excreted unchanged in the urine, while an additional 8 to 15 percent appears in the form of metabolites. The main path of metabolism appears to be an initial oxidation of the alcohol to an aldehydic intermediate, followed by conversion to a dicarboxylic acid. From 20 to 22 percent of the initial dose is excreted in the feces as unchanged drug. No drug accumulation has been observed with consecutive single daily doses of 25 mg/kg in patients with normal kidney function, although marked accumulation has been demonstrated in patients with renal insufficiency.
MYAMBUTOL diffuses into actively growing *mycobacterium* cells such as tubercle bacilli. MYAMBUTOL appears to inhibit the synthesis of one or more metabolites, thus causing impairment of cell metabolism, arrest of multiplication, and cell death. No cross resistance with other available antimycobacterial agents has been demonstrated.
MYAMBUTOL has been shown to be effective against strains of *Mycobacterium tuberculosis* but does not seem to be active against fungi, viruses, or other bacteria. *Mycobacterium tuberculosis* strains previously unexposed to MYAMBUTOL have been uniformly sensitive to concentrations of 8 or less micrograms/mL, depending on the nature of the culture media. When MYAMBUTOL has been used alone for treatment of tuberculosis, tubercle bacilli from these patients have developed resistance to MYAMBUTOL ethambutol hydrochloride by *in vitro* susceptibility tests; the development of resistance has been unpredictable and appears to occur in a step-like manner. No cross resistance between MYAMBUTOL and other antituberculous drugs has been reported. MYAMBUTOL has reduced the incidence of the emergence of mycobacterial resistance to isoniazid when both drugs have been used concurrently.
An agar diffusion microbiologic assay, based upon inhibition of *Mycobacterium smegmatis* (ATCC 607) may be used to determine concentrations of MYAMBUTOL in serum and urine. This technique has not been published, but further information can be obtained upon inquiry to Lederle Laboratories.

ANIMAL PHARMACOLOGY

Toxicological studies in dogs on high prolonged doses produced evidence of myocardial damage and failure, and depigmentation of the tapetum lucidum of the eyes, the significance of which is not known. Degenerative changes in the central nervous system, apparently not dose-related, have also been noted in dogs receiving ethambutol hydrochloride over a prolonged period.
In the rhesus monkey, neurological signs appeared after treatment with high doses given daily over a period of several months. These were correlated with specific serum levels of ethambutol hydrochloride and with definite neuroanatomical changes in the central nervous system. Focal interstitial carditis was also noted in monkeys which received ethambutol hydrochloride in high doses for a prolonged period.
When pregnant mice or rabbits were treated with high doses of ethambutol hydrochloride, fetal mortality was slightly but not significantly (P>0.05) increased. Female rats treated with ethambutol hydrochloride displayed slight but insignificant (P>0.05) decreases in fertility and litter size.
In fetuses born of mice treated with high doses of MYAMBUTOL during pregnancy, a low incidence of cleft palate, exencephaly and abnormality of the vertebral column were observed. Minor abnormalities of the cervical vertebra were seen in the newborn of rats treated with high doses of ethambutol hydrochloride during pregnancy. Rabbits receiving high doses of MYAMBUTOL during pregnancy gave birth to two fetuses with monophthalmia, one with a shortened right forearm accompanied by bilateral wrist-joint contracture and one with hare lip and cleft palate.

INDICATIONS

MYAMBUTOL is indicated for the treatment of pulmonary tuberculosis. It should not be used as the sole antituberculous drug, but should be used in conjunction with at least one other antituberculous drug. Selection of the companion drug should be based on clinical experience, considerations of comparative safety and appropriate *in vitro* susceptibility studies. In patients who have not received previous antituberculous therapy, ie, initial treatment, the most frequently used regimens have been the following:

MYAMBUTOL plus isoniazid
MYAMBUTOL plus isoniazid plus streptomycin.

In patients who have received previous antituberculous therapy, mycobacterial resistance to other drugs used in initial therapy is frequent. Consequently, in such retreatment patients, MYAMBUTOL should be combined with at least one of the second line drugs not previously administered to the patient and to which bacterial susceptibility has been indicated by appropriate *in vitro* studies. Antituberculous drugs used with MYAMBUTOL have included cycloserine, ethionamide, pyrazinamide, viomycin, and other drugs. Isoniazid, aminosalicylic acid, and streptomycin have also been used in multiple drug regimens. Alternating drug regimens have also been utilized.

CONTRAINDICATIONS

MYAMBUTOL is contraindicated in patients who are known to be hypersensitive to this drug. It is also contraindicated in patients with known optic neuritis unless clinical judgment determines that it may be used.

PRECAUTIONS

The effects of combinations of MYAMBUTOL ethambutol hydrochloride with other antituberculous drugs on the fetus is not known. While administration of this drug to pregnant human patients has produced no detectable effect upon the fetus, the possible teratogenic potential in women capable of bearing children should be weighed carefully against the benefits of therapy. There are published reports of five women who received the drug during pregnancy without apparent adverse effect upon the fetus.
MYAMBUTOL is not recommended for use in children under 13 years of age since safe conditions for use have not been established.
Patients with decreased renal function need the dosage reduced as determined by serum levels of MYAMBUTOL, since the main path of excretion of this drug is by the kidneys.
Because this drug may have adverse effects on vision, physical examination should include ophthalmoscopy, finger perimetry, and testing of color discrimination. In patients with visual defects such as cataracts, recurrent inflammatory

Continued on next page

Myambutol—Cont.

conditions of the eye, optic neuritis, and diabetic retinopathy, the evaluation of changes in visual acuity is more difficult, and care should be taken to be sure the variations in vision are not due to the underlying disease conditions. In such patients, consideration should be given to relationship between benefits expected and possible visual deterioration since evaluation of visual changes is difficult. (For recommended procedures, see next paragraphs under **ADVERSE REACTIONS.**)
As with any potent drug, periodic assessment of organ system functions, including renal, hepatic, and hematopoietic, should be made during long-term therapy.

ADVERSE REACTIONS

MYAMBUTOL may produce decreases in visual acuity which appear to be due to optic neuritis and to be related to dose and duration of treatment. The effects are generally reversible when administration of the drug is discontinued promptly. In rare cases recovery may be delayed for up to 1 year or more and the effect may possibly be irreversible in these cases.
Patients should be advised to report promptly to their physician any change of visual acuity.
The change in visual acuity may be unilateral or bilateral and hence *each eye must be tested separately and both eyes tested together.* Testing of visual acuity should be performed before beginning MYAMBUTOL therapy and periodically during drug administration, except that it should be done monthly when a patient is on a dosage of more than 15 mg per kilogram per day. Snellen eye charts are recommended for testing of visual acuity. Studies have shown that there are definite fluctuations of one or two lines of the Snellen chart in the visual acuity of many tuberculous patients *not* receiving MYAMBUTOL.
The following table may be useful in interpreting possible changes in visual acuity attributable to MYAMBUTOL.
[See table below]
In general, changes in visual acuity less than those indicated under "Significant Number of Lines" and "Decrease-Number of Points," may be due to chance variation, limitations of the testing method or physiologic variability. Conversely, changes in visual acuity equaling or exceeding those under "Significant Number of Lines" and "Decrease-Number of Points" indicate need for retesting and careful evaluation of the patient's visual status. If careful evaluation confirms the magnitude of visual change and fails to reveal another cause, MYAMBUTOL should be discontinued and the patient reevaluated at frequent intervals. Progressive decreases in visual acuity during therapy must be considered to be due to MYAMBUTOL.
If corrective glasses are used prior to treatment, these must be worn during visual acuity testing. During 1 to 2 years of therapy, a refractive error may develop which must be corrected in order to obtain accurate test results. Testing the visual acuity through a pinhole eliminates refractive error.
Patients developing visual abnormality during MYAMBUTOL treatment may show subjective visual symptoms before, or simultaneously with, the demonstration of decreases in visual acuity, and all patients receiving MYAMBUTOL should be questioned periodically about blurred vision and other subjective eye symptoms.
Recovery of visual acuity generally occurs over a period of weeks to months after the drug has been discontinued. Patients have then received MYAMBUTOL ethambutol hydrochloride again without recurrence of loss of visual acuity.
Other adverse reactions reported include: anaphylactoid reactions, dermatitis pruritus and joint pain; anorexia, nausea, vomiting, gastrointestinal upset, abdominal pain; fever, malaise, headache, and dizziness; mental confusion, disorientation and possible hallucinations. Numbness and tingling of the extremities due to peripheral neuritis have been reported infrequently.
Elevated serum uric acid levels occur and precipitation of acute gout has been reported. Pulmonary infiltrates and eosinophilia have also been reported during MYAMBUTOL therapy. Transient impairment of liver function as indicated by abnormal liver function tests is not an unusual finding. Since MYAMBUTOL is recommended for therapy in conjunction with one or more other antituberculous drugs, these changes may be related to the concurrent therapy.

DOSAGE AND ADMINISTRATION

MYAMBUTOL should not be used alone, in initial treatment or in retreatment. MYAMBUTOL should be administered on a once every 24-hour basis only. Absorption is not significantly altered by administration with food. Therapy, in general, should be continued until bacteriological conversion has become permanent and maximal clinical improvement has occurred.
MYAMBUTOL is not recommended for use in children under thirteen years of age since safe conditions for use have not been established.
Initial Treatment: In patients who have not received previous antituberculous therapy, administer MYAMBUTOL 15 mg per kilogram (7 mg per pound) of body weight, as a single oral dose once every 24 hours. In the more recent studies, isoniazid has been administered concurrently in a single, daily, oral dose.
Retreatment: In patients who have received previous antituberculous therapy, administer MYAMBUTOL 25 mg per kilogram (11 mg per pound) of body weight, as a single oral dose once every 24 hours. Concurrently administer at least one other antituberculous drug to which the organisms have been demonstrated to be susceptible by appropriate *in vitro* tests. Suitable drugs usually consist of those not previously used in the treatment of the patient. After 60 days of MYAMBUTOL administration, decrease the dose to 15 mg per kilogram (7 mg per pound) of body weight, and administer as a single oral dose once every 24 hours.
During the period when a patient is on a daily dose of 25 mg/kg, monthly eye examinations are advised.
See Table for easy selection of proper weight-dose tablet(s).

Weight-Dose Table

Weight Range Pounds	Weight Range Kilograms	Daily Dose In mg
15 mg/kg (7 mg/lb) Schedule		
Under 85 lbs	Under 37 kg	500
85–94.5	37–43	600
95–109.5	43–50	700
110–124.5	50–57	800
125–139.5	57–64	900
140–154.5	64–71	1000
155–169.5	71–79	1100
170–184.5	79–84	1200
185–199.5	84–90	1300
200–214.5	90–97	1400
215 and Over	Over 97	1500
25 mg/kg (11 mg/lb) Schedule		
Under 85 lbs	Under 38 kg	900
85–92.5	38–42	1000
93–101.5	42–45.5	1100
102–109.5	45.5–50	1200
110–118.5	50–54	1300
119–128.5	54–58	1400
129–136.5	58–62	1500
137–146.5	62–67	1600
147–155.5	67–71	1700
156–164.5	71–75	1800
165–173.5	75–79	1900
174–182.5	79–83	2000
183–191.5	83–87	2100
192–199.5	87–91	2200
200–209.5	91–95	2300
210–218.5	95–99	2400
219 and Over	Over 99	2500

HOW SUPPLIED

MYAMBUTOL® ethambutol hydrochloride Tablets
100 mg—round, convex, white, film coated tablets engraved M6 on one side and LL on the other, are supplied as follows:
NDC 0005-5015-23 - Bottle of 100
400 mg—round, convex, white, scored, film coated tablets engraved with LL on one side and M to the left and 7 to the right of the score on the other side, are supplied as follows:
NDC 0005-5084-62 - Unit-of-Issue 100s with CRC
NDC 0005-5084-34 - Bottle of 1000
NDC 0005-5084-60 - Unit Dose 10 (2 × 5) Strips
Store at Controlled Room Temperature 15–30°C (59–86°F).
Manufactured by:
LEDERLE PHARMACEUTICAL DIVISION
American Cyanamid Company
Pearl River, NY 10965
Shown in Product Identification Guide, page 319

Initial Snellen Reading	Reading Indicating Significant Decrease	Significant Number of Lines	Decrease Number of Points
20/13	20/25	3	12
20/15	20/25	2	10
20/20	20/30	2	10
20/25	20/40	2	15
20/30	20/50	2	20
20/40	20/70	2	30
20/50	20/70	1	20

NEPTAZANE® ℞

[*nĕp-ta-zāne*]
methazolamide
Tablets, USP

(For full prescribing information, please refer to the 1999 PDR for Ophthalmology.)

POLIOVIRUS VACCINE LIVE ORAL TRIVALENT ℞

ORIMUNE®
[*or-ĭ-mūn*]
SABIN STRAINS TYPES 1, 2 and 3

DESCRIPTION

Manufacture and Composition: Poliovirus Vaccine Live Oral Trivalent ORIMUNE is a mixture of three types of Sabin strain attenuated polioviruses — type 1 (Strain LS - c-2ab), type 2 (Strain P712 - Ch, 2ab), and type 3 (Strain Leon - $12a_1$b-RSO+1) — that have been propagated in *Cercopithecus aethiops* monkey kidney cell culture. The cells are grown in the presence of Eagle's basal medium consisting of Earle's balanced salt solution containing amino acids, antibiotics (streptomycin and neomycin), and calf serum. After cell growth, the medium is removed and replaced with fresh medium containing the inoculating virus but no calf serum. The inoculated cultures are maintained at a specific temperature during the course of viral propagation. Forty-eight to seventy-two hours post inoculation, the cell culture fluid from the kidneys of one monkey is harvested aseptically into a common container and stored frozen. The poliovirus harvest fluids from one or more monkeys are thawed and combined in a common container to form a poliovirus monovalent pool. Measured quantities of monovalent pools of each poliovirus Types 1, 2, and 3 are combined and diluted to form the final vaccine. The final vaccine is diluted with a buffered salt solution containing 0.5% lactalbumin and sorbitol. Each dose (0.5 mL) contains less than 25 micrograms of each of the antibiotics, streptomycin and neomycin, and less than 0.002%, by calculation, of calf serum.
Potency of the vaccine is expressed in terms of the amount of virus ($\log_{10}$) contained in the recommended dose as tissue culture infective doses ($TCID_{50}$). The human dose of vaccine containing all three virus types shall be constituted to have infectivity titers in the final container material of $10^{5.4}$ to $10^{6.4}$ for Type 1, $10^{4.5}$ to $10^{5.5}$ for Type 2, and $10^{5.2}$ to $10^{6.2}$ for Type 3, when the primary monkey kidney tube titration method is used.[1] If the more sensitive HEp-2 microtitration procedure is employed to determine the infectivity titers in each human dose, then equivalent vaccine is achieved with numerical infectivity titers of $10^{6.0}$ to $10^{7.0}$ for Type 1, $10^{5.1}$ to $10^{6.1}$ for Type 2, and $10^{5.8}$ to $10^{6.8}$ for Type 3.[2]
The vaccine is a clear liquid usually pink in color, although some containers of vaccine, shipped or stored in dry ice, may exhibit a yellow coloration due to the very low temperature or possible absorption of carbon dioxide. The color of the vaccine prior to use (red-orange-pink-yellow) has no effect on the virus or efficacy of the vaccine. This vaccine contains no preservative.
ORIMUNE is administered orally using a disposable pipette containing a single dose of 0.5 mL.

CLINICAL PHARMACOLOGY

Polioviruses are enteroviruses, in the picornavirus family of single-stranded RNA viruses. Three distinct serotypes (types 1, 2, and 3) are known to exist.[3]
Poliovirus replicates in the intestinal tract and adjacent lymphoid tissue. Manifestations of infection by polioviruses can range from inapparent illness to severe paralysis or death. Paralytic poliomyelitis results from spread of virus to the gray matter of the brain and spinal cord. Necrosis of these neurons leads to paralysis of the corresponding affected muscles.[3]
In 1954, prior to the introduction of poliovirus vaccines, over 18,000 cases of paralytic polio were reported. With widespread use of the inactivated (Salk) vaccine beginning in 1955, and replaced by the oral (Sabin) vaccine in 1962, wild poliomyelitis has virtually been eradicated in the United States.[4]
Administration of attenuated, live oral poliovirus vaccine (OPV) simulates natural infection, inducing active systemic and mucosal immunity without producing symptoms of disease. Three doses of OPV induce serum neutralizing antibodies in 98% to 100% of infants.[5,6] In one recent study in the US, 70% to 80% of 23 OPV recipients developed nasopharyngeal neutralizing antibodies after three doses, and 100% had detectable levels of nasopharyngeal IgA antibodies to each of the three poliovirus types.[5] For optimal mucosal immunity to occur, it is necessary for the viruses to multiply in the intestinal tract. A primary series of three doses of trivalent vaccine is designed to produce an antibody response to poliovirus Types 1, 2, and 3. This response is comparable to the immunity induced by the natural disease. The antibodies thus formed help protect the individual against clinical poliomyelitis infection by any of the three

types of poliovirus. Multiple sequential doses of OPV are administered to ensure that immunity to all three types of poliovirus has been achieved.[7] Serologic surveys indicate that, in a well-immunized population, >90% of school-age children, adolescents, and young adults have detectable antibody to poliovirus types 1 and 2, and >85% have antibody to type 3.[8,9] After complete primary vaccination with three doses of OPV, ≥95% of recipients develop long-lasting (probably life-long) immunity to all three poliovirus types.[10]

INDICATIONS AND USAGE

This vaccine is indicated for use in the prevention of poliomyelitis caused by poliovirus Types 1, 2, and 3.

Use in Infants, Children, and Adolescents

Infants beginning at 6 to 12 weeks of age, and *all unimmunized children and adolescents* up to age 18 are the usual candidates for routine prophylaxis.

The Advisory Committee on Immunization Practices (ACIP), the American Academy of Pediatrics (AAP) and the American Academy of Family Physicians (AAFP) state that any of three polio vaccination schedules are acceptable: a) a sequential schedule of 2 doses of enhanced inactivated poliovirus vaccine (eIPV) followed by 2 doses of OPV; b) an OPV-only schedule (4 doses); and c) an eIPV only schedule (4 doses).[10–13] (See **DOSAGE AND ADMINISTRATION**). The ACIP recommends the sequential IPV-OPV schedule. The AAP and the AAFP recommend that parents and caregivers be informed of the advantages and disadvantages of each of the three schedules, and after discussion with their children's health care professionals, may choose a schedule appropriate for their own family.

Efficacy of OPV-containing schedules: The OPV-only schedule is effective in preventing poliomyelitis. From the experience of limited studies of IPV-OPV schedules and from the experience of several countries which have implemented other IPV-OPV schedules not the same as the specific sequential schedule recommended in the US, general conclusions to support the specific US recommended sequential schedule have been drawn by the ACIP as follows:

1. Serum neutralizing antibodies — It is expected that the US sequential IPV-OPV schedule will induce detectable levels of serum neutralizing antibody against poliovirus types 1, 2, and 3 in at least 90% of recipients.
2. Secretory antibody for intestinal mucosal immunity — Studies conducted to date with other sequential schedules support the expectation that the US sequential IPV-OPV schedule will induce higher levels of secretory antibody in the intestinal tract than with an IPV-only schedule.
3. Potential reduction in recipient cases of vaccine-associated paralytic poliomyelitis (VAPP) — It is expected, but as yet unproven with the US sequential schedule, that the risk of recipient VAPP will be lower when compared to an OPV-only schedule.
4. The effect of the sequential schedule on the occurrence of rare contact cases of VAPP from exposure to OPV recipients is unknown. However, the risk of contact-associated VAPP is expected to be somewhat lower.
5. Persistence of serum neutralizing antibody — It is expected, but not yet proven, that long-term antibody protection will be comparable to that provided by OPV-only or IPV-only schedules.

OPV induces intestinal immunity, is simple to administer, is well accepted by patients, results in immunization of some unvaccinated contacts of a vaccinated person, and has a record of having eliminated disease associated with wild poliovirus in this country.[10] OPV is also recommended for control of epidemic poliomyelitis. The ACIP recommends that OPV alone be used when the vaccination series is started after 6 months of age, when parents decline additional injections, when there is a concern a child will not return on time for future vaccinations, or when a child is likely to travel to a polio-endemic country. In addition, the AAP suggests that OPV may be preferred in populations with low immunization rates.[12]

IPV alone is recommended for immunocompromised persons and their family contacts (see **CONTRAINDICATIONS** and **INDICATIONS AND USAGE: Use in Adults** for details).[10,12,13]

Prior to immunization, the parent, guardian, or adult patient should be informed of the two types of poliovirus vaccines available, the risks and benefits of each of the three vaccination schedules to the individual and to the community, and the reasons why recommendations are made for giving specific vaccines under certain circumstances.

Past history of clinical poliomyelitis or prior vaccination with IPV in otherwise healthy individuals does not preclude the administration of OPV when otherwise indicated to insure immunity against all three poliovirus serotypes. Thus, an immunization series started with IPV can be completed with OPV.

Prior administration of non-enhanced IPV has not always offered protection against rare occurrences of VAPP (see **ADVERSE REACTIONS**). Cases of VAPP were reported in individuals who had received OPV after receiving a non-enhanced IPV vaccine.[14,15] There have been no reported cases of VAPP in the limited number of children routinely immunized with enhanced inactivated poliovirus vaccine (eIPV) prior to receipt of OPV, although US experience with this sequential schedule is very limited.

Genetic sequencing studies suggest that reversion of Sabin poliovirus strains to potentially more neurovirulent phenotypes can occur after OPV administration.[16,17] However, findings of three studies indicate that the use of IPV followed by OPV may not reduce the frequency of excretion of revertant virus (as measured by specific base changes).[18–21]

Viremia due to vaccine virus has been reported to occur following ingestion of OPV. Viremia is more likely to occur in triple antibody negative infants than in individuals who are poliovirus antibody positive.[22–24]

Administration of Immune Globulin (IG), if necessary, within 7 days prior to immunization with OPV does not reduce the antibody response to OPV based on a study conducted in Peace Corps volunteers.[25] However, it is not known whether antibody response to trivalent OPV might be affected by concurrent intravenous (IV) administration of IG (IGIV). If OPV has been given, during a period in which IGIV has been administered, physicians may wish to consider giving a booster dose of OPV 3 or 4 months after the last dose of IGIV administration in order to ensure immunity by OPV.

As with any vaccine, ORIMUNE may not protect 100% of the individuals receiving the vacine.

Use in Adults

ACIP states that routine primary poliovirus immunization of adults (generally those 18 years of age or older), residing in the US, is not necessary. Immunization *is* recommended by the ACIP for certain adults who are at greater risk of exposure to wild polioviruses than the general population, including travelers to areas where poliomyelitis is endemic or epidemic, members of communities or specific population groups with disease caused by wild polioviruses, laboratory workers handling specimens that may contain polioviruses, and health care workers in close contact with patients who might be excreting wild polioviruses, and unvaccinated adults whose children will be receiving OPV as follows:

Unimmunized adults - primary immunization with enhanced-potency IPV is recommended. However, if less than 1 month is available before protection is needed, a single dose of either OPV or enhanced-potency IPV is recommended, with the remaining doses given later if the person remains at increased risk. *Incompletely immunized adults* who have had (1) at least one dose of OPV, (2) fewer than 3 doses of conventional IPV, or (3) a combination of conventional IPV and OPV totaling fewer than 3 doses, should receive at least 1 dose of OPV or enhanced-potency IPV. Additional doses needed to complete a primary series should be given prior to exposure, if time permits. *Adults who have completed a primary series* with any one or a combination of polio vaccines may be given a dose of OPV or enhanced-potency IPV.[10]

Immunization with IPV may be undertaken in unimmunized or inadequately immunized adults in households in which children are to be given OPV (see **ADVERSE REACTIONS**).[10]

Epidemic Control

Poliovirus Vaccine Live Oral Trivalent has been recommended for epidemic control. Within an epidemic area, OPV should be provided for all persons over 6 weeks of age who have not been completely immunized or whose immunization status is unknown, with the exceptions noted under immunodeficiency[7,10] (see **CONTRAINDICATIONS**).

In certain tropical endemic areas, where poliomyelitis is still endemic, the physician may wish to administer OPV to the infant at birth. Because successful immunization is less likely in newborn infants, a complete series of OPV should follow the neonatal dose beginning when the infants are 2 months old.[7] If the physician elects to immunize the infant at birth, it may be prudent to wait until the child is 3 days old, and to recommend abstention from breast-feeding for 2 to 3 hours before and after oral immunization to minimize exposure of the vaccine viruses to colostrum and to permit the establishment of the vaccine viruses in the gut.[26]

CONTRAINDICATIONS

Hypersensitivity to any component of the vaccine, including streptomycin and neomycin, is a contraindication.

OPV should not be administered to persons who have experienced an anaphylactic reaction within 24 hours of a previous dose of OPV.[16]

ORIMUNE *must not* be administered to patients with immune deficiency diseases such as combined immunodeficiency, hypogammaglobulinemia, and agammaglobulinemia. Further, ORIMUNE *must not* be administered to patients with altered immune states, such as those occurring in human immunodeficiency virus (HIV) infection, thymic abnormalities, leukemia, lymphoma, generalized malignancy, or advanced debilitating conditions, or by lowered resistance from therapy with corticosteroids, alkylating drugs, antimetabolites, or radiation. Because vaccine viruses are excreted by the vaccinee, and may spread to contacts, ORIMUNE should not be used in families with immunodeficient members.[7,10]

Recipients of the vaccine should avoid close household-type contact with all persons with altered immune status for at least 6 to 8 weeks.

Because of the possibility of immunodeficiency in other children born to a family, OPV should not be given to a member of a household in which there is a family history of immunodeficiency until the immune status of the intended recipient and other children in the family is determined to be normal.[7]

Immunization of all persons in the above-described circumstances should be with IPV.

WARNINGS

Under no circumstances should this vaccine be administered parenterally.

The decision to administer or delay vaccination because of a current or recent febrile illness depends largely on the severity of the symptoms and their etiology. Although a moderate or severe febrile illness is sufficient reason to postpone vaccination, minor illnesses such as a mild upper respiratory infection with or without low grade fever are not contraindications.[10] In addition, immunization should be deferred in the presence of persistent vomiting or diarrhea, or suspected gastroenteritis infection. Other natural disease viruses (including poliovirus and other enteroviruses) may compromise the desired response to this vaccine, since their presence in the intestinal tract may interfere with replication of the attenuated strains of poliovirus.

The decision to administer ORIMUNE to individuals with allergy to antibiotics (i.e., streptomycin and neomycin) should be made on an individual basis considering the potential risks and benefits.

IPV should be used instead of OPV when the intended recipient or household contacts are immunodeficient or immunosuppressed (see CONTRAINDICATIONS).

It is known and expected that subjects receiving OPV may shed revertant virus, regardless of whether they may have received IPV previously.[19,20,27]

In 1993, the Institute of Medicine (IOM) conducted a review of adverse events associated with childhood vaccines, including OPV.[28] The IOM concluded that there is a causal relationship between OPV and paralytic poliomyelitis, which is known to occur on rare occasions in vaccinees and their close contacts.[7,10,28–31] In addition, the IOM concluded that OPV, very rarely, has caused fatal paralytic poliomyelitis in immunocompromised persons.[28] (See **ADVERSE REACTIONS**.)

The IOM also concluded that there is adequate evidence to accept or reject a causal relationship between OPV administration and transverse myelitis, death from Sudden Infant Death Syndrome (SIDS) or death from causes other than paralytic poliomyelitis.[28] (See **ADVERSE REACTIONS**.)

PRECAUTIONS

General

Under no circumstances should this vaccine be administered parenterally.

Care is to be taken by the health care provider for the safe and effective use of this product. Prior to administration of ORIMUNE, the patient or the parent or guardian should be asked about the personal history, family history, and recent health status of the patient. The health care provider should ascertain previous immunization history and current health status, including immune status of patient and family members, to determine the existene of any contraindications to immunization with ORIMUNE. The health care provider should question patient, parent, or guardian about reactions to a previous dose of ORIMUNE.

As with any biological, before administration of ORIMUNE, the physician should take all known precautions for prevention of allergic or any other reactions. This includes a review of the patient's history for possible sensitivity (including sensitivity to streptomycin or neomycin, which are found in trace amounts in ORIMUNE), the ready availability of epinephrine (1:1000) and other appropriate agents used for control of immediate allergic reactions, and a knowledge of the recent literature pertaining to the use of the biological concerned, including the nature of side effects and adverse reactions which may follow its use.

The vaccine is not effective in modifying or preventing cases of existing and/or incubating poliomyelitis.

Information for Patients

Prior to administration of this vaccine, health care personnel should inform the patient, or the parent, guardian, or other responsible adult, of the benefits and risks to the patient, the availability of IPV and the circumstances under which each type of vaccine is recommended, and the importance of completing the immunization series. Patients, parents, or guardians should be instructed to report any serious adverse reactions to their health care provider. The health care provider is required to provide vaccine information pamphlets (available from the Centers for Disease Control and Prevention) at the time of each vaccination, as stated in the National Childhood Vaccine Injury Act.[32,33]

Continued on next page

Orimune—Cont.

Drug Interactions
ORIMUNE *must not* be administered to patients with altered immune states, such as those occurring from therapy with corticosteroids, alkylating drugs, antimetabolites, or radiation (see **CONTRAINDICATIONS**). Typhoid Vaccine Live Oral should not be given concurrently with OPV.
Carcinogenesis, Mutagenesis, Impairment of Fertility
ORIMUNE has not been evaluated for its carcinogenic, mutagenic potential or for impairment of fertility.
Use in Pregnancy
Pregnancy Category C. Animal reproduction studies have not been conducted with Poliovirus Vaccine Live Oral Trivalent. It is also not known whether OPV can cause fetal harm when administered to a pregnant woman or can affect reproduction capacity.
Although there is no convincing evidence documenting adverse effects of either OPV or IPV on the developing fetus or pregnant women, it is prudent on theoretical grounds to avoid vaccinating pregnant women. However, if immediate protection against poliomyelitis is needed, she may be administered OPV or IPV in accordance with the recommended schedules for adults[7,10] (see **CONTRAINDICATIONS** and **ADVERSE REACTIONS**).
Use in Nursing Mothers
It is not known if this product is excreted in human milk. Because many drugs are excreted in human milk, caution should be exercised when ORIMUNE is administered to a nursing woman.
Pediatric Use
OPV has been shown to be usually well-tolerated and highly immunogenic in infants and children of all ages. See **DOSAGE AND ADMINISTRATION** for the recommended pediatric dosage.

ADVERSE REACTIONS

In 1993, the IOM conducted a review of adverse events associated with childhood vaccines, including OPV.[28] The IOM concluded that there is a causal relationship between OPV and paralytic poliomyelitis, which is known to occur on rare occasions in vaccinees and their close contacts.[7,10,28–31] In addition, the IOM concluded that OPV, very rarely, has caused fatal paralytic poliomyelitis in immunocompromised persons.[28] Vaccine viruses are shed in the vaccinee's stools for up to 6 to 8 weeks as well as via the pharyngeal route for one or two weeks after administration.
The available evidence indicates that administration of OPV does not measurably increase the risk for Guillain-Barré syndrome.[10] Preliminary findings from the two studies in Finland led to a contrary conclusion in a review conducted by the IOM in 1993.[27] After the IOM review was completed, however, these data were reanalyzed and an observational study was completed in the US. Neither the reanalysis nor the results from this completed study provided evidence of a causal relationship between OPV administration and Guillain-Barré syndrome.[34]
A review by the IOM found inadequate evidence to accept or reject a causal relationship between OPV administration and transverse myelitis, death from Sudden Infant Death Syndrome (SIDS), or death from causes other than paralytic poliomyelitis.[28]
Prior to administration of the vaccine, the attending physician should warn or specifically direct personnel acting under their authority to convey the warnings to the vaccinee, parent, guardian or other responsible person of the risks and benefits of the vaccine, including the possibility of vaccine-associated paralysis, particularly to the recipient, susceptible family members, and other close personal contacts.[7,10]
The Centers for Disease Control and Prevention (CDC) report that during the years 1980 through 1994 approximately 303 million OPV doses were distributed in the US. During the same period, 133 confirmed cases of paralytic poliomyelitis were reported, of which 125 were vaccine-associated cases (1 case per 2.4 million doses distributed), six were classified as imported, and two were classified as indeterminate. Of these 125 cases, 49 occurred in vaccine recipients (1 case per 6.2 million doses distributed), 40 occurred in household and nonhousehold contacts of vaccinees (1 case per 7.6 million doses distributed), 30 occurred in immunodeficient recipients or contacts (1 case per 10.1 million doses distributed), and 6 occurred in persons with no history of vaccine exposure, from whom vaccine-like viruses were isolated.[10,31]
Forty (82%) of the recipient cases, 26 (65%) of the contact cases, and 11 (36%) of the immune deficient cases were associated with the recipient's first dose of OPV. Because the majority of cases of vaccine-associated paralysis have occurred in association with the first dose, the CDC has estimated the likelihood of paralysis in association with first *v* subsequent doses of OPV, using the number of births during 1980–1994 to estimate the number of first doses distributed, and subtracting this from the total distribution to estimate the number of subsequent doses distributed. This method estimates a frequency of paralysis for recipients of one case per 1.4 million first doses *v* one case per 27.2 million subsequent doses; for contacts, one case per 2.2 million first doses *v* one case per 17.5 million subsequent doses; and an overall frequency of one case per 750,000 first doses *v* one case per 5.1 million subsequent doses.[10,31]
Other methods of estimating the likelihood of paralysis in association with OPV have been described. Because the number of susceptible vaccine recipients or contacts of recipients is not known, the true risk of vaccine-associated poliomyelitis is impossible to determine precisely.[29]
Previous immunization with IPV may not prevent all cases of VAPP. In the 2 1/2 year period after the introduction of OPV (December 1961 through June 1964), 17 cases of VAPP were reported in individuals who received OPV following prior immunization with first generation, non-enhanced IPV. Most (11/17) were at least 15 years of age.[14] However, the first generation, non-enhanced inactivated poliovirus vaccines have not been used since 1988. There have been no reported cases of VAPP in the limited number of children routinely immunized with eIPV prior to receipt of OPV, although US experience with this sequential schedule is very limited.
Adults who have been inadequately immunized against poliomyelitis are at a minimal risk for developing VAPP when OPV is administered to the children in their households. According to the ACIP, "Because of the overriding importance of ensuring prompt and complete immunization, sequential IPV-OPV vaccination of children should begin regardless of the poliovirus vaccine status of adult household contacts. If unvaccinated or inadequately vaccinated persons are known to reside in the child's household, IPV alone should be used to complete the child's vaccination, thereby reducing the already minimal risk for VAPP among household contacts."[10]
ADVERSE EVENT REPORTING
Any adverse reactions following immunization should be reported by the health care provider to the US Department of Health and Human Services (DHHS). The **National Childhood Vaccine Injury Act** requires that the manufacturer and lot number of the vaccine administered be recorded by the health care provider in the vaccine recipient's permanent medical record (or in a permanent office log or file), along with the date of administration of the vaccine and the name, address, and title of the person administering the vaccine. The Act further requires that the health care provider report to the Secretary of the DHHS, the occurrence following immunization of any event set forth in the Vaccine Injury Table, including; paralytic poliomyelitis — (in a non-immunodeficient recipient, within 30 days of vaccination; in an immunodeficient recipient, within 6 months of vaccination); — any vaccine-associated community case of paralytic poliomyelitis; or any acute complication or sequela (including death) of above events.[32,33] The US DHHS has established the Vaccine Adverse Event Reporting System (VAERS) to accept all reports of suspected adverse events after administration of any vaccine including, but not limited to, the reporting of events required by the National Childhood Vaccine Injury Act of 1986.[32,33] The VAERS toll-free number for VAERS forms and information is 800-822-7967.

DOSAGE AND ADMINISTRATION

ORIMUNE® is to be administered *orally; under the supervision of a physician. Under no circumstances should this vaccine be administered parenterally.* For convenience, the vaccine is supplied in a disposable pipette containing a single dose of 0.5 mL which should be administered directly into the mouth of the vaccinee. Breast feeding does not interfere with successful immunization when OPV is administered according to the following schedule.[10]
Primary Series: The primary series consists of three doses.
Infants:
For the full OPV-only schedule, the ACIP and AAP advise that the first dose of OPV should be given at approximately 2 months (6 to 12 weeks) of age, and the second dose 6 to 8 weeks later, commonly at 4 months of age. A third dose is recommended at 6 to 18 months of age to complete the primary series. A supplemental dose should be given before the child enters school, ie, 4 to 6 years of age.[10–12]
If utilizing the sequential IPV/OPV schedule, the ACIP advises that eIPV be administered at 2 months and at 4 months of age as the first two doses, followed by a third dose of OPV at 12 to 18 months of age and a subsequent OPV dose at 4 to 6 years of age.[10–12]
Accelerated Schedule:
Both the ACIP and AAP recommend an OPV-only schedule for infants and children who start vaccination late (i.e., 6 months of age or older) or for whom accelerated protection against poliomyelitis is required.[10–12] The minimum interval between doses of OPV under an accelerated schedule is 4 weeks.[10] According to the ACIP, incompletely vaccinated children who are at increased risk of exposure to poliovirus should be administered the remaining doses, or administered at least a single dose of either vaccine if time is a limiting factor.[10]
Interruption of the recommended schedules with a delay between doses does not interfere with the final immunity achieved; nor does it necessitate starting the series over again regardless of the length of time elapsed between doses.[35]
Adults:
For unvaccinated adults, primary vaccination with IPV is recommended. For adults who have had a primary series of OPV or IPV and who are at increased risk of exposure to poliovirus, a booster dose of either OPV or IPV should be administered.[10] See **INDICATIONS AND USAGE: Use in Adults.**
Supplemental Doses:
The requirements for supplemental vaccination at school entry will vary depending on the child's primary polio schedule, the child's age, and the child's vaccination history. Children who followed a sequential IPV/OPV schedule should receive a second dose of OPV, regardless of the age at which the series was begun. Children who are immunized according to an OPV-only schedule should receive a fourth dose unless the third dose was administered on or after the fourth birthday.[10]
SIMULTANEOUS ADMINISTRATION WITH OTHER VACCINES
Routine simultaneous administration of OPV, diphtheria and tetanus toxoids and whole-cell or acellular pertussis vaccine (DTP or DTaP), Haemophilus b conjugate vaccine, hepatitis B vaccine, varicella vaccine, and measles-mumps-rubella vaccine (MMR) may be given to children who are the recommended age to receive these vaccines and for whom no specific contraindications exist at the time of the visit.[10,35] Typhoid Vaccine Live Oral should not be given concurrently with OPV.

STORAGE

To maintain the potency of ORIMUNE, it is necessary to store this vaccine at a temperature that will maintain ice continuously in a solid state (below 0°C or 32°F). However, since the vaccine contains sorbitol it may remain fluid at temperatures above -14°C (+7°F). Ice cubes that remain frozen continuously when stored in the same freezer compartment will confirm that the temperature is appropriate for storage of ORIMUNE. If frozen, the vaccine must be completely thawed prior to use. A container of vaccine that has been frozen and then is thawed may be carried through a maximum of 10 freeze-thaw cycles, provided the temperature does not exceed 8°C (46°F) during the periods of thaw, and provided the total cumulative duration of thaw does not exceed 24 hours. If the 24-hour period is exceeded, the vaccine must then be used within 30 days, during which time it must be stored at a temperature between 2°C to 8°C (36°F to 46°F). Ideally, an ORIMUNE DISPETTE should be removed from the freezer and thawed immediately prior to use.
Color Change: This vaccine contains phenol red as a pH indicator. The usual color of the vaccine is pink, although some containers of vaccine, shipped or stored in dry ice, may exhibit a yellow coloration due to the very low temperature or possible absorption of carbon dioxide. The color of the vaccine prior to use (red-orange-pink-yellow) has no effect on the virus or efficacy of the vaccine.
DIRECTIONS FOR USE: Pull off the protective cap and squeeze the DISPETTE to expel contents into the vaccinee's mouth.

HOW SUPPLIED

NDC 0005-2084-08—10 (0.5 mL) DISPETTE
NDC 0005-2084-12—50 (0.5 mL) DISPETTE

REFERENCES

1. *Code of Federal Regulations.* 21 CFR:630.17[c], page 94, revised April 1, 1989.
2. Albrecht P, Enterline JC, Boone EJ, et al. Poliovirus and polio antibody assay in HEp-2 and Vero cell cultures. *J Biol Stand.* 1983; 11:91–97.
3. Mandell GL, Douglas RG, Bennett JE, *Principles and Practice of Infectious Diseases.* 3rd ed. New York, NY: Churchill Livingston: 1990: 1360.
4. Kim-Farley RJ, Bart KJ, Schonberger LB, et al. Poliomyelitis in the USA: virtual elimination of disease caused by wild virus. *Lancet.* 1984;2:1315–1317.
5. Faden H, Modin JF, Thoms ML, et al. Comparative evaluation of immunization with live attenuated and enhanced-potency inactivated trivalent poliovirus vaccines in childhood: systemic and local immune response. *J Infect Dis.* 1990;162:1291–1297.
6. Modlin JF, Halsey NA, Thoms ML, et al. Humoral and mucosal immunity in infants induced by three sequential inactivated poliovirus vaccine-live attenuated poliovirus vaccine immunization schedules. *J Infect Dis.* 1997;175(suppl 1):S228–234.
7. American Academy of Pediatrics. *Report of the Committee on Infectious Diseases.* 24th ed. Elk Grove Village, Ill: American Academy of Pediatrics;1997:424–433.
8. Kelley PW, Petruccelli BP, Stehr-Green P, et al. The susceptibility of young adult Americans to vaccine-preventable infections: a national serosurvey of US army recruits. *JAMA.* 1991, 266:2724–2729.

9. Orenstein WA, Wassilak, SGF, Deforest, A, et al. Sero-prevalence of polio virus antibodies among Massachusetts schoolchildren (abstract). In: Program and Abstracts of the 28th Interscience Conference on Antimicrobial Agents and Chemotherapy. Washington, DC: American Society of Microbiology; 1988.
10. Recommendations of the Advisory Committee on Immunization Practices (ACIP). Poliomyelitis prevention in the United States: introduction of a sequential vaccination schedule of inactivated poliovirus vaccine followed by oral poliovirus vaccine. *MMWR*. 1997;46(No. RR-3):1–25.
11. CDC. Recommended Childhood Immunization Schedule — United States, 1998. *MMWR*. 1998;47(1):8–12.
12. American Academy of Pediatrics, Committee on Infectious Disease. Poliomyelitis prevention: recommendations for use of inactivated poliovirus vaccine and live oral poliovirus vaccine. *Pediatrics*. 1997;99(2):300–305.
13. Zimmerman RK. AAFP, AAP and ACIP release 1997 childhood immunization schedule. *Am Fam Physician*. 1997;55(1):342–346.
14. Henderson DA, Witte JJ, Morris L, et al. Paralytic disease associated with oral polio vaccines. *JAMA* 1964;190(1):41–48.
15. von Magnus H, Peterson I. Vaccination with inactivated poliovirus vaccine and oral poliovirus vaccine in Denmark. *Rev Infect Dis*. 1984;6(suppl):S471–474.
16. Minor PD, John A, Ferguson M, et al. Antigenic and molecular evolution of the vaccine strain of type 3 poliovirus during the period of excretion by a primary vaccine. *J Gen Virol*. 1986;67:693–706.
17. Kew OM, Nottay BK, Hatch MH, et al. Multiple genetic changes can occur in the oral poliovaccines upon replication in humans. *J Gen Virol*. 1981;56:337–347.
18. Lepow ML, Robbins FC, Woods WA. Influence of vaccination with formalin inactivated vaccine upon gastrointestinal infection with polioviruses. *AJPH*. 1960:50(4):531–542.
19. Ogra PL, Faden HS, Abraham R, et al. Effect of prior immunity on the shedding of virulent revertant virus in feces after oral immunization with live attenuated polio vaccine. *J Infect Dis*. 1991;164:191–194.
20. Abraham, R. Minor P, Dunn G, et al. Shedding of virulent poliovirus revertants during immunization with oral poliovirus vaccine after prior immunization with inactivated polio vaccine. *J Infect Dis*. 1993;168:1105–1109.
21. Murdin AD, Barreto L, Plotkin S. Inactivated poliovirus vaccine; past and present experience. *Vaccine*. 1996; 14: 735–746.
22. Melnick JL, et al. Free and bound virus in serum after administration of oral poliovirus vaccine. *Amer J Epidem*. 1966;84:329–342.
23. Horstmann DM, Opton EM, Klemperer R, et al. Viremia in infants vaccinated with oral poliovirus vaccine (Sabin) *Am J Hyg*. 1964;79:47–63.
24. McKay HW, Fodor AR, Kokko UP. Viremia following the administration of live poliovirus vaccine. *AJPH*. 1963;53(2):274–285.
25. Kaplan JE, Nelson DB, Schonberger LB, et al. The effect of immune globulin on the response to trivalent oral poliovirus and yellow fever vaccinations. *Bull WHO*. 1984; 62(4):585–590.
26. Welsh JH, May JT. Anti-infective properties of breast milk. *J Pediatr*. 1979:94(1):1–9.
27. Evans DMA. Dunn G, Minor PD, et al. Increased neurovirulence associated with a single nucleotide change in a noncoding region of the Sabin type 3 poliovirus genome. *Nature*. 1985;314:548–550.
28. Institute of Medicine. Stratton KR, Howe CJ, Johnston RB, eds. Adverse events associated with childhood vaccines: evidence bearing on causality. Washington, DC: National Academy Press. 1994:187–210.
29. Prevots DR, Sutter RW, Strebel PM, et al. Completeness of reporting for paralytic poliomyelitis, United States, 1980 through 1991. *Arch Pediatr Adolesc Med*. 1994;148:479–485.
30. Esteves K. Safety of oral poliomyelitis vaccine: results of a WHO enquiry. *Bull WHO*. 1988;66(6):739–746.
31. CDC. Paralytic Poliomyelitis — United States, 1980 – 1994. *MMWR*. 1997;46(4):79–83.
32. *Federal Register Notice*. National vaccine injury compensation program revision of the vaccine injury table; final rule. 1995;66(26):7677–7696.
33. CDC. Vaccine Adverse Event Reporting System — United States. *MMWR*. 1990;39(41):730–733.
34. Rantala H, Cherry JD, Shields, WD, et al. Epidemiology of Guillain-Barré syndrome in children: relationship of oral polio vaccine administration to occurrence. *J Pediatr*. 1994;124:220–223.
35. Recommendations of the Advisory Committee on Immunization Practices (ACIP). General recommendations on immunization. *MMWR*. 1994;43(RR-1):12.

Manufactured by:
LEDERLE LABORATORIES

Division American Cyanamid Company
Pearl River, NY 10965
US Gov't. License No. 17
Marketed by:
WYETH-LEDERLE VACCINES
Wyeth-Ayerst Laboratories
Philadelphia, PA 19101

Shown in Product Identification Guide, page 319

PIPRACIL®

℞

[pĭp-ră-sĭl]
piperacillin sodium
For Intravenous and Intramuscular Use

DESCRIPTION

PIPRACIL® piperacillin sodium is a semisynthetic broad-spectrum penicillin for parenteral use derived from D(-)α-aminobenzylpenicillin. The chemical name of piperacillin sodium is 4-Thia-1-azabicyclo [3.2.0] heptane-2-carboxylic acid, 6-[[[[(4-ethyl-2,3-dioxo-1-piperazinyl)carbonyl]amino]phenylacetyl]amino]-3,3-dimethyl-7-oxo-, monosodium salt, [2S-[2α, 5α, 6β(S*)]].

PIPRACIL is a white to off-white solid having the characteristic appearance of products prepared by freeze-drying. Freely soluble in water and in alcohol. The pH of the aqueous solution is 5.5 to 7.5. One g contains 1.85 mEq (42.5 mg) of sodium (Na⁺).

CLINICAL PHARMACOLOGY

Intravenous Administration. In healthy adult volunteers, mean serum levels immediately after a two to three minute intravenous injection of 2, 4, or 6 g were 305, 412, and 775 mcg/mL. Serum levels lack dose proportionality.
[See table at bottom of next page]

Intramuscular Administration. PIPRACIL is rapidly absorbed after intramuscular injection. In healthy volunteers, the mean peak serum concentration occurs approximately 30 minutes after a single dose of 2 g and is about 36 mcg/mL. The oral administration of 1 g probenecid before injection produces an increase in piperacillin peak serum level of about 30%. The area under the curve (AUC) is increased by approximately 60%.

General

PIPRACIL is not absorbed when given orally. Peak serum concentrations are attained approximately 30 minutes after intramuscular injections and immediately after completion of intravenous injection or infusion. The serum half-life in healthy volunteers ranges from 36 minutes to one hour and 12 minutes. The mean elimination half-life of PIPRACIL in healthy adult volunteers is 54 minutes following administration of 2 g and 63 minutes following 6 g. As with other penicillins, PIPRACIL is eliminated primarily by glomerular filtration and tubular secretion; it is excreted rapidly as unchanged drug in high concentrations in the urine. Approximately 60% to 80% of the administered dose is excreted in the urine in the first 24 hours. Piperacillin urine concentrations, determined by microbioassay, were as high as 14,100 mcg/mL following a 6 g intravenous dose and 8,500 mcg/mL following a 4 g intravenous dose. These urine drug concentrations remained well above 1,000 mcg/mL throughout the dosing interval. The elimination half-life is increased twofold in mild to moderate renal impairment and fivefold to sixfold in severe impairment.

PIPRACIL binding to human serum proteins is 16%. The drug is widely distributed in human tissues and body fluids, including bone, prostate, and heart and reaches high concentrations in bile. After a 4 g bolus, maximum biliary concentrations averaged 3,205 mcg/mL. It penetrates into the cerebrospinal fluid in the presence of inflamed meninges. Because PIPRACIL is excreted by the biliary route as well as by the renal route, it can be used safely in appropriate dosage (see **DOSAGE AND ADMINISTRATION**) in patients with severely restricted kidney function, and can be used effectively in treatment of hepatobiliary infections.

Microbiology

PIPRACIL is an antibiotic which exerts its bactericidal activity by inhibiting both septum and cell wall synthesis. It is active against a variety of gram-positive and gram-negative aerobic and anaerobic bacteria. *In vitro*, piperacillin is active against most strains of clinical isolates of the following microorganisms:

Aerobic and facultatively anaerobic organisms
  Gram-negative bacteria
  Escherichia coli
  Proteus mirabilis
  Proteus vulgaris
  Morganella morganii (formerly *Proteus morganii*)
  Providencia rettgeri (formerly *Proteus rettgeri*)
  Serratia species including *S marcescens* and *S liquefaciens*
  Klebsiella pneumoniae
  Klebsiella species
  Enterobacter species including *E aerogenes* and *E cloacae*
  Citrobacter species including *C freundii* and *C diversus*

  Salmonella species*
  Shigella species*
  Pseudomonas aeruginosa
  Pseudomonas species including *P cepacia,* *P maltophilia,* and *P fluorescens*
  Acinetobacter species (formerly *Mima-Herellea*)
  Haemophilus influenzae (non-β-lactamase-producing strains)
  Neisseria gonorrhoeae
  Neisseria meningitidis
  Moraxella species*
  Yersinia species* (formerly *Pasteurella*)
Gram-positive bacteria
  Group D streptococci including
    Enterococci (*Streptococcus faecalis, S faecium*)
    Non-enterococci*
  β-hemolytic streptococci including
    Group A *Streptococcus* (*S pyogenes*)
    Group B *Streptococcus* (*S agalactiae*)
  Streptococcus pneumoniae
  Streptococcus viridans
  Staphylococcus aureus (non-penicillinase-producing)*
  Staphylococcus epidermidis (non-penicillinase-producing)*
Anaerobic bacteria
  Actinomyces species*
  Bacteroides species including
    B fragilis group (*B fragilis, B vulgatus*)
    Non-*B fragilis* group (*B melaninogenicus*)
    B asaccharolyticus
  Clostridium species including
    C perfringens and *C difficile*
  Eubacterium species
  Fusobacterium species including *F nucleatum* and *F necrophorum*
  Peptococcus species
  Peptostreptococcus species
  Veillonella species

*Piperacillin has been shown to be active *in vitro* against these organisms; however, clinical efficacy has not yet been established.

In vitro, PIPRACIL is inactivated by staphylococcal β-lactamases, and β-lactamases produced by gram-negative bacteria. However, it is active against β-lactamase-producing gonococci.

Many strains of gram-negative organisms resistant to certain antibiotics have been found to be susceptible to PIPRACIL.

PIPRACIL has excellent activity against gram-positive organisms, including enterococci (*S faecalis*). It is active against obligate anaerobes such as *Bacteroides* species and also against *C difficile* (which has been associated with pseudomembranous colitis).

Piperacillin is active against many gram-negative bacteria including *Enterobacteriaceae, Klebsiella, Serratia, Pseudomonas, E coli, Proteus,* and *Citrobacter,* and, in addition, it is active against anaerobes and enterococci.

In vitro tests show piperacillin to act synergistically with aminoglycoside antibiotics against most isolates of *P aeruginosa.*

Susceptibility Testing

The use of a 100 mcg piperacillin antibiotic disk with susceptibility test methods which measure zone diameter gives an accurate estimation of susceptibility of organisms to PIPRACIL. The following standard procedure[†] has been recommended for use with disks for testing antimicrobials.

[†] NCCLS Approved Standard; M2-A2 (Formerly ASM-2) Performance Standards for Antimicrobic Disk Susceptibility Tests, Second Edition, available from the National Committee of Clinical Laboratory Standards.

With this type of procedure, a report of "susceptible" from the laboratory indicates that the infecting organism is likely to respond to therapy. A report of "intermediate susceptibility" suggests that the organism would be susceptible if high dosage is used or if the infection is confined to tissue and fluids (eg, urine) in which high antibiotic levels are obtained. A report of "resistant" indicates that the infecting organism is not likely to respond to therapy. With the piperacillin disk, a zone of 18 mm or greater indicates susceptibility, zone sizes of 14 mm or less indicate resistance, and zone sizes of 15 to 17 mm indicate intermediate susceptibility.

Haemophilus and *Neisseria* species which give zones of ≥29 mm are susceptible; resistant strains give zones of ≤28 mm. The above interpretive criteria are based on the use of the standardized procedure. Antibiotic susceptibility testing requires carefully prescribed procedures. Susceptibility tests are biased to a considerable degree when different methods are used.

Continued on next page

Pipracil—Cont.

The standardized procedure requires the use of control organisms. The 100 mcg piperacillin disk should give zone diameters between 24 and 30 mm for *E coli* ATCC No. 25922 and between 25 and 33 mm for *Pseudomonas aeruginosa* ATCC No. 27853.

Dilution methods such as those described in the International Collaborative Study[‡] have been used to determine susceptibility of organisms to PIPRACIL.

‡*Acta Pathol Microbiol Scand* [B] 1971; suppl 217.

Enterobacteriaceae, Pseudomonas species and *Acinetobacter* sp are considered susceptible if the minimal inhibitory concentration (MIC) of piperacillin is no greater than 64 mcg/mL and are considered resistant if the MIC is greater than 128 mcg/mL.

Haemophilus and *Neisseria* species are considered susceptible if the MIC of piperacillin is ≤ to 1 mcg/mL.

When anaerobic organisms are isolated from infection sites, it is recommended that other tests such as the modified Broth-Disk Method[§] be used to determine the antibiotic susceptibility of these slowly growing organisms.

§ Wilkins TD and Thiel T. *Antimicrob Agents Chemother* 1973;3:350–356.

INDICATIONS AND USAGE

Therapeutic. PIPRACIL is indicated for the treatment of serious infections caused by susceptible strains of the designated organisms in the conditions as listed below.

Intra-Abdominal Infections including hepatobiliary and surgical infections caused by *E coli, P aeruginosa,* enterococci, *Clostridium* sp, anaerobic cocci, and *Bacteroides* sp, including *B fragilis.*

Urinary Tract Infections caused by *E coli, Klebsiella* sp, *P aeruginosa, Proteus* sp, including *P mirabilis,* and enterococci.

Gynecologic Infections including endometritis, pelvic inflammatory disease, pelvic cellulitis caused by *Bacteroides* sp including *B fragilis,* anaerobic cocci, *Neisseria gonorrhoeae,* and enterococci *(S faecalis).*

Septicemia including bacteremia caused by *E coli, Klebsiella* sp, *Enterobacter* sp, *Serratia* sp, *P mirabilis, S pneumoniae,* enterococci, *P aeruginosa, Bacteroides* sp, and anaerobic cocci.

Lower Respiratory Tract Infections caused by *E coli, Klebsiella* sp, *Enterobacter* sp, *Pseudomonas aeruginosa, Serratia* sp, *H influenzae, Bacteroides* sp, and anaerobic cocci. Although improvement has been noted in patients with cystic fibrosis, lasting bacterial eradication may not necessarily be achieved.

Skin and Skin Structure Infections caused by *E coli, Klebsiella* sp, *Serratia* sp, *Acinetobacter* sp, *Enterobacter* sp, *Pseudomonas aeruginosa,* indole-positive *Proteus* sp, *Proteus mirabilis, Bacteroides* sp, including *B fragilis,* anaerobic cocci, and enterococci.

Bone and Joint Infections caused by *P aeruginosa,* enterococci, *Bacteroides* sp, and anaerobic cocci.

Gonococcal Infections. PIPRACIL has been effective in the treatment of uncomplicated gonococcal urethritis.

PIPRACIL has also been shown to be clinically effective for the treatment of infections at various sites caused by *Streptococcus* species including Group A β-hemolytic *Streptococcus* and *S pneumoniae;* however, infections caused by these organisms are ordinarily treated with more narrow spectrum penicillins. Because of its broad spectrum of bactericidal activity against gram-positive and gram-negative aerobic and anaerobic bacteria, PIPRACIL is particularly useful for the treatment of mixed infections and presumptive therapy prior to the identification of the causative organisms.

Also, PIPRACIL may be administered as single drug therapy in some situations where normally two antibiotics might be employed.

Piperacillin has been successfully used with aminoglycosides, especially in patients with impaired host defenses. Both drugs should be used in full therapeutic doses.

Appropriate cultures should be made for susceptibility testing before initiating therapy and therapy adjusted, if appropriate, once the results are known.

Prophylaxis: PIPRACIL is indicated for prophylactic use in surgery including intra-abdominal (gastrointestinal and biliary) procedures, vaginal hysterectomy, abdominal hysterectomy, and cesarean section. Effective prophylactic use depends on the time of administration, and PIPRACIL should be given one-half to one hour before the operation so that effective levels can be achieved in the site prior to the procedure.

The prophylactic use of piperacillin should be stopped within 24 hours, since continuing administration of any antibiotic increases the possibility of adverse reactions, but in the majority of surgical procedures, does not reduce the incidence of subsequent infections. If there are signs of infection, specimens for culture should be obtained for identification of the causative organism so that appropriate therapy can be instituted.

CONTRAINDICATIONS

A history of allergic reactions to any of the penicillins and/or cephalosporins.

WARNINGS

Serious and occasionally fatal hypersensitivity (anaphylactic) reactions have been reported in patients receiving therapy with penicillins. These reactions are more apt to occur in persons with a history of sensitivity to multiple allergens. There have been reports of patients with a history of penicillin hypersensitivity who have experienced severe hypersensitivity reactions when treated with a cephalosporin. Before initiating therapy with PIPRACIL, careful inquiry should be made concerning previous hypersensitivity reactions to penicillins, cephalosporins, and other allergens. If an allergic reaction occurs during therapy with PIPRACIL, the antibiotic should be discontinued. The usual agents (antihistamines, pressor amines, and corticosteroids) should be readily available. SERIOUS ANAPHYLACTOID REACTIONS REQUIRE IMMEDIATE EMERGENCY TREATMENT WITH EPINEPHRINE. OXYGEN AND INTRAVENOUS CORTICOSTEROIDS AND AIRWAY MANAGEMENT INCLUDING INTUBATION SHOULD ALSO BE ADMINISTERED AS NECESSARY.

PRECAUTIONS

General

While piperacillin possesses the characteristic low toxicity of the penicillin group of antibiotics, periodic assessment of organ system functions, including renal, hepatic, and hematopoietic, during prolonged therapy is advisable.

Bleeding manifestations have occurred in some patients receiving β-lactam antibiotics, including piperacillin. These reactions have sometimes been associated with abnormalities of coagulation tests such as clotting time, platelet aggregation and prothrombin time and are more likely to occur in patients with renal failure.

If bleeding manifestations occur, the antibiotic should be discontinued and appropriate therapy instituted.

The possibility of the emergence of resistant organisms which might cause superinfections should be kept in mind, particularly during prolonged treatment. If this occurs, appropriate measures should be taken.

As with other penicillins, patients may experience neuromuscular excitability or convulsions if higher than recommended doses are given intravenously.

PIPRACIL® is a monosodium salt containing 1.85 mEq of Na^+ per g. This should be considered when treating patients requiring restricted salt intake. Periodic electrolyte determinations should be made in patients with low potassium reserves, and the possibility of hypokalemia should be kept in mind with patients who have potentially low potassium reserves and who are receiving cytotoxic therapy or diuretics.

Antimicrobials used in high doses for short periods to treat gonorrhea may mask or delay the symptoms of incubating syphilis. Therefore, prior to treatment, patients with gonorrhea should also be evaluated for syphilis. Specimens for darkfield examination should be obtained from patients with any suspected primary lesion, and serologic tests should be performed. In all cases where concomitant syphilis is suspected, monthly serological tests should be made for a minimum of 4 months.

As with other semisynthetic penicillins, PIPRACIL therapy has been associated with an increased incidence of fever and rash in cystic fibrosis patients.

Drug Interactions

The mixing of piperacillin with an aminoglycoside *in vitro* can result in substantial inactivation of the aminoglycosides.

Piperacillin when used concomitantly with vecuronium has been implicated in the prolongation of the neuromuscular blockage of vecuronium. Due to their similar mechanism of action, it is expected that the neuromuscular blockade produced by any of the non-depolarizing muscle relaxants could be prolonged in the presence of piperacillin. (See package insert for vecuronium bromide.)

Pregnancy–Pregnancy Category B

Although reproduction studies in mice and rats performed at doses up to 4 times the human dose have shown no evidence of impaired fertility or harm to the fetus, safety of PIPRACIL use in pregnant women has not been determined by adequate and well-controlled studies. Because animal reproduction studies are not always predictive of human response, this drug should be used during pregnancy only if clearly needed. It has been found to cross the placenta in rats.

Nursing Mothers

Caution should be exercised when PIPRACIL is administered to nursing mothers. It is excreted in low concentrations in milk.

Pediatric Use

Dosages for children under the age of 12 have not been established. The safety of PIPRACIL in neonates is not known. In dog neonates, dilated renal tubules and peritubular hyalinization occurred following administration of PIPRACIL.

ADVERSE EFFECTS

PIPRACIL is generally well tolerated. The most common adverse reactions have been local in nature, following intravenous or intramuscular injection. The following adverse reactions may occur.

Local Reactions. In clinical trials thrombophlebitis was noted in 4% of patients. Pain, erythema, and/or induration at the injection site occurred in 2% of patients. Less frequent reactions including ecchymosis, deep vein thrombosis and hematomas have also occurred.

Gastrointestinal. Diarrhea and loose stools were noted in 2% of patients. Other less frequent reactions included vomiting, nausea, increases in liver enzymes (LDH, SGOT, SGPT), hyperbilirubinemia, cholestatic hepatitis, bloody diarrhea and, rarely, pseudomembranous colitis.

Hypersensitivity Reactions: Anaphylactoid Reactions, see **WARNINGS.**

Rash was noted in 1% of patients. Other less frequent findings included pruritus, vesicular eruptions, positive Coombs tests.

Other dermatologic manifestations such as erythema multiforme and Stevens-Johnson syndrome have been reported rarely.

Renal. Elevations of creatinine or BUN, and, rarely, interstitial nephritis.

PIPERACILLIN SERUM LEVELS IN ADULTS (mcg/mL) AFTER A TWO- TO THREE-MINUTE IV INJECTION

DOSE	0	10 min	20 min	30 min	1 h	1.5 h	2 h	3 h	4 h	6 h	8 h
2	305 (159–615)	202 (164–225)	156 (52–165)	67 (41–88)	40 (25–57)	24 (18–31)	20 (14–24)	8 (3–11)	3 (2–4)	2 (<0.6–3)	—
4	412 (389–484)	344 (315–379)	295 (269–330)	117 (98–138)	93 (78–110)	60 (50–67)	36 (26–51)	20 (17–24)	8 (7–11)	4 (3.7–4.1)	0.9 (0.7–1)
6	775 (695–849)	609 (530–670)	563 (492–630)	325 (292–363)	208 (180–239)	138 (115–175)	90 (71–113)	38 (29–53)	33 (25–44)	8 (3–19)	3.2 (<2–6)

PIPERACILLIN SERUM LEVELS IN ADULTS (mcg/mL) AFTER A 30-MINUTE IV INFUSION

DOSE	0	5 min	10 min	15 min	30 min	45 min	1 h	1.5 h	2 h	4 h	6 h	7.5 h
4	244 (155–298)	215 (169–247)	186 (140–209)	177 (142–213)	141 (122–156)	146 (110–265)	105 (85–133)	72 (53–105)	53 (36–69)	15 (6–24)	4 (1–9)	2 (0.5–3)
6	353 (324–371)	298 (242–339)	298 (232–331)	272 (219–314)	229 (185–249)	180 (144–209)	149 (117–171)	104 (89–113)	73 (66–94)	22 (12–39)	16 (5–49)	— —

A 30-minute infusion of 6 g every 6 h gave, on the fourth day, a mean peak serum concentration of 420 mcg/mL.

Central Nervous System. Headache, dizziness, fatigue.
Hemic and Lymphatic. Reversible leukopenia, neutropenia, thrombocytopenia and/or eosinophilia have been reported. As with other β-lactam antibiotics, reversible leukopenia (neutropenia) is more apt to occur in patients receiving prolonged therapy at high dosages or in association with drugs known to cause this reaction.
Serum Electrolytes. Individuals with liver disease or individuals receiving cytotoxic therapy or diuretics were reported rarely to demonstrate a decrease in serum potassium concentrations with high doses of piperacillin.
Skeletal. Rarely, prolonged muscle relaxation.
Other. Superinfection, including candidiasis. Hemorrhagic manifestations.

DOSAGE AND ADMINISTRATION

PIPRACIL may be administered by the intramuscular route (see NOTE) or intravenously or given in a three- to five-minute intravenous injection. The usual dosage of PIPRACIL for serious infections is 3- to 4-g given every four to six hours as a 20- to 30-minute infusion. For serious infections, the intravenous route should be used.
PIPRACIL should not be mixed with an aminoglycoside in a syringe or infusion bottle since this can result in inactivation of the aminoglycoside.
The maximum daily dose for adults is usually 24 g/day, although higher doses have been used.
Intramuscular injections (See NOTE) should be limited to 2 g per injection site. This route of administration has been used primarily in the treatment of patients with uncomplicated gonorrhea and urinary tract infections.
NOTE: THE ADD-VANTAGE VIAL IS *NOT* FOR IM USE.

DOSAGE RECOMMENDATIONS

Type of Infection	Usual Total Daily Dose
Serious infections such as septicemia, nosocomial pneumonia, intra-abdominal infections, aerobic and anaerobic gynecologic infections, and skin and soft tissue infections	12–18 g/d IV (200 to 300 mg/kg/d) in divided doses every 4 to 6 h
Complicated urinary tract infections	8–16 g/d IV (125–200 mg/kg/d) in divided doses every 6 to 8 h
Uncomplicated urinary tract infections and most community-acquired pneumonia	6–8 g/d IM or IV (100 to 125 mg/kg/d) in divided doses every 6 to 12 h
Uncomplicated gonorrhea infections	2 g IM″ as a one-time dose

″ One g of probenecid given orally one-half hour prior to injection.

The average duration of PIPRACIL treatment is from seven to ten days, except in the treatment of gynecologic infections, in which it is from 3 to 10 days; the duration should be guided by the patient's clinical and bacteriological progress. For most acute infections, treatment should be continued for at least 48 to 72 hours after the patient becomes asymptomatic. Antibiotic therapy for Group A β-hemolytic streptococcal infections should be maintained for at least ten days to reduce the risk of rheumatic fever or glomerulonephritis.
When PIPRACIL is given concurrently with aminoglycosides, both drugs should be used in full therapeutic doses.

Renal Impairment

Dosage in Renal Impairment

Creatinine Clearance mL/min	Urinary Tract Infection (uncomplicated)	Urinary Tract Infection (complicated)	Serious Systemic Infection
>40	No dosage adjustment necessary		
20–40	No dosage adjustment necessary	9 g/day 3 g every 8 h	12 g/day 4 g every 8 h
<20	6 g/day 3 g every 12 h	6 g/day 3 g every 12 h	8 g/day 4 g every 12 h

For patients on hemodialysis the maximum daily dose is 6 g/day (2 g every 8 hours). In addition, because hemodialysis removes 30%–50% of piperacillin in 4 hours, 1 g additional dose should be administered following each dialysis period.

For patients with renal failure and hepatic insufficiency, measurement of serum levels of PIPRACIL will provide additional guidance for adjusting dosage.

Prophylaxis
When possible, PIPRACIL should be administered as a 20- to 30-minute infusion just prior to anesthesia. Administration while the patient is awake will facilitate identification of possible adverse reactions during drug infusion.

INDICATION	1st Dose	2nd Dose	3rd Dose
Intra-abdominal Surgery	2 g IV just prior to surgery	2 g during surgery	2 g every 6 h Post-Op for no more than 24 h
Vaginal Hysterectomy	2 g IV just prior to surgery	2 g 6 h after 1st dose	2 g 12 h after 1st dose
Cesarean Section	2 g IV after cord is clamped	2 g 4 h after 1st dose	2 g 8 h after 1st dose
Abdominal Hysterectomy	2 g IV just prior to surgery	2 g on return to recovery room	2 g after 6 h

Infants and Children: Dosages in infants and children under 12 years of age have not been established.

PRODUCT RECONSTITUTION/DOSAGE PREPARATION

Conventional Vials:
Diluents for Reconstitution
Sterile Water for Injection
Bacteriostatic¹ Water for Injection
Sodium Chloride Injection
Bacteriostatic¹ Sodium Chloride Injection
Dextrose 5% in Water
Dextrose 5% and 0.9% Sodium Chloride
#Lidocaine HCl 0.5% to 1% (without epinephrine)

¹ Either Parabens or Benzyl Alcohol
For Intramuscular Use Only. Lidocaine is contraindicated in patients with a known history of hypersensitivity to local anesthetics of the amide type.

Conventional Vials:
Intravenous Solutions
Dextrose 5% in Water
0.9% Sodium Chloride
Dextrose 5% and 0.9% Sodium Chloride
Lactated Ringer's Injection††
Dextran 6% in 0.9% Sodium Chloride

†† When PIPRACIL® is further diluted with Lactated Ringer's Injection, the diluted solution must be administered within 2 hours.

Intravenous Admixtures
Normal Saline [+ KCl 40 mEq]
5% Dextrose in Water [+ KCl 40 mEq]
5% Dextrose/Normal Saline [+ KCl 40 mEq]
Ringer's Injection [+ KCl 40 mEq]
Lactated Ringer's Injection [+ KCl 40 mEq]††

†† When PIPRACIL® is further diluted with Lactated Ringer's Injection, the diluted solution must be administered within 2 hours.

ADD-Vantage Vials:**
ADD-Vantage System Admixtures
Dextrose 5% in Water (50 or 100 mL)
0.9% Sodium Chloride (50 or 100 mL)

** (ADD-Vantage is the registered trademark of Abbott Laboratories.)

INTRAVENOUS ADMINISTRATION
Reconstitution Directions for Conventional Vials: Reconstitute each gram of PIPRACIL with at least 5 mL of a suitable diluent (except Lidocaine HCl 0.5% to 1% without epinephrine) listed above. Shake well until dissolved. Reconstituted solution may be further diluted to the desired volume (eg, 50 or 100 mL) in the above listed intravenous solutions and admixtures.
Reconstitution Directions for ADD-Vantage Vials: See Instruction Sheet provided in box.
Reconstitution Directions for PHARMACY BULK VIAL: Reconstitute the 40 g vial with 172 mL of a suitable diluent (except Lidocaine HCl 0.5% to 1% without epinephrine) listed above to achieve a concentration of 1 g per 5 mL.
Directions for Administration:
Intermittent IV Infusion
Infuse diluted solution over a period of about 30 minutes. During infusion it is desirable to discontinue the primary intravenous solution.

Intravenous Injection (Bolus)
Reconstituted solution should be injected slowly over a 3- to 5-minute period to help avoid vein irritation.
INTRAMUSCULAR ADMINISTRATION (CONVENTIONAL VIALS ONLY)
Reconstitution Directions: Reconstitute each gram of PIPRACIL with 2 mL of a suitable diluent listed above to achieve a concentration of 1 g per 2.5 mL. Shake well until dissolved.
Directions for Administration
When indicated by clinical and bacteriological findings, intramuscular administration of 6 to 8 g daily of PIPRACIL, in divided doses, may be utilized for initiation of therapy. In addition, intramuscular administration of the drug may be considered for maintenance therapy after clinical and bacteriologic improvement has been obtained with intravenous piperacillin sodium treatment. Intramuscular administration should not exceed 2 g per injection at any one site.
The preferred site is the upper outer quadrant of the buttock (ie, *gluteus maximus*).
The deltoid area should be used only if well-developed, and then only with caution to avoid radial nerve injury. Intramuscular injections should not be made into the lower or mid-third of the upper arm.
Stability of PIPRACIL Following Reconstitution
PIPRACIL is stable in both glass and plastic containers when reconstituted with recommended diluents and when diluted with the intravenous solutions and intravenous admixtures indicated above.
Extensive stability studies have demonstrated chemical stability (potency, pH, and clarity) through 24 hours at room temperature, up to one week refrigerated, and up to one month frozen (−10° to −20°C). (Note: The 40 g Pharmacy Bulk Vial should not be frozen after reconstitution.) Appropriate consideration of aseptic technique and individual hospital policy, however, may recommend discarding unused portions after storage for 48 hours under refrigeration and discarding after 24 hours storage at room temperature.
ADD-Vantage System
Stability studies with the ad-mixed ADD-Vantage system have demonstrated chemical stability (potency, pH, and clarity) through 24 hours at room temperature. (Note: The admixed ADD-Vantage should not be refrigerated or frozen after reconstitution.)
Additional stability data available upon request.

HOW SUPPLIED
PIPRACIL® piperacillin sodium is available in vials containing sterile freeze-dried piperacillin sodium powder equivalent to two, three, four and 40 g of piperacillin. One g of piperacillin (as a monosodium salt) contains 1.85 mEq (42.5 mg) of sodium.
Product Numbers
2 gram/Vial—10 per box—NDC 0206-3879-16
3 gram/Vial—10 per box—NDC 0206-3882-55
4 gram/Vial—10 per box—NDC 0206-3880-25
3 gram infusion Bottle—10 per box—NDC 0206-3882-65
4 gram infusion Bottle—10 per box—NDC 0206-3880-66
2 gram ADD-Vantage Vial—10 per box—NDC 0206-3879-27
3 gram ADD-Vantage Vial—10 per box—NDC 0206-3882-28
4 gram ADD-Vantage Vial—10 per box—NDC 0206-3880-29
40 gram Pharmacy Bulk Vial—NDC 0206-3877-60
This product should be stored at controlled room temperature 15°–30°C (59°–86°F).
Caution: Federal law prohibits dispensing without prescription.
Manufactured by:
LEDERLE PIPERACILLIN, INC.
Carolina, Puerto Rico 00987
Shown in Product Identification Guide, page 319

PNEUMOCOCCAL VACCINE POLYVALENT
PNU–IMUNE® 23   ℞
[new-ĭ-mūne]

DESCRIPTION
Pneumococcal Vaccine Polyvalent PNU-IMUNE 23 is a sterile preparation intended for intramuscular or subcutaneous use. PNU-IMUNE 23 is indicated for immunization against infections caused by the 23 most prevalent types of *Streptococcus pneumoniae* (pneumococci) which are responsible for approximately 90% of serious pneumococcal disease in the United States and worldwide.[1-5] PNU-IMUNE 23 consists of a mixture of purified capsular polysaccharides from 23 types of *S pneumoniae*.
[See table at top of next page]
Each of the pneumococcal polysaccharide types is produced separately to assure a high degree of purity. After an individual pneumococcal type is grown, the polysaccharide is separated from the cell and purified by a series of steps including ethanol fractionation. The vaccine is formulated to contain 25 μg of each of the 23 purified polysaccharide types

Continued on next page

Pnu-Imune 23—Cont.

per 0.5 mL dose of vaccine. Thimerosal (a mercury derivative) at a final concentration of 0.01% is added as a preservative.

The vaccine is a clear, colorless liquid.

CLINICAL PHARMACOLOGY

Disease caused by *S pneumoniae* remains an important cause of morbidity and mortality in the US, particularly in the very young, the elderly, and persons with certain high-risk conditions. Pneumococcal pneumonia accounts for 10% to 25% of all pneumonias and an estimated 40,000 deaths annually.[2]

Studies suggest annual rates of bacteremia of 15 to 19/100,000 for the total population, and 50/100,000 for persons 65 and older. Certain population groups, eg, Native Americans may have considerably higher disease rates.[2]

Mortality from pneumococcal disease is highest in patients with bacteremia or meningitis, patients with underlying medical conditions, and older persons. In some high-risk patients, mortality has been reported to be over 40% for bacteremic disease and 55% for meningitis, despite appropriate antimicrobial therapy.[2]

In addition to the very young and persons 65 years of age or older, patients with certain chronic conditions are at increased risk of developing pneumococcal infection and severe pneumococcal illness. Patients with chronic cardiovascular or pulmonary disease, diabetes mellitus, alcoholism, and cirrhosis are generally immunocompetent but have increased risk. Other patients at greater risk because of decreased responsiveness to polysaccharide antigens or more rapid decline in serum antibody include those with functional or anatomic asplenia (eg, sickle-cell disease or splenectomy), Hodgkin's disease, lymphoma, multiple myeloma, chronic renal failure, nephrotic syndrome, and organ transplantation. Studies indicate that patients with acquired immunodeficiency syndrome (AIDS) are also at increased risk of pneumococcal disease.[6,7] Recurrent pneumococcal meningitis may occur in patients with cerebrospinal fluid leakage that complicates skull fractures or neurologic procedures.

The polysaccharide capsules of pneumococci give these organisms resistance to the phagocytic action of polymorphonuclear leukocytes and monocytes. However, type-specific antibody facilitates their destruction in the body by the mechanism of complement-mediated lysis.

Most healthy adults, including the elderly, demonstrate at least a two-fold rise in type-specific antibodies within two to three weeks of immunization. Similar antibody responses have been reported in patients with alcoholic cirrhosis and diabetes mellitus. In contrast, elderly individuals with chronic pulmonary disease failed to mount a comparable immune response.[8] In immunocompromised patients, the response to immunization may also be lower. Children under two years of age respond poorly to most capsular polysaccharide types. Further, response to some pneumococcal types (eg, 6A and 14) important in pediatric infection is decreased in children less than 5 years of age.[9]

In clinical studies with PNU-IMUNE 23, more than 90% of all adults showed two-fold or greater increase in geometric mean antibody titer for each capsular type contained in the vaccine.[10]

Patients over the age of 2 years, with anatomical or functional asplenia and otherwise intact lymphoid function, generally respond to pneumococcal vaccines with a serological conversion comparable to that observed in healthy individuals of the same age.[11]

Patients with acquired immunodeficiency syndrome (AIDS) may have an impaired antibody response to pneumococcal vaccine.[7,12] However, asymptomatic human immunodeficiency virus (HIV)-infected patients, or those with generalized lymphadenopathy, respond to the 23-valent pneumococcal vaccine.[13]

Following immunization of healthy adults, antibody levels remain elevated for at least 5 years, but in some individuals these may fall to preimmunization levels within 10 years.[14,15] A more rapid decline in antibodies may occur in children, particularly those who have undergone a splenectomy and those with sickle-cell disease, in whom antibodies for some types can fall to preimmunization levels 3 to 5 years after immunization.[16,17] Similar rates of decline can occur in children with nephrotic syndrome.[18]

Controlled clinical trials in South Africa involving 12,000 gold miners have shown a 6-valent and a 13-valent pneumococcal vaccine to be 78.5% effective in preventing type-specific pneumococcal pneumonia and 82.3% effective in preventing pneumococcal bacteremia with the types contained in the vaccine.[19] In a preliminary study of an 8-valent polysaccharide vaccine in a group consisting of 77 patients with sickle-cell disease and 19 asplenic persons, there were no pneumococcal infections in the immunized patients within two years of immunization. There were eight cases of pneumococcal infection in 106 unimmunized, age-matched patients with sickle-cell disease. Antibody response of the asplenic patients was comparable to that of normal controls.[20]

Nomenclature

													Pneumococcal Types												
Danish	1	2	3	4	5	6B	7F	8	9N	9V	10A	11A	12F	14	15B	17F	18C	19F	19A	20	22F	23F	33F
US	1	2	3	4	5	26	51	8	9	68	34	43	12	14	54	17	56	19	57	20	22	23	70

In a study carried out by Austrian and colleagues with 13-valent pneumococcal vaccines prepared for the National Institute of Allergy and Infectious Disease, the reduction in pneumonias caused by the capsular types present in the vaccines was 79%. Reduction in type-specific pneumococcal bacteremia was 82%.[19]

In a double-blind study of a 14-valent pneumococcal vaccine carried out in Papua, New Guinea, pneumococcal infection was 84% lower in the immunized group and mortality from pneumonia 44% lower.[21]

Five case-control studies in the US have evaluated the efficacy of pneumococcal vaccine in the prevention of serious pneumococcal disease. Four of these studies showed the vaccine to be efficacious, with point estimates of efficacy ranging from 61% to 70%.[22-25] One study failed to show efficacy in preventing pneumococcal bacteremia.[26] This study was judged inadequate in determination of vaccination status, and the selection of controls was considered potentially biased.[2]

A prospective study failed to demonstrate efficacy against pneumococcal pneumonia and bronchitis;[8] this study has been criticized for methodological flaws.[2] In contrast, a prospective French study found pneumococcal vaccine to be 77% effective in reducing the incidence of pneumonia among nursing home residents.[27]

Despite conflicting findings, the data continue to support the use of pneumococcal vaccine for certain well-defined groups at risk.[2]

INDICATIONS AND USAGE

PNU-IMUNE 23 is indicated for immunization against pneumococcal disease caused by those pneumococcal types included in the vaccine.

Adults

1. All adults 65 or older,[2] with emphasis on immunization of the older adult while in good health.
2. Immunocompetent adults who are at increased risk of pneumococcal disease or its complications because of chronic illnesses (eg, cardiovascular or pulmonary disease, diabetes mellitus, alcoholism, cirrhosis, or cerebrospinal fluid leaks).[2]
3. Immunocompromised adults at increased risk of pneumococcal disease or its complications (eg, splenic dysfunction or anatomic asplenia, Hodgkin's disease, lymphoma, multiple myeloma, chronic renal failure, nephrotic syndrome, or conditions such as organ transplantation associated with immunosuppression).[2]

Children

1. Children 2 years of age or older with chronic illnesses specifically associated with increased risk of pneumococcal disease or its complications (eg, anatomic or functional asplenia [including sickle-cell disease], nephrotic syndrome, cerebrospinal fluid leaks, and conditions associated with immunosuppression).[2]

Special Groups

1. Persons living in special environments or social settings with an identified increased risk of pneumococcal disease or its complications.[2]
2. Patients with acquired immunodeficiency syndrome (AIDS) have been shown to have an impaired antibody response to pneumococcal vaccine. However, asymptomatic or symptomatic human immunodeficiency virus (HIV)-infected patients or those with persistent generalized lymphadenopathy respond to the 23-valent vaccine.[2]

Timing of Immunization

When elective splenectomy is being considered, pneumococcal vaccine should be given at least two weeks before surgery, if possible.[2]

For planning cancer chemotherapy or other immunosuppressive therapy, the interval between immunization and initiation of chemotherapy or immunosuppression should be at least two weeks.[2]

CONTRAINDICATIONS

HYPERSENSITIVITY TO ANY COMPONENT OF THE VACCINE, INCLUDING THIMEROSAL, A MERCURY DERIVATIVE, IS A CONTRAINDICATION TO THE USE OF THE PRODUCT.

THE OCCURRENCE OF ANY TYPE OF NEUROLOGICAL SYMPTOMS OR SIGNS FOLLOWING ADMINISTRATION OF THIS PRODUCT IS A CONTRAINDICATION TO FURTHER USE.

THE VACCINE SHOULD NOT BE ADMINISTERED TO PERSONS WITH ACUTE FEBRILE ILLNESSES UNTIL THEIR TEMPORARY SYMPTOMS AND/OR SIGNS HAVE ABATED.

The clinical judgment of the attending physician should prevail at all times.

WARNINGS

PNU-IMUNE 23 is not an effective agent for prophylaxis against pneumococcal disease caused by types not present in the vaccine.

PNU-IMUNE 23 is not indicated for children under two years of age, since antibody response to most capsular polysaccharide types is poor in this age group.[2]

Patients with impaired immune responsiveness whether due to the use of immunosuppressive therapy, a genetic defect, human immunodeficiency virus (HIV) infection, or other causes may have a reduced antibody response to active immunization procedures.[2]

Patients who have received extensive chemotherapy and/or splenectomy for the treatment of Hodgkin's disease have been shown to have an impaired serum antibody response to pneumococcal vaccine.[28,29]

In one study, administration of the vaccine to patients on immunosuppressive drugs and/or irradiation for Hodgkin's disease resulted in reduction of preexisting antibody levels in several patients.[28] It is unclear whether this effect was due to the vaccine or to the effects of irradiation and/or chemotherapy.

At least two weeks should elapse between immunization and the initiation of chemotherapy or immunosuppressive therapy.[2]

Routine reimmunization with this vaccine is not recommended. For reimmunization recommendations (including recommendations regarding reimmunization of individuals at highest risk of fatal pneumococcal infection) see **DOSAGE AND ADMINISTRATION.**

In one study, local reactions after reimmunization were more severe than after initial immunization when the interval between immunizations was 13 months.[30]

Patients who have had episodes of pneumococcal pneumonia or other pneumococcal infection may have high levels of preexisting pneumococcal antibodies that may result in increased reactions to PNU-IMUNE 23, mostly local, but occasionally systemic.[31] Caution should be exercised if such patients are considered for immunization with PNU-IMUNE 23.

Do not administer the vaccine intradermally since severe reactions may occur.

PRECAUTIONS

General

1. This product should not be used in children under 2 years of age.
2. PRIOR TO ADMINISTRATION OF ANY DOSE OF PNU-IMUNE 23, THE PARENT, GUARDIAN, OR ADULT PATIENT SHOULD BE ASKED ABOUT THE RECENT HEALTH STATUS, MEDICAL AND IMMUNIZATION HISTORY OF THE PATIENT TO BE IMMUNIZED TO DETERMINE THE EXISTENCE OF ANY CONTRAINDICATION TO IMMUNIZATION WITH PNEUMOCOCCAL VACCINE (SEE **CONTRAINDICATIONS, WARNINGS).**
3. BEFORE ADMINISTRATION OF ANY BIOLOGICAL, THE PHYSICIAN SHOULD TAKE ALL KNOWN PRECAUTIONS FOR PREVENTION OF ALLERGIC OR ANY OTHER REACTIONS. This includes: a review of the patient's history regarding possible sensitivity, the ready availability of epinephrine 1:1,000 and other appropriate agents used for control of immediate allergic reactions, and a knowledge of the recent literature pertaining to use of the biological concerned, including the nature of side effects and adverse reactions that may follow its use.
4. A separate sterile syringe and needle or a sterile disposable unit should be used for each individual patient to prevent transmission of infectious agents from one person to another.

PRIOR TO ADMINISTRATION OF THIS VACCINE, HEALTH CARE PERSONNEL SHOULD INFORM THE PARENT, GUARDIAN, OR ADULT PATIENT OF THE BENEFITS AND RISKS OF IMMUNIZATION WITH PNEUMOCOCCAL VACCINE.

Pregnancy Category C: Animal reproduction studies have not been conducted with PNU-IMUNE 23. It is also not known whether PNU-IMUNE 23 can cause fetal harm when administered to a pregnant woman or affect reproduction capacity. PNU-IMUNE 23 is not recommended for use in pregnant women.

It is not known whether the drug is excreted in human milk. Because many drugs are excreted in human milk, caution should be exercised when PNU-IMUNE 23 is administered to a nursing woman.

ADVERSE REACTIONS

Pneumococcal Vaccine Polyvalent PNU-IMUNE 23 is associated with a relatively low incidence of adverse reactions. The adverse reactivity observed in clinical studies was of short duration and not serious.

In a study of 32 individuals who received PNU-IMUNE 23, 23 (72%) experienced local reaction characterized by soreness at the injection site within 3 days after immunization.[10]

Low grade fever (less than 37.8°C [100°F]) and mild myalgia occur occasionally and are usually confined to the 24-hour period following immunization. Rash and arthralgia have been reported infrequently.

Although rare, fever over 38.9°C (102°F) and marked local swelling have been reported with pneumococcal polysaccharide vaccine. Rash, urticaria, arthritis, arthralgia, and adenitis have been reported rarely.

Patients with otherwise stabilized idiopathic thrombocytopenic purpura have, on rare occasions, experienced a relapse in their thrombocytopenia, occurring 2 to 14 days after immunization, and lasting up to 2 weeks.[32]

Reactions of greater severity, or extent are unusual. Rarely, anaphylactoid reactions have been reported.

Temporal association of neurological disorders such as paresthesias and acute radiculoneuropathy, including Guillain-Barré syndrome, have been reported following parenteral injections of biological products including pneumococcal vaccine.

DOSAGE AND ADMINISTRATION

The immunization schedule consists of a single 0.5 mL dose given intramuscularly or subcutaneously. Intradermal administration should be avoided. *Do not inject intravenously.* Parenteral drug products should be inspected visually for particulate matter and discoloration prior to administration (see **DESCRIPTION**).

Before injection, the skin at the injection site should be cleansed with a suitable germicide. After insertion of the needle, aspirate to help avoid inadvertent injection into a blood vessel.

Simultaneous Administration with Other Vaccines

Many patients who receive pneumococcal vaccine should also be immunized with influenza vaccine which may be given simultaneously at a different site. In contrast to pneumococcal vaccine, influenza vaccine is recommended annually.[2]

Reimmunization

The incidence of local reactions after reimmunization were found to be more severe than after initial immunization when the interval between immunizations was 13 months.[29] Reports of reimmunization after longer intervals in children and adults, including a large group of elderly persons reimmunized at least 4 years after primary immunization, suggest a similar incidence of such reactions.[2] The Immunization Practices Advisory Committee (ACIP) recommendations regarding reimmunization are as follows: Persons who receive the 14-valent vaccine should not *routinely* be reimmunized with the 23-valent vaccine. However, reimmunization with 23-valent vaccine should be strongly considered for persons who received the 14-valent vaccine *if they are at highest risk* of fatal pneumococcal infection (eg, asplenic patients). Reimmunization should also be carefully considered for adults at high risk who received the 23-valent vaccine more than 6 years before and for those shown to have a rapid decline in antibody levels (eg, patients with nephrotic syndrome, renal failure, or transplant patients). Reimmunization should be carefully considered after 3 to 5 years for children with nephrotic syndrome, asplenia, or sickle-cell anemia who would be 10 years old or younger at the time of reimmunization.[2]

HOW SUPPLIED

PNU-IMUNE 23 is supplied as follows:
NDC 0005-2309-31 2.5 mL Vial, for use with syringe only.
NDC 0005-2309-33 5 × One Dose (0.5 mL) LEDERJECT® Disposable Syringes.

STORAGE

DO NOT FREEZE. STORE REFRIGERATED, AWAY FROM FREEZER COMPARTMENT AT 2°C TO 8°C (36°F TO 46°F).

Directions for Use of the LEDERJECT Disposable Syringe:

1. Twist the plunger rod clockwise to be sure the rod is secure to rubber plunger base.

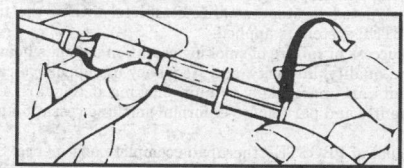

2. Hold needle shield in place with index finger and thumb of one hand while, with the other thumb, exert light pressure on plunger rod until the plunger base has been freed and demonstrates slight movement when pressure is applied.

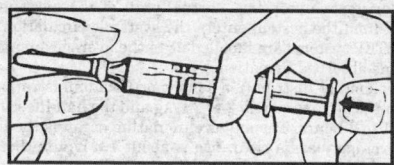

3. Grasp the rubber needle shield at its base; twist and pull to remove.

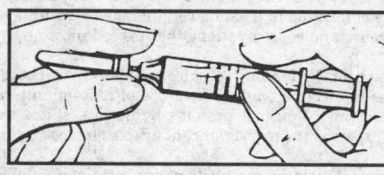

4. To prevent needle-stick injuries, needles should not be recapped, purposely bent, or broken by hand.

REFERENCES

1. Austrian R. Surveillance of pneumococcal infection for field trials of polyvalent vaccines. *Annual Contract Prog Report to the Nat Inst of Allerg and Inf Dis* 1975; Update to Dec. 1977, personal communication.
2. Immunization Practices Advisory Committee. Pneumococcal polysaccharide vaccine—recommendations of the ACIP. *MMWR.* 1989;38(5):64–76. Recommendations also published in: *JAMA.* 1989;261(9):1265–1267.
3. Lund E. Distribution of pneumococcal types at different times and different areas. In: Finland M, Marget W, Bartman K eds. *Bayer-Symposium III Bacterial Infections.* New York, NY:Springer-Verlag, 1971:49.
4. Mufson MA, Kruss DM, Wasil RE, et al. Capsular types and outcome of bacteremic pneumococcal disease in the antibiotic era. *Arch Int Med.* 1974;134:505–510.
5. Robbins JB, Austrian R, Lee CJ, et al. Consideration for formulating the second generation pneumococcal capsular polysaccharide vaccine with emphasis on the cross-reactive types within groups. *J Infec Dis.* 1983; 148(6):1136–1159.
6. Lane CH, Masur H, Edgar LC, et al. Abnormalities of B-cell activation and immunoregulation in patients with the acquired immunodeficiency syndrome. *N Engl J Med.* 1983;309:453–458.
7. Ammann AJ, Schiffman G, Abrams D, et al. B-cell immunodeficiency in acquired immune deficiency syndrome. *JAMA.* 1984;251:1447–1449.
8. Simberkoff MS, Cross AP, Al-Ibrahim M, et al. Efficacy of pneumococcal vaccine in high-risk patients: results of a Veterans Administration cooperative study. *N Eng J Med.* 1986;315:1318–1327.
9. Douglas RM, Paton JC, Duncan SJ, et al. Antibody response to pneumococcal vaccination in children younger than five years of age. *J Infect Dis.* 1983;148:131–137.
10. Data on file, Lederle Laboratories.
11. Sullivan JL, Ochs HD, Schiffman G, et al. Immune response after splenectomy. *Lancet.* 1978;1:178–181.
12. Ballet J-J, Sulcebe G, Couderc L-J, et al. Impaired antipneumococcal antibody response in patients with AIDS-related persistent generalized lymphadenopathy. *Clin Exp Immunol.* 1987;68:479–487.
13. Huang K-L, Ruben FL, Rinaldo CR Jr, et al. Antibody responses after influenza and pneumococcal immunization in HIV-infected homosexual men. *JAMA.* 1987; 257:2047–2050.
14. Mufson MA, Krause HE, Schiffman G. Long term persistence of antibodies following immunization with pneumococcal polysaccharide vaccine. *Proc Soc Exp Bio Med.* 1983;173:270–275.
15. Mufson MA, Krause HE, Schiffman G, et al. Pneumococcal antibody levels one decade after immunization of healthy adults. *Am J Med Sci.* 1987;293:279–284.
16. Giebiuk GS, Le CT, Schiffman G. Decline of serum antibody in splenectomized children after vaccination with pneumococcal capsular polysaccharides. *J Pediatr.* 1984;105:576–582.
17. Weintrub PS, Schiffman G, Addiego JE Jr, et al. Long-term follow-up and booster immunization with polyvalent pneumococcal polysaccharide in patient with sickle cell anemia. *J Pediatr.* 1984;105:261–263.
18. Spika JS, Halsey NA, Le CT, et al. Decline of vaccine-induced antipneumococcal antibody in children with nephrotic syndrome. *Am J Kidney Dis.* 1986;7:466–470.
19. Austrian R, Douglas RM, Schiffman G, et al. Prevention of pneumococcal pneumonia by vaccination. *Trans Assoc Am Phys.* 1976;89:184–194.
20. Ammann AJ, Addiego K, Wara DW, et al. Polyvalent pneumococcal-polysaccharide immunization of patients with sickle-cell anemia and patients with splenectomy. *N Engl J Med.* 1977;297:897–900.
21. Riley ID, Tarr PI, Andrews M, et al. Immunisation with a polyvalent pneumococcal vaccine: reduction of adult respiratory mortality in a New Guinea Highlands community. *Lancet.* 1977;1:1338–1341.
22. Shapiro ED, Clemens JD. A controlled evaluation of the protective efficacy of pneumococcal vaccine for patients at high risk of serious pneumococcal infections. *Ann Intern Med.* 1984;101:325–330.
23. Shapiro ED, Austrian R, Adair RK, et al. The protective efficacy of pneumococcal vaccine (Abstract). *Clin Res.* 1988;36:470A.
24. Sims RV, Steinmann WC, McConville JH, et al. The clinical effectiveness of pneumococcal vaccine in the elderly. *Ann Intern Med.* 1988;108:653–657.
25. Bolan G, Broome CV, Facklam RR, et al. Pneumococcal vaccine efficacy in selected populations in the United States. *Ann Intern Med.* 1986;104:1–6.
26. Forrester HL, Jahnigen DW, LaForce FM. Inefficacy of pneumococcal vaccine in a high-risk population. *Am J Med.* 1987;83:425–430.
27. Gaillat J, Zmirou D, Mallaret MR, et al. Essai clinique du vaccin antipneumococcique chez des personnes agées vivant en institution. *Rev Epidémiol Santé Publique.* 1985;33:437–444.
28. Siber GR, Weitzman SA, Aisenberg AC, et al. Impaired antibody response to pneumococcal vaccine after treatment for Hodgkin's disease. *N Eng J Med.* 1978;299:442–448.
29. Siber GR, Gorham C, Martin P, et al. Antibody response to pretreatment immunization and post-treatment boosting with bacterial polysaccharide vaccines in patients with Hodgkin's disease. *Ann Intern Med.* 1986;104:467–475.
30. Borgono JM, McLean AA, Vella PP, et al. Vaccination and revaccination with polyvalent pneumococcal polysaccharide vaccines in adults and infants. *Proc Soc Exper Biol Med.* 1978;157:148–154.
31. Ponka A, Leinonen M: Adverse reactions to polyvalent pneumococcal vaccine. *Scand J Infect Dis.* 1982;14:67–71.
32. Kelton JG. Vaccination-associated relapse of immune thrombocytopenia. *JAMA.* 1981;245(4):369–371.

Manufactured by:
LEDERLE LABORATORIES
Division American Cyanamid Company
Pearl River, NY 10965
US Gov't. License No. 17
Marketed by:
WYETH-LEDERLE VACCINES
Wyeth-Ayerst Laboratories
Philadelphia, PA 19101

Shown in Product Identification Guide, page 319

PROSTEP®
(nicotine transdermal system)
Systemic delivery of 22 or 11 mg/day over 24 hours

℞

DESCRIPTION

PROSTEP is a transdermal system that provides systemic delivery of nicotine following its application to intact skin. Nicotine is a tertiary amine composed of a pyridine and a pyrrolidine ring. It is a colorless to pale yellow, freely water-soluble, strongly alkaline, oily, volatile, hygroscopic liquid obtained from the tobacco plant. Nicotine has a characteristic pungent odor and turns brown on exposure to air or light. Of its two stereoisomers, *S* (-)-nicotine is the more active. It is the prevalent form in tobacco, and is the form in the PROSTEP system. The free alkaloid is absorbed rapidly through the skin and respiratory tract.

Chemical Name:
 S - 3 - (1-methyl-2-pyrrolidinyl)pyridine
Molecular Formula: $C_{10}H_{14}N_2$
Molecular Weight: 162.23
Ionization Constants: $pK_{a1}=7.84$, $pK_{a2}=3.04$
Octanol-Water Partition Coefficient: 15.1 at pH 7

The PROSTEP system is a round, flat adhesive pad with a round well in the center containing nicotine (the active agent) in a hydrogel matrix. Proceeding from the visible outer surface toward the inner surface attached to the skin are: (1) a beige-colored foam tape and pressure-sensitive acrylate adhesive; (2) backing foil, gelatin and low density polyethylene; (3) nicotine-gel matrix; (4) protective foil with well and (5) release liner which overlies the adhesive layer and must be removed prior to use. PROSTEP systems are packaged in child-resistant pouches.

Continued on next page

Prostep—Cont.

STICKY SIDE:
APPLY TO SKIN

NON-STICKY SIDE:
DISCARD

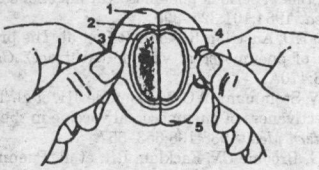

1 = FOAM TAPE AND ACRYLATE ADHESIVE
2 = BACKING FOIL, GELATIN AND LOW DENSITY POLYETHYLENE COATING
3 = NICOTINE-GEL MATRIX
4 = PROTECTIVE FOIL WITH WELL
5 = RELEASE LINER

Nicotine is the active ingredient; other components of the system are pharmacologically inactive.
The amount of nicotine delivered to the patient from each system (130 mcg/cm^2-h) is proportional to the surface area of the nicotine-gel matrix. About 27% of the total amount of nicotine remains in the system 24 hours after application. PROSTEP systems are labelled with the average dose absorbed by the patient. The dose of nicotine absorbed from a PROSTEP system represents 98% of the amount released from the system in 24 hours.

Dose Absorbed in 24 hrs (mg/day)	System Surface Area (cm^2)	Total Nicotine Content (mg)	Residual Nicotine after 24 hrs (mg)
22	7	30	8
11	3.5	15	4

CLINICAL PHARMACOLOGY
Pharmacologic Action
Nicotine, the chief alkaloid in tobacco products, binds stereoselectively to acetylcholine receptors at the autonomic ganglia, in the adrenal medulla, at neuromuscular junctions, and in the brain. Two types of central nervous system effects are believed to be the basis of nicotine's positively reinforcing properties. A stimulating effect, exerted mainly in the cortex via the locus ceruleus, produces increased alertness and cognitive performance. A "reward" effect via the "pleasure system" in the brain is exerted in the limbic system. At low doses the stimulant effects predominate while at high doses the reward effects predominate. Intermittent intravenous administration of nicotine activates neurohormonal pathways, releasing acetylcholine, norepinephrine, dopamine, serotonin, vasopressin, beta-endorphin, growth hormone, and ACTH.
Pharmacodynamics
The cardiovascular effects of nicotine include peripheral vasoconstriction, tachycardia, and elevated blood pressure. Acute and chronic tolerance to nicotine develops from smoking tobacco or ingesting nicotine preparations. Acute tolerance (a reduction in response for a given dose) develops rapidly (less than 1 hour) but not at the same rate for different physiologic effects (skin temperature, heart rate, subjective effects). Withdrawal symptoms, such as cigarette craving, can be reduced in some individuals by plasma nicotine levels lower than those from smoking.
Withdrawal from nicotine in addicted individuals is characterized by craving, nervousness, restlessness, irritability, mood lability, anxiety, drowsiness, sleep disturbances, impaired concentration, increased appetite, minor somatic complaints (headache, myalgia, constipation, fatigue), and weight gain. Nicotine toxicity is characterized by nausea, abdominal pain, vomiting, diarrhea, diaphoresis, flushing, dizziness, disturbed hearing and vision, confusion, weakness, palpitations, altered respirations and hypotension.
The cardiovascular effects of PROSTEP 22 mg/day systems include slight increase in heart rate and blood pressure. The cardiovascular effects of applying one or two PROSTEP 22 mg/day systems used continuously for 24 hours were compared to placebo for 7 days. Changes in heart rate (increased 4 beats/min), systolic blood pressure (increased 4 mmHg) and diastolic blood pressure (increased by 3 mmHg) were observed.
Both smoking and nicotine can increase circulating cortisol and catecholamines, and tolerance does not develop to the catecholamine-releasing effects of nicotine. Changes in the response to a concomitantly administered adrenergic agonist or antagonist should be watched for when nicotine intake is altered during nicotine replacement therapy with PROSTEP systems (see **Drug Interactions**).

Pharmacokinetics
Following application of the PROSTEP system to the upper body or upper outer arm, virtually all of the nicotine released from the system enters the systemic circulation. All PROSTEP systems are labelled as to the average amount of nicotine absorbed by patients.
The volume of distribution following IV administration of nicotine is approximately 2 to 3 L/kg and the half-life ranges from 1 to 2 hours. The major eliminating organ is the liver, and average plasma clearance is about 1.2 L/min; the kidney and lung also metabolize nicotine. There is no significant skin metabolism of nicotine. More than 20 metabolites of nicotine have been identified, all of which are believed to be less active than the parent compound. The primary metabolite of nicotine in plasma, cotinine, has a half-life of 15 to 20 hours and concentrations that exceed nicotine by 10-fold.
Plasma protein binding of nicotine is <5%. Therefore changes in nicotine binding from use of concomitant drugs or alterations of plasma proteins by disease states would not be expected to have significant effects on nicotine kinetics.
The primary urinary metabolites are cotinine (15% of the dose) and trans-3-hydroxycotinine (45% of the dose). Usually about 10% of nicotine is excreted unchanged in the urine. As much as 30% may be excreted unchanged in the urine with high urine flow rates and acidification below pH 5.
The pharmacokinetic model which best fits the plasma nicotine concentrations from PROSTEP systems is an open, two compartment model with a skin depot through which nicotine enters the central disposition compartment.
The PROSTEP system gel matrix contacts the skin directly and acts as a reservoir from which nicotine is absorbed slowly over the 24 hours.

Steady-State Plasma Nicotine Concentrations for Two Consecutive Applications of PROSTEP 22 mg/day (Mean ± 2 SD, N=22)

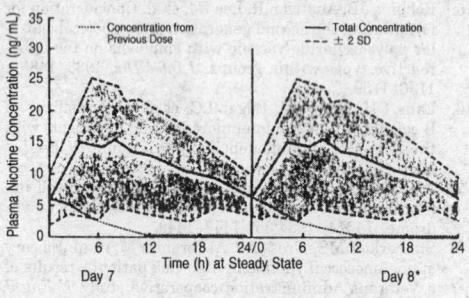

*Day 8 is a reproduction of Day 7 data to represent steady-state dosing.

Following application of a system, nicotine concentrations increase to a peak between 4 and 12 hours and then decrease gradually (see graph). Steady state for nicotine is attained within 2 days of initiating PROSTEP treatment and plasma nicotine concentrations average 23% higher compared to single-dose application. Plasma nicotine concentrations are proportional to dose (i.e., linear kinetics are observed) for the two dosages of PROSTEP systems. Nicotine kinetics are similar for all sites of application on the upper torso and upper outer arm.
Following removal of PROSTEP systems, plasma nicotine concentrations decline in an exponential fashion with an apparent mean half-life of 3–4 hours due to continued absorption from the skin depot (see dotted line in figure) in contrast to a half-life of 1–2 hours following IV administration. Most nonsmoking patients will have nondetectable nicotine concentrations in 10 to 12 hours after patch removal.

Steady State Nicotine Pharmacokinetic Parameters for 22 mg/day PROSTEP Systems (mean, std dev, range)

Parameter (units)	22 mg/day (N=22)		
	Mean	SD	Range
C_{max} (ng/mL)	16	6	7–31
C_{avg} (ng/mL)	11	3	6–17
C_{min} (ng/mL)	5	1	3–9
T_{max} (hrs)	9	5	4–24

C_{max}: maximum observed plasma concentration
C_{avg}: average plasma concentration
C_{min}: minimum observed plasma concentration
T_{max}: time of maximum plasma concentration

CLINICAL TRIALS
The efficacy of PROSTEP treatment as an aid to smoking cessation was demonstrated in two placebo-controlled, double-blind trials in otherwise healthy patients smoking at least one pack per day (N=516). In one of these trials, PROSTEP therapy was combined with concomitant individual patient counseling (10 minutes each visit) and in the other trial PROSTEP therapy was used with group counseling (1 hour each visit). In both trials, patients were treated for 8 weeks with a fixed dosage of 22 mg/day or placebo followed by abrupt cessation of PROSTEP treatment and decrease in support therapy. Patients in these two trials received prestudy counseling at two visits before beginning treatment. Two earlier trials (N=409) were carried out without prestudy counseling with treatment for 6 weeks and weaning to the 11 mg/day patch in one of them (N=329). In all four trials quitting was defined as total abstinence from smoking as measured by patient diary and verified by expired carbon monoxide. The "quit rates" are the proportions of all persons initially enrolled who abstained after week 2.

Quit Rates by Treatment After Week 2 (range by clinics)*

Nicotine Treatment	Number of Patients	After 6 Weeks	After 6 Months
PROSTEP (22 mg/day)	259	10%–57%	0%–37%
Placebo	257	3%–30%	0%–20%

* Trial involved 7 clinics, number of patients per treatment ranged from 29 to 60.

The two trials with prestudy counseling demonstrated that with concomitant support, fixed dosage therapy with PROSTEP therapy was more effective than placebo after 6 weeks and data from these 2 studies are combined in the quit rate table. At 8 weeks, just prior to abrupt termination of PROSTEP treatment (no weaning), quit rates were 6%–50%. At follow-up, three to five days later, quit rates were 3%–50%. In the two other studies without prestudy counseling, quit rates of 0%–46% with PROSTEP 22 mg/day and 3%–31% with placebo were observed at 6 weeks. In each of the four studies, there was a large variation in quit rates among clinics for each treatment.
Patients using PROSTEP systems dropped out of the trials significantly less frequently than did patients receiving placebo (26% vs 34%). The quit rate for 30 patients over age 60 was comparable to the quit rate for 486 patients aged 60 and under.
Patients who used the 22 mg/day PROSTEP treatment in clinical trials had a significant reduction in craving for cigarettes (desire to smoke), a major nicotine withdrawal symptom, as compared to placebo-treated patients (see figure). Reduction in craving, as with quit rate, is quite variable. This variability from clinic to clinic is presumed to be due to inherent differences in patient populations, e.g., patient motivation, concomitant illnesses, number of cigarettes smoked per day, number of years smoking, exposure to other smokers, socioeconomic status, etc., as well as differences among the clinics.

Severity of Craving by Treatment from Clinical Trials (N=516)

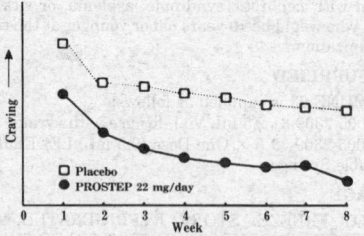

Individualization of Dosage
It is important to make sure that patients read the instructions made available to them and have their questions answered. They should clearly understand the directions for applying and disposing of PROSTEP systems. They should be instructed to stop smoking completely when the first PROSTEP system is applied.
The success or failure of smoking cessation depends heavily on the quality, intensity, and frequency of supportive care. Patients are more likely to quit smoking if they are seen frequently and participate in formal smoking cessation programs.
The goal of PROSTEP therapy is complete abstinence. Significant health benefits have not been demonstrated for reduction of smoking. If a patient is unable to stop smoking by the fourth week of therapy, treatment should probably be discontinued. Patients who have not stopped smoking after four weeks of PROSTEP therapy are unlikely to quit on that attempt.

Patients who fail to quit on any attempt may benefit from interventions to improve their chances for success on subsequent attempts. Patients who were unsuccessful should be counseled to determine why they failed. Patients should then probably be given a "therapy holiday" before the next attempt. A new quit attempt should be encouraged when the factors that contributed to failure can be eliminated or reduced, and conditions are more favorable.

Based on the clinical trials, a reasonable approach to assisting patients in their attempt to quit smoking is to initiate therapy with PROSTEP 22 mg/day except for small patients less than 100 pounds (see **DOSING SCHEDULE** below). The need for dose adjustment should be assessed during the first 2 weeks. The symptoms of nicotine withdrawal and toxicity overlap (see **Pharmacodynamics** and **ADVERSE REACTION** sections). Since patients using PROSTEP treatment may also smoke intermittently, it may be difficult to determine if patients are experiencing nicotine withdrawal or nicotine excess.

The controlled clinical trials using PROSTEP therapy suggest that sweating, abdominal pain, and somnolence are more often symptoms of nicotine excess while irritability is more often a symptom of nicotine withdrawal.

Patients should continue the dose selected with counseling and support over the following month. Those who have successfully stopped smoking during that time can stop PROSTEP treatment or may be weaned (reduction to 11 mg/day) over 4 weeks, after which treatment should be terminated.

May Require a Decrease in Dose at Cessation of Smoking	Possible Mechanism
acetaminophen, caffeine, imipramine, oxazepam, pentazocine, propranolol, theophylline	Deinduction of hepatic enzymes on smoking cessation.
insulin	Increase of subcutaneous insulin absorption with smoking cessation.
adrenergic antagonists (e.g., prazosin, labetalol)	Decrease in circulating catecholamines with smoking cessation.

May Require an Increase in Dose at Cessation of Smoking	Possible Mechanism
adrenergic agonists (e.g., isoproterenol, phenylephrine)	Decrease in circulating catecholamines with smoking cessation.

DOSING SCHEDULE

	Patients ≥100 lbs.	Patients <100 lbs.
Initial/Starting Dose	22 mg/day	11 mg/day
Duration of Treatment	4–8 weeks	4–8 weeks
Optional Weaning Dose	11 mg/day	off
Duration of Treatment	2–4 weeks	

INDICATIONS AND USAGE

PROSTEP treatment is indicated as an aid to smoking cessation for the relief of nicotine withdrawal symptoms. PROSTEP treatment should be used as a part of a comprehensive behavioral smoking cessation program.

The use of PROSTEP systems for longer than 3 months has not been studied.

CONTRAINDICATIONS

Use of PROSTEP systems is contraindicated in patients with hypersensitivity or allergy to nicotine or to any of the components of the therapeutic system.

WARNINGS

Nicotine from any source can be toxic and addictive. Smoking causes lung cancer, heart disease, emphysema, and may adversely affect the fetus and the pregnant woman. For any smoker, with or without concomitant disease or pregnancy, the risk of nicotine replacement in a smoking-cessation program should be weighed against the hazard of continued smoking while using PROSTEP systems, and the likelihood of achieving cessation of smoking without nicotine replacement.

Pregnancy Warning

Tobacco smoke, which has been shown to be harmful to the fetus, contains nicotine, hydrogen cyanide, and carbon monoxide. Nicotine has been shown in animal studies to cause fetal harm. It is therefore presumed that PROSTEP treatment can cause fetal harm when administered to a pregnant woman. The effect of nicotine delivery by PROSTEP systems has not been examined in pregnancy (see **PRECAUTIONS**). Therefore pregnant smokers should be encouraged to attempt cessation using educational and behavioral interventions before using pharmacological approaches. If PROSTEP therapy is used during pregnancy, or if the patient becomes pregnant while using PROSTEP treatment, the patient should be apprised of the potential hazard to the fetus.

Safety Note Concerning Children

The amounts of nicotine that are tolerated by adult smokers can produce symptoms of poisoning and could prove fatal if PROSTEP systems are applied or ingested by children or pets. Used 22 mg/day systems contain about 27% (8 mg) of their initial drug content. Therefore, patients should be cautioned to keep both used and unused PROSTEP systems out of the reach of children and pets.

PRECAUTIONS

The patient should be urged to stop smoking completely when initiating PROSTEP therapy (see **DOSAGE AND ADMINISTRATION**). Patients should be informed that if they continue to smoke while using PROSTEP systems, they may experience adverse effects due to peak nicotine levels higher than those experienced from smoking alone. If there is a clinically significant increase in cardiovascular or other effects attributable to nicotine, the PROSTEP dose should be reduced or PROSTEP treatment discontinued (see **WARNINGS**). Physicians should anticipate that concomitant medications may need dosage adjustment (see **Drug Interactions**).

The use of PROSTEP systems beyond 3 months by patients who stop smoking should be discouraged because the chronic consumption of nicotine by any route can be harmful and addicting.

Allergic Reactions

In a 3-week open-label dermal irritation and sensitization study of PROSTEP systems, 16 of 205 patients (8%) exhibited definite erythema at 24 hours after system removal. None of those patients exhibited contact allergy. In the first 4 weeks of the efficacy trials, moderate erythema following system removal was seen in 22% of patients, some edema in 8%, and dropouts due to skin reactions occurred in 7% of 459 patients using the 22 mg/day system. Patients who develop contact sensitization should be cautioned that a serious reaction could occur from exposure to other nicotine-containing products or smoking.

Patients should be instructed to promptly discontinue the PROSTEP treatment and contact their physician if they experience severe or persistent local skin reactions at the site of application (e.g., severe erythema, pruritus or edema) or a generalized skin reaction (e.g., urticaria, hives, or generalized rash).

Skin Disease

PROSTEP systems are usually well tolerated by patients with normal skin, but may be irritating for patients with some skin disorders (atopic or eczematous dermatitis).

Cardiovascular or Peripheral Vascular Diseases

The risks of nicotine replacement in patients with certain cardiovascular and peripheral vascular diseases should be weighed against the benefits of including nicotine replacement in a smoking cessation program for them. Specifically, patients with coronary heart disease (history of myocardial infarction and/or angina pectoris), serious cardiac arrhythmias, or vasospastic diseases (Buerger's disease, Prinzmetal's variant angina) should be carefully screened and evaluated before nicotine replacement is prescribed.

Tachycardia occurring in association with the use of PROSTEP treatment was reported occasionally. If serious cardiovascular symptoms occur with PROSTEP treatment, it should be discontinued.

PROSTEP treatment should generally not be used in patients during the immediate post-myocardial infarction period, patients with serious arrhythmias, and patients with severe or worsening angina pectoris.

Renal or Hepatic Insufficiency

The pharmacokinetics of nicotine have not been studied in the elderly or patients with renal or hepatic impairment. However, given that nicotine is extensively metabolized and that its total system clearance is dependent on liver blood flow, some influence of hepatic impairment on drug kinetics (reduced clearance) should be anticipated. Only severe renal impairment would be expected to affect the clearance of nicotine or its metabolites from the circulation (see **Pharmacokinetics**).

Endocrine Diseases

PROSTEP treatment should be used with caution in patients with hyperthyroidism, pheochromocytoma, or insulin-dependent diabetes since nicotine causes the release of catecholamines by the adrenal medulla.

Peptic Ulcer Disease

Nicotine delays healing in peptic ulcer disease; therefore, PROSTEP treatment should be used with caution in patients with active peptic ulcers and only when the benefits of including nicotine replacement in a smoking cessation program outweigh the risks.

Accelerated Hypertension

Nicotine constitutes a risk factor for development of malignant hypertension in patients with accelerated hypertension; therefore, PROSTEP treatment should be used with caution in these patients and only when the benefits of including nicotine replacement in a smoking cessation program outweigh the risks.

Information for Patient

A patient instruction sheet is included in the package of PROSTEP systems dispensed to the patient. It contains important information and instructions on how to use and dispose of PROSTEP systems properly. Patients should be encouraged to ask questions of the physician and pharmacist. Patients must be advised to keep both used and unused systems out of the reach of children and pets.

Drug Interactions

Smoking cessation, with or without nicotine replacement, may alter the pharmacokinetics of certain concomitant medications.

[See table above]

Carcinogenesis, Mutagenesis, Impairment of Fertility

Nicotine itself does not appear to be a carcinogen in laboratory animals. However, nicotine and its metabolites increased the incidences of tumors in the cheek pouches of hamsters and forestomach of F344 rats, respectively, when given in combination with tumor-initiators. One study, which could not be replicated, suggested that cotinine, the primary metabolite of nicotine, may cause lymphoreticular sarcoma in the large intestine in rats.

Neither nicotine nor cotinine were mutagenic in the Ames' *Salmonella* test. Nicotine induced repairable DNA damage in an *E. coli* test system. Nicotine was shown to be genotoxic in a test system using Chinese hamster ovary cells. In rats and rabbits, implantation can be delayed or inhibited by a reduction in DNA synthesis that appears to be caused by nicotine. Studies have shown a decrease in litter size in rats treated with nicotine during gestation.

PREGNANCY

Pregnancy Category D (see WARNINGS section)

The harmful effects of cigarette smoking on maternal and fetal health are clearly established. These include low birth weight, an increased risk of spontaneous abortion, and increased perinatal mortality. The specific effects of PROSTEP treatment on fetal development are unknown. Therefore pregnant smokers should be encouraged to attempt cessation using educational and behavioral interventions before using pharmacological approaches.

Spontaneous abortion during nicotine replacement therapy has been reported; as with smoking, nicotine as a contributing factor cannot be excluded.

PROSTEP treatment should be used during pregnancy only if the likelihood of smoking cessation justifies the potential risk of use of nicotine replacement by the patient, who may continue to smoke.

Teratogenicity

Animal Studies: Nicotine was shown to produce skeletal abnormalities in the offspring of mice when given doses toxic to the dams (25 mg/kg IP or SC).

Human Studies: Nicotine teratogenicity has not been studied in humans except as a component of cigarette smoke (each cigarette smoked delivers about 1 mg of nicotine). It has not been possible to conclude whether cigarette smoking is teratogenic to humans.

Other Effects

Animal Studies: A nicotine bolus (up to 2 mg/kg) to pregnant rhesus monkeys caused acidosis, hypercarbia, and hy-

Continued on next page

Prostep—Cont.

potension (fetal and maternal concentrations were about 20 times those achieved after smoking one cigarette in 5 minutes). Fetal breathing movements were reduced in the fetal lamb after intravenous injection of 0.25 mg/kg nicotine to the ewe (equivalent to smoking 1 cigarette every 20 seconds for 5 minutes). Uterine blood flow was reduced about 30% after infusion of 0.1 mg/kg/min nicotine for 20 minutes to pregnant rhesus monkeys (equivalent to smoking about six cigarettes every minute for 20 minutes).

Human Experience: Cigarette smoking during pregnancy is associated with an increased risk of spontaneous abortion, low birth weight infants and perinatal mortality. Nicotine and carbon monoxide are considered the most likely mediators of these outcomes. The effects of cigarette smoking on fetal cardiovascular parameters have been studied near term. Cigarettes increased fetal aortic blood flow and heart rate and decreased uterine blood flow and fetal breathing movements. PROSTEP treatment has not been studied in pregnant humans.

Labor and Delivery
PROSTEP systems are not recommended to be left on during labor and delivery. The effects of nicotine on the mother or the fetus during labor are unknown.

Use in Nursing Mothers
Caution should be exercised when PROSTEP therapy is administered to nursing women. The safety of PROSTEP treatment in nursing infants has not been examined. Nicotine passes freely into breast milk; the milk to plasma ratio averages 2.9. Nicotine is absorbed orally. An infant has the ability to clear nicotine by hepatic first pass clearance; however the efficiency of removal is probably lowest at birth. The nicotine concentrations in milk can be expected to be lower with PROSTEP treatment when used as directed than with cigarette smoking, as maternal plasma nicotine concentrations are generally reduced with nicotine replacement. The risk of exposure of the infant to nicotine from PROSTEP systems should be weighed against the risks associated with the infant's exposure to nicotine from continued smoking by the mother (passive smoke exposure and contamination of breast milk with other components of tobacco smoke) and from PROSTEP systems alone or in combination with continued smoking.

Pediatric Use
PROSTEP systems are not recommended for use in children because the safety and effectiveness of PROSTEP treatment in children and adolescents who smoke have not been evaluated.

Geriatric Use
Thirty patients over the age of 60 participated in clinical trials of PROSTEP therapy. PROSTEP therapy appeared to be as effective in this age group as in younger smokers.

ADVERSE REACTIONS
Assessment of adverse events in the 903 patients who participated in controlled clinical trials is complicated by the occurrence of GI and CNS effects of nicotine withdrawal as well as nicotine excess. The actual incidences of both are confounded by concurrent smoking by many of the patients. In the trials, when reporting adverse events, the investigators did not attempt to identify the cause of the symptom.

Topical Adverse Events
The most common adverse event associated with topical nicotine is a mild short-lived erythema, pruritus, or burning at the application site, which was seen at least once in 54% of patients (N=459) on PROSTEP treatment in the 6–8 week clinical trials. Local erythema after system removal was noted at least once in 22% of patients and local edema in 8%. Erythema generally resolved within 24 hours. Cutaneous hypersensitivity (contact sensitization) occurred in 3% of patients on PROSTEP treatment (see **PRECAUTIONS, Allergic Reactions**). Skin discoloration at application sites has been rarely reported.

Probably Causally Related
The following adverse events were reported more frequently in PROSTEP-treated patients than in placebo-treated patients or exhibited a dose response in clinical trials. The reports of awakening at night were collected as one of the expected withdrawal symptoms.
Digestive system—Abdominal pain[†], diarrhea[‡].
Nervous system—Somnolence*.
Skin—Rash,[†] sweating[†].
The following adverse events were reported in PROSTEP- and placebo-treated patients at about the same frequency in clinical trials and have also been reported post-marketing.
Digestive system—Nausea[†]

Frequencies for 22 mg/day system
* Reported in 3% to 9% of patients.
[†] Reported in 1% to 3% of patients.
[‡] Spontaneous reports only, not seen in clinical trials.
Unmarked if reported in <1% of patients.

Causal Relationship UNKNOWN
Adverse events reported in PROSTEP and placebo-treated patients at about the same frequency in clinical trials are listed below. The clinical significance of the association between PROSTEP treatment and these events is unknown, but they are reported as alerting information for the clinician.
Body as a Whole—Back pain,[†] pain*.
Digestive system—Constipation,[†] dyspepsia.
Musculoskeletal system—Myalgia[†].
Nervous system—Dizziness,[†] headache (11%), insomnia*, abnormal dreams[‡].
Respiratory system—Pharyngitis,* sinusitis*.
Urogenital system—Dysmenorrhea[†].

Frequencies for 22 mg/day system
* Reported in 3% to 9% of patients.
[†] Reported in 1% to 3% of patients.
[‡] Spontaneous reports only, not seen in clinical trials.
Unmarked if reported in <1% of patients.

DRUG ABUSE AND DEPENDENCE
PROSTEP systems are likely to have a low abuse potential based on differences between it and cigarettes in four characteristics commonly considered important in contributing to abuse: much slower absorption, much smaller fluctuations in blood levels, lower blood levels of nicotine, and less frequent use (i.e., once daily).
The abuse potential of PROSTEP systems was examined in a prospective, randomized trial of 10 smokers (5 drug abusers and 5 non-abusers). "Liking" scores for either one (22 mg/day) or two systems (44 mg/day) were no different from placebo. No abuse potential was observed in that study.
Dependence on nicotine polacrilex chewing gum replacement therapy has been reported and such dependence might also occur from transference to PROSTEP systems of tobacco-based nicotine dependence. The use of the system beyond 3 months has not been evaluated and should be discouraged.
PROSTEP therapy has been evaluated in both a gradual and abrupt discontinuation of treatment. If gradual withdrawal is desirable, patients using the 22 mg/day PROSTEP treatment should use the 11 mg/day dosage for 2 to 4 weeks (see **Individualization of Dosage** and **DOSAGE AND ADMINISTRATION**).

OVERDOSAGE
The effects of applying several PROSTEP systems simultaneously or of swallowing unused PROSTEP systems are unknown (see **WARNINGS, Safety Note Concerning Children**). The oral LD$_{50}$ for nicotine in rodents varies with the species but is in excess of 24 mg/kg; death is due to respiratory paralysis. The oral minimum lethal dose of nicotine in dogs is greater than 5 mg/kg. The oral minimum acute lethal dose for nicotine in human adults is reported to be 40 to 60 mg (<1 mg/kg).
PROSTEP gels containing 8 mg of nicotine were ingested by 12 adult smokers with an average weight of 74 kg (range 62–93 kg). Peak nicotine serum levels were 9.5 ng/mL (range 3–18 ng/mL) and occurred at 2 hours (1–2 hours) and declined to baseline levels by 8 hours after ingestion. Some gastrointestinal effects (burning on ingestion and nausea) were reported.
Signs and symptoms of an overdose of PROSTEP systems would be expected to be the same as those of acute nicotine poisoning including: pallor, cold sweat, nausea, salivation, vomiting, abdominal pain, diarrhea, headache, dizziness, disturbed hearing and vision, tremor, mental confusion, and weakness. Prostration, hypotension, and respiratory failure may ensue with large overdoses. Lethal doses produce convulsions quickly and death follows as a result of peripheral or central respiratory paralysis or, less frequently, cardiac failure.

Overdose from Topical Exposure
The PROSTEP system should be removed immediately if the patient shows signs of overdosage and the patient should seek immediate medical care. The skin surface may be flushed with water and dried. No soap should be used since it may increase nicotine absorption. Nicotine will continue to be delivered into the bloodstream for several hours (see **Pharmacokinetics**) after removal of the system because of a depot of nicotine in the skin.

Overdose from Ingestion
Ingestion of a 22 mg/day PROSTEP system containing 30 mg of nicotine is potentially more harmful than ingestion of a used system which contains about 8 mg after 24 hours use. Persons ingesting PROSTEP systems should be referred to a health care facility for management. Due to the possibility of nicotine-induced seizures, activated charcoal should be administered. In unconscious patients with a secure airway, instill activated charcoal via nasogastric tube. A saline cathartic or sorbitol added to the first dose of activated charcoal may speed gastrointestinal passage of the system. Repeated doses of activated charcoal should be administered as long as the system remains in the gastrointestinal tract since it will continue to release nicotine for many hours.

Management of Nicotine Poisoning
Other supportive measures include diazepam or barbiturates for seizures, atropine for excessive bronchial secretions or diarrhea, respiratory support for respiratory failure, and vigorous fluid support for hypotension and cardiovascular collapse.

DOSAGE AND ADMINISTRATION
Patients must desire to stop smoking and should be instructed to *stop smoking immediately* as they begin using PROSTEP therapy. The patient should read the patient instruction sheet on PROSTEP treatment and be encouraged to ask any questions. Treatment should be initiated with PROSTEP 22 mg/day except for patients who weigh less than 100 pounds. They may start with PROSTEP 11 mg/day and the dose increased as appropriate (see **Individualization of Dosage**). Once the appropriate dosage is selected the patient should begin 4–8 weeks of therapy at that dosage. The patient should stop smoking cigarettes completely during this period. If the patient is unable to stop cigarette smoking within 4 weeks, PROSTEP should probably be stopped, since few additional patients in clinical trials were able to quit after this time.
Those who have successfully stopped smoking during that time may have PROSTEP therapy discontinued. If a gradual reduction is desired, patients may be treated for an additional 2 to 4 weeks, after which treatment should be terminated.
The entire course of nicotine substitution should take 6–12 weeks. The use of PROSTEP systems beyond 3 months has not been studied and should be discouraged.
The PROSTEP system should be applied promptly upon its removal from the protective pouch to prevent evaporative loss of nicotine from the system. PROSTEP systems should be used only when the pouch is intact to assure that the product has not been tampered with.
PROSTEP systems should be applied only once a day to a non-hairy, clean, and dry skin site on the upper trunk or upper outer arm. After 24 hours, the used PROSTEP system should be removed and a new system applied to an alternate skin site. Skin sites should not be reused for at least a week. Patients should be cautioned not to continue to use the same system for more than 24 hours.

SAFETY AND HANDLING
PROSTEP systems can be a dermal irritant and can cause contact sensitization. Although exposure of health care workers to nicotine from PROSTEP systems should be minimal, care should be taken to avoid unnecessary contact with active systems. If you do handle active systems, wash with water alone, since soap may increase nicotine absorption. Do not touch your eyes.

Disposal
When the used system is removed from the skin, it should be folded over with the adhesive sides together and placed in the protective pouch which contained the new system. The used system should be immediately disposed of in such a way as to prevent its access by children or pets. See patient information for further directions for handling and disposal.

HOW SUPPLIED
[See table below]
How to Store
Do not store above 25°C (77°F) because PROSTEP systems are sensitive to heat. A slight discoloration of the system is not significant.
Do not store unpouched. Once removed from the protective pouch, PROSTEP systems should be applied promptly since nicotine is volatile and the system may lose strength.
CAUTION: Federal law prohibits dispensing without prescription.
© 1996
Manufactured for
LEDERLE PHARMACEUTICAL DIVISION
Pearl River, New York 10965
by
élan pharma Ltd.
Athlone, County Westmeath
Ireland
Using Elan's DERMAFLEX® transdermal system.
Shown in Product Identification Guide, page 320

Nicotine Delivery Rate (in vivo)	Nicotine in System	System Size	Package Size	NDC Number
22 mg/day	30 mg	7.0 cm²	7 systems	0005-2402-90
11 mg/day	15 mg	3.5 cm²	7 systems	0005-2401-90

PYRAZINAMIDE TABLETS, USP
500 mg

℞

DESCRIPTION

Pyrazinamide, the pyrazine analogue of nicotinamide, is an antituberculous agent. It is a white crystalline powder, stable at room temperature, and sparingly soluble in water. Pyrazinamide has the following chemical formula: $C_5H_5N_3O$, and the following molecular weight: 123.11.

Each Pyrazinamide tablet for oral administration contains 500 mg of pyrazinamide and the following inactive ingredients: Corn Starch, Magnesium Stearate, Modified Food Starch and Stearic Acid.

CLINICAL PHARMACOLOGY

Pyrazinamide is well absorbed from the GI tract and attains peak plasma concentrations within 2 hours. Plasma concentrations generally range from 30 to 50 mcg/mL with doses of 20 to 25 mg/kg. It is widely distributed in body tissues and fluids including the liver, lungs and cerebrospinal fluid (CSF). The CSF concentration is approximately equal to concurrent steady-state plasma concentrations in patients with inflamed meninges.[1] Pyrazinamide is approximately 10% bound to plasma proteins.[2]

The half-life (t1/2) of pyrazinamide is 9 to 10 hours in patients with normal renal and hepatic function. The plasma half-life may be prolonged in patients with impaired renal or hepatic function. Pyrazinamide is hydrolyzed in the liver to its major active metabolite, pyrazinoic acid. Pyrazinoic acid is hydroxylated to the main excretory product, 5-hydroxypyrazinoic acid.[3]

Approximately 70% of an oral dose is excreted in urine, mainly by glomerular filtration within 24 hours.[3]

Pyrazinamide may be bacteriostatic or bactericidal against *Mycobacterium tuberculosis* depending on the concentration of the drug attained at the site of infection. The mechanism of action is unknown. *In vitro* and *in vivo* the drug is active only at a slightly acidic pH.

INDICATIONS AND USAGE

Pyrazinamide is indicated for the initial treatment of active tuberculosis in adults and children when combined with other antituberculous agents. (The current recommendation of the CDC for drug-susceptible disease is to use a six-month regimen for initial treatment of active tuberculosis, consisting of isoniazid, rifampin and pyrazinamide given for 2 months, followed by isoniazid and rifampin for 4 months.*[4])

(Patients with drug-resistant disease should be treated with regimens individualized to their situation. Pyrazinamide frequently will be an important component of such therapy.) (In patients with concomitant HIV infection, the physician should be aware of current recommendations of CDC. It is possible these patients may require a longer course of treatment.)

It is also indicated after treatment failure with other primary drugs in any form of active tuberculosis.

Pyrazinamide should only be used in conjunction with other effective antituberculous agents.

*See recommendations of Center for Disease Control (CDC) and American Thoracic Society for complete regimen and dosage recommendations.[4]

CONTRAINDICATIONS

Pyrazinamide is contraindicated in persons:
- with severe hepatic damage.
- who have shown hypersensitivity to it.
- with acute gout.

WARNINGS

Patients started on pyrazinamide should have baseline serum uric acid and liver function determinations. Those patients with preexisting liver disease or those at increased risk for drug related hepatitis (e.g., alcohol abusers) should be followed closely.

Pyrazinamide should be discontinued and not be resumed if signs of hepatocellular damage or hyperuricemia accompanied by an acute gouty arthritis appear.

PRECAUTIONS
General

Pyrazinamide inhibits renal excretion of urates, frequently resulting in hyperuricemia which is usually asymptomatic. If hyperuricemia is accompanied by acute gouty arthritis, pyrazinamide should be discontinued.

Pyrazinamide should be used with caution in patients with a history of diabetes mellitus, as management may be more difficult.

Primary resistance of *M. tuberculosis* to pyrazinamide is uncommon. In cases with known or suspected drug resistance, *in vitro* susceptibility tests with recent cultures of *M. tuberculosis* against pyrazinamide and the usual primary drugs should be performed. There are few reliable *in vitro* tests for pyrazinamide resistance. A reference laboratory capable of performing these studies must be employed.

Recommended Drugs for the Initial Treatment of Tuberculosis in Children and Adults

Drug	Daily Dose*		Maximal Daily Dose in Children and Adults	Twice Weekly Dose	
	Children	Adults		Children	Adults
Isoniazid	10 to 20 mg/kg PO or IM	5 mg/kg PO or IM	300 mg	20 to 40 mg/kg Max. 900 mg	15 mg/kg Max. 900 mg
Rifampin	10 to 20 mg/kg PO	10 mg/kg PO	600 mg	10 to 20 mg/kg Max. 600 mg	10 mg/kg Max. 600 mg
Pyrazinamide	15 to 30 mg/kg PO	15 to 30 mg/kg PO	2 g	50 to 70 mg/kg	50 to 70 mg/kg
Streptomycin	20 to 40 mg/kg IM	15 mg/kg** IM	1 g**	25 to 30 mg/kg IM	25 to 30 mg/kg IM
Ethambutol	15 to 25 mg/kg PO	15 to 25 mg/kg PO	2.5 g	50 mg/kg	50 mg/kg

Definition of abbreviations: PO = perorally; IM = intramuscularly.

* Doses based on weight should be adjusted as weight changes.

** In persons older than 60 yrs of age the daily dose of streptomycin should be limited to 10 mg/kg with a maximal dose of 750 mg.

Information for Patients

Patients should be instructed to notify their physicians promptly if they experience any of the following: fever, loss of appetite, malaise, nausea and vomiting, darkened urine, yellowish discoloration of the skin and eyes, pain or swelling of the joints.

Compliance with the full course of therapy must be emphasized, and the importance of not missing any doses must be stressed.

Laboratory Tests

Baseline liver function studies [especially ALT (SGPT), AST (SGOT) determinations] and uric acid levels should be determined prior to therapy. Appropriate laboratory testing should be performed at periodic intervals and if any clinical signs or symptoms occur during therapy.

Drug/Laboratory Test Interactions

Pyrazinamide has been reported to interfere with ACE-TEST® and KETOSTIX® urine tests to produce a pink-brown color.[5]

Carcinogenicity, Mutagenicity, Impairment of Fertility[6,7,8]

In lifetime bioassays in rats and mice, pyrazinamide was administered in the diet at concentrations of up to 10,000 ppm. This resulted in estimated daily doses for the mouse of 2 g/kg, or 40 times the maximum human dose, and for the rat of 0.5 g/kg, or 10 times the maximum human dose. Pyrazinamide was not carcinogenic in rats or male mice and no conclusion was possible for female mice due to insufficient numbers of surviving control mice.

Pyrazinamide was not mutagenic in the Ames bacterial test, but induced chromosomal aberrations in human lymphocyte cell cultures.

Pregnancy: Teratogenic Effects—Pregnancy Category C

Animal reproduction studies have not been conducted with pyrazinamide. It is also not known whether pyrazinamide can cause fetal harm when administered to a pregnant woman or can affect reproduction capacity. Pyrazinamide should be given to a pregnant woman only if clearly needed.

Nursing Mothers

Pyrazinamide has been found in small amounts in breast milk. Therefore, it is advised the pyrazinamide be used with caution in nursing mothers taking into account the risk-benefit of this therapy.[9]

Usage in Children

Pyrazinamide regimens employed in adults are probably equally effective in children.[4,10,11] Pyrazinamide appears to be well tolerated in children.

Geriatric Use[12]

Clinical studies of pyrazinamide did not include sufficient numbers of patients aged 65 and over to determine whether they respond differently from younger patients. Other reported clinical experience has not identified differences in responses between the elderly and younger patients. In general, dose selection for an elderly patient should be cautious, usually starting at the low end of the dosing range, reflecting the greater frequency of decreased hepatic or renal function, and of concomitant disease or other drug therapy.

It does not appear that patients with impaired renal function require a reduction in dose. It may be prudent to select doses at the low end of the dosing range, however.[13]

ADVERSE REACTIONS
General

Fever, porphyria and dysuria have rarely been reported. Gout (see PRECAUTIONS).

Gastrointestinal

The principal adverse effect is a hepatic reaction (see WARNINGS). Hepatotoxicity appears to be dose related, and may appear at any time during therapy. GI disturbances including nausea, vomiting and anorexia have also been reported.

Hematologic and Lymphatic

Thrombocytopenia and sideroblastic anemia with erythroid hyperplasia, vacuolation of erythrocytes and increased serum iron concentration have occurred rarely with this drug. Adverse effects on blood clotting mechanisms have also been rarely reported.

Other

Mild arthralgia and myalgia have been reported frequently. Hypersensitivity reactions including rashes, urticaria, and pruritus have been reported. Fever, acne, photosensitivity, porphyria, dysuria and interstitial nephritis have been reported rarely.

OVERDOSAGE

Overdosage experience is limited. In one case report of overdose, abnormal liver function tests developed. These spontaneously reverted to normal when the drug was stopped. Clinical monitoring and supportive therapy should be employed. Pyrazinamide is dialyzable.[13]

DOSAGE AND ADMINISTRATION

Pyrazinamide should always be administered with other effective antituberculous drugs. It is administered for the initial 2 months of a 6-month or longer treatment regimen for drug-susceptible patients. Patients who are known or suspected to have drug-resistant disease should be treated with regimens individualized to their situation. Pyrazinamide frequently will be an important component of such therapy. Patients with concomitant HIV infection may require longer courses of therapy. Physicians treating such patients should be alert to any revised recommendations from CDC for this group of patients.

Usual dose: Pyrazinamide is administered orally, 15 to 30 mg/kg once daily. Older regimens employed 3 to 4 divided doses daily, but most current recommendations are for once a day. Three grams per day should not be exceeded. The CDC recommendations do not exceed 2 g per day when given as a daily regimen (see table).

Alternatively, a twice weekly dosing regimen (50 to 70 mg/kg twice weekly based on lean body weight) has been developed to promote patient compliance with a regimen on an outpatient basis. In studies evaluating the twice weekly regimen, doses of pyrazinamide in excess of 3 g twice weekly have been administered. This exceeds the recommended maximum 3 g/daily dose. However, an increased incidence of adverse reactions has not been reported.

The table is taken from the CDC-American Thoracic Society joint recommendations:[4]

[See table above]

HOW SUPPLIED

Pyrazinamide Tablets, USP 500 mg are round, white, scored tablets, engraved P36 on the scored side, and LL on the other side, supplied as:

NDC 0005-5093-23 - Bottle of 100
NDC 0005-5093-31 - Bottle of 500

Store in a well-closed container at controlled room temperature 15°–30°C (59°–86°F).

Caution: Federal law prohibits dispensing without prescription.

Manufactured by:
LEDERLE PHARMACEUTICAL DIVISION
American Cyanamid Company
Pearl River, NY 10965

REFERENCES

1. *Drug Information, American Hospital Formulary Service.* American Society of Hospital Pharmacists. Bethesda, Md. 1991.

Continued on next page

Pyrazinamide—Cont.

2. *USPDI, Drug Information for the Health Care Professional.* United States Pharmacopeial Convention, Inc. Rockville, Md. 1991:1B:2226–2227.
3. Goodman-Gilman A, Rall TW, Nies AS, Taylor P. *The Pharmacological Basis of Therapeutics,* ed 8. New York, Pergamon Press. 1990;1154.
4. Treatment of tuberculosis and tuberculosis infection in adults and children. *Am Rev Respir Dis.* 1986;134:363–368.
5. Reynolds JEF, Parfitt K, Parsons AV, Sweetman SC. *Martindale The Extra Pharmacopeia,* ed 29. London, The Pharmaceutical Press. 1989;569-570.
6. Bioassay of pyrazinamide for possible carcinogenicity. National Cancer Institute Carcinogenesis Technical Report Series No. 48, 1978.
7. Zerger E, Anderson B, Haworth S, Lawlor T, Mortelmans K, Speck W. Salmonella mutagenicity tests: III. Results from the testing of 255 chemicals. *Environ Mutagen.* 1987;9(Suppl 9):1–109.
8. Roman IC, Georgian L. Cytogenetic effects of some antituberculosis drugs in vitro. *Mutation Research.* 1977;48:215–224.
9. Holdiness M. Antituberculosis drugs and breast-feeding. *Arch Intern Med.* 1984;144:1888.
10. Turcios N, Evans H. Preventing and managing tuberculosis in children. *J Resp Dis.* 1989;10(6)(Jun):23.
11. Starke JR. Multidrug therapy for tuberculosis in children. *Pediatr Infec Dis J.* 1990;9:785–793.
12. Specific requirements on content and format of labeling for human prescription drugs; proposed addition of "geriatric use" subsection in the labeling. *Federal Register.* 1990;55(212) (Nov 1):46134–46137.
13. Stamathakis G, Montes C, Trouvin JH, et al. Pyrazinamide and pyrazinoic acid pharmacokinetics in patients with chronic renal failure. *Clinical Nephrology.* 1988;30:230–234.

RHEUMATREX® Dose Pack   ℞
Methotrexate 2.5 mg Tablets

Please see page 1397 for full Prescribing Information for Methotrexate.

Shown in Product Identification Guide, page 320

SUPRAX®   ℞
Cefixime
Oral

DESCRIPTION

SUPRAX (cefixime) is a semisynthetic, cephalosporin antibiotic for oral administration. Chemically, it is (6R,7R)-7-[2-(2-Amino-4-thiazolyl)glyoxylamido]-8-oxo-3-vinyl-5-thia-1-azabicyclo[4.2.0]oct-2-ene-2-carboxylic acid, 7^2-(Z)-[O-(carboxymethyl)oxime]trihydrate. Molecular weight = 507.50 as the trihydrate.
SUPRAX is available in scored 200 mg and 400 mg film coated tablets and in a powder for oral suspension which when reconstituted provides 100 mg/5 mL.
Inactive ingredients contained in the 200 mg and 400 mg tablets are: dibasic calcium phosphate, hydroxypropyl methylcellulose 2910, light mineral oil, magnesium stearate, microcrystalline cellulose, pregelatinized starch, sodium lauryl sulfate, and titanium dioxide. The powder for oral suspension is strawberry flavored and contains sodium benzoate, sucrose, and xanthan gum.

CLINICAL PHARMACOLOGY

SUPRAX, given orally, is about 40% to 50% absorbed whether administered with or without food; however, time to maximal absorption is increased approximately 0.8 hours when administered with food. A single 200 mg tablet of SUPRAX produces an average peak serum concentration of approximately 2 mcg/mL (range 1 to 4 mcg/mL); a single 400 mg tablet produces an average peak concentration of approximately 3.7 mcg/mL (range 1.3 to 7.7 mcg/mL). The oral suspension produces average peak concentrations approximately 25%–50% higher than the tablets, when tested in normal *adult* volunteers. Two hundred and 400 mg doses of oral suspension produce average peak concentrations of 3 mcg/mL (range 1 to 4.5 mcg/mL) and 4.6 mcg/mL (range 1.9 to 7.7 mcg/mL), respectively, when tested in normal *adult* volunteers. The area under the time versus concentration curve is greater by approximately 10%–25% with the oral suspension than with the tablet after doses of 100 to 400 mg, when tested in normal *adult* volunteers. This increased absorption should be taken into consideration if the oral suspension is to be substituted for the tablet. Because of the lack of bioequivalence, tablets should not be substituted for oral suspension in the treatment of otitis media. (See **DOSAGE AND ADMINISTRATION.**) Cross-over studies of tablet versus suspension have not been performed in children.
Peak serum concentrations occur between 2 and 6 hours following oral administration of a single 200 mg tablet, a single 400 mg tablet, or 400 mg of suspension of SUPRAX. Peak serum concentrations occur between 2 and 5 hours following a single administration of 200 mg of suspension.

TABLE

Serum Levels of Cefixime
After Administration of Tablets (mcg/mL)

DOSE	1h	2h	4h	6h	8h	12h	24h
100 mg	0.3	0.8	1.0	0.7	0.4	0.2	0.02
200 mg	0.7	1.4	2.0	1.5	1.0	0.4	0.03
400 mg	1.2	2.5	3.5	2.7	1.7	0.6	0.04

Serum Levels of Cefixime
After Administration of Oral Suspension (mcg/mL)

DOSE	1h	2h	4h	6h	8h	12h	24h
100 mg	0.7	1.1	1.3	0.9	0.6	0.2	0.02
200 mg	1.2	2.1	2.8	2.0	1.3	0.5	0.07
400 mg	1.8	3.3	4.4	3.3	2.2	0.8	0.07

Approximately 50% of the absorbed dose is excreted unchanged in the urine in 24 hours. In animal studies, it was noted that cefixime is also excreted in the bile in excess of 10% of the administered dose. Serum protein binding is concentration independent with a bound fraction of approximately 65%. In a multiple dose study conducted with a research formulation which is less bioavailable than the tablet or suspension, there was little accumulation of drug in serum or urine after dosing for 14 days.
The serum half-life of cefixime in healthy subjects is independent of dosage form and averages 3.0–4.0 hours but may range up to 9 hours in some normal volunteers. Average AUCs at steady state in elderly patients are approximately 40% higher than average AUCs in other healthy adults.
In subjects with moderate impairment of renal function (20 to 40mL/min creatinine clearance), the average serum half-life of cefixime is prolonged to 6.4 hours. In severe renal impairment (5 to 20 mL/min creatinine clearance), the half-life increased to an average of 11.5 hours. The drug is not cleared significantly from the blood by hemodialysis or peritoneal dialysis. However, a study indicated that with doses of 400 mg, patients undergoing hemodialysis have similar blood profiles as subjects with creatinine clearances of 21–60 mL/min. There is no evidence of metabolism of cefixime *in vivo*.
Adequate data on CSF levels of cefixime are not available.

MICROBIOLOGY

As with other cephalosporins, bactericidal action of SUPRAX results from inhibition of cell-wall synthesis. SUPRAX is highly stable in the presence of beta-lactamase enzymes. As a result, many organisms resistant to penicillins and some cephalosporins due to the presence of beta-lactamases, may be susceptible to cefixime. SUPRAX has been shown to be active against most strains of the following organisms both *in vitro* and in clinical infections (see **INDICATIONS AND USAGE**):
Gram-positive Organisms.
  Streptococcus pneumoniae,
  Streptococcus pyogenes,
Gram-negative Organisms.
  Haemophilus influenzae (beta-lactamase positive and negative strains),
  Moraxella (Branhamella) catarrhalis (most of which are beta-lactamase positive),
  Escherichia coli,
  Proteus mirabilis.

Neisseria gonorrhoeae (including penicillinase- and non-penicillinase-producing strains).
SUPRAX has been shown to be active *in vitro* against most strains of the following organisms; however, clinical efficacy has not been established.
Gram-positive Organisms.
  Streptococcus agalactiae.
Gram-negative Organisms.
  Haemophilus parainfluenzae (beta-lactamase positive and negative strains),
  Proteus vulgaris,
  Klebsiella pneumoniae,
  Klebsiella oxytoca,
  Pasteurella multocida,
  Providencia species,
  Salmonella species,
  Shigella species,
  Citrobacter amalonaticus,
  Citrobacter diversus,
  Serratia marcescens.
Note: *Pseudomonas* species, strains of group D streptococci (including enterococci), *Listeria monocytogenes*, most strains of staphylococci (including methicillin-resistant strains) and most strains of *Enterobacter* are resistant to SUPRAX. In addition, most strains of *Bacteroides fragilis* and *Clostridia* are resistant to SUPRAX.

SUSCEPTIBILITY TESTING

SUSCEPTIBILITY TESTS: DIFFUSION TECHNIQUES
Quantitative methods that require measurement of zone diameters give an estimate of antibiotic susceptibility. One such procedure[1–3] has been recommended for use with disks to test susceptibility to cefixime. Interpretation involves correlation of the diameters obtained in the disk test with minimum inhibitory concentration (MIC) for cefixime.
Reports from the laboratory giving results of the standard single-disk susceptibility test with a 5-mcg cefixime disk should be interpreted according to the following criteria:
[See table at bottom of page]
A report of "Susceptible" indicates that the pathogen is likely to be inhibited by generally achievable blood levels. A report of "Moderately Susceptible" indicates that inhibitory concentrations of the antibiotic may well be achieved if high dosage is used or if the infection is confined to tissues and fluids (eg, urine) in which high antibiotic levels are attained. A report of "Resistant" indicates that achievable concentrations of the antibiotic are unlikely to be inhibitory and other therapy should be selected.
Standardized procedures require the use of laboratory control organisms. The 5-mcg disk should give the following zone diameter:

Organism	Zone diameter (mm)
E. coli ATCC 25922	23–27
N. gonorrhoeae ATCC 49226[a]	37–45

[a] Using GC Agar Base with a defined 1% supplement with cysteine.

The class disk for cephalosporin susceptibility testing (the cephalothin disk) is not appropriate because of spectrum differences with cefixime. The 5-mcg cefixime disk should be used for all *in vitro* testing of isolates.
Dilution Techniques: Broth or agar dilution methods can be used to determine the minimum inhibitory concentration (MIC) value for susceptibility of bacterial isolates to cefixime. The recommended susceptibility breakpoints are as follows:
[See table at top of next page]
As with standard diffusion methods, dilution procedures require the use of laboratory control organisms. Standard cefixime powder should give the following MIC ranges in daily testing of quality control organisms:

Organism	MIC Range (µg/mL)
E. coli ATCC 25922	0.25 –1
S. aureus ATCC 29213	8–32
N. gonorrhoeae ATCC 49226[a]	0.008-0.03

[a] Using GC Agar Base with a defined 1% supplement without cysteine.

INDICATIONS AND USAGE

SUPRAX (cefixime) is indicated in the treatment of the following infections when caused by susceptible strains of the designated microorganisms:
Uncomplicated Urinary Tract Infections caused by *Escherichia coli* and *Proteus mirabilis.*
Otitis Media caused by *Haemophilus influenzae* (beta-lactamase positive and negative strains), *Moraxella (Branhamella) catarrhalis,* (most of which are beta-lactamase positive) and *S. pyogenes.**

SUPRAX®   Recommended Susceptibility Ranges: Agar Disk Diffusion

Organisms	Resistant	Moderately Susceptible	Susceptible
Neisseria gonorrhoeae[a]	—	—	≥31 mm
All other organisms	≤ 15 mm	16–18 mm	≥19 mm

[a] Using GC Agar Base with a defined 1% supplement without cysteine.

Note: For information on otitis media caused by *Streptococcus pneumoniae,* see **CLINICAL STUDIES** section.

Pharyngitis and Tonsillitis, caused by *S. pyogenes.*

Note: Penicillin is the usual drug of choice in the treatment of *S. pyogenes* infections, including the prophylaxis of rheumatic fever. SUPRAX is generally effective in the eradication of *S. pyogenes* from the nasopharynx; however, data establishing the efficacy of SUPRAX in the subsequent prevention of rheumatic fever are not available.

Acute Bronchitis and Acute Exacerbations of Chronic Bronchitis, caused by *Streptococcus pneumoniae* and *Haemophilus influenzae* (beta-lactamase positive and negative strains).

Uncomplicated Gonorrhea (cervical/urethral), caused by *Neisseria gonorrhoeae* (penicillinase- and nonpenicillinase-producing strains).

Appropriate cultures and susceptibility studies should be performed to determine the causative organism and its susceptibility to SUPRAX; however, therapy may be started while awaiting the results of these studies. Therapy should be adjusted, if necessary, once these results are known.

* Efficacy for this organism in this organ system was studied in fewer than 10 infections.

CLINICAL STUDIES

In clinical trials of otitis media in nearly 400 children between the ages of 6 months to 10 years, *Streptococcus pneumoniae* was isolated from 47% of the patients, *Haemophilus influenzae* from 34%, *Moraxella (Branhamella) catarrhalis* from 15%, and *S. pyogenes* from 4%.

The overall response rate of *Streptococcus pneumoniae* to cefixime was approximately 10% lower and that of *Haemophilus influenzae* or *Moraxella (Branhamella) catarrhalis* approximately 7% higher (12% when beta-lactamase positive strains of *H. influenzae* are included) than the response rates of these organisms to the active control drugs.

In these studies, patients were randomized and treated with either cefixime at dose regimens of 4 mg/kg BID or 8 mg/kg QD, or with a standard antibiotic regimen. Sixty-nine to 70% of the patients in each group had resolution of signs and symptoms of otitis media when evaluated 2 to 4 weeks posttreatment, but persistent effusion was found in 15% of the patients. When evaluated at the completion of therapy, 17% of patients receiving cefixime and 14% of patients receiving effective comparative drugs (18% including those patients who had *Haemophilus influenzae* resistant to the control drug and who received the control antibiotic) were considered to be treatment failures. By the 2 to 4 week follow-up, a total of 30%–31% of patients had evidence of either treatment failure or recurrent disease.

[See second table above]

CONTRAINDICATIONS

SUPRAX is contraindicated in patients with known allergy to the cephalosporin group of antibiotics.

WARNINGS

BEFORE THERAPY WITH SUPRAX IS INSTITUTED, CAREFUL INQUIRY SHOULD BE MADE TO DETERMINE WHETHER THE PATIENT HAS HAD PREVIOUS HYPERSENSITIVITY REACTIONS TO CEPHALOSPORINS, PENICILLINS, OR OTHER DRUGS. IF THIS PRODUCT IS TO BE GIVEN TO PENICILLIN-SENSITIVE PATIENTS, CAUTION SHOULD BE EXERCISED BECAUSE CROSS-HYPERSENSITIVITY AMONG BETA-LACTAM ANTIBIOTICS HAS BEEN CLEARLY DOCUMENTED AND MAY OCCUR IN UP TO 10% OF PATIENTS WITH A HISTORY OF PENICILLIN ALLERGY. IF AN ALLERGIC REACTION TO SUPRAX OCCURS, DISCONTINUE THE DRUG. SERIOUS ACUTE HYPERSENSITIVITY REACTIONS MAY REQUIRE TREATMENT WITH EPINEPHRINE AND OTHER EMERGENCY MEASURES, INCLUDING OXYGEN, INTRAVENOUS FLUIDS, INTRAVENOUS ANTIHISTAMINES, CORTICOSTEROIDS, PRESSOR AMINES AND AIRWAY MANAGEMENT, AS CLINICALLY INDICATED.

Antibiotics, including SUPRAX, should be administered cautiously to any patient who has demonstrated some form of allergy, particularly to drugs.

Treatment with broad-spectrum antibiotics, including SUPRAX, alters the normal flora of the colon and may permit overgrowth of clostridia. Studies indicate that a toxin produced by *Clostridium difficile* is a primary cause of severe antibiotic-associated diarrhea, including pseudomembranous colitis.

Pseudomembranous colitis has been reported with the use of SUPRAX and other broad-spectrum antibiotics (including macrolides, semisynthetic penicillins, and cephalosporins); therefore, it is important to consider this diagnosis in patients who develop diarrhea in association with the use of antibiotics. Symptoms of pseudomembranous colitis may occur during or after antibiotic treatment and may range in severity from mild to life- threatening. Mild cases of pseudomembranous colitis usually respond to drug discontinuation alone. In moderate to severe cases, management should include fluids, electrolytes, and protein supplementation. If the colitis does not improve after the drug has been discontinued, or if the symptoms are severe, oral vancomycin is the drug of choice for antibiotic-associated pseudomembranous colitis produced by *C difficile.* Other causes of colitis should be excluded.

MIC Interpretive Standards (μg/mL)

Organisms	Resistant	Moderately Susceptible	Susceptible
Neisseria gonorrhoeae[a]	—	—	≤ 0.25
All other organisms	≥ 4	2	≤ 1

Bacteriological Outcome of Otitis Media at Two to Four Weeks Post-Therapy Based on Repeat Middle Ear Fluid Culture or Extrapolation from Clinical Outcome

Organism	Cefixime[(a)] 4 mg/kg BID		Cefixime[(a)] 8 mg/kg QD		Control[(a)] drugs	
Streptococcus pneumoniae	48/70	(69%)	18/22	(82%)	82/100	(82%)
Haemophilus influenzae beta-lactamase negative	24/34	(71%)	13/17	(76%)	23/34	(68%)
Haemophilus influenzae beta-lactamase positive	17/22	(77%)	9/12	(75%)	1/1[(b)]	
Moraxella (Branhamella) catarrhalis	26/31	(84%)	5/5		18/24	(75%)
S. pyogenes	5/5		3/3		6/7	
All Isolates	120/162	(74%)	48/59	(81%)	130/166	(78%)

(a) Number eradicated/number isolated.

(b) An additional 20 beta-lactamase positive strains of *Haemophilus influenzae* were isolated, but were excluded from this analysis because they were resistant to the control antibiotic. In nineteen of these, the clinical course could be assessed, and a favorable outcome occurred in 10. When these cases are included in the overall bacteriological evaluation of therapy with the control drugs, 140/185 (76%) of pathogens were considered to be eradicated.

PRECAUTIONS

GENERAL

The possibility of the emergence of resistant organisms, which might result in overgrowth should be kept in mind, particularly during prolonged treatment. In such use, careful observation of the patient is essential. If superinfection occurs during therapy, appropriate measures should be taken.

The dose of SUPRAX should be adjusted in patients with renal impairment as well as those undergoing continuous ambulatory peritoneal dialysis (CAPD) and hemodialysis (HD). Patients on dialysis should be monitored carefully. (See **DOSAGE AND ADMINISTRATION**.)

SUPRAX should be prescribed with caution in individuals with a history of gastrointestinal disease, particularly colitis.

DRUG INTERACTIONS

Carbamazepine: Elevated carbamazepine levels have been reported when SUPRAX is administered concomitantly. Drug monitoring may be of assistance in detecting alterations in carbamazepine plasma concentrations.

DRUG/LABORATORY TEST INTERACTIONS

A false-positive reaction for ketones in the urine may occur with tests using nitroprusside but not with those using nitroferricyanide.

The administration of SUPRAX may result in a false-positive reaction for glucose in the urine using Clinitest®,** Benedict's solution, or Fehling's solution. It is recommended that glucose tests based on enzymatic glucose oxidase reactions (such as Clinistix®** or Tes-Tape®**) be used.

A false-positive direct Coombs test has been reported during treatment with other cephalosporin antibiotics; therefore, it should be recognized that a positive Coombs test may be due to the drug.

CARCINOGENESIS, MUTAGENESIS, IMPAIRMENT OF FERTILITY

Lifetime studies in animals to evaluate carcinogenic potential have not been conducted. SUPRAX did not cause point mutations in bacteria or mammalian cells, DNA damage, or chromosome damage *in vitro* and did not exhibit clastogenic potential *in vivo* in the mouse micronucleus test. In rats, fertility and reproductive performance were not affected by cefixime at doses up to 125 times the adult therapeutic dose.

USAGE IN PREGNANCY

Pregnancy Category B: Reproduction studies have been performed in mice and rats at doses up to 400 times the human dose and have revealed no evidence of harm to the fetus due to SUPRAX. There are no adequate and well-controlled studies in pregnant women. Because animal reproduction studies are not always predictive of human response, this drug should be used during pregnancy only if clearly needed.

LABOR AND DELIVERY

SUPRAX has not been studied for use during labor and delivery. Treatment should only be given if clearly needed.

NURSING MOTHERS

It is not known whether SUPRAX is excreted in human milk. Consideration should be given to discontinuing nursing temporarily during treatment with this drug.

PEDIATRIC USE

Safety and effectiveness of SUPRAX in children aged less than 6 months old have not been established.

The incidence of gastrointestinal adverse reactions, including diarrhea and loose stools, in the pediatric patients receiving the suspension, was comparable to the incidence seen in adult patients receiving tablets.

ADVERSE REACTIONS

Most of the adverse reactions observed in clinical trials were of a mild and transient nature. Five percent (5%) of patients in the US trials discontinued therapy because of drug-related adverse reactions. The most commonly seen adverse reactions in US trials of the tablet formulation were gastrointestinal events, which were reported in 30% of adult patients on either the BID or the QD regimen. Clinically mild gastrointestinal side effects occurred in 20% of all patients, moderate events occurred in 9% of all patients, and severe adverse reactions occurred in 2% of all patients. Individual event rates included diarrhea 16%, loose or frequent stools 6%, abdominal pain 3%, nausea 7%, dyspepsia 3%, and flatulence 4%. The incidence of gastrointestinal adverse reactions, including diarrhea and loose stools, in pediatric patients receiving the suspension was comparable to the incidence seen in adult patients receiving tablets.

These symptoms usually responded to symptomatic therapy or ceased when SUPRAX was discontinued.

Several patients developed severe diarrhea and/or documented pseudomembranous colitis, and a few required hospitalization.

The following adverse reactions have been reported following the use of SUPRAX. Incidence rates were less than 1 in 50 (less than 2%), except as noted above for gastrointestinal events.

Gastrointestinal (See Above): Diarrhea, loose stools, abdominal pain, dyspepsia, nausea, and vomiting. Several cases of documented pseudomembranous colitis were identified during the studies. The onset of pseudomembranous colitis symptoms may occur during or after therapy.

Hypersensitivity Reactions: Skin rashes, urticaria, drug fever, and pruritus. Erythema multiforme, Stevens-Johnson syndrome, and serum sickness-like reactions have been reported.

Hepatic: Transient elevations in SGPT, SGOT, and alkaline phosphatase.

Renal: Transient elevations in BUN or creatinine.

Central Nervous System: Headaches or dizziness.

Hemic and Lymphatic Systems: Transient thrombocytopenia, leukopenia, and eosinophilia. Prolongation in prothrombin time was seen rarely.

Other: Genital pruritus, vaginitis, candidiasis.

In addition to the adverse reactions listed above, which have been observed in patients treated with SUPRAX, the following adverse reactions and altered laboratory tests have been reported for cephalosporin-class antibiotics:

Adverse reactions: Allergic reactions including anaphylaxis, toxic epidermal necrolysis, superinfection, renal dysfunction, toxic nephropathy, hepatic dysfunction including cholestasis, aplastic anemia, hemolytic anemia, hemorrhage, and colitis.

Several cephalosporins have been implicated in triggering seizures, particularly in patients with renal impairment when the dosage was not reduced. (See **DOSAGE AND ADMINISTRATION** and **OVERDOSAGE**.) If sei-

Continued on next page

Suprax—Cont.

zures associated with drug therapy occur, the drug should be discontinued. Anticonvulsant therapy can be given if clinically indicated.

Abnormal Laboratory Tests: Positive direct Coombs test, elevated bilirubin, elevated LDH, pancytopenia, neutropenia, agranulocytosis.

OVERDOSAGE

Gastric lavage may be indicated; otherwise, no specific antidote exists. Cefixime is not removed in significant quantities from the circulation by hemodialysis or peritoneal dialysis. Adverse reactions in small numbers of healthy adult volunteers receiving single doses up to 2 g of SUPRAX did not differ from the profile seen in patients treated at the recommended doses.

DOSAGE AND ADMINISTRATION

Adults: The recommended dose of SUPRAX is 400 mg daily. This may be given as a 400 mg tablet daily or as 200 mg tablet every 12 hours.

For the treatment of uncomplicated cervical/urethral gonococcal infections, a single oral dose of 400 mg is recommended.

Children: The recommended dose is 8 mg/kg/day of the suspension. This may be administered as a single daily dose or may be given in two divided doses, as 4 mg/kg every 12 hours.

PEDIATRIC DOSAGE CHART

Patient Weight (kg)	Dose/Day mg	Dose/Day mL	Dose/Day tsp of suspension
6.25	50	2.5	$\frac{1}{2}$
12.5	100	5.0	1
18.75	150	7.5	$1\frac{1}{2}$
25.0	200	10.0	2
31.25	250	12.5	$2\frac{1}{2}$
37.5	300	15.0	3

Children weighing more than 50 kg or older than 12 years should be treated with the recommended adult dose.

Otitis media should be treated with the suspension. Clinical studies of otitis media were conducted with the suspension, and the suspension results in higher peak blood levels than the tablet when administered at the same dose. Therefore, the tablet should not be substituted for the suspension in the treatment of otitis media. (See **CLINICAL PHARMACOLOGY**.)

Efficacy and safety in infants aged less than six months have not been established.

In the treatment of infections due to *S. pyogenes*, a therapeutic dosage of SUPRAX should be administered for at least 10 days.

RENAL IMPAIRMENT

SUPRAX may be administered in the presence of impaired renal function. Normal dose and schedule may be employed in patients with creatinine clearances of 60 mL/min or greater. Patients whose clearance is between 21 and 60 mL/min or patients who are on renal hemodialysis may be given 75% of the standard dosage at the standard dosing interval (ie, 300 mg daily). Patients whose clearance is < 20 mL/min, or patients who are on continuous ambulatory peritoneal dialysis may be given half the standard dosage at the standard dosing interval (ie, 200 mg daily). Neither hemodialysis nor peritoneal dialysis removes significant amounts of drug from the body.

RECONSTITUTION DIRECTIONS FOR ORAL SUSPENSION

Bottle Size	Reconstitution Directions
100 mL	To reconstitute, suspend with **69 mL water**. Method: Tap the bottle several times to loosen powder contents prior to reconstitution. Add approximately half the total amount of water for reconstitution and shake well. Add the remainder of water and shake well.
75 mL	To reconstitute, suspend with **52 mL water**. Method: Tap the bottle several times to loosen powder contents prior to reconstitution. Add approximately half the total amount of water for reconstitution and shake well. Add the remainder of water and shake well.
50 mL	To reconstitute, suspend with **36 mL water**. Method: Tap the bottle several times to loosen powder contents prior to reconstitution. Add approximately half the total amount of water for reconstitution and shake well. Add the remainder of water and shake well.

After reconstitution, the suspension may be kept for 14 days either at room temperature, or under refrigeration, without significant loss of potency. Keep tightly closed. Shake well before using. Discard unused portion after 14 days.

HOW SUPPLIED

SUPRAX® (cefixime) Tablets, 200 mg, are convex, rectangular, white, film-coated tablets with rounded corners and beveled edges and a divided break line on each side, engraved with SUPRAX across one side and LL to the left and 200 to the right on the other side, supplied as follows:

NDC 0005-3899-23—Bottle of 100

Store at Controlled Room Temperature 15°–30°C (59°–86°F).

SUPRAX® (cefixime) Tablets, 400 mg, are convex, rectangular, white, film-coated tablets with rounded corners and beveled edges and a divided break line on each side, engraved with SUPRAX across one side and LL to the left and 400 to the right on the other side, supplied as follows:

NDC 0005-3897-94—Unit-of-Issue 10s with CRC
NDC 0005-3897-18—Bottle of 50
NDC 0005-3897-33—Bottle of 100
NDC 0005-3897-60—10 (2 × 5) Strips

Store at Controlled Room Temperature 15°–30°C (59°–86°F).

SUPRAX® (cefixime) for Oral Suspension is an off-white to cream-colored powder which when reconstituted as directed contains cefixime 100 mg/5 mL, supplied as follows:

NDC 0005-3898-40—50 mL Bottle
NDC 0005-3898-42—75 mL Bottle
NDC 0005-3898-46—100 mL Bottle

Prior to Reconstitution: Store at Controlled Room Temperature 15°–30°C (59°–86°F).

REFERENCES

1. Bauer AW, Kirby WMM, Sherris JC, et al.: Antibiotic susceptibility testing by a standard single disk method. *Am J Clin Pathol* 1966;45:493.
2. National Committee for Clinical Laboratory Standards, Approved Standard: Performance Standards for Antimicrobial Disk Susceptibility Tests (M2-A3), December 1984.
3. Standardized disk susceptibility test. *Federal Register.* 1974;39(May 30): 19182–19184.

**Clinitest® and Clinistix® are registered trademarks of Ames Division, Miles Laboratories, Inc. Tes-Tape® is a registered trademark of Eli Lilly and Company.

Manufactured by:
LEDERLE PHARMACEUTICAL DIVISION
American Cyanamid Company,
Pearl River, NY 10965
Under License of
Fujisawa Pharmaceutical Co., Ltd.
Osaka, Japan

Shown in Product Identification Guide, page 320

TETANUS AND DIPHTHERIA TOXOIDS ADSORBED ℞
FOR ADULT USE
Aluminum Phosphate-Adsorbed
PUROGENATED®

DESCRIPTION

Tetanus and Diphtheria Toxoids Adsorbed For Adult Use, aluminum phosphate-adsorbed PUROGENATED® is a sterile combination of refined tetanus and diphtheria toxoids for intramuscular use only. After shaking, the vaccine is a homogeneous white suspension.

The tetanus and diphtheria toxins are produced according to the method of Mueller and Miller,[1,2] and are detoxified by use of formaldehyde. The toxoids are refined by the Pillemer alcohol fractionation method[3] and are diluted with a solution containing sodium phosphate monobasic, sodium phosphate dibasic, aluminum phosphate, glycine and thimerosal (mercury derivative) as a preservative. The final concentration of thimerosal in the combined vaccine is 1:10,000. The aluminum content of the final product does not exceed 0.80 mg per 0.5 mL dose.

Each 0.5 mL dose is formulated to contain 5 Lf units of tetanus toxoid and 2 Lf units of diphtheria toxoid.

CLINICAL PHARMACOLOGY

Tetanus is an intoxication manifested primarily by neuromuscular dysfunction, caused by a potent exotoxin elaborated by *Clostridium tetani*. The incidence of tetanus in the

U.S. has dropped dramatically with the routine use of tetanus toxoid, remaining relatively constant over the last decade at about 90 cases reported annually.[4] Spores of *C tetani* are ubiquitous, and there is essentially no natural immunity to tetanus toxin. Thus, universal primary immunization with tetanus toxoid, and subsequent maintenance of adequate antitoxin levels by means of timed boosters, is necessary to protect all age groups.[4] Tetanus toxoid is a highly effective antigen, and a completed primary series generally induces protective levels of serum antitoxin that persist for at least 10 years.[4]

Diphtheria is primarily a localized and generalized intoxication caused by diphtheria toxin, an extracellular protein metabolite of toxinogenic strains of *Corynebacterium diphtheriae*. While the incidence of diphtheria in the U.S. has decreased from over 200,000 cases reported in 1921 before the general use of diphtheria toxoid to only 15 cases reported from 1980 to 1983, the ratio of fatalities to attack rate has remained constant at about 5% to 10%.[4] The highest case fatality rates are in the very young and the elderly. Following adequate immunization with diphtheria toxoid, which induces antitoxin, it is thought that protection lasts for at least 10 years.[4] This significantly reduces both the risk of developing diphtheria and the severity of clinical illness. It does not, however, eliminate carriage of *C diphtheriae* in the pharynx or on the skin.[4]

INDICATIONS AND USAGE

Tetanus and Diphtheria Toxoids For Adult Use, aluminum phosphate-adsorbed PUROGENATED® (Td) is indicated for active immunization against tetanus and diphtheria in adults and children 7 years of age and older.[4,5]

The Immunization Practices Advisory Committee (ACIP) of the U.S. Public Health Service recommends the use of the combined toxoids vaccine rather than single component vaccines for both primary and booster injections, including active tetanus immunization in wound management.[4]

Persons recovering from tetanus or diphtheria. Tetanus or diphtheria infection may not confer immunity; therefore, initiation or completion of active immunization is indicated at the time of recovery from these infections.[4]

Neonatal tetanus prevention. There is no evidence that tetanus and diphtheria toxoids are teratogenic. A previously unimmunized pregnant woman, who may deliver her child under nonhygienic circumstances and/or surroundings, should receive two properly spaced doses of Td before delivery, preferably during the last two trimesters. Incompletely immunized pregnant women should complete the three-dose series. Those immunized more than 10 years previously should have a booster dose.[4] (See also pregnancy information under **PRECAUTIONS.**)

CONTRAINDICATIONS

HYPERSENSITIVITY TO ANY COMPONENT OF THE VACCINE, INCLUDING THIMEROSAL, A MERCURY DERIVATIVE, IS A CONTRAINDICATION.

THE OCCURRENCE OF ANY NEUROLOGICAL SYMPTOMS OR SIGNS FOLLOWING ADMINISTRATION OF THIS PRODUCT IS A CONTRAINDICATION TO FURTHER USE.

IMMUNIZATION SHOULD BE DEFERRED DURING THE COURSE OF ANY FEBRILE ILLNESS OR ACUTE INFECTION. A MINOR AFEBRILE ILLNESS SUCH AS A MILD UPPER RESPIRATORY INFECTION IS NOT USUALLY REASON TO DEFER IMMUNIZATION.[4]

The clinical judgment of the attending physician should prevail at all times.

Routine immunization should be deferred during an outbreak of poliomyelitis, providing the patient has not sustained an injury that increases the risk of tetanus and providing an outbreak of diphtheria does not occur simultaneously.

WARNINGS

THIS PRODUCT IS NOT RECOMMENDED FOR IMMUNIZING PERSONS LESS THAN 7 YEARS OF AGE. The concentration of diphtheria toxoid in preparations intended for use in persons 7 years of age or older is lower than that of the pediatric formulation (Diphtheria and Tetanus Toxoids Adsorbed, for pediatric use, [DT]): a lower dosage of diphtheria toxoid is recommended for persons 7 years of age or older because adverse reactions to the diphtheria component are thought to be related to both dose and age.[4]

THE OCCURRENCE OF A NEUROLOGICAL OR SEVERE HYPERSENSITIVITY REACTION FOLLOWING A PREVIOUS DOSE IS A CONTRAINDICATION TO FURTHER USE OF THIS PRODUCT.[4]

THE ADMINISTRATION OF BOOSTER DOSES MORE FREQUENTLY THAN RECOMMENDED (see **DOSAGE AND ADMINISTRATION**) MAY BE ASSOCIATED WITH INCREASED INCIDENCE AND SEVERITY OF REACTIONS.[4]

Persons who experience Arthus-type hypersensitivity reactions or temperature greater than 39.4°C (103°F), after a previous dose of tetanus toxoid usually have very high serum antitoxin levels and should not be given even

emergency doses of Td more frequently than every 10 years, even if they have a wound that is neither clean nor minor.[4] If a contraindication to using tetanus toxoid-containing preparations exists in a person who has not completed a primary immunizing course of tetanus toxoid, and other than a clean, minor wound is sustained, only passive immunization should be given using human Tetanus Immune Globulin (TIG).[4]

Td should not be given to individuals with thrombocytopenia or any coagulation disorder that would contraindicate intramuscular injection unless the potential benefits clearly outweigh the risk of administration.

Patients with impaired immune responsiveness, whether due to the use of immunosuppressive therapy (including irradiation, corticosteroids, antimetabolites, alkylating agents, and cytotoxic agents), a genetic defect, human immunodeficiency virus (HIV) infection, or other causes, may have a reduced antibody response to active immunization procedures.[4-6] Deferral of administration of vaccine may be considered in individuals receiving immunosuppressive therapy.[4,5]

Special care should be taken to prevent injection into a blood vessel.

PRECAUTIONS

General

1. **THIS PRODUCT SHOULD BE USED FOR INDIVIDUALS 7 YEARS OF AGE OR OLDER.**
2. PRIOR TO ADMINISTRATION OF ANY DOSE OF Td, THE PARENT, GUARDIAN, OR ADULT PATIENT SHOULD BE ASKED ABOUT THE RECENT HEALTH STATUS AND IMMUNIZATION HISTORY OF THE PATIENT TO BE IMMUNIZED IN ORDER TO DETERMINE THE EXISTENCE OF ANY CONTRAINDICATION TO IMMUNIZATION WITH Td (SEE **CONTRAINDICATIONS, WARNINGS**).
3. WHEN THE PATIENT RETURNS FOR THE NEXT DOSE IN A SERIES, THE PARENT, GUARDIAN, OR ADULT PATIENT SHOULD BE QUESTIONED CONCERNING OCCURRENCE OF ANY SYMPTOM AND/OR SIGN OF AN ADVERSE REACTION AFTER THE PREVIOUS DOSE (SEE **CONTRAINDICATIONS, ADVERSE REACTIONS**).
4. BEFORE THE INJECTION OF ANY BIOLOGICAL, THE PHYSICIAN SHOULD TAKE ALL PRECAUTIONS KNOWN FOR PREVENTION OF ALLERGIC OR ANY OTHER SIDE REACTIONS. This should include: a review of the patient's history regarding possible sensitivity; the ready availability of epinephrine 1:1,000 and other appropriate agents used for control of immediate allergic reactions; and a knowledge of the recent literature pertaining to use of the biological concerned, including the nature of side effects and adverse reactions that may follow its use.
5. A separate sterile syringe and needle or a sterile disposable unit should be used for each individual patient to prevent transmission of hepatitis or other infectious agents from one person to another.
6. *Shake vigorously before withdrawing each dose to resuspend the contents of the vial or syringe.*
7. NATIONAL CHILDHOOD VACCINE INJURY ACT OF 1986 (AS AMENDED IN 1987) This Act requires that the manufacturer and lot number of the vaccine administered be recorded by the health care provider in the vaccine recipient's permanent medical record, along with the date of administration of the vaccine and the name, address and title of the person administering the vaccine. The Act further requires the health care provider to report to a health department or to the FDA the occurrence following immunization of any event set forth in the Vaccine Injury Table including: anaphylaxis or anaphylactic shock within 24 hours, encephalopathy or encephalitis within 7 days, residual seizure disorder, any acute complication or sequelae (including death) of above events, or any event that would contraindicate further doses of vaccine, according to this package insert.[7]

Information for the Patient

PRIOR TO ADMINISTRATION OF THIS VACCINE, HEALTH CARE PERSONNEL SHOULD INFORM THE PARENT, GUARDIAN, OR ADULT PATIENT OF THE BENEFITS AND RISKS OF VACCINATION AGAINST TETANUS AND DIPHTHERIA.

Use in Pregnancy

Pregnancy Category C.

Animal reproductive studies have not been conducted with this product. There is no evidence that tetanus and diphtheria toxoids are teratogenic. Td should be given to inadequately immunized pregnant women because it affords protection against neonatal tetanus.[8] Waiting until the second trimester is a reasonable precaution to minimize any theoretical concern.[4] Maintenance of adequate immunization by routine boosters in non-pregnant women of child-bearing age (see **DOSAGE AND ADMINISTRATION**) can obviate the need to vaccinate women during pregnancy.

ADVERSE REACTIONS

Local reactions, such as erythema, induration, and tenderness, are common after the administration of Td.[9,10,11,12]

Such local reactions are usually self-limited and require no therapy. Nodule,[13] sterile abscess formation, or subcutaneous atrophy may occur at the site of injection. Systemic reactions, such as fever, chills, myalgias, and headaches, also may occur.[9,10,11,12]

Arthus-type hypersensitivity reactions, or high fever, may occur in persons who have very high serum antitoxin antibodies due to overly frequent injections of toxoid (See **WARNINGS**).

NEUROLOGICAL COMPLICATIONS,[14] SUCH AS CONVULSIONS,[15] ENCEPHALOPATHY,[15,16] AND VARIOUS MONO- AND POLYNEUROPATHIES,[16-22] INCLUDING GUILLAIN-BARRÉ SYNDROME,[23,24] HAVE BEEN REPORTED FOLLOWING ADMINISTRATION OF PREPARATIONS CONTAINING TETANUS AND/OR DIPHTHERIA ANTIGENS.

URTICARIA, ERYTHEMA MULTIFORME OR OTHER RASH, ARTHRALGIAS,[15] AND, MORE RARELY, A SEVERE ANAPHYLACTIC REACTION (IE, URTICARIA WITH SWELLING OF THE MOUTH, DIFFICULTY BREATHING, HYPOTENSION, OR SHOCK) HAVE BEEN REPORTED FOLLOWING ADMINISTRATION OF PREPARATIONS CONTAINING TETANUS AND/OR DIPHTHERIA ANTIGENS.

DOSAGE AND ADMINISTRATION

For Intramuscular Use Only

Shake vigorously before withdrawing each dose to resuspend the contents of the vial or syringe.

Parenteral drug products should be inspected visually for particulate matter and discoloration prior to administration. (See **DESCRIPTION**.)

The vaccine should be injected intramuscularly, preferably into the deltoid muscle, with care to avoid major peripheral nerve trunks. Before injection, the skin at the injection site should be cleansed and prepared with a suitable germicide. After insertion of the needle, aspirate to help avoid inadvertent injection into a blood vessel.

The primary immunizing course for unimmunized individuals 7 years of age or older consists of two doses of 0.5 mL each, 4 to 8 weeks apart, followed by a third (reinforcing) dose of 0.5 mL 6 to 12 months after the second dose. The reinforcing dose is an integral part of the primary immunizing course.[4]

Interruption of the recommended schedule with a delay between doses does not interfere with the final immunity achieved, nor does it necessitate starting the series over again, regardless of the length of time elapsed between doses.[4]

A booster dose of 0.5 mL of Td is given 10 years after completion of primary immunization and every 10 years thereafter. If a dose is given sooner than 10 years, as part of wound management or on exposure to diphtheria, the next booster is not needed for 10 years thereafter. MORE FREQUENT BOOSTER DOSES ARE NOT INDICATED AND MAY BE ASSOCIATED WITH INCREASED INCIDENCE AND SEVERITY OF REACTIONS.[4] (See **WARNINGS**.)

Diphtheria Prophylaxis for Case Contacts

All case contacts, household and others, who have previously received fewer than three doses of diphtheria toxoid, should receive an immediate dose of an appropriate diphtheria toxoid-containing preparation and should complete the series according to schedule. Case contacts who have previously received three or more doses, but who have not received a dose of a preparation containing diphtheria toxoid within the previous five years, should receive a booster dose of a diphtheria toxoid-containing preparation appropriate for their age.[4] Td is an appropriate preparation in these circumstances for persons 7 years of age or older.

Tetanus Prophylaxis in Wound Management

The need for active immunization with a tetanus toxoid-containing preparation, with or without passive immunization with human Tetanus Immune Globulin (TIG) depends on both the condition of the wound and the patient's immunization history. Tetanus has rarely occurred among persons with a documented primary series of tetanus toxoid injections. A thorough attempt must be made to determine whether a patient has completed primary immunization.[4]

Individuals who have completed primary immunization against tetanus, and who sustain wounds which are minor and uncontaminated, should receive a booster dose of a tetanus-toxoid preparation only if they have not received tetanus toxoid within the preceding 10 years. For other wounds, a booster is appropriate if the patient has not received tetanus toxoid within the preceding 5 years. Antitoxin antibodies develop rapidly in persons who have previously received at least two doses of tetanus toxoid.[4]

Individuals who have not completed primary immunization against tetanus, or whose immunization history is unknown or uncertain, should be immunized with a tetanus toxoid-containing product. Completion of primary immunization thereafter should be ensured. In addition, if these individuals have sustained a tetanus-prone wound, the use of human Tetanus Immune Globulin (TIG) is recommended. A separate syringe and site of administration should be used.[4]

SUMMARY GUIDE TO TETANUS PROPHYLAXIS IN ROUTINE WOUND MANAGEMENT[4]*

History of tetanus toxoid (doses)	Clean, minor wounds		All other wounds†	
	Td	TIG	Td	TIG
Unknown <three	Yes	No	Yes	Yes
≥three¶	No**	No	No††	No

* Important details are in the text.
† Such as, but not limited to, wounds contaminated with dirt, feces, soil, saliva, etc.; puncture wounds; avulsions; and wounds resulting from missiles, crushing, burns, and frostbite.
¶ If only three doses of *fluid* toxoid have been received, a fourth dose of toxoid, preferably an adsorbed toxoid, should be given.
** Yes, if more than 10 years since last dose.
†† Yes, if more than 5 years since last dose. (More frequent boosters are not needed and can accentuate side effects.)

Td is the preferred preparation for active tetanus immunization in wound management of patients 7 years of age or older. This is to enhance diphtheria protection, since a large proportion of adults are susceptible. Thus, by taking advantage of acute health care visits for wound management, some patients can be protected who otherwise would remain susceptible.[4]

HOW SUPPLIED

NDC 0005-1875-31   5.0 mL vial
NDC 0005-1875-47   10 (0.5 mL) LEDERJECT® disposable syringes. For directions on use of LEDERJECT® disposable syringe, please see package insert accompanying product.

STORAGE

DO NOT FREEZE. STORE REFRIGERATED, AWAY FROM FREEZER COMPARTMENT, AT 2°C to 8°C (36°F to 46°F).

REFERENCES

1. Mueller JH, Miller PA: Factors influencing the production of tetanal toxin. *J Immunol* 1947;56:143–147.
2. Mueller JH, Miller PA: Production of diphtheria toxin of high potency (100Lf) on a reproducible medium. *J Immunol* 1941;40:21–32.
3. Pillemer L, Grossberg DB, Wittler RG: The immunochemistry of toxins and toxoids. II. The preparation and immunological evaluation of purified tetanal toxoid. *J Immunol* 1946;54:213–224.
4. Recommendation of the Immunization Practices Advisory Committee (ACIP): Diphtheria, tetanus and pertussis: Guidelines for vaccine prophylaxis and other preventive measures. *MMWR* 1985;34:405–426.
5. Committee on Immunization, Council of Medical Societies American College of Physicians: Guide for Adult Immunization, 1st Edition 1985; Philadelphia, PA.
6. Recommendation of the ACIP: Immunization of children infected with Human T-Lymphotrophic Virus Type III/ Lymphadenopathy associated virus. *MMWR* 1986;35(38):595–606.
7. National Childhood Vaccine Injury Act: Requirements for permanent vaccination records and for reporting of selected events after vaccination. *MMWR* 1988;37(13): 197–200.
8. Recommendations of the ACIP: General recommendations on immunization. *MMWR* 1983;32(1):1–17.
9. Deacon SP, et al: A comparative clinical study of adsorbed tetanus vaccine and adult-type tetanus-diphtheria vaccine. *J Hyg (Cambridge)* 1982;89:513–519.
10. Macko MB, Powell CE: Comparison of the morbidity of tetanus toxoid boosters with tetanus-diphtheria toxoid boosters. *Ann Emerg Med* 1985;14(1):33–35.
11. Myers MG, et al: Primary immunization with tetanus and diphtheria toxoids. *JAMA* 1982;248(19):2478–2480.
12. Sisk CW, et al: Reactions to tetanus-diphtheria toxoid (adult). *Arch Environ Health* 1965;11:34–36.
13. Fawcett HA, Smith NP: Injection-site granuloma due to aluminum. *Arch Dermatol* 1984;120:1318–1322.
14. Rutledge SL, Snead OC: Neurological complications of immunizations. *J Pediatr* 1986;109:917–924.
15. Adverse Events Following Immunization. *MMWR* 1985;34(3):43–47.
16. Schlenska GK: Unusual neurological complications following tetanus toxoid administration. *J Neurol* 1977;215:299–302.
17. Blumstein GI, Kreithen H: Peripheral neuropathy following tetanus toxoid administration. *JAMA* 1966;198: 1030–1031.
18. Reinstein L, Pargament JM, Goodman JS: Peripheral neuropathy after multiple tetanus toxoid injections. *Arch Phys Med Rehabil* 1982;63:332–334.

Continued on next page

Tetanus & Diphtheria Toxoids—Cont.

19. Tsairis P, Duck PJ, Mulder DW: Natural history of brachial plexus neuropathy. *Arch Neurol* 1972;27:109–117.
20. Quast U, Hennessen W, Widmark RM: Mono- and polyneuritis after tetanus vaccination. *Devel Bio Stand* 1979;43:25–32.
21. Holliday PL, Bauer RB: Polyradiculoneuritis secondary to immunization with tetanus and diphtheria toxoids. *Arch Neurol* 1983;40:56–67.
22. Fenichel GM: Neurological complications of tetanus toxoid. *Arch Neurol* 1983;40:390.
23. Pollard JD, Selby G: Relapsing neuropathy due to tetanus toxoid. *J Neurol Sci* 1978;37:113–125.
24. Newton N, Janati A: Guillain-Barré syndrome after vaccination with purified tetanus toxoid. *S Med J* 1987;80: 1053–1054.

Manufactured by:
LEDERLE LABORATORIES
Division American Cyanamid Company
Pearl River, NY 10965
US Gov't. License No. 17
Marketed by:
WYETH-LEDERLE VACCINES
Wyeth-Ayerst Laboratories
Philadelphia, PA 19101

TETANUS TOXOID ADSORBED ℞

Tetanus Toxoid Aluminum Phosphate-Adsorbed
PUROGENATED®

DESCRIPTION

Tetanus Toxoid Adsorbed, aluminum phosphate-adsorbed, PUROGENATED is a sterile preparation of refined tetanus toxoid for intramuscular use only. After shaking, the product is a homogenous white suspension.

The tetanus toxin is produced according to the method of Mueller and Miller[1] and is detoxified by use of formaldehyde. The toxoid is refined by the Pillemer alcohol fractionation method[2] and is diluted with a solution containing sodium phosphate dibasic, sodium phosphate monobasic, glycine, sodium chloride and thimerosal (mercury derivative) in a final concentration of 1:10,000 as a preservative and aluminum phosphate as adjuvant. The aluminum content does not exceed 0.80 mg per 0.5 mL dose.

Each 0.5 mL dose is formulated to contain 5 Lf units of tetanus toxoid.

CLINICAL PHARMACOLOGY

Tetanus is an intoxication manifested primarily by neuromuscular dysfunction caused by a potent exotoxin elaborated by *Clostridium tetani.* The incidence of tetanus in the U.S. has dropped dramatically with the routine use of tetanus toxoid, remaining relatively constant over the last decade at about 90 cases reported annually.[3] Spores of *C tetani* are ubiquitous and there is essentially no natural immunity to tetanus toxin. Thus, universal primary immunization with tetanus toxoid, and subsequent maintenance of adequate antitoxin levels by means of timed boosters, is necessary to protect all age groups.[3] Tetanus toxoid is a highly effective antigen, and a completed primary series generally induces protective levels of serum antitoxin that persist for at least 10 years.[3]

INDICATIONS AND USAGE

Tetanus Toxoid Adsorbed is indicated for active immunization against tetanus in adults and children 2 months of age or older.

Immunization of persons 7 years of age or older may be accomplished by the use of Tetanus and Diphtheria Toxoids Adsorbed, for Adult Use (Td), Tetanus Toxoid Adsorbed, or Tetanus Toxoid Fluid. The Immunization Practices Advisory Committee (ACIP) of the U.S. Public Health Service recommends the use of the combined toxoids vaccine rather than single component vaccines for both primary and booster injections, including active tetanus immunization in wound management.[3] Individuals for whom the use of a vaccine containing diphtheria toxoid is contraindicated should receive a single-component tetanus toxoid-containing vaccine.

Immunization of infants and children 2 months of age up to the seventh birthday is usually accomplished by the use of Diphtheria and Tetanus Toxoids and Pertussis Vaccine Adsorbed (DTP) or Diphtheria and Tetanus Toxoids Adsorbed, for pediatric use (DT). Tetanus Toxoid Adsorbed may be used for immunizing infants and children for whom the use of a vaccine containing diphtheria toxoid and pertussis antigen is contraindicated.

Comparative tests have shown that the adsorbed toxoids are superior to the fluid toxoids in antibody titers produced and in the durability of protection achieved. The promptness of antibody response to booster doses of either fluid or adsorbed toxoid is not sufficiently different to be of clinical importance. When Tetanus Immune Globulin (TIG) is to be administered at the same visit as tetanus toxoid, the adsorbed toxoid should be used.[3,4]

Persons recovering from tetanus. Tetanus infection may not confer immunity; therefore, initiation or completion of active immunization is indicated at the time of recovery from this infection.[3]

Neonatal tetanus prevention. There is no evidence that tetanus toxoid is teratogenic. A previously unimmunized pregnant woman who may deliver her child under nonhygienic circumstances and/or surroundings should receive two properly spaced doses of a tetanus toxoid-containing preparation before delivery, preferably during the last two trimesters. Incompletely immunized pregnant women should complete the three-dose series. Those immunized more than 10 years previously should have a booster dose.[3] (See also pregnancy information under **PRECAUTIONS**.)

CONTRAINDICATIONS

HYPERSENSITIVITY TO ANY COMPONENT OF THE VACCINE, INCLUDING THIMEROSAL, A MERCURY DERIVATIVE, IS A CONTRAINDICATION.

THE OCCURRENCE OF ANY TYPE OF NEUROLOGICAL SYMPTOMS OR SIGNS FOLLOWING ADMINISTRATION OF THIS PRODUCT IS A CONTRAINDICATION TO FURTHER USE.

IMMUNIZATION SHOULD BE DEFERRED DURING THE COURSE OF ANY FEBRILE ILLNESS OR ACUTE INFECTION. A MINOR AFEBRILE ILLNESS SUCH AS A MILD UPPER RESPIRATORY INFECTION IS NOT USUALLY REASON TO DEFER IMMUNIZATION.[3]

The clinical judgment of the attending physician should prevail at all times.

Routine immunization should be deferred during an outbreak of poliomyelitis providing the patient has not sustained an injury that increases the risk of tetanus.

WARNINGS

THE OCCURRENCE OF A NEUROLOGIC OR SEVERE HYPERSENSITIVITY REACTION FOLLOWING A PREVIOUS DOSE IS A CONTRAINDICATION TO FURTHER USE OF THIS PRODUCT.[3]

THE ADMINISTRATION OF BOOSTER DOSES MORE FREQUENTLY THAN RECOMMENDED (See **DOSAGE AND ADMINISTRATION**) MAY BE ASSOCIATED WITH INCREASED INCIDENCE AND SEVERITY OF REACTIONS.[3]

Persons who experience Arthus-type hypersensitivity reactions or temperature greater than 39.4°C (103°F) after a previous dose of tetanus toxoid usually have very high serum tetanus antitoxin levels and should not be given even emergency doses of tetanus toxoid more frequently than every 10 years, even if they have a wound that is neither clean nor minor.[3]

If a contraindication to using tetanus toxoid exists in a person who has not completed a primary immunizing course of tetanus toxoid, and other than a clean, minor wound is sustained, only passive immunization should be given using human Tetanus Immune Globulin (TIG).[3]

Tetanus Toxoid Adsorbed should not be given to individuals with thrombocytopenia or any coagulation disorder that would contraindicate intramuscular injection, unless the potential benefit clearly outweighs the risk of administration.

Patients with impaired immune responsiveness, whether due to the use of immunosuppressive therapy (including irradiation, corticosteroids, antimetabolites, alkylating agents, and cytotoxic agents), a genetic defect, human immunodeficiency virus (HIV) infection, or other causes, may have a reduced antibody response to active immunization procedures.[3–5] Deferral of administration of vaccine may be considered in individuals receiving immunosuppressive therapy.[3,4]

Special care should be taken to prevent injection into a blood vessel.

PRECAUTIONS

General

1. PRIOR TO ADMINISTRATION OF ANY DOSE OF VACCINE THE PARENT, GUARDIAN, OR ADULT PATIENT SHOULD BE ASKED ABOUT THE RECENT HEALTH STATUS AND IMMUNIZATION HISTORY OF THE PATIENT TO BE IMMUNIZED IN ORDER TO DETERMINE THE EXISTENCE OF ANY CONTRAINDICATIONS TO IMMUNIZATION (SEE **CONTRAINDICATIONS, WARNINGS**).
2. WHEN THE PATIENT RETURNS FOR THE NEXT DOSE IN A SERIES, THE PARENT, GUARDIAN, OR ADULT PATIENT SHOULD BE QUESTIONED CONCERNING OCCURRENCE OF ANY SYMPTOM AND/OR SIGN OF AN ADVERSE REACTION AFTER THE PREVIOUS DOSE (SEE **CONTRAINDICATIONS, ADVERSE REACTIONS**).
3. BEFORE THE INJECTION OF ANY BIOLOGICAL, THE PHYSICIAN SHOULD TAKE ALL PRECAUTIONS KNOWN FOR PREVENTION OF ALLERGIC OR ANY OTHER SIDE REACTIONS. This should include: a review of the patient's history regarding possible sensitivity; the ready availability of epinephrine 1:1,000 and other appropriate agents used for control of immediate allergic reactions; and a knowledge of the recent literature pertaining to use of the biological concerned, including the nature of side effects and adverse reactions that may follow its use.
4. A separate sterile syringe and needle or a sterile disposable unit should be used for each individual patient to prevent transmission of hepatitis or other infectious agents from one person to another.
5. *Shake vigorously before withdrawing each dose to resuspend the contents of the vial.*
6. NATIONAL CHILDHOOD VACCINE INJURY ACT OF 1986 (AS AMENDED IN 1987)
   This Act requires that the manufacturer and lot number of the vaccine administered be recorded by the health care provider in the vaccine recipient's permanent record, along with the date of administration of the vaccine and the name, address and title of the person administering the vaccine.
   The Act further requires the health care provider to report to a health department or to the FDA the occurrence following immunization of any event set forth in the Vaccine Injury Table including: anaphylaxis or anaphylactic shock within 24 hours, encephalopathy or encephalitis within 7 days, residual seizure disorder, any acute complication or sequelae (including death) of above events, or any event that would contraindicate further doses of vaccine, according to this package insert.[6]

Information for the Patient

PRIOR TO ADMINISTRATION OF THIS VACCINE, HEALTH CARE PERSONNEL SHOULD INFORM THE PARENT, GUARDIAN, OR ADULT PATIENT OF THE BENEFITS AND RISKS OF VACCINATION AGAINST TETANUS.

Use in Pregnancy

Pregnancy Category C.

Animal reproductive studies have not been conducted with this product. There is no evidence that tetanus toxoid is teratogenic. An appropriate tetanus toxoid-containing preparation (usually Td) should be given to inadequately immunized women because it affords protection against neonatal tetanus.[7] Waiting until the second trimester is a reasonable precaution to minimize any theoretical concern.[4] Maintenance of adequate immunization by routine boosters in non-pregnant women of child-bearing age (see **DOSAGE AND ADMINISTRATION**) can obviate the need to vaccinate women during pregnancy.

ADVERSE REACTIONS

Local reactions, such as erythema, induration and tenderness, are common after the administration of tetanus toxoid.[8,9,10] Such local reactions are usually self-limiting and require no therapy. Nodule,[11] sterile abscess formation, or subcutaneous atrophy may occur at the site of injection. Systemic reactions such as fever, chills, myalgia, and headaches also may occur.[8,9,10]

Arthus-type hypersensitivity reactions, or high fever, may occur in persons who have very high serum antitoxin antibodies due to overly frequent injections of toxoid.[3] (See **WARNINGS**.)

NEUROLOGICAL COMPLICATIONS[12] SUCH AS CONVULSIONS,[13] ENCEPHALOPATHY,[13,14] AND VARIOUS MONO- AND POLYNEUROPATHIES,[14–20] INCLUDING GUILLAIN-BARRÉ SYNDROME,[21,22] HAVE BEEN REPORTED FOLLOWING ADMINISTRATION OF PREPARATIONS CONTAINING TETANUS ANTIGEN.

URTICARIA, ERYTHEMA MULTIFORME OR OTHER RASH, ARTHRALGIAS[13] AND, MORE RARELY, A SEVERE ANAPHYLACTIC REACTION (I.E., URTICARIA WITH SWELLING OF THE MOUTH, DIFFICULTY BREATHING, HYPOTENSION OR SHOCK) HAVE BEEN REPORTED FOLLOWING ADMINISTRATION OF PREPARATIONS CONTAINING TETANUS ANTIGEN.

DOSAGE AND ADMINISTRATION

For Intramuscular Use Only

Shake vigorously before withdrawing each dose to resuspend the contents of the vial or syringe.

Parenteral drug products should be inspected visually for particulate matter and discoloration prior to administration. (See **DESCRIPTION.**)

Preferred injection sites for intramuscular injection include the anterolateral aspect of the upper thigh and the deltoid area of the upper arm. Care should be taken to avoid major peripheral nerve trunks.

Before injection, the skin at the injection site should be cleansed and prepared with a suitable germicide.

After insertion of the needle, aspirate to help avoid inadvertent injection into a blood vessel.

The primary immunizing course for unimmunized individuals one year of age or older consists of *two* doses of 0.5 mL each, 4 to 8 weeks apart, followed by a *third* (reinforcing) dose of 0.5 mL, 6 to 12 months after the second dose. The reinforcing dose is an integral part of the primary immunizing course.

If, after beginning combined immunization against diphtheria, tetanus, and pertussis, further doses of vaccine containing pertussis and diphtheria antigens become contraindicated, Tetanus Toxoid Adsorbed may be substituted for each of the remaining doses.

When immunization with Tetanus Toxoid Adsorbed is begun in the first year of life, the primary series consists of *three* doses of 0.5 mL each, 4 to 8 weeks apart, followed by a *fourth* (reinforcing) dose of 0.5 mL, 6 to 12 months after the third dose.

Interruption of the recommended schedule with a delay between doses does not interfere with the final immunity achieved with Tetanus Toxoid Adsorbed. There is no need to start the series over again, regardless of the length of time elapsed between doses.[3]

Booster Doses

A single injection of 0.5 mL of Tetanus Toxoid Adsorbed is given 10 years after completion of primary immunization and every 10 years thereafter. If a dose is given sooner as part of wound management, the next booster is not needed for 10 years thereafter. MORE FREQUENT BOOSTER DOSES ARE NOT INDICATED AND MAY BE ASSOCIATED WITH INCREASED INCIDENCE AND SEVERITY OF REACTIONS.[3]

Tetanus Prophylaxis in Wound Management

The need for active immunization with a tetanus toxoid-containing preparation, with or without passive immunization with human Tetanus Immune Globulin (TIG) depends on both the condition of the wound and the patient's immunization history. Tetanus has rarely occurred among persons with a documented primary series of toxoid injections. A thorough attempt must be made to determine whether a patient has completed primary immunization.[3]

Individuals who have completed primary immunization against tetanus, and who sustain wounds which are minor and uncontaminated, should receive a booster dose of the appropriate tetanus toxoid-containing preparation (see **INDICATIONS AND USAGE**) only if they have not received tetanus toxoid within the preceding 10 years. For other wounds, a booster is appropriate if the patient has not received tetanus toxoid within the preceding 5 years. Antitoxin antibodies develop rapidly in persons who have previously received at least two doses of tetanus toxoid.[3]

Individuals who have not completed primary immunization against tetanus, or whose immunization history is unknown or uncertain, should be immunized with the appropriate tetanus toxoid-containing product (see **INDICATIONS AND USAGE**). Completion of primary immunization thereafter should be ensured. In addition, if these individuals have sustained a tetanus-prone wound, the use of human Tetanus Immune Globulin (TIG) is recommended. A separate syringe and site of administration should be used. When TIG is to be administered at the same visit as tetanus toxoid, an adsorbed tetanus toxoid-containing preparation should be used.[3]

SUMMARY GUIDE TO TETANUS PROPHYLAXIS IN ROUTINE WOUND MANAGEMENT[3]*

History of tetanus toxoid (doses)	Clean, minor wounds		All other wounds†	
	Td§	TIG	Td§	TIG
Unknown or <three	Yes	No	Yes	Yes
≥three¶	No**	No	No††	No

* Important details are in the text.
† Such as, but not limited to, wounds contaminated with dirt, feces, soil, saliva, etc.; puncture wounds; avulsions; and wounds resulting from missiles, crushing, burns and frostbite.
§ For children under 7 years old DTP (DT, if pertussis vaccine is contraindicated) is preferred to tetanus toxoid alone. For persons 7 years and older, Td is preferred to tetanus toxoid alone.
¶ If only three doses of *fluid* toxoid have been received, a fourth dose of toxoid, preferably an adsorbed toxoid, should be given.
** Yes, if more than 10 years since last dose.
†† Yes, if more than 5 years since last dose. (More frequent boosters are not needed and can accentuate side effects.)

In order to enhance diphtheria protection in the population, the ACIP recommends Tetanus and Diphtheria Toxoids For Adult Use as the preferred preparation for active tetanus immunization in wound management of patients 7 years of age or older.[3]

HOW SUPPLIED

NDC 0005-1938-31 5.0 mL vial
NDC 0005-1938-47 10×0.5 mL LEDERJECT® disposable syringe. For directions on use of LEDERJECT® disposable syringe, please see package insert accompanying product.

STORAGE

DO NOT FREEZE. STORE REFRIGERATED, AWAY FROM FREEZER COMPARTMENT, AT 2°C to 8°C (36°F to 46°F).

REFERENCES

1. Mueller JH, Miller PA: Factors influencing the production of tetanal toxin. *J Immunol* 1947;56:143–147.
2. Pillemer L, Grossberg DB, Wittler RG: The immunochemistry of toxins and toxoids. II. The preparation and immunological evaluation of purified tetanal toxoid. *J Immunol* 1946;54:213–224.
3. Recommendation of the Immunization Practices Advisory Committee (ACIP): Diphtheria, tetanus and pertussis: Guidelines for vaccine prophylaxis and other preventive measures. *MMWR* 1985;34:405–426.
4. Committee on Immunization, Council of Medical Societies, American College of Physicians: Guide for Adult Immunization, 1st Edition 1985; Philadelphia, PA.
5. Recommendation of the ACIP: Immunization of children infected with Human T-Lymphotrophic Virus Type III/Lymphadenopathy associated virus. *MMWR* 1986;35(38):595–606.
6. National Childhood Vaccine Injury Act: Requirements for permanent vaccination records and for reporting of selected events after vaccination. *MMWR* 1988;37(13):197–200.
7. Recommendations of the ACIP: General recommendations on immunization. *MMWR* 1983;32(1):1–17.
8. Macko MB, Powell CE: Comparison of the morbidity of tetanus toxoid boosters with tetanus-diphtheria toxoid boosters. *Ann Emerg Med* 1985;14:(1)33–35.
9. Deacon SP, et al: A comparative clinical study of adsorbed tetanus vaccine and adult-type tetanus-diphtheria vaccine. *J Hyg (Cambridge)* 1982;89:513–519.
10. Jacobs RL, et al: Adverse reactions to tetanus toxoid. *JAMA* 1982;247(1):40–42.
11. Fawcett HA, Smith N: Injection-site granuloma due to aluminum. *Arch Dermatol* 1984;120:1318–1322.
12. Rutledge SL, Snead OC: Neurologic complications of immunizations. *J Pediatr* 1986;109:917–924.
13. Adverse Events Following Immunization. *MMWR* 1985;34(3):43–47.
14. Schlenska GK: Unusual neurological complications following tetanus toxoid administration. *J Neurol* 1977;215:299–302.
15. Blumstein GI, Kreithen H: Peripheral neuropathy following tetanus toxoid administration. *JAMA* 1966;198:1030–1031.
16. Reinstein L, Pargament JM, Goodman JS: Peripheral neuropathy after multiple tetanus toxoid injections. *Arch Phys Med Rehabil* 1982;63:332–334.
17. Tsairis P, Duck PJ, Mulder DW: Natural history of brachial plexus neuropathy. *Arch Neurol* 1972;27:109–117.
18. Quast U, Hennessen W, Widmark RM: Mono- and polyneuritis after tetanus vaccination. *Devel Bio Stand* 1979;43:25–32.
19. Holliday PL, Bauer RB: Polyradiculoneuritis secondary to immunization with tetanus and diphtheria toxoids. *Arch Neurol* 1983;40:56–57.
20. Fenichel GM: Neurological complications of tetanus toxoid. *Arch Neurol* 1983;40:390.
21. Pollard JD, Selby G: Relapsing neuropathy due to tetanus toxoid. *J Neurol Sci* 1978;37:113–125.
22. Newton N, Janati A: Guillain-Barré syndrome after vaccination with purified tetanus toxoid. *S Med J* 1987;80:1053–1054.

Manufactured by:
LEDERLE LABORATORIES
Division American Cyanamid Company
Pearl River, NY 10965
US Gov't. License No. 17
Marketed by:
WYETH-LEDERLE VACCINES
Wyeth-Ayerst Laboratories
Philadelphia, PA 19101

DIPHTHERIA AND TETANUS TOXOIDS AND PERTUSSIS VACCINE ADSORBED AND HAEMOPHILUS b CONJUGATE VACCINE (DIPHTHERIA CRM₁₉₇ PROTEIN CONJUGATE) TETRAMUNE®   ℞

[tet 'rə-myoon]

DESCRIPTION

Diphtheria and Tetanus Toxoids and Pertussis Vaccine Adsorbed and Haemophilus b Conjugate Vaccine (Diphtheria CRM₁₉₇ Protein Conjugate) TETRAMUNE, (DTP-HbOC), is a sterile combination of PUROGENATED® Diphtheria Toxoid aluminum phosphate-adsorbed, PUROGENATED® Tetanus Toxoid aluminum phosphate-adsorbed, Pertussis Vaccine (DTP), and a conjugate of oligosaccharides of the capsular antigen of *Haemophilus influenzae* type b and diphtheria CRM₁₉₇ protein (HbOC), manufactured by Lederle Laboratories. These are antigenic components of TRI-IMMUNOL® and HibTITER®. TETRAMUNE is for intramuscular use only. After shaking, the vaccine is a homogeneous white suspension.

The diphtheria and tetanus toxoids are derived from *Corynebacterium diphtheriae* and *Clostridium tetani*, respectively, which are grown in media according to the method of Mueller and Miller.[1,2] *C. diphtheriae* is grown in a defined medium containing casamino acids and *C. tetani* in a medium containing beef heart infusion. They are detoxified by use of formaldehyde. The toxoids are refined by the Pillemer alcohol fractionation method[3] and are diluted with a solution containing sodium phosphate monobasic, sodium phosphate dibasic, glycine, and thimerosal (mercury derivative) as a preservative.

Pertussis Vaccine is prepared by growing Phase I *Bordetella pertussis* in a modified Cohen-Wheeler broth containing acid hydrolysate of casein. The *B. pertussis* is inactivated with thimerosal, harvested, and then suspended in a solution containing potassium phosphate monobasic, sodium phosphate dibasic, sodium chloride, and thimerosal (mercury derivative) as a preservative.

The oligosaccharides for the Haemophilus b conjugate component are derived from highly purified capsular polysaccharide, polyribosylribitol phosphate, isolated from *Haemophilus influenzae* type b (Haemophilus b) grown in a chemically defined medium (a mixture of mineral salts, amino acids, and cofactors). The oligosaccharides are purified and sized by diafiltrations through a series of ultrafiltration membranes, and coupled by reductive amination directly to highly purified CRM₁₉₇.[4,5] CRM₁₉₇ is a nontoxic variant of diphtheria toxin isolated from cultures of *C. diphtheriae* C7 (β 197) grown in a casamino acids and yeast extract-based medium. The conjugate is purified through ultrafiltration, ammonium sulfate precipitation, and ion-exchange chromatography to high purity.

The Haemophilus b conjugate component is combined with the diphtheria and tetanus toxoids and pertussis vaccine adsorbed to produce the final vaccine. As a preservative, thimerosal (mercury derivative) is added to the combination vaccine to a final concentration of 1:10,000. The aluminum content (from aluminum phosphate adjuvant) of the final product does not exceed 0.85 mg per 0.5 mL dose as determined by assay. The residual-free formaldehyde content by assay is ≤0.02%.

Each single dose of 0.5 mL of TETRAMUNE is formulated to contain 12.5 Lf of diphtheria toxoid, 5 Lf of tetanus toxoid (both toxoids induce not less than 2 units of antitoxin per mL in the guinea pig potency test), 10 μg of purified Haemophilus b saccharide, and approximately 25 μg of CRM₁₉₇ protein. Each 0.5 mL dose of vaccine is formulated to contain less than 16 OPUs of inactivated pertussis cells. The total human immunizing dose (the first three 0.5 mL doses given) contains an estimate of 12 units of pertussis vaccine with an estimate of 4 protective units per single human dose, as determined by the mouse pertussis potency test. The potency for the Haemophilus b conjugate component of TETRAMUNE is determined by gas chromatography assay for total saccharide. Each component of the vaccine—diphtheria, tetanus, pertussis, and Haemophilus b conjugate—meets the required potency standards, and contains no other active ingredients.

CLINICAL PHARMACOLOGY

Simultaneous immunization against diphtheria, tetanus, and pertussis during infancy and childhood has been a routine practice in the United States since the late 1940s, and immunization against Haemophilus b has been a routine practice since 1985. These immunizations have played a major role in markedly reducing the incidence of cases and deaths from each of these diseases.

Diphtheria is primarily a localized and generalized intoxication caused by diphtheria toxin, an extracellular protein metabolite of toxinogenic strains of *C. diphtheriae*. While the incidence of diphtheria in the US has decreased from over 200,000 cases reported in 1921, before the general use of diphtheria toxoid, to only 15 cases reported from 1980 to 1983,[6] the case fatality rate has remained constant at about 5% to 10%. The highest case fatality rates are in the very young and in the elderly.

Following adequate immunization with diphtheria toxoid, it is thought that protection lasts for at least 10 years.[6] Antitoxin levels of at least 0.01 antitoxin units/mL are generally regarded as protective.[7] This significantly reduces both the risk of developing diphtheria and the severity of clinical illness. It does not, however, eliminate carriage of *C. diphtheriae* in the pharynx or on the skin.[6]

Tetanus is an intoxication manifested primarily by neuromuscular dysfunction caused by a potent exotoxin elaborated by *C. tetani*. The incidence of tetanus in the US has dropped dramatically with the routine use of tetanus toxoid, remaining relatively constant over the last decade at about 90 cases reported annually. Spores of *C. tetani* are ubiquitous, and there is essentially no natural immunity to tetanus toxin.

Continued on next page

Tetramune—Cont.

Thus, universal primary immunization with tetanus toxoid with subsequent maintenance of adequate antitoxin levels, by means of timed boosters, is recommended to protect all age groups.[6] Tetanus toxoid is a highly effective antigen and a completed primary series generally induces serum antitoxin levels of at least 0.01 antitoxin units, a level that has been reported to be protective.[8] It is thought that protection persists for at least 10 years.[6]

The toxoids of tetanus and diphtheria induce neutralizing antibodies to the toxins produced by the infecting organism. In clinical studies with Lederle-produced diphtheria and tetanus toxoids, administered in combination with pertussis vaccine, serum antitoxin levels have been shown to be greater than 0.01 antitoxin units/mL in 97% to 100% of 372 infants following three doses.[9,10] These levels are generally regarded to be protective.[7,8]

Pertussis (whooping cough) is a disease of the respiratory tract caused by *B. pertussis*. This gram-negative coccobacillus produces a variety of active components including endotoxin and a number of other substances that have been defined primarily on the basis of their biological activity in animals. These active components, have been associated with a number of effects, such as lymphocytosis, leukocytosis, sensitivity to histamine, changes in glucose and/or insulin levels, possible neurological effects, and adjuvant activity.[11] The roles of each of the different components in either the pathogenesis of, or immunity to, pertussis are not well understood.

Pertussis (whooping cough) is a highly communicable disease of the respiratory tract. Attack rates of over 90% have been reported in unimmunized household contacts.[12] Since immunization against pertussis (whooping cough) became widespread, the number of reported cases and associated mortality in the US has declined from about 120,000 cases and 1,100 deaths in 1950,[13] to an annual average of about 3,500 cases and 10 fatalities in recent years.[6,14] Precise data do not exist since bacteriological confirmation of pertussis can be obtained in less than half of the suspected cases. Most reported illness from *B. pertussis* occurs in infants and young children; two thirds of reported deaths occur in children less than 1 year old. Older children and adults, in whom classic signs are often absent, may go undiagnosed and serve as reservoirs of disease.[6,15]

The potency of the pertussis component of the vaccine is measured and shown to be acceptable in the mouse potency test. Previously, serum agglutinin titers of pertussis vaccines have been correlated with clinical protection in the Medical Research Council trials.[8] The pertussis component induces immunity against pertussis disease in humans.

Haemophilus influenzae type b was the most common cause of invasive bacterial disease, including meningitis, in young children in the US prior to licensure of vaccines for this disease. Although nonencapsulated *H. influenzae* are common and six capsular polysaccharide types are known, strains with the type b capsule caused most of the invasive Haemophilus diseases prior to the introduction of Haemophilus b conjugate vaccines.[16]

Prior to routine immunization, Haemophilus b disease occurred primarily in children under 5 years of age. In the US, the incidence of invasive Haemophilus b disease peaked between 6 months and 1 year of age, and approximately 55% of disease occurred between 6 and 18 months of age.[16] The cumulative risk of developing invasive Haemophilus b disease during the first 5 years of life was about 1 in 200 prior to the introduction of Haemophilus b conjugate vaccines. Approximately 60% of cases were meningitis. Cellulitis, epiglottitis, pericarditis, pneumonia, sepsis, or septic arthritis made up the remaining 40%. An estimated 12,000 cases of Haemophilus b meningitis occurred annually prior to the routine use of conjugate vaccines in infants and toddlers.[16,17] The mortality rate can be 5%, and neurologic sequelae have been observed in up to 38% of survivors.[18]

The incidence of invasive Haemophilus b disease is increased in certain children, such as those who are native Americans, black, or from lower socioeconomic status and those with medical conditions such as asplenia, sickle cell disease, malignancies associated with immunosuppression, and antibody deficiency syndromes.[16,17,19]

The protective activity of antibody to Haemophilus b polysaccharide was demonstrated by the efficacy study of Haemophilus b polysaccharide (HbPs) vaccine.[20] Data from passive antibody studies indicate that a preexisting titer of antibody to HbPs of 0.15 µg/mL correlates with protection.[21] Data from a Finnish field trial in children 18 to 71 months of age indicate that a titer of >1.0 µg/mL 3 weeks after vaccination is associated with long-term protection.[22,23]

Linkage of Haemophilus b saccharides to a protein such as CRM_{197} converts the saccharide (HbO) to a T-dependent (HbOC) antigen, and results in an enhanced antibody response to the saccharide in young infants that primes for an anamnestic response and is predominantly of the IgG class.[24] Laboratory evidence indicates that the native state of the CRM_{197} protein and the use of oligosaccharides in the formulation of HibTITER Haemophilus b Conjugate Vaccine (Diphtheria CRM_{197} Protein Conjugate) (HbOC), enhances its immunogenicity.[25–27] NO PUBLISHED DATA ARE AVAILABLE TO SUPPORT THE INTERCHANGEABILITY OF HbOC AND OTHER HAEMOPHILUS b CONJUGATE VACCINES WITH ONE ANOTHER FOR PRIMARY IMMUNIZATION.

HbOC was shown to be effective in a large-scale controlled clinical trial in a multiethnic population in northern California carried out between February 1988 and June 1990.[28,29] It should be noted that DTP was administered simultaneously with HbOC but at a separate site. There were no (0) vaccine failures in infants who received three doses of HbOC and 12 cases of Haemophilus b disease (6 cases of meningitis) in the control group. The estimate of efficacy is 100% (P=.0002) with 95% confidence intervals of 68% to 100%. Through the end of 1991, with an additional 49,000 person-years of follow-up, there were still no cases of Haemophilus b disease in fully vaccinated infants less than 2 years of age.[10,30] Person-years may be defined as the number of individuals receiving the appropriate number of doses times the average number of years of follow-up for all of the individuals. One case of disease has been reported in a $3^1/_2$-year-old child who did not receive the recommended booster dose.

Evidence of efficacy postlicensure of Haemophilus b conjugate vaccines in the US is indicated by reports of significant reductions (71% to 94%) in Haemophilus b disease that are closely associated with increases in the net doses of Haemophilus b conjugate vaccines distributed.[30,31] Occasional cases of vaccine failures have, however, been reported to the US Department of Health and Human Services through the Vaccine Adverse Event Reporting System (VAERS) since licensure of Haemophilus b conjugate vaccines.

TETRAMUNE has been given to 6,793 children as part of a series of studies to test the safety and immunogenicity of this combined product when compared to separate administration of DTP and HbOC. The vaccines were given at 2, 4, and 6 months of age or at 15 to 18 months of age. Local reactions and systemic events after vaccination were generally comparable between the groups that received the combination product or separate injections. (It should be noted that comparison of local reactions was done by comparing the combined product to the separate injection site that gave the largest reactions or to the DTP injection site.) Scattered reactions occurred more frequently (P <.05) in the combination group for some doses (swelling and drowsiness after the first dose; irritability and restless sleep after the second dose; injection site warmth and irritability after the third dose; injection site swelling, warmth, tenderness, irritability after the toddler dose). Rash was seen more commonly in the separate group. There was no consistent or identifiable pattern to these group differences across studies or doses. The large trial with 6,497 infants receiving TETRAMUNE allowed analysis of rare adverse events, including SIDS (sudden infant death syndrome), hospitalizations, and emergency room visits, following vaccination. No differences were found between the cohorts (see **ADVERSE REACTIONS**).[10] Taken together, the safety studies conducted in infants and in toddlers indicate that this vaccine is safe and that there was no consistent pattern of enhanced adverse events following combined vaccine (TETRAMUNE) as compared to separate injections.

The antibody response to each of the components of TETRAMUNE was measured (n=189) and compared to separate administration of the DTP and HbOC vaccines (n=189). After three doses, the antibody response to TETRAMUNE was equal to or higher for all four components: tetanus (IU/mL), diphtheria (IU/mL), pertussis (microagglutination), and *H. influenzae* b polysaccharide (µg IgG/mL as per ELISA). In addition, responses to specific pertussis antigens (ie, pertussis toxin, FHA, and 69K protein) were found to be as high or higher in the TETRAMUNE product compared to separate administration of DTP. Therefore, the immunogenicity of the combined vaccine is at least as good as the two vaccines given separately.[10]

INDICATIONS AND USAGE

Diphtheria and Tetanus Toxoids and Pertussis Vaccine Adsorbed and Haemophilus b Conjugate Vaccine (Diphtheria CRM_{197} Protein Conjugate) TETRAMUNE is indicated for the active immunization of children 2 months of age to 5 years of age for protection against diphtheria, tetanus, pertussis, and Haemophilus b disease when indications for immunization with DTP vaccine and Haemophilus b Conjugate Vaccine coincide. Typically, this is at 2, 4, 6, and 15 months of age.

Children who have recovered from culture-confirmed pertussis need not receive further doses of a vaccine containing pertussis.[6] However, these children should receive additional doses of Diphtheria and Tetanus Toxoids Adsorbed, for Pediatric Use (DT) as well as Haemophilus b Conjugate Vaccine as appropriate to complete the series.

The American Academy of Pediatrics (AAP) has recommended that children who have experienced invasive Haemophilus b disease when <24 months of age should continue immunization against Haemophilus b, but that children whose disease occurred at ≥24 months need not receive further doses of Haemophilus b Conjugate Vaccine.[32] However, these children should receive additional doses of DTP (or if pertussis is contraindicated, DT should be used) as appropriate to complete the series.

TETRAMUNE is intended for active immunization against diphtheria, tetanus, pertussis, and Haemophilus type b diseases and is not to be used for treatment of actual infection.

TETRAMUNE is not routinely recommended for immunization of persons older than 5 years of age. Under certain circumstances, TETRAMUNE may be used beyond age 5 years. Because TETRAMUNE contains pediatric DTP vaccine, it is not recommended for use beyond the seventh birthday.

As with any vaccine, TETRAMUNE may not protect 100% of individuals receiving the vaccine.

If passive immunization is needed, Tetanus Immune Globulin (human TIG) and/or Diphtheria Antitoxin are recommended for tetanus and diphtheria, respectively (see **DOSAGE AND ADMINISTRATION**).[6]

CONTRAINDICATIONS

HYPERSENSITIVITY TO ANY COMPONENT OF THE VACCINE, INCLUDING THIMEROSAL, A MERCURY DERIVATIVE, IS A CONTRAINDICATION.

IMMUNIZATION SHOULD BE DEFERRED DURING THE COURSE OF ANY FEBRILE ILLNESS OR ACUTE INFECTION. THE IMMUNIZATION PRACTICES ADVISORY COMMITTEE (ACIP) HAS STATED THAT "...MINOR ILLNESSES SUCH AS MILD UPPER RESPIRATORY INFECTIONS WITH OR WITHOUT LOW GRADE FEVER ARE NOT CONTRAINDICATIONS."[6,33]

IMMUNIZATION WITH TETRAMUNE IS CONTRAINDICATED IF THE CHILD HAS EXPERIENCED ANY EVENT FOLLOWING PREVIOUS IMMUNIZATION WITH A PERTUSSIS-CONTAINING VACCINE, WHICH IS CONSIDERED BY THE AAP OR ACIP TO BE A CONTRAINDICATION TO FURTHER DOSES OF PERTUSSIS VACCINE. THESE EVENTS INCLUDE:

- AN IMMEDIATE ANAPHYLACTIC REACTION.
- ENCEPHALOPATHY OCCURRING WITHIN 7 DAYS FOLLOWING VACCINATION. THIS IS DEFINED AS AN ACUTE, SEVERE CENTRAL-NERVOUS-SYSTEM DISORDER OCCURRING WITHIN 7 DAYS FOLLOWING VACCINATION, AND GENERALLY CONSISTING OF MAJOR ALTERATIONS IN CONSCIOUSNESS, UNRESPONSIVENESS, GENERALIZED OR FOCAL SEIZURES THAT PERSIST MORE THAN A FEW HOURS, WITH FAILURE TO RECOVER WITHIN 24 HOURS.[6,33]

THE OCCURRENCE OF ANY TYPE OF NEUROLOGICAL SYMPTOMS OR SIGNS, INCLUDING ONE OR MORE CONVULSIONS (SEIZURES) FOLLOWING ADMINISTRATION OF TETRAMUNE, IS GENERALLY A CONTRAINDICATION TO FURTHER USE. ANY DECISION TO ADMINISTER SUBSEQUENT DOSES OF A VACCINE CONTAINING DIPHTHERIA, TETANUS, OR PERTUSSIS ANTIGENS SHOULD BE DELAYED UNTIL THE PATIENT'S NEUROLOGICAL STATUS IS BETTER DEFINED.[6]

THE PRESENCE OF ANY EVOLVING OR CHANGING DISORDER AFFECTING THE CENTRAL NERVOUS SYSTEM IS A CONTRAINDICATION TO ADMINISTRATION OF A PERTUSSIS-CONTAINING VACCINE, SUCH AS TETRAMUNE, REGARDLESS OF WHETHER THE SUSPECTED NEUROLOGICAL DISORDER IS ASSOCIATED WITH OCCURRENCE OF SEIZURE ACTIVITY OF ANY TYPE.[6,33]

STUDIES HAVE INDICATED THAT A PERSONAL OR FAMILY HISTORY OF SEIZURES IS ASSOCIATED WITH INCREASED FREQUENCY OF SEIZURES FOLLOWING PERTUSSIS IMMUNIZATION.[34–36]

The ACIP and the AAP recognize certain circumstances in which children with stable central nervous system disorders, including well-controlled seizures or satisfactorily explained single seizures, may receive pertussis vaccine. The ACIP and AAP do not consider a family history of seizures to be a contraindication to pertussis vaccine despite the increased risk of seizures in these individuals.[6,33,34]

The decision to administer a pertussis-containing vaccine to children must be made by the physician on an individual basis, with consideration of all relevant factors, and assessment of potential risks and benefits for that individual. The physician should review the full text of ACIP and AAP guidelines prior to considering vaccination for children.[6,33,34] The parent or guardian should be advised of the increased risk involved.

There are no data on whether the prophylactic use of antipyretics can decrease the risk of febrile convulsions. However, data suggest that acetaminophen will reduce the incidence of postvaccination fever.[37] The ACIP and AAP suggest administering acetaminophen at age-appropriate doses at the time of vaccination and every 4 to 6 hours to children at higher risk for seizures than the general population.[6,33,34]

TETRAMUNE is not routinely recommended for immunization of persons older than 5 years of age. Under certain cir-

cumstances, TETRAMUNE may be used beyond age 5 years. Because TETRAMUNE contains pediatric DTP vaccine, it is not recommended for use beyond the seventh birthday.

ROUTINE IMMUNIZATION SHOULD BE DEFERRED DURING AN OUTBREAK OF POLIOMYELITIS PROVIDING THE PATIENT HAS NOT SUSTAINED AN INJURY THAT INCREASES THE RISK OF TETANUS AND PROVIDING AN OUTBREAK OF DIPHTHERIA OR PERTUSSIS DOES NOT OCCUR SIMULTANEOUSLY.[38]

The clinical judgment of the attending physician should prevail at all times.

WARNINGS

THE ACIP STATES THAT IF ANY OF THE FOLLOWING EVENTS OCCUR IN TEMPORAL RELATION TO RECEIPT OF DTP, THE DECISION TO GIVE SUBSEQUENT DOSES OF VACCINE CONTAINING THE PERTUSSIS COMPONENT SHOULD BE CAREFULLY CONSIDERED.

TEMPERATURE OF ≥40.5°C (105°F) WITHIN 48 HOURS NOT DUE TO IDENTIFIABLE CAUSE.

COLLAPSE OR SHOCK-LIKE STATE (HYPOTONIC-HYPORESPONSIVE EPISODE) WITHIN 48 HOURS.

PERSISTENT, INCONSOLABLE CRYING LASTING ≥3 HOURS, OCCURRING WITHIN 48 HOURS.

CONVULSIONS WITH OR WITHOUT FEVER OCCURRING WITHIN 3 DAYS.

"ALTHOUGH THESE EVENTS WERE CONSIDERED ABSOLUTE CONTRAINDICATIONS IN PREVIOUS ACIP RECOMMENDATIONS, THERE MAY BE CIRCUMSTANCES, SUCH AS A HIGH INCIDENCE OF PERTUSSIS, IN WHICH THE POTENTIAL BENEFITS OUTWEIGH POSSIBLE RISKS, PARTICULARLY BECAUSE THESE EVENTS ARE NOT ASSOCIATED WITH PERMANENT SEQUELAE."[6]

IF A CONTRAINDICATION TO ANY OF THE COMPONENTS OF THIS COMBINATION VACCINE EXISTS (SEE **CONTRAINDICATIONS** SECTION), THEN TETRAMUNE SHOULD NOT BE USED. FOR EXAMPLE, IF THERE IS A CONTRAINDICATION AGAINST THE USE OF A PERTUSSIS VACCINE COMPONENT, THEN DIPHTHERIA AND TETANUS TOXOIDS ADSORBED, FOR PEDIATRIC USE (DT), AND HAEMOPHILUS b CONJUGATE VACCINE (DIPHTHERIA CRM₁₉₇ PROTEIN CONJUGATE) HibTITER, AS SEPARATE INJECTIONS, SHOULD BE SUBSTITUTED FOR EACH OF THE REMAINING DOSES.

THE OCCURRENCE OF SUDDEN INFANT DEATH SYNDROME (SIDS) HAS BEEN REPORTED FOLLOWING ADMINISTRATION OF DTP.[39-41] HOWEVER, A LARGE CASE-CONTROL STUDY IN THE US REVEALED NO CAUSAL RELATIONSHIP BETWEEN RECEIPT OF DTP VACCINE AND SIDS.[42] A RECENT STUDY OF 6,497 INFANTS IN NORTHERN CALIFORNIA FOUND NO INCREASE IN THE RATE OF SIDS AMONG TETRAMUNE RECIPIENTS.[10]

AS WITH ANY INTRAMUSCULAR INJECTION, TETRAMUNE SHOULD BE GIVEN WITH CAUTION TO INFANTS OR CHILDREN WITH THROMBOCYTOPENIA OR ANY COAGULATION DISORDER THAT WOULD CONTRAINDICATE INTRAMUSCULAR INJECTION (SEE **DRUG INTERACTIONS**).

As reported with Haemophilus b polysaccharide vaccine, cases of Haemophilus type b disease may occur prior to the onset of the protective effect of this vaccine.[16,43]

TETRAMUNE WILL NOT PROTECT AGAINST *H. INFLUENZAE* OTHER THAN TYPE b STRAINS.

ANTIGENURIA HAS BEEN DETECTED FOLLOWING RECEIPT OF HAEMOPHILUS b CONJUGATE VACCINE[44] AND, THEREFORE ANTIGEN DETECTION IN URINE MAY NOT HAVE DIAGNOSTIC VALUE IN SUSPECTED HAEMOPHILUS b DISEASE WITHIN 2 WEEKS OF IMMUNIZATION.

PRECAUTIONS

GENERAL

CARE IS TO BE TAKEN BY THE HEALTH CARE PROVIDER FOR SAFE AND EFFECTIVE USE OF THIS PRODUCT.

1. TETRAMUNE is not routinely recommended for immunization of persons older than 5 years of age. Under certain circumstances, TETRAMUNE may be used beyond age 5 years. Because TETRAMUNE contains pediatric DTP vaccine, it is not recommended for use beyond the seventh birthday.

2. PRIOR TO ADMINISTRATION OF ANY DOSE OF TETRAMUNE, THE PARENT OR GUARDIAN SHOULD BE ASKED ABOUT THE PERSONAL HISTORY, FAMILY HISTORY, AND RECENT HEALTH STATUS OF THE VACCINE RECIPIENT. THE HEALTH CARE PROVIDER SHOULD ASCERTAIN PREVIOUS IMMUNIZATION HISTORY, CURRENT HEALTH STATUS, AND OCCURRENCE OF ANY SYMPTOMS AND/OR SIGNS OF AN ADVERSE EVENT AFTER PREVIOUS IMMUNIZATIONS, IN THE CHILD TO BE IMMUNIZED, IN ORDER TO DETERMINE THE EXISTENCE OF ANY

CONTRAINDICATION TO IMMUNIZATION WITH TETRAMUNE AND TO ALLOW AN ASSESSMENT OF BENEFITS AND RISKS.

3. BEFORE THE INJECTION OF ANY BIOLOGICAL, THE HEALTH CARE PROVIDER SHOULD TAKE ALL PRECAUTIONS KNOWN FOR THE PREVENTION OF ALLERGIC OR ANY OTHER SIDE REACTIONS. This should include: a review of the patient's history regarding possible sensitivity; the ready availability of epinephrine 1:1,000 and other appropriate agents used for control of immediate allergic reactions; and a knowledge of the recent literature pertaining to use of the biological concerned, including the nature of side effects and adverse reactions that may follow its use.

4. Children with impaired immune responsiveness, whether due to the use of immunosuppressive therapy (including irradiation, corticosteroids, antimetabolites, alkylating agents, and cytotoxic agents), a genetic defect, human immunodeficiency virus (HIV) infection, or other causes, may have reduced antibody response to active immunization procedures.[6,33,45] Deferral of administration of vaccine may be considered in individuals receiving immunosuppressive therapy.[6,33] Other groups should receive this vaccine according to the usual recommended schedule.[6,33,45,46] (See **DRUG INTERACTIONS**.)

5. This product is not contraindicated based on the presence of human immunodeficiency virus infection.[47]

6. *Since this product is a suspension containing an adjuvant, shake vigorously to obtain a uniform suspension prior to withdrawing each dose from the multiple dose vial.*

7. A separate sterile syringe and needle or a sterile disposable unit should be used for each individual patient to prevent transmission of infectious agents from one person to another. Needles should be disposed of properly and should not be recapped.

8. Special care should be taken to prevent injection into a blood vessel.

NATIONAL CHILDHOOD VACCINE INJURY ACT

This Act requires that the manufacturer and lot number of the vaccine administered be recorded by the health care provider in the vaccine recipient's permanent medical record (or in a permanent office log or file), along with the date of administration of the vaccine and the name, address, and title of the person administering the vaccine.

The Act further requires the health care provider to report to the Secretary of the Department of Health and Human Services through the Vaccine Adverse Event Reporting System (VAERS) the occurrence following immunization of any event set forth in the Vaccine Injury Table, including: anaphylaxis or anaphylactic shock within 24 hours; encephalopathy or encephalitis within 7 days; shock-collapse or hypotonic-hyporesponsive collapse within 7 days; residual seizure disorder; any acute complication or sequelae (including death) of above events, or any event that would contraindicate further doses of vaccine, according to this TETRAMUNE package insert.

The US Department of Health and Human Services has established VAERS to accept all reports of suspected adverse events after the administration of any vaccine, including but not limited to the reporting of events required by the National Childhood Vaccine Injury Act of 1986.[48] The VAERS toll-free number for VAERS forms and information is 800-822-7967.

INFORMATION FOR PATIENT

PRIOR TO ADMINISTRATION OF TETRAMUNE, HEALTH CARE PERSONNEL SHOULD INFORM THE PARENT, GUARDIAN, OR OTHER RESPONSIBLE ADULT OF THE RECOMMENDED IMMUNIZATION SCHEDULE FOR PROTECTION AGAINST DIPHTHERIA, TETANUS, PERTUSSIS, AND HAEMOPHILUS b DISEASE AND THE BENEFITS AND RISKS TO THE CHILD RECEIVING THIS VACCINE. GUIDANCE SHOULD BE PROVIDED ON MEASURES TO BE TAKEN SHOULD ADVERSE EVENTS OCCUR, SUCH AS ANTIPYRETIC MEASURES FOR ELEVATED TEMPERATURES AND THE NEED TO REPORT ADVERSE EVENTS TO THE HEALTH CARE PROVIDER. PARENTS SHOULD BE PROVIDED WITH VACCINE INFORMATION PAMPHLETS AT THE TIME OF EACH VACCINATION, AS STATED IN THE NATIONAL CHILDHOOD VACCINE INJURY ACT.[48]

THE HEALTH CARE PROVIDER SHOULD INFORM THE PATIENT, PARENT, OR GUARDIAN OF THE IMPORTANCE OF COMPLETING THE IMMUNIZATION SERIES.

PATIENTS, PARENTS, OR GUARDIANS SHOULD BE INSTRUCTED TO REPORT ANY SERIOUS ADVERSE REACTIONS TO THEIR HEALTH CARE PROVIDER.

DRUG INTERACTIONS

Children receiving immunosuppressive therapy may have a reduced response to active immunization procedures.[6,33,45] As with other intramuscular injections, TETRAMUNE should be given with caution to children on anticoagulant therapy.

Tetanus Immune Globulin or Diphtheria Antitoxin, if used, should be given in a separate site with a separate needle and syringe.

The AAP recommends that influenza virus vaccine should not be administered within 3 days of immunization with a pertussis-containing vaccine since both vaccines may cause febrile reactions in young children.[33]

Data are not yet available concerning adverse reactions that may occur when TETRAMUNE is given simultaneously with Oral Poliovirus Vaccine (OPV), Measles-Mumps-Rubella (MMR), or Hepatitis B (HB) vaccine at separate sites. Also, data are not available concerning the effects on immune response of OPV, MMR, or HB vaccine when TETRAMUNE is given simultaneously. Clinical studies with TETRAMUNE did, however, allow for the administration of OPV according to the routine immunization schedule for OPV.[10]

CARCINOGENESIS, MUTAGENESIS, IMPAIRMENT OF FERTILITY

TETRAMUNE has not been evaluated for its carcinogenic, mutagenic potential, or for impairment of fertility.

PREGNANCY

Pregnancy Category C.

Animal reproduction studies have not been conducted with TETRAMUNE. This product is not recommended for use in individuals 7 years of age or older.

PEDIATRIC USE

The safety and effectiveness of TETRAMUNE in children below the age of 6 weeks have not been established.

For immunization of children 7 years of age or older, Tetanus and Diphtheria Toxoids Adsorbed for Adult Use (Td) is recommended.[6,33] If contraindication to the pertussis component exists, Diphtheria and Tetanus Toxoids Adsorbed, for Pediatric Use (DT) should be substituted in children who have not reached their seventh birthday.

Full protection against the indicated diseases (tetanus, diphtheria, pertussis, and Haemophilus type b disease) is based on a full course of immunization.

ADVERSE REACTIONS

The safety of TETRAMUNE has been evaluated in 6,793 children at 2, 4, and 6 months of age or at 15 to 18 months of age in three separate sites. The percent of doses administered associated with injection site reactions within 72 hours, or common systemic symptoms within 4 days, is summarized below:

[See table at top of next page]

Based on review of the Kaiser-Permanente Medical Care Program utilization data base of hospitalizations (within 60 days) and emergency room visits (within 30 days of immunization) in 6,497 infants who received TETRAMUNE, the most common reasons for seeking care include: trauma, viral illness, and respiratory illnesses (eg, upper respiratory infection, otitis media, bronchitis/bronchiolitis, and pneumonia). One child who received TETRAMUNE became transiently pale and tremulous without loss of responsiveness 4 hours after immunization and was hospitalized with a diagnosis of seizure. No other hospital visits for seizure or hypotonic, hyporesponsive episodes were reported within 72 hours of immunization. These results were not different from those observed in 3,935 infants who received DTP and HbOC at separate injection sites.

As with other aluminum-containing vaccines,[49] a nodule may occasionally be palpable at the injection site for several weeks. Although not seen in studies with TETRAMUNE, sterile abscess formation or subcutaneous atrophy at the injection site may also occur.

The following significant adverse events have occurred following administration of DTP vaccines: persistent, inconsolable crying ≥3 hours (1/100 doses), high-pitched, unusual crying (1/1,000 doses), fever ≥40.5°C (105°F) (1/330 doses), transient shock-like (hypotonic, hyporesponsive) episode (1/1,750 doses), convulsions (1/1,750 doses).[6,33]

The ACIP states: "Although DTP may rarely produce symptoms that some have classified as acute encephalopathy, a causal relation between DTP vaccine and permanent brain damage has not been demonstrated. If the vaccine ever causes brain damage, the occurrence of such an event must be exceedingly rare. A similar conclusion has been reached by the Committee on Infectious Diseases of the American Academy of Pediatrics, the Child Neurology Society, the Canadian National Advisory Committee on Immunization, the British Joint Committee on Vaccination and Immunization, the British Pediatric Association, and the Institute of Medicine."[6]

The occurrence of sudden infant death syndrome (SIDS) has been reported following administration of DTP.[39-41] However, a large case-control study in the US revealed no causal relationship between receipt of DTP vaccine and SIDS.[42] A recent study of 6,497 infants in northern California found no increase in the rate of SIDS among TETRAMUNE recipients.[10]

Continued on next page

Tetramune—Cont.

Onset of infantile spasms has occurred in infants who have recently received DTP or DT. Analysis of data from the National Childhood Encephalopathy Study on children with infantile spasms showed that receipt of preparations containing diphtheria, tetanus, and/or pertussis antigens was not causally related to infantile spasms.[50] The incidence of onset of infantile spasms increases at 3 to 9 months of age, the time period in which the second and third doses of DTP are generally given. Therefore, some cases of infantile spasms can be expected to be related by chance alone to recent receipt of vaccines containing DTP.[6]

Bulging fontanel[51–53] has been reported after DTP immunization, although no cause and effect relationship has been established.

Cardiac effects[54–56] and respiratory difficulties, including apnea, have been reported rarely following DTP immunization.

Other events that have been reported following administration of vaccines containing diphtheria, tetanus, pertussis, or Haemophilus b antigens include: urticaria, erythema multiforme or other rash, arthralgias,[57] and, more rarely, a severe anaphylactic reaction (eg, urticaria with swelling of the mouth, difficulty breathing, hypotension, or shock) and neurological complications,[58] such as convulsions,[57,59] encephalopathy,[57,60] and various mono- and polyneuropathies,[60–66] including Guillain-Barré syndrome.[67–69] Permanent neurological disability and death have also been reported rarely in temporal relation to immunization although a causal relationship has not been established.

DOSAGE AND ADMINISTRATION

For Intramuscular Use Only

For infants beginning at 2 months of age, the immunization series for TETRAMUNE consists of three doses of 0.5 mL each at approximately 2-month intervals, followed by a fourth dose of 0.5 mL at approximately 15 months of age. TETRAMUNE may be substituted for DTP and HibTITER administered separately, whenever the recommended schedules for use of these two vaccines coincide (see DTP and HibTITER recommended dosage schedules).[6,32,33,70] However, no published data are available to support the interchangeability of the Haemophilus b conjugate vaccine in TETRAMUNE and HibTITER with other Haemophilus b conjugate vaccines for the primary series. Therefore, it is recommended that the same conjugate vaccine be used throughout the primary series, consistent with the data supporting licensure of the vaccine.[32]

RECOMMENDED IMMUNIZATION SCHEDULES

For Previously Unvaccinated *Younger* Children

Dose	Age	Immunization
1	2 months	TETRAMUNE
2	4 months	TETRAMUNE
3	6 months	TETRAMUNE
4	15–18 months	TETRAMUNE*
5	4–6 years	DTP or DTaP

* Children 15 to 18 months of age may receive DTaP plus a Haemophilus b conjugate vaccine as separate injections.

For Previously Unvaccinated *Older* Children[33]

Immunization schedules should be considered on an individual basis for children not vaccinated according to the recommended schedule. Three doses of a product containing DTP, given at approximately 2-month intervals, are required, followed by a fourth dose of a product containing DTP or DTaP approximately 12 months later, and a fifth dose of a product containing DTP or DTaP at 4 to 6 years of age. If the fourth dose of a pertussis-containing vaccine is not given until after the fourth birthday, no further doses of a pertussis-containing vaccine are necessary.

The number of doses of an HbOC-containing product indicated depends on the age that immunization is begun. A child 7 to 11 months of age should receive 3 doses of a product containing HbOC. A child 12 to 14 months of age should receive 2 doses of a product containing HbOC. A child 15 to 59 months of age should receive 1 dose of a product containing HbOC.

As indicated previously, TETRAMUNE may be substituted for DTP and HibTITER administered separately, whenever the recommended schedule for use of these two vaccines coincides.

Preterm infants should be vaccinated with TETRAMUNE according to their chronological age, from birth.[6]

Interruption of the recommended schedules with a delay between doses does not interfere with the final immunity achieved; nor does it necessitate starting the series over again, regardless of the length of time elapsed between doses.[6,33]

If a contraindication to the pertussis vaccine component occurs, Diphtheria and Tetanus Toxoids Adsorbed, for Pediat-

ric Use (DT), and Haemophilus b Conjugate Vaccine HibTITER, as separate injections, should be substituted for each of the remaining doses.

The use of reduced volume (fractional doses) is not recommended. The effect of such practices on the frequency of serious adverse events and on protection against disease has not been determined.

Shake vigorously to obtain a uniform suspension prior to withdrawing each dose from the multiple dose vial. The vaccine should not be used if it cannot be resuspended.

Parenteral drug products should be inspected visually for particulate matter and discoloration prior to administration whenever solution and container permit. (See **DESCRIPTION.**)

The vaccine should be injected intramuscularly. The preferred sites are the anterolateral aspect of the thigh or the deltoid muscle of the upper arm. The vaccine should not be injected in the gluteal area or areas where there may be a major nerve trunk. Before injection, the skin at the injection site should be cleansed and prepared with a suitable germicide.

After insertion of the needle, aspirate to help avoid inadvertent injection into a blood vessel.

For either primary or booster immunization against tetanus and diphtheria of individuals 7 years of age and older, the use of Tetanus and Diphtheria Toxoids Adsorbed for Adult Use (Td) is recommended.[6,33]

For passive immunization against tetanus and diphtheria, human TIG, and/or Diphtheria Antitoxin are recommended.[6] A separate syringe and site of injection should be used.

HOW SUPPLIED

NDC 0005-1960-31 5.0 mL vial

STORAGE

DO NOT FREEZE. STORE REFRIGERATED, AWAY FROM FREEZER COMPARTMENT, AT 2°C TO 8°C (36°F TO 46°F).

% of Doses Associated with Symptoms[10]

	Infants‡ (542 doses)	Infants§ (7269 doses)	Toddlers (107 doses)
Local*			
Erythema	34	19	40
Pain/Tenderness	21	30	65
Swelling	20	20	43
Warmth	16	—	35
Systemic†			
Fever ≥38.0°C	24	40''	33
Irritability	42	54	49
Drowsiness	26	—	9
Restless Sleep	—	28	—
Loss of Appetite	—	4	—
Vomiting	5	2	1
Diarrhea	9	1	10
Rash	3	—	0

* Within 72 hours of immunization.
† Within 4 days of immunization.
‡ A separate multicenter safety and immunogenicity study, not a subset of the 7,269 infant Kaiser study.
§ Data for this study all collected within 24 hours of immunization (percentages calculated from a range of 7269 to 7500 doses) in the Kaiser Permanente Safety and Immunogenicity Study.
'' Perceived fever.

REFERENCES

1. Mueller JH, Miller PA. Production of diphtheria toxin of high potency (100 Lf) on a reproducible medium. *J Immunol.* 1941;40:21–32.
2. Mueller JH, Miller PA. Factors influencing the production of tetanal toxin. *J Immunol.* 1947;56:143–147.
3. Pillemer L, Grossberg DB, Wittler RG. The immunochemistry of toxins and toxoids, II. The preparation and immunologic evaluation of purified tetanal toxoid. *J Immunol.* 1946;54:213–224.
4. United States Patent Number 4,902,506 by Anderson PW, Eby RJ filed May 5, 1986 issued February 20, 1990.
5. Seid RC Jr, Boykins RA, Liu DF, et al. Chemical evidence for covalent linkage of a semi-synthetic glycoconjugate vaccine for *Haemophilus influenzae* type b disease. *Glycoconjugate J.* 1989;6:489–498.
6. Diphtheria, tetanus and pertussis: Recommendations for vaccine use and other preventive measures—recommendations of the Immunization Practices Advisory Committee (ACIP). *MMWR.* 1991;40/No. RR-10.
7. Pappenheimer AM Jr. Diphtheria. In: Germanier R, ed. *Bacterial Vaccines.* New York, NY: Academic Press Inc; 1984:1–36.
8. *Federal Register Notice,* Friday, December 13, 1985, Vol. 50, No. 240.
9. Blumberg DA, Mink CM, Cherry JD, et al. Comparison of acellular and whole-cell pertussis-component diphtheria-tetanus-pertussis vaccines in infants. *J Pediatr.* 1991; 119:194–204.
10. Unpublished data available from Lederle Laboratories.
11. Manclark CR, Cowell JL. Pertussis Vaccine. In: Germanier R, ed. *Bacterial Vaccines.* New York, NY: Academic Press Inc; 1984:69–106.
12. Kendrick PL. Secondary familial attack rates from pertussis in vaccinated and unvaccinated children. *Am J Hygiene.* 1940;32:89–91.
13. Reported incidence of notifiable diseases in the United States. *MMWR.* 1970;19(53):44.
14. Pertussis surveillance—United States, 1986–1988. *MMWR.* 1990;39(4):57–66.
15. Mortimer EA Jr. Pertussis and its prevention: a family affair. *J Infect Dis.* 1990;161:437–479.
16. Wenger JD, Ward JL, Broome CV. Prevention of *Haemophilus influenzae* type b disease: vaccines and passive prophylaxis. In: Remington JS, Swartz MS, eds. *Current Clinical Topics in Infectious Diseases.* New York, NY: McGraw-Hill Inc; 1989;10:306–339.
17. Recommendation of the Immunization Practices Advisory Committee (ACIP). Polysaccharide vaccine for prevention of *Haemophilus influenzae* type b disease. *MMWR.* 1985;34:201–205.
18. Sell SH. Long term sequelae of bacterial meningitis in children. *Pediatr Infect Dis J.* 1983;2:90–93.
19. Broome CV. Epidemiology of *Haemophilus influenzae* type b infections in the United States. *Pediatr Infect Dis J.* 1987;6:779–782.
20. Peltola H, Kayhty H, Sivonen A. *Haemophilus influenzae* type b capsular polysaccharide vaccine in children: a double-blind field study of 100,000 vaccines 3 months to 5 years of age in Finland. *Pediatrics.* 1977;60:730–737.
21. Robbins JB, Parke JC, Schneerson R. Quantitative measurement of "natural" and immunization-induced *Haemophilus influenzae* type b capsular polysaccharide antibodies. *Pediatr Res.* 1973;7:103–110.
22. Kayhty H, Peltola H, Karanko V, et al. The protective level of serum antibodies to the capsular polysaccharide of *Haemophilus influenzae* type b. *J Infect Dis.* 1983;147:1100.
23. Kayhty H, Karanko V, Peltola H, et al. Serum antibodies after vaccination with *Haemophilus influenzae* type b capsular polysaccharide and responses to reimmunization: no evidence of immunologic tolerance or memory. *Pediatrics.* 1984;74:857-865.
24. Weinberg GA, Granoff DM. Polysaccharide-protein conjugate vaccines for the prevention of *Haemophilus influenzae* type b disease. *J Pediatr.* 1988;113:621–631.
25. Makela O, Péterfy F, Outshoorn IG, et al. Immunogenic properties of a (1–6) dextran, its protein conjugates, and conjugates of its breakdown products in mice. *Scand J Immunol.* 1984;19:541–550.
26. Anderson P, Pichichero ME, Insel RA. Immunogens consisting of oligosaccharides from *Haemophilus influenzae* type b coupled to diphtheria toxoid or the toxin protein CRM$_{197}$. *J Clin Invest.* 1985;76:52–59.
27. Madore DV, Phipps DC, Eby R, et al. Immune response of young children vaccinated with *Haemophilus influenzae* type b conjugate vaccines. In: Cruse JM, Lewis RE, eds. *Contributions to Microbiology and Immunology: Conjugate Vaccines.* New York, NY: Karger Medical and Scientific Publishers; 1989;10:125–150.
28. Black SB, Shinefield HR, Lampert D, et al. Safety and immunogenicity of oligosaccharide conjugate *Haemophilus influenzae* type b (HbOC) vaccine in infancy. *Pediatr Infect Dis J.* 1991;10:92–96.
29. Black SB, Shinefield HR, Fireman B, et al. Efficacy in infancy of oligosaccharide conjugate *Haemophilus influenzae* type b (HbOC) vaccine in a United States population of 61,080 children. *Pediatr Infect Dis J.* 1991;10:97–104.

30. Black SB, Shinefield HR, The Kaiser Permanente Pediatric Vaccine Study Group. Immunization with oligosaccharide conjugate *Haemophilus influenzae* type b (HbOC) vaccine on a large health maintenance organization population: extended follow-up and impact on *Haemophilus influenzae* disease epidemiology. *Pediatr Infect Dis J.* 1992;11:610–613.
31. Adams WG, Deaver KA, Cochi SL, et al. Decline of childhood *Haemophilus influenzae* type b (Hib) disease in the Hib vaccine era. *JAMA.* 1993;269:221–226.
32. Recommendations of the AAP: *Haemophilus influenzae* type b conjugate vaccine: recommendations for immunization of infants and children 2 months of age and older: update. *Pediatrics.* 1991;88:169–172.
33. American Academy of Pediatrics: Report of the Committee on Infectious Diseases. 22nd ed. Elk Grove Village, Ill: American Academy of Pediatrics; 1991.
34. Pertussis immunization: family history of convulsions and use of antipyretics—supplementary ACIP statement. *MMWR.* 1987;36(18):281–282.
35. Stetler HC, Orenstein WA, Bart KJ, et al. History of convulsions and use of pertussis vaccine. *J Pediatr.* 1985;107(2):175–179.
36. Hirtz DG, Nelson KB, Ellenberg JH. Seizures following childhood immunizations. *J Pediatr.* 1983; 102(1):14–18.
37. Ipp MM, Gold R, Greenberg S, et al. Acetaminophen prophylaxis of adverse reactions following vaccination of infants with diphtheria-pertussis-tetanus toxoids-polio vaccine. *Pediatr Infect Dis J.* 1987;6:721–725.
38. Sutter RW, Patriarca PA, Suleiman AJM, et al. Attributable risk of DTP (Diphtheria and Tetanus Toxoids and Pertussis Vaccine) injection in provoking paralytic poliomyelitis during a large outbreak in Oman. *J Infect Dis.* 1992;165:444–449.
39. Bernier R, Frank JA, Dondero TJ, et al. Diphtheria-tetanus toxoids, pertussis vaccination and sudden infant deaths in Tennessee. *J Pediatr.* 1982;101:419–421.
40. Baraff L, Ablon WJ, Weiss RC. Possible temporal association between diptheria-tetanus toxoid, pertussis vaccination and sudden infant death syndrome. *Pediatr Inf Dis.* 1983;2:7–11.
41. Walker AM, Jick H, Perera DR, et al. Diphtheria-tetanus-pertussis immunization and sudden infant death. *AJPH.* 1987;77(8):945–951.
42. Hoffman HJ, Hunter JC, Damus K, et al. Diphtheria-tetanus-pertussis immunization and sudden infant death: results of the National Institute of Child Health and Human Development cooperative study of sudden infant death syndrome risk factors. *Pediatrics.* 1987; 79(4):598–611.
43. Mortimer EA. Efficacy of Haemophilus b polysaccharide vaccine: an enigma. *JAMA.* 1988;260:1454–1455.
44. Scheifele D, Bjornsen GLG, Arcand T, et al. Antigenuria after receipt of Haemophilus b Diphtheria Toxoid Conjugate Vaccine. *Pediatr Infect Dis J.* 1989;8:887–888.
45. Recommendation of the ACIP—Immunization of children infected with human T-lymphotrophic virus type III/lymphadenopathy-associated virus. *MMWR.* 1986; 35(38):595–606.
46. Immunization of children infected with human immunodeficiency virus—supplementary ACIP statement. *MMWR.* 1988;37(12):181–183.
47. General Recommendations on Immunization—recommendations of the Immunization Practices Advisory Committee (ACIP). *MMWR.* 1989;38(13):221.
48. CDC. Vaccine Adverse Event Reporting System—United States. *MMWR.* 1990;39:730–733.
49. Fawcett HA, Smith NP. Injection-site granuloma due to aluminum. *Arch Dermatol.* 1984;120:1318–1322.
50. Bellman MH, Ross EM, Miller DL. Infantile spasms and pertussis immunization. *Lancet.* 1983;1:1031–1034.
51. Mathur R, Kumari S. Bulging fontanel following triple vaccine (letter). *Indian Pediatrics.* 1981;18(6):417–418.
52. Shendurnikar N, Gandhi DJ, Patel J, et al. Bulging fontanel following DTP vaccine (letter). *Indian Pediatrics.* 1986;23(11):960.
53. Jacob J, Mannino F. Increased intracranial pressure after diphtheria, tetanus, and pertussis immunization. *Am J Dis Child.* 1979;133:217–218.
54. Leung A. Congenital heart disease and DTP vaccination. *Can Med Assoc J.* 1984;131:541.
55. Park JM, Ledbetter EO, South MA, et al. Paroxysmal supraventricular tachycardia precipitated by pertussis vaccine. *Pediatrics.* 1983;102(6):883–885.
56. Amsel SG, Hanukoglu A, Fried D, et al. Myocarditis after triple immunization. *Arch Dis Child.* 1986; 61:403–404.
57. CDC. Adverse events following immunization. *MMWR.* 1985;34:43–47.
58. Rutledge SL, Snead OC. Neurologic complications of immunizations. *J Pediatr.* 1986;109:917–924.
59. Milstein JB, Gross TP, Kuritsky JN. Adverse reactions reported following receipt of *Haemophilus influenzae* type b vaccine: an analysis after one year of marketing. *Pediatrics.* 1987;80:270–274.
60. Schlenska GK. Unusual neurological complications following tetanus toxoid administration. *J Neurol.* 1977; 215:299–302.
61. Blumstein GI, Kreithen H. Peripheral neuropathy following tetanus toxoid administration. *JAMA.* 1966; 198: 1030–1031.
62. Reinstein L, Pargament JM, Goodman JS. Peripheral neuropathy after multiple tetanus toxoid injections. *Arch Phys Med Rehabil.* 1982;63:332–334.
63. Tsairis P, Dyck PJ, Mulder DW. Natural history of brachial plexus neuropathy. *Arch Neurol.* 1972; 27:109–117.
64. Quast U, Hennessen W, Widmark RM. Mono- and polyneuritis after tetanus vaccination. *Devel Bio Stand.* 1979; 43:25–32.
65. Holliday PL, Bauer RB. Polyradiculoneuritis secondary to immunization with tetanus and diphtheria toxoids. *Arch Neurol.* 1983;40:56–57.
66. Fenichel GM. Neurological complications of tetanus toxoid. *Arch Neurol.* 1983;40:390.
67. Pollard JD, Selby G. Relapsing neuropathy due to tetanus toxoid. *J Neurol Sci.* 1978;37:113–125.
68. Newton N, Janati A. Guillain-Barré syndrome after vaccination with purified tetanus toxoid. *S Med J.* 1987; 80: 1053–1054.
69. D'Cruz DF, Shapiro ED, Spiegelman KN, et al. Acute inflammatory demyelinating polyradiculoneuropathy (Guillain-Barré syndrome) after immunization with *Haemophilus influenzae* type b conjugate vaccine. *J Pediatr.* 1989;115:743–746.
70. Recommendation of the ACIP: Haemophilus b conjugate vaccines for prevention of *Haemophilus influenzae* type b disease among infants and children two months of age and older. *MMWR.* 1991;40:1–7.

Manufactured by:
LEDERLE LABORATORIES
Division American Cyanamid Company
Pearl River, NY 10965
US Gov't. License No. 17
Marketed by:
WYETH-LEDERLE VACCINES
Philadelphia, PA 19101
Wyeth-Ayerst Laboratories

Shown in Product Identification Guide, page 320

VERELAN® ℞

[vĕr'ă-lăn]
Verapamil HCl
Sustained-Release Pellet Filled Capsules

DESCRIPTION

VERELAN (verapamil hydrochloride capsules) is a calcium ion influx inhibitor (slow channel blocker or calcium ion antagonist). VERELAN is available for oral administration as a 360 mg hard gelatin capsule (lavender cap/yellow body), a 240 mg hard gelatin capsule (dark blue cap/yellow body), a 180 mg hard gelatin capsule (light grey cap/yellow body), and a 120 mg hard gelatin capsule (yellow cap/yellow body). These pellet filled capsules provide a sustained-release of the drug in the gastrointestinal tract.

Chemical name: Benzeneacetonitrile, α-[3-[[2-(3,4-dimethoxyphenyl)-ethyl]methylamino]propyl]-3,4-dimethoxy-α-(1-methylethyl) monohydrochloride.

Verapamil HCl is an almost white, crystalline powder, practically free of odor, with a bitter taste. It is soluble in water, chloroform, and methanol. Verapamil HCl is not structurally related to other cardioactive drugs.

In addition to verapamil HCl the VERELAN capsule contains the following inactive ingredients: fumaric acid, talc, sugar spheres, povidone, shellac, gelatin, FD&C red #40, yellow iron oxide, titanium dioxide, methylparaben, propylparaben, silicon dioxide, and sodium lauryl sulfate. In addition, the VERELAN 240 mg and 360 mg capsules contain FD&C blue #1 and D&C red #28; and the VERELAN 180 mg capsule contains black iron oxide.

CLINICAL PHARMACOLOGY

VERELAN is a calcium ion influx inhibitor (slow channel blocker or calcium ion antagonist) which exerts its pharmacologic effects by modulating the influx of ionic calcium across the cell membrane of the arterial smooth muscle as well as in conductile and contractile myocardial cells.

Normal sinus rhythm is usually not affected by verapamil HCl. However in patients with sick sinus syndrome, verapamil HCl may interfere with sinus node impulse generation and may induce sinus arrest or sinoatrial block. Atrioventricular block can occur in patients without preexisting conduction defects. (See **WARNINGS.**) Verapamil HCl does not alter the normal atrial action potential or intraventricular conduction time, but depresses amplitude, velocity of depolarization and conduction in depressed atrial fibers. Verapamil HCl may shorten the antegrade effective refractory period of accessory bypass tracts. Acceleration of ventricular rate and/or ventricular fibrillation has been reported in patients with atrial flutter or atrial fibrillation and a coexisting accessory AV pathway following administration of verapamil. (See **WARNINGS.**)

Verapamil HCl has a local anesthetic action that is 1.6 times that of procaine on an equimolar basis. It is not known whether this action is important at the doses used in man.

Mechanism of Action

Essential Hypertension

Verapamil HCl exerts antihypertensive effects by decreasing systemic vascular resistance, usually without orthostatic decreases in blood pressure or reflex tachycardia; bradycardia (rate less than 50 beats/minute is uncommon). Verapamil HCl regularly reduces arterial pressure at rest and at a given level of exercise by dilating peripheral arterioles and reducing the total peripheral resistance (afterload) against which the heart works.

Pharmacokinetics and Metabolism

With the immediate release formulations, more than 90% of the orally administered dose is absorbed, and peak plasma concentrations of verapamil are observed 1 to 2 hours after dosing. Because of rapid biotransformation of verapamil during its first pass through the portal circulation, the absolute bioavailability ranges from 20% to 35%. Chronic oral administration of the highest recommended dose (120 mg every 6 hours) resulted in plasma verapamil levels ranging from 125 to 400 ng/mL with higher values reported occasionally. A nonlinear correlation between the verapamil HCl dose administered and verapamil plasma levels does exist. During initial dose titration with verapamil a relationship exists between verapamil plasma concentrations and the prolongation of the PR interval. However, during chronic administration this relationship may disappear. The quantitative relationship between plasma verapamil concentrations and blood pressure reduction has not been fully characterized.

In a multiple dose pharmacokinetic study, peak concentrations for a single daily dose of VERELAN 240 mg were approximately 65% of those obtained with an 80 mg t.i.d. dose of the conventional immediate-release tablets, and the 24-hour post-dose concentrations were approximately 30% higher. At a total daily dose of 240 mg, VERELAN was shown to have a similar extent of verapamil bioavailability based on the AUC-24 as that obtained with the conventional immediate-release tablets. In this same study VERELAN doses of 120 mg, 240 mg and 360 mg once daily were compared after multiple doses. The ratios of the verapamil and norverapamil AUCs for the VERELAN 120 mg, 240 mg, and 360 mg once daily doses are 1 (565 ng·hr/mL):3 (1660 ng·hr/mL):5 (2729 ng·hr/mL) and 1 (621 ng·hr/mL):3 (1614 ng·hr/mL):4 (2535 ng·hr/mL), respectively, indicating that the AUC increased non-proportionately with increasing doses.

Food does not affect the extent or rate of the absorption of verapamil from the controlled release VERELAN capsule. The VERELAN 240 mg capsule when administered with food had a C_{max} of 77 ng/mL which occurred 9.0 hours after dosing, and an AUC(0-inf) of 1387 ng·hr/mL. VERELAN 240 mg under fasting conditions had a C_{max} of 77 ng/mL which occurred 9.8 hours after dosing, and an AUC(0-inf) of 1541 ng·hr/mL.

The bioequivalence of VERELAN 240 mg, administered as the pellets sprinkled on applesauce and as the intact capsule, was demonstrated in a single-dose, cross-over study in 32 healthy adults. Comparative ratios (sprinkled/intact) of verapamil were 0.95, 1.02, and 1.01 for C_{max}, T_{max}, and AUC (O-inf) respectively. Similar results were observed with norverapamil.

The time to reach maximum verapamil concentrations (T_{max}) with VERELAN has been found to be approximately 7–9 hours in each of the single dose (fasting), single dose (fed), the multiple dose (steady state) studies, and dose proportionality pharmacokinetic studies. Similarly the apparent half-life ($t_{1/2}$) has been found to be approximately 12 hours independent of dose. Aging may affect the pharmacokinetics of verapamil. Elimination half-life may be prolonged in the elderly.

In healthy man, orally administered verapamil HCl undergoes extensive metabolism in the liver. Twelve metabolites have been identified in plasma; all except norverapamil are present in trace amounts only. Norverapamil can reach steady-state plasma concentrations approximately equal to those of verapamil itself. The biologic activity of norverapamil appears to be approximately 20% that of verapamil. Approximately 70% of an administered dose of verapamil HCl is excreted as metabolites in the urine and 16% or more in the feces within 5 days. About 3% to 4% is excreted in the urine as unchanged drug. Approximately 90% is bound to plasma proteins. In patients with hepatic insufficiency, metabolism is delayed and elimination half-life prolonged up to 14 to 16 hours (see **PRECAUTIONS**), the volume of distribution is increased and plasma clearance reduced to about 30% of normal. Verapamil clearance values suggest that patients with liver dysfunction may attain therapeutic verapamil plasma concentrations with one-third of the oral daily dose required for patients with normal liver function.

Continued on next page

Verelan—Cont.

After four weeks of oral dosing (120 mg q.i.d.), verapamil and norverapamil levels were noted in the cerebrospinal fluid with estimated partition coefficient of 0.06 for verapamil and 0.04 for norverapamil.

In 10 healthy males, administration of oral verapamil (80 mg every 8 hours for 6 days) and a single oral dose of ethanol (0.8 g/kg), resulted in a 17% increase in mean peak ethanol concentrations (106.45 ± 21.40 to 124.23 ± 24.74 mg/dL) compared with placebo. (See **PRECAUTIONS, Drug Interactions.**)

The area under the blood ethanol concentration versus time curve (AUC over 12 hours) increased by 30% (365.67 ± 93.52 to 475.07 ± 97.24 mg·hr/dL). Verapamil AUCs were positively correlated (r=0.71) to increased ethanol blood AUC values.

Hemodynamics and Myocardial Metabolism

Verapamil HCl reduces afterload and myocardial contractility. Improved left ventricular diastolic function in patients with IHSS and those with coronary heart disease has also been observed with verapamil HCl therapy. In most patients, including those with organic cardiac disease, the negative inotropic action of verapamil HCl is countered by reduction of afterload and cardiac index is usually not reduced. In patients with severe left ventricular dysfunction however, (e.g., pulmonary wedge pressure above 20 mmHg or ejection fraction lower than 30%), or in patients on beta-adrenergic blocking agents or other cardiodepressant drugs, deterioration of ventricular function may occur. (See **DRUG INTERACTIONS.**)

Pulmonary Function

Verapamil HCl does not induce broncho-constriction and hence, does not impair ventilatory function.

INDICATIONS AND USAGE

VERELAN (verapamil HCl) is indicated for the management of essential hypertension.

CONTRAINDICATIONS

Verapamil HCl is contraindicated in:
1. Severe left ventricular dysfunction. (See **WARNINGS**.)
2. Hypotension (less than 90 mm Hg systolic pressure) or cardiogenic shock.
3. Sick sinus syndrome (except in patients with a functioning artificial ventricular pacemaker).
4. Second- or third-degree AV block (except in patients with a functioning artificial ventricular pacemaker).
5. Patients with atrial flutter or atrial fibrillation and an accessory bypass tract (e.g., Wolff-Parkinson-White, Lown-Ganong-Levine syndromes). (See **WARNINGS**.)
6. Patients with known hypersensitivity to verapamil hydrochloride.

WARNINGS

Heart Failure

Verapamil has a negative inotropic effect which, in most patients, is compensated by its afterload reduction (decreased systemic vascular resistance) properties without a net impairment of ventricular performance. In clinical experience with 4,954 patients, 87 (1.8%) developed congestive heart failure or pulmonary edema. Verapamil should be avoided in patients with severe left ventricular dysfunction (e.g., ejection fraction less than 30% or moderate to severe symptoms of cardiac failure) and in patients with any degree of ventricular dysfunction if they are receiving a beta-adrenergic blocker. (See **Drug Interactions**.) Patients with milder ventricular dysfunction should, if possible, be controlled with optimum doses of digitalis and/or diuretics before verapamil treatment (note interactions with digoxin under: **PRECAUTIONS**).

Hypotension

Occasionally, the pharmacologic action of verapamil may produce a decrease in blood pressure below normal levels which may result in dizziness or symptomatic hypotension. The incidence of hypotension observed in 4,954 patients enrolled in clinical trials was 2.5%. In hypertensive patients, decreases in blood pressure below normal are unusual. Tilt table testing (60 degrees) was not able to induce orthostatic hypotension.

Elevated Liver Enzymes

Elevations of transaminases with and without concomitant elevations in alkaline phosphatase and bilirubin have been reported. Such elevations have sometimes been transient and may disappear even in the face of continued verapamil treatment. Several cases of hepatocellular injury related to verapamil have been proven by rechallenge; half of these had clinical symptoms (malaise, fever, and/or right upper quadrant pain) in addition to elevations of SGOT, SGPT, and alkaline phosphatase. Periodic monitoring of liver function in patients receiving verapamil is therefore prudent.

Accessory Bypass Tract (Wolff-Parkinson-White or Lown-Ganong-Levine)

Some patients with paroxysmal and/or chronic atrial flutter or atrial fibrillation and a coexisting accessory AV pathway have developed increased antegrade conduction across the accessory pathway bypassing the AV node, producing a very

rapid ventricular response or ventricular fibrillation after receiving intravenous verapamil (or digitalis). Although a risk of this occurring with oral verapamil has not been established, such patients receiving oral verapamil may be at risk and its use in these patients is contraindicated. (See **CONTRAINDICATIONS**.)

Treatment is usually DC-cardioversion. Cardioversion has been used safely and effectively after oral verapamil.

Atrioventricular Block

The effect of verapamil on AV conduction and the SA node may lead to asymptomatic first-degree AV block and transient bradycardia, sometimes accompanied by nodal escape rhythms. PR interval prolongation is correlated with verapamil plasma concentrations, especially during the early titration phase of therapy. Higher degrees of AV block, however, were infrequently (0.8%) observed.

Marked first-degree block or progressive development to second- or third-degree AV block requires a reduction in dosage or, in rare instances, discontinuation of verapamil HCl and institution of appropriate therapy depending upon the clinical situation.

Patients with Hypertrophic Cardiomyopathy (IHSS)

In 120 patients with hypertrophic cardiomyopathy (most of them refractory or intolerant to propranolol) who received therapy with verapamil at doses up to 720 mg/day, a variety of serious adverse effects were seen. Three patients died in pulmonary edema; all had severe left ventricular outflow obstruction and a past history of left ventricular dysfunction. Eight other patients had pulmonary edema and/or severe hypotension; abnormally high (over 20 mm Hg) capillary wedge pressure and a marked left ventricular outflow obstruction were present in most of these patients. Concomitant administration of quinidine (see **Drug Interactions**) preceded the severe hypotension in 3 of the 8 patients (2 of whom developed pulmonary edema). Sinus bradycardia occurred in 11% of the patients, second-degree AV block in 4% and sinus arrest in 2%. It must be appreciated that this group of patients had a serious disease with a high mortality rate. Most adverse effects responded well to dose reduction and only rarely did verapamil have to be discontinued.

PRECAUTIONS

THE CONTENTS OF THE VERELAN CAPSULE SHOULD NOT BE CRUSHED OR CHEWED.

General

Use in Patients with Impaired Hepatic Function

Since verapamil is highly metabolized by the liver, it should be administered cautiously to patients with impaired hepatic function. Severe liver dysfunction prolongs the elimination half-life of immediate-release verapamil to about 14 to 16 hours; hence, approximately 30% of the dose given to patients with normal liver function should be administered to these patients. Careful monitoring for abnormal prolongation of the PR interval or other signs of excessive pharmacologic effects (see **OVERDOSAGE**) should be carried out.

Use in Patients with Attenuated (Decreased) Neuromuscular Transmission

It has been reported that verapamil decreases neuromuscular transmission in patients with Duchenne's muscular dystrophy, and that verapamil prolongs recovery from the neuromuscular blocking agent, vecuronium. It may be necessary to decrease the dosage of verapamil when it is administered to patients with attenuated neuromuscular transmission.

Use in Patients with Impaired Renal Function

About 70% of an administered dose of verapamil is excreted as metabolites in the urine. Until further data are available, verapamil should be administered cautiously to patients with impaired renal function. These patients should be carefully monitored for abnormal prolongation of the PR interval or other signs of overdosage (see **OVERDOSAGE**).

Information for Patients

When the sprinkle method of administration is prescribed, details of the proper technique should be explained to the patient. (See **DOSAGE AND ADMINISTRATION**.)

Drug Interactions

Beta Blockers

Concomitant therapy with beta-adrenergic blockers and verapamil may result in additive negative effects on heart rate, atrioventricular conduction, and/or cardiac contractility. The combination of sustained-release verapamil and beta-adrenergic blocking agents has not been studied. However, there have been reports of excess bradycardia and AV block, including complete heart block, when the combination has been used for the treatment of hypertension.

For hypertensive patients, the risk of combined therapy may outweigh the potential benefits. The combination should be used only with caution and close monitoring.

Asymptomatic bradycardia (36 beats/min) with a wandering atrial pacemaker has been observed in a patient receiving concomitant timolol (a beta-adrenergic blocker) eyedrops and oral verapamil.

A decrease in metoprolol clearance has been reported when verapamil and metoprolol were administered together. A similar effect has not been observed when verapamil and atenolol are given together.

Digitalis

Clinical use of verapamil in digitalized patients has shown the combination to be well tolerated if digoxin doses are properly adjusted. Chronic verapamil treatment can increase serum digoxin levels by 50% to 75% during the first week of therapy, and this can result in digitalis toxicity. In patients with hepatic cirrhosis the influence of verapamil on digoxin kinetics is magnified. Maintenance digitalis doses should be reduced when verapamil is administered, and the patient should be carefully monitored to avoid over- or underdigitalization. Whenever overdigitalization is suspected, the daily dose of digoxin should be reduced or temporarily discontinued. Upon discontinuation of verapamil HCl, the patient should be reassessed to avoid underdigitalization.

Antihypertensive Agents

Verapamil administered concomitantly with oral antihypertensive agents (e.g., vasodilators, angiotensin-converting enzyme inhibitors, diuretics, beta blockers) will usually have an additive effect on lowering blood pressure. Patients receiving these combinations should be appropriately monitored. Concomitant use of agents that attenuate alpha-adrenergic function with verapamil may result in reduction in blood pressure that is excessive in some patients. Such an effect was observed in one study following the concomitant administration of verapamil and prazosin.

Antiarrhythmic Agents

Disopyramide: Until data on possible interactions between verapamil and disopyramide phosphate are obtained, disopyramide should not be administered within 48 hours before or 24 hours after verapamil administration.

Flecainide: A study in healthy volunteers showed that the concomitant administration of flecainide and verapamil may have additive effects on myocardial contractility, AV conduction, and repolarization. Concomitant therapy with flecainide and verapamil may result in additive negative inotropic effect and prolongation of atrioventricular conduction.

Quinidine: In a small number of patients with hypertrophic cardiomyopathy (IHSS), concomitant use of verapamil and quinidine resulted in significant hypotension. Until further data are obtained, combined therapy of verapamil and quinidine in patients with hypertrophic cardiomyopathy should probably be avoided.

The electrophysiological effects of quinidine and verapamil on AV conduction were studied in 8 patients. Verapamil significantly counteracted the effects of quinidine on AV conduction. There has been a report of increased quinidine levels during verapamil therapy.

Nitrates: Verapamil has been given concomitantly with short- and long-acting nitrates without any undesirable drug interactions. The pharmacologic profile of both drugs and the clinical experience suggest beneficial interactions.

Alcohol: Verapamil has been found to significantly inhibit ethanol elimination resulting in elevated blood ethanol concentrations that may prolong the intoxicating effects of alcohol. (See **CLINICAL PHARMACOLOGY, Pharmacokinetics and Metabolism**.)

Other

Cimetidine: The interaction between cimetidine and chronically administered verapamil has not been studied. Variable results on clearance have been obtained in acute studies of healthy volunteers; clearance of verapamil was either reduced or unchanged.

Lithium: Pharmacokinetic and pharmacodynamic interactions between oral verapamil and lithium have been reported. The former may result in a lowering of serum lithium levels in patients receiving chronic stable oral lithium therapy. The latter may result in an increased sensitivity to the effects of lithium. Patients receiving both drugs must be monitored carefully.

Carbamazepine: Verapamil therapy may increase carbamazepine concentrations during combined therapy. This may produce carbamazepine side effects such as diplopia, headache, ataxia, or dizziness.

Rifampin: Therapy with rifampin may markedly reduce oral verapamil bioavailability.

Phenobarbital: Phenobarbital therapy may increase verapamil clearance.

Cyclosporine: Verapamil therapy may increase serum levels of cyclosporine.

Inhalation Anesthetics: Animal experiments have shown that inhalation anesthetics depress cardiovascular activity by decreasing the inward movement of calcium ions. When used concomitantly, inhalation anesthetics and calcium antagonists, such as verapamil, should be titrated carefully to avoid excessive cardiovascular depression.

Neuromuscular Blocking Agents: Clinical data and animal studies suggest that verapamil may potentiate the activity of neuromuscular blocking agents (curare-like and depolarizing). It may be necessary to decrease the dose of verapamil and/or the dose of the neuromuscular blocking agent when the drugs are used concomitantly.

Carcinogenesis, Mutagenesis, Impairment of Fertility

An 18-month toxicity study in rats, at a low multiple (6-fold) of the maximum recommended human dose, and not the maximum tolerated dose, did not suggest a tumorigenic potential. There was no evidence of a carcinogenic potential of verapamil administered in the diet of rats for 2 years at doses of 10, 35 and 120 mg/kg per day or approximately 1x, 3.5x, and 12x, respectively, the maximum recommended human daily dose (480 mg per day or 9.6 mg/kg/day).

Verapamil was not mutagenic in the Ames test in 5 test strains at 3 mg per plate, with or without metabolic activation.

Studies in female rats at daily dietary doses up to 5.5 times (55 mg/kg/day) the maximum recommended human dose did not show impaired fertility. Effects on male fertility have not been determined.

Pregnancy

Pregnancy Category C. Reproduction studies have been performed in rabbits and rats at oral doses up to 1.5 (15 mg/kg/day) and 6 (60 mg/kg/day) times the maximum recommended human daily dose, respectively, and have revealed no evidence of teratogenicity. In the rat, however, this multiple of the human dose was embryocidal and retarded fetal growth and development, probably because of adverse maternal effects reflected in reduced weight gains of the dams. This oral dose has also been shown to cause hypotension in rats. There are no adequate and well-controlled studies in pregnant women. Because animal reproduction studies are not always predictive of human response, this drug should be used during pregnancy only if clearly needed. Verapamil crosses the placental barrier and can be detected in umbilical vein blood at delivery.

Labor and Delivery

It is not known whether the use of verapamil during labor or delivery has immediate or delayed adverse effects on the fetus, or whether it prolongs the duration of labor or increases the need for forceps delivery or other obstetric intervention. Such adverse experiences have not been reported in the literature, despite a long history of use of verapamil HCl in Europe in the treatment of cardiac side effects of beta-adrenergic agonist agents used to treat premature labor.

Nursing Mothers

Verapamil is excreted in human milk. Because of the potential for adverse reactions in nursing infants from verapamil, nursing should be discontinued while verapamil is administered.

Pediatric Use

Safety and efficacy of verapamil in children below the age of 18 years have not been established.

Animal Pharmacology and/or Animal Toxicology

In chronic animal toxicology studies verapamil causes lenticular and/or suture line changes at 30 mg/kg/day or greater and frank cataracts at 62.5 mg/kg/day or greater in the beagle dog but not the rat. Development of cataracts due to verapamil has not been reported in man.

ADVERSE REACTIONS

Serious adverse reactions are uncommon when verapamil HCl therapy is initiated with upward dose titration within the recommended single and total daily dose. See **WARNINGS** for discussion of heart failure, hypotension, elevated liver enzymes, AV block, and rapid ventricular response. Reversible (upon discontinuation of verapamil) non-obstructive, paralytic ileus has been infrequently reported in association with the use of verapamil.

In clinical trials involving 285 hypertensive patients on VERELAN for greater than 1 week the following adverse reactions were reported in greater than 1.0% of the patients:

Constipation	7.4%
Headache	5.3%
Dizziness	4.2%
Lethargy	3.2%
Dyspepsia	2.5%
Rash	1.4%
Ankle Edema	1.4%
Sleep Disturbance	1.4%
Myalgia	1.1%

In clinical trials of other formulations of verapamil HCl (N=4,954) the following reactions have occurred at rates greater than 1.0%:

Constipation	7.3%
Dizziness	3.3%
Nausea	2.7%
Hypotension	2.5%
Edema	1.9%
Headache	2.2%
Rash	1.2%
CHF/Pulmonary Edema	1.8%
Fatigue	1.7%
Bradycardia (HR<50/min)	1.4%
AV block-total	
1°, 2°, 3°	1.2%
2° and 3°	0.8%
Flushing	0.6%
Elevated Liver Enzymes (see WARNINGS)	

In clinical trials related to the control of ventricular response in digitalized patients who had atrial fibrillation or atrial flutter, ventricular rate below 50/min at rest occurred in 15% of patients and asymptomatic hypotension occurred in 5% of patients.

The following reactions, reported in 1.0% or less of patients, occurred under conditions (open trials, marketing experience) where a causal relationship is uncertain; they are listed to alert the physician to a possible relationship:

Cardiovascular: angina pectoris, atrioventricular dissociation, chest pain, claudication, myocardial infarction, palpitations, purpura (vasculitis), syncope.

Digestive System: diarrhea, dry mouth, gastrointestinal distress, gingival hyperplasia.

Hemic and Lymphatic: ecchymosis or bruising.

Nervous System: cerebrovascular accident, confusion, equilibrium disorders, insomnia, muscle cramps, paresthesia, psychotic symptoms, shakiness, somnolence.

Respiratory: dyspnea.

Skin: arthralgia and rash, exanthema, hair loss, hyperkeratosis, maculae, sweating, urticaria, Stevens-Johnson syndrome, erythema multiforme.

Special Senses: blurred vision, tinnitus.

Urogenital: gynecomastia, impotence, increased urination, spotty menstruation.

Treatment of Acute Cardiovascular Adverse Reactions

The frequency of cardiovascular adverse reactions which require therapy is rare; hence, experience with their treatment is limited. Whenever severe hypotension or complete AV block occurs following oral administration of verapamil, the appropriate emergency measures should be applied immediately, e.g., intravenously administered isoproterenol HCl, levarterenol bitartrate, atropine (all in the usual doses), or calcium gluconate (10% solution). In patients with hypertrophic cardiomyopathy (IHSS), alpha-adrenergic agents (phenylephrine, metaraminol bitartrate or methoxamine) should be used to maintain blood pressure, and isoproterenol and levarterenol should be avoided. If further support is necessary, inotropic agents (dopamine or dobutamine) may be administered. Actual treatment and dosage should depend on the severity and the clinical situation and the judgment and experience of the treating physician.

OVERDOSAGE

Treatment of overdosage should be supportive. Beta-adrenergic stimulation or parenteral administration of calcium solutions may increase calcium ion flux across the slow channel, and have been used effectively in treatment of deliberate overdosage with verapamil. Verapamil cannot be removed by hemodialysis. Clinically significant hypotensive reactions or high degree AV block should be treated with vasopressor agents or cardiac pacing, respectively. Asystole should be handled by the usual measures including cardiopulmonary resuscitation.

DOSAGE AND ADMINISTRATION

Essential Hypertension

The dose of VERELAN should be individualized by titration. The usual daily dose of sustained-release verapamil, VERELAN, in clinical trials has been 240 mg given by mouth once daily in the morning. However, initial doses of 120 mg a day may be warranted in patients who may have an increased response to verapamil (e.g., elderly, small people, etc). Upward titration should be based on therapeutic efficacy and safety evaluated approximately 24 hours after dosing. The antihypertensive effects of VERELAN are evident within the first week of therapy.

If adequate response is not obtained with 120 mg of VERELAN, the dose may be titrated upward in the following manner:

(a) 180 mg in the morning
(b) 240 mg in the morning
(c) 360 mg in the morning
(d) 480 mg in the morning

VERELAN sustained-release capsules are for once-a-day administration. When switching from immediate-release verapamil to VERELAN capsules, the same total daily dose of VERELAN capsules can be used.

As with immediate-release verapamil, dosages of VERELAN capsules should be individualized and titration may be needed in some patients.

Sprinkling the Capsule Contents on Food

VERELAN Pellet Filled Capsules may also be administered by carefully opening the capsule and sprinkling the pellets on a spoonful of applesauce. The applesauce should be swallowed immediately without chewing and followed with a glass of cool water to ensure complete swallowing of the pellets. The applesauce used should not be hot, and it should be soft enough to be swallowed without chewing. Any pellet/applesauce mixture should be used immediately and not stored for future use. Subdividing the contents of a VERELAN capsule is not recommended.

HOW SUPPLIED

VERELAN® verapamil HCl sustained-release pellet filled capsules are supplied in four dosage strengths:

120 mg—Two-piece, size 2 hard gelatin capsule (yellow cap/yellow body), printed with Lederle above V8 on left and VERELAN above 120 mg on right side of the capsule in black ink, supplied as follows:
NDC 0005-2490-23—Bottle of 100s

180 mg—Two-piece, size 1 elongated hard gelatin capsule (light grey cap/yellow body), printed with Lederle above V7 on left and VERELAN above 180 mg on right side of the capsule in black ink, supplied as follows:
NDC 0005-2489-23—Bottle of 100s

240 mg—Two-piece, size 0 hard gelatin capsule (dark blue cap/yellow body), printed with Lederle above V9 on left and VERELAN above 240 mg on right side of the capsule in black ink, supplied as follows:
NDC 0005-2491-23—Bottle of 100s

360 mg—Two-piece, size 00 hard gelatin capsule (lavender cap/yellow body), printed with Lederle above V6 on left and VERELAN above 360 mg on right side of the capsule in black ink, supplied as follows:
NDC 0005-2495-23—Bottle of 100s.

Store at controlled room temperature 20°–25°C (68°–77°F) [See USP]. Avoid excessive heat. Brief digressions above 25°C, while not detrimental, should be avoided. Protect from moisture.

Dispense in tight, light-resistant container as defined in USP.

Manufactured for
LEDERLE PHARMACEUTICAL DIVISION
American Cyanamid Company
Pearl River, NY 10965
by

ELAN PHARMA, INC.
Pharmaceutical Division
Gainesville, GA 30504
Shown in Product Identification Guide, page 320

ZEBETA®   ℞
[zē-bā-tə]
(Bisoprolol Fumarate)
Tablets

DESCRIPTION

ZEBETA (bisoprolol fumarate) is a synthetic beta$_1$-selective (cardioselective) adrenoceptor blocking agent. The chemical name for bisoprolol fumarate is (±)-1-[4-[[2-(1-Methylethoxy) ethoxy]methyl]phenoxy]-3-[(1-methylethyl)amino]-2-propanol (E) -2-butenedioate (2:1) (salt). It possesses an asymmetric carbon atom in its structure and is provided as a racemic mixture. The S(-) enantiomer is responsible for most of the beta-blocking activity. Its empirical formula is $(C_{18}H_{31}NO_4)_2 \cdot C_4H_4O_4$.

Bisoprolol fumarate has a molecular weight of 766.97. It is a white crystalline powder which is approximately equally hydrophilic and lipophilic, and is readily soluble in water, methanol, ethanol, and chloroform.

ZEBETA is available as 5 and 10 mg tablets for oral administration.

Inactive ingredients include Colloidal Silicon Dioxide, Corn Starch, Crospovidone, Diabasic Calcium Phosphate, Hydroxypropyl Methylcellulose, Magnesium Stearate, Microcrystalline Cellulose, Polyethylene Glycol, Polysorbate 80, and Titanium Dioxide. The 5 mg tablets also contain Red and Yellow Iron Oxide.

CLINICAL PHARMACOLOGY

ZEBETA is a beta$_1$-selective (cardioselective) adrenoceptor blocking agent without significant membrane stabilizing activity or intrinsic sympathomimetic activity in its therapeutic dosage range. Cardioselectivity is not absolute, however, and at higher doses (≥ 20 mg) bisoprolol fumarate also inhibits beta$_2$-adrenoceptors, chiefly located in the bronchial and vascular musculature; to retain selectivity, it is therefore important to use the lowest effective dose.

Pharmacokinetics and Metabolism

The absolute bioavailability after a 10 mg oral dose of bisoprolol fumarate is about 80%. Absorption is not affected by the presence of food. The first pass metabolism of bisoprolol fumarate is about 20%.

Binding to serum proteins is approximately 30%. Peak plasma concentrations occur within 2–4 hours of dosing with 5 to 20 mg, and mean peak values range from 16 ng/mL at 5 mg to 70 ng/mL at 20 mg. Once daily dosing with bisoprolol fumarate results in less than twofold intersubject variation in peak plasma levels. The plasma elimination half-life is 9–12 hours and is slightly longer in elderly patients, in part because of decreased renal function in that population. Steady state is attained within 5 days of once daily dosing. In both young and elderly populations, plasma accumulation is low; the accumulation factor ranges from 1.1 to 1.3, and is what would be expected from the first order kinetics and once daily dosing. Plasma concentrations are

Continued on next page

Zebeta—Cont.

proportional to the administered dose in the range of 5 to 20 mg. Pharmacokinetic characteristics of the two enantiomers are similar.

Bisoprolol fumarate is eliminated equally by renal and non-renal pathways with about 50% of the dose appearing unchanged in the urine and the remainder appearing in the form of inactive metabolites. In humans, the known metabolites are labile or have no known pharmacologic activity. Less than 2% of the dose is excreted in the feces. Bisoprolol fumarate is not metabolized by cytochrome P450 II D6 (debrisoquin hydroxylase).

In subjects with creatinine clearance less than 40 mL/min, the plasma half-life is increased approximately threefold compared to healthy subjects.

In patients with cirrhosis of the liver, the elimination of ZEBETA (bisoprolol fumarate) is more variable in rate and significantly slower than that in healthy subjects, with plasma half-life ranging from 8.3 to 21.7 hours.

Pharmacodynamics

The most prominent effect of ZEBETA is the negative chronotropic effect, resulting in a reduction in resting and exercise heart rate. There is a fall in resting and exercise cardiac output with little observed change in stroke volume, and only a small increase in right atrial pressure or pulmonary capillary wedge pressure at rest or during exercise.

Findings in short-term clinical hemodynamics studies with ZEBETA are similar to those observed with other beta-blocking agents.

The mechanism of action of its antihypertensive effects has not been completely established. Factors which may be involved include:

1) Decreased cardiac output,
2) Inhibition of renin release by the kidneys,
3) Diminution of tonic sympathetic outflow from the vasomotor centers in the brain.

In normal volunteers, ZEBETA therapy resulted in a reduction of exercise- and isoproterenol-induced tachycardia. The maximal effect occurred within 1–4 hours post-dosing. Effects persisted for 24 hours at doses equal to or greater than 5 mg.

Electrophysiology studies in man have demonstrated that ZEBETA significantly decreases heart rate, increases sinus node recovery time, prolongs AV node refractory periods, and, with rapid atrial stimulation, prolongs AV nodal conduction.

Beta₁-selectivity of ZEBETA has been demonstrated in both animal and human studies. No effects at therapeutic doses on beta₂-adrenoceptor density have been observed. Pulmonary function studies have been conducted in healthy volunteers, asthmatics, and patients with chronic obstructive pulmonary disease (COPD). Doses of ZEBETA ranged from 5 to 60 mg, atenolol from 50 to 200 mg, metoprolol from 100 to 200 mg, and propranolol from 40 to 80 mg. In some studies, slight, asymptomatic increases in airways resistance (AWR) and decreases in forced expiratory volume (FEV₁) were observed with doses of bisoprolol fumarate 20 mg and higher, similar to the small increases in AWR also noted with the other cardioselective beta-blockers. The changes induced by beta-blockade with all agents were reversed by bronchodilator therapy.

ZEBETA had minimal effect on serum lipids during antihypertensive studies. In U.S. placebo-controlled trials, changes in total cholesterol averaged +0.8% for bisoprolol fumarate-treated patients, and +0.7% for placebo. Changes in triglycerides averaged +19% for bisoprolol fumarate-treated patients, and +17% for placebo.

ZEBETA has also been given concomitantly with thiazide diuretics. Even very low doses of hydrochlorothiazide (6.25 mg) were found to be additive with bisoprolol fumarate in lowering blood pressure in patients with mild-to-moderate hypertension.

CLINICAL STUDIES

In two randomized double-blind placebo-controlled trials conducted in the U.S., reductions in systolic and diastolic blood pressure and heart rate 24 hours after dosing in patients with mild-to-moderate hypertension are shown below. In both studies, mean systolic/diastolic blood pressures at baseline were approximately 150/100 mm Hg, and mean heart rate was 76 bpm. Drug effect is calculated by subtracting the placebo effect from the overall change in blood pressure and heart rate.

[See table below]

Blood pressure responses were seen within one week of treatment and changed little thereafter. They were sustained for 12 weeks and for over a year in studies of longer duration. Blood pressure returned to baseline when bisoprolol fumarate was tapered over two weeks in a long-term study.

Overall, significantly greater blood pressure reductions were observed on bisoprolol fumarate than on placebo, regardless of race, age, or gender. There were no significant differences in response between black and nonblack patients.

INDICATIONS AND USAGE

ZEBETA is indicated in the management of hypertension. It may be used alone or in combination with other antihypertensive agents.

CONTRAINDICATIONS

ZEBETA is contraindicated in patients with cardiogenic shock, overt cardiac failure, second or third degree AV block, and marked sinus bradycardia.

WARNINGS

Cardiac Failure

Sympathetic stimulation is a vital component supporting circulatory function in the setting of congestive heart failure, and beta-blockade may result in further depression of myocardial contractility and precipitate more severe failure. In general, beta-blocking agents should be avoided in patients with overt congestive failure. However, in some patients with compensated cardiac failure it may be necessary to utilize them. In such a situation, they must be used cautiously.

In Patients Without a History of Cardiac Failure

Continued depression of the myocardium with beta-blockers can, in some patients, precipitate cardiac failure. At the first signs or symptoms of heart failure, discontinuation of ZEBETA should be considered. In some cases, beta-blocker therapy can be continued while heart failure is treated with other drugs.

Abrupt Cessation of Therapy

Exacerbation of angina pectoris, and, in some instances, myocardial infarction or ventricular arrhythmia, have been observed in patients with coronary artery disease following abrupt cessation of therapy with beta-blockers. Such patients should, therefore, be cautioned against interruption or discontinuation of therapy without the physician's advice. Even in patients without overt coronary artery disease, it may be advisable to taper therapy with ZEBETA over approximately one week with the patient under careful observation. If withdrawal symptoms occur, ZEBETA therapy should be reinstituted, at least temporarily.

Peripheral Vascular Disease

Beta-blockers can precipitate or aggravate symptoms of arterial insufficiency in patients with peripheral vascular disease. Caution should be exercised in such individuals.

Bronchospastic Disease

PATIENTS WITH BRONCHOSPASTIC DISEASE SHOULD, IN GENERAL, NOT RECEIVE BETA-BLOCKERS. Because of its relative beta₁-selectivity, however, ZEBETA may be used with caution in patients with bronchospastic disease who do not respond to, or who cannot tolerate other antihypertensive treatment. Since beta₁-selectivity is not absolute, the lowest possible dose of ZEBETA should be used, with therapy starting at 2.5 mg. A beta₂ agonist (bronchodilator) should be made available.

Anesthesia and Major Surgery

If ZEBETA treatment is to be continued perioperatively, particular care should be taken when anesthetic agents which depress myocardial function, such as ether, cyclopropane, and trichloroethylene, are used. See OVERDOSAGE for information on treatment of bradycardia and hypertension.

Diabetes and Hypoglycemia

Beta-blockers may mask some of the manifestations of hypoglycemia, particularly tachycardia. Nonselective beta-blockers may potentiate insulin-induced hypoglycemia and delay recovery of serum glucose levels. Because of its beta₁-selectivity, this is less likely with ZEBETA. However, patients subject to spontaneous hypoglycemia, or diabetic patients receiving insulin or oral hypoglycemic agents, should be cautioned about these possibilities and bisoprolol fumarate should be used with caution.

Thyrotoxicosis

Beta-adrenergic blockade may mask clinical signs of hyperthyroidism, such as tachycardia. Abrupt withdrawal of beta-blockade may be followed by an exacerbation of the symptoms of hyperthyroidism or may precipitate thyroid storm.

PRECAUTIONS

Impaired Renal or Hepatic Function

Use caution in adjusting the dose of ZEBETA in patients with renal or hepatic impairment (see CLINICAL PHARMACOLOGY and DOSAGE AND ADMINISTRATION).

Drug Interactions

ZEBETA should not be combined with other beta-blocking agents. Patients receiving catecholamine-depleting drugs, such as reserpine or guanethidine, should be closely monitored, because the added beta-adrenergic blocking action of ZEBETA may produce excessive reduction of sympathetic activity. In patients receiving concurrent therapy with clonidine, if therapy is to be discontinued, it is suggested that ZEBETA be discontinued for several days before the withdrawal of clonidine.

ZEBETA should be used with care when myocardial depressants or inhibitors of AV conduction, such as certain calcium antagonists [particularly of the phenylalkylamine (verapamil) and benzothiazepine (diltiazem) classes], or antiarrhythmic agents, such as disopyramide, are used concurrently.

Concurrent use of rifampin increases the metabolic clearance of ZEBETA, resulting in a shortened elimination half-life of ZEBETA. However, initial dose modification is generally not necessary. Pharmacokinetic studies document no clinically relevant interactions with other agents given concomitantly, including thiazide diuretics, digoxin and cimetidine. There was no effect of ZEBETA on prothrombin time in patients on stable doses of warfarin.

Risk of Anaphylactic Reaction: While taking beta-blockers, patients with a history of severe anaphylactic reaction to a variety of allergens may be more reactive to repeated challenge, either accidental, diagnostic, or therapeutic. Such patients may be unresponsive to the usual doses of epinephrine used to treat allergic reactions.

Information for Patients

Patients, especially those with coronary artery disease, should be warned about discontinuing use of ZEBETA without a physician's supervision. Patients should also be advised to consult a physician if any difficulty in breathing occurs, or if they develop signs or symptoms of congestive heart failure or excessive bradycardia.

Patients subject to spontaneous hypoglycemia, or diabetic patients receiving insulin or oral hypoglycemic agents, should be cautioned that beta-blockers may mask some of the manifestations of hypoglycemia, particularly tachycardia, and bisoprolol fumarate should be used with caution.

Patients should know how they react to this medicine before they operate automobiles and machinery or engage in other tasks requiring alertness.

Carcinogenesis, Mutagenesis, Impairment of Fertility

Long-term studies were conducted with oral bisoprolol fumarate administered in the feed of mice (20 and 24 months) and rats (26 months). No evidence of carcinogenic potential was seen in mice dosed up to 250 mg/kg/day or rats dosed up to 125 mg/kg/day. On a body-weight basis, these doses are 625 and 312 times, respectively, the maximum recommended human dose (MRHD) of 20 mg, (or 0.4 mg/kg/day based on a 50 kg individual); on a body-surface-area-basis, these doses are 59 times (mice) and 64 times (rats) the MRHD. The mutagenic potential of bisoprolol fumarate was evaluated in the microbial mutagenicity (Ames) test, the point mutation and chromosome aberration assays in Chinese hamster V79 cells, the unscheduled DNA synthesis test,

---

Sitting Systolic/Diastolic Pressure (BP) and Heart Rate (HR)
Mean Decrease (Δ) After 3 to 4 Weeks

Study A

	Placebo	Bisoprolol Fumarate		
		5 mg	10 mg	20 mg
n=	61	61	61	61
Total ΔBP (mm Hg)	5.4/3.2	10.4/8.0	11.2/10.9	12.8/11.9
Drug Effect[a]	—	5.0/4.8	5.8/7.7	7.4/8.7
Total ΔHR (bpm)	0.5	7.2	8.7	11.3
Drug Effect[a]	—	6.7	8.2	10.8

Study B

	Placebo	Bisoprolol Fumarate	
		2.5 mg	10 mg
n=	56	59	62
Total ΔBP (mm Hg)	3.0/3.7	7.6/8.1	13.5/11.2
Drug Effect[a]	—	4.6/4.4	10.5/7.5
Total ΔHR (bpm)	1.6	3.8	10.7
Drug Effect[a]	—	2.2	9.1

[a] Observed total change from baseline minus placebo.

the micronucleus test in mice, and the cytogenetics assay in rats. There was no evidence of mutagenic potential in these *in vitro* and *in vivo* assays.

Reproduction studies in rats did not show any impairment of fertility at doses up to 150 mg/kg/day of bisoprolol fumarate, or 375 and 77 times the MRHD on the basis of body-weight and body-surface-area, respectively.

Pregnancy Category C

In rats, bisoprolol fumarate was not teratogenic at doses up to 150 mg/kg/day which is 375 and 77 times the MRHD on the basis of body-weight and body-surface-area, respectively. Bisoprolol fumarate was fetotoxic (increased late resorptions) at 50 mg/kg/day and maternotoxic (decreased food intake and body-weight gain) at 150 mg/kg/day. The fetotoxicity in rats occurred at 125 times the MRHD on a body-weight-basis and 26 times the MRHD on the basis of body-surface-area. The maternotoxicity occurred at 375 times the MRHD on a body-weight basis and 77 times the MRHD on the basis of body-surface-area. In rabbits, bisoprolol fumarate was not teratogenic at doses up to 12.5 mg/kg/day, which is 31 and 12 times the MRHD based on body-weight and body-surface-area, respectively, but was embryolethal (increased early resorptions) at 12.5 mg/kg/day. There are no adequate and well-controlled studies in pregnant women. ZEBETA should be used during pregnancy only if the potential benefit justifies the potential risk to the fetus.

Nursing Mothers

Small amounts of bisoprolol fumarate (<2% of the dose) have been detected in the milk of lactating rats. It is not known whether this drug is excreted in human milk. Because many drugs are excreted in human milk caution should be exercised when bisoprolol fumarate is administered to nursing women.

Use in Elderly Patients

ZEBETA has been used in elderly patients with hypertension. Response rates and mean decreases in systolic and diastolic blood pressure were similar to the decreases in younger patients in the U.S. clinical studies. Although no dose response study was conducted in elderly patients, there was a tendency for older patients to be maintained on higher doses of bisoprolol fumarate.

Observed reductions in heart rate were slightly greater in the elderly than in the young and tended to increase with increasing dose. In general, no disparity in adverse experience reports or dropouts for safety reasons was observed between older and younger patients. Dose adjustment based on age is not necessary.

Pediatric Use

Safety and effectiveness in children have not been established.

ADVERSE REACTIONS

Safety data are available in more than 30,000 patients or volunteers. Frequency estimates and rates of withdrawal of therapy for adverse events were derived from two U.S. placebo-controlled studies.

In Study A, doses of 5, 10 and 20 mg bisoprolol fumarate were administered for 4 weeks. In Study B, doses of 2.5, 10 and 40 mg of bisoprolol fumarate were administered for 12 weeks. A total of 273 patients were treated with 5–20 mg of bisoprolol fumarate; 132 received placebo.

Withdrawal of therapy for adverse events was 3.3% for patients receiving bisoprolol fumarate and 6.8% for patients on placebo. Withdrawals were less than 1% for either bradycardia or fatigue/lack of energy.

The following table presents adverse experiences, whether or not considered drug related, reported in at least 1% of patients in these studies, for all patients studied in placebo controlled clinical trials (2.5–40 mg), as well as for a subgroup that was treated with doses within the recommended dosage range (5–20 mg). Of the adverse events listed in the table, bradycardia, diarrhea, asthenia, fatigue and sinusitis appear to be dose related.

[See table above]

The following is a comprehensive list of adverse experiences reported with bisoprolol fumarate in worldwide studies, or in post marketing experience (in italics):

Central Nervous System: Dizziness, vertigo, headache, paresthesia, hypoaesthesia, somnolence, anxiety/restlessness, decreased concentration/memory.

Autonomic Nervous System: Dry mouth.

Cardiovascular: Bradycardia, palpitations and other rhythm disturbances, cold extremities, claudication, hypotension, orthostatic hypotension, chest pain, congestive heart failure, dyspnea on exertion.

Psychiatric: Vivid dreams, insomnia, depression.

Gastrointestinal: Gastric/epigastric/abdominal pain, gastritis, dyspepsia, nausea, vomiting, diarrhea, constipation.

Musculoskeletal: Muscle/joint pain, back/neck pain, muscle cramps, twitching/tremor.

Skin: Rash, acne, eczema, skin irritation, pruritus, flushing, sweating, alopecia, *angioedema, exfoliative dermatitis,* cutaneous vasculitis.

Body System/Adverse Experience	All Adverse Experiences (% [a])		
		Bisoprolol Fumarate	
	Placebo (n = 132)	5–20 mg (n = 273)	2.5–40 mg (n = 404)
	%	%	%
Skin			
increased sweating	1.5	0.7	1.0
Musculo-skeletal			
arthralgia	2.3	2.2	2.7
Central Nervous System			
dizziness	3.8	2.9	3.5
headache	11.4	8.8	10.9
hypoaesthesia	0.8	1.1	1.5
Autonomic Nervous System			
dry mouth	1.5	0.7	1.3
Heart Rate/Rhythm			
bradycardia	0	0.4	0.5
Psychiatric			
vivid dreams	0	0	0
insomnia	2.3	1.5	2.5
depression	0.8	0	0.2
Gastrointestinal			
diarrhea	1.5	2.6	3.5
nausea	1.5	1.5	2.2
vomiting	0	1.1	1.5
Respiratory			
bronchospasm		0	0
cough	4.5	2.6	3.5
dyspnea	0.8	1.1	1.5
pharyngitis	2.3	2.2	2.2
rhinitis	3.0	2.9	4.0
sinusitis	1.5	2.2	2.2
URI	3.8	4.8	5.0
Body as a Whole			
asthenia	0	0.4	1.5
chest pain	0.8	1.1	1.5
fatigue	1.5	6.6	8.2
edema (peripheral)	3.8	3.7	3.0

[a] percentage of patients with event.

Special Senses: Visual disturbances, ocular pain/pressure, abnormal lacrimation, tinnitus, earache, taste abnormalities.

Metabolic: Gout.

Respiratory: Asthma/bronchospasm, bronchitis, coughing, dyspnea, pharyngitis, rhinitis, sinusitis, URI.

Genito-urinary: Decreased libido/impotence, *Peyronie's disease,* cystitis, renal colic.

Hematologic: Purpura.

General: Fatigue, asthenia, chest pain, malaise, edema, weight gain.

In addition, a variety of adverse effects have been reported with other beta-adrenergic blocking agents and should be considered potential adverse effects of ZEBETA:

Central Nervous System: Reversible mental depression progressing to catatonia, hallucinations, an acute reversible syndrome characterized by disorientation to time and place, emotional lability, slightly clouded sensorium.

Allergic: Fever, combined with aching and sore throat, laryngospasm, respiratory distress.

Hematologic: Agranulocytosis, thrombocytopenia, thrombocytopenic purpura.

Gastrointestinal: Mesenteric arterial thrombosis, ischemic colitis.

Miscellaneous: The oculomucocutaneous syndrome associated with the beta-blocker practolol has not been reported with ZEBETA during investigational use or extensive foreign marketing experience.

LABORATORY ABNORMALITIES: In clinical trials, the most frequently reported laboratory change was an increase in serum triglycerides, but this was not a consistent finding. Sporadic liver test abnormalities have been reported. In the U.S. controlled trials experience with bisoprolol fumarate treatment for 4–12 weeks, the incidence of concomitant elevations in SGOT and SGPT of between 1–2 times normal was 3.9%, compared to 2.5% for placebo. No patient had concomitant elevations greater than twice normal.

In the long-term, uncontrolled experience with bisoprolol fumarate treatment for 6–18 months, the incidence of one or more concomitant elevations in SGOT and SGPT of between 1–2 times normal was 6.2%. The incidence of multiple occurrences was 1.9%. For concomitant elevations in SGOT and SGPT of greater than twice normal, the incidence was 1.5%. The incidence of multiple occurrences was 0.3%. In many cases these elevations were attributed to underlying disorders, or resolved during continued treatment with bisoprolol fumarate.

Other laboratory changes included small increases in uric acid, creatinine, BUN, serum potassium, glucose, and phosphorus and decreases in WBC and platelets. These were generally not of clinical importance and rarely resulted in discontinuation of bisoprolol fumarate.

As with other beta-blockers, ANA conversions have also been reported on bisoprolol fumarate. About 15% of patients in long-term studies converted to a positive titer, although about one-third of these patients subsequently reconverted to a negative titer while on continued therapy.

OVERDOSAGE

The most common signs expected with overdosage of a beta-blocker are bradycardia, hypotension, congestive heart failure, bronchospasm, and hypoglycemia. To date, a few cases of overdose (maximum: 2000 mg) with bisoprolol fumarate have been reported. Bradycardia and/or hypotension were noted. Sympathomimetic agents were given in some cases, and all patients recovered.

In general, if overdose occurs, ZEBETA therapy should be stopped and supportive and symptomatic treatment should be provided. Limited data suggest that bisoprolol fumarate is not dialyzable. Based on the expected pharmacologic actions and recommendations for other beta-blockers, the following general measures should be considered when clinically warranted:

Bradycardia

Administer IV atropine. If the response is inadequate, isoproterenol or another agent with positive chronotropic properties may be given cautiously. Under some circumstances, transvenous pacemaker insertion may be necessary.

Hypotension

IV fluids and vasopressors should be administered. Intravenous glucagon may be useful.

Heart Block (Second or Third Degree)

Patients should be carefully monitored and treated with isoproterenol infusion or transvenous cardiac pacemaker insertion, as appropriate.

Congestive Heart Failure

Initiate conventional therapy (ie, digitalis, diuretics, inotropic agents, vasodilating agents).

Bronchospasm

Administer bronchodilator therapy such as isoproterenol and/or aminophylline.

Hypoglycemia

Administer IV glucose.

DOSAGE AND ADMINISTRATION

The dose of ZEBETA must be individualized to the needs of the patient. The usual starting dose is 5 mg once daily. In some patients, 2.5 mg may be an appropriate starting dose (see Bronchospastic Disease in WARNINGS). If the antihypertensive effect of 5 mg is inadequate, the dose may be increased to 10 mg and then, if necessary, to 20 mg once daily.

Patients with Renal or Hepatic Impairment

In patients with hepatic impairment (hepatitis or cirrhosis) or renal dysfunction (creatinine clearance less than 40 mL/min), the initial daily dose should be 2.5 mg and caution should be used in dose-titration. Since limited data suggest that bisoprolol fumarate is not dialyzable, drug replacement is not necessary in patients undergoing dialysis.

Continued on next page

Zebeta—Cont.

Elderly Patients

It is not necessary to adjust the dose in the elderly, unless there is also significant renal or hepatic dysfunction (see above and **Use in Elderly Patients** in **PRECAUTIONS**).

Children

There is no pediatric experience with ZEBETA.

HOW SUPPLIED

ZEBETA® (bisoprolol fumarate) is supplied as 5 mg and 10 mg tablets.

The 5 mg tablet is pink, heart-shaped, biconvex, film-coated, and vertically scored in half on both sides, with an engraved B1 on one side and LL on the reverse side, supplied as follows:

NDC 0005-3816-38—Bottle of 30 with CRC

The 10 mg tablet is white, heart-shaped, biconvex, film-coated, with an engraved B3 on one side and LL on the reverse side, supplied as follows:

NDC 0005-3817-38—Bottle of 30 with CRC

Store at controlled room temperature 20°–25°C (68°– 77°F), protected from moisture.

Dispense in tight containers as defined in the USP.

Manufactured by:

LEDERLE PHARMACEUTICAL DIVISION
American Cyanamid Company
Pearl River, NY 10965
Under License of E. MERCK
Darmstadt, Germany

Shown in Product Identification Guide, page 320

ZIAC®

[zī 'ăk]

(Bisoprolol Fumarate and Hydrochlorothiazide) Tablets

℞

DESCRIPTION

ZIAC (bisoprolol fumarate and hydrochlorothiazide) is indicated for the treatment of hypertension. It combines two antihypertensive agents in a once-daily dosage: a synthetic beta$_1$-selective (cardioselective) adrenoceptor blocking agent (bisoprolol fumarate) and a benzothiadiazine diuretic (hydrochlorothiazide).

Bisoprolol fumarate is chemically described as (±)-1-[4-[[2-(1-methylethoxy)ethoxy]methyl]phenoxy]-3-[(1-methylethyl) amino]-2-propanol(E)-2-butenedioate (2:1) (salt). It possesses an asymmetric carbon atom in its structure and is provided as a racemic mixture. The S(-) enantiomer is responsible for most of the beta-blocking activity. Its empirical formula is $(C_{18}H_{31}NO_4)_2 \cdot C_4H_4O_4$ and it has a molecular weight of 766.97.

Bisoprolol fumarate is a white crystalline powder, approximately equally hydrophilic and lipophilic, and readily soluble in water, methanol, ethanol, and chloroform.

Hydrochlorothiazide (HCTZ) is 6-Chloro-3,4-dihydro-2H-1,2,4-benzothiadiazine-7-sulfonamide 1,1-dioxide. It is a white, or practically white, practically odorless crystalline powder. It is slightly soluble in water, sparingly soluble in dilute sodium hydroxide solution, freely soluble in n-butylamine and dimethylformamide, soluble in methanol, and insoluble in ether, chloroform, and dilute mineral acids. Its empirical formula is $C_7H_8ClN_3O_4S_2$ and it has a molecular weight of 297.73.

Each ZIAC®-2.5 mg/6.25 mg tablet for oral administration contains:

Bisoprolol fumarate .... 2.5 mg
Hydrochlorothiazide .... 6.25 mg

Each ZIAC®-5 mg/6.25 mg tablet for oral administration contains:

Bisoprolol fumarate .... 5 mg
Hydrochlorothiazide .... 6.25 mg

Each ZIAC®-10 mg/6.25 mg tablet for oral administration contains:

Bisoprolol fumarate .... 10 mg
Hydrochlorothiazide .... 6.25 mg

Inactive ingredients include Colloidal Silicon Dioxide, Corn Starch, Dibasic Calcium Phosphate, Hydroxypropyl Methylcellulose, Magnesium Stearate, Microcrystalline Cellulose, Polyethylene Glycol, Polysorbate 80, and Titanium Dioxide. The 5 mg/6.25 mg tablet also contains Red and Yellow Iron Oxide. The 2.5 mg/6.25 mg tablet also contains Crospovidone, Pregelatinized Starch and Yellow Iron Oxide.

CLINICAL PHARMACOLOGY

Bisoprolol fumarate and HCTZ have been used individually and in combination for the treatment of hypertension. The antihypertensive effects of these agents are additive; HCTZ 6.25 mg significantly increases the antihypertensive effect of bisoprolol fumarate. The incidence of hypokalemia with the bisoprolol fumarate and HCTZ 6.25 mg combination (B/H) is significantly lower than with HCTZ 25 mg. In clinical trials of ZIAC (bisoprolol fumarate and hydrochlorothi-

azide), mean changes in serum potassium for patients treated with ZIAC 2.5/6.25 mg, 5/6.25 mg or 10/6.25 mg or placebo were less than ± 0.1 mEq/L. Mean changes in serum potassium for patients treated with any dose of bisoprolol in combination with HCTZ 25 mg ranged from –0.1 to –0.3 mEq/L.

Bisoprolol fumarate is a beta$_1$-selective (cardioselective) adrenoceptor blocking agent without significant membrane stabilizing or intrinsic sympathomimetic activities in its therapeutic dose range. At higher doses ($\geq$ 20 mg) bisoprolol fumarate also inhibits beta$_2$-adrenoreceptors located in bronchial and vascular musculature. To retain relative selectivity, it is important to use the lowest effective dose. Hydrochlorothiazide is a benzothiadiazine diuretic. Thiazides affect renal tubular mechanisms of electrolyte reabsorption and increase excretion of sodium and chloride in approximately equivalent amounts. Natriuresis causes a secondary loss of potassium.

Pharmacokinetics and Metabolism

ZIAC

In healthy volunteers, both bisoprolol fumarate and hydrochlorothiazide are well absorbed following oral administration of ZIAC. No change is observed in the bioavailability of either agent when given together in a single tablet. Absorption is not affected whether ZIAC is taken with or without food. Mean peak bisoprolol fumarate plasma concentrations of about 9.0 ng/mL, 19 ng/mL and 36 ng/mL occur approximately 3 hours after the administration of the 2.5 mg/6.25 mg, 5 mg/6.25 mg and 10 mg/6.25 mg combination tablets, respectively. Mean peak plasma hydrochlorothiazide concentrations of 30 ng/mL occur approximately 2.5 hours following the administration of the combination. Dose proportional increases in plasma bisoprolol concentrations are observed between the 2.5 and 5, as well as between the 5 and 10 mg doses. The elimination T$_{1/2}$ of bisoprolol ranges from 7 to 15 hours and of hydrochlorothiazide ranges from 4 to 10 hours. The percent of dose excreted unchanged in urine is about 55% for bisoprolol and about 60% for hydrochlorothiazide.

Bisoprolol Fumarate

The absolute bioavailability after a 10 mg oral dose of bisoprolol fumarate is about 80%. The first pass metabolism of bisoprolol fumarate is about 20%.

The pharmacokinetic profile of bisoprolol fumarate has been examined following single doses and at steady state. Binding to serum proteins is approximately 30%. Peak plasma concentrations occur within 2–4 hours of dosing with 2.5 to 20 mg, and mean peak values range from 9.0 ng/mL at 2.5 mg to 70 ng/mL at 20 mg. Once-daily dosing with bisoprolol fumarate results in less than twofold intersubject variation in peak plasma concentrations. Plasma concentrations are proportional to the administered dose in the range of 2.5 to 20 mg. The plasma elimination half-life is 9–12 hours and is slightly longer in elderly patients, in part because of decreased renal function. Steady state is attained within 5 days with once-daily dosing. In both young and elderly populations, plasma accumulation is low; the accumulation factor ranges from 1.1 to 1.3, and is what would be expected from the half-life and once-daily dosing. Bisoprolol is eliminated equally by renal and nonrenal pathways with about 50% of the dose appearing unchanged in the urine and the remainder in the form of inactive metabolites. In humans, the known metabolites are labile or have no known pharmacologic activity. Less than 2% of the dose is excreted in the feces. The pharmacokinetic characteristics of the two enantiomers are similar. Bisoprolol is not metabolized by cytochrome P450 II D6 (debrisoquin hydroxylase).

In subjects with creatinine clearance less than 40 mL/min, the plasma half-life is increased approximately threefold compared to healthy subjects.

In patients with liver cirrhosis, the rate of elimination of bisoprolol is more variable and significantly slower than that in healthy subjects, with a plasma half-life ranging from 8 to 22 hours.

In elderly subjects, mean plasma concentrations at steady state are increased, in part attributed to lower creatinine clearance. However, no significant differences in the degree of bisoprolol accumulation is found between young and elderly populations.

Hydrochlorothiazide

Hydrochlorothiazide is well absorbed (65%–75%) following oral administration. Absorption of hydrochlorothiazide is reduced in patients with congestive heart failure.

Peak plasma concentrations are observed within 1–5 hours of dosing, and range from 70–490 ng/mL following oral doses of 12.5–100 mg. Plasma concentrations are linearly related to the administered dose. Concentrations of hydrochlorothiazide are 1.6–1.8 times higher in whole blood than in plasma. Binding to serum proteins has been reported to be approximately 40% to 68%. The plasma elimination half-life has been reported to be 6–15 hours. Hydrochlorothiazide is eliminated primarily by renal pathways. Following oral doses of 12.5–100 mg, 55%–77% of the administered dose appears in urine and greater than 95% of the absorbed dose is excreted in urine as unchanged drug. Plasma con-

centrations of hydrochlorothiazide are increased and the elimination half-life is prolonged in patients with renal disease.

Pharmacodynamics

Bisoprolol Fumarate

Findings in clinical hemodynamics studies with bisoprolol fumarate are similar to those observed with other beta-blockers. The most prominent effect is the negative chronotropic effect, giving a reduction in resting and exercise heart rate. There is a fall in resting and exercise cardiac output with little observed change in stroke volume, and only a small increase in right atrial pressure, or pulmonary capillary wedge pressure at rest or during exercise.

In normal volunteers, bisoprolol fumarate therapy resulted in a reduction of exercise- and isoproterenol-induced tachycardia. The maximal effect occurred within 1–4 hours postdosing. Effects generally persisted for 24 hours at doses of 5 mg or greater.

In controlled clinical trials, bisoprolol fumarate given as a single daily dose has been shown to be an effective antihypertensive agent when used alone or concomitantly with thiazide diuretics (see **CLINICAL STUDIES**).

The mechanism of bisoprolol fumarate's antihypertensive effect has not been completely established. Factors that may be involved include:

1) Decreased cardiac output
2) Inhibition of renin release by the kidneys
3) Diminution of tonic sympathetic outflow from vasomotor centers in the brain

Beta$_1$-selectivity of bisoprolol fumarate has been demonstrated in both animal and human studies. No effects at therapeutic doses on beta$_2$-adrenoreceptor density have been observed. Pulmonary function studies have been conducted in healthy volunteers, asthmatics, and patients with chronic obstructive pulmonary disease (COPD). Doses of bisoprolol fumarate ranged from 5 to 60 mg, atenolol from 50 to 200 mg, metoprolol from 100 to 200 mg, and propranolol from 40 to 80 mg. In some studies, slight, asymptomatic increases in airway resistance (AWR) and decreases in forced expiratory volume (FEV$_1$) were observed with doses of bisoprolol fumarate 20 mg and higher, similar to the small increases in AWR noted with other cardioselective beta-blocking agents. The changes induced by beta-blockade with all agents were reversed by bronchodilator therapy.

Electrophysiology studies in man have demonstrated that bisoprolol fumarate significantly decreases heart rate, increases sinus node recovery time, prolongs AV node refractory periods, and, with rapid atrial stimulation, prolongs AV nodal conduction.

Hydrochlorothiazide

Acute effects of thiazides are thought to result from a reduction in blood volume and cardiac output, secondary to a natriuretic effect, although a direct vasodilatory mechanism has also been proposed. With chronic administration, plasma volume returns toward normal, but peripheral vascular resistance is decreased.

Thiazides do not affect normal blood pressure. Onset of action occurs within 2 hours of dosing, peak effect is observed at about 4 hours, and activity persists for up to 24 hours.

CLINICAL STUDIES

In controlled clinical trials, bisoprolol fumarate/hydrochlorothiazide 6.25 mg has been shown to reduce systolic and diastolic blood pressure throughout a 24-hour period when administered once daily. The effects on systolic and diastolic blood pressure reduction of the combination of bisoprolol fumarate and hydrochlorothiazide were additive. Further, treatment effects were consistent across age groups (<60, $\geq$60 years), racial groups (black, nonblack), and gender (male, female).

In two randomized, double-blind, placebo-controlled trials conducted in the U.S., reductions in systolic and diastolic blood pressure and heart rate 24 hours after dosing in patients with mild-to-moderate hypertension are shown below. In both studies mean systolic/diastolic blood pressure and heart rate at baseline were approximately 151/101 mm Hg and 77 bpm.

[See table at bottom of next page]

Blood pressure responses were seen within 1 week of treatment but the maximum effect was apparent after 2 to 3 weeks of treatment. Overall, significantly greater blood pressure reductions were observed on ZIAC than on placebo. Further, blood pressure reductions were significantly greater for each of the bisoprolol fumarate plus hydrochlorothiazide combinations than for either of the components used alone regardless of race, age, or gender. There were no significant differences in response between black and nonblack patients.

INDICATIONS AND USAGE

ZIAC is indicated in the management of hypertension.

CONTRAINDICATIONS

ZIAC is contraindicated in patients in cardiogenic shock, overt cardiac failure (see **WARNINGS**), second or third de-

gree AV block, marked sinus bradycardia, anuria, and hypersensitivity to either component of this product or to other sulfonamide-derived drugs.

WARNINGS

Cardiac Failure: In general, beta-blocking agents should be avoided in patients with overt congestive failure. However, in some patients with compensated cardiac failure, it may be necessary to utilize these agents. In such situations, they must be used cautiously.

Patients Without a History of Cardiac Failure: Continued depression of the myocardium with beta-blockers can, in some patients, precipitate cardiac failure. At the first signs or symptoms of heart failure, discontinuation of ZIAC should be considered. In some cases ZIAC therapy can be continued while heart failure is treated with other drugs.

Abrupt Cessation of Therapy: Exacerbations of angina pectoris and, in some instances, myocardial infarction or ventricular arrhythmia, have been observed in patients with coronary artery disease following abrupt cessation of therapy with beta-blockers. Such patients should, therefore, be cautioned against interruption or discontinuation of therapy without the physician's advice. Even in patients without overt coronary artery disease, it may be advisable to taper therapy with ZIAC over approximately 1 week with the patient under careful observation. If withdrawal symptoms occur, beta-blocking agent therapy should be reinstituted, at least temporarily.

Peripheral Vascular Disease: Beta-blockers can precipitate or aggravate symptoms of arterial insufficiency in patients with peripheral vascular disease. Caution should be exercised in such individuals.

Bronchospastic Disease: PATIENTS WITH BRONCHOSPASTIC PULMONARY DISEASE SHOULD, IN GENERAL, NOT RECEIVE BETA-BLOCKERS. Because of the relative $beta_1$-selectivity of bisoprolol fumarate, ZIAC may be used with caution in patients with bronchospastic disease who do not respond to, or who cannot tolerate other antihypertensive treatment. Since $beta_1$-selectivity is not absolute, the lowest possible dose of ZIAC should be used. A $beta_2$ agonist (bronchodilator) should be made available.

Anesthesia and Major Surgery: If ZIAC treatment is to be continued perioperatively, particular care should be taken when anesthetic agents that depress myocardial function, such as ether, cyclopropane, and trichloroethylene, are used. See **OVERDOSAGE** for information on treatment of bradycardia and hypotension.

Diabetes and Hypoglycemia: Beta-blockers may mask some of the manifestations of hypoglycemia, particularly tachycardia. Nonselective beta-blockers may potentiate insulin-induced hypoglycemia and delay recovery of serum glucose levels. Because of its $beta_1$-selectivity, this is less likely with bisoprolol fumarate. However, patients subject to spontaneous hypoglycemia, or diabetic patients receiving insulin or oral hypoglycemic agents, should be cautioned about these possibilities. Also, latent diabetes mellitus may become manifest and diabetic patients given thiazides may require adjustment of their insulin dose. Because of the very low dose of HCTZ employed, this may be less likely with ZIAC.

Thyrotoxicosis: Beta-adrenergic blockade may mask clinical signs of hyperthyroidism, such as tachycardia. Abrupt withdrawal of beta-blockade may be followed by an exacerbation of the symptoms of hyperthyroidism or may precipitate thyroid storm.

Renal Disease: Cumulative effects of the thiazides may develop in patients with impaired renal function. In such patients, thiazides may precipitate azotemia. In subjects with creatinine clearance less than 40 mL/min, the plasma half-life of bisoprolol fumarate is increased up to threefold, as compared to healthy subjects. If progressive renal impairment becomes apparent, ZIAC should be discontinued. (See **Pharmacokinetics and Metabolism.**)

Hepatic Disease: ZIAC should be used with caution in patients with impaired hepatic function or progressive liver disease. Thiazides may alter fluid and electrolyte balance, which may precipitate hepatic coma. Also, elimination of bisoprolol fumarate is significantly slower in patients with cirrhosis than in healthy subjects. (See **Pharmacokinetics and Metabolism.**)

PRECAUTIONS

General

Electrolyte and Fluid Balance Status: Although the probability of developing hypokalemia is reduced with ZIAC because of the very low dose of HCTZ employed, periodic determination of serum electrolytes should be performed, and patients should be observed for signs of fluid or electrolyte disturbances, ie, hyponatremia, hypochloremic alkalosis, and hypokalemia and hypomagnesemia. Thiazides have been shown to increase the urinary excretion of magnesium; this may result in hypomagnesemia.

Warning signs or symptoms of fluid and electrolyte imbalance include dryness of mouth, thirst, weakness, lethargy, drowsiness, restlessness, muscle pains or cramps, muscular fatigue, hypotension, oliguria, tachycardia, and gastrointestinal disturbances such as nausea and vomiting.

Hypokalemia may develop, especially with brisk diuresis when severe cirrhosis is present, during concomitant use of corticosteroids or adrenocorticotropic hormone (ACTH) or after prolonged therapy. Interference with adequate oral electrolyte intake will also contribute to hypokalemia. Hypokalemia and hypomagnesemia can provoke ventricular arrhythmias or sensitize or exaggerate the response of the heart to the toxic effects of digitalis. Hypokalemia may be avoided or treated by potassium supplementation or increased intake of potassium-rich foods.

Dilutional hyponatremia may occur in edematous patients in hot weather; appropriate therapy is water restriction rather than salt administration, except in rare instances when the hyponatremia is life-threatening. In actual salt depletion, appropriate replacement is the therapy of choice.

Parathyroid Disease: Calcium excretion is decreased by thiazides, and pathologic changes in the parathyroid glands, with hypercalcemia and hypophosphatemia, have been observed in a few patients on prolonged thiazide therapy.

Hyperuricemia: Hyperuricemia or acute gout may be precipitated in certain patients receiving thiazide diuretics. Bisoprolol fumarate, alone or in combination with HCTZ, has been associated with increases in uric acid. However, in U.S. clinical trials, the incidence of treatment-related increases in uric acid was higher during therapy with HCTZ 25 mg (25%) than with B/H 6.25 mg (10%). Because of the very low dose of HCTZ employed, hyperuricemia may be less likely with ZIAC.

Drug Interactions: ZIAC may potentiate the action of other antihypertensive agents used concomitantly. ZIAC should not be combined with other beta-blocking agents. Patients receiving catecholamine-depleting drugs, such as reserpine or guanethidine, should be closely monitored because the added beta-adrenergic blocking action of bisoprolol fumarate may produce excessive reduction of sympathetic activity. In patients receiving concurrent therapy with clonidine, if therapy is to be discontinued, it is suggested that ZIAC be discontinued for several days before the withdrawal of clonidine.

ZIAC should be used with caution when myocardial depressants or inhibitors of AV conduction, such as certain calcium antagonists (particularly of the phenylalkylamine [verapamil] and benzothiazepine [diltiazem] classes), or antiarrhythmic agents, such as disopyramide, are used concurrently.

Bisoprolol Fumarate

Concurrent use of rifampin increases the metabolic clearance of bisoprolol fumarate, shortening its elimination half-life. However, initial dose modification is generally not necessary. Pharmacokinetic studies document no clinically relevant interactions with other agents given concomitantly, including thiazide diuretics, digoxin and cimetidine. There was no effect of bisoprolol fumarate on prothrombin times in patients on stable doses of warfarin.

Risk of Anaphylactic Reaction: While taking beta-blockers, patients with a history of severe anaphylactic reaction to a variety of allergens may be more reactive to repeated challenge, either accidental, diagnostic, or therapeutic. Such patients may be unresponsive to the usual doses of epinephrine used to treat allergic reactions.

Hydrochlorothiazide

When given concurrently the following drugs may interact with thiazide diuretics.

Alcohol, barbiturates, or narcotics—potentiation of orthostatic hypotension may occur.

Antidiabetic drugs (oral agents and insulin)—dosage adjustment of the antidiabetic drug may be required.

Other antihypertensive drugs—additive effect or potentiation.

Cholestyramine and colestipol resins—absorption of hydrochlorothiazide is impaired in the presence of anionic exchange resins. Single doses of cholestyramine and colestipol resins bind the hydrochlorothiazide and reduce its absorption in the gastrointestinal tract by up to 85 percent and 43 percent, respectively.

Corticosteroids, ACTH—intensified electrolyte depletion, particularly hypokalemia.

Pressor amines (eg, norepinephrine)—possible decreased response to pressor amines but not sufficient to preclude their use.

Skeletal muscle relaxants, nondepolarizing (eg, tubocurarine)—possible increased responsiveness to the muscle relaxant.

Lithium—generally should not be given with diuretics. Diuretic agents reduce the renal clearance of lithium and add a high risk of lithium toxicity. Refer to the package insert for lithium preparations before use of such preparations with ZIAC.

Nonsteroidal anti-inflammatory drugs—in some patients, the administration of a nonsteroidal anti-inflammatory agent can reduce the diuretic, natriuretic, and antihypertensive effects of loop, potassium-sparing and thiazide diuretics. Therefore, when ZIAC and nonsteroidal anti-inflammatory agents are used concomitantly, the patient should be observed closely to determine if the desired effect of the diuretic is obtained.

In patients receiving thiazides, sensitivity reactions may occur with or without a history of allergy or bronchial asthma. Photosensitivity reactions and possible exacerbation or activation of systemic lupus erythematosus have been reported in patients receiving thiazides. The antihypertensive effects of thiazides may be enhanced in the post-sympathectomy patient.

Laboratory Test Interactions: Based on reports involving thiazides, ZIAC may decrease serum levels of protein-bound iodine without signs of thyroid disturbance.

Because it includes a thiazide, ZIAC should be discontinued before carrying out tests for parathyroid function (see **PRECAUTIONS—Parathyroid Disease**).

INFORMATION FOR PATIENTS

Patients, especially those with coronary artery disease, should be warned against discontinuing use of ZIAC without a physician's supervision. Patients should also be advised to consult a physician if any difficulty in breathing occurs, or if they develop other signs or symptoms of congestive heart failure or excessive bradycardia.

Patients subject to spontaneous hypoglycemia, or diabetic patients receiving insulin or oral hypoglycemic agents, should be cautioned that beta-blockers may mask some of the manifestations of hypoglycemia, particularly tachycardia, and bisoprolol fumarate should be used with caution.

Patients should know how they react to this medicine before they operate automobiles and machinery or engage in other tasks requiring alertness. Patients should be advised that photosensitivity reactions have been reported with thiazides.

Carcinogenesis, Mutagenesis, Impairment of Fertility:

Carcinogenesis

ZIAC: Long-term studies have not been conducted with the bisoprolol fumarate/hydrochlorothiazide combination.

Bisoprolol Fumarate: Long-term studies were conducted with oral bisoprolol fumarate administered in the feed of mice (20 and 24 months) and rats (26 months). No evidence of carcinogenic potential was seen in mice dosed up to 250 mg/kg/day or rats dosed up to 125 mg/kg/day. On a body-weight basis, these doses are 625 and 312 times, respectively, the maximum recommended human dose (MRHD) of 20 mg, or 0.4 mg/kg/day, based on 50 kg individuals; on a body-surface-area basis, these doses are 59 times (mice) and 64 times (rats) the MRHD.

Hydrochlorothiazide: Two-year feeding studies in mice and rats, conducted under the auspices of the National Toxicology Program (NTP), treated mice and rats with doses of hydrochlorothiazide up to 600 and 100 mg/kg/day, respectively. On a body-weight basis, these doses are 2400 times (in mice) and 400 times (in rats) the MRHD of hydrochlorothiazide (12.5 mg/day) in ZIAC (bisoprolol fumarate and hydrochlorothiazide). On a body-surface-area basis, these doses are 226 times (in mice) and 82 times (in rats) the MRHD. These studies uncovered no evidence of carcino-

Continued on next page

Sitting Systolic/Diastolic Pressure (BP) and Heart Rate (HR)
Mean Decrease (Δ) After 3–4 weeks

	Study 1			Study 2		
	Placebo	B5/H6.25 mg	Placebo	H6.25 mg	B2.5/H6.25 mg	B10/H6.25 mg
n=	75	150	56	23	28	25
Total ΔBP (mm Hg)	–2.9/–3.9	–15.8/–12.6	–3.0/–3.7	–6.6/–5.8	–14.1/–10.5	–15.3/–14.3
Drug Effect[a]	—/—	–12.9/–8.7	—/—	–3.6/–2.1	–11.1/–6.8	–12.3/–10.6
Total ΔHR (bpm)	–0.3	–6.9	–1.6	–0.8	–3.7	–9.8
Drug Effect[a]	—	–6.6	—	+0.8	–2.1	–8.2

[a] Observed mean change from baseline minus placebo.

Ziac—Cont.

genic potential of hydrochlorothiazide in rats or female mice, but there was equivocal evidence of hepatocarcinogenicity in male mice.

Mutagenesis

ZIAC: The mutagenic potential of the bisoprolol fumarate/hydrochlorothiazide combination was evaluated in the microbial mutagenicity (Ames) test, the point mutation and chromosomal aberration assays in Chinese hamster V79 cells, and the micronucleus test in mice. There was no evidence of mutagenic potential in these *in vitro* and *in vivo* assays.

Bisoprolol Fumarate: The mutagenic potential of bisoprolol fumarate was evaluated in the microbial mutagenicity (Ames) test, the point mutation and chromosome aberration assays in Chinese hamster V79 cells, the unscheduled DNA synthesis test, the micronucleus test in mice, and the cytogenetics assay in rats. There was no evidence of mutagenic potential in these *in vitro* and *in vivo* assays.

Hydrochlorothiazide: Hydrochlorothiazide was not genotoxic in *in vitro* assays using strains TA 98, TA 100, TA 1535, TA 1537 and TA 1538 of *Salmonella typhimurium* (the Ames test); in the Chinese Hamster Ovary (CHO) test for chromosomal aberrations; or in *in vivo* assays using mouse germinal cell chromosomes, Chinese hamster bone marrow chromosomes, and the *Drosophila* sex-linked recessive lethal trait gene. Positive test results were obtained in the *in vitro* CHO Sister Chromatid Exchange (clastogenicity) test and in the mouse Lymphoma Cell (mutagenicity) assays, using concentrations of hydrochlorothiazide of 43 to 1300 µg/mL. Positive test results were also obtained in the *Aspergillus nidulans* nondisjunction assay, using an unspecified concentration of hydrochlorothiazide.

Impairment of Fertility

ZIAC: Reproduction studies in rats did not show any impairment of fertility with the bisoprolol fumarate/hydrochlorothiazide combination doses containing up to 30 mg/kg/day of bisoprolol fumarate in combination with 75 mg/kg/day of hydrochlorothiazide. On a body-weight basis, these doses are 75 and 300 times, respectively, the MRHD of bisoprolol fumarate and hydrochlorothiazide. On a body-surface-area basis, these study doses are 15 and 62 times, respectively, the MRHD.

Bisoprolol Fumarate: Reproduction studies in rats did not show any impairment of fertility at doses up to 150 mg/kg/day of bisoprolol fumarate, or 375 and 77 times the MRHD on the basis of body-weight and body-surface-area, respectively.

Hydrochlorothiazide: Hydrochlorothiazide had no adverse effects on the fertility of mice and rats of either sex in studies wherein these species were exposed, via their diet, to doses of up to 100 and 4 mg/kg/day, respectively, prior to mating and throughout gestation. Corresponding multiples of maximum recommended human doses are 400 (mice) and 16 (rats) on the basis of body-weight and 38 (mice) and 3.3 (rats) on the basis of body-surface-area.

Pregnancy: Teratogenic Effects-Pregnancy Category C:

ZIAC: In rats, the bisoprolol fumarate/hydrochlorothiazide (B/H) combination was not teratogenic at doses up to 51.4 mg/kg/day of bisoprolol fumarate in combination with 128.6 mg/kg/day of hydrochlorothiazide. Bisoprolol fumarate and hydrochlorothiazide doses used in the rat study are, as multiples of the MRHD in the combination, 129 and 514 times greater, respectively, on a body-weight basis, and 26 and 106 times greater, respectively, on the basis of body-surface-area. The drug combination was maternotoxic (decreased body weight and food consumption) at B5.7/H14.3 (mg/kg/day) and higher, and fetotoxic (increased late resorptions) at B17.1/H42.9 (mg/kg/day) and higher. Maternotoxicity was present at 14/57 times the MRHD of B/H, respectively, on a body-weight basis, and 3/12 times the MRHD of B/H doses, respectively, on the basis of body-surface-area. Fetotoxicity was present at 43/172 times the MRHD of B/H, respectively, on a body-weight basis, and 9/35 times the MRHD of B/H doses, respectively, on the basis of body-surface-area. In rabbits, the B/H combination was not teratogenic at doses of B10/H25 (mg/kg/day). Bisoprolol fumarate and hydrochlorothiazide used in the rabbit study were not teratogenic at 25/100 times the B/H MRHD, respectively, on a body-weight basis, and 10/40 times the B/H MRHD, respectively, on the basis of body-surface-area. The drug combination was maternotoxic (decreased body weight) at B1/H2.5 (mg/kg/day) and higher, and fetotoxic (increased resorptions) at B10/H25 (mg/kg/day). The multiples of the MRHD for the B/H combination that were maternotoxic were, respectively, 2.5/10 (on the basis of body-weight) and 1/4 (on the basis of body-surface-area), and for fetotoxicity were, respectively, 25/100 (on the basis of body-weight) and 10/40 (on the basis of body-surface-area).

There are no adequate and well-controlled studies with ZIAC in pregnant women. ZIAC should be used during pregnancy only if the potential benefit justifies the risk to the fetus.

Bisoprolol Fumarate: In rats, bisoprolol fumarate was not teratogenic at doses up to 150 mg/kg/day, which were 375 and 77 times the MRHD on the basis of body-weight and body-surface-area, respectively. Bisoprolol fumarate was fetotoxic (increased late resorptions) at 50 mg/kg/day and maternotoxic (decreased food intake and body-weight gain) at 150 mg/kg/day. The fetotoxicity in rats occurred at 125 times the MRHD on a body-weight basis and 26 times the MRHD on the basis of body-surface-area. The maternotoxicity occurred at 375 times the MRHD on a body-weight basis and 77 times the MRHD on the basis of body-surface-area. In rabbits, bisoprolol fumarate was not teratogenic at doses up to 12.5 mg/kg/day, which is 31 and 12 times the MRHD based on body-weight and body-surface-area, respectively, but was embryolethal (increased early resorptions) at 12.5 mg/kg/day.

Body System/ Adverse Experience	% of Patients with Adverse Experiences* All Adverse Experiences		Drug Related Adverse Experiences	
	Placebo† (n=144) %	B2.5–40/H6.25† (n=252) %	Placebo† (n=144) %	B2.5–10/H6.25† (n=221) %
Cardiovascular				
bradycardia	0.7	1.1	0.7	0.9
arrhythmia	1.4	0.4	0.0	0.0
peripheral ischemia	0.9	0.7	0.9	0.4
chest pain	0.7	1.8	0.7	0.9
Respiratory				
bronchospasm	0.0	0.0	0.0	0.0
cough	1.0	2.2	0.7	1.5
rhinitis	2.0	0.7	0.7	0.9
URI	2.3	2.1	0.0	0.0
Body as a Whole				
asthenia	0.0	0.0	0.0	0.0
fatigue	2.7	4.6	1.7	3.0
peripheral edema	0.7	1.1	0.7	0.9
Central Nervous System				
dizziness	1.8	5.1	1.8	3.2
headache	4.7	4.5	2.7	0.4
Musculoskeletal				
muscle cramps	0.7	1.2	0.7	1.1
myalgia	1.4	2.4	0.0	0.0
Psychiatric				
insomnia	2.4	1.1	2.0	1.2
somnolence	0.7	1.1	0.7	0.9
loss of libido	1.2	0.4	1.2	0.4
impotence	0.7	1.1	0.7	1.1
Gastrointestinal				
diarrhea	1.4	4.3	1.2	1.1
nausea	0.9	1.1	0.9	0.9
dyspepsia	0.7	1.2	0.7	0.9

* Averages adjusted to combine across studies.
† Combined across studies.

Hydrochlorothiazide: Hydrochlorothiazide was orally administered to pregnant mice and rats during respective periods of major organogenesis at doses up to 3000 and 1000 mg/kg/day, respectively. At these doses, which are multiples of the MRHD equal to 12,000 for mice and 4000 for rats, based on body-weight, and equal to 1129 for mice and 824 for rats, based on body-surface-area, there was no evidence of harm to the fetus. There are, however, no adequate and well-controlled studies in pregnant women. Because animal reproduction studies are not always predictive of human response, this drug should be used during pregnancy only if clearly needed.

Nonteratogenic Effects: Thiazides cross the placental barrier and appear in the cord blood. The use of thiazides in pregnant women requires that the anticipated benefit be weighed against possible hazards to the fetus. These hazards include fetal or neonatal jaundice, pancreatitis, thrombocytopenia, and possibly other adverse reactions which have occurred in the adult.

Nursing Mothers: Bisoprolol fumarate alone or in combination with HCTZ has not been studied in nursing mothers. Thiazides are excreted in human breast milk. Small amounts of bisoprolol fumarate (<2% of the dose) have been detected in the milk of lactating rats. Because of the potential for serious adverse reactions in nursing infants, a decision should be made whether to discontinue nursing or to discontinue the drug, taking into account the importance of the drug to the mother.

Use in Elderly Patients: In clinical trials, at least 270 patients treated with bisoprolol fumarate plus HCTZ were 60 years of age or older. HCTZ added significantly to the antihypertensive effect of bisoprolol in elderly hypertensive patients. No overall differences in effectiveness or safety were observed between these patients and younger patients. Other reported clinical experience has not identified differences in responses between the elderly and younger patients, but greater sensitivity of some older individuals cannot be ruled out.

Pediatric Use: Safety and effectiveness of ZIAC in children have not been established.

ADVERSE REACTIONS

ZIAC:

Bisoprolol fumarate/H6.25 mg is well tolerated in most patients. Most adverse effects (AEs) have been mild and transient. In more than 65,000 patients treated worldwide with bisoprolol fumarate, occurrences of bronchospasm have been rare. Discontinuation rates for AEs were similar for B/H6.25 mg and placebo-treated patients.

In the United States, 252 patients received bisoprolol fumarate (2.5, 5, 10, or 40 mg)/H6.25 mg and 144 patients received placebo in two controlled trials. In Study 1, bisoprolol fumarate 5/H6.25 mg was administered for 4 weeks. In Study 2, bisoprolol fumarate 2.5, 10 or 40/H6.25 mg was administered for 12 weeks. All adverse experiences, whether drug related or not, and drug related adverse experiences in patients treated with B2.5–10/H6.25 mg, reported during comparable, 4 week treatment periods by at least 2% of bisoprolol fumarate/H6.25 mg-treated patients (plus additional selected adverse experiences) are presented in the following table:

[See table at left]

Other adverse experiences that have been reported with the individual components are listed below.

Bisoprolol Fumarate

In clinical trials worldwide, a variety of other AEs, in addition to those listed above, have been reported. While in many cases it is not known whether a causal relationship exists between bisoprolol and these AEs, they are listed to alert the physician to a possible relationship.

Central Nervous System: Unsteadiness, vertigo, syncope, paresthesia, hyperesthesia, sleep disturbance/vivid dreams, depression, anxiety/restlessness, decreased concentration/memory.

Cardiovascular: Palpitations and other rhythm disturbances, cold extremities, claudication, hypotension, orthostatic hypotension, chest pain, congestive heart failure.

Gastrointestinal: Gastric/epigastric/abdominal pain, peptic ulcer, gastritis, vomiting, constipation, dry mouth.

Musculoskeletal: Arthralgia, muscle/joint pain, back/neck pain, twitching/tremor.

Skin: Rash, acne, eczema, psoriasis, skin irritation, pruritus, purpura, flushing, sweating, alopecia, dermatitis, exfoliative dermatitis (very rarely), cutaneous vasculitis.

Special Senses: Visual disturbances, ocular pain/pressure, abnormal lacrimation, tinnitus, decreased hearing, earache, taste abnormalities.

Metabolic: Gout.

Respiratory: Asthma, bronchitis, dyspnea, pharyngitis, sinusitis.

Genito-urinary: Peyronie's disease (very rarely), cystitis, renal colic, polyuria.

General: Malaise, edema, weight gain, angioedema.

In addition, a variety of adverse effects have been reported with other beta-adrenergic blocking agents and should be considered potential adverse effects:

Central Nervous System: Reversible mental depression progressing to catatonia, hallucinations, an acute reversible syndrome characterized by disorientation to time and place, emotional lability, slightly clouded sensorium.
Allergic: Fever, combined with aching and sore throat, laryngospasm, and respiratory distress.
Hematologic: Agranulocytosis, thrombocytopenia.
Gastrointestinal: Mesenteric arterial thrombosis and ischemic colitis.
Miscellaneous: The oculomucocutaneous syndrome associated with the beta-blocker practolol has not been reported with bisoprolol fumarate during investigational use or extensive foreign marketing experience.

Hydrochlorothiazide

The following adverse experiences, in addition to those listed in the above table, have been reported with hydrochlorothiazide (generally with doses of 25 mg or greater).
General: Weakness.
Central Nervous System: Vertigo, paresthesia, restlessness.
Cardiovascular: Orthostatic hypotension (may be potentiated by alcohol, barbiturates, or narcotics).
Gastrointestinal: Anorexia, gastric irritation, cramping, constipation, jaundice (intrahepatic cholestatic jaundice), pancreatitis, cholecystitis, sialadenitis, dry mouth.
Musculoskeletal: Muscle spasm.
Hypersensitive Reactions: Purpura, photosensitivity, rash, urticaria, necrotizing angiitis (vasculitis and cutaneous vasculitis), fever, respiratory distress including pneumonitis and pulmonary edema, anaphylactic reactions.
Special Senses: Transient blurred vision, xanthopsia.
Metabolic: Gout.
Genitourinary: Sexual dysfunction, renal failure, renal dysfunction, interstitial nephritis.

LABORATORY ABNORMALITIES:

ZIAC:

Because of the low dose of hydrochlorothiazide in ZIAC, adverse metabolic effects with B/H6.25 mg are less frequent and of smaller magnitude than with HCTZ 25 mg. Laboratory data on serum potassium from the U.S. placebo-controlled trials are shown in the following table:
[See table above]

Serum Potassium Data from U.S. Placebo Controlled Studies

	Placebo† (n = 130*)	B2.5/H6.25 mg (n = 28*)	B5/H6.25 mg (n = 149*)	B10/H6.25 mg (n = 28*)	HCTZ25 mg† (n = 142*)
Potassium					
Mean Change[a] (mEq/L)	+0.04	+0.11	−0.08	0.00	−0.30
% Hypokalemia[b]	0.0%	0.0%	0.7%	0.0%	5.5%

* Patients with normal serum potassium at baseline.
[a] Mean change from baseline at Week 4.
[b] Percentage of patients with abnormality at Week 4.
† Combined across studies.

Treatment with both beta blockers and thiazide diuretics is associated with increases in uric acid. However, the magnitude of the change in patients treated with B/H6.25 mg was smaller than in patients treated with HCTZ 25 mg. Mean increases in serum triglycerides were observed in patients treated with bisoprolol fumarate and hydrochlorothiazide 6.25 mg. Total cholesterol was generally unaffected, but small decreases in HDL cholesterol were noted.
Other laboratory abnormalities that have been reported with the individual components are listed below.

Bisoprolol Fumarate: In clinical trials, the most frequently reported laboratory change was an increase in serum triglycerides, but this was not a consistent finding.
Sporadic liver test abnormalities have been reported. In the U.S. controlled trials experience with bisoprolol fumarate treatment for 4 to 12 weeks, the incidence of concomitant elevations in SGOT and SGPT of between 1 and 2 times normal was 3.9%, compared to 2.5% for placebo. No patient had concomitant elevations greater than twice normal.
In the long-term, uncontrolled experience with bisoprolol fumarate treatment for 6 to 18 months, the incidence of one or more concomitant elevations in SGOT and SGPT of between 1 and 2 times normal was 6.2%. The incidence of multiple occurrence was 1.9%. For concomitant elevations in SGOT and SGPT of greater than twice normal, the incidence was 1.5%. The incidence of multiple occurrences was 0.3%. In many cases these elevations were attributed to underlying disorders, or resolved during continued treatment with bisoprolol fumarate.
Other laboratory changes included small increases in uric acid, creatinine, BUN, serum potassium, glucose, and phosphorus and decreases in WBC and platelets. There have been occasional reports of eosinophilia. These were generally not of clinical importance and rarely resulted in discontinuation of bisoprolol fumarate.
As with other beta-blockers, ANA conversions have also been reported on bisoprolol fumarate. About 15% of patients in long-term studies converted to a positive titer, although about one-third of these patients subsequently reconverted to a negative titer while on continued therapy.

Hydrochlorothiazide: Hyperglycemia, glycosuria, hyperuricemia, hypokalemia and other electrolyte imbalances (see **PRECAUTIONS**), hyperlipidemia, hypercalcemia, leukopenia, agranulocytosis, thrombocytopenia, aplastic anemia, and hemolytic anemia have been associated with HCTZ therapy.

OVERDOSAGE

There are limited data on overdose with ZIAC. However, several cases of overdose with bisoprolol fumarate have been reported (maximum: 2000 mg). Bradycardia and/or hypotension were noted. Sympathomimetic agents were given in some cases, and all patients recovered.
The most frequently observed signs expected with overdosage of a beta-blocker are bradycardia and hypotension. Lethargy is also common, and with severe overdoses, delirium, coma, convulsions, and respiratory arrest have been reported to occur. Congestive heart failure, bronchospasm, and hypoglycemia may occur, particularly in patients with underlying conditions. With thiazide diuretics, acute intoxication is rare. The most prominent feature of overdose is acute loss of fluid and electrolytes. Signs and symptoms include cardiovascular (tachycardia, hypotension, shock), neuromuscular (weakness, confusion, dizziness, cramps of the calf muscles, paresthesia, fatigue, impairment of consciousness), gastrointestinal (nausea, vomiting, thirst), renal (polyuria, oliguria, or anuria [due to hemoconcentration]), and laboratory findings (hypokalemia, hyponatremia, hypochloremia, alkalosis, increased BUN [especially in patients with renal insufficiency]).
If overdosage of ZIAC is suspected, therapy with ZIAC should be discontinued and the patient observed closely. Treatment is symptomatic and supportive; there is no specific antidote. Limited data suggest bisoprolol fumarate is not dialyzable; similarly, there is no indication that hydrochlorothiazide is dialyzable. Suggested general measures include induction of emesis and/or gastric lavage, administration of activated charcoal, respiratory support, correction of fluid and electrolyte imbalance, and treatment of convulsions. Based on the expected pharmacologic actions and recommendations for other beta-blockers and hydrochlorothiazide, the following measures should be considered when clinically warranted:
Bradycardia: Administer IV atropine. If the response is inadequate, isoproterenol or another agent with positive chronotropic properties may be given cautiously. Under some circumstances, transvenous pacemaker insertion may be necessary.
Hypotension, Shock: The patient's legs should be elevated. IV fluids should be administered and lost electrolytes (potassium, sodium) replaced. Intravenous glucagon may be useful. Vasopressors should be considered.
Heart Block (second or third degree): Patients should be carefully monitored and treated with isoproterenol infusion or transvenous cardiac pacemaker insertion, as appropriate.
Congestive Heart Failure: Initiate conventional therapy (ie, digitalis, diuretics, vasodilating agents, inotropic agents).
Bronchospasm: Administer a bronchodilator such as isoproterenol and/or aminophylline.
Hypoglycemia: Administer IV glucose.
Surveillance: Fluid and electrolyte balance (especially serum potassium) and renal function should be monitored until normalized.

DOSAGE AND ADMINISTRATION

Bisoprolol is an effective treatment of hypertension in once-daily doses of 2.5 to 40 mg, while hydrochlorothiazide is effective in doses of 12.5 to 50 mg. In clinical trials of bisoprolol/hydrochlorothiazide combination therapy using bisoprolol doses of 2.5–20 mg and hydrochlorothiazide doses of 6.25–25 mg, the antihypertensive effects increased with increasing doses of either component.
The adverse effects (see **WARNINGS**) of bisoprolol are a mixture of dose-dependent phenomena (primarily bradycardia, diarrhea, asthenia and fatigue) and dose-independent phenomena (eg, occasional rash); those of hydrochlorothiazide are a mixture of dose-dependent phenomena (primarily hypokalemia) and dose-independent phenomena (eg, possibly pancreatitis); the dose-dependent phenomena for each being much more common than the dose-independent phenomena. The latter consist of those few that are truly idiosyncratic in nature or those that occur with such low frequency that a dose relationship may be difficult to discern. Therapy with a combination of bisoprolol and hydrochlorothiazide will be associated with both sets of dose-independent adverse effects, and to minimize these, it may be appropriate to begin combination therapy only after a patient has failed to achieve the desired effect with monotherapy. On the other hand, regimens that combine low doses of bisoprolol and hydrochlorothiazide should produce minimal dose-dependent adverse effects, eg, bradycardia, diarrhea, asthenia and fatigue, and minimal dose-dependent adverse metabolic effects, ie, decreases in serum potassium (see **CLINICAL PHARMACOLOGY**).

Therapy Guided by Clinical Effect: A patient whose blood pressure is not adequately controlled with 2.5–20 mg bisoprolol daily may instead be given ZIAC (bisoprolol fumarate and hydrochlorothiazide). Patients whose blood pressures are adequately controlled with 50 mg of hydrochlorothiazide daily, but who experience significant potassium loss with this regimen, may achieve similar blood pressure control without electrolyte disturbance if they are switched to ZIAC.

Initial Therapy: Antihypertensive therapy may be initiated with the lowest dose of ZIAC, one 2.5/6.25 mg tablet once daily. Subsequent titration (14 day intervals) may be carried out with ZIAC tablets up to the maximum recommended dose 20/12.5 mg (two 10/6.25 mg tablets) once daily, as appropriate.

Replacement Therapy: The combination may be substituted for the titrated individual components.

Cessation of Therapy: If withdrawal of ZIAC therapy is planned, it should be achieved gradually over a period of about 2 weeks. Patients should be carefully observed.

Patients with Renal or Hepatic Impairment: As noted in the **WARNINGS** section, caution must be used in dosing/titrating patients with hepatic impairment or renal dysfunction. Since there is no indication that hydrochlorothiazide is dialyzable, and limited data suggest that bisoprolol is not dialyzable, drug replacement is not necessary in patients undergoing dialysis.

Elderly Patients: Dosage adjustment on the basis of age is not usually necessary, unless there is also significant renal or hepatic dysfunction (see above and **WARNINGS** section).

Children: There is no pediatric experience with ZIAC.

HOW SUPPLIED

ZIAC®-2.5 mg/6.25 mg Tablets (bisoprolol fumarate 2.5 mg and hydrochlorothiazide 6.25 mg) are yellow, round, convex, film coated tablets, engraved with a script "LL" within an engraved heart shape on one side and "B" above "12" on the other; approximately 1/4" in diameter, supplied as follows:
NDC 0005-3238-38—Bottle of 30 with child resistant closure
NDC 0005-3238-23—Bottle of 100
ZIAC®-5 mg/6.25 mg Tablets (bisoprolol fumarate 5 mg and hydrochlorothiazide 6.25 mg) are pink, round, convex, film coated tablets, engraved with a script "LL" within an engraved heart shape on one side and "B" above "13" on the other; approximately 9/32" in diameter, supplied as follows:
NDC 0005-3234-38—Bottle of 30 with child resistant closure
NDC 0005-3234-23—Bottle of 100
ZIAC®-10 mg/6.25 mg Tablets (bisoprolol fumarate 10 mg and hydrochlorothiazide 6.25 mg) are white, round, convex, film coated tablets, engraved with a script "LL" within an engraved heart shape on one side and "B" above "14" on the other; approximately 9/32" in diameter, supplied as follows:
NDC 0005-3235-38—Bottle of 30 with child resistant closure
Store at Controlled Room Temperature 15°–30°C (59°–86°F) in a well-closed container.
Manufactured by:
LEDERLE PHARMACEUTICAL DIVISION
American Cyanamid Company
Pearl River, NY 10965
Under License of E. MERCK
Darmstadt, Germany

Shown in Product Identification Guide, page 320

ZOSYN® ℞

[zō ′sĭn]

(Sterile Piperacillin Sodium and Tazobactam Sodium)

DESCRIPTION

Zosyn in an injectable antibacterial combination product consisting of the semisynthetic antibiotic piperacillin sodium and the β-lactamase inhibitor tazobactam sodium for intravenous administration.
Piperacillin sodium is derived from D(-)-α-aminobenzylpenicillin. The chemical name of piperacillin sodium is sodium (2*S*,5*R*,6*R*)-6-[(*R*)-2-(4-ethyl-2,3-dioxo-1-piperazine-

Continued on next page

Zosyn—Cont.

carboxamido)-2-phenylacetamido]-3,3-dimethyl-7-oxo-4-thia-1-azabicyclo[3.2.0] heptane-2-carboxylate. The chemical formula is $C_{23}H_{26}N_5NaO_7S$ and the molecular weight is 539.6.

Tazobactam sodium, a derivative of the penicillin nucleus, is a penicillanic acid sulfone. Its chemical name is sodium $(2S,3S,5R)$-3-methyl-7-oxo-3-$(1H$-1,2,3-triazol-1-ylmethyl)-4-thia-1-azabicyclo[3.2.0]heptane-2-carboxylate-4,4-dioxide. The chemical formula is $C_{10}H_{11}N_4NaO_5S$ and the molecular weight is 322.3.

Zosyn, piperacillin/tazobactam parenteral combination, is a white to off-white sterile, cryodesiccated powder consisting of piperacillin and tazobactam as their sodium salts packaged in glass vials. The product does not contain excipients or preservatives.

Each Zosyn 2.25 g single dose vial or ADD-Vantage® vial contains an amount of drug sufficient for withdrawal of piperacillin sodium equivalent to 2 grams of piperacillin and tazobactam sodium equivalent to 0.25 g of tazobactam.

Each Zosyn 3.375 g single dose vial or ADD-Vantage® vial contains an amount of drug sufficient for withdrawal of piperacillin sodium equivalent to 3 grams of piperacillin and tazobactam sodium equivalent to 0.375 g of tazobactam.

Each Zosyn 4.5 g single dose vial or ADD-Vantage® vial contains an amount of drug sufficient for withdrawal of piperacillin sodium equivalent to 4 grams of piperacillin and tazobactam sodium equivalent to 0.5 g of tazobactam.

Zosyn is a monosodium salt of piperacillin and a monosodium salt of tazobactam containing a total of 2.35 mEq (54 mg) of Na+ per gram of piperacillin in the combination product.

CLINICAL PHARMACOLOGY

Peak plasma concentrations of piperacillin and tazobactam are attained immediately after completion of an intravenous infusion of Zosyn. Piperacillin plasma concentrations, following a 30-minute infusion of Zosyn, were similar to those attained when equivalent doses of piperacillin were administered alone, with mean peak plasma concentrations of approximately 134, 242, and 298 μg/mL for the 2.25 g, 3.375 g, and 4.5 g Zosyn (piperacillin/tazobactam) doses, respectively. The corresponding mean peak plasma concentrations of tazobactam were 15, 24, and 34 μg/mL, respectively. Following a 30-minute I.V. infusion of 3.375 g Zosyn every 6 hours, steady-state plasma concentrations of piperacillin and tazobactam were similar to those attained after the first dose. In like manner, steady-state plasma concentrations were not different from those attained after the first dose when 2.25 g or 4.5 g doses of Zosyn were administered via 30-minute infusions every 6 hours. Steady-state plasma concentrations after 30-minute infusions every 6 hours are provided in Table 1.

Following single or multiple Zosyn doses to healthy subjects, the plasma half-life of piperacillin and of tazobactam ranged from 0.7 to 1.2 hours and was unaffected by dose or duration of infusion.

Piperacillin is metabolized to a minor microbiologically active desethyl metabolite. Tazobactam is metabolized to a single metabolite that lacks pharmacological and antibacterial activities. Both piperacillin and tazobactam are eliminated via the kidney by glomerular filtration and tubular secretion. Piperacillin is excreted rapidly as unchanged drug with 68% of the administered dose excreted in the urine. Tazobactam and its metabolite are eliminated primarily by renal excretion with 80% of the administered dose excreted as unchanged drug and the remainder as the single metabolite. Piperacillin, tazobactam, and desethyl piperacillin are also secreted into the bile.

Both piperacillin and tazobactam are approximately 30% bound to plasma proteins. The protein binding of either piperacillin or tazobactam is unaffected by the presence of the other compound. Protein binding of the tazobactam metabolite is negligible.

Piperacillin and tazobactam are widely distributed into tissues and body fluids including intestinal mucosa, gallbladder, lung, female reproductive tissues (uterus, ovary, and fallopian tube), interstitial fluid, and bile. Mean tissue concentrations are generally 50 to 100% of those in plasma. Distribution of piperacillin and tazobactam into cerebrospinal fluid is low in subjects with non-inflamed meninges, as with other penicillins.

After the administration of single doses of piperacillin/tazobactam to subjects with renal impairment, the half-life of piperacillin and of tazobactam increases with decreasing creatinine clearance. At creatinine clearance below 20 mL/min, the increase in half-life is twofold for piperacillin and fourfold for tazobactam compared to subjects with normal renal function. Dosage adjustments for Zosyn are recommended when creatinine clearance is below 40 mL/min in patients receiving the usual recommended daily dose of Zosyn. (See **Dosage and Administration** section for specific recommendations for the treatment of patients with renal insufficiency.)

Hemodialysis removes 30 to 40% of a piperacillin/tazobactam dose with an additional 5% of the tazobactam dose removed as the tazobactam metabolite. Peritoneal dialysis removes approximately 6% and 21% of the piperacillin and tazobactam doses, respectively, with up to 16% of the tazobactam dose removed as the tazobactam metabolite. For dosage recommendations for patients undergoing hemodialysis, see **Dosage and Administration** section.

The half-life of piperacillin and of tazobactam increases by approximately 25% and 18%, respectively, in patients with hepatic cirrhosis compared to healthy subjects. However, this difference does not warrant dosage adjustment of Zosyn due to hepatic cirrhosis.

[See table below]

Microbiology

Piperacillin sodium exerts bactericidal activity by inhibiting septum formation and cell wall synthesis. *In vitro*, piperacillin is active against a variety of gram-positive and gram-negative aerobic and anaerobic bacteria. Tazobactam sodium has very little intrinsic microbiologic activity due to its very low level binding to penicillin-binding proteins; however, it is a beta-lactamase inhibitor of the Richmond-Sykes class III (Bush class 2b & 2b') penicillinases and cephalosporinases. It varies in its ability to inhibit class II and IV (2a & 4) penicillinases. Tazobactam does not induce chromosomally-mediated β-lactamases at tazobactam levels achieved with the recommended dosage regimen. Piperacillin/tazobactam has been shown to be active against most strains of the following piperacillin-resistant, β-lactamase producing microorganisms both *in vitro* and in clinical infections as described in the **Indications and Usage** section.

Gram-positive aerobes:
Staphylococcus aureus (NOT methicillin/oxacillin-resistant strains)
Gram-negative aerobes:
Escherichia coli
Haemophilus influenzae (NOT β-lactamase negative, ampicillin-resistant strains)
Gram-negative anaerobes:
Bacteroides fragilis group (*B. fragilis, B. ovatus, B. thetaiotaomicron,* or *B. vulgatus*)
The following *in vitro* data are available; **but their clinical significance is unknown.**
Piperacillin/tazobactam exhibits *in vitro* minimum inhibitory concentrations (MICs) of 16.0 μg/mL or less against most (≥90%) strains of *Enterobacteriaceae*, MICs of 1.0 μg/mL or less against most (≥90%) strains of *Haemophilus* species, MICs of 8.0 μg/mL or less against most (≥90%) strains of *Staphylococcus* species, and MICs of 16.0 μg/mL or less against most (≥90%) strains of *Bacteroides* species. Beta-lactamase negative strains should be tested against piperacillin alone; piperacillin break points should be used in evaluation of these results. However, the safey and efficacy of piperacillin/tazobactam in treating clinical infections due to these microorganisms have not been established in adequate and well-controlled clinical trials.
Gram-positive aerobes:
Enterococcus faecalis (piperacillin susceptible)
Staphylococcus epidermidis (NOT methicillin/oxacillin-resistant strains)
Streptococcus agalactiae†
Streptococcus pneumoniae†
Streptococcus pyogenes†
Viridans group streptococci†
Gram-negative aerobes:
Klebsiella oxytoca
Klebsiella pneumoniae
Moraxella catarrhalis
Morganella morganii
Neisseria gonorrhoeae
Neisseria meningitidis†
Proteus mirabilis
Proteus vulgaris
Pseudomonas aeruginosa (piperacillin susceptible)
Serratia marcescens
Gram-positive anaerobes:
Clostridium perfringens
Gram-negative anaerobes:
Bacteroides distasonis
Fusobacterium nucleatum
Prevotella melaninogenica (formerly *Bacteroides melaninogenicus*)
†These are not β-lactamase producing strains and, therefore, are susceptible to piperacillin alone.

Susceptibility Tests

Dilution Techniques

Quantitative methods are used to determine minimum inhibitory concentrations (MICs). These MICs provide estimates of the susceptibility of bacteria to antimicrobial compounds. The MICs should be determined using a standardized procedure. Standardized procedures are based on a dilution method (broth or agar) or equivalent with standardized inoculum concentrations and standardized concentrations of piperacillin and tazobactam powders.[1] MIC values should be determined using serial dilutions of piperacillin combined with a fixed concentration of 4 μg/mL tazobactam. The MIC values obtained should be interpreted according to the following criteria:

For *Enterobacteriaceae*:

MIC (μg/mL)	Interpretation
≤16	Susceptible (S)
32–64	Intermediate (I)
≥128	Resistant (R)

For *Haemophilus* species:

MIC (μg/mL)	Interpretation
≤1	Susceptible (S)
≥2	Resistant (R)

For *Staphylococcus* species:

MIC (μg/mL)	Interpretation
≤8	Susceptible (S)
≥16	Resistant (R)

A report of "Susceptible" indicates that the pathogen is likely to be inhibited if the antimicrobial compound in the blood reaches the concentrations usually achievable. A report of "Intermediate" indicates that the result should be considered equivocal, and, if the microorganism is not fully

TABLE 1
STEADY STATE MEAN PLASMA CONCENTRATIONS IN ADULTS AFTER 30-MINUTE INTRAVENOUS INFUSION OF PIPERACILLIN/TAZOBACTAM EVERY 6 HOURS
PIPERACILLIN

Piperacillin/ Tazobactam Dose[a]	No. of Evaluable Subjects	Plasma Concentrations** (μg/mL)						AUC[a] (μg·hr/mL)
		30 min	1 hr	2 hr	3 hr	4 hr	6 hr	AUC$_{0-6}$
2.25 g	8	134 (14)	57 (14)	17.1 (23)	5.2 (32)	2.5 (35)	0.9 (14)[b]	131 (14)
3.375 g	6	242 (12)	106 (8)	34.6 (20)	11.5 (19)	5.1 (22)	1.0 (10)	242 (10)
4.5 g	8	298 (14)	141 (19)	46.6 (28)	16.4 (29)	6.9 (29)	1.4 (30)	322 (16)

TAZOBACTAM

Piperacillin/ Tazobactam Dose[a]	No. of Evaluable Subjects	Plasma Concentrations** (mcg/mL)						AUC** (mcg·hr/mL)
		30 min	1 hr	2 hr	3 hr	4 hr	6 hr	AUC$_{0-6}$
2.25 g	8	14.8 (14)	7.2 (22)	2.6 (30)	1.1 (35)	0.7 (6)[c]	<0.5	16.0 (21)
3.375 g	6	24.2 (14)	10.7 (7)	4.0 (18)	1.4 (21)	0.7 (16)[b]	<0.5	25.0 (8)
4.5 g	8	33.8 (12)	17.3 (16)	6.8 (24)	2.8 (25)	1.3 (30)	<0.5	39.8 (15)

** Numbers in parentheses are coefficients of variation (CV%).
a: Piperacillin and tazobactam were given in combination.
b: N = 4
c: N = 3

susceptible to alternative, clinically feasible drugs, the test should be repeated. This category implies possible clinical applicability in body sites where the drug is physiologically concentrated or in situations where high dosage of drug can be used. This category also provides a buffer zone which prevents small uncontrolled technical factors from causing major discrepancies in interpretation. A report of "Resistant" indicates that the pathogen is not likely to be inhibited if the antimicrobial compound in the blood reaches the concentrations usually achievable; other therapy should be selected.

Standardized susceptibility test procedures require the use of laboratory control microorganisms to control the technical aspects of the laboratory procedures.

Laboratory control microorganisms are specific strains of microbiological assay organisms with intrinsic biological properties relating to resistance mechanisms and their genetic expression within bacteria; the specific strains are not clinically significant in their current microbiological status. Standard piperacillin and tazobactam powders should provide the following MIC values when tested against the designated quality control strains:

Microorganism	MIC (µg/mL)
Escherichia coli ATCC 25922	1–4
Escherichia coli ATCC 35218	0.5–2
Haemophilus influenzae ATCC 49247	0.06–0.5
Staphylococcus aureus ATCC 29213	0.25–2

Anaerobic Techniques

For anaerobic bacteria, the susceptibility to piperacillin/tazobactam can be determined by the reference agar dilution method or by alternate standardized test methods.[2]

For Bacteroides species, the dilution values should be interpreted as follows:

MIC (µg/mL)	Interpretation
≤16	Susceptible (S)
≥32	Resistant (R)

Serial dilutions of piperacillin combined with a fixed concentration of 4 µg/mL tazobactam should provide the following MIC values:

Microorganism	MIC (µg/mL)
Bacteroides fragilis ATCC 25285	0.12–0.5
Bacteroides thetaiotaomicron ATCC 29741	4–16

Diffusion Techniques

Quantitative methods that require measurement of zone diameters also provide reproducible estimates of the susceptibility of bacteria to antimicrobial compounds. One such standardized procedure requires the use of standardized inoculum concentrations.[3] This procedure uses paper disks impregnated with 100 µg of piperacillin and 10 µg of tazobactam to test the susceptibility of microorganisms to piperacillin/tazobactam. Interpretation is identical to that stated above for results using dilution techniques.

Reports from the laboratory providing results of the standard single-disk-susceptibility test with a 100/10-µg piperacillin/tazobactam disk should be interpreted according to the following criteria:

For Enterobacteriaceae:

Zone Diameter (mm)	Interpretation
≥21	Susceptible (S)
18–20	Intermediate (I)
≤17	Resistant (R)

For Staphylococcus species:

Zone Diameter (mm)	Interpretation
≥20	Susceptible (S)
≤19	Resistant (R)

As with standardized dilution techniques, diffusion methods require the use of laboratory control microorganisms to control the technical aspects of the laboratory procedures. Laboratory control microorganisms are specific strains of microbiological assay organisms with intrinsic biological properties relating to resistance mechanisms and their genetic expression within bacteria; the specific strains are not clinically significant in their current microbiological status. For the diffusion technique, the 100/10-µg piperacillin/tazobactam disk should provide the following zone diameters in these laboratory test quality control strains:

Microorganism	Zone Diameter (mm)
Escherichia coli ATCC 25922	24–30
Escherichia coli ATCC 35218	24–30
Staphylococcus aureus ATCC 25923	27–36

INDICATIONS AND USAGE

Zosyn is indicated for the treatment of patients with moderate to severe infections caused by piperacillin-resistant, piperacillin/tazobactam-susceptible, β-lactamase producing strains of the designated microorganisms in the specified conditions listed below:

Appendicitis (complicated by rupture or abscess) and peritonitis caused by piperacillin-resistant, β-lactamase producing strains of Escherichia coli or the following members of the Bacteroides fragilis group: B. fragilis, B. ovatus, B. thetaiotamicron, or B. vulgatus. The individual members of this group were studied in less than 10 cases.

Uncomplicated and complicated skin and skin structure infections, including cellulitis, cutaneous abscesses and ischemic/diabetic foot infections caused by piperacillin-resistant, β-lactamase producing strains of Staphylococcus aureus.

Postpartum endometritis or pelvic inflammatory disease caused by piperacillin-resistant, β-lactamase producing strains of Escherichia coli.

Community-acquired pneumonia (moderate severity only) caused by piperacillin-resistant, β-lactamase producing strains of Haemophilius influenzae.

Nosocomial pneumonia (moderate to severe) caused by piperacillin-resistant, β-lactamase producing strains of Staphylococcus aureus.

Initial presumptive treatment of patients with nosocomial pneumonia should start with Zosyn at a dosage of 3.375 g every 4 hours plus an aminoglycoside. Treatment with the aminoglycoside should be continued in patients from whom Pseudomonas aeruginosa is isolated. If Pseudomonas aeruginosa is not isolated, the aminoglycoside may be discontinued at the discretion of the treating physician. (See **Dosage and Administration**.)

A study for the treatment of nosocomial lower respiratory tract infection was initiated with Zosyn as monotherapy at 3.375 g every 6 hours. This study was terminated because of an unacceptable level of efficacy at this dosage. However, another multicenter study conducted in North America, used Zosyn at a dosing regimen of 3.375 g every 4 hours in combination with an aminoglycoside in the treatment of patients with nosocomial lower respiratory tract infections. In this study, Zosyn (in combination with varying durations of aminoglycoside therapy) demonstrated acceptable rates of overall clinical and microbiologic success in the treatment of nosocomial pneumonia. There was an insufficient number of nosocomial bronchitis cases to prove efficacy in this condition.

Clinical trial data for the treatment of complicated urinary tract infections demonstrated inadequate efficacy at the dosage regimen of Zosyn studied (i.e., 3.375 g every 8 hours). There are no other adequate and well-controlled trial data to support the use of this product in the treatment of complicated urinary tract infections.

As a combination product, Zosyn is indicated only for the specified conditions listed above. Infections caused by piperacillin-susceptible organisms, for which piperacillin has been shown to be effective, are also amenable to Zosyn treatment due to its piperacillin content. The tazobactam component of this combination product does not decrease the activity of the piperacillin component against piperacillin-susceptible organisms. Therefore, the treatment of mixed infections caused by piperacillin-susceptible organisms and piperacillin-resistant, β-lactamase producing organisms susceptible to Zosyn should not require the addition of another antibiotic. An exception is in the treatment of Pseudomonas aeruginosa in nosocomial pneumonia which should be in combination with an aminoglycoside.

Zosyn is useful as presumptive therapy in the indicated conditions prior to the identification of causative organisms because of its broad spectrum of bactericidal activity against gram-positive and gram-negative aerobic and anaerobic organisms.

Appropriate cultures should usually be performed before initiating antimicrobial treatment in order to isolate and identify the organisms causing infection and to determine their susceptibility to Zosyn. Antimicrobial therapy should be adjusted, if appropriate, once the results of culture(s) and antimicrobial testing are known.

CONTRAINDICATIONS

Zosyn is contraindicated in patients with a history of allergic reactions to any of the penicillins, cephalosporins, or β-lactamase inhibitors.

WARNINGS

SERIOUS AND OCCASIONALLY FATAL HYPERSENSITIVITY (ANAPHYLACTIC) REACTIONS HAVE BEEN REPORTED IN PATIENTS ON PENICILLIN THERAPY. THESE REACTIONS ARE MORE LIKELY TO OCCUR IN INDIVIDUALS WITH A HISTORY OF PENICILLIN HYPERSENSITIVITY OR A HISTORY OF SENSITIVITY TO MULTIPLE ALLERGENS. THERE HAVE BEEN REPORTS OF INDIVIDUALS WITH A HISTORY OF PENICILLIN HYPERSENSITIVITY WHO HAVE EXPERIENCED SEVERE REACTIONS WHEN TREATED WITH CEPHALOSPORINS. BEFORE INITIATING THERAPY WITH ZOSYN, CAREFUL INQUIRY SHOULD BE MADE CONCERNING PREVIOUS HYPERSENSITIVITY REACTIONS TO PENICILLINS, CEPHALOSPORINS, OR OTHER ALLERGENS. IF AN ALLERGIC REACTION OCCURS, ZOSYN SHOULD BE DISCONTINUED AND APPROPRIATE THERAPY INSTITUTED. SERIOUS ANAPHYLACTIC REACTIONS REQUIRE IMMEDIATE EMERGENCY TREATMENT WITH EPINEPHRINE. OXYGEN, INTRAVENOUS STEROIDS AND AIRWAY MANAGEMENT, INCLUDING INTUBATION, SHOULD ALSO BE ADMINISTERED AS INDICATED.

Pseudomembranous colitis has been reported with nearly all antibacterial agents, including piperacillin/tazobactam, and may range in severity from mild to life-threatening. Therefore, it is important to consider this diagnosis in patients who present with diarrhea subsequent to the administration of antibacterial agents.

Treatment with antibacterial agents alters the normal flora of the colon and may permit overgrowth of clostridia. Studies indicate that a toxin produced by Clostridium difficile is one primary cause of "antibiotic-associated colitis."

After the diagnosis of pseudomembranous colitis has been established, therapeutic measures should be initiated. Mild cases of pseudomembranous colitis usually respond to drug discontinuation alone. In moderate to severe cases, consideration should be given to management with fluids and electrolytes, protein supplementation, and treatment with an antibacterial drug clinically effective against Clostridium difficile colitis.

PRECAUTIONS

General

Bleeding manifestations have occurred in some patients receiving β-lactam antibiotics, including piperacillin. These reactions have sometimes been associated with abnormalities of coagulation tests such as clotting time, platelet aggregation, and prothrombin time, and are more likely to occur in patients with renal failure. If bleeding manifestations occur, Zosyn should be discontinued and appropriate therapy instituted.

The possibility of the emergence of resistant organisms that might cause superinfections should be kept in mind. If this occurs, appropriate measures should be taken.

As with other penicillins, patients may experience neuromuscular excitability or convulsions if higher than recommended doses are given intravenously (particularly in the presence of renal failure).

Zosyn is a monosodium salt of piperacillin and a monosodium salt of tazobactam and contains a total of 2.35 mEq (54 mg) of Na⁺ per gram of piperacillin in the combination product. This should be considered when treating patients requiring restricted salt intake. Periodic electrolyte determinations should be performed in patients with low potassium reserves, and the possibility of hypokalemia should be kept in mind with patients who have potentially low potassium reserves and who are receiving cytotoxic therapy or diuretics.

As with other semisynthetic penicillins, piperacillin therapy has been associated with an increased incidence of fever and rash in cystic fibrosis patients.

Laboratory Tests

Periodic assessment of hematopoietic function should be performed, especially with prolonged therapy, i.e., ≥21 days. (See **Adverse Reactions—Adverse Laboratory Events**.)

Drug Interactions

Aminoglycosides

The mixing of Zosyn with an aminoglycoside in vitro can result in substantial inactivation of the aminoglycoside. (See **Dosage and Administration**—COMPATIBLE INTRAVENOUS DILUENT SOLUTIONS.)

When Zosyn is co-administered with tobramycin, the area under the curve, renal clearance, and urinary recovery of tobramycin were decreased by 11%, 32% and 38%, respectively. The alterations in the pharmacokinetics of tobramycin when administered in combination with piperacillin/tazobactam may be due to in vivo and in vitro inactivation of tobramycin in the presence of piperacillin/tazobactam. The inactivation of aminoglycosides in the presence of penicillin-class drugs has been recognized. It has been postulated that penicillin-aminoglycoside complexes form; these complexes are microbiologically inactive and of unknown toxicity. In patients with severe renal dysfunction (i.e., chronic hemodialysis patients), the pharmacokinetics of tobramycin are significantly altered when tobramycin is administered in combination with piperacillin.[4] The alteration of tobramycin pharmacokinetics and the potential toxicity of the penicillin-aminoglycoside complexes in patients with mild to moderate renal dysfunction who are administered an aminoglycoside in combination with piperacillin/tazobactam is unknown.

Probenecid

Probenecid administered concomitantly with Zosyn prolongs the half-life of piperacillin by 21% and that of tazobactam by 71%.

Continued on next page

Zosyn—Cont.

Vancomycin
No pharmacokinetic interactions have been noted between Zosyn and vancomycin.
Heparin
Coagulation parameters should be tested more frequently and monitored regularly during simultaneous administration of high doses of heparin, oral anticoagulants, or other drugs that may affect the blood coagulation system or the thrombocyte function.
Vecuronium
Piperacillin when used concomitantly with vecuronium has been implicated in the prolongation of the neuromuscular blockade of vecuronium. Zosyn (piperacillin/tazobactam) could produce the same phenomenon if given along with vecuronium. Due to their similar mechanism of action, it is expected that the neuromuscular blockade produced by any of the non-depolarizing muscle relaxants could be prolonged in the presence of piperacillin. (See package insert for vecuronium bromide.)

Drug/Laboratory Test Interactions
As with other penicillins, the administration of Zosyn may result in a false-positive reaction for glucose in the urine using a copper-reduction method (CLINITEST®). It is recommended that glucose tests based on enzymatic glucose oxidase reactions (such as DIASTIX® or TES-TAPE®) be used.

Carcinogenesis, Mutagenesis, Impairment of Fertility
Long term carcinogenicity studies in animals have not been conducted with piperacillin/tazobactam, piperacillin, or tazobactam.
Piperacillin/tazobactam was negative in microbial mutagenicity assays at concentrations up to 14.84/1.86 µg/plate. Piperacillin/tazobactam was negative in the unscheduled DNA synthesis (UDS) test at concentrations up to 5689/711 µg/mL. Piperacillin/tazobactam was negative in a mammalian point mutation (Chinese hamster ovary cell HPRT) assay at concentrations up to 8000/1000 µg/mL. Piperacillin/tazobactam was negative in a mammalian cell (BALB/c-3T3) transformation assay at concentrations up to 8/1 µg/mL. *In vivo,* piperacillin/tazobactam did not induce chromosomal aberrations in rats dosed I.V. with 1500/187.5 mg/kg; this dose is similar to the maximum recommended human daily dose on a body-surface-area basis (mg/m^2).
Piperacillin was negative in microbial mutagenicity assays at concentrations up to 50 µg/plate. There was no DNA damage in bacteria (Rec assay) exposed to piperacillin at concentrations up to 200 µg/disk. Piperacillin was negative in the UDS test at concentrations up to 10,000 µg/mL.
In a mammalian point mutation (mouse lymphoma cells) assay, piperacillin was positive at concentrations ≥2500 µg/mL. Piperacillin was negative in a cell (BALB/c-3T3) transformation assay at concentrations up to 3000 µg/mL. *In vivo,* piperacillin did not induce chromosomal aberrations in mice at I.V. doses up to 2000 mg/kg/day or rats at I.V. doses up to 1500 mg/kg/day. These doses are half (mice) or similar (rats) to the maximum recommended human daily dose based on body-surface area (mg/m^2). In another *in vivo* test, there was no dominant lethal effect when piperacillin was administered to rats at I.V. doses up to 2000 mg/kg/day, which is similar to the maximum recommended human daily dose based on body-surface area (mg/m^2). When mice were administered piperacillin at I.V. doses up to 2000 mg/kg/day, which is half the maximum recommended human daily dose based on body-surface area (mg/m^2), urine from these animals was not mutagenic when tested in a microbial mutagenicity assay. Bacteria injected into the peritoneal cavity of mice administered piperacillin at I.V. doses up to 2000 mg/kg/day did not show increased mutation frequencies.
Tazobactam was negative in microbial mutagenicity assays at concentrations up to 333 µg/plate. Tazobactam was negative in the UDS test at concentrations up to 2000 µg/mL. Tazobactam was negative in a mammalian point mutation (Chinese hamster ovary cell HPRT) assay at concentrations up to 5000 µg/mL. In another mammalian point mutation (mouse lymphoma cells) assay, tazobactam was positive at concentrations ≥3000 µg/mL. Tazobactam was negative in a cell (BALB/c-3T3) transformation assay at concentrations up to 900 µg/mL. In an *in vitro* cytogenetics (Chinese hamster lung cells) assay, tazobactam was negative at concentrations up to 3000 µg/mL. *In vivo,* tazobactam did not induce chromosomal aberrations in rats at I.V. doses up to 5000 mg/kg, which is 23 times the maximum recommended human daily dose based on body-surface area (mg/m^2).

Pregnancy
Teratogenic effects—Pregnancy Category B
Piperacillin/tazobactam
Reproduction studies have been performed in rats and have revealed no evidence of impaired fertility due to piperacillin/tazobactam administered up to a dose which is similar to the maximum recommended human daily dose based on body-surface area (mg/m^2).
Teratology studies have been performed in mice and rats and have revealed no evidence of harm to the fetus due to piperacillin/tazobactam administered up to a dose which is 1 to 2 times and 2 to 3 times the human dose of piperacillin and tazobactam, respectively, based on body-surface area (mg/m^2).
Piperacillin
Reproduction and teratology studies have been performed in mice and rats and have revealed no evidence of impaired fertility or harm to the fetus due to piperacillin administered up to a dose which is half (mice) or similar (rats) to the maximum recommended human daily dose based on body-surface area (mg/m^2).
Tazobactam
Reproduction studies have been performed in rats and have revealed no evidence of impaired fertility due to tazobactam administered at doses up to 3 times the maximum recommended human daily dose based on body-surface area (mg/m^2).
Teratology studies have been performed in mice and rats and have revealed no evidence of harm to the fetus due to tazobactam administered at doses up to 6 and 14 times, respectively, the human dose based on body-surface area (mg/m^2). In rats, tazobactam crosses the placenta. Concentrations in the fetus are less than or equal to 10% of those found in maternal plasma.
There are, however, no adequate and well-controlled studies with the piperacillin/tazobactam combination or with piperacillin or tazobactam alone in pregnant women. Because animal reproduction studies are not always predictive of the human response, this drug should be used during pregnancy only if clearly needed.

Nursing Mothers
Piperacillin is excreted in low concentrations in human milk; tazobactam concentrations in human milk have not been studied. Caution should be exercised when Zosyn is administered to a nursing woman.

Pediatric Use
Safety and efficacy in pediatric patients have not been established.

Geriatric Use
Patients over 65 years are **not** at an increased risk of developing adverse effects solely because of age. However, dosage should be adjusted in the presence of renal insufficiency. (See **Dosage and Administration.**)

ADVERSE REACTIONS

During the initial clinical investigations, 2621 patients worldwide were treated with Zosyn in phase 3 trials. In the key North American clinical trials (n=830 patients), 90% of the adverse events reported were mild to moderate in severity and transient in nature. However, in 3.2% of the patients treated worldwide, Zosyn was discontinued because of adverse events primarily involving the skin (1.3%), including rash and pruritis; the gastrointestinal system (0.9%), including diarrhea, nausea, and vomiting; and allergic reactions (0.5%).
Adverse local reactions that were reported, irrespective of relationship to therapy with Zosyn, were phlebitis (1.3%), injection site reaction (0.5%), pain (0.2%), inflammation (0.2%), thrombophlebitis (0.2%), and edema (0.1%).
In the completed study of nosocomial lower respiratory tract infections, 155 patients were treated with Zosyn in a dosing regimen of 3.375 g every 4 hours in combination with an aminoglycoside. In this trial, 88.5% of the adverse experiences reported were mild to moderate in severity and transient in nature. However, in this trial, therapy with Zosyn was discontinued in four patients (2.6%) due to adverse experiences.
Irrespective of drug relationship or degree of severity, the adverse experiences which led to the discontinuation of Zosyn in these four patients were: thrombocytopenia and pancreatitis in one patient; fever in one patient; fever and eosinophilia in another patient; and diarrhea and elevated liver enzymes in the fourth patient.

Adverse Clinical Events
Based on patients from the North American trials (n=1063), the events with the highest incidence in patients, irrespective of relationship to Zosyn therapy, were diarrhea (11.3%); headache (7.7%); constipation (7.7%); nausea (6.9%); insomnia (6.6%); rash (4.2%), including maculopapular, bullous, urticarial, and eczematoid; vomiting (3.3%); dyspepsia (3.3%); pruritis (3.1%); stool changes (2.4%); fever (2.4%); agitation (2.1%); pain (1.7%); moniliasis (1.6%); hypertension (1.6%); dizziness (1.4%); abdominal pain (1.3%); chest pain (1.3%); edema (1.2%); anxiety (1.2%); rhinitis (1.2%); and dyspnea (1.1%).
Based on patients in the completed study of nosocomial lower respiratory tract infections (n=155), using every 4 hour dosing and aminoglycoside therapy, the events with the highest incidence in patients, irrespective of relationship to Zosyn and aminoglycoside therapy were: diarrhea (20%); constipation (8.4%); agitation (7.1%); nausea (5.8%); headache (4.5%); insomnia (4.5%); oral thrush (3.9%); erythematous rash (3.9%); anxiety (3.2%); fever (3.2%); pain (3.2%); pruritis (3.2%); hiccough (2.6%); vomiting (2.6%); dyspepsia (1.9%); edema (1.9%); fluid overload (1.9%); stool changes (1.9%); anorexia (1.3%); cardiac arrest (1.3%); confusion (1.3%); diaphoresis (1.3%); duodenal ulcer (1.3%); flatulence (1.3%); hypertension (1.3%); hypotension (1.3%); inflammation at injection site (1.3%); pleural effusion (1.3%); pneumothorax (1.3%); rash, not otherwise specified (1.3%); supraventricular tachycardia (1.3%); thrombophlebitis (1.3%); and urinary incontinence (1.3%).
Additional adverse systemic clinical events reported in 1.0% or less of the patients in the initial North American trials and/or in the patients administered Zosyn 3.375 g every 4 hours plus an aminoglycoside in the study of nosocomial lower respiratory tract are listed below within each body system (bracketed events occurred only in the nosocomial pneumonia trial);
Autonomic nervous system—hypotension, ileus, syncope
Body as a whole—rigors, back pain, malaise, [asthenia, chest pain]
Cardiovascular—tachycardia, including supraventricular and ventricular; bradycardia; arrhythmia, including atrial fibrillation, ventricular fibrillation, cardiac arrest, cardiac failure, circulatory failure, myocardial infarction, [angina]
Central nervous system—tremor, convulsions, vertigo, [aggressive reaction (combative)]
Gastrointestinal—melena, flatulence, hemorrhage, gastritis, hiccough, ulcerative stomatitis, [fecal incontinence, gastric ulcer, pancreatitis]
Pseudomembranous colitis was reported in one patient during the clinical trials. The onset of pseudomembranous colitis symptoms may occur during or after antibacterial treatment. (See **Warnings.**)
Hearing and Vestibular System—tinnitus, [deafness, earache]
Hypersensitivity—anaphylaxis
Metabolic and Nutritional—symptomatic hypoglycemia, thirst, [gout, vitamin B_{12} deficiency anemia]
Musculoskeletal—myalgia, arthralgia
Platelet, Bleeding, Clotting—mesenteric embolism, purpura, epistaxis, pulmonary embolism, [ecchymosis, hemoptysis] (See **Precautions—General.**)
Psychiatric—confusion, hallucination, depression
Reproductive, Female—leukorrhea, vaginitis, [perineal irritation/pain]
Reproductive, Male—[balanoposthitis]
Respiratory—pharyngitis, pulmonary edema, bronchospasm, coughing, [atelectasis, dyspnea, hypoxia]
Skin and Appendages—genital pruritus, diaphoresis, [conjunctivitis, xerosis]
Special senses—taste perversion
Urinary—retention, dysuria, oliguria, hematuria, incontinence, [urinary tract infection with trichomonas, yeast in urine]
Vision—photophobia
Vascular (extracardiac)—flushing, [cerebrovascular accident]
Additional adverse events reported from worldwide marketing experience with Zosyn, occurring under circumstances where causal relationship to Zosyn is uncertain:
Renal—rarely, interstitial nephritis

Adverse Laboratory Events (Seen During Clinical Trials)
Of the studies reported, including that of nosocomial lower respiratory tract infections in which a higher dose of Zosyn was used in combination with an aminoglycoside, changes in laboratory parameters, without regard to drug relationship include:
Hematologic—decreases in hemoglobin and hematocrit, thrombocytopenia, increases in platelet count, eosinophilia, leukopenia, neutropenia. The leukopenia/neutropenia associated with Zosyn administration appears to be reversible and most frequently associated with prolonged administration, i.e., ≥21 days of therapy. These patients were withdrawn from therapy; some had accompanying systemic symptoms (e.g., fever, rigors, chills).
Coagulation—positive direct Coombs' test, prolonged prothrombin time, prolonged partial thromboplastin time
Hepatic—transient elevations of AST (SGOT), ALT (SGPT), alkaline phosphatase, bilirubin
Renal—increases in serum creatinine, blood urea nitrogen
Urinalysis—proteinuria, hematuria, pyuria
Additional laboratory events include abnormalities in electrolytes (i.e., increases and decreases in sodium, potassium, and calcium), hyperglycemia, decreases in total protein or albumin.
The following adverse reactions have also been reported for PIPRACIL® (sterile piperacillin sodium):
Skin and Appendages—Erythema multiforme and Stevens-Johnson syndrome, rarely reported
Gastrointestinal—Cholestatic hepatitis
Skeletal—Prolonged muscle relaxation (See **Precautions—Drug Interactions.**)

OVERDOSAGE

Information on overdosage of Zosyn in humans is not available.
Excessive serum levels of either piperacillin or tazobactam may be reduced by hemodialysis. (See **Clinical Pharma-**

cology.) No specific antidote is known. As with other penicillins, neuromuscular excitability or convulsions have occurred following large intravenous doses, primarily in patients with impaired renal function.

In the case of motor excitability or convulsions, general supportive measures, including administration of anticonvulsive agents (e.g., diazepam or barbiturates) may be considered.

DOSAGE AND ADMINISTRATION

Zosyn should be administered by intravenous infusion over 30 minutes

Normal Renal Function (Creatinine Clearance ≥90 mL/min)
The usual total dose of Zosyn for adults is 12 g/1.5 g, given 3.375 g every six hours.

Treatment of patients with nosocomial pneumonia should start with Zosyn at a dosage of 3.375 g every four hours **plus** an aminoglycoside. This gives a total dose of piperacillin/tazobactam of 18 g/2.25 g in twenty-four hours. Treatment with the aminoglycoside should be continued in patients from whom *Pseudomonas aeruginosa* is isolated. If *Pseudomonas aeruginosa* is not isolated, the aminoglycoside may be discontinued at the discretion of the treating physician as guided by the severity of the infection and the patient's clinical and bacteriological progress.

Renal Insufficiency
In patients with renal insufficiency (Creatinine Clearance <90 mL/min), the intravenous dose of Zosyn should be adjusted to the degree of actual renal function impairment. In patients with nosocomial pneumonia receiving concomitant aminoglycoside therapy, the aminoglycoside dosage should be adjusted according to the recommendations of the manufacturer. The recommended daily doses of Zosyn® for patients with renal insufficiency are as follows:

Zosyn Dosage Recommendations For All Indications
Including Nosocomial Pneumonia

Creatinine Clearance (mL/min)	Recommended Dosage Regimen
>40–90	12 g/1.5 g/day in divided doses of 3.375 g q 6 h
20–40	8 g/1.0 g/day in divided doses of 2.25 g q 6 h
<20	6 g/0.75 g/day in divided doses of 2.25 g q 6 h

For patients on hemodialysis, irrespective of the condition under treatment, the maximum dose is 2.25 g Zosyn q eight hours. In addition, because hemodialysis removes 30% to 40% of a Zosyn dose in four hours, one additional dose of 0.75 g Zosyn should be administered following each dialysis period. For patients with renal failure, measurement of serum levels of piperacillin and tazobactam will provide additional guidance for adjusting dosage.

Duration of Therapy
The usual duration of Zosyn treatment is from seven to ten days. However, the recommended duration of Zosyn treatment of nosocomial pneumonia is seven to fourteen days. In all conditions, the duration of therapy should be guided by the severity of the infection and the patient's clinical and bacteriological progress.

Intravenous Administration
For conventional vials, reconstitute Zosyn per gram of piperacillin with 5 mL of a compatible reconstitution diluent from the list provided below. Shake well until dissolved. Single dose vials should be used immediately after reconstitution. Discard any unused portion after 24 hours if stored at room temperature, or after 48 hours if stored at refrigerated temperature (2° to 8°C [36° to 46°F]).

Compatible Reconstitution Diluents
0.9% Sodium Chloride for Injection
Sterile Water for Injection
Dextrose 5%
Bacteriostatic Saline/Parabens
Bacteriostatic Water/Parabens
Bacteriostatic Saline/Benzyl Alcohol
Bacteriostatic Water/Benzyl Alcohol
Reconstituted Zosyn solution should be further diluted (recommended volume per dose of 50 mL to 150 mL) in a compatible intravenous diluent solution listed below.
Administer by infusion over a period of at least 30 minutes. During the infusion it is desirable to discontinue the primary infusion solution.

Compatible Intravenous Diluent Solutions
0.9% Sodium Chloride for Injection
Sterile Water for Injection‡
Dextrose 5%
Dextran 6% in Saline
‡ Maximum recommended volume per dose of Sterile Water for Injection is 50 mL.

Add-Vantage® System Admixtures
Dextrose 5% in Water (50 or 100 mL)
0.9% Sodium Chloride (50 or 100 mL)

For ADD-VANTAGE® vials reconstitution directions, see *INSTRUCTIONS FOR USE* sheet provided in the box.

LACTATED RINGERS SOLUTION IS NOT COMPATIBLE WITH ZOSYN.

When concomitant therapy with aminoglycosides is indicated, Zosyn and the aminoglycoside should be reconstituted and administered separately, due to the *in vitro* inactivation of the aminoglycoside by the penicillin. (See Precautions–DRUG INTERACTIONS.)

Zosyn can be used in ambulatory intravenous infusion pumps.

Stability Of Zosyn Following Reconstitution
Zosyn is stable in glass and plastic containers (plastic syringes, I.V. bags, and tubing) when used with compatible diluents.

Stability studies in the I.V. bags have demonstrated chemical stability (potency, pH of reconstituted solution, and clarity of solution) for up to 24 hours at room temperature and up to one week at refrigerated temperature. Zosyn contains no preservatives. Appropriate consideration of aseptic technique should be used.

Stability of Zosyn in an ambulatory intravenous infusion pump has been demonstrated for a period of 12 hours at room temperature. Each dose was reconstituted and diluted to a volume of 37.5 mL or 25 mL. One-day supplies of dosing solution were aseptically transferred into the medication reservoir (I.V. bags or cartridge). The reservoir was fitted to a preprogrammed ambulatory intravenous infusion pump per the manufacturer's instructions. Stability of Zosyn is not affected when administered using an ambulatory intravenous infusion pump.

Stability studies with the ad-mixed ADD-Vantage® system have demonstrated chemical stability (potency, pH and clarity) through 24 hours at room temperature. (Note: The ad-mixed ADD-Vantage® should not be refrigerated or frozen after reconstitution.)

Parenteral drug products should be inspected visually for particulate matter and discoloration prior to administration, whenever solution and container permit.

HOW SUPPLIED

Zosyn® (sterile piperacillin sodium and tazobactam sodium) is supplied in the following sizes:

Each Zosyn 2.25 g vial provides piperacillin sodium equivalent to 2 grams of piperacillin and tazobactam sodium equivalent to 0.25 gram of tazobactam. Each vial contains 4.69 mEq (108 mg) of sodium.

Supplied 10 per box–NDC 0206-8452-16

Each Zosyn 3.375 g vial provides piperacillin sodium equivalent to 3 grams of piperacillin and tazobactam sodium equivalent to 0.375 gram of tazobactam. Each vial contains 7.04 mEq (162 mg) of sodium.

Supplied 10 per box–NDC 0206-8454-55

Each Zosyn 4.5 g vial provides piperacillin sodium equivalent to 4 grams of piperacillin and tazobactam sodium equivalent to 0.5 gram of tazobactam. Each vial contains 9.39 mEq (216 mg) of sodium.

Supplied 10 per box–NDC 0206-8455-25

Each Zosyn 2.25 g ADD-Vantage® vial provides piperacillin sodium equivalent to 2 grams of piperacillin and tazobactam sodium equivalent to 0.25 grams of tazobactam. Each ADD-VANTAGE® vial contains 4.69 mEq (108 mg) of sodium.

Supplied 10 per box—NDC 0206-8452-17

Each Zosyn 3.375 g ADD-Vantage® vial provides piperacillin sodium equivalent to 3 grams of piperacillin and tazobactam sodium equivalent to 0.375 grams of tazobactam. Each ADD-Vantage® vial contains 7.04 mEq (162 mg) of sodium.

Supplied 10 per box—NDC 0206-8454-17

Each Zosyn 4.5 g ADD-Vantage® vial provides piperacillin sodium equivalent to 4 grams of piperacillin and tazobactam sodium equivalent to 0.5 grams of tazobactam. Each ADD-VANTAGE® vial contains 9.39 mEq (216 mg) of sodium.

Supplied 10 per box—NDC 0206-8455-17

Zosyn conventional and ADD-Vantage® vials should be stored at controlled room temperature 15° to 30°C (59° to 86°F) prior to reconstitution.

ALSO AVAILABLE
Zosyn is also supplied as follows:
40.5 g pharmacy bulk vial containing 36 grams of piperacillin and 4.5 grams of tazobactam. Each pharmacy bulk vial contains 84.5 mEq (1,944 mg) of sodium.
NDC 0206-8620-11

Also Available
Zosyn® (piperacillin sodium and tazobactam sodium injection) in Galaxy® Container (PL 2040 Plastic) is supplied as a frozen, iso-osmotic, sterile, nonpyrognic solution in single-dose plastic containers as follows:

2.25 g (2 g piperacillin/0.25 g tazobactam) in 50 mL. Each container has 5.7 mEq (131 mg) of sodium.
Supplied 24/box—NDC 0206-8820-02

3.375 g (3 g piperacillin/0.375 g tazobactam) in 50 mL. Each container has 8.6 mEq (197 mg) of sodium.
Supplied 24/box—NDC 0206-8821-02

4.5 g (4 g piperacillin/0.5 g tazobactam) in 100 mL. Each container has 11.4 mEq (263 mg) of sodium.
Supplied 12/box—NDC 0206-88202-02
Store at or below -20°C (-4°F).

REFERENCES

1. National Committee for Clinical Laboratory Standards, Methods for Dilution Antimicrobial Susceptibility Tests for Bacteria that Grow Aerobically–Third Edition. Approved Standard NCCLS Document M7-A3, Vol. 13, No. 25, NCCLS, Villanova, PA, December, 1993.
2. National Committee for Clinical Laboratory Standards, Methods for Antimicrobial Susceptibility Testing for Anaerobic Bacteria–Third Edition. Approved Standard NCCLS Document M11-A3, Vol. 13, No. 26, NCCLS, Villanova, PA, December, 1993.
3. National Committee for Clinical Laboratory Standards. Performance Standard for Antimicrobial Disk Susceptibility Tests–Fifth Edition. Approved Standard NCCLS Document M2-A5, Vol. 13, No. 24, NCCLS, Villanova, PA, December, 1993.
4. Halstenson CE, Hirata CAI, Heim-Duthoy KL, Abraham PA, and Matzke GR. Effect of concomitant administraton of piperacillin on the dispositions of netilmicin and tobramycin in patients with end-stage renal disease. Antimicrob Agents Chemother 34(1):128-133, 1990.

CLINITEST® and DIASTIX® are registered trademarks of Ames Division, Miles Laboratories, Inc.

TES-TAPE® is a registered trademark of Eli Lilly and Company.

ADD-VANTAGE is a registered trademark of Abbott Laboratories

Manufactured by:
LEDERLE PIPERACILLIN, INC.
Carolina, Puerto Rico 00987

Shown in Product Identification Guide, page 320

ZOSYN®   ℞
(Sterile Piperacillin Sodium and Tazobactam Sodium)

> **Pharmacy Bulk Package**
> **Not for Direct Infusion**

RECONSTITUTED STOCK SOLUTION MUST BE TRANSFERRED AND FURTHER DILUTED FOR I.V. INFUSION

PACKAGE DESCRIPTION

The PHARMACY BULK VIAL is a container of sterile preparation which contains many single doses for parenteral use. The contents are intended for use in a pharmacy admixture program and are restricted to the preparation of admixtures for intravenous infusion.

PRODUCT DESCRIPTION

ZOSYN is an injectable antibacterial combination product consisting of the semisynthetic antibiotic piperacillin sodium and the beta-lactamase inhibitor tazobactam sodium for intravenous administration.

Piperacillin sodium is derived from D(-)-α-aminobenzylpenicillin. The chemical name of piperacillin sodium is sodium (2S, 5R, 6R)-6-[(R)-2-(4-ethyl-2,3-dioxo-1-piperazinecarboxamido) -2- phenylacetamido] -3,3- dimethyl -7- oxo-4-thia-1-azabicyclo[3.2.0]heptane-2-carboxylate. The chemical formula is $C_{23}H_{26}N_5NaO_7S$ and the molecular weight is 539.5.

Tazobactam sodium, a derivative of the penicillin nucleus, is a penicillanic acid sulfone. Its chemical name is sodium (2S, 3S, 5R)-3-methyl-7-oxo-3-(1H-1, 2, 3-triazol-1-ylmethyl)-4-thia-1-azabicyclo[3.2.0]heptane-2-carboxylate-4, 4-dioxide. The chemical formula is $C_{10}H_{11}N_4NaO_5S$ and the molecular weight is 322.3.

ZOSYN, piperacillin/tazobactam parenteral combination, is a white to off-white sterile, cryodesiccated powder consisting of piperacillin and tazobactam as their sodium salts packaged in glass vials. The product does not contain excipients or preservatives.

Each ZOSYN 40.5 g pharmacy bulk vial contains piperacillin sodium equivalent to 36 grams of piperacillin and tazobactam sodium equivalent to 4.5 g of tazobactam sufficient for delivery of multiple doses.

ZOSYN is a monosodium salt of piperacillin and a monosodium salt of tazobactam containing a total of 2.35 mEq (54 mg) of Na⁺ per gram of piperacillin in the combination product.

HOW SUPPLIED

ZOSYN® (sterile piperacillin sodium and tazobactam sodium) is supplied as a powder in the pharmacy bulk vial as follows:

Each ZOSYN 40.5 g pharmacy bulk vial contains piperacillin sodium equivalent to 36 grams of piperacillin and tazo-

Continued on next page

Zosyn Pharmacy Bulk —Cont.

bactam sodium equivalent to 4.5 grams tazobactam. Each pharmacy bulk vial contains 84.5 mEq (1,944 mg) of sodium.

  NDC 0206-8620-11

ZOSYN pharmacy bulk vials should be stored at controlled room temperature 15 to 30°C (59 to 86°F) prior to reconstitution.

For prescribing information write to Professional Service, Wyeth-Ayerst Laboratories, P.O. Box 8299, Philadelphia, PA 19101.

  Shown in Product Identification Guide, page 320

Lederle Standard Products
Pearl River, NY 10965

The following list of Lederle Standard Products includes the alphanumeric LEDERMARK® codes which provide quick and positive identification of Lederle Standard Products capsules and tablets:

Product Identity Code No.	Product
A3	Tetracycline HCl Capsules, 250mg
A5	Tetracycline HCl Capsules, 500mg
A7	Atenolol Tablets, 25mg
A31	Ampicillin Trihydrate Capsules, USP, 250mg
A32	Ampicillin Trihydrate Capsules, USP, 500mg
—	Ampicillin Trihydrate for Oral Suspension, USP, 125mg/5mL
—	Ampicillin Trihydrate for Oral Suspension, USP, 250mg/5mL
A45	Albuterol Sulfate Tablets, 2mg
A46	Albuterol Sulfate Tablets, 4mg
A49	Atenolol Tablets, 50mg
A51	Alprazolam Tablets, USP, 0.25mg
A52	Alprazolam Tablets, USP, 0.5mg
A53	Alprazolam Tablets, USP, 1mg
A54	Alprazolam Tablets, USP, 2mg
A71	Atenolol Tablets, 100mg
C42	Clonidine HCl Tablets, USP, 0.1mg
C43	Clonidine HCl Tablets, USP, 0.2mg
C44	Clonidine HCl Tablets, USP, 0.3mg
C64	Cephalexin Capsules, USP, 250mg
C65	Cephalexin Capsules, USP, 500mg
CB300	Cimetidine Tablets, USP, 300mg
CB400	Cimetidine Tablets, USP, 400mg
CB800	Cimetidine Tablets, USP, 800mg
D44	Dipyridamole Tablets, 25mg
D45	Dipyridamole Tablets, 50mg
D46	Dipyridamole Tablets, 75mg
D51	Diazepam Tablets, USP, 2mg
D52	Diazepam Tablets, USP, 5mg
D53	Diazepam Tablets, USP, 10mg
D71	Diltiazem HCl Tablets, 30mg
D72	Diltiazem HCl Tablets, 60mg
D75	Diltiazem HCl Tablets, 90mg
D77	Diltiazem HCl Tablets, 120mg
—	Erythromycin Ethylsuccinate/Sulfisoxazole Acetyl for Oral Suspension, 200mg/600mg/5mL
—	Sterile Erythromycin Lactobionate for Injection, USP, 500mg/5 x 10mL vials
—	Sterile Erythromycin Lactobionate for Injection, USP, 1g/5 x 20mL vials
—	Folic Acid Injection, USP, 5mg/mL
F22	Fenoprofen Calcium Tablets, USP, 600mg
H11	Hydralazine HCl Tablets, USP, 25mg
H12	Hydralazine HCl Tablets, USP, 50mg
H14	Hydrochlorothiazide Tablets, USP, 25mg
H15	Hydrochlorothiazide Tablets, USP, 50mg
J1	Methazolamide Tablets, USP, 25mg
J2	Methazolamide Tablets, USP, 50mg
K1	Ketoprofen Capsules, 25mg
K2	Ketoprofen Capsules, 50mg
K3	Ketoprofen Capsules, 75mg
M20	Methocarbamol Tablets, USP, 750mg
M22	Methyldopa Tablets, USP, 250mg
M23	Methyldopa Tablets, USP, 500mg
M36	Methyldopa and Hydrochlorothiazide Tablets, USP, 250mg/15mg
M37	Methyldopa and Hydrochlorothiazide Tablets, USP, 250mg/25mg
N11	Naproxen Tablets, USP, 250mg
N17	Naproxen Tablets, USP, 375mg
N77	Naproxen Tablets, USP, 500mg
—	Nystatin Oral Suspension, 100,000 units/mL
—	Nystatin Powder, USP
P33	Propylthiouracil Tablets, USP, 50mg
P36	Pyrazinamide Tablets, 500mg
P69	Prazosin HCl Capsules, USP, 1mg
P70	Prazosin HCl Capsules, USP, 2mg
P71	Prazosin HCl Capsules, USP, 5mg
Q11	Quinidine Sulfate Tablets, USP, 200mg
S16	Sulindac Tablets, USP, 150mg
S17	Sulindac Tablets, USP, 200mg
T13	Tobramycin Sulfate Injection, USP, 40mg/mL
T13	Sulfamethoxazole and Trimethoprim Tablets, USP, 400mg/80mg
T16	Sulfamethoxazole and Trimethoprim Tablets, USP, 800mg/160mg
—	Vancomycin HCl, USP, 500mg vial
—	Vancomycin HCl, USP, 1g vial
—	Vancomycin HCl, USP, 5g vial

  Shown in Product Identification Guide, page 320

Eli Lilly and Company
LILLY CORPORATE CENTER
INDIANAPOLIS, IN 46285

Direct Inquiries to:
Lilly Corporate Center
Indianapolis, IN 46285
(317) 276-2000
For Medical Information Contact:
Lilly Research Laboratories
Lilly Corporate Center
Indianapolis, IN 46285
(800) 545-5979

LEGEND

ADD-Vantage®—*Vials and Diluent Containers, Abbott*
Gelseal®—*Filled Elastic Capsule, Lilly*
Identi-Code®—*Formula Identification Code, Lilly*
Identi-Dose®—*Unit Dose Medication, Lilly*
Pulvule®—*Filled Gelatin Capsule, Lilly*
℞Pak—*Prescription Package, Lilly*
Solvet®—*Soluble Tablet, Lilly*
Traypak®—*Multivial Carton, Lilly*

IDENTI-CODE® Index
(formula identification code, Lilly)
Provides Positive Product Identification

A letter-number symbol, a 4-digit number, the name of the product, the strength of the product, or a combination of these appears on each Lilly capsule and most tablets and on each label of pediatric liquids, and powders for oral suspension. The letter/number or 4-digit number identifies the product.

Identi-Code®	Product Name
Coated Tablets	
C51	**Darvocet-N® 50** Composition (Each Coated Tablet): Propoxyphene napsylate, 50 mg; acetaminophen, 325 mg (USP)
C53	**Darvon-N®** Composition (Each Coated Tablet): Propoxyphene Napsylate, USP, 100 mg
C63	**Darvocet-N® 100** Composition (Each Coated Tablet): Propoxyphene napsylate, 100 mg; acetaminophen, 650 mg (USP)
Pulvules®	
H03	**Darvon®** Composition (Each Pulvule®): Propoxyphene Hydrochloride, USP, 65 mg
H17	**Aventyl® HCl** Composition (Each Pulvule®): Nortriptyline Hydrochloride, USP, 10 mg (equiv. to base)
H19	**Aventyl® HCl** Composition (Each Pulvule®): Nortriptyline Hydrochloride, USP, 25 mg (equiv. to base)
3061	**Ceclor®** Composition (Each Pulvule®): Cefaclor, USP, 250 mg
3062	**Ceclor®** Composition (Each Pulvule®): Cefaclor, USP, 500 mg
3111	**Darvon® Compound-65** Composition (Each Pulvule®): Propoxyphene hydrochloride, 65 mg; aspirin, 389 mg; caffeine, 32.4 mg
3125	**Vancocin® HCl** Composition (Each Pulvule®): Vancomycin hydrochloride, 125 mg
3126	**Vancocin® HCl** Composition (Each Pulvule®): Vancomycin hydrochloride, 250 mg
3144	**Axid®** Composition (Each Pulvule®): Nizatidine, 150 mg
3145	**Axid®** Composition (Each Pulvule®): Nizatidine, 300 mg
3170	**Lorabid®** Composition (Each Pulvule®): Loracarbef, 200 mg
3171	**Lorabid®** Composition (Each Pulvule®): Loracarbef, 400 mg
Compressed Tablets	
T24	**Sodium Chloride** Composition (Each Compressed Tablet): Sodium Chloride, USP, 1 g
T29	**Sodium Bicarbonate** Composition (Each Compressed Tablet): Sodium Bicarbonate, USP, 10 grs (648 mg)
T35	**Calcium Carbonate** Composition (Each Compressed Tablet): Calcium Carbonate, USP, Aromatic, 10 grs (648 mg)
U03	**Dymelor®** Composition (Each Compressed Tablet): Acetohexamide, USP, 250 mg
U07	**Dymelor®** Composition (Each Compressed Tablet): Acetohexamide, USP, 500 mg
4165	**Evista®** Composition (Each Compressed Tablet): Raloxifene Hydrochloride, 60 mg
4112	**Zyprexa®** Composition (Each Compressed Tablet): Olanzapine, USP, 2.5 mg
4115	**Zyprexa®** Composition (Each Compressed Tablet): Olanzapine, USP, 5 mg
4116	**Zyprexa®** Composition (Each Compressed Tablet): Olanzapine, USP, 7.5 mg
4117	**Zyprexa®** Composition (Each Compressed Tablet): Olanzapine, USP, 10 mg

UNIT-DOSE PACKAGING

Identi-Dose® (unit dose medication, Lilly)
Reverse-Numbered Package
Closed-circuit control of medication from pharmacy to nurse to patient and return. Simplifies counting and dispensing whether in single-unit or prescription-size quantities. Fits into any dispensing system for ready identification and legibility, better inventory control, protection from contamination, easier handling and recording under Medicare, prevention of drug loss through pilferage or spilling, better control of Federal Controlled Substances, and less chance of medication errors.

The following products are available through normal channels of supply:

Identi-Dose® (ID100)
Pulvules® No.
℞365 Darvon®, 65 mg
℞369 Darvon® Compound-65
3061 Ceclor®, 250 mg
Tablets No.
℞1883 Darvon-N®, 100 mg
℞1893 Darvocet-N® 100
Reverse-Numbered Package (RN500)
Pulvules® No.
Tablets No.
℞1893 Darvocet-N® 100
Single-Cut Identi-Dose® (ID500)
Tablets No.
℞1893 Darvocet-N® 100

℃, ℃, ℞ Federal Controlled Substances.

AXID®
[ak'sid]
(nizatidine capsules, USP)

DESCRIPTION

Axid® (Nizatidine, USP) is a histamine H_2-receptor antagonist. Chemically, it is N-[2-[[[2-[(dimethylamino)methyl]-4-thiazolyl] methyl]thio]ethyl]-N'-methyl-2-nitro-1,1-ethenediamine.

The structural formula is as follows:

Nizatidine

Nizatidine has the empirical formula $C_{12}H_{21}N_5O_2S_2$ representing a molecular weight of 331.47. It is an off-white to buff crystalline solid that is soluble in water. Nizatidine has a bitter taste and mild sulfur-like odor. Each Pulvule® (capsule) contains for oral administration gelatin, pregelatinized starch, dimethicone, starch, titanium dioxide, yellow iron oxide, 150 mg (0.45 mmol) or 300 mg (0.91 mmol) of nizatidine, and other inactive ingredients. The 150-mg Pulvule also contains magnesium stearate, and the 300-mg Pulvule also contains croscarmellose sodium, povidone, red iron oxide, and talc.

CLINICAL PHARMACOLOGY

Axid is a competitive, reversible inhibitor of histamine at the histamine H_2-receptors, particularly those in the gastric parietal cells.

Antisecretory Activity —1. <u>Effects</u> on <u>Acid</u> <u>Secretion</u>: Axid significantly inhibited nocturnal gastric acid secretion for up to 12 hours. Axid also significantly inhibited gastric acid secretion stimulated by food, caffeine, betazole, and pentagastrin (Table 1).

Table 1
Effect of Oral Axid on Gastric Acid Secretion

	Time After Dose (h)	% Inhibition of Gastric Acid Output by Dose (mg)				
		20-50	75	100	150	300
Nocturnal	Up to 10	57		73		90
Betazole	Up to 3		93		100	99
Pentagastrin	Up to 6		25		64	67
Meal	Up to 4	41	64		98	97
Caffeine	Up to 3		73		85	96

2. <u>Effects</u> on <u>Other</u> <u>Gastrointestinal</u> <u>Secretions</u>—Pepsin: Oral administration of 75 to 300 mg of Axid did not affect pepsin activity in gastric secretions. Total pepsin output was reduced in proportion to the reduced volume of gastric secretions.

<u>Intrinsic Factor</u>: Oral administration of 75 to 300 mg of Axid increased betazole-stimulated secretion of intrinsic factor.

<u>Serum Gastrin</u>: Axid had no effect on basal serum gastrin. No rebound of gastrin secretion was observed when food was ingested 12 hours after administration of Axid.

3. Other Pharmacologic Actions—
a. Hormones: Axid was not shown to affect the serum concentrations of gonadotropins, prolactin, growth hormone, antidiuretic hormone, cortisol, triiodothyronine, thyroxin, testosterone, 5α-dihydrotestosterone, androstenedione, or estradiol.
b. Axid had no demonstrable antiandrogenic action.

4. Pharmacokinetics—The absolute oral bioavailability of nizatidine exceeds 70%. Peak plasma concentrations (700 to 1,800 µg/L for a 150-mg dose and 1,400 to 3,600 µg/L for a 300-mg dose) occur from 0.5 to 3 hours following the dose. A concentration of 1,000 µg/L is equivalent to 3 µmol/L; a dose of 300 mg is equivalent to 905 µmoles. Plasma concentrations 12 hours after administration are less than 10 µg/L. The elimination half-life is 1 to 2 hours, plasma clearance is 40 to 60 L/h, and the volume of distribution is 0.8 to 1.5 L/kg. Because of the short half-life and rapid clearance of nizatidine, accumulation of the drug would not be expected in individuals with normal renal function who take either 300 mg once daily at bedtime or 150 mg twice daily. Axid exhibits dose proportionality over the recommended dose range.

The oral bioavailability of nizatidine is unaffected by concomitant ingestion of propantheline. Antacids consisting of aluminum and magnesium hydroxides with simethicone decrease the absorption of nizatidine by about 10%. With food, the AUC and C_{max} increase by approximately 10%.

In humans, less than 7% of an oral dose is metabolized as N2-monodesmethylnizatidine, an H_2-receptor antagonist, which is the principal metabolite excreted in the urine. Other likely metabolites are the N2-oxide (less than 5% of the dose) and the S-oxide (less than 6% of the dose).

More than 90% of an oral dose of nizatidine is excreted in the urine within 12 hours. About 60% of an oral dose is excreted as unchanged drug. Renal clearance is about 500 mL/min, which indicates excretion by active tubular secretion. Less than 6% of an administered dose is eliminated in the feces.

Moderate to severe renal impairment significantly prolongs the half-life and decreases the clearance of nizatidine. In individuals who are functionally anephric, the half-life is 3.5 to 11 hours, and the plasma clearance is 7 to 14 L/h. To avoid accumulation of the drug in individuals with clinically significant renal impairment, the amount and/or frequency of doses of Axid should be reduced in proportion to the severity of dysfunction (*see* Dosage and Administration).

Approximately 35% of nizatidine is bound to plasma protein, mainly to $α_1$-acid glycoprotein. Warfarin, diazepam, acetaminophen, propantheline, phenobarbital, and propranolol did not affect plasma protein binding of nizatidine in vitro.

Clinical Trials —1. <u>Active</u> <u>Duodenal</u> <u>Ulcer</u>: In multicenter, double-blind, placebo-controlled studies in the United States, endoscopically diagnosed duodenal ulcers healed more rapidly following administration of Axid, 300 mg h.s. or 150 mg b.i.d., than with placebo (Table 2). Lower doses, such as 100 mg h.s., had slightly lower effectiveness.
[See table 2 above]

2. <u>Maintenance</u> of <u>Healed</u> <u>Duodenal</u> <u>Ulcer</u>:
Treatment with a reduced dose of Axid has been shown to be effective as maintenance therapy following healing of active duodenal ulcers. In multicenter, double-blind, placebo-controlled studies conducted in the United States, 150 mg of Axid taken at bedtime resulted in a significantly lower incidence of duodenal ulcer recurrence in patients treated for up to 1 year (Table 3).

Table 3
Percentage of Ulcers Recurring by 3, 6, and 12 Months in Double-Blind Studies Conducted in the United States

Month	Axid, 150 mg h.s.	Placebo
3	13% (28/208)*	40% (82/204)
6	24% (45/188)*	57% (106/187)
12	34% (57/166)*	64% (112/175)

* $P < 0.001$ as compared with placebo.

3. <u>Gastroesophageal</u> <u>Reflux</u> <u>Disease</u> <u>(GERD)</u>:
In 2 multicenter, double-blind, placebo-controlled clinical trials performed in the United States and Canada, Axid was more effective than placebo in improving endoscopically diagnosed esophagitis and in healing erosive and ulcerative esophagitis.

In patients with erosive or ulcerative esophagitis, 150 mg b.i.d. of Axid given to 88 patients compared with placebo in 98 patients in Study 1 yielded a higher healing rate at 3 weeks (16% vs 7%) and at 6 weeks (32% vs 16%, $P<0.05$). Of 99 patients on Axid and 94 patients on placebo, Study 2 at the same dosage yielded similar results at 6 weeks (21% vs 11%, $P<0.05$) and at 12 weeks (29% vs 13%, $P<0.01$).

In addition, relief of associated heartburn was greater in patients treated with Axid. Patients treated with Axid consumed fewer antacids than did patients treated with placebo.

4. <u>Active</u> <u>Benign</u> <u>Gastric</u> <u>Ulcer</u>:
In a multicenter, double-blind, placebo-controlled study conducted in the United States and Canada, endoscopically diagnosed benign gastric ulcers healed significantly more rapidly following administration of nizatidine than of placebo (Table 4).

Table 4

Week	Treatment	Healing Rate	vs. Placebo p-value*
4	Niz 300 mg h.s.	52/153 (34%)	0.342
	Niz 150 mg b.i.d.	65/151 (43%)	0.022
	Placebo	48/151 (32%)	
8	Niz 300 mg h.s.	99/153 (65%)	0.011
	Niz 150 mg b.i.d.	105/151 (70%)	<0.001
	Placebo	78/151 (52%)	

* P-values are one-sided, obtained by Chi-square test, and not adjusted for multiple comparisons.

In a multicenter, double-blind, comparator-controlled study in Europe, healing rates for patients receiving nizatidine (300 mg h.s. or 150 mg b.i.d.) were equivalent to rates for patients receiving a comparator drug, and statistically superior to historical placebo control rates.

INDICATIONS AND USAGE

Axid is indicated for up to 8 weeks for the treatment of active duodenal ulcer. In most patients, the ulcer will heal within 4 weeks.

Axid is indicated for maintenance therapy for duodenal ulcer patients, at a reduced dosage of 150 mg h.s. after healing of an active duodenal ulcer. The consequences of continuous therapy with Axid for longer than 1 year are not known.

Axid is indicated for up to 12 weeks for the treatment of endoscopically diagnosed esophagitis, including erosive and ulcerative esophagitis, and associated heartburn due to GERD.

Axid is indicated for up to 8 weeks for the treatment of active benign gastric ulcer. Before initiating therapy, care should be taken to exclude the possibility of malignant gastric ulceration.

CONTRAINDICATION

Axid is contraindicated in patients with known hypersensitivity to the drug. Because cross sensitivity in this class of compounds has been observed, H_2-receptor antagonists, including Axid, should not be administered to patients with a history of hypersensitivity to other H_2-receptor antagonists.

PRECAUTIONS

General —1. Symptomatic response to nizatidine therapy does not preclude the presence of gastric malignancy.
2. Because nizatidine is excreted primarily by the kidney, dosage should be reduced in patients with moderate to severe renal insufficiency (*see* Dosage and Administration).
3. Pharmacokinetic studies in patients with hepatorenal syndrome have not been done. Part of the dose of nizatidine is metabolized in the liver. In patients with normal renal function and uncomplicated hepatic dysfunction, the disposition of nizatidine is similar to that in normal subjects.
Laboratory Tests —False-positive tests for urobilinogen with Multistix® may occur during therapy with nizatidine.
Drug Interactions —No interactions have been observed between Axid and theophylline, chlordiazepoxide, lorazepam, lidocaine, phenytoin, and warfarin. Axid does not inhibit the cytochrome P-450-linked drug-metabolizing enzyme system; therefore, drug interactions mediated by inhibition of hepatic metabolism are not expected to occur. In patients given very high doses (3,900 mg) of aspirin daily, increases in serum salicylate levels were seen when nizatidine, 150 mg b.i.d., was administered concurrently.
Carcinogenesis, Mutagenesis, Impairment of Fertility —A 2-year oral carcinogenicity study in rats with doses as high as 500 mg/kg/day (about 80 times the recommended therapeutic dose) showed no evidence of a carcinogenic ef-

Table 2
Healing Response of Ulcers to Axid

AXID						
	300 mg h.s.		150 mg b.i.d.		Placebo	
	Number Entered	Healed/ Evaluable	Number Entered	Healed/ Evaluable	Number Entered	Healed/ Evaluable
STUDY 1						
Week 2			276	93/265 (35%)*	279	55/260 (21%)
Week 4				198/259 (76%)*		95/243 (39%)
STUDY 2						
Week 2	108	24/103 (23%)*	106	27/101 (27%)*	101	9/93 (10%)
Week 4		65/97 (67%)*		66/97 (68%)*		24/84 (29%)
STUDY 3						
Week 2	92	22/90 (24%)†			98	13/92 (14%)
Week 4		52/85 (61%)*				29/88 (33%)
Week 8		68/83 (82%)*				39/79 (49%)

* $P < 0.01$ as compared with placebo.
† $P < 0.05$ as compared with placebo.

Continued on next page

* Identi-Code® symbol. This product information was prepared in June 1998. Current information on these and other products of Eli Lilly and Company may be obtained by direct inquiry to Lilly Research Laboratories, Lilly Corporate Center, Indianapolis, Indiana 46285, (800) 545-5979.

Axid—Cont.

fect. There was a dose-related increase in the density of enterochromaffin-like (ECL) cells in the gastric oxyntic mucosa. In a 2-year study in mice, there was no evidence of a carcinogenic effect in male mice; although hyperplastic nodules of the liver were increased in the high-dose males as compared with placebo. Female mice given the high dose of Axid (2,000 mg/kg/day, about 330 times the human dose) showed marginally statistically significant increases in hepatic carcinoma and hepatic nodular hyperplasia with no numerical increase seen in any of the other dose groups. The rate of hepatic carcinoma in the high-dose animals was within the historical control limits seen for the strain of mice used. The female mice were given a dose larger than the maximum tolerated dose, as indicated by excessive (30%) weight decrement as compared with concurrent controls and evidence of mild liver injury (transaminase elevations). The occurrence of a marginal finding at high dose only in animals given an excessive and somewhat hepatotoxic dose, with no evidence of a carcinogenic effect in rats, male mice, and female mice (given up to 360 mg/kg/day, about 60 times the human dose), and a negative mutagenicity battery are not considered evidence of a carcinogenic potential for Axid.

Axid was not mutagenic in a battery of tests performed to evaluate its potential genetic toxicity, including bacterial mutation tests, unscheduled DNA synthesis, sister chromatid exchange, the mouse lymphoma assay, chromosome aberration tests, and a micronucleus test.

In a 2-generation, perinatal and postnatal fertility study in rats, doses of nizatidine up to 650 mg/kg/day produced no adverse effects on the reproductive performance of parental animals or their progeny.

Pregnancy—Teratogenic Effects—Pregnancy Category B—Oral reproduction studies in pregnant rats at doses up to 1500 mg/kg/day (9000 mg/m^2/day, 40.5 times the recommended human dose based on body surface area) and in pregnant rabbits at doses up to 275 mg/kg/day (3245 mg/m^2/day, 14.6 times the recommended human dose based on body surface area) have revealed no evidence of impaired fertility or harm to the fetus due to nizatidine. There are, however, no adequate and well-controlled studies in pregnant women. Because animal reproduction studies are not always predictive of human response, this drug should be used during pregnancy only if clearly needed.

Nursing Mothers—Studies conducted in lactating women have shown that 0.1% of the administered oral dose of nizatidine is secreted in human milk in proportion to plasma concentrations. Because of the growth depression in pups reared by lactating rats treated with nizatidine, a decision should be made whether to discontinue nursing or discontinue the drug, taking into account the importance of the drug to the mother.

Use in Pediatric Patients—Safety and effectiveness in pediatric patients have not been established.

Use in Elderly Patients—Ulcer healing rates in elderly patients are similar to those in younger age groups. The incidence rates of adverse events and laboratory test abnormalities are also similar to those seen in other age groups. Age alone may not be an important factor in the disposition of nizatidine. Elderly patients may have reduced renal function (*see* Dosage and Administration).

ADVERSE REACTIONS

Worldwide, controlled clinical trials of nizatidine included over 6,000 patients given nizatidine in studies of varying durations. Placebo-controlled trials in the United States and Canada included over 2,600 patients given nizatidine and over 1,700 given placebo. Among the adverse events in these placebo-controlled trials, anemia (0.2% vs 0%) and urticaria (0.5% vs 0.1%) were significantly more common in the nizatidine group.

Incidence in Placebo-Controlled Clinical Trials in the United States and Canada—Table 5 lists adverse events that occurred at a frequency of 1% or more among nizatidine-treated patients who participated in placebo-controlled trials. The cited figures provide some basis for estimating the relative contribution of drug and nondrug factors to the side effect incidence rate in the population studied.

Table 5
Incidence of Treatment-Emergent
Adverse Events in Placebo-Controlled
Clinical Trials
In The United States and Canada

Body System/Adverse Event*	Percentage of Patients Reporting Event	
	Nizatidine (N=2,694)	Placebo (N=1,729)
Body as a Whole		
Headache	16.6	15.6
Abdominal pain	7.5	12.5
Pain	4.2	3.8
Asthenia	3.1	2.9
Back pain	2.4	2.6
Chest pain	2.3	2.1
Infection	1.7	1.1
Fever	1.6	2.3
Surgical procedure	1.4	1.5
Injury, accident	1.2	0.9
Digestive		
Diarrhea	7.2	6.9
Nausea	5.4	7.4
Flatulence	4.9	5.4
Vomiting	3.6	5.6
Dyspepsia	3.6	4.4
Constipation	2.5	3.8
Dry mouth	1.4	1.3
Nausea and vomiting	1.2	1.9
Anorexia	1.2	1.6
Gastrointestinal disorder	1.1	1.2
Tooth disorder	1.0	0.8
Musculoskeletal		
Myalgia	1.7	1.5
Nervous		
Dizziness	4.6	3.8
Insomnia	2.7	3.4
Abnormal dreams	1.9	1.9
Somnolence	1.9	1.6
Anxiety	1.6	1.4
Nervousness	1.1	0.8
Respiratory		
Rhinitis	9.8	9.6
Pharyngitis	3.3	3.1
Sinusitis	2.4	2.1
Cough, increased	2.0	2.0
Skin and Appendages		
Rash	1.9	2.1
Pruritus	1.7	1.3
Special Senses		
Amblyopia	1.0	0.9

*Events reported by at least 1% of nizatidine-treated patients are included.

A variety of less common events were also reported; it was not possible to determine whether these were caused by nizatidine.

Hepatic—Hepatocellular injury, evidenced by elevated liver enzyme tests (SGOT [AST], SGPT [ALT], or alkaline phosphatase), occurred in some patients and was possibly or probably related to nizatidine. In some cases there was marked elevation of SGOT, SGPT enzymes (greater than 500 IU/L) and, in a single instance, SGPT was greater than 2,000 IU/L. The overall rate of occurrences of elevated liver enzymes and elevations to 3 times the upper limit of normal, however, did not significantly differ from the rate of liver enzyme abnormalities in placebo-treated patients. All abnormalities were reversible after discontinuation of Axid. Since market introduction, hepatitis and jaundice have been reported. Rare cases of cholestatic or mixed hepatocellular and cholestatic injury with jaundice have been reported with reversal of the abnormalities after discontinuation of Axid.

Cardiovascular—In clinical pharmacology studies, short episodes of asymptomatic ventricular tachycardia occurred in 2 individuals administered Axid and in 3 untreated subjects.

CNS—Rare cases of reversible mental confusion have been reported.

Endocrine—Clinical pharmacology studies and controlled clinical trials showed no evidence of antiandrogenic activity due to Axid. Impotence and decreased libido were reported with similar frequency by patients who received Axid and by those given placebo. Rare reports of gynecomastia occurred.

Hematologic—Anemia was reported significantly more frequently in nizatidine- than in placebo-treated patients. Fatal thrombocytopenia was reported in a patient who was treated with Axid and another H$_2$-receptor antagonist. On previous occasions, this patient had experienced thrombocytopenia while taking other drugs. Rare cases of thrombocytopenic purpura have been reported.

Integumental—Sweating and urticaria were reported significantly more frequently in nizatidine- than in placebo-treated patients. Rash and exfoliative dermatitis were also reported. Vasculitis has been reported rarely.

Hypersensitivity—As with other H$_2$-receptor antagonists, rare cases of anaphylaxis following administration of nizatidine have been reported. Rare episodes of hypersensitivity reactions (eg, bronchospasm, laryngeal edema, rash, and eosinophilia) have been reported.

Body as a Whole—Serum sickness-like reactions have occurred rarely in conjunction with nizatidine use.

Genitourinary—Reports of impotence have occurred.

Other—Hyperuricemia unassociated with gout or nephrolithiasis was reported. Eosinophilia, fever, and nausea related to nizatidine administration have been reported.

OVERDOSAGE

Overdoses of Axid have been reported rarely. The following is provided to serve as a guide should such an overdose be encountered.

Signs and Symptoms—There is little clinical experience with overdosage of Axid in humans. Test animals that received large doses of nizatidine have exhibited cholinergic-type effects, including lacrimation, salivation, emesis, miosis, and diarrhea. Single oral doses of 800 mg/kg in dogs and of 1,200 mg/kg in monkeys were not lethal. Intravenous median lethal doses in the rat and mouse were 301 mg/kg and 232 mg/kg respectively.

Treatment—To obtain up-to-date information about the treatment of overdose, a good resource is your certified Regional Poison Control Center. Telephone numbers of certified poison control centers are listed in the *Physicians' Desk Reference (PDR)*. In managing overdosage, consider the possibility of multiple drug overdoses, interaction among drugs, and unusual drug kinetics in your patient.

If overdosage occurs, use of activated charcoal, emesis, or lavage should be considered along with clinical monitoring and supportive therapy. The ability of hemodialysis to remove nizatidine from the body has not been conclusively demonstrated; however, due to its large volume of distribution, nizatidine is not expected to be efficiently removed from the body by this method.

DOSAGE AND ADMINISTRATION

Active Duodenal Ulcer—The recommended oral dosage for adults is 300 mg once daily at bedtime. An alternative dosage regimen is 150 mg twice daily.

Maintenance of Healed Duodenal Ulcer—The recommended oral dosage for adults is 150 mg once daily at bedtime.

Gastroesophageal Reflux Disease—The recommended oral dosage in adults for the treatment of erosions, ulcerations, and associated heartburn is 150 mg twice daily.

Active Benign Gastric Ulcer—The recommended oral dosage is 300 mg given either as 150 mg twice daily or 300 mg once daily at bedtime. Prior to treatment, care should be taken to exclude the possibility of malignant gastric ulceration.

Dosage Adjustment for Patients With Moderate to Severe Renal Insufficiency—The dose for patients with renal dysfunction should be reduced as follows:

Active Duodenal Ulcer, GERD and Benign Gastric Ulcer

C$_{cr}$	Dose
20–50 mL/min	150 mg daily
<20 mL/min	150 mg every other day

Maintenance Therapy

C$_{cr}$	Dose
20–50 mL/min	150 mg every other day
<20 mL/min	150 mg every 3 days

Some elderly patients may have creatinine clearances of less than 50 mL/min, and, based on pharmacokinetic data in patients with renal impairment, the dose for such patients should be reduced accordingly. The clinical effects of this dosage reduction in patients with renal failure have not been evaluated.

HOW SUPPLIED

Axid® Pulvules®* are available in:
The 150-mg Pulvules are imprinted with script "Lilly" and "3144" on the opaque dark yellow cap and "AXID 150 mg" on the opaque pale yellow body, using black ink. They are available as follows:

Bottles of 60†	NDC 0002-3144-60 (PU3144)	
Bottles of 500	NDC 0002-3144-03 (PU3144)	
ID‡100	NDC 0002-3144-33 (PU3144)	
	(10 strips of 10 Pulvules)	
ID‡620§	NDC 0002-3144-82 (PU3144)	
	(20 cards of 31 Pulvules)	

The 300-mg Pulvules are imprinted with script "Lilly" and "3145" on the opaque brown cap and "AXID 300 mg" on the opaque pale yellow body, using black ink. They are available as follows:

Bottles of 30†	NDC 0002-3145-30 (PU3145)

* Pulvules® (filled gelatin capsules, Lilly)
† RxPak (prescription package, Lilly)
‡ Identi-Dose® (unit dose medication, Lilly)
§FlexPak (flexible blister card, Lilly)
Store at controlled room temperature-, 20° to 25°C (68° to 77°F) in a tightly closed container [see USP].
The USP defines controlled room temperature as: A temperature maintained thermostatically that encompasses the usual and customary working environment of 20° to 25°C (68° to 77°F); that results in a mean kinetic temperature calculated to be not more than 25°C; and that allows for excursions between 15° and 30°C (59° and 86°F) that are experienced in pharmacies, hospitals, and warehouses.
CAUTION-Federal (USA) law prohibits dispensing without prescription.
Literature revised August 22, 1996   [082296]
PV 2099AMP
Shown in Product Identification Guide, page 320

CECLOR® ℞

[sē 'klôr]
cefaclor, USP

DESCRIPTION

Ceclor® (Cefaclor, USP) is a semisynthetic cephalosporin antibiotic for oral administration. It is chemically designated as 3-chloro-7-D- (2-phenylglycinamido)-3-cephem-4-carboxylic acid monohydrate. The chemical formula for cefaclor is $C_{15}H_{14}ClN_3O_4S \bullet H_2O$ and the molecular weight is 385.82.

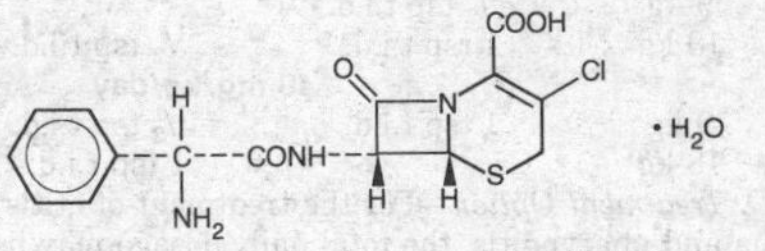

Each Pulvule® contains cefaclor monohydrate equivalent to 250 mg (0.68 mmol) or 500 mg (1.36 mmol) anhydrous cefaclor. The Pulvules also contain cornstarch, F D & C Blue No. 1, F D & C Red No. 3, gelatin, magnesium stearate, silicone, titanium dioxide, and other inactive ingredients. The 500-mg Pulvule also contains iron oxide.
After mixing, each 5 mL of Ceclor for Oral Suspension will contain cefaclor monohydrate equivalent to 125 mg (0.34 mmol), 187 mg (0.51 mmol), 250 mg (0.68 mmol), or 375 mg (1.0 mmol) anhydrous cefaclor. The suspensions also contain cellulose, cornstarch, F D & C Red No. 40, flavors, silicone, sodium lauryl sulfate, sucrose, and xanthan gum.

CLINICAL PHARMACOLOGY

Cefaclor is well absorbed after oral administration to fasting subjects. Total absorption is the same whether the drug is given with or without food; however, when it is taken with food, the peak concentration achieved is 50% to 75% of that observed when the drug is administered to fasting subjects and generally appears from three fourths to 1 hour later. Following administration of 250-mg, 500-mg, and 1-g doses to fasting subjects, average peak serum levels of approximately 7, 13, and 23 µg/mL respectively were obtained within 30 to 60 minutes. Approximately 60% to 85% of the drug is excreted unchanged in the urine within 8 hours, the greater portion being excreted within the first 2 hours. During this 8-hour period, peak urine concentrations following the 250-mg, 500-mg, and 1-g doses were approximately 600, 900, and 1,900 µg/mL respectively. The serum half-life in normal subjects is 0.6 to 0.9 hours. In patients with reduced renal function, the serum half-life of cefaclor is slightly prolonged. In those with complete absence of renal function, the plasma half-life of the intact molecule is 2.3 to 2.8 hours. Excretion pathways in patients with markedly impaired renal function have not been determined. Hemodialysis shortens the half-life by 25% to 30%.
Microbiology—In vitro tests demonstrate that the bactericidal action of cephalosporins results from inhibition of cell-wall synthesis. Cefaclor has been shown to be active against most strains of the following microorganisms, both *in vitro* and in clinical infections as described in the INDICATIONS AND USAGE section.

Aerobes, Gram-positive
Staphylococcus aureus, including β-lactamase-producing strains
Staphylococcus epidermidis, including β-lactamase-producing strains
Streptococcus pneumoniae
Streptococcus pyogenes
Aerobes, Gram-negative
Escherichia coli
Haemophilus influenzae, including β-lactamase-producing, ampicillin-resistant strains
Klebsiella spp
Proteus mirabilis

The following *in vitro* data are available, **but their clinical significance is unknown.**
Cefaclor exhibits *in vitro* minimal inhibitory concentrations (MICs) of ≤8 µg/mL or less against most (≥90%) strains of the following microorganisms; however, the safety and effectiveness of cefaclor in treating clinical infections due to these microorganisms have not been established in adequate and well-controlled clinical trials.

Aerobes, Gram-negative
Citrobacter diversus
Moraxella (Branhamella) catarrhalis
Neisseria gonorrhoeae
Anaerobes, Gram-positive
Bacteroides spp (excluding *Bacteroides fragilis*)
Peptococcus niger
Peptostreptococcus spp
Propionibacterium acnes

Note: Pseudomonas spp. *Acinetobacter calcoaceticus* (formerly *Mima* spp and *Herellea* spp), and most strains of enterococci (*Enterococcus faecalis* [formerly *Streptococcus faecalis*], group D streptococci), *Enterobacter* spp, indole-positive *Proteus*, and *Serratia* spp are resistant to cefaclor. When tested by in vitro methods, staphylococci exhibit cross-resistance between cefaclor and methicillin-type antibiotics.
Disk Susceptibility Tests—
Diffusion techniques—Quantitative methods that require measurement of zone diameters provide reproducible estimates of the susceptibility of bacteria to antimicrobial compounds. One such standardized procedure[1] that has been recommended for use with disks to test the susceptibility of microorganisms to cefaclor uses the 30-µg cefaclor disk. Interpretation involves correlation of the diameter obtained in the disk test with the MIC for cefaclor. With this procedure, a report from the laboratory of "resistant" indicates that the infecting organism is not likely to respond to therapy. A report of "intermediate susceptibility" suggests that the organism would be susceptible if the infection is confined to tissues and fluids (eg, urine) in which high antibiotic levels can be obtained or if high dosage is used.
Reports from the laboratory providing results of the standard single-disk susceptibility test with a 30-µg cefaclor disk should be interpreted according to the following criteria:

Zone Diameter (mm)	Interpretation
≥18	Susceptible (S)
15–17	Intermediate (I)
≤14	Resistant (R)

When Testing H. *influenzae**

Zone Diameter (mm)	Interpretation
≥20	Susceptible (S)
17–19	Intermediate (I)
≤16	Resistant (R)

*Disk susceptibility tests performed using Haemophilus Test Medium (HTM)[1]

A report of "Susceptible" indicates that the pathogen is likely to be inhibited by usually achievable concentrations of the antimicrobial compound in blood. A report of "Intermediate" indicates that the result should be considered equivocal, and, if the microorganism is not fully susceptible to alternative, clinically feasible drugs, the test should be repeated. This category implies possible clinical applicability in body sites where the drug is physiologically concentrated or in situations where high dosage of drug can be used. This category also provides a buffer zone that prevents small uncontrolled technical factors from causing major discrepancies in interpretation. A report of "Resistant" indicates that usually achievable concentrations of the antimicrobial compound in the blood are unlikely to be inhibitory and that other therapy should be selected.
Measurement of MIC or MBC and achieved antimicrobial compound concentrations may be appropriate to guide therapy in some infections. (*See* CLINICAL PHARMACOLOGY section for further information on drug concentrations achieved in infected body sites and other pharmacokinetic properties of this antimicrobial drug product.)
Standardized susceptibility test procedures require the use of laboratory control microorganisms. The 30-µg cefaclor disk should provide the following zone diameters in these laboratory test quality control strains:

Microorganisms	Zone Diameter (mm)
E. coli ATCC 25922	23–27
S. aureus ATCC 25923	27–31

When Testing *H. influenzae**

Microorganisms	Zone Diameter (mm)
H. influenzae ATCC 49766	25–31

*Disk susceptibility tests performed using Haemophilus Test Medium (HTM)[1]

Dilution techniques—Quantitative methods that are used to determine minimum inhibitory concentrations provide reproducible estimates of the susceptibility of bacteria to antimicrobial compounds. One such standardized procedure uses a standardized dilution method[2] (broth, agar, microdilution) or equivalent with cefaclor powder. The MIC values obtained should be interpreted according to the following criteria:

MIC (µg/mL)	Interpretation
≤8	Susceptible (S)
16	Intermediate (I)
≥32	Resistant (R)

Interpretation should be as stated above for results using diffusion techniques.
As with standard diffusion techniques, dilution methods require the use of laboratory control microorganisms. Standard cefaclor powder should provide the following MIC values:

Microorganism	MIC (µg/mL)
E. coli ATCC 25922	1–4
E. faecalis ATCC 29212	>32
S. aureus ATCC 29213	1–4

When Testing *H. Influenzae**

Microorganism	MIC (µg/mL)
H. influenzae ATCC 49766	1–4

*Broth microdilution tests performed using Haemophilus Test Medium (HTM)[2]

INDICATIONS AND USAGE

Ceclor is indicated in the treatment of the following infections when caused by susceptible strains of the designated microorganisms.
Otitis media caused by *Streptococcus pneumoniae, Haemophilus influenzae*, staphylococci, and *Streptococcus pyogenes*
Lower respiratory tract infections, including pneumonia, caused by *Streptococcus pneumoniae, Haemophilus influenzae,* and *Streptococcus pyogenes*
Pharyngitis and Tonsillitis, caused by *Streptococcus pyogenes*
Note: Penicillin is the usual drug of choice in the treatment and prevention of streptococcal infections, including the prophylaxis of rheumatic fever. Ceclor is generally effective in the eradication of streptococci from the nasopharynx; however, substantial data establishing the efficacy of Ceclor in the subsequent prevention of rheumatic fever are not available at present.
Urinary tract infections, including pyelonephritis and cystitis, caused by *Escherichia coli, Proteus mirabilis, Klebsiella* spp, and coagulase-negative staphylococci
Skin and skin structure infections caused by *Staphylococcus aureus* and *Streptococcus pyogenes*
Appropriate culture and susceptibility studies should be performed to determine susceptibility of the causative organism to cefaclor.

CONTRAINDICATION

Ceclor is contraindicated in patients with known allergy to the cephalosporin group of antibiotics.

WARNINGS

BEFORE THERAPY WITH CECLOR IS INSTITUTED, CAREFUL INQUIRY SHOULD BE MADE TO DETERMINE WHETHER THE PATIENT HAS HAD PREVIOUS HYPERSENSITIVITY REACTIONS TO CEFACLOR, CEPHALOSPORINS, PENICILLINS, OR OTHER DRUGS. IF THIS PRODUCT IS TO BE GIVEN TO PENICILLIN-SENSITIVE PATIENTS, CAUTION SHOULD BE EXERCISED BECAUSE CROSS-HYPERSENSITIVITY AMONG β-LACTAM ANTIBIOTICS HAS BEEN CLEARLY DOCUMENTED AND MAY OCCUR IN UP TO 10% OF PATIENTS WITH A HISTORY OF PENICILLIN ALLERGY.
IF AN ALLERGIC REACTION TO CECLOR OCCURS, DISCONTINUE THE DRUG. SERIOUS ACUTE HYPERSENSITIVITY REACTIONS MAY REQUIRE TREATMENT WITH EPINEPHRINE AND OTHER EMERGENCY MEASURES, INCLUDING OXYGEN, INTRAVENOUS FLUIDS, INTRAVENOUS ANTIHISTAMINES, CORTICOSTEROIDS, PRESSOR AMINES, AND AIRWAY MANAGEMENT, AS CLINICALLY INDICATED.
Antibiotics, including Ceclor, should be administered cautiously to any patient who has demonstrated some form of allergy, particularly to drugs.
Pseudomembranous colitis has been reported with nearly all antibacterial agents, including cefaclor, and has ranged in severity from mild to life-threatening. Therefore, it is important to consider this diagnosis in patients who present with diarrhea subsequent to the administration of antibacterial agents.
Treatment with antibacterial agents alters the normal flora of the colon and may permit overgrowth of clostridia. Studies indicate that a toxin produced by *Clostridium difficile* is one primary cause of antibiotic-associated colitis.
After the diagnosis of pseudomembranous colitis has been established, therapeutic measures should be initiated. Mild cases of pseudomembranous colitis usually respond to drug discontinuation alone. In moderate to severe cases, consideration should be given to management with fluids and electrolytes, protein supplementation and treatment with an antibacterial drug effective against *C. difficile*.

PRECAUTIONS

General—Prolonged use of Ceclor may result in the overgrowth of nonsusceptible organisms. Careful observation of

Continued on next page

*** Identi-Code® symbol. This product information was prepared in June 1998. Current information on these and other products of Eli Lilly and Company may be obtained by direct inquiry to Lilly Research Laboratories, Lilly Corporate Center, Indianapolis, Indiana 46285, (800) 545-5979.**

Ceclor—Cont.

the patient is essential. If superinfection occurs during therapy, appropriate measures should be taken.

Positive direct Coombs' tests have been reported during treatment with the cephalosporin antibiotics. It should be recognized that a positive Coombs' test may be due to the drug, eg, in hematologic studies or in transfusion cross-matching procedures when antiglobulin tests are performed on the minor side or in Coombs' testing of newborns whose mothers have received cephalosporin antibiotics before parturition.

Ceclor should be administered with caution in the presence of markedly impaired renal function. Since the half-life of cefaclor in anuria is 2.3 to 2.8 hours, dosage adjustments for patients with moderate or severe renal impairment are usually not required. Clinical experience with cefaclor under such conditions is limited; therefore, careful clinical observation and laboratory studies should be made.

As with other β-lactam antibiotics, the renal excretion of cefaclor is inhibited by probenecid.

Antibiotics, including cephalosporins, should be prescribed with caution in individuals with a history of gastrointestinal disease, particularly colitis.

Drug/Laboratory Test Interactions—Patients receiving Ceclor may show a false-positive reaction for glucose in the urine with tests that use Benedict's and Fehling's solutions and also with Clinitest® tablets.

There have been reports of increased anticoagulant effect when Ceclor and oral anticoagulants were administered concomitantly.

Carcinogenesis, Mutagenesis, Impairment of Fertility—Studies have not been performed to determine potential for carcinogenicity, mutagenicity, or impairment of fertility.

Pregnancy—Teratogenic Effects—Pregnancy Category B—Reproduction studies have been performed in mice and rats at doses up to 12 times the human dose and in ferrets given 3 times the maximum human dose and have revealed no harm to the fetus due to Ceclor. There are, however, no adequate and well-controlled studies in pregnant women. Because animal reproduction studies are not always predictive of human response, this drug should be used during pregnancy only if clearly needed.

Labor and Delivery—The effect of Ceclor on labor and delivery is unknown.

Nursing Mothers—Small amounts of Ceclor have been detected in mother's milk following administration of single 500-mg doses. Average levels were 0.18, 0.20, 0.21, and 0.16 µg/mL at 2, 3, 4, and 5 hours respectively. Trace amounts were detected at 1 hour. The effect on nursing infants is not known. Caution should be exercised when Ceclor is administered to a nursing woman.

Pediatric Use—Safety and effectiveness of this product for use in infants less than 1 month of age have not been established.

ADVERSE REACTIONS

Adverse effects considered to be related to therapy with Ceclor are listed below:

Hypersensitivity reactions have been reported in about 1.5% of patients and include morbilliform eruptions (1 in 100). Pruritus, urticaria, and positive Coombs' tests each occur in less than 1 in 200 patients.

Cases of **serum-sickness-like** reactions have been reported with the use of Ceclor. These are characterized by findings of erythema multiforme, rashes, and other skin manifestations accompanied by arthritis/arthralgia, with or without fever, and differ from classic serum sickness in that there is infrequently associated lymphadenopathy and proteinuria, no circulating immune complexes, and no evidence to date of sequelae of the reaction. Occasionally, solitary symptoms may occur, but do not represent a **serum-sickness-like** reaction. While further investigation is ongoing, **serum-sickness-like** reactions appear to be due to hypersensitivity and more often occur during or following a second (or subsequent) course of therapy with Ceclor. Such reactions have been reported more frequently in pediatric patients than in adults with an overall occurrence ranging from 1 in 200 (0.5%) in one focused trial to 2 in 8,346 (0.024%) in overall clinical trials (with an incidence in pediatric patients in clinical trials of 0.055%) to 1 in 38,000 (0.003%) in spontaneous event reports. Signs and symptoms usually occur a few days after initiation of therapy and subside within a few days after cessation of therapy; occasionally these reactions have resulted in hospitalization, usually of short duration (median hospitalization = 2 to 3 days, based on postmarketing surveillance studies). In those requiring hospitalization, the symptoms have ranged from mild to severe at the time of admission with more of the severe reactions occurring in pediatric patients. Antihistamines and glucocorticoids appear to enhance resolution of the signs and symptoms. No serious sequelae have been reported.

More severe hypersensitivity reactions, including Stevens-Johnson syndrome, toxic epidermal necrolysis, and anaphylaxis have been reported rarely. Anaphylactoid events may be manifested by solitary symptoms, including angioedema, asthenia, edema (including face and limbs), dyspnea, paresthesias, syncope, hypotension, or vasodilatation. Anaphylaxis may be more common in patients with a history of penicillin allergy.

Rarely, hypersensitivity symptoms may persist for several months.

Gastrointestinal symptoms occur in about 2.5% of patients and include diarrhea (1 in 70).

Onset of pseudomembranous colitis symptoms may occur during or after antibiotic treatment. (*see* **WARNINGS**) Nausea and vomiting have been reported rarely. As with some penicillins and some other cephalosporins, transient hepatitis and cholestatic jaundice have been reported rarely.

Other effects considered related to therapy included eosinophilia (1 in 50 patients), genital pruritus or vaginitis (less than 1 in 100 patients), and, rarely, thrombocytopenia or reversible interstitial nephritis.

Causal Relationship Uncertain —

CNS —Rarely, reversible hyperactivity, agitation, nervousness, insomnia, confusion, hypertonia, dizziness, hallucinations, and somnolence have been reported.

Transitory abnormalities in clinical laboratory test results have been reported. Although they were of uncertain etiology, they are listed below to serve as alerting information for the physician.

Hepatic —Slight elevations of AST, ALT, or alkaline phosphatase values (1 in 40).

Hematopoietic —As has also been reported with other β-lactam antibiotics, transient lymphocytosis, leukopenia, and, rarely, hemolytic anemia, aplastic anemia, agranulocytosis, and reversible neutropenia of possible clinical significance.

There have been rare reports of increased prothrombin time with or without clinical bleeding in patients receiving Ceclor and Coumadin® concomitantly.

Renal —Slight elevations in BUN or serum creatinine (less than 1 in 500) or abnormal urinalysis (less than 1 in 200).

Cephalosporin-class Adverse Reactions

In addition to the adverse reactions listed above that have been observed in patients treated with cefaclor, the following adverse reactions and altered laboratory tests have been reported for cephalosporin-class antibiotics: fever, abdominal pain, superinfection, renal dysfunction, toxic nephropathy, hemorrhage, false positive test for urinary glucose, elevated bilirubin, elevated LDH, and pancytopenia.

Several cephalosporins have been implicated in triggering seizures, particularly in patients with renal impairment when the dosage was not reduced. If seizures associated with drug therapy occur, the drug should be discontinued. Anticonvulsant therapy can be given if clinically indicated (*see* **DOSAGE AND ADMINISTRATION** and **OVERDOSAGE** sections).

OVERDOSAGE

Signs and Symptoms —The toxic symptoms following an overdose of cefaclor may include nausea, vomiting, epigastric distress, and diarrhea. The severity of the epigastric distress and the diarrhea are dose related. If other symptoms are present, it is probable that they are secondary to an underlying disease state, an allergic reaction, or the effects of other intoxication.

Treatment —To obtain up-to-date information about the treatment of overdose, a good resource is your certified Regional Poison Control Center. Telephone numbers of certified poison control centers are listed in the *Physicians' Desk Reference* (*PDR*). In managing overdosage, consider the possibility of multiple drug overdoses, interaction among drugs, and unusual drug kinetics in your patient.

Unless 5 times the normal dose of cefaclor has been ingested, gastrointestinal decontamination will not be necessary.

Protect the patient's airway and support ventilation and perfusion. Meticulously monitor and maintain, within acceptable limits, the patient's vital signs, blood gases, serum electrolytes, etc. Absorption of drugs from the gastrointestinal tract may be decreased by giving activated charcoal, which, in many cases, is more effective than emesis or lavage; consider charcoal instead of or in addition to gastric emptying. Repeated doses of charcoal over time may hasten elimination of some drugs that have been absorbed. Safeguard the patient's airway when employing gastric emptying or charcoal.

Forced diuresis, peritoneal dialysis, hemodialysis, or charcoal hemoperfusion have not been established as beneficial for an overdose of cefaclor.

DOSAGE AND ADMINISTRATION

Ceclor is administered orally.

Adults —The usual adult dosage is 250 mg every 8 hours. For more severe infections (such as pneumonia) or those caused by less susceptible organisms, doses may be doubled.

Pediatric Patients —The usual recommended daily dosage for pediatric patients is 20 mg/kg/day in divided doses every 8 hours. In more serious infections, otitis media, and infections caused by less susceptible organisms, 40 mg/kg/day are recommended, with a maximum dosage of 1 g/day.

Ceclor Suspension

Weight	125 mg/5 mL	250 mg/5 mL
20 mg/kg/day		
9 kg	$^1/_2$ tsp t.i.d.	
18 kg	1 tsp t.i.d.	$^1/_2$ tsp t.i.d.
40 mg/kg/day		
9 kg	1 tsp t.i.d.	$^1/_2$ tsp t.i.d.
18 kg		1 tsp t.i.d.

B.I.D. Treatment Option—For the treatment of otitis media and pharyngitis, the total daily dosage may be divided and administered every 12 hours.

Ceclor Suspension

Weight	187 mg/5 mL	375 mg/5 mL
20 mg/kg/day (Pharyngitis)		
9 kg	$^1/_2$ tsp b.i.d.	
18 kg	1 tsp b.i.d.	$^1/_2$ tsp b.i.d.
40 mg/kg/day (Otitis Media)		
9 kg	1 tsp b.i.d.	$^1/_2$ tsp b.i.d.
18 kg		1 tsp b.i.d.

Ceclor may be administered in the presence of impaired renal function. Under such a condition, the dosage usually is unchanged (*see* **PRECAUTIONS**).

In the treatment of β-hemolytic streptococcal infections, a therapeutic dosage of Ceclor should be administered for at least 10 days.

HOW SUPPLIED

Pulvules:

250 mg, purple and white (No. 3061)—(RxPak* of 15) NDC 0002-3061-15; (100s) NDC 0002-3061-02; (ID†100) NDC 0002-3061-33

500 mg, purple and gray (No. 3062)—(RxPak of 15) NDC 0002-3062-15; (100s) NDC 0002-3062-02; (ID100) NDC 0002-3062-33

For Oral Suspension:

125 mg/5 mL, strawberry flavor (M-5057‡)—(75-mL size) NDC 0002-5057-18; (150-mL size) NDC 0002-5057-68

187 mg/5 mL, strawberry flavor (M-5130‡)—(50-mL size) NDC 0002-5130-87; (100-mL size) NDC 0002-5130-48

250 mg/5 mL, strawberry flavor (M-5058‡)—(75-mL size) NDC 0002-5058-18; (150-mL size) NDC 0002-5058-68

375 mg/5 mL, strawberry flavor (M-5132‡)—(50-mL size) NDC 0002-5132-87; (100-mL size) NDC 0002-5132-48

* All RxPaks (prescription packages, Lilly) have safety closures.

† Identi-Dose® (unit dose medication, Lilly).

‡ After mixing, store in a refrigerator. Shake well before using. Keep tightly closed. The mixture may be kept for 14 days without significant loss of potency. Discard unused portion after 14 days.

Store at controlled room temperature, 59° to 86°F (15° to 30°C).

REFERENCES

1. National Committee for Clinical Laboratory Standards. Performance Standards for Antimicrobial Disk Susceptibility Tests—Fifth Edition, Approved Standard NCCLS Document M2-A5, Vol. 13, No. 24, NCCLS, Villanova, PA, December, 1993.
2. National Committee for Clinical Laboratory Standards. Methods for Dilution Antimicrobial Susceptibility Tests for Bacteria that Grow Aerobically—Third Edition. Approved Standard NCCLS Document M7-A3, Vol. 13, No. 25, NCCLS, Villanova, PA, December, 1993.

Literature revised January 13, 1998

PV 0709 AMP [011398]

CEFACLOR, *see* Ceclor® (Cefaclor, USP). ℞

CEFAMANDOLE NAFATE, *see* Mandol® (Cefamandole Nafate, USP). ℞

CEFAZOLIN SODIUM, *see* Kefzol® (Cefazolin Sodium, USP). ℞

CEFTAZIDIME, *see* Tazidime® (Ceftazidime, USP). ℞

CEFUROXIME SODIUM, *see* Kefurox® (Cefuroxime Sodium, USP). ℞

DARVOCET–N® 50 Ⓒ

[*dăr 'vō-sĕt ĕn*]

and

DARVOCET–N® 100

(propoxyphene napsylate and acetaminophen tablets, USP)

DESCRIPTION

Darvon-N® (Propoxyphene Napsylate, USP) is an odorless, white crystalline powder with a bitter taste. It is very slightly soluble in water and soluble in methanol, ethanol, chloroform, and acetone. Chemically, it is (αS,1R)-α-[2-(Dimethylamino) -1 -methylethyl]- α -phenylphenethyl propionate compound with 2-naphthalenesulfonic acid (1:1) monohydrate, which can be represented by the accompanying structural formula. Its molecular weight is 565.72.

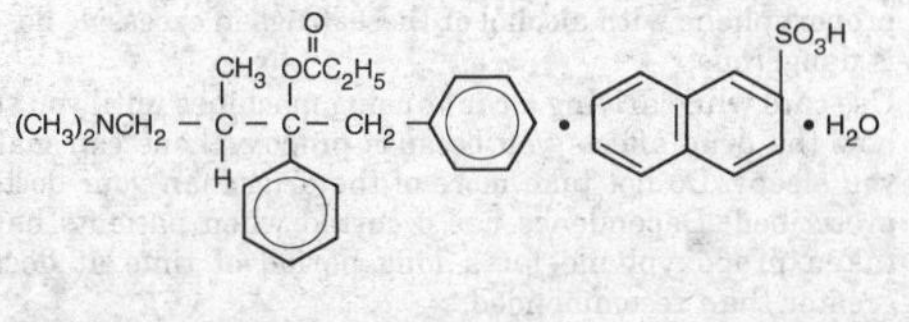

Propoxyphene napsylate differs from propoxyphene hydrochloride in that it allows more stable liquid dosage forms and tablet formulations. Because of differences in molecular weight, a dose of 100 mg (176.8 µmol) of propoxyphene napsylate is required to supply an amount of propoxyphene equivalent to that present in 65 mg (172.9 µmol) of propoxyphene hydrochloride.

Each tablet of Darvocet-N 50 contains 50 mg (88.4 µmol) propoxyphene napsylate and 325 mg (2,150 µmol) acetaminophen.

Each tablet of Darvocet-N 100 contains 100 mg (176.8 µmol) propopoxyphene napsylate and 650 mg (4,300 µmol) acetaminophen.

Each tablet also contains amberlite, cellulose, F D & C Yellow No. 6, magnesium stearate, stearic acid, titanium dioxide, and other inactive ingredients.

CLINICAL PHARMACOLOGY

Propoxyphene is a centrally acting narcotic analgesic agent. Equimolar doses of propoxyphene hydrochloride or napsylate provide similar plasma concentrations. Following administration of 65, 130, or 195 mg of propoxyphene hydrochloride, the bioavailability of propoxyphene is equivalent to that of 100, 200, or 300 mg respectively of propoxyphene napsylate. Peak plasma concentrations of propoxyphene are reached in 2 to 2 $^1/_2$ hours. After a 100-mg oral dose of propoxyphene napsylate, peak plasma levels of 0.05 to 0.1 µg/mL are achieved. As shown in Figure 1, the napsylate salt tends to be absorbed more slowly than the hydrochloride. At or near therapeutic doses, this absorption difference is small when compared with that among subjects and among doses.

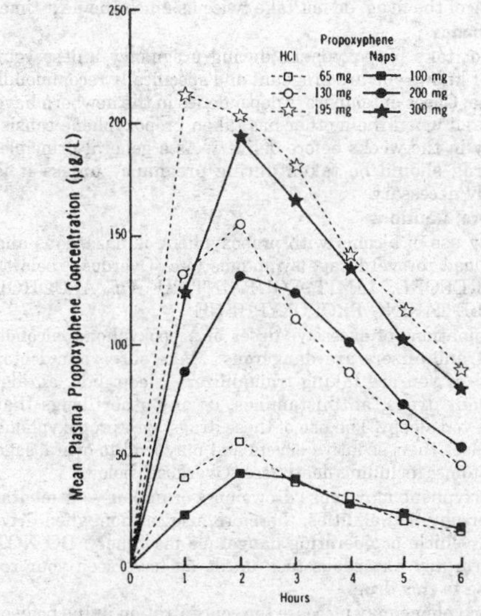

Figure 1. Mean plasma concentrations of propoxyphene in 8 human subjects following oral administration of 65 and 130 mg of the hydrochloride salt and 100 and 200 mg of the napsylate salt and in 7 given 195 mg of the hydrochloride and 300 mg of the napsylate salt.

Because of this several hundredfold difference in solubility, the absorption rate of very large doses of the napsylate salt is significantly lower than that of equimolar doses of the hydrochloride.

Repeated doses of propoxyphene at 6-hour intervals lead to increasing plasma concentrations, with a plateau after the ninth dose at 48 hours.

Propoxyphene is metabolized in the liver to yield norpropoxyphene. Propoxyphene has a half-life of 6 to 12 hours, whereas that of norpropoxyphene is 30 to 36 hours.

Norpropoxyphene has substantially less central-nervous-system-depressant effect than propoxyphene but a greater local anesthetic effect, which is similar to that of amitriptyline and antiarrhythmic agents, such as lidocaine and quinidine.

In animal studies in which propoxyphene and norpropoxyphene were continuously infused in large amounts, intracardiac conduction time (PR and QRS intervals) was prolonged. Any intracardiac conduction delay attributable to high concentrations of norpropoxyphene may be of relatively long duration.

ACTIONS

Propoxyphene is a mild narcotic analgesic structurally related to methadone. The potency of propoxyphene napsylate is from two-thirds to equal that of codeine.

Darvocet-N 50 and Darvocet-N 100 provide the analgesic activity of propoxyphene napsylate and the antipyretic-analgesic activity of acetaminophen.

The combination of propoxyphene and acetaminophen produces greater analgesia than that produced by either propoxyphene or acetaminophen administered alone.

INDICATION

These products are indicated for the relief of mild to moderate pain, either when pain is present alone or when it is accompanied by fever.

CONTRAINDICATIONS

Hypersensitivity to propoxyphene or acetaminophen

WARNINGS

- **Do not prescribe propoxyphene for patients who are suicidal or addiction-prone.**
- **Prescribe propoxyphene with caution for patients taking tranquilizers or antidepressant drugs and patients who use alcohol in excess.**
- **Tell your patients not to exceed the recommended dose and to limit their intake of alcohol.**

Propoxyphene products in excessive doses, either alone or in combination with other CNS depressants, including alcohol, are a major cause of drug-related deaths. Fatalities within the first hour of overdosage are not uncommon. In a survey of deaths due to overdosage conducted in 1975, in approximately 20% of the fatal cases, death occurred within the first hour (5% occurred within 15 minutes). Propoxyphene should not be taken in doses higher than those recommended by the physician. The judicious prescribing of propoxyphene is essential to the safe use of this drug. With patients who are depressed or suicidal, consideration should be given to the use of non-narcotic analgesics. Patients should be cautioned about the concomitant use of propoxyphene products and alcohol because of potentially serious CNS-additive effects of these agents. Because of its added depressant effects, propoxyphene should be prescribed with caution for those patients whose medical condition requires the concomitant administration of sedatives, tranquilizers, muscle relaxants, antidepressants, or other CNS-depressant drugs. Patients should be advised of the additive depressant effects of these combinations.

Many of the propoxyphene-related deaths have occurred in patients with previous histories of emotional disturbances or suicidal ideation or attempts as well as histories of misuse of tranquilizers, alcohol, and other CNS-active drugs. Some deaths have occurred as a consequence of the accidental ingestion of excessive quantities of propoxyphene alone or in combination with other drugs. Patients taking propoxyphene should be warned not to exceed the dosage recommended by the physician.

Drug Dependence —Propoxyphene, when taken in higher-than-recommended doses over long periods of time, can produce drug dependence characterized by psychic dependence and, less frequently, physical dependence and tolerance. Propoxyphene will only partially suppress the withdrawal syndrome in individuals physically dependent on morphine or other narcotics. The abuse liability of propoxyphene is qualitatively similar to that of codeine although quantitatively less, and propoxyphene should be prescribed with the same degree of caution appropriate to the use of codeine.

Usage in Ambulatory Patients —Propoxyphene may impair the mental and/or physical abilities required for the performance of potentially hazardous tasks, such as driving a car or operating machinery. The patient should be cautioned accordingly.

PRECAUTIONS

General —Propoxyphene should be administered with caution to patients with hepatic or renal impairment since higher serum concentrations or delayed elimination may occur.

Drug Interactions —The CNS-depressant effect of propoxyphene is additive with that of other CNS depressants, including alcohol.

As is the case with many medicinal agents, propoxyphene may slow the metabolism of a concomitantly administered drug. Should this occur, the higher serum concentrations of that drug may result in increased pharmacologic or adverse effects of that drug. Such occurrences have been reported when propoxyphene was administered to patients on antidepressants, anticonvulsants, or warfarin-like drugs. Severe neurologic signs, including coma, have occurred with concurrent use of carbamazepine.

Usage in Pregnancy —Safe use in pregnancy has not been established relative to possible adverse effects on fetal development. Instances of withdrawal symptoms in the neonate have been reported following usage during pregnancy. Therefore, propoxyphene should not be used in pregnant women unless, in the judgment of the physician, the potential benefits outweigh the possible hazards.

Usage in Nursing Mothers —Low levels of propoxyphene have been detected in human milk. In postpartum studies involving nursing mothers who were given propoxyphene, no adverse effects were noted in infants receiving mother's milk.

Usage in Pediatric Patients —Safety and effectiveness in pediatric patients have not been established.

Usage in the Elderly —The rate of propoxyphene metabolism may be reduced in some patients. Increased dosing interval should be considered.

A Patient Information Sheet is available for this product. See text following "How Supplied" section below.

ADVERSE REACTIONS

In a survey conducted in hospitalized patients, less than 1% of patients taking propoxyphene hydrochloride at recommended doses experienced side effects. The most frequently reported were dizziness, sedation, nausea, and vomiting. Some of these adverse reactions may be alleviated if the patient lies down.

Other adverse reactions include constipation, abdominal pain, skin rashes, lightheadedness, headache, weakness, euphoria, dysphoria, hallucinations, and minor visual disturbances.

Liver dysfunction has been reported in association with both active components of Darvocet-N 50 and Darvocet-N 100. Propoxyphene therapy has been associated with abnormal liver function tests and, more rarely, with instances of reversible jaundice (including cholestatic jaundice). Hepatic necrosis may result from acute overdose of acetaminophen (*see* Management of Overdosage). In chronic ethanol abusers, this has been reported rarely with short-term use of acetaminophen dosages of 2.5 to 10 g/day. Fatalities have occurred.

Renal papillary necrosis may result from chronic acetaminophen use, particularly when the dosage is greater than recommended and when combined with aspirin.

Subacute painful myopathy has occurred following chronic propoxyphene overdosage.

DOSAGE AND ADMINISTRATION

These products are given orally. The usual dosage is 100 mg propoxyphene napsylate and 650 mg acetaminophen every 4 hours as needed for pain. The maximum recommended dose of propoxyphene napsylate is 600 mg per day.

Consideration should be given to a reduced total daily dosage in patients with hepatic or renal impairment.

MANAGEMENT OF OVERDOSAGE

In all cases of suspected overdosage, call your regional Poison Control Center to obtain the most up-to-date information about the treatment of overdose. This recommendation is made because, in general, information regarding the treatment of overdosage may change more rapidly than do package inserts.

Initial consideration should be given to the management of the CNS effects of propoxyphene overdosage. Resuscitative measures should be initiated promptly.

Symptoms of Propoxyphene Overdosage —The manifestations of acute overdosage with propoxyphene are those of narcotic overdosage. The patient is usually somnolent but may be stuporous or comatose and convulsing. Respiratory depression is characteristic. The ventilatory rate and/or tidal volume is decreased, which results in cyanosis and hypoxia. Pupils, initially pinpoint, may become dilated as hypoxia increases. Cheyne-Stokes respiration and apnea may occur. Blood pressure and heart rate are usually normal initially, but blood pressure falls and cardiac performance deteriorates, which ultimately results in pulmonary

Continued on next page

*** Identi-Code® symbol. This product information was prepared in June 1998. Current information on these and other products of Eli Lilly and Company may be obtained by direct inquiry to Lilly Research Laboratories, Lilly Corporate Center, Indianapolis, Indiana 46285, (800) 545-5979.**

Darvocet N—Cont.

edema and circulatory collapse, unless the respiratory depression is corrected and adequate ventilation is restored promptly. Cardiac arrhythmias and conduction delay may be present. A combined respiratory-metabolic acidosis occurs owing to retained CO_2 (hypercapnia) and to lactic acid formed during anaerobic glycolysis. Acidosis may be severe if large amounts of salicylates have also been ingested. Death may occur.

Treatment of Propoxyphene Overdosage — Attention should be directed first to establishing a patent airway and to restoring ventilation. Mechanically assisted ventilation, with or without oxygen, may be required, and positive pressure respiration may be desirable if pulmonary edema is present. The narcotic antagonist naloxone will markedly reduce the degree of respiratory depression, and 0.4 to 2 mg should be administered promptly, preferably intravenously. If the desired degree of counteraction with improvement in respiratory functions is not obtained, naloxone should be repeated at 2- to 3-minute intervals. The duration of action of the antagonist may be brief. If no response is observed after 10 mg of naloxone have been administered, the diagnosis of propoxyphene toxicity should be questioned. Naloxone may also be administered by continuous intravenous infusion.

Treatment of Propoxyphene Overdosage in Pediatric Patients —The usual initial dose of naloxone in pediatric patients is 0.01 mg/kg body weight given intravenously. If this dose does not result in the desired degree of clinical improvement, a subsequent increased dose of 0.1 mg/kg body weight may be administered. If an IV route of administration is not available, naloxone may be administered IM or subcutaneously in divided doses. If necessary, naloxone can be diluted with Sterile Water for Injection.

Blood gases, pH, and electrolytes should be monitored in order that acidosis and any electrolyte disturbance present may be corrected promptly. Acidosis, hypoxia, and generalized CNS depression predispose to the development of cardiac arrhythmias. Ventricular fibrillation or cardiac arrest may occur and necessitate the full complement of cardiopulmonary resuscitation (CPR) measures. Respiratory acidosis rapidly subsides as ventilation is restored and hypercapnia eliminated, but lactic acidosis may require intravenous bicarbonate for prompt correction.

Electrocardiographic monitoring is essential. Prompt correction of hypoxia, acidosis, and electrolyte disturbance (when present) will help prevent these cardiac complications and will increase the effectiveness of agents administered to restore normal cardiac function.

In addition to the use of a narcotic antagonist, the patient may require careful titration with an anticonvulsant to control convulsions. Analeptic drugs (for example, caffeine or amphetamine) should not be used because of their tendency to precipitate convulsions.

General supportive measures, in addition to oxygen, include, when necessary, intravenous fluids, vasopressor-inotropic compounds, and, when infection is likely, anti-infective agents. Gastric lavage may be useful, and activated charcoal can adsorb a significant amount of ingested propoxyphene. Dialysis is of little value in poisoning due to propoxyphene. Efforts should be made to determine whether other agents, such as alcohol, barbiturates, tranquilizers, or other CNS depressants, were also ingested, since these increase CNS depression as well as cause specific toxic effects.

Symptoms of Acetaminophen Overdosage — Shortly after oral ingestion of an overdose of acetaminophen and for the next 24 hours, anorexia, nausea, vomiting, diaphoresis, general malaise, and abdominal pain have been noted. The patient may then present no symptoms, but evidence of liver dysfunction may become apparent up to 72 hours after ingestion, with elevated serum transaminase and lactic dehydrogenase levels, an increase in serum bilirubin concentrations, and a prolonged prothrombin time. Death from hepatic failure may result 3 to 7 days after overdosage.

Acute renal failure may accompany the hepatic dysfunction and has been noted in patients who do not exhibit signs of fulminant hepatic failure. Typically, renal impairment is more apparent 6 to 9 days after ingestion of the overdose.

Treatment of Acetaminophen Overdosage —Acetaminophen in massive overdosage may cause hepatic toxicity in some patients. *In all cases of suspected overdose, immediately call your regional poison center or the Rocky Mountain Poison Center's toll-free number* (800-525-6115) for assistance in diagnosis and for directions in the use of N-acetylcysteine as an antidote.

In adults, hepatic toxicity has rarely been reported with acute overdoses of less than 10 g and fatalities with less than 15 g. Importantly, young children seem to be more resistant than adults to the hepatotoxic effect of an acetaminophen overdose. Despite this, the measures outlined below should be initiated in any adult or pediatric patient suspected of having ingested an acetaminophen overdose.

Because clinical and laboratory evidence of hepatic toxicity may not be apparent until 48 to 72 hours postingestion, liver function studies should be obtained initially and repeated at 24-hour intervals.

Consider emptying the stomach promptly by lavage or by induction of emesis with syrup of ipecac. Patients' estimates of the quantity of a drug ingested are notoriously unreliable. Therefore, if an acetaminophen overdose is suspected, a serum acetaminophen assay should be obtained as early as possible, but no sooner than 4 hours following ingestion. The antidote, N-acetylcysteine, should be administered as early as possible, and within 16 hours of the overdose ingestion for optimal results. Following recovery, there are no residual, structural, or functional hepatic abnormalities.

ANIMAL TOXICOLOGY

The acute lethal doses of the hydrochloride and napsylate salts of propoxyphene were determined in 4 species. The results shown in Figure 2 indicate that, on a molar basis, the napsylate salt is less toxic than the hydrochloride. This may be due to the relative insolubility and retarded absorption of propoxyphene napsylate.

Figure 2. Acute oral toxicity of propoxyphene

$\frac{LD_{50}\ (mg/kg) \pm SE}{LD_{50}\ (mmol/kg)}$

Species	Propoxyphene Hydrochloride	Propoxyphene Napsylate
Mouse	282 ± 39 / 0.75	915 ± 163 / 1.62
Rat	230 ± 44 / 0.61	647 ± 95 / 1.14
Rabbit	*ca*82 / 0.22	>183 / >0.32
Dog	*ca* 100 / 0.27	>183 / >0.32

Some indication of the relative insolubility and retarded absorption of propoxyphene napsylate was obtained by measuring plasma propoxyphene levels in 2 groups of 4 dogs following oral administration of equimolar doses of the 2 salts. As shown in Figure 3, the peak plasma concentration observed with propoxyphene hydrochloride was much higher than that obtained after administration of the napsylate salt.

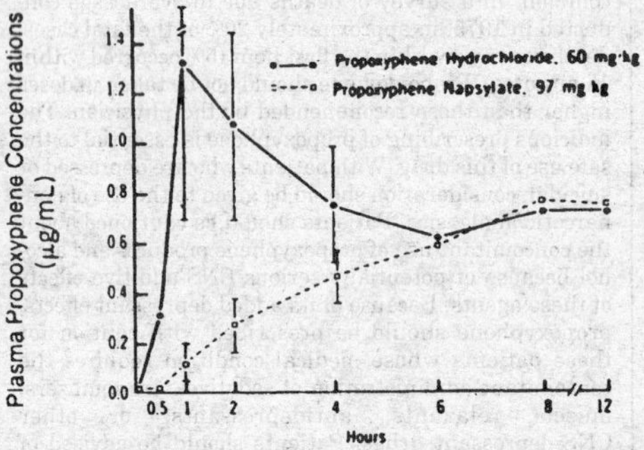

Figure 3. Plasma propoxyphene concentrations in dogs following large doses of the hydrochloride and napsylate salts.

Although none of the animals in this experiment died, 3 of the 4 dogs given propoxyphene hydrochloride exhibited convulsive seizures during the time interval corresponding to the peak plasma levels. The 4 animals receiving the napsylate salt were mildly ataxic but not acutely ill.

HOW SUPPLIED

Darvocet-N® Tablets (No. 1890) are available in:

The 50 mg tablets are dark orange, capsule shaped, film coated, and imprinted with the script "Lilly" and "Darvocet-N 50" on one side of the tablet, using edible black ink. They are available as follows:

Bottles of 100 (RxPak*)	NDC 0002-0351-02 (TA1890)

Darvocet-N® Tablets (No. 1893) are available in:

The 100 mg tablets are dark orange, capsule shaped, film coated, and imprinted with the script "Lilly" on one side and "Darvocet-N 100" on the other side of the tablet, using edible black ink. They are available as follows:

Bottles of 100 (RxPak*)	NDC 0002-0363-02 (TA1893)
Bottles of 500	NDC 0002-0363-03 (TA1893)
ID† 100	NDC 0002-0363-33 (TA1893)
ID† 500	NDC 0002-0363-43 (TA1893)
RN‡ 500	NDC 0002-0363-46 (TA1893)

* All RxPaks (prescription packages, Lilly) have safety closures.
† Identi-Dose® (unit dose medication, Lilly).
‡ Reverse-numbered package.

Store at controlled room temperature, 59° to 86°F (15° to 30°C).

CAUTION — Federal (USA) law prohibits dispensing without prescription.

The following information, including description of dosage forms and the maximum daily dosage of each, is available to patients receiving Darvon products.

Patient Information Sheet

YOUR PRESCRIPTION FOR A DARVON® (PROPOXYPHENE) PRODUCT ©IV

Summary

Products containing Darvon are used to relieve pain.

LIMIT YOUR INTAKE OF ALCOHOL WHILE TAKING THIS DRUG. Make sure your doctor knows if you are taking tranquilizers, sleep aids, antidepressants, antihistamines, or any other drugs that make you sleepy. Combining propoxyphene with alcohol or these drugs in excessive doses is dangerous.

Use care while driving a car or using machines until you see how the drug affects you because propoxyphene can make you sleepy. Do not take more of the drug than your doctor prescribed. Dependence has occurred when patients have taken propoxyphene for a long period of time at doses greater than recommended.

The rest of this leaflet gives you more information about propoxyphene. Please read it and keep it for future use.

Uses of Darvon

Products containing Darvon are used for the relief of mild to moderate pain. Products that contain Darvon plus aspirin or acetaminophen are prescribed for the relief of pain or pain associated with fever.

Before Taking Darvon

Make sure your doctor knows if you have ever had an allergic reaction to propoxyphene, aspirin, or acetaminophen. Some forms of propoxyphene products contain aspirin to help relieve the pain. Your doctor should be advised if you have a history of ulcers or if your are taking an anticoagulant ("blood thinner"). The aspirin may irritate the stomach lining and may cause bleeding, particularly if an ulcer is present. Also, bleeding may occur if you are taking an anticoagulant. In a small group of people, aspirin may cause an asthma attack. If you are one of these people, be sure your drug does not contain aspirin.

The effect of propoxyphene in pediatric patients under 12 has not been studied. Therefore, use of the drug in this age group is not recommended.

Also, due to the possible association between aspirin and Reye Syndrome, those propoxyphene products containing aspirin should not be given to children, including teenagers, with chicken pox or flu unless prescribed by a physician.

The following propoxyphene product contains aspirin:

Darvon® Compound-65 (Propoxyphene Hydrochloride, Aspirin, and Caffeine, USP)

How to Take Darvon

Follow your doctor's directions exactly. Do not increase the amount you take without your doctor's approval. If you miss a dose of the drug, do not take twice as much the next time.

Pregnancy

Do not take propoxyphene during pregnancy unless your doctor knows you are pregnant and specifically recommends its use. Cases of temporary dependence in the newborn have occurred when the mother has taken propoxyphene consistently in the weeks before delivery. As a general principle, no drug should be taken during pregnancy unless it is clearly necessary.

General Cautions

Heavy use of alcohol with propoxyphene is hazardous and may lead to overdosage symptoms (*see* "Overdose" below). THEREFORE, LIMIT YOUR INTAKE OF ALCOHOL WHILE TAKING PROPOXYPHENE.

Combinations of excessive doses of propoxyphene, alcohol, and tranquilizers are dangerous. Make sure your doctor knows if you are taking tranquilizers, sleep aids, antidepressant drugs, antihistamines, or any other drugs that make you sleepy. The use of these drugs with propoxyphene increases their sedative effects and may lead to overdosage symptoms, including death (*see* "Overdose" below).

Propoxyphene may cause drowsiness or impair your mental and/or physical abilities; therefore, use caution when driving a vehicle or operating dangerous machinery. DO NOT perform any hazardous task until you have seen your response to this drug.

Propoxyphene may increase the concentration in the body of medications, such as anticoagulants ("blood thinners"), antidepressants, or drugs used for epilepsy. The result may be excessive or adverse effects of these medications. Make sure your doctor knows if you are taking any of these medications.

Dependence

You can become dependent on propoxyphene if you take it in higher than recommended doses over a long period of time. Dependence is a feeling of need for the drug and a feeling that you cannot perform normally without it.

Overdose

An overdose of Darvon, alone or in combination with other drugs, including alcohol, may cause weakness, difficulty in breathing, confusion, anxiety, and more severe drowsiness and dizziness. Extreme overdosage may lead to unconsciousness and death.

If the propoxyphene product contains acetaminophen, the overdosage symptoms include nausea, vomiting, lack of appetite, and abdominal pain. Liver damage may occur even after symptoms disappear. Death can occur days later.

When the propoxyphene product contains aspirin, symptoms of taking too much of the drug are headache, dizziness, ringing in the ears, difficulty in hearing, dim vision, confusion, drowsiness, sweating, thirst, rapid breathing, nausea, vomiting, and, occasionally, diarrhea.

In any suspected overdosage situation, contact your doctor or nearest hospital emergency room. GET EMERGENCY HELP IMMEDIATELY.

KEEP THIS DRUG AND ALL DRUGS OUT OF THE REACH OF THE PEDIATRIC POPULATION.

Possible Side Effects

When propoxyphene is taken as directed, side effects are infrequent. Among those reported are drowsiness, dizziness, nausea, and vomiting. If these effects occur, it may help if you lie down and rest.

Less frequently reported side effects are constipation, abdominal pain, skin rashes, lightheadedness, headache, weakness, hallucinations, minor visual disturbances, and feelings of elation or discomfort.

If side effects occur and concern you, contact your doctor.

Other Information

The safe and effective use of propoxyphene depends on your taking it exactly as directed. This drug has been prescribed specifically for you and your present condition. Do not give this drug to others who may have similar symptoms. Do not use it for any other reason.

If you would like more information about propoxyphene, ask your doctor or pharmacist. They have a more technical leaflet (professional labeling) you may read.

Selected Darvon Products

Maximum Daily Dosage		
6	Dark Orange, Capsule Shaped, Film Coated Tablets Imprinted with Script "Lilly" on the one side and "Darvocet-N 100" on the other, using edible black ink	DARVOCET-N® 100 CIV Propoxyphene Napsylate and Acetaminophen Tablets
6	Parobolic-Shaped Capsules Imprinted with Script "Lilly" and "3111" on the opaque gray cap and "Darvon Comp 65" on the opaque red body, using edible black ink	DARVON® COMPOUND-65 CIV Propoxyphene Hydrochloride, Aspirin, and Caffeine Pulvules®
6	Parabolic-Shaped Capsules Imprinted with Script "Lilly" and "H03" on the opaque pink cap and "Darvon" on the opaque pink body, using edible black ink	DARVON® CIV Propoxyphene Hydrochloride Pulvules, 65 mg

Literature revised November 11, 1997

RV1517AMP [111197]

Shown in Product Identification Guide, page 320

DARVON® CIV

[där 'von]

(propoxyphene hydrochloride)

Capsules, USP

DESCRIPTION

Darvon® (Propoxyphene Hydrochloride, USP) is an odorless, white crystalline powder with a bitter taste. It is freely soluble in water. Chemically, it is (*2S, 3R*)-(+)-4-(Dimethylamino)-3-methyl-1,2-diphenyl-2-butanol propionate (ester) hydrochloride, which can be represented by the accompanying structural formula. Its molecular weight is 375.94.

[See chemical structure at top of next column]

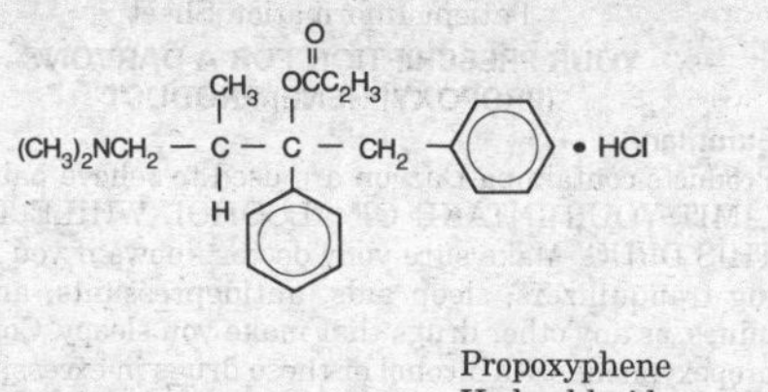

Propoxyphene Hydrochloride

Each Pulvule® contains 65 mg (172.9 µmol) propoxyphene hydrochloride. It also contains D & C Red No. 33, F D & C Yellow No. 6, gelatin, magnesium stearate, silicone, starch, titanium dioxide, and other inactive ingredients.

CLINICAL PHARMACOLOGY

Propoxyphene is a centrally acting narcotic analgesic agent. Equimolar doses of propoxyphene hydrochloride or napsylate provide similar plasma concentrations. Following administration of 65, 130, or 195 mg of propoxyphene hydrochloride, the bioavailability of propoxyphene is equivalent to that of 100, 200, or 300 mg respectively of propoxyphene napsylate. Peak plasma concentrations of propoxyphene are reached in 2 to 2 $^1/_2$ hours. After a 65-mg oral dose of propoxyphene hydrochloride, peak plasma levels of 0.05 to 0.1 µg/mL are achieved.

Repeated doses of propoxyphene at 6-hour intervals lead to increasing plasma concentrations, with a plateau after the ninth dose at 48 hours.

Propoxyphene is metabolized in the liver to yield norpropoxyphene. Propoxyphene has a half-life of 6 to 12 hours, whereas that of norpropoxyphene is 30 to 36 hours.

Norpropoxyphene has substantially less central-nervous-system-depressant effect than propoxyphene but a greater local anesthetic effect, which is similar to that of amitriptyline and antiarrhythmic agents, such as lidocaine and quinidine.

In animal studies in which propoxyphene and norpropoxyphene were continuously infused in large amounts, intracardiac conduction time (PR and QRS intervals) was prolonged. Any intracardiac conduction delay attributable to high concentrations of norpropoxyphene may be of relatively long duration.

ACTIONS

Propoxyphene is a mild narcotic analgesic structurally related to methadone. The potency of propoxyphene hydrochloride is from two-thirds to equal that of codeine.

The combination of propoxyphene with a mixture of aspirin and caffeine produces greater analgesia than that produced by either propoxyphene or aspirin and caffeine administered alone.

INDICATION

For the relief of mild to moderate pain.

CONTRAINDICATION

Hypersensitivity to propoxyphene.

WARNINGS

- **Do not prescribe propoxyphene for patients who are suicidal or addiction-prone.**
- **Prescribe propoxyphene with caution for patients taking tranquilizers or antidepressant drugs and patients who use alcohol in excess.**
- **Tell your patients not to exceed the recommended dose and to limit their intake of alcohol.**

Propoxyphene products in excessive doses, either alone or in combination with other CNS depressants, including alcohol, are a major cause of drug-related deaths. Fatalities within the first hour of overdosage are not uncommon. In a survey of deaths due to overdosage conducted in 1975, in approximately 20% of the fatal cases, death occurred within the first hour (5% occurred within 15 minutes). Propoxyphene should not be taken in doses higher than those recommended by the physician. The judicious prescribing of propoxyphene is essential to the safe use of this drug. With patients who are depressed or suicidal, consideration should be given to the use of non-narcotic analgesics. Patients should be cautioned about the concomitant use of propoxyphene products and alcohol because of potentially serious CNS-additive effects of these agents. Because of its added depressant effects, propoxyphene should be prescribed with caution for those patients whose medical condition requires the concomitant administration of sedatives, tranquilizers, muscle relaxants, antidepressants, or other CNS-depressant drugs. Patients should be advised of the additive depressant effects of these combinations.

Many of the propoxyphene-related deaths have occurred in patients with previous histories of emotional disturbances or suicidal ideation or attempts as well as histories of misuse of tranquilizers, alcohol, and other CNS-active drugs. Some deaths have occurred as a consequence of the accidental ingestion of excessive quantities of propoxyphene alone or in combination with other drugs. Patients taking propoxyphene should be warned not to exceed the dosage recommended by the physician.

Drug Dependence —Propoxyphene, when taken in higher-than-recommended doses over long periods of time, can produce drug dependence characterized by psychic dependence and, less frequently, physical dependence and tolerance. Propoxyphene will only partially suppress the withdrawal syndrome in individuals physically dependent on morphine or other narcotics. The abuse liability of propoxyphene is qualitatively similar to that of codeine although quantitatively less, and propoxyphene should be prescribed with the same degree of caution appropriate to the use of codeine.

Usage in Ambulatory Patients —Propoxyphene may impair the mental and/or physical abilities required for the performance of potentially hazardous tasks, such as driving a car or operating machinery. The patient should be cautioned accordingly.

PRECAUTIONS

General —Propoxyphene should be administered with caution to patients with hepatic or renal impairment since higher serum concentrations or delayed elimination may occur.

Drug Interactions —The CNS-depressant effect of propoxyphene is additive with that of other CNS depressants, including alcohol.

As is the case with medicinal agents, propoxyphene may slow the metabolism of a concomitantly administered drug. Should this occur, the higher serum concentrations of that drug may result in increased pharmacologic or adverse effects of that drug. Such occurrences have been reported when propoxyphene was administered to patients on antidepressants, anticonvulsants, or warfarin-like drugs. Severe neurologic signs, including coma, have occurred with concurrent use of carbamazepine.

Usage in Pregnancy —Safe use in pregnancy has not been established relative to possible adverse effects on fetal development. Instances of withdrawal symptoms in the neonate have been reported following usage during pregnancy. Therefore, propoxyphene should not be used in pregnant women unless, in the judgment of the physician, the potential benefits outweigh the possible hazards.

Usage in Nursing Mothers —Low levels of propoxyphene have been detected in human milk. In postpartum studies involving nursing mothers who were given propoxyphene, no adverse effects were noted in infants receiving mother's milk.

Usage in Pediatric Patients —Safety and effectiveness in pediatric patients have not been established.

Usage in the Elderly —The rate of propoxyphene metabolism may be reduced in some patients. Increased dosing interval should be considered.

A Patient Information Sheet is available for this product. See text following "How Supplied" section below.

ADVERSE REACTIONS

In a survey conducted in hospitalized patients, less than 1% of patients taking propoxyphene hydrochloride at recommended doses experienced side effects. The most frequently reported were dizziness, sedation, nausea, and vomiting. Some of these adverse reactions may be alleviated if the patient lies down.

Other adverse reactions include constipation, abdominal pain, skin rashes, lightheadedness, headache, weakness, euphoria, dysphoria, hallucinations, and minor visual disturbances.

Propoxyphene therapy has been associated with abnormal liver function tests and, more rarely, with instances of reversible jaundice (including cholestatic jaundice).

Subacute painful myopathy has occurred following chronic propoxyphene overdosage.

DOSAGE AND ADMINISTRATION

Darvon is given orally. The usual dosage is 65 mg propoxyphene hydrochloride every 4 hours as needed for pain. The maximum recommended dose of propoxyphene hydrochloride is 390 mg/day.

Consideration should be given to a reduced total daily dosage in patients with hepatic or renal impairment.

MANAGEMENT OF OVERDOSAGE

In all cases of suspected overdosage, call your regional Poison Control Center to obtain the most up-to-date information about the treatment of overdose. This recommendation is made because, in general, information regarding the treatment of overdosage may change more rapidly than do package inserts.

Initial consideration should be given to the management of the CNS effects of propoxyphene overdosage. Resuscitative measures should be initiated promptly.

Continued on next page

*** Identi-Code® symbol. This product information was prepared in June 1998. Current information on these and other products of Eli Lilly and Company may be obtained by direct inquiry to Lilly Research Laboratories, Lilly Corporate Center, Indianapolis, Indiana 46285, (800) 545-5979.**

Darvon—Cont.

Symptoms of Propoxyphene Overdosage—The manifestations of acute overdosage with propoxyphene are those of narcotic overdosage. The patient is usually somnolent but may be stuporous or comatose and convulsing. Respiratory depression is characteristic. The ventilatory rate and/or tidal volume is decreased, which results in cyanosis and hypoxia. Pupils, initially pinpoint, may become dilated as hypoxia increases. Cheyne-Stokes respiration and apnea may occur. Blood pressure and heart rate are usually normal initially, but blood pressure falls and cardiac performance deteriorates, which ultimately results in pulmonary edema and circulatory collapse, unless the respiratory depression is corrected and adequate ventilation is restored promptly. Cardiac arrhythmias and conduction delay may be present. A combined respiratory-metabolic acidosis occurs owing to retained CO_2 (hypercapnia) and to lactic acid formed during anaerobic glycolysis. Acidosis may be severe if large amounts of salicylates have also been ingested. Death may occur.

Treatment of Propoxyphene Overdosage—Attention should be directed first to establishing a patent airway and to restoring ventilation. Mechanically assisted ventilation, with or without oxygen, may be required, and positive pressure respiration may be desirable if pulmonary edema is present. The narcotic antagonist naloxone will markedly reduce the degree of respiratory depression, and 0.4 to 2 mg should be administered promptly, preferably intravenously. If the desired degree of counteraction with improvement in respiratory functions is not obtained, naloxone should be repeated at 2- to 3-minute intervals. The duration of action of the antagonist may be brief. If no response is observed after 10 mg of naloxone have been administered, the diagnosis of propoxyphene toxicity should be questioned. Naloxone may also be administered by continuous intravenous infusion.

Treatment of Propoxyphene Overdosage in Pediatric Patients—The usual initial dose of naloxone in pediatric patients is 0.01 mg/kg body weight given intravenously. If this dose does not result in the desired degree of clinical improvement, a subsequent increased dose of 0.1 mg/kg body weight may be administered. If an IV route of administration is not available, naloxone may be administered IM or subcutaneously in divided doses. If necessary, naloxone can be diluted with Sterile Water for Injection.

Blood gases, pH, and electrolytes should be monitored in order that acidosis and any electrolyte disturbance present may be corrected promptly. Acidosis, hypoxia, and generalized CNS depression predispose to the development of cardiac arrhythmias. Ventricular fibrillation or cardiac arrest may occur and necessitate the full complement of cardiopulmonary resuscitation (CPR) measures. Respiratory acidosis rapidly subsides as ventilation is restored and hypercapnia eliminated, but lactic acidosis may require intravenous bicarbonate for prompt correction.

Electrocardiographic monitoring is essential. Prompt correction of hypoxia, acidosis, and electrolyte disturbance (when present) will help prevent these cardiac complications and will increase the effectiveness of agents administered to restore normal cardiac function.

In addition to the use of a narcotic antagonist, the patient may require careful titration with an anticonvulsant to control convulsions. Analeptic drugs (for example, caffeine or amphetamine) should not be used because of their tendency to precipitate convulsions.

General supportive measures, in addition to oxygen, include, when necessary, intravenous fluids, vasopressor-inotropic compounds, and, when infection is likely, anti-infective agents. Gastric lavage may be useful and activated charcoal can adsorb a significant amount of ingested propoxyphene. Dialysis is of little value in poisoning due to propoxyphene. Efforts should be made to determine whether other agents, such as alcohol, barbiturates, tranquilizers, or other CNS depressants, were also ingested, since these increase CNS depression as well as cause specific toxic effects.

HOW SUPPLIED

Darvon® Pulvules® (No. 365) are available in:

The 65 mg parabolic-shaped capsules are imprinted with the script "Lilly" and "H03" on the opaque pink cap and "Darvon" on the opaque pink body, using edible black ink. They are available as follows:

Bottles of 100 (RxPak*)	NDC 0002-0803-02 (PU0365)
Bottles of 500	NDC 0002-0803-03 (PU0365)
ID†100	NDC 0002-0803-33 (PU0365)

* All RxPaks (prescription packages, Lilly) have safety closures.

† Identi-Dose® (unit dose medication, Lilly)

Store at controlled room temperature, 59° to 86°F (15° to 30°C).

CAUTION—Federal (USA) law prohibits dispensing without prescription.

The following information, including description of dosage forms and the maximum daily dosage of each, is available to patients receiving Darvon products.

Patient Information Sheet

YOUR PRESCRIPTION FOR A DARVON® (PROPOXYPHENE) PRODUCT

Summary

Products containing Darvon are used to relieve pain.

LIMIT YOUR INTAKE OF ALCOHOL WHILE TAKING THIS DRUG. Make sure your doctor knows if you are taking tranquilizers, sleep aids, antidepressants, antihistamines, or any other drugs that make you sleepy. Combining propoxyphene with alcohol or these drugs in excessive doses is dangerous.

Use care while driving a car or using machines until you see how the drug affects you because propoxyphene can make you sleepy. Do not take more of the drug than your doctor prescribed. Dependence has occurred when patients have taken propoxyphene for a long period of time at doses greater than recommended.

The rest of this leaflet gives you more information about propoxyphene. Please read it and keep it for future use.

Uses of Darvon

Products containing Darvon are used for the relief of mild to moderate pain. Products that contain Darvon plus aspirin or acetaminophen are prescribed for the relief of pain or pain associated with fever.

Before Taking Darvon

Make sure your doctor knows if you have ever had an allergic reaction to propoxyphene, aspirin, or acetaminophen. Some forms of propoxyphene products contain aspirin to help relieve the pain. Your doctor should be advised if you have a history of ulcers or if you are taking an anticoagulant ("blood thinner"). The aspirin may irritate the stomach lining and may cause bleeding, particularly if an ulcer is present. Also, bleeding may occur if you are taking an anticoagulant. In a small group of people, aspirin may cause an asthma attack. If you are one of these people, be sure your drug does not contain aspirin.

The effect of propoxyphene in pediatric patients under 12 has not been studied. Therefore, use of the drug in this age group is not recommended.

Also, due to the possible association between aspirin and Reye Syndrome, those propoxyphene products containing aspirin should not be given to children, including teenagers, with chicken pox or flu unless prescribed by a physician.

The following propoxyphene product contains aspirin: Darvon® Compound-65 (Propoxyphene Hydrochloride, Aspirin, and Caffeine, USP)

How to Take Darvon

Follow your doctor's directions exactly. Do not increase the amount you take without your doctor's approval. If you miss a dose of the drug, do not take twice as much the next time.

Pregnancy

Do not take propoxyphene during pregnancy unless your doctor knows you are pregnant and specifically recommends its use. Cases of temporary dependence in the newborn have occurred when the mother has taken propoxyphene consistently in the weeks before delivery. As a general principle, no drug should be taken during pregnancy unless it is clearly necessary.

General Cautions

Heavy use of alcohol with propoxyphene is hazardous and may lead to overdosage symptoms (*see* "Overdose" below). THEREFORE, LIMIT YOUR INTAKE OF ALCOHOL WHILE TAKING PROPOXYPHENE.

Combinations of excessive doses of propoxyphene, alcohol, and tranquilizers are dangerous. Make sure your doctor knows if you are taking tranquilizers, sleep aids, antidepressant drugs, antihistamines, or any other drugs that make you sleepy. The use of these drugs with propoxyphene increases their sedative effects and may lead to overdosage symptoms, including death (*see* "Overdose" below).

Propoxyphene may cause drowsiness or impair your mental and/or physical abilities; therefore, use caution when driving a vehicle or operating dangerous machinery. DO NOT perform any hazardous task until you have seen your response to this drug.

Propoxyphene may increase the concentration in the body of medications such as anticoagulants ("blood thinners"), antidepressants, or drugs used for epilepsy. The result may be excessive or adverse effects of these medications. Make sure your doctor knows if you are taking any of these medications.

Dependence

You can become dependent on propoxyphene if you take it in higher than recommended doses over a long period of time. Dependence is a feeling of need for the drug and a feeling that you cannot perform normally without it.

Overdose

An overdose of Darvon, alone or in combination with other drugs, including alcohol, may cause weakness, difficulty in breathing, confusion, anxiety, and more severe drowsiness and dizziness. Extreme overdosage may lead to unconsciousness and death.

If the propoxyphene product contains acetaminophen, the overdosage symptoms include nausea, vomiting, lack of appetite, and abdominal pain. Liver damage may occur.

When the propoxyphene product contains aspirin, symptoms of taking too much of the drug are headache, dizziness, ringing in the ears, difficulty in hearing, dim vision, confusion, drowsiness, sweating, thirst, rapid breathing, nausea, vomiting, and, occasionally, diarrhea.

In any suspected overdosage situation, contact your doctor or nearest hospital emergency room. GET EMERGENCY HELP IMMEDIATELY.

KEEP THIS DRUG AND ALL DRUGS OUT OF THE REACH OF THE PEDIATRIC POPULATION.

Possible Side Effects

When propoxyphene is taken as directed, side effects are infrequent. Among those reported are drowsiness, dizziness, nausea, and vomiting. If these effects occur, it may help if you lie down and rest.

Less frequently reported side effects are constipation, abdominal pain, skin rashes, lightheadedness, headache, weakness, hallucinations, minor visual disturbances, and feelings of elation or discomfort.

If side effects occur and concern you, contact your doctor.

Other Information

The safe and effective use of propoxyphene depends on your taking it exactly as directed. This drug has been prescribed specifically for you and your present condition. Do not give this drug to others who may have similar symptoms. Do not use it for any other reason.

If you would like more information about propoxyphene, ask your doctor or pharmacist. They have a more technical leaflet (professional labeling) you may read.

Selected Darvon Products

Maximum Daily Dosage		
6	Dark Orange, Capsule Shaped, Film Coated Tablets Imprinted with Script "Lilly" on the one side and "Darvocet-N 100" on the other, using edible black ink	DARVOCET-N® 100 CIV Propoxyphene Napsylate and Acetaminophen Tablets
6	Parabolic-Shaped Capsules Imprinted with Script "Lilly" and "3111" on the opaque gray cap and "Darvon Comp 65" on the opaque red body, using edible black ink	DARVON® COMPOUND-65 CIV Propoxyphene Hydrochloride, Aspirin, and Caffeine Pulvules®
6	Parabolic-Shaped Capsules Imprinted with Script "Lilly" and "H03" on the opaque pink cap and "Darvon" on the opaque pink body, using edible black ink	DARVON® CIV Propoxyphene Hydrochloride Pulvules, 65 mg

Literature issued January 27, 1997

PV 3000 AMP [012797]

DARVON® COMPOUND-65 CIV

[*där 'vŏn kŏm 'pound*]

(propoxyphene hydrochloride, aspirin and caffeine capsules, USP)

DESCRIPTION

Darvon® (Propoxyphene Hydrochloride, USP) is an odorless, white crystalline powder with a bitter taste. It is freely soluble in water. Chemically, it is (2*S*,3*R*)-(+)-4-(Dimethylamino)-3-methyl-1,2-diphenyl-2-butanol propionate (ester) hydrochloride, which can be represented by the accompanying structural formula. Its molecular weight is 375.94.

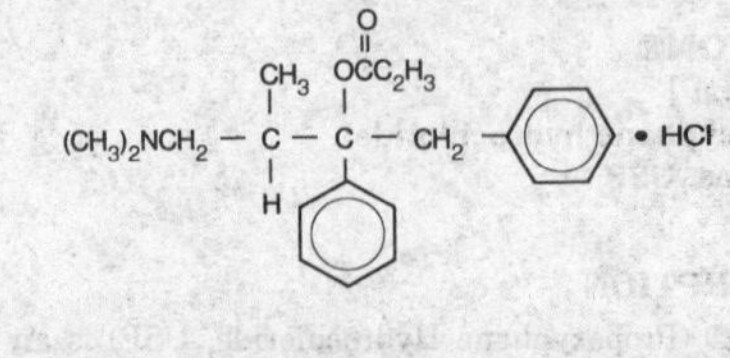

Each Pulvule® contains 65 mg (172.9 µmol) propoxyphene hydrochloride, 389 mg (2,159 µmol) aspirin, and 32.4 mg (166.8 µmol) caffeine.

It also contains F D & C Red No. 3, F D & C Yellow No. 6, gelatin, glutamic acid hydrochloride, iron oxide, kaolin, silicone, titanium dioxide, and other inactive ingredients.

CLINICAL PHARMACOLOGY

Propoxyphene is a centrally acting narcotic analgesic agent. Equimolar doses of propoxyphene hydrochloride or napsylate provide similar plasma concentrations. Following administration of 65, 130, or 195 mg of propoxyphene hydrochloride, the bioavailability of propoxyphene is equivalent to that of 100, 200, or 300 mg respectively of propoxyphene napsylate. Peak plasma concentrations of propoxyphene are reached in 2 to 2 1/2 hours. After a 65-mg oral dose of propoxyphene hydrochloride, peak plasma levels of 0.05 to 0.1 µg/mL are achieved.

Repeated doses of propoxyphene at 6-hour intervals lead to increasing plasma concentrations, with a plateau after the ninth dose at 48 hours.

Propoxyphene is metabolized in the liver to yield norpropoxyphene.

Propoxyphene has a half-life of 6 to 12 hours, whereas that of norpropoxyphene is 30 to 36 hours.

Norpropoxyphene has substantially less central-nervous-system-depressant effect than propoxyphene but a greater local anesthetic effect, which is similar to that of amitriptyline and antiarrhythmic agents, such as lidocaine and quinidine.

In animal studies in which propoxyphene and norpropoxyphene were continuously infused in large amounts, intracardiac conduction time (PR and QRS intervals) was prolonged. Any intracardiac conduction delay attributable to high concentrations of norpropoxyphene may be of relatively long duration.

ACTIONS

Propoxyphene is a mild narcotic analgesic structurally related to methadone. The potency of propoxyphene hydrochloride is from two thirds to equal that of codeine.

The combination of propoxyphene with a mixture of aspirin and caffeine produces greater analgesia than that produced by either propoxyphene or aspirin and caffeine administered alone.

INDICATION

This product is indicated for the relief of mild to moderate pain, either when pain is present alone or when it is accompanied by fever.

CONTRAINDICATION

Hypersensitivity to propoxyphene, aspirin, or caffeine.

WARNINGS

- **Do not prescribe propoxyphene for patients who are suicidal or addiction-prone.**
- **Prescribe propoxyphene with caution for patients taking tranquilizers or antidepressant drugs and patients who use alcohol in excess.**
- **Tell your patients not to exceed the recommended dose and to limit their intake of alcohol.**

Propoxyphene products in excessive doses, either alone or in combination with other CNS depressants, including alcohol, are a major cause of drug-related deaths. Fatalities within the first hour of overdosage are not uncommon. In a survey of deaths due to overdosage conducted in 1975, in approximately 20% of the fatal cases, death occurred within the first hour (5% occurred within 15 minutes). Propoxyphene should not be taken in doses higher than those recommended by the physician. The judicious prescribing of propoxyphene is essential to the safe use of this drug. With patients who are depressed or suicidal, consideration should be given to the use of nonnarcotic analgesics. Patients should be cautioned about the concomitant use of propoxyphene products and alcohol because of potentially serious CNS-additive effects of these agents. Because of its added depressant effects, propoxyphene should be prescribed with caution for those patients whose medical condition requires the concomitant administration of sedatives, tranquilizers, muscle relaxants, antidepressants, or other CNS-depressant drugs. Patients should be advised of the additive depressant effects of these combinations.

Many of the propoxyphene-related deaths have occurred in patients with previous histories of emotional disturbances or suicidal ideation or attempts as well as histories of misuse of tranquilizers, alcohol, and other CNS-active drugs. Some deaths have occurred as a consequence of the accidental ingestion of excessive quantities of propoxyphene alone or in combination with other drugs. Patients taking propoxyphene should be warned not to exceed the dosage recommended by the physician.

Drug Dependence—Propoxyphene, when taken in higher-than-recommended doses over long periods of time, can produce drug dependence characterized by psychic dependence and, less frequently, physical dependence and tolerance. Propoxyphene will only partially suppress the withdrawal syndrome in individuals physically dependent on morphine or other narcotics. The abuse liability of propoxyphene is qualitatively similar to that of codeine although quantitatively less, and propoxyphene should be prescribed with the same degree of caution appropriate to the use of codeine.

Usage in Ambulatory Patients—Propoxyphene may impair the mental and/or physical abilities required for the performance of potentially hazardous tasks, such as driving a car or operating machinery. The patient should be cautioned accordingly.

Warning: Reye Syndrome is a rare but serious disease which can follow flu or chicken pox in children and teenagers. While the cause of Reye Syndrome is unknown, some reports claim aspirin (or salicylates) may increase the risk of developing this disease.

PRECAUTIONS

General—Salicylates should be used with extreme caution in the presence of peptic ulcer or coagulation abnormalities. Propoxyphene should be administered with caution to patients with hepatic or renal impairment since higher serum concentrations or delayed elimination may occur.

Drug Interactions—The CNS-depressant effect of propoxyphene is additive with that of other CNS depressants, including alcohol.

Salicylates may enhance the effect of anticoagulants and inhibit the uricosuric effect of uricosuric agents.

As is the case with medicinal agents, propoxyphene may slow the metabolism of a concomitantly administered drug. Should this occur, the higher serum concentrations of that drug may result in increased pharmacologic or adverse effects of that drug. Such occurrences have been reported when propoxyphene was administered to patients on antidepressants, anticonvulsants, or warfarin-like drugs. Severe neurologic signs, including coma, have occurred with concurrent use of carbamazepine.

Usage in Pregnancy—Safe use in pregnancy has not been established relative to possible adverse effects on fetal development. Instances of withdrawal symptoms in the neonate have been reported following usage during pregnancy. Therefore, propoxyphene should not be used in pregnant women unless, in the judgment of the physician, the potential benefits outweigh the possible hazards. Aspirin does not appear to have teratogenic effects. However, prolonged pregnancy and labor with increased bleeding before and after delivery, decreased birth weight, and increased rate of stillbirth were reported with high blood salicylate levels. Because of possible adverse effects on the neonate and the potential for increased maternal blood loss, aspirin should be avoided during the last 3 months of pregnancy.

Usage in Nursing Mothers—Low levels of propoxyphene have been detected in human milk. In postpartum studies involving nursing mothers who were given propoxyphene, no adverse effects were noted in infants receiving mother's milk.

Usage in Pediatric Patients—Safety and effectiveness in pediatric patients have not been established.

Usage in the Elderly—The rate of propoxyphene metabolism may be reduced in some patients. Increased dosing interval should be considered.

A Patient Information Sheet is available for this product. See text following "How Supplied" section below.

ADVERSE REACTIONS

In a survey conducted in hospitalized patients, less than 1% of patients taking propoxyphene hydrochloride at recommended doses experienced side effects. The most frequently reported were dizziness, sedation, nausea, and vomiting. Some of these adverse reactions may be alleviated if the patient lies down.

Other adverse reactions include constipation, abdominal pain, skin rashes, lightheadedness, headache, weakness, euphoria, dysphoria, hallucinations, and minor visual disturbances.

Propoxyphene therapy has been associated with abnormal liver function tests and, more rarely, with instances of reversible jaundice (including cholestatic jaundice).

Renal papillary necrosis may result from chronic aspirin use, particularly when the dosage is greater than recommended and when combined with acetaminophen.

Subacute painful myopathy has occurred following chronic propoxyphene overdosage.

DOSAGE AND ADMINISTRATION

This product is given orally. The usual dosage is 65 mg propoxyphene hydrochloride, 389 mg aspirin, and 32.4 mg caffeine every 4 hours as needed for pain.

The maximum recommended dose of propoxyphene hydrochloride is 390 mg/day.

Consideration should be given to a reduced total daily dosage in patients with hepatic or renal impairment.

MANAGEMENT OF OVERDOSAGE

In all cases of suspected overdosage, call your regional Poison Control Center to obtain the most up-to-date information about the treatment of overdose. This recommendation is made because, in general, information regarding the treatment of overdosage may change more rapidly than do package inserts.

Initial consideration should be given to the management of the CNS effects of propoxyphene overdosage. Resuscitative measures should be initiated promptly.

Symptoms of Propoxyphene Overdosage—The manifestations of acute overdosage with propoxyphene are those of narcotic overdosage. The patient is usually somnolent but may be stuporous or comatose and convulsing. Respiratory depression is characteristic. The ventilatory rate and/or tidal volume is decreased, which results in cyanosis and hypoxia. Pupils, initially pinpoint, may become dilated as hypoxia increases. Cheyne-Stokes respiration and apnea may occur. Blood pressure and heart rate are usually normal initially, but blood pressure falls and cardiac performance deteriorates, which ultimately results in pulmonary edema and circulatory collapse, unless the respiratory depression is corrected and adequate ventilation is restored promptly. Cardiac arrhythmias and conduction delay may be present. A combined respiratory-metabolic acidosis occurs owing to retained CO_2 (hypercapnia) and to lactic acid formed during anaerobic glycolysis. Acidosis may be severe if large amounts of salicylates have also been ingested. Death may occur.

Treatment of Propoxyphene Overdosage—Attention should be directed first to establishing a patent airway and to restoring ventilation. Mechanically assisted ventilation, with or without oxygen, may be required, and positive pressure respiration may be desirable if pulmonary edema is present. The narcotic antagonist naloxone will markedly reduce the degree of respiratory depression, and 0.4 to 2 mg should be administered promptly, preferably intravenously. If the desired degree of counteraction with improvement in respiratory functions is not obtained, naloxone should be repeated at 2- to 3-minute intervals. The duration of action of the antagonist may be brief. If no response is observed after 10 mg of naloxone have been administered, the diagnosis of propoxyphene toxicity should be questioned. Naloxone may also be administered by continuous intravenous infusion.

Treatment of Propoxyphene Overdosage in Pediatric Patients—The usual initial dose of naloxone in pediatric patients is 0.01 mg/kg body weight given intravenously. If this dose does not result in the desired degree of clinical improvement, a subsequent increased dose of 0.1 mg/kg body weight may be administered. If an IV route of administration is not available, naloxone may be administered IM or subcutaneously in divided doses. If necessary, naloxone can be diluted with Sterile Water for Injection.

Blood gases, pH, and electrolytes should be monitored in order that acidosis and any electrolyte disturbance present may be corrected promptly. Acidosis, hypoxia, and generalized CNS depression predispose to the development of cardiac arrhythmias. Ventricular fibrillation or cardiac arrest may occur and necessitate the full complement of cardiopulmonary resuscitation (CPR) measures. Respiratory acidosis rapidly subsides as ventilation is restored and hypercapnia eliminated, but lactic acidosis may require intravenous bicarbonate for prompt correction.

Electrocardiographic monitoring is essential. Prompt correction of hypoxia, acidosis, and electrolyte disturbance (when present) will help prevent these cardiac complications and will increase the effectiveness of agents administered to restore normal cardiac function.

In addition to the use of a narcotic antagonist, the patient may require careful titration with an anticonvulsant to control convulsions. Analeptic drugs (for example, caffeine or amphetamine) should not be used because of their tendency to precipitate convulsions.

General supportive measures, in addition to oxygen, include, when necessary, intravenous fluids, vasopressor-inotropic compounds, and, when infection is likely, anti-infective agents. Gastric lavage may be useful and activated charcoal can adsorb a significant amount of ingested propoxyphene. Dialysis is of little value in poisoning due to propoxyphene. Efforts should be made to determine whether other agents, such as alcohol, barbiturates, tranquilizers, or other CNS depressants, were also ingested, since these increase CNS depression as well as cause specific toxic effects.

Symptoms of Salicylate Overdosage—Such symptoms include central nausea and vomiting, tinnitus and deafness, vertigo and headaches, mental dullness and confusion, diaphoresis, rapid pulse, and increased respiration and respiratory alkalosis.

Treatment of Salicylate Overdosage—When Darvon Compound-65 has been ingested, the clinical picture may be complicated by salicylism.

The treatment of acute salicylate intoxication includes minimizing drug absorption, promoting elimination through the

Continued on next page

---

* **Identi-Code® symbol. This product information was prepared in June 1998. Current information on these and other products of Eli Lilly and Company may be obtained by direct inquiry to Lilly Research Laboratories, Lilly Corporate Center, Indianapolis, Indiana 46285, (800) 545-5979.**

Darvon Compound-65—Cont.

kidneys, and correcting metabolic derangements affecting body temperature, hydration, acid-base balance, and electrolyte balance. The technique to be employed for eliminating salicylate from the bloodstream depends on the degree of drug intoxication.

If the patient is seen within 4 hours of ingestion, the stomach should be emptied by inducing vomiting or by gastric lavage as soon as possible.

The nomogram of Done is a useful prognostic guide in which the expected severity of salicylate intoxication is based on serum salicylate levels and the time interval between ingestion and taking the blood sample.

Exchange transfusion is most feasible for a small infant. Intermittent peritoneal dialysis is useful for cases of moderate severity in adults. Intravenous fluids alkalinized by the addition of sodium bicarbonate or potassium citrate are helpful. Hemodialysis with the artificial kidney is the most effective means of removing salicylate and is indicated for the very severe cases of salicylate intoxication.

HOW SUPPLIED

Darvon® Compound-65 Pulvules® (No. 369) are available in:

The 65 mg parabolic-shaped capsules are imprinted with the script "Lilly" and "3111" on the opaque gray cap and "Darvon Comp 65" on the opaque red body, using edible black ink. They are available as follows:

Bottles of 100 (RxPak*)   NDC 0002-3111-02 (PU0369)
Bottles of 500   NDC 0002-3111-03 (PU0369)

*All RxPaks (prescription packages, Lilly) have safety closures.

Store at controlled room temperature, 59° to 86°F (15° to 30°C).

CAUTION—Federal (USA) law prohibits dispensing without prescription.

The following information, including description of dosage forms and the maximum daily dosage of each, is available to patients receiving Darvon products.

Patient Information Sheet   ℞
YOUR PRESCRIPTION FOR A DARVON® (PROPOXYPHENE) PRODUCT

Summary

Products containing Darvon are used to relieve pain.
LIMIT YOUR INTAKE OF ALCOHOL WHILE TAKING THIS DRUG. Make sure your doctor knows if you are taking tranquilizers, sleep aids, antidepressants, antihistamines, or any other drugs that make you sleepy. Combining propoxyphene with alcohol or these drugs in excessive doses is dangerous.

Use care while driving a car or using machines until you see how the drug affects you because propoxyphene can make you sleepy. Do not take more of the drug than your doctor prescribed. Dependence has occurred when patients have taken propoxyphene for a long period of time at doses greater than recommended.

The rest of this leaflet gives you more information about propoxyphene. Please read it and keep it for future use.

Uses of Darvon

Products containing Darvon are used for the relief of mild to moderate pain. Products that contain Darvon plus aspirin or acetaminophen are prescribed for the relief of pain or pain associated with fever.

Before Taking Darvon

Make sure your doctor knows if you have ever had an allergic reaction to propoxyphene, aspirin, or acetaminophen. Some forms of propoxyphene products contain aspirin to help relieve the pain. Your doctor should be advised if you have a history of ulcers or if you are taking an anticoagulant ("blood thinner"). The aspirin may irritate the stomach lining and may cause bleeding, particularly if an ulcer is present. Also, bleeding may occur if you are taking an anticoagulant. In a small group of people, aspirin may cause an asthma attack. If you are one of these people, be sure your drug does not contain aspirin.

The effect of propoxyphene in pediatric patients under 12 has not been studied. Therefore, use of the drug in this age group is not recommended.

Also, due to the possible association between aspirin and Reye Syndrome, those propoxyphene products containing aspirin should not be given to children, including teenagers, with chicken pox or flu unless prescribed by a physician. The following propoxyphene product contains aspirin:

Darvon® Compound-65 (Propoxyphene Hydrochloride, Aspirin, and Caffeine, USP)

How to Take Darvon

Follow your doctor's directions exactly. Do not increase the amount you take without your doctor's approval. If you miss a dose of the drug, do not take twice as much the next time.

Pregnancy

Do not take propoxyphene during pregnancy unless your doctor knows you are pregnant and specifically recommends its use. Cases of temporary dependence in the newborn have occurred when the mother has taken propoxyphene consistently in the weeks before delivery. IT IS ESPECIALLY IMPORTANT NOT TO USE DARVON COMPOUND-65 DURING THE LAST 3 MONTHS OF PREGNANCY UNLESS SPECIFICALLY DIRECTED TO DO SO BY A DOCTOR BECAUSE ASPIRIN MAY CAUSE PROBLEMS IN THE UNBORN CHILD OR COMPLICATIONS DURING DELIVERY. As a general principle, no drug should be taken during pregnancy unless it is clearly necessary.

General Cautions

Heavy use of alcohol with propoxyphene is hazardous and may lead to overdosage symptoms (see "Overdose" below). THEREFORE, LIMIT YOUR INTAKE OF ALCOHOL WHILE TAKING PROPOXYPHENE.

Combinations of excessive doses of propoxyphene, alcohol, and tranquilizers are dangerous. Make sure your doctor knows if you are taking tranquilizers, sleep aids, antidepressant drugs, antihistamines, or any other drugs that make you sleepy. The use of these drugs with propoxyphene increases their sedative effects and may lead to overdosage symptoms, including death (see "Overdose" below).

Propoxyphene may cause drowsiness or impair your mental and/or physical abilities; therefore, use caution when driving a vehicle or operating dangerous machinery. DO NOT perform any hazardous task until you have seen your response to this drug.

Propoxyphene may increase the concentration in the body of medications such as anticoagulants ("blood thinners"), antidepressants, or drugs used for epilepsy. The result may be excessive or adverse effects of these medications. Make sure your doctor knows if you are taking any of these medications.

Dependence

You can become dependent on propoxyphene if you take it in higher than recommended doses over a long period of time. Dependence is a feeling of need for the drug and a feeling that you cannot perform normally without it.

Overdose

An overdose of Darvon, alone or in combination with other drugs, including alcohol, may cause weakness, difficulty in breathing, confusion, anxiety, and more severe drowsiness and dizziness. Extreme overdosage may lead to unconsciousness and death.

If the propoxyphene product contains acetaminophen, the overdosage symptoms include nausea, vomiting, lack of appetite, and abdominal pain. Liver damage may occur.

When the propoxyphene product contains aspirin, symptoms of taking too much of the drug are headache, dizziness, ringing in the ears, difficulty in hearing, dim vision, confusion, drowsiness, sweating, thirst, rapid breathing, nausea, vomiting, and, occasionally, diarrhea.

In any suspected overdosage situation, contact your doctor or nearest hospital emergency room. GET EMERGENCY HELP IMMEDIATELY.

KEEP THIS DRUG AND ALL DRUGS OUT OF THE REACH OF THE PEDIATRIC POPULATION.

Possible Side Effects

When propoxyphene is taken as directed, side effects are infrequent. Among those reported are drowsiness, dizziness, nausea, and vomiting. If these effects occur, it may help if you lie down and rest.

Less frequently reported side effects are constipation, abdominal pain, skin rashes, lightheadedness, headache, weakness, hallucinations, minor visual disturbances, and feelings of elation or discomfort.

If side effects occur and concern you, contact your doctor.

Other Information

The safe and effective use of propoxyphene depends on your taking it exactly as directed. This drug has been prescribed specifically for you and your present condition. Do not give this drug to others who may have similar symptoms. Do not use it for any other reason.

If you would like more information about propoxyphene, ask your doctor or pharmacist. They have a more technical leaflet (professional labeling) you may read.

[See table below]

Literature revised July 18, 1996
PA 6242 AMP   [071896]

DARVON-N® TABLETS   ℞
[där 'vŏn]
(propoxyphene napsylate tablets, USP)

DESCRIPTION

Darvon-N® (Propoxyphene Napsylate, USP) is an odorless, white crystalline powder with a bitter taste. It is very slightly soluble in water and soluble in methanol, ethanol, chloroform, and acetone. Chemically, it is $(\alpha S,1R)$-α-[2-(Dimethylamino)-1-methylethyl]-α-phenylphenethyl propionate compound with 2-naphthalenesulfonic acid (1:1) monohydrate, which can be represented by the accompanying structural formula. Its molecular weight is 565.72.

Propoxyphene napsylate differs from propoxyphene hydrochloride in that it allows more stable liquid dosage forms and tablet formulations. Because of differences in molecular weight, a dose of 100 mg (176.8 μmol) of propoxyphene napsylate is required to supply an amount of propoxyphene equivalent to that present in 65 mg (172.9 μmol) of propoxyphene hydrochloride.

Each tablet of Darvon-N contains 100 mg (176.8 μmol) propoxyphene napsylate. The tablet also contains cellulose, cornstarch, iron oxides, lactose, magnesium stearate, silicon dioxide, stearic acid, and titanium dioxide.

CLINICAL PHARMACOLOGY

Propoxyphene is a centrally acting narcotic analgesic agent. Equimolar doses of propoxyphene hydrochloride or napsylate provide similar plasma concentrations. Following administration of 65, 130, or 195 mg of propoxyphene hydrochloride, the bioavailability of propoxyphene is equivalent to that of 100, 200, or 300 mg respectively of propoxyphene napsylate. Peak plasma concentrations of propoxyphene are reached in 2 to 2 1/2 hours. After a 100-mg oral dose of propoxyphene napsylate, peak plasma levels of 0.05 to 0.1 μg/mL are achieved. As shown in Figure 1, the napsylate salt tends to be absorbed more slowly than the hydrochloride. At or near therapeutic doses, this difference is small when compared with that among subjects and among doses.
[See figure at top of next column]

Selected Darvon Products

Maximum Daily Dosage		
6	Dark, Orange, Capsule Shaped, Film Coated Tablets Imprinted with Script "Lilly" on one side and "Darvocet-N 100" on the other, using edible black ink	DARVOCET-N® 100 ℞ Propoxyphene Napsylate and Acetaminophen Tablets
6	Parabolic-Shaped Capsules Imprinted with Script "Lilly" and "3111" on the opaque gray cap and "Darvon Comp 65" on the opaque red body, using edible black ink	DARVON® COMPOUND-65 ℞ Propoxyphene Hydrochloride, Aspirin, and Caffeine Pulvules®
6	Parabolic-Shaped Capsules Imprinted with Script "Lilly" and "H03" on the opaque pink cap and "Darvon" on the opaque pink body, using edible black ink	DARVON® ℞ Propoxyphene Hydrochloride Pulvules, 65 mg

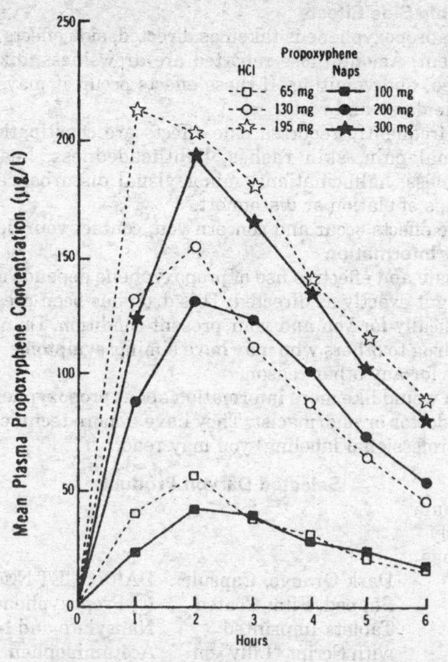

Figure 1. Mean plasma concentrations of propoxyphene in 8 human subjects following oral administration of 65 and 130 mg of the hydrochloride sale and 100 and 200 mg of the napsylate salt and in 7 given 195 mg of the hydrochloride and 300 mg of the napsylate salt.

Because of this several hundredfold difference in solubility, the absorption rate of very large doses of the napsylate salt is significantly lower than that of equimolar doses of the hydrochloride.

Repeated doses of propoxyphene at 6-hour intervals lead to increasing plasma concentrations, with a plateau after the ninth dose at 48 hours.

Propoxyphene is metabolized in the liver to yield norpropoxyphene. Propoxyphene has a half-life of 6 to 12 hours, whereas that of norpropoxyphene is 30 to 36 hours.

Norpropoxyphene has substantially less central-nervous-system-depressant effect than propoxyphene but a greater local anesthetic effect, which is similar to that of amitriptyline and antiarrhythmic agents, such as lidocaine and quinidine.

In animal studies in which propoxyphene and norpropoxyphene were continuously infused in large amounts, intracardiac conduction time (PR and QRS intervals) was prolonged. Any intracardiac conduction delay attributable to high concentrations of norpropoxyphene may be of relatively long duration.

ACTIONS

Propoxyphene is a mild narcotic analgesic structurally related to methadone. The potency of propoxyphene napsylate is from two thirds to equal that of codeine.

INDICATION

For the relief of mild to moderate pain.

CONTRAINDICATION

Hypersensitivity to propoxyphene.

WARNINGS

- **Do not prescribe propoxyphene for patients who are suicidal or addiction-prone.**
- **Prescribe propoxyphene with caution for patients taking tranquilizers or antidepressant drugs and patients who use alcohol in excess.**
- **Tell your patients not to exceed the recommended dose and to limit their intake of alcohol.**

Propoxyphene products in excessive doses, either alone or in combination with other CNS depressants, including alcohol, are a major cause of drug-related deaths. Fatalities within the first hour of overdosage are not uncommon. In a survey of deaths due to overdosage conducted in 1975, in approximately 20% of the fatal cases, death occurred within the first hour (5% occurred within 15 minutes). Propoxyphene should not be taken in doses higher than those recommended by the physician. The judicious prescribing of propoxyphene is essential to the safe use of this drug. With patients who are depressed or suicidal, consideration should be given to the use of non-narcotic analgesics. Patients should be cautioned about the concomitant use of propoxyphene products and alcohol because of potentially serious CNS-additive effects of these agents. Because of its added depressant effects, propoxyphene should be prescribed with caution for those patients whose medical condition requires the concomitant administration of sedatives, tranquilizers, muscle relaxants, antidepressants, or other CNS-depressant drugs. Patients should be advised of the additive depressant effects of these combinations.

Many of the propoxyphene-related deaths have occurred in patients with previous histories of emotional disturbances or suicidal ideation or attempts as well as histories of misuse of tranquilizers, alcohol, and other CNS-active drugs. Some deaths have occurred as a consequence of the accidental ingestion of excessive quantities of propoxyphene alone or in combination with other drugs. Patients taking propoxyphene should be warned not to exceed the dosage recommended by the physician.

Drug Dependence—Propoxyphene, when taken in higher-than-recommended doses over long periods of time, can produce drug dependence characterized by psychic dependence and, less frequently, physical dependence and tolerance. Propoxyphene will only partially suppress the withdrawal syndrome in individuals physically dependent on morphine or other narcotics. The abuse liability of propoxyphene is qualitatively similar to that of codeine although quantitatively less, and propoxyphene should be prescribed with the same degree of caution appropriate to the use of codeine.

Usage in Ambulatory Patients—Propoxyphene may impair the mental and/or physical abilities required for the performance of potentially hazardous tasks, such as driving a car or operating machinery. The patient should be cautioned accordingly.

PRECAUTIONS

General—Propoxyphene should be administered with caution to patients with hepatic or renal impairment since higher serum concentrations or delayed elimination may occur.

Drug Interactions—The CNS-depressant effect of propoxyphene is additive with that of other CNS depressants, including alcohol.

As is the case with many medicinal agents, propoxyphene may slow the metabolism of a concomitantly administered drug. Should this occur, the higher serum concentrations of that drug may result in increased pharmacologic or adverse effects of that drug. Such occurrences have been reported when propoxyphene was administered to patients on antidepressants, anticonvulsants, or warfarin-like drugs. Severe neurologic signs, including coma, have occurred with concurrent use of carbamazepine.

Usage in Pregnancy—Safe use in pregnancy has not been established relative to possible adverse effects on fetal development. Instances of withdrawal symptoms in the neonate have been reported following usage during pregnancy. Therefore, propoxyphene should not be used in pregnant women unless, in the judgment of the physician, the potential benefits outweigh the possible hazards.

Usage in Nursing Mothers—Low levels of propoxyphene have been detected in human milk. In postpartum studies involving nursing mothers who were given propoxyphene, no adverse effects were noted in infants receiving mother's milk.

Usage in Pediatric Patients— Safety and effectiveness in pediatric patients have not been established.

Usage in the Elderly—The rate of propoxyphene metabolism may be reduced in some patients. Increased dosing interval should be considered.

A Patient Information Sheet is available for this product. See text following "How Supplied" section below.

ADVERSE REACTIONS

In a survey conducted in hospitalized patients, less than 1% of patients taking propoxyphene hydrochloride at recommended doses experienced side effects. The most frequently reported were dizziness, sedation, nausea, and vomiting. Some of these adverse reactions may be alleviated if the patient lies down.

Other adverse reactions include constipation, abdominal pain, skin rashes, lightheadedness, headache, weakness, euphoria, dysphoria, hallucinations, and minor visual disturbances.

Propoxyphene therapy has been associated with abnormal liver function tests and, more rarely, with instances of reversible jaundice (including cholestatic jaundice).

Subacute painful myopathy has occurred following chronic propoxyphene overdosage.

DOSAGE AND ADMINISTRATION

Darvon-N is given orally. The usual dosage is 100 mg propoxyphene napsylate every 4 hours as needed for pain. The maximum recommended dose of propoxyphene napsylate is 600 mg per day.

Consideration should be given to a reduced total daily dosage in patients with hepatic or renal impairment.

MANAGEMENT OF OVERDOSAGE

In all cases of suspected overdosage, call your regional Poison Control Center to obtain the most up-to-date information about the treatment of overdose. This recommendation is made because, in general, information regarding the treatment of overdosage may change more rapidly than do package inserts.

Initial consideration should be given to the management of the CNS effects of propoxyphene overdosage. Resuscitative measures should be initiated promptly.

Symptoms of Propoxyphene Overdosage—The manifestations of acute overdosage with propoxyphene are those of narcotic overdosage. The patient is usually somnolent but may be stuporous or comatose and convulsing. Respiratory depression is characteristic. The ventilatory rate and/or tidal volume is decreased, which results in cyanosis and hypoxia. Pupils, initially pinpoint, may become dilated as hypoxia increases. Cheyne-Stokes respiration and apnea may occur. Blood pressure and heart rate are usually normal initially, but blood pressure falls and cardiac performance deteriorates, which ultimately results in pulmonary edema and circulatory collapse, unless the respiratory depression is corrected and adequate ventilation is restored promptly. Cardiac arrhythmias and conduction delay may be present. A combined respiratory-metabolic acidosis occurs owing to retained CO_2 (hypercapnia) and to lactic acid formed during anaerobic glycolysis. Acidosis may be severe if large amounts of salicylates have also been ingested. Death may occur.

Treatment of Propoxyphene Overdosage—Attention should be directed first to establishing a patent airway and to restoring ventilation. Mechanically assisted ventilation, with or without oxygen, may be required, and positive pressure respiration may be desirable if pulmonary edema is present. The narcotic antagonist naloxone will markedly reduce the degree of respiratory depression, and 0.4 to 2 mg should be administered promptly, preferably intravenously. If the desired degree of counteraction with improvement in respiratory functions is not obtained, naloxone should be repeated at 2- to 3-minute intervals. The duration of action of the antagonist may be brief. If no response is observed after 10 mg of naloxone have been administered, the diagnosis of propoxyphene toxicity should be questioned. Naloxone may also be administered by continuous intravenous infusion.

Treatment of Propoxyphene Overdosage in Pediatric Patients—The usual initial dose of naloxone in pediatric patients is 0.01 mg/kg body weight given intravenously. If this dose does not result in the desired degree of clinical improvement, a subsequent increased dose of 0.1 mg/kg body weight may be administered. If an IV route of administration is not available, naloxone may be administered IM or subcutaneously in divided doses. If necessary, naloxone can be diluted with Sterile Water for Injection.

Blood gases, pH, and electrolytes should be monitored in order that acidosis and any electrolyte disturbance present may be corrected promptly. Acidosis, hypoxia, and generalized CNS depression predispose to the development of cardiac arrhythmias. Ventricular fibrillation or cardiac arrest may occur and necessitate the full complement of cardiopulmonary resuscitation (CPR) measures. Respiratory acidosis rapidly subsides as ventilation is restored and hypercapnia eliminated, but lactic acidosis may require intravenous bicarbonate for prompt correction.

Electrocardiographic monitoring is essential. Prompt correction of hypoxia, acidosis, and electrolyte disturbance (when present) will help prevent these cardiac complications and will increase the effectiveness of agents administered to restore normal cardiac function.

In addition to the use of a narcotic antagonist, the patient may require careful titration with an anticonvulsant to control convulsions. Analeptic drugs (for example, caffeine or amphetamine) should not be used because of their tendency to precipitate convulsions.

General supportive measures, in addition to oxygen, include, when necessary, intravenous fluids, vasopressor-inotropic compounds, and, when infection is likely, anti-infective agents. Gastric lavage may be useful, and activated charcoal can adsorb a significant amount of ingested propoxyphene. Dialysis is of little value in poisoning due to propoxyphene. Efforts should be made to determine whether other agents, such as alcohol, barbiturates, tranquilizers, or other CNS depressants, were also ingested, since these increase CNS depression as well as cause specific toxic effects.

ANIMAL TOXICOLOGY

The acute lethal doses of the hydrochloride and napsylate salts of propoxyphene were determined in 4 species. The results shown in Figure 2 indicate that, on a molar basis, the napsylate salt is less toxic than the hydrochloride. This may be due to the relative insolubility and retarded absorption of propoxyphene napsylate.

Continued on next page

*** Identi-Code® symbol. This product information was prepared in June 1998. Current information on these and other products of Eli Lilly and Company may be obtained by direct inquiry to Lilly Research Laboratories, Lilly Corporate Center, Indianapolis, Indiana 46285, (800) 545-5979.**

Darvon-N—Cont.

Figure 2. Acute oral toxicity of propoxyphene

Species	$\frac{LD_{50}\ (mg/kg) \pm SE}{LD_{50}(mmol/kg)}$	
	Propoxyphene Hydrochloride	Propoxyphene Napsylate
Mouse	$\frac{282 \pm 39}{0.75}$	$\frac{915 \pm 163}{1.62}$
Rat	$\frac{230 \pm 44}{0.61}$	$\frac{647 \pm 95}{1.14}$
Rabbit	$\frac{ca82}{0.22}$	$\frac{>183}{>0.32}$
Dog	$\frac{ca\ 100}{0.27}$	$\frac{>183}{>0.32}$

Some indication of the relative insolubility and retarded absorption of propoxyphene napsylate was obtained by measuring plasma propoxyphene levels in 2 groups of 4 dogs following oral administration of equimolar doses of the 2 salts. As shown in Figure 3, the peak plasma concentration observed with propoxyphene hydrochloride was much higher than that obtained after administration of the napsylate salt.

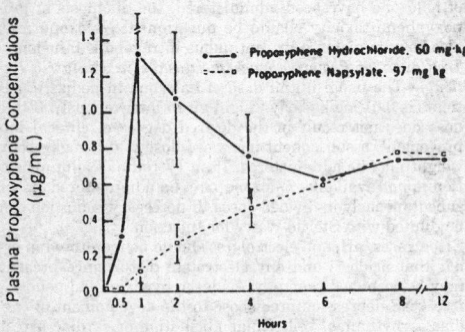

Figure 3. Plasma propoxyphene concentrations in dogs following large doses of the hydrochloride and napsylate salts

Although none of the animals in this experiment died, 3 of the 4 dogs given propoxyphene hydrochloride exhibited convulsive seizures during the time interval corresponding to the peak plasma levels. The 4 animals receiving the napsylate salt were mildly ataxic but not acutely ill.

HOW SUPPLIED

Darvon-N® Tablets (No. 1883) are available in:
The 100 mg tablets are buff colored, elliptical shaped, film coated, and imprinted with the script "Lilly" and "Darvon-N 100" on one side of the tablet, using edible black ink. They are available as follows:

Bottles of 100 (RxPak*)   NDC 0002-0353-02 (TA1883)
Bottles of 500   NDC 0002-0353-03 (TA1883)
ID†100   NDC 0002-0353-33 (TA1883)

*All RxPaks (prescription packages, Lilly) have safety closures.
†Identi-Dose® (unit dose medication, Lilly).
Store at controlled room temperature, 59° to 86°F (15° to 30°C).
CAUTION—Federal (USA) law prohibits dispensing without prescription.
The following information, including description of dosage forms and the maximum daily dosage of each, is available to patients receiving Darvon products.

Patient Information Sheet   Ⓝ

YOUR PRESCRIPTION FOR A DARVON® (PROPOXYPHENE) PRODUCT

Summary

Products containing Darvon are used to relieve pain. LIMIT YOUR INTAKE OF ALCOHOL WHILE TAKING THIS DRUG. Make sure your doctor knows if you are taking tranquilizers, sleep aids, antidepressants, antihistamines, or any other drugs that make you sleepy. Combining propoxyphene with alcohol or these drugs in excessive doses is dangerous.

Use care while driving a car or using machines until you see how the drug affects you because propoxyphene can make you sleepy. Do not take more of the drug than your doctor prescribed. Dependence has occurred when patients have taken propoxyphene for a long period of time at doses greater than recommended.
The rest of this leaflet gives you more information about propoxyphene. Please read it and keep it for future use.

Uses of Darvon

Products containing Darvon are used for the relief of mild to moderate pain. Products that contain Darvon plus aspirin or acetaminophen are prescribed for the relief of pain or pain associated with fever.

Before Taking Darvon

Make sure your doctor knows if you have ever had an allergic reaction to propoxyphene, aspirin, or acetaminophen. Some forms of propoxyphene products contain aspirin to help relieve the pain. Your doctor should be advised if you have a history of ulcers or if you are taking an anticoagulant ("blood thinner"). The aspirin may irritate the stomach lining and may cause bleeding, particularly if an ulcer is present. Also, bleeding may occur if you are taking an anticoagulant. In a small group of people, aspirin may cause an asthma attack. If you are one of these people, be sure your drug does not contain aspirin.
The effect of propoxyphene in pediatric patients under 12 has not been studied. Therefore, use of the drug in this age group is not recommended.
Also, due to the possible association between aspirin and Reye Syndrome, those propoxyphene products containing aspirin should not be given to children, including teenagers, with chicken pox or flu unless prescribed by a physician. The following propoxyphene product contains aspirin:
Darvon® Compound-65 (Propoxyphene Hydrochloride, Aspirin, and Caffeine, USP)

How to Take Darvon

Follow your doctor's directions exactly. Do not increase the amount you take without your doctor's approval. If you miss a dose of the drug, do not take twice as much the next time.

Pregnancy

Do not take propoxyphene during pregnancy unless your doctor knows you are pregnant and specifically recommends its use. Cases of temporary dependence in the newborn have occurred when the mother has taken propoxyphene consistently in the weeks before delivery. As a general principle, no drug should be taken during pregnancy unless it is clearly necessary.

General Cautions

Heavy use of alcohol with propoxyphene is hazardous and may lead to overdosage symptoms (see "Overdose" below). THEREFORE, LIMIT YOUR INTAKE OF ALCOHOL WHILE TAKING PROPOXYPHENE.
Combinations of excessive doses of propoxyphene, alcohol, and tranquilizers are dangerous. Make sure your doctor knows if you are taking tranquilizers, sleep aids, antidepressant drugs, antihistamines, or any other drugs that make you sleepy. The use of these drugs with propoxyphene increases their sedative effects and may lead to overdosage symptoms, including death (see "Overdose" below).
Propoxyphene may cause drowsiness or impair your mental and/or physical abilities; therefore, use caution when driving a vehicle or operating dangerous machinery. DO NOT perform any hazardous task until you have seen your response to this drug.
Propoxyphene may increase the concentration in the body of medications, such as anticoagulants ("blood thinners"), antidepressants, or drugs used for epilepsy. The result may be excessive or adverse effects of these medications. Make sure your doctor knows if you are taking any of these medications.

Dependence

You can become dependent on propoxyphene if you take it in higher than recommended doses over a long period of time. Dependence is a feeling of need for the drug and a feeling that you cannot perform normally without it.

Overdose

An overdose of Darvon, alone or in combination with other drugs, including alcohol, may cause weakness, difficulty in breathing, confusion, anxiety, and more severe drowsiness and dizziness. Extreme overdosage may lead to unconsciousness and death.
If the propoxyphene product contains acetaminophen, the overdosage symptoms include nausea, vomiting, lack of appetite, and abdominal pain. Liver damage may occur.
When the propoxyphene product contains aspirin, symptoms of taking too much of the drug are headache, dizziness, ringing in the ears, difficulty in hearing, dim vision, confusion, drowsiness, sweating, thirst, rapid breathing, nausea, vomiting, and, occasionally, diarrhea.
In any suspected overdose situation, contact your doctor or nearest hospital emergency room. GET EMERGENCY HELP IMMEDIATELY.
KEEP THIS DRUG AND ALL DRUGS OUT OF THE REACH OF THE PEDIATRIC POPULATION.

Possible Side Effects

When propoxyphene is taken as directed, side effects are infrequent. Among those reported are drowsiness, dizziness, nausea, and vomiting. If these effects occur, it may help if you lie down and rest.
Less frequently reported side effects are constipation, abdominal pain, skin rashes, lightheadedness, headache, weakness, hallucinations, minor visual disturbances, and feelings of elation or discomfort.
If side effects occur and concern you, contact your doctor.

Other Information

The safe and effective use of propoxyphene depends on your taking it exactly as directed. This drug has been prescribed specifically for you and your present condition. Do not give this drug to others who may have similar symptoms. Do not use it for any other reason.
If you would like more information about propoxyphene, ask your doctor or pharmacist. They have a more technical leaflet (professional labeling) you may read.

Selected Darvon Products

Maximum Daily Dosage		
6	Dark Orange, Capsule Shaped, Film Coated Tablets Imprinted with Script "Lilly" on the one side and "Darvocet-N 100"on the other, using edible black ink	DARVOCET-N® 100 Ⓝ Propoxyphene Napsylate and Acetaminophen Tablets
6	Parabolic-Shaped Capsules Imprinted with Script "Lilly" and "3111" on the opaque gray cap and "Darvon Comp 65" on the opaque red body, using edible black ink	DARVON® COMPOUND-65 Ⓝ Propoxyphene Hydrochloride, Aspirin, and Caffeine Pulvules®
6	Parabolic-Shaped Capsules Imprinted with Script "Lilly" and "H03" on the opaque pink cap and "Darvon" on the opaque pink body, using edible black ink	DARVON® Ⓝ Propoxyphene Hydrochloride Pulvules, 65 mg

Literature revised July 18, 1996
PA 8872 AMP   [071896]

DOBUTREX® SOLUTION   ℞
[dō ′bū-trĕks]
(dobutamine injection, USP)

DESCRIPTION

Dobutrex® Solution (Dobutamine Injection, USP) is 1, 2-benzenediol, 4-[2-[[3-(4-hydroxyphenyl)-1-methylpropyl]amino]ethyl]-, hydrochloride, (±)-. It is a synthetic catecholamine.

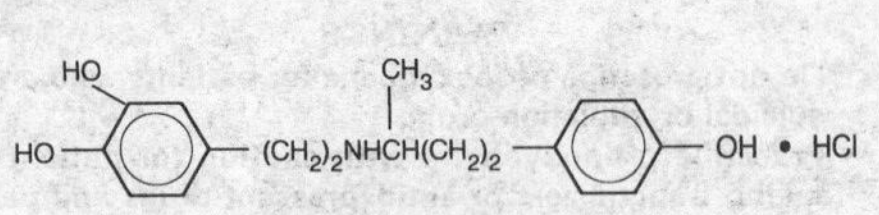

Molecular Formula: $C_{18}H_{23}NO_3 \cdot HCl$
Molecular Weight: 337.85

The clinical formulation is supplied in a sterile form for intravenous use only. Each mL contains 12.5 mg (41.5 µmol) dobutamine hydrochloride, 0.24 mg sodium bisulfite (added during manufacture), and water for injection, q.s. Hydrochloric acid and/or sodium hydroxide may have been added during manufacture to adjust the pH.

CLINICAL PHARMACOLOGY

Dobutrex Solution is a direct-acting inotropic agent whose primary activity results from stimulation of the β receptors of the heart while producing comparatively mild chronotropic, hypertensive, arrhythmogenic, and vasodilative effects. It does not cause the release of endogenous norepinephrine, as does dopamine. In animal studies, dobutamine hydrochloride produces less increase in heart rate and less decrease in peripheral vascular resistance for a given inotropic effect than does isoproterenol.
In patients with depressed cardiac function, both dobutamine hydrochloride and isoproterenol increase the cardiac output to a similar degree. In the case of dobutamine hydrochloride, this increase is usually not accompanied by marked increases in heart rate (although tachycardia is oc-

casionally observed), and the cardiac stroke volume is usually increased. In contrast, isoproterenol increases the cardiac index primarily by increasing the heart rate while stroke volume changes little or declines.

Facilitation of atrioventricular conduction has been observed in human electrophysiologic studies and in patients with atrial fibrillation.

Systemic vascular resistance is usually decreased with administration of dobutamine hydrochloride. Occasionally, minimum vasoconstriction has been observed.

Most clinical experience with dobutamine hydrochloride is short-term—not more than several hours in duration. In the limited number of patients who were studied for 24, 48, and 72 hours, a persistent increase in cardiac output occurred in some, whereas output returned toward baseline values in others.

The onset of action of Dobutrex Solution is within 1 to 2 minutes; however, as much as 10 minutes may be required to obtain the peak effect of a particular infusion rate.

The plasma half-life of dobutamine hydrochloride in humans is 2 minutes. The principal routes of metabolism are methylation of the catechol and conjugation. In human urine, the major excretion products are the conjugates of dobutamine and 3-O-methyl dobutamine. The 3-O-methyl derivative of dobutamine is inactive.

Alteration of synaptic concentrations of catecholamines with either reserpine or tricyclic antidepressants does not alter the actions of dobutamine in animals, which indicates that the actions of dobutamine hydrochloride are not dependent on presynaptic mechanisms.

INDICATIONS AND USAGE

Dobutrex Solution is indicated when parenteral therapy is necessary for inotropic support in the short-term treatment of adults with cardiac decompensation due to depressed contractility resulting either from organic heart disease or from cardiac surgical procedures.

In patients who have atrial fibrillation with rapid ventricular response, a digitalis preparation should be used prior to institution of therapy with Dobutrex Solution.

CONTRAINDICATIONS

Dobutrex Solution is contraindicated in patients with idiopathic hypertrophic subaortic stenosis and in patients who have shown previous manifestations of hypersensitivity to Dobutrex Solution.

WARNINGS

1. *Increase in Heart Rate or Blood Pressure*—Dobutrex Solution may cause a marked increase in heart rate or blood pressure, especially systolic pressure. Approximately 10% of patients in clinical studies have had rate increases of 30 beats/minute or more, and about 7.5% have had a 50 mm Hg or greater increase in systolic pressure. Usually, reduction of dosage promptly reverses these effects. Because dobutamine hydrochloride facilitates atrioventricular conduction, patients with atrial fibrillation are at risk of developing rapid ventricular response. Patients with preexisting hypertension appear to face an increased risk of developing an exaggerated pressor response.

2. *Ectopic Activity*—Dobutrex Solution may precipitate or exacerbate ventricular ectopic activity, but it rarely has caused ventricular tachycardia.

3. *Hypersensitivity* —Reactions suggestive of hypersensitivity associated with administration of Dobutrex Solution, including skin rash, fever, eosinophilia, and bronchospasm, have been reported occasionally.

4. Dobutrex Solution contains sodium bisulfite, a sulfite that may cause allergic-type reactions, including anaphylactic symptoms and life-threatening or less severe asthmatic episodes, in certain susceptible people. The overall prevalence of sulfite sensitivity in the general population is unknown and probably low. Sulfite sensitivity is seen more frequently in asthmatic than in nonasthmatic people.

PRECAUTIONS

General—**1. During the administration of Dobutrex Solution, as with any adrenergic agent, ECG and blood pressure should be continuously monitored. In addition, pulmonary wedge pressure and cardiac output should be monitored whenever possible to aid in the safe and effective infusion of Dobutrex Solution.**

2. Hypovolemia should be corrected with suitable volume expanders before treatment with Dobutrex Solution is instituted.

3. No improvement may be observed in the presence of marked mechanical obstruction, such as severe valvular aortic stenosis.

Usage Following Acute Myocardial Infarction—Clinical experience with Dobutrex Solution following myocardial infarction has been insufficient to establish the safety of the drug for this use. There is concern that any agent that increases contractile force and heart rate may increase the size of an infarction by intensifying ischemia, but it is not known whether dobutamine hydrochloride does so.

Table 1
Dobutrex Solution Infusion Rate (mL/kg/min)
for Concentrations of 250, 500, and 1,000 μg/mL

Drug Delivery Rate (μg/kg/min)	Infusion Delivery Rate 250 μg/mL* (mL/kg/min)	500 μg/mL† (mL/kg/min)	1,000 μg/mL‡ (mL/kg/min)
2.5	0.01	0.005	0.0025
5	0.02	0.01	0.005
7.5	0.03	0.015	0.0075
10	0.04	0.02	0.01
12.5	0.05	0.025	0.0125
15	0.06	0.03	0.015

*250 μg/mL of diluent
†500 μg/mL or 250 mg/500 mL of diluent
‡1,000 μg/mL or 250 mg/250 mL of diluent

Laboratory Tests—Dobutamine, like other β_2-agonists, can produce a mild reduction in serum potassium concentration, rarely to hypokalemic levels. Accordingly, consideration should be given to monitoring serum potassium.

Drug Interactions—Animal studies indicate that dobutamine may be ineffective if the patient has recently received a β-blocking drug. In such a case, the peripheral vascular resistance may increase.

Preliminary studies indicate that the concomitant use of dobutamine hydrochloride and nitroprusside results in a higher cardiac output and, usually, a lower pulmonary wedge pressure than when either drug is used alone.

There was no evidence of drug interactions in clinical studies in which Dobutrex Solution was administered concurrently with other drugs, including digitalis preparations, furosemide, spironolactone, lidocaine, glyceryl trinitrate, isosorbide dinitrate, morphine, atropine, heparin, protamine, potassium chloride, folic acid, and acetaminophen.

Carcinogenesis, Mutagenesis, Impairment of Fertility—Studies to evaluate the carcinogenic or mutagenic potential of dobutamine, or its potential to affect fertility, have not been conducted.

Pregnancy—Teratogenic Effects—Pregnancy Category-B—Reproduction studies performed in rats at doses up to the normal human dose (10 μg/kg/min for 24 h, total daily dose of 14.4 mg/kg) and in rabbits at doses up to twice the normal human dose, have revealed no evidence of harm to the fetus due to dobutamine. There are, however, no adequate and well-controlled studies in pregnant women. Because animal reproduction studies are not always predictive of human response, this drug should be used during pregnancy only if clearly needed.

Labor and Delivery—The effect of Dobutrex Solution on labor and delivery is unknown.

Nursing Mothers—It is not known whether this drug is excreted in human milk. Because many drugs are excreted in human milk, caution should be exercised when Dobutrex Solution is administered to a nursing woman. If a mother requires Dobutrex Solution treatment, breast-feeding should be discontinued for the duration of the treatment.

Pediatric Use—The safety and effectiveness of Dobutrex Solution for use in children have not been studied.

ADVERSE REACTIONS

Increased Heart Rate, Blood Pressure, and Ventricular Ectopic Activity—A 10- to 20-mm increase in systolic blood pressure and an increase in heart rate of 5 to 15 beats/minute have been noted in most patients (*see* Warnings regarding exaggerated chronotropic and pressor effects). Approximately 5% of patients have had increased premature ventricular beats during infusions. These effects are dose related.

Hypotension —Precipitous decreases in blood pressure have occasionally been described in association with Dobutrex Solution therapy. Decreasing the dose or discontinuing the infusion typically results in rapid return of blood pressure to baseline values. In rare cases, however, intervention may be required and reversibility may not be immediate.

Reactions at Sites of Intravenous Infusion—Phlebitis has occasionally been reported. Local inflammatory changes have been described following inadvertent infiltration. Isolated cases of cutaneous necrosis (destruction of skin tissue) have been reported.

Miscellaneous Uncommon Effects—The following adverse effects have been reported in 1% to 3% of patients: nausea, headache, anginal pain, nonspecific chest pain, palpitations, and shortness of breath.

Isolated cases of thrombocytopenia have been reported.

Administration of Dobutrex Solution, like other catecholamines, can produce a mild reduction in serum potassium concentration, rarely to hypokalemic levels (*see* Precautions).

Longer-Term Safety—Infusions of up to 72 hours have revealed no adverse effects other than those seen with shorter infusions.

OVERDOSAGE

Overdoses of Dobutrex Solution have been reported rarely. The following is provided to serve as a guide if such an overdose is encountered.

Signs and Symptoms —Toxicity from Dobutrex Solution is usually due to excessive cardiac β-receptor stimulation. The duration of action of Dobutrex Solution is generally short ($T_{1/2}$ = 2 minutes) because it is rapidly metabolized by catechol-O-methyltransferase. The symptoms of toxicity may include anorexia, nausea, vomiting, tremor, anxiety, palpitations, headache, shortness of breath, and anginal and nonspecific chest pain. The positive inotropic and chronotropic effects of Dobutrex Solution on the myocardium may cause hypertension, tachyarrhythmias, myocardial ischemia, and ventricular fibrillation. Hypotension may result from vasodilation.

Treatment —To obtain up-to-date information about the treatment of overdose, a good resource is your certified Regional Poison Control Center. Telephone numbers of certified poison control centers are listed in the *Physicians' Desk Reference (PDR)*. In managing overdosage, consider the possibility of multiple drug overdoses, interaction among drugs, and unusual drug kinetics in your patient.

The initial actions to be taken in a Dobutrex Solution overdose are discontinuing administration, establishing an airway, and ensuring oxygenation and ventilation. Resuscitative measures should be initiated promptly. Severe ventricular tachyarrhythmias may be successfully treated with propranolol or lidocaine. Hypertension usually responds to a reduction in dose or discontinuation of therapy.

Protect the patient's airway and support ventilation and perfusion. If needed, meticulously monitor and maintain, within acceptable limits, the patient's vital signs, blood gases, serum electrolytes, etc.

If the product is ingested, unpredictable absorption may occur from the mouth and the gastrointestinal tract. Absorption of drugs from the gastrointestinal tract may be decreased by giving activated charcoal, which, in many cases, is more effective than emesis or lavage; consider charcoal instead of or in addition to gastric emptying. Repeated doses of charcoal over time may hasten elimination of some drugs that have been absorbed. Safeguard the patient's airway when employing gastric emptying or charcoal.

Forced diuresis, peritoneal dialysis, hemodialysis, or charcoal hemoperfusion have not been established as beneficial for an overdose of Dobutrex Solution.

DOSAGE AND ADMINISTRATION

Note —Do not add Dobutrex Solution to 5% Sodium Bicarbonate Injection or to any other strongly alkaline solution. Because of potential physicial incompatibilities, it is recommended that Dobutrex Solution not be mixed with other drugs in the same solution. Dobutrex Solution should not be used in conjunction with other agents or diluents containing both sodium bisulfite and ethanol.

Preparation and Stability —At the time of administration, Dobutrex Solution must be further diluted in an IV container to at least a 50-mL solution using one of the following intravenous solutions as a diluent: 5% Dextrose Injection, 5% Dextrose and 0.45% Sodium Chloride Injection, 5% Dextrose and 0.9% Sodium Chloride Injection, 10% Dextrose Injection, Isolyte® M with 5% Dextrose Injection, Lactated Ringer's Injection, 5% Dextrose in Lactated Ringer's Injection, Normosol®-M in D5-W, 20% Osmitrol® in Water for Injection, 0.9% Sodium Chloride Injection, or Sodium Lactate Injection. Intravenous solutions should be used within 24 hours.

Continued on next page

*** Identi-Code® symbol. This product information was prepared in June 1998. Current information on these and other products of Eli Lilly and Company may be obtained by direct inquiry to Lilly Research Laboratories, Lilly Corporate Center, Indianapolis, Indiana 46285, (800) 545-5979.**

Dobutrex—Cont.

Recommended Dosage—The rate of infusion needed to increase cardiac output usually ranged from 2.5 to 15 µg/kg/min (see Table 1). On rare occasions, infusion rates up to 40 µg/kg/min have been required to obtain the desired effect.
[See table 1 at top of previous page]
Rates of infusion in mL/h for Dobutrex Solution concentrations of 500 µg/mL, 1,000 µg/mL, and 2,000 µg/mL are given in Table 2.

Table 2
Dobutrex Solution Infusion Rate (mL/h) for 500 µg/mL concentration

Drug Delivery Rate (µg/kg/min)	Patient Body Weight (kg)								
	30	40	50	60	70	80	90	100	110
2.5	9	12	15	18	21	24	27	30	33
5	18	24	30	36	42	48	54	60	66
7.5	27	36	45	54	63	72	81	90	99
10	36	48	60	72	84	96	108	120	132
12.5	45	60	75	90	105	120	135	150	165
15	54	72	90	108	126	144	162	180	198

Dobutrex Solution Infusion Rate (mL/h) for 1,000 µg/mL concentration

Drug Delivery Rate (µg/kg/min)	Patient Body Weight (kg)								
	30	40	50	60	70	80	90	100	110
2.5	4.5	6	7.5	9	10.5	12	13.5	15	16.5
5	9	12	15	18	21	24	27	30	33
7.5	13.5	18	22.5	27	31.5	36	40.5	45	49.5
10	18	24	30	36	42	48	54	60	66
12.5	22.5	30	37.5	45	52.5	60	67.5	75	82.5
15	27	36	45	54	63	72	81	90	99

Dobutrex Solution Infusion Rate (mL/h) for 2,000 µg/mL concentration

Drug Delivery Rate (µg/kg/min)	Patient Body Weight (kg)								
	30	40	50	60	70	80	90	100	110
2.5	2	3	4	4.5	5	6	7	7.5	8
5	4.5	6	7.5	9	10.5	12	13.5	15	16.5
7.5	7	9	11	13.5	16	18	20	22.5	25
10	9	12	15	18	21	24	27	30	33
12.5	11	15	19	22.5	26	30	34	37.5	41
15	13.5	18	22.5	27	31.5	36	40.5	45	49.5

The rate of administration and the duration of therapy should be adjusted according to the patient's response as determined by heart rate, presence of ectopic activity, blood pressure, urine flow, and, whenever possible, measurement of central venous or pulmonary wedge pressure and cardiac output.
Concentrations up to 5,000 µg/mL have been administered to humans (250 mg/50 mL). The final volume administered should be determined by the fluid requirements of the patient.
Intravenous drug products should be inspected visually and should not be used if particulate matter or discoloration is present.

HOW SUPPLIED

Vials:
250 mg,* 20-mL size
NDC 0002-7175-01 (No. 7175)—1s
NDC 0002-7175-10 (No. 7175)—(Traypak† of 10)

---

* Equivalent to dobutamine hydrochloride.
† Traypak™ (multivial carton, Lilly)
Store at controlled room temperature, 59° to 86°F (15° to 30°C).
CAUTION—Federal (USA) law prohibits dispensing without prescription.
Literature revised September 2, 1997
PA7366AMP   [090297]

EVISTA®   ℞
Raloxifene Hydrochloride
60 mg Tablets

DESCRIPTION

EVISTA® (raloxifene hydrochloride) is a selective estrogen receptor modulator (SERM) that belongs to the benzothiophene class of compounds. The chemical structure is:
[See chemical structure at top of next column]

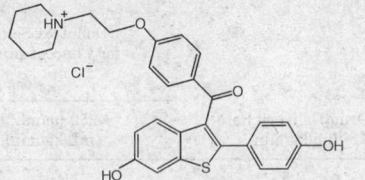

The chemical designation is methanone, [6-hydroxy-2-(4-hydroxyphenyl)benzo[*b*]thien-3-yl]-[4-[2-(1-piperidinyl)ethoxy]phenyl]-, hydrochloride. Raloxifene hydrochloride (HCl) has the empirical formula $C_{28}H_{27}NO_4S \cdot HCl$, which corresponds to a molecular weight of 510.05. Raloxifene HCl is an off-white to pale-yellow solid that is very slightly soluble in water.
EVISTA is supplied in a tablet dosage form for oral administration. Each EVISTA tablet contains 60 mg of raloxifene HCl, which is the molar equivalent of 55.71 mg of free base. Inactive ingredients include anhydrous lactose, carnauba wax, crospovidone, F D & C Blue No. 2 aluminum lake, hydroxypropyl methylcellulose, lactose monohydrate, magnesium stearate, modified pharmaceutical glaze, polyethylene glycol, polysorbate 80, povidone, propylene glycol, and titanium dioxide.

CLINICAL PHARMACOLOGY
Mechanism of Action
Decreases in estrogen levels after oophorectomy or menopause lead to increases in bone resorption and bone loss. Bone is initially lost rapidly because the compensatory increase in bone formation is inadequate to offset resorptive losses. This imbalance between resorption and formation is related to loss of estrogen, and may also involve age-related impairment of osteoblasts or their precursors.
Raloxifene reduces resorption of bone and decreases overall bone turnover. These effects on bone are manifested as reductions in the serum and urine levels of bone turnover markers, evidence from radiocalcium kinetics studies for decreased bone resorption and increases in bone mineral density (BMD).
Raloxifene's biological actions, like those of estrogen, are mediated through binding to estrogen receptors. This binding results in differential expression of multiple estrogen-regulated genes in different tissues. Recent data suggest that the estrogen receptor can regulate gene expression by at least two distinct pathways which are ligand-, tissue-, and/or gene-specific.
Clinical data indicate that raloxifene, a selective estrogen receptor modulator (SERM), has estrogen-like effects on bone (increase in BMD) and on lipid (decrease in total and LDL cholesterol levels) metabolism. Preclinical data demonstrate that raloxifene is an estrogen antagonist in uterine and breast tissues. Preliminary clinical data (through 30 months) suggest EVISTA lacks estrogen-like effects on uterus and breast tissue.

Pharmacokinetics
The disposition of raloxifene has been evaluated in 276 postmenopausal women in conventional clinical pharmacology studies and in more than 1300 postmenopausal women in selected raloxifene trials. Raloxifene exhibits high within-subject variability (approximately 30% coefficient of variation) of most pharmacokinetic parameters. Table 1 summarizes the pharmacokinetic parameters of raloxifene.

Absorption
Raloxifene is absorbed rapidly after oral administration. Approximately 60% of an oral dose is absorbed, but presystemic glucuronide conjugation is extensive. Absolute bioavailability of raloxifene is 2.0%. The time to reach average maximum plasma concentration and bioavailability are functions of systemic interconversion and enterohepatic cycling of raloxifene and its glucuronide metabolites.

Administration of raloxifene HCl with a standardized, high-fat meal increases the absorption of raloxifene (C_{max} 28% and AUC 16%), but does not lead to clinically meaningful changes in systemic exposure. EVISTA can be administered without regard to meals.

Distribution
Following oral administration of single doses ranging from 30 to 150 mg of raloxifene HCl, the apparent volume of distribution is 2348 L/kg and is not dose dependent.
Raloxifene and the monoglucuronide conjugates are highly bound to plasma proteins. Raloxifene binds to both albumin and α1-acid glycoprotein, but not to sex steroid binding globulin. In vitro, raloxifene did not interact with the binding of warfarin, phenytoin, or tamoxifen to plasma proteins.

Metabolism
Biotransformation and disposition of raloxifene in humans have been determined following oral administration of ^{14}C-labeled raloxifene. Raloxifene undergoes extensive first-pass metabolism to the glucuronide conjugates: raloxifene-4'-glucuronide, raloxifene-6-glucuronide, and raloxifene-6,4'-diglucuronide. No other metabolites have been detected, providing strong evidence that raloxifene is not metabolized by cytochrome P450 pathways. Unconjugated raloxifene comprises less than 1% of the total radiolabeled material in plasma. The terminal log-linear portions of the plasma concentration curves for raloxifene and the glucuronides are generally parallel. This is consistent with interconversion of raloxifene and the glucuronide metabolites.
Following intravenous administration, raloxifene is cleared at a rate approximating hepatic blood flow. Apparent oral clearance is 44.1 L/kg • hr. Raloxifene and its glucuronide conjugates are interconverted by reversible systemic metabolism and enterohepatic cycling, thereby prolonging its plasma elimination half-life to 27.7 hours after oral dosing. Results from single oral doses of raloxifene predict multiple-dose pharmacokinetics. Following chronic dosing, clearance ranges from 40 to 60 L/kg • hr. Increasing doses of raloxifene HCl (ranging from 30 to 150 mg) result in slightly less than a proportional increase in the area under the plasma time concentration curve (AUC).

Excretion
Raloxifene is primarily excreted in feces, and less than 0.2% is excreted unchanged in urine. Less than 6% of the raloxifene dose is eliminated in urine as glucuronide conjugates. In the osteoporosis prevention trials, raloxifene and metabolite concentrations are similar for women with estimated creatinine clearance as low as 23 mL/min.
[See table 1 below]

Special Populations
Geriatric—No differences in raloxifene pharmacokinetics were detected with regard to age (range 42 to 84 years).
Pediatric—The pharmacokinetics of raloxifene have not been evaluated in a pediatric population.
Gender—Total extent of exposure and oral clearance, normalized for lean body weight, are not significantly different between age-matched female and male volunteers.
Race—Pharmacokinetic differences due to race have been studied on a limited basis in 1053 women consisting of 93.5% Caucasian, 4.3% Hispanic, 1.2% Asian, and 0.5% Black in the osteoporosis prevention trials. There were no discernible differences in raloxifene plasma concentrations among these groups; however, the influence of race cannot be effectively determined.
Renal Insufficiency—Since negligible amounts of raloxifene are eliminated in urine, a study in patients with renal insufficiency was not conducted.
Hepatic Dysfunction—Raloxifene was studied, as a single dose, in Child-Pugh Class A patients with cirrhosis and total serum bilirubin ranging from 0.6 to 2.0 mg/dL. Plasma raloxifene concentrations were approximately 2.5 times higher than in controls and correlated with bilirubin

Table 1.   Summary of raloxifene pharmacokinetic parameters in the healthy postmenopausal woman

	C_{max}[a] (ng/mL)/ (mg/kg)	$t_{1/2}$ (hr)	$AUC_{0-\infty}$[a] (ng • hr/mL)/ (mg/kg)	CL/F (L/kg • hr)	V/F (L/kg)
Single Dose					
Mean	0.50	27.7	27.2	44.1	2348
CV (%)	52	10.7 to 273[b]	44	46	52
Multiple Dose					
Mean	1.36	32.5	24.2	47.4	2853
CV (%)	37	15.8 to 86.6[b]	36	41	56

Abbreviations: C_{max} = maximum plasma concentration, $t_{1/2}$ = half-life, AUC = area under the curve, CL = clearance, V = volume of distribution, F = bioavailability, CV = coefficient of variation.

[a] Data normalized for dose in mg and body weight in kg.
[b] Range of observed half-life.

concentrations. Safety and efficacy have not been evaluated further in patients with hepatic insufficiency (see WARNINGS).

Drug-Drug Interactions
Clinically significant drug-drug interactions are discussed in PRECAUTIONS.

Ampicillin—Peak concentrations of raloxifene and the overall extent of absorption are reduced 28% and 14%, respectively, with coadministration of ampicillin. These reductions are consistent with decreased-enterohepatic cycling associated with antibiotic reduction of enteric bacteria. However, the systemic exposure and the elimination rate of raloxifene were not affected. Therefore, EVISTA can be concurrently administered with ampicillin.

Antacids—Concurrent administration of calcium carbonate or aluminum and magnesium hydroxide-containing antacids does not affect the systemic exposure of raloxifene.

Corticosteroids—The coadministration of EVISTA with corticosteroids has not been evaluated.

Cyclosporine—The coadministration of EVISTA with cyclosporine has not been evaluated.

Digoxin—Raloxifene has no effect on the pharmacokinetics of digoxin.

Animal Pharmacology
The skeletal effects of raloxifene treatment were assessed in ovariectomized rats and monkeys. In rats, raloxifene prevented increased bone resorption and bone loss after ovariectomy. There were positive effects of raloxifene on bone strength, but the effects varied with time. Cynomolgus monkeys were treated with raloxifene or conjugated estrogens for 2 years, equivalent at the bone level to approximately 6 years in humans. Raloxifene and estrogen increased BMD, but variability among animals obscured the ability to detect effects of either treatment on biomechanical strength. However, bone strength was positively correlated to BMD in both raloxifene- and estrogen-treated monkeys, indicating that BMD is a reasonable marker for bone strength. Histologic examination of bone from rats and monkeys treated with raloxifene showed no evidence of woven bone, marrow fibrosis, or mineralization defects.

These results are consistent with data from human studies of radiocalcium kinetics and markers of bone metabolism, and are consistent with EVISTA's action as a skeletal antiresorptive agent.

Clinical Studies
Effects on Total Body and Regional Bone Mineral Density
In postmenopausal women, EVISTA preserves bone mass and increases BMD relative to calcium alone at 24 months. The effect on hip bone mass is similar to that for the spine. The relationships of BMD changes to skeletal fracture rates have not yet been established in EVISTA-treated women.

The effects of EVISTA on BMD in postmenopausal women were examined in three large randomized, placebo-controlled, double-blind osteoporosis prevention trials: (1) a North American trial enrolled 544 women; (2) a European trial, 601 women; and (3) an international trial, 619 women who had undergone hysterectomy. In these trials, all women received calcium supplementation (400 to 600 mg/day). Women enrolled in these studies had a median age of 54 years and a median time since menopause of 5 years (less than 1 year up to 15 years postmenopause). The majority of the women were Caucasian (93.5%). Women were included if they had spine bone mineral density between 2.5 standard deviations below and 2 standard deviations above the mean value for healthy young women. The mean T scores (number of standard deviations above or below the mean in healthy young women) for the 3 studies ranged from −1.01 to −0.74 for spine BMD and included women both with normal and low BMD. EVISTA, 60 mg administered once daily, produced increases in bone mass versus calcium supplementation alone, as reflected by dual-energy x-ray absorptiometric (DXA) measurements of hip, spine, and total body BMD. Compared with placebo, the increases in BMD for each of the 3 studies were statistically significant at 12 months and were maintained at 24 months (Table 2). The calcium-supplemented placebo groups lost approximately 1% of BMD over 24 months. (See figures below for total hip results.)

Table 2. EVISTA (60 mg once daily) related increases in BMD for the three osteoporosis prevention studies expressed as mean percentage increase versus calcium-supplemented placebo at 24 months[a]

	Study		
Site	NA %	EU %	INT[b] %
Total Hip	2.0	2.4	1.3
Femoral Neck	2.1	2.5	1.6
Trochanter	2.2	2.7	1.3
Intertrochanter	2.3	2.4	1.3
Lumbar Spine	2.0	2.4	1.8

Abbreviations: NA = North American, EU = European, INT = International.
[a] Intent-to-treat analysis; last observation carried forward.
[b] All women in the study had previously undergone hysterectomy.

EVISTA also increased BMD compared with placebo in the total body by 1.3% to 2.0% and in Ward's Triangle (hip) by 3.1% to 4.0%. The effects of EVISTA on forearm BMD were inconsistent between studies. In Study EU, EVISTA prevented bone loss at the ultradistal radius, whereas in Study NA, it did not.

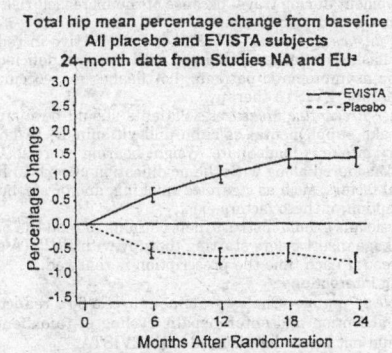

Total hip mean percentage change from baseline
All placebo and EVISTA subjects
24-month data from Studies NA and EU[a]

* Intent to treat analysis, last observation carried forward

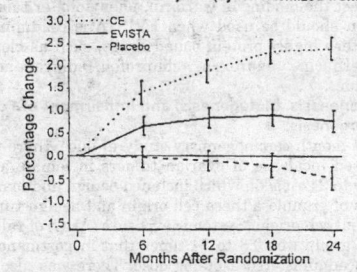

Total hip mean percentage change from baseline
All placebo, EVISTA, and CE subjects
24-month data from Study INT (hysterectomized women)[a]

CE = conjugated estrogens 0.625 mg/day
[a] Intent to treat analysis, last observation carried forward

Assessments of Bone Turnover
In a 31-week open-label radiocalcium kinetics study, 33 early postmenopausal women were randomized to treatment with once-daily EVISTA 60 mg, cyclic estrogen/progestin (0.625 mg conjugated estrogens daily with 5 mg medroxyprogesterone acetate daily for the first two weeks of each month [HRT]), or no treatment. Treatment with either EVISTA or HRT was associated with reduced bone resorption and a positive shift in calcium balance (−82 mg Ca/day and +60 mg Ca/day, respectively for EVISTA and −162 mg Ca/day and +91 mg Ca/day, respectively for HRT).

In the osteoporosis prevention trials, EVISTA therapy resulted in consistent, statistically significant suppression of bone resorption and bone formation, as reflected by changes in serum and urine markers of bone turnover (e.g., bone-specific alkaline phosphatase, osteocalcin, and collagen breakdown products). The suppression of bone turnover markers was evident by 3 months and persisted throughout the 24-month observation period.

Bone Histomorphometry
The tissue- and cellular-level effects of raloxifene were assessed by histomorphometric evaluation of human iliac crest bone biopsies taken after administration of a fluorochrome substance to label areas of mineralizing bone. The effects of EVISTA on bone histomorphometry were determined by pre- and post-treatment biopsies in a 6-month study of Caucasian postmenopausal women who received once-daily doses of EVISTA 60 mg or 0.625 mg conjugated estrogens. Ten raloxifene-treated and 8 estrogen-treated women had evaluable bone biopsies at baseline and after 6 months of therapy. Bone formation rate/bone volume and activation frequency, the primary efficacy parameters, decreased to a greater extent with conjugated estrogen treatment versus EVISTA treatment, although the differences were not statistically significant. Bone in EVISTA- and estrogen-treated women showed no evidence of mineralization defects, woven bone, or marrow fibrosis. In a blinded ongoing study, light microscopic evaluation of transiliac biopsies taken at baseline and after 2 years of therapy in 59 postmenopausal women receiving placebo, 60 mg-, or 120

mg-raloxifene hydrochloride showed no osteomalacia, osteocyte damage, woven bone, marrow fibrosis, or other abnormalities.

Effects on Lipid Metabolism
The effects of EVISTA on selected lipid fractions and clotting factors were evaluated in a 6-month study of 390 postmenopausal women. EVISTA was compared with oral continuous combined estrogen/progestin (0.625 mg conjugated estrogens plus 2.5 mg medroxyprogesterone acetate, [HRT]) and placebo (Table 3). EVISTA decreased serum total and LDL cholesterol without effects on serum total HDL cholesterol or triglycerides. In addition, EVISTA significantly decreased serum fibrinogen and lipoprotein (a).

Table 3. EVISTA (60 mg once daily) and oral HRT effects on selected lipid fractions and clotting factors in a 6-month study—Median percentage change from baseline

	Treatment Group		
Endpoint	EVISTA (N=95) %	HRT (N=96) %	PLACEBO (N=98) %
Total Cholesterol	−6.6[a]	−4.4[a]	0.9
LDL Cholesterol	−10.9[a]	−12.7[a]	1.0
HDL Cholesterol	0.7[b]	10.6[a]	0.9
HDL-2 Cholesterol	15.4[b]	33.3[a]	0.0
HDL-3 Cholesterol	−2.5[ab]	2.7	0.0
Fibrinogen	−12.2[ab]	−2.8	−2.1
Lipoprotein (a)	−4.1[ab]	−16.3[a]	3.3
Triglycerides	−4.1[b]	20.0[a]	−0.3
Plasminogen Activator Inhibitor-1	−2.1[b]	−29.0[a]	−9.4

Abbreviations: HRT = continuous combined estrogen/progestin (0.625 mg conjugated estrogens plus 2.5 mg medroxyprogesterone acetate).
[a] Significantly different from placebo (p<0.05).
[b] Significantly different from HRT (p<0.05).

In the osteoporosis prevention studies (N=1764), 24-month data were consistent with results from the 6-month study. Compared with placebo, EVISTA significantly decreased serum total and LDL cholesterol by approximately 5% and 8% respectively, but did not affect HDL cholesterol or triglycerides.

Effects on the Uterus
In placebo-controlled osteoporosis prevention trials, endometrial thickness was evaluated every 6 months (for 24 months) by transvaginal ultrasonography (TVU). A total of 2978 TVU measurements were collected from 831 women in all dose groups. Endometrial thickness measurements in raloxifene-treated women were indistinguishable from placebo. There were no differences between the raloxifene and placebo groups with respect to the incidence of reported vaginal bleeding.

In a 6-month study of 18 postmenopausal women that compared EVISTA to conjugated estrogens (0.625 mg/day [ERT]), endpoint endometrial biopsies demonstrated stimulatory effects of ERT, which were not observed for EVISTA. All samples from EVISTA-treated women showed nonproliferative endometria.

A 12-month study of uterine effects compared a higher dose of raloxifene HCl (150 mg/day) with HRT. At baseline, 43 raloxifene-treated postmenopausal women and 37 HRT-treated women had a nonproliferative endometrium. At study completion, endometria in all of the raloxifene-treated women remained nonproliferative whereas 13 HRT-treated women had developed proliferative changes. Also, HRT significantly increased uterine volume; raloxifene did not increase uterine volume. Thus, no stimulatory effect of raloxifene on the endometrium was detected at more than twice the recommended dose.

Effects on the Breast
Across all placebo-controlled trials, EVISTA was indistinguishable from placebo with regard to frequency and severity of breast pain and tenderness. EVISTA was associated with significantly less breast pain and tenderness than reported by women receiving estrogens with or without added progestin (see ADVERSE REACTIONS and Table 5).

INDICATIONS AND USAGE

EVISTA is indicated for the prevention of osteoporosis in postmenopausal women.

The effects of EVISTA on fracture risk are not yet known. Supplemental calcium should be added to the diet if daily intake is inadequate.

No single clinical finding or test result can quantify risk of postmenopausal osteoporosis with certainty. However, clin-

Continued on next page

* Identi-Code® symbol. This product information was prepared in June 1998. Current information on these and other products of Eli Lilly and Company may be obtained by direct inquiry to Lilly Research Laboratories, Lilly Corporate Center, Indianapolis, Indiana 46285, (800) 545-5979.

Evista—Cont.

ical assessment can help to identify women at increased risk. Widely accepted risk factors include Caucasian or Asian descent, slender body build, early estrogen deficiency, smoking, alcohol consumption, low calcium diet, sedentary lifestyle, and family history of osteoporosis. Evidence of increased bone turnover from serum and urine markers and low bone mass (e.g., at least 1 standard deviation below the mean for healthy, young adult women) as determined by densitometric techniques are also predictive. The greater the number of clinical risk factors, the greater the probability of developing postmenopausal osteoporosis.

CONTRAINDICATIONS

EVISTA is contraindicated in women who are or may become pregnant. EVISTA may cause fetal harm when administered to a pregnant woman. In rabbit studies, abortion and a low rate of fetal heart anomalies (ventricular septal defects) occurred in rabbits at doses ≥0.1 mg/kg (≥0.04 times the human dose based on surface area, mg/m^2), and hydrocephaly was observed in fetuses at doses ≥10 mg/kg (≥4 times the human dose based on surface area, mg/m^2). In rat studies, retardation of fetal development and developmental abnormalities (wavy ribs, kidney cavitation) occurred at doses ≥1 mg/kg (≥0.2 times the human dose based on surface area, mg/m^2). Treatment of rats at doses of 0.1 to 10 mg/kg (0.02 to 1.6 times the human dose based on surface area, mg/m^2) during gestation and lactation produced effects that included delayed and disrupted parturition; decreased neonatal survival and altered physical development; sex- and age-specific reductions in growth and changes in pituitary hormone content; and decreased lymphoid compartment size in offspring. At 10 mg/kg, raloxifene disrupted parturition which resulted in maternal and progeny death and morbidity. Effects in adult offspring (4 months of age) included uterine hypoplasia and reduced fertility; however, no ovarian or vaginal pathology was observed. The patient should be apprised of the potential hazard to the fetus if this drug is used during pregnancy, or if the patient becomes pregnant while taking this drug.

EVISTA is contraindicated in women with active or past history of venous thromboembolic events, including deep vein thrombosis, pulmonary embolism, and retinal vein thrombosis.

EVISTA is contraindicated in women known to be hypersensitive to raloxifene or other constituents of the tablets.

WARNINGS

Venous Thromboembolic Events—An analysis of EVISTA-treated women across all placebo-controlled clinical trials showed an increased risk of venous thromboembolic events defined as deep vein thrombosis, pulmonary embolism, and retinal vein thrombosis. The greatest risk for thromboembolic events occurs during the first 4 months of treatment. EVISTA should be discontinued at least 72 hours prior to and during prolonged immobilization (e.g., post-surgical recovery, prolonged bed rest), and EVISTA therapy should be resumed only after the patient is fully ambulatory. Patients should be advised to avoid prolonged restrictions of movement during travel. The risk-benefit balance should be considered in women at risk of thromboembolic disease for other reasons, such as congestive heart failure and active malignancy.

Premenopausal Use—There is no indication for premenopausal use of EVISTA. Safety of EVISTA in premenopausal women has not been established and its use is not recommended (see CONTRAINDICATIONS).

Hepatic Dysfunction—Raloxifene was studied, as a single dose, in Child-Pugh Class A patients with cirrhosis and serum total bilirubin ranging from 0.6 to 2.0 mg/dL. Plasma raloxifene concentrations were approximately 2.5 times higher than in controls and correlated with total bilirubin concentrations. Safety and efficacy have not been evaluated further in patients with severe hepatic insufficiency.

PRECAUTIONS

General

Concurrent Estrogen Therapy—The concurrent use of EVISTA and systemic estrogen or hormone replacement therapy (ERT or HRT) has not been studied in prospective clinical trials and therefore concomitant use of EVISTA with systemic estrogens is not recommended.

Lipid Metabolism—EVISTA lowers serum total and LDL cholesterol by 6% to 11%, but does not affect serum concentrations of total HDL cholesterol or triglycerides.

These effects should be taken into account in therapeutic decisions for patients who may require therapy for hyperlipidemia.

Concurrent use of EVISTA and lipid-lowering agents has not been studied.

Endometrium—EVISTA has not been associated with endometrial proliferation (see **Clinical Studies** and ADVERSE REACTIONS). Unexplained uterine bleeding should be investigated as clinically indicated.

Breast—EVISTA has not been associated with breast enlargement, breast pain, or an increased risk of breast cancer (see **Clinical Studies** and ADVERSE REACTIONS). Any unexplained breast abnormality occurring during EVISTA therapy should be investigated.

History of Breast Cancer—EVISTA has not been adequately studied in women with a prior history of breast cancer.

Use in Men—Safety and efficacy have not been evaluated in men.

Information for Patients

For safe and effective use of EVISTA, the physician should inform patients about the following:

Patient Immobilization—EVISTA should be discontinued at least 72 hours prior to and during prolonged immobilization (e.g., post-surgical recovery, prolonged bed rest), and patients should be advised to avoid prolonged restrictions of movement during travel because of the increased risk of venous thromboembolic events.

Hot flashes or flushes—EVISTA is not effective in reducing hot flashes or flushes associated with estrogen deficiency. In some asymptomatic patients, hot flashes may occur upon beginning EVISTA therapy.

Other Preventive Measures—Patients should be instructed to take supplemental calcium and vitamin D, if daily dietary intake is inadequate. Weight-bearing exercise should be considered along with the modification of certain behavioral factors, such as cigarette smoking, and/or alcohol consumption, if these factors exist.

Physicians should instruct their patients to read the patient package insert before starting therapy with EVISTA and to re-read it each time the prescription is renewed.

Drug Interactions

Cholestyramine—Cholestyramine causes a 60% reduction in the abortion and enterohepatic cycling of raloxifene and should not be coadministered with EVISTA.

Warfarin—The coadministration of EVISTA and warfarin has not been assessed under chronic conditions. However, 10% decreases in prothrombin time have been observed in single-dose studies. If EVISTA is given concurrently with warfarin, prothrombin time should be monitored.

Other Highly Protein-Bound Drugs—Raloxifene is more than 95% bound to plasma proteins. In vitro, raloxifene did not affect the binding of warfarin, phenytoin, or tamoxifen. Caution should be used when EVISTA is coadministered with other highly protein-bound drugs, such as clofibrate, indomethacin, naproxen, ibuprofen, diazepam, and diazoxide.

Carcinogenesis, Mutagenesis, and Impairment of Fertility

Carcinogenesis:

In a 21-month carcinogenicity study in mice, there was an increased incidence of ovarian tumors in female animals given 9 to 242 mg/kg, which included benign and malignant tumors of granulosa/theca cell origin and benign tumors of epithelial cell origin. Systemic exposure (AUC) of raloxifene in this group was 0.3 to 34 times that in postmenopausal women administered a 60-mg dose. There was also an increased incidence of testicular interstitial cell tumors and prostatic adenomas and adenocarcinomas in males given 41 or 210 mg/kg (4.7 or 24 times the AUC in humans), and prostatic leiomyoblastoma in males given 210 mg/kg.

In a 2-year carcinogenicity study in rats, an increased incidence in ovarian tumors of granulosa/theca cell origin was observed in females given 279 mg/kg (approximately 400 times the AUC in humans). The female rodents in these studies were treated during their reproductive lives when their ovaries were functional and responsive to hormonal stimulation. The clinical relevance of these tumor findings is not known.

Mutagenesis:

Raloxifene HCl was not genotoxic in any of the following test systems: the Ames test for bacterial mutagenesis with and without metabolic activation, the unscheduled DNA synthesis assay in rat hepatocytes, the mouse lymphoma assay for mammalian cell mutation, the chromosomal aberration assay in Chinese hamster ovary cells, the in vivo sister chromatid exchange assay in Chinese hamsters, and the in vivo micronucleus test in mice.

Impairment of Fertility:

When male and female rats were given daily doses ≥5 mg/kg (≥0.8 times the human dose based on surface area, mg/m^2) prior to and during mating, no pregnancies occurred. In male rats, daily doses up to 100 mg/kg (16 times the human dose based on surface area, mg/m^2) for at least 2 weeks did not affect sperm production or quality, or reproductive performance. In female rats, at doses of 0.1 to 10 mg/kg/day (0.02 to 1.6 times the human dose based on surface area, mg/m^2), raloxifene disrupted estrous cycles and inhibited ovulation. These effects of raloxifene were reversible. In another study in rats in which raloxifene was given during the preimplantation period at doses ≥0.1 mg/kg (≥0.02 times the human dose based on surface area, mg/m^2), raloxifene delayed and disrupted embryo implantation resulting in prolonged gestation and reduced litter size. The reproductive and developmental effects observed in animals are consistent with the estrogen receptor activity of raloxifene.

Pregnancy

Pregnancy Category X—EVISTA should not be used in women who are or may become pregnant (see CONTRAINDICATIONS).

Nursing Mothers—EVISTA should not be used by lactating women (see CONTRAINDICATIONS). It is not known whether raloxifene is excreted in human milk.

Pediatric Use—EVISTA should not be used in pediatric patients.

ADVERSE REACTIONS

The safety of raloxifene has been assessed primarily in 12 Phase 2 and Phase 3 studies with placebo, estrogen, and estrogen-progestin replacement therapy (HRT) control groups. The duration of treatment ranged from 2 to 30 months and 2036 women were exposed to raloxifene (371 patients received 10 to 50 mg/day, 828 received 60 mg/day, and 837 received from 120 to 600 mg/day).

The majority of adverse events occurring during clinical trials were mild and generally did not require discontinuation of therapy.

Therapy was discontinued due to an adverse event in 11.4% of 581 EVISTA-treated women and 12.2% of 584 placebo-treated women. Common adverse events considered to be drug-related were hot flashes and leg cramps (see Table 4). The first occurrence of hot flashes was most commonly reported during the first 6 months of treatment. Discontinuation rates due to hot flashes did not differ significantly between EVISTA and placebo groups (1.7% and 2.2%, respectively).

Adverse Events in Placebo-Controlled Clinical Trials

Table 4 lists adverse events occurring in the placebo-controlled clinical trial database at a frequency ≥2.0% in either group and in more EVISTA-treated women than in placebo-treated women. Adverse events are shown without attribution of causality.

Table 4. Adverse events occurring in placebo-controlled clinical trials at a frequency of ≥2.0% and in more EVISTA-treated (60 mg once daily) women than placebo-treated women

Body System	EVISTA N=581 %	Placebo N=584 %
Body as a Whole		
Infection	15.1	14.6
Flu Syndrome	14.6	13.5
Leg Cramps	5.9	1.9
Chest Pain	4.0	3.6
Fever	3.1	2.6
Cardiovascular		
Hot Flashes	24.6	18.3
Migraine	2.4	2.1
Digestive		
Nausea	8.8	8.6
Dyspepsia	5.9	5.8
Vomiting	3.4	3.3
Flatulence	3.1	2.4
Gastrointestinal Disorder	3.3	2.1
Gastroenteritis	2.6	2.1
Metabolic and Nutritional		
Weight Gain	8.8	6.8
Peripheral Edema	3.3	1.9
Musculoskeletal		
Arthralgia	10.7	10.1
Myalgia	7.7	6.2
Arthritis	4.0	3.6
Nervous		
Depression	6.4	6.0
Insomnia	5.5	4.3
Respiratory		
Sinusitis	10.3	6.5
Pharyngitis	7.6	7.2
Cough Increased	6.0	5.7
Pneumonia	2.6	1.5
Laryngitis	2.2	1.4
Skin and Appendages		
Rash	5.5	3.8
Sweating	3.1	1.7
Urogenital		
Vaginitis	4.3	3.6
Urinary Tract Infection	4.0	3.9
Cystitis	3.3	3.1
Leukorrhea	3.3	1.7
Endometrial Disorder[a]	3.1	1.9

[a] Treatment-emergent uterine-related adverse event, including only patients with an intact uterus: EVISTA, N=354, Placebo, n=364.

Comparison of EVISTA and Hormone Replacement Therapy Adverse Events

EVISTA was compared with estrogen-progestin replacement therapy (HRT) in 3 clinical trials. Table 5 shows adverse events occurring more frequently in one treatment group and at an incidence ≥2.0% in any group. Adverse events are shown without attribution of causality.

Table 5. Adverse events reported in clinical trials with EVISTA (60 mg once daily) and continuous combined or cyclic estrogen plus progestin (HRT) at an incidence ≥2.0% in any treatment group[a]

Adverse Event	EVISTA (N=317) %	HRT-Continuous Combined (N=96) %	HRT-Cyclic (N=219) %
Urogenital			
Breast Pain	4.4	37.5	29.7
Vaginal Bleeding[b]	6.2	64.2	88.5
Digestive			
Flatulence	1.6	12.5	6.4
Cardiovascular			
Hot Flashes	28.7	3.1	5.9
Body as a Whole			
Infection	11.0	0	6.8
Abdominal Pain	6.6	10.4	18.7
Chest Pain	2.8	0	0.5

[a] These data are from both blinded and open-label studies.
[b] Treatment-emergent uterine-related adverse event, including only patients with an intact uterus: EVISTA, n=290, HRT-Continuous Combined, n=67, HRT-Cyclic, n=217.
Continuous Combined HRT = 0.625 mg conjugated estrogens plus 2.5 mg medroxyprogesterone acetate.
Cyclic HRT = 0.625 mg conjugated estrogens for 28 days with concomitant 5 mg medroxyprogesterone acetate or 0.15 mg norgestrel on days 1 through 14 or 17 through 28.

Laboratory Changes
The following changes in analyte concentrations are commonly observed during EVISTA therapy: increased apolipoprotein A1; and reduced serum total cholesterol, LDL cholesterol, fibrinogen, apolipoprotein B, and lipoprotein (a). EVISTA modestly increases hormone-binding globulin concentrations, including sex steroid-binding globulin, thyroxine-binding globulin, and corticosteroid-binding globulin with corresponding increases in measured total hormone concentrations. There is no evidence that these changes in hormone-binding globulin concentrations affect concentrations of the corresponding free hormones.
There were small decreases in serum total calcium, inorganic phosphate, total protein, and albumin which were generally of lesser magnitude than decreases observed during ERT/HRT. Platelet count was also decreased slightly and was not different from ERT.
Additional Safety Information
Incidences of estrogen-dependent carcinoma of the endometrium and breast are being evaluated across all completed and ongoing clinical trials involving 12,802 patients, of which approximately 8300 women have received at least one dose of raloxifene. The duration of exposure has been up to 39 months.
Endometrium—Compared to placebo, raloxifene did not increase the risk of endometrial cancer.
Breast—Compared to placebo, raloxifene did not increase the risk of breast cancer.

OVERDOSAGE

Incidents of overdose in humans have not been reported. In an 8-week study of 63 postmenopausal women, a dose of raloxifene HCl 600 mg/day was safely tolerated. No mortality was seen after a single oral dose in rats or mice at 5000 mg/kg (810 times the human dose for rats and 405 times the human dose for mice based on surface area, mg/m^2) or in monkeys at 1000 mg/kg (80 times the AUC in humans). There is no specific antidote for raloxifene.

DOSAGE AND ADMINISTRATION

The recommended dosage is one 60-mg EVISTA tablet daily which may be administered any time of day without regard to meals. The effect of EVISTA on BMD beyond two years of treatment is not known at this time, but is being evaluated in ongoing clinical trials.

HOW SUPPLIED

EVISTA 60-mg tablets are white, elliptical, and film coated. They are imprinted on one side with LILLY and the tablet code 4165 in edible blue ink. They are available as follows:

Bottle (count)	NDC Number
30 (unit of use)	NDC - 0002-4165-30
100 (unit of use)	NDC - 0002-4165-02
2000	NDC - 0002-4165-07

Store at controlled room temperature, 20° to 25°C (68° to 77°F) [see USP]. The USP defines controlled room temperature as a temperature maintained thermostatically that encompasses the usual and customary working environment of 20° to 25°C (68° to 77°F); that results in a mean kinetic temperature calculated to be not more than 25°C; and that allows for excursions between 15° and 30°C (59° and 86°F) that are experienced in pharmacies, hospitals, and warehouses.
CAUTION—Federal (USA) law prohibits dispensing without prescription.
Literature issued December 11, 1997
Printed in USA
PV 3080 AMP [121197]

FLUOXETINE HYDROCHLORIDE, ℞
see Prozac® (Fluoxetine Hydrochloride).

GEMZAR® ℞
(GEMCITABINE HCl) FOR INJECTION

DESCRIPTION

Gemzar® (gemcitabine HCl) is a nucleoside analogue that exhibits antitumor activity. Gemcitabine HCl is 2′-deoxy-2′,2′- difluorocytidine monohydrochloride (β-isomer).
The structural formula is as follows:

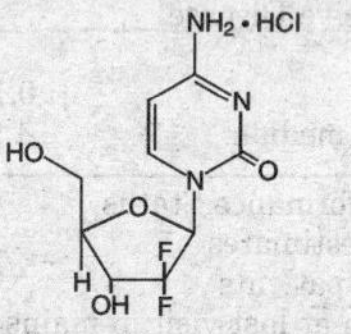

The empirical formula for gemcitabine HCl is $C_9H_{11}F_2N_3O_4$•HCl. It has a molecular weight of 299.66.
Gemcitabine HCl is a white to off-white solid. It is soluble in water, slightly soluble in methanol, and practically insoluble in ethanol and polar organic solvents.
The clinical formulation is supplied in a sterile form for intravenous use only. Vials of Gemzar contain either 200 mg or 1 g of gemcitabine HCl (expressed as free base) formulated with mannitol (200 mg or 1 g, respectively) and sodium acetate (12.5 mg or 62.5 mg, respectively) as a sterile lyophilized powder. Hydrochloric acid and/or sodium hydroxide may have been added for pH adjustment.

CLINICAL PHARMACOLOGY

Gemcitabine exhibits cell phase specificity, primarily killing cells undergoing DNA synthesis (S-phase) and also blocking the progression of cells through the G1/S-phase boundary. Gemcitabine is metabolized intracellularly by nucleoside kinases to the active diphosphate (dFdCDP) and triphosphate (dFdCTP) nucleosides. The cytotoxic effect of gemcitabine is attributed to a combination of two actions of the diphosphate and the triphosphate nucleosides, which leads to inhibition of DNA synthesis. First, gemcitabine diphosphate inhibits ribonucleotide reductase, which is responsible for catalyzing the reactions that generate the deoxynucleoside triphosphates for DNA synthesis. Inhibition of this enzyme by the diphosphate nucleoside causes a reduction in the concentrations of deoxynucleotides, including dCTP. Second, gemcitabine triphosphate competes with dCTP for incorporation into DNA. The reduction in the intracellular concentration of dCTP (by the action of the diphosphate) enhances the incorporation of gemcitabine triphosphate into DNA (self-potentiation). After the gemcitabine nucleotide is incorporated into DNA, only one additional nucleotide is added to the growing DNA strands. After this addition, there is inhibition of further DNA synthesis. DNA polymerase epsilon is unable to remove the gemcitabine nucleotide and repair the growing DNA strands (masked chain termination). In CEM T lymphoblastoid cells, gemcitabine induces internucleosomal DNA fragmentation, one of the characteristics of programmed cell death.
Human Pharmacokinetics—Gemcitabine disposition was studied in five patients who received a single 1000 mg/m^2/30 minute infusion of radiolabeled drug. Within one (1) week, 92% to 98% of the dose was recovered, almost entirely in the urine. Gemcitabine (<10%) and the inactive uracil metabolite, 2′-deoxy-2′,2′-difluorouridine (dFdU), accounted for 99% of the excreted dose. The metabolite dFdU is also found in plasma. Gemcitabine plasma protein binding is negligible.
The pharmacokinetics of gemcitabine were examined in 353 patients, about 2/3 men, with various solid tumors. Pharmacokinetic parameters were derived using data from patients treated for varying durations of therapy given weekly with periodic rest weeks and using both short infusions (<70 minutes) and long infusions (70 to 285 minutes). The total Gemzar dose varied from 500 to 3600 mg/m^2.
Gemcitabine pharmacokinetics are linear and are described by a 2-compartment model. Population pharmacokinetic analyses of combined single and multiple dose studies showed that the volume of distribution of gemcitabine was significantly influenced by duration of infusion and gender. Clearance was affected by age and gender. Differences in either clearance or volume of distribution based on patient characteristics or the duration of infusion result in changes in half-life and plasma concentrations. Table 1 shows plasma clearance and half-life of gemcitabine following short infusions for typical patients by age and gender.

Table 1
Gemcitabine Clearance and Half-Life for the "Typical" Patient

Age	Clearance Men (L/hr/m^2)	Clearance Women (L/hr/m^2)	Half-Life[a] Men (min)	Half-Life[a] Women (min)
29	92.2	69.4	42	49
45	75.7	57.0	48	57
65	55.1	41.5	61	73
79	40.7	30.7	79	94

[a]Half-life for patients receiving a short infusion (<70 min)

Gemcitabine half-life for short infusions ranged from 32 to 94 minutes, and the value for long infusions varied from 245 to 638 minutes, depending on age and gender, reflecting a greatly increased volume of distribution with longer infusions. The lower clearance in women and the elderly results in higher concentrations of gemcitabine for any given dose. The volume of distribution was increased with infusion length. Volume of distribution of gemcitabine was 50 L/m^2 following infusions lasting <70 minutes, indicating that gemcitabine, after short infusions, is not extensively distributed into tissues. For long infusions, the volume of distribution rose to 370 L/m^2, reflecting slow equilibration of gemcitabine within the tissue compartment.
The maximum plasma concentrations of dFdU (inactive metabolite) were achieved up to 30 minutes after discontinuation of the infusions and the metabolite is excreted in urine without undergoing further biotransformation. The metabolite did not accumulate with weekly dosing, but its elimination is dependent on renal excretion, and could accumulate with decreased renal function.
The effects of significant renal or hepatic insufficiency on the disposition of gemcitabine have not been assessed.
The active metabolite, gemcitabine triphosphate, can be extracted from peripheral blood mononuclear cells. The half-life of the terminal phase for gemcitabine triphosphate from mononuclear cells ranges from 1.7 to 19.4 hours.

CLINICAL STUDIES

Data from two clinical trials evaluated the use of Gemzar in patients with locally advanced or metastatic pancreatic cancer. The first trial compared Gemzar to 5-Fluorouracil (5-FU) in patients who had received no prior chemotherapy. A second trial studied the use of Gemzar in pancreatic cancer patients previously treated with 5-FU or a 5-FU-containing regimen. In both studies, the first cycle of Gemzar was administered intravenously at a dose of 1000 mg/m^2 over 30 minutes once weekly for up to 7 weeks (or until toxicity necessitated holding a dose) followed by a week of rest from treatment with Gemzar. Subsequent cycles consisted of injections once weekly for 3 consecutive weeks out of every 4 weeks.
The primary efficacy parameter in these studies was "clinical benefit response", which is a measure of clinical improvement based on analgesic consumption, pain intensity, performance status, and weight change. Definitions for improvement in these variables were formulated prospectively during the design of the two trials. A patient was considered a clinical benefit responder if either:

i) the patient showed a ≥50% reduction in pain intensity (Memorial Pain Assessment Card) or analgesic consumption, or a twenty point or greater improvement in performance status (Karnofsky Performance Scale) for a period of at least four consecutive weeks, without showing any sustained worsening in any of the other parameters. Sustained worsening was defined as four consecutive weeks with either any increase in pain intensity or analgesic consumption or a 20 point decrease in performance status occurring during the first 12 weeks of therapy.

OR:

ii) the patient was stable on all of the aforementioned parameters, and showed a marked, sustained weight gain (≥7% increase maintained for ≥4 weeks) not due to fluid accumulation.

Continued on next page

*** Identi-Code® symbol. This product information was prepared in June 1998. Current information on these and other products of Eli Lilly and Company may be obtained by direct inquiry to Lilly Research Laboratories, Lilly Corporate Center, Indianapolis, Indiana 46285, (800) 545-5979.**

Gemzar—Cont.

The first study was a multicenter (17 sites in US and Canada), prospective, single-blinded, two-arm, randomized comparison of Gemzar and 5-FU in patients with locally advanced or metastatic pancreatic cancer who had received no prior treatment with chemotherapy. 5-FU was administered intravenously at a weekly dose of 600 mg/m² for 30 minutes. The results from this randomized trial are shown in Table 2. Patients treated with Gemzar had statistically significant increases in clinical benefit response, survival, and time to progressive disease compared to 5-FU. The Kaplan-Meier curve for survival is shown in Figure 1. No confirmed objective tumor responses were observed with either treatment. [See table 2 above]

Figure 1
Kaplan-Meier Survival Curve

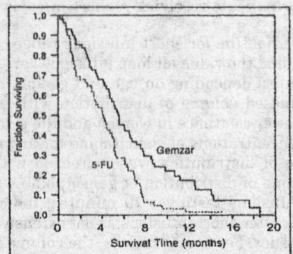

Clinical benefit response was achieved by 14 patients treated with Gemzar and 3 patients treated with 5-FU. One patient on the Gemzar arm showed improvement in all three primary parameters (pain intensity, analgesic consumption, and performance status). Eleven patients on the Gemzar arm and two patients on the 5-FU arm showed improvement in analgesic consumption and/or pain intensity with stable performance status. Two patients on the Gemzar arm showed improvement in analgesic consumption or pain intensity with improvement in performance status. One patient on the 5-FU arm was stable with regard to pain intensity and analgesic consumption, with improvement in performance status. No patient on either arm achieved a clinical benefit response based on weight gain. The second trial was a multicenter (17 US and Canadian centers), open-label study of Gemzar in 63 patients with advanced pancreatic cancer previously treated with 5-FU or a 5-FU-containing regimen. The study showed a clinical benefit response rate of 27% and median survival of 3.9 months. When Gemzar was administered more frequently than once weekly or with infusions longer than 60 minutes, increased toxicity was observed. Results of a Phase 1 study of Gemzar to assess the maximum tolerated dose (MTD) on a daily × 5 schedule showed that patients developed significant hypotension and severe flu-like symptoms that were intolerable at doses above 10 mg/m². The incidence and severity of these events were dose-related. Other Phase 1 studies using a twice-weekly schedule reached MTDs of only 65 mg/m² (30-minute infusion) and 150 mg/m² (5-minute bolus). The dose-limiting toxicities were thrombocytopenia and flu-like symptoms, particularly asthenia. In a Phase 1 study to assess the maximum tolerated infusion time, clinically significant toxicity, defined as myelosuppression, was seen with weekly doses of 300 mg/m² at or above a 270-minute infusion time. The half-life of gemcitabine is influenced by the length of the infusion (see Clinical Pharmacology) and the toxicity appears to be increased if Gemzar is administered more frequently than once weekly or with infusions longer than 60 minutes (see Warnings).

In a single trial where Gemzar at a dose of 1000 mg/m² was administered for up to six (6) consecutive weeks concurrently with therapeutic thoracic radiation to patients with NSCLC, significant toxicity in the form of severe, and potentially life-threatening, esophagitis and pneumonitis was observed, particularly in patients receiving large volumes of radiotherapy. The optimum regimen for safe administration of Gemzar with therapeutic doses of radiation has not yet been determined (see Precautions).

INDICATIONS AND USAGE

Therapeutic Indication—Gemzar is indicated as first-line treatment for patients with locally advanced (nonresectable Stage II or Stage III) or metastatic (Stage IV) adenocarcinoma of the pancreas. Gemzar is indicated for patients previously treated with 5-FU.

CONTRAINDICATION

Gemzar is contraindicated in those patients with a known hypersensitivity to the drug (see Adverse Reactions—Allergic).

Table 2
Gemzar Versus 5-FU in Pancreatic Cancer

	Gemzar	5-FU	
Number of Patients	63	63	
Male	34	34	
Female	29	29	
Median Age	62 years	61 years	
Range	37 to 79	36 to 77	
Stage IV Disease	71.4%	76.2%	
Baseline KPS[a] ≤70	69.8%	68.3%	
Clinical benefit response	22.2% (N[c] = 14)	4.8% (N = 3)	p = 0.004
Survival			p = 0.0009
Median	5.7 months	4.2 months	
6-month probability[b]	(N = 30) 46%	(N = 19) 29%	
9-month probability[b]	(N = 14) 24%	(N = 4) 5%	
1-year probability[b]	(N = 9) 18%	(N = 2) 2%	
Range	0.2 to 18.6 months	0.4 to 15.1+ months	
95% C.I. of the median	4.7 to 6.9 months	3.1 to 5.1 months	
Time to Progressive Disease			p = 0.0013
Median	2.1 months	0.9 months	
Range	0.1+to 9.4 months	0.1 to 12.0+months	
95% C.I. of the median	1.9 to 3.4 months	0.9 to 1.1 months	

[a] Karnofsky Performance Status
[b] Kaplan-Meier estimates
[c] N = number of patients
+ No progression at last visit; remains alive.
The p-value for clinical benefit response was calculated using the 2-sided test for difference in binomial proportions. All other p-values were calculated using the Log Rank test for difference in overall time to an event.

Table 3
Selected WHO-Graded Adverse Events in Patients Receiving Gemzar

	All Patients[a]			Pancreatic Cancer Patients[b]			Discontinuations(%)[c]
	All Grades	Grade 3	Grade 4	All Grades	Grade 3	Grade 4	All Patients
Laboratory[d]							
Hematologic							
Anemia	68	7	1	73	8	2	<1
Leukopenia	62	9	<1	64	8	1	<1
Neutropenia	63	19	6	61	17	7	—
Thrombocytopenia	24	4	1	36	7	<1	<1
Hepatic							<1
ALT	68	8	2	72	10	1	
AST	67	6	2	78	12	5	
Alkaline Phosphatase	55	7	2	77	16	4	
Bilirubin	13	2	<1	26	6	2	
Renal							<1
Proteinuria	45	<1	0	32	<1	0	
Hematuria	35	<1	0	23	0	0	
BUN	16	0	0	15	0	0	
Creatinine	8	<1	0	6	0	0	
Nonlaboratory[e]							
Nausea and Vomiting	69	13	1	71	10	2	<1
Pain	48	9	<1	42	6	<1	<1
Fever	41	2	0	38	2	0	<1
Rash	30	<1	0	28	<1	0	<1
Dyspnea	23	3	<1	10	0	<1	<1
Constipation	23	1	<1	31	3	<1	0
Diarrhea	19	1	0	30	3	0	0
Hemorrhage	17	<1	<1	4	2	<1	<1
Infection	16	1	<1	10	2	<1	<1
Alopecia	15	<1	0	16	0	0	0
Stomatitis	11	<1	0	10	<1	0	<1
Somnolence	11	<1	<1	11	2	<1	<1
Paresthesias	10	<1	0	10	<1	0	0

Grade based on criteria from the World Health Organization (WHO)

[a]N = 699–974; all patients with data
[b]N = 161–241; all pancreatic cancer patients with data
[c]N = 979
[d]Regardless of causality
[e] Table includes nonlaboratory data with incidence for all patients ≥10%. For approximately 60% of the patients, nonlaboratory events were graded only if assessed to be possibly drug related.

WARNINGS

Caution—Prolongation of the infusion time beyond 60 minutes and more frequent than weekly dosing have been shown to increase toxicity (see Clinical Studies).
Gemzar can suppress bone marrow function as manifested by leukopenia, thrombocytopenia, and anemia (see Adverse Reactions), and myelosuppression is usually the dose-limiting toxicity. Patients should be monitored for myelosuppression during therapy. See Dosage and Administration for recommended dose adjustments.

Table 4
Selected WHO-Graded Adverse Events from Comparative Trial of Gemzar and 5-FU
WHO Grades (% incidence)

	Gemzar[a]			5-FU[b]		
	All Grades	Grade 3	Grade 4	All Grades	Grade 3	Grade 4
Laboratory[c]						
Hematologic						
Anemia	65	7	3	45	0	0
Leukopenia	71	10	0	15	2	0
Neutropenia	62	19	7	18	2	3
Thrombocytopenia	47	10	0	15	2	0
Hepatic						
ALT	72	8	2	38	0	0
AST	72	10	2	52	2	0
Alkaline Phosphatase	71	16	0	64	10	3
Bilirubin	16	2	2	25	6	3
Renal						
Proteinuria	10	0	0	2	0	0
Hematuria	13	0	0	0	0	0
BUN	8	0	0	10	0	0
Creatinine	2	0	0	0	0	0
Nonlaboratory[d]						
Nausea and Vomiting	64	10	3	58	5	0
Pain	10	2	0	7	0	0
Fever	30	0	0	16	0	0
Rash	24	0	0	13	0	0
Dyspnea	6	0	0	3	0	0
Constipation	10	3	0	11	2	0
Diarrhea	24	2	0	31	5	0
Hemorrhage	0	0	0	2	0	0
Infection	8	0	0	3	2	0
Alopecia	18	0	0	16	0	0
Stomatitis	14	0	0	15	0	0
Somnolence	5	2	0	7	2	0
Paresthesias	2	0	0	2	0	0

Grade based on criteria from the World Health Organization (WHO)

[a]N = 58–63; all Gemzar patients with data
[b]N = 61–63; all 5-FU patients with data
[c]Regardless of causality
[d]Nonlaboratory events were graded only if assessed to be possibly drug-related.

Hemolytic-Uremic Syndrome (HUS) has been reported rarely with the use of Gemzar. (*see* Adverse Reactions—Renal)

Pregnancy—Pregnancy Category D. Gemzar can cause fetal harm when administered to a pregnant woman. Gemcitabine is embryotoxic causing fetal malformations (cleft palate, incomplete ossification) at doses of 1.5 mg/kg/day in mice (about $^1/_{200}$ the recommended human dose on a mg/m^2 basis). Gemcitabine is fetotoxic causing fetal malformations (fused pulmonary artery, absence of gall bladder) at doses of 0.1 mg/kg/day in rabbits (about $^1/_{600}$ the recommended human dose on a mg/m^2 basis). Embryotoxicity was characterized by decreased fetal viability, reduced live litter sizes, and developmental delays. There are no studies of Gemzar in pregnant women. If Gemzar is used during pregnancy, or if the patient becomes pregnant while taking Gemzar, the patient should be apprised of the potential hazard to the fetus.

PRECAUTIONS

General—Patients receiving therapy with Gemzar should be monitored closely by a physician experienced in the use of cancer chemotherapeutic agents. Most adverse events are reversible and do not need to result in discontinuation, although doses may need to be withheld or reduced. There was a greater tendency in women, especially older women, not to proceed to the next cycle.

Laboratory Tests—Patients receiving Gemzar should be monitored prior to each dose with a complete blood count (CBC), including differential and platelet count. Suspension or modification of therapy should be considered when marrow suppression is detected (*see* Dosage and Administration).

Laboratory evaluation of renal and hepatic function should be performed prior to initiation of therapy and periodically thereafter.

Carcinogenesis, Mutagenesis, Impairment of Fertility—Long-term animal studies to evaluate the carcinogenic potential of Gemzar have not been conducted. Gemcitabine induced forward mutations *in vitro* in a mouse lymphoma (L5178Y) assay and was clastogenic in an *in vivo* mouse micronucleus assay. Gemcitabine was negative when tested using the Ames, *in vivo* sister chromatid exchange, and *in vitro* chromosomal aberration assays, and did not cause unscheduled DNA synthesis *in vitro*. Gemcitabine I.P. doses of 0.5 mg/kg/day (about $^1/_{700}$ the human dose on a mg/m^2 basis) in male mice had an effect on fertility with moderate to severe hypospermatogenesis, decreased fertility, and decreased implantations. In female mice, fertility was not af-

fected but, maternal toxicities were observed at 1.5 mg/kg/day I.V. (about $^1/_{200}$ the human dose on a mg/m^2 basis) and fetotoxicity or embryolethality was observed at 0.25 mg/kg/day I.V. (about $^1/_{1300}$ the human dose on a mg/m^2 basis).

Pregnancy—Category D. *See* Warnings.

Nursing Mothers—It is not known whether Gemzar or its metabolites are excreted in human milk. Because many drugs are excreted in human milk and because of the potential for serious adverse reactions from Gemzar in nursing infants, the mother should be warned and a decision should be made whether to discontinue nursing or to discontinue the drug, taking into account the importance of the drug to the mother and the potential risk to the infant.

Elderly Patients—Gemzar clearance is affected by age (*see* Clinical Pharmacology). There is no evidence, however, that unusual dose adjustments, (ie, other than those already recommended in the Dosage and Administration section) are necessary in patients over 65, and, in general adverse reaction rates were similar in patients above and below 65. Grade 3/4 thrombocytopenia was more common in the elderly.

Gender—Gemzar clearance is affected by gender (*see* Clinical Pharmacology). There is no evidence, however, that unusual dose adjustments (ie, other than those already recommended in the Dosage and Administration section) are necessary in women. In general, adverse reaction rates were similar in men and women but women, especially older women were more likely not to proceed to a subsequent cycle and to experience grade 3/4 neutropenia and thrombocytopenia.

Pediatric Patients—Gemzar has not been studied in pediatric patients. Safety and effectiveness in pediatric patients have not been established.

Patients with Renal or Hepatic Impairment—Gemzar should be used with caution in patients with preexisting renal impairment or hepatic insufficiency. Gemzar has not been studied in patients with significant renal or hepatic impairment.

Drug Interactions—No confirmed interactions have been reported with the use of Gemzar. No specific drug interaction studies have been conducted.

Combination Therapy—Safe and effective regimens for the administration of Gemzar with therapeutic doses of radiation have not yet been determined (*See* Clinical Studies).

ADVERSE REACTIONS

Myelosuppression is the principal dose-limiting factor with Gemzar therapy. Dosage adjustments for hematologic toxicity are frequently needed and are described in the Dosage and Administration section.

Data in Table 3 are based on 22 clinical studies (N = 979) of Gemzar administered as a single agent, using starting doses in the range of 800 to 1250 mg/m^2 administered weekly as a 30-minute infusion for treatment of a wide variety of malignancies. Data are also shown for the subset of patients with pancreatic cancer treated in 5 clinical studies. The frequency of all grades and severe (WHO Grade 3 or 4) adverse events were generally similar for the overall safety database and the subset of patients with pancreatic cancer. Adverse reactions reported in the overall database resulted in discontinuation of Gemzar therapy in about 10% of patients. In the comparative trial, the discontinuation rate for adverse reactions was 14.3% for the gemcitabine arm and 4.8% for the 5-FU arm.

All WHO-graded laboratory events are listed in Table 3, regardless of causality. Nonlaboratory adverse events listed in Table 3 or discussed below were those reported, regardless of causality, for at least 10% of all patients, except the categories of Extravasation, Allergic, and Cardiovascular and certain specific events under the Renal, Pulmonary, and Infection categories. Table 4 presents the data from the comparative trial of Gemzar and 5-FU for the same adverse events as Table 3, regardless of incidence.

[See table 3 at top of previous page]
[See table 4 above]

Hematologic—Myelosuppression is the dose-limiting toxicity with Gemzar, but <1% of patients discontinued therapy for either anemia, leukopenia, or thrombocytopenia. Red blood cell transfusions were required by 19% of patients. The incidence of sepsis was less than 1%. Petechiae or mild blood loss (hemorrhage), from any cause, were reported in 16% of patients; less than 1% of patients required platelet transfusions. Patients should be monitored for myelosuppression during Gemzar therapy and dosage modified or suspended according to the degree of hematologic toxicity (*see* Dosage and Administration).

Gastrointestinal—Nausea and vomiting were commonly reported (69%) but were usually mild to moderate. Severe nausea and vomiting (WHO Grade 3/4) occurred in <15% of patients. Diarrhea was reported by 19% of patients, and stomatitis by 11% of patients.

Hepatic—Gemzar was associated with transient elevations of serum transaminases in approximately two-thirds of patients, but there was no evidence of increasing hepatic toxicity with either longer duration of exposure to Gemzar or with greater total cumulative dose.

Renal—Mild proteinuria and hematuria were commonly reported. Clinical findings consistent with the hemolytic uremic syndrome (HUS) were reported in 6 of 2429 patients (0.25%) receiving Gemzar in clinical trials. Four patients developed HUS on Gemzar therapy, two immediately posttherapy. Renal failure may not be reversible even with discontinuation of therapy, and dialysis may be required.

Fever—The overall incidence of fever was 41%. This is in contrast to the incidence of infection (16%) and indicates that Gemzar may cause fever in the absence of clinical infection. Fever was frequently associated with other flu-like symptoms and was usually mild and clinically manageable.

Rash—Rash was reported in 30% of patients. The rash was typically a macular or finely granular maculopapular pruritic eruption of mild to moderate severity involving the trunk and extremities. Pruritus was reported for 13% of patients.

Pulmonary—Dyspnea was reported in 23% of patients, severe dyspnea in 3%. Dyspnea may be due to underlying disease such as lung cancer (40% of study population) or pulmonary manifestations of other malignancies. Dyspnea was occasionally accompanied by bronchospasm (<2% of patients.) Rare reports of parenchymal lung toxicity consistent with drug induced pneumonitis have been associated with the use of Gemzar.

Edema—Edema (13%), peripheral edema (20%), and generalized edema (<1%) were reported. Less than 1% of patients discontinued due to edema.

Flu-like Symptoms—"Flu syndrome" was reported for 19% of patients. Individual symptoms of fewer, asthenia, anorexia, headache, cough, chills, and myalgia were commonly reported. Fever and asthenia were also reported frequently as isolated symptoms. Insomia, rhinitis, sweating, and malaise were reported infrequently. Less than 1% of patients discontinued due to flu-like symptoms.

Infection—Infections were reported for 16% of patients. Sepsis was rarely reported (<1%).

Alopecia—Hair loss, usually minimal, was reported by 15% of patients.

Neurotoxicity—There was a 10% incidence of mild paresthesias and a <1% rate of severe paresthesias.

Continued on next page

---

* Identi-Code® symbol. This product information was prepared in June 1998. Current information on these and other products of Eli Lilly and Company may be obtained by direct inquiry to Lilly Research Laboratories, Lilly Corporate Center, Indianapolis, Indiana 46285, (800) 545-5979.

Gemzar—Cont.

Extravasation—Injection-site related events were reported for 4% of patients. There were no reports of injection site necrosis. Gemzar is not a vesicant.
Allergic—Bronchospasm was reported for less than 2% of patients. Anaphylactoid reaction has been reported rarely. Gemzar should not be administered to patients with a known hypersensitivity to this drug (*see* Contraindication).
Cardiovascular—Two percent of patients discontinued therapy with Gemzar due to cardiovascular events such as myocardial infarction, cerebrovascular accident, arrhythmia, and hypertension. Many of these patients had a prior history of cardiovascular disease.

OVERDOSAGE

There is no known antidote for overdoses of Gemzar. Myelosuppression, paresthesias and severe rash were the principal toxicities seen when a single dose as high as 5700 mg/m^2 was administered by IV infusion over 30 minutes every 2 weeks to several patients in a Phase 1 study. In the event of suspected overdose, the patient should be monitored with appropriate blood counts and should receive supportive therapy, as necessary.

DOSAGE AND ADMINISTRATION

Gemzar is for intravenous use only.
Adults—Gemzar should be administered by intravenous infusion at a dose of 1000 mg/m^2 over 30 minutes once weekly for up to 7 weeks (or until toxicity necessitates reducing or holding a dose), followed by a week of rest from treatment. Subsequent cycles should consist of infusions once weekly for 3 consecutive weeks out of every 4 weeks. Dosage adjustment is based upon the degree of hematologic toxicity experienced by the patient (*see* Warnings). Clearance in women and the elderly is reduced and women were somewhat less able to progress to subsequent cycles (*see* Human Pharmacokinetics and Precautions).
Patients receiving Gemzar should be monitored prior to each dose with a complete blood count (CBC), including differential and platelet count. If marrow suppression is detected, therapy should be modified or suspended according to the guidelines in Table 5.

Table 5
Dosage Reduction Guidelines

Absolute granulocyte count ($\times 10^6$/L)		Platelet count ($\times 10^6$/L)	% of full dose
≥1,000	and	≥100,000	100
500–999	or	50,000–99,000	75
<500	or	<50,000	hold

Laboratory evaluation of renal and hepatic function, including transaminases and serum creatinine, should be performed prior to initiation of therapy and periodically thereafter. Gemzar should be administered with caution in patients with evidence of significant renal or hepatic impairment.
Patients who complete an entire 7 week initial cycle of Gemzar therapy or a subsequent 3 week cycle at a dose of 1000 mg/m^2 may have the dose for subsequent cycles increased by 25% (to 1250 mg/m^2), provided that the absolute granulocyte count (AGC) and platelet nadirs exceed 1500 $\times$ 10^6/L and 100,000 $\times$ 10^6/L, respectively, and if nonhematologic toxicity has not been greater than WHO Grade 1. If patients tolerate the subsequent course of Gemzar at a dose of 1250 mg/m^2, the dose for the next cycle can be increased to 1500 mg/m^2, provided again that the AGC and platelet nadirs exceed 1500 $\times$ 10^6/L and 100,000 $\times$ 10^6/L, respectively, and again, if nonhematologic toxicity has not been greater than WHO Grade 1.
Gemzar may be administered on an outpatient basis.
Instructions for Use/Handling—The recommended diluent for reconstitution of Gemzar is 0.9% Sodium Chloride Injection without preservatives. Due to solubility considerations, the maximum concentration for Gemzar upon reconstitution is 40 mg/mL. Reconstitution at concentrations greater than 40 mg/mL may result in incomplete dissolution, and should be avoided.
To reconstitute, add 5 mL of 0.9% Sodium Chloride Injection to the 200 mg vial or 25 mL of 0.9% Sodium Chloride Injection to the 1 g vial. Shake to dissolve. These dilutions each yield a gemcitabine concentration of 38 mg/mL which includes accounting for the displacement volume of the lyophilized powder (0.26 mL for the 200 mg vial or 1.3 mL for the 1 g vial). The total volume upon reconstitution will be 5.26 mL or 26.3 mL, respectively. Complete withdrawal of the vial contents will provide 200 mg or 1 g of gemcitabine, respectively. The appropriate amount of drug may be administered as prepared or further diluted with 0.9% Sodium Chloride Injection to concentrations as low as 0.1 mg/mL.
Reconstituted Gemzar is a clear, colorless to light straw-colored solution. After reconstitution with 0.9% Sodium Chloride Injection, the pH of the resulting solution lies in the range of 2.7 to 3.3. The solution should be inspected visually for particulate matter and discoloration, prior to administration, whenever solution or container permit. If particulate matter or discoloration is found, do not administer.
When prepared as directed, Gemzar solutions are stable for 24 hours at controlled room temperature 20° to 25°C (68° to 77°F) [*See* USP]. Discard unused portion. Solutions of reconstituted Gemzar should not be refrigerated, as crystallization may occur.
The compatibility of Gemzar with other drugs has not been studied. No incompatibilities have been observed with infusion bottles or polyvinyl chloride bags and administration sets.
Unopened vials of Gemzar are stable until the expiration date indicated on the package when stored at controlled room temperature 20° to 25°C (68° to 77°F) [*See* USP].
Caution should be exercised in handling and preparing Gemzar solutions. The use of gloves is recommended. If Gemzar solution contacts the skin or mucosa, immediately wash the skin thoroughly with soap and water or rinse the mucosa with copious amounts of water. Although acute dermal irritation has not been observed in animal studies, two of three rabbits exhibited drug-related systemic toxicities (death, hypoactivity, nasal discharge, shallow breathing) due to dermal absorption.
Procedures for proper handling and disposal of anti-cancer drugs should be considered. Several guidelines on this subject have been published.[1–7] There is no general agreement that all of the procedures recommended in the guidelines are necessary or appropriate.

HOW SUPPLIED

Vials:
200 mg white, lyophilized powder in a 10-mL size sterile single use vial (No. 7501) NDC 0002-7501-01
1 g white, lyophilized powder in a 50-mL size sterile single use vial (No. 7502) NDC 0002-7502-01
Store at controlled room temperature (20° to 25°C) (68° to 77°F). The USP has defined controlled room temperature as "A temperature maintained thermostatically that encompasses the usual and customary working environment of 20° to 25°C (68° to 77°F); that results in a mean kinetic temperature calculated to be not more than 25°C; and that allows for excursions between 15° and 30°C (59° and 86°F) that are experienced in pharmacies, hospitals, and warehouses."
CAUTION—Federal (USA) law prohibits dispensing without prescription.

REFERENCES

1. Recommendations for the safe handling of parenteral antineoplastic drugs. NIH publication No. 83-2621. US Government Printing Office, Washington, DC 20402.
2. Council on Scientific Affairs: Guidelines for handling parenteral antineoplastics. *JAMA* 1985;253:1590.
3. National Study Commission on Cytotoxic Exposure—Recommendations for handling cytotoxic agents, 1987. Available from Louis P Jeffrey, ScD, Director of Pharmacy Services, Rhode Island Hospital, 593 Eddy Street, Providence, Rhode Island 02902.
4. Clinical Oncological Society of Australia: Guidelines and recommendations for safe handling of antineoplastic agents. *Med J Aust* 1983;1:426.
5. Jones RB, et al. Safe handling of chemotherapeutic agents: A report from the Mount Sinai Medical Center. *CA* 1983;33(Sept/Oct):258.
6. American Society of Hospital Pharmacists: Technical assistance bulletin on handling cytotoxic drugs in hospitals. *AM J Hosp Pharm* 1990;47:1033.
7. Yodaiken RE, Bennet D, OSHA work-practice guidelines for personnel dealing with cytotoxic (antineoplastic) drugs. *Am J Hosp Pharm* 1988;43:1193-1204.

Literature issued May 14, 1997
PA 1632 AMP [051497]

GLUCAGON FOR INJECTION ℞

[glōō 'ka-gŏn]
USP

DESCRIPTION

Glucagon, manufactured by Eli Lilly and Company, is extracted from beef and pork pancreas.
Chemically unrelated to insulin, glucagon is a single-chain polypeptide containing 29 amino acid residues and having a molecular weight of 3,483.
The empirical formula is $C_{153}H_{225}N_{43}O_{49}S$. The structure of glucagon is shown below.

His-Ser-Gln-Gly-Thr-Phe-Thr-Ser-Asp-Tyr-Ser-Lys-Tyr-Leu-Asp-Ser-
1 2 3 4 5 6 7 8 9 10 11 12 13 14 15 16

Arg-Arg-Ala-Gln-Asp-Phe-Val-Gln-Trp-Leu-Met-Asn-Thr
17 18 19 20 21 22 23 24 25 26 27 28 29

Crystalline glucagon is a white powder containing less than 0.05% zinc. It is relatively insoluble in water but is soluble at a pH of less than 3 or more than 9.5. Glucagon is stable in lyophilized form at room temperatures.
Glucagon for Injection contains glucagon as the hydrochloride. The 1-mg vials contain 1 mg (1 unit) of glucagon and 49 mg of lactose. One USP unit of glucagon is equivalent to 1 International Unit of glucagon and also to about 1 mg of glucagon.[1] The diluent contains glycerin, 1.2%, Hydrochloric acid may have been added during manufacture to adjust the pH.

CLINICAL PHARMACOLOGY

Glucagon causes an increase in blood glucose concentration and is used in the treatment of hypoglycemia. It is effective in small doses, and no evidence of toxicity has been reported with its use. Glucagon acts only on liver glycogen, converting it to glucose.
Parenteral administration of glucagon produces relaxation of the smooth muscle of the stomach, duodenum, small bowel, and colon.
The half-life of glucagon in plasma is approximately 3 to 6 minutes, which is similar to that of insulin.

INDICATIONS AND USAGE

For the treatment of hypoglycemia:
Glucagon is useful in counteracting severe hypoglycemic reactions.
The patient with type I diabetes does not have as great a response in blood glucose levels as does the stable type II diabetes patient. Therefore, supplementary carbohydrate should be given as soon as possible, especially to the pediatric patient.
For use as a diagnostic aid:
Glucagon is indicated as a diagnostic aid in the radiologic examination of the stomach, duodenum, small bowel, and colon when a hypotonic state would be advantageous.
Glucagon is as effective for this examination as are the anticholinergic drugs, but it has fewer side effects. When glucagon is administered concomitantly with an anticholinergic agent, the response is not significantly greater than when either drug is used alone. However, the addition of the anticholinergic agent results in increased side effects.

CONTRAINDICATIONS

Glucagon is contraindicated in patients with known hypersensitivity to it or in patients with pheochromocytoma.

WARNINGS

Glucagon should be administered cautiously to patients with a history suggestive of insulinoma and/or pheochromocytoma. In patients with insulinoma, intravenous administration of glucagon will produce an initial increase in blood glucose; however, because of glucagon's insulin-releasing effect, it may cause the insulinoma to release its insulin and subsequently cause hypoglycemia. A patient developing symptoms of hypoglycemia after a dose of glucagon should be given glucose orally, intravenously, or by gavage, whichever is more appropriate.
Exogenous glucagon also stimulates the release of catecholamines. In the presence of pheochromocytoma, glucagon can cause the tumor to release catecholamines, which results in a sudden and marked increase in blood pressure. If a patient suddenly develops a marked increase in blood pressure, 5 to 10 mg of phentolamine mesylate may be administered intravenously in an attempt to control the blood pressure.
Generalized allergic reactions, including urticaria, respiratory distress, and hypotension, have been reported in patients who received glucagon by injection.

PRECAUTIONS

General —Glucagon is helpful in hypoglycemia only if liver glycogen is available. Because glucagon is of little or no help in states of starvation, adrenal insufficiency, or chronic hypoglycemia, glucose should be considered for the treatment of hypoglycemia.
Laboratory Tests —Blood glucose determinations may be obtained to follow the patient in hypoglycemic shock until he or she is asymptomatic.
Carcinogenesis, Mutagenesis, Impairment of Fertility —Because glucagon is usually given in a single dose and has a very short half-life (3 to 6 minutes), no studies have been done regarding carcinogenesis.
Reproduction studies have been performed in rats at doses up to 2 mg/kg b.i.d. (up 120 times the human dose) and have revealed no evidence of impaired fertility.
Usage in Pregnancy —Pregnancy Category B —Reproduction studies have been performed in rats at doses up to 2 mg/kg b.i.d. (up to 120 times the human dose), and have revealed no evidence of harm to the fetus due to glucagon. There are, however, no adequate and well-controlled studies in pregnant women. Because animal reproduction studies are not always predictive of human response, this drug should be used during pregnancy only if clearly needed.
Nursing Mothers —It is not known whether this drug is excreted in human milk. Because many drugs are excreted in human milk, caution should be exercised when glucagon is administered to a nursing woman. If the drug is excreted in human milk during its short half-life, it will be handled like any other polypeptide, ie, it will be hydrolyzed and absorbed. Glucagon is not active when taken orally because it is destroyed in the gastrointestinal tract before it can be absorbed.

Usage in pediatric patients—For the treatment of hypoglycemia: The use of glucagon in pediatric patients has been reported to be safe and effective.[2-6]

For use as a diagnostic aid: Effectiveness has not been established in pediatric patients.

ADVERSE REACTIONS

Glucagon is relatively free of adverse reactions except for occasional nausea and vomiting, which may also occur with hypoglycemia. Generalized allergic reactions have been reported (*see* Warnings).

OVERDOSAGE

Signs and Symptoms —No cases of human overdosage of glucagon have been reported. Glucagon is generally well tolerated. If overdosage occurred, it would not be expected to cause consequential toxicity but would be expected to be associated with nausea, vomiting, gastric hypotonicity, and diarrhea.

Intravenous administration of glucagon has been shown to have a positive inotropic and chronotropic effect. A transient increment in both blood pressure and pulse rate may occur following the administration of glucagon. Patients taking β-blockers might be expected to have a greater increment in both pulse and blood pressure. This increase will be transient because of glucagon's short half-life. The increase in blood pressure and pulse rate may require therapy in patients with pheochromocytoma or coronary artery disease. When glucagon was given in large doses to cardiac patients, investigators reported a positive inotropic effect. These investigators administered glucagon in doses of 0.5 to 16 mg/hour by continuous infusion for periods of 5 to 166 hours. Total doses ranged from 25 to 996 mg, and a 21-month-old infant received approximately 8.25 mg in 165 hours. Side effects included nausea, vomiting, and decreasing serum potassium concentration. Serum potassium concentration could be maintained within normal limits with supplemental potassium.

The intravenous median lethal dose for glucagon in mice is approximately 300 mg/kg.

Because glucagon is a polypeptide, it would be rapidly destroyed in the gastrointestinal tract if it were to be accidentally ingested.

Treatment —To obtain up-to-date information about the treatment of overdose, a good resource is your certified Regional Poison Control Center. Telephone numbers of certified poison control centers are listed in the *Physicians' Desk Reference (PDR)*. In managing overdosage, consider the possibility of multiple drug overdoses, interaction among drugs, and unusual drug kinetics in your patient.

In view of the extremely short half-life of glucagon and its prompt destruction and excretion, the treatment of overdosage is symptomatic, primarily for nausea, vomiting, and possible hypokalemia.

If the patient develops a dramatic increase in blood pressure, 5 to 10 mg of phentolamine has been shown to be effective in lowering blood pressure for the short time that control would be needed.

Forced diuresis, peritoneal dialysis, hemodialysis, or charcoal hemoperfusion have not been established as beneficial for an overdose of glucagon; it is extremely unlikely that one of these procedures would ever be indicated.

DOSAGE AND ADMINISTRATION

For the treatment of hypoglycemia:

The diluent is provided for use only in the preparation of glucagon for *intermittent* parenteral injection and for no other use.

Glucagon reconstituted with the supplied diluting solution should be used immediately. **Discard any unused portion.**

If glucagon is to be given at doses higher than 2 mg, it should be reconstituted with Sterile Water for Injection instead of the supplied diluting solution and used immediately.

Directions for Use of Glucagon —1. Dissolve the lyophilized glucagon in the accompanying diluent.

2. Glucagon should not be used at concentrations greater than 1 mg (1 unit/mL).

3. Glucagon solutions should not be used unless they are clear and of a water-like consistency.

4. For adults and for pediatric patients weighing more than 20 kg, give 1 mg (1 unit) by subcutaneous, intramuscular, or intravenous injection.

5. For pediatric patients weighing less than 20 kg, give 0.5 mg (0.5 unit) or a dose equivalent to 20–30 µg/kg.[2-6]

6. The patient will usually awaken within 15 minutes. If the response is delayed, there is no contraindication to the administration of 1 or 2 additional doses of glucagon; however, in view of the deleterious effects of cerebral hypoglycemia and depending on the duration and depth of coma, the use of parenteral glucose *must* be considered by the physician.

7. Intravenous glucose *must* be given if the patient fails to respond to glucagon.

8. When the patient responds, give supplemental carbohydrate to restore the liver glycogen and prevent secondary hypoglycemia.

Instructions to the Family —Instructions describing the method of using this preparation are included in the literature that accompanies the patient's package. It is advisable for the patient and family members to become familiar with the technique of preparing Glucagon for Injection before an emergency arises. Patients are instructed to use 1 mg (1 unit) for adults and, if recommended by a doctor, $^1/_2$ the adult dose (0.5 mg) [0.5 unit] for pediatric patients weighing less than 44 lb (20 kg).

General Management of Hypoglycemia —The following are helpful measures in the prevention of hypoglycemic reactions due to insulin:

1. Reasonable uniformity from day to day with regard to diet, insulin, and exercise.

2. Careful adjustment of the insulin program so that the type (or types) of insulin, dose, and time (or times) of administration are suited to the individual patient.

3. Frequent testing of the blood or urine for glucose so that a change in insulin requirements can be foreseen.

4. Routine carrying of sugar, candy, or other readily absorbable carbohydrate by the patient so that it may be taken at the first warning of an oncoming reaction.

If the patient is unaware of the symptoms of hypoglycemia, he/she may lapse into insulin shock; therefore, the physician should instruct the patient in this regard when feasible.

It is important that the patient be aroused as quickly as possible, because prolonged hypoglycemic reactions may result in cortical damage. Glucagon or intravenous glucose will awaken the patient sufficiently so that oral carbohydrates may be taken.

CAUTION—Although the patient may use glucagon for the treatment of hypoglycemia during an emergency, the physician must still be notified when hypoglycemic reactions occur so that the treatment regimen may be adjusted if necessary.

For use as a diagnostic aid:

Dissolve the lyophilized glucagon in the accompanying diluting solution.

Reconstituted Glucagon should be used immediately. **Discard any unused portion.**

Glucagon should not be used at concentrations greater than 1 mg (1 unit/mL).

The following doses may be administered for relaxation of the stomach, duodenum, and small bowel, depending on the time of onset of action and the duration of effect required for the examination. Since the stomach is less sensitive to the effect of glucagon, 0.5 mg (0.5 units) IV or 2 mg (2 units) IM are recommended.

[See table above]

For examination of the colon, it is recommended that a 2-mg (2 units) dose be administered intramuscularly approximately 10 minutes prior to initiation of the procedure. Relaxation of the colon and reduction of discomfort to the patient will allow the radiologist to perform a more satisfactory examination.

HOW SUPPLIED

Glucagon Emergency Kit (MS8009):

1 mg (1 unit)—(VL7519), with 1-mL vial of diluting solution (Hyporet* HY7530)

   (1s) NDC 0002-8009-01

Glucagon for Injection, USP (MS8239):

1 mg (1 unit)—(VL7519), with 1-mL of diluting solution (Hyporet* HY7530)

   (1s) NDC 0002-8239-01

* Hyporet® (disposable syringe, Lilly).

Stability and Storage:

Before Reconstitution—Vials of Glucagon as well as the Diluting Solution for Glucagon for Injection, USP, may be stored at controlled room temperature, 20° to 25°C (68° to 77°F) [see USP].

The USP defines controlled room temperature as: A temperature maintained thermostatically that encompasses the usual and customary working environment of 20° to 25°C (68° to 77°F); that results in a mean kinetic temperature calculated to be not more than 25°C; and that allows for excursions between 15° and 30°C (59° and 86°F) that are experienced in pharmacies, hospitals, and warehouses.

After Reconstitution—Glucagon for Injection should be used immediately.

Discard any unused portion.

Dose	Route of Administration	Time of Onset of Action	Approximate Duration of Effect
0.25–0.5 mg	IV	1 minute	9–17 minutes
1 mg	IM	8–10 minutes	12–27 minutes
2 mg*	IV	1 minute	22–25 minutes
2 mg*	IM	4–7 minutes	21–32 minutes

*Administration of 2-mg (2 units) doses produces a higher incidence of nausea and vomiting than do lower doses.

REFERENCES

1. *Drug Information for the Health Care Professional*. 11th ed. Rockville, Maryland: The United States Pharmacopeial Convention, Inc; 1991;IA:1380.
2. Gibbs et al: Use of Glucagon to terminate insulin reactions in diabetic children. *Nebr Med J* 1958;43:56–57.
3. Cornblath M, et al: Studies of carbohydrate metabolism in the newborn: Effect of glucagon on concentration of sugar in capillary blood of newborn infant. *Pediatrics* 1958;21:885–892.
4. Carson MJ, Koch R, Clinical studies with glucagon in children. *J Pediatr* 1955;47:167–170.
5. Shipp JC, et al; Treatment of insulin hypoglycemia in diabetic campers. *Diabetes* 1964;13:645–648.
6. Aman J, Wranne L: Hypoglycemia in childhood diabetes II: Effect of subcutaneous or intramuscular injection of different doses of glucagon. *Acta Pediatr Scand* 1988;77: 548–553.

CAUTION—Federal (USA) law prohibits dispensing without prescription.

Literature revised January 9, 1998

PA 1120 AMP   [010998]

HEPARIN SODIUM   ℞

[hĕp 'ă-rŭn sō 'dē-ŭm]

Injection, USP

WARNING—This is a potent drug, and serious consequences may result if used without constant medical supervision.

DESCRIPTION

Heparin is a heterogenous group of straight-chain anionic mucopolysaccharides, called glycosaminoglycans, having anticoagulant properties. Although others may be present, the main sugars in heparin are: (1) α-L-iduronic acid 2-sulfate, (2) 2-deoxy-2-sulfamino-α-glucose 6-sulfate, (3) β-D-glucuronic acid, (4) 2-acetamido-2-deoxy-α-D-glucose, and (5) α-L-iduronic acid. These sugars are present in decreasing amounts, usually in the order (2)>(1)>(4)>(3)>(5), and are joined by glycosidic linkages, forming polymers of varying sizes. Heparin is strongly acidic because of its covalently linked sulfate and carboxylic acid groups. In heparin sodium, the acidic protons of the sulfate units are partially replaced by sodium ions.

Structure of Heparin Sodium (representative subunits):

Heparin Sodium Injection, USP, is a sterile solution of heparin sodium derived from porcine intestinal mucosa, which is standardized for anticoagulant activity. It is to be administered by intravenous or deep subcutaneous routes. The potency is determined by a biological assay using a USP reference standard based on units of heparin activity per milligram.

Each mL of Vial No. 520 contains 10,000 USP heparin units (derived from porcine intestinal mucosa) and sodium chloride, 0.1%.

During manufacture, 1% benzyl alcohol is added as a preservative to each vial of heparin sodium. Sodium hydroxide and/or hydrochloric acid may be added during manufacture to adjust the pH.

Continued on next page

* Identi-Code® symbol. This product information was prepared in June 1998. Current information on these and other products of Eli Lilly and Company may be obtained by direct inquiry to Lilly Research Laboratories, Lilly Corporate Center, Indianapolis, Indiana 46285, (800) 545-5979.

Heparin Sodium—Cont.

CLINICAL PHARMACOLOGY

Heparin inhibits reactions that lead to the clotting of blood and the formation of fibrin clots both in vitro and in vivo. Heparin acts at multiple sites in the normal coagulation system. Small amounts of heparin in combination with antithrombin III (heparin cofactor) can inhibit thrombosis by inactivating activated Factor X and inhibiting the conversion of prothrombin to thrombin. Once active thrombosis has developed, larger amounts of heparin can inhibit further coagulation by inactivating thrombin and preventing the conversion of fibrinogen to fibrin. Heparin also prevents the formation of a stable fibrin clot by inhibiting the activation of the fibrin stabilizing factor.

Bleeding time is usually unaffected by heparin. Clotting time is prolonged by full therapeutic doses of heparin; in most cases, it is not measurably affected by low doses.

Peak plasma levels of heparin are achieved 2 to 4 hours following subcutaneous administration, although there are considerable individual variations. Log linear plots of heparin plasma concentrations with time for a wide range of dose levels are linear, which suggests the absence of zero order processes. The liver and the reticuloendothelial system are the sites of biotransformation. The biphasic elimination curve, a rapidly declining α phase ($t_{1/2}$ = 10') and, after the age of 40, a slower β phase indicate uptake in organs. The absence of a relationship between anticoagulant half-life and concentration half-life may reflect factors such as protein binding of heparin.

Heparin does not have fibrinolytic activity; therefore, it will not lyse existing clots.

INDICATIONS AND USAGE

Heparin sodium is indicated for:

Anticoagulant therapy in prophylaxis and treatment of venous thrombosis and its extension

Prevention (in a low-dose regimen) of postoperative deep venous thrombosis and pulmonary embolism in patients undergoing major abdominothoracic surgery or who, for other reasons, are at risk of developing thromboembolic disease (*see* Dosage and Administration)

Prophylaxis and treatment of pulmonary embolism

Atrial fibrillation with embolization

Diagnosis and treatment of acute and chronic consumption coagulopathies (eg, disseminated intravascular coagulation)

Prevention of clotting in arterial and heart surgery

Prophylaxis and treatment of peripheral arterial embolism

As an anticoagulant in blood transfusions, extracorporeal circulation, and dialysis procedures and in blood samples for laboratory purposes

CONTRAINDICATIONS

Heparin sodium should not be used in patients with severe thrombocytopenia or patients for whom suitable blood coagulation tests (eg, tests for whole-blood clotting time and partial thromboplastin time) cannot be performed at appropriate intervals. (This restriction refers to full-dose administration of heparin; it is usually unnecessary to monitor coagulation parameters in patients receiving low-dose heparin). In addition, heparin sodium should not be administered to patients in an uncontrollable active bleeding state (*see* Warnings), except when this condition is the result of disseminated intravascular coagulation.

WARNINGS

Heparin is not intended for intramuscular use.

Hypersensitivity —Patients with documented hypersensitivity to heparin should be given the drug only in clearly life-threatening situations.

Hemorrhage —Hemorrhage can occur at virtually any site in patients receiving heparin. An unexplained fall in hematocrit, a fall in blood pressure, or any other unexplained symptom warrants consideration of a hemorrhagic event.

Heparin sodium should be used with extreme caution in disease states in which there is increased danger of hemorrhage. Some of the conditions in which this danger exists are as follows:

Cardiovascular —Subacute bacterial endocarditis. Severe hypertension.

Surgical —During and immediately following (a) a spinal tap or spinal anesthesia or (b) major surgery, especially involving the brain, spinal cord, or eye.

Hematologic —Conditions associated with increased bleeding tendencies, such as hemophilia, thrombocytopenia, and some vascular purpuras.

Gastrointestinal —Ulcerative lesions and continuous tube drainage of the stomach or small intestine.

Other —Menstruation and liver disease with impaired hemostasis.

Coagulation Testing —When heparin sodium is administered in therapeutic amounts, its dosage should be regulated by frequent blood coagulation tests. If the coagulation test result is unduly prolonged or if hemorrhage occurs, heparin sodium should be discontinued promptly (*see* Overdosage).

Thrombocytopenia —Thrombocytopenia occurs in patients receiving heparin with a reported incidence of 0% to 30%. Mild thrombocytopenia (count greater than 100,000/mm^3) may remain stable or reverse, even if heparin is continued. However, thrombocytopenia of any degree should be monitored closely. If the count falls below 100,000/mm^3 or if recurrent thrombosis develops (*see* Precautions, *White-Clot Syndrome*), the heparin product should be discontinued. If continued heparin therapy is essential, utilize heparin from a different organ source and reinstitute therapy with caution.

Miscellaneous —This product contains benzyl alcohol as a preservative. Benzyl alcohol has been reported to be associated with a fatal "gasping syndrome" in premature infants.

PRECAUTIONS

General —White-Clot Syndrome —It has been reported that patients taking heparin may develop new thrombus formation in association with thrombocytopenia. This development is the result of the irreversible aggregation of platelets induced by heparin, ie, the so-called "white-clot syndrome." The process may lead to severe thromboembolic complications such as skin necrosis, gangrene of the extremities that may lead to amputation, myocardial infarction, pulmonary embolism, stroke, and possibly death. Therefore, heparin administration should be promptly discontinued if a patient develops new thrombosis in association with thrombocytopenia.

Heparin Resistance —Increased resistance to heparin is frequently encountered in cases involving fever, thrombosis, thrombophlebitis, infections with thrombosing tendencies, myocardial infarction, and cancer. Increased resistance can also occur in postsurgical patients.

Increased Risk in Older Women —A higher incidence of bleeding has been reported in women over 60 years of age.

Laboratory Tests —Periodic platelet counts, hematocrit determinations, and tests for occult blood in the stool are recommended during the entire course of heparin therapy, regardless of the route of administration (*see* Dosage and Administration).

Drug Interactions —Oral anticoagulants: Heparin sodium may prolong the one-stage prothrombin time. Therefore, if a valid prothrombin time is to be obtained when heparin sodium is given with dicumarol or warfarin sodium, a period of at least 5 hours after the last intravenous dose or 24 hours after the last subcutaneous dose should elapse before blood is drawn.

Platelet inhibitors: Drugs such as acetylsalicylic acid, dextran, phenylbutazone, ibuprofen, indomethacin, dipyridamole, hydroxychloroquine, and others that interfere with platelet-aggregation reactions (the main hemostatic defense of heparinized patients) may induce bleeding and should be used with caution in patients receiving heparin sodium.

Other interactions: Digitalis, tetracyclines, nicotine, or antihistamines may partially counteract the anticoagulant action of heparin sodium.

Intravenous nitroglycerin administered to heparinized patients may result in a decrease of the partial thromboplastin time with subsequent rebound effect upon discontinuation of nitroglycerin. Careful monitoring of partial thromboplastin time and adjustment of heparin dosage are recommended during coadministration of heparin and intravenous nitroglycerin.

When clinical circumstances require reversal of heparinization, consult the labeling of Protamine Sulfate Injection, USP.

Drug/Laboratory Test Interactions —Hyperaminotransferasemia. Significant elevations of aminotransferase (SGOT and SGPT) levels have occurred in a high percentage of patients (and healthy subjects) who have received heparin. Since aminotransferase determinations are important in the differential diagnosis of myocardial infarction, liver disease, and pulmonary emboli, increases that might be caused by drugs (eg, heparin) should be interpreted with caution.

Carcinogenesis, Mutagenesis, Impairment of Fertility —No long-term studies in animals have been performed to evaluate the carcinogenic potential of heparin. Also, no reproduction studies in animals have been performed concerning mutagenesis or impairment of fertility.

Pregnancy —Teratogenic Effects: Pregnancy Category C —Animal reproduction studies have not been conducted with heparin sodium. It is also not known whether heparin sodium can cause fetal harm when administered to a pregnant woman or can affect reproduction capacity. Heparin sodium should be given to a pregnant woman only if clearly needed.

Nonteratogenic Effects: Heparin does not cross the placental barrier.

Nursing Mothers —Heparin is not excreted in human milk.

Pediatric Use —*See* Dosage and Administration.

ADVERSE REACTIONS

Hemorrhage —Hemorrhage is the chief complication that may result from heparin therapy (*see* Warnings). An overly prolonged clotting time or minor bleeding during therapy can usually be controlled by withdrawing the drug (*see* Overdosage). *Gastrointestinal or urinary tract bleeding during anticoagulant therapy may indicate the presence of an underlying occult lesion.* Bleeding can occur at any site, but certain specific hemorrhagic complications may be difficult to detect:

Adrenal hemorrhage, with resultant acute adrenal insufficiency, has occurred during anticoagulant therapy. Therefore, such treatment should be discontinued in patients who develop signs and symptoms of acute adrenal hemorrhage and insufficiency. Initiation of corrective therapy should not be delayed for laboratory confirmation of the diagnosis, since any delay in an acute situation may result in the patient's death.

Ovarian (corpus luteum) hemorrhage developed in a number of women of reproductive age receiving short- or long-term anticoagulant therapy. If unrecognized, this complication may be fatal.

Retroperitoneal hemorrhage has occurred.

Local Irritation —Local irritation, erythema, mild pain, hematoma, or ulceration may follow deep subcutaneous (intrafat) injection of heparin sodium. These complications are much more common after intramuscular use; therefore, such use is not recommended.

Hypersensitivity —Generalized hypersensitivity reactions have been reported, with chills, fever, and urticaria as the most common manifestations; asthma, rhinitis, lacrimation, headache, nausea and vomiting, and anaphylactoid reactions (including shock) have occurred more rarely. Itching and burning, especially on the plantar site of the feet, may occur.

The occurrence of thrombocytopenia has been reported in patients receiving heparin, with an incidence of 0% to 30%. Although often mild and of no obvious clinical significance, such thrombocytopenia can be accompanied by severe thromboembolic complications, such as skin necrosis, gangrene of the extremities that may lead to amputation, myocardial infarction, pulmonary embolism, stroke, and possibly death (*see* Warnings *and* Precautions).

Certain episodes of painful, ischemic, and cyanosed limbs have, in the past, been attributed to allergic vasospastic reactions. Whether these are, in fact, identical to the thrombocytopenia-associated complications remains to be determined.

Miscellaneous —Osteoporosis following long-term administration of high doses of heparin, cutaneous necrosis after systemic administration, suppression of aldosterone synthesis, delayed transient alopecia, priapism, and rebound hyperlipemia occurring after discontinuation of heparin sodium have also been reported.

Significant elevations of aminotransferase (SGOT and SGPT) levels have occurred in a high percentage of patients (and healthy subjects) who have received heparin.

OVERDOSAGE

Signs and Symptoms —Overdose of heparin may follow parenteral administration, but oral heparin has little systemic effect. Bleeding is the chief sign of heparin overdosage. Excessive heparin effect also increases whole-blood clotting time and activated partial thromboplastin time (APTT). The half-life of heparin ranges from 0.5 to 2.5 hours and may vary widely in cases involving an overdose.

The intravenous median lethal dose in mice is 1,500 mg/kg.

Treatment —To obtain up-to-date information about the treatment of overdose, a good resource is your certified Regional Poison Control Center. Telephone numbers of certified poison control centers are listed in the *Physicians' Desk Reference (PDR)*. In managing overdosage, consider the possibility of multiple drug overdoses, interaction among drugs, and unusual drug kinetics in your patient.

Minor bleeding occurring during therapy with heparin can often be treated by reducing the dose or increasing the dosing interval.

For major bleeding episodes, heparin may be neutralized by protamine; 1 mg of protamine will neutralize approximately 115 units of heparin of porcine intestinal mucosal origin. Protamine dosage may be guided by determining the amount of time by which clotting is shortened in vitro or by the results of other hematologic tests. Note that protamine may cause anaphylactoid reactions that may be life threatening. (See the protamine label for additional information.) The administration of whole blood or fresh frozen plasma should be considered for patients with significant blood losses. Vitamin K will not reverse the activity of heparin.

DOSAGE AND ADMINISTRATION

Parenteral drug products should be inspected visually for particulate matter and discoloration prior to administration if solution and container permit. Slight discoloration does not alter potency.

When heparin is added to an infusion solution for continuous intravenous administration, the container should be inverted at least 6 times to ensure adequate mixing and prevent pooling of the heparin in the solution.

Heparin sodium is not effective by oral administration and should be given by intermittent intravenous injection, intravenous infusion, or deep subcutaneous (intrafat, ie, above the iliac crest or abdominal fat layer) injection. *The intra-*

Method of Administration	Frequency	Recommended Dose*
Deep Subcutaneous (Intrafat) Injection (A different site should be used for each injection to prevent the development of massive hematoma)	Initial dose	5,000 units by IV injection, followed by 10,000–20,000 units of a concentrated solution, subcutaneously
	Every 8 hours or	8,000–10,000 units of a concentrated solution
	Every 12 hours	15,000–20,000 units of a concentrated solution
Intermittent Intravenous Injection	Initial dose	10,000 units, either undiluted or in 50–100 mL of 0.9% Sodium Chloride Injection, USP
	Every 4 to 6 hours	5,000–10,000 units, either undiluted or in 50–100 mL of 0.9% Sodium Chloride Injection, USP
Continuous Intravenous Infusion	Initial dose	5,000 units by IV injection
	Continuous Infusion	20,000–40,000 units/24 hours in 1,000 mL of 0.9% Sodium-Chloride Injection, USP (or in any compatible solution) for infusion

* Based on 150-lb (68-kg) patient.

muscular route of administration should be avoided because of the frequent occurrence of hematoma at the injection site. The dosage of heparin sodium should be adjusted according to the patient's coagulation test results. When heparin is given by continuous intravenous infusion, the coagulation time should be determined approximately every 4 hours in the early stages of treatment. When the drug is administered intermittently by intravenous injection, coagulation tests should be performed before each injection during the early stages of treatment and at appropriate intervals thereafter. Dosage is considered adequate when the APTT is 1.5 to 2 times normal or when the whole-blood clotting time is elevated approximately 2.5 to 3 times the control value. After deep subcutaneous (intrafat) injections, tests for adequacy of dosage are best performed on samples drawn 4 to 6 hours after the injections.

Periodic platelet counts, hematocrit determinations, and tests for occult blood in the stool are recommended during the entire course of heparin therapy, regardless of the route of administration.

Converting to Oral Anticoagulant —When an oral anticoagulant of the coumarin (or similar) type is to be administered in patients already receiving heparin sodium, baseline and subsequent tests of prothrombin activity must be determined at times during which heparin activity is too low to affect the prothrombin time. Such a time usually occurs about 5 hours after the last IV bolus and 24 hours after the last subcutaneous dose. If heparin is continuously infused by IV, prothrombin time can usually be measured at any time.

In converting from heparin to an oral anticoagulant, the oral anticoagulant should be given in the usual initial amount; thereafter, prothrombin time should be determined at the usual intervals. To ensure continuous anticoagulation, it is advisable to continue full heparin therapy for several days after the prothrombin time has reached the limit of the therapeutic range. Heparin therapy may then be discontinued without tapering.

Therapeutic Anticoagulant Effect With Full-Dose Heparin—Although dosage must be adjusted for the individual patient according to the results of appropriate laboratory tests, the following dosage schedule may be used as a guideline:

[See table above]

Pediatric Use —Follow recommendations of appropriate pediatric reference texts. In general, the following dosage schedule may be used as a guideline:

Initial Dose: 50 units/kg (IV, drip)

Maintenance Dose: 100 units/kg (IV, drip) every 4 hours, or 20,000 units/m^2/24 hours, infused continuously

Surgery of the Heart and Blood Vessel —Patients undergoing total body perfusion for open heart surgery should receive an initial dose of not less than 150 units of heparin sodium per kg of body weight. Frequently, a dose of 300 units/ kg is used for procedures estimated to last less than 60 minutes; a dose of 400 units/kg is often used for those procedures likely to last longer than 60 minutes.

Low-Dose Prophylaxis of Postoperative Thromboembolism—A number of well-controlled clinical trials have demonstrated that low-dose heparin prophylaxis, given prior to and after surgery, will reduce the incidences of postoperative deep-vein thrombosis in the legs (as measured by the I-125 fibrinogen technique and venography) and of clinical pulmonary embolism. The most widely used dosage is 5,000 units given 2 hours before surgery and 5,000 units given every 8 to 12 hours thereafter for 7 days or until the patient is fully ambulatory, whichever is longer. The heparin is given by deep subcutaneous (intrafat, ie, above the iliac crest or abdominal fat layer, arm, or thigh) injection with a fine (25- to 26-gauge) needle to minimize tissue trauma. A concentrated solution of heparin sodium is recommended. Such prophylaxis should be reserved for patients over the age of 40 who are undergoing major surgery. Patients with bleeding disorders and those having brain or spinal-cord surgery, spinal anesthesia, eye surgery, or potentially sanguineous operations should be excluded from this treatment, as should patients receiving oral anticoagulants or platelet-active drugs (*see* Warnings). The value of such prophylaxis in hip surgery has not been established. The possibility of increased bleeding during surgery or postoperatively should be borne in mind. If such bleeding occurs, discontinuance of heparin and neutralization with protamine sulfate are advisable. If clinical evidence of thromboembolism develops despite low-dose prophylaxis, full therapeutic doses of anticoagulants should be given unless contraindicated. Prior to initiating heparinization, the physician should rule out the probability of bleeding disorders by taking a thorough history and performing the appropriate laboratory tests. Appropriate coagulation tests should be repeated just prior to surgery. Coagulation test values should be normal or only slightly elevated at these times.

Extracorporeal Dialysis —Follow equipment manufacturers' operating directions carefully.

Blood Transfusion —The addition of 400 to 600 USP units to each 100 mL of whole blood for transfusion is usually employed to prevent coagulation. Usually, 7,500 USP units of heparin sodium are mixed with 100 mL of 0.9% Sodium Chloride Injection, USP (or 75,000 USP units/1,000 mL of 0.9% Sodium Chloride Injection, USP); 6 to 8 mL of this sterile solution is then added to each 100 mL of whole blood used.

Laboratory Samples —70 to 150 units of heparin sodium are usually added per 10- to 20-mL sample of whole blood to prevent coagulation of the sample. Leukocyte counts should be performed on heparinized blood within 2 hours after the addition of the heparin. Heparinized blood should not be used for isoagglutinin, complement, or erythrocyte fragility tests or for taking platelet counts.

Clearing Intermittent Infusion (Heparin Lock) Sets —To prevent clot formation in a heparin lock set following its proper insertion, dilute heparin solution (*see* USP monograph for Heparin Lock Flush Solution, USP) should be injected via the injection hub in a quantity sufficient to fill the entire set to the needle tip. This solution should be replaced each time the heparin lock is used. Aspirate before administering any solution via the lock in order to confirm the patency and location of the needle or catheter tip. If the drug to be administered is incompatible with heparin, the entire heparin lock set should be flushed with sterile water or normal saline before and after the medication is administered; following the second cleansing flush, the dilute heparin solution may be reinstilled in the set. The set manufacturer's instructions should be consulted for specifics concerning the heparin lock set being used at a given time.

NOTE: Since repeated injections of small doses of heparin can alter tests for activated partial thromboplastin time (APTT), a baseline value for APTT should be obtained prior to insertion of a heparin lock set.

HOW SUPPLIED

Multiple-Dose Vials:

10,000 USP heparin units/mL, 5 mL (No. 520)—(1s) NDC 0002-7217-01

Protect from light. Store at controlled room temperature, 59° to 86°F (15° to 30°C).

CAUTION—Federal (USA) law prohibits dispensing without prescription.

Text revised April 2, 1992

Literature revised July 19, 1996 [071996]

PA 0710 AMP

HUMALOG® ℞

INSULIN LISPRO INJECTION
(rDNA ORIGIN)

DESCRIPTION

Humalog® (insulin lispro, rDNA origin) is a human insulin analog that is a rapid-acting, parenteral blood glucose-lowering agent. Chemically, it is Lys(B28), Pro(B29) human insulin analog, created when the amino acids at positions 28 and 29 on the insulin B-chain are reversed. Humalog is synthesized in a special non-pathogenic laboratory strain of *Escherichia coli* bacteria that has been genetically altered by the addition of the gene for insulin lispro.

Humalog has the following primary structure:

Figure 1

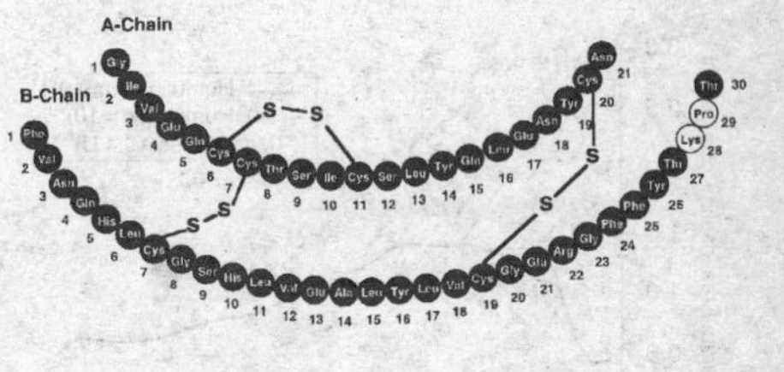

Humalog has the empirical formula $C_{257}H_{383}N_{65}O_{77}S_6$ and a molecular weight of 5808, both identical to that of human insulin.

The vials and cartridges contain a sterile solution of Humalog for use as an injection. Humalog injection consists of zinc-insulin lispro crystals dissolved in a clear aqueous fluid.

Each milliliter of Humalog injection contains insulin lispro 100 Units, 16 mg glycerin, 1.88 mg dibasic sodium phosphate, 3.15 mg *m*-cresol, zinc oxide content adjusted to provide 0.0197 mg zinc ion, trace amounts of phenol, and water for injection. Insulin lispro has a pH of 7.0-7.8. Hydrochloric acid 10% and/or sodium hydroxide 10% may be added to adjust pH.

CLINICAL PHARMACOLOGY

Antidiabetic Activity—The primary activity of insulin, including Humalog, is the regulation of glucose metabolism. In addition, all insulins have several anabolic and anti-catabolic actions on many tissues in the body. In muscle and other tissues (except the brain), insulin causes rapid transport of glucose and amino acids intracellularly, promotes anabolism, and inhibits protein catabolism. In the liver, insulin promotes the uptake and storage of glucose in the form of glycogen, inhibits gluconeogenesis, and promotes the conversion of excess glucose into fat.

Humalog has been shown to be equipotent to human insulin on a molar basis. One unit of Humalog has the same glucose-lowering effect as one unit of human regular insulin, but its effect is more rapid and of shorter duration. The glucose-lowering activity of Humalog and human regular insulin is comparable when administered to normal volunteers by the intravenous route.

Pharmacokinetics—

Absorption and Bioavailability—Humalog is as bioavailable as human regular insulin, with absolute bioavailability ranging between 55%–77% with doses between 0.1–0.2 U/kg, inclusive. Studies in normal volunteers and patients with type I (insulin-dependent) diabetes demonstrated that Humalog is absorbed faster than human regular insulin (U100) (Figure 2). In normal volunteers given subcutaneous doses of Humalog ranging from 0.1–0.4 U/kg, peak serum levels were seen 30–90 minutes after dosing. When normal volunteers received equivalent doses of human regular insulin, peak insulin doses occurred between 50–120 minutes after dosing. Similar results were seen in patients with type I diabetes. The pharmacokinetic profiles of Humalog and human regular insulin are comparable to one another when administered to normal volunteers by the intravenous route. Humalog was absorbed at a consistently faster rate than human regular insulin in healthy male volunteers given 0.2 U/kg human regular insulin or Humalog at abdominal, deltoid, or femoral sites, the three sites often used by patients with diabetes. After abdominal administration of Humalog, serum drug levels are higher and the duration of action is slightly shorter than after deltoid or thigh administration (*see* DOSAGE AND ADMINISTRATION section). Humalog has less intra- and inter-patient variability compared to human regular insulin.

[See figure 2 at top of next column]

Distribution—The volume of distribution for Humalog is identical to that of human regular insulin, with a range of 0.26–0.36 L/kg.

Metabolism—Human metabolism studies have not been conducted. However, animal studies indicate that the metabolism of Humalog is identical to that of human regular insulin.

Continued on next page

*** Identi-Code® symbol. This product information was prepared in June 1998. Current information on these and other products of Eli Lilly and Company may be obtained by direct inquiry to Lilly Research Laboratories, Lilly Corporate Center, Indianapolis, Indiana 46285, (800) 545-5979.**

Humalog—Cont.

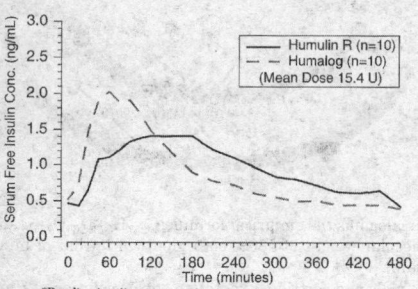

Figure 2
Serum Humalog and Insulin levels after subcutaneous injection of human regular insulin or Humalog (0.2 U/kg) immediately before a high carbohydrate meal in 10 patients with Type I diabetes.*

*Baseline insulin concentration was maintained by infusion of 0.2 mU/min/kg human insulin.

Elimination—When Humalog is given subcutaneously, its $t_{1/2}$ is shorter than that of human regular insulin (1 vs 1.5 hours, respectively). When given intravenously, Humalog and human regular insulin show identical dose-dependent elimination, with a $t_{1/2}$ of 26 and 52 minutes at 0.1 U/kg and 0.2 U/kg, respectively.

Pharmacodynamics—Studies in normal volunteers and patients with diabetes demonstrated that Humalog has a more rapid onset of glucose-lowering activity, an earlier peak for glucose lowering, and a shorter duration of glucose-lowering activity than human regular insulin (Figure 3). The earlier onset of activity of Humalog is directly related to its more rapid rate of absorption. The time course of action of insulin and insulin analogs such as Humalog may vary considerably in different individuals or within the same individual. The parameters of Humalog activity (time of onset, peak time, and duration) as designated in Figure 3 should be considered only as general guidelines. The rate of insulin absorption and consequently the onset of activity is known to be affected by the site of injection, exercise, and other variables (see PRECAUTIONS, Absorption and Bioavailability sub-section).

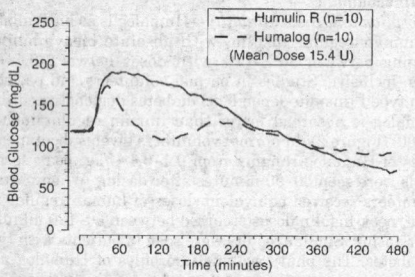

Figure 3
Blood glucose levels after subcutaneous injection of human regular insulin or Humalog (0.2 U/kg) immediately before a high carbohydrate meal in 10 patients with Type I diabetes.*

*Baseline insulin concentration was maintained by infusion of 0.2 mU/min/kg human insulin.

In open-label, crossover studies of 1008 patients with type I diabetes and 722 patients with type II (non-insulin-dependent) diabetes, Humalog reduced postprandial glucose compared with human regular insulin (see Table). The clinical significance of improvement in postprandial hyperglycemia has not been established.

Comparison of Means of Glycemic Parameters at the End of Combined Treatment Periods. All Randomized Patients in Cross-over Studies (3 months for each treatment)

Type I, N=1008 Glycemic Parameter, (mmol/L)†	Humalog [a]	Humulin® R[a*]	p-value
Premeal Blood			
Glucose	11.64 ± 5.09	11.34 ± 4.96	.274
1-Hour			
Postprandial	12.91 ± 5.43	13.89 ± 5.37	<.001
2-Hour			
Postprandial	11.16 ± 5.30	12.87 ± 5.77	<.001
HbA1c (%)	8.24 ± 1.49	8.17 ± 1.46	.089

Type II, N=722 Glycemic Parameter, (mmol/L)†	Humalog [a]	Humulin R[a]	p-value
Premeal Blood			
Glucose	10.67 ± 3.77	10.17 ± 3.67	.002
1-Hour			
Postprandial	13.23 ± 4.43	13.89 ± 4.18	<.001
2-Hour			
Postprandial	12.08 ± 4.62	13.14 ± 4.48	<.001
HbA1c (%)	8.18 ± 1.30	8.18 ± 1.38	.924

[a] Mean ± Standard Deviation
*Humulin® (Regular insulin human injection, USP, [recombinant DNA origin])
† mg/dL = mmol/L × 18.0

In 12-month parallel studies of type I and type II patients, hemoglobin A_{1c} did not differ between patients treated with human regular insulin and those treated with Humalog. While the overall rate of hypoglycemia did not differ between patients with type I and type II diabetes treated with Humalog compared with human regular insulin, patients with type I diabetes treated with Humalog had fewer hypoglycemic episodes between midnight and 6 a.m. The lower rate of hypoglycemia in the Humalog-treated group may have been related to higher nocturnal blood glucose levels, as reflected by a small increase in mean fasting blood glucose levels.

Special Populations—
Age and Gender—Information on the effect of age and gender on the pharmacokinetics of Humalog is unavailable. However, in large clinical trials, subgroup analysis based on age and gender did not indicate any difference in postprandial glucose parameters between Humalog and human regular insulin.

Smoking—The effect of smoking on the pharmacokinetics and glucodynamics of Humalog has not been studied.

Pregnancy—The effect of pregnancy on the pharmacokinetics and glucodynamics of Humalog has not been studied.

Obesity—The effect of obesity and/or subcutaneous fat thickness on the pharmacokinetics and glucodynamics of Humalog has not been studied. In large clinical trials, which included patients with Body-Mass-Index up to and including 35 kg/m², no consistent differences were seen between Humalog and Humulin R with respect to postprandial glucose parameters.

Renal Impairment—Some studies with human insulin have shown increased circulating levels of insulin in patients with renal failure. Information on the effect of renal impairment on the pharmacokinetics of Humalog is limited. Careful glucose monitoring and dose adjustments of insulin, including Humalog, may be necessary in patients with renal dysfunction.

Hepatic Impairment—Some studies with human insulin have shown increased circulating levels of insulin in patients with hepatic failure. Careful glucose monitoring and dose adjustments of insulin, including Humalog, may be necessary in patients with hepatic dysfunction.

INDICATIONS AND USAGE

Humalog is an insulin analog that is indicated in the treatment of patients with diabetes mellitus for the control of hyperglycemia. Humalog has a more rapid onset and a shorter duration of action than human regular insulin. Therefore, Humalog should be used in regimens including a longer-acting insulin.

CONTRAINDICATIONS

Humalog is contraindicated during episodes of hypoglycemia and in patients sensitive to Humalog or one of its excipients.

WARNINGS

This human insulin analog differs from human regular insulin by its rapid onset of action as well as a shorter duration of activity. When used as a mealtime insulin, the dose of Humalog should be given within 15 minutes before the meal. Because of the short duration of action of Humalog, patients with type I diabetes also require a longer-acting insulin to maintain glucose control.

Hypoglycemia is the most common adverse effect of insulins, including Humalog. As with all insulins, the timing of hypoglycemia may differ among various insulin formulations. Glucose monitoring is recommended for all patients with diabetes[1].

Any change of insulin should be made cautiously and only under medical supervision. Changes in insulin strength, manufacturer, type (e.g., regular, NPH, analog), species (animal, human), or method of manufacture (rDNA versus animal-source insulin) may result in the need for a change in dosage.

PRECAUTIONS

General—Hypoglycemia and hypokalemia are among the potential clinical adverse effects associated with the use of all insulins. Because of differences in the action of Humalog and other insulins, care should be taken in patients in whom such potential side effects might be clinically relevant (e.g., patients who are fasting, have autonomic neuropathy, or are using potassium-lowering drugs). Lipodystrophy and hypersensitivity are among other potential clinical adverse effects associated with the use of all insulins.

As with all insulin preparations, the time course of Humalog action may vary in different individuals or at different times in the same individual and is dependent on site of injection, blood supply, temperature, and physical activity. Adjustment of dosage of any insulin may be necessary if patients change their physical activity or their usual meal plan. Insulin requirements may be altered during illness, emotional disturbances, or other stress.

Hypoglycemia—As with all insulin preparations, hypoglycemic reactions may be associated with the administration of Humalog. Rapid changes in serum glucose levels may induce symptoms of hypoglycemia in persons with diabetes, regardless of the glucose value. Early warning symptoms of hypoglycemia may be different or less pronounced under certain conditions, such as long duration of diabetes, diabetic nerve disease, use of medications such as beta-blockers, or intensified diabetes control.

Renal Impairment—Although there are no specific data in patients with diabetes, Humalog requirements may be reduced in the presence of renal impairment, similar to observations found with other insulins.

Hepatic Impairment—Although studies have not been performed in diabetes patients with hepatic disease, Humalog requirements may be reduced in the presence of impaired hepatic function, similar to observations found with other insulins.

Allergy—Local Allergy—As with any insulin therapy, patients may experience redness, swelling, or itching at the site of injection. These minor reactions usually resolve in a few days to a few weeks. In some instances, these reactions may be related to factors other than insulin, such as irritants in a skin cleansing agent or poor injection technique. Systemic Allergy—Less common, but potentially more serious, is generalized allergy to insulin, which may cause rash (including pruritus) over the whole body, shortness of breath, wheezing, reduction in blood pressure, rapid pulse, or sweating. Severe cases of generalized allergy, including anaphylactic reaction, may be life threatening. In controlled clinical trials, pruritus (with or without rash) was seen in 17 patients receiving Humulin R (N=2969) and 30 patients receiving Humalog (N=2944) (p=.053). Localized reactions and generalized myalgias have been reported with the use of cresol as an injectable excipient.

Antibody Production—In large clinical trials, antibodies that cross react with human insulin and insulin lispro were observed in both Humulin R- and Humalog-treatment groups. As expected, the largest increase in the antibody levels during the 12-month clinical trials was observed with patients new to insulin therapy.

Information for Patients—Patients should be informed of the potential risks and advantages of Humalog and alternative therapies. Patients should also be informed about the importance of proper insulin storage, injection technique, timing of dosage, adherence to meal planning, regular physical activity, regular blood glucose monitoring, periodic glycosylated hemoglobin testing, recognition and management of hypo- and hyperglycemia, and periodic assessment for diabetes complications.

Patients should be advised to inform their physician if they are pregnant or intend to become pregnant.

Refer patients to the Information for the Patient circular for information on proper injection technique, timing of Humalog dosing (≤15 minutes before a meal), storing and mixing insulin, and common adverse effects.

Laboratory Tests—As with all insulins, the therapeutic response to Humalog should be monitored by periodic blood glucose tests. Periodic measurement of glycosylated hemoglobin is recommended for the monitoring of long-term glycemic control.

Drug Interactions—(see CLINICAL PHARMACOLOGY) Insulin requirements may be increased by medications with hyperglycemic activity such as corticosteroids, isoniazid, certain lipid-lowering drugs (e.g., niacin), estrogens, oral contraceptives, phenothiazines, and thyroid replacement therapy.

Insulin requirements may be decreased in the presence of drugs with hypoglycemic activity, such as oral hypoglycemic agents, salicylates, sulfa antibiotics, and certain antidepressants (monoamine oxidase inhibitors), certain angiotensin-converting-enzyme inhibitors, beta-adrenergic blockers, inhibitors of pancreatic function (e.g., octreotide), and alcohol. Beta-adrenergic blockers may mask the symptoms of hypoglycemia in some patients.

Mixing of Insulins—Care should be taken when mixing all insulins as a change in peak action may occur. The American Diabetes Association warns in its Position Statement on Insulin Administration, "On mixing, physiochemical changes in the mixture may occur (either immediately or over time). As a result, the physiological response to the insulin mixture may differ from that of the injection of the

insulins separately."[1] A decrease in the absorption rate, but not total bioavailability, was seen when Humalog was mixed with Humulin N. This decrease in absorption rate was not seen when Humalog was mixed with Humulin U (Figure 4). When Humalog is mixed with either Humulin U or Humulin N, the mixture should be given within 15 minutes before a meal.

Figure 4
Effect of Mixing Humalog and Longer-acting Insulins*

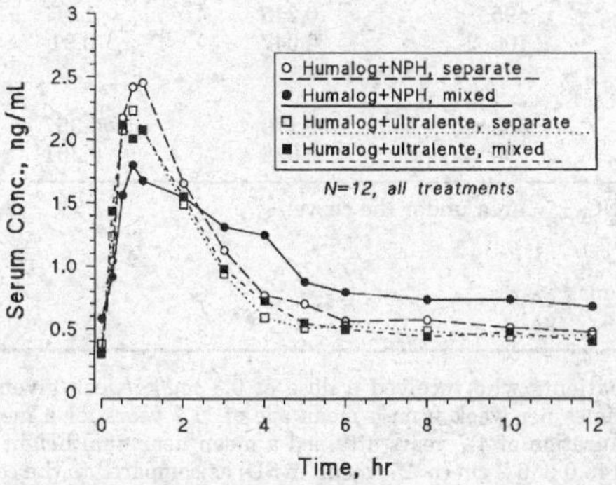

*Humalog and NPH or ultralente insulins were either injected from separate syringes or mixed in the same syringe and injected together.

The effects of mixing Humalog with insulins of animal source or insulin preparations produced by other manufacturers have not been studied (*see* WARNINGS).
If Humalog is mixed with a longer-acting insulin, Humalog should be drawn into the syringe first to prevent clouding of the Humalog by the longer-acting insulin. Injection should be made immediately after mixing. Mixtures should not be administered intravenously.
Carcinogenesis, Mutagenesis, Impairment of Fertility—Long-term studies in animals have not been performed to evaluate the carcinogenic potential of Humalog. Humalog was not mutagenic in a battery of *in vitro* and *in vivo* genetic toxicity assays (bacterial mutation tests, unscheduled DNA synthesis, mouse lymphoma assay, chromosomal aberration tests, and a micronucleus test). There is no evidence from animal studies of Humalog-induced impairment of fertility.
Pregnancy—Teratogenic Effects—Pregnancy Category B—Reproduction studies have been performed in pregnant rats and rabbits at parenteral doses up to 4 and 0.3 times, respectively, the average human dose (40 units/day) based on body surface area. The results have revealed no evidence of impaired fertility or harm to the fetus due to Humalog. There are, however, no adequate and well-controlled studies in pregnant women. Because animal reproduction studies are not always predictive of human response, this drug should be used during pregnancy only if clearly needed.
Although there are no clinical studies of the use of Humalog in pregnancy, published studies with human insulins suggest that optimizing overall glycemic control, including postprandial control, before conception and during pregnancy improves fetal outcome. Although the fetal complications of maternal hyperglycemia have been well documented, fetal toxicity also has been reported with maternal hypoglycemia. Insulin requirements usually fall during the first trimester and increase during the second and third trimesters. Careful monitoring of the patient is required throughout pregnancy. During the perinatal period, careful monitoring of infants born to mothers with diabetes is warranted.
Nursing Mothers—It is unknown whether Humalog is excreted in significant amounts in human milk. Many drugs, including human insulin, are excreted in human milk. For this reason, caution should be exercised when Humalog is administered to a nursing woman. Patients with diabetes who are lactating may require adjustments in Humalog dose, meal plan, or both.
Pediatric Use--Safety and effectiveness in patients less than 12 years of age have not been established.

ADVERSE REACTIONS

Clinical studies comparing Humalog with human regular insulin did not demonstrate a difference in frequency of adverse events between the two treatments.
Adverse events commonly associated with human insulin therapy include the following:
Body as a Whole—allergic reactions (*see* PRECAUTIONS)
Skin and Appendages—injection site reaction, lipodystrophy, pruritus, rash
Other—hypoglycemia (see WARNINGS *and* PRECAUTIONS)

OVERDOSAGE

Hypoglycemia may occur as a result of an excess of insulin relative to food intake, energy expenditure, or both. Mild episodes of hypoglycemia usually can be treated with oral glucose. Adjustments in drug dosage, meal patterns, or exercise, may be needed. More severe episodes with coma, seizure, or neurologic impairment may be treated with intramuscular/subcutaneous glucagon or concentrated intravenous glucose. Sustained carbohydrate intake and observation may be necessary because hypoglycemia may recur after apparent clinical recovery.

DOSAGE AND ADMINISTRATION

Humalog is intended for subcutaneous administration. Dosage regimens of Humalog will vary among patients and should be determined by the health care professional familiar with the patient's metabolic needs, eating habits, and other lifestyle variables. Pharmacokinetic and pharmacodynamic studies showed Humalog to be equipotent to human regular insulin (i.e., one unit of Humalog has the same glucose-lowering capability as one unit of human regular insulin), but with more rapid activity. The quicker glucose-lowering effect of Humalog is related to the more rapid absorption rate from subcutaneous tissue. An adjustment of dose or schedule of basal insulin may be needed when a patient changes from other insulins to Humalog, particularly to prevent pre-meal hyperglycemia.
When used as a meal-time insulin, Humalog should be given within 15 minutes before a meal. Human regular insulin is best given 30–60 minutes before a meal. To achieve optimal glucose control, the amount of longer-acting insulin being given may need to be adjusted when using Humalog.
The rate of insulin absorption and consequently the onset of activity is known to be affected by the site of injection, exercise, and other variables. Humalog was absorbed at a consistently faster rate than human regular insulin in healthy male volunteers given 0.2 U/kg human regular insulin or Humalog at abdominal, deltoid, or femoral sites, the three sites often used by patients with diabetes. When not mixed in the same syringe with other insulins, Humalog maintains its rapid onset of action and has less variability in its onset of action among injection sites compared with human regular insulin (*see* PRECAUTIONS). After abdominal administration, Humalog concentrations are higher than those following deltoid or thigh injections. Also, the duration of action of Humalog is slightly shorter following abdominal injection, compared with deltoid and femoral injections. As with all insulin preparations, the time course of action of Humalog may vary considerably in different individuals or within the same individual. Patients must be educated to use proper injection techniques.
Parenteral drug products should be inspected visually prior to administration whenever the solution and the container permit. If the solution is cloudy, contains particulate matter, is thickened, or is discolored, the contents must not be injected. Humalog should not be used after its expiration date.

HOW SUPPLIED

Humalog (insulin lispro injection) is available in the following package sizes:
100 units per mL (U 100)

10 mL vials	NDC 0002-7510-01 (VL-7510)
5–1.5 mL cartridges*	NDC 0002-7515-59 (VL-7515)

*Cartridges are for use in Becton Dickinson and Company's B-D®† Pen and Novo Nordisk A/S's NovoPen®‡, NovolinPen®‡, and NovoPen®‡ 1.5 insulin delivery devices.
Storage—Humalog should be stored in a refrigerator (2° to 8°C [36° to 46°F]), but not in the freezer. If refrigeration is impossible, the vial or cartridge of Humalog in use can be unrefrigerated for up to 28 days, as long as it is kept as cool as possible (not greater than 86°F [30°C]) and away from direct heat and light. Unrefrigerated vials and cartridges must be used within this time period or be discarded. Do not use Humalog if it has been frozen.
CAUTION—Federal (USA) law prohibits dispensing without prescription.

REFERENCES

1. American Diabetes Association: Clinical Practice Recommendations 1996, Insulin Administration. *Diabetes Care*, 1996; 19(Supp 1):31-34.

†B-D® is a registered trademark of Becton Dickinson and Company
‡NovolinPen® and NovoPen® are registered trademarks of Novo Nordisk A/S.
Literature revised July 30, 1997
PA 9122 FSAMP [073097]

HUMATROPE® ℞

[*hū 'ma-trōp*]
somatropin (rDNA origin) for injection

DESCRIPTION

Humatrope® (Somatropin, rDNA Origin, for Injection) is a polypeptide hormone of recombinant DNA origin. Humatrope has 191 amino acid residues and a molecular weight of about 22,125 daltons. The amino acid sequence of the product is identical to that of human growth hormone of pituitary origin. Humatrope is synthesized in a strain of *Escherichia coli* that has been modified by the addition of the gene for human growth hormone.
Humatrope is a sterile, white, lyophilized powder intended for subcutaneous or intramuscular administration after reconstitution. Each vial of Humatrope contains 5 mg somatropin (15 IU* or 225 nanomoles); 25 mg mannitol; 5 mg glycine; and 1.13 mg dibasic sodium phosphate. Phosphoric acid and/or sodium hydroxide may have been added at the time of manufacture to adjust the pH. This product is oxygen sensitive. Each vial is supplied in a combination package with an accompanying 5-mL vial of diluting solution. The diluent contains water for injection with 0.3% *m*-cresol as a preservative and 1.7% glycerin added at the time of manufacture.
Humatrope is a highly purified preparation. The 1.7% glycerin content makes the reconstituted product nearly isotonic at a concentration of 2 mg of Humatrope/mL diluent. Reconstituted solutions have a pH of approximately 7.5.

*The units per vial of Humatrope have changed from approximately 13 IU to 15 IU. This does not represent a change in product purity or the quantity (mg) of somatropin per vial. The change in units is a result of harmonizing the defined specific activity of the current reference standard with the international WHO (World Health Organization) reference standard. The specific activity of the International Standard for somatropin is defined as 3 International Units per mg of protein (previously designated as approximately 2.67 IU/mg). Humatrope is now labeled based on a specific activity of 3 IU/mg. This change in reference standard activity does not affect the recommended weekly dosage of 0.18 mg of somatropin per kg of body weight for pediatric patients. However, due to the reference standard change the weekly units administered will be measured as 0.54 IU/kg of body weight (previously approximately 0.48 IU/kg of body weight).

CLINICAL PHARMACOLOGY

General: *Linear Growth*—Humatrope stimulates linear growth in pediatric patients who lack adequate normal endogenous growth hormone. In vitro, preclinical, and clinical testing have demonstrated that Humatrope is therapeutically equivalent to human growth hormone of pituitary origin and achieves equivalent pharmacokinetic profiles in normal adults. Treatment of growth hormone-deficient pediatric patients and patients with Turner syndrome with Humatrope produces increased growth rate and IGF-I (Insulin-like Growth Factor-I/Somatomedin-C) concentrations similar to those seen after therapy with human growth hormone of pituitary origin.
In addition, the following actions have been demonstrated for Humatrope and/or human growth hormone of pituitary origin.
A. *Tissue Growth*—1. Skeletal Growth: Humatrope stimulates skeletal growth in pediatric patients with growth hormone deficiency. The measurable increase in body length after administration of either Humatrope or human growth hormone of pituitary origin results from an effect on the growth plates of long bones. Concentrations of IGF-I, which may play a role in skeletal growth, are low in the serum of growth hormone-deficient pediatric patients but increase during treatment with Humatrope. Elevations in mean serum alkaline phosphatase concentrations are also seen. 2. Cell Growth: It has been shown that there are fewer skeletal muscle cells in short-statured pediatric patients who lack endogenous growth hormone as compared with normal pediatric populations. Treatment with human growth hormone of pituitary origin results in an increase in both the number and size of muscle cells.
B. *Protein Metabolism*—Linear growth is facilitated in part by increased cellular protein synthesis. Nitrogen retention, as demonstrated by decreased urinary nitrogen excretion and serum urea nitrogen, follows the initiation of therapy with human growth hormone of pituitary origin. Treatment with Humatrope results in a similar decrease in serum urea nitrogen.
C. *Carbohydrate Metabolism*—Pediatric patients with hypopituitarism sometimes experience fasting hypoglycemia that is improved by treatment with Humatrope. Large doses of human growth hormone may impair glucose tolerance. Untreated patients with Turner syndrome have an increased incidence of glucose intolerance. Administration of human growth hormone to normal adults or patients with

Continued on next page

*** Identi-Code® symbol. This product information was prepared in June 1998. Current information on these and other products of Eli Lilly and Company may be obtained by direct inquiry to Lilly Research Laboratories, Lilly Corporate Center, Indianapolis, Indiana 46285, (800) 545-5979.**

Humatrope—Cont.

Turner syndrome resulted in increases in mean serum fasting and postprandial insulin levels although mean values remained in the normal range. In addition, mean fasting and postprandial glucose and hemoglobin A_{1C} levels remained in the normal range.

D. *Lipid Metabolism*—In growth hormone-deficient patients, administration of human growth hormone of pituitary origin has resulted in lipid mobilization, reduction in body fat stores, and increased plasma fatty acids.

E. *Mineral Metabolism*—Retention of sodium, potassium, and phosphorus is induced by human growth hormone of pituitary origin. Serum concentrations of inorganic phosphate increased in patients with growth hormone deficiency after therapy with Humatrope or human growth hormone of pituitary origin. Serum calcium is not significantly altered in patients treated with either human growth hormone of pituitary origin or Humatrope.

PHARMACOKINETICS: *Absorption*—Humatrope has been studied following intramuscular, subcutaneous, and intravenous administration in adult volunteers. The absolute bioavailability of somatropin is 75% and 63% after subcutaneous and intramuscular administration, respectively.

Distribution—The volume of distribution of somatropin after intravenous injection is about 0.07 L/kg.

Metabolism—Extensive metabolism studies have not been conducted. The metabolic fate of somatropin involves classical protein catabolism in both the liver and kidneys. In renal cells, at least a portion of the breakdown products of growth hormone is returned to the systemic circulation. In normal volunteers, mean clearance is 0.14 L/hr/kg. The mean half-life of intravenous somatropin is 0.36 hours, whereas subcutaneously and intramuscularly administered somatropin have mean half-lives of 3.8 and 4.9 hours, respectively. The longer half-life observed after subcutaneous or intramuscular administration is due to slow absorption from the injection site.

Excretion—Urinary excretion of intact Humatrope has not been measured. Small amounts of somatropin have been detected in the urine of pediatric patients following replacement therapy.

Special Populations

Geriatric—The pharmacokinetics of Humatrope has not been studied in patients greater than 60 years of age.

Pediatric—The pharmacokinetics of Humatrope in pediatric patients is similar to adults.

Gender—No studies have been performed with Humatrope. The available literature indicates that the pharmacokinetics of growth hormone is similar in both men and women.

Race—No data are available.

Renal, Hepatic insufficiency—No studies have been performed with Humatrope.

[See table 1 above]

Single Dose Average Plasma Concentrations vs Time in Normal Adult Volunteers

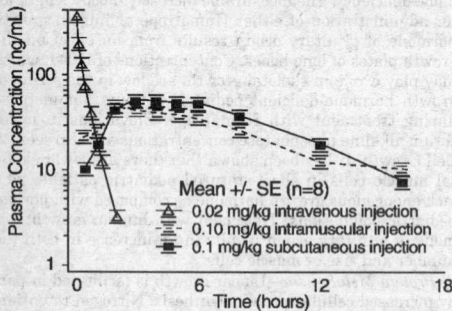

Effects of Humatrope treatment in adults with somatotropin deficiency

Two multicenter trials in adult onset somatotropin deficiency (n=98) and two studies in childhood onset somatotropin deficiency (n=67) were designed to assess the effects of replacement therapy with Humatrope. The primary efficacy measures were body composition (lean body mass and fat mass), lipid parameters, and the Nottingham Health Profile. The Nottingham Health Profile is a general health-related quality of life questionnaire. These four studies each included a 6-month randomized, blinded, placebo-controlled phase followed by 12 months of open-label therapy for all patients. The Humatrope dosages for all studies were identical: one month of therapy at 0.00625 mg/kg/day followed by the proposed maintenance dose of 0.0125 mg/kg/day. Adult onset patients and childhood onset patients differed by diagnosis (organic versus idiopathic pituitary disease), body size (normal versus small for mean height and weight), and age (mean = 44 versus 29 years). Lean body mass was determined by bioelectrical impedance analysis (BIA), vali-

dated with potassium 40. Body fat was assessed by BIA and sum of skinfold thickness. Lipid subfractions were analyzed by standard assay methods in a central laboratory.

Humatrope-treated adult onset patients, as compared to placebo, experienced an increase in lean body mass (2.59 versus -0.22 kg, p<0.001) and a decrease in body fat (-3.27 versus 0.56 kg, p<0.001). Similar changes were seen in childhood onset somatotropin deficient patients. These significant changes in lean body mass persisted throughout the 18 month period as compared to baseline for both groups, and for fat mass in the childhood onset group. Total cholesterol decreased short term (first 3 months) although the changes did not persist. However, the low HDL cholesterol levels observed at baseline (mean = 30.1 mg/mL and 33.9 mg/mL in adult onset and childhood onset patients) normalized by the end of 18 months of therapy (a change of 13.7 and 11.1 mg/dL for the adult onset and childhood onset groups, p<0.001). Adult onset patients reported significant improvements as compared to placebo in the following 2 of 6 possible health related domains: physical mobility and social isolation (Table 2). Patients with childhood onset disease failed to demonstrate improvements in Nottingham Health Profile outcomes.

Two additional studies on the effect of Humatrope on exercise capacity were also conducted. Improved physical function was documented by increased exercise capacity (VO$_2$ max, p<0.005) and work performance (Watts, p<0.01) (J Clin Endocrinol Metab 1995; 80:552-557).

Table 2
Changes[a] in Nottingham Health Profile Scores[b] in Adult Onset Somatotropin Deficient Patients

Outcome Measure	Placebo (6 Months)	Humatrope Therapy (6 Months)	Significance
Energy Level	−11.4	−15.5	NS
Physical Mobility	−3.1	−10.5	p <0.01
Social Isolation	0.5	−4.7	p <0.01
Emotional Reactions	−4.5	−5.4	NS
Sleep	−6.4	−3.7	NS
Pain	−2.8	−2.9	NS

[a]=An improvement in score is indicated by a more negative change in the score.

[b]=To account for multiple analyses, appropriate statistical methods were applied and the required level of significance is 0.01.

NS = not significant

Effects of growth hormone treatment in patients with Turner syndrome

One long-term, randomized, open-label multicenter concurrently controlled study, two long-term, open-label multicenter, historically controlled studies and one long-term, randomized, dose-response study were conducted to evaluate the efficacy of growth hormone for the treatment of patients with short stature due to Turner syndrome.

In the randomized study, GDCT, comparing growth hormone-treated patients to a concurrent control group who received no growth hormone, the growth hormone-treated

patients who received a dose of 0.3 mg/kg/week given 6 times per week from a mean age of 11.7 years for a mean duration of 4.7 years attained a mean near final height of 146.0 ± 6.2 cm (n=27, mean ± SD) as compared to the control group who attained a near final height of 142.1 ± 4.8 cm (n=19). By analysis of covariance†, the effect of growth hormone therapy was a mean height increase of 5.4 cm (p = 0.001).

†Analysis of covariance includes adjustments for baseline height relative to age and for mid-parental height.

In two of the studies (85-023 and 85-044), the effect of long-term growth hormone treatment (0.375 mg/kg/week given either 3 times per week or daily) on adult height was determined by comparing adult heights in the treated patients with those of age-matched historical controls with Turner syndrome who never received any growth-promoting therapy. The greatest improvement in adult height was observed in patients who received early growth hormone treatment and estrogen after age 14 years. In Study 85-023, this resulted in a mean adult height gain of 7.4 cm (mean duration of GH therapy of 7.6 years) vs. matched historical controls by analysis of covariance.

In Study 85-044, patients treated with early growth hormone therapy were randomized to receive estrogen replacement therapy (conjugated estrogens, 0.3 mg escalating to 0.625 mg daily) at either age 12 or 15 years. Compared with matched historical controls, early GH therapy (mean duration of GH therapy 5.6 years) combined with estrogen replacement at age 12 years resulted in an adult height gain of 5.9 cm (n=26), whereas patients who initiated estrogen at age 15 years (mean duration of GH therapy 6.1 years) had a mean adult height gain of 8.3 cm (n=29). Patients who initiated GH therapy after age 11 (mean age 12.7 years; mean duration of GH therapy 3.8 years) had a mean adult height gain of 5.0 cm (n=51).

In a randomized blinded dose-response study, GDCI, patients were treated from a mean age of 11.1 years for a mean duration of 5.3 years with a weekly dose of either 0.27 mg/kg or 0.36 mg/kg administered 3 or 6 times weekly. The mean near final height of patients receiving growth hormone was 148.7 ±6.5 cm (n=31). When compared to historical control data, the mean gain in adult height was approximately 5 cm.

In some studies, Turner syndrome patients (n=181) treated to final adult height achieved statistically significant average height gains ranging from 5.0 - 8.3 cm.

[See table 3 at top of next page]

INDICATIONS AND USAGE

Pediatric Patients—Humatrope is indicated for the long-term treatment of pediatric patients who have growth failure due to an inadequate secretion of normal endogenous growth hormone.

Humatrope is indicated for the treatment of short stature associated with Turner syndrome in patients whose epiphyses are not closed.

Adult Patients—Humatrope is indicated for replacement of endogenous somatropin in adults with somatropin deficiency syndrome who meet both of the following two criteria:

1. Adult Onset: Patients who have somatropin deficiency syndrome, either alone or with multiple hormone deficiencies (hypopituitarism), as a result of pituitary disease, hypothalamic disease, surgery, radiation therapy, or trauma; **or**

Childhood Onset: Patients who were growth hormone-deficient during childhood who have somatropin deficiency syndrome confirmed as an adult before replacement therapy with Humatrope is started.

and

Table 1
Summary of Somatropin Parameters in the Normal Population

	C_{max} (ng/mL)	$t_{1/2}$ (hr)	$AUC_{0-\infty}$ (ng•hr/mL)	Cls (L/kg•hr)	Vβ (L/kg)
0.02 mg (0.05 IU*)/kg iv					
MEAN	415	0.363	156	0.135	0.0703
SD	75	0.053	33	0.029	0.0173
0.1 mg (0.27 IU*)/kg im					
MEAN	53.2	4.93	495	0.215	1.55
SD	25.9	2.66	106	0.047	0.91
0.1 mg (0.27 IU*)/kg sc					
MEAN	63.3	3.81	585	0.179	0.957
SD	18.2	1.40	90	0.028	0.301

Abbreviations: C_{max} = maximum concentration: $t_{1/2}$ = half-life; $AUC_{0-\infty}$ = area under the curve;
   Cls = systemic clearance;
   Vβ = volume distribution; iv = intravenous;
   SD = standard deviation; im = intramuscular; sc = subcutaneous.
* Based on previous International Standard of 2.7 IU = 1 mg

Table 3
Summary Table of Efficacy Results

Study/ Group	Study Design[a]	N at Adult Height	GH Age (yr)	Estrogen Age (yr)	GH Duration (yr)	Adult Height Gain (cm)[b]
GDCT	RCT	27	11.7	13	4.7	5.4
85-023	MHT	17	9.1	15.2	7.6	7.4
85-044: A*	MHT	29	9.4	15	6.1	8.3
B*		26	9.6	12.3	5.6	5.9
C*		51	12.7	13.7	3.8	5
GDCI	RDT	31	11.1	8–13.5	5.3	~5[c]

[a] RCT: randomized controlled trial; MHT: method historical controlled trial; RDT: randomized dose-response trial.
[b] Analysis of covariance vs controls
[c] Compared with historical data
* A: GH age <11 yr, estrogen age 15 yr
  B: GH age <11 yr, estrogen age 12 yr
  C: GH age >11 yr, estrogen at month 12

Table 4
Treatment-Emergent Events of Special Interest by Treatment Group in Turner Syndrome

Adverse Event	Treatment Group			
	Overall	hGH[1]	Untreated[2]	Significance
Total Number of Patients	136	74	62	
Surgical Procedure	50 (36.8%)	33 (44.6%)	17 (27.4%)	p≤0.05
Otitis Media	48 (35.3%)	32 (43.2%)	16 (25.8%)	p≤0.05
Ear Disorders	16 (11.8%)	13 (17.6%)	3 (4.8%)	p≤0.05
Bone Disorder	13 (9.6%)	6 (8.1%)	7 (11.3%)	NS
Edema				
Conjunctival	1 (0.7%)	0	1 (1.6%)	NS
Non-specific	3 (2.2%)	2 (2.7%)	1 (1.6%)	NS
Facial	1 (0.7%)	1 (1.4%)	0	NS
Peripheral	6 (4.4%)	5 (6.8%)	1 (1.6%)	NS
Hyperglycemia	0	0	0	NS
Hypothyroidism	15 (11.0%)	10 (13.5%)	5 (8.1%)	NS
Increased Nevi[3]	10 (7.4%)	8 (10.8%)	2 (3.2%)	NS
Lymphedema	0	0	0	NS

[1] Dose = 0.3 mg/kg/week
[2] Open label study
[3] Includes any nevi coded to the following preferred terms: melanosis, skin hypertrophy, or skin benign neoplasm.
NS = not significant

Table 5
Treatment-Emergent Adverse Events with ≥5% Overall Incidence in Adult Onset Patients Treated with Humatrope for 18 Months as Compared with 6 Month Placebo and 12 Month Humatrope Exposure

Adverse Event	18 Months Exposure [Placebo (6 Months)/hGH (12 Months)] (N=46)		18 Months hGH Exposure (N=52)	
	n	%	n	%
Edema[a]	7	15.2	11	21.2
Arthralgia	7	15.2	9	17.3
Paresthesia	6	13.0	9	17.3
Myalgia	6	13.0	7	13.5
Pain	6	13.0	7	13.5
Rhinitis	5	10.9	7	13.5
Peripheral Edema[b]	8	17.4	6	11.5
Back Pain	5	10.9	5	9.6
Headache	5	10.9	4	7.7
Hypertension	2	4.3	4	7.7
Acne	0	0	3	5.8
Joint Disorder	1	2.2	3	5.8
Surgical Procedure	1	2.2	3	5.8
Flu Syndrome	3	6.5	2	3.9

Abbreviations: hGH = Humatrope; N = number of patients receiving treatment in the period stated; n = number of patients reporting each treatment-emergent adverse event.
[a] p = 0.04 as compared to placebo (6 months)
[b] p = 0.02 as compared to placebo (6 months)

2. Biochemical diagnosis of somatotropin deficiency syndrome, by means of a negative response to a standard growth hormone stimulation test [maximum peak < 5 ng/mL when measured by RIA (polyclonal antibody) or < 2.5 ng/mL when measured by IRMA (monoclonal antibody)].

CONTRAINDICATIONS
Humatrope should not be used for growth promotion in pediatric patients with closed epiphyses.
Humatrope should not be used or should be discontinued when there is any evidence of active malignancy. Antimalignancy treatment must be complete with evidence of remission prior to the institution of therapy.
Humatrope should not be reconstituted with the supplied Diluent for Humatrope by patients with a known sensitivity to either *m*-cresol or glycerin.

WARNING
If sensitivity to the diluent should occur, the vials may be reconstituted with Bacteriostatic Water for Injection, USP or, Sterile Water for Injection, USP. When Humatrope is used with Bacteriostatic Water (Benzyl Alcohol preserved), the solution should be kept refrigerated at 36° to 46°F (2° to 8°C) and used within 14 days. **Benzyl alcohol as a preservative in Bacteriostatic Water for Injection, USP has been associated with toxicity in newborns.** When administering Humatrope to newborns, use the Humatrope diluent provided or if the patient is sensitive to the diluent, use Sterile Water, USP. When Humatrope is reconstituted with Sterile Water, USP in this manner, use only one dose per Humatrope vial and discard the unused portion. If the solution is not used immediately, it must be refrigerated (36° to 46°F [2° to 8°C]) and used within 24 hours.

PRECAUTIONS
General—Therapy with Humatrope should be directed by physicians who are experienced in the diagnosis and management of patients with growth hormone deficiency, Turner syndrome or adult patients with either childhood-onset or adult-onset somatotropin deficiency.
Patients with preexisting tumors or with growth hormone deficiency secondary to an intracranial lesion should be examined routinely for progression or recurrence of the underlying disease process. In pediatric patients, clinical literature has demonstrated no relationship between somatropin replacement therapy and CNS tumor recurrence. In adults, it is unknown whether there is any relationship between somatropin replacement therapy and CNS tumor recurrence. Patients should be monitored carefully for any malignant transformation of skin lesions.
For patients with diabetes mellitus, the insulin dose may require adjustment when somatropin therapy is instituted. Because human growth hormone may induce a state of insulin resistance, patients should be observed for evidence of glucose intolerance. Patients with diabetes or glucose intolerance should be monitored closely during somatropin therapy.
In patients with hypopituitarism (multiple hormonal deficiencies) standard hormonal replacement therapy should be monitored closely when somatropin therapy is administered. Hypothyroidism may develop during treatment with somatropin, and inadequate treatment of hypothyroidism may prevent optimal response to somatropin.
Pediatric Patients (*see* General Precautions)—Pediatric patients with endocrine disorders, including growth hormone deficiency, may develop slipped capital epiphyses more frequently. Any pediatric patient with the onset of a limp during growth hormone therapy should be evaluated.
Growth hormone has not been shown to increase the incidence of scoliosis. Progression of scoliosis can occur in children who experience rapid growth. Because growth hormone increases growth rate, patients with a history of scoliosis who are treated with growth hormone should be monitored for progression of scoliosis. Skeletal abnormalities including scoliosis are commonly seen in untreated Turner syndrome patients.
Patients with Turner syndrome should be evaluated carefully for otitis media and other ear disorders since these patients have an increased risk of ear or hearing disorders (see Adverse Reactions). Patients with Turner syndrome are at risk for cardiovascular disorders (e.g. stroke, aortic aneurysm, hypertension) and these conditions should be monitored closely.
Patients with Turner syndrome have an inherently increased risk of developing autoimmune thyroid disease. Therefore, patients should have periodic thyroid function tests and be treated as indicated (*see* General Precautions).
Intracranial hypertension (IH) with papilledema, visual changes, headache, nausea and/or vomiting has been reported in a small number of pediatric patients treated with growth hormone products. Symptoms usually occurred within the first eight (8) weeks of the initiation of growth hormone therapy. In all reported cases, IH-associated signs and symptoms resolved after termination of therapy or a reduction of the growth hormone dose. Funduscopic examination of patients is recommended at the initiation and periodically during the course of growth hormone therapy. Patients with Turner syndrome may be at increased risk for development of IH.
Adult Patients (*see* General Precautions)—Patients with epiphyseal closure who were treated with growth hormone replacement therapy in childhood should be re-evaluated according to the criteria in *INDICATIONS AND USAGE* before continuation of somatropin therapy at the reduced dose level recommended for somatropin-deficient adults.
Experience in patients above 60 years is lacking.
Experience with prolonged treatment in adults is limited.
Drug Interactions—Excessive glucocorticoid therapy may prevent optimal response to somatropin. If glucocorticoid replacement therapy is required, the glucocorticoid dosage and compliance should be monitored carefully to avoid either adrenal insufficiency or inhibition of growth promoting effects.
Limited published data indicate that growth hormone (GH) treatment increases cytochrome P450 (CP450) mediated antipyrine clearance in man. These data suggest that GH administration may alter the clearance of compounds known to be metabolized by CP450 liver enzymes (e.g., corticosteroids, sex steroids, anticonvulsants, cyclosporin). Careful

Continued on next page

* Identi-Code® symbol. This product information was prepared in June 1998. Current information on these and other products of Eli Lilly and Company may be obtained by direct inquiry to Lilly Research Laboratories, Lilly Corporate Center, Indianapolis, Indiana 46285, (800) 545-5979.

Humatrope—Cont.

monitoring is advisable when GH is administered in combination with other drugs known to be metabolized by CP450 liver enzymes.

Carcinogenesis, Mutagenesis, Impairment of Fertility—Long-term animal studies for carcinogenicity and impairment of fertility with this human growth hormone (Humatrope) have not been performed. There has been no evidence to date of Humatrope-induced mutagenicity.

Pregnancy—Pregnancy Category C—Animal reproduction studies have not been conducted with Humatrope. It is not known whether Humatrope can cause fetal harm when administered to a pregnant woman or can affect reproduction capacity. Humatrope should be given to a pregnant woman only if clearly needed.

Nursing Mothers—There have been no studies conducted with Humatrope in nursing mothers. It is not known whether this drug is excreted in human milk. Because many drugs are excreted in human milk, caution should be exercised when Humatrope is administered to a nursing woman.

Information for Patients—Patients being treated with growth hormone and/or their parents should be informed of the potential benefits and risks associated with treatment. If home use is determined to be desirable by the physician, instructions on appropriate use should be given, including a review of the contents of the patient information insert. This information is intended to aid in the safe and effective administration of the medication. It is not a disclosure of all possible adverse or intended effects.

If home use is prescribed, a puncture resistant container for the disposal of used syringes and needles should be recommended to the patient. Patients and/or parents should be thoroughly instructed in the importance of proper needle disposal and cautioned against any reuse of needles and syringes (*see* Information for the Patient insert).

ADVERSE REACTIONS

Growth-Hormone Deficient Pediatric Patients—As with all protein pharmaceuticals, a small percentage of patients may develop antibodies to the protein. During the first six months of Humatrope therapy in 314 naive patients, only 1.6% developed specific antibodies to Humatrope (binding capacity ≥ 0.02 mg/L). None had antibody concentrations which exceeded 2 mg/L. Throughout 8 years of this same study, 2 patients (0.6%) had binding capacity >2 mg/L. Neither patient demonstrated a decrease in growth velocity at or near the time of increased antibody production. It has been reported that growth attenuation from pituitary-derived growth hormone may occur when antibody concentrations are >1.5 mg/L.

In addition to an evaluation of compliance with the treatment program and of thyroid status, testing for antibodies to human growth hormone should be carried out in any patient who fails to respond to therapy.

In studies with growth hormone-deficient pediatric patients, injection site pain was reported infrequently. A mild and transient edema, which appeared in 2.5% of patients, was observed early during the course of treatment.

Leukemia has been reported in a small number of pediatric patients who have been treated with growth hormone, including growth hormone of pituitary origin as well as of recombinant DNA origin (somatrem and somatropin). The relationship, if any, between leukemia and growth hormone therapy is uncertain.

Turner Syndrome Patients—In a randomized, concurrent controlled trial, there was a statistically significant increase, as compared to untreated controls, in otitis media (43% vs 26%), ear disorders (18% vs 5%) and surgical procedures (45% vs 27%) in patients receiving Humatrope (Table 4). Other adverse events of special interest to Turner syndrome patients were not significantly different between treatment groups (Table 4). A similar increase in otitis media was observed in an 18 month placebo-controlled trial.
[See table 4 on previous page]

Adult Patients—In clinical studies in which high doses of Humatrope were administered to healthy adult volunteers, the following events occurred infrequently: headache, localized muscle pain, weakness, mild hyperglycemia, and glucosuria.

In the first 6 months of controlled blinded trials, adult onset somatotropin-deficient adults experienced a statistically significant increase in edema (Humatrope 17.3% vs. placebo 4.4%, p=0.043) and peripheral edema (11.5% vs. 0% respectively, p=0.017). In patients with adult onset somatotropin deficiency syndrome, edema, muscle pain, joint pain, and joint disorder were reported early in therapy and tended to be transient or responsive to dosage titration.

Two out of 113 adult onset patients developed carpal tunnel syndrome after beginning maintenance therapy without a low dose (0.00625 mg/kg/day) lead-in phase. Symptoms abated in these patients after dosage reduction.

All treatment-emergent overall adverse events with $\geq$5% overall incidence during 12 or 18 months of replacement therapy with Humatrope are shown in Table 5 (adult onset patients) and in Table 6 (childhood onset patients).

Adult patients treated with Humatrope who had been diagnosed with growth hormone deficiency in childhood reported side effects less frequently than those with adult onset somatotropin deficiency.
[See table 5 on previous page]
[See table 6 below]

Other adverse drug events that have been reported in growth hormone-treated patients include the following:
1) Metabolic: Infrequent, mild and transient peripheral or generalized edema. 2) Musculoskeletal: Rare carpal tunnel syndrome. 3) Skin: Rare increased growth of pre-existing nevi. Patients should be monitored carefully for malignant transformation. 4) Endocrine: Rare gynecomastia. Rare pancreatitis.

OVERDOSAGE

Acute overdosage could lead initially to hypoglycemia and subsequently to hyperglycemia. Long-term overdosage could result in signs and symptoms of gigantism/acromegaly consistent with the known effects of excess human growth hormone. (See recommended and maximal dosage instructions given below.)

DOSAGE AND ADMINISTRATION

Pediatric Patients—The Humatrope dosage and administration schedule should be individualized for each patient. Therapy should not be continued if epiphyseal fusion has occurred. Response to growth hormone therapy tends to decrease with time.

However, failure to increase growth rate, particularly during the first year of therapy, should require close assessment of compliance and evaluation of other causes of growth failure such as hypothyroidism, under-nutrition and advanced bone age.

Growth hormone-deficient pediatric patients—The recommended weekly dosage is 0.18 mg/kg (0.54 IU/kg) of body weight. The maximal replacement weekly dosage is 0.3 mg/kg (0.90 IU/kg) of body weight. It should be divided into equal doses given either on 3 alternate days, 6 times per week or daily. The subcutaneous route of administration is preferable; intramuscular injection is also acceptable. The dosage and administration schedule for Humatrope should be individualized for each patient.

Turner Syndrome—A weekly dosage of up to 0.375 mg/kg (1.125 IU/kg) of body weight administered by subcutaneous injection is recommended. It should be divided into equal doses given either daily or on 3 alternate days.

Adult Patients—

Somatotropin-deficient adult patients—The recommended dosage at the start of therapy is not more than 0.006 mg/kg/day (0.018 IU/kg/day) given as a daily subcutaneous injection. The dose may be increased according to individual patient requirements to a maximum of 0.0125 mg/kg/day (0.0375 IU/kg/day).

During therapy, dosage should be titrated if required by the occurrence of side effects or to maintain the IGF-I response below the upper limit of normal IGF-I levels, matched for age and sex. To minimize the occurrence of adverse events in patients with increasing age or excessive body weight, dose reductions may be necessary.

Each 5-mg vial of Humatrope should be reconstituted with 1.5 to 5 mL of Diluent for Humatrope. The diluent should be injected into the vial of Humatrope by aiming the stream of liquid against the glass wall. Following reconstitution, the vial should be swirled with a GENTLE rotary motion until the contents are completely dissolved. DO NOT SHAKE. The resulting solution should be inspected for clarity. It should be clear. If the solution is cloudy or contains particulate matter, the contents MUST NOT be injected.

Before and after injection, the septum of the vial should be wiped with rubbing alcohol or an alcoholic antiseptic solution to prevent contamination of the contents by repeated needle insertions. Sterile disposable syringes and/or needles should be used for administration of Humatrope. The volume of the syringe should be small enough so that the prescribed dose can be withdrawn from the vial with reasonable accuracy.

STABILITY AND STORAGE

Before Reconstitution—Vials of Humatrope as well as the Diluent for Humatrope are stable when refrigerated (36° to 46°F [2° to 8°C]). Avoid freezing Diluent for Humatrope. Expiration dates are stated on the labels.

After Reconstitution—Vials of Humatrope are stable for up to 14 days when reconstituted with Diluent for Humatrope or Bacteriostatic Water for Injection, USP and stored in a refrigerator at 36° to 46°F (2° to 8°C). Avoid freezing the reconstituted vial of Humatrope.

After Reconstitution with Sterile Water, USP—Use only one dose per Humatrope vial and discard the unused portion. If the solution is not used immediately, it must be refrigerated (36° to 46°F [2° to 8°C]) and used within 24 hours.

HOW SUPPLIED

Vials:
  5 mg (No. 7335)—(6s) NDC 0002-7335-16, and 5-mL vials of Diluent for Humatrope (No. 7336).
CAUTION—Federal (USA) law prohibits dispensing without prescription.
Literature revised September 8, 1997
PA 1646 AMP   [090897]

HUMULIN® 50/50®   **OTC**
[*hŭ 'mŭ-lĭn*]
(50% Human Insulin
Isophane Suspension
and
50% Human Insulin Injection
[rDNA Origin])

INFORMATION FOR THE PATIENT
WARNINGS
THIS LILLY HUMAN INSULIN PRODUCT DIFFERS FROM ANIMAL-SOURCE INSULINS BECAUSE IT IS STRUCTURALLY IDENTICAL TO THE INSULIN PRODUCED BY YOUR BODY'S PANCREAS AND BECAUSE OF ITS UNIQUE MANUFACTURING PROCESS.
ANY CHANGE OF INSULIN SHOULD BE MADE CAUTIOUSLY AND ONLY UNDER MEDICAL SUPERVISION. CHANGES IN STRENGTH, MANUFACTURER, TYPE (E.G., REGULAR, NPH, LENTE®), SPECIES (BEEF, PORK, BEEF-PORK, HUMAN), OR METHOD OF MANUFACTURE (rDNA VERSUS ANIMAL-SOURCE INSULIN) MAY RESULT IN THE NEED FOR A CHANGE IN DOSAGE.
SOME PATIENTS TAKING HUMULIN® (HUMAN INSULIN, rDNA ORIGIN) MAY REQUIRE A CHANGE IN DOSAGE FROM THAT USED WITH ANIMAL-SOURCE INSULINS. IF AN ADJUSTMENT IS NEEDED, IT MAY OCCUR WITH THE FIRST DOSE OR DURING THE FIRST SEVERAL WEEKS OR MONTHS.

Table 6
Treatment-Emergent Adverse Events with ≥5% Overall Incidence in Childhood Onset Patients Treated with Humatrope for 18 Months as Compared with 6 Month Placebo and 12 Month Humatrope Exposure

Adverse Event	18 Months Exposure [Placebo (6 Months)/hGH (12 Months)] (N=35)		18 Months hGH Exposure (N=32)	
	n	%	n	%
Flu Syndrome	8	22.9	5	15.6
AST Increased[a]	2	5.7	4	12.5
Headache	4	11.4	3	9.4
Asthenia	1	2.9	2	6.3
Cough Increased	0	0	2	6.3
Edema	3	8.6	2	6.3
Hypesthesia	0	0	2	6.3
Myalgia	2	5.7	2	6.3
Pain	3	8.6	2	6.3
Rhinitis	2	5.7	2	6.3
ALT Increased	2	5.7	2	6.3
Respiratory Disorder	2	5.7	1	3.1
Gastritis	2	5.7	0	0
Pharyngitis	5	14.3	1	3.1

Abbreviations: hGH = Humatrope; N = number of patients receiving treatment in the period stated; n = number of patients reporting each treatment-emergent adverse event; ALT = alanine amino transferase, formerly SGPT; AST = aspartate amino transferase, formerly SGOT.
[a]p = 0.03 as compared to placebo (6 months)

DIABETES

Insulin is a hormone produced by the pancreas, a large gland that lies near the stomach. This hormone is necessary for the body's correct use of food, especially sugar. Diabetes occurs when the pancreas does not make enough insulin to meet your body's needs.

To control your diabetes, your doctor has prescribed injections of insulin to keep your blood glucose at a nearly normal level. Proper control of your diabetes requires close and constant cooperation with your doctor. In spite of diabetes, you can lead an active, healthy, and useful life if you eat a balanced diet daily, exercise regularly, and take your insulin injections as prescribed.

You have been instructed to test your blood and/or your urine regularly for glucose. If your blood tests consistently show above- or below-normal glucose levels or your urine tests consistently show the presence of glucose, your diabetes is not properly controlled and you must let your doctor know.

Always keep an extra supply of insulin as well as a spare syringe and needle on hand. Always wear diabetic identification so that appropriate treatment can be given if complications occur away from home.

50/50 HUMAN INSULIN
Description
Humulin is synthesized in a non-disease-producing special laboratory strain of *Escherichia coli* bacteria that has been genetically altered by the addition of the gene for human insulin production. Humulin 50/50 is a mixture of 50% Human Insulin Isophane Suspension and 50% Human Insulin Injection. It is an intermediate-acting insulin combined with the more rapid onset of action of regular insulin. The duration of activity may last up to 24 hours following injection. The time course of action of any insulin may vary considerably in different individuals or at different times in the same individual. As with all insulin preparations, the duration of action of Humulin 50/50 is dependent on dose, site of injection, blood supply, temperature, and physical activity. Humulin 50/50 is a sterile suspension and is for subcutaneous injection only. It should not be used intravenously or intramuscularly. The concentration of Humulin 50/50 is 100 units/mL (U-100).

Identification
Human insulin manufactured by Eli Lilly and Company has the trademark Humulin and is available in 6 formulations—Regular (**R**), NPH (**N**), Lente (**L**), Ultralente® (**U**), 50% Human Insulin Isophane Suspension [NPH]/50% Human Insulin Injection [buffered regular] (**50/50**) and 70% Human Insulin Isophane Suspension [NPH]/30% Human Insulin Injection [buffered regular] (**70/30**). Your doctor has prescribed the type of insulin that he/she believes is best for you. **DO NOT USE ANY OTHER INSULIN EXCEPT ON HIS/ HER ADVICE AND DIRECTION.**

Always check the carton and the bottle label for the name and letter designation of the insulin you receive from your pharmacy to make sure it is the same as that your doctor has prescribed. Humulin 50/50 can be identified as follows: [See graphic below]

Always examine the appearance of your bottle of insulin before withdrawing each dose. A bottle of Humulin 50/50 must be carefully shaken or rotated before each injection so that the contents are uniformly mixed. Humulin 50/50 should look uniformly cloudy or milky after mixing. Do not use it if the insulin substance (the white material) remains at the bottom of the bottle after mixing. Do not use a bottle of Humulin 50/50 if there are clumps in the insulin after mixing (Figure 1). Do not use a bottle of Humulin 50/50 if solid white particles stick to the bottom or wall of the bottle, giving it a frosted appearance (Figure 2). Always check the appearance of your bottle of insulin before using, and if you note anything unusual in the appearance of your insulin or notice your insulin requirements changing markedly, consult your doctor.

[See figures 1 & 2 at top of next column]

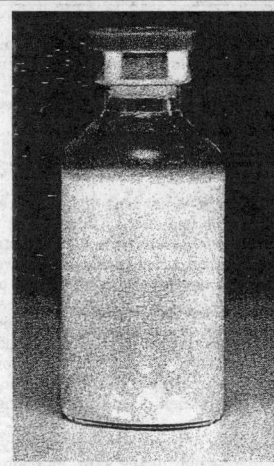

Fig. 1.—Do not use if there are clumps in the insulin after mixing.

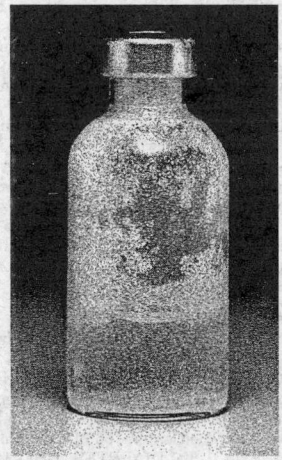

Fig. 2.—Do not use if particles on the bottom or wall give the bottle a frosted appearance

Storage
Insulin should be stored in a refrigerator but not in the freezer. If refrigeration is not possible, the bottle of insulin that you are currently using can be kept unrefrigerated as long as it is kept as cool as possible (below 86°F [30°C]) and away from heat and light. Do not use insulin if it has been frozen. Do not use a bottle of insulin after the expiration date stamped on the label.

INJECTION PROCEDURES
Correct Syringe
Doses of insulin are measured in **units**. U-100 insulin contains 100 units/mL (1 mL = 1 cc). With Humulin 50/50, it is important to use a syringe that is marked for U-100 insulin preparations. Failure to use the proper syringe can lead to a mistake in dosage, causing serious problems for you, such as a blood glucose level that is too low or too high.

Syringe Use
To help avoid contamination and possible infection, follow these instructions exactly.

Disposable syringes and needles should be used only once and then discarded. **NEEDLES AND SYRINGES MUST NOT BE SHARED.**

Reusable syringes and needles must be sterilized before each injection. **Follow the package directions supplied with your syringe.** Described below are 2 methods of sterilizing.
Boiling
1. Put syringe, plunger, and needle in strainer, place in saucepan, and cover with water. Boil for 5 minutes.
2. Remove articles from water. When they have cooled, insert plunger into barrel, and fasten needle to syringe with a slight twist.
3. Push plunger in and out several times until water is completely removed.

Isopropyl Alcohol
If the syringe, plunger, and needle cannot be boiled, as when you are traveling, they may be sterilized by immersion for at least 5 minutes in Isopropyl Alcohol, 91%. Do not use bathing, rubbing, or medicated alcohol for this sterilization. If the syringe is sterilized with alcohol, it must be absolutely dry before use.

Preparing the Dose
1. Wash your hands.
2. Carefully shake or rotate the insulin bottle several times to completely mix the insulin.
3. Inspect the insulin. Humulin 50/50 should look uniformly cloudy or milky. Do not use it if you notice anything unusual in the appearance.
4. If using a new bottle, flip off the plastic protective cap, but **do not** remove the stopper. When using a new bottle, wipe the top of the bottle with an alcohol swab.
5. Draw air into the syringe equal to your insulin dose. Put the needle through rubber top of the insulin bottle and inject the air into the bottle.
6. Turn the bottle and syringe upside down. Hold the bottle and syringe firmly in 1 hand and shake gently.
7. Making sure the tip of the needle is in the insulin, withdraw the correct dose of insulin into the syringe.
8. Before removing the needle from the bottle, check your syringe for air bubbles which reduce the amount of insulin in it. If bubbles are present, hold the syringe straight up and tap its side until the bubbles float to the top. Push them out with the plunger and withdraw the correct dose.
9. Remove the needle from the bottle and lay the syringe down so that the needle does not touch anything.

Injection
Cleanse the skin with alcohol where the injection is to be made. Stabilize the skin by spreading it or pinching up a large area. Insert the needle as instructed by your doctor. Push the plunger in as far as it will go. Pull the needle out and apply gentle pressure over the injection site for several seconds. **Do not rub the area.** To avoid tissue damage, give the next injection at a site at least $\frac{1}{2}$" from the previous site.

DOSAGE
Your doctor has told you which insulin to use, how much, and when and how often to inject it. Because each patient's case of diabetes is different, this schedule has been individualized for you.

Your usual insulin dose may be affected by changes in your food, activity, or work schedule. Carefully follow your doctor's instructions to allow for these changes. Other things that may affect your insulin dose are:
Illness
Illness, especially with nausea and vomiting, may cause your insulin requirements to change. Even if you are not eating, you will still require insulin. You and your doctor should establish a sick day plan for you to use in case of illness. When you are sick, test your blood/urine frequently and call your doctor as instructed.
Pregnancy
Good control of diabetes is especially important for you and your unborn baby. Pregnancy may make managing your diabetes more difficult. If you are planning to have a baby, are pregnant, or are nursing a baby, consult your doctor.
Medication
Insulin requirements may be increased if you are taking other drugs with hyperglycemic activity, such as oral contraceptives, corticosteroids, or thyroid replacement therapy. Insulin requirements may be reduced in the presence of drugs with hypoglycemic activity, such as oral hypoglycemics, salicylates (for example, aspirin), sulfa antibiotics, and certain antidepressants. Always discuss any medications you are taking with your doctor.
Exercise
Exercise may lower your body's need for insulin during and for some time after the activity. Exercise may also speed up the effect of an insulin dose, especially if the exercise in-

Continued on next page

* **Identi-Code® symbol. This product information was prepared in June 1998. Current information on these and other products of Eli Lilly and Company may be obtained by direct inquiry to Lilly Research Laboratories, Lilly Corporate Center, Indianapolis, Indiana 46285, (800) 545-5979.**

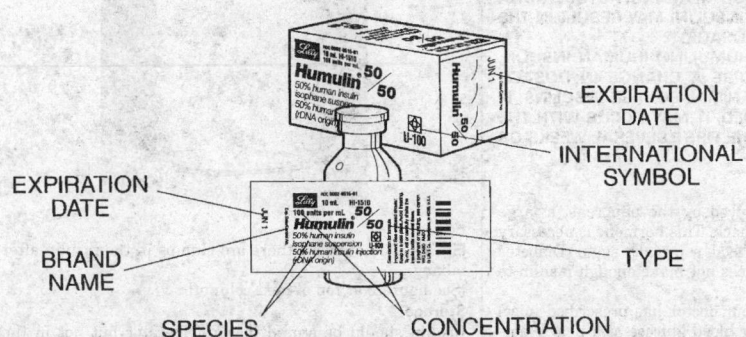

EXPIRATION DATE

INTERNATIONAL SYMBOL

EXPIRATION DATE

BRAND NAME

TYPE

SPECIES

CONCENTRATION

Humulin 50/50—Cont.

volves the area of injection site (for example, the leg should not be used for injection just prior to running). Discuss with your doctor how you should adjust your regimen to accommodate exercise.

Travel

Persons traveling across more than 2 time zones should consult their doctor concerning adjustments in their insulin schedule.

COMMON PROBLEMS OF DIABETES

Hypoglycemia (Insulin Reaction)

Hypoglycemia (too little glucose in the blood) is one of the most frequent adverse events experienced by insulin users. It can be brought about by:

1. Taking too much insulin
2. Missing or delaying meals
3. Exercising or working more than usual
4. An infection or illness (especially with diarrhea or vomiting)
5. A change in the body's need for insulin
6. Diseases of the adrenal, pituitary, or thyroid gland, or progression of kidney or liver disease
7. Interactions with other drugs that lower blood glucose, such as oral hypoglycemics, salicylates (for example, aspirin), sulfa antibiotics, and certain antidepressants
8. Consumption of alcoholic beverages

Symptoms of mild to moderate hypoglycemia may occur suddenly and can include:

- sweating
- dizziness
- palpitation
- tremor
- hunger
- restlessness
- tingling in the hands, feet, lips, or tongue
- lightheadedness
- inability to concentrate
- headache
- drowsiness
- sleep disturbances
- anxiety
- blurred vision
- slurred speech
- depressed mood
- irritability
- abnormal behavior
- unsteady movement
- personality changes

Signs of severe hypoglycemia can include:

- disorientation
- unconsciousness
- seizures
- death

Therefore, it is important that assistance be obtained immediately.

Early warning symptoms of hypoglycemia may be different or less pronounced under certain conditions, such as long duration of diabetes, diabetic nerve disease, medications such as beta-blockers, change in insulin preparations, or intensified control (3 or more insulin injections per day) of diabetes.

A few patients who have experienced hypoglycemic reactions after transfer from animal-source insulin to human insulin have reported that the early warning symptoms of hypoglycemia were less pronounced or different from those experienced with their previous insulin.

Without recognition of early warning symptoms, you may not be able to take steps to avoid more serious hypoglycemia. Be alert for all of the various types of symptoms that may indicate hypoglycemia. Patients who experience hypoglycemia without early warning symptoms should monitor their blood glucose frequently, especially prior to activities such as driving. If the blood glucose is below your normal fasting glucose, you should consider eating or drinking sugar-containing foods to treat your hypoglycemia.

Mild to moderate hypoglycemia may be treated by eating foods or drinks that contain sugar. Patients should always carry a quick source of sugar, such as candy mints or glucose tablets. More severe hypoglycemia may require the assistance of another person. Patients who are unable to take sugar orally or who are unconscious require an injection of glucagon or should be treated with intravenous administration of glucose at a medical facility.

You should learn to recognize your own symptoms of hypoglycemia. If you are uncertain about these symptoms, you should monitor your blood glucose frequently to help you learn to recognize the symptoms that you experience with hypoglycemia.

If you have frequent episodes of hypoglycemia or experience difficulty in recognizing the symptoms, you should consult your doctor to discuss possible changes in therapy, meal plans, and/or exercise programs to help you avoid hypoglycemia.

Hyperglycemia and Diabetic Acidosis

Hyperglycemia (too much glucose in the blood) may develop if your body has too little insulin. Hyperglycemia can be brought about by:

1. Omitting your insulin or taking less than the doctor has prescribed
2. Eating significantly more than your meal plan suggests
3. Developing a fever, infection, or other significant stressful situation

In patients with insulin-dependent diabetes, prolonged hyperglycemia can result in diabetic acidosis. The first symptoms of diabetic acidosis usually come on gradually, over a period of hours or days, and include a drowsy feeling, flushed face, thirst, loss of appetite, and fruity odor on the breath. With acidosis, urine tests show large amounts of glucose and acetone. Heavy breathing and a rapid pulse are more severe symptoms. If uncorrected, prolonged hyperglycemia or diabetic acidosis can lead to nausea, vomiting, dehydration, loss of consciousness or death. Therefore, it is important that you obtain medical assistance immediately.

Lipodystrophy

Rarely, administration of insulin subcutaneously can result in lipoatrophy (depression in the skin) or lipohypertrophy (enlargement or thickening of tissue). If you notice either of these conditions, consult your doctor. A change in your injection technique may help alleviate the problem.

Allergy to Insulin

Local Allergy —Patients occasionally experience redness, swelling, and itching at the site of injection of insulin. This condition, called local allergy, usually clears up in a few days to a few weeks. In some instances, this condition may be related to factors other than insulin, such as irritants in the skin cleansing agent or poor injection technique. If you have local reactions, contact your doctor.

Systemic Allergy —Less common, but potentially more serious, is generalized allergy to insulin, which may cause rash over the whole body, shortness of breath, wheezing, reduction in blood pressure, fast pulse, or sweating. Severe cases of generalized allergy may be life threatening. If you think you are having a generalized allergic reaction to insulin, notify a doctor immediately.

ADDITIONAL INFORMATION

Additional information about diabetes may be obtained from your diabetes educator.

DIABETES FORECAST is a national magazine designed especially for patients with diabetes and their families and is available by subscription from the American Diabetes Association, National Service Center, 1660 Duke Street, Alexandria, Virginia 22314, 1-800-DIABETES (1-800-342-2383).

Another publication, **DIABETES COUNTDOWN**, is available from the Juvenile Diabetes Foundation, 432 Park Avenue South, New York, New York 10016-8013, 1-800-JDF-CURE (1-800-533-2873).

Additional information about Humulin can be obtained by calling 1-888-88-LILLY (1-888-88-4559).

Literature revised March 26, 1997
PA 6052 AMP   [032697]

HUMULIN® 70/30   OTC
[hū 'mŭ-lĭn]
(70% Human Insulin Isophane Suspension and 30% Human Insulin Injection [rDNA origin])

INFORMATION FOR THE PATIENT
WARNINGS

THIS LILLY HUMAN INSULIN PRODUCT DIFFERS FROM ANIMAL-SOURCE INSULINS BECAUSE IT IS STRUCTURALLY IDENTICAL TO THE INSULIN PRODUCED BY YOUR BODY'S PANCREAS AND BECAUSE OF ITS UNIQUE MANUFACTURING PROCESS.

ANY CHANGE OF INSULIN SHOULD BE MADE CAUTIOUSLY AND ONLY UNDER MEDICAL SUPERVISION. CHANGES IN STRENGTH, MANUFACTURER, TYPE (E.G., REGULAR, NPH, LENTE®), SPECIES (BEEF, PORK, BEEF-PORK, HUMAN), OR METHOD OF MANUFACTURE (rDNA VERSUS ANIMAL-SOURCE INSULIN) MAY RESULT IN THE NEED FOR A CHANGE IN DOSAGE.

SOME PATIENTS TAKING HUMULIN® (HUMAN INSULIN, rDNA ORIGIN) MAY REQUIRE A CHANGE IN DOSAGE FROM THAT USED WITH ANIMAL-SOURCE INSULINS. IF AN ADJUSTMENT IS NEEDED, IT MAY OCCUR WITH THE FIRST DOSE OR DURING THE FIRST SEVERAL WEEKS OR MONTHS.

DIABETES

Insulin is a hormone produced by the pancreas, a large gland that lies near the stomach. This hormone is necessary for the body's correct use of food, especially sugar. Diabetes occurs when the pancreas does not make enough insulin to meet your body's needs.

To control your diabetes, your doctor has prescribed injections of insulin to keep your blood glucose at a nearly normal level. Proper control of your diabetes requires close and constant cooperation with your doctor. In spite of diabetes,

you can lead an active, healthy, and useful life if you eat a balanced diet daily, exercise regularly, and take your insulin injections as prescribed.

You have been instructed to test your blood and/or your urine regularly for glucose. If your blood tests consistently show above- or below-normal glucose levels or your urine tests consistently show the presence of glucose, your diabetes is not properly controlled and you must let your doctor know.

Always keep an extra supply of insulin as well as a spare syringe and needle on hand. Always wear diabetic identification so that appropriate treatment can be given if complications occur away from home.

70/30 HUMAN INSULIN

Description

Humulin is synthesized in a non-disease-producing special laboratory strain of *Escherichia coli* bacteria that has been genetically altered by the addition of the gene for human insulin production. Humulin 70/30 is a mixture of 70% Human Insulin Isophane Suspension and 30% Human Insulin Injection. It is an intermediate-acting insulin combined with the more rapid onset of action of regular insulin. The duration of activity may last up to 24 hours following injection. The time course of action of any insulin may vary considerably in different individuals or at different times in the same individual. As with all insulin preparations, the duration of action of Humulin 70/30 is dependent on dose, site of injection, blood supply, temperature, and physical activity. Humulin 70/30 is a sterile suspension and is for subcutaneous injection only. It should not be used intravenously or intramuscularly. The concentration of Humulin 70/30 is 100 units/mL (U-100).

Identification

Human insulin manufactured by Eli Lilly and Company has the trademark Humulin and is available in 6 formulations—Regular (**R**), NPH (**N**), Lente (**L**), Ultralente® (**U**), 50% Human Insulin Isophane Suspension [NPH]/50% Human Insulin Injection [buffered regular] (**50/50**), and 70% Human Insulin Isophane Suspension [NPH]/30% Human Insulin Injection [buffered regular] (**70/30**). Your doctor has prescribed the type of insulin that he/she believes is best for you. **DO NOT USE ANY OTHER INSULIN EXCEPT ON HIS/ HER ADVICE AND DIRECTION.**

Always check the carton and the bottle label for the name and letter designation of the insulin you receive from your pharmacy to make sure it is the same as that your doctor has prescribed. Humulin 70/30 can be identified as follows: Always examine the appearance of your bottle of insulin before withdrawing each dose. A bottle of Humulin 70/30 must be carefully shaken or rotated before each injection so that the contents are uniformly mixed. Humulin 70/30 should look uniformly cloudy or milky after mixing. Do not use it if the insulin substance (the white material) remains at the bottom of the bottle after mixing. Do not use a bottle of Humulin 70/30 if there are clumps in the insulin after mixing (Figure 1). Do not use a bottle of Humulin 70/30 if solid white particles stick to the bottom or wall of the bottle, giving it a frosted appearance (Figure 2). Always check the appearance of your bottle of insulin before using, and if you note anything unusual in the appearance of your insulin or notice your insulin requirements changing markedly, consult your doctor.

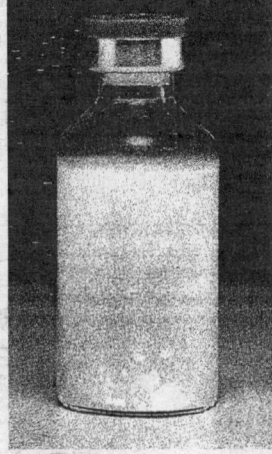

Fig. 1.—Do not use if there are clumps in the insulin after mixing.
[See figure 2 at top of next column]

Storage

Insulin should be stored in a refrigerator but not in the freezer. If refrigeration is not possible, the bottle of insulin that you are currently using can be kept unrefrigerated as

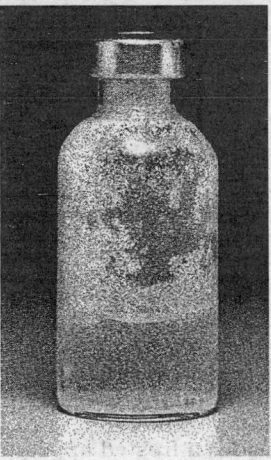

Fig. 2.—Do not use if particles on the bottom or wall give the bottle a frosted appearance.

long as it is kept as cool as possible (below 86°F [30°C]) and away from heat and light. Do not use insulin if it has been frozen. Do not use a bottle of insulin after the expiration date stamped on the label.

INJECTION PROCEDURES

Correct Syringe

Doses of insulin are measured in **units.** U-100 insulin contains 100 units/mL (1 mL=1 cc). With Humulin 70/30, it is important to use a syringe that is marked for U-100 insulin preparations. Failure to use the proper syringe can lead to a mistake in dosage, causing serious problems for you, such as a blood glucose level that is too low or too high.

Syringe Use

To help avoid contamination and possible infection, follow these instructions exactly.

Disposable syringes and needles should be used only once and then discarded. **NEEDLES AND SYRINGES MUST NOT BE SHARED.**

Reusable syringes and needles must be sterilized before each injection. **Follow the package directions supplied with your syringe.** Described below are 2 methods of sterilizing.

Boiling

1. Put syringe, plunger, and needle in strainer, place in saucepan, and cover with water. Boil for 5 minutes.
2. Remove articles from water. When they have cooled, insert plunger into barrel, and fasten needle to syringe with a slight twist.
3. Push plunger in and out several times until water is completely removed.

Isopropyl Alcohol

If the syringe, plunger, and needle cannot be boiled, as when you are traveling, they may be sterilized by immersion for at least 5 minutes in Isopropyl Alcohol, 91%. Do not use bathing, rubbing, or medicated alcohol for this sterilization. If the syringe is sterilized with alcohol, it must be absolutely dry before use.

Preparing the Dose

1. Wash your hands.
2. Carefully shake or rotate the insulin bottle several times to completely mix the insulin.
3. Inspect the insulin. Humulin 70/30 should look uniformly cloudy or milky. Do not use it if you notice anything unusual in the appearance.
4. If using a new bottle, flip off the plastic protective cap, but **do not** remove the stopper. When using a new bottle, wipe the top of the bottle with an alcohol swab.
5. Draw air into the syringe equal to your insulin dose. Put the needle through rubber top of the insulin bottle and inject the air into the bottle.
6. Turn the bottle and syringe upside down. Hold the bottle and syringe firmly in 1 hand and shake gently.
7. Making sure the tip of the needle is in the insulin, withdraw the correct dose of insulin into the syringe.
8. Before removing the needle from the bottle, check your syringe for air bubbles which reduce the amount of insulin in it. If bubbles are present, hold the syringe straight up and tap its side until the bubbles float to the top. Push them out with the plunger and withdraw the correct dose.
9. Remove the needle from the bottle and lay the syringe down so that the needle does not touch anything.

Injection

Cleanse the skin with alcohol where the injection is to be made. Stabilize the skin by spreading it or pinching up a large area. Insert the needle as instructed by your doctor. Push the plunger in as far as it will go. Pull the needle out and apply gentle pressure over the injection site for several seconds. **Do not rub the area.** To avoid tissue damage, give the next injection at a site at least $\frac{1}{2}''$ from the previous site.

DOSAGE

Your doctor has told you which insulin to use, how much, and when and how often to inject it. Because each patient's case of diabetes is different, this schedule has been individualized for you.

Your usual insulin dose may be affected by changes in your food, activity, or work schedule. Carefully follow your doctor's instructions to allow for these changes. Other things that may affect your insulin dose are:

Illness

Illness, especially with nausea and vomiting, may cause your insulin requirements to change. Even if you are not eating, you will still require insulin. You and your doctor should establish a sick day plan for you to use in case of illness. When you are sick, test your blood/urine frequently and call your doctor as instructed.

Pregnancy

Good control of diabetes is especially important for you and your unborn baby. Pregnancy may make managing your diabetes more difficult. If you are planning to have a baby, are pregnant, or are nursing a baby, consult your doctor.

Medication

Insulin requirements may be increased if you are taking other drugs with hyperglycemic activity, such as oral contraceptives, corticosteroids, or thyroid replacement therapy. Insulin requirements may be reduced in the presence of drugs with hypoglycemic activity, such as oral hypoglycemics, salicylates (for example, aspirin), sulfa antibiotics, and certain antidepressants. Always discuss any medications you are taking with your doctor.

Exercise

Exercise may lower your body's need for insulin during and for some time after the activity. Exercise may also speed up the effect of an insulin dose, especially if the exercise involves the area of injection site (for example, the leg should not be used for injection just prior to running). Discuss with your doctor how you should adjust your regimen to accommodate exercise.

Travel

Persons traveling across more than 2 time zones should consult their doctor concerning adjustments in their insulin schedule.

COMMON PROBLEMS OF DIABETES

Hypoglycemia (Insulin Reaction)

Hypoglycemia (too little glucose in the blood) is one of the most frequent adverse events experienced by insulin users. It can be brought about by:

1. Taking too much insulin
2. Missing or delaying meals
3. Exercising or working more than usual
4. An infection or illness (especially with diarrhea or vomiting)
5. A change in the body's need for insulin
6. Diseases of the adrenal, pituitary, or thyroid gland, or progression of kidney or liver disease
7. Interactions with other drugs that lower blood glucose, such as oral hypoglycemics, salicylates (for example, aspirin), sulfa antibiotics, and certain antidepressants
8. Consumption of alcoholic beverages

Symptoms of mild to moderate hypoglycemia may occur suddenly and can include:

- sweating
- dizziness
- palpitation
- tremor
- hunger
- restlessness
- tingling in the hands, feet, lips, or tongue
- lightheadedness
- inability to concentrate
- headache
- drowsiness
- sleep disturbances
- anxiety
- blurred vision
- slurred speech
- depressed mood
- irritability
- abnormal behavior
- unsteady movement
- personality changes

Signs of severe hypoglycemia can include:

- disorientation
- unconsciousness
- seizures
- death

Therefore, it is important that assistance be obtained immediately.

Early warning symptoms of hypoglycemia may be different or less pronounced under certain conditions, such as long duration of diabetes, diabetic nerve disease, medications such as beta-blockers, change in insulin preparations, or intensified control (3 or more insulin injections per day) of diabetes.

A few patients who have experienced hypoglycemic reactions after transfer from animal-source insulin to human insulin have reported that the early warning symptoms of hypoglycemia were less pronounced or different from those experienced with their previous insulin.

Without recognition of early warning symptoms, you may not be able to take steps to avoid more serious hypoglycemia. Be alert for all of the various types of symptoms that may indicate hypoglycemia. Patients who experience hypoglycemia without early warning symptoms should monitor their blood glucose frequently, especially prior to activities such as driving. If the blood glucose is below your normal fasting glucose, you should consider eating or drinking sugar-containing foods to treat your hypoglycemia.

Mild to moderate hypoglycemia may be treated by eating foods or drinks that contain sugar. Patients should always carry a quick source of sugar, such as candy mints or glucose tablets. More severe hypoglycemia may require the assistance of another person. Patients who are unable to take sugar orally or who are unconscious require an injection of glucagon or should be treated with intravenous administration of glucose at a medical facility.

You should learn to recognize your own symptoms of hypoglycemia. If you are uncertain about these symptoms, you should monitor your blood glucose frequently to help you learn to recognize the symptoms that you experience with hypoglycemia.

If you have frequent episodes of hypoglycemia or experience difficulty in recognizing the symptoms, you should consult your doctor to discuss possible changes in therapy, meal plans, and/or exercise programs to help you avoid hypoglycemia.

Hyperglycemia and Diabetic Acidosis

Hyperglycemia (too much glucose in the blood) may develop if your body has too little insulin. Hyperglycemia can be brought about by:

1. Omitting your insulin or taking less than the doctor has prescribed
2. Eating significantly more than your meal plan suggests
3. Developing a fever, infection, or other significant stressful situation

In patients with insulin-dependent diabetes, prolonged hyperglycemia can result in diabetic acidosis. The first symptoms of diabetic acidosis usually come on gradually, over a period of hours or days, and include a drowsy feeling, flushed face, thirst, loss of appetite, and fruity odor on the breath. With acidosis, urine tests show large amounts of glucose and acetone. Heavy breathing and a rapid pulse are more severe symptoms. If uncorrected, prolonged hyperglycemia or diabetic acidosis can lead to nausea, vomiting, dehydration, loss of consciousness or death. Therefore, it is important that you obtain medical assistance immediately.

Lipodystrophy

Rarely, administration of insulin subcutaneously can result in lipoatrophy (depression in the skin) or lipohypertrophy (enlargement or thickening of tissue). If you notice either of these conditions, consult your doctor. A change in your injection technique may help alleviate the problem.

Allergy to Insulin

Local Allergy—Patients occasionally experience redness, swelling, and itching at the site of injection of insulin. This condition, called local allergy, usually clears up in a few days to a few weeks. In some instances, this condition may be related to factors other than insulin, such as irritants in the skin cleansing agent or poor injection technique. If you have local reactions, contact your doctor.

Systemic Allergy—Less common, but potentially more serious, is generalized allergy to insulin, which may cause rash over the whole body, shortness of breath, wheezing, reduction in blood pressure, fast pulse, or sweating. Severe cases of generalized allergy may be life threatening. If you think you are having a generalized allergic reaction to insulin, notify a doctor immediately.

ADDITIONAL INFORMATION

Additional information about diabetes may be obtained from your diabetes educator.

DIABETES FORECAST is a national magazine designed especially for patients with diabetes and their families and is available by subscription from the American Diabetes Association, National Service Center, 1660 Duke Street, Alexandria, Virginia 22314, 1-800-DIABETES (1-800-342-2383).

Another publication, **DIABETES COUNTDOWN,** is available from the Juvenile Diabetes Foundation, 432 Park Avenue South, New York, New York 10016-8013, 1-800-JDF-CURE (1-800-533-2873).

Continued on next page

* Identi-Code® symbol. This product information was prepared in June 1998. Current information on these and other products of Eli Lilly and Company may be obtained by direct inquiry to Lilly Research Laboratories, Lilly Corporate Center, Indianapolis, Indiana 46285, (800) 545-5979.

Humulin 70/30—Cont.

Additional information about Humulin can be obtained by calling 1-888-88-LILLY (1-888-885-4559).
Literature revised March 26, 1997
PA6376AMP   [032697]

HUMULIN® 70/30   OTC
[hū 'mŭ-lĭn]
Cartridge
(70% Human Insulin Isophane Suspension and
30% Human Insulin Injection [rDNA origin]
1.5 mL Cartridge)

For use in Becton Dickinson and Company's B-D®* Pen and Novo Nordisk A/S's NovoPen®†, NovolinPen®†, and NovoPen®† 1.5 insulin delivery devices.

INFORMATION FOR THE PATIENT

                        WARNINGS
THIS LILLY HUMAN INSULIN PRODUCT DIFFERS FROM ANIMAL-SOURCE INSULINS BECAUSE IT IS STRUCTURALLY IDENTICAL TO THE INSULIN PRODUCED BY YOUR BODY'S PANCREAS AND BECAUSE OF ITS UNIQUE MANUFACTURING PROCESS.
ANY CHANGE OF INSULIN SHOULD BE MADE CAUTIOUSLY AND ONLY UNDER MEDICAL SUPERVISION. CHANGES IN STRENGTH, MANUFACTURER, TYPE (E.G., REGULAR, NPH, LENTE, ETC), SPECIES (BEEF, PORK, BEEF-PORK, HUMAN), OR METHOD OF MANUFACTURE (rDNA VERSUS ANIMAL-SOURCE INSULIN) MAY RESULT IN THE NEED FOR A CHANGE IN DOSAGE.
SOME PATIENTS TAKING HUMULIN® (HUMAN INSULIN, rDNA ORIGIN) MAY REQUIRE A CHANGE IN DOSAGE FROM THAT USED WITH ANIMAL-SOURCE INSULINS. IF AN ADJUSTMENT IS NEEDED, IT MAY OCCUR WITH THE FIRST DOSE OR DURING THE FIRST SEVERAL WEEKS OR MONTHS.
TO OBTAIN AN ACCURATE DOSE, CAREFULLY READ AND FOLLOW THE INSULIN DELIVERY DEVICE ("INSULIN PEN") MANUFACTURER'S INSTRUCTIONS AND THIS INFORMATION FOR THE PATIENT INSERT BEFORE USING THIS PRODUCT IN AN INSULIN PEN. (*see* INSTRUCTIONS FOR USE section)

DIABETES
Insulin is a hormone produced by the pancreas, a large gland that lies near the stomach. This hormone is necessary for the body's correct use of food, especially sugar. Diabetes occurs when the pancreas does not make enough insulin to meet your body's needs.
To control your diabetes, your doctor has prescribed injections of insulin to keep your blood glucose at a nearly normal level. Proper control of your diabetes requires close and constant cooperation with your doctor. In spite of diabetes, you can lead an active, healthy, and useful life if you eat a balanced diet daily, exercise regularly, and take your insulin injections as prescribed.
You have been instructed to test your blood and/or your urine regularly for glucose. If your blood tests consistently show above- or below-normal glucose levels or your urine tests consistently show the presence of glucose, your diabetes is not properly controlled and you must let your doctor know.
Always keep an extra supply of insulin as well as a spare syringe and needle on hand. Always wear diabetic identification so that appropriate treatment can be given if complications occur away from home.

70/30 HUMAN INSULIN
Description
Humulin is synthesized in a non-disease-producing special laboratory strain of *Escherichia coli* bacteria that has been genetically altered by the addition of the human gene for insulin production. Humulin® 70/30 is a mixture of 70% Human Insulin Isophane Suspension and 30% Human Insulin Injection. It is an intermediate-acting insulin combined with the more rapid onset of action of regular insulin. The duration of activity may last up to 24 hours following injection. The time course of action of any insulin may vary considerably in different individuals or at different times in the same individual. As with all insulin preparations, the duration of action of Humulin 70/30 is dependent on dose, site of injection, blood supply, temperature, and physical activity. Humulin 70/30 is a sterile suspension and is for subcutaneous injection only. It should not be used intravenously or intramuscularly. The concentration of Humulin 70/30 in cartridges is 100 units/mL (U-100).

Identification
Cartridges of Humulin manufactured by Eli Lilly and Company are available in 3 formulations—Regular, NPH, and 70/30.
Your doctor has prescribed the type of insulin that he/she believes is best for you. **DO NOT USE ANY OTHER INSULIN EXCEPT ON HIS/HER ADVICE AND DIRECTION.**

Cartridges of Humulin 70/30, 1.5 mL, are available in boxes of 5. The cartridge containing Humulin 70/30 is not designed to allow any other insulin to be mixed in the cartridge or for the cartridge to be reused.
1.5 mL Cartridge
Humulin® 70/30 1.5 mL cartridges are for use in Becton Dickinson and Company's B-D® Pen and Novo Nordisk A/S's NovoPen®, NovolinPen®, and NovoPen® 1.5 insulin delivery devices.
Always examine the appearance of a cartridge of insulin before administering a dose. A cartridge of Humulin 70/30 contains a small glass bead to assist in mixing. A cartridge of Humulin 70/30 must be rolled between the palms 10 times and inverted 180° 10 times before each injection so that the contents are uniformly mixed (see Figures 1 and 2). Before inserting it in the insulin pen, inspect the cartridge for uniform mixing and repeat the above steps as necessary.

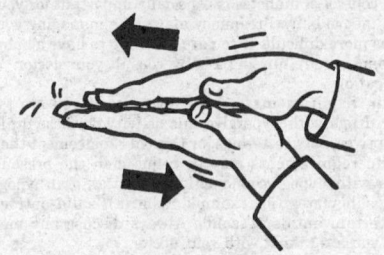

Figure 1.

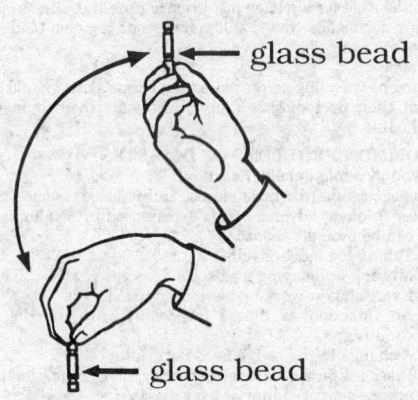

glass bead

glass bead

Figure 2.

Humulin 70/30 should look uniformly cloudy or milky after mixing. Do not use if the insulin substance (the white material) remains visibly separated from the liquid after mixing. Do not use a cartridge of Humulin 70/30 if there are clumps in the insulin after mixing (see Figure 3). Do not use a cartridge of Humulin 70/30 if solid white particles stick to the walls of the cartridge, giving it a frosted appearance (see Figure 4).
Always check the appearance of the cartridge before using, and if you note anything unusual in the appearance of your insulin or notice your insulin requirements changing markedly, consult your doctor.

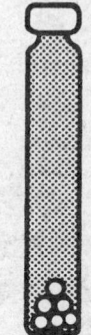

Figure 3.-- Do not use
if there are clumps
in the insulin after
mixing.

[See figure at top of next column]

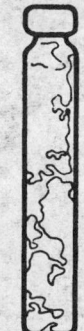

Figure 4.-- Do not use if
particles on the bottom
or wall give the
cartridge a frosted appearance.

Storage
Insulin cartridges should be stored in a refrigerator but not in the freezer. The insulin pen and cartridge of insulin that you are currently using should not be refrigerated but should be kept as cool as possible (below 86°F [30°C]) and away from heat and light. Do not use insulin if it has been frozen. Unrefrigerated 1.5 mL cartridges **must be discarded after 1 week**, even if they still contain insulin. **Do not use a cartridge of Humulin 70/30 after the expiration date stamped on the label.**

INSTRUCTIONS FOR USE
Pens for insulin delivery differ in their operation. It is important to read, understand, and follow the instructions for use of the particular insulin pen you are using.
NEVER SHARE INSULIN PENS, CARTRIDGES, OR NEEDLES.
PREPARING FOR AN INJECTION:
1. Roll the cartridge between the palms 10 times (see Figure 1 above).
2. Holding the cartridge by one end, invert it 180° slowly 10 times to allow the glass bead to travel the full length of the cartridge with each inversion (see Figure 2 above).
3. Inspect the appearance of the Humulin 70/30 before you insert the cartridge into the insulin pen. Humulin 70/30 should look uniformly cloudy or milky. If not, repeat the above steps until the contents are mixed. Do not use a cartridge of Humulin 70/30 if there are clumps in the insulin or if solid white particles stick to the walls of the cartridge (see Figures 3 and 4 above).
4. Follow the insulin pen manufacturer's instructions carefully for loading the cartridge into the insulin pen and for use of the insulin pen.
5. Use an alcohol swab to wipe the exposed rubber surface on the metal cap end of the cartridge.
6. Follow the insulin needle manufacturer's instructions for attaching and changing the needle.
7. Insulin cartridges may contain an air bubble(s) which must be removed from the cartridge and needle by proper priming prior to injection.
8. Once the cartridge is in use in an insulin pen, the insulin must be mixed and inspected before each injection. Roll the insulin pen, containing the cartridge, between the palms 10 times, and invert the insulin pen 180° slowly 10 times to mix the insulin. Do not use a cartridge of Humulin 70/30 if there are clumps in the insulin or if solid white particles stick to the walls of the cartridge (see Figures 3 and 4 above).

GENERAL INJECTION INSTRUCTIONS:
1. Wash your hands.
2. To avoid tissue damage, choose a site for each injection that is at least 1/2 inch from the previous injection site. The usual sites of injection are abdomen, thighs, and arms.
3. Cleanse the skin with alcohol where the injection is to be made.
4. With one hand, stabilize the skin by spreading it or pinching up a large area.
5. Insert the needle as instructed by your doctor.
6. After dispensing a dose, pull the needle out and apply gentle pressure over the injection site for several seconds. **Do not rub the area.**
7. Immediately after an injection, remove the needle from the insulin pen. Doing so will guard against contamination, leakage, reentry of air, and needle clogs. **Do not reuse needles. Dispose of needles in a responsible manner.**
8. *1.5 mL cartridge* - Once the cartridge is in use, do not continue to use it if the leading edge of the plunger is beyond the black band on the cartridge. If a dose is started when the leading edge of the plunger is beyond the black band, an appropriate dose may not be delivered. Use the gauge on the side of the cartridge to help you

judge how much Humulin 70/30 remains. The distance between each mark on the 1.5 mL cartridge is about 10 units.

DOSAGE

Your doctor has told you which insulin to use, how much, and when and how often to inject it. Because each patient's case of diabetes is different, this schedule has been individualized for you.

Your usual insulin dose may be affected by changes in your food, activity, or work schedule. Carefully follow your doctor's instructions to allow for these changes. Other things that may affect your insulin dose are:

Illness

Illness, especially with nausea and vomiting, may cause your insulin requirements to change. Even if you are not eating, you will still require insulin. You and your doctor should establish a sick day plan for you to use in case of illness. When you are sick, test your blood glucose/urine glucose and ketones frequently and call your doctor as instructed.

Pregnancy

Good control of diabetes is especially important for you and your unborn baby. Pregnancy may make managing your diabetes more difficult. If you are planning to have a baby, are pregnant, or are nursing a baby, consult your doctor.

Medication

Insulin requirements may be increased if you are taking other drugs with hyperglycemic activity, such as oral contraceptives, corticosteroids, or thyroid replacement therapy. Insulin requirements may be reduced in the presence of drugs with hypoglycemic activity, such as oral hypoglycemics, salicylates (for example, aspirin), sulfa antibiotics, and certain antidepressants. Always discuss any medications you are taking with your doctor.

Exercise

Exercise may lower your body's need for insulin during and for some time after the activity. Exercise may also speed up the effect of an insulin dose, especially if the exercise involves the area of injection site (for example, the leg should not be used for injection just prior to running). Discuss with your doctor how you should adjust your regimen to accommodate exercise.

Travel

Persons traveling across more than 2 time zones should consult their doctor concerning adjustments in their insulin schedule.

COMMON PROBLEMS OF DIABETES

Hypoglycemia (Insulin Reaction)

Hypoglycemia (too little glucose in the blood) is one of the most frequent adverse events experienced by insulin users. It can be brought about by:

1. Taking too much insulin
2. Missing or delaying meals
3. Exercising or working more than usual
4. An infection or illness (especially with diarrhea or vomiting)
5. A change in the body's need for insulin
6. Diseases of the adrenal, pituitary or thyroid gland, or progression of kidney or liver disease
7. Interactions with other drugs that lower blood glucose, such as oral hypoglycemics, salicylates (for example, aspirin), sulfa antibiotics, and certain antidepressants
8. Consumption of alcoholic beverages

Symptoms of mild to moderate hypoglycemia may occur suddenly and can include:

- sweating
- dizziness
- palpitation
- tremor
- hunger
- restlessness
- tingling in the hands, feet, lips, or tongue
- lightheadedness
- inability to concentrate
- headache
- drowsiness
- sleep disturbances
- anxiety
- blurred vision
- slurred speech
- depressed mood
- irritability
- abnormal behavior
- unsteady movement
- personality changes

Signs of severe hypoglycemia can include:

- disorientation
- unconsciousness
- seizures
- death

Therefore, it is important that assistance be obtained immediately.

Early warning symptoms of hypoglycemia may be different or less pronounced under certain conditions, such as long duration of diabetes, diabetic nerve disease, medications such as beta-blockers, change in insulin preparations, or intensified control (3 or more insulin injections per day) of diabetes.

A few patients who have experienced hypoglycemic reactions after transfer from animal-source insulin to human insulin have reported that the early warning symptoms of hypoglycemia were less pronounced or different from those experienced with their previous insulin.

Without recognition of early warning symptoms, you may not be able to take steps to avoid more serious hypoglycemia. Be alert for all of the various types of symptoms that may indicate hypoglycemia. Patients who experience hypoglycemia without early warning symptoms should monitor their blood glucose frequently, especially prior to activities such as driving. If the blood glucose is below your normal fasting glucose, you should consider eating or drinking sugar-containing foods to treat your hypoglycemia.

Mild to moderate hypoglycemia may be treated by eating foods or drinks that contain sugar. Patients should always carry a quick source of sugar, such as candy mints or glucose tablets. More severe hypoglycemia may require the assistance of another person. Patients who are unable to take sugar orally or who are unconscious require an injection of glucagon or should be treated with intravenous administration of glucose at a medical facility.

You should learn to recognize your own symptoms of hypoglycemia. If you are uncertain about these symptoms, you should monitor your blood glucose frequently to help you learn to recognize the symptoms that you experience with hypoglycemia.

If you have frequent episodes of hypoglycemia or experience difficulty in recognizing the symptoms, you should consult your doctor to discuss possible changes in therapy, meal plans, and/or exercise programs to help you avoid hypoglycemia.

Hyperglycemia and Diabetic Acidosis

Hyperglycemia (too much glucose in the blood) may develop if your body has too little insulin. Hyperglycemia can be brought about by:

1. Omitting your insulin or taking less than the doctor has prescribed
2. Eating significantly more than your meal plan suggests
3. Developing a fever, infection, or other significant stressful situation

In patients with insulin-dependent diabetes, prolonged hyperglycemia can result in diabetic acidosis. The first symptoms of diabetic acidosis usually come on gradually, over a period of hours or days, and include a drowsy feeling, flushed face, thirst, loss of appetite, and fruity odor on the breath. With acidosis, urine tests show large amounts of glucose and acetone. Heavy breathing and a rapid pulse are more severe symptoms. If uncorrected, prolonged hyperglycemia or diabetic acidosis can lead to nausea, vomiting, dehydration, loss of consciousness or death. Therefore, it is important that you obtain medical assistance immediately.

Lipodystrophy

Rarely, administration of insulin subcutaneously can result in lipoatrophy (depression in the skin) or lipohypertrophy (enlargement or thickening of tissue). If you notice either of these conditions, consult your doctor. A change in your injection technique may help alleviate the problem.

Allergy to Insulin

Local Allergy—Patients occasionally experience redness, swelling, and itching at the site of injection of insulin. This condition, called local allergy, usually clears up in a few days to a few weeks. In some instances, this condition may be related to factors other than insulin, such as irritants in the skin cleansing agent or poor injection technique. If you have local reactions, contact your doctor.

Systemic Allergy—Less common, but potentially more serious, is generalized allergy to insulin, which may cause rash over the whole body, shortness of breath, wheezing, reduction in blood pressure, fast pulse, or sweating. Severe cases of generalized allergy may be life threatening. If you think you are having a generalized allergic reaction to insulin, notify a doctor immediately.

ADDITIONAL INFORMATION

Additional information about diabetes may be obtained from your diabetes educator.

DIABETES FORECAST is a national magazine designed especially for patients with diabetes and their families and is available on subscription from the American Diabetes Association, National Service Center, 1660 Duke Street, Alexandria, Virginia 22314, 1-800-DIABETES (1-800-342-2383).

Another publication, **DIABETES COUNTDOWN**, is available from the Juvenile Diabetes Foundation, 432 Park Avenue South, New York, New York 10016-8013, 1-800-JDF-CURE (1-800-533-2873).

Additional information about Humulin can be obtained by calling 1-888-88-LILLY (1-888-885-4559).

Literature revised March 17, 1998

PA 9076 FSAMP [031798]

* B-D® is a registered trademark of Becton Dickinson and Company.

†NovolinPen® and NovoPen® are registered trademarks of Novo Nordisk A/S.

HUMULIN® L OTC

[*hū 'mŭ-lĭn ĕl*]

Lente®

(human insulin [rDNA origin] zinc suspension)

INFORMATION FOR THE PATIENT

WARNINGS

THIS LILLY HUMAN INSULIN PRODUCT DIFFERS FROM ANIMAL-SOURCE INSULINS BECAUSE IT IS STRUCTURALLY IDENTICAL TO THE INSULIN PRODUCED BY YOUR BODY'S PANCREAS AND BECAUSE OF ITS UNIQUE MANUFACTURING PROCESS.

ANY CHANGE OF INSULIN SHOULD BE MADE CAUTIOUSLY AND ONLY UNDER MEDICAL SUPERVISION. CHANGES IN STRENGTH, MANUFACTURER, TYPE (E.G., REGULAR, NPH, LENTE®), SPECIES (BEEF, PORK, BEEF-PORK, HUMAN), OR METHOD OF MANUFACTURE (rDNA VERSUS ANIMAL-SOURCE INSULIN) MAY RESULT IN THE NEED FOR A CHANGE IN DOSAGE.

SOME PATIENTS TAKING HUMULIN® (HUMAN INSULIN, rDNA ORIGIN) MAY REQUIRE A CHANGE IN DOSAGE FROM THAT USED WITH ANIMAL-SOURCE INSULINS. IF AN ADJUSTMENT IS NEEDED, IT MAY OCCUR WITH THE FIRST DOSE OR DURING THE FIRST SEVERAL WEEKS OR MONTHS.

DIABETES

Insulin is a hormone produced by the pancreas, a large gland that lies near the stomach. This hormone is necessary for the body's correct use of food, especially sugar. Diabetes occurs when the pancreas does not make enough insulin to meet your body's needs.

To control your diabetes, your doctor has prescribed injections of insulin to keep your blood glucose at a nearly normal level. Proper control of your diabetes requires close and constant cooperation with your doctor. In spite of diabetes, you can lead an active, healthy, and useful life if you eat a balanced diet daily, exercise regularly, and take your insulin injections as prescribed.

You have been instructed to test your blood and/or your urine regularly for glucose. If your blood tests consistently show above- or below-normal glucose levels or your urine tests consistently show the presence of glucose, your diabetes is not properly controlled and you must let your doctor know.

Always keep an extra supply of insulin as well as a spare syringe and needle on hand. Always wear diabetic identification so that appropriate treatment can be given if complications occur away from home.

LENTE HUMAN INSULIN

Description

Humulin is synthesized in a special non-disease-producing laboratory strain of *Escherichia coli* bacteria that has been genetically altered by the addition of the gene for human insulin production. Humulin L is an amorphous and crystalline suspension of human insulin with zinc providing an intermediate-acting insulin with a slower onset and a longer duration of activity (up to 24 hours) than regular insulin. The time course of action of any insulin may vary considerably in different individuals or at different times in the same individual. As with all insulin preparations, the duration of action of Humulin L is dependent on dose, site of injection, blood supply, temperature, and physical activity. Humulin L is a sterile suspension and is for subcutaneous injection only. It should not be used intravenously or intramuscularly. The concentration of Humulin L is 100 units/mL (U-100).

Identification

Human insulin manufactured by Eli Lilly and Company has the trademark Humulin and is available in 6 formulations—Regular (**R**), NPH (**N**), Lente (**L**), Ultralente® (**U**), 50% Human Insulin Isophane Suspension [NPH]/50% Human Insulin Injection [buffered regular] (**50/50**), and 70% Human Insulin Isophane Suspension [NPH]/30% Human Insulin Injection [buffered regular] (**70/30**). Your doctor has prescribed the type of insulin that he/she believes is best for you. **DO NOT USE ANY OTHER INSULIN EXCEPT ON HIS/HER ADVICE AND DIRECTION.**

Continued on next page

*** Identi-Code® symbol. This product information was prepared in June 1998. Current information on these and other products of Eli Lilly and Company may be obtained by direct inquiry to Lilly Research Laboratories, Lilly Corporate Center, Indianapolis, Indiana 46285, (800) 545-5979.**

Humulin L—Cont.

Always check the carton and the bottle label for the name and letter designation of the insulin you receive from your pharmacy to make sure it is the same as that your doctor has prescribed. Humulin L can be identified as follows:
[See graphic at bottom of page]

Always examine the appearance of your bottle of insulin before withdrawing each dose. A bottle of Humulin L must be carefully shaken or rotated before each injection so that the contents are uniformly mixed. Humulin L should look uniformly cloudy or milky after mixing. Do not use it if the insulin substance (the white material) remains at the bottom of the bottle after mixing (Figure 1). Do not use a bottle of Humulin L if there are clumps in the insulin after mixing (Figure 2). Always check the appearance of your bottle of insulin before using, and if you note anything unusual in the appearance of your insulin or notice your insulin requirements changing markedly, consult your doctor.

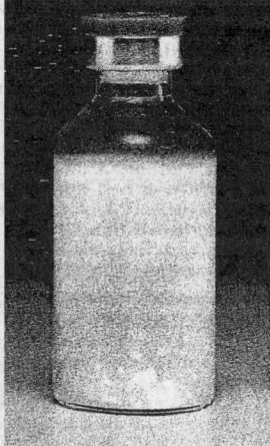

Fig. 1.—Do not use if the insulin material remains at the bottom of the bottle after mixing.

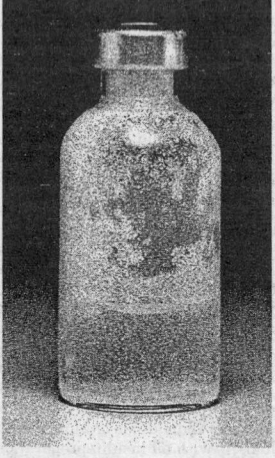

Fig. 2.—Do not use if there are clumps in the insulin after mixing.

Storage

Insulin should be stored in a refrigerator but not in the freezer. If refrigeration is not possible, the bottle of insulin that you are currently using can be kept unrefrigerated as long as it is kept as cool as possible (below 86°F [30°C]) and away from heat and light. Do not use insulin if it has been frozen. Do not use a bottle of insulin after the expiration date stamped on the label.

INJECTION PROCEDURES

Correct Syringe

Doses of insulin are measured in **units**. U-100 insulin contains 100 units/mL (1 mL=1 cc). With Humulin L, it is important to use a syringe that is marked for U-100 insulin preparations. Failure to use the proper syringe can lead to a mistake in dosage, causing serious problems for you, such as a blood glucose level that is too low or too high.

Syringe Use

To help avoid contamination and possible infection, follow these instructions exactly.

Disposable syringes and needles should be used only once and then discarded. **NEEDLES AND SYRINGES MUST NOT BE SHARED.**

Reusable syringes and needles must be sterilized before each injection. **Follow the package directions supplied with your syringe.** Described below are 2 methods of sterilizing.

Boiling

1. Put syringe, plunger, and needle in strainer, place in saucepan, and cover with water. Boil for 5 minutes.
2. Remove articles from water. When they have cooled, insert plunger into barrel, and fasten needle to syringe with a slight twist.
3. Push plunger in and out several times until water is completely removed.

Isopropyl Alcohol

If the syringe, plunger, and needle cannot be boiled, as when you are traveling, they may be sterilized by immersion for at least 5 minutes in Isopropyl Alcohol, 91%. Do not use bathing, rubbing, or medicated alcohol for this sterilization. If the syringe is sterilized with alcohol, it must be absolutely dry before use.

Preparing the Dose

1. Wash your hands.
2. Carefully shake or rotate the insulin bottle several times to completely mix the insulin.
3. Inspect the insulin. Humulin L should look uniformly cloudy or milky. Do not use it if you notice anything unusual in the appearance.
4. If using a new bottle, flip off the plastic protective cap, but **do not** remove the stopper. When using a new bottle, wipe the top of the bottle with an alcohol swab.
5. If you are mixing insulins, refer to the instructions for mixing that follow.
6. Draw air into the syringe equal to your insulin dose. Put the needle through rubber top of the insulin bottle and inject the air into the bottle.
7. Turn the bottle and syringe upside down. Hold the bottle and syringe firmly in 1 hand and shake gently.
8. Making sure the tip of the needle is in the insulin, withdraw the correct dose of insulin into the syringe.
9. Before removing the needle from the bottle, check your syringe for air bubbles which reduce the amount of insulin in it. If bubbles are present, hold the syringe straight up and tap its side until the bubbles float to the top. Push them out with the plunger and withdraw the correct dose.
10. Remove the needle from the bottle and lay the syringe down so that the needle does not touch anything.

Mixing Humulin L with Regular or Ultralente Human Insulin

1. Lente human insulin should be mixed with regular or Ultralente human insulin only on the advice of your doctor.
2. Draw air into your syringe equal to the amount of Humulin L you are taking. Insert the needle into the Humulin L bottle and inject the air. Withdraw the needle.
3. Now inject air into your regular or Ultralente human insulin bottle in the same manner, but **do not** withdraw the needle.
4. Turn the bottle and syringe upside down.
5. Making sure the tip of the needle is in the insulin, withdraw the correct dose of regular or Ultralente insulin into the syringe.

6. Before removing the needle from the bottle, check your syringe for air bubbles which reduce the amount of insulin in it. If bubbles are present, hold the syringe straight up and tap its side until the bubbles float to the top. Push them out with the plunger and withdraw the correct dose.
7. Remove the needle from the bottle of regular or Ultralente insulin and insert it into the bottle of Humulin L. Turn the bottle and syringe upside down. Hold the bottle and syringe firmly in 1 hand and shake gently. Making sure the tip of the needle is in the insulin, withdraw your dose of Humulin L.
8. Remove the needle and lay the syringe down so that the needle does not touch anything.

Follow your doctor's instructions on whether to mix your insulins ahead of time or just before giving your injection. It is important to be consistent in your method.

Syringes from different manufacturers may vary in the amount of space between the bottom line and the needle. Because of this, do not change:
• the sequence of mixing, or
• the model and brand of syringe or needle that the doctor has prescribed.

Injection

Cleanse the skin with alcohol where the injection is to be made. Stabilize the skin by spreading it or pinching up a large area. Insert the needle as instructed by your doctor. Push the plunger in as far as it will go. Pull the needle out and apply gentle pressure over the injection site for several seconds. **Do not rub the area.** To avoid tissue damage, give the next injection at a site at least $\frac{1}{2}$" from the previous site.

DOSAGE

Your doctor has told you which insulin to use, how much, and when and how often to inject it. Because each patient's case of diabetes is different, this schedule has been individualized for you.

Your usual insulin dose may be affected by changes in your food, activity, or work schedule. Carefully follow your doctor's instructions to allow for these changes. Other things that may affect your insulin dose are:

Illness

Illness, especially with nausea and vomiting, may cause your insulin requirements to change. Even if you are not eating, you will still require insulin. You and your doctor should establish a sick day plan for you to use in case of illness. When you are sick, test your blood/urine frequently and call your doctor as instructed.

Pregnancy

Good control of diabetes is especially important for you and your unborn baby. Pregnancy may make managing your diabetes more difficult. If you are planning to have a baby, are pregnant, or are nursing a baby, consult your doctor.

Medication

Insulin requirements may be increased if you are taking other drugs with hyperglycemic activity, such as oral contraceptives, corticosteroids, or thyroid replacement therapy. Insulin requirements may be reduced in the presence of drugs with hypoglycemic activity, such as oral hypoglycemics, salicylates (for example, aspirin), sulfa antibiotics, and certain antidepressants. Always discuss any medications you are taking with your doctor.

Exercise

Exercise may lower your body's need for insulin during and for some time after the activity. Exercise may also speed up the effect of an insulin dose, especially if the exercise involves the area of injection site (for example, the leg should not be used for injection just prior to running). Discuss with your doctor how you should adjust your regimen to accommodate exercise.

Travel

Persons traveling across more than 2 time zones should consult their doctor concerning adjustments in their insulin schedule.

COMMON PROBLEMS OF DIABETES

Hypoglycemia (Insulin Reaction)

Hypoglycemia (too little glucose in the blood) is one of the most frequent adverse events experienced by insulin users. It can be brought about by:
1. Taking too much insulin
2. Missing or delaying meals
3. Exercising or working more than usual
4. An infection or illness (especially with diarrhea or vomiting)
5. A change in the body's need for insulin
6. Diseases of the adrenal, pituitary, or thyroid gland, or progression of kidney or liver disease
7. Interactions with other drugs that lower blood glucose, such as oral hypoglycemics, salicylates (for example, aspirin), sulfa antibiotics, and certain antidepressants
8. Consumption of alcoholic beverages

Symptoms of mild to moderate hypoglycemia may occur suddenly and can include:
• sweating
• dizziness
• palpitation
• tremor
• hunger
• restlessness
• tingling in the hands, feet, lips, or tongue

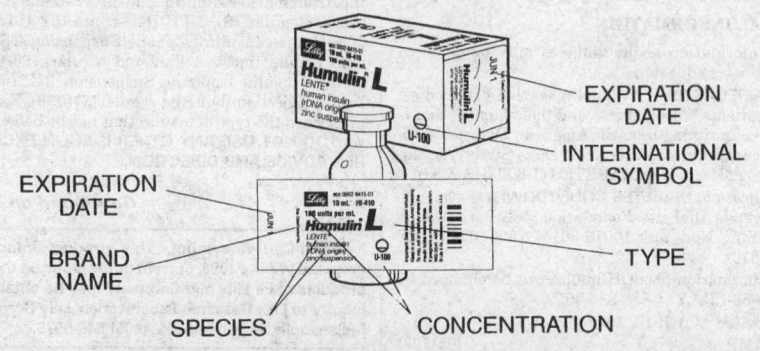

- lightheadedness
- inability to concentrate
- headache
- drowsiness
- sleep disturbances
- anxiety
- blurred vision
- slurred speech
- depressed mood
- irritability
- abnormal behavior
- unsteady movement
- personality changes

Signs of severe hypoglycemia can include:
- disorientation
- unconsciousness
- seizures
- death

Therefore, it is important that assistance be obtained immediately.

Early warning symptoms of hypoglycemia may be different or less pronounced under certain conditions, such as long duration of diabetes, diabetic nerve disease, medications such as beta-blockers, change in insulin preparations, or intensified control (3 or more insulin injections per day) of diabetes.

A few patients who have experienced hypoglycemic reactions after transfer from animal-source insulin to human insulin have reported that the early warning symptoms of hypoglycemia were less pronounced or different from those experienced with their previous insulin.

Without recognition of early warning symptoms, you may not be able to take steps to avoid more serious hypoglycemia. Be alert for all of the various types of symptoms that may indicate hypoglycemia. Patients who experience hypoglycemia without early warning symptoms should monitor their blood glucose frequently, especially prior to activities such as driving. If the blood glucose is below your normal fasting glucose, you should consider eating or drinking sugar-containing foods to treat your hypoglycemia.

Mild to moderate hypoglycemia may be treated by eating foods or drinks that contain sugar. Patients should always carry a quick source of sugar, such as candy mints or glucose tablets. More severe hypoglycemia may require the assistance of another person. Patients who are unable to take sugar orally or who are unconscious require an injection of glucagon or should be treated with intravenous administration of glucose at a medical facility.

You should learn to recognize your own symptoms of hypoglycemia. If you are uncertain about these symptoms, you should monitor your blood glucose frequently to help you learn to recognize the symptoms that you experience with hypoglycemia.

If you have frequent episodes of hypoglycemia or experience difficulty in recognizing the symptoms, you should consult your doctor to discuss possible changes in therapy, meal plans, and/or exercise programs to help you avoid hypoglycemia.

Hyperglycemia and Diabetic Acidosis

Hyperglycemia (too much glucose in the blood) may develop if your body has too little insulin. Hyperglycemia can be brought about by:
1. Omitting your insulin or taking less than the doctor has prescribed
2. Eating significantly more than your meal plan suggests
3. Developing a fever, infection, or other significant stressful situation

In patients with insulin-dependent diabetes, prolonged hyperglycemia can result in diabetic acidosis. The first symptoms of diabetic acidosis usually come on gradually, over a period of hours or days, and include a drowsy feeling, flushed face, thirst, loss of appetite, and fruity odor on the breath. With acidosis, urine tests show large amounts of glucose and acetone. Heavy breathing and a rapid pulse are more severe symptoms. If uncorrected, prolonged hyperglycemia or diabetic acidosis can lead to nausea, vomiting, dehydration, loss of consciousness or death. Therefore, it is important that you obtain medical assistance immediately.

Lipodystrophy

Rarely, administration of insulin subcutaneously can result in lipoatrophy (depression in the skin) or lipohypertrophy (enlargement or thickening of tissue). If you notice either of these conditions, consult your doctor. A change in your injection technique may help alleviate the problem.

Allergy to Insulin

Local Allergy —Patients occasionally experience redness, swelling, and itching at the site of injection of insulin. This condition, called local allergy, usually clears up in a few days to a few weeks. In some instances, this condition may be related to factors other than insulin, such as irritants in the skin cleansing agent or poor injection technique. If you have local reactions, contact your doctor.

Systemic Allergy —Less common, but potentially more serious, is generalized allergy to insulin, which may cause rash over the whole body, shortness of breath, wheezing, reduction in blood pressure, fast pulse, or sweating. Severe cases

of generalized allergy may be life threatening. If you think you are having a generalized allergic reaction to insulin, notify a doctor immediately.

ADDITIONAL INFORMATION

Additional information about diabetes may be obtained from your diabetes educator.

DIABETES FORECAST is a national magazine designed especially for patients with diabetes and their families and is available by subscription from the American Diabetes Association, National Service Center, 1660 Duke Street, Alexandria, Virginia 22314, 1-800-DIABETES (1-800-342-2383).

Another publication, **DIABETES COUNTDOWN**, is available from the Juvenile Diabetes Foundation, 432 Park Avenue South, New York, New York 10016–8013, 1-800-JDF-CURE (1-800-533-2873).

Additional information about Humulin can be obtained by calling 1-888-88-LILLY (1-888-885-4559).

Literature revised March 26, 1997

PA 6354 AMP   [032697]

HUMULIN® N   OTC

[*hū 'mŭ-lĭn ĕn*]

NPH

(human insulin [rDNA origin]

isophane suspension)

INFORMATION FOR THE PATIENT
WARNINGS

THIS LILLY HUMAN INSULIN PRODUCT DIFFERS FROM ANIMAL-SOURCE INSULINS BECAUSE IT IS STRUCTURALLY IDENTICAL TO THE INSULIN PRODUCED BY YOUR BODY'S PANCREAS AND BECAUSE OF ITS UNIQUE MANUFACTURING PROCESS.

ANY CHANGE OF INSULIN SHOULD BE MADE CAUTIOUSLY AND ONLY UNDER MEDICAL SUPERVISION. CHANGES IN STRENGTH, MANUFACTURER, TYPE (E.G., REGULAR, NPH, LENTE®), SPECIES (BEEF, PORK, BEEF-PORK, HUMAN), OR METHOD OF MANUFACTURE (rDNA VERSUS ANIMAL-SOURCE INSULIN) MAY RESULT IN THE NEED FOR A CHANGE IN DOSAGE.

SOME PATIENTS TAKING HUMULIN® (HUMAN INSULIN, rDNA ORIGIN) MAY REQUIRE A CHANGE IN DOSAGE FROM THAT USED WITH ANIMAL-SOURCE INSULINS. IF AN ADJUSTMENT IS NEEDED, IT MAY OCCUR WITH THE FIRST DOSE OR DURING THE FIRST SEVERAL WEEKS OR MONTHS.

DIABETES

Insulin is a hormone produced by the pancreas, a large gland that lies near the stomach. This hormone is necessary for the body's correct use of food, especially sugar. Diabetes occurs when the pancreas does not make enough insulin to meet your body's needs.

To control your diabetes, your doctor has prescribed injections of insulin to keep your blood glucose at a nearly normal level. Proper control of your diabetes requires close and constant cooperation with your doctor. In spite of diabetes, you can lead an active, healthy, and useful life if you eat a balanced diet daily, exercise regularly, and take your insulin injections as prescribed.

You have been instructed to test your blood and/or your urine regularly for glucose. If your blood tests consistently show above- or below-normal glucose levels or your urine tests consistently show the presence of glucose, your diabetes is not properly controlled and you must let your doctor know.

Always keep an extra supply of insulin as well as a spare syringe and needle on hand. Always wear diabetic identification so that appropriate treatment can be given if complications occur away from home.

NPH HUMAN INSULIN

Description

Humulin is synthesized in a special non-disease-producing laboratory strain of *Escherichia coli* bacteria that has been genetically altered by the addition of the gene for human insulin production. Humulin N is a crystalline suspension of human insulin with protamine and zinc providing an intermediate-acting insulin with a slower onset of action and a longer duration of activity (up to 24 hours) than that of regular insulin. The time course of action of any insulin may vary considerably in different individuals or at different times in the same individual. As with all insulin preparations, the duration of action of Humulin N is dependent on dose, site of injection, blood supply, temperature, and physical activity. Humulin N is a sterile suspension and is for subcutaneous injection only. It should not be used intravenously or intramuscularly. The concentration of Humulin N is 100 units/mL (U-100).

Identification

Human insulin manufactured by Eli Lilly and Company has the trademark Humulin and is available in 6 formulations—Regular (**R**), NPH (**N**), Lente (**L**), Ultralente® (**U**), 50% Human Insulin Isophane Suspension [NPH]/50% Human Insulin Injection [buffered regular] (**50/50**), and 70% Human Insulin Isophane Suspension [NPH]/30% Human

Insulin Injection [buffered regular] (**70/30**). Your doctor has prescribed the type of insulin that he/she believes is best for you. **DO NOT USE ANY OTHER INSULIN EXCEPT ON HIS/ HER ADVICE AND DIRECTION.**

Always check the carton and the bottle label for the name and letter designation of the insulin you receive from your pharmacy to make sure it is the same as that your doctor has prescribed. Humulin N can be identified as follows: [See graphic at bottom of next page]

Always examine the appearance of your bottle of insulin before withdrawing each dose. A bottle of Humulin N must be carefully shaken or rotated before each injection so that the contents are uniformly mixed. Humulin N should look uniformly cloudy or milky after mixing. Do not use it if the insulin substance (the white material) remains at the bottom of the bottle after mixing. Do not use a bottle of Humulin N if there are clumps in the insulin after mixing (Figure 1). Do not use a bottle of Humulin N if solid white particles stick to the bottom or wall of the bottle, giving it a frosted appearance (Figure 2). Always check the appearance of your bottle of insulin before using, and if you note anything unusual in the appearance of your insulin or notice your insulin requirements changing markedly, consult your doctor.

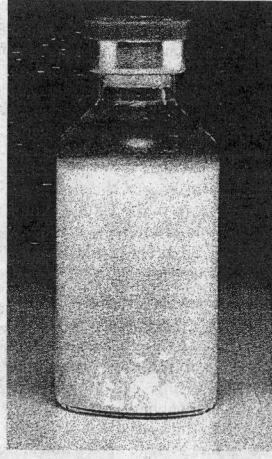

Fig. 1.—Do not use if there are clumps in the insulin after mixing.

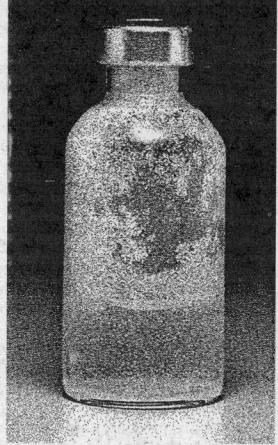

Fig. 2.—Do not use if particles on the bottom or wall give the bottle a frosted appearance.

Storage

Insulin should be stored in a refrigerator but not in the freezer. If refrigeration is not possible, the bottle of insulin that you are currently using can be kept unrefrigerated as long as it is kept as cool as possible (below 86°F [30°C]) and away from heat and light. Do not use insulin if it has been frozen. Do not use a bottle of insulin after the expiration date stamped on the label.

INJECTION PROCEDURES

Correct Syringe

Doses of insulin are measured in **units**. U-100 insulin contains 100 units/mL (1 mL = 1 cc). With Humulin N, it is

Continued on next page

---

* **Identi-Code® symbol. This product information was prepared in June 1998. Current information on these and other products of Eli Lilly and Company may be obtained by direct inquiry to Lilly Research Laboratories, Lilly Corporate Center, Indianapolis, Indiana 46285, (800) 545-5979.**

Consult 1999 PDR® supplements and future editions for revisions

Humulin N—Cont.

important to use a syringe that is marked for U-100 insulin preparations. Failure to use the proper syringe can lead to a mistake in dosage, causing serious problems for you, such as a blood glucose level that is too low or too high.

Syringe Use

To help avoid contamination and possible infection, follow these instructions exactly.

Disposable syringes and needles should be used only once and then discarded. **NEEDLES AND SYRINGES MUST NOT BE SHARED.**

Reusable syringes and needles must be sterilized before each injection. **Follow the package directions supplied with your syringe.** Described below are 2 methods of sterilizing.

Boiling

1. Put syringe, plunger, and needle in strainer, place in saucepan, and cover with water. Boil for 5 minutes.
2. Remove articles from water. When they have cooled, insert plunger into barrel, and fasten needle to syringe with a slight twist.
3. Push plunger in and out several times until water is completely removed.

Isopropyl Alcohol

If the syringe, plunger, and needle cannot be boiled, as when you are traveling, they may be sterilized by immersion for at least 5 minutes in Isopropyl Alcohol, 91%. Do not use bathing, rubbing, or medicated alcohol for this sterilization. If the syringe is sterilized with alcohol, it must be absolutely dry before use.

Preparing the Dose

1. Wash your hands.
2. Carefully shake or rotate the insulin bottle several times to completely mix the insulin.
3. Inspect the insulin. Humulin N should look uniformly cloudy or milky. Do not use it if you notice anything unusual in the appearance.
4. If using a new bottle, flip off the plastic protective cap, but **do not** remove the stopper. When using a new bottle, wipe the top of the bottle with an alcohol swab.
5. If you are mixing insulins, refer to the instructions for mixing that follow.
6. Draw air into the syringe equal to your insulin dose. Put the needle through rubber top of the insulin bottle and inject the air into the bottle.
7. Turn the bottle and syringe upside down. Hold the bottle and syringe firmly in 1 hand and shake gently.
8. Making sure the tip of the needle is in the insulin, withdraw the correct dose of insulin into the syringe.
9. Before removing the needle from the bottle, check your syringe for air bubbles which reduce the amount of insulin in it. If bubbles are present, hold the syringe straight up and tap its side until the bubbles float to the top. Push them out with the plunger and withdraw the correct dose.
10. Remove the needle from the bottle and lay the syringe down so that the needle does not touch anything.

Mixing Humulin N and Regular Human Insulin

1. NPH human insulin should be mixed only with regular human insulin.
2. Draw air into your syringe equal to the amount of Humulin N you are taking. Insert the needle into the Humulin N bottle and inject the air. Withdraw the needle.
3. Now inject air into your regular human insulin bottle in the same manner, but **do not** withdraw the needle.
4. Turn the bottle and syringe upside down.
5. Making sure the tip of the needle is in the insulin, withdraw the correct dose of regular insulin into the syringe.
6. Before removing the needle from the bottle, check your syringe for air bubbles which reduce the amount of insulin in it. If bubbles are present, hold the syringe straight up and tap its side until the bubbles float to the top. Push them out with the plunger and withdraw the correct dose.
7. Remove the needle from the bottle of regular insulin and insert it into the bottle of Humulin N. Turn the bottle and syringe upside down. Hold the bottle and syringe firmly in 1 hand and shake gently. Making sure the tip

of the needle is in the insulin, withdraw your dose of Humulin N.
8. Remove the needle and lay the syringe down so that the needle does not touch anything.

Follow your doctor's instructions on whether to mix your insulins ahead of time or just before giving your injection. It is important to be consistent in your method.

Syringes from different manufacturers may vary in the amount of space between the bottom line and the needle. Because of this, do not change:

- the sequence of mixing, or
- the model and brand of syringe or needle that the doctor has prescribed.

Injection

Cleanse the skin with alcohol where the injection is to be made. Stabilize the skin by spreading it or pinching up a large area. Insert the needle as instructed by your doctor. Push the plunger in as far as it will go. Pull the needle out and apply gentle pressure over the injection site for several seconds. **Do not rub the area.** To avoid tissue damage, give the next injection at a site at least $1/2$" from the previous site.

DOSAGE

Your doctor has told you which insulin to use, how much, and when and how often to inject it. Because each patient's case of diabetes is different, this schedule has been individualized for you.

Your usual insulin dose may be affected by changes in your food, activity, or work schedule. Carefully follow your doctor's instructions to allow for these changes. Other things that may affect your insulin dose are:

Illness

Illness, especially with nausea and vomiting, may cause your insulin requirements to change. Even if you are not eating, you will still require insulin. You and your doctor should establish a sick day plan for you to use in case of illness. When you are sick, test your blood/urine frequently and call your doctor as instructed.

Pregnancy

Good control of diabetes is especially important for you and your unborn baby. Pregnancy may make managing your diabetes more difficult. If you are planning to have a baby, are pregnant, or are nursing a baby, consult your doctor.

Medication

Insulin requirements may be increased if you are taking other drugs with hyperglycemic activity, such as oral contraceptives, corticosteroids, or thyroid replacement therapy. Insulin requirements may be reduced in the presence of drugs with hypoglycemic activity, such as oral hypoglycemics, salicylates (for example, aspirin), sulfa antibiotics, and certain antidepressants. Always discuss any medications you are taking with your doctor.

Exercise

Exercise may lower your body's need for insulin during and for some time after the activity. Exercise may also speed up the effect of an insulin dose, especially if the exercise involves the area of injection site (for example, the leg should not be used for injection just prior to running). Discuss with your doctor how you should adjust your regimen to accomodate exercise.

Travel

Persons traveling across more than 2 time zones should consult their doctor concerning adjustments in their insulin schedule.

COMMON PROBLEMS OF DIABETES

Hypoglycemia (Insulin Reaction)

Hypoglycemia (too little glucose in the blood) is one of the most frequent adverse events experienced by insulin users. It can be brought about by:

1. Taking too much insulin
2. Missing or delaying meals
3. Exercising or working more than usual
4. An infection or illness (especially with diarrhea or vomiting)
5. A change in the body's need for insulin
6. Diseases of the adrenal, pituitary, or thyroid gland, or progression of kidney or liver disease

7. Interactions with other drugs that lower blood glucose, such as oral hypoglycemics, salicylates (for example, aspirin), sulfa antibiotics, and certain antidepressants
8. Consumption of alcoholic beverages

Symptoms of mild to moderate hypoglycemia may occur suddenly and can include:

- sweating
- dizziness
- palpitation
- tremor
- hunger
- restlessness
- tingling in the hands, feet, lips, or tongue
- lightheadedness
- inability to concentrate
- headache
- drowsiness
- sleep disturbances
- anxiety
- blurred vision
- slurred speech
- depressed mood
- irritability
- abnormal behavior
- unsteady movement
- personality changes

Signs of severe hypoglycemia can include:

- disorientation
- unconsciousness
- seizures
- death

Therefore, it is important that assistance be obtained immediately.

Early warning symptoms of hypoglycemia may be different or less pronounced under certain conditions, such as long duration of diabetes, diabetic nerve disease, medications such as beta-blockers, change in insulin preparations, or intensified control (3 or more insulin injections per day) of diabetes.

A few patients who have experienced hypoglycemic reactions after transfer from animal-source insulin to human insulin have reported that the early warning symptoms of hypoglycemia were less pronounced or different from those experienced with their previous insulin.

Without recognition of early warning symptoms, you may not be able to take steps to avoid more serious hypoglycemia. Be alert for all of the various types of symptoms that may indicate hypoglycemia. Patients who experience hypoglycemia without early warning symptoms should monitor their blood glucose frequently, especially prior to activities such as driving. If the blood glucose is below your normal fasting glucose, you should consider eating or drinking sugar-containing foods to treat your hypoglycemia.

Mild to moderate hypoglycemia may be treated by eating foods or drinks that contain sugar. Patients should always carry a quick source of sugar, such as candy mints or glucose tablets. More severe hypoglycemia may require the assistance of another person. Patients who are unable to take sugar orally or who are unconscious require an injection of glucagon or should be treated with intravenous administration of glucose at a medical facility.

You should learn to recognize your own symptoms of hypoglycemia. If you are uncertain about these symptoms, you should monitor your blood glucose frequently to help you learn to recognize the symptoms that you experience with hypoglycemia.

If you have frequent episodes of hypoglycemia or experience difficulty in recognizing the symptoms, you should consult your doctor to discuss possible changes in therapy, meal plans, and/or exercise programs to help you avoid hypoglycemia.

Hyperglycemia and Diabetic Acidosis

Hyperglycemia (too much glucose in the blood) may develop if your body has too little insulin. Hyperglycemia can be brought about by:

1. Omitting your insulin or taking less than the doctor has prescribed
2. Eating significantly more than your meal plan suggests
3. Developing a fever, infection, or other significant stressful situation

In patients with insulin-dependent diabetes, prolonged hyperglycemia can result in diabetic acidosis. The first symptoms of diabetic acidosis usually come on gradually, over a period of hours or days, and include a drowsy feeling, flushed face, thirst, loss of appetite, and fruity odor on the breath. With acidosis, urine tests show large amounts of glucose and acetone. Heavy breathing and a rapid pulse are more severe symptoms. If uncorrected, prolonged hyperglycemia or diabetic acidosis can lead to nausea, vomiting, dehydration, loss of consciousness or death. Therefore, it is important that you obtain medical assistance immediately.

Lipodystrophy

Rarely, administration of insulin subcutaneously can result in lipoatrophy (depression in the skin) or lipohypertrophy (enlargement or thickening of tissue). If you notice either of these conditions, consult your doctor. A change in your injection technique may help alleviate the problem.

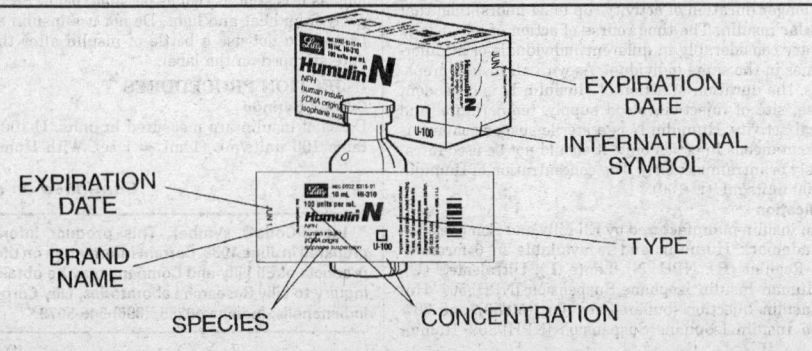

EXPIRATION DATE

INTERNATIONAL SYMBOL

EXPIRATION DATE

BRAND NAME

SPECIES

CONCENTRATION

TYPE

Allergy to Insulin

Local Allergy —Patients occasionally experience redness, swelling, and itching at the site of injection of insulin. This condition, called local allergy, usually clears up in a few days to a few weeks. In some instances, this condition may be related to factors other than insulin, such as irritants in the skin cleansing agent or poor injection technique. If you have local reactions, contact your doctor.

Systemic Allergy —Less common, but potentially more serious, is generalized allergy to insulin, which may cause rash over the whole body, shortness of breath, wheezing, reduction in blood pressure, fast pulse, or sweating. Severe cases of generalized allergy may be life threatening. If you think you are having a generalized allergic reaction to insulin, notify a doctor immediately.

ADDITIONAL INFORMATION

Additional information about diabetes may be obtained from your diabetes educator.

DIABETES FORECAST is a national magazine designed especially for patients with diabetes and their families and is available by subscription from the American Diabetes Association, National Service Center, 1660 Duke Street, Alexandria, Virginia 22314, 1-800-DIABETES (1-800-342-2383). Another publication, **DIABETES COUNTDOWN**, is available from the Juvenile Diabetes Foundation, 432 Park Avenue South, New York, New York 10016–8013, 1-800-JDF-CURE (1-800-533-2873).

Additional information about Humulin can be obtained by calling 1-888-88-LILLY (1-888-885-4559).

Literature revised March 26, 1997

PA 6345 AMP   [032697]

HUMULIN® N
NPH

[hū 'mŭ-lĭn ĕn]
(human insulin [rDNA origin] isophane suspension)
1.5 mL cartridge

CARTRIDGE

For use in Becton Dickinson and Company's B-D®* Pen and Novo Nordisk A/S's NovoPen®†, NovolinPen®†, and NovoPen®† 1.5 insulin delivery devices.

INFORMATION FOR THE PATIENT

WARNINGS

THIS LILLY HUMAN INSULIN PRODUCT DIFFERS FROM ANIMAL-SOURCE INSULINS BECAUSE IT IS STRUCTURALLY IDENTICAL TO THE INSULIN PRODUCED BY YOUR BODY'S PANCREAS AND BECAUSE OF ITS UNIQUE MANUFACTURING PROCESS.

ANY CHANGE OF INSULIN SHOULD BE MADE CAUTIOUSLY AND ONLY UNDER MEDICAL SUPERVISION. CHANGES IN STRENGTH, MANUFACTURER, TYPE (E.G., REGULAR, NPH, LENTE, ETC), SPECIES (BEEF, PORK, BEEF-PORK, HUMAN), OR METHOD OF MANUFACTURE (rDNA VERSUS ANIMAL-SOURCE INSULIN) MAY RESULT IN THE NEED FOR A CHANGE IN DOSAGE.

SOME PATIENTS TAKING HUMULIN® (HUMAN INSULIN, rDNA ORIGIN) MAY REQUIRE A CHANGE IN DOSAGE FROM THAT USED WITH ANIMAL-SOURCE INSULINS. IF AN ADJUSTMENT IS NEEDED, IT MAY OCCUR WITH THE FIRST DOSE OR DURING THE FIRST SEVERAL WEEKS OR MONTHS.

TO OBTAIN AN ACCURATE DOSE, CAREFULLY READ AND FOLLOW THE INSULIN DELIVERY DEVICE ("INSULIN PEN") MANUFACTURER'S INSTRUCTIONS AND THIS INFORMATION FOR THE PATIENT INSERT BEFORE USING THIS PRODUCT IN AN INSULIN PEN. (see INSTRUCTIONS FOR USE section)

DIABETES

Insulin is a hormone produced by the pancreas, a large gland that lies near the stomach. This hormone is necessary for the body's correct use of food, especially sugar. Diabetes occurs when the pancreas does not make enough insulin to meet your body's needs.

To control your diabetes, your doctor has prescribed injections of insulin to keep your blood glucose at a nearly normal level. Proper control of your diabetes requires close and constant cooperation with your doctor. In spite of diabetes, you can lead an active, healthy, and useful life if you eat a balanced diet daily, exercise regularly, and take your insulin injections as prescribed.

You have been instructed to test your blood and/or your urine regularly for glucose. If your blood tests consistently show above- or below-normal glucose levels or your urine tests consistently show the presence of glucose, your diabetes is not properly controlled and you must let your doctor know.

Always keep an extra supply of insulin as well as a spare syringe and needle on hand. Always wear diabetic identification so that appropriate treatment can be given if complications occur away from home.

NPH HUMAN INSULIN
Description

Humulin is synthesized in a non-disease-producing special laboratory strain of *Escherichia coli* bacteria that has been genetically altered by the addition of the human gene for insulin production. Humulin® N is a crystalline suspension of human insulin with protamine and zinc providing an intermediate-acting insulin with a slower onset of action and a longer duration of activity (up to 24 hours) than that of regular insulin. The time course of action of any insulin may vary considerably in different individuals or at different times in the same individual. As with all insulin preparations, the duration of action of Humulin N is dependent on dose, site of injection, blood supply, temperature, and physical activity. Humulin N is a sterile suspension and is for subcutaneous injection only. It should not be used intravenously or intramuscularly. The concentration of Humulin N in cartridges is 100 units/mL (U-100).

Identification

Cartridges of Humulin manufactured by Eli Lilly and Company are available in 3 formulations—Regular, NPH, and 70/30.

Your doctor has prescribed the type of insulin that he/she believes is best for you. **DO NOT USE ANY OTHER INSULIN EXCEPT ON HIS/HER ADVICE AND DIRECTION.**

Cartridges of Humulin N, 1.5 mL, are available in boxes of 5. The cartridge containing Humulin N is not designed to allow any other insulin to be mixed in the cartridge or for the cartridge to be reused.

1.5 mL Cartridge

Humulin® N 1.5 mL cartridges are for use in Becton Dickinson and Company's B-D® Pen and Novo Nordisk A/S's NovoPen®, NovolinPen®, and NovoPen® 1.5 insulin delivery devices.

Always examine the appearance of a cartridge of insulin before administering a dose. A cartridge of Humulin N contains a small glass bead to assist in mixing. A cartridge of Humulin N must be rolled between the palms 10 times and inverted 180° 10 times before each injection so that the contents are uniformly mixed (*see* Figures 1 and 2). Before inserting it in the insulin pen, inspect the cartridge for uniform mixing and repeat the above steps as necessary.

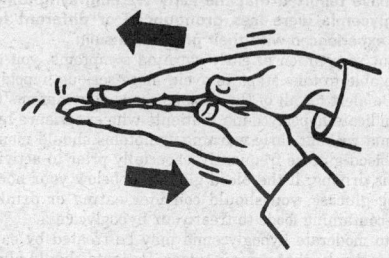

Figure 1.

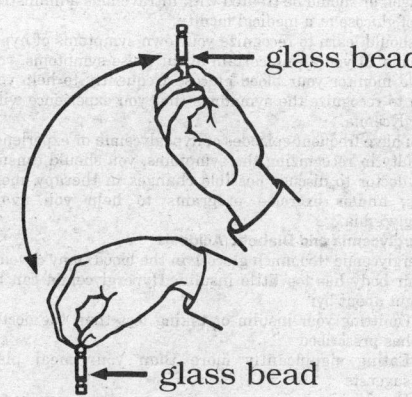

glass bead

glass bead

Figure 2.

Humulin N should look uniformly cloudy or milky after mixing. Do not use if the insulin substance (the white material) remains visibly separated from the liquid after mixing. Do not use a cartridge of Humulin N if there are clumps in the insulin after mixing (*see* Figure 3). Do not use a cartridge of Humulin N if solid white particles stick to the walls of the cartridge, giving it a frosted appearance (*see* Figure 4).

Always check the appearance of the cartridge before using, and if you note anything unusual in the appearance of your insulin or notice your insulin requirements changing markedly, consult your doctor.

[See figures 3 & 4 at top of next column]

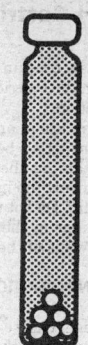

Figure 3.-- Do not use if there are clumps in the insulin after mixing.

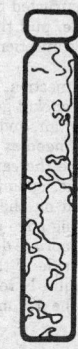

Figure 4.-- Do not use if particles on the bottom or wall give the cartridge a frosted appearance.

Storage

Insulin cartridges should be stored in a refrigerator but not in the freezer. The insulin pen and cartridge of insulin that you are currently using should not be refrigerated but should be kept as cool as possible (below 86°F [30°C]) and away from heat and light. Do not use insulin if it has been frozen.

Unrefrigerated 1.5 mL cartridges **must be discarded after 1 week,** even if they still contain insulin. **Do not use a cartridge of Humulin N after the expiration date stamped on the label.**

INSTRUCTIONS FOR USE

Pens for insulin delivery differ in their operation. It is important to read, understand, and follow the instructions for use of the particular insulin pen you are using.

NEVER SHARE INSULIN PENS, CARTRIDGES, OR NEEDLES.

PREPARING FOR AN INJECTION:

1. Roll the cartridge between the palms 10 times (*see* Figure 1 above).
2. Holding the cartridge by one end, invert it 180° slowly 10 times to allow the glass bead to travel the full length of the cartridge with each inversion (*see* Figure 2 above).
3. Inspect the appearance of the Humulin N before you insert the cartridge into the insulin pen. Humulin N should look uniformly cloudy or milky. If not, repeat the above steps until the contents are mixed. Do not use a cartridge of Humulin N if there are clumps in the insulin or if solid white particles stick to the walls of the cartridge (*see* Figures 3 and 4 above).
4. Follow the insulin pen manufacturer's instructions carefully for loading the cartridge into the insulin pen and for use of the insulin pen.
5. Use an alcohol swab to wipe the exposed rubber surface on the metal cap end of the cartridge.
6. Follow the insulin needle manufacturer's instructions for attaching and changing the needle.

Continued on next page

---

* Identi-Code® symbol. This product information was prepared in June 1998. Current information on these and other products of Eli Lilly and Company may be obtained by direct inquiry to Lilly Research Laboratories, Lilly Corporate Center, Indianapolis, Indiana 46285, (800) 545-5979.

Humulin N NPH Cartridge—Cont.

7. Insulin cartridges may contain an air bubble(s) which must be removed from the cartridge and needle by proper priming prior to injection.

8. Once the cartridge is in use in an insulin pen, the insulin must be mixed and inspected before each injection. Roll the insulin pen, containing the cartridge, between the palms 10 times, and invert the insulin pen 180° slowly 10 times to mix the insulin. Do not use a cartridge of Humulin N if there are clumps in the insulin or if solid white particles stick to the walls of the cartridge (*see* Figures 3 and 4 above).

GENERAL INJECTION INSTRUCTIONS:

1. Wash your hands.

2. To avoid tissue damage, choose a site for each injection that is at least 1/2 inch from the previous injection site. The usual sites of injection are abdomen, thighs, and arms.

3. Cleanse the skin with alcohol where the injection is to be made.

4. With one hand, stabilize the skin by spreading it or pinching up a large area.

5. Insert the needle as instructed by your doctor.

6. After dispensing a dose, pull the needle out and apply gentle pressure over the injection site for several seconds. **Do not rub the area.**

7. Immediately after an injection, remove the needle from the insulin pen. Doing so will guard against contamination, leakage, reentry of air, and needle clogs. **Do not reuse needles. Dispose of needles in a responsible manner.**

8. *1.5 mL cartridge* - Once the cartridge is in use, do not continue to use it if the leading edge of the plunger is beyond the black band on the cartridge. If a dose is started when the leading edge of the plunger is beyond the black band, an appropriate dose may not be delivered. Use the gauge on the side of the cartridge to help you judge how much Humulin N remains. The distance between each mark on the 1.5 mL cartridge is about 10 units.

DOSAGE

Your doctor has told you which insulin to use, how much, and when and how often to inject it. Because each patient's case of diabetes is different, this schedule has been individualized for you.

Your usual insulin dose may be affected by changes in your food, activity, or work schedule. Carefully follow your doctor's instructions to allow for these changes. Other things that may affect your insulin dose are:

Illness

Illness, especially with nausea and vomiting, may cause your insulin requirements to change. Even if you are not eating, you will still require insulin. You and your doctor should establish a sick day plan for you to use in case of illness. When you are sick, test your blood glucose/urine glucose and ketones frequently and call your doctor as instructed.

Pregnancy

Good control of diabetes is especially important for you and your unborn baby. Pregnancy may make managing your diabetes more difficult. If you are planning to have a baby, are pregnant, or are nursing a baby, consult your doctor.

Medication

Insulin requirements may be increased if you are taking other drugs with hyperglycemic activity, such as oral contraceptives, corticosteroids, or thyroid replacement therapy. Insulin requirements may be reduced in the presence of drugs with hypoglycemic activity, such as oral hypoglycemics, salicylates (for example, aspirin), sulfa antibiotics, and certain antidepressants. Always discuss any medications you are taking with your doctor.

Exercise

Exercise may lower your body's need for insulin during and for some time after the activity. Exercise may also speed up the effect of an insulin dose, especially if the exercise involves the area of injection site (for example, the leg should not be used for injection just prior to running). Discuss with your doctor how you should adjust your regimen to accommodate exercise.

Travel

Persons traveling across more than 2 time zones should consult their doctor concerning adjustments in their insulin schedule.

COMMON PROBLEMS OF DIABETES

Hypoglycemia (Insulin Reaction)

Hypoglycemia (too little glucose in the blood) is one of the most frequent adverse events experienced by insulin users. It can be brought about by:

1. Taking too much insulin

2. Missing or delaying meals

3. Exercising or working more than usual

4. An infection or illness (especially with diarrhea or vomiting)

5. A change in the body's need for insulin

6. Diseases of the adrenal, pituitary or thyroid gland, or progression of kidney or liver disease

7. Interactions with other drugs that lower blood glucose, such as oral hypoglycemics, salicylates (for example, aspirin), sulfa antibiotics, and certain antidepressants

8. Consumption of alcoholic beverages

Symptoms of mild to moderate hypoglycemia may occur suddenly and can include:

- sweating
- dizziness
- palpitation
- tremor
- hunger
- restlessness
- tingling in the hands, feet, lips, or tongue
- lightheadedness
- inability to concentrate
- headache
- drowsiness
- sleep disturbances
- anxiety
- blurred vision
- slurred speech
- depressed mood
- irritability
- abnormal behavior
- unsteady movement
- personality changes

Signs of severe hypoglycemia can include:

- disorientation
- unconsciousness
- seizures
- death

Therefore, it is important that assistance be obtained immediately.

Early warning symptoms of hypoglycemia may be different or less pronounced under certain conditions, such as long duration of diabetes, diabetic nerve disease, medications such as beta-blockers, change in insulin preparations, or intensified control (3 or more insulin injections per day) of diabetes.

A few patients who have experienced hypoglycemic reactions after transfer from animal-source insulin to human insulin have reported that the early warning symptoms of hypoglycemia were less pronounced or different from those experienced with their previous insulin.

Without recognition of early warning symptoms, you may not be able to take steps to avoid more serious hypoglycemia. Be alert for all of the various types of symptoms that may indicate hypoglycemia. Patients who experience hypoglycemia without early warning symptoms should monitor their blood glucose frequently, especially prior to activities such as driving. If the blood glucose is below your normal fasting glucose, you should consider eating or drinking sugar-containing foods to treat your hypoglycemia.

Mild to moderate hypoglycemia may be treated by eating foods or drinks that contain sugar. Patients should always carry a quick source of sugar, such as candy mints or glucose tablets. More severe hypoglycemia may require the assistance of another person. Patients who are unable to take sugar orally or who are unconscious require an injection of glucagon or should be treated with intravenous administration of glucose at a medical facility.

You should learn to recognize your own symptoms of hypoglycemia. If you are uncertain about these symptoms, you should monitor your blood glucose frequently to help you learn to recognize the symptoms that you experience with hypoglycemia.

If you have frequent episodes of hypoglycemia or experience difficulty in recognizing the symptoms, you should consult your doctor to discuss possible changes in therapy, meal plans, and/or exercise programs to help you avoid hypoglycemia.

Hyperglycemia and Diabetic Acidosis

Hyperglycemia (too much glucose in the blood) may develop if your body has too little insulin. Hyperglycemia can be brought about by:

1. Omitting your insulin or taking less than the doctor has prescribed

2. Eating significantly more than your meal plan suggests

3. Developing a fever, infection, or other significant stressful situation

In patients with insulin-dependent diabetes, prolonged hyperglycemia can result in diabetic acidosis. The first symptoms of diabetic acidosis usually come on gradually, over a period of hours or days, and include a drowsy feeling, flushed face, thirst, loss of appetite, and fruity odor on the breath. With acidosis, urine tests show large amounts of glucose and acetone. Heavy breathing and a rapid pulse are more severe symptoms. If uncorrected, prolonged hyperglycemia or diabetic acidosis can lead to nausea, vomiting, dehydration, loss of consciousness or death. Therefore, it is important that you obtain medical assistance immediately.

Lipodystrophy

Rarely, administration of insulin subcutaneously can result in lipoatrophy (depression in the skin) or lipohypertrophy (enlargement or thickening of tissue). If you notice either of these conditions, consult your doctor. A change in your injection technique may help alleviate the problem.

Allergy to Insulin

Local Allergy—Patients occasionally experience redness, swelling, and itching at the site of injection of insulin. This condition, called local allergy, usually clears up in a few days to a few weeks. In some instances, this condition may be related to factors other than insulin, such as irritants in the skin cleansing agent or poor injection technique. If you have local reactions, contact your doctor.

Systemic Allergy—Less common, but potentially more serious, is generalized allergy to insulin, which may cause rash over the whole body, shortness of breath, wheezing, reduction in blood pressure, fast pulse, or sweating. Severe cases of generalized allergy may be life threatening. If you think you are having a generalized allergic reaction to insulin, notify a doctor immediately.

ADDITIONAL INFORMATION

Additional information about diabetes may be obtained from your diabetes educator.

DIABETES FORECAST is a national magazine designed especially for patients with diabetes and their families and is available on subscription from the American Diabetes Association, National Service Center, 1660 Duke Street, Alexandria, Virginia 22314, 1-800-DIABETES (1-800-342-2383).

Another publication, **DIABETES COUNTDOWN**, is available from the Juvenile Diabetes Foundation, 432 Park Avenue South, New York, New York 10016-8013, 1-800-JDF-CURE (1-800-533-2873).

Additional information about Humulin can be obtained by calling 1-888-88-LILLY (1-888-885-4559).

Literature revised March 17, 1998

PA 9066 FSAMP   [031798]

---

* B-D® is a registered trademark of Becton Dickinson and Company.

† NovolinPen® and NovoPen® are registered trademarks of Novo Nordisk A/S.

HUMULIN® R   OTC

[hū 'mū-lĭn är]

**Regular
(insulin human injection, USP [rDNA origin])**

INFORMATION FOR THE PATIENT
WARNINGS
**THIS LILLY HUMAN INSULIN PRODUCT DIFFERS FROM ANIMAL-SOURCE INSULINS BECAUSE IT IS STRUCTURALLY IDENTICAL TO THE INSULIN PRODUCED BY YOUR BODY'S PANCREAS AND BECAUSE OF ITS UNIQUE MANUFACTURING PROCESS.
ANY CHANGE OF INSULIN SHOULD BE MADE CAUTIOUSLY AND ONLY UNDER MEDICAL SUPERVISION. CHANGES IN STRENGTH, MANUFACTURER, TYPE (E.G., REGULAR, NPH, LENTE®), SPECIES (BEEF, PORK, BEEF-PORK, HUMAN), OR METHOD OF MANUFACTURE (rDNA VERSUS ANIMAL-SOURCE INSULIN) MAY RESULT IN THE NEED FOR A CHANGE IN DOSAGE.
SOME PATIENTS TAKING HUMULIN® (HUMAN INSULIN, rDNA ORIGIN) MAY REQUIRE A CHANGE IN DOSAGE FROM THAT USED WITH ANIMAL-SOURCE INSULINS. IF AN ADJUSTMENT IS NEEDED, IT MAY OCCUR WITH THE FIRST DOSE OR DURING THE FIRST SEVERAL WEEKS OR MONTHS.**

DIABETES

Insulin is a hormone produced by the pancreas, a large gland that lies near the stomach. This hormone is necessary for the body's correct use of food, especially sugar. Diabetes occurs when the pancreas does not make enough insulin to meet your body's needs.

To control your diabetes, your doctor has prescribed injections of insulin to keep your blood glucose at a nearly normal level. Proper control of your diabetes requires close and constant cooperation with your doctor. In spite of diabetes, you can lead an active, healthy, and useful life if you eat a balanced diet daily, exercise regularly, and take your insulin injections as prescribed.

You have been instructed to test your blood and/or your urine regularly for glucose. If your blood tests consistently show above- or below-normal glucose levels or your urine tests consistently show the presence of glucose, your diabetes is not properly controlled and you must let your doctor know.

Always keep an extra supply of insulin as well as a spare syringe and needle on hand. Always wear diabetic identification so that appropriate treatment can be given if complications occur away from home.

REGULAR HUMAN INSULIN
Description

Humulin is synthesized in a special non-disease-producing laboratory strain of *Escherichia coli* bacteria that has been

genetically altered by the addition of the gene for human insulin production. Humulin R consists of zinc-insulin crystals dissolved in a clear fluid. Humulin R has had nothing added to change the speed or length of its action. It takes effect rapidly and has a relatively short duration of activity (4 to 12 hours) as compared with other insulins. The time course of action of any insulin may vary considerably in different individuals or at different times in the same individual. As with all insulin preparations, the duration of action of Humulin R is dependent on dose, site of injection, blood supply, temperature, and physical activity. Humulin R is a sterile solution and is for subcutaneous injection. It should not be used intramuscularly. The concentration of Humulin R is 100 units/mL (U-100).

Identification

Human insulin manufactured by Eli Lilly and Company has the trademark Humulin and is available in 6 formulations—Regular (**R**), NPH (**N**), Lente (**L**), Ultralente® (**U**), 50% Human Insulin Isophane Suspension [NPH]/50% Human Insulin Injection [buffered regular] (**50/50**), and 70% Human Insulin Isophane Suspension [NPH]/30% Human Insulin Injection [buffered regular] (**70/30**). Your doctor has prescribed the type of insulin that he/she believes is best for you. **DO NOT USE ANY OTHER INSULIN EXCEPT ON HIS/HER ADVICE AND DIRECTION.**

Always check the carton and the bottle label for the name and letter designation of the insulin you receive from your pharmacy to make sure it is the same as that your doctor has prescribed. Humulin R can be identified as follows: [See graphic below]

Always examine the appearance of your bottle of insulin before withdrawing each dose. Humulin R is a clear and colorless liquid with a water-like appearance and consistency. Do not use if it appears cloudy, thickened, or slightly colored or if solid particles are visible. Always check the appearance of your bottle of insulin before using, and if you note anything unusual in the appearance of your insulin or notice your insulin requirements changing markedly, consult your doctor.

Storage

Insulin should be stored in a refrigerator but not in the freezer. If refrigeration is not possible, the bottle of insulin that you are currently using can be kept unrefrigerated as long as it is kept as cool as possible (below 86°F [30°C]) and away from heat and light. Do not use insulin if it has been frozen. Do not use a bottle of insulin after the expiration date stamped on the label.

INJECTION PROCEDURES

Correct Syringe

Doses of insulin are measured in **units**. U-100 insulin contains 100 units/mL (1 mL = 1 cc). With Humulin R, it is important to use a syringe that is marked for U-100 insulin preparations. Failure to use the proper syringe can lead to a mistake in dosage, causing serious problems for you, such as a blood glucose level that is too low or too high.

Syringe Use

To help avoid contamination and possible infection, follow these instructions exactly.

Disposable syringes and needles should be used only once and then discarded. **NEEDLES AND SYRINGES MUST NOT BE SHARED.**

Reusable syringes and needles must be sterilized before each injection.

Follow the package directions supplied with your syringe. Described below are 2 methods of sterilizing.

Boiling

1. Put syringe, plunger, and needle in strainer, place in saucepan, and cover with water. Boil for 5 minutes.
2. Remove articles from water. When they have cooled, insert plunger into barrel, and fasten needle to syringe with a slight twist.
3. Push plunger in and out several times until water is completely removed.

Isopropyl Alcohol

If the syringe, plunger, and needle cannot be boiled, as when you are traveling, they may be sterilized by immersion for at least 5 minutes in Isopropyl Alcohol, 91%. Do not use bathing, rubbing, or medicated alcohol for this sterilization. If the syringe is sterilized with alcohol, it must be absolutely dry before use.

Preparing the Dose

1. Wash your hands.
2. Inspect the insulin. Humulin R should look clear and colorless. Do not use Humulin R if it appears cloudy, thickened, or slightly colored or if solid particles are visible.
3. If using a new bottle, flip off the plastic protective cap, but **do not** remove the stopper. When using a new bottle, wipe the top of the bottle with an alcohol swab.
4. If you are mixing insulins, refer to instructions for mixing that follow.
5. Draw air into the syringe equal to your insulin dose. Put the needle through rubber top of the insulin bottle and inject the air into the bottle.
6. Turn the bottle and syringe upside down. Hold the bottle and syringe firmly in 1 hand.
7. Making sure the tip of the needle is in the insulin, withdraw the correct dose of insulin into the syringe.
8. Before removing the needle from the bottle, check your syringe for air bubbles which reduce the amount of insulin in it. If bubbles are present, hold the syringe straight up and tap its side until the bubbles float to the top. Push them out with the plunger and withdraw the correct dose.
9. Remove the needle from the bottle and lay the syringe down so that the needle dose not touch anything.

Mixing Humulin R with Longer-acting Human Insulins

1. Regular human insulin should be mixed with longer-acting human insulins only on the advice of your doctor.
2. Draw air into your syringe equal to the amount of longer-acting insulin you are taking. Insert the needle into the longer-acting insulin bottle and inject the air. Withdraw the needle.
3. Now inject air into your regular human insulin bottle in the same manner, but **do not** withdraw the needle.
4. Turn the bottle and syringe upside down.
5. Making sure the tip of the needle is in the insulin, withdraw the correct dose of regular insulin into the syringe.
6. Before removing the needle from the bottle, check your syringe for air bubbles which reduce the amount of insulin in it. If bubbles are present, hold the syringe straight up and tap its side until the bubbles float to the top. Push them out with the plunger and withdraw the correct dose.
7. Remove the needle from the bottle of regular insulin and insert it into the bottle of the longer-acting insulin. Turn the bottle and syringe upside down. Hold the bottle and syringe firmly in 1 hand and shake gently. Making sure the tip of the needle is in the insulin, withdraw your dose of longer-acting insulin.
8. Remove the needle and lay the syringe down so that the needle does not touch anything.

Follow your doctor's instructions on whether to mix your insulins ahead of time or just before giving your injection. It is important to be consistent in your method.

Syringes from different manufacturers may vary in the amount of space between the bottom line and the needle. Because of this, do not change:
- the sequence of mixing, or
- the model and brand of syringe or needle that the doctor has prescribed.

Injection

Cleanse the skin with alcohol where the injection is to be made. Stabilize the skin by spreading it or pinching up a large area. Insert the needle as instructed by your doctor. Push the plunger in as far as it will go. Pull the needle out and apply gentle pressure over the injection site for several seconds. **Do not rub the area**. To avoid tissue damage, give the next injection at a site at least $1/2''$ from the previous site.

DOSAGE

Your doctor has told you which insulin to use, how much, and when and how often to inject it. Because each patient's case of diabetes is different, this schedule has been individualized for you.

Your usual insulin dose may be affected by changes in your food, activity, or work schedule. Carefully follow your doctor's instructions to allow for these changes. Other things that may affect your insulin dose are:

Illness

Illness, especially with nausea and vomiting, may cause your insulin requirements to change. Even if you are not eating, you will still require insulin. You and your doctor should establish a sick day plan for you to use in case of illness. When you are sick, test your blood/urine frequently and call your doctor as instructed.

Pregnancy

Good control of diabetes is especially important for you and your unborn baby. Pregnancy may make managing your diabetes more difficult. If you are planning to have a baby, are pregnant, or are nursing a baby, consult your doctor.

Medication

Insulin requirements may be increased if you are taking other drugs with hyperglycemic activity, such as oral contraceptives, corticosteroids, or thyroid replacement therapy. Insulin requirements may be reduced in the presence of drugs with hypoglycemic activity, such as oral hypoglycemics, salicylates (for example, aspirin), sulfa antibiotics, and certain antidepressants. Always discuss any medications you are taking with your doctor.

Exercise

Exercise may lower your body's need for insulin during and for some time after the activity. Exercise may also speed up the effect of an insulin dose, especially if the exercise involves the area of injection site (for example, the leg should not be used for injection just prior to running). Discuss with your doctor how you should adjust your regimen to accommodate exercise.

Travel

Persons traveling across more than 2 time zones should consult their doctor concerning adjustments in their insulin schedule.

COMMON PROBLEMS OF DIABETES

Hypoglycemia (Insulin Reaction)

Hypoglycemia (too little glucose in the blood) is one of the most frequent adverse events experienced by insulin users. It can be brought about by:

1. Taking too much insulin
2. Missing or delaying meals
3. Exercising or working more than usual
4. An infection or illness (especially with diarrhea or vomiting)
5. A change in the body's need for insulin
6. Diseases of the adrenal, pituitary, or thyroid gland, or progression of kidney or liver disease
7. Interactions with other drugs that lower blood glucose, such as oral hypoglycemics, salicylates (for example, aspirin), sulfa antibiotics, and certain antidepressants
8. Consumption of alcoholic beverages

Symptoms of mild to moderate hypoglycemia may occur suddenly and can include:
- sweating
- dizziness
- palpitation
- tremor
- hunger
- restlessness
- tingling in the hands, feet, lips, or tongue
- lightheadedness
- inability to concentrate
- headache
- drowsiness
- sleep disturbances
- anxiety
- blurred vision
- slurred speech
- depressed mood
- irritability
- abnormal behavior
- unsteady movement
- personality changes

Signs of severe hypoglycemia can include:
- disorientation
- unconsciousness
- seizures
- death

Therefore, it is important that assistance be obtained immediately.

Early warning symptoms of hypoglycemia may be different or less pronounced under certain conditions, such as long duration of diabetes, diabetic nerve disease, medications such as beta-blockers, change in insulin preparations, or intensified control (3 or more insulin injections per day) of diabetes.

Continued on next page

* Identi-Code® symbol. This product information was prepared in June 1998. Current information on these and other products of Eli Lilly and Company may be obtained by direct inquiry to Lilly Research Laboratories, Lilly Corporate Center, Indianapolis, Indiana 46285, (800) 545-5979.

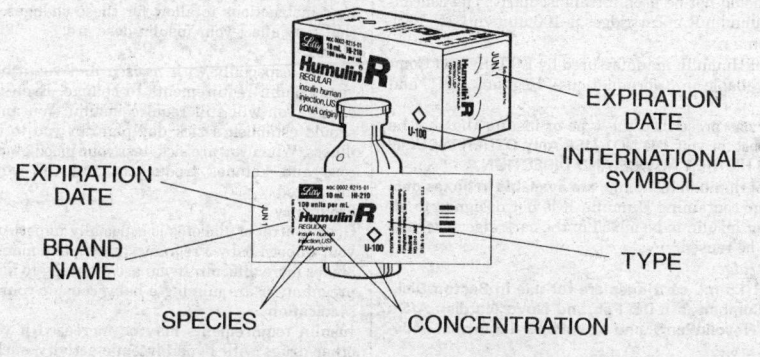

EXPIRATION DATE

INTERNATIONAL SYMBOL

EXPIRATION DATE

BRAND NAME

SPECIES

CONCENTRATION

TYPE

Humulin R Regular—Cont.

A few patients who have experienced hypoglycemic reactions after transfer from animal-source insulin to human insulin have reported that the early warning symptoms of hypoglycemia were less pronounced or different from those experienced with their previous insulin.

Without recognition of early warning symptoms, you may not be able to take steps to avoid more serious hypoglycemia. Be alert for all of the various types of symptoms that may indicate hypoglycemia. Patients who experience hypoglycemia without early warning symptoms should monitor their blood glucose frequently, especially prior to activities such as driving. If the blood glucose is below your normal fasting glucose, you should consider eating or drinking sugar-containing foods to treat your hypoglycemia.

Mild to moderate hypoglycemia may be treated by eating foods or drinks that contain sugar. Patients should always carry a quick source of sugar, such as candy mints or glucose tablets. More severe hypoglycemia may require the assistance of another person. Patients who are unable to take sugar orally or who are unconscious require an injection of glucagon or should be treated with intravenous administration of glucose at a medical facility.

You should learn to recognize your own symptoms of hypoglycemia. If you are uncertain about these symptoms, you should monitor your blood glucose frequently to help you learn to recognize the symptoms that you experience with hypoglycemia.

If you have frequent episodes of hypoglycemia or experience difficulty in recognizing the symptoms, you should consult your doctor to discuss possible changes in therapy, meal plans, and/or exercise programs to help you avoid hypoglycemia.

Hyperglycemia and Diabetic Acidosis

Hyperglycemia (too much glucose in the blood) may develop if your body has too little insulin. Hyperglycemia can be brought about by:

1. Omitting your insulin or taking less than the doctor has prescribed
2. Eating significantly more than your meal plan suggests
3. Developing a fever, infection, or other significant stressful situation

In patients with insulin-dependent diabetes, prolonged hyperglycemia can result in diabetic acidosis. The first symptoms of diabetic acidosis usually come on gradually, over a period of hours or days, and include a drowsy feeling, flushed face, thirst, loss of appetite, and fruity odor on the breath. With acidosis, urine tests show large amounts of glucose and acetone. Heavy breathing and a rapid pulse are more severe symptoms. If uncorrected, prolonged hyperglycemia or diabetic acidosis can lead to nausea, vomiting, dehydration, loss of consciousness or death. Therefore, it is important that you obtain medical assistance immediately.

Lipodystrophy

Rarely, administration of insulin subcutaneously can result in lipoatrophy (depression in the skin) or lipohypertrophy (enlargement or thickening of tissue). If you notice either of these conditions, consult your doctor. A change in your injection technique may help alleviate the problem.

Allergy to Insulin

Local Allergy—Patients occasionally experience redness, swelling, and itching at the site of injection of insulin. This condition, called local allergy, usually clears up in a few days to a few weeks. In some instances, this condition may be related to factors other than insulin, such as irritants in the skin cleansing agent or poor injection technique. If you have local reactions, contact your doctor.

Systemic Allergy—Less common, but potentially more serious, is generalized allergy to insulin, which may cause rash over the whole body, shortness of breath, wheezing, reduction in blood pressure, fast pulse, or sweating. Severe cases of generalized allergy may be life threatening. If you think you are having a generalized allergic reaction to insulin, notify a doctor immediately.

ADDITIONAL INFORMATION

Additional information about diabetes may be obtained from your diabetes educator.

DIABETES FORECAST is a national magazine designed especially for patients with diabetes and their families and is available by subscription from the American Diabetes Association, National Service Center, 1660 Duke Street, Alexandria, Virginia 22314, 1-800-DIABETES (1-800-342-2383). Another publication, **DIABETES COUNTDOWN**, is available from the Juvenile Diabetes Foundation, 432 Park Avenue South, New York, New York 10016-8013, 1-800-JDF-CURE (1-800-533-2873).

Additional information about Humulin can be obtained by calling 1-888-88-LILLY (1-888-885-4559).

Literature revised March 26, 1997

PA 6325 AMP   [032697]

HUMULIN® R   OTC
[hū 'mū-lĭ är]

Regular
Cartridge
(insulin human injection, USP
[rDNA origin])
1.5 ML CARTRIDGE

For use in Becton Dickinson and Company's B-D®* Pen and Novo Nordisk A/S's NovoPen®†, NovolinPen®†, and NovoPen®† 1.5 insulin delivery devices.

INFORMATION FOR THE PATIENT
WARNINGS

THIS LILLY HUMAN INSULIN PRODUCT DIFFERS FROM ANIMAL-SOURCE INSULINS BECAUSE IT IS STRUCTURALLY IDENTICAL TO THE INSULIN PRODUCED BY YOUR BODY'S PANCREAS AND BECAUSE OF ITS UNIQUE MANUFACTURING PROCESS.

ANY CHANGE OF INSULIN SHOULD BE MADE CAUTIOUSLY AND ONLY UNDER MEDICAL SUPERVISION. CHANGES IN STRENGTH, MANUFACTURER, TYPE (E.G., REGULAR, NPH, LENTE, ETC), SPECIES (BEEF, PORK, BEEF-PORK, HUMAN), OR METHOD OF MANUFACTURE (rDNA VERSUS ANIMAL-SOURCE INSULIN) MAY RESULT IN THE NEED FOR A CHANGE IN DOSAGE.

SOME PATIENTS TAKING HUMULIN® (HUMAN INSULIN, rDNA ORIGIN) MAY REQUIRE A CHANGE IN DOSAGE FROM THAT USED WITH ANIMAL-SOURCE INSULINS. IF AN ADJUSTMENT IS NEEDED, IT MAY OCCUR WITH THE FIRST DOSE OR DURING THE FIRST SEVERAL WEEKS OR MONTHS.

TO OBTAIN AN ACCURATE DOSE, CAREFULLY READ AND FOLLOW THE INSULIN DELIVERY DEVICE ("INSULIN PEN") MANUFACTURER'S INSTRUCTIONS AND THIS INFORMATION FOR THE PATIENT INSERT BEFORE USING THIS PRODUCT IN AN INSULIN PEN. (*see* INSTRUCTIONS FOR USE section)

DIABETES

Insulin is a hormone produced by the pancreas, a large gland that lies near the stomach. This hormone is necessary for the body's correct use of food, especially sugar. Diabetes occurs when the pancreas does not make enough insulin to meet your body's needs.

To control your diabetes, your doctor has prescribed injections of insulin to keep your blood glucose at a nearly normal level. Proper control of your diabetes requires close and constant cooperation with your doctor. In spite of diabetes, you can lead an active, healthy, and useful life if you eat a balanced diet daily, exercise regularly, and take your insulin injections as prescribed.

You have been instructed to test your blood and/or your urine regularly for glucose. If your blood tests consistently show above- or below-normal glucose levels or your urine tests consistently show the presence of glucose, your diabetes is not properly controlled and you must let your doctor know.

Always keep an extra supply of insulin as well as a spare syringe and needle on hand. Always wear diabetic identification so that appropriate treatment can be given if complications occur away from home.

REGULAR HUMAN INSULIN
Description

Humulin is synthesized in a non-disease-producing special laboratory strain of *Escherichia coli* bacteria that has been genetically altered by the addition of the human gene for insulin production. Humulin® R consists of zinc-insulin crystals dissolved in a clear fluid. Humulin R has had nothing added to change the speed or length of its action. It takes effect rapidly and has a relatively short duration of activity (4 to 12 hours) as compared with other insulins. The time course of action of any insulin may vary considerably in different individuals or at different times in the same individual. As with all insulin preparations, the duration of action of Humulin R is dependent on dose, site of injection, blood supply, temperature, and physical activity.

Humulin R is a sterile solution and is for subcutaneous injection. It should not be used intramuscularly. The concentration of Humulin R in cartridges is 100 units/mL (U-100).

Identification

Cartridges of Humulin manufactured by Eli Lilly and Company are available in 3 formulations—Regular, NPH, and 70/30.

Your doctor has prescribed the type of insulin that he/she believes is best for you. **DO NOT USE ANY OTHER INSULIN EXCEPT ON HIS/HER ADVICE AND DIRECTION.**

Cartridges of Humulin R, 1.5 mL, are available in boxes of 5. The cartridge containing Humulin R is not designed to allow any other insulin to be mixed in the cartridge or for the cartridge to be reused.

1.5 mL Cartridge

Humulin® R 1.5 mL cartridges are for use in Becton Dickinson and Company's B-D® Pen and Novo Nordisk A/S's NovoPen®, NovolinPen®, and NovoPen® 1.5 insulin delivery devices.

Always examine the appearance of a cartridge of insulin before administering a dose. Humulin R is a clear and colorless liquid with a water-like appearance and consistency. Do not use if it appears cloudy, thickened, or slightly colored, or if solid particles are visible.

Always check the appearance of the cartridge before using, and if you note anything unusual in the appearance of your insulin or notice your insulin requirements changing markedly, consult your doctor.

Storage

Insulin cartridges should be stored in a refrigerator but not in the freezer. The insulin pen and cartridge of insulin that you are currently using should not be refrigerated but should be kept as cool as possible (below 86°F [30°C]) and away from heat and light. Do not use insulin if it has been frozen. Unrefrigerated 1.5 mL cartridges **must be discarded after 28 days**, even if they still contain insulin. **Do not use a cartridge of Humulin R after the expiration date stamped on the label.**

INSTRUCTIONS FOR USE

Pens for insulin delivery differ in their operation. It is important to read, understand, and follow the instructions for use of the particular insulin pen you are using.
NEVER SHARE INSULIN PENS, CARTRIDGES, OR NEEDLES.

PREPARING FOR AN INJECTION:

1. Inspect the Humulin R before you insert the cartridge into the insulin pen. Humulin R should look clear and colorless. Do not use a cartridge of Humulin R if it appears cloudy, thickened, slightly colored, or if solid particles are visible. Once the cartridge is in use, inspect the insulin in the insulin pen before each injection.
2. Follow the insulin pen manufacturer's instructions carefully for loading the cartridge into the insulin pen and for use of the insulin pen.
3. Use an alcohol swab to wipe the exposed rubber surface on the metal cap end of the cartridge.
4. Follow the insulin needle manufacturer's instructions for attaching and changing the needle.
5. Insulin cartridges may contain an air bubble(s) which must be removed from the cartridge and needle by proper priming prior to injection.

GENERAL INJECTION INSTRUCTIONS:

1. Wash your hands.
2. To avoid tissue damage, choose a site for each injection that is at least 1/2 inch from the previous injection site. The usual sites of injection are abdomen, thighs, and arms.
3. Cleanse the skin with alcohol where the injection is to be made.
4. With one hand, stabilize the skin by spreading it or pinching up a large area.
5. Insert the needle as instructed by your doctor.
6. After dispensing a dose, pull the needle out and apply gentle pressure over the injection site for several seconds. **Do not rub the area.**
7. Immediately after an injection, remove the needle from the insulin pen. Doing so will guard against contamination, leakage, reentry of air, and needle clogs. **Do not reuse needles. Dispose of needles in a responsible manner.**
8. *1.5 mL cartridge*—Once the cartridge is in use, do not continue to use it if the leading edge of the plunger is beyond the black band on the cartridge. If a dose is started when the leading edge of the plunger is beyond the black band, an appropriate dose may not be delivered. Use the gauge on the side of the cartridge to help you judge how much Humulin R remains. The distance between each mark on the 1.5 mL cartridge is about 10 units.

DOSAGE

Your doctor has told you which insulin to use, how much, and when and how often to inject it. Because each patient's case of diabetes is different, this schedule has been individualized for you.

Your usual insulin dose may be affected by changes in your food, activity, or work schedule. Carefully follow your doctor's instructions to allow for these changes. Other things that may affect your insulin dose are:

Illness

Illness, especially with nausea and vomiting, may cause your insulin requirements to change. Even if you are not eating, you will still require insulin. You and your doctor should establish a sick day plan for you to use in case of illness. When you are sick, test your blood glucose/urine glucose and ketones frequently and call your doctor as instructed.

Pregnancy

Good control of diabetes is especially important for you and your unborn baby. Pregnancy may make managing your diabetes more difficult. If you are planning to have a baby, are pregnant, or are nursing a baby, consult your doctor.

Medication

Insulin requirements may be increased if you are taking other drugs with hyperglycemic activity, such as oral con-

traceptives, corticosteroids, or thyroid replacement therapy. Insulin requirements may be reduced in the presence of drugs with hypoglycemic activity, such as oral hypoglycemics, salicylates (for example, aspirin), sulfa antibiotics, and certain antidepressants. Always discuss any medications you are taking with your doctor.

Exercise

Exercise may lower your body's need for insulin during and for some time after the activity. Exercise may also speed up the effect of an insulin dose, especially if the exercise involves the area of injection site (for example, the leg should not be used for injection just prior to running). Discuss with your doctor how you should adjust your regimen to accommodate exercise.

Travel

Persons traveling across more than 2 time zones should consult their doctor concerning adjustments in their insulin schedule.

COMMON PROBLEMS OF DIABETES

Hypoglycemia (Insulin Reaction)

Hypoglycemia (too little glucose in the blood) is one of the most frequent adverse events experienced by insulin users. It can be brought about by:

1. Taking too much insulin
2. Missing or delaying meals
3. Exercising or working more than usual
4. An infection or illness (especially with diarrhea or vomiting)
5. A change in the body's need for insulin
6. Diseases of the adrenal, pituitary or thyroid gland, or progression of kidney or liver disease
7. Interactions with other drugs that lower blood glucose, such as oral hypoglycemics, salicylates (for example, aspirin), sulfa antibiotics, and certain antidepressants
8. Consumption of alcoholic beverages

Symptoms of mild to moderate hypoglycemia may occur suddenly and can include:

- sweating
- dizziness
- palpitation
- tremor
- hunger
- restlessness
- tingling in the hands, feet, lips, or tongue
- lightheadedness
- inability to concentrate
- headache
- drowsiness
- sleep disturbances
- anxiety
- blurred vision
- slurred speech
- depressed mood
- irritability
- abnormal behavior
- unsteady movement
- personality changes

Signs of severe hypoglycemia can include:

- disorientation
- unconsciousness
- seizures
- death

Therefore, it is important that assistance be obtained immediately.

Early warning symptoms of hypoglycemia may be different or less pronounced under certain conditions, such as long duration of diabetes, diabetic nerve disease, medications such as beta-blockers, change in insulin preparations, or intensified control (3 or more insulin injections per day) of diabetes.

A few patients who have experienced hypoglycemic reactions after transfer from animal-source insulin to human insulin have reported that the early warning symptoms of hypoglycemia were less pronounced or different from those experienced with their previous insulin.

Without recognition of early warning symptoms, you may not be able to take steps to avoid more serious hypoglycemia. Be alert for all of the various types of symptoms that may indicate hypoglycemia. Patients who experience hypoglycemia without early warning symptoms should monitor their blood glucose frequently, especially prior to activities such as driving. If the blood glucose is below your normal fasting glucose, you should consider eating or drinking sugar-containing foods to treat your hypoglycemia.

Mild to moderate hypoglycemia may be treated by eating foods or drinks that contain sugar. Patients should always carry a quick source of sugar, such as candy mints or glucose tablets. More severe hypoglycemia may require the assistance of another person. Patients who are unable to take sugar orally or who are unconscious require an injection of glucagon or should be treated with intravenous administration of glucose at a medical facility.

You should learn to recognize your own symptoms of hypoglycemia. If you are uncertain about these symptoms, you

should monitor your blood glucose frequently to help you learn to recognize the symptoms that you experience with hypoglycemia.

If you have frequent episodes of hypoglycemia or experience difficulty in recognizing the symptoms, you should consult your doctor to discuss possible changes in therapy, meal plans, and/or exercise programs to help you avoid hypoglycemia.

Hyperglycemia and Diabetic Acidosis

Hyperglycemia (too much glucose in the blood) may develop if your body has too little insulin. Hyperglycemia can be brought about by:

1. Omitting your insulin or taking less than the doctor has prescribed
2. Eating significantly more than your meal plan suggests
3. Developing a fever, infection, or other significant stressful situation

In patients with insulin-dependent diabetes, prolonged hyperglycemia can result in diabetic acidosis. The first symptoms of diabetic acidosis usually come on gradually, over a period of hours or days, and include a drowsy feeling, flushed face, thirst, loss of appetite, and fruity odor on the breath. With acidosis, urine tests show large amounts of glucose and acetone. Heavy breathing and a rapid pulse are more severe symptoms. If uncorrected, prolonged hyperglycemia or diabetic acidosis can lead to nausea, vomiting, dehydration, loss of consciousness or death. Therefore, it is important that you obtain medical assistance immediately.

Lipodystrophy

Rarely, administration of insulin subcutaneously can result in lipoatrophy (depression in the skin) or lipohypertrophy (enlargement or thickening of tissue). If you notice either of these conditions, consult your doctor. A change in your injection technique may help alleviate the problem.

Allergy to Insulin

Local Allergy—Patients occasionally experience redness, swelling, and itching at the site of injection of insulin. This condition, called local allergy, usually clears up in a few days to a few weeks. In some instances, this condition may be related to factors other than insulin, such as irritants in the skin cleansing agent or poor injection technique. If you have local reactions, contact your doctor.

Systemic Allergy—Less common, but potentially more serious, is generalized allergy to insulin, which may cause rash over the whole body, shortness of breath, wheezing, reduction in blood pressure, fast pulse, or sweating. Severe cases of generalized allergy may be life threatening. If you think you are having a generalized allergic reaction to insulin, notify a doctor immediately.

ADDITIONAL INFORMATION

Additional information about diabetes may be obtained from your diabetes educator.

DIABETES FORECAST is a national magazine designed especially for patients with diabetes and their families and is available on subscription from the American Diabetes Association, National Service Center, 1660 Duke Street, Alexandria, Virginia 22314, 1-800-DIABETES (1-800-342-2383).

Another publication, **DIABETES COUNTDOWN**, is available from the Juvenile Diabetes Foundation, 432 Park Avenue South, New York, New York 10016-8013, 1-800-JDF-CURE (1-800-533-2873).

Additional information about Humulin can be obtained by calling 1-888-88-LILLY (1-888-885-4559).

Literature revised March 17, 1998

PA 9056 FSAMP   [031798]

---

* B-D® is a registered trademark of Becton Dickinson and Company.

† NovolinPen® and NovoPen® are registered trademarks of Novo Nordisk A/S.

HUMULIN® R   ℞

[hū 'mū-lĭn är]

Regular U-500 (CONCENTRATED)
(insulin human injection, USP
[recombinant DNA origin])

WARNINGS

THIS LILLY HUMAN INSULIN PRODUCT DIFFERS FROM ANIMAL-SOURCE INSULINS BECAUSE IT IS STRUCTURALLY IDENTICAL TO THE INSULIN PRODUCED BY YOUR BODY'S PANCREAS AND BECAUSE OF ITS UNIQUE MANUFACTURING PROCESS.

ANY CHANGE OF INSULIN BE MADE CAUTIOUSLY AND ONLY UNDER MEDICAL SUPERVISION. CHANGES IN PURITY, STRENGTH, BRAND (MANUFACTURER), TYPE (REGULAR, NPH, LENTE®, ETC), SPECIES (BEEF, PORK, BEEF-PORK, HUMAN), AND/OR METHOD OF MANUFACTURE (RECOMBINANT DNA VERSUS ANIMAL-SOURCE INSULIN) MAY RESULT IN THE NEED FOR A CHANGE IN DOSAGE.

SOME PATIENTS TAKING HUMULIN® (HUMAN INSULIN, RECOMBINANT DNA ORIGIN, LILLY) MAY REQUIRE A

CHANGE IN DOSAGE FROM THAT USED WITH ANIMAL-SOURCE INSULINS. IF AN ADJUSTMENT IS NEEDED, IT MAY OCCUR WITH THE FIRST DOSE OR DURING THE FIRST SEVERAL WEEKS OR MONTHS.

This insulin preparation contains 500 units of insulin in each milliliter. Extreme caution must be observed in the measurement of dosage because inadvertent overdose may result in irreversible insulin shock. Serious consequences may result if it is used other than under constant medical supervision.

DESCRIPTION

Humulin is synthesized in a special non-disease-producing laboratory strain of *Escherichia coli* bacteria that has been genetically altered by the addition of the gene for human insulin production. Humulin R (U-500) consists of zinc-insulin crystals dissolved in a clear fluid. Humulin R (U-500) is a sterile solution and is for subcutaneous injection. It should not be used intravenously or intramuscularly. The concentration of Humulin R (U-500) is 500 units/mL.

Each milliliter contains 500 units of biosynthetic human insulin, 16 mg glycerin, 2.5 mg *m*-cresol as a preservative, and zinc-oxide calculated to supplement endogenous zinc to obtain a total zinc content of 0.017 mg/100 units. Sodium hydroxide and hydrochloride acid are added during manufacture to adjust the pH.

CLINICAL PHARMACOLOGY

Adequate insulin dosage permits the diabetic patient to utilize carbohydrates and fats in a comparatively satisfactory manner. Regardless of concentration, the action of insulin is basically the same: to enable carbohydrate metabolism to occur and thus to prevent the production of ketone bodies by the liver. Although, under usual circumstances, diabetes can be controlled with doses in the vicinity of 40 to 60 units or less, an occasional patient develops such resistance or becomes so unresponsive to the effect of insulin that daily doses of several hundred, or even several thousand, units are required. Patients who require doses in excess of 300 to 500 units daily usually have impaired insulin receptor function.

Occasionally, a cause of the insulin resistance can be found (such as hemochromatosis, cirrhosis of the liver, some complicating disease of the endocrine glands other than the pancreas, allergy, or infection), but in other cases, no cause of the high insulin requirement can be determined.

Humulin R (U-500) is unmodified by any agent that might prolong its action; however, clinical experience has shown that it frequently has a time action similar to a repository insulin preparation. It takes effect rapidly but has a relatively long duration of activity following a single dose (up to 24 hours) as compared with other Regular insulins. This effect has been credited to the high concentration of the preparation. The time course of action of any insulin may vary considerably in different individuals or at different times in the same individual. As with all insulin preparations, the duration of action of Humulin R (U-500) is dependent on dose, site of injection, blood supply, temperature, and physical activity.

INDICATIONS AND USAGE

Humulin R (U-500) is especially useful for the treatment of diabetic patients with marked insulin resistance (daily requirements more than 200 units), since a large dose may be administered subcutaneously in a reasonable volume.

CONTRAINDICATIONS

Humulin R (U-500) is contraindicated in hypoglycemia.

PRECAUTIONS

General—Every patient exhibiting insulin resistance who requires Humulin R (U-500) for control of diabetes should be under close observation until appropriate dosage is established. The response will vary among patients. Some patients can be controlled with a single dose daily; others may require 2 or 3 injections per day. Most patients will show a "tolerance" to insulin, so that minor variations in dosage can occur without the development of untoward symptoms of insulin shock.

Insulin resistance is frequently self-limited; after several weeks or months during which high dosage is required, responsiveness to the pharmacologic effect of insulin may be regained and dosage can be reduced.

Information for Patients—Patients should be instructed regarding their dosage and should be reminded that this formulation requires the administration of a smaller volume of solution than is the case with less concentrated formulations.

Continued on next page

Humulin R Reg. U-500—Cont.

Laboratory Tests—Blood and urine glucose, glycohemoglobin, and urine ketones should be monitored frequently.
Drug Interactions—The concurrent use of oral hypoglycemic agents with Humulin R (U-500) is not recommended since there are no data to support such use.
Pregnancy-Teratogenic Effects—No reproduction studies have been conducted in animals, and there are no adequate and well-controlled studies in pregnant women. It would be anticipated that the benefits of this insulin preparation would outweigh any risk to the developing fetus.
Nonteratogenic Effects—Insulin does not cross the placenta as does glucose.
Labor and Delivery—Careful monitoring of the patient is required, since the insulin requirement may decrease following delivery.
Nursing Mothers—It is not known whether insulin is excreted in significant amounts in human milk. Because many drugs are excreted in human milk, caution should be exercised when Humulin R (U-500) insulin injection is administered to a nursing woman.
Pediatric Use—There are no special precautions relating to the use of this insulin formulation in the pediatric age group.

ADVERSE REACTIONS

As with other human insulin preparations, hypoglycemic reactions may be associated with the administration of Humulin R (U-500). However, deep secondary hypoglycemic reactions may develop 18 to 24 hours after the original injection of Humulin R (U-500). Consequently, patients should be carefully observed, and prompt treatment of such reactions should be initiated with glucagon injections and/or with glucose by intravenous injection or gavage.

Hypoglycemia

Hypoglycemia is one of the most frequent adverse events experienced by insulin users.
Symptoms of mild to moderate hypoglycemia may occur suddenly and can include:

- sweating
- dizziness
- palpitation
- tremor
- hunger
- restlessness
- tingling in the hands, feet, lips, or tongue
- lightheadedness
- inability to concentrate
- headache
- drowsiness
- sleep disturbances
- anxiety
- blurred vision
- slurred speech
- depressive mood
- irritability
- abnormal behavior
- unsteady movement
- personality changes

Signs of severe hypoglycemia can include:

- disorientation
- unconsciousness
- seizures
- death

Early warning symptoms of hypoglycemia may be different or less pronounced under certain conditions, such as long duration of diabetes, diabetic nerve disease, medications such as beta-blockers, change in insulin preparations, or intensified control (3 or more insulin injections per day) of diabetes.
A few patients who have experienced hypoglycemic reactions after transfer from animal-source insulin to human insulin have reported that the early warning symptoms of hypoglycemia were less pronounced or different from those experienced with their previous insulin.
Without recognition of early warning symptoms, the patient may not be able to take steps to avoid more serious hypoglycemia. Patients who experience hypoglycemia without early warning symptoms should monitor their blood glucose frequently, especially prior to activities such as driving.
Mild to moderate hypoglycemia may be treated by eating foods or taking drinks that contain sugar. Patients should always carry a quick source of sugar, such as candy mints or glucose tablets.
Hypoglycemia when using Humulin R (U-500) can be prolonged and severe.

Lipodystrophy

Rarely, administration of insulin subcutaneously can result in lipoatrophy (depression in the skin) or lipohypertrophy (enlargement or thickening of tissue).

Allergy to Insulin

Local Allergy—Patients occasionally experience erythema, local edema, and pruritus at the site of injection of insulin. This condition usually is self-limiting. In some instances, this condition may be related to factors other than insulin, such as irritants in the skin cleansing agent or poor injection technique.
Systemic Allergy—Less common, but potentially more serious, is generalized allergy to insulin, which may cause rash over the whole body, shortness of breath, wheezing, reduction in blood pressure, fast pulse, or sweating. Severe cases of generalized allergy (anaphylaxis) may be life threatening.

DOSAGE AND ADMINISTRATION

Humulin R (U-500) should only be administered subcutaneously. It is inadvisable to inject Humulin R (U-500) intravenously because of possible inadvertent overdosage.
It is recommended that an insulin syringe or tuberculin-type syringe be used for the measurement of dosage. Variations in dosage are frequently possible in the insulin-resistant patient, since the individual is unresponsive to the pharmacologic effect of the insulin. Nevertheless, accuracy of measurement is to be encouraged because of the potential danger of the preparation.

STORAGE

Insulin should be kept in a cold place, preferably in a refrigerator, but must not be frozen.
Do not inject insulin that is not water-clear. Discoloration, turbidity, or unusual viscosity indicates deterioration or contamination.
Use of a package of insulin should not be started after the expiration date stamped on it.

HOW SUPPLIED

Vials, 500 units/mL, 20 mL (HI-500) (1s), NDC 0002-8501-01
CAUTION—Federal (USA) law prohibits dispensing without prescription.
Literature issued November 18, 1996
PA 2660 AMP [111896]

HUMULIN® R

[hū 'mū-lĭn är]
Regular U-500
(Concentrated)
(insulin human injection, usp [recombinant DNA origin])

INFORMATION FOR THE PATIENT

WARNINGS

THIS LILLY HUMAN INSULIN PRODUCT DIFFERS FROM ANIMAL-SOURCE INSULINS BECAUSE IT IS STRUCTURALLY IDENTICAL TO THE INSULIN PRODUCED BY YOUR BODY'S PANCREAS AND BECAUSE OF ITS UNIQUE MANUFACTURING PROCESS.
ANY CHANGE OF INSULIN SHOULD BE MADE CAUTIOUSLY AND ONLY UNDER MEDICAL SUPERVISION. CHANGES IN PURITY, STRENGTH, BRAND (MANUFACTURER), TYPE (REGULAR, NPH, LENTE®, ETC), SPECIES (BEEF, PORK, BEEF-PORK, HUMAN), AND/OR METHOD OF MANUFACTURE (RECOMBINANT DNA VERSUS ANIMAL-SOURCE INSULIN) MAY RESULT IN THE NEED FOR A CHANGE IN DOSAGE.
SOME PATIENTS TAKING HUMULIN® (HUMAN INSULIN, RECOMBINANT DNA ORIGIN, LILLY) MAY REQUIRE A CHANGE IN DOSAGE FROM THAT USED WITH ANIMAL-SOURCE INSULINS. IF AN ADJUSTMENT IS NEEDED, IT MAY OCCUR WITH THE FIRST DOSE OR DURING THE FIRST SEVERAL WEEKS OR MONTHS.
This insulin preparation contains 500 units of insulin in each milliliter. Extreme caution must be observed in the measurement of dosage because inadvertent overdose may result in irreversible insulin shock. Serious consequences may result if it is used other than under constant medical supervision.

DIABETES

Insulin is a hormone produced by the pancreas, a large gland that lies near the stomach. This hormone is necessary for the body's correct use of food, especially sugar. Diabetes occurs when the pancreas does not make enough insulin to meet your body's needs.
To control your diabetes, your doctor has prescribed injections of insulin to keep your blood glucose at a nearly normal level. Proper control of your diabetes requires close and constant cooperation with your doctor. In spite of diabetes, you can lead an active, healthy, and useful life if you eat a balanced diet daily, exercise regularly, and take your insulin injections as prescribed.
You have been instructed to test your blood and/or your urine regularly for glucose. If your blood tests consistently show above- or below-normal glucose levels or your urine tests consistently show the presence of glucose, your diabetes is not properly controlled and you must let your doctor know.
Always keep an extra supply of insulin as well as a spare syringe and needle on hand. Always wear diabetic identification so that appropriate treatment can be given if complications occur away from home.

REGULAR HUMAN INSULIN

Description

Humulin is synthesized in a special non-disease-producing laboratory strain of *Escherichia coli* bacteria that has been genetically altered by the addition of the gene for human insulin production. Humulin R (U-500) consists of zinc-insulin crystals dissolved in a clear fluid. Humulin R (U-500) has had nothing added to change the speed or length of its action. It takes effect rapidly but has a relatively long duration of activity (up to 24 hours) as compared with other Regular insulins. The time course of action of any insulin may vary considerably in different individuals or at different times in the same individual. As with all insulin preparations, the duration of action of Humulin R (U-500) is dependent on dose, site of injection, blood supply, temperature, and physical activity. Humulin R (U-500), is a sterile solution and should only be administered subcutaneously. It should not be used intravenously or intramuscularly. The concentration of Humulin R (U-500) is 500 units/mL.

Identification

Human insulin manufactured by Eli Lilly and Company has the trademark Humulin and is available in 6 formulations—Regular (**R**), NPH (**N**), Lente (**L**), Ultralente® (**U**), 50% Human Insulin Isophane Suspension [NPH]/50% Human Insulin Injection [buffered regular] (**50/50**), and 70% Human Insulin Isophane Suspension [NPH]/30% Human Insulin Injection [buffered regular] (**70/30**). Humulin R (U-500) is the only human insulin manufactured by Eli Lilly and Company that has a concentration of 500 units/mL. Your doctor has prescribed this type of insulin because he/she believes it is best for you. **DO NOT USE ANY OTHER INSULIN EXCEPT ON HIS/HER ADVICE AND DIRECTION.**
Always check the carton and the bottle label for the name and letter designation of the insulin you receive from your pharmacy to make sure it is the same as that your doctor has prescribed. Humulin R (U-500) can be identified as follows:
Always examine the appearance of your bottle of insulin before withdrawing each dose. Humulin R (U-500) is a clear and colorless liquid with a water-like appearance and consistency. Do not use if it appears cloudy, thickened, or slightly colored or if solid particles are visible. Always check the appearance of your bottle of insulin before using, and if you note anything unusual in the appearance of your insulin or notice your insulin requirements changing markedly, consult your doctor.

Storage

Insulin should be stored in a refrigerator but not in the freezer. If refrigeration is not possible, the bottle of insulin that you are currently using can be kept unrefrigerated as long as it is kept as cool as possible (below 86°F [30°C]) and away from heat and light. Do not use insulin if it has been frozen. Do not use a bottle of insulin after the expiration date stamped on the label.

INJECTION PROCEDURES

Correct Syringe

Doses of insulin are measured in **units**. U-500 insulin contains 500 units/mL (1 mL = 1 cc). With Humulin R (U-500), it is important to use a tuberculin (or similar) syringe as instructed by your doctor. Failure to use the syringe properly can lead to a mistake in dosage, potentially causing serious problems for you, such as a blood glucose level that is too low or too high.

Syringe Use

To help avoid contamination and possible spread of infection, follow these instructions exactly.
Disposable syringes and needles should be used only once and then discarded. **NEEDLES AND SYRINGES MUST NOT BE SHARED.**
Reusable syringes and needles must be sterilized before each injection. **Follow the package directions supplied with your syringe.** Described below are 2 methods of sterilizing.

Boiling

1. Put syringe, plunger, and needle in strainer, place in saucepan, and cover with water. Boil for 5 minutes.
2. Remove articles from water. When they have cooled, insert plunger into barrel, and fasten needle to syringe with a slight twist.
3. Push plunger in and out several times until water is completely removed.

Isopropyl Alcohol

If the syringe, plunger, and needle cannot be boiled, as when you are traveling, they may be sterilized by immersion for at least 5 minutes in Isopropyl Alcohol, 91%. Do not use bathing, rubbing, or medicated alcohol for this sterilization. If the syringe is sterilized with alcohol, it must be absolutely dry before use.

Preparing the Dose

1. Wash your hands.
2. Inspect the insulin. Humulin R (U-500) should look clear and colorless. Do not use Humulin R (U-500) if it appears cloudy, thickened, or slightly colored or if solid particles are visible.
3. If using a new bottle, flip off the plastic protective cap, but **do not** remove the stopper. When using a new bottle, wipe the top of the bottle with an alcohol swab.
4. Draw air into the syringe equal to your insulin dose. Put the needle through the rubber top of the insulin bottle and inject the air into the bottle.

5. Turn the bottle and syringe upside down. Hold the bottle and syringe firmly in 1 hand.
6. Making sure the tip of the needle is in the insulin, withdraw the correct dose of insulin into the syringe.
7. Before removing the needle from the bottle, check your syringe for air bubbles which reduce the amount of insulin in it. If bubbles are present, hold the syringe straight up and tap its side until the bubbles float to the top. Push them out with the plunger and withdraw the correct dose.
8. Remove the needle from the bottle and lay the syringe down so that the needle does not touch anything.

Injection

Cleanse the skin with alcohol where the injection is to be made. Stabilize the skin by spreading it or pinching up a large area. Insert the needle as instructed by your doctor. Push the plunger in as far as it will go. Pull the needle out and apply gentle pressure over the injection site for several seconds. **Do not rub the area.** To avoid tissue damage, give the next injection at a site at least 1/2″ from the previous site.

DOSAGE

Your doctor has told you which insulin to use, how much, and when and how often to inject it. Because each patient's case of diabetes is different, this schedule has been individualized for you.

Your usual insulin dose may be affected by changes in your food, activity, or work schedule. Carefully follow your doctor's instructions to allow for these changes. Other things that may affect your insulin dose are:

Illness

Illness, especially with nausea and vomiting, may cause your insulin requirements to change. Even if you are not eating, you will still require insulin. You and your doctor should establish a sick day plan for you to use in case of illness. When you are sick, test your blood/urine frequently and call your doctor as instructed.

Pregnancy

Good control of diabetes is especially important for you and your unborn baby. Pregnancy may make managing your diabetes more difficult. If you are planning to have a baby, are pregnant, or are nursing a baby, consult your doctor.

Medication

Insulin requirements may be increased if you are taking other drugs with hyperglycemic activity, such as oral contraceptives, corticosteroids, or thyroid replacement therapy. Insulin requirements may be reduced in the presence of drugs with hypoglycemic activity, such as oral hypoglycemics, salicylates (for example, aspirin), sulfa antibiotics, and certain antidepressants. Always discuss any medications you are taking with your doctor.

Exercise

Exercise may lower your body's need for insulin during and for some time after the activity. Exercise may also speed up the effect of an insulin dose, especially if the exercise involves the area of injection site (for example, the leg should not be used for injection just prior to running). Discuss with your doctor how you should adjust your regimen to accommodate exercise.

Travel

Persons traveling across more than 2 time zones should consult their doctor concerning adjustments in their insulin schedule.

COMMON PROBLEMS OF DIABETES

Hypoglycemia (Insulin Reaction)

Hypoglycemia (too little glucose in the blood) is one of the most frequent adverse events experienced by insulin users. It can be brought about by:

1. Taking too much insulin
2. Missing or delaying meals
3. Exercising or working more than usual
4. An infection or illness (especially with diarrhea or vomiting)
5. A change in the body's need for insulin
6. Diseases of the adrenal, pituitary, or thyroid gland, or progression of kidney or liver disease
7. Interactions with other drugs that lower blood glucose, such as oral hypoglycemics, salicylates (for example, aspirin), sulfa antibiotics, and certain antidepressants
8. Consumption of alcoholic beverages

Symptoms of mild to moderate hypoglycemia may occur suddenly and can include:
- sweating
- dizziness
- palpitation
- tremor
- hunger
- restlessness
- tingling in the hands, feet, lips, or tongue
- lightheadedness
- inability to concentrate
- headache
- drowsiness
- sleep disturbances
- anxiety

- blurred vision
- slurred speech
- depressive mood
- irritability
- abnormal behavior
- unsteady movement
- personality changes

Signs of severe hypoglycemia can include:
- disorientation
- unconsciousness
- seizures
- death

Therefore, it is important that assistance be obtained immediately.

Early warning symptoms of hypoglycemia may be different or less pronounced under certain conditions, such as long duration of diabetes, diabetic nerve disease, medications such as beta-blockers, change in insulin preparations, or intensified control (3 or more insulin injections per day) of diabetes.

A few patients who have experienced hypoglycemic reactions after transfer from animal-source insulin to human insulin have reported that the early warning symptoms of hypoglycemia were less pronounced or different from those experienced with their previous insulin.

Without recognition of early warning symptoms, you may not be able to take steps to avoid more serious hypoglycemia. Be alert for all of the various types of symptoms that may indicate hypoglycemia. Patients who experience hypoglycemia without early warning symptoms should monitor their blood glucose frequently, especially prior to activities such as driving. If the blood glucose is below your normal fasting glucose, you should consider eating or drinking sugar-containing foods to treat your hypoglycemia.

Mild to moderate hypoglycemia may be treated by eating foods or taking drinks that contain sugar. Patients should always carry a quick source of sugar, such as candy mints or glucose tablets. More severe hypoglycemia may require the assistance of another person. Patients who are unable to take sugar orally or who are unconscious require an injection of glucagon or should be treated with intravenous administration of glucose at a medical facility.

Hypoglycemia when using Humulin R (U-500) can be prolonged and severe. All hypoglycemic episodes should be reported to your doctor.

You should learn to recognize your own symptoms of hypoglycemia. If you are uncertain about these symptoms, you should monitor your blood glucose frequently to help you learn to recognize the symptoms that you experience with hypoglycemia.

If you have frequent episodes of hypoglycemia or experience difficulty in recognizing the symptoms, you should consult your doctor to discuss possible changes in therapy, meal plans, and/or exercise programs to help you avoid hypoglycemia.

Hyperglycemia and Diabetic Acidosis

Hyperglycemia (too much glucose in the blood) may develop if your body has too little insulin. Hyperglycemia can be brought about by:

1. Omitting your insulin or taking less than the doctor has prescribed
2. Eating significantly more than your meal plan suggests
3. Developing a fever, infection, or other significant stressful situation

In patients with insulin-dependent diabetes, prolonged hyperglycemia can result in diabetic acidosis. The first symptoms of diabetic acidosis usually come on gradually, over a period of hours or days, and include a drowsy feeling, flushed face, thirst, loss of appetite, and fruity odor on the breath. With acidosis, urine tests show large amounts of glucose and acetone. Heavy breathing and a rapid pulse are more severe symptoms. If uncorrected, prolonged hyperglycemia or diabetic acidosis can lead to nausea, vomiting, dehydration, loss of consciousness or death. Therefore, it is important that you obtain medical assistance immediately.

Lipodystrophy

Rarely, administration of insulin subcutaneously can result in lipoatrophy (depression in the skin) or lipohypertrophy (enlargement or thickening of tissue). If you notice either of these conditions, consult your doctor. A change in your injection technique may help alleviate the problem.

Allergy to Insulin

Local Allergy—Patients occasionally experience redness, swelling, and itching at the site of injection of insulin. This condition, called local allergy, usually clears up in a few days to a few weeks. In some instances, this condition may be related to factors other than insulin, such as irritants in the skin cleansing agent or poor injection technique. If you have local reactions, contact your doctor.

Systemic Allergy—Less common, but potentially more serious, is generalized allergy to insulin, which may cause rash over the whole body, shortness of breath, wheezing, reduction in blood pressure, fast pulse, or sweating. Severe cases of generalized allergy may be life threatening. If you think you are having a generalized allergic reaction to insulin, notify a doctor immediately.

ADDITIONAL INFORMATION

Additional information about diabetes may be obtained from your diabetes educator.

DIABETES FORECAST is a national magazine designed especially for patients with diabetes and their families and is available by subscription from the American Diabetes Association, National Service Center, 1660 Duke Street, Alexandria, Virginia 22314.

Another publication, **DIABETES COUNTDOWN**, is available from the Juvenile Diabetes Foundation, 432 Park Avenue South, New York, New York 10016-8013.

Literature issued November 18, 1996

PA 2670 AMP   [111896]

HUMULIN® U   OTC
[hū ′mŭ-lĭn ū]
Ultralente®
(human Insulin [rDNA origin]
extended zinc suspension)

INFORMATION FOR THE PATIENT

WARNINGS

THIS LILLY HUMAN INSULIN PRODUCT DIFFERS FROM ANIMAL-SOURCE INSULINS BECAUSE IT IS STRUCTURALLY IDENTICAL TO THE INSULIN PRODUCED BY YOUR BODY'S PANCREAS AND BECAUSE OF ITS UNIQUE MANUFACTURING PROCESS.

ANY CHANGE OF INSULIN SHOULD BE MADE CAUTIOUSLY AND ONLY UNDER MEDICAL SUPERVISION. CHANGES IN STRENGTH, MANUFACTURER, TYPE (E.G., REGULAR, NPH, LENTE®, ETC), SPECIES (BEEF, PORK, BEEF-PORK, HUMAN), OR METHOD OF MANUFACTURE (rDNA VERSUS ANIMAL-SOURCE INSULIN) MAY RESULT IN THE NEED FOR A CHANGE IN DOSAGE.

SOME PATIENTS TAKING HUMULIN® (HUMAN INSULIN, rDNA ORIGIN) MAY REQUIRE A CHANGE IN DOSAGE FROM THAT USED WITH ANIMAL-SOURCE INSULINS. IF AN ADJUSTMENT IS NEEDED, IT MAY OCCUR WITH THE FIRST DOSE OR DURING THE FIRST SEVERAL WEEKS OR MONTHS.

DIABETES

Insulin is a hormone produced by the pancreas, a large gland that lies near the stomach. This hormone is necessary for the body's correct use of food, especially sugar. Diabetes occurs when the pancreas does not make enough insulin to meet your body's needs.

To control your diabetes, your doctor has prescribed injections of insulin to keep your blood glucose at a nearly normal level. Proper control of your diabetes requires close and constant cooperation with your doctor. In spite of diabetes, you can lead an active, healthy, and useful life if you eat a balanced diet daily, exercise regularly, and take your insulin injections as prescribed.

You have been instructed to test your blood and/or your urine regularly for glucose. If your blood tests consistently show above- or below-normal glucose levels or your urine tests consistently show the presence of glucose, your diabetes is not properly controlled and you must let your doctor know.

Always keep an extra supply of insulin as well as a spare syringe and needle on hand. Always wear diabetic identification so that appropriate treatment can be given if complications occur away from home.

ULTRALENTE HUMAN INSULIN

Description

Humulin is synthesized in a special non-disease-producing laboratory strain of *Escherichia coli* bacteria that has been genetically altered by the addition of the gene for human insulin production. Humulin U is a crystalline suspension of human insulin with zinc providing a slower onset and a longer and less intense duration of activity (up to 28 hours) than regular insulin or the intermediate-acting insulins (NPH and Lente). The time course of action of any insulin may vary considerably in different individuals or at different times in the same individual. As with all insulin preparations, the duration of action of Humulin U is dependent on dose, site of injection, blood supply, temperature, and physical activity. Humulin U is a sterile suspension and is for subcutaneous injection only. It should not be used intravenously or intramuscularly. The concentration of Humulin U is 100 units/mL (U-100).

Identification

Human insulin manufactured by Eli Lilly and Company has the trademark Humulin and is available in 6 formula-

Continued on next page

* Identi-Code® symbol. This product information was prepared in June 1998. Current information on these and other products of Eli Lilly and Company may be obtained by direct inquiry to Lilly Research Laboratories, Lilly Corporate Center, Indianapolis, Indiana 46285, (800) 545-5979.

Humulin U—Cont.

tions—Regular (**R**), NPH (**N**), Lente (**L**), Ultralente (**U**), 50% Human Insulin Isophane Suspension [NPH]/50% Human Insulin Injection [buffered regular] (**50/50**), and 70% Human Insulin Isophane Suspension [NPH]/30% Human Insulin Injection [buffered regular] (**70/30**). Your doctor has prescribed the type of insulin that he/she believes is best for you. **DO NOT USE ANY OTHER INSULIN EXCEPT ON HIS/HER ADVICE AND DIRECTION.**

Always check the carton and the bottle label for the name and letter designation of the insulin you receive from your pharmacy to make sure it is the same as that your doctor has prescribed. Humulin U can be identified as follows: [See graphic at right]

Always examine the appearance of your bottle of insulin before withdrawing each dose. A bottle of Humulin U must be carefully shaken or rotated before each injection so that the contents are uniformly mixed. Humulin U should look uniformly cloudy or milky after mixing. Do not use it if the insulin substance (the white material) remains at the bottom of the bottle after mixing (Figure 1). Do not use a bottle of Humulin U if there are clumps in the insulin after mixing (Figure 2). Always check the appearance of your bottle of insulin before using, and if you note anything unusual in the appearance of your insulin or notice your insulin requirements changing markedly, consult your doctor.

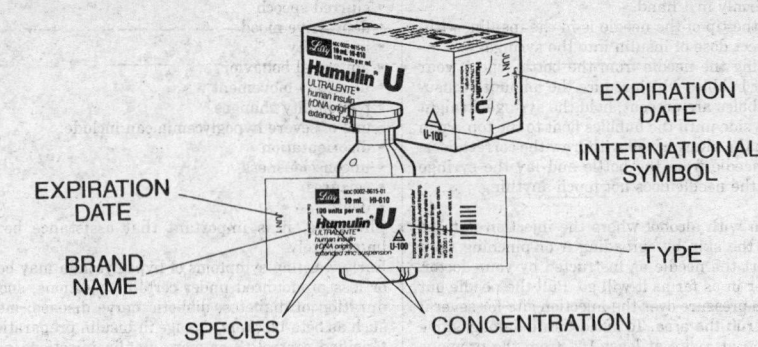

EXPIRATION DATE

INTERNATIONAL SYMBOL

TYPE

CONCENTRATION

EXPIRATION DATE

BRAND NAME

SPECIES

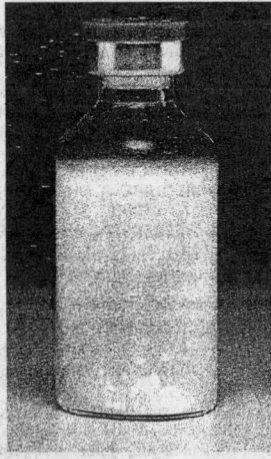

Fig 1.—Do not use if the insulin material remains at the bottom of the bottle after mixing.

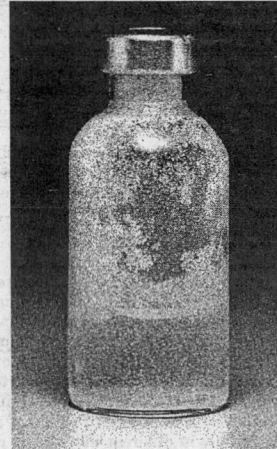

Fig 2.—Do not use if there are clumps in the insulin after mixing.

Storage

Insulin should be stored in a refrigerator but not in the freezer. If refrigeration is not possible, the bottle of insulin that you are currently using can be kept unrefrigerated as long as it is kept as cool as possible (below 86°F [30°C]) and away from heat and light. Do not use insulin if it has been frozen. Do not use a bottle of insulin after the expiration date stamped on the label.

INJECTION PROCEDURES

Correct Syringe

Doses of insulin are measured in **units**. U-100 insulin contains 100 units/mL (1 mL = 1 cc). With Humulin U, it is important to use a syringe that is marked for U-100 insulin preparations. Failure to use the proper syringe can lead to a mistake in dosage, causing serious problems for you, such as a blood glucose level that is too low or too high.

Syringe Use

To help avoid contamination and possible infection, follow these instructions exactly.

Disposable syringes and needles should be used only once and then discarded. **NEEDLES AND SYRINGES MUST NOT BE SHARED.**

Reusable syringes and needles must be sterilized before each injection. **Follow the package directions supplied with your syringe.** Described below are 2 methods of sterilizing.

Boiling

1. Put syringe, plunger, and needle in strainer, place in saucepan, and cover with water. Boil for 5 minutes.
2. Remove articles from water. When they have cooled, insert plunger into barrel, and fasten needle to syringe with a slight twist.
3. Push plunger in and out several times until water is completely removed.

Isopropyl Alcohol

If the syringe, plunger, and needle cannot be boiled, as when you are traveling, they may be sterilized by immersion for at least 5 minutes in Isopropyl Alcohol, 91%. Do not use bathing, rubbing, or medicated alcohol for this sterilization. If the syringe is sterilized with alcohol, it must be absolutely dry before use.

Preparing the Dose

1. Wash your hands.
2. Carefully shake or rotate the insulin bottle several times to completely mix the insulin.
3. Inspect the insulin. Humulin U should look uniformly cloudy or milky. Do not use it if you notice anything unusual in the appearance.
4. If using a new bottle, flip off the plastic protective cap, but **do not** remove the stopper. When using a new bottle, wipe the top of the bottle with an alcohol swab.
5. If you are mixing insulins, refer to the instructions for mixing that follow.
6. Draw air into the syringe equal to your insulin dose. Put the needle through rubber top of the insulin bottle and inject the air into the bottle.
7. Turn the bottle and syringe upside down. Hold the bottle and syringe firmly in 1 hand and shake gently.
8. Making sure the tip of the needle is in the insulin, withdraw the correct dose of insulin into the syringe.
9. Before removing the needle from the bottle, check your syringe for air bubbles which reduce the amount of insulin in it. If bubbles are present, hold the syringe straight up and tap its side until the bubbles float to the top. Push them out with the plunger and withdraw the correct dose.
10. Remove the needle from the bottle and lay the syringe down so that the needle does not touch anything.

Mixing Humulin U with Regular or Lente Human Insulin

1. Ultralente human insulin should be mixed with regular or Lente human insulin only on the advice of your doctor.
2. Draw air into your syringe equal to the amount of Humulin U you are taking. Insert the needle into the Humulin U bottle and inject the air. Withdraw the needle.
3. Now inject air into your regular or Lente human insulin bottle in the same manner, but **do not** withdraw the needle.
4. Turn the bottle and syringe upside down.
5. Making sure the tip of the needle is in the insulin, withdraw the correct dose of regular or Lente insulin into the syringe.
6. Before removing the needle from the bottle, check your syringe for air bubbles which reduce the amount of insulin in it. If bubbles are present, hold the syringe straight up and tap its side until the bubbles float to the top. Push them out with the plunger and withdraw the correct dose.
7. Remove the needle from the bottle of regular or Lente insulin and insert it into the bottle of Humulin U. Turn the bottle and syringe upside down. Hold the bottle and syringe firmly in 1 hand and shake gently. Making sure the tip of the needle is in the insulin, withdraw your dose of Humulin U.

8. Remove the needle and lay the syringe down so that the needle does not touch anything.

Follow your doctor's instructions on whether to mix your insulins ahead of time or just before giving your injection. It is important to be consistent in your method.

Syringes from different manufacturers may vary in the amount of space between the bottom line and the needle. Because of this, do not change:

- the sequence of mixing, or
- the model and brand of syringe or needle that the doctor has prescribed.

Injection

Cleanse the skin with alcohol where the injection is to be made. Stabilize the skin by spreading it or pinching up a large area. Insert the needle as instructed by your doctor. Push the plunger in as far as it will go. Pull the needle out and apply gentle pressure over the injection site for several seconds. **Do not rub the area.** To avoid tissue damage, give the next injection at a site at least $1/2''$ from the previous site.

DOSAGE

Your doctor has told you which insulin to use, how much, and when and how often to inject it. Because each patient's case of diabetes is different, this schedule has been individualized for you.

Your usual insulin dose may be affected by changes in your food, activity, or work schedule. Carefully follow your doctor's instructions to allow for these changes. Other things that may affect your insulin dose are:

Illness

Illness, especially with nausea and vomiting, may cause your insulin requirements to change. Even if you are not eating, you will still require insulin. You and your doctor should establish a sick day plan for you to use in case of illness. When you are sick, test your blood/urine frequently and call your doctor as instructed.

Pregnancy

Good control of diabetes is especially important for you and your unborn baby. Pregnancy may make managing your diabetes more difficult. If you are planning to have a baby, are pregnant, or are nursing a baby, consult your doctor.

Medication

Insulin requirements may be increased if you are taking other drugs with hyperglycemic activity, such as oral contraceptives, corticosteroids, or thyroid replacement therapy. Insulin requirements may be reduced in the presence of drugs with hypoglycemic activity, such as oral hypoglycemics, salicylates (for example, aspirin), sulfa antibiotics, and certain antidepressants. Always discuss any medications you are taking with your doctor.

Exercise

Exercise may lower your body's need for insulin during and for some time after the activity. Exercise may also speed up the effect of an insulin dose, especially if the exercise involves the area of injection site (for example, the leg should not be used for injection just prior to running). Discuss with your doctor how you should adjust your regimen to accommodate exercise.

Travel

Persons traveling across more than 2 time zones should consult their doctor concerning adjustments in their insulin schedule.

COMMON PROBLEMS OF DIABETES

Hypoglycemia (Insulin Reaction)

Hypoglycemia (too little glucose in the blood) is one of the most frequent adverse events experienced by insulin users. It can be brought about by:

1. Taking too much insulin
2. Missing or delaying meals
3. Exercising or working more than usual
4. An infection or illness (especially with diarrhea or vomiting)
5. A change in the body's need for insulin

6. Diseases of the adrenal, pituitary, or thyroid gland, or progression of kidney or liver disease

7. Interactions with other drugs that lower blood glucose, such as oral hypoglycemics, salicylates (for example, aspirin) sulfa antibiotics, and certain antidepressants

8. Consumption of alcoholic beverages

Symptoms of mild to moderate hypoglycemia may occur suddenly and can include:

• sweating
• dizziness
• palpitation
• tremor
• hunger
• restlessness
• tingling in the hands, feet, lips, or tongue
• lightheadedness
• inability to concentrate
• headache
• drowsiness
• sleep disturbances
• anxiety
• blurred vision
• slurred speech
• depressed mood
• irritability
• abnormal behavior
• unsteady movement
• personality changes

Signs of severe hypoglycemia can include:

• disorientation
• unconsciousness
• seizures
• death

Therefore, it is important that assistance be obtained immediately.

Early warning symptoms of hypoglycemia may be different or less pronounced under certain conditions, such as long duration of diabetes, diabetic nerve disease, medications such as beta-blockers, change in insulin preparations, or intensified control (3 or more insulin injections per day) of diabetes.

A few patients who have experienced hypoglycemic reactions after transfer from animal-source insulin to human insulin have reported that the early warning symptoms of hypoglycemia were less pronounced or different from those experienced with their previous insulin.

Without recognition of early warning symptoms, you may not be able to take steps to avoid more serious hypoglycemia. Be alert for all of the various types of symptoms that may indicate hypoglycemia. Patients who experience hypoglycemia without early warning symptoms should monitor their blood glucose frequently, especially prior to activities such as driving. If the blood glucose is below your normal fasting glucose, you should consider eating or drinking sugar-containing foods to treat your hypoglycemia.

Mild to moderate hypoglycemia may be treated by eating foods or drinks that contain sugar. Patients should always carry a quick source of sugar, such as candy mints or glucose tablets. More severe hypoglycemia may require the assistance of another person. Patients who are unable to take sugar orally or who are unconscious require an injection of glucagon or should be treated with intravenous administration of glucose at a medical facility.

You should learn to recognize your own symptoms of hypoglycemia. If you are uncertain about these symptoms, you should monitor your blood glucose frequently to help you learn to recognize the symptoms that you experience with hypoglycemia.

If you have frequent episodes of hypoglycemia or experience difficulty in recognizing the symptoms, you should consult your doctor to discuss possible changes in therapy, meal plans, and/or exercise programs to help you avoid hypoglycemia.

Hyperglycemia and Diabetic Acidosis

Hyperglycemia (too much glucose in the blood) may develop if your body has too little insulin. Hyperglycemia can be brought about by:

1. Omitting your insulin or taking less than the doctor has prescribed
2. Eating significantly more than your meal plan suggests
3. Developing a fever, infection, or other significant stressful situation

In patients with insulin-dependent diabetes, prolonged hyperglycemia can result in diabetic acidosis. The first symptoms of diabetic acidosis usually come on gradually, over a period of hours or days, and include a drowsy feeling, flushed face, thirst, loss of appetite, and fruity odor on the breath. With acidosis, urine tests show large amounts of glucose and acetone. Heavy breathing and a rapid pulse are more severe symptoms. If uncorrected, prolonged hyperglycemia or diabetic acidosis can lead to nausea, vomiting, dehydration, loss of consciousness or death. Therefore, it is important that you obtain medical assistance immediately.

Lipodystrophy

Rarely, administration of insulin subcutaneously can result in lipoatrophy (depression in the skin) or lipohypertrophy

(enlargement or thickening of tissue). If you notice either of these conditions, consult your doctor. A change in your injection technique may help alleviate the problem.

Allergy to Insulin

Local Allergy—Patients occasionally experience redness, swelling, and itching at the site of injection of insulin. This condition, called local allergy, usually clears up in a few days to a few weeks. In some instances, this condition may be related to factors other than insulin, such as irritants in the skin cleansing agent or poor injection technique. If you have local reactions, contact your doctor.

Systemic Allergy—Less common, but potentially more serious, is generalized allergy to insulin, which may cause rash over the whole body, shortness of breath, wheezing, reduction in blood pressure, fast pulse, or sweating. Severe cases of generalized allergy may be life threatening. If you think you are having a generalized allergic reaction to insulin, notify a doctor immediately.

ADDITIONAL INFORMATION

Additional information about diabetes may be obtained from your diabetes educator.

DIABETES FORECAST is a national magazine designed especially for patients with diabetes and their families and is available by subscription from the American Diabetes Association, National Service Center, 1660 Duke Street, Alexandria, Virginia 22314, 1-800-DIABETES (1-800-342-2383).

Another publication, **DIABETES COUNTDOWN**, is available from the Juvenile Diabetes Foundation, 432 Park Avenue South, New York, New York 10016-8013, 1-800-JDF-CURE (1-800-533-2873).

Additional information about Humulin can be obtained by calling 1-888-88-LILLY (1-888-885-4559).

Literature revised March 26, 1997

PA 6364 AMP   [032697]

LENTE® ILETIN® II   OTC

[lĕn-tā ī 'lĕ-tĭn]

(Insulin Zinc Suspension, USP, purified pork)

INFORMATION FOR THE PATIENT
WARNINGS

ANY CHANGE OF INSULIN SHOULD BE MADE CAUTIOUSLY AND ONLY UNDER MEDICAL SUPERVISION. CHANGES IN PURITY, STRENGTH, BRAND (MANUFACTURER), TYPE (REGULAR, NPH, LENTE®), SPECIES (BEEF, PORK, BEEF-PORK, HUMAN), AND/OR METHOD OF MANUFACTURE (RECOMBINANT DNA VERSUS ANIMAL-SOURCE INSULIN) MAY RESULT IN THE NEED FOR A CHANGE IN DOSAGE. IF AN ADJUSTMENT IS NEEDED, IT MAY OCCUR WITH THE FIRST DOSE OR DURING THE FIRST SEVERAL WEEKS OR MONTHS.

DIABETES

Insulin is a hormone produced by the pancreas, a large gland that lies near the stomach. This hormone is necessary for the body's correct use of food, especially sugar. Diabetes occurs when the pancreas does not make enough insulin to meet your body's needs.

To control your diabetes, your doctor has prescribed injections of insulin to keep your blood glucose at a nearly normal level. Proper control of your diabetes requires close and constant cooperation with your doctor. In spite of diabetes, you can lead an active, healthy, and useful life if you eat a balanced diet daily, exercise regularly, and take your insulin injections as prescribed.

You have been instructed to test your blood and/or your urine regularly for glucose. If your blood tests consistently show above- or below-normal glucose levels or your urine tests consistently show the presence of glucose, your diabetes is not properly controlled and you must let your doctor know.

Always keep an extra supply of insulin as well as a spare syringe and needle on hand. Always wear diabetic identification so that appropriate treatment can be given if complications occur away from home.

LENTE PORK INSULIN

Description

Lente pork insulin is obtained from pork pancreas. Lente® Iletin® II (purified insulin, Lilly) is an amorphous and crystalline suspension of insulin with zinc providing an intermediate-acting insulin with a slower onset and a longer duration of activity (slightly more than 24 hours) than regular insulin. The time course of action of any insulin may vary considerably in different individuals or at different times in the same individual. As with all insulin preparations, the duration of action of Lente Iletin II is dependent on dose, site of injection, blood supply, temperature, and physical activity. Lente Iletin II is a sterile suspension and is for subcutaneous injection only. It should not be used intravenously or intramuscularly. The concentration of Lente Iletin II is 100 units/mL (U-100).

Identification

This insulin, manufactured by Eli Lilly and Company, has the trademark Iletin II and is available in various types—Regular, NPH, and Lente. Your doctor has prescribed the type of insulin that he/she believes is best for you. **DO NOT USE ANY OTHER INSULIN EXCEPT ON HIS/HER ADVICE AND DIRECTION.**

Always check the carton and the bottle label for the name and letter designation of the insulin you receive from your pharmacy to make sure it is the same as that your doctor has prescribed.

Always examine the appearance of your bottle of insulin before withdrawing each dose. A bottle of Lente Iletin II must be carefully shaken or rotated before each injection so that the contents are uniformly mixed. Lente Iletin II should look uniformly cloudy or milky after mixing. Do not use it if the insulin substance (the white material) remains at the bottom of the bottle after mixing. Do not use a bottle of Lente Iletin II if there are clumps in the insulin after mixing. Always check the appearance of your bottle of insulin before using, and if you note anything unusual in the appearance of your insulin or notice your insulin requirements changing markedly, consult your doctor.

Storage

Insulin should be stored in a refrigerator but not in the freezer. If refrigeration is not possible, the bottle of insulin that you are currently using can be kept unrefrigerated as long as it is kept as cool as possible (below 86°F [30°C]) and away from heat and light. Do not use insulin if it has been frozen. Do not use a bottle of insulin after the expiration date stamped on the label.

INJECTION PROCEDURES

Correct Syringe

Doses of insulin are measured in **units**. U-100 insulin contains 100 units/mL (1 mL = 1 cc). With Lente Iletin II, it is important to use a syringe that is marked for U-100 insulin preparations. Failure to use the proper syringe can lead to a mistake in dosage, causing serious problems for you, such as a blood glucose level that is too low or too high.

Syringe Use

To help avoid contamination and possible infection, follow these instructions exactly.

Disposable syringes and needles should be used only once and then discarded. **NEEDLES AND SYRINGES MUST NOT BE SHARED.**

Reusable syringes and needles must be sterilized before each injection.

Follow the package directions supplied with your syringe. Described below are 2 methods of sterilizing.

Boiling

1. Put syringe, plunger, and needle in strainer, place in saucepan, and cover with water. Boil for 5 minutes.
2. Remove articles from water. When they have cooled, insert plunger into barrel, and fasten needle to syringe with a slight twist.
3. Push plunger in and out several times until water is completely removed.

Isopropyl Alcohol

If the syringe, plunger, and needle cannot be boiled, as when you are traveling, they may be sterilized by immersion for at least 5 minutes in Isopropyl Alcohol, 91%. Do not use bathing, rubbing, or medicated alcohol for this sterilization. If the syringe is sterilized with alcohol, it must be absolutely dry before use.

Preparing the Dose

1. Wash your hands.
2. Carefully shake or rotate the insulin bottle several times to completely mix the insulin.
3. Inspect the insulin. Lente Iletin II should look uniformly cloudy or milky. Do not use it if you notice anything unusual in the appearance.
4. If using a new bottle, flip off the plastic protective cap, but **do not** remove the stopper. When using a new bottle, wipe the top of the bottle with an alcohol swab.
5. If you are mixing insulins, refer to the Warnings below.
6. Draw air into the syringe equal to your insulin dose. Put the needle through rubber top of the insulin bottle and inject the air into the bottle.
7. Turn the bottle and syringe upside down. Hold the bottle and syringe firmly in 1 hand and shake gently.
8. Making sure the tip of the needle is in the insulin, withdraw the correct dose of insulin into the syringe.
9. Before removing the needle from the bottle, check your syringe for air bubbles which reduce the amount of insulin in it. If bubbles are present, hold the sy-

Continued on next page

---

* **Identi-Code® symbol. This product information was prepared in June 1998. Current information on these and other products of Eli Lilly and Company may be obtained by direct inquiry to Lilly Research Laboratories, Lilly Corporate Center, Indianapolis, Indiana 46285, (800) 545-5979.**

Lente Iletin II (Pork)—Cont.

ringe straight up and tap its side until the bubbles float to the top. Push them out with the plunger and withdraw the correct dose.
10. Remove the needle from the bottle and lay the syringe down so that the needle does not touch anything.

WARNINGS—SEE ADDITIONAL WARNINGS ABOVE

Patients who have been directed by their doctors to mix 2 types of insulin should be aware that insulin hypodermic syringes of different manufacturers may vary in the amount of space between the bottom line and the needle.
Because of this, do not change:
1. The order of mixing that the doctor has prescribed or
2. The model and brand of syringe or needle without first consulting your doctor.

The mixing should be done immediately prior to injection. Failure to heed this warning could result in a dosage error.

Injection

Cleanse the skin with alcohol where the injection is to be made. Stabilize the skin by spreading it or pinching up a large area. Insert the needle as instructed by your doctor. Push the plunger in as far as it will go. Pull the needle out and apply gentle pressure over the injection site for several seconds. **Do not rub the area.** To avoid tissue damage, give the next injection at a side at least 1/2" from the previous site.

DOSAGE

Your doctor has told you which insulin to use, how much, and when and how often to inject it. Because each patient's case of diabetes is different, this schedule has been individualized for you.
Your usual insulin dose may be affected by changes in your food, activity, or work schedule. Carefully follow your doctor's instructions to allow for these changes. Other things that may affect your insulin dose are:

Illness

Illness, especially with nausea and vomiting, may cause your insulin requirements to change. Even if you are not eating, you will still require insulin. You and your doctor should establish a sick day plan for you to use in case of illness. When you are sick, test your blood/urine frequently and call your doctor as instructed.

Pregnancy

Good control of diabetes is especially important for you and your unborn baby. Pregnancy may make managing your diabetes more difficult. If you are planning to have a baby, are pregnant, or are nursing a baby, consult your doctor.

Medication

Insulin requirements may be increased if you are taking other drugs with hyperglycemic activity, such as oral contraceptives, corticosteroids, or thyroid replacement therapy. Insulin requirements may be reduced in the presence of drugs with hypoglycemic activity, such as oral hypoglycemics, salicylates (for example, aspirin), sulfa antibiotics, and certain antidepressants. Always discuss any medications you are taking with your doctor.

Exercise

Exercise may lower your body's need for insulin during and for some time after the activity. Exercise may also speed up the effect of an insulin dose, especially if the exercise involves the area of injection site (for example, the leg should not be used for injection just prior to running). Discuss with your doctor how you should adjust your regimen to accommodate exercise.

Travel

Persons traveling across more than 2 time zones should consult their doctor concerning adjustments in their insulin schedule.

COMMON PROBLEMS OF DIABETES

Hypoglycemia (Insulin Reaction)

Hypoglycemia (too little glucose in the blood) is one of the most frequent adverse events experienced by insulin users. It can be brought about by:
1. Taking too much insulin
2. Missing or delaying meals
3. Exercising or working more than usual
4. An infection or illness (especially with diarrhea or vomiting)
5. A change in the body's need for insulin
6. Diseases of the adrenal, pituitary, or thyroid gland, or progression of kidney or liver disease
7. Interactions with other drugs that lower blood glucose, such as oral hypoglycemics, salicylates (for example, aspirin), sulfa antibiotics, and certain antidepressants
8. Consumption of alcoholic beverages

Symptoms of mild to moderate hypoglycemia may occur suddenly and can include:
- sweating
- dizziness
- palpitation
- tremor
- hunger
- restlessness
- tingling in the hands, feet, lips, or tongue
- lightheadedness
- inability to concentrate
- headache
- drowsiness
- sleep disturbances
- anxiety
- blurred vision
- slurred speech
- depressive mood
- irritability
- abnormal behavior
- unsteady movement
- personality changes

Signs of severe hypoglycemia can include:
- disorientation
- unconsciousness
- seizures
- death

Therefore, it is important that assistance be obtained immediately.
Early warning symptoms of hypoglycemia may be different or less pronounced under certain conditions, such as long duration of diabetes, diabetic nerve disease, medications such as beta-blockers, change in insulin preparations, or intensified control (3 or more insulin injections per day) of diabetes.
Without recognition of early warning symptoms, you may not be able to take steps to avoid more serious hypoglycemia. Be alert for all of the various types of symptoms that may indicate hypoglycemia. Patients who experience hypoglycemia without early warning symptoms should monitor their blood glucose frequently, especially prior to activities such as driving. If the blood glucose is below your normal fasting glucose, you should consider eating or drinking sugar-containing foods to treat your hypoglycemia.
Mild to moderate hypoglycemia may be treated by eating foods or taking drinks that contain sugar. Patients should always carry a quick source of sugar, such as candy mints or glucose tablets. More severe hypoglycemia may require the assistance of another person. Patients who are unable to take sugar orally or who are unconscious require an injection of glucagon or should be treated with intravenous administration of glucose at a medical facility.
You should learn to recognize your own symptoms of hypoglycemia. If you are uncertain about these symptoms, you should monitor your blood glucose frequently to help you learn to recognize the symptoms that you experience with hypoglycemia.
If you have frequent episodes of hypoglycemia or experience difficulty in recognizing the symptoms, you should consult your doctor to discuss possible changes in therapy, meal plans, and/or exercise programs to help you avoid hypoglycemia.

Hyperglycemia and Diabetic Acidosis

Hyperglycemia (too little glucose in the blood) may develop if your body has too little insulin. Hyperglycemia can be brought about by:
1. Omitting your insulin or taking less than the doctor has prescribed
2. Eating significantly more than your meal plan suggests
3. Developing a fever or infection

In patients with insulin-dependent diabetes, prolonged hyperglycemia can result in diabetic acidosis. The first symptoms of diabetic acidosis usually come on gradually, over a period of hours or days, and include a drowsy feeling, flushed face, thirst, loss of appetite, and fruity odor on the breath. With acidosis, urine tests show large amounts of glucose and acetone. Heavy breathing and a rapid pulse are more severe symptoms. If uncorrected, prolonged hyperglycemia or diabetic acidosis can result in loss of consciousness or death. Therefore, it is important that you obtain medical assistance immediately.

Lipodystrophy

Rarely, administration of insulin subcutaneously can result in lipoatrophy (depression in the skin) or lipohypertrophy (enlargement or thickening of tissue). If you notice either of these conditions, consult your doctor. A change in your injection technique may help alleviate the problem.

Allergy to Insulin

Local Allergy—Patients occasionally experience redness, swelling, and itching at the site of injection of insulin. This condition, called local allergy, usually clears up in a few days to a few weeks. In some instances, this condition may be related to factors other than insulin, such as irritants in the skin cleansing agent or poor injection technique. If you have local reactions, contact your doctor.
Systemic Allergy—Less common, but potentially more serious, is generalized allergy to insulin, which may cause rash over the whole body, shortness of breath, wheezing, reduction in blood pressure, fast pulse, or sweating. Severe cases of generalized allergy may be life threatening. If you think you are having a generalized allergic reaction to insulin, notify a doctor immediately.

ADDITIONAL INFORMATION

Additional information about diabetes may be obtained from your diabetes educator.
DIABETES FORECAST is a national magazine designed especially for patients with diabetes and their families and is available by subscription from the American Diabetes Association, National Service Center, 1660 Duke Street, Alexandria, Virginia 22314.
Another publication, **DIABETES COUNTDOWN**, is available from the Juvenile Diabetes Foundation, 432 Park Avenue South, New York, New York 10016–8013.
Literature revised May 23, 1995
PA8548AMP [052395]

NPH ILETIN® II **OTC**
[*ĕn 'pē-āch ī 'lĕ-tĭn*]
(Isophane Insulin Suspension, USP, purified pork)

INFORMATION FOR THE PATIENT

WARNINGS

ANY CHANGE OF INSULIN SHOULD BE MADE CAUTIOUSLY AND ONLY UNDER MEDICAL SUPERVISION. CHANGES IN PURITY, STRENGTH, BRAND (MANUFACTURER), TYPE (REGULAR, NPH, LENTE®), SPECIES (BEEF, PORK, BEEF-PORK, HUMAN), AND/OR METHOD OF MANUFACTURE (RECOMBINANT DNA VERSUS ANIMAL-SOURCE INSULIN) MAY RESULT IN THE NEED FOR A CHANGE IN DOSAGE. IF AN ADJUSTMENT IS NEEDED, IT MAY OCCUR WITH THE FIRST DOSE OR DURING THE FIRST SEVERAL WEEKS OR MONTHS.

DIABETES

Insulin is a hormone produced by the pancreas, a large gland that lies near the stomach. This hormone is necessary for the body's correct use of food, especially sugar. Diabetes occurs when the pancreas does not make enough insulin to meet your body's needs.
To control your diabetes, your doctor has prescribed injections of insulin to keep your blood glucose at a nearly normal level. Proper control of your diabetes requires close and constant cooperation with your doctor. In spite of diabetes, you can lead an active, healthy, and useful life if you eat a balanced diet daily, exercise regularly, and take your insulin injections as prescribed.
You have been instructed to test your blood and/or your urine regularly for glucose. If your blood tests consistently show above- or below-normal glucose levels or your urine tests consistently show the presence of glucose, your diabetes is not properly controlled and you must let your doctor know.
Always keep an extra supply of insulin as well as a spare syringe and needle on hand. Always wear diabetic identification so that appropriate treatment can be given if complications occur away from home.

NPH PORK INSULIN

Description

NPH pork insulin is obtained from pork pancreas.
NPH Iletin® II (purified insulin, Lilly) is a crystalline suspension of insulin with protamine and zinc providing an intermediate-acting insulin with a slower onset of action and a longer duration of activity (slightly more than 24 hours) than that of regular insulin. The time course of action of any insulin may vary considerably in different individuals or at different times in the same individual. As with all insulin preparations, the duration of action of NPH Iletin II is dependent on dose, site of injection, blood supply, temperature, and physical activity. NPH Iletin II is a sterile suspension and is for subcutaneous injection only. It should not be used intravenously or intramuscularly. The concentration of NPH Iletin II is 100 units/mL (U-100).

Identification

This insulin, manufactured by Eli Lilly and Company, has the trademark Iletin II and is available in various types—Regular, NPH, and Lente. Your doctor has prescribed the type of insulin that he/she believes is best for you. **DO NOT USE ANY OTHER INSULIN EXCEPT ON HIS/HER ADVICE AND DIRECTION.**
Always check the carton and the bottle label for the name and letter designation of the insulin you receive from your pharmacy to make sure it is the same as that your doctor has prescribed.
Always examine the appearance of your bottle of insulin before withdrawing each dose. A bottle of NPH Iletin II must be carefully shaken or rotated before each injection so that the contents are uniformly mixed. NPH Iletin II should look uniformly cloudy or milky after mixing. Do not use it if the insulin substance (the white material) remains at the bottom of the bottle after mixing. Do not use a bottle of NPH Iletin II if there are clumps in the insulin after mixing. Always check the appearance of your bottle of insulin before using, and if you note anything unusual in the appearance of your insulin or notice your insulin requirements changing markedly, consult your doctor.

Storage

Insulin should be stored in a refrigerator but not in the freezer. If refrigeration is not possible, the bottle of insulin that you are currently using can be kept unrefrigerated as long as it is kept as cool as possible (below 86°F [30°C]) and away from heat and light. Do not use insulin if it has been frozen. Do not use a bottle of insulin after the expiration date stamped on the label.

INJECTION PROCEDURES

Correct Syringe

Doses of insulin are measured in **units**. U-100 insulin contains 100 units/mL (1 mL = 1 cc). With NPH Iletin II, it is important to use a syringe that is marked for U-100 insulin preparations. Failure to use the proper syringe can lead to a mistake in dosage, causing serious problems for you, such as a blood glucose level that is too low or too high.

Syringe Use

To help avoid contamination and possible infection, follow these instructions exactly.

Disposable syringes and needles should be used only once and then discarded. **NEEDLES AND SYRINGES MUST NOT BE SHARED.**

Reusable syringes and needles must be sterilized before each injection.

Follow the package directions supplied with your syringe. Described below are 2 methods of sterilizing.

Boiling

1. Put syringe, plunger, and needle in strainer, place in saucepan, and cover with water. Boil for 5 minutes.
2. Remove articles from water. When they have cooled, insert plunger into barrel, and fasten needle to syringe with a slight twist.
3. Push plunger in and out several times until water is completely removed.

Isopropyl Alcohol

If the syringe, plunger, and needle cannot be boiled, as when you are traveling, they may be sterilized by immersion for at least 5 minutes in Isopropyl Alcohol, 91%. Do not use bathing, rubbing, or medicated alcohol for this sterilization. If the syringe is sterilized with alcohol, it must be absolutely dry before use.

Preparing the Dose

1. Wash your hands.
2. Carefully shake or rotate the insulin bottle several times to completely mix the insulin.
3. Inspect the insulin. NPH Iletin II should look uniformly cloudy or milky. Do not use it if you notice anything unusual in the appearance.
4. If using a new bottle, flip off the plastic protective cap, but **do not** remove the stopper. When using a new bottle, wipe the top of the bottle with an alcohol swab.
5. If you are mixing insulins, refer to the Warnings below.
6. Draw air into the syringe equal to your insulin dose. Put the needle through rubber top of the insulin bottle and inject the air into the bottle.
7. Turn the bottle and syringe upside down. Hold the bottle and syringe firmly in 1 hand and shake gently.
8. Making sure the tip of the needle is in the insulin, withdraw the correct dose of insulin into the syringe.
9. Before removing the needle from the bottle, check your syringe for air bubbles which reduce the amount of insulin in it. If bubbles are present, hold the syringe straight up and tap its side until the bubbles float to the top. Push them out with the plunger and withdraw the correct dose.
10. Remove the needle from the bottle and lay the syringe down so that the needle does not touch anything.

WARNINGS—SEE ADDITIONAL WARNINGS ABOVE

Patients who have been directed by their doctors to mix 2 types of insulin should be aware that insulin hypodermic syringes of different manufacturers may vary in the amount of space between the bottom line and the needle.

Because of this, do not change:

1. The order of mixing that the doctor has prescribed or
2. The model and brand of syringe or needle without first consulting your doctor.

The mixing should be done immediately prior to injection. Failure to heed this warning could result in a dosage error.

Injection

Cleanse the skin with alcohol where the injection is to be made. Stabilize the skin by spreading it or pinching up a large area. Insert the needle as instructed by your doctor. Push the plunger in as far as it will go. Pull the needle out and apply gentle pressure over the injection site for several seconds. **Do not rub the area.** To avoid tissue damage, give the next tissue damage, give the next injection at a site at least ¹/₂″ from the previous site.

DOSAGE

Your doctor has told you which insulin to use, how much, and when and how often to inject it. Because each patient's case of diabetes is different, this schedule has been individualized for you.

Your usual insulin dose may be affected by changes in your food, activity, or work schedule. Carefully follow your doctor's instructions to allow for these changes. Other things that may affect your insulin dose are:

Illness

Illness, especially with nausea and vomiting, may cause your insulin requirements to change. Even if you are not eating, you will still require insulin. You and your doctor should establish a sick day plan for you to use in case of illness. When you are sick, test your blood/urine frequently and call your doctor as instructed.

Pregnancy

Good control of diabetes is especially important for you and your unborn baby. Pregnancy may make managing your diabetes more difficult. If you are planning to have a baby, are pregnant, or are nursing a baby, consult your doctor.

Medication

Insulin requirements may be increased if you are taking other drugs with hyperglycemic activity, such as oral contraceptives, corticosteroids, or thyroid replacement therapy. Insulin requirements may be reduced in the presence of drugs with hypoglycemic activity, such as oral hypoglycemics, salicylates (for example, aspirin), sulfa antibiotics, and certain antidepressants. Always discuss any medications you are taking with your doctor.

Exercise

Exercise may lower your body's need for insulin during and for some time after the activity. Exercise may also speed up the effect of an insulin dose, especially if the exercise involves the area of injection site (for example, the leg should not be used for injection prior to running). Discuss with your doctor how you should adjust your regimen to accommodate exercise.

Travel

Persons traveling across more than 2 times zones should consult their doctor concerning adjustments in their insulin schedule.

COMMON PROBLEMS OF DIABETES

Hypoglycemia (Insulin Reaction)

Hypoglycemia (too little glucose in the blood) is one of the most frequent adverse events experienced by insulin users. It can be brought about by:

1. Taking too much insulin
2. Missing or delaying meals
3. Exercising or working more than usual
4. An infection or illness (especially with diarrhea or vomiting)
5. A change in the body's need for insulin
6. Diseases of the adrenal, pituitary, or thyroid gland, or progression of kidney or liver disease
7. Interactions with other drugs that lower blood glucose, such as oral hypoglycemics, salicylates (for example, aspirin), sulfa antibiotics, and certain antidepressants
8. Consumption of alcoholic beverages

Symptoms of mild to moderate hypoglycemia may occur suddenly and can include:

- sweating
- dizziness
- palpitation
- tremor
- hunger
- restlessness
- tingling in the hands, feet, lips, or tongue
- lightheadedness
- inability to concentrate
- headache
- drowsiness
- sleep disturbances
- anxiety
- blurred vision
- slurred speech
- depressive mood
- irritability
- abnormal behavior
- unsteady movement
- personality changes

Signs of severe hypoglycemia can include:

- disorientation
- unconsciousness
- seizures
- death

Therefore, it is important that assistance be obtained immediately

Early warning symptoms of hypoglycemia may be different or less pronounced under certain conditions, such as long duration of diabetes, diabetic nerve disease, medications such as beta-blockers, change in insulin preparations, or intensified control (3 or more insulin injections per day) of diabetes.

Without recognition of early warning symptoms, you may not be able to take steps to avoid more serious hypoglycemia. Be alert for all of the various types of symptoms that may indicate hypoglycemia. Patients who experience hypoglycemia without early warning symptoms should monitor their blood glucose frequently, especially prior to activities

such as driving. If the blood glucose is below your normal fasting glucose, you should consider eating or drinking sugar-containing foods to treat your hypoglycemia.

Mild to moderate hypoglycemia may be treated by eating foods or taking drinks that contain sugar. Patients should always carry a quick source of sugar, such as candy mints or glucose tablets. More severe hypoglycemia may require the assistance of another person. Patients who are unable to take sugar orally or who are unconscious require an injection of glucagon or should be treated with intravenous administration of glucose at a medical facility.

You should learn to recognize your own symptoms of hypoglycemia. If you are uncertain about these symptoms, you should monitor your blood glucose frequently to help you learn to recognize the symptoms that you experience with hypoglycemia.

If you have frequent episodes of hypoglycemia or experience difficulty in recognizing the symptoms, you should consult your doctor to discuss possible changes in therapy, meal plans, and/or exercise programs to help you avoid hypoglycemia.

Hyperglycemia and Diabetic Acidosis

Hyperglycemia (too much glucose in the blood) may develop if your body has too little insulin. Hyperglycemia can be brought about by:

1. Omitting your insulin or taking less than the doctor has prescribed
2. Eating significantly more than your meal plan suggests
3. Developing a fever or infection

In patients with insulin-dependent diabetes, prolonged hyperglycemia can result in diabetic acidosis. The first symptoms of diabetic acidosis usually come on gradually, over a period of hours or days, and include a drowsy feeling, flushed face, thirst, loss of appetite, and fruity odor on the breath. With acidosis, urine tests show large amounts of glucose and acetone. Heavy breathing and a rapid pulse are more severe symptoms. If uncorrected, prolonged hyperglycemia or diabetic acidosis can result in loss of consciousness or death. Therefore, it is important that you obtain medical assistance immediately.

Lipodystrophy

Rarely, administration of insulin subcutaneously can result in lipoatrophy (depression in the skin) or lipohypertrophy (enlargement or thickening of tissue). If you notice either of these conditions, consult your doctor. A change in your injection technique may help alleviate the problem.

Allergy to Insulin

Local Allergy—Patients occasionally experience redness, swelling, and itching at the site of injection of insulin. This condition, called local allergy, usually clears up in a few days to a few weeks. In some instances, this condition may be related to factors other than insulin, such as irritants in the skin cleansing agent or poor injection technique. If you have local reactions, contact your doctor.

Systemic Allergy—Less common, but potentially more serious, is generalized allergy to insulin, which may cause rash over the whole body, shortness of breath, wheezing, reduction in blood pressure, fast pulse, or sweating. Severe cases of generalized allergy may be life threatening. If you think you are having a generalized allergic reaction to insulin, notify a doctor immediately.

ADDITIONAL INFORMATION

Additional information about diabetes may be obtained from your diabetes educator.

DIABETES FORECAST is a national magazine designed especially for patients with diabetes and their families and is available by subscription from the American Diabetes Association, National Service Center, 1660 Duke Street, Alexandria, Virginia 22314.

Another publication, **DIABETES COUNTDOWN**, is available from the Juvenile Diabetes Foundation, 432 Park Avenue South, New York, New York 10016–8013.

Literature revised October 28, 1992
PA8516AMP   [102892]

REGULAR ILETIN® II   **OTC**
[rĕg-ū-lĕr ī 'lĕ-tĭn]
(Insulin Injection, USP, purified pork)

INFORMATION FOR THE PATIENT
WARNINGS

ANY CHANGE OF INSULIN SHOULD BE MADE CAUTIOUSLY AND ONLY UNDER MEDICAL SUPERVISION. CHANGES IN PURITY, STRENGTH, BRAND (MANUFAC-

Continued on next page

Regular Iletin II (Pork)—Cont.

TURER), TYPE (REGULAR, NPH, LENTE®), SPECIES (BEEF, PORK, BEEF-PORK, HUMAN), AND/OR METHOD OF MANUFACTURE (RECOMBINANT DNA VERSUS ANIMAL-SOURCE INSULIN) MAY RESULT IN THE NEED FOR A CHANGE IN DOSAGE. IF AN ADJUSTMENT IS NEEDED, IT MAY OCCUR WITH THE FIRST DOSE OR DURING THE FIRST SEVERAL WEEKS OR MONTHS.

DIABETES

Insulin is a hormone produced by the pancreas, a large gland that lies near the stomach. This hormone is necessary for the body's correct use of food, especially sugar. Diabetes occurs when the pancreas does not make enough insulin to meet your body's needs.

To control your diabetes, your doctor has prescribed injections of insulin to keep your blood glucose at a nearly normal level. Proper control of your diabetes requires close and constant cooperation with your doctor. In spite of diabetes, you can lead an active, healthy, and useful life if you eat a balanced diet daily, exercise regularly, and take your insulin injections as prescribed.

You have been instructed to test your blood and/or your urine regularly for glucose. If your blood tests consistently show above- or below-normal glucose levels or your urine tests consistently show the presence of glucose, your diabetes is not properly controlled and you must let your doctor know.

Always keep an extra supply of insulin as well as a spare syringe and needle on hand. Always wear diabetic identification so that appropriate treatment can be given if complications occur away from home.

REGULAR PORK INSULIN
Description

Regular pork insulin is obtained from pork pancreas. Regular Iletin® II (purified insulin, Lilly) consists of zinc-insulin crystals dissolved in a clear fluid. Regular Iletin II has had nothing added to change the speed or length of its action. It takes effect rapidly and has a relatively short duration of activity (4 to 12 hours) as compared with other insulins. The time course of action of any insulin may vary considerably in different individuals or at different times in the same individual. As with all insulin preparations, the duration of action of Regular Iletin II is dependent on dose, site of injection, blood supply, temperature, and physical activity. Regular Iletin II is a sterile solution and is for subcutaneous injection. It should not be used intramuscularly. The concentration of Regular Iletin II is 100 units/mL (U-100).

Identification

This insulin, manufactured by Eli Lilly and Company, has the trademark Iletin II and is available in various types—Regular, NPH, and Lente. Your doctor has prescribed the type of insulin that he/she believes is best for you. **DO NOT USE ANY OTHER INSULIN EXCEPT ON HIS/HER ADVICE AND DIRECTION.**

Always check the carton and the bottle label for the name and letter designation of the insulin you receive from your pharmacy to make sure it is the same as that your doctor has prescribed.

Always examine the appearance of your bottle of insulin before withdrawing each dose. Regular Iletin II is a clear and colorless liquid with a water-like appearance and consistency. Do not use if it appears cloudy, thickened, or slightly colored or if solid particles are visible. Always check the appearance of your bottle of insulin before using, and if you note anything unusual in the appearance of your insulin or notice your insulin requirements changing markedly, consult your doctor.

Storage

Insulin should be stored in a refrigerator but not in the freezer. If refrigeration is not possible, the bottle of insulin that you are currently using can be kept unrefrigerated as long as it is kept as cool as possible (below 86°F [30°C]) and away from heat and light. Do not use insulin if it has been frozen. Do not use a bottle of insulin after the expiration date stamped on the label.

INJECTION PROCEDURES
Correct Syringe

Doses of insulin are measured in **units.** U-100 insulin contains 100 units/mL (1 mL=1 cc). With Regular Iletin II, it is important to use a syringe that is marked for U-100 insulin preparations. Failure to use the proper syringe can lead to a mistake in dosage, causing serious problems for you, such as a blood glucose level that is too low or too high.

Syringe Use

To help avoid contamination and possible infection, follow these instructions exactly.

Disposable syringes and needles should be used only once and then discarded. **NEEDLES AND SYRINGES MUST NOT BE SHARED.**

Reusable syringes and needles must be sterilized before each injection. **Follow the package directions supplied with your syringe.** Described below are 2 methods of sterilizing.

Boiling

1. Put syringe, plunger, and needle in strainer, place in saucepan, and cover with water. Boil for 5 minutes.
2. Remove articles from water. When they have cooled, insert plunger into barrel, and fasten needle to syringe with a slight twist.
3. Push plunger in and out several times until water is completely removed.

Isopropyl Alcohol

If the syringe, plunger, and needle cannot be boiled, as when you are traveling, they may be sterilized by immersion for at least 5 minutes in Isopropyl Alcohol, 91%. Do not use bathing, rubbing, or medicated alcohol for this sterilization. If the syringe is sterilized with alcohol, it must be absolutely dry before use.

Preparing the Dose

1. Wash your hands.
2. Inspect the insulin. Regular Iletin II should look clear and colorless. Do not use Regular Iletin II if it appears cloudy, thickened, or slightly colored or if solid particles are visible.
3. If using a new bottle, flip off the plastic protective cap, but **do not** remove the stopper. When using a new bottle, wipe the top of the bottle with an alcohol swab.
4. If you are mixing insulins, refer to the Warnings below.
5. Draw air into the syringe equal to your insulin dose. Put the needle through rubber top of the insulin bottle and inject the air into the bottle.
6. Turn the bottle and syringe upside down. Hold the bottle and syringe firmly in 1 hand.
7. Making sure the tip of the needle is in the insulin, withdraw the correct dose of insulin into the syringe.
8. Before removing the needle from the bottle, check your syringe for air bubbles which reduce the amount of insulin in it. If bubbles are present, hold the syringe straight up and tap its side until the bubbles float to the top. Push them out with the plunger and withdraw the correct dose.
9. Remove the needle from the bottle and lay the syringe down so that the needle does not touch anything.

WARNINGS—SEE ADDITIONAL WARNINGS ABOVE

Patients who have been directed by their doctors to mix 2 types of insulin should be aware that insulin hypodermic syringes of different manufacturers may vary in the amount of space between the bottom line and the needle.

Because of this, do not change:
1. The order of mixing that the doctor has prescribed or
2. The model and brand of syringe or needle without first consulting your doctor.

The mixing should be done immediately prior to injection. Failure to heed this warning could result in a dosage error.

Injection

Cleanse the skin with alcohol where the injection is to be made. Stabilize the skin by spreading it or pinching up a large area. Insert the needle as instructed by your doctor. Push the plunger in as far as it will go. Pull the needle out and apply gentle pressure over the injection site for several seconds. **Do not rub the area.** To avoid tissue damage, give the next injection at a site at least $\frac{1}{2}''$ from the previous site.

DOSAGE

Your doctor has told you which insulin to use, how much, and when and how often to inject it. Because each patient's case of diabetes is different, this schedule has been individualized for you.

Your usual insulin dose may be affected by changes in your food, activity, or work schedule. Carefully follow your doctor's instructions to allow for these changes. Other things that may affect your insulin dose are:

Illness

Illness, especially with nausea and vomiting, may cause your insulin requirements to change. Even if you are not eating, you will still require insulin. You and your doctor should establish a sick day plan for you to use in case of illness. When you are sick, test your blood/urine frequently and call your doctor as instructed.

Pregnancy

Good control of diabetes is especially important for you and your unborn baby. Pregnancy may make managing your diabetes more difficult. If you are planning to have a baby, are pregnant, or are nursing a baby, consult your doctor.

Medication

Insulin requirements may be increased if you are taking other drugs with hyperglycemic activity, such as oral contraceptives, corticosteroids, or thyroid replacement therapy. Insulin requirements may be reduced in the presence of drugs with hypoglycemic activity, such as oral hypoglycemics, salicylates (for example, aspirin), sulfa antibiotics, and certain antidepressants. Always discuss any medications you are taking with your doctor.

Exercise

Exercise may lower your body's need for insulin during and for some time after the activity. Exercise may also speed up the effect of an insulin dose, especially if the exercise involves the area of injection site (for example, the leg should not be used for injection just prior to running). Discuss with your doctor how you should adjust your regimen to accommodate exercise.

Travel

Persons traveling across more than 2 time zones should consult their doctor concerning adjustments in their insulin schedule.

COMMON PROBLEMS OF DIABETES
Hypoglycemia (Insulin Reaction)

Hypoglycemia (too little glucose in the blood) is one of the most frequent adverse events experienced by insulin users. It can be brought about by:
1. Taking too much insulin
2. Missing or delaying meals
3. Exercising or working more than usual
4. An infection or illness (especially with diarrhea or vomiting)
5. A change in the body's need for insulin
6. Diseases of the adrenal, pituitary, or thyroid gland, or progression of kidney or liver disease
7. Interactions with other drugs that lower blood glucose, such as oral hypoglycemics, salicylates (for example, aspirin), sulfa antibiotics, and certain antidepressants
8. Consumption of alcoholic beverages

Symptoms of mild to moderate hypoglycemia may occur suddenly and can include:
- sweating
- dizziness
- palpitation
- tremor
- hunger
- restlessness
- tingling in the hands, feet, lips, or tongue
- lightheadedness
- inability to concentrate
- headache
- drowsiness
- sleep disturbances
- anxiety
- blurred vision
- slurred speech
- depressive mood
- irritability
- abnormal behavior
- unsteady movement
- personality changes

Signs of severe hypoglycemia can include:
- disorientation
- unconsciousness
- seizures
- death

Therefore, it is important that assistance be obtained immediately.

Early warning symptoms of hypoglycemia may be different or less pronounced under certain conditions, such as long duration of diabetes, diabetic nerve disease, medications such as beta-blockers, change in insulin preparations, or intensified control (3 or more insulin injections per day) of diabetes.

Without recognition of early warning symptoms, you may not be able to take steps to avoid more serious hypoglycemia. Be alert for all of the various types of symptoms that may indicate hypoglycemia. Patients who experience hypoglycemia without early warning symptoms should monitor their blood glucose frequently, especially prior to activities such as driving. If the blood glucose is below your normal fasting glucose, you should consider eating or drinking sugar-containing foods to treat your hypoglycemia.

Mild to moderate hypoglycemia may be treated by eating foods or taking drinks that contain sugar. Patients should always carry a quick source of sugar, such as candy mints or glucose tablets. More severe hypoglycemia may require the assistance of another person. Patients who are unable to take sugar orally or who are unconscious require an injection of glucagon or should be treated with intravenous administration of glucose at a medical facility.

You should learn to recognize your own symptoms of hypoglycemia. If you are uncertain about these symptoms, you should monitor your blood glucose frequently to help you learn to recognize the symptoms that you experience with hypoglycemia.

If you have frequent episodes of hypoglycemia or experience difficulty in recognizing the symptoms, you should consult your doctor to discuss possible changes in therapy, meal plans, and/or exercise programs to help you avoid hypoglycemia.

Hyperglycemia and Diabetic Acidosis

Hyperglycemia (too much glucose in the blood) may develop if your body has too little insulin. Hyperglycemia can be brought about by:
1. Omitting your insulin or taking less than the doctor has prescribed
2. Eating significantly more than your meal plan suggests
3. Developing a fever or infection

In patients with insulin-dependent diabetes, prolonged hyperglycemia can result in diabetic acidosis. The first symptoms of diabetic acidosis usually come on gradually, over a period of hours or days, and include a drowsy feeling, flushed face, thirst, loss of appetite, and fruity odor on the breath. With acidosis, urine tests show large amounts of glucose and acetone. Heavy breathing and a rapid pulse are more severe symptoms. If uncorrected, prolonged hyperglycemia or diabetic acidosis can result in loss of consciousness or death. Therefore, it is important that you obtain medical assistance immediately.

Lipodystrophy

Rarely, administration of insulin subcutaneously can result in lipoatrophy (depression in the skin) or lipohypertrophy (enlargement or thickening of tissue). If you notice either of these conditions, consult your doctor. A change in your injection technique may help alleviate the problem.

Allergy to Insulin

Local Allergy —Patients occasionally experience redness, swelling, and itching at the site of injection of insulin. This condition, called local allergy, usually clears up in a few days to a few weeks. In some instances, this condition may be related to factors other than insulin, such as irritants in the skin cleansing agent or poor injection technique. If you have local reactions, contact your doctor.

Systemic Allergy —Less common, but potentially serious, is generalized allergy to insulin, which may cause rash over the whole body, shortness of breath, wheezing, reduction in blood pressure, fast pulse, or sweating. Severe cases of generalized allergy may be life threatening. If you think you are having a generalized allergic reaction to insulin, notify a doctor immediately.

ADDITIONAL INFORMATION

Additional information about diabetes may be obtained from your diabetes educator.

DIABETES FORECAST is a national magazine designed especially for patients with diabetes and their families and is available by subscription from the American Diabetes Association, National Service Center, 1660 Duke Street, Alexandria, Virginia 22314.

Another publication, **DIABETES COUNTDOWN**, is available from the Juvenile Diabetes Foundation, 432 Park Avenue South, New York, New York 10016–8013.

Literature revised October 28, 1992

PA 8486 AMP [102892]

KEFUROX® ℞

[*kĕf 'yū-rŏeks*]

(sterile cefuroxime sodium)

USP

DESCRIPTION

Cefuroxime is a semisynthetic, broad spectrum cephalosporin antibiotic for intravenous administration. It is the sodium salt of (6R.7R) 3-carbamoyloxymethyl-7-[Z-2-methoxyimino-2-(fur-2-yl)acetamiodo]ceph-3-em-4-carboxylate, and it has the following structural formula:

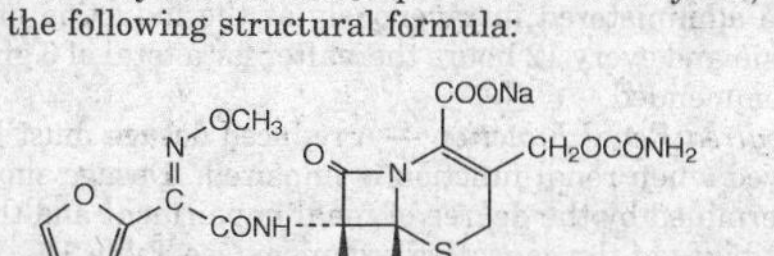

The chemical formula is $C_{16}H_{15}N_4NaO_8S$, and the molecular weight is 446.37.

Kefurox contains approximately 54.2 mg (2.4 mEq) of sodium per gram of cefuroxime activity.

Kefurox in sterile crystalline form is supplied in vials equivalent to 750 mg. 1.5 g. or 7.5 g of cefuroxime as cefuroxime sodium. Solutions of Kefurox range in color from light yellow to amber, depending on the concentration and diluent used. The pH of freshly constituted solutions usually ranges from 4.5–8.5.

CLINICAL PHARMACOLOGY

Following IV doses of 750 mg and 1.5 g, serum concentrations were approximately 50 and 100 mcg/mL, respectively, at 15 minutes. Therapeutic serum concentrations of approximately 2 mcg/mL or more were maintained for 5.3 hours and 8 hours or more, respectively. There was no evidence of accumulation of cefuroxime in the serum following IV administration of 1.5-g doses every 8 hours to normal volunteers. The serum half-life after IV injections is approximately 80 minutes.

Approximately 89% of a dose of cefuroxime is excreted by the kidneys over an 8-hour period, resulting in high urinary concentrations.

Intravenous doses of 750 mg and 1.5 g produced urinary levels averaging 1,150 and 2,500 mcg/mL, respectively, during the first 8-hour period.

The concomitant oral administration of probenecid with cefuroxime slows tubular secretion, decreases renal clearance by approximately 40%, increases the peak serum level by approximately 30%, and increases the serum half-life by approximately 30%. Cefuroxime is detectable in therapeutic concentrations in pleural fluid, joint fluid, bile, sputum, bone, cerebrospinal fluid (in patients with meningitis), and aqueous humor.

Cefuroxime is approximately 50% bound to serum protein.

Microbiology: Cefuroxime has *in vitro* activity against a wide range of gram-positive and gram-negative organisms, and it is highly stable in the presence of beta-lactamases of certain gram-negative bacteria. The bactericidal action of cefuroxime results from inhibition of cell-wall synthesis.

Cefuroxime is usually active against the following organisms *in vitro*.

Aerobes, Gram-positive: *Staphylococcus aureus; Staphylococcus epidermidis; Streptococcus pneumoniae;* and *Streptococcus pyogenes* (and other streptococci).

NOTE: Most strains of enterococci, e.g., *Enterococcus faecalis* (formerly *Streptococcus faecalis*), are resistant to cefuroxime Methicillin-resistant staphylococci and *Listeria monocytogenes* are resistant to cefuroxime.

Aerobes, Gram-negative: *Citrobacter* spp. *Enterobacter* spp., *Escherichia coli; Haemophilus influenzae* (including ampicillin-resistant strains); *Haemophilus parainfluenzae; Klebsiella* spp. (including *Klebsiella pneumoniae); Moraxella (Branhamella) catarrhalis* (including ampicillin- and cephalothin-resistant strains); *Morganella morganii* (formerly *Proteus morganii*); *Neisseria gonorrhoeae* (including penicillinase- and non-penicillinase-producing strains); *Neisseria meningitidis; Proteus mirabilis; Providencia rettgeri* (formerly *Proteus rettgeri*); *Salmonella* spp.; and *Shigella* spp.

NOTE: Some strains of *Morganella morganii, Enterobacter cloacae*, and *Citrobacter* spp. have been shown by *in vitro* tests to be resistant to cefuroxime and other cephalosporins. *Pseudomonas* and *Campylobacter* spp., *Acinetobacter calcoaceticus*, and most strains of *Serratia* spp. and *Proteus vulgaris* are resistant to most first- and second-generation cephalosporins.

Anaerobes: Gram-positive and gram-negative cocci (including *Peptococcus* and *Peptostreptococcus* spp); gram-positive bacilli (including *Clostridium* spp); gram-negative bacilli (including *Bacteroides* and *Fusobacterium* spp).

NOTE: *Clostridium difficile* and most strains of *Bacteroides fragilis* are resistant to cefuroxime.

Susceptibility Tests: ***Diffusion Techniques:*** Quantitative methods that require measurement of zone diameters give an estimate of antibiotic susceptibility. One such standard procedure[1] that has been recommended for use with disks to test susceptibility of organisms to cefuroxime uses the 30-mcg cefuroxime disk. Interpretation involves the correlation of the diameters obtained in the disk test with minimum inhibitory concentration (MIC) for cefuroxime.

A report of "Susceptible" indicates that the pathogen is likely to be inhibited by generally achievable blood levels. A report of "Moderately Susceptible" suggests that the organism would be susceptible if high dosage is used or if the infection is confined to tissues and fluids in which high antibiotic levels are attained. A report of "Intermediate" suggests an equivocable or indeterminate result. A report of "Resistant" indicates that achievable concentrations of the antibiotic are unlikely to be inhibitory and other therapy should be selected.

Reports from the laboratory giving results of the standard single-disk susceptibility test for organisms other than *Haemophilus* spp. and *Neisseria gonorrhoeae* with a 30-mcg cefuroxime disk should be interpreted according to the following criteria:

Zone Diameter (mm)	Interpretation
≥ 18	(S) Susceptible
15-17	(MS) Moderately Susceptible
≤ 14	(R) Resistant

Results for *Haemophilus* spp. should be interpreted according to the following criteria:

Zone Diameter (mm)	Interpretation
≥ 24	(S) Susceptible
21-23	(I) Intermediate
≤ 20	(R) Resistant

Results for *Neisseria gonorrhoeae* should be interpreted according to the following criteria:

Zone Diameter (mm)	Interpretation
≥ 31	(S) Susceptible
26-30	(MS) Moderately Susceptible
≤ 25	(R) Resistant

Organisms should be tested with the cefuroxime disk since cefuroxime has been shown by *in vitro* tests to be active against certain strains found resistant when other beta-lactam disks are used. The cefuroxime disk should not be used for testing susceptibility to other cephalosporins.

Standardized procedures require the use of laboratory control organisms. The 30-mcg cefuroxime disk should give the following zone diameters

1. Testing for organisms other than *Haemophilus* ssp. and *Neisseria gonorrhoeae:*

Organism	Zone Diameter (mm)
Staphylococcus aureus ATCC 25923	27-35
Escherichia coli ATCC 25922	20-26

2. Testing for *Haemophilus* spp.:

Organism	Zone Diameter (mm)
Haemophilus influenzae ATCC 49766	28-36

3. Testing for *Neisseria gonorrhoeae:*

Organism	Zone Diameter (mm)
Neisseria gonorrhoeae ATCC 49226	33-41
Staphylococcus aureus ATCC 25923	29-33

Dilution Techniques: Use a standardized dilution method[1] (broth, agar, microdilution) or equivalent with cefuroxime powder. The MIC values obtained for bacterial isolates other than *Haemophilus* spp. and *Neisseria gonorrhoeae* should be interpreted according to the following criteria:

MIC (mcg/mL)	Interpretation
≤ 8	(S) Susceptible
16	(MS) Moderately Susceptible
≥ 32	(R) Resistant

MIC values obtained for *Haemophilus* spp. should be interpreted according to the following criteria:

MIC (mcg/mL)	Interpretation
≤ 4	(S) Susceptible
8	(I) Intermediate
≥ 16	(R) Resistant

MIC values obtained for *Neisseria gonorrhoeae* should be interpreted according to the following criteria:

MIC (mcg/mL)	Interpretation
≤ 1	(S) Susceptible
2	(MS) Moderately Susceptible
≥ 4	(R) Resistant

As with standard diffusion techniques, dilution methods require the use of laboratory control organisms. Standard cefuroxime powder should provide the following MIC values.

1. For organisms other than *Haemophilus* spp. and *Neisseria gonorrhoeae:*

Organism	MIC (mcg/mL)
Staphylococcus aureus ATCC 29213	0.5-2.0
Escherichia coli ATCC 25922	2.0-8.0

2. For *Haemophilus* spp.:

Organism	MIC (mcg/mL)
Haemophilus influenzae ATCC 49766	0.25-1.0

3. For *Neisseria gonorrhoeae:*

Organism	MIC (mcg/mL)
Neisseria gonorrhoeae ATCC 49226	0.25-1.0
Staphylococcus aureus ATCC 29213	0.25-1.0

INDICATIONS AND USAGE

Kefurox is indicated for the treatment of patients with infections caused by susceptible strains of the designated organisms in the following diseases:

1. **Lower Respiratory Tract Infections**, including pneumonia, caused by *Streptococcus pneumoniae, Haemophilus influenzae* (including ampicillin-resistant strains), *Klebsiella* spp., *Staphylococcus aureus*, (penicillinase- and non-penicillinase-producing strains). *Streptococcus pyogenes*, and *Escherichia coli*.
2. **Urinary Tract Infections** caused by *Escherichia coli* and *Klebsiella* spp.
3. **Skin and Skin Structure Infections** caused by *Staphylococcus aureus* (penicillinase- and non-penicillinase-producing strains) *Streptococcus pyogenes, Escherichia coli, Klebsiella* spp., and *Enterobacter* spp.

Continued on next page

*** Identi-Code® symbol. This product information was prepared in June 1998. Current information on these and other products of Eli Lilly and Company may be obtained by direct inquiry to Lilly Research Laboratories, Lilly Corporate Center, Indianapolis, Indiana 46285, (800) 545-5979.**

Kefurox—Cont.

4. **Septicemia** caused by *Staphylococcus aureus* (penicillinase- and non-penicillinase-producing strains). *Streptococcus pneumoniae, Escherichia coli, Haemophilus influenzae* (including ampicillin-resistant strains), and *Klebsiella* spp.
5. **Meningitis** caused by *Streptococcus pneumoniae, Haemophilus influenzae* (including ampicillin-resistant strains). *Neisseria meningitidis*, and *Staphylococcus aureus* (penicillinase- and non-penicillinase-producing strains) (See PRECAUTIONS).
6. **Gonorrhea**—Uncomplicated and disseminated gonococcal infections due to *Neisseria gonorrhoeae* (penicillinase- and non-penicillinase-producing strains) in both males and females.
7. **Bone and Joint Infections** caused by *Staphylococcus aureus* (penicillinase- and non-penicillinase-producing strains).

Clinical microbiological studies in skin and skin structure infections frequently reveal the growth of susceptible strains of both aerobic and anaerobic organisms. Kefurox has been used successfully in these mixed infections in which several organisms have been isolated. Appropriate cultures and susceptibility studies should be performed to determine the susceptibility of the causative organisms to Kefurox (sterile cefuroxime sodium).

Therapy may be started while awaiting the results of these studies; however, once these results become available, the antibiotic treatment should be adjusted accordingly. In certain cases of confirmed or suspected gram-positive or gram-negative sepsis or in patients with other serious infections in which the causative organism has not been identified, Kefurox may be used concomitantly with an aminoglycoside (see PRECAUTIONS). The recommended doses of both antibiotics may be given depending on the severity of the infection and the patient's condition.

Prevention: The preoperative prophylactic administration of Kefurox may prevent the growth of susceptible disease-causing bacteria and, thereby, may reduce the incidence of certain postoperative infections in patients undergoing surgical procedures (e.g., vaginal hysterectomy) that are classified as clean-contaminated or potentially contaminated procedures. Effective prophylactic use of antibiotics in surgery depends on the time of administration. Kefurox should usually be given one-half to 1 hour before the operation to allow sufficient time to achieve effective antibiotic concentrations in the wound tissues during the procedure. The dose should be repeated intraoperatively if the surgical procedure is lengthy.

Prophylactic administration is usually not required after the surgical procedure ends and should be stopped within 24 hours. In the majority of surgical procedures, continuing prophylactic administration of any antibiotic does not reduce the incidence of subsequent infections but will increase the possibility of adverse reactions and the development of bacterial resistance.

The perioperative use of Kefurox has also been effective during open heart surgery for surgical patients in whom infections at the operative site would present a serious risk. For these patients, it is recommended that Kefurox therapy be continued for at least 48 hours after the surgical procedure ends. If an infection is present, specimens for culture should be obtained for the identification of the causative organism and appropriate antimicrobial therapy should be instituted.

CONTRAINDICATIONS

Kefurox is contraindicated in patients with known allergy to the cephalosporin group of antibiotics.

WARNINGS

BEFORE THERAPY WITH KEFUROX IS INSTITUTED, CAREFUL INQUIRY SHOULD BE MADE TO DETERMINE WHETHER THE PATIENT HAS HAD PREVIOUS HYPERSENSITIVITY REACTIONS TO CEPHALOSPORINS, PENICILLINS, OR OTHER DRUGS. THIS PRODUCT SHOULD BE GIVEN CAUTIOUSLY TO PENICILLIN-SENSITIVE PATIENTS. ANTIBIOTICS SHOULD BE ADMINISTERED WITH CAUTION TO ANY PATIENT WHO HAS DEMONSTRATED SOME FORM OF ALLERGY, PARTICULARLY TO DRUGS. IF AN ALLERGIC REACTION TO KEFUROX (STERILE CEFUROXIME SODIUM) OCCURS, DISCONTINUE THE DRUG. SERIOUS ACUTE HYPERSENSITIVITY REACTIONS MAY REQUIRE EPINEPHRINE AND OTHER EMERGENCY MEASURES.

Pseudomembranous colitis has been reported with the use of cephalosporins (and other broad-spectrum antibiotics); therefore, it is important to consider its diagnosis in patients who develop diarrhea in association with antibiotic use.

Treatment with broad-spectrum antibiotics alters the normal flora of the colon and may permit overgrowth of clostridia. Studies indicate a toxin produced by *Clostridium difficile* is one primary cause of antibiotic-associated colitis. Cholestyramine and colestipol resins have been shown to bind the toxin *in vitro*.

Mild cases of colitis may respond to drug discontinuation alone. Moderate to severe cases should be managed with fluid, electrolyte, and protein supplementation as indicated. When the colitis is not relieved by drug discontinuation or when it is severe, oral vancomycin is the treatment of choice for antibiotic-associated pseudomembranous colitis produced by *Clostridium difficile.* Other causes of colitis should also be considered.

PRECAUTIONS

General: Although Kefurox rarely produces alterations in kidney function, evaluation of renal status during therapy is recommended, especially in seriously ill patients receiving the maximum doses. Cephalosporins should be given with caution to patients receiving concurrent treatment with potent diuretics as these regimens are suspected of adversely affecting renal function.

The total daily dose of Kefurox should be reduced in patients with transient or persistent renal insufficiency (*see* DOSAGE AND ADMINISTRATION) because high and prolonged serum antibiotic concentrations can occur in such individuals from usual doses.

As with other antibiotics, prolonged use of Kefurox may result in overgrowth of nonsusceptible organisms. Careful observation of the patient is essential. If superinfection occurs during therapy, appropriate measures should be taken.

Broad-spectrum antibiotics should be prescribed with caution in individuals with a history of gastrointestinal disease, particularly colitis.

Nephrotoxicity has been reported following concomitant administration of aminoglycoside antibiotics and cephalosporins.

As with other therapeutic regimens used in the treatment of meningitis, mild-to-moderate hearing loss has been reported in some pediatric patients treated with cefuroxime sodium. Persistence of positive CSF (cerebrospinal fluid) cultures at 18 to 36 hours, particularly in patients with *Haemophilus influenzae* isolates, has also been noted; however, the precise clinical impact of this is unknown.

Drug/Laboratory Test Interactions: A false-positive reaction for glucose in the urine may occur with copper reduction tests (Benedict's or Fehling's solution or with Clinitest® tablets) but not with enzyme-based tests for glycosuria (e.g., Tes-Tape®, Glucose Enzymatic Test Strips, USP). As a false-negative result may occur in the ferricyanide test, it is recommended that either the glucose oxidase or hexokinase method be used to determine blood plasma glucose levels in patients receiving Kefurox.

Cefuroxime does not interfere with the assay of serum and urine creatinine by the the alkaline picrate method.

Carcinogenesis, Mutagenesis, and Impairment of Fertility—Although no long-term studies in animals have been performed to evaluate carcinogenic potential, no mutagenic potential of cefuroxime was found in standard laboratory tests.

Reproductive studies revealed no impairment of fertility in animals.

Pregnancy: Teratogenic Effects—Pregnancy Category B —Reproduction studies have been performed in mice and rabbits at doses up to 60 times the human dose and have revealed no evidence of impaired fertility or harm to the fetus due to cefuroxime. There are, however, no adequate well-controlled studies in pregnant women. Because animal reproduction studies are not always predictive of human response, this drug should be used during pregnancy only if clearly needed.

Nursing Mothers —Since Kefurox is excreted in human milk, caution should be exercised when Kefurox (sterile cefuroxime sodium) is administered to a nursing woman.

Pediatric Use —Safety and effectiveness in pediatric patients below the age of 3 months have not been established. Accumulation of other members of the cephalosporin class in newborn infants (with resulting prolongation of drug half-life) has been reported.

ADVERSE REACTIONS

Kefurox is generally well tolerated. The most common adverse effects have been local reactions following IV administration. Other adverse reactions have been encountered only rarely.

Local Reactions —Thrombophlebitis has occurred with IV administration in 1 in 60 patients.

Gastrointestinal —Gastrointestinal symptoms occurred in 1 in 150 patients and included diarrhea (1 in 220 patients) and nausea (1 in 440 patients). Onset of pseudomembranous colitis symptoms may occur during or after antibiotic treatment. (see WARNINGS).

Hypersensitivity Reactions —Hypersensitivity reactions have been reported in fewer than 1% of the patients treated with Kefurox and include rash (1 in 125). Pruritus and urticaria and positive Coombs' test each occurred in less than 1 in 250 patients, and, as with other cephalosporins, rare cases of anaphylaxis, drug fever, erthema multiforme, toxic epidermal necrolysis, and Stevens-Johnson syndrome have occurred.

Blood —A decrease in hemoglobin and hematocrit has been observed in 1 in 10 patients and transient eosinophilia in 1 in 14 patients. Less common reactions seen were transient neutropenia (fewer than 1 in 100 patients) and leukopenia (1 in 750 patients). A similar pattern and incidence were seen with other cephalosporins used in controlled studies. As with other cephalosporins, there have been rare reports of thrombocytopenia.

Hepatic —Transient rise in AST (SGOT) and ALT (SGPT) (1 in 25 patients), alkaline phosphatase (1 in 50 patients), LDH (1 in 75 patients), and bilirubin (1 in 500 patients) levels has been noted.

Kidney —Elevations in serum creatinine and/or blood urea nitrogen and a decreased creatinine clearance have been observed, but their relationship to cefuroxime is unknown.

In addition to the adverse reactions listed above that have been observed in patients treated with cefuroxime, the following adverse reactions and altered laboratory tests have been reported for cephalosporin-class antibiotics:

Adverse Reactions: vomiting, abdominal pain, colitis, vaginitis including vaginal candidiasis, toxic nephropathy, hepatic dysfunction including cholestasis, aplastic anemia, hemolytic anemia, hemorrhage.

Several cephalosporins have been implicated in triggering seizures, particularly in patients with renal impairment when the dosage was not reduced (see DOSAGE AND ADMINISTRATION). If seizures associated with drug therapy should occur, the drug should be discontinued. Anticonvulsant therapy can be given if clinically indicated.

Altered Laboratory Tests: Prolonged prothrombin time, pancytopenia, agranulocytosis.

OVERDOSAGE

Overdosage of cephalosporins can cause cerebral irritation leading to convulsions. Serum levels of cefuroxime can be reduced by hemodialysis and peritoneal dialysis.

DOSAGE AND ADMINISTRATION

DOSAGE: Adults—The usual adult dosage range for Kefurox (sterile cefuroxime sodium) is 750 mg to 1.5 grams every 8 hours, usually for 5 to 10 days. In uncomplicated urinary tract infections, skin and skin structure infections, disseminated gonococcal infections, and uncomplicated pneumonia, a 750-mg dose every 8 hours is recommended. In severe or complicated infections, a 1.5-g dose every 8 hours is recommended.

In bone and joint infections, a dosage of 1.5 gram dose every 8 hours is recommended. In clinical trials, surgical intervention was performed, when indicated as an adjunct to Kefurox therapy. A course of oral antibiotics was administered when appropriate following the completion of parenteral administration of Kefurox.

In life-threatening infections or infections due to less susceptible organisms, 1.5 grams every 6 hours may be required. In bacterial meningitis, the dose should not exceed 3 grams every 8 hours. For preventive use for clean-contaminated or potentially contaminated surgical procedures, a 1.5-gram dose administered intravenously just before surgery (approximately one-half to 1 hour before the initial incision) is recommended. Thereafter, give 750 mg intravenously every 8 hours when the procedure is prolonged.

For preventive use during open heart surgery, a 1.5-gram dose administered intravenously at the induction of anesthesia and every 12 hours thereafter for a total of 6 grams is recommended.

Impaired Renal Function — A reduced dosage must be employed when renal function is impaired,. Dosage should be determined by the degree of renal impairment and the susceptibility of the causative organism (see Table 1).

TABLE 1: Dosage of Kefurox in Adults With Reduced Renal Function

Creatinine Clearance (mL/min)	Dose	Frequency
>20	750 mg–1.5 g	q 8 h
10–20	750 mg	q 12 h
<10	750 mg	q 24 h*

* Since Kefurox is dialyzable, patients on hemodialysis should be given a further dose at the end of the dialysis.

When only serum creatinine is available, the following formula[2] (based on sex, weight, and age of the patient) may be used to convert this value into creatinine clearance. The serum creatinine should represent a steady state of renal function.

$$\text{Males: Creatinine Clearance (mL/min)} = \frac{\text{Weight (kg)} \times (140 - \text{age})}{72 \times \text{serum creatinine (mg/dL)}}$$

Females: 0.85 × male value

Note: As with antibiotic therapy in general, administration of Kefurox should be continued for a minimum of 48 to 72 hours after the patient becomes asymptomatic or after evidence of bacterial eradication has been obtained; a minimum of 10 days of treatment is recommended in infections

TABLE 2: Preparation of Solution

Strength	Amount of Diluent to Be Added (mL)		Volume to Be Withdrawn (mL)	Approximate Concentration (mg/mL)
750 mg/10 mL vial	7	(IV)	Total	100
1.5 g/20 mL vial	14	(IV)	Total	100
750 mg/100 mL bottle	50	(IV)	—	15
750 mg/100 mL bottle	100	(IV)	—	7.5
1.5 g/100 mL bottle	50	(IV)	—	30
1.5 g/100 mL bottle	100	(IV)	—	15
750 mg/ADD-Vantage	50	(IV)	—	15
750 mg/ADD-Vantage	100	(IV)	—	7.5
1.5 g/ADD-Vantage	50	(IV)	—	30
1.5 g/ADD-Vantage	100	(IV)	—	15

caused by *Streptococcus pyogenes* in order to guard against the risk of rheumatic fever or glomerulonephritis; frequent bacteriologic and clinical appraisal is necessary during therapy of chronic urinary tract infection and may be required for several months after therapy has been completed; persistent infections may require treatment for several weeks; and doses smaller than those indicated above should not be used. In staphylococcal and other infections involving a collection of pus, surgical drainage should be carried out where indicated.

Infants and Children Above 3 Months of Age —Administration of 50 to 100 mg/kg/day in equally divided doses, every 6 to 8 hours, has been successful for most infections susceptible to cefuroxime. The higher dose of 100 mg/kg/day (not to exceed the maximum adult dosage) should be used for the more severe or serious infections.

In bone and joint infections, 150 mg/kg per day (not to exceed the maximum adult dose) is recommended in equally divided doses every 8 hours. In clinical trials, a course of oral antibiotics was administered to children following the completion of parenteral administration of Kefurox.

In cases of bacterial meningitis, a larger dosage of Kefurox is recommended, 200 to 240 mg/kg per day intravenously in divided doses every 6 to 8 hours.

In children with renal insufficiency, the frequency of dosage should be modified to be consistent with the recommendations for adults.

Preparation of Solution: The directions for preparing Kefurox (sterile cefuroxime sodium) for IV use is summarized in Table 2.

For Intravenous Use: Each 750-mg vial/10-mL should be constituted with 7 mL of sterile water for injection. Withdraw completely the resulting solution for injection.

Each 1.5-g vial should be constituted with 14 mL of sterile water for injection, and the solution should be completely withdrawn for injection.

[See table 2 above]

Administration: After constitution, Kefurox may be given intravenously.

Intravenous Administration —The IV route may be preferable for patients with bacterial septicemia or other severe or life-threatening infections or for patients who may be poor risks because of lowered resistance, particularly if shock is present or impending.

For Direct Intermittent IV Administration —Slowly inject the solution into a vein over a period of 3 to 5 minutes or give it through the tubing system by which the patient is also receiving IV solutions.

For Intermittent IV Infusion with a Y-Type Administration Set —Dosing can be accomplished through the tubing system by which the patient may be receiving other IV solutions.

However, during infusion of the solution containing Kefurox, it is advisable to temporarily discontinue administration of any other solutions at the same site.

ADD-Vantage® vials are to be constituted only with 50 or 100 mL of 5% dextrose injection, 0.9% sodium chloride injection, or 0.45% sodium chloride injection in Abbott ADD-Vantage flexible diluent containers (see Instructions for Constitution). ADD-Vantage vials that have been joined to Abbott ADD-Vantage diluent containers and activated to dissolve the drug are stable for 24 hours at room temperature or for 7 days under refrigeration. Joined vials that have not been activated may be used within a 14-day period; this period corresponds to that for use of Abbott ADD-Vantage containers following removal of the outer packaging (overwrap).

Freezing solutions of Kefurox in the ADD-Vantage system is not recommended.

DIRECTIONS FOR USE OF KEFUROX (sterile cefuroxime sodium) IN ADD-VANTAGE® VIALS

To Open Diluent Container:

Peel overwrap at corner and remove solution container. Some opacity of the plastic due to moisture absorption during the sterilization process may be observed. This is normal and does not affect the solution quality or safety. The opacity will diminish gradually.

To Assemble Vial and Flexible Diluent Container: (Use Aseptic Technique)

1. Remove the protective covers from the top of the vial and the vial port on the diluent container as follows:
   a. To remove the breakaway vial cap, swing the pull ring over the top of the vial and pull down far enough to start the opening (SEE FIGURE 1), then pull straight up to remove the cap. (SEE FIGURE 2.)
   NOTE: Do not access vial with syringe.
   b. To remove the vial port cover, grasp the tab on the pull ring, pull up to break the 3 tie strings, then pull back to remove the cover. (SEE FIGURE 3.)

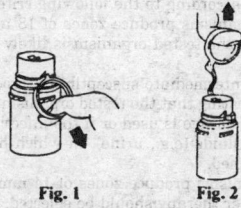

Fig. 1   Fig. 2

2. Screw the vial into the vial port until it will go no further. THE VIAL MUST BE SCREWED IN TIGHTLY TO ASSURE A SEAL. This occurs approximately ½ turn (180°) after the first audible click. (SEE FIGURE 4.) The clicking sound does not assure a seal; the vial must be turned as far as it will go.
   NOTE: Once vial is sealed, do not attempt to remove. (SEE FIGURE 4.)
3. Recheck the vial to assure that it is tight by trying to turn it further in the direction of assembly.
4. Label appropriately

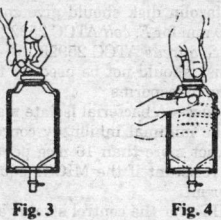

Fig. 3   Fig. 4

To Reconstitute the Drug:

1. Squeeze the bottom of the diluent container gently to inflate the portion of the container surrounding the end of the drug vial.
2. With the other hand, push the drug vial down into the container telescoping the walls of the container. Grasp the inner cap of the vial through the walls of the container. (SEE FIGURE 5.)
3. Pull the inner cap from the drug vial. (SEE FIGURE 6.) Verify that the rubber stopper has been pulled out, allowing the drug and diluent to mix.
4. Mix container contents throroughly and use within the specified time.

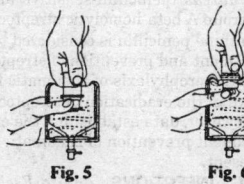

Fig. 5   Fig. 6

For Continuous IV Infusion —A solution of Kefurox may be added to an IV bottle containing one of the following fluids: 0.9% sodium chloride injection, 5% dextrose injection, 10% dextrose injection, 5% dextrose and 0.9% sodium chloride injection, 5% dextrose and 0.45% sodium chloride injection, or 1/6 M sodium lactate injection

Solutions of Kefurox, like those of most beta-lactam antibiotics, should not be added to solutions of aminoglycoside antibiotics because of potential interaction.

However, if concurrent therapy with Kefurox (sterile cefuroxime sodium) and an aminoglycoside is indicated, each of these antibiotics can be administered separately to the same patient.

Compatibility and Stability —Intravenous—When the 750-mg and 1.5-g vials are constituted as directed with sterile water for injection, the Kefurox solutions for IV administration maintain satisfactory potency for 24 hours at room temperature and for 48 hours (750-mg and 1.5-g vials under refrigeration (5°C). More dilute solutions, such as 750 mg or 1.5 g plus 100 mL of sterile water for injection, 5% dextrose injection, or 0.9% sodium chloride injection, also maintain satisfactory potency for 24 hours at room temperature and for 7 days under refrigeration.

These solutions may be further diluted to concentrations of between 1 and 30 mg/mL in the following solutions and will lose not more than 10% activity for 24 hours at room temperature or for at least 7 days under refrigeration: 0.9% sodium chloride injection, 1/6 M sodium lactate injection, ringer's injection, USP; lactated ringer's injection, USP, 5% dextrose and 0.9% sodium chloride injection; 5% dextrose injection; 5% dextrose and 0.45% sodium chloride injection; 5% dextrose and 0.225% sodium chloride injection; 10% dextrose injection; and 10% invert sugar in water for injection. Unused solutions should be discarded after the time periods mentioned above.

Kefurox has also been found compatible for 24 hours at room temperature when admixed in IV infusion with the following: Heparin (10 and 50 units/mL) in 0.9% sodium chloride injection, or potassium chloride (10 and 40 mEq/L) in 0.9% sodium chloride injection. Sodium bicarbonate injection, USP, is not recommended for the dilution of Kefurox.

The 750-mg and 1.5-g Kefurox ADD-Vantage vials, when diluted in 50 or 100 mL of 5% dextrose injection, 0.9% sodium chloride injection, or 0.45% sodium chloride injection, may be stored for up to 24 hours at room temperature or for 7 days under refrigeration.

Frozen Stability: Constitute the 750-mg and 1.5-g vial as directed for IV administration in Table 2. Immediately withdraw the total contents of the 750-mg or 1.5-g vial and add to a Viaflex® Mini-bag™ containing 50 or 100 mL of 0.9% sodium chloride injection or 5% dextrose injection and freeze. Frozen solutions are stable for 6 months when stored at –20 C. Frozen solutions should be thawed at room temperature and not refrozen. Do not force thaw by immersion in water baths or by microwave irradiation. Thawed solutions may be stored for up to 24 hours at room temperature or for 7 days in a refrigerator.

Note: Parenteral drug products should be inspected visually for particulate matter and discoloration before administration whenever solution and container permit.

As with other cephalosporins, Kefurox powder as well as solutions and suspensions tend to darken, depending on storage conditions, without adversely affecting product potency.

HOW SUPPLIED

Kefurox (sterile cefuroxime sodium) in the dry state should be stored between 15° and 30° C (59° and 86° F) and protected from light. Kefurox is a dry, white to off-white powder supplied in vials as follows:

Vials:
   750 mg,‡ 10-mL size (No. 7271)—(Traypak§ of 25) NDC 0002-7271-25
   1.5 g,‡ 20-mL size (No. 7272)—(Traypak of 10) NDC 0002-7272-10
   750 mg,‡ 100-mL size (No. 7273)—(Traypak of 10) NDC 0002-7273-10
   1.5 g,‡ 100-mL size (No. 7274)—(Traypak of 10) NDC 0002-7274-10

ADD-Vantage‖ Vials:
   750 mg,‡ (No. 7278)—(Traypak of 25) NDC 0002-7278-25
   1.5 g,‡ (No. 7279)—(Traypak of 10) NDC 0002-7279-10

The above ADD-Vantage Vials are to be used only with Abbott Laboratories' ADD-Vantage Antibiotic Diluent Container.

Also available:

Pharmacy Bulk Package:
   7.5 g,‡ 100-mL size (No. 7275)—(Traypak of 6) NDC 0002-7275-16

‡ Equivalent to cefuroxime.

§ Traypak™ (multivial carton, Lilly).

‖ ADD-Vantage® (vials and diluent containers, Abbott).

Continued on next page

* **Identi-Code® symbol. This product information was prepared in June 1998. Current information on these and other products of Eli Lilly and Company may be obtained by direct inquiry to Lilly Research Laboratories, Lilly Corporate Center, Indianapolis, Indiana 46285, (800) 545-5979.**

Kefurox—Cont.

REFERENCES:

1. National Committee for Clinical Laboratory Standards, *Performance Standards for Antimicrobial Susceptibility Testing* Third Informational Supplement. NCCLS Document M100–S3, Vol. 11, No. 17 Villanova, Pa NCCCLS: 1991.
2. Cockcroft DW, Gault MH Prediction of creatinine clearance from serum creatinine Nephron 1976:16:31–41.

CAUTION Federal (USA) law prohibits dispensing without prescription.
Literature issued Oct. 1, 1996.
Manufactured for **ELI LILLY AND COMPANY,**
Indianapolis, IN 46285, USA.
by BMH Limited, Philadelphia, PA 19101
KX:1.3

KEFZOL® ℞

[*kĕf 'zōl*]
CEFAZOLIN FOR INJECTION, USP

DESCRIPTION

Kefzol® (cefazolin for injection, USP) is a semi-synthetic cephalosporin for parenteral administration. It is the sodium salt of 3-{[(5-methyl-1,3,4-thiadiazol-2-yl)thio] methyl}-8-oxo-7-[2-(1*H*-tetrazol-1-yl)acetamido]-5-thia-1-azabicyclo[4.2.0]oct-2-ene-2-caboxylic acid.
Structural Formula:

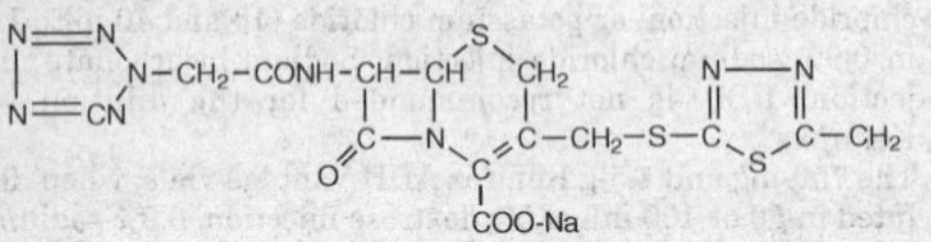

The sodium content is 46 mg per gram of cefazolin.
Kefzol in lyophilized form is supplied in vials equivalent to 500 mg or 1 gram of cefazolin: in "Piggyback" Vials for intravenous admixture equivalent to 1 gram of cefazolin; and in Pharmacy Bulk Vials equivalent to 10 grams of cefazolin.

CLINICAL PHARMACOLOGY

Human Pharmacology: After intramuscular administration of *Kefzol* to normal volunteers, the mean serum concentrations were 37 mcg/mL at one hour and 3 mcg/mL at eight hours following a 500 mg dose, and 64 mcg/mL at one hour and 7 mcg/mL at eight hours following a 1 gram dose.
Studies have shown that the following intravenous administration of *Kefzol* to normal volunteers, mean serum concentrations peaked at approximately 185 mcg/mL and were approximately 4 mcg/mL at eight hours for a 1 gram dose.
The serum half-life for *Kefzol* is approximately 1.8 hours following I.V. administration and approximately 2.0 hours following I.M. administration.
In a study (using normal volunteers) of constant intravenous infusion with dosages of 3.5 mg/kg for one hour (approximately 250 mg) and 1.5 mg/kg the next two hours (approximately 100 mg). *Kefzol* produced a steady serum level at the third hour of approximately 28 mcg/mL.
Studies in patients hospitalized with infections indicated that Kefzol (cefazolin for injection) produces mean peak serum levels approximately equivalent to those seen in normal volunteers.
Bile levels in patients without obstructive biliary disease can reach or exceed serum levels by up to five times; however, in patients with obstructive biliary disease, bile levels of *Kefzol* are considerably lower than serum levels (<1.0 mcg/mL).
In synovial fluid, the *Kefzol* level becomes comparable to that reached in serum at about four hours after drug administration.
Studies of cord blood show prompt transfer of *Kefzol* across the placenta. *Kefzol* is present in very low concentrations in the milk of nursing mothers.
Kefzol is excreted unchanged in the urine. In the first six hours approximately 60% of the drug is excreted in the urine and this increases to 70%–80% within 24 hours. *Kefzol* achieves peak urine concentrations of approximately 2400 mcg/mL and 4000 mcg/mL respectively following 500 mg and 1 gram intramuscular doses.
In patients undergoing peritoneal dialysis (2 L/hr.), *Kefzol* produced mean serum levels of approximately 10 and 30 mcg/mL after 24 hours' instillation of a dialyzing solution containing 50 mg/L and 150 mg/L, respectively. Mean peak levels were 29 mcg/mL (range 13–44 mcg/mL) with 50 mg/L (three patients), and 72 mcg/mL (range 26–142 mcg/mL) with 150 mg/L (six patients). Intraperitoneal administration of *Kefzol* is usually well tolerated.
Controlled studies on adult normal volunteers, receiving 1 gram 4 times a day for 10 days, monitoring CBC, SGOT, SGPT, bilirubin, alkaline, phosphatase, BUN, creatinine and urinalysis, indicated no clinically significant changes attributed to *Kefzol.*

Microbiology: *In vitro* tests demonstrate that the bactericidal action of cephalosporins results from inhibition of cell wall synthesis. Kefzol (cefazolin for injection) is active against the following organisms *in vitro* and in clinical infections:
Staphylococcus aureus (including penicillinase-producing strains)
Staphylococcus epidermidis
Methicillin-resistant staphylococci are uniformly resistant to cefazolin
Group A beta-hemolytic streptococci and other strains of streptococci (many strains of enterococci are resistant)

Streptococcus pneumoniae	*Enterobacter aerogenes*
Escherichia coli	*Haemophilus influenzae*
Proteus mirabilis	
Klebsiella species	

Most strains of indole-positive *Proteus (Proteus vulgaris), Enterobacter cloacae, Morganella morganii* and *Providencia rettgeri* are resistant.
Serratia, Pseudomonas, Mima, Herellea species are almost uniformly resistant to cefazolin.

Disk Susceptibility Tests

Disk diffusion technique—Quantitative methods that require measurement of zone diameters give the most precise estimates of antibiotic susceptibility. One such procedure[1] has been recommended for use with disks to test susceptibility to cefazolin.
Reports from a laboratory using the standardized single-disk susceptibility test[1] with a 30 mcg cefazolin disk should be interpreted according to the following criteria:
Susceptible organisms produce zones of 18 mm or greater, indicating that the tested organism is likely to respond to therapy.
Organisms of intermediate susceptibility produce zones 15 to 17 mm, indicating that the tested organism would be susceptible if high dosage is used or if the infection is confined to tissues and fluids (e.g., urine), in which high antibiotic levels are attained.
Resistant organisms produce zones of 14 mm or less, indicating that other therapy should be selected.
For gram-positive isolates, a zone of 18 mm is indicative of a cefazolin-susceptible organism when tested with either the cephalosporin-class disk (30 mcg cephalothin) or the cefazolin disk (30 mcg cefazolin).
Gram-negative organisms should be tested with the cefazolin disk (using the above criteria), since cefazolin has been shown by *in vitro* tests to have activity against certain strains of Enterobacteriaceae found resistant when tested with the cephalothin disk. Gram-negative organisms having zones of less than 18 mm around the cephalothin disk may be susceptible to cefazolin.
Standardized procedures require use of control organisms. The 30 mcg cefazolin disk should give zone diameter between 23 and 29 mm for *E. coli* ATCC 25922 and between 29 and 35 mm for *S. aureus* ATCC 25923.
The cefazolin disk should not be used for testing susceptibility to other cephalosporins

Dilution Techniques—A bacterial isolate may be considered susceptible if the minimal inhibitory concentration (MIC) for cefazolin is not more than 16 mcg per mL. Organisms are considered resistant if the MIC is equal to or greater than 64 mcg per mL.
The range of MIC's for the control strains are as follows:
S. aureus ATCC 25923, 0.25–1.0 mcg/mL
E. coli ATCC 25922, 1.0–4.0 mcg/mL

[1] Bauer, A.W.; Kirby, W.M.M.; Sherris, J.C., and Turck, M.: Antibiotic Testing by a Standardized Single Disc Method, Am J. Clin. Path. 45:493, 1966. Standardized Disc Susceptibility Test, Federal Register 39:19182-19184, 1974.

INDICATIONS AND USAGE

Kefzol (cefazolin for injection) is indicated in the treatment of the following serious infections due to susceptible organisms:

RESPIRATORY TRACT INFECTIONS due to *Streptococcus pneumoniae, Klebsiella* species *Haemophilus influenzae, Staphylococcus aureus* (penicillin-sensitive and penicillin-resistant) and group A beta-hemolytic streptococci.
Injectable benzathine penicillin is considered to be the drug of choice in treatment and prevention of streptococcal infections, including the prophylaxis of rheumatic fever.
Kefzol is effective in the eradication of streptococci from the nasopharynx, however, data establishing the efficacy of *Kefzol* in the subsequent prevention of rheumatic fever are not available at present.

URINARY TRACT INFECTIONS due to *Escherichia coli, Proteus mirabilis, Klebsiella* species and some strains of enterobacter and enterococci.

SKIN AND SKIN STRUCTURE INFECTIONS due to *Staphylococcus aureus* (penicillin-sensitive and penicillin-resistant), group A beta hemolytic streptococci and other strains of streptococci.

BILIARY TRACT INFECTIONS due to *Escherichia coli*, various strains of streptococci *Proteus mirabilis, Klebsiella* species and *Staphylococcus aureus.*

BONE AND JOINT INFECTIONS due to *Staphylococcus aureus.*

GENITAL INFECTIONS (i.e., prostatitis epididymitis) due to *Escherichia coli, Proteus mirabilis, Klebsiella* species and some strains of enterococci.

SEPTICEMIA due to *Streptococcus neumoniae, Staphylococcus aureus* (penicillin sensitive and penicillin-resistant). *Proteus mirabilis, Escherichia coli* and *Klebsiella* species.

ENDOCARDITIS due to *Staphylococcus aureus* (penicillin-sensitive and penicillin-resistant and group A beta-hemolytic streptococci.
Appropriate culture and susceptible studies should be performed to determine susceptibility of the causative organism to *Kefzol*.

PERIOPERATIVE PROPHYLAXIS: The prophylactic administration of *Kefzol* preoperatively, intraoperatively and postoperatively may reduce the incidence of certain postoperative infections in patients undergoing surgical procedures that are classified as contaminated or potentially contaminated (e.g., vaginal hysterectomy, and cholecystectomy in high-risk patients such as those over 70 year of age, with acute cholecystitis, obstructive jaundice or common duct bile stones).
The perioperative use of *Kefzol* may also be effective in surgical patients in whom infection at the operative site would present a serious risk (e.g., during open-heart surgery and prosthetic arthroplasty).
The prophylactic administration of *Kefzol* should usually be discontinued within a 24-hour period after the surgical procedure. In surgery where the occurrence of infection may be particularly devastating (e.g., open-heart surgery and prosthetic arthroplasty), the prophylactic administration of *Kefzol* may be continued for 3 to 5 days following the completion of surgery.
If there are signs of infection, specimens for cultures should be obtained for the identification of the causative organism so that appropriate therapy may be instituted.
(See DOSAGE AND ADMINISTRATION.)

CONTRAINDICATIONS

KEFZOL (CEFAZOLIN FOR INJECTION) IS CONTRAINDICATED IN PATIENTS WITH KNOWN ALLERGY TO THE CEPHALOSPORIN GROUP OF ANTIBIOTICS.

WARNINGS

SERIOUS AND OCCASIONALLY FATAL HYPERSENSITIVITY (anaphylactic) REACTIONS HAVE BEEN REPORTED IN PATIENTS ON PENICILLIN THERAPY. THESE REACTIONS ARE MORE LIKELY TO OCCUR IN INDIVIDUALS WITH A HISTORY OF PENICILLIN HYPERSENSITIVITY AND/OR A HISTORY OF SENSITIVITY TO MULTIPLE ALLERGENS. THERE HAVE BEEN REPORTS OF INDIVIDUALS WITH A HISTORY OF PENICILLIN HYPERSENSITIVITY WHO HAVE EXPERIENCED SEVERE REACTIONS WHEN TREATED WITH CEPHALOSPORINS, BEFORE INITIATING THERAPY WITH *KEFZOL*. CAREFUL INQUIRY SHOULD BE MADE CONCERNING PREVIOUS HYPERSENSITIVITY REACTIONS TO PENICILLINS, CEPHALOSPORINS OR OTHER ALLERGENS. IF AN ALLERGIC REACTION OCCURS, *KEFZOL* SHOULD BE DISCONTINUED AND APPROPRIATE THERAPY SHOULD BE INSTITUTED. **SERIOUS ANAPHYLACTIC REACTIONS REQUIRE IMMEDIATE EMERGENCY TREATMENT WITH EPINEPHRINE. OXYGEN, INTRAVENOUS STEROIDS AND AIRWAY MANAGEMENT, INCLUDING INTUBATION, SHOULD ALSO BE ADMINISTERED AS INDICATED.**

Pseudomembranous colitis has been reported with nearly all antibacterial agents, including *Kefzol*, and may range in severity from mild to life-threatening. Therefore, it is important to consider this diagnosis in patients who present with diarrhea subsequent to the administration of antibacterial agents.

Treatment with antibacterial agents alters the normal flora of the colon and may permit overgrowth of clostridia. Studies indicate that a toxin produced by *Clostridium difficile* is one primary cause of "antibiotic-associated colitis."
After the diagnosis of pseudomembranous colitis has been established, therapeutic measures should be initiated. Mild cases of pseudomembranous colitis usually respond to drug discontinuation alone. In moderate to severe cases, consideration should be given to management with fluids and electrolytes, protein supplementation and treatment with an antibacterial drug clinically effective against *C. difficile* colitis.

PRECAUTIONS

General—Prolonged use of Kefzol (cefazolin for injection) may result in the overgrowth of nonsusceptible organisms. Careful clinical observation of the patient is essential.
When *Kefzol* is administered to patients with low urinary output because of impaired renal function, lower daily dosage is required (see DOSAGE AND ADMINISTRATION).

As with other beta-lactam antibiotics, seizures may occur if inappropriately high doses are administered to patients with impaired renal function (see DOSAGE AND ADMINISTRATION).

Kefzol, as with all cephalosporins, should be prescribed with caution in individuals with a history of gastrointestinal disease, particularly colitis.

Drug Interactions—Probenecid may decrease renal tubular secretion of cephalosporins when used concurrently, resulting in increased and more prolonged cephalosporin blood levels.

Drug/Laboratory Test Interactions—A false positive reaction for glucose in the urine may occur with Benedict's solution. Fehling's solution, or with Clinitest® tablets, but not with enzyme-based tests such as Clinistix® and Tes-Tape®. Positive direct and indirect antiglobulin (Coombs) tests have occurred; these may also occur in neonates whose mothers received cephalosporins before delivery.

Carcinogenesis/Mutagenesis—Mutagenicity studies and long-term studies in animals to determine the carcinogenic potential of Kefzol (cefazolin for injection) have not been performed.

Pregnancy—Teratogenic Effects—Pregnancy Category B. Reproduction studies have been performed in rats, mice and rabbits at doses up to 25 times the human dose and have revealed no evidence of impaired fertility or harm to the fetus due to *Kefzol*. There are, however, no adequate and well-controlled studies in pregnant women. Because animal reproduction studies are not always predictive of human response, this drug should be used during pregnancy only if clearly needed.

Labor and Delivery—When cefazolin has been administered prior to caesarean section, drug levels in cord blood have been approximately one quarter to one third of maternal drug levels. The drug appears to have no adverse effect on the fetus.

Nursing Mothers—*Kefzol* is present in very low concentrations in the milk of nursing mothers. Caution should be exercised when Kefzol (cefazolin for injection) is administered to a nursing woman.

Pediatric Use—Safety and effectiveness for use in prematures and infants under one month of age have not been established. See DOSAGE AND ADMINISTRATION for recommended dosage in children over one month.

ADVERSE REACTIONS

The following reactions have been reported:

Gastrointestinal: Diarrhea, oral candidiasis (oral thrush), vomiting, nausea, stomach cramps, anorexia and pseudomembranous colitis. Onset of pseudomembranous colitis symptoms may occur during or after antibiotic treatment (see WARNINGS). Nausea and vomiting have been reported rarely.

Allergic: Anaphylaxis, eosinophilia, itching, drug fever, skin rash, Stevens-Johnson syndrome.

Hematologic: Neutropenia, leukopenia, thrombocytopenia, thrombocythemia.

Hepatic and Renal: Transient rise in SGOT, SGPT, BUN and alkaline phosphatase levels has been observed without clinical evidence of renal or hepatic impairment.

Local Reactions: Rare instances of phlebitis have been reported at site of injection. Pain at the site of injection after intramuscular administration has occurred infrequently. Some induration has occurred.

Other Reactions: Genital and anal pruritus (including vulvar pruritus, genital moniliasis and vaginitis).

DOSAGE AND ADMINISTRATION

Usual Adult Dosage

Type of Infection	Dose	Frequency
Moderate to severe infections	500 mg to 1 gram	every 6 to 8 hrs.
Mild infections caused by susceptible gram + cocci	250 mg to 500 mg	every 8 hours
Acute, uncomplicated urinary tract infections	1 gram	every 12 hours
Pneumococcal pneumonia	500 mg	every 12 hours
Severe, life-threatening infections (e.g., endocarditis, septicemia)*	1 gram to 1.5 grams	every 6 hours

*In rare instances, doses up to 12 grams of *Kefzol* per day have been used.

PEDIATRIC DOSAGE GUIDE

Weight		25 mg/kg/Day Divided Into 3 Doses		25 mg/kg/Day Divided Into 4 Doses	
Lbs	Kg	Approximate Single Dose mg/q8h	Vol. (mL) needed with dilution of 125 mg/mL	Approximate Single Dose mg/q6h	Vol. (mL) needed with dilution of 125 mg/mL
10	4.5	40 mg	0.35 mL	30 mg	0.25 mL
20	9.0	75 mg	0.60 mL	55 mg	0.45 mL
30	13.6	115 mg	0.90 mL	85 mg	0.70 mL
40	18.1	150 mg	1.20 mL	115 mg	0.90 mL
50	22.7	190 mg	1.50 mL	140 mg	1.10 mL

PEDIATRIC DOSAGE GUIDE

Weight		50 mg/kg/Day Divided Into 3 Doses		50 mg/kg/Day Divided Into 4 Doses	
Lbs	Kg	Approximate Single Dose mg/q8h	Vol. (mL) needed with dilution of 225 mg/mL	Approximate Single Dose mg/q6h	Vol. (mL) needed with dilution of 225 mg/mL
10	4.5	75 mg	0.35 mL	55 mg	0.25 mL
20	9.0	150 mg	0.70 mL	110 mg	0.50 mL
30	13.6	225 mg	1.00 mL	170 mg	0.75 mL
40	18.1	300 mg	1.35 mL	225 mg	1.00 mL
50	22.7	375 mg	1.70 mL	285 mg	1.25 mL

Perioperative Prophylactic Use

To prevent postoperative infection in contaminated or potentially contaminated surgery, recommended doses are:

a. 1 gram I.V. or I.M. administered 1/2 hour to 1 hour prior to the start of surgery.

b. For lengthy operative procedures (e.g., 2 hours or longer), 500 mg to 1 gram I.V. or I.M. during surgery (administration modified depending on the duration of the operative procedure).

c. 500 mg to 1 gram I.V. or I.M. every 6 to 8 hours for 24 hours postoperatively.

It is important that (1) the preoperative dose be given just (1/2 hour to 1 hour) prior to the start of surgery so that adequate antibiotic levels are present in the serum and tissues at the time of the initial surgical incision; and (2) *Kefzol* be administered, if necessary, at appropriate intervals during surgery to provide sufficient levels of the antibiotic at the anticipated moments of greatest exposure to infective organisms.

In surgery where the occurrence of infection may be particularly devastating (e.g., open-heart surgery and prosthetic arthroplasty), the prophylactic administration of Kefzol (cefazolin for injection) may be continued for 3 to 5 days following the completion of surgery.

Dosage Adjustment for Patients With Reduced Renal Function

Kefzol may be used in patients with reduced renal function with the following dosage adjustments: Patients with a creatinine clearance of 55 mL/min, or greater or a serum creatinine of 1.5 mg % or less can be given full doses. Patients with creatinine clearance rates of 35 to 54 mL/min, or serum creatinine of 1.6 to 3.0 mg % can also be given full doses but dosage should be restricted to at least 8 hour intervals. Patients with creatinine clearance rates of 11 to 34 mL/min, or serum creatinine of 3.1 to 4.5 mg % should be given 1/2 the usual dose every 12 hours. Patients with creatinine clearance rates of 10 mL/min, or less or serum creatinine of 4.6 mg % or greater should be given 1/2 the usual dose every 18 to 24 hours. All reduced dosage recommendations apply after an initial loading dose appropriate to the severity of the infection. Patients undergoing peritoneal dialysis: see Human Pharmacology.

Pediatric Dosage

In children, a total daily dosage of 25 to 50 mg per kg (approximately 10 to 20 mg per pound) of body weight, divided into three or four equal doses, is effective for most mild to moderately severe infections. Total daily dosage may be increased to 100 mg per kg (45 mg per pound) of body weight for severe infections. Since safety for use in premature infants and infants under one month has not been established, the use of Kefzol (cefazolin for injection) in these patients is not recommended.

[See first table at top of page]
[See second table at top of page]

In children with mild to moderate renal impairment (creatinine clearance of 70 to 40 mL/min.), 60% of the normal daily dose given in equally divided doses every 12 hours should be sufficient. In patients with moderate impairment (creatinine clearance of 40 to 20 mL/min.), 25% of the normal daily dose given in equally divided doses every 12 hours should be adequate. Children with severe renal impairment (creatinine clearance of 20 to 5 mL/min.) may be given 10% of the normal daily dose every 24 hours. All dosage recommendations apply after an initial loading dose.

RECONSTITUTION

Preparation of Parenteral Solution

Parenteral drug products should be SHAKEN WELL when reconstituted, and inspected visually for particulate matter prior to administration. If particulate matter is evident in reconstituted fluids, the drug solution should be discarded. When reconstituted or diluted according to the instructions below, Kefzol (cefazolin for injection) is stable for 24 hours at room temperature or for 10 days if stored under refrigeration (5°C or 41°F). Reconstituted solutions may range in color from pale yellow to yellow without a change in potency.

Single-Dose Vials

For I.M. injection, I.V. direct (bolus) injection or I.V. infusion, reconstitute with Sterile Water for Injection according to the following table. SHAKE WELL.

Vial Size	Amount of Diluent	Approximate Concentration	Approximate Available Volume
500 mg	2.0 mL	225 mg/mL	2.2 mL
1 gram	2.5 mL	330 mg/mL	3.0 mL

Pharmacy Bulk Vials

Add Sterile Water for Injection, Bacteriostatic Water for Injection or Sodium Chloride Injection according to the table below. SHAKE WELL.

Vial Size	Amount of Diluent	Approximate Concentration	Approximate Available Volume
10 grams	45 mL	1 gram/5 mL	51 mL
	96 mL	1 gram/10 mL	102 mL

Continued on next page

* Identi-Code® symbol. This product information was prepared in June 1998. Current information on these and other products of Eli Lilly and Company may be obtained by direct inquiry to Lilly Research Laboratories, Lilly Corporate Center, Indianapolis, Indiana 46285, (800) 545-5979.

Kefzol—Cont.

"Piggyback" Vials

Reconstitute with 50 to 100 mL of Sodium Chloride Injection or other I.V. solution listed under ADMINISTRATION. When adding diluent to vial, allow air to escape by using a small vent needle or by pumping the syringe. SHAKE WELL. Administer with primary I.V. fluids, as a single dose.

ADMINISTRATION

Intramuscular Administration—Reconstitute vials with Sterile Water for Injection according to the dilution table above. Shake well until dissolved. *Kefzol* should be injected into a large muscle mass. Pain on injection is infrequent in *Kefzol*.

Intravenous Administration—Direct (bolus) injection: Following reconstitution according to the above table, further dilute vials with approximately 5 mL Sterile Water for Injection. Inject the solution slowly over 3 to 5 minutes, directly or through tubing for patients receiving parenteral fluids (see list below).

Intermittent or continuous infusion. Dilute reconstituted *Kefzol* in 50 to 100 mL of one of the following solutions:
Sodium Chloride Injection, USP
5% or 10% Dextrose Injection, USP
5% Dextrose in Lactated Ringer's Injection, USP
5% Dextrose and 0.9% Sodium Chloride Injection, USP
5% Dextrose and 0.45% Sodium Chloride Injection, USP
5% Dextrose and 0.2% Sodium Chloride Injection, USP
Lactated Ringer's Injection, USP
Invert Sugar 5% or 10% in Sterile Water for Injection
Ringer's Injection, USP
5% Sodium Bicarbonate Injection, USP

HOW SUPPLIED

Kefzol (cefazolin for injection)—supplied in vials equivalent to 500 mg or 1 gram of cefazolin in "Piggyback" Vials for intravenous admixture equivalent to 1 gram of cefazolin; and in Pharmacy Bulk vials equivalent to 10 grams of cefazolin.

Vials:
500 mg, 10-mL size (No. 767)—(Traypak* of 25) NDC 0002-1497-25
1 gram, 10-mL size (No. 768)—(Traypak of 25) NDC 0002-1498-25
1 gram, 100-mL size (No. 7011)†—(Traypak of 10) NDC 0002-7011-10

Pharmacy Bulk Vials:
10 gram, 100-mL size (No. 7014)—(Traypak of 6) NDC 0002-7014-16

Also Available:

Faspak‡:
1 gram (No. 7202)†—(Faspak of 96) NDC 0002-7202-74

ADD-Vantage§ Vials:
500 mg (No. 7265)—(Traypak of 25) NDC 0002-7265-25
1 gram (No. 7266)—(Traypak of 25) NDC 0002-7266-25
The above ADD-Vantage Vials are to be used *only* with Abbott Laboratories' 50-mL or 100-mL Flexible Diluent Containers containing 0.9% Sodium Chloride Injection or 5% Dextrose Injection.
Instructions for use of the ADD-Vantage Vials are enclosed in the package.

---

*Traypak™ (multivial carton. Lilly).
†For IV use
‡Faspak® (flexible plastic bag. Lilly)

§ADD-Vantage® (vials and diluent containers, Abbott).

As with other cephalosporins, *Kefzol* tends to darken depending on storage conditions; within the stated recommendations, however, product potency is not adversely affected.
Before reconstitution protect from light and store between 15° and 30°C (59° and 86°F)
CAUTION—Federal (USA) law prohibits dispensing without prescription.
Literature revised November 1997.

Manufactured for
ELI LILLY AND COMPANY
Indianapolis, IN 46285, USA
by
BMH Limited
Philadelphia, PA 19101

LENTE® ILETIN® II   **OTC**
(insulin zinc suspension, Lilly)
See under Iletin® (insulin)

LORABID®   ℞
[lōr´ă-bĭd]
(Loracarbef, USP)

DESCRIPTION

LORABID® (loracarbef, USP) is a synthetic β-lactam antibiotic of the carbacephem class for oral administration.

Chemically, carbacephems differ from cephalosporin-class antibiotics in the dihydrothiazine ring where a methylene group has been substituted for a sulfur atom.
The chemical name for loracarbef is (6R, 7S)-7-[(R)-2-amino-2-phenylacetamido]-3-chloro-8-oxo-1-azabicyclo[4.2.0] oct-2-ene-2-carboxylic acid, monohydrate. It is a white to off-white solid with a molecular weight of 367.8. The empirical formula is $C_{16}H_{16}ClN_3O_4 \cdot H_2O$. The structural formula is:

Lorabid Pulvules® (loracarbef capsules, USP) and Lorabid for Oral Suspension (loracarbef for oral suspension, USP) are intended for oral administration only.
Each Pulvule contains loracarbef equivalent to 200 mg (0.57 mmol) or 400 mg (1.14 mmol) anhydrous loracarbef activity. They also contain cornstarch, dimethicone, F D & C Blue No. 2, gelatin, iron oxides, magnesium stearate, titanium dioxide, and other inactive ingredients.
After reconstitution, each 5 mL of Lorabid for Oral Suspension contains loracarbef equivalent to 100 mg (0.286 mmol) or 200 mg (0.57 mmol) anhydrous loracarbef activity. The suspensions also contain cellulose, F D & C Red No. 40, flavors, methylparaben, propylparaben, simethicone emulsion, sodium carboxymethylcellulose, sucrose, and xanthan gum.

CLINICAL PHARMACOLOGY

Loracarbef, after oral administration, was approximately 90% absorbed from the gastrointestinal tract. When capsules were taken with food, peak plasma concentrations were 50% to 60% of those achieved when the drug was administered to fasting subjects and occurred from 30 to 60 minutes later. Total absorption, as measured by urinary recovery and area under the plasma concentration versus time curve (AUC), was unchanged. The effect of food on the rate and extent of absorption of the suspension formulation has not been studied to date.
The pharmacokinetics of loracarbef were linear over the recommended dosage range of 200 to 400 mg, with no accumulation of the drug noted when it was given twice daily.
Average peak plasma concentrations after administration of 200-mg or 400-mg single doses of loracarbef as capsules to fasting subjects were approximately 8 and 14 µg/mL, respectively, and were obtained within 1.2 hours after dosing. The average peak plasma concentration in adults following a 400-mg single dose of suspension was 17 µg/mL and was obtained within 0.8 hour after dosing (see Table).

Dosage (mg)	Mean Plasma Loracarbef Concentrations (µg/mL)	
	Peak C_{max}	Time to Peak T_{max}
Capsule (single dose)		
200 mg	8	1.2 h
400 mg	14	1.2 h
Suspension (single dose)		
400 mg (adult)	17	0.8 h
7.5 mg/kg (pediatric)	13	0.8 h
15 mg/kg (pediatric)	19	0.8 h

Following administration of 7.5 and 15 mg/kg single doses of oral suspension to children, average peak plasma concentrations were 13 and 19 µg/mL, respectively, and were obtained within 40 to 60 minutes.
This increased rate of absorption (suspension > capsule) should be taken into consideration if the oral suspension is to be substituted for the capsule, and capsules should not be substituted for the oral suspension in the treatment of otitis media (see DOSAGE AND ADMINISTRATION).
The elimination half-life was an average of 1.0 h in patients with normal renal function. Concomitant administration of probenecid decreased the rate of urinary excretion and increased the half-life to 1.5 hours.
In subjects with moderate impairment of renal function (creatinine clearance 10 to 50 mL/min/1.73 m²), following a single 400-mg dose, the plasma half-life was prolonged to approximately 5.6 hours. In subjects with severe renal impairment (creatinine clearance <10 mL/min/1.73 m²), the half-life was increased to approximately 32 hours. During hemodialysis the half-life was approximately 4 hours. In patients with severe renal impairment, the C_{max} increased from 15.4 µg/mL to 23 µg/mL (see PRECAUTIONS and DOSAGE AND ADMINISTRATION).
In single-dose studies, plasma half-life and AUC were not significantly altered in healthy elderly subjects with normal renal function.
There is no evidence of metabolism of loracarbef in humans. Approximately 25% of circulating loracarbef is bound to plasma proteins.

Middle-ear fluid concentrations of loracarbef were approximately 48% of the plasma concentration 2 hours after drug administration in pediatric patients. The peak concentration of loracarbef in blister fluid was approximately half that obtained in plasma. Adequate data on CSF levels of loracarbef are not available.
Microbiology—Loracarbef exerts its bactericidal action by binding to essential target proteins of the bacterial cell wall, leading to inhibition of cell-wall synthesis. It is stable in the presence of some bacterial β-lactamases. Loracarbef has been shown to be active against most strains of the following organisms both *in vitro* and in clinical infections (see **INDICATIONS AND USAGE**):

Gram-positive aerobes:
 Staphylococcus aureus (including penicillinase-producing strains)
  NOTE: Loracarbef (like most β-lactam antimicrobials) is inactive against methicillin-resistant staphylococci.
 Staphylococcus saprophyticus
 Streptococcus pneumoniae
 Streptococcus pyogenes
Gram-negative aerobes:
 Escherichia coli
 Haemophilus influenzae (including β-lactamase-producing strains)
 Moraxella (Branhamella) catarrhalis (including β-lactamase-producing strains)
The following *in vitro* data are available: however, their clinical significance is unknown.
Loracarbef exhibits *in vitro* minimum inhibitory concentrations (MIC) of 8 µg/mL or less against most strains of the following organisms; however, the safety and efficacy of loracarbef in treating clinical infections due to these organisms have not been established in adequate and well-controlled trials.
Gram-positive aerobes:
 Staphylococcus epidermidis
 Streptococcus agalactiae (group B streptococci)
 Streptococcus bovis
 Streptococci, groups C, F, and G
 viridans group streptococci
Gram-negative aerobes:
 Citrobacter diversus
 Haemophilus parainfluenzae
 Klebsiella pneumoniae
 Neisseria gonorrhoeae (including penicillinase-producing strains)
 Pasteurella multocida
 Proteus mirabilis
 Salmonella species
 Shigella species
 Yersinia enterocolitica
NOTE: Loracarbef is inactive against most strains of *Acinetobacter, Enterobacter, Morganella morganii, Proteus vulgaris, Providencia, Pseudomonas,* and *Serratia.*
Anaerobic organisms:
 Clostridium perfringens
 Fusobacterium necrophorum
 Peptococcus niger
 Peptostreptococcus intermedius
 Propionibacterium acnes
Susceptibility Testing

Diffusion Techniques—Quantitative methods that require measurement of zone diameters give the most precise estimate of the susceptibility of bacteria to antimicrobial agents. One such standardized method[1] has been recommended for use with the 30-µg loracarbef disk. Interpretation involves the correlation of the diameter obtained in the disk test with MIC for loracarbef.
Reports from the laboratory giving results of the standard single-disk susceptibility test with a 30-µg loracarbef disk should be interpreted according to the following criteria:

Zone Diameter (mm)	Interpretation
≥ 18	(S) Susceptible
15–17	(MS) Moderately Susceptible
≤ 14	(R) Resistant

A report of "susceptible" implies that the pathogen is likely to be inhibited by generally achievable blood concentrations. A report of "moderately susceptible" indicates that inhibitory concentrations of the antibiotic may be achieved if high dosage is used or if the infection is confined to tissues and fluids (e.g., urine) in which high antibiotic concentrations are attained. A report of "resistant" indicates that achievable concentrations of the antibiotic are unlikely to be inhibitory and other therapy should be selected.
Standardized procedures require the use of laboratory control organisms. The 30-µg loracarbef disk should give the following zone diameters with the NCCLS approved procedure:

Organism	Zone Diameter (mm)
E. coli ATCC 25922	23–29
S. aureus ATCC 25923	23–31

Dilution Techniques—Use a standardized dilution method[2] (broth, agar, or microdilution) or equivalent with loracarbef powder. The MIC values obtained should be interpreted according to the following criteria:

MIC (µg/mL)	Interpretation
≤8	(S) Susceptible
16	(MS) Moderately Susceptible
≥32	(R) Resistant

As with standard diffusion methods, dilution procedures require the use of laboratory control organisms. Standard loracarbef powder should give the following MIC values with the NCCLS approved procedure:

Organism	MIC Range (µg/mL)
E. coli ATCC 25922	0.5–2
S. aureus ATCC 29213	0.5–2

INDICATIONS AND USAGE

Lorabid is indicated in the treatment of patients with mild to moderate infections caused by susceptible strains of the designated microorganisms in the conditions listed below. (As recommended dosages, durations of therapy, and applicable patient populations vary among these infections, please see **DOSAGE AND ADMINISTRATION** for specific recommendations.)

Lower Respiratory Tract

Secondary Bacterial Infection of Acute Bronchitis caused by S. pneumoniae, H. influenzae (including β-lactamase-producing strains), or M. catarrhalis (including β-lactamase-producing strains).

Acute Bacterial Exacerbations of Chronic Bronchitis caused by S. pneumoniae, H. influenzae (including β-lactamase-producing strains), or M. catarrhalis (including β-lactamase-producing strains).

Pneumonia caused by S. pneumoniae or H. influenzae (non-β-lactamase-producing strains only). Data are insufficient at this time to establish efficacy in patients with pneumonia caused by β-lactamase-producing strains of H. influenzae.

Upper Respiratory Tract

Otitis Media† caused by S. pneumoniae, H. influenzae (including β-lactamase-producing strains), M. catarrhalis (including β-lactamase-producing strains), or S. pyogenes.

Acute Maxillary Sinusitis † caused by S. pneumoniae, H. influenzae (non-β-lactamase-producing strains only), or M. catarrhalis (including β-lactamase-producing strains). Data are insufficient at this time to establish efficacy in patients with acute maxillary sinusitis caused by β-lactamase-producing strains of H. influenzae.

†NOTE: In a patient population with significant numbers of β-lactamase-producing organisms, loracarbef's clinical cure and bacteriological eradication rates were somewhat less than those observed with a product containing a β-lactamase inhibitor. Lorabid's decreased potential for toxicity compared to products containing β-lactamase inhibitors along with the susceptibility patterns of the common microbes in a given geographic area should be taken into account when considering the use of an antimicrobial (see **CLINICAL STUDIES** section). For information on use in pediatric patients, see **PRECAUTIONS—Pediatric Use**.

Pharyngitis and Tonsillitis caused by S. pyogenes. (The usual drug of choice in the treatment and prevention of streptococcal infections, including the prophylaxis of rheumatic fever, is penicillin administered by the intramuscular route. Lorabid is generally effective in the eradication of S. pyogenes from the nasopharynx; however, data establishing the efficacy of Lorabid in the subsequent prevention of rheumatic fever are not available at present.)

Skin and Skin Structure

Uncomplicated Skin and Skin Structure Infections caused by S. aureus (including penicillinase-producing strains) or S. pyogenes. Abscesses should be surgically drained as clinically indicated.

Urinary Tract

Uncomplicated Urinary Tract Infections (cystitis) caused by E. coli or S. saprophyticus*.

NOTE: In considering the use of Lorabid in the treatment of cystitis, Lorabid's lower bacterial eradication rates and lower potential for toxicity should be weighed against the increased eradication rates and increased potential for toxicity demonstrated by some other classes of approved agents (see **CLINICAL STUDIES** section).

Uncomplicated Pyelonephritis caused by E. coli.

*Although treatment of infections due to this organism in this organ system demonstrated a clinically acceptable overall outcome, efficacy was studied in fewer than 10 infections.

Culture and susceptibility testing should be performed when appropriate to determine the causative organism and its susceptibility to loracarbef. Therapy may be started while awaiting the results of these studies. Once these results become available, antimicrobial therapy should be adjusted accordingly.

CONTRAINDICATION

Lorabid is contraindicated in patients with known allergy to loracarbef or cephalosporin-class antibiotics.

WARNINGS

BEFORE THERAPY WITH LORABID IS INSTITUTED, CAREFUL INQUIRY SHOULD BE MADE TO DETERMINE WHETHER THE PATIENT HAS HAD PREVIOUS HYPERSENSITIVITY REACTIONS TO LORACARBEF, CEPHALOSPORINS, PENICILLINS, OR OTHER DRUGS. IF THIS PRODUCT IS TO BE GIVEN TO PENICILLIN-SENSITIVE PATIENTS, CAUTION SHOULD BE EXERCISED BECAUSE CROSS-HYPERSENSITIVITY AMONG β-LACTAM ANTIBIOTICS HAS BEEN CLEARLY DOCUMENTED AND MAY OCCUR IN UP TO 10% OF PATIENTS WITH A HISTORY OF PENICILLIN ALLERGY. IF AN ALLERGIC REACTION TO LORABID OCCURS, DISCONTINUE THE DRUG. SERIOUS ACUTE HYPERSENSITIVITY REACTIONS MAY REQUIRE THE USE OF EPINEPHRINE AND OTHER EMERGENCY MEASURES, INCLUDING OXYGEN, INTRAVENOUS FLUIDS, INTRAVENOUS ANTIHISTAMINES, CORTICOSTEROIDS, PRESSOR AMINES, AND AIRWAY MANAGEMENT, AS CLINICALLY INDICATED.

Pseudomembranous colitis has been reported with nearly all antibacterial agents and may range from mild to life-threatening. Therefore, it is important to consider this diagnosis in patients who present with diarrhea subsequent to the administration of antibacterial agents.

Treatment with broad-spectrum antibiotics alters the normal flora of the colon and may permit overgrowth of clostridia. Studies indicate that a toxin produced by Clostridium difficile is a primary cause of "antibiotic-associated colitis."

After the diagnosis of pseudomembranous colitis has been established, therapeutic measures should be initiated. Mild cases of pseudomembranous colitis usually respond to discontinuation of drug alone. In moderate to severe cases, consideration should be given to management with fluids and electrolytes, protein supplementation, and treatment with an antibacterial drug effective against C. difficile-associated colitis.

PRECAUTIONS

General —In patients with known or suspected renal impairment (see **DOSAGE AND ADMINISTRATION**), careful clinical observation and appropriate laboratory studies should be performed prior to and during therapy. The total daily dose of loracarbef should be reduced in these patients because high and/or prolonged plasma antibiotic concentrations can occur in such individuals administered the usual doses. Loracarbef, like cephalosporins, should be given with caution to patients receiving concurrent treatment with potent diuretics because these diuretics are suspected of adversely affecting renal function.

As with other broad-spectrum antimicrobials, prolonged use of loracarbef may result in the overgrowth of nonsusceptible organisms. Careful observation of the patient is essential. If superinfection occurs during therapy, appropriate measures should be taken.

Loracarbef, as with other broad-spectrum antimicrobials, should be prescribed with caution in individuals with a history of colitis.

Information for Patients —Lorabid should be taken either at least 1 hour prior to eating or at least 2 hours after eating a meal.

Drug Interactions —

Probenecid: As with other β-lactam antibiotics, renal excretion of loracarbef is inhibited by probenecid and resulted in an approximate 80% increase in the AUC for loracarbef (see **CLINICAL PHARMACOLOGY**).

Carcinogenesis, Mutagenesis, Impairment of Fertility —Although lifetime studies in animals have not been performed to evaluate carcinogenic potential, no mutagenic potential was found for loracarbef in standard tests of genotoxicity, which included bacterial mutation tests and *in vitro* and *in vivo* mammalian systems. In rats, fertility and reproductive performance were not affected by loracarbef at doses up to 33 times the maximum human exposure in mg/kg (10 times the exposure based on mg/m²).

Usage in Pregnancy—Pregnancy Category B —Reproduction studies have been performed in mice, rats, and rabbits at doses up to 33 times the maximum human exposure in mg/kg (4, 10, and 4 times the exposure, respectively, based on mg/m²) and have revealed no evidence of impaired fertility or harm to the fetus due to loracarbef. There are, however, no adequate and well-controlled studies in pregnant women. Because animal reproduction studies are not always predictive of human response, this drug should be used during pregnancy only if clearly needed.

Labor and Delivery —Lorabid has not been studied for use during labor and delivery. Treatment should be given only if clearly needed.

Nursing Mothers —It is not known whether this drug is excreted in human milk. Because many drugs are excreted in human milk, caution should be exercised when Lorabid is administered to a nursing woman.

Pediatric Use —The safety and efficacy of Lorabid have been established for children aged six months to twelve years for acute maxillary sinusitis based upon its approval in adults. Use of Lorabid in pediatric patients is supported by pharmacokinetic and safety data in adults and children, and by clinical and microbiologic data from adequate and well-controlled studies of the treatment of acute maxillary sinusitis in adults and of acute otitis media with effusion in children. It is also supported by post-marketing adverse events surveillance. (See **CLINICAL PHARMACOLOGY, INDICATIONS AND USAGE, ADVERSE REACTIONS, DOSAGE AND ADMINISTRATION**, and **CLINICAL STUDIES** sections).

Geriatric Use —Healthy geriatric volunteers (≥65 years old) with normal renal function who received a single 400-mg dose of loracarbef had no significant differences in AUC or clearance when compared to healthy adult volunteers 20 to 40 years of age. In clinical studies, when geriatric patients received the usual recommended adult doses, clinical efficacy and safety were comparable to results in nongeriatric adult patients. Because significant numbers of elderly patients have decreased renal function, evaluation of renal function in this population is recommended (see **DOSAGE AND ADMINISTRATION**).

ADVERSE REACTIONS

The nature of adverse reactions to loracarbef are similar to those observed with orally administered β-lactam antimicrobials. The majority of adverse reactions observed in clinical trials were of a mild and transient nature; 1.5% of patients discontinued therapy because of drug-related adverse reactions. No one reaction requiring discontinuation accounted for >0.03% of the total patient population; however, of those reactions resulting in discontinuation, gastrointestinal events (diarrhea and abdominal pain) and skin rashes predominated.

All Patients

The following adverse events, irrespective of relationship to drug, have been reported following the use of Lorabid in clinical trials. Incidence rates (combined for all dosing regimens and dosage forms) were less than 1% for the total patient population, except as otherwise noted:

Gastrointestinal: The most commonly observed adverse reactions were related to the gastrointestinal system. The incidence of gastrointestinal adverse reactions increased in patients treated with higher doses. Individual event rates included diarrhea, 4.1%; nausea, 1.9%; vomiting, 1.4%; abdominal pain, 1.4%; and anorexia.

Hypersensitivity: Hypersensitivity reactions including, skin rashes (1.2%), urticaria, pruritus, and erythema multiforme.

Central Nervous System: Headache (2.9%), somnolence, nervousness, insomnia, and dizziness.

Hemic and Lymphatic Systems: Transient thrombocytopenia, leukopenia, and eosinophilia.

Hepatic: Transient elevations in AST (SGOT), ALT (SGPT), and alkaline phosphatase.

Renal: Transient elevations in BUN and creatinine.

Cardiovascular System: Vasodilatation.

Genitourinary: Vaginitis (1.3%), vaginal moniliasis (1.1%).

As with other β-lactam antibiotics, the following potentially severe adverse experiences have been reported rarely with loracarbef in worldwide post-marketing surveillance: anaphylaxis, hepatic dysfunction including cholestasis, prolongation of the prothrombin time with clinical bleeding in patients taking anticoagulants, and Stevens-Johnson syndrome.

Pediatric Patients

The incidences of several adverse events, irrespective of relationship to drug, following treatment with Lorabid were significantly different in the pediatric population and the adult population as follows:

Event	Pediatric	Adult
Diarrhea	5.8%	3.6%
Headache	0.9%	3.2%
Rhinitis	6.3%	1.6%
Nausea	0.0%	2.5%
Rash	2.9%	0.7%
Vomiting	3.3%	0.5%
Somnolence	2.1%	0.4%
Anorexia	2.3%	0.3%

Continued on next page

* Identi-Code® symbol. This product information was prepared in June 1998. Current information on these and other products of Eli Lilly and Company may be obtained by direct inquiry to Lilly Research Laboratories, Lilly Corporate Center, Indianapolis, Indiana 46285, (800) 545-5979.

Lorabid—Cont.

β-Lactam Antimicrobial Class Labeling:
The following adverse reactions and altered laboratory test results have been reported in patients treated with β-lactam antibiotics:

Adverse Reactions —Allergic reactions, aplastic anemia, hemolytic anemia, hemorrhage, agranulocytosis, toxic epidermal necrolysis, renal dysfunction, and toxic nephropathy. As with other β-lactam antibiotics, serum sickness-like reactions have been reported rarely with loracarbef.

Several β-lactam antibiotics have been implicated in triggering seizures, particularly in patients with renal impairment when the dosage was not reduced. If seizures associated with drug therapy should occur, the drug should be discontinued. Anticonvulsant therapy can be given if clinically indicated.

Altered Laboratory Tests —Increased prothrombin time, positive direct Coombs' test, elevated LDH, pancytopenia, and neutropenia.

OVERDOSAGE

Signs and Symptoms —The toxic symptoms following an overdose of β-lactams may include nausea, vomiting, epigastric distress, and diarrhea.

Loracarbef is eliminated primarily by the kidneys. Forced diuresis, peritoneal dialysis, hemodialysis, or hemoperfusion have not been established as beneficial for an overdose of loracarbef. Hemodialysis has been shown to be effective in hastening the elimination of loracarbef from plasma in patients with chronic renal failure.

DOSAGE AND ADMINISTRATION

Lorabid is administered orally either at least 1 hour prior to eating or at least 2 hours after eating. The recommended dosages, durations of treatment, and applicable patient populations are described in the following chart:

Population/Infection	Dosage (mg)	Duration (days)
ADULTS (13 years and older)		
Lower Respiratory Tract		
Secondary Bacterial Infection of Acute Bronchitis	200–400 q12h	7
Acute Bacterial Exacerbation of Chronic Bronchitis	400 q12h	7
Pneumonia	400 q12h	14
Upper Respiratory Tract		
Pharyngitis/Tonsillitis	200 q12h	10[a]
Sinusitis	400 q12h	10
(See CLINICAL STUDIES and INDICATIONS AND USAGE for further information.)		
Skin and Skin Structure		
Uncomplicated Skin and Skin Structure Infections	200 q12h	7
Urinary Tract		
Uncomplicated cystitis	200 q24h	7
(See CLINICAL STUDIES and INDICATIONS AND USAGE for further information.)		
Uncomplicated pyelonephritis	400 q12h	14
PEDIATRIC PATIENTS (6 months to 12 years)		
Upper Respiratory Tract		
Acute Otitis Media[b]	30 mg/kg/day in divided doses q12h	10

PEDIATRIC DOSAGE CHART
DAILY DOSE 15 mg/kg/day

		100 mg/5 mL Suspension		200 mg/5 mL Suspension	
Weight		Dose given twice daily		Dose given twice daily	
lb	kg	mL	tsp	mL	tsp
15	7	2.6	0.5	—	—
29	13	4.9	1.0	2.5	0.5
44	20	7.5	1.5	3.8	0.75
57	26	9.8	2.0	4.9	1.0

PEDIATRIC DOSAGE CHART
DAILY DOSE 30 mg/kg/day

		100 mg/5 mL Suspension		200 mg/5 mL Suspension	
Weight		Dose given twice daily		Dose given twice daily	
lb	kg	mL	tsp	mL	tsp
15	7	5.2	1.0	2.6	0.5
29	13	9.8	2.0	4.9	1.0
44	20	—	—	7.5	1.5
57	26	—	—	9.8	2.0

(See CLINICAL STUDIES and INDICATIONS AND USAGE for further information.)

Acute maxillary sinusitis	30 mg/kg/day in divided doses q12h	10

(See CLINICAL STUDIES and INDICATIONS AND USAGE for further information.)

Pharyngitis/Tonsillitis	15 mg/kg/day in divided doses q12h	10[a]

Skin and Skin Structure

Impetigo	15 mg/kg/day in divided doses q12h	7

[a] In the treatment of infections due to *S. pyogenes*, Lorabid should be administered for at least 10 days.

[b] Otitis media should be treated with the suspension. Clinical studies of otitis media were conducted with the suspension formulation only. The suspension is more rapidly absorbed than the capsules, resulting in higher peak plasma concentrations when administered at the same dose. Therefore, the capsule should not be substituted for the suspension in the treatment of otitis media (see CLINICAL PHARMACOLOGY).

[See first table at bottom of page]
[See second table at bottom of page]

Renal Impairment: Lorabid may be administered to patients with impaired renal function. The usual dose and schedule may be employed in patients with creatinine clearance levels of 50 mL/min or greater. Patients with creatinine clearance between 10 and 49 mL/min may be given half of the recommended dose at the usual dosage interval, or the normal recommended dose at twice the usual dosage interval. Patients with creatinine clearance levels less than 10 mL/min may be treated with the recommended dose given every 3 to 5 days; patients on hemodialysis should receive another dose following dialysis.

When only the serum creatinine is available, the following formula (based on sex, weight, and age of the patient) may be used to convert this value into creatinine clearance (CL_{cr}, mL/min). The equation assumes the patient's renal function is stable.

$$\text{Males} = \frac{(\text{weight in kg}) \times (140 - \text{age})}{(72) \times \text{serum creatinine (mg/100 mL)}}$$

$$\text{Females} = (0.85) \times (\text{above value})$$

Reconstitution Directions for Oral Suspension

Bottle Size	Reconstitution Directions
50 mL	Add 30 mL of water in 2 portions to the dry mixture in the bottle. Shake well after each addition.
75 mL	Add 45 mL of water in 2 portions to the dry mixture in the bottle. Shake well after each addition.
100 mL	Add 60 mL of water in 2 portions to the dry mixture in the bottle. Shake well after each addition.

After mixing, the suspension may be kept at room temperature, 59° to 86°F (15° to 30°C), for 14 days without significant loss of potency. Keep tightly closed. Discard unused portion after 14 days.

HOW SUPPLIED

Pulvules:
200 mg, (blue and gray) (No. 3170) (Identi-Code* 3170) (30s) NDC 0002-3170-30
400 mg, (blue and pink) (No. 3171) (Identi-Code 3171) (30s) NDC 0002-3171-30
Keep tightly closed. Store at controlled room temperature, 59° to 86°F (15° to 30°C). Protect from heat.
For Oral Suspension (strawberry bubble gum flavor):
100 mg/5 mL, (M-5135) (50-mL size) NDC 0002-5135-87; (100-mL size) NDC 0002-5135-48
200 mg/5 mL, (M-5136) (50-mL size) NDC 0002-5136-87; (75-mL size) NDC 0002-5136-48; (100-mL size) NDC 0002-5136-48

*Identi-Code® (formula identification code, Lilly).

Clinical Studies:

Acute Otitis Media

Study 1 In a controlled clinical study of acute otitis media performed in the United States where significant rates of β-lactamase-producing organisms were found, loracarbef was compared to an oral antimicrobial agent that contained a specific β-lactamase inhibitor. In this study, using very strict evaluability criteria and microbiologic and clinical response criteria at the 10- to 16-day post therapy follow-up, the following presumptive bacterial eradication/clinical cure outcomes (ie, clinical success) and safety results were obtained:

US Acute Otitis Media Study
Loracarbef vs β-lactamase inhibitor-containing control drug
Efficacy:

Pathogen	% of Cases With Pathogens (n=204)	Outcome
S. pneumoniae	42.6%	Loracarbef equivalent to control
H. influenzae	30.4%	Loracarbef success rate 9% less than control
M. catarrhalis	20.6%	Loracarbef success rate 19% less than control
S. pyogenes	6.4%	Loracarbef equivalent to control
Overall	100.0%	Loracarbef success rate 12% less than control

Safety: The incidences of the following adverse events were clinically and statistically significantly higher in the control arm versus the loracarbef arm.

Event	Loracarbef	Control
Diarrhea	15%	26%
Rash*	8%	15%

*The majority of these involved the diaper area in young pediatric patients.

Study 2 In a controlled clinical study of acute otitis media performed in Europe, loracarbef was compared to amoxicillin. As expected in a European population, this study population had a lower incidence of β-lactamase-producing organisms than usually seen in US trials. In this study, using very strict evaluability criteria and microbiologic and clinical response criteria at the 10- to 16-day post therapy follow-up, the following presumptive bacterial eradication/clinical cure outcomes (ie, clinical success) were obtained:

European Acute Otitis Media Study
Loracarbef vs Amoxicillin
Efficacy:

Pathogen	% of Cases With Pathogens (n=291)	Outcome
S. pneumoniae	51.5%	Loracarbef equivalent to amoxicillin
H. influenzae	29.2%	Loracarbef success rate 14% greater than amoxicillin
M. catarrhalis	15.8%	Loracarbef success rate 31% greater than amoxicillin
S. pyogenes	3.4%	Loracarbef equivalent to amoxicillin
Overall	100.0%	Loracarbef equivalent to amoxicillin

Acute Maxilliary Sinusitis

In a controlled clinical study of acute maxillary sinusitis performed in Europe, loracarbef was compared to doxycycline. In this study, there were 210 sinus-puncture evaluable patients. As expected in a European population, this study population had a lower incidence of β-lactamase-producing organisms than usually seen in US trials. In this study, using very strict evaluability criteria and microbio-

logic and clinical response criteria at the 1- to 2-week post therapy follow-up, the following presumptive bacterial eradication/clinical cure outcomes (ie, clinical success) were obtained:

European Acute Maxillary Sinusitis Study
Loracarbef vs Doxycycline

Efficacy:

Pathogen	% of Cases With Pathogens (n=210)	Outcome
S. pneumoniae	47.6%	Loracarbef equivalent to doxycycline
H. influenzae	41.4%	Loracarbef equivalent to doxycycline
M. catarrhalis	11.0%	Loracarbef equivalent to doxycycline
Overall	100.0%	Loracarbef equivalent to doxycycline

CYSTITIS

Study 1 In a controlled clinical study of cystitis performed in the United States, loracarbef was compared to cefaclor. In this study, using very strict evaluability criteria and microbiologic and clinical response criteria at the 5- to 9-day post therapy follow-up, the following bacterial eradication rates were obtained:

U.S. Uncomplicated Cystitis Study
Loracarbef vs Cefaclor

Efficacy:

Pathogen	% of Cases With Pathogens (n=186)	Outcome
E. coli	77.4%	Loracarbef eradication rate 4% greater than cefaclor (loracarbef eradication rate 80%)
Other major *Enterobacteriaceae*	12.5%	Loracarbef equivalent to cefaclor (loracarbef eradication rate 61%)
S. saprophyticus	3.8%	Loracarbef equivalent to cefaclor

Study 2 In a second controlled clinical study of cystitis, performed in Europe, loracarbef was compared to an oral quinolone. In this study, using very strict evaluability criteria and microbiologic and clinical response criteria at the 5- to 9-day post therapy follow-up, the following bacterial eradication rates were obtained:

European Uncomplicated Cystitis Study
Loracarbef vs Quinolone

Efficacy:

Pathogen	% of Cases With Pathogens (n=189)	Outcome
E. coli	82.0%	Loracarbef eradication rate 7% less than quinolone (loracarbef eradication rate 81%)
Other major *Enterobacteriaceae*	10.1%	Loracarbef eradication rate 32% less than quinolone (loracarbef eradication rate 50%)

REFERENCES

1. National Committee for Clinical Laboratory Standards, M2-A4 performance standards for antimicrobial disk susceptibility tests, ed 4, Villanova, PA, April, 1990.
2. National Committee for Clinical Laboratory Standards, M7-A2 methods for dilution antimicrobial susceptibility tests for bacteria that grow aerobically, ed 2, Villanova, PA, April, 1990.

CAUTION—Federal (USA) law prohibits dispensing without prescription.

Literature revised Nevermber 11, 1997

PV 2731 AMP [111197]

Shown in Product Identification Guide, page 320

MANDOL® ℞

[măn 'dōl]

(Cefamandole Nafate for Injection, USP)

DESCRIPTION

Mandol® (Cefamandole Nafate for Injection, USP) is a semisynthetic broad-spectrum cephalosporin antibiotic for parenteral administration. It is 5-thia-1-azabicyclo[4.2.0]oct-2-ene-2-carboxylic acid, 7-[[(formyloxy)phenylacetyl]amino]-3-[[(1-methyl-1*H*-tetrazol-5-yl)thio]methyl]-8-oxo-,mono-sodium salt, [6*R*-[6α,7β(*R**)]]. Cefamandole has the empirical formula $C_{19}H_{17}N_6NaO_6S_2$ representing a molecular weight of 512.49. Mandol also contains 63 mg sodium carbonate/g of cefamandole activity. The total sodium content is approximately 77 mg (3.3 mEq sodium ion) per g of cefamandole activity. After addition of diluent, cefamandole nafate rapidly hydrolyzes to cefamandole, and both compounds have microbiologic activity in vivo. Solutions of Mandol range from light-yellow to amber, depending on concentration and diluent used. The pH of freshly reconstituted solutions usually ranges from 6.0 to 8.5. The structural formula is as follows:

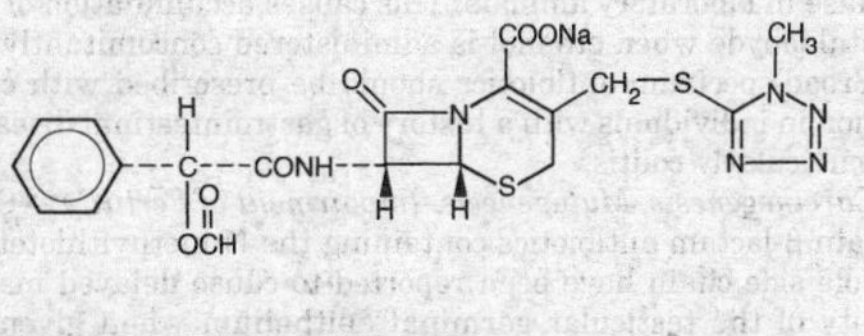

CLINICAL PHARMACOLOGY

After intramuscular administration of a 500-mg dose of cefamandole to normal volunteers, the mean peak serum concentration was 13 µg/mL. After a 1-g dose, the mean peak concentration was 25 µg/mL. These peaks occurred at 30 to 120 minutes. Following intravenous doses of 1, 2, and 3 g, serum concentrations were 139, 240, and 533 µg/mL respectively at 10 minutes. These concentrations declined to 0.8, 2.2, and 2.9 µg/mL at 4 hours. Intravenous administration of 4-g doses every 6 hours produced no evidence of accumulation in the serum. The half-life after an intravenous dose is 32 minutes; after intramuscular administration, the half-life is 60 minutes.

Sixty-five percent to 85% of cefamandole is excreted by the kidneys over an 8-hour period, resulting in high urinary concentrations. Following intramuscular doses of 500 mg and 1 g, urinary concentrations averaged 254 and 1,357 µg/mL respectively. Intravenous doses of 1 and 2 g produced urinary levels averaging 750 and 1,380 µg/mL respectively. Probenecid slows tubular excretion and doubles the peak serum level and the duration of measurable serum concentrations.

The antibiotic reaches therapeutic levels in pleural and joint fluids and in bile and bone.

Microbiology—The bactericidal action of cefamandole results from inhibition of cell-wall synthesis. Cephalosporins have in vitro activity against a wide range of gram-positive and gram-negative organisms. Cefamandole is usually active against the following organisms in vitro and in clinical infections:

Gram-positive
- *Staphylococcus aureus,* including penicillinase- and non-penicillinase-producing strains
- *Staphylococcus epidermidis*
- β-hemolytic and other streptococci (Most strains of enterococci, eg, *Enterococcus faecalis* [formerly *Streptococcus faecalis*], are resistant.)
- *Streptococcus pneumoniae*

Gram-negative
- *Escherichia coli*
- *Klebsiella* sp
- *Enterobacter* sp (Initially susceptible organisms occasionally may become resistant during therapy.)
- *Haemophilus influenzae*
- *Proteus mirabilis*
- *Providencia rettgeri (formerly Proteus rettgeri)*
- *Morganella morganii (formerly Proteus morganii)*
- *Proteus vulgaris* (Some strains of *P. vulgaris* have been shown by in vitro tests to be resistant to cefamandole and other cephalosporins.)

Anaerobic organisms
- Gram-positive and gram-negative cocci (including *Peptococcus* and *Peptostreptococcus* sp)
- Gram-positive bacilli (including *Clostridium* sp)
- Gram-negative bacilli (including *Bacteroides* and *Fusobacterium* sp). Most strains of *Bacteroides fragilis* are resistant.

Pseudomonas, Acinetobacter calcoaceticus (formerly *Mima* and *Herellea* sp), and most *Serratia* strains are resistant to cefamandole and certain other cephalosporins. Cefamandole is resistant to degradation by β-lactamases from certain members of the *Enterobacteriaceae.*

Susceptibility Tests —Quantitative methods that require measurement of zone diameters give the most precise estimates of antibiotic susceptibility. One such procedure[1] has been recommended for use with disks to test susceptibility to cefamandole. Interpretation involves correlation of the diameters obtained in the disk test with minimal inhibitory concentration (MIC) values for cefamandole.

Reports from the laboratory giving results of the standardized single-disk susceptibility test[1] using a 30-µg cefamandole disk should be interpreted according to the following criteria:

Susceptible organisms produce zones of 18 mm or greater, indicating that the tested organism is likely to respond to therapy.

Organisms of intermediate susceptibility produce zones of 15 to 17 mm, indicating that the tested organism would be susceptible if high dosage is used or if the infection is confined to tissues and fluids (eg, urine) in which high antibiotic levels are attained.

Resistant organisms produce zones of 14 mm or less, indicating that other therapy should be selected.

For gram-positive isolates, the test may be performed with either the cephalosporin-class disk (30 µg cephalothin) or the cefamandole disk (30 µg cefamandole), and a zone of 18 mm is indicative of a cefamandole-susceptible organism.

Gram-negative organisms should be tested with the cefamandole disk (using the above criteria), since cefamandole has been shown by in vitro tests to have activity against certain strains of *Enterobacteriaceae* found resistant when tested with the cephalosporin-class disk. Gram-negative organisms having zones of less than 18 mm around the cephalothin disk are not necessarily of intermediate susceptibility or resistant to cefamandole.

The cefamandole disk should not be used for testing susceptibility to other cephalosporins.

A bacterial isolate may be considered susceptible if the MIC value for cefamandole[2] is not more than 16 µg/mL. Organisms are considered resistant if the MIC is greater than 32 µg/mL.

INDICATIONS AND USAGE

Mandol is indicated for the treatment of serious infections caused by susceptible strains of the designated microorganisms in the diseases listed below:

Lower respiratory infections, including pneumonia, caused by *S. pneumoniae, H. influenzae, Klebsiella* sp, *S. aureus* (penicillinase- and non-penicillinase-producing), β-hemolytic streptococci, and *P. mirabilis*

Urinary tract infections caused by *E. coli, Proteus* sp (both indole-negative and indole-positive), *Enterobacter* sp, *Klebsiella* sp, group D streptococci (Note: Most enterococci, eg, *E. faecalis,* are resistant), and *S. epidermidis*

Peritonitis caused by *E. coli* and *Enterobacter* sp.

Septicemia caused by *E. coli, S. aureus* (penicillinase- and non-penicillinase-producing), *S. pneumoniae, S. pyogenes* (group A β-hemolytic streptococci), *H. influenzae,* and *Klebsiella* sp

Skin and skin structure infections caused by *S. aureus* (penicillinase- and non-penicillinase-producing), *S. pyogenes* (group A β-hemolytic streptococci), *H. influenzae, E. coli, Enterobacter* sp, and *P. mirabilis*

Bone and joint infections caused by *S. aureus* (penicillinase- and non-penicillinase-producing)

Clinical microbiologic studies in nongonococcal pelvic inflammatory disease in females, lower respiratory infections, and skin infections frequently reveal the growth of susceptible strains of both aerobic and anaerobic organisms. Mandol has been used successfully in those infections in which several organisms have been isolated. Most strains of *B. fragilis* are resistant in vitro; however, infections caused by susceptible strains have been treated successfully.

Specimens for bacteriologic cultures should be obtained in order to isolate and identify causative organisms and to determine their susceptibilities to cefamandole. Therapy may be instituted before results of susceptibility studies are known; however, once these results become available, the antibiotic treatment should be adjusted accordingly.

In certain cases of confirmed or suspected gram-positive or gram-negative sepsis or in patients with other serious infections in which the causative organism has not been identified, Mandol may be used concomitantly with an aminoglycoside (*see* Precautions). The recommended doses of both antibiotics may be given, depending on the severity of the infection and the patient's condition. The renal function of the patient should be carefully monitored, especially if higher dosages of the antibiotics are to be administered.

Antibiotic therapy of β-hemolytic streptococcal infections should continue for at least 10 days.

Preventive Therapy —The administration of Mandol preoperatively, intraoperatively, and postoperatively may reduce the incidence of certain postoperative infections in patients undergoing surgical procedures that are classified as contaminated or potentially contaminated (eg, gastrointestinal surgery, cesarean section, vaginal hysterectomy, or cholecystectomy in high-risk patients such as those with acute cholecystitis, obstructive jaundice, or common-bile-duct stones).

In major surgery in which the risk of postoperative infection is low but serious (cardiovascular surgery, neurosurgery, or prosthetic arthroplasty), Mandol may be effective in preventing such infections.

Continued on next page

*** Identi-Code® symbol. This product information was prepared in June 1998. Current information on these and other products of Eli Lilly and Company may be obtained by direct inquiry to Lilly Research Laboratories, Lilly Corporate Center, Indianapolis, Indiana 46285, (800) 545-5979.**

Mandol—Cont.

If signs of infection occur, specimens for culture should be obtained for identification of the causative organism so that appropriate antibiotic therapy may be instituted.

CONTRAINDICATION

Mandol is contraindicated in patients with known allergy to the cephalosporin group of antibiotics.

WARNINGS

BEFORE THERAPY WITH MANDOL IS INSTITUTED, CAREFUL INQUIRY SHOULD BE MADE TO DETERMINE WHETHER THE PATIENT HAS HAD PREVIOUS HYPERSENSITIVITY REACTIONS TO CEPHALOSPORINS, PENICILLINS, OR OTHER DRUGS. THIS PRODUCT SHOULD BE GIVEN CAUTIOUSLY TO PENICILLIN-SENSITIVE PATIENTS. ANTIBIOTICS SHOULD BE ADMINISTERED WITH CAUTION TO ANY PATIENT WHO HAS DEMONSTRATED SOME FORM OF ALLERGY, PARTICULARLY TO DRUGS. SERIOUS ACUTE HYPERSENSITIVITY REACTIONS MAY REQUIRE EPINEPHRINE AND OTHER EMERGENCY MEASURES.

In neonates, accumulation of other cephalosporin-class antibiotics (with resulting prolongation of drug half-life) has been reported.

Pseudomembranous colitis has been reported with virtually all broad-spectrum antibiotics (including macrolides, semisynthetic penicillins, and cephalosporins); therefore, it is important to consider its diagnosis in patients who develop diarrhea in association with the use of antibiotics. Such colitis may range in severity from mild to life threatening.

Treatment with broad-spectrum antibiotics alters the normal flora of the colon and may permit overgrowth of clostridia. Studies indicate that a toxin produced by *Clostridium difficile* is a primary cause of antibiotic-associated colitis.

Mild cases of pseudomembranous colitis usually respond to drug discontinuance alone. In moderate to severe cases, management should include sigmoidoscopy, appropriate bacteriologic studies, and fluid, electrolyte, and protein supplementation. When the colitis does not improve after the drug has been discontinued, or when it is severe, oral vancomycin is the drug of choice for antibiotic-associated pseudomembranous colitis produced by *C. difficile*. Other causes of colitis should be ruled out.

PRECAUTIONS

General —Although Mandol rarely produces alteration in kidney function, evaluation of renal status is recommended, especially in seriously ill patients receiving maximum doses.

Prolonged use of Mandol may result in the overgrowth of nonsusceptible organisms. Careful observation of the patient is essential. If superinfection occurs during therapy, appropriate measures should be taken.

Nephrotoxicity has been reported following concomitant administration of aminoglycoside antibiotics and cephalosporins.

A false-positive reaction for glucose in the urine may occur with Benedict's or Fehling's solution or with Clinitest® tablets. There may be a false-positive test for proteinuria with acid and denaturization-precipitation tests.

As with other broad-spectrum antibiotics, hypoprothrombinemia, with or without bleeding, has been reported rarely, but it has been promptly reversed by administration of vitamin K. Such episodes usually have occurred in elderly, debilitated, or otherwise compromised patients with deficient stores of vitamin K. Treatment of such individuals with antibiotics possessing significant gram-negative and/or anaerobic activity is thought to alter the number and/or type of intestinal bacterial flora, with consequent reduction in synthesis of vitamin K. Prophylactic administration of vitamin K may be indicated in such patients, especially when intestinal sterilization and surgical procedures are performed.

In a few patients receiving Mandol, nausea, vomiting, and vasomotor instability with hypotension and peripheral vasodilatation occurred following the ingestion of ethanol. Cefamandole inhibits the enzyme acetaldehyde dehydrogenase in laboratory animals. This causes accumulation of acetaldehyde when ethanol is administered concomitantly.

Broad-spectrum antibiotics should be prescribed with caution in individuals with a history of gastrointestinal disease, particularly colitis.

Carcinogenesis, Mutagenesis, Impairment of Fertility —Certain β-lactam antibiotics containing the N-methylthiotetrazole side chain have been reported to cause delayed maturity of the testicular germinal epithelium when given to neonatal rats during initial spermatogenic development (6 to 36 days of age). In animals that were treated from 6 to 36 days of age with 1,000 mg/kg/day of cefamandole (approximately 5 times the maximum clinical dose), the delayed maturity was pronounced and was associated with decreased testicular weights and a reduced number of germinal cells in the leading waves of spermatogenic development. The effect was slight in rats given 50 or 100 mg/kg/day. Some animals that were given 1,000 mg/kg/day during days 6 to 36 were infertile after becoming sexually mature. No adverse effects have been observed in rats exposed in utero, in neonatal rats (4 days of age or younger) treated prior to the initiation of spermatogenesis, or in older rats (more than 36 days of age) after exposure for up to 6 months. The significance to humans of these findings in rats is unknown because of differences in the time of initiation of spermatogenesis, rate of spermatogenic development, and duration of puberty.

Usage in Pregnancy —Pregnancy Category B —Reproduction studies have been performed in rats given doses of 500 or 1,000 mg/kg/day and have revealed no evidence of impaired fertility or harm to the fetus due to Mandol. There are, however, no adequate and well-controlled studies in pregnant women. Because animal reproduction studies are not always predictive of human response, this drug should be used during pregnancy only if clearly needed.

Nursing Mothers —Caution should be exercised when Mandol is administered to a nursing woman.

Usage in Infancy—Mandol has been effectively used in this age group, but all laboratory parameters have not been extensively studied in infants between 1 and 6 months of age; safety of this product has not been established in premature infants and term neonates under 1 month of age. Therefore, if Mandol is administered to infants, the physician should determine whether the potential benefits outweigh the possible risks involved.

ADVERSE REACTIONS

Gastrointestinal —Symptoms of pseudomembranous colitis may appear either during or after antibiotic treatment. Nausea and vomiting have been reported rarely. As with some penicillins and some other cephalosporins, transient hepatitis and cholestatic jaundice have been reported rarely.

Hypersensitivity —Anaphylaxis, maculopapular rash, urticaria, eosinophilia, and drug fever have been reported. These reactions are more likely to occur in patients with a history of allergy, particularly to penicillin.

Blood —Thrombocytopenia has been reported rarely. Neutropenia has been reported, especially in long courses of treatment. Some individuals have developed positive direct Coombs' tests during treatment with the cephalosporin antibiotics.

Liver —Transient rise in SGOT, SGPT, and alkaline phosphatase levels has been noted.

Kidney —Decreased creatinine clearance has been reported in patients with prior renal impairment. As with some other cephalosporins, transitory elevations of BUN have occasionally been observed with Mandol; their frequency increases in patients over 50 years of age. In some of these cases, there was also a mild increase in serum creatinine.

Local Reactions —Pain on intramuscular injection is infrequent. Thrombophlebitis occurs rarely.

OVERDOSAGE

The administration of inappropriately large doses of parenteral cephalosporins may cause seizures, particularly in patients with renal impairment. Dosage reduction is necessary when renal function is impaired (*see* Dosage and Administration). If seizures occur, the drug should be promptly discontinued; anticonvulsant therapy may be administered if clinically indicated. Hemodialysis may be considered in cases of overwhelming overdosage.

DOSAGE AND ADMINISTRATION

Dosage—Adults: The usual dosage range for cefamandole is 500 mg to 1 g every 4 to 8 hours.

In infections of skin structures and in uncomplicated pneumonia, a dosage of 500 mg every 6 hours is adequate.

In uncomplicated urinary tract infections, a dosage of 500 mg every 8 hours is sufficient. In more serious urinary tract infections, a dosage of 1 g every 8 hours may be needed.

In severe infections, 1-g doses may be given at 4 to 6-hour intervals.

In life-threatening infections or infections due to less susceptible organisms, doses up to 2 g every 4 hours (ie, 12 g/day) may be needed.

Infants and Children: Administration of 50 to 100 mg/kg/day in equally divided doses every 4 to 8 hours has been effective for most infections susceptible to Mandol. This may be increased to a total daily dose of 150 mg/kg (not to exceed the maximum adult dose) for severe infections. (*See* recommendations regarding this age group in Warnings *and* Precautions.)

Note: As with antibiotic therapy in general, administration of Mandol should be continued for a minimum of 48 to 72 hours after the patient becomes asymptomatic or after evidence of bacterial eradication has been obtained; a minimum of 10 days of treatment is recommended in infections caused by group A β-hemolytic streptococci in order to guard against the risk of rheumatic fever or glomerulonephritis; frequent bacteriologic and clinical appraisal is necessary during therapy of chronic urinary tract infection and may be required for several months after therapy has been completed; persistent infections may require treatment for several weeks; and doses smaller than those indicated above should not be used.

For perioperative use of Mandol, the following dosages are recommended:

Adults —1 or 2 g intravenously or intramuscularly $^1/_2$ to 1 hour prior to the surgical incision followed by 1 or 2 g every 6 hours for 24 to 48 hours.

Pediatric Patients (3 months of age and older) —50 to 100 mg/kg/day in equally divided doses by the routes and schedule designated above.

Note: In patients undergoing prosthetic arthroplasty, administration is recommended for as long as 72 hours.

In patients undergoing cesarean section, the initial dose may be administered just prior to surgery or immediately after the cord has been clamped.

Impaired Renal Function —When renal function is impaired, a reduced dosage must be employed and the serum levels closely monitored. After an initial dose of 1 to 2 g (depending on the severity of infection), a maintenance dosage schedule should be followed (see chart). Continued dosage should be determined by degree of renal impairment, severity of infection, and susceptibility of the causative organism. [See table at left]

MAINTENANCE DOSAGE GUIDE FOR PATIENTS WITH RENAL IMPAIRMENT

Creatinine Clearance (mL/min/1.73 m^2)	Renal Function	Life-Threatening Infections—Maximum Dosage	Less Severe Infections
>80	Normal	2 g q4h	1–2 g q6h
80–50	Mild Impairment	1.5 g q4h OR 2 g q6h	0.75–1.5 g q6h
50–25	Moderate Impairment	1.5 g q6h OR 2 g q8h	0.75–1.5 g q8h
25–10	Severe Impairment	1 g q6h OR 1.25 g q8h	0.5–1 g q8h
10–2	Marked Impairment	0.67 g q8h OR 1 g q12h	0.5–0.75 g q12h
<2	None	0.5 g q8h OR 0.75 g q12h	0.25–0.5 g q12h

When only serum creatinine is available, the following formula (based on sex, weight, and age of the patient) may be used to convert this value into creatinine clearance. The serum creatinine should represent a steady state of renal function.

$$\text{Males: } \frac{\text{Weight (kg)} \times (140 - \text{age})}{72 \times \text{serum creatinine}}$$

$$\text{Females: } 0.9 \times \text{above value}$$

Modes of Administration —Mandol may be given intravenously or by deep intramuscular injection into a large muscle mass (such as the gluteus or lateral part of the thigh) to minimize pain.

Intramuscular Administration —Each g of Mandol should be diluted with 3 mL of 1 of the following diluents: Sterile

Water for Injection, Bacteriostatic Water for Injection, 0.9% Sodium Chloride Injection, or Bacteriostatic Sodium Chloride Injection. Shake well until dissolved.

Intravenous Administration—The intravenous route may be preferable for patients with bacterial septicemia, localized parenchymal abscesses (such as intra-abdominal abscess), peritonitis, or other severe or life-threatening infections when they may be poor risks because of lowered resistance. In those with normal renal function, the intravenous dosage for such infections is 3 to 12 g of Mandol daily. In conditions such as bacterial septicemia, 6 to 12 g/day may be given initially by the intravenous route for several days, and dosage may then be gradually reduced according to clinical response and laboratory findings.

If combination therapy with Mandol and an aminoglycoside is indicated, each of these antibiotics should be administered in different sites. *Do not mix an aminoglycoside with Mandol in the same intravenous fluid container.*

A SOLUTION OF 1 G OF MANDOL IN 22 ML OF STERILE WATER FOR INJECTION IS ISOTONIC.

The choice of saline, dextrose, or electrolyte solution and the volume to be employed are dictated by fluid and electrolyte management.

For direct intermittent intravenous administration, each g of cefamandole should be reconstituted with 10 mL of Sterile Water for Injection, 5% Dextrose Injection, or 0.9% Sodium Chloride Injection. Slowly inject the solution into the vein over a period of 3 to 5 minutes, or give it through the tubing of an administration set while the patient is also receiving 1 of the following intravenous fluids: 0.9% Sodium Chloride Injection; 5% Dextrose Injection; 10% Dextrose Injection; 5% Dextrose and 0.9% Sodium Chloride Injection; 5% Dextrose and 0.45% Sodium Chloride Injection; 5% Dextrose and 0.2% Sodium Chloride Injection; or Sodium Lactate Injection (M/6).

Intermittent intravenous infusion with a Y-type administration set or volume control set can also be accomplished while any of the above-mentioned intravenous fluids are being infused. However, during infusion of the solution containing Mandol, it is desirable to discontinue the other solution. When this technique is employed, careful attention should be paid to the volume of the solution containing Mandol so that the calculated dose will be infused. When a Y-tube hookup is used, 100 mL of the appropriate diluent should be added to the 1- or 2-g piggyback (100-mL) vial. If Sterile Water for Injection is used as the diluent, reconstitute with approximately 20 mL/g to avoid a hypotonic solution.

For continuous intravenous infusion, each g of cefamandole should be diluted with 10 mL of Sterile Water for Injection. An appropriate quantity of the resulting solution may be added to an IV bottle containing 1 of the following fluids: 0.9% Sodium Chloride Injection; 5% Dextrose Injection; 10% Dextrose Injection; 5% Dextrose and 0.9% Sodium Chloride Injection; 5% Dextrose and 0.45% Sodium Chloride Injection; 5% Dextrose and 0.2% Sodium Chloride Injection; or Sodium Lactate Injection (M/6).

STABILITY

Reconstituted Mandol is stable for 24 hours at room temperature (25°C) and for 96 hours if stored under refrigeration (5°C). *During storage at room temperature, carbon dioxide develops inside the vial after reconstitution. This pressure may be dissipated prior to withdrawal of the vial contents, or it may be used to aid withdrawal if the vial is inverted over the syringe needle and the contents are allowed to flow into the syringe.*

Solutions of Mandol in Sterile Water for Injection, 5% Dextrose Injection, or 0.9% Sodium Chloride Injection that are frozen immediately after reconstitution in the conventional vials in which the drugs are supplied are stable for 6 months when stored at −20°C. **If the product is warmed (to a maximum of 37°C), care should be taken to avoid heating it after the thawing is complete. Once thawed, the solution should not be refrozen.**

HOW SUPPLIED

Vials (Dry Powder):

1 g,* 10-mL size (No. 7061)—(Traypak of 25) NDC 0002-7061-25

1 g,* 100-mL size (No. 7068)—(Traypak of 10) NDC 0002-7068-10

2 g,* 20-mL size (No. 7064)—(Traypak of 10) NDC 0002-7064-10

2 g,* 100-mL size (No. 7069)—(Traypak of 10) NDC 0002-7069-10

ADD-Vantage§ Vials:

1 g* (No. 7268)—(Traypak of 25) NDC 0002-7268-25

2 g* (No. 7269)—(Traypak of 10) NDC 0002-7269-10

The above ADD-Vantage Vials are to be used only with Abbott Laboratories' ADD-Vantage Diluent Containers.

Instructions for use of the ADD-Vantage Vials are enclosed in the package.

Also Available:

Pharmacy Bulk Package:

10 g,* 100-mL size (No. 7072)—(Traypak of 6) NDC 0002-7072-16

CAUTION—Federal (USA) law prohibits dispensing without prescription.

---

* Equivalent to cefamandole activity.

† Traypak™ (multivial carton, Lilly).

§ ADD-Vantage® (vials and diluent containers, Abbott).

Literature revised October 1, 1996

PA 6921 ITAMP [100196]

---

1. Bauer AW, Kirby WMM, et al: Antibiotic susceptibility testing by a standardized single disk method. *Am J Clin Pathol* 1966;45:493. Standardized disk susceptibility test. *Federal Register* 1974;39:19182–19184. National Committee for Clinical Laboratory Standards. Approved Standard: M2-A3 Performance standards for antimicrobial disk susceptibility tests—Fourth Edition, December, 1988.
2. Determined by the ICS agar-dilution method (Ericsson HM, Sherris JC: *Acta Pathol Microbiol Scand* 1971;[suppl 217]: B), or any other method that has been shown to give equivalent results.

NEBCIN® ℞

[*nĕb 'sĭn*]

(Tobramycin Sulfate Injection, USP)

WARNINGS

Patients treated with Nebcin® (Tobramycin Sulfate Injection, USP) and other aminoglycosides should be under close clinical observation, because these drugs have an inherent potential for causing ototoxicity and nephrotoxicity.

Neurotoxicity, manifested as both auditory and vestibular ototoxicity, can occur. The auditory changes are irreversible, are usually bilateral, and may be partial or total. Eighth-nerve impairment and nephrotoxicity may develop, primarily in patients having preexisting renal damage and in those with normal renal function to whom aminoglycosides are administered for longer periods or in higher doses than those recommended. Other manifestations of neurotoxicity may include numbness, skin tingling, muscle twitching, and convulsions. The risk of aminoglycoside-induced hearing loss increases with the degree of exposure to either high peak or high trough serum concentrations. Patients who develop cochlear damage may not have symptoms during therapy to warn them of eighth-nerve toxicity, and partial or total irreversible bilateral deafness may continue to develop after the drug has been discontinued.

Rarely, nephrotoxicity may not become apparent until the first few days after cessation of therapy. Aminoglycoside-induced nephrotoxicity usually is reversible.

Renal and eighth-nerve function should be closely monitored in patients with known or suspected renal impairment and also in those whose renal function is initially normal but who develop signs of renal dysfunction during therapy. Peak and trough serum concentrations of aminoglycosides should be monitored periodically during therapy to assure adequate levels and to avoid potentially toxic levels. Prolonged serum concentrations above 12 µg/mL should be avoided. Rising trough levels (above 2 µg/mL) may indicate tissue accumulation. Such accumulation, excessive peak concentrations, advanced age, and cumulative dose may contribute to ototoxicity and nephrotoxicity (*see* **PRECAUTIONS**). Urine should be examined for decreased specific gravity and increased excretion of protein, cells, and casts. Blood urea nitrogen, serum creatinine, and creatinine clearance should be measured periodically. When feasible, it is recommended that serial audiograms be obtained in patients old enough to be tested, particularly high-risk patients. Evidence of impairment of renal, vestibular, or auditory function requires discontinuation of the drug or dosage adjustment.

Nebcin should be used with caution in premature and neonatal infants because of their renal immaturity and the resulting prolongation of serum half-life of the drug.

Concurrent and sequential use of other neurotoxic and/or nephrotoxic antibiotics, particularly other aminoglycosides (eg, amikacin, streptomycin, neomycin, kanamycin, gentamicin, and paromomycin), cephaloridine, viomycin, polymyxin B, colistin, cisplatin, and vancomycin, should be avoided. Other factors that may increase patient risk are advanced age and dehydration.

Aminoglycosides should not be given concurrently with potent diuretics, such as ethacrynic acid and furosemide. Some diuretics themselves cause ototoxicity, and intravenously administered diuretics enhance aminoglycoside toxicity by altering antibiotic concentrations in serum and tissue.

Aminoglycosides can cause fetal harm when administered to a pregnant woman (*see* **PRECAUTIONS**).

DESCRIPTION

Tobramycin sulfate, a water-soluble antibiotic of the aminoglycoside group, is derived from the actinomycete *Streptomyces tenebrarius.* Nebcin, Injection, is a clear and colorless sterile aqueous solution for parenteral administration.

Tobramycin sulfate is *O*-3-amino-3-deoxy-α-D-glucopyranosyl-(1→4)-*O*-[2,6-diamino-2,3,6-trideoxy-α-D-*ribo*-hexopyranosyl-(1→6)]-2-deoxy-L-streptamine, sulfate (2:5)(salt) and has the chemical formula $(C_{18}H_{37}N_5O_9)_2 \cdot 5H_2SO_4$. The molecular weight is 1425.45. The structural formula for tobramycin is as follows:

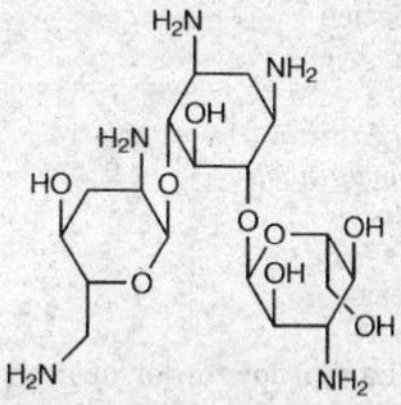

Each mL also contains phenol as a preservative (5 mg, multiple-dose vials; 1.25 mg, ADD-Vantage® vials), sodium bisulfite (3.2 mg, multiple-dose vials; 1.6 mg, ADD-Vantage vials), 0.1 mg edetate disodium, and water for injection, qs. Sulfuric acid and/or sodium hydroxide may have been added to adjust the pH.

CLINICAL PHARMACOLOGY

Tobramycin is rapidly absorbed following intramuscular administration. Peak serum concentrations of tobramycin occur between 30 and 90 minutes after intramuscular administration. Following an intramuscular dose of 1 mg/kg of body weight, maximum serum concentrations reach about 4 µg/mL, and measurable levels persist for as long as 8 hours. Therapeutic serum levels are generally considered to range from 4 to 6 µg/mL. When Nebcin is administered by intravenous infusion over a 1-hour period, the serum concentrations are similar to those obtained by intramuscular administration. Nebcin is poorly absorbed from the gastrointestinal tract.

In patients with normal renal function, except neonates, Nebcin administered every 8 hours does not accumulate in the serum. However, in those patients with reduced renal function and in neonates, the serum concentration of the antibiotic is usually higher and can be measured for longer periods of time than in normal adults. Dosage for such patients must, therefore, be adjusted accordingly (*see* **DOSAGE AND ADMINISTRATION**).

Following parenteral administration, little, if any, metabolic transformation occurs, and tobramycin is eliminated almost exclusively by glomerular filtration. Renal clearance is similar to that of endogenous creatinine. Ultrafiltration studies demonstrate that practically no serum protein binding occurs. In patients with normal renal function, up to 84% of the dose is recoverable from the urine in 8 hours and up to 93% in 24 hours.

Peak urine concentrations ranging from 75 to 100 µg/mL have been observed following the intramuscular injection of a single dose of 1 mg/kg. After several days of treatment, the amount of tobramycin excreted in the urine approaches the daily dose administered. When renal function is impaired, excretion of Nebcin is slowed, and accumulation of the drug may cause toxic blood levels.

The serum half-life in normal individuals is 2 hours. An inverse relationship exists between serum half-life and creatinine clearance, and the dosage schedule should be adjusted according to the degree of renal impairment (*see* **DOSAGE AND ADMINISTRATION**). In patients undergoing dialysis, 25% to 70% of the administered dose may be removed, depending on the duration and type of dialysis.

Tobramycin can be detected in tissues and body fluids after parenteral administration. Concentrations in bile and stools ordinarily have been low, which suggests minimum biliary excretion. Tobramycin has appeared in low concentration in the cerebrospinal fluid following parenteral administration, and concentrations are dependent on dose, rate of penetration, and degree of meningeal inflammation. It has also been found in sputum, peritoneal fluid, synovial fluid, and abscess fluids, and it crosses the placental membranes. Concentrations in the renal cortex are several times higher than the usual serum levels.

Continued on next page

*** Identi-Code® symbol. This product information was prepared in June 1998. Current information on these and other products of Eli Lilly and Company may be obtained by direct inquiry to Lilly Research Laboratories, Lilly Corporate Center, Indianapolis, Indiana 46285, (800) 545-5979.**

Nebcin—Cont.

Probenecid does not affect the renal tubular transport of tobramycin.

Microbiology – Tobramycin acts by inhibiting synthesis of protein in bacterial cells. *In vitro* tests demonstrate that tobramycin is bactericidal.

Tobramycin has been shown to be active against most strains of the following organisms both *in vitro* and in clinical infections as described in the Indications and Usage section:

Aerobic Gram-positive microorganisms
  Staphylococcus aureus
Aerobic Gram-negative microorganisms
  Citrobacter species
  Enterobacter species
  Escherichia coli
  Klebsiella species
  Morganella morganii
  Pseudomonas aeruginosa
  Proteus mirabilis
  Proteus vulgaris
  Providencia species
  Serratia species

Aminoglycosides have a low order of activity against most gram-positive organisms, including *Streptococcus pyogenes*, *Streptococcus pneumoniae*, and enterococci.

Although most strains of enterococci demonstrate *in vitro* resistance, some strains in this group are susceptible. *In vitro* studies have shown that an aminoglycoside combined with an antibiotic that interferes with cell-wall synthesis affects some enterococcal strains synergistically. The combination of penicillin G and tobramycin results in a synergistic bactericidal effect *in vitro* against certain strains of *Enterococcus faecalis*. However, this combination is not synergistic against other closely related organisms, eg, *Enterococcus faecium*. Speciation of enterococci alone cannot be used to predict susceptibility. Susceptibility testing and tests for antibiotic synergism are emphasized.

Cross resistance between aminoglycosides may occur.
Susceptibility Tests —
Diffusion techniques: Quantitative methods that require measurement of zone diameters give the most precise estimates of susceptibility of bacteria to antimicrobial agents. One such procedure is the National Committee for Clinical Laboratory Standards (NCCLS)-approved procedure.[1] This method has been recommended for use with disks to test susceptibility to tobramycin. Interpretation involves correlation of the diameters obtained in the disk test with minimum inhibitory concentrations (MIC) for tobramycin.

Reports from the laboratory giving results of the standard single-disk susceptibility test with a 10-μg tobramycin disk should be interpreted according to the following criteria:

Zone Diameter (mm)	Interpretation
≥15	(S) Susceptible
13–14	(I) Intermediate
≤12	(R) Resistant

A report of "Susceptible" indicates that the pathogen is likely to be inhibited by generally achievable blood levels. A report of "Intermediate" suggests that the organism would be susceptible if high dosage is used or if the infection is confined to tissues and fluids in which high antimicrobial levels are obtained. A report of "Resistant" indicates that achievable concentrations are unlikely to be inhibitory and other therapy should be selected.

Standardized procedures require the use of laboratory control organisms. The 10-μg tobramycin disk should give the following zone diameters:

Organism	Zone Diameter (mm)
E. coli ATCC 25922	18–26
P. aeruginosa ATCC 27853	19–25
S. aureus ATCC 25923	19–29

Dilution techniques: Broth and agar dilution methods, such as those recommended by the NCCLS,[2] may be used to determine MICs of tobramycin. MIC test results should be interpreted according to the following criteria:

MIC (μg/mL)	Interpretation
≤4	(S) Susceptible
8	(I) Intermediate
≥16	(R) Resistant

As with standard diffusion methods, dilution procedures require the use of laboratory control organisms. Tobramycin laboratory reagent should give the following MIC values:

Organism	MIC Range (μg/mL)
E. faecalis ATCC 29212	8.0–32.0
E. coli ATCC 25922	0.25–1
P. aeruginosa ATCC 27853	0.12–2
S. aureus ATCC 29213	0.12–1

INDICATIONS AND USAGE

Nebcin is indicated for the treatment of serious bacterial infections caused by susceptible strains of the designated microorganisms in the diseases listed below:

Septicemia in the pediatric patient and adult caused by *P. aeruginosa*, *E. coli*, and *Klebsiella* spp

Lower respiratory tract infections caused by *P. aeruginosa*, *Klebsiella* spp, *Enterobacter* spp, *Serratia* spp, *E. coli*, and *S. aureus* (penicillinase- and non-penicillinase-producing strains)

Serious central-nervous-system infections (meningitis) caused by susceptible organisms

Intra-abdominal infections, including peritonitis, caused by *E. coli*, *Klebsiella* spp, and *Enterobacter* spp

Skin, bone, and skin structure infections caused by *P. aeruginosa*, *Proteus* spp, *E. coli*, *Klebsiella* spp, *Enterobacter* spp, and *S. aureus*

Complicated and recurrent urinary tract infections caused by *P. aeruginosa*, *Proteus* spp (indole-positive and indole-negative), *E. coli*, *Klebsiella* spp, *Enterobacter* spp, *Serratia* spp, *S. aureus*, *Providencia* spp, and *Citrobacter* spp

Aminoglycosides, including Nebcin, are not indicated in uncomplicated initial episodes of urinary tract infections unless the causative organisms are not susceptible to antibiotics having less potential toxicity. Nebcin may be considered in serious staphylococcal infections when penicillin or other potentially less toxic drugs are contraindicated and when bacterial susceptibility testing and clinical judgment indicate its use.

Bacterial cultures should be obtained prior to and during treatment to isolate and identify etiologic organisms and to test their susceptibility to tobramycin. If susceptibility tests show that the causative organisms are resistant to tobramycin, other appropriate therapy should be instituted. In patients in whom a serious life-threatening gram-negative infection is suspected, including those in whom concurrent therapy with a penicillin or cephalosporin and an aminoglycoside may be indicated, treatment with Nebcin may be initiated before the results of susceptibility studies are obtained. The decision to continue therapy with Nebcin should be based on the results of susceptibility studies, the severity of the infection, and the important additional concepts discussed in the WARNINGS box above.

CONTRAINDICATIONS

A hypersensitivity to any aminoglycoside is a contraindication to the use of tobramycin. A history of hypersensitivity or serious toxic reactions to aminoglycosides may also contraindicate the use of any other aminoglycoside because of the known cross-sensitivity of patients to drugs in this class.

WARNINGS

See **WARNINGS** box above.

Nebcin contains sodium bisulfite, a sulfite that may cause allergic-type reactions, including anaphylactic symptoms and life-threatening or less severe asthmatic episodes, in certain susceptible people. The overall prevalence of sulfite sensitivity in the general population is unknown and probably low. Sulfite sensitivity is seen more frequently in asthmatic than in nonasthmatic people.

Serious allergic reactions including anaphylaxis and dermatologic reactions including exfoliative dermatitis, toxic epidermal necrolysis, erythema multiforme, and Stevens-Johnson Syndrome have been reported rarely in patients on tobramycin therapy. Although rare, fatalities have been reported. (*See* **CONTRAINDICATIONS**.)

If an allergic reaction occurs, the drug should be discontinued and appropriate therapy instituted.

PRECAUTIONS

Serum and urine specimens for examination should be collected during therapy, as recommended in the WARNINGS box. Serum calcium, magnesium, and sodium should be monitored.

Peak and trough serum levels should be measured periodically during therapy. Prolonged concentrations above 12 μg/mL should be avoided. Rising trough levels (above 2 μg/mL) may indicate tissue accumulation. Such accumulation, advanced age, and cumulative dosage may contribute to ototoxicity and nephrotoxicity. It is particularly important to monitor serum levels closely in patients with known renal impairment.

A useful guideline would be to perform serum level assays after 2 or 3 doses, so that the dosage could be adjusted if necessary, and at 3- to 4-day intervals during therapy. In the event of changing renal function, more frequent serum levels should be obtained and the dosage or dosage interval adjusted according to the guidelines provided in the Dosage and Administration section.

In order to measure the peak level, a serum sample should be drawn about 30 minutes following intravenous infusion or 1 hour after an intramuscular injection. Trough levels are measured by obtaining serum samples at 8 hours or just prior to the next dose of Nebcin. These suggested time intervals are intended only as guidelines and may vary ac-

cording to institutional practices. It is important, however, that there be consistency within the individual patient program unless computerized pharmacokinetic dosing programs are available in the institution. These serum-level assays may be especially useful for monitoring the treatment of severely ill patients with changing renal function or of those infected with less susceptible organisms or those receiving maximum dosage.

Neuromuscular blockade and respiratory paralysis have been reported in cats receiving very high doses of tobramycin (40 mg/kg). The possibility of prolonged or secondary apnea should be considered if tobramycin is administered to anesthetized patients who are also receiving neuromuscular blocking agents, such as succinylcholine, tubocurarine, or decamethonium, or to patients receiving massive transfusions of citrated blood. If neuromuscular blockade occurs, it may be reversed by the administration of calcium salts.

Cross-allergenicity among aminoglycosides has been demonstrated.

In patients with extensive burns, or cystic fibrosis, altered pharmacokinetics may result in reduced serum concentrations of aminoglycosides. In such patients treated with Nebcin, measurement of serum concentration is especially important as a basis for determination of appropriate dosage. Elderly patients may have reduced renal function that may not be evident in the results of routine screening tests, such as BUN or serum creatinine. A creatinine clearance determination may be more useful. Monitoring of renal function during treatment with aminoglycosides is particularly important in such patients.

An increased incidence of nephrotoxicity has been reported following concomitant administration of aminoglycoside antibiotics and cephalosporins.

Aminoglycosides should be used with caution in patients with muscular disorders, such as myasthenia gravis or parkinsonism, since these drugs may aggravate muscle weakness because of their potential curare-like effect on neuromuscular function.

Aminoglycosides may be absorbed in significant quantities from body surfaces after local irrigation or application and may cause neurotoxicity and nephrotoxicity.

Aminoglycosides have not been approved for intraocular and/or subconjunctival use. Physicians are advised that macular necrosis has been reported following administration of aminoglycosides, including tobramycin, by these routes.

See **WARNINGS** box regarding concurrent use of potent diuretics and concurrent and sequential use of other neurotoxic or nephrotoxic drugs.

The inactivation of tobramycin and other aminoglycosides by β-lactam-type antibiotics (penicillins or cephalosporins) has been demonstrated *in vitro* and in patients with severe renal impairment. Such inactivation has not been found in patients with normal renal function who have been given the drugs by separate routes of administration.

Therapy with tobramycin may result in overgrowth of nonsusceptible organisms. If overgrowth of nonsusceptible organisms occurs, appropriate therapy should be initiated.

*Pregnancy Category D —*Aminoglycosides can cause fetal harm when administered to a pregnant woman. Aminoglycoside antibiotics cross the placenta, and there have been several reports of total irreversible bilateral congenital deafness in children whose mothers received streptomycin during pregnancy. Serious side effects to mother, fetus, or newborn have not been reported in the treatment of pregnant women with other aminoglycosides. If tobramycin is used during pregnancy or if the patient becomes pregnant while taking tobramycin, she should be apprised of the potential hazard to the fetus.

Pediatric Use —See **INDICATIONS AND USAGE** *and* **DOSAGE AND ADMINISTRATION**.

ADVERSE REACTIONS

*Neurotoxicity —*Adverse effects on both the vestibular and auditory branches of the eighth nerve have been noted, especially in patients receiving high doses or prolonged therapy, in those given previous courses of therapy with an ototoxin, and in cases of dehydration. Symptoms include dizziness, vertigo, tinnitus, roaring in the ears, and hearing loss. Hearing loss is usually irreversible and is manifested initially by diminution of high-tone acuity. Tobramycin and gentamicin sulfates closely parallel each other in regard to ototoxic potential.

*Nephrotoxicity —*Renal function changes, as shown by rising BUN, NPN, and serum creatinine and by oliguria, cylindruria, and increased proteinuria, have been reported, especially in patients with a history of renal impairment who are treated for longer periods or with higher doses than those recommended. Adverse renal effects can occur in patients with initially normal renal function.

Clinical studies and studies in experimental animals have been conducted to compare the nephrotoxic potential of tobramycin and gentamicin. In some of the clinical studies and in the animal studies, tobramycin caused nephrotoxicity significantly less frequently than gentamicin. In some

TABLE 1. DOSAGE SCHEDULE GUIDE FOR ADULTS WITH NORMAL RENAL FUNCTION
(Dosage at 8-Hour Intervals)

For Patient Weighing		Usual Dose for Serious Infections		Maximum Dose for Life-Threatening Infections (Reduce as soon as possible)	
		1 mg/kg q8h (Total, 3 mg/kg/day)		1.66 mg/kg q8h (Total, 5 mg/kg/day)	
kg	lb	mg/dose q8h	mL/dose*	mg/dose q8h	mL/dose*
120	264	120 mg	3 mL	200 mg	5 mL
115	253	115 mg	2.9 mL	191 mg	4.75 mL
110	242	110 mg	2.75 mL	183 mg	4.5 mL
105	231	105 mg	2.6 mL	175 mg	4.4 mL
100	220	100 mg	2.5 mL	166 mg	4.2 mL
95	209	95 mg	2.4 mL	158 mg	4 mL
90	198	90 mg	2.25 mL	150 mg	3.75 mL
85	187	85 mg	2.1 mL	141 mg	3.5 mL
80	176	80 mg	2 mL	133 mg	3.3 mL
75	165	75 mg	1.9 mL	125 mg	3.1 mL
70	154	70 mg	1.75 mL	116 mg	2.9 mL
65	143	65 mg	1.6 mL	108 mg	2.7 mL
60	132	60 mg	1.5 mL	100 mg	2.5 mL
55	121	55 mg	1.4 mL	91 mg	2.25 mL
50	110	50 mg	1.25 mL	83 mg	2.1 mL
45	99	45 mg	1.1 mL	75 mg	1.9 mL
40	88	40 mg	1 mL	66 mg	1.6 mL

*Applicable to all product forms except Nebcin, Pediatric, Injection (see How Supplied).

other clinical studies, no significant difference in the incidence of nephrotoxicity between tobramycin and gentamicin was found.

Other reported adverse reactions possibly related to Nebcin include anemia, granulocytopenia, and thrombocytopenia; and fever, rash, exfoliative dermatitis, itching, urticaria, nausea, vomiting, diarrhea, headache, lethargy, pain at the injection site, mental confusion, and disorientation. Laboratory abnormalities possibly related to Nebcin include increased serum transaminases (AST, ALT); increased serum LDH and bilirubin; decreased serum calcium, magnesium, sodium, and potassium; and leukopenia, leukocytosis, and eosinophilia.

OVERDOSAGE

Signs and Symptoms —The severity of the signs and symptoms following a tobramycin overdose are dependent on the dose administered, the patient's renal function, state of hydration, and age and whether or not other medications with similar toxicities are being administered concurrently. Toxicity may occur in patients treated more than 10 days, in adults given more than 5 mg/kg/day, in pediatric patients given more than 7.5 mg/kg/day, or in patients with reduced renal function where dose has not been appropriately adjusted.

Nephrotoxicity following the parenteral administration of an aminoglycoside is most closely related to the area under the curve of the serum concentration versus time graph. Nephrotoxicity is more likely if trough blood concentrations fail to fall below 2 µg/mL and is also proportional to the average blood concentration. Patients who are elderly, have abnormal renal function, are receiving other nephrotoxic drugs, or are volume depleted are at greater risk for developing acute tubular necrosis. Auditory and vestibular toxicities have been associated with aminoglycoside overdose. These toxicities occur in patients treated longer than 10 days, in patients with abnormal renal function, in dehydrated patients, or in patients receiving medications with additive auditory toxicities. These patients may not have signs or symptoms or may experience dizziness, tinnitus, vertigo, and a loss of high-tone acuity as ototoxicity progresses. Ototoxicity signs and symptoms may not begin to occur until long after the drug has been discontinued.

Neuromuscular blockade or respiratory paralysis may occur following administration of aminoglycosides. Neuromuscular blockade, respiratory failure, and prolonged respiratory paralysis may occur more commonly in patients with myasthenia gravis or Parkinson's disease. Prolonged respiratory paralysis may also occur in patients receiving decamethonium, tubocurarine, or succinylcholine. If neuromuscular blockade occurs, it may be reversed by the administration of calcium salts but mechanical assistance may be necessary. If tobramycin were ingested, toxicity would be less likely because aminoglycosides are poorly absorbed from an intact gastrointestinal tract.

Treatment —In all cases of suspected overdosage, call your Regional Poison Control Center to obtain the most up-to-date information on the treatment of overdose. This recommendation is made because, in general, information regarding the treatment of overdose may change more rapidly than the package insert. In managing overdosage, consider the possibility of multiple drug overdoses, interaction among drugs, and unusual drug kinetics in your patient.

The initial intervention in a tobramycin overdose is to establish an airway and ensure oxygenation and ventilation. Resuscitative measures should be initiated promptly if respiratory paralysis occurs.

Patients who have received an overdose of tobramycin and who have normal renal function should be adequately hydrated to maintain a urine output of 3 to 5 mL/kg/hr. Fluid balance, creatinine clearance, and tobramycin plasma levels should be carefully monitored until the serum tobramycin level falls below 2 µg/mL.

Patients in whom the elimination half-life is greater than 2 hours or whose renal function is abnormal may require more aggressive therapy. In such patients, hemodialysis may be beneficial.

DOSAGE AND ADMINISTRATION

Nebcin may be given intramuscularly or intravenously. ADD-Vantage vials are not for intramuscular administration. Recommended dosages are the same for both routes. The patient's pretreatment body weight should be obtained for calculation of correct dosage. It is desirable to measure both peak and trough serum concentrations (see **WARNINGS** box *and* **PRECAUTIONS**).

Administration for Patients With Normal Renal Function —Adults With Serious Infections: 3 mg/kg/day in 3 equal doses every 8 hours (see Table 1).

Adults With Life-Threatening Infections: Up to 5 mg/kg/day may be administered in 3 or 4 equal doses (see Table 1). The dosage should be reduced to 3 mg/kg/day as soon as clinically indicated. To prevent increased toxicity due to excessive blood levels, dosage should not exceed 5 mg/kg/day unless serum levels are monitored (see **WARNINGS** box *and* **PRECAUTIONS**).
[See table 1 above]

Pediatric Patients: 6 to 7.5 mg/kg/day in 3 or 4 equally divided doses (2 to 2.5 mg/kg every 8 hours or 1.5 to 1.89 mg/kg every 6 hours).

Premature or Full-Term Neonates 1 Week of Age or Less: Up to 4 mg/kg/day may be administered in 2 equal doses every 12 hours.

It is desirable to limit treatment to a short term. The usual duration of treatment is 7 to 10 days. A longer course of therapy may be necessary in difficult and complicated infections. In such cases, monitoring of renal, auditory, and vestibular functions is advised, because neurotoxicity is more likely to occur when treatment is extended longer than 10 days.

Dosage in Patients with Cystic Fibrosis—In patients with cystic fibrosis, altered pharmacokinetics may result in reduced serum concentrations of aminoglycosides. Measurement of tobramycin serum concentration during treatment is especially important as a basis for determining appropriate dose. In patients with severe cystic fibrosis, an initial dosing regimen of 10 mg/kg/day in 4 equally divided doses is recommended. This dosing regimen is suggested only as a guide. The serum levels of tobramycin should be measured directly during treatment due to wide interpatient variability.

Administration for Patients With Impaired Renal Function—Whenever possible, serum tobramycin concentrations should be monitored during therapy.

Following a loading dose of 1 mg/kg, subsequent dosage in these patients must be adjusted, either with reduced doses administered at 8-hour intervals or with normal doses given at prolonged intervals. Both of these methods are suggested as guides to be used when serum levels of tobramycin cannot be measured directly. They are based on either the creatinine clearance level or the serum creatinine level of the patient because these values correlate with the half-life of tobramycin. The dosage schedule derived from either method should be used in conjunction with careful clinical and laboratory observations of the patient and should be modified as necessary. Neither method should be used when dialysis is being performed.

Reduced dosage at 8-hour intervals: When the creatinine clearance rate is 70 mL or less per minute or when the serum creatinine value is known, the amount of the reduced dose can be determined by multiplying the normal dose from Table 1 by the percent of normal dose from the accompanying nomogram.

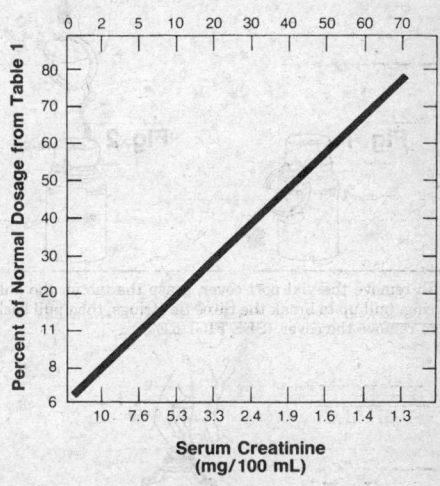

REDUCED DOSAGE NOMOGRAM*
Creatinine Clearance (mL/min/1.73 m²)

Serum Creatinine
(mg/100 mL)

***Scales have been adjusted to
facilitate dosage calculations.**

An alternate rough guide for determining reduced dosage at 8-hour intervals (for patients whose steady-state serum creatinine values are known) is to divide the normally recommended dose by the patient's serum creatinine.

Normal dosage at prolonged intervals: If the creatinine clearance rate is not available and the patient's condition is stable, a dosage frequency *in hours* for the dosage given in Table 1 can be determined by multiplying the patient's serum creatinine by 6.

Dosage in Obese Patients —The appropriate dose may be calculated by using the patient's estimated lean body weight plus 40% of the excess as the basic weight on which to figure mg/kg.

Intramuscular Administration —Nebcin may be administered by withdrawing the appropriate dose directly from a vial or by using a prefilled Hypuret®. ADD-Vantage vials are not for intramuscular administration.

Intravenous Administration—For intravenous administration, the usual volume of diluent (0.9% Sodium Chloride Injection or 5% Dextrose Injection) is 50 to 100 mL for adult doses. For pediatric patients, the volume of diluent should be proportionately less than that for adults. The diluted solution usually should be infused over a period of 20 to 60 minutes. Infusion periods of less than 20 minutes are not recommended, because peak serum levels may exceed 12 µg/mL (see **WARNINGS** box).

Use of ADD-Vantage Nebcin Vials —ADD-Vantage Nebcin vials are not intended for multiple use and should not be used with a syringe in the conventional way. These products are intended for use only with Abbott ADD-Vantage diluent containers and in those instances in which the physician's order specified 60-mg or 80-mg doses. Use within 24 hours after activation.

Nebcin should not be physically premixed with other drugs but should be administered separately according to the recommended dose and route.

Prior to administration, parenteral drug products should be inspected visually for particulate matter and discoloration whenever solution and container permit.

Continued on next page

* **Identi-Code® symbol. This product information was prepared in June 1998. Current information on these and other products of Eli Lilly and Company may be obtained by direct inquiry to Lilly Research Laboratories, Lilly Corporate Center, Indianapolis, Indiana 46285, (800) 545-5979.**

Consult 1999 PDR® supplements and future editions for revisions

Nebcin—Cont.

INSTRUCTIONS FOR USE-*ADD-Vantage®* Vial

To Open:

Peel overwrap from the corner and remove container. Some opacity of the plastic due to moisture absorption during the sterilization process may be observed. This is normal and does not affect the solution quality or safety. The opacity will diminish gradually.

To Assemble Vial and Flexible Diluent Container: USE ASEPTIC TECHNIQUE

1. Remove the protective covers from the top of the vial and the vial port on the diluent container as follows:

a. To remove the breakaway vial cap, swing the pull ring over the top of the vial and pull down far enough to start the opening (SEE FIGURE 1.), then pull straight up to remove the cap. (SEE FIGURE 2.) NOTE: Do not access vial with syringe.

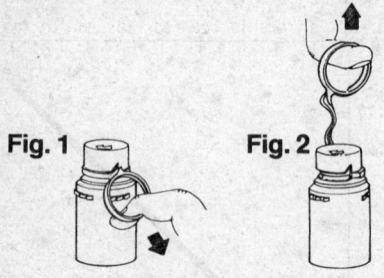

Fig. 1   **Fig. 2**

b. To remove the vial port cover, grasp the tab on the pull ring, pull up to break the three tie strings, then pull back to remove the cover. (SEE FIGURE 3.)

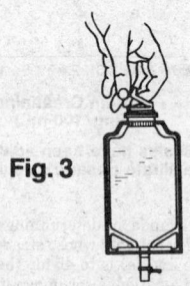

Fig. 3

2. Screw the vial into the vial port until it will go no further. THE VIAL MUST BE SCREWED IN TIGHTLY TO ASSURE A SEAL. This occurs approximately 1/2 turn (180°) after the first audible click. (SEE FIGURE 4.) The clicking sound does not assure a seal; the vial must be turned as far as it will go. NOTE: Once vial is seated, do not attempt to remove. (SEE FIGURE 4.)

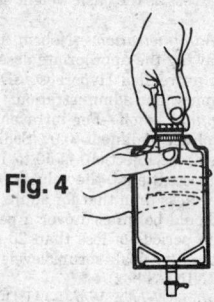

Fig. 4

3. Recheck the vial to assure that it is tight by trying to turn it further in the direction of assembly.
4. Label appropriately.

To Mix the Drug:

1. Squeeze the bottom of the diluent container gently to inflate the portion of the container surrounding the end of the drug vial.
2. With the other hand, push the drug vial down into the container telescoping the walls of the container. Grasp the inner cap of the vial through the walls of the container. (SEE FIGURE 5.)
   [See figure 5 at top of next column]
3. Pull the inner cap from the drug vial (SEE FIGURE 6.) Verify that the rubber stopper has been pulled out, allowing the drug and diluent to mix.
   [See figure 6 at top of next column]
4. Mix container contents thoroughly and use within the specified time.
5. Immediately prior to administration, confirm that the contents of the vial have been mixed by observing the inner cap/stopper in the flexible container.

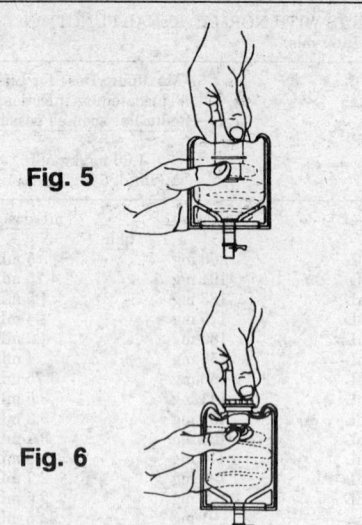

Fig. 5

Fig. 6

HOW SUPPLIED

Multiple-Dose Vials:
   80 mg*/2 mL, 2 mL (No. 781)—(1s) NDC 0002-1499-01; (Traypak† of 25) NDC 0002-1499-25
   Pediatric, 20 mg*/2 mL, 2 mL (No. 782)—(1s) NDC 0002-0501-01
   40 mg*/mL, 1.2 g/30 mL (No. 7090)—(Traypak of 6) NDC 0002-7090-10

Hyporets®‡, each scored with a 10-mg (0.25-mL) fractional dose scale:
   60 mg*/1.5 mL, 1.5 mL (No. 55)—(24s) NDC 0002-0509-24
   80 mg*/2 mL, 2 mL (No. 42)—(24s) NDC 0002-0503-24

ADD-Vantage§ Vials:
   60 mg*/6 mL, 6 mL (No. 7293)—(Traypak of 25) NDC 0002-7293-25
   80 mg*/8 mL, 8 mL (No. 7294)—(Traypak of 25) NDC 0002-7294-25

The above ADD-Vantage vials are to be used only with Abbott Laboratories' diluent containers.

Instructions for the use of ADD-Vantage vials are described above. (*See* **DOSAGE AND ADMINISTRATION**.)

Also Available:
Pharmacy Bulk Vial:
1.2 g* (Dry Powder) (40-mL size) (No. 7040)—(Traypak of 6) NDC 0002-7040-16

Store at controlled room temperature 59° to 86°F (15° to 30°C).

---

* Equivalent to tobramycin.
† Traypak™ (multivial carton, Lilly).
‡ Hyporet® (disposable syringe, Lilly).
§ ADD-Vantage® (vials and diluent containers, Abbott).

REFERENCES

1. National Committee for Clinical Laboratory Standards, Performance standards for antimicrobial disk susceptibility tests—5th ed. Approved Standard NCCLS Document M2-A5, Vol 13, No 24, NCCLS, Villanova, PA, 1993.
2. National Committee for Clinical Laboratory Standards, Methods for dilution antimicrobial susceptibility tests for bacteria that grow aerobically—3rd ed. Approved Standard NCCLS Document M7-A3, Vol 13, No 25, NCCLS, Villanova, PA, 1993.

CAUTION—Federal (USA) law prohibits dispensing without prescription.
Literature revised October 21, 1997
PA 2011 AMP   [102197]

NPH ILETIN® II   **OTC**
(isophane insulin suspension, Lilly) See Under Iletin®
(insulin)

ONCOVIN®   ℞
[ŏn ′kō-vĭn]
(Vincristine Sulfate Injection, USP)
Solution

WARNINGS

Caution—This preparation should be administered by individuals experienced in the administration of Oncovin. It is extremely important that the intravenous

needle or catheter be properly positioned before any vincristine is injected. Leakage into surrounding tissue during intravenous administration of Oncovin may cause considerable irritation. If extravasation occurs, the injection should be discontinued immediately, and any remaining portion of the dose should then be introduced into another vein. Local injection of hyaluronidase and the application of moderate heat to the area of leakage help disperse the drug and are thought to minimize discomfort and the possibility of cellulitis. **FATAL IF GIVEN INTRATHECALLY. FOR INTRAVENOUS USE ONLY.** *See Warnings section for the treatment of patients given intrathecal Oncovin.*

DESCRIPTION

Oncovin® (Vincristine Sulfate, USP) is vincaleukoblastine, 22-oxo-, sulfate (1:1) (salt). It is the salt of an alkaloid obtained from a common flowering herb, the periwinkle plant (*Vinca rosea* Linn). Originally known as leurocristine, it has also been referred to as LCR and VCR. The empirical formula for vincristine sulfate is $C_{46}H_{56}N_4O_{10} \cdot H_2SO_4$. It has a molecular weight of 923.04. The structural formula is as follows:

Vincristine sulfate is a white to off-white powder. It is soluble in methanol, freely soluble in water, but only slightly soluble in 95% ethanol.

Each mL contains vincristine sulfate, 1 mg (1.08 μmol); mannitol, 100 mg; methylparaben, 1.3 mg; propylparaben, 0.2 mg; and water for injection, qs. Acetic acid and sodium acetate have been added for pH control. The pH of Oncovin Solution ranges from 3.5 to 5.5. This product is a sterile solution for cancer/oncolytic use.

CLINICAL PHARMACOLOGY

The mechanisms of action of Oncovin remain under investigation. The mechanism of action of Oncovin has been related to the inhibition of microtubule formation in the mitotic spindle, resulting in an arrest of dividing cells at the metaphase stage.

Central nervous system leukemia has been reported in patients undergoing otherwise successful therapy with Oncovin. This suggests that Oncovin does not penetrate well into the cerebrospinal fluid.

Pharmacokinetic studies in patients with cancer have shown a triphasic serum decay pattern following rapid intravenous injection. The initial, middle, and terminal half-lives are 5 minutes, 2.3 hours, and 85 hours respectively; however, the range of the terminal half-life in humans is from 19 to 155 hours. The liver is the major excretory organ in humans and animals. The metabolism of vinca alkaloids has been shown to be mediated by hepatic cytochrome P450 isoenzymes in the CYP 3A subfamily. This metabolic pathway may be impaired in patients with hepatic dysfunction or who are taking concomitant potent inhibitors of these isoenzymes (*see* Precautions). About 80% of an injected dose of Oncovin appears in the feces and 10% to 20% can be found in the urine. Within 15 to 30 minutes after injection, over 90% of the drug is distributed from the blood into tissue, where it remains tightly, but not irreversibly, bound.

Current principles of cancer chemotherapy involve the simultaneous use of several agents. Generally, each agent used has a unique toxicity and mechanism of action so that therapeutic enhancement occurs without additive toxicity. It is rarely possible to achieve equally good results with single-agent methods of treatment. Thus, Oncovin is often chosen as part of polychemotherapy because of lack of significant bone-marrow suppression (at recommended doses) and of unique clinical toxicity (neuropathy). *See* Dosage and Administration for possible increased toxicity when used in combination therapy.

INDICATIONS AND USAGE

Oncovin is indicated in acute leukemia.

Oncovin has also been shown to be useful in combination with other oncolytic agents in Hodgkin's disease, non-Hodgkin's malignant lymphomas (lymphocytic, mixed-cell, histiocytic, undifferentiated, nodular, and diffuse types), rhabdomyosarcoma, neuroblastoma, and Wilms' tumor.

CONTRAINDICATIONS

Patients with the demyelinating form of Charcot-Marie-Tooth syndrome should not be given Oncovin. Careful attention should be given to those conditions listed under Warnings *and* Precautions.

WARNINGS

This preparation is for intravenous use only. It should be administered by individuals experienced in the administration of Oncovin. The intrathecal administration of Oncovin usually results in death. Syringes containing this product should be labeled, using the auxiliary sticker provided, to state "FATAL IF GIVEN INTRATHECALLY. FOR INTRAVENOUS USE ONLY."

Extemporaneously prepared syringes containing this product must be packaged in an overwrap which is labeled "DO NOT REMOVE COVERING UNTIL MOMENT OF INJECTION. FATAL IF GIVEN INTRATHECALLY. FOR INTRAVENOUS USE ONLY."

Treatment of patients following intrathecal administration of Oncovin has included immediate removal of spinal fluid and flushing with Lactated Ringer's , as well as other solutions and has not prevented ascending paralysis and death. In one case, progressive paralysis in an adult was arrested by the following treatment **initiated immediately after the intrathecal injection:**

1. As much spinal fluid was removed as could be safely done through lumbar access.
2. The subarachnoid space was flushed with Lactated Ringer's solution infused continuously through a catheter in a cerebral lateral ventricle at the rate of 150 mL/h. The fluid was removed through a lumbar access.
3. As soon as fresh frozen plasma became available, the fresh frozen plasma, 25 mL, diluted in 1 L of Lactated Ringer's solution was infused through the cerebral ventricular catheter at the rate of 75 mL/h with removal through the lumbar access. The rate of infusion was adjusted to maintain a protein level in the spinal fluid of 150 mg/dL.
4. Glutamic acid, 10 g, was given intravenously over 24 hours followed by 500 mg 3 times daily by mouth for 1 month or until neurological dysfunction stabilized. The role of glutamic acid in this treatment is not certain and may not be essential.

Pregnancy Category D —Oncovin can cause fetal harm when administered to a pregnant woman. When pregnant mice and hamsters were given doses of Oncovin that caused the resorption of 23% to 85% of fetuses, fetal malformations were produced in those that survived. Five monkeys were given single doses of Oncovin between days 27 and 34 of their pregnancies; 3 of the fetuses were normal at term, and 2 viable fetuses had grossly evident malformations at term. In several animal species, Oncovin can induce teratogenesis as well as embryo death at doses that are nontoxic to the pregnant animal. There are no adequate and well-controlled studies in pregnant women. If this drug is used during pregnancy or if the patient becomes pregnant while receiving this drug, she should be apprised of the potential hazard to the fetus. Women of childbearing potential should be advised to avoid becoming pregnant.

PRECAUTIONS

General—Acute uric acid nephropathy, which may occur after the administration of oncolytic agents, has also been reported with Oncovin. In the presence of leukopenia or a complicating infection, administration of the next dose of Oncovin warrants careful consideration.

If central nervous system leukemia is diagnosed, additional agents may be required because Oncovin does not appear to cross the blood-brain barrier in adequate amounts.

Particular attention should be given to dosage and neurologic side effects if Oncovin is administered to patients with preexisting neuromuscular disease and when other drugs with neurotoxic potential are also being used.

Acute shortness of breath and severe bronchospasm have been reported following the administration of vinca alkaloids. These reactions have been encountered most frequently when the vinca alkaloid was used in combination with mitomycin C and may require aggressive treatment, particularly when there is preexisting pulmonary dysfunction. The onset of these reactions may occur minutes to several hours after the vinca alkaloid is injected and may occur up to 2 weeks following the dose of mitomycin. Progressive dyspnea requiring chronic therapy may occur. Oncovin should not be readministered.

Care must be taken to avoid contamination of the eye with concentrations of Oncovin used clinically. If accidental contamination occurs, severe irritation (or, if the drug was delivered under pressure, even corneal ulceration) may result. The eye should be washed immediately and thoroughly.

Laboratory Tests —Because dose-limiting clinical toxicity is manifested as neurotoxicity, clinical evaluation (eg, history, physical examination) is necessary to detect the need for dosage modification. Following administration of Oncovin, some individuals may have a fall in the white-blood-cell count or platelet count, particularly when previous therapy or the disease itself has reduced bone-marrow function. Therefore, a complete blood count should be done before administration of each dose. Acute elevation of serum uric acid may also occur during induction of remission in acute leukemia; thus, such levels should be determined frequently during the first 3 to 4 weeks of treatment or appropriate measures taken to prevent uric acid nephropathy. The laboratory performing these tests should be consulted for its range of normal values.

Drug Interaction —The simultaneous oral or intravenous administration of phenytoin and antineoplastic chemotherapy combinations that included vincristine sulfate has been reported to reduce blood levels of the anticonvulsant and to increase seizure activity. Dosage adjustment should be based on serial blood level monitoring. The contribution of vincristine sulfate to this interaction is not certain. The interaction may result from reduced absorption of phenytoin and an increase in the rate of its metabolism and elimination.

Caution should be exercised in patients concurrently taking drugs known to inhibit drug metabolism by hepatic cytochrome P450 isoenzymes in the CYP 3A subfamily, or in patients with hepatic dysfunction. Concurrent administration of vincristine sulfate with itraconazole (a known inhibitor of the metabolic pathway) has been reported to cause an earlier onset and/or an increased severity of neuromuscular side effects (*see* Adverse Reactions). This interaction is presumed to be related to inhibition of the metabolism of vincristine.

Carcinogenesis, Mutagenesis, Impairment of Fertility —Neither in vivo nor in vitro laboratory tests have conclusively demonstrated the mutagenicity of this product. Fertility following treatment with Oncovin alone for malignant disease has not been studied in humans. Clinical reports of both male and female patients who received multiple-agent chemotherapy that included Oncovin indicate that azoospermia and amenorrhea can occur in postpubertal patients. Recovery occurred many months after completion of chemotherapy in some but not all patients. When the same treatment is administered to prepubertal patients, permanent azoospermia and amenorrhea are much less likely. Patients who received chemotherapy with Oncovin in combination with anticancer drugs known to be carcinogenic have developed second malignancies. The contributing role of Oncovin in this development has not been determined. No evidence of carcinogenicity was found following intraperitoneal administration of Oncovin in rats and mice, although this study was limited.

Usage in Pregnancy —Pregnancy Category D —See Warnings.

Nursing Mothers —It is not known whether this drug is excreted in human milk. Because many drugs are excreted in human milk and because of the potential for serious adverse reactions due to Oncovin in nursing infants, a decision should be made either to discontinue nursing or the drug, taking into account the importance of the drug to the mother.

Pediatric —See Dosage and Administration section.

ADVERSE REACTIONS

Prior to the use of this drug, patients and/or their parents/guardian should be advised of the possibility of untoward symptoms.

In general, adverse reactions are reversible and are related to dosage. The most common adverse reaction is hair loss; the most troublesome adverse reactions are neuromuscular in origin.

When single, weekly doses of the drug are employed, the adverse reactions of leukopenia, neuritic pain, and constipation occur but are usually of short duration (ie, less than 7 days). When the dosage is reduced, these reactions may lessen or disappear. The severity of such reactions seems to increase when the calculated amount of drug is given in divided doses. Other adverse reactions, such as hair loss, sensory loss, paresthesia, difficulty in walking, slapping gait, loss of deep-tendon reflexes, and muscle wasting, may persist for at least as long as therapy is continued. Generalized sensorimotor dysfunction may become progressively more severe with continued treatment. Although most such symptoms usually disappear by about the sixth week after discontinuance of treatment, some neuromuscular difficulties may persist for prolonged periods in some patients. Regrowth of hair may occur while maintenance therapy continues.

The following adverse reactions have been reported:

Hypersensitivity —Rare cases of allergic-type reactions, such as anaphylaxis, rash, and edema, that are temporally related to vincristine therapy have been reported in patients receiving vincristine as a part of multidrug chemotherapy regimens.

Gastrointestinal —Constipation, abdominal cramps, weight loss, nausea, vomiting, oral ulceration, diarrhea, paralytic ileus, intestinal necrosis and/or perforation, and anorexia have occurred. Constipation may take the form of upper-colon impaction, and, on physical examination, the rectum may be empty. Colicky abdominal pain coupled with an empty rectum may mislead the physician. A flat film of the abdomen is useful in demonstrating this condition. All cases have responded to high enemas and laxatives. A routine prophylactic regimen against constipation is recommended for all patients receiving Oncovin.

Paralytic ileus (which mimics the "surgical abdomen") may occur, particularly in young pediatric patients. The ileus will reverse itself with temporary discontinuance of Oncovin and with symptomatic care.

Genitourinary —Polyuria, dysuria, and urinary retention due to bladder atony have occurred. Other drugs known to cause urinary retention (particularly in the elderly) should, if possible, be discontinued for the first few days following administration of Oncovin.

Cardiovascular —Hypertension and hypotension have occurred. Chemotherapy combinations that have included vincristine sulfate, when given to patients previously treated with mediastinal radiation, have been associated with coronary artery disease and myocardial infarction. Causality has not been established.

Neurologic —Frequently, there is a sequence to the development of neuromuscular side effects. Initially, only sensory impairment and paresthesia may be encountered. With continued treatment, neuritic pain and, later, motor difficulties may occur. There have been no reports of any agent that can reverse the neuromuscular manifestations that may accompany therapy with Oncovin.

Loss of deep-tendon reflexes, foot drop, ataxia, and paralysis have been reported with continued administration. Cranial nerve manifestations, such as isolated paresis and/or paralysis of muscles controlled by cranial motor nerves, including potentially life-threatening bilateral vocal cord paralysis, may occur in the absence of motor impairment elsewhere; extraocular and laryngeal muscles are those most commonly involved. Jaw pain, pharyngeal pain, parotid gland pain, bone pain, back pain, limb pain, and myalgias have been reported; pain in these areas may be severe. Convulsions, frequently with hypertension, have been reported in a few patients receiving Oncovin. Several instances of convulsions followed by coma have been reported in pediatric patients. Transient cortical blindness and optic atrophy with blindness have been reported. Treatment with vinca alkaloids has resulted rarely in both vestibular and auditory damage to the eighth cranial nerve. Manifestations include partial or total deafness which may be temporary or permanent, and difficulties with balance including dizziness, nystagmus, and vertigo. Particular caution is warranted when Oncovin is used in combination with other agents known to be ototoxic such as the platinum-containing oncolytics.

Pulmonary—See Precautions.

Endocrine —Rare occurrences of a syndrome attributable to inappropriate antidiuretic hormone secretion have been observed in patients treated with Oncovin. This syndrome is characterized by high urinary sodium excretion in the presence of hyponatremia; renal or adrenal disease, hypotension, dehydration, azotemia, and clinical edema are absent. With fluid deprivation, improvement occurs in the hyponatremia and in the renal loss of sodium.

Hematologic —Oncovin does not appear to have any constant or significant effect on platelets or red blood cells. Serious bone-marrow depression is usually not a major dose-limiting event. However, anemia, leukopenia, and thrombocytopenia have been reported. Thrombocytopenia, if present when therapy with Oncovin is begun, may actually improve before the appearance of marrow remission.

Skin —Alopecia and rash have been reported.

Other —Fever and headache have occurred.

OVERDOSAGE

Side effects following the use of Oncovin are dose related. In pediatric patients under 13 years of age, death has occurred following doses of Oncovin that were 10 times those recommended for therapy. Severe symptoms may occur in this patient group following dosages of 3 to 4 mg/m^2. Adults can be expected to experience severe symptoms after single doses of 3 mg/m^2 or more (*see* Adverse Reactions). Therefore, following administration of doses higher than those recommended, patients can be expected to experience exaggerated side effects. Supportive care should include the following: (1) prevention of side effects resulting from the syndrome of inappropriate antidiuretic hormone secretion (preventive treatment would include restriction of fluid intake and perhaps the administration of a diuretic affecting the function of Henle's loop and the distal tubule); (2) administration of

Continued on next page

---

* Identi-Code® symbol. This product information was prepared in June 1998. Current information on these and other products of Eli Lilly and Company may be obtained by direct inquiry to Lilly Research Laboratories, Lilly Corporate Center, Indianapolis, Indiana 46285, (800) 545-5979.

Oncovin—Cont.

anticonvulsants; (3) use of enemas or cathartics to prevent ileus (in some instances, decompression of the gastrointestinal tract may be necessary); (4) monitoring the cardiovascular system; and (5) determining daily blood counts for guidance in transfusion requirements.

Folinic acid has been observed to have a protective effect in normal mice that were administered lethal doses of Oncovin (*Cancer Res* 1963; 23:1390). Isolated case reports suggest that folinic acid may be helpful in treating humans who have received an overdose of Oncovin. It is suggested that 100 mg of folinic acid be administered intravenously every 3 hours for 24 hours and then every 6 hours for at least 48 hours. Theoretically (based on pharmacokinetic data), tissue levels of Oncovin can be expected to remain significantly elevated for at least 72 hours. Treatment with folinic acid does not eliminate the need for the above-mentioned supportive measures.

Most of an intravenous dose of Oncovin is excreted into the bile after rapid tissue binding (*see* Clinical Pharmacology). Because only very small amounts of the drug appear in dialysate, hemodialysis is not likely to be helpful in cases of overdosage. An increase in the severity of side effects may be experienced by patients with liver disease that is severe enough to decrease biliary excretion.

Enhanced fecal excretion of parenterally administered vincristine has been demonstrated in dogs pretreated with cholestyramine. There are no published clinical data on the use of cholestyramine as an antidote in humans.

There are no published clinical data on the consequences of oral ingestion of vincristine. Should oral ingestion occur, the stomach should be evacuated. Evacuation should be followed by oral administration of activated charcoal and a cathartic.

DOSAGE AND ADMINISTRATION

This preparation is for intravenous use only (see Warnings). *Neurotoxicity appears to be dose related. Extreme care must be used in calculating and administering the dose of Oncovin since overdosage may have a very serious or fatal outcome.*

Special Dispensing Information—WHEN DISPENSING VINCRISTINE IN OTHER THAN THE ORIGINAL CONTAINER, IT IS IMPERATIVE THAT IT BE PACKAGED IN THE PROVIDED OVERWRAP WHICH BEARS THE FOLLOWING STATEMENT: "DO NOT REMOVE COVERING UNTIL MOMENT OF INJECTION. FATAL IF GIVEN INTRATHECALLY. FOR INTRAVENOUS USE ONLY". (*see* Warnings) A syringe containing a specific dose must be labeled, using the auxiliary sticker provided, to state: "FATAL IF GIVEN INTRATHECALLY. FOR INTRAVENOUS USE ONLY."

The concentration of vincristine contained in all vials and Hyporets® of Oncovin is 1 mg/mL. Do not add extra fluid to the vial prior to removal of the dose. Withdraw the solution of Oncovin into an accurate dry syringe, measuring the dose carefully. Do not add extra fluid to the vial in an attempt to empty it completely.

Caution—*It is extremely important that the intravenous needle or catheter be properly positioned before any vincristine is injected. Leakage into surrounding tissue during intravenous administration of Oncovin may cause considerable irritation. If extravasation occurs, the injection should be discontinued immediately, and any remaining portion of the dose should then be introduced into another vein. Local injection of hyaluronidase and the application of moderate heat to the area of leakage will help disperse the drug and may minimize discomfort and the possibility of cellulitis.*

Oncovin must be administered via an intact, free-flowing intravenous needle or catheter. Care should be taken that there is no leakage or swelling occurring during administration (*see* boxed Warnings).

The solution may be injected either directly into a vein or into the tubing of a running intravenous infusion (*see* Drug Interactions below). Injection of Oncovin should be accomplished within 1 minute.

The drug is administered intravenously *at weekly intervals.* The usual dose of Oncovin for pediatric patients is 1.5–2 mg/m². For pediatric patients weighing 10 kg or less, the starting dose should be 0.05 mg/kg, administered once a week. The usual dose of Oncovin for adults is 1.4 mg/m². A 50% reduction in the dose of Oncovin is recommended for patients having a direct serum bilirubin value above 3 mg/100 mL.

Oncovin should not be given to patients while they are receiving radiation therapy through ports that include the liver. When Oncovin is used in combination with L-asparaginase, Oncovin should be given 12 to 24 hours before administration of the enzyme in order to minimize toxicity; administering L-asparaginase before Oncovin may reduce hepatic clearance of Oncovin.

Drug Incompatibilities—Oncovin should not be diluted in solutions that raise or lower the pH outside the range of 3.5 to 5.5. It should not be mixed with anything other than normal saline or glucose in water.

Whenever solution and container permit, parenteral drug products should be inspected visually for particulate matter and discoloration prior to administration.

Procedures for proper handling and disposal of anticancer drugs should be considered. Several guidelines on this subject have been published.[1–7] There is no general agreement that all of the procedures recommended in the guidelines are necessary or appropriate.

HOW SUPPLIED

Multiple-Dose Vials:
1 mg/1 mL, 1 mL (No. 7194)—(1s) NDC 0002-7194-01
2 mg/2 mL, 2 mL (No. 7195)—(1s) NDC 0002-7195-01
5 mg/5 mL, 5 mL (No. 7196)—(1s) NDC 0002-7196-01
Hyporets,* each marked with a 0.1-mg (0.1 mL) fractional dose scale:
1 mg/1 mL, 1 mL (No. 7198)—(3s) NDC 0002-7198-09
2 mg/2 mL, 2 mL (No. 7199)—(3s) NDC 0002-7199-09
*Hyporet® (disposable syringe, Lilly)
This product should be refrigerated.
CAUTION—Federal (USA) law prohibits dispensing without prescription.

REFERENCES

1. Recommendations for the Safe Handling of Parenteral Antineoplastic Drugs, NIH Publication No. 83-2621. For sale by the Superintendent of Documents, U.S. Government Printing Office, Washington, DC 20402.
2. AMA Council Report, Guidelines for Handling Parenteral Antineoplastics. JAMA, 1985;253(11):1590–1592.
3. National Study Commission on Cytotoxic Exposure—Recommendations for Handling Cytotoxic Agents. Available from Louis P. Jeffrey, ScD., Chairman, National Study Commission on Cytotoxic Exposure, Massachusetts College of Pharmacy and Allied Health Sciences, 179 Longwood Avenue, Boston, Massachusetts 02115.
4. Clinical Oncological Society of Australia, Guidelines and Recommendations for Safe Handling of Antineoplastic Agents. Med J Australia, 1983;1:426–428.
5. Jones RB, et al: Safe Handling of Chemotherapeutic Agents: A Report from the Mount Sinai Medical Center. CA—A Cancer Journal for Clinicians, 1983; (Sept/Oct)258–263.
6. American Society of Hospital Pharmacists Technical Assistance Bulletin on Handling Cytotoxic and Hazardous Drugs. Am J Hosp Pharm, 1990;47:1033–1049.
7. OSHA Work-Practice Guidelines for Personnel Dealing with Cytotoxic (Antineoplastic) Drugs. Am J Hosp Pharm, 1986;43:1193–1204.

Literature revised October 2, 1997
PA 0102 AMP   [100297]

PROTAMINE SULFATE   ℞
[prō 'ta-mēn sŭl 'fāt]
Injection, USP

DESCRIPTION

Protamines are simple proteins of low molecular weight that are rich in arginine and strongly basic. They occur in the sperm of salmon and certain other species of fish.

Protamine sulfate occurs as fine white or off-white amorphous or crystalline powder. It is sparingly soluble in water. The pH is between 6 and 7. The cationic hydrogenated protamine at a pH of 6.8 to 7.1 reacts with anionic heparin at a pH of 5.0 to 7.5 to form an inactive complex.

Protamine Sulfate Injection, USP, is a sterile, isotonic solution of protamine sulfate. It acts as a heparin antagonist. It is also a weak anticoagulant.

Each 25-mL vial contains protamine sulfate equivalent to 250 mg of activity. Product also contains 0.9% Sodium Chloride Reagent in Water for Injection, USP. Sodium phosphate and/or sulfuric acid may have been added during manufacture to adjust the pH. Contains no preservative.

Protamine sulfate is administered intravenously.

CLINICAL PHARMACOLOGY

When administered alone, protamine has an anticoagulant effect. However, when it is given in the presence of heparin (which is strongly acidic), a stable salt is formed and the anticoagulant activity of both drugs is lost.

Protamine sulfate has a rapid onset of action. Neutralization of heparin occurs within 5 minutes after intravenous administration of an appropriate dose of protamine sulfate. Although the metabolic fate of the heparin-protamine complex has not been elucidated, it has been postulated that protamine sulfate in the heparin-protamine complex may be partially metabolized or may be attacked by fibrinolysin, thus freeing heparin.

INDICATIONS AND USAGE

Protamine sulfate is indicated in the treatment of heparin overdosage.

CONTRAINDICATION

Protamine sulfate is contraindicated in patients who have shown previous intolerance to the drug.

WARNINGS

Hyperheparinemia or bleeding has been reported in experimental animals and in some patients 30 minutes to 18 hours after cardiac surgery (under cardiopulmonary bypass) in spite of complete neutralization of heparin by adequate doses of protamine sulfate at the end of the operation. It is important to keep the patient under close observation after cardiac surgery. Additional doses of protamine sulfate should be administered if indicated by coagulation studies, such as the heparin titration test with protamine and the determination of plasma thrombin time.

Too-rapid administration of protamine sulfate can cause severe hypotensive and anaphylactoid reactions (see Dosage and Administration). Facilities to treat shock should be available.

PRECAUTIONS

General—Because of the anticoagulant effect of protamine, it is unwise to give more than 50 mg over a short period unless a larger dose is clearly needed.

Patients with a history of allergy to fish may develop hypersensitivity reactions to protamine, although to date no relationship has been established between allergic reactions to protamine and fish allergy.

Previous exposure to protamine can induce a humoral immune response and predispose susceptible individuals to the development of untoward reactions from the subsequent use of this drug. Patients exposed to protamine through the use of protamine-containing insulin or during heparin neutralization may experience life-threatening reactions and fatal anaphylaxis upon receiving large doses of protamine intravenously. Severe reactions to intravenous protamine can occur in the absence of local or systemic allergic reactions to subcutaneous injection of protamine-containing insulin. Reports of the presence of antiprotamine antibodies in the sera of infertile or vasectomized men suggest that some of these individuals may react to use of protamine sulfate.

Fatal anaphylaxis has been reported in one patient with no prior history of allergies.

Drug Interactions—Protamine sulfate has been shown to be incompatible with certain antibiotics, including several of the cephalosporins and penicillins (*see* Dosage and Administration).

Carcinogenesis, Mutagenesis, Impairment of Fertility—Studies have not been performed to determine potential for carcinogenicity, mutagenicity, or impairment of fertility.

Pregnancy—Pregnancy Category C—Animal reproduction studies have not been conducted with protamine sulfate. It is also not known whether protamine sulfate can cause fetal harm when administered to a pregnant woman or can affect reproduction capacity. Protamine sulfate should be given to a pregnant woman only if clearly needed.

Nursing Mothers—It is not known whether this drug is excreted in human milk. Because many drugs are excreted in human milk, caution should be exercised when protamine sulfate is administered to a nursing woman.

Pediatric Use—Safety and effectiveness in pediatric patients have not been established.

ADVERSE REACTIONS

The intravenous administration of protamine sulfate may cause a sudden fall in blood pressure and bradycardia. Other reactions include transitory flushing and feeling of warmth, dyspnea, nausea, vomiting, and lassitude. Back pain has been reported in conscious patients undergoing such procedures as cardiac catheterization.

Severe adverse reactions have been reported including: (1) Anaphylaxis that resulted in severe respiratory distress, circulatory collapse, and capillary leak (*see* Precautions). Fatal anaphylaxis has been reported in one patient with no prior history of allergies; (2) Anaphylactoid reactions with circulatory collapse, capillary leak, and noncardiogenic pulmonary edema; acute pulmonary hypertension.

Complement activation by the heparin-protamine complexes, release of lysosomal enzymes from neutrophils, and prostaglandin and thromboxane generation have been associated with the development of anaphylactoid reactions.

Severe and potentially irreversible circulatory collapse associated with myocardial failure and reduced cardiac output can also occur. The mechanism(s) of this reaction and the role played by concurrent factors are unclear.

High-protein, noncardiogenic pulmonary edema associated with the use of protamine has been reported in patients on cardiopulmonary bypass who are undergoing cardiovascular surgery. The etiologic role of protamine in the pathogenesis of this condition is uncertain, and multiple factors have been present in most cases. The condition has been reported in association with administration of certain blood products, other drugs, cardiopulmonary bypass alone, and other etiologic factors. It is difficult to treat, and it can be life threatening. Because fatal anaphylactic and anaphylactoid reactions have been reported after the administration of protamine sulfate, the drug should be given only when resuscitation techniques and treatment of anaphylactic and anaphylactoid shock are readily available.

OVERDOSAGE

Signs and Symptoms—Overdose of protamine sulfate may cause bleeding. Protamine has a weak anticoagulant effect due to an interaction with platelets and with many proteins including fibrinogen. This effect should be distinguished from the rebound anticoagulation that may occur 30 minutes to 18 hours following the reversal of heparin with protamine.

Rapid administration of protamine is more likely to result in bradycardia, dyspnea, a sensation of warmth, flushing, and severe hypotension. Hypertension has also occurred.

The median lethal intravenous dose of protamine sulfate is 50 mg/kg in mice. Serum concentrations of protamine sulfate are not clinically useful. Information is not available on the amount of drug in a single dose that is associated with overdosage or is likely to be life threatening.

Treatment—To obtain up-to-date information about the treatment of overdose, a good resource is your certified Regional Poison Control Center. Telephone numbers of certified poison control centers are listed in the *Physicians' Desk Reference (PDR)*. In managing overdosage, consider the possibility of multiple drug overdoses, interaction among drugs, and unusual drug kinetics in your patient.

Replace blood loss with blood transfusions or fresh frozen plasma.

If the patient is hypotensive, consider fluids, epinephrine, dobutamine, or dopamine.

DOSAGE AND ADMINISTRATION

Each mg of protamine sulfate neutralizes approximately 90 USP units of heparin activity derived from lung tissue or about 115 USP units of heparin activity derived from intestinal mucosa.

Protamine Sulfate Injection should be given by very slow intravenous injection over a 10-minute period in doses not to exceed 50 mg (*see* Warnings).

Protamine sulfate is intended for injection without further dilution; however, if further dilution is desired, D5-W or normal saline may be used. Diluted solutions should not be stored since they contain no preservative.

Protamine sulfate should not be mixed with other drugs without knowledge of their compatibility, because protamine sulfate has been shown to be incompatible with certain antibiotics, including several of the cephalosporins and penicillins.

Because heparin disappears rapidly from the circulation, the dose of protamine sulfate required also decreases rapidly with the time elapsed following intravenous injection of heparin. For example, if the protamine sulfate is administered 30 minutes after the heparin, one half the usual dose may be sufficient.

The dosage of protamine sulfate should be guided by blood coagulation studies (*see* Warnings).

Parenteral drug products should be inspected visually for particulate matter and discoloration prior to administration whenever solution and container permit.

HOW SUPPLIED

Vials:

25 mL (No. 735)—(1s) NDC 0002-1462-01

Vials should be stored in the refrigerator between 2° and 8°C (35.6° and 46.4°F).

CAUTION—The total dose of protamine sulfate contained in Vials No. 735 is 250 mg of activity in 25 mL.

The large-size vials (No. 735) are designed for antiheparin treatment only when large doses of heparin have been given during surgery and are to be neutralized by large doses of protamine sulfate after surgical procedures.

CAUTION—Federal (USA) law prohibits dispensing without prespcription.

PA8182AMP [080696]

REGULAR ILETIN® II — OTC

(insulin injection, Lilly) See under Iletin® (insulin)

REOPRO® — ℞

Abciximab

For intravenous administration

DESCRIPTION

Abciximab, ReoPro®, is the Fab fragment of the chimeric human-murine monoclonal antibody 7E3. Abciximab binds to the glycoprotein (GP) IIb/IIIa ($\alpha_{IIb}\beta_3$) receptor of human platelets and inhibits platelet aggregation. Abciximab also binds to the vitronectin ($\alpha_v\beta_3$) receptor found on platelets and vessel wall endothelial and smooth muscle cells.

The chimeric 7E3 antibody is produced by continuous perfusion in mammalian cell culture. The 47,615 dalton Fab fragment is purified from cell culture supernatant by a series of steps involving specific viral inactivation and removal procedures, digestion with papain and column chromatography.

ReoPro® is a clear, colorless, sterile, non-pyrogenic solution for intravenous (IV) use. Each single use vial contains 2 mg/mL of Abciximab in a buffered solution (pH 7.2) of 0.01 M sodium phosphate, 0.15 M sodium chloride and 0.001% polysorbate 80 in Water for Injection. No preservatives are added.

CLINICAL PHARMACOLOGY

General: Abciximab binds to the intact platelet GPIIb/IIIa receptor, which is a member of the integrin family of adhesion receptors and the major platelet surface receptor involved in platelet aggregation. Abciximab inhibits platelet aggregation by preventing the binding of fibrinogen, von Willebrand factor, and other adhesive molecules to GPIIb/IIIa receptor sites on activated platelets. The mechanism of action is thought to involve steric hindrance and/or conformational effects to block access of large molecules to the receptor rather than direct interaction with the RGD (arginine-glycine-aspartic acid) binding site of GPIIb/IIIa.

Abciximab binds with similar affinity to the vitronectin receptor, also known as the $\alpha_v\beta_3$ integrin. The vitronectin receptor mediates the procoagulant properties of platelets and the proliferative properties of vascular endothelial and smooth muscle cells. In *in vitro* studies using a model cell line derived from melanoma cells, Abciximab blocked $\alpha_v\beta_3$-mediated effects including cell adhesion (IC_{50}=0.34 μg/mL). At concentrations which, *in vitro*, provide >80% GPIIb/IIIa receptor blockade, but above the *in vivo* therapeutic range, Abciximab more effectively blocked the burst of thrombin generation that followed platelet activation than select comparator antibodies which inhibit GPIIb/IIIa alone(1). The relationship of these *in vitro* data to clinical efficacy is uncertain.

Pre-clinical experience: Maximal inhibition of platelet aggregation was observed when ≥ 80% of GPIIb/IIIa receptors were blocked by Abciximab. In non-human primates, Abciximab bolus doses of 0.25 mg/kg generally achieved a blockade of at least 80% of platelet receptors and fully inhibited platelet aggregation. Inhibition of platelet function was temporary following a bolus dose, but receptor blockade could be sustained at ≥ 80% by continuous intravenous infusion. The inhibitory effects of Abciximab were substantially reversed by the transfusion of platelets in monkeys. The antithrombotic efficacy of prototype antibodies [murine 7E3 Fab and $F(ab')_2$] and Abciximab was evaluated in dog, monkey and baboon models of coronary, carotid, and femoral artery thrombosis. Doses of the murine version of 7E3 or Abciximab sufficient to produce high-grade (≥ 80%) GPIIb/IIIa receptor blockade prevented acute thrombosis and yielded lower rates of thrombosis compared with aspirin and/or heparin.

Pharmacokinetics: Following intravenous bolus administration, free plasma concentrations of Abciximab decrease rapidly with an initial half-life of less than 10 minutes and a second phase half-life of about 30 minutes, probably related to rapid binding to the platelet GPIIb/IIIa receptors. Platelet function generally recovers over the course of 48 hours (2,3), although Abciximab remains in the circulation for 15 days or more in a platelet-bound state. Intravenous administration of a 0.25 mg/kg bolus dose of Abciximab followed by continuous infusion of 10 μg/min (or a weight-adjusted infusion of 0.125 μg/kg/min to a maximum of 10 μg/min) produces approximately constant free plasma concentrations throughout the infusion. At the termination of the infusion period, free plasma concentrations fall rapidly for approximately six hours then decline at a slower rate.

Pharmacodynamics: Intravenous administration in humans of single bolus doses of Abciximab from 0.15 mg/kg to 0.30 mg/kg produced rapid dose-dependent inhibition of platelet function as measured by *ex vivo* platelet aggregation in response to adenosine diphosphate (ADP) or by prolongation of bleeding time. At the two highest doses (0.25 and 0.30 mg/kg) at two hours post injection, over 80% of the GPIIb/IIIa receptors were blocked and platelet aggregation in response to 20 μM ADP was almost abolished. The median bleeding time increased to over 30 minutes at both doses compared with a baseline value of approximately five minutes.

Intravenous administration in humans of a single bolus dose of 0.25 mg/kg followed by a continuous infusion of 10 μg/min for periods of 12 to 96 hours produced sustained high-grade GPIIb/IIIa receptor blockade (≥ 80%) and inhibition of platelet function (*ex vivo* platelet aggregation in response to 5 μM or 20 μM ADP less than 20% of baseline and bleeding time greater than 30 minutes) for the duration of the infusion in most patients. Similar results were obtained when a weight-adjusted infusion dose (0.125 μg/kg/min to a maximum of 10 μg/min) was used in patients weighing up to 80 kg. Results in patients who received the 0.25 mg/kg bolus followed by a 5 μg/min infusion for 24 hours showed a similar initial receptor blockade and inhibition of platelet aggregation, but the response was not maintained throughout the infusion period.

Low levels of GPIIb/IIIa receptor blockade are present for more than 10 days following cessation of the infusion. After discontinuation of Abciximab infusion, platelet function returns gradually to normal. Bleeding time returned to ≤ 12 minutes within 12 hours following the end of infusion in 15 of 20 patients (75%), and within 24 hours in 18 of 20 patients (90%). *Ex vivo* platelet aggregation in response to 5 μM ADP returned to ≥ 50% of baseline within 24 hours following the end of infusion in 11 of 32 patients (34%) and within 48 hours in 23 of 32 patients (72%). In response to 20 μM ADP, *ex vivo* platelet aggregation returned to ≥ 50% of baseline within 24 hours in 20 of 32 patients (62%) and within 48 hours in 28 of 32 patients (88%).

CLINICAL STUDIES

Abciximab has been studied in three Phase 3 clinical trials, all of which evaluated the effect of Abciximab in patients undergoing percutaneous coronary intervention: in patients at high risk for abrupt closure of the treated coronary vessel (EPIC), in a broader group of patients (EPILOG), and in unstable angina patients not responding to conventional medical therapy (CAPTURE). Percutaneous intervention included balloon angioplasty, atherectomy, or stent placement. All trials involved the use of various, concomitant heparin dose regimens and, unless contraindicated, aspirin (325 mg) was administered orally two hours prior to the planned procedure and then once daily.

EPIC was a multicenter, double-blind, placebo-controlled trial of Abciximab in patients undergoing percutaneous transluminal coronary angioplasty or atherectomy (4). In the EPIC trial, 2099 patients between 26 and 83 years of age who were at high risk for abrupt closure of the treated coronary vessel were randomly allocated to one of three treatments: 1) an Abciximab bolus (0.25 mg/kg) followed by an Abciximab infusion (10 μg/min) for 12 hours (bolus plus infusion group); 2) an Abciximab bolus (0.25 mg/kg) followed by a placebo infusion (bolus group), or; 3) a placebo bolus followed by a placebo infusion (placebo group). Patients at high risk during or following percutaneous coronary intervention were defined as those with unstable angina or non-Q wave myocardial infarction (n=489), those with an acute Q-wave myocardial infarction within 12 hours of symptom onset (n=66), and those who were at high risk because of coronary morphology and/or clinical characteristics (n=1544). Treatment with study agent in each of the three arms was initiated 10–60 minutes before the onset of percutaneous coronary intervention. All patients initially received an intravenous heparin bolus (10,000 to 12,000

Continued on next page

Table 1
PRIMARY ENDPOINT EVENT RATE AT 30 DAYS - EPIC TRIAL

	Placebo (n=696)	Abciximab Bolus (n=695)	Abciximab Bolus + Infusion (n=708)
		Number of Patients (%)	
Death, MI, or urgent intervention[a]	89 (12.8)	79 (11.5)	59 (8.3)
p-value vs. placebo		0.428	0.008
Components of Primary Endpoint[b]			
Death	12 (1.7)	9 (1.3)	12 (1.7)
Acute myocardial infarctions in surviving patients	55 (7.9)	40 (5.8)	31 (4.4)
Urgent intervention in surviving patients without an acute MI	22 (3.2)	30 (4.4)	16 (2.2)

[a]Patients who experienced more than one event in the first 30 days are counted only once.
[b]Patients are counted only once under the most serious component (death > acute MI > urgent intervention).

*** Identi-Code® symbol. This product information was prepared in June 1998. Current information on these and other products of Eli Lilly and Company may be obtained by direct inquiry to Lilly Research Laboratories, Lilly Corporate Center, Indianapolis, Indiana 46285, (800) 545-5979.**

ReoPro—Cont.

units) and boluses of up to 3,000 units thereafter to a maximum of 20,000 units during percutaneous coronary intervention. Heparin infusion was continued for 12 hours to maintain a therapeutic elevation of activated partial thromboplastin time (APTT, 1.5–2.5 times normal).

The primary endpoint was the occurrence of any of the following events within 30 days of percutaneous coronary intervention: death, myocardial infarction (MI), or the need for urgent intervention for recurrent ischemia [i.e., urgent percutaneous transluminal coronary angioplasty, urgent coronary artery bypass graft (CABG) surgery, a coronary stent, or an intra-aortic balloon pump]. The 30-day (Kaplan-Meier) primary endpoint event rates for each treatment group by intention-to-treat analysis of all randomized patients are shown in Table 1. The 4.5% lower incidence of the primary endpoint rates in the bolus plus infusion treatment group, compared with the placebo group, was statistically significant, whereas the 1.3% lower incidence in the bolus treatment group was not. A lower incidence of the primary endpoint was observed in the bolus plus infusion treatment arm for all three high-risk subgroups: patients with unstable angina, patients presenting within 12 hours of the onset of symptoms of an acute myocardial infarction, and patients with other high-risk clinical and/or morphologic characteristics (4). The treatment effect was largest in the first two subgroups and smallest in the third subgroup.

[See table 1 at top of previous page]

The primary endpoint event rates in the bolus plus infusion treatment group were reduced mostly in the first 48 hours and this benefit was sustained through blinded evaluations at 30 days(4), six months(5) and three years(6). At the six-month follow-up visit this event rate remained lower in the bolus infusion arm (12.3%) than in the placebo arm (17.6%) (p=0.006 vs. placebo). Median long-term follow up was 3.1 years (99% of patients had follow up between 2.5 and 3.5 years). Using Kaplan-Meier estimates, at 3 years the absolute reduction in events was maintained with an event rate of 19.6% in the bolus plus infusion arm and 24.4% in the placebo arm (p=0.027 vs. placebo).

EPILOG was a randomized, double-blind, multicenter, placebo-controlled trial which evaluated Abciximab in a broad population of patients undergoing percutaneous coronary intervention (excluding patients with myocardial infarction and unstable angina meeting the EPIC high risk criteria)(7). EPILOG tested the hypothesis that use of a low-dose, weight-adjusted heparin regimen, early femoral arterial sheath removal, improved access site management and weight-adjustment of the Abciximab infusion dose could significantly lower the bleeding rate yet maintain the efficacy seen in the EPIC trial. EPILOG was a three treatment-arm trial: Abciximab plus standard dose, weight-adjusted heparin[1]; Abciximab plus low dose, weight-adjusted heparin[2]; and placebo plus standard dose, weight-adjusted heparin. The Abciximab bolus dose was the same as that used in the EPIC trial (0.25 mg/kg), but the continuous infusion dose was weight adjusted in patients up to 80 kg[3] (0.125 µg/kg/min). Specific patient and access site management procedures as well as a strong recommendation for early sheath removal were also incorporated into the trial as described in PRECAUTIONS. The EPILOG trial achieved the objective of lowering the bleeding rate while maintaining efficacy: in the Abciximab treatment arms major bleeding was not significantly different from that in the placebo arm (see ADVERSE REACTIONS: Bleeding).

[1] Bolus administration of 100 U/kg weight-adjusted heparin to achieve an activated clotting time (ACT) of 300 seconds (maximum initial bolus 10,000 units).

[2] Bolus administration of 70 U/kg weight-adjusted heparin to achieve an activated clotting time (ACT) of 200 seconds (maximum initial bolus 7,000 units).

[3] Bolus administration of 0.25 mg/kg Abciximab 10 to 60 minutes before percutaneous coronary intervention immediately followed by a 0.125 µg/kg/min infusion (maximum 10 µg/min) for 12 hours.

The primary endpoint of the EPILOG trial was the composite of death or MI occurring within 30 days of percutaneous coronary intervention. The composite of death, MI, or urgent intervention was an important secondary endpoint. As seen in the EPIC trial, the endpoint events in the Abciximab treatment group were reduced mostly in the first 48 hours and this benefit was sustained through blinded evaluations at 30 days and six months. The (Kaplan-Meier) endpoint event rates at 30 days are shown in Table 2 for each treatment group by intention-to-treat analysis of all 2792 randomized patients. At the six-month follow-up visit, the event rate for death, MI, or repeat (urgent or non-urgent) intervention remained lower in the Abciximab treatment arms (22.3% and 22.8%, respectively, for the standard- and low-dose heparin arms) than in the placebo arm (25.8%) and the event rate for death, MI, or urgent intervention was substantially lower in the Abciximab treatment arms (8.3% and 8.4%, respectively, for the standard- and low-dose hep-

Table 2
ENDPOINT EVENT RATES AT 30 DAYS - EPILOG TRIAL

	Placebo + Standard Dose Heparin (n=939)	Abciximab + Standard Dose Heparin (n=918)	Abciximab + Low Dose Heparin (n=935)
	Number of Patients (%)		
Death or MI[a]	85 (9.1)	38 (4.2)	35 (3.8)
p-value vs. placebo		<0.001	<0.001
Death, MI, or urgent intervention[a]	109 (11.7)	49 (5.4)	48 (5.2)
p-value vs. placebo		<0.001	<0.001
Components of Composite Endpoints[b]			
Death	7 (0.8)	4 (0.4)	3 (0.3)
Acute myocardial infarctions in surviving patients	78 (8.4)	34 (3.7)	32 (3.4)
Urgent intervention in surviving patients without an acute MI	24 (2.6)	11 (1.2)	13 (1.4)

[a]Patients who experienced more than one event in the first 30 days are counted only once.
[b]Patients are counted only once under the most serious component (death > acute MI > urgent intervention).

Table 3
PRIMARY ENDPOINT EVENT RATE AT 30 DAYS - CAPTURE TRIAL

	Placebo (n=635)	Abciximab (n=630)
	Number of Patients (%)	
Death, MI, or urgent intervention[a]	101 (15.9)	71 (11.3)
p-value vs. placebo		0.012
Components of Primary Endpoint[b]		
Death	8 (1.3)	6 (1.0)
MI in surviving patients	49 (7.7)	24 (3.8)
Urgent intervention in surviving patients without acute MI	44 (6.9)	41 (6.6)

[a] Patients who experienced more than one event in the first 30 days are counted only once. Urgent interventions included any unplanned percutaneous coronary intervention after the planned intervention, as well as any stent placement for immediate patency and any unplanned CABG or use of an intra-aortic balloon pump.
[b] Patients are counted only once under the most serious component (death>acute MI>urgent intervention).

arin arms) than in the placebo arm (14.7%). The proportionate reductions in endpoint event rates were similar irrespective of the type of coronary intervention used (balloon angioplasty, atherectomy, or stent placement). Risk assessment using the American College of Cardiology/American Heart Association clinical/morphological criteria had large inter-observer variability. Consequently, a low risk subgroup could not be reproducibly identified in which to evaluate efficacy.

[See table 2 above]

CAPTURE was a randomized, double-blind, multicenter, placebo-controlled trial of the use of Abciximab in unstable angina patients not responding to conventional medical therapy for whom percutaneous coronary intervention was planned, but not immediately performed(8) In contrast to the EPIC and EPILOG trials, the CAPTURE trial involved the administration of placebo or Abciximab starting 18 to 24 hours prior to percutaneous coronary intervention and continuing until one hour after completion of the intervention. Patients were assessed as having unstable angina not responding to conventional medical therapy if they had at least one episode of myocardial ischemia despite bed rest and at least two hours of therapy with intravenous heparin and oral or intravenous nitrates. These patients were enrolled into the CAPTURE trial, if during a screening angiogram, they were determined to have a coronary lesion amenable to percutaneous coronary intervention. Patients received a bolus dose and intravenous infusion of placebo or Abciximab for 18 to 24 hours. At the end of the infusion period, the intervention was performed. The Abciximab or placebo infusion was discontinued one hour following the intervention. Patients were treated with intravenous heparin and oral or intravenous nitrates throughout the 18 to 24-hour Abciximab infusion period prior to the percutaneous coronary intervention.

The Abciximab dose was a 0.25 mg/kg bolus followed by a continuous infusion at a rate of 10 µg/min. The CAPTURE trial incorporated weight adjustment of the standard heparin dose only during the performance of the intervention, but did not investigate the effect of a lower heparin dose, and arterial sheaths were left in place for approximately 40 hours. The primary endpoint of the CAPTURE trial was the occurrence of any of the following events within 30 days of percutaneous coronary intervention: death, MI, or urgent intervention. The 30-day (Kaplan-Meier) primary endpoint event rates for each treatment group by intention-to-treat analysis of all 1265 randomized patients are shown in Table 3.

[See table 3 above]

The 30-day results are consistent with EPIC results, with the greatest effects on the myocardial infarction and urgent intervention components of the composite endpoint. As secondary endpoints, the components of the composite end-

point were analyzed separately for the period prior to the percutaneous coronary intervention and the period from the beginning of the intervention through Day 30. The greatest difference in MI occurred in the post-intervention period: the rates of MI were lower in the Abciximab group compared with placebo (Abciximab 3.6%, placebo 6.1%). There was also a reduction in MI occurring prior to the percutaneous coronary intervention (Abciximab 0.6%, placebo 2.0%). An Abciximab-associated reduction in the incidence of urgent intervention occurred in the post-intervention period. No effect on mortality was observed in either period. At six months of follow up, the composite endpoint of death, MI, or repeat intervention (urgent or non-urgent) was not different between the Abciximab and placebo groups (Abciximab 31.0%, placebo 30.8%, p=0.77).

Mortality was uncommon in all three trials, EPIC, EPILOG and CAPTURE. Similar mortality rates were observed in all arms within each trial. In all three trials, the rates of acute MI were significantly lower in the groups treated with Abciximab. Urgent intervention rates were also lower in Abciximab-treated groups in these trials.

Anticoagulation: Due to the incidence of bleeding seen in the EPIC trial, the dosing regimens of concomitant heparin and the target levels for anticoagulation were successively varied in the CAPTURE and EPILOG trials. These modified dosing regimens combined with other measures for patient management were associated with reduced bleeding rates (see ADVERSE REACTIONS: Bleeding)

EPILOG trial: Heparin was weight adjusted in all treatment arms. A baseline ACT was determined prior to percutaneous coronary intervention. In the low-dose heparin arm of the trial, heparin was administered as follows: The initial heparin bolus was based upon the results of the baseline ACT, according to the following regimen:

ACT < 150 seconds: administer 70 U/kg heparin
ACT 150 - 199 seconds: administer 50 U/kg heparin
ACT ≥ 200 seconds: administer no heparin

Additional 20 U/kg heparin boluses were given to achieve and maintain an ACT of 200 seconds during the procedure.

Discontinuation of heparin immediately after the procedure and removal of the arterial sheath within six hours were strongly recommended in the trial. If prolonged heparin therapy or delayed sheath removal was clinically indicated, heparin was adjusted to keep the APTT at a target of 60 to 85 seconds.

CAPTURE trial: Anticoagulation was initiated prior to the administration of Abciximab. Anticoagulation was initiated with an intravenous heparin infusion to achieve a target APTT of 60 to 85 seconds. The heparin infusion was not uniformly weight adjusted in this trial. The heparin infusion was maintained during the Abciximab infusion and was adjusted to achieve an ACT of 300 seconds

Table 4
NON-CABG BLEEDING IN THE EPIC, EPILOG AND CAPTURE TRIALS
Number of Patients with Bleeds (%)

EPIC:

	Placebo (n = 696)	Abciximab (Bolus + Infusion) (n = 708)
Major[a]	23 (3.3)	75 (10.6)
Minor	64 (9.2)	119 (16.8)
Requiring Transfusion[b]	14 (2.0)	55 (7.8)

CAPTURE:

	Placebo (n = 635)	Abciximab (n = 630)
Major[a]	12 (1.9)	24 (3.8)
Minor	13 (2.0)	30 (4.8)
Requiring Transfusion[b]	9 (1.4)	15 (2.4)

EPILOG:

	Placebo (n = 939)	Abciximab + Standard-dose Heparin (n = 918)	Abciximab + Low-dose Heparin (n = 935)
Major[a]	10 (1.1)	17 (1.9)	10 (1.1)
Minor	32 (3.4)	70 (7.6)	37 (4.0)
Requiring Transfusion[b]	10 (1.1)	7 (0.8)	6 (0.6)

[a] Patients who had bleeding in more than one classification are counted only once according to the most severe classification. Patients with multiple bleeding events of the same classification are also counted once within that classification.
[b] Packed red blood cells or whole blood

or an APTT of 70 seconds during the percutaneous coronary intervention. Following the intervention, heparin management was as outlined above for the EPILOG trial.

INDICATIONS AND USAGE

Abciximab is indicated as an adjunct to percutaneous coronary intervention for the prevention of cardiac ischemic complications.
- in patients undergoing percutaneous coronary intervention
- in patients with unstable angina not responding to conventional medical therapy when percutaneous coronary intervention is planned within 24 hours

Abciximab use in patients not undergoing percutaneous coronary intervention has not been studied.

Abciximab is intended for use with aspirin and heparin and has been studied only in that setting, as described in CLINICAL STUDIES.

CONTRAINDICATIONS

Because Abciximab may increase the risk of bleeding, Abciximab is contraindicated in the following clinical situations:
- Active internal bleeding
- Recent (within six weeks) gastrointestinal (GI) or genitourinary (GU) bleeding of clinical significance
- History of cerebrovascular accident (CVA) within two years, or CVA with a significant residual neurological deficit
- Bleeding diathesis
- Administration of oral anticoagulants within seven days unless prothrombin time is ≤ 1.2 times control
- Thrombocytopenia (< 100,000 cells/µL)
- Recent (within six weeks) major surgery or trauma
- Intracranial neoplasm, arteriovenous malformation, or aneurysm
- Severe uncontrolled hypertension
- Presumed or documented history of vasculitis
- Use of intravenous dextran before percutaneous coronary intervention, or intent to use it during an intervention

Abciximab is also contraindicated in patients with known hypersensitivity to any component of this product or to murine proteins.

WARNINGS

Abciximab has the potential to increase the risk of bleeding, particularly in the presence of anticoagulation, e.g., from heparin, other anticoagulants, or thrombolytics (see ADVERSE REACTIONS: Bleeding).

The risk of major bleeds due to Abciximab therapy may be increased in patients receiving thrombolytics and should be weighed against the anticipated benefits.

Should serious bleeding occur that is not controllable with pressure, the infusion of Abciximab and any concomitant heparin should be stopped.

PRECAUTIONS

Bleeding Precautions: Results of the EPILOG trial show that bleeding can be reduced by the use of low-dose, weight-adjusted heparin regimens, adherence to stricter anticoagulation guidelines, early femoral arterial sheath removal, careful patient and access site management and weight-adjustment of the Abciximab infusion dose.

Therapy with Abciximab requires careful attention to all potential bleeding sites (including catheter insertion sites, arterial and venous puncture sites, cutdown sites, needle puncture sites, and gastrointestinal, genitourinary, and retroperitoneal sites).

Arterial and venous punctures, intramuscular injections, and use of urinary catheters, nasotracheal intubation, nasogastric tubes and automatic blood pressure cuffs should be minimized. When obtaining intravenous access, non-compressible sites (e.g., subclavian or jugular veins) should be avoided. Saline or heparin locks should be considered for blood drawing. Vascular puncture sites should be documented and monitored. Gentle care should be provided when removing dressings.

Femoral artery access site:

Arterial access site care is important to prevent bleeding. Care should be taken when attempting vascular access that only the anterior wall of the femoral artery is punctured, avoiding a Seldinger (through and through) technique for obtaining sheath access. Femoral vein sheath placement should be avoided unless needed. While the vascular sheath is in place, patients should be maintained on complete bed rest with the head of the bed ≤30° and the affected limb restrained in a straight position. Patients may be medicated for back/groin pain as necessary.

Discontinuation of heparin immediately upon completion of the procedure and removal of the arterial sheath within six hours is strongly recommended if APTT ≤ 50 sec or ACT ≤ 175 sec (See PRECAUTIONS: Laboratory Tests). In all circumstances, heparin should be discontinued at least two hours prior to arterial sheath removal.

Following sheath removal, pressure should be applied to the femoral artery for at least 30 minutes using either manual compression or a mechanical device for hemostasis. A pressure dressing should be applied following hemostasis. The patient should be maintained on bed rest for six to eight hours following sheath removal or discontinuation of Abciximab, or four hours following discontinuation of heparin, whichever is later. The pressure dressing should be removed prior to ambulation. The sheath insertion site and distal pulses of affected leg(s) should be frequently checked while the femoral artery sheath is in place and for six hours after femoral artery sheath removal. Any hematoma should be measured and monitored for enlargement.

The following conditions have been associated with an increased risk of bleeding and may be additive with the effect of Abciximab in the angioplasty setting: percutaneous coronary intervention within 12 hours of the onset of symptoms for acute myocardial infarction, prolonged percutaneous coronary intervention (lasting more than 70 minutes) and failed percutaneous coronary intervention.

Use of Thrombolytics, Anticoagulants and Other Antiplatelet Agents: In the EPIC, EPILOG and CAPTURE trials, Abciximab was used concomitantly with heparin and aspirin. For details of the anticoagulation algorithms used in these clinical trials, see CLINICAL STUDIES: Anticoagulation. Because Abciximab inhibits platelet aggregation, caution should be employed when it is used with other drugs that affect hemostasis, including thrombolytics, oral anticoagulants, non-steroidal anti-inflammatory drugs, dipyridamole, and ticlopidine.

In the EPIC trial, there was limited experience with the administration of Abciximab with low molecular weight dextran. Low molecular weight dextran was usually given for the deployment of a coronary stent, for which oral anticoagulants were also given. In the 11 patients who received low molecular weight dextran with Abciximab, five had major bleeding events and four had minor bleeding events. None of the five placebo patients treated with low molecular weight dextran had a major or minor bleeding event (see CONTRAINDICATIONS).

There are limited data on the use of Abciximab in patients receiving thrombolytic agents. Because of concern about synergistic effects on bleeding, systemic thrombolytic therapy should be used judiciously.

Thrombocytopenia: Platelet counts should be monitored prior to treatment, two to four hours following the bolus dose of Abciximab and at 24 hours or prior to discharge, whichever is first. If a patient experiences an acute platelet decrease (e.g., a platelet decrease to less than 100,000 cells/µL and a decrease of at least 25% from pre-treatment value), additional platelet counts should be determined. These platelet counts should be drawn in three separate tubes containing ethylenediaminetetraacetic acid (EDTA), citrate and heparin, respectively, to exclude pseudothrombocytopenia due to *in vitro* anticoagulant interaction. If true thrombocytopenia is verified, Abciximab should be immediately discontinued and the condition appropriately monitored and treated. For patients with thrombocytopenia in the clinical trials, a daily platelet count was obtained until it returned to normal. If a patient's platelet count dropped to 60,000 cells/µL, heparin and aspirin were discontinued. If a patient's platelet count dropped below 50,000 cells/µL, platelets were transfused. Most cases of severe thrombocytopenia (<50,000 cells/µL) occurred within the first 24 hours of Abciximab administration.

Restoration of Platelet Function: In the event of serious uncontrolled bleeding or the need for emergency surgery, Abciximab should be discontinued. If platelet function does not return to normal, it may be restored, at least in part, with platelet transfusion.

Laboratory Tests: Before infusion of Abciximab, platelet count, prothrombin time, ACT and APTT should be measured to identify pre-existing hemostatic abnormalities.

Based on an integrated analysis of data from all studies, the following guidelines may be utilized to minimize the risk for bleeding:

When Abciximab is initiated 18 to 24 hours before percutaneous coronary intervention, the APTT should be maintained between 60 and 85 seconds during the Abciximab and heparin infusion period.

During percutaneous coronary intervention the ACT should be maintained between 200 and 300 seconds.

If anticoagulation is continued in these patients following percutaneous coronary intervention, the APTT should be maintained between 60 and 85 seconds.

The APTT or ACT should be checked prior to arterial sheath removal. The sheath should not be removed unless APTT ≤ 50 seconds or ACT ≤ 175 seconds.

Readministration: Administration of Abciximab may result in human anti-chimeric antibody (HACA) formation that could potentially cause allergic or hypersensitivity reactions (including anaphylaxis), thrombocytopenia or diminished benefit upon readministration of Abciximab. In the EPIC, EPILOG, and CAPTURE trials, positive HACA responses occurred in approximately 5.8% of the Abciximab-treated patients. There was no excess of hypersensitivity or allergic reactions related to Abciximab treatment.

Readministration of Abciximab to 29 healthy volunteers who had not developed a HACA response after first administration has not led to any change in Abciximab pharmacokinetics or to any reduction in antiplatelet potency. However, results in this small group of patients suggest that the incidence of HACA response may be increased after readministration. Readministration to patients who have developed a positive HACA response after initial administration has not been evaluated in clinical trials.

Allergic Reactions: Anaphylaxis has not been reported for Abciximab-treated patients in any of the Phase 3 clinical trials. However, anaphylaxis may occur. If it does, administration of Abciximab should be immediately stopped and standard appropriate resuscitative measures should be initiated.

Drug Interactions: Although drug interactions with Abciximab have not been studied systematically, Abciximab has been administered to patients with ischemic heart disease treated concomitantly with a broad range of medications used in the treatment of angina, myocardial infarction and hypertension. These medications have included heparin, warfarin, beta-adrenergic receptor blockers, calcium channel antagonists, angiotensin converting enzyme inhibitors, intravenous and oral nitrates, and aspirin. Heparin, other anticoagulants, thrombolytics, and antiplatelet agents may be associated with an increase in bleeding. Patients with

Continued on next page

* **Identi-Code® symbol. This product information was prepared in June 1998. Current information on these and other products of Eli Lilly and Company may be obtained by direct inquiry to Lilly Research Laboratories, Lilly Corporate Center, Indianapolis, Indiana 46285, (800) 545-5979.**

ReoPro—Cont.

HACA titers may have allergic or hypersensitivity reactions when treated with other diagnostic or therapeutic monoclonal antibodies.

Carcinogenesis, Mutagenesis and Impairment of Fertility: *In vitro* and *in vivo* mutagenicity studies have not demonstrated any mutagenic effect. Long-term studies in animals have not been performed to evaluate the carcinogenic potential or effects on fertility in male or female animals.

Pregnancy Category C: Animal reproduction studies have not been conducted with Abciximab. It is also not known whether Abciximab can cause fetal harm when administered to a pregnant woman or can affect reproduction capacity. Abciximab should be given to a pregnant woman only if clearly needed.

Nursing Mothers: It is not known whether this drug is excreted in human milk or absorbed systemically after ingestion. Because many drugs are excreted in human milk, caution should be exercised when Abciximab is administered to a nursing woman.

Pediatric Use: Safety and effectiveness in pediatric patients have not been studied.

ADVERSE REACTIONS

Bleeding: Abciximab has the potential to increase the risk of bleeding, particularly in the presence of anticoagulation, e.g. from heparin, other anticoagulants or thrombolytics. Bleeding in the Phase 3 trials was classified as major, minor or insignificant by the criteria of the Thrombolysis in Myocardial Infarction study group(9). Major bleeding events were defined as either an intracranial hemorrhage or a decrease in hemoglobin greater than 5 g/dL. Minor bleeding events included spontaneous gross hematuria, spontaneous hematemesis, observed blood loss with a hemoglobin decrease of more than 3 g/dL, or a decrease in hemoglobin of at least 4 g/dL without an identified bleeding site. Insignificant bleeding events were defined as a decrease in hemoglobin of less than 3 g/dL or a decrease in hemoglobin between 3–4 g/dL without observed bleeding. In patients who received transfusions, the number of units of blood lost was esti-

mated through an adaptation of the method of Landefeld, et al.(10).

In the EPIC trial, in which a non-weight-adjusted, standard heparin dose regimen was used, the most common complication during Abciximab therapy was bleeding during the first 36 hours. The incidences of major bleeding, minor bleeding and transfusion of blood products were significantly increased. Approximately 70% of Abciximab-treated patients with major bleeding had bleeding at the arterial access site in the groin. Abciximab-treated patients also had a higher incidence of major bleeding events from gastrointestinal, genitourinary, retroperitoneal, and other sites. Bleeding rates were reduced in the CAPTURE trial, and further reduced in the EPILOG trial by use of modified dosing regimens and specific patient management techniques. In EPILOG, using the heparin and Abciximab dosing, sheath removal and arterial access site guidelines described under PRECAUTIONS, the incidence of major bleeding in patients treated with Abciximab and low-dose, weight-adjusted heparin was not significantly different from that in patients receiving placebo.

Subgroup analyses in the EPIC and CAPTURE trials showed that non-CABG major bleeding was more common in Abciximab patients weighing ≤ 75 kg. In the EPILOG trial which used weight-adjusted heparin dosing, the non-CABG major bleeding rates for Abciximab-treated patients did not differ substantially by weight subgroup.

Although data are limited, Abciximab treatment was not associated with excess major bleeding in patients who underwent CABG surgery. (The range among all treatment arms was 3–5% in EPIC and 1–2% in the CAPTURE and EPILOG trials.) Some patients with prolonged bleeding times received platelet transfusions to correct the bleeding time prior to surgery. (See PRECAUTIONS: Restoration of Platelet Function.)

The rates of major bleeding, minor bleeding and bleeding events requiring transfusions in the EPIC, CAPTURE and EPILOG trials are shown in Table 4. The rates of insignificant bleeding events are not included in Table 4.

[See table 4 at top of previous page]

Intracranial Hemorrhage and Stroke: The total incidence of intracranial hemorrhage and non-hemorrhagic stroke

across all three trials was not significantly different, 7/2225 for placebo patients and 10/3112 for Abciximab treated patients. The incidence of intracranial hemorrhage was 3/2225 for placebo patients and 6/3112 for Abciximab patients.

Thrombocytopenia: In the clinical trials, patients treated with Abciximab were more likely than patients treated with placebo to experience decreases in platelet counts. The rates of thrombocytopenia and transfusions were lower in the subsequent CAPTURE and EPILOG trials (Table 5).

[See table 5 below]

Other Adverse Reactions: Table 6 shows adverse events other than bleeding and thrombocytopenia from the combined EPIC, EPILOG and CAPTURE trials which occurred in patients in the bolus plus infusion arm at an incidence of more than 0.5% higher than in those treated with placebo.

[See table 6 below]

The following additional adverse events from the EPIC, EPILOG and CAPTURE trials were reported by investigators for patients treated with a bolus plus infusion of Abciximab at incidences which were less than 0.5% higher than for patients in the placebo arm.

Cardiovascular System—ventricular tachycardia (1.4%), pseudoaneurysm (0.8%), palpitation (0.5%), arteriovenous fistula (0.4%), incomplete AV block (0.3%), nodal arrhythmia (0.2%), complete AV block (0.1%), embolism (limb)(0.1%); thrombophlebitis (0.1%);

Gastrointestinal System—dyspepsia (2.1%), diarrhea (1.1%), ileus (0.1%), gastroesophageal reflux (0.1%);

Hemic and Lymphatic System—anemia (1.3%), leukocytosis (0.5%), petechiae (0.2%);

Nervous System—dizziness (2.9%), anxiety (1.7%), abnormal thinking (1.3%), agitation (0.7%), hypesthesia (0.6%), confusion (0.5%), muscle contractions (0.4%), coma (0.2%), hypertonia (0.2%), diplopia (0.1%);

Respiratory System—pneumonia (0.4%), rales (0.4%), pleural effusion (0.3%), bronchitis (0.3%) bronchospasm (0.3%), pleurisy (0.2%), pulmonary embolism (0.2%), rhonchi (0.1%);

Musculoskeletal System—myalgia (0.2%);

Urogenital System—urinary retention (0.7%), dysuria (0.4%), abnormal renal function (0.4%), frequent micturition (0.1%), cystalgia (0.1%), urinary incontinence (0.1%), prostatitis (0.1%);

Miscellaneous—pain (5.4%), sweating increased (1.0%), asthenia (0.7%), incisional pain (0.6%), pruritus (0.5%), abnormal vision (0.3%), edema (0.3%), wound (0.2%), abscess (0.2%), cellulitis (0.2%), peripheral coldness (0.2%), injection site pain (0.1%), dry mouth (0.1%), pallor (0.1%), diabetes mellitus (0.1%), hyperkalemia (0.1%), enlarged abdomen (0.1%), bullous eruption (0.1%), inflammation (0.1%), drug toxicity (0.1%).

OVERDOSAGE

There has been no experience of overdosage in human clinical trials.

DOSAGE AND ADMINISTRATION

The safety and efficacy of Abciximab have only been investigated with concomitant administration of heparin and aspirin as described in CLINICAL STUDIES.

In patients with failed percutaneous coronary interventions, the continuous infusion of Abciximab should be stopped because there is no evidence for Abciximab efficacy in that setting.

In the event of serious bleeding that cannot be controlled by compression, Abciximab and heparin should be discontinued immediately.

The recommended dosage of Abciximab in adults is a 0.25 mg/kg intravenous bolus administered 10–60 minutes before the start of percutaneous coronary intervention, followed by a continuous intravenous infusion of 0.125 µg/kg/min (to a maximum of 10 µg/min) for 12 hours.

Patients with unstable angina not responding to conventional medical therapy and who are planned to undergo percutaneous coronary intervention within 24 hours may be treated with an Abciximab 0.25 mg/kg intravenous bolus followed by an 18 to 24-hour intravenous infusion of 10 µg/min, concluding one hour after the percutaneous coronary intervention.

Instructions for Administration

1. Parenteral drug products should be inspected visually for particulate matter prior to administration. Preparations of Abciximab containing visibly opaque particles should NOT be used.

2. Hypersensitivity reactions should be anticipated whenever protein solutions such as Abciximab are administered. Epinephrine, dopamine, theophylline, antihistamines, and corticosteroids should be available for immediate use. If symptoms of an allergic reaction or anaphylaxis appear, the infusion should be stopped and appropriate treatment given.

3. As with all parenteral drug products, aseptic procedures should be used during the administration of Abciximab.

Table 5
THROMBOCYTOPENIA AND PLATELET TRANSFUSIONS[a]

	Placebo + Standard-dose Heparin	Abciximab + Standard-dose Heparin	Abciximab + Low-dose Heparin
	Total number of patients enrolled		
EPIC	n = 696	n = 708	—
CAPTURE	n = 635	n = 630	—
EPILOG	n = 939	n = 918	n = 935
Patients with decrease of platelets to <50,000 cells/µL[a]	% of patients with events		
EPIC	0.7	1.6	—
CAPTURE	0.3	1.7	—
EPILOG	0.4	0.9	0.4
Patients with decrease of platelets to <100,000 cells/µL[a]			
EPIC	3.4	5.2	—
CAPTURE	1.3	5.6	—
EPILOG	1.5	2.6	2.5
Patients who received platelet tranfusions[b]			
EPIC	2.6	5.5	—
CAPTURE	0.3	2.1	—
EPILOG	1.1	1.6	0.9

[a] Patients with a platelet count of <50,000 cells/µL are also included in the category of patients with a platelet count of <100,000 cells/µL.
[b] Includes patients receiving platelet transfusions for thrombocytopenia or any other reason.

Table 6
ADVERSE EVENTS AMONG TREATED PATIENTS IN THE EPIC, EPILOG AND CAPTURE TRIALS

Event	Placebo (n = 2226)	Bolus + Infusion (n = 3111)
	Number of Patients (%)	
Cardiovascular System		
Hypotension	230 (10.3)	447 (14.4)
Bradycardia	79 (3.5)	140 (4.5)
Gastrointestinal System		
Nausea	255 (11.5)	423 (13.6)
Vomiting	152 (6.8)	226 (7.3)
Abdominal Pain	49 (2.2)	97 (3.1)
Miscellaneous		
Back Pain	304 (13.7)	546 (17.6)
Chest Pain	208 (9.3)	356 (11.4)
Headache	122 (5.5)	200 (6.4)
Puncture Site Pain	58 (2.6)	113 (3.6)
Peripheral Edema	25 (1.1)	49 (1.6)

4. Withdraw the necessary amount of Abciximab for bolus injection into a syringe. Filter the bolus injection using a sterile, non-pyrogenic, low protein-binding 0.2 or 0.22 µm filter (Millipore SLGV025LS or equivalent).
5. Withdraw the necessary amount of Abciximab for the continuous infusion into a syringe. Inject into an appropriate container of sterile 0.9% saline or 5% dextrose and infuse at the calculated rate via a continuous infusion pump. The continuous infusion should be filtered either upon admixture using a sterile, non-pyrogenic, low protein-binding 0.2 or 0.22 µm syringe filter (Millipore SLGV025LS or equivalent) or upon administration using an in-line, sterile, non-pyrogenic, low protein-binding 0.2 or 0.22 µm filter (Abbott #4524 or equivalent). Discard the unused portion at the end of the infusion.
6. No incompatibilities have been shown with intravenous infusion fluids or commonly used cardiovascular drugs. Nevertheless, Abciximab should be administered in a separate intravenous line whenever possible and not mixed with other medications.
7. No incompatibilities have been observed with glass bottles or polyvinyl chloride bags and administration sets.

HOW SUPPLIED

Abciximab (ReoPro®) 2 mg/mL is supplied in 5 mL vials containing 10 mg (NDC 0002-7140-01).
Vials should be stored at 2 to 8°C (36 to 46°F). Do not freeze. Do not shake. Do not use beyond the expiration date. Discard any unused portion left in the vial.

REFERENCES

1. Reverter JC, Beguin S, Kessels H, Kumar R, Hemmer HC, Coller BS. Inhibition of platelet-mediated, tissue-factor-induced thrombin generation by the mouse/human chimeric 7E3 antibody; potential implications for the effect of c7E3 Fab treatment on acute thrombosis and "clinical restenosis". *J Clin Invest.* 1996;**98**:863–874.
2. Tcheng J, Ellis SG, George BS. Pharmacodynamics of chimeric glycoprotein IIb/IIIa integrin antiplatelet antibody Fab 7E3 in high risk coronary angioplasty. *Circulation.* 1994;**90**:1757–1764.
3. Simoons ML, de Boer MJ, van der Brand MJBM, et al. Randomized trial of a GPIIb/IIIa platelet receptor blocker in refractory unstable angina. *Circulation.* 1994;**89**:596–603.
4. EPIC Investigators. Use of a monoclonal antibody directed against the platelet glycoprotein IIb/IIIa receptor in high-risk coronary angioplasty. *N Engl J Med* 1994.**330**:956–961.
5. Topol EJ, Califf RM, Weisman HF, et al. Randomised trial of coronary intervention with antibody against platelet IIb/IIIa integrin for reduction of clinical restenosis: results at six months. *Lancet.* 1994;**343**:881–886.
6. Topol EJ, Ferguson JJ, Weisman HF, et al. for the EPIC Investigators. Long term protection from myocardial ischemic events in a randomized trial of brief integrin blockade with percutaneous coronary intervention. *JAMA.* 1997;**278**:479–484.
7. EPILOG Investigators. Platelet glycoprotein IIb/IIIa receptor blockade and low dose heparin during percutaneous coronary revascularization. *N Eng J Med.* 1997;**336**:1689–1696.
8. CAPTURE Investigators. Randomised placebo-controlled trial of abciximab before and during coronary intervention in refractory unstable angina: the CAPTURE study. *Lancet.* 1997;**349**;1429–1435.
9. Rao AK, Pratt C, Berke A, et al. Thrombolysis in Myocardial Infarction (TIMI) Trial – Phase I: Hemorrhagic manifestations and changes in plasma fibrinogen and the fibrinolytic system in patients treated with recombinant tissue plasminogen activator and streptokinase. *J Am Coll Cardiol.* 1988;**11**:1–11.
10. Landefeld CS, Cook EF, Flatley M, et al. Identification and preliminary validation of predictors of major bleeding in hospitalized patients starting anticoagulant therapy. *Am J Med.* 1987;**82**:703–713.

Revision Date: February 12, 1998

Manufactured by:
Centocor B.V.
Leiden, The Netherlands
U.S. License Number: 1178

Distributed by:
Eli Lilly and Company
Indianapolis, IN 46285

Shown in Product Identification Guide, page 320

TAZIDIME® ℞

[*tă ′zī-dēm*]
brand of
(ceftazidime) for injection, USP
for intravenous or intramuscular use

DESCRIPTION

Ceftazidime is a semisynthetic, broad-spectrum, beta-lactam antibiotic for parenteral administration. It is the pentahydrate of Pyridinium, 1-[[7-[[(2-amino-4-thiazolyl) [(1-carboxy-1-methylethoxy) imino]acetyl]amino]-2-carboxy-8-oxo-5-thia-1-azabicyclo(4.2.0)oct-2-en-3-yl] methyl]-, hydroxide, inner salt, [6R-[6α,7β(Z)]]. It has the following structure:

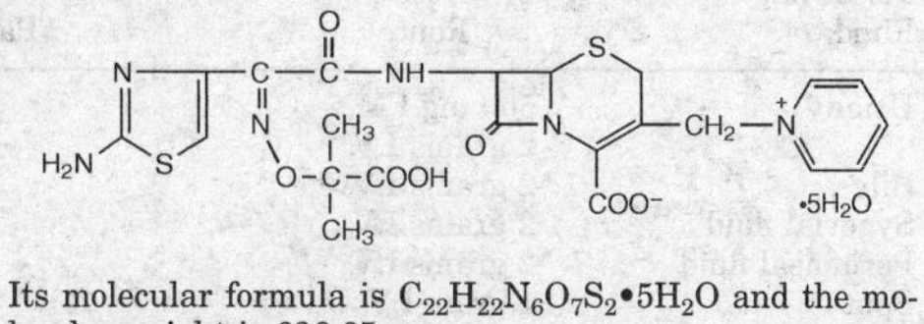

Its molecular formula is $C_{22}H_{22}N_6O_7S_2 \bullet 5H_2O$ and the molecular weight is 636.65.
Tazidime® (ceftazidime for injection, USP) is a sterile, dry powdered mixture of ceftazidime pentahydrate and sodium carbonate. The sodium carbonate at a concentration of 118 mg/gram of ceftazidime activity has been admixed to facilitate dissolution. The total sodium content of the mixture is approximately 54 mg (2.3 mEq)/gram of ceftazidime activity. Solutions of *Tazidime* range in color from light yellow to amber, depending on the diluent and volume used. The pH of freshly reconstituted solutions usually ranges from 5.0 to 8.0.

CLINICAL PHARMACOLOGY

After intravenous administration of 500 mg and 1 gram doses of ceftazidime over five minutes to normal adult male volunteers, mean peak serum concentrations of 45 mcg/mL and 90 mcg/mL, respectively, were achieved. After intravenous infusion of 500 mg, 1 gram and 2 gram doses of ceftazidime over 20 to 30 minutes to normal adult male volunteers, mean peak serum concentrations of 42 mcg/mL, 69 mcg/mL and 170 mcg/mL, respectively, were achieved. The average serum concentrations following intravenous infusion of 500 mg, 1 gram and 2 gram doses to these volunteers over an eight-hour interval are given in Table 1.

Table 1

Ceftazidime	Serum Concentrations (mcg/mL)				
I.V. Dosage	0.5 hr.	1 hr.	2 hr.	4 hr.	8 hr.
500 mg	42	25	12	6	2
1 gram	60	39	23	11	3
2 grams	129	75	42	13	5

The absorption and elimination of ceftazidime were directly proportional to the size of the dose. The half-life following intravenous administration was approximately 1.9 hours. Less than 10% of ceftazidime was protein bound. The degree of protein binding was independent of concentration. There was no evidence of accumulation of ceftazidime in the serum in individuals with normal renal function following multiple intravenous doses of 1 gram and 2 grams every eight hours for ten days.
Following intramuscular administration of 500 mg and 1 gram doses of ceftazidime to normal adult volunteers, the mean peak serum concentrations were 17 mcg/mL and 39 mcg/mL, respectively, at approximately one hour. Serum concentrations remained above 4 mcg/mL for six and eight hours after the intramuscular administration of 500 mg and 1 gram doses, respectively. The half-life of ceftazidime in these volunteers was approximately two hours.
The presence of hepatic dysfunction had no effect on the pharmacokinetics of ceftazidime in individuals administered 2 grams intravenously every eight hours for five days. Therefore, a dosage adjustment from the normal recommended dosage is not required for patients with hepatic dysfunction, provided renal function is not impaired.
Approximately 80%–90% of an intramuscular or intravenous dose of ceftazidime is excreted unchanged by the kidneys over a 24-hour period. After the intravenous administration of single 500 mg or 1 gram doses, approximately 50% of the dose appeared in the urine in the first two hours. An additional 20% was excreted between two and four hours after dosing, and approximately another 12% of the dose appeared in the urine between four and eight hours later. The elimination of ceftazidime by the kidneys resulted in high therapeutic concentrations in the urine.
The mean renal clearance of ceftazidime was approximately 100 mL/min. The calculated plasma clearance of approximately 115 mL/min, indicated nearly complete elimination of ceftazidime by the renal route. Administration of probenecid prior to dosing had no effect on the elimination kinetics of ceftazidime. This suggests that ceftazidime is eliminated by glomerular filtration and is not actively secreted by renal tubular mechanisms.
Since ceftazidime is eliminated almost solely by the kidneys, its serum half-life is significantly prolonged in patients with impaired renal function. Consequently, dosage adjustments to such patients as described in the DOSAGE AND ADMINISTRATION section are suggested.
Therapeutic concentrations of ceftazidime are achieved in the following body tissues and fluid.
[See table 2 at top of next page]

Microbiology

Ceftazidime is bactericidal in action, exerting its effect by inhibition of enzymes responsible for cell-wall synthesis. A wide range of gram-negative organisms is susceptible to ceftazidime *in vitro*, including strains resistant to gentamicin and other aminoglycosides. In addition, ceftazidime has been shown to be active against gram-positive organisms. It is highly stable to most clinically important beta-lactamases, plasmid or chromosomal, which are produced by both gram-negative and gram-positive organisms, and consequently is active against many strains resistant to ampicillin and other cephalosporins.
Ceftazidime has been shown to be active against the following organisms both *in vitro* and in clinical infections (see INDICATIONS AND USAGE).
Aerobes, Gram-Negative: *Citrobacter* species (including *Citrobacter freundii* and *Citrobacter diversus*): *Enterobacter* species (including *Enterobacter cloacae* and *Enterobacter aerogenes*). *Escherichia coli; Haemophilus influenzae,* including ampicillin-resistant strains; *Klebsiella* species (including *Klebsiella pneumoniae*); *Neisseria meningitidis; Proteus mirabilis; Proteus vulgaris; Pseudomonas* species (including *Pseudomonas aeruginosa*); and *Serratia* species.
Aerobes, Gram-Positive: *Staphylococcus aureus,* including penicillinase- and non-penicillinase-producing strains; *Streptococcus agalactiae* (group B streptococci); *Streptococcus pneumoniae;* and *Streptococcus progenes* (group A beta-hemolytic streptococci).
Anaerobes: *Bacteroides* species (NOTE: Many strains of *Bacteroides fragilis* are resistant).
Ceftazidime has also been shown to demonstrate *in vitro* activity against the following microorganisms, although the clinical significance of these data is unknown. *Acinetobacter* species; *Clostridium* species (not including *Clostridium difficile*); *Haemophilus parainfluenzae; Morganella morganii* (formerly *Proteus morganii*); *Neisseria gonorrhoeae; Peptococcus* species; *Peptostreptococcus* species *Providencia* species (including *Providencia rettgeri,* formerly *Proteus rettgeri*); *Salmonella* species; *Shigella* species; *Staphylococcus epidermidis;* and *Yersinia enterocolitica.*
Ceftazidime and the aminoglycosides have been shown to be synergistic *in vitro* against Enterobacteriaceae and *Pseudomonas aeruginosa.* Ceftazidime and carbenicillin have also been shown to be synergistic *in vitro* against *P. aeruginosa.*
Ceftazidime is not active *in vitro* against *Campylobacter* species; *Clostridium difficle; Listeria monocytogenes;* methicillin–resistant staphylococci; or *Streptococcus faecalis* and many other enterococci.

Susceptibility Tests

Diffusion Techniques

Quantitative methods that require measurement of zone diameters give the most precise estimate of antibiotic susceptibility. One such procedure[1–3] has been recommended for use with disks to test susceptibility to ceftazidime.
Reports from the laboratory giving results of the standard single-disk susceptibility test with a 30 mcg ceftazidime disk should be interpreted according to the following criteria:
Susceptible organisms produce zones of 18 mm or greater, indicating that the test organism is likely to respond to therapy.
Organisms that produce zones of 15 mm to 17 mm are expected to be susceptible if high dosage is used or if the infection is confined to tissues and fluids (e.g., urine) in which high antibiotic levels are attained.
Resistant organisms produce zones of 14 mm or less, indicating that other therapy should be selected.
Organisms should be tested with the ceftazidime disk, since ceftazidime has been shown by *in vitro* tests to be active against certain strains found resistant when other beta-lactam disks are used.
Standardized procedures require the use of laboratory control organisms. The 30 mcg ceftazidime disk should give zone diameters between 25 mm and 32 mm for *E. coli.* ATCC 25922. For *P. aeruginosa* ATCC 27853, the zone diameters should be between 22 mm and 29 mm. For *S. aureus* ATCC 25923, the zone diameters should be between 16 mm and 20 mm.

Dilution Techniques

In other susceptibility testing procedures, e.g., the ICS agar dilution or the equivalent, bacterial isolate may be considered susceptible if the MIC value for ceftazidime is not more than 16 mcg/mL. Organisms are considered resistant to

Continued on next page

*** Identi-Code® symbol. This product information was prepared in June 1998. Current information on these and other products of Eli Lilly and Company may be obtained by direct inquiry to Lilly Research Laboratories, Lilly Corporate Center, Indianapolis, Indiana 46285, (800) 545-5979.**

Tazidime—Cont.

ceftazidime if the MIC is equal to or greater than 64 mcg/mL. Organisms having an MIC value of less than 64 mcg/mL but greater than 16 mcg/mL are expected to be susceptible if high dosage is used or if the infection is confined to tissues and fluids (e.g., urine) in which high antibiotic levels are attained.

As with standard diffusion methods, dilution procedures require the use of laboratory control organisms. Standard ceftazidime powder should give MIC values in the range of 4 mcg/mL and 16 mcg/mL for *S. aureus* ATCC 25923. For *E. coli* ATCC 25922, the MIC range should be between 0.125 mcg/mL and 0.5 mcg/mL. For *P. aeruginosa* ATCC 27853, the MIC range should be between 0.5 mcg/mL and 2 mcg/mL.

INDICATIONS AND USAGE

Tazidime (ceftazidime for injection) is indicated for the treatment of patients with infections caused by susceptible strains of the designated organisms in the diseases listed below:

LOWER RESPIRATORY TRACT INFECTIONS, including pneumonia, caused by *P. aeruginosa* and other *Pseudomonas* species; *H. influenzae, including* ampicillin-resistant strains; *Klebsiella* species; *Enterobacter* species; *P. mirabilis; E. coli; Serratia* species; *Citrobacter* species; *S. pneumoniae;* and *S. aureus* (methicillin-susceptible strains).

SKIN AND SKIN STRUCTURE INFECTIONS, caused by *P. aeruginosa, Klebsiella* species; *E. coli; Proteus* species including *P. mirabilis* and indole-positive *Proteus, Enterobacter* species; *Serratia* species; *S. aureus* (methicillin-susceptible strains) and *S. progenes* (group A beta-hemolytic streptococci).

URINARY TRACT INFECTIONS, both complicated and uncomplicated, caused by *P. aeruginosa; Enterobacter* species; *Proteus* species, including *P. mirabilis* and indole-positive *Proteus; Klebsiella* species and *E. coli.*

BACTERIAL SEPTICEMIA caused by *P. aeruginosa, Klebsiella* species; *H. influenzae, E. coli, Serratia* species, *S. pneumoniae* and *S. aureus* (methicillin-susceptible strains).

BONE AND JOINT INFECTIONS, caused by *P. aeruginosa; Klebsiella* species; *Enterobacter* species; and *S. aureus* (methicillin-susceptible strains).

GYNECOLOGICAL INFECTIONS, including endometritis, pelvic cellulitis and other infections of the female genital tract caused by *E. coli.*

INTRA-ABDOMINAL INFECTIONS, including peritonitis caused by *E. coli, Klebsiella* species; *S. aureus* (methicillin-susceptible strains), and polymicrobial infections caused by aerobic and anaerobic organisms, and *Bacteroides* species (many strains of *B. fragilis* are resistant).

CENTRAL NERVOUS SYSTEM INFECTIONS, including meningitis caused by *H. influenzae* and *Neisseria meningitidis.* Ceftazidime has also been used successfully in a limited number of cases of meningitis due to *P. aeruginosa* and *S. pneumoniae.*

Specimens for bacterial cultures should be obtained prior to therapy in order to isolate and identify causative organisms and to determine their susceptibility to ceftazidime. Therapy may be instituted before results of susceptibility studies are known; however, once these results become available, the antibiotic treatment should be adjusted accordingly.

Tazidime (ceftazidime for injection) may be used alone in cases of confirmed or suspected sepsis. Ceftazidime has been used successfully in clinical trials as empiric therapy in cases where various concomitant therapies with other antibiotics have been used.

Tazidime may also be used concomitantly with other antibiotics, such as aminoglycosides, vancomycin and clindamycin, in severe and life-threatening infections and in the immunocompromised patient. When such concomitant treatment is appropriate, prescribing information in the labeling for the other antibiotics should be followed. The dose depends on the severity of the infection and the patient's condition.

CONTRAINDICATION

Tazidime is contraindicated in patients who have shown hypersensitivity to ceftazidime or the cephalosporin group of antibiotics.

WARNINGS

SERIOUS AND OCCASIONALLY FATAL HYPERSENSITIVITY (anaphylactic) REACTIONS HAVE BEEN REPORTED IN PATIENTS ON PENICILLIN THERAPY. THESE REACTIONS ARE MORE LIKELY TO OCCUR IN INDIVIDUALS WITH A HISTORY OF PENICILLIN HYPERSENSITIVITY AND/OR A HISTORY OF SENSITIVITY TO MULTIPLE ALLERGENS. THERE HAVE BEEN REPORTS OF INDIVIDUALS WITH A HISTORY OF PENICILLIN HYPERSENSITIVITY WHO HAVE EXPERIENCED SEVERE REACTIONS WHEN TREATED WITH CEPHALOSPORINS. BEFORE INITIATING THERAPY WITH *TAZIDIME*, CAREFUL INQUIRY SHOULD BE MADE CONCERNING PREVIOUS HYPERSENSITIVITY REACTIONS TO PENICILLINS, CEPHALOSPORINS OR OTHER ALLERGENS. IF AN ALLERGIC REACTION OCCURS, *TAZIDIME* SHOULD BE DISCONTINUED AND APPROPRIATE THERAPY SHOULD BE INSTITUTED, **SERIOUS ANAPHYLACTIC REACTIONS REQUIRE IMMEDIATE EMERGENCY TREATMENT WITH EPINEPHRINE, OXYGEN, INTRAVENOUS STEROIDS AND AIRWAY MANAGEMENT, INCLUDING INTUBATION, SHOULD ALSO BE ADMINISTERED AS INDICATED.**

Pseudomembranous colitis has been reported with nearly all antibacterial agents, including *Tazidime,* and may range in severity from mild to life-threatening. Therefore, it is important to consider this diagnosis in patients who present with diarrhea subsequent to the administration of antibacterial agents.

Treatment with antibacterial agents alters the normal flora of the colon and may permit overgrowth of clostridia. Studies indicate that a toxin produced by *Clostridium difficile* is a primary cause of "antibiotic-associated colitis."

After the diagnosis of pseudomembranous colitis has been established, therapeutic measures should be initiated. Mild cases of pseudomembranous colitis usually respond to drug discontinuation alone. In moderate to severe cases, consideration should be given to management with fluids and electrolytes, protein supplementation and treatment with an antibacterial drug clinically effective against *C. difficile* colitis.

Elevated levels of ceftazidime in patients with renal insufficiency can lead to seizures, encephalopathy, asterixis and neuromuscular excitability (see PRECAUTIONS).

Table 2. Ceftazidime Concentrations in Body Tissues and Fluids

Tissue or Fluid	Dose/ Route	No. Patients	Time of Sample Post-Dose	Average Tissue or Fluid Level (mcg/mL)
Urine	500 mg I.M.	6	0–2 hours	2,100
	2 grams I.V.	6	0–2 hours	12,000
Bile	2 grams I.V.	3	90 min.	36.4
Synovial fluid	2 grams I.V.	13	2 hours	25.6
Peritoneal fluid	2 grams I.V.	8	2 hours	48.6
Sputum	1 gram I.V.	8	1 hour	9
Cerebrospinal fluid	2 grams q8h I.V.	5	120 min.	9.8
(inflamed meninges)	2 grams q8h I.V.	6	180 min.	9.4
Aqueous humor	2 grams I.V.	13	1–3 hours	11
Blister fluid	1 gram I.V.	7	2–3 hours	19.7
Lymphatic fluid	1 gram I.V.	7	2–3 hours	23.4
Bone	2 grams I.V.	8	0.67 hour	31.1
Heart muscle	2 grams I.V.	35	30–280 min.	12.7
Skin	2 grams I.V.	22	30–180 min.	6.6
Skeletal muscle	2 grams I.V.	35	30–280 min.	9.4
Myometrium	2 grams I.V.	31	1–2 hours	18.7

PRECAUTIONS

General: Ceftazidime has not been shown to be nephrotoxic; however, because high and prolonged serum antibiotic concentrations can occur from usual doses in patients with transient or persistent reduction of urinary output because of renal insufficiency, the total daily dosage should be reduced when ceftazidime is administered to such patients (see DOSAGE AND ADMINISTRATION). Continued dosage should be determined by degree of renal impairment, severity of infection and susceptibility of the causative organisms.

As with other antibiotics, prolonged use of Tazidime (ceftazidime for injection) may result in overgrowth of nonsusceptible organisms. Repeated evaluation of the patient's condition is essential. If superinfection occurs during therapy, appropriate measures should be taken.

Cephalosporins may be associated with a fall in prothrombin activity. Those at risk include patients with renal or hepatic impairment, or poor nutritional state, as well as patients receiving a protracted course of antimicrobial therapy. Prothrombin time should be monitored in patients at risk and exogenous vitamin K administered as indicated.

Tazidime should be prescribed with caution in individuals with a history of gastrointestinal disease, particularly colitis.

Drug Interactions: Nephrotoxicity has been reported following concomitant administration of cephalosporins with aminoglycoside antibiotics or potent diuretics, such as furosemide. Renal function should be carefully monitored, especially if higher dosages of the aminoglycosides are to be administered or if therapy is prolonged because of the potential nephrotoxicity and ototoxicity of aminoglycoside antibiotics. Nephrotoxicity and ototoxicity were not noted when ceftazidime was given alone in clinical trials. Chloramphenicol in combination with cephalosporins, including ceftazidime, has been shown to be antagonistic *in vitro.* Due to the possibility of antagonism *in vivo,* this combination should be avoided.

Drug/Laboratory Test Interactions: The administration of ceftazidime may result in a false-positive reaction for glucose in the urine when using Clinitest® tablets. Benedict's solution or Fehling's solution. It is recommended that glucose tests based on enzymatic glucose oxidase reactions (such as Clinistix® or Tes-Tape® [Glucose Enzymatic Test Strip USP]) be used.

Carcinogenesis, Mutagenesis, Impairment of Fertility: Long-term studies in animals have not been performed to evaluate carcinogenic potential. However, a mouse micronucleus test and an Ames test were both negative for mutagenic effects.

Usage in Pregnancy: Teratogenic Effects: Pregnancy Category B. Reproduction studies have been performed in mice and rats at doses up to 40 times the human dose and have revealed no evidence of impaired fertility or harm to the fetus due to ceftazidime. There are, however, no adequate and well-controlled studies in pregnant women. Because animal reproduction studies are not always predictive of human response, this drug should be used during pregnancy only if clearly needed.

Nursing Mothers: Ceftazidime is excreted in human milk in low concentrations. Caution should be exercised when *Tazidime* is administered to a nursing woman.

Pediatric Use: See DOSAGE AND ADMINISTRATION.

ADVERSE REACTIONS

Ceftazidime is generally well tolerated. The incidence of adverse reactions associated with the administration of ceftazidime was low in clinical trials. The most common were local reactions following intravenous injection, and allergic and gastrointestinal reactions. Other adverse reactions were encountered infrequently. No disulfiram-like reactions were reported. The following adverse effects from premarketing clinical trials were considered to be either related to ceftazidime therapy or were of uncertain etiology.

Local Effects, reported in less than 2% of patients, were phlebitis and inflammation at the site of injection (1 in 69 patients).

Hypersensitivity Reactions, reported in 2% of patients, were pruritus, rash and fever. Immediate reactions, generally manifested by rash and/or pruritus, occurred in 1 in 285 patients.

Gastrointestinal Symptoms, reported in less than 2% of patients, were diarrhea (1 in 78), nausea (1 in 156), vomiting (1 in 500) and abdominal pain (1 in 416).

Symptoms of pseudomembranous colitis can appear during or after antibiotic treatment (See WARNINGS section).

Central Nervous System Reactions (fewer than 1%) include headache, dizziness and paresthesia. Seizures have been reported with several cephalosporins, including ceftazidime. In addition, encephalopathy, asterixis and neuromuscular excitability have been reported in renally impaired patients treated with unadjusted dosage regimens of ceftazidime (see PRECAUTIONS: General).

Less Frequent Adverse Events (less than 1%) were candidiasis and vaginitis: central nervous system events which included headache, dizziness and paresthesia.

Laboratory Test Changes noted during Tazidime (ceftazidime for injection) clinical trials were transient and included: eosinophilia (1 in 13), positive Coombs' test without hemolysis (1 in 23), thrombocytosis (1 in 45), and slight elevations in one or more of the hepatic enzymes, aspartate aminotransferase (AST, SGOT) (1 in 16), alanine aminotransferase (ALT, SGPT) (1 in 15), LDH (1 in 18). GGT (1 in 19) and alkaline phosphatase (1 in 23). As with some other cephalosporins, transient elevations of blood urea, blood urea nitrogen and/or serum creatinine were observed occasionally. Transient leukopenia, neutropenia, agranulocytosis, thrombocytopenia and lymphocytosis were seen very rarely.

In addition to the adverse reactions listed above that have been observed with ceftazidime, the following adverse reactions and altered laboratory tests have been reported for cephalosporin-class antibiotics:

Adverse Reactions: Urticaria, Stevens-Johnson syndrome, erythema multiforme, toxic epidermal necrolysis, colitis, renal dysfunction, toxic nephropathy, hepatic dysfunction including cholestasis, aplastic anemia, hemolytic anemia, hemorrhage.

Altered Laboratory Tests: Prolonged prothrombin time, false-positive test for urinary glucose, elevated bilirubin, pancytopenia.

OVERDOSAGE

Ceftazidime overdosage has occurred in patients with renal failure. Reactions have included seizure activity, encephalopathy, asterixis and neuromuscular excitability. Patients who receive an acute overdosage should be carefully observed and given supportive treatment. In the presence of renal insufficiency, hemodialysis or peritoneal dialysis may aid in the removal of ceftazidime from the body.

DOSAGE AND ADMINISTRATION

Dosage: The usual adult dosage is 1 gram administered intravenously or intramuscularly every eight or 12 hours. The dosage and route should be determined by the susceptibility of the causative organisms, the severity of infection and the condition and renal function of the patient.

The guidelines for dosage of *Tazidime* are listed in Table 3. The following dosage schedule is recommended.

[See table 3 above]

Impaired Hepatic Function: No adjustment in dosage is required for patients with hepatic dysfunction.

Impaired Renal Function: Ceftazidime is excreted by the kidneys almost exclusively by glomerular filtration. Therefore, in patients with impaired renal function (GFR <50 mL/min.), it is recommended that the dosage of ceftazidime be reduced to compensate for its slower excretion. In patients with suspected renal insufficiency, an initial loading dose of 1 gram of ceftazidime may be given. An estimate of GFR should be made to determine the appropriate maintenance dose. The recommended dosage is presented in Table 4.

Table 4. Recommended Maintenance Doses of Tazidime (ceftazidime for injection) in Renal Insufficiency

NOTE: IF THE DOSE RECOMMENDED IN TABLE 3 ABOVE IS LOWER THAN THAT RECOMMENDED FOR PATIENTS WITH RENAL INSUFFICIENCY AS OUTLINED IN TABLE 4, THE LOWER DOSE SHOULD BE USED.

Creatinine Clearance (mL/min.)	Recommended Unit Dose of Ceftazidime	Frequency of Dosing
50–31	1 gram	q12h
30–16	1 gram	q24h
15–6	500 mg	q24h
<5	500 mg	q48h

When only serum creatinine is available, the following formula (Cockroft's equation)[4] may be used to estimate creatinine clearance. The serum creatinine should represent a steady state of renal function:

$$\text{Males: Creatinine clearance (mL/min.)} = \frac{\text{Weight (kg)} \times (140 - \text{age})}{72 \times \text{serum creatinine (mg/dL)}}$$

Females: $0.85 \times$ above value

In patients with severe infections who would normally receive 6 grams of ceftazidime daily were it not for renal insufficiency, the unit dose given in the table above may be increased by 50% or the dosing frequency increased appropriately. Further dosing should be determined by therapeutic monitoring, severity of the infection and susceptibility of the causative organism.

In children as for adults, the creatinine clearance should be adjusted for body surface area or lean body mass and the dosing frequency reduced in cases of renal insufficiency.

In patients undergoing hemodialysis, a loading dose of 1 gram is recommended, followed by 1 gram after each hemodialysis period.

Tazidime (ceftazidime for injection) can also be used in patients undergoing intra-peritoneal dialysis (IPD) and continuous ambulatory peritoneal dialysis (CAPD). In such patients, a loading dose of *Tazidime* 1 gram may be given, followed by 500 mg every 24 hours. In addition to intravenous use, *Tazidime* can be incorporated in the dialysis fluid at a concentration of 250 mg for 2 liters of dialysis fluid.

NOTE: Generally, *Tazidime* should be continued for two days after the signs and symptoms of infection have disappeared, but in complicated infections longer therapy may be required.

Administration: *Tazidime* may be given intravenously or by deep intramuscular injection into a large muscle mass such as the upper outer quadrant of the gluteus maximus or lateral part of the thigh.

NOTE: Ceftazidime for injection in ADD-Vantage® vials is not intended for direct intravenous or intramuscular injection.

Table 3. Recommended Dosage Schedule

	Dose	Frequency
Adults		
Usual recommended dose	1 gram I.V. or I.M.	q8–12h
Uncomplicated urinary tract infections	250 mg I.V. or I.M.	q12h
Bone and joint infections	2 grams I.V.	q12
Complicated urinary tract infections	500 mg I.V. or I.M.	q8–12h
Uncomplicated pneumonia; mild skin and skin structure infections	500 mg-1 gram I.V. or I.M.	q8h
Serious gynecological and intra-abdominal infections	2 grams I.V.	q8h
Meningitis	2 grams I.V.	q8h
Very severe life-threatening infections especially in immuno-compromised patients	2 grams I.V.	q8h
Lung infections caused by *Pseudomonas* species in patients with cystic fibrosis with normal renal function*	30–50 mg/kg I.V. to a maximum of 6 grams/day	q8h
Neonates (0–4 weeks)	30 mg/kg I.V.	q12h
Infants and children (1 month–12 years)	30–50 mg/kg I.V. to a maximum of 6 grams/day†	q8h

*Although clinical improvement has been shown, bacteriological cures cannot be expected in patients with chronic respiratory disease and cystic fibrosis.

†The higher dose should be reserved for immunocompromised children or children with cystic fibrosis or meningitis.

Intramuscular Administration: For intramuscular administration. *Tazidime* should be reconstituted with Sterile Water for Injection Refer to Table 5.

Intravenous Administration: The I.V. route is preferable for patients with bacterial septicemia, bacterial meningitis, peritonitis, or other severe or life-threatening infections, or for patients who may be poor risks because of lowered resistance resulting from such debilitating conditions as malnutrition, trauma, surgery, diabetes, heart failure or malignancy, particularly if shock is present or pending.

For direct intermittent intravenous administration, reconstitute *Tazidime* as directed in Table 5 with Sterile Water for Injection. Slowly inject directly into the vein over a period of three to five minutes or give through the tubing of an administration set while the patient is also receiving one of the compatible intravenous fluids (See COMPATIBILITY AND STABILITY).

For intravenous infusion, reconstitute the 1 or 2 gram piggyback vial with 100 mL of Sodium Chloride Injection or one of the compatible intravenous fluids listed in the COMPATIBILITY AND STABILITY section. Alternatively, reconstitute the 1 gram or 2 gram vial and add an appropriate quantity of the resulting solution to an I.V. container with one of the compatible intravenous fluids.

Intermittent intravenous infusion with a Y-type administration set can be accomplished with compatible solutions. However, during infusion of a solution containing *Tazidime* it is advisable to discontinue the other solution.

All vials of *Tazidime* as supplied are under reduced pressure. When *Tazidime* is dissolved, carbon dioxide is released and a positive pressure develops. See RECONSTITUTION.

Solutions of *Tazidime*, like those of most beta-lactam antibiotics should not be added to solutions of aminoglycoside antibiotics because of potential interaction.

However, if concurrent therapy with *Tazidime* and an aminoglycoside is indicated, each of these antibiotics can be administered separately to the same patient.

TAZIDIME INJECTION IN ADD-VANTAGE® VIALS

NOTE: Tazidime (ceftazidime for injection) in the ADD-Vantage® vial is intended to be administered as a single-dose intravenous infusion with the ADD-Vantage® flexible diluent container.

Tazidime in single-dose ADD-Vantage® vials should be prepared as directed (see RECONSTITUTION, for ADD-Vantage® Vials) with either 0.9% Sodium Chloride Injection in the 50 mL or 100 mL flexible diluent containers, 0.45% Sodium Chloride Injection in the 50 mL container or 5% Dextrose Injection in the 50 mL or 100 mL containers.

RECONSTITUTION

Single Dose Vials:

For I.M. Injection, I.V. direct (bolus) injection, or I.V. infusion, reconstitute with Sterile Water for Injection according to the following table. The vacuum may assist entry of the diluent. SHAKE WELL.

Table 5

Vial Size	Diluent to Be Added	Approx. Avail. Volume	Approx. Avg. Concentration
Intramuscular or Intravenous Direct (bolus) Injection			
1 gram	3.0 mL	3.6 mL	280 mg/mL
Intravenous Infusion			
1 gram	10 mL	10.6 mL	95 mg/mL
2 gram	10 mL	11.2 mL	180 mg/mL

Withdraw the total volume of solution into the syringe (the pressure in the vial may aid withdrawal). The withdrawn solution may contain some bubbles of carbon dioxide.

NOTE: As with the administration of all parenteral products, accumulated gases should be expressed from the syringe immediately before injection of *Tazidime*.

These solutions of *Tazidime* are stable for 24 hours at room temperature or seven days if refrigerated (5°C). Slight yellowing does not affect potency.

For I.V. infusion, dilute reconstituted solution in 50 to 100 mL of one of the parenteral fluids listed under COMPATIBILITY AND STABILITY.

Pharmacy Bulk Vials:

Reconstitute with Sterile Water for Injection according to the following table.

Continued on next page

* Identi-Code® symbol. This product information was prepared in June 1998. Current information on these and other products of Eli Lilly and Company may be obtained by direct inquiry to Lilly Research Laboratories, Lilly Corporate Center, Indianapolis, Indiana 46285, (800) 545-5979.

Tazidime—Cont.

Table 6

Diluent to Be Added	Approx. Avail. Volume	Approx. Avg. Concentration
26 mL	30 mL	1 gram/5 mL
56 mL	60 mL	1 gram/10 mL

The vacuum may assist entry of the diluent. SHAKE WELL.

Insert a gas relief needle through the vial closure to relieve the internal pressure. Remove the gas relief needle before extracting any solution.

NOTE: **To preserve product sterility, it is important that a gas relief needle is not inserted through the vial closure before the product has dissolved.**

These solutions of *Tazidime* are stable for 24 hours at room temperature or seven days if refrigerated (5°C). Slight yellowing does not affect potency. For I.V. infusion add to one of the parenteral fluids listed under COMPATIBILITY AND STABILITY.

"Piggyback" Vials:

For I.V. infusion, reconstitute with 10 mL of Sodium Chloride Injection according to the following table. The vacuum may assist entry of the diluent. SHAKE WELL.

Table 7

Vial Size	Diluent to Be Added	Approx. Avail. Volume	Approx. Avg. Concentration
1 gram	100 mL*	100 mL	10 mg/mL
2 gram	100 mL*	100 mL	20 mg/mL

*Addition should be in two stages.

Insert a gas relief needle through the vial closure to relieve the internal pressure. With the gas relief needle in position, add the remaining 90 mL of Sodium Chloride Injection. Remove the gas relief needle and syringe needle; shake the vial and set up for infusion in the normal way.

NOTE: **To preserve product sterility, it is important that a gas relief needle is not inserted through the vial closure before the product has dissolved.**

These solutions of *Tazidime* (ceftazidime for injection) are stable for 24 hours at room temperature or seven days if refrigerated (5°C). Slight yellowing does not affect potency.

ADD-Vantage® Vials: ADD-Vantage® vials of *Tazidime* are to be reconstituted only with 0.9% Sodium Chloride Injection or 5% Dextrose Injection in the 50 mL or 100 mL flexible diluent containers, or with 0.45% Sodium Chloride Injection in the 50 mL container.

DIRECTIONS FOR USE OF TAZIDIME (ceftazidime for injection, USP) IN ADD-VANTAGE® VIALS

To Open Diluent Container:

Peel overwrap at corner and remove solution container. Some opacity of the plastic due to moisture absorption during the sterilization process may be observed. This is normal and does not affect the solution quality or safety. The opacity will diminish gradually.

To Assemble Vial and Flexible Diluent Container:
(Use Aseptic Technique)

1. Remove the protective covers from the top of the vial and the vial port on the diluent container as follows:

   a. To remove the breakaway vial cap, swing the pull ring over the top of the vial and pull down far enough to start the opening (SEE FIGURE 1), then pull straight up to remove the cap. (SEE FIGURE 2.)
   NOTE: Do no access vial with syringe.

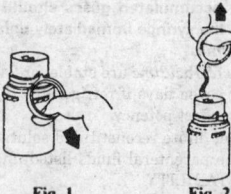

Fig. 1   **Fig. 2**

   b. To remove the vial port cover, grasp the tab on the pull ring, pull up to break the 3 tie strings, then pull back to remove the cover. (SEE FIGURE 3.)
2. Screw the vial into the vial port until it will go no further. THE VIAL MUST BE SCREWED IN TIGHTLY TO ASSURE A SEAL. This occurs approximately 1/2 turn (180°) after the first audible click. (SEE FIGURE 4.) The clicking sound does not assure a seal; the vial must be turned as far as it will go.
   NOTE: Once vial is sealed, do not attempt to remove. (SEE FIGURE 4.)

3. Recheck the vial to assure that it is tight by trying to turn it further in the direction of assembly.
4. Label appropriately.

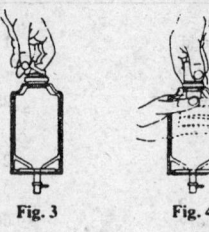

Fig. 3   **Fig. 4**

To Reconstitute the Drug:

1. Squeeze the bottom of the diluent container gently to inflate the portion of the container surrounding the end of the drug vial.
2. With the other hand, push the drug vial down into the container telescoping the walls of the container. Grasp the inner cap of the vial through the walls of the container. (SEE FIGURE 5.)
3. Pull the inner cap from the drug vial. (SEE FIGURE 6.) Verify that the rubber stopper has been pulled out, allowing the drug and diluent to mix.
4. Mix container contents thoroughly and use within the specified time.

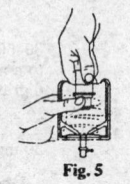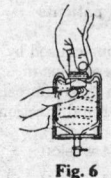

Fig. 5   **Fig. 6**

Preparation for Administration:
(Use Aseptic Technique)

1. Confirm the activation and admixture of vial contents.
2. Check for leaks by squeezing container firmly. If leaks are found discard unit as sterility may be impaired.
3. Close flow control clamp of administration set.
4. Remove cover from outlet port at bottom of container.
5. Insert piercing pin of administration set into port with a twisting motion until the pin is firmly seated. **NOTE:** See full directions on administration set carton.
6. Lift the free end of the hanger loop on the bottom of the vial, breaking the 2 tie strings. Bend the loop outward to lock it in the upright position, then suspend container from hanger.
7. Squeeze and release drip chamber to establish proper fluid level in chamber.
8. Open flow control clamp and clear air from set. Close clamp.
9. Attach set to venipuncture device. If device is not indwelling, prime and make venipuncture.
10. Regulate rate of administration with flow control clamp.

WARNING: Do not use flexible container in series connections.

COMPATIBILITY AND STABILITY

Intramuscular: *Tazidime*, when reconstituted as directed with Sterile Water for Injection, maintains satisfactory potency for 24 hours at room temperature or for seven days under refrigeration (5°C). Solutions in Sterile Water for Injection that are frozen immediately after reconstitution in the original container are stable for three months when stored at –20°C. Once thawed, solutions should not be refrozen. Thawed solutions may be stored for up to eight hours at room temperature or for four days in a refrigerator (5°C).

Intravenous: Tazidime (ceftazidime for injection) when reconstituted as directed with Sterile Water for Injection, maintains satisfactory potency for 24 hours at room temperature or for seven days under refrigeration (5°C). Solutions in Sterile Water for Injection in the original container or in 0.9% Sodium Chloride Injection in small volume containers that are frozen immediately after reconstitution are stable for three months when stored at –20°C. For larger volumes where it may be necessary to warm the frozen product (to a maximum of 40°C), care should be taken to avoid heating after thawing is complete. Once thawed, solutions should not be refrozen. Thawed solutions may be stored for up to eight hours at room temperature or for four days in a refrigerator (5°C).

Tazidime is compatible with the more commonly used intravenous infusion fluids. Solutions at concentrations between 1 mg/mL and 40 mg/mL in the following infusion fluids may be stored for up to 24 hours at room temperature or for seven days if refrigerated: 0.9% Sodium Chloride Injection; Ringer's Injection USP; Lactated Ringer's Injection USP; 5% Dextrose Injection; 5% Dextrose and 0.225% Sodium Chloride Injection; 5% Dextrose and 0.45% Sodium Chloride Injection; 5% Dextrose and 0.9% Sodium Chloride Injection; 10% Dextrose Injection.

Tazidime is less stable in Sodium Bicarbonate Injection than in other intravenous fluids. It is not recommended as a diluent Solutions of *Tazidime* in 5% Dextrose and 0.9% Sodium Chloride Injection are stable for at least six hours at room temperature in plastic tubing, drip chambers and volume control devices of common intravenous infusion sets. Ceftazidime at a concentration of 20 mg/mL has been found physically compatible for 24 hours at room temperature or seven days under refrigeration in Sterile Water for Injection when admixed with: cefazolin sodium 330 mg/mL; heparin 1000 units/mL; and cimetidine HCl 150 mg/mL.

Ceftazidime at a concentration of 20 mg/mL has been found physically compatible for 24 hours at room temperature or seven days under refrigeration in 5% Dextrose Injection when admixed with potassium chloride 40 mEq/l.

Vancomycin solution exhibits a physical incompatibility when mixed with a number of drugs, including ceftazidime. The likelihood of precipitation with ceftazidime is dependent on the concentrations of vancomycin and ceftazidime present. It is therefore recommended, when both drugs are to be administered by intermittent IV infusion, that they be given separately, flushing the IV lines (with one of the compatible IV fluids) between the administration of these two agents.

ADD-Vantage®* Vials: Ordinarily. ADD-Vantage® vials should be reconstituted only when it is certain that the patient is ready to receive the drug. However, *Tazidime* in ADD-Vantage® vials is stable for 24 hours at room temperature when reconstituted as directed (see RECONSTITUTION, ADD-Vantage® Vials and DIRECTIONS FOR USE OF TAZIDIME® INJECTION IN ADD-VANTAGE® VIALS).

Note: Parenteral drug products should be inspected visually for particulate matter prior to administration wherever solution and container permit.

As with other cephalosporins, *Tazidime* powder, as well as solutions, tend to darken depending on storage conditions; within the stated recommendations, however, product potency is not adversely affected.

HOW SUPPLIED

Before reconstitution protect from light and store between 15°–30°C (59°–86°F).

Tazidime (ceftazidime for injection, USP) is supplied in vials equivalent to 1 gram and 2 grams of ceftazidime: in "Piggyback" Vials for I.V. admixture equivalent to 1 gram and 2 grams of ceftazidime; and in ADD-Vantage®* Vials containing ceftazidime pentahydrate equivalent to 1 gram and 2 grams of ceftazidime.

1g† (No. 7290)—(Traypak of 25) NDC 0002-7290-25
2g† (No. 7291)—(Traypak of 10) NDC 0002-7291-10
The above ADD-Vantage® Vials are to be used only with Abbott Laboratories' ADD-Vantage® Diluent Containers.
Vials (Dry Powder):
500 mg,† 10-mL size (No. 7230)—(Traypak‡ of 25)
NDC 0002-7230-25
1g,† 20-mL size (No. 7231)—(Traypak of 25)
NDC 0002-7231-25
1g,† 100-mL size (No. 7238)—(Traypak of 10)
NDC 0002-7238-10
2g,† 60-mL size (No. 7234)—(Traypak of 10)
NDC 0002-7234-10
2g,† 100-mL size (No. 7239)—(Traypak of 10)
NDC 0002-7239-10
Also available:
Faspak§:
1 g† (No. 7245)—(Faspak of 24) NDC 0002-7245-24
2 g† (No. 7246)—(Faspak of 24) NDC 0002-7246-24
Pharmacy Bulk Package:
6g,† 100-mL size (No. 7241)—(Traypak of 6)
NDC 0002-7241-16

*ADD-Vantage® (vials and diluent containers. Abbott).
†Equivalent to ceftazidime activity.
‡Traypak™ (multivial carton, Lilly).
§Faspak® (flexible plastic bag, Lilly).

REFERENCES

1. Bauer, A.W.; Kirby, W.M.M., and Sherris, J.C., et al.: Antibiotic susceptibility testing by a standardized single disc method, Am. J. Clin. Pathol. 45:493, 1966. 2. National Committee for Clinical Laboratory Standards, Approved Standard: Performance Standards for Antimicrobial Disc Susceptibility Tests (M2–A3), December, 1984. 3. Standardized disc susceptibility test. Federal Register 39:19182–19184, 1974. 4. Cockcroft, D.W., and Gault, M.H.: Prediction of creatinine clearance from serum creatinine, Nephron 16:31–41, 1976.

DATE OF ISSUANCE AUG. 1995

Manufactured for
ELI LILLY AND COMPANY
Indianapolis, IN 46285, USA
by
BMH Limited
Philadelphia, PA 19101

TD:L4

TOBRAMYCIN SULFATE ℞
See Nebcin® (Tobramycin Sulfate Injection, USP).

VANCOCIN® HCl ℞
[*văn ′kō-sĭn ăch ′sē-ĕl*]
(Sterile Vancomycin Hydrochloride, USP)
IntraVenous

VIALS

DESCRIPTION

Vancocin® HCl (Sterile Vancomycin Hydrochloride, USP), IntraVenous, is a chromatographically purified, tricyclic glycopeptide antibiotic derived from *Amycolatopsis orientalis* (formerly *Nocardia orientalis*) and has the chemical formula $C_{66}H_{75}Cl_2H_9O_{24}$ • HCl. The molecular weight is 1,485.73; 500 mg of the base is equivalent to 0.34 mmol.
Vancomycin hydrochloride has the following structural formula:

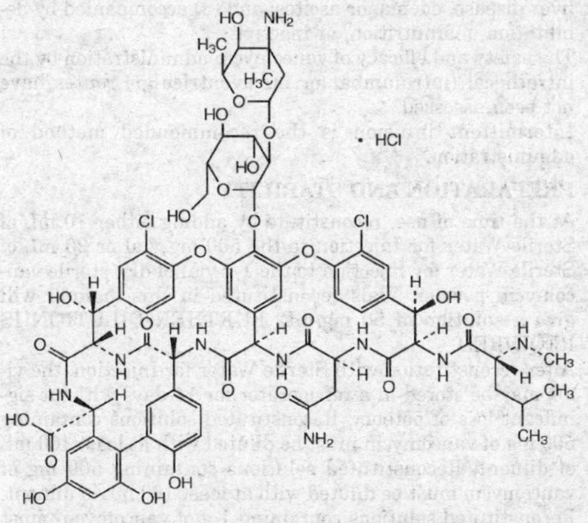

The vials contain sterile vancomycin hydrochloride equivalent to either 500 mg or 1 g vancomycin activity. Vancomycin hydrochloride is an off-white lyophilized plug. When reconstituted in water, it forms a clear solution with a pH range of 2.5 to 4.5. This product is oxygen sensitive.

CLINICAL PHARMACOLOGY

Vancomycin is poorly absorbed after oral administration; it is given intravenously for therapy of systemic infections. Intramuscular injection is painful.
In subjects with normal kidney function, multiple intravenous dosing of 1 g of vancomycin (15 mg/kg) infused over 60 minutes produces mean plasma concentrations of approximately 63 µg/mL immediately after the completion of infusion, mean plasma concentrations of approximately 23 µg/mL 2 hours after infusion, and mean plasma concentrations of approximately 8 µg/mL 11 hours after the end of the infusion. Multiple dosing of 500 mg infused over 30 minutes produces mean plasma concentrations of about 49 µg/mL at the completion of infusion, mean plasma concentrations of about 19 µg/mL 2 hours after infusion, and mean plasma concentrations of about 10 µg/mL 6 hours after infusion. The plasma concentrations during multiple dosing are similar to those after a single dose.
The mean elimination half-life of vancomycin from plasma is 4 to 6 hours in subjects with normal renal function. In the first 24 hours, about 75% of an administered dose of vancomycin is excreted in urine by glomerular filtration. Mean plasma clearance is about 0.058 L/kg/h, and mean renal clearance is about 0.048 L/kg/h. Renal dysfunction slows excretion of vancomycin. In anephric patients, the average half-life of elimination is 7.5 days. The distribution coefficient is from 0.3 to 0.43 L/kg. There is no apparent metabolism of the drug. About 60% of an intraperitoneal dose of vancomycin administered during peritoneal dialysis is absorbed systemically in 6 hours. Serum concentrations of about 10 µg/mL are achieved by intraperitoneal injection of 30 mg/kg of vancomycin. Although vancomycin is not effectively removed by either hemodialysis or peritoneal dialysis, there have been reports of increased vancomycin clearance with hemoperfusion and hemofiltration.
Total systemic and renal clearance of vancomycin may be reduced in the elderly.
Vancomycin is approximately 55% serum protein bound as measured by ultrafiltration at vancomycin serum concentrations of 10 to 100 µg/mL. After IV administration of Vancocin HCl, inhibitory concentrations are present in pleural, pericardial, ascitic, and synovial fluids; in urine; in peritoneal dialysis fluid; and in atrial appendage tissue. Vancocin HCl does not readily diffuse across normal meninges into the spinal fluid; but, when the meninges are inflamed, penetration into the spinal fluid occurs.
Microbiology —The bactericidal action of vancomycin results primarily from inhibition of cell-wall biosynthesis. In addition, vancomycin alters bacterial-cell-membrane permeability and RNA synthesis. There is no cross-resistance between vancomycin and other antibiotics. Vancomycin is active against staphylococci, including *Staphylococcus aureus* and *Staphylococcus epidermidis* (including heterogeneous methicillin-resistant strains); streptococci, including *Streptococcus pyogenes, Streptococcus pneumoniae* (including penicillin-resistant strains), *Streptococcus agalactiae,* the viridans group, *Streptococcus bovis,* and enterococci (eg, *Enterococcus faecalis* [formerly *Streptococcus faecalis*]); *Clostridium difficile* (eg, toxigenic strains implicated in pseudomembranous enterocolitis); and diphtheroids. Other organisms that are susceptible to vancomycin in vitro include *Listeria monocytogenes, Lactobacillus* species, *Actinomyces* species, *Clostridium* species, and *Bacillus* species.
Vancomycin is not active in vitro against gram-negative bacilli, mycobacteria, or fungi.
Synergy —The combination of vancomycin and an aminoglycoside acts synergistically in vitro against many strains of *S. aureus,* nonenterococcal group D streptococci, enterococci, and *Streptococcus* species (viridans group).
Disk Susceptibility Tests —The standardized disk method described by the National Committee for Clinical Laboratory Standards has been recommended to test susceptibility to vancomycin. Results of standard susceptibility tests with a 30-µg vancomycin hydrochloride disk should be interpreted according to the following criteria: Susceptible organisms produce zones greater than or equal to 12 mm, indicating that the test organism is likely to respond to therapy. Organisms that produce zones of 10 or 11 mm are considered to be of intermediate susceptibility. Organisms in this category are likely to respond if the infection is confined to tissues or fluids in which high antibiotic concentrations are attained. Resistant organisms produce zones of 9 mm or less, indicating that other therapy should be selected.
Using a standardized dilution method, a bacterial isolate may be considered susceptible if the MIC value for vancomycin is 4 µg/mL or less. Organisms are considered resistant to vancomycin if the MIC is greater than or equal to 16 µg/mL. Organisms having an MIC value of less than 16 µg/mL but greater than 4 µg/mL are considered to be of intermediate susceptibility.[1-2]
Standardized procedures require the use of laboratory control organisms. The 30-µg vancomycin disk should give zone diameters between 15 and 19 mm for *S. aureus* ATCC 25923. As with the standard diffusion methods, dilution procedures require the use of laboratory control organisms. Standard vancomycin powder should give MIC values in the range of 0.5 µg/mL to 2.0 µg/mL for *S. aureus* ATCC 29213. For *E. faecalis* ATCC 29212, the MIC range should be 1.0 to 4.0 µg/mL.

INDICATIONS AND USAGE

Vancocin HCl is indicated for the treatment of serious or severe infections caused by susceptible strains of methicillin-resistant (beta-lactam-resistant) staphylococci. It is indicated for penicillin-allergic patients, for patients who cannot receive or who have failed to respond to other drugs, including the penicillins or cephalosporins, and for infections caused by vancomycin-susceptible organisms that are resistant to other antimicrobial drugs. Vancocin HCl is indicated for initial therapy when methicillin-resistant staphylococci are suspected, but after susceptibility data are available, therapy should be adjusted accordingly.
Vancocin HCl is effective in the treatment of staphylococcal endocarditis. Its effectiveness has been documented in other infections due to staphylococci, including septicemia, bone infections, lower respiratory tract infections, and skin and skin structure infections. When staphylococcal infections are localized and purulent, antibiotics are used as adjuncts to appropriate surgical measures.
Vancocin HCl has been reported to be effective alone or in combination with an aminoglycoside for endocarditis caused by *Streptococcus viridans* or *S. bovis.* For endocarditis caused by enterococci (eg, *E. faecalis*), Vancocin HCl has been reported to be effective only in combination with an aminoglycoside.
Vancocin HCl has been reported to be effective for the treatment of diphtheroid endocarditis. Vancocin HCl has been used successfully in combination with either rifampin, an aminoglycoside, or both in early-onset prosthetic valve endocarditis caused by *S. epidermidis* or diphtheroids.
Specimens for bacteriologic cultures should be obtained in order to isolate and identify causative organisms and to determine their susceptibilities to Vancocin HCl.
The parenteral form of Vancocin HCl may be administered orally for treatment of antibiotic-associated pseudomembranous colitis caused by *C. difficile* and for staphylococcal enterocolitis. Parenteral administration of Vancocin HCl alone is of unproven benefit for these indications. **Vancocin HCl is not effective by the oral route for other types of infection.**
Although no controlled clinical efficacy studies have been conducted, intravenous vancomycin has been suggested by the American Heart Association and the American Dental Association as prophylaxis against bacterial endocarditis in penicillin-allergic patients who have congenital heart disease or rheumatic or other acquired valvular heart disease when these patients undergo dental procedures or surgical procedures of the upper respiratory tract.
Note: When selecting antibiotics for the prevention of bacterial endocarditis, the physician or dentist should read the full joint statement of the American Heart Association and the American Dental Association.[3]

CONTRAINDICATION

Vancocin HCl is contraindicated in patients with known hypersensitivity to this antibiotic.

WARNINGS

Rapid bolus administration (eg, over several minutes) may be associated with exaggerated hypotension, and, rarely, cardiac arrest.
Vancocin HCl should be administered in a dilute solution over a period of not less than 60 minutes to avoid rapid-infusion-related reactions. Stopping the infusion usually results in prompt cessation of these reactions.
Ototoxicity has occurred in patients receiving Vancocin HCl. It may be transient or permanent. It has been reported mostly in patients who have been given excessive doses, who have an underlying hearing loss, or who are receiving concomitant therapy with another ototoxic agent, such as an aminoglycoside. Vancomycin should be used with caution in patients with renal insufficiency because the risk of toxicity is appreciably increased by high, prolonged blood concentrations.
Dosage of Vancocin HCl must be adjusted for patients with renal dysfunction (*see* PRECAUTIONS *and* DOSAGE AND ADMINISTRATION).
Pseudomembranous colitis has been reported with nearly all antibacterial agents, including vancomycin, and may range in severity from mild to life-threatening. Therefore, it is important to consider this diagnosis in patients who present with diarrhea subsequent to the administration of antibacterial agents.
Treatment with antibacterial agents alters the normal flora of the colon and may permit overgrowth of clostridia. Studies indicate that a toxin produced by *Clostridium difficile* is a primary cause of "antibiotic-associated colitis." After the diagnosis of pseudomembranous colitis has been established, therapeutic measures should be initiated. Mild cases of pseudomembranous colitis usually respond to drug discontinuation alone. In moderate to severe cases, consideration should be given to management with fluids and electrolytes, protein supplementation, and treatment with an antibacterial drug clinically effective against *C. difficile* colitis.

PRECAUTIONS

General —Clinically significant serum concentrations have been reported in some patients who have taken multiple oral doses of vancomycin for active *C. difficile*-induced pseudomembranous colitis.
Prolonged use of Vancocin HCl may result in the overgrowth of nonsusceptible organisms. Careful observation of the patient is essential. If superinfection occurs during therapy, appropriate measures should be taken.
In order to minimize the risk of nephrotoxicity when treating patients with underlying renal dysfunction or patients receiving concomitant therapy with an aminoglycoside, serial monitoring of renal function should be performed and particular care should be taken in following appropriate dosing schedules (*see* DOSAGE AND ADMINISTRATION).
Serial tests of auditory function may be helpful in order to minimize the risk of ototoxicity.
Reversible neutropenia has been reported in patients receiving Vancocin HCl (*see* ADVERSE REACTIONS). Patients who will undergo prolonged therapy with Vancocin HCl or those who are receiving concomitant drugs that may cause neutropenia should have periodic monitoring of the leukocyte count.
Vancocin HCl is irritating to tissue and must be given by a secure intravenous route of administration. Pain, tenderness, and necrosis occur with intramuscular injection of Vancocin HCl or with inadvertent extravasation. Thrombophlebitis may occur, the frequency and severity of which can be minimized by administering the drug slowly as a dilute solution (2.5 to 5 g/L) and by rotating the sites of infusion.
There have been reports that the frequency of infusion-related events (including hypotension, flushing, erythema, urticaria, and pruritus) increases with the concomitant administration of anesthetic agents. Infusion-related events may be minimized by the administration of Vancocin HCl as a 60-minute infusion prior to anesthetic induction.

Continued on next page

*** Identi-Code® symbol. This product information was prepared in June 1998. Current information on these and other products of Eli Lilly and Company may be obtained by direct inquiry to Lilly Research Laboratories, Lilly Corporate Center, Indianapolis, Indiana 46285, (800) 545-5979.**

Vancocin HCl Intravenous—Cont.

The safety and efficacy of vancomycin administration by the intrathecal (intralumbar or intraventricular) routes have not been assessed.

Reports have revealed that administration of sterile vancomycin HCl by the intraperitoneal route during continuous ambulatory peritoneal dialysis (CAPD) has resulted in a syndrome of chemical peritonitis. To date, this syndrome has ranged from a cloudy dialysate alone to a cloudy dialysate accompanied by variable degrees of abdominal pain and fever. This syndrome appears to be short-lived after discontinuation of intraperitoneal vancomycin.

Drug Interactions—Concomitant administration of vancomycin and anesthetic agents has been associated with erythema and histamine-like flushing (*see* USAGE IN PEDIATRICS *under* PRECAUTIONS) and anaphylactoid reactions (*see* ADVERSE REACTIONS).

Concurrent and/or sequential systemic or topical use of other potentially neurotoxic and/or nephrotoxic drugs, such as amphotericin B, aminoglycosides, bacitracin, polymyxin B, colistin, viomycin, or cisplatin, when indicated, requires careful monitoring.

Usage in Pregnancy—*Pregnancy Category C*—Animal reproduction studies have not been conducted with Vancocin HCl. It is not known whether Vancocin HCl can affect reproduction capacity. In a controlled clinical study, the potential ototoxic and nephrotoxic effects of Vancocin HCl on infants were evaluated when the drug was administered to pregnant women for serious staphylococcal infections complicating intravenous drug abuse. Vancocin HCl was found in cord blood. No sensorineural hearing loss or nephrotoxicity attributable to Vancocin HCl was noted. One infant whose mother received Vancocin HCl in the third trimester experienced conductive hearing loss that was not attributed to the administration of Vancocin HCl. Because the number of patients treated in this study was limited and Vancocin HCl was administered only in the second and third trimesters, it is not known whether Vancocin HCl causes fetal harm. Vancocin HCl should be given to a pregnant woman only if clearly needed.

Nursing Mothers—Vancocin HCl is excreted in human milk. Caution should be exercised when Vancocin HCl is administered to a nursing woman. Because of the potential for adverse events, a decision should be made whether to discontinue nursing or to discontinue the drug, taking into account the importance of the drug to the mother.

Usage in Pediatrics—In premature neonates and young infants, it may be appropriate to confirm desired vancomycin serum concentrations. Concomitant administration of vancomycin and anesthetic agents has been associated with erythema and histamine-like flushing in children (*see* ADVERSE REACTIONS).

Geriatrics—The natural decrement of glomerular filtration with increasing age may lead to elevated vancomycin serum concentrations if dosage is not adjusted. Vancomycin dosage schedules should be adjusted in elderly patients (*see* DOSAGE AND ADMINISTRATION).

ADVERSE REACTIONS

Infusion-Related Events—During or soon after rapid infusion of Vancocin HCl, patients may develop anaphylactoid reactions, including hypotension (*see* ANIMAL PHARMACOLOGY), wheezing, dyspnea, urticaria, or pruritus. Rapid infusion may also cause flushing of the upper body ("Red Man Syndrome") or pain and muscle spasm of the chest and back. These reactions usually resolve within 20 minutes but may persist for several hours. Such events are infrequent if Vancocin HCl is given by a slow infusion over 60 minutes. In studies of normal volunteers, infusion-related events did not occur when Vancocin HCl was administered at a rate of 10 mg/min or less.

Nephrotoxicity—Rarely, renal failure, principally manifested by increased serum creatinine or BUN concentrations, especially in patients given large doses of Vancocin HCl, has been reported. Rare cases of interstitial nephritis have been reported. Most of these have occurred in patients who were given aminoglycosides concomitantly or who had preexisting kidney dysfunction. When Vancocin HCl was discontinued, azotemia resolved in most patients.

Gastrointestinal—Onset of pseudomembranous colitis symptoms may occur during or after antibiotic treatment (*see* WARNINGS).

Ototoxicity—A few dozen cases of hearing loss associated with Vancocin HCl have been reported. Most of these patients had kidney dysfunction or a preexisting hearing loss or were receiving concomitant treatment with an ototoxic drug. Vertigo, dizziness, and tinnitus have been reported rarely.

Hematopoietic—Reversible neutropenia, usually starting 1 week or more after onset of therapy with Vancocin HCl or after a total dosage of more than 25 g, has been reported for several dozen patients. Neutropenia appears to be promptly reversible when Vancocin HCl is discontinued. Thrombocytopenia has rarely been reported.

Although a causal relationship has not been established, reversible agranulocytosis (granulocytes $<500/mm^3$) has been reported rarely.

Phlebitis—Inflammation at the injection site has been reported.

Miscellaneous—Infrequently, patients have been reported to have had anaphylaxis, drug fever, nausea, chills, eosinophilia, rashes (including exfoliative dermatitis), Stevens-Johnson syndrome, toxic epidermal necrolysis, and rare cases of vasculitis in association with administration of Vancocin HCl.

Chemical peritonitis has been reported following intraperitoneal administration of vancomycin (*see* PRECAUTIONS).

OVERDOSAGE

Supportive care is advised, with maintenance of glomerular filtration. Vancomycin is poorly removed by dialysis. Hemofiltration and hemoperfusion with polysulfone resin have been reported to result in increased vancomycin clearance. The median lethal intravenous dose is 319 mg/kg in rats and 400 mg/kg in mice.

To obtain up-to-date information about the treatment of overdose, a good resource is your certified Regional Poison Control Center. Telephone numbers of certified poison control centers are listed in the *Physicians' Desk Reference (PDR)*. In managing overdosage, consider the possibility of multiple drug overdoses, interaction among drugs, and unusual drug kinetics in your patient.

DOSAGE AND ADMINISTRATION

Infusion-related events are related to both concentration and rate of administration of vancomycin. Concentrations of no more than 5 mg/mL and rates of no more than 10 mg/min are recommended in adults (see also age-specific recommendations). In selected patients in need of fluid restriction, a concentration up to 10 mg/mL may be used; use of such higher concentrations may increase the risk of infusion-related events. Infusion-related events may occur, however, at any rate or concentration.

Patients With Normal Renal Function

Adults—The usual daily intravenous dose is 2 g divided either as 500 mg every 6 hours or 1 g every 12 hours. Each dose should be administered at no more than 10 mg/min or over a period of at least 60 minutes, whichever is longer. Other patient factors, such as age or obesity, may call for modification of the usual intravenous daily dose.

Children—The usual intravenous dosage of Vancocin HCl is 10 mg/kg per dose given every 6 hours. Each dose should be administered over a period of at least 60 minutes.

Infants and Neonates—In neonates and young infants, the total daily intravenous dosage may be lower. In both neonates and infants, an initial dose of 15 mg/kg is suggested, followed by 10 mg/kg every 12 hours for neonates in the 1st week of life and every 8 hours thereafter up to the age of 1 month. Each dose should be administered over 60 minutes. Close monitoring of serum concentrations of vancomycin may be warranted in these patients.

Patients With Impaired Renal Function and Elderly Patients

Dosage adjustment must be made in patients with impaired renal function. In premature infants and the elderly, greater dosage reductions than expected may be necessary because of decreased renal function. Measurement of vancomycin serum concentrations can be helpful in optimizing therapy, especially in seriously ill patients with changing renal function. Vancomycin serum concentrations can be determined by use of microbiologic assay, radioimmunoassay, fluorescence polarization immunoassay, fluorescence immunoassay, or high-pressure liquid chromatography.

If creatinine clearance can be measured or estimated accurately, the dosage for most patients with renal impairment can be calculated using the following table. The dosage of Vancocin HCl per day in mg is about 15 times the glomerular filtration rate in mL/min:

DOSAGE TABLE FOR VANCOMYCIN
IN PATIENTS WITH IMPAIRED RENAL FUNCTION
(Adapted from Moellering et al)[4]

Creatinine Clearance mL/min	Vancomycin Dose mg/24 h
100	1,545
90	1,390
80	1,235
70	1,080
60	925
50	770
40	620
30	465
20	310
10	155

The initial dose should be no less than 15 mg/kg, even in patients with mild to moderate renal insufficiency.

The table is not valid for functionally anephric patients. For such patients, an initial dose of 15 mg/kg of body weight should be given to achieve prompt therapeutic serum concentrations. The dose required to maintain stable concen-

trations is 1.9 mg/kg/24 h. In patients with marked renal inpairment, it may be more convenient to give maintenance doses of 250 to 1,000 mg once every several days rather than administering the drug on a daily basis. In anuria, a dose of 1,000 mg every 7 to 10 days has been recommended.

When only the serum creatinine concentration is known, the following formula (based on sex, weight, and age of the patient) may be used to calculate creatinine clearance. Calculated creatinine clearances (mL/min) are only estimates. The creatinine clearance should be measured promptly.

Men: $\dfrac{\text{Weight (kg)} \times (140 - \text{age in years})}{72 \times \text{serum creatinine concentration (mg/dL)}}$

Women: $0.85 \times$ above value

The serum creatinine must represent a steady state of renal function. Otherwise, the estimated value for creatinine clearance is not valid. Such a calculated clearance is an overestimate of actual clearance in patients with conditions: (1) characterized by decreasing renal function, such as shock, severe heart failure, or oliguria; (2) in which a normal relationship between muscle mass and total body weight is not present, such as obese patients or those with liver disease, edema, or ascites; and (3) accompanied by debilitation, malnutrition, or inactivity.

The safety and efficacy of vancomycin administration by the intrathecal (intralumbar or intraventricular) routes have not been assessed.

Intermittent infusion is the recommended method of administration.

PREPARATION AND STABILITY

At the time of use, reconstitute by adding either 10 mL of Sterile Water for Injection to the 500-mg vial or 20 mL of Sterile Water for Injection to the 1-g vial of dry, sterile vancomycin powder. Vials reconstituted in this manner will give a solution of 50 mg/mL. FURTHER DILUTION IS REQUIRED.

After reconstitution with Sterile Water for Injection, the vials may be stored in a refrigerator for 14 days without significant loss of potency. Reconstituted solutions containing 500 mg of vancomycin must be diluted with at least 100 mL of diluent. Reconstituted solutions containing 500 mg of vancomycin must be diluted with at least 100 mL of diluent. Reconstituted solutions containing 1 g of vancomycin must be diluted with at least 200 mL of diluent. The desired dose, diluted in this manner, should be administered by intermittent intravenous infusion over a period of at least 60 minutes.

Compatibility With Intravenous Fluids—Solutions that are diluted with 5% Dextrose Injection or 0.9% Sodium Chloride Injection may be stored in a refrigerator for 14 days without significant loss of potency. Solutions that are diluted with the following infusion fluids may be stored in a refrigerator for 96 hours:

5% Dextrose Injection and 0.9% Sodium Chloride Injection, USP
Lactated Ringer's Injection, USP
Lactated Ringer's and 5% Dextrose Injection, USP
Normosol®-M* and 5% Dextrose
Isolyte® E**
Acetated Ringer's Injection

Vancomycin solution has a low pH and may cause chemical or physical instability when it is mixed with other compounds.

Prior to administration, parenteral drug products should be inspected visually for particulate matter and discoloration whenever solution or container permits.

For Oral Administration—Oral Vancocin HCl is used in treating antibiotic-associated pseudomembranous colitis caused by *C. difficile* and for staphylococcal enterocolitis. Vancocin HCl is not effective by the oral route for other types of infections. The usual adult total daily dosage is 500 mg to 2 g given in 3 or 4 divided doses for 7 to 10 days. The total daily dosage in children is 40 mg/kg of body weight in 3 or 4 divided doses for 7 to 10 days. The total daily dosage should not exceed 2 g. The appropriate dose may be diluted in 1 oz of water and given to the patient to drink. Common flavoring syrups may be added to the solution to improve the taste for oral administration. The diluted solution may be administered via a nasogastric tube.

*Normosol®-M, Abbott Hospital Products
   (Division of Abbott Laboratories)
**Isolyte® E, McGaw, Inc.

HOW SUPPLIED

Vancocin® HCl Vials (or Sterile Vancomycin Hydrochloride, USP) are available in:
The 500 mg,* 10-mL vials are available as follows:
   10-mL vials   NDC 0002-1444-01 (VL 657)
   Traypak† of 25   NDC 0002-1444-25 (VL 657)
The 1 g,* 20-mL vials are available as follows:
   Traypak of 25   NDC 0002-7321-25 (VL 7321)
Also available:
Vancocin-HCl ADD-Vantage‡ Vials (or Sterile Vancomycin Hydrochloride, USP) are available in:
The 500 mg,* 15-mL vials are available as follows:
   Traypak of 10   NDC 0002-7297-10 (VL 7297)

The 1 g,* 15-mL vials are available as follows:
Traypak of 10 NDC 0002-7298-10 (VL 7298)
Vancocin HCl Pharmacy Bulk Package (or Vancomycin Hydrochloride for Injection, USP) are available in:
The 10 g,* 100-mL vials are available as follows:
100-mL vial NDC 0002-7355-01 (VL 7355)
Prior to reconstitution, the vials may be stored at room temperature, 59° to 86°F (15° to 30°C).

*Equivalent to vancomycin.
†Traypak™ (multivial carton, Lilly).
‡ADD-Vantage® (vials and diluent containers, Abbott).
CAUTION—Federal (USA) law prohibits dispensing without prescription.

ANIMAL PHARMACOLOGY

In animal studies, hypotension and bradycardia occurred in dogs receiving an intravenous infusion of vancomycin hydrochloride, 25 mg/kg, at a concentration of 25 mg/mL and an infusion rate of 13.3 mL/min.

REFERENCES

1. National Committee for Clinical Laboratory Standards. Performance Standards for Antimicrobial Disk Susceptibility Tests–Fifth Edition. Approved Standard NCCLS Document M2-A5, Vol. 13, No. 24, NCCLS, Villanova, PA, December, 1993.
2. National Committee for Clinical Laboratory Standards. Methods for Dilution Antimicrobial Susceptibility Tests for Bacteria that Grow Aerobically–Third Edition. Approved Standard NCCLS Document M7-A3, Vol. 13, No. 25, NCCLS, Villanova, PA, December, 1993.
3. Dajani, Adnan S, et al: Prevention of bacterial endocarditis. Recommendations by the American Heart Association. *JAMA* 264 (22):2919–2922, December 12, 1990.
4. Moellering RC, Krogstad DJ, Greenblatt DJ: Vancomycin therapy in patients with impaired renal function: A nomogram for dosage. *Ann Intern Med* 1981;94:343.

Literature revised June 13, 1997
PA 1856 AMP [061397]

VANCOCIN® HCl ℞

[*văn 'kō-sĭn ăch 'sē-ĕl*]
(vancomycin hydrochloride)
For Oral Solution, USP

This preparation for the treatment of colitis is for oral use only and is not systemically absorbed. Vancocin® HCl must be given orally for treatment of staphylococcal enterocolitis and antibiotic-associated pseudomembranous colitis caused by *Clostridium difficile*. Orally administered Vancocin HCl is *not* effective for other types of infection.

Parenteral administration of Vancocin HCl is not effective for treatment of staphylococcal enterocolitis and antibiotic-associated pseudomembranous colitis caused by *C. difficile*. If parenteral vancomycin therapy is desired, use Vancocin® HCl (Sterile Vancomycin Hydrochloride, USP), IntraVenous, and consult package insert accompanying that preparation.

DESCRIPTION

Vancocin® HCl for Oral Solution (Vancomycin Hydrochloride for Oral Solution, USP), contains chromatographically purified vancomycin hydrochloride, a tricyclic glycopeptide antibiotic derived from *Amycolatopsis orientalis* (formerly *Nocardia orientalis*), which has the chemical formula $C_{66}H_{75}Cl_2N_9O_{24}$ • HCl. The molecular weight of vancomycin hydrochloride is 1,485.73; 500 mg of the base is equivalent to 0.34 mmol.

Vancocin HCl for Oral Solution contains vancomycin hydrochloride equivalent to 10 g (6.7 mmol) or 1 g (0.67 mmol) vancomycin. Calcium disodium edetate, equivalent to 0.2 mg edetate per gram of vancomycin, is added at the time of manufacture. The 10-g bottle may contain up to 40 mg of ethanol per gram of vancomycin.

Vancomycin hydrochloride has the following structure:
[See chemical structure at top of next column]

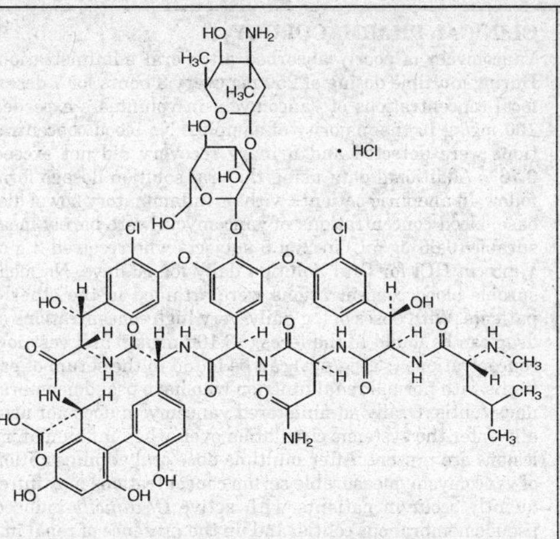

CLINICAL PHARMACOLOGY

Vancomycin is poorly absorbed after oral administration. During multiple dosing of 250 mg every 8 hours for 7 doses, fecal concentrations of vancomycin in volunteers exceeded 100 mg/kg in the majority of samples. No blood concentrations were detected and urinary recovery did not exceed 0.76%. In anephric patients with no inflammatory bowel disease, blood concentrations of vancomycin were barely measurable (0.66 µg/mL) in 2 of 5 subjects who received 2 g of Vancocin HCl for Oral Solution daily for 16 days. No measurable blood concentrations were attained in the other 3 patients. With doses of 2 g daily, very high concentrations of drug can be found in the feces (>3,100 mg/kg) and very low concentrations (<1 µg/mL) can be found in the serum of patients with normal renal function who have pseudomembranous colitis. Orally administered vancomycin does not usually enter the systemic circulation even when inflammatory lesions are present. After multiple-dose oral administration of vancomycin, measurable serum concentrations may infrequently occur in patients with active *C. difficile*-induced pseudomembranous colitis, and, in the presence of renal impairment, the possibility of accumulation exists.

Microbiology —The bactericidal action of vancomycin results primarily from inhibition of cell-wall biosynthesis. In addition, vancomycin alters bacterial-cell-membrane permeability and RNA synthesis. There is no cross-resistance between vancomycin and other antibiotics. Vancomycin is active against *C. difficile* (eg, toxigenic strains implicated in pseudomembranous enterocolitis). It is also active against staphylococci, including *Staphylococcus aureus.*

For further information, see prescribing information for Vancocin HCl, IntraVenous.

Vancomycin is not active in vitro against gram-negative bacilli, mycobacteria, or fungi.

Disk Susceptibility Tests —The standardized disk and/or dilution methods described by the National Committee for Clinical Laboratory Standards have been recommended to test susceptibility to vancomycin.

INDICATIONS AND USAGE

Vancocin HCl for Oral Solution is administered orally for treatment of staphylococcal enterocolitis and antibiotic-associated pseudomembranous colitis caused by *C. difficile.* Parenteral administration of Vancocin HCl is not effective for the above indications; therefore, Vancocin HCl must be given orally for these indications. **Orally administered Vancocin HCl is not effective for other types of infection.**

CONTRAINDICATION

Vancocin HCl is contraindicated in patients with known hypersensitivity to this antibiotic.

PRECAUTIONS

General —Clinically significant serum concentrations have been reported in some patients who have taken multiple oral doses of vancomycin for active *C. difficile*-induced pseudomembranous colitis; therefore, monitoring of serum concentrations may be appropriate.

Some patients with inflammatory disorders of the intestinal mucosa may have significant systemic absorption of vancomycin and, therefore, may be at risk for the development of adverse reactions associated with the parenteral administration of vancomycin (See package insert accompanying the intravenous preparation.) The risk is greater if renal impairment is present. It should be noted that the total systemic and renal clearances of vancomycin are reduced in the elderly.

Ototoxicity has occurred in patients receiving Vancocin HCl. It may be transient or permanent. It has been reported mostly in patients who have been given excessive intravenous doses, who have an underlying hearing loss, or who are receiving concomitant therapy with another ototoxic agent, such as an aminoglycoside. Serial tests of auditory function may be helpful in order to minimize the risk of ototoxicity.

When patients with underlying renal dysfunction or those receiving concomitant therapy with an aminoglycoside are being treated, serial monitoring of renal function should be performed.

Usage in Pregnancy —Pregnancy Category C —Animal reproduction studies have not been conducted with Vancocin HCl. It is not known whether Vancocin HCl can affect reproduction capacity. In a controlled clinical study, the potential ototoxic and nephrotoxic effects of Vancocin HCl on infants were evaluated when the drug was administered intravenously to pregnant women for serious staphylococcal infections complicating intravenous drug abuse. Vancocin HCl was found in cord blood. No sensorineural hearing loss or nephrotoxicity attributable to Vancocin HCl was noted. One infant whose mother received Vancocin HCl in the third trimester experienced conductive hearing loss that was not attributed to the administration of Vancocin HCl. Because the number of patients treated in this study was limited and Vancocin HCl was administered only in the second and third trimesters, it is not known whether Vancocin HCl causes fetal harm. Vancocin HCl should be given to a pregnant woman only if clearly needed.

Nursing Mothers —Vancocin HCl is excreted in human milk based on information obtained with the intravenous administration of Vancocin HCl. Blood concentrations achieved with oral administration are very low (*see* CLINICAL PHARMACOLOGY). Caution should be exercised when Vancocin HCl is administered to a nursing woman. Because of the potential for adverse events, a decision should be made whether to discontinue nursing or discontinue the drug, taking into account the importance of the drug to the mother.

ADVERSE REACTIONS

Nephrotoxicity —Rarely, renal failure, principally manifested by increased serum creatinine or BUN concentrations, especially in patients given large doses of intravenously administered Vancocin HCl, has been reported. Rare cases of interstitial nephritis have been reported. Most of these have occurred in patients who were given aminoglycosides concomitantly or who had preexisting kidney dysfunction. When Vancocin HCl was discontinued, azotemia resolved in most patients.

Ototoxicity —A few dozen cases of hearing loss associated with intravenously administered Vancocin HCl have been reported. Most of these patients had kidney dysfunction or a preexisting hearing loss or were receiving concomitant treatment with an ototoxic drug. Vertigo, dizziness, and tinnitus have been reported rarely.

Hematopoietic —Reversible neutropenia, usually starting 1 week or more after onset of intravenous therapy with Vancocin HCl or after a total dosage of more than 25 g, has been reported for several dozen patients. Neutropenia appears to be promptly reversible when Vancocin HCl is discontinued. Thrombocytopenia has rarely been reported.

Miscellaneous —Infrequently, patients have been reported to have had anaphylaxis, drug fever, chills, nausea, eosinophilia, rashes (including exfoliative dermatitis), Stevens-Johnson syndrome, toxic epidermal necrolysis, and rare cases of vasculitis in association with the administration of Vancocin HCl.

A condition has been reported that is similar to the IV-induced syndrome with symptoms consistent with anaphylactoid reactions, including hypotension, wheezing, dyspnea, urticaria, pruritus, flushing of the upper body ("Red Man Syndrome"), pain and muscle spasm of the chest and back. These reactions usually resolve within 20 minutes but may persist for several hours.

OVERDOSAGE

Supportive care is advised, with maintenance of glomerular filtration. Vancomycin is poorly removed by dialysis. Hemofiltration and hemoperfusion with polysulfone resin have been reported to result in increased vancomycin clearance.

Treatment —To obtain up-to-date information about the treatment of overdose, a good resource is your certified Regional Poison Control Center. Telephone numbers of certified poison control centers are listed in the *Physicians' Desk Reference (PDR).* In managing overdosage, consider the possibility of multiple drug overdoses, interaction among drugs, and unusual drug kinetics in your patient.

DOSAGE AND ADMINISTRATION

Adults —Oral Vancocin HCl is used in treating antibiotic-associated pseudomembranous colitis caused by *C. difficile* and staphylococcal enterocolitis. Vancocin HCl is not effective by the oral route for other types of infections. The usual adult total daily dosage is 500 mg to 2 g administered orally in 3 or 4 divided doses for 7 to 10 days.

Pediatric Patients —The usual daily dosage is 40 mg/kg in 3 or 4 divided doses for 7 to 10 days. The total daily dosage should not exceed 2 g.

PREPARATION AND STABILITY

The contents of the 10-g bottle may be mixed with distilled or deionized water (115 mL) for oral administration. When mixed with 115 mL of water, each 6 mL provides approximately 500 mg of vancomycin. The contents of the 1-g bottle may be mixed with distilled or deionized water (20 mL). When reconstituted with 20 mL, each 5 mL contains approximately 250 mg of vancomycin. Mix thoroughly to dissolve. These mixtures may be kept for 2 weeks in a refrigerator without significant loss of potency.

The appropriate oral solution dose may be diluted in 1 oz of water and given to the patient to drink. Common flavoring syrups may be added to the solution to improve the taste for

Continued on next page

*** Identi-Code® symbol. This product information was prepared in June 1998. Current information on these and other products of Eli Lilly and Company may be obtained by direct inquiry to Lilly Research Laboratories, Lilly Corporate Center, Indianapolis, Indiana 46285, (800) 545-5979.**

Vancocin HCl for Oral Sol.—Cont.

oral administration. The diluted material may be administered via nasogastric tube.

HOW SUPPLIED

Vancocin® HCl For Oral Solution (or Vancomycin Hydrochloride for Oral Solution, USP) is available in:
The 10 g* per 50 mL Oral Solution, in a screw-cap bottle, is available as follows:
10-g Bottle NDC 0002-2372-37 (M-206)
The 1 g* per 10 mL Oral Solution, in a screw-cap bottle, is available as follows:
Traypak† of 6 NDC 0002-5105-16 (M-5105)
Prior to reconstitution, store at controlled room temperature, 59° to 86°F (15° to 30°C).
Also available:
Vancocin HCl Pulvules® (or Vancomycin Hydrochloride Capsules, USP) are available in:
The 125 mg* Pulvules have an opaque blue cap and opaque brown body imprinted with "3125" on the cap and "VANCOCIN HCL 125 MG" on the body in white ink. They are available in:
ID‡20 NDC 0002-3125-42 (PU3125)
The 250 mg* Pulvules have an opaque blue cap and opaque lavender body imprinted with "3126" on the cap and "VANCOCIN HCL 250 MG" on the body in white ink. They are available in:
ID20 NDC 0002-3126-42 (PU3126)

*Equivalent to vancomycin.
†Traypak™ (multivial carton, Lilly).
‡Identi-Dose® (unit dose medication, Lilly).
CAUTION —Federal (USA) law prohibits dispensing without prescription.
Literature revised June 13, 1997
PA 0559 AMP [061397]

VANCOCIN® HCl ℞

[*văn 'kō-sĭn*]
(vancomycin hydrochloride)
Capsules, USP
Pulvules®

This preparation for the treatment of colitis is for oral use only and is not systemically absorbed. Vancocin® HCl must be given orally for treatment of staphylococcal enterocolitis and antibiotic-associated pseudomembranous colitis caused by *Clostridium difficile.* Orally administered Vancocin HCl is *not* effective for other types of infection.
Parenteral administration of Vancocin HCl is not effective for treatment of staphylococcal enterocolitis and antibiotic-associated pseudomembranous colitis caused by *C. difficile.* If parenteral vancomycin therapy is desired, use Vancocin® HCl (Sterile Vancomycin Hydrochloride, USP), IntraVenous, and consult package insert accompanying that preparation.

DESCRIPTION

Pulvules® Vancocin® HCl (Vancomycin Hydrochloride Capsules, USP) contain chromatographically purified vancomycin hydrochloride, a tricyclic glycopeptide antibiotic derived from *Amycolatopsis orientalis* (formerly *Nocardia orientalis*), which has the chemical formula $C_{66}H_{75}Cl_2N_9O_{24}$•HCl. The molecular weight of vancomycin hydrochloride is 1,485.73; 500 mg of the base is equivalent to 0.34 mmol.
The Pulvules contain vancomycin hydrochloride equivalent to 125 mg (0.08 mmol) or 250 mg (0.17 mmol) vancomycin. The Pulvules also contain F D & C Blue No. 2, gelatin, iron oxide, polyethylene glycol, titanium dioxide, and other inactive ingredients.
Vancomycin hydrochloride has the following structural formula:

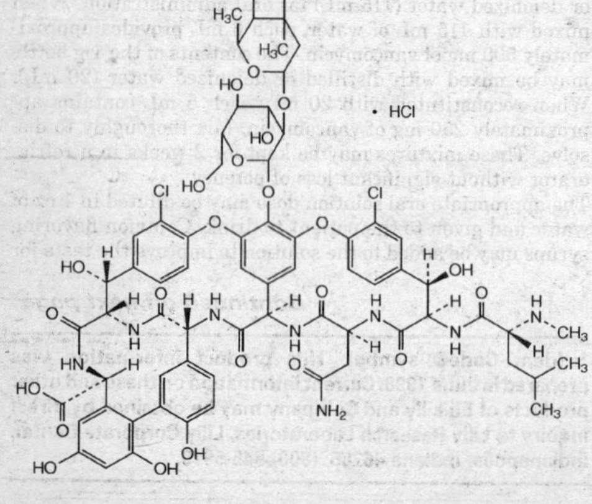

CLINICAL PHARMACOLOGY

Vancomycin is poorly absorbed after oral administration. During multiple dosing of 250 mg every 8 hours for 7 doses, fecal concentrations of vancomycin in volunteers exceeded 100 mg/kg in the majority of samples. No blood concentrations were detected and urinary recovery did not exceed 0.76%. Additional data using the oral solution dosage form follow. In anephric patients with no inflammatory bowel disease, blood concentrations of vancomycin were barely measurable (0.66 µg/mL) in 2 of 5 subjects who received 2 g of Vancocin HCl for Oral Solution daily for 16 days. No measurable blood concentrations were attained in the other 3 patients. With doses of 2 g daily, very high concentrations of drug can be found in the feces (>3,100 mg/kg) and very low concentrations (<1 µg/mL) can be found in the serum of patients with normal renal function who have pseudomembranous colitis. Orally administered vancomycin does not usually enter the systemic circulation even when inflammatory lesions are present. After multiple-dose oral administration of vancomycin, measurable serum concentrations may infrequently occur in patients with active *C. difficile*-induced pseudomembranous colitis, and, in the presence of renal impairment, the possibility of accumulation exists.
Microbiology—The bactericidal action of vancomycin results primarily from inhibition of cell-wall biosynthesis. In addition, vancomycin alters bacterial-cell-membrane permeability and RNA synthesis. There is no cross-resistance between vancomycin and other antibiotics. Vancomycin is active against *C. difficile* (eg, toxigenic strains implicated in pseudomembranous enterocolitis). It is also active against staphylococci, including *Staphylococcus aureus.*
For further information, see prescribing information for Vancocin HCl, IntraVenous.
Vancomycin is not active in vitro against gram-negative bacilli, mycobacteria, or fungi.
Disk Susceptibility Tests—The standardized disk and/or dilution methods described by the National Committee for Clinical Laboratory Standards have been recommended to test susceptibility to vancomycin.

INDICATIONS AND USAGE

Pulvules Vancocin HCl may be administered orally for treatment of staphylococcal enterocolitis and antibiotic-associated pseudomembranous colitis caused by *C. difficile.* Parenteral administration of Vancocin HCl is not effective for the above indications; therefore, Vancocin HCl must be given orally for these indications. **Orally administered Vancocin HCl is not effective for other types of infection.**

CONTRAINDICATION

Vancocin HCl is contraindicated in patients with known hypersensitivity to this antibiotic.

PRECAUTIONS

General—Clinically significant serum concentrations have been reported in some patients who have taken multiple oral doses of vancomycin for active *C. difficile*-induced pseudomembranous colitis; therefore, monitoring of serum concentrations may be appropriate in some instances, eg, in patients with renal insufficiency and/or colitis.
Some patients with inflammatory disorders of the intestinal mucosa may have significant systemic absorption of vancomycin and, therefore, may be at risk for the development of adverse reactions associated with the parenteral administration of vancomycin. (See package insert accompanying the intravenous preparation.) The risk is greater if renal impairment is present. It should be noted that the total systemic and renal clearances of vancomycin are reduced in the elderly.
Ototoxicity has occurred in patients receiving Vancocin HCl. It may be transient or permanent. It has been reported mostly in patients who have been given excessive intravenous doses, who have an underlying hearing loss, or who are receiving concomitant therapy with another ototoxic agent, such as an aminoglycoside. Serial tests of auditory function may be helpful in order to minimize the risk of ototoxicity.
When patients with underlying renal dysfunction or those receiving concomitant therapy with an aminoglycoside are being treated, serial monitoring of renal function should be performed.
Carcinogenesis, Mutagenesis, Impairment of Fertility—No long-term carcinogenesis studies in animals have been conducted.
At concentrations up to 1,000 µg/mL, vancomycin had no mutagenic effect *in vitro* in the mouse lymphoma forward mutation assay or the primary rat hepatocyte unscheduled DNA synthesis assay. The concentrations tested *in vitro* were above the peak plasma vancomycin concentrations of 20 to 40 µg/mL usually achieved in humans after slow infusion of the maximum recommended dose of 1 g. Vancomycin had no mutagenic effect *in vivo* in the Chinese hamster sister chromatid exchange assay (400 mg/kg IP) or the mouse micronucleus assay (800 mg/kg IP).
No definitive fertility studies have been conducted.
Pregnancy—Teratogenic Effects—Pregnancy Category B—The highest doses of vancomycin tested were not teratogenic in rats given up to 200 mg/kg/day IV (1,180 mg/m² or 1 times the recommended maximum human dose based on a mg/m² basis) or in rabbits given up to 120 mg/kg/day IV (1,320 mg/m² or 1.1 times the recommended maximum human dose based on a mg/m² basis). No effects on fetal weight or development were seen in rats at the highest dose tested or in rabbits given 80 mg/kg/day (880 mg/m² or 0.74 times the recommended maximum human dose based on mg/m²).
In a controlled clinical study, the potential ototoxic and nephrotoxic effects of Vancocin HCl on infants were evaluated when the drug was administered intravenously to pregnant women for serious staphylococcal infections complicating intravenous drug abuse. Vancocin HCl was found in cord blood. No sensorineural hearing loss or nephrotoxicity attributable to Vancocin HCl was noted. One infant whose mother received Vancocin HCl in the third trimester experienced conductive hearing loss that was not attributed to the administration of Vancocin HCl. Because the number of patients treated in this study was limited and Vancocin HCl was administered only in the second and third trimesters, it is not known whether Vancocin HCl causes fetal harm. Because animal reproduction studies are not always predictive of human response, Vancocin HCl should be given to a pregnant woman only if clearly needed.
Nursing Mothers—Vancocin HCl is excreted in human milk based on information obtained with the intravenous administration of Vancocin HCl. Blood concentrations achieved with oral administration are very low (*see* CLINICAL PHARMACOLOGY). It is not known whether oral vancomycin is excreted in human milk, as no studies of vancomycin concentration in human milk after oral administration have been done. Caution should be exercised when Vancocin HCl is administered to a nursing woman. Because of the potential for adverse events, a decision should be made whether to discontinue nursing or discontinue the drug, taking into account the importance of the drug to the mother.
Pediatric Use—Safety and effectiveness in pediatric patients have not been established.

ADVERSE REACTIONS

Nephrotoxicity—Rarely, renal failure, principally manifested by increased serum creatinine or BUN concentrations, especially in patients given large doses of intravenously administered Vancocin HCl has been reported. Rare cases of interstitial nephritis have been reported. Most of these have occurred in patients who were given aminoglycosides concomitantly or who had preexisting kidney dysfunction. When Vancocin HCl was discontinued, azotemia resolved in most patients.
Ototoxicity—A few dozen cases of hearing loss associated with intravenously administered Vancocin HCl have been reported. Most of these patients had kidney dysfunction or a preexisting hearing loss or were receiving concomitant treatment with an ototoxic drug. Vertigo, dizziness, and tinnitus have been reported rarely.
Hematopoietic—Reversible neutropenia, usually starting 1 week or more after onset of intravenous therapy with Vancocin HCl or after a total dose of more than 25 g, has been reported for several dozen patients. Neutropenia appears to be promptly reversible when Vancocin HCl is discontinued. Thrombocytopenia has rarely been reported.
Miscellaneous—Infrequently, patients have been reported to have had anaphylaxis, drug fever, chills, nausea, eosinophilia, rashes (including exfoliative dermatitis), Stevens-Johnson syndrome, toxic epidermal necrolysis, and rare cases of vasculitis in association with the administration of Vancocin HCl.
A condition has been reported that is similar to the IV-induced syndrome with symptoms consistent with anaphylactoid reactions, including hypotension, wheezing, dyspnea, urticaria, pruritus, flushing of the upper body ("Red Man Syndrome"), pain and muscle spasm of the chest and back. These reactions usually resolve within 20 minutes but may persist for several hours.

OVERDOSAGE

Supportive care is advised, with maintenance of glomerular filtration. Vancomycin is poorly removed by dialysis. Hemofiltration and hemoperfusion with polysulfone resin have been reported to result in increased vancomycin clearance.
Treatment—To obtain up-to-date information about the treatment of overdose, a good resource is your certified Regional Poison Control Center. Telephone numbers of certified poison control centers are listed in the *Physicians' Desk Reference (PDR).* In managing overdosage, consider the possibility of multiple drug overdoses, interaction among drugs, and unusual drug kinetics in your patient.

DOSAGE AND ADMINISTRATION

Adults—Oral Vancocin HCl is used in treating antibiotic-associated pseudomembranous colitis caused by *C. difficile* and staphylococcal enterocolitis. Vancocin HCl is not effective by the oral route for other types of infections. The usual adult total daily dosage is 500 mg to 2 g administered orally in 3 or 4 divided doses for 7 to 10 days.

Pediatric Patients—The usual daily dosage is 40 mg/kg in 3 or 4 divided doses for 7 to 10 days. The total daily dosage should not exceed 2 g.

HOW SUPPLIED

Vancocin® HCl Pulvules® (or Vancomycin Hydrochloride Capsules, USP) are available in:

The 125 mg* Pulvules have an opaque blue cap and opaque brown body imprinted with "3125" on the cap and "VANCOCIN HCL 125 MG" on the body in white ink. They are available in:

ID†20 NDC 0002-3125-42 (PU3125)

The 250 mg* Pulvules have an opaque blue cap and opaque lavender body imprinted with "3126" on the cap and "VANCOCIN HCL 250 MG" on the body in white ink. They are available in:

ID†20 NDC 0002-3126-42 (PU3126)

Also Available:

Vancocin HCl For Oral Solution (or Vancomycin Hydrochloride for Oral Solution, USP) is available in:

The 10 g* per 50 mL Oral Solution, in a screw-cap bottle, is available as follows:

10-g Bottle NDC 0002-2372-37 (M-206)

The 1 g* per 10 mL Oral Solution, in a screw-cap bottle, is available as follows:

Traypak‡ of 6 NDC 0002-5105-16 (M-5105)

Store at controlled room temperature, 59° to 86°F (15° to 30°C).

*Equivalent to vancomycin.
†Identi-Dose® (unit dose medication, Lilly).
‡Traypak™ (multivial carton, Lilly).

CAUTION—Federal (USA) law prohibits dispensing without prescription.

Literature revised June 13, 1997
PV 1981 AMP [061397]

VANCOMYCIN HYDROCHLORIDE ℞
See Vancocin® HCl (Vancomycin Hydrochloride, USP).

VELBAN® ℞
[*vĕl 'băn*]
(vinblastine sulfate for Injection, USP)

WARNINGS

Caution—This preparation should be administered by individuals experienced in the administration of Velban. It is extremely important that the needle be properly positioned in the vein before this product is injected. If leakage into surrounding tissue should occur during intravenous administration of Velban, it may cause considerable irritation. The injection should be discontinued immediately, and any remaining portion of the dose should then be introduced into another vein. Local injection of hyaluronidase and the application of moderate heat to the area of leakage help disperse the drug and are thought to minimize discomfort and the possibility of cellulitis.

FATAL IF GIVEN INTRATHECALLY. FOR INTRAVENOUS USE ONLY. *See Warnings section for the treatment of patients given intrathecal Velban.*

DESCRIPTION

Velban® (Vinblastine Sulfate for Injection, USP) is vincaleukoblastine, sulfate (1:1) (salt). It is the salt of an alkaloid extracted from *Vinca rosea* Linn, a common flowering herb known as the periwinkle (more properly known as *Catharanthus roseus* G. Don). Previously, the generic name was vincaleukoblastine, abbreviated VLB. It is a stathmokinetic oncolytic agent. When treated in vitro with this preparation, growing cells are arrested in metaphase.

Chemical and physical evidence indicate that Velban has the empirical formula $C_{46}H_{58}N_4O_9 \bullet H_2SO_4$ and that it is a dimeric alkaloid containing both indole and dihydroindole moieties. It has a molecular weight of 909.07. The structural formula is as follows:

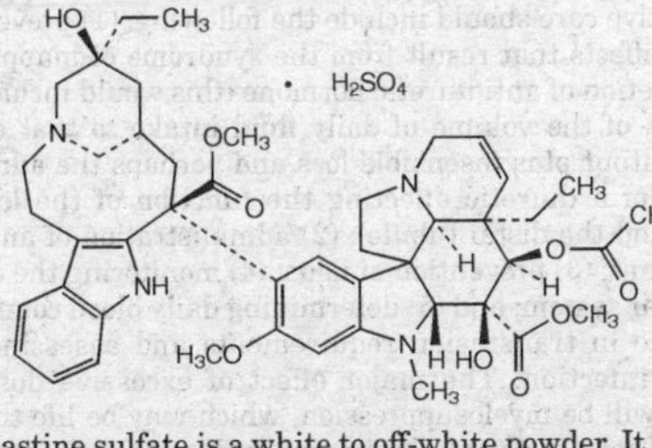

Vinblastine sulfate is a white to off-white powder. It is freely soluble in water, soluble in methanol, and slightly soluble in ethanol. It is insoluble in benzene, ether, and naphtha.

The clinical formulation is supplied in a sterile form for intravenous use only. Vials of Velban contain 10 mg (0.011 mmol) of vinblastine sulfate, in the form of a white, amorphous, solid lyophilized plug, without excipients. After reconstitution with sodium chloride solution, the pH of the resulting solution lies in the range of 3.5 to 5.

CLINICAL PHARMACOLOGY

Experimental data indicate that the action of Velban is different from that of other recognized antineoplastic agents. Tissue-culture studies suggest an interference with metabolic pathways of amino acids leading from glutamic acid to the citric acid cycle and to urea. In vivo experiments tend to confirm the in vitro results. A number of studies in vitro and in vivo have demonstrated that Velban produces a stathmokinetic effect and various atypical mitotic figures. The therapeutic responses, however, are not fully explained by the cytologic changes, since these changes are sometimes observed clinically and experimentally in the absence of any oncolytic effects.

Reversal of the antitumor effect of Velban by glutamic acid or tryptophan has been observed. In addition, glutamic acid and aspartic acid have protected mice from lethal doses of Velban. Aspartic acid was relatively ineffective in reversing the antitumor effect.

Other studies indicate that Velban has an effect on cell-energy production required for mitosis and interferes with nucleic acid synthesis. The mechanism of action of Velban has been related to the inhibition of microtubule formation in the mitotic spindle, resulting in an arrest of dividing cells at the metaphase stage.

Pharmacokinetic studies in patients with cancer have shown a triphasic serum decay pattern following rapid intravenous injection. The initial, middle, and terminal half-lives are 3.7 minutes, 1.6 hours, and 24.8 hours respectively. The volume of the central compartment is 70% of body weight, probably reflecting very rapid tissue binding to formed elements of the blood. Extensive reversible tissue binding occurs. Low body stores are present at 48 and 72 hours after injection. Since the major route of excretion may be through the biliary system, toxicity from this drug may be increased when there is hepatic excretory insufficiency. The metabolism of vinca alkaloids has been shown to be mediated by hepatic cytochrome P450 isoenzymes in the CYP 3A subfamily. This metabolic pathway may be impaired in patients with hepatic dysfunction or who are taking concomitant potent inhibitors of these isoenzymes such as erythromicin. Enhanced toxicity has been reported in patients receiving concomitant erythromycin (See PRECAUTIONS). Following injection of tritiated vinblastine in the human cancer patient, 10% of the radioactivity was found in the feces and 14% in the urine; the remaining activity was not accounted for. Similar studies in dogs demonstrated that, over 9 days, 30% to 36% of radioactivity was found in the bile and 12% to 17% in the urine. A similar study in the rat demonstrated that the highest concentrations of radioactivity were found in the lung, liver, spleen, and kidney 2 hours after injection.

Hematologic Effects—Clinically, leukopenia is an expected effect of Velban, and the level of the leukocyte count is an important guide to therapy with this drug. In general, the larger the dose employed, the more profound and longer lasting the leukopenia will be. The fact that the white-blood-cell count returns to normal levels after drug-induced leukopenia is an indication that the white-cell-producing mechanism is not permanently depressed. Usually, the white count has completely returned to normal after the virtual disappearance of white cells from the peripheral blood. Following therapy with Velban, the nadir in white-blood-cell count may be expected to occur 5 to 10 days after the last day of drug administration. Recovery of the white blood count is fairly rapid thereafter and is usually complete within another 7 to 14 days. With the smaller doses employed for maintenance therapy, leukopenia may not be a problem.

Although the thrombocyte count ordinarily is not significantly lowered by therapy with Velban, patients whose bone marrow has been recently impaired by prior therapy with radiation or with other oncolytic drugs may show thrombocytopenia (less than 200,000 platelets/mm^3). When other chemotherapy or radiation has not been employed previously, thrombocyte reduction below the level of 200,000/mm^3 is rarely encountered, even when Velban may be causing significant leukopenia. Rapid recovery from thrombocytopenia within a few days is the rule.

The effect of Velban upon the red-cell count and hemoglobin is usually insignificant when other therapy does not complicate the picture. It should be remembered, however, that patients with malignant disease may exhibit anemia even in the absence of any therapy.

INDICATIONS AND USAGE

Vinblastine sulfate is indicated in the palliative treatment of the following:

I. Frequently Responsive Malignancies—
Generalized Hodgkin's disease (Stages III and IV, Ann Arbor modification of Rye staging system)
Lymphocytic lymphoma (nodular and diffuse, poorly and well differentiated)
Histiocytic lymphoma
Mycosis fungoides (advanced stages)
Advanced carcinoma of the testis
Kaposi's sarcoma
Letterer-Siwe disease (histiocytosis X)

II. Less Frequently Responsive Malignancies—
Choriocarcinoma resistant to other chemotherapeutic agents
Carcinoma of the breast, unresponsive to appropriate endocrine surgery and hormonal therapy

Current principles of chemotherapy for many types of cancer include the concurrent administration of several antineoplastic agents. For enhanced therapeutic effect without additive toxicity, agents with different dose-limiting clinical toxicities and different mechanisms of action are generally selected. Therefore, although Velban is effective as a single agent in the aforementioned indications, it is usually administered in combination with other antineoplastic drugs. Such combination therapy produces a greater percentage of response than does a single-agent regimen. These principles have been applied, for example, in the chemotherapy of Hodgkin's disease.

Hodgkin's Disease—Velban has been shown to be one of the most effective single agents for the treatment of Hodgkin's disease. Advanced Hodgkin's disease has also been successfully treated with several multiple-drug regimens that included Velban. Patients who had relapses after treatment with the MOPP program—mechlorethamine hydrochloride (nitrogen mustard), vincristine sulfate (Oncovin [Vincristine Sulfate Injection]), prednisone, and procarbazine—have likewise responded to combination-drug therapy that included Velban. A protocol using cyclophosphamide in place of nitrogen mustard and Velban instead of Oncovin is an alternative therapy for previously untreated patients with advanced Hodgkin's disease.

Advanced testicular germinal-cell cancers (embryonal carcinoma, teratocarcinoma, and choriocarcinoma) are sensitive to Velban alone, but better clinical results are achieved when Velban is administered concomitantly with other antineoplastic agents. The effect of bleomycin is significantly enhanced if Velban is administered 6 to 8 hours prior to the administration of bleomycin; this schedule permits more cells to be arrested during metaphase, the stage of the cell cycle in which bleomycin is active.

CONTRAINDICATIONS

Velban is contraindicated in patients who have significant granulocytopenia unless this is a result of the disease being treated. It should not be used in the presence of bacterial infections. Such infections must be brought under control prior to the initiation of therapy with Velban.

WARNINGS

This product is for intravenous use only. It should be administered by individuals experienced in the administration of Velban. The intrathecal administration of Velban has resulted in death. Syringes containing this product should be labeled "WARNING—FOR IV USE ONLY."

Extemporaneously prepared syringes containing this product must be packaged in an overwrap that is labeled "DO NOT REMOVE COVERING UNTIL MOMENT OF INJECTION. FATAL IF GIVEN INTRATHECALLY. FOR INTRAVENOUS USE ONLY."

The following treatment successfully arrested progressive paralysis in a single patient mistakenly given the related vinca alkaloid, vincristine sulfate, intrathecally. If Velban is mistakenly administered intrathecally, this treatment is recommended and should be initiated immediately after the intrathecal injection.

1. Remove as much spinal fluid as can be safely done through the lumbar access.
2. Insert a catheter in a lateral cerebral ventricle for the purpose of flushing the subarachnoid space from above with removal through a lumbar access.
3. Initiate flushing through the cerebral catheter with lactated Ringer's solution infused at the rate of 150 mL/h.
4. As soon as fresh frozen plasma becomes available, infuse fresh frozen plasma, 25 mL, diluted in 1 L of Lactated Ringer's solution through the cerebral ventricular catheter at the rate of 75 mL/h with removal through the lumbar access. The rate of infusion should be adjusted to maintain a protein level in the spinal fluid of 150 mg/dL.

Continued on next page

*** Identi-Code® symbol. This product information was prepared in June 1998. Current information on these and other products of Eli Lilly and Company may be obtained by direct inquiry to Lilly Research Laboratories, Lilly Corporate Center, Indianapolis, Indiana 46285, (800) 545-5979.**

Velban—Cont.

5. Administer 10 g of glutamic acid intravenously over 24 hours followed by 500 mg 3 times daily by mouth for 1 month or until neurological dysfunction stabilizes. The role of glutamic acid in this treatment is not certain and may not be essential.

The use of this treatment has not been reported following intrathecal vinblastine sulfate.

Usage in Pregnancy —Caution is necessary with the administration of all oncolytic drugs during pregnancy. Information on the use of Velban during human pregnancy is very limited. Animal studies with Velban suggest that teratogenic effects may occur. Vinblastine sulfate can cause fetal harm when administered to a pregnant woman. Laboratory animals given this drug early in pregnancy suffer resorption of the conceptus: surviving fetuses demonstrate gross deformities. There are no adequate and well-controlled studies in pregnant women. If this drug is used during pregnancy, or if the patient becomes pregnant while receiving this drug, she should be apprised of the potential hazard to the fetus. Women of childbearing potential should be advised to avoid becoming pregnant.

Aspermia has been reported in man. Animal studies show metaphase arrest and degenerative changes in germ cells. Leukopenia (granulocytopenia) may reach dangerously low levels following administration of the higher recommended doses. It is therefore important to follow the dosage technique recommended under the Dosage and Administration section. Stomatitis and neurologic toxicity, although not common or permanent, can be disabling.

PRECAUTIONS

General—Toxicity may be enhanced in the presence of hepatic insufficiency.

If leukopenia with less than 2,000 white blood cells/mm^3 occurs following a dose of Velban, the patient should be watched carefully for evidence of infection until the white-blood-cell count has returned to a safe level.

When cachexia or ulcerated areas of the skin surface are present, there may be a more profound leukopenic response to the drug; therefore, its use should be avoided in older persons suffering from either of these conditions.

In patients with malignant-cell infiltration of the bone marrow, the leukocyte and platelet counts have sometimes fallen precipitously after moderate doses of Velban. Further use of the drug in such patients is inadvisable.

Acute shortness of breath and severe bronchospasm have been reported following the administration of vinca alkaloids. These reactions have been encountered most frequently when the vinca alkaloid was used in combination with mitomycin C and may require aggressive treatment, particularly when there is pre-existing pulmonary dysfunction. The onset may be within minutes or several hours after the vinca is injected and may occur up to 2 weeks following a dose of mitomycin. Progressive dyspnea requiring chronic therapy may occur. Velban should not be readministered.

The use of small amounts of Velban daily for long periods is not advised, even though the resulting total weekly dosage may be similar to that recommended. Little or no added therapeutic effect has been demonstrated when such regimens have been used. *Strict adherence to the recommended dosage schedule is very important.* When amounts equal to several times the recommended weekly dosage were given in 7 daily installments for long periods, convulsions, severe and permanent central-nervous-system damage, and even death occurred.

Care must be taken to avoid contamination of the eye with concentrations of Velban used clinically. If accidental contamination occurs, severe irritation (or, if the drug was delivered under pressure, even corneal ulceration) may result. The eye should be washed with water immediately and thoroughly.

It is not necessary to use preservative-containing solvents if unused portions of the remaining solutions are discarded immediately. Unused preservative-containing solutions should be refrigerated for future use.

Information for Patients —The patient should be warned to report immediately the appearance of sore throat, fever, chills, or sore mouth. Advice should be given to avoid constipation, and the patient should be made aware that alopecia may occur and that jaw pain and pain in the organs containing tumor tissue may occur. The latter is thought possibly to result from swelling of tumor tissue during its response to treatment. Scalp hair will regrow to its pretreatment extent even with continued treatment with Velban. Nausea and vomiting, although not common, may occur. Any other serious medical event should be reported to the physician.

Laboratory Tests —Since dose-limiting clinical toxicity is the result of depression of the white-blood-cell count, it is imperative that this count be obtained just before the planned dose of Velban. Following administration of Velban, a fall in the white-blood-cell count may occur. The nadir of this fall is observed from 5 to 10 days following a dose. Recovery to pretreatment levels is usually observed from 7 to 14 days after treatment. These effects will be exaggerated when preexisting bone marrow damage is present and also with the higher recommended doses (*see* Dosage and Administration). The presence of this drug or its metabolites in blood or body tissues is not known to interfere with clinical laboratory tests.

Drug Interactions —Solutions should be made with normal saline (with or without preservative) and should not be combined in the same container with any other chemical. Unused portions of the remaining solutions that do not contain preservatives should be discarded immediately.

The simultaneous oral or intravenous administration of phenytoin and antineoplastic chemotherapy combinations that included vinblastine sulfate has been reported to have reduced blood levels of the anticonvulsant and to have increased seizure activity. Dosage adjustment should be based on serial blood level monitoring. The contribution of vinblastine sulfate to this interaction is not certain. The interaction may result from either reduced absorption of phenytoin or an increase in the rate of its metabolism and elimination.

Caution should be exercised in patients concurrently taking drugs known to inhibit drug metabolism by hepatic cytochrome P450 isoenzymes in the CYP 3A subfamily, or in patients with hepatic dysfunction. Concurrent administration of vinblastine sulfate with an inhibitor of this metabolic pathway may cause an earlier onset and/or an increased severity of side effects. Enhanced toxicity has been reported in patients receiving cocomitant erythromycin (*see* Adverse Reactions).

Carcinogenesis, Mutagenesis, Impairment of Fertility —Aspermia has been reported in man. Animal studies suggest that teratogenic effects may occur. *See* Warnings regarding impaired fertility. Animal studies have shown metaphase arrest and degenerative changes in germ cells. Amenorrhea has occurred in some patients treated with the combination consisting of an alkylating agent, procarbazine, prednisone, and Velban. Its occurrence was related to the total dose of these 4 agents used. Recovery of menses was frequent. The same combination of drugs given to male patients produced azoospermia; if spermatogenesis did return, it was not likely to do so with less than 2 years of unmaintained remission.

Mutagenicity —Tests in *Salmonella typhimurium* and with the dominant lethal assay in mice failed to demonstrate mutagenicity. Sperm abnormalities have been noted in mice. Velban has produced an increase in micronuclei formation in bone marrow cells of mice; however, since Velban inhibits mitotic spindle formation, it cannot be concluded that this is evidence of mutagenicity. Additional studies in mice demonstrated no reduction in fertility of males. Chromosomal translocations did occur in male mice. First-generation male offspring of these mice were not heterozygous translocation carriers.

In vitro tests using hamster lung cells in culture have produced chromosomal changes, including chromatid breaks and exchanges, whereas tests using another type of hamster cell failed to demonstrate mutation. Breaks and aberrations were not observed on chromosome analysis of marrow cells from patients being treated with this drug.

It is not clear from the literature how this drug affects synthesis of DNA and RNA. Some believe that there is no interference. Others believe that vinblastine interferes with nucleic acid metabolism but may not do so by direct effect but possibly as the result of biochemical disturbance in some other part of the molecular organization of the cell. No inhibition of RNA synthesis occurred in rat hepatoma cells exposed in culture to noncytotoxic levels of vinblastine. Conflicting results have been noted by others regarding interference with DNA synthesis.

Carcinogenesis —There is no currently available evidence to indicate that Velban itself has been carcinogenic in humans since the inception of its clinical use in the late 1950s. Patients treated for Hodgkin's disease have developed leukemia following radiation therapy and administration of Velban in combination with other chemotherapy including agents known to intercalate with DNA. It is not known to what extent Velban may have contributed to the appearance of leukemia. Available data in rats and mice have failed to demonstrate clearly evidence of carcinogenesis when the animals were treated with the maximum tolerated dose and with one half that dose for 6 months. This testing system demonstrated that other agents were clearly carcinogenic, whereas Velban was in the group of drugs causing slightly increased or the same tumor incidence as controls in one study and 1.5 to twofold increase in tumor incidence over controls in another study.

Usage in Pregnancy —Pregnancy Category D (*see* Warnings). Velban should be given to a pregnant woman only if clearly needed. Animal studies suggest that teratogenic effects may occur.

Pediatric Use —The dosage schedule for pediatric patients is indicated under Dosage and Administration.

Nursing Mothers —It is not known whether this drug is excreted in human milk. Because many drugs are excreted in human milk and because of the potential for serious adverse reactions from Velban in nursing infants, a decision should be made whether to discontinue nursing or the drug, taking into account the importance of the drug to the mother.

ADVERSE REACTIONS

Prior to the use of the drug, patients should be advised of the possibility of untoward symptoms.

In general, the incidence of adverse reactions attending the use of Velban appears to be related to the size of the dose employed. With the exception of epilation, leukopenia, and neurologic side effects, adverse reactions generally have not persisted for longer than 24 hours. Neurologic side effects are not common; but when they do occur, they often last for more than 24 hours. Leukopenia, the most common adverse reaction, is usually the dose-limiting factor.

The following are manifestations that have been reported as adverse reactions, in decreasing order of frequency. The most common adverse reactions are underlined:

Hematologic —Leukopenia (granulocytopenia), anemia, thrombocytopenia (myelosuppression).

Dermatologic —Alopecia is common. A single case of light sensitivity associated with this product has been reported.

Gastrointestinal —Constipation, anorexia, nausea, vomiting, abdominal pain, ileus, vesiculation of the mouth, pharyngitis, diarrhea, hemorrhagic enterocolitis, bleeding from an old peptic ulcer, rectal bleeding.

Neurologic —Numbness of digits (paresthesias), loss of deep tendon reflexes, peripheral neuritis, mental depression, headache, convulsions.

Treatment with vinca alkaloids has resulted rarely in both vestibular and auditory damage to the eighth cranial nerve. Manifestations include partial or total deafness which may be temporary or permanent, and difficulties with balance including dizziness, nystagmus, and vertigo. Particular caution is warranted when vinblastine sulfate is used in combination with other agents known to be ototoxic such as the platinum-containing oncolytics.

Cardiovascular —Hypertension. Cases of unexpected myocardial infarction and cerebrovascular accidents have occurred in patients undergoing combination chemotherapy with vinblastine, bleomycin, and cisplatin. Raynaud's phenomenon has also been reported with this combination.

Pulmonary —See Precautions.

Miscellaneous —Malaise, bone pain, weakness, pain in tumor-containing tissue, dizziness, jaw pain, skin vesiculation, hypertension, Raynaud's phenomenon when patients are being treated with Velban in combination with bleomycin and cis-platinum for testicular cancer. The syndrome of inappropriate secretion of antidiuretic hormone has occurred with higher than recommended doses.

Nausea and vomiting usually may be controlled with ease by antiemetic agents. When epilation develops, it frequently is not total; and, in some cases, hair regrows while maintenance therapy continues.

Extravasation during intravenous injection may lead to cellulitis and phlebitis. If the amount of extravasation is great, sloughing may occur.

OVERDOSAGE

Signs and Symptoms—Side effects following the use of Velban are dose related. Therefore, following administration of more than the recommended dose, patients can be expected to experience these effects in an exaggerated fashion. (*See* Clinical Pharmacology, Contraindications, Warnings, Precautions, and Adverse Reactions.) There is no specific antidote. In addition, neurotoxicity similar to that with Oncovin may be observed. Since the major route of excretion may be through the biliary system, toxicity from this drug may be increased when there is hepatic insufficiency.

Treatment—To obtain up-to-date information about the treatment of overdose, a good resource is your certified Regional Poison Control Center. Telephone numbers of certified poison control centers are listed in the *Physicians' Desk Reference (PDR)*. In managing overdosage, consider the possibility of multiple drug overdoses, interaction among drugs, and unusual drug kinetics in your patient. Overdoses of Velban have been reported rarely. The following is provided to serve as a guide should such an overdose be encountered.

Supportive care should include the following: (1) prevention of side effects that result from the syndrome of inappropriate secretion of antidiuretic hormone (this would include restriction of the volume of daily fluid intake to that of the urine output plus insensible loss and perhaps the administration of a diuretic affecting the function of the loop of Henle and the distal tubule); (2) administration of an anticonvulsant; (3) prevention of ileus; (4) monitoring the cardiovascular system; and (5) determining daily blood counts for guidance in transfusion requirements and assessing the risk of infection. The major effect of excessive doses of Velban will be myelosuppression, which may be life threatening. There is no information regarding the effectiveness of dialysis nor of cholestyramine for the treatment of overdosage.

Velban in the dry state is irregularly and unpredictably absorbed from the gastrointestinal tract following oral administration. Absorption of the solution has not been studied. If vinblastine is swallowed, activated charcoal in a water slurry may be given by mouth along with a cathartic. The use of cholestyramine in this situation has not been reported.

Symptoms of overdose will appear when greater-than-recommended doses are given. Any dose of Velban that results in elimination of platelets and neutrophils from blood and marrow and their precursors from marrow should be considered life threatening. The exact dose that will do this in all patients is unknown. Overdoses occurring during prolonged, consecutive-day infusions may be more toxic than the same total dose given by rapid intravenous injection. The intravenous median lethal dose in mice is 10 mg/kg body weight; in rats, it is 2.9 mg/kg. The oral median lethal dose in rats is 7 mg/kg.

Protect the patient's airway and support ventilation and perfusion. Meticulously monitor and maintain, within acceptable limits, the patient's vital signs, blood gases, serum electrolytes, etc. Absorption of drugs from the gastrointestinal tract may be decreased by giving activated charcoal, which, in many cases, is more effective than emesis or lavage; consider charcoal instead of or in addition to gastric emptying if the drug has been swallowed. Repeated doses of charcoal over time may hasten elimination of some drugs that have been absorbed. Safeguard the patient's airway when employing gastric emptying or charcoal.

DOSAGE AND ADMINISTRATION

***Caution*—It is extremely important that the needle be properly positioned in the vein before this product is injected.**

If leakage into surrounding tissue should occur during intravenous administration of Velban, it may cause considerable irritation. The injection should be discontinued immediately, and any remaining portion of the dose should then be introduced into another vein. Local injection of hyaluronidase and the application of moderate heat to the area of leakage help disperse the drug and are thought to minimize discomfort and the possibility of cellulitis.

There are variations in the depth of the leukopenic response that follows therapy with Velban. For this reason, it is recommended that the drug be given no more frequently than *once every 7 days.*

Adult Patients—It is wise to initiate therapy for adults by administering a single intravenous dose of 3.7 mg/m^2 of body surface area (bsa). Thereafter, white-blood-cell counts should be made to determine the patient's sensitivity to Velban.

A simplified and conservative incremental approach to dosage *at weekly intervals* may be outlined as follows:

First dose	3.7	mg/m^2 bsa
Second dose	5.5	mg/m^2 bsa
Third dose	7.4	mg/m^2 bsa
Fourth dose	9.25	mg/m^2 bsa
Fifth dose	11.1	mg/m^2 bsa

The above mentioned increases may be used until a maximum dose not exceeding 18.5 mg/m^2 bsa for adults is reached. The dose should not be increased after that dose which reduces the white-cell count to approximately 3,000 $cells/mm^3$. In some adults, 3.7 mg/m^2 bsa may produce this leukopenia; other adults may require more than 11.1 mg/m^2 bsa; and, very rarely, as much as 18.5 mg/m^2 bsa may be necessary. For most adult patients, however, the weekly dose will prove to be 5.5 to 7.4 mg/m^2 bsa.

When the dose of Velban which will produce the above degree of leukopenia has been established, a dose of *1 increment smaller* than this should be administered at weekly intervals for maintenance. Thus, the patient is receiving the maximum dose that does not cause leukopenia. *It should be emphasized that, even though 7 days have elapsed, the next dose of Velban should not be given until the white-cell count has returned to at least 4,000/mm³.* In some cases, oncolytic activity may be encountered before leukopenic effect. When this occurs, there is no need to increase the size of subsequent doses (*see* Precautions).

Pediatric Patients—A review of published literature from 1993 to 1995 showed that initial doses of Velban in pediatric patients varied depending on the schedule used and whether Velban was administered as a single agent or incorporated within a particular chemotherapeutic regimen. As a single agent for Letterer-Siwe disease (histiocytosis X), the initial dose of Velban was reported as 6.5 mg/m^2. When Velban was used in combination with other chemotherapeutic agents for the treatment of Hodgkin's disease, the initial dose was reported as 6 mg/m^2. For testicular germ cell carcinomas, the initial dose of Velban was reported as 3 mg/m^2 in a combination regimen. Dose modifications should be guided by hematologic tolerance.

Patients with Renal or Hepatic Impairment—A reduction of 50% in the dose of Velban is recommended for patients having a direct serum bilirubin value above 3 mg/100 mL. Since metabolism and excretion are primarily hepatic, no modification is recommended for patients with impaired renal function.

The duration of maintenance therapy varies according to the disease being treated and the combination of antineoplastic agents being used. There are differences of opinion regarding the duration of maintenance therapy with the same protocol for a particular disease; for example, various durations have been used with the MOPP program in treating Hodgkin's disease. Prolonged chemotherapy for maintaining remissions involves several risks, among which are life-threatening infectious diseases, sterility, and possibly the appearance of other cancers through suppression of immune surveillance.

In some disorders, survival following complete remission may not be as prolonged as that achieved with shorter periods of maintenance therapy. On the other hand, failure to provide maintenance therapy in some patients may lead to unnecessary relapse; complete remissions in patients with testicular cancer, unless maintained for at least 2 years, often result in early relapse.

To prepare a solution containing 1 mg of Velban/mL, add 10 mL of Bacteriostatic Sodium Chloride Injection (preserved with benzyl alcohol) or 10 mL of Sodium Chloride Injection (unpreserved) to the 10 mg of Velban in the sterile vial. Do not use other solutions. The drug dissolves instantly to give a clear solution.

Parenteral drug products should be inspected visually for particulate matter and discoloration prior to administration, whenever solution and container permit.

Unused portions of the remaining solutions made with normal saline that do not contain preservatives should be discarded immediately. Unused preservative-containing solutions made with normal saline may be stored in a refrigerator for future use for a maximum of 28 days.

The dose of Velban (calculated to provide the desired amount) may be injected either into the tubing of a running intravenous infusion or directly into a vein. The latter procedure is readily adaptable to outpatient therapy. In either case, the injection may be completed in about 1 minute. If care is taken to insure that the needle is securely within the vein and that no solution containing Velban is spilled extravascularly, cellulitis and/or phlebitis will not occur. To minimize further the possibility of extravascular spillage, it is suggested that the syringe and needle be rinsed with venous blood before withdrawal of the needle. The dose should not be diluted in large volumes of diluent (ie, 100 to 250 mL) or given intravenously for prolonged periods (ranging from 30 to 60 minutes or more), since this frequently results in irritation of the vein and increases the chance of extravasation.

Because of the enhanced possibility of thrombosis, it is considered inadvisable to inject a solution of Velban into an extremity in which the circulation is impaired or potentially impaired by such conditions as compressing or invading neoplasm, phlebitis, or varicosity.

Procedures for proper handling and disposal of anticancer drugs should be considered. Several guidelines on this subject have been published. There is no general agreement that all of the procedures recommended in the guidelines are necessary or appropriate.

Special Dispensing Information—When dispensing Velban in other than the original container, eg, a syringe containing a specific dose, it is imperative that it be packaged in an overwrap bearing the statement: "DO NOT REMOVE COVERING UNTIL MOMENT OF INJECTION. FATAL IF GIVEN INTRATHECALLY. FOR INTRAVENOUS USE ONLY" (*see* Warnings).

HOW SUPPLIED

Vials, 10 mg, 10-mL size (No. 687)—(1s) NDC 0002-1452-01. The vials should be stored in a refrigerator (2° to 8°C, or 36° to 46°F) to assure extended stability.

CAUTION—Federal (USA) law prohibits dispensing without prescription.

REFERENCES

1. Recommendations for the Safe Handling of Parenteral Antineoplastic Drugs, NIH Publication No. 83-2621. For sale by the Superintendent of Documents, U.S. Government Printing Office, Washington, DC 20402.
2. AMA Council Report, Guidelines for Handling Parenteral Antineoplastics. JAMA, 1985;253(11):1590-1592.
3. National Study Commission on Cytotoxic Exposure–Recommendations for Handling Cytotoxic Agents. Available from Louis P. Jeffrey, ScD., Chairman, National Study Commission on Cytotoxic Exposure, Massachusetts College of Pharmacy and Allied Health Sciences, 179 Longwood Avenue, Boston, Massachusetts 02115.
4. Clinical Oncological Society of Australia, Guidelines and Recommendations for Safe Handling of Antineoplastic Agents. Med J Australia, 1983;1:426-428.
5. Jones RB, et al: Safe Handling of Chemotherapeutic Agents: A Report from the Mount Sinai Medical Center. CA–A Cancer Journal for Clinicians, 1983; (Sept/Oct)258-263.
6. American Society of Hospital Pharmacists Technical Assistance Bulletin on Handling Cytotoxic and Hazardous Drugs. Am J Hosp Pharm, 1990;47:1033-1049.
7. OSHA Work-Practice Guidelines for Personnel Dealing with Cytotoxic (Antineoplastic) Drugs. Am J Hosp Pharm, 1986;43:1193-1204.

Text revised October 2, 1997

PA 2564 AMP [100297]

ZINC-INSULIN CRYSTALS **OTC**

See under Iletin® (insulin).

ZYPREXA® ℞

[zī-prex-ah]

(Olanzapine)

DESCRIPTION

ZYPREXA® (olanzapine) is an antipsychotic agent that belongs to the thienobenzodiazepine class. The chemical designation is 2-methyl-4-(4-methyl-1-piperazinyl)-10*H*-thieno[2,3-*b*] [1,5]benzodiazepine. The molecular formula is $C_{17}H_{20}N_4S$, which corresponds to a molecular weight of 312.44. The chemical structure is:

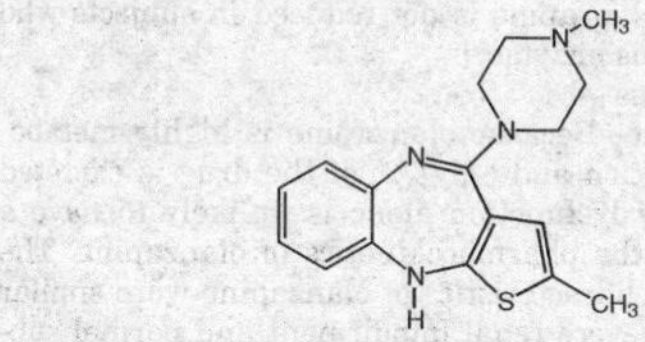

Olanzapine is a yellow crystalline solid, which is practically insoluble in water.

ZYPREXA tablets are intended for oral administration only. Each tablet contains olanzapine equivalent to 2.5 mg (8 μmol), 5 mg (16 μmol), 7.5 mg (24 μmol), or 10 mg (32 μmol). Inactive ingredients are carnauba wax, color mixture white, crospovidone, FD&C Blue No. 2 Aluminum Lake, hydroxypropyl cellulose, hydroxypropyl methylcellulose, lactose, magnesium stearate, microcrystalline cellulose, and other inactive ingredients.

CLINICAL PHARMACOLOGY

Pharmacodynamics:

Olanzapine is a selective monoaminergic antagonist with high affinity binding to the following receptors: serotonin $5HT_{2A/2C}$ (K_i=4 and 11 nM, respectively), dopamine D_{1-4} (K_i=11–31 nM), muscarinic M_{1-5} (K_i=1.9–25 nM), histamine H_1 (K_i=7 nM), and adrenergic α_1 receptors (K_i=19 nM). Olanzapine binds weakly to $GABA_A$, BZD, and β adrenergic receptors (K_i > 10 μM).

The mechanism of action of olanzapine, as with other antipsychotic drugs, is unknown. However, it has been proposed that this drug's antipsychotic activity is mediated through a combination of dopamine and serotonin type 2 ($5HT_2$) antagonism. Antagonism at receptors other than dopamine and $5HT_2$ with similar receptor affinities may explain some of the other therapeutic and side effects of olanzapine. Olanzapine's antagonism of muscarinic M_{1-5} receptors may explain its anticholinergic effects. Olanzapine's antagonism of histamine H_1 receptors may explain the somnolence observed with this drug. Olanzapine's antagonism of adrenergic α_1 receptors may explain the orthostatic hypotension observed with this drug.

Pharmacokinetics:

Olanzapine is well absorbed and reaches peak concentrations in approximately 6 hours following an oral dose. It is eliminated extensively by first pass metabolism, with approximately 40% of the dose metabolized before reaching the systemic circulation. Food does not affect the rate or extent of olanzapine absorption.

Olanzapine displays linear kinetics over the clinical dosing range. Its half-life ranges from 21 to 54 hours (5th to 95th percentile; mean of 30 hr), and apparent plasma clearance ranges from 12 to 47 L/hr (5th to 95th percentile; mean of 25 L/hr).

Administration of olanzapine once daily leads to steady-state concentrations in about one week that are approximately twice the concentrations after single doses. Plasma concentrations, half-life, and clearance of olanzapine may vary between individuals on the basis of smoking status, gender and age (*see* Special Populations).

Continued on next page

*** Identi-Code® symbol. This product information was prepared in June 1998. Current information on these and other products of Eli Lilly and Company may be obtained by direct inquiry to Lilly Research Laboratories, Lilly Corporate Center, Indianapolis, Indiana 46285, (800) 545-5979.**

Zyprexa—Cont.

Olanzapine is extensively distributed throughout the body, with a volume of distribution of approximately 1000 L. It is 93% bound to plasma proteins over the concentration range of 7 to 1100 ng/mL, binding primarily to albumin and α_1-acid glycoprotein.

Metabolism and Elimination—Following a single oral dose of ^{14}C labeled olanzapine, 7% of the dose of olanzapine was recovered in the urine as unchanged drug, indicating that olanzapine is highly metabolized. Approximately 57% and 30% of the dose was recovered in the urine and feces, respectively. In the plasma, olanzapine accounted for only 12% of the AUC for total radioactivity, indicating significant exposure to metabolites. After multiple dosing, the major circulating metabolites were the 10-N-glucuronide, present at steady state at 44% of the concentration of olanzapine, and 4′-N-desmethyl olanzapine, present at steady state at 31% of the concentration of olanzapine. Both metabolites lack pharmacological activity at the concentrations observed.

Direct glucuronidation and cytochrome P450 (CYP) mediated oxidation are the primary metabolic pathways for olanzapine. In vitro studies suggest that CYPs 1A2 and 2D6, and the flavin-containing monooxygenase system are involved in olanzapine oxidation. CYP2D6 mediated oxidation appears to be a minor metabolic pathway in vivo, because the clearance of olanzapine is not reduced in subjects who are deficient in this enzyme.

Special Populations—

Renal Impairment—Because olanzapine is highly metabolized before excretion and only 7% of the drug is excreted unchanged, renal dysfunction alone is unlikely to have a major impact on the pharmacokinetics of olanzapine. The pharmacokinetic characteristics of olanzapine were similar in patients with severe renal impairment and normal subjects, indicating that dosage adjustment based upon the degree of renal impairment is not required. In addition, olanzapine is not removed by dialysis. The effect of renal impairment on metabolite elimination has not been studied.

Hepatic Impairment—Although the presence of hepatic impairment may be expected to reduce the clearance of olanzapine, a study of the effect of impaired liver function in subjects (n=6) with clinically significant (Childs Pugh Classification A and B) cirrhosis revealed little effect on the pharmacokinetics of olanzapine.

Age—In a study involving 24 healthy subjects, the mean elimination half-life of olanzapine was about 1.5 times greater in elderly (>65 years) than in non-elderly subjects (≤65 years). Caution should be used in dosing the elderly, especially if there are other factors that might additively influence drug metabolism and/or pharmacodynamic sensitivity (*see* DOSAGE AND ADMINISTRATION).

Gender—Clearance of olanzapine is approximately 30% lower in women than in men. There were, however, no apparent differences between men and women in effectiveness or adverse effects. Dosage modifications based on gender should not be needed.

Smoking Status—Olanzapine clearance is about 40% higher in smokers than in nonsmokers, although dosage modifications are not routinely recommended.

Race—No specific pharmacokinetic study was conducted to investigate the effects of race. A cross-study comparison between data obtained in Japan and data obtained in the US suggests that exposure to olanzapine may be about 2-fold greater in the Japanese when equivalent doses are administered. Clinical trial safety and efficacy data, however, did not suggest clinically significant differences among Caucasian patients, patients of African descent, and a third pooled category including Asian and Hispanic patients. Dosage modifications for race are, therefore, not recommended.

Combined Effects—The combined effects of age, smoking, and gender could lead to substantial pharmacokinetic differences in populations. The clearance in young smoking males, for example, may be 3 times higher than that in elderly nonsmoking females. Dosing modification may be necessary in patients who exhibit a combination of factors that may result in slower metabolism of olanzapine (*see* DOSAGE AND ADMINISTRATION).

Clinical Efficacy Data:

The efficacy of olanzapine in the management of the manifestations of psychotic disorders was established in 2 short-term (6-week) controlled trials of psychotic inpatients who met DSM III-R criteria for schizophrenia. A single haloperidol arm was included as a comparative treatment in one of the two trials, but this trial did not compare these two drugs on the full range of clinically relevant doses for both.

Several instruments were used for assessing psychiatric signs and symptoms in these studies, among them the Brief Psychiatric Rating Scale (BPRS), a multi-item inventory of general psychopathology traditionally used to evaluate the effects of drug treatment in psychosis. The BPRS psychosis cluster (conceptual disorganization, hallucinatory behavior, suspiciousness, and unusual though content) is considered a particularly useful subset for assessing actively psychotic schizophrenic patients. A second traditional assessment, the Clinical Global Impression (CGI), reflects the impression of a skilled observer, fully familiar with the manifestations of schizophrenia, about the overall clinical state of the patient. In addition, two more recently developed but less well evaluated scales were employed; these included the 30-item Positive and Negative Symptoms Scale (PANSS), in which is embedded the 18 items of the BPRS, and the Scale for Assessing Negative Symptoms (SANS). The trial summaries below focus on the following outcomes: PANSS total and/or BPRS total; BPRS psychosis cluster; PANSS negative subscale or SANS; and CGI Severity. The results of the trials follow:

(1) In a 6-week, placebo-controlled trial (n=149) involving two fixed olanzapine doses of 1 and 10 mg/day (once daily schedule), olanzapine, at 10 mg/day (but not at 1 mg/day), was superior to placebo on the PANSS total score (also on the extracted BPRS total), on the BPRS psychosis cluster, on the PANSS Negative subscale, and on CGI Severity.

(2) In a 6-week, placebo-controlled trial (n=253) involving 3 fixed dose ranges of olanzapine (5.0±2.5 mg/day, 10.0±2.5 mg/day, and 15.0±2.5 mg/day) on a once daily schedule, the two highest olanzapine dose groups (actual mean doses of 12 and 16 mg/day, respectively) were superior to placebo on BPRS total score, BPRS psychosis cluster, and CGI severity score; the highest olanzapine dose group was superior to placebo on the SANS. There was no clear advantage for the high dose group over the medium dose group.

Examination of population subsets (race and gender) did not reveal any differential responsiveness on the basis of these subgroupings.

INDICATIONS AND USAGE

ZYPREXA is indicated for the management of the manifestations of psychotic disorders.

The antipsychotic efficacy of ZYPREXA was established in short-term (6-week) controlled trials of schizophrenic inpatients (*see* CLINICAL PHARMACOLOGY).

The effectiveness of ZYPREXA in long-term use, that is, for more than 6 weeks, has not been systematically evaluated in controlled trials. Therefore, the physician who elects to use ZYPREXA for extended periods should periodically re-evaluate the long-term usefulness of the drug for the individual patient (*see* DOSAGE AND ADMINISTRATION).

CONTRAINDICATIONS

ZYPREXA is contraindicated in patients with a known hypersensitivity to the product.

WARNINGS

Neuroleptic Malignant Syndrome (NMS)—A potentially fatal symptom complex sometimes referred to as Neuroleptic Malignant Syndrome (NMS) has been reported in association with administration of antipsychotic drugs. Clinical manifestations of NMS are hyperpyrexia, muscle rigidity, altered mental status and evidence of autonomic instability (irregular pulse or blood pressure, tachycardia, diaphoresis and cardiac dysrhythmia). Additional signs may include elevated creatinine phosphokinase, myoglobinuria (rhabdomyolysis), and acute renal failure.

The diagnostic evaluation of patients with this syndrome is complicated. In arriving at a diagnosis, it is important to exclude cases where the clinical presentation includes both serious medical illness (e.g., pneumonia, systemic infection, etc.) and untreated or inadequately treated extrapyramidal signs and symptoms (EPS). Other important considerations in the differential diagnosis include central anticholinergic toxicity, heat stroke, drug fever, and primary central nervous system pathology.

The management of NMS should include: 1) immediate discontinuation of antipsychotic drugs and other drugs not essential to concurrent therapy; 2) intensive symptomatic treatment and medical monitoring; and 3) treatment of any concomitant serious medical problems for which specific treatments are available. There is no general agreement about specific pharmacological treatment regimens for NMS.

If a patient requires antipsychotic drug treatment after recovery from NMS, the potential reintroduction of drug therapy should be carefully considered. The patient should be carefully monitored, since recurrences of NMS have been reported.

Tardive Dyskinesia—A syndrome of potentially irreversible, involuntary, dyskinetic movements may develop in patients treated with antipsychotic drugs. Although the prevalence of the syndrome appears to be highest among the elderly, especially elderly women, it is impossible to rely upon prevalence estimates to predict, at the inception of antipsychotic treatment, which patients are likely to develop the syndrome. Whether antipsychotic drug products differ in their potential to cause tardive dyskinesia is unknown.

The risk of developing tardive dyskinesia and the likelihood that it will become irreversible are believed to increase as the duration of treatment and the total cumulative dose of antipsychotic drugs administered to the patient increase. However, the syndrome can develop, although much less commonly, after relatively brief treatment periods at low doses.

There is no known treatment for established cases of tardive dyskinesia, although the syndrome may remit, partially or completely, if antipsychotic treatment is withdrawn. Antipsychotic treatment, itself, however, may suppress (or partially suppress) the signs and symptoms of the syndrome and thereby may possibly mask the underlying process. The effect that symptomatic suppression has upon the long-term course of the syndrome is unknown.

Given these considerations, olanzapine should be prescribed in a manner that is most likely to minimize the occurrence of tardive dyskinesia. Chronic antipsychotic treatment should generally be reserved for patients (1) who suffer from a chronic illness that is known to respond to antipsychotic drugs, and (2) for whom alternative, equally effective, but potentially less harmful treatments are not available or appropriate. In patients who do require chronic treatment, the smallest dose and the shortest duration of treatment producing a satisfactory clinical response should be sought. The need for continued treatment should be reassessed periodically.

If signs and symptoms of tardive dyskinesia appear in a patient on olanzapine, drug discontinuation should be considered. However, some patients may require treatment with olanzapine despite the presence of the syndrome.

PRECAUTIONS

General

Orthostatic Hypotension—Olanzapine may induce orthostatic hypotension associated with dizziness, tachycardia, and in some patients, syncope, especially during the initial dose-titration period, probably reflecting its α_1-adrenergic antagonistic properties. Syncope was reported in 0.6% (15/2500) of olanzapine-treated patients in phase 2-3 studies. The risk of orthostatic hypotension and syncope may be minimized by initiating therapy with 5 mg QD (*see* DOSAGE AND ADMINISTRATION). A more gradual titration to the target dose should be considered if hypotension occurs. Olanzapine should be used with particular caution in patients with known cardiovascular disease (history of myocardial infarction or ischemia, heart failure, or conduction abnormalities), cerebrovascular disease, and conditions which would predispose patients to hypotension (dehydration, hypovolemia, and treatment with antihypertensive medications).

Seizures—During premarketing testing, seizures occurred in 0.9% (22/2500) of olanzapine-treated patients. There were confounding factors that may have contributed to the occurrence of seizures in many of these cases. Olanzapine should be used cautiously in patients with a history of seizures or with conditions that potentially lower the seizure threshold, e.g., Alzheimer's dementia. Conditions that lower the seizure threshold may be more prevalent in a population of 65 years or older.

Hyperprolactinemia—As with other drugs that antagonize dopamine D_2 receptors, olanzapine elevates prolactin levels, and a modest elevation persists during chronic administration. Tissue culture experiments indicate that approximately one-third of human breast cancers are prolactin dependent in vitro, a factor of potential importance if the prescription of these drugs is contemplated in a patient with previously detected breast cancer of this type. Although disturbances such as galactorrhea, amenorrhea, gynecomastia, and impotence have been reported with prolactin-elevating compounds, the clinical significance of elevated serum prolactin levels is unknown for most patients. As is common with compounds which increase prolactin release, an increase in mammary gland neoplasia was observed in the olanzapine carcinogenicity studies conducted in mice and rats (*see* Carcinogenesis). However, neither clinical studies nor epidemiologic studies have shown an association between chronic administration of this class of drugs and tumorigenesis in humans; the available evidence is considered too limited to be conclusive.

Transaminase Elevations—In placebo-controlled studies, clinically significant ALT (SGPT) elevations (≥3 times the upper limit of the normal range) were observed in 2% (6/243) of patients exposed to olanzapine compared to none (0/115) of the placebo patients. None of these patients experienced jaundice. In two of these patients, liver enzymes decreased toward normal despite continued treatment and in two others, enzymes decreased upon discontinuation of olanzapine. In the remaining two patients, one, seropositive for hepatitis C, had persistent enzyme elevation for four months after discontinuation, and the other had insufficient follow-up to determine if enzymes normalized.

Within the larger premarketing database of about 2400 patients with baseline SGPT ≤90 IU/L, the incidence of SGPT elevation to >200 IU/L was 2% (50/2381). Again, none of these patients experienced jaundice or other symptoms attributable to liver impairment and most had transient changes that tended to normalize while olanzapine treatment was continued.

Among all 2500 patients in clinical trials, about 1% (23/2500) discontinued treatment due to transaminase increases.

Caution should be exercised in patients with signs and symptoms of hepatic impairment, in patients with pre-existing conditions associated with limited hepatic functional reserve, and in patients who are being treated with potentially hepatotoxic drugs. Periodic assessment of transaminases is recommended in patients with significant hepatic disease (*see* Laboratory Tests).

Potential for Cognitive and Motor Impairment—Somnolence was a commonly reported adverse event associated with olanzapine treatment, occurring at an incidence of 26% in olanzapine patients compared to 15% in placebo patients. This adverse event was also dose related. Somnolence led to discontinuation in 0.4% (9/2500) of patients in the premarketing database.

Since olanzapine has the potential to impair judgment, thinking, or motor skills, patients should be cautioned about operating hazardous machinery, including automobiles, until they are reasonably certain that olanzapine therapy does not affect them adversely.

Body Temperature Regulation—Disruption of the body's ability to reduce core body temperature has been attributed to antipsychotic agents. Appropriate care is advised when prescribing olanzapine for patients who will be experiencing conditions which may contribute to an elevation in core body temperature, e.g., exercising strenuously, exposure to extreme heat, receiving concomitant medication with anticholinergic activity, or being subject to dehydration.

Dysphagia—Esophageal dysmotility and aspiration have been associated with antipsychotic drug use. Two olanzapine-treated patients in a study of olanzapine in Alzheimer's dementia died from aspiration pneumonia. One of these patients had experienced dysphagia prior to the development of aspiration pneumonia. Aspiration pneumonia is a common cause of morbidity and mortality in patients with advanced Alzheimer's dementia. Olanzapine and other antipsychotic drugs should be used cautiously in patients at risk for aspiration pneumonia.

Suicide—The possibility of a suicide attempt is inherent in schizophrenia, and close supervision of high-risk patients should accompany drug therapy. Prescriptions for olanzapine should be written for the smallest quantity of tablets consistent with good patient management, in order to reduce the risk of overdose.

Use in Patients with Concomitant Illness—Clinical experience with olanzapine in patients with certain concomitant systemic illnesses (*see* Renal Impairment and Hepatic Impairment *under* CLINICAL PHARMACOLOGY, Special Populations) is limited.

Olanzapine exhibits in vitro muscarinic receptor affinity. In premarketing clinical trials with olanzapine, olanzapine was associated with constipation, dry mouth, and tachycardia, all adverse events possibly related to cholinergic antagonism. Such adverse events were not often the basis for discontinuations from olanzapine, but olanzapine should be used with caution in patients with clinically significant prostatic hypertrophy, narrow angle glaucoma, or a history of paralytic ileus.

Olanzapine has not been evaluated or used to any appreciable extent in patients with a recent history of myocardial infarction or unstable heart disease. Patients with these diagnoses were excluded from premarketing clinical studies. Because of the risk of orthostatic hypotension with olanzapine, caution should be observed in cardiac patients (*see* Orthostatic Hypotension).

Information for Patients—Physicians are advised to discuss the following issues with patients for whom they prescribe olanzapine:

Orthostatic Hypotension—Patients should be advised of the risk of orthostatic hypotension, especially during the period of initial dose titration and in association with the use of concomitant drugs that may potentiate the orthostatic effect of olanzapine, e.g., diazepam or alcohol (*see* Drug Interactions).

Interference with Cognitive and Motor Performance—Because olanzapine has the potential to impair judgment, thinking, or motor skills, patients should be cautioned about operating hazardous machinery, including automobiles, until they are reasonably certain that olanzapine therapy does not affect them adversely.

Pregnancy—Patients should be advised to notify their physician if they become pregnant or intend to become pregnant during therapy with olanzapine.

Nursing—Patients should be advised not to breast-feed an infant if they are taking olanzapine.

Concomitant Medication—Patients should be advised to inform their physicians if they are taking, or plan to take, any prescription or over-the-counter drugs, since there is a potential for interactions.

Alcohol—Patients should be advised to avoid alcohol while taking olanzapine.

Heat Exposure and Dehydration—Patients should be advised regarding appropriate care in avoiding overheating and dehydration.

Laboratory Tests—Periodic assessment of transaminases is recommended in patients with significant hepatic disease (*see* Transaminase Elevations).

Drug Interactions—The risks of using olanzapine in combination with other drugs have not been extensively evaluated in systematic studies. Given the primary CNS effects of olanzapine, caution should be used when olanzapine is taken in combination with other centrally acting drugs and alcohol.

Because of its potential for inducing hypotension, olanzapine may enhance the effects of certain antihypertensive agents.

Olanzapine may antagonize the effects of levodopa and dopamine agonists.

The Effect of Other Drugs on Olanzapine—Agents that induce CYP1A2 or glucuronyl transferase enzymes, such as omeprazole and rifampin, may cause an increase in olanzapine clearance. Inhibitors of CYP1A2 (e.g., fluvoxamine) could potentially inhibit olanzapine elimination. Because olanzapine is metabolized by multiple enzyme systems, inhibition of a single enzyme may not appreciably decrease olanzapine clearance.

Charcoal—The administration of activated charcoal (1 g) reduced the Cmax and AUC of olanzapine by about 60%. As peak olanzapine levels are not typically obtained until about 6 hours after dosing, charcoal may be a useful treatment for olanzapine overdose.

Cimetidine and Antacids—Single doses of cimetidine (800 mg) or aluminum- and magnesium-containing antacids did not affect the oral bioavailability of olanzapine.

Carbamazepine—Carbamazepine therapy (200 mg bid) causes an approximately 50% increase in the clearance of olanzapine. This increase is likely due to the fact that carbamazepine is a potent inducer of CYP1A2 activity. Higher daily doses of carbamazepine may cause an even greater increase in olanzapine clearance.

Ethanol—Ethanol (45 mg/70 kg single dose) did not have an effect on olanzapine pharmacokinetics.

Warfarin—Warfarin (20 mg single dose) did not affect olanzapine pharmacokinetics.

Effect of Olanzapine on Other Drugs—In vitro studies utilizing human liver microsomes suggest that olanzapine has little potential to inhibit CYP1A2, CYP2C9, CYP2C19, CYP2D6, and CYP3A. Thus, olanzapine is unlikely to cause clinically important drug interactions mediated by these enzymes.

Single doses of olanzapine did not affect the pharmacokinetics of imipramine or its active metabolite desipramine, and warfarin. Multiple doses of olanzapine did not influence the kinetics of diazepam and its active metabolite N-desmethyldiazepam, lithium, ethanol, or biperiden. However, the coadministration of either diazepam or ethanol with olanzapine potentiated the orthostatic hypotension observed with olanzapine. Multiple doses of olanzapine did not affect the pharmacokinetics of theophylline or its metabolites.

Carcinogenesis, Mutagenesis, Impairment of Fertility—

Carcinogenesis—Oral carcinogenicity studies were conducted in mice and rats. Olanzapine was administered to mice in two 78-week studies at doses of 3, 10, 30/20 mg/kg/day (equivalent to 0.8-5 times the maximum recommended human daily dose on a mg/m^2 basis) and 0.25, 2, 8 mg/kg/day (equivalent to 0.06-2 times the maximum recommended human daily dose on a mg/m^2 basis). Rats were dosed for 2 years at doses of 0.25, 1, 2.5, 4 mg/kg/day (males) and 0.25, 1, 4, 8 mg/kg/day (females) (equivalent to 0.13-2 and 0.13-4 times the maximum recommended human daily dose on a mg/m^2 basis, respectively). The incidence of liver hemangiomas and hemangiosarcomas was significantly increased in one mouse study in female mice dosed at 8 mg/kg/day (2 times the maximum recommended human daily dose on a mg/m^2 basis). These tumors were not increased in another mouse study in females dosed at 10 or 30/20 mg/kg/day (2-5 times the maximum recommended human daily dose on a mg/m^2 basis); in this study, there was a high incidence of early mortalities in males of the 30/20 mg/kg/day group. The incidence of mammary gland adenomas and adenocarcinomas was significantly increased in female mice dosed at ≥ 2 mg/kg/day and in female rats dosed at ≥ 4 mg/kg/day (0.5 and 2 times the maximum recommended human daily dose on a mg/m^2 basis, respectively). Antipsychotic drugs have been shown to chronically elevate prolactin levels in rodents. Serum prolactin levels were not measured during the olanzapine carcinogenicity studies; however, measurements during subchronic toxicity studies showed that olanzapine elevated serum prolactin levels up to 4-fold in rats at the same doses used in the carcinogenicity study. An increase in mammary gland neoplasms has been found in rodents after chronic administration of other antipsychotic drugs and is considered to be prolactin mediated. The relevance for human risk of the finding of prolactin mediated endocrine tumors in rodents is unknown (*see* Hyperprolactinemia *under* PRECAUTIONS, General).

Mutagenesis—No evidence of mutagenic potential for olanzapine was found in the Ames reverse mutation test, in vivo micronucleus test in mice, the chromosomal aberration test in Chinese hamster ovary cells, unscheduled DNA synthesis test in rat hepatocytes, induction of forward mutation test in mouse lymphoma cells, or in vivo sister chromatid exchange test in bone marrow of Chinese hamsters.

Impairment of Fertility—In a fertility and reproductive performance study in rats, male mating performance, but not fertility, was impaired at a dose of 22.4 mg/kg/day and female fertility was decreased at a dose of 3 mg/kg/day (11 and 1.5 times the maximum recommended human daily dose on a mg/m^2 basis, respectively). Discontinuance of olanzapine treatment reversed the effects on male mating performance. In female rats, the precoital period was increased and the mating index reduced at 5 mg/kg/day (2.5 times the maximum recommended human daily dose on a mg/m^2 basis). Diestrous was prolonged and estrous delayed at 1.1 mg/kg/day (0.6 times the maximum recommended human daily dose on a mg/m^2 basis); therefore olanzapine may produce a delay in ovulation.

Pregnancy—

Pregnancy Category C—In reproduction studies in rats at doses up to 18 mg/kg/day and in rabbits at doses up to 30 mg/kg/day (9 and 30 times the maximum recommended human daily dose on a mg/m^2 basis, respectively) no evidence of teratogenicity was observed. In a rat teratology study, early resorptions and increased numbers of nonviable fetuses were observed at a dose of 18 mg/kg/day (9 times the maximum recommended human daily dose on a mg/m^2 basis). Gestation was prolonged at 10 mg/kg/day (5 times the maximum recommended human daily dose on a mg/m^2 basis). In a rabbit teratology study, fetal toxicity (manifested as increased resorptions and decreased fetal weight) occurred at a maternally toxic dose of 30 mg/kg/day (30 times the maximum recommended human daily dose on a mg/m^2 basis).

Placental transfer of olanzapine occurs in rat pups.

There are no adequate and well-controlled trials with olanzapine in pregnant females. Seven pregnancies were observed during clinical trials with olanzapine, including 2 resulting in normal births, 1 resulting in neonatal death due to a cardiovascular defect, 3 therapeutic abortions, and 1 spontaneous abortion. Because animal reproduction studies are not always predictive of human response, this drug should be used during pregnancy only if the potential benefit justifies the potential risk to the fetus.

Labor and Delivery—Parturition in rats was not affected by olanzapine. The effect of olanzapine on labor and delivery in humans is unknown.

Nursing Mothers—Olanzapine was excreted in milk of treated rats during lactation. It is not known if olanzapine is excreted in human milk. It is recommended that women receiving olanzapine should not breast-feed.

Pediatric Use—Safety and effectiveness in pediatric patients have not been established.

Geriatric Use—Of the 2500 patients in clinical studies with olanzapine, 11% (263) were 65 years of age or over. In general, there was no indication of any different tolerability of olanzapine in the elderly compared to younger adults. Nevertheless, the presence of factors that might decrease pharmacokinetic clearance or increase the pharmacodynamic response to olanzapine should lead to consideration of a lower starting dose (*see* PRECAUTIONS and DOSAGE AND ADMINISTRATION).

ADVERSE REACTIONS

The premarketing development program for olanzapine included over 3100 patients and/or normal subjects exposed to 1 or more doses of olanzapine. Of these 3100 subjects, 2500 were patients who participated in multiple-dose effectiveness trials, and their experience corresponded to approximately 1122 patient-years. The conditions and duration of treatment with olanzapine varied greatly and included (in overlapping categories) open-label and double-blind phases of studies, inpatients and outpatients, fixed-dose and dose-titration studies, and short-term or longer-term exposure. Adverse reactions were assessed by collecting adverse events, results of physical examinations, vital signs, weights, laboratory analytes, ECGs, chest-x-rays, and results of ophthalmologic examinations.

Adverse events during exposure were obtained by spontaneous report and recorded by clinical investigators using terminology of their own choosing. Consequently, it is not possible to provide a meaningful estimate of the proportion of individuals experiencing adverse events without first grouping similar types of events into a smaller number of standardized event categories. In the tables and tabulations that follow, standard COSTART dictionary terminology has been used to classify reported adverse events.

The stated frequencies of adverse events represent the proportion of individuals who experienced, at least once, a treatment-emergent adverse event of the type listed. An

Continued on next page

*** Identi-Code® symbol. This product information was prepared in June 1998. Current information on these and other products of Eli Lilly and Company may be obtained by direct inquiry to Lilly Research Laboratories, Lilly Corporate Center, Indianapolis, Indiana 46285, (800) 545-5979.**

Zyprexa—Cont.

event was considered treatment emergent if it occurred for the first time or worsened while receiving therapy following baseline evaluation.

Adverse Findings Observed in Short-Term, Placebo-Controlled Trials—The following findings are based on a pool of two 6-week, placebo-controlled trials in which mean olanzapine doses ranged from 7-16 mg/day.

Adverse Events Associated with Discontinuation of Treatment in Short-Term, Placebo-Controlled Trials—Overall, there was no difference in the incidence of discontinuation due to adverse events (5% for olanzapine vs 6% for placebo). However, discontinuations due to increases in SGPT were considered to be drug related (2% for olanzapine vs 0% for placebo) (see PRECAUTIONS).

Adverse Events Occurring at an Incidence of 1% or More Among Olanzapine-Treated Patients in Short-Term, Placebo-Controlled Trials—Table 1 enumerates the incidence, rounded to the nearest percent, of treatment-emergent adverse events that occurred during acute therapy (up to 6 weeks) of schizophrenia in 1% or more of patients treated with olanzapine (doses ≥2.5 mg/day) where the incidence in patients treated with olanzapine was greater than the incidence in placebo-treated patients.

The prescriber should be aware that the figures in the tables and tabulations cannot be used to predict the incidence of side effects in the course of usual medical practice where patient characteristics and other factors differ from those that prevailed in the clinical trials. Similarly, the cited frequencies cannot be compared with figures obtained from other clinical investigations involving different treatments, uses, and investigators. The cited figures, however, do provide the prescribing physician with some basis for estimating the relative contribution of drug and nondrug factors to the side effect incidence in the population studied.

Table 1
Treatment-Emergent Adverse Event Incidence in 6-Week Placebo-Controlled Clinical Trials[1]

Body System/Adverse Event	Percentage of Patients Reporting Event Olanzapine (N=248)	Placebo (N=118)
Body as a Whole		
Headache	17	15
Fever	5	3
Abdominal pain	4	2
Back pain	4	3
Chest pain	4	2
Neck rigidity	2	1
Intentional injury	1	0
Cardiovascular System		
Postural hypotension	5	2
Tachycardia	4	1
Hypotension	2	1
Digestive System		
Constipation	9	3
Dry mouth	7	4
Increased appetite	2	1
Metabolic and Nutritional Disorders		
Weight gain	6	1
Peripheral edema	2	0
Lower extremity edema	1	0
Musculoskeletal System		
Joint pain	5	3
Extremity pain (other than joint)	4	3
Twitching	2	1
Nervous System		
Somnolence	26	15
Agitation	23	17
Insomnia	20	19
Nervousness	16	14
Hostility	15	14
Dizziness	11	4
Anxiety	9	8
Personality disorder[2]	8	4
Akathisia	5	1
Hypertonia	4	3
Tremor	4	3
Amnesia	2	0
Articulation impairment	2	0
Euphoria	2	0
Stuttering	2	0
Respiratory System		
Rhinitis	10	6
Cough increased	5	3
Pharyngitis	5	3

Skin and Appendages		
Vesiculobullous rash	2	1
Special Senses		
Amblyopia	5	4
Blepharitis	2	1
Corneal lesion	1	0
Urogenital System		
Premenstrual syndrome[3]	2	0

[1] Events reported by at least 1% of patients treated with olanzapine, except the following events which had an incidence equal to or less than placebo: abnormal dreams, accidental injury, anorexia, apathy, asthenia, cogwheel rigidity, confusion, conjunctivitis, dental pain, diarrhea, depression, dysmenorrhea[3], dyspepsia, ecchymosis, emotional lability, hallucinations, hyperkinesia, hypertension, hypokinesia, joint stiffness, libido increased, myalgia, nausea, paranoid reaction, paresthesia, pruritus, rash, schizophrenic reaction, sweating, thinking abnormal, tooth caries, vaginitis[3], vomiting.
[2] Personality disorder is the COSTART term for designating non-aggressive objectionable behavior.
[3] Denominator used was for females only (olanzapine, N=41; placebo, N=23).

Commonly Observed Adverse Events in Short-Term, Placebo-Controlled Trials—The most commonly observed adverse events associated with the use of olanzapine (incidence of 5% or greater) and not observed at an equivalent incidence among placebo-treated patients (olanzapine incidence at least twice that for placebo) were:

Common Treatment-Emergent Adverse Events Associated with the Use of Olanzapine in 6-Week Trials

Adverse Event	Percentage of Patients Reporting Event	
	Olanzapine (N=248)	Placebo (N=118)
Postural hypotension	5	2
Constipation	9	3
Weight gain	6	1
Dizziness	11	4
Personality disorder[1]	8	4
Akathisia	5	1

[1] Personality disorder is the COSTART term for designating non-aggressive objectionable behavior.

Dose Dependency of Adverse Events in Short-Term, Placebo-Controlled Trials—

Extrapyramidal Symptoms: The following table enumerates the percentage of patients with treatment-emergent extrapyramidal symptoms as assessed by categorical analyses of formal rating scales during acute therapy in a controlled clinical trial comparing olanzapine at 3 fixed doses with placebo in the treatment of schizophrenia.

TREATMENT-EMERGENT EXTRAPYRAMIDAL SYMPTOMS ASSESSED BY RATING SCALES INCIDENCE IN A FIXED DOSAGE RANGE, PLACEBO-CONTROLLED CLINICAL TRIAL—ACUTE PHASE*

	Percentage of Patients		
	Placebo	Olanzapine 5 ± 2.5 mg/day	Olanzapine 10 ± 2.5 mg/day	Olanzapine 15 ± 2.5 mg/day
Parkinsonism[1]	15	14	12	14
Akathisia[2]	23	16	19	27

* No statistically significant differences.
[1] Percentage of patients with a Simpson-Angus Scale total score >3.
[2] Percentage of patients with a Barnes Akathisia Scale global score ≥2.

The following table enumerates the percentage of patients with treatment-emergent extrapyramidal symptoms as assessed by spontaneously reported adverse events during acute therapy in the same controlled clinical trial comparing olanzapine at 3 fixed doses with placebo in the treatment of schizophrenia.

TREATMENT-EMERGENT EXTRAPYRAMIDAL SYMPTOMS ASSESSED BY ADVERSE EVENTS INCIDENCE IN A FIXED DOSAGE RANGE, PLACEBO-CONTROLLED CLINICAL TRIAL—ACUTE PHASE

	Percentage of Patients Reporting Event			
	Placebo (N=68)	Olanzapine 5±2.5 mg/day (N=65)	Olanzapine 10±2.5 mg/day (N=64)	Olanzapine 15±2.5 mg/day (N=69)
Dystonic events[1]	1	3	2	3
Parkinsonism events[2]	10	8	14	20
Akathisia events[3]	1	5	11*	10*
Dyskinetic events[4]	4	0	2	1
Residual events[5]	1	2	5	1
Any extrapyramidal event	16	15	25	32*

* Statistically significantly different from placebo.
[1] Patients with the following COSTART terms were counted in this category: dystonia, generalized spasm, neck rigidity, oculogyric crisis, opisthotonos, torticollis.
[2] Patients with the following COSTART terms were counted in this category: akinesia, cogwheel rigidity, extrapyramidal syndrome, hypertonia, hypokinesia, masked facies, tremor.
[3] Patients with the following COSTART terms were counted in this category: akathisia, hyperkinesia.
[4] Patients with the following COSTART terms were counted in this category: buccoglossal syndrome, choreoathetosis, dyskinesia, tardive dyskinesia.
[5] Patients with the following COSTART terms were counted in this category: movement disorder, myoclonus, twitching.

Other Adverse Events: The following table addresses dose relatedness for other adverse events using data from a trial involving fixed dosage ranges. It enumerates the percentage of patients with treatment-emergent adverse events for the three fixed-dose range groups and placebo. The data were analyzed using the Cochran-Armitage test, excluding the placebo group, and the table includes only those adverse events for which there was a statistically significant trend.

	Percentage of Patients Reporting Event			
Adverse Event	Placebo (N=68)	Olanzapine 5±2.5 mg/day (N=65)	Olanzapine 10±2.5 mg/day (N=64)	Olanzapine 15±2.5 mg/day (N=69)
Asthenia	15	8	9	20
Dry mouth	4	3	5	13
Nausea	9	0	2	9
Somnolence	16	20	30	39
Tremor	3	0	5	7

Vital Sign Changes—Olanzapine is associated with orthostatic hypotension and tachycardia (see PRECAUTIONS).

Weight Gain—In placebo-controlled, 6-week studies, weight gain was reported in 5.6% of olanzapine patients compared to 0.8% of placebo patients. Olanzapine patients gained an average of 2.8 kg, compared to an average 0.4 kg weight loss in placebo patients; 29% of olanzapine patients gained greater than 7% of their baseline weight, compared to 3% of placebo patients. A categorization of patients at baseline on the basis of body mass index (BMI) revealed a significantly greater effect in patients with low BMI compared to normal or overweight patients; nevertheless, weight gain was greater in all 3 olanzapine groups compared to the placebo group. During long-term continuation therapy with olanzapine (238 median days of exposure), 56% of olanzapine patients met the criterion for having gained greater than 7% of their baseline weight. Average weight gain during long-term therapy was 5.4 kg.

Laboratory Changes—An assessment of the premarketing experience for olanzapine revealed an association with asymptomatic increases in SGPT, SGOT, and GGT (see PRECAUTIONS). Olanzapine administration was also as-

sociated with increases in serum prolactin (*see* PRECAUTIONS), with an asymptomatic elevation of the eosinophil in 0.3% of patients, and with an increase in CPK.

Given the concern about neutropenia associated with other psychotropic compounds and the finding of leukopenia associated with the administration of olanzapine in several animal models (*see* ANIMAL TOXICOLOGY), careful attention was given to examination of hematologic parameters in premarketing studies with olanzapine. There was no indication of a risk of clinically significant neutropenia associated with olanzapine treatment in the premarketing database for this drug.

ECG Changes—Between-group comparisons for pooled placebo-controlled trials revealed no statistically significant olanzapine/placebo differences in the proportions of patients experiencing potentially important changes in ECG parameters, including QT, QTc, and PR intervals. Olanzapine use was associated with a mean increase in heart rate of 2.4 beats per minute compared to no change among placebo patients. This slight tendency to tachycardia may be related to olanzapine's potential for inducing orthostatic changes (*see* PRECAUTIONS).

Other Adverse Events Observed During the Premarketing Evaluation of Olanzapine—Following is a list of COSTART terms that reflect treatment-emergent adverse events as defined in the introduction to the ADVERSE REACTIONS section reported by patients treated with olanzapine at multiple doses ≥1 mg/day during any phase of a trial within the database of 2500 patients. All reported events are included except those already listed in Table 1 or elsewhere in labeling, those events for which a drug cause was remote, those event terms which were so general as to be uninformative, and events reported only once and which did not have a substantial probability of being acutely life-threatening. It is important to emphasize that, although the events reported occurred during treatment with olanzapine, they were not necessarily caused by it.

Events are further categorized by body system and listed in order of decreasing frequency according to the following definitions: frequent adverse events are those occurring in at least 1/100 patients (only those not already listed in the tabulated results from placebo-controlled trials appear in this listing); infrequent adverse events are those occurring in 1/100 to 1/1000 patients; rare events are those occurring in fewer than 1/1000 patients.

Body as a Whole—*Frequent:* flu syndrome and suicide attempt; *Infrequent:* chills, chills and fever, face edema, hangover effect, malaise, moniliasis, neck pain, pelvic pain, and photosensitivity reaction; *Rare:* abdomen enlarged and sudden death.

Cardiovascular System—*Infrequent:* cerebrovascular accident, hemorrhage, migraine, palpitation, vasodilatation, and ventricular extrasystoles; *Rare:* heart arrest.

Digestive System—*Frequent:* increased salivation, nausea and vomiting, and thirst; *Infrequent:* aphthous stomatitis, dysphagia, eructation, esophagitis, fecal incontinence, flatulence, gastritis, gastroenteritis, gingivitis, glossitis, hepatitis, melena, mouth ulceration, oral moniliasis, peridontal abscess, rectal hemorrhage, stomatitis, and tongue edema; *Rare:* enteritis, esophageal ulcer, and tongue discoloration.

Endocrine System—*Infrequent:* diabetes mellitus and goiter; *Rare:* diabetic acidosis.

Hemic and Lymphatic System—*Infrequent:* cyanosis, leukocytosis, lymphadenopathy, and thrombocythemia.

Metabolic and Nutritional Disorders—*Frequent:* weight loss; *Infrequent:* alkaline phosphatase increased, bilirubinemia, dehydration, hyperglycemia, hyperkalemia, hyperuricemia, hypoglycemia, hypokalemia, hyponatremia, ketosis, and water intoxication; *Rare:* hypercholesteremia and hyperlipemia.

Musculoskeletal System—*Infrequent:* arthritis, back and hip pain, bursitis, leg cramps, myasthenia, and rheumatoid arthritis; *Rare:* bone pain and myopathy.

Nervous System—*Frequent:* tardive dyskinesia; *Infrequent:* abnormal gait, alcohol misuse, antisocial reaction, ataxia, CNS stimulation, coma, delirium, depersonalization, hypesthesia, hypotonia, incoordination, libido decreased, obsessive compulsive symptoms, phobias, somatization, stimulant misuse, stupor, vertigo, and withdrawal syndrome; *Rare:* facial paralysis, neuralgia, nystagmus, and subarachnoid hemorrhage.

Respiratory System—*Frequent:* dyspnea; *Infrequent:* apnea, asthma, epistaxis, hemoptysis, hyperventilation, and voice alteration; *Rare:* laryngitis.

Skin and Appendages—*Infrequent:* alopecia, contact dermatitis, dry skin, eczema, hirsutism, seborrhea, skin ulcer, and urticaria; *Rare:* maculopapular rash and skin discoloration.

Special Senses—*Infrequent:* cataract, deafness, diplopia, dry eyes, ear pain, eye hemorrhage, eye inflammation, eye pain, ocular muscle abnormality, taste perversion, and tinnitus; *Rare:* abnormality of accommodation, glaucoma, keratoconjunctivitis, macular hypopigmentation, mydriasis, and pigment deposits lens.

Urogenital System—*Frequent:* hematuria, metrorrhagia*, urinary incontinence, and urinary tract infection; *Infrequent:* abnormal ejaculation*, amenorrhea*, breast pain, cystitis, decreased menstruation*, dysuria, increased menstruation*, female lactation, impotence*, menorrhagia*, polyuria, pyuria, urinary retention, urinary frequency, urination impaired, and uterine fibroids enlarged*; *Rare:* albuminuria.

*Adjusted for gender.

DRUG ABUSE AND DEPENDENCE

Controlled Substance Class—Olanzapine is not a controlled substance.

Physical and Psychological Dependence—In studies prospectively designed to assess abuse and dependence potential, olanzapine was shown to have acute depressive CNS effects but little or no potential of abuse or physical dependence in rats administered oral doses up to 15 times the maximum recommended human daily dose (20 mg) and rhesus monkeys administered oral doses up to 8 times the maximum recommended human daily dose on a mg/m^2 basis.

Olanzapine has not been systematically studied in humans for its potential for abuse, tolerance, or physical dependence. While the clinical trials did not reveal any tendency for any drug-seeking behavior, these observations were not systematic, and it is not possible to predict on the basis of this limited experience the extent to which a CNS-active drug will be misused, diverted, and/or abused once marketed. Consequently, patients should be evaluated carefully for a history of drug abuse, and such patients should be observed closely for signs of misuse or abuse of olanzapine (e.g., development of tolerance, increases in dose, drug-seeking behavior).

OVERDOSAGE

Human Experience—In premarketing trials involving more than 3100 patients and/or normal subjects, accidental or intentional acute overdosage of olanzapine was identified in 67 patients. In the patient taking the largest identified amount, 300 mg, the only symptoms reported were drowsiness and slurred speech. In the limited number of patients who were evaluated in hospitals, including the patient taking 300 mg, there were no observations indicating an adverse change in laboratory analytes or ECG. Vital signs were usually within normal limits following overdoses.

Overdosage Management—The possibility of multiple drug involvement should be considered. In case of acute overdosage, establish and maintain an airway and ensure adequate oxygenation and ventilation. Gastric lavage (after intubation, if patient is unconscious) and administration of activated charcoal together with a laxative should be considered. The possibility of obtundation, seizures, or dystonic reaction of the head and neck following overdose may create a risk of aspiration with induced emesis. Cardiovascular monitoring should commence immediately and should include continuous electrocardiographic monitoring to detect possible arrhythmias.

There is no specific antidote to olanzapine. Therefore, appropriate supportive measures should be initiated. Hypotension and circulatory collapse should be treated with appropriate measures such as intravenous fluids and/or sympathomimetic agents. (Do not use epinephrine, dopamine, or other sympathomimetics with beta-agonist activity, since beta stimulation may worsen hypotension in the setting of olanzapine-induced alpha blockade.) Close medical supervision and monitoring should continue until the patient recovers.

DOSAGE AND ADMINISTRATION

Usual Dose—Olanzapine should be administered on a once-a-day schedule without regard to meals, generally beginning with 5 to 10 mg initially, with a target dose of 10 mg/day within several days. Further dosage adjustments, if indicated, should generally occur at intervals of not less than 1 week, since steady state for olanzapine would not be achieved for approximately 1 week in the typical patient. When dosage adjustments are necessary, dose increments/decrements of 5 mg QD are recommended.

Antipsychotic efficacy was demonstrated in a dose range of 10 to 15 mg/day in clinical trials. However, doses above 10 mg/day were not demonstrated to be more efficacious than the 10 mg/day dose. An increase to a dose greater than the target dose of 10 mg/day (i.e., to a dose of 15 mg/day or greater) is recommended only after clinical assessment. The safety of doses above 20 mg/day has not been evaluated in clinical trials.

Dosing in Special Populations—The recommended starting dose is 5 mg in patients who are debilitated, who have a predisposition to hypotensive reactions, who otherwise exhibit a combination of factors that may result in slower metabolism of olanzapine (e.g., nonsmoking female patients ≥65 years of age), or who may be more pharmacodynamically sensitive to olanzapine (*see* CLINICAL PHARMACOLOGY; also *see* Use in Patients with Concomitant Illness and Drug Interactions *under* PRECAUTIONS). When indicated, dose escalation should be performed with caution in these patients.

Maintenance Treatment—While there is no body of evidence available to answer the question of how long the patient treated with olanzapine should remain on it, the effectiveness of maintenance treatment is well established for many other antipsychotic drugs. It is recommended that responding patients be continued on olanzapine, but at the lowest dose needed to maintain remission. Patients should be periodically reassessed to determine the need for maintenance treatment.

HOW SUPPLIED

All tablets are white, round, film-coated, and imprinted in blue ink with LILLY and the tablet number. They are available as:

	TABLET STRENGTH			
	2.5 mg	5 mg	7.5 mg	10 mg
Tablet No.	4112	4115	4116	4117
Imprint	LILLY 4112	LILLY 4115	LILLY 4116	LILLY 4117
NDC Codes:				
Bottles 60	NDC-0002-4112-60	NDC-0002-4115-60	NDC-0002-4116-60	NDC-0002-4117-60
Blisters-ID* 100	—	NDC-0002-4115-33	NDC-0002-4116-33	NDC-0002-4117-33

∗Identi-Dose® (unit dose medication, Lilly)

Store at controlled room temperature, 20° to 25°C (68° to 77°F) [*see* USP]. The USP defines controlled room temperature as a temperature maintained thermostatically that encompasses the usual and customary working environment of 20° to 25°C (68° to 77°F); that results in a mean kinetic temperature calculated to be not more than 25°C; and that allows for excursions between 15° and 30°C (59° and 86°F) that are experienced in pharmacies, hospitals, and warehouses.

Protect from light and moisture.

ANIMAL TOXICOLOGY

In animal studies with olanzapine, the principal hematologic findings were reversible peripheral cytopenias in individual dogs dosed at 10 mg/kg (17 times the maximum recommended human daily dose on a mg/m^2 basis), dose-related decreases in lymphocytes and neutrophils in mice, and lymphopenia in rats. A few dogs treated with 10 mg/kg developed reversible neutropenia and/or reversible hemolytic anemia between 1 and 10 months of treatment. Dose-related decreases in lymphocytes and neutrophils were seen in mice given doses of 10 mg/kg (equal to 2 times the maximum recommended human daily dose on a mg/m^2 basis) in studies of 3 months' duration. Nonspecific lymphopenia, consistent with decreased body weight gain, occurred in rats receiving 22.5 mg/kg (11 times the maximum recommended human daily dose on a mg/m^2 basis) for 3 months or 16 mg/kg (8 times the maximum recommended human daily dose on a mg/m^2 basis) for 6 or 12 months. No evidence of bone marrow cytotoxicity was found in any of the species examined. Bone marrows were normocellular or hypercellular, indicating that the reductions in circulating blood cells were probably due to peripheral (non-marrow) factors.

CAUTION—Federal (USA) law prohibits dispensing without prescription.

Literature revised August 11, 1997

Manufactured by **Eli Lilly Industries, Inc.**

Carolina, Puerto Rico 00985, a subsidiary of

Eli Lilly and Company, Indianapolis, IN, USA

PV 2963 AMP [081197]

EDUCATIONAL MATERIAL

Diabetes Patient Education Materials

Managing Your Diabetes Patient Education System

- Comprehensive book on self-care & basic facts
- Topical brochures (eg, insulin and travel)
- Meal planning, gestational diabetes, injecting-insulin 5 part video series
- Self-monitoring records
- Meal plans
- Spanish and English versions

Professional Education Materials and Services

CE programs

Speaker programs

Professional slide series

Diabetes patient management software

For information on these and other educational materials, see your Lilly sales representative.

*** Identi-Code® symbol. This product information was prepared in June 1998. Current information on these and other products of Eli Lilly and Company may be obtained by direct inquiry to Lilly Research Laboratories, Lilly Corporate Center, Indianapolis, Indiana 46285, (800) 545-5979.**

The Liposome Company, Inc.
ONE RESEARCH WAY
PRINCETON, NJ 08540-6619

Direct Inquiries to:
Professional Services
(800) 335-5476
FAX: (800) 236-4507

For Medical Information Contact:
Professional Services
Director Clinical Research
(609) 452-7060 or
(800) 335-5476
FAX: (609) 452–8512

ABELCET®
['ā-bəl-"set]
(Amphotericin B Lipid Complex Injection)

℞

DESCRIPTION
ABELCET® is a sterile, pyrogen-free suspension for intravenous infusion. ABELCET® consists of amphotericin B complexed with two phospholipids in a 1:1 drug-to-lipid molar ratio. The two phospholipids, L-α-dimyristoylphosphatidylcholine (DMPC) and L-α-dimyristoylphosphatidylglycerol (DMPG), are present in a 7:3 molar ratio. ABELCET® is yellow and opaque in appearance, with a pH of 5–7.

NOTE: Liposomal encapsulation or incorporation in a lipid complex can substantially affect a drug's functional properties relative to those of the unencapsulated or nonlipid-associated drug. In addition, different liposomal or lipid-complexed products with a common active ingredient may vary from one another in the chemical composition and physical form of the lipid component. Such differences may affect functional properties of these drug products.

Amphotericin B is a polyene, antifungal antibiotic produced from a strain of *Streptomyces nodosus*. Amphotericin B is designated chemically as [1R-(1R*, 3S*, 5R*, 6R*, 9R*, 11R*, 15S*, 16R*, 17R*, 18S*, 19E, 21E, 23E, 25E, 27E, 29E, 31E, 33R*, 35S*, 36R*, 37S*)]-33-[(3-Amino-3, 6-dideoxy-β-D-mannopyranosyl) oxy]-1,3,5,6,9,11,17,37-octahydroxy-15,16,18-trimethyl-13-oxo-14,39-dioxabicyclo[33.3.1] nonatriaconta-19,21,23,25,27,29,31-heptaene-36-carboxylic acid.

It has a molecular weight of 924.09 and a molecular formula of $C_{47}H_{73}NO_{17}$. The structural formula is:

ABELCET® is provided as a sterile, opaque suspension in 20 mL glass, single-use vials. Each vial of ABELCET® contains 100 mg of amphotericin B (see DOSAGE AND ADMINISTRATION), and each mL of ABELCET® contains:

Amphotericin B USP	5 mg
L-α-dimyristoylphosphatidylcholine (DMPC)	3 . 4 mg
L-α-dimyristoylphosphatidylglycerol (DMPG)	1 . 5 mg
Sodium Chloride USP	9 mg
Water for Injection USP, q.s. 1 mL	

MICROBIOLOGY
Mechanism of Action
The active component of ABELCET®, amphotericin B, acts by binding to sterols in the cell membrane of susceptible fungi, with a resultant change in the permeability of the membrane. Mammalian cell membranes also contain sterols, and damage to human cells is believed to occur through the same mechanism of action.

Activity *in vitro* and *in vivo*
ABELCET® shows *in vitro* activity against *Aspergillus* sp. (n=3) and *Candida* sp. (n=10), with MICs generally <1 μg/mL. Depending upon the species and strain of *Aspergillus* and *Candida* tested, significant *in vitro* differences in susceptibility to amphotericin B have been reported (MICs ranging from 0.1 to >10 μg/mL). However, standardized techniques for susceptibility testing for antifungal agents have not been established, and results of susceptibility studies do not necessarily correlate with clinical outcome. ABELCET® is active in animal models against *Aspergillus fumigatus*, *Candida albicans*, *C. guillermondii*, *C. stellatoideae*, and *C. tropicalis*, *Cryptococcus* sp., *Coccidioidomyces sp.*, *Histoplasma sp.*, *and Blastomyces sp.* in which endpoints were clearance of microorganisms from target organ(s) and/or prolonged survival of infected animals.

Drug Resistance
Fungal species with decreased susceptibility to amphotericin B have been isolated after serial passage in culture media containing the drug, and from some patients receiving prolonged therapy. Although the relevance of drug resistance to clinical outcome has not been established, fungal species which are resistant to amphotericin B may also be resistant to ABELCET®.

CLINICAL PHARMACOLOGY
Pharmacokinetics
The assay used to measure amphotericin B in the blood after the administration of ABELCET® does not distinguish amphotericin B that is complexed with the phospholipids of ABELCET® from amphotericin B that is uncomplexed.

The pharmacokinetics of amphotericin B after the administration of ABELCET® are nonlinear. Volume of distribution and clearance from blood increase with increasing dose of ABELCET®, resulting in less than proportional increases in blood concentrations of amphotericin B over a dose range of 0.6–5 mg/kg/day. The pharmacokinetics of amphotericin B in whole blood after the administration of ABELCET® and amphotericin B desoxycholate are:
[See table at bottom of page]
The large volume of distribution and high clearance from blood of amphotericin B after the administration of ABELCET® probably reflect uptake by tissues. The long terminal elimination half-life probably reflects a slow redistribution from tissues. Although amphotericin B is excreted slowly, there is little accumulation in the blood after repeated dosing. AUC of amphotericin B increased approximately 34% from day 1 after the administration of ABELCET® 5 mg/kg/day for 7 days. The effect of gender or ethnicity on the pharmacokinetics of ABELCET® has not been studied.
Tissue concentrations of amphotericin B have been obtained at autopsy from one heart transplant patient who received three doses of ABELCET® at 5.3 mg/kg/day:

Concentration in Human Tissues

Organ	Amphotericin B Tissue Concentration (μg/g)
Spleen	290
Lung	222
Liver	196
Lymph Node	7.6
Kidney	6.9
Heart	5
Brain	1.6

This pattern of distribution is consistent with that observed in preclinical studies in dogs in which greatest concentrations of amphotericin B after ABELCET® administration were observed in the liver, spleen, and lung; however, the relationship of tissue concentrations of amphotericin B to its biological activity when administered as ABELCET® is unknown.

Special Populations
Hepatic Impairment: The effect of hepatic impairment on the disposition of ABELCET® is not known.
Renal Impairment: The effect of renal impairment on the disposition of ABELCET® is not known. The effect of dialysis on the elimination of ABELCET® has not been studied; however, amphotericin B is not removed by hemodialysis when administered as amphotericin B desoxycholate.
Pediatric and Elderly Patients: The pharmacokinetics and pharmacodynamics of pediatric patients (≤16 years of age) and elderly patients (≥65 years of age) have not been studied.

INDICATIONS AND USAGE
ABELCET® is indicated for the treatment of invasive fungal infections in patients who are refractory to or intolerant of conventional amphotericin B therapy. This is based on open-label treatment of patients judged by their physicians to be intolerant to or failing conventional amphotericin B therapy (See DESCRIPTION OF CLINICAL STUDIES).

DESCRIPTION OF CLINICAL STUDIES
Fungal Infections
Data from 473 patients were pooled from three open-label studies in which ABELCET® was provided for the treatment of patients with invasive fungal infections who were judged by their physicians to be refractory to or intolerant of conventional amphotericin B, or who had preexisting nephrotoxicity. Results of these studies demonstrated effectiveness of ABELCET® in the treatment of invasive fungal infections as a second line therapy.
Patients were defined by their individual physician as being refractory to or failing conventional amphotericin B therapy based on overall clinical judgement after receiving a minimum total dose of 500 mg of amphotericin B. Nephrotoxicity was defined as a serum creatinine that had increased to >2.5 mg/dL in adults and >1.5 mg/dL in pediatric patients, or a creatinine clearance of <25 mL/min while receiving conventional amphotericin B therapy.
Of the 473 patients, four were enrolled more than once; each enrollment contributed separately to the denominator. The median age was 39 years (range of <1 to 93 years); 307 patients were male and 166 female. Patients were Caucasian (381, 81%), African-American (41, 9%), Hispanic (27, 6%), Asian (10, 2%), and various other races (14, 3%). The median baseline neutrophil count was 4,000 PMN/mm³; of these, 101 (21%) had a baseline neutrophil count <500/mm³.
Two-hundred eighty-two patients of the 473 patients were considered evaluable for response to therapy; the other 191 patients were excluded on the basis of unconfirmed diagnosis, confounding factors, concomitant systemic antifungal therapy, or receiving 4 doses or less of ABELCET®. For evaluable patients, the following fungal infections were treated (n=282): aspergillosis (n=111), candidiasis (n=87), zygomycosis (n=25), cryptococcosis (n=16), and fusariosis (n=11). There were fewer than 10 evaluable patients for each of several other fungal species treated.
For each type of fungal infection listed above there were some patients successfully treated. However, in the absence of controlled studies it is unknown how response would have compared to either continuing conventional amphotericin B therapy or the use of alternative antifungal agents.
Renal Function: Patients with aspergillosis who initiated treatment with ABELCET® when serum creatinine was above 2.5 mg/dL experienced a decline in serum creatinine during treatment (Figure 1). Serum creatinine levels were also lower during treatment with ABELCET® when compared to the serum creatinine levels of patients treated with conventional amphotericin B in a retrospective historical control study. Meaningful statistical testing of the differences between these two groups is precluded since these data were obtained from two separate studies.
[See figure 1 at top of next column]
[See figure 2 at top of next column]
In a randomized study of ABELCET® for the treatment of invasive candidiasis in patients with normal baseline renal function, the incidence of nephrotoxicity was significantly less for ABELCET® at a dose of 5 mg/kg/day than for conventional amphotericin B at a dose of 0.7 mg/kg/day.
Despite generally less nephrotoxicity of ABELCET® observed at a dose of 5 mg/kg/day compared with conventional amphotericin B therapy at a dose range of 0.6–1 mg/kg/day,

Pharmacokinetic Parameters of Amphotericin B in Whole Blood in Patients Administered Multiple Doses of ABELCET® or Amphotericin B Desoxycholate

Pharmacokinetic Parameter	ABELCET® 5 mg/kg/day for 5–7 days Mean ± SD	Amphotericin B 0.6 mg/kg/day for 42 days[a] Mean ± SD
Peak Concentration (μg/mL)	1.7 ± 0.8 (n=10)[b]	1.1 ± 0.2 (n=5)
Concentration at End of Dosing Interval (μg/mL)	0.6 ± 0.3 (n=10)[b]	0.4 ± 0.2 (n=5)
Area Under Blood Concentration-Time Curve (AUC$_{0-24h}$) (μg*h/mL)	14 ± 7 (n=14)[b,c]	17.1 ± 5 (n=5)
Clearance (mL/h*kg)	436 ± 188.5 (n=14)[b,c]	38 ± 15 (n=5)
Apparent Volume of Distribution (Vd$_{area}$) (L/kg)	131 ± 57.7 (n=8)[c]	5 ± 2.8 (n=5)
Terminal Elimination Half-Life (h)	173.4 ± 78 (n=8)[c]	91.1 ± 40.9 (n=5)
Amount Excreted in Urine Over 24 h After Last Dose (% of dose)[d]	0.9 ± 0.4 (n=8)[c]	9.6 ± 2.5 (n=8)

[a] Data from patients with mucocutaneous leishmaniasis. Infusion rate was 0.25 mg/kg/h.
[b] Data from studies in patients with cytologically proven cancer being treated with chemotherapy or neutropenic patients with presumed or proven fungal infection. Infusion rate was 2.5 mg/kg/h.
[c] Data from patients with mucocutaneous leishmaniasis. Infusion rate was 4 mg/kg/h.
[d] Percentage of dose excreted in 24 hours after last dose.

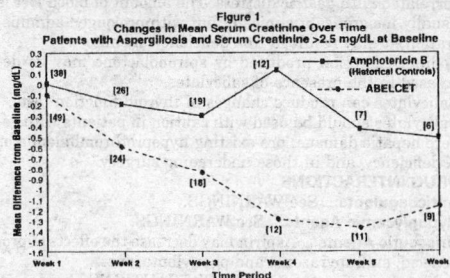

Figure 1
Changes in Mean Serum Creatinine Over Time
Patients with Aspergillosis and Serum Creatinine >2.5 mg/dL at Baseline

[ ]= Number of patients at each time point.
Note: These curves do not represent the clinical course of a given patient, but that of an open-label cohort of patients.

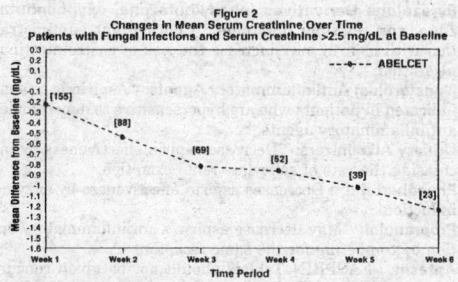

Figure 2
Changes in Mean Serum Creatinine Over Time
Patients with Fungal Infections and Serum Creatinine >2.5 mg/dL at Baseline

[ ]= Number of patients at each time point.
Note: These curves do not represent the clinical course of a given patient, but that of an open-label cohort of patients.

dose-limiting renal toxicity may still be observed with ABELCET®. Renal toxicity of doses greater than 5 mg/kg/ day of ABELCET® has not been formally studied.

CONTRAINDICATIONS
ABELCET® is contraindicated in patients who have shown hypersensitivity to amphotericin B or any other component in the formulation.

WARNINGS
Anaphylaxis has been reported with amphotericin B desoxycholate and other amphotericin B-containing drugs. Anaphylaxis has been reported with ABELCET® with an incidence rate of <0.1%. If severe respiratory distress occurs, the infusion should be immediately discontinued. The patient should not receive further infusions of ABELCET®.

PRECAUTIONS
General: As with any amphotericin B-containing product, during the initial dosing of ABELCET®, the drug should be administered under close clinical observation by medically trained personnel.
Acute reactions including fever and chills may occur 1 to 2 hours after starting an intravenous infusion of ABELCET®. These reactions are usually more common with the first few doses of ABELCET® and generally diminish with subsequent doses. Infusion has been rarely associated with hypotension, bronchospasm, arrhythmias, and shock.
Laboratory Tests: Serum creatinine should be monitored frequently during ABELCET® therapy (see ADVERSE REACTIONS). It is also advisable to regularly monitor liver function, serum electrolytes (particularly magnesium and potassium), and complete blood counts.
Drug Interactions: No formal clinical studies of drug interactions have been conducted with ABELCET®. However, when administered concomitantly, the following drugs are known to interact with amphotericin B; therefore, the following drugs may interact with ABELCET®:
Antineoplastic agents: Concurrent use of antineoplastic agents and amphotericin B may enhance the potential for renal toxicity, bronchospasm, and hypotension. Antineoplastic agents should be given concomitantly with ABELCET® with great caution.
Corticosteroids and corticotropin (ACTH): Concurrent use of corticosteroids and corticotropin (ACTH) with amphotericin B may potentiate hypokalemia which could predispose the patient to cardiac dysfunction if used concomitantly with ABELCET®, serum electrolytes and cardiac function should be closely monitored.
Cyclosporin A: Data from a prospective study of prophylactic ABELCET® in 22 patients undergoing bone marrow transplantation suggested that concurrent initiation of cyclosporin A and ABELCET® within several days of bone marrow ablation may be associated with increased nephrotoxicity.
Digitalis glycosides: Concurrent use of amphotericin B may induce hypokalemia and may potentiate digitalis toxicity. When administered concomitantly with ABELCET®, serum potassium levels should be closely monitored.
Flucytosine: Concurrent use of flucytosine with amphotericin B-containing preparations may increase the toxicity of flucytosine by possibly increasing its cellular uptake and/or impairing its renal excretion. Flucytosine should be given concomitantly with ABELCET® with caution.
Imidazoles (e.g., ketoconazole, miconazole, clotrimazole, fluconazole, etc): Antagonism between amphotericin B and imidazole derivatives such as miconazole and ketoconazole, which inhibit ergosterol synthesis, has been reported in both *in vitro* and *in vivo* animal studies. The clinical significance of these findings has not been determined.
Leukocyte transfusions: Acute pulmonary toxicity has been reported in patients receiving intravenous amphotericin B and leukocyte transfusions. Leukocyte transfusions and ABELCET® should not be given concurrently.
Other nephrotoxic medications: Concurrent use of amphotericin B and agents such as aminoglycosides and pentamidine may enhance the potential for drug-induced renal toxicity. Aminoglycosides and pentamidine should be used concomitantly with ABELCET® only with great caution. Intensive monitoring of renal function is recommended in patients requiring any combination of nephrotoxic medications.
Skeletal muscle relaxants: Amphotericin B-induced hypokalemia may enhance the curariform effect of skeletal muscle relaxants (e.g., tubocurarine) due to hypokalemia. When administered concomitantly with ABELCET®, serum potassium levels should be closely monitored.
Zidovudine: Increased myelotoxicity and nephrotoxicity were observed in dogs when either ABELCET® (at doses of 0.16 or 0.5 times the recommended human dose) or amphotericin B desoxycholate (at 0.5 times the recommended human dose) were administered concomitantly with zidovudine for 30 days. If zidovudine is used concomitantly with ABELCET®, renal hematologic function should be closely monitored.

Carcinogenesis, Mutagenesis, and Impairment of Fertility: No long-term studies in animals have been performed to evaluate the carcinogenic potential of ABELCET®. The following *in vitro* (with and without metabolic activation) and *in vivo* studies to assess ABELCET® for mutagenic potential were conducted: bacterial reverse mutation assay, mouse lymphoma forward mutation assay, chromosomal aberration assay in CHO cells, and *in vivo* mouse micronucleus assay. ABELCET® was found to be without mutagenic effects in all assay systems. Studies demonstrated that ABELCET® had no impact on fertility in male and female rats at doses up to 0.32 times the recommended human dose (based on body surface area considerations).
Pregnancy: There are no reports of pregnant women having been treated with ABELCET®. Teratogenic Effects. Pregnancy Category B: Reproductive studies in rats and rabbits at doses of ABELCET® up to 0.64 times the human dose revealed no harm to the fetus. Because animal reproductive studies are not always predictive of human response, and adequate and well-controlled studies have not been conducted in pregnant women, ABELCET® should be used during pregnancy only after taking into account the importance of the drug to the mother.
Nursing Mothers: It is not known whether ABELCET® is excreted in human milk. Because many drugs are excreted in human milk, and because of the potential for serious adverse reactions in breast-fed infants from ABELCET®, a decision should be made whether to discontinue nursing or to discontinue the drug, taking into account the importance of the drug to the mother.
Pediatric Use: One hundred eleven children (2 were enrolled twice and counted as separate patients), age 16 years and under, of whom 11 were less than 1 year, have been treated with ABELCET® at 5 mg/kg/day in two open-label studies and one small, prospective, single-arm study. In one single-center study, 5 children with hepatosplenic candidiasis were effectively treated with 2.5 mg/kg/day of ABELCET®. No serious unexpected adverse events have been reported.
Geriatric Use: Forty-nine elderly patients, age 65 years or over, have been treated with ABELCET® at 5 mg/kg/day in two open-label studies and one small, prospective, single-arm study. No serious unexpected adverse events have been reported.

ADVERSE REACTIONS
The total safety data base is composed of 921 patients treated with ABELCET® (5 patients were enrolled twice and counted as separate patients), of whom 775 were treated with 5 mg/kg/day. Of these 775 patients, 194 patients were treated in four comparative studies; 25 were treated in open-label, non-comparative studies; and 556 patients were treated in an open-label, emergency-use program. Most had underlying hematologic neoplasms, and many were receiving multiple concomitant medications. Of the 556 patients treated with ABELCET®, 9% discontinued treatment due to adverse events regardless of presumed relationship to study drug.
In general, the adverse events most commonly reported with ABELCET® were transient chills and/or fever during infusion of the drug.

Adverse Events[a] with an Incidence of ≥3% (N=556)

Adverse Event	Percentage (%) of Patients
Chills	18
Fever	14
Increased Serum Creatinine	11
Multiple Organ Failure	11
Nausea	9
Hypotension	8
Respiratory Failure	8
Vomiting	8
Dyspnea	7
Sepsis	7
Diarrhea	6
Headache	6
Heart Arrest	6
Hypertension	5
Hypokalemia	5
Infection	5
Kidney Failure	5
Pain	5
Thrombocytopenia	5
Abdominal Pain	4
Anemia	4
Bilirubinemia	4
Gastrointestinal Hemorrhage	4
Leukopenia	4
Rash	4
Respiratory Disorder	4
Chest Pain	3
Nausea and Vomiting	3

[a] The causal association between these adverse events and ABELCET® is uncertain.

The following adverse events have also been reported in patients using ABELCET® in open-label, uncontrolled clinical studies. The causal association between these adverse events and ABELCET® is uncertain.
Body as a whole: malaise, weight loss, deafness, injection site reaction including inflammation
Allergic: bronchospasm, wheezing, asthma, anaphylactoid and other allergic reactions
Cardiopulmonary: cardiac failure, pulmonary edema, shock, myocardial infarction, hemoptysis, tachypnea, thrombophlebitis, pulmonary embolus, cardiomyopathy, pleural effusion, arrhythmias including ventricular fibrillation
Dermatological: maculopapular rash, pruritus, exfoliative dermatitis, erythema multiforme
Gastrointestinal: acute liver failure, hepatitis, jaundice, melena, anorexia, dyspepsia, cramping, epigastric pain, veno-occlusive liver disease, diarrhea, hepatomegaly, cholangitis, cholecystitis
Hematologic: coagulation defects, leukocytosis, blood dyscrasias including eosinophilia
Musculoskeletal: myasthenia, including bone, muscle, and joint pains
Neurologic: convulsions, tinnitus, visual impairment, hearing loss, peripheral neuropathy, transient vertigo, diplopia, encephalopathy, cerebral vascular accident, extrapyramidal syndrome and other neurologic symptoms
Urogenital: oliguria, decreased renal function, anuria, renal tubular acidosis, impotence, dysuria
Serum electrolyte abnormalities: hypomagnesemia, hyperkalemia, hypocalcemia, hypercalcemia
Liver function test abnormalities: increased AST, ALT, alkaline phosphatase, LDH
Renal function test abnormalities: increased BUN
Other test abnormalities: acidosis, hyperamylasemia, hypoglycemia, hyperglycemia, hyperuricemia, hypophosphatemia

OVERDOSAGE
Amphotericin B desoxycholate overdose has been reported to result in cardio-respiratory arrest. Fifteen patients have been reported to have received one or more doses of ABELCET® between 7–13 mg/kg. None of these patients had a serious acute reaction to ABELCET®. If an overdose is suspected, discontinue therapy, monitor the patient's clinical status, and administer supportive therapy as required. ABELCET® is not hemodialyzable.

DOSAGE AND ADMINISTRATION
The recommended daily dosage for adults and children is 5 mg/kg given as a single infusion. ABELCET® should be administered by intravenous infusion at a rate of 2.5 mg/kg/h. If the infusion time exceeds 2 hours, mix the contents by shaking the infusion bag every 2 hours.
Renal toxicity of ABELCET®, as measured by serum creatinine levels, has been shown to be dose dependent. Deci-

Continued on next page

Abelcet—Cont.

sions about dose adjustments should be made only after taking into account the overall clinical condition of the patient.

Preparation of Admixture for Infusion: Shake the vial gently until there is no evidence of any yellow sediment at the bottom. Withdraw the appropriate dose of ABELCET® from the required number of vials into one or more sterile 20 mL syringes using an 18-gauge needle. Remove the needle from each syringe filled with ABELCET® and replace with the 5-micron filter needle supplied with each vial. Each filter needle may be used to filter the contents of up to four vials. Insert the filter needle of the syringe into an IV bag containing 5% Dextrose Injection USP, and empty the contents of the syringe into the bag. The final infusion concentration should be 1 mg/mL. For pediatric patients and patients with cardiovascular disease the drug may be diluted with 5% Dextrose Injection to a final infusion concentration of 2 mg/mL. Before infusion, shake the bag until the contents are thoroughly mixed. Do not use the admixture after dilution with 5% Dextrose Injection if there is any evidence of foreign matter. Vials are for single use. Unused material should be discarded. Aseptic technique must be strictly observed throughout handling of ABELCET®, since no bacteriostatic agent or preservative is present.

DO NOT DILUTE WITH SALINE SOLUTIONS OR MIX WITH OTHER DRUGS OR ELECTROLYTES as the compatibility of ABELCET® with these materials has not been established. An existing intravenous line should be flushed with 5% Dextrose Injection before infusion of ABELCET®, or a separate infusion line should be used. DO NOT USE AN IN-LINE FILTER.

The diluted ready-for-use admixture is stable for up to 48 hours at 2° to 8°C (36° to 46°F) and an additional 6 hours at room temperature.

HOW SUPPLIED

Each vial contains 100 mg of ABELCET® in 20 mL of suspension. Single-use vials along with 5-micron filter needles are individually packaged. NDC 61799-101-41.

STORAGE

Prior to admixture, ABELCET® should be stored at 2° to 8°C (36° to 46°F) and protected from exposure to light. Do not freeze. ABELCET® should be retained in the carton until time of use.

The admixed ABELCET® and 5% Dextrose Injection may be stored for up to 48 hours at 2° to 8° (36° to 46°F) and an additional 6 hours at room temperature. Do not freeze. Any unused material should be discarded.

U.S. Patent Nos. 4,973,465
5,616,334

The Liposome Company, Inc. 5/98
Princeton, NJ, USA I-101-41-US-G

Shown in Product Identification Guide, page 321

Lotus Biochemical Corporation

P.O. BOX 3586
RADFORD, VA 24143

Direct Inquiries to:
Iain Speirs
(800) 455-5525
FAX: (800) 962-2200

For Medical Information Contact:
In Emergencies:
Lawrence P. Olon
(423) 989-9190
FAX: (423) 989-3532

EASPRIN® ℞

[ē-ăsprin]
(Aspirin Delayed-release Tablets, USP)
Enteric Coated Tablets

DESCRIPTION

Easprin®, (Aspirin Delayed-release Tablets, USP, enteric coated (E/C) contain 975 mg (15 grains) aspirin for oral administration. The enteric coating is designed to prevent the release of aspirin in the stomach and thereby reduce gastric irritation and total occult blood loss. The pharmacologic effects of aspirin include analgesia, antipyresis, antiinflammatory activity, and antirheumatic activity. The structural formula of aspirin (salicylic acid acetate) is:

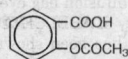

$C_9H_8O_4$
MOL. WT. 180.16

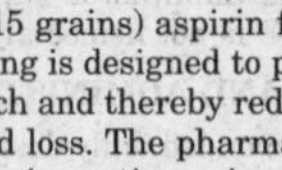

INACTIVE INGREDIENTS

Microcrystalline cellulose, starch, croscarmellose sodium, silicon dioxide, talc, shellac, titanium dioxide, hydropropyl methylcellulose phthalate, polyvinyl acetate phthalate, cellulose acetate phthalate.

CLINICAL PHARMACOLOGY

Aspirin is a salicylate that has demonstrated antiinflammatory, analgesic, antipyretic, and antirheumatic activity.

Aspirin's mode of action as an antiinflammatory and antirheumatic agent may be due to inhibition of synthesis and release of prostaglandins.

Aspirin appears to produce analgesia by virtue of both a peripheral and CNS effect. Peripherally, aspirin acts by inhibiting the synthesis and release of prostaglandins. Acting centrally, it would appear to produce analgesia at a hypothalamic site in the brain, although the mode of action is not known.

Aspirin also acts on the hypothalamus to produce antipyresis; heat dissipation is increased as a result of vasodilation and increased peripheral blood flow. Aspirin's antipyretic activity may also be related to inhibition of synthesis and release of prostaglandins.

EASPRIN tablets are enteric coated. This coating acts to prevent the release of aspirin in the stomach but permits the tablet to dissolve with resultant absorption in the upper portion of the small intestine. This reduces any gastric irritation that may occur with uncoated aspirin but does delay the onset of action. Aspirin is rapidly hydrolyzed primarily in the liver to salicylic acid, which is conjugated with glycine (forming salicyluric acid) and glucuronic acid and excreted largely in the urine. As a result of the rapid hydrolysis, plasma concentrations of aspirin are always low and rarely exceed 20 mcg/mL at ordinary therapeutic doses. The peak salicylate level for uncoated aspirin occurs in about 2 hours, however, with enteric coated aspirin tablets this is delayed. A direct correlation between salicylate plasma levels and clinical analgesic effectiveness has not been definitely established, but effective analgesia is usually achieved at plasma levels of 15 to 30 mg per 100 ml. Effective antiinflammatory activity is usually achieved at salicylate plasma levels of 20 to 30 mg per 100 mL. There is also poor correlation between toxic symptoms and plasma salicylate concentrations, but most patients exhibit symptoms of salicylism at plasma salicylate levels of 35 mg per 100 ml. The plasma half-life for aspirin is approximately 15 minutes; that for salicylate lengthens as the dose increases. Doses of 300 to 600 mg have a half-life of 3.1 to 3.2 hours, with doses of 1 gram, the half-life is increased to 5 hours and with 2 grams it is increased to about 9 hours.

Salicylates are excreted mainly by the kidney. Studies in man indicate that salicylate is excreted in the urine as free salicylic acid (10%), salicyluric acid (75%), salicylic phenolic (10%), and acyl (5%) glucuronides and gentisic acid.

INDICATIONS AND USAGE

EASPRIN Tablet indicated in patients who need the higher 975 mg dose of aspirin in the long-term palliative treatment of mild to moderate pain and inflammation of arthritic and other inflammatory conditions.

CONTRAINDICATIONS

EASPRIN Tablet should not be used in patients who have previously exhibited hypersensitivity to aspirin and/or nonsteroidal antiinflammatory agents.

EASPRIN Tablets should not be given to patients with a recent history of gastrointestinal bleeding or in patients with bleeding disorders (eg, hemophilia).

WARNINGS

EASPRIN Tablets should be used with caution when anticoagulants are prescribed concurrently, for aspirin may depress the concentration of prothrombin in plasma and thereby increase bleeding time. Large doses of salicylates have a hypoglycemic action and may enhance the effect of the oral hypoglycemics. Consequently, they should not be given concomitantly; if however, this is necessary, the dosage of the hypoglycemic agent must be reduced while the salicylate is given. This hypoglycemic action may also effect the insulin requirements of diabetics.

Although salicylates in large doses are uricosuric agents, smaller amounts may decrease the uricosuric effects of probenecid, sulfinpyrazone, and phenylbutazone.

PRECAUTIONS

General: EASPRIN Tablets should be administered with caution to patients with asthma, nasal polyps, or nasal allergies.

In patients receiving large doses of aspirin and/or prolonged therapy mild salicylate intoxication (salicyslism) may develop that may be reversed by reduction in dosage.

Although the fecal blood loss with EASPRIN Tablets is less than that with uncoated aspirin tablets, EASPRIN Tablets should be administered with caution to patients with a history of gastric distress, ulcer, or bleeding problems. Occult gastrointestinal bleeding occurs in many patients but is not correlated with gastric distress. The amount of blood lost is usually insignificant clinically, but with prolonged administration, it may result in iron deficiency anemia.

Sodium excretion produced by spironolactone may be decreased in the presence of salicylates.

Salicylates can produce changes in thyroid function tests.

Salicylates should be used with caution in patients with severe hepatic damage, pre-existing hypoprothrombinemia or K deficiency, and in those undergoing surgery.

DRUG INTERACTIONS

Anticoagulants: See WARNINGS.

Hypoglycemic Agents: See WARNINGS.

Uricosuric Agents: Aspirin may decrease the effects of probenecid, sulfinpyrazone, and phenylbutazone.

Spironolactone: See General PRECAUTIONS above.

Alcohol: Has a synergistic effect with aspirin in causing gastrointestinal bleeding.

Corticosteroids: Concomitant administration with aspirin may increase the risk of gastrointestinal ulceration.

Pyrazolone Derivatives (phenylbutazone, oxyphenbutazone, and possibly dipyrone): Concomitant administration with aspirin may increase the risk of gastrointestinal ulceration.

Nonsteroidal Antiinflammatory Agents: Aspirin is contraindicated in patients who are hypersensitive to nonsteroidal antiinflammatory agents.

Urinary Alkalinizers: Decrease aspirin effectiveness by increasing the rate of salicylate renal excretion.

Phenobarbital: Decreases aspirin effectiveness by enzyme induction.

Propranolol: May decrease aspirin's antiinflammatory action by competing for the same receptors.

Antacid: EASPRIN Tablets should not be given concurrently with antacids, since an increase in the pH of the stomach may effect the enteric coating of the tablets.

Usage in Pregnancy: Aspirin does not appear to have any teratogenic effects. However, it has been reported that adverse effects were increased in the mother and fetus following chronic ingestion of aspirin. Prolonged pregnancy and labor with increased bleeding before and after delivery, as well as decreased birth weight and increased risk of stillbirth were correlated with high blood salicylate levels. Because of possible adverse effects on the neonate and the potential for increased maternal blood loss, aspirin should be avoided during the last three months of pregnancy.

ADVERSE REACTIONS

Gastrointestinal: Dyspepsia, nausea, vomiting, diarrhea, gastrointestinal bleeding, and/or ulceration.

Ear: Tinnitus, vertigo, reversible hearing loss.

Hematologic: Prolongation of bleeding time, leukopenia, thrombocytopenia, purpura, decreased plasma iron concentration and shortened erythrocyte survival time.

Dermatologic and Hypersensitivity: Urticaria, angioedema, pruritus, various skin eruptions, asthma, and anaphylaxis.

Miscellaneous: Acute reversible hepatotoxicity, mental confusion, drowsiness, sweating, dizziness, headache, fever, thirst, and dimness of vision.

OVERDOSAGE

Overdosage of 200 to 500 mg/kg is in the fatal range. Early symptoms are CNS stimulation with vomiting, hyperpnea, hyperactivity, and possibly convulsions. This progresses quickly to depression, coma, respiratory failure, and collapse. These symptoms are accompanied by severe electrolyte disturbances.

In the treatment of salicylate overdosage, intensive supportive therapy should be instituted immediately. Plasma salicylate levels should be measured in order to determine the severity of the poisoning and to provide a guide for therapy. Emptying the stomach should be accomplished as soon as possible with ipecac syrup unless the patient is depressed. In depressed patients, use airway protected gastric lavage. Delay absorption with activated charcoal and give a saline cathartic. Proceed according to Standard Reference Procedures for Salicylate intoxication.

DOSAGE AND ADMINISTRATION

Usual Adult Dosage: One tablet 3 to 4 times daily.

Patients who have displayed no significant adverse effects on a long term qid regimen and who receive a total daily dosage of aspirin no greater than 3.9 grams may be considered for a bid regimen (2 EASPRIN Tablets twice daily). Patients on the bid regimen should be closely monitored for serum salicylate levels, increased incidence of CNS-related adverse effects, increased fecal blood loss, or any other signs or symptoms suggestive of significant blood loss.

If necessary, dosage may be increased until relief is obtained, but dosages should be maintained slightly below that which produces tinnitus. Plasma salicylate levels may also be helpful in determining proper dosage (see Clinical Pharmacology section).

HOW SUPPLIED

EASPRIN Tablets, white, imprinted, each containing 975 mg (15 grains) aspirin are available in bottles of 100's (NDC 59417-975-71).

Storage: Store at controlled room temperatures 15°–30°C (59°–86°F).
Rx only
Manufactured for:
LOTUS BIOCHEMICAL CORPORATION
Radford, VA 24143, USA
By:
Time-Cap Labs, Inc.
Farmingdale, NY 11735, USA
©Lotus Biochemical Corporation
All Rights Reserved

Rev. 07/98

ERGOMAR® Sublingual Tablets, 2 mg ℞
[er 'go-mar"]
(ergotamine tartrate tablets, USP)

DESCRIPTION

Each sublingual tablet of ERGOMAR contains 2 mg ergotamine tartrate, USP.
Inactive Ingredients: Corn starch, D & C Yellow No. 10, FD & C Blue No. 1, lactose monohydrate NF, magnesium stearate, peppermint oil, saccharin sodium.
Pharmacological Category: Vasoconstrictor, uterine stimulant, alpha adrenoreceptor antagonist.
Therapeutic Class: Anti-migraine.
Chemical Name: Ergotaman-3',6', 18-trione, 12'-hydroxy-2'-methyl-5'-(phenyl-methyl)-,(5'α)-,[R-(R*,R*)]-2, 3-dihydroxybutanedioate(2:1)(tartrate).
Structural Formula:

CLINICAL PHARMACOLOGY

The pharmacological properties of ergotamine are extremely complex; some of its actions are unrelated to each other, and even mutually antagonistic. The drug has partial agonist and/or antagonist activity against tryptaminergic, dopaminergic and alpha adrenergic receptors depending upon their site, and it is a highly active uterine stimulant. It causes constriction of peripheral and cranial blood vessels and produces depression of central vasomotor centers. The pain of a migraine attack is believed to be due to greatly increased amplitude of pulsations in the cranial arteries, especially the meningeal branches of the external carotid artery. Ergotamine reduces extracranial blood flow, causes a decline in the amplitude of pulsation in the cranial arteries, and decreases hyperperfusion of the territory of the basilar artery. It does not reduce cerebral hemispheric blood flow. Long term usage has established the fact that ergotamine tartrate is effective in controlling up to 70% of acute migraine attacks, so that it is now considered specific for the treatment of this headache syndrome. Ergotamine produces constriction of both arteries and veins. In doses used in the treatment of vascular headaches, ergotamine usually produces only small increases in blood pressure but it does increase peripheral resistance and decrease blood flow in various organs. Small doses of the drug increase the force and frequency of uterine contraction; larger doses increase the resting tone of the uterus also. The gravid uterus is particularly sensitive to these effects of ergotamine. Although specific teratogenic effects attributable to ergotamine have not been found, the fetus suffers if ergotamine is given to the mother. Retarded fetal growth and an increase in intrauterine death and resorption have been seen in animals. These are thought to result from ergotamine induced increases in uterine motility and vasoconstriction in the placental vascular bed.
The bioavailability of sublingually administered ergotamine has not been determined.
Ergotamine is metabolized by the liver by largely undefined pathways, and 90% of the metabolites are excreted in the bile. The unmetabolized drug is erratically secreted in the saliva, and only traces of unmetabolized drug appear in the urine and feces. Ergotamine is secreted in breast milk. The elimination half-life of ergotamine from plasma is about 2 hours, but the drug may be stored in some tissues, which would account for its long lasting therapeutic and toxic actions.

INDICATIONS AND USAGE

ERGOMAR is indicated as therapy to abort or prevent vascular headache, e.g., migraine, migraine variants, or so called "histaminic cephalalgia."

CONTRAINDICATIONS

ERGOMAR is contraindicated in peripheral vascular disease (thromboangitis obliterans, luetic arteritis, severe arteriosclerosis, thrombophlebitis, Raynaud's disease), coronary heart disease, hypertension, impaired hepatic or renal function, severe pruritis, and sepsis. It is also contraindicated in patients who are hypersensitive to any of its components. ERGOMAR may cause fetal harm when administered to a pregnant woman by virtue of its powerful uterine stimulant actions. ERGOMAR is contraindicated in women who are, or may become, pregnant.

PRECAUTIONS

General: Although signs and symptoms of ergotism rarely develop even after long term intermittent use of ergotamine, care should be exercised to remain within the limits of recommended dosage.
Drug Interactions: The effects of ERGOMAR may be potentiated by triacetyloleandomycin which inhibits the metabolism of ergotamine. The pressor effects of ERGOMAR and other vasoconstrictor drugs can combine to cause dangerous hypertension.
Carcinogenesis: No studies have been performed to investigate ERGOMAR for carcinogenic effects.
Pregnancy: Pregnancy Category X—See CONTRAINDICATIONS section.
Nursing Mothers: Ergotamine is secreted into human milk. It can reach the breast-fed infant by this route and exert pharmacologic effects in it. Caution should be exercised when ERGOMAR is administered to a nursing woman. Excessive dosing or prolonged administration of ergotamine may inhibit lactation.

ADVERSE REACTIONS

Nausea and vomiting occur in up to 10% of patients after ingestion of therapeutic doses of ergotamine. Weakness of the legs and pain in limb muscles are also frequent complaints. Numbness and tingling of the fingers and toes, precordial pain, transient changes in heart rate and localized edema and itching may also occur, particularly in patients who are sensitive to the drug.

DRUG ABUSE AND DEPENDENCE

Patients who take ergotamine for extended periods of time may become dependent upon it and require progressively increasing doses for relief of vascular headaches, and for prevention of dysphoric effects which follow withdrawal of the drug.

OVERDOSAGE

Overdosage with ergotamine causes nausea, vomiting, weakness of the legs, pain in limb muscles, numbness and tingling of the fingers and toes, precordial pain, tachycardia or bradycardia, hypertension or hypotension and localized edema and itching together with signs and symptoms of ischemia due to vasoconstriction of peripheral arteries and arterioles. The feet and hands become cold, pale and numb. Muscle pain occurs while walking and later at rest also. Gangrene may ensue. Confusion, depression, drowsiness and convulsions are occasional signs of ergotamine toxicity. Overdosage is particularly likely to occur in patients with sepsis or impaired renal or hepatic function. Patients with peripheral vascular disease are specially at risk of developing peripheral ischemia following treatment with ergotamine. Some cases of ergotamine poisoning have been reported in patients who have taken less than 5 mg of the drug. Usually, however, toxicity is seen in doses of ergotamine tartrate in excess of about 15 mg in 24 hours or 40 mg in a few days.
Treatment of ergotamine overdosage consists of the withdrawal of the drug followed by symptomatic measures including attempts to maintain an adequate circulation in the affected parts. Anticoagulant drugs, low molecular weight dextran and potent vasodilator drugs may all be beneficial. Intravenous infusion of sodium nitroprusside has also been reported to be successful. Vasodilators must be used with special care in the presence of hypotension.
Nausea and vomiting may be relieved by atropine or antiemetic compounds of the phenothiazine group. Ergotamine is dialyzable.

DOSAGE AND ADMINISTRATION

All efforts should be made to initiate therapy as soon as possible after the first symptoms of the attack are noted, since success is proportional to rapidity of treatment, and lower dosages will be effective. At the first sign of an attack or to relieve symptoms after onset of an attack one 2 mg tablet is placed under the tongue. Another tablet should be taken at half-hour intervals thereafter, if necessary, but dosage must not exceed three tablets in any 24 hour period. Dosage should be limited to not more than five tablets (10mg) in any one week.

HOW SUPPLIED

20 tablets (green) each containing 2 mg ergotamine tartrate, supplied in foil strips in a plastic child resistant container. Each tablet is debossed with the following product identification code: LB 2. Protect from light and heat. Keep out of the reach of children.
NDC 59417-120-20 Containers of 20.
Rx only
Manufactured for:
LOTUS BIOCHEMICAL CORPORATION
Radford, VA 24143, USA
By: Schwarz Pharma, Inc.
©Lotus Biochemical Corporation
All Rights Reserved

REV. 6/98

Lunsco, Inc.
ROUTE 2, BOX 62
PULASKI, VA 24301

Direct Inquiries to:
(540) 980-4358

For Medical Information Contact:
In Emergencies:
(540) 980-4358

ANABAR ℞

COMPOSITION
Each capsule contains
Acetaminophen 300 mg.
Salicylamide 200 mg.
Phenyltoloxamine citrate 20 mg.
SUPPLIED
Bottles of 100

DYLIX ELIXIR ℞
[dī-lĭx elixir]

COMPOSITION
Ea. 15 ml. (one tablespoonful) contains dyphylline - 100 mg, alcohol (by volume) 20%
SUPPLIED
Pints (16 fl. oz. (473 ml)

DYTUSS OTC

COMPOSITION
Ea. Teaspoonful (5mL) contains:
Diphenhydramine HCl 12.5 mg.
Alcohol 5%.
SUPPLIED
Pint.

FETRIN ℞

COMPOSITION
Each sustained-release capsule contains: Ferrous Fumarate (Equivalent to 66 mg. Elemental Iron) 200 mg., Ascorbic Acid 60 mg., Cyanocobalamin 5 mcg with Intrinsic Factor.
SUPPLIED
Bottles of 100.

PACAPS ℞

COMPOSITION
Each capsule represents: Butalbital 50 mg., Caffeine 40 mg., Acetaminophen 325 mg.
SUPPLIED
Bottles of 100.

PROTID ℞

COMPOSITION
Each tablet represents: Acetaminophen 500 mg., Chlorpheniramine Maleate 8 mg., Phenylephrine HCl 40 mg.
SUPPLIED
Bottles of 100.

MDR Fitness Corp.

MEDICAL DOCTORS' RESEARCH
14101 NW 4th STREET
SUNRISE, FL 33325

Direct Inquiries to:
1-800-637-8227 ext 5277

MDR FITNESS TABS FOR MEN OTC
MDR FITNESS TABS FOR WOMEN

DESCRIPTION

MDR Fitness Tabs are formulated by Medical Doctors Research based on a two tablet per day system to allow enhanced absorption of nutrients. The A.M. and P.M. dosage allows more absorption of the water soluble vitamins (B-complex and C) which are not readily stored by the body. The AM tablet provides more micronutrients required for energy producing reactions when physical activity is greater. The MDR formulas are free of dyes, yeast, preservatives, fillers, soy, wheat gluten, lactose and other sugars.

INDICATIONS AND USAGE

MDR Fitness Tabs are designed for the maintenance of good health and nutrition for men and women, 11 years of age or older, whenever a multi-vitamin, mineral supplement is indicated to help provide nutrients missing from the diet or to replace nutrient loss from oral contraceptives, antacids, excessive alcohol, smoking, physical or emotional stress, exercise, weight loss diets, or illness. Daily use of MDR Fitness Tabs may also play a protective role for good health by assuring adequate intake of essential nutrients, including antioxidant nutrients shown in recent research to enhance the body's natural defenses.

Directions: After the first meal of the day, take one "AM" Fitness Tab. After lunch or dinner, take one "PM" Fitness Tab. Swallow Fitness Tab with a full glass of water.

PRECAUTIONS

Not recommended for persons with severe kidney disease or those undergoing renal dialysis, unless under a physician's supervision. Diabetics may need to adjust insulin dosage and should be monitored. Not recommended for those suffering from pernicious anemia, or Parkinson patients on levodopa therapy, due to the presence of vitamin B-6 which may decrease levodopa's efficacy. Pregnant and lactating women may need additional supplementation.

Note: MDR also provides a Stress Defense supplement to be taken with MDR Fitness Tabs when higher dosages are indicated.

Also available: Nite-Cal Calcium, Children's Chewable, Arthritis, (MDR) and Fibromyalgia Nutritional Support.

For Samples, Product or Order Information Call
1-800-MDR-TABS ext. 5277 or fax (954) 845-9505
or write: (MDR) Medical Doctors' Research
14101 NW 4th Street
SUNRISE, FL 33325

MGI PHARMA, Inc.

SUITE 300 E, OPUS CENTER
9900 BREN ROAD EAST
MINNETONKA, MN 55343-9667

For Medical Information Contact:
Generally:
Medical Affairs
(800) 644-4811
FAX: (612) 935-0468

In Emergencies:
Medical Affairs
(800) 562-5580
FAX: (612) 935-0468

DIDRONEL® I.V. INFUSION ℞
(etidronate disodium)
DILUTE BEFORE USE

DESCRIPTION

Didronel I.V. Infusion is a clear, colorless, sterile solution of etidronate disodium, the disodium salt of (1-hydroxyethylidene) diphosphonic acid. Each 6-ml ampule contains a 5% solution of 300 mg etidronate disodium in water for injection for slow intravenous infusion. Etidronate disodium is a white powder, highly soluble in water, with a molecular weight of 250 and the following structural formula:
[See chemical structure at top of next column]

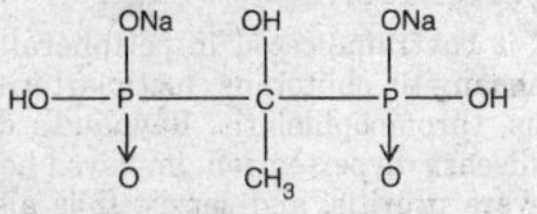

CLINICAL PHARMACOLOGY

Didronel acts primarily on bone. Its major pharmacologic action is the reduction of normal and abnormal bone resorption. Secondarily, it reduces bone formation since formation is coupled to resorption. This reduces bone turnover, but the reduction of bone turnover, *per se,* is not the important action in the reduction of hypercalcemia.

Didronel's reduction of abnormal bone resorption is responsible for its therapeutic benefit in hypercalcemia. The antiresorptive action of Didronel has been demonstrated under a variety of conditions, although the exact mechanism(s) is not fully understood. It may be related to the drug's inhibition of hydroxyapatite crystal dissolution and/or its action on bone resorbing cells. The number of osteoclasts in active bone turnover sites is substantially reduced after Didronel therapy is administered. Didronel also can inhibit the formation and growth of hydroxyapatite crystals and their amorphous precursors at concentrations in excess of those required to inhibit crystal dissolution.

Etidronate disodium is not metabolized. A large fraction of the infused dose is excreted rapidly and unchanged in the urine. The mean residence time in the exchangeable pool is approximately 8.7 ± 1.0 hours. The mean volume of distribution at steady-state in normal humans is 1370 ± 203 ml/kg while the plasma half-life ($t_{1/2}$) is 6.0 ± 0.7 hours. In these same subjects, nonrenal clearance from the exchangeable pool amounts to 30–50% of the infused dose. This nonrenal clearance is considered to be due to uptake of the drug by bone; subsequently the drug is slowly eliminated through bone turnover. The half-life of the dose on bone is in excess of 90 days.

Hyperphosphatemia, which is often observed in association with oral Didronel medication at doses of 10–20 mg/kg/day, occurs less frequently, in association with intravenous medication of patients with hypercalcemia of malignancy.

Hyperphosphatemia is apparently due to increased tubular reabsorption of phosphate by the kidney. No adverse effects have been associated with Didronel-related hyperphosphatemia and its occurrence is not a contraindication to therapy. Serum phosphate elevations usually return to normal 2–4 weeks after medication is discontinued.

The responsiveness of animal tumors susceptible to four commonly employed classes or subclasses of chemotherapeutic agents, antitumor antibiotics (doxorubicin), a classic alkylating agent (cyclophosphamide), a nitrosourea (carmustine), and a pyrimidine antagonist (5-fluorouracil), were not adversely altered by the concurrent administration of intravenous Didronel.

Hypercalcemia of Malignancy: Hypercalcemia of malignancy is usually related to increased bone resorption associated with the presence of neoplastic tissue. It occurs in 8 to 20% of patients with malignant disease. Whereas hypercalcemia is more often seen in patients with demonstrable osteolytic, osteoblastic, or mixed metastatic tumors in bone, discrete skeletal lesions cannot be demonstrated in at least 30% of patients.

Patients with certain types of neoplasms, such as carcinoma of the breast, bronchogenic carcinoma, renal cell carcinoma, cancers of the head and neck, lymphomas, and multiple myeloma, are especially prone to developing hypercalcemia.

As hypercalcemia of malignancy evolves, the renal tubules develop a diminished capacity to concentrate urine. The resultant polyuria and nocturia decrease the extracellular fluid volume. This decrease may be aggravated by vomiting and reduced fluid intake. Thus, the ability of the kidney to eliminate excess calcium is compromised. Renal impairment can eventually cause nitrogen retention, acidosis, renal failure, and further decrease in excretion of calcium. Didronel I.V. Infusion, by inhibiting excessive bone resorption, interrupts this process. Salt loading and use of "high ceiling" or "loop" diuretics may be used to promote calcium excretion, because the rate of renal calcium excretion is directly related to the rate of sodium excretion.

The physiologic derangements induced by excessive serum calcium are due to increased levels of ionized calcium. The pathophysiologic effects of excessive serum calcium are heightened by reductions in serum albumin which normally binds a fraction (about 40%) of the total serum calcium. In patients with hypercalcemia of malignancy, serum albumin is often reduced and this tends to mask the magnitude of the increase in the level of ionized calcium. By reducing the flow of calcium from resorbing bone, Didronel I.V. Infusion effectively reduces total and ionized serum calcium.

In the principal clinical study of Didronel for hypercalcemia of malignancy, patients with elevated calcium levels (10.1–17.4 mg/dl) were treated simultaneously with daily administrations of intravenous Didronel over a 3-day period and up to 3000 ml of saline and 80 mg of loop diuretic. The response to treatment for these patients was compared with that from patients treated with saline and loop diuretics alone. In terms of total serum calcium changes, 88% of patients treated with Didronel I.V. Infusion as described, had reductions of serum calcium of 1 mg/dl or more. Total serum calcium returned to normal in 63% of patients within 7 days compared to 33% of patients treated with hydration alone. Reductions in urinary calcium excretion, which accompany reductions in excessive bone resorption, became apparent after 24 hours. This was accompanied or followed by maximum decreases in serum calcium which were observed, most frequently, 72 hours after the first infusion.

The physiologically important component of serum calcium is the ionized portion. In most institutions, this cannot be measured directly. It is important to recognize that factors influencing the ratio of free and bound calcium such as serum proteins, particularly albumin, may complicate the interpretation of total serum calcium measurements. If indicated, a corrected serum calcium value should be calculated using an established algorithm.

When the total serum calcium values are adjusted for serum albumin levels, there was a return to normocalcemia in 24% of Didronel-treated patients and in 7% of patients treated with saline infusion. Eighty-seven percent of patients receiving Didronel and 67% of patients on saline had albumin-adjusted serum calcium levels returned to normal or reduced by at least 1 mg/dl.

In the above mentioned study, a second course of Didronel I.V. Infusion was tried in a small number of patients who had a recurrence of hypercalcemia following an initial response to a 3-day infusion of the drug. All patients who received a second 3-day course of Didronel I.V. Infusion showed a decrease of total serum calcium of at least 1 mg/dl. Normalization of total serum calcium occurred in 11 out of 14 patients.

In another small study of Didronel I.V. Infusion, patients with elevated albumin-adjusted calcium levels received a single 24-hour infusion of 25 mg/kg body weight (13 patients: mean baseline adjusted calcium 13.3 ± 0.3 mg/dl) or 30 mg/kg body weight (12 patients: 13.8 ± 0.4 mg/dl). Following treatment, mean nadir adjusted calcium levels were 10.9 ± 0.4 mg/dl and 10.5 ± 0.3 mg/dl for the two doses respectively.

Didronel I.V. Infusion does not appear to alter renal tubular reabsorption of calcium, and does not affect hypercalcemia in patients with hyperparathyroidism where increased calcium reabsorption may be a factor in the hypercalcemia.

Limited clinical study results suggest that continuation of Didronel therapy with oral tablets may maintain clinically acceptable serum calcium levels and prolong normocalcemia.

INDICATIONS AND USAGE

Didronel I.V. Infusion, together with achievement and maintenance of adequate hydration, is indicated for the treatment of hypercalcemia of malignancy inadequately managed by dietary modification and/or oral hydration.

In the treatment of hypercalcemia of malignancy, it is important to initiate rehydration with saline together with "high ceiling" or "loop" diuretics if indicated to restore urine output. This also is intended to increase the renal excretion of calcium and initiate a reduction in serum calcium. Since increased bone resorption is usually the underlying cause of an increased flux of calcium into the vascular compartment, concurrent therapy with Didronel I.V. Infusion is recommended as soon as there is a restoration of urine output. Since Didronel is excreted by the kidney, it is important to know that renal function is adequate to handle not only the increased fluid load but also the excretion of the drug itself. (See WARNINGS.)

Didronel I.V. Infusion is also indicated for the treatment of hypercalcemia of malignancy which persists after adequate hydration has been restored. Patients with and without metastases and with a variety of tumors have been responsive to treatment with Didronel I.V. Infusion. Adequate hydration of patients should be maintained, but in aged patients and in those with cardiac failure, care must be taken to avoid overhydration.

CONTRAINDICATIONS

In patients with Class Dc and higher renal functional impairment (serum creatinine greater than 5.0 mg/dl) Didronel I.V. Infusion should be withheld.

WARNINGS

Occasional mild to moderate abnormalities in renal function (elevated BUN and/or serum creatinine) have been observed when Didronel I.V. Infusion was given as directed to patients with hypercalcemia of malignancy. These changes were reversible or remained stable, without worsening, after completion of the course of Didronel I.V. Infusion. In some patients with pre-existing renal impairment or in those who had received potentially nephrotoxic drugs, further depression of renal function was sometimes seen. This

suggests that Didronel I.V. Infusion may produce or aggravate the depression of renal function in approximately 8 of 203 treatment courses when used to treat hypercalcemia of malignancy. In a study of Didronel I.V. Infusion administered in a 24-hour infusion, one patient with evidence of pre-existing renal insufficiency developed anuria 18 hours after initiation of the 30 mg/kg dose. (See PRECAUTIONS)
A possible relationship of acute renal failure in this patient to intravenous administration of Didronel cannot be ruled out. Therefore, it is recommended that appropriate monitoring of renal function with serum creatinine and/or BUN be carried out with Didronel I.V. Infusion treatment.
The effects of Didronel I.V. Infusion administration on renal function in patients with serum creatinine greater than 2.5 mg/dl (Class Cc and higher, Classification of Renal Functional Impairment, Council on the Kidney in Cardiovascular Disease, American Heart Association, Ann. Int. Med. 75:251–52, 1971) has not been systematically examined in controlled trials.
Since Didronel is excreted by the kidney, it is important to know that renal function is adequate to handle not only the increased fluid load but also the excretion of the drug itself. Since these capacities are impaired in patients with underlying renal disease and since experience with Didronel I.V. Infusion in patients with serum creatinine >2.5 mg/dl is limited, the use of Didronel I.V. Infusion in such patients should occur only after a careful assessment of renal status or potential risks and potential benefits. (See WARNINGS.)
Reduction of the dose of Didronel I.V. Infusion, if used at all, may be advisable in Class Cc renal functional impairment (serum creatinine 2.5 to 4.9 mg/dl); and, Didronel I.V. Infusion be used only if the potential benefit of hypercalcemia correction will substantially exceed the potential for worsening of renal function. In patients with Class Dc and higher renal functional impairment (serum creatinine greater than 5.0 mg/dl) Didronel I.V. Infusion should be withheld.
Following infusion of Didronel, renal function should be evaluated with standard laboratory measurements every few days for the first 2 weeks.

PRECAUTIONS

General: Hypercalcemia may cause or exacerbate impaired renal function. In clinical trials, while elevations of serum creatinine or blood urea nitrogen were seen in patients with hypercalcemia of malignancy prior to treatment with Didronel I.V. Infusion, these measurements improved in some patients or remained unchanged in most patients. Nevertheless, elevations in serum creatinine during treatment with Didronel I.V. Infusion have been observed in approximately 10% of patients.
Rare cases of acute renal failure have been reported in association with the use of Didronel I.V. Infusion (See also WARNINGS). Concomitant use of non-steroidal anti-inflammatory drugs and diuretics in these patients may have contributed to the renal failure.
In animal preclinical studies, administration of Didronel I.V. Infusion in amounts or at rates in excess of those recommended produced transient hypocalcemia or induced proximal renal tubular damage.
In the principal clinical trial of Didronel I.V. Infusion, 33 of 185 patients (18%) treated one or more times with Didronel I.V. Infusion had serum calcium values below the lower limits of normal. When adjusted for levels of reduced serum albumin, less than 1% of the 185 patients are estimated to have hypocalcemic ionized serum calcium levels. No adverse effects have been traced to hypocalcemia.
The hypercalcemia of hyperparathyroidism is refractory to Didronel I.V. Infusion. It is possible for this disease to coexist in patients with malignancy.
Carcinogenesis, Mutagenesis, Impairment of Fertility: Long-term studies in rats indicate that Didronel is not carcinogenic.
Pregnancy: Teratogenic Effects: Pregnancy Category C. Animal reproduction studies have not been conducted with Didronel I.V. Infusion. It is also not known whether Didronel I.V. Infusion can cause fetal harm when administered to a pregnant woman or can affect reproduction capacity. Didronel I.V. Infusion should be given to a pregnant woman only if clearly needed.
Nursing Mothers: It is not known whether this drug is excreted in human milk. Because many drugs are excreted in human milk, caution should be exercised when Didronel I.V. Infusion is administered to a nursing woman.
Pediatric Use: Safety and effectiveness in pediatric patinets have not been established.

ADVERSE REACTIONS

Hypercalcemia of malignancy is frequently associated with abnormal elevations of serum creatinine and BUN. One-third of the patients participating in multiclinic trials had such elevations before receiving Didronel I.V. Infusion. In these trials, the elevations of BUN or serum creatinine improved in some patients, or remained unchanged in most patients; however, in approximately 10% of patients, occasional mild to moderate abnormalities in renal function (increases of >0.5 mg/dl serum creatinine) were observed during or immediately after treatment. The possibility that Didronel I.V. Infusion contributed to these changes cannot be excluded (see WARNINGS).
Of patients who participated in the controlled hypercalcemia trials, 10 of 221 (5%) treatment courses reported a metallic or altered taste, or loss of taste, which usually disappeared within hours, during and/or shortly after Didronel I.V. Infusion. A few patients with Paget's Disease of bone have reported allergic skin rashes in association with oral Didronel medication.

OVERDOSAGE

Rapid intravenous administration of Didronel at doses above 27 mg/kg has produced ECG changes and bleeding problems in animals. These abnormalities are probably related to marked and/or rapid decreases in ionized calcium levels in blood and tissue fluids. They are thought to be due to chelation of calcium by massive amounts of diphosphonate. These abnormalities have been shown to be reversible in animal studies by the administration of ionizable calcium salts.
Similar problems are not expected to occur in humans treated with Didronel I.V. Infusion used as recommended (see DOSAGE AND ADMINISTRATION). Moreover, signs and symptoms of hypocalcemia such as paresthesias and carpopedal spasms have not been reported. The chelation effects of the diphosphonate, should they occur in man, should be reversible with the intravenous administration of calcium gluconate.
A dose of 30 mg/kg body weight per day of Didronel I.V. Infusion was continuously administered for 72 hours in one patient (total dose 90 mg/kg). No adverse experiences associated with the infusion were reported. Another patient with one kidney and slowly rising creatinine prior to therapy received 30 mg/kg body weight per day of Didronel I.V. Infusion for 48 hours (total dose 60 mg/kg). This patient reported altered taste and a further gradual increase in serum creatinine from 2.1 mg/dl to 2.7 mg/dl during the week after therapy was observed. (See PRECAUTIONS).
Administration of intravenous etidronate disodium at doses and possibly at rates in excess of those recommended has been reported to be associated with renal insufficiency.

DOSAGE AND ADMINISTRATION

Didronel I.V. Infusion: The recommended dose of Didronel I.V. Infusion is 7.5 mg/kg body weight/day infused over at least two hours on three successive days. Infusions may be continued for up to seven days if necessary. **This daily dose must be diluted in at least 250 ml of sterile normal saline and may be added to volumes of fluid greater than 250 ml when this is convenient.** Single (one day) 24 hour infusions of 25–30 mg/kg body weight were administered to only a limited number of patients, and are NOT recommended for initial treatment. This single dose must be diluted in at least 1000 ml of sterile normal saline. Stability studies show that diluted solution stored at controlled room temperature (59°F to 86°F or 15°C to 30°C) shows no loss of drug for a 48-hour period.
THE DILUTED DOSE OF DIDRONEL I.V. INFUSION SHOULD BE ADMINISTERED INTRAVENOUSLY OVER A PERIOD OF AT LEAST 2 HOURS.
REGARDLESS OF THE VOLUME OF SOLUTION IN WHICH DIDRONEL I.V. INFUSION IS DILUTED, SLOW INFUSION IS IMPORTANT TO SAFETY. The minimum infusion time of two hours at the recommended dose (7.5 mg/kg body weight) or smaller doses, should be observed. The usual course of treatment is one infusion of 7.5 mg/kg body weight/day on each of 3 consecutive days but some patients have been treated for up to 7 days. When patients are treated for more than 3 days, there may be an increased possibility of producing hypocalcemia.
Retreatment with Didronel I.V. Infusion may be appropriate if hypercalcemia recurs. There should be at least a seven-day interval between courses of treatment with Didronel I.V. Infusion. The dose and manner of retreatment is the same as that for initial treatment. Retreatment with 7.5 mg/kg body weight for more than three days has not been adequately studied. The safety and efficacy of more than two courses of therapy with Didronel I.V. Infusion have not been studied. In the presence of renal impairment, reduction of the dose may be advisable.
Parenteral drug products should be inspected visually for particulate matter and discoloration prior to administration whenever solution and container permit.
Didronel Oral Tablets: Didronel (etidronate disodium) tablets may be started on the day following the last dose of Didronel I.V. Infusion. The recommended oral dose of Didronel for patients who have had hypercalcemia is 20 mg/kg body weight/day for 30 days. If serum calcium levels remain normal or at clinically acceptable levels, treatment may be extended. Treatment for more than 90 days has not been adequately studied and is not recommended. Please consult the package insert pertaining to oral Didronel tablets for additional prescribing information.

HOW SUPPLIED

Didronel I.V. Infusion is supplied in 6 ml ampules as a 5% solution containing 300 mg etidronate disodium.
NDC 58063-457-01 carton of 6 ampules.
Avoid excessive heat (over 104°F or 40°C) for undiluted product.
Address medical inquiries to **MGI PHARMA, INC.** Medical Department, Suite 300E, Opus Center, 9900 Bren Road East, Minnetonka, MN 55343-9667.
CAUTION: Federal law prohibits dispensing without prescription.
Didronel® is a registered trademark of Procter & Gamble Pharmaceuticals, Inc.
Manufactured by
Taylor Pharmaceuticals
Decatur, Illinois 62525
for **MGI PHARMA, INC.**
Minnetonka, Minnesota 55343–9667
January 1998

Shown in Product Identification Guide, page 321

SALAGEN® TABLETS ℞

[sal 'ə jən]
(pilocarpine hydrochloride)

DESCRIPTION

SALAGEN® Tablets contain pilocarpine hydrochloride, a cholinergic agonist for oral use. Pilocarpine hydrochloride is a hygroscopic, odorless, bitter tasting white crystal or powder which is soluble in water and alcohol and virtually insoluble in most non-polar solvents. Pilocarpine hydrochloride, with a chemical name of (3*S*-*cis*)-2(3*H*)-Furanone, 3-ethyldihydro-4-[(1-methyl-1*H*-imidazol-5-yl)methyl] monohydrochloride, has a molecular weight of 244.72.

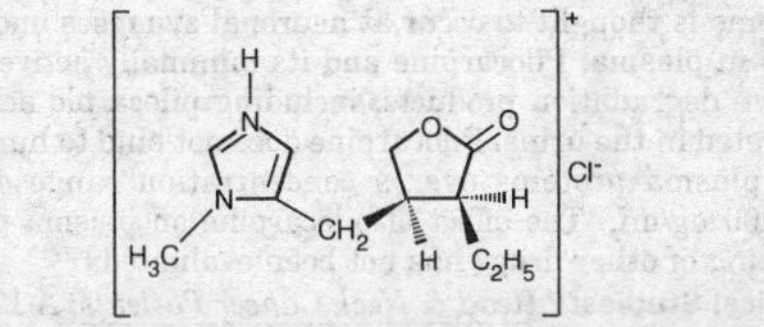

Each SALAGEN® Tablet for oral administration contains 5 mg of pilocarpine hydrochloride. Inactive ingredients in the tablet, the tablet's film coating, polishing, and branding are: carnauba wax, hydroxypropyl methylcellulose, iron oxide, microcrystalline cellulose, stearic acid, titanium dioxide and other ingredients.

CLINICAL PHARMACOLOGY

Pharmacodynamics: Pilocarpine is a cholinergic parasympathomimetic agent exerting a broad spectrum of pharmacologic effects with predominant muscarinic action. Pilocarpine, in appropriate dosage, can increase secretion by the exocrine glands. The sweat, salivary, lacrimal, gastric, pancreatic, and intestinal glands and the mucous cells of the respiratory tract may be stimulated. When applied topically to the eye as a single dose it causes miosis, spasm of accommodation, and may cause a transitory rise in intraocular pressure followed by a more persistent fall. Dose-related smooth muscle stimulation of the intestinal tract may cause increased tone, increased motility, spasm, and tenesmus. Bronchial smooth muscle tone may increase. The tone and motility of urinary tract, gallbladder, and biliary duct smooth muscle may be enhanced. Pilocarpine may have paradoxical effects on the cardiovascular system. The expected effect of a muscarinic agonist is vasodepression, but administration of pilocarpine may produce hypertension after a brief episode of hypotension. Bradycardia and tachycardia have both been reported with use of pilocarpine.
In a study of 12 healthy male volunteers there was a dose-related increase in unstimulated salivary flow following single 5 and 10 mg oral doses of SALAGEN® Tablets. This effect of pilocarpine on salivary flow was time-related with an onset at 20 minutes and a peak effect at 1 hour with a duration of 3 to 5 hours (See **Pharmacokinetics** section).
Head and Neck Cancer Patients: In a 12 week randomized, double-blind, placebo-controlled study in 207 patients (placebo, N=65; 5 mg, N=73; 10 mg, N=69), increases from baseline (means 0.072 and 0.112 mL/min, ranges −0.690 to 0.728 and −0.380 to 1.689) of whole saliva flow for the 5 mg (63%) and 10 mg (90%) tablet, respectively, were seen 1 hour after the first dose of SALAGEN® Tablets. Increases in unstimulated parotid flow were seen following the first dose (means 0.025 and 0.046 mL/min, ranges 0 to 0.414 and −0.070 to 1.002 mL/min for the 5 and 10 mg dose, respectively). In this study, no correlation existed between the amount of increase in salivary flow and the degree of symptomatic relief.
Sjögren's Syndrome Patients: In two 12 week randomized, double-blind, placebo-controlled studies in 629 patients (placebo, n=253; 2.5 mg, n=121; 5 mg, n=255; 5-7.5 mg,

Continued on next page

Salagen—Cont.

n=114), the ability of SALAGEN® Tablets to stimulate saliva production was assessed. In these trials using varying doses of SALAGEN® Tablets (2.5–7.5 mg), the rate of saliva production was plotted against time. An Area Under the Curve (AUC) representing the total amount of saliva produced during the observation interval was calculated. Relative to placebo, an increase in the amount of saliva being produced was observed following the first dose of SALAGEN® Tablets and was maintained throughout the duration (12 weeks) of the trials in an approximate dose response fashion (See Clinical Studies section).

Pharmacokinetics: In a multiple-dose pharmacokinetic study in male volunteers following 2 days of 5 or 10 mg of oral pilocarpine hydrochloride tablets given at 8 a.m., noontime, and 6 p.m., the mean elimination half-life was 0.76 hours for the 5 mg dose and 1.35 hours for the 10 mg dose. T_{max} values were 1.25 hours and 0.85 hours. C_{max} values were 15 ng/mL and 41 ng/mL. The AUC trapezoidal values were 33 h(ng/mL) and 108 h(ng/mL), respectively, for the 5 and 10 mg doses following the last 6 hour dose.

Pharmacokinetics in elderly male volunteers (n=11) were comparable to those in younger men. In five healthy elderly female volunteers, the mean C_{max} and AUC were approximately twice that of elderly males and young normal male volunteers.

When taken with a high fat meal by 12 healthy male volunteers, there was a decrease in the rate of absorption of pilocarpine from SALAGEN® Tablets. Mean $T_{max's}$ were 1.47 and 0.87 hours, and mean $C_{max's}$ were 51.8 and 59.2 ng/mL for fed and fasted, respectively.

Limited information is available about the metabolism and elimination of pilocarpine in humans. Inactivation of pilocarpine is thought to occur at neuronal synapses and probably in plasma. Pilocarpine and its minimally active or inactive degradation products, including pilocarpic acid, are excreted in the urine. Pilocarpine does not bind to human or rat plasma proteins over a concentration range of 5 to 25,000 ng/mL. The effect of pilocarpine on plasma protein binding of other drugs has not been evaluated.

Clinical Studies: *Head & Neck Cancer Patients:* A 12 week randomized, double-blind, placebo-controlled study in 207 patients (142 men, 65 women) was conducted in patients whose mean age was 58.5 years with a range of 19 to 77; the racial distribution was Caucasian 95%, Black 4%, and other 1%. In this population, a statistically significant improvement in mouth dryness occurred in the 5 and 10 mg SALAGEN® Tablet treated patients compared to placebo treated patients. The 5 and 10 mg treated patients could not be distinguished. (See Pharmacodynamics section for flow study details.)

Another 12 week, double-blind, randomized, placebo-controlled study was conducted in 162 patients whose mean age was 57.8 years with a range of 27 to 80; the racial distribution was Caucasian 88%, Black 10%, and other 2%. The effects of placebo were compared to 2.5 mg three times a day of SALAGEN® Tablets for 4 weeks followed by titration to 5 mg three times a day and 10 mg three times a day. Lowering of the dose was necessary because of adverse events in 3 of 67 patients treated with 5 mg of SALAGEN® Tablets and in 7 of 66 patients treated with 10 mg of SALAGEN® Tablets. After 4 weeks of treatment, 2.5 mg of SALAGEN® Tablets three times a day was comparable to placebo in relieving dryness. In patients treated with 5 mg and 10 mg of SALAGEN® Tablets, the greatest improvement in dryness was noted in patients with no measurable salivary flow at baseline.

In both studies, some patients noted improvement in the global assessment of their dry mouth, speaking without liquids, and a reduced need for supplemental oral comfort agents.

In the two placebo-controlled clinical trials, the most common adverse events related to drug, and increasing in rate as dose increases, were sweating, nausea, rhinitis, diarrhea, chills, flushing, urinary frequency, dizziness, and asthenia. The most common adverse experience causing withdrawal from treatment was sweating (5 mg t.i.d. ≤ 1%; 10 mg t.i.d.=12%).

Sjögren's Syndrome Patients: Two separate studies were conducted in patients with primary or secondary Sjögren's Syndrome. In both studies, the majority of patients best fit the European criteria for having primary Sjögren's Syndrome. ["Criteria for the Classification of Sjögren's Syndrome" (Vitali C, Bombardieri S, Moutsopoulos HM, et al: Preliminary criteria for the classification of Sjögren's syndrome. Arthritis Rheum 36:340–347, 1993.)]

A 12-week, randomized, double-blind, parallel-group, placebo-controlled study was conducted in 256 patients (14 men, 242 women) whose mean age was 57 years with a range of 24 to 85 years. The racial distribution was as follows: Caucasian 91%, Black 6%, and other 3%.

The effects of placebo were compared with those of SALAGEN® Tablets 5 mg four times a day (20 mg/day) for 6 weeks. At 6 weeks, the patients' dosage was increased from

5 mg SALAGEN® Tablets q.i.d. to 7.5 mg q.i.d. The data collected during the first 6 weeks of the trial were evaluated for safety and efficacy, and the data of the second 6 weeks of the trial were used to provide additional evidence of safety. After 6 weeks of treatment, statistically significant global improvement of dry mouth was observed compared to placebo. "Global improvement" is defined as a score of 55 mm or more on a 100 mm visual analogue scale in response to the question, "Please rate your present condition of dry mouth (xerostomia) compared with your condition at the start of this study. Consider the changes to your dry mouth and other symptoms related to your dry mouth that have occurred since you have taken this medication." Patients' assessments of specific dry mouth symptoms such as severity of dry mouth, mouth discomfort, ability to speak without water, ability to sleep without drinking water, ability to swallow food without drinking, and a decreased use of saliva substitutes were found to be consistent with the significant global improvement described.

Another 12 week randomized, double-blind, parallel-group, placebo-controlled study was conducted in 373 patients (16 men, 357 women) whose mean age was 55 years with a range of 21 to 84. The racial distribution was Caucasian 80%, Oriental 14%, Black 2%, and 4% of other origin. The treatment groups were 2.5 mg pilocarpine tablets, 5 mg SALAGEN® Tablets, and placebo. All treatments were administered on a four times a day regimen.

After 12 weeks of treatment, statistically significant global improvement of dry mouth was observed at a dose of 5 mg compared with placebo. The 2.5 mg (10mg/day) group was not significantly different than placebo. However, a subgroup of patients with rheumatoid arthritis tended to improve in global assessments at both the 2.5 mg q.i.d (9 patients) and 5 mg q.i.d. (16 patients) dose (10–20 mg/day). The clinical significance of this finding is unknown.

Patients' assessments of specific dry mouth symptoms such as severity of dry mouth, mouth discomfort, ability to sleep without drinking water, and decreased use of saliva substitutes were also found to be consistent with the significant global improvement described when measured after 6 weeks and 12 weeks of SALAGEN® Tablets use.

INDICATIONS AND USAGE

SALAGEN® Tablets are indicated for 1) the treatment of symptoms of dry mouth from salivary gland hypofunction caused by radiotherapy for cancer of the head and neck; and 2) the treatment of symptoms of dry mouth in patients with Sjögren's syndrome.

CONTRAINDICATIONS

SALAGEN® Tablets are contraindicated in patients with uncontrolled asthma, known hypersensitivity to pilocarpine, and when miosis is undesirable, e.g., in acute iritis and in narrow-angle (angle closure) glaucoma.

WARNINGS

Cardiovascular Disease: Patients with significant cardiovascular disease may be unable to compensate for transient changes in hemodynamics or rhythm induced by pilocarpine. Pulmonary edema has been reported as a complication of pilocarpine toxicity from high ocular doses given for acute angle-closure glaucoma. Pilocarpine should be administered with caution in and under close medical supervision of patients with significant cardiovascular disease.

Ocular: Ocular formulations of pilocarpine have been reported to cause visual blurring which may result in decreased visual acuity, especially at night and in patients with central lens changes, and to cause impairment of depth perception. Caution should be advised while driving at night or performing hazardous activities in reduced lighting.

Pulmonary Disease: Pilocarpine has been reported to increase airway resistance, bronchial smooth muscle tone, and bronchial secretions. Pilocarpine hydrochloride should be administered with caution to and under close medical supervision in patients with controlled asthma, chronic bronchitis, or chronic obstructive pulmonary disease requiring pharmacotherapy.

PRECAUTIONS

General: Pilocarpine toxicity is characterized by an exaggeration of its parasympathomimetic effects. These may include: headache, visual disturbance, lacrimation, sweating, respiratory distress, gastrointestinal spasm, nausea, vomiting, diarrhea, atrioventricular block, tachycardia, bradycardia, hypotension, hypertension, shock, mental confusion, cardiac arrhythmia, and tremors.

The dose-related cardiovascular pharmacologic effects of pilocarpine include hypotension, hypertension, bradycardia, and tachycardia.

Pilocarpine should be administered with caution to patients with known or suspected cholelithiasis or biliary tract disease. Contractions of the gallbladder or biliary smooth muscle could precipitate complications including cholecystitis, cholangitis, and biliary obstruction.

Pilocarpine may increase ureteral smooth muscle tone and could theoretically precipitate renal colic (or "ureteral reflux"), particularly in patients with nephrolithiasis.

Cholinergic agonists may have dose-related central nervous system effects. This should be considered when treating patients with underlying cognitive or psychiatric disturbances.

Renal Insufficiency: The pharmacokinetics of orally administered pilocarpine in patients with renal and hepatic disease is not known.

Information for Patients: Patients should be informed that pilocarpine may cause visual disturbances, especially at night, that could impair their ability to drive safely.

If a patient sweats excessively while taking pilocarpine hydrochloride and cannot drink enough liquid, the patient should consult a physician. Dehydration may develop.

Drug Interactions: Pilocarpine should be administered with caution to patients taking beta adrenergic antagonists because of the possibility of conduction disturbances. Drugs with parasympathomimetic effects administered concurrently with pilocarpine would be expected to result in additive pharmacologic effects. Pilocarpine might antagonize the anticholinergic effects of drugs used concomitantly. These effects should be considered when anticholinergic properties may be contributing to the therapeutic effect of concomitant medication (e.g., atropine, inhaled ipratropium).

While no formal drug interaction studies have been performed, the following concomitant drugs were used in at least 10% of patients in either or both Sjögren's efficacy studies: acetylsalicylic acid, artificial tears, calcium, conjugated estrogens, hydroxychloroquine sulfate, ibuprofen, levothyroxine sodium, medroxyprogesterone acetate, methotrexate, multivitamins, naproxen, omeprazole, paracetamol, and prednisone.

Carcinogenesis, Mutagenesis, Impairment of Fertility: No definitive long term animal studies have evaluated the carcinogenic potential of pilocarpine. No evidence that pilocarpine has the potential to cause genetic toxicity was obtained in a series of studies that included: 1) bacterial assays (Salmonella and E. coli) for reverse gene mutations; 2) an *in vitro* chromosome aberration assay in a Chinese hamster ovary cell line; 3) an *in vivo* chromosome aberration assay (micronucleus test) in mice; and 4) a primary DNA damage assay (unscheduled DNA synthesis) in rat hepatocyte primary cultures.

Oral administration of pilocarpine to male and female rats at a dosage of 18 mg/kg/day (approximately 5 times the maximum recommended dose for a 50 kg human when compared on the basis of body surface area (mg/m^2) estimates) resulted in impaired reproductive function, including reduced fertility, decreased sperm motility, and morphologic evidence of abnormal sperm. It is unclear whether the reduction in fertility was due to effects on male animals, female animals, or both males and females. In dogs, exposure to pilocarpine at a dosage of 3 mg/kg/day (approximately 3 times the maximum recommended dose for a 50 kg human when compared on the basis of body surface area (mg/m^2) estimates) for six months resulted in evidence of impaired spermatogenesis. The data obtained in these studies suggest that pilocarpine may impair the fertility of male and female humans.

SALAGEN® Tablets should be administered to individuals who are attempting to conceive a child only if the potential benefit justifies potential impairment of fertility.

Pregnancy: Teratogenic effects

Pregnancy Category C: Pilocarpine was associated with a reduction in the mean fetal body weight and an increase in the incidence of skeletal variations when given to pregnant rats at a dosage of 90 mg/kg/day (approximately 26 times the maximum recommended dose for a 50 kg human when compared on the basis of body surface area (mg/m^2) estimates). These effects may have been secondary to maternal toxicity. In another study, oral administration of pilocarpine to female rats during gestation and lactation at a dosage of 36 mg/kg/day (approximately 10 times the maximum recommended dose for a 50 kg human when compared on the basis of body surface area (mg/m^2) estimates) resulted in an increased incidence of stillbirths; decreased neonatal survival and reduced mean body weight of pups were observed at dosages of 18 mg/kg/day (approximately 5 times the maximum recommended dose for a 50 kg human when compared on the basis of body surface area (mg/m^2) estimates) and above. There are no adequate and well-controlled studies in pregnant women. SALAGEN® Tablets should be used during pregnancy only if the potential benefit justifies the potential risk to the fetus.

Nursing Mothers: It is not known whether this drug is excreted in human milk. Because many drugs are excreted in human milk and because of the potential for serious adverse reactions in nursing infants from SALAGEN® Tablets, a decision should be made whether to discontinue nursing or to discontinue the drug, taking into account the importance of the drug to the mother.

Pediatric Use: Safety and effectiveness in pediatric patients have not been established.

Geriatric Use: *Head and Neck Cancer Patients:* In the placebo-controlled clinical trials (see Clinical Studies section) the mean age of patients was approximately 58 years (range 19 to 80). Of these patients, 97/369 (61/217 receiving pilo-

carpine) were over the age of 65 years. In the healthy volunteer studies, 15/150 subjects were over the age of 65 years. In both study populations, the adverse events reported by those over 65 years and those 65 years and younger were comparable. Of the 15 elderly volunteers (5 women, 10 men), the 5 women had higher C_{max}'s and AUC's than the men. (See **Pharmacokinetics** section.)

Sjögren's Syndrome Patients: In the placebo-controlled clinical trials (see **Clinical Studies** section), the mean age of patients was approximately 55 years (range 21 to 85). The adverse events reported by those over 65 years and those 65 years and younger were comparable except for notable trends for urinary frequency, diarrhea, and dizziness (see **ADVERSE REACTIONS** section).

ADVERSE REACTIONS

Head & Neck Cancer Patients: In controlled studies, 217 patients received pilocarpine, of whom 68% were men and 32% were women. Race distribution was 91% Caucasian, 8% Black, and 1% of other origin. Mean age was approximately 58 years. The majority of patients were between 50 and 64 years (51%), 33% were 65 years and older and 16% were younger than 50 years of age.

The most frequent adverse experiences associated with SALAGEN® Tablets were a consequence of the expected pharmacologic effects of pilocarpine.

Adverse Event	10 mg t.i.d. (30mg/day) n=121	5mg t.i.d. (15mg/day) n=141	Placebo (t.i.d.) n=152
Sweating	68%	29%	9%
Nausea	15	6	4
Rhinitis	14	5	7
Diarrhea	7	4	5
Chills	15	3	<1
Flushing	13	8	3
Urinary Frequency	12	9	7
Dizziness	12	5	4
Asthenia	12	6	3

In addition, the following adverse events (≥3% incidence) were reported at dosages of 15–30 mg/day in the controlled clinical trials:

Adverse Event	Pilocarpine HCl 5-10 mg t.i.d. (15-30 mg/day) n=212	Placebo (t.i.d.) n=152
Headache	11%	8%
Dyspepsia	7	5
Lacrimation	6	8
Edema	5	4
Abdominal Pain	4	4
Amblyopia	4	2
Vomiting	4	1
Pharyngitis	3	8
Hypertension	3	1

The following events were reported with treated head and neck cancer patients at incidences of 1% to 2% at dosages of 7.5 to 30 mg/day: abnormal vision, conjunctivitis, dysphagia, epistaxis, myalgias, pruritus, rash, sinusitis, tachycardia, taste perversion, tremor, voice alteration.

The following events were reported rarely in treated head and neck cancer patients (<1%): Causal relation is unknown.

Body as a whole: body odor, hypothermia, mucous membrane abnormality

Cardiovascular: bradycardia, ECG abnormality, palpitations, syncope

Digestive: anorexia, increased appetite, esophagitis, gastrointestinal disorder, tongue disorder

Hematologic: leukopenia, lymphadenopathy

Nervous: anxiety, confusion, depression, abnormal dreams, hyperkinesia, hypesthesia, nervousness, paresthesias, speech disorder, twitching

Respiratory: increased sputum, stridor, yawning

Skin: seborrhea

Special senses: deafness, eye pain, glaucoma

Urogenital: dysuria, metrorrhagia, urinary impairment

In long-term treatment were two patients with underlying cardiovascular disease of whom one experienced a myocardial infarct and another an episode of syncope. The association with drug is uncertain.

Sjögren's Syndrome Patients: In controlled studies, 376 patients received pilocarpine, of whom 5% were men and 95% were women. Race distribution was 84% Caucasian, 9% Oriental, 3% Black, and 4% of other origin. Mean age was 55 years. The majority of patients were between 40 and 69 years (70%), 16% were 70 years and older and 14% were younger than 40 years of age. Of these patients, 161/629 (89/376 receiving pilocarpine) were over the age of 65 years. The adverse events reported by those over 65 years and those 65 years and younger were comparable except for notable trends for urinary frequency, diarrhea, and dizziness.

The incidences of urinary frequency and diarrhea in the elderly were about double those in the non-elderly. The incidence of dizziness was about three times as high in the elderly as in the non-elderly. These adverse experiences were not considered to be serious. In the 2 placebo-controlled studies, the most common adverse events related to drug use were sweating, urinary frequency, chills, and vasodilatation (flushing). The most commonly reported reason for patient discontinuation of treatment was sweating. Expected pharmacologic effects of pilocarpine include the following adverse experiences associated with SALAGEN® Tablets:

Adverse Event	5 mg q.i.d. (20 mg/day) n=255	Placebo (q.i.d.) n=253
Sweating	40%	7%
Urinary Frequency	10	4
Nausea	9	9
Flushing	9	2
Rhinitis	7	8
Diarrhea	6	7
Chills	4	2
Increased Salivation	3	0
Asthenia	2	2

In addition, the following adverse events (≥3% incidence) were reported at dosing of 20 mg/day in the controlled clinical trials:

Adverse Event	Pilocarpine HCl 5 mg q.i.d. (20 mg/day) n=255	Placebo (q.i.d.) n=253
Headache	13%	19%
Flu Syndrome	9	9
Dyspepsia	7	7
Dizziness	6	7
Pain	4	2
Sinusitis	4	5
Abdominal Pain	3	4
Pharyngitis	2	5
Rash	2	3
Infection	2	6

The following events were reported in Sjögren's patients at incidences of 1% to 2% at dosing of 20 mg/day: accidental injury, allergic reaction, back pain, blurred vision, constipation, increased cough, edema, epistaxis, face edema, fever, flatulence, glossitis, lab test abnormalities, including chemistry, hematology, and urinalysis, myalgia, palpitation, pruritis, somnolence, stomatitis, tachycardia, tinnitus, urinary incontinence, urinary tract infection, vaginitis, vomiting.

The following events were reported rarely in treated Sjögren's patients (<1%): Causal relation is unknown.

Body as a whole: chest pain, cyst, death, moniliasis, neck pain, neck rigidity, photosensitivity reaction

Cardiovascular: angina pectoris, arrhythmia, ECG abnormality, hypotension, hypertension, intracranial hemorrhage, migraine, myocardial infarction

Digestive: anorexia, bilirubinemia, cholelithiasis, colitis, dry mouth, eructation, gastritis, gastroenteritis, gastrointestinal disorder, gingivitis, hepatitis, abnormal liver function tests, melena, nausea & vomiting, pancreatitis, parotid gland enlargement, salivary gland enlargement, sputum increased, taste loss, tongue disorder, tooth disorder

Hematologic: hematuria, lymphadenopathy, abnormal platelets, thrombocythemia, thrombocytopenia, thrombosis, abnormal WBC

Metabolic and Nutritional: peripheral edema, hypoglycemia

Musculoskeletal: arthralgia, arthritis, bone disorder, spontaneous bone fracture, pathological fracture, myasthenia, tendon disorder, tenosynovitis

Nervous: aphasia, confusion, depression, abnormal dreams, emotional lability, hyperkinesia, hypesthesia, insomnia, leg cramps, nervousness, paresthesias, abnormal thinking, tremor

Respiratory: bronchitis, dyspnea, hiccup, laryngismus, laryngitis, pneumonia, viral infection, voice alteration

Skin: alopecia, contact dermatitis, dry skin, eczema, erythema nodosum, exfoliative dermatitis, herpes simplex, skin ulcer, vesiculobullous rash

Special senses: cataract, conjunctivitis, dry eyes, ear disorder, ear pain, eye disorder, eye hemorrhage, glaucoma, lacrimation disorder, retinal disorder, taste perversion, abnormal vision

Urogenital: breast pain, dysuria, mastitis, menorrhagia, metrorrhagia, ovarian disorder, pyuria, salpingitis, urethral pain, urinary urgency, vaginal hemorrhage, vaginal moniliasis

The following adverse experiences have been reported rarely with ocular pilocarpine: A-V block, agitation, ciliary congestion, confusion, delusion, depression, dermatitis, middle ear disturbance, eyelid twitching, malignant glaucoma, iris cysts, macular hole, shock, and visual hallucination.

MANAGEMENT OF OVERDOSE

Fatal overdosage with pilocarpine has been reported in the scientific literature at doses presumed to be greater than 100 mg in two hospitalized patients. 100 mg of pilocarpine is considered potentially fatal. Overdosage should be treated with atropine titration (0.5 mg to 1.0 mg given subcutaneously or intravenously) and supportive measures to maintain respiration and circulation. Epinephrine (0.3 mg to 1.0 mg, subcutaneously or intramuscularly) may also be of value in the presence of severe cardiovascular depression or bronchoconstriction. It is not known if pilocarpine is dialyzable.

DOSAGE AND ADMINISTRATION

Head & Neck Cancer Patients:
The recommended initial dose of SALAGEN® Tablets is one tablet (5 mg) taken three times a day. Dosage should be titrated according to therapeutic response and tolerance. The usual dosage range is up to 3–6 tablets or 15–30 mg per day. (Not to exceed 2 tablets per dose.) Although early improvement may be realized, at least 12 weeks of uninterrupted therapy with SALAGEN® Tablets may be necessary to assess whether a beneficial response will be achieved. The incidence of the most common adverse events increases with dose. The lowest dose that is tolerated and effective should be used for maintenance.

Sjögren's Syndrome Patients:
The recommended dose of SALAGEN® Tablets is one tablet (5 mg) taken four times a day. Efficacy was established by 6 weeks of use.

HOW SUPPLIED

SALAGEN® Tablets, 5 mg, are white, film coated, round tablets, coded MGI 705. Each tablet contains 5 mg pilocarpine hydrochloride. They are supplied as follows:
NDC 58063-705-10 bottles of 100
Store at Controlled Room Temperature 15°–30°C (59°–86°F).
Manufactured by:
Boehringer Ingelheim Pharmaceuticals, Inc., Ridgefield, CT 06877
For: MGI PHARMA, INC., Minnetonka, MN 55343–9667
© 1998 MGI PHARMA, INC.   February 1998
Salagen® is a registered trademark of MGI PHARMA, INC.
Shown in Product Identification Guide, page 321

3M Pharmaceuticals
3M CENTER 275-3W-01
P.O. BOX 33275
ST. PAUL, MN 55133-3275

Commercial Customers:
Orders, Returns, Accounting
(800) 447-4537

Trade and Government:
(800) 328-6523

For Medical Matters Contact:
Medical Services Department
3M Pharmaceuticals
3M Center, Bldg. 275-2E-13
PO Box 33275
St. Paul MN, 55133-3275
(800) 328-0255

In Emergencies:
(651) 736-4930 (all hours)

Website:
www.3M.com/pharma

ALDARA™   ℞
[al dar 'a]
(imiquimod)
Cream, 5%
For Dermatologic Use Only -
Not for Ophthalmic Use

DESCRIPTION

Aldara™ is the brand name for imiquimod which is an immune response modifier. Each gram of the 5% cream contains 50 mg of imiquimod in an off-white oil-in-water vanishing cream base consisting of isostearic acid, cetyl alcohol, stearyl alcohol, white petrolatum, polysorbate 60, sorbitan monostearate, glycerin, xanthan gum, purified water, benzyl alcohol, methylparaben, and propylparaben.

Chemically, imiquimod is 1-(2-methylpropyl)-1*H*-imidazo[4,5-c]quinolin-4-amine. Imiquimod has a molecular formula of $C_{14}H_{16}N_4$ and a molecular weight of 240.3. Its structural formula is:
[See chemical structure at top of next column]

Continued on next page

Aldara—Cont.

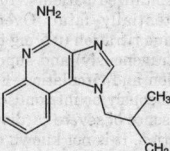

CLINICAL PHARMACOLOGY

Pharmacodynamics

The mechanism of action of imiquimod in treating genital/perianal warts is unknown. Imiquimod has no direct antiviral activity in cell culture. Mouse skin studies suggest that imiquimod induces cytokines including interferon-α. However, the clinical relevance of these findings is unknown.

Pharmacokinetics

Percutaneous absorption of [^{14}C] imiquimod was minimal in a study involving 6 healthy subjects treated with a single topical application (5 mg) of [^{14}C] imiquimod cream formulation. No radioactivity was detected in the serum (lower limit of quantitation: 1 ng/mL) and <0.9% of the radiolabelled dose was excreted in the urine and feces following topical application.

CLINICAL STUDIES

In a double-blind, placebo-controlled clinical trial, 209 otherwise healthy patients 18 years of age and older with genital/perianal warts were treated with Aldara 5% cream or vehicle control 3X/week for a maximum of 16 weeks. The median baseline wart area was 69 mm^2 (range 8 to 5525 mm^2). Patient accountability is shown in the figure below.
[See graphic at top right of page]
Data on complete clearance are listed in the table below. The median time to complete wart clearance was 10 weeks. [See second table at right]

INDICATIONS AND USAGE

Aldara 5% cream is indicated for the treatment of external genital and perianal warts/condyloma acuminata in adults.

CONTRAINDICATIONS

None known

WARNINGS

Aldara cream has not been evaluated for the treatment of urethral, intra-vaginal, cervical, rectal, or intra-anal human papilloma viral disease and is not recommended for these conditions.

PRECAUTIONS

General

Local skin reactions such as erythema, erosion, excoriation/flaking, and edema are common. Should severe local skin reaction occur, the cream should be removed by washing the treatment area with mild soap and water. Treatment with Aldara cream can be resumed after the skin reaction has subsided. There is no clinical experience with Aldara cream therapy immediately following the treatment of genital/perianal warts with other cutaneously applied drugs; therefore, Aldara cream administration is not recommended until genital/perianal tissue is healed from any previous drug or surgical treatment. Aldara has the potential to exacerbate inflammatory conditions of the skin.

Information for Patients

Patients using Aldara 5% cream should receive the following information and instructions: The effect of Aldara 5% cream on the transmission of genital/perianal warts is unknown. Aldara 5% cream may weaken condoms and vaginal diaphragms. Therefore, concurrent use is not recommended.
1. This medication is to be used as directed by a physician. It is for external use only. Eye contact should be avoided.
2. The treatment area should not be bandaged or otherwise covered or wrapped as to be occlusive.

3. Sexual (genital, anal, oral) contact should be avoided while the cream is on the skin.
4. It is recommended that 6–10 hours following Aldara 5% cream application the treatment area be washed with mild soap and water.
5. It is common for patients to experience local skin reactions such as erythema, erosion, excoriation/flaking, and edema at the site of application or surrounding areas. Most skin reactions are mild to moderate. Severe skin reactions can occur and should be reported promptly to the prescribing physician.
6. Uncircumcised males treating warts under the foreskin should retract the foreskin and clean the area daily.
7. Patients should be aware that new warts may develop during therapy, as Aldara is not a cure.

Carcinogenicity, Mutagenesis, and Impairment of Fertility

Rodent carcinogenicity data are not available. Imiquimod was without effect in a series of eight different mutagenicity assays including Ames, mouse lymphoma, CHO chromosome aberration, human lymphocyte chromosome aberration, SHE cell transformation, rat and hamster bone marrow cytogenetics, and mouse dominant lethal test. Daily oral administration of imiquimod to rats, at doses up to 8 times the recommended human dose on a mg/m^2 basis throughout mating, gestation, parturition and lactation, demonstrated no impairment of reproduction.

Pregnancy

Pregnancy Category B: There are no adequate and well-controlled studies in pregnant women. Imiquimod was not found to be teratogenic in rat or rabbit teratology studies. In rats at a high maternally toxic dose (28 times human dose on a mg/m^2 basis), reduced pup weights and delayed ossification were observed. In developmental studies with offspring of pregnant rats treated with imiquimod (8 times human dose), no adverse effects were demonstrated.

Nursing Mothers

It is not known whether topically applied imiquimod is excreted in breast milk.

Pediatric Use

Safety and efficacy in patients below the age of 18 years have not been established.

ADVERSE REACTIONS

In controlled clinical trials, the most frequently reported adverse reactions were those of local skin and application site reactions; some patients also reported systemic reactions. These reactions were usually mild to moderate in intensity; however, severe reactions were reported with 3X/week application. **These reactions were more frequent and more intense with daily application than with 3X/week application.** Overall, in the 3X/week application clinical studies, 1.2% (4/327) of the patients discontinued due to local skin/application site reactions. The incidence and severity of local skin reactions during controlled clinical trials are shown in the following table.
[See table below]
Remote site skin reactions were also reported in female and male patients treated 3X/week with imiquimod 5% cream. The severe remote site skin reactions reported for females were erythema (3%), ulceration (2%), and edema (1%); and for males, erosion (2%), and erythema, edema, induration, and excoriation/flaking (each 1%).

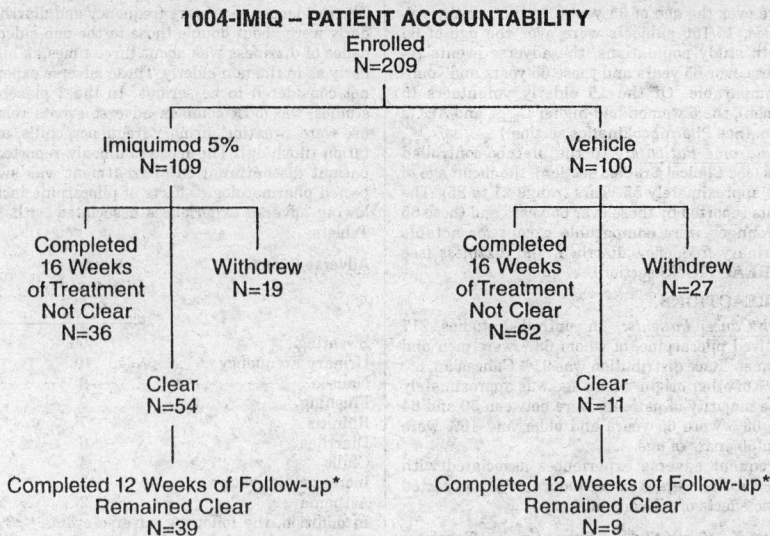

1004-IMIQ – PATIENT ACCOUNTABILITY

Enrolled N=209
- Imiquimod 5% N=109
  - Completed 16 Weeks of Treatment Not Clear N=36
  - Withdrew N=19
  - Clear N=54
    - Completed 12 Weeks of Follow-up* Remained Clear N=39
- Vehicle N=100
  - Completed 16 Weeks of Treatment Not Clear N=62
  - Withdrew N=27
  - Clear N=11
    - Completed 12 Weeks of Follow-up* Remained Clear N=9

*The other patients were either lost to follow-up or experienced recurrences.

CLEARANCE—STUDY 1004			
Treatment	Patients with Complete Clearance of Warts	Patients Without Follow-up	Patients with Warts Remaining at Week 16
Overall			
imiquimod 5% (N =109)	50%	17%	33%
vehicle (N =100)	11%	27%	62%
Females			
imiquimod 5% (N =46)	72%	11%	17%
vehicle (N =40)	20%	33%	48%
Males			
imiquimod 5% (N =63)	33%	22%	44%
vehicle (N =60)	5%	23%	72%

3X/WEEK APPLICATION
Wart Site Reaction As Assessed By Investigator

	Mild/Moderate				Severe			
	Females		Males		Females		Males	
	5% Imiquimod N=114	Vehicle N=99	5% Imiquimod N=156	Vehicle N=157	5% Imiquimod N=114	Vehicle N=99	5% Imiquimod N=156	Vehicle N=157
Erythema	61%	21%	54%	22%	4%	0%	4%	0%
Erosion	30%	8%	29%	6%	1%	0%	1%	0%
Excoriation/Flaking	18%	8%	25%	8%	0%	0%	1%	0%
Edema	17%	5%	12%	1%	1%	0%	0%	0%
Induration	5%	2%	7%	2%	0%	0%	0%	0%
Ulceration	5%	1%	4%	1%	3%	0%	0%	0%
Scabbing	4%	0%	13%	3%	0%	0%	0%	0%
Vesicles	3%	0%	2%	0%	0%	0%	0%	0%

| | 3X/WEEK APPLICATION | | | |
| | Females | | Males | |
	5% Imiquimod (N=117)	Vehicle (N=103)	5% Imiquimod (N=156)	Vehicle (N=158)
Application Site Disorders:				
Application Site Reactions				
Wart Site:				
Itching	32%	20%	22%	10%
Burning	26%	12%	9%	5%
Pain	8%	2%	2%	1%
Soreness	3%	0%	0%	1%
Fungal Infection[a]	11%	3%	2%	1%
Systemic Reactions:				
Headache	4%	3%	5%	2%
Influenza-like symptoms	3%	2%	1%	0%
Myalgia	1%	0%	1%	1%

[a] Incidences reported without regard to causality with Aldara.

Adverse events judged to be probably or possibly related to Aldara reported by more than 5% of patients are listed below; also included are soreness, influenza-like symptoms and myalgia.
[See table above]
Adverse events judged to be possibly or probably related to Aldara and reported by more than 1% of patients include: **Application Site Disorders: Wart Site Reactions** (burning, hypopigmentation, irritation, itching, pain, rash, sensitivity, soreness, stinging, tenderness); **Remote Site Reactions** (bleeding, burning, itching, pain, tenderness, tinea cruris); **Body as a Whole:** fatigue, fever, influenza-like symptoms; **Central and Peripheral Nervous System Disorders:** headache; **Gastro-Intestinal System Disorders:** diarrhea; **Musculo-Skeletal System Disorders:** myalgia.

OVERDOSAGE

Overdosage of Aldara 5% cream in humans is unlikely due to minimal percutaneous absorption. Animal studies reveal a rabbit dermal lethal imiquimod dose of greater than 1600 mg/m^2. Persistent topical overdosing of Aldara 5% cream could result in severe local skin reactions. The most clinically serious adverse event reported following multiple oral imiquimod doses of >200 mg was hypotension which resolved following oral or intravenous fluid administration.

DOSAGE AND ADMINISTRATION

Aldara cream is to be applied 3 times per week, prior to normal sleeping hours, and left on the skin for 6–10 hours. Following the treatment period cream should be removed by washing the treated area with mild soap and water. Examples of 3 times per week application schedules are: Monday, Wednesday, Friday; or Tuesday, Thursday, Saturday application prior to sleeping hours. Aldara treatment should continue until there is total clearance of the genital/perianal warts or for a maximum of 16 weeks. Local skin reactions (erythema) at the treatment site are common. A rest period of several days may be taken if required by the patient's discomfort or severity of the local skin reaction. Treatment may resume once the reaction subsides. Non-occlusive dressings such as cotton gauze or cotton underwear may be used in the management of skin reactions. The technique for proper dose administration should be demonstrated by the prescriber to maximize the benefit of Aldara therapy. Handwashing before and after cream application is recommended. Aldara 5% cream is packaged in single-use packets which contain sufficient cream to cover a wart area of up to 20 cm^2; use of excessive amounts of cream should be avoided. Patients should be instructed to apply Aldara cream to external genital/perianal warts. A thin layer is applied to the wart area and rubbed in until the cream is no longer visible. The application site is not to be occluded.

HOW SUPPLIED

Aldara (imiquimod) cream, 5%, is supplied in single-use packets which contain 250 mg of the cream. Available as: box of 12 packets NDC 0089-0610-12. Store below 25°C (77°F). Avoid freezing.
Rx only
Distributed by
3M Pharmaceuticals
Northridge, CA 91324
3/98   614500
Shown in Product Identification Guide, page 321

ALU-TAB™ Tablets   OTC
(aluminum hydroxide)
and
ALU-CAP™ Capsules
(aluminum hydroxide)

For indications, actions, warnings, dosage, and precautions see container label or call 800-328-0255 for a copy.

HOW SUPPLIED

Bottles of 250 green film-coated Alu-Tab tablets (NDC 0089-0107-25). Bottles of 100 red and green Alu-Cap capsules (NDC 0089-0105-10).

CALCIUM DISODIUM VERSENATE   ℞
(edetate calcium disodium injection, USP)

> **WARNINGS**
> Calcium Disodium Versenate is capable of producing toxic effects which can be fatal. Lead encephalopathy is relatively rare in adults, but occurs more often in pediatric patients in whom it may be incipient and thus overlooked. The mortality rate in pediatric patients has been high. Patients with lead encephalopathy and cerebral edema may experience a lethal increase in intracranial pressure following intravenous infusion; the intramuscular route is preferred for these patients. In cases where the intravenous route is necessary, avoid rapid infusion. The dosage schedule should be followed and at no time should the recommended daily dose be exceeded.

DESCRIPTION

Calcium Disodium Versenate (edetate calcium disodium injection, USP) is a sterile, injectable, chelating agent in concentrated solution for intravenous infusion or intramuscular injection. Each 5 ml ampul contains 1000 mg of edetate calcium disodium (equivalent to 200 mg/ml) in water for injection. Chemically, this product is called [[N,N'-1,2-ethanediylbis[N-(carboxymethyl)-glycinato]](4-)-N,N',O,O',O^N,O^N]-,disodium, hydrate, (OC-6-21)-Calciate(2-).

Structural Formula:

$$C_{10}H_{10}CaN_2Na_2O_8 \cdot xH_2O$$
Molecular weight 374.27 (anhydrous)

CLINICAL PHARMACOLOGY

The pharmacologic effects of edetate calcium disodium are due to the formation of chelates with divalent and trivalent metals. A stable chelate will form with any metal that has the ability to displace calcium from the molecule, a feature shared by lead, zinc, cadmium, manganese, iron and mercury. The amounts of manganese and iron mobilized are not significant. Copper[1] is not mobilized and mercury is unavailable for chelation because it is too tightly bound to body ligands or it is stored in inaccessible body compartments. The excretion of calcium by the body is not increased following intravenous administration of edetate calcium disodium, but the excretion of zinc is considerably increased.[1] Edetate calcium disodium is poorly absorbed from the gastrointestinal tract. In blood, all the drug is found in the plasma. Edetate calcium disodium does not appear to penetrate cells; it is distributed primarily in the extracellular fluid with only about 5% of the plasma concentration found in spinal fluid.
The half life of edetate calcium disodium is 20 to 60 minutes. It is excreted primarily by the kidney, with about 50% excreted in one hour and over 95% within 24 hours.[2] Almost none of the compound is metabolized.
The primary source of lead chelated by Calcium Disodium Versenate is from bone; subsequently, soft-tissue lead is redistributed to bone when chelation is stopped.[3,4] There is also some reduction in kidney lead levels following chelation therapy.

It has been shown in animals that following a single dose of Calcium Disodium Versenate urinary lead output increases, blood lead concentration decreases, but brain lead is significantly increased due to internal redistribution of lead.[5] (See **WARNINGS.**) These data are in agreement with the recent results of others in experimental animals showing that after a five day course of treatment there is no net reduction in brain lead.[6]

INDICATIONS AND USAGE

Edetate calcium disodium is indicated for the reduction of blood levels and depot stores of lead in lead poisoning (acute and chronic) and lead encephalopathy, in both pediatric populations and adults.
Chelation therapy should not replace effective measures to eliminate or reduce further exposure to lead.

CONTRAINDICATIONS

Edetate calcium disodium should not be given during periods of anuria, nor to patients with active renal disease or hepatitis.

WARNINGS

See boxed warning.

PRECAUTIONS

General Precautions: Edetate calcium disodium may produce the same renal damage as lead poisoning, such as proteinuria and microscopic hematuria. Treatment-induced nephrotoxicity is dose-dependent and may be reduced by assuring adequate diuresis before therapy begins. Urine flow must be monitored throughout therapy which must be stopped if anuria or severe oliguria develop. The proximal tubule hydropic degeneration usually recovers upon cessation of therapy. Edetate calcium disodium must be used in reduced doses in patients with pre-existing mild renal disease.
Patients should be monitored for cardiac rhythm irregularities and other ECG changes during intravenous therapy.
Information for patients: Patients should be instructed to immediately inform their physician if urine output stops for a period of 12 hours.
Laboratory Tests: Urinarlysis and urine sediment, renal and hepatic function and serum electrolyte levels should be checked before each course of therapy and then be monitored daily during therapy in severe cases, and in less serious cases after the second and fifth day of therapy. Therapy must be discontinued at the first sign of renal toxicity. The presence of large renal epithelial cells or increasing number of red blood cells in urinary sediment or greater proteinuria call for immediate stopping of edetate calcium disodium administration. Alkaline phosphatase values are frequently depressed (possibly due to decreased serum zinc levels), but return to normal within 48 hours after cessation of therapy. Elevated erythrocyte protoporphyrin levels (>35 mcg/dl of whole blood) indicate the need to perform a venous blood lead determination. If the whole blood lead concentration is between 25–55 mcg/dl a mobilization test can be considered.[7,8] (See **Diagnostic Test.**) An elevation of urinary coproporphyrin (adults: >250 mcg/day; pediatric patients under 80 lbs: >75 mcg/day) and elevation of urinary delta aminolevulinic acid (ALA) (adults: >4 mg/day; pediatric patients: >3 mg/m^2/day) are associated with blood lead levels >40 mcg/dl. Urinary coproporphyrin may be falsely negative in terminal patients and in severely iron-depleted pediatric patients who are not regenerating heme.[9] In growing pediatric patients long bone x-rays showing lead lines and abdominal x-rays showing radio-opaque material in the abdomen may be of help in estimating the level of exposure to lead.

Drug Interactions: There is no known drug interference with standard clinical laboratory tests. Steroids enhance the renal toxicity of edetate calcium disodium in animals.[7] Edetate calcium disodium interferes with the action of zinc insulin preparations by chelating the zinc.[7]
Carcinogenesis, Mutagenesis, Impairment of Fertility: Long term animal studies have not been conducted with edetate calcium disodium to evaluate its carcinogenic potential, mutagenic potential or its effect on fertility.
Pregnancy: Category B: One reproduction study was performed in rats at doses up to 13 times the human dose and revealed no evidence of impaired fertility or harm to the fetus due to Caclium Disodium Versenate.[10] Another reproduction study performed in rats at doses up to about 25 to 40 times the human dose revealed evidence of fetal malformations due to Calcium Disodium Versenate, which were prevented by simultaneous supplementation of dietary zinc.[11] There are, however, no adequate and well-controlled studies in pregnant women. Because animal reproduction studies are not always predictive of human response, this drug should be used during pregnancy only if clearly needed.
Labor and Delivery: Calcium Disodium Versenate has no recognized use during labor and delivery, and its effects during these processes are unknown.

Continued on next page

Calcium Disodium Versenate—Cont.

Nursing Mothers: It is not known whether this drug is excreted in human milk. Because many drugs are excreted in human milk, caution should be exercised when Calcium Disodium Versenate is administered to a nursing woman.

Pediatric Use: Since lead poisoning occurs in pediatric populations and adults but is frequently more severe in pediatric patients, Calcium Disodium Versenate is used in patients of all ages. The intramuscular route is preferred by some for young pediatric patients. In cases where the intravenous route is necessary, avoid rapid infusion (See **WARNINGS.**) Urine flow must be monitored throughout therapy; Calcium Disodium Versenate therapy must be stopped if anuria or severe oliguria develops. (See **General Precautions.**) At no time should the recommended daily dosage be exceeded (See **DOSAGE AND ADMINISTRATION.**)

ADVERSE REACTIONS

The following adverse effects have been associated with the use of edetate calcium disodium:

Body as a Whole: pain at intramuscular injection site, fever, chills, malaise, fatigue, myalgia, arthralgia.

Cardiovascular: hypotension, cardiac rhythm irregularities.

Renal: acute necrosis of proximal tubules (which may result in fatal nephrosis), infrequent changes in distal tubules and glomeruli.

Urinary: glycosuria, proteinuria, microscopic hematuria and large epithelial cells in urinary sediment.

Nervous System: tremors, headache, numbness, tingling.

Gastrointestinal: cheilosis, nausea, vomiting, anorexia, excessive thirst.

Hepatic: mild increases in SGOT and SGPT are common, and return to normal within 48 hours after cessation of therapy.

Immunogenic: histamine-like reactions (sneezing, nasal congestion, lacrimation), rash.

Hematopoietic: transient bone marrow depression, anemia.

Metabolic: zinc deficiency, hypercalcemia.

OVERDOSAGE

Symptoms: Inadvertent administration of 5 times the recommended dose, infused intravenously over a 24 hour period, to an asymptomatic 16 month old patient with a blood lead content of 56 mcg/dl did not cause any ill effects. Edetate calcium disodium can aggravate the symptoms of severe lead poisoning, therefore, most toxic effects (cerebral edema, renal tubular necrosis) appear to be associated with lead poisoning.

Because of cerebral edema, a therapeutic dose may be lethal to an adult or a pediatric patient with lead encephalopathy. Higher dosage of edetate calcium disodium may produce a more severe zinc deficiency.

Treatment: Cerebral edema should be treated with repeated doses of mannitol. Steroids enhance the renal toxicity of edetate calcium disodium in animals and, therefore, are no longer recommended.[7] Zinc levels must be monitored. Good urinary output must be maintained because diuresis will enhance drug elimination. It is not known if edetate calcium disodium is dialyzable.

DOSAGE AND ADMINISTRATION

When a source for the lead intoxication has been identified, the patient should be removed from the source, if possible. The recommended dose of Calcium Disodium Versenate for asymptomatic adults and pediatric patients whose blood lead level is <70 mcg/dl but >20 mcg/dl (World Health Organization recommended upper allowable level) is 1000 mg/m²/day whether given intravenously or intramuscularly. (See Surface Area Nomogram.)

[See figure at top of next column]

For adults with lead nephropathy, the following dosing regimen has been suggested: 500 mg/m² every 24 hours for 5 days for patients with serum creatinine levels of 2–3 mg/dl, every 48 hours for 3 doses for patients with creatinine levels of 3–4 mg/dl, and once weekly for patients with creatinine levels above 4 mg/dl. These regimens may be repeated at one month intervals.[12]

Calcium Disodium Versenate, used alone, may aggravate symptoms in patients with very high blood lead levels. When the blood lead level is >70 mcg/dl or clinical symptoms consistent with lead poisoning are present, it is recommended that Calcium Disodium Versenate be used in conjunction with BAL (dimercaprol). Please consult published protocols and specialized references for dosage recommendations of combination therapy.[14–18]

Therapy of lead poisoning in adults and pediatric patients with Calcium Disodium Versenate is continued over a period of five days. Therapy is then interrupted for 2 to 4 days to allow redistribution of the lead and to prevent severe depletion of zinc and other essential metals. Two courses of treatment are usually employed; however, it depends on severity of the lead toxicity and the patient's tolerance of the drug.

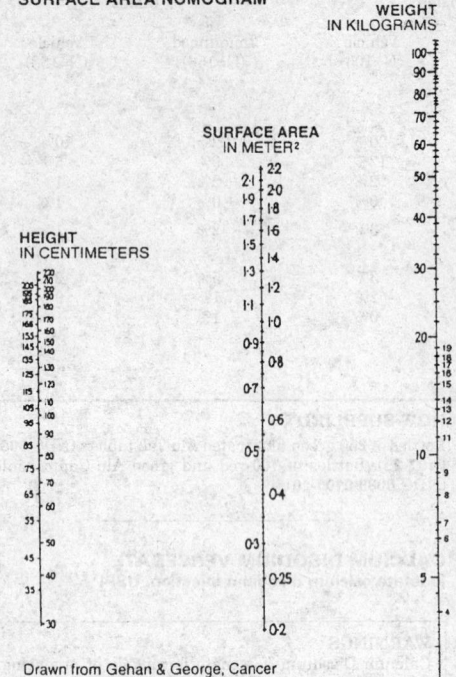

SURFACE AREA NOMOGRAM

Drawn from Gehan & George, Cancer Chemotherapy Reports 54:225, 1970.

Calcium Disodium Versenate is equally effective whether administered intravenously or intramuscularly. The intramuscular route is used for all patients with overt lead encephalopathy and this route is preferred by some for young pediatric patients.

Acutely ill individuals may be dehydrated from vomiting. Since edetate calcium disodium is excreted almost exclusively in the urine, it is very important to establish urine flow with intravenous fluid administration before the first dose of the chelating agent is given; however, excessive fluid must be avoided in patients with encephalopathy. Once urine flow is established, further intravenous fluid is restricted to basal water and electrolyte requirements. Administration of Calcium Disodium Versenate should be stopped whenever there is cessation of urine flow in order to avoid unduly high tissue levels of the drug. Edetate calcium disodium must be used in reduced doses in patients with pre-existing mild renal disease.

Intravenous Administration: Add the total daily dose of Calcium Disodium Versenate (1000 mg/m²/day) to 250–500 ml of 5% dextrose or 0.9% sodium chloride injection. The total daily dose should be infused over a period of 8–12 hours. Calcium Disodium Versenate injection is incompatible with 10% dextrose, 10% invert sugar in 0.9% sodium chloride, lactate Ringer's, Ringer's, one-sixth molar sodium lactate injections, and with injectable amphotericin B and hydralazine hydrochloride.

Intramuscular Administration: The total daily dosage (1000 mg/m²/day) should be divided into equal doses spaced 8–12 hours apart. Lidocaine or procaine should be added to the Calcium Disodium Versenate injection to minimize pain at the injection site. The final lidocaine or procaine concentration of 5 mg/ml (0.5%) can be obtained as follows: 0.25 ml of 10% lidocaine solution per 5 ml (entire content of ampul) concentrated Calcium Disodium Versenate; 1 ml of 1% lidocaine or procaine solution per ml of concentrated Calcium Disodium Versenate. When used alone, regardless of method of administration, Calcium Disodium Versenate should not be given at doses larger than those recommended.

Diagnostic Test: Several methods have been described for lead mobilization tests using edetate calcium disodium to assess body stores.[7,9,12,13,18]

These procedures have advantages and disadvantages that should be reviewed in current references. Edetate calcium disodium mobilization test should not be performed in symptomatic patients and in patients with blood lead levels above 55 mcg/dl for whom appropriate therapy is indicated. Parenteral drug should be inspected visually for particulate matter and discoloration prior to administration, whenever solution and container permit.

HOW SUPPLIED

Calcium Disodium Versenate injection, 5 ml ampul containing 200 mg of edetate calcium disodium per ml (1 g per ampul), in boxes containing 6 ampuls (NDC 0089-0510-06).

Store at controlled room temperature 15°–30°C (59°–86°F).

CAUTION

Federal law prohibits dispensing without prescription.

REFERENCES

1. Thomas DJ, Chisolm JJ. Lead, zinc and copper decorporation during calcium disodium ethylenediamine tetraacetate treatment of lead-poisoned children. J Pharmacol Exp Therapeu 1986; 239:829-835.
2. The Pharmacological Basis of Therapeutics, 7th edition, Goodman and Gilman, editors. Macmillan Publishing Company, New York, 1985, pp. 1619–1622.
3. Hammond PB, Aronson AL, Olson WC. The mechanism of mobilization of lead by ethylenediaminetetraacetate. J Pharmacol Exp Therapeu 1967; 157:196-206.
4. Van deVyver FL, D'Haese PC, Visser WJ, et al. Bone lead in dialysis patients. Kidney Intl 1988; 33:601-607.
5. Cory-Slecta DA, Weiss B, Cox C. Mobilization and redistribution of lead over the course of calcium disodium ethylenediamine tetraacetate chelation therapy. J Pharmacol Exp Therapeu 1987; 243:804-813.
6. Chisolm JJ. Mobilization of lead by calcium disodium edetate. Am J Dis Child 1987; 141:1256-1257.
7. Drug Evaluations, 6th Edition, American Medical Association, Saunders, Philadelphia, 1986, pp. 1637–1639.
8. Centers for Disease Control: Preventing lead poisoning in young children. Atlanta, GA, Department of Health and Human Services, 1985 Jan.
9. Finberg L, Rajagopal V. Diagnosis and treatment of lead poisoning in children. J Family Med 1985 April: 3–12.
10. Schardein JL, Sakowski R, Petrere J, et al. Teratogenesis studies with EDTA and its salts in rats. Toxicol Appl Pharmacol 1981; 61:423-428.
11. Swenerton H, Hurley LS. Teratogenic effects of a chelating agent and their prevention by zinc. Science 1971; 173:62-64.
12. American Hospital Formulary Service, Drug Information, 1988, pp. 1695–1698.
13. Markowitz ME, Rosen JF. Assessment of lead stores in children: Validation of an 8-hour CaNa₂ EDTA (Calcium Disodium Versenate) provocative test. J Pediatrics 1984; 104:337-341.
14. Piomelli S, Rosen JF, Chisolm JJ, et al. Management of childhood lead poisoning. J Pediatrics 1984; 105:523-532.
15. Sachs HK, Blanksma LA, Murray EF, et al. Ambulatory treatment of lead poisoning: Report of 1,155 cases. Pediatrics 1970; 46:389.
16. Chisolm JJ. The use of chelating agents in the treatment of acute and chronic lead intoxication in childhood. J Pediatrics 1968; 73:1.
17. Coffin R, Phillips JL, Staples WI, et al. Treatment of lead encephalopathy in children. J Pediatrics 1966; 69:198-206.
18. Chisolm JJ. Increased lead absorption and acute lead poisoning. Current Pediatric Therapy 12, Gillis and Kagan, editors, WB Saunders, Philadelphia, 1986, pp. 667–671.

Distributed by:
3M Pharmaceuticals
Northridge, CA 91324
994002   AUGUST 1997

DISALCID™   ℞
(salsalate)
Tablets and Capsules

DESCRIPTION

DISALCID (salsalate) is a nonsteroidal anti-inflammatory agent for oral administration. Chemically, salsalate (salicylsalicylic acid or 2-hydroxybenzoic acid, 2-carboxyphenyl ester) is a dimer of salicylic acid; its structural formula is shown below.

Chemical Structure:

salsalate

Each DISALCID capsule contains 500 mg salsalate and also contains colloidal silicon dioxide, gelatin, magnesium stearate, pregelatinized starch, corn starch, titanium dioxide, FD&C blue #1, and D&C yellow #10.

Each DISALCID tablet contains 500 or 750 mg salsalate and also contains croscarmellose sodium, hydroxypropyl

methylcellulose, magnesium stearate, microcrystalline cellulose, polyethylene glycol, polysorbate 80, propylene glycol, talc, titanium dioxide, FD&C blue #1, and D&C yellow #10. (See HOW SUPPLIED.)

CLINICAL PHARMACOLOGY

DISALCID is insoluble in acid gastric fluids (<0.1 mg/ml at pH 1.0), but readily soluble in the small intestine where it is partially hydrolyzed to two molecules of salicylic acid. A significant portion of the parent compound is absorbed unchanged and undergoes rapid esterase hydrolysis in the body; its half-life is about one hour. About 13% is excreted through the kidneys as a glucuronide conjugate of the parent compound, the remainder as salicylic acid and its metabolites. Thus, the amount of salicylic acid available from DISALCID is about 15% less than from aspirin, when the two drugs are administered on a salicylic acid molar equivalent basis (3.6 g salsalate/5 g aspirin). Salicylic acid biotransformation is saturated at anti-inflammatory doses of DISALCID. Such capacity-limited biotransformation results in an increase in the half-life of salicylic acid from 3.5 to 16 or more hours. Thus, dosing with DISALCID twice a day will satisfactorily maintain blood levels within the desired therapeutic range (10 to 30 mg/100 ml) throughout the 12-hour intervals. Therapeutic blood levels continue for up to 16 hours after the last dose. The parent compound does not show capacity-limited biotransformation, nor does it accumulate in the plasma on multiple dosing. Food slows the absorption of all salicylates including DISALCID.

The mode of anti-inflammatory action of DISALCID and other nonsteroidal anti-inflammatory drugs is not fully defined. Although salicylic acid (the primary metabolite of DISALCID) is a weak inhibitor of prostaglandin synthesis **in vitro**, DISALCID appears to selectively inhibit prostaglandin synthesis **in vivo**,[1] providing anti-inflammatory activity equivalent to aspirin[2] and indomethacin.[3] Unlike aspirin, DISALCID does not inhibit platelet aggregation.[4]

The usefulness of salicylic acid, the active **in vivo** product of DISALCID, in the treatment of arthritic disorders has been established.[5,6] In contrast to aspirin, DISALCID causes no greater fecal gastrointestinal blood loss than placebo.[7]

INDICATIONS AND USAGE

DISALCID is indicated for relief of the signs and symptoms of rheumatoid arthritis, osteoarthritis and related rheumatic disorders.

CONTRAINDICATIONS

DISALCID is contraindicated in patients hypersensitive to salsalate.

WARNINGS

Reye's Syndrome may develop in individuals who have chicken pox, influenza, or flu symptoms. Some studies suggest a possible association between the development of Reye's Syndrome and the use of medicines containing salicylate or apirin. DISALCID contains a salicylate and therefore is not recommended for use in patients with chicken pox, influenza, or flu symptoms.

PRECAUTIONS

General Precautions: Patients on treatment with DISALCID should be warned not to take other salicylates so as to avoid potentially toxic concentrations. Great care should be exercised when DISALCID is prescribed in the presence of chronic renal insufficiency or peptic ulcer disease. Protein binding of salicylic acid can be influenced by nutritional status, competitive binding of other drugs, and fluctuations in serum proteins caused by disease (rheumatoid arthritis, etc.).

Although cross reactivity, including bronchospasm, has been reported occasionally with non-acetylated salicylates, including salsalate, in aspirin-sensitive patients,[8,9] salsalate is less likely than aspirin to induce asthma in such patients.[10]

Laboratory Tests: Plasma salicylic acid concentrations should be periodically monitored during long-term treatment with DISALCID to aid maintenance of therapeutically effective levels: 10 to 30 mg/100 ml. Toxic manifestations are not usually seen until plasma concentrations exceed 30 mg/100 ml (see OVERDOSAGE). Urinary pH should also be regularly monitored: sudden acidification, as from pH 6.5 to 5.5, can double the plasma level, resulting in toxicity.

Drug Interactions: Salicylates antagonize the uricosuric action of drugs used to treat gout. ASPIRIN AND OTHER SALICYLATE DRUGS WILL BE ADDITIVE TO DISALCID AND MAY INCREASE PLASMA CONCENTRATIONS OF SALICYLIC ACID TO TOXIC LEVELS. Drugs and foods that raise urine pH will increase renal clearance and urinary excretion of salicylic acid, thus lowering plasma levels; acidifying drugs or foods will decrease urinary excretion and increase plasma levels. Salicylates given concomitantly with anticoagulant drugs may predispose to systemic bleeding. Salicylates may enhance the hypoglycemic effect of oral anti-diabetic drugs of the sulfonylurea class. Salicylate competes with a number of drugs for protein binding sites, notably penicillin, thiopental, thyroxine, triiodothyronine,

phenytoin, sulfinpyrazone, naproxen, warfarin, methotrexate, and possibly corticosteroids.

Drug/Laboratory Test Interactions: Salicylate competes with thyroid hormone for binding to plasma proteins, which may be reflected in a depressed plasma T_4 value in some patients; thyroid function and basal metabolism are unaffected.

Carcinogenesis: No long-term animal studies have been performed with DISALCID to evaluate its carcinogenic potential.

Use in Pregnancy: Pregnancy Category C: Salsalate and salicylic acid have been shown to be teratogenic and embryocidal in rats when given in doses 4 to 5 times the usual human dose. These effects were not observed at doses twice as great as the usual human dose. There are no adequate and well-controlled studies in pregnant women. DISALCID should be used during pregnancy only if the potential benefit justifies the potential risk to the fetus.

Labor and Delivery: There exist no adequate and well-controlled studies in pregnant women. Although adverse effects on mother or infant have not been reported with DISALCID use during labor, caution is advised when anti-inflammatory dosage is involved. However, other salicylates have been associated with prolonged gestation and labor, maternal and neonatal bleeding sequelae, potentiation of narcotic and barbiturate effects (respiratory or cardiac arrest in the mother), delivery problems and stillbirth.

Nursing Mothers: It is not known whether salsalate per se is excreted in human milk; salicylic acid, the primary metabolite of DISALCID, has been shown to appear in human milk in concentrations approximating the maternal blood level. Thus, the infant of a mother on DISALCID therapy might ingest in mother's milk 30 to 80% as much salicylate per kg body weight as the mother is taking. Accordingly, caution should be exercised when DISALCID is administered to a nursing woman.

Pediatric Use: Safety and effectiveness in pediatric patients have not been established. (See WARNINGS section.)

ADVERSE REACTIONS

In two well-controlled clinical trials (n=280 patients), the following reversible adverse experiences characteristic of salicylates were most commonly reported with DISALCID, listed in descending order of frequency: tinnitus, nausea, hearing impairment, rash, and vertigo. These common symptoms of salicylates, i.e., tinnitus or reversible hearing impairment, are often used as a guide to therapy.

Although cause-and-effect relationships have not been established, spontaneous reports over a ten-year period have included the following additional medically significant adverse experiences: abdominal pain, abnormal hepatic function, anaphylactic shock, angioedema, bronchospasm, decreased creatinine clearance, diarrhea, G.I. bleeding, hepatitis, hypotension, nephritis and urticaria.

DRUG ABUSE AND DEPENDENCE

Drug abuse and dependence have not been reported with DISALCID.

OVERDOSAGE

Death has followed ingestion of 10 to 30 g of salicylates in adults, but much larger amounts have been ingested without fatal outcome.

Symptoms: The usual symptoms of salicylism—tinnitus, vertigo, headache, confusion, drowsiness, sweating, hyperventilation, vomiting and diarrhea—will occur. More severe intoxication will lead to disruption of electrolyte balance and blood pH, and hyperthermia and dehydration.

Treatment: Further absorption of DISALCID from the G.I. tract should be prevented by emesis (syrup of ipecac) and, if necessary, by gastric lavage.

Fluid and electrolyte imbalance should be corrected by the administration of appropriate I.V. therapy. Adequate renal function should be maintained. Hemodialysis or peritoneal dialysis may be required in extreme cases.

DOSAGE AND ADMINISTRATION

Adults: The usual dosage is 3000 mg daily, given in divided doses as follows: 1) two doses of two 750 mg tablets; 2) two doses of three 500 mg tablets/capsules; or 3) three doses of two 500 mg tablets/capsules. Some patients, e.g., the elderly, may require a lower dosage to achieve therapeutic blood concentrations and to avoid the more common side effects such as auditory.

Alleviation of symptoms is gradual, and full benefit may not be evident for 3 to 4 days, when plasma salicylate levels have achieved steady state. There is no evidence for development of tissue tolerance (tachyphylaxis) but salicylate therapy may induce increased activity of metabolizing liver enzymes, causing a greater rate of salicyluric acid production and excretion, with a resultant increase in dosage requirement for maintenance of therapeutic serum salicylate levels.

Children: Dosage recommendations and indications for DISALCID use in children have not been established.

HOW SUPPLIED

Each DISALCID 500 mg aqua/white capsule printed with Disalcid/3M is available in:
Bottles of 100 (NDC #0089-0148-10)
Each DISALCID 500 mg aqua, film coated, round, bisected tablet embossed with DISALCID on one side and 3M on the other side is available in:
Bottles of 100 (NDC #0089-0149-10)
Bottles of 500 (NDC #0089-0149-50)
Each DISALCID 750 mg aqua, film coated, capsule shaped, bisected tablet embossed with DISALCID 750 on one side and 3M on the other side is available in:
Bottles of 100 (NDC #0089-0151-10)
Bottles of 500 (NDC #0089-0151-50)
Store at controlled room temperature 15°-30°C (59°-86°F).
CAUTION: Federal law prohibits dispensing without prescription.

REFERENCES

1. Morris HG, et al. Effects of salsalate (non-acetylated salicylate) and aspirin on serum prostaglandins in humans. Thera Drug Mon 1985;7:435–438.
2. April PA, et al. Does the acetyl group of aspirin contribute to the anti-inflammatory efficacy of salicylic acid in the treatment of rheumatoid arthritis? Sem Arth & Rheum 1990;19:(4)2:20–28.
3. Deodhar SD, et al. A short term comparative trial of salsalate and indomethacin in rheumatoid arthritis. Curr Med Res Opin 1977;5:185–188.
4. Estes D, Kaplan K. Lack of platelet effect with the aspirin analog, salsalate. Arth & Rheum 1980;23:1303–1307.
5. Dick C, et al. Effect of anti-inflammatory drug therapy on clearance of ^{133}Xe from knee joints of patients with rheumatoid arthritis. Br Med J 1969;3:278–280.
6. Dick WC, et al. Indices of inflammatory activity. Ann of Rheum Dis 1970;29:643–648.
7. Cohen A, Fecal blood loss and plasma salicylate study of salicylsalicylic acid and aspirin. J Clin Pharmacol 1979;19:242–247.
8. Chudwin DS, et al. Sensitivity to non-acetylated salicylates in a patient with asthma, nasal polyps, and rheumatoid arthritis. Ann of Allergy 1986;57:133–134.
9. Spector SL, et al. Aspirin and concomitant idiosyncrasies in adult asthmatic patients. J Allergy Clin Immunol 1979;64:500–506.
10. Stevenson DD, et al. Salsalate cross sensitivity in aspirin-sensitive asthmatics. J Allergy Clin Immunol 1990;86:749–758.

622502   October 1996
3M Pharmaceuticals
Northridge, CA 91324

MAXAIR™ Autohaler™ ℞
(pirbuterol acetate inhalation aerosol)

Patient's Instructions for Use

Questions? Call our Patient Assistance Line at 1-(800)-841-3885, 8:30 a.m.—5:00 p.m. EST (Weekdays).
IMPORTANT NOTE:
Use Maxair Autohaler according to the instructions given to you by your physician, who will advise you on the number of puffs to take. If you have previously been using a "press-and-breathe" inhaler, you should take the same number of puffs through your Maxair Autohaler as you did through the "press-and-breathe" inhaler.

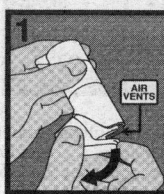

Remove mouthpiece cover by pulling down lip on **back** of cover.
Inspect mouthpiece for foreign objects.
Locate "Up" arrows on Maxair Autohaler.
Locate air vents at bottom of Maxair Autohaler.

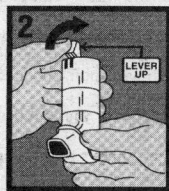

Hold Maxair Autohaler **upright** as shown in figure 2. The arrows should point up.

Continued on next page

Maxair Autohaler—Cont.

Maxair Autohaler must be held upright while raising lever.
Raise lever so that it stays up. It will "snap" into place.
Do not lower lever until step 6.

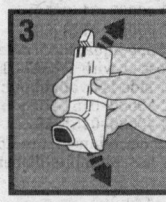

Hold Maxair Autohaler around the middle as shown in figure 3.
Shake Maxair Autohaler gently several times.

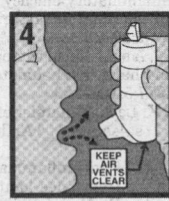

Continue to hold Maxair Autohaler **upright** as shown in figure 4.
Do not block air vents at bottom of Maxair Autohaler.
Exhale normally before use.

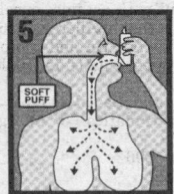

Seal your lips tightly around mouthpiece as shown in figure 5.
Inhale deeply through mouthpiece with **steady, moderate force.** You will hear a "click" and feel a **soft** puff when your inhaling triggers the release of medicine.
Do not stop when you hear and feel the puff. Continue to take a **full, deep breath.**
Take Maxair Autohaler away from your mouth when done inhaling.
Hold your breath for 10 seconds, then exhale slowly.

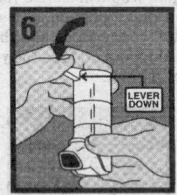

Continue to hold Maxair Autohaler upright while lowering the lever as shown in figure 6. Lower lever after each puff.
If your physician has prescribed additional puffs, wait one minute then repeat steps 2 through 6.
Following use, make sure lever is down and replace mouthpiece cover.

General Information about Maxair Autohaler
Your Maxair Autohaler is a new type of inhaler designed to be very easy to use. Maxair Autohaler automatically releases a puff of medicine when you inhale.

What will I feel when I use Maxair Autohaler?
Maxair Autohaler provides a **soft spray** of medicine. It is designed to automatically deliver a precisely measured dose of your medicine with each puff, so you can be assured of a consistent dose of medicine.
When medicine is delivered, you will hear a "click" and feel a **soft** puff.

How will I know when there's no more medicine in Maxair Autohaler?
The Maxair Autohaler you receive from the pharmacy contains 400 puffs (the Maxair Autohaler sample contains 80 puffs and says "SAMPLE" on the back; the Maxair Autohaler hospital unit also contains 80 puffs and says "Hospital Pack" on the back). You can estimate how many days it will

last by dividing 80 or 400 (total puffs in a unit) by the number of puffs you normally use in a day. The chart below can help you calculate about how long your 400 puff Maxair Autohaler will last. Acutal usage may vary depending on how many puffs you use each day. A total daily dose of 12 puffs should not be exceeded. Discard your Maxair Autohaler when there is no more medicine remaining.

Average Number of Puffs Per Day	Approximate Days of Therapy Available
2 puffs/day	200 days
4 puffs/day	100 days
6 puffs/day	65 days
8 puffs/day	50 days

How to clean and care for Maxair Autohaler.

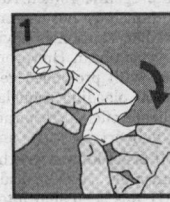

Remove mouthpiece cover by pulling down lip on **back** of cover.

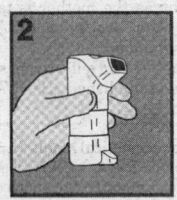

Turn Maxair Autohaler upside down.
Wipe mouthpiece with a clean dry cloth.

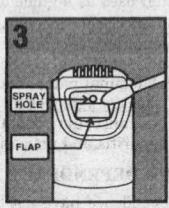

Gently tap back of Maxair Autohaler so flap comes down and spray hole can be seen. With white flap down as shown in the picture, clean the surface of the flap with a dry cotton swab.

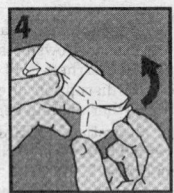

Replace mouthpiece cover. When you are not using Maxair Autohaler, make sure lever is down and mouthpiece cover is in place.
Repeat cleaning instructions weekly or as often as required.

Important Information:
Caution: Contents of canister under pressure. Do not puncture. Do not use near heat or open flame. Exposure to temperatures above 120°F may cause bursting. Store between 15° and 30° C (59° to 86° F). Avoid spraying in eyes.
Caution: Federal law prohibits dispensing without a prescription.
Use Maxair Autohaler only as prescribed by your physician.
Handle with care.
DO NOT USE WITH OTHER CANISTERS OR MOUTHPIECES.
For information on the drug, refer to your doctor or pharmacist.
Keep out of reach of children.

MAXAIR™ AUTOHALER™   Rx
(pirbuterol acetate inhalation aerosol)
Bronchodilator Aerosol
For Inhalation Only

DESCRIPTION
The active component of MAXAIR AUTOHALER (pirbuterol acetate) is (R,S) α^6-{[(1,1-dimethylethyl)amino]methyl}-3-hydroxy-2,6-pyridinedimethanol monoacetate salt, a beta-2 adrenergic bronchodilator, having the following chemical structure:

$$\text{HO} \quad \text{HO—CH}_2 \quad \text{N} \quad \text{CH—CH}_2\text{—NH—C—CH}_3 \cdot \text{CH}_3\text{COOH}$$
$$\text{OH} \quad \quad \text{CH}_3$$

Pirbuterol acetate is a white, crystalline racemic mixture of two optically active isomers. It is a powder, freely soluble in water, with a molecular weight of 300.3 and empirical formula of $C_{12}H_{20}N_2O_3 \cdot C_2H_4O_2$.

MAXAIR AUTOHALER is a metered dose aerosol unit for oral inhalation. It provides a fine–particle suspension of pirbuterol acetate in the propellant mixture of trichloromonofluoromethane and dichlorodifluoromethane, with sorbitan trioleate. Each actuation delivers from the mouthpiece pirbuterol acetate equivalent to 0.2 mg of pirbuterol with the majority of particles less than 5 microns in diameter. The unit is breath-actuated such that the medication is delivered automatically during inspiration without the need for the patient to coordinate actuation with inspiration.

CLINICAL PHARMACOLOGY
In vitro studies and *in vivo* pharmacologic studies have demonstrated that MAXAIR has a preferential effect on beta-2 adrenergic receptors compared with isoproterenol. While it is recognized that beta-2 adrenergic receptors are the predominant receptors in bronchial smooth muscle, recent data indicate that there is a population of beta-2 receptors in the human heart, existing in a concentration between 10–50%. The precise function of these, however, is not yet established (see WARNINGS section).

The pharmacologic effects of beta adrenergic agonist drugs, including pirbuterol, are at least in part attributable to stimulation through beta adrenergic receptors of intracellular adenyl cyclase, the enzyme which catalyzes the conversion of adenosine triphosphate (ATP) to cyclic-3',5'-adenosine monophosphate (c-AMP). Increased c-AMP levels are associated with relaxation of bronchial smooth muscle and inhibition of release of mediators of immediate hypersensitivity from cells, especially from mast cells.

Bronchodilator activity of MAXAIR was manifested clinically by an improvement in various pulmonary function parameters (FEV_1, MMF, PEFR, airway resistance [RAW] and conductance [GA/V_{tgl}]).

In controlled double-blind single dose clinical trials, the onset of improvement in pulmonary function occurred within 5 minutes in most patients as determined by forced expiratory volume in one second (FEV_1). FEV_1 and MMF measurements also showed that maximum improvement in pulmonary function generally occurred 30–60 minutes following one (1) or two (2) inhalations of pirbuterol (0.2–0.4 mg). The duration of action of MAXAIR is maintained for 5 hours (the time at which the last observations were made) in a substantial number of patients, based on a 15% or greater increase in FEV_1. In controlled repetitive dose studies of 12 weeks' duration, 74% of 156 patients on pirbuterol and 62% of 141 patients on metaproterenol showed a clinically significant improvement based on a 15% or greater increase in FEV_1 on at least half of the days. Onset and duration were equivalent to that seen in single dose studies. Continued effectiveness was demonstrated over the 12-week period in the majority (94%) of responding patients; however, chronic dosing was associated with the development of tachyphylaxis (tolerance) to the bronchodilator effect in some patients in both treatment groups.

A placebo-controlled double-blind single dose study (24 patients per treatment group), utilizing continuous Holter monitoring for 5 hours after drug administration, showed no significant difference in ectopic activity between the pla-

cebo control group and MAXAIR at the recommended dose (0.2–0.4 mg), and twice the recommended dose (0.8 mg). As with other inhaled beta adrenergic agonists, supraventricular and ventricular ectopic beats have been seen with MAXAIR (see WARNINGS).
Recent studies in laboratory animals (minipigs, rodents, and dogs) recorded the occurrence of cardiac arrhythmias and sudden death (with histologic evidence of myocardial necrosis) when beta agonists and methylxanthines were administered concurrently. The significance of these findings when applied to humans is currently unknown.
Two randomized, double-blind, cross-over studies in a total of 97 patients, have compared the clinical effects of either one inhalation or two inhalations of the pirbuterol formulations in the Autohaler actuator and the conventional inhaler and demonstrated no significant difference between the formulations for the means of peak changes in FEV_1, time to peak FEV_1, onset, duration, or area under the FEV_1 curve.

Pharmacokinetics

As expected by extrapolation from oral data, systemic blood levels of pirbuterol are below the limit of assay sensitivity (2–5 ng/ml) following inhalation of doses up to 0.8 mg (twice the maximum recommended dose). A mean of 51% of the dose is recovered in urine as pirbuterol plus its sulfate conjugate following administration by aerosol. Pirbuterol is not metabolized by catechol-O-methyltransferase.
The percent of administered dose recovered as pirbuterol plus its sulfate conjugate does not change significantly over the dose range of 0.4 mg to 0.8 mg and is not significantly different from that after oral administration of pirbuterol. The plasma half-life measured after oral administration is about two hours.

INDICATIONS AND USAGE

MAXAIR AUTOHALER is indicated for the prevention and reversal of bronchospasm in patients with reversible bronchospasm including asthma. It may be used with or without concurrent theophylline and/or steroid therapy.

CONTRAINDICATIONS

MAXAIR is contraindicated in patients with a history of hypersensitivity to any of its ingredients.

WARNINGS

As with other beta adrenergic aerosols, MAXAIR should not be used in excess. Controlled clinical studies and other clinical experience have shown that MAXAIR like other inhaled beta adrenergic agonists can produce a significant cardiovascular effect in some patients, as measured by pulse rate, blood pressure, symptoms, and/or ECG changes. As with other beta adrenergic aerosols, the potential for paradoxical bronchospasm (which can be life threatening) should be kept in mind. If it occurs, the preparation should be discontinued immediately and alternative therapy instituted.
Fatalities have been reported in association with excessive use of inhaled sympathomimetic drugs.
The contents of MAXAIR AUTOHALER are under pressure. Do not puncture. Do not use or store near heat or open flame. Exposure to temperature above 120°F may cause bursting. Never throw container into fire or incinerator. Keep out of reach of children.

PRECAUTIONS

General

Since pirbuterol is a sympathomimetic amine, it should be used with caution in patients with cardiovascular disorders, including ischemic heart disease, hypertension, or cardiac arrhythmias, in patients with hyperthyroidism or diabetes mellitus, and in patients who are unusually responsive to sympathomimetic amines or who have convulsive disorders. Significant changes in systolic and diastolic blood pressure could be expected to occur in some patients after use of any beta adrenergic aerosol bronchodilator.

Information for Patients

MAXAIR effects may last up to five hours or longer. It should not be used more often than recommended and the patient should not increase the number of inhalations or frequency of use without first asking the physician. If symptoms of asthma get worse, adverse reactions occur, or the patient does not respond to the usual dose, the patient should be instructed to contact the physician immediately. The patient should be advised to see the Illustrated Patient's Instructions for Use.
The Autohaler actuator should not be used with any other inhalation aerosol canister. In addition, canisters for use with MAXAIR AUTOHALER should not be utilized with any other actuator.

Drug Interactions

Other beta adrenergic aerosol bronchodilators should not be used concomitantly with MAXAIR because they may have additive effects. Beta adrenergic agonists should be administered with caution to patients being treated with monoamine oxidase inhibitors or tricyclic antidepressants, since the action of beta adrenergic agonists on the vascular system may be potentiated.

Carcinogenesis, Mutagenesis and Impairment of Fertility

Pirbuterol hydrochloride administered in the diet to rats for 24 months and to mice for 18 months was free of carcinogenic activity at doses corresponding to 200 times the maximum human inhalation dose. In addition, the intragastric intubation of the drug at doses corresponding to 6250 times the maximum recommended human daily inhalation dose resulted in no increase in tumors in a 12-month rat study. Studies with pirbuterol revealed no evidence of mutagenesis. Reproduction studies in rats revealed no evidence of impaired fertility.

Teratogenic Effects—Pregnancy Category C

Reproduction studies have been performed in rats and rabbits by the inhalation route at doses up to 12 times (rat) and 16 times (rabbit) the maximum human inhalation dose and have revealed no significant findings. Animal reproduction studies in rats at *oral doses* up to 300 mg/kg and in rabbits at oral doses up to 100 mg/kg have shown no adverse effect on reproductive behavior, fertility, litter size, peri- and postnatal viability or fetal development. In rabbits at the highest dose level given, 300 mg/kg, abortions and fetal mortality were observed. There are no adequate and well controlled studies in pregnant women and MAXAIR should be used during pregnancy only if the potential benefit justifies the potential risk to the fetus.

Nursing Mothers

It is not known whether MAXAIR is excreted in human milk. Therefore, MAXAIR should be used during nursing only if the potential benefit justifies the possible risk to the newborn.

Pediatric Use

MAXAIR AUTOHALER is not recommended for patients under the age of 12 years because of insufficient clinical data to establish safety and effectiveness.

ADVERSE REACTIONS

The following rates of adverse reactions to pirbuterol are based on single and multiple dose clinical trials involving 761 patients, 400 of whom received multiple doses (mean duration of treatment was 2.5 months and maximum was 19 months).
The following were the adverse reactions reported more frequently than 1 in 100 patients:
CNS: nervousness (6.9%), tremor (6.0%), headache (2.0%), dizziness (1.2%).
Cardiovascular: palpitations (1.7%), tachycardia (1.2%).
Respiratory: cough (1.2%).
Gastrointestinal: nausea (1.7%).
The following adverse reactions occurred less frequently than 1 in 100 patients and there may be a causal relationship with pirbuterol:
CNS: depression, anxiety, confusion, insomnia, weakness, hyperkinesia, syncope.
Cardiovascular: hypotension, skipped beats, chest pain.
Gastrointestinal: dry mouth, glossitis, abdominal pain/cramps, anorexia, diarrhea, stomatitis, nausea and vomiting.
Ear, Nose and Throat: smell/taste changes, sore throat.
Dermatological: rash, pruritus.
Other: numbness in extremities, alopecia, bruising, fatigue, edema, weight gain, flushing.
Other adverse reactions were reported with a frequency of less than 1 in 100 patients but a causal relationship between pirbuterol and the reaction could not be determined: migraine, productive cough, wheezing, and dermatitis.
The following rates of adverse reactions during three-month controlled clinical trials involving 310 patients are noted. The table does not include mild reactions.

PERCENT OF PATIENTS WITH MODERATE TO SEVERE ADVERSE REACTIONS

Reaction	Pirbuterol N=157	Metaproterenol N=153
Central Nervous System		
tremors	1.3%	3.3%
nervousness	4.5%	2.6%
headache	1.3%	2.0%
weakness	.0%	1.3%
drowsiness	.0%	0.7%
dizziness	0.6%	.0%
Cardiovascular		
palpitations	1.3%	1.3%
tachycardia	1.3%	2.0%
Respiratory		
chest pain/tightness	1.3%	.0%
cough	.0%	0.7%
Gastrointestinal		
nausea	1.3%	2.0%
diarrhea	1.3%	0.7%
dry mouth	1.3%	1.3%
vomiting	.0%	0.7%
Dermatological		
skin reaction	.0%	0.7%
rash	.0%	1.3%
Other		
bruising	0.6%	.0%
smell/taste change	0.6%	.0%
backache	.0%	0.7%
fatigue	.0%	0.7%
hoarseness	.0%	0.7%
nasal congestion	.0%	0.7%

OVERDOSAGE

The expected symptoms with overdosage are those of excessive beta-stimulation and/or any of the symptoms listed under adverse reactions, e.g., angina, hypertension or hypotension, arrhythmias, nervousness, headache, tremor, dry mouth, palpitation, nausea, dizziness, fatigue, malaise, and insomnia.
Treatment consists of discontinuation of pirbuterol together with appropriate symptomatic therapy.
The oral acute lethal dose in male and female rats and mice was greater than 2000 mg base/kg. The aerosol acute lethal dose was not determined.

DOSAGE AND ADMINISTRATION

The usual dose for adults and children 12 years and older is two inhalations (0.4 mg) repeated every 4–6 hours. One inhalation (0.2 mg) repeated every 4–6 hours may be sufficient for some patients.
A total daily dose of 12 inhalations should not be exceeded.
If a previously effective dosage regimen fails to provide the usual relief, medical advice should be sought immediately as this is often a sign of seriously worsening asthma which would require reassessment of therapy.

HOW SUPPLIED

MAXAIR AUTOHALER is supplied in a pressurized aluminum canister with a light blue plastic breath-activated actuator. DO NOT USE WITH OTHER CANISTERS OR MOUTHPIECES. Each actuation delivers pirbuterol acetate equivalent to 0.2 mg of pirbuterol from the mouthpiece. Canister with breath-activated Autohaler actuator. Net content weight 14 g, a minimum of 400 inhalations (NDC **0089-0815-21**) and net content weight 2.8 g, a minimum of 80 inhalations (Hospital Pack: NDC **0089-0817-10**, Sample Pack: NDC **0089-0815-08**).
Note: The indented statement below is required by the Federal goverment's Clean Air Act for all products containing or manufactured with chlorofluorocarbons (CFC's).

> **WARNING:** Contains trichloromonofluoromethane and dichlorodifluoromethane, substances which harm public health and environment by destroying ozone in the upper atmosphere.

A notice similar to the above WARNING has been placed in the "Patient's Instructions for Use" of this product pursuant to EPA regulations.

CAUTION

Federal law prohibits dispensing without prescription.
Store between 15° and 30°C (59° to 86°F).

3M

3M Pharmaceuticals
Northridge, CA 91324

609903 JUNE 1996

Shown in Product Identification Guide, page 321

MAXAIR™ Inhaler ℞

(pirbuterol acetate inhalation aerosol)
Bronchodilator Aerosol
For Inhalation Only

DESCRIPTION

The active component of MAXAIR Inhaler is (R,S)α^6-[[(1,1-dimethylethyl) amino]methyl]-3-hydroxy-2,6-pyridine-dimethanol monoacetate salt, a beta-2 adrenergic bronchodilator, having the following chemical structure:

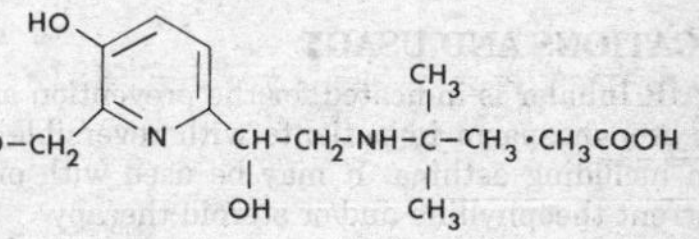

Pirbuterol acetate is a white, crystalline racemic mixture of two optically active isomers. It is a powder, freely soluble in water, with a molecular weight of 300.3 and empirical formula of $C_{12}H_{20}N_2O_3 \cdot C_2H_4O_2$.
MAXAIR Inhaler is a metered dose aerosol unit for oral inhalation. It provides a fine-particle suspension of pirbuterol acetate in the propellant mixture of trichloromonofluoromethane and dichlorodifluoromethane, with sorbitan trioleate. Each actuation delivers from the mouthpiece pirbuterol acetate equivalent to 0.2 mg of pirbuterol with the majority of particles less than 5 microns in diameter. Each canister provides at least 300 inhalations.

Continued on next page

Maxair Inhaler—Cont.

CLINICAL PHARMACOLOGY

In vitro studies and *in vivo* pharmacologic studies have demonstrated that MAXAIR has a preferential effect on beta-2 adrenergic receptors compared with isoproterenol. While it is recognized that beta-2 adrenergic receptors are the predominant receptors in bronchial smooth muscle, recent data indicate that there is a population of beta-2 receptors in the human heart, existing in a concentration between 10–50%. The precise function of these, however, is not yet established (see WARNINGS section).

The pharmacologic effects of beta adrenergic agonist drugs, including pirbuterol, are at least in part attributable to stimulation through beta adrenergic receptors of intracellular adenyl cyclase, the enzyme which catalyzes the conversion of adenosine triphosphate (ATP) to cyclic-3',5'-adenosine monophosphate (c-AMP). Increased c-AMP levels are associated with relaxation of bronchial smooth muscle and inhibition of release of mediators of immediate hypersensitivity from cells, especially from mast cells.

Bronchodilator activity of MAXAIR was manifested clinically by an improvement in various pulmonary function parameters (FEV_1, MMF, PEFR, airway resistance [RAW] and conductance [GA/V_{tg}]).

In controlled double-blind single dose clinical trials, the onset of improvement in pulmonary function occurred within 5 minutes in most patients as determined by forced expiratory volume in one second (FEV_1). FEV_1 and MMF measurements also showed that maximum improvement in pulmonary function generally occurred 30–60 minutes following one (1) or two (2) inhalations of pirbuterol (0.2–0.4 mg). The duration of action of MAXAIR is maintained for 5 hours (the time at which the last observations were made) in a substantial number of patients, based on a 15% or greater increase in FEV_1. In controlled repetitive dose studies of 12 weeks' duration, 74% of 156 patients on pirbuterol and 62% of 141 patients on metaproterenol showed a clinically significant improvement based on a 15% or greater increase in FEV_1 on at least half of the days. Onset and duration were equivalent to that seen in single dose studies. Continued effectiveness was demonstrated over the 12-week period in the majority (94%) of responding patients; however, chronic dosing was associated with the development of tachyphylaxis (tolerance) to the bronchodilator effect in some patients in both treatment groups.

A placebo-controlled double-blind single dose study (24 patients per treatment group), utilizing continuous Holter monitoring for 5 hours after drug administration, showed no significant difference in ectopic activity between the placebo control group and MAXAIR at the recommended dose (0.2–0.4 mg), and twice the recommended dose (0.8 mg). As with other inhaled beta adrenergic agonists, supraventricular and ventricular ectopic beats have been seen with MAXAIR (see WARNINGS).

Recent studies in laboratory animals (minipigs, rodents, and dogs) recorded the occurrence of cardiac arrhythmias and sudden death (with histologic evidence of myocardial necrosis) when beta agonists and methylxanthines were administered concurrently. The significance of these findings when applied to humans is currently unknown.

Pharmacokinetics

As expected by extrapolation from oral data, systemic blood levels of pirbuterol are below the limit of assay sensitivity (2–5 ng/ml) following inhalation of doses up to 0.8 mg (twice the maximum recommended dose). A mean of 51% of the dose is recovered in urine as pirbuterol plus its sulfate conjugate following administration by aerosol. Pirbuterol is not metabolized by catechol-O-methyltransferase. The percent of administered dose recovered as pirbuterol plus its sulfate conjugate does not change significantly over the dose range of 0.4 mg to 0.8 mg and is not significantly different from that after oral administration of pirbuterol. The plasma half-life measured after oral administration is about two hours.

INDICATIONS AND USAGE

MAXAIR Inhaler is indicated for the prevention and reversal of bronchospasm in patients with reversible bronchospasm including asthma. It may be used with or without concurrent theophylline and/or steroid therapy.

CONTRAINDICATIONS

MAXAIR is contraindicated in patients with a history of hypersensitivity to any of its ingredients.

WARNINGS

As with other beta adrenergic aerosols, MAXAIR should not be used in excess. Controlled clinical studies and other clinical experience have shown that MAXAIR like other inhaled beta adrenergic agonists can produce a significant cardiovascular effect in some patients, as measured by pulse rate, blood pressure, symptoms, and/or ECG changes. As with other beta adrenergic aerosols, the potential for paradoxical bronchospasm (which can be life threatening) should be kept in mind. If it occurs, the preparation should be discontinued immediately and alternative therapy instituted.

Fatalities have been reported in association with excessive use of inhaled sympathomimetic drugs.

The contents of MAXAIR Inhaler are under pressure. Do not puncture. Do not use or store near heat or open flame. Exposure to temperature above 120°F may cause bursting. Never throw container into fire or incinerator. Keep out of reach of children.

PRECAUTIONS

General

Since pirbuterol is a sympathomimetic amine, it should be used with caution in patients with cardiovascular disorders, including ischemic heart disease, hypertension, or cardiac arrhythmias, in patients with hyperthyroidism or diabetes mellitus, and in patients who are unusually responsive to sympathomimetic amines or who have convulsive disorders. Significant changes in systolic and diastolic blood pressure could be expected to occur in some patients after use of any beta adrenergic aerosol bronchodilator.

Information for Patients

MAXAIR effects may last up to five hours or longer. It should not be used more often than recommended and the patient should not increase the number of inhalations or frequency of use without first asking the physician. If symptoms of asthma get worse, adverse reactions occur, or the patient does not respond to the usual dose, the patient should be instructed to contact the physician immediately. The patient should be advised to see the Illustrated Directions for Use.

Drug Interactions

Other beta adrenergic aerosol bronchodilators should not be used concomitantly with MAXAIR because they may have additive effects. Beta adrenergic agonists should be administered with caution to patients being treated with monoamine oxidase inhibitors or tricyclic antidepressants, since the action of beta adrenergic agonists on the vascular system may be potentiated.

Carcinogenesis, Mutagenesis and Impairment of Fertility

Pirbuterol hydrochloride administered in the diet to rats for 24 months and to mice for 18 months was free of carcinogenic activity at doses corresponding to 200 times the maximum human inhalation dose. In addition, the intragastric intubation of the drug at doses corresponding to 6250 times the maximum recommended human daily inhalation dose resulted in no increase in tumors in a 12-month rat study. Studies with pirbuterol revealed no evidence of mutagenesis. Reproduction studies in rats revealed no evidence of impaired fertility.

Teratogenic Effects—Pregnancy Category C

Reproduction studies have been performed in rats and rabbits by the inhalation route at doses up to 12 times (rat) and 16 times (rabbit) the maximum human inhalation dose and have revealed no significant findings. Animal reproduction studies in rats at *oral doses* up to 300 mg/kg and in rabbits at oral doses up to 100 mg/kg have shown no adverse effect on reproductive behavior, fertility, litter size, peri- and postnatal viability or fetal development. In rabbits at the highest dose level given, 300 mg/kg, abortions and fetal mortality were observed. There are no adequate and well controlled studies in pregnant women and MAXAIR should be used during pregnancy only if the potential benefit justifies the potential risk to the fetus.

Nursing Mothers

It is not known whether MAXAIR is excreted in human milk. Therefore, MAXAIR should be used during nursing only if the potential benefit justifies the possible risk to the newborn.

Pediatric Use

MAXAIR Inhaler is not recommended for patients under the age of 12 years because of insufficient clinical data to establish safety and effectiveness.

ADVERSE REACTIONS

The following rates of adverse reactions to pirbuterol are based on single and multiple dose clinical trials involving 761 patients, 400 of whom received multiple doses (mean duration of treatment was 2.5 months and maximum was 19 months).

The following were the adverse reactions reported more frequently than 1 in 100 patients:

CNS: nervousness (6.9%), tremor (6.0%), headache (2.0%), dizziness (1.2%).

Cardiovascular: palpitations (1.7%), tachycardia (1.2%).

Respiratory: cough (1.2%).

Gastrointestinal: nausea (1.7%).

The following adverse reactions occurred less frequently than 1 in 100 patients and there may be a causal relationship with pirbuterol:

CNS: depression, anxiety, confusion, insomnia, weakness, hyperkinesia, syncope.

Cardiovascular: hypotension, skipped beats, chest pain.

Gastrointestinal: dry mouth, glossitis, abdominal pain/cramps, anorexia, diarrhea, stomatitis, nausea and vomiting.

Ear, Nose and Throat: smell/taste changes, sore throat.

Dermatological: rash, pruritus.

Other: numbness in extremities, alopecia, bruising, fatigue, edema, weight gain, flushing.

Other adverse reactions were reported with a frequency of less than 1 in 100 patients but a causal relationship between pirbuterol and the reaction could not be determined: migraine, productive cough, wheezing, and dermatitis.

The following rates of adverse reactions during three-month controlled clinical trials involving 310 patients are noted. The table does not include mild reactions.

PERCENT OF PATIENTS WITH MODERATE TO SEVERE ADVERSE REACTIONS

Reaction	Pirbuterol N=157	Metaproterenol N=153
Central Nervous System		
tremors	1.3%	3.3%
nervousness	4.5%	2.6%
headache	1.3%	2.0%
weakness	.0%	1.3%
drowsiness	.0%	0.7%
dizziness	0.6%	.0%
Cardiovascular		
palpitations	1.3%	1.3%
tachycardia	1.3%	2.0%
Respiratory		
chest pain/tightness	1.3%	.0%
cough	.0%	0.7%
Gastrointestinal		
nausea	1.3%	2.0%
diarrhea	1.3%	0.7%
dry mouth	1.3%	1.3%
vomiting	.0%	0.7%
Dermatological		
skin reaction	.0%	0.7%
rash	.0%	1.3%
Other		
bruising	0.6%	.0%
smell/taste change	0.6%	.0%
backache	.0%	0.7%
fatigue	.0%	0.7%
hoarseness	.0%	0.7%
nasal congestion	.0%	0.7%

OVERDOSAGE

The expected symptoms with overdosage are those of excessive beta-stimulation and/or any of the symptoms listed under adverse reactions, e.g., angina, hypertension or hypotension, arrhythmias, nervousness, headache, tremor, dry mouth, palpitation, nausea, dizziness, fatigue, malaise, and insomnia.

Treatment consists of discontinuation of pirbuterol together with appropriate symptomatic therapy.

The oral acute lethal dose in male and female rats and mice was greater than 2000 mg base/kg. The aerosol acute lethal dose was not determined.

DOSAGE AND ADMINISTRATION

The usual dose for adults and children 12 years and older is two inhalations (0.4 mg) repeated every 4–6 hours. One inhalation (0.2 mg) repeated every 4–6 hours may be sufficient for some patients.

A total daily dose of 12 inhalations should not be exceeded. If a previously effective dosage regimen fails to provide the usual relief, medical advice should be sought immediately as this is often a sign of seriously worsening asthma which would require reassessment of therapy.

HOW SUPPLIED

MAXAIR Inhaler is supplied in a pressurized aluminum canister with a light-blue plastic actuator and attached white mouthpiece. Each actuation delivers pirbuterol acetate equivalent to 0.2 mg of pirbuterol from the mouthpiece. Net content weight 25.6 g, a minimum of 300 actuations (NDC 0089-0790-21).

Note: The indented statement below is required by the Federal government's Clean Air Act for all products containing or manufactured with chlorofluorocarbons (CFC's).

> **WARNING:** Contains trichloromonofluoromethane and dichlorodifluoromethane, substances which harm public health and environment by destroying ozone in the upper atmosphere.

A notice similar to the above WARNING has been placed in the "Patient's Instructions for Use" of this product pursuant to EPA regulations.

CAUTION

Federal law prohibits dispensing without prescription.
Store between 15° and 30°C (59° to 86°F).

3M Pharmaceuticals
Northridge, CA 91324
610000   JUNE 1995
Shown in Product Identification Guide, page 321

MEDIHALER-ISO™ ℞
(isoproterenol sulfate)
Inhalation Aerosol

For full prescribing information see leaflet accompanying product or call 800-328-0255 for a copy.

HOW SUPPLIED
MEDIHALER-ISO is an aerosol device which delivers 0.08 mg isoproterenol sulfate through the oral adapter with each depression of the valve.
15-ml and oral adapter containing 21.0 gm, a minimum of 300 actuations (NDC **0089-0785-21**).
15-ml refill vial only, containing 21.0 gm, a minimum of 300 actuations (NDC **0089-0785-11**)

METROGEL-VAGINAL® ℞
(metronidazole vaginal gel)
0.75% Vaginal Gel
FOR INTRAVAGINAL USE ONLY
NOT FOR OPHTHALMIC, DERMAL, OR ORAL USE

DESCRIPTION
METROGEL-VAGINAL is the intravaginal dosage form of the synthetic antibacterial agent, metronidazole, USP at a concentration of 0.75%. Metronidazole is a member of the imidazole class of antibacterial agents and is classified therapeutically as an anti-protozoal and anti-bacterial agent. Chemically, metronidazole is a 2-methyl-5-nitroimidazole-1-ethanol. It has a chemical formula of $C_6H_9N_3O_3$, a molecular weight of 171.16, and has the following structure:

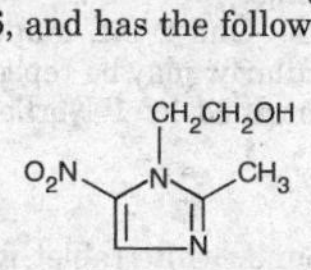

METROGEL-VAGINAL is a gelled, purified water solution, containing metronidazole at a concentration of 7.5 mg/g (0.75%). The gel is formulated at pH 4.0. The gel also contains carbomer 934P, edetate disodium, methylparaben, propylparaben, propylene glycol, and sodium hydroxide. Each applicator full of 5 grams of vaginal gel contains approximately 37.5 mg of metronidazole.

CLINICAL PHARMACOLOGY
Normal Subjects:
Following a single, intravaginal 5 gram dose of metronidazole vaginal gel (equivalent to 37.5 mg of metronidazole) to 12 normal subjects, a mean maximum serum metronidazole concentration of 237 ng/mL was reported (range: 152 to 368 ng/mL). This is approximately 2% of the mean maximum serum metronidazole concentration reported in the same subjects administered a single, oral 500 mg dose of metronidazole (mean C_{max} = 12,785 ng/mL, range: 10,013 to 17,400 ng/mL). These peak concentrations were obtained in 6 to 12 hours after dosing with metronidazole vaginal gel and 1 to 3 hours after dosing with oral metronidazole.
The extent of exposure [area under the curve (AUC)] of metronidazole, when administered as a single intravaginal 5 gram dose of metronidazole vaginal gel (equivalent to 37.5 mg of metronidazole), was approximately 4% of the AUC of a single oral 500 mg dose of metronidazole (4977 ng-hr/mL and approximately 125,000 ng-hr/mL, respectively).
Dose-adjusted comparisons of AUCs demonstrated that, on a mg to mg comparison basis, the absorption of metronidazole, when administered vaginally, was approximately half that of an equivalent oral dosage.
Patients with Bacterial Vaginosis:
Following single and multiple 5 gram doses of metronidazole vaginal gel to 4 patients with bacterial vaginosis, a mean maximum serum metronidazole concentration of 214 ng/mL on day 1 and 294 ng/mL (range: 228 to 349 ng/mL) on day five were reported. Steady-state metronidazole serum concentrations following oral dosages of 400 to 500 mg BID have been reported to range from 6,000 to 20,000 ng/mL.
Microbiology:
The intracellular targets of action of metronidazole on anaerobes are largely unknown. The 5-nitro group of metronidazole is reduced by metabolically active anaerobes, and studies have demonstrated that the reduced form of the drug interacts with bacterial DNA. However, it is not clear whether interaction with DNA alone is an important component in the bactericidal action of metronidazole on anaerobic organisms.
Culture and sensitivity testing of bacteria are not routinely performed to establish the diagnosis of bacterial vaginosis. (See **INDICATIONS AND USAGE.**)
Standard methodology for the susceptibility testing of the potential bacterial vaginosis pathogens, *Gardnerella vaginalis, Mobiluncus* spp., and *Mycoplasma hominis*, has not been defined. Nonetheless, metronidazole is an antimicrobial agent active *in vitro* against most strains of the following organisms that have been reported to be associated with bacterial vaginosis:
Bacteroides spp.
Gardnerella vaginalis
Mobiluncus spp.
Peptostreptococcus spp.

INDICATIONS AND USAGE
METROGEL-VAGINAL is indicated in the treatment of bacterial vaginosis (formerly referred to as *Haemophilus* vaginitis, *Gardnerella* vaginitis, nonspecific vaginitis, *Corynebacterium* vaginitis, or anaerobic vaginosis).
NOTE: For purposes of this indication, a clinical diagnosis of bacterial vaginosis is usually defined by the presence of a homogeneous vaginal discharge that (a) has a pH of greater than 4.5, (b) emits a "fishy" amine odor when mixed with a 10% KOH solution, and (c) contains clue cells on microscopic examination. Gram's stain results consistent with a diagnosis of bacterial vaginosis include (a) markedly reduced or absent *Lactobacillus* morphology, (b) predominance of *Gardnerella* morphotype, and (c) absent or few white blood cells. Other pathogens commonly associated with vulvovaginitis, e.g., *Trichomonas vaginalis, Chlamydia trachomatis, N. gonorrhoeae, Candida albicans*, and *Herpes simplex* virus should be ruled out.

CONTRAINDICATIONS
METROGEL-VAGINAL is contraindicated in patients with a prior history of hypersensitivity to metronidazole, parabens, other ingredients of the formulation, or other nitroimidazole derivatives.

WARNINGS
Convulsive Seizures and Peripheral Neuropathy:
Convulsive seizures and peripheral neuropathy, the latter characterized mainly by numbness or paresthesia of an extremity, have been reported in patients treated with oral or intravenous metronidazole. The appearance of abnormal neurologic signs demands the prompt discontinuation of metronidazole vaginal gel therapy. Metronidazole vaginal gel should be administered with caution to patients with central nervous system diseases.
Psychotic Reactions:
Psychotic reactions have been reported in alcoholic patients who were using oral metronidazole and disulfiram concurrently. Metronidazole vaginal gel should not be administered to patients who have taken disulfiram within the last two weeks.

PRECAUTIONS
METROGEL-VAGINAL affords minimal peak serum levels and systemic exposure (AUCs) of metronidazole compared to 500 mg oral metronidazole dosing. Although these lower levels of exposure are less likely to produce the common reactions seen with oral metronidazole, the possibility of these and other reactions cannot be excluded presently. Data from well-controlled trials directly comparing metronidazole administered orally to metronidazole administered vaginally are not available.
General: Patients with severe hepatic disease metabolize metronidazole slowly. This results in the accumulation of metronidazole and its metabolites in the plasma. Accordingly, for such patients, metronidazole vaginal gel should be administered cautiously.
Known or previously unrecognized vaginal candidiasis may present more prominent symptoms during therapy with metronidazole vaginal gel. Approximately 6–10% of patients treated with METROGEL-VAGINAL developed symptomatic *Candida* vaginitis during or immediately after therapy.
Disulfiram-like reaction to alcohol has been reported with oral metronidazole, thus the possibility of such a reaction occurring while on metronidazole vaginal gel therapy cannot be excluded.
METROGEL-VAGINAL contains ingredients that may cause burning and irritation of the eye. In the event of accidental contact with the eye, rinse the eye with copious amounts of cool tap water.
Information for the Patient: The patient should be cautioned about drinking alcohol while being treated with metronidazole vaginal gel. While blood levels are significantly lower with METROGEL-VAGINAL than with usual doses of oral metronidazole, a possible interaction with alcohol cannot be excluded.
The patient should be instructed not to engage in vaginal intercourse during treatment with this product.
Drug Interactions: Oral metronidazole has been reported to potentiate the anticoagulant effect of warfarin and other coumarin anticoagulants, resulting in a prolongation of prothrombin time. This possible drug interaction should be considered when metronidazole vaginal gel is prescribed for patients on this type of anticoagulant therapy.
In patients stabilized on relatively high doses of lithium, short-term oral metronidazole therapy has been associated with elevation of serum lithium levels and, in a few cases, signs of lithium toxicity.
Use of cimetidine with oral metronidazole may prolong the half-life and decrease plasma clearance of metronidazole.
Drug/Laboratory Test Interactions: Metronidazole may interfere with certain types of determinations of serum chemistry values, such as aspartate aminotransferase (AST, SGOT), alanine aminotransferase (ALT, SGPT), lactate dehydrogenase (LDH), triglycerides, and glucose hexokinase. Values of zero may be observed. All of the assays in which interference has been reported involve enzymatic coupling of the assay to oxidation-reduction of nicotinamide-adenine dinucleotides (NAD+NADH). Interference is due to the similarity in absorbance peaks of NADH (340 nm) and metronidazole (322 nm) at pH 7.
Carcinogenesis, Mutagenesis, Impairment of Fertility: Metronidazole has shown evidence of carcinogenic activity in a number of studies involving chronic oral administration in mice and rats. Prominent among the effects in the mouse was the promotion of pulmonary tumorigenesis. This has been observed in all six reported studies in that species, including one study in which the animals were dosed on an intermittent schedule (administration during every fourth week only). At very high dose levels (approx. 500 mg/kg/day), there was a statistically significant increase in the incidence of malignant liver tumors in males. Also, the published results of one of the mouse studies indicate an increase in the incidence of malignant lymphomas as well as pulmonary neoplasms associated with lifetime feeding of the drug. All these effects are statistically significant. Several long-term oral dosing studies in the rat have been completed. There were statistically significant increases in the incidence of various neoplasms, particularly in mammary and hepatic tumors, among female rats administered metronidazole over those noted in the concurrent female control groups. Two lifetime tumorigenicity studies in hamsters have been performed and reported to be negative.
These studies have not been conducted with 0.75% metronidazole vaginal gel, which would result in significantly lower systemic blood levels than those obtained with oral formulations.
Although metronidazole has shown mutagenic activity in a number of *in vitro* assay systems, studies in mammals (*in vivo*) have failed to demonstrate a potential for genetic damage.
Fertility studies have been performed in mice up to six times the recommended human oral dose (based on mg/m^2) and have revealed no evidence of impaired fertility.
Pregnancy: Teratogenic Effects Pregnancy Category B
There has been no experience to date with the use of METROGEL-VAGINAL in pregnant patients. Metronidazole crosses the placental barrier and enters the fetal circulation rapidly. No fetotoxicity or teratogenicity was observed when metronidazole was administered orally to pregnant mice at six times the recommended human dose (based on mg/m^2); however, in a single small study where the drug was administered intraperitoneally, some intrauterine deaths were observed. The relationship of these findings to the drug is unknown.
There are, however, no adequate and well-controlled studies in pregnant women. Because animal reproduction studies are not always predictive of human response, and because metronidazole is a carcinogen in rodents, this drug should be used during pregnancy only if clearly needed.
Nursing mothers: Specific studies of metronidazole levels in human milk following intravaginally administered metronidazole have not been performed. However, metronidazole is secreted in human milk in concentrations similar to those found in plasma following oral administration of metronidazole.
Because of the potential for tumorigenicity shown for metronidazole in mouse and rat studies, a decision should be made whether to discontinue nursing or to discontinue the drug, taking into account the importance of the drug to the mother.
Pediatric use: Safety and effectiveness in children have not been established.

ADVERSE EVENTS
Clinical Trials:
There were no deaths or serious adverse events related to drug therapy in clinical trials involving 800 non-pregnant women who received METROGEL-VAGINAL.
In a randomized, single-blind clinical trial of 505 non-pregnant women who received METROGEL-VAGINAL once or twice a day, 2 patients (1 from each regimen) discontinued therapy early due to drug-related adverse events. One patient discontinued drug because of moderate abdominal cramping and loose stools, while the other patient discontinued drug because of mild vaginal burning. These symptoms resolved after discontinuation of drug.
Medical events judged to be related, probably related, or possibly related to administration of METROGEL-VAGINAL once or twice a day were reported for 195/505 (39%) patients. The incidence of individual adverse reactions were not significantly different between the two regimens. Unless percentages are otherwise stipulated, the incidence of individual adverse reactions listed below was less than 1%:
Reproductive: Vaginal discharge (12%), symptomatic *Candida* cervicitis/vaginitis (10%), vulva/vaginal irritative symptoms (9%), pelvic discomfort (3%).

Continued on next page

Metrogel—Cont.

Gastrointestinal: Gastrointestinal discomfort (7%), nausea and/or vomiting (4%), unusual taste (2%), diarrhea/loose stools (1%), decreased appetite (1%), abdominal bloating/gas; thirsty, dry mouth. *Neurologic:* Headache (5%), dizziness (2%), depression. *Dermatologic:* Generalized itching or rash. *Other:* Unspecified cramping (1%), fatigue, darkened urine.

In previous clinical trials submitted for approved labeling of MetroGel-Vaginal the following was also reported: *Laboratory:* Increased/decreased white blood cell counts (1.7%).

Other Metronidazole Formulations: Other effects that have been reported in association with the use of **topical (dermal)** formulations of metronidazole include skin irritation, transient skin erythema, and mild skin dryness and burning. None of these adverse events exceeded an incidence of 2% of patients.

METROGEL-VAGINAL affords minimal peak serum levels and systemic exposure (AUC) of metronidazole compared to 500 mg oral metronidazole dosing. Although these lower levels of exposure are less likely to produce the common reactions seen with oral metronidazole, the possibility of these and other reactions cannot be excluded presently.

The following adverse reactions and altered laboratory tests have been reported with the **oral or parenteral** use of metronidazole:

Cardiovascular: Flattening of the T-wave may be seen in electrocardiographic tracings.

Central Nervous System: (See **WARNINGS**). Headache, dizziness, syncope, ataxia, confusion, convulsive seizures, peripheral neuropathy, vertigo, incoordination, irritability, depression, weakness, insomnia.

Gastrointestinal: Abdominal discomfort; nausea; vomiting; diarrhea; an unpleasant metallic taste; anorexia; epigastric distress; abdominal cramping; constipation; "furry" tongue; glossitis; stomatitis; pancreatitis; and modification of taste of alcoholic beverages.

Genitourinary: Overgrowth of *Candida* in the vagina, dyspareunia, decreased libido, proctitis.

Hematopoietic: Reversible neutropenia, reversible thrombocytopenia.

Hypersensitivity Reactions: Urticaria; erythematous rash; flushing; nasal congestion; dryness of the mouth, vagina, or vulva; fever; pruritus; fleeting joint pains.

Renal: Dysuria, cystitis, polyuria, incontinence, a sense of pelvic pressure, darkened urine.

OVERDOSAGE

There is no human experience with overdosage of metronidazole vaginal gel. Vaginally applied metronidazole gel, 0.75% could be absorbed in sufficient amounts to produce systemic effects.
(See **WARNINGS**.)

DOSAGE AND ADMINISTRATION

The recommended dose is one applicator full of METROGEL-VAGINAL (approximately 5 grams containing approximately 37.5 mg of metronidazole) intravaginally once or twice a day for 5 days. For once a day dosing, MetroGel-Vaginal should be administered at bedtime.

HOW SUPPLIED

METROGEL-VAGINAL (metronidazole vaginal gel, 0.75%) 0.75% Vaginal Gel is supplied in a 70 gram tube and packaged with 5 vaginal applicators. NDC number for the 70 gram tube is 0089-0200-25. Store at controlled room temperature 15° to 30°C (59° to 86°F). Protect from freezing.

Clinical Studies

In a randomized, single-blind, clinical trial of non-pregnant women with bacterial vaginosis who received MetroGel-Vaginal daily for 5 days, the clinical cure rates for evaluable patients, determined at 4 weeks after completion of therapy for the QD and BID regimens were 98/185 (53%) and 109/190 (57%), respectively.

Rx only
620700 March 1998

Manufactured for
3M Pharmaceuticals
Northridge, CA 91324
Manufactured by
DPT Laboratories, Inc.
San Antonio, TX, 78215
Shown in Product Identification Guide, page 321

MINITRAN™　℞
(nitroglycerin)
Transdermal Delivery System

For full prescribing information see leaflet accompanying product or call 800-328-0255 for a copy.

HOW SUPPLIED
[See table below]

NORFLEX™　℞
(orphenadrine citrate)
Extended-release
Tablets and Injection

DESCRIPTION

Orphenadrine citrate is the citrate salt of orphenadrine (2-dimethylaminoethyl 2-methylbenzhydryl ether citrate). It occurs as a white, crystalline powder having a bitter taste. It is practically odorless; sparingly soluble in water, slightly soluble in alcohol.

Each Norflex Extended-release tablet contains 100 mg orphenadrine citrate. Norflex Extended-release tablets also contain: calcium stearate, ethylcellulose, and lactose. Norflex Injection contains 60 mg of orphenadrine citrate in aqueous solution in each ampul. Norflex Injection also contains: sodium bisulfite NF, 2.0 mg; sodium chloride USP, 5.8 mg; sodium hydroxide, to adjust pH; and water for injection USP, q.s. to 2 mL.

ACTIONS

The mode of therapeutic action has not been clearly identified, but may be related to its analgesic properties. Orphenadrine citrate also possesses anticholinergic actions.

INDICATIONS

Orphenadrine citrate is indicated as an adjunct to rest, physical therapy, and other measures for the relief of discomfort associated with acute painful musculoskeletal conditions. The mode of action of the drug has not been clearly identified, but may be related to its analgesic properties. Orphenadrine citrate does not directly relax tense skeletal muscles in man.

CONTRAINDICATIONS

Contraindicated in patients with glaucoma, pyloric or duodenal obstruction, stenosing peptic ulcers, prostatic hypertrophy or obstruction of the bladder neck, cardio-spasm (megaesophagus) and myasthenia gravis. Contraindicated in patients who have demonstrated a previous hypersensitivity to the drug.

WARNINGS

Some patients may experience transient episodes of light-headedness, dizziness or syncope. Norflex may impair the ability of the patient to engage in potentially hazardous activities such as operating machinery or driving a motor vehicle; ambulatory patients should therefore be cautioned accordingly.

Norflex Injection contains sodium bisulfite, a sulfite that may cause allergic-type reactions including anaphylactic symptoms and life-threatening or less severe asthmatic episodes in certain susceptible people. The overall prevalence of sulfite sensitivity in the general population is unknown and probably low. Sulfite sensitivity is seen more frequently in asthmatic than nonasthmatic people.

PREGNANCY

Pregnancy Category C. Animal reproduction studies have not been conducted with Norflex. It is also not known whether Norflex can cause fetal harm when administered to a pregnant woman or can affect reproduction capacity. Norflex should be given to a pregnant woman only if clearly needed.

PEDIATRIC USE

Safety and effectiveness in pediatric patients have not been established.

PRECAUTIONS

Confusion, anxiety and tremors have been reported in few patients receiving propoxyphene and orphenadrine concomitantly. As these symptoms may be simply due to an additive effect, reduction of dosage and/or discontinuation of one or both agents is recommended in such cases.

Orphenadrine citrate should be used with caution in patients with tachycardia, cardiac decompensation, coronary insufficiency, cardiac arrhythmias.

Safety of continuous long-term therapy with orphenadrine has not been established. Therefore, if orphenadrine is prescribed for prolonged use, periodic monitoring of blood, urine and liver function values is recommended.

ADVERSE REACTIONS

Adverse reactions of orphenadrine are mainly due to the mild anticholinergic action of orphenadrine, and are usually associated with higher dosage. Dryness of the mouth is usually the first adverse effect to appear. When the daily dose is increased, possible adverse effects include: tachycardia, palpitation, urinary hesitancy or retention, blurred vision, dilatation of pupils, increased ocular tension, weakness, nausea, vomiting, headache, dizziness, constipation, drowsiness, hypersensitivity reactions, pruritus, hallucinations, agitation, tremor, gastric irritation, and rarely urticaria and other dermatoses. Infrequently, an elderly patient may experience some degree of mental confusion. These adverse reactions can usually be eliminated by reduction in dosage. Very rare cases of aplastic anemia associated with the use of orphenadrine tablets have been reported. No causal relationship has been established.

Rare instances of anaphylactic reaction have been reported associated with the intramuscular injection of Norflex Injection.

DOSAGE AND ADMINISTRATION

TABLETS: Adults—Two tablets per day; one in the morning and one in the evening.

INJECTION: Adults—One 2 mL ampul (60 mg) intravenously or intramuscularly; may be repeated every 12 hours. Relief may be maintained by 1 Norflex Extended-release tablet twice daily.

HOW SUPPLIED

TABLETS: Each round, white tablet imprinted with "3M" on one side and "221" on the other. Bottles of 100 (NDC **0089-0221-10**) and 500 (NDC **0089-0221-50**). Each tablet contains 100 mg of orphenadrine citrate.

INJECTION: Boxes of 6 (NDC **0089-0540-06**) 2 mL ampuls, each ampul containing 60 mg of orphenadrine citrate in aqueous solution.

Store at controlled room temperature, 15°–30°C (59°–86°F).

CAUTION: Federal law prohibits dispensing without prescription.

994101 　　　　　　　　　　　　　　　AUGUST 1997
Tablets Manufactured by　　　　Injection Manufactured for
3M Pharmaceuticals　　　　　　**3M Pharmaceuticals**
Northridge, CA 91324　　　　　　Northridge, CA 91324
　　　　　　　　　　　　　　　　By Abbott Laboratories
　　　　　　　　　　　　　　　　North Chicago, IL 60064
Shown in Product Identification Guide, page 321

NORGESIC™　℞
and
NORGESIC™ FORTE　℞
Tablets

ACTIONS

Orphenadrine citrate is a centrally acting (brain stem) compound which in animals selectively blocks facilitatory functions of the reticular formation. Orphenadrine does not produce myoneural block, nor does it affect crossed extensor reflexes. Orphenadrine prevents nicotine-induced convulsions but not those produced by strychnine.

Chronic administration of Norgesic to dogs and rats has revealed no drug-related toxicity. No blood or urine changes were observed, nor were there any macroscopic or microscopic pathological changes detected. Extensive experience with combinations containing aspirin and caffeine has established them as safe agents. The addition of orphenadrine citrate does not alter the toxicity of aspirin and caffeine.

The mode of therapeutic action of orphenadrine has not been clearly identified, but may be related to its analgesic properties. Orphenadrine citrate also possesses anticholinergic actions.

INDICATIONS

1. Symptomatic relief of mild to moderate pain of acute musculoskeletal disorders.
2. The orphenadrine component is indicated as an adjunct to rest, physical therapy, and other measures for the relief of discomfort associated with acute painful musculoskeletal conditions.

The mode of action of orphenadrine has not been clearly identified, but may be related to its analgesic properties. Norgesic and Norgesic Forte do not directly relax tense skeletal muscles in man.

CONTRAINDICATIONS

Because of the mild anticholinergic effect of orphenadrine, Norgesic or Norgesic Forte should not be used in patients

---

MINITRAN System Rated Release In Vivo	System Size	Total Nitroglycerin in System	NDC Number (30 per carton)
0.1 mg/hr	3.3 cm²	9 mg	NDC-0089-0301-02
0.2 mg/hr	6.7 cm²	18 mg	NDC-0089-0302-02
0.4 mg/hr	13.3 cm²	36 mg	NDC-0089-0303-02
0.6 mg/hr	20.0 cm²	54 mg	NDC-0089-0304-02

with glaucoma, pyloric or duodenal obstruction, achalasia, prostatic hypertrophy or obstructions at the bladder neck. Norgesic or Norgesic Forte is also contraindicated in patients with myasthenia gravis and in patients known to be sensitive to aspirin or caffeine.

The drug is contraindicated in patients who have demonstrated a previous hypersensitivity to the drug.

WARNINGS

Reye's Syndrome may develop in individuals who have chicken pox, influenza, or flu symptoms. Some studies suggest a possible association between the development of Reye's Syndrome and the use of medicines containing salicylate or aspirin. Norgesic and Norgesic Forte contain aspirin and therefore are not recommended for use in patients with chicken pox, influenza, or flu symptoms.

Norgesic and Norgesic Forte may impair the ability of the patient to engage in potentially hazardous activities such as operating machinery or driving a motor vehicle; ambulatory patients should therefore be cautioned accordingly.

Aspirin should be used with extreme caution in the presence of peptic ulcers and coagulation abnormalities.

USAGE IN PREGNANCY

Since safety of the use of this preparation in pregnancy, during lactation, or in the childbearing age has not been established, use of the drug in such patients requires that the potential benefits of the drug be weighed against its possible hazard to the mother and child.

PEDIATRIC USE

Safety and effectiveness in pediatric patients have not been established.

PRECAUTIONS

Confusion, anxiety and tremors have been reported in a few patients receiving propoxyphene and orphenadrine concomitantly. As these symptoms may be simply due to an additive effect, reduction of dosage and/or discontinuation of one or both agents is recommended in such cases.

Safety of continuous long term therapy with Norgesic or Norgesic Forte has not been established; therefore, if Norgesic or Norgesic Forte is prescribed for prolonged use, periodic monitoring of blood, urine and liver function values is recommended.

ADVERSE REACTIONS

Side effects of Norgesic or Norgesic Forte are those seen with aspirin and caffeine or those usually associated with mild anticholinergic agents. These may include tachycardia, palpitation, urinary hesitancy or retention, dry mouth, blurred vision, dilatation of the pupil, increased intraocular tension, weakness, nausea, vomiting, headache, dizziness, constipation, drowsiness, and rarely, urticaria and other dermatoses. Infrequently, an elderly patient may experience some degree of confusion. Mild central excitation and occasional hallucinations may be observed. These mild side effects can usually be eliminated by reduction in dosage. One case of aplastic anemia associated with the use of Norgesic has been reported. No causal relationship has been established. Rare G.I. hemorrhage due to aspirin content may be associated with the administration of Norgesic or Norgesic Forte. Some patients may experience transient episodes of light-headedness, dizziness or syncope.

DOSAGE AND ADMINISTRATION

Norgesic: Adults 1 to 2 tablets 3 to 4 times daily.

Norgesic Forte: Adults $^1/_2$ to 1 tablet 3 to 4 times daily.

HOW SUPPLIED

Norgesic tablets can be identified by their two layers colored white and yellow. Each round tablet is embossed "NORGESIC" on one side and "3M" on the other and contains orphenadrine citrate (2-dimethylaminoethyl 2-methylbenzhydryl ether citrate) 25 mg, aspirin 385 mg, and caffeine 30 mg.

Norgesic Forte tablets are exactly twice the strength of Norgesic. They are identified by their scored capsule shape and by their two layers colored white and yellow. Each capsule shaped tablet is embossed "NORGESIC FORTE" on one side and "3M" on the other and contains orphenadrine citrate 50 mg, aspirin 770 mg, and caffeine 60 mg.

Norgesic and Norgesic Forte also contain: lactose, polyethylene glycol, povidone, starch, sucrose, zinc stearate, and D&C yellow #10.

Norgesic: Bottles of 100 tablets (NDC **0089-0231-10**) and 500 tablets (NDC **0089-0231-50**).

Norgesic Forte: Bottles of 100 tablets (NDC **0089-0233-10**) and 500 tablets (NDC **0089-0233-50**).

Store below 30°C (86°F).

CAUTION

Federal law prohibits dispensing without prescription.

603500 January 1997

3M Pharmaceuticals

Northridge, CA 91324

Shown in Product Identification Guide, page 321

TAMBOCOR™ ℞

[*tăm-ba-kōr*]

(flecainide acetate)

Tablets

DESCRIPTION

TAMBOCOR™ (flecainide acetate) is an antiarrhythmic drug available in tablets of 50, 100 or 150 mg for oral administration.

Flecainide acetate is benzamide, N-(2-piperidinylmethyl)-2,5-bis(2,2,2-trifluoroethoxy)-monoacetate. The structural formula is given below.

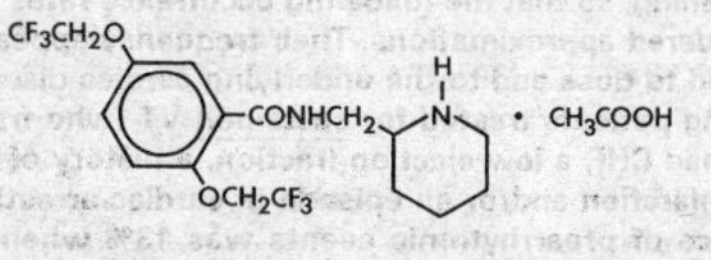

Flecainide acetate is a white crystalline substance with a pK_a of 9.3. It has an aqueous solubility of 48.4 mg/mL at 37°C.

TAMBOCOR tablets also contain: croscarmellose sodium, hydrogenated vegetable oil, magnesium stearate, microcrystalline cellulose and starch.

CLINICAL PHARMACOLOGY

TAMBOCOR has local anesthetic activity and belongs to the membrane stabilizing (Class 1) group of antiarrhythmic agents; it has electrophysiologic effects characteristic of the IC class of antiarrhythmics.

Electrophysiology. In man, TAMBOCOR produces a dose-related decrease in intracardiac conduction in all parts of the heart with the greatest effect on the His-Purkinje system (H-V conduction). Effects upon atrioventricular (AV) nodal conduction time and intra-atrial conduction times, although present, are less pronounced than those on ventricular conduction velocity. Significant effects on refractory periods were observed only in the ventricle. Sinus node recovery times (corrected) following pacing and spontaneous cycle lengths are somewhat increased. This latter effect may become significant in patients with sinus node dysfunction. (See Warnings.)

TAMBOCOR causes a dose-related and plasma-level related decrease in single and multiple PVCs and can suppress recurrence of ventricular tachycardia. In limited studies of patients with a history of ventricular tachycardia, TAMBOCOR has been successful 30–40% of the time in fully suppressing the inducibility of arrhythmias by programmed electrical stimulation. Based on PVC suppression, it appears that plasma levels of 0.2 to 1.0 µg/mL may be needed to obtain the maximal therapeutic effect. It is more difficult to assess the dose needed to suppress serious arrhythmias, but trough plasma levels in patients successfully treated for recurrent ventricular tachycardia were between 0.2 and 1.0 µg/mL. Plasma levels above 0.7–1.0 µg/mL are associated with a higher rate of cardiac adverse experiences such as conduction defects or bradycardia. The relation of plasma levels to proarrhythmic events is not established, but dose reduction in clinical trials of patients with ventricular tachycardia appears to have led to a reduced frequency and severity of such events.

Hemodynamics. TAMBOCOR does not usually alter heart rate, although bradycardia and tachycardia have been reported occasionally.

In animals and isolated myocardium, a negative inotropic effect of flecainide has been demonstrated. Decreases in ejection fraction, consistent with a negative inotropic effect, have been observed after single administration of 200 to 250 mg of the drug in man; both increases and decreases in ejection fraction have been encountered during multidose therapy in patients at usual therapeutic doses. (See Warnings.)

Metabolism in Humans. Following oral administration, the absorption of TAMBOCOR is nearly complete. Peak plasma levels are attained at about three hours in most individuals (range, 1 to 6 hours). Flecainide does not undergo any consequential presystemic biotransformation (first-pass effect). Food or antacid do not affect absorption. Milk, however, may inhibit absorption in infants. A reduction in TAMBOCOR dosage should be considered when milk is removed from the diet of infants.

The apparent plasma half-life averages about 20 hours and is quite variable (range, 12 to 27 hours) after multiple oral doses in patients with premature ventricular contractions (PVCs). With multiple dosing, plasma levels increase because of its long half-life with steady-state levels approached in 3 to 5 days; once at steady-state, no additional (or unexpected) accumulation of drug in plasma occurs during chronic therapy. Over the usual therapeutic range, data suggest that plasma levels in an individual are approximately proportional to dose, deviating upwards from linearity only slightly (about 10 to 15% per 100 mg on average).

In healthy subjects, about 30% of a single oral dose (range, 10 to 50%) is excreted in urine as unchanged drug. The two major urinary metabolites are meta-O-dealkylated flecainide (active, but about one-fifth as potent) and the meta-O-dealkylated lactam of flecainide (non-active metabolite). These two metabolites (primarily conjugated) account for most of the remaining portion of the dose. Several minor metabolites (3% of the dose or less) are also found in urine; only 5% of an oral dose is excreted in feces. In patients, free (unconjugated) plasma levels of the two major metabolites are very low (less than 0.05 µg/mL).

In vitro metabolic studies have confirmed that cytochrome P450IID6 is involved in the metabolism of flecainide.

When urinary pH is very alkaline (8 or higher), as may occur in rare conditions (e.g., renal tubular acidosis, strict vegetarian diet), flecainide elimination from plasma is much slower.

The elimination of flecainide from the body depends on renal function (i.e., 10 to 50% appears in urine as unchanged drug). With increasing renal impairment, the extent of unchanged drug excretion in urine is reduced and the plasma half-life of flecainide is prolonged. Since flecainide is also extensively metabolized, there is no simple relationship between creatinine clearance and the rate of flecanide elimination from plasma. (See Dosage and Administration.)

In patients with NYHA class III congestive heart failure (CHF), the rate of flecainide elimination from plasma (mean half-life, 19 hours) is moderately slower than for healthy subjects (mean half-life, 14 hours), but similar to the rate for patients with PVCs without CHF. The extent of excretion of unchanged drug in urine is also similar. (See Dosage and Administration.)

Under one year of age, currently available data are limited but suggest that the half-life at birth may be as long as 29 hours, decreasing to 11–12 hours by three months of age and 6 hours by one year of age. The pharmacokinetics in hydropic infants have not been studied, but case reports suggest prolonged elimination. In children aged 1 year to 12 years the half-life is approximately 8 hours. In adolescents (age 12 to 15) the plasma elimination half-life is approximately 11–12 hours. Since milk may inhibit absorption in infants, a reduction in TAMBOCOR dosage should be considered when milk is removed from the diet (e.g., gastroenteritis, weaning). Plasma trough flecainide levels should be monitored during major changes in dietary milk intake.

From age 20 to 80, plasma levels are only slightly higher with advancing age; flecainide elimination from plasma is somewhat slower in elderly subjects than in younger subjects. Patients up to age 80+ have been safely treated with usual dosages.

The extent of flecainide binding to human plasma proteins is about 40% and is independent of plasma drug level over the range of 0.015 to about 3.4 µg/mL. Thus, clinically significant drug interactions based on protein binding effects would not be expected.

Hemodialysis removes only about 1% of an oral dose as unchanged flecainide.

Small increases in plasma digoxin levels are seen during coadministration of TAMBOCOR with digoxin. Small increases in both flecainide and propranolol plasma levels are seen during coadministration of these two drugs. (See Precautions, Drug Interactions.)

Clinical Trials. In two randomized, crossover, placebo-controlled clinical trials of 16 weeks double-blind duration, 79% of patients with paroxysmal supraventricular tachycardia (PSVT) receiving flecainide were attack free, whereas 15% of patients receiving placebo remained attack free. The median time-before-recurrence of PSVT in patients receiving placebo was 11 to 12 days, whereas over 85% of patients receiving flecainide had no recurrence at 60 days.

In two randomized, crossover, placebo-controlled clinical trials of 16 weeks double-blind duration, 31% of patients with paroxysmal atrial fibrillation/flutter (PAF) receiving flecainide were attack free, whereas 8% receiving placebo remained attack free. The median time-before-recurrence of PAF in patients receiving placebo was about 2 to 3 days, whereas for those receiving flecainide the median time-before-recurrence was 15 days.

INDICATIONS AND USAGE

In patients without structural heart disease, TAMBOCOR is indicated for the prevention of

— paroxysmal supraventricular tachycardias (PSVT), including atrioventricular nodal reentrant tachycardia, atrioventricular reentrant tachycardia and other supraventricular tachycardias of unspecified mechanism associated with disabling symptoms

— paroxysmal atrial fibrillation/flutter (PAF) associated with disabling symptoms

TAMBOCOR is also indicated for the prevention of

— documented ventricular arrhythmias, such as sustained ventricular tachycardia (sustained VT), that in the judgment of the physician are life-threatening.

Use of TAMBOCOR for the treatment of sustained VT, like other antiarrhythmics, should be initiated in the hospital.

Continued on next page

Tambocor—Cont.

The use of TAMBOCOR is not recommended in patients with less severe ventricular arrhythmias even if the patients are symptomatic.

Because of the proarrhythmic effects of TAMBOCOR, its use should be reserved for patients in whom, in the opinion of the physician, the benefits of treatment outweigh the risks. TAMBOCOR should not be used in patients with recent myocardial infarction. (See Boxed Warnings.)

Use of TAMBOCOR in chronic atrial fibrillation has not been adequately studied and is not recommended. (See Boxed Warnings.)

As is the case for other antiarrhythmic agents, there is no evidence from controlled trials that the use of TAMBOCOR favorably affects survival or the incidence of sudden death.

CONTRAINDICATIONS

TAMBOCOR is contraindicated in patients with pre-existing second- or third-degree AV block, or with right bundle branch block when associated with a left hemiblock (bifascicular block), unless a pacemaker is present to sustain the cardiac rhythm should complete heart block occur. TAMBOCOR is also contraindicated in the presence of cardiogenic shock or known hypersensitivity to the drug.

WARNINGS

Mortality. TAMBOCOR was included in the National Heart Lung and Blood Institute's Cardiac Arrhythmia Suppression Trial (CAST), a long-term, multicenter, randomized, double-blind study in patients with asymptomatic non-life-threatening ventricular arrhythmias who had a myocardial infarction more than six days but less than two years previously. An excessive mortality or non-fatal cardiac arrest rate was seen in patients treated with TAMBOCOR compared with that seen in patients assigned to a carefully matched placebo-treated group. This rate was 16/315 (5.1%) for TAMBOCOR and 7/309 (2.3%) for the matched placebo. The average duration of treatment with TAMBOCOR in this study was ten months.

The applicability of the CAST results to other populations (e.g., those without recent myocardial infarction) is uncertain, but at present, it is prudent to consider the risks of Class IC agents (including TAMBOCOR), coupled with the lack of any evidence of improved survival, generally unacceptable in patients without life-threatening ventricular arrhythmias, even if the patients are experiencing unpleasant, but not life-threatening, symptoms or signs.

Ventricular Pro-arrhythmic Effects in Patients with Atrial Fibrillation/Flutter. A review of the world literature revealed reports of 568 patients treated with oral TAMBOCOR for paroxysmal atrial fibrillation/flutter (PAF). Ventricular tachycardia was experienced in 0.4% (2/568) of these patients. Of 19 patients in the literature with chronic atrial fibrillation (CAF), 10.5% (2) experienced VT or VF. FLECAINIDE IS NOT RECOMMENDED FOR USE IN PATIENTS WITH CHRONIC ATRIAL FIBRILLATION. Case reports of ventricular proarrhythmic effects in patients treated with TAMBOCOR for atrial fibrillation/flutter have included increased PVCs, VT, ventricular fibrillation (VF), and death.

As with other Class I agents, patients treated with TAMBOCOR for atrial flutter have been reported with 1:1 atrioventricular conduction due to slowing the atrial rate. A paradoxical increase in the ventricular rate also may occur in patients with atrial fibrillation who receive TAMBOCOR. Concomitant negative chronotropic therapy such as digoxin or beta-blockers may lower the risk of this complication.

PROARRHYTHMIC EFFECTS

TAMBOCOR, like other antiarrhythmic agents, can cause new or worsened supraventricular or ventricular arrhythmias. Ventricular proarrhythmic effects range from an increase in frequency of PVCs to the development of more severe ventricular tachycardia, e.g., tachycardia that is more sustained or more resistant to conversion to sinus rhythm, with potentially fatal consequences. In studies of ventricular arrhythmia patients treated with TAMBOCOR, three-fourths of proarrhythmic events were new or worsened ventricular tachyarrhythmias, the remainder being increased frequency of PVCs or new supraventricular arrhythmias. In patients treated with flecainide for sustained ventricular tachycardia, 80% (51/64) of proarrhythmic events occurred within 14 days of the onset of therapy. In studies of 225 patients with supraventricular arrhythmia (108 with paroxysmal supraventricular tachycardia and 117 with paroxysmal atrial fibrillation), there were 9 (4%) proarrhythmic events, 8 of them in patients with paroxysmal atrial fibrillation. Of the 9, 7 (including the one in a PSVT patient) were exacerbations of supraventricular arrhythmias (longer duration, more rapid rate, harder to reverse) while 2 were ventricular arrhythmias, including one fatal case of VT/VF and one wide complex VT (the patient showed inducible VT, however, after withdrawal of flecainide), both in patients with paroxysmal atrial fibrillation and known coronary artery disease.

It is uncertain if TAMBOCOR's risk of proarrhythmia is exaggerated in patients with chronic atrial fibrillation (CAF), high ventricular rate, and/or exercise. Wide complex tachycardia and ventricular fibrillation have been reported in two of 12 CAF patients undergoing maximal exercise tolerance testing.

In patients with complex ventricular arrhythmias, it is often difficult to distinguish a spontaneous variation in the patient's underlying rhythm disorder from drug-induced worsening, so that the following occurrence rates must be considered approximations. Their frequency appears to be related to dose and to the underlying cardiac disease.

Among patients treated for sustained VT (who frequently also had CHF, a low ejection fraction, a history of myocardial infarction and/or an episode of cardiac arrest), the incidence of proarrhythmic events was 13% when dosage was initiated at 200 mg/day with slow upward titration, and did not exceed 300 mg/day in most patients. In early studies in patients with sustained VT utilizing a higher initial dose (400 mg/day) the incidence of proarrhythmic events was 26%; moreover, in about 10% of the patients treated proarrhythmic events resulted in death, despite prompt medical attention. With lower initial doses, the incidence of proarrhythmic events resulting in death decreased to 0.5% of these patients. Accordingly, it is extremely important to follow the recommended dosage schedule. (See Dosage and Administration.)

The relatively high frequency of proarrhythmic events in patients with sustained VT and serious underlying heart disease, and the need for careful titration and monitoring, requires that therapy of patients with sustained VT be started in the hospital. (See Dosage and Administration.)

HEART FAILURE

TAMBOCOR has a negative inotropic effect and may cause or worsen CHF, particularly in patients with cardiomyopathy, preexisting severe heart failure (NYHA functional class III or IV) or low ejection fractions (less than 30%). In patients with supraventricular arrhythmias new or worsened CHF developed in 0.4% (1/225) of patients. In patients with sustained ventricular tachycardia during a mean duration of 7.9 months of TAMBOCOR therapy, 6.3% (20/317) developed new CHF. In patients with sustained ventricular tachycardia and a history of CHF, during a mean duration of 5.4 months of TAMBOCOR therapy, 25.7% (78/304) developed worsened CHF. Exacerbation of preexisting CHF occurred more commonly in studies which included patients with class III or IV failure than in studies which excluded such patients. TAMBOCOR should be used cautiously in patients who are known to have a history of CHF or myocardial dysfunction. The initial dosage in such patients should be no more than 100 mg bid (see Dosage and Administration) and patients should be monitored carefully. Close attention must be given to maintenance of cardiac function, including optimization of digitalis, diuretic, or other therapy. In cases where CHF has developed or worsened during treatment with TAMBOCOR, the time of onset has ranged from a few hours to several months after starting therapy. Some patients who develop evidence of reduced myocardial function while on TAMBOCOR can continue on TAMBOCOR with adjustment of digitalis or diuretics, others may require dosage reduction or discontinuation of TAMBOCOR. When feasible, it is recommended that plasma flecainide levels be monitored. Attempts should be made to keep trough plasma levels below 0.7 to 1.0 µg/mL.

Effects on Cardiac Conduction. TAMBOCOR slows cardiac conduction in most patients to produce dose-related increases in PR, QRS, and QT intervals.

PR interval increases on average about 25% (0.04 seconds) and as much as 118% in some patients. Approximately one-third of patients may develop new first-degree AV heart block (PR interval ≥ 0.20 seconds). The QRS complex increases on average about 25% (0.02 seconds) and as much as 150% in some patients. Many patients develop QRS complexes with a duration of 0.12 seconds or more. In one study, 4% of patients developed new bundle branch block while on TAMBOCOR. The degree of lengthening of PR and QRS intervals does not predict either efficacy or the development of cardiac adverse effects. In clinical trials, it was unusual for PR intervals to increase to 0.30 seconds or more, or for QRS intervals to increase to 0.18 seconds or more. Thus, caution should be used when such intervals occur, and dose reductions may be considered. The QT interval widens about 8%, but most of this widening (about 60% to 90%) is due to widening of the QRS duration. The JT interval (QT minus QRS) only widens about 4% on the average. Significant JT prolongation occurs in less than 2% of patients. There have been rare cases of Torsade de Pointes-type arrhythmia associated with TAMBOCOR therapy.

Clinically significant conduction changes have been observed at these rates: sinus node dysfunction such as sinus pause, sinus arrest and symptomatic bradycardia (1.2%), second-degree AV block (0.5%) and third-degree AV block (0.4%). An attempt should be made to manage the patient on the lowest effective dose in an effort to minimize these effects. (See Dosage and Administration.) If second- or third-degree AV block, or right bundle branch block associated with a left hemiblock occur, TAMBOCOR therapy should be discontinued unless a temporary or implanted ventricular pacemaker is in place to ensure an adequate ventricular rate.

Sick Sinus Syndrome (Bradycardia-Tachycardia Syndrome). TAMBOCOR should be used only with extreme caution in patients with sick sinus syndrome because it may cause sinus bradycardia, sinus pause, or sinus arrest.

Effects on Pacemaker Thresholds. TAMBOCOR is known to increase endocardial pacing thresholds and may suppress ventricular escape rhythms. These effects are reversible if flecainide is discontinued. It should be used with caution in patients with permanent pacemakers or temporary pacing electrodes and should not be administered to patients with existing poor thresholds or nonprogrammable pacemakers unless suitable pacing rescue is available.

The pacing threshold in patients with pacemakers should be determined prior to instituting therapy with TAMBOCOR, again after one week of administration and at regular intervals thereafter. Generally threshold changes are within the range of multiprogrammable pacemakers and, when these occur, a doubling of either voltage or pulse width is usually sufficient to regain capture.

Electrolyte Disturbances. Hypokalemia or hyperkalemia may alter the effects of Class I antiarrhythmic drugs. Pre-existing hypokalemia or hyperkalemia should be corrected before administration of TAMBOCOR.

Pediatric Use. The safety and efficacy of TAMBOCOR in the fetus, infant, or child have not been established in double-blind, randomized, placebo-controlled trials. The proarrhythmic effects of TAMBOCOR, as described previously, apply also to children. In pediatric patients with structural heart disease, TAMBOCOR has been associated with cardiac arrest and sudden death. TAMBOCOR should be started in the hospital with rhythm monitoring. Any use of TAMBOCOR in children should be directly supervised by a cardiologist skilled in the treatment of arrhythmias in children.

PRECAUTIONS

Drug Interactions. TAMBOCOR has been administered to patients receiving **digitalis** preparations or **beta-adrenergic blocking agents** without adverse effects. During administration of multiple oral doses of TAMBOCOR to healthy subjects stabilized on a maintenance dose of **digoxin**, a 13%–19% increase in plasma **digoxin** levels occurred at six hours postdose.

In a study involving healthy subjects receiving TAMBOCOR and **propranolol** concurrently, plasma flecainide levels were increased about 20% and **propranolol** levels were increased about 30% compared to control values. In this formal interaction study, TAMBOCOR and **propranolol** were each found to have negative inotropic effects; when the drugs were administered together, the effects were additive. The effects of concomitant administration of TAMBOCOR and **propranolol** on the PR interval were less than additive. In TAMBOCOR clinical trials, patients who were receiving **beta blockers** concurrently did not experience an increased incidence of side effects. Nevertheless, the possibility of additive negative inotropic effects of **beta blockers** and flecainide should be recognized.

Flecainide is not extensively bound to plasma proteins. In vitro studies with several drugs which may be administered concomitantly showed that the extent of flecainide binding to human plasma proteins is either unchanged or only slightly less. Consequently, interactions with other drugs which are highly protein bound (e.g., **anticoagulants**) would not be expected. TAMBOCOR has been used in a large number of patients receiving **diuretics** without apparent interaction. Limited data in patients receiving known enzyme inducers (**phenytoin, phenobarbital, carbamazepine**) indicate only a 30% increase in the rate of flecainide elimination. In healthy subjects receiving **cimetidine** (1 gm daily) for one week, plasma flecainide levels increased by about 30% and half-life increased by about 10%.

When **amiodarone** is added to flecainide therapy, plasma flecainide levels may increase two-fold or more in some patients, if flecainide dosage is not reduced. (See Dosage and Administration.)

Drugs that inhibit cytochrome P450IID6, such as **quinidine**, might increase the plasma concentrations of flecainide in patients that are on chronic flecainide therapy; especially if these patients are extensive metabolizers.

There has been little experience with the coadministration of TAMBOCOR and either **disopyramide** or **verapamil**. Because both of these drugs have negative inotropic properties and the effects of coadministration with TAMBOCOR are unknown, neither **disopyramide** nor **verapamil** should be administered concurrently with TAMBOCOR unless, in the judgment of the physician, the benefits of this combination

outweigh the risks. There has been too little experience with the coadministration of TAMBOCOR with **nifedipine** or **diltiazem** to recommend concomitant use.

Carcinogenesis, Mutagenesis, Impairment of Fertility. Long-term studies with flecainide in rats and mice at doses up to 60 mg/kg/day have not revealed any compound-related carcinogenic effects. Mutagenicity studies (Ames test, mouse lymphoma and in vivo cytogenetics) did not reveal any mutagenic effects. A rat reproduction study at doses up to 50 mg/kg/day (seven times the usual human dose) did not reveal any adverse effect on male or female fertility.

Pregnancy. Pregnancy Category C. Flecainide has been shown to have teratogenic effects (club paws, sternebrae and vertebrae abnormalities, pale hearts with contracted ventricular septum) and an embryotoxic effect (increased resorptions) in one breed of rabbit (New Zealand White) when given doses of 30 and 35 mg/kg/day, but not in another breed of rabbit (Dutch Belted) when given doses up to 30 mg/kg/day. No teratogenic effects were observed in rats and mice given doses up to 50 and 80 mg/kg/day, respectively; however, delayed sternebral and vertebral ossification was observed at the high dose in rats. Because there are no adequate and well-controlled studies in pregnant women, TAMBOCOR should be used during pregnancy only if the potential benefit justifies the potential risk to the fetus.

Labor and Delivery. It is not known whether the use of TAMBOCOR during labor or delivery has immediate or delayed adverse effects on the mother or fetus, affects the duration of labor or delivery, or increases the possibility of forceps delivery or other obstetrical intervention.

Nursing Mothers. Results from a multiple dose study conducted in mothers soon after delivery indicates that flecainide is excreted in human breast milk in concentrations as high as 4 times (with average levels about 2.5 times) corresponding plasma levels; assuming a maternal plasma level at the top of the therapeutic range (1 μg/mL), the calculated daily dose to a nursing infant (assuming about 700 mL breast milk over 24 hours) would be less than 3 mg.

Pediatric Use. The safety and efficacy of TAMBOCOR in the fetus, infant, or child have not been established in double-blind, randomized, placebo-controlled trials (see CLINICAL PHARMACOLOGY, WARNINGS, and DOSAGE AND ADMINISTRATION).

Hepatic Impairment. Since flecainide elimination from plasma can be markedly slower in patients with significant hepatic impairment, TAMBOCOR should not be used in such patients unless the potential benefits clearly outweigh the risks. If used, frequent and early plasma level monitoring is required to guide dosage (see Plasma Level Monitoring); dosage increases should be made very cautiously when plasma levels have plateaued (after more than four days).

ADVERSE REACTIONS

In post-myocardial infarction patients with asymptomatic PVCs and non-sustained ventricular tachycardia, TAMBOCOR therapy was found to be associated with a 5.1% rate of death and non-fatal cardiac arrest, compared with a 2.3% rate in a matched placebo group. (See Warnings.)

Adverse effects reported for TAMBOCOR, described in detail in the Warnings section, were new or worsened arrhythmias which occurred in 1% of 108 patients with PSVT and in 7% of 117 patients with PAF; and new or exacerbated ventricular arrhythmias which occurred in 7% of 1330 patients with PVCs, non-sustained or sustained VT. In patients treated with flecainide for sustained VT, 80% (51/64) of proarrhythmic events occurred within 14 days of the onset of therapy. 198 patients with sustained VT experienced a 13% incidence of new or exacerbated ventricular arrhythmias when dosage was initiated at 200 mg/day with slow upward titration, and did not exceed 300 mg/day in most patients. In some patients, TAMBOCOR treatment has been associated with episodes of unresuscitatable VT or ventricular fibrillation (cardiac arrest). (See Warnings.)

New or worsened CHF occurred in 6.3% of 1046 patients with PVCs, non-sustained or sustained VT. Of 297 patients with sustained VT, 9.1% experienced new or worsened CHF. New or worsened CHF was reported in 0.4% of 225 patients with supraventricular arrhythmias. There have also been instances of second- (0.5%) or third-degree (0.4%) AV block. Patients have developed sinus bradycardia, sinus pause, or sinus arrest, about 1.2% altogether (see Warnings). The frequency of most of these serious adverse events probably increases with higher trough plasma levels, especially when these trough levels exceed 1.0 μg/mL.

There have been rare reports of isolated elevations of serum alkaline phosphatase and isolated elevations of serum transaminase levels. These elevations have been asymptomatic and no cause and effect relationship with TAMBOCOR has been established. In foreign postmarketing surveillance studies, there have been rare reports of hepatic dysfunction including reports of cholestasis and hepatic failure, and extremely rare reports of blood dyscrasias. Although no cause and effect relationship has been established, it is advisable to discontinue TAMBOCOR in patients who develop unexplained jaundice or signs of hepatic dysfunction or blood dyscrasias in order to eliminate TAMBOCOR as the possible causative agent.

Table 1
Most Common Non-Cardiac Adverse Effects in Ventricular Arrhythmia Patients Treated with
TAMBOCOR in the Multicenter Study

Adverse Effect	Incidence All 429 Patients at Any Dose	Incidence By Dose During Upward Titration 200 mg/Day (N=426)	300 mg/Day (N=293)	400 mg/Day (N=100)
Dizziness*	18.9%	11.0%	10.6%	13.0%
Visual Disturbances†	15.9%	5.4%	12.3%	18.0%
Dyspnea	10.3%	5.2%	7.5%	4.0%
Headache	9.6%	4.5%	6.1%	9.0%
Nausea	8.9%	4.9%	4.8%	6.0%
Fatigue	7.7%	4.5%	4.4%	3.0%
Palpitation	6.1%	3.5%	2.4%	7.0%
Chest Pain	5.4%	3.1%	3.8%	1.0%
Asthenia	4.9%	2.6%	2.0%	4.0%
Tremor	4.7%	2.4%	3.4%	2.0%
Constipation	4.4%	2.8%	2.1%	1.0%
Edema	3.5%	1.9%	1.4%	2.0%
Abdominal pain	3.3%	1.9%	2.4%	1.0%

---

* Dizziness includes reports of dizziness, lightheadedness, faintness, unsteadiness, near syncope, etc.
† Visual disturbance includes reports of blurred vision, difficulty in focusing, spots before eyes, etc.

Incidence figures for other adverse effects in patients with ventricular arrhythmias are based on a multicenter efficacy study, utilizing starting doses of 200 mg/day with gradual upward titration to 400 mg/day. Patients were treated for an average of 4.7 months, with some receiving up to 22 months of therapy. In this trial, 5.4% of patients discontinued due to non-cardiac adverse effects.

[See table 1 above]

The following additional adverse experiences, possibly related to TAMBOCOR therapy and occurring in 1% to less than 3% of patients, have been reported in acute and chronic studies: *Body as a Whole* —malaise, fever; *Cardiovascular* —tachycardia, sinus pause or arrest; *Gastrointestinal* —vomiting, diarrhea, dyspepsia, anorexia; *Skin* —rash; *Visual* —diplopia; *Nervous System* —hypoesthesia, paresthesia, paresis, ataxia, flushing, increased sweating, vertigo, syncope, somnolence, tinnitus; *Psychiatric* —anxiety, insomnia, depression.

The following additional adverse experiences, possibly related to TAMBOCOR, have been reported in less than 1% of patients: *Body as a Whole* —swollen lips, tongue and mouth; arthralgia, bronchospasm, myalgia; *Cardiovascular* —angina pectoris, second-degree and third-degree AV block, bradycardia, hypertension, hypotension; *Gastrointestinal* —flatulence; *Urinary System* —polyuria, urinary retention; *Hematologic* —leukopenia, granulocytopenia, thrombocytopenia; *Skin* —urticaria, exfoliative dermatitis, pruritus, alopecia; *Visual* —eye pain or irritation, photophobia, nystagmus; *Nervous System* —twitching, weakness, change in taste, dry mouth, convulsions, impotence, speech disorder, stupor, neuropathy; *Respiratory* —pneumonitis/pulmonary infiltration possibly due to chronic flecainide treatment; *Psychiatric* —amnesia, confusion, decreased libido, depersonalization, euphoria, morbid dreams, apathy.

For patients with supraventricular arrhythmias, the most commonly reported noncardiac adverse experiences remain consistent with those known for patients treated with TAMBOCOR for ventricular arrhythmias. Dizziness is possibly more frequent in PAF patients.

OVERDOSAGE

No specific antidote has been identified for the treatment of TAMBOCOR overdosage. Overdoses ranging up to 8000 mg have been survived, with peak plasma flecainide concentrations as high as 5.3 μg/mL. Untoward effects in these cases included nausea and vomiting, convulsions, hypotension, bradycardia, syncope, extreme widening of the QRS complex, widening of the QT interval, widening of the PR interval, ventricular tachycardia, AV nodal block, asystole, bundle branch block, cardiac failure, and cardiac arrest. The spectrum of events observed in fatal cases was much the same as that seen in the non-fatal cases. Death has resulted following ingestion of as little as 1000 mg; concomitant overdose of other drugs and/or alcohol in many instances undoubtedly contributed to the fatal outcome. Treatment of overdosage should be supportive and may include the following: removal of unabsorbed drug from the gastrointestinal tract, administration of inotropic agents or cardiac stimulants such as dopamine, dobutamine or isoproterenol; mechanically assisted respiration; circulatory assists such as intra-aortic balloon pumping; and transvenous pacing in the event of conduction block. Because of the long plasma half-life of flecainide (12 to 27 hours in patients receiving usual doses), and the possibility of markedly non-linear elimination kinetics at very high doses, these supportive treatments may need to be continued for extended periods of time.

Hemodialysis is not an effective means of removing flecainide from the body. Since flecainide elimination is much slower when urine is very alkaline (pH 8 or higher), theoretically, acidification of urine to promote drug excretion may be beneficial in overdose cases with very alkaline urine. There is no evidence that acidification from normal urinary pH increases excretion.

DOSAGE AND ADMINISTRATION

For patients with sustained VT, no matter what their cardiac status, TAMBOCOR, like other antiarrhythmics, should be initiated in-hospital with rhythm monitoring.

Flecainide has a long half-life (12 to 27 hours in patients). Steady-state plasma levels, in patients with normal renal and hepatic function, may not be achieved until the patient has received 3 to 5 days of therapy at a given dose. Therefore, **increases in dosage should be made no more frequently than once every four days,** since during the first 2 to 3 days of therapy the optimal effect of a given dose may not be achieved.

For patients with PSVT and patients with PAF the recommended starting dose is 50 mg every 12 hours. TAMBOCOR doses may be increased in increments of 50 mg bid every four days until efficacy is achieved. For PAF patients, a substantial increase in efficacy without a substantial increase in discontinuations for adverse experiences may be achieved by increasing the TAMBOCOR dose from 50 mg to 100 mg bid. The maximum recommended dose for patients with paroxysmal supraventricular arrhythmias is 300 mg/day.

For sustained VT the recommended starting dose is 100 mg every 12 hours. This dose may be increased in increments of 50 mg bid every four days until efficacy is achieved. Most patients with sustained VT do not require more than 150 mg every 12 hours (300 mg/day), and the maximum dose recommended is 400 mg/day.

In patients with sustained VT, use of higher initial doses and more rapid dosage adjustments have resulted in an increased incidence of proarrhythmic events and CHF, particularly during the first few days of dosing (see Warnings). Therefore, a loading dose is not recommended.

Intravenous lidocaine has been used occasionally with TAMBOCOR while awaiting the therapeutic effect of TAMBOCOR. No adverse drug interactions were apparent. However, no formal studies have been performed to demonstrate the usefulness of this regimen.

An occasional patient not adequately controlled by (or intolerant to) a dose given at 12-hour intervals may be dosed at eight-hour intervals.

Once adequate control of the arrhythmia has been achieved, it may be possible in some patients to reduce the dose as necessary to minimize side effects or effects on conduction. In such patients, efficacy at the lower dose should be evaluated.

TAMBOCOR should be used cautiously in patients with a history of CHF or myocardial dysfunction (see Warnings).

Any use of TAMBOCOR in children should be directly supervised by a cardiologist skilled in the treatment of arrhythmias in children. Because of the evolving nature of information in this area, specialized literature should be consulted. Under six months of age, the initial starting dose of TAMBOCOR in children is approximately 50 mg/M² body surface area daily, divided into two or three equally spaced doses. Over six months of age, the initial starting dose may be increased to 100 mg/M² per day. The maximum recommended dose is 200 mg/M² per day. This dose should not be exceeded. In some children on higher doses, despite previously low plasma levels, the level has increased rapidly to far above therapeutic values while taking the same dose. Small changes in dose may also lead to disproportionate increases in plasma levels. Plasma trough (less than one hour pre-dose) flecainide levels and electrocardiograms should be obtained at presumed steady state (after at least five doses) either after initiation or change in TAMBOCOR dose,

Continued on next page

Tambocor—Cont.

whether the dose was increased for lack of effectiveness, or increased growth of the patient. For the first year on therapy, whenever the patient is seen for reasons of clinical follow-up, it is suggested that a 12-lead electrocardiogram and plasma trough flecainide level are obtained. The usual therapeutic level of flecainide in children is 200–500 ng/mL. In some cases, levels as high as 800 ng/mL may be required for control.

In patients with severe renal impairment (creatinine clearance of 35 mL/min/1.73 square meters or less), the initial dosage should be 100 mg once daily (or 50 mg bid); when used in such patients, frequent plasma level monitoring is required to guide dosage adjustments (see Plasma Level Monitoring). In patients with less severe renal disease, the initial dosage should be 100 mg every 12 hours; plasma level monitoring may also be useful in these patients during dosage adjustment. In both groups of patients, dosage increases should be made very cautiously when plasma levels have plateaued (after more than four days), observing the patient closely for signs of adverse cardiac effects or other toxicity. It should be borne in mind that in these patients it may take longer than four days before a new steady-state plasma level is reached following a dosage change.

Based on theoretical considerations, rather than experimental data, the following suggestion is made: when transferring patients from another antiarrhythmic drug to TAMBOCOR allow at least two to four plasma half-lives to elapse for the drug being discontinued before starting TAMBOCOR at the usual dosage. In patients where withdrawal of a previous antiarrhythmic agent is likely to produce life-threatening arrhythmias, the physician should consider hospitalizing the patient.

When flecainide is given in the presence of amiodarone, reduce the usual flecainide dose by 50% and monitor the patient closely for adverse effects. Plasma level monitoring is strongly recommended to guide dosage with such combination therapy (see below).

Plasma Level Monitoring. The large majority of patients successfully treated with TAMBOCOR were found to have trough plasma levels between 0.2 and 1.0 µg/mL. The probability of adverse experiences, especially cardiac, may increase with higher trough plasma levels, especially when these exceed 1.0 µg/mL. Periodic monitoring of trough plasma levels may be useful in patient management. Plasma level monitoring is required in patients with severe renal failure or severe hepatic disease, since elimination of flecainide from plasma may be markedly slower. Monitoring of plasma levels is strongly recommended in patients on concurrent amiodarone therapy and may also be helpful in patients with CHF and in patients with moderate renal disease.

HOW SUPPLIED

All tablets are embossed with 3M on one side and TR 50, TR 100 or TR 150 on the other side.

Tambocor, 50 mg per white, round tablet, is available in
Bottles of 100—NDC #0089-0305-10.
Boxes of 100 in unit dose blister strips—NDC #0089-0305-16.

Tambocor, 100 mg per white, round, scored tablet, is available in
Bottles of 100—NDC #0089-0307-10.
Boxes of 100 in unit dose blister strips—NDC #0089-0307-16.

Tambocor, 150 mg per white, oval, scored tablet, is available in
Bottles of 100—NDC #0089-0314-10.

Store at controlled room temperature 15°–30°C (59°–86°F) in a tight, light-resistant container.

CAUTION: Federal law prohibits dispensing without prescription.
602600   July 1996
Manufactured by
3M Pharmaceuticals
Northridge, CA 91324
Shown in Product Identification Guide, page 321

THEOLAIR™   ℞
(theophylline tablets USP)
TABLETS

For full prescribing information see leaflet accompanying product or call 800-328-0255 for a copy.

HOW SUPPLIED
THEOLAIR™ Tablets:
125 mg tablets—Each round, white, scored tablet imprinted with "3M" on one side and "342" on the other. Bottles of 100 (NDC 0089-0342-10).
250 mg tablets—Each capsule-shaped, white, scored tablet imprinted with "3M" on one side and "THEOLAIR 250" on the other. Bottles of 100 (NDC 0089-0344-10).

THEOLAIR™–SR   ℞
(anhydrous theophylline,
sustained-release)
TABLETS

For full prescribing information see leaflet accompanying product or call 800-328-0255 for a copy.

HOW SUPPLIED
THEOLAIR-SR Tablets:
200 mg sustained-release tablets—Each round, white, scored tablet imprinted with "3M" on one side and "SR 200" on the other. Bottles of 100 (NDC 0089-0341-10) and 1000 (NDC 0089-0341-80).
250 mg sustained-release tablets—Each round, white, scored tablet imprinted with "3M" on one side and "SR 250" on the other. Bottles of 100 (NDC 0089-0345-10).
300 mg sustained-release tablets—Each oval, white, scored tablet imprinted with "3M" on one side and "SR 300" on the other. Bottles of 100 (NDC 0089-0343-10) and 1000 (NDC 0089-0343-80).
500 mg sustained-release tablets—Each capsule-shaped, white, scored tablet imprinted with "3M" on one side and "SR 500" on the other. Bottles of 100 (NDC 0089-0347-10).

UREX™   ℞
(methenamine hippurate)

For full prescribing information see leaflet accompanying product or call 800-328-0255 for a copy.

HOW SUPPLIED
UREX Tablets are capsule-shaped, scored, white, imprinted "3M" on one side, and "UREX" on the other. Each tablet contains methenamine hippurate 1 g.
Bottles of 100 tablets (NDC **0089-0371-10**).

Marlyn Health Care
**14851 N. SCOTTSDALE RD.
SCOTTSDALE, AZ 85254**

Direct Inquiries to:
Stephen Collins
14851 North Scottsdale Road
Scottsdale, AZ 85254
(800) 4-MARLYN
In AZ: (602) 991-0200
EMAIL info@marlyn.com

HEP–FORTE®   OTC
[hep-for 'tay]

DESCRIPTION
Hep Forte is a comprehensive formulation of protein, B factors and other nutritional factors which can be important as a dietary supplement for maintenance and support of normal hepatic function.

COMPOSITION
Each capsule contains:
Vitamin A (Palmitate)	1,200 I.U.
Vitamin E (d-Alpha Tocopherol)	10 I.U.
Vitamin C (Ascorbic Acid)	10 mg.
Folic Acid	0.06 mg.
Vitamin B1 (Thiamine Mononitrate)	1 mg.
Vitamin B2 (Riboflavin)	1 mg.
Niacinamide	10 mg.
Vitamin B6 (Pyridoxine HCl)	0.5 mg.
Vitamin B12 (Cobalamin)	1 mcg.
Biotin	3.3 mcg.
Pantothenic Acid	2 mg.
Choline Bitartrate	21 mg.
Zinc (Zinc Sulfate)	2 mg.
Desiccated Liver	194.4 mg.
Liver Concentrate	64.8 mg.
Liver Fraction Number 2	64.8 mg.
Yeast (Dried)	64.8 mg.
dl-Methionine	10 mg.
Inositol	10 mg.

INDICATIONS
Hep Forte is a balanced formulation of vitamins, minerals, lipotropic factors, and vitamin-protein supplements. It is of value as a nutritional supplement for persons who are receiving professional treatment for alcoholism, hepatic dysfunction due to hepatotoxic drugs and liver poisons, male and female infertility due to hormonal imbalance caused by hepatic dysfunction, and for nutritional supplementation after treatment.

CONTRAINDICATIONS
There are no known contraindications to Hep Forte.

DOSAGE
Three to six capsules daily.

HOW SUPPLIED
Bottles of 100, 300 or 500 capsules.
Literature Available.

MARLYN FORMULA 50®   OTC

PRODUCT OVERVIEW

KEY FACTS
MARLYN FORMULA 50 is a dietary supplement providing a combination of amino acids and B6 in a gelatin capsule which provides protein "building blocks" important to growth and development of all protein containing tissue including nails, hair, and skin.

MAJOR USES
Dermatologists recommend Formula 50 for splitting, peeling nails. Since splitting and peeling nails are often associated with nail fungus, Formula 50 may be recommended in conjunction with drug therapy for nail fungus in order to provide protein necessary to growth and development of nails. OB-Gyn's recommend it for help in controlling excessive hair fall-out after child birth.

SAFETY INFORMATION
There are no known contraindications or adverse reactions.

PRESCRIBING INFORMATION
MARLYN FORMULA 50®

COMPOSITION
Each capsule contains:
Amino Acids	0.3 Gm*
Vitamin B6 (pyridoxine HCl)	1.0 mg.

*Approximate analysis of the amino acids: indispensable amino acids (lysine, tryptophan, phenylalanine, methionine, threonine, leucine, isoleucine, valine), 35.30%; semi-dispensable amino acids (arginine, histidine, tyrosine, cystine, glycine), 19.18%; dispensable amino acids (glutamic acid, alanine, aspartic acid, serine, proline), 45.56%.
Amino acids: Protein "building blocks" important to growth and development of all protein containing tissue including nails, hair, and skin.

DOSAGE AND ADMINISTRATION
The recommended daily dose is 6 capsules daily.

SUPPLY
Bottles of 100, 250 and 500 capsules.

Mayor Pharmaceutical Laboratories
**KareMor International
2401 S. 24TH ST.
PHOENIX, AZ 85034**

Direct Inquiries to:
Medical Director
(602) 244-8899

VITAMIST® Intra-Oral Spray   OTC
[vit '-ə-mĭst]
Dietary Supplements

DESCRIPTION
Vitamist® products are patented, intra-oral sprays for the delivery of vitamins, minerals, and other nutritional supplements, directly into the oral cavity. A 55 microliter spray delivers high concentrations of nutrients directly onto the mouth's sensitive tissue. The buccal mucosa transfers the nutrients into the bloodstream, bypassing the G.I. tract. (U.S. Patent 4,525,341—Foreign patents pending.)
[See figure at top of next column]
Benefits:
• Spray supplementation provides an absorption rate approximately nine times greater than that of pills.
• Once the formula is sprayed into the mouth, the nutrients reach the bloodstream within minutes.
• No fillers or binders are added; the body receives only pure ingredients.
• An alternative method of supplementation for those that cannot take pills, or simply do not enjoy swallowing pills.
• Convenient administration; no water needed.

PRODUCT OVERVIEW
Multiple: vitamins and minerals in three separate formulations: adult, children's, and prenatal.

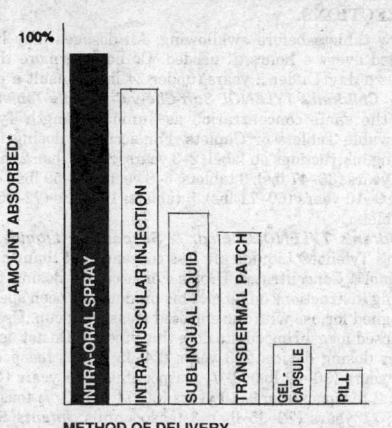

100%

AMOUNT ABSORBED*

INTRA-ORAL SPRAY
INTRA-MUSCULAR INJECTION
SUBLINGUAL LIQUID
TRANSDERMAL PATCH
GEL-CAPSULE
PILL

METHOD OF DELIVERY

*Representative of the product class.

C+Zinc: with vitamin E and the amino acids L-lysine and glycine.

B12: contains 1000% of the US RDI of vitamin B12.

Stress: herbal formula with B vitamins.

VitaZac™: St. John's wort extract with vitamin B12, ginkgo biloba, kava kava and folic acid.

E+Selenium: contains vitamin E and selenomethionine.

Anti-Oxidant: with vitamins A, C, E, niacin, folate, and beta-carotene.

VitaSight™: with vitamins A, C and E, beta-carotene, zinc, selenium, bilberry, lutein, and ginkgo biloba.

Colloidal Minerals: more than 70 trace and essential minerals from natural sources.

Smoke-Less™: herbal combination with additional nutrients designed to reduce cravings.

PMS and Lady Mate: supplementation for the nutritional needs of pre-menstrual syndrome.

Folacin: vitamins B6 and B12 added to folate (folic acid).

Slender-Mist®: dietary snack supplements containing a combination of B vitamins, hydroxy-citric acid, L-carnitine and chromium. Four different flavors.

Blue-Green Sea Spray: spirulina extract, additional omega 3 fatty acids from flaxseed oil, and vitamin E.

Herbal Re-Leaf: a blend of more than 10 herbs that are recommended for minor discomfort, anxiety, and stress.

Herbal OsteoCalMag: herbal supplement with additional vitamin D, calcium and magnesium.

Pro-Bio Mist PB and GS: proanthocyanidins from pine bark (PB) and grape seed (GS) source, with essential B vitamins.

Extend, Renew, Advance™: three performance sprays designed for the needs of physical activity.

CardioCare™: with vitamins C and E, the amino acids L-lysine and L-proline, coenzyme Q10 and additional herbal extracts.

Melatonin: a natural hormone that is effective in re-establishing sleep patterns.

DHEA: dehydroepiandrosterone in both men's and women's formulations.

Revitalizer®: high levels of B vitamins, as well as vitamins A and E, the amino acids L-cysteine and glycine, and selenium.

GinkgoMist™: with ginkgo biloba, vitamin B12, acetyl-L-carnitine, choline, inositol, phosphatidylserine and niacin.

ArthriFlex™: with chondroitin sulfate, glucosamine sulfate, vitamins C and D, calcium, manganese, boron and dong quai.

VitaMotion-S™: dimenhydrinate with ginger and vitamin B6.

VitaMinophen™: acetaminophen and B vitamins combined.

HOW SUPPLIED

Vitamist dietary supplements are supplied in sealed containers fitted with a natural pump. Each container provides a 30-day supply.

RECOMMENDED DOSAGE

Two sprays, four times per day, for a total dosage of eight sprays per day.

For EMERGENCY telephone numbers, consult the **Manufacturers' Index.**

McNeil Consumer Products Company

Division of McNeil-PPC, Inc.
FORT WASHINGTON, PA 19034

Direct Inquiries to:
Consumer Affairs Department
Fort Washington, PA 19034
(215) 233-7000

Children's MOTRIN®   OTC
Ibuprofen Oral Suspension, Concentrated Drops and Chewable Tablets

DESCRIPTION

Children's MOTRIN® Ibuprofen Oral Suspension and *Children's MOTRIN® Concentrated Drops* are alcohol-free, berry-flavored liquid especially developed for children. Each 5 mL (teaspoon) of *Children's MOTRIN® Ibuprofen Oral Suspension* contains ibuprofen 100 mg. Each 1.25 mL (dropperful) of *Children's MOTRIN® Concentrated Drops* contains ibuprofen 50 mg. Each *Children's MOTRIN® Ibuprofen Chewable Tablet* contains 50 mg of ibuprofen in an orange-flavored chewable tablet.

USES

Children's MOTRIN® Ibuprofen Oral Suspension, Children's MOTRIN® Concentrated Drops and Children's MOTRIN® Ibuprofen Chewable Tablets are indicated for temporary reduction of fever and relief of minor aches and pains due to colds, flu, sore throat, headaches and toothaches. One dose lasts 6–8 hours.

DIRECTIONS

Repeat dose every 6–8 hours, if needed. Do not use more than 4 times a day. If possible, use weight to dose; otherwise use age. If stomach upset occurs while taking this product, give with food or milk. *Children's MOTRIN® Ibuprofen Oral Suspension:* Shake well before using. Only use enclosed measuring cup for accurate dosing. Replace original bottle cap to maintain child resistance. 2–3 years (24–35 lbs): 1 tsp; 4–5 years (36–47 lbs): 1½ tsp; 6–8 years (48–59 lbs): 2 tsp; 9–10 years (60–71 lbs): 2½ tsp; 11 years (72–95 lbs): 3 tsp. Under 2 years (under 24 lbs), consult a physician. *Children's MOTRIN® Concentrated Drops:* Shake well before using. Only use enclosed dropper; fill to prescribed level and dispense liquid slowly into child's mouth, toward inner cheek. 2–3 years (24–35 lbs): 2 dropperfuls (2 × 1.25 mL). Under 2 years (under 24 lbs), consult a physician. *Children's MOTRIN® Ibuprofen Chewable Tablets:* 4–5 years (36–47 lbs): 3 tablets; 6–8 years (48–59 lbs): 4 tablets; 9–10 years (60–71 lbs): 5 tablets; 11 years (72–95 lbs): 6 tablets. Under 4 years (under 36 lbs), consult a physician.

WARNINGS

ALLERGIC REACTIONS: Children's Motrin may cause a severe allergic reaction which may include: wheezing (asthma), shortness of breath, hives, swelling of the face, fast, irregular pulse or heartbeat, changing color of the skin (shock).

ASPIRIN SENSITIVE PATIENTS: Although Children's Motrin does not contain aspirin, it may cause a severe reaction, similar to that listed above, in people allergic to aspirin or other pain relievers/fever reducers.

Any of these reactions could be serious. Stop using this product and get emergency medical help immediately. These reactions can occur after taking a single dose or any subsequent dose in persons both with, and without, prior reaction to Children's Motrin or other pain relievers/fever reducers.

CALL YOUR DOCTOR IF:
• Your child is under a doctor's care for any serious condition or is taking any other drug.
• Your child has problems or serious side effects from taking fever reducers or pain relievers.
• Your child does not get any relief within first day (24 hours) of treatment, or pain or fever gets worse.
• Stomach upset gets worse or lasts.
• Redness or swelling is present in the painful area.
• Sore throat is severe, lasts for more than 2 days or occurs with fever, headache, rash, nausea or vomiting.
• Any new symptoms appear.

DO NOT USE:
• With any other product that contains ibuprofen, or other pain reliever/fever reducer, unless directed by a doctor.
• For more than **3 days** for fever or pain unless directed by a doctor.
• For stomach pain unless directed by a doctor.
• If your child is dehydrated (significant fluid loss) due to continued vomiting, diarrhea or lack of fluid intake.

IMPORTANT:
Do not exceed recommended dose. Taking more than the recommended dose (overdose) may not provide more relief and could cause serious health problems. **Keep this and all drugs out of the reach of children. In case of accidental overdose, seek professional assistance or contact a poison control center immediately.**
NOTE: In addition to the above:
Children's MOTRIN® Ibuprofen Oral Suspension:
• If plastic carton wrap or bottle wrap imprinted "Safety Seal®", is broken or missing.
Children's MOTRIN® Concentrated Drops:
• If plastic bottle wrap imprinted with "Safety Seal®" and "Use With Enclosed Dropper Only" is broken or missing.
Children's MOTRIN® Ibuprofen Oral Suspension:
• If blister unit is broken or open.
WHEN USING THIS PRODUCT:
• Mouth or throat burning may occur; give with water or food.
• Phenylketonurics: Contains phenylalanine 3 mg per tablet.

PROFESSIONAL INFORMATION
OVERDOSAGE INFORMATION

The *toxicity of ibuprofen overdose* is dependent upon the amount of drug ingested and the time elapsed since ingestion, though individual response may vary, which makes it necessary to evaluate each case individually. Although uncommon, serious toxicity and death have been reported in the medical literature with ibuprofen overdosage. The most frequently reported symptoms of ibuprofen overdose include abdominal pain, nausea, vomiting, lethargy and drowsiness. Other central nervous system symptoms include headache, tinnitus, CNS depression and seizures. Metabolic acidosis, coma, acute renal failure and apnea (primarily in very young children) may rarely occur. Cardiovascular toxicity, including hypotension, bradycardia, tachycardia and atrial fibrillation, also have been reported.

The *treatment of acute ibuprofen overdose* is primarily supportive. Management of hypotension, acidosis and gastrointestinal bleeding may be necessary. In cases of acute overdose, the stomach should be emptied through ipecac-induced emesis or lavage. Emesis is most effective if initiated within 30 minutes of ingestion. Orally administered activated charcoal may help in reducing the absorption and reabsorption of ibuprofen.

In children, the estimated amount of ibuprofen ingested per body weight may be helpful to predict the potential for development of toxicity although each case must be evaluated. Ingestion of less than 100 mg/kg is unlikely to produce toxicity. Children ingesting 100 to 200 mg/kg may be managed with induced emesis and a minimal observation time of four hours. Children ingesting 200 to 400 mg/kg of ibuprofen should have immediate gastric emptying and at least four hours observation in a health care facility. Children ingesting greater than 400 mg/kg require immediate medical referral, careful observation and appropriate supportive therapy. Ipecac-induced emesis is not recommended in overdoses greater than 400 mg/kg because of the risk of convulsions and the potential for aspiration of gastric contents.

In adult patients the history of the dose reportedly ingested does not appear to be predictive of toxicity. The need for referral and follow-up must be judged by the circumstances at the time of the overdose ingestion. Symptomatic adults should be admitted to a health care facility for observation.

INACTIVE INGREDIENTS

Children's MOTRIN® Ibuprofen Oral Suspension: Citric acid, cornstarch, D&C Yellow #10, FD&C Red #40, artificial flavors, glycerin, polysorbate 80, purified water, sodium benzoate, sucrose, xanthan gum.

Children's MOTRIN® Concentrated Drops: Citric acid, cornstarch, FD&C Red #40, artificial flavors, glycerin, polysorbate 80, purified water, sodium benzoate, sorbitol, sucrose, xanthan gum.

Children's MOTRIN® Ibuprofen Chewable Tablets: Aspartame, citric acid, FD&C Yellow #6, natural and artificial flavors, hydroxyethyl cellulose, hydroxypropyl methylcellulose, magnesium stearate, mannitol, microcrystalline cellulose, povidone, sodium lauryl sulfate, sodium starch glycolate.

HOW SUPPLIED

Children's MOTRIN® Ibuprofen Oral Suspension: Orange colored liquid in tamper-resistant bottles of 2 and 4 fl. oz.
Children's MOTRIN® Concentrated Drops: Pink colored liquid in ½ fl. oz. bottles.
Children's MOTRIN® Ibuprofen Chewable Tablets: Orange colored tablets available in 24 count blister pack.
Store at room temperature 15°-30°C (59°-86°F).

Shown in Product Identification Guide, page 321

Children's TYLENOL®   OTC
ALLERGY-D Chewable Tablets and Liquid

DESCRIPTION

Children's TYLENOL® ALLERGY-D Chewable Tablets are bubble gum flavored and each tablet contains acetamino-

Continued on next page

Children's Tylenol Allergy-D—Cont.

phen 80 mg, diphenhydramine HCl 6.25 mg and pseudoephedrine HCl 7.5 mg. ***Children's TYLENOL® ALLERGY-D Liquid*** is bubble gum flavored and contains no alcohol or aspirin. Each teaspoon (5 mL) contains acetaminophen 160 mg, diphenhydramine HCl 12.5 mg and pseudoephedrine HCl 15 mg.

ACTIONS

Children's TYLENOL® ALLERGY-D Liquid and **Chewable Tablets** combine the analgesic-antipyretic acetaminophen with the antihistamine diphenhydramine hydrochloride and the decongestant pseudoephedrine hydrochloride to provide fast, effective, temporary relief of all your child's symptoms associated with hay fever and other respiratory allergies including sneezing, sore throat, itchy throat, itchy/watery eyes, runny nose, stuffy nose and nasal congestion. Acetaminophen is equal to aspirin in analgesic and antipyretic effectiveness and it is unlikely to produce the side effects often associated with aspirin or aspirin-containing products.

USES

For the reduction of fever. For the temporary relief of these hay fever and other upper respiratory allergy symptoms: sneezing, itchy/watery eyes, nasal congestion, sore throat, runny nose, itchy throat and stuffy nose.

DIRECTIONS

All doses may be repeated every 4-6 hours, if needed. Do not use more than 4 times in 24 hours. Under 6 years (under 48 lbs), consult a physician. An Accudose™ measuring cup is provided for accurate dosing. ***Children's TYLENOL® ALLERGY-D Chewable Tablets:*** 6-11 years (48–95 lbs): 4 tablets. ***Children's TYLENOL® ALLERGY-D Liquid:*** 6-11 years (48–95 lbs): 2 teaspoonfuls.

WARNINGS

Do not take for pain for more than 5 days or for fever for more than 3 days unless directed by a doctor. If pain or fever persists, or gets worse, if new symptoms occur, or if redness or swelling is present, consult a doctor because these could be signs of a serious condition. If sore throat is severe, persists for more than 2 days, is accompanied or followed by fever, headache, rash, nausea or vomiting, consult a doctor promptly. **Do not exceed recommended dosage.** If nervousness, dizziness or sleeplessness occur, discontinue use and consult a doctor. May cause excitability especially in children. Do not give this product to children who have a breathing problem such as chronic bronchitis, or who have glaucoma, heart disease, high blood pressure, thyroid disease, or diabetes without first consulting the child's doctor. May cause marked drowsiness; sedatives and tranquilizers may increase the drowsiness effect. Do not give this product to children who are taking sedatives or tranquilizers without first consulting the child's doctor. **Do not exceed recommended dose.** Taking more than the recommended dose (overdose) may not provide more relief and could cause serious health problems. Keep this and all drugs out of the reach of children. In case of accidental overdose, contact a doctor or poison control center immediately. Prompt medical attention is critical for adults as well as for children even if you do not notice any signs or symptoms. Do not use with other products containing acetaminophen.

NOTE: In addition to the above:

Children's TYLENOL® ALLERGY-D Chewable Tablets: DO NOT USE IF CARTON IS OPENED OR IF BLISTER UNIT IS BROKEN. Phenylketonurics: Contains Phenylalanine 5.4 mg per tablet.

Children's TYLENOL® ALLERGY-D Liquid: DO NOT USE IF PLASTIC CARTON WRAP, BOTTLE WRAP, OR FOIL INNER SEAL IMPRINTED "SAFETY SEAL®" IS BROKEN OR MISSING.

DRUG INTERACTION PRECAUTIONS

Do not give this product to a child who is taking a prescription monoamine oxidase inhibitor (MAOI) (certain drugs for depression, psychiatric or emotional conditions), or for 2 weeks after stopping the MAOI drug. If you are uncertain whether your child's prescription drug contains an MAOI, consult a health professional before giving this product.

PROFESSIONAL INFORMATION

OVERDOSAGE INFORMATION Acetaminophen in massive overdosage may cause hepatic toxicity in some patients. In adults and adolescents, hepatic toxicity has rarely been reported following ingestion of acute overdosage of less than 7.5 to 10 grams. Fatalities are infrequent (less than 3–4% of untreated cases) and have rarely been reported with overdoses of less than 15 grams. In children, an acute overdosage of less than 150 mg/kg has not been associated with hepatic toxicity.

Early symptoms following a potentially hepatotoxic overdose may include: nausea, vomiting, diaphoresis and general malaise. Clinical and laboratory evidence of hepatic toxicity may not be apparent until 48 to 72 hours postingestion. In adults and adolescents, regardless of the quantity of acetaminophen reported to have been ingested, administer acetylcysteine immediately if 24 hours or less have elapsed from the reported time of ingestion. For full prescribing information, refer to the acetylcysteine package insert. Do not await the results of assays for acetaminophen levels before initiating treatment with acetylcysteine. The following additional procedures are recommended: Promptly initiate gastric decontamination of the stomach. A plasma acetaminophen assay should be obtained as early as possible, but no sooner than four hours following ingestion. If plasma level falls above the lower treatment line on the acetaminophen overdose nomogram, acetylcysteine therapy should be continued. Liver function studies should be obtained initially and repeated at 24-hour intervals. Serious toxicity or fatalities are extremely infrequent in children, possibly due to differences in the way they metabolize acetaminophen. In children, the maximum potential amount ingested can be more easily estimated. If more than 150 mg/kg or an unknown amount was ingested, obtain a plasma acetaminophen level. The plasma acetaminophen level should be obtained as soon as possible, but no sooner than 4 hours following ingestion. If plasma level falls above the lower treatment line on the acetaminophen overdose nomogram, the acetylcysteine therapy should be initiated and continued for a full course of therapy. If plasma acetaminophen assay capability is not available, and the estimated acetaminophen ingestion exceeds 150 mg/kg, acetylcysteine therapy should be initiated and continued for a full course of therapy.

For additional emergency information, call your regional poison center or call the Rocky Mountain Poison Center toll-free (1–800–525–6115).

Diphenhydramine toxicity should be treated as you would an antihistamine/anticholinergic overdose and is likely to be present within a few hours after acute ingestion.

Symptoms from pseudoephedrine overdose consist most often of mild anxiety, tachycardia and/or mild hypertension. Symptoms usually appear within 4 to 8 hours of ingestion and are transient usually requiring no treatment.

INACTIVE INGREDIENTS

Tablets: Aspartame, Cellulose, Cellulose Acetate, Flavors, Magnesium Stearate, Mannitol, Polymethacrylate, Povidone and Red #7.

Liquid: Benzoic Acid, Citric Acid, Corn Syrup, D&C Red #33, FD&C Red #40, Flavors, Polyethylene Glycol, Propylene Glycol, Purified Water, Sodium Benzoate, and Sorbitol.

HOW SUPPLIED

Tablets: Pink colored chewable tablets in blister packs of 24.

Liquid:

Pinkish-red colored liquid in child resistant bottles 4 fl. oz.

Shown in Product Identification Guide, page 322

Children's TYLENOL® OTC
acetaminophen
Soft-Chew Chewable Tablets, Elixir, and Suspension Liquid
Infants' TYLENOL®
acetaminophen
Concentrated Drops

DESCRIPTION

Infants' TYLENOL® Grape Concentrated Drops are stable, alcohol-free, grape-flavored and purple in color. ***Infants' TYLENOL® Cherry Concentrated Drops*** are stable, alcohol-free, cherry-flavored and red in color. Each 0.8 mL (one calibrated dropperful) contains 80 mg acetaminophen. ***Children's TYLENOL® Elixir*** is stable and alcohol-free, cherry-flavored, and red in color. ***Children's TYLENOL® Suspension Liquid*** is stable, alcohol-free, cherry-flavored, and red in color, or bubble gum flavored, and pink in color or grape flavored and purple in color. Each 5 mL (one teaspoonful) contains 160 mg acetaminophen. Each ***Children's TYLENOL® Soft-Chew Chewable Tablet*** contains 80 mg acetaminophen in a grape, bubble gum, or fruit flavor.

ACTIONS

Acetaminophen is a clinically proven analgesic/antipyretic. Acetaminophen produces analgesia by elevation of the pain threshold and antipyresis through action on the hypothalamic heat regulating center. Acetaminophen is equal to aspirin in analgesic and antipyretic effectiveness and it is unlikely to produce many of the side effects associated with aspirin and aspirin containing products.

USES

Children's TYLENOL® Soft-Chew Chewable Tablets, Elixir, Suspension Liquid and ***Infants' TYLENOL® Concentrated Drops:*** For the reduction of fever. For the temporary relief of minor aches and pains associated with a cold, flu, headache, sore throat, immunizations, toothache.

PRECAUTIONS

If a rare sensitivity reaction occurs, the drug should be stopped.

DIRECTIONS

Chew tablets before swallowing. All dosages may be repeated every 4 hours, if needed. Do not use more than 5 times a day. Under 2 years (under 24 lbs), consult a physician. ***Children's TYLENOL Soft-Chew Chewable Tablets*** are not the same concentration as Junior Strength Tylenol Chewable Tablets or Caplets. For accurate dosing follow dosing instructions on label. 2–3 years (24–35 lbs): 2 tablets; 4–5 years (36–47 lbs): 3 tablets; 6–8 years (48–59 lbs): 4 tablets; 9–10 years (60–71 lbs): 5 tablets; 11 years (72–95 lbs): 6 tablets.

Children's TYLENOL® Elixir & Suspension Liquid: Children's Tylenol® Liquids are less concentrated than Infants' Tylenol® Concentrated Drops. For accurate dosing follow dosing instructions on label. This product has been specially designed for use with the enclosed measuring cup. Use only enclosed measuring cup to dose this product. Do not use any other dosing device. 2–3 years (24–35 lbs): 1 teaspoonful; 4–5 years (36–47 lbs): 1 $^{1}/_{2}$ teaspoonfuls; 6–8 years (48–59 lbs): 2 teaspoonfuls; 9–10 years (60–71 lbs): 2 $^{1}/_{2}$ teaspoonfuls; 11 years (72–95 lbs): 3 teaspoonfuls. ***Infants' TYLENOL® Concentrated Drops:*** Infants' Tylenol® Drops are more concentrated than Children's Tylenol® Liquids. For accurate dosing follow dosing instructions on label. This product has been specially designed for use only with enclosed dropper. Do not use any other dosing device with this product. 2–3 years (24–35 lbs): 2 dropperfuls (2 × 0.8 mL).

Professional Dosage Schedule: ***Children's TYLENOL® Elixir & Suspension Liquid:*** Children's Tylenol® Liquids are less concentrated than Infants' Tylenol® Concentrated Drops. For accurate dosing follow dosing instructions on label. This product has been specially designed for use with the enclosed measuring cup. Use only enclosed measuring cup to dose this product. Do not use any other dosing device. 4–11 months (12–17 lbs): $^{1}/_{2}$ teaspoonful; 12–23 months (18–23 lbs): $^{3}/_{4}$ teaspoonful. ***Infants' TYLENOL® Concentrated Drops:*** Infants' Tylenol® Drops are more concentrated than Children's Tylenol® Liquids. For accurate dosing follow dosing instructions on label. This product has been specially designed for use only with enclosed dropper. Do not use any other dosing device with this product. 0–3 months (6–11 lbs): 0.4 mL; 4–11 months (12–17 lbs): 0.8 mL; 12–23 months (18–23 lbs): 1.2 mL. All dosages may be repeated every 4 hours, if needed. Do not use more than 5 times a day.

WARNINGS

Children's TYLENOL® Soft-Chew Chewable Tablets, Elixir, Suspension Liquid and Infants' TYLENOL® Concentrated Drops:

Do Not Use:

- with any other products containing acetaminophen.
- for more than 3 days for fever unless directed by a doctor.
- for more than 5 days for pain unless directed by a doctor.

Stop Using This Product and Ask a Doctor if:

- symptoms do not improve.
- new symptoms occur.
- pain or fever persists or gets worse.
- redness or swelling is present.
- sore throat is severe, lasts for more than 2 days or occurs with fever, headache, rash, nausea or vomiting.

Do not exceed recommended dose. Taking more than the recommended dose (overdose) may not provide more relief and could cause serious health problems. Keep this and all drugs out of the reach of children. In case of accidental overdose, contact a physician or poison control center immediately. Prompt medical attention is critical even if you do not notice any signs or symptoms.

NOTE: In addition to the above:

Infants' TYLENOL® Concentrated Drops: Do not use if plastic carton wrap or bottle wrap imprinted "Safety Seal®" is broken or missing.

Children's TYLENOL® Elixir and Suspension Liquid: Do not use if plastic carton wrap, bottle wrap, or foil inner seal imprinted "Safety Seal®" is broken or missing. Not a USP elixir.

Children's TYLENOL® Soft-Chew Chewable Tablets: Do not use if carton is opened or if neck wrap or foil inner seal imprinted "Safety Seal®" is broken or missing. Phenylketonurics: grape contains phenylalanine 5 mg per tablet, bubble gum contains 6 mg per tablet, fruit contains 6 mg per tablet.

PROFESSIONAL INFORMATION

OVERDOSAGE INFORMATION Acetaminophen in massive overdosage may cause hepatic toxicity in some patients. In adults and adolescents, hepatic toxicity has rarely been reported following ingestion of acute overdoses of less than 7.5 to 10 grams. Fatalities are infrequent (less than 3–4% of untreated cases) and have rarely been reported with overdoses of less than 15 grams. In children, an acute overdosage of less than 150 mg/kg has not been associated with hepatic toxicity.

Early symptoms following a potentially hepatotoxic overdose may include: nausea, vomiting, diaphoresis and general malaise. Clinical and laboratory evidence of hepatic toxicity may not be apparent until 48 to 72 hours postingestion.

In adults and adolescents, regardless of the quantity of acetaminophen reported to have been ingested, administer acetylcysteine immediately if 24 hours or less have elapsed from the reported time of ingestion. For full prescribing information, refer to the acetylcysteine package insert. Do not await results of assays for acetaminophen levels before initiating treatment with acetylcysteine. The following additional procedures are recommended: Promptly initiate gastric decontamination of the stomach. A plasma acetaminophen assay should be obtained as early as possible, but no sooner than four hours following ingestion. If plasma level falls above the lower treatment line on the acetaminophen overdose nomogram, acetylcysteine therapy should be continued. Liver function studies should be obtained initially and repeated at 24-hour intervals.

Serious toxicity or fatalities are extremely infrequent in children, possibly due to differences in the way they metabolize acetaminophen. In children, the maximum potential amount ingested can be more easily estimated. If more than 150 mg/kg or an unknown amount was ingested, obtain a plasma acetaminophen level. The plasma acetaminophen level should be obtained as soon as possible, but no sooner than 4 hours following ingestion. If plasma level falls above the lower treatment line on the acetaminophen overdose nomogram, the acetylcysteine therapy should be initiated and continued for a full course of therapy. If plasma acetaminophen assay capability is not available, and the estimated acetaminophen ingestion exceeds 150 mg/kg, acetylcysteine therapy should be initiated and continued for a full course of therapy.

For additional emergency information, call your regional poison center or call the Rocky Mountain Poison Center toll free, (1-800-525-6115).

INACTIVE INGREDIENTS

Children's TYLENOL® Soft-Chew Fruit Flavored Chewable Tablets: Aspartame, Cellulose, Corn Starch, D&C Red #7 Flavors, Magnesium Stearate, and Mannitol. May contain Ethylcellulose or Cellulose Acetate and Povidone.

Children's TYLENOL® Soft-Chew Grape Flavored Chewable Tablets: Aspartame, Cellulose, Citric Acid, Corn Starch, FD&C Blue #1, D&C Red #7, D&C Red #30, Flavors, Magnesium Stearate, and Mannitol. May contain Ethylcellulose or Cellulose Acetate and Povidone.

Children's TYLENOL® Soft-Chew Bubble Gum Flavored Chewable Tablets: Aspartame, Cellulose, Corn Starch, D&C Red #7, Flavors, Magnesium Stearate, and Mannitol. May contain Ethylcellulose or Cellulose Acetate and Povidone.

Children's TYLENOL® Elixir: Benzoic Acid, Citric Acid, Flavors, Glycerin, Polyethylene Glycol, Propylene Glycol, Sodium Benzoate, Sorbitol, Sucrose, Purified Water, Red #33, Red #40.

Children's TYLENOL® Suspension Liquid: Butylparaben, Cellulose, Citric Acid, Corn Syrup, Flavors, Glycerin, Propylene Glycol, Purified Water, Sodium Benzoate, Sorbitol, Xanthan Gum. In addition to the above ingredients cherry flavored suspension contains FD&C Red #40, bubble gum flavored suspension contains D&C Red #33, and FD&C Red #40, and grape flavored suspension contains D&C Blue #1 and D&C Red #33.

Infants' TYLENOL® Cherry Concentrated Drops: Butylparaben, Cellulose, Citric Acid, Corn Syrup, Flavors, Glycerin, Propylene Glycol, Purified Water, Sodium Benzoate, Sorbitol, Xanthan Gum, FD&C Red #40.

Infants' TYLENOL® Grape Concentrated Drops: Butylparaben, Cellulose, Citric Acid, Corn Syrup, Flavors, Glycerin, Propylene Glycol, Purified Water, Sodium Benzoate, Sorbitol, Xanthan Gum, D&C Red #33, and FD&C Blue #1.

HOW SUPPLIED

Soft-Chew Chewable Tablets (pink colored fruit, purple colored grape, pink colored bubble gum, scored, imprinted "TY80"): Bottles of 30 and also blister packaged 60's and 96's. (fruit). **Elixir** (cherry colored red): bottles of 2 and 4 fl. oz. **Suspension liquid** (cherry colored red): bottles of 2 and 4 fl. oz. (bubble gum flavored colored pink and grape flavored colored purple): bottle of 4 fl. oz. **Concentrated drops** (grape colored purple): bottles of $^{1}/_{2}$ oz (15 mL) (cherry colored red): bottles of $^{1}/_{2}$ oz and 1 oz, each with calibrated plastic dropper.

All packages listed above have child-resistant safety caps or blisters.

Shown in Product Identification Guide, page 322

Children's TYLENOL® COLD Multi Symptom Chewable Tablets and Liquid — OTC

DESCRIPTION

Each ***Children's TYLENOL® COLD Multi Symptom Chewable Grape-Flavored Tablet*** contains acetaminophen 80 mg, chlorpheniramine maleate 0.5 mg and pseudoephedrine hydrochloride 7.5 mg. ***Children's TYLENOL® COLD Multi Symptom Liquid*** is grape flavored and contains no alcohol. Each teaspoon (5 mL) contains acetaminophen 160 mg, chlorpheniramine maleate 1 mg, and pseudoephedrine hydrochloride 15 mg.

ACTIONS

Children's TYLENOL® COLD Multi Symptom Chewable Tablets and Liquid combine the analgesic-antipyretic acetaminophen with the decongestant pseudoephedrine hydrochloride and the antihistamine chlorpheniramine maleate to help relieve nasal congestion, dry runny noses and prevent sneezing as well as to relieve the fever, aches, pains and general discomfort associated with colds and upper respiratory infections.

Acetaminophen is equal to aspirin in analgesic and antipyretic effectiveness and it is unlikely to produce the side effects often associated with aspirin or aspirin-containing products.

USES

For temporary relief of these cold symptoms: nasal congestion, runny nose, sore throat, sneezing, minor aches and pains, headaches and fever.

PRECAUTIONS

If a rare sensitivity reaction occurs, the drug should be stopped.

DIRECTIONS

All doses may be repeated every 4–6 hours, if needed. Do not use more than 4 times in 24 hours. Under 6 years (under 48 lbs), consult a physician. ***Children's TYLENOL® COLD Chewable Tablets:*** 6–11 years (48–95 lbs): 4 tablets. ***Children's TYLENOL® COLD Liquid Formula:*** An Accudose™ measuring cup is provided and marked for accurate dosing. 6–11 years (48–95 lbs): 2 teaspoonfuls.

Professional Dosage Schedule: ***Children's TYLENOL® COLD Chewable Tablets:*** 2–5 years (24–47 lbs): 2 tablets. ***Children's TYLENOL® COLD Liquid:*** 2–5 years (24–47 lbs): 1 teaspoonful. All doses may be repeated every 4–6 hours, if needed. Do not use more than 4 times in 24 hours.

WARNINGS

Do not take for pain for more than 5 days or for fever for more than 3 days unless directed by a doctor. If pain or fever persists, or gets worse, if new symptoms occur, or if redness or swelling is present, consult a doctor because these could be signs of a serious condition. If sore throat is severe, persists for more than 2 days, is accompanied or followed by fever, headache, rash, nausea, or vomiting, consult a doctor promptly. **Do not exceed recommended dosage.** If nervousness, dizziness, or sleeplessness occur, discontinue use and consult a doctor. May cause excitability especially in children. Do not give this product to children who have a breathing problem such as chronic bronchitis, or who have glaucoma, heart disease, high blood pressure, thyroid disease, or diabetes without first consulting the child's doctor. May cause drowsiness. Sedatives and tranquilizers may increase the drowsiness effect. Do not give this product to children who are taking sedatives or tranquilizers, without first consulting the child's doctor. **Do not exceed recommended dose.** Taking more than the recommended dose (overdose) may not provide more relief and could cause serious health problems. Keep this and all drugs out of the reach of children. In case of accidental overdose, contact a doctor or poison control center immediately. Prompt medical attention is critical even if you do not notice any signs or symptoms. Do not use with other products containing acetaminophen.

NOTE: In addition to the above:

Children's TYLENOL® COLD Chewable Tablets: DO NOT USE IF CARTON IS OPENED OR IF BLISTER UNIT IS BROKEN. Phenylketonurics: contains phenylalanine 6 mg per tablet.

Children's TYLENOL® COLD Liquid: DO NOT USE IF PLASTIC CARTON WRAP, BOTTLE WRAP OR FOIL IMPRINTED "SAFETY SEAL®" IS BROKEN OR MISSING.

DRUG INTERACTION PRECAUTION

Do not give this product to a child who is taking a prescription monamine omidase inhibitor (MAOI) (certain drugs for depression, psychiatric or emotional conditions), or for 2 weeks after stopping the MAOI drug. If you are uncertain whether your child's prescription drug contains an MAOI, consult a health professional before giving this product.

PROFESSIONAL INFORMATION

OVERDOSAGE INFORMATION

Acetaminophen in massive overdosage may cause hepatic toxicity in some patients. In adults and adolescents, hepatic toxicity has rarely been reported following ingestion of acute overdoses of less than 7.5 to 10 grams. Fatalities are infrequent (less than 3–4% of untreated cases) and have rarely been reported with overdoses of less than 15 grams. In children, an acute overdosage of less than 150 mg/kg has not been associated with hepatic toxicity.

Early symptoms following a potentially hepatotoxic overdose may include: nausea, vomiting, diaphoresis and general malaise. Clinical and laboratory evidence of hepatic toxicity may not be apparent until 48 to 72 hours postingestion.

In adults and adolescents, regardless of the quantity of acetaminophen reported to have been ingested, administer acetylcysteine immediately if 24 hours or less have elapsed from the reported time of ingestion. For full prescribing information, refer to the acetylcysteine package insert. Do not await the results of assays for acetaminophen levels before initiating treatment with acetylcysteine. The following additional procedures are recommended: Promptly initiate gastric decontamination of the stomach. A plasma acetaminophen assay should be obtained as early as possible, but no sooner than four hours following ingestion. If plasma level falls above the lower treatment line on the acetaminophen overdose nomogram, acetylcysteine therapy should be continued. Liver function studies should be obtained initially and repeated at 24-hour intervals.

Serious toxicity or fatalities are extremely infrequent in children, possibly due to differences in the way they metabolize acetaminophen. In children, the maximum potential amount ingested can be more easily estimated. If more than 150 mg/kg or an unknown amount was ingested, obtain a plasma acetaminophen level. The plasma acetaminophen level should be obtained as soon as possible, but no sooner than 4 hours following ingestion. If plasma level falls above the lower treatment line on the acetaminophen overdose nomogram, the acetylcysteine therapy should be initiated and continued for a full course of therapy. If plasma acetaminophen assay capability is not available, and the estimated acetaminophen ingestion exceeds 150 mg/kg, acetylcysteine therapy should be initiated and continued for a full course of therapy.

For additional emergency information, call your regional poison center or call the Rocky Mountain Poison Center toll-free, (1-800-525-6115).

Chlorpheniramine toxicity should be treated as you would an antihistamine/anticholinergic overdose and is likely to be present within a few hours after acute ingestion.

Symptoms from pseudoephedrine overdose consist most often of mild anxiety, tachycardia and/or mild hypertension. Symptoms usually appear within 4 to 8 hours of ingestion and are transient, usually requiring no treatment.

INACTIVE INGREDIENTS

Chewable Tablets: Aspartame, Basic Polymethacrylate, Cellulose Acetate, Citric Acid, D&C Red #7, FD&C Blue #1, Flavors, Hydroxypropyl Methylcellulose, Magnesium Stearate, Mannitol, and Microcrystalline Cellulose.

Liquid: Benzoic Acid, Citric Acid, FD&C Blue #1, FD&C Red #40, Flavors, Glycerin, Malic Acid, Polyethylene Glycol, Propylene Glycol, Purified Water, Sodium Benzoate, Sorbitol, and Sucrose.

HOW SUPPLIED

Chewable Tablets (colored purple, scored, imprinted "Tylenol Cold") on one side and "TC" on opposite side—Blisters of 24. **Liquid Formula**—bottles (colored purple) of 4 fl. oz.

Shown in Product Identification Guide, page 322

Children's TYLENOL® COLD Multi Symptom PLUS COUGH Chewable Tablets and Liquid — OTC

DESCRIPTION

Each ***Children's TYLENOL® COLD Multi Symptom Plus Cough Chewable Cherry-Flavored Tablet*** contains: acetaminophen 80 mg, chlorpheniramine maleate 0.5 mg, dextromethorphan hydrobromide 2.5 mg, and pseudoephedrine hydrochloride 7.5 mg.

Children's TYLENOL® COLD Multi Symptom Plus Cough Liquid is cherry flavored and contains no alcohol. Each teaspoon (5 mL) contains acetaminophen 160 mg, chlorpheniramine maleate 1 mg, dextromethorphan hydrobromide 5 mg and pseudoephedrine hydrochloride 15 mg.

ACTIONS

Children's TYLENOL® COLD Multi Symptom Plus Cough Chewable Tablets and ***Liquid*** combines the analgesic-antipyretic acetaminophen with the decongestant pseudoephedrine hydrochloride, the cough suppressant dextromethorphan hydrobromide, and the antihistamine chlorpheniramine maleate to help relieve coughs, nasal congestion, and sore throat, dry runny noses, and prevent sneezing as well as to relieve the fever, aches, pains and general discomfort associated with colds and upper respiratory infections.

Acetaminophen is equal to aspirin in analgesic and antipyretic effectiveness and it is unlikely to produce the side effects often associated with aspirin or aspirin-containing products.

USES

For the temporary relief of these cold symptoms: minor aches and pains, headaches, sore throat, nasal congestion, runny nose, coughs, sneezing and fever.

Continued on next page

Children's Tylenol Cold/Cough—Cont.

PRECAUTION

If a rare sensitivity reaction occurs, the drug should be stopped.

DIRECTIONS

All doses may be repeated every 4–6 hours, if needed. Do not use more than 4 times in 24 hours. Under 6 years (under 48 lbs), consult a doctor.

Children's TYLENOL® COLD Plus Cough Chewable Tablets: 6–11 years (48–95 lbs): 4 tablets. ***Children's TYLENOL® COLD Plus Cough Liquid:*** An Accudose™ measurig cup is provided and marked for accurate dosing, 6–11 years (48–95 lbs): 2 teaspoonfuls.

Professional Dosage Schedule: ***Children's TYLENOL® COLD Plus Cough Chewable Tablets:*** 2–5 years (24–47 lbs): 2 tablets. ***Children's TYLENOL® COLD Plus Cough Liquid:*** 2–5 years (24–47 lbs): 1 teaspoonful. All doses may be repeated every 4–6 hours, if needed. Do not use more than 4 times in 24 hours.

WARNINGS

Do not take for pain for more than 5 days or for fever for more than 3 days unless directed by a doctor. If pain or fever persists, or gets worse, if new symptoms occur, or if redness or swelling is present, consult a doctor because these could be signs of a serious condition. If sore throat is severe, persists for more than 2 days, is accompanied or followed by fever, headache, rash, nausea or vomiting, consult a doctor promptly. **Do not exceed recommended dosage.** If nervousness, dizziness, or sleeplessness occur, discontinue use and consult a doctor. May cause excitability especially in children. Do not give this product to children who have a breathing problem such as chronic bronchitis, or who have glaucoma, heart disease, high blood pressure, thyroid disease, or diabetes, without first consulting the child's doctor. May cause drowsiness. Sedatives and tranquilizers may increase the drowsiness effect. Do not give this product to children who are taking sedatives or tranquilizers, without first consulting the child's doctor. A persistent cough may be a sign of a serious condition. If cough persists for more than 1 week, tends to recur, or is accompanied by fever, rash or persistent headache, consult a doctor. Do not give this product for persistent or chronic cough such as occurs with asthma or if cough is accompanied by excessive phlegm (mucus) unless directed by a doctor. **Do not exceed recommended dose.** Taking more than the recommended dose (overdose) may not provide more relief and could cause serious health problems. Keep this and all drugs out of the reach of children. In case of accidental overdose, contact a doctor or poison control center immediately. Prompt medical attention is critical even if you do not notice any signs or symptoms. Do not use with other products containing acetaminophen.

NOTE: In addition to the above:

Chewable Tablets: DO NOT USE IF CARTON IS OPENED OR IF BLISTER UNIT IS BROKEN. Phenylketonurics: contains phenylalanine 4 mg per tablet.

Liquid: DO NOT USE IF PLASTIC CARTON WRAP, BOTTLE WRAP, OR FOIL INNER SEAL IMPRINTED "SAFETY SEAL®" IS BROKEN OR MISSING.

DRUG INTERACTION PRECAUTION

Do not give this product to a child who is taking a prescription monoamine oxidase inhibitor (MAOI) (certain drugs for depression, psychiatric or emotional conditions), or for 2 weeks after stopping the MAOI drug. If you are uncertain whether your child's prescription drug contains an MAOI, consult a health professional before giving this product.

PROFESSIONAL INFORMATION

OVERDOSAGE INFORMATION

Acetaminophen in massive overdosage may cause hepatic toxicity in some patients. In adults and adolescents, hepatic toxicity has rarely been reported following ingestion of acute overdoses of less than 7.5 to 10 grams. Fatalities are infrequent (less than 3–4% of untreated cases) and have rarely been reported with overdoses of less than 15 grams. In children, an acute overdosage of less than 150 mg/kg has not been associated with hepatic toxicity.

Early symptoms following a potentially hepatotoxic overdose may include: nausea, vomiting, diaphoresis and general malaise. Clinical and laboratory evidence of hepatic toxicity may not be apparent until 48 to 72 hours postingestion.

In adults and adolescents, regardless of the quantity of acetaminophen reported to have been ingested, administer acetylcysteine immediately if 24 hours or less have elapsed from the reported time of ingestion. For full prescribing information, refer to the acetylcysteine package insert. Do not await the results of assays for plasma acetaminophen levels before initiating treatment with acetylcysteine. The following additional procedures are recommended: Promptly initiate gastric decontamination of the stomach. A plasma acetaminophen assay should be obtained as early as possible, but no sooner than four hours following ingestion. If plasma level falls above the lower treatment line on the acetaminophen overdose nomogram, acetylcysteine therapy should be continued. Liver function studies should be obtained initially and repeated at 24-hour intervals.

Serious toxicity or fatalities are extremely infrequent in children, possibly due to differences in the way they metabolize acetaminophen. In children, the maximum potential amount ingested can be more easily estimated. If more than 150 mg/kg or an unknown amount was ingested, obtain a plasma acetaminophen level. The plasma acetaminophen level should be obtained as soon as possible, but no sooner than 4 hours following the ingestion. If plasma level falls above the lower treatment line on the acetaminophen overdose nomogram, the acetylcysteine therapy should be initiated and continued for a full course of therapy. If plasma acetaminophen assay capability is not available, and the estimated acetaminophen ingestion exceeds 150 mg/kg, acetylcysteine therapy should be initiated and continued for a full course of therapy.

For additional emergency information, call your regional poison center or call the Rocky Mountain Poison Center toll-free, (1-800-525-6115).

Chlorpheniramine toxicity should be treated as you would an antihistamine/anticholinergic overdose and is likely to be present within a few hours after acute ingestion.

Symptoms from pseudoephedrine overdose consist most often of mild anxiety, tachycardia and/or mild hypertension. Symptoms usually appear within 4 to 8 hours of ingestion and are transient, usually requiring no treatment.

Acute dextromethorphan overdose usually does not result in serious signs and symptoms unless massive amounts have been ingested. Signs and symptoms of a substantial overdose may include nausea and vomiting, visual disturbances, CNS disturbances, and urinary retention.

INACTIVE INGREDIENTS

Chewable Tablets: Aspartame, Basic Polymethacrylate, Cellulose Acetate, D&C Red #7, Flavors, Hydroxypropyl Methylcellulose, Magnesium Stearate, Mannitol, and Microcrystalline Cellulose.

Liquid: Citric Acid, Corn Syrup, D&C Red #33, FD&C Red #40, Flavors, Polyethylene Glycol, Propylene Glycol, Purified Water, Sodium Benzoate, Sodium Carboxymethylcellulose, and Sorbitol.

HOW SUPPLIED

Chewable Tablets (colored pink, imprinted "TYLENOL C/C" on one side and "TC/C" on the opposite side)—Blisters of 24.

Liquid Formula—(red colored) bottles of 4 fl. oz.

Shown in Product Identification Guide, page 322

Children's TYLENOL® FLU Liquid — OTC

DESCRIPTION

Children's TYLENOL® FLU Liquid is bubble-gum flavored and contains no alcohol or aspirin. Each teaspoon (5 mL) contains acetaminophen 160 mg, pseudoephedrine HCl 15 mg, dextromethorphan HBr 7.5 mg, and chlorpheniramine maleate 1 mg.

ACTIONS

Children's TYLENOL® FLU Liquid combines the analgesic-antipyretic acetaminophen with the decongestant pseudoephedrine hydrochloride, the cough suppressant dextromethorphan hydrobromide and the antihistamine chlorpheniramine maleate to provide fast, effective, temporary relief of all your child's symptoms associated with flu including fever, body aches, headache, stuffy nose, runny nose, sore throat and coughs.

Acetaminophen is equal to aspirin in analgesic and antipyretic effectiveness and it is unlikely to produce the side effects often associated with aspirin or aspirin-containing products.

USES

For the temporary relief of these cold or flu symptoms: fever, minor aches and pains, headaches, sore throat, nasal congestion, runny nose and coughs.

DIRECTIONS

All doses may be repeated every 6–8 hours, if needed. Do not use more than 4 times in 24 hours. Under 6 years (under 48 lbs), consult a physician. An Accudose™ measuring cup is provided for accurate dosing. ***Children's TYLENOL® FLU Liquid.*** 6–11 years (48–95 lbs): 2 teaspoonfuls.

Professional Dosage Schedule: 2-5 years (24–47 lbs): 1 teaspoonful. All doses may be repeated every 6–8 hours, if needed. Do not use more than 4 times in 24 hours.

WARNINGS

DO NOT USE IF PLASTIC CARTON WRAP, BOTTLE WRAP, OR FOIL INNER SEAL IMPRINTED "SAFETY SEAL"® IS BROKEN OR MISSING. Do not take for pain for more than 5 days or for fever for more than 3 days unless directed by a doctor. If pain or fever persists, or gets worse, if new symptoms occur, or if redness or swelling is present, consult a doctor because these could be signs of a serious condition. If sore throat is severe, persists for more than 2 days, is accompanied or followed by fever, headache, rash, nausea or vomiting, consult a doctor promptly. **Do not exceed recommended dosage.** If nervousness, dizziness or sleeplessness occur, discontinue use and consult a doctor. May cause excitability especially in children. Do not give this product to children who have a breathing problem such as chronic bronchitis, or who have glaucoma, heart disease, high blood pressure, thyroid disease or diabetes without first consulting the child's doctor. May cause drowsiness. Sedatives and tranquilizers may increase the drowsiness effect. Do not give this product to children who are taking sedatives or tranquilizers without first consulting the child's doctor. A persistent cough may be a sign of a serious condition. If cough persists for more than 1 week, tends to recur, or is accompanied by fever, rash, or persistent headache, consult a doctor. Do not give this product for persistent or chronic cough such as occurs with asthma or if cough is accompanied by excessive phlegm (mucus) unless directed by a doctor. **Do not exceed recommended dose.** Taking more than the recommended dose (overdose) may not provide more relief and could cause serious health problems. Keep this and all drugs out of the reach of children. In case of accidental overdose, contact a doctor or poison control center immediately. Prompt medical attention is critical even if you do not notice any signs or symptoms. Do not use with other products containing acetaminophen.

DRUG INTERACTION PRECAUTION

Do not give this product to a child who is taking a prescription monoamine oxidase inhibitor (MAOI) (certain drugs for depression, psychiatric or emotional conditions) or for 2 weeks after stopping the MAOI drug. If you are uncertain whether your child's prescription drug contains an MAOI, consult a health professional before giving this product.

PROFESSIONAL INFORMATION

OVERDOSAGE INFORMATION

Acetaminophen in massive overdosage may cause hepatic toxicity in some patients. In adults and adolescents, hepatic toxicity has rarely been reported following ingestion of acute overdoses of less than 7.5 to 10 grams. Fatalities are infrequent (less than 3–4% of untreated cases) and have rarely been reported with overdoses of less than 15 grams. In children, an acute overdosage of less than 150 mg/kg has not been associated with hepatic toxicity.

Early symptoms following a potentially hepatotoxic overdose may include: nausea, vomiting, diaphoresis and general malaise. Clinical and laboratory evidence of hepatic toxicity may not be apparent until 48 to 72 hours postingestion.

In adults and adolescents, regardless of the quantity of acetaminophen reported to have been ingested, administer acetylcysteine immediately if 24 hours or less have elapsed from the reported time of ingestion. For full prescribing information, refer to the acetylcysteine package insert. Do not await the results of assays for plasma acetaminophen levels before initiating treatment with acetylcysteine. The following additional procedures are recommended: Promptly initiate gastric decontamination of the stomach. A plasma acetaminophen assay should be obtained as early as possible, but no sooner than four hours following ingestion. If plasma level falls above the lower treatment line on the acetaminophen overdose nomogram, acetylcysteine therapy should be continued. Liver function studies should be obtained initially and repeated at 24–hour intervals.

Serious toxicity or fatalities are extremely infrequent in children, possibly due to differences in the way they metabolize acetaminophen. In children, the maximum potential amount ingested can be more easily estimated. If more than 150 mg/kg or an unknown amount was ingested, obtain a plasma acetaminophen level. The plasma acetaminophen level should be obtained as soon as possible, but no sooner than 4 hours following ingestion. If plasma level falls above the lower treatment line on the acetaminophen overdose nomogram, the acetylcysteine therapy should be initiated and continued for a full course of therapy. If plasma acetaminophen assay capability is not available, and the estimated acetaminophen ingestion exceeds 150 mg/kg, acetylcysteine therapy should be initiated and continued for a full course of therapy.

For additional emergency information, call your regional poison center or call the Rocky Mountain Poison Center toll-free, (1-800-525-6115).

Chlorpheniramine toxicity should be treated as you would an antihistamine/anticholinergic overdose and is likely to be present within a few hours after acute ingestion.

Symptoms from pseudoephedrine overdose consist most often of mild anxiety, tachycardia, and/or mild hypertension. Symptoms usually appear within 4 to 8 hours of ingestion and are transient, usually requiring no treatment.

Acute dextromethorphan overdose usually does not result in serious signs and symptoms unless massive amounts have

been ingested. Signs and symptoms of a substantial overdose may include nausea and vomiting, visual disturbances, CNS disturbances, and urinary retention.

INACTIVE INGREDIENTS

Citric Acid, Corn Syrup, D&C Red #33, FD&C Red #40 Flavors, Polyethylene Glycol, Propylene Glycol, Purified Water, Sodium Benzoate, Sodium Carboxymethylcellulose and Sorbitol.

HOW SUPPLIED

Pinkish-red colored liquid in child resistant bottles of 4 fl. oz.

Shown in Product Identification Guide, page 322

Children's TYLENOL® SINUS Chewable Tablets and Liquid — OTC

DESCRIPTION

Children's TYLENOL® SINUS Chewable Tablets are fruit flavored and each tablet contains acetaminophen 80 mg and pseudoephedrine HCl 7.5 mg. ***Children's TYLENOL® SINUS Liquid*** is fruit flavored and contains no alcohol or aspirin. Each teaspoon (5 mL) contains acetaminophen 160 mg and pseudoephedrine HCl 15 mg.

ACTIONS

Children's TYLENOL® SINUS Chewable Tablets and Liquid combine the analgesic-antipyretic acetaminophen with the decongestant pseudoephedrine hydrochloride to provide fast, effective, temporary relief of all your child's sinus symptoms including stuffy nose, sinus headache, sinus pressure, sinus pain, and nasal congestion. Acetaminophen is equal to aspirin in analgesic and antipyretic effectiveness and is unlikely to produce the side effects often associated with aspirin or aspirin-containing products.

INDICATIONS

For the reduction of fever. For the temporary relief of minor aches, pains and headaches, sinus congestion, stuffy nose and sinus pressure.

DIRECTIONS

All doses may be repeated every 4–6 hours, if needed. Do not use more than 4 times in 24 hours. Under 2 years (under 24 lbs), consult a physician. An Accudose™ measuring cup is provided for accurate dosing. ***Children's TYLENOL® SINUS Chewable Tablets:*** 2–5 years (24–47 lbs) 2 tablets; 6–11 years (48–95 lbs): 4 tablets. ***Children's TYLENOL® SINUS Liquid:*** 2–5 years (24–47 lbs): 1 teaspoonful; 6–11 years (48–95 lbs): 2 teaspoonfuls.

WARNINGS

Do not take for pain for more than 5 days or for fever for more than 3 days unless directed by a doctor. If pain or fever persists, or gets worse, if new symptoms occur, or if redness or swelling is present, consult a doctor because these could be signs of a serious condition. **Do not exceed recommended dosage.** If nervousness, dizziness or sleeplessness occur, discontinue use and consult a doctor. Do not give this product to a child who has heart disease, high blood pressure, thyroid disease, or diabetes without first consulting the child's doctor. **Do not exceed recommended dose.** Taking more than the recommended dose (overdose) may not provide more relief and could cause serious health problems. Keep this and all drugs out of the reach of children. In case of accidental overdose, contact a doctor or poison control center immediately. Prompt medical attention is critical for adults as for children even if you do not notice any signs or symptoms. Do not use with other products containing acetaminophen.

NOTE: In addition to the above:

Children's TYLENOL® SINUS Chewable Tablets: DO NOT USE IF CARTON IS OPENED OR IF BLISTER UNIT IS BROKEN. Phenylketonurics: contains phenylalanine 5.4 mg per tablet.

Children's TYLENOL® SINUS Liquid: DO NOT USE IF PLASTIC CARTON WRAP, BOTTLE WRAP, OR FOIL INNER SEAL IMPRINTED "SAFETY SEAL®" IS BROKEN OR MISSING.

DRUG INTERACTION PRECAUTION

Do not give this product to a child who is taking a prescription monoamine oxidase inhibitor (MAOI) (certain drugs for depression, psychiatric or emotional conditions), or for 2 weeks after stopping the MAOI drug. If you are uncertain whether your child's prescription drug contains an MAOI, consult a health professional before giving this product.

PROFESSIONAL INFORMATION

OVERDOSAGE INFORMATION

Acetaminophen in massive overdosage may cause hepatic toxicity in some patients. In adults and adolescents, hepatic toxicity has rarely been reported following ingestion of acute overdosage of less than 7.5 to 10 grams. Fatalities are infrequent (less than 3–4% of untreated cases) and have rarely been reported with overdoses of less than 15 grams. In children an acute overdosage of less than 150 mg/kg has not been associated with hepatic toxicity.

Early symptoms following a potentially hepatotoxic overdose may include: nausea, vomiting, diaphoresis and general malaise. Clinical and laboratory evidence of hepatic toxicity may not be apparent until 48 to 72 hours postingestion. In adults and adolescents, regardless of the quantity of acetaminophen reported to have been ingested, administer acetylcysteine immediately if 24 hours or less have elapsed from the reported time of ingestion. For full prescribing information, refer to the acetylcysteine package insert. Do not await the results of assays for acetaminophen levels before initiating treatment with acetylcysteine. The following additional procedures are recommended: Promptly initiate gastric decontamination of the stomach. A plasma acetaminophen assay should be obtained as early as possible, but no sooner than 4 hours following ingestion. If plasma level falls above the lower treatment line on the acetaminophen overdose nomogram, acetylcysteine therapy should be continued. Liver function studies should be obtained initially and repeated at 24–hour intervals. Serious toxicity or fatalities are extremely infrequent in children, possibly due to differences in the way they metabolize acetaminophen. In children, the maximal potential amount ingested can be more easily estimated. If more than 150 mg/kg or an unknown amount was ingested, obtain a plasma acetaminophen level. The plasma acetaminophen level should be obtained as soon as possible, but no sooner than 4 hours following ingestion. If plasma level falls above the lower treatment line on the acetaminophen overdose nomogram, the acetylcysteine therapy should be initiated and continued for a full course of therapy. If plasma acetaminophen assay capability is not available, and the estimated acetaminophen ingestion exceeds 150 mg/kg, acetylcysteine therapy should be initiated and continued for a full course of therapy.

For additional emergency information, call your regional poison center or call the Rocky Mountain Poison Center toll-free, (1–800–525–6115).

Symptoms from pseudoephedrine overdose consist most often of mild anxiety, tachycardia and/or mild hypertension. Symptoms usually appear within 4 to 8 hours of ingestion and are transient, usually requiring no treatment.

INACTIVE INGREDIENTS

Tablets: Aspartame, Cellulose, Cellulose Acetate, Citric Acid, Flavor, Magnesium Stearate, Mannitol, Polymethacrylate, Povidone, and Red #7.

Liquid: Acesulfame Potassium, Benzoic Acid, Citric Acid, Corn Syrup, D&C Red #33, FD&C Red #40, Flavors, Polyethylene Glycol, Propylene Glycol, Purified Water, Sodium Benzoate, and Sorbitol.

HOW SUPPLIED

Tablets: Pink colored tablets in blister packs of 24.

Liquid: Red colored liquid in child resistant bottles 4 fl oz.

Shown in Product Identification Guide, page 322

IMODIUM® A–D (loperamide hydrochloride) — OTC

DESCRIPTION

Each 5 mL (teaspoon) of ***IMODIUM® A-D*** liquid contains loperamide hydrochloride 1 mg. ***IMODIUM® A-D*** liquid is stable, cherry-mint flavored, and clear in color.

Each caplet of ***IMODIUM® A-D*** contains 2 mg of loperamide and is scored and colored green.

ACTIONS

IMODIUM® A-D contains a clinically proven antidiarrheal medication. Loperamide HCl acts by slowing intestinal motility and by affecting water and electrolyte movement through the bowel.

INDICATIONS

IMODIUM® A-D is indicated for the control and symptomatic relief of acute nonspecific diarrhea, including Travelers' Diarrhea.

DIRECTIONS

Adults and children 12 years of age and older: Take four teaspoonfuls or two caplets after first loose bowel movement. If needed, take two teaspoonfuls or one caplet after each subsequent loose bowel movement. Do not exceed eight teaspoonfuls or four caplets in any 24 hour period, unless directed by a physician.

Children 9–11 years old (60–95 lbs.): Two teaspoonfuls or one caplet after first loose bowel movement, followed by one teaspoonful or one-half caplet after each subsequent loose bowel movement. Do not exceed six teaspoonfuls or three caplets a day.

Children 6–8 years old (48–59 lbs.): Two teaspoonfuls or one caplet after first loose bowel movement, followed by one teaspoonful or one-half caplet after each subsequent loose bowel movement. Do not exceed four teaspoonfuls or two caplets a day.

Professional Dosage Schedule for children 2–5 years old (24–47 lbs): One teaspoon after first loose bowel movement, followed by one after each subsequent loose bowel movement. Do not exceed three teaspoonfuls a day.

WARNINGS

KEEP THIS AND ALL DRUGS OUT OF THE REACH OF CHILDREN. Do not use for more than two days unless directed by a physician. DO NOT USE IF DIARRHEA IS ACCOMPANIED BY HIGH FEVER (GREATER THAN 101°F), OR IF BLOOD OR MUCUS IS PRESENT IN THE STOOL, OR IF YOU HAVE HAD A RASH OR OTHER ALLERGIC REACTION TO LOPERAMIDE HCl. If you are taking antibiotics or have a history of liver disease, consult a physician before using this product. As with any drug, if you are pregnant or nursing a baby, seek the advice of a health professional before using this product. In case of accidental overdose, seek professional assistance or contact a poison control center immediately.

PROFESSIONAL INFORMATION

OVERDOSAGE INFORMATION

Overdosage of loperamide HCl in man may result in constipation, CNS depression and nausea. A slurry of activated charcoal administered promptly after ingestion of loperamide hydrochloride can reduce the amount of drug which is absorbed. If vomiting occurs spontaneously upon ingestion, a slurry of 100 grams of activated charcoal should be administered orally as soon as fluids can be retained. If vomiting has not occurred, and CNS depression is evident, gastric lavage should be performed followed by administration of 100 gms of the activated charcoal slurry through the gastric tube. In the event of overdosage, patients should be monitored for signs of CNS depression for at least 24 hours. Children may be more sensitive to central nervous system effects than adults. If CNS depression is observed, naloxone may be administered. If responsive to naloxone, vital signs must be monitored carefully for recurrence of symptoms of drug overdose for at least 24 hours after the last dose of naloxone.

INACTIVE INGREDIENTS

Liquid: Benzoic acid, citric acid, flavors, glycerin, propylene glycol, purified water, sodium benzoate, sorbitol, sucrose, contains 0.5% alcohol.

Caplets: Dibasic calcium phosphate, magnesium stearate, microcrystalline cellulose, colloidal silicon dioxide, FD&C Blue #1 and D&C Yellow #10.

HOW SUPPLIED

Liquid: Cherry-mint flavored liquid (clear) 2 fl. oz., and 4 fl. oz. tamper evident bottles with child resistant safety caps and special dosage cups.

Caplets: Green scored caplets in 6's and 12's, 18's and 24's blister packaging which is tamper evident and child resistant.

Shown in Product Identification Guide, page 321

IMODIUM® ADVANCED Chewable Tablets (loperamide HCl/simethicone) — OTC

DESCRIPTION

Each chewable tablet of ***Imodium® Advanced*** contains loperamide HCl 2 mg/simethicone 125 mg.

ACTIONS

Imodium® Advanced combines original prescription strength Imodium® to control the symptoms of diarrhea plus simethicone to relieve bloating, pressure and cramps commonly referred to as gas.

Loperamide HCl acts by slowing intestinal motility and by affecting water and electrolyte movement through the bowel. Simethicone acts in the stomach and intestines by altering the surface tension of gas bubbles enabling them to coalesce, thereby freeing and eliminating the gas more easily by belching or passing flatus.

INDICATIONS

Imodium® Advanced is indicated for the control of symptoms of diarrhea plus bloating, pressure and cramps commonly referred to as gas.

DIRECTIONS

Chew the first dose and take with water after the first loose stool. If needed, chew the next dose and take with water after the next loose stool. Drink plenty of clear liquids to prevent dehydration.

Continued on next page

Imodium Advanced—Cont.

Adults aged 12 years and older: Chew 2 tablets and take with water after the first loose stool. If needed, chew 1 tablet and take with water after the next loose stool. Do not exceed 4 tablets a day.

Children 9-11 years (60-95 lbs): Chew 1 tablet and take with water after the first loose stool. If needed, chew 1/2 tablet and take with water after the next loose stool. Do not exceed 3 tablets a day.

Children 6-8 years (48-59 lbs): Chew 1 tablet and take with water after the first loose stool. If needed, chew 1/2 tablet and take with water after the next loose stool. Do not exceed 2 tablets a day.

Children under 6 years old (up to 47 lbs): Consult a physician. Not intended for use in children under 6 years old.

WARNINGS

Do Not Use if:
- You have a high fever (over 101° F)
- Blood or mucus is in your stool
- You have had a rash or other allergic reaction to Loperamide HCl

Do Not Use Without Asking A Doctor:
- For more than 2 days
- If you are taking antibiotics
- If you have a history of liver disease

As with any drug, If you are pregnant or nursing a baby, seek the advice of a health professional before using this product.
- **Keep this and all drugs out of the reach of children.**
- In case of accidental overdose, seek professional assistance or call a poison control center immediately.

Store at 15–30°C (59–86°F).

PROFESSIONAL INFORMATION
OVERDOSAGE INFORMATION

Overdosage of loperamide HCl in man may result in constipation, CNS depression and nausea. A slurry of activated charcoal administered promptly after ingestion of loperamide hydrochloride can reduce the amount of drug which is absorbed. If vomiting occurs spontaneously upon ingestion, a slurry of 100 grams of activated charcoal should be administered orally as soon as fluids can be retained. If vomiting has not occurred, and CNS depression is evident, gastric lavage should be performed followed by administration of 100 gms of the activated charcoal slurry through the gastric tube. In the event of overdosage, patients should be monitored for signs of CNS depression for at least 24 hours. Children may be more sensitive to central nervous system effects than adults. If CNS depression is observed, naloxone may be administered. If responsive to naloxone, vital signs must be monitored carefully for recurrence of symptoms of drug overdose for at least 24 hours after the last dose of naloxone. No treatment is necessary for the simethicone ingestion in this circumstance.

INACTIVE INGREDIENTS

cellulose acetate, corn starch, dextrates, flavors, microcrystalline cellulose, polymethacrylates, saccharin sodium, sorbitol, stearic acid, sucrose, tribasic calcium phosphate, FD&C Blue No.1, D&C Yellow No.10

HOW SUPPLIED

Vanilla mint chewable tablets in 6's, 12's, 18's and 30's blister packaging which is tamper evident and child resistant. Each Imodium® Advanced tablet is round, light green in color and has "IMODIUM" embossed on one side and "2/125" on the other side.

Shown in Product Identification Guide, page 321

Infants' TYLENOL® COLD   OTC
Decongestant & Fever Reducer Concentrated Drops

DESCRIPTION

Infants' TYLENOL® COLD Decongestant & Fever Reducer Concentrated Drops are alcohol-free, bubble gum flavored and red in color. Each 1.6 mL (2 dropperfuls) contains acetaminophen 160 mg and pseudoephedrine HCl 15 mg.

ACTIONS

Acetaminophen is a clinically proven analgesic/antipyretic. Acetaminophen produces analgesia by elevation of the pain threshold and antipyresis through action on the hypothalamic heat regulating center. Acetaminophen is equal to aspirin in analgesic and antipyretic effectiveness and it is unlikely to produce many of the side effects associated with aspirin and aspirin containing products. Pseudoephedrine hydrochloride is a sympathomimetic amine which provides temporary relief of nasal congestion.

USES

For the reduction of fever. For the temporary relief of these cold symptoms: minor aches and pains, headaches and nasal congestion.

PRECAUTIONS

If a rare sensitivity reaction occurs, the drug should be stopped.

DIRECTIONS

Infants' TYLENOL® Cold Drops are more concentrated than Children's TYLENOL® Cold Liquid Products. For accurate dosing follow the dosing instructions on the label. All dosages may be repeated every 4–6 hours, if needed. Do not use more than 4 times in 24 hours. Under 2 years (under 24 lbs), consult a physician. A calibrated dropper is provided for accurate dosing. Attention: This product has been specially designed for use only with the enclosed dropper. Do not use any other dosing device with this product.
Infants' TYLENOL® COLD Decongestant & Fever Reducer Concentrated Drops: 2–3 years (24–35 lbs): 2 dropperfuls (2 ×0.8 mL).

Professional Dosage Schedule: 0–3 months (6-11 lbs): 0.4 mL; 4–11 months (12–17 lbs): 0.8 mL; 12–23 months (18–23 lbs); 1.2 mL. All dosages may be repeated every 4–6 hours, if needed. Do not use more than 4 times in 24 hours.

WARNINGS

Do not use if plastic carton wrap or bottle wrap imprinted "safety seal®" is broken or missing. Do not take for pain for more than 5 days or for fever for more than 3 days unless directed by a doctor. If pain or fever persists or gets worse, if new symptoms occur, or if redness or swelling is present, consult a doctor because these could be signs of a serious condition. **Do not exceed recommended dosage.** If nervousness, dizziness or sleeplessness occur, discontinue use and consult a doctor. Do not give this product to children who have heart disease, high blood pressure, thyroid disease, or diabetes unless directed by a doctor. **Do not exceed recommended dose.** Taking more than the recommended dose (overdose) may not provide more relief and could cause serious health problems. Keep this and all drugs out of the reach of children. In case of accidental overdose, contact a doctor or poison control center immediately. Prompt medical attention is critical even if you do not notice any signs or symptoms. Do not use with other products containing acetaminophen.

DRUG INTERACTION PRECAUTION

Do not give this product to a child who is taking a prescription monoamine oxidase inhibitor (MAOI) (certain drugs for depression, psychiatric or emotional conditions), or for 2 weeks after stopping the MAOI drug. If you are uncertain whether your child's prescription drug contains an MAOI, consult a health professional before giving this product.

PROFESSIONAL INFORMATION
OVERDOSAGE INFORMATION

Acetaminophen in massive overdosage may cause hepatic toxicity in some patients. In adults and adolescents, hepatic toxicity has rarely been reported following ingestion of acute overdoses of less than 7.5 to 10 grams. Fatalities are infrequent (less than 3–4% of untreated cases) and have rarely been reported with overdoses of less than 15 grams. In children, an acute overdosage of less than 150 mg/kg has not been associated with hepatic toxicity.

Early symptoms following a potentially hepatotoxic overdose may include: nausea, vomiting, diaphoresis and general malaise. Clinical and laboratory evidence of hepatic toxicity may not be apparent until 48 to 72 hours postingestion. In adults and adolescents, regardless of the quantity of acetaminophen reported to have been ingested, administer acetylcysteine immediately if 24 hours or less have elapsed from the reported time of ingestion. For full prescribing information, refer to the acetylcysteine package insert. Do not await results of assays for plasma acetaminophen levels before initiating treatment with acetylcysteine. The following additional procedures are recommended: Promptly initiate gastric decontamination of the stomach. A plasma acetaminophen assay should be obtained as early as possible, but no sooner than four hours following ingestion. If plasma level falls above the lower treatment line on the acetaminophen overdose nomogram, acetylcysteine therapy should be continued. Liver function studies should be obtained initially and repeated at 24-hour intervals.

Serious toxicity or fatalities are extremely infrequent in children, possibly due to differences in the way they metabolize acetaminophen. In children, the maximum potential amount ingested can be more easily estimated. If more than 150 mg/kg or an unknown amount was ingested, obtain a plasma acetaminophen level. The plasma acetaminophen level should be obtained as soon as possible, but no sooner than 4 hours following ingestion. If plasma level falls above the lower treatment line on the acetaminophen overdose nomogram, the acetylcysteine therapy should be initiated and continued for a full course of therapy. If plasma acetaminophen assay capability is not available, and the estimated acetaminophen ingestion exceeds 150 mg/kg, acetylcysteine therapy should be initiated and continued for a full course of therapy.

For additional emergency information, call your regional poison center or call the Rocky Mountain Poison Center toll-free, (1-800-525-6115).

Symptoms from pseudoephedrine overdose consist most often of mild anxiety, tachycardia and/or mild hypertension. Symptoms usually appear within 4 to 8 hours of ingestion and are transient, usually requiring no treatment.

INACTIVE INGREDIENTS

Citric Acid, Corn Syrup, Flavors, Polyethylene Glycol, Propylene Glycol, Purified Water, Red #40, Saccharin and Sodium Benzoate.

HOW SUPPLIED

Red-colored drops in bottles of 1/2 fl. oz.
Shown in Product Identification Guide, page 321

INFANT'S TYLENOL® COLD
PLUS COUGH   OTC
Decongestant & Fever Reducer Concentrated Drops

DESCRIPTION

Infants' TYLENOL® COLD PLUS COUGH Decongestant & Fever Reducer Concentrated Drops are alcohol-free, cherry flavored and red in color. Each 1.6 mL (2 dropperfuls) contains acetaminophen 160 mg, pseudoephedrine HCl 15 mg, and dextromethorphan HBr 5 mg.

ACTIONS

Acetaminophen is a clinically proven analgesic/antipyretic. Acetaminophen produces analgesia by elevation of the pain threshold and antipyresis through action on the hypothalamic heat regulating center. Acetaminophen is equal to aspirin in analgesic and antipyretic effectiveness and it is unlikely to produce many of the side effects associated with aspirin and aspirin containing products. Pseudoephedrine Hydrochloride is a sympathomimetic amine which provides temporary relief of nasal congestion. Dextromethorphan hydrobromide is a cough suppressant which helps relieve coughs.

USES

For the reduction of fever. For the temporary relief of these cold symptoms: coughs, sore throat, nasal congestion, headaches and minor aches and pains.

PRECAUTIONS

If a rare sensitivity reaction occurs, the drug should be stopped.

DIRECTIONS

Infants' TYLENOL® Cold Drops are more concentrated than Children's TYLENOL® Cold Liquid Products. For accurate dosing, follow the dosing instructions on the label. All dosages may be repeated every 4–6 hours, if needed. Do not use more than 4 times in 24 hours. Under 2 years (under 24 lbs), consult a physician. A calibrated dropper is provided for accurate dosing. Attention: This product has been specially designed for use only with the enclosed dropper. Do not use any other dosing device with this product.
Infant's TYLENOL® COLD PLUS COUGH Decongestant & Fever Reducer Concentrated Drops: 2–3 years (24–35 lbs) 2 dropperfuls (2 × 0.8 mL).

WARNINGS

Do not use if plastic carton wrap or bottle wrap imprinted "Safety Seal®" is broken or missing. Do not take for pain for more than 5 days or for fever for more than 3 days unless directed by a doctor. If pain or fever persists, or gets worse, if new symptoms occur, or if redness or swelling is present, consult a doctor because these could be signs of a serious condition. If sore throat is severe, persists for more than 2 days, is accompanied or followed by fever, headache, rash, nausea, or vomiting, consult a doctor promptly. **Do not exceed recommended dosage.** If nervousness, dizziness or sleeplessness occur, discontinue use and consult a doctor. Do not give this product to children who have heart disease, high blood pressure, thyroid disease, or diabetes without first consulting the child's doctor. A persistent cough may be a sign of a serious condition. If cough persists for more than 1 week, tends to recur or is accompanied by fever, rash or persistent headache, consult a doctor. Do not give this product for persistent or chronic cough such as occurs with asthma or if cough is accompanied by excessive phlegm (mucus) unless directed by a doctor. **Do not exceed recommended dose.** Taking more than the recommended dose (overdose) may not provide more relief and could cause serious health problems. Keep this and all drugs out of the reach of children. In case of accidental overdose, contact a doctor or poison control center immediately. Prompt medical attention is critical even if you do not notice any signs or symptoms. Do not use with other products containing acetaminophen.

DRUG INTERACTION PRECAUTION

Do not give this product to a child who is taking a prescription monoamine oxidase inhibitor (MAOI) (certain drugs for depression, psychiatric or emotional conditions), or for 2

weeks after stopping the MAOI drug. If you are uncertain whether your child's prescription drug contains an MAOI, consult a health professional before giving this product.

PROFESSIONAL INFORMATION
OVERDOSAGE INFORMATION

Acetaminophen in massive overdosage may cause hepatic toxicity in some patients. In adults and adolescents, hepatic toxicity has rarely been reported following ingestion of acute overdoses of less than 7.5 to 10 grams. Fatalities are infrequent (less than 3–4% of untreated cases) and have rarely been reported with overdoses of less than 15 grams. In children, an acute overdosage of less than 150 mg/kg has not been associated with hepatic toxicity.

Early symptoms following a potentially hepatotoxic overdose may include: nausea, vomiting, diaphoresis and general malaise. Clinical and laboratory evidence of hepatic toxicity may not be apparent until 48 to 72 hours postingestion. In adults and adolescents, regardless of the quantity of acetaminophen reported to have been ingested, administer acetylcysteine immediately if 24 hours or less have elapsed from the reported time of ingestion. For full prescribing information, refer to the acetylcysteine package insert. Do not await results of assays for plasma acetaminophen levels before initiating treatment with acetylcysteine. The following additional procedures are recommended: Promptly initiate gastric decontamination of the stomach. A plasma acetaminophen assay should be obtained as early as possible, but no sooner than four hours following ingestion. If plasma level falls above the lower treatment line on the acetaminophen overdose nomogram, acetylcysteine therapy should be continued. Liver function studies should be obtained initially and repeated at 24-hour intervals.

Serious toxicity or fatalities are extremely infrequent in children, possibly due to differences in the way they metabolize acetaminophen. In children, the maximum potential amount ingested can be more easily estimated. If more than 150 mg/kg or an unknown amount was ingested, obtain a plasma acetaminophen level. The plasma acetaminophen level should be obtained as soon as possible, but no sooner than 4 hours following ingestion. If plasma level falls above the lower treatment line on the acetaminophen overdose nomogram, the acetylcysteine therapy should be initiated and continued for a full course of therapy. If plasma acetaminophen assay capability is not available, and the estimated acetaminophen ingestion exceeds 150 mg/kg, acetylcysteine therapy should be initiated and continued for a full course of therapy.

For additional emergency information, call your regional poison center or call the Rocky Mountain Poison Center toll-free, (1-800-525-6115).

Symptoms from pseudoephedrine overdose consist most often of mild anxiety, tachycardia and/or mild hypertension. Symptoms usually appear within 4 to 8 hours of ingestion and are transient, usually requiring no treatment.

Acute dextromethorphan overdose usually does not result in serious signs and symptoms unless massive amounts have been ingested. Signs and symptoms of a substantial overdose may include nausea and vomiting, visual disturbances, CNS disturbances and urinary retention.

INACTIVE INGREDIENTS

Acesulfame Potassium, Citric Acid, Corn Syrup, Flavors, Polyethylene Glycol, Propylene Glycol, Purified Water, Red #40, Sodium Benzoate.

HOW SUPPLIED

Red-colored drops in bottles of ½ fl. oz.
Shown in Product Identification Guide, page 321

Junior Strength MOTRIN®   OTC
Ibuprofen Caplets and Chewable Tablets

DESCRIPTION

Each *Junior Strength MOTRIN® Ibuprofen Caplet or Chewable Tablet* contains 100 mg ibuprofen in an easy-to-swallow caplet (capsule shaped tablet) or orange-flavored chewable tablet.

INDICATIONS

Junior Strength MOTRIN® Ibuprofen Caplets and Junior Strength MOTRIN® Ibuprofen Chewable Tablets are indicated for temporary reduction of fever and relief of minor aches and pains due to colds, flu, sore throat, headaches and toothaches.

DIRECTIONS

Repeat dose every 6–8 hours if needed. Do not use more than 4 times a day. Under 6 (under 48 lbs), consult a physician. If possible, use weight to dose; otherwise use age. If stomach upset occurs while taking this product, give with food or milk.

Junior Strength MOTRIN® Ibuprofen Caplets and Chewable Tablets: 6–8 years (48–59 lbs): 2 caplets or tablets; 9–10 years (60–71 lbs): 2 1/2 caplets or tablets; 11 years (72–95 lbs): 3 caplets or tablets.

WARNINGS

ALLERGIC REACTIONS: Junior Strength Motrin may cause a severe allergic reaction which may include: wheezing (asthma), shortness of breath, hives, swelling of the face, fast, irregular pulse or heartbeat, changing color of the skin (shock).

ASPIRIN-SENSITIVE PATIENTS: Although Junior Strength Motrin does not contain aspirin, it may cause a severe reaction, similar to that listed above in people allergic to aspirin or other pain relievers/fever reducers.

Any of these reactions could be serious. Stop using this product and get emergency medical help immediately. These reactions can occur after taking a single dose or any subsequent dose in persons both with, and without, prior reaction to Junior Strength Motrin or other pain relievers/fever reducers.

CALL YOUR DOCTOR IF:
- Your child is under a doctor's care for any serious condition or is taking any other drug.
- Your child has problems or serious side effects from taking fever reducers or pain relievers.
- Your child does not get any relief within first day (24 hours) of treatment, or pain or fever gets worse.
- Stomach upset gets worse or lasts.
- Redness or swelling is present in the painful area.
- Sore throat is severe, lasts for more than 2 days or occurs with fever, headache, rash, nausea or vomiting.
- Any new symptoms appear.

DO NOT USE:
- With any other product that contains ibuprofen, or any other pain reliever/fever reducer, unless directed by a doctor.
- For more than **3 days** for fever or pain unless directed by a doctor.
- For stomach pain unless directed by a doctor.
- If your child is dehydrated (significant fluid loss) due to continued vomiting, diarrhea or lack of fluid intake.
- If blister unit is broken or open.

IMPORTANT:
Do not exceed recommended dose. Taking more than the recommended dose (overdose) may not provide more relief and could cause serious health problems. **Keep this and all drugs out of the reach of children. In case of accidental overdose, seek professional assistance or contact a poison control center immediately.**
NOTE: In addition to the above:
Junior Strength MOTRIN® Ibuprofen Chewable Tablets:
Phenylketonurics: Contains phenylalanine 6 mg per tablet.
WHEN USING THIS PRODUCT:
- Mouth or throat burning may occur; give with water or food.

PROFESSIONAL INFORMATION
OVERDOSAGE INFORMATION

The *toxicity of ibuprofen overdose* is dependent upon the amount of drug ingested and the time elapsed since ingestion, though individual response may vary, which makes it necessary to evaluate each case individually. Although uncommon, serious toxicity and death have been reported in the medical literature with ibuprofen overdosage. The most frequently reported symptoms of ibuprofen overdose include abdominal pain, nausea, vomiting, lethargy and drowsiness. Other central nervous system symptoms include headache, tinnitus, CNS depression and seizures. Metabolic acidosis, coma, acute renal failure and apnea (primarily in very young children) may rarely occur. Cardiovascular toxicity, including hypotension, bradycardia, tachycardia and atrial fibrillation, also have been reported.

The *treatment of acute ibuprofen overdose* is primarily supportive. Management of hypotension, acidosis and gastrointestinal bleeding may be necessary. In cases of acute overdose, the stomach should be emptied through ipecac-induced emesis or lavage. Emesis is most effective if initiated within 30 minutes of ingestion. Orally administered activated charcoal may help in reducing the absorption and reabsorption of ibuprofen.

In children, the estimated amount of ibuprofen ingested per body weight may be helpful to predict the potential for development of toxicity although each case must be evaluated. Ingestion of less than 100 mg/kg is unlikely to produce toxicity. Children ingesting 100 to 200 mg/kg may be managed with induced emesis and a minimal observation time of four hours. Children ingesting 200 to 400 mg/kg of ibuprofen should have immediate gastric emptying and at least four hours observation in a health care facility. Children ingesting greater than 400 mg/kg require immediate medical referral, careful observation and appropriate supportive therapy. Ipecac-induced emesis is not recommended in overdoses greater than 400 mg/kg because of the risk for convulsions and the potential for aspiration of gastric contents.

In adult patients the history of the dose reportedly ingested does not appear to be predictive of toxicity. The need for referral and follow-up must be judged by the circumstances at the time of the overdose ingestion. Symptomatic adults should be admitted to a health care facility for observation.

INACTIVE INGREDIENTS

Junior Strength MOTRIN® Ibuprofen Caplets: Carnauba wax, colloidal silicon dioxide, cornstarch, D&C Yellow #10, FD&C Yellow #6, hydroxypropyl methylcellulose, microcrystalline cellulose, polydextrose, polyethylene glycol, propylene glycol, sodium starch glycolate, titanium dioxide, triacetin.
Junior Strength MOTRIN® Ibuprofen Chewable Tablets: Aspartame, citric acid, FD&C Yellow # 6, natural and artificial flavors, hydroxyethyl cellulose, hydroxypropyl methylcellulose, magnesium stearate, mannitol, microcrystalline cellulose, povidone, sodium lauryl sulfate, sodium starch glycolate.

HOW SUPPLIED

Junior Strength MOTRIN® Ibuprofen Caplets: (white, imprinted "M 100" in orange) in blister packs of 24
Junior Strength MOTRIN® Ibuprofen Chewable Tablets: Orange-colored, round tablets available in blister packs of 24.
Store at room temperature 15°–30°C (59°–86°F).
Shown in Product Identification Guide, page 321

Junior Strength TYLENOL®   OTC
acetaminophen
Coated Caplets and Chewable Tablets

DESCRIPTION

Each *Junior Strength TYLENOL® Coated Caplet or Chewable Tablet* contains 160 mg acetaminophen in a small, coated, capsule shaped tablet or grape or fruit flavored chewable tablet.

ACTIONS

Acetaminophen is a clinically proven analgesic/antipyretic. Acetaminophen produces analgesia by elevation of the pain threshold and antipyresis through action on the hypothalamic heat-regulating center. Acetaminophen is equal to aspirin in analgesic and antipyretic effectiveness and it is unlikely to produce many of the side effects associated with aspirin and aspirin-containing products.

USES

Junior Strength TYLENOL® Caplets are designed for easy swallowability in older children and young adults. Both *Junior Strength TYLENOL® Caplets and Junior Strength TYLENOL® Chewable Tablets* provide fast, effective temporary relief of minor aches and pains associated with a cold, flu, headache, muscle aches, sprains, overexertion and for the reduction of fever.

PRECAUTIONS

If a rare sensitivity reaction occurs, the drug should be stopped.

DIRECTIONS

Caplets should be taken with liquid. Chewable tablets should be well chewed. All dosages may be repeated every 4 hours, if needed. Do not use more than 5 times a day. Under 6 years (under 48 lbs), consult a physician. *Junior Strength TYLENOL® Caplets and Chewable Tablets:* 6–8 years (48–59 lbs): 2 caplets or tablets; 9–10 years (60–71 lbs): 2 ¹/₂ caplets or tablets; 11 years (72–95 lbs): 3 caplets or tablets; 12 years (96 lbs and over): 4 caplets or tablets.

WARNINGS

Do not use if carton is opened or if blister unit is broken.
Do Not Use:
- with any other products containing acetaminophen.
- for more than 3 days for fever unless directed by a doctor.
- for more than 5 days for pain unless directed by a doctor.
Stop Using This Product and Ask a Doctor If:
- symptoms do not improve.
- new symptoms occur.
- pain or fever persists or gets worse.
- redness or swelling is present.
Do not exceed recommended dose. Taking more than the recommended dose (overdose) may not provide more relief and could cause serious health problems. Keep this and all drugs out of the reach of children. In case of accidental overdose, contact a physician or poison control center immediately. Prompt medical attention is critical even if you do not notice any signs or symptoms.
NOTE: In addition to the above: The Grape and Fruit Flavored Chewable Tablet packages state: Phenylketonurics:

Continued on next page

Junior Strength Tylenol—Cont.

Contains phenylalanine 6 mg per tablet. The caplet package states: Not for children who have difficulty swallowing tablets.

PROFESSIONAL INFORMATION

OVERDOSAGE INFORMATION

Acetaminophen in massive overdosage may cause hepatic toxicity in some patients. In adults and adolescents, hepatic toxicity has rarely been reported following ingestion of acute overdosage of less than 7.5 to 10 grams. Fatalities are infrequent (less than 3–4% of untreated cases) and have rarely been reported with overdoses of less than 15 grams. In children, an acute overdosage of less than 150 mg/kg has not been associated with hepatic toxicity.
Early symptoms following a potentially hepatotoxic overdose may include: nausea, vomiting, diaphoresis and general malaise. Clinical and laboratory evidence of hepatic toxicity may not be apparent until 48 to 72 hours postingestion.
In adults and adolescents, regardless of the quantity of acetaminophen reported to have been ingested, administer acetylcysteine immediately if 24 hours or less have elapsed from the reported time of ingestion. For full prescribing information, refer to the acetylcysteine package insert. Do not await the results of assays for acetaminophen levels before initiating treatment with acetylcysteine. The following additional procedures are recommended: Promptly initiate gastric decontamination of the stomach. A plasma acetaminophen assay should be obtained as early as possible, but no sooner than four hours following ingestion. If plasma level falls above the lower treatment line on the acetaminophen overdose nomogram, acetylcysteine therapy should be continued. Liver function studies should be obtained initially and repeated at 24-hour intervals.
Serious toxicity or fatalities are extremely infrequent in children, possibly due to differences in the way they metabolize acetaminophen. In children, the maximum potential amount ingested can be more easily estimated. If more than 150 mg/kg or an unknown amount was ingested, obtain a plasma acetaminophen level. The plasma acetaminophen level should be obtained as soon as possible, but no sooner than 4 hours following ingestion. If plasma level falls above the lower treatment line on the acetaminophen overdose nomogram, the acetylcysteine therapy should be initiated and continued for a full course of therapy. If plasma acetaminophen assay capability is not available, and the estimated acetaminophen ingestion exceeds 150 mg/kg, acetylcysteine therapy should be initiated and continued for a full course of therapy.
For additional emergency information, call your regional poison center or call the Rocky Mountain Poison Center toll-free, (1-800-525-6115).

INACTIVE INGREDIENTS

Junior Strength Caplets: Cellulose, Corn Starch, Ethylcellulose, Magnesium Stearate, Sodium Lauryl Sulfate, and Sodium Starch Glycolate.
Junior Strength Fruit Flavored Chewable Tablets: Aspartame, Cellulose, Citric Acid, Corn Starch, D&C Red #7, Flavors, Magnesium Stearate, and Mannitol. May contain Ethylcellulose or Cellulose Acetate and Povidone.
Junior Strength Grape Flavored Chewable Tablets: Aspartame, Cellulose, Citric Acid, Corn Starch, D&C Red #7, D&C Red #30, FD&C Blue #1, Flavors, Magnesium Stearate and Mannitol. May contain Ethylcellulose or Cellulose Acetate and Povidone.

HOW SUPPLIED

Coated Caplets, (colored white, coated, scored, imprinted "TYLENOL 160") Package of 30.
Chewable Tablets (colored purple or pink, imprinted "TYLENOL 160") Package of 24. All packages are safety sealed and use child resistant blister packaging.

Shown in Product Identification Guide, page 322

LACTAID® Drops OTC
(lactase enzyme)

DESCRIPTION

LACTAID® is the original dairy digestive supplement that makes milk more digestible. ***LACTAID®*** lactase enzyme hydrolyzes lactose into two digestible simple sugars: glucose and galactose. ***LACTAID® Drops*** are added to milk for *in vitro* hydrolysis of lactose.
LACTAID® Drops contain sufficient lactase enzyme (derived from *Kluyveromyces lactis*) to hydrolyze lactose in milk.

ACTIONS

LACTAID® Drops are a liquid form of the natural lactase enzyme that makes milk more digestible. The lactase enzyme hydrolyzes the lactose sugar (a double sugar) into its simple sugar components, glucose and galactose.

INDICATIONS

Lactose intolerance, suspected from gastrointestinal discomfort (ie; gas, bloating, cramps, and diarrhea) after drinking milk.

DIRECTIONS

LACTAID® Drops are a liquid form of the natural lactase enzyme that makes milk more digestible. To use, add ***LACTAID® Drops*** to a quart of milk, shake gently and refrigerate for 24 hours. We recommend starting with 5–7 drops per quart of milk but because sensitivity to lactose can vary, you may have to adjust the number of drops you use. If you are still experiencing discomfort after consuming milk with 5–7 ***LACTAID® Drops*** per quart, you may want to add 10 drops per quart or even 15 drops per quart. 15 drops per quart should remove nearly all of the lactose in the milk. Lactaid can be used with any kind of milk: whole, 1%, 2%, non-fat, skim, powdered and chocolate milk.

WARNINGS:

If you experience any symptoms which are unusual or seem unrelated to the condition for which you took this product, consult a doctor before taking any more of it. Do not use if carton is opened or if printed plastic bodywrap is broken.

INGREDIENTS

Glycerin, Water, Lactase Enzyme

HOW SUPPLIED

LACTAID® Drops are available in .22 fl. oz. (7 mL), (30 quart supply). Store at or below room temperature (below 77°F). Refrigerate after opening.
Lactaid Drops are certified kosher from the Orthodox Union.
Also available: 70% lactose reduced Lactaid Milk and 100% lactose-free Lactaid Milk.

Shown in Product Identification Guide, page 321

LACTAID® Original Strength Caplets OTC
(lactase enzyme)

LACTAID® Extra Strength Caplets
(lactase enzyme)

LACTAID® ULTRA Caplets
(lactase enzyme)

DESCRIPTION

Each ***LACTAID® Original Strength Caplet*** contains 3000 FCC (Food Chemical Codex) units of lactase enzyme (derived from *Aspergillus oryzae*).
Each ***LACTAID® Extra Strength Caplet*** contains 4500 FCC units of lactase enzyme (derived from *Aspergillus oryzae*).
Each ***LACTAID® ULTRA Caplet*** contains 9000 FCC units of lactase enzyme (derived from *Aspergillus oryzae*).
LACTAID® is the original lactase dietary supplement that makes milk and dairy foods more digestible. ***LACTAID®*** lactase enzyme hydrolyzes lactose into two digestible simple sugars: glucose and galactose. ***LACTAID® Caplets*** are taken orally for *in vivo* hydrolysis of lactose.

ACTIONS

LACTAID® Caplets work to naturally replenish lactase enzyme that aids in dairy food digestion. Lactase enzyme hydrolyzes lactose sugar (a double sugar) into its simple sugar components, glucose and galactose.

INDICATIONS

Lactose intolerance, suspected from gastrointestinal discomfort (ie, gas, bloating, flatulence, cramps, and diarrhea) after drinking milk or ingesting other dairy foods such as cheese and ice cream.

DIRECTIONS

These convenient, portable caplets are easy to swallow or chew and can be used with milk or any dairy food. **Original Strength:** Swallow or chew 3 caplets with the first bite of dairy food. For best results, you may have to adjust the number of caplets up or down. Take no more than 6 caplets at a time. **Extra Strength:** Swallow or chew 2 caplets with first bite of dairy food. For best results, you may have to adjust the number of caplets up or down. Take no more than 4 caplets at a time. **Ultra:** Swallow 1 caplet with the first bite of dairy food. For best results, you may have to adjust the number of caplets up or down. Take no more than 2 caplets at a time. Don't be discouraged if at first Lactaid does not work to your satisfaction. Because the degree of enzyme deficiency naturally varies from person to person and from food to food, you may have to adjust the number of caplets up or down to find your own level of comfort. Since Lactaid Caplets work only on the food as you eat it, use them every time you enjoy dairy foods.

WARNINGS

Consult your doctor: If you experience any symptoms which are unusual or seem unrelated to the condition for which you took this product. Do not use if carton is open or if printed plastic neckwrap is broken or if single serve packet is open.

INGREDIENTS

LACTAID® Original Strength Caplets: Mannitol, Cellulose, Lactase Enzyme (3,000 FCC Lactase units/Caplet), Magnesium Stearate, Dextrose, Sodium Citrate.
LACTAID® Extra Strength Caplets: Lactase Enzyme (4,500 FCC Lactase units/Caplet), Mannitol, Cellulose, Dextrose, Sodium Citrate, Magnesium Stearate.
LACTAID® ULTRA Caplets: Cellulose, Lactase Enzyme (9,000 FCC Lactase units/Caplet), Dextrose, Sodium Citrate, Magnesium Stearate, Colloidal Silicon Dioxide.

HOW SUPPLIED

LACTAID® Original Strength Caplets are available in bottles of 60, and 120 counts. ***LACTAID® Extra Strength Caplets*** are available in bottles of 24, and 50 counts. ***LACTAID® ULTRA Caplets*** are available in single serve packets of 12, 32 and 60 counts. Store at or below room temperature (below 77°F) but do not refrigerate. Keep away from heat.
LACTAID® Caplets are certified kosher from the Orthodox Union.
Also available: 70% lactose reduced Lactaid Milk and 100% lactose-free Lactaid Milk.

Shown in Product Identification Guide, page 321

MOTRIN® IB Pain Reliever Tablets, Caplets and Gelcaps OTC

DESCRIPTION

Each ***Motrin® IB Pain Reliever Tablet, Caplet and Gelcap*** contains ibuprofen 200 mg.

INDICATIONS

Motrin® IB Pain Reliever Tablets, Caplets and Gelcaps are indicated for the temporary relief of headache, muscular aches, the minor pain of arthritis, toothache, backache, minor aches and pains associated with the common cold, the pain of menstrual cramps, and for reduction of fever.

DIRECTIONS

Adults: Take 1 tablet, caplet or gelcap every 4 to 6 hours while symptoms persist. If pain or fever does not respond to 1 tablet, caplet or gelcap, 2 tablets, caplets or gelcaps may be used, but do not exceed 6 tablets, caplets or gelcaps in 24 hours, unless directed by a doctor. The smallest effective dose should be used. Take with food or milk if occasional and mild heartburn, upset stomach or stomach pain occurs with use. Consult a doctor if these symptoms are more than mild or if they persist. **Children:** Do not give this product to children under 12 except under the advice and supervision of a doctor.

WARNINGS

Do not take for pain for more than 10 days or for fever for more than 3 days unless directed by a doctor. If pain or fever persists or gets worse, if new symptoms occur, or if the painful area is red or swollen, consult a doctor. These could be signs of a serious illness. If you are under a doctor's care for any serious condition, consult a doctor before taking this product. As with aspirin and acetaminophen, if you have any condition which requires you to take prescription drugs, or if you have had any problems or serious side effects from taking any non-prescription pain reliever, do not take Motrin® IB without first discussing it with your doctor. If you experience any symptoms which are unusual or seem unrelated to the condition for which you took ibuprofen, consult a doctor before taking any more of it. Although ibuprofen is indicated for the same conditions as aspirin and acetaminophen, it should not be taken with them except under a doctor's direction. Do not combine this product with any other ibuprofen-containing product. **Do not exceed recommended dose.** Keep this and all drugs out of the reach of children. In case of accidental overdose, seek professional assistance or contact a poison control center immediately. As with any drug, if you are pregnant or nursing a baby, seek the advice of a health professional before using this product. IT IS ESPECIALLY IMPORTANT NOT TO USE IBUPROFEN DURING THE LAST 3 MONTHS OF PREGNANCY UNLESS SPECIFICALLY DIRECTED TO DO SO BY A DOCTOR BECAUSE IT MAY CAUSE PROBLEMS IN THE UNBORN CHILD OR COMPLICATIONS DURING DELIVERY.
ALLERGIC REACTIONS: Motrin® IB may cause a severe allergic reaction which may include: wheezing (asthma), shortness of breath, hives, swelling of the face, fast irregular pulse or heartbeat, changing color of the skin (shock).
ASPIRIN SENSITIVE PATIENTS: Although Motrin® IB does not contain aspirin, it may cause a severe reaction, similar to that listed above, in people allergic to aspirin or other pain relievers/fever reducers.
Any of these reactions could be serious. Stop using this product and get emergency help immediately.

These reactions can occur after taking a single dose or any subsequent dose in persons both with, and without, prior reaction to Motrin® IB or other pain relievers/fever reducers.

ALCOHOL WARNING

If you drink 3 or more alcoholic beverages daily, ask your doctor whether you should take Motrin® IB or other pain relievers. Motrin® IB may increase your risk of stomach bleeding.

Store at room temperature. Avoid excessive heat 40°C (104°F).

PROFESSIONAL INFORMATION

OVERDOSAGE INFORMATION

The *toxicity of ibuprofen overdose* is dependent upon the amount of drug ingested and the time elapsed since ingestion, though individual response may vary, which makes it necessary to evaluate each case individually. Although uncommon, serious toxicity and death have been reported in the medical literature with ibuprofen overdosage. The most frequently reported symptoms of ibuprofen overdose include abdominal pain, nausea, vomiting, lethargy and drowsiness. Other central nervous system symptoms include headache, tinnitus, CNS depression and seizures. Metabolic acidosis, coma, acute renal failure and apnea (primarily in very young children) may rarely occur. Cardiovascular toxicity, including hypotension, bradycardia, tachycardia and atrial fibrillation, also have been reported.

The *treatment of acute ibuprofen overdose* is primarily supportive. Management of hypotension, acidosis and gastrointestinal bleeding may be necessary. In cases of acute overdose, the stomach should be emptied through ipecac-induced emesis or lavage. Emesis is most effective if initiated within 30 minutes of ingestion. Orally administered activated charcoal may help in reducing the absorption and reabsorption of ibuprofen. In children, the estimated amount of ibuprofen ingested per body weight may be helpful to predict the potential for development of toxicity although each case must be evaluated. Ingestion of less than 100 mg/kg is unlikely to produce toxicity. Children ingesting 100 to 200 mg/kg may be managed with induced emesis and a minimal observation time of four hours. Children ingesting 200 to 400 mg/kg of ibuprofen should have immediate gastric emptying and at least four hours observation in a health care facility. Children ingesting greater than 400 mg/kg require immediate medical referral, careful observation and appropriate supportive therapy. Ipecac-induced emesis is not recommended in overdoses greater than 400 mg/kg because of the risk of convulsions and the potential for aspiration of gastric contents.

In adult patients the history of the dose reportedly ingested does not appear to be predictive of toxicity. The need for referral and follow-up must be judged by the circumstances at the time of the overdose ingestion. Symptomatic adults should be admitted to a health care facility for observation.

INACTIVE INGREDIENTS

Tablets and Caplets: Carnauba wax, cornstarch, hydroxypropyl methylcellulose, iron oxide black, pregelatanized starch, propylene glycol, silicon dioxide, stearic acid, titanium dioxide.

Gelcaps: Benzyl alcohol, butylparaben, butyl alcohol, castor oil, colloidal silicon dioxide, edetate calcium disodium, FDC Yellow No. 6, gelatin, hydroxypropyl methylcellulose, iron oxide black, magnesium stearate, methylparaben, microcrystalline cellulose, povidone, pregelatinized starch, propylene glycol, propylparaben, SDA 3A alcohol, sodium lauryl sulfate, sodium propionate, sodium starch glycolate, starch and titanium dioxide.

HOW SUPPLIED

Tablets: (white, printed "Motrin IB" in black) in tamper evident packaging of 24, 50, 100, 130, 135, and 165.

Caplets: (white, printed "Motrin IB" in black) in tamper evident packaging of 24, 50, 60, 100, 130, 135, 165, 250 and 500.

Gelcaps: (colored orange and white, printed "Motrin IB" in black) in tamper evident packaging of 24 and 50.

Shown in Product Identification Guide, page 321

MOTRIN® IB SINUS Pain Reliever/Fever Reducer/Nasal Decongestant Tablets and Caplets OTC

DESCRIPTION

Each ***Motrin® IB Sinus Tablet and Caplet*** contains ibuprofen 200 mg and pseudoephedrine HCl 30 mg

INDICATIONS

Motrin® IB Sinus Tablets and Caplets are indicated for the temporary relief of symptoms associated with sinusitis, the common cold or flu including nasal congestion, headache, body aches, pains and fever.

DIRECTIONS

Adults and children 12 years of age and older: Take 1 tablet or caplet every 4 to 6 hours while symptoms persist. If symptoms do not respond to 1 tablet or caplet, 2 tablets or caplets may be used but do not exceed 6 tablets or caplets in 24 hours, unless directed by a doctor. The smallest effective dose should be used. Take with food or milk if occasional and mild heartburn, upset stomach, or stomach pain occurs with use. Consult a doctor if these symptoms are more than mild or if they persist. Children: Do not give this product to children under 12 years of age except under the advice and supervision of a doctor.

WARNINGS

Do not take for more than 7 days. If symptoms do not improve or are accompanied by fever that persists for more than 3 days, or if new symptoms occur, consult a doctor. These could be signs of a serious illness. As with aspirin and acetaminophen, if you have any condition which requires you to take prescription drugs or if you have had any problems or serious side effects from taking any non-prescription pain reliever, do not take this product without first discussing it with your doctor. IF YOU EXPERIENCE ANY SYMPTOMS WHICH ARE UNUSUAL OR SEEM UNRELATED TO THE CONDITION FOR WHICH YOU TOOK THIS PRODUCT CONSULT A DOCTOR BEFORE TAKING ANY MORE OF IT. If you are under a doctor's care for any serious condition, consult a doctor before taking this product. **Do not exceed recommended dosage.** If nervousness, dizziness, or sleeplessness occur, discontinue use and consult a doctor. Do not take this product if you have heart disease, high blood pressure, thyroid disease, diabetes, or difficulty in urination due to enlargement of the prostate gland, unless directed by a doctor. Do not combine this product with other non-prescription pain relievers. Do not combine this product with any other ibuprofen-containing product. Keep this and all drugs out of the reach of children. In case of accidental overdose, seek professional assistance or contact a poison control center immediately.

As with any drug, if you are pregnant or nursing a baby, seek the advice of a health professional before using this product. IT IS ESPECIALLY IMPORTANT NOT TO USE THIS PRODUCT DURING THE LAST 3 MONTHS OF PREGNANCY UNLESS SPECIFICALLY DIRECTED TO DO SO BY A DOCTOR BECAUSE IT MAY CAUSE PROBLEMS IN THE UNBORN CHILD OR COMPLICATIONS DURING DELIVERY.

ALLERGIC REACTIONS: Motrin® IB Sinus may cause a severe allergic reaction which may include: wheezing (asthma), shortness of breath, hives, swelling of the face, fast, irregular pulse or heartbeat, changing color of the skin (shock).

ASPIRIN-SENSITIVE PATIENTS: Although Motrin® IB Sinus does not contain aspirin, it may cause a severe reaction, similar to that listed above, in people allergic to aspirin or other pain relievers/fever reducers. **Any of these reactions could be serious. Stop using this product and get emergency medical help immediately.** These reactions can occur after taking a single dose or any subsequent dose in persons both with, and without, prior reaction to Motrin® IB Sinus or other pain relievers/fever reducers.

Store at room temperature, 15–30°C (59–86°F).

ALCOHOL WARNING

If you drink 3 or more alcoholic beverages daily, ask your doctor whether you should take Motrin® IB Sinus or other pain relievers. Motrin® IB Sinus may increase your risk of stomach bleeding.

DRUG INTERACTION PRECAUTION

Do not use this product if you are now taking a prescription monoamine oxidase inhibitor (MAOI) (certain drugs for depression, psychiatric or emotional conditions, or Parkinson's disease), or for 2 weeks after stopping the MAOI drug. If you are uncertain whether your drug contains an MAOI, consult a health professional before taking this product.

PROFESSIONAL INFORMATION

OVERDOSAGE INFORMATION

The *toxicity of ibuprofen overdose* is dependent upon the amount of drug ingested and the time elapsed since ingestion, though individual response may vary, which makes it necessary to evaluate each case individually. Although uncommon, serious toxicity and death have been reported in the medical literature with ibuprofen overdosage. The most frequently reported symptoms of ibuprofen overdose include abdominal pain, nausea, vomiting, lethargy and drowsiness. Other central nervous system symptoms include headache, tinnitus, CNS depression and seizures. Metabolic acidosis, coma, acute renal failure and apnea (primarily in very young children) may rarely occur. Cardiovascular toxicity, including hypotension, bradycardia, tachycardia and atrial fibrillation, also have been reported.

The *treatment of acute ibuprofen overdose* is primarily supportive. Management of hypotension, acidosis and gastrointestinal bleeding may be necessary. In cases of acute overdose, the stomach should be emptied through ipecac-induced emesis or lavage. Emesis is most effective if initiated within 30 minutes of ingestion. Orally administered activated charcoal may help in reducing the absorption and reabsorption of ibuprofen. In children, the estimated amount of ibuprofen ingested per body weight may be helpful to predict the potential for development of toxicity although each case must be evaluated. Ingestion of less than 100 mg/kg is unlikely to produce toxicity. Children ingesting 100 to 200 mg/kg may be managed with induced emesis and a minimal observation time of four hours. Children ingesting 200 to 400 mg/kg of ibuprofen should have immediate gastric emptying and at least four hours observation in a health care facility. Children ingesting greater than 400 mg/kg require immediate medical referral, careful observation and appropriate supportive therapy. Ipecac-induced emesis is not recommended in overdoses greater than 400 mg/kg because of the risk of convulsions and the potential for aspiration of gastric contents.

In adult patients the history of the dose reportedly ingested does not appear to be predictive of toxicity. The need for referral and follow-up must be judged by the circumstances at the time of the overdose ingestion. Symptomatic adults should be admitted to a health care facility for observation. Symptoms from pseudoephedrine overdose consist most often of mild anxiety, tachycardia and/or hypertension. Symptoms usually appear within 4 to 8 hours of ingestion and are transient, usually requiring no treatment.

INACTIVE INGREDIENTS:

Tablets and Caplets: Cellulose, Corn Starch, Glyceryl Triacetate, Hydroxypropyl Methylcellulose, Silicon Dioxide, Sodium Lauryl Sulfate, Sodium Starch Glycolate, Stearic Acid, Titanium Dioxide, Red #40 Aluminum Lake.

HOW SUPPLIED

Tablets: (white, printed "Motrin IB Sinus" in orange) in blister packs of 20 and 30.

Caplets: (white, printed "Motrin IB Sinus" in orange) in blister packs of 20 and 30.

Shown in Product Identification Guide, page 321

MOTRIN® Ibuprofen Suspension ℞
100 mg/5 mL

MOTRIN® Ibuprofen Oral Drops ℞
40 mg/mL

MOTRIN® Ibuprofen Chewable Tablets ℞
50 mg and 100 mg

MOTRIN® Ibuprofen Caplets ℞
100 mg

DESCRIPTION

The active ingredient in MOTRIN is ibuprofen, which is a member of the propionic acid group of nonsteroidal anti-inflammatory drugs (NSAIDs). Ibuprofen is a racemic mixture of [+]S- and [−]R-enantiomers. It is a white to off-white crystalline powder, with a melting point of 74° to 77°C. It is practically insoluble in water (<0.1 mg/mL), but readily soluble in organic solvents such as ethanol and acetone. Ibuprofen has a pKa of 4.43 ± 0.03 and an n-octanol/water partition coefficient of 11.7 at pH 7.4. The chemical name for ibuprofen is (±)-2-(p-isobutylphenyl) propionic acid. The molecular weight of ibuprofen is 206.28. Its molecular formula is $C_{13}H_{18}O_2$ and it has the following structural formula:

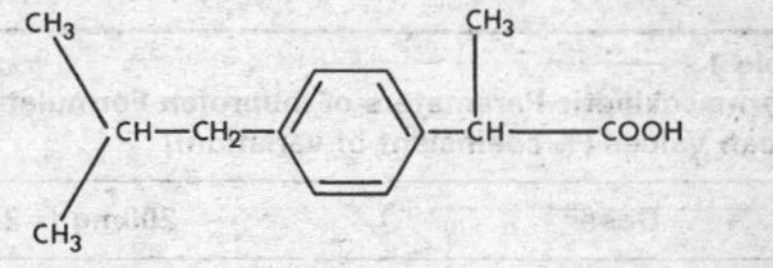

MOTRIN Suspension is a sucrose-sweetened, orange-colored, berry-flavored liquid suspension containing 100 mg of ibuprofen in 5 mL (20 mg/mL). Inactive ingredients include citric acid, glycerin, polysorbate 80, pregelatinized starch, purified water, sodium benzoate, sucrose, xanthan gum, D&C Yellow #10 and FD&C Red #40, and artificial flavors.

MOTRIN Oral Drops (intended for pediatric use only) is a sucrose-sweetened, pink-colored, berry-flavored liquid suspension containing 40 mg of ibuprofen per mL. Inactive ingredients include citric acid, glycerin, polysorbate 80, pregelatinized starch, purified water, sodium benzoate, sorbitol, sucrose, xanthan gum, FD&C Red #40, and artificial flavors.

MOTRIN Chewable Tablets are aspartame-sweetened, citrus-tasting, orange-colored tablets, that contain 50 mg or 100 mg of ibuprofen per tablet. Inactive ingredients include aspartame, citric acid, hydroxyethyl cellulose, hydroxypropyl methylcellulose, magnesium stearate, mannitol, micro-

Continued on next page

Motrin—Cont.

crystalline cellulose, povidone, sodium lauryl sulfate, sodium starch glycolate, FD&C Yellow #6, and artificial flavors.

MOTRIN Caplets are unsweetened, white-colored, unflavored, film-coated, capsule-shaped tablets, containing 100 mg of ibuprofen per tablet. Inactive ingredients include carnauba wax, colloidal silicone dioxide, cornstarch, hydroxypropyl methylcellulose, microcrystalline cellulose, polydextrose, polyethylene glycol, pregelatinized starch, propylene glycol, sodium starch glycolate, titanium dioxide, triacetin, D&C Yellow #10, and FD&C Yellow #6.

CLINICAL PHARMACOLOGY

Pharmacodynamics—Ibuprofen is a nonsteroidal anti-inflammatory drug (NSAID) that possesses anti-inflammatory, analgesic and antipyretic activity. Its mode of action, like that of other NSAIDs, is not completely understood, but may be related to prostaglandin synthetase inhibition. After absorption of the racemic ibuprofen, the [−]R-enantiomer undergoes interconversion to the [+]S-form. The biological activities of ibuprofen are associated with the [+]S-enantiomer.

In clinical studies in adult patients with rheumatoid arthritis and osteoarthritis, ibuprofen has been shown to be comparable to aspirin in controlling pain and inflammation, though causing fewer of the mild gastrointestinal side effects (see ADVERSE REACTIONS). MOTRIN may be well tolerated in some patients who have had gastrointestinal side effects with aspirin, but these patients, when treated with MOTRIN, should be carefully followed for signs and symptoms of gastrointestinal ulceration and bleeding. Although it is not definitely known whether ibuprofen causes less peptic ulceration than aspirin, in one study involving 885 adult patients with rheumatoid arthritis treated for up to one year (438 patients on ibuprofen and 447 patients on aspirin), there were no reports of gastric ulceration with ibuprofen whereas frank ulceration was reported in 13 patients in the aspirin group (statistically significant p<.001).

Gastroscopic studies at varying doses of ibuprofen showed an increased tendency toward endoscopic lesions at higher doses. However, at clinically comparable doses (2,400 mg of ibuprofen vs. 3,600 mg of aspirin), endoscopic lesions were approximately half that seen with aspirin. Studies using ^{51}Cr-tagged red cells indicate that fecal blood loss associated with ibuprofen in doses up to 2400 mg daily did not exceed the range of normal, and was significantly less than that seen in aspirin-treated patients. The clinical significance of these findings is unknown.

Pharmacokinetics—As noted in the DESCRIPTION section, ibuprofen is a racemic mixture of [−]R-and [+]S-isomers. *In vivo* and *in vitro* studies indicate that the [+]S-isomer is responsible for clinial activity. The [−]R-form, while thought to be pharmacologically inactive, is slowly and incompletely (60%) interconverted into the active [+]S species in adults. The degree of interconversion in children is unknown, but is thought to be similar. The [−]R-isomer serves as a circulating reservoir to maintain levels of active drug. Ibuprofen is well absorbed orally, with less than 1% being excreted in the urine unchanged. It has a biphasic elimination time curve with a plasma half-life of approximately 2 hours. Studies in febrile children have established the dose-proportionality of 5 and 10 mg/kg doses of ibuprofen. Studies in adults have established the dose-proportionality of ibuprofen as a single oral dose from 50 to 600 mg for total drug and up to 1200 mg for free drug.

Absorption—*In vivo* studies indicate that ibuprofen is well absorbed orally from the suspension, drops, caplet and chewable tablet formulations, with peak plasma levels usually occurring within 1 to 2 hours. The pharmacokinetic differences between the products in adults (see Table 1) are due to differences in the rate of absorption of ibuprofen from the various dosage forms. The observed differences in the table between adults and children, in terms of AUC and C_{max}, are due to both differences in dose per body weight and age-or fever-related change in volume of distribution (Vd/F). All of the formulations are equally bioavailable in terms of peak plasma levels (C_{max}) and extent of absorption (AUC), however, the time-to-peak (T_{max}) is different between the products. Clinically, this has been shown to have no effect on either onset or peak fever reduction in children.

[See table 1 below]

*Antacid—*A bioavailability study in adults has shown that there was no interference with the absorption of ibuprofen when given in conjunction with an antacid containing both aluminum hydroxide and magnesium hydroxide.

*Food Effects—*Absorption is most rapid when MOTRIN is given under fasting conditions. Administration of MOTRIN Suspension, MOTRIN Oral Drops, MOTRIN Chewable Tablets and MOTRIN Caplets with food affects the rate but not the extent of absorption. When taken with food, T_{max} is delayed by approximately 30 to 60 minutes, and peak levels are reduced by approximately 30 to 50%.

Distribution—Ibuprofen, like most other drugs of its class, is highly protein bound (>99% bound at 20 μg/mL). Protein binding is saturable and at concentrations >20 μg/mL binding is non-linear. Based on oral dosing data there is an age-or fever-related change in volume of distribution for ibuprofen. Febrile children <11 years old have a volume of approximately 0.2 L/kg while adults have a volume of approximately 0.12 L/kg. The clinical significance of these findings is unknown.

Metabolism—Following oral administration, the majority of the dose was recovered in the urine within 24 hours as the hydroxy-(25%) and carboxypropyl-(37%) phenylpropionic acid metabolites. The percentages of free and conjugated ibuprofen found in the urine were approximately 1% and 14%, respectively. The remainder of the drug was found in the stool as both metabolites and unabsorbed drug.

Elimination—Ibuprofen is rapidly metabolized and eliminated in the urine. The excretion of ibuprofen is virtually complete 24 hours after the last dose. It has a biphasic plasma elimination time curve with a half-life of approximately 2.0 hours. There is no difference in the observed terminal elimination rate or half-life between children and adults; however, there is an age-or fever-related change in total clearance. This suggests that the observed change in clearance is due to changes in the volume of distribution of ibuprofen (see Table 1 for Cl/F values).

Clinical Studies—Controlled clinical trials comparing doses of 5 and 10 mg/kg ibuprofen suspension and 10-15 mg/kg of acetaminophen elixir have been conducted in children 6 months to 12 years of age with fever primarily do to viral illnesses. In these studies there were no differences between treatment in fever reduction for the first hour and maximum fever reduction occurred between 2 and 4 hours. Response after 1 hour was dependent on both the level of temperature elevation as well as the treatment. In children with baseline temperatures at or below 102.5°F both ibuprofen doses and acetaminophen were equally effective in their maximum effect. In children with temperatures above 102.5°F, the ibuprofen 10 mg/kg dose was more effective. By 6 hours, children treated with ibuprofen 5mg/kg tended to have recurrence in fever, whereas children treated with ibuprofen 10 mg/kg still had significant fever reduction at 8 hours. In control groups treated with 10 mg/kg acetaminophen, fever reduction resembled that seen in children treated with 5 mg/kg of ibuprofen, with the exception that temperature elevation tended to return 1-2 hours earlier.

A comparison of MOTRIN Chewable Tablets and MOTRIN Suspension in febrile children showed similar antipyretic effects of the two formulations, lasting between 6 and 8 hours. No clinical studies of fever reduction in children have been performed with MOTRIN Caplets or MOTRIN Oral Drops.

Controlled single-dose clinical analgesia trials comparing doses of 5 and 10 mg/kg ibuprofen suspension with acetaminophen suspension 12.5 mg/kg and placebo, have been conducted in children 5 to 12 years of age, with sore throat pain due to an infectious agent, or ear pain due to acute otitis media. Onset of pain relief provided by ibuprofen was similar to that of acetaminophen, occurring within the first hour, usually around the half-hour mark. All active treatments showed significant pain relief verus placebo, and the 10 mg/kg dose of ibuprofen had a duration of analgesic effect of 6 to 8 hours. Ibuprofen 10 mg/kg provided more overall pain relief than the 5 mg/kg dose.

Controlled studies have demonstrated that ibuprofen is a more effective analgesic than propoxyphene for the relief of episiotomy pain, pain following dental extraction procedures, and for the relief of the symptoms of primary dysmenorrhea.

In patients with primary dysmenorrhea, ibuprofen has been shown to reduce elevated levels of prostaglandin activity in the menstrual fluid and to reduce resting and active intrauterine pressure, as well as the frequency of uterine contractions. The probable mechanism of action is to inhibit prostaglandin synthesis rather than simply to provide analgesia.

In clinical studies in adult patients with rheumatoid arthritis, ibuprofen has been shown to be comparable to indomethacin in controlling the signs and symptoms of disease activity, with a lower incidence of milder gastrointestinal and CNS side effects than indomethacin.

MOTRIN may be used in combination with gold salts and/or corticosteroids.

INDICATIONS AND USAGE

In Children

MOTRIN is indicated:

- For the reduction of fever in patients aged 6 months and older.
- For relief of mild to moderate pain in patients aged 6 months and older.
- For relief of signs and symptoms of juvenille arthritis.

In Adults

MOTRIN is indicated:

- For relief of mild to moderate pain.
- For treatment of primary dysmenorrhea.
- For relief of the signs and symptoms of rheumatoid arthritis and osteoarthritis.

Since there have been no controlled trials to demonstrate whether there is any beneficial effect or harmful interaction with the use of ibuprofen in conjuction with aspirin, the combination cannot be recommended (see PRECAUTIONS—Drug Interactions).

CONTRAINDICATIONS

MOTRIN should not be used in patients with previously demonstrated hypersensitivity to ibuprofen, or in individuals with a history of allergic manifestations to aspirin or other NSAIDs. Severe anaphylactic-like reactions to ibuprofen have been reported in such patients, some with fatal outcome.

WARNINGS

Risk of GI Ulceration, Bleeding and Perforation with NSAID Therapy. Serious gastrointestinal toxicity such as bleeding, ulceration, and perforation, can occur at any time, with or without warning symptoms, in patients treated chronically with NSAID therapy. Although minor upper gastrointestinal problems, such as dyspepsia, are common, usually developing early in therapy, physicians should remain alert for ulceration and bleeding in patients treated chronically with NSAIDs even in the absence of previous GI tract symptoms. In patients observed in clinical trials of several months to two years duration, symptomatic upper GI ulcers, gross bleeding or perforation appear to occur in approximately 1% of patients treated for 3–6 months, and in about 2–4% of patients treated for one year. Physicians should inform patients about the signs and/or symptoms of serious GI toxicity and what steps to take if they occur.

Studies to date have not identified any subset of patients not at risk of developing peptic ulceration and bleeding. Except for a prior history of serious GI events and other risk factors known to be associated with peptic ulcer disease, such as alcoholism, smoking, etc., no risk factors (e.g., age, sex) have been associated with increased risk. Elderly or debilitated patients seem to tolerate ulceration or bleeding less well than other individuals and most spontaneous reports of fatal GI events are in this population. Studies to date are inconclusive concerning the relative risk of various NSAIDs in causing such reactions. High doses of any NSAID probably carry a greater risk of these reactions, al-

Table 1
Pharmacokinetic Parameters of Ibuprofen Formulations
[Mean Values (% coefficient of variation)]

Dose	200mg (=2.8 mg/kg) in Adults				10 mg/kg in Febrile Children	
Formulation	Suspension	Drops	Caplet	Chewable Tablet	Suspension	Chewable Tablet
Number of Patients	24	24	25	24	18	18
AUCinf (μg·h/mL)	64 (27%)	74 (19%)	60 (19%)	66 (22%)	155 (24%)	176 (25%)
Cmax (μg/mL)	19 (22%)	24 (21%)	20 (18%)	15 (24%)	55 (23%)	43 (39%)
Tmax (h)	0.79 (69%)	1.0 (60%)	1.04 (50%)	2.0 (56%)	0.97 (57%)	1.43 (69%)
Cl/F (mL/h/kg)	45.6 (22%)	43.4 (18%)	45.0 (19%)	42.8 (18%)	68.6 (22%)	60.9 (27%)

Legend: AUCinf = Area-under-the-curve to infinity
Tmax = Time-to-peak plasma concentration
Cmax = Peak plasma concentration
Cl/F = Clearance divided by fraction at drug absorbed

though controlled clinical trials showing this do not exist in most cases. In considering the use of relatively large doses (within the recommended dosage range), sufficient benefit should be anticipated to offset the potential increased risk of GI toxicity.

Anaphylactoid Reactions: Anaphylactoid reactions may occur even in patients without prior exposure to ibuprofen. Extreme caution should be exercised when giving MOTRIN to patients with bronchospastic reactivity (e.g., asthma), nasal polyps, or those with a history of angiodema. Emergency help should be sought in case such anaphylactoid reaction occurs.

Advanced Renal Disease: In cases with advanced kidney disease, treatment with MOTRIN should not be initiated; if MOTRIN is used in such cases, close monitoring of the patient's kidney functions is advisable (see PRECAUTIONS—Renal Effects).

PRECAUTIONS

Renal Effects: Caution should be used when initiating treatment with MOTRIN in patients with considerable dehydration. It is advisable to rehydrate patients first and then start therapy with MOTRIN. Caution is also recommended in patients with pre-existing kidney disease (see WARNINGS—Advanced Renal Disease).

As with other NSAIDs, long-term administration of ibuprofen to animals has resulted in renal papillary necrosis and other abnormal renal pathology. In humans, there have been reports of acute interstitial nephritis with hematuria, proteinuria, and occasionally nephrotic syndrome.

A second form of renal toxicity has been seen in patients with prerenal conditions leading to a reduction in renal blood flow or blood volume, where the renal prostaglandins have a supportive role in the maintenance of renal perfusion. In these patients, administration of an NSAID may cause a dose-dependent reduction in prostaglandin formation and may precipitate overt renal decompensation. Patients at greatest risk of this reaction are those with impaired renal function, heart failure, liver dysfunction, those taking diuretics and the elderly. Discontinuation of NSAID therapy is typically followed by recovery to the pre-treatment state.

Those patients at high risk, who chronically take ibuprofen, should have renal function monitored if they have signs or symptoms which may be consistent with mild azotemia, such as malaise, fatigue, loss of appetite, etc. Occasional patients may develop some elevation of serum creatinine and BUN levels without signs or symptoms.

Since ibuprofen is eliminated primarily by the kidneys, patients with significantly impaired renal function should be closely monitored and a reduction in dosage should be anticipated to avoid drug accumulation. Prospective studies on the safety of ibuprofen in patients with chronic renal failure have not been conducted.

Fluid Retention: Fluid retention and edema have been reported in association with ibuprofen, therefore, the drug should be used with caution in patients with a history of cardiac decompensation or hypertension.

Hematologic Effects: MOTRIN can inhibit platelet aggregation but, unlike aspirin, its effect on platelet function is reversible, quantitatively less, and of shorter duration. Because this prolonged bleeding effect may be exaggerated in patients with underlying hemostatic defects, MOTRIN should be used with caution in persons with intrinsic coagulation defects and those on anticoagulant therapy.

Hepatic Effects: As with other nonsteroidal anti-inflammatory drugs, borderline elevations of one or more liver laboratory tests may occur in up to 15% of patients. These abnormalities may progress, may remain essentially unchanged, or may be transient with continued therapy. The ALT (SGPT) test is probably the most sensitive indicator of liver dysfunction. Meaningful (3 times the upper limit of normal) elevations of ALT and AST (SGOT) occurred in controlled clinical trials in less than 1% of patients. A patient with symptoms and/or signs suggesting liver dysfunction, or in whom an abnormal liver test has occurred, should be evaluated for evidence of the development of more severe hepatic reactions while on therapy with MOTRIN. Severe hepatic reactions, including jaundice and cases of fatal hepatitis, have been reported with ibuprofen as with other nonsteroidal anti-inflammatory drugs. Although such reactions are rare, if abnormal liver tests persist or worsen, if clinical signs and symptoms consistent with liver disease develop, or if systemic manifestations occur (e.g., eosinophilia, rash, etc.), treatment with MOTRIN should be discontinued.

Aseptic Meningitis: Aseptic meningitis, with fever and coma, has been observed on rare occasions in patients on ibuprofen therapy. Although it is probably more likely to occur in patients with systemic lupus erythematosus and related connective tissue diseases, it has been reported in patients who do not have an underlying chronic disease. If signs or symptoms of meningitis develop in a patient receiving MOTRIN, the possibility of its being related to ibuprofen should be considered.

Other Precautions—The pharmacological activity of MOTRIN may induce fever reduction and inflammation, thus diminishing their utility as diagnostic signs in detecting underlying conditions.

In order to avoid exacerbation of manifestations of adrenal insufficiency, patients who have been on prolonged corticosteroid therapy should have their therapy tapered slowly rather than discontinued abruptly when ibuprofen is added to the treatment program.

Blurred and/or diminished vision, scotomata, and/or changes in color vision have been reported. If a patient develops such complaints while receiving MOTRIN Chewable Tablets, the drug should be discontinued and the patient should have an ophthalmologic examination which includes central visual fields and color vision testing.

Phenylketonurics: MOTRIN Chewable Tablets 50 mg contain phenylalanine 3 mg per tablet, and the 100 mg tablets contain phenylalanine 6 mg per tablet.

Diabetics: MOTRIN Suspension and MOTRIN Oral Drops contain 0.3 g sucrose and 1.6 calories per mL, or 1.5 g sucrose and 8 calories per teaspoon, which should be taken into consideration when treating diabetic patients with this product.

Information for Patients—MOTRIN, like other drugs of its class, is not free of side effects. The side effects of these drugs can cause discomfort and, rarely, there are more serious side effects, such as gastrointestinal bleeding, which may result in hospitalization and even fatal outcomes.

NSAIDs are often essential agents in the management of arthritis, pain and fever, but they also may be commonly employed for conditions which are less serious.

Physicians may wish to discuss with their patients the potential risks (see WARNINGS, PRECAUTIONS, and ADVERSE REACTIONS) and likely benefits of NSAID treatment, particularly when the drugs are used for less serious conditions where treatment without NSAIDs may represent an acceptable alternative to both the patient and physician.

Patients on MOTRIN should report to their physicians signs or symptoms of gastrointestinal ulceration or bleeding, blurred vision or other eye symptoms, skin rash, weight gain, or edema.

Because serious GI tract ulceration and bleeding can occur without warning symptoms, physicians should follow chronically treated patients for the signs and symptoms of ulceration and bleeding and should inform them of the importance of this follow-up (see WARNINGS).

Patients should also be instructed to seek medical emergency help in case of an occurrence of an anaphylactoid reaction (see WARNINGS).

LABORATORY TESTS

Hemoglobin Levels: In cross-study comparisons, in adults, with doses ranging from 1200 mg to 3200 mg daily for several weeks, a slight dose-response decrease in hemoglobin/hematocrit was noted. This has been observed with other nonsteroidal anit-inflammatory drugs; the mechanism is unknown. However, even with daily doses of 3200 mg, the total decrease in hemoglobin usually does not exceed 1 g/dL; if there are no signs of bleeding, it is probably not clinically important.

In two postmarketing clinical studies with ibuprofen, the incidence of a decreased hemoglobin level was greater than previously reported. Decrease in hemoglobin of 1 g/dL or more was observed in 17.1% of 193 patients on 1600 mg ibuprofen daily (osteoarthritis), and 22.8% of 189 patients taking 2400mg of ibuprofen daily (rheumatoid arthritis). Positive stool occult blood tests and elevated serum creatinine levels were also observed in these studies.

DRUG INTERACTIONS

Coumarin-type anticoagulants: Several short-term controlled studies failed to show that iburprofen significantly affected prothrombin times or a variety of other clotting factors administered to individuals on coumarin-type anticoagulants. Because bleeding has been reported when ibuprofen and other nonsteroidal anti-inflammatory agents have been administered to patients on coumarin-type anticoagulants, the physician should be cautious when administering MOTRIN to patients on anticoagulants.

Aspirin: Animal studies show that aspirin given with NSAIDs, including ibuprofen, yields a net decrease in anti-inflammatory activity with lowered blood levels of the non-aspirin drug. Single-dose bioavailability studies in normal volunteers have failed to show an effect of aspirin on ibuprofen blood levels. Correlative clinical studies have not been done.

Methotrexate: Ibuprofen, as well as other NSAIDs, has been reported to competitively inhibit methotrexate accumulation in rabbit kidney slices. This may indicate that ibuprofen could enhance the toxicity of methotrexate. Caution should be used, therefore, if MOTRIN is administered concomitantly with methotrexate.

H-2 Antagonists: In studies with human volunteers, coadministration of cimetidine or ranitidine with ibuprofen had no substantive effect on ibuprofen serum concentrations.

ACE-inhibitors: Reports suggest that NSAIDs, including ibuprofen, may diminish the antihypertensive effect of ACE-inhibitors. This interaction should be given consideration in patients taking MOTRIN concomitantly with ACE-inhibitors.

Furosemide: Clinical studies, as well as random observations, have shown that ibuprofen can reduce the natriuretic effect of furosemide and thiazides in some patients. This response has been attributed to inhibition of renal prostaglandin synthesis. During concomitant therapy with MOTRIN, the patient should be observed closely for signs of renal failure (see PRECAUTIONS, Renal Effects), as well as to assure diuretic efficacy.

Lithium: Ibuprofen produced an elevation of plasma lithium levels and a reduction in renal lithium clearance in a study of eleven normal volunteers. The mean minimum lithium concentration increased 15% and the renal clearance of lithium was decreased by 19% during this period of concomitant drug administration. This effect has been attributed to inhibition of renal prostaglandin synthesis by ibuprofen. Thus, when MOTRIN and lithium are administered concurrently, subjects should be observed carefully for signs of lithium toxicity. (Read circulars for lithium preparation before use of such concurrent therapy.)

Teratogenic Effects—Pregnancy Category B: Reproductive studies conducted in rats and rabbits at doses somewhat less than the maximal clinical dose did not demonstrate evidence of developmental abnormalities. However, animal reproduction studies are not always predictive of human response. As there are no adequate and well-controlled studies in pregnant women, this drug should be used during pregnancy only if clearly needed. Because of the known effects of nonsteroidal anti-inflammatory drugs on the fetal cardiovascular system (closure of ductus arteriosus), use during late pregnancy should be avoided. Administration of MOTRIN is not recommended during pregnancy.

Labor and Delivery: As with other drugs known to inhibit prostaglandin synthesis, an increased incidence of dystocia and delayed parturition occurred in rats. Administration of MOTRIN is not recommended during labor and delivery.

Nursing Mothers: In limited studies, an assay capable of detecting 1 µg/mL did not demonstrate ibuprofen in the milk of lactating mothers. Because of the limited nature of these studies, however, and the possible adverse effects of prostaglandin inhibiting drugs on neonates, MOTRIN is not recommended for use in nursing mothers.

Pediatric Use: Safety and efficacy of MOTRIN in children below the age of 6 months has not been established (see CLINICAL PHARMACOLOGY-Clinical Studies). There is no evidence of age-dependent kinetics in patients 2 to 11 years old (see CLINICAL PHARMACOLOGY-Pharmacokinetics). Dosing of MOTRIN in children 6 months or older should be guided by their body weight (see DOSAGE AND ADMINISTRATION).

ADVERSE REACTIONS

The most frequent type of adverse reaction occurring with ibuprofen is gastrointestinal. In controlled clinical trials, the percentage of adult patients reporting one or more gastrointestinal complaints ranged from 4% to 16%.

In controlled studies in adults, when ibuprofen was compared to aspirin and indomethacin in equally effective doses, the overall incidence of gastrointestinal complaints was about half that seen in either the aspirin- or indomethacin-treated patients.

Adverse reactions observed during controlled clinical trials in adults at an incidence greater than 1% are listed in the chart. Those reactions listed under the heading "Incidence Greater than 1% (but less than 3%) Probable Causal Relationship," encompass observations in approximately 3,000 patients. More than 500 of these patients were treated for periods of at least 54 weeks.

Still other reactions, occurring less frequently than 1 in 100, were reported in controlled clinical trials and from marketing experience. These reactions have been divided into two categories: "Incidence less than 1%—Probable Causal Relationships," lists reactions with Ibuprofen therapy for which the probability of a causal relationship exists; this category was completed over time with postmarketing serious adverse reactions. "Incidence less than 1% —Causal Relationship Unknown," lists reactions with ibuprofen therapy for which a causal relationship has not been established, but are presented as alerting information for physicians.

INCIDENCE OF 1% OR GREATER

Probable Causal Relationship

*Incidence between 3 and 9%=ADR marked with**

Incidence between 1 and <3%=unmarked ADR

Cardiovascular system: Edema, fluid retention (generally responds promptly to drug discontinuation) (See PRECAUTIONS).

Digestive system: Nausea*, epigastric pain*, heartburn*, diarrhea, abdominal distress, nausea and vomiting, indigestion, constipation, abdominal cramps or pain, fullness of Gl tract (bloating and flatulence).

Nervous system: Dizziness*, headache, nervousness.

Skin and appendages: Rash* (including maculopapular type), pruritus

Specal senses: Tinnitus.

Continued on next page

Motrin—Cont.

INCIDENCE LESS THAN 1%

Probable Causal Relationship: The following adverse reactions were reported in clinical trials at an incidence of less than 1%, or were reported from postmarketing or foreign experience. The probability exists between the drug and these adverse reactions.

Body as a whole: Anaphylaxis and anaphylactoid reactions (see WARNINGS).

Cardiovascular system: Cerebrovascular accident, hypotension, congestive heart failure in patients with marginal cardiac function, elevated blood pressure, palpitations.

Digestive system: Gastric or duodenal ulcer with bleeding and/or perforation, gastrointestinal hemorrhage, pancreatitis, melena, gastritis, duodenitis, esophagitis, hematemesis, hepatorenal syndrome, liver necrosis, liver failure, hepatitis, jaundice, abnormal liver tests.

Hematologic system: Neutropenia, agranulocytosis, aplastic anemia, hemolytic anemia (sometimes Coombs positive), thrombocytopenia with or without purpura, eosinophilia, decrease in hemoglobin and hematocrit (see PRECAUTIONS), pancytopenia.

Nervous system: Depression, insomia, confusion, emotional liability, somnolence, convulsions, aseptic meningitis with fever and coma (see PRECAUTIONS).

Respiratory: Bronchospasm, dyspnea, apnea.

Skin and appendages: Vesiculobullous eruptions, urticaria, erythema multiforme, Stevens-Johnson syndrome, alopecia, exfoliative dermatitis, Lyell's syndrome (toxic epidermal necrolysis), photosensitivity reactions.

Special senses: Hearing loss, amblyopia (blurred and/or diminished vision, scotomata and/or changes in color vision) (see PRECAUTIONS—Other Precautions).

Urogenital system: Acute renal failure in patients with pre-existing significantly impaired renal function (see PRECAUTIONS), renal papillary necrosis, tubular necrosis, glomerulitis, decreased creatinine clearance, polyuria, azotemia, cystitis, hematuria.

Miscellaneous: Dry eyes and mouth, gingival ulcer, rhinitis.

INCIDENCE LESS THAN 1%

Causal Relationship Unknown: The following adverse reactions occurred at an incidence of less than 1% in clinical trials, or were suggested by marketing experience under circumstances where a causal relationship could not be definitely established. They are listed as alerting information for the physician.

Allergic: Serum sickness, lupus erythematosus syndrome, Henoch-Schönlein vasculitis, angioedema.

Cardivascular system: Arrhythmias (sinus tachycardia, sinus bradycardia).

Hematologic system: Bleeding episodes (e.g., epistaxis, menorrhagia).

Metabolic/endocrine: Gynecomastia, hypoglycemic reaction, acidosis.

Nervous system: Paresthesias, hallucinations, dream abnormalities, pseudo-tumor cerebri.

Special senses: Conjunctivitis, diplopia, optic neuritis, cataracts.

OVERDOSAGE

The *toxicity of ibuprofen overdose* is dependent upon the amount of drug ingested and the time elapsed since ingestion, though individual response may vary, which makes it necessary to evaluate each case individually. Although uncommon, serious toxicity and death have been reported in the medical literature with ibuprofen overdosage. The most frequently reported symptoms of ibuprofen overdose include abdominal pain, nausea, vomiting, lethargy and drowsiness. Other central nervous system symptoms include headache, tinnitus, CNS depression and seizures. Metabolic acidosis, coma, acute renal failure and apnea (primarily in very young children) may rarely occur. Cardiovascular toxicity, including hypotension, bradycardia, tachycardia and atrial fibrillation, also have been reported.

The *treatment of acute ibuprofen overdose* is primarily supportive. Management hypotension acidosis and gastrointestinal bleeding may be necessary. In cases of acute overdose, the stomach should be emptied through ipecac-induced emesis or lavage. Emesis is most effective if initiated within 30 mintues of ingestion. Orally administered activated charcoal may help in reducing the absorption and reabsorption of ibuprofen.

In children, the estimated amount of ibuprofen ingested per body weight may be helpful to predict the potential for development of toxicity although each case must be evaluated. Ingestion of less than 100 mg/kg is unlikely to produce toxicity. Children ingesting 100 to 200 mg/kg may be managed with induced emesis and a minimal observation time of four hours. Children ingesting 200 to 400 mg/kg of ibuprofen should have immediate gastric emptying and at least four hours observation in a health care facility. Children ingesting greater than 400 mg/kg require immediate medical referral, careful observation and appropriate supportive therapy. Ipecac-induced emesis is not recommended in overdoses greater than 400 mg/kg because of the risk for convulsions and the potential for aspiration of gastric contents.

In adult patients the history of the dose reportedly ingested does not appear to be predictive of toxicity. The need for referral and follow-up must be judged by the circumstances at the time of the overdose ingestion. Symptomatic adults should be admitted to a health care facility for observation.

DOSAGE AND ADMINISTRATION

CHILDREN

Fever reduction: For reduction of fever in children, 6 months to 12 years of age, the dosage should be adjusted on the basis of the initial temperature level (see CLINICAL PHARMACOLOGY). The recommended dose is 5 mg/kg if the baseline temperature is less than 102.5°F, or 10 mg/kg if the baseline temperature is 102.5°F or greater. The duration of fever reduction is generally 6 to 8 hours. The recommended maximum daily dose is 40 mg/kg.

Analgesia: For relief of mild to moderate pain in children, 6 months to 12 years of age, the recommended dosage is 10 mg/kg, every 6 to 8 hours. The recommended maximum daily dose is 40 mg/kg. Doses should be given so as not to disturb the child's sleep pattern. Taking fluids after chewing MOTRIN Chewable Tablets may help to promote absorption of the drug (see CLINICAL PHARMACOLOGY—Pharmacokinetics, and "Individualization of Dosage" in this section).

Juvenile Arthritis: The recommended dose is 30 to 40 mg/kg/day divided into three to four doses (see Individualization of Dosage). Patients with milder disease may be adequately treated with 20 mg/kg/day.

ADULTS

Analgesia: 400 mg every 4 to 6 hours as necessary for the relief of mild to moderate pain in adults. In controlled analgesic clincial trials, doses of MOTRIN greater than 400 mg were no more effective than the 400 mg dose.

Primary Dysmenorrhea: For the treatment of primary dysmenorrhea, beginning with the earliest onset of such pain, MOTRIN should be given in a dose of 400 mg every 4 hours, as necessary, for the relief of pain.

Rheumatoid arthritis and osteoarthritis, including flare-ups of chronic disease: Suggested dosage: 1200-3200 mg daily (300 mg q.i.d or 400 mg, 600 mg or 800 mg t.i.d. or q.i.d). Individual patients may show a better response to 3200 mg daily, as compared with 2400 mg, although in well-controlled clinical trials patients on 3200 mg did not show a better mean response in terms of efficacy. Therefore, when treating patients with 3200 mg/day, the physician should observe sufficient increased clincial benefits to offset potential increased risk.

Individualization of Dosage The dose of MOTRIN should be tailored to each patient, and may be lowered or raised from the suggested doses depending on the severity of symptoms either at time of initiating drug therapy or as the patient responds or fails to respond.

One fever study showed that, after the initial dose of MOTRIN, subsequent doses may be lowered and still provide adequate fever control.

In a situation when low fever would require the MOTRIN 5 mg/kg dose in a child with pain, the dose that will effectively treat the predominant symptom should be chosen.

In chronic conditions, a therapeutic response to MOTRIN therapy is sometimes seen in a few days to a week, but most often is observed by two weeks. After a satisfactory response has been achieved, the patient's dose should be reviewed and adjusted as required.

In patients with juvenile arthritis, doses above 50 mg/kg/day are not recommended because they have not been studied and doses exceeding the upper recommended dose of 40 mg/kg/day may increase the risk of causing serious adverse events. The therapeutic response may require from a few days to several weeks to be achieved. Once a clincial effect is obtained, the dosage should be lowered to the smallest dose of MOTRIN needed to maintain adequate control of symptoms.

In general, patients with rheumatoid arthritis seem to require higher doses than do patients with osteoarthritis. The smallest dose of MOTRIN that yields acceptable control should be employed.

HOW SUPPLIED

MOTRIN® (ibuprofen) Suspension 100 mg/5 mL

Orange-colored, berry-flavored suspension

–Bottles of 120 mL—NDC 0045-0448-04

–Bottles of 480 mL—NDC 0045-0448-16

Shake well before using. Store at controlled room temperature [15° to 30°C (59° to 86°F)]

MOTRIN® (ibuprofen) Oral Drops, 40mg/mL

(intended for pediatric use only)

Pink-colored, berry flavored suspension

–Bottles of 15 ml—NDC 0045-0446-15

Shake well before using. Store at controlled room temperature [15° to 30°C (59° to 86°F)].

MOTRIN® (ibuprofen) Chewable Tablets, 50 mg

Round, orange-colored, citrus-tasting, scored tablet, debossed "MOTRIN 50"

–Bottles of 100 Chewable Tablets—NDC 0045-0361-10

Store at controlled room temperature [15° to 30°C (59° to 86°F)]

MOTRIN® (ibuprofen) Chewable Tablets, 100 mg

Round, orange-colored, citrus-tasting, scored tablet, debossed "MOTRIN 100"

–Bottles of 100 Chewable Tablets—NDC 0045-0431-10

Store at controlled room temperature [15° to 30°C (59° to 86°F)]

MOTRIN® (ibuprofen) Caplets, 100 mg

White-colored, scored capsule-shaped tablet, imprinted "M 100"

–Bottles of 100 Caplets—NDC 0045-0445-10

Store at controlled room temperature [15° to 30°C (59° to 86°F)]

Caution: Federal Law prohibits dispensing without prescription.

McNEIL CONSUMER PRODUCTS CO.
DIVISION OF McNEIL-PPC, INC.
FORT WASHINGTON, PA 19034-USA
DECEMBER 1994

Shown in Product Identification Guide, page 321

NICOTROL® INHALER ℞

(nicotine inhalation system) 10 mg/cartridge (4 mg delivered)

DESCRIPTION

NICOTROL® Inhaler (nicotine inhalation system) consists of a mouthpiece and a plastic cartridge delivering 4 mg of nicotine from a porous plug containing 10 mg nicotine. The cartridge is inserted into the mouthpiece prior to use.

Nicotine is a tertiary amine composed of a pyridine and a pyrrolidine ring. It is a colorless to pale yellow, freely water-soluble, strongly alkaline, oily, volatile, hygroscopic liquid obtained from the tobacco plant. Nicotine has a characteristic pungent odor and turns brown on exposure to air or light. Of its two stereoisomers, S(-)nicotine is the more active. It is the prevalent form in tobacco, and is the form in the NICOTROL Inhaler. The free alkaloid is absorbed rapidly through the skin, mucous membranes, and respiratory tract.

Structural formula:

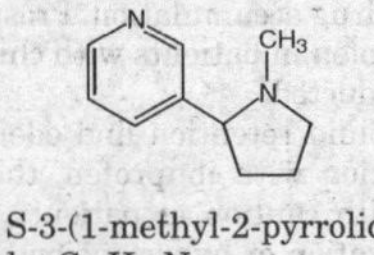

Chemical Name: S-3-(1-methyl-2-pyrrolidinyl) pyridine

Molecular Formula: $C_{10}H_{14}N_2$

Molecular Weight: 162.23

Ionization Constants: $pKa_1 = 7.84$, $pKa_2 = 3.04$ at 15°C

Octanol-Water Partition Coefficient: 15:1 at pH 7

Nicotine is the active ingredient; inactive components of the product are menthol and a porous plug which are pharmacologically inactive. Nicotine is released when air is inhaled through the Inhaler.

CLINICAL PHARMACOLOGY

Pharmacologic Action

Nicotine, the chief alkaloid in tobacco products, binds stereo-selectively to nicotinic-cholinergic receptors at the autonomic ganglia, in the adrenal medulla, at neuromuscular junctions, and in the brain. Two types of central nervous system effects are believed to be the basis of nicotine's positively reinforcing properties. A stimulating effect is exerted mainly in the cortex via the locus ceruleus and a reward effect is exerted in the limbic system. At low doses the stimulant effects predominate while at high doses the reward effects predominate. Intermittent intravenous administration of nicotine activates neurohormonal pathways, releasing acetylcholine, norepinephrine, dopamine, serotonin, vasopressin, beta-endorphin, growth hormone, and ACTH.

Pharmacodynamics

The cardiovascular effects of nicotine include peripheral vasoconstriction, tachycardia, and elevated blood pressure. Acute and chronic tolerance to nicotine develops from smoking tobacco or ingesting nicotine preparations. Acute tolerance (a reduction in response for a given dose) develops rapidly (less than 1 hour), but not at the same rate for different physiologic effects (skin temperature, heart rate, subjective effects). Withdrawal symptoms such as cigarette craving can be reduced in most individuals by plasma nicotine levels lower than those from smoking.

Withdrawal from nicotine in addicted individuals can be characterized by craving, nervousness, restlessness, irritability, mood lability, anxiety, drowsiness, sleep disturbances, impaired concentration, increased appetite, minor somatic complaints (headache, myalgia, constipation, fatigue), and weight gain. Nicotine toxicity is characterized by nausea,

abdominal pain, vomiting, diarrhea, diaphoresis, flushing, dizziness, disturbed hearing and vision, confusion, weakness, palpitations, altered respiration and hypotension. Both smoking and nicotine can increase circulating cortisol and catecholamines, and tolerance does not develop to the catecholamine-releasing effects of nicotine. Changes in the response to a concomitantly administered adrenergic agonist or antagonist should be watched for when nicotine intake is altered during NICOTROL Inhaler therapy and/or smoking cessation (See PRECAUTIONS, Drug Interactions).

PHARMACOKINETICS

Absorption

Most of the nicotine released from the NICOTROL Inhaler is deposited in the mouth. Only a fraction of the dose released, less than 5%, reaches the lower respiratory tract. An intensive inhalation regimen (80 deep inhalations over 20 minutes) releases on the average 4 mg of the nicotine content of each cartridge of which about 2 mg is systemically absorbed. Peak plasma concentrations are typically reached within 15 minutes of the end of inhalation.

Absorption of nicotine through the buccal mucosa is relatively slow and the high and rapid rise followed by the decline in nicotine arterial plasma concentrations seen with cigarette smoking are not achieved with the inhaler. After use of the single inhaler the arterial nicotine concentrations rise slowly to an average of 6 ng/mL in contrast to those of a cigarette, which increase rapidly and reach a mean C_{max} of approximately 49 ng/mL within 5 minutes.

The temperature dependency of nicotine release from the NICOTROL Inhaler was studied between 68°F and 104°F in eighteen patients. Average achievable steady state plasma levels after 20 minutes of an intensive inhalation regimen each hour at ambient room temperature are on the order of 23 ng/mL. The corresponding nicotine plasma levels achievable at 86°F and 104°F are on the order of 30 and 34 ng/mL. Nicotine peak plasma concentration (C_{max}) at steady-state, after 20 minutes of an intensive inhalation regimen per hour, for 10 hours.

	C_{max} (ng/mL)		
	20°C/68°F	30°C/86°F	40°C/104°F
	N = 18	N = 18	N = 18
Mean	22.5	29.7	34.0
S.D.	7.7	8.3	6.9
Min	11.1	17.6	24.1
Max	40.4	47.2	48.6

Ad libitum use of the NICOTROL Inhaler typically produces nicotine plasma levels of 6-8 ng/mL, corresponding to about 1/3 of those achieved with cigarette smoking.

Distribution

The volume of distribution following IV administration of nicotine is approximately 2 to 3 L/kg. Plasma protein binding of nicotine is <5%. Therefore, changes in nicotine binding from use of concomitant drugs or alterations of plasma proteins by disease states would not be expected to have significant effects on nicotine kinetics.

Metabolism

More than 20 metabolites of nicotine have been identified, all of which are less active than the parent compound. The primary urinary metabolites are cotinine (15% of the dose) and trans-3-hydroxycotinine (45% of the dose). Cotinine has a half-life of 15 to 20 hours and concentrations that exceed nicotine by 10–fold. The major site for the metabolism of nicotine is the liver. The kidney and lung are also sites of nicotine metabolism.

Elimination

About 10% of the nicotine absorbed is excreted unchanged in the urine. This may be increased to up to 30% with high urine flow rates and urinary acidification below pH 5. The average plasma clearance is about 1.2 L/min in a healthy adult smoker. The apparent elimination half-life of nicotine is 1 to 2 hours.

Gender Differences

Intersubject variability coefficients of variation (C.V.) for the pharmacokinetic parameters (AUC and C_{max}) were approximately 40% and 30%, respectively, for males and females. There were no medically significant differences between females and males in the kinetics of NICOTROL Inhaler.

CLINICAL TRIALS

The efficacy of NICOTROL Inhaler therapy as an aid to smoking cessation was demonstrated in two single-center, placebo-controlled, double-blind trials with a total of 445 healthy patients. The number of Nicotrol Inhaler cartridges used was a minimum dose of 4 cartridges/day and a maximum dose of 20 cartridges/day.

In both studies, the recommended duration of treatment was 3 months; however, the patients were permitted to continue to use the product for up to 6 months, if they wished. The quit rates are the percentage of all persons initially enrolled who continuously abstained after week 2. NICOTROL Inhaler was more effective than placebo at 6 weeks, 3 months and 6 months. The efficacy is shown in the following table.

		Quit Rates by Treatment (N = 445 Patients in 2 Studies)			
Group	Number of Patients	At 6 Weeks	At 3 Months	At 6 Months	At 12 Months*
Nicotrol Inhaler	223	44-45%	31-32%	20-21%	11-13%
Placebo	222	14-23%	8-15%	6-11%	5-10%

* Follow-up, patients not on treatment.

Patients who used NICOTROL Inhaler had a significant reduction in the "urge to smoke", a major nicotine withdrawal symptom, compared with placebo-treated patients throughout the first week, (see Figure 1).

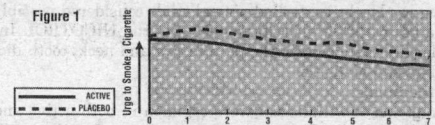

Figure 1

ACTIVE
PLACEBO

INDICATIONS AND USAGE

NICOTROL Inhaler is indicated as an aid to smoking cessation for the relief of nicotine withdrawal symptoms. NICOTROL Inhaler therapy is recommended for use as part of a comprehensive behavioral smoking cessation program.

CONTRAINDICATIONS

Use of NICOTROL Inhaler therapy is contraindicated in patients with known hypersensitivity or allergy to nicotine or to menthol.

WARNINGS

Nicotine from any source can be toxic and addictive. Smoking causes lung disease, cancer and heart disease, and may adversely affect pregnant women or the fetus. For any smoker, with or without concomitant disease or pregnancy, the risk of nicotine replacement in a smoking cessation program should be weighed against the hazard of continued smoking, and the likelihood of achieving cessation of smoking without nicotine replacement.

Pregnancy, Warning

Tobacco smoke, which has been shown to be harmful to the fetus, contains nicotine, hydrogen cyanide, and carbon monoxide. The Nicotrol Inhaler does not deliver hydrogen cyanide and carbon monoxide. However, nicotine has been shown in animal studies to cause fetal harm. It is therefore presumed that NICOTROL Inhaler can cause fetal harm when administered to a pregnant woman. The effect of nicotine delivery by NICOTROL Inhaler has not been examined in pregnancy (See PRECAUTIONS). **Therefore, pregnant smokers should be encouraged to attempt cessation using educational and behavioral interventions before using pharmacological approaches.** If NICOTROL Inhaler is used during pregnancy, or if the patient becomes pregnant while using it, the patient should be apprised of the potential hazard to the fetus.

Safety Note Concerning Children

This product contains nicotine and should be kept out of the reach of children and pets. The amounts of nicotine that are tolerated by adult smokers can produce symptoms of poisoning and could prove fatal if the nicotine from the Nicotrol Inhaler is inhaled, ingested or buccally absorbed by children or pets. A cartridge contains about 60% of its initial drug content when it is discarded, which is about 6 mg. Patients should be cautioned to keep both the used and unused cartridges of NICOTROL Inhaler out of the reach of children and pets.

All components of the NICOTROL Inhaler system should also be kept out of the reach of children and pets to avoid accidental swallowing and choking.

PRECAUTIONS

General

The patient should be urged to stop smoking completely when initiating NICOTROL Inhaler therapy (See DOSAGE AND ADMINISTRATION). Patients should be informed that if they continue to smoke while using the product, they may experience adverse effects due to peak nicotine levels higher than those experienced from smoking alone. If there is a clinically significant increase in cardiovascular or other effects attributable to nicotine, the treatment should be dis-

continued (See WARNINGS). Physicians should anticipate that concomitant medications may need dosage adjustment (See Drug Interactions). Sustained use (beyond 6 months) of NICOTROL Inhaler by patients who stop smoking has not been studied and is not recommended.(See DRUG ABUSE AND DEPENDENCE).

Bronchospastic Disease

Nicotrol Inhaler has not been specifically studied in asthma or chronic pulmonary disease. Nicotine is an airway irritant and might cause bronchospasm. Nicotrol Inhaler should be used with caution in patients with bronchospastic disease. Other forms of nicotine replacement might be preferable in patients with severe bronchospastic airway disease.

Cardiovascular or Peripheral Vascular Diseases

The risks of nicotine replacement in patients with cardiovascular and peripheral vascular diseases should be weighed against the benefits of including nicotine replacement in a smoking cessation program for them. Specifically, patients with coronary heart disease (history of myocardial infarction and/or angina pectoris), serious cardiac arrhythmias, or vasospastic diseases (Buerger's disease, Prinzmetal's variant angina and Raynaud's phenomena) should be evaluated carefully before nicotine replacement is prescribed.

Tachycardia and palpitations have been reported occasionally with the use of NICOTROL Inhaler as well as with other nicotine replacement therapies. No serious cardiovascular events were reported in clinical studies with NICOTROL Inhaler, but if such symptoms occur, its use should be discontinued.

NICOTROL Inhaler generally should not be used in patients during the immediate post-myocardial infarction period, nor in patients with serious arrhythmias, or with severe or worsening angina.

Renal or Hepatic Insufficiency

The pharmacokinetics of nicotine have not been studied in the elderly or in patients with renal or hepatic impairment. However, given that nicotine is extensively metabolized and that its total system clearance is dependent on liver blood flow, some influence of hepatic impairment on drug kinetics (reduced clearance) should be anticipated. Only severe renal impairment would be expected to affect the clearance of nicotine or its metabolites from the circulation (See PHARMACOKINETICS).

Endocrine Diseases

NICOTROL Inhaler therapy should be used with caution in patients with hyperthyroidism, pheochromocytoma or insulin-dependent diabetes, since nicotine causes the release of catecholamines by the adrenal medulla.

Peptic Ulcer Disease

Nicotine delays healing in peptic ulcer disease; therefore, NICOTROL Inhaler therapy should be used with caution in patients with active peptic ulcers and only when the benefits of including nicotine replacement in a smoking cessation program outweigh the risks.

Accelerated Hypertension

Nicotine therapy constitutes a risk factor for development of malignant hypertension in patients with accelerated hypertension; therefore, NICOTROL Inhaler therapy should be used with caution in these patients and only when the benefits of including nicotine replacement in a smoking cessation program outweigh the risks.

Information for Patient

A patient information sheet is included in the package of NICOTROL Inhaler cartridges dispensed to the patient. Patients should be encouraged to read the information sheet carefully and to ask their physician and pharmacist about the proper use of the product (See DOSAGE AND ADMINISTRATION). Patients must be advised to keep both used and unused cartridges out of the reach of children and pets.

Drug Interactions

Physiological changes resulting from smoking cessation, with or without nicotine replacement, may alter the pharmacokinetics of certain concomitant medications, such as tricyclic antidepressants and theophylline. Doses of these and perhaps other medications may need to be adjusted in patients who successfully quit smoking.

Carcinogenesis, Mutagenesis, Impairment of Fertility

Nicotine itself does not appear to be a carcinogen in laboratory animals. However, nicotine and its metabolites increased the incidences of tumors in the cheek pouches of hamsters and forestomach of F344 rats, respectively when given in combination with tumor initiators. One study, which could not be replicated, suggested that cotinine, the primary metabolite of nicotine, may cause lymphoreticular sarcoma in the large intestine of rats.

Neither nicotine nor cotinine was mutagenic in the Ames salmonella test. Nicotine induced reparable DNA damage in an E. coli test system. Nicotine was shown to be genotoxic in a test system using Chinese hamster ovary cells. In rats and rabbits, implantation can be delayed or inhibited by a reduction in DNA synthesis that appears to be caused by nicotine. Studies have shown a decrease in litter size in rats treated with nicotine during gestation.

Continued on next page

Nicotrol Inhaler—Cont.

PREGNANCY

Pregnancy Category D (See **WARNINGS** sections).

The harmful effects of cigarette smoking on maternal and fetal health are clearly established. These include low birth weight, an increased risk of spontaneous abortion, and increased perinatal mortality. The specific effects of NICOTROL Inhaler therapy on fetal development are unknown. Therefore pregnant smokers should be encouraged to attempt cessation using educational and behavioral interventions before using pharmacological approaches.

Spontaneous abortion during nicotine replacement therapy has been reported; as with smoking, nicotine as a contributing factor cannot be excluded.

NICOTROL Inhaler therapy should be used during pregnancy only if the likelihood of smoking cessation justifies the potential risk of using it by the pregnant patient, who might continue to smoke.

Teratogenicity

Animal Studies: Nicotine was shown to produce skeletal abnormalitites in the offspring of mice when toxic doses were given to the dams (25 mg/kg IP or SC).

Human Studies: Nicotine teratogenicity has not been studied in humans except as a component of cigarette smoke (each cigarette smoked delivers about 1 mg of nicotine). It has not been possible to conclude whether cigarette smoking is teratogenic to humans.

Other Effects

Animal Studies: A nicotine bolus (up to 2 mg/kg) to pregnant rhesus monkeys caused acidosis, hypercarbia, and hypotension (fetal and maternal concentrations were about 20 times those achieved after smoking one cigarette in 5 minutes). Fetal breathing movements were reduced in the fetal lamb after intravenous injection of 0.25 mg/kg nicotine to the ewe (equivalent to smoking 1 cigarette every 20 seconds for 5 minutes). Uterine blood flow was reduced about 30% after infusion of 0.1 μg/kg/min nicotine to pregnant rhesus monkeys (equivalent to smoking about six cigarettes every minute for 20 minutes).

Human Experience: Cigarette smoking during pregnancy is associated with an increased risk of spontaneous abortion, low birth weight infants and perinatal mortality. Nicotine and carbon monoxide are considered the most likely mediators of these outcomes. The effects of cigarette smoking on fetal cardiovascular parameters have been studied near term. Cigarettes increased fetal aortic blood flow and heart rate and decreased uterine blood flow and fetal breathing movements. NICOTROL Inhaler has not been studied in pregnant women.

Labor and Delivery

NICOTROL Inhaler is not recommended for use during labor and delivery. The effect of nicotine on a mother or the fetus during labor is unknown.

Use in Nursing Mothers

Caution should be exercised when the NICOTROL Inhaler is administered to nursing mothers. The safety of NICOTROL Inhaler therapy in nursing infants has not been examined. Nicotine passes freely into breast milk; the milk to plasma ratio averages 2.9. Nicotine is absorbed orally. An infant has the ability to clear nicotine by hepatic first-pass clearance; however, the efficiency of removal is probably lowest at birth. Nicotine concentrations in milk can be expected to be lower with NICOTROL Inhaler when used as recommended than with cigarette smoking, as maternal plasma nicotine concentrations are generally reduced with nicotine replacement. The risk of exposure of the infant to nicotine from NICOTROL Inhaler therapy should be weighed against the risks associated with the infant's exposure to nicotine from continued smoking by the mother (passive smoke exposure and contamination of breast milk with other components of tobacco smoke) and from NICOTROL Inhaler alone, or in combination with continued smoking.

Pediatric Use

Safety and effectiveness in pediatric and adolescent patients below the age of 18 years have not been established for any nicotine replacement product. However, no specific medical risk is known or expected in nicotine dependent adolescents. Nicotrol Inhaler should be used for the treatment of tobacco dependence in the older adolescent only if the potential benefit justifies the potential risk.

Geriatric Use

One hundred and thirty-two patients aged 60 or more participated in clinical trials of NICOTROL Inhaler. Nicotrol Inhaler appeared to be as effective in this age group as in younger smokers. Because medical conditions that are precautions to nicotine use are more common in the elderly, physicians should use care in prescribing this product to these patients.

ADVERSE REACTIONS

Assessment of adverse events in the 1,439 patients (730 on active drug) who participated in controlled clinical trials (including three dose finding studies) is complicated by the occurrence of signs and symptoms of nicotine withdrawal in some patients and nicotine excess in others. The incidence of adverse events is confounded by: (1) the many minor complaints that smokers commonly have, (2) continued smoking by many patients (3) the local irritation from both the active drug and the placebo.

Local Irritation

NICOTROL Inhaler and the placebo were both associated with local irritant side effects. Local irritation in mouth and throat was reported by 40% of patients on active drug as compared to 18% of patients on placebo. Irritant effects were higher in the two pivotal trials with higher doses, being 66% on active drug and 42% on placebo. Coughing (32% active versus 12% placebo) and rhinitis (23% active versus 16% placebo) were also higher on active drug. The majority of patients rated these symptoms as mild.

The frequency of cough and mouth and throat irritation declined with continued use of NICOTROL Inhaler. Other adverse events that occurred in over 3% of patients on active drug in placebo controlled pivotal trials considered possibly related to the local irritant effects of the NICOTROL Inhaler are taste comments, pain in jaw and neck, tooth disorders and sinusitis.

Withdrawal

Symptoms of withdrawal were common in both active and placebo groups. Common withdrawal symptoms seen in over 3% of patients on active drug included: dizziness, anxiety, sleep disorder, depression, withdrawal syndrome, drug dependence, fatigue and myalgia.

Nicotine Related Adverse Events

The most common nicotine-related adverse event was dyspepsia. This was present in 18% of patients in the active group compared to 9% of patients in the placebo group. Other nicotine related events present in greater than 3% of patients on active drug include nausea, diarrhea, and hiccup.

Smoking Related Adverse Events

Smoking related adverse events present in greater than 3% of patients on active drug include chest discomfort, bronchitis, and hypertension.

Other Adverse Events

Adverse events of unknown relationship to nicotine occurring in greater than 3% of patients on active drug include headache (26% of patients on active drug and 15% of patients on placebo), influenza-like symptoms, pain, backpain, allergy, paraesthesias, flatulence and fever.

DRUG ABUSE AND DEPENDENCE

The NICOTROL Inhaler is likely to have a low abuse potential based on differences between the product and cigarettes in three characteristics commonly considered important in contributing to abuse: slower absorption, smaller fluctuations in blood levels and lower blood levels of nicotine. NICOTROL Inhaler, like many other nicotine-based smoking cessation therapies, does not produce arterial concentrations similar to cigarettes. However, nicotine withdrawal symptoms were noted in clinical trials at the time of NICOTROL Inhaler tapering and after NICOTROL Inhaler discontinuation.

Dependence might occur from transference of tobacco-related nicotine dependence to the NICOTROL Inhaler. The use of the inhaler beyond 6 months has not been evaluated in clinical trials and is not recommended. To minimize the risk of dependence, patients should be encouraged to withdraw gradually from NICOTROL Inhaler therapy after 3 months of usage (See **DOSAGE AND ADMINISTRATION**). If necessary, dose reduction can be achieved by gradual reduction of the dose over a 6 to 12 week period.

OVERDOSAGE

Signs and Symptoms of Nicotine Toxicity

Signs and symptoms of an overdose of the NICOTROL Inhaler would be expected to be the same as those of acute nicotine poisoning including: pallor, cold sweat, nausea, salivation, vomiting, abdominal pain, diarrhea, headache, dizziness, disturbed hearing and vision, tremor, mental confusion, and weakness. Prostration, hypotension, and respiratory failure may ensue with large overdoses. Lethal doses produce convulsions quickly and death follows as a result of peripheral or central respiratory paralysis or, less frequently, cardiac failure.

Overdose from Inhalation

The oral LD_{50} for nicotine is >5 mg/kg in dogs and >24 mg/kg in rodents. Death is due to respiratory paralysis. The oral minimum acute lethal dose for nicotine in adult humans is reported to be 40 to 60 mg (<1 mg/kg). The effects of using several cartridges in rapid succession are unknown (See **WARNINGS, Safety Note Concerning Children**).

One cartridge of NICOTROL Inhaler contains 10 mg nicotine, of which, approximately 4 mg is delivered nicotine. It is unlikely that an excessive nicotine overdose will occur via inhalation. Should such an overdose occur, however, with signs of nicotine poisoning, the patient should be instructed to contact his/her physician immediately. For additional emergency information, call your regional poison center or call the National Capital Poison Center toll free (1-800-498-8666).

Overdose from Ingestion

Persons ingesting NICOTROL Inhaler cartridges should be referred to a health care facility for management. In unconscious patients with a secure airway, instill activated charcoal via a nasogastric tube. A saline cathartic or sorbitol may be added to the first dose of activated charcoal. Repeated doses of activated charcoal should be administered as long as the cartridge remains in the gastrointestinal tract since it will continue to release nicotine for many hours. The NICOTROL Inhaler cartridges can be identified with a radiogram.

Management of Nicotine Poisoning

Other supportive measures include diazepam or barbiturates for seizures, atropine for excessive bronchial secretions or dairrhea, respiratory support for respiratory failure, and vigorous fluid support for hypotension and cardiovascular collapse.

DOSAGE AND ADMINISTRATION

Patients must desire to stop smoking and should be instructed to ***stop smoking completely*** as they begin using NICOTROL Inhaler. It is important that patients understand the instructions, and have their questions answered. They should clearly understand the directions for using the NICOTROL Inhaler and safely disposing of the used cartridges.

The initial dosage of NICOTROL Inhaler is individualized. Patients may self-titrate to the level of nicotine they require. Most successful patients in the clinical trials used between 6 and 16 cartridges a day. Best effect was achieved by frequent continuous puffing (20 minutes). The recommended duration of treatment is 3 months, after which patients may be weaned from the NICOTROL Inhaler by gradual reduction of the daily dose over the following 6 to 12 weeks. The safety and efficacy of the continued use of NICOTROL Inhaler for periods longer than 6 months have not been studied and such use is not recommeded.

Dosing recommendations are summarized in the table below.

[See table below]

Initial Treatment (Up to 12 Weeks)

For best results, patients should be encouraged to use at least 6 cartridges per day at least for the first 3 to 6 weeks of treatment. In clinical trials, the average daily dose was >6 (range 3 to 18) cartridges for patients who successfully quit smoking. Additional doses may be needed to control the urge to smoke with a maximum of 16 cartridges daily for up to 12 weeks. Regular use of NICOTROL Inhaler during the first week of treatment may help patients adapt to the irritant effects of the product. Some patients may exhibit signs or symptoms of nicotine withdrawal or excess which will require an adjustment of the dosage (see **Individualization of Dosage**).

Gradual Reduction of Dose (Up to 12 Weeks)

Most patients will need to gradually discontinue use of the NICOTROL Inhaler after the initial treatment period. Gradual reduction of dose may begin after twelve weeks of initial treatment and may last for up to twelve weeks. Recommended strategies for discontinuing use include suggesting to patients that they use the product less frequently, keep a tally of daily usage, try to meet a steadily reducing target or set a planned quit date for stopping use of the product.

Individualization of Dosage

The Nicotrol Inhaler provides the smoker with adequate amounts of nicotine to reduce the urge to smoke, and may provide some degree of comfort by providing a hand-to-mouth ritual similar to smoking, although the importance of such an effect in smoking cessation is, as yet, unknown. The success or failure of smoking cessation is influenced by the quality, intensity and frequency of supportive care. Patients are more likely to quit smoking if they are seen frequently and participate in formal smoking cessation programs.

RECOMMENDED DOSING

Duration	Recommended Cartridges/day	
INITIAL TREATMENT	Up to 12 weeks	6-16
Gradual Reduction (if needed)	6-12 weeks	No tapering strategy has been shown to be superior to any other in clinical studies.

The goal of NICOTROL Inhaler therapy is complete abstinence. If a patient is unable to stop smoking by the fourth week of therapy, treatment should probably be discontinued.

Patients who fail to quit on any attempt may benefit from interventions to improve their chances for success on subsequent attempts. Patients who were unsuccessful should be counseled and should then probably be given a therapeutic holiday before the next attempt. A new quit attempt should be encouraged when conditions are more favorable.

Based on the clinical trials, a reasonable approach to assisting patients in their attempt to quit smoking is to begin initial treatment, using the recommended dosage (See **DOSAGE AND ADMINISTRATION**). Dosage can then be adjusted in those patients with signs or symptoms of nicotine withdrawal or excess. Patients who are successfully abstinent on NICOTROL Inhaler should be treated at the selected dosage for up to 12 weeks, after which use of the Inhaler should be gradually reduced over the next 6 to 12 weeks. Some patients may not require gradual reduction of dosage and may abruptly stop treatment successfully. The safe use of this product for longer than six months has not been established.

The symptoms of nicotine withdrawal overlap those of nicotine excess (See **Pharmacodynamics** and **ADVERSE REACTION** sections). Since patients using NICOTROL Inhaler may also smoke intermittently, it is sometimes difficult to determine if they are experiencing nicotine withdrawal or nicotine excess. Controlled clinical trials of nicotine products suggest that palpitations, nausea and sweating are more often symptoms of nicotine excess, whereas anxiety, nervousness and irritability are more often symptoms of nicotine withdrawal.

SAFETY AND HANDLING
Disposal
See patient information sheet for instructions on handling and disposal. After using the NICOTROL Inhaler, carefully separate the mouthpiece, remove the used cartridge and throw it away, out of the reach of children and pets. Store the mouthpiece in the plastic storage case for further use. The mouthpiece is reusable and should be cleaned regularly with soap and water. The NICOTROL Inhaler cartridges can be detected on a radiogram.

HOW SUPPLIED
NDC 0045–0901–01
NICOTROL INHALER (nicotine inhalation system) is supplied as 42 cartridges each containing 10 mg (4 mg is delivered) nicotine. Each unit consists of 1 mouthpiece, 7 storage trays each containing 6 cartridges and 1 plastic storage case. A patient information leaflet is enclosed with the package.
Store at room temperatue not to exceed 30°C (86°F). Protect cartridges from light.
CAUTION: Federal law prohibits dispensing without a prescription.
Manufactured by: Pharmacia & Upjohn AB, Sweden
Distributed by: McNEIL Consumer Products Co.
                 Division of McNEIL-PPC, Inc.
                 Fort Washington, PA 19034 USA
                 ©McN-PPC, Inc. '97
                 MADE IN SWEDEN
                 U.S. Patent No. 5,400,808
Shown in Product Identification Guide, page 321

NICOTROL® NS   ℞
(nicotine nasal spray)
10 mg/mL

DESCRIPTION
Nicotrol® NS (nicotine nasal spray) is an aqueous solution of nicotine intended for administration as a metered spray to the nasal mucosa.
Nicotine is a tertiary amine composed of pyridine and a pyrrolidine ring. It is a colorless to pale yellow, freely water-soluble, strongly alkaline, oily, volatile, hygroscopic liquid obtained from the tobacco plant. Nicotine has a characteristic pungent odor and turns brown on exposure to air or light. Of its two stereoisomers, S(-)nicotine is the more active. It is the prevalent form in tobacco, and is the form in NICOTROL NS. The free alkaloid is absorbed rapidly through skin, mucous membranes, and the respiratory tract.
Chemical Name: S-3-(1-methyl-2-pyrrolidinyl) pyridine
Molecular Formula $C_{10}H_{14}N_2$
Molecular Weight: 162.23
Ionization Constants: pKa_1 =7.84, pKa_2 =3.04 at 15°C
Octanol-Water Partition Coefficient: 15:1 at pH 7
[See chemical structure at top of next column]
Each 10 mL spray bottle contains 100 mg nicotine (10 mg/mL) in an inactive vehicle containing disodium phosphate, sodium dihydrogen phosphate, citric acid, methylparaben,

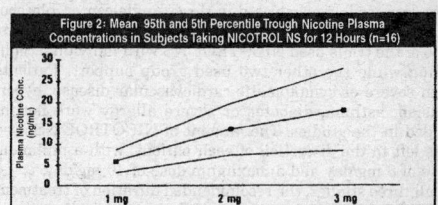

propylparaben, edetate disodium, sodium chloride, polysorbate 80, aroma and water. The solution is isotonic with a pH of 7. It contains no chlorofluorocarbons.
After priming the delivery system for NICOTROL NS, each actuation of the unit delivers a metered dose spray containing approximately 0.5 mg of nicotine. The size of the droplets produced by the unit is in excess of 8 microns. One NICOTROL NS unit delivers approximately 200 applications.

CLINICAL PHARMACOLOGY
Pharmacologic Action
Nicotine, the chief alkaloid in tobacco products, binds stereo-selectively to nicotinic-cholinergic receptors at the autonomic ganglia, in the adrenal medulla, at neuromuscular junctions, and in the brain. Two types of central nervous system effects are believed to be the basis of nicotine's positively reinforcing properties. A stimulating effect is exerted mainly in the cortex via the locus ceruleus and a reward effect is exerted in the limbic system. At low doses, the stimulant effects predominate while at high doses the reward effects predominate. Intermittent intravenous administration of nicotine activates neurohormonal pathways, releasing acetylcholine, norepinephrine, dopamine, serotonin, vasopressin, beta-endorphin, growth hormone, and ACTH.

Pharmacodynamics
The cardiovascular effects of nicotine include peripheral vasoconstriction, tachycardia and elevated blood pressure. Acute and chronic tolerance to nicotine develops from smoking tobacco or ingesting nicotine preparations. Acute tolerance (a reduction in response for a given dose) develops rapidly (less than 1 hour), but not at the same rate for different physiologic effects (skin temperature, heart rate, subjective effects). Withdrawal symptoms such as cigarette craving can be reduced in most individuals by plasma nicotine levels lower than those from smoking.
Withdrawal from nicotine in addicted individuals can be characterized by craving, nervousness, restlessness, irritability, mood lability, anxiety, drowsiness, sleep disturbances, impaired concentration, increased appetite, minor somatic complaints (headache, myalgia, constipation, fatigue), and weight gain. Nicotine toxicity is characterized by nausea, abdominal pain, vomiting, diarrhea, diaphoresis, flushing, dizziness, disturbed hearing and vision, confusion, weakness, palpitations, altered respiration and hypotension.
Both smoking and nicotine can increase circulating cortisol and catecholamines, and tolerance does not develop to the catecholamine-releasing effects of nicotine. Changes in the response to a concomitantly administered adrenergic agonist or antagonist should be watched for when nicotine intake is altered during NICOTROL NS therapy and/or smoking cessation (See **PRECAUTIONS**, **Drug Interactions**).

PHARMACOKINETICS
Each actuation of NICOTROL NS delivers a metered 50 microliter spray containing approximately 0.5 mg of nicotine. One dose is considered 1 mg of nicotine (2 sprays, one in each nostril).
Absorption
Following administration of 2 sprays of NICOTROL NS approximately 53% ±16% (Mean ±SD) enters the systemic circulation. No significant difference in rate or extent of absorption could be seen due to the deposition of nicotine on different parts of the nasal mucosa. Plasma concentrations of nicotine obtained from 1 dose (1 mg nicotine) of NICOTROL NS rise rapidly, reaching maximum venous concentrations of 2–12 ng/mL in 4–15 minutes. The apparent absorption half-life of nicotine is approximately 3 minutes. There is wide variation among subjects in their plasma nicotine concentrations from the spray. As a result, after a 1 mg dose of spray approximately 20% of the subjects reached peak nicotine concentrations similar to those seen after smoking one cigarette (7–17 ng/mL) (See **DRUG ABUSE AND DEPENDENCE** Section). Figure 1 below plots the mean and 5th and 95th percentile nicotine concentrations after a 1 mg single dose of the nasal spray (n=30).

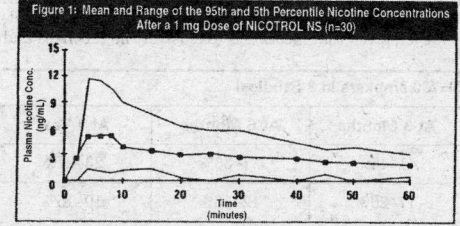

Figure 1: Mean and Range of the 95th and 5th Percentile Nicotine Concentrations After a 1 mg Dose of NICOTROL NS (n=30)

Table 1: Trough Plasma Nicotine Concentrations after 11 Hours of Dosing With 1 mg, 2 mg and 3 mg of NICOTROL NS per hour (n=16)

Dose	Mean (ng/mL) ±SD	(Range)
1 mg every 60 minutes (1 mg/hr)	6 ± 3	(1.7–12)
1 mg every 30 minutes (2 mg/hr)	14 ± 6	(1.5–24)
1 mg every 20 minutes (3 mg/hr)	18 ± 10	(1.2–35)

The data from Table 1 is derived from a three-way crossover study of repeated applications of NICOTROL NS in sixteen smokers (8 male, 8 female) ranging in age from 18 to 48 years. There is a slight deviation from dose-concentration proportionality from one dose to three doses of NICOTROL NS per hour as shown in Figure 2.

Figure 2: Mean 95th and 5th Percentile Trough Nicotine Plasma Concentrations in Subjects Taking NICOTROL NS for 12 Hours (n=16)

Sixteen smokers (7 males and 9 females) ranging in age from 22 to 44 years were dosed with 1 mg of NICOTROL NS every hour for 10 hours. The pharmacokinetic parameters that were obtained are presented in Table 2.

Table 2 Nicotine Pharmacokinetic Parameters at Steady-State for 1 mg hour of NICOTROL NS Administered Hourly for Ten Hours (Mean ± SD and Range) (n=16)

Parameter	1 mg (2 sprays)	(Range)
Cavg (ng/mL)	8 ± 3	(2.5–12)
Cmax (ng/mL)	9 ± 3	(3.1–14)
Tmax (minutes)	13 ± 5	(10–20)

Cavg: average plasma nicotine concentration for the dosing interval of 10–11 hours
Cmax: maximum measured plasma concentration after last dose administration
Tmax: time of maximum plasma concentration after last dose administration

Distribution
The volume of distribution following IV administration of nicotine is approximately 2 to 3 L/kg. Plasma protein binding of nicotine is <5%. Therefore, changes in nicotine binding from use of concomitant drugs or alterations of plasma proteins by disease states would not be expected to have significant effects on nicotine kinetics.

Metabolism
More than 20 metabolites of nicotine have been identified, all of which are less active than the parent compound. The primary urinary metabolites are cotinine (15% of the dose) and trans-3-hydroxycotinine (45% of the dose). Cotinine has a half-life of 15 to 20 hours and concentrations that exceed nicotine by 10-fold. The major site for the metabolism of nicotine is the liver. The kidney and lung are also sites of nicotine metabolism.

Elimination
About 10% of the nicotine absorbed is excreted unchanged in the urine. This may be increased to up to 30% with high urine flow rates and urinary acidification below pH 5. The average plasma clearance is about 1.2 L/min in a healthy adult smoker. The apparent elimination half-life of nicotine from NICOTROL NS is 1 to 2 hours.

Pharmacokinetic Model
The data were well described by a two-compartment model with first-order input.
Based on individual fits (N=18) the following parameters were derived after the administration of a 1 mg dose: Absorption rate constant Ka =14.4 ±7.3 hr⁻¹ (Mean ±SD). Elimination rate constant (Ke) =0.60 ±0.53 hr⁻¹. Distribution rate constants K_{12}=4.84 ±2.57 hr⁻¹, (K_{21}) =4.35 ±2.30 hr⁻¹. Volume of distribution over fraction absorbed (V/F) =2.73 ±0.82 L/kg in 8 female and 10 male adults weighing 76 ±15 kg.

Continued on next page

Nicotrol NS—Cont.

Gender Differences
Intersubject variability (50% coefficient of variation) among the pharmacokinetic parameters (AUC, C_{max} and Clearance/kg) were observed for both genders. There were no differences between females or males in the kinetics of NICOTROL NS.

Drug/Drug Interactions
The extent of absorption is slightly reduced (approximately 10%) in patients with the common cold/rhinitis. In patients with rhinitis the peak plasma concentration is reduced by approximately 20% (concentrations are lower by 1.5 ng/mL on average) and the time to peak concentration prolonged by approximately 30% (delayed by 7 minutes on average). The use of a nasal vasoconstrictor such as xylometazoline in patients with rhinitis will further prolong the time to peak by approximately 40% (delayed by 15 minutes on average), but the peak plasma concentration remains on average the same as those with rhinitis.

CLINICAL TRIALS
The efficacy of NICOTROL NS therapy as an aid to smoking cessation was demonstrated in three single-center, placebo-controlled, double-blind trials with a total of 730 patients. One of the trials used NICOTROL NS with individual counseling while the other two used group support. Patients with severe or symptomatic cardiovascular disease, hypertension, asthma, diabetes or severe allergy were not included in the studies. The amount of NICOTROL NS used was left to the discretion of each patient, with a minimum dose of 8 mg/day and a maximum dose of 40 mg/day.
In all three studies, the recommended duration of treatment was 3 months; however in two of these trials, 241 patients were permitted to continue to use the product for up to 1 year, if they wished. Among the 64 patients abstinent from cigarettes at the end of a year, 23 (36%) were still using the spray, and probable dependence on the spray was seen in several patients. (See **DRUG ABUSE AND DEPENDENCE**).
Quitting was defined as *total abstinence* from smoking for at least 4 weeks. The "quit rates" are the percentage of all persons initially enrolled who continuously abstained after week 2 or 4.
In all three studies, NICOTROL NS was more effective than placebo at 6 weeks, 3 months, 6 months, and 1 year. The two studies where NICOTROL NS could be used for more than 6 months did not have a better outcome at 1 year than the study in which NICOTROL NS was discontinued at 6 months.
[See table 3 below]
Patients treated with NICOTROL NS had more relief of the urge to smoke and withdrawal symptoms compared with placebo-treated patients.
NICOTROL NS allows the patient to vary the dose of nicotine on a short-term basis. As with other variable dose smoking cessation products, NICOTROL NS may be useful in the management of highly dependent smokers.

INDICATIONS AND USAGE
NICOTROL NS is indicated as an aid to smoking cessation for the relief of nicotine withdrawal symptoms. NICOTROL NS therapy should be used as a part of a comprehensive behavioral smoking cessation program.
The safety and efficacy of the continued use of NICOTROL NS for periods longer than 6 months have not been adequately studied and such use is not recommended.

CONTRAINDICATIONS
Use of NICOTROL NS therapy is contraindicated in patients with known hypersensitivity or allergy to nicotine or to any component of the product.

WARNINGS
Nicotine from any source can be toxic and addictive. Smoking causes lung disease, cancer, and heart disease and may adversely affect pregnant women or the fetus. For any smoker, with or without concomitant disease or pregnancy, the risk of nicotine replacement in a smoking cessation program should be weighed against the hazard of continued smoking, and the likelihood of achieving cessation of smoking without nicotine replacement.

Pregnancy, Warning
Tobacco smoke, which has been shown to be harmful to the fetus, contains nicotine, hydrogen cyanide, and carbon monoxide. Nicotine has been shown in animal studies to cause fetal harm. It is therefore presumed that NICOTROL NS can cause fetal harm when administered to a pregnant

woman. The effect of nicotine delivery by NICOTROL NS has not been examined in pregnancy (See **PRECAUTIONS**). Therefore, pregnant smokers should be encouraged to attempt cessation using educational and behavioral interventions before using pharmacological approaches. If NICOTROL NS is used during pregnancy, or if the patient becomes pregnant while using it, the patient should be apprised of the potential hazard to the fetus.

Safety Note Concerning Children
The amounts of nicotine that are tolerated by adult smokers can produce symptoms of poisoning and could prove fatal if NICOTROL NS is used or ingested by children or pets. A full bottle of NICOTROL NS contains 100 mg of nicotine, some of which will still be in the bottle when it is discarded. Therefore, patients should be cautioned to keep both used and unused containers of NICOTROL NS out of the reach of children and pets.

PRECAUTIONS
General
The patient should be urged to stop smoking completely when initiating NICOTROL NS therapy (See **DOSAGE AND ADMINISTRATION**). Patients should be informed that if they continue to smoke while using the product, they may experience adverse effects due to peak nicotine levels higher than those experienced from smoking alone. If there is a clinically significant increase in cardiovascular or other effects attributable to nicotine, the treatment should be discontinued (See **WARNINGS**). Physicians should anticipate that concomitant medications may need dosage adjustment (See **Drug Interactions**).
Sustained use (beyond 6 months) of NICOTROL NS by patients who stop smoking is not recommended and should be discouraged (See **DRUG ABUSE AND DEPENDENCE**).
Use of NICOTROL NS is not recommended in patients with known chronic nasal disorders (e.g. allergy, rhinitis, nasal polyps and sinusitis) since such use has not been adequately studied.

Asthma, Bronchospasm and Reactive Airway Disease
Exacerbation of bronchospasm in patients with pre-existing asthma has been reported. Use of NICOTROL NS in patients with severe reactive airway disease is not recommended.

Effect of NICOTROL NS on the Nasal Mucosa
Topical application of either nicotine or tobacco products is irritating to the nasal mucosa and physicians should consider both the risks and benefits to the patient before initiating or continuing NICOTROL NS therapy.
The effect of NICOTROL NS on the nasal mucosa was studied in 39 cigarette smokers who used NICOTROL NS for 1 month. When compared to baseline, random biopsies taken after four weeks of treatment revealed 1 patient with persistence of pre-existing dysplasia and 1 patient with a newly found dysplasia. In both, dysplasia was not seen after a recovery period of eight weeks.
Forty-two patients who used NICOTROL NS for more than 6 months underwent follow-up ear, nose and throat examinations 1 to 3 months after discontinuing the use of the spray. Many reported local irritant effects of the spray during spray use, but none showed persistent mucosal injury that the examining physician could attribute to use of the product.
The clinical significance of these findings is not known, but extended use of the product beyond six months is not recommended.

Cardiovascular or Peripheral Vascular Diseases
The risks of nicotine replacement in patients with cardiovascular and peripheral vascular diseases should be weighed against the benefits of including nicotine replacement in a smoking cessation program for them. Specifically, patients with coronary heart disease (history of myocardial infarction and/or angina pectoris), serious cardiac arrhythmias, or vasospastic diseases (Buerger's disease, Prinzmetal's variant angina and Raynaud's phenomena) should be evaluated carefully before nicotine replacement is prescribed.
Tachycardia occurring in association with nicotine replacement therapy has been reported. No serious cardiovascular events were reported in clinical studies with NICOTROL NS, but if symptoms occur, its use should be discontinued. NICOTROL NS generally should not be used in patients during the immediate post-myocardial infarction period, nor in patients with serious arrhythmias, or with severe or worsening angina.

Renal or Hepatic Insufficiency
The pharmacokinetics of nicotine have not been studied in the elderly or in patients with renal or hepatic impairment. However, given that nicotine is extensively metabolized and

that its total system clearance is dependent on liver blood flow, some influence of hepatic impairment on drug kinetics (reduced clearance) should be anticipated. Only severe renal impairment would be expected to affect the clearance of nicotine or its metabolites from the circulation (See **PHARMACOKINETICS**).

Endocrine Diseases
NICOTROL NS therapy should be used with caution in patients with hyperthyroidism, pheochromocytoma or insulin-dependent diabetes, since nicotine causes the release of catecholamines by the adrenal medula.

Peptic Ulcer Disease
Nicotine delays healing in peptic ulcer disease, therefore, NICOTROL NS therapy should be used with caution in patients with active peptic ulcers and only when the benefits of including nicotine replacement in a smoking cessation program outweigh the risks.

Accelerated Hypertension
Nicotine therapy constitutes a risk factor for development of malignant hypertension in patients with accelerated hypertension; therefore, NICOTROL NS therapy should be used with caution in these patients and only when the benefits of including nicotine replacement in a smoking cessation program outweigh the risks.

Information to Patient
A patient instruction sheet is included in the package of NICOTROL NS dispensed to the patient. Patients should be encouraged to read the instruction sheet carefully and to ask their physician and pharmacist about the proper use of the product (See **DOSAGE AND ADMINISTRATION**).
It should be explained to patients that they are likely to experience nasal irritation, which may become less bothersome with continued use.
Patients must be advised to keep both used and unused containers out of the reach of children and pets.

Drug Interactions
The extent of absorption and peak plasma concentration is slightly reduced in patients with the common cold/rhinitis. In addition, the time to peak concentration is prolonged. The use of a nasal vasoconstrictor such as xylometazoline in patients with rhinitis will further prolong the time to peak (See **PHARMACOKINETICS**). Smoking cessation, with or without nicotine replacement, may alter the pharmacokinetics of certain concomitant medications.

May Require a Decrease in Dose at Cessation of Smoking	Possible Mechanism
Acetaminophen caffeine imipramine, oxazepam, pentazocine, propranolol, or other beta-blockers, theophylline	Deinduction of hepatic enzymes or smoking cessation
Insulin	Increase of subcutaneous insulin absorption with smoking cessation
Adrenergic antagonists (e.g. prazosin labetalol)	Decrease in circulating catecholamines with smoking cessation
May Require an Increase in Dose at Cessation of Smoking	**Possible Mechanism**
Adrenergic agonists (e.g. isoproterenol, phenylephrine)	Decrease in circulating catecholamines with smoking cessation

Carcinogenesis, Mutagenesis, Impairment of Fertility
Nicotine itself does not appear to be a carcinogen in laboratory animals. However, nicotine and its metabolites increased the incidence of tumors in the cheek pouches of hamsters and forestomach of F344 rats, respectively, when given in combination with tumor-initiators. One study, which could not be replicated, suggested that cotinine, the primary metabolite of nicotine, may cause lymphoreticular sarcoma in the large intestine of rats.
Neither nicotine nor cotinine were mutagenic in the Ames salmonella test. Nicotine induced repairable DNA damage in an E. coli test system. Nicotine was shown to be genotoxic in a test system using Chinese hamster ovary cells. In rats and rabbits, implantation can be delayed or inhibited by a reduction in DNA synthesis that appears to be caused by nicotine. Studies have shown a decrease in litter size in rats treated with nicotine during gestation.

PREGNANCY
Pregnancy Category D (See **WARNINGS** sections).
The harmful effects of cigarette smoking on maternal and fetal health are clearly established. These include low birth weight, an increased risk of spontaneous abortion, and increased perinatal mortality. The specific effects of NICOTROL NS on fetal development are unknown. There-

Table 3 Quit Rates by Treatment (N=730 smokers in 3 Studies)

Group	Size (n)	At 6 Weeks	At 3 Months	At 6 Months	At 1 Year
NICOTROL NS	369	49–58%	41–45%	31–35%	23–27%
Placebo	361	21–32%	17–20%	12–15%	10–15%

fore pregnant smokers should be encouraged to attempt cessation using educational and behavioral interventions before using pharmacological approaches.
Spontaneous abortion during nicotine replacement therapy has been reported; as with smoking, nicotine as a contributing factor cannot be excluded.
NICOTROL NS should be used during pregnancy only if the likelihood of smoking cessation justifies the potential risk of using it by the pregnant patient, who might continue to smoke.

Teratogenicity

Animal Studies Nicotine was shown to produce skeletal abnormalities in the offspring of mice when toxic doses were given to the dams (25 mg/kg IP or SC).
Human Studies Nicotine teratogenicity has not been studied in humans except as a component of cigarette smoke (each cigarette smoked delivers about 1 mg of nicotine). It has not been possible to conclude whether cigarette smoking is teratogenic to humans.

Other Effects

Animal Studies A nicotine bolus (up to 2 mg/kg) to pregnant rhesus monkeys caused acidosis, hypercarbia, and hypotension (fetal and maternal concentrations were about 20 times those achieved after smoking one cigarette in 5 minutes). Fetal breathing movements were reduced in the fetal lamb after intravenous injection of 0.25 mg/kg nicotine to the ewe (equivalent to smoking 1 cigarette every 20 seconds for 5 minutes). Uterine blood flow was reduced about 30% after infusion of 0.1 μg/kg/min nicotine to pregnant rhesus monkeys (equivalent to smoking about six cigarettes every minute for 20 minutes)
Human Experience Cigarette smoking during pregnancy is associated with an increased risk of spontaneous abortion, low birth weight infants and perinatal mortality. Nicotine and carbon monoxide are considered the most likely mediators of these outcomes. The effects of cigarette smoking on fetal cardiovascular parameters have been studied near term. Cigarettes increased fetal aortic blood flow and heart rate and decreased uterine blood flow and fetal breathing movements. NICOTROL NS has not been studied in pregnant women.

Labor and Delivery

NICOTROL NS is not recommended for use during labor and delivery. The effect of nicotine on a mother or the fetus during labor is unknown.

Use in Nursing Mothers

Caution should be exercised when NICOTROL NS is administered to nursing mothers. The safety of NICOTROL NS therapy in nursing infants has not been examined. Nicotine passes freely into breast milk; the milk to plasma ratio averages 2.9. Nicotine is absorbed orally. An infant has the ability to clear nicotine by hepatic first-pass clearance; however, the efficiency of removal is probably lowest at birth. Nicotine concentrations in milk can be expected to be lower with NICOTROL NS when used as recommended than with cigarette smoking, as maternal plasma nicotine concentrations are generally reduced with nicotine replacement. The risk of exposure of the infant to nicotine from NICOTROL NS therapy should be weighed against the risks associated with the infant's exposure to nicotine from continued smoking by the mother (passive smoke exposure and contamination of breast milk with other components of tobacco smoke) and from NICOTROL NS alone, or in combination with continued smoking.

Pediatric Use

NICOTROL NS therapy is not recommended for use in the pediatric population because its safety and effectiveness in children and adolescents who smoke have not been evaluated.

Geriatric Use

Forty-one patients over the age of 60 participated in clinical trials of NICOTROL NS. The spray appeared to be as effective in this age group as in younger smokers. Because medical conditions that are precautions to nicotine use are more common in the elderly, physicians should use care in prescribing this product to these patients.

ADVERSE REACTIONS

Assessment of adverse events in the 730 patients who participated in controlled clinical trials is complicated by the occurrence of signs and symptoms of nicotine withdrawal in some patients and nicotine excess in others. The incidence of adverse events is confounded by the many minor complaints that smokers commonly have, by continued smoking by many patients and the local irritation from both active drug and the pepper placebo. No serious adverse events were reported during the trials.
Common Smoker's Complaints
Common complaints experienced by the smokers in the study (users of both active and placebo spray) include, chest tightness, dyspepsia, paraesthesia (tingling) in limbs, constipation, and stomatitis.
Tobacco Withdrawal Symptoms
Symptoms of tobacco withdrawal were frequent in users of both active and placebo sprays. Common withdrawal symptoms seen in over 5% of patients included: anxiety, irritability, restlessness, cravings, dizziness, impaired concentration, weight increase, emotional lability, somnolence and fatigue, increased sweating, and insomnia. Less frequently seen probable withdrawal symptoms (under 5%) included: confusion, depression, apathy, tremor, increased appetite, incoordination and increased dreaming.
Anxiety, irritability, restlessness and tobacco cravings occurred about equally in both groups, while other symptoms tended to be slightly more common on placebo spray.
Effects of the Spray
NICOTROL NS and the pepper-containing placebo were both associated with irritant side effects on the nasopharyngeal and ocular tissues. During the first 2 days of treatment, nasal irritation was reported by nearly all (94%) of the patients, the majority of whom rated it as either moderate or severe. Both the frequency and severity of nasal irritation declined with continued use of NICOTROL NS but was still experienced by most (81%) of the patients after 3 weeks of treatment, with most patients rating it as moderate or mild. Other common side-effects for both active and placebo groups were runny nose, throat irritation, watering eyes, sneezing, and cough.
The following local events were reported somewhat more commonly for active than for placebo spray: nasal congestion, subjective comments related to the taste or use of the dosage form, sinus irritation, transient epistaxis, eye irritation, transient changes in sense of smell, pharyngitis, paraesthesias of the nose, mouth or head, numbness of the nose, or mouth, burning of the nose or eyes, earache, facial flushing, transient changes in sense of taste, hoarseness, nasal ulcer or blister.
Effects of Nicotine
Feelings of dependence on the spray were reported by more patients on active spray than placebo. Drug-like effects such as calming were also more frequent on active spray. (See **DRUG ABUSE AND DEPENDENCE**)
Other Adverse Effects
Adverse events which could not be classified and listed above and which were reported by >1% of patients on active spray are listed in the following table

Adverse Events Not Attributable to Intercurrent Illness

Adverse Event	Active	Placebo
HEADACHE	18%	15%
BACK PAIN	6%	4%
DYSPNEA	5%	6%
NAUSEA	5%	5%
ARTHRALGIA	5%	1%
MENSTRUAL DISORDER	4%	4%
PALPITATION	4%	4%
FLATULENCE	4%	3%
TOOTH DISORDER	4%	1%
GUM PROBLEMS	4%	1%
MYALGIA	3%	4%
ABDOMINAL PAIN	3%	3%
CONFUSION	3%	3%
ACNE	3%	1%
DYSMENORRHEA	3%	0%
PRURITUS	2%	3%

Adverse events reported with a frequency of <1% among active spray users are listed below:
Body as a Whole: edema peripheral, pain, numbness, allergy
Gastrointestinal: dry mouth, hiccup, diarrhea
Hematologic: purpura
Neurological: aphasia, amnesia, migraine, numbness
Respiratory: bronchitis, bronchospasm, sputum increased
Skin and appendages: rash, purpura
Special Senses: vision abnormal

DRUG ABUSE AND DEPENDENCE

NICOTROL NS has a dependence potential intermediate between other nicotine-based therapies and cigarettes. This is the result of differences between cigarettes, NICOTROL NS, nicotine gum and nicotine patches in pharmacokinetic and dosing characteristics commonly associated with abuse and dependence. NICOTROL NS is distinct from other nicotine-based smoking cessation therapies in its greater speed of onset, greater capacity for self-titration of dose, and frequent and rapid fluctuations in plasma nicotine concentration.
Dependence on nicotine nasal spray occurred in the clinical trials. Feelings of dependency on the spray were reported by 32% of active spray users and 13% of placebo spray users. Such dependence may represent transference of tobacco-related nicotine dependence to NICOTROL NS.
Fifteen to 20% of patients used the active spray for longer periods than recommended (6 months to 1 year) and 5% used the spray at a higher dose than recommended. Some of these patients experienced anxiety about stopping the spray and some reported craving for the spray rather than for cigarettes.

OVERDOSAGE

The oral LD_{50} for nicotine is >5 mg/kg in dogs and >24 mg/kg in rodents. Death is due to respiratory paralysis. The oral minimum acute lethal dose for nicotine in adult humans is reported to be 40 to 60 mg (<1 mg/kg). A full bottle of NICOTROL NS contains 100 mg of nicotine.
NICOTROL NS would be expected to be irritating if sprayed in the eyes, mouth or ears. Eye exposure should be treated with copious irrigation with water for 20 minutes. Large oral nicotine ingestions cause vomiting, and the consequences of an overdose will vary; should this occur, patients should contact their physician immediately. For additional emergency information, call your regional poison center or call the National Capital Poison Center toll-free (1-800-498-8666).

Signs and Symptoms of Nicotine Toxicity

Signs and symptoms of an overdose of NICOTROL NS would be expected to be the same as those of acute nicotine poisoning including: pallor, cold sweat, nausea, salivation, vomiting, abdominal pain, diarrhea, headache, dizziness, disturbed hearing and vision, tremor, mental confusion, and weakness. Prostration, hypotension, and respiratory failure may ensue with large overdoses. Lethal doses produce convulsions quickly and death follows as a result of peripheral or central respiratory paralysis or, less frequently, cardiac failure.

Overdose from Ingestion

If emesis has not occurred, it should be induced in conscious patients with a suitable emetic followed by an appropriate dose of activated charcoal. In unconscious patients with a secure airway, instill activated charcoal via a nasogastric tube. A saline cathartic or sorbitol may be added to the first dose of activated charcoal.

Management of Nicotine Poisoning

Other supportive measures include diazepam or barbiturates for seizures, atropine for excessive bronchial secretions or diarrhea, respiratory support for respiratory failure, and vigorous fluid support for hypotension and cardiovascular collapse.

DOSAGE AND ADMINISTRATION

It is important that patients understand the instructions for use of NICOTROL NS, and have their questions answered. They should clearly understand the directions for using NICOTROL NS and safely disposing of the used container. They should be instructed to stop smoking completely when they begin using the product.
Patients should be instructed not to sniff, swallow or inhale through the nose as the spray is being administered. They should also be advised to administer the spray with the head tilted back slightly.
The dose of NICOTROL NS, should be **individualized** on the basis of each patient's nicotine dependence and the occurrence of symptoms of nicotine excess (See Individualization of Dosage).
Each actuation of NICOTROL NS delivers a metered 50 microliter spray containing 0.5 mg of nicotine. One dose is 1 mg of nicotine (2 sprays, one in each nostril).
Patients should be started with 1 or 2 doses per hour, which may be increased up to a maximum recommended dose of 40 mg (80 sprays, somewhat less than 1/2 bottle) per day. For best results, patients should be encouraged to use at least the recommended minimum of 8 doses per day, as less is unlikely to be effective. In clinicals trials, the patients who successfully quit smoking used the product heavily when nicotine withdrawal was at its peak, sometimes up to the recommended maximum of 40 doses per day (in heavier smokers). Dosing recommendations are summarized in Table 4.
[See table 4 above]

Table 4

Maximum Recommended Duration of Treatment	Recommended Doses per Hour	Maximum Doses per Hour	Maximum Doses per Day
3 months	1–2*	5	40

* One dose = 2 sprays (one in each nostril). One dose delivers 1 mg of nicotine to the nasal mucosa.

No tapering strategy has been shown to be optimal in clinical studies. Many patients simply stopped using the spray at their last clinic visit.
Recommended strategies for discontinuation of use include suggesting that patients: use only 1/2 a dose (1 spray) at a time, use the spray less frequently, keep a tally of daily usage, try to meet a steadily reducing usage target, skip a dose by not medicating every hour, or set a planned "quit date" for stopping use of the spray.

Continued on next page

Nicotrol NS—Cont.

Individualization of Dosage

The success or failure of smoking cessation is influenced by the quality, intensity and frequency of supportive care. Patients are more likely to quit smoking if they are seen frequently and participate in formal smoking cessation programs.

The goal of NICOTROL NS therapy is complete abstinence. If a patient is unable to stop smoking by the fourth week of therapy, treatment should probably be discontinued.

Patients who fail to quit on any attempt may benefit from interventions to improve their chances for success on subsequent attempts. Patients who were unsuccessful should be counseled and should then probably be given a "therapy holiday" before the next attempt. A new quit attempt should be encouraged when conditions are more favorable.

Based on the clinical trials, a reasonable approach to assisting patients in their attempt to quit smoking is to begin initial treatment, using the recommended dosage (See **DOSAGE AND ADMINISTRATION**). Regular use of the spray during the first week of treatment may help patients adapt to the irritant effects of the spray. Dosage can then be adjusted in those subjects with signs or symptoms of nicotine withdrawal or excess. Patients who are successfully abstinent on NICOTROL NS should be treated at the selected dosage for up to 8 weeks, following which use of the spray should be discontinued over the next 4 to 6 weeks. Some patients may not require gradual reduction of dosage and may abruptly stop treatment successfully. Treatment with NICOTROL NS for longer periods has not been shown to improve outcome, and the safety of use for periods longer than 6 months has not been established.

The symptoms of nicotine withdrawal overlap those of nicotine excess (See **Pharmacodynamics and ADVERSE REACTIONS** sections). Since patients using NICOTROL NS may also smoke intermittently, it is sometimes difficult to determine if patients are experiencing nicotine withdrawal or nicotine excess. Controlled clinical trials of nicotine products suggest that palpitations, nausea and sweating are more often symptoms of nicotine excess, whereas anxiety, nervousness and irritability are more often symptoms of nicotine withdrawal

SAFETY AND HANDLING

As with all medicines, especially ones in liquid form, care should be taken in handling NICOTROL NS during periods of opening and closing the container (See **WARNINGS and Safety Note Concerning Children**). If it is dropped it may break. If this occurs, the spill should be cleaned up immediately with an absorbent cloth/paper towel. Care should be taken to avoid contact of the solution with the skin. Broken glass should be picked up carefully, using a broom. The area of the spill should be washed several times. Absorbent material may be disposed of as any other household waste. Should even a small amount of NICOTROL NS come in contact with the skin, lips, mouth, eyes or ears, the affected area(s) should be immediately rinsed with water only.

Disposal

Used bottles of NICOTROL NS should be disposed of with their child-resistant caps in place. Used bottles should be disposed of in such a way as to prevent access by children or pets. See patient information for further information on handling and disposal.

HOW SUPPLIED

NDC 0045-0899-01

Nicotrol® NS (nicotine nasal spray) 10 mg/mL, is supplied in individual 10 mL bottles.

Each unit consists of a glass container, mounted with a metered spray pump

A patient information leaflet is enclosed with the package

Store at room temperature not to exceed 30°C/86°F.

CAUTION: Federal law prohibits dispensing without prescription.

Manufactured by Pharmacia and Upjohn AB, Sweden

Shown in Product Identification Guide, page 321

NICOTROL®   OTC
NICOTINE TRANSDERMAL SYSTEM

DESCRIPTION

NICOTROL® (nicotine transdermal system) is a multilayered, rectangular, thin film laminated unit containing nicotine as the active ingredient. **NICOTROL®** Patch provides systemic delivery of 15 mg of nicotine over 16 hours.

ACTIONS

NICOTROL® (nicotine transdermal system) Patch helps smokers quit by reducing nicotine withdrawal symptoms. Many **NICOTROL®** Patch users will be able to stop smoking

for a few days but often will start smoking again. Most smokers have to try to quit several times before they completely stop.

Your own chances of quitting smoking depend on how much you want to quit, how strongly you are addicted to nicotine and how closely you follow a quitting program like the **PATHWAYS TO CHANGE®** Program that comes with the **NICOTROL®** Patch.

If you find you cannot stop or if you start smoking again after using **NICOTROL®** Patch, please talk to a health care professional who can help you find a program that may work better for you. Remember that breaking this addiction doesn't happen overnight.

Because the **NICOTROL®** Patch provides some nicotine, the **NICOTROL®** Patch will help you stop smoking by reducing nicotine withdrawal symptoms such as nicotine cravings, nervousness and irritability.

INDICATIONS

NICOTROL® Patch is indicated as a stop smoking aid to reduce withdrawal symptoms, including nicotine craving, associated with quitting smoking. **NICOTROL®** Patch is for people who smoke over 10 cigarettes a day.

DIRECTIONS

- Stop smoking completely when you begin using the **NICOTROL®** Patch.
- Refer to enclosed patient information leaflet before using this product.
- Use one **NICOTROL®** Patch every day for six weeks. Remove backing from the patch and immediately press onto clean dry hairless skin. Hold for ten seconds. Wash hands.
- The **NICOTROL®** Patch should be worn during awake hours and removed prior to sleep.

For Best Results In Quitting Smoking:

1. Firmly commit to quitting smoking.
2. Use enclosed support materials.
3. Use the **NICOTROL®** Patches for six weeks.
4. Stop using **NICOTROL®** Patches at the end of week six. If you still feel the need for **NICOTROL®** Patches talk to your doctor.

WARNINGS

- Keep this and all medication out of reach of children and pets. Even used patches have enough nicotine to poison children and pets. Be sure to fold sticky ends together and throw away out of reach of children and pets. In case of accidental overdose, seek professional assistance or contact a poison control center immediately.
- Nicotine can increase your baby's heart rate. First try to stop smoking without the nicotine patch. As with any drug, if you are pregnant or nursing a baby, seek the advice of a health professional before using this product.
- Do not smoke even when you are not wearing the patch. The nicotine in your skin will still be entering your bloodstream for several hours after you take the patch off.
- If you forget to remove the patch at bedtime you may have vivid dreams or other sleep disruptions.

Do Not Use if You:

- Continue to smoke, chew tobacco, use snuff, or use a nicotine gum or other nicotine containing products.

Ask Your Doctor Before Use if You:

- Are under 18 years of age.
- Have heart disease, recent heart attack or irregular heartbeat. Nicotine can increase your heart rate.
- Have high blood pressure not controlled with medication. Nicotine can increase blood pressure.
- Take prescription medicine for depression or asthma. Your prescription dose may need to be adjusted.
- Are allergic to adhesive tape or have skin problems, because you are more likely to get rashes.

Stop Use and See Your Doctor if You Have:

- Skin redness caused by the patch that does not go away after four days, or if your skin swells or you get a rash.
- Irregular heartbeat or palpitations.
- Symptoms of nicotine overdose such as nausea, vomiting, dizziness, weakness and rapid heartbeat.

INACTIVE INGREDIENTS

Non-woven polyester, pigmented aluminized polyester, polybutene, polyisobutylenes, siliconized polyester.

HOW SUPPLIED

Starter Kit-7 and 14 patches, Refill Kit-7 and 14 patches. DO NOT USE IF POUCH IS DAMAGED OR OPEN. Do not Store above 86°F (30°C)

- **Not for sale to those under 18 years of age.**
- **Proof of age required.**
- **Not for sale in vending machines or from any source where proof of age cannot be verified.**

Shown in Product Identification Guide, page 321

Maximum Strength   OTC
SINE-AID® Sinus Medication Gelcaps, Caplets and Tablets

DESCRIPTION

Each **Maximum Strength SINE-AID® Gelcap, Caplet** or **Tablet** contains acetaminophen 500 mg and pseudoephedrine HCl 30 mg.

ACTIONS

Maximum Strength SINE-AID® Gelcaps, Caplets and **Tablets** contain a clinically proven analgesic-antipyretic and a decongestant. Maximum allowable non-prescription levels of acetaminophen and pseudoephedrine provide temporary relief of sinus congestion and pain. Acetaminophen is equal to aspirin in analgesic and antipyretic effectiveness and it is unlikely to produce many of the side effects associated with aspirin and aspirin-containing products. Acetaminophen produces analgesia by elevation of the pain threshold and antipyresis through action on the hypothalamic heat-regulating center. Pseudoephedrine hydrochloride is a sympathomimetic amine that promotes sinus cavity drainage by reducing nasopharyngeal mucosal congestion.

INDICATIONS

Maximum Strength SINE-AID® Gelcaps, Caplets and **Tablets** provide effective symptomatic relief from sinus headache pain and congestion. **SINE-AID®** is particularly well-suited in patients with aspirin allergy, hemostatic disturbances (including anticoagulant therapy), and bleeding diatheses (e.g. hemophilia) and upper gastrointestinal disease (e.g. ulcer, gastritis, hiatus hernia).

PRECAUTIONS

If a rare sensitivity occurs, the drug should be discontinued. Although pseudoephedrine is virtually without pressor effect in normotensive patients, it should be used with caution in hypertensives.

DIRECTIONS

Adults & children 12 years of age and older: Two gelcaps, caplets or tablets every 4 to 6 hours. Do not exceed eight gelcaps, caplets or tablets in any 24 hour period. Not for use in children under 12 years of age.

WARNINGS

Do not use if carton is open or if blister unit is broken.

Do not take for pain for more than 7 days or for fever for more than 3 days unless directed by a doctor. If pain or fever persists, or gets worse, if new symptoms occur, or if redness or swelling is present, consult a doctor because these could be signs of a serious condition. **Do not exceed recommended dosage.** If nervousness, dizziness or sleeplessness occur, discontinue use and consult a doctor. Do not take this product if you have heart disease, high blood pressure, thyroid disease, diabetes or difficulty in urination due to enlargement of the prostate gland unless directed by a doctor. As with any drug, if you are pregnant or nursing a baby, seek the advice of a health professional before using this product. Keep this and all drugs out of the reach of children. In case of accidental overdose, contact a doctor or poison control center immediately. Prompt medical attention is critical for adults as well as for children even if you do not notice any signs or symptoms. Do not use with other products containing acetaminophen.

ALCOHOL WARNING

For this and all other pain relievers, including aspirin, ibuprofen, ketoprofen and naproxen sodium, if you generally consume 3 or more alcohol-containing drinks per day, you should consult your physician for advice on when and how you should take pain relievers.

DRUG INTERACTION PRECAUTION

Do not use this product if you are now taking a prescription monoamine oxidase inhibitor (MAOI) (certain drugs for depression, psychiatric or emotional conditions, or Parkinson's disease), or for 2 weeks after stopping the MAOI drug. If you are uncertain whether your prescription drug contains an MAOI, consult a health professional before taking this product.

PROFESSIONAL INFORMATION

OVERDOSAGE INFORMATION

Acetaminophen in massive overdosage may cause hepatic toxicity in some patients. In adults and adolescents, hepatic toxicity has rarely been reported following ingestion of acute overdoses of less than 7.5 to 10 grams. Fatalities are infrequent (less than 3–4% of untreated cases) and have rarely been reported with overdoses of less than 15 grams. In children, an acute overdosage of less than 150 mg/kg has not been associated with hepatic toxicity. Early symptoms following a potentially hepatotoxic overdose may include: nausea, vomiting, diaphoresis and general malaise. Clinical and laboratory evidence of hepatic toxicity may not be apparent until 48 to 72 hours postingestion.

In adults and adolescents, regardless of the quantity of acetaminophen reported to have been ingested, administer acetylcysteine immediately if 24 hours or less have elapsed from the reported time of ingestion. For full prescribing information, refer to the acetylcysteine package insert. Do not await results of assays for plasma acetaminophen levels before initiating treatment with acetylcysteine. The following additional procedures are recommended: Promptly initiate gastric decontamination of the stomach. A plasma acetaminophen assay should be obtained as early as possible, but no sooner than four hours following ingestion. If plasma level

falls above the lower treatment line on the acetaminophen overdose nomogram, acetylcysteine therapy should be continued. Liver function studies should be obtained initially and repeated at 24-hour intervals.

Serious toxicity or fatalities are extremely infrequent in children, possibly due to differences in the way they metabolize acetaminophen. In children, the maximum potential amount ingested can be more easily estimated. If more than 150 mg/kg or an unknown amount was ingested, obtain a plasma acetaminophen level. The plasma acetaminophen level should be obtained as soon as possible, but no sooner than 4 hours following ingestion. If plasma level falls above the lower treatment line on the acetaminophen overdose nomogram, the acetylcysteine therapy should be initiated and continued for a full course of therapy. If plasma acetaminophen assay capability is not available, and the estimated acetaminophen ingestion exceeds 150 mg/kg, acetylcysteine therapy should be initiated and continued for a full course of therapy.

For additional emergency information, call your regional poison center or call the Rocky Mountain Poison Center toll-free, (1-800-525-6115).

Symptoms from pseudoephedrine overdose consist most often of mild anxiety, tachycardia and/or mild hypertension. Symptoms usually appear within 4 to 8 hours of ingestion and are transient, usually requiring no treatment.

ALCOHOL INFORMATION

Chronic heavy alcohol abusers may be at increased risk of liver toxicity from excessive acetaminophen use, although reports of this event are rare. Reports usually involve cases of severe chronic alcoholics and the dosages of acetaminophen most often exceed recommended doses and often involve substantial overdose. Professionals should alert their patients who regularly consume large amounts of alcohol not to exceed recommended doses of acetaminophen.

INACTIVE INGREDIENTS

Gelcaps: Benzyl Alcohol, Butylparaben, Castor Oil, Cellulose, Corn Starch, Edetate Calcium Disodium, Gelatin, Hydroxypropyl Methylcellulose, Iron Oxide Black, Magnesium Stearate, Methylparaben, Propylparaben, Sodium Lauryl Sulfate, Sodium Propionate, Sodium Starch Glycolate, Titanium Dioxide, FD&C Red #40.

Caplets: Cellulose, Corn Starch, Hydroxypropyl Methylcellulose, Magnesium Stearate, Polyethylene Glycol, Sodium Starch Glycolate, Titanium Dioxide, Blue #1 and Red #40.

Tablets: Cellulose, Corn Starch, Magnesium Stearate and Sodium Starch Glycolate.

HOW SUPPLIED

Gelcaps (colored red and white imprinted "SINE-AID")—blister package of 20.

Caplets (colored white imprinted "Maximum SINE-AID")—blister package of 24.

Tablets (colored white embossed "SINE-AID")—blister package of 24.

Shown in Product Identification Guide, page 322

Extra Strength **OTC**
TYLENOL® acetaminophen
Gelcaps, Geltabs, Caplets, Tablets

Extra Strength
TYLENOL® acetaminophen
Adult Liquid Pain Reliever

Regular Strength
TYLENOL® acetaminophen
Caplets and Tablets

TYLENOL® Arthritis Extended Relief Caplets
acetaminophen extended release
Caplets

Product information for all dosage forms of Adult TYLENOL acetaminophen have been combined under this heading.

DESCRIPTION

Each ***Extra Strength TYLENOL® Gelcap, Geltab, Caplet, or Tablet*** contains acetaminophen 500 mg.

Each 15 mL ($^1/_2$ fl oz or one tablespoonful) of ***Extra Strength TYLENOL® acetaminophen Adult Liquid Pain Reliever*** contains 500 mg acetaminophen (alcohol 7%).

Each ***Regular Strength TYLENOL® Caplet or Tablet*** contains acetaminophen 325 mg.

Each ***TYLENOL® Arthritis Extended Relief Caplet*** contains acetaminophen 650 mg.

ACTIONS

Acetaminophen is a clinically proven analgesic and antipyretic. Acetaminophen produces analgesia by elevation of the pain threshold and antipyresis through action on the hypothalamic heat-regulating center. Acetaminophen is equal to aspirin in analgesic and antipyretic effectiveness and it is unlikely to produce many of the side effects associated with aspirin and aspirin-containing products.

Tylenol Arthritis Extended Relief uses a unique, patented bilayer caplet. The first layer dissolves quickly to provide prompt relief while the second layer is time released to provide up to 8 hours of relief.

USES

For the temporary relief of minor aches and pains associated with headache, muscular aches, backache, minor arthritis pain, common cold, toothache, menstrual cramps and for the reduction of fever.

DIRECTIONS

Extra Strength TYLENOL® Gelcaps, Geltabs, Caplets, or Tablets: Adults and Children 12 years of Age and Older: Take two gelcaps, geltabs, caplets, or tablets every 4 to 6 hours as needed. Do not take more than 8 gelcaps, geltabs, caplets or tablets in 24 hours, or as directed by a doctor.

Children under 12 years:

Do not use this adult Extra Strength product in children under 12 years of age. This will provide more than the recommended dose (overdose) of TYLENOL® and could cause serious health problems.

Extra Strength TYLENOL® Adult Liquid Pain Reliever: Adults and children 12 years of age and older: Take 2 Tablespoons (tbsp.) in dose cup provided every 4 to 6 hours as needed. Do not take more than 8 Tablespoons in 24 hours, or as directed by a doctor.

Children under 12 years: Do not use this adult Extra Strength product in children under 12 years of age. This will provide more than the recommended dose (overdose) of TYLENOL® and could cause serious health problems.

Regular Strength TYLENOL® Caplets or Tablets: Adults and Children 12 years of Age and Older: Take two caplets or tablets every 4 to 6 hours as needed. Do not take more than 12 caplets or tablets in 24 hours, or as directed by a doctor.

Children 6–11 years of age. Take 1 caplet or tablet every 4 to 6 hours as needed. Do not take more than 5 caplets or tablets in 24 hours.

Children under 6 years of age: Do not use this adult Regular Strength product in children under 6 years of age. This will provide more than the recommended dose (overdose) of TYLENOL® and could cause serious health problems.

TYLENOL® Arthritis Extended Relief Caplets: Adults and Children 12 years of Age and Older: Take two caplets every 8 hours, not to exceed 6 caplets in any 24-hour period. TAKE TWO CAPLETS WITH WATER, SWALLOW EACH CAPLET WHOLE. DO NOT CRUSH, CHEW, OR DISSOLVE THE CAPLET. Not for use in children under 12 years of age.

PRECAUTIONS

If a rare sensitivity reaction occurs, the drug should be discontinued.

WARNINGS

Extra Strength TYLENOL® Gelcaps, Geltabs, Caplets, or Tablets, Extra Strength TYLENOL® Adult Liquid Pain Reliever, Regular Strength TYLENOL® Caplets or Tablets: Do not use if carton is opened or red neck wrap or foil seal imprinted with "SAFETY SEAL®" is broken.

Do not Use:

- with any other product containing acetaminophen
- for more than 10 days for pain unless directed by a doctor.
- for more than 3 days for fever unless directed by a doctor.

Stop Using and Ask a Doctor if:

- symptoms do not improve
- new symptoms occur
- pain or fever persists or gets worse
- redness or swelling is present

Do not exceed recommended dose. Keep this and all drugs out of the reach of children. In case of accidental overdose, contact a physician or poison control center immediately. Prompt medical attention is critical for adults as well as for children even if you do not notice any signs or symptoms. As with any drug, if you are pregnant or nursing a baby, seek the advice of a health professional before using this product.

TYLENOL® Arthritis Extended Relief Caplets: Do not use if carton is open or red neck wrap or foil inner seal imprinted with "Safety Seal®" is broken. Do not take for pain for more than 10 days or for fever for more than 3 days unless directed by a physician. If pain or fever persists, or gets worse, if new symptoms occur, or if redness or swelling is present, consult a physician because these could be signs of a serious condition. As with any drug, if you are pregnant or nursing a baby, seek the advice of a health professional before using this product. Keep this and all drugs out of the reach of children. In case of accidental overdose, contact a physician or poison control center immediately. Prompt medical attention is critical for adults as well as for children even if you do not notice any signs or symptoms. Do not use with other products containing acetaminophen.

ALCOHOL WARNING

Extra Strength TYLENOL® Gelcaps, Geltabs, Caplets and Tablets, Extra Strength TYLENOL® Adult Liquid Pain Reliever, Regular Strength TYLENOL® Caplets and Tablets: If you drink 3 or more alcoholic beverages everyday, ask your doctor if you should take TYLENOL or other pain relievers. Chronic heavy alcohol users may be at increased risk of liver damage when taking more than the recommended dose (overdose) of TYLENOL.

TYLENOL® Arthritis Extended Relief Caplets: If you generally consume 3 or more alcohol-containing drinks per day, you should consult your physician for advice on when and how you should take TYLENOL® Arthritis Extended Relief and other pain relievers.

PROFESSIONAL INFORMATION

OVERDOSAGE INFORMATION

Acetaminophen in massive overdosage may cause hepatic toxicity in some patients. In adults and adolescents, hepatic toxicity has rarely been reported following ingestion of acute overdoses of less than 7.5 to 10 grams. Fatalities are infrequent (less than 3–4% of untreated cases) and have rarely been reported with overdoses of less than 15 grams. In children, an acute overdosage of less than 150 mg/kg has not been associated with hepatic toxicity.

Early symptoms following a potentially hepatotoxic overdose may include: nausea, vomiting, diaphoresis and general malaise. Clinical and laboratory evidence of hepatic toxicity may not be apparent until 48 to 72 hours postingestion. In adults and adolescents, regardless of the quantity of acetaminophen reported to have been ingested, administer acetylcysteine immediately if 24 hours or less have elapsed from the reported time of ingestion. For full prescribing information, refer to the acetylcysteine package insert. Do not await results of assays for plasma acetaminophen levels before initiating treatment with acetylcysteine. The following additional procedures are recommended: Promptly initiate gastric decontamination of the stomach. A plasma acetaminophen assay should be obtained as early as possible, but no sooner than four hours following ingestion. If an acetaminophen extended release product is involved, it may be appropriate to obtain an additional plasma acetaminophen level 4–6 hours following the initial plasma acetaminophen level. If either plasma level falls above the lower treatment line on the acetaminophen overdose nomogram, acetylcysteine therapy should be continued. Liver function studies should be obtained initially and repeated at 24-hour intervals.

Serious toxicity or fatalities are extremely infrequent in children, possibly due to differences in the way they metabolize acetaminophen. In children, the maximum potential amount ingested can be more easily estimated. If more than 150 mg/kg or an unknown amount was ingested, obtain a plasma acetaminophen level. The plasma acetaminophen level should be obtained as soon as possible, but no sooner than 4 hours following ingestion. If an acetaminophen *extended release* product is involved, it may be appropriate to obtain an additional plasma acetaminophen level 4–6 hours following the initial plasma acetaminophen level. If either plasma level falls above the lower treatment line on the acetaminophen overdose nomogram, the acetylcysteine therapy should be initiated and continued for a full course of therapy. If plasma acetaminophen assay capability is not available, and the estimated acetaminophen ingestion exceeds 150 mg/kg, acetylcysteine therapy should be initiated and continued for a full course of therapy.

For additional emergency information, call your regional poison center or call the Rocky Mountain Poison Center toll-free, (1-800-525-6115).

ALCOHOL INFORMATION

Chronic heavy alcohol abusers may be at increased risk of liver toxicity from excessive acetaminophen use, although reports of this event are rare. Reports usually involve cases of severe chronic alcoholics and the dosages of acetaminophen most often exceed recommended doses and often involve substantial overdose. Professionals should alert their patients who regularly consume large amounts of alcohol not to exceed recommended doses of acetaminophen.

INACTIVE INGREDIENTS

Extra Strength TYLENOL®: **Tablets:** Magnesium Stearate, Cellulose, Sodium Starch Glycolate and Starch. **Caplets:** Cellulose, Cornstarch, Hydroxypropyl Methylcellulose, Magnesium Stearate, Polyethylene Glycol, Sodium Starch Glycolate, and Red #40. **Gelcaps:** Benzyl Alcohol, Butylparaben, Castor Oil, Cellulose, Edetate Calcium Disodium, Gelatin, Hydroxypropyl Methylcellulose, Magnesium Stearate, Methylparaben, Propylparaben, Sodium Lauryl Sulfate, Sodium Propionate, Sodium Starch Glycolate, Starch, Titanium Dioxide, Blue #1 and #2, Red #40, and Yellow #10. **Geltabs:** Benzyl Alcohol, Butylparaben, Castor Oil, Cellulose, Corn Starch, Edetate Calcium Disodium, Gelatin, Hydroxypropyl Methylcellulose, Magnesium Stearate, Methylparaben, Propylparaben, Sodium Lauryl Sulfate, Sodium Propionate, Sodium Starch Glycolate, Titanium Dioxide, Blue #1 and #2, Red #40, and Yellow #10.

Extra Strength TYLENOL® Adult Liquid Pain Reliever: Alcohol (7%), Citric Acid, Flavors, Glycerin, Polyethylene Glycol, Purified Water, Sodium Benzoate, Sorbitol, Sucrose, Yellow #6 (Sunset Yellow), Yellow #10 and Blue #1.

Continued on next page

Tylenol—Cont.

Regular Strength TYLENOL®: **Tablets:** Magnesium Stearate, Cellulose, Sodium Starch Glycolate and Starch. **Caplets:** Cellulose, Hydroxypropyl Methylcellulose, Magnesium Stearate, Polyethylene Glycol, Sodium Starch Glycolate, Starch and Red #40.
TYLENOL® Arthritis Extended Relief Caplets: Corn Starch, Hydroxyethyl Cellulose, Hydroxypropyl Methylcellulose, Magnesium Stearate, Microcrystalline Cellulose, Povidone, Powdered Cellulose, Pregelatinized Starch, Sodium Starch Glycolate, Titanium Dioxide, Triacetin.

HOW SUPPLIED

Extra Strength TYLENOL®: **Tablets** (colored white, imprinted "TYLENOL" and "500")—vials of 10, and tamper-resistant bottles of 30, 60, 100, and 200. **Caplets** (colored white, imprinted "TYLENOL 500 mg")—vials of 10, 10 blister packs, and tamper-resistant bottles of 24, 50, 100, 175, and 250 and FastCap package of 72. **Gelcaps** (colored yellow and red, imprinted "Tylenol 500") vials of 10 and tamper-resistant bottles of 24, 50, 100, and 225 and FastCap package of 72. **Geltabs** (colored yellow and red, imprinted "Tylenol 500") tamper-resistant bottles of 24, 50, and 100.
Extra Strength TYLENOL® Adult Liquid Pain Reliever: Mint-flavored liquid (colored green) 8 fl. oz. tamper-resistant bottle with child resistant safety cap and special dosage cup.
Regular Strength TYLENOL®: **Tablets** (colored white, scored, imprinted "TYLENOL" and "325")—tamper-evident bottles of 24, 50, 100 and 200. **Caplets** (colored white, "TYLENOL 325")—tamper-evident bottles of 24, 50, 100.
TYLENOL® Arthritis Extended Relief Caplets: (colored white, engraved "TYLENOL ER") tamper-evident bottles of 24, 50, and 100's.

Shown in Product Identification Guide, page 321

TYLENOL® SEVERE ALLERGY OTC
Medication Caplets
Maximum Strength

TYLENOL® ALLERGY SINUS NIGHTTIME
Caplets
Maximum Strength

TYLENOL® ALLERGY SINUS
Caplets, Gelcaps and Geltabs

Product information for all dosage forms of TYLENOL ALLERGY have been combined under this heading.

DESCRIPTION

Each ***TYLENOL® SEVERE ALLERGY Caplet*** contains acetaminophen 500 mg, and diphenhydramine HCl 12.5 mg. Each ***Maximum Strength TYLENOL® ALLERGY SINUS NightTime Caplet*** contains acetaminophen 500 mg, pseudoephedrine HCl 30 mg, and diphenhydramine HCl 25 mg. Each ***Maximum Strength TYLENOL® ALLERGY SINUS Caplet Gelcap and Geltab*** contains acetaminophen 500 mg, chlorpheniramine maleate 2 mg, and pseudoephedrine HCl 30 mg.

ACTIONS

TYLENOL® SEVERE ALLERGY Caplets contain a clinically proven analgesic-antipyretic and antihistamine. Acetaminophen produces analgesia by elevation of the pain threshold and antipyresis through action on the hypothalamic heat-regulating center. Acetaminophen is equal to aspirin in analgesic and antipyretic effectiveness, and it is unlikely to produce many of the side effects associated with aspirin and aspirin-containing products.
Diphenhydramine is an antihistamine which helps provide temporary relief of itchy, watery eyes, runny nose, sneezing, itching of the nose or throat due to hay fever or other respiratory allergies.
Maximum Strength TYLENOL® ALLERGY SINUS NightTime Caplets contain, in addition to the above ingredients, a decongestant, pseudoephedrine. Pseudoephedrine is a sympathomimetic amine which provides temporary relief of nasal and sinus congestion.
Maximum Strength TYLENOL® ALLERGY SINUS Caplets, Gelcaps and Geltabs contain acetaminophen, pseudoephedrine and the antihistamine, chlorpheniramine. Chlorpheniramine is an antihistamine which helps provide temporary relief of runny nose, sneezing and watery and itchy eyes.

INDICATIONS

TYLENOL® SEVERE ALLERGY provides effective temporary relief of itchy, watery eyes, runny nose, sneezing, sore or scratchy throat and itching of the nose or throat due to hay fever or other upper respiratory allergies.
TYLENOL® ALLERGY SINUS NightTime *and* ***TYLENOL® ALLERGY SINUS*** provide effective temporary relief of runny nose, sneezing, itching of the nose or throat, and itchy, watery eyes due to hay fever or other upper respiratory allergies, nasal and sinus congestion, and sinus pain and headaches.

PRECAUTIONS

TYLENOL® SEVERE ALLERGY: If a rare sensitivity reaction occurs, the drug should be stopped.
TYLENOL® ALLERGY SINUS NightTime and ***TYLENOL® ALLERGY SINUS:*** If a rare sensitivity reaction occurs, the drug should be stopped. Although pseudoephedrine is virtually without pressor effect in normotensive patients, it should be used with caution in hypertensives.

DIRECTIONS

TYLENOL® SEVERE ALLERGY: Adults and children 12 years of age and older: Two caplets every four to six hours. Do not exceed 8 caplets in any 24 hour period. Not for use in children under 12 years of age.
TYLENOL® ALLERGY SINUS NightTime: Adults and children 12 years of age and older: Two caplets at bedtime. Not for use in children under 12 years of age.
TYLENOL® ALLERGY SINUS: Adults and children 12 years of age and older: Two caplets, gelcaps or geltabs every six hours. Do not exceed 8 caplets, gelcaps, or geltabs in any 24 hour period. Not for use in children under 12 years of age.

WARNINGS

TYLENOL® SEVERE ALLERGY: **DO NOT USE IF CARTON IS OPEN OR IF A BLISTER UNIT IS BROKEN.** Do not take for pain for more than 10 days or for fever for more than 3 days unless directed by a doctor. If pain or fever persists, or gets worse, if new symptoms occur, or if redness or swelling is present, consult a doctor because these could be signs of a serious condition. If sore throat is severe, persists for more than 2 days, is accompanied or followed by fever, headache, rash, nausea or vomiting, consult a doctor promptly. May cause excitability especially in children. Do not take this product, unless directed by a doctor, if you have a breathing problem such as emphysema or chronic bronchitis, or if you have glaucoma or difficulty in urination due to enlargement of the prostate gland. May cause marked drowsiness; alcohol, sedatives and tranquilizers may increase the drowsiness effect.
Avoid alcoholic beverages while taking this product. Do not take this product if you are taking sedatives or tranquilizers without first consulting your doctor. Use caution while driving a motor vehicle or operating machinery. As with any drug, if you are pregnant or nursing a baby, seek the advice of a health professional before using this product. Keep this and all drugs out of the reach of children. In case of accidental overdose, contact a doctor or poison control center immediately. Prompt medical attention is critical for adults as well as for children even if you do not notice any signs or symptoms. Do not use with other products containing acetaminophen.
TYLENOL® ALLERGY SINUS NightTime and TYLENOL® ALLERGY SINUS: **Do not use if carton is open or if a blister unit is broken.** Do not take for pain for more than 7 days or for fever for more than 3 days unless directed by a doctor. If pain or fever persists, or gets worse, if new symptoms occur, or if redness or swelling is present, consult a doctor because these could be signs of a serious condition. **Do not exceed recommended dosage.** If nervousness, dizziness or sleeplessness occur, discontinue use and consult a doctor.
May cause excitability, especially in children. Do not take this product unless directed by a doctor, if you have a breathing problem such as emphysema or chronic bronchitis, or if you have glaucoma or difficulty in urination due to enlargement of the prostate gland. Do not take this product if you have heart disease, high blood pressure, thyroid disease or diabetes unless directed by a doctor. May cause marked drowsiness; alcohol, sedatives and tranquilizers may increase the drowsiness effect. Avoid alcoholic beverages while taking this product. Do not take this product if you are taking sedatives or tranquilizers without first consulting your doctor.
Use caution when driving a motor vehicle or operating machinery. As with any drug, if you are pregnant or nursing a baby, seek the advice of a health professional before using this product. Keep this and all drugs out of the reach of children. In case of accidental overdose, contact a doctor or poison control center immediately. Prompt medical attention is critical for adults as well as for children even if you do not notice any signs or symptoms. Do not use with other products containing acetaminophen.

ALCOHOL WARNING

For this and all other pain relievers, including aspirin, ibuprofen, ketoprofen and naproxen sodium. if you generally consume 3 or more alcohol-containing drinks per day, you should consult your physician for advice on when and how you should take pain relievers.

DRUG INTERACTION PRECAUTION

TYLENOL® ALLERGY SINUS NightTime and TYLENOL® ALLERGY SINUS: Do not use this product if you are now taking a prescription monamine oxidase inhibitor (MAOI) (certain drugs for depression, psychiatric or emotional condition, or Parkinson's disease), or for 2 weeks after stopping the MAOI drug. If you are uncertain whether your prescription drug contains an MAOI, consult a health professional before taking this product.

PROFESSIONAL INFORMATION
OVERDOSAGE INFORMATION

Acetaminophen in massive overdosage may cause hepatic toxicity in some patients. In adults and adolescents, hepatic toxicity has rarely been reported following ingestion of acute overdoses of less than 7.5 to 10 grams. Fatalities are infrequent (less than 3–4% of untreated cases) and have rarely been reported with overdoses of less than 15 grams. In children, an acute overdosage of less than 150 mg/kg has not been associated with hepatic toxicity.
Early symptoms following a potentially hepatotoxic overdose may include: nausea, vomiting, diaphoresis and general malaise. Clinical and laboratory evidence of hepatic toxicity may not be apparent until 48 to 72 hours postingestion. In adults and adolescents, regardless of the quantity of acetaminophen reported to have been ingested, administer acetylcysteine immediately if 24 hours or less have elapsed from the reported time of ingestion. For full prescribing information, refer to the acetylcysteine package insert. Do not await results of assays for plasma acetaminophen levels before initiating treatment with acetylcysteine. The following additional procedures are recommended: Promptly initiate gastric decontamination of the stomach. A plasma acetaminophen assay should be obtained as early as possible, but no sooner than four hours following ingestion. If plasma level falls above the lower treatment line on the acetaminophen overdose nomogram, acetylcysteine therapy should be continued. Liver function studies should be obtained initially and repeated at 24-hour intervals.
Serious toxicity or fatalities are extremely infrequent in children, possibly due to differences in the way they metabolize acetaminophen. In children, the maximum potential amount ingested can be more easily estimated. If more than 150 mg/kg or an unknown amount was ingested, obtain a plasma acetaminophen level. The plasma acetaminophen level should be obtained as soon as possible, but no sooner than 4 hours following ingestion. If plasma level falls above the lower treatment line on the acetaminophen overdose nomogram, the acetylcysteine therapy should be initiated and continued for a full course of therapy. If plasma acetaminiophen assay capability is not available, and the estimated acetaminophen ingestion exceeds 150 mg/kg, acetylcysteine therapy should be initiated and continued for a full course of therapy.
For additional emergency information, call your regional poison center or call the Rocky Mountain Poison Center toll-free (1–800–525–6115).
Symptoms for pseudoephedrine overdose consist most often of mild anxiety, tachycardia and/or hypertension. Symptoms usually appear within 4 to 8 hours of ingestion and are transient, usually requiring no treatment.
Diphenhydramine and chlorpheniramine toxicity should be treated as you would an antihistamine/anticholinergic overdose and is likely to be present within a few hours after acute ingestion.

ALCOHOL INFORMATION

Chronic heavy alcohol abusers may be at increased risk of liver toxicity from excessive acetaminophen use, although reports of this event are rare. Reports usually involve cases of severe chronic alcoholics and the dosages of acetaminophen most often exceed recommended doses and often involve substantial overdose. Professionals should alert their patients who regularly consume large amounts of alcohol not to exceed recommended doses of acetaminophen.

INACTIVE INGREDIENTS

TYLENOL® SEVERE ALLERGY Caplets: Cellulose, Corn Starch, Hydroxpropyl Cellulose, Hydroxypropyl Methylcellulose, Iron Oxide Black, Magnesium Stearate, Polyethylene Glycol, Sodium Citrate, Sodium Starch Glycolate, Titanium Dioxide, Yellow #6 and Yellow #10.
TYLENOL® ALLERGY SINUS NightTime Caplets: Cellulose, Corn Starch, Hydroxypropyl Methylcellulose, Iron Oxide Black, Magnesium Stearate, Polyethylene Glycol, Polysorbate 80, Sodium Citrate, Sodium Starch Glycolate, Titanium Dioxide, Blue #1, and Yellow #10.
TYLENOL® ALLERGY SINUS: **Caplets:** Carnauba Wax, Cellulose, Cornstarch, Hydroxypropyl Cellulose, Hydroxypropyl Methylcellulose, Iron Oxide Black, Magnesium Stearate, Polyethylene Glycol, Sodium Starch Glycolate, Titanium Dioxide, Blue #1, Yellow #6, and Yellow #10. **Gelcaps and Geltabs:** Benzyl Alcohol, Butylparaben, Castor Oil, Cellulose, Cornstarch, Edetate Calcium Disodium, Gelatin, Hydroxypropyl Methylcellulose, Magnesium Stearate, Methylparaben, Propylparaben, Sodium Lauryl Sulfate, Sodium Propionate, Sodium Starch Glycolate, Titanium Dioxide, Blue #1, Blue #2 and Yellow #10.

HOW SUPPLIED

TYLENOL® SEVERE ALLERGY: **Caplets** (dark yellow, imprinted "TYLENOL Severe Allergy") blister packs of 12 and 24.

TYLENOL® ALLERGY SINUS NightTime: Caplets (light blue, imprinted "TYLENOL A/S NightTime") child-resistant blister packs of 24.

TYLENOL® ALLERGY SINUS: Caplets: (dark yellow, imprinted "TYLENOL Allergy Sinus") Blister packs of 24 and 48.

Gelcaps and Geltabs: (dark green and dark yellow, imprinted "TYLENOL A/S") Blister packs of 24 and 48.

Shown in Product Identification Guide, page 322

TYLENOL® COLD ® Medication   OTC
No Drowsiness Formula
Caplets and Gelcaps

Multi-Symptom Formula
TYLENOL® COLD Medication
Tablets and Caplets

TYLENOL® COLD Multi-Symptom
Hot Medication Liquid Packets

Product information for all dosage forms of TYLENOL COLD have been combined under this heading.

DESCRIPTION
Each **TYLENOL COLD Medication No Drowsiness Formula Caplet and Gelcap** contains acetaminophen 325 mg, pseudoephedrine HCl 30 mg, and dextromethorphan HBr 15 mg.

Each **Multi-Symptom Formula TYLENOL® COLD Tablet or Caplet** contains acetaminophen 325 mg, chlorpheniramine maleate 2 mg, pseudoephedrine HCl 30 mg, and dextromethorphan HBr 15 mg.

Each packet of **TYLENOL® COLD Multi-Symptom Hot Medication** contains acetaminophen 650 mg, chlorpheniramine maleate 4 mg, pseudoephedrine HCl 60 mg, and dextromethorphan HBr 30 mg.

ACTIONS
TYLENOL® COLD Medication No Drowsiness Formula contains a clinically proven analgesic-antipyretic, decongestant and cough suppressant. Acetaminophen produces analgesia by elevation of the pain threshold and antipyresis through action on the hypothalamic heat-regulating center. Acetaminophen is equal to aspirin in analgesic and antipyretic effectiveness and it is unlikely to produce many of the side effects associated with aspirin and aspirin-containing products. Pseudoephedrine is a sympathomimetic amine which provides temporary relief of nasal congestion. Dextromethorphan is a cough suppressant which provides temporary relief of coughs due to minor throat irritations that may occur with the common cold.

Multi-Symptom Formula TYLENOL® COLD Medication and TYLENOL® COLD Multi-Symptom Hot Medication contain, in addition to the above ingredients, an antihistamine. Chlorpheniramine is an antihistamine which helps provide temporary relief of runny nose, sneezing and watery and itchy eyes.

INDICATIONS
TYLENOL® COLD Medication No Drowsiness Formula provides effective temporary symptom relief of nasal congestion, coughing, sore throat, headaches, body aches and fever.

Multi-Symptom Formula TYLENOL® COLD Medication and TYLENOL® COLD Multi-Symptom Hot Medication provide effective temporary symptom relief of nasal congestion, runny nose, sneezing, watery and itchy eyes, coughing, sore throat, headaches, body aches and fever.

DIRECTIONS
TYLENOL® COLD No Drowsiness Formula and Multi-Symptom Formula TYLENOL® COLD Medication: Adults (12 years and older): Two every 6 hours, not to exceed 8 in 24 hours. **Children (6–11 years):** One every 6 hours, not to exceed 4 in 24 hours. Not for use in children under 6 years of age.

TYLENOL® COLD Multi-Symptom Hot Medication: Adults (12 years and older): Dissolve one packet in 6 oz. cup of hot water. Sip while hot. Sweeten to taste, if desired. May repeat every 6 hours, not to exceed 4 doses in 24 hours. Not for use in children under 12 years of age.

PRECAUTIONS
TYLENOL® COLD Medication No Drowsiness Formula, Multi-Symptom Formula TYLENOL® COLD Medication and TYLENOL® COLD Multi-Symptom Hot Medication: If a rare sensitivity reaction occurs, the drug should be stopped. Although pseudoephedrine is virtually without pressor effect in normotensive patients, it should be used with caution in hypertensives.

WARNINGS
TYLENOL® COLD Medication No Drowsiness Formula: Do not use if carton is opened or if a blister unit is broken. Do not take for pain for more than 7 days or for fever for more than 3 days unless directed by a doctor. If pain or fever persists, or gets worse, if new symptoms occur, or if redness or swelling is present, consult a doctor because these could be signs of a serious condition. If sore throat is severe, persists for more than 2 days, is accompanied or followed by fever, headache, rash, nausea or vomiting, consult a doctor promptly. A persistent cough may be a sign of a serious condition. If cough persists for more than 1 week, tends to recur or is accompanied by fever, rash or persistent headache, consult a doctor. Do not take this product for persistent or chronic cough such as occurs with smoking, asthma, emphysema or if cough is accompanied by excessive phlegm (mucus) unless directed by a doctor. **Do not exceed recommended dosage** If nervousness, dizziness or sleeplessness occur, discontinue use and consult a doctor. Do not take this product if you have heart disease, high blood pressure, thyroid disease, diabetes or difficulty in urination due to enlargement of the prostate gland unless directed by a doctor. As with any drug, if you are pregnant or nursing a baby, seek the advice of a health professional before using this product. Keep this and all drugs out of the reach of children. In case of accidental overdose, contact a doctor or poison control center immediately. Prompt medical attention is critical for adults as well as for children even if you do not notice any signs or symptoms. Do not use with other products containing acetaminophen.

Multi-Symptom Formula TYLENOL® COLD Medication: Do not use if carton is opened or if a blister unit is broken Do not take for pain for more than 7 days or for fever for more than 3 days unless directed by a doctor. If pain or fever persists, or gets worse, if new symptoms occur, or if redness or swelling is present, consult a doctor because these could be signs of a serious condition. If sore throat is severe, persists for more than 2 days, is accompanied or followed by fever, headache, rash, nausea or vomiting, consult a doctor promptly. A persistent cough may be a sign of a serious condition. If cough persists for more than 1 week, tends to recur or is accompanied by fever, rash or persistent headache, consult a doctor. Do not take this product for persistent or chronic cough such as occurs with smoking, asthma, emphysema or if cough is accompanied by excessive phlegm (mucus) unless directed by a doctor. **Do not exceed recommended dosage.** If nervousness, dizziness or sleeplessness occur, discontinue use and consult a doctor. May cause excitability especially in children. Do not take this product unless directed by a doctor, if you have a breathing problem such as emphysema or chronic bronchitis, or if you have glaucoma or difficulty in urination due to enlargement of the prostate gland. Do not take this product if you have heart disease, high blood pressure, thyroid disease or diabetes unless directed by a doctor. May cause drowsiness; alcohol, sedatives and tranquilizers may increase the drowsiness effect. Avoid alcoholic beverages while taking this product. Do not take this product if you are taking sedatives or tranquilizers without first consulting your doctor. Use caution when driving a motor vehicle or operating machinery. As with any drug, if you are pregnant or nursing a baby, seek the advice of a health professional before using this product. Keep this and all drugs out of the reach of children. In case of accidental overdose, contact a doctor or poison control center immediately. Prompt medical attention is critical for adults as well as for children even if you do not notice any signs or symptoms. Do not use with other products containing acetaminophen.

TYLENOL® COLD Multi-Symptom Hot Medication: Do not use if carton is opened or if foil packet is torn or broken. Do not take for pain for more than 7 days or for fever for more than 3 days unless directed by a doctor. If pain or fever persists, or gets worse, if new symptoms occur, or if redness or swelling is present, consult a doctor because these could be signs of a serious condition. If sore throat is severe, persists for more than 2 days, is accompanied or followed by fever, headache, rash, nausea or vomiting, consult a doctor promptly. A persistent cough may be a sign of a serious condition. If cough persists for more than 1 week, tends to recur or is accompanied by fever, rash or persistent headache, consult a doctor. Do not take this product for persistent or chronic cough such as occurs with smoking, asthma, emphysema or if cough is accompanied by excessive phlegm (mucus) unless directed by a doctor. **Do not exceed recommended dosage.** If nervousness, dizziness or sleeplessness occur, discontinue use and consult a doctor. May cause excitability especially in children. Do not take this product, unless directed by a doctor, if you have a breathing problem such as emphysema or chronic bronchitis, or if you have glaucoma or difficulty in urination due to enlargement of the prostate gland. Do not take this product if you have heart disease, high blood pressure, thyroid disease or diabetes unless directed by a doctor. May cause drowsiness; alcohol, sedatives and tranquilizers may increase the drowsiness effect. Avoid alcoholic beverages while taking this product. Do not take this product if you are taking sedatives or tranquilizers without first consulting your doctor. Use caution when driving a motor vehicle or operating machinery. As with any drug, if you are pregnant or nursing a baby, seek the advice of a health professional before using this product. Keep this and all drugs out of the reach of children. In case of accidental overdose, contact a doctor or poison control center immediately. Prompt medical attention is critical for adults as well as for children even if you do not notice any signs or symptoms. Do not use with other products containing acetaminophen.

PHENYLKETONURICS: CONTAINS PHENYLALANINE 11 MG PER PACKET.

ALCOHOL WARNING
TYLENOL® COLD Medication No Drowsiness Formula, Multi-Symptom Formula TYLENOL® COLD Medication and TYLENOL® COLD Multi-Symptom Hot Medication: For this and all other pain relievers, including aspirin, ibuprofen, ketoprofen and naproxen sodium, if you generally consume 3 or more alcohol-containing drinks per day, you should consult your physician for advice on when and how you should take pain relievers.

DRUG INTERACTION PRECAUTION
TYLENOL® COLD Medication No Drowsiness Formula, Multi-Symptom Formula TYLENOL® COLD Medication and TYLENOL® COLD Multi-Symptom Hot Medication: Do not use this product if you are now taking a prescription monoamine oxidase inhibitor (MAOI) (certain drugs for depression, psychiatric or emotional conditions, or Parkinson's disease), or for 2 weeks after stopping the MAOI drug. If you are uncertain whether your prescription drug contains an MAOI, consult a health professional before taking this product.

PROFESSIONAL INFORMATION
OVERDOSAGE INFORMATION
TYLENOL® COLD Medication No Drowsiness Formula, Multi-Symptom Formula TYLENOL® COLD Medication and TYLENOL® COLD Multi-Symptom Hot Medication: Acetaminophen in massive overdosage may cause hepatic toxicity in some patients. In adults and adolescents, hepatic toxicity has rarely been reported following ingestion of acute overdoses of less than 7.5 to 10 grams. Fatalities are infrequent (less than 3–4% of untreated cases) and have rarely been reported with overdoses of less than 15 grams. In children, an acute overdosage of less than 150 mg/kg has not been associated with hepatic toxicity.

Early symptoms following a potentially hepatotoxic overdose may include: nausea, vomiting, diaphoresis and general malaise. Clinical and laboratory evidence of hepatic toxicity may not be apparent until 48 to 72 hours postingestion. In adults and adolescents, regardless of the quantity of acetaminophen reported to have been ingested, administer acetylcysteine immediately if 24 hours or less have elapsed from the reported time of ingestion. For full prescribing information, refer to the acetylcysteine package insert. Do not await results of assays for plasma acetaminophen levels before initiating treatment with acetylcysteine. The following additional procedures are recommended: Promptly initiate gastric decontamination of the stomach. A plasma acetaminophen assay should be obtained as early as possible, but no sooner than four hours following ingestion. If plasma level falls above the lower treatment line on the acetaminophen overdose nomogram, acetylcysteine therapy should be continued. Liver function studies should be obtained initially and repeated at 24-hour intervals.

Serious toxicity or fatalities are extremely infrequent in children, possibly due to differences in the way they metabolize acetaminophen. In children, the maximum potential amount ingested can be more easily estimated. If more than 150 mg/kg or an unknown amount was ingested, obtain a plasma acetaminophen level. The plasma acetaminophen level should be obtained as soon as possible, but no sooner than 4 hours following ingestion. If plasma level falls above the lower treatment line on the acetaminophen overdose nomogram, the acetylcysteine therapy should be initiated and continued for a full course of therapy. If plasma acetaminophen assay capability is not available, and the estimated acetaminophen ingestion exceeds 150 mg/kg, acetylcysteine therapy should be initiated and continued for a full course of therapy.

For additional emergency information, call your regional poison center or call the Rocky Mountain Poison Center toll-free, (1-800-525-6115).

Symptoms from pseudoephedrine overdose consist most often of mild anxiety, tachycardia and/or mild hypertension. Symptoms usually appear within 4 to 8 hours of ingestion and are transient, usually requiring no treatment.

Acute dextromethorphan overdose usually does not result in serious signs and symptoms unless massive amounts have been ingested. Signs and symptoms of a substantial overdose may include nausea and vomiting, visual disturbances, CNS disturbances, and urinary retention.

Chlorpheniramine toxicity should be treated as you would an antihistamine/anticholinergic overdose and is likely to be present within a few hours after acute ingestion.

ALCOHOL INFORMATION
TYLENOL® COLD Medication No Drowsiness Formula, Multi-symptom Formula TYLENOL® COLD Medication and

Continued on next page

Tylenol Cold—Cont.

TYLENOL® COLD Multi-Symptom Hot Medication: Chronic heavy alcohol abusers may be at increased risk of liver toxicity from excessive acetaminophen use, although reports of this event are rare. Reports usually involve cases of severe chronic alcoholics and the dosages of acetaminophen most often exceed recommended doses and often involve substantial overdose. Professionals should alert their patients who regularly consume large amounts of alcohol not to exceed recommended doses of acetaminophen.

INACTIVE INGREDIENTS

TYLENOL® COLD No Drowsiness Formula: Caplets: Cellulose, Corn Starch, Glyceryl Triacetate, Hydroxypropyl Methylcellulose, Iron Oxide Black, Magnesium Stearate, Sodium Starch Glycolate, Titanium Dioxide, Blue #1 and Yellow #10. **Gelcaps:** Benzyl Alcohol, Butylparaben, Castor Oil, Cellulose, Corn Starch, Edetate Calcium Disodium, Gelatin, Hydroxypropyl Methylcellulose, Magnesium Stearate, Methylparaben, Propylparaben, Sodium Propionate, Sodium Lauryl Sulfate, Sodium Starch Glycolate, Titanium Dioxide, Red #40 and Yellow #10.
Multi-Symptom Formula TYLENOL® COLD Medication: Tablets: Cellulose, Corn starch, Magnesium Stearate, Sodium Starch Glycolate Yellow #6 and Yellow #10. **Caplets:** Cellulose, Corn Starch, Glyceryl Triacetate, Hydroxypropyl Methylcellulose, Iron Oxide Black, Magnesium Stearate, Sodium Starch Glycolate, Titanium Dioxide, Blue #1 and Yellow #6 and #10.
TYLENOL® COLD Multi-Symptom Hot Medication: Aspartame, Citric Acid, Corn Starch, Flavors, Sodium Citrate, Sucrose, Red #40 and Yellow #10.

HOW SUPPLIED

TYLENOL® COLD No Drowsiness Formula: Caplets (colored white, imprinted "TYLENOL COLD") blister packs of 24. **Gelcaps** (colored red and tan, imprinted "TYLENOL COLD") blister packs of 24.
Multi-Symptom Formula TYLENOL® COLD Medication: Tablets (colored yellow, imprinted "TYLENOL Cold") blister packs of 24. **Caplets** (light yellow, imprinted "TYLENOL Cold") blister packs of 24.
TYLENOL® COLD Multi-Symptom Hot Medication: Packets of powder (yellow colored) in cartons of 6 tamper-evident foil packets.

Shown in Product Identification Guide, page 322

MULTI-SYMPTOM OTC
TYLENOL® COLD
SEVERE CONGESTION

DESCRIPTION

EACH CAPLET contains acetaminophen 325 mg, pseudoephedrine HCl 30 mg, guaifenesin 200 mg and dextromethorphan HBr 15 mg.

ACTIONS

Multi-Symptom ***TYLENOL® COLD SEVERE CONGESTION Caplets*** contains a clinically proven analgesic-antipyretic, decongestant, expectorant and cough suppressant. Acetaminophen produces analgesia by elevation of the pain threshold and antipyresis through action on the hypothalamic heat-regulating center. Acetaminophen is equal to aspirin in analgesic and antipyretic effectiveness and is unlikely to produce many of the side effects associated with aspirin and aspirin-containing products. Pseudoephedrine is a sympathomimetic amine which provides temporary relief of nasal congestion. Guaifenesin is an expectorant which helps loosen phlegm (mucus) and thin bronchial secretions to make coughs more productive. Dextromethorphan is a cough suppressant which provides temporary relief of coughs due to minor throat irritations that may occur with the common cold.

INDICATIONS

Multi-Symptom ***TYLENOL® COLD SEVERE CONGESTION Caplets*** provide temporary symptom relief without drowsiness of nasal congestion, chest congestion, coughing, sore throat, headaches, body aches and fever.

DIRECTIONS

Adults and Children 12 years of Age and older: Take two caplets every 6–8 hours, not to exceed 8 caplets in any 24 hour period.
Children 6 to 11 years of age: One caplet every 6–8 hours not to exceed 4 caplets in any 24 hour period. Not for use in children under 6 years of age.

PRECAUTIONS

If a rare sensitivity reaction occurs, the drug should be discontinued. Although pseudoephedrine is virtually without pressor effect in normotensive patients, it should be used with caution in hypertensives.

WARNINGS

DO NOT USE IF CARTON IS OPENED OR IF A BLISTER UNIT IS BROKEN. Do not take for pain for more than 7 days or for fever for more than 3 days unless directed by a doctor. If pain or fever persists, or gets worse, if new symptoms occur, or if redness or swelling is present, consult a doctor because these could be signs of a serious condition. If sore throat is severe, persists for more than 2 days, is accompanied or followed by fever, headache, rash, nausea or vomiting, consult a doctor promptly. A persistent cough may be a sign of a serious condition. If cough persists for more than 1 week, tends to recur or is accompanied by fever, rash or persistent headache, consult a doctor. Do not take this product for persistent or chronic cough such as occurs with smoking, asthma, emphysema or if cough is accompanied by excessive phlegm (mucus) unless directed by a doctor. **Do not exceed recommended dosage.** If nervousness, dizziness, or sleeplessness occur, discontinue use and consult a doctor. Do not take this product if you have heart disease, high blood pressure, thyroid disease, diabetes or difficulty in urination due to enlargement of the prostate gland unless directed by a doctor. As with any drug, if you are pregnant or nursing a baby, seek the advice of a health professional before using this product. Keep this and all drugs out of the reach of children. In case of accidental overdose, contact a doctor or poison control center immediately. Prompt medical attention is critical for adults as well as for children even if you do not notice any signs or symptoms. Do not use with other products containing acetaminophen.

ALCOHOL WARNING

For this and all other pain relievers, including aspirin, ibuprofen, ketoprofen and naproxen sodium, if you generally consume 3 or more alcohol-containing drinks per day you should consult your physician for advice on when and how you should take pain relievers.

DRUG INTERACTION PRECAUTION

Do not use this product if you are now taking a prescription monoamine oxidase inhibitor (MAOI) (certain drugs for depression, psychiatric or emotional conditions, or Parkinson's disease), or for 2 weeks after stoppping the MAOI drug. If you are uncertain whether your prescription drug contains an MAOI, consult a health professional before taking this product.

PROFESSIONAL INFORMATION
OVERDOSAGE INFORMATION

Acetaminophen in massive overdosage may cause hepatic toxicity in some patients. In adults and adolescents, hepatic toxicity has rarely been reported following ingestion of acute overdoses of less than 7.5 to 10 grams. Fatalities are infrequent (less than 3–4% of untreated cases) and have rarely been reported with overdoses of less than 15 grams. In children, an acute overdosage of less than 150 mg/kg has not been associated with hepatic toxicity.
Early symptoms following a potentially hepatotoxic overdose may include: nausea, vomiting, diaphoresis and general malaise. Clinical and laboratory evidence of hepatic toxicity may not be apparent until 48 to 72 hours postingestion. In adults and adolescents, regardless of the quantity of acetaminophen reported to have been ingested, administer acetylcysteine immediately if 24 hours or less have elapsed from the reported time of ingestion. For full prescribing information, refer to the acetylcysteine package insert. Do not await results of assays for plasma acetaminophen levels before initiating treatment with acetylcysteine. The following additional procedures are recommended: Promptly initiate gastric decontamination of the stomach. A plasma acetaminophen assay should be obtained as early as possible, but no sooner than four hours following ingestion. If plasma level falls above the lower treatment line on the acetaminophen overdose nomogram, acetylcysteine therapy should be continued. Liver function studies should be obtained initially and repeated at 24-hour intervals.
Serious toxicity or fatalities are extremely infrequent in children, possibly due to differences in the way they metabolize acetaminophen. In children, the maximum potential amount ingested can be more easily estimated. If more than 150 mg/kg or an unknown amount was ingested, obtain a plasma acetaminophen level. The plasma acetaminophen level should be obtained as soon as possible, but no sooner than 4 hours following ingestion. If plasma level falls above the lower treatment line on the acetaminophen overdose nomogram, the acetylcysteine therapy should be initiated and continued for a full course of therapy. If plasma acetaminophen assay capability is not available, and the estimated acetaminophen ingestion exceeds 150 mg/kg, acetylcysteine therapy should be initiated and continued for a full course of therapy.
For additional emergency information, call your regional poison center or call the Rocky Mountain Poison Center toll-free, (1-800-525-6115).
Symptoms from pseudoephedrine overdose consist most often of mild anxiety, tachycardia and/or mild hypertension. Symptoms usually appear within 4 to 8 hours of ingestion and are transient, usually requiring no treatment.

Acute dextromethorphan overdose usually does not result in serious signs and symptoms unless massive amounts have been ingested. Signs and symptoms of a substantial overdose may include nausea and vomiting, visual disturbance, CNS disturbances, and urinary retention.
Chlorpheniramine toxicity should be treated as you would an antihistamine/anticholinergic overdose and is likely to be present within a few hours after acute ingestion. Guaifenesin should be treated as a non-toxic ingestion.

ALCOHOL INFORMATION

Chronic heavy alcohol abusers may be at increased risk of liver toxicity from excessive acetaminophen use, although reports of this event are rare. Reports usually involve cases of severe chronic alcoholics and the dosages of acetaminophen most often exceed recommended doses and often involve substantial overdose. Professionals should alert their patients who regularly consume large amounts of alcohol not to exceed recommended doses of acetaminophen.

INACTIVE INGREDIENTS

Carnauba Wax, Cellulose, Colloidal Silicon Dioxide, Corn Starch, Hydroxypropyl Methylcellulose, Iron Oxide, Povidone, Pregelatinized Starch, Propylene Glycol, Sodium Starch Glycolate, Stearic Acid, Titanium Dioxide, Triacetin, Blue #1, Yellow #6 and Yellow #10.

HOW SUPPLIED

Caplets (colored buttery-tan, with green imprinted "TYLENOL COLD SC") in blister packs of 12 and 24.
©McN-PPC, Inc. '96   8702830
Shown in Product Identification Guide, page 322

Multi-Symptom
TYLENOL® COUGH Medication OTC
Multi-Symptom
TYLENOL® COUGH Medication
with Decongestant

Product information for all dosage forms of TYLENOL COUGH have been combined under this heading.

DESCRIPTION

Each 15 mL (3 tsp.) adult dose of **Multi-Symptom TYLENOL® COUGH Medication** contains dextromethorphan HBr 30 mg, and acetaminophen 650 mg.
Each 15 mL (3 tsp.) adult dose of **Multi-Symptom TYLENOL® COUGH Medication with Decongestant** contains dextromethorphan HBr 30 mg, acetaminophen 650 mg, and pseudoephedrine HCl 60 mg.

ACTIONS

Multi-Symptom TYLENOL® COUGH Medication contains a clinically proven cough suppressant, and an analgesic-antipyretic. Acetaminophen produces analgesia by elevation of the pain threshold and antipyresis through action on the hypothalamic heat-regulating center. Dextromethorphan is a cough suppressant which provides temporary relief of coughs due to minor throat irritations that may occur with the common cold.
Multi-Symptom TYLENOL® COUGH Medication with Decongestant contains, in addition to the above ingredients, a sympathomimetic amine, pseudoephedrine HCl, which provides temporary relief of nasal congestion.

INDICATIONS

Multi-Symptom TYLENOL® COUGH Medication provides effective, temporary relief of coughing, and the aches, pains and sore throat that may accompany a cough due to a cold.
Multi-Symptom TYLENOL® COUGH Medication with Decongestant provides effective, temporary relief of coughing, nasal congestion and the aches, pains and sore throat that may accompany a cough due to a cold.

DIRECTIONS

Multi-Symptom TYLENOL® COUGH Medication and Multi-Symptom TYLENOL® COUGH Medication with Decongestant: Adults (12 years and older): Take 1 tablespoon or 3 teaspoons every 6–8 hours, not to exceed 4 doses in 24 hours.
Children: (ages 6–11) Take 1½ teaspoons every 6–8 hours, not to exceed 4 doses in 24 hours. Consult a physician for use in children under 6 years of age.

PRECAUTIONS

Multi-Symptom TYLENOL® COUGH Medication: If a rare sensitivity reaction occurs, the drug should be discontinued.
Multi-Symptom TYLENOL® COUGH Medication with Decongestant: If a rare sensitivity reaction occurs, the drug should be discontinued. Although pseudoephedrine is virtually without pressor effect in normotensive patients, it should be used with caution in hypertensives.

WARNINGS

Multi-Symptom TYLENOL® COUGH Medication: **Do not use if carton is opened, or if bottle wrap or foil inner seal imprinted "Safety Seal®" is broken or missing.** Do not take for pain for more than 10 days or for fever for more than 3

days unless directed by a physician. If pain or fever persists, or gets worse, if new symptoms occur, or if redness or swelling is present, consult a doctor because these could be signs of a serious condition. If sore throat is severe, persists for more than 2 days, is accompanied or followed by fever, headache, rash, nausea, or vomiting, consult a doctor promptly. A persistent cough may be a sign of a serious condition. If cough persists for more than 1 week, tends to recur or is accompanied by fever, rash or persistent headache, consult a doctor. Do not take this product for persistent or chronic cough such as occurs with smoking, asthma, emphysema, or if cough is accompanied by excessive phlegm (mucus) unless directed by a doctor.
As with any drug, if you are pregnant or nursing a baby, seek the advice of a health professional before using this product. Keep this and all drugs out of the reach of children. In case of accidental overdose, contact a doctor or poison control center immediately. Prompt medical attention is critical for adults as well as for children even if you do not notice any signs or symptoms. Do not use with other products containing acetaminophen.
Multi-Symptom TYLENOL® COUGH Medication with Decongestant: **Do not use if carton is opened, or if bottle wrap or foil inner seal imprinted "Safety Seal®" is broken or missing.** Do not take for pain for more than 7 days or for fever for more than 3 days unless directed by a doctor. If pain or fever persists, or gets worse, if new symptoms occur, or if redness or swelling is present, consult a doctor because these could be signs of a serious condition. If sore throat is severe, persists for more than 2 days, is accompanied or followed by fever, headache, rash, nausea or vomiting, consult a doctor promptly. A persistent cough may be a sign of a serious condition. If cough persists for more than 1 week, tends to recur or is accompanied by fever, rash or persistent headache, consult a doctor. Do not take this product for persistent or chronic cough such as occurs with smoking, asthma, emphysema, or if cough is accompanied by excessive phlegm (mucus) unless directed by a doctor. **Do not exceed the recommended dosage.** If nervousness, dizziness or sleeplessness occur, discontinue use and consult a doctor. Do not take this product if you have heart disease, high blood pressure, thyroid disease, diabetes or difficulty in urination due to enlargement of the prostate gland unless directed by a doctor.
As with any drug, if you are pregnant or nursing a baby, seek the advice of a health professional before using this product. Keep this and all drugs out of the reach of children. In case of accidental overdose, contact a doctor or poison control center immediately. Prompt medical attention is critical for adults as well as for children even if you do not notice any signs or symptoms. Do not use with other products containing acetaminophen.

ALCOHOL WARNING

Multi-Symptom TYLENOL® COUGH Medication and Multi-Symptom TYLENOL® COUGH Medication with Decongestant: For this and all other pain relievers, including aspirin, ibuprofen, ketoprofen and naproxen sodium; if you generally consume 3 or more alcohol-containing drinks per day, you should consult your physician for advice on when and how you should take pain relievers.

DRUG INTERACTION PRECAUTION

Multi-Symptom TYLENOL® COUGH Medication and Multi-Symptom TYLENOL® COUGH Medication with Decongestant: Do not use this product if you are now taking a prescription monoamine oxidase inhibitor (MAOI) (certain drugs for depression or psychiatric or emotional conditions, or Parkinson's Disease), or for 2 weeks after stopping the MAOI drug. If you are uncertain whether your prescription drug contains an MAOI, consult a health professional before taking this product.

PROFESSIONAL INFORMATION

OVERDOSAGE INFORMATION

Multi-Symptom TYLENOL® COUGH Medication and Multi-Symptom TYLENOL® COUGH Medication with Decongestant: Acetaminophen in massive overdosage may cause hepatic toxicity in some patients. In adults and adolescents, hepatic toxicity has rarely been reported following ingestion of acute overdoses of less than 7.5 to 10 grams. Fatalities are infrequent (less than 3–4% of untreated cases) and have rarely been reported with overdoses of less than 15 grams. In children, an acute overdosage of less than 150 mg/kg has not been associated with hepatic toxicity.
Early symptoms following a potentially hepatotoxic overdose may include: nausea, vomiting, diaphoresis and general malaise. Clinical and laboratory evidence of hepatic toxicity may not be apparent until 48 to 72 hours postingestion. In adults and adolescents, regardless of the quantity of acetaminophen reported to have been ingested, administer acetylcysteine immediately if 24 hours or less have elapsed from the reported time of ingestion. For full prescribing information, refer to the acetylcysteine package insert. Do not await results of assays for plasma acetaminophen levels before initiating treatment with acetylcysteine. The following additional procedures are recommended: Promptly initiate gastric decontamination of the stomach. A plasma acetaminophen assay should be obtained as early as possible, but no sooner than four hours following ingestion. If plasma level falls above the lower treatment line on the acetaminophen overdose nomogram, acetylcysteine therapy should be continued. Liver function studies should be obtained initially and repeated at 24-hour intervals.
Serious toxicity or fatalities are extremely infrequent in children, possibly due to differences in the way they metabolize acetaminophen. In children, the maximum potential amount ingested can be more easily estimated. If more than 150 mg/kg or an unknown amount was ingested, obtain a plasma acetaminophen level. The plasma acetaminophen level should be obtained as soon as possible, but no sooner than 4 hours following ingestion. If the plasma level falls above the lower treatment line on the acetaminophen overdose nomogram, the acetylcysteine therapy should be initiated and continued for a full course of therapy. If plasma acetaminophen assay capability is not available, and the estimated acetaminophen ingestion exceeds 150 mg/kg, acetylcysteine therapy should be initiated and continued for a full course of therapy.
For additional emergency information, call your regional poison center or call the Rocky Mountain Poison Center toll-free, (1-800-525-6115).
Acute dextromethorphan overdose usually does not result in serious signs and symptoms unless massive amounts have been ingested. Signs and symptoms of a substantial overdose may include nausea and vomiting, visual disturbances, CNS disturbances, and urinary retention.
Symptoms from pseudoephedrine overdose consist most often of mild anxiety, tachycardia and/or mild hypertension. Symptoms usually appear within 4 to 8 hours of ingestion and are transient, usually requiring no treatment.

ALCOHOL INFORMATION

Multi-Symptom TYLENOL® COUGH Medication and Multi-Symptom TYLENOL® COUGH Medication with Decongestant: Chronic heavy alcohol abusers may be at increased risk of liver toxicity from excessive acetaminophen use, although reports of this event are rare. Reports usually involve cases of severe chronic alcoholics and the dosages of acetaminophen most often exceed recommended doses and often involve substantial overdose. Professionals should alert their patients who regularly consume large amounts of alcohol not to exceed recommended doses of acetaminophen.

INACTIVE INGREDIENTS

Multi-Symptom TYLENOL® COUGH Medication: Alcohol (5%), Citric Acid, Flavors, High Fructose Corn Syrup, Polyethylene Glycol, Propylene Glycol, Purified Water, Sodium Benzoate, Sodium Carboxymethylcellulose, Sodium Saccharin, Sorbitol, Red #40.
Multi-Symptom TYLENOL® COUGH Medication with Decongestant: Alcohol (5%), Citric Acid, Flavors, High Fructose Corn Syrup, Polyethylene Glycol, Propylene Glycol, Purified Water, Sodium Benzoate, Sodium Carboxymethylcellulose, Sodium Saccharin, Sorbitol, Blue #1, Red #40.

HOW SUPPLIED

Multi-Symptom TYLENOL® COUGH Medication is available in a 4 oz. bottle with child resistant safety cap and tamper evident packaging.
Multi-Symptom TYLENOL® COUGH Medication with Decongestant is available in a 4 oz. bottle with child resistant safety cap, and tamper evident packaging.

Shown in Product Identification Guide, page 322

Maximum Strength
TYLENOL® FLU Medication **OTC**
No Drowsiness Formula Gelcaps

Maximum Strength
TYLENOL® FLU NightTime
Medication Gelcaps

Maximum Strength
TYLENOL® FLU NightTime
Hot Medication Packets

Maximum Strength
TYLENOL® FLU NightTime
Liquid

Product information for all dosage forms of TYLENOL FLU have been combined under this heading.

DESCRIPTION

Each ***Maximum Strength TYLENOL® FLU Medication No Drowsiness Formula Gelcap*** contains acetaminophen 500 mg, pseudoephedrine hydrochloride 30 mg, and dextromethorphan hydrobromide 15 mg.
Each ***Maximum Strength TYLENOL® FLU NightTime Medication Gelcap*** contains acetaminophen 500 mg, pseudoephedrine hydrochloride 30 mg, and diphenhydramine hydrochloride 25 mg.
Each packet of ***Maximum Strength TYLENOL FLU NightTime Hot Medication*** contains acetaminophen 1000 mg, pseudoephedrine hydrochloride 60 mg and diphenhydramine hydrochloride 50 mg. Each 30 mL (2 tablespoonsful) contains acetaminophen 1000 mg, dextromethorphan HBr 30 mg, doxylamine succinate 12.5 mg, and pseudoephedrine HCl 60 mg.

ACTIONS

Maximum Strength TYLENOL® FLU Medication No Drowsiness Formula contains a clinically proven analgesic-antipyretic, decongestant and cough suppressant. Acetaminophen produces analgesia by elevation of the pain threshold and antipyresis through action on the hypothalamic heat-regulating center. Acetaminophen is equal to aspirin in analgesic and antipyretic effectiveness and it is unlikely to produce many of the side effects associated with aspirin and aspirin-containing products. Pseudoephedrine hydrochloride is a sympathomimetic amine which provides temporary relief of nasal congestion. Dextromethorphan is a cough suppressant which provides temporary relief of coughs due to minor throat irritations that may occur with the common cold.
Maximum Strength TYLENOL® FLU NightTime Medication and ***Maximum Strength TYLENOL® FLU NightTime Hot Medication*** contains the same clinically proven analgesic-antipyretic and decongestant as Maximum Strength TYLENOL FLU Medication No Drowsiness Formula along with an antihistamine. Diphenhydramine is an antihistamine which helps provide temporary relief of runny nose and sneezing. ***Maximum Strength TYLENOL® FLU NightTime Liquid*** contains the same clinically proven analgesic-antipyretic and decongestant as Maximum Strength TYLENOL FLU Medication No Drowsiness Formula along with an antihistamine. Doxylamine succinate is an antihistamine which helps provide temporary relief of runny nose and sneezing.

INDICATIONS

Maximum Strength TYLENOL® FLU Medication No Drowsiness Formula provides temporary symptom relief without drowsiness of body aches, headaches, fever, sore throat, coughing and nasal congestion.
Maximum Strength TYLENOL® FLU NightTime Medication and ***Maximum Strength TYLENOL® FLU NightTime Hot Medication*** provide temporary symptom relief so you can rest of body aches, headaches, fever, sore throat, nasal congestion, and runny nose/sneezing ***Maximum Strength TYLENOL® FLU NightTime Liquid:*** for the temporary relief of: body aches and headache, coughing, nasal congestion, sore throat, runny nose/sneezing, and for the reduction of fever.

DIRECTIONS

Maximum Strength TYLENOL® FLU Medication No Drowsiness Formula: **Adults (12 years and older):** Take two gelcaps every 6 hours, not to exceed 8 gelcaps in 24 hours. Not for use in children under 12 years of age.
Maximum Strength TYLENOL® FLU NightTime Medication: **Adults (12 years and older):** Take two gelcaps at bedtime. May repeat every 6 hours, not to exceed 8 gelcaps in 24 hours. Not for use in children under 12 years of age.
Maximum Strength TYLENOL® FLU NightTime Hot Medication: **Adults (12 years and older):** Dissolve one packet in 6 oz. cup of hot water. Sip while hot. Sweeten to taste, if desired. May repeat every 6 hours, not to exceed 4 doses in 24 hours. Not for use in children under 12 years of age.
Maximum Strength TYLENOL® FLU NightTime Liquid: **Adults and Children 12 years of Age and Older:** Take 2 Tablespoons (tbsp) in dose cup provided. May repeat every 6 hours. Do not use more than 4 times in 24 hours or as directed by a doctor.
Children under 12 years of Age: Do not use this adult product in children under 12 years of age. This will provide more than the recommended dose (overdose) and could cause serious health problems.

PRECAUTIONS

Maximum Strength TYLENOL® FLU Medication No Drowsiness Formula, Maximum Strength TYLENOL® FLU NightTime Medication, and Maximum Strength TYLENOL® FLU NightTime Hot Medication: If a rare sensitivity reaction occurs, the drug should be stopped. Although pseudoephedrine is virtually without pressor effect in normotensive patients, it should be used with caution in hypertensives.

WARNINGS

Maximum Strength TYLENOL® FLU Medication No Drowsiness Formula: **Do not use if carton is opened or if a blister unit is broken.** Do not take for pain for more than 7 days or for fever for more than 3 days unless directed by a doctor. If pain or fever persists, or gets worse, if new symptoms occur, or if redness or swelling is present, consult a doctor because these could be signs of a serious condition. If sore throat is severe, persists for more than 2 days, is accompanied or followed by fever, headache, rash, nausea or vomiting, consult a doctor promptly. A persistent cough may be a sign of a serious condition. If cough persists for more than 1 week,

Continued on next page

Tylenol Flu—Cont.

tends to recur or is accompanied by fever, rash or persistent headache, consult a doctor. Do not take this product for persistent or chronic cough such as occurs with smoking, asthma, emphysema or if cough is accompanied by excessive phlegm (mucus) unless directed by a doctor. **Do not exceed recommended dosage.** If nervousness, dizziness or sleeplessness occur, discontinue use and consult a doctor. Do not take this product if you have heart disease, high blood pressure, thyroid disease, diabetes, or difficulty in urination due to enlargement of the prostate gland unless directed by a doctor.

As with any drug, if you are pregnant or nursing a baby, seek the advice of a health professional before using this product. Keep this and all drugs out of the reach of children. In case of accidental overdose, contact a doctor or poison control center immediately. Prompt medical attention is critical for adults as well as for children even if you do not notice any signs or symptoms. Do not use with other products containing acetaminophen.

Maximum Strength TYLENOL® FLU NightTime Medication Gelcaps: Do not use if carton is opened or if a blister unit is broken. Do not take for pain for more than 7 days or for fever for more than 3 days unless directed by a doctor. If pain or fever persists, or gets worse, if new symptoms occur, or if redness or swelling is present, consult a doctor because these could be signs of a serious condition. If sore throat is severe, persists for more than 2 days, is accompanied by fever, headache, rash, nausea or vomiting, consult a doctor promptly. **Do not exceed recommended dosage.** If nervousness, dizziness, or sleeplessness occur, discontinue use and consult a doctor. May cause excitability, especially in children. Do not take this product, unless directed by a doctor, if you have a breathing problem such as emphysema or chronic bronchitis, or if you have glaucoma or difficulty in urination due to enlargement of the prostate gland. Do not take this product if you have heart disease, high blood pressure, thyroid disease, or diabetes unless directed by a doctor. May cause marked drowsiness; alcohol, sedatives and tranquilizers may increase the drowsiness effect. Avoid alcoholic beverages while taking this product. Do not take this product if you are taking sedatives or tranquilizers without first consulting your doctor. Use caution when driving a motor vehicle or operating machinery.

As with any drug, if you are pregnant or nursing a baby, seek the advice of a health professional before using this product. Keep this and all drugs out of the reach of children. In case of accidental overdose, contact a doctor or poison control center immediately. Prompt medical attention is critical for adults as well as for children even if you do not notice any signs or symptoms. Do not use with other products containing acetaminophen.

Maximum Strength TYLENOL® FLU NightTime Hot Medication: Do not use if carton is opened or if foil packet is torn or broken. Do not take for pain for more than 7 days or for fever for more than 3 days unless directed by a doctor. If pain or fever persists, or gets worse, if new symptoms occur, or if redness or swelling is present, consult a doctor because these could be signs of a serious condition. If sore throat is severe, persists for more than 2 days, is accompanied or followed by fever, headache, rash, nausea or vomiting, consult a doctor promptly. **Do not exceed recommended dosage.** If nervousness, dizziness, or sleeplessness occur, discontinue use and consult a doctor. May cause excitability especially in children. Do not take this product, unless directed by a doctor, if you have a breathing problem such as emphysema or chronic bronchitis, or if you have glaucoma or difficulty in urination due to enlargement of the prostate gland. Do not take this product if you have heart disease, high blood pressure, thyroid disease or diabetes unless directed by a doctor. May cause marked drowsiness; alcohol, sedatives and tranquilizers may increase the drowsiness effect. Avoid alcoholic beverages while taking this product. Do not take this product if you are taking sedatives or tranquilizers without first consulting your doctor. Use caution when driving a motor vehicle or operating machinery.

As with any drug, if you are pregnant or nursing a baby, seek the advice of a health professional before using this product. Keep this and all drugs out of the reach of children. In case of accidental overdose, contact a doctor or poison control center immediately. Prompt medical attention is critical for adults as well as for children even if you do not notice any signs or symptoms. Do not use with other products containing acetaminophen.

PHENYLKETONURICS: CONTAINS PHENYLALANINE 67 MG PER PACKET.

Maximum Strength TYLENOL® FLU NightTime Liquid:
Do not take for pain for more than 7 days or for fever for more than 3 days unless directed by a doctor. If pain or fever persists, or gets worse, if new symptoms occur, or if redness or swelling is present, consult a doctor because these could be signs of a serious condition. If sore throat is severe, persists for more than 2 days, is accompanied or followed by fever, headache, rash, nausea or vomiting, consult a doctor

promptly. A persistent cough may be a sign of a serious condition. If cough persists for more than 1 week, tends to recur or is accompanied by fever, rash or persistent headache, consult a doctor. Do not take this product for persistent or chronic cough such as occurs with smoking, asthma, or emphysema or if cough is accompanied by excessive phlegm (mucus) unless directed by a doctor.

Do not exceed recommended dosage. If nervousness, dizziness or sleeplessness occur, discontinue use and consult a doctor. May cause excitability especially in children.

Do not take this product, unless directed by a doctor, if you have a breathing problem such as emphysema or chronic bronchitis, or if you have glaucoma or difficulty in urination due to enlargement of the prostate gland. Do not take this product if you have heart disease, high blood pressure, thyroid disease or diabetes unless directed by a doctor.

May cause marked drowsiness; alcohol, sedatives and tranquilizers may increase the drowsiness effect. Avoid alcoholic beverages while taking this product. Do not take this product if you are taking sedatives or tranquilizers, without first consulting your doctor. Use caution when driving a motor vehicle or operating machinery.

Keep this and all drugs out of the reach of children. In case of accidental overdose, contact a doctor or poison control center immediately. Prompt medical attention is critical for adults as well as for children even if you do not notice any signs or symptoms. As with any drug, if you are pregnant or nursing a baby, seek the advice of a health professional before using this product. Do not use with other products containing acetaminophen.

DO NOT USE IF CARTON IS OPENED OR IF BOTTLE WRAP OR FOIL INNER SEAL IMPRINTED "SAFETY SEAL®" IS BROKEN OR MISSING.

ALCOHOL WARNING

Maximum Strength TYLENOL® FLU Medication No Drowsiness Formula, Maximum Strength TYLENOL® FLU NightTime Medication, and Maximum Strength TYLENOL® FLU NightTime Hot Medication: For this and all other pain relievers, including aspirin, ibuprofen, ketoprofen and naproxen sodium, if you generally consume 3 or more alcohol-containing drinks per day, you should consult your physician for advice on when and how you should take pain relievers.

Maximum Strength TYLENOL® FLU NightTime Liquid: If you drink 3 or more alcoholic beverages every day, ask your doctor if you should take Tylenol Flu NightTime Liquid or other products containing acetaminophen or other pain relievers. Chronic heavy alcohol users may be at increased risk of liver damage when taking more than the recommended dose (overdose) of acetaminophen.

DRUG INTERACTION PRECAUTION

Maximum Strength TYLENOL® FLU Medication No Drowsiness Formula, Maximum Strength TYLENOL® FLU NightTime Medication, and Maximum Strength TYLENOL® FLU NightTime Hot Medication: Do not use this product if you are now taking a prescription monoamine oxidase inhibitor (MAOI) (certain drugs for depression, psychiatric or emotional conditions, or Parkinson's disease), or for 2 weeks after stopping the MAOI drug. If you are uncertain whether your prescription drug contains an MAOI, consult a health professional before taking this product.

PROFESSIONAL INFORMATION
OVERDOSAGE INFORMATION

Maximum Strength TYLENOL® FLU Medication No Drowsiness Formula, Maximum Strength TYLENOL® FLU NightTime Medication, Maximum Strength TYLENOL® FLU NightTime Hot Medication and Maximum Strength TYLENOL® FLU NightTime Liquid: Acetaminophen in massive overdosage may cause hepatic toxicity in some patients. In adults and adolescents, hepatic toxicity has rarely been reported following ingestion of acute overdoses of less than 7.5 to 10 grams. Fatalities are infrequent (less than 3–4% of untreated cases) and have rarely been reported with overdosage of less than 15 grams. In children, an acute overdosage of less than 150 mg/kg has not been associated with hepatic toxicity.

Early symptoms following a potentially hepatotoxic overdose may include: nausea, vomiting, diaphoresis and general malaise. Clinical and laboratory evidence of hepatic toxicity may not be apparent until 48 to 72 hours postingestion. In adults and adolescents, regardless of the quantity of acetaminophen reported to have been ingested, administer acetylcysteine immediately if 24 hours or less have elapsed from the reported time of ingestion. For full prescribing information, refer to the acetylcysteine package insert. Do not await results of assays for plasma acetaminophen levels before initiating treatment with acetylcysteine. The following additional procedures are recommended: Promptly initiate gastric decontamination of the stomach. A plasma acetaminophen assay should be obtained as early as possible, but not sooner than four hours following ingestion. If plasma level falls above the lower treatment line on the acetamino-

phen overdose nomogram, acetylcysteine therapy should be continued. Liver function studies should be obtained initially and repeated at 24-hour intervals.

Serious toxicity or fatalities are extremely infrequent in children, possibly due to differences in the way they metabolize acetaminophen. In children, the maximum potential amount ingested can be more easily estimated. If more than 150 mg/kg or an unknown amount was ingested, obtain an plasma acetaminophen level. The plasma acetaminophen level should be obtained as soon as possible, but no sooner than 4 hours following ingestion. If plasma level falls above the lower treatment line on the acetaminophen overdose nomogram, the acetylcysteine therapy should be initiated and continued for a full course of therapy. If plasma acetaminophen assay capability is not available, and the estimated acetaminophen ingestion exceeds 150 mg/kg, acetylcysteine therapy should be initiated and continued for a full course of therapy.

For additional emergency information, call your regional poison center or call the Rocky Mountain Poison Center tollfree, (1-800-525-6115).

Symptoms from pseudoephedrine overdose consist most often of mild anxiety, tachycardia and/or mild hypertension. Symptoms usually appear within 4 to 8 hours of ingestion and are transient, usually requiring no treatment.

Acute dextromethorphan overdose usually does not result in serious signs and symptoms unless massive amounts have been ingested. Signs and symptoms of a substantial overdose may include nausea and vomiting, visual disturbances, CNS disturbances, and urinary retention.

Diphenhydramine and doxylamine toxicity should be treated as you would an antihistamine/anticholinergic overdose and is likely to be present within a few hours after acute ingestion.

ALCOHOL INFORMATION

Maximum Strength TYLENOL® FLU Medication No Drowsiness Formula, Maximum Strength TYLENOL® FLU NightTime Medication, Maximum Strength TYLENOL® FLU NightTime Hot Medication, and Maximum Strength TYLENOL® FLU NightTime Liquid: Chronic heavy alcohol abusers may be at increased risk of liver toxicity from excessive acetaminophen use, although reports of this event are rare. Reports usually involve cases of severe chronic alcoholics and the dosages of acetaminophen most often exceed recommended doses and often involve substantial overdose. Professionals should alert their patients who regularly consume large amounts of alcohol not to exceed recommended doses of acetaminophen.

INACTIVE INGREDIENTS

Maximum Strength TYLENOL® FLU Medication No Drowsiness Formula Gelcaps: Benzyl Alcohol, Butylparaben, Castor Oil, Cellulose, Corn Starch Edetate Calcium Disodium, Gelatin, Hydroxypropyl Methylcellulose, Iron Oxide Black, Magnesium Stearate, Methylparaben, Propylparaben, Sodium Lauryl Sulfate, Sodium Propionate, Sodium Starch Glycolate, Titanium Dioxide, Red #40 and Blue #1.

Maximum Strength TYLENOL® FLU NightTime Medication Gelcaps: Benzyl Alcohol, Butylparaben, Castor Oil, Cellulose, Corn Starch, Edetate Calcium Disodium, Gelatin, Hydroxypropyl Methylcellulose, Iron Oxide Black, Magnesium Stearate, Methylparaben, Propylparaben, Sodium Citrate, Sodium Lauryl Sulfate, Sodium Propionate, Sodium Starch Glycolate, Titanium Dioxide, D&C Red #28 and FD&C Blue #1.

Maximum Strength TYLENOL® FLU Hot Medication Packets: Ascorbic Acid (Vitamin C), Aspartame, Citric Acid, Flavors, Sodium Citrate, Sucrose, Yellow #10, Blue #1, Red #40, and Yellow #6. May Also Contain: Silicon Dioxide.

Maximum Strength TYLENOL® FLU NightTime Liquid: Citric Acid, Corn Syrup, D&C Red #33, FD&C Red #40, Flavors, High Fructose Corn Syrup, Polyethylene Glycol, Propylene Glycol, Purified Water, Saccharin Sodium, Sodium Benzoate, Sorbitol.

HOW SUPPLIED

Maximum Strength TYLENOL® FLU Medication No Drowsiness Formula: Gelcaps (colored burgundy and white, imprinted "TYLENOL FLU") in blister packs of 10 and 20.

Maximum Strength TYLENOL® FLU NightTime Medication: Gelcaps (colored blue and white, imprinted "TYLENOL FLU NT") in blister packs of 10 and 20.

Maximum Strength TYLENOL® FLU Hot Medication Packets: Packets of powder (yellow colored) in cartons of 6 tamper-evident foil packets.

Maximum Strength TYLENOL® FLU NightTime Liquid: red-colored liquid in 8 oz bottle with child resistant safety cap and tamper evident packaging.

Shown in Product Identification Guide, page 322

Extra Strength   OTC
TYLENOL® PM
Pain Reliever/Sleep Aid Caplets,
Geltabs and Gelcaps

DESCRIPTION

Each *Extra Strength TYLENOL® PM Caplet, Geltab* or *Gelcap* contains acetaminophen 500 mg and diphenhydramine HCl 25 mg.

ACTIONS

Extra Strength TYLENOL® PM Caplets, Geltabs and ***Gelcaps*** contain a clinically proven analgesic-antipyretic and an antihistamine. Maximum allowable non-prescription levels of acetaminophen and diphenhydramine provide temporary relief of occasional headaches and minor aches and pains accompanying sleeplessness. Acetaminophen is equal to aspirin in analgesic and antipyretic effectiveness and it is unlikely to produce many of the side effects associated with aspirin containing products. Acetaminophen produces analgesia by elevation of the pain threshold. Diphenhydramine HCl is an antihistamine with sedative properties.

USES

Extra Strength TYLENOL® PM Caplets, Geltabs and ***Gelcaps*** provide temporary relief of occasional headaches and minor aches and pains with accompanying sleeplessness.

PRECAUTIONS

If a rare sensitivity reaction occurs, the drug should be discontinued.

DIRECTIONS

Adults and Children 12 years of Age and Older: Take Two caplets, geltabs or gelcaps at bedtime or as directed by doctor. Children under 12 years of age: Do not use this adult product in children under 12 years of age. This will provide more than the recommended dose (overdose) and could cause serious health problems.

WARNINGS

Do not use if carton is opened or neck wrap or foil inner seal imprinted with "Safety Seal®" is broken. If sleeplessness persists continuously for more than 2 weeks, consult your doctor. Insomnia may be a symptom of serious underlying medical illness. Do not take for pain for more than 10 days or for fever for more than 3 days unless directed by a doctor. If pain or fever persists, or gets worse, if new symptoms occur, or if redness or swelling is present, consult a doctor because these could be signs of a serious condition. Do not take this product, unless directed by a doctor, if you have a breathing problem such as emphysema or chronic bronchitis, or if you have glaucoma or difficulty in urination due to enlargement of the prostate gland. Avoid alcoholic beverages while taking this product. Do not take this product if your are taking sedatives or tranquilizers without first consulting your doctor.

Do not exceed recommended dose. Keep this and all drugs out of the reach of children. In case of accidental overdose, contact a doctor or poison control center immediately. Prompt medical attention is critical for adults as well as for children even if you do not notice any signs or symptoms. As with any drug, if you are pregnant or nursing a baby, seek the advice of a health professional before using this product. Do not use with other products containing acetaminophen.

ALCOHOL WARNING

If you drink 3 or more alcoholic beverages every day, ask your doctor if you should take TYLENOL® PM or other products containing acetaminophen or other pain relievers. Chronic heavy alcohol users may be at increased risk of liver damage when taking more than the recommended dose (overdose) of acetaminophen.

Caution: This product will cause drowsiness. Do not drive a motor vehicle or operate machinery after use.

PROFESSIONAL INFORMATION

OVERDOSAGE INFORMATION

Acetaminophen in massive overdosage may cause hepatic toxicity in some patients. In adults and adolescents, hepatic toxicity has rarely been reported following ingestion of acute overdoses of less than 7.5 to 10 grams. Fatalities are infrequent (less than 3–4% of untreated cases) and have rarely been reported with overdoses of less than 15 grams. In children, an acute overdosage of less than 150 mg/kg has not been associated with hepatic toxicity.

Early symptoms following a potentially hepatotoxic overdose may include: nausea, vomiting, diaphoresis and general malaise. Clinical and laboratory evidence of hepatic toxicity may not be apparent until 48 to 72 hours postingestion.

In adults and adolescents, regardless of the quantity of acetaminophen reported to have been ingested, administer acetylcysteine immediately if 24 hours or less have elapsed from the reported time of ingestion. For full prescribing information, refer to the acetylcysteine package insert. Do not await results of assays for plasma acetaminophen levels before initiating treatment with acetylcysteine. The following additional procedures are recommended: Promptly initiate gastric decontamination of the stomach. A plasma acetaminophen assay should be obtained as early as possible, but no sooner than four hours following ingestion. If plasma level falls above the lower treatment line on the acetaminophen overdose nomogram, acetylcysteine therapy should be continued. Liver function studies should be obtained initially and repeated at 24-hour intervals.

Serious toxicity or fatalities are extremely infrequent in children, possibly due to differences in the way they metabolize acetaminophen. In children, the maximum potential amount ingested can be more easily estimated. If more than 150 mg/kg or an unknown amount was ingested, obtain a plasma acetaminophen level. The plasma acetaminophen level should be obtained as soon as possible, but no sooner than 4 hours following ingestion. If the plasma level falls above the lower treatment line on the acetaminophen overdose nomogram, the acetylcysteine therapy should be initiated and continued for a full course of therapy. If plasma acetaminophen assay capability is not available, and the estimated acetaminophen ingestion exceeds 150 mg/kg, acetylcysteine therapy should be initiated and continued for a full course of therapy.

For additional emergency information, call your regional poison center or call the Rocky Mountain Poison Center toll-free, (1-800-525-6115).

Diphenhydramine toxicity should be treated as you would an antihistamine/anticholinergic overdose and is likely to be present within a few hours after acute ingestion.

ALCOHOL INFORMATION

Chronic heavy alcohol abusers may be at increased risk of liver toxicity from excessive acetaminophen use, although reports of this event are rare. Reports usually involve cases of severe chronic alcoholics and the dosages of acetaminophen most often exceed recommended doses and often involve substantial overdose. Professionals should alert their patients who regularly consume large amounts of alcohol not to exceed recommended doses of acetaminophen.

INACTIVE INGREDIENTS

Caplets: Cellulose, Cornstarch, Hydroxypropyl Methylcellulose, Magnesium Stearate or Stearic Acid and Colloidal Silicon Dioxide, Polyethylene Glycol, Polysorbate 80, Sodium Citrate, Sodium Starch Glycolate, Titanium Dioxide, Blue #1 and Blue #2.

Geltabs/Gelcaps: Benzyl Alcohol, Butylparaben, Castor Oil, Cellulose, Cornstarch, Sodium Citrate, D&C Red #28, Edetate Calcium Disodium, FD&C Blue #1, Gelatin, Hydroxypropyl Methylcellulose, Magnesium Stearate, Methylparaben, Propylparaben, Sodium Lauryl Sulfate, Sodium Propionate, Sodium Starch Glycolate, Titanium Dioxide.

HOW SUPPLIED

Caplets (colored light blue imprinted "Tylenol PM") tamper-evident bottles of 24, 50, 100, and 150.

Gelcaps (colored blue and white imprinted "TYLENOL PM") tamper-evident bottles of 24 and 50.

Geltabs (colored blue and white imprinted "TYLENOL PM") tamper-evident bottles of 24, 50, and 100.

Shown in Product Identification Guide, page 322

Maximum Strength **OTC**

TYLENOL® SINUS
Geltabs, Gelcaps, Caplets and Tablets

DESCRIPTION

Each ***Maximum Strength TYLENOL® SINUS Geltab, Gelcap, Caplet or Tablet*** contains acetaminophen 500 mg and pseudoephedrine hydrochloride 30 mg.

ACTIONS

Maximum Strength TYLENOL® SINUS contains a clinically proven analgesic-antipyretic and a decongestant. Maximum allowable non-prescription levels of acetaminophen and pseudoephedrine provide temporary relief of sinus headache and congestion. Acetaminophen is equal to aspirin in analgesic and antipyretic effectiveness and it is unlikely to produce many of the side effects associated with aspirin and aspirin-containing products.

Acetaminophen produces analgesia by elevation of the pain threshold and antipyresis through action on the hypothalamic heat-regulating center. Pseudoephedrine hydrochloride is a sympathomimetic amine which promotes sinus cavity drainage by reducing nasopharyngeal mucosal congestion.

INDICATIONS

Maximum Strength TYLENOL® SINUS provides for the temporary relief of nasal and sinus congestion and sinus pain and headaches. ***Maximum Strength TYLENOL® SINUS*** is particularly well-suited in patients with aspirin allergy, hemostatic disturbances (including anticoagulant therapy), and bleeding diatheses (e.g., hemophilia) and upper gastrointestinal disease (e.g., ulcer, gastritis, hiatus hernia).

PRECAUTIONS

If a rare sensitivity occurs, the drug should be discontinued. Although pseudoephedrine is virtually without pressor effect in normotensive patients, it should be used with caution in hypertensives.

DIRECTIONS

Adults and Children 12 years of Age and Older: Two Geltabs, Gelcaps, Caplets, or Tablets every 4–6 hours. Do not exceed eight Geltabs, Gelcaps, Caplets or Tablets in any 24-hour period. Not for use in children under 12 years of age.

WARNINGS

Do not use if carton is opened or if blister unit is broken. Do not take for pain for more than 7 days or for fever for more than 3 days unless directed by a doctor. If pain or fever persists, or gets worse, if new symptoms occur, or if redness or swelling is present, consult a doctor because these could be signs of a serious condition. **Do not exceed recommended dosage.** If nervousness, dizziness or sleeplessness occur, discontinue use and consult a doctor. Do not take this product if you have heart disease, high blood pressure, thyroid disease, diabetes, or difficulty in urination due to enlargement of the prostate gland unless directed by a doctor.

As with any drug, if you are pregnant or nursing a baby, seek the advice of a health professional before using this product. Keep this and all drugs out of the reach of children. In case of accidental overdose, contact a doctor or poison control center immediately. Prompt medical attention is critical for adults as well as for children even if you do not notice any signs or symptoms. Do not use with other products containing acetaminophen.

ALCOHOL WARNING

For this and all other pain relievers, including aspirin, ibuprofen, ketoprofen and naproxen sodium, if you generally consume 3 or more alcohol-containing drinks per day, you should consult your physician for advice on when and how you should take pain relievers.

DRUG INTERACTIONS PRECAUTION

Do not use this product if you are now taking a prescription monoamine oxidase inhibitor (MAOI) (certain drugs for depression, psychiatric or emotional conditions, or Parkinson's disease), or for 2 weeks after stopping the MAOI drug. If you are uncertain whether your prescription drug contains an MAOI, consult a health professional before taking this product.

PROFESSIONAL INFORMATION

OVERDOSAGE INFORMATION

Acetaminophen in massive overdosage may cause hepatic toxicity in some patients. In adults and adolescents, hepatic toxicity has rarely been reported following ingestion of acute overdoses of less than 7.5 to 10 grams. Fatalities are infrequent (less than 3–4% of untreated cases) and have rarely been reported with overdoses of less than 15 grams. In children, an acute overdosage of less than 150 mg/kg has not been associated with hepatic toxicity.

Early symptoms following a potentially hepatotoxic overdose may include: nausea, vomiting, diaphoresis and general malaise. Clinical and laboratory evidence of hepatic toxicity may not be apparent until 48 to 72 hours postingestion.

In adults and adolescents, regardless of the quantity of acetaminophen reported to have been ingested, administer acetylcysteine immediately if 24 hours or less have elapsed from the reported time of ingestion. For full prescribing information, refer to the acetylcysteine package insert. Do not await results of assays for plasma acetaminophen levels before initiating treatment with acetylcysteine. The following additional procedures are recommended: Promptly initiate gastric decontamination of the stomach. A plasma acetaminophen assay should be obtained as early as possible, but no sooner than four hours following ingestion. If plasma level falls above the lower treatment line on the acetaminophen overdose nomogram, acetylcysteine therapy should be continued. Liver function studies should be obtained initially and repeated at 24-hour intervals.

Serious toxicity or fatalities are extremely infrequent in children, possibly due to differences in the way they metabolize acetaminophen. In children, the maximum potential amount ingested can be more easily estimated. If more than 150 mg/kg or an unknown amount was ingested, obtain a plasma acetaminophen level. The plasma acetaminophen level should be obtained as soon as possible, but no sooner than 4 hours following ingestion. If plasma level falls above the lower treatment line on the acetaminophen overdose nomogram, the acetylcysteine therapy should be initiated and continued for a full course of therapy. If plasma acetaminophen assay capability is not available, and the estimated acetaminophen ingestion exceeds 150 mg/kg, acetylcysteine therapy should be initiated and continued for a full course of therapy.

For additional emergency information, call your regional poison center or call the Rocky Mountain Poison Center toll-free (1-800-525-6115).

Symptoms from pseudoephedrine overdose consist most often of mild anxiety, tachycardia and/or mild hypertension. Symptoms usually appear within 4 to 8 hours after ingestion and are transient, usually requiring no treatment.

Continued on next page

Tylenol Sinus—Cont.

ALCOHOL INFORMATION

Chronic heavy alcohol abusers may be at increased risk of liver toxicity from excessive acetaminophen use, although reports of this event are rare. Reports usually involve cases of severe chronic alcoholics and the dosages of acetaminophen most often exceed recommended doses and often involve substantial overdose. Professionals should alert their patients who regularly consume large amounts of alcohol not to exceed recommended doses of acetaminophen.

INACTIVE INGREDIENTS

Caplets: Carnauba Wax, Cellulose, Corn Starch, Hydroxypropyl Methylcellulose, Magnesium Stearate, Polyethylene Glycol, Polysorbate 80, Sodium Starch Glycolate, Titanium Dioxide, Blue #1, Red #40, Yellow #10.

Tablets: Cellulose, Corn Starch, Magnesium Stearate, Sodium Starch Glycolate,. Blue #1, Yellow #6, and Yellow #10.

Gelcaps: Benzyl Alcohol, Butylparaben, Castor Oil, Cellulose, Corn Starch, Edetate Calcium Disodium, Gelatin, Hydroxypropyl Methylcellulose, Iron Oxide Black, Magnesium Stearate, Methylparaben, Propylparaben, Sodium Lauryl Sulfate, Sodium Propionate, Sodium Starch Glycolate, Titanium Dioxide, Blue #1 and Yellow #10.

Geltabs: Benzyl Alcohol, Butylparaben, Castor Oil, Cellulose, Corn Starch, Edetate Calcium Disodium, Gelatin, Hydroxypropyl Methylcellulose, Iron Oxide Black, Magnesium Stearate, Methylparaben, Propylparaben, Sodium Lauryl Sulfate, Sodium Propionate, Sodium Starch Glycolate, Titanium Dioxide, D&C Yellow #10, FD&C Blue #1

HOW SUPPLIED

Tablets: (colored light green, imprinted "Maximum Strength TYLENOL SINUS")—in blister packs of 24.

Caplets: (light green coating, printed "TYLENOL SINUS" in dark green) in blister packs of 24 and 48.

Gelcaps: (colored green and white), printed "TYLENOL SINUS" in blister packs of 24 and 48.

Geltabs: (colored green and white), printed "TYLENOL SINUS" in blister packs of 24 and 48.

Shown in Product Identification Guide, page 322

McNeil Pharmaceutical

see Ortho-McNeil Pharmaceutical

Mead Johnson Nutritionals
Mead Johnson & Company

**2400 W. LLOYD EXPRESSWAY
EVANSVILLE, INDIANA 47721-0001**

Direct Inquiries to:
Medical Services Department
(812) 429-5599

ENFAMIL®
NATALINS® RX

[nā-tă-lins]

Multivitamin and multimineral supplement with beta-carotene, 1 mg Folic Acid and 54 mg Iron per 2 Tablet Dose

DESCRIPTION

Natalins Rx tablets provide twelve vitamins and five minerals to supplement the diet during pregnancy or lactation. Each Natalins Rx dose supplies:

Supplement Facts

Dosage Size 2 Tablets Daily

Amount Per 2 Tablets	% Daily Value for pregnant or lactating women
Vitamin A 4000 IU	50%
33% as beta-carotene	
Vitamin C 80 mg	133%
Vitamin D 400 IU	100%
Vitamin E 15 IU	50%
Thiamin 1.5 mg	88%
Riboflavin 1.6 mg	80%
Niacin 17 mg	85%
Vitamin B6 4 mg	160%
Folic Acid 1 mg	125%
Vitamin B12 2.5 mcg	31%
Biotin 30 mcg	10%
Pantothenic Acid 7 mg	70%
Calcium 200 mg	15%
Iron 54 mg	300%
Magnesium 100 mg	22%
Zinc 25 mg	167%
Copper 3 mg	150%

Active Ingredient: Each dose (2 tablets) contains 1 mg folic acid.

Other Ingredients: Beta-carotene, biotin, calcium carbonate, calcium pantothenate, cupric oxide, ferrous fumarate, hydroxypropyl methylcellulose, magnesium hydroxide, magnesium stearate, microcrystalline cellulose, niacinamide, polacrilin potassium, polyethylene glycol, povidone, riboflavin, silicon dioxide, sodium ascorbate, stearic acid, thiamin mononitrate, titanium dioxide, vitamin A acetate, vitamin B6 hydrochloride, vitamin B12, vitamin D3, vitamin E acetate, zinc oxide.

INDICATIONS AND USAGE

Natalins Rx tablets help assure an adequate intake of the vitamins and minerals listed above. Folic acid helps prevent the development of megaloblastic anemia during pregnancy.

CONTRAINDICATIONS

Supplemental vitamins and minerals should not be prescribed for patients with hemochromatosis or Wilson's disease.

> WARNING: Accidental overdose of iron-containing products is a leading cause of fatal poisoning in children under 6. Keep this product out of reach of children. In case of accidental overdose, call a doctor or poison control center immediately.

PRECAUTIONS

Folic acid above 0.1 mg daily may obscure pernicious anemia (hematologic remission may occur while neurological manifestations remain progressive). Do not exceed the prescribed dose.

ADVERSE REACTIONS

No adverse reactions or undesirable side effects have been attributed to the use of Natalins Rx tablets.

DOSAGE AND ADMINISTRATION

Two tablets daily, or as prescribed.

HOW SUPPLIED

NDC 0087-0702-49 Bottles of 200

P4757-05/P9735-00

Medeva Pharmaceuticals, Inc.

**P.O. Box 1710
ROCHESTER, NY 14603**

Direct Inquiries to:
Customer Service Department
P.O. Box 1766
Rochester, NY 14603
(716) 274-5300
(888) 9-MEDEVA
In Emergencies:
(800) 932-1950 (24 hours)

AIRET™
**Albuterol Sulfate Inhalation
Solution 0.083%***
(*Potency expressed as albuterol)

PRESCRIBING INFORMATION

DESCRIPTION

Albuterol sulfate inhalation solution is a relatively selective beta2-adrenergic bronchodilator (see **CLINICAL PHARMACOLOGY** section below). Albuterol sulfate, the racemic form of albuterol, has the chemical name α^1-[(tert-butylamino)methyl]-4-hydroxy-m-xylene-α,α'-diol sulfate (2:1) (salt), and the following chemical structure:

$$\left[HOCH_2 - \underset{HO}{\bigcirc} - CHCH_2NHC(CH_3)_3 \atop OH \right]_2 \cdot H_2SO_4$$

Albuterol sulfate has a molecular weight of 576.7 and the molecular formula $(C_{13}H_{21}NO_3)_2 \cdot H_2SO_4$. Albuterol sulfate is a white or practically white powder, freely soluble in water and slightly soluble in alcohol.

The World Health Organization recommended name for albuterol base is salbutamol.

Albuterol sulfate inhalation solution 0.083% requires no dilution before administration.

Each mL of albuterol sulfate inhalation solution (0.083%) contains 0.83 mg of albuterol (as 1 mg of albuterol sulfate)

in an isotonic, sterile, aqueous solution containing sodium chloride, edetate disodium, sodium citrate, and hydrochloric acid to adjust the pH between 3 and 5. Albuterol sulfate inhalation solution (0.083%) contains no sulfiting agents. It is supplied in 3 mL unit dose vials.

Albuterol sulfate inhalation solution is a clear, colorless to light yellow solution.

CLINICAL PHARMACOLOGY

The prime action of beta-adrenergic drugs is to stimulate adenyl cyclase, the enzyme which catalyzes the formation of cyclic-3′,5′-adenosine monophosphate (cyclic AMP) from adenosine triphosphate (ATP). The cyclic AMP thus formed mediates the cellular responses. *In vitro* studies and *in vivo* pharmacologic studies have demonstrated that albuterol has a preferential effect on beta2-adrenergic receptors compared with isoproterenol. While it is recognized that beta2-adrenergic receptors are the predominant receptors in bronchial smooth muscle, recent data indicate that 10 to 50% of the beta-receptors in the human heart may be beta2-receptors. The precise function of these receptors, however, is not yet established. Albuterol has been shown in most controlled clinical trials to have more effect on the respiratory tract in the form of bronchial smooth muscle relaxation than isoproterenol at comparable doses while producing fewer cardiovascular effects. Controlled clinical studies and other clinical experience have shown that inhaled albuterol, like other beta-adrenergic agonist drugs, can produce a significant cardiovascular effect in some patients, as measured by pulse rate, blood pressure, symptoms, and/or electrocardiographic changes.

Albuterol is longer acting than isoproterenol in most patients by any route of administration because it is not a substrate for the cellular uptake processes for catecholamines nor for catechol-O-methyl transferase.

Studies in asthmatic patients have shown that less than 20% of a single albuterol dose was absorbed following the IPPB or nebulizer administration; the remaining amount was recovered from the nebulizer and apparatus and expired air. Most of the absorbed dose was recovered in the urine 24 hours after drug administration. There was a significant dose-related response in FEV1 (forced expiratory volume in one second) and peak flow rate (PFR). It has been demonstrated that following oral administration of 4 mg albuterol, the elimination half-life was five to six hours.

Animal studies show that albuterol does not pass the blood-brain barrier. Recent studies in laboratory animals (minipigs, rodents, and dogs) recorded the occurrence of cardiac arrhythmias and sudden death (with histologic evidence of myocardial necrosis) when beta-agonists and methylxanthines were administered concurrently. The significance of these findings when applied to humans is currently unknown.

In controlled clinical trials, most patients exhibited an onset of improvement in pulmonary function within 5 minutes as determined by FEV1. FEV1 measurements also showed that the maximum average improvement in pulmonary function usually occurred at approximately 1 hour following inhalation of 2.5 mg of albuterol by compressor-nebulizer, and remained close to peak for 2 hours. Clinically significant improvement in pulmonary function (defined as maintenance of a 15% or more increase in FEV1 over baseline values) continued for 3 to 4 hours in most patients and in some patients continued up to 6 hours.

In repetitive dose studies, continued effectiveness was demonstrated throughout the three-month period of treatment in some patients.

INDICATIONS AND USAGE

Albuterol sulfate inhalation solution is indicated for the relief of bronchospasm in patients with reversible obstructive airway disease and acute attacks of bronchospasm.

CONTRAINDICATIONS

Albuterol sulfate inhalation solution is contraindicated in patients with a history of hypersensitivity to any of its components.

WARNINGS

As with other inhaled beta-adrenergic agonists, albuterol sulfate inhalation solution can produce paradoxical bronchospasm, which can be life threatening. If occurs, the preparation should be discontinued immediately and alternative therapy instituted.

Fatalities have been reported in association with excessive use of inhaled sympathomimetic drugs and with the home use of nebulizers. It is, therefore, essential that the physician instruct the patient in the need for further evaluation if his/her asthma becomes worse. In individual patients, any beta2-adrenergic agonist, including albuterol solution for inhalation, may have a clinically significant cardiac effect. Immediate hypersensitivity reactions may occur after administration of albuterol as demonstrated by rare cases of urticaria, angioedema, rash, bronchospasm, and oropharyngeal edema.

PRECAUTIONS

General: Albuterol, as with all sympathomimetic amines, should be used with caution in patients with cardiovascular disorders, especially coronary insufficiency, cardiac arrhythmias and hypertension, in patients with convulsive disorders, hyperthyroidism or diabetes mellitus and in patients who are unusually responsive to sympathomimetic amines. Large doses of intravenous albuterol have been reported to aggravate preexisting diabetes mellitus and ketoacidosis. As with other beta-agonists, inhaled and intravenous albuterol may produce a significant hypokalemia in some patients, possibly through intracellular shunting, which has the potential to produce adverse cardiovascular effects. The decrease is usually transient, not required supplementation.

Information for Patients: The action of albuterol sulfate inhalation solution may last up to six hours, and therefore it should not be used more frequently than recommended. Do not increase the dose or frequency of medication without medical consultation. If symptoms get worse, medical consultation should be sought promptly. While taking albuterol sulfate inhalation solution, other anti-asthma medicines should not be used unless prescribed.
See illustrated Patient's Instructions for Use.

Drug Interactions: Other sympathomimetic aerosol bronchodilators or epinephrine should not be used concomitantly with albuterol.
Albuterol should be administered with extreme caution to patients being treated with monoamine oxidase inhibitors or tricyclic antidepressants, since the action of albuterol on the vascular system may be potentiated.
Beta-receptor blocking agents and albuterol inhibit the effect of each other.

Carcinogenesis, Mutagenesis, and Impairment of Fertility: Albuterol sulfate caused a significant dose-related increase in the incidence of benign leiomyomas of the mesovarium in a 2-year study in the rat at oral doses of 2, 10, and 50 mg/kg, corresponding to 10, 50 and 250 times, respectively, the maximum nebulization dose for a 50 kg human. In another study, this effect was blocked by the coadministration of propranolol. The relevance of these findings to humans is not known. An 18-month study in mice and a lifetime study in hamsters revealed no evidence of tumorigenicity. Studies with albuterol revealed no evidence of mutagenesis. Reproduction studies in rats revealed no evidence of impaired fertility.

Pregnancy: Teratogenetic Effects: Pregnancy Category C: Albuterol has been shown to be teratogenic in mice when given subcutaneously in doses corresponding to the human nebulization dose. There are no adequate and well-controlled studies in pregnant women. Albuterol should be used during pregnancy only if the potential benefit justifies the potential risk to the fetus.
A reproduction study in CD-1 mice given albuterol subcutaneously (0.025, 0.25, and 2.5 mg/kg, corresponding to 0.125, 1.25 and 12.5 times, respectively, the maximum nebulization dose for a 50 kg human) showed cleft palate formation in 5 of 111 (4.5%) of fetuses at 0.25 mg/kg and in 10 of 108 (9.3%) of fetuses at 2.5 mg/kg. None were observed at 0.025 mg/kg. Cleft palate also occurred in 22 of 72 (30.5%) fetuses treated with 2.5 mg/kg isoproterenol (positive control). A reproduction study in Stride Dutch rabbits revealed cranioschisis in 7 of 19 (37%) of fetuses at 50 mg/kg, corresponding to 250 times the maximum human nebulization dose.
During worldwide marketing experience, various congenital anomalies, including cleft palate and limb defects, have been rarely reported in the offspring of patients being treated with albuterol. Some of the mothers were taking multiple medications during their pregnancies. No consistent pattern of defects can be discerned, and a relationship between albuterol use and congenital anomalies has not been established.

Labor and Delivery: Oral albuterol has been shown to delay preterm labor in some reports. There are presently no well controlled studies that demonstrate that it will stop preterm labor or prevent labor at term. Therefore, cautious use of albuterol sulfate inhalation solution is required in pregnant patients when given for relief of bronchospasm so as to avoid interference with uterine contractibility.

Nursing Mothers: It is not known whether this drug is excreted in human milk. Because of the potential for tumorigenicity shown for albuterol in some animal studies, a decision should be made whether to discontinue nursing or to discontinue the drug, taking into accord the importance of the drug to the mother.

Pediatric Use: Safety and effectiveness of albuterol solution for inhalation in pediatric patients below the age of 12 years have not been established.

ADVERSE REACTION

The results of clinical trials with albuterol sulfate inhalation solution in 135 patients showed the following side effects which were considered probably or possibly drug related:
Central Nervous System: tremors (20%), dizziness (7%), nervousness (4%), headache (3%), insomnia (1%).

Gastrointestinal: nausea (4%), dyspepsia (1%).
Ear, Nose and Throat: pharyngitis (<1%), nasal congestion (1%).
Cardiovascular: tachycardia (1%), hypertension (1%).
Respiratory: bronchospasm (8%), cough (4%), bronchitis (4%), wheezing (1%).
No clinically relevant laboratory abnormalities related to albuterol sulfate inhalation solution administration were determined in these studies.
In comparing the adverse reactions reported for patients treated with albuterol sulfate inhalation solution with those of patients treated with isoproterenol during clinical trials of three months, the following moderate to severe reactions, as judged by the investigators, were reported. This table does not include mild reactions.

Percent Incidence of Moderate to Severe Adverse Reactions

Reaction	Albuterol N = 65	Isoproterenol N = 65
Central Nervous System		
Tremors	10.7%	13.8%
Headache	3.1%	1.5%
Insomnia	3.1%	1.5%
Cardiovascular		
Hypertension	3.1%	3.1%
Arrhythmias	0%	3%
* Palpitation	0%	22%
Respiratory		
**Bronchospasm	15.4%	18%
Cough	3.1%	5%
Bronchitis	1.5%	5%
Wheeze	1.5%	1.5%
Sputum Increase	1.5%	1.5%
Dyspnea	1.5%	1.5%
Gastrointestinal		
Nausea	3.1%	0%
Dyspepsia	1.5%	0%
Systemic		
Malaise	1.5%	0%

* The finding of no arrhythmias and no palpitations after albuterol administration in this clinical study should not be interpreted as indicating that these adverse effects can not occur after the administration of inhaled albuterol.

** In most cases of bronchospasm, this term was generally used to describe exacerbations in the underlying pulmonary disease.

Rare cases of urticaria, angioedema, rash, bronchospasm and oropharyngeal edema have been reported after the use of inhaled albuterol.

OVERDOSAGE

Manifestations of overdosage may include seizures, anginal pain, hypertension, hypokalemia, tachycardia with rates up to 200 beats per minute, and exaggeration of the pharmacological effects listed in **ADVERSE REACTIONS**.
The oral LD_{50} in rats and mice was greater than 2,000 mg/kg. The inhalational LD_{50} could not be determined.
There is insufficient evidence to determine if dialysis is beneficial for overdosage of albuterol.

DOSAGE AND ADMINISTRATION

The usual dosage for adults and children 12 years and older is 2.5 mg of albuterol administered 3 to 4 times daily by nebulization. More frequent administration or high doses is not recommended. To administer 2.5 mg of albuterol, use the entire contents of one unit-dose vial (3 mL of 0.083% inhalation solution) by nebulization. The flow rate is regulated to suit the particular nebulizer so that the albuterol sulfate inhalation solution will be delivered over approximately 5 to 15 minutes. (A 2.5 mg dose of albuterol is equivalent to 0.5 mL of a 0.5% solution.)
The use of albuterol sulfate inhalation solution can be continued as medically indicated to control recurring bouts of bronchospasm. During this time most patients gain optimum benefit from regular use of the inhalation solution.
If a previously effective dosage regimen fails to provide the usual relief, medical advice should be sought immediately, as this is often a sign of seriously worsening asthma which would require reassessment of therapy.

HOW SUPPLIED

Unit-dose plastic vial containing AIRET™ Albuterol Sulfate Inhalation Solution 0.083%, 2.5 mg/3 mL* (*potency expressed as albuterol). Equivalent to 0.5 mL albuterol (as the sulfate) 0.5% (2.5 mg albuterol) diluted to 3 mL. Supplied in cartons as listed below.
NDC 53014-075-25   Twenty-five vials per carton.
NDC 53014-075-60   Sixty vials per carton.
Storage: PROTECT FROM LIGHT. RETAIN IN CARTON UNTIL TIME OF USE.
Store between 2° and 25°C (36° and 77°F).

CAUTION: Federal law prohibits dispensing without prescription.
Manufactured for:
Medeva Pharmaceuticals, Inc.
Rochester, NY 14623 USA
By: Dey Laboratories, Napa CA 94558
03-272-07
754/1196   Revised:
35750003   Nov 1996

Patient's Instructions for Use

AIRET™ Albuterol Sulfate Inhalation Solution 0.083%*
*Potency expressed as albuterol
Note: This is a unit-dose vial. No dilution is required.
Read complete instructions carefully before using.
1. Twist the cap completely off the vial and squeeze the contents into the nebulizer reservoir (Figure 1).

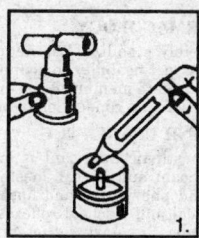

2. Connect the nebulizer reservoir to the mouthpiece or face mask (Figure 2).

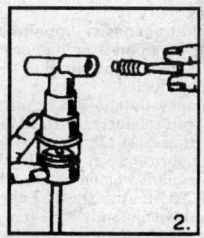

3. Connect the nebulizer to the compressor.
4. Sit in a comfortable, upright position; place the mouthpiece in your mouth (Figure 3) (or put on the face mask); and turn on the compressor.

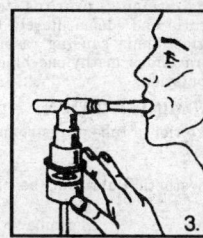

5. **Breathe as calmly, deeply and evenly** as possible until no more mist is formed in the nebulizer chamber (about 5–15 minutes). At this point, the treatment is finished.
6. Clean the nebulizer (see manufacturer's instructions).
Note: Use only as directed by your physician. More frequent administration or higher doses are not recommended.
Store Albuterol Sulfate Inhalation Solution 0.083%* between 2° and 25°C (36° and 77°F).
ADDITIONAL INSTRUCTIONS:
_____
_____

Manufactured for:
Medeva Pharmaceuticals, Inc.
Rochester, NY 14623 USA
By: Dey Laboratories, Napa CA 94558

Continued on next page

Information on the Medeva Pharmaceuticals, Inc. products listed on these pages contains the full prescribing information from product circulars in use as of July 1998. For further information, please consult the package insert currently accompanying the product.

AMERICAINE®
ANESTHETIC LUBRICANT
[uh-mer 'i-kān "]
(benzocaine)
R238C
Rev. 7/96

℞

DESCRIPTION

AMERICAINE Anesthetic Lubricant contains benzocaine 20% with benzethonium chloride 0.1% as a preservative in a water soluble base of polyethylene glycol 300 and 3350. Benzocaine, a local anesthetic, is chemically ethyl p -aminobenzoate, $C_9H_{11}NO_2$, with a molecular weight of 165.19 and has the following structural formula:

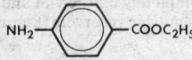

CLINICAL PHARMACOLOGY

Benzocaine reversibly stabilizes the neuronal membrane which decreases its permeability to sodium ions. Depolarization of the neuronal membrane is inhibited thereby blocking the initiation and conduction of nerve impulses.

INDICATIONS AND USAGE

AMERICAINE Anesthetic Lubricant is indicated for general use as a lubricant and topical anesthetic on intratracheal catheters and pharyngeal and nasal airways to obtund the pharyngeal and tracheal reflexes; on nasogastric and endoscopic tubes; urinary catheters; laryngoscopes; proctoscopes; sigmoidoscopes and vaginal specula.

CONTRAINDICATIONS

Known allergy or hypersensitivity to benzocaine.

PRECAUTIONS

General: Medication should be discontinued if sensitivity or irritation occurs.
Carcinogenesis, Mutagenesis, Impairment of Fertility: Long-term studies in animals or humans to evaluate the carcinogenic and mutagenic potential or the effect on fertility have not been conducted.
Pregnancy: Pregnancy Category C. Animal reproduction studies have not been conducted with AMERICAINE Anesthetic Lubricant. It is also not known whether AMERICAINE Anesthetic Lubricant can cause fetal harm when administered to a pregnant woman or can affect reproduction capacity. AMERICAINE Anesthetic Lubricant should be given to a pregnant woman only if clearly needed.
Nursing Mothers: It is not known whether this drug is excreted in human milk. Because many drugs are excreted in human milk, caution should be exercised when AMERICAINE Anesthetic Lubricant is administered to a nursing woman.
Pediatric Use: Do not use in infants under 1 year of age.

ADVERSE REACTIONS

Contact dermatitis and/or hypersensitivity to benzocaine can cause burning, stinging, pruritus, tenderness, erythema, rash, urticaria and edema. Rarely, benzocaine may induce methemoglobinemia causing respiratory distress and cyanosis. Intravenous methylene blue is the specific therapy for this condition.

DOSAGE AND ADMINISTRATION

Apply evenly to exterior of tube or instrument prior to use.

HOW SUPPLIED

AMERICAINE Anesthetic Lubricant (benzocaine) is available in:

NDC 53014-376-16   28 g tube
NDC 53014-376-62   2.5 g unit dose foil packs, 144 per carton

Store at 15°–25°C (59°–77°F).
CAUTION: Federal law prohibits dispensing without prescription.
MEDEVA PHARMACEUTICALS
Medeva Pharmaceuticals, Inc.
Rochester, NY 14623 USA
®Ciba-Geigy Corporation
©1996, Medeva Pharmaceuticals Manufacturing, Inc.
Rev. 7/96
R238C

AMERICAINE® OTIC
[uh-mer 'i-kān "]
(benzocaine)
Topical Anesthetic Ear Drops
Rev. 7/96
R239C

℞

DESCRIPTION

AMERICAINE Otic, topical anesthetic ear drops, contains benzocaine 20% (w/w) in a water soluble base of glycerin 1% (w/w) and polyethylene glycol 300 with benzethonium chloride 0.1% as a preservative.

Benzocaine, a local anesthetic, is chemically ethyl p -aminobenzoate, $C_9H_{11}NO_2$, with a molecular weight of 165.19 and has the following structural formula:

$$NH_2 \langle \rangle COOC_2H_5$$

CLINICAL PHARMACOLOGY

Benzocaine reversibly stabilizes the neuronal membrane which decreases its permeability to sodium ions. Depolarization of the neuronal membrane is inhibited thereby blocking the initiation and conduction of nerve impulses.

INDICATIONS AND USAGE

AMERICAINE Otic is indicated for relief of pain and pruritus in acute congestive and serous otitis media, acute swimmer's ear, and other forms of otitis externa.

CONTRAINDICATIONS

In the presence of a perforated tympanic membrane or ear discharge.
Known allergy or hypersensitivity to benzocaine.

WARNINGS

Indiscriminate use of anesthetic ear drops may mask symptoms of fulminating infection of the middle ear.

PRECAUTIONS

General: Medication should be discontinued if sensitivity or irritation occurs.
Carcinogenesis, Mutagenesis, Impairment of Fertility: Long-term studies in animals or humans to evaluate the carcinogenic and mutagenic potential or the effect on fertility have not been conducted.
Pregnancy: Pregnancy Category C. Animal reproduction studies have not been conducted with AMERICAINE Otic. It is also not known whether AMERICAINE Otic can cause fetal harm when administered to a pregnant woman or can affect reproduction capacity. AMERICAINE Otic should be given to a pregnant woman only if clearly needed.
Nursing Mothers: It is not known whether this drug is excreted in human milk. Because many drugs are excreted in human milk, caution should be exercised when AMERICAINE Otic is administered to a nursing woman.
Pediatric Use: Do not use in infants under 1 year of age.

ADVERSE REACTIONS

Contact dermatitis and/or hypersensitivity to benzocaine can cause burning, stinging, pruritus, tenderness, erythema, rash, urticaria and edema. Rarely, benzocaine may induce methemoglobinemia causing respiratory distress and cyanosis. Intravenous methylene blue is the specific therapy for this condition.

DOSAGE AND ADMINISTRATION

Instill 4–5 drops of AMERICAINE Otic in the external auditory canal, then insert a cotton pledget into the meatus. Application may be repeated every one to two hours if necessary.

HOW SUPPLIED

AMERICAINE Otic (benzocaine), topical anesthetic ear drops, is available in dropper-top bottles.
NDC 53014-377-51   15 mL bottle
Keep bottle tightly closed. Store at 15°–30°C (59°–86°F). Keep out of the reach of children.
CAUTION: Federal law prohibits dispensing without prescription.
Marketed by:
MEDEVA PHARMACEUTICALS
Medeva Pharmaceuticals, Inc.
Rochester, NY 14623 USA
Manufactured by:
Akorn Manufacturing, Inc.
Decatur, IL 62525
® Ciba-Geigy Corporation
© 1996, Medeva Pharmaceuticals Manufacturing, Inc.
Rev. 7/96
R239C

ATROHIST® PEDIATRIC
Capsules
(chlorpheniramine maleate and pseudoephedrine HCl)

℞

DESCRIPTION:

Each extended-release capsule contains:
Chlorpheniramine maleate .... 4 mg
Pseudoephedrine hydrochloride .... 60 mg
in a specially prepared base to provide prolonged action. This product contains ingredients of the following therapeutic classes; antihistamine and nasal decongestant.

Inactive Ingredients: dibutyl sebacate, ethylcellulose, fumed silica, hydroxypropyl methylcellulose, methacrylic acid, oleic acid, propylene glycol, sugar spheres NF, and talc NF.

CLINICAL PHARMACOLOGY

Chlorpheniramine maleate is an alkylamine type antihistamine. This group of antihistamines is among the most active histamine antagonists and are generally effective in relatively low doses. The drugs are not so prone to produce drowsiness and are among the most suitable agents for day time use; but again, a significant proportion of patients do experience this effect. Pseudoephedrine hydrochloride is a sympathomimetic which acts predominantly on alpha receptors and has little action on beta receptors. It therefore functions as an oral nasal decongestant with minimal CNS stimulation.

INDICATIONS AND USAGE

For the temporary relief of symptoms of the common cold, allergic rhinitis (hay fever) and sinusitis.

CONTRAINDICATIONS

Hypersensitivity to any of the ingredients. Also contraindicated in patients with severe hypertension, severe coronary artery disease, patients on monoamine oxidase inhibitor (MAOI) therapy or for 14 days after stopping MAOI therapy (See **Drug Interactions**), patients with narrow-angle glaucoma, urinary retention, peptic ulcer and during an asthmatic attack.
Should not be used in nursing mothers.

WARNINGS

Considerable caution should be exercised in patients with hypertension, diabetes mellitus, ischemic heart disease, hyperthyroidism, increased intraocular pressure and prostatic hypertrophy. The elderly (60 years or older) are more likely to exhibit adverse reactions.
Antihistamines may cause excitability, especially in pediatric patients. At dosages higher than the recommended dose, nervousness, dizziness or sleeplessness may occur.

PRECAUTIONS

General: Caution should be exercised in patients with high blood pressure, heart disease, diabetes or thyroid disease. The antihistamine in this product may exhibit additive effects with CNS depressants, including alcohol.
Information for Patients: Antihistamine may cause drowsiness and ambulatory patients who operate machinery or motor vehicles should be cautioned accordingly.
Drug Interactions: Do not prescribe this product for use in patients that are now taking a prescription MAOI (certain drugs for depression, psychiatric or emotional conditions, or Parkinson's disease), or for 14 days after stopping the MAOI drug therapy. MAOI and beta adrenergic blockers increase the effects of sympathomimetics. Sympathomimetics may reduce the antihypertensive effects of methyldopa, macamylamine, reserpine and veratrum alkaloids. Concomitant use of antihistamines with alcohol and other CNS depressants may have an additive effect.
Pregnancy: Category C: Animal reproduction studies have not been conducted with Atrohist® Pediatric Capsules. It is also not known whether Atrohist Pediatric Capsules can cause fetal harm when administered to a pregnant woman or can affect reproduction capacity. Atrohist® Pediatric Capsules should be given to a pregnant woman only if clearly needed.
Pediatric Use: Safety and effectiveness of Atrohist Pediatric Capsules in pediatric patients under the age of 12 years have not been established.

ADVERSE REACTIONS

Adverse reactions include drowsiness, lassitude, nausea, giddiness, dryness of mouth, blurred vision, cardiac palpitations, flushing, increased irritability or excitement (especially in pediatric patients).

OVERDOSAGE

Acute overdosage with Atrohist® Pediatric Capsules may produce clinical signs of CNS stimulation and variable cardiovascular effects. Pressor amines should be used with great caution in the presence of pseudoephedrine. Patients with signs of stimulation should be treated conservatively.

DOSAGE AND ADMINISTRATION

Adolescents 12 years and older: Two capsules every 12 hours; Children 6 to under 12 years of age: One capsule every 12 hours; Children 2 to under 6 years of age: As determined and directed by physician.

HOW SUPPLIED

NDC 53014-400-10
Bottle of 100 white and yellow Capsules, imprinted "MEDEVA" on the yellow cap and "400" on the white body of the capsule shell.
CAUTION: Federal law prohibits dispensing without prescription.
DISPENSE IN A TIGHT CONTAINER AS DEFINED IN THE USP/NF, WITH A CHILD-RESISTANT CLOSURE.

Keep out of reach of pediatric population.
STORE AT CONTROLLED ROOM TEMPERATURE 15° – 30°C (59° – 86°F).
Medeva Pharmaceuticals, Inc.
Rochester, NY 14623 USA

ATROHIST®
Pediatric Suspension
DYE-FREE

℞

DESCRIPTION

ATROHIST is an antihistamic/decongestant combination available for oral administration as Pediatric Suspension.

Each 5 mL (teaspoonful) of the Pediatric Suspension contains:

Phenylephrine Tannate	5 mg
Chlorpheniramine Tannate	2 mg
Pyrilamine Tannate	12.5 mg

Other ingredients: Citric acid, disodium edta, flavors, glycerin, magnesium aluminum silicate, methylparaben, purified water, sodium benzoate, sodium citrate, sodium saccharin, sorbitol, sucrose, xanthan gum.

CLINICAL PHARMACOLOGY

ATROHIST combines the sympathomimetic decongestant effect of phenylephrine with the antihistaminic actions of chlorpheniramine and pyrilamine.

INDICATIONS AND USAGE

ATROHIST is indicated for symptomatic relief of the coryza and nasal congestion associated with the common cold, sinusitis, allergic rhinitis and other upper respiratory tract conditions. Appropriate therapy should be provided for the primary disease.

CONTRAINDICATIONS

ATROHIST is contraindicated for neonates, nursing mothers and patients sensitive to any of the ingredients or related compounds.

WARNINGS

Use with caution in patients with hypertension, cardiovascular disease, hyperthyroidism, diabetes, narrow angle glaucoma or prostatic hypertrophy. Use with caution or avoid use in patients taking monoamine oxidase inhibitors (MAOI). This product contains antihistamines which may cause drowsiness and may have additive central nervous system (CNS) effects with alcohol or other CNS depressants (e.g., hypnotics, sedatives, tranquilizers).

PRECAUTIONS

General: Antihistamines are more likely to cause dizziness, sedation and hypotension in elderly patients. Antihistamines may cause excitation, particularly in pediatric patients, but their combination may cause either mild stimulation or mild sedation.
Information for Patients: Caution patients against drinking alcoholic beverages or engaging in potentially hazardous activities requiring alertness, such as driving a car or operating machinery while using this product.
Drug Interactions: Do not prescribe this product for use in patients that are now taking a prescription MAOI (certain drugs for depression, psychiatric or emotional conditions, or Parkinson's disease), or for 14 days after stopping the MAOI drug therapy. MAOI may prolong and intensify the anticholinergic effects of antihistamines and the overall effects of sympathomimetic agents.
Carcinogenesis, Mutagenesis, Impairment of Fertility: No long term animal studies have been performed with ATROHIST.
Pregnancy: Teratogenic Effects: Pregnancy Category C. Animal reproduction studies have not been conducted with ATROHIST. It is also not known whether ATROHIST can cause fetal harm when administered to a pregnant woman or can affect reproduction capacity. ATROHIST should be given to a pregnant woman only if clearly needed.
Nursing Mothers: ATROHIST should not be administered to a nursing mother.

ADVERSE REACTIONS

Adverse effects associated with ATROHIST at recommended doses have been minimal. The most common have been drowsiness, sedation, dryness of mucous membranes, and gastrointestinal effects. Serious side effects with oral antihistamines or sympathomimetics have been rare.

OVERDOSAGE

Signs and Symptoms: May vary from CNS depression to stimulation (restlessness to convulsions). Antihistamine overdosage in pediatric patients may lead to convulsions and death. Atropine-like signs and symptoms may be prominent.
Treatment: Induce vomiting if it has not occurred spontaneously. Precautions must be taken against aspiration especially in the pediatric population and comatose patients. If gastric lavage is indicated, isotonic or half-isotonic saline solution is preferred. Stimulants should not be used. If hypotension is a problem, vasopressor agents may be considered.

DOSAGE AND ADMINISTRATION

Administer the recommended dose every 12 hours.
ATROHIST Pediatric Suspension:
Pediatric patients over six years of age – 5 to 10 mL (1 to 2 teaspoonfuls);
Pediatric patients two to six years of age – 2.5 to 5 mL(1/2 to 1 teaspoonful);
Pediatric patients under two years of age – Titrate dose individually.

HOW SUPPLIED

ATROHIST Pediatric Suspension - Dye Free: Light beige to brown, viscous suspension with raspberry flavor, in a 4 fl oz unit-of-use container (NDC 53014-503-12) and in pint bottles (NDC 53014-503-47).
Storage:
Store at controlled room temperature, 15°C - 25°C (59°F - 77°F). Protect from freezing.
MG #11883
5034/996   35503003
Mfd. for:
Medeva Pharmaceuticals, Inc.
Rochester, NY 14623 USA
by: Copley Pharmaceuticals, Inc.
Canton, MA 02021
LEA501102

ATROHIST® PLUS Tablets

℞

DESCRIPTION

Each yellow, scored Atrohist PLUS Tablet provides: 25 mg phenylephrine hydrochloride, 50 mg phenylpropanolamine hydrochloride, 8 mg chlorpheniramine maleate, 0.19 mg hyoscyamine sulfate, 0.04 mg atropine sulfate and 0.01 mg scopolamine hydrobromide in a sustained-release formulation. Atrohist PLUS Tablets are intended for oral administration.

Atrohist PLUS Tablets are an antihistaminic, nasal decongestant and anti-secretory preparation. Inactive ingredients: colloidal silicon dioxide NF, D & C yellow #10 lake, glycerin USP, hydroxypropyl methylcellulose USP, lactose NF, magnesium stearate NF.

INDICATIONS AND USAGE

Atrohist PLUS Tablets provide relief of the symptoms resulting from irritation of sinus, nasal and upper respiratory tract tissues. Phenylephrine and phenylpropanolamine combine to exert a vasoconstrictive and decongestive action while chlorpheniramine maleate decreases the symptoms of watering eyes, post nasal drip and sneezing which may be associated with an allergic-like response. The belladonna alkaloids, hyoscyamine, atropine and scopolamine further augment the anti-secretory activity of Atrohist PLUS Tablets.

CONTRAINDICATIONS

This product is contraindicated in patients with hypersensitivity to antihistamines or sympathomimetics. Atrohist PLUS Tablets are contraindicated in pediatric patients under 12 years of age and in patients with glaucoma, bronchial asthma and women who are pregnant. Concomitant use of monamine oxidase inhibitors (MAOI) is contraindicated. (See **Drug Interactions** section).

WARNINGS

Atrohist PLUS Tablets may cause drowsiness. Patients should be warned of possible additive effects caused by taking antihistamines with alcohol, hypnotics or tranquilizers.

PRECAUTIONS

Atrohist PLUS Tablets contain belladonna alkaloids, and must be administered with care to those patients with urinary bladder neck obstruction. Caution should be exercised when Atrohist PLUS Tablets are given to patients with hypertension cardiac or peripheral vascular disease or hyperthyroidism. Patients should avoid driving a motor vehicle or operating dangerous machinery. (See **WARNINGS**.)
Drug Interactions: Do not prescribe this product for use in patients that are now taking a prescription MAOI (certain drugs for depression, psychiatric or emotional conditions, or Parkinson's disease), or for 14 days after stopping the MAOI drug therapy.
Pediatric Use: Safety and effectiveness of Atrohist PLUS tablets in pediatric patients under the age of 12 years have not been established.

ADVERSE REACTIONS

Hypersensitivity reactions such as rash, urticaria, leukopenia, agranulocytosis, and thrombocytopenia may occur. Large overdoses may cause tachypnea, delirium, fever, stupor, coma and respiratory failure.
Gastrointestinal: nausea, vomiting, diarrhea, constipation, epigastric distress.
Genitourinary System: urinary frequency and dysuria.
Cardiovascular: tightness of the chest, palpitation, tachycardia, hypotension/hypertension.
Central Nervous System: drowsiness, giddiness, faintness, dizziness, headache, incoordination, mydriasis, hyper-irritability, nervousness, and insomnia.
Metabolic/Endocrine: lassitude, anorexia.
Miscellaneous: dryness of mucous membranes, xerostomia.
Respiratory: thickening of bronchial secretions.
Special Senses: tinnitus, visual disturbances, blurred vision.
Pregnancy: Category C: Animal reproduction studies have not been conducted with Atrohist Plus. It is also not known whether Atrohist Plus can cause fetal harm when administered to a pregnant woman or can affect reproduction capacity. Atrohist Plus should be given to a pregnant woman only if clearly needed.

OVERDOSAGE

Since the action of sustained release products may continue for as long as 12 hours, treatment of overdoses directed at reversing the effects of the drug and supporting the patient should be maintained for at least that length of time. In pediatric patients, antihistamine overdosage may produce convulsions or death.

DOSAGE AND ADMINISTRATION

Adults and adolescents over 12 years of age: One tablet every 12 hours not to exceed 2 tablets in 24 hours. Not recommended for use in pediatric patients under 12 years of age. Tablets are to be swallowed whole.

HOW SUPPLIED

Bottles of 100 tablets (NDC 53014-024-10) and 500 tablets (NDC 53014-024-50). Scored, yellow tablets are embossed with "Medeva" on one side and "0" to the left of the score and "24" to the right of the score on the other side. Store at controlled room temperature 15° C – 30° C (59° F – 86° F). Dispense in tight, light-resistant containers.
CAUTION: Federal law prohibits dispensing without prescription.
Keep out of reach of pediatric population.
Manufactured by: Vintage Pharmaceuticals, Inc.
Charlotte, NC 28206
For: Medeva Pharmaceuticals, Inc.
        Rochester, NY 14623 USA
35240006   0244/996
IN-129   R3

DECONSAL® II Tablets
(pseudoephedrine HCl + guaifenesin)

℞

DESCRIPTION

Each scored, dark blue DECONSAL® II Tablet provides 60 mg pseudoephedrine hydrochloride and 600 mg guaifenesin in a sustained-release formulation intended for oral administration. Inactive ingredients: Stearic acid, dibasic calcium phosphate, FD & C Blue #1 Lake, sodium lauryl sulfate, ethylcellulose, magnesium stearate.

Pseudoephedrine hydrochloride is a nasal decongestant. Chemically, it is $[S-(R^*,R^*)]-\alpha-[1-(methylamino)\ ethyl]$ benzenemethanol hydrochloride and has the following structural formula:

$C_{10}H_{15}NO \cdot HCl$ MW = 201.70

Guaifenesin is an expectorant. Chemically, it is 3-(2-methoxyphenoxy)-1, 2-propanediol and has the following structural formula:
[See chemical structure at top of next column]

Continued on next page

Information on the Medeva Pharmaceuticals, Inc. products listed on these pages contains the full prescribing information from product circulars in use as of July 1998. For further information, please consult the package insert currently accompanying the product.

Deconsal II—Cont.

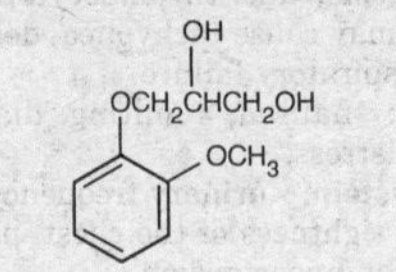

$C_{10}H_{14}O_4$ MW = 198.22

CLINICAL PHARMACOLOGY

Pseudoephedrine hydrochloride is an orally indirect acting sympathomimetic amine and exerts a decongestant action on the nasal mucosa. It does this by vasoconstriction which results in reduction of tissue hyperemia, edema, nasal congestion, and an increase in nasal airway patency. The vasoconstriction action of pseudoephedrine is similar to that of ephedrine. In the usual dose it has minimal vasopressor effects. Pseudoephedrine is rapidly and almost completely absorbed from the gastrointestinal tract. It has a plasma half-life of 6 to 8 hours. Alkaline urine is associated with slower elimination of the drug. The drug is distributed to body tissues and fluids, including the central nervous sytem (CNS). Approximately 50% to 75% of the administered dose is excreted unchanged in the urine; the remainder is apparently metabolized in the liver to inactive compounds by N-demethylation, parahydroxylation and oxidative deamination. Guaifenesin is an expectorant which increases respiratory tract fluid secretions and helps to loosen phlegm and bronchial secretions. By reducing the viscosity of secretions, guaifenesin increases the efficiency of the mucociliary mechanism in removing accumulated secretions from the upper and lower airway. Guaifenesin is readily absorbed from the gastrointestinal tract and is rapidly metabolized and excreted in the urine. Guaifenesin has a plasma half-life of one hour. The major urinary metabolite is β-(2-methoxyphenoxy) lactic acid.

INDICATIONS AND USAGE

DECONSAL® II Tablets are indicated for the temporary relief of nasal congestion and cough associated with respiratory tract infections and related conditions such as sinusitis, pharyngitis, bronchitis, and asthma, when these conditions are complicated by tenacious mucus and/or mucus plugs and congestion. The product is effective in productive as well as non-productive cough, but is of particular value in dry, non-productive cough which tends to injure the mucous membrane of the air passages.

CONTRAINDICATIONS

This product is contraindicated in patients with hypersensitivity to guaifenesin, or with hypersensitivity or idiosyncrasy to sympathomimetic amines which may be manifested by insomnia, dizziness, weakness, tremor or arrhythmias. Sympathomimetic amines are contraindicated in patients with severe hypertension, severe coronary artery disease and patients on monoamine oxidase inhibitor (MAOI) therapy and for 14 days after stopping MAOI therapy (see Drug Interactions section).

WARNINGS

Sympathomimetic amines should be used with caution in patients with hypertension, ischemic heart disease, diabetes mellitus, increased intraocular pressure, hyperthyroidism, or prostatic hypertophy. Sympathomimetics may produce central nervous system stimulation with convulsions or cardiovascular collapse with accompanying hypotension.
Do not exceed recommended dosage.
Hypertensive crises can occur with concurrent use of pseudoephedrine and MAOI, and for 14 days after stopping MAOI therapy, indomethacin, or with beta-blockers and methyldopa. If a hypertensive crisis occurs, these drugs should be discontinued immediately and therapy to lower blood pressure should be instituted. Fever should be managed by means of external cooling.

PRECAUTIONS

General: Use with caution in patients with diabetes, hypertension, cardiovascular disease and intolerance to ephedrine.
Before prescribing medication to suppress or modify cough, it is important to ascertain that the underlying cause of cough is identified, that modification of cough does not increase the risk of clinical or physiologic complications, and that appropriate therapy for the primary disease is instituted.
Information for Patients: Patients should be instructed to check with physician if symptoms do not improve within 5 days or if fever is present.
Pediatric Use: This product is not recommended for use in pediatric patients under 2 years of age.
Use in Elderly: The elderly (60 years and older) are more likely to experience adverse reactions to sypathomimetics. Overdosage of sympathomimetics in this age group may cause hallucinations, convulsions, CNS depression, and death.
Drug Interactions: Do not prescribe this product for use in patients that are now taking a prescription MAOI (certain drugs for depression, psychiatric or emotional conditions, or Parkinson's disease), or for 14 days after stopping the MAOI drug therapy. Beta-adrenergic blockers and MAOI may potentiate the pressor effect of pseudoephedrine (see **WARNINGS**). Concurrent use of digitalis glycosides may increase the possibility of cardiac arrhythmias. Sympathomimetics may reduce the hypotensive effects of guanethidine, mecamylamine, methyldopa, reserpine and veratrum alkaloids. Concurrent use of tricyclic antidepressants may antagonize the effects of pseudoephedrine.
Drug/Laboratory Test Interactions: Guaifenesin may increase renal clearance for urate and thereby lower serum uric acid levels. Guaifenesin may produce an increase in urinary 5-hydroxyindoleacetic acid and may therefore interfere with the interpretation of this test for the diagnosis of carcinoid syndrome. It may also falsely elevate the VMA test for catechols. Administration of this drug should be discontinued 48 hours prior to the collection of urine specimens for such tests.
Carcinogenesis, Mutagenesis, Impairment of Fertility: No data are available on the long-term potential of the components of this product for carcinogenesis, mutagenesis, or impairment of fertility in animals or humans.
Pregnancy: Category C: Animal reproduction studies have not been conducted with DECONSAL® II Tablets. It is also not known whether DECONSAL® II Tablets can cause fetal harm when administered to a pregnant woman or can affect reproduction capacity. DECONSAL® II Tablets should be given to a pregnant woman only if clearly needed.
Nursing Mothers: Pseudoephedrine is excreted in breast milk. Use of this product by nursing mothers is not recommended because of the higher than usual risk for infants from sypathomimetic amines.

ADVERSE REACTIONS

Hyper-reactive individuals may display ephedrine-like reactions such as tachycardia, palpitations, headache, dizziness, or nausea. Sympathomimetics have been associated with certain untoward reactions including fear, anxiety, nervousness, restlessness, tremor, weakness, pallor, respiratory difficulty, dysuria, insomnia, hallucinations, convulsions, CNS depression, arrhythmias, and cardiovascular collapse with hypotension. No serious side effects have been reported with the use of guaifenesin.

OVERDOSAGE

Since DECONSAL® II Tablets contain two pharmacologically different compounds, treatment of overdosage should be based upon the symptomatology of the patient as it relates to the individual ingredients. Treatment of acute overdosage would probably be based upon treating the patient for pseudoephedrine toxicity which may manifest itself as excessive CNS stimulation resulting in excitement, tremor, restlessness, and insomnia. Other effects may include tachycardia, hypertension, pallor, mydriasis, hyperglycemia and urinary retention. Severe overdosage may cause tachypnea or hyperpnea, hallucinations, convulsions or delirium, but in some individuals there may be CNS depression with somnolence, stupor or respiratory depression. Arrhythmias (including ventricular fibrillation) may lead to hypotension and circulatory collapse. Severe hypokalemia can occur, probably due to a compartmental shift rather than a depletion of potassium. No organ damage or significant metabolic derangement is associated with pseudoephedrine overdosage. Overdosage with guaifenesin is unlikely to produce toxic effects since its toxicity is much lower than that of pseudoephedrine. In severe cases of overdose, it is recommended to monitor the patient in an intensive care setting. The LD_{50} of pseudoephedrine (single oral dose) has been reported to be 726 mg/kg in the mouse, 2206 mg/kg in the rat and 1177 mg/kg in the rabbit. The toxic and lethal concentrations in human biologic fluids are not known. Urinary excretion increases with acidification and decreases with alkalinization of the urine. There are few published reports of toxicity due to pseudoephedrine and no case of fatal overdosage has been reported. Guaifenesin, when administered by stomach tube to test animals in doses up to 5 grams/kg. produced no signs of toxicity.
Since the action of sustained release products may continue for as long as 12 hours, treatment of overdosage should be directed toward reducing further absorption and supporting the patient for at least that length of time. Gastric emptying (Syrup of Ipecac) and/or lavage is recommended as soon as possible after ingestion, even if the patient has vomited spontaneously. Either isotonic or half-isotonic saline may be used for lavage. Administration of an activated charcoal slurry is beneficial after lavage and/or emesis if less than 4 hours have passed since ingestion. Saline cathartics, such as Milk of Magnesia, are useful for hastening the evacuation of unreleased medication.
Adrenergic receptor blocking agents are antidotes to pseudoephedrine. In practice, the most useful is the beta-blocker propranolol, which is indicated when there are signs of cardiac toxicity. Theoretically, pseudoephedrine is dialyzable but procedures have not been clinically established.

DOSAGE AND ADMINISTRATION

Adults and adolescents over 12 years of age: One or two tablets every 12 hours not to exceed 4 tablets in 24 hours. **Children 6 to 12 years:** 1 tablet every 12 hours not to exceed 2 tablets in 24 hours. **Children 2 to 6 years:** 1/2 tablet every 12 hours not to exceed 1 tablet in 24 hours.

HOW SUPPLIED

Bottles of 100 tablets (NDC 53014-017-10) and 500 tablets (NDC 53014-017-50). Scored, dark blue tablets are embossed with "MEDEVA" on one side, and "017" to the right of the score on the other side. Store at controlled room temperature between 15° C and 30° C (59° F and 86° F). Dispense in tight containers.
Keep out of reach of pediatric population.
CAUTION: Federal law prohibits dispensing without prescription.
Medeva Pharmaceuticals, Inc.
Rochester, NY 14623 USA

DEXACORT™ Phosphate ℞
(dexamethasone sodium phosphate)
in TURBINAIRE® (dispenser)
Aerosol for Intranasal Application

DESCRIPTION

DEXACORT™ Phosphate (dexamethasone sodium phosphate) in TURBINAIRE® (Dispenser) is an aerosol for intranasal application. The inactive ingredients are chlorofluorocarbons† as propellants and alcohol 2%. One cartridge delivers an amount sufficient to ensure delivery of 170 metered sprays, each containing dexamethasone sodium phosphate equivalent to approximately 0.1 mg dexamethasone phosphate or to approximately 0.084 mg dexamethasone. Twelve sprays deliver a theoretical maximum of 1.0 mg dexamethasone.
Dexamethasone sodium phosphate, a synthetic adrenocortical steroid, is a white or slightly yellow, crystalline powder. It is freely soluble in water and is exceedingly hygroscopic. The molecular weight is 516.41. It is designated chemically as 9-fluoro-11β, 17-dihydroxy-16α-methyl-21-(phosphonooxy) pregna-1,4-diene-3, 20-dione disodium salt. The empirical formula is $C_{22}H_{28}FNa_2O_8P$ and the structural formula is:

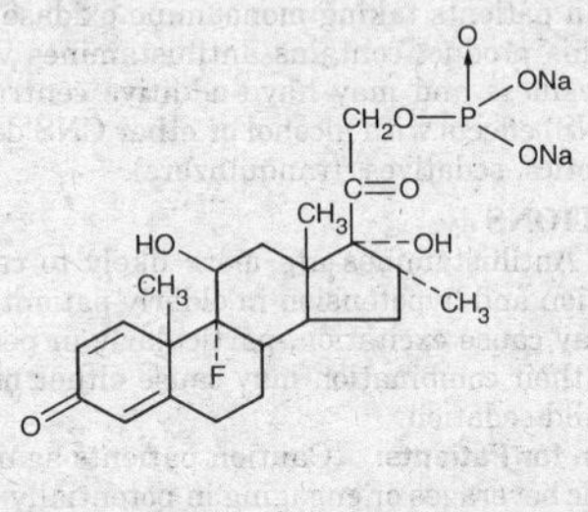

ACTION

Inhibition of inflammatory response to inciting agents of mechanical, chemical or immunological nature.

† WARNING: Chlorofluorocarbons (CFCs) are substances which harm public health and environment by destroying ozone in the upper atmosphere.

INDICATIONS

Allergic or inflammatory nasal conditions, and nasal polyps (excluding polyps originating within the sinuses).

CONTRAINDICATIONS

Systemic fungal infections.
Hypersensitivity to components.
Tuberculous, viral and fungal nasal conditions, ocular herpes simplex.

WARNINGS

In patients on therapy with DEXACORT Phosphate in TURBINAIRE subjected to unusual stress, increased dosage of rapidly acting corticosteroids before, during, and after the stressful situation is indicated.
Drug-induced secondary adrenocortical insufficiency may result from too rapid withdrawal of corticosteroids and may be minimized by gradual reduction of dosage. This type of relative insufficiency may persist for months after discontinuation of therapy; therefore, in any situation of stress occurring during that period, hormone therapy should be reinstituted. If the patient is receiving steroids already, dosage may have to be increased. Since mineralocorticoid secretion may by impaired, salt and/or a mineralocorticoid should be administered concurrently.
Dexamethasone may mask some signs of infection, and new infections may appear during its use. There may be decreased resistance and inability to localize infection when

corticosteroids are used. Therefore, patients with bacterial infections should also be given appropriate antibiotic therapy if DEXACORT Phosphate in TURBINAIRE is used. Moreover, dexamethasone may affect the nitrobluetetrazolium test for bacterial infection and produce false negative results.

Corticosteroids may activate latent amebiasis. Therefore, it is recommended that latent or active amebiasis be ruled out before initiating corticosteroid therapy in any patient who has spent time in the tropics or any patient with unexplained diarrhea.

Prolonged use of DEXACORT Phosphate in TURBINAIRE may produce posterior subcapsular cataracts, glaucoma with possible damage to the optic nerves, and may enhance the establishment of secondary ocular infections due to fungi or viruses.

Usage in pregnancy: Since adequate human reproduction studies have not been done with DEXACORT Phosphate in TURBINAIRE, use of this drug in pregnancy or in women of childbearing potential requires that the anticipated benefits be weighed against the possible hazards to the mother and embryo or fetus. Infants born of mothers who have received substantial doses of dexamethasone during pregnancy, should be carefully observed for signs of hypoadrenalism.

Dexamethasone appears in breast milk and could suppress growth, interfere with endogenous corticosteroid production, or cause other unwanted effects. Mothers taking pharmacologic doses of dexamethasone should be advised not to nurse.

Average and large doses of hydrocortisone or cortisone can cause elevation of blood pressure, salt and water retention, and increased excretion of potassium. These effects are less likely to occur with the synthetic derivatives and with DEXACORT Phosphate in TURBINAIRE, except when used in large doses. Dietary salt restriction and potassium supplementation may be necessary. All corticosteroids increase calcium excretion.

Administration of live virus vaccines, including smallpox, is contraindicated in individuals receiving immunosuppressive doses of corticosteroids. If inactivated viral or bacterial vaccines are administered to individuals receiving immunosuppressive doses of corticosteroids, the expected serum antibody response may not be obtained.

Patients who are on drugs which suppress the immune system are more susceptible to infections than healthy individuals. Chickenpox and measles, for example can have a more serious or even fatal course in non-immune children (see PRECAUTIONS regarding use of this product in children) or adults on corticosteroids. In such children or adults who have not had these diseases, particular care should be taken to avoid exposure. The risk of developing a disseminated infection varies among individuals and can be related to the dose, route and duration of corticosteroid administration as well as to the underlying disease. If exposed to chickenpox, prophylaxis with varicella zoster immune globulin (VZIG) may be indicated. If chickenpox develops, treatment with antiviral agents may be considered. If exposed to measles, prophylaxis with immune globulin (IG) may be indicated. (See the respective package inserts for VZIG and IG for complete prescribing information.)

If DEXACORT Phosphate in TURBINAIRE is indicated in patients with latent tuberculosis or tuberculin reactivity, close observation is necessary as reactivation of the disease may occur. During prolonged therapy with DEXACORT Phosphate in TURBINAIRE, these patients should receive chemoprophylaxis.

Literature reports suggest an apparent association between use of corticosteroids and left ventricular free wall rupture after a recent myocardial infarction; therefore, therapy with corticosteroids should be used with great caution in these patients.

Keep out of reach of children.

PRECAUTIONS

During local corticosteroid therapy, the possibility of pharyngeal candidiasis should be kept in mind.

Although systemic absorption is low when DEXACORT Phosphate in TURBINAIRE is used in the recommended dosage, adrenal suppression may occur. In addition, other systemic effects of steroid administration must be considered as a possibility.

Following prolonged therapy, withdrawal of corticosteroids may result in symptoms of the corticosteroid withdrawal syndrome including fever, myalgia, arthralgia, and malaise. This may occur in patients even without evidence of adrenal insufficiency. Replacement of systemic steroid with DEXACORT Phosphate in TURBINAIRE should be gradual and carefully monitored by the physician.

There is an enhanced effect of dexamethasone in patients with hypothyroidism and in those with cirrhosis.

DEXACORT Phosphate in TURBINAIRE should be used cautiously in patients with ocular herpes simplex for fear of corneal perforation.

The lowest possible dose of DEXACORT Phosphate in TURBINAIRE should be used to control the condition under treatment, and when reduction in dosage is possible, the re-

duction must be gradual. If beneficial effect is not evident within 7 days after initiation of therapy, the patient should be re-evaluated.

Psychic derangements may appear when dexamethasone is used, ranging from euphoria, insomnia, mood swings, personality changes, and severe depression, to frank psychotic manifestations. Also, existing emotional instability or psychotic tendencies may be aggravated.

Aspirin should be used cautiously in conjunction with DEXACORT Phosphate in TURBINAIRE in hypoprothrombinemia.

DEXACORT Phosphate in TURBINAIRE should be used with caution in patients with nonspecific ulcerative colitis, if there is a probability of impending perforation, abscess or other pyogenic infection; also in diverticulitis; fresh intestinal anastomoses; active or latent peptic ulcer; renal insufficiency; hypertension; osteoporosis; and myasthenia gravis. Signs of peritoneal irritation following gastrointestinal perforation in patients receiving large doses of corticosteroids may be minimal or absent. Fat embolism has been reported as a possible complication of hypercortisonism.

Because clinical studies have not been done, the use of this product in children under the age of 6 years is not recommended. Growth and development of children 6 years of age or older on prolonged therapy with DEXACORT Phosphate in TURBINAIRE should be carefully followed.

Dexamethasone may increase or decrease motility and number of spermatozoa in some patients.

Phenytoin, phenobarbital, ephedrine and rifampin may enhance the metabolic clearance of dexamethasone, resulting in decreased blood levels and lessened physiologic activity, thus requiring adjustment in dexamethasone dosage.

The prothrombin time should be checked frequently in patients who are receiving DEXACORT Phosphate in TURBINAIRE and coumarin anticoagulants at the same time because of reports that corticosteroids have altered the response to these anticoagulants. Studies have shown that the usual effect produced by adding corticosteroids is inhibition of response to coumarins, although there have been some conflicting reports of potentiation, not substantiated by studies.

When DEXACORT Phosphate in TURBINAIRE is used concomitantly with potassium-depleting diuretics, patients should be observed closely for development of hypokalemia. Since the contents of DEXACORT Phosphate in TURBINAIRE are under pressure, the container should not be broken, stored in extreme heat, or incinerated. It should be stored at a temperature below 120°F.

Information for Patients

Susceptible patients who are on immunuosuppressant doses of corticosteroids should be warned to avoid exposure to chickenpox or measles. Patients should also be advised that if they are exposed, medical advice should be sought without delay.

ADVERSE REACTIONS

Nasal irritation and dryness are the most common adverse reactions. The following have been reported: headache, lightheadedness, urticaria, nausea, epistaxis, rebound congestion, bronchial asthma, perforation of the nasal septum, and anosmia. Signs of adrenal hypercorticism may occur in some patients, especially with overdosage.

Systemic effects from therapy with DEXACORT Phosphate in TURBINAIRE are less likely to occur than with oral or parenteral corticosteroid therapy because of a lower total dose administered. Nevertheless, patients should be observed for the hormonal effects described below because of absorption of dexamethasone from the nasal mucosa.

Fluid and Electrolyte Disturbances
Sodium retention
Fluid retention
Congestive heart failure in susceptible patients
Potassium loss
Hypokalemic alkalosis
Hypertension
Musculoskeletal
Muscle weakness
Steroid myopathy
Loss of muscle mass
Osteoporosis
Vertebral compression fractures
Aseptic necrosis of femoral and humeral heads
Pathologic fracture of long bones
Tendon rupture
Gastrointestinal
Peptic ulcer with possible subsequent perforation and hemorrhage
Perforation of the small and large bowel, particularly in patients with inflammatory bowel disease
Pancreatitis
Abdominal distention
Ulcerative esophagitis
Dermatologic
Impaired wound healing
Thin fragile skin
Petechiae and ecchymoses

Erythema
Increased sweating
May suppress reactions to skin tests
Other cutaneous reactions, such as allergic dermatitis, urticaria, angioneurotic edema
Neurologic
Convulsions
Increased intracranial pressure with papilledema (pseudotumor cerebri) usually after treatment.
Vertigo
Headache
Psychic disturbances
Endocrine
Menstrual irregularities
Development of cushingoid state
Suppression of growth in children
Secondary adrenocortical and pituitary unresponsiveness, particularly in times of stress, as in trauma, surgery, or illness.
Decreased carbohydrate tolerance
Manifestations of latent diabetics mellitus
Increased requirements for insulin or oral hypoglycemic agents in diabetics
Hirsutism
Ophthalmic
Posterior subcapsular cataracts
Increased intraocular pressure
Glaucoma
Exophthalmos
Metabolic
Negative nitrogen balance due to protein catabolism
Cardiovascular
Myocardial rupture following recent myocardial infarction (see WARNINGS).
Other
Hypersensitivity
Thromboembolism
Weight gain
Increased appetite
Nausea
Malaise
Hiccups

OVERDOSAGE

Reports of acute toxicity and/or death following overdosage of glucocorticoids are rare. In the event of overdosage, no specific antidote is available; treatment is supportive and symptomatic.

Significant lethality was observed in female mice at single oral doses of 3630 mg/m^2 (1210 mg/kg) and single intravenous doses of 2382 mg/m^2 (794 mg/kg).

DOSAGE AND ADMINISTRATION

DO NOT EXCEED THE RECOMMENDED DOSAGE.
The usual initial dosage of DEXACORT Phosphate in TURBINAIRE is:
Adults—2 sprays in each nostril 2 or 3 times a day.
Children (6 to 12 years of age)—1 or 2 sprays in each nostril 2 times a day depending on age.
See accompanying instructions on the proper use of TURBINAIRE.
When improvement occurs the dosage should be gradually reduced. Some patients will be symptom-free on one spray in each nostril 2 times a day. The maximum daily dosage for adults is 12 sprays, and for children, 8 sprays. Therapy should be discontinued as soon as feasible. It may be reinstituted if recurrence of symptoms occurs.

HOW SUPPLIED

DEXACORT Phosphate in TURBINAIRE, aerosol for intranasal application, is supplied as follows: NDC 53014-201-13 in a pressurized container and includes a plastic adapter, 12.6 grams, 170 metered doses.
Storage
Store at a temperature below 49°C (120°F).
35201003   2014/1094

GASTROCROM®   ℞
[gas 'tro-krōm]
(cromolyn sodium, USP)
Oral Concentrate
For Oral Use Only—Not for Inhalation or Injection
Rev. 7/96
R081B

DESCRIPTION

Each 5 mL ampule of GASTROCROM contains 100 mg cromolyn sodium, USP, in purified water. Cromolyn sodium is a

Continued on next page

Gastrocrom—Cont.

hygroscopic, white powder having little odor. It may leave a slightly bitter aftertaste. GASTROCROM (cromolyn sodium, USP) Oral Concentrate is clear, colorless, and sterile. It is intended for oral use.

Chemically, cromolyn sodium is disodium 5,5'-[(2- hydroxytrimethylene)dioxy]bis[4-oxo-4H-1-benzopyran-2- carboxylate]. The empirical formula is $C_{23}H_{14}Na_2O_{11}$: the molecular weight is 512.34. Its chemical structure is:

Pharmacologic Category: Mast cell stabilizer
Therapeutic Category: Antiallergic

CLINICAL PHARMACOLOGY

In vitro and *in vivo* animal studies have shown that cromolyn sodium inhibits the release of mediators from sensitized mast cells. Cromolyn sodium acts by inhibiting the release of histamine and leukotrienes (SRS-A) from the mast cell.

Cromolyn sodium has no intrinsic vasoconstrictor, antihistamine, or glucocorticoid activity.

Cromolyn sodium is poorly absorbed from the gastrointestinal tract. No more the 1% of an administered dose is absorbed by humans after oral administration, the remainder being excreted in the feces. Very little absorption of cromolyn sodium was seen after oral administration of 500 mg by mouth to each of 12 volunteers. From 0.28 to 0.50% of the administered dose was recovered in the first 24 hours of urinary excretion in 3 subjects. The mean urinary excretion of an administered dose over 24 hours in the remaining 9 subjects was 0.45%.

CLINICAL STUDIES

Four randomized, controlled clinical trials were conducted with GASTROCROM in patients with either cutaneous or systemic mastocytosis, two of which utilized a placebo-controlled crossover design, one utilized an active-controlled (chlorpheniramine plus cimetidine) crossover design, and one utilized a placebo-controlled parallel group design. Due to the rare nature of this disease, only 36 patients qualified for study entry, of whom 32 were considered evaluable. Consequently, formal statistical analyses were not performed. Clinically significant improvement in gastrointestinal symptoms (diarrhea, abdominal pain) were seen in the majority of patients with some improvement also seen for cutaneous manifestations (urticaria, pruritus, flushing) and cognitive function. The benefit seen with GASTROCROM 200 mg QID was similar to chlorpheniramine (4 mg QID) plus cimetidine (300 mg QID) for both cutaneous and systemic symptoms of mastocytosis.

Clinical improvement occurred within 2–6 weeks of treatment initiation and persisted for 2–3 weeks after treatment withdrawal. GASTROCROM did not affect urinary histamine levels or peripheral eosinophilia, although neither of these variables appeared to correlate with disease severity. Positive clinical benefits were also reported for 37 of 51 patients who received GASTROCROM in United States and foreign humanitarian programs.

INDICATIONS AND USAGE

GASTROCROM is indicated in the management of patients with mastocytosis. Use of this product has been associated with improvement in diarrhea, flushing, headaches, vomiting, urticaria, abdominal pain, nausea, and itching in some patients.

CONTRAINDICATIONS

GASTROCROM is contraindicated in those patients who have shown hypersensitivity to cromolyn sodium.

WARNINGS

The recommended dosage should be decreased in patients with decreased renal or hepatic function. Severe anaphylactic reactions may occur rarely in association with cromolyn sodium administration.

PRECAUTIONS

In view of the biliary and renal routes of excretion of GASTROCROM, consideration should be given to decreasing the dosage of the drug in patients with impaired renal or hepatic function.

Carcinogenesis, Mutagenesis, and Impairment of Fertility: Long term studies of cromolyn sodium in mice (12 months intraperitoneal administration at doses up to 150 mg/kg three days per week), hamsters, (intraperitoneal administration at doses up to 52.6 mg/kg three days per week for 15 weeks followed by 17.5 mg/kg three days per week for 37 weeks), and rats (18 months subcutaneous administration at doses up to 75 mg/kg six days per week) showed no neoplastic effects. The average daily maximum dose levels administered in these studies were 192.9 mg/m^2 for mice, 47.2 mg/m^2 for hamsters and 385.8 mg/m^2 for rats. These doses correspond to 13%, 3.2%, and 26% of the maximum daily human dose of 1480 mg/m^2.

Cromolyn sodium showed no mutagenic potential in Ames Salmonella/microsome plate assays, mitotic gene conversion in *Saccharomyces cerevisiae* and in an *in vitro* cytogenetic study in human peripheral lymphocytes.

No evidence of impaired fertility was shown in laboratory reproduction studies conducted subcutaneously in rats at the highest doses tested, 175 mg/kg/day (1050 mg/m^2) in males and 100 mg/kg/day (600 mg/m^2) in females. These doses are approximately 71% and 41% of the maximum daily human dose, respectively, based on mg/m^2.

Pregnancy: Pregnancy Category B. Reproduction studies with cromolyn sodium administered subcutaneously to pregnant mice and rats at maximum daily dose of 540 mg/kg (1620 mg/m^2) and 164 mg/kg (984 mg/m^2), respectively, and intravenously to rabbits at a maximum daily doses of 485 mg/kg (5820 mg/m^2) produced no evidence of fetal malformations. These doses represent 109%, 66% and 393%, respectively, of the maximum daily human dose on a mg/m^2 basis. Adverse fetal effects (increased resorption and decreased fetal weight) were noted only at very high parenteral doses that produced maternal toxicity. There are, however, no adequate and well controlled studies in pregnant women.

Because animal reproduction studies are not always predictive of human response, this drug should be used during pregnancy only if clearly needed.

Drug Interaction During Pregnancy: Cromolyn sodium and isoproterenol were studied following subcutaneous injections in pregnant mice. Cromolyn sodium alone in doses of 60 to 540 mg/kg (38 to 338 times the human dose) did not cause significant increases in resorptions or major malformations. Isoproterenol alone at a dose of 2.7 mg/kg (90 times the human dose) increased both resorptions and malformations. The addition of cromolyn sodium (338 times the human dose) to isoproterenol (90 times the human dose) appears to have increased the incidence of both resorptions and malformations.

Nursing Mothers: It is not known whether this drug is excreted in human milk. Because many drugs are excreted in human milk, caution should be exercised when GASTROCROM is administered to a nursing woman.

Pediatric Use: Animal studies suggest increased risk of toxicity in premature animals when given doses much higher than clinically recommended. In term infants up to six months of age, available clinical data suggest that the dose should not exceed 20 mg/day. The use of this product in pediatric patients less than two years of age should be reserved for patients with severe disease in which the potential benefits clearly outweigh the risks.

ADVERSE REACTIONS

Most of the adverse events reported in mastocytosis patients have been transient and could represent symptoms of the disease. The most frequently reported adverse events in mastocytosis patients who have received GASTROCROM during clinical studies were headache and diarrhea, each of which occurred in 4 of the 87 patients. Pruritus, nausea, and myalgia were each reported in 3 patients and abdominal pain, rash, and irritability in 2 patients each. One report of malaise was also recorded.

Other Adverse Events: Additional adverse events have been reported during studies in other clinical conditions and from worldwide postmarketing experience. In most cases the available information is incomplete and attribution to the drug cannot be determined. The majority of these reports involve the gastrointestinal system and include: diarrhea, nausea, abdominal pain, constipation, dyspepsia, flatulence, glossitis, stomatitis, vomiting, dysphagia, esophagospasm.

Other less commonly reported events (the majority representing only a single report) include the following:

Skin:	pruritus, rash, urticaria/angioedema, erythema/burning, photosensitivity
Musculoskeletal:	arthralgia, myalgia, stiffness/weakness of legs
Neurologic:	headache, dizziness, hypoesthesia, paresthesia, migraine, convulsions, flushing
Psychiatric:	psychosis, anxiety, depression, hallucinations, behavior change, insomnia, nervousness
Heart Rate:	tachycardia, premature ventricular contractions (PVCs), palpitations
Respiratory:	pharyngitis, dyspnea
Miscellaneous:	fatigue, edema, unpleasant taste, chest pain, postprandial lightheadedness and lethargy, dysuria, urinary frequency, purpura, hepatic function test abnormal, polycythemia, neutropenia, pancytopenia, tinnitus, lupus erythematosus (LE) syndrome

DOSAGE AND ADMINISTRATION

NOT FOR INHALATION OR INJECTION. SEE DIRECTIONS FOR USE.

The usual starting dose is as follows:

Adults (13 Years and Older): Two ampules four times daily, taken one-half hour before meals and at bedtime.

Children 2–12 Years: One ampule four times daily, taken one-half hour before meals and at bedtime.

Pediatric Patients Under 2 Years: Not recommended.

If satisfactory control of symptoms is not achieved within two to three weeks, the dosage may be increased but should not exceed 40 mg/kg/day.

Patients should be advised that the effect of GASTROCROM therapy is dependent upon its administration at regular intervals, as directed.

Maintenance Dose: Once a therapeutic response has been achieved, the dose may be reduced to the minimum required to maintain the patient with a lower degree of symptomatology. To prevent relapses, the dosage should be maintained.

Administration: GASTROCROM should be administered as a solution at least $^1/_2$ hour before meals and at bedtime after preparation according to the following directions:

1. Break open ampule(s) and squeeze liquid contents of ampule(s) into a glass of water.
2. Stir solution.
3. Drink all of the liquid.

HOW SUPPLIED

GASTROCROM Oral Concentrate is an unpreserved, colorless solution supplied in a low density polyethylene plastic unit dose ampule with 8 ampules per foil pouch. Each 5 mL ampule contains 100 mg cromolyn sodium, USP, in purified water.

NDC 53014-678-70 96 ampules × 5 mL

GASTROCROM Oral Concentrate should be stored between 15°–30°C (59°–86°F) and protected from light. Do not use if it contains a precipitate or becomes discolored. Keep out of the reach of children.

Store ampules in foil pouch until ready for use.

CAUTION: Federal law prohibits dispensing without prescription.

Marketed by:

MEDEVA PHARMACEUTICALS

Medeva Pharmaceuticals, Inc.
Rochester, NY 14623 USA

Manufactured by:

Automatic Liquid Packaging, Inc.
Woodstock, IL 60098 USA
®FISONS plc

7/96
R081B

©1996, Medeva Pharmaceuticals Manufacturing, Inc.

HUMIBID® L.A. Tablets ℞
(guaifenesin)

DESCRIPTION

Each light green, capsule shaped, scored tablet provides 600 mg guaifenesin in a sustained-released formulation intended for oral administration. Inactive ingredients: Dibasic calcium phosphate, ethylcellulose, FD & C Blue #1 Lake, D & C Yellow #10 Lake, magnesium stearate, sodium lauryl sulfate, stearic acid.

Chemically, guaifenesin is 3-(2-methoxyphenoxy)-1, 2-propanediol and has the following structural formula:

$C_{10}H_{14}O_4$ MW = 198.22

CLINICAL PHARMACOLOGY

Guaifenesin is an expectorant which increases respiratory tract fluid secretions and helps to loosen phlegm and bronchial secretions. By reducing the viscosity of secretions, guaifenesin increases the efficiency of the mucociliary mechanism in removing accumulated secretions from the upper and lower airway. Guaifenesin is readily absorbed from the

gastrointestinal tract and is rapidly metabolized and excreted in the urine. Guaifenesin has a plasma half-life of one hour. The major urinary metabolite is β-(2-methoxyphenoxy) lactic acid.

INDICATIONS AND USAGE

HUMIBID® L.A. Tablets are indicated for the temporary relief of coughs associated with respiratory tract infections and related conditions such as sinusitis, pharyngitis, bronchitis, and asthma, when these conditions are complicated by tenacious mucus and/or mucus plugs and congestion. The drug is effective in productive as well as non-productive cough, but is of particular value in dry, non-productive cough which tends to injure the mucous membrane of the air passages.

CONTRAINDICATIONS

This product is contraindicated in patients with hypersensitivity to guaifenesin.

PRECAUTIONS

General: Before prescribing medication to suppress or modify cough, it is important to ascertain that the underlying cause of cough is identified, that modification of cough does not increase the risk of clinical or physiologic complications, and that appropriate therapy for the primary disease is instituted.

Drug/Laboratory Test Interactions:
Guaifenesin may increase renal clearance for urate and thereby lower serum uric acid levels. Guaifenesin may produce an increase in urinary 5-hydroxyindoleacetic acid and may therefore interfere with the interpretation of this test for the diagnosis of carcinoid syndrome. It may also falsely elevate the VMA test for catechols. Administration of this drug should be discontinued 48 hours prior to the collection of urine specimens for such tests.

Carcinogenesis, Mutagenesis, Impairment of Fertility: No data are available on the long-term potential for carcinogenesis, mutagenesis, or impairment of fertility in animals or humans.

Pregnancy: Category C: Animal reproduction studies have not been conducted with HUMIBID® L.A. Tablets. It is also not known whether HUMIBID® L.A. Tablets can cause fetal harm when administered to a pregnant woman or can affect reproduction capacity. HUMIBID® L.A. Tablets should be given to a pregnant woman only if clearly needed.

Nursing Mothers: It is not known whether guaifenesin is excreted in human milk. Because many drugs are excreted in human milk, caution should be exercised when guaifenesin is administered to a nursing mother and a decision should be made whether to discontinue nursing or to discontinue the drug, taking into account the importance of the drug to the mother.

ADVERSE REACTIONS

No serious side effects from guaifenesin have been reported.

OVERDOSAGE

Overdosage with guaifenesin is unlikely to produce toxic effects since its toxicity is low. Guaifenesin, when administered by stomach tube to test animals in doses up to 5 grams/kg, produced no signs of toxicity. In severe cases of overdosage, treatment should be aimed at reducing further absorption of the drug. Gastric emptying (Syrup of lpecac) and/or lavage is recommended as soon as possible after ingestion.

DOSAGE AND ADMINISTRATION

Adults and adolescents over 12 years of age: One or two tablets every 12 hours not to exceed 4 tablets (2400 mg) in 24 hours. **Children 6 to 12 years:** One tablet every 12 hours not to exceed 2 tablets (1200 mg) in 24 hours. **Children 2 to 6 years:** 1/2 tablet every 12 hours not to exceed 1 tablet (600 mg) in 24 hours.

HOW SUPPLIED

Bottles of 100 tablets (NDC 53014-012-10) and 500 tablets (NDC 53014-012-50). Light green, capsule shaped, scored tablets are embossed with "MEDEVA" on one side, and "012" to the right of the score on the other side. Store at controlled room temperature between 15° C and 30 C (59° F and 86° F). Dispense in tight containers.

Keep out of reach of pediatric population.

CAUTION: Federal law prohibits dispensing without prescription.

Medeva Pharmaceuticals, Inc.
Rochester, NY 14623 USA

HYLOREL®Tablets ℞
[hi 'lō-rel"]
(guanadrel sulfate tablets, USP)
Rev. 7/96
R253A
814 438 105

DESCRIPTION

HYLOREL Tablets for oral administration contain guanadrel sulfate, an antihypertensive agent belonging to the class of adrenergic neuron blocking drugs. Guanadrel sulfate is (1,4-Dioxaspiro[4.5] dec-2-ylmethyl) guanidine sulfate with a molecular weight of 524.63. The empirical formula is $(C_{10}H_{19}N_3O_2)_2 \cdot H_2SO_4$. It is a white to off-white crystalline powder, which melts with decomposition at about 235°C. It is soluble in water to the extent of 76 mg/mL.
The structural formula is:

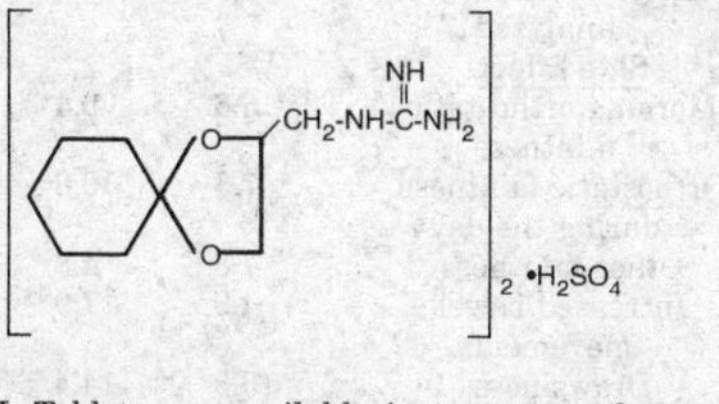

HYLOREL Tablets are available in two strengths: 10 mg and 25 mg. Inactive ingredients: colloidal silicon dioxide, corn starch, lactose monohydrate, magnesium stearate, microcrystalline cellulose and talc. The 10 mg tablet also contains FD&C Yellow No. 6.

CLINICAL PHARMACOLOGY

Guanadrel sulfate is an orally effective antihypertensive agent that lowers both systolic and diastolic arterial blood pressures. Guanadrel sulfate inhibits sympathetic vasoconstriction by inhibiting norepinephrine release from neuronal storage sites in response to stimulation of the nerve and also causes depletion of norepinephrine from the nerve ending. This results in relaxation of vascular smooth muscle which decreases total peripheral resistance, and decreases venous return, both of which reduce the ability to maintain blood pressure in the upright position. The result is a hypotensive effect that is greater in the standing than in the supine position by about 10 mmHg systolic and 3.5 mmHg diastolic, on the average. Heart rate is also decreased usually by about 5 beats/minute. Fluid retention occurs during treatment with guanadrel, particularly when it is not accompanied by a diuretic. The drug does not inhibit parasympathetic nerve function nor does it enter the central nervous system.

Guanadrel sulfate is rapidly absorbed after oral administration. Plasma concentrations generally peak $1^1/_2$ to 2 hours after ingestion. The half-life is about 10 hours, but individual variability is great. Approximately 85% of the drug is eliminated in the urine. Urinary excretion is approximately 85% complete within 24 hours after administration; about 40% of the dose is excreted as unchanged drug. The disposition of guanadrel sulfate is significantly altered in patients with impaired renal function. A study in such patients has shown that as renal function (measured as creatinine clearance) declines, apparent total blody clearance, renal and apparent nonrenal clearances decrease, and the terminal elimination half-life is prolonged. Dosage adjustments may be necessary, especially in patients with creatinine clearances of less than 60 mL/min (see DOSAGE AND ADMINISTRATION).

Guanadrel sulfate begins to decrease blood pressure within two hours and produces maximal decreases in four to six hours. No significant change in cardiac output accompanies the blood pressure decline in normal individuals.

Because drugs of the adrenergic neuron blocking class are transported into the neuron by the "norepinephrine pump", drugs that compete for the pump may block their effects. Tricyclic antidepressants have been shown to block the norepinephrine-depleting effect of guanadrel sulfate in rats and monkeys, and the blood pressure lowering effect of guanadrel sulfate in monkeys. Similar effects have been seen with guanethidine and inhibition of the antihypertensive effects of guanadrel sulfate by tricyclic antidepressants in humans should be presumed.

Therefore caution is recommended if guanadrel sulfate and a tricyclic antidepressant are used concomitantly. Should patients be on both a tricyclic antidepressant and guanadrel sulfate, caution is advised upon discontinuation of the tricyclic antidepressant, especially if discontinued abruptly, as an enhanced effect of guanadrel sulfate may occur.

Chlorpromazine seems to have a similar effect on guanethidine and may affect guanadrel as well. Indirectly acting adrenergic amines are transported into the neuron by the "norepinephrine pump" and may interfere with uptake or may displace blocking agents. Ephedrine rapidly reverses the effects of guanadrel but other agents have not been studied.

Agents of the guanethidine class cause increased sensitivity to circulating norepinephrine, probably by preventing uptake of norepinephrine by adrenergic neurons, the usual mechanism for terminating norepinephrine effects. Agents of this class are thus dangerous in the presence of excess norepinephrine, e.g., in the presence of a pheochromocytoma.

In controlled clinical studies comparing guanadrel to guanethidine and methyldopa, involving about 2000 patients exposed to guanadrel, patients with initial supine blood pressures averaging 160–170/105–110 mmHg had decreases in blood pressure of 20–25/15–20 mmHg in the standing position. The decreases in supine blood pressure were less than the decreases in standing blood pressure by 6–10/2–7 mmHg in different studies. Guanethidine and guanadrel were very similar in effectiveness while methyldopa had a larger effect on supine systolic pressure. Side effects of guanadrel and guanethidine were generally similar in type (see ADVERSE REACTIONS) while methyldopa had more central nervous system effects (depression, drowsiness) but fewer orthostatic effects and less diarrhea.

INDICATIONS AND USAGE

HYLOREL Tablets are indicated for the treatment of hypertension in patients not responding adequately to a thiazide type diuretic. HYLOREL should be added to a diuretic regimen for optimum blood pressure control.

CONTRAINDICATIONS

HYLOREL Tablets are contraindicated in known or suspected pheochromocytoma.

HYLOREL should not be used concurrently with, or within one week of, monoamine oxidase inhibitors.

HYLOREL should not be used in patients hypersensitive to the drug.

HYLOREL should not be used in patients with frank congestive heart failure.

WARNINGS

a. *Orthostatic Hypotension*

Orthostatic hypotension and its consequences (dizziness and weakness) are frequent in people treated with HYLOREL Tablets. Rarely, fainting upon standing or exercise is seen. Careful instructions to the patient can minimize these symptoms, as can recognition by the physician that the supine blood pressure does not constitute an adequate assessment of the effects of this drug. Patients with known regional vascular disease (cerebral, coronary) are at particular risk from marked orthostatic hypotension and HYLOREL should be avoided in them unless drugs with lesser degrees of orthostatic hypotension are ineffective or unacceptable. In such patients hypotensive episodes should be avoided, even if this requires accepting a poorer degree of blood pressure control.

Instructions to patients: Patients should be advised about the risk of orthostatic hypotension and told to sit or lie down immediately at the onset of dizziness or weakness so that they can prevent loss of consciousness. They should be told that postural hypotension is worst in the morning and upon arising, and may be exaggerated by alcohol, fever, hot weather, prolonged standing, or exercise.

Surgery: To reduce the possibility of vascular collapse during anesthesia, guanadrel should be discontinued 48–72 hours before elective surgery. If emergency surgery is required, the anesthesiologist should be made aware that the patient has been taking HYLOREL and that preanesthetic and anesthetic agents should be administered cautiously in reduced dosage. If vasopressors are needed they must be used cautiously, as guanadrel can enhance the pressor response to such agents and increase their arrhythmogenicity.

b. *Drug Interactions*

As discussed above (CLINICAL PHARMACOLOGY), tricyclic antidepressants and indirect-acting sympathomimetics such as ephedrine or phenylpropanolamine, and possibly phenothiazines, can reverse the effects of neuronal blocking agents. IN VIEW OF THE PRESENCE OF SYMPATHOMIMETIC AMINES IN MANY NON-PRESCRIPTION DRUGS FOR THE TREATMENT OF COLDS, ALLERGY, OR ASTHMA, PATIENTS GIVEN GUANADREL SHOULD BE SPECIFICALLY WARNED NOT TO USE SUCH PREPARATIONS WITHOUT THEIR PHYSICIAN'S ADVICE.

Guanadrel enhances the activity of direct-acting sympathomimetics, like norepinephrine, by blocking neuronal uptake.

Drugs that affect the adrenergic response by the same or other mechanisms would be expected to potentiate the effects of guanadrel, causing excessive postural hypotension and bradycardia. These include alpha- or beta-adrenergic blocking agents and reserpine. There is no clinical experience with the combination of HYLOREL with alpha-adrenergic blocking agents or reserpine.

When HYLOREL was added to the treatment regimen in hypertensive patients inadequately controlled with a diuretic and propranolol, no significant adverse effects, including bradycardia, were reported in the 26 patients treated concomitantly with the three drugs.

Continued on next page

Information on the Medeva Pharmaceuticals, Inc. products listed on these pages contains the full prescribing information from product circulars in use as of July 1998. For further information, please consult the package insert currently accompanying the product.

Hylorel—Cont.

The use of HYLOREL with vasodilators has not been adequately studied and is not generally recommended because concomitant use may increase the potential for symptomatic orthostatic hypotension.

c. Asthmatic patients

Special care is needed in patients with bronchial asthma, as their condition may be aggravated by catecholamine depletion and sympathomimetic amines may interfere with the hypotensive effect of guanadrel.

PRECAUTIONS

General: Salt and water retention may occur with the use of HYLOREL Tablets. In clinical studies major problems did not arise because of concomitant diuretic use. Patients with heart failure have not been studied on HYLOREL, but guanadrel could interfere with the adrenergic mechanisms that maintain compensation.

In patients with a history of peptic ulcer, which could be aggravated by a relative increase in parasympathetic tone, HYLOREL should be used cautiously.

In patients with compromised renal function, decreases in renal and nonrenal clearances and an increase in the elimination half-life of guanadrel sulfate have been found. This could possibly lead to an increased incidence of side effects if standard doses are used in these patients. Titration of dose based on the blood pressure response is necessary because of marked interpatient variability (see DOSAGE AND ADMINISTRATION).

A transient increase in blood pressure has been observed in some patients.

Information for patients
See WARNINGS section.

Drug Interactions
See WARNINGS section.

Carcinogenesis, mutagenesis, impairment of fertility: No evidence of carcinogenic potential appeared in a 2-year mouse study of guanadrel sulfate. In a 2-year rat study, an increased number of benign testicular interstitial cell tumors was observed at dosages of 100 mg/kg/day and 400 mg/kg/day. These are common spontaneous tumors in aged rats and their significance to therapy with HYLOREL in man is unknown. Salmonella testing (Ames test) showed no evidence of mutagenic activity.

A reproduction study was performed in male and female rats at dosages of 0, 10, 30 and 100 mg/kg/day. Suppressed libido and reduced fertility were noted at 100 mg/kg/day (12 times the maximum human dose in a 50 kg subject) and libido was suppressed to a lesser extent at 30 mg/kg/day.

Pregnancy Category B
Teratology studies performed in rats and rabbits at doses up to 12 times the maximum recommended human dose (in a 50 kg subject) revealed no significant harm to the fetus due to guanadrel sulfate. There are, however, no adequate and well-controlled studies in pregnant women. Because animal reproduction studies are not always predictive, HYLOREL should be used in pregnant women only when the potential benefit outweighs the potential risk to mother and infant.

Nursing mothers: Whether guanadrel sulfate is excreted in human milk is not known, but because many drugs are excreted in human milk and because of the potential for serious adverse reactions in nursing infants from guanadrel, a decision should be made whether to discontinue nursing or discontinue the drug, taking into account the importance of the drug to the mother.

Pediatric Use: Safety and effectiveness in pediatric patients have not been established.

ADVERSE REACTIONS

The adverse reaction data for guanadrel is derived principally from comparative long-term (6 months to 3 years) studies with methyldopa and guanethidine in which side effects were assessed through use of periodic questionnaires, a method that tends to give high adverse reaction rates. In the tables that follow, some of the adverse effects reported may not be drug-related, but in the absence of a placebo-treated group, these cannot be readily distinguished. Comparative results with two well-known drugs, methyldopa and guanethidine should aid in interpretation of these adverse reaction rates.

The following table displays the frequency of side effects which are believed to be related to sympathetic blocking agents: orthostatic faintness, increased bowel movements and ejaculation disturbances for peripherally acting drugs such as guanadrel and drowsiness for centrally acting drugs such as methyldopa. The frequencies observed were generally higher during the first 8 weeks of therapy. Week 0 frequencies, which were recorded just prior to administration of the antihypertensive drugs while the patients were receiving diuretics, serve as a reference point. Frequency while on therapy is shown for the first 8 weeks and for weeks 9 to 52.

FREQUENCY OF SIDE EFFECTS
Percent of Clinic Visits in Which Side Effect was Reported

Guanadrel

	Pre Drug		
Week	0	1–8	9–52
Number of clinic visits analyzed	470	3003	4260
Side Effect			
Morning orthostatic faintness	6.6	9.4	6.8
Orthostatic faintness during the day	7.5	10.8	8.5
Other faintness	7.8	4.8	4.5
Increased bowel movements	4.9	7.9	6.1
Drowsiness	15.3	14.4	8.7
Fatigue	25.7	26.6	23.7
Ejaculation disturbance	7.0	17.5	12.0

Methyldopa

	Pre Drug		
Week	0	1–8	9–52
Number of clinic visits analyzed	266	1610	2216
Side Effect			
Morning orthostatic faintness	6.8	8.1	7.4
Orthostatic faintness during the day	7.5	8.0	7.8
Other faintness	6.2	3.7	3.8
Increased bowel movements	4.9	5.9	3.8
Drowsiness	13.2	21.2	18.6
Fatigue	32.9	22.6	27.6
Ejaculation disturbance	10.3	13.4	11.5

Guanethidine

	Pre Drug		
Week	0	1–8	9–52
Number of clinic visits analyzed	215	1421	2009
Side Effect			
Morning orthostatic faintness	4.6	10.7	7.9
Orthostatic faintness during the day	5.6	8.9	6.3
Other faintness	5.9	2.7	2.0
Increased bowel movements	3.7	7.9	9.4
Drowsiness	10.2	10.3	6.4
Fatigue	21.4	20.5	17.5
Ejaculation disturbance	6.9	16.6	18.2

The frequency of side effects over time may be reduced by the discontinuation of drugs in patients who experience intolerable side effects. Reasons for discontinuation of therapy with guanadrel are shown in the following table.

PERCENT OF PATIENTS WHO DISCONTINUED

	Guana-drel	Methyl-dopa	Guane-thidine
Orthostatic faintness	0.6	0.7	6.0*
Syncope	0.4	0.3	2.0
Other faintness	1.2	0.0	0.0
Increased bowel movements	0.8	0.7	1.4
Drowsiness	0.0	1.9 *	0.0
Fatigue	0.2	2.6 *	0.0
Ejaculation disturbances	0.4	0.0	0.0

---

* significantly greater than HYLOREL, p<0.003

The following paragraph shows the incidence of reactions often associated with adrenergic neuron blockers as the percent of patients who reported the event at least once over the treatment periods of 6 months to 3 years. For such long-term studies these incidence rates of side effects, which are found often in untreated patients, tend to be high and accumulate with time. The incidence rates for two well-known comparison drugs, methyldopa and guanethidine should aid in interpreting the high rates. It can be seen that the serious consequences of the orthostatic effect of guanadrel, such as syncope, were very uncommon.

1544 guanadrel, 743 methyldopa and 330 guanethidine patients were evaluated in comparison studies. The observed incidence rates of major drug related side effects for guanadrel, methyldopa and guanethidine, respectively, are as follows: orthostatic faintness: 49%, 41%, 48%; other faintness: 47%, 46%, 45%; increased bowel movements: 31%, 28%, 36%; ejaculation disturbances: 18%, 21%, 22%; impotence: 5.1%, 12.2%, 7.2%; syncope: 0.4%, 0.3%, 2%; urine retention: 0.2%, 0%, 0%.

Apart from these adverse effects, many others were reported. Relationship to therapy is less clear, although some (such as peripheral edema with all three drugs, depression with methyldopa) are in part drug related. All adverse effects reported in at least 1% of guanadrel patients are listed in the following table:

Drug No. pts. treated Event	Guanadrel 1544 %	Methyl-dopa 743 %	Guanethi-dine 330 %
Cardiovascular-Respiratory			
Chest Pain	27.9	37.4	27.3
Coughing	26.9	36.2	21.5
Palpitations	29.5	35.0	24.5
Shortness of breath at rest	18.3	22.3	17.0
Shortness of breath on exertion	45.9	53.2	48.8
Central Nervous System-Special Senses			
Confusion	14.8	22.6	10.9
Depression	1.9	3.9	1.8
Drowsiness	44.6	64.1	28.5
Headache	58.1	69.0	49.7
Paresthesias	25.1	35.1	16.4
Psychological problems	3.8	4.8	3.9
Sleep disorders	2.1	2.3	2.7
Visual disturbances	29.2	35.3	26.1
Gastrointestinal			
Abdominal distress or pain	1.7	1.9	1.5
Anorexia	18.7	23.0	17.6
Constipation	21.0	29.1	20.3
Dry mouth, dry throat	1.7	4.0	0.6
Gas pain	32.0	39.7	29.4
Glossitis	8.4	10.8	4.8
Indigestion	23.7	30.8	18.5
Nausea and/or vomiting	3.9	4.8	3.6
Genitourinary			
Hematuria	2.3	4.2	2.1
Nocturia	48.4	52.4	41.5
Peripheral edema	28.6	37.4	22.7
Urinary urgency or frequency	33.6	39.8	27.6
Miscellaneous			
Excessive weight gain	44.3	53.7	42.4
Excessive weight loss	42.2	51.1	41.5
Fatigue	63.6	76.2	57.0
Musculoskeletal			
Aching limbs	42.9	51.7	33.9
Backache or neckache	1.5	1.1	1.8
Joint pain or inflammation	1.7	2.0	2.4
Leg cramps during the day	21.1	26.0	20.0
Leg cramps during the night	25.6	32.6	21.2

OVERDOSAGE

Overdosage usually produces marked dizziness and blurred vision related to postural hypotension and may progress to syncope on standing. The patient should lie down until these symptoms subside.

If excessive hypotension occurs and persists despite conservative treatment, intensive therapy may be needed to support vital functions. A vasoconstrictor such as phenylephrine will ameliorate the effect of HYLOREL Tablets, but great care must be used because patients may be hypersensitive to such agents.

DOSAGE AND ADMINISTRATION

As with other sympathetic suppressant drugs, the dose response to HYLOREL Tablets varies widely and must be adjusted for each patient until the therapeutic goal is achieved. With long-term therapy, some tolerance may occur and the dosage may have to be increased.

Because HYLOREL has a substantial orthostatic effect, monitoring both supine and standing pressures is essential, especially while dosage is being adjusted.

HYLOREL should be administered in divided doses. The usual starting dosage for treating hypertension is 10 mg per day, which can be given as 5 mg b.i.d. by breaking the 10 mg tablet. The dosage should be adjusted weekly or monthly until blood pressure is controlled. Most patients will require daily dosage in the range of 20 to 75 mg usually in twice daily doses. For larger doses 3 or 4 times daily dosing may be needed. A dosage of more than 400 mg/day is rarely required.

Dosage should be adjusted for patients with impaired renal function (see CLINICAL PHARMACOLOGY and PRECAUTIONS). As a general guideline, it is recommended that initial therapy with HYLOREL in patients with creatinine clearances of 30 to 60 mL/min be reduced to 5 mg every 24

hours. In patients with creatinine clearances less than 30 mL/min, the dosing interval should be increased to 48 hours. The time to achieve steady state will be increased. Dosage increases should be made cautiously at intervals not less than 7 days in patients with moderate renal insufficiency and not less than 14 days in patients with severe renal insufficiency. These recommendations are based upon human pharmacokinetic data and not clinical experience.

HOW SUPPLIED

HYLOREL Tablets are available as follows:
10 mg, scored elliptical tablets (light orange)
  Bottles of 100—NDC 53014-787-71
25 mg, scored elliptical tablets (white)
  Bottles of 100—NDC 53014-788-71
Store at controlled room temperature 15°–30° C (59°–86°F). Keep out of the reach of children.
CAUTION: Federal law prohibits dispensing without prescription.
Marketed by:
MEDEVA PHARMACEUTICALS
Medeva Pharmaceuticals, Inc.
Rochester, NY 14623 USA
Manufactured by: Rev. 7/96
Pharmacia & Upjohn Company   R253A
Kalamazoo, MI 49001, USA   814 438 105
® Fisons Intelmark Holdings, Inc.
                                                      691015
© 1996, Medeva Pharmaceuticals Manufacturing, Inc.

IONAMIN® Capsules   C IV R
(phentermine resin)

DESCRIPTION

IONAMIN '15' and IONAMIN '30' contain 15 mg and 30 mg respectively of phentermine as the cationic exchange resin complex. Phentermine is α, α-dimethyl phenethylamine (phenyl-tertiary-butylamine).
Inactive Ingredients: D&C Yellow No. 10, dibasic calcium phosphate, FD&C Yellow No. 6, gelatin, iron oxides (15 mg capsules only), lactose, magnesium stearate, titanium dioxide.

ACTIONS

IONAMIN is a sympathomimetic amine with pharmacologic activity similar to the prototype drug of this class used in obesity, amphetamine (d- and d/-amphetamine). Actions include central nervous system stimulation and elevation of blood pressure. Tachyphylaxis and tolerance have been demonstrated with all drugs of this class in which these phenomena have been looked for.
Drugs of this class used in obesity are commonly known as "anorectics" or "anorexigenics." It has not been established, however, that the action of such drugs in treating obesity is primarily one of appetite suppression. Other central nervous system actions, or metabolic effects may be involved. Adult obese subjects instructed in dietary management and treated with "anorectic" drugs, lose more weight on the average than those treated with placebo and diet, as determined in relatively short-term clinical trials.
The magnitude of increased weight loss of drug-treated patients over placebo-treated patients is only a fraction of a pound a week. The rate of weight loss is greatest in the first weeks of therapy for both drug and placebo subjects and tends to decrease in succeeding weeks. The possible origins of the increased weight loss due to the various drug effects are not established. The amount of weight loss associated with the use of an "anorectic" drug varies from trial to trial, and the increased weight loss appears to be related in part to variables other than the drugs prescribed, such as the physician-investigator, the population treated, and the diet prescribed. Studies do not permit conclusions as to the relative importance of the drug and non-drug factors on weight loss.
The natural history of obesity is measured in years, whereas the studies cited are restricted to a few weeks' or months' duration; thus, the total impact of drug-induced weight loss over that of diet alone must be considered clinically limited.
The bioavailability of IONAMIN has been studied in humans in which blood levels of phentermine were measured by a gas chromatography method. Blood levels obtained with the 15 mg and 30 mg resin complex formulations indicated slower absorption with a reduced but prolonged peak concentration and without a significant difference in prolongation of blood levels when compared with the same doses of phentermine hydrochloride. The clinical significance of these differences is not known. In clinical trials establishing the efficacy of IONAMIN, a single daily dose produced an effect comparable to that produced by other regimens of "anorectic" drug therapy.

INDICATION

IONAMIN Capsules are indicated as a short-term (a few weeks) adjunct in a regimen of weight reduction based on

| | BODY MASS INDEX (BMI), kg/m² | | | | | |
| | Height (feet, inches) | | | | | |
Weight (pounds)	5'0"	5'3"	5'6"	5'9"	6'0"	6'3"
140	27	25	23	21	19	18
150	29	27	24	22	20	19
160	31	28	26	24	22	20
170	33	30	28	25	23	21
180	35	32	29	27	25	23
190	37	34	31	28	26	24
200	39	36	32	30	27	25
210	41	37	34	31	29	26
220	43	39	36	33	30	28
230	45	41	37	34	31	29
240	47	43	39	36	33	30
250	49	44	40	37	34	31

exercise, behavioral modification, and caloric restriction in the management of exogenous obesity for patients with an initial body mass index ≥30 kg/m², or ≥27 kg/m² in the presence of other risk factors (e.g., hypertension, diabetes, hyperlipidemia).
Below is a chart of Body Mass Index (BMI) based on various heights and weights.
BMI is calculated by taking the patient's weight, in kilograms (kg), divided by the patient's height, in meters (m), squared. Metric conversions are as follows: pounds ÷ 2.2 = kg; inches × 0.0254 = meters.
[See table above]
The limited usefulness of agents of this class (see ACTIONS) should be measured against possible risk factors inherent in their use such as those described below.

CONTRAINDICATIONS

Advanced arteriosclerosis, cardiovascular disease, moderate to severe hypertension, hyperthyroidism, known hypersensitivity, or idiosyncrasy to the sympathomimetic amines, glaucoma.
Agitated states.
Patients with a history of drug abuse.
During or within 14 days following the administration of monoamine oxidase inhibitors (hypertensive crises may result).

WARNINGS

IONAMIN Capsules are indicated only as short-term monotherapy for the management of exogenous obesity. The safety and efficacy of combination therapy with phentermine and any other drug products for weight loss, including selective serotonin reuptake inhibitors (e.g., fluoxetine, sertraline, fluvoxamine, paroxetine), have not been established. Therefore, the coadministration of these drug products for weight loss is not recommended.
Primary Pulmonary Hypertension (PPH)—a rare, frequently fatal disease of the lungs—has been reported to occur in patients receiving a combination of phentermine with fenfluramine or dexfenfluramine. The possibility of an association between PPH and the use of phentermine alone cannot be ruled out. The initial symptom of PPH is usually dyspnea. Other initial symptoms include: angina pectoris, syncope, or lower extremity edema. Patients should be advised to report immediately any deterioration in exercise tolerance. Treatment should be discontinued in patients who develop new, unexplained symptoms of dyspnea, angina pectoris, syncope, or lower extremity edema.
Valvular Heart Disease: Serious regurgitant cardiac valvular disease, primarily affecting the mitral, aortic and/or tricuspid valves, has been reported in otherwise healthy persons who had taken a combination of phentermine with fenfluramine or dexfenfluramine for weight loss. The etiology of these valvulopathies has not been established and their course in individuals after the drugs are stopped is not known.
If tolerance to the "anorectic" effect develops, the recommended dose should not be exceeded in an attempt to increase the effect: rather, the drug should be discontinued.
IONAMIN may impair the ability of the patient to engage in potentially hazardous activities such as operating machinery or driving a motor vehicle; the patient should therefore be cautioned accordingly.
When using CNS active agents, consideration must always be given to the possibility of adverse interactions with alcohol.
Drug Dependence: IONAMIN is related chemically and pharmacologically to amphetamine (d- and d/-amphet-

amine) and other stimulant drugs that have been extensively abused. The possibility of abuse of IONAMIN should be kept in mind when evaluating the desirability of including a drug as part of a weight reduction program. Abuse of amphetamine (d- and d/-amphetamine) and related drugs may be associated with intense psychological dependence and severe social dysfunction. There are reports of patients who have increased the dosage of some of these drugs to many times that recommended. Abrupt cessation following prolonged high dosage administration results in extreme fatigue and mental depression; changes are also noted on the sleep EEG. Manifestations of chronic intoxication with anorectic drugs include severe dermatoses, marked insomnia, irritability, hyperactivity, and personality changes. The most severe manifestation of chronic intoxications is psychosis, often clinically indistinguishable from schizophrenia.
Usage in Pregnancy: Safe use in pregnancy has not been established. Use of IONAMIN by women who are or may become pregnant requires that the potential benefit be weighed against the possible hazard to mother and infant.
Pediatric Use: IONAMIN Capsules (phentermine resin) are not recommended for use in pediatric patients under 16 years of age.

PRECAUTIONS

Caution is to be exercised in prescribing IONAMIN for patients with even mild hypertension. Insulin requirements in diabetes mellitus may be altered in association with the use of IONAMIN and the concomitant dietary regimen.
IONAMIN may decrease the hypotensive effect of adrenergic neuron blocking drugs.
The least amount feasible should be prescribed or dispensed at one time in order to minimize the possibility of overdosage.

ADVERSE REACTIONS

Cardiovascular: Primary pulmonary hypertension (see WARNINGS), palpitation, tachycardia, elevation of blood pressure.
Central Nervous System: Overstimulation, restlessness, dizziness, insomnia, euphoria, dysphoria, tremor, headache; rarely psychotic episodes at recommended doses with some drugs in this class.
Gastrointestinal: Dryness of the mouth, unpleasant taste, diarrhea, constipation, other gastrointestinal disturbances.
Allergic: Urticaria.
Endocrine: Impotence, changes in libido.

DOSAGE AND ADMINISTRATION

One capsule daily, before breakfast or 10–14 hours before retiring. For individuals exhibiting greater drug responsiveness, IONAMIN '15' will usually suffice.
IONAMIN '30' is recommended for less responsive patients. IONAMIN is not recommended for use in pediatric patients under 16 years of age.
IONAMIN Capsules should be swallowed whole.

Continued on next page

Information on the Medeva Pharmaceuticals, Inc. products listed on these pages contains the full prescribing information from product circulars in use as of July 1998. For further information, please consult the package insert currently accompanying the product.

Ionamin—Cont.

OVERDOSAGE

Manifestations of acute overdosage may include restlessness, tremor, hyperreflexia, rapid respiration, confusion, assaultiveness, hallucinations, panic states.

Fatigue and depression usually follow the central stimulation.

Cardiovascular effects include arrhythmias, hypertension, or hypotension and circulatory collapse.

Gastrointestinal symptoms include nausea, vomiting, diarrhea, and abdominal cramps. Overdosage of pharmacologically similar compounds has resulted in fatal poisoning, usually terminating in convulsions and coma.

Management of acute IONAMIN intoxication is largely symptomatic and includes lavage and sedation with a barbiturate. Experience with hemodialysis or peritoneal dialysis is inadequate to permit recommendation in this regard. Intravenous phentolamine (Regitine) has been suggested on pharmacologic grounds for possible acute, severe hypertension, if this complicates overdosage.

HOW SUPPLIED

IONAMIN Capsules (phentermine resin) are available in two strengths:

15 mg, yellow/grey capsules, imprinted with "IONAMIN 15."

NDC 53014-903-71 Bottle of 100's
NDC 53014-903-84 Bottle of 400's

30 mg, yellow/yellow capsules, imprinted with "IONAMIN 30."

NDC 53014-904-71 Bottle of 100's
NDC 53014-904-84 Bottle of 400's

Dispense in a tight container. Store at room temperature. Keep out of the reach of children.

CAUTION: Federal law prohibits dispensing without prescription.

MEDEVA PHARMACEUTICALS

Medeva Pharmaceuticals, Inc.
Rochester, NY 14623 USA
©1997 Medeva Pharmaceuticals Manufacturing, Inc.

Rev. 12/97

®Fisons BV   R195F

MYKROX® TABLETS   ℞
[mī ′krahks]
(metolazone tablets, USP)
R156G
Rev. 7/96

DO NOT INTERCHANGE

MYKROX TABLETS ARE A RAPIDLY AVAILABLE FORMULATION OF METOLAZONE FOR ORAL ADMINISTRATION. MYKROX TABLETS AND OTHER FORMULATIONS OF METOLAZONE THAT SHARE ITS MORE RAPID AND COMPLETE BIOAVAILABILITY ARE NOT THERAPEUTICALLY EQUIVALENT TO ZAROXOLYN® TABLETS AND OTHER FORMULATIONS OF METOLAZONE THAT SHARE ITS SLOW AND INCOMPLETE BIOAVAILABILITY. FORMULATIONS BIOEQUIVALENT TO MYKROX AND FORMULATIONS BIOEQUIVALENT TO ZAROXOLYN SHOULD NOT BE INTERCHANGED FOR ONE ANOTHER.

DESCRIPTION

MYKROX Tablets (metolazone tablets, USP) for oral administration contain $1/2$ mg of metolazone, USP, a diuretic/saluretic/antihypertensive drug of the quinazoline class. Metolazone has the molecular formula $C_{16}H_{16}ClN_3O_3S$, the chemical name 7-chloro-1,2,3,4-tetrahydro-2-methyl-3-(2-methylphenyl)-4-oxo-6-quinazolinesulfonamide, and a molecular weight of 365.83. The structural formula is:

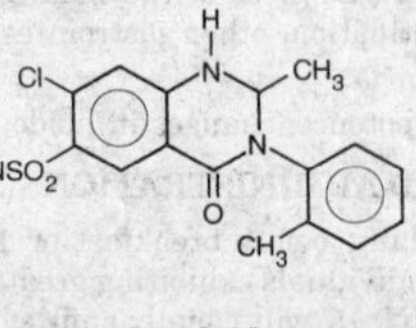

Metolazone is only sparingly soluble in water, but more soluble in plasma, blood, alkali and organic solvents.

Inactive Ingredients: Dibasic calcium phosphate, magnesium stearate, microcrystalline cellulose, pregelatinized starch, sodium starch glycolate.

CLINICAL PHARMACOLOGY

MYKROX (metolazone) is a quinazoline diuretic, with properties generally similar to the thiazide diuretics. The actions of MYKROX result from interference with the renal tubular mechanism of electrolyte reabsorption. MYKROX acts primarily to inhibit sodium reabsorption at the cortical diluting site and to a lesser extent in the proximal convoluted tubule. Sodium and chloride ions are excreted in approximately equivalent amounts. The increased delivery of sodium to the distal tubular exchange site results in increased potassium excretion. MYKROX does not inhibit carbonic anhydrase. A proximal action of metolazone has been shown in humans by increased excretion of phosphate and magnesium ions and by a markedly increased fractional excretion of sodium in patients with severely compromised glomerular filtration. This action has been demonstrated in animals by micropuncture studies.

The antihypertensive mechanism of action of metolazone is not fully understood but is presumed to be related to its saluretic and diuretic properties.

In two double-blind, controlled clinical trials of MYKROX Tablets, the maximum effect on mean blood pressure was achieved within 2 weeks of treatment and showed some evidence of an increased response at 1 mg compared to $1/2$ mg. There was no indication of an increased response with 2 mg. After six weeks of treatment, the mean fall in serum potassium was 0.42 mEq/L at $1/2$ mg, 0.66 mEq/L at 1 mg and 0.7 mEq/L at 2 mg. Serum uric acid increased by 1.1 to 1.4 mg/dL at increasing doses. There were small falls in serum sodium and chloride and a 1.3–2.1 mg/dL increase in BUN at increasing doses.

The rate and extent of absorption of metolazone from MYKROX Tablets were equivalent to those from an oral solution of metolazone. Peak blood levels are obtained within 2 to 4 hours of oral administration with an elimination half-life of approximately 14 hours. MYKROX Tablets have been shown to produce blood levels that are dose proportional between $1/2$–2 mg. Steady state blood levels are usually reached in 4–5 days.

In contrast, other formulations of metolazone produce peak blood concentrations approximately 8 hours following oral administration; absorption continues for an additional 12 hours.

INDICATIONS AND USAGE

MYKROX Tablets are indicated for the treatment of hypertension, alone or in combination with other antihypertensive drugs of a different class.

MYKROX TABLETS HAVE NOT BEEN EVALUATED FOR THE TREATMENT OF CONGESTIVE HEART FAILURE OR FLUID RETENTION DUE TO RENAL OR HEPATIC DISEASE AND THE CORRECT DOSAGE FOR THESE CONDITIONS AND OTHER EDEMA STATES HAS NOT BEEN ESTABLISHED. SINCE A SAFE AND EFFECTIVE DIURETIC DOSE HAS NOT BEEN ESTABLISHED, MYKROX TABLETS SHOULD NOT BE USED WHEN DIURESIS IS DESIRED.

Usage in Pregnancy

The routine use of diuretics in an otherwise healthy woman is inappropriate and exposes mother and fetus to unnecessary hazard. Diuretics do not prevent development of toxemia of pregnancy, and there is no evidence that they are useful in the treatment of developed toxemia (see PRECAUTIONS).

Edema during pregnancy may arise from pathologic causes or from the physiologic and mechanical consequences of pregnancy. MYKROX is not indicated for the treatment of edema in pregnancy. Dependent edema in pregnancy resulting from restriction of venous return by the expanded uterus is properly treated through elevation of the lower extremities and use of support hose; use of diuretics to lower intravascular volume in this case is illogical and unnecessary. There is hypervolemia during normal pregnancy which is harmful to neither the fetus nor the mother (in the absence of cardiovascular disease), but which is associated with edema, including generalized edema, in the majority of pregnant women. If this edema produces discomfort, increased recumbency will often provide relief. In rare instances, this edema may cause extreme discomfort which is not relieved by rest. In these cases, a short course of diuretics may be appropriate.

CONTRAINDICATIONS

Anuria, hepatic coma or precoma, known allergy or hypersensitivity to metolazone.

WARNINGS

Rapid Onset Hyponatremia

Rarely, the rapid onset of severe hyponatremia and/or hypokalemia has been reported following initial doses of thiazide and non-thiazide diuretics. When symptoms consistent with severe electrolyte imbalance appear rapidly, drug should be discontinued and supportive measures should be initiated immediately. Parenteral electrolytes may be required. Appropriateness of therapy with this class of drugs should be carefully reevaluated.

Hypokalemia

Hypokalemia may occur, with consequent weakness, cramps, and cardiac dysrhythmias. Serum potassium should be determined at regular intervals, and dose reduction, potassium supplementation or addition of a potassium sparing diuretic instituted whenever indicated. Hypokalemia is a particular hazard in patients who are digitalized or who have or have had a ventricular arrhythmia; dangerous or fatal arrhythmias may be precipitated. Hypokalemia is dose related.

In controlled clinical trials, 1.5% of patients taking $1/2$ mg and 3.1% of patients taking 1 mg of MYKROX daily developed clinical hypokalemia (defined as hypokalemia accompanied by signs or symptoms); 21% of the patients taking $1/2$ mg and 30% of the patients taking 1 mg of MYKROX daily developed hypokalemia (defined as a serum potassium concentration below 3.5 mEq/L); in another controlled clinical trial in which the patients started therapy with a serum potassium level greater than 4.0 mEq/L, 8% of patients taking $1/2$ mg of MYKROX daily developed hypokalemia (defined as a serum potassium concentration below 3.5 mEq/L).

Concomitant Therapy

Lithium

In general, diuretics should not be given concomitantly with lithium because they reduce its renal clearance and add a high risk of lithium toxicity. Read prescribing information for lithium preparations before use of such concomitant therapy.

Furosemide: Unusually large or prolonged losses of fluids and electrolytes may result when metolazone is administered concomitantly to patients receiving furosemide (see PRECAUTIONS, DRUG INTERACTIONS).

Other Antihypertensive Drugs: When MYKROX Tablets are used with other antihypertensive drugs, particular care must be taken to avoid excessive reduction of blood pressure, especially during initial therapy.

Cross-Allergy

Cross-allergy, while not reported to date, theoretically may occur when MYKROX Tablets are given to patients known to be allergic to sulfonamide-derived drugs, thiazides, or quinethazone.

Sensitivity Reactions

Sensitivity reactions (e.g., angioedema, bronchospasm) may occur with or without a history of allergy or bronchial asthma and may occur with the first dose of MYKROX.

PRECAUTIONS

DO NOT INTERCHANGE

MYKROX TABLETS ARE A RAPIDLY AVAILABLE FORMULATION OF METOLAZONE FOR ORAL ADMINISTRATION. MYKROX TABLETS AND OTHER FORMULATIONS OF METOLAZONE THAT SHARE ITS MORE RAPID AND COMPLETE BIOAVAILABILITY ARE NOT THERAPEUTICALLY EQUIVALENT TO ZAROXOLYN TABLETS AND OTHER FORMULATIONS OF METOLAZONE THAT SHARE ITS SLOW AND INCOMPLETE BIOAVAILABILITY. FORMULATIONS BIOEQUIVALENT TO MYKROX AND FORMULATIONS BIOEQUIVALENT TO ZAROXOLYN SHOULD NOT BE INTERCHANGED FOR ONE ANOTHER.

GENERAL:

Fluid and Electrolytes

All patients receiving therapy with MYKROX Tablets should have serum electrolyte measurements done at appropriate intervals and be observed for clinical signs of fluid and/or electrolyte imbalance: namely, hyponatremia, hypochloremic alkalosis, and hypokalemia. In patients with severe edema accompanying cardiac failure or renal disease, a low-salt syndrome may be produced, especially with hot weather and a low-salt diet. Serum and urine electrolyte determinations are particularly important when the patient has protracted vomiting, severe diarrhea, or is receiving parenteral fluids. Warning signs of imbalance are: dryness of mouth, thirst, weakness, lethargy, drowsiness, restlessness, muscle pains or cramps, muscle fatigue, hypotension, oliguria, tachycardia, and gastrointestinal disturbances such as nausea and vomiting. Hyponatremia may occur at any time during long term therapy and, on rare occasions, may be life threatening.

The risk of hypokalemia is increased when larger doses are used, when diuresis is rapid, when severe liver disease is present, when corticosteroids are given concomitantly, when oral intake is inadequate or when excess potassium is being lost extrarenally, such as with vomiting or diarrhea.

Thiazide-like diuretics have been shown to increase the urinary excretion of magnesium; this may result in hypomagnesemia.

Glucose Tolerance

Metolazone may raise blood glucose concentrations possibly causing hyperglycemia and glycosuria in patients with diabetes or latent diabetes.

Hyperuricemia

MYKROX regularly causes an increase in serum uric acid and can occasionally precipitate gouty attacks even in patients without a prior history of them.

Azotemia

Azotemia, presumably prerenal azotemia, may be precipitated during the administration of MYKROX Tablets. If azotemia and oliguria worsen during treatment of patients with severe renal disease, MYKROX Tablets should be discontinued.

Renal Impairment

Use caution when administering MYKROX Tablets to patients with severely impaired renal function. As most of the drug is excreted by the renal route, accumulation may occur.

Orthostatic Hypotension
Orthostatic hypotension may occur; this may be potentiated by alcohol, barbiturates, narcotics, or concurrent therapy with other antihypertensive drugs. In controlled clinical trials, 1.4% of patients treated with MYKROX Tablets (1/2 mg) had orthostatic hypotension; this effect was not reported in the placebo group.
Hypercalcemia
Hypercalcemia may infrequently occur with metolazone, especially in patients taking high doses of vitamin D or with high bone turnover states, and may signify hidden hyperparathyroidism. Metolazone should be discontinued before tests for parathyroid function are performed.
Systemic Lupus Erythematosus
Thiazide diuretics have exacerbated or activated systemic lupus erythematosus and this possibility should be considered with MYKROX Tablets.
INFORMATION FOR PATIENTS: Patients should be informed of possible adverse effects, advised to take the medication as directed and promptly report any possible adverse reactions to the treating physician.
DRUG INTERACTIONS:
Diuretics
Furosemide and probably other loop diuretics given concomitantly with metolazone can cause unusually large or prolonged losses of fluid and electrolytes (see WARNINGS).
Other Antihypertensives
When MYKROX Tablets are used with other antihypertensive drugs, care must be taken, especially during initial therapy. Dosage adjustments of other antihypertensives may be necessary.
Alcohol, Barbiturates, and Narcotics
The hypotensive effects of these drugs may be potentiated by the volume contraction that may be associated with metolazone therapy.
Digitalis Glycosides
Diuretic-induced hypokalemia can increase the sensitivity of the myocardium to digitalis. Serious arrhythmias can result.
Corticosteroids or ACTH
May increase the risk of hypokalemia and increase salt and water retention.
Lithium
Serum lithium levels may increase (see WARNINGS).
Curariform Drugs
Diuretic-induced hypokalemia may enhance neuromuscular blocking effects of curariform drugs (such as tubocurarine)—the most serious effect would be respiratory depression which could proceed to apnea. Accordingly, it may be advisable to discontinue MYKROX Tablets three days before elective surgery.
Salicylates and Other Non-Steroidal Anti-Inflammatory Drugs
May decrease the antihypertensive effects of MYKROX Tablets.
Sympathomimetics
Metolazone may decrease arterial responsiveness to norepinephrine, but this diminution is not sufficient to preclude effectiveness of the pressor agent for therapeutic use.
Insulin and Oral Antidiabetic Agents
See Glucose Tolerance under PRECAUTIONS, GENERAL.
Methenamine
Efficacy may be decreased due to urinary alkalizing effect of metolazone.
Anticoagulants
Metolazone, as well as other thiazide-like diuretics, may affect the hypoprothrombinemic response to anticoagulants; dosage adjustments may be necessary.
DRUG/LABORATORY TEST INTERACTIONS: None reported.
CARCINOGENESIS, MUTAGENESIS, IMPAIRMENT OF FERTILITY: Mice and rats administered metolazone 5 days/week for up to 18 and 24 months, respectively, at daily doses of 2, 10 and 50 mg/kg, exhibited no evidence of a tumorigenic effect of the drug. The small number of animals examined histologically and poor survival in the mice limit the conclusions that can be reached from these studies.
Metolazone was not mutagenic *in vitro* in the Ames Test using Salmonella typhimurium strains TA-97, TA-98, TA-100, TA-102 and TA-1535.
Reproductive performance has been evaluated in mice and rats. There is no evidence that metolazone possesses the potential for altering reproductive capacity in mice. In a rat study, in which males were treated orally with metolazone at doses of 2, 10 and 50 mg/kg for 127 days prior to mating with untreated females, an increased number of resorption sites was observed in dams mated with males from the 50 mg/kg group. In addition, the birth weight of offspring was decreased and the pregnancy rate was reduced in dams mated with males from the 10 and 50 mg/kg groups.
PREGNANCY
Teratogenic Effects—Pregnancy Category B.
Reproduction studies performed in mice, rabbits and rats treated during the appropriate periods of gestation at doses up to 50 mg/kg/day have revealed no evidence of harm to the fetus due to metolazone. There are, however, no adequate and well-controlled studies in pregnant women. Because animal reproduction studies are not always predictive of human response, MYKROX Tablets should be used during pregnancy only if clearly needed. Metolazone crosses the placental barrier and appears in cord blood.
Non-Teratogenic Effects
The use of MYKROX Tablets in pregnant women requires that the anticipated benefit be weighed against possible hazards to the fetus. These hazards include fetal or neonatal jaundice, thrombocytopenia, and possibly other adverse reactions which have occurred in the adult. It is not known what effect the use of the drug during pregnancy has on the later growth, development and functional maturation of the child. No such effects have been reported with metolazone.
LABOR AND DELIVERY: Based on clinical studies in which women received metolazone in late pregnancy until the time of delivery, there is no evidence that the drug has any adverse effects on the normal course of labor or delivery.
NURSING MOTHERS: Metolazone appears in breast milk. Because of the potential for serious adverse reactions in nursing infants from metolazone, a decision should be made whether to discontinue nursing or to discontinue the drug, taking into account the importance of the drug to the mother.
PEDIATRIC USE: Safety and effectiveness of MYKROX Tablets in pediatric patients have not been established, and such use is not recommended.

ADVERSE REACTIONS

Adverse experience information is available from more than 14 years of accumulated marketing experience with other formulations of metolazone for which reliable quantitative information is lacking and from controlled clinical trials with MYKROX from which incidences can be calculated.
In controlled clinical trials with MYKROX, adverse experiences resulted in discontinuation of therapy in 6.7–6.8% of patients given 1/2 to 1 mg of MYKROX.
Adverse experiences occurring in controlled clinical trials with MYKROX with an incidence of > 2%, whether or not considered drug-related, are summarized in the following table.

Incidence of Adverse Experiences Volunteered or Elicited (by Patient in Percent)*

	MYKROX n=226†
Dizziness (lightheadedness)	10.2
Headaches	9.3
Muscle Cramps	5.8
Fatigue (malaise, lethargy, lassitude)	4.4
Joint Pain, swelling	3.1
Chest Pain (precordial discomfort)	2.7

* Percent of patients reporting an adverse experience one or more times.
† All doses combined (1/2, 1 and 2 mg).

Some of the adverse effects reported in association with MYKROX also occur frequently in untreated hypertensive patients, such as headache and dizziness, which occurred in 14.8 and 7.4% of patients in a smaller parallel placebo group.
The following adverse effects were reported in less than 2% of the MYKROX treated patients.
Cardiovascular: Cold extremities, edema, orthostatic hypotension, palpitations.
Central and Peripheral Nervous System: Anxiety, depression, dry mouth, impotence, nervousness, neuropathy, weakness, "weird" feeling.
Dermatological: Pruritus, rash, skin dryness.
Eyes, Ears, Nose, Throat: Cough, epistaxis, eye itching, sinus congestion, sore throat, tinnitus.
Gastrointestinal: Abdominal discomfort (pain, bloating), bitter taste, constipation, diarrhea, nausea, vomiting.
Genitourinary: Nocturia.
Musculoskeletal: Back pain.
Other Adverse Experiences:
Adverse experiences reported with other marketed metolazone formulations and most thiazide diuretics, for which quantitative data are not available, are listed in decreasing order of severity within body systems. Several are single or rare occurrences.
Cardiovascular: excessive volume depletion, hemoconcentration, venous thrombosis.
Central and Peripheral Nervous System: syncope, paresthesias, drowsiness, restlessness (sometimes resulting in insomnia).
Dermatologic/Hypersensitivity: necrotizing angiitis (cutaneous vasculitis), purpura, dermatitis, photosensitivity, urticaria.
Gastrointestinal: hepatitis, intrahepatic cholestatic jaundice, pancreatitis, anorexia.
Hematologic: aplastic (hypoplastic) anemia, agranulocytosis, leukopenia.
Metabolic: hypokalemia (see WARNINGS, Hypokalemia), hyponatremia, hyperuricemia, hypochloremia, hypochloremic alkalosis, hyperglycemia, glycosuria, increase in serum urea nitrogen (BUN) or creatinine, hypophosphatemia, hypomagnesemia, hypercalcemia.
Musculoskeletal: acute gouty attacks.
Other: transient blurred vision, chills.
In addition, rare adverse experiences reported in association with similar anti-hypertensive-diuretics but not reported to date for metolazone include: sialadenitis, xanthopsia, respiratory distress (including pneumonitis), thrombocytopenia, and anaphylactic reactions. These experiences could occur with clinical use of metolazone.

OVERDOSAGE

Intentional overdosage has been reported rarely with metolazone and similar diuretic drugs.
Signs and Symptoms
Orthostatic hypotension, dizziness, drowsiness, syncope, electrolyte abnormalities, hemoconcentration and hemodynamic changes due to plasma volume depletion may occur. In some instances depressed respiration may be observed. At high doses, lethargy of varying degree may progress to coma within a few hours. The mechanism of CNS depression with thiazide overdosage is unknown. Also, GI irritation and hypermotility may occur. Temporary elevation of BUN has been reported, especially in patients with impairment of renal function. Serum electrolyte changes and cardiovascular and renal function should be closely monitored.
Treatment
There is no specific antidote available but immediate evacuation of stomach contents is advised. Dialysis is not likely to be effective. Care should be taken when evacuating the gastric contents to prevent aspiration, especially in the stuporous or comatose patient. Supportive measures should be initiated as required to maintain hydration, electrolyte balance, respiration and cardiovascular and renal function.

DOSAGE AND ADMINISTRATION

Therapy should be individualized according to patient response.
For initial treatment of mild to moderate hypertension, the recommended dose is one MYKROX Tablet (1/2 mg) once daily, usually in the morning. If patients are inadequately controlled with one 1/2 mg tablet, the dose can be increased to two MYKROX Tablets (1 mg) once a day. An increase in hypokalemia may occur. Doses larger than 1 mg do not give increased effectiveness.
The same dose titration is necessary if MYKROX Tablets are to be substituted for other dosage forms of metolazone in the treatment of hypertension.
If blood pressure is not adequately controlled with two MYKROX Tablets alone, the dose should not be increased; rather, another antihypertensive agent with a different mechanism of action should be added to therapy with MYKROX Tablets.

HOW SUPPLIED

MYKROX Tablets (metolazone tablets, USP), 1/2 mg are white, flat-faced, round tablets, debossed "MYKROX" on one side, and "1/2" on reverse side.
NDC 53014-847-71 Bottle of 100's
Store at room temperature. Dispense in a tight, light-resistant container. Keep out of the reach of children.
CAUTION: Federal law prohibits dispensing without prescription.
MEDEVA PHARMACEUTICALS
Medeva Pharmaceuticals, Inc.
Rochester, NY 14623 USA
®Fisons BV

Rev. 7/96
R156G

PEDIAPRED® ℞

[*pēd 'ē-uh-pred*]
(prednisolone sodium phosphate, USP)
ORAL SOLUTION
R024H
Rev. 8/96

DESCRIPTION

PEDIAPRED (prednisolone sodium phosphate, USP) Oral Solution is a dye free, colorless to light straw colored, rasp-

Continued on next page

Information on the Medeva Pharmaceuticals, Inc. products listed on these pages contains the full prescribing information from product circulars in use as of July 1998. For further information, please consult the package insert currently accompanying the product.

Pediapred—Cont.

berry flavored solution. Each 5 mL (teaspoonful) of PEDIAPRED contains 6.7 mg prednisolone sodium phosphate (5 mg prednisolone base) in a palatable, aqueous vehicle.
Inactive Ingredients: Dibasic sodium phosphate, edetate disodium, methylparaben, purified water, sodium biphosphate, sorbitol, natural and artificial raspberry flavor.
Prednisolone sodium phosphate occurs as white or slightly yellow, friable granules or powder. It is freely soluble in water; soluble in methanol; slightly soluble in alcohol and in chloroform; and very slightly soluble in acetone and in dioxane. The chemical name of prednisolone sodium phosphate is pregna -1,4- diene-3,20-dione, 11,17-dihydroxy -21-(phosphonooxy)-, disodium salt, (11β)-. The empirical formula is $C_{21}H_{27}Na_2O_8P$; the molecular weight is 484.39. Its chemical structure is:

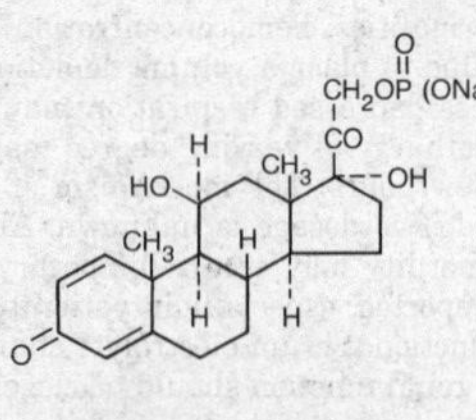

Pharmacological Category: Glucocorticoid

CLINICAL PHARMACOLOGY

Prednisolone is a synthetic adrenocortical steroid drug with predominantly glucocorticoid properties. Some of these properties reproduce the physiological actions of endogenous glucocorticosteroids, but others do not necessarily reflect any of the adrenal hormones' normal functions; they are seen only after administration of large therapeutic doses of the drug. The pharmacological effects of prednisolone which are due to its glucocorticoid properties include: promotion of gluconeogenesis; increased deposition of glycogen in the liver; inhibition of the utilization of glucose; anti-insulin activity; increased catabolism of protein; increased lipolysis; stimulation of fat synthesis and storage; increased glomerular filtration rate and resulting increase in urinary excretion of urate (creatinine excretion remains unchanged); and increased calcium excretion.
Depressed production of eosinophils and lymphocytes occurs, but erythropoiesis and production of polymorphonuclear leukocytes are stimulated. Anti-inflammatory processes (edema, fibrin deposition, capillary dilatation, migration of leukocytes and phagocytosis) and the later stages of wound healing (capillary proliferation, deposition of collagen, cicatrization) are inhibited. Prednisolone can stimulate secretion of various components of gastric juice. Stimulation of the production of corticotropin may lead to suppression of endogenous corticosteroids. Prednisolone has slight mineralocorticoid activity, whereby entry of sodium into cells and loss of intracellular potassium is stimulated. This is particularly evident in the kidney, where rapid ion exchange leads to sodium retention and hypertension.
Prednisolone is rapidly and well absorbed from the gastrointestinal tract following oral administration. PEDIAPRED Oral Liquid produces a 20% higher peak plasma level of prednisolone which occurs approximately 15 minutes earlier than the peak seen with tablet formulations. Prednisolone is 70–90% protein-bound in the plasma and it is eliminated from the plasma with a half-life of 2 to 4 hours. It is metabolized mainly in the liver and excreted in the urine as sulfate and glucuronide conjugates.

INDICATIONS AND USAGE

PEDIAPRED Oral Solution is indicated in the following conditions:

1. Endocrine Disorders
Primary or secondary adrenocortical insufficiency (hydrocortisone or cortisone is the first choice; synthetic analogs may be used in conjunction with mineralocorticoids where applicable; in infancy mineralocorticoid supplementation is of particular importance); congenital adrenal hyperplasia; hypercalcemia associated with cancer; nonsuppurative thyroiditis.

2. Rheumatic Disorders
As adjunctive therapy for short term administration (to tide the patient over an acute episode or exacerbation) in: psoriatic arthritis; rheumatoid arthritis, including juvenile rheumatoid arthritis (selected cases may require low dose maintenance therapy); ankylosing spondylitis; acute and subacute bursitis; acute nonspecific tenosynovitis; acute gouty arthritis; post-traumatic osteoarthritis; synovitis of osteoarthritis; epicondylitis.

3. Collagen Diseases
During an exacerbation or as maintenance therapy in selected cases of: systemic lupus erythematosus; systemic dermatomyositis (polymyositis); acute rheumatic carditis.

4. Dermatologic Diseases
Pemphigus; bullous dermatitis herpetiformis; severe erythema multiforme (Stevens-Johnson syndrome); exfoliative dermatitis; mycosis fungoides; severe psoriasis; severe seborrheic dermatitis.

5. Allergic States
Control of severe or incapacitating allergic conditions intractable to adequate trials of conventional treatment in: seasonal or perennial allergic rhinitis; bronchial asthma; contact dermatitis; atopic dermatitis; serum sickness; drug hypersensitivity reactions.

6. Ophthalmic Diseases
Severe acute and chronic allergic and inflammatory processes involving the eye and its adnexa such as: allergic conjunctivitis; keratitis; allergic corneal marginal ulcers; herpes zoster ophthalmicus; iritis and iridocyclitis; chorioretinitis; anterior segment inflammation; diffuse posterior uveitis and choroiditis; optic neuritis; sympathetic ophthalmia.

7. Respiratory Diseases
Symptomatic sarcoidosis; Loeffler's syndrome not manageable by other means; berylliosis; fulminating or disseminated pulmonary tuberculosis when used concurrently with appropriate antituberculous chemotherapy; aspiration pneumonitis.

8. Hematologic Disorders
Idiopathic thrombocytopenic purpura in adults; secondary thrombocytopenia in adults; acquired (autoimmune) hemolytic anemia; erythroblastopenia (RBC anemia); congenital (erythroid) hypoplastic anemia.

9. Neoplastic Diseases
For palliative management of: leukemias and lymphomas in adults; acute leukemia of childhood.

10. Edematous States
To induce a diuresis or remission of proteinuria in the nephrotic syndrome, without uremia, of the idiopathic type or that due to lupus erythematosus.

11. Gastrointestinal Diseases
To tide the patient over a critical period of the disease in: ulcerative colitis; regional enteritis.

12. Nervous System
Acute exacerbations of multiple sclerosis.

13. Miscellaneous
Tuberculous meningitis with subarachnoid block or impending block when used concurrently with appropriate antituberculous chemotherapy; trichinosis with neurologic or myocardial involvement.

CONTRAINDICATIONS

Systemic fungal infections.

WARNINGS

In patients on corticosteroid therapy subjected to unusual stress, increased dosage of rapidly acting corticosteroids before, during and after the stressful situation is indicated.
Corticosteroids may mask some signs of infection, and new infections may appear during their use. There may be decreased resistance and inability to localize infection when corticosteroids are used.
Prolonged use of corticosteroids may produce posterior subcapsular cataracts, glaucoma with possible damage to the optic nerves, and may enhance the establishment of secondary ocular infections due to fungi or viruses.
Average and large doses of hydrocortisone or cortisone can cause elevation of blood pressure, salt and water retention, and increased excretion of potassium. These effects are less likely to occur with the synthetic derivatives except when used in large doses. Dietary salt restriction and potassium supplementation may be necessary. All corticosteroids increase calcium excretion. **While on corticosteroid therapy patients should not be vaccinated against smallpox. Other immunization procedures should not be undertaken in patients who are on corticosteroids, especially on high doses, because of possible hazards of neurological complications and a lack of antibody response.**
The use of prednisolone in active tuberculosis should be restricted to those cases of fulminating or disseminated tuberculosis in which the corticosteroid is used for the management of the disease in conjunction with an appropriate antituberculous regimen.
If corticosteroids are indicated in patients with latent tuberculosis or tuberculin reactivity, close observation is necessary as reactivation of the disease may occur. During prolonged corticosteroid therapy these patients should receive chemoprophylaxis.
Persons who are on drugs which suppress the immune system are more susceptible to infections than healthy individuals. Chicken pox and measles, for example, can have a more serious or even fatal course in non-immune children or adults on corticosteroids. In such children or adults who have not had these diseases, particular care should be taken to avoid exposure. How the dose, route and duration of corticosteroid administration affects the risk of developing a disseminated infection is not known. The contribution of the underlying disease and/or prior corticosteroid treatment to the risk is also not known. If exposed to chicken pox, prophylaxis with varicella zoster immune globulin (VZIG) may be indicated. If exposed to measles, prophylaxis with pooled intramuscular immunoglobulin (IG) may be indicated. (See the respective package inserts for complete VZIG and IG prescribing information). If chicken pox develops, treatment with antiviral agents may be considered.
Similarly, corticosteroids should be used with great care in patients with known or suspected Strongyloides (threadworm) infestation. In such patients, corticosteroid-induced immunosuppression may lead to Strongyloides hyperinfection and dissemination with widespread larval migration, often accompanied by severe enterocolitis and potentially fatal gram-negative septicemia.

PRECAUTIONS

General: Drug-induced secondary adrenocortical insufficiency may be minimized by gradual reduction of dosage. This type of relative insufficiency may persist for months after discontinuation of therapy; therefore, in any situation of stress occurring during that period, hormone therapy should be reinstituted. Since mineralocorticoid secretion may be impaired, salt and/or a mineralocorticoid should be administered concurrently.
There is an enhanced effect of corticosteroids in patients with hypothyroidism and in those with cirrhosis.
Corticosteroids should be used cautiously in patients with ocular herpes simplex because of possible corneal perforation.
The lowest possible dose of corticosteroid should be used to control the condition under treatment, and when reduction in dosage is possible, the reduction should be gradual.
Psychic derangements may appear when corticosteroids are used, ranging from euphoria, insomnia, mood swings, personality changes, and severe depression, to frank psychotic manifestations. Also, existing emotional instability or psychotic tendencies may be aggravated by corticosteroids.
Aspirin should be used cautiously in conjunction with corticosteroids in hypoprothrombinemia.
Steroids should be used with caution in nonspecific ulcerative colitis, if there is a probability of impending perforation, abscess or other pyogenic infection; diverticulitis; fresh intestinal anastomoses; active or latent peptic ulcer; renal insufficiency; hypertension; osteoporosis; and myasthenia gravis.
Growth and development of infants and children on prolonged corticosteroid therapy should be carefully observed.
Although controlled clinical trials have shown corticosteroids to be effective in speeding the resolution of acute exacerbations of multiple sclerosis, they do not show that they affect the ultimate outcome or natural history of the disease. The studies do show that relatively high doses of corticosteroids are necessary to demonstrate a significant effect. (See DOSAGE AND ADMINISTRATION.)
Since complications of treatment with glucocorticoids are dependent on the size of the dose and the duration of treatment, a risk/benefit decision must be made in each individual case as to dose and duration of treatment and as to whether daily or intermittent therapy should be used.
Information for Patients: Patients should be warned not to discontinue the use of PEDIAPRED abruptly or without medical supervision, to advise any medical attendants that they are taking PEDIAPRED and to seek medical advice at once should they develop fever or other signs of infection.
Persons who are on immunosuppressant doses of corticosteroids should be warned to avoid exposure to chicken pox or measles. Patients should also be advised that if they are exposed, medical advice should be sought without delay.
Drug Interactions: Drugs such as barbiturates which induce hepatic microsomal drug metabolizing enzyme activity may enhance metabolism of prednisolone and require that the dosage of PEDIAPRED be increased.
Pregnancy: Pregnancy Category C—Prednisolone has been shown to be teratogenic in many species when given in doses equivalent to the human dose. There are no adequate and well controlled studies in pregnant women. PEDIAPRED should be used during pregnancy only if the potential benefit justifies the potential risk to the fetus. Animal studies in which prednisolone has been given to pregnant mice, rats and rabbits have yielded an increased incidence of cleft palate in the offspring.
Nursing Mothers: Prednisolone is excreted in breast milk, but only to a small (less than 1% of the administered dose) and probably clinically insignificant extent. Caution should be exercised when PEDIAPRED is administered to a nursing woman.

ADVERSE REACTIONS

Fluid and Electrolyte Disturbances
Sodium retention; fluid retention; congestive heart failure in susceptible patients; potassium loss; hypokalemic alkalosis; hypertension.

Musculoskeletal
Muscle weakness; steroid myopathy; loss of muscle mass; osteoporosis; vertebral compression fractures; aseptic necrosis of femoral and humeral heads; pathologic fracture of long bones.

Gastrointestinal
Peptic ulcer with possible perforation and hemorrhage; pancreatitis; abdominal distention; ulcerative esophagitis.

Dermatologic
Impaired wound healing; thin fragile skin; petechiae and ecchymoses; facial erythema; increased sweating; may suppress reactions to skin tests.

Metabolic
Negative nitrogen balance due to protein catabolism.

Neurological
Convulsions; increased intracranial pressure with papilledema (pseudotumor cerebri) usually after treatment; vertigo; headache.

Endocrine
Menstrual irregularities; development of cushingoid state; secondary adrenocortical and pituitary unresponsiveness, particularly in times of stress, as in trauma, surgery or illness; suppression of growth in children; decreased carbohydrate tolerance; manifestations of latent diabetes mellitus; increased requirements for insulin or oral hypoglycemic agents in diabetes.

Ophthalmic
Posterior subcapsular cataracts; increased intraocular pressure; glaucoma; exophthalmos.

OVERDOSAGE

The effects of accidental ingestion of large quantities of prednisolone over a very short period of time have not been reported, but prolonged use of the drug can produce mental symptoms, moon face, abnormal fat deposits, fluid retention, excessive appetite, weight gain, hypertrichosis, acne, striae, ecchymosis, increased sweating, pigmentation, dry scaly skin, thinning scalp hair, increased blood pressure, tachycardia, thrombophlebitis, decreased resistance to infection, negative nitrogen balance with delayed bone and wound healing, headache, weakness, menstrual disorders, accentuated menopausal symptoms, neuropathy, fractures, osteoporosis, peptic ulcer, decreased glucose tolerance, hypokalemia, and adrenal insufficiency. Hepatomegaly and abdominal distention have been observed in children.

Treatment of acute overdosage is by immediate gastric lavage or emesis. For chronic overdosage in the face of severe disease requiring continuous steroid therapy the dosage of prednisolone may be reduced only temporarily, or alternate day treatment may be introduced.

DOSAGE AND ADMINISTRATION

The initial dosage of PEDIAPRED may vary from 5 mL to 60 mL (5 to 60 mg prednisolone base) per day depending on the specific disease entity being treated. In situations of less severity lower doses will generally suffice while in selected patients higher initial doses may be required. The initial dosage should be maintained or adjusted until a satisfactory response is noted. If after a reasonable period of time there is a lack of satisfactory clinical response, PEDIAPRED should be discontinued and the patient transferred to other appropriate therapy. **IT SHOULD BE EMPHASIZED THAT DOSAGE REQUIREMENTS ARE VARIABLE AND MUST BE INDIVIDUALIZED ON THE BASIS OF THE DISEASE UNDER TREATMENT AND THE RESPONSE OF THE PATIENT.** After a favorable response is noted, the proper maintenance dosage should be determined by decreasing the initial drug dosage in small decrements at appropriate time intervals until the lowest dosage which will maintain an adequate clinical response is reached. It should be kept in mind that constant monitoring is needed in regard to drug dosage. Included in the situations which may make dosage adjustments necessary are changes in clinical status secondary to remissions or exacerbations in the disease process, the patient's individual drug responsiveness, and the effect of patient exposure to stressful situations not directly related to the disease entity under treatment; in this latter situation it may be necessary to increase the dosage of PEDIAPRED for a period of time consistent with the patient's condition. If after long term therapy the drug is to be stopped, it is recommended that it be withdrawn gradually rather than abruptly.

In the treatment of acute exacerbations of multiple sclerosis daily doses of 200 mg of prednisolone for a week followed by 80 mg every other day or 4 to 8 mg dexamethasone every other day for one month have been shown to be effective.

For the purpose of comparison, the following is the equivalent milligram dosage of the various glucocorticoids: cortisone, 25; hydrocortisone, 20; prednisolone, 5; prednisone, 5; methylprednisolone, 4; triamcinolone, 4; paramethasone, 2; betamethasone, 0.75; dexamethasone, 0.75. These dose relationships apply only to oral or intravenous administration of these compounds. When these substances or their derivatives are injected intramuscularly or into joint spaces, their relative properties may be greatly altered.

HOW SUPPLIED

PEDIAPRED (prednisolone sodium phosphate, USP) Oral Solution is a colorless to light straw colored solution containing 6.7 mg prednisolone sodium phosphate (5 mg prednisolone base) per 5 mL (teaspoonful).
NDC 53014-250-01   120 mL bottle

Store at 4°–25°C (39°–77°F). May be refrigerated. Keep tightly closed and out of the reach of children.
CAUTION: Federal law prohibits dispensing without prescription.

MEDEVA PHARMACEUTICALS
Medeva Pharmaceuticals, Inc.
Rochester, NY 14623 USA   8/96
® Fisons Corp.   R024H
© 1996, Medeva Pharmaceuticals Manufacturing, Inc.

SEMPREX®-D CAPSULES   ℞
[sĕm-prĕx]
(acrivastine and pseudoephedrine hydrochloride)

DESCRIPTION

SEMPREX-D Capsules (acrivastine and pseudoephedrine hydrochloride) are a fixed combination product formulated for oral administration. Acrivastine is an antihistamine and pseudoephedrine is a decongestant. Each capsule contains 8 mg acrivastine and 60 mg pseudoephedrine hydrochloride and the inactive ingredients: lactose, magnesium stearate and sodium starch glycolate. The green and white capsule shell consists of gelatin, D&C Yellow No. 10, FD&C Green No. 3, and titanium dioxide. The yellow band around the capsule consists of gelatin and D&C Yellow No. 10. The capsules may contain one or more parabens and are printed with edible black and white inks.

The chemical name of acrivastine is (E,E)-3-[6-[1-(4-methylphenyl)-3-(1-pyrrolidinyl)-1-propenyl]-2-pyridinyl]-2-propenoic acid; the molecular formula is $C_{22}H_{24}N_2O_2$. As an analog of triprolidine hydrochloride, acrivastine is classified as an alkylamine antihistamine. Acrivastine is an odorless, white to pale cream crystalline powder that is soluble in chloroform and alcohol and slightly soluble in water.

The chemical name of pseudoephedrine hydrochloride is $[S$-$(R^*,R^*)]$-α-[1-(methylamino)ethyl]benzenemethanol hydrochloride; the molecular formula is $C_{10}H_{15}NO \cdot HCl$. Pseudoephedrine is one of the naturally occurring dextrorotatory diastereoisomers of ephedrine and is classified as an indirect sympathomimetic amine. Pseudoephedrine hydrochloride occurs as odorless, fine white to off-white crystals or powder; the drug is soluble in water, alcohol and chloroform. Structural formulae for the active ingredients of SEMPREX-D Capsules are as follows:

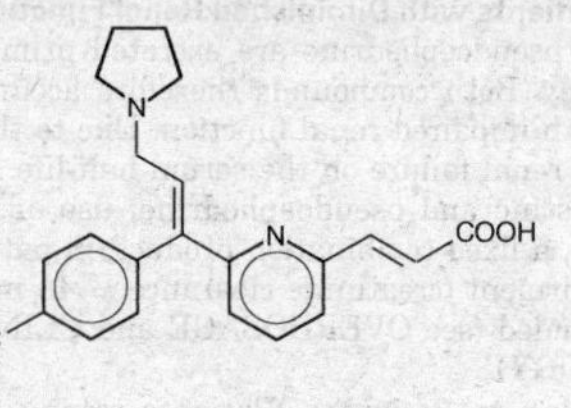

(a) Acrivastine
    (Molecular Weight = 348.44)

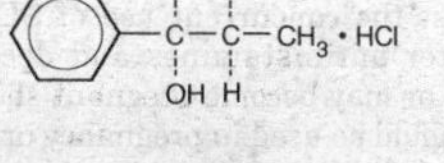

(b) Pseudoephedrine hydrochloride
    (Molecular Weight = 201.70)

CLINICAL PHARMACOLOGY

Acrivastine, a structural analog of triprolidine hydrochloride, exhibits H_1-antihistaminic activity in isolated tissues, animals, and humans, and has sedative effects in humans (see PRECAUTIONS). The propionic acid derivative of acrivastine is a metabolite in several animal species (as well as in man) and also exhibits H_1-antihistaminic activity.

Pseudoephedrine hydrochloride is an indirect sympathomimetic agent; that is, it releases norepinephrine from adrenergic nerves.

In vitro tests and in vivo studies in animals of acrivastine and pseudoephedrine in combination failed to demonstrate evidence of any beneficial or deleterious pharmacologic interaction between the two agents.

Pharmacokinetics and Metabolism

Acrivastine was absorbed rapidly from the combination capsule following oral administration and was as bioavailable as a solution of acrivastine. After administration of SEMPREX-D Capsules, maximum plasma acrivastine concentrations were achieved at 1.14 ± 0.23 hours. A mass balance study in seven healthy volunteers showed that acrivastine is primarily eliminated by the kidneys. Over a 72-hour collection period, about 84% of the administered total radioactivity was recovered in urine and about 13% in feces, for a combined recovery of about 97%. Further, 67% of the admin-

istered radioactive dose was recovered in urine as the unchanged drug, 11% as the propionic acid metabolite, and 6% as other unknown metabolites.

Acrivastine exhibits linear kinetics over dosages ranging from 2 to 32 mg t.i.d. The mean ± SD terminal half-life for acrivastine was 1.9 ± 0.3 hours following single oral doses and increased to 3.5 ± 1.9 hours at steady state. The terminal half-life for the propionic acid metabolite was 3.8 ± 1.4 hours. Because of the short half-lives of both acrivastine and its metabolites, accumulation in the plasma following multiple dosing is not expected.

The steady-state maximum acrivastine plasma concentration was 227 ± 47 ng/mL. The oral clearance and apparent volume of distribution were 2.9 ± 0.7 mL/min/kg and 0.46 ± 0.05 L/kg, respectively, following a single oral dose; oral clearance did not change at steady state (2.86 ± 0.75 mL/min/kg). The apparent volume of distribution increased to 0.82 ± 0.6 L/kg to parallel the increase in the elimination half-life of the drug.

Acrivastine binding to human plasma proteins was 50 ± 2.0% and was concentration-independent over the range of 5 to 1000 ng/mL. The main binding protein was serum albumin although the drug was slightly bound to α1-acid glycoprotein. No displacement interaction was observed between acrivastine and either phenytoin or theophylline. The binding of acrivastine was not affected by the presence of pseudoephedrine.

Pseudoephedrine hydrochloride was also rapidly absorbed from the combination capsule, and the capsule was as bioavailable as a solution of pseudoephedrine. Steady state maximum plasma concentration for pseudoephedrine was 498 ± 129 ng/mL. The terminal half-life, oral clearance and apparent volume of distribution were 6.2 ± 1.8 hours, 5.9 ± 1.7 mL/min/kg, and 3.0 ± 0.4 L/kg, respectively. Elimination of pseudoephedrine is primarily through the renal route as 55% to 75% of an administered dose appears unchanged in the urine. Pseudoephedrine elimination, however, is highly dependent upon urine pH; the plasma half-life decreased to about 4 hours at pH 5 and increased to 13 hours at pH 8. Pseudoephedrine did not bind to human plasma proteins over the concentration range of 50 to 2000 ng/mL.

Acrivastine and pseudoephedrine do not influence the pharmacokinetics of the other drug when administered concomitantly.

Special Populations

A single dose pharmacokinetic study showed that the elimination half-lives of acrivastine, the propionic acid metabolite of acrivastine, and pseudoephedrine were prolonged in patients with chronic renal insufficiency. Compared to normal volunteers, the elimination half-life of acrivastine was about 50% increased in patients with mild renal insufficiency (creatinine clearance = 26 to 48 mL/min) and was increased by about 130% in patients with moderate (creatinine clearance = 12 to 17 mL/min) or severe (creatinine clearance 6 to 10 mL/min) renal insufficiency. Oral clearance of acrivastine was diminished by the same magnitude as the half-life was prolonged in each of the three renally impaired groups. The elimination half-life of the propionic acid metabolite of acrivastine was about 140% increased in patients with mild renal insufficiency and about 5 times increased in patients with moderate or severe renal insufficiency.

Compared to normal volunteers, the elimination half-life of pseudoephedrine was about 3 times increased in patients with mild renal insufficiency, about 7 times increased in patients with moderate renal insufficiency, and about 10 times increased in patients with severe renal insufficiency. Oral clearance of pseudoephedrine was diminished by about the same magnitude as the half-life was prolonged in each of the three renally impaired groups (see PRECAUTIONS: Use in Patients with Diminished Renal Function).

The total body load removed by dialysis is approximately 20%, 27%, and 38% for acrivastine, the propionic acid metabolite of acrivastine, and pseudoephedrine, respectively, and therefore, a supplemental dose after a dialysis session is not required.

Based on a multiple dose cross study comparison, the apparent volume of distribution for acrivastine was 44% lower in elderly (n = 36, 65–75 yr) than in young volunteers (n = 16, 19–33 yr). This difference could be attributed to the decrease in total body water that occurs with aging. Despite this difference, no appreciable differences in plasma acrivastine concentrations were seen in the elderly compared to the young, and no appreciable accumulation of acrivastine occurred in plasma at steady-state. The elimination half-life for pseudoephedrine was 18% longer in elderly (7.9 hours)

Continued on next page

Semprex-D—Cont.

than in younger subjects (6.7 hours), presumably due to the decline in average renal function that occurs with aging. Despite this difference, clearance of pseudoephedrine was not appreciably different in elderly and younger subjects. Elderly patients should therefore be given the same dosage as younger patients. SEMPREX-D Capsules are not recommended, however, in patients with renal impairment (see PRECAUTIONS: Use in Patients with Diminished Renal Function).

The effect of age and sex on the pharmacokinetic parameters of acrivastine and pseudoephedrine was determined in 93 healthy volunteers who participated in various studies. All of the 93 volunteers were Caucasian (81 males and 12 females); 57 were between the ages of 18 and 38 years and 36 were between the ages of 65 and 75 years. There were no age- or sex-related differences in the pharmacokinetic parameters of either acrivastine or pseudoephedrine.

The effect of race on acrivastine and pseudoephedrine pharmacokinetics was examined by screening data obtained from 1035 patients, age 12 to 71 years, who participated in the eight safety and efficacy studies. No race-related differences were observed in the pharmacokinetics of either acrivastine or pseudoephedrine.

Clinical Studies

In healthy volunteers, histamine-induced wheal and flare areas were significantly reduced relative to placebo at 30 minutes after administration of a single dose of acrivastine 8 mg. Maximum reductions of wheal and flare occurred by 1 to 2 hours and significant reductions relative to placebo persisted for up to 6 hours after a single oral dose of acrivastine 8 mg. No additional reductions of wheal and flare were observed following single doses of acrivastine up to 24 mg. The exact correlation between responses on skin testing and clinical efficacy is not established.

Five randomized, placebo- and/or active-controlled trials compared SEMPREX-D with its acrivastine and pseudoephedrine components for the symptomatic relief of seasonal allergic rhinitis. In these studies, 696 patients received four daily doses of acrivastine 8 mg plus pseudoephedrine hydrochloride 60 mg (i.e., SEMPREX-D Capsules or bioequivalent formulations administered concurrently) or the same doses of the components for 14 days. The combination reduced the intensity of sneezing, rhinorrhea, pruritus, and lacrimation more than pseudoephedrine and reduced the intensity of nasal congestion more than acrivastine, demonstrating a contribution of each of the components. The onset of antihistaminic and nasal decongestant actions occurred within one or two hours after the first dose of SEMPREX-D Capsules. Somnolence occurred in about 12% of patients given SEMPREX-D compared with about 6% on placebo.

INDICATIONS AND USAGE

SEMPREX-D Capsules are indicated for relief of symptoms associated with seasonal allergic rhinitis such as sneezing, rhinorrhea, pruritus, lacrimation, and nasal congestion. SEMPREX-D Capsules should be administered when both the antihistaminic activity of acrivastine and the nasal decongestant activity of pseudoephedrine are desired (see CLINICAL PHARMACOLOGY). The efficacy of SEMPREX-D Capsules beyond 14 days of continuous treatment in patients with seasonal allergic rhinitis has not been adequately investigated in clinical trials.

SEMPREX-D Capsules have not been adequately studied for effectiveness in relieving the symptoms of the common cold.

CONTRAINDICATIONS

SEMPREX-D Capsules are contraindicated in patients with a known sensitivity to acrivastine, other alkylamine antihistamines (e.g., triprolidine), pseudoephedrine, other sympathomimetic amines (e.g., phenylpropanolamine), or any other components of the formulation. SEMPREX-D Capsules are contraindicated in patients with severe hypertension or severe coronary artery disease. SEMPREX-D Capsules are contraindicated in patients taking monoamine oxidase (MAO) inhibitors and for two weeks after stopping use of an MAO inhibitor (see Drug Interactions).

WARNINGS

SEMPREX-D Capsules should be used with caution in patients with hypertension, diabetes mellitus, ischemic heart disease, increased intraocular pressure, hyperthyroidism, prostatic hypertrophy, stenosing peptic ulcer, or pyloroduodenal obstruction. Overdose of sympathomimetic amines may produce CNS stimulation with convulsions or cardiovascular collapse with accompanying hypotension. The elderly are more likely to have adverse reactions to sympathomimetic amines.

PRECAUTIONS

General: Acrivastine is sedating in some patients. In controlled clinical trials, somnolence (i.e., drowsiness, sedation, sleepiness) was more common with SEMPREX-D Capsules (by an average of 6%) than with placebo (see ADVERSE EXPERIENCES).

ADVERSE EVENTS REPORTED IN CLINICAL TRIALS* (PERCENT OF PATIENTS REPORTING)†

	Controlled Studies			
	Placebo (n = 1767)	Acrivastine (n = 1935)	Pseudoephedrine (n = 887)	Acrivastine plus Pseudoephedrine (n = 1650)
CNS				
Somnolence‡	6	12	8	12
Headache	18	19	19	19
Dizziness	2	3	3	3
Nervousness‡	1	2	4	3
Insomnia‡	1	1	6	4
MISCELLANEOUS				
Nausea	2	3	3	2
Dry Mouth‡	2	3	5	7
Asthenia	2	3	2	2
Dyspepsia	1	1	2	2
Pharyngitis	2	1	1	3
Cough Increase	1	2	1	2
Dysmenorrhea	1	2	3	2

* Includes all events regardless of causal relationship to treatment.
† Includes all adverse events with a reported frequency of >1% for the acrivastine plus pseudoephedrine treatment group.
‡ SEMPREX-D demonstrates a statistically higher frequency of events than placebo, P ≤0.05.

Patients should be advised to assess their individual responses to SEMPREX-D Capsules before engaging in any activity requiring mental alertness, such as driving a motor vehicle or operating machinery. Concurrent use of SEMPREX-D Capsules with alcohol or other CNS depressants may cause additional reductions in alertness and impairment of CNS performance and should be avoided (see Drug Interactions).

Use in Patients with Diminished Renal Function: Acrivastine and pseudoephedrine are excreted primarily through the kidney. Both compounds therefore accumulate in patients with impaired renal function. Due to the differential effects of renal failure on the serum half-life and clearance of acrivastine and pseudoephedrine, use of SEMPREX-D Capsules, a fixed combination product, in patients with renal impairment (creatinine clearance ≤ 48 mL/min) is not recommended (see OVERDOSAGE and CLINICAL PHARMACOLOGY).

Information to Patients: Patients taking SEMPREX-D Capsules should receive the following information. SEMPREX-D Capsules are prescribed to reduce symptoms associated with seasonal allergic rhinitis. Patients should be instructed to take SEMPREX-D Capsules only as prescribed and not to exceed the prescribed dose. Patients should be advised against the concurrent use of SEMPREX-D with over-the-counter antihistamines and decongestants. Patients who are or may become pregnant should be told that this product should be used in pregnancy or during lactation only if the potential benefit justifies the potential risks to the fetus or nursing infant. Due to the risk of hypertensive crisis, patients should be instructed not to take SEMPREX-D Capsules if they are presently taking a monoamine oxidase inhibitor or for two weeks after stopping use of an MAO inhibitor. Patients should be advised to assess their individual responses to SEMPREX-D Capsules before engaging in any activity requiring mental alertness, such as driving a car or operating machinery. Patients should be advised that the concurrent use of SEMPREX-D Capsules with alcohol and other CNS depressants may lead to additional reductions in alertness and impairment of CNS performance and should be avoided.

Use in the Elderly (Approximately 60 Years or Older): Elderly patients who participated in clinical trials did not differ in effectiveness or adverse effects from younger patients. Antihistamines, however, as a pharmaceutical class, are more likely to cause dizziness, sedation, bladder-neck obstruction, and hypotension in elderly patients. The elderly are also more likely to have adverse reactions to sympathomimetics such as pseudoephedrine (see CLINICAL PHARMACOLOGY and WARNINGS).

Drug Interactions: MAO inhibitors and beta-adrenergic agonists increase the effects of sympathomimetic amines. Concomitant use of sympathomimetic amines with MAO inhibitors can result in a hypertensive crisis (see CONTRAINDICATIONS). Because MAO inhibitors are long-acting, SEMPREX-D Capsules should not be taken with an MAO

inhibitor or for two weeks after stopping use of an MAO inhibitor.

Because of their pseudoephedrine content, SEMPREX-D Capsules may reduce the antihypertensive effects of drugs that interfere with sympathetic activity. Care should be taken in the administration of SEMPREX-D Capsules concomitantly with other sympathomimetic amines because the combined effects on the cardiovascular system may be harmful to the patient.

Concomitant administration of SEMPREX-D Capsules with alcohol and other CNS depressants may result in additional reductions in alertness and impairment of CNS performance and should be avoided.

No formal drug interaction studies between SEMPREX-D Capsules and other possibly co-administered drugs have been performed.

Carcinogenesis, Mutagenesis, and Impairment of Fertility: Carcinogenicity studies with the combination of acrivastine and pseudoephedrine have not been performed. Oral doses of acrivastine alone at levels up to 40 mg/kg/day (236 mg/m²/day or 10 times the recommended human daily dose) for 20 to 22 months in rats and up to 250 mg/kg/day (750 mg/m²/day or 32 times the recommended human daily dose) for 20 to 24 months in mice revealed no evidence of carcinogenic potential. No evidence of mutagenicity (with or without metabolic activation) was observed in the Ames Salmonella mutagenicity assay or in the L5178Y/tk$^{+/-}$ mouse lymphoma assay. In an in vitro cytogenetic study performed in cultured human lymphocytes, acrivastine induced structural chromosomal abnormalities in the absence of metabolic activation, but not in its presence. In an in vivo cytogenetic study in rats given single oral doses of acrivastine up to 1000 mg/kg (5900 mg/m² or 249 times the recommended human daily dose) there were no structural chromosomal alterations.

Reproduction-fertility studies in rats given acrivastine alone at levels up to 200 mg/kg/day (1180 mg/m²/day or 50 times the recommended human daily dose) had no effect on male or female fertility. Similarly no effect on fertility was seen in male rats given acrivastine 20 mg/kg/day and pseudoephedrine 100 mg/kg/day (118 and 590 mg/m²/day or 5 and 3 times the recommended human daily doses, respectively) or in female rats given acrivastine 4 mg/kg/day and pseudoephedrine 20 mg/kg/day (23.6 and 118 mg/m²/day or 1 and 0.7 times the recommended human daily doses, respectively).

Pregnancy: Pregnancy Category B:
Teratogenic Effects: No evidence of teratogenicity was seen in rats and rabbits given acrivastine 1000 and 400 mg/kg/day, respectively (5900 and 4720 mg/m²/day or 249 and 200 times the recommended human daily dose). No evidence of teratogenicity was seen in rats given a combination of acrivastine 30 mg/kg/day and pseudoephedrine 150 mg/kg/day (177 and 885 mg/m²/day or 8 and 5 times the recommended human daily dose, respectively). Similarly, no evidence of teratogenicity was observed in rabbits given acrivastine 20

mg/kg/day and pseudoephedrine 100 mg/kg/day (236 and 1180 mg/m^2/day or 10 and 7 times the recommended human daily doses, respectively). There are, however, no adequate and well-controlled studies in pregnant women. Because animal teratology studies are not always predictive of human responses, SEMPREX-D Capsules should be used during pregnancy only if the potential benefit justifies the potential risks to the fetus.

Nonteratogenic Effects: In a perinatal-postnatal study in rats, acrivastine given alone at levels up to 500 mg/kg/day (2950 mg/m^2/day or 124 times the recommended human daily dose) was associated with maternal and neonatal mortality at the maximum dose level. Neonatal survival was decreased in rats given a combination of acrivastine 20 mg/kg/day and pseudoephedrine 100 mg/kg/day (118 and 590 mg/m^2/day or 5 and 3 times the human dose, respectively).

Nursing Mothers: It is not known whether acrivastine is excreted in human milk; pseudoephedrine is excreted in human milk. SEMPREX-D Capsules should only be used in nursing mothers when the potential benefit justifies the potential risks to the nursing infant.

Pediatric Use: Safety and effectiveness of SEMPREX-D Capsules in pediatric patients under the age of 12 years have not been established.

ADVERSE EXPERIENCES

Information on the incidence of adverse events in clinical investigations conducted in the U.S. was obtained from 33 controlled and 15 uncontrolled clinical studies in which 2499 patients received acrivastine and 2631 patients received acrivastine plus pseudoephedrine hydrochloride for treatment periods ranging from one day to one year. The majority of patients in clinical trials were exposed to acrivastine or acrivastine plus pseudoephedrine for less than 90 days. Acrivastine dosages ranged from 3 to 96 mg/day; 1336 patients received dosages equal to or greater than acrivastine 24 mg/day. Acrivastine plus pseudoephedrine hydrochloride dosages ranged from acrivastine 8 to 48 mg/day plus pseudoephedrine hydrochloride 60 to 240 mg/day. A total of 2335 patients received three or four daily doses of acrivastine 8 mg plus pseudoephedrine hydrochloride 60 mg. In controlled clinical trials, only 12 spontaneously elicited adverse events were reported with frequencies greater than 1% in the acrivastine plus pseudoephedrine hydrochloride treatment group (see table).

[See table at top of previous page]

The nature and overall frequencies of adverse events from international clinical trials (35 studies involving approximately 1600 patients) were similar to the results obtained in the U.S. studies.

Post-marketing clinical experience reports with acrivastine and acrivastine plus pseudoephedrine have included rare serious hypersensitivity reactions manifested by anaphylaxis, angioedema, bronchospasm, and erythema multiforme. No deaths associated with use of acrivastine or acrivastine plus pseudoephedrine have been reported.

Pseudoephedrine may cause ephedrine-like reactions such as tachycardia, palpitations, headache, dizziness, or nausea (see WARNINGS and OVERDOSAGE).

OVERDOSAGE

There have been no reports of overdosage with SEMPREX-D Capsules. In the clinical trial program and in international post-marketing experience, there have been two reported overdoses with acrivastine. Doses were 72 mg and 322 mg. Both patients recovered without sequelae. Adverse events included trembling, stridor, loss of consciousness and possible convulsions in the first patient and somnolence in the second.

Since acrivastine and pseudoephedrine have pharmacologically different actions, it is difficult to predict how an individual will respond to overdosage with SEMPREX-D Capsules. However, acute overdosage with SEMPREX-D Capsules may produce clinical signs of either CNS stimulation or depression. Overdosage of sympathomimetics has been associated with the following events: fear, anxiety, tenseness, restlessness, tremor, weakness, pallor, respiratory difficulty, dysuria, insomnia, hallucinations, convulsions. CNS depression, arrhythmias, and cardiovascular collapse with hypotension. Treatment for overdosage with SEMPREX-D Capsules should follow general symptomatic and supportive principles.

In a placebo-controlled, double-blind clinical trial in 18 healthy male subjects, single doses of acrivastine up to 400 mg (50 times the recommended antihistaminic dose) produced only a weak vagolytic effect, manifested as an increase in heart rate, and did not cause cardiac repolarization delays (i.e., increased QTc). Daily doses of acrivastine up to 2400 mg (75 times the recommended antihistamine dose) in an uncontrolled study in 38 cancer patients produced a 15–beats-per-minute increase in mean heart rate and occasional episodes of nausea and vomiting. The effects of acrivastine plus pseudoephedrine at single or multiple doses higher than the recommended daily dose of SEMPREX-D Capsules (i.e., 32 mg acrivastine plus 240 mg pseudoephedrine) on heart rate and cardiac repolarization have not been investigated in clinical trials.

The mean LD_{50} (single, oral dose) of acrivastine is greater than 4000 mg/kg (23600 mg/m^2 or 1000 times the recommended human daily dose) in rats and greater than 1200 mg/kg (3600 mg/m^2 or 153 times the recommended human daily dose) in mice. The mean LD_{50} (single, oral dose) of pseudoephedrine hydrochloride is 2206 mg/kg (13015 mg/m^2 or 73 times the recommended daily dose) in rats and 726 mg/kg (2178 mg/m^2 or 12 times the recommended human daily dose) in mice. The toxic and lethal concentrations of acrivastine and pseudoephedrine in human biologic fluids are not known. Based upon pharmacokinetic screening data from clinical trials, the maximum plasma acrivastine concentration after dosing with acrivastine 8 mg was 393 ng/mL and the maximum plasma pseudoephedrine concentration after dosing with pseudoephedrine hydrochloride 60 mg was 1308 ng/mL.

DOSAGE AND ADMINISTRATION

The recommended dosage for adults and children 12 years and older is one capsule administered orally, every 4 to 6 hours four times a day.

HOW SUPPLIED

SEMPREX-D Capsules (dark green opaque cap and white opaque body with a yellow band) contain acrivastine 8 mg and pseudoephedrine hydrochloride 60 mg. The cap is printed with "Medeva" in white ink, and the body is printed with "SEMPREX-D" in black ink.

Bottles of 100 (NDC 53014-404-10).

The capsules should be stored at 15° to 25°C (59° to 77°F) in a dry place and protected from light.

U.S. Patents Nos. 4501893 and 4650807

Rx Only

Marketed by:
Medeva Pharmaceuticals, Inc.
Rochester, NY 14623 USA
Manufactured by:
Catalytica Pharmaceuticals, Inc.
Greenville, NC 27834 USA
U.S. Patent Nos. 4501893 and 4650807
® Medeva California, Inc.
© 1998, Medeva Pharmaceuticals
Manufacturing Inc. Rev. 3/98
R314
466051

SYN™-Rx Tablets ℞
A.M. (pseudoephedrine HCl + guaifenesin)
P.M. (guaifenesin)
14 Day Treatment Regimen

DESCRIPTION

Each Syn™-Rx Tablets 14 Day Treatment Regimen pack of 56 tablets consists of two different drug treatment phases as follows: an **A.M. Treatment Phase** comprised of 28 dark blue scored controlled-release tablets, each containing 60 mg pseudoephedrine HCl and 600 mg guaifenesin, embossed with "MEDEVA" on one side and "017" to the right of the score on the other side, and a **P.M. Treatment Phase** comprised of 28 light green scored controlled-release tablets, each containing 600 mg guaifenesin, embossed with "MEDEVA" on one side and "012" to the right of the score on the other side.

Syn™-Rx Tablets 14 Day Treatment Regimen contains ingredients of two therapeutic classes: nasal decongestant and expectorant.

Pseudoephedrine hydrochloride is a nasal decongestant. Chemically, it is [S-(R,R')]-α-[1-(methylamino)ethyl] benzenemethanol hydrochloride and has the following structural formula:

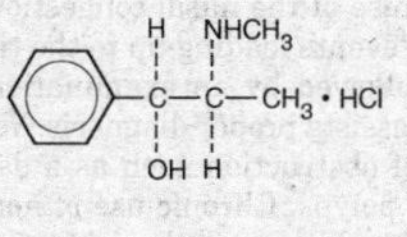

Molecular weight = 201.70 chemical formula = $C_{10}H_{15}NO{\cdot}HCl$

Guaifenesin is an expectorant. Chemically, it is 3-(2-methoxyphenoxy)-1, 2–propanediol and has the following structural formula:

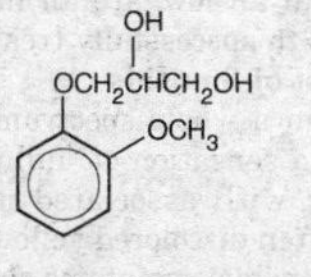

Molecular weight = 198.22 chemical formula = $C_{10}H_{14}O_4$

Inactive Ingredients: Each dark blue A.M. tablet and light green P.M. tablet contains dibasic calcium phosphate, ethylcellulose, FD&C Blue #1 Lake, magnesium stearate, sodium lauryl sulfate, stearic acid; each light green P.M. tablet also contains D & C Yellow #10 Lake.

CLINICAL PHARMACOLOGY

Pseudoephedrine hydrochloride is an orally indirect acting sympathomimetic amine and exerts a decongestant action on the nasal mucosa. It does this by vasoconstriction which results in reduction of tissue hyperemia, edema, nasal congestion, and an increase in nasal airway patency. In the usual dose it has minimal vasopressor effects. Pseudoephedrine is rapidly and almost completely absorbed from the gastrointestinal tract. It has a plasma half-life of 6 to 8 hours. Alkaline urine is associated with slower elimination of the drug. The drug is distributed to body tissues and fluids, including the central nervous system (CNS). Approximately 50% to 75% of the administered dose is excreted unchanged in the urine; the remainder is apparently metabolized in the liver to inactive compounds by N-demethylation, parahydroxylation and oxidative deamination.

Guaifenesin is an expectorant which increases respiratory tract fluid secretions and helps to loosen phlegm, bronchial and nasal secretions. By reducing the viscosity of secretions, guaifenesin increases the efficiency of the mucociliary mechanism in removing accumulated secretions from the upper and lower airway. Guaifenesin is readily absorbed from the gastrointestinal tract and is rapidly metabolized and excreted in the urine. Guaifenesin has a plasma half-life of one hour. The major urinary metabolite is β-(2-methoxyphenoxy) lactic acid.

INDICATIONS AND USAGE

Syn™-Rx Tablets 14 Day Treatment Regimen is indicated for the temporary relief of nasal congestion associated with respiratory tract infections and related conditions such as sinusitis, bronchitis, and asthma, when these conditions are complicated by tenacious mucus, and/or mucus plugs and congestion. In the treatment of bacterial sinusitis this treatment regimen may be used concomitantly with appropriate antibiotic therapy.

CONTRAINDICATIONS

This product is contraindicated in patients with hypersensitivity to guaifenesin or pseudoephedrine HCl, or with hypersensitivity or idiosyncrasy to sympathomimetic amines which may be manifested by insomnia, dizziness, weakness, tremor or arrhythmias.

Sympathomimetic amines are contraindicated in patients with severe hypertension, severe coronary artery disease and patients on monoamine oxidase inhibitor (MAOI) therapy and for 14 days after stopping MAOI therapy. (see **Drug Interactions** section).

WARNINGS

Sympathomimetic amines should be used in caution in patients with hypertension, ischemic heart disease, diabetes mellitus, increased intraocular pressure, hyperthyroidism, or prostatic hypertrophy. Sympathomimetics may produce central nervous system stimulation with convulsions or cardiovascular collapse with accompanying hypotension. **Do not exceed recommended dosage.**

Hypertensive crises can occur with concurrent use of pseudoephedrine and monoamine oxidase inhibitors (MAOI), and for 14 days after stopping the MAOI drug therapy, indomethacin, or with beta-blockers and methyldopa. If a hypertensive crisis occurs, these drugs should be discontinued immediately and therapy to lower blood pressure should be instituted. Fever should be managed by means of external cooling.

PRECAUTIONS

General: Use with caution in patients with diabetes, hypertension, cardiovascular disease and intolerence to ephedrine.

Failure of symptoms to completely resolve should alert the patient and physician that further diagnostic studies are indicated.

Pediatric Use: Safety and effectiveness of Syn™-Rx Tablets in pediatric patients under 12 years of age have not been established.

Use In Elderly: The elderly (60 years and older) are more likely to experience adverse reactions to sympathomimetics. Overdosage of sympathomimetics in this age group may cause hallucinations, convulsions, CNS depression, and death.

Drug Interactions: Do not prescribe this product for use in patients that are now taking a monoamine oxidase inhibitor

Continued on next page

Information on the Medeva Pharmaceuticals, Inc. products listed on these pages contains the full prescribing information from product circulars in use as of July 1998. For further information, please consult the package insert currently accompanying the product.

Syn-Rx—Cont.

(MAOI) drug (certain drugs for depression, psychiatric or emotional conditions, or Parkinson's disease) or for 14 days after stopping the MAOI drug therapy. Beta-adrenergic blockers and inhibitors (MAOI) may potentiate the pressor effect of pseudoephedrine. Concurrent use of digitalis glycosides may increase the possibility of cardiac arrhythmias. Sympathomimetics may reduce the hypotensive effects of guanethidine, mecamylamine, methyldopa, reserpine and veratrum alkaloids. Concurrent use of tricyclic antidepressants may antagonize the effects of pseudoephedrine.

Drug/Laboratory Test Interactions: Guaifenesin may increase renal clearance for urate and thereby lower serum uric acid levels. Guaifenesin may produce an increase in urinary 5-hydroxyindoleacetic acid and may therefore interfere with the interpretation of this test for the diagnosis of carcinoid syndrome. It may also falsely elevate the VMA test for catechols. Administration of this drug should be discontinued 48 hours prior to the collection of urine specimens for such tests.

Carcinogenesis, Mutagenesis, Impairment of Fertility: No data are available on the long-term potential of the components of this product for carcinogenesis, mutagenesis, or impairment of fertility in animals or humans.

Pregnancy Category C: Animal reproduction studies have not been conducted with Syn™-Rx Tablets. It is also not known whether Syn™-Rx Tablets can cause fetal harm when administered to a pregnant woman or can affect reproduction capacity. Syn™-Rx Tablets should be given to a pregnant woman only if clearly needed.

Nursing Mothers: Pseudoephedrine is excreted in breast milk. Use of this product by nursing mothers is not recommended because of the higher than usual risk for pediatric patients from sympathomimetic amines.

ADVERSE REACTIONS

Some individuals may display sympathomimetic amine effects such as tachycardia, palpitations, headache, dizziness or nausea. Sympathomimetics have been associated with certain untoward reactions including fear, anxiety, nervousness, restlessness, tremor, weakness, pallor, respiratory difficulty, dysuria, insomnia, hallucinations, convulsions, CNS depression, arrhythmias, and cardiovascular collapse with hypotension. No serious side effects have been reported with the use of guaifenesin.

OVERDOSAGE

Since Syn™-Rx Tablets 14 Day Treatment Regimen contains two pharmacologically different compounds, treatment of overdosage should be based upon the symptomatology of the patient as it relates to the individual ingredients. Treatment of acute overdosage would probably be based upon treating the patient for pseudoephedrine toxicity which may manifest itself as excessive CNS stimulation resulting in excitement, tremor, restlessness, and insomnia. Other effects may include tachycardia, hypertension, pallor, mydriasis, hyperglycemia and urinary retention. Severe overdosage may cause tachypnea or hyperpnea, hallucinations, convulsions or delirium, but in some individuals there may be CNS depression with somnolence, stupor or respiratory depression. Arrhythmias (including ventricular fibrillation) may lead to hypotension and circulatory collapse. Severe hypokalemia can occur, probably due to a compartmental shift rather than a depletion of potassium. No organ damage or significant metabolic derangement is associated with pseudoephedrine overdosage. Overdosage with guaifenesin is unlikely to produce toxic effects since its toxicity is much lower than that of pseudoephedrine. In severe cases of overdosage, it is recommended to monitor the patient in an intensive care setting.

The LD_{50} of pseudoephedrine (single oral dose) has been reported to be 726 mg/kg in the mouse, 2206 mg/kg in the rat and 1177 mg/kg in the rabbit. The toxic and lethal concentrations in human biologic fluids are not known. Urinary excretion increases with acidification and decreases with alkalinization of the urine. There are few published reports of toxicity due to pseudoephedrine and no case of fatal overdosage has been reported. Guaifenesin, when administered by stomach tube to test animals in doses up to 5 grams/kg, produced no signs of toxicity.

Since the action of sustained release products may continue for as long as 12 hours, treatment of overdosage should be directed toward reducing further absorption and supporting the patient for at least that length of time. Gastric emptying (Syrup of Ipecac) and/or lavage is recommended as soon as possible after ingestion, even if the patient has vomited spontaneously. Either isotonic or half-isotonic saline may be used for lavage. Administration of an activated charcoal slurry is beneficial after lavage and/or emesis if less than 4 hours have passed since ingestion. Saline cathartics, such as Milk of Magnesia, are useful for hastening the evacuation of unreleased medication.

Adrenergic receptor blocking agents are antidotes to pseudoephedrine. In practice, the most useful is the beta-blocker propranolol which is indicated when there are signs of cardiac toxicity. Theoretically, pseudoephedrine is dialyzable but procedures have not been clinically established.

DOSAGE AND ADMINISTRATION

Adults and adolescents over 12 years of age: 1 or 2 dark blue A.M. tablet(s) in the morning and 1 or 2 light green P.M. tablet(s) 12 hours later. Repeat A.M. and P.M. dosing cycle every 12 hours for 14 days.

Do not crush or chew tablets prior to swallowing.

HOW SUPPLIED

NDC 53014-308-14 SYN™-Rx Tablets 14 Day Treatment Regimen, containing 56 controlled-release tablets as follows:

NDC 53014-017, 28 dark blue elongated and scored A.M. tablets embossed with "MEDEVA" on one side and "017" to the right of the score on the other side, each containing 60 mg pseudoephedrine HCl and 600 mg guaifenesin;

NDC 53014-012, 28 light green elongated and scored P.M. tablets embossed with "MEDEVA" on one side and "012" to the right of the score on the other side, each containing 600 mg guaifenesin.

Store at controlled room temperature between 15°C and 30°C (59°F and 86°F).

Dispense as a complete 14 day pack.

Keep out of reach of pediatric population.

Caution: Federal law prohibits dispensing without prescription.

Medeva Pharmaceuticals, Inc.
Fort Worth, TX 76155–2645

PATIENT INFORMATION
SINUSITIS

Sinusitis is an inflammation of the membranes that line the sinuses. Sinusitis can be a self-limited condition in association with a routine upper respiratory infection or it can become chronic and persistent, lasting months or years. While infection is a very common cause of sinusitis, other factors need to be considered such as allergies, mechanical obstruction in the nasal cavity from a deviated septum, seasonal activities of swimming or diving, inadvertent overuse of non-prescription nasal sprays, irritation from tobacco smoke or other chemical irritants, and disorders of the immune system. Nasal polyps may result in some individuals who suffer with persistent sinusitis. Treating patients with nasal polyps requires an ongoing effort to control the inflammatory process.

Location of the Sinuses

The sinuses are air-filled cavities lined with a mucous membrane and located within the bones of the skull and face (Figure 1). When pain occurs with sinusitis, it can occur over the affected area or it can radiate to an adjacent area making exact diagnosis more difficult.

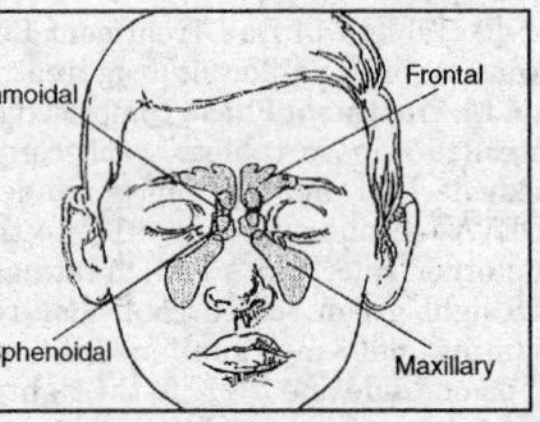

Nasal Congestion Can Lead to Blockage of the Sinus Opening

When the nasal airway becomes congested without relief, a sinus opening may not function normally and obstruction occurs. Mucus within the sinus cavity, which is normally cleared through the sinus opening, is then trapped within the sinus and infection may occur. It is important, therefore, that through communications with your physician, you understand the cause of the nasal congestion.

A history of the events leading up to the time of the onset of the sinusitis, followed by an examination of that area by your physician assists proper diagnosis. Your physician may look for signs of obstruction such as a deviated septum or the presence of polyps. Chronic use of non-prescription nasal sprays might alert your physician to another cause of nasal congestion. Your doctor may recommend against swimming or diving when you have sinusitis. Flying will require your physician's approval if you have sinusitis.

Understanding the importance of obstruction of the nasal airway as a factor in sinusitis, and managing nasal congestion through efforts aimed to "decongest" the nasal airway and restore normal airflow, are an important part of your physician's efforts to successfully treat sinusitis.

Symptoms Typical of Sinusitis

Sinusitis results in a whole spectrum of symptoms. There may be pain and a sensation of "fullness or pressure" over the affected area with associated nasal congestion and draining mucus often discolored yellow or green. Contrarily, there may be only vague symptoms such as a dull headache or decreased energy level. If the sinus opening is totally obstructed, drainage will be limited. Fever may or may not occur even with an infection. When sinusitis is chronic, a cough may be the primary cause for your physician's consideration of sinusitis.

X-ray is an Important Diagnostic Tool

When sinusitis is persistent, a routine x-ray examination may be requested by your physician to pinpoint the affected areas. A CAT scan (computerized axial tomography) to locate affected areas may be needed in your physician's judgement. Your physician will look for signs of inflammation such as thickening of the membranes and fluid in the cavities, plus evidence of obstruction on the x-ray exam.

Treatment of Sinusitis

A common approach to sinusitis therapy is to:

1) Eliminate or control the cause of the inflammation within the nasal and sinus airways.
2) Eliminate primary or secondary infection.
3) Promote normal drainage through elimination of congestion and associated obstruction.
4) Correct obstruction caused by factors such as nasal polyps or septal deviation.

Syn™-Rx Tablets: 14 Day Treatment Regimen

Syn™-Rx Tablets are formulated to help thin nasal and sinus secretions, decongest nasal and sinus tissues and promote drainage. The Syn™-Rx Tablets package contains two separate medications. The dark blue A.M. tablets contain medication to decongest the swollen tissue and thin the thickened secretions and are taken each morning. The light green P.M. tablets, taken each evening, contain medication which continues to thin the secretions, yet will not cause sleeplessness.

Syn™-Rx Tablets Can be Used with Antibiotics and Steroid Nasal Spray

Depending on your physician's assessment and the presence or absence of inflammation and/or infection, Syn™-Rx Tablets may be prescribed to be taken alone or along with antibiotics or topical steroid nasal sprays in the treatment of sinusitis.

Sinusitis Should not be Ignored

Untreated prolonged sinusitis can result in serious complications well known to your physician. Sinus infections may require prompt diagnosis to prevent the development of chronic sinusitis. Always seek your physician's advice concerning suspicion of new symptoms or lingering symptoms of sinusitis.

SYN™-Rx DM Tablets ℞

A.M. (pseudoephedrine HCl + guaifenesin)
P.M. (dextromethorphan HBr + guaifenesin)
14 Day Treatment Regimen

DESCRIPTION

Each SYN™-Rx DM Tablets 14 Day Treatment Regimen pack of 56 tablets consists of two different drug treatment phases as follows: an **A.M. Treatment Phase** comprised of 28 light blue scored controlled-release tablets, each containing 60 mg pseudoephedrine HCl and 600 mg guaifenesin embossed with "MEDEVA" on one side and "310" to the right of the score on the other side; and a **P.M. Treatment Phase** comprised of 28 yellow scored controlled-release tablets each containing 30 mg dextromethorphan hydrobromide and 600 mg guaifenesin, embossed with "MEDEVA" on one side and "309" to the right of the score on the other side.

SYN™-Rx DM Tablets 14 Day Treatment Regimen contains ingredients of three therapeutic classes: nasal decongestant, antitussive, and expectorant.

Pseudoephedrine hydrochloride is a nasal decongestant. Chemically, it is [S-(R*,R*)]-α-[1-(methylamino)ethyl] benzenemethanol hydrochloride and has the following structural formula:

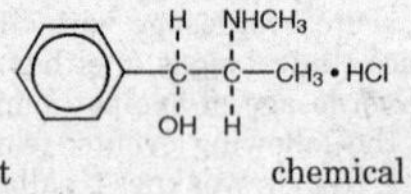

Molecular weight = 201.70 chemical formula = $C_{10}H_{15}NO \cdot HCl$

Dextromethorphan hydrobromide is a salt of the methyl ether of the dextrorotatory isomer of levorphanol, a narcotic analgesic. Chemically, it is 3-methoxy-17-methyl-9α, 13α, 14α - morphinan hydrobromide monohydrate and has the following structural formula:

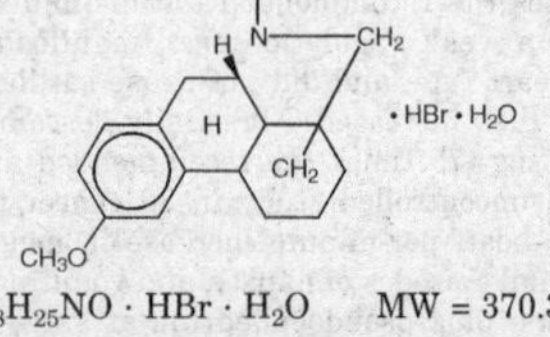

$C_{18}H_{25}NO \cdot HBr \cdot H_2O$ MW = 370.33

Guaifenesin is an expectorant. Chemically, it is 3-(2-methoxyphenoxy)-1,2-propanediol and has the following structural formula:

[See chemical structure at top of next column]

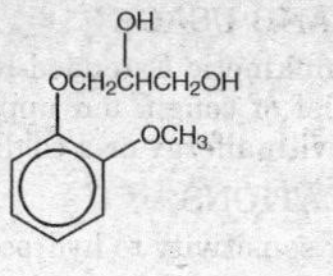
OH
OCH2CHCH2OH
OCH3

Molecular weight = 198.22 chemical formula = $C_{10}H_{14}O_4$

Inactive Ingredients: Each light blue A.M. tablet and yellow P.M. tablet contains dibasic calcium phosphate, ethylcellulose, magnesium stearate, sodium lauryl sulfate, stearic acid. Each light blue A.M. tablet also contains FD&C Blue #1 Aluminum Lake. Each yellow P.M. tablet also contains D & C Yellow #10 Lake.

CLINICAL PHARMACOLOGY

Pseudoephedrine hydrochloride is an orally indirect acting sympathomimetic amine and exerts a decongestant action on the nasal mucosa. It does this by vasoconstriction which results in reduction of tissue hyperemia, edema, nasal congestion, and an increase in nasal airway patency. In the usual dose it has minimal vasopressor effects. Pseudoephedrine is rapidly and almost completely absorbed from the gastrointestinal tract. It has a plasma half-life of 6 to 8 hours. Alkaline urine is associated with slower elimination of the drug. The drug is distributed to body tissues and fluids, including the central nervous system (CNS). Approximately 50% to 75% of the administered dose is excreted unchanged in the urine; the remainder is apparently metabolized in the liver to inactive compounds by N-demethylation, parahydroxylation and oxidative deamination.

Dextromethorphan is an antitussive agent which, unlike the isomeric levorphanol, has no analgesic or addictive properties. The drug acts centrally and elevates the threshold for coughing. It is about equal to codeine in depressing the cough reflex. In therapeutic dosage, dextromethorphan does not inhibit ciliary activity. Dextromethorphan is rapidly absorbed from the gastrointestinal tract, metabolized by the liver and excreted primarily in the urine.

Guaifenesin is an expectorant which increases respiratory tract fluid secretions and helps to loosen phlegm, bronchial and nasal secretions. By reducing the viscosity of secretions, guaifenesin increases the efficiency of the mucociliary mechanism in removing accumulated secretions from the upper and lower airway. Guaifenesin is readily absorbed from the gastrointestinal tract and is rapidly metabolized and excreted in the urine. Guaifenesin has a plasma half-life of one hour. The major urinary metabolite is β-(2-methoxyphenoxy) lactic acid.

INDICATIONS AND USAGE

SYN™-Rx DM Tablets 14 Day Treatment Regimen is indicated for the temporary relief of nasal congestion and cough associated with respiratory tract infections and related conditions such as sinusitis, bronchitis, and asthma, when these conditions are complicated by tenacious mucus, and/or mucus plugs and congestion. In the treatment of bacterial sinusitis this treatment regimen may be used concomitantly with appropriate antibiotic therapy. The product is effective in productive as well as nonproductive cough, but is of particular value in dry, nonproductive cough which tends to injure the mucous membrane of the air passages.

CONTRAINDICATIONS

This product is contraindicated in patients with hypersensitivity to guaifenesin, dextromethorphan HBr, or pseudoephedrine HCl, or with hypersensitivity or idiosyncrasy to sympathomimetic amines which may be manifested by insomnia, dizziness, weakness, tremor or arrhythmias.

Sympathomimetic amines are contraindicated in patients with severe hypertension and severe coronary artery disease.

The product is contraindicated in patients on monoamine oxidase inhibitor (MAOI) therapy and for 14 days after stopping MAOI therapy. (see **Drug Interaction** section).

WARNINGS

Sympathomimetic amines should be used with caution in patients with hypertension, ischemic heart disease, diabetes mellitus, increased intraocular pressure, hyperthyroidism, or prostatic hypertrophy. Sympathomimetics may produce central nervous system stimulation with convulsions or cardiovascular collapse with accompanying hypotension.

Do not exceed recommended dosage.

Do not prescribe this product for use in patients that are now taking a prescription MAOI (certain drugs for depression, psychiatric or emotional conditions, or Parkinson's disease), or for 14 days after stopping the MAOI drug therapy. Hypertensive crises can occur with concurrent use of pseudoephedrine and monoamine oxidase inhibitors (MAOI), and for 14 days after stopping the MAOI drug therapy, indomethacin, or with beta-blockers and methyldopa. If a hypertensive crisis occurs, these drugs should be discontinued immediately and therapy to lower blood pressure should be instituted. Fever should be managed by means of external cooling.

PRECAUTIONS

General: Use with caution in patients with diabetes, hypertension, cardiovascular disease and intolerence to ephedrine.

Before prescribing medication to suppress or modify cough, it is important that the underlying cause of cough is identified, that modification of cough does not increase the risk of clinical or physiological complications, and that appropriate therapy for the primary disease is instituted.

Dextromethorphan should be used with caution in sedated or debilitated patients, and in patients confined to the supine position.

Failure of symptoms to completely resolve should alert the patient and physician that further diagnostic studies are indicated.

Pediatric Use: The safety and effectiveness of Syn™-Rx DM Tablets in pediatric patients under 12 years of age have not been established.

Use in Elderly: The elderly (60 years and older) are more likely to experience adverse reactions to sympathomimetics. Ovedosage of sympathomimetics in this age group may cause hallucinations, convulsions, CNS depression, and death.

Drug Interactions: Do not prescribe this product for use in patients that are now taking a monoamine oxidase inhibitor (MAOI) drug (certain drugs for depression, psychiatric or emotional conditions, or Parkinson's disease) or for 14 days after stopping the MAOI drug therapy. Beta-adrenergic blockers and inhibitors (MAOI) may potentiate the pressor effect of pseudoephedrine. Concurrent use of digitalis glycosides may increase the possibility of cardiac arrhythmias. Sympathomimetics may reduce the hypotensive effects of guanethidine, mecamylamine, methyldopa, reserpine and veratrum alkaloids. Concurrent use of tricyclic antidepressants may antagonize the effects of pseudoephedrine.

Drug/Laboratory Test Interactions: Guaifenesin may increase renal clearance for urate and thereby lower serum uric acid levels. Guaifenesin may produce an increase in urinary 5-hydroxyindoleacetic acid and may therefore interfere with the interpretation of this test for the diagnosis of carcinoid syndrome. It may also falsely elevate the VMA test for catechols. Administration of this drug should be discontinued 48 hours prior to the collection of urine specimens for such tests.

Carcinogenesis, Mutagenesis, Impairment of Fertility: No data are available on the long-term potential of the components of this product for carcinogenesis, mutagenesis, or impairment of fertility in animals or humans.

Pregnancy Category C: Animal reproduction studies have not been conducted with Syn™-Rx DM Tablets. It is also not known whether Syn™-Rx DM Tablets can cause fetal harm when administered to a pregnant woman or can affect reproduction capacity. Syn™-Rx DM Tablets should be given to a pregnant woman only if clearly needed.

Nursing Mothers: Pseudoephedrine is excreted in breast milk. Use of this product by nursing mothers is not recommended because of the higher than usual risk for pediatric patients from sympathomimetic amines.

ADVERSE REACTIONS

Some individuals may display sympathomimetic amine effects such as tachycardia, palpitations, headache, dizziness or nausea. Sympathomimetics have been associated with certain untoward reactions including fear, anxiety, nervousness, restlessness, tremor, weakness, pallor, respiratory difficulty, dysuria, insomnia, hallucinations, convulsions, CNS depression, arrhythmias, and cardiovascular collapse with hypotension. No serious side effects have been reported with the use of guaifenesin or dextromethorphan HBr.

OVERDOSAGE

Since SYN™-Rx DM Tablets 14 Day Treatment Regimen contains three pharmacologically different compounds, treatment of overdosage should be based upon the symptomatology of the patient as it relates to the individual ingredients. Treatment of acute overdosage would probably be based upon treating the patient for pseudoephedrine toxicity which may manifest itself as excessive CNS stimulation resulting in excitement, tremor, restlessness, and insomnia. Other effects may include tachycardia, hypertension, pallor, mydriasis, hyperglycemia and urinary retention. Severe overdosage may cause tachypnea or hyperpnea, hallucinations, convulsions or delirium, but in some individuals there may be CNS depression with somnolence, stupor or respiratory depression. Arrhythmias (including ventricular fibrillation) may lead to hypotension and circulatory collapse. Severe hypokalemia can occur, probably due to a compartmental shift rather than a depletion of potassium. No organ damage or significant metabolic derangement is associated with pseudoephedrine overdosage. Overdosage with guaifenesin is unlikely to produce toxic effects since its toxicity is much lower than that of pseudoephedrine. In severe cases of overdosage, it is recommended to monitor the patient in an intensive care setting.

The LD_{50} of pseudoephedrine (single oral dose) has been reported to be 726 mg/kg in the mouse, 2206 mg/kg in the rat and 1177 mg/kg in the rabbit. The toxic and lethal concentrations in human biologic fluids are not known. Urinary excretion increases with acidification and decreases with alkalinization of the urine. There are few published reports of toxicity due to pseudoephedrine and no case of fatal overdosage has been reported. Guaifenesin, when administered by stomach tube to test animals in doses up to 5 grams/kg, produced no signs of toxicity.

Overdosage with dextromethorphan may produce central excitement and mental confusion. Very high doses may produce respiratory depression. One case of toxic psychosis (hyperactivity, marked visual and auditory hallucinations) after ingestion of a single 300 mg dose of dextromethorphan has been reported.

Since the action of sustained release products may continue for as long as 12 hours, treatment of overdosage should be directed toward reducing further absorption and supporting the patient for at least that length of time. Gastric emptying (Syrup of Ipecac) and/or lavage is recommended as soon as possible after ingestion, even if the patient has vomited spontaneously. Either isotonic or half-isotonic saline may be used for lavage. Administration of an activated charcoal slurry is beneficial after lavage and/or emesis if less than 4 hours have passed since ingestion. Saline cathartics, such as Milk of Magnesia, are useful for hastening the evacuation of unreleased medication.

Adrenergic receptor blocking agents are antidotes to pseudoephedrine. In practice, the most useful is the beta-blocker propranolol which is indicated when there are signs of cardiac toxicity. Theoretically, pseudoephedrine is dialyzable but procedures have not been clinically established.

DOSAGE AND ADMINISTRATION

Adults and adolescents over 12 years of age: 1 or 2 light blue A.M. tablets in the morning and 1 or 2 yellow P.M. tablets 12 hours later. Repeat A.M. and P.M. dosing cycle every 12 hours for 14 days. **Do not crush or chew tablets prior to swallowing.**

HOW SUPPLIED

NDC 53014-311-14 SYN™-Rx DM Tablets 14 Day Treatment Regimen, containing 56 controlled-release tablets as follows:

NDC 53014-310, 28 light blue elongated and scored A.M. tablets embossed with "MEDEVA" on one side and "310" to the right of the score on the other side, each containing 60 mg pseudoephedrine HCl and 600 mg guaifenesin;

NDC 53014-309, 28 yellow elongated and scored P.M. tablets embossed with "MEDEVA" on one side and "309" to the right of the score on the other side, each containing 30 mg dextromethorphan HBr and 600 mg guaifenesin

Store at controlled room temperature between 15°C and 30°C (59°F and 86°F).

Dispense as a complete 14 day pack.

Keep out of reach of pediatric population.

Caution: Federal law prohibits dispensing without prescription.

Medeva Pharmaceuticals, Inc.
Fort Worth, TX 76155–2645

PATIENT INFORMATION

SINUSITIS

Sinusitis is an inflammation of the membranes that line the sinuses. Sinusitis can be a self-limited condition in association with a routine upper respiratory infection or it can become chronic and persistent, lasting months or years. While infection is a very common cause of sinusitis, other factors need to be considered such as allergies, mechanical obstruction in the nasal cavity from a deviated septum, seasonal activities of swimming or diving, inadvertent overuse of non-prescription nasal sprays, irritation from tobacco smoke or other chemical irritants, and disorders of the immune system. Nasal polyps may result in some individuals who suffer with persistent sinusitis. Treating patients with nasal polyps requires an ongoing effort to control the inflammatory process.

Location of the Sinuses

The sinuses are air-filled cavities lined with a mucous membrane and located within the bones of the skull and face (Figure 1). When pain occurs with sinusitis, it can occur over the affected area or it can radiate to an adjacent area making exact diagnosis more difficult.

[See figure at top of next column]

Nasal Congestion Can Lead to Blockage of the Sinus Opening

When the nasal airway becomes congested without relief, a sinus opening may not function normally and obstruction occurs. Mucus within the sinus cavity, which is normally

Continued on next page

Information on the Medeva Pharmaceuticals, Inc. products listed on these pages contains the full prescribing information from product circulars in use as of July 1998. For further information, please consult the package insert currently accompanying the product.

Syn-Rx DM—Cont.

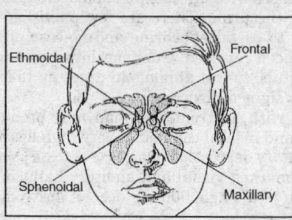

cleared through the sinus opening, is then trapped within the sinus and infection may occur. It is important, therefore, that through communications with your physician, you understand the cause of the nasal congestion.

A history of the events leading up to the time of the onset of the sinusitis, followed by an examination of that area by your physician assists proper diagnosis. Your physician may look for signs of obstruction such as a deviated septum or the presence of polyps. Chronic use of non-prescription nasal sprays might alert your physician to another cause of nasal congestion. Your doctor may recommend against swimming or diving when you have sinusitis. Flying will require your physician's approval if you have sinusitis.

Understanding the importance of obstruction of the nasal airway as a factor in sinusitis, and managing nasal congestion through efforts aimed to "decongest" the nasal airway and restore normal airflow, are an important part of your physician's efforts to successfully treat sinusitis.

Symptoms Typical of Sinusitis

Sinusitis results in a whole spectrum of symptoms. There may be pain and a sensation of "fullness or pressure" over the affected area with associated nasal congestion and draining mucus often discolored yellow or green. Contrarily, there may be only vague symptoms such as a dull headache or decreased energy level. If the sinus opening is totally obstructed, drainage will be limited. Fever may or may not occur even with an infection. When sinusitis is chronic, a cough may be the primary cause for your physician's consideration of sinusitis.

X-ray is an Important Diagnostic Tool

When sinusitis is persistent, a routine x-ray examination may be requested by your physician to pinpoint the affected areas. A CAT scan (computerized axial tomography) to locate affected areas may be needed in your physician's judgement. Your physician will look for signs of inflammation such as thickening of the membranes and fluid in the cavities, plus evidence of obstruction on the x-ray exam.

Treatment of Sinusitis

A common approach to sinusitis therapy is to:
1) Eliminate or control the cause of the inflammation within the nasal and sinus airways.
2) Eliminate primary or secondary infection.
3) Promote normal drainage through elimination of congestion and associated obstruction.
4) Correct obstruction caused by factors such as nasal polyps or septal deviation.

Syn™-Rx DM Tablets: 14-Day Treatment Regimen

Syn™-Rx DM Tablets are formulated for the temporary relief of nasal congestion and coughs associated with respiratory tract infections and related conditions such as sinusitis, bronchitis, and asthma. The Syn™-Rx DM Tablets package contains two separate medications. The light blue A.M. tablets contain medication to decongest the swollen tissue and thin the thickened secretions and are taken each morning. The yellow P.M. tablets, taken each evening, contain medication for coughs and continue to thin the secretions, yet will not cause sleeplessness.

Syn™-Rx DM Tablets May be Used with Antibiotics and Steroid Nasal Spray

Depending on your physician's assessment and the presence or absence of inflammation and/or infection, Syn™-Rx DM Tablets may be prescribed to be taken alone or along with antibiotics or topical steroid nasal sprays in the treatment of sinusitis.

Sinusitis Should not be Ignored

Untreated prolonged sinusitis can result in serious complications well known to your physician. Sinus infections may require prompt diagnosis to prevent the development of chronic sinusitis. Always seek your physician's advice concerning suspicion of new symptoms or lingering symptoms of sinusitis.

TUSSIONEX®

[tus´e-uh-nex]   Ⓒ Ⓡ
Pennkinetic® Extended Release Suspension
(hydrocodone polistirex
and chlorpheniramine polistirex)
R240F
Rev. 9/96

DESCRIPTION

Each teaspoonful (5 mL) of TUSSIONEX Pennkinetic Extended-Release Suspension contains hydrocodone polistirex equivalent to 10 mg of hydrocodone bitartrate (Warning: May be habit forming) and chlorpheniramine polistirex equivalent to 8 mg of chlorpheniramine maleate. TUSSIONEX Pennkinetic Extended-Release Suspension provides up to 12-hour relief per dose. Hydrocodone is a centrally-acting narcotic antitussive. Chlorpheniramine is an antihistamine. TUSSIONEX Pennkinetic Extended-Release Suspension is for oral use only.

Hydrocodone Polistirex: sulfonated styrenedivinylbenzene copolymer complex with 4,5α epoxy-3-methoxy-17-methylmorphinan-6-one.

Chlorpheniramine Polistirex: sulfonated styrene-divinylbenzene copolymer complex with 2-[p-chloro-α-[2-(dimethylamino)ethyl]-benzyl]pyridine.

Inactive Ingredients: Ascorbic acid, D&C Yellow No. 10, ethylcellulose, FD&C Yellow No. 6, flavor, high fructose corn syrup, methylparaben, polyethylene glycol 3350, polysorbate 80, pregelatinized starch, propylene glycol, propylparaben, purified water, sucrose, vegetable oil, xanthan gum.

CLINICAL PHARMACOLOGY

Hydrocodone is a semisynthetic narcotic antitussive and analgesic with multiple actions qualitatively similar to those of codeine. The precise mechanism of action of hydrocodone and other opiates is not known; however, hydrocodone is believed to act directly on the cough center. In excessive doses, hydrocodone, like other opium derivatives, will depress respiration. The effects of hydrocodone in therapeutic doses on the cardiovascular system are insignificant. Hydrocodone can produce miosis, euphoria, physical and psychological dependence.

Chlorpheniramine is an antihistamine drug (H₁ receptor antagonist) that also possesses anticholinergic and sedative activity. It prevents released histamine from dilating capillaries and causing edema of the respiratory mucosa.

Hydrocodone release from TUSSIONEX Pennkinetic Extended-Release Suspension is controlled by the Pennkinetic System, an extended-release drug delivery system which combines an ion-exchange polymer matrix with a diffusion rate-limiting permeable coating. Chlorpheniramine release is prolonged by use of an ion-exchange polymer system.

Following multiple dosing with TUSSIONEX Pennkinetic Extended-Release Suspension, hydrocodone mean (S.D.) peak plasma concentrations of 22.8 (5.9) ng/mL occurred at 3.4 hours. Chlorpheniramine mean (S.D.) peak plasma concentrations of 58.4 (14.7) ng/mL occurred at 6.3 hours following multiple dosing. Peak plasma levels obtained with an immediate-release syrup occurred at approximately 1.5 hours for hydrocodone and 2.8 hours for chlorpheniramine. The plasma half-lives of hydrocodone and chlorpheniramine have been reported to be approximately 4 and 16 hours, respectively.

INDICATIONS AND USAGE

TUSSIONEX Pennkinetic Extended-Release Suspension is indicated for relief of cough and upper respiratory symptoms associated with allergy or a cold.

CONTRAINDICATIONS

Known allergy or sensitivity to hydrocodone or chlorpheniramine.

WARNINGS

Respiratory Depression: As with all narcotics, TUSSIONEX Pennkinetic Extended-Release Suspension produces dose-related respiratory depression by directly acting on brain stem respiratory centers. Hydrocodone affects the center that controls respiratory rhythm, and may produce irregular and periodic breathing. Caution should be exercised when TUSSIONEX Pennkinetic Extended-Release Suspension is used postoperatively and in patients with pulmonary disease or whenever ventilatory function is depressed. If respiratory depression occurs, it may be antagonized by the use of naloxone hydrochloride and other supportive measures when indicated (see OVERDOSAGE).

Head Injury and Increased Intracranial Pressure: The respiratory depressant effects of narcotics and their capacity to elevate cerebrospinal fluid pressure may be markedly exaggerated in the presence of head injury, other intracranial lesions or a pre-existing increase in intracranial pressure. Furthermore, narcotics produce adverse reactions which may obscure the clinical course of patients with head injuries.

Acute Abdominal Conditions: The administration of narcotics may obscure the diagnosis or clinical course of patients with acute abdominal conditions.

Obstructive Bowel Disease: Chronic use of narcotics may result in obstructive bowel disease especially in patients with underlying intestinal motility disorder.

Pediatric Use: In pediatric patients, as well as adults, the respiratory center is sensitive to the depressant action of narcotic cough suppressants in a dose-dependent manner. Benefit to risk ratio should be carefully considered especially in pediatric patients with respiratory embarrassment (e.g., croup) (see PRECAUTIONS).

PRECAUTIONS

General: Caution is advised when prescribing this drug to patients with narrow-angle glaucoma, asthma or prostatic hypertrophy.

Special Risk Patients: As with any narcotic agent, TUSSIONEX Pennkinetic Extended-Release Suspension should be used with caution in elderly or debilitated patients and those with severe impairment of hepatic or renal function, hypothyroidism. Addison's disease, prostatic hypertrophy or urethral stricture. The usual precautions should be observed and the possibility of respiratory depression should be kept in mind.

Information for Patients: As with all narcotics, TUSSIONEX Pennkinetic Extended-Release Suspension may produce marked drowsiness and impair the mental and/or physical abilities required for the performance of potentially hazardous tasks such as driving a car or operating machinery; patients should be cautioned accordingly. TUSSIONEX Pennkinetic Extended-Release Suspension must not be diluted with fluids or mixed with other drugs as this may alter the resin-binding and change the absorption rate, possibly increasing the toxicity.

Keep out of the reach of children.

Cough Reflex: Hydrocodone suppresses the cough reflex; as with all narcotics, caution should be exercised when TUSSIONEX Pennkinetic Extended-Release Suspension is used postoperatively, and in patients with pulmonary disease.

Drug Interactions: Patients receiving narcotics, antihistaminics, antipsychotics, antianxiety agents or other CNS depressants (including alcohol) concomitantly with TUSSIONEX Pennkinetic Extended-Release Suspension may exhibit an additive CNS depression. When combined therapy is contemplated, the dose of one or both agents should be reduced.

The use of MAO inhibitors or tricyclic antidepressants with hydrocodone preparations may increase the effect of either the antidepressant or hydrocodone.

The concurrent use of other anticholinergics with hydrocodone may produce paralytic ileus.

Carcinogenesis, Mutagenesis, Impairment of Fertility: Carcinogenicity, mutagenicity and reproductive studies have not been conducted with TUSSIONEX Pennkinetic Extended-Release Suspension.

Pregnancy: Teratogenic Effects – Pregnancy Category C. Hydrocodone has been shown to be teratogenic in hamsters when given in doses 700 times the human dose. There are no adequate and well-controlled studies in pregnant women. TUSSIONEX Pennkinetic Extended-Release Suspension should be used during pregnancy only if the potential benefit justifies the potential risk to the fetus.

Nonteratogenic Effects: Babies born to mothers who have been taking opioids regularly prior to delivery will be physically dependent. The withdrawal signs include irritability and excessive crying, tremors, hyperactive reflexes, in-

creased respiratory rate, increased stools, sneezing, yawning, vomiting and fever. The intensity of the syndrome does not always correlate with the duration of maternal opioid use or dose.

Labor and Delivery: As with all narcotics, administration of TUSSIONEX Pennkinetic Extended-Release Suspension to the mother shortly before delivery may result in some degree of respiratory depression in the newborn, especially if higher doses are used.

Nursing Mothers: It is not known whether this drug is excreted in human milk. Because many drugs are excreted in human milk and because of the potential for serious adverse reactions in nursing infants from TUSSIONEX Pennkinetic Extended-Release Suspension, a decision should be made whether to discontinue nursing or to discontinue the drug, taking into account the importance of the drug to the mother.

Pediatric Use: Safety and effectiveness of TUSSIONEX Pennkinetic Extended-Release Suspension in pediatric patients under six have not been established.

ADVERSE REACTIONS

Central Nervous System: Sedation, drowsiness, mental clouding, lethargy, impairment of mental and physical performance, anxiety, fear, dysphoria, euphoria, dizziness, psychic dependence, mood changes.

Dermatologic System: Rash, pruritus.

Gastrointestinal System: Nausea and vomiting may occur; they are more frequent in ambulatory than in recumbent patients. Prolonged administration of TUSSIONEX Pennkinetic Extended-Release Suspension may produce constipation.

Genitourinary System: Ureteral spasm, spasm of vesicle sphincters and urinary retention have been reported with opiates.

Respiratory Depression: TUSSIONEX Pennkinetic Extended-Release Suspension may produce dose-related respiratory depression by acting directly on brain stem respiratory centers (see OVERDOSAGE).

Respiratory System: Dryness of the pharynx, occasional tightness of the chest.

DRUG ABUSE AND DEPENDENCE

TUSSIONEX Pennkinetic Extended-Release Suspension is a Schedule III narcotic. Psychic dependence, physical dependence and tolerance may develop upon repeated administration of narcotics; therefore, TUSSIONEX Pennkinetic Extended-Release Suspension should be prescribed and administered with caution. However, psychic dependence is unlikely to develop when TUSSIONEX Pennkinetic Extended-Release Suspension is used for a short time for the treatment of cough. Physical dependence, the condition in which continued administration of the drug is required to prevent the appearance of a withdrawal syndrome, assumes clinically significant proportions only after several weeks of continued oral narcotic use, although some mild degree of physical dependence may develop after a few days of narcotic therapy.

OVERDOSAGE

Signs and Symptoms: Serious overdosage with hydrocodone is characterized by respiratory depression (a decrease in respiratory rate and/or tidal volume, Cheyne-Stokes respiration, cyanosis), extreme somnolence progressing to stupor or coma, skeletal muscle flaccidity, cold and clammy skin, and sometimes bradycardia and hypotension. Although miosis is characteristic of narcotic overdose, mydriasis may occur in terminal narcosis or severe hypoxia. In severe overdosage apnea, circulatory collapse, cardiac arrest and death may occur. The manifestations of chlorpheniramine overdosage may vary from central nervous system depression to stimulation.

Treatment: Primary attention should be given to the reestablishment of adequate respiratory exchange through provision of a patient airway and the institution of assisted or controlled ventilation. The narcotic antagonist naloxone hydrochloride is a specific antidote for respiratory depression which may result from overdosage or unusual sensitivity to narcotics including hydrocodone. Therefore, an appropriate dose of naloxone hydrochloride should be administered, preferably by the intravenous route, simultaneously with efforts at respiratory resuscitation. Since the duration of action of hydrocodone in this formulation may exceed that of the antagonist, the patient should be kept under continued surveillance and repeated doses of the antagonist should be administered as needed to maintain adequate respiration. For further information, see full prescribing information for naloxone hydrochloride. An antagonist should not be adminisetered in the absence of clinically significant respiratory depression. Oxygen, intravenous fluids, vasopressors and other supportive measures should be employed as indicated. Gastric emptying may be useful in removing unabsorbed drug.

DOSAGE AND ADMINISTRATION

Shake well before using.

Adults: 1 teaspoonful (5 mL) every 12 hours; do not exceed 2 teaspoonfuls in 24 hours.

Children 6–12: 1/2 teaspoonful every 12 hours; **do not exceed 1 teaspoonfuls in 24 hours.**

Not recommended for children under 6 years of age (see PRECAUTIONS).

HOW SUPPLIED

TUSSIONEX Pennkinetic (hydrocodone polistirex and chlorpheniramine polistirex) Extended-Release Suspension is a gold-colored suspension.

NDC 53014-548-67 473 mL bottle
NDC 53014-548-91 900 mL bottle

Shake well. Dispense in a well-closed container. Store at 59°–86°F (15°–30°C).

CAUTION: Federal law prohibits dispensing without prescription.

MEDEVA PHARMACEUTICALS
Medeva Pharmaceuticals, Inc.
Rochester, NY 14623 USA
® Fisons BV
© 1996, Medeva Pharmaceuticals
Manufacturing, Inc.

Rev. 9/96
R240F

ZAROXOLYN® TABLETS ℞

[zar″ ox ′ uh-lin]
(metolazone tablets, USP)
R 241G
Rev. 4/97

DO NOT INTERCHANGE

DO NOT INTERCHANGE ZAROXOLYN TABLETS AND OTHER FORMULATIONS OF METOLAZONE THAT SHARE ITS SLOW AND INCOMPLETE BIOAVAILABILITY AND ARE NOT THERAPEUTICALLY EQUIVALENT AT THE SAME DOSES TO MYKROX® TABLETS, A MORE RAPIDLY AVAILABLE AND COMPLETELY BIOAVAILABLE METOLAZONE PRODUCT. FORMULATIONS BIOEQUIVALENT TO ZAROXOLYN AND FORMULATIONS BIOEQUIVALENT TO MYKROX SHOULD NOT BE INTERCHANGED FOR ONE ANOTHER.

DESCRIPTION

ZAROXOLYN Tablets (metolazone tablets, USP) for oral administration contain $2^1/_2$, 5 or 10 mg of metolazone, USP, a diuretic/saluretic/antihypertensive drug of the quinazoline class.

Metolazone has the molecular formula $C_{16}H_{16}ClN_3O_3S$, the chemical name 7-chloro-1,2,3,4-tetrahydro-2-methyl-3-(2-methylphenyl)-4-oxo-6- quinazolinesulfonamide and a molecular weight of 365.83. The structural formula is:

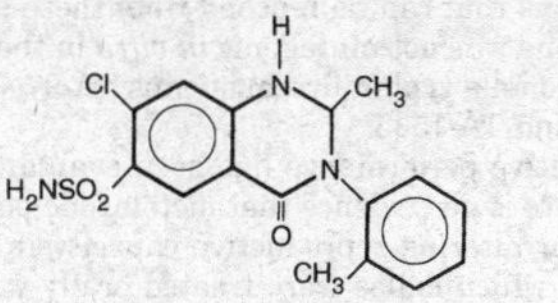

Metolazone is only sparingly soluble in water, but more soluble in plasma, blood, alkali and organic solvents.

Inactive Ingredients: magnesium stearate, microcrystalline cellulose and dye: $2^1/_2$ mg-D&C Red No. 33; 5 mg-FD&C Blue No. 2; 10 mg-D&C Yellow No. 10 and FD&C Yellow No. 6.

CLINICAL PHARMACOLOGY

ZAROXOLYN (metolazone) is a quinazoline diuretic, with properties generally similar to the thiazide diuretics. The actions of ZAROXOLYN result from interference with the renal tubular mechanism of electrolyte reabsorption. ZAROXOLYN acts primarily to inhibit sodium reabsorption at the cortical diluting site and to a lesser extent in the proximal convoluted tubule. Sodium and chloride ions are excreted in approximately equivalent amounts. The increased delivery of sodium to the distal tubular exchange site results in increased potassium excretion. ZAROXOLYN does not inhibit carbonic anhydrase. A proximal action of metolazone has been shown in humans by increased excretion of phosphate and magnesium ions and by a markedly increased fractional excretion of sodium in patients with severely compromised glomerular filtration. This action has been demonstrated in animals by micropuncture studies.

When ZAROXOLYN Tablets are given, diuresis and saluresis usually begin within one hour and may persist for 24 hours or more. For most patients, the duration of effect can be varied by adjusting the daily dose. High doses may prolong the effect. A single daily dose is recommended. When a desired therapeutic effect has been obtained, it may be possible to reduce dosage to a lower maintenance level.

The diuretic potency of ZAROXOLYN at maximum therapeutic dosage is approximately equal to thiazide diuretics. However, unlike thiazides, ZAROXOLYN may produce diuresis in patients with glomerular filtration rates below 20 mL/min.

ZAROXOLYN and furosemide administered concurrently have produced marked diuresis in some patients where edema or ascites was refractory to treatment with maximum recommended doses of these or other diuretics administered alone. The mechanism of this interaction is unknown (see WARNINGS and PRECAUTIONS, DRUG INTERACTIONS).

Maximum blood levels of metolazone are found approximately eight hours after dosing. A small fraction of metolazone is metabolized. Most of the drug is excreted in the unconverted form in the urine.

INDICATIONS AND USAGE

ZAROXOLYN is indicated for the treatment of salt and water retention including:

—edema accompanying congestive heart failure;

—edema accompanying renal diseases, including the nephrotic syndrome and states of diminished renal function.

ZAROXOLYN is also indicated for the treatment of hypertension, alone or in combination with other antihypertensive drugs of a different class. MYKROX Tablets, a more rapidly available form of metolazone, are intended for the treatment of new patients with mild to moderate hypertension. A dose titration is necessary if MYKROX Tablets are to be substituted for ZAROXOLYN in the treatment of hypertension. See package circular for MYKROX Tablets (Medeva).

Usage in Pregnancy

The routine use of diuretics in an otherwise healthy woman is inappropriate and exposes mother and fetus to unnecessary hazard. Diuretics do not prevent development of toxemia of pregnancy, and there is no evidence that they are useful in the treatment of developed toxemia.

Edema during pregnancy may arise from pathologic causes or from the physiologic and mechanical consequences of pregnancy. ZAROXOLYN is indicated in pregnancy when edema is due to pathologic causes, just as it is in the absence of pregnancy (see PRECAUTIONS). Dependent edema in pregnancy resulting from restriction of venous return by the expanded uterus is properly treated through elevation of the lower extremities and use of support hose; use of diuretics to lower intravascular volume in this case is illogical and unnecessary. There is hypervolemia during normal pregnancy which is harmful to neither the fetus nor the mother (in the absence of cardiovascular disease), but which is associated with edema, including generalized edema, in the majority of pregnant women. If this edema produces discomfort, increased recumbency will often provide relief. In rare instances, this edema may cause extreme discomfort which is not relieved by rest. In these cases, a short course of diuretics may be appropriate.

CONTRAINDICATIONS

Anuria, hepatic coma or precoma, known allergy or hypersensitivity to metolazone.

WARNINGS

Rapid Onset Hyponatremia

Rarely, the rapid onset of severe hyponatremia and/or hypokalemia has been reported following initial doses of thiazide and non-thiazide diuretics. When symptoms consistent with severe electrolyte imbalance appear rapidly, drug should be discontinued and supportive measures should be initiated immediately. Parenteral electrolytes may be required. Appropriateness of therapy with this class of drugs should be carefully reevaluated.

Hypokalemia

Hypokalemia may occur with consequent weakness, cramps, and cardiac dysrhythmias. Serum potassium should be determined at regular intervals, and dose reduction, potassium supplementation or addition of a potassium-sparing diuretic instituted whenever indicated. Hypokalemia is a particular hazard in patients who are digitalized or who have or have had a ventricular arrhythmia; dangerous or fatal arrhythmias may be precipitated. Hypokalemia is dose related.

Concomitant Therapy

Lithium

In general, diuretics should not be given concomitantly with lithium because they reduce its renal clearance and add a high risk of lithium toxicity. Read prescribing information for lithium preparations before use of such concomitant therapy.

Continued on next page

Information on the Medeva Pharmaceuticals, Inc. products listed on these pages contains the full prescribing information from product circulars in use as of July 1998. For further information, please consult the package insert currently accompanying the product.

Zaroxolyn—Cont.

Furosemide: Unusually large or prolonged losses of fluids and electrolytes may result when ZAROXOLYN is administered concomitantly to patients receiving furosemide (see PRECAUTIONS, DRUG INTERACTIONS).

Other Antihypertensive Drugs: When ZAROXOLYN is used with other antihypertensive drugs, particular care must be taken to avoid excessive reduction of blood pressure, especially during initial therapy.

Cross-Allergy

Cross-allergy, while not reported to date, theoretically may occur when ZAROXOLYN is given to patients known to be allergic to sulfonamide-derived drugs, thiazides, or quinethazone.

Sensitivity Reactions: Sensitivity reactions (e.g., angioedema, bronchospasm) may occur with or without a history of allergy or bronchial asthma and may occur with the first dose of ZAROXOLYN.

PRECAUTIONS

DO NOT INTERCHANGE

DO NOT INTERCHANGE ZAROXOLYN TABLETS AND OTHER FORMULATIONS OF METOLAZONE THAT SHARE ITS SLOW AND INCOMPLETE BIOAVAILABILITY AND ARE NOT THERAPEUTICALLY EQUIVALENT AT THE SAME DOSES TO MYKROX TABLETS, A MORE RAPIDLY AVAILABLE AND COMPLETELY BIOAVAILABLE METOLAZONE PRODUCT. FORMULATIONS BIOEQUIVALENT TO ZAROXOLYN AND FORMULATIONS BIOEQUIVALENT TO MYKROX SHOULD NOT BE INTERCHANGED FOR ONE ANOTHER.

GENERAL:

Fluid and Electrolytes

All patients receiving therapy with ZAROXOLYN Tablets should have serum electrolyte measurements done at appropriate intervals and be observed for clinical signs of fluid and/or electrolyte imbalance: namely, hyponatremia, hypochloremic alkalosis, and hypokalemia. In patients with severe edema accompanying cardiac failure or renal disease, a low-salt syndrome may be produced, especially with hot weather and a low-salt diet. Serum and urine electrolyte determinations are particularly important when the patient has protracted vomiting, severe diarrhea, or is receiving parenteral fluids. Warning signs of imbalance are: dryness of mouth, thirst, weakness, lethargy, drowsiness, restlessness, muscle pains or cramps, muscle fatigue, hypotension, oliguria, tachycardia, and gastrointestinal disturbances such as nausea and vomiting. Hyponatremia may occur at any time during long term therapy and, on rare occasions, may be life threatening.

The risk of hypokalemia is increased when larger doses are used, when diuresis is rapid, when severe liver disease is present, when corticosteroids are given concomitantly, when oral intake is inadequate or when excess potassium is being lost extrarenally, such as with vomiting or diarrhea.

Thiazide-like diuretics have been shown to increase the urinary excretion of magnesium; this may result in hypomagnesemia.

Glucose Tolerance

Metolazone may raise blood glucose concentrations possibly causing hyperglycemia and glycosuria in patients with diabetes or latent diabetes.

Hyperuricemia

ZAROXOLYN regularly causes an increase in serum uric acid and can occasionally precipitate gouty attacks even in patients without a prior history of them.

Azotemia

Azotemia, presumably prerenal azotemia, may be precipitated during the administration of ZAROXOLYN. If azotemia and oliguria worsen during treatment of patients with severe renal disease, ZAROXOLYN should be discontinued.

Renal Impairment

Use caution when administering ZAROXOLYN Tablets to patients with severely impaired renal function. As most of the drug is excreted by the renal route, accumulation may occur.

Orthostatic Hypotension

Orthostatic hypotension may occur; this may be potentiated by alcohol, barbiturates, narcotics, or concurrent therapy with other antihypertensive drugs.

Hypercalcemia

Hypercalcemia may infrequently occur with metolazone, especially in patients taking high doses of vitamin D or with high bone turnover states, and may signify hidden hyperparathyroidism. Metolazone should be discontinued before tests for parathyroid function are performed.

Systemic Lupus Erythematosus

Thiazide diuretics have exacerbated or activated systemic lupus erythematosus and this possibility should be considered with ZAROXOLYN Tablets.

INFORMATION FOR PATIENTS: Patients should be informed of possible adverse effects, advised to take the medication as directed and promptly report any possible adverse reactions to the treating physician.

DRUG INTERACTIONS:

Diuretics

Furosemide and probably other loop diuretics given concomitantly with metolazone can cause unusually large or prolonged losses of fluid and electrolytes (see WARNINGS).

Other Antihypertensives

When ZAROXOLYN Tablets are used with other antihypertensive drugs, care must be taken, especially during initial therapy. Dosage adjustments of other antihypertensives may be necessary.

Alcohol, Barbiturates, and Narcotics

The hypotensive effects of these drugs may be potentiated by the volume contraction that may be associated with metolazone therapy.

Digitalis Glycosides

Diuretic-induced hypokalemia can increase the sensitivity of the myocardium to digitialis. Serious arrhythmias can result.

Corticosteroids or ACTH

May increase the risk of hypokalemia and increase salt and water retention.

Lithium

Serum lithium levels may increase (see WARNINGS).

Curariform Drugs

Diuretic-induced hypokalemia may enhance neuromuscular blocking effects of curariform drugs (such as tubocurarine) — the most serious effect would be respiratory depression which could proceed to apnea. Accordingly, it may be advisable to discontinue ZAROXOLYN Tablets three days before elective surgery.

Salicylates and Other Non-Steroidal Anti-Inflammatory Drugs

May decrease the antihypertensive effects of ZAROXOLYN Tablets.

Sympathomimetics

Metolazone may decrease arterial responsiveness to norepinephrine, but this diminution is not sufficient to preclude effectiveness of the pressor agent for therapeutic use.

Insulin and Oral Antidiabetic Agents

See Glucose Tolerance under PRECAUTIONS, GENERAL.

Methenamine

Efficacy may be decreased due to urinary alkalizing effect of metolazone.

Anticoagulants: Metolazone, as well as other thiazide-like diuretics, may affect the hypoprothrombinemic response to anticoagulants; dosage adjustments may be necessary.

DRUG/LABORATORY TEST INTERACTIONS: None reported.

CARCINOGENESIS, MUTAGENESIS, IMPAIRMENT OF FERTILITY: Mice and rats administered metolazone 5 days/week for up to 18 and 24 months, respectively, at daily doses of 2, 10 and 50 mg/kg, exhibited no evidence of a tumorigenic effect of the drug. The small number of animals examined histologically and poor survival in the mice limit the conclusions that can be reached from these studies.

Metolazone was not mutagenic *in vitro* in the Ames Test using Salmonella typhimurium strains TA-97, TA-98, TA-100, TA-102 and TA-1535.

Reproductive performance has been evaluated in mice and rats. There is no evidence that metolazone possesses the potential for altering reproductive capacity in mice. In a rat study, in which males were treated orally with metolazone at doses of 2, 10 and 50 mg/kg for 127 days prior to mating with untreated females, an increased number of resorption sites was observed in dams mated with males from the 50 mg/kg group. In addition, the birth weight of offspring was decreased and the pregnancy rate was reduced in dams mated with males from the 10 and 50 mg/kg groups.

PREGNANCY:

Teratogenic Effects—Pregnancy Category B.

Reproduction studies performed in mice, rabbits and rats treated during the appropriate period of gestation at doses up to 50 mg/kg/day have revealed no evidence of harm to the fetus due to metolazone. There are, however, no adequate and well-controlled studies in pregnant women. Because animal reproduction studies are not always predictive of human response, ZAROXOLYN Tablets should be used during pregnancy only if clearly needed. Metolazone crosses the placental barrier and appears in cord blood.

Non-Teratogenic Effects

The use of ZAROXOLYN Tablets in pregnant women requires that the anticipated benefit be weighed against possible hazards to the fetus. These hazards include fetal or neonatal jaundice, thrombocytopenia, and possibly other adverse reactions which have occurred in the adult. It is not known what effect the use of the drug during pregnancy has on the later growth, development and functional maturation of the child. No such effects have been reported with metolazone.

LABOR AND DELIVERY: Based on clinical studies in which women received metolazone in late pregnancy until the time of delivery, there is no evidence that the drug has any adverse effects on the normal course of labor or delivery.

NURSING MOTHERS: Metolazone appears in breast milk. Because of the potential for serious adverse reactions in nursing infants from metolazone, a decision should be made whether to discontinue nursing or to discontinue the drug, taking into account the importance of the drug to the mother.

PEDIATRIC USE: Safety and effectiveness in pediatric patients have not been established and such use is not recommended.

ADVERSE REACTIONS

ZAROXOLYN is usually well tolerated, and most reported adverse reactions have been mild and transient. Many ZAROXOLYN related adverse reactions represent extensions of its expected pharmacologic activity and can be attributed to either its antihypertensive action or its renal/ metabolic actions. The following adverse reactions have been reported. Several are single or comparably rare occurrences. Adverse reactions are listed in decreasing order of severity within body systems.

Cardiovascular: Chest pain/discomfort, orthostatic hypotension, excessive volume depletion, hemoconcentration, venous thrombosis, palpitations.

Central and Peripheral Nervous System: Syncope, neuropathy, vertigo, paresthesias, psychotic depression, impotence, dizziness/light-headedness, drowsiness, fatigue, weakness, restlessness (sometimes resulting in insomnia), headache.

Dermatologic/Hypersensitivity: Necrotizing angiitis (cutaneous vasculitis), purpura, dermatitis (photosensitivity), urticaria and skin rashes.

Gastrointestinal: Hepatitis, intrahepatic cholestatic jaundice, pancreatitis, vomiting, nausea, epigastric distress, diarrhea, constipation, anorexia, abdominal bloating.

Hematologic: Aplastic/hypoplastic anemia, agranulocytosis, leukopenia.

Metabolic: Hypokalemia, hyponatremia, hyperuricemia, hypochloremia, hypochloremic alkalosis, hyperglycemia, glycosuria, increase in serum urea nitrogen (BUN) or creatinine, hypophosphatemia, hypomagnesemia, hypercalcemia.

Musculoskeletal: Joint pain, acute gouty attacks, muscle cramps or spasm.

Other: Transient blurred vision, chills.

In addition, adverse reactions reported with similar antihypertensive-diuretics, but which have not been reported to date for ZAROXOLYN include: bitter taste, dry mouth, sialadenitis, xanthopsia, respiratory distress (including pneumonitis), thrombocytopenia and anaphylactic reactions. These reactions should be considered as possible occurrences with clinical usage of ZAROXOLYN.

Whenever adverse reactions are moderate or severe, ZAROXOLYN dosage should be reduced or therapy withdrawn.

OVERDOSAGE

Intentional overdosage has been reported rarely with metolazone and similar diuretic drugs.

Signs and Symptoms

Orthostatic hypotension, dizziness, drowsiness, syncope, electrolyte abnormalities, hemoconcentration and hemodynamic changes due to plasma volume depletion may occur. In some instances depressed respiration may be observed. At high doses, lethargy of varying degree may progress to coma within a few hours. The mechanism of CNS depression with thiazide overdosage is unknown. Also, GI irritation and hypermotility may occur. Temporary elevation of BUN has been reported, especially in patients with impairment of renal function. Serum electrolyte changes and cardiovascular and renal function should be closely monitored.

Treatment

There is no specific antidote available but immediate evacuation of stomach contents is advised. Dialysis is not likely to be effective. Care should be taken when evacuating the gastric contents to prevent aspiration, especially in the stuporous or comatose patient. Supportive measures should be initiated as required to maintain hydration, electrolyte balance, respiration, and cardiovascular and renal function.

DOSAGE AND ADMINISTRATION

Effective dosage of ZAROXOLYN should be individualized according to indication and patient response. A single daily dose is recommended. Therapy with ZAROXOLYN should be titrated to gain an initial therapeutic response and to determine the minimal dose possible to maintain the desired therapeutic response.

Usual Single Daily Dosage Schedules

Suitable initial dosages will usually fall in the ranges given.

Edema of cardiac failure:

ZAROXOLYN 5 to 20 mg once daily.

Edema of renal disease:

ZAROXOLYN 5 to 20 mg once daily.

Mild to moderate essential hypertension:

ZAROXOLYN $2^1/_2$ to 5 mg once daily.

New patients—MYKROX Tablets (metolazone tablets, USP) (see MYKROX package circular). If considered desirable to switch patients currently on ZAROXOLYN to MYKROX, the dose should be determined by titration starting at one tablet ($^1/_2$ mg) once daily and increasing to two tablets (1 mg) once daily if needed.

Treatment of Edematous States

The time interval required for the initial dosage to produce an effect may vary. Diuresis and saluresis usually begin within one hour and persist for 24 hours or longer. When a desired therapeutic effect has been obtained, it may be advisable to reduce the dose if possible. The daily dose depends on the severity of the patient's condition, sodium intake and responsiveness. A decision to change the daily dose should be based on the results of thorough clinical and laboratory evaluations. If antihypertensive drugs or diuretics are given concurrently with ZAROXOLYN, more careful dosage adjustment may be necessary. For patients who tend to experience paroxysmal nocturnal dyspnea, it may be advisable to employ a larger dose to ensure prolongation of diuresis and saluresis for a full 24-hour period.

Treatment of Hypertension

The time interval required for the initial dosage regimen to show effect may vary from three or four days to three to six weeks in the treatment of elevated blood pressure. Doses should be adjusted at appropriate intervals to achieve maximum therapeutic effect.

HOW SUPPLIED

ZAROXOLYN TABLETS (metolazone tablets, USP) are shallow biconvex, round tablets, and are available in three strengths: $2^1/_2$ mg, pink, debossed "ZAROXOLYN" on one side, and "$2^1/_2$" on reverse side.

NDC 53014-975-71	Bottle of 100's
NDC 53014-975-90	Bottle of 1000's
NDC 53014-975-72	Carton of 100's, unit dose

5 mg. blue, debossed "ZAROXOLYN" on one side, and "5" on reverse side.

NDC 53014-850-71	Bottle of 100's
NDC 53014-850-90	Bottle of 1000's
NDC 53014-850-72	Carton of 100's, unit dose

10 mg, yellow, debossed "ZAROXOLYN" on one side, and "10" on reverse side.

NDC 53014-835-71	Bottle of 100's
NDC 53014-835-90	Bottle of 1000's
NDC 53014-835-72	Carton of 100's, unit dose

Store at room temperature. Dispense in a tight, light-resistant container. Keep out of the reach of children.

CAUTION: Federal law prohibits dispensing without prescription.

MEDEVA PHARMACEUTICALS
Medeva Pharmaceuticals, Inc.
Rochester, NY 14623 USA
® Fisons Investments Inc.
© 1997, Medeva Pharmaceuticals Manufacturing, Inc.

Rev. 4/97
R 241G

EDUCATIONAL MATERIAL

For educational information, please write to Medeva Pharmaceuticals, Inc., PO Box 1766, Rochester, NY 14603.

MEDICIS THE DERMATOLOGY COMPANY®

**4343 EAST CAMELBACK RD
PHOENIX, AZ 85018**

For Medical Information Contact:
Generally:
Medical Affairs Department
(602) 808-8800
FAX: (602) 808-0822

In Emergencies:
(602) 808-8800

BENZASHAVE® 5%
**Benzoyl Peroxide, USP 5%
Medicated Shave Cream**

℞

BENZASHAVE® 10%
**Benzoyl Peroxide, USP 10%
Medicated Shave Cream**

℞

DESCRIPTION

BENZASHAVE 5% and BENZASHAVE 10% Benzoyl Peroxide, USP (5% and 10%) are topical shave cream preparations for use in the treatment of pseudofolliculitis (*p. barbae;* ingrown hairs, razor bumps) and acne vulgaris associated with shaving. Benzoyl peroxide is an oxidizing agent which possesses antibacterial properties and is classified as a keratolytic agent. Benzoyl peroxide ($C_{14}H_{10}O_4$) is represented by the following chemical structure:

INGREDIENTS

BENZASHAVE 5% & 10% contain: ACTIVES: Benzoyl Peroxide, USP, 5% or 10%; INACTIVES: Stearic Acid, Mineral Oil, Triethanolamine, Diisopropyl Dimerate, PEG-15 Cocamine, Carbomer 940, Aloe Vera, Purified Water; PRESERVATIVES: Diazolidinyl Urea, Methylparaben and Propylparaben.

CLINICAL PHARMACOLOGY

The mechanism of action of benzoyl peroxide has not been determined but may be related to its antibacterial activity against *Propionibacterium acnes* and its ability to cause drying and peeling. Benzoyl peroxide reduces the concentration of free fatty acids in the sebum. Little is known about the percutaneous penetration, metabolism and excretion of benzoyl peroxide, although it is likely that benzoic acid is a major metabolite. There is no evidence of systemic toxicity caused by benzoyl peroxide in humans.

INDICATIONS AND USAGE

These products are indicated for the topical treatment of acne vulgaris.

CONTRAINDICATIONS

These products are contraindicated in patients with a history of hypersensitivity to any of the components of the preparations.

PRECAUTIONS

General: For external use only. Not for ophthalmic use. If severe irritation develops, discontinue use and institute appropriate therapy. After the reaction clears, treatment may often be resumed with less frequent application. This preparation should not be used in or near the eyes or on mucous membranes.

Information for Patients: Avoid contact with eyes, eyelids, lips and mucous membranes. If accidental contact occurs, rinse with water. May bleach hair and colored fabrics. If excessive irritation develops, discontinue use and consult your physician.

Carcinogensis, Mutagenesis, Impairment of Fertility: Data from several studies using mice known to be highly susceptible to cancer suggest that benzoyl peroxide acts as a tumor promotor. The clinical significance of these findings to humans is unknown.

Pregnancy: *Pregnancy Category C:* Animal reproduction studies have not been conducted with benzoyl peroxide. It is also *not* known whether benzoyl peroxide can cause fetal harm when administered to a pregnant woman or can affect reproduction capacity. Benzoyl peroxide should be used by a pregnant woman only if clearly needed. There are no data available on the effect of benzoyl peroxide on the growth, development and functional maturation of the unborn child.

Nursing Mothers: It is not known whether this drug is excreted in human milk. Because many drugs are excreted in human milk, caution should be exercised when benzoyl peroxide is administered to a nursing woman.

Pediatric Use: Safety and effectiveness in children have not been established.

ADVERSE REACTIONS

Allergic contact dermatitis has been reported with topical benzoyl peroxide therapy.

DOSAGE AND ADMINISTRATION

Wet area to be shaved. Apply a small amount of BENZASHAVE with fingertips. Gently rub over entire area and shave.

HOW SUPPLIED

BENZASHAVE® Benzoyl Peroxide, USP (5%), 4 oz (113.4 g) tube, NDC 99207-530-04.
BENZASHAVE® Benzoyl Peroxide, USP (10%), 4 oz (113.4 g) tube, NDC 99207-540-04.
Keep out of reach of children.
Store at Controlled Room Temperature 15°–30°C (59°–86°F).
For external use only. Not for ophthalmic use.
Lot number and expiration date on package.

CAUTION

Federal law prohibits dispensing without prescription.
Manufactured specially for:
MEDICIS THE DERMATOLOGY COMPANY®
Phoenix, AZ 85018
by: Zenith Goldline Dermatologicals, Inc.
Syosset, NY 11791

DYNACIN®

℞

[dī 'nă-cən]
**(MINOCYCLINE
HCl CAPSULES, USP)**

DESCRIPTION

Minocycline hydrochloride, a semisynthetic derivative of tetracycline, is [4S-(4α, 4aα, 5aα, 12aα)]-4,7-bis(dimethylamino) -1,4,4a,5,5a,6,11,12a -octahydro -3,10,12,12a -tetrahydroxy-1,11-dioxo-2-naphthacenecarboxamide monohydrochloride. The structural formula is represented below:

$C_{23}H_{27}N_3O_7 \cdot HCl$ M.W. 493.94

Each minocycline hydrochloride capsule for oral administration contains the equivalent of 50 mg or 100 mg of minocycline. In addition each capsule contains the following inactive ingredients: magnesium stearate and starch (corn). The 50 mg and 100 mg capsule shells contain: gelatin, silicon dioxide, sodium lauryl sulfate and titanium dioxide. The 100 mg capsule shell also contains: black iron oxide.

CLINICAL PHARMACOLOGY

Following oral administration of minocycline hydrochloride capsules, absorption from the gastrointestinal tract is rapid. Maximum serum concentrations following a single dose of minocycline hydrochloride to normal fasting adult volunteers were attained in 1 to 4 hours. The serum half-life in normal volunteers ranges from approximately 11 hours to 22 hours.

When minocycline hydrochloride capsules were given concomitantly with a meal which included dairy products, the extent of absorption of minocycline hydrochloride capsules was not noticably influenced. The peak plasma concentrations were slightly decreased and delayed by one hour when administered with food, compared to dosing under fasting conditions.

In previous studies with other minocycline dosage forms, the minocycline serum half-life ranged from 11 to 16 hours in 7 patients with hepatic dysfunction, and from 18 to 69 hours in 5 patients with renal dysfunction. The urinary and fecal recovery of minocycline when administered to 12 normal volunteers is one-half to one-third that of other tetracyclines.

Microbiology: The tetracyclines are primarily bacteriostatic and are thought to exert their antimicrobial effect by the inhibition of protein synthesis. The tetracyclines, including minocycline, have similar antimicrobial spectra of activity against a wide range of gram-positive and gram-negative organisms. Cross-resistance of these organisms to tetracyclines is common.

While *in vitro* studies have demonstrated the susceptibility of most strains of the following microorganisms, clinical efficacy for infections other than those included in the **INDICATIONS AND USAGE** section has not been documented.

Gram-Negative Bacteria
Bartonella bacilliformis
Brucella species
Campylobacter fetus
Francisella tularensis
Haemophilus ducreyi
Haemophilus influenzae
Listeria monocytogenes
Neisseria gonorrhoeae
Vibrio cholerae
Yersinia pestis

Because many strains of the following groups of gram-negative microorganisms have been shown to be resistant to tetracyclines, culture and susceptibility tests are especially recommended:

Acinetobacter species
Bacteroides species
Enterobacter aerogenes
Escherichia coli
Klebsiella species
Shigella species

Gram-Positive Bacteria
Because many strains of the following groups of gram-positive microorganisms have been shown to be resistant to tet-

Continued on next page

Dynacin—Cont.

racyclines, culture and susceptibility testing are especially recommended. Up to 44 percent of *Streptococcus pyogenes* strains have been found to be resistant to tetracycline drugs. Therefore, tetracyclines should not be used for streptococcal disease unless the organism has been demonstrated to be susceptible.

Alpha-hemolytic streptococci (viridans group)
Streptococcus pneumoniae
Streptococcus pyogenes

Other Microorganisms
Actinomyces species
Bacillus anthracis
Balantidium coli
Borrelia recurrentis
Chlamydia psittaci
Chlamydia trachomatis
Clostridium species
Entamoeba species
Fusobacterium fusiforme
Propionibacterium acnes
Treponema pallidum
Treponema pertenue
Ureaplasma urealyticum

Susceptibility Tests: *Diffusion Techniques:* The use of antibiotic disk susceptibility test methods which measure zone diameter give an accurate estimation of susceptibility of microorganisms to minocycline. One such standard procedure[1] has been recommended for use with disks for testing antimicrobials. Either the 30 mcg tetracycline-class disk or the 30 mcg minocycline disk should be used for the determination of the susceptibility of microorganisms to minocycline. With this type of procedure a report of "susceptible" from the laboratory indicates that the infecting organism is likely to respond to therapy. A report of "intermediate susceptibility" suggests that the organism would be susceptible if a high dosage is used or if the infection is confined to tissues and fluids (e.g., urine) in which high antibiotic levels are attained. A report of "resistant" indicates that the infecting organism is not likely to respond to therapy. With either the tetracycline-class disk or the minocycline disk, zone sizes of 19 mm or greater indicate susceptibility, zone sizes of 14 mm or less indicate resistance, and zone sizes of 15 to 18 mm indicate intermediate susceptibility.

Standardized procedures require the use of laboratory control organisms. The 30 mcg tetracycline disk should give zone diameters between 19 and 28 mm for *Staphylococcus aureus* ATCC 25923 and between 18 and 25 mm for *Escherichia coli* ATCC 25922. The 30 mcg minocycline disk should give zone diameters between 25 and 30 mm for *S aureus* ATCC 25923 and between 19 and 25 mm for *E coli* ATCC 25922.

Dilution Techniques: When using the NCCLS agar dilution or broth dilution (including microdilution) method[2] or equivalent, a bacterial isolate may be considered susceptible if the MIC (minimal inhibitory concentration) of minocycline is 4 mcg/mL or less. Organisms are considered resistant if the MIC is 16 mcg/mL or greater. Organisms with an MIC value of less than 16 mcg/mL but greater than 4 mcg/mL are expected to be susceptible if a high dosage is used or if the infection is confined to tissues and fluids (e.g., urine) in which high antibiotic levels are attained.

As with standard diffusion methods, dilution procedures require the use of laboratory control organisms. Standard tetracycline or minocycline powder should give MIC values of 0.25 mcg/mL to 1.0 mcg/mL for *S aureus* ATCC 25923, and 1.0 mcg/mL to 4.0 mcg/mL for *E coli* ATCC 25922.

INDICATIONS AND USAGE

Minocycline Hydrochloride Capsules are indicated in the treatment of the following infections due to susceptible strains of the designated microorganisms:

Rocky Mountain spotted fever, typhus fever and the typhus group, Q fever, rickettsialpox and tick fevers caused by Rickettsiae

Respiratory tract infections caused by *Mycoplasma pneumoniae*

Lymphogranuloma venereum caused by *Chlamydia trachomatis*

Psittacosis (Ornithosis) due to *Chlamydia psittaci*

Trachoma caused by *Chlamydia trachomatis,* although the infectious agent is not always eliminated, as judged by immunofluorescence

Inclusion conjunctivitis caused by *Chlamydia trachomatis*

Nongonococcal urethritis in adults caused by *Ureaplasma urealyticum* or *Chlamydia trachomatis*

Relapsing fever due to *Borrelia recurrentis*

Chancroid caused by *Haemophilus ducreyi*

Plague due to *Yersinia pestis*

Tularemia due to *Francisella tularensis*

Cholera caused by *Vibrio cholerae*

Campylobacter fetus infections caused by *Campylobacter fetus*

Brucellosis due to *Brucella* species (in conjunction with streptomycin)

Bartonellosis due to *Bartonella bacilliformis*

Granuloma inguinale caused by *Calymmatobacterium granulomatis*

Minocycline is indicated for treatment of infections caused by the following gram-negative microorganisms, when bacteriologic testing indicates appropriate susceptibility to the drug:
Escherichia coli
Enterobacter aerogenes
Shigella species
Acinetobacter species

Respiratory tract infections caused by *Haemophilus influenzae*

Respiratory tract and urinary tract infections caused by *Klebsiella* species

Minocycline hydrochloride capsules are indicated for the treatment of infections caused by the following gram-positive microorganisms when bacteriologic testing indicates appropriate susceptibility to the drug:

Upper respiratory tract infections caused by *Streptococcus pneumoniae*

Skin and skin structure infections caused by *Staphylococcus aureus.* (Note: Minocycline is not the drug of choice in the treatment of any type of staphylococcal infection.)

Uncomplicated urethritis in men due to *Neisseria gonorrhoeae* and for the treatment of other gonococcal infections when penicillin is contraindicated .

When penicillin is contraindicated, minocycline is an alternative drug in the treatment of the following infections:

Infections in women caused by *Neisseria gonorrhoeae*

Syphilis caused by *Treponema pallidum*

Yaws caused by *Treponema pertenue*

Listeriosis due to *Listeria monocytogenes*

Anthrax due to *Bacillus anthracis*

Vincent's infection caused by *Fusobacterium fusiforme*

Actinomycosis caused by *Actinomyces israelii*

Infections caused by *Clostridium* species

In *acute intestinal amebiasis,* minocycline may be a useful adjunct to amebicides.

In severe acne, minocycline may be useful adjunctive therapy.

Oral minocycline is indicated in the treatment of asymptomatic carriers of *Neisseria meningitidis* to eliminate meningococci from the nasopharynx. In order to preserve the usefulness of minocycline in the treatment of asymptomatic meningococcal carrier, diagnostic laboratory procedures, including serotyping and susceptibility testing, should be performed to establish the carrier state and the correct treatment. It is recommended that the prophylactic use of minocycline be reserved for situations in which the risk of meningococcal meningitis is high.

Oral minocycline is not indicated for the treatment of meningococcal infection.

Although no controlled clinical efficacy studies have been conducted, limited clinical data show that oral minocycline hydrochloride has been used successfully in the treatment of infections caused by *Mycobacterium marinum.*

CONTRAINDICATIONS

This drug is contraindicated in persons who have shown hypersensitivity to any of the tetracyclines.

WARNINGS

MINOCYCLINE, LIKE OTHER TETRACYCLINE-CLASS ANTIBIOTICS, CAN CAUSE FETAL HARM WHEN ADMINISTERED TO A PREGNANT WOMAN. IF ANY TETRACYCLINE IS USED DURING PREGNANCY OR IF THE PATIENT BECOMES PREGNANT WHILE TAKING THESE DRUGS, THE PATIENT SHOULD BE APPRISED OF THE POTENTIAL HAZARD TO THE FETUS. THE USE OF DRUGS OF THE TETRACYCLINE CLASS DURING TOOTH DEVELOPMENT (LAST HALF OF PREGNANCY, INFANCY, AND CHILDHOOD TO THE AGE OF 8 YEARS) MAY CAUSE PERMANENT DISCOLORATION OF THE TEETH (YELLOW-GRAY-BROWN).

This adverse reaction is more common during long-term use of the drug but has been observed following repeated short-term courses. Enamel hypoplasia has also been reported. TETRACYCLINE DRUGS, THEREFORE, SHOULD NOT BE USED DURING TOOTH DEVELOPMENT UNLESS OTHER DRUGS ARE NOT LIKELY TO BE EFFECTIVE OR ARE CONTRAINDICATED.

All tetracyclines form a stable calcium complex in any bone-forming tissue. A decrease in fibula growth rate has been observed in young animals (rats and rabbits) given oral tetracycline in doses of 25 mg/kg every six hours. This reaction was shown to be reversible when the drug was discontinued. Results of animal studies indicate that tetracyclines cross the placenta, are found in fetal tissues, and can have toxic effects on the developing fetus (often related to retardation of skeletal development). Evidence of embryotoxicity has been noted in animals treated early in pregnancy.

The anti-anabolic action of the tetracyclines may cause an increase in BUN. While this is not a problem in those with normal renal function, in patients with significantly impaired function, higher serum levels of tetracycline may lead to azotemia, hyperphosphatemia, and acidosis. If renal impairment exists, even usual oral or parenteral doses may lead to excessive systemic accumulations of the drug and possible liver toxicity. Under such conditions, lower than usual total doses are indicated, and if therapy is prolonged, serum level determinations of the drug may be advisable.

Photosensitivity manifested by an exaggerated sunburn reaction has been observed in some individuals taking tetracyclines. This has been reported rarely with minocycline. Central nervous system side effects including lightheadedness, dizziness, or vertigo have been reported with minocycline therapy.

Patients who experience these symptoms should be cautioned about driving vehicles or using hazardous machinery while on minocycline therapy. These symptoms may disappear during therapy and usually disappear rapidly when the drug is discontinued.

PRECAUTIONS

General: As with other antibiotic preparations, use of this drug may result in overgrowth of nonsusceptible organisms, including fungi. If superinfection occurs, the antibiotic should be discontinued and appropriate therapy instituted.

Pseudotumor cerebri (benign intracranial hypertension) in adults has been associated with the use of tetracyclines. The usual clinical manifestations are headache and blurred vision. Bulging fontanels have been associated with the use of tetracyclines in infants. While both of these conditions and related symptoms usually resolve after discontinuation of tetracycline, the possibility for permanent sequelae exists. Incision and drainage or other surgical procedures should be performed in conjunction with antibiotic therapy when indicated.

Information for Patients: Photosensitivity manifested by an exaggerated sunburn reaction has been observed in some individuals taking tetracyclines. Patients apt to be exposed to direct sunlight or ultraviolet light should be advised that this reaction can occur with tetracycline drugs, and treatment should be discontinued at the first evidence of skin erythema. This reaction has been reported rarely with use of minocycline.

Patients who experience central nervous system symptoms (see **WARNINGS**) should be cautioned about driving vehicles or using hazardous machinery while on minocycline therapy.

Concurrent use of tetracycline may render oral contraceptives less effective (see **Drug Interactions**).

Laboratory Tests: In venereal disease when coexistent syphilis is suspected, a dark-field examination should be done before treatment is started and the blood serology repeated monthly for at least four months.

In long-term therapy, periodic laboratory evaluations of organ systems, including hematopoietic, renal, and hepatic studies should be performed.

Drug Interactions: Because tetracyclines have been shown to depress plasma prothrombin activity, patients who are on anticoagulant therapy may require downward adjustment of their anticoagulant dosage.

Since bacteriostatic drugs may interfere with the bactericidal action of penicillin, it is advisable to avoid giving tetracycline-class drugs in conjunction with penicillin.

Absorption of tetracyclines is impaired by antacids containing aluminum, calcium or magnesium, and iron-containing preparations. The concurrent use of tetracycline and methoxyflurane has been reported to result in fatal renal toxicity.

Concurrent use of tetracyclines may render oral contraceptives less effective.

Drug/Laboratory Test Interactions: False elevations of urinary catecholamine levels may occur due to interference with the fluorescence test.

Carcinogenesis, Mutagenesis, Impairment of Fertility: Dietary administration of minocycline in long-term tumorigenicity studies in rats resulted in evidence of thyroid tumor production. Minocycline has also been found to produce thyroid hyperplasia in rats and dogs. In addition, there has been evidence of oncogenic activity in rats in studies with a related antibiotic, oxytetracycline (i.e., adrenal and pituitary tumors). Likewise, although mutagenicity studies of minocycline have not been conducted, positive results in *in vitro* mammalian cell assays (i.e., mouse lymphoma and Chinese hamster lung cells) have been reported for related antibiotics (tetracycline hydrochloride and oxytetracycline). Segment I (fertility and general reproduction) studies have provided evidence that minocycline impairs fertility in male rats.

Teratogenic Effects: *Pregnancy:* Pregnancy Category D (See **WARNINGS**.)

Labor and Delivery: The effect of tetracyclines on labor and delivery is unknown.

Nursing Mothers: Tetracyclines are excreted in human milk. Because of the potential for serious adverse reactions in nursing infants from the tetracyclines, a decision should be made whether to discontinue nursing or discontinue the drug, taking into account the importance of the drug to the mother (See **WARNINGS**).

Pediatric Use: (See **WARNINGS**).

ADVERSE REACTIONS

Due to oral minocycline's virtually complete absorption, side effects to the lower bowel, particularly diarrhea, have been infrequent. The following adverse reactions have been observed in patients receiving tetracyclines.

Gastrointestinal: Anorexia, nausea, vomiting, diarrhea, glossitis, dysphagia, enterocolitis, pancreatitis, and inflammatory lesions (with monilial overgrowth) in the anogenital region, increases in liver enzymes. Rarely, hepatitis and liver failure have been reported. Rare instances of esophagitis and esophageal ulcerations have been reported in patients taking the tetracycline-class anitibiotics in capsule and tablet form. Most of these patients took the medication immediately before going to bed (see **DOSAGE AND ADMINISTRATION**).

Skin: Maculopapular and erythematous rashes. Exfoliative dermatitis has been reported but is uncommon. Fixed drug eruptions, including balanitis, have been rarely reported. Erythema multiforme and rarely Stevens-Johnson syndrome have been reported. Photosensitivity is discussed above (see **WARNINGS**). Pigmentation of the skin and mucous membranes has been reported.

Renal toxicity: Elevations in BUN have been reported and are apparently dose related (See **WARNINGS**).

Hypersensitivity reactions: Urticaria, angioneurotic edema, anaphylaxis, anaphylactoid purpura, pericarditis, exacerbation of systemic lupus erythematosus and rarely pulmonary infiltrates with eosinophilia have been reported. A transient, lupus-like syndrome has also been reported.

Blood: Hemolytic anemia, thrombocytopenia, neutropenia, and eosinophilia have been reported.

Central Nervous System: Bulging fontanels in infants and benign intracranial hypertension (Pseudotumor cerebri) in adults (see **PRECAUTIONS-General**) have been reported. Headache has also been reported.

Other: When given over prolonged periods, tetracyclines have been reported to produce brown-black microscopic discoloration of the thyroid glands. Very rare cases of abnormal thyroid function have been reported. Decreased hearing has been rarely reported in patients on minocycline hydrochloride.

Tooth discoloration in children less than 8 years of age (see **WARNINGS**) and also, rarely, in adults have been reported.

OVERDOSAGE

In case of overdosage, discontinue medication, treat symptomatically and institute supportive measures.

DOSAGE AND ADMINISTRATION

THE USUAL DOSAGE AND FREQUENCY OF ADMINISTRATION OF MINOCYCLINE DIFFERS FROM THAT OF THE OTHER TETRACYCLINES. EXCEEDING THE RECOMMENDED DOSAGE MAY RESULT IN AN INCREASED INCIDENCE OF SIDE EFFECTS.

Minocycline hydrochloride capsules may be taken with or without food. (See **CLINICAL PHARMACOLOGY**.)

Adults: The usual dosage of minocycline hydrochloride is 200 mg initially followed by 100 mg every 12 hours. Alternatively, if more frequent doses are preferrred, two or four 50 mg capsules may be given initially followed by one 50 mg capsule four times daily.

For children above 8 years of age: The usual dosage of minocycline hydrochloride is 4 mg/kg initially followed by 2 mg/kg every 12 hours.

Uncomplicated gonococcal infections other than urethritis and anorectal infections in men: 200 mg initially, followed by 100 mg every 12 hours for a minimum of four days, with post-therapy cultures within 2 to 3 days.

In the treatment of uncomplicated gonococcal urethritis in men, 100 mg every 12 hours for five days is recommended.

For the treatment of syphilis, the usual dosage of minocycline should be administered over a period of 10 to 15 days. Close follow-up, including laboratory tests, is recommended.

In the treatment of meningococcal carrier state, the recommended dosage is 100 mg every 12 hours for five days.

Mycobacterium marinum infections: Although optimal doses have not been established, 100 mg every 12 hours for 6 to 8 weeks have been used successfully in a limited number of cases.

Uncomplicated nongonococcal urethral infection in adults caused by *Chlamydia trachomatis* or *Ureaplasma urealyticum:* 100 mg orally, every 12 hours for at least seven days.

Ingestion of adequate amounts of fluids along with capsule forms of drugs in the tetracycline-class is recommended to reduce the risk of esophageal irritation and ulceration.

In patients with renal impairment (see **WARNINGS**), the total dosage should be decreased by either reducing the recommended individual doses and/or extending the time intervals between doses.

HOW SUPPLIED

DYNACIN® (Minocycline Hydrochloride Capsules, USP) equivalent to 50 mg minocycline are opaque white capsules imprinted "0497" and "DYNACIN 50 mg" supplied in bottles of 100 and 500.

DYNACIN® (Minocycline Hydrochloride Capsules, USP) equivalent to 100 mg minocycline are opaque dark gray and opaque white capsules imprinted "0498" and "DYNACIN 100 mg" supplied in bottles of 50 and 500.

Dispense in tight, light-resistant container with child-resistant closure.

Store at controlled room temperature, 15°–30°C (59°–86°F).

Protect from light, moisture and excessive heat.

CAUTION

Federal law prohibits dispensing without prescription.

ANIMAL PHARMACOLOGY AND TOXICOLOGY: Minocycline hydrochloride has been observed to cause a dark discoloration of the thyroid in experimental animals (rats, minipigs, dogs and monkeys). In the rat, chronic treatment with minocycline hydrochloride has resulted in goiter accompanied by elevated radioactive iodine uptake, and evidence of thyroid tumor production. Minocycline hydrochloride has also been found to produce thyroid hyperplasia in rats and dogs.

REFERENCES

1. National Committee for Clinical Laboratory Standards, Approved Standard: *Performance Standards for Antimicrobial Disk Susceptibility Tests,* 3rd Edition, Vol. 4(16): M2-A3, Villanova, PA, December 1984.
2. National Committee for Clinical Laboratory Standards, Approved Standard: *Methods for Dilution Antimicrobial Susceptibility Tests for Bacteria that Grow Aerobically,* 2nd Edition, Vol. 5(22):M7-A, Villanova, PA, December 1985.

Manufactured specially for:
MEDICIS THE DERMATOLOGY COMPANY®
Phoenix, AZ 85018
by: DANBURY PHARMACAL INC.
Danbury, CT 06810

MG6432

LIDEX® ℞
[li 'dex]
(fluocinonide)
Cream 0.05%
Gel 0.05%
Ointment 0.05%
Topical Solution 0.05%

LIDEX–E® ℞
(fluocinonide)
Cream 0.05%

SYNALAR® ℞
[sin 'ă-lahr]
(fluocinolone acetonide)
Cream 0.025%
Ointment 0.025%
Topical Solution 0.01%

SYNEMOL® ℞
[sin 'ĕ-mol]
(fluocinolone acetonide)
Cream 0.025%

DESCRIPTION

These preparations are all intended for topical administration.

LIDEX preparations have as their active component the corticosteroid fluocinonide, which is the 21-acetate ester of fluocinolone acetonide and has the chemical name pregna-1,4-diene-3,20-dione, 21- (acetyloxy) -6,9-difluoro-11-hydroxy-16,17-[(1-methylethylidene)bis(oxy)]-, (6α,11β, 16α)-.

LIDEX cream contains fluocinonide 0.5 mg/g in FAPG® cream, a specially formulated cream base consisting of citric acid, 1,2,6-hexanetriol, polyethylene glycol 8000, propylene glycol and stearyl alcohol. This white cream vehicle is greaseless, non-staining, anhydrous and completely water miscible. The base provides emollient and hydrophilic properties. In this formulation the active ingredient is totally in solution.

LIDEX gel contains fluocinonide 0.5 mg/g in a specially formulated gel base consisting of carbomer 940, edetate disodium, propyl gallate, propylene glycol, sodium hydroxide and/or hydrochloric acid (to adjust the pH), and water (purified). This clear, colorless thixotropic vehicle is greaseless, non-staining and completely water miscible. In this formulation the active ingredient is totally in solution.

LIDEX ointment contains fluocinonide 0.5 mg/g in a specially formulated ointment base consisting of glyceryl monostearate, white petrolatum, propylene carbonate, propylene glycol, and white wax. It provides the occlusive and emollient effects desirable in an ointment. In this formulation the active ingredient is totally in solution.

LIDEX topical solution contains fluocinonide 0.5 mg/mL in a solution of alcohol (35%), citric acid, diisopropyl adipate, and propylene glycol. In this formulation the active ingredient is totally in solution.

LIDEX-E cream contains fluocinonide 0.5 mg/g in a water-washable aqueous emollient base of cetyl alcohol, citric acid, mineral oil, polysorbate 60, propylene glycol, sorbitan monostearate, stearyl alcohol, and water (purified).

SYNALAR preparations have as their active component the corticosteroid fluocinolone acetonide, which has the chemical name pregna-1,4-diene-3,20-dione,6,9-difluoro-11,21-dihydroxy-16,17-[(1-methylethylidene)bis(oxy)]-,(6α,11β, 16α)-.

SYNALAR cream contains fluocinolone acetonide 0.25 mg/g in a water-washable aqueous base of stearyl alcohol, propylene glycol, cetyl alcohol, polyoxyl 20 cetostearyl ether, mineral oil, white wax, simethicone, butylated hydroxytoluene, edetate disodium, citric acid, and purified water, with methylparaben and propylparaben as preservatives.

SYNALAR ointment contains fluocinolone acetonide 0.25 mg/g in white petrolatum U.S.P.

SYNALAR solution contains fluocinolone acetonide 0.1 mg/mL in a water-washable base of citric acid and propylene glycol.

SYNEMOL cream contains fluocinolone acetonide 0.25 mg/g in an emollient base of cetyl alcohol, citric acid, mineral oil, polysorbate 60, propylene glycol, sorbitan monostearate, stearyl alcohol, and water (purified).

CLINICAL PHARMACOLOGY

Topical corticosteroids share anti-inflammatory, anti- pruritic and vasoconstrictive actions.

The mechanism of anti-inflammatory activity of the topical corticosteroids is unclear. Various laboratory methods, including vasoconstrictor assays, are used to compare and predict potencies and/or clinical efficacies of the topical corticosteroids. There is some evidence to suggest that a recognizable correlation exists between vasoconstrictor potency and therapeutic efficacy in man.

Pharmacokinetics: The extent of percutaneous absorption of topical corticosteroids is determined by many factors including the vehicle, the integrity of the epidermal barrier, and the use of occlusive dressings. A significantly greater amount of fluocinonide is absorbed from the solution than from the cream or gel formulations.

Topical corticosteroids can be absorbed from normal intact skin. Inflammation and/or other disease processes in the skin increase percutaneous absorption. Occlusive dressings substantially increase the percutaneous absorption of topical corticosteroids. Thus, occlusive dressings may be a valuable therapeutic adjunct for treatment of resistant dermatoses. (See DOSAGE AND ADMINISTRATION).

Once absorbed through the skin, topical corticosteroids are handled through pharmacokinetic pathways similar to systemically administered corticosteroids. Corticosteroids are bound to plasma proteins in varying degrees. Corticosteroids are metabolized primarily in the liver and are then excreted by the kidneys. Some of the topical corticosteroids and their metabolites are also excreted into the bile.

INDICATIONS AND USAGE

These products are indicated for the relief of the inflammatory and pruritic manifestations of corticosteroid-responsive dermatoses.

CONTRAINDICATIONS

Topical corticosteroids are contraindicated in those patients with a history of hypersensitivity to any of the components of the preparation.

PRECAUTIONS

General: Systemic absorption of topical corticosteroids has produced reversible hypothalamic-pituitary-adrenal (HPA) axis suppression, manifestations of Cushing's syndrome, hyperglycemia, and glucosuria in some patients. Conditions which augment systemic absorption include the application of the more potent steroids, use over large surface areas, prolonged use and the addition of occlusive dressings.

Therefore, patients receiving a large dose of a potent topical steroid applied to a large surface area or under an occlusive dressing should be evaluated periodically for evidence of HPA axis suppression by using the urinary free cortisol and ACTH stimulation tests. If HPA axis suppression is noted, an attempt should be made to withdraw the drug, to reduce the frequency of application, or to substitute a less potent steroid.

Recovery of HPA axis function is generally prompt and complete upon discontinuation of the drug. Infrequently, signs and symptoms of steroid withdrawal may occur, requiring supplemental systemic corticosteroids.

Pediatric patients may absorb proportionally larger amounts of topical corticosteroids and thus be more susceptible to systemic toxicity. (See PRECAUTIONS—Pediatric Use).

Not for ophthalmic use. Severe irritation is possible if fluocinonide solution contacts the eye. If that should occur, immediate flushing of the eye with a large volume of water is recommended.

Continued on next page

Lidex—Cont.

If irritation develops, topical corticosteroids should be discontinued and appropriate therapy instituted.
As with any topical corticosteroid product, prolonged use may produce atrophy of the skin and subcutaneous tissues. When used on intertriginous or flexor areas, or on the face, this may occur even with short-term use.
In the presence of dermatological infections, the use of an appropriate antifungal or antibacterial agent should be instituted. If a favorable response does not occur promptly, the corticosteroid should be discontinued until the infection has been adequately controlled.
Information for the Patient: Patients using topical corticosteroids should receive the following information and instructions:

1. This medication is to be used as directed by the physician. It is for external use only. Avoid contact with the eyes. If there is contact with the eyes and severe irritation occurs, immediately flush with a large volume of water.
2. Patients should be advised not to use this medication for any disorder other than for which it was prescribed.
3. The treated skin area should not be bandaged or otherwise covered or wrapped as to be occlusive unless directed by the physician.
4. Patients should report any signs of local adverse reactions especially under occlusive dressing.
5. Parents of pediatric patients should be advised not to use tight-fitting diapers or plastic pants on a child being treated in the diaper area, as these garments may constitute occlusive dressings.

Laboratory Tests: The following tests may be helpful in evaluating HPA axis suppression: Urinary free cortisol test and ACTH stimulation test.
Carcinogenesis, Mutagenesis, and Impairment of Fertility: Long-term animal studies have not been performed to evaluate the carcinogenic potential or the effect on fertility of topical corticosteroids.
Studies to determine mutagenicity with prednisolone and hydrocortisone have revealed negative results.
Pregnancy Category C: Corticosteroids are generally teratogenic in laboratory animals when administered systemically at relatively low dosage levels. The more potent corticosteroids have been shown to be teratogenic after dermal application in laboratory animals. There are no adequate and well-controlled studies in pregnant women on teratogenic effects from topically applied corticosteroids. Therefore, topical corticosteroids should be used during pregnancy only if the potential benefit justifies the potential risk to the fetus. Drugs of this class should not be used extensively on pregnant patients, in large amounts, or for prolonged periods of time.
Nursing Mothers: It is not known whether topical administration of corticosteroids could result in sufficient systemic absorption to produce detectable quantities in breast milk. Systemically administered corticosteroids are secreted into breast milk in quantities *not* likely to have a deleterious effect on the infant. Nevertheless, caution should be exercised when topical corticosteroids are administered to a nursing woman.
Pediatric Use: Pediatric patients may demonstrate greater susceptibility to topical corticosteroid-induced HPA axis suppression and Cushing's syndrome than mature patients because of a larger skin surface area to body weight ratio.
Parents of pediatric patients should be advised not to use tight-fitting diapers or plastic pants on a child being treated in the diaper area as these garments may constitute occlusive dressings.
Hypothalamic-pituitary-adrenal (HPA) axis suppression, Cushing's syndrome, and intracranial hypertension have been reported in children receiving topical corticosteroids. Manifestations of adrenal suppression in children include linear growth retardation, delayed weight gain, low plasma cortisol levels, and absence of response to ACTH stimulation. Manifestations of intracranial hypertension include bulging fontanelles, headaches, and bilateral papilledema. Administration of topical corticosteroids to children should be limited to the least amount compatible with an effective therapeutic regimen. Chronic corticosteroid therapy may interfere with the growth and development of children.

ADVERSE REACTIONS

The following local adverse reactions are reported infrequently with topical corticosteroids, but may occur more frequently with the use of occlusive dressings. These reactions are listed in an approximate decreasing order of occurrence: burning, itching, irritation, dryness, folliculitis, hypertrichosis, acneiform eruptions, hypopigmentation, perioral dermatitis, allergic contact dermatitis, maceration of the skin, secondary infection, skin atrophy, striae, miliaria.

OVERDOSAGE

Topically applied corticosteroids can be absorbed in sufficient amounts to produce systemic effects (See PRECAUTIONS).

DOSAGE AND ADMINISTRATION

Topical corticosteroids are generally applied to the affected area as a thin film from two to four times daily depending on the severity of the condition. In hairy sites, the hair should be parted to allow direct contact with the lesion.
Occlusive dressings may be used for the management of psoriasis or recalcitrant conditions. Some plastic films may be flammable and due care should be exercised in their use. Similarly, caution should be employed when such films are used on children or left in their proximity, to avoid the possibility of accidental suffocation.
If an infection develops, the use of occlusive dressings should be discontinued and appropriate antimicrobial therapy instituted.

HOW SUPPLIED

LIDEX Cream 0.05%—15 g Tube (NDC 99207-511-13), 30 g Tube (NDC 99207-511-14), 60 g Tube (NDC 99207-511-17), 120 g Tube (NDC 99207-511-22). Store at 59° to 86°F (15° to 30°C). Avoid excessive heat, above 104°F (40°C).
LIDEX Gel 0.05%—15 g Tube (NDC 99207-507-13), 30 g Tube (NDC 99207-507-14), 60 g Tube (NDC 99207-507-17). Store at 59° to 86°F (15° to 30°C).
LIDEX Ointment 0.05%—15 g Tube (NDC 99207-514-13), 30 g Tube (NDC 99207-514-14), 60 g Tube (NDC 99207-514-17), 120 g Tube (NDC 99207-514-22). Store at 59° to 86°F (15° to 30°C). Avoid temperature above 86°F (30°C).
LIDEX Topical Solution 0.05%—Plastic squeeze bottles: 20cc (NDC 99207-517-44), 60cc (NDC 99207-517-46). Store at 59° to 86°F (15° to 30°C). Avoid excessive heat, above 104°F (40°C).
LIDEX-E Cream 0.05%—15 g Tube (NDC 99207-513-13), 30 g Tube (NDC 99207-513-14), 60 g Tube (NDC 99207-513-17). Store at 59° to 86°F (15° to 30°C). Avoid excessive heat, above 104°F (40°C).
SYNALAR Cream 0.025%—15 g Tube (NDC 99207-501-13), 60 g Tube (NDC 99207-501-17). Store at 59° to 86°F (15° to 30°C). Avoid excessive heat, above 104°F (40°C).
SYNALAR Topical Solution 0.01%—20cc (NDC 99207-506-44), 60cc (NDC 99207-506-46). Store at 59° to 86°F (15° to 30°C). Avoid freezing.
SYNALAR Ointment 0.025%—60 g Tube (NDC 99207-504-17). Store at 59° to 86°F (15° to 30°C). Avoid excessive heat, above 104°F (40°C).
SYNEMOL Cream 0.025%—60 g Tube (NDC 99207-509-17). Store at 59° to 86°F (15° to 30°C). Avoid excessive heat, above 104°F (40°C).
Manufactured specially for:
MEDICIS THE DERMATOLOGY COMPANY®
Phoenix, AZ 85018
by: Patheon, Inc.
Mississauga, Ontario
CANADA L5N 7K9

LUSTRA™ ℞

[*lŭs' tră*]
(HYDROQUINONE USP 4%)

DESCRIPTION

Hydroquinone is 1,4-benzenediol. Hydroquinone is structurally related to monobenzone. Hydroquinone occurs as fine, white needles. The drug is freely soluble in water and in alcohol and has a pKa of 9.96. Chemically, hydroquinone is designated as p-dihydroxybenzene; the empirical formula is $C_6H_6O_2$; molecular weight 110.1. The structural formula is:

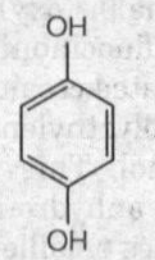

$C_6H_6O_2$

Each gram of LUSTRA contains 40 mg of Hydroquinone USP in a base of Purified Water, Phenyl Trimethicone, Glycerin, Alcohol, Cetyl Alcohol, Linoleic Acid, Glycolic Acid, Glyceryl Stearate, PEG-100 Stearate, Polydimethylcyclosiloxane, Ascorbyl Palmitate, Triethanolamine, Ceteary1 Alcohol, Ceteareth-20, Tocopheryl Acetate, Laureth-7, Polyacrylamide, C13-14 Isoparaffin, Benzyl Alcohol, Lecithin, Sodium Metabisulfite, Polysilicone-11, Disodium EDTA, Ascorbic Acid, Vitamin E, BHA, Fragrance.

CLINICAL PHARMACOLOGY

Topical application of hydroquinone produces a reversible depigmentation of the skin by inhibition of the enzymatic oxidation of tyrosine to 3-(3,4-dihydroxyphenyl) alanine (dopa)[1] and suppression of other melanocyte metabolic processes.[2]

INDICATIONS AND USAGE

LUSTRA is indicated for the gradual treatment of ultraviolet induced dyschromia and discoloration resulting from the use of oral contraceptives, pregnancy, hormone replacement therapy, or skin trauma.

DOSAGE AND ADMINISTRATION

LUSTRA should be applied to the affected areas twice daily, morning and before bedtime, or as directed by a physician. During and after the use of LUSTRA sun exposure should be limited, and a sunscreen agent or sun-protective clothing should be used to cover the treated areas, to prevent repigmentation. There is no recommended dosage for pediatric patients under 12 years of age except under the advice and supervision of a physician.

CONTRAINDICATIONS

LUSTRA is contraindicated in any patient that has a prior history of hypersensitivity or allergic reaction to hydroquinone or any of the other ingredients. The safety of topical hydroquinone use during pregnancy or on children (12 years and under) has not been established.

WARNINGS

A. CAUTION: Hydroquinone is a depigmenting agent which may produce unwanted cosmetic effects if not used as directed. The physician should be familiar with the contents of this insert before prescribing or dispensing this medication.
B. Test for skin sensitivity before using LUSTRA by applying a small amount to an unbroken patch of skin and check within 24 hours. Minor redness is not a contraindication, but where there is itching, vesicle formation, or excessive inflammatory response further treatment is not advised. Close patient supervision is recommended. Contact with the eyes should be avoided. If no lightening effect is noted after two months of treatment, LUSTRA should be discontinued.
C. Sunscreen use is an essential aspect of hydroquinone therapy, because even minimal sunlight sustains melanocytic activity. During treatment and maintenance therapy, sun exposure should be avoided on treated skin by application of a broad spectrum sunscreen (SPF 15 or greater) or by use of protective clothing to prevent repigmentation. Although LUSTRA has an antioxidant system in its vehicle, there are no sunblocking or sunscreening agents in LUSTRA.
D. Keep this and all medications out of the reach of children. In case of accidental ingestion, contact a physician or a poison control center immediately.
E. WARNING: Contains sodium metabisulfite, a sulfite which may cause serious allergic reactions (e.g., hives, itching, wheezing, anaphylaxis, severe asthma attack) in certain susceptible persons.

PRECAUTIONS

SEE WARNINGS
A. Pregnancy *Category C:* Animal reproduction studies have not been conducted with topical hydroquinone. It is also not known whether hydroquinone can cause fetal harm when used topically on a pregnant woman or can affect reproductive capacity. It is not known to what degree, if any, topical hydroquinone is absorbed systemically. Topical hydroquinone should be used in pregnant women only where clearly indicated.
B. Nursing mothers: It is not known whether topical hydroquinone is absorbed or excreted in human milk. Caution is advised when hydroquinone is used by a nursing mother.
C. Pediatric usage: Safety and effectiveness in pediatric patients below the age of 12 years have not been established.

ADVERSE REACTIONS

No systemic reactions have been reported. Occasional cutaneous hypersensitivity (localized contact dermatitis) may occur, in which case the medication should be discontinued and the physician notified immediately.

OVERDOSAGE

There have been no systemic reactions reported from the use of topical hydroquinone. However, treatment should be limited to relatively small areas of the body at one time, since some patients experience a transient skin reddening and a mild burning sensation which does not preclude treatment.

HOW SUPPLIED

LUSTRA is available as follows:
1.0 ounce jar (28.4 g) NDC 99207-250-10
1/8 ounce jar (3.5 g) NDC 99207-250-01

REFERENCES

1. Denton, C., A.B. Lerner, and T.B. Fitzpatrick, "Inhibition of Melanin Formation by Chemical Agents." *Journal of Investigative Dermatology.* 1952;18:119–135.
2. Jimbow, K., H. Obata, M. Pathak, and T.B. Fitzpatrick. "Mechanism of Depigmentation by Hydroquinone." *Journal of Investigative Dermatology.* 1974;62:436–449.

LUSTRA should be stored at controlled room temperature: 15°–30°C (59°–86°F).
Patent pending.

Manufactured specially for:
MEDICIS THE DERMATOLOGY COMPANY®
by: Contract Pharmaceuticals Limited, Mississauga, Ontario CANADA L5N 2B8

25010–08A

NOVACET® LOTION ℞

[*nov 'a set*]
(sodium sulfacetamide 10% and sulfur 5%)

DESCRIPTION

Each gram of NOVACET Lotion (sodium sulfacetamide 10% and sulfur 5%) contains 100 mg of sodium sulfacetamide and 50 mg of sulfur in a lotion containing propylene glycol, isopropyl myristate, propylene glycol stearate, cetyl alcohol, PEG-8 stearate, benzyl alcohol, sodium thiosulfate, EDTA disodium, buffering agent, emulsifying wax, and purified water.

Sodium sulfacetamide is a sulfonamide with antibacterial activity while sulfur acts as a keratolytic agent. Chemically sodium sulfacetamide is N'-[(4-aminophenyl) sulfonyl]-acetamide, monosodium salt, monohydrate. The structural formula is:

$$NH_2 - C_6H_4 - SO_2NCOCH_3 \cdot H_2O \quad (Na)$$

CLINICAL PHARMACOLOGY

The most widely accepted mechanism of action of sulfonamides is the Woods-Fildes theory which is based on the fact that sulfonamides act as competitive antagonists to para-aminobenzoic acid (PABA), an essential component for bacterial growth. While absorption through intact skin has not been determined, sodium sulfacetamide is readily absorbed from the gastrointestinal tract when taken orally and excreted in the urine, largely unchanged. The biological half-life has variously been reported as 7 to 12.8 hours.

The exact mode of action of sulfur in the treatment of acne is unknown, but it has been reported that it inhibits the growth of *P. acnes* and the formation of free fatty acids.

INDICATIONS

NOVACET Lotion is indicated in the topical control of acne vulgaris, acne rosacea and seborrheic dermatitis.

CONTRAINDICATIONS

NOVACET Lotion is contraindicated for use by patients having known hypersensitivity to sulfonamides, sulfur or any other component of this preparation. NOVACET Lotion is not to be used by patients with kidney disease.

WARNINGS

Although rare, sensitivity to sodium sulfacetamide may occur. Therefore, caution and careful supervision should be observed when prescribing this drug for patients who may be prone to hypersensitivity to topical sulfonamides. Systemic toxic reactions such as agranulocytosis, acute hemolytic anemia, purpura hemorrhagica, drug fever, jaundice, and contact dermatitis indicate hypersensitivity to sulfonamides. Particular caution should be employed if areas of denuded or abraded skin are involved.

PRECAUTIONS

General—If irritation develops, use of the product should be discontinued and appropriate therapy instituted. For external use only. Keep away from eyes. Patients should be carefully observed for possible local irritation or sensitization during long-term therapy. The object of this therapy is to achieve desquamation without irritation, but sodium sulfacetamide and sulfur can cause reddening and scaling of epidermis. These side effects are not unusual in the treatment of acne vulgaris, but patients should be cautioned about the possibility. Keep out of the reach of children.

Carcinogenesis, Mutagenesis and Impairment of Fertility—Long-term studies in animals have not been performed to evaluate carcinogenic potential.

Pregnancy—*Category C.* Animal reproduction studies have not been conducted with NOVACET Lotion. It is also not known whether NOVACET Lotion can cause fetal harm when administered to a pregnant woman or can affect reproduction capacity.

NOVACET Lotion should be given to a pregnant woman only if clearly needed.

Nursing Mothers—It is not known whether sodium sulfacetamide is excreted in the human milk following topical use of NOVACET Lotion. However, small amounts of orally administered sulfonamides have been reported to be eliminated in human milk. In view of this and because many drugs are excreted in human milk, caution should be exercised when NOVACET Lotion is administered to a nursing woman.

Pediatric Use—Safety and effectiveness in children under the age of 12 have not been established.

ADVERSE REACTIONS

Although rare, sodium sulfacetamide may cause local irritation.

DOSAGE AND ADMINISTRATION

Apply a thin film of NOVACET Lotion to affected areas 1 to 3 times daily.

HOW SUPPLIED

30 g tubes (NDC 99207-740-30) and 60 g tubes (NDC 99207-740-60)

Store at controlled room temperature 15°–30°C (59°–86°F).

CAUTION

Federal law prohibits dispensing without prescription.

Manufactured specially for:
MEDICIS THE DERMATOLOGY COMPANY®
Phoenix, Arizona 85018
by: DPT Laboratories, Inc.
San Antonio, TX 78215

SYNALAR® ℞

(fluocinolone acetonide)
Cream 0.025%
Ointment 0.025%
Topical Solution 0.01%

Refer to entry under LIDEX® (fluocinonide)

SYNEMOL® ℞

(fluocinolone acetonide)
Cream 0.025%

Refer to entry under LIDEX® (fluocinonide)

THERAMYCIN Z® ℞
ERYTHROMYCIN
TOPICAL SOLUTION 2%

DESCRIPTION

THERAMYCIN Z (Erythromycin Topical Solution 2%) is an antibiotic produced from a strain of *Streptomyces erythraeus*. It is basic and readily forms salts with acids. The active ingredient is represented by the following structure:

CONTENTS

Each mL of THERAMYCIN Z (Erythromycin Topical Solution 2%) Contains: ACTIVE: Erythromycin, USP, 20mg in a clear solution vehicle of; INACTIVES: SD Alcohol 40B 81% (by weight) equivalent to Absolute Alcohol 86% (by volume), Propylene Glycol, Lauramide DEA, Hydroxypropyl Cellulose, Fragrance, and Zinc Acetate.

CLINICAL PHARMACOLOGY

Although the mechanism by which Erythromycin Topical Solution 2% acts in reducing inflammatory lesions of acne vulgaris is unknown, it is presumably due to its antibiotic action.

INDICATIONS AND USAGE

Erythromycin Topical Solution 2% is indicated for the topical control of acne vulgaris.

CONTRAINDICATIONS

Erythromycin Topical Solution 2% is contraindicated in persons who have shown hypersensitivity to erythromycin or any of the other listed ingredients.

WARNING

The safe use of Erythromycin Topical Solution 2% during pregnancy or lactation has *not* been established.

PRECAUTIONS

General—The use of antibiotic agents may be associated with the overgrowth of antibiotic-resistant organisms. If this occurs, administration of this drug should be discontinued and appropriate measures taken.

Information for Patients—Erythromycin Topical Solution 2% is for external use only and should be kept away from the eyes, nose, mouth and other mucous membranes. Concomitant topical acne therapy should be used with caution because a cumulative irritant effect may occur, especially with the use of peeling, desquamating, or abrasive agents.

Carcinogenesis, Mutagenesis, Impairment of Fertility—Long-term animal studies to evaluate carcinogenic potential, mutagenicity, or the effect on fertility of erythromycin have *not* been performed.

Pregnancy—*Pregnancy Category C.* Animal reproduction studies have *not* been conducted with erythromycin. It is also *not* known whether erythromycin can cause fetal harm when administered to a pregnant woman or can affect reproduction capacity. Erythromycin should be given to a pregnant woman only if clearly needed.

Nursing Mothers—Erythromycin is excreted in breast milk. Caution should be exercised when erythromycin is administered to a nursing mother.

ADVERSE REACTIONS

Adverse conditions reported include dryness, pruritus, desquamation, erythema, oiliness, and burning sensation. Irritation of the eyes has also been reported. A case of generalized urticarial reaction, possibly related to the drug, which required the use of systemic steroid therapy has been reported.

DOSAGE AND ADMINISTRATION

THERAMYCIN Z (Erythromycin Topical Solution 2%) should be applied (ball type applicator should be rubbed) twice a day, once in the morning and once in the evening, to areas usually affected by acne. These areas should be washed with warm water and soap and patted dry before applying THERAMYCIN Z. Acne lesions on the face, neck, shoulder, chest, and back may be treated in this manner. Shake well before using and close tightly after each use.

HOW SUPPLIED

THERAMYCIN Z (Erythromycin Topical Solution 2%), 2 fl oz (59.14 mL) in a 60 mL plastic bottle with applicator attached—NDC 99207-550-02.

STORAGE

THERAMYCIN Z (Erythromycin Topical Solution 2%) should be stored at Controlled Room Temperature 15°–30°C (59°–86°F). Preserve in a light-resistant container.

INSTRUCTIONS FOR INSTALLING APPLICATOR

1. Remove and discard temporary shipping cap.
2. Push applicator firmly into bottle using white cap as holder.
3. Screw cap down to seat applicator.

WARNINGS: Contains Alcohol—Do not use near open flame.

For external use only. Not for ophthalmic use.

Keep out of reach of children.

CAUTION: Federal law prohibits dispensing without prescription.

Manufactured specially for:
MEDICIS THE DERMATOLOGY COMPANY®
Phoenix, AZ 85018
by: Zenith Goldline Dermatologicals, Inc.
Syosset, NY 11791

TRIAZ® ℞

[*trī 'ăz*]
(benzoyl peroxide)
Gel 6%
Gel 9%
Gel 10%
Cleanser 6%
Cleanser 10%

DESCRIPTION

TRIAZ 6%, 9% and 10% Gels and TRIAZ 6% and 10% Cleansers are topical, gel-based, benzoyl peroxide containing preparations for use in the treatment of acne vulgaris. Benzoyl peroxide is an oxidizing agent that possesses antibacterial properties and is classified as a keratolytic. Benzoyl peroxide ($C_{14}H_{10}O_4$) is represented by the following chemical structure:

TRIAZ 6% and TRIAZ 10% Gels contain, respectively, Benzoyl Peroxide 6% and 10% as the active ingredient in a gel-based formulation consisting of: Water, C12-15 Alkyl Benzoate, Glycerin, Cetyl Stearyl Alcohol, Glycolic Acid, Polyacrylamide (and) C13-14 Isoparaffin (and) Laureth-7, Glyceryl Stearate (and) PEG-100 Stearate, Steareth S-2, Sodium Hydroxide, Steareth S-20, Dimethicone, Zinc Lactate, Disodium EDTA.

TRIAZ 9% Gel contains Benzoyl Peroxide 9% as the active ingredient in a gel-based formulation consisting of: Water,

Continued on next page

Triaz—Cont.

C12-15 Alkyl benzoate, Glycolic Acid, Polyacrylamide (and) C13-14 Isoparaffin (and) Laureth-7, Cetyl Stearyl Alcohol, Glyceryl Stearate (and) PEG-100 Stearate, Glycerin, Steareth S-2, Sodium Hydroxide, Steareth S-20, Dimethicone, Zinc Lactate, Special Petrolatum Fraction.
TRIAZ 6% and TRIAZ 10% Cleansers contain, respectively, Benzoyl Peroxide 6% and 10% as the active ingredient in a vehicle consisting of: Glycerin, Petrolatum, C12-15 Alkyl Benzoate, Sodium Cocoyl Isethionate, Water, Special Petrolatum Fraction, Sodium C14-16 Olefin Sulfonate, Zinc Lactate, Carbomer, Potassium Polymetaphosphate, Titanium Dioxide Triethanolamine, Glycolic Acid, Lavender Extract, Menthol.

CLINICAL PHARMACOLOGY

The mechanism of action of benzoyl peroxide is not totally understood but its antibacterial activity against *Propionibacterium acnes* is thought to be a major mode of action. In addition, patients treated with benzoyl peroxide show a reduction in lipids and free fatty acids and mild desquamation (drying and peeling activity) with simultaneous reduction in comedones and acne lesions.
Little is known about the percutaneous penetration, metabolism, and excretion of benzoyl peroxide, although it has been shown that benzoyl peroxide absorbed by the skin is metabolized to benzoic acid and then excreted as benzoate in the urine. There is no evidence of systemic toxicity caused by benzoyl peroxide in humans.

INDICATIONS AND USAGE

TRIAZ 6%, 9% and 10% Gels and TRIAZ 6% and 10% Cleansers are indicated for the topical treatment of acne vulgaris.

CONTRAINDICATIONS

These preparations are contraindicated in patients with a history of hypersensitivity to any of their components.

WARNINGS

When using this product, avoid unnecessary sun exposure and use a sunscreen.

PRECAUTIONS

General: For external use only. If severe irritation develops, discontinue use and institute appropriate therapy. After reaction clears, treatment may often be resumed with less frequent application. These preparations should not be used in or near the eyes or on mucous membranes.
Information for patients: Avoid contact with eyes, eyelids, lips and mucous membranes. If accidental contact occurs, rinse with water. Contact with any colored material (including hair and fabric) may result in bleaching or discoloration. If excessive irritation develops, discontinue use and consult your physician.
Carcinogenesis, Mutagenesis, Impairment of Fertility: Data from several studies employing a strain of mice that are highly susceptible to developing cancer suggest that benzoyl peroxide acts as a tumor promoter. The clinical significance of these findings to humans is unknown. Benzoyl peroxide has not been found to be mutagenic (Ames Test) and there are no published data indicating it impairs fertility.
Pregnancy: Teratogenic Effects: *Pregnancy Category C:* Animal reproduction studies have not been conducted with benzoyl peroxide. It is not known whether benzoyl peroxide can cause fetal harm when administered to a pregnant woman or can affect reproduction capacity. Benzoyl peroxide should be used by a pregnant woman only if clearly needed. There are no available data on the effect of benzoyl peroxide on the later growth, development and functional maturation of the unborn child.
Nursing Mothers: It is not known whether this drug is excreted in human milk. Because many drugs are excreted in human milk, caution should be exercised when benzoyl peroxide is administered to a nursing woman.
Pediatric Use: Safety and effectiveness in children have not been established.

ADVERSE REACTIONS

Allergic contact dermatitis and dryness have been reported with topical benzoyl peroxide therapy.

OVERDOSAGE

If excessive scaling, erythema or edema occurs, the use of this preparation should be discontinued. To hasten resolution of the adverse effects, cool compresses may be used. After symptoms and signs subside, a reduced dosage schedule may be cautiously tried if the reaction is judged to be due to excessive use and not allergenicity.

DOSAGE AND ADMINISTRATION

TRIAZ Gels: Apply once or twice daily to cover affected areas, or as directed by your dermatologist. Use after washing with a mild cleanser, such as one of the TRIAZ Cleansers, and water.
TRIAZ Cleansers: Wash affected areas once or twice daily, or as directed by your dermatologist. Avoid contact with eyes or mucous membranes. Wet skin and liberally apply to areas to be cleansed, massage gently into skin for 10–20 seconds working into a full lather, rinse thoroughly and pat dry. If drying occurs, it may be controlled by rinsing cleanser off sooner or using less often.

HOW SUPPLIED

TRIAZ 6% Gel—1.5 oz. (42.5 g) tube, NDC 99207-051-01.
TRIAZ 9% Gel—1.5 oz. (42.5 g) tube, NDC 99207-209-01.
TRIAZ 10% Gel—1.5 oz. (42.5 g) tube, NDC 99207-210-01.
TRIAZ 6% Cleanser—6 oz. (170.3 g) tube, NDC 99207-116-12.
TRIAZ 10% Cleanser—3 oz. (85.1 g) tube, NDC 99207-106-02.
TRIAZ 10% Cleanser—6 oz. (170.3 g) tube, NDC 99207-106-12.
Caution: Federal law prohibits dispensing without prescription. Store at controlled room temperature 15°–30°C (59°–86°F).
Covered by US Patents: 5,648,389; 5,254,334; 5,409,706; and 5,632,996.
Manufactured specially for:
MEDICIS THE DERMATOLOGY COMPANY®
Phoenix, AZ 85018
by: Contract Pharmaceuticals Limited,
Mississauga, Ontario CANADA L5N2B8

ZONALON® CREAM ℞

[zŏn a lon]
(doxepin hydrochloride cream), 5%
FOR TOPICAL DERMATOLOGIC USE ONLY—
NOT FOR OPHTHALMIC, ORAL, OR INTRAVAGINAL USE.

DESCRIPTION

ZONALON CREAM (doxepin hydrochloride cream) is a topical antipruritic cream. Each gram contains: 50 mg of doxepin hydrochloride (equivalent to 44.3 mg of doxepin).
Doxepin hydrochloride is one of a class of agents known as dibenzoxepin tricyclic compounds. It is an isomeric mixture of

N,N-Dimethyldibenz[b,e]oxepin-$\Delta^{11(6H),\gamma}$-propylamine hydrochloride

Doxepin hydrochloride has an empirical formula of $C_{19}H_{21}NO \cdot HCl$ and a molecular weight of 316.
The base is a cream of pH 3.5 to 5.5 that includes the inactive ingredients: sorbitol, cetyl alcohol, isopropyl myristate, glyceryl stearate, PEG-100 stearate, petrolatum, benzyl alcohol, titanium dioxide, and purified water.

CLINICAL PHARMACOLOGY

The exact mechanism by which doxepin exerts its antipruritic effect is unknown. Doxepin HCl does have potent H1 and potent H2 receptor blocking actions. Histamine-blocking drugs appear to compete at histamine receptor sites and inhibit the biological activation of histamine receptors. In addition, doxepin produces drowsiness in significant numbers of patients. Sedation may have an effect on certain pruritic symptoms. In 19 pruritic eczema patients treated with ZONALON CREAM, PLASMA doxepin concentrations ranged from nondetectable to 47 ng/mL from percutaneous absorption. Target therapeutic plasma levels of ORAL doxepin HCl for the treatment of depression range from 30 to 150 ng/mL.
Once absorbed into the systemic circulation, doxepin undergoes hepatic metabolism that results in conversion to pharmacologically-active desmethyldoxepin. Further glucuronidation results in urinary excretion of the parent drug and its metabolites. Desmethyldoxepin has a half life reportedly that ranges from 28 to 52 hours and is not affected by multiple dosing. Plasma levels of both doxepin and desmethyldoxepin are highly variable and are poorly correlated with dosage. Wide distribution occurs in body tissues including lungs, heart, brain, and liver. Renal disease, genetic factors, age, and other medications affect the metabolism and subsequent elimination of doxepin. (See **Precautions—Drug Interactions**.)

INDICATIONS AND USAGE

ZONALON CREAM is indicated for the short-term (up to 8 days) management of moderate pruritus in adult patients with the following forms of eczematous dermatitis: atopic dermatitis and lichen simplex chronicus. (See **Dosage and Administration**.)

CONTRAINDICATIONS

Because doxepin HCl has an anticholinergic effect and because significant plasma levels of doxepin are detectable after topical ZONALON CREAM application, the use of ZONALON CREAM is contraindicated in patients with untreated narrow angle glaucoma or a tendency to urinary retention.
ZONALON CREAM is contraindicated in individuals who have shown previous sensitivity to any of its components.

WARNINGS

Drowsiness occurs in over 20% of patients treated with ZONALON CREAM, especially in patients receiving treatment to greater than 10% of their body surface area. Patients should be warned of this possibility and cautioned against driving a motor vehicle or operating hazardous machinery while being treated with ZONALON CREAM.
Patients should also be warned that the effects of alcoholic beverages can be potentiated when using ZONALON CREAM.
If excessive drowsiness occurs it may be necessary to reduce the number of applications, the amount of cream applied, and/or the percentage of body surface area treated, or discontinue the drug.
Keep this product away from the eyes.

PRECAUTIONS

Drug Interactions
Studies have not been performed examining drug interactions with ZONALON CREAM. However, data are available regarding potentially significant drug interactions regarding doxepin. As plasma levels of doxepin similar to therapeutic ranges for antidepressant therapy can be obtained following topical application of ZONALON CREAM, it would not be unexpected for the following drug interactions to be possible following topical ZONALON CREAM application.
MAO Inhibitors
Serious side effects and even death have been reported following the concomitant use of certain orally administered drugs chemically related to doxepin and MAO inhibitors. Therefore, MAO inhibitors should be discontinued at least two weeks prior to the initiation of treatment with ZONALON CREAM.
Cimetidine
Cimetidine has been reported to produce clinically significant fluctuations in steady-state serum concentrations of various tricyclic antidepressants. Serious anticholinergic symptoms have been associated with elevations in the serum levels of tricyclic antidepressants when cimetidine therapy is initiated. Additionally, higher than expected tricyclic antidepressant levels have been observed in patients already taking cimetidine. In patients who have been reported to be well-controlled on tricyclic antidepressants receiving concurrent cimetidine therapy, discontinuation of cimetidine has been reported to decrease established steady-state serum tricyclic antidepressant levels and compromise their therapeutic effects.
Alcohol
Alcohol ingestion may exacerbate the potential sedative effects of ZONALON CREAM.
Drugs Metabolized by $P_{450}IID6$
A subset (3% to 10%) of the population has reduced activity of certain drug metabolizing enzymes such as the cytochrome P_{450} isozyme $P_{450}IID6$. Such individuals are referred to as "poor metabolizers" of drug such as debrisoquin, dextromethorphan, and the tricyclic antidepressants. These individuals may have higher than expected plasma concentrations of tricyclic antidepressant when given usual doses. In addition, certain drugs that are metabolized by this isozyme, including many antidepressants (tricyclic antidepressants, selective serotonin reuptake inhibitors, and others), may inhibit the activity of this isozyme, and thus may make normal metabolizers resemble poor metabolizers with regard to concomitant therapy with other drugs metabolized by this enzyme system, leading to drug interactions. Concomitant use of tricyclic antidepressants with other drugs metabolized by cytochrome $P_{450}IID6$ may require lower doses than usually prescribed for either the tricyclic antidepressant or the other drug. Therefore, co-administration of tricyclic antidepressants with other drugs that are metabolized by this isoenzyme, including other antidepressants, phenothiazines, carbamazepine, and Type 1C antiarrhythmics (e.g., propafenone, flecainide and encainide), or that inhibit this enzyme (e.g., quinidine), should be approached with caution. Concomitant use of ZONALON CREAM with drugs metabolized by cytochrome $P_{450}IID6$ has not been formally studied.
Carcinogenesis, Mutagenesis, Impairment of Fertility
Carcinogenesis, mutagenesis, and impairment of fertility studies have not been conducted with doxepin hydrochloride.
Pregnancy Pregnancy Category B:
Teratology studies have been performed in rats and rabbits at oral doses up to 8 times the topical human dose (based on a mg/kg basis) and have revealed no evidence of impaired fertility or harm to the fetus due to doxepin. There are, however, no adequate and well-controlled studies in pregnant women. Because animal reproduction studies are not always predictive of human response, this drug should be used during pregnancy only if clearly needed.
Nursing Mothers
Doxepin is excreted in human milk after oral administration. There have been no studies conducted to date to determine if doxepin is excreted in human milk after topical administration; however, it is known that significant systemic

levels of doxepin are obtained after topical administration. It is therefore possible that doxepin could be secreted in human milk following topical administration.

One case has been reported of apnea and drowsiness in a nursing infant whose mother was taking an oral dosage form of doxepin HCl.

Because of the potential for serious adverse reactions in nursing infants from doxepin, a decision should be made whether to discontinue nursing or to discontinue the drug, taking into account the importance of the drug to the mother.

Pediatric Use

Safety and effectiveness of ZONALON CREAM in children have not been established.

ADVERSE REACTIONS

CONTROLLED CLINICAL TRIALS:

Systemic Adverse Effects:

In controlled clinical trials of patients treated with ZONALON CREAM, the most common systemic adverse effect reported was drowsiness. Drowsiness occurred in 22% of patients treated with ZONALON CREAM (and 2% of patients treated with placebo cream) and resulted in the premature discontinuation of the drug in approximately 5% of patients treated.

Other systemic adverse effects reported in approximately 1 to 10% of these patients included:

Dry mouth, dry lips, thirst, headache, fatigue, dizziness, emotional changes, and taste changes.

Other systemic adverse effects reported in less than 1% of these patients included:

Nausea, anxiety, and fever.

Local Site Adverse Effects:

In controlled clinical trials of patients treated with ZONALON CREAM, the most common local site adverse effect reported was burning and/or stinging at the site of application. These occurred in approximately 21% of these patients. Most of these reactions were categorized as "mild"; however, approximately 25% of patients who reported burning and/or stinging reported the reaction as "severe". Four patients treated with ZONALON CREAM withdrew from the study because of the burning and/or stinging.

Other local site adverse effects reported in approximately 1 to 10% of these patients included:

Pruritus exacerbation, eczema exacerbation, dryness and tightness to skin, paresthesias, and edema.

Other local site adverse effects reported in less than 1% of these patients included:

Irritation, tingling, scaling, and cracking.

OVERDOSAGE

Overdosage with a topical product is unlikely, should it occur, the signs and symptoms include:

Mild: Drowsiness, stupor, blurred vision, excessive dryness of mouth.

Severe: Respiratory depression, hypotension, coma, convulsions, cardiac arrhythmias and tachycardias. Also, urinary retention (bladder atony), decreased gastrointestinal motility (paralytic ileus), hyperthermia (or hypothermia), hypertension, dilated pupils, hyperactive reflexes.

Management and Treatment

Mild: Observation and supportive therapy is all that is usually necessary. It may be necessary to reduce the percent of body surface area treated or the frequency of application or apply a thinner layer of cream.

Severe: Medical management of severe doxepin overdosage consists of aggressive supportive therapy. The area covered with doxepin HCl cream should be thoroughly washed. An adequate airway should be established in comatose patients and assisted ventilation used if necessary. EKG monitoring may be required for several days, because relapse after apparent recovery has been reported with oral doxepin HCl. Arrhythmias should be treated with the appropriate antiarrhythmic agent. It has been reported that many of the cardiovascular and CNS symptoms of tricyclic antidepressant poisoning in adults may be reversed by the slow intravenous administration of 1 mg to 3 mg of physostigmine salicylate. Because physostigmine is rapidly metabolized, the dosage should be repeated as required. Convulsions may respond to standard anticonvulsant therapy; however, **barbiturates may potentiate any respiratory depression.**

Dialysis and forced diuresis generally are not of value in the management of overdosage due to high tissue and protein binding of doxepin HCl.

DOSAGE AND ADMINISTRATION

A thin film of ZONALON CREAM should be applied four times each day with at least a 3 to 4 hour interval between applications. There are no data to establish the safety and effectivness of ZONALON CREAM when used for greater than 8 days. Chronic use beyond eight days may result in higher systemic levels.

Clinical experience has shown that **drowsiness is significantly more common in patients applying ZONALON CREAM to over 10% of body surface area;** therefore, patients with greater than 10% of body surface area affected should be particularly cautioned concerning possible drowsiness and other systemic adverse effects of doxepin. If excessive drowsiness occurs it may be necessary to do one or more of the following: reduce the body surface area treated, reduce the number of applications per day, reduce the amount of cream applied, or discontinue the drug.

Occlusive dressings may increase absorption of most topical drugs; therefore, occlusive dressings with ZONALON CREAM should not be utilized.

HOW SUPPLIED

ZONALON CREAM is available in 30g (NDC 99207-523-30) and 45g (NDC 99207-523-45) aluminum tubes. Store at or below 27°C (80°F).

CAUTION

Federal law prohibits dispensing without prescription.

Manufactured specially for:

MEDICIS THE DERMATOLOGY COMPANY®

Phoenix, Arizona 85018

by: DPT Laboratories, Inc.

San Antonio, TX 78215

MedImmune, Inc.

35 WEST WATKINS MILL ROAD
GAITHERSBURG, MD 20878

For Medical Information Contact:
(800) 949-3789

Adverse Drug Experience:
(800) 949-3789

In Emergencies:
24-hour emergency
(800) 949-3789

Sales and Ordering/Customer Service:
(800) 527-7130

CYTOMEGALOVIRUS ℞

IMMUNE GLOBULIN INTRAVENOUS (HUMAN)

CYTOGAM® Liquid Formulation Solvent Detergent Treated

DESCRIPTION

CytoGam®, Cytomegalovirus Immune Globulin Intravenous (Human) (CMV-IGIV), is an immunoglobulin G (IgG) containing a standardized amount of antibody to Cytomegalovirus (CMV). CMV-IGIV is formulated in final vial as a sterile liquid. The globulin is stabilized with 5% sucrose and 1% Albumin (Human). CytoGam® contains no preservative. The purified immunoglobulin is derived from pooled adult human plasma selected for high titers of antibody for Cytomegalovirus (CMV).[1] Source material for fractionation may be obtained from another U.S. licensed manufacturer. Pooled plasma was fractionated by ethanol precipitation of the proteins according to Cohn Methods 6 and 9, modified to yield a product suitable for intravenous administration. A widely utilized solvent-detergent viral inactivation process is also.[2] Certain manufacturing operations may be performed by other firms. Each milliliter contains: 50 ± 10 mg of immunoglobulin, primarily IgG, and trace amounts of IgA and IgM; 50 mg of sucrose; 10 mg of Albumin (Human). The sodium content is 20–30 mEq per liter; i.e. 0.4–0.6 mEq per 20 ml or 1.0–1.5 mEq per 50 ml. The solution should appear colorless and translucent.

CLINICAL PHARMACOLOGY

CytoGam® contains IgG antibodies representative of the large number of normal persons who contributed to the plasma pools from which the product was derived. The globulin contains a relatively high concentration of antibodies directed against Cytomegalovirus (CMV). In the case of persons who may be exposed to CMV, CytoGam® can raise the relevant antibodies to levels sufficient to attenuate or reduce the incidence of serious CMV disease.

In two separate clinical trials, CytoGam® was shown to provide effective prophylaxis in renal-transplant recipients at risk for primary CMV disease. In the first randomized trial,[3] the incidence of virologically confirmed CMV-associated syndromes was reduced from 60% in controls (n=35) to 21% in recipients of CMV immune globulin (n=24) ($P<0.01$); marked leukopenia was reduced from 37% in controls to 4% in globulin recipients ($P<0.01$); and fungal or parasite superinfections were not seen in globulin recipients but occurred in 20% of controls. ($P = 0.05$). Serious CMV disease was reduced from 46% to 13%. There was a concomitant but not statistically significant reduction in the incidence of CMV pneumonia (17% of controls is as compared with 4% of globulin recipients). There was no effect on rates of viral isolation or seroconversion although the rate of viremia was less in CytoGam® recipients. In a subsequent nonrandomized trial in renal transplant recipients (n=36),[4] the incidence of virologically confirmed CMV-associated syndrome was reduced to 36% in the globulin recipients. The rates of CMV-associated pneumonia, CMV-associated hepatitis, and concomitant fungal and parasitic superinfection were similar to those in the first trial.

INDICATIONS AND USAGE

Cytomegalovirus Immune Globulin Intravenous (Human) is indicated for the attenuation of primary (1°) Cytomegalovirus disease associated with kidney transplantation. Specifically, the product is indicated for kidney transplant recipients who are seronegative for CMV and who receive a kidney from a CMV seropositive donor. In a population of seronegative recipients of seropositive kidneys approximately 75% of the untreated recipients would be expected to develop CMV disease.[1,5] Clinical studies have shown a 50% reduction in 1° CMV disease in renal transplant patients given Cytomegalovirus Immune Globulin Intravenous (Human).[3,4,6]

CONTRAINDICATIONS

CytoGam® should not be used in individuals with a history of a prior severe reaction associated with the administration of this or other human immunoglobulin preparations. Persons with selective immunoglobulin A deficiency have the potential for developing antibodies to immunoglobulin A and could have anaphylactic reactions to subsequent administration of blood products that contain immunoglobulin A, including CytoGam®.

WARNINGS

During administration, the patient's vital signs should be monitored continuously and careful observation made for any symptoms throughout the infusion. Epinephrine should be available for the treatment of an acute anaphylactic reaction (see PRECAUTIONS section).

PRECAUTIONS

Although systemic allergic reactions are rare (see ADVERSE REACTIONS section), epinephrine and diphenhydramine should be available for treatment of acute allergic symptoms. If hypertension or anaphylaxis occur, the administration of the immunoglobulin should be discontinued immediately and an antidote should be given as noted above.

An aseptic meningitis syndrome (AMS) has been reported to occur infrequently in association with immune Globulin Intravenous (Human) (IGIV) treatment (7–10). The syndrome usually begins within several hours to two days following IGIV treatment. It is characterized by symptoms and signs including severe headache, nuchal rigidity, drowsiness, fever, photophobia, painful eye movements, and nausea and vomiting. Cerebrospinal fluid studies are frequently positive with pleocytosis up to several thousand cells per cu.mm., predominantly from the granulocytic series, and elevated protein levels up to several hundred mg/dl. Patients exhibiting such symptoms and signs should receive a thorough neurological examination, including CSF studies, to rule out other causes of meningitis. AMS may occur more frequently in association with high dose (2 g/kg) IGIV treatment. Discontinuation of IGIV treatment has resulted in remission of AMS within several days without sequelae.

CMV-IGIV is made from human plasma and, like other plasma products, carries the possibility for transmission of blood-borne vial agents. The risk of transmission of recognized blood-borne viruses is considered to be low because of the viral inactivation and removal properties in the Cohn-Oncley cold ethanol precipitation procedure used for purification of immune globulin products (11–13). Until 1993, cold ethanol manufactured immune globulins licensed in the United States had not been documented to transmit any viral agent. However, during a brief period in late 1993 to early 1994, intravenous immune globulin made by one U.S. manufacturer was associated with transmission of Hepatitis C virus (14). To further guard against possible transmission of blood-borne viruses, including Hepatitis C, CMV-IGIV is treated with a solvent detergent viral inactivation procedure (2) known to inactivate a wide spectrum of lipid enveloped viruses, including HIV-1, HIV-2, Hepatitis B, and Hepatitis C (15). However, because new blood-borne viruses may yet emerge, some of which may not be inactivated by the manufacturing process or by solvent detergent treatment, CMV-IGIV, like any other blood product, should be given only if a benefit is expected.

CytoGam® does not contain a preservative. The vial should be entered only once for administration purposes and the infusion should begin within 6 hours. The infusion schedule should be adhered to closely (see INFUSION section). Do not use if the solution is turbid.

Drug Interaction: Antibodies present in immune globulin preparations may interfere with the immune response to live virus vaccines such as measles, mumps, and rubella; therefore, vaccination with live virus vaccines should be deferred until approximately three months after administration of CytoGam®. If such vaccinations were given shortly after CytoGam®, a revaccination may be necessary. Admixtures of CytoGam® with other drugs have not been evalu-

Continued on next page

CytoGam—Cont.

ated. It is recommended that CytoGam® be administered separately from other drugs or medications which the patient may be receiving (see ADMINISTRATION section).
Pregnancy Category C: Animal reproduction studies have not been conducted with Cytomegalovirus Immune Globulin Intravenous (Human). It is also not known whether Cytomegalovirus Immune Globulin Intravenous (Human) can cause fetal harm when administered to a pregnant woman or can affect reproduction capacity. Cytomegalovirus Immune Globulin Intravenous (Human) should be given to a pregnant woman only if clearly needed.

ADVERSE REACTIONS

Minor reactions such as flushing, chills, muscle cramps, back pain, fever, nausea, vomiting, arthralgia, and wheezing were the most frequent adverse reactions observed during the clinical trials of CytoGam®. The incidence of these reactions during the clinical trials was less than 5.0% of all infusions and were most often related to infusion rates. A potential side reaction might be hypotension but this has not been observed in over 200 infusions. If a patient develops a minor side effect, slow the rate immediately or temporarily interrupt the infusion.
Severe reactions such as angioneurotic edema and anaphylactic shock, although not observed during clinical trials, are a possibility. Clinical anaphylaxis may occur even when the patient is not known to be sensitized to immune globulin products. A reaction may be related to the rate of infusion; therefore, carefully adhere to the infusion rates as outlined under "DOSAGE AND ADMINISTRATION." If anaphylaxis or drop in blood pressure occurs, *discontinue infusion* and use antidote such as diphenhydramine and adrenalin.

OVERDOSAGE

Although little data are available, clinical experience with other immunoglobulin preparations suggests that the major manifestations would be those related to volume overload.

DOSAGE AND ADMINISTRATION

The maximum recommended total dosage per infusion is 150 mg/kg, administered according to the following schedule:

Within:	72 hours of transplant:	150 mg/kg
	2 weeks post transplant:	100 mg/kg
	4 weeks post transplant:	100 mg/kg
	6 weeks post transplant:	100 mg/kg
	8 weeks post transplant:	100 mg/kg
	12 weeks post transplant:	50 mg/kg
	16 weeks post transplant:	50 mg/kg

Preparation for Administration. Remove the tab portion of the vial cap and clean the rubber stopper with 70% alcohol or equivalent. DO NOT SHAKE VIAL; AVOID FOAMING.
Parenteral drug products should be inspected visually for particulate matter and discoloration prior to administration whenever solution and container permit. Infuse the solution only if it is colorless, free of particulate matter and not turbid.
Infusion. Infusion should begin within 6 hours after entering the vial and should be complete within 12 hours of entering the vial. Vital signs should be taken preinfusion, mid-way and post-infusion as well as before any rate increase. CytoGam® should be administered through an intravenous line using a constant infusion pump (i.e., IVAC pump or equivalent). Pre-dilution of CytoGam® before infusion is not recommended. CytoGam® should be administered through a separate intravenous line. If this is not possible, CytoGam® may be "piggybacked" into a pre-existing line if that line contains either Sodium Chloride, Injection, USP, or one of the following dextrose solutions (with or without NaCl added): 2.5% dextrose in water, 5% dextrose in water, 10% dextrose in water, 20% dextrose in water. If a preexisting line must be used, the CytoGam® should not be diluted more than 1:2 with any of the above-named solutions. Admixtures of CytoGam® with any other solutions have not been evaluated. While filters are not necessary, and in-line filter may be used for the infusion of CytoGam®.
Initial Dose. Administer Intravenously at 15 mg per kg body weight per hour. If no adverse reactions occur after 30 minutes, the rate may be increased to 30 mg/kg/hr; If no adverse reactions occur after a subsequent 30 minutes, then the Infusion may be increased to 60 mg/kg/hr (volume not to exceed 75 ml/hour). DO NOT EXCEED THIS RATE OF ADMINISTRATION. The patient should be monitored closely during and after each rate change.
Subsequent Doses. Administer at 15 mg/kg/hr for 15 minutes. If no adverse reactions occur, increase to 30 mg/kg/hr for 15 minutes and then increase to a maximum rate of 60 mg/kg/hr (volume not to exceed 75 ml/hour). DO NOT EXCEED THIS RATE OF ADMINISTRATION. The patient should be monitored closely during each rate change.
Potential adverse reactions are: flushing, chills, muscle cramps, back pain, fever, nausea, vomiting, wheezing, drop in blood pressure. Minor adverse reactions have been infusion rate related-if the patient develops a minor side effect (i.e., nausea, back pain, flushing), slow the rate or temporarily interrupt the infusion. If anaphylaxis or drop in blood pressure occurs, discontinue infusion and use antidote such as diphenhydramine and adrenalin.
To prevent the transmission of hepatitis viruses or other infectious agents from one person to another, sterile disposable syringes and needles should be used. The syringes and needles should not be reused.

HOW SUPPLIED

CytoGam®, Cytomegalovirus Immune Globulin Intravenous (Human), is supplied in two single-dose vial forms:

NDC No.	Total Quantity of Immunoglobulin	Volume	Concentration
60574-3102-1	1000 mg ± 200 mg	20 ml	50 ± 10 mg/ml
60574-3101-1	2500 mg ± 500 mg	50 ml	50 ± 10 mg/ml

STORAGE

CytoGam® should be stored between 2°C and 8°C (35.6°F and 46.4°F), and used within 6 hours after entering the vial.

REFERENCES

1. Snydman, D.R., McIver, J., Leszczynski, J., Cho, S.I., Werner, B.G., Berardi, V.P., LoGerfo, F., HeinzeLacey, B., Grady, G.F. A Pilot Trial of a Novel Cytomegalovirus Immune Globulin in Renal Transplant Recipients. Transplantation 38(5):553–557, 1984.
2. Horowitz, B., Wiebe, M.E., Lippin, A. et al. Inactivation of Viruses in Labile Blood Derivatives. Transfusion; 25: 516–522, 1985.
3. Snydman, D.R., Werner, B.G., and Heinze-Lacey, B.H., et al. Use of Cytomegalovirus Immune Globulin to Prevent Cytomegalovirus Disease in Renal Transplant Recipients. NEJM 317:1049–1054, 1987.
4. Snydman, D.R., Werner, B.G., and Tilney, N.L., et al. A Final Analysis of Primary Cytomegalovirus Disease Prevention in Renal Transplant Recipient with a Cytomegalovirus Immune Globulin:Comparison of Randomized and Open-Label Trials. Transplant. Proceed. 23(1):1357–1360, 1991.
5. Ho, M., Suwansirikul, S., Dowling, J.N., et al. The Transplant Kidney as a Source of Cytomegalovirus Infection. NEJM 293 (2):1109–1112, 1975.
6. Werner, B.G., Snydman, D.R., Freeman, R., et al. Cytomegalovirus Immune Globulin for the Prevention of Primary CMV Disease in Renal Transplant Patients: Analysis of Usage Under Treatment IND Status. Transplant. Proceed. 25(1):1441–1443, 1993.
7. Sekul E, Culper E. Dalaks M. Aseptic meningitis associated with high-dose intravenous immunoglobulin therapy: Frequency and risk factors. Ann Int Med; 123:259–262, 1994.
8. Kato E, Shindo S, Eto Y, Hashimoto N, Yamamoto M, Sakata Y, Hiyoshi Y, Administration of immune globulin associated with aseptic meningitis. JAMA; 3269–3270, 1988.
9. Casteels Van Daele M, Wijndaele L, Hunnick K, Gillis P. Intravenous immunoglobulin and acute aseptic meningitis. N Engl J Med; 323(9):614–615, 1990.
10. Scribner C, Kapit R, Philips E, Rickels N. Aseptic meningitis and intravenous immunoglobulin therapy. Ann Intern Med; 121:305–306, 1994.
11. Bossell, et al. Safety of therapeutic immune globulin preparations with respect to transmission of human T-lymphotropic virus type III/lymphodenopathy-associated virus infection MMWR vol. 35 (14):231–233, April 11, 1986.
12. Wells MA, Wittek AE, Epstein JS, et al. Inactivation and partition of human T-cell lymphotropic virus, type III, during ethanol fractionation of plasma. Transfusion 26: 210–213, 1986.
13. McIver, J. Grady, G. Immunoglobulin preparations. In: Churchill WH and Kurtz SR, (ed): Transfusion Medicine. Boston: Blackwell; 1988.
14. Schneider L, Geha R. Outbreak of Hepatitis C associated with intravenous immunoglobulin administration-United States, October 1993–June 1994. MMWR vol. 43 (28):505–509, July 22, 1994.
15. Edwards CA, Piet MP J, China S. Horowitz B. Tri(n Butyl) phosphate detergent treatment of licensed therapeutic and experimental blood derivatives. Vox Sang 52: 53–59, 1987.

For additional information concerning Cytomegalovirus Immune Globulin Intravenous (Human) contact:
Professional Services
Medimmune, Inc.
35 West Watkins Mill Road
Gaithersburg, MD 20878, USA
1-800-949-3789

Manufactured by:
MASSACHUSETTS PUBLIC HEALTH
BIOLOGICAL LABORATORIES
Boston, Massachusetts 02130, USA
U.S. Govt. License No. 64
Marketed by:
MedImmune, Inc.
35 West Watkins Mill Road
Gaithersburg, MD 20878, USA
3AA1201
Product Information as of June, 1996 Ed.003
2754

SYNAGIS™ ℞
(palivizumab)
for Intramuscular Administration

DESCRIPTION

Synagis™, palivizumab, is a humanized monoclonal antibody (IgG1κ) produced by recombinant DNA technology, directed to an epitope in the A antigenic site of the F protein of respiratory syncytial virus (RSV). Palivizumab is a composite human (95%) and murine (5%) antibody sequences. The human heavy chain sequence was derived from the constant domains of human IgG1 and the variable framework regions of the V_H genes Cor (1) and Cess (2). The human light chain sequence was derived from the constant domain of Cκ and the variable framework regions of the V_L gene K104 with Jκ -4 (3). The murine sequences were derived from a murine monoclonal antibody, Mab 1129 (4), in a process which involved the grafting of the murine complementarity determining regions into the human antibody frameworks. Synagis™ is composed of two heavy chains and two light chains and has a molecular weight of approximately 148,000 Daltons.
Synagis™ is supplied as a sterile lyophilized product for reconstitution with sterile water for injection. Reconstituted Synagis™ is to be administered by intramuscular injection only. Upon reconstitution, Synagis™ contains the following excipients: 47 mM histidine, 3.0 mM glycine and 5.6% mannitol and the active ingredient, palivizumab, at a concentration of 100 milligrams per vial. The reconstituted solution should appear clear or slightly opalescent.

CLINICAL PHARMACOLOGY

Mechanism of Action: Synagis™ exhibits neutralizing and fusion-inhibitory activity against RSV. These activities inhibit RSV replication in laboratory experiments. Although resistant RSV strains may be isolated in laboratory studies, a panel of 57 clinical RSV isolates were all neutralized by Synagis™ (5). Synagis™ serum concentrations of ≥ 40 μg/ml have been shown to reduce pulmonary RSV replication in the cotton rat model of RSV infection by 100-fold (5). The *in vivo* neutralizing activity of the active ingredient in Synagis™ (palivizumab) was assessed in a randomized, placebo-controlled study of 35 pediatric patients tracheally intubated because of RSV disease. In these patients, palivizumab significantly reduced the quantity of RSV in the lower respiratory tract compared to control patients (6).
Pharmacokinetics: In studies in adult volunteers Synagis™ had a pharmacokinetic profile similar to a human IgG1 antibody in regard to the volume of distribution and the half-life (mean 18 days). In pediatric patients less than 24 months of age, the mean half-life of Synagis™ was 20 days and monthly intramuscular doses of 15 mg/kg achieved mean ±SD 30 day trough serum drug concentrations of 37 ±21 μg/mL after the first injection, 57 ±41 μg/mL after the second injection 68 ±51 μg/mL after the third injection and 72 ±50 μg/mL after the fourth injection (7). In pediatric patients given Synagis™ for a second season, the mean ±SD serum concentrations following the first and fourth injections were 61 ±17 μg/mL and 86 ±31 μg/mL, respectively.

CLINICAL STUDIES

The safety and efficacy of Synagis™ were assessed in a randomized, double-blind, placebo-controlled trial (IMpact-RSV Trial) of RSV disease prophylaxis among high-risk pediatric patients (7). This trial, conducted at 139 centers in the United States, Canada and the United Kingdom, studied patients ≤ 24 months of age with bronchopulmonary dysplasia (BPD) and patients with premature birth (≤ 35 weeks gestation) who were ≤ 6 months of age at study entry. Patients with uncorrected congenital heart disease were excluded from enrollment. In this trial, 500 patients were randomized to receive five monthly placebo injections and 1,002 patients were randomized to receive five monthly injections of 15 mg/kg of Synagis™. Subjects were randomized into the study from November 15, to December 13, 1996, and were followed for safety and efficacy for 150 days. Ninety-nine percent of all subjects completed the study and 93% received all five injections. The primary endpoint was the incidence of RSV hospitalization.
RSV hospitalizations occurred among 53 of 500 (10.6%) patients in the placebo group and 48 of 1002 (4.8%) patients in the Synagis™ group, a 55% reduction ($p<0.001$). The reduction of RSV hospitalization was observed both in patients

enrolled with a diagnosis of BPD (34/266 [12.8%] placebo vs 39/496 [7.9%] Synagis™) and patients enrolled with a diagnosis of prematurity without BPD (19/234 [8.1%] placebo vs 9/506 [1.8%] Synagis™). The reduction of RSV hospitalization was observed throughout the course of the RSV season. Among secondary endpoints, the incidence of ICU admission during hospitalization for RSV infection was lower among subjects receiving Synagis™ (1.3%) than among those receiving placebo (3.0%), but there was no difference in the mean duration of ICU care between the two groups for patients requiring ICU care. Overall, the data do not suggest that RSV illness was less severe among patients who received Synagis™ and who required hospitalization due to RSV infection than among placebo patients who required hospitalization due to RSV infection. Synagis™ did not alter the incidence and mean duration of hospitalization for non-RSV respiratory illness or the incidence of otitis media.

INDICATIONS AND USAGE

Synagis™ (palivizumab) is indicated for the prevention of serious lower respiratory tract disease caused by respiratory virus (RSV) in pediatric patients at high risk of RSV disease. Safety and efficacy were established in infants with bronchopulmonary dysplasia (BPD) and infants with a history of prematurity (≤ 35 weeks gestational age). See *Clinical Studies* section.

CONTRAINDICATIONS

Synagis™ should not be used in pediatric patients with a history of a severe prior reaction to Synagis™ or other components of this product.

WARNINGS

Anaphylactoid reactions following the administration of Synagis™ have not been observed but can occur following the administration of proteins. **If anaphylaxis or severe allergic reaction occurs, administer epinephrine (1:1000) and provide supportive care as required.**

PRECAUTIONS

General: Synagis™ is for intramuscular use only. As with any intramuscular injection, Synagis™ should be given with caution to patients with thrombocytopenia or any coagulation disorder.

The safety and efficacy of Synagis™ have been demonstrated for treatment of established RSV disease.

The single-use vial of Synagis™ does not contain a preservative. Injections should be given within 6 hours after reconstitution.

Immunogenicity: In the IMpact-RSV trial, the incidence of anti-humanized antibody following the fourth injection was 1.1% in the placebo group and 0.7% in the Synagis™ group. In pediatric patients receiving Synagis™ for a second season, one of fifty-six patients had transient, low titer reactivity. This reactivity was not associated with adverse events or alteration in Synagis™ serum concentrations.

Drug Interactions: No formal drug-drug interaction studies were conducted. In the IMpact-RSV trial, the proportions of patients in the placebo and Synagis™ groups who received routine childhood vaccines, influenza vaccine, bronchodilators or corticosteroids were similar and no incremental increase in adverse reactions was observed among patients receiving these agents.

Carcinogenesis, Mutagenesis, Impairment of Fertility: Carcinogenesis, mutagenesis and reproductive toxicity studies have not been performed.

Pregnancy: Pregnancy Category C: Synagis™ is not indicated for adult usage and animal reproduction studies have not been conducted. It is also not known whether Synagis™ can cause fetal harm when administered to a pregnant woman or could affect reproductive capacity.

ADVERSE REACTIONS

In the combined pediatric prophylaxis studies of pediatric patients with BPD or prematurity involving 520 subjects receiving placebo and 1168 subjects receiving Synagis™, the proportions of subjects in the placebo and Synagis™ groups who experienced any adverse event or any serious adverse event were similar.

Most of the safety information was derived from the IMpact-RSV trial. In this study, Synagis™ was discontinued in five patients: two because of vomiting and diarrhea, one because of erythema and moderate induration at the site of the fourth injection, and two because of pre-existing medical conditions which required management (one with congenital anemia and one with pulmonary venous stenosis requiring cardiac surgery). Deaths in study patients occurred in five of 500 placebo recipients and four of 1002 Synagis™ recipients. Sudden infant death syndrome was responsible for two of these deaths in the placebo group and one death in the Synagis™ group. Adverse events which occurred in more than 1% of patients receiving Synagis™ in the IMpact-RSV study for which the incidence in the Synagis™ group was 1% greater than in the placebo group are shown in Table 1.

Table 1. Adverse Events Occurring in IMpact-RSV Study at Greater Frequency in the Synagis™ Group

% of patients with:	Placebo n = 500	Synagis™ n = 1002
upper respiratory infection	49.0%	52.6%
otitis media	40.0%	41.9%
rhinitis	23.4%	28.7%
rash	22.4%	25.6%
pain	6.8%	8.5%
hernia	5.0%	6.3%
SGOT increased	3.8%	4.9%
pharyngitis	1.4%	2.6%

Other adverse events reported in more than 1% of the Synagis™ group included: cough, wheeze, bronchiolitis, pneumonia, bronchitis, asthma, croup, dyspnea, sinusitis, apnea, failure to thrive, nervousness, diarrhea, vomiting, and gastroenteritis, SGPT increase, liver function abnormality, study drug injections site reaction, conjunctivitis, viral infection, oral monilia, fungal dermatitis, eczema, seborrhea, anemia and flu syndrome. The incidence of these adverse events was similar between the Synagis™ and placebo groups.

OVERDOSAGE

No data from clinical studies are available on overdosage. No toxicity was observed in rabbits administered a single intramuscular or subcutaneous injection of Synagis™ at a dose of 50 mg/kg. No data are available from human subjects who have received more than 5 monthly Synagis™ doses during a single RSV season.

DOSAGE AND ADMINISTRATION

The recommended dose of Synagis™ is 15 mg/kg of body weight. Patients, including those who develop an RSV infection, should receive monthly doses throughout the RSV season. The first dose should be administered prior to commencement of the RSV season. In the northern hemisphere, the RSV season typically commences in November and lasts through April, but it may begin earlier or persist later in certain communities.

Synagis™ should be administered in a dose of 15 mg/kg intramuscularly using aseptic technique, preferably in the anterolateral aspect of the thigh. The gluteal muscle should not be used routinely as an injection site because of the risk of damage to the sciatic nerve. The dose per month = [patient weight (kg) × 15 mg/kg ÷ 100 mg/mL of Synagis™]. Injection volumes over 1 mL should be given as a divided dose.

Preparation for Administration

- To reconstitute, remove the tab portion of the vial cap and clean the rubber stopper with 70% ethanol or equivalent.
- Slowly add 1.0 mL of sterile water for injection to a 100 mg vial. The vial should be gently swirled for 30 seconds to avoid foaming. DO NOT SHAKE VIAL.
- Reconstituted Synagis™ should stand at room temperature for a minimum of 20 minutes until the solution clarifies.
- Reconstituted Synagis™ does not contain a preservative and should be administered within 6 hours of reconstitution

To prevent the transmission of hepatitis viruses or other infectious agents from one person to another, sterile disposable syringes and needles should be used. Do not reuse syringes and needles.

HOW SUPPLIED

Synagis™ is supplied in a single use vial containing 100 mg lyophilized product.

NDC 60574-4111-1 100 mg vial

Upon receipt and until reconstitution for use, Synagis™ should be stored between 2 and 8°C (35.6° and 46.4°F) in its original container. Do not freeze. Do not use beyond the expiration date.

REFERENCES

1. Press E, and Hogg N. The amino acid sequences of the Fd Fragments of Two Human gamma-1 heavy chains. Biochem. J. 1970;117:641–660.
2. Takahashi N, Noma T, and Honjo T. Rearranged immunoglobulin heavy chain variable region (V_H) psuedogene that deletes the second complimentary-determining region. Proc. Nat. Acad. Sci. USA 1984;81:5194–5198.
3. Bently D, and Rabbitts T. Human immunoglobulin variable region genes – DNA sequences of two V_k genes and a pseudogene. Nature 1980;288:730–733.
4. Beeler JA and Van Wyke Coelingh K. Neutralization epitopes of the F Protein of Respiratory Syncytial Virus: Effect of mutation upon fusion function. J. Virology 1989;63:2941–2950

5. Johnson S, Oliver C, Prince GA, et al. Development of a humanized monoclonal antibody (MEDI-493) with potent in vitro and in vivo activity against respiratory syncytial virus. J. Infect. Dis. 1997; 176:1215–1224.
6. DeVincenzo, JP, Malley R, Ramilo O, et al. Viral Concentration in Upper and Lower Respiratory Secretions from Respiratory Syncytial Virus (RSV) Infected Children Treated with RSV Monoclonal Antibody (MEDI-493). Pediatric Research 1998; 43: 144A [Abstract 830].
7. The IMpact RSV Study Group, Palivizumab, a Humanized Respiratory Syncytial Virus Monoclonal Antibody, Reduces Hospitalization From Respiratory Syncytial Virus Infection in High-risk Infants. *Pediatrics in press.*

Manufactured by:
MedImmune, Inc.
Gaithersburg, MD 20878
(1-800-949-3789)
Co-Marketed by:
Ross Products Division
Abbott Laboratories, Inc.
Columbus, OH 43215
Rev. date: June 19, 1998

Merck & Co., Inc.
WEST POINT, PA 19486

For Medical Information Contact:
Generally:
Product and service information:
Call the Merck National Service Center, 8:00 AM to 7:00 PM (ET), Monday through Friday:
(800) NSC-MERCK
(800) 672-6372
FAX: (800) MERCK-68
FAX: (800) 637-2568
Adverse Drug Experiences:
Call the Merck National Service Center, 8:00 AM to 7:00 PM (ET), Monday through Friday:
(800) NSC-MERCK
(800) 672-6372
In Emergencies:
24-hour emergency information for healthcare professionals:
(800) NSC-MERCK
(800) 672-6372

Sales and Ordering:
For product orders and direct account inquiries only, call the Order Management Center,
8:00 AM to 7:00 PM (ET), Monday through Friday:
(800) MERCK RX
(800) 637-2579

AGGRASTAT® ℞
(tirofiban hydrochloride injection premixed)
AGGRASTAT®
(tirofiban hydrochloride injection)

DESCRIPTION

AGGRASTAT* (tirofiban hydrochloride), a non-peptide antagonist of the platelet glycoprotein (GP) llb/llla receptor, inhibits platelet aggregation.

Tiroban hydrochloride monohydrate, a non-peptide molecule, is chemically described as *N*-(butylsulfonyl)-*O*-[4-(4-piperidinyl)butyl]-L-tyrosine monohydrochloride monohydrate.

Its molecular formula is $C_{22}H_{36}N_2O_5S \cdot HCl \cdot H_2O$ and its structural formula is:

Tirofiban hydrochloride monohydrate is a white to off-white, non-hygroscopic, free-flowing powder, with a molecular weight of 495.08. It is very slightly soluble in water.
AGGRASTAT Injection Premixed is supplied as a sterile solution in water for injection, for intravenous use only, in plastic containers. Each 500 mL of the premixed, iso-osmotic intravenous injection contains 28.09 mg tirofiban hydrochloride monohydrate equivalent to 25 mg tirofiban (50

Continued on next page

Aggrastat—Cont.

µg/mL) and the following inactive ingredients: 4.5 g sodium chloride, 270 mg sodium citrate dihydrate, and 16 mg citric acid anhydrous. The pH ranges from 5.5 to 6.5 and may have been adjusted with hydrochloric acid and/or sodium hydroxide.

The flexible container is manufactured from a specially designed multilayer plastic (PL2408). Solutions in contact with the plastic container leach out certain chemical components from the plastic in very small amounts; however, biological testing was supportive of the safety of the plastic container materials.

AGGRASTAT Injection is a sterile concentrated solution for intravenous infusion after dilution and is supplied in a 50 mL vial. Each mL of the solution contains 0.281 mg of tirofiban hydrochloride monohydrate equivalent to 0.25 mg of tirofiban and the following inactive ingredients: 0.16 mg citric acid anhydrous, 2.7 mg sodium citrate dihydrate, 8 mg sodium chloride, and water for injection. The pH ranges from 5.5 to 6.5 and may have been adjusted with hydrochloric acid and/or sodium hydroxide.

---

*Registered trademark of MERCK & CO., Inc.

CLINICAL PHARMACOLOGY

Mechanism of Action

AGGRASTAT is a reversible antagonist of fibrinogen binding to the GP llb/llla receptor, the major platelet surface receptor involved in platelet aggregation. When administered intravenously, AGGRASTAT inhibits *ex vivo* platelet aggregation in a dose- and concentration-dependent manner. When given according to the recommended regimen, >90% inhibition is attained by the end of the 30-minute infusion. Platelet aggregation inhibition is reversible following cessation of the infusion of AGGRASTAT.

Pharmacokinetics

Tirofiban has a half-life of approximately 2 hours. It is cleared from the plasma largely by renal excretion, with about 65% of an administered dose appearing in urine and about 25% in feces, both largely as unchanged tirofiban. Metabolism appears to be limited.

Tirofiban is not highly bound to plasma proteins and protein binding is concentration independent over the range of 0.01 to 25 µg/mL. Unbound fraction in human plasma is 35%. The steady state volume of distribution of tirofiban ranges from 22 to 42 liters.

In healthy subjects, the plasma clearance of tirofiban ranges from 213 to 314 mL/min. Renal clearance accounts for 39 to 69% of plasma clearance. The recommended regimen of a loading infusion followed by a maintenance infusion produces a peak tirofiban plasma concentration that is similar to the steady state concentration during the infusion. In patients with coronary artery disease, the plasma clearance of tirofiban ranges from 152 to 267 mL/min; renal clearance accounts for 39% of plasma clearance.

Special Populations

Gender

Plasma clearance of tirofiban in patients with coronary artery disease is similar in males and females.

Elderly

Plasma clearance of tirofiban is about 19 to 26% lower in elderly (>65 years) patients with coronary artery disease than in younger (≤65 years) patients.

Race

No difference in plasma clearance was detected in patients of different races.

Hepatic Insufficiency

In patients with mild to moderate hepatic insufficiency, plasma clearance of tirofiban is not significantly different from clearance in healthy subjects.

Renal Insufficiency

Plasma clearance of tirofiban is significantly decreased (>50%) in patients with creatinine clearance <30 mL/min, including patients requiring hemodialysis (see DOSAGE AND ADMINISTRATION, *Recommended Dosage*). Tirofiban is removed by hemodialysis.

Pharmacodynamics

AGGRASTAT inhibits platelet function, as demonstrated by its ability to inhibit *ex vivo* adenosine phosphate (ADP)-induced platelet aggregation and prolong bleeding time in healthy subjects and patients with coronary artery disease. The time course of inhibition parallels the plasma concentration profile of the drug. Following discontinuation of an infusion of AGGRASTAT, 0.10 µg/kg/min, *ex vivo* platelet aggregation returns to near baseline in approximately 90% of patients with coronary artery disease in 4 to 8 hours. The addition of heparin to this regimen does not significantly alter the percentage of subjects with >70% inhibition of platelet aggregation (IPA), but does increase the average bleeding time, as well as the number of patients with bleeding times prolonged to >30 minutes.

In patients with unstable angina, a two-staged intravenous infusion regimen of AGGRASTAT (loading infusion of 0.4 µg/kg/min for 30 minutes followed by 0.1 µg/kg/min for up to 48 hours in the presence of heparin and aspirin), produces approximately 90% inhibition of *ex vivo* ADP-induced platelet aggregation with a 2.9-fold prolongation of bleeding time during the loading infusion. Inhibition persists over the duration of the maintenance infusion.

Clinical Trials

Three large-scale clinical studies were conducted to study the efficacy and safety of AGGRASTAT in the management of patients with Acute Coronary Syndrome (unstable angina/non-Q-wave myocardial infarction). Acute Coronary Syndrome is characterized by prolonged (≥10 minutes) or repetitive symptoms of cardiac ischemia occurring at rest or with minimal exertion, associated with either ischemic ST-T wave changes on electrocardiogram (ECG) or elevated cardiac enzymes. The definition includes "unstable angina" and "non-Q-wave myocardial infarction" but excludes myocardial infarction that is associated with Q-waves or non-transient ST-segment elevation. The three studies examined AGGRASTAT alone and as an addition to heparin, prior to and after angioplasty (if indicated) (PRISM-PLUS), in comparison to heparin in a similar population (PRISM), and in addition to heparin in patients undergoing percutaneous transluminal coronary angioplasty (PTCA) or atherectomy (RESTORE). These trials are discussed in detail below.

PRISM-PLUS (Platelet Receptor Inhibition for Ischemic Syndrome Management–Patients Limited by Unstable Signs and Symptoms)

In the multi-center, randomized, parallel, double-blind PRISM-PLUS trial, the use of AGGRASTAT in combination with heparin (n=773) was compared to heparin alone (n=797) in patients with documented unstable angina/non-Q-wave myocardial infarction within 12 hours of entry into the study and initiation of treatment. All patients with unstable angina/non-Q-wave myocardial infarction had cardiac ischemia documented by ECG or had elevated cardiac enzymes. Patients who were medically managed or who subsequently underwent revascularization procedures were studied. The mean age of the population was 63 years; 32% of patients were female and approximately half of the population presented with non-Q-wave myocardial infarction. Exclusions included contraindications to anticoagulation (see CONTRAINDICATIONS), decompensated heart failure, platelet count <150,000/mm^3, and creatinine >2.5 mg/dL. In this study, patients were randomized to either AGGRASTAT (30 minute loading infusion of 0.4 µg/kg/min followed by a maintenance infusion of 0.10 µg/kg/min) and heparin (bolus of 5,000 units (U) followed by an infusion of 1,000 U/hr titrated to maintain an activated partial thromboplastin time (APTT) of approximately 2 times control), or heparin alone (bolus of 5,000 U followed by an infusion of 1,000 U/hr titrated to maintain an APTT of approximately 2 times control). All patients received concomitant aspirin unless contraindicated. Patients underwent 48 hours of medical stabilization on study drug therapy, and they were to undergo angiography before 96 hours (and, if indicated, angioplasty/atherectomy, while continuing on AGGRASTAT and heparin for 12–24 hours after the procedure). Some patients went on to coronary artery bypass grafting (CABG) after cessation of drug therapy. AGGRASTAT and heparin could be continued for up to 108 hours. On average, patients received AGGRASTAT for 71.3 hours. A third group of patients was initially randomized to AGGRASTAT alone (no heparin). This arm was stopped when the group was found, at an interim look, to have greater mortality than the other two groups. Note, however, that a direct comparison of heparin and tirofiban alone in the PRISM study (see below) did not show excess mortality

The primary endpoint of the study was a composite of refractory ischemia, new myocardial infarction and death at 7 days after initiation of AGGRASTAT and heparin. At the primary endpoint, there was a 32% risk reduction in the overall composite. The components of the composite were examined separately (they total more than the composite because a patient could have more than one, e.g., by dying after having a new infarction). There was a 47% risk reduction in myocardial infarction and a 30% risk reduction in refractory ischemia. The results are shown in Table 1.

[See table 1 below]

The benefit seen at 7 days was maintained over time. At 30 days, the risk of the composite endpoint was reduced by 22% (p=0.029) and there was a 30% reduction in the composite of myocardial infarction and death (p=0.027). At 6 months, the risk of the composite endpoint was reduced by 19% (p=0.024). The risk reduction in the composite endpoint at 30 days and 6 months is shown in the Kaplan-Meier curve below.

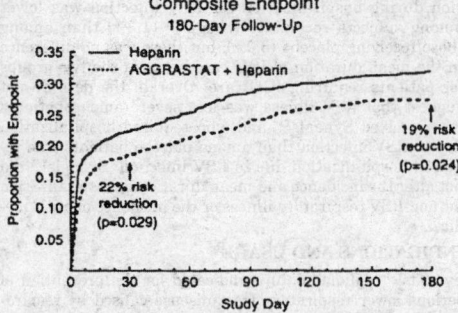

PRISM-PLUS was not designed to provide definitive results in subsets of the overall population. Nonetheless, results were examined for demographic (age, gender, race) subsets and for people who did and did not receive PTCA, atherectomy, or CABG.

In PRISM-PLUS, there was a consistent treatment effect in patients either greater or less than 65 years old, and in men and women. Too few non-Caucasians were enrolled to make a definite statement about racial differences in treatment effect.

Approximately 90% of patients in the PRISM-PLUS study underwent coronary angiography and 30% underwent angioplasty/atherectomy during the first 30 days of the study. The majority of these patients continued on study drug throughout these procedures. AGGRASTAT was continued for 12-24 hours (average 15 hours) after angioplasty/atherectomy. The effects of AGGRASTAT at Day 30 did not appear to differ among the sub-populations that did or did not receive PTCA or CABG, both prior to and after the procedure.

A sub-study in PRISM-PLUS of angiograms after 48 to 96 hours found that there was a significant decrease in the extent of angiographically apparent thrombus in patients treated with AGGRASTAT in combination with heparin compared to heparin alone. In addition, flow in the affected coronary artery was significantly improved.

PRISM (Platelet Receptor Inhibition for Ischemic Syndrome Management)

In the PRISM study, a randomized, parallel, double-blind, active control study, AGGRASTAT alone (n=1616) was compared to heparin (n=1616) alone as medical management in patients with unstable angina/non-Q-wave myocardial infarction. In this study, the drug was started within 24 hours of the time the patient experienced chest pain. The mean age of the population was 62 years; 32% of the population was female and 25% had non-Q-wave myocardial infraction on presentation. Thirty percent had no ECG evidence of cardiac ischemia. Exclusion criteria were similar to PRISM-PLUS. The primary, prospectively identified endpoint was the composite endpoint of refractory ischemia, myocardial infarction or death after a 48-hour drug infusion with AGGRASTAT. The results are shown in Table 2.

[See table 2 at top of next page]

In the PRISM study, no adverse effect of AGGRASTAT on mortality at either 7 or 30 days was detected. This result is in conflict with the PRISM-PLUS study, where the arm that included AGGRASTAT without heparin (n=345) was dropped at an interim analysis by the Data Safety Monitoring Committee due to increased mortality at 7 days. A pooled analysis of the data from these two trials (PRISM and PRISM-PLUS) demonstrated that the effect of AGGRASTAT alone on mortality (at 7 and 30 days) was comparable to that of heparin alone.

RESTORE (Randomized Efficacy Study of Tirofiban for Outcomes and Restenosis)

The RESTORE study (n=2141) was a randomized, placebo-controlled comparison of AGGRASTAT and placebo, each added to heparin, in patients undergoing PTCA or atherectomy within 72 hours of presentation with unstable angina

Table 1
Cardiac Ischemic Events (7 Days)

Endpoint	AGGRASTAT+ Heparin (n=773)	Heparin (n=797)	Risk Reduction	p-value
Composite Endpoint	12.9%	17.9%	32%	0.004
Components				
Myocardial Infarction and Death	4.9%	8.3%	43%	0.006
Myocardial Infarction	3.9%	7.0%	47%	0.006
Death	1.9%	1.9%	—	—
Refractory Ischemia	9.3%	12.7%	30%	0.023

Table 2
Cardiac Ischemic Events

Composite Endpoint	AGGRASTAT (n=1616)	Heparin (n=1616)	Risk Reduction	p-value
2 Days	3.8%	5.6%	33%	0.015
7 Days	10.3%	11.3%	10%	0.33
30 Days	15.9%	17.1%	8%	0.34

Table 3
Cardiac Ischemic Events

Composite Endpoint	AGGRASTAT (n=1071)	Placebo (n=1070)	Risk Reduction	p-value
2 Days	5.4%	8.7%	38%	0.004
7 Days	7.6%	10.4%	28%	0.023
30 Days	10.3%	12.2%	17%	0.17

or acute myocardial infarction. The mean age of the population was 59 years; 27% were female. Two-thirds of patients underwent angioplasty for unstable angina and the remainder in association with acute myocardial infarction. Exclusions included anatomy not amenable to angioplasty, contraindications to anticoagulation (see CONTRAINDICATIONS), platelet count <150,000/mm³, and creatinine >2.0 mg/dL. AGGRASTAT (with heparin) was initiated immediately prior to the angioplasty/atherectomy at a dose of 10 µg/kg bolus (over 3 minutes) followed by an infusion of 0.15 µg/kg/min along with a heparin bolus (bolus of 10,000 U, or 150 U/kg for patients <70 kg). The infusion dose of AGGRASTAT is 50% higher than the dose used in the PRISM-PLUS trial. AGGRASTAT was administered for a total of 36 hours. In general, heparin was to be discontinued at the conclusion of the angioplasty/atherectomy. Reasons for continued heparin included: imperfect outcome (e.g., large tear, intraluminal filling defect, or residual stenosis >40%), large thrombus load, continuing rest angina through the procedure, abrupt closure or very active artery during the procedure, or side branch occlusion. The primary endpoint was the composite of all deaths, non-fatal myocardial infarctions, and all repeat revascularization procedures at 30 days. For results see Table 3. A sub-study in RESTORE of angiograms after approximately 6 months found that AGGRASTAT had no significant effect on the extent of coronary artery restenosis following angioplasty.

[See Table 3 above]

The risk reduction in the composite endpoint at 180 days is shown in the Kaplan-Meier curve below.

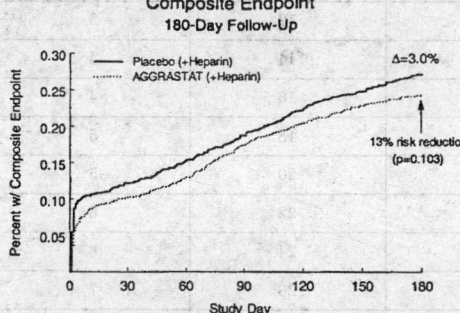

Composite Endpoint
180-Day Follow-Up

INDICATIONS AND USAGE

AGGRASTAT, in combination with heparin, is indicated for the treatment of acute coronary syndrome, including patients who are to be managed medically and those undergoing PTCA or atherectomy. In this setting, AGGRASTAT has been shown to decrease the rate of a combined endpoint of death, new myocardial infarction or refractory ischemia/repeat cardiac procedure (for discussion of trial results and for definition of acute coronary syndrome see CLINICAL PHARMACOLOGY, *Clinical Trials*).

AGGRASTAT has been studied in a setting, as described in *Clinical Trials*, that included aspirin and heparin.

CONTRAINDICATIONS

AGGRASTAT is contraindicated in patients with:
- known hypersensitivity to any component of the product
- active internal bleeding or a history of bleeding diathesis within the previous 30 days
- a history of intracranial hemorrhage, intracranial neoplasm, arteriovenous malformation, or aneurysm
- a history of thrombocytopenia following prior exposure to AGGRASTAT
- history of stroke within 30 days or any history of hemorrhagic stroke

- major surgical procedure or severe physical trauma within the previous month
- history, symptoms, or findings suggestive of aortic dissection
- severe hypertension (systolic blood pressure >180 mmHg and/or diastolic blood pressure >110 mmHg)
- concomitant use of another parenteral GP IIb/IIIa inhibitor
- acute pericarditis

WARNINGS

Bleeding is the most common complication encountered during therapy with AGGRASTAT. Administration of AGGRASTAT is associated with an increase in bleeding events classified as both major and minor bleeding events by criteria developed by the Thrombolysis in Myocardial Infarction Study group (TIMI).** Most major bleeding associated with AGGRASTAT occurs at the arterial access site for cardiac catheterization.

AGGRASTAT should be used with caution in patients with platelet count <150,000/mm³ and in patients with hemorrhagic retinopathy.

Because AGGRASTAT inhibits platelet aggregation, caution should be employed when it is used with other drugs that affect hemostasis. The safety of AGGRASTAT when used in combination with thrombolytic agents has not been established.

During therapy with AGGRASTAT, patients should be monitored for potential bleeding. When bleeding cannot be controlled with pressure, infusion of AGGRASTAT and heparin should be discontinued.

** Bovill, E.G.; et al.: Hemorrhagic Events during Therapy with Recombinant Tissue-Type Plasminogen Activator, Heparin, and Aspirin for Acute Myocardial Infarction, Results of the Thrombolysis in Myocardial Infarction (TIMI) Phase II Trial, Annals of Internal Medicine, *115*(4):256-265, 1991.

PRECAUTIONS

Bleeding Precautions
Percutaneous Coronary Intervention—Care of the femoral artery access site: Therapy with AGGRASTAT is associated with increases in bleeding rates particularly at the site of arterial access for femoral sheath placement. Care should be taken when attempting vascular access that only the anterior wall of the femoral artery is punctured. Prior to pulling the sheath, heparin should be discontinued for 3-4 hours and activated clotting time (ACT) <180 seconds or APTT <45 seconds should be documented. Care should be taken to obtain proper hemostasis after removal of the sheaths using standard compressive techniques followed by close observation. While the vascular sheath is in place, patients should be maintained on complete bed rest with the head of the bed elevated 30° and the affected limb restrained in a straight position. Sheath hemostasis should be achieved at least 4 hours before hospital discharge.

Minimize Vascular and Other Trauma: Other arterial and venous punctures, intramuscular injections, and the use of urinary catheters, nasotracheal intubation and nasogastric tubes should be minimized. When obtaining intravenous access, non-compressible sites (e.g., subclavian or jugular veins) should be avoided.

Laboratory Monitoring: Platelet counts, and hemoglobin and hematocrit should be monitored prior to treatment, within 6 hours following the loading infusion, and at least daily thereafter during therapy with AGGRASTAT (or more frequently if there is evidence of significant decline). If the patient experiences a platelet decrease to <90,000/mm³, additional platelet counts should be performed to exclude pseudothrombocytopenia. If thrombocytopenia is confirmed, AGGRASTAT and heparin should be discontinued and the condition appropriately monitored and treated.

To monitor unfractionated heparin, APTT should be monitored 6 hours after the start of the heparin infusion; heparin should be adjusted to maintain APTT at approximately 2 times control.

Severe Renal Insufficiency
In clinical studies, patients with severe renal insufficiency (creatinine clearance <30 mL/min) showed decreased plasma clearance of AGGRASTAT. The dosage of AGGRASTAT should be reduced in these patients (see DOSAGE AND ADMINISTRATION and CLINICAL PHARMACOLOGY, *Clinical Trials*).

Drug Interactions
AGGRASTAT has been studied on a background of aspirin and heparin.

The use of AGGRASTAT, in combination with heparin and aspirin, has been associated with an increase in bleeding compared to heparin and aspirin alone (see ADVERSE REACTIONS). Caution should be employed when AGGRASTAT is used with other drugs that affect hemostasis (e.g., warfarin). No information is available about the concomitant use of AGGRASTAT with thrombolytic agents (see PRECAUTIONS, *Bleeding Precautions*).

In a sub-set of patients (n=762) in the PRISM study, the plasma clearance of tirofiban in patients receiving one of the following drugs was compared to that in patients not receiving that drug. There were no clinically significant effects of co-administration of these drugs on the plasma clearance of tirofiban: acebutolol, acetaminophen, alprazolam, amlodipine, aspirin preparations, atenolol, bromazepam, captopril, diazepam, digoxin, diltiazem, docusate sodium, enalapril, furosemide, glyburide, heparin, insulin, isosorbide, lorazepam, lovastatin, metoclopramide, metoprolol, morphine, nifedipine, nitrate preparations, oxazepam, potassium chloride, propranolol, ranitidine, simvastatin, sucralfate and temazepam. Patients who received levothyroxine or omeprazole along with AGGRASTAT had a higher rate of clearance of AGGRASTAT. The clinical significance of this is unknown.

Carcinogenesis, Mutagenesis, Impairment of Fertility
The carcinogenic potential of AGGRASTAT has not been evaluated.

Tirofiban HCl was negative in the *in vitro* microbial mutagenesis and V-79 mammalian cell mutagenesis assays. In addition, there was no evidence of direct genotoxicity in the *in vitro* alkaline elution and *in vitro* chromosomal aberration assays. There was no induction of chromosomal aberrations in bone marrow cells of male mice after the administration of intravenous doses up to 5 mg tirofiban/kg (about 3 times the maximum recommended daily human dose when compared on a body surface area basis).

Fertility and reproductive performance were not affected in studies with male and female rats given intravenous doses of tirofiban hydrochloride up to 5 mg/kg/day (about 5 times the maximum recommended daily human dose when compared on a body surface area basis).

Pregnancy
Pregnancy Category B
Tirofiban has been shown to cross the placenta in pregnant rats and rabbits. Studies with tirofiban HCl at intravenous doses up to 5 mg/kg/day (about 5 and 13 times the maximum recommended daily human dose for rat and rabbit, respectively, when compared on a body surface area basis) have revealed no harm to the fetus. There are, however, no adequate and well-controlled studies in pregnant women. Because animal reproduction studies are not always predictive of human response, this drug should be used during pregnancy only if clearly needed.

Nursing Mothers
It is not known whether tirofiban is excreted in human milk. However, significant levels of tirofiban were shown to be present in rat milk. Because many drugs are excreted in human milk, and because of the potential for adverse effects on the nursing infant, a decision should be made whether to discontinue nursing or discontinue the drug, taking into account the importance of the drug to the mother.

Pediatric Use
Safety and effectiveness of AGGRASTAT in pediatric patients (<18 years old) have not been established.

Use in the Elderly
Of the total number of patients in controlled clinical studies of AGGRASTAT, 42.8% were 65 years and over, while 11.7% were 75 and over. With respect to efficacy, the effect of AGGRASTAT in the elderly (≥65 years) appeared similar to that seen in younger patients (<65 years). Elderly patients receiving AGGRASTAT with heparin or heparin alone had a higher incidence of bleeding complications than younger patients, but the incremental risk of bleeding in patients treated with AGGRASTAT in combination with heparin compared to the risk in patients treated with heparin alone was similar regardless of age. The overall incidence of non-bleeding adverse events was higher in older patients (compared to younger patients) but this was true both for AGGRASTAT with heparin and heparin alone. No dose adjust-

Continued on next page

Aggrastat—Cont.

ment is recommended for the elderly population (see DOSAGE AND ADMINISTRATION, *Recommended Dosage*).

ADVERSE REACTIONS

In clinical trials, 1946 patients received AGGRASTAT in combination with heparin and 2002 patients received AGGRASTAT alone. Duration of exposure was up to 116 hours. 43% of the population was >65 years of age and approximately 30% of patients were female.

BLEEDING

The most common drug-related adverse event reported during therapy with AGGRASTAT when used concomitantly with heparin and aspirin, was bleeding (usually reported by the investigators as oozing or mild). The incidences of major and minor bleeding using the TIMI criteria in the PRISM-PLUS and RESTORE studies are shown below.

[See first table above]

There were no reports of intracranial bleeding in the PRISM-PLUS study for AGGRASTAT in combination with heparin or in the heparin control group. The incidence of intracranial bleeding in the RESTORE study was 0.1% for AGGRASTAT in combination with heparin and 0.3% for the control group (which received heparin). In the PRISM-PLUS study, the incidences of retroperitoneal bleeding reported for AGGRASTAT in combination with heparin, and for the heparin control group were 0.0% and 0.1%, respectively. In the RESTORE study, the incidences of retroperitoneal bleeding reported for AGGRASTAT in combination with heparin, and the control group were 0.6% and 0.3%, respectively. The incidences of TIMI major gastrointestinal and genitourinary bleeding for AGGRASTAT in combination with heparin in the PRISM-PLUS study were 0.1% and 0.1%, respectively; the incidences in the RESTORE study for AGGRASTAT in combination with heparin were 0.2% and 0.0%, respectively.

The incidence rates of TIMI major bleeding in patients undergoing percutaneous procedures in PRISM-PLUS are shown below.

[See second table above]

The incidence rates of TIMI major bleeding (in some cases possibly reflecting hemodilution rather than actual bleeding) in patients undergoing CABG in the PRISM-PLUS and RESTORE studies within one day of discontinuation of AGGRASTAT are shown below.

[See third table above]

Female patients and elderly patients receiving AGGRASTAT with heparin or heparin alone had a higher incidence of bleeding complications than male patients or younger patients. The incremental risk of bleeding in patients treated with AGGRASTAT in combination with heparin over the risk in patients treated with heparin alone was comparable regardless of age or gender. No dose adjustment is recommended for these populations (see DOSAGE AND ADMINISTRATION, *Recommended Dosage*).

NON-BLEEDING

The incidences of non-bleeding adverse events that occurred at an incidence of >1% and numerically higher than control, regardless of drug relationship, are shown below:

	AGGRASTAT+ Heparin (n=1953) %	Heparin (n=1887) %
Body as a Whole		
Edema/swelling	2	1
Pain, pelvic	6	5
Reaction, vasovagal	2	1
Cardiovascular System		
Bradycardia	4	3
Dissection, coronary artery	5	4
Musculoskeletal System		
Pain, leg	3	2
Nervous System / Psychiatric		
Dizziness	3	2
Skin and Skin Appendage		
Sweating	2	1

Other non-bleeding side effects (considered at least possibly related to treatment) reported at a >1% rate with AGGRASTAT administered concomitantly with heparin were nausea, fever, and headache; these side effects were reported at a similar rate in the heparin group.

In clinical studies, the incidences of adverse events were generally similar among different races, patients with or without hypertension, patients with or without diabetes mellitus, and patients with or without hypercholesteremia. The overall incidence of non-bleeding adverse events was higher in female patients (compared to male patients) and older patients (compared to younger patients). However, the incidences of non-bleeding adverse events in these patients

Bleeding	PRISM-PLUS* (UAP/Non-Q-Wave MI Study)		RESTORE* (Angioplasty/Atherectomy Study)	
	AGGRASTAT** + Heparin*** (n=773) % (n)	Heparin*** (n=797) % (n)	AGGRASTAT† + Heparin†† (n=1071) % (n)	Heparin†† (n=1070) % (n)
Major Bleeding (TIMI Criteria)‡	1.4 (11)	0.8 (6)	2.2 (24)	1.6 (17)
Minor Bleeding (TIMI Criteria)§	10.5 (81)	8.0 (64)	12.0 (129)	6.3 (67)
Transfusions	4.0 (31)	2.8 (22)	4.3 (46)	2.5 (27)

* Patients received aspirin unless contraindicated.
** 0.4 µg/kg/min loading infusion; 0.10 µg/kg/min maintenance infusion.
*** 5,000 U bolus followed by 1,000 U/hr titrated to maintain an APTT of approximately 2 times control.
† 10 µg/kg bolus followed by infusion of 0.15 µg/kg/min.
†† Bolus of 10,000 U or 150 U/kg for patients <70 kg followed by administration as necessary to maintain ACT in approximate range of 300 to 400 seconds during procedure.
‡ Hemoglobin drop of >50 g/L with or without an identified site, intracranial hemorrhage, or cardiac tamponade.
§ Hemoglobin drop of >30 g/L with bleeding from a known site, spontaneous gross hematuria, hematemesis or hemoptysis.

	AGGRASTAT + Heparin		Heparin	
	n	%	n	%
Prior to Procedures	2/773	0.3	1/797	0.1
Following Angiography	9/697	1.3	5/708	0.7
Following PTCA	6/239	2.5	5/236	2.2

	AGGRASTAT + Heparin		Heparin	
	n	%	n	%
PRISM-PLUS	5/29	17.2	11/31	35.4
RESTORE	3/12	25.0	6/16	37.5

Patient Weight (kg)	Most Patients		Severe Renal Impairment	
	30 Min Loading Infusion Rate (mL/hr)	Maintenance Infusion Rate (mL/hr)	30 Min Loading Infusion Rate (mL/hr)	Maintenance Infusion Rate (mL/hr)
30–37	16	4	8	2
38–45	20	5	10	3
46–54	24	6	12	3
55–62	28	7	14	4
63–70	32	8	16	4
71–79	36	9	18	5
80–87	40	10	20	5
88–95	44	11	22	6
96–104	48	12	24	6
105–112	52	13	26	7
113–120	56	14	28	7
121–128	60	15	30	8
129–137	64	16	32	8
138–145	68	17	34	9
146–153	72	18	36	9

were comparable between the AGGRASTAT with heparin and the heparin alone groups. (See above for bleeding adverse events.)

Allergic Reactions / Readministration

No patients in the clinical database developed anaphylaxis and/or hives requiring discontinuation of the infusion of tirofiban. No information is available regarding the development of antibodies to tirofiban; very few patients received tirofiban twice.

Laboratory Findings

The most frequently observed laboratory adverse events in patients receiving AGGRASTAT concomitantly with heparin were related to bleeding. Decreases in hemoglobin (2.1%) and hematocrit (2.2%) were observed in the group receiving AGGRASTAT compared to 3.1% and 2.6%, respectively, in the heparin group. Increases in the presence of urine and fecal occult blood were also observed (10.7% and

18.3%, respectively) in the group receiving AGGRASTAT compared to 7.8% and 12.2%, respectively, in the heparin group.

Patients treated with AGGRASTAT, with heparin, were more likely to experience decreases in platelet counts than the control group. These decreases were reversible upon discontinuation of AGGRASTAT. The percentage of patients with a decrease of platelets to <90,000/mm^3 was 1.5%, compared with 0.6% in the patients who received heparin alone. The percentage of patients with a decrease of platelets to <50,000/mm^3 was 0.3%, compared with 0.1% of the patients who received heparin alone.

OVERDOSAGE

In clinical trials, inadvertent overdosage with AGGRASTAT occurred in doses up to 5 times and 2 times the recom-

mended dose for bolus administration and loading infusion, respectively. Inadvertent overdosage occurred in doses up to 9.8 times the 0.15 µg/kg/min maintenance infusion rate. The most frequently reported manifestation of overdosage was bleeding, primarily minor mucocutaneous bleeding events and minor bleeding at the sites of cardiac catheterization (see PRECAUTIONS, *Bleeding Precautions*). Overdosage of AGGRASTAT should be treated by assessment of the patient's clinical condition and cessation or adjustment of the drug infusion as appropriate. AGGRASTAT can be removed by hemodialysis.

DOSAGE AND ADMINISTRATION

AGGRASTAT Injection must first be diluted to the same strength as AGGRASTAT Injection Premixed, as noted under *Directions for Use*.

Use with Aspirin and Heparin
In the clinical studies, patients received aspirin, unless it was contraindicated, and heparin. AGGRASTAT and heparin can be administered through the same intravenous catheter.

Precautions
AGGRASTAT is intended for intravenous delivery using sterile equipment and technique. Do not add other drugs or remove solution directly from the bag with a syringe. Do not use plastic containers in series connections; such use can result in air embolism by drawing air from the first container if it is empty of solution. Discard unused solution 24 hours following the start of infusion.

Directions for Use
AGGRASTAT Injection is first diluted to the same strength as AGGRASTAT Injection Premixed as follows: withdraw and discard 100 mL from a 500 mL bag of sterile 0.9% sodium chloride or 5% dextrose in water and replace this volume with 100 mL of AGGRASTAT Injection (from two 50 mL vials) or withdraw and discard 50 mL from a 250 mL bag of sterile 0.9% sodium chloride of 5% dextrose in water and replace this volume with 50 mL of AGGRASTAT Injection (from one 50 mL vial), to achieve a final concentration of 50 µg/mL. Mix well prior to administration.
AGGRASTAT Injection Premixed is supplied as 500 mL of 0.9% sodium chloride containing tirofiban hydrochloride 50 µg/mL. It is supplied in IntraVia *** containers (PL 2408 plastic). To open the IntraVia™ container, first tear off its dust cover. The plastic may be somewhat opaque because of moisture absorption during sterilization; the opacity will diminish gradually. Check for leaks by squeezing the inner bag firmly; if any leaks are found, the sterility is suspect and the solution should be discarded. Do not use unless the solution is clear and the seal is intact. Suspend the container from its eyelet support, remove the plastic protector from the outlet port, and attach a conventional administration set.

Recommended Dosage
In most patients, AGGRASTAT should be administered intravenously, at an initial rate of 0.4 µg/kg/min for 30 minutes and then continued at 0.1 µg/kg/min. Patients with severe renal insufficiency (creatinine clearance <30 mL/min) should receive half the usual rate of infusion (see PRECAUTIONS, *Severe Renal Insufficiency* and CLINICAL PHARMACOLOGY, *Pharmacokinetics, Special Populations, Renal Insufficiency*). The table below is provided as a guide to dosage adjustment by weight.
[See fourth table on previous page]
No dosage adjustment is recommended for elderly or female patients (see PRECAUTIONS, *Use in the Elderly*). In PRISM-PLUS, AGGRASTAT was administered in combination with heparin for 48 to 108 hours. The infusion should be continued through angiography and for 12 to 24 hours after angioplasty or atherectomy.

*** Trademark of Baxter International, Inc.

HOW SUPPLIED

FOR INTRAVENOUS USE ONLY
No. 3713—AGGRASTAT Injection 12.5 mg per 50 mL (250 µg per mL) is a non-preserved, clear, colorless concentrated sterile solution for intravenous infusion after dilution and is supplied as follows:
NDC 0006-3713-50, 50 mL vials.
No. 3739—AGGRASTAT Injection Premixed 25 mg per 500 mL (50 µg per mL) is a clear, non-preserved, sterile solution premixed in a vehicle made iso-osmotic with sodium chloride, and is supplied as follows:
NDC 0006-3739-43, 500 mL single-dose IntraVia™ containers (PL 2408 Plastic).
Storage
AGGRASTAT Injection
Store at 25°C (77°F) with excursions permitted between 15–30°C (59–86°F) (see USP Controlled Room Temperature). Do not freeze. Protect from light during storage.
AGGRASTAT Injection Premixed
Store at 25°C (77°F) with excursions permitted between 15–30°C (59–86°F) (see USP Controlled Room Temperature). Do not freeze. Protect from light during storage.

AGGRASTAT (Tirofiban Hydrochloride Injection Premixed) is manufactured by:
MERCK & CO., INC., West Point, PA 19486, USA
by:
BAXTER HEALTHCARE CORPORATION
Deerfield, Illinois 60015 USA
AGGRASTAT (Tirofiban Hydrochloride Injection) is manufactured for:
MERCK & Co., INC., West Point, PA 19486, USA
by:
BEN VENUE LABORATORIES
Bedford, Ohio 44146 USA
9123301 Issued May 1998
COPYRIGHT © MERCK & CO., Inc., 1998
All rights reserved

ALDOCLOR® Tablets ℞
(Methyldopa-Chlorothiazide), U.S.P.

WARNING

This fixed combination drug is not indicated for initial therapy of hypertension. Hypertension requires therapy titrated to the individual patient. If the fixed combination represents the dosage so determined, its use may be more convenient in patient management. The treatment of hypertension is not static, but must be re-evaluated as conditions in each patient warrant.

DESCRIPTION

ALDOCLOR* (Methyldopa-Chlorothiazide) combines two antihypertensives: methyldopa and chlorothiazide.

Methyldopa
Methyldopa is an antihypertensive and is the *L* - isomer of alpha-methyldopa. It is levo-3-(3,4-dihydroxyphenyl)-2- methylalanine. Its empirical formula is $C_{10}H_{13}NO_4$, with a molecular weight of 211.22, and its structural formula is:

Methyldopa is a white to yellowish white, odorless fine powder, and is soluble in water.

Chlorothiazide
Chlorothiazide is a diuretic and antihypertensive. It is 6-chloro-2*H* -1, 2, 4-benzothiadiazine-7-sulfonamide 1, 1-dioxide. Its empirical formula is $C_7H_6ClN_3O_4S_2$ and its structural formula is:

It is a white, or practically white crystalline powder with a molecular weight of 295.73, which is very slightly soluble in water, but readily soluble in dilute aqueous sodium hydroxide. It is soluble in urine to the extent of about 150 mg per 100 mL at pH 7.
ALDOCLOR is supplied as tablets for oral use, each containing 250 mg of methyldopa and 250 mg of chlorothiazide. Each tablet contains the following inactive ingredients: calcium disodium edetate, cellulose, citric acid, D&C Yellow 10 aluminum lake, ethylcellulose, FD&C Yellow 6 aluminum lake, gelatin, glycerin, guar gum, hydroxypropyl methylcellulose, magnesium stearate, starch, talc, titanium dioxide, and FD&C Blue 2 aluminum lake.

*Registered trademark of MERCK & CO., Inc.

CLINICAL PHARMACOLOGY

Methyldopa
Methyldopa is an aromatic-amino-acid decarboxylase inhibitor in animals and in man. Although the mechanism of action has yet to be conclusively demonstrated, the antihypertensive effect of methyldopa probably is due to its metabolism to alpha-methylnorepinephrine, which then lowers arterial pressure by stimulation of central inhibitory alpha-adrenergic receptors, false neurotransmission, and/or reduction of plasma renin activity. Methyldopa has been shown to cause a net reduction in the tissue concentration of serotonin, dopamine, norepinephrine, and epinephrine.
Only methyldopa, the *L* -isomer of alpha-methyldopa, has the ability to inhibit dopa decarboxylase and to deplete animal tissues of norepinephrine. In man, the antihyperten-

sive activity appears to be due solely to the *L* -isomer. About twice the dose of the racemate (*DL* -alpha-methyldopa) is required for equal antihypertensive effect.
Methyldopa has no direct effect on cardiac function and usually does not reduce glomerular filtration rate, renal blood flow, or filtration fraction. Cardiac output usually is maintained without cardiac acceleration. In some patients the heart rate is slowed.
Normal or elevated plasma renin activity may decrease in the course of methyldopa therapy.
Methyldopa reduces both supine and standing blood pressure. It usually produces highly effective lowering of the supine pressure with infrequent symptomatic postural hypotension. Exercise hypotension and diurnal blood pressure variations rarely occur.
Chlorothiazide
The mechanism of the antihypertensive effect of thiazides is unknown. Chlorothiazide does not usually affect normal blood pressure.
Chlorothiazide affects the distal renal tubular mechanism of electrolyte reabsorption. At maximal therapeutic dosage all thiazides are approximately equal in their diuretic efficacy.
Chlorothiazide increases excretion of sodium and chloride in approximately equivalent amounts. Natriuresis may be accompanied by some loss of potassium and bicarbonate. After oral use diuresis begins within 2 hours, peaks in about 4 hours and lasts about 6 to 12 hours.
Pharmacokinetics and Metabolism
Methyldopa
The maximum decrease in blood pressure occurs four to six hours after oral dosage. After withdrawal, blood pressure usually returns to pretreatment levels within 24–48 hours. Methyldopa is extensively metabolized. The known urinary metabolites are: α-methyldopa mono-0-sulfate; 3-0 methyl-α- methyldopa; 3,4,-dihydroxyphenylacetone; α-methyldopamine; 3-0-methyl-α-methyldopamine and their conjugates.
Approximately 70 percent of the drug which is absorbed is excreted in the urine as methyldopa and its mono-0-sulfate conjugate. The renal clearance is about 130 mL/min in normal subjects and is diminished in renal insufficiency. The plasma half-life of methyldopa is 105 minutes. After oral doses, excretion is essentially complete in 36 hours.
Methyldopa crosses the placental barrier, appears in cord blood, and appears in breast milk.
Chlorothiazide
Chlorothiazide is not metabolized but is eliminated rapidly by the kidney. The plasma half-life is 45–120 minutes. After oral doses, 20–24 percent of the dose is excreted unchanged in the urine. Chlorothiazide crosses the placental but not the blood-brain barrier and is excreted in breast milk.

INDICATION AND USAGE

Hypertension (see box warning).

CONTRAINDICATIONS

ALDOCLOR is contraindicated in patients:
— with active hepatic disease, such as acute hepatitis and active cirrhosis
— with liver disorders previously associated with methyldopa therapy (see WARNINGS)
— with anuria
— with hypersensitivity to methyldopa, or to chlorothiazide or other sulfonamide-derived drugs
— on therapy with monoamine oxidase (MAO) inhibitors.

WARNINGS

Methyldopa
It is important to recognize that a positive Coombs test, hemolytic anemia, and liver disorders may occur with methyldopa therapy. The rare occurrences of hemolytic anemia or liver disorders could lead to potentially fatal complications unless properly recognized and managed. Read this section carefully to understand these reactions.
With prolonged methyldopa therapy, 10 to 20 percent of patients develop a positive direct Coombs test which usually occurs between 6 and 12 months of methyldopa therapy. Lowest incidence is at daily dosage of 1 g or less. This on rare occasions may be associated with hemolytic anemia, which could lead to potentially fatal complications. One cannot predict which patients with a positive direct Coombs test may develop hemolytic anemia.
Prior existence or development of a positive direct Coombs test is not in itself a contraindication to use of methyldopa.

Continued on next page

Aldoclor—Cont.

If a positive Coombs test develops during methyldopa therapy, the physician should determine whether hemolytic anemia exists and whether the positive Coombs test may be a problem. For example, in addition to a positive direct Coombs test there is less often a positive indirect Coombs test which may interfere with cross matching of blood.

Before treatment is started, it is desirable to do a blood count (hematocrit, hemoglobin, or red cell count) for a baseline or to establish whether there is anemia. Periodic blood counts should be done during therapy to detect hemolytic anemia. It may be useful to do a direct Coombs test before therapy and at 6 and 12 months after the start of therapy. If Coombs-positive hemolytic anemia occurs, the cause may be methyldopa and the drug should be discontinued. Usually the anemia remits promptly. If not, corticosteroids may be given and other causes of anemia should be considered. If the hemolytic anemia is related to methyldopa, the drug should not be reinstituted.

When methyldopa causes Coombs positivity alone or with hemolytic anemia, the red cell is usually coated with gamma globulin of the IgG (gamma G) class only. The positive Coombs test may not revert to normal until weeks to months after methyldopa is stopped.

Should the need for transfusion arise in a patient receiving methyldopa, both a direct and an indirect Coombs test should be performed. In the absence of hemolytic anemia, usually only the direct Coombs test will be positive. A positive direct Coombs test alone will not interfere with typing or cross matching. If the indirect Coombs test is also positive, problems may arise in the major cross match and the assistance of a hematologist or transfusion expert will be needed.

Occasionally, fever has occurred within the first three weeks of methyldopa therapy, associated in some cases with eosinophilia or abnormalities in one or more liver function tests, such as serum alkaline phosphatase, serum transaminases (SGOT, SGPT), bilirubin, and prothrombin time. Jaundice, with or without fever, may occur with onset usually within the first two to three months of therapy. In some patients the findings are consistent with those of cholestasis. In others the findings are consistent with hepatitis and hepatocellular injury.

Rarely, fatal hepatic necrosis has been reported after use of methyldopa. These hepatic changes may represent hypersensitivity reactions. Periodic determination of hepatic function should be done particularly during the first 6 to 12 weeks of therapy or whenever an unexplained fever occurs. If fever, abnormalities in liver function tests, or jaundice appear, stop therapy with methyldopa. If caused by methyldopa, the temperature and abnormalities in liver function characteristically have reverted to normal when the drug was discontinued. Methyldopa should not be reinstituted in such patients.

Rarely, a reversible reduction of the white blood cell count with a primary effect on the granulocytes has been seen. The granulocyte count returned promptly to normal on discontinuance of the drug. Rare cases of granulocytopenia have been reported. In each instance, upon stopping the drug, the white cell count returned to normal. Reversible thrombocytopenia has occurred rarely.

Chlorothiazide

Use with caution in severe renal disease. In patients with renal disease, thiazides may precipitate azotemia. Cumulative effects of the drug may develop in patients with impaired renal function.

Thiazides should be used with caution in patients with impaired hepatic function or progressive liver disease, since minor alterations of fluid and electrolyte balance may precipitate hepatic coma.

Thiazides may add to or potentiate the action of other antihypertensive drugs.

Sensitivity reactions may occur in patients with or without a history of allergy or bronchial asthma.

The possibility of exacerbation or activation of systemic lupus erythematosus has been reported.

Lithium generally should not be given with diuretics (see PRECAUTIONS, *Drug Interactions*).

PRECAUTIONS

General
Methyldopa

Methyldopa should be used with caution in patients with a history of previous liver disease or dysfunction (see WARNINGS).

Some patients taking methyldopa experience clinical edema or weight gain which may be controlled by use of a diuretic. Methyldopa should not be continued if edema progresses or signs of heart failure appear.

Hypertension has recurred occasionally after dialysis in patients given methyldopa because the drug is removed by this procedure.

Rarely, involuntary choreoathetotic movements have been observed during therapy with methyldopa in patients with severe bilateral cerebrovascular disease. Should these movements occur, stop therapy.

Chlorothiazide

All patients receiving diuretic therapy should be observed for evidence of fluid or electrolyte imbalance: namely, hyponatremia, hypochloremic alkalosis, and hypokalemia. Serum and urine electrolyte determinations are particularly important when the patient is vomiting excessively or receiving parenteral fluids. Warning signs or symptoms of fluid and electrolyte imbalance, irrespective of cause include dryness of mouth, thirst, weakness, lethargy, drowsiness, restlessness, confusion, seizures, muscle pains or cramps, muscular fatigue, hypotension, oliguria, tachycardia, and gastrointestinal disturbances such as nausea and vomiting. Hypokalemia may develop, especially after prolonged therapy or when severe cirrhosis is present (see CONTRAINDICATIONS and WARNINGS).

Interference with adequate oral electrolyte intake will also contribute to hypokalemia. Hypokalemia may cause cardiac arrhythmia and may also sensitize or exaggerate the response of the heart to the toxic effects of digitalis (e.g., increased ventricular irritability). Hypokalemia may be avoided or treated by use of potassium sparing diuretics or potassium supplements such as foods with a high potassium content.

Although any chloride deficit is generally mild and usually does not require specific treatment except under extraordinary circumstances (as in liver disease or renal disease), chloride replacement may be required in the treatment of metabolic alkalosis.

Dilutional hyponatremia may occur in edematous patients in hot weather; appropriate therapy is water restriction, rather than administration of salt, except in rare instances when the hyponatremia is life threatening. In actual salt depletion, appropriate replacement is the therapy of choice. Hyperuricemia may occur or acute gout may be precipitated in certain patients receiving thiazides.

In diabetic patients dosage adjustments of insulin or oral hypoglycemic agents may be required. Hyperglycemia may occur with thiazide diuretics. Thus latent diabetes mellitus may become manifest during thiazide therapy.

The antihypertensive effects of the drug may be enhanced in the postsympathectomy patient.

If progressive renal impairment becomes evident, consider withholding or discontinuing diuretic therapy.

Thiazides have been shown to increase the urinary excretion of magnesium; this may result in hypomagnesemia.

Thiazides may decrease urinary calcium excretion. Thiazides may cause intermittent and slight elevation of serum calcium in the absence of known disorders of calcium metabolism. Marked hypercalcemia may be evidence of hidden hyperparathyroidism. Thiazides should be discontinued before carrying out tests for parathyroid function.

Increases in cholesterol and triglyceride levels may be associated with thiazide diuretic therapy.

Laboratory Tests
Methyldopa

Blood count, Coombs test and liver function tests are recommended before initiating therapy and at periodic intervals (see WARNINGS).

Chlorothiazide

Periodic determination of serum electrolytes to detect possible electrolyte imbalance should be done at appropriate intervals.

Drug Interactions
Methyldopa

When methyldopa is used with other antihypertensive drugs, potentiation of antihypertensive effect may occur. Patients should be followed carefully to detect side reactions or unusual manifestations of drug idiosyncrasy.

Patients may require reduced doses of anesthetics when on methyldopa. If hypotension does occur during anesthesia, it usually can be controlled by vasopressors. The adrenergic receptors remain sensitive during treatment with methyldopa.

Monoamine oxidase (MAO) inhibitors: See CONTRAINDICATIONS.

Chlorothiazide

When given concurrently the following drugs may interact with thiazide diuretics.

Alcohol, barbiturates, or narcotics —potentiation of orthostatic hypotension may occur.

Antidiabetic drugs (oral agents and insulin)—dosage adjustment of the antidiabetic drug may be required.

Other antihypertensive drugs —additive effect or potentiation.

Cholestyramine and colestipol resins —Both cholestyramine and colestipol resins have the potential of binding thiazide diuretics and reducing diuretic absorption from the gastrointestinal tract.

Corticosteroids, ACTH —intensified electrolyte depletion, particularly hypokalemia.

Pressor amines (e.g., norepinephrine) —possible decreased response to pressor amines but not sufficient to preclude their use.

Skeletal muscle relaxants, nondepolarizing (e.g., tubocurarine) —possible increased responsiveness to the muscle relaxant.

Lithium —generally should not be given with diuretics. Diuretic agents reduce the renal clearance of lithium and add a high risk of lithium toxicity. Refer to the package insert for lithium preparations before use of such preparations with ALDOCLOR.

Non-steroidal Anti-inflammatory Drugs —In some patients, the administration of a non-steroidal anti-inflammatory agent can reduce the diuretic, natriuretic, and antihypertensive effects of loop, potassium-sparing and thiazide diuretics. Therefore, when ALDOCLOR and non-steroidal anti-inflammatory agents are used concomitantly, the patient should be observed closely to determine if the desired effect of the diuretic is obtained.

Drug / Laboratory Test Interactions
Methyldopa

Methyldopa may interfere with measurement of: urinary uric acid by the phosphotungstate method, serum creatinine by the alkaline picrate method, and SGOT by colorimetric methods. Interference with spectrophotometric methods for SGOT analysis has not been reported.

Since methyldopa causes fluorescence in urine samples at the same wave lengths as catecholamines, falsely high levels of urinary catecholamines may be reported. This will interfere with the diagnosis of pheochromocytoma. It is important to recognize this phenomenon before a patient with a possible pheochromocytoma is subjected to surgery. Methyldopa does not interfere with measurement of VMA (vanillylmandelic acid), a test for pheochromocytoma, by those methods which convert VMA to vanillin. Methyldopa is not recommended for the treatment of patients with pheochromocytoma. Rarely, when urine is exposed to air after voiding, it may darken because of breakdown of methyldopa or its metabolites.

Chlorothiazide

Thiazides should be discontinued before carrying out tests for parathyroid function (see PRECAUTIONS, *General*).

Carcinogenesis, Mutagenesis, Impairment of Fertility

Studies to evaluate the carcinogenic or mutagenic potential of the methyldopa-chlorothiazide combination, or the effects of this combination on fertility have not been performed.

Methyldopa

No evidence of a tumorigenic effect was seen when methyldopa was given for two years to mice at doses up to 1800 mg/kg/day or to rats at doses up to 240 mg/kg/day (30 and 4 times the maximum recommended human dose in mice and rats, respectively, when compared on the basis of body weight; 2.5 and 0.6 times the maximum recommended human dose in mice and rats, respectively, when compared on the basis of body surface area; calculations assume a patient weight of 50 kg).

Methyldopa was not mutagenic in the Ames Test and did not increase chromosomal aberration or sister chromatid exchanges in Chinese hamster ovary cells. These *in vitro* studies were carried out both with and without exogenous metabolic activation.

Fertility was unaffected when methyldopa was given to male and female rats at 100 mg/kg/day (1.7 times the maximum daily human dose when compared on the basis of body weight; 0.2 times the maximum daily human dose when compared on the basis of body surface area). Methyldopa decreased sperm count, sperm motility, the number of late spermatids and the male fertility index when given to male rats of 200 and 400 mg/kg/day (3.3 and 6 times the maximum daily human dose when compared on the basis of body weight; 0.5 and 1 times the maximum daily human dose when compared on the basis of body surface area).

Chlorothiazide

Carcinogenicity studies have not been done with chlorothiazide.

Chlorothiazide was not mutagenic *in vitro* in the Ames microbial mutagen test (using a maximum concentration of 5 mg/plate and *Salmonella typhimurium* strains TA 98 and TA 100) and was not mutagenic and did not induce miotic nondis junction to diploid-strains of *Aspergillus nidulans*.

Chlorothiazide had no adverse effects on fertility in female rats at doses up to 60/mg/kg/day and no adverse effects on fertility in male rats at doses up to 40 mg/kg/day. These doses are 1.5 and 1.0 times* the recommended maximum human dose, respectively, when compared on a body weight basis.

*Calculations based on a human body weight of 50 kg.

Pregnancy
Use of diuretics during normal pregnancy is inappropriate and exposes mother and fetus to unnecessary hazard. Diuretics do not prevent development of toxemia of pregnancy and there is no satisfactory evidence that they are useful in treatment of toxemia.
Teratogenic Effects—Pregnancy Category C: Reproduction studies in the rat, at doses up to 40 mg/kg/day (3–4 times the maximum recommended human dose), did not impair fertility or cause abnormalities of the fetus due to ALDOCLOR.
There are no adequate and well-controlled studies with ALDOCLOR in pregnant women. Because animal reproduction studies are not always predictive of human response, this drug should be used during pregnancy only if clearly needed.
Chlorothiazide: Thiazides cross the placental barrier and appear in cord blood.
Although reproduction studies performed with chlorothiazide doses of 50 mg/kg/day in rabbits, 60 mg/kg/day in rats and 500 mg/kg/day in mice revealed no external abnormalities or impairment of neonatal growth and survival due to chlorothiazide, such studies did not include complete visceral and skeletal examinations.
Methyldopa: Reproduction studies performed with methyldopa at oral doses up to 1000 mg/kg in mice, 200 mg/kg in rabbits, and 100 mg/kg in rats revealed no evidence of harm to the fetus. These doses are 16.6 times, 3.3 times and 1.7 times, respectively, the maximum daily human dose when compared on the basis of body weight: 1.4 times, 1.1 times and 0.2 times, respectively, when compared on the basis of body surface area: calculations assume a patient weight of 50 kg. There are, however, no adequate and well-controlled studies in pregnant women in the first trimester of pregnancy. Because animal reproduction studies are not always predictive of human response, methyldopa should be used during pregnancy only if clearly needed.
Published reports of the use of methyldopa during all trimesters indicate that if this drug is used during pregnancy the possibility of fetal harm appears remote. In five studies, three of which were controlled, involving 332 pregnant hypertensive women, treatment with methyldopa was associated with an improved fetal outcome. The majority of these women were in the third trimester when methyldopa therapy was begun.
In one study, women who had begun methyldopa treatment between weeks 16 and 20 of pregnancy gave birth to infants whose average head circumference was reduced by a small amount (34.2 ± 1.7 cm vs. 34.6 ± 1.3 cm [mean ± 1 S.D.]). Long-term follow up of 195 (97.5%) of the children born to methyldopa-treated pregnant women (including those who began treatment between weeks 16 and 20) failed to uncover any significant adverse effect on the children. At four years of age, the developmental delay commonly seen in children born to hypertensive mothers was less evident in those whose mothers were treated with methyldopa during pregnancy than those whose mothers were untreated. The children of the treated group scored consistently higher than the children of the untreated group on five major indices of intellectual and motor development. At age seven and one-half developmental scores and intelligence indices showed no significant differences in children of treated or untreated hypertensive women.
Nonteratogenic Effects: These may include fetal or neonatal jaundice, thrombocytopenia, and possibly other adverse reactions which have occurred in the adult.
Nursing Mothers
Methyldopa and thiazides appear in breast milk. Therefore, because of the potential for serious adverse reactions in nursing infants from chlorothiazide, a decision should be made whether to discontinue nursing or to discontinue the drug, taking into account the importance of the drug to the mother.
Pediatric Use
Safety and effectiveness of ALDOCLOR in pediatric patients have not been established.

ADVERSE REACTIONS

The following adverse reactions have been reported and, within each category, are listed in order of decreasing severity.
Methyldopa
Sedation, usually transient, may occur during the initial period of therapy or whenever the dose is increased. Headache, asthenia, or weakness may be noted as early and transient symptoms. However, significant adverse effects due to methyldopa have been infrequent and this agent usually is well tolerated.
Cardiovascular: Aggravation of angina pectoris, congestive heart failure, prolonged carotid sinus hypersensitivity, orthostatic hypotension (decrease daily dosage), edema or weight gain, bradycardia.
Digestive: Pancreatitis, colitis, vomiting, diarrhea, sialadenitis, sore or "black" tongue, nausea, constipation, distension, flatus, dryness of mouth.
Endocrine: Hyperprolactinemia.
Hematologic: Bone marrow depression, leukopenia, granulocytopenia, thrombocytopenia, hemolytic anemia; positive tests for antinuclear antibody, LE cells, and rheumatoid factor, positive Coombs test.
Hepatic: Liver disorders including hepatitis, jaundice, abnormal liver function tests (see WARNINGS).
Hypersensitivity: Myocarditis, pericarditis, vasculitis, lupus-like syndrome, drug-related fever, eosinophilia.
Nervous System/Psychiatric: Parkinsonism, Bell's palsy, decreased mental acuity, involuntary choreoathetotic movements, symptoms of cerebrovascular insufficiency, psychic disturbances including nightmares and reversible mild psychoses or depression, headache, sedation, asthenia or weakness, dizziness, lightheadedness, paresthesias.
Metabolic: Rise in BUN.
Musculoskeletal: Arthralgia, with or without joint swelling; myalgia.
Respiratory: Nasal stuffiness.
Skin: Toxic epidermal necrolysis, rash.
Urogenital: Amenorrhea, breast enlargement, gynecomastia, lactation, impotence, decreased libido.
Chlorothiazide
Body as a Whole: Weakness.
Cardiovascular: Hypotension including orthostatic hypotension (may be aggravated by alcohol, barbiturates, narcotics or antihypertensive drugs).
Digestive: Pancreatitis, jaundice (intrahepatic cholestatic jaundice), diarrhea, vomiting, sialadenitis, cramping, constipation, gastric irritation, nausea, anorexia.
Hematologic: Aplastic anemia, agranulocytosis, leukopenia, hemolytic anemia, thrombocytopenia.
Hypersensitivity: Anaphylactic reactions, necrotizing angiitis (vasculitis and cutaneous vasculitis), respiratory distress including pneumonitis and pulmonary edema, photosensitivity, fever, urticaria, rash, purpura.
Metabolic: Electrolyte imbalance (see PRECAUTIONS), hyperglycemia, glycosuria, hyperuricemia.
Musculoskeletal: Muscle spasm.
Nervous System/Psychiatric: Vertigo, paresthesias, dizziness, headache, restlessness.
Renal: Renal failure, renal dysfunction, interstitial nephritis. (See WARNINGS.)
Skin: Erythema multiforme including Stevens-Johnson syndrome, exfoliative dermatitis including toxic epidermal necrolysis, alopecia.
Special Senses: Transient blurred vision, xanthopsia.
Urogenital: Impotence.

OVERDOSAGE

Acute overdosage may produce acute hypotension with other responses attributable to brain and gastrointestinal malfunction (excessive sedation, weakness, bradycardia, dizziness, lightheadedness, constipation, distention, flatus, diarrhea, nausea, vomiting).
In the event of overdosage, symptomatic and supportive measures should be employed. When ingestion is recent, gastric lavage or emesis may reduce absorption. Otherwise, management includes special attention to cardiac rate and output, blood volume, electrolyte imbalance, paralytic ileus, urinary function and cerebral activity.
Sympathomimetic drugs [e.g., levarterenol, epinephrine, ARAMINE* (Metaraminol Bitartrate)] may be indicated. Methyldopa is dialyzable. The degree to which chlorothiazide is removed by hemodialysis has not been established. The oral LD_{50} of methyldopa is greater than 1.5 g/kg in both the mouse and the rat. The oral LD_{50} of chlorothiazide is 8.5 g/kg, greater than 10 g/kg, and greater than 1 g/kg in the mouse, rat, and dog respectively.

*Registered trademark of MERCK & CO., INC.

DOSAGE AND ADMINISTRATION

DOSAGE MUST BE INDIVIDUALIZED, AS DETERMINED BY TITRATION OF THE INDIVIDUAL COMPONENTS (see box warning). Once the patient has been successfully titrated, ALDOCLOR may be substituted if the previously determined titrated doses are the same as in the combination. The usual starting dosage is one tablet of ALDOCLOR 250 two or three times a day.
When administered individually, the usual daily dosage of chlorothiazide is 0.5 g to 1.0 g in single or divided doses and that of methyldopa is 500 mg to 2 g. To minimize the sedation associated with methyldopa, start dosage increases in the evening.
Occasionally tolerance to methyldopa may occur, usually between the second and third month of therapy. Additional separate doses of methyldopa or replacement of ALDOCLOR with single entity agents is necessary until the new effective dose ratio is re-established by titration. The maximum recommended daily dose of methyldopa is 3 g. When ALDOCLOR 250 is used to provide 1 g of methyldopa, 1 g of chlorothiazide is delivered. It is prudent, if greater than 1 g of methyldopa per day is required, to provide the additional methyldopa as methyldopa alone.
If ALDOCLOR does not adequately control blood pressure, additional doses of other agents may be given. When ALDOCLOR is given with antihypertensives other than thiazides, the initial dosage of methyldopa should be limited to 500 mg daily in divided doses and the dose of these other agents may need to be adjusted to effect a smooth transition. Since both components of ALDOCLOR have a relatively short duration of action, withdrawal is followed by return of hypertension usually within 48 hours. This is not complicated by an overshoot of blood pressure.
Since methyldopa is largely excreted by the kidney, patients with impaired renal function may respond to smaller doses. Syncope in older patients may be related to an increased sensitivity and advanced arteriosclerotic vascular disease. This may be avoided by lower doses.

HOW SUPPLIED

No. 3319—Tablets ALDOCLOR 250 are green, oval, film coated tablets coded MSD 634 on one side and ALDOCLOR on the other. Each tablet contains 250 mg of methyldopa and 250 mg of chlorothiazide. They are supplied as follows:
NDC 0006-0634-68 bottles of 100.
Shown in Product Identification Guide, page 322
Storage
Keep container tightly closed. Protect from moisture, light, and freezing, −20°C (−4°F) and store at room temperature, 15–30°C (59–86°F).
7899645 Issued February 1997
COPYRIGHT © MERCK & CO., INC., 1986, 1992
All rights reserved

ALDOMET® Tablets ℞
(Methyldopa), U.S.P.

ALDOMET® Oral Suspension ℞
(Methyldopa), U.S.P.

DESCRIPTION

ALDOMET* (Methyldopa) is an antihypertensive drug.
Methyldopa, the *L*-isomer of alpha-methyldopa is levo-3-(3,4 - dihydroxyphenyl) -2-methylalanine. Its empirical formula is $C_{10}H_{13}NO_4$, with a molecular weight of 211.22, and its structural formula is:

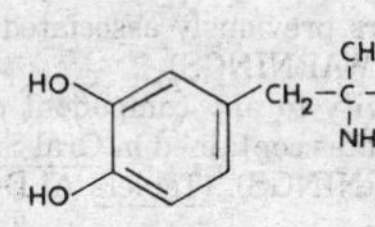

Methyldopa is a white to yellowish white, odorless fine powder, and is soluble in water.
ALDOMET is supplied as tablets, for oral use, in three strengths: 125 mg, 250 mg, or 500 mg of methyldopa per tablet. Inactive ingredients in the tablets are: calcium disodium edetate, cellulose, citric acid, colloidal silicon dioxide, D&C Yellow 10, ethylcellulose, guar gum, hydroxypropyl methylcellulose, iron oxide, magnesium stearate, propylene glycol, talc, and titanium dioxide.
Oral Suspension ALDOMET is supplied as a white to off-white preparation; each 5 mL contains 250 mg of methyldopa and alcohol 1 percent, with benzoic acid 0.1 percent and sodium bisulfite 0.2 percent added as preservatives. Inactive ingredients in the oral suspension are: artificial and natural flavors, cellulose, citric acid, confectioner's sugar, disodium edetate, glycerin, polysorbate, purified water, and sodium carboxymethylcellulose.

*Registered trademark of MERCK & CO., INC.

CLINICAL PHARMACOLOGY

ALDOMET is an aromatic-amino-acid decarboxylase inhibitor in animals and in man. Although the mechanism of action has yet to be conclusively demonstrated, the antihypertensive effect of methyldopa probably is due to its metabolism to alpha-methylnorepinephrine, which then lowers arterial pressure by stimulation of central inhibitory alpha-adrenergic receptors, false neurotransmission, and/or reduction of plasma renin activity. Methyldopa has been shown to cause a net reduction in the tissue concentration of serotonin, dopamine, norepinephrine, and epinephrine.
Only methyldopa, the *L*-isomer of alpha-methyldopa, has the ability to inhibit dopa decarboxylase and to deplete an-

Continued on next page

Information on the Merck & Co., Inc. products listed on these pages is the full prescribing information from product circulars in use August 31, 1998. For information, please call 1-800-NSC MERCK [1-800-672-6372].

Aldomet—Cont.

imal tissues of norepinephrine. In man the antihypertensive activity appears to be due solely to the *L*-isomer. About twice the dose of the racemate (*DL*-alpha-methyldopa) is required for equal antihypertensive effect.
Methyldopa has no direct effect on cardiac function and usually does not reduce glomerular filtration rate, renal blood flow, or filtration fraction. Cardiac output usually is maintained without cardiac acceleration. In some patients the heart rate is slowed.
Normal or elevated plasma renin activity may decrease in the course of methyldopa therapy.
ALDOMET reduces both supine and standing blood pressure. Methyldopa usually produces highly effective lowering of the supine pressure with infrequent symptomatic postural hypotension. Exercise hypotension and diurnal blood pressure variations rarely occur.

Pharmacokinetics and Metabolism

The maximum decrease in blood pressure occurs four to six hours after oral dosage. Once an effective dosage level is attained, a smooth blood pressure response occurs in most patients in 12 to 24 hours. After withdrawal, blood pressure usually returns to pretreatment levels within 24–48 hours.
Methyldopa is extensively metabolized. The known urinary metabolites are: α-methyldopa mono-0-sulfate; 3-0-methyl-α-methyldopa; 3,4-dihydroxyphenylacetone; α-methyldopamine; 3-0-methyl-α-methyldopamine and their conjugates.
Approximately 70% of the drug which is absorbed is excreted in the urine as methyldopa and its mono-0-sulfate conjugate. The renal clearance is about 130 mL/min in normal subjects and is diminished in renal insufficiency. The plasma half-life of methyldopa is 105 minutes. After oral doses, excretion is essentially complete in 36 hours.
Methyldopa crosses the placental barrier, appears in cord blood, and appears in breast milk.

INDICATION AND USAGE

Hypertension.

CONTRAINDICATIONS

ALDOMET is contraindicated in patients:
— with active hepatic disease, such as acute hepatitis and active cirrhosis
— with liver disorders previously associated with methyldopa therapy (see WARNINGS)
— with hypersensitivity to any component of these products, including sulfites contained in Oral Suspension ALDOMET (see WARNINGS). (Tablets ALDOMET do not contain sulfites.)
— on therapy with monoamine oxidase (MAO) inhibitors.

WARNINGS

It is important to recognize that a positive Coombs test, hemolytic anemia, and liver disorders may occur with methyldopa therapy. The rare occurrences of hemolytic anemia or liver disorders could lead to potentially fatal complications unless properly recognized and managed. Read this section carefully to understand these reactions.
With prolonged methyldopa therapy, 10 to 20 percent of patients develop a positive direct Coombs test which usually occurs between 6 and 12 months of methyldopa therapy. Lowest incidence is at daily dosage of 1 g or less. This on rare occasions may be associated with hemolytic anemia, which could lead to potentially fatal complications. One cannot predict which patients with a positive direct Coombs test may develop hemolytic anemia.
Prior existence or development of a positive direct Coombs test is not in itself a contraindication to use of methyldopa. If a positive Coombs test develops during methyldopa therapy, the physician should determine whether hemolytic anemia exists and whether the positive Coombs test may be a problem. For example, in addition to a positive direct Coombs test there is less often a positive indirect Coombs test which may interfere with cross matching of blood.
Before treatment is started, it is desirable to do a blood count (hematocrit, hemoglobin, or red cell count) for a baseline or to establish whether there is anemia. Periodic blood counts should be done during therapy to detect hemolytic anemia. It may be useful to do a direct Coombs test before therapy and at 6 and 12 months after the start of therapy.
If Coombs-positive hemolytic anemia occurs, the cause may be methyldopa and the drug should be discontinued. Usually the anemia remits promptly. If not, corticosteroids may be given and other causes of anemia should be considered. If the hemolytic anemia is related to methyldopa, the drug should not be reinstituted.
When methyldopa causes Coombs positivity alone or with hemolytic anemia, the red cell is usually coated with gamma globulin of the IgG (gamma G) class only. The positive Coombs test may not revert to normal until weeks to months after methyldopa is stopped.
Should the need for transfusion arise in a patient receiving methyldopa, both a direct and an indirect Coombs test should be performed. In the absence of hemolytic anemia, usually only the direct Coombs test will be positive. A positive direct Coombs test alone will not interfere with typing or cross matching. If the indirect Coombs test is also positive, problems may arise in the major cross match and the assistance of a hematologist or transfusion expert will be needed.
Occasionally, fever has occurred within the first 3 weeks of methyldopa therapy, associated in some cases with eosinophilia or abnormalities in one or more liver function tests, such as serum alkaline phosphatase, serum transaminases (SGOT, SGPT), bilirubin, and prothrombin time. Jaundice, with or without fever, may occur with onset usually within the first 2 to 3 months of therapy. In some patients the findings are consistent with those of cholestasis. In others the findings are consistent with hepatitis and hepatocellular injury.
Rarely, fatal hepatic necrosis has been reported after use of methyldopa. These hepatic changes may represent hypersensitivity reactions. Periodic determinations of hepatic function should be done particularly during the first 6 to 12 weeks of therapy or whenever an unexplained fever occurs. If fever, abnormalities in liver function tests, or jaundice appear, stop therapy with methyldopa. If caused by methyldopa, the temperature and abnormalities in liver function characteristically have reverted to normal when the drug was discontinued. Methyldopa should not be reinstituted in such patients.
Rarely, a reversible reduction of the white blood cell count with a primary effect on the granulocytes has been seen. The granulocyte count returned promptly to normal on discontinuance of the drug. Rare cases of granulocytopenia have been reported. In each instance, upon stopping the drug, the white cell count returned to normal. Reversible thrombocytopenia has occurred rarely.
Oral Suspension ALDOMET (but not Tablets ALDOMET) contains sodium bisulfite, a sulfite that may cause allergic-type reactions including anaphylactic symptoms and life-threatening or less severe asthmatic episodes in certain susceptible people. The overall prevalence of sulfite sensitivity in the general population is unknown and probably low. Sulfite sensitivity is seen more frequently in asthmatic than in nonasthmatic people.

PRECAUTIONS

General

Methyldopa should be used with caution in patients with a history of previous liver disease or dysfunction (see WARNINGS).
Some patients taking methyldopa experience clinical edema or weight gain which may be controlled by use of a diuretic. Methyldopa should not be continued if edema progresses or signs of heart failure appear.
Hypertension has recurred occasionally after dialysis in patients given methyldopa because the drug is removed by this procedure.
Rarely involuntary choreoathetotic movements have been observed during therapy with methyldopa in patients with severe bilateral cerebrovascular disease. Should these movements occur, stop therapy.

Laboratory Tests

Blood count, Coombs test, and liver function tests are recommended before initiating therapy and at periodic intervals (see WARNINGS).

Drug Interactions

When methyldopa is used with other antihypertensive drugs, potentiation of antihypertensive effect may occur. Patients should be followed carefully to detect side reactions or unusual manifestations of drug idiosyncrasy.
Patients may require reduced doses of anesthetics when on methyldopa. If hypotension does occur during anesthesia, it usually can be controlled by vasopressors. The adrenergic receptors remain sensitive during treatment with methyldopa.
When methyldopa and lithium are given concomitantly the patient should be carefully monitored for symptoms of lithium toxicity. Read the circular for lithium preparations.
Monoamine oxidase (MAO) inhibitors: see CONTRAINDICATIONS.

Drug/Laboratory Test Interactions

Methyldopa may interfere with measurement of: urinary uric acid by the phosphotungstate method, serum creatinine by the alkaline picrate method, and SGOT by colorimetric methods. Interference with spectrophotometric methods for SGOT analysis has not been reported.
Since methyldopa causes fluorescence in urine samples at the same wave lengths as catecholamines, falsely high levels of urinary catecholamines may be reported. This will interfere with the diagnosis of pheochromocytoma. It is important to recognize this phenomenon before a patient with a possible pheochromocytoma is subjected to surgery. Methyldopa does not interfere with measurement of VMA (vanillylmandelic acid), a test for pheochromocytoma, by those methods which convert VMA to vanillin. Methyldopa is not recommended for the treatment of patients with pheochromocytoma. Rarely, when urine is exposed to air after voiding, it may darken because of breakdown of methyldopa or its metabolites.

Carcinogenesis, Mutagenesis, Impairment of Fertility

No evidence of a tumorigenic effect was seen when methyldopa was given for two years to mice at doses up to 1800 mg/kg/day or to rats at doses up to 240 mg/kg/day (30 and 4 times the maximum recommended human dose in mice and rats, respectively, when compared on the basis of body weight; 2.5 and 0.6 times the maximum recommended human dose in mice and rats, respectively, when compared on the basis of body surface area; calculations assume a patient weight of 50 kg).
Methyldopa was not mutagenic in the Ames Test and did not increase chromosomal aberration or sister chromatid exchanges in Chinese hamster ovary cells. These *in vitro* studies were carried out both with and without exogenous metabolic activation.
Fertility was unaffected when methyldopa was given to male and female rats at 100 mg/kg/day (1.7 times the maximum daily human dose when compared on the basis of body weight; 0.2 times the maximum daily human dose when compared on the basis of body surface area). Methyldopa decreased sperm count, sperm motility, the number of late spermatids and the male fertility index when given to male rats at 200 and 400 mg/kg/day (3.3 and 6.7 times the maximum daily human dose when compared on the basis of body weight; 0.5 and 1 times the maximum daily human dose when compared on the basis of body surface area).

Pregnancy

Pregnancy Category B. Reproduction studies performed with methyldopa at oral doses up to 1000 mg/kg in mice, 200 mg/kg in rabbits and 100 mg/kg in rats revealed no evidence of harm to the fetus. These doses are 16.6 times, 3.3 times and 1.7 times, respectively, the maximum daily human dose when compared on the basis of body weight; 1.4 times, 1.1 times and 0.2 times, respectively, when compared on the basis of body surface area; calculations assume a patient weight of 50 kg. There are, however, no adequate and well-controlled studies in pregnant women in the first trimester of pregnancy. Because animal reproduction studies are not always predictive of human response, ALDOMET should be used during pregnancy only if clearly needed.
Published reports of the use of methyldopa during all trimesters indicate that if this drug is used during pregnancy the possibility of fetal harm appears remote. In five studies, three of which were controlled, involving 332 pregnant hypertensive women, treatment with ALDOMET was associated with an improved fetal outcome. The majority of these women were in the third trimester when methyldopa therapy was begun.
In one study, women who had begun methyldopa treatment between weeks 16 and 20 of pregnancy gave birth to infants whose average head circumference was reduced by a small amount (34.2 ± 1.7 cm vs. 34.6 ± 1.3 cm [mean ± 1 S.D.]). Long-term follow up of 195 (97.5%) of the children born to methyldopa-treated pregnant women (including those who began treatment between weeks 16 and 20) failed to uncover any significant adverse effect on the children. At four years of age, the developmental delay commonly seen in children born to hypertensive mothers was less evident in those whose mothers were treated with methyldopa during pregnancy than those whose mothers were untreated. The children of the treated group scored consistently higher than the children of the untreated group on five major indices of intellectual and motor development. At age seven and one-half developmental scores and intelligence indices showed no significant differences in children of treated or untreated hypertensive women.

Nursing Mothers

Methyldopa appears in breast milk. Therefore, caution should be exercised when methyldopa is given to a nursing woman.

Pediatric Use

There are no well-controlled clinical trials in pediatric patients. Information on dosing in pediatric patients is supported by evidence from published literature regarding the treatment of hypertension in pediatric patients. (See DOSAGE AND ADMINISTRATION.)

ADVERSE REACTIONS

Sedation, usually transient, may occur during the initial period of therapy or whenever the dose is increased. Headache, asthenia, or weakness may be noted as early and transient symptoms. However, significant adverse effects due to ALDOMET have been infrequent and this agent usually is well tolerated.
The following adverse reactions have been reported and, within each category, are listed in order of decreasing severity.

Cardiovascular: Aggravation of angina pectoris, congestive heart failure, prolonged carotid sinus hypersensitivity, orthostatic hypotension (decrease daily dosage), edema or weight gain, bradycardia.
Digestive: Pancreatitis, colitis, vomiting, diarrhea, sialadenitis, sore or "black" tongue, nausea, constipation, distension, flatus, dryness of mouth.
Endocrine: Hyperprolactinemia.
Hematologic: Bone marrow depression, leukopenia, granulocytopenia, thrombocytopenia, hemolytic anemia; positive tests for antinuclear antibody, LE cells, and rheumatoid factor, positive Coombs test.
Hepatic: Liver disorders including hepatitis, jaundice, abnormal liver function tests (see WARNINGS).
Hypersensitivity: Myocarditis, pericarditis, vasculitis, lupus-like syndrome, drug-related fever, eosinophilia.
Nervous System/Psychiatric: Parkinsonism, Bell's palsy, decreased mental acuity, involuntary choreoathetotic movements, symptoms of cerebrovascular insufficiency, psychic disturbances including nightmares and reversible mild psychoses or depression, headache, sedation, asthenia or weakness, dizziness, lightheadedness, paresthesias.
Metabolic: Rise in BUN.
Musculoskeletal: Arthralgia, with or without joint swelling; myalgia.
Respiratory: Nasal stuffiness.
Skin: Toxic epidermal necrolysis, rash.
Urogenital: Amenorrhea, breast enlargement, gynecomastia, lactation, impotence, decreased libido.

OVERDOSAGE

Acute overdosage may produce acute hypotension with other responses attributable to brain and gastrointestinal malfunction (excessive sedation, weakness, bradycardia, dizziness, lightheadedness, constipation, distention, flatus, diarrhea, nausea, vomiting).
In the event of overdosage, symptomatic and supportive measures should be employed. When ingestion is recent, gastric lavage or emesis may reduce absorption. When ingestion has been earlier, infusions may be helpful to promote urinary excretion. Otherwise, management includes special attention to cardiac rate and output, blood volume, electrolyte balance, paralytic ileus, urinary function and cerebral activity.
Sympathomimetic drugs [e.g., levarterenol, epinephrine, ARAMINE* (Metaraminol Bitartrate)] may be indicated. Methyldopa is dialyzable.
The oral LD_{50} of methyldopa is greater than 1.5 g/kg in both the mouse and the rat.

*Registered trademark of MERCK & CO., INC.

DOSAGE AND ADMINISTRATION

ADULTS

Initiation of Therapy
The usual starting dosage of ALDOMET is 250 mg two or three times a day in the first 48 hours. The daily dosage then may be increased or decreased, preferably at intervals of not less than two days, until an adequate response is achieved. To minimize the sedation, start dosage increases in the evening. By adjustment of dosage, morning hypotension may be prevented without sacrificing control of afternoon blood pressure.
When methyldopa is given to patients on other antihypertensives, the dose of these agents may need to be adjusted to effect a smooth transition. When ALDOMET is given with antihypertensives other than thiazides, the initial dosage of ALDOMET should be limited to 500 mg daily in divided doses; when ALDOMET is added to a thiazide, the dosage of thiazide need not be changed.
Maintenance Therapy
The usual daily dosage of ALDOMET is 500 mg to 2 g in two to four doses. Although occasional patients have responded to higher doses, the maximum recommended daily dosage is 3 g. Once an effective dosage range is attained, a smooth blood pressure response occurs in most patients in 12 to 24 hours. Since methyldopa has a relatively short duration of action, withdrawal is followed by return of hypertension usually within 48 hours. This is not complicated by an overshoot of blood pressure.
Occasionally tolerance may occur, usually between the second and third month of therapy. Adding a diuretic or increasing the dosage of methyldopa frequently will restore effective control of blood pressure. A thiazide may be added at any time during methyldopa therapy and is recommended if therapy has not been started with a thiazide or if effective control of blood pressure cannot be maintained on 2 g of methyldopa daily.
Methyldopa is largely excreted by the kidney and patients with impaired renal function may respond to smaller doses. Syncope in older patients may be related to an increased sensitivity and advanced arteriosclerotic vascular disease. This may be avoided by lower doses.

PEDIATRIC PATIENTS

Initial dosage is based on 10 mg/kg of body weight daily in two to four doses. The daily dosage then is increased or decreased until an adequate response is achieved. The maximum dosage is 65 mg/kg or 3 g daily, whichever is less. (See **PRECAUTIONS**, *Pediatric Use*.)

HOW SUPPLIED

No. 3341—Tablets ALDOMET, 125 mg, are yellow, film coated, round tablets, coded MSD 135 on one side and ALDOMET on the other. They are supplied as follows:
NDC 0006-0135-68 bottles of 100.
Shown in Product Identification Guide, page 322
No. 3290—Tablets ALDOMET, 250 mg, are yellow, film coated, round tablets, coded MSD 401 on one side and ALDOMET on the other. They are supplied as follows:
NDC 0006-0401-68 bottles of 100
(6505-00-890-1856, 250 mg 100's)
NDC 0006-0401-78 unit of use bottles of 100
NDC 0006-0401-82 bottles of 1000
(6505-00-931-6646, 250 mg 1000's).
Shown in Product Identification Guide, page 322
No. 3292—Tablets ALDOMET, 500 mg, are yellow, film coated, round tablets, coded MSD 516 on one side and ALDOMET on the other. They are supplied as follows:
NDC 0006-0516-68 bottles of 100
(6505-01-003-4119, 500 mg 100's)
NDC 0006-0516-74 bottles of 500
(6505-01-199-8339, 500 mg 500's).
Shown in Product Identification Guide, page 322
No. 3382—Oral Suspension ALDOMET, 250 mg per 5 mL, is an off-white, creamy suspension with a citric orange-pineapple flavor. It is supplied as follows:
NDC 0006-3382-74 bottles of 473 mL.
Storage
Store Tablets ALDOMET in a well-closed container at controlled room temperature [15–30°C (59–86°F)].
Store Oral Suspension ALDOMET below 26°C (78°F) in a tight, light-resistant container. Protect from freezing.
7843430 Issued February 1997
COPYRIGHT © MERCK & CO., INC., 1985
All rights reserved

ALDOMET® Ester HCl Injection (Methyldopate HCl), U.S.P. ℞

DESCRIPTION

Injection ALDOMET* Ester Hydrochloride (Methyldopate HCl) is an antihypertensive agent for intravenous use.
Methyldopate hydrochloride [levo-3-(3,4-dihydroxyphenyl)-2-methylalanine, ethyl ester hydrochloride]is the ethyl ester of methyldopa, supplied as the hydrochloride salt with a molecular weight of 275.73. Methyldopate hydrochloride is more soluble and stable in solution than methyldopa and is the preferred form for intravenous use.
The empirical formula for methyldopate hydrochloride is $C_{12}H_{17}NO_4 \cdot HCl$ and its structural formula is:

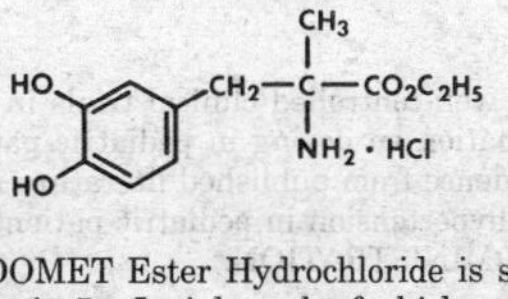

Injection ALDOMET Ester Hydrochloride is supplied as a sterile solution in 5 mL vials each of which contains:

Methyldopate hydrochloride	250.0 mg
Inactive ingredients:	
Citric acid anhydrous	25.0 mg
Disodium edetate	2.5 mg
Monothioglycerol	10.0 mg
Sodium hydroxide to adjust pH	
Water for Injection, q.s. to 5 mL	

Methylparaben 7.5 mg, propylparaben 1 mg, and sodium bisulfite 16 mg added as preservatives.

*Registered trademark of MERCK & CO., INC.

CLINICAL PHARMACOLOGY

ALDOMET (Methyldopa), an antihypertensive, is an aromatic-amino-acid decarboxylase inhibitor in animals and in man. Although the mechanism of action has yet to be conclusively demonstrated, the antihypertensive effect of methyldopa probably is due to its metabolism to alpha-methyl-norepinephrine, which then lowers arterial pressure by stimulation of central inhibitory alpha-adrenergic receptors, false neurotransmission, and/or reduction of plasma renin activity. Methyldopa has been shown to cause a net reduction in the tissue concentration of serotonin, dopamine, norepinephrine, and epinephrine.
Only methyldopa, the *L*-isomer of alpha-methyldopa, has the ability to inhibit dopa decarboxylase and to deplete animal tissues of norepinephrine. In man the antihypertensive activity appears to be due solely to the *L*-isomer. About twice the dose of the racemate (*DL*-alpha-methyldopa) is required for equal antihypertensive effect.
Methyldopa has no direct effect on cardiac function and usually does not reduce glomerular filtration rate, renal blood flow, or filtration fraction. Cardiac output usually is maintained without cardiac acceleration. In some patients the heart rate is slowed.
Normal or elevated plasma renin activity may decrease in the course of methyldopa therapy.
Methyldopa reduces both supine and standing blood pressure. It usually produces highly effective lowering of the supine pressure with infrequent symptomatic postural hypotension. Exercise hypotension and diurnal blood pressure variations rarely occur.
Pharmacokinetics and Metabolism
Methyldopate hydrochloride is the ethyl ester of methyldopa hydrochloride and possesses the same pharmacologic attributes.
Methyldopa is extensively metabolized. The known urinary metabolites are: α-methyldopa mono-0-sulfate; 3-0-methyl-α-methyldopa; 3,4-dihydroxyphenylacetone; α-methyldopamine; 3-0-methyl-α-methyldopamine and their conjugates.
Following intravenous administration of methyldopate hydrochloride a decrease in blood pressure may occur in four to six hours and last 10 to 16 hours.
Approximately 49 percent of the dose of methyldopate hydrochloride is excreted in the urine as methyldopa and its mono-0-sulfate. The renal clearance of methyldopa following methyldopate hydrochloride is about 156 mL/min in normal subjects and is diminished in renal insufficiency. Following methyldopate hydrochloride injection the plasma half-life of methyldopa is 90–127 mins. Approximately 17 percent of a dose of methyldopate hydrochloride given to normal subjects appears in plasma as free methyldopa.
Methyldopa crosses the placental barrier, appears in cord blood, and appears in breast milk.

INDICATION AND USAGE

Hypertension, when parenteral medication is indicated.
The treatment of hypertensive crises may be initiated with Injection ALDOMET Ester Hydrochloride.

CONTRAINDICATIONS

Injection ALDOMET Ester Hydrochloride is contraindicated in patients:
— with active hepatic disease, such as acute hepatitis and active cirrhosis
— with liver disorders previously associated with methyldopa therapy (see WARNINGS)
— with hypersensitivity to any component of this product, including sulfites (see WARNINGS)
— on therapy with monoamine oxidase (MAO) inhibitors.

WARNINGS

It is important to recognize that a positive Coombs test, hemolytic anemia, and liver disorders may occur with methyldopa therapy. The rare occurrences of hemolytic anemia or liver disorders could lead to potentially fatal complications unless properly recognized and managed. Read this section carefully to understand these reactions.
With prolonged methyldopa therapy, 10 to 20 percent of patients develop a positive direct Coombs test which usually occurs between 6 and 12 months of methyldopa therapy. Lowest incidence is at daily dosage of 1 g or less. This on rare occasions may be associated with hemolytic anemia, which could lead to potentially fatal complications. One cannot predict which patients with a positive direct Coombs test may develop hemolytic anemia.
Prior existence or development of a positive direct Coombs test is not in itself a contraindication to use of methyldopa. If a positive Coombs test develops during methyldopa therapy, the physician should determine whether hemolytic anemia exists and whether the positive Coombs test may be a problem. For example, in addition to a positive direct Coombs test there is less often a positive indirect Coombs test which may interfere with cross matching of blood.
Before treatment is started, it is desirable to do a blood count (hematocrit, hemoglobin, or red cell count) for a baseline or to establish whether there is anemia. Periodic blood counts should be done during therapy to detect hemolytic anemia. It may be useful to do a direct Coombs test before therapy and at 6 and 12 months after the start of therapy.

Continued on next page

Information on the Merck & Co., Inc. products listed on these pages is the full prescribing information from product circulars in use August 31, 1998. For information, please call 1-800-NSC MERCK [1-800-672-6372].

Aldomet Ester HCl—Cont.

If Coombs-positive hemolytic anemia occurs, the cause may be methyldopa and the drug should be discontinued. Usually the anemia remits promptly. If not, corticosteroids may be given and other causes of anemia should be considered. If the hemolytic anemia is related to methyldopa, the drug should not be reinstituted.

When methyldopa causes Coombs positivity alone or with hemolytic anemia, the red cell is usually coated with gamma globulin of the IgG (gamma G) class only. The positive Coombs test may not revert to normal until weeks to months after methyldopa is stopped.

Should the need for transfusion arise in a patient receiving methyldopa, both a direct and an indirect Coombs test should be performed. In the absence of hemolytic anemia, usually only the direct Coombs test will be positive. A positive direct Coombs test alone will not interfere with typing or cross matching. If the indirect Coombs test is also positive, problems may arise in the major cross match and the assistance of a hematologist or transfusion expert will be needed.

Occasionally, fever has occurred within the first three weeks of methyldopa therapy, associated in some cases with eosinophilia or abnormalities in one or more liver function tests, such as serum alkaline phosphatase, serum transaminases (SGOT, SGPT), bilirubin and prothrombin time. Jaundice, with or without fever, may occur with onset usually within the first two to three months of therapy. In some patients the findings are consistent with those of cholestasis. In others the findings are consistent with hepatitis and hepatocellular injury.

Rarely fatal hepatic necrosis has been reported after use of methyldopa. These hepatic changes may represent hypersensitivity reactions. Periodic determination of hepatic function should be done particularly during the first 6 to 12 weeks of therapy or whenever an unexplained fever occurs. If fever, abnormalities in liver function tests, or jaundice appear, stop therapy with methyldopa. If caused by methyldopa, the temperature and abnormalities in liver function characteristically have reverted to normal when the drug was discontinued. Methyldopa should not be reinstituted in such patients.

Rarely, a reversible reduction of the white blood cell count with a primary effect on the granulocytes has been seen. The granulocyte count returned promptly to normal on discontinuance of the drug. Rare cases of granulocytopenia have been reported. In each instance, upon stopping the drug, the white cell count returned to normal. Reversible thrombocytopenia has occurred rarely.

Injection ALDOMET Ester Hydrochloride contains sodium bisulfite, a sulfite that may cause allergic-type reactions including anaphylactic symptoms and life-threatening or less severe asthmatic episodes in certain susceptible people. The overall prevalence of sulfite sensitivity in the general population is unknown and probably low. Sulfite sensitivity is seen more frequently in asthmatic than in nonasthmatic people.

PRECAUTIONS

General

Methyldopa should be used with caution in patients with a history of previous liver disease or dysfunction (see WARNINGS).

Some patients taking methyldopa experience clinical edema or weight gain which may be controlled by use of a diuretic. Methyldopa should not be continued if edema progresses or signs of heart failure appear.

A paradoxical pressor response has been reported with intravenous administration of ALDOMET Ester Hydrochloride.

Hypertension has recurred occasionally after dialysis in patients given methyldopa because the drug is removed by this procedure.

Rarely involuntary choreoathetotic movements have been observed during therapy with methyldopa in patients with severe bilateral cerebrovascular disease. Should these movements occur, stop therapy.

Laboratory Tests

Blood count, Coombs test, and liver function tests are recommended before initiating therapy and at periodic intervals (see WARNINGS).

Drug Interactions

When methyldopa is used with other antihypertensive drugs, potentiation of antihypertensive effect may occur. Patients should be followed carefully to detect side reactions or unusual manifestations of drug idiosyncrasy.

Patients may require reduced doses of anesthetics when on methyldopa. If hypotension does occur during anesthesia, it usually can be controlled by vasopressors. The adrenergic receptors remain sensitive during treatment with methyldopa.

When methyldopa and lithium are given concomitantly the patient should be carefully monitored for symptoms of lithium toxicity. Read the circular for lithium preparations.

Monoamine oxidase (MAO) inhibitors: See CONTRAINDICATIONS.

Drug/Laboratory Test Interactions

Methyldopa may interfere with measurement of: urinary uric acid by the phosphotungstate method, serum creatinine by the alkaline picrate method, and SGOT by colorimetric methods. Interference with spectrophotometric methods for SGOT analysis has not been reported.

Since methyldopa causes fluorescence in urine samples at the same wave lengths as catecholamines, falsely high levels of urinary catecholamines may be reported. This will interfere with the diagnosis of pheochromocytoma. It is important to recognize this phenomenon before a patient with a possible pheochromocytoma is subjected to surgery. Methyldopa does not interfere with measurement of VMA (vanillylmandelic acid), a test for pheochromocytoma, by those methods which convert VMA to vanillin. Methyldopa is not recommended for the treatment of patients with pheochromocytoma. Rarely, when urine is exposed to air after voiding, it may darken because of breakdown of methyldopa or its metabolites.

Carcinogenesis, Mutagenesis, Impairment of Fertility

No evidence of a tumorigenic effect was seen when methyldopa was given for two years to mice at doses up to 1800 mg/kg/day or to rats at doses up to 240 mg/kg/day (30 and 4 times the maximum recommended human dose in mice and rats, respectively, when compared on the basis of body weight; 2.5 and 0.6 times the maximum recommended human dose in mice and rats, respectively, when compared on the basis of body surface area; calculations assume a patient weight of 50 kg).

Methyldopa was not mutagenic in the Ames Test and did not increase chromosomal aberration or sister chromatid exchanges in Chinese hamster ovary cells. These in vitro studies were carried out both with and without exogenous metabolic activation.

Fertility was unaffected when methyldopa was given to male and female rats at 100 mg/kg/day (1.7 times the maximum daily human dose when compared on the basis of body weight; 0.2 times the maximum daily human dose when compared on the basis of body surface area). Methyldopa decreased sperm count, sperm motility, the number of late spermatids and the male fertility index when given to male rats at 200 and 400 mg/kg/day (3.3 and 6.7 times the maximum daily human dose when compared on the basis of body weight; 0.5 and 1 times the maximum daily human dose when compared on the basis of body surface area).

Long-term studies in animals have not been performed to evaluate the carcinogenic potential of methyldopate hydrochloride; nor have evaluations of this ester's mutagenic potential or potential to affect fertility been carried out.

Pregnancy

Pregnancy Category C. Animal reproduction studies have not been conducted with ALDOMET Ester Hydrochloride. It is also not known whether ALDOMET Ester Hydrochloride can affect reproduction capacity or can cause fetal harm when given to a pregnant woman. ALDOMET Ester Hydrochloride should be given to a pregnant woman only if clearly needed.

Nursing Mothers

Methyldopa appears in breast milk. Therefore, caution should be exercised when methyldopa is given to a nursing woman.

Pediatric Use

There are no well-controlled clinical trials in pediatric patients. Information on dosing in pediatric patients is supported by evidence from published literature regarding the treatment of hypertension in pediatric patients. (See DOSAGE AND ADMINISTRATION.)

ADVERSE REACTIONS

Sedation, usually transient, may occur during the initial period of therapy or whenever the dose is increased. Headache, asthenia, or weakness may be noted as early and transient symptoms. However, significant adverse effects due to methyldopa have been infrequent and this agent usually is well tolerated.

The following adverse reactions have been reported and, within each category, are listed in order of decreasing severity.

Cardiovascular: Aggravation of angina pectoris, congestive heart failure, prolonged carotid sinus hypersensitivity, paradoxical pressor response with intravenous use, orthostatic hypotension (decrease daily dosage), edema or weight gain, bradycardia.

Digestive: Pancreatitis, colitis, vomiting, diarrhea, sialadenitis, sore or "black" tongue, nausea, constipation, distension, flatus, dryness of mouth.

Endocrine: Hyperprolactinemia.

Hematologic: Bone marrow depression, leukopenia, granulocytopenia, thrombocytopenia, hemolytic anemia; positive tests for antinuclear antibody, LE cells, and rheumatoid factor, positive Coombs tests.

Hepatic: Liver disorders including hepatitis, jaundice, abnormal liver function tests (see WARNINGS).

Hypersensitivity: Myocarditis, pericarditis, vasculitis, lupus-like syndrome, drug-related fever, eosinophilia.

Nervous System/Psychiatric: Parkinsonism, Bell's palsy, decreased mental acuity, involuntary choreoathetotic movements, symptoms of cerebrovascular insufficiency, psychic disturbances including nightmares and reversible mild psychoses or depression, headache, sedation, asthenia or weakness, dizziness, lightheadedness, paresthesias.

Metabolic: Rise in BUN.

Musculoskeletal: Arthralgia, with or without joint swelling; myalgia.

Respiratory: Nasal stuffiness.

Skin: Toxic epidermal necrolysis, rash.

Urogenital: Amenorrhea, breast enlargement, gynecomastia, lactation, impotence, decreased libido.

OVERDOSAGE

Acute overdosage may produce acute hypotension with other responses attributable to brain and gastrointestinal malfunction (excessive sedation, weakness, bradycardia, dizziness, lightheadedness, constipation, distention, flatus, diarrhea, nausea, vomiting).

In the event of overdosage, symptomatic and supportive measures should be employed. Management includes special attention to cardiac rate and output, blood volume, electrolyte balance, paralytic ileus, urinary function and cerebral activity.

Sympathomimetic drugs [e.g. levarterenol, epinephrine, ARAMINE* (Metaraminol Bitartrate)] may be indicated.

The acute intravenous LD_{50} of ALDOMET Ester Hydrochloride in the mouse is 321 mg/kg.

*Registered trademark of MERCK & CO., INC.

DOSAGE AND ADMINISTRATION

Injection ALDOMET Ester Hydrochloride, when given intravenously in effective doses, causes a decline in blood pressure that may begin in four to six hours and last 10 to 16 hours after injection.

Add the desired dose of Injection ALDOMET Ester Hydrochloride to 100 mL of 5 percent Dextrose Injection USP. Alternatively the desired dose may be given in 5% dextrose in water in a concentration of 100 mg / 10 mL. Give this intravenous infusion slowly over a period of 30 to 60 minutes.

The vial containing Injection ALDOMET Ester Hydrochloride should be inspected visually for particulate matter and discoloration before use whenever solution and container permit.

ADULTS

The usual adult dosage intravenously is 250 to 500 mg at six hour intervals as required. The maximum recommended intravenous dose is 1 g every six hours.

When control has been obtained, oral therapy with Tablets ALDOMET (Methyldopa) may be substituted for intravenous therapy, starting with the same dosage schedule used for the parenteral route. The effectiveness and anticipated responses are described in the circular for Tablets ALDOMET (Methyldopa).

Since methyldopa has a relatively short duration of action, withdrawal is followed by return of hypertension usually within 48 hours. This is not complicated by an overshoot of blood pressure.

Occasionally tolerance may occur, usually between the second and third month of therapy. Adding a diuretic or increasing the dosage of methyldopa frequently will restore effective control of blood pressure. A thiazide may be added at any time during methyldopa therapy and is recommended if therapy has not been started with a thiazide or if effective control of blood pressure cannot be maintained on 2 g of methyldopa daily.

Methyldopa is largely excreted by the kidney and patients with impaired renal function may respond to smaller doses. Syncope in older patients may be related to an increased sensitivity and advanced arteriosclerotic vascular disease. This may be avoided by lower doses.

PEDIATRIC PATIENTS

The recommended daily dosage is 20 to 40 mg/kg of body weight in divided doses every six hours. The maximum dosage is 65 mg/kg or 3 g daily, whichever is less. When the blood pressure is under control, continue with oral therapy using Tablets ALDOMET (Methyldopa) in the same dosage as for the parenteral route. (See PRECAUTIONS, Pediatric Use.)

HOW SUPPLIED

No. 3293—Injection ALDOMET Ester Hydrochloride, 250 mg per 5 mL, is a clear, colorless solution and is supplied as follows:

NDC 0006-3293-05 in 5 mL vials (6505-01-096-2735, 5 mL vial).

Storage

Store below 30°C (86°F).

Protect from freezing.

7900438 Issued February 1997
COPYRIGHT © MERCK & CO., INC., 1989
All rights reserved

ALDORIL® Tablets ℞
(Methyldopa-Hydrochlorothiazide), U.S.P.

WARNING
This fixed combination drug is not indicated for initial therapy of hypertension. Hypertension requires therapy titrated to the individual patient. If the fixed combination represents the dosage so determined, its use may be more convenient in patient management. The treatment of hypertension is not static, but must be reevaluated as conditions in each patient warrant.

DESCRIPTION

ALDORIL* (Methyldopa-Hydrochlorothiazide) combines two antihypertensives: methyldopa and hydrochlorothiazide.

Methyldopa
Methyldopa is an antihypertensive and is the *L*-isomer of alphamethyldopa. It is levo-3-(3,4-dihydroxyphenyl)-2-methylalanine. Its empirical formula is $C_{10}H_{13}NO_4$, with a molecular weight of 211.22, and its structural formula is:

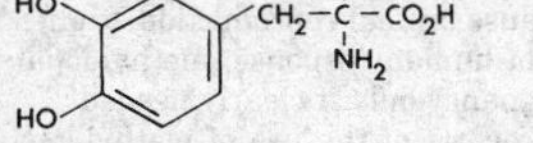

Methyldopa is a white to yellowish white, odorless fine powder, and is soluble in water.
Hydrochlorothiazide
Hydrochlorothiazide is a diuretic and antihypertensive. It is the 3,4-dihydro derivative of chlorothiazide. Its chemical name is 6-chloro-3,4-dihydro-2*H*-1,2,4-benzothiadiazine-7-sulfonamide 1,1-dioxide. Its empirical formula is $C_7H_8ClN_3O_4S_2$ and its structural formula is:

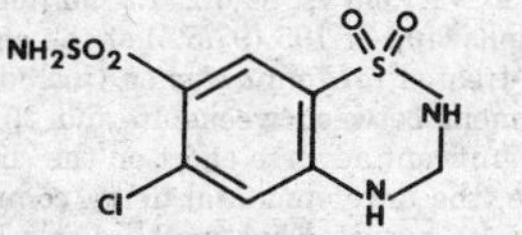

Hydrochlorothiazide is a white, or practically white, crystalline powder with a molecular weight of 297.74, which is slightly soluble in water, but freely soluble in sodium hydroxide solution.
ALDORIL is supplied as tablets in four strengths for oral use:
ALDORIL 15, contains 250 mg of methyldopa and 15 mg of hydrochlorothiazide.
ALDORIL 25, contains 250 mg of methyldopa and 25 mg of hydrochlorothiazide.
ALDORIL D30, contains 500 mg of methyldopa and 30 mg of hydrochlorothiazide.
ALDORIL D50, contains 500 mg of methyldopa and 50 mg of hydrochlorothiazide.
Each tablet contains the following inactive ingredients: calcium disodium edetate, calcium phosphate, cellulose, citric acid, colloidal silicon dioxide, ethylcellulose, guar gum, hydroxypropyl methylcellulose, magnesium stearate, propylene glycol, talc, and titanium dioxide. ALDORIL 15 and ALDORIL D30 also contain iron oxide.

*Registered trademark of MERCK & CO., INC.

CLINICAL PHARMACOLOGY

Methyldopa
Methyldopa is an aromatic-amino-acid decarboxylase inhibitor in animals and in man. Although the mechanism of action has yet to be conclusively demonstrated, the antihypertensive effect of methyldopa probably is due to its metabolism to alpha-methylnorepinephrine, which then lowers arterial pressure by stimulation of central inhibitory alpha-adrenergic receptors, false neurotransmission, and/or reduction of plasma renin activity. Methyldopa has been shown to cause a net reduction in the tissue concentration of serotonin, dopamine, norepinephrine, and epinephrine.
Only methyldopa, the *L*-isomer of alpha-methyldopa, has the ability to inhibit dopa decarboxylase and to deplete animal tissues of norepinephrine. In man, the antihypertensive activity appears to be due solely to the *L*-isomer. About twice the dose of the racemate (*DL*-alpha-methyldopa) is required for equal antihypertensive effect.
Methyldopa has no direct effect on cardiac function and usually does not reduce glomerular filtration rate, renal blood flow, or filtration fraction. Cardiac output usually is maintained without cardiac acceleration. In some patients the heart rate is slowed.
Normal or elevated plasma renin activity may decrease in the course of methyldopa therapy.
Methyldopa reduces both supine and standing blood pressure. It usually produces highly effective lowering of the supine pressure with infrequent symptomatic postural hypotension. Exercise hypotension and diurnal blood pressure variations rarely occur.
Hydrochlorothiazide
The mechanism of the antihypertensive effect of thiazides is unknown. Hydrochlorothiazide does not usually affect normal blood pressure.
Hydrochlorothiazide affects the distal renal tubular mechanism of electrolyte reabsorption. At maximal therapeutic dosage all thiazides are approximately equal in their diuretic efficacy.
Hydrochlorothiazide increases excretion of sodium and chloride in approximately equivalent amounts. Natriuresis may be accompanied by some loss of potassium and bicarbonate.
After oral use diuresis begins within 2 hours, peaks in about 4 hours and lasts about 6 to 12 hours.
Pharmacokinetics and Metabolism
Methyldopa
The maximum decrease in blood pressure occurs four to six hours after oral dosage. Once an effective dosage level is attained, a smooth blood pressure response occurs in most patients in 12 to 24 hours. After withdrawal, blood pressure usually returns to pretreatment levels within 24–48 hours.
Methyldopa is extensively metabolized. The known urinary metabolites are: α-methyldopa mono-0-sulfate; 3-0-methyl-α-methyldopa; 3,4-dihydroxyphenylacetone; α-methyldopamine; 3-0-methyl-α-methyldopamine and their conjugates.
Approximately 70 percent of the drug which is absorbed is excreted in the urine as methyldopa and its mono-0-sulfate conjugate. The renal clearance is about 130 mL/min in normal subjects and is diminished in renal insufficiency. The plasma half-life of methyldopa is 105 minutes. After oral doses, excretion is essentially complete in 36 hours.
Methyldopa crosses the placental barrier, appears in cord blood, and appears in breast milk.
Hydrochlorothiazide
Hydrochlorothiazide is not metabolized but is eliminated rapidly by the kidney. When plasma levels have been followed for at least 24 hours, the plasma half-life has been observed to vary between 5.6 and 14.8 hours. At least 61 percent of the oral dose is eliminated unchanged within 24 hours. Hydrochlorothiazide crosses the placental but not the blood-brain barrier and is excreted in breast milk.

INDICATION AND USAGE

Hypertension (see box warning).

CONTRAINDICATIONS

ALDORIL is contraindicated in patients:
— with active hepatic disease, such as acute hepatitis and active cirrhosis
— with liver disorders previously associated with methyldopa therapy (see WARNINGS)
— with anuria
— with hypersensitivity to methyldopa, or to hydrochlorothiazide or other sulfonamide-derived drugs
— on therapy with monoamine oxidase (MAO) inhibitors.

WARNINGS

Methyldopa
It is important to recognize that a positive Coombs test, hemolytic anemia, and liver disorders may occur with methyldopa therapy. The rare occurrences of hemolytic anemia or liver disorders could lead to potentially fatal complications unless properly recognized and managed. Read this section carefully to understand these reactions.
With prolonged methyldopa therapy, 10 to 20 percent of patients develop a positive direct Coombs test which usually occurs between 6 and 12 months of methyldopa therapy. Lowest incidence is at daily dosage of 1 g or less. This on rare occasions may be associated with hemolytic anemia, which could lead to potentially fatal complications. One cannot predict which patients with a positive direct Coombs test may develop hemolytic anemia.
Prior existence or development of a positive direct Coombs test is not in itself a contraindication to use of methyldopa. If a positive Coombs test develops during methyldopa therapy, the physician should determine whether hemolytic anemia exists and whether the positive Coombs test may be a problem. For example, in addition to a positive direct Coombs test there is less often a positive indirect Coombs test which may interfere with cross matching of blood.
Before treatment is started it is desirable to do a blood count (hematocrit, hemoglobin, or red cell count) for a baseline or to establish whether there is anemia. Periodic blood counts should be done during therapy to detect hemolytic anemia. It may be useful to do a direct Coombs test before therapy and at 6 and 12 months after the start of therapy.
If Coombs-positive hemolytic anemia occurs, the cause may be methyldopa and the drug should be discontinued. Usually the anemia remits promptly. If not, corticosteroids may be given and other causes of anemia should be considered. If the hemolytic anemia is related to methyldopa, the drug should not be reinstituted.
When methyldopa causes Coombs positivity alone or with hemolytic anemia, the red cell is usually coated with gamma globulin of the IgG (gamma G) class only. The positive Coombs test may not revert to normal until weeks to months after methyldopa is stopped.
Should the need for transfusion arise in a patient receiving methyldopa, both a direct and an indirect Coombs test should be performed. In the absence of hemolytic anemia, usually only the direct Coombs test will be positive. A positive direct Coombs test alone will not interfere with typing or cross matching. If the indirect Coombs test is also positive, problems may arise in the major cross match and the assistance of a hematologist or transfusion expert will be needed.
Occasionally, fever has occurred within the first three weeks of methyldopa therapy, associated in some cases with eosinophilia or abnormalities in one or more liver function tests, such as serum alkaline phosphatase, serum transaminases (SGOT, SGPT), bilirubin, and prothrombin time. Jaundice, with or without fever, may occur with onset usually within the first two to three months of therapy. In some patients the findings are consistent with those of cholestasis. In others the findings are consistent with hepatitis and hepatocellular injury.
Rarely, fatal hepatic necrosis has been reported after use of methyldopa. These hepatic changes may represent hypersensitivity reactions. Periodic determination of hepatic function should be done particularly during the first 6 to 12 weeks of therapy or whenever an unexplained fever occurs.
If fever, abnormalities in liver function tests, or jaundice appear, stop therapy with methyldopa. If caused by methyldopa, the temperature and abnormalities in liver function characteristically have reverted to normal when the drug was discontinued. Methyldopa should not be reinstituted in such patients.
Rarely, a reversible reduction of the white blood cell count with a primary effect on the granulocytes has been seen. The granulocyte count returned promptly to normal on discontinuance of the drug. Rare cases of granulocytopenia have been reported. In each instance, upon stopping the drug, the white cell count returned to normal. Reversible thrombocytopenia has occurred rarely.
Hydrochlorothiazide
Use with caution in severe renal disease. In patients with renal disease, thiazides may precipitate azotemia. Cumulative effects of the drug may develop in patients with impaired renal function.
Thiazides should be used with caution in patients with impaired hepatic function or progressive liver disease, since minor alterations of fluid and electrolyte balance may precipitate hepatic coma.
Thiazides may add to or potentiate the action of other antihypertensive drugs.
Sensitivity reactions may occur in patients with or without a history of allergy or bronchial asthma.
The possibility of exacerbation or activation of systemic lupus erythematosus has been reported.
Lithium generally should not be given with diuretics (see PRECAUTIONS, *Drug Interactions*).

PRECAUTIONS

General
Methyldopa
Methyldopa should be used with caution in patients with a history of previous liver disease or dysfunction (see WARNINGS).
Some patients taking methyldopa experience clinical edema or weight gain which may be controlled by use of a diuretic. Methyldopa should not be continued if edema progresses or signs of heart failure appear.
Hypertension has recurred occasionally after dialysis in patients given methyldopa because the drug is removed by this procedure.
Rarely, involuntary choreoathetotic movements have been observed during therapy with methyldopa in patients with severe bilateral cerebrovascular disease. Should these movements occur, stop therapy.

Continued on next page

Information on the Merck & Co., Inc. products listed on these pages is the full prescribing information from product circulars in use August 31, 1998. For information, please call 1-800-NSC MERCK [1-800-672-6372].

Aldoril Tablets—Cont.

Hydrochlorothiazide

All patients receiving diuretic therapy should be observed for evidence of fluid or electrolyte imbalance: namely; hyponatremia, hypochloremic alkalosis, and hypokalemia. Serum and urine electrolyte determinations are particularly important when the patient is vomiting excessively or receiving parenteral fluids. Warning signs or symptoms of fluid and electrolyte imbalance, irrespective of cause, include dryness of mouth, thirst, weakness, lethargy, drowsiness, restlessness, confusion, seizures, muscle pains or cramps, muscular fatigue, hypotension, oliguria, tachycardia, and gastrointestinal disturbances such as nausea and vomiting.

Hypokalemia may develop especially after prolonged therapy or when severe cirrhosis is present (see CONTRAINDICATIONS and WARNINGS).

Interference with adequate oral electrolyte intake will also contribute to hypokalemia. Hypokalemia may cause cardiac arrhythmia and may also sensitize or exaggerate the response of the heart to the toxic effects of digitalis (e.g., increased ventricular irritability). Hypokalemia may be avoided or treated by use of potassium sparing diuretics or potassium supplements such as foods with a high potassium content.

Although any chloride deficit is generally mild and usually does not require specific treatment except under extraordinary circumstances (as in liver disease or renal disease), chloride replacement may be required in the treatment of metabolic alkalosis.

Dilutional hyponatremia may occur in edematous patients in hot weather; appropriate therapy is water restriction, rather than administration of salt, except in rare instances when the hyponatremia is life threatening. In actual salt depletion, appropriate replacement is the therapy of choice.

Hyperuricemia may occur or acute gout may be precipitated in certain patients receiving thiazides.

In diabetic patients dosage adjustment of insulin or oral hypoglycemic agents may be required. Hyperglycemia may occur with thiazide diuretics. Thus latent diabetes mellitus may become manifest during thiazide therapy.

The antihypertensive effects of the drug may be enhanced in the postsympathectomy patient.

If progressive renal impairment becomes evident, consider withholding or discontinuing diuretic therapy.

Thiazides have been shown to increase the urinary excretion of magnesium; this may result in hypomagnesemia.

Thiazides may decrease urinary calcium excretion. Thiazides may cause intermittent and slight elevation of serum calcium in the absence of known disorders of calcium metabolism. Marked hypercalcemia may be evidence of hidden hyperparathyroidism. Thiazides should be discontinued before carrying out tests for parathyroid function.

Increases in cholesterol and triglyceride levels may be associated with thiazide diuretic therapy.

Laboratory Tests

Methyldopa

Blood count, Coombs test and liver function test, are recommended before initiating therapy and at periodic intervals (see WARNINGS).

Hydrochlorothiazide

Periodic determination of serum electrolytes to detect possible electrolyte imbalance should be done at appropriate intervals.

Drug Interactions

Methyldopa

When methyldopa is used with other antihypertensive drugs, potentiation of antihypertensive effect may occur. Patients should be followed carefully to detect side reactions or unusual manifestations of drug idiosyncrasy.

Patients may require reduced doses of anesthetics when on methyldopa. If hypotension does occur during anesthesia, it usually can be controlled by vasopressors. The adrenergic receptors remain sensitive during treatment with methyldopa.

Monoamine oxidase (MAO) inhibitors: see CONTRAINDICATIONS.

Hydrochlorothiazide

When given concurrently the following drugs may interact with thiazide diuretics.

Alcohol, barbiturates, or narcotics —potentiation of orthostatic hypotension may occur.

Antidiabetic drugs (oral agents and insulin) —dosage adjustment of the antidiabetic drug may be required.

Other antihypertensive drugs —additive effect or potentiation.

Cholestyramine and colestipol resins—Absorption of hydrochlorothiazide is impaired in the presence of anionic exchange resins. Single doses of either cholestyramine or colestipol resins bind the hydrochlorothiazide and reduce its absorption from the gastrointestinal tract by up to 85 and 43 percent, respectively.

Corticosteroids, ACTH —intensified electrolyte depletion, particularly hypokalemia.

Pressor amines (e.g., norepinephrine) —possible decreased response to pressor amines but not sufficient to preclude their use.

Skeletal muscle relaxants, nondepolarizing (e.g., tubocurarine) —possible increased responsiveness to the muscle relaxant.

Lithium —generally should not be given with diuretics. Diuretic agents reduce the renal clearance of lithium and add a high risk of lithium toxicity. Refer to the package insert for lithium preparations before use of such preparations with ALDORIL.

Non-steroidal Anti-inflammatory Drugs —In some patients, the administration of a non-steroidal anti-inflammatory agent can reduce the diuretic, natriuretic, and antihypertensive effects of loop, potassium-sparing and thiazide diuretics. Therefore, when ALDORIL and non-steroidal anti-inflammatory agents are used concomitantly, the patient should be observed closely to determine if the desired effect of the diuretic is obtained.

Drug/Laboratory Test Interactions

Methyldopa

Methyldopa may interfere with measurement of: urinary uric acid by the phosphotungstate method, serum creatinine by the alkaline picrate method, and SGOT by colorimetric methods. Interference with spectrophotometric methods for SGOT analysis has not been reported.

Since methyldopa causes fluorescence in urine samples at the same wave lengths as catecholamines, falsely high levels of urinary catecholamines may be reported. This will interfere with the diagnosis of pheochromocytoma. It is important to recognize this phenomenon before a patient with a possible pheochromocytoma is subjected to surgery. Methyldopa does not interfere with measurement of VMA (vanillylmandelic acid), a test for pheochromocytoma, by those methods which convert VMA to vanillin. Methyldopa is not recommended for the treatment of patients with pheochromocytoma. Rarely, when urine is exposed to air after voiding, it may darken because of breakdown of methyldopa or its metabolites.

Hydrochlorothiazide

Thiazides should be discontinued before carrying out tests for parathyroid function (see PRECAUTIONS, *General*).

Carcinogenesis, Mutagenesis,

Impairment of Fertility

Long-term studies in animals have not been performed to evaluate the effects upon fertility, mutagenic or carcinogenic potential of the combination.

Methyldopa

No evidence of a tumorigenic effect was seen when methyldopa was given for two years to mice at doses up to 1800 mg/kg/day or to rats at doses up to 240 mg/kg/day (30 and 4 times the maximum recommended human dose in mice and rats, respectively, when compared on the basis of body weight; 2.5 and 0.6 times the maximum recommended human dose in mice and rats, respectively, when compared on the basis of body surface area; calculations assume a patient weight of 50 kg).

Methyldopa was not mutagenic in the Ames Test and did not increase chromosomal aberration or sister chromatid exchanges in Chinese hamster ovary cells. These *in vitro* studies were carried out both with and without exogenous metabolic activation.

Fertility was unaffected when methyldopa was given to male and female rats at 100 mg/kg/day (1.7 times the maximum daily human dose when compared on the basis of body weight; 0.2 times the maximum daily human dose when compared on the basis of body surface area). Methyldopa decreased sperm count, sperm motility, the number of late spermatids and the male fertility index when given to male rats at 200 and 400 mg/kg/day (3.3 and 6.7 times the maximum daily human dose when compared on the basis of body weight; 0.5 and 1 times the maximum daily human dose when compared on the basis of body surface area).

Hydrochlorothiazide

Two-year feeding studies in mice and rats conducted under the auspices of the National Toxicology Program (NTP) uncovered no evidence of a carcinogenic potential of hydrochlorothiazide in female mice (at doses of up to approximately 600 mg/kg/day) or in male and female rats (at doses of up to approximately 100 mg/kg/day). The NTP, however, found equivocal evidence for hepatocarcinogenicity in male mice. Hydrochlorothiazide was not genotoxic *in vitro* in the Ames mutagenicity assay of *Salmonella typhimurium* strains TA 98, TA 100, TA 1535, TA 1537, and TA 1538 and in the Chinese Hamster Ovary (CHO) test for chromosomal aberrations, or *in vivo* in assays using mouse germinal cell chromosomes, Chinese hamster bone marrow chromosomes, and the *Drosophila* sex-linked recessive lethal trait gene. Positive test results were obtained only in the *in vitro* CHO Sister Chromatid Exchange (clastogenicity) and in the Mouse Lymphoma Cell (mutagenicity) assays, using concentrations of hydrochlorothiazide from 43 to 1300 μg/mL, and in the *Aspergillus nidulans* non-disjunction assay at an unspecified concentration.

Hydrochlorothiazide had no adverse effects on the fertility of mice and rats of either sex in studies wherein these spe-

cies were exposed, via their diet, to doses of up to 100 and 4 mg/kg, respectively, prior to conception and throughout gestation.

Pregnancy

Use of diuretics during normal pregnancy is inappropriate and exposes mother and fetus to unnecessary hazard. Diuretics do not prevent development of toxemia of pregnancy and there is no satisfactory evidence that they are useful in the treatment of toxemia.

Teratogenic Effects—Pregnancy Category C: Animal reproduction studies have not been conducted with ALDORIL. It is also not known whether ALDORIL can affect reproduction capacity or can cause fetal harm when given to a pregnant woman. ALDORIL should be given to a pregnant woman only if clearly needed.

Hydrochlorothiazide: Studies in which hydrochlorothiazide was orally administered to pregnant mice and rats during their respective periods of major organogenesis at doses up to 3000 and 1000 mg hydrochlorothiazide/kg, respectively, provided no evidence of harm to the fetus. There are, however, no adequate and well-controlled studies in pregnant women.

Methyldopa: Reproduction studies performed with methyldopa at oral doses up to 1000 mg/kg in mice, 200 mg/kg in rabbits and 100 mg/kg in rats revealed no evidence of harm to the fetus. These doses are 16.6 times, 3.3 times and 1.7 times, respectively, the maximum daily human dose when compared on the basis of body weight; 1.4 times, 1.1 times and 0.2 times, respectively, when compared on the basis of body surface area; calculations assume a patient weight of 50 kg. There are, however, no adequate and well-controlled studies in pregnant women in the first trimester of pregnancy. Because animal reproduction studies are not always predictive of human response, methyldopa should be used during pregnancy only if clearly needed.

Published reports of the use of methyldopa during all trimesters indicate that if this drug is used during pregnancy the possibility of fetal harm appears remote. In five studies, three of which were controlled, involving 332 pregnant hypertensive women, treatment with methyldopa was associated with an improved fetal outcome. The majority of these women were in the third trimester when methyldopa therapy was begun.

In one study, women who had begun methyldopa treatment between weeks 16 and 20 of pregnancy gave birth to infants whose average head circumference was reduced by a small amount (34.2 ± 1.7 cm vs. 34.6 ± 1.3 cm [mean ± 1 S.D.]). Long term follow-up of 195 (97.5%) of the children born to methyldopa-treated pregnant women (including those who began treatment between weeks 16 and 20) failed to uncover any significant adverse effect on the children. At four years of age, the developmental delay commonly seen in children born to hypertensive mothers was less evident in those whose mothers were treated with methyldopa during pregnancy than those whose mothers were untreated. The children of the treated group scored consistently higher than the children of the untreated group on five major indices of intellectual and motor development. At age 7 and one-half developmental scores and intelligence indices showed no significant differences in children of treated or untreated hypertensive women.

Nonteratogenic Effects: Thiazides cross the placental barrier and appear in cord blood. There is a risk of fetal or neonatal jaundice, thrombocytopenia, and possibly other adverse reactions that have occurred in adults.

Nursing Mothers

Methyldopa and thiazides appear in breast milk. Therefore, because of the potential for serious adverse reactions in nursing infants from hydrochlorothiazide, a decision should be made whether to discontinue nursing or to discontinue the drug, taking into account the importance of the drug to the mother.

Pediatric Use

Safety and effectiveness of ALDORIL in pediatric patients have not been established.

ADVERSE REACTIONS

The following adverse reactions have been reported and, within each category, are listed in order of decreasing severity.

Methyldopa

Sedation, usually transient, may occur during the initial period of therapy or whenever the dose is increased. Headache, asthenia, or weakness may be noted as early and transient symptoms. However, significant adverse effects due to methyldopa have been infrequent and this agent usually is well tolerated.

Cardiovascular: Aggravation of angina pectoris, congestive heart failure, prolonged carotid sinus hypersensitivity, orthostatic hypotension (decrease daily dosage), edema or weight gain, bradycardia.

Digestive: Pancreatitis, colitis, vomiting, diarrhea, sialadenitis, sore or "black" tongue, nausea, constipation, distention, flatus, dryness of mouth.

Endocrine: Hyperprolactinemia.

Hematologic: Bone marrow depression, leukopenia, granulocytopenia, thrombocytopenia, hemolytic anemia; positive tests for antinuclear antibody, LE cells, and rheumatoid factor, positive Coombs test.
Hepatic: Liver disorders including hepatitis, jaundice, abnormal liver function tests (see WARNINGS).
Hypersensitivity: Myocarditis, pericarditis, vasculitis, lupus-like syndrome, drug-related fever, eosinophilia.
Nervous System/Psychiatric: Parkinsonism, Bell's palsy, decreased mental acuity, involuntary choreoathetotic movements, symptoms of cerebrovascular insufficiency, psychic disturbances including nightmares and reversible mild psychoses or depression, headache, sedation, asthenia or weakness, dizziness, lightheadedness, paresthesias.
Metabolic: Rise in BUN.
Musculoskeletal: Arthralgia, with or without joint swelling; myalgia.
Respiratory: Nasal stuffiness.
Skin: Toxic epidermal necrolysis, rash.
Urogenital: Amenorrhea, breast enlargement, gynecomastia, lactation, impotence, decreased libido.
Hydrochlorothiazide
Body as a Whole: Weakness.
Cardiovascular: Hypotension including orthostatic hypotension (may be aggravated by alcohol, barbiturates, narcotics or antihypertensive drugs).
Digestive: Pancreatitis, jaundice (intrahepatic cholestatic jaundice), diarrhea, vomiting, sialadenitis, cramping, constipation, gastric irritation, nausea, anorexia.
Hematologic: Aplastic anemia, agranulocytosis, leukopenia, hemolytic anemia, thrombocytopenia.
Hypersensitivity: Anaphylactic reactions, necrotizing angiitis (vasculitis and cutaneous vasculitis), respiratory distress including pneumonitis and pulmonary edema, photosensitivity, fever, urticaria, rash, purpura.
Metabolic: Electrolyte imbalance (see PRECAUTIONS), hyperglycemia, glycosuria, hyperuricemia.
Musculoskeletal: Muscle spasm.
Nervous System/Psychiatric: Vertigo, paresthesias, dizziness, headache, restlessness.
Renal: Renal failure, renal dysfunction, interstitial nephritis. (See WARNINGS.)
Skin: Erythema multiforme including Stevens-Johnson syndrome, exfoliative dermatitis including toxic epidermal necrolysis, alopecia.
Special Senses: Transient blurred vision, xanthopsia.
Urogenital: Impotence.

OVERDOSAGE

Acute overdosage may produce acute hypotension with other responses attributable to brain and gastrointestinal malfunction (excessive sedation, weakness, bradycardia, dizziness, lightheadedness, constipation, distention, flatus, diarrhea, nausea, vomiting).
In the event of overdosage, symptomatic and supportive measures should be employed. When ingestion is recent, gastric lavage or emesis may reduce absorption. When ingestion has been earlier, infusions may be helpful to promote urinary excretion. Otherwise, management includes special attention to cardiac rate and output, blood volume, electrolyte balance, paralytic ileus, urinary function and cerebral activity.
Sympathomimetic drugs [e.g., levarterenol, epinephrine, ARAMINE* (Metaraminol Bitartrate)] may be indicated.
Methyldopa is dialyzable. The degree to which hydrochlorothiazide is removed by hemodialysis has not been established.
The oral LD_{50} of methyldopa is greater than 1.5 g/kg in both the mouse and the rat. The oral LD_{50} of hydrochlorothiazide is greater than 10 g/kg in the mouse and rat.

---

*Registered trademark of MERCK & CO., INC.

DOSAGE AND ADMINISTRATION

DOSAGE MUST BE INDIVIDUALIZED, AS DETERMINED BY TITRATION OF THE INDIVIDUAL COMPONENTS (see box warning). Once the patient has been successfully titrated, ALDORIL may be substituted if the previously determined titrated doses are the same as in the combination. The usual starting dosage is one tablet of ALDORIL 15 two or three times a day or one tablet of ALDORIL 25 two times a day. For those patients requiring higher doses, one tablet of ALDORIL D30 or ALDORIL D50 two times a day may be used.
Patients usually do not require doses of hydrochlorothiazide in excess of 50 mg daily when combined with other antihypertensive agents. The usual daily dosage of methyldopa is 500 mg to 2 g. To minimize the sedation associated with methyldopa, start dosage increases in the evening.
Occasionally tolerance to methyldopa may occur, usually between the second and third month of therapy. Additional separate doses of methyldopa or replacement of ALDORIL with single entity agents is necessary until the new effective dose ratio is re-established by titration. The maximum recommended daily dose of methyldopa is 3 g and of hydrochlorothiazide is 200 mg.
If ALDORIL does not adequately control blood pressure, additional doses of other agents may be given. When ALDORIL is given with antihypertensives other than thiazides, the initial dosage of methyldopa should be limited to 500 mg daily in divided doses and the dose of these other agents may need to be adjusted to effect a smooth transition.
Since both components of ALDORIL have a relatively short duration of action, withdrawal is followed by return of hypertension usually within 48 hours. This is not complicated by an overshoot of blood pressure.
Since methyldopa is largely excreted by the kidney, patients with impaired renal function may respond to smaller doses. Syncope in older patients may be related to an increased sensitivity and advanced arteriosclerotic vascular disease. This may be avoided by lower doses.

HOW SUPPLIED

No. 3294—Tablets ALDORIL 15 are salmon, round, film coated tablets, coded MSD 423 on one side and ALDORIL on the other. Each tablet contains 250 mg of methyldopa and 15 mg of hydrochlorothiazide. They are supplied as follows:
NDC 0006-0423-68 bottles of 100
NDC 0006-0423-82 bottles of 1000.
Shown in Product Identification Guide, page 322
No. 3295—Tablets ALDORIL 25 are white, round, film coated tablets, coded MSD 456 on one side and ALDORIL on the other. Each tablet contains 250 mg of methyldopa and 25 mg of hydrochlorothiazide. They are supplied as follows:
NDC 0006-0456-68 bottles of 100
NDC 0006-0456-82 bottles of 1000.
Shown in Product Identification Guide, page 322
No. 3362—Tablets ALDORIL D30 are salmon, oval, film coated tablets, coded MSD 694 on one side and ALDORIL on the other. Each tablet contains 500 mg of methyldopa and 30 mg of hydrochlorothiazide. They are supplied as follows:
NDC 0006-0694-68 bottles of 100.
Shown in Product Identification Guide, page 322
No. 3363—Tablets ALDORIL D50 are white, oval, film coated tablets, coded MSD 935 on one side and ALDORIL on the other. Each tablet contains 500 mg of methyldopa and 50 mg of hydrochlorothiazide. They are supplied as follows:
NDC 0006-0935-68 bottles of 100.
Shown in Product Identification Guide, page 322
Storage
Keep container tightly closed. Protect from light, moisture, freezing, −20°C (−4°F) and store at controlled room temperature, 15–30°C (59–86°F).
7843552 Issued February 1997

AMINOHIPPURATE SODIUM "PAH" ℞
Injection, U.S.P.

DESCRIPTION

Aminohippurate sodium* is an agent to measure effective renal plasma flow (ERPF). It is the sodium salt of para-aminohippuric acid, commonly abbreviated "PAH."It is water soluble, lipid-insoluble, and has a pKa of 3.83. The empirical formula of the anhydrous salt is $C_9H_9N_2NaO_3$ and its structural formula is:

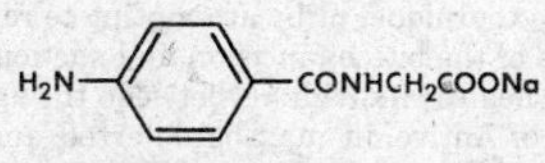
H₂N
CONHCH₂COONa

It is provided as a sterile, non-preserved 20 percent aqueous solution for injection, with a pH of 6.7 to 7.6. Each 10 mL contains: Aminohippurate sodium 2 g. Inactive ingredients: Sodium hydroxide to adjust pH, water for injection, q.s.

---

*Formerly referred to as Sodium para-Aminohippurate.

CLINICAL PHARMACOLOGY

PAH is filtered by the glomeruli and is actively secreted by the proximal tubules. At low plasma concentrations (1.0 to 2.0 mg/100 mL), an average of 90 percent of PAH is cleared by the kidneys from the renal blood stream in a single circulation. It is ideally suited for measurement of ERPF since it has a high clearance, is essentially nontoxic at the plasma concentrations reached with recommended doses and its analytical determination is relatively simple and accurate.
PAH is also used to measure the functional capacity of the renal tubular secretory mechanism or transport maximum (Tm_{PAH}). This is accomplished by elevating the plasma concentration to levels (40–60 mg/100 mL) sufficient to saturate the maximal capacity of the tubular cells to secrete PAH.
Inulin clearance is generally measured during Tm_{PAH} determinations since glomerular filtration rate (GFR) must be known before calculations of secretory Tm measurements can be done (See *Calculations*).

INDICATIONS AND USAGE

Estimation of effective renal plasma flow.
Measurement of the functional capacity of the renal tubular secretory mechanism.

CONTRAINDICATIONS

Hypersensitivity to this product or to its components.

PRECAUTIONS

General
Intravenous solutions must be given with caution to patients with low cardiac reserve, since a rapid increase in plasma volume can precipitate congestive heart failure.
For measurement of ERPF, small doses of PAH are used. However, in research procedures to measure Tm_{PAH}, high plasma levels are required to saturate the capacity of the tubular cells. During these procedures the intravenous administration of PAH solutions should be carried out slowly and with caution. The patient should be continuously observed for any adverse reactions.
Drug Interactions
Renal clearance measurements of PAH cannot be made with any significant accuracy in patients receiving sulfonamides, procaine, or thiazolesulfone. These compounds interfere with chemical color development essential to the analytical procedures.
Probenecid depresses tubular secretion of certain weak acids such as PAH. Therefore, patients receiving probenecid will have erroneously low ERPF and Tm_{PAH} values.
Carcinogenesis, Mutagenesis, Impairment of Fertility
Long-term studies in animals have not been done to evaluate any effects upon fertility or carcinogenic potential of PAH.
Pregnancy
Pregnancy Category C. Animal reproduction studies have not been done with PAH. It is also not known whether PAH can cause fetal harm when given to a pregnant woman or can affect reproduction capacity. PAH should be given to a pregnant woman only if clearly needed.
Nursing Mothers
It is not known whether this drug is excreted in human milk. Because many drugs are excreted in human milk, caution should be exercised when PAH is administered to a nursing woman.
Pediatric Use
Safety and effectiveness in pediatric patients have not been established.

ADVERSE REACTIONS

Vasomotor disturbances, flushing, tingling, nausea, vomiting, and cramps may occur.
Patients may have a sensation of warmth or the desire to defecate or urinate during or shortly following initiation of infusion.

OVERDOSAGE

The intravenous LD_{50} in female mice is 7.22 g/kg.

DOSAGE AND ADMINISTRATION

For intravenous use only
Clearance measurements using single injection technics are generally inaccurate, particularly in the measurement of ERPF. For this reason, intravenous infusions at fixed rates are used to sustain the plasma PAH concentration at the desired level.
To measure ERPF, the concentration of PAH in the plasma should be maintained at 2 mg per 100 mL, which can be achieved with a priming dose of 6 to 10 mg/kg and an infusion dose of 10 to 24 mg/min.
As a research procedure for the measurement of Tm_{PAH}, the plasma level of PAH must be sufficient to saturate the capacity of the tubular secretory cells. Concentrations of from 40 to 60 mg per 100 mL are usually necessary.
Technical details of these tests may be found in Smith[1]; Wesson[2]; Bauer[3]; Pitts[4]; and Schnurr.[5]
Parenteral drug products should be inspected visually for particulate matter and discoloration prior to use, whenever solution and container permit. NOTE: The normal color range for this product is a colorless to yellow/brown solution. The efficacy is not affected by color changes within this range.

Continued on next page

Information on the Merck & Co., Inc. products listed on these pages is the full prescribing information from product circulars in use August 31, 1998. For information, please call 1-800-NSC MERCK [1-800-672-6372].

Aminohippurate Sodium—Cont.

Calculations
Effective Renal Plasma Flow (ERPF)
The clearance of PAH, which is extracted almost completely from the plasma during its passage through the renal circulation, constitutes a measure of ERPF. Hence:

$$ERPF \quad \frac{U_{PAH}V}{P_{PAH}}$$

Where U_{PAH} = concentration of PAH (mg/mL) in the urine
V = rate of urine excretion (mL/min), and
P_{PAH} = plasma concentration of PAH (mg/mL).

Example: U_{PAH} = 8.0 mg/mL
V = 1.5 mL/min
P_{PAH} = 0.02 mg/mL

$$ERPF = \frac{8.0 \times 1.5}{0.02} = 600 \text{ mL/min.}$$

Based on PAH clearance studies, the normal values for ERPF are:

men	675 ± 150 mL/min
women	595 ± 125 mL/min.

Maximum Tubular Secretory Mechanism (Tm_{PAH})
The quantity of PAH, secreted by the tubules (Tm_{PAH}) is given by the difference between the total rate of excretion ($U_{PAH}V$) and the quantity filtered by the glomeruli (GFR × P_{PAH}). Hence:

$$Tm_{PAH} = U_{PAH}V - (GFR \times P_{PAH} \times 0.83)$$

The factor, 0.83, corrects for that portion of PAH which is bound to plasma protein and hence is unfilterable.

Example: U_{PAH} = 9.55 mg/mL
V = 16.68 mL/min
GFR = 120 mL/min
P_{PAH} = 0.60 mg/mL

Then $Tm_{PAH} = 9.55 \times 16.68 - (120 \times 0.60 \times 0.83) = 100$ mg/min.
Average normal values of Tm_{PAH} are 80–90 mg/min.
The value of the expression $U_{PAH}V$, used in calculations of ERPF and Tm_{PAH}, may be found by determining the amount of PAH in a measured volume of urine excreted within a specific period of time.
These calculations are based on a body surface area of 1.73 m^2. Corrections for variations in surface area are made by multiplying the values obtained for ERPF and Tm_{PAH} by 1.73/A, where A is the subject surface area.

HOW SUPPLIED

No. 95—Aminohippurate Sodium, 20 percent sterile solution for intravenous injection, is supplied as follows:
NDC 0006-3395-11 in 10 mL vials.
Storage
Avoid storage at temperatures below −20°C (−4°F) and above 40°C (104°F).

REFERENCES

1. Smith, H. W.: Lectures on the kidney, University Extension Division, University of Kansas, Lawrence, Kansas, 1943.
2. Wesson, L. G., Jr.: "Physiology of the Human Kidney," New York, Grune & Stratton, 1969, pp. 632–655.
3. Bauer, J. D.; Ackermann, P. G.; Toro, G.: "Brays Clinical Laboratory Methods," ed. 7, St. Louis, Mosby, 1968.
4. Pitts, R. F.: "Physiology of the Kidney and Body Fluids," ed. 2, Chicago, Year Book Medical Publishers, 1968.
5. Schnurr, E., Lahme, W., Kuppers, H.: Measurement of renal clearance of inulin and PAH in the steady state without urine collection; Clinical Nephrology, *13* (1): (26–29), 1980.

7470621 Issued September 1996

ANTIVENIN ℞
(Latrodectus mactans), U.S.P.
(Black Widow Spider Antivenin)
Equine Origin

DESCRIPTION

Antivenin (Latrodectus mactans) is a sterile, non-pyrogenic preparation derived by drying a frozen solution of specific venom-neutralizing globulins obtained from the blood serum of healthy horses immunized against venom of black widow spiders (Latrodectus mactans). It is standardized by biological assay on mice, in terms of one dose of antivenin neutralizing the venom in not less than 6000 mouse LD_{50} of Latrodectus mactans. Thimerosal (mercury derivative) 1:10,000 is added as a preservative. When constituted as specified, it is opalescent, ranging in color from light (straw) to very dark (iced tea), and contains not more than 20.0 percent of solids.
Each vial contains not less than 6000 Antivenin units. One unit of Antivenin will neutralize one average mouse lethal dose of black widow spider venom when the Antivenin and the venom are injected simultaneously in mice under suitable conditions.

CLINICAL PHARMACOLOGY

The pharmacological mode of action is unknown and metabolic and pharmacokinetic data in humans are unavailable.

INDICATIONS AND USAGE

Antivenin (Latrodectus mactans) is used to treat patients with symptoms due to bites by the black widow spider (Latrodectus mactans). Early use of the Antivenin is emphasized for prompt relief.
Local muscular cramps begin from 15 minutes to several hours after the bite which usually produces a sharp pain similar to that caused by puncture with a needle. The exact sequence of symptoms depends somewhat on the location of the bite. The venom acts on the myoneural junctions or on the nerve endings, causing an ascending motor paralysis or destruction of the peripheral nerve endings. The groups of muscles most frequently affected at first are those of the thigh, shoulder, and back. After a varying length of time, the pain becomes more severe, spreading to the abdomen, and weakness and tremor usually develop. The abdominal muscles assume a boardlike rigidity, but tenderness is slight. Respiration is thoracic. The patient is restless and anxious. Feeble pulse, cold, clammy skin, labored breathing and speech, light stupor, and delirium may occur. Convulsions also may occur, particularly in small children. The temperature may be normal or slightly elevated. Urinary retention, shock, cyanosis, nausea and vomiting, insomnia, and cold sweats also have been reported. The syndrome following the bite of the black widow spider may be confused easily with any medical or surgical condition with acute abdominal symptoms.
The symptoms of black widow spider bite increase in severity for several hours, perhaps a day, and then very slowly become less severe, gradually passing off in the course of two or three days except in fatal cases. Residual symptoms such as general weakness, tingling, nervousness, and transient muscle spasm may persist for weeks or months after recovery from the acute stage.
If possible, the patient should be hospitalized. Other additional measures giving greatest relief are prolonged warm baths and intravenous injection of 10 mL of 10 percent solution of calcium gluconate repeated as necessary to control muscle pain. Morphine also may be required to control pain. Barbiturates may be used for extreme restlessness. However, as the venom is a neurotoxin, it can cause respiratory paralysis. This must be borne in mind when considering use of morphine or a barbiturate. Adrenocorticosteroids have been used with varying degrees of success. Supportive therapy is indicated by the condition of the patient. Local treatment of the site of the bite is of no value. Nothing is gained by applying a tourniquet or by attempting to remove venom from the site of the bite by incision and suction.
In otherwise healthy individuals between the ages of 16 and 60, the use of Antivenin may be deferred and treatment with muscle relaxants may be considered.

WARNINGS

Prior to treatment with any product prepared from horse serum, a careful review of the patient's history should be taken emphasizing prior exposure to horse serum or any allergies. Serious sickness and even death could result from the use of horse serum in a sensitive patient. A skin or conjunctival test should be performed prior to administration of Antivenin.
Skin test: Inject into (not under) the skin not more than 0.02 mL of the test material (1:10 dilution of normal horse serum in physiologic saline). Evaluate result in 10 minutes. A positive reaction is an urticarial wheal surrounded by a zone of erythema. A control test using Sodium Chloride Injection facilitates interpretation of the results.
Conjunctival test: For adults instill into the conjunctival sac one drop of a 1:10 dilution of horse serum and for children one drop of 1:100 dilution. Itching of the eye and reddening of the conjunctiva indicate a positive reaction, usually within 10 minutes.
Patients should be observed for serum sickness for an average of 8 to 12 days following administration of Antivenin.
Desensitization should be attempted only when the administration of Antivenin is considered necessary to save life. Epinephrine must be available in case of untoward reaction.
Desensitization: If the history is positive or the results of the sensitivity tests are mildly or quetionably positive, Antivenin should be administered as follows to reduce the risk of an immediate severe allergic reaction:

1. In separate sterile vials or syringes prepare 1:10 or 1:100 dilutions of Antivenin in Sodium Chloride for Injection.
2. Allow at least 15 but preferably 30 minutes between injections and only proceed with the next dose if no reactions occurred following the previous dose.
3. Using a tuberculin syringe, inject subcutaneously 0.1, 0.2 and 0.5 mL of the 1:100 dilution at 15 or 30 minute intervals; repeat with the 1:10 dilution, and finally the undiluted Antivenin.
4. If there is a reaction after any of the injections, place a tourniquet proximal to the sites of injection and administer epinephrine, 1:1000 (0.3 to 1.0 mL subcutaneously, 0.05 to 0.1 mL intravenously), proximal to the tourniquet or into another extremity. Wait at least 30 minutes before giving another injection of Antivenin, the amount of which should be the same as the last one not evoking a reaction.
5. If no reaction has occurred after 0.5 mL of undiluted Antivenin has been given, it is probably safe to continue the dose at 15 minute intervals until the entire dose has been injected.

PRECAUTIONS

Carcinogenesis, Mutagenesis, Impairment of Fertility
No long term studies in animals have been performed to evaluate the potential for carcinogenesis, mutagenesis, or impairment of fertility.
Pregnancy
Pregnancy Category C. Animal reproduction studies have not been conducted with Black Widow Spider Antivenin. It is also not known whether Black Widow Spider Antivenin can cause fetal harm when administered to a pregnant woman or can affect reproduction capacity. Black Widow Spider Antivenin should be given to a pregnant woman only if clearly needed.
Nursing Mothers
It is not known whether this drug is excreted in human milk. Because many drugs are excreted in human milk, caution should be exercised when Black Widow Spider Antivenin is administered to a nursing woman.
Pediatric Use
Controlled clinical studies for safety and effectiveness in children have not been conducted; however, there have been virtually no adverse effects reported in those children who have received the product.

ADVERSE REACTIONS

Anaphylaxis and serum sickness have been reported following use of Antivenin.

DOSAGE AND ADMINISTRATION

Using a sterile syringe, remove from the accompanying vial 2.5 mL of Sterile Diluent for Antivenin and inject into the vial of Antivenin. With the needle still in the rubber stopper, shake the vial to dissolve the contents completely.
Parenteral drug products should be inspected visually for particulate matter prior to administration, whenever solution and container permit (see DESCRIPTION).
The dose for adults and children is the entire contents of a restored vial (2.5 mL) of Antivenin. It may be given intramuscularly, preferably in the region of the anterolateral thigh so that a tourniquet may be applied in the event of a systemic reaction. Symptoms usually subside in 1 to 3 hours. Although one dose of Antivenin usually is adequate, a second dose may be necessary in some cases.
Antivenin also may be given intravenously in 10 to 50 mL of saline solution over a 15 minute period. It is the preferred route in severe cases, or when the patient is under 12, or in shock. One restored vial usually is enough.

HOW SUPPLIED

No. 4084—Antivenin (Latrodectus mactans) equine origin is a white to grey crystalline powder, each vial containing not less than 6000 Antivenin units. Thimerosal (mercury derivative) 1:10,000 is added as preservative, **NDC** 0006-4084-00. A 2.5 mL vial of Sterile Diluent for Antivenin is included. Also supplied is a 1 mL vial of normal horse serum (1:10 dilution) for sensitivity testing. Thimerosal (mercury derivative) 1:10,000 is added as preservative.
Storage
Antivenin must be stored and shipped at 2–8°C (36–46°F). When reconstituted as directed, the color of Antivenin ranges from light (straw) to very dark (iced tea), but the color has no effect on potency. *Do not freeze.*

A.H.F.S. Category: 80:04
7972114 Issued March 1995

AquaMEPHYTON® Injection ℞
(Phytonadione), U.S.P.
Aqueous Colloidal Solution of Vitamin K₁

AquaMEPHYTON
Summary of Dosage Guidelines
(See circular text for details)

Newborns	Dosage
Hemorrhagic Disease of the Newborn	
Prophylaxis	0.5–1 mg IM within 1 hour of birth
Treatment	1 mg SC or IM (Higher doses may be necessary if the mother has been receiving oral anticoagulants)

Adults	Initial Dosage
Anticoagulant-Induced Prothrombin Deficiency (caused by coumarin or indanedione derivatives)	2.5 mg–10 mg or up to 25 mg (rarely 50 mg)
Hypoprothrombinemia due to other causes (Antibiotics; Salicylates or other drugs; Factors limiting absorption or synthesis)	2.5 mg–25 mg or more (rarely up to 50 mg)

WARNING—INTRAVENOUS USE

Severe reactions, including fatalities, have occurred during and immediately after INTRAVENOUS injection of AquaMEPHYTON* (Phytonadione), even when precautions have been taken to dilute the AquaMEPHYTON and to avoid rapid infusion. Typically these severe reactions have resembled hypersensitivity or anaphylaxis, including shock and cardiac and/or respiratory arrest. Some patients have exhibited these severe reactions on receiving AquaMEPHYTON for the first time. Therefore the INTRAVENOUS route should be restricted to those situations where other routes are not feasible and the serious risk involved is considered justified.

---

*Registered trademark of MERCK & CO., INC.

DESCRIPTION

Phytonadione is a vitamin, which is a clear, yellow to amber, viscous, odorless or nearly odorless liquid. It is insoluble in water, soluble in chloroform and slightly soluble in ethanol. It has a molecular weight of 450.70.

Phytonadione is 2-methyl-3-phytyl-1,4-naphthoquinone. Its empirical formula is $C_{31}H_{46}O_2$ and its structural formula is:

AquaMEPHYTON injection is a yellow, sterile, aqueous colloidal solution of vitamin K₁, with a pH of 5.0 to 7.0, available for injection by the intravenous, intramuscular, and subcutaneous routes. Each milliliter contains:

Phytonadione	2 mg or 10 mg
Inactive ingredients:	
Polyoxyethylated fatty acid derivative	70 mg
Dextrose	37.5 mg
Water for Injection, q.s.	1 mL
Added as preservative:	
Benzyl alcohol	0.9%

CLINICAL PHARMACOLOGY

AquaMEPHYTON aqueous colloidal solution of vitamin K₁ for parenteral injection, possesses the same type and degree of activity as does naturally-occurring vitamin K, which is necessary for the production via the liver of active prothrombin (factor II), proconvertin (factor VII), plasma thromboplastin component (factor IX), and Stuart factor (factor X). The prothrombin test is sensitive to the levels of three of these four factors—II, VII, and X. Vitamin K is an essential cofactor for a microsomal enzyme that catalyzes the post-translational carboxylation of multiple, specific, peptide-bound glutamic acid residues in inactive hepatic precursors of factors II, VII, IX, and X. The resulting gamma-carboxyglutamic acid residues convert the precursors into active coagulation factors that are subsequently secreted by liver cells into the blood.

Phytonadione is readily absorbed following intramuscular administration. After absorption, phytonadione is initially concentrated in the liver, but the concentration declines rapidly. Very little vitamin K accumulates in tissues. Little is known about the metabolic fate of vitamin K. Almost no free unmetabolized vitamin K appears in bile or urine.

In normal animals and humans, phytonadione is virtually devoid of pharmacodynamic activity. However, in animals and humans deficient in vitamin K, the pharmacological action of vitamin K is related to its normal physiological function, that is, to promote the hepatic biosynthesis of vitamin K dependent clotting factors.

The action of the aqueous colloidal solution, when administered intravenously, is generally detectable within an hour or two and hemorrhage is usually controlled within 3 to 6 hours. A normal prothrombin level may often be obtained in 12 to 14 hours.

In the prophylaxis and treatment of hemorrhagic disease of the newborn, phytonadione has demonstrated a greater margin of safety than that of the water-soluble vitamin K analogues.

INDICATIONS AND USAGE

AquaMEPHYTON is indicated in the following coagulation disorders which are due to faulty formation of factors II, VII, IX and X when caused by vitamin K deficiency or interference with vitamin K activity.

AquaMEPHYTON injection is indicated in:
— anticoagulant-induced prothrombin deficiency caused by coumarin or indanedione derivatives;
— prophylaxis and therapy of hemorrhagic disease of the newborn;
— hypoprothrombinemia due to antibacterial therapy;
— hypoprothrombinemia secondary to factors limiting absorption or synthesis of vitamin K, e.g., obstructive jaundice, biliary fistula, sprue, ulcerative colitis, celiac disease, intestinal resection, cystic fibrosis of the pancreas, and regional enteritis;
— other drug-induced hypoprothrombinemia where it is definitely shown that the result is due to interference with vitamin K metabolism, e.g., salicylates.

CONTRAINDICATION

Hypersensitivity to any component of this medication.

WARNINGS

Benzyl alcohol as a preservative in Bacteriostatic Sodium Chloride Injection has been associated with toxicity in newborns. Data are unavailable on the toxicity of other preservatives in this age group. There is no evidence to suggest that the small amount of benzyl alcohol contained in AquaMEPHYTON, when used as recommended, is associated with toxicity.

An immediate coagulant effect should not be expected after administration of phytonadione. It takes a minimum of 1 to 2 hours for measurable improvement in the prothrombin time. Whole blood or component therapy may also be necessary if bleeding is severe.

Phytonadione will not counteract the anticoagulant action of heparin.

When vitamin K₁ is used to correct excessive anticoagulant-induced hypoprothrombinemia, anticoagulant therapy still being indicated, the patient is again faced with the clotting hazards existing prior to starting the anticoagulant therapy. Phytonadione is not a clotting agent, but overzealous therapy with vitamin K₁ may restore conditions which originally permitted thromboembolic phenomena. Dosage should be kept as low as possible, and prothrombin time should be checked regularly as clinical conditions indicate.

Repeated large doses of vitamin K are not warranted in liver disease if the response to initial use of the vitamin is unsatisfactory. Failure to respond to vitamin K may indicate that the condition being treated is inherently unresponsive to vitamin K.

PRECAUTIONS

Drug Interactions
Temporary resistance to prothrombin-depressing anticoagulants may result, especially when larger doses of phytonadione are used. If relatively large doses have been employed, it may be necessary when reinstituting anticoagulant therapy to use somewhat larger doses of the prothrombin-depressing anticoagulant, or to use one which acts on a different principle, such as heparin sodium.

Laboratory Tests
Prothrombin time should be checked regularly as clinical conditions indicate.

Carcinogenesis, Mutagenesis, Impairment of Fertility
Studies of carcinogenicity, mutagenesis or impairment of fertility have not been conducted with AquaMEPHYTON.

Pregnancy
Pregnancy Category C: Animal reproduction studies have not been conducted with AquaMEPHYTON. It is also not known whether AquaMEPHYTON can cause fetal harm when administered to a pregnant woman or can affect reproduction capacity. AquaMEPHYTON should be given to a pregnant woman only if clearly needed.

Nursing Mothers
It is not known whether this drug is excreted in human milk. Because many drugs are excreted in human milk, caution should be exercised when AquaMEPHYTON is administered to a nursing woman.

Pediatric Use
Hemolysis, jaundice, and hyperbilirubinemia in newborns, particularly in premature infants, may be related to the dose of AquaMEPHYTON. Therefore, the recommended dose should not be exceeded (see ADVERSE REACTIONS and DOSAGE AND ADMINISTRATION).

ADVERSE REACTIONS

Deaths have occurred after intravenous administration. (See Box Warning at beginning of circular.)

Transient "flushing sensations" and "peculiar" sensations of taste have been observed, as well as rare instances of dizziness, rapid and weak pulse, profuse sweating, brief hypotension, dyspnea, and cyanosis.

Pain, swelling, and tenderness at the injection site may occur.

The possibility of allergic sensitivity, including an anaphylactoid reaction, should be kept in mind.

Infrequently, usually after repeated injection, erythematous, indurated, pruritic plaques have occurred; rarely, these have progressed to sclerodermalike lesions that have persisted for long periods. In other cases, these lesions have resembled erythema perstans.

Hyperbilirubinemia has been observed in the newborn following administration of phytonadione. This has occurred rarely and primarily with doses above those recommended. (See PRECAUTIONS, *Pediatric Use.*)

OVERDOSAGE

The intravenous LD₅₀ of AquaMEPHYTON in the mouse is 41.5 and 52 mL/kg for the 0.2% and 1% concentrations respectively.

DOSAGE AND ADMINISTRATION

Whenever possible, AquaMEPHYTON should be given by the subcutaneous or intramuscular route. When intravenous administration is considered unavoidable, the drug should be injected very slowly, not exceeding 1 mg per minute.

Protect from light at all times.

Parenteral drug products should be inspected visually for particulate matter and discoloration prior to administration, whenever solution and container permit.

Directions for Dilution
AquaMEPHYTON may be diluted with 0.9% Sodium Chloride Injection, 5% Dextrose Injection, or 5% Dextrose and Sodium Chloride Injection. Benzyl alcohol as a preservative has been associated with toxicity in newborns. *Therefore, all*

Continued on next page

Information on the Merck & Co., Inc. products listed on these pages is the full prescribing information from product circulars in use August 31, 1998. For information, please call 1-800-NSC MERCK [1-800-672-6372].

AquaMephyton—Cont.

of the above diluents should be preservative-free (see WARNINGS). *Other diluents should not be used.* When dilutions are indicated, administration should be started immediately after mixture with the diluent, and unused portions of the dilution should be discarded, as well as unused contents of the ampul.

Prophylaxis of Hemorrhagic Disease of the Newborn

The American Academy of Pediatrics recommends that vitamin K_1 be given to the newborn. A single intramuscular dose of AquaMEPHYTON 0.5 to 1 mg within one hour of birth is recommended.

Treatment of Hemorrhagic Disease of the Newborn

Empiric administration of vitamin K_1 should not replace proper laboratory evaluation of the coagulation mechanism. A prompt response (shortening of the prothrombin time in 2 to 4 hours) following administration of vitamin K_1 is usually diagnostic of hemorrhagic disease of the newborn, and failure to respond indicates another diagnosis or coagulation disorder.

AquaMEPHYTON 1 mg should be given either subcutaneously or intramuscularly. Higher doses may be necessary if the mother has been receiving oral anticoagulants.

[See table at top of previous page]

Whole blood or component therapy may be indicated if bleeding is excessive. This therapy, however, does not correct the underlying disorder and AquaMEPHYTON should be given concurrently.

Anticoagulant-Induced Prothrombin Deficiency in Adults

To correct excessively prolonged prothrombin time caused by oral anticoagulant therapy—2.5 to 10 mg or up to 25 mg initially is recommended. In rare instances 50 mg may be required. Frequency and amount of subsequent doses should be determined by prothrombin time response or clinical condition (see WARNINGS). If in 6 to 8 hours after parenteral administration the prothrombin time has not been shortened satisfactorily, the dose should be repeated.

In the event of shock or excessive blood loss, the use of whole blood or component therapy is indicated.

Hypoprothrombinemia Due to Other Causes in Adults

A dosage of 2.5 to 25 mg or more (rarely up to 50 mg) is recommended, the amount and route of administration depending upon the severity of the condition and response obtained.

If possible, discontinuation or reduction of the dosage of drugs interfering with coagulation mechanisms (such as salicylates, antibiotics) is suggested as an alternative to administering concurrent AquaMEPHYTON. The severity of the coagulation disorder should determine whether the immediate administration of AquaMEPHYTON is required in addition to discontinuation or reduction of interfering drugs.

HOW SUPPLIED

Injection AquaMEPHYTON is a yellow, sterile, aqueous colloidal solution and is supplied in the following concentrations:

No. 7780—10 mg of vitamin K_1 per mL
NDC 0006-7780-64 boxes of 6 × 1 mL ampuls
(6505-00-854-2499 10 mg 1 mL 6's)
NDC 0006-7780-66 boxes of 25 × 1 mL ampuls.
No. 7782—10 mg of vitamin K_1 per mL
NDC 0006-7782-30 in 2.5 mL multiple dose vials
NDC 0006-7782-03 in 5 mL multiple dose vials.
No. 7784—1 mg of vitamin K_1 per 0.5 mL
NDC 0006-7784-33 boxes of 25 × 0.5 mL ampuls
(6505-00-180-6372 1 mg 0.5 mL 25's).

Storage

Store in a dark place.

9073021 Issued September 1997

ARAMINE® Injection (Metaraminol Bitartrate), U.S.P. ℞

DESCRIPTION

Metaraminol bitartrate is a potent sympathomimetic amine that increases both systolic and diastolic blood pressure.

Metaraminol bitartrate is [*R*-(*R**,*S**)]-α-(1-aminoethyl)-3-hydroxybenzenemethanol [*R*-(*R**,*R**)]-2,3-dihydroxybutanedioate (1:1) (salt), which is levorotatory. Its empirical formula is $C_9H_{13}NO_2 \cdot C_4H_6O_6$ and its structural formula is:

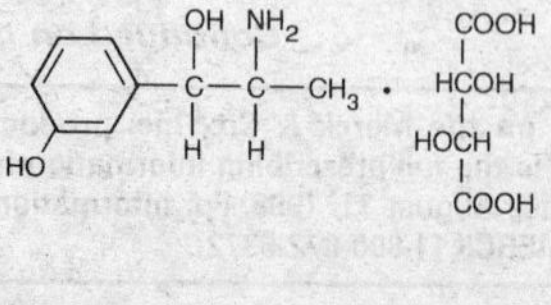

Metaraminol bitartrate is a white, crystalline powder with a molecular weight of 317.29, is freely soluble in water, slightly soluble in alcohol, and practically insoluble in chloroform and in ether.

Injection ARAMINE* (Metaraminol Bitartrate) is a sterile solution. Each mL contains:

Metaraminol bitartrate equivalent to metaraminol	10 mg
Inactive ingredients:	
Sodium chloride	4.4 mg
Water for Injection q.s. ad	1 mL
Methylparaben 0.15%, propylparaben 0.02%, and sodium bisulfite 0.2% added as preservatives.	

*Registered trademark of MERCK & CO., INC.

CLINICAL PHARMACOLOGY

The pressor effect of ARAMINE begins in 1 to 2 minutes after intravenous infusion, in about 10 minutes after intramuscular injection, and in 5 to 20 minutes after subcutaneous injection. The effect lasts from about 20 minutes to one hour. ARAMINE has a positive inotropic effect on the heart and a peripheral vasoconstrictor action.

Renal, coronary, and cerebral blood flow are a function of perfusion pressure and regional resistance. In patients with insufficient or failing vasoconstriction, there is additional advantage to the peripheral action of ARAMINE, but in most patients with shock, vasoconstriction is adequate and any further increase is unnecessary. Blood flow to vital organs may decrease with ARAMINE if regional resistance increases excessively.

The pressor effect of ARAMINE is decreased but not reversed by alpha-adrenergic blocking agents. Primary or secondary fall in blood pressure and tachyphylactic response to repeated use are uncommon.

INDICATIONS AND USAGE

ARAMINE is indicated for prevention and treatment of the acute hypotensive state occurring with spinal anesthesia. It is also indicated as adjunctive treatment of hypotension due to hemorrhage, reactions to medications, surgical complications, and shock associated with brain damage due to trauma or tumor.

CONTRAINDICATIONS

Use of ARAMINE with cyclopropane or halothane anesthesia should be avoided, unless clinical circumstances demand such use.

Hypersensitivity to any component of this product, including sulfites (see WARNINGS).

WARNINGS

Use of sympathomimetic amines with monoamine oxidase inhibitors or tricyclic antidepressants may result in potentiation of the pressor effect. (See PRECAUTIONS, *Drug Interactions.*)

ARAMINE contains sodium bisulfite, a sulfite that may cause allergic-type reactions including anaphylactic symptoms and life-threatening or less severe asthmatic episodes in certain susceptible people. The overall prevalence of sulfite sensitivity in the general population is unknown and probably low. Sulfite sensitivity is seen more frequently in asthmatic than in nonasthmatic people.

PRECAUTIONS

General

Caution should be used to avoid excessive blood pressure response. Rapidly induced hypertensive responses have been reported to cause acute pulmonary edema, arrhythmias, cerebral hemorrhage, or cardiac arrest.

Patients with cirrhosis should be treated with caution, with adequate restoration of electrolytes if diuresis ensues. Fatal ventricular arrhythmia was reported in one patient with Laennec's cirrhosis while receiving metaraminol bitartrate.

In several instances, ventricular extrasystoles that appeared during infusion of this vasopressor subsided promptly when the rate of infusion was reduced.

With the prolonged action of ARAMINE, a cumulative effect is possible. If there is an excessive vasopressor response there may be a prolonged elevation of blood pressure even after discontinuation of therapy.

When vasopressor amines are used for long periods, the resulting vasoconstriction may prevent adequate expansion of circulating volume and may cause perpetuation of shock. There is evidence that plasma volume may be reduced in all types of shock, and that the measurement of central venous pressure is useful in assessing the adequacy of the circulating blood volume. Therefore, blood or plasma volume expanders should be used when the principal reason for hypotension or shock is decreased circulating volume.

Because of its vasoconstrictor effect ARAMINE should be given with caution in heart or thyroid disease, hypertension, or diabetes. Sympathomimetic amines may provoke a relapse in patients with a history of malaria.

Drug Interactions

ARAMINE should be used with caution in digitalized patients, since the combination of digitalis and sympathomimetic amines may cause ectopic arrhythmias.

Monoamine oxidase inhibitors or tricyclic antidepressants may potentiate the action of sympathomimetic amines. Therefore, when initiating pressor therapy in patients receiving these drugs, the initial dose should be small and given with caution. (See WARNINGS.)

Carcinogenesis, Mutagenesis, Impairment of Fertility

Studies in animals have not been performed to evaluate the mutagenic or carcinogenic potential of ARAMINE or its potential to affect fertility.

Pregnancy

Pregnancy Category C. Animal reproduction studies have not been conducted with ARAMINE. It is not known whether ARAMINE can cause fetal harm when given to a pregnant woman or can affect reproduction capacity. ARAMINE should be given to a pregnant woman only if clearly needed.

Nursing Mothers

It is not known whether this drug is secreted in human milk. Because many drugs are secreted in human milk, caution should be exercised when ARAMINE is given to a nursing woman.

Pediatric Use

Safety and effectiveness in pediatric patients have not been established.

ADVERSE REACTIONS

Sympathomimetic amines, including ARAMINE, may cause sinus or ventricular tachycardia, or other arrhythmias, especially in patients with myocardial infarction. (See PRECAUTIONS.)

In patients with a history of malaria, these compounds may provoke a relapse.

Abscess formation, tissue necrosis, or sloughing rarely may follow the use of ARAMINE. In choosing the site of injection, it is important to avoid those areas recognized as *not* suitable for use of any pressor agent and to discontinue the infusion immediately if infiltration or thrombosis occurs. Although the physician may be forced by the urgent nature of the patient's condition to choose injection sites that are not recognized as suitable, he should, when possible, use the preferred areas of injection. The larger veins of the antecubital fossa or the thigh are preferred to veins in the dorsum of the hand or ankle veins, particularly in patients with peripheral vascular disease, diabetes mellitus, Buerger's disease, or conditions with coexistent hypercoagulability.

OVERDOSAGE

Overdosage may result in severe hypertension accompanied by headache, constricting sensation in the chest, nausea, vomiting, euphoria, diaphoresis, pulmonary edema, tachycardia, bradycardia, sinus arrhythmia, atrial or ventricular arrhythmias, cerebral hemorrhage, myocardial infarction, cardiac arrest or convulsions.

Should an excessive elevation of blood pressure occur, it may be immediately relieved by a sympatholytic agent, e.g. phentolamine. An appropriate antiarrhythmic agent may also be required.

The oral LD_{50} in the rat and mouse is 240 mg/kg and 99 mg/kg, respectively.

DOSAGE AND ADMINISTRATION

ARAMINE may be given intramuscularly, subcutaneously, or intravenously, the route depending on the nature and severity of the indication.

Parenteral drug products should be inspected visually for particulate matter and discoloration prior to use, whenever solution and container permit.

Allow at least 10 minutes to elapse before increasing the dose because the maximum effect is not immediately apparent. When the vasopressor is discontinued, observe the patient carefully as the effect of the drug tapers off, so that therapy can be reinitiated promptly if the blood pressure falls too rapidly. The response to vasopressors may be poor in patients with coexistent shock and acidosis. When indicated, established methods of shock management should be used, such as blood or fluid replacement.

Intramuscular or Subcutaneous Injection (for prevention of hypotension—see INDICATIONS): The recommended dose is 2 to 10 mg (0.2 to 1 mL). As with other agents given subcutaneously, only the preferred sites of injection, as set forth in standard texts, should be used.

Intravenous Infusion (for adjunctive treatment of hypotension—see INDICATIONS): The recommended dose is 15 to

100 mg (1.5 to 10 mL) in 500 mL of Sodium Chloride Injection or 5% Dextrose Injection, adjusting the rate of infusion to maintain the blood pressure at the desired level. Higher concentrations of ARAMINE, 150 to 500 mg per 500 mL of infusion fluid, have been used.

If the patient needs more saline or dextrose solution at a rate of flow that would provide an excessive dose of the vasopressor, the recommended volume of infusion fluid (500 mL) should be increased accordingly. ARAMINE may also be added to *less* than 500 mL of infusion fluid if a smaller volume is desired.

Compatibility Information

In addition to Sodium Chloride Injection and Dextrose Injection 5%, the following infusion solutions were found physically and chemically compatible with Injection ARAMINE when 5 mL of Injection ARAMINE, 10 mg/mL (metaraminol equivalent), was added to 500 mL of infusion solution: Ringer's Injection, Lactated Ringer's Injection, Dextran 6% in Saline†, Normosol®-R pH 7.4†, and Normosol®-M in D5-W†.

When Injection ARAMINE is mixed with an infusion solution, sterile precautions should be observed. Since infusion solutions generally do not contain preservatives, mixtures should be used within 24 hours.

Direct Intravenous Injection: In severe shock, when time is of great importance, this agent should be given by direct intravenous injection. The suggested dose is 0.5 to 5 mg (0.05 to 0.5 mL), followed by an infusion of 15 to 100 mg (1.5 to 10 mL) in 500 mL of infusion fluid as described previously.

Vials may be sterilized by autoclaving or by immersion in a sterilizing solution.

† Product of Abbott Laboratories

HOW SUPPLIED

No. 3222X—Injection ARAMINE 1%, containing metaraminol bitartrate equivalent to 10 mg of metaraminol per mL, is a clear, colorless solution and is supplied as follows:

NDC 0006-3222-10 in 10 mL vials
(6505-00-753-9601 10 mL vial).

Storage

Protect from light. Store container in carton until contents have been used.

Avoid storage at temperatures below -20°C (-4°F) and above 40°C (104°F).

7348524 Issued September 1996

COPYRIGHT © MERCK & CO., INC., 1987
All rights reserved

ATTENUVAX® ℞

(Measles Virus Vaccine Live), U.S.P.
(More Attenuated Enders' Strain)

DESCRIPTION

ATTENUVAX* (Measles Virus Vaccine Live) is a live virus vaccine for immunization against measles (rubeola).

ATTENUVAX is a sterile lyophilized preparation of a more attenuated line of measles virus derived from Enders' attenuated Edmonston strain. The further modification of the virus in ATTENUVAX was achieved in the Merck Institute for Therapeutic Research by multiple passage of Edmonston strain virus in cell cultures of chick embryo at low temperature.

The reconstituted vaccine is for subcutaneous administration. When reconstituted as directed, the dose for injection is 0.5 mL and contains not less than the equivalent of 1,000 $TCID_{50}$ (tissue culture infectious doses) of the U.S. Reference Measles Virus. Each dose also contains approximately 25 mcg of neomycin. The product contains no preservative. Sorbitol and hydrolized gelatin are added as stabilizers.

*Registered trademark of MERCK & CO., INC.

CLINICAL PHARMACOLOGY

ATTENUVAX produces a modified measles infection in susceptible persons. Fever and rash may appear. Extensive clinical trials have demonstrated that ATTENUVAX is highly immunogenic and generally well tolerated. A single injection of the vaccine has been shown to induce measles hemagglutination-inhibiting (HI) antibodies in 97 percent or more of susceptible persons. Vaccine-induced antibody levels have been shown to persist for at least 13 years without substantial decline. Continued surveillance will be necessary to determine further duration of antibody persistence.

INDICATIONS AND USAGE

ATTENUVAX is indicated for immunization against measles (rubeola) in persons 15 months of age or older. A second dose of ATTENUVAX is recommended (see *Revaccination*). Infants who are less than 15 months of age may fail to respond to the vaccine due to presence in the circulation of residual measles antibody of maternal origin; the younger the infant, the lower the likelihood of seroconversion. In geographically isolated or other relatively inaccessible populations for whom immunization programs are logistically difficult, and in population groups in which natural measles infection may occur in a significant proportion of infants before 15 months of age, it may be desirable to give the vaccine to infants at an earlier age. Infants vaccinated under these conditions at less than 12 months of age should be revaccinated after reaching 15 months of age. There is some evidence to suggest that infants immunized at less than one year of age may not develop sustained antibody levels when later reimmunized. The advantage of early protection must be weighed against the chance for failure to respond adequately on reimmunization.

According to ACIP recommendations, most persons born in 1956 or earlier are likely to have been infected naturally and generally need not be considered susceptible. All children, adolescents, and adults born after 1956 are considered susceptible and should be vaccinated, if there are no contraindications. This includes persons who may be immune to measles but who lack adequate documentation of immunity as evidenced by: (1) physician-diagnosed measles, (2) laboratory evidence of measles immunity, or (3) adequate immunization with live measles vaccine on or after the first birthday.

ATTENUVAX given immediately after exposure to natural measles may provide some protection. If, however, the vaccine is given a few days before exposure, substantial protection may be provided.

Individuals planning travel outside the United States, if not immune, can acquire measles, mumps or rubella and import these diseases to the United States. Therefore, prior to International travel, individuals known to be susceptible to one or more of these diseases can receive either a single antigen vaccine (measles, mumps or rubella), or a combined antigen vaccine as appropriate. However, M-M-R* II (Measles, Mumps, and Rubella Virus Vaccine Live) is preferred for persons likely to be susceptible to mumps and rubella; and if single-antigen measles vaccine is not readily available, travelers should receive M-M-R II (Measles, Mumps, and Rubella Virus Vaccine Live) regardless of their immune status to mumps or rubella.

Revaccination: Children first vaccinated when younger than 12 months of age should be revaccinated at 15 months of age, particularly if vaccine was administered with immune serum globulin or measles immune globulin, a standardized globulin preparation.

The American Academy of Pediatrics (AAP), the Immunization Practices Advisory Committee (ACIP), and some state and local health agencies have recommended guidelines for routine measles revaccination and to help control measles outbreaks.**

Vaccines available for revaccination include monovalent measles vaccine (ATTENUVAX) and polyvalent vaccines containing measles [e.g., M-M-R II (Measles, Mumps, and Rubella Virus Vaccine Live), M-R-VAX* II (Measles and Rubella Virus Vaccine Live)]. If the prevention of sporadic measles outbreaks is the sole objective, revaccination with a monovalent measles vaccine should be considered (see appropriate product circular). If concern also exists about immune status regarding mumps or rubella, revaccination with appropriate monovalent or polyvalent vaccines should be considered after consulting the appropriate product circulars. Unnecessary doses of a vaccine are best avoided by ensuring that written documentation of vaccination is preserved and a copy given to each vaccinee's parent or guardian.

Despite the risk of reactions (see ADVERSE REACTIONS), persons born since 1956 who have previously been given inactivated vaccine alone or followed by live vaccine within 3 months should be revaccinated with live vaccine to reduce the risk of the severe atypical form of natural measles that may occur.

Use with other Vaccines

Routine administration of DTP (diphtheria, tetanus, pertussis) and/or OPV (oral poliovirus vaccine) concomitantly with measles, mumps and rubella vaccines is not recommended because there are insufficient data relating to the simultaneous administration of these antigens. However, the American Academy of Pediatrics has noted that in some circumstances, particularly when the patient may not return, some practitioners prefer to administer all these antigens on a single day. If done, separate sites and syringes should be used for DTP and ATTENUVAX.

ATTENUVAX should not be given less than one month before or after administration of other virus vaccines.

* Registered trademark of MERCK & CO., INC.

** NOTE: A primary difference among these recommendations is the timing of revaccination: the ACIP recommends routine revaccination at entry into kindergarten or first grade, whereas the AAP recommends routine revaccination at entrance to middle school or junior high school. In addition, some public health jurisdictions mandate the age for revaccination. The complete text of applicable guidelines should be consulted.

CONTRAINDICATIONS

Do not give ATTENUVAX to pregnant females; the possible effects of the vaccine on fetal development are unknown at this time. If vaccination of postpubertal females is undertaken, pregnancy should be avoided for three months following vaccination (see PRECAUTIONS, *Pregnancy*).

Anaphylactic or anaphylactoid reactions to neomycin (each dose of reconstituted vaccine contains approximately 25 mcg of neomycin).

History of anaphylactic or anaphylactoid reactions to eggs (see HYPERSENSITIVITY TO EGGS below).

Any febrile respiratory illness or other active febrile infection.

Active untreated tuberculosis.

Patients receiving immunosuppressive therapy. This contraindication does not apply to patients who are receiving corticosteroids as replacement therapy, e.g., for Addison's disease.

Individuals with blood dyscrasias, leukemia, lymphomas of any type, or other malignant neoplasms affecting the bone marrow or lymphatic systems.

Primary and acquired immunodeficiency states, including patients who are immunosuppressed in association with AIDS or other clinical manifestations of infection with human immunodeficiency viruses; cellular immune deficiencies; and hypogammaglobulinemic and dysgammaglobulinemic states.

Individuals with a family history of congenital or hereditary immunodeficiency, until the immune competence of the potential vaccine recipient is demonstrated.

HYPERSENSITIVITY TO EGGS

Live measles vaccine is produced in chick embryo cell culture. Persons with a history of anaphylactic, anaphylactoid or other immediate reactions (e.g., hives, swelling of the mouth and throat, difficulty breathing, hypotension and shock) subsequent to egg ingestion should not be vaccinated. Evidence indicates that persons are not at increased risk if they have egg allergies that are not anaphylactic or anaphylactoid in nature. Such persons should be vaccinated in the usual manner. There is no evidence to indicate that persons with allergies to chickens or feathers are at increased risk of reaction to the vaccine.

PRECAUTIONS

General

Adequate treatment provisions including epinephrine, should be available for immediate use should an anaphylactic or anaphylactoid reaction occur.

Due caution should be employed in administration of measles vaccine to persons with a history of cerebral injury, individual or family histories of convulsions, or of any other condition in which stress due to fever should be avoided. The physician should be alert to the temperature elevation which may occur following vaccination. (See ADVERSE REACTIONS.)

Children and young adults who are known to be infected with human immunodeficiency viruses but without overt clinical manifestations of immunosuppression may be vaccinated; however, the vaccinees should be monitored closely for vaccine-preventable diseases because immunization may be less effective than for uninfected persons.

Vaccination should be deferred for at least 3 months following blood or plasma transfusions, or administration of human immune serum globulin.

There are no reports of transmission of live attenuated measles virus from vaccinees to susceptible contacts.

It has been reported that attenuated measles virus vaccine, live, may result in a temporary depression of tuberculin skin sensitivity. Therefore, if a tuberculin test is to be done, it should be administered either before or simultaneously with ATTENUVAX.

Children under treatment for tuberculosis have not experienced exacerbation of the disease when immunized with live measles virus vaccine; no studies have been reported to date of the effect of measles virus vaccines on untreated tuberculous children.

As for any vaccine, vaccination with ATTENUVAX may not result in seroconversion in 100% of susceptible persons given the vaccine.

Continued on next page

Information on the Merck & Co., Inc. products listed on these pages is the full prescribing information from product circulars in use August 31, 1998. For information, please call 1-800-NSC MERCK [1-800-672-6372].

Attenuvax—Cont.

Pregnancy
Pregnancy Category C
Animal reproduction studies have not been conducted with ATTENUVAX. It is also not known whether ATTENUVAX can cause fetal harm when administered to a pregnant woman or can affect reproduction capacity. Therefore, the vaccine should not be administered to pregnant females; furthermore, pregnancy should be avoided for three months following vaccination (see CONTRAINDICATIONS).
Reports have indicated that contracting of natural measles during pregnancy enhances fetal risk. Increased rates of spontaneous abortion, stillbirth, congenital defects and prematurity have been observed subsequent to natural measles during pregnancy. There are no adequate studies of the attenuated (vaccine) strain of measles virus in pregnancy. However, it would be prudent to assume that the vaccine strain of virus is also capable of inducing adverse fetal effects for up to three months following vaccination.
Vaccine administration to postpubertal females entails a potential for inadvertent immunization during pregnancy. Theoretical risks involved should be weighed against the risks that measles poses to the unimmunized adolescent or adult. Advisory committees reviewing this matter have recommended vaccination of postpubertal females who are presumed to be susceptible to measles and not known to be pregnant. If a measles exposure occurs during pregnancy, one should consider the possibility of providing temporary passive immunity through the administration of immune globulin (human).
Nursing Mothers
It is not known whether measles vaccine virus is secreted in human milk. Therefore, because many drugs are excreted in human milk, caution should be exercised when ATTENUVAX is administered to a nursing woman.

ADVERSE REACTIONS

Burning and/or stinging of short duration at the injection site have been reported.
Anaphylaxis and anaphylactoid reactions have been reported.
Occasional
Moderate fever [101–102.9°F (38.3–39.4°C)] may occur during the month after vaccination. Generally, fever, rash, or both appear between the 5th and the 12th days. Cough and rhinitis have also been reported. Rash, when it occurs, is usually minimal, but rarely may be generalized. Erythema multiforme has also been reported rarely.
Less Common
High fever [over 103°F (39.4°C)].
Mild lymphadenopathy has been reported.
Rare
Reactions at injection site. Allergic reactions such as wheal and flare at the injection site or urticaria have been reported.
Diarrhea has been reported after vaccination with measles-containing vaccines.
Children developing fever may, on rare occasions, exhibit febrile convulsions. Afebrile convulsions or seizures have occurred rarely following vaccination with live attenuated measles vaccine. Syncope, particularly at the time of mass vaccination, has been reported.
Thrombocytopenia and purpura have occurred rarely.
Vasculitis has been reported rarely.
Forms of optic neuritis, including retrobulbar neuritis, papillitis, and retinitis may infrequently follow viral infections, and have been reported to occur 1 to 3 weeks following inoculation with some live virus vaccines.
Experience from more than 80 million doses of all live measles vaccines given in the U.S. through 1975 indicates that significant central nervous system reactions such as encephalitis and encephalopathy, occurring within 30 days after vaccination, have been temporally associated with measles vaccine very rarely. In no case has it been shown that reactions were actually caused by vaccine. The Center for Disease Control has pointed out that "a certain number of cases of encephalitis may be expected to occur in a large childhood population in a defined period of time even when no vaccines are administered". However, the data suggest the possibility that some of these cases may have been caused by measles vaccines. The risk of such serious neurological disorders following live measles virus vaccine administration remains far less than that for encephalitis and encephalopathy with natural measles (one per two thousand reported cases).
There have been rare reports of ocular palsies, Guillain-Barré syndrome, or ataxia occurring after immunization with vaccines containing live attenuated measles virus. The ocular palsies have occurred approximately 3–24 days following vaccination. No definite causal relationship has been established between either of these events and vaccination.
There have been reports of subacute sclerosing panencephalitis (SSPE) in children who did not have a history of natural measles but did receive measles vaccine. Some of these cases may have resulted from unrecognized measles in the first year of life or possibly from the measles vaccination. Based on estimated nationwide measles vaccine distribution, the association of SSPE cases to measles vaccination is about one case per million vaccine doses distributed. This is far less than the association with natural measles, 6–22 cases of SSPE per million cases of measles. The results of a retrospective case-controlled study conducted by the Center for Disease Control suggest that the overall effect of measles vaccine has been to protect against SSPE by preventing measles with its inherent higher risk of SSPE.
Local reactions characterized by marked swelling, redness and vesiculation at the injection site of attenuated live virus measles vaccines, and systemic reactions including atypical measles, have occurred in persons who have previously received killed measles vaccine. Rarely, more severe reactions that require hospitalization, including prolonged high fevers, panniculitis, and extensive local reactions, have been reported.

DOSAGE AND ADMINISTRATION

FOR SUBCUTANEOUS ADMINISTRATION
Do not inject intravenously
The dosage of vaccine is the same for all persons. Inject the total volume of the single dose vial (about 0.5 mL) or 0.5 mL of the multiple dose vial of reconstituted vaccine subcutaneously, preferably into the outer aspect of upper arm. *Do not give immune globulin (IG) concurrently with* ATTENUVAX.
During shipment, to insure that there is no loss of potency, the vaccine must be maintained at a temperature of 10°C (50°F) or less.
Before reconstitution, store ATTENUVAX at 2–8°C (36–46°F). *Protect from light.*
CAUTION: A sterile syringe free of preservatives, antiseptics, and detergents should be used for each injection and/or reconstitution of the vaccine because these substances may inactivate the live virus vaccine. A 25 gauge, 5/8" needle is recommended.
To reconstitute, use only the diluent supplied, since it is free of preservatives or other antiviral substances which might inactivate the vaccine.
Single Dose Vial —First withdraw the entire volume of diluent into the syringe to be used for reconstitution. Inject all the diluent in the syringe into the vial of lyophilized vaccine, and agitate to mix thoroughly. Withdraw the entire contents into a syringe and inject the total volume of restored vaccine subcutaneously.
It is important to use a separate sterile syringe and needle for each individual patient to prevent transmission of hepatitis B and other infectious agents from one person to another.
10 Dose Vial (available only to government agencies / institutions) — Withdraw the entire contents (7 mL) of the diluent vial into the sterile syringe to be used for reconstitution, and introduce into the 10 dose vial of lyophilized vaccine. Agitate to ensure thorough mixing. The outer labeling suggests "For Jet Injector or Syringe Use". Use with separate sterile syringes is permitted for containers of 10 doses or less. The vaccine and diluent do not contain preservatives; therefore, the user must recognize the potential contamination hazards and exercise special precautions to protect the sterility and potency of the product. The use of aseptic techniques and proper storage prior to and after restoration of the vaccine and subsequent withdrawal of the individual doses is essential. Use 0.5 mL of the reconstituted vaccine for subcutaneous injection.
It is important to use a separate sterile syringe and needle for each individual patient to prevent transmission of hepatitis B and other infectious agents from one person to another.
50 Dose Vial (available only to government agencies / institutions) —Withdraw the entire contents (30 mL) of diluent vial into the sterile syringe to be used for reconstitution and introduce into the 50 dose vial of lyophilized vaccine. Agitate to ensure thorough mixing. With full aseptic precautions, attach the vial to the sterilized multidose jet injector apparatus. Use 0.5 mL of the reconstituted vaccine for subcutaneous injection.
Each dose of ATTENUVAX contains not less than 1,000 $TCID_{50}$ (tissue culture infectious doses) of measles virus vaccine expressed in terms of the assigned titer of the U.S. Reference Measles Virus.
Parenteral drug products should be inspected visually for particulate matter and discoloration prior to administration. ATTENUVAX, when reconstituted, is clear yellow.

HOW SUPPLIED

No. 4709—ATTENUVAX is supplied as a single-dose vial of lyophilized vaccine, **NDC** 0006-4709-00, and a vial of diluent.
No. 4589X/4309—ATTENUVAX is supplied as follows: (1) a box of 10 single-dose vials of lyophilized vaccine (package A), **NDC** 0006-4589-00; and (2) a box of 10 vials of diluent (package B). To conserve refrigerator space, the diluent may be stored separately at room temperature
(6505-01-038-0794, Ten Pack).
Available only to government agencies / institutions:
No. 4614X—ATTENUVAX is supplied as one 10 dose vial of lyophilized vaccine, **NDC** 0006-4614-00, and one 7 mL vial of diluent.
No. 4591X—ATTENUVAX is supplied as one 50 dose vial of lyophilized vaccine, **NDC** 0006-4591-00, and one 30 mL vial of diluent
(6505-01-222-6467, 50 Dose).
Storage
It is recommended that the vaccine be used as soon as possible after reconstitution. Protect vaccine from light at all times, since such exposure may inactivate the virus. Store reconstituted vaccine in the vaccine vial in a dark place at 2–8°C (36–46°F) and discard if not used within 8 hours.

A.H.F.S. Category: 80:12
7680014 Issued March 1995
COPYRIGHT © MERCK & CO., INC., 1990
All rights reserved

BENEMID® Tablets (Probenecid), U.S.P. ℞

DESCRIPTION

BENEMID* (Probenecid) is a uricosuric and renal tubular transport blocking agent.
Probenecid is the generic name for 4-[(dipropylamino-)sulfonyl] benzoic acid (molecular weight 285.36). It has the following structural formula:

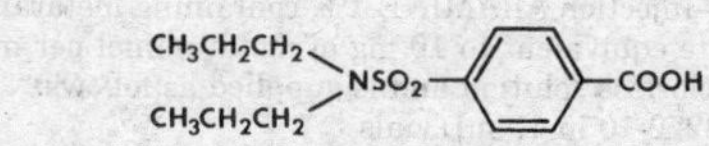
CH3CH2CH2
NSO2
COOH
CH3CH2CH2

Probenecid is a white or nearly white, fine, crystalline powder. Probenecid is soluble in dilute alkali, in alcohol, in chloroform, and in acetone; it is practically insoluble in water and in dilute acids.
Each tablet contains 0.5 g probenecid and the following inactive ingredients: calcium stearate, D&C Yellow 10, gelatin, hydroxypropyl methylcellulose, iron oxide, magnesium carbonate, polyethylene glycol, starch, talc, and titanium dioxide.

*Registered trademark of MERCK & CO., INC.

ACTIONS

BENEMID is a uricosuric and renal tubular blocking agent. It inhibits the tubular reabsorption of urate, thus increasing the urinary excretion of uric acid and decreasing serum urate levels. Effective uricosuria reduces the miscible urate pool, retards urate deposition, and promotes resorption of urate deposits.
BENEMID inhibits the tubular secretion of penicillin and usually increases penicillin plasma levels by any route the antibiotic is given. A 2-fold to 4-fold elevation has been demonstrated for various penicillins.
BENEMID also has been reported to inhibit the renal transport of many other compounds including aminohippuric acid (PAH), aminosalicylic acid (PAS), indomethacin, sodium iodomethamate and related iodinated organic acids, 17-ketosteroids, pantothenic acid, phenolsulfonphthalein (PSP), sulfonamides, and sulfonylureas. See also DRUG INTERACTIONS.
BENEMID decreases both hepatic and renal excretion of sulfobromophthalein (BSP). The tubular reabsorption of phosphorus is inhibited in hypoparathyroid but not in euparathyroid individuals.
BENEMID does not influence plasma concentrations of salicylates, nor the excretion of streptomycin, chloramphenicol, chlortetracycline, oxytetracycline, or neomycin.

INDICATIONS

For treatment of the hyperuricemia associated with gout and gouty arthritis.
As an adjuvant to therapy with penicillin or with ampicillin, methicillin, oxacillin, cloxacillin, or nafcillin, for elevation and prolongation of plasma levels by whatever route the antibiotic is given.

CONTRAINDICATIONS

Hypersensitivity to this product.
Children under 2 years of age.
Not recommended in persons with known blood dyscrasias or uric acid kidney stones.

BENEMID® (Probenecid) Penicillin Therapy (Gonorrhea)*

	Recommended Regimens**	Remarks
Uncomplicated gonococcal infection in men and women (urethral, cervical, rectal)	4.8 million units of aqueous procaine penicillin G† I.M., in at least 2 doses injected at different sites at one visit + 1 g of BENEMID (Probenecid) orally just before injections *or* 3.5 g of ampicillin† orally + 1 g of BENEMID orally given simultaneously.	Follow-up: Obtain urethral and other appropriate cultures from men, and cervical, anal, and other appropriate cultures from women, 7 to 14 days after completion of treatment. Treatment of sexual partners: Persons with known recent exposure to gonorrhea should receive same treatment as those known to have gonorrhea. Examination and treatment of male sex partners of persons with gonorrhea are essential because of high prevalence of nonsymptomatic urethral gonococcal infection in such men.
Pharyngeal gonococcal infection in men and women	4.8 million units of aqueous procaine penicillin G† I.M., in at least 2 doses injected at different sites at one visit + 1 g of BENEMID orally just before injections	Pharyngeal gonococcal infections may be more difficult to treat than anogenital gonorrhea. Posttreatment cultures are essential.
Uncomplicated gonorrhea in pregnant patients	4.8 million units of aqueous procaine penicillin G†I.M., in at least 2 doses injected at different sites at one visit *or* 3.5 g of ampicillin† orally + 1 g of BENEMID orally given simultaneously	
Acute gonococcal salpingitis	*Outpatients:* Aqueous procaine penicillin G† or ampicillin† with BENEMID as for gonorrhea in pregnancy, followed by 500 mg of ampicillin 4 times a day for 10 days *Hospitalized patients:* See details in CDC recommendations	Follow-up of patients with acute salpingitis is essential. All patients should receive repeat pelvic examinations and cultures for *Neisseria gonorrhoeae* after treatment. Examination and appropriate treatment of male sex partners are essential because of high prevalence of nonsymptomatic urethral gonorrhea in such men.
Disseminated gonococcal infection (arthritis-dermatitis syndrome)	10 million units of aqueous crystalline penicillin G† I.V. a day for 3 days or till significant clinical improvement occurs. May be followed with 500 mg of ampicillin† 4 times a day orally to complete 7 days of treatment *or* 3.5 g of ampicillin† orally with 1 g of BENEMID, followed by 500 mg of ampicillin† 4 times a day for at least 7 days	
Gonococcal infection in children	For postpubertal children and/or those weighing over 45 kg (100 lb) use the dosage regimens given above for adults Uncomplicated vulvovaginitis and urethritis: aqueous procaine penicillin G†75,000—100,000 units/kg I.M., with BENEMID 23 mg/kg orally	See CDC recommendations for detailed information about prevention and treatment of neonatal gonococcal infection and gonococcal ophthalmia.

Note: Before treating gonococcal infections in patients with suspected primary or secondary syphilis, perform proper diagnostic procedures including darkfield examinations. If concomitant syphilis is suspected, perform monthly serological tests for at least 4 months.

* Recommended by Venereal Disease Control Advisory Committee, Center for Disease Control, U.S. Department of Health, Education, and Welfare, Public Health Service (Morbidity and Mortality Weekly Report, Vol. *23*: 341, 342, 347, 348, Oct. 11, 1974).

** See CDC recommendations for definition of regimens of choice, alternative regimens, treatment of hypersensitive patients, and other aspects of therapy.

† See package circulars of manufacturers for detailed information about contraindications, warnings, precautions, and adverse reactions.

Therapy with BENEMID should not be started until an acute gouty attack has subsided.

WARNINGS

Exacerbation of gout following therapy with BENEMID may occur; in such cases colchicine or other appropriate therapy is advisable.

BENEMID increases plasma concentrations of methotrexate in both animals and humans. In animal studies, increased methotrexate toxicity has been reported. If BENEMID is given with methotrexate, the dosage of methotrexate should be reduced and serum levels may need to be monitored.

In patients on BENEMID the use of salicylates in either small or large doses is contraindicated because it antagonizes the uricosuric action of BENEMID. The biphasic action of salicylates in the renal tubules accounts for the so-called "paradoxical effect" of uricosuric agents. In patients on BENEMID who require a mild analgesic agent the use of acetaminophen rather than small doses of salicylates would be preferred.

Rarely, severe allergic reactions and anaphylaxis have been reported with the use of BENEMID. Most of these have been reported to occur within several hours after readministration following prior usage of the drug.

The appearance of hypersensitivity reactions requires cessation of therapy with BENEMID.

Use in Pregnancy: BENEMID crosses the placental barrier and appears in cord blood. The use of any drug in women of childbearing potential requires that the anticipated benefit be weighed against possible hazards.

PRECAUTIONS

General

Hematuria, renal colic, costovertebral pain, and formation of uric acid stones associated with the use of BENEMID in gouty patients may be prevented by alkalization of the urine and a liberal fluid intake (*see* DOSAGE AND ADMINISTRATION). In these cases when alkali is administered, the acid-base balance of the patient should be watched.

Use with caution in patients with a history of peptic ulcer. BENEMID has been used in patients with some renal impairment but dosage requirements may be increased. BENEMID may not be effective in chronic renal insufficiency particularly when the glomerular filtration rate is 30 mL/minute or less. Because of its mechanism of action, BENEMID is not recommended in conjunction with a penicillin in the presence of *known* renal impairment.

A reducing substance may appear in the urine of patients receiving BENEMID. This disappears with discontinuance of therapy. Suspected glycosuria should be confirmed by using a test specific for glucose.

Drug Interactions

When BENEMID is used to elevate plasma concentrations of penicillin or other beta-lactams, or when such drugs are given to patients taking BENEMID therapeutically, high plasma concentrations of the other drug may increase the incidence of adverse reactions associated with that drug. In the case of penicillin or other beta-lactams, psychic disturbances have been reported.

The use of salicylates antagonizes the uricosuric action of BENEMID (*see* WARNINGS). The uricosuric action of BENEMID is also antagonized by pyrazinamide.

BENEMID produces an insignificant increase in free sulfonamide plasma concentrations but a significant increase in total sulfonamide plasma levels. Since BENEMID decreases the renal excretion of conjugated sulfonamides, plasma concentrations of the latter should be determined from time to time when a sulfonamide and BENEMID are coadministered for prolonged periods. BENEMID may prolong or enhance the action of oral sulfonylureas and thereby increase the risk of hypoglycemia.

It has been reported that patients receiving BENEMID require significantly less thiopental for induction of anesthesia. In addition, ketamine and thiopental anesthesia were significantly prolonged in rats receiving probenecid.

The concomitant administration of probenecid increases the mean plasma elimination half-life of a number of drugs which can lead to increased plasma concentrations. These include agents such as indomethacin, acetaminophen, naproxen, ketoprofen, meclofenamate, lorazepam, and rifampin. Although the clinical significance of this observation has not been established, a lower dosage of the drug may be required to produce a therapeutic effect, and increases in dosage of the drug in question should be made cautiously and in small increments when probenecid is being co-administered. Although specific instances of toxicity due to this potential interaction have not been observed to date physicians should be alert to this possibility.

Probenecid given concomitantly with sulindac had only a slight effect on plasma sulfide levels, while plasma levels of sulindac and sulfone were increased. Sulindac was shown to produce a modest reduction in the uricosuric action of probenecid, which probably is not significant under most circumstances.

In animals and in humans, BENEMID has been reported to increase plasma concentrations of methotrexate (*see* WARNINGS).

Falsely high readings for theophylline have been reported in an *in vitro* study, using the Schack and Waxler technic, when therapeutic concentrations of theophylline and BENEMID were added to human plasma.

ADVERSE REACTIONS

The following adverse reactions have been observed and within each category are listed in order of decreasing severity.

Central Nervous System: headache, dizziness.

Metabolic: precipitation of acute gouty arthritis.

Gastrointestinal: hepatic necrosis, vomiting, nausea, anorexia, sore gums.

Genitourinary: nephrotic syndrome, uric acid stones with or without hematuria, renal colic, costovertebral pain, urinary frequency.

Continued on next page

Information on the Merck & Co., Inc. products listed on these pages is the full prescribing information from product circulars in use August 31, 1998. For information, please call 1-800-NSC MERCK [1-800-672-6372].

Benemid—Cont.

Hypersensitivity: anaphylaxis, fever, urticaria, pruritus.
Hematologic: aplastic anemia, leukopenia, hemolytic anemia which in some patients could be related to genetic deficiency of glucose -6- phosphate dehydrogenase in red blood cells, anemia.
Integumentary: dermatitis, alopecia, flushing.

DOSAGE AND ADMINISTRATION

Gout

Therapy with BENEMID should not be *started* until an acute gouty attack has subsided. However, if an acute attack is precipitated *during* therapy, BENEMID may be continued without changing the dosage, and full therapeutic dosage of colchicine or other appropriate therapy should be given to control the acute attack.

The recommended adult dosage is 0.25 g ($^1/_2$ tablet of BENEMID) twice a day for one week, followed by 0.5 g (1 tablet) twice a day thereafter.

Some degree of renal impairment may be present in patients with gout. A daily dosage of 1 g may be adequate. However, if necessary, the daily dosage may be increased by 0.5 g increments every 4 weeks within tolerance (and usually not above 2 g per day) if symptoms of gouty arthritis are not controlled or the 24 hour uric acid excretion is not above 700 mg. As noted, BENEMID may not be effective in chronic renal insufficiency particularly when the glomerular filtration rate is 30 mL/minute or less.

Gastric intolerance may be indicative of overdosage, and may be corrected by decreasing the dosage.

As uric acid tends to crystallize out of an acid urine, a liberal fluid intake is recommended, as well as sufficient sodium bicarbonate (3 to 7.5 g daily) or potassium citrate (7.5 g daily) to maintain an alkaline urine (*see* PRECAUTIONS). Alkalization of the urine is recommended until the serum urate level returns to normal limits and tophaceous deposits disappear, i.e., during the period when urinary excretion of uric acid is at a high level. Thereafter, alkalization of the urine and the usual restriction of purine-producing foods may be somewhat relaxed.

BENEMID should be continued at the dosage that will maintain normal serum urate levels. When acute attacks have been absent for 6 months or more and serum urate levels remain within normal limits, the daily dosage may be decreased by 0.5 g every 6 months. The maintenance dosage should not be reduced to the point where serum urate levels tend to rise.

BENEMID *and Penicillin Therapy (General)*
Adults:
The recommended dosage is 2 g (4 tablets of BENEMID) daily in divided doses. This dosage should be reduced in older patients in whom renal impairment may be present.
Children 2-14 years of age:
Initial dose: 25 mg/kg body weight (*or* 0.7 g/square meter body surface).
Maintenance dose: 40 mg/kg body weight (*or* 1.2 g/square meter body surface) per day, divided into 4 doses.
For children weighing more than 50 kg (110 lb) the adult dosage is recommended.
BENEMID is contraindicated in children under 2 years of age.
The PSP excretion test may be used to determine the effectiveness of BENEMID in retarding penicillin excretion and maintaining therapeutic levels. The renal clearance of PSP is reduced to about one-fifth the normal rate when dosage of BENEMID is adequate.
Penicillin Therapy (Gonorrhea)
[See table at top of previous page]

HOW SUPPLIED

No. 3337—Tablets BENEMID, 0.5 g, are yellow, capsule shaped, scored, film coated tablets, coded MSD 501. They are supplied as follows:
NDC 0006-0501-68 bottles of 100
(6505-00-527-6885 100's)
NDC 0006-0501-28 unit dose packages of 100
NDC 0006-0501-82 bottles of 1000
(6505-00-181-8387 1000's).
Shown in Product Identification Guide, page 322
7876122   Issued August 1988

BIAVAX®II   ℞
(Rubella and Mumps Virus Vaccine Live), U.S.P.

DESCRIPTION

BIAVAX* II (Rubella and Mumps Virus Vaccine Live) is a live virus vaccine for immunization against rubella (German measles) and mumps.
BIAVAX II is a sterile lyophilized preparation of the Wistar RA 27/3 strain of live attenuated rubella virus grown in hu-

man diploid cell (WI-38) culture; and the Jeryl Lynn (B level) strain of mumps virus grown in cell cultures of chick embryo. The vaccine viruses are the same as those used in the manufacture of MERUVAX* II (Rubella Virus Vaccine Live) and MUMPSVAX* (Mumps Virus Vaccine Live). The two viruses are mixed before being lyophilized.
The reconstituted vaccine is for subcutaneous administration. When reconstituted as directed, the dose for injection is 0.5 mL and contains not less than the equivalent of 1,000 TCID$_{50}$ of the U.S. Reference Rubella Virus and 20,000 TCID$_{50}$ of the U.S. Reference Mumps Virus. Each dose contains approximately 25 mcg of neomycin. The product contains no preservative. Sorbitol and hydrolized gelatin are added as stabilizers.

*Registered trademark of MERCK & CO., INC.

CLINICAL PHARMACOLOGY

Clinical studies of 73 double seronegative children 12 months to 2 years of age demonstrated that BIAVAX II is highly immunogenic and generally well tolerated. In these studies, a single injection of the vaccine induced rubella hemagglutination-inhibition (HI) antibodies in 100 percent, and mumps neutralizing antibodies in 97 percent of the susceptible children.
The RA 27/3 rubella strain in BIAVAX II elicits higher immediate post-vaccination HI, complement-fixing and neutralizing antibody levels than other strains of rubella vaccine and has been shown to induce a broader profile of circulating antibodies including anti-theta and anti-iota precipitating antibodies. The RA 27/3 rubella strain immunologically simulates natural infection more closely than other rubella vaccine viruses. The increased levels and broader profile of antibodies produced by RA 27/3 strain rubella virus vaccine appear to correlate with greater resistance to subclinical reinfection with the wild virus, and provide greater confidence for lasting immunity.
Vaccine induced antibody levels following administration of BIAVAX II have been shown to persist for at least two years without substantial decline. Antibody levels after immunization with BIAVAX (Rubella and Mumps Virus Vaccine Live), containing the HPV-77 strain of rubella, have persisted for 10.5 years without substantial decline. If the present pattern continues, it will provide a basis for the expectation that immunity following vaccination will be permanent. However, continued surveillance will be required to demonstrate this point.

INDICATIONS AND USAGE

BIAVAX II is indicated for simultaneous immunization against rubella and mumps in persons 12 months of age or older. A booster is not needed.
The vaccine is not recommended for infants younger than 12 months because they may retain maternal rubella and mumps neutralizing antibodies which may interfere with the immune response.
Previously unimmunized children of susceptible pregnant women should receive live attenuated rubella vaccine, because an immunized child will be less likely to acquire natural rubella and introduce the virus into the household.
Individuals planning travel outside the United States, if not immune, can acquire measles, mumps or rubella and import these diseases to the United States. Therefore, prior to International travel, individuals known to be susceptible to one or more of these diseases can receive either a single antigen vaccine (measles, mumps, or rubella), or a combined antigen vaccine as appropriate. However, M-M-R* II (Measles, Mumps, and Rubella Virus Vaccine Live) is preferred for persons likely to be susceptible to mumps and rubella; and if single-antigen measles vaccine is not readily available, travelers should receive M-M-R II (Measles, Mumps, and Rubella Virus Vaccine Live) regardless of their immune status to mumps or rubella.
Non-Pregnant Adolescent and Adult Females
Immunization of susceptible non-pregnant adolescent and adult females of childbearing age with live attenuated rubella virus vaccine is indicated if certain precautions are observed (see below and PRECAUTIONS). Vaccinating susceptible postpubertal females confers individual protection against subsequently acquiring rubella infection during pregnancy, which in turn prevents infection of the fetus and consequent congenital rubella injury.
Women of childbearing age should be advised not to become pregnant for three months after vaccination and should be informed of the reasons for this precaution.**
It is recommended that rubella susceptibility be determined by serologic testing prior to immunization.***
If immune, as evidenced by a specific rubella antibody titer of 1:8 or greater (hemagglutination-inhibition test), vaccination is unnecessary. Congenital malformations do occur in up to seven percent of all live births. Their chance appearance after vaccination could lead to misinterpretation of the cause, particularly if the prior rubella-immune status of vaccinees is unknown.

Postpubertal females should be informed of the frequent occurrence of generally self-limited arthralgia and/or arthritis beginning 2 to 4 weeks after vaccination (see ADVERSE REACTIONS).
Postpartum Women
It has been found convenient in many instances to vaccinate rubella-susceptible women in the immediate postpartum period. (See *Nursing Mothers*).
Revaccination: Children vaccinated when younger than 12 months of age should be revaccinated. Based on available evidence, there is no reason to routinely revaccinate persons who were vaccinated originally when 12 months of age or older. However, persons should be revaccinated if there is evidence to suggest that initial immunization was ineffective.
Use with other Vaccines
Routine administration of DTP (diphtheria, tetanus, pertussis) and/or OPV (oral poliovirus vaccine) concomitantly with measles, mumps and rubella vaccines is not recommended because there are insufficient data relating to the simultaneous administration of these antigens. However, the American Academy of Pediatrics has noted that in some circumstances, particularly when the patient may not return, some practitioners prefer to administer all these antigens on a single day. If done, separate sites and syringes should be used for DTP and BIAVAX II.
BIAVAX II should not be given less than one month before or after administration of other virus vaccines.

---

* Registered trademark of MERCK & CO., INC.
** NOTE: The Immunization Practices Advisory Committee (ACIP) has recommended "In view of the importance of protecting this age group against rubella, reasonable precautions in a rubella immunization program include asking females if they are pregnant, excluding those who say they are, and explaining the theoretical risks to the others."
*** NOTE: The Immunization Practices Advisory Committee (ACIP) has stated "When practical, and when reliable laboratory services are available, potential vaccinees of childbearing age can have serologic tests to determine susceptibility to rubella. . . . However, routinely performing serologic tests for all females of childbearing age to determine susceptibility so that vaccine is given only to proven susceptibles is expensive and has been ineffective in some areas. Accordingly, the ACIP believes that rubella vaccination of a woman who is not known to be pregnant and has no history of vaccination is justifiable without serologic testing."

CONTRAINDICATIONS

Do not give BIAVAX II to pregnant females; the possible effects of the vaccine on fetal development are unknown at this time. If vaccination of postpubertal females is undertaken, pregnancy should be avoided for three months following vaccination. (See PRECAUTIONS, *Pregnancy*).
Anaphylactic or anaphylactoid reactions to neomycin (each dose of reconstituted vaccine contains approximately 25 mcg of neomycin).
History of anaphylactic or anaphylactoid reactions to eggs (see HYPERSENSITIVITY TO EGGS below).
Any febrile respiratory illness or other active febrile infection.
Active untreated tuberculosis.
Patients receiving immunosuppressive therapy. This contraindication does not apply to patients who are receiving corticosteroids as replacement therapy, e.g., for Addison's disease.
Individuals with blood dyscrasias, leukemia, lymphomas of any type, or other malignant neoplasms affecting the bone marrow or lymphatic systems.
Primary and acquired immunodeficiency states, including patients who are immunosuppressed in association with AIDS or other clinical manifestations of infection with human immunodeficiency viruses; cellular immune deficiencies; and hypogammaglobulinemic and dysgammaglobulinemic states.
Individuals with a family history of congenital or hereditary immunodeficiency, until the immune competence of the potential vaccine recipient is demonstrated.

HYPERSENSITIVITY TO EGGS

Live mumps vaccine is produced in chick embryo cell culture. Persons with a history of anaphylactic, anaphylactoid, or other immediate reactions (e.g., hives, swelling of the mouth and throat, difficulty breathing, hypotension, or shock) subsequent to egg ingestion should not be vaccinated. Evidence indicates that persons are not at increased

risk if they have egg allergies that are not anaphylactic or anaphylactoid in nature. Such persons may be vaccinated in the usual manner. There is no evidence to indicate that persons with allergies to chickens or feathers are at increased risk of reaction to the vaccine.

PRECAUTIONS

General

Adequate treatment provisions including epinephrine, should be available for immediate use should an anaphylactic or anaphylactoid reaction occur.

Children and young adults who are known to be infected with human immunodeficiency viruses but without overt clinical manifestations of immunosuppression may be vaccinated; however, the vaccinees should be monitored closely for vaccine-preventable diseases because immunization may be less effective than for uninfected persons.

Vaccination should be deferred for at least 3 months following blood or plasma transfusions, or administration of human immune serum globulin.

Excretion of small amounts of the live attenuated rubella virus from the nose and throat has occurred in the majority of susceptible individuals 7–28 days after vaccination. There is no confirmed evidence to indicate that such virus is transmitted to susceptible persons who are in contact with the vaccinated individuals. Consequently, transmission through close personal contact, while accepted as a theoretical possibility, is not regarded as a significant risk. However, transmission of the rubella vaccine virus to infants via breast milk has been documented (see *Nursing Mothers*).

There are no reports of transmission of live attenuated mumps virus from vaccinees to susceptible contacts.

It has been reported that live attenuated rubella and mumps virus vaccines given individually may result in a temporary depression of tuberculin skin sensitivity. Therefore, if a tuberculin test is to be done, it should be administered either before or simultaneously with BIAVAX II.

As for any vaccine, vaccination with BIAVAX II may not result in seroconversion in 100% of susceptible persons given the vaccine.

Pregnancy

Pregnancy Category C

Animal reproduction studies have not been conducted with BIAVAX II. It is also not known whether BIAVAX II can cause fetal harm when administered to a pregnant woman or can affect reproduction capacity. Therefore, the vaccine should not be administered to pregnant females; furthermore, pregnancy should be avoided for three months following vaccination (see CONTRAINDICATIONS).

In counseling women who are inadvertently vaccinated when pregnant or who become pregnant within 3 months of vaccination, the physician should be aware of the following: (1) In a 10 year survey involving over 700 pregnant women who received rubella vaccine within 3 months before or after conception, (of whom 189 received the Wistar RA 27/3 strain) none of the newborns had abnormalities compatible with congenital rubella syndrome; and (2) although mumps virus is capable of infecting the placenta and fetus, there is no good evidence that it causes congenital malformations in humans. Mumps vaccine virus also has been shown to infect the placenta, but the virus has not been isolated from the fetal tissues from susceptible women who were vaccinated and underwent elective abortions.

Nursing Mothers

It is not known whether mumps vaccine virus is secreted in human milk. Recent studies have shown that lactating postpartum women immunized with live attenuated rubella vaccine may secrete the virus in breast milk and transmit it to breast-fed infants. In the infants with serological evidence of rubella infection, none exhibited severe disease; however, one exhibited mild clinical illness typical of acquired rubella. Caution should be exercised when BIAVAX II is administered to a nursing woman.

ADVERSE REACTIONS

Burning and/or stinging of short duration at the injection site have been reported.

The adverse clinical reactions associated with the use of BIAVAX II are those expected to follow administration of the monovalent vaccines given separately. These may include malaise, sore throat, cough, rhinitis, headache, dizziness, fever, rash, nausea, vomiting or diarrhea; mild local reactions such as erythema, induration, tenderness and regional lymphadenopathy; parotitis, orchitis, nerve deafness, thrombocytopenia and purpura; allergic reactions such as wheal and flare at the injection site or urticaria; polyneuritis; and arthralgia and/or arthritis (usually transient and rarely chronic).

Anaphylaxis and anaphylactoid reactions have been reported.

Vasculitis has been reported rarely.

Moderate fever [101–102.9°F (38.3–39.4°C)] occurs occasionally, and high fever [above 103°F (39.4°C)] occurs less commonly. On rare occasions, children developing fever may exhibit febrile convulsions. Syncope, particularly at the time of mass vaccination, has been reported. Rash occurs infrequently and is usually minimal, but rarely may be generalized. Erythema multiforme has also been reported rarely.

Forms of optic neuritis, including retrobulbar neuritis and papillitis may infrequently follow viral infections, and have been reported to occur 1 to 3 weeks following inoculation with some live virus vaccines.

Isolated reports of polyneuropathy including Guillain-Barré syndrome have been reported after immunization with rubella-containing vaccines.

Clinical experience with live attenuated rubella and mumps virus vaccines given individually indicates that encephalitis and other nervous system reactions have occurred very rarely. These might occur also with BIAVAX II.

Arthralgia and/or arthritis (usually transient and rarely chronic), and polyneuritis are features of natural rubella and vary in frequency and severity with age and sex, being greatest in adult females and least in prepubertal children. This type of involvement as well as myalgia and paresthesia have also been reported following administration of MERUVAX II (Rubella Virus Vaccine Live).

Chronic arthritis has been associated with natural rubella infection and has been related to persistent virus and/or viral antigen isolated from body tissues. Only rarely have vaccine recipients developed chronic joint symptoms.

Following vaccination in children, reactions in joints are uncommon and generally of brief duration. In women, incidence rates for arthritis and arthralgia are generally higher than those seen in children (children: 0–3%; women: 12–20%), and the reactions tend to be more marked and of longer duration. Symptoms may persist for a matter of months or on rare occasions for years. In adolescent girls, the reactions appear to be intermediate in incidence between those seen in children and in adult women. Even in older women (35–45 years), these reactions are generally well tolerated and rarely interfere with normal activities.

DOSAGE AND ADMINISTRATION

FOR SUBCUTANEOUS ADMINISTRATION

Do not inject intravenously.

The dosage of vaccine is the same for all persons. Inject the total volume (about 0.5 mL) of reconstituted vaccine subcutaneously, preferably into the outer aspect of upper arm. *Do not give immune globulin (IG) concurrently with* BIAVAX II.

During shipment, to insure that there is no loss of potency, the vaccine must be maintained at a temperature of 10°C (50°F) or less.

Before reconstitution, store BIAVAX II at 2–8°C (36–46°F).

Protect from light.

CAUTION: A sterile syringe free of preservatives, antiseptics, and detergents should be used for each injection of the vaccine because these substances may inactivate the live virus vaccine. A 25 gauge, $^{5}/_{8}$" needle is recommended.

To reconstitute, use only the diluent supplied, since it is free of preservatives or other antiviral substances which might inactivate the vaccine. First withdraw the entire volume of diluent into the syringe to be used for reconstitution. Inject all the diluent in the syringe into the vial of lyophilized vaccine, and agitate to mix thoroughly. Withdraw the entire contents into a syringe and inject the total volume of restored vaccine subcutaneously.

It is important to use a separate sterile syringe and needle for each individual patient to prevent transmission of hepatitis B virus and other infectious agents from one person to another.

Each dose of BIAVAX II contains not less than the equivalent of 1,000 $TCID_{50}$ of the U.S. Reference Rubella Virus and 20,000 $TCID_{50}$ of the U.S. Reference Mumps Virus.

Parenteral drug products should be inspected visually for particulate matter and discoloration prior to administration. BIAVAX II, when reconstituted, is clear yellow.

HOW SUPPLIED

No. 4746—BIAVAX II is supplied as a single-dose vial of lyophilized vaccine, **NDC** 0006-4746-00, and a vial of diluent.

No. 4669/4309—BIAVAX II is supplied as follows: (1) a box of 10 single-dose vials of lyophilized vaccine (package A), **NDC** 0006-4669-00; and (2) a box of 10 vials of diluent (package B). To conserve refrigerator space, the diluent may be stored separately at room temperature.

Storage

It is recommended that the vaccine be used as soon as possible after reconstitution. Protect the vaccine from light at all times, since such exposure may inactivate the virus. Store reconstituted vaccine in the vaccine vial in a dark place at 2–8°C (36–46°F) and discard if not used within eight hours.

A.H.F.S. Category: 80:12

7680116 Issued March 1995

BLOCADREN® Tablets (Timolol Maleate), U.S.P. ℞

DESCRIPTION

BLOCADREN* (Timolol Maleate) is a non-selective beta-adrenergic receptor blocking agent. The chemical name for timolol maleate is (*S*)-1-[(1,1-dimethylethyl)amino] -3-[[4-(4-morpholinyl)-1,2,5-thiadiazol-3-yl]oxy]-2-propanol (*Z*)-2-butenedioate (1:1) salt. It possesses an asymmetric carbon atom in its structure and is provided as the levo isomer. Its empirical formula is $C_{13}H_{24}N_4O_3S{\cdot}C_4H_4O_4$ and its structural formula is:

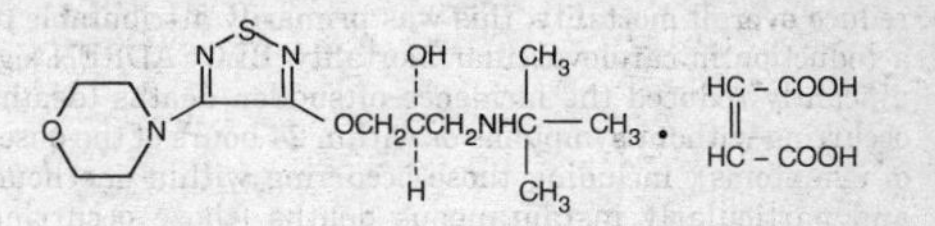

Timolol maleate has a molecular weight of 432.50. It is a white, odorless, crystalline powder which is soluble in water, methanol, and alcohol.

BLOCADREN is supplied as tablets in three strengths containing 5 mg, 10 mg or 20 mg timolol maleate for oral administration. Inactive ingredients are cellulose, FD&C Blue 2, magnesium stearate, and starch.

*Registered trademark of MERCK & CO., INC.

CLINICAL PHARMACOLOGY

BLOCADREN is a $beta_1$ and $beta_2$ (non-selective) adrenergic receptor blocking agent that does not have significant intrinsic sympathomimetic, direct myocardial depressant, or local anesthetic activity.

Pharmacodynamics

Clinical pharmacology studies have confirmed the beta-adrenergic blocking activity as shown by (1) changes in resting heart rate and response of heart rate to changes in posture; (2) inhibition of isoproterenol-induced tachycardia; (3) alteration of the response to the Valsalva maneuver and amyl nitrite administration; and (4) reduction of heart rate and blood pressure changes on exercise.

BLOCADREN decreases the positive chronotropic, positive inotropic, bronchodilator, and vasodilator responses caused by beta-adrenergic receptor agonists. The magnitude of this decreased response is proportional to the existing sympathetic tone and the concentration of BLOCADREN at receptor sites.

In normal volunteers, the reduction in heart rate response to a standard exercise was dose dependent over the test range of 0.5 to 20 mg, with a peak reduction at 2 hours of approximately 30% at higher doses.

Beta-adrenergic receptor blockade reduces cardiac output in both healthy subjects and patients with heart disease. In patients with severe impairment of myocardial function beta-adrenergic receptor blockade may inhibit the stimulatory effect of the sympathetic nervous system necessary to maintain adequate cardiac function.

Beta-adrenergic receptor blockade in the bronchi and bronchioles results in increased airway resistance from unopposed parasympathetic activity. Such an effect in patients with asthma or other bronchospastic conditions is potentially dangerous.

Clinical studies indicate that BLOCADREN at a dosage of 20–60 mg/day reduces blood pressure without causing postural hypotension in most patients with essential hypertension. Administration of BLOCADREN to patients with hypertension results initially in a decrease in cardiac output, little immediate change in blood pressure, and an increase in calculated peripheral resistance. With continued administration of BLOCADREN, blood pressure decreases within a few days, cardiac output usually remains reduced, and peripheral resistance falls toward pretreatment levels. Plasma volume may decrease or remain unchanged during therapy with BLOCADREN. In the majority of patients with hypertension BLOCADREN also decreases plasma renin activity. Dosage adjustment to achieve optimal antihypertensive effect may require a few weeks. When therapy with BLOCADREN is discontinued, the blood pressure tends to return to pretreatment levels gradually. In most patients the antihypertensive activity of BLOCADREN is maintained with long-term therapy and is well tolerated.

The mechanism of the antihypertensive effects of beta-adrenergic receptor blocking agents is not established at this

Continued on next page

Information on the Merck & Co., Inc. products listed on these pages is the full prescribing information from product circulars in use August 31, 1998. For information, please call 1-800-NSC MERCK [1-800-672-6372].

Blocadren—Cont.

time. Possible mechanisms of action include reduction in cardiac output, reduction in plasma renin activity, and a central nervous system sympatholytic action.

A Norwegian multi-center, double-blind study compared the effects of timolol maleate with placebo in 1,884 patients who had survived the acute phase of a myocardial infarction. Patients with systolic blood pressure below 100 mm Hg, sick sinus syndrome and contraindications to beta blockers, including uncontrolled heart failure, second or third degree AV block and bradycardia (<50 beats per minute), were excluded from the multi-center trial. Therapy with BLOCADREN, begun 7 to 28 days following infarction, was shown to reduce overall mortality; this was primarily attributable to a reduction in cardiovascular mortality. BLOCADREN significantly reduced the incidence of sudden deaths (deaths occurring without symptoms or within 24 hours of the onset of symptoms), including those occurring within one hour, and particularly instantaneous deaths (those occurring without preceding symptoms). The protective effect of BLOCADREN was consistent regardless of age, sex or site of infarction. The effect was clearest in patients with a first infarction who were considered at a high risk of dying, defined as those with one or more of the following characteristics during the acute phase: transient left ventricular failure, cardiomegaly, newly appearing atrial fibrillation or flutter, systolic hypotension, or SGOT (ASAT) levels greater than four times the upper limit of normal. Therapy with BLOCADREN also reduced the incidence of non-fatal reinfarction. The mechanism of the protective effect of BLOCADREN is unknown.

BLOCADREN was studied for the prophylactic treatment of migraine headache in placebo-controlled clinical trials involving 400 patients, mostly women between the ages of 18 and 66 years. Common migraine was the most frequent diagnosis. All patients had at least two headaches per month at baseline. Approximately 50 percent of patients who received BLOCADREN had a reduction in the frequency of migraine headache of at least 50 percent, compared to a similar decrease in frequency in 30 percent of patients receiving placebo. The most common cardiovascular adverse effect was bradycardia (5%).

Pharmacokinetics and Metabolism
BLOCADREN is rapidly and nearly completely absorbed (about 90%) following oral ingestion. Detectable plasma levels of timolol occur within one-half hour and peak plasma levels occur in about one to two hours. The drug half-life in plasma is approximately 4 hours and this is essentially unchanged in patients with moderate renal insufficiency. Timolol is partially metabolized by the liver and timolol and its metabolites are excreted by the kidney. Timolol is not extensively bound to plasma proteins; i.e., <10% by equilibrium dialysis and approximately 60% by ultrafiltration. An in vitro hemodialysis study, using ^{14}C timolol added to human plasma or whole blood, showed that timolol was readily dialyzed from these fluids; however, a study of patients with renal failure showed that timolol did not dialyze readily. Plasma levels following oral administration are about half those following intravenous administration indicating approximately 50% first pass metabolism. The level of beta sympathetic activity varies widely among individuals, and no simple correlation exists between the dose or plasma level of timolol maleate and its therapeutic activity. Therefore, objective clinical measurements such as reduction of heart rate and/or blood pressure should be used as guides in determining the optimal dosage for each patient.

INDICATIONS AND USAGE

Hypertension
BLOCADREN is indicated for the treatment of hypertension. It may be used alone or in combination with other antihypertensive agents, especially thiazide-type diuretics.

Myocardial Infarction
BLOCADREN is indicated in patients who have survived the acute phase of a myocardial infarction, and are clinically stable, to reduce cardiovascular mortality and the risk of reinfarction.

Migraine
BLOCADREN is indicated for the prophylaxis of migraine headache.

CONTRAINDICATIONS
BLOCADREN is contraindicated in patients with bronchial asthma or with a history of bronchial asthma, or severe chronic obstructive pulmonary disease (see WARNINGS); sinus bradycardia; second and third degree atrioventricular block; overt cardiac failure (see WARNINGS); cardiogenic shock; hypersensitivity to this product.

WARNINGS

Cardiac Failure
Sympathetic stimulation may be essential for support of the circulation in individuals with diminished myocardial con-

tractility, and its inhibition by beta-adrenergic receptor blockade may precipitate more severe failure. Although beta blockers should be avoided in overt congestive heart failure, they can be used, if necessary, with caution in patients with a history of failure who are well-compensated, usually with digitalis and diuretics. Both digitalis and timolol maleate slow AV conduction. If cardiac failure persists, therapy with BLOCADREN should be withdrawn.

In Patients Without a History of Cardiac Failure continued depression of the myocardium with beta-blocking agents over a period of time can, in some cases, lead to cardiac failure. At the first sign or symptom of cardiac failure, patients receiving BLOCADREN should be digitalized and/or be given a diuretic, and the response observed closely. If cardiac failure continues, despite adequate digitalization and diuretic therapy, BLOCADREN should be withdrawn.

Exacerbation of Ischemic Heart Disease Following Abrupt Withdrawal —Hypersensitivity to catecholamines has been observed in patients withdrawn from beta blocker therapy; exacerbation of angina and, in some cases, myocardial infarction have occurred after *abrupt* discontinuation of such therapy. When discontinuing chronically administered timolol maleate, particularly in patients with ischemic heart disease, the dosage should be gradually reduced over a period of one to two weeks and the patient should be carefully monitored. If angina markedly worsens or acute coronary insufficiency develops, timolol maleate administration should be reinstituted promptly, at least temporarily, and other measures appropriate for the management of unstable angina should be taken. Patients should be warned against interruption or discontinuation of therapy without the physician's advice. Because coronary artery disease is common and may be unrecognized, it may be prudent not to discontinue timolol maleate therapy abruptly even in patients treated only for hypertension.

Obstructive Pulmonary Disease
PATIENTS WITH CHRONIC OBSTRUCTIVE PULMONARY DISEASE (e.g., CHRONIC BRONCHITIS, EMPHYSEMA) OF MILD OR MODERATE SEVERITY, BRONCHOSPASTIC DISEASE OR A HISTORY OF BRONCHOSPASTIC DISEASE (OTHER THAN BRONCHIAL ASTHMA OR A HISTORY OF BRONCHIAL ASTHMA, IN WHICH 'BLOCADREN' IS CONTRAINDICATED, see CONTRAINDICATIONS), SHOULD IN GENERAL NOT RECEIVE BETA BLOCKERS, INCLUDING 'BLOCADREN'. However, if BLOCADREN is necessary in such patients, then the drug should be administered with caution since it may block bronchodilation produced by endogenous and exogenous catecholamine stimulation of beta$_2$ receptors.

Major Surgery
The necessity or desirability of withdrawal of beta-blocking therapy prior to major surgery is controversial. Beta-adrenergic receptor blockade impairs the ability of the heart to respond to beta-adrenergically mediated reflex stimuli. This may augment the risk of general anesthesia in surgical procedures. Some patients receiving beta-adrenergic receptor blocking agents have been subject to protracted severe hypotension during anesthesia. Difficulty in restarting and maintaining the heartbeat has also been reported. For these reasons, in patients undergoing elective surgery, some authorities recommend gradual withdrawal of beta-adrenergic receptor blocking agents.

If necessary during surgery, the effects of beta-adrenergic blocking agents may be reversed by sufficient doses of such agonists as isoproterenol, dopamine, dobutamine or levarterenol (see OVERDOSAGE).

Diabetes Mellitus
BLOCADREN should be administered with caution in patients subject to spontaneous hypoglycemia or to diabetic patients (especially those with labile diabetes) who are receiving insulin or oral hypoglycemic agents. Beta-adrenergic receptor blocking agents may mask the signs and symptoms of acute hypoglycemia.

Thyrotoxicosis
Beta-adrenergic blockade may mask certain clinical signs (e.g., tachycardia) of hyperthyroidism. Patients suspected of developing thyrotoxicosis should be managed carefully to avoid abrupt withdrawal of beta blockade which might precipitate a thyroid storm.

PRECAUTIONS

General
Impaired Hepatic or Renal Function: Since BLOCADREN is partially metabolized in the liver and excreted mainly by the kidneys, dosage reductions may be necessary when hepatic and/or renal insufficiency is present.
Dosing in the Presence of Marked Renal Failure: Although the pharmacokinetics of BLOCADREN are not greatly altered by renal impairment, marked hypotensive responses

have been seen in patients with marked renal impairment undergoing dialysis after 20 mg doses. Dosing in such patients should therefore be especially cautious.
Muscle Weakness: Beta-adrenergic blockade has been reported to potentiate muscle weakness consistent with certain myasthenic symptoms (e.g., diplopia, ptosis, and generalized weakness). Timolol has been reported rarely to increase muscle weakness in some patients with myasthenia gravis or myasthenic symptoms.
Cerebrovascular Insufficiency: Because of potential effects of beta-adrenergic blocking agents relative to blood pressure and pulse, these agents should be used with caution in patients with cerebrovascular insufficiency. If signs or symptoms suggesting reduced cerebral blood flow are observed, consideration should be given to discontinuing these agents.

Drug Interactions
Catecholamine-depleting drugs: Close observation of the patient is recommended when BLOCADREN is administered to patients receiving catecholamine-depleting drugs such as reserpine, because of possible additive effects and the production of hypotension and/or marked bradycardia, which may produce vertigo, syncope, or postural hypotension.
Non-steroidal anti-inflammatory drugs: Blunting of the antihypertensive effect of beta-adrenoceptor blocking agents by non-steroidal anti-inflammatory drugs has been reported. When using these agents concomitantly, patients should be observed carefully to confirm that the desired therapeutic effect has been obtained.
Calcium antagonists: Literature reports suggest that oral calcium antagonists may be used in combination with beta-adrenergic blocking agents when heart function is normal, but should be avoided in patients with impaired cardiac function. Hypotension, AV conduction disturbances, and left ventricular failure have been reported in some patients receiving beta-adrenergic blocking agents when an oral calcium antagonist was added to the treatment regimen. Hypotension was more likely to occur if the calcium antagonist were a dihydropyridine derivative, e.g., nifedipine, while left ventricular failure and AV conduction disturbances were more likely to occur with either verapamil or diltiazem.
Intravenous calcium antagonists should be used with caution in patients receiving beta-adrenergic blocking agents.
Digitalis and either diltiazem or verapamil: The concomitant use of beta-adrenergic blocking agents with digitalis and either diltiazem or verapamil may have additive effects in prolonging AV conduction time.
Quinidine: Potentiated systemic beta-blockade (e.g., decreased heart rate) has been reported during combined treatment with quinidine and timolol, possibly because quinidine inhibits the metabolism of timolol via the P-450 enzyme, CYP2D6.
Clonidine: Beta adrenergic blocking agents may exacerbate the rebound hypertension which can follow the withdrawal of clonidine. If the two drugs are coadministered, the beta adrenergic blocking agent should be withdrawn several days before the gradual withdrawal of clonidine. If replacing clonidine by beta-blocker therapy, the introduction of beta adrenergic blocking agents should be delayed for several days after clonidine administration has stopped.
Risk from Anaphylactic Reaction: While taking beta-blockers, patients with a history of atopy or a history of severe anaphylactic reaction to a variety of allergens may be more reactive to repeated accidental, diagnostic, or therapeutic challenge with such allergens. Such patients may be unresponsive to the usual doses of epinephrine used to treat anaphylactic reactions.

Carcinogenesis, Mutagenesis, Impairment of Fertility
In a two-year study of timolol maleate in rats, there was a statistically significant increase in the incidence of adrenal pheochromocytomas in male rats administered 300 mg/kg/day (250 times* the maximum recommended human dose). Similar differences were not observed in rats administered doses equivalent to approximately 20 or 80 times* the maximum recommended human dose.
In a lifetime study in mice, there were statistically significant increases in the incidence of benign and malignant pulmonary tumors, benign uterine polyps and mammary adenocarcinoma in female mice at 500 mg/kg/day (approximately 400 times* the maximum recommended human dose), but not at 5 or 50 mg/kg/day. In a subsequent study in female mice, in which post-mortem examinations were limited to uterus and lungs, a statistically significant increase in the incidence of pulmonary tumors was again observed at 500 mg/kg/day.
The increased occurrence of mammary adenocarcinoma was associated with elevations in serum prolactin that occurred in female mice administered timolol at 500 mg/kg/day, but not at doses of 5 or 50 mg/kg/day. An increased incidence of mammary adenocarcinomas in rodents has been associated with administration of several other therapeutic agents which elevate serum prolactin, but no correlation between serum prolactin levels and mammary tumors has been established in man. Furthermore, in adult human female subjects who received oral dosages of up to 60 mg of timolol

maleate, the maximum recommended human oral dosage, there were no clinically meaningful changes in serum prolactin.

Timolol maleate was devoid of mutagenic potential when evaluated *in vivo* (mouse) in the micronucleus test and cytogenetic assay (doses up to 800 mg/kg) and *in vitro* in a neoplastic cell transformation assay (up to 100 μg/mL). In Ames tests the highest concentrations of timolol employed, 5000 or 10,000 μg/plate, were associated with statistically significant elevations of revertants observed with tester strain TA100 (in seven replicate assays), but not in three additional strains. In the assays with tester strain TA100, no consistent dose response relationship was observed, nor did the ratio of test to control revertants reach 2. A ratio of 2 is usually considered the criterion for a positive Ames test. Reproduction and fertility studies in rats showed no adverse effect on male or female fertility at doses up to 125 times* the maximum recommended human dose.

*Based on patient weight of 50 kg
Pregnancy
Pregnancy Category C. Teratogenicity studies with timolol in mice, rats and rabbits at doses up to 50 mg/kg/day (approximately 40 times* the maximum recommended daily human dose) showed no evidence of fetal malformations. Although delayed fetal ossification was observed at this dose in rats, there were no adverse effects on postnatal development of offspring. Doses of 1000 mg/kg/day (approximately 830 times* the maximum recommended daily human dose) were maternotoxic in mice and resulted in an increased number of fetal resorptions. Increased fetal resorptions were also seen in rabbits at doses of approximately 40 times* the maximum recommended daily human dose, in this case without apparent maternotoxicity. There are no adequate and well-controlled studies in pregnant women. BLOCADREN should be used during pregnancy only if the potential benefit justifies the potential risk to the fetus.

*Based on patient weight of 50 kg
Nursing Mothers
Timolol maleate has been detected in human milk. Because of the potential for serious adverse reactions from timolol in nursing infants, a decision should be made whether to discontinue nursing or to discontinue the drug, taking into account the importance of the drug to the mother.
Pediatric Use
Safety and effectiveness in pediatric patients have not been established.

ADVERSE REACTIONS

BLOCADREN is usually well tolerated in properly selected patients. Most adverse effects have been mild and transient. In a multicenter (12-week) clinical trial comparing timolol maleate and placebo in hypertensive patients, the following adverse reactions were reported spontaneously and considered to be causally related to timolol maleate:

	Timolol Maleate (n = 176) %	Placebo (n = 168) %
BODY AS A WHOLE		
fatigue/tiredness	3.4	0.6
headache	1.7	1.8
chest pain	0.6	0
asthenia	0.6	0
CARDIOVASCULAR		
bradycardia	9.1	0
arrhythmia	1.1	0.6
syncope	0.6	0
edema	0.6	1.2
DIGESTIVE		
dyspepsia	0.6	0.6
nausea	0.6	0
SKIN		
pruritus	1.1	0
NERVOUS SYSTEM		
dizziness	2.3	1.2
vertigo	0.6	0
paresthesia	0.6	0
PSYCHIATRIC		
decreased libido	0.6	0
RESPIRATORY		
dyspnea	1.7	0.6
bronchial spasm	0.6	0
rales	0.6	0
SPECIAL SENSES		
eye irritation	1.1	0.6
tinnitus	0.6	0

These data are representative of the incidence of adverse effects that may be observed in properly selected patients treated with BLOCADREN, i.e., excluding patients with bronchospastic disease, congestive heart failure or other contraindications to beta blocker therapy.

BLOCADREN	Adverse Reaction†		Withdrawal‡	
	Timolol (n = 945) %	Placebo (n = 939) %	Timolol (n = 945) %	Placebo (n = 939) %
Asthenia or Fatigue	5	1	<1	<1
Heart Rate <40 beats/minute	5	<1	4	<1
Cardiac Failure—Nonfatal	8	7	3	2
Hypotension	3	2	3	1
Pulmonary Edema—Nonfatal	2	<1	<1	<1
Claudication	3	3	1	<1
AV Block 2nd or 3rd degree	<1	<1	<1	<1
Sinoatrial Block	<1	<1	<1	<1
Cold Hands and Feet	8	<1	<1	0
Nausea or Digestive Disorders	8	6	1	<1
Dizziness	6	4	1	0
Bronchial Obstruction	2	<1	1	<1

† When an adverse reaction recurred in a patient, it is listed only once.
‡ Only principal reason for withdrawal in each patient is listed.
These adverse reactions can also occur in patients treated for hypertension.

In patients with migraine the incidence of bradycardia was 5 percent.
In a coronary artery disease population studied in the Norwegian multi-center trial (see CLINICAL PHARMACOLOGY), the frequency of the principal adverse reactions and the frequency with which these resulted in discontinuation of therapy in the timolol and placebo groups were:
[See table above]
The following additional adverse effects have been reported in clinical experience with the drug: *Body as a Whole:* extremity pain, decreased exercise tolerance, weight loss, fever; *Cardiovascular:* cardiac arrest, cardiac failure, cerebrovascular accident, worsening of angina pectoris, worsening of arterial insufficiency, Raynaud's phenomenon, palpitations, vasodilatation; *Digestive:* gastrointestinal pain, hepatomegaly, vomiting, diarrhea, dyspepsia; *Hematologic:* nonthrombocytopenic purpura; *Endocrine:* hyperglycemia, hypoglycemia; *Skin:* rash, skin irritation, increased pigmentation, sweating, alopecia; *Musculoskeletal:* arthralgia; *Nervous System:* local weakness, increase in signs and symptoms of myasthenia gravis; *Psychiatric:* depression, nightmares, somnolence, insomnia, nervousness, diminished concentration, hallucinations; *Respiratory:* cough; *Special Senses:* visual disturbances, diplopia, ptosis, dry eyes; *Urogenital:* impotence, urination difficulties.
There have been reports of retroperitoneal fibrosis in patients receiving timolol maleate and in patients receiving other beta-adrenergic blocking agents. A causal relationship between this condition and therapy with beta-adrenergic blocking agents has not been established.
Potential Adverse Effects: In addition, a variety of adverse effects not observed in clinical trials with BLOCADREN, but reported with other beta-adrenergic blocking agents, should be considered potential adverse effects of BLOCADREN: *Nervous System:* Reversible mental depression progressing to catatonia; an acute reversible syndrome characterized by disorientation for time and place, short-term memory loss, emotional lability, slightly clouded sensorium, and decreased performance on neuropsychometrics; *Cardiovascular:* Intensification of AV block (see CONTRAINDICATIONS); *Digestive:* Mesenteric arterial thrombosis, ischemic colitis; *Hematologic:* Agranulocytosis, thrombocytopenic purpura; *Allergic:* Erythematous rash, fever combined with aching and sore throat, laryngospasm with respiratory distress; *Miscellaneous:* Peyronie's disease.
There have been reports of a syndrome comprising psoriasiform skin rash, conjunctivitis sicca, otitis, and sclerosing serositis attributed to the beta-adrenergic receptor blocking agent, practolol. This syndrome has not been reported with BLOCADREN.
Clinical Laboratory Test Findings: Clinically important changes in standard laboratory parameters were rarely associated with the administration of BLOCADREN. Slight increases in blood urea nitrogen, serum potassium, uric acid, and triglycerides, and slight decreases in hemoglobin, hematocrit and HDL cholesterol occurred, but were not progressive or associated with clinical manifestations. Increases in liver function tests have been reported.

OVERDOSAGE

Overdosage has been reported with Tablets BLOCADREN. A 30-year-old female ingested 650 mg of BLOCADREN (maximum recommended daily dose—60 mg) and experienced second and third degree heart block. She recovered without treatment but approximately two months later developed irregular heartbeat, hypertension, dizziness, tinnitus, faintness, increased pulse rate and borderline first degree heart block.
The oral LD$_{50}$ of the drug is 1190 and 900 mg/kg in female mice and female rats, respectively.

An *in vitro* hemodialysis study, using ^{14}C timolol added to human plasma or whole blood, showed that timolol was readily dialyzed from these fluids; however, a study of patients with renal failure showed that timolol did not dialyze readily.
The most common signs and symptoms to be expected with overdosage with a beta-adrenergic receptor blocking agent are symptomatic bradycardia, hypotension, bronchospasm, and acute cardiac failure. Therapy with BLOCADREN should be discontinued and the patient observed closely. The following additional therapeutic measures should be considered:
(1) *Gastric lavage*
(2) *Symptomatic bradycardia:* Use atropine sulfate intravenously in a dosage of 0.25 mg to 2 mg to induce vagal blockade. If bradycardia persists, intravenous isoproterenol hydrochloride should be administered cautiously. In refractory cases the use of a transvenous cardiac pacemaker may be considered.
(3) *Hypotension:* Use sympathomimetic pressor drug therapy, such as dopamine, dobutamine or levarterenol. In refractory cases the use of glucagon hydrochloride has been reported to be useful.
(4) *Bronchospasm:* Use isoproterenol hydrochloride. Additional therapy with aminophylline may be considered.
(5) *Acute cardiac failure:* Conventional therapy with digitalis, diuretics, and oxygen should be instituted immediately. In refractory cases the use of intravenous aminophylline is suggested. This may be followed if necessary by glucagon hydrochloride which has been reported to be useful.
(6) *Heart block (second or third degree):* Use isoproterenol hydrochloride or a transvenous cardiac pacemaker.

DOSAGE AND ADMINISTRATION

Hypertension
The usual initial dosage of BLOCADREN is 10 mg twice a day, whether used alone or added to diuretic therapy. Dosage may be increased or decreased depending on heart rate and blood pressure response. The usual total maintenance dosage is 20–40 mg per day. Increases in dosage to a maximum of 60 mg per day divided into two doses may be necessary. There should be an interval of at least seven days between increases in dosages.
BLOCADREN may be used with a thiazide diuretic or with other antihypertensive agents. Patients should be observed carefully during initiation of such concomitant therapy.
Myocardial Infarction
The recommended dosage for long-term prophylactic use in patients who have survived the acute phase of a myocardial infarction is 10 mg given twice daily (see CLINICAL PHARMACOLOGY).
Migraine
The usual initial dosage of BLOCADREN is 10 mg twice a day. During maintenance therapy the 20 mg daily dosage may be administered as a single dose. Total daily dosage may be increased to a maximum of 30 mg, given in divided doses, or decreased to 10 mg once per day, depending on clinical response and tolerability. If a satisfactory response is not obtained after 6-8 weeks use of the maximum daily dosage, therapy with BLOCADREN should be discontinued.

Continued on next page

Information on the Merck & Co., Inc. products listed on these pages is the full prescribing information from product circulars in use August 31, 1998. For information, please call 1-800-NSC MERCK [1-800-672-6372].

Consult 1999 PDR® supplements and future editions for revisions

Blocadren—Cont.

HOW SUPPLIED

No. 3343—Tablets BLOCADREN, 5 mg, are light blue, round, compressed tablets, with code MSD 59 on one side and BLOCADREN on the other. They are supplied as follows:

NDC 0006-0059-68 bottles of 100.
Shown in Product Identification Guide, page 322
No. 3344—Tablets BLOCADREN, 10 mg, are light blue, round, scored, compressed tablets, with code MSD 136 on one side and BLOCADREN on the other. They are supplied as follows:

NDC 0006-0136-68 bottles of 100.
(6505-01-132-0651, 10 mg 100's)
Shown in Product Identification Guide, page 322
No. 3371—Tablets BLOCADREN, 20 mg, are light blue, capsule shaped, scored, compressed tablets, with code MSD 437 on one side and BLOCADREN on the other. They are supplied as follows:

NDC 0006-0437-68 bottles of 100
(6505-01-132-0652, 20 mg 100's)
Shown in Product Identification Guide, page 322
Storage
Store at controlled room temperature. 15–30°C (59–86°F).
Keep container tightly closed. Protect from light.
7901231 Issued November 1997
COPYRIGHT © MERCK & CO., INC., 1985
All rights reserved

CHIBROXIN®
(Norfloxacin)
Sterile Ophthalmic Solution

℞

DESCRIPTION

CHIBROXIN* (Norfloxacin) Ophthalmic Solution is a synthetic broad-spectrum antibacterial agent supplied as a sterile isotonic solution for topical ophthalmic use. Norfloxacin, a fluoroquinolone, is 1-ethyl-6-fluoro-1,4-dihydro-4-oxo-7-(1-piperazinyl) -3- quinoline-carboxylic acid. Its empirical formula is $C_{16}H_{18}FN_3O_3$ and the structural formula is:

Norfloxacin is a white to pale yellow crystalline powder with a molecular weight of 319.34 and a melting point of about 221°C. It is freely soluble in glacial acetic acid and very slightly soluble in ethanol, methanol and water.
CHIBROXIN Ophthalmic Solution 0.3% is supplied as a sterile isotonic solution. Each mL contains 3 mg norfloxacin. Inactive ingredients: disodium edetate, sodium acetate, sodium chloride, hydrochloric acid (to adjust pH) and water for injection, Benzalkonium chloride 0.0025% is added as preservative. The pH of CHIBROXIN is approximately 5.2 and the osmolarity is approximately 285 mOsmol/liter.
Norfloxacin, a fluoroquinolone, differs from quinolones by having a fluorine atom at the 6 position and a piperazine moiety at the 7 position.

---

*Registered trademark of MERCK & CO., INC.

CLINICAL PHARMACOLOGY

Microbiology
Norfloxacin has *in vitro* activity against a broad spectrum of gram-positive and gram-negative aerobic bacteria. The fluorine atom at the 6 position provides increased potency against gram-negative organisms and the piperazine moiety at the 7 position is responsible for anti-pseudomonal activity.
Norfloxacin inhibits bacterial deoxyribonucleic acid synthesis and is bactericidal. At the molecular level three specific events are attributed to CHIBROXIN in *E. coli* cells:
1) inhibition of the ATP-dependent DNA supercoiling reaction catalyzed by DNA gyrase;
2) inhibition of the relaxation of supercoiled DNA;
3) promotion of double-stranded DNA breakage.
There is generally no cross-resistance between norfloxacin and other classes of antibacterial agents. Therefore, norfloxacin generally demonstrates activity against indicated organisms resistant to some other antimicrobial agents. When such cross-resistance does occur, it is probably due to decreased entry of the drugs into the bacterial cells. Antagonism has been demonstrated *in vitro* between norfloxacin and nitrofurantoin.
Norfloxacin has been shown to be active against most strains of the following organisms both *in vitro* and clinically in ophthalmic infections (see INDICATIONS AND USAGE):

Gram-positive bacteria including:
Staphylococcus aureus
Staphylococcus epidermidis
Staphylococcus warnerii
Streptococcus pneumoniae
Gram-negative bacteria including:
Acinetobacter calcoaceticus
Aeromonas hydrophila
Haemophilus influenzae
Proteus mirabilis
Pseudomonas aeruginosa
Serratia marcescens
Norfloxacin has been shown to be active *in vitro* against most strains of the following organisms; however, *the clinical significance of these data in ophthalmic infections is unknown.*
Gram-positive bacteria:
Bacillus cereus
Enterococcus faecalis (formerly *Streptococcus faecalis*)
Staphylococcus saprophyticus
Gram-negative bacteria:
Citrobacter diversus
Citrobacter freundii
Edwardsiella tarda
Enterobacter aerogenes
Enterobacter cloacae
Escherichia coli
Hafnia alvei
Haemophilus aegyptius (Koch-Weeks bacillus)
Klebsiella oxytoca
Klebsiella pneumoniae
Klebsiella rhinoscleromatis
Morganella morganii
Neisseria gonorrhoeae
Proteus vulgaris
Providencia alcalifaciens
Providencia rettgeri
Providencia stuartii
Salmonella typhi
Vibrio cholerae
Vibrio parahemolyticus
Yersinia enterocolitica
Other:
Ureaplasma urealyticum
Norfloxacin is not active against obligate anaerobes.
Clinical Studies
Clinical studies were conducted comparing CHIBROXIN Ophthalmic Solution (n=152) with ophthalmic solutions of tobramycin, gentamicin, and chloramphenicol (n=158) in patients with conjunctivitis and positive bacterial cultures. After seven days of therapy with CHIBROXIN Ophthalmic Solution, 72 percent of patients were clinically cured. Of those cured, 85 percent had all their pathogens eradicated. Eradication was also achieved in 62 percent (23/37) of patients whose clinical outcome was not completely cured by day seven. These results were similar among all treatment groups.
Another clinical study compared CHIBROXIN Ophthalmic Solution with placebo in patients with conjunctivitis and positive bacterial cultures. Placebo in this study was the liquid vehicle for CHIBROXIN Ophthalmic Solution and contained the preservative. After five days of therapy, 64 percent (36/56) of patients on CHIBROXIN Ophthalmic Solution were clinically cured compared to 50 percent (23/46) of patients receiving placebo. Of those cured, 78 percent had all their pathogens eradicated. Eradication was also achieved in 50 percent (10/20) of patients whose clinical outcome was not completely cured. The response to CHIBROXIN Ophthalmic Solution was statistically significantly better than the response to placebo.

INDICATIONS AND USAGE

CHIBROXIN Ophthalmic Solution is indicated for the treatment of conjunctivitis when caused by susceptible strains of the following bacteria:
*Acinetobacter calcoaceticus**
*Aeromonas hydrophila**
Haemophilus influenzae
*Proteus mirabilis**
*Pseudomonas aeruginosa**
*Serratia marcescens**
Staphylococcus aureus
Staphylococcus epidermidis
*Staphylococcus warnerii**
Streptococcus pneumoniae
Appropriate monitoring of bacterial response to topical antibiotic therapy should accompany the use of CHIBROXIN Ophthalmic Solution.

---

*Efficacy for this organism was studied in fewer than 10 infections.

CONTRAINDICATIONS

CHIBROXIN Ophthalmic Solution is contraindicated in patients with a history of hypersensitivity to norfloxacin, or the other members of the quinolone group of antibacterial agents or any other component of this medication.

WARNINGS

NOT FOR INJECTION INTO THE EYE.
Serious and occasionally fatal hypersensitivity (anaphylactoid or anaphylactic) reactions, some following the first dose, have been reported in patients receiving systemic quinolone therapy. Some reactions were accompanied by cardiovascular collapse, loss of consciousness, tingling, pharyngeal or facial edema, dyspnea, urticaria, and itching. Only a few patients had a history of hypersensitivity reactions. Serious anaphylactoid or anaphylactic reactions require immediate emergency treatment with epinephrine. Oxygen, intravenous steroids and airway management, including intubation, should be administered as indicated.

PRECAUTIONS

General
As with other antibiotic preparations, prolonged use may result in overgrowth of nonsusceptible organisms, including fungi. If superinfection occurs, appropriate measures should be initiated. Whenever clinical judgment dictates, the patient should be examined with the aid of magnification, such as slit lamp biomicroscopy and, where appropriate, fluorescein staining.
Information For Patients
Patients should be instructed to avoid allowing the tip of the dispensing container to contact the eye or surrounding structures.
Patients should be advised that norfloxacin may be associated with hypersensitivity reactions, even following a single dose, and to discontinue the drug at the first sign of a skin rash or other allergic reaction.
Patients being treated for bacterial conjunctivitis generally should not wear contact lenses. However, if the physician considers the use of contact lenses appropriate, patients should be instructed to wait at least 15 minutes after instilling CHIBROXIN Ophthalmic Solution before inserting their lenses because the preservative in CHIBROXIN Ophthalmic Solution, benzalkonium chloride, may be absorbed by contact lenses.
Drug Interactions
Specific drug interaction studies have not been conducted with norfloxacin ophthalmic solution. However, the systemic administration of some quinolones has been shown to elevate plasma concentrations of theophylline, interfere with the metabolism of caffeine, and enhance the effects of the oral anticoagulant warfarin and its derivatives. Elevated serum levels of cyclosporine have been reported with concomitant use of cyclosporine with norfloxacin. Therefore, cyclosporine serum levels should be monitored and appropriate cyclosporine dosage adjustments made when these drugs are used concomitantly.
Carcinogenesis, Mutagenesis, Impairment of Fertility
No increase in neoplastic changes was observed with norfloxacin as compared to controls in a study in rats, lasting up to 96 weeks at doses eight to nine times the usual human oral dose*.
Norfloxacin was tested for mutagenic activity in a number of *in vivo* and *in vitro* tests. Norfloxacin had no mutagenic effect in the dominant lethal test in mice and did not cause chromosomal aberrations in hamsters or rats at doses 30 to 60 times the usual oral dose*. Norfloxacin had no mutagenic activity *in vitro* in the Ames microbial mutagen test, Chinese hamster fibroblasts and V-79 mammalian cell assay. Although norfloxacin was weakly positive in the Rec-assay for DNA repair, all other mutagenic assays were negative including a more sensitive test (V-79).
Norfloxacin did not adversely affect the fertility of male and female mice at oral doses up to 33 times the usual human oral dose*.
Pregnancy
Pregnancy Category C: Norfloxacin has been shown to produce embryonic loss in monkeys when given in doses 10 times the maximum human oral dose* (400 mg b.i.d.), with peak plasma levels that are two to three times those obtained in humans. There has been no evidence of a teratogenic effect in any of the animal species tested (rat, rabbit, mouse, monkey) at 6 to 50 times the human oral dose. There are no adequate and well-controlled studies in pregnant women. CHIBROXIN Ophthalmic Solution should be used during pregnancy only if the potential benefit justifies the potential risk to the fetus.
Nursing Mothers
It is not known whether norfloxacin is excreted in human milk following ocular administration. Because many drugs are excreted in human milk, and because of the potential for serious adverse reactions in nursing infants from norfloxacin, a decision should be made to discontinue nursing or to

discontinue the drug, taking into account the importance of the drug to the mother (see ANIMAL PHARMACOLOGY).

Pediatric Use

Safety and effectiveness in infants below the age of one year have not been established.

Although quinolones including norfloxacin have been shown to cause arthropathy in immature animals after oral administration, topical ocular administration of other quinolones to immature animals has not shown any arthropathy and there is no evidence that the ophthalmic dosage form of those quinolones has any effects on the weight-bearing joints.

---

*All factors are based on a standard patient weight of 50 kg. The usual oral dose of norfloxacin is 800 mg daily. One drop of CHIBROXIN Ophthalmic Solution 0.3% contains about 1/6,666 of this dose (0.12 mg).

ADVERSE REACTIONS

In clinical trials, the most frequently reported drug-related adverse reaction was local burning or discomfort. Other drug-related adverse reactions were conjunctival hyperemia, chemosis, photophobia and a bitter taste following instillation.

DOSAGE AND ADMINISTRATION

The recommended dose in adults and pediatric patients (one year and older) is one or two drops of CHIBROXIN Ophthalmic Solution applied topically to the affected eye(s) four times daily for up to seven days. Depending on the severity of the infection, the dosage for the first day of therapy may be one or two drops every two hours during the waking hours.

HOW SUPPLIED

CHIBROXIN Ophthalmic Solution is a clear, colorless to light yellow solution.

No. 3526—CHIBROXIN Ophthalmic Solution 0.3% is supplied in a white, opaque, plastic OCUMETER* ophthalmic dispenser with a controlled drop tip as follows:

NDC 0006-3526-03, 5 mL.

Storage

Store CHIBROXIN Ophthalmic Solution at room temperature, 15°–30°C (59°–86°F). Protect from light.

---

*Registered trademark of MERCK & CO., INC.

ANIMAL PHARMACOLOGY

The oral administration of single doses of norfloxacin, six times the recommended human oral dose**, caused lameness in immature dogs. Histologic examination of the weight-bearing joints of these dogs revealed permanent lesions of the cartilage. Related drugs also produced erosions of the cartilage in weight-bearing joints and other signs of arthropathy in immature animals of various species.

**All factors are based on a standard patient weight of 50 kg. The usual oral dose of norfloxacin is 800 mg daily. One drop of CHIBROXIN Ophthalmic Solution 0.3% contains about 1/6,666 of this dose (0.12 mg).

ADDITIONAL CAUTIONARY INFORMATION

Norfloxacin is available as an oral dosage form in addition to the ophthalmic dosage form. The following adverse effects, while they have not been reported with the ophthalmic dosage form, have been reported with the oral dosage form. However, it should be noted that the usual dosage of oral norfloxacin (800 mg/day) contains 6,666 times the amount in one drop of CHIBROXIN Ophthalmic Solution 0.3% (0.12 mg).

Convulsions have been reported in patients receiving oral norfloxacin. Convulsions, increased intracranial pressure, and toxic psychoses have been reported with other drugs in this class. Orally administered quinolones may also cause central nervous system (CNS) stimulation which may lead to tremors, restlessness, lightheadedness, confusion and hallucinations. If these reactions occur in patients receiving norfloxacin, the drug should be discontinued and appropriate measures instituted.

The effects of norfloxacin on brain function or on the electrical activity of the brain have not been tested. Therefore, as with all quinolones, norfloxacin should be used with caution in patients with known or suspected CNS disorders, such as severe cerebral arteriosclerosis, epilepsy, and other factors which predispose to seizures.

The following adverse effects have been reported with Tablets NOROXIN* (Norfloxacin). *Hypersensitivity Reactions:* Hypersensitivity reactions including anaphylactoid reactions, angioedema, dyspnea, vasculitis, urticaria, arthritis, arthralgia, myalgia; *Gastrointestinal:* Pseudomembranous

colitis, hepatitis, jaundice, including cholestatic jaundice, pancreatitis; *Hematologic:* Neutropenia, leukopenia, thrombocytopenia; *Nervous System/Psychiatric:* CNS effects characterized as generalized seizures and myoclonus; neurological changes such as ataxia, diplopia and possible exacerbation of myasthenia gravis; psychic disturbances including psychotic reactions and confusion, depression; *Renal:* Interstitial nephritis, renal failure; *Skin:* Toxic epidermal necrolysis, Stevens-Johnson syndrome and erythema multiforme, exfoliative dermatitis, rash, photosensitivity; *Special Senses:* Transient hearing loss.

Abnormal laboratory values observed with oral norfloxacin included elevation of ALT (SGPT) and AST (SGOT), alkaline phosphatase, BUN, serum creatinine, and LDH.

Please consult the package circular for Tablets NOROXIN (Norfloxacin) for additional information concerning these and other adverse effects and other cautionary information.

---

*Registered trademark of MERCK & CO., INC.

9011205   Issued October 1996

COPYRIGHT © MERCK & CO., INC., 1991

All rights reserved

CLINORIL® Tablets   ℞
(Sulindac), U.S.P.

DESCRIPTION

Sulindac is a non-steroidal, anti-inflammatory indene derivative designated chemically as (Z)- 5-fluoro-2-methyl - 1 - [[p - (methylsulfinyl) phenyl]methylene]-1H-indene-3-acetic acid. It is not a salicylate, pyrazolone or propionic acid derivative. Its empirical formula is $C_{20}H_{17}FO_3S$, with a molecular weight of 356.42. Sulindac, a yellow crystalline compound, is a weak organic acid practically insoluble in water below pH 4.5, but very soluble as the sodium salt or in buffers of pH 6 or higher.

CLINORIL* (Sulindac) is available in 150 and 200 mg tablets for oral administration. Each tablet contains the following inactive ingredients: cellulose, magnesium stearate, starch.

Following absorption, sulindac undergoes two major biotransformations—reversible reduction to the sulfide metabolite, and irreversible oxidation to the sulfone metabolite. Available evidence indicates that the biological activity resides with the sulfide metabolite.

The structural formulas of sulindac and its metabolites are:

---

*Registered trademark of MERCK & CO., INC.

CLINICAL PHARMACOLOGY

CLINORIL is a non-steroidal anti-inflammatory drug, also possessing analgesic and antipyretic activities. Its mode of action, like that of other non-steroidal, anti-inflammatory agents, is not known; however, its therapeutic action is not due to pituitary-adrenal stimulation. Inhibition of prostaglandin synthesis by the sulfide metabolite may be involved in the anti-inflammatory action of CLINORIL.

Sulindac is approximately 90% absorbed in man after oral administration. The peak plasma concentrations of the biologically active sulfide metabolite are achieved in about two hours when sulindac is administered in the fasting state, and in about three to four hours when sulindac is adminis-

tered with food. The mean half-life of sulindac is 7.8 hours while the mean half-life of the sulfide metabolite is 16.4 hours. Sustained plasma levels of the sulfide metabolite are consistent with a prolonged anti-inflammatory action which is the rationale for a twice per day dosage schedule.

Sulindac and its sulfone metabolite undergo extensive enterohepatic circulation relative to the sulfide metabolite in animals. Studies in man have also demonstrated that recirculation of the parent drug, sulindac, and its sulfone metabolite, is more extensive than that of the active sulfide metabolite. The active sulfide metabolite accounts for less than six percent of the total intestinal exposure to sulindac and its metabolites.

The primary route of excretion in man is via the urine as both sulindac and its sulfone metabolite (free and glucuronide conjugates). Approximately 50% of the administered dose is excreted in the urine, with the conjugated sulfone metabolite accounting for the major portion. Less than 1% of the administered dose of sulindac appears in the urine as the sulfide metabolite. Approximately 25% is found in the feces, primarily as the sulfone and sulfide metabolites.

The bioavailability of sulindac, as assessed by urinary excretion, was not changed by concomitant administration of an antacid containing magnesium hydroxide 200 mg and aluminum hydroxide 225 mg per 5 mL.

Because CLINORIL is excreted in the urine primarily as biologically inactive forms, it may possibly affect renal function to a lesser extent than other non-steroidal anti-inflammatory drugs, however, renal adverse experiences have been reported with CLINORIL (see ADVERSE REACTIONS). In a study of patients with chronic glomerular disease treated with therapeutic doses of CLINORIL, no effect was demonstrated on renal blood flow, glomerular filtration rate, or urinary excretion of prostaglandin E_2 and the primary metabolite of prostacyclin, 6-keto-PGF$_1\alpha$. However, in other studies in healthy volunteers and patients with liver disease, CLINORIL was found to blunt the renal responses to intravenous furosemide, i.e., the diuresis, natriuresis, increments in plasma renin activity and urinary excretion of prostaglandins. These observations may represent a differentiation of the effects of CLINORIL on renal functions based on differences in pathogenesis of the renal prostaglandin dependence associated with differing dose-response relationships of different NSAIDs to the various renal functions influenced by prostaglandins. These observations need further clarification and in the interim, sulindac should be used with caution in patients whose renal function may be impaired (see PRECAUTIONS).

In healthy men, the average fecal blood loss, measured over a two-week period during administration of 400 mg per day of CLINORIL, was similar to that for placebo, and was statistically significantly less than that resulting from 4800 mg per day of aspirin.

In controlled clinical studies CLINORIL was evaluated in the following five conditions:

1. Osteoarthritis

In patients with osteoarthritis of the hip and knee, the anti-inflammatory and analgesic activity of CLINORIL was demonstrated by clinical measurements that included: assessments by both patient and investigator of overall response; decrease in disease activity as assessed by both patient and investigator; improvement in ARA Functional Class; relief of night pain; improvement in overall evaluation of pain, including pain on weight bearing and pain on active and passive motion; improvement in joint mobility, range of motion, and functional activities; decreased swelling and tenderness; and decreased duration of stiffness following prolonged inactivity.

In clinical studies in which dosages were adjusted according to patient needs, CLINORIL 200 to 400 mg daily was shown to be comparable in effectiveness to aspirin 2400 to 4800 mg daily. CLINORIL was generally well tolerated, and patients on it had a lower overall incidence of total adverse effects, of milder gastrointestinal reactions, and of tinnitus than did patients on aspirin. (See ADVERSE REACTIONS.)

2. Rheumatoid Arthritis

In patients with rheumatoid arthritis, the anti-inflammatory and analgesic activity of CLINORIL was demonstrated by clinical measurements that included: assessments by both patient and investigator of overall response; decrease in disease activity as assessed by both patient and investigator; reduction in overall joint pain; reduction in duration and severity of morning stiffness; reduction in day and night pain; decrease in time required to walk 50 feet; decrease in general pain as measured on a visual analog scale; improvement in the Ritchie articular index; decrease in proximal interphalangeal joint size; improvement in ARA Functional Class; increase in grip strength; reduction in

Continued on next page

Clinoril—Cont.

painful joint count and score; reduction in swollen joint count and score; and increased flexion and extension of the wrist.

In clinical studies in which dosages were adjusted according to patient needs, CLINORIL 300 to 400 mg daily was shown to be comparable in effectiveness to aspirin 3600 to 4800 mg daily. CLINORIL was generally well tolerated, and patients on it had a lower overall incidence of total adverse effects, of milder gastrointestinal reactions, and of tinnitus than did patients on aspirin. (See ADVERSE REACTIONS.)

In patients with rheumatoid arthritis, CLINORIL may be used in combination with gold salts at usual dosage levels. In clinical studies, CLINORIL added to the regimen of gold salts usually resulted in additional symptomatic relief but did not alter the course of the underlying disease.

3. Ankylosing spondylitis

In patients with ankylosing spondylitis, the anti-inflammatory and analgesic activity of CLINORIL was demonstrated by clinical measurements that included: assessments by both patient and investigator of overall response; decrease in disease activity as assessed by both patient and investigator; improvement in ARA Functional Class; improvement in patient and investigator evaluation of spinal pain, tenderness and/or spasm; reduction in the duration of morning stiffness; increase in the time to onset of fatigue; relief of night pain; increase in chest expansion; and increase in spinal mobility evaluated by fingers-to-floor distance, occiput to wall distance, the Schober Test, and the Wright Modification of the Schober Test. In a clinical study in which dosages were adjusted according to patient need, CLINORIL 200 to 400 mg daily was as effective as indomethacin 75 to 150 mg daily. In a second study, CLINORIL 300 to 400 mg daily was comparable in effectiveness to phenylbutazone 400 to 600 mg daily. CLINORIL was better tolerated than phenylbutazone. (See ADVERSE REACTIONS.)

4. Acute painful shoulder (Acute subacromial bursitis/supraspinatus tendinitis)

In patients with acute painful shoulder (acute subacromial bursitis/supraspinatus tendinitis), the anti-inflammatory and analgesic activity of CLINORIL was demonstrated by clinical measurements that included: assessments by both patient and investigator of overall response; relief of night pain, spontaneous pain, and pain on active motion; decrease in local tenderness; and improvement in range of motion measured by abduction, and internal and external rotation. In clinical studies in acute painful shoulder, CLINORIL 300 to 400 mg daily and oxyphenbutazone 400 to 600 mg daily were shown to be equally effective and well tolerated.

5. Acute gouty arthritis

In patients with acute gouty arthritis, the anti-inflammatory and analgesic activity of CLINORIL was demonstrated by clinical measurements that included: assessments by both the patient and investigator of overall response; relief of weight-bearing pain; relief of pain at rest and on active and passive motion; decrease in tenderness; reduction in warmth and swelling; increase in range of motion; and improvement in ability to function. In clinical studies, CLINORIL at 400 mg daily and phenylbutazone at 600 mg daily were shown to be equally effective. In these short-term studies in which reduction of dosage was permitted according to response, both drugs were equally well tolerated.

INDICATIONS AND USAGE

CLINORIL is indicated for acute or long-term use in the relief of signs and symptoms of the following:
1. Osteoarthritis
2. Rheumatoid arthritis*
3. Ankylosing spondylitis
4. Acute painful shoulder (Acute subacromial bursitis/supraspinatus tendinitis)
5. Acute gouty arthritis

---

*The safety and effectiveness of CLINORIL have not been established in rheumatoid arthritis patients who are designated in the American Rheumatism Association classification as Functional Class IV (incapacitated, largely or wholly bedridden, or confined to wheelchair; little or no self-care).

CONTRAINDICATIONS

CLINORIL should not be used in:
Patients who are hypersensitive to this product.
Patients in whom acute asthmatic attacks, urticaria, or rhinitis are precipitated by aspirin or other non-steroidal anti-inflammatory agents.

WARNINGS

Gastrointestinal Effects

Peptic ulceration and gastrointestinal bleeding have been reported in patients receiving CLINORIL. Fatalities have

occurred. Gastrointestinal bleeding is associated with higher morbidity and mortality in patients acutely ill with other conditions, the elderly and patients with hemorrhagic disorders. In patients with active gastrointestinal bleeding or an active peptic ulcer, an appropriate ulcer regimen should be instituted, and the physician must weigh the benefits of therapy with CLINORIL against possible hazards, and carefully monitor the patient's progress. When CLINORIL is given to patients with a history of either upper or lower gastrointestinal tract disease, it should be given under close supervision and only after consulting the ADVERSE REACTIONS section.

Risk of GI Ulcerations, Bleeding and Perforation with NSAID Therapy

Serious gastrointestinal toxicity such as bleeding, ulceration, and perforation, can occur at any time, with or without warning symptoms, in patients treated chronically with NSAID therapy. Although minor upper gastrointestinal problems, such as dyspepsia, are common, usually developing early in therapy, physicians should remain alert for ulceration and bleeding in patients treated chronically with NSAIDs even in the absence of previous GI tract symptoms. In patients observed in clinical trials of several months to two years duration, symptomatic upper GI ulcers, gross bleeding or perforation appear to occur in approximately 1% of patients treated for 3-6 months, and in about 2-4% of patients treated for one year. Physicians should inform patients about the signs and/or symptoms of serious GI toxicity and what steps to take if they occur.

Studies to date have not identified any subset of patients not at risk of developing peptic ulceration and bleeding. Except for a prior history of serious GI events and other risk factors known to be associated with peptic ulcer disease, such as alcoholism, smoking, etc., no risk factors (e.g., age, sex) have been associated with increased risk. Elderly or debilitated patients seem to tolerate ulceration or bleeding less well than other individuals and most spontaneous reports of fatal GI events are in this population. Studies to date are inconclusive concerning the relative risk of various NSAIDs in causing such reactions. High doses of any NSAID probably carry a greater risk of these reactions, although controlled clinical trials showing this do not exist in most cases. In considering the use of relatively large doses (within the recommended dosage range), sufficient benefit should be anticipated to offset the potential increased risk of GI toxicity.

Hypersensitivity

Rarely, fever and other evidence of hypersensitivity (see ADVERSE REACTIONS) including abnormalities in one or more liver function tests and severe skin reactions have occurred during therapy with CLINORIL. Fatalities have occurred in these patients. Hepatitis, jaundice, or both, with or without fever, may occur usually within the first one to three months of therapy. Determinations of liver function should be considered whenever a patient on therapy with CLINORIL develops unexplained fever, rash or other dermatologic reactions or constitutional symptoms. If unexplained fever or other evidence of hypersensitivity occurs, therapy with CLINORIL should be discontinued. The elevated temperature and abnormalities in liver function caused by CLINORIL characteristically have reverted to normal after discontinuation of therapy. Administration of CLINORIL should not be reinstituted in such patients.

Hepatic Effects

In addition to hypersensitivity reactions involving the liver, in some patients the findings are consistent with those of cholestatic hepatitis. As with other non-steroidal anti-inflammatory drugs, borderline elevations of one or more liver tests without any other signs and symptoms may occur in up to 15% of patients. These abnormalities may progress, may remain essentially unchanged, or may be transient with continued therapy. The SGPT (ALT) test is probably the most sensitive indicator of liver dysfunction. Meaningful (3 times the upper limit of normal) elevations of SGPT or SGOT (AST) occurred in controlled clinical trials in less than 1% of patients. A patient with symptoms and/or signs suggesting liver dysfunction, or in whom an abnormal liver test has occurred, should be evaluated for evidence of the development of more severe hepatic reaction while on therapy with CLINORIL. Although such reactions as described above are rare, if abnormal liver tests persist or worsen, if clinical signs and symptoms consistent with liver disease develop, or if systemic manifestations occur (e.g. eosinophilia, rash, etc.), CLINORIL should be discontinued.

In clinical trials with CLINORIL, the use of doses of 600 mg/day has been associated with an increased incidence of mild liver test abnormalities (see DOSAGE AND ADMINISTRATION for maximum dosage recommendation).

PRECAUTIONS

General

Non-steroidal anti-inflammatory drugs, including CLINORIL, may mask the usual signs and symptoms of infection. Therefore, the physician must be continually on the alert for this and should use the drug with extra care in the presence of existing infection.

Although CLINORIL has less effect on platelet function and bleeding time than aspirin, it is an inhibitor of platelet function; therefore, patients who may be adversely affected should be carefully observed when CLINORIL is administered.

Pancreatitis has been reported in patients receiving CLINORIL (see ADVERSE REACTIONS). Should pancreatitis be suspected, the drug should be discontinued and not restarted, supportive medical therapy instituted, and the patient monitored closely with appropriate laboratory studies (e.g., serum and urine amylase, amylase/creatinine clearance ratio, electrolytes, serum calcium, glucose, lipase, etc.). A search for other causes of pancreatitis as well as those conditions which mimic pancreatitis should be conducted.

Because of reports of adverse eye findings with non-steroidal anti-inflammatory agents, it is recommended that patients who develop eye complaints during treatment with CLINORIL have ophthalmologic studies.

In patients with poor liver function, delayed, elevated and prolonged circulating levels of the sulfide and sulfone metabolites may occur. Such patients should be monitored closely; a reduction of daily dosage may be required.

Edema has been observed in some patients taking CLINORIL. Therefore, as with other non-steroidal anti-inflammatory drugs, CLINORIL should be used with caution in patients with compromised cardiac function, hypertension, or other conditions predisposing to fluid retention. CLINORIL may allow a reduction in dosage or the elimination of chronic corticosteroid therapy in some patients with rheumatoid arthritis. However, it is generally necessary to reduce corticosteroids gradually over several months in order to avoid an exacerbation of disease or signs and symptoms of adrenal insufficiency. Abrupt withdrawal of chronic corticosteroid treatment is generally not recommended even when patients have had a serious complication of chronic corticosteroid therapy.

Renal Effects

As with other non-steroidal anti-inflammatory drugs, long term administration of sulindac to animals has resulted in renal papillary necrosis and other abnormal renal pathology. In humans, there have been reports of acute interstitial nephritis with hematuria, proteinuria, and occasionally nephrotic syndrome.

A second form of renal toxicity has been seen in patients with prerenal and renal conditions leading to a reduction in renal blood flow or blood volume, where the renal prostaglandins have a supportive role in the maintenance of renal perfusion. In these patients administration of an NSAID may cause a dose dependent reduction in prostaglandin formation and may precipitate overt renal decompensation. CLINORIL may affect renal function less than other NSAIDs in patients with chronic glomerular renal disease (see CLINICAL PHARMACOLOGY). Until these observations are better understood and clarified, however, and because renal adverse experiences have been reported with CLINORIL (see ADVERSE REACTIONS), caution should be exercised when administering the drug to patients with conditions associated with increased risk of the effects of non-steroidal anti-inflammatory drugs on renal function, such as those with renal or hepatic dysfunction, diabetes mellitus, advanced age, extracellular volume depletion from any cause, congestive heart failure, septicemia, pyelonephritis, or concomitant use of any nephrotoxic drug. Discontinuation of NSAID therapy is typically followed by recovery to the pretreatment state.

Since CLINORIL is eliminated primarily by the kidneys, patients with significantly impaired renal function should be closely monitored; a lower daily dosage should be anticipated to avoid excessive drug accumulation.

Sulindac metabolites have been reported rarely as the major or a minor component in renal stones in association with other calculus components. CLINORIL should be used with caution in patients with a history of renal lithiasis, and they should be kept well hydrated while receiving CLINORIL.

Information for Patients

CLINORIL, like other drugs of its class, is not free of side effects. The side effects of these drugs can cause discomfort and, rarely, there are more serious side effects such as gastrointestinal bleeding, which may result in hospitalization and even fatal outcomes.

NSAIDs (Non-steroidal Anti-inflammatory Drugs) are often essential agents in the management of arthritis, but they also may be commonly employed for conditions which are less serious.

Physicians may wish to discuss with their patients the potential risks (see WARNINGS, PRECAUTIONS and ADVERSE REACTIONS) and likely benefits of NSAID treatment, particularly when the drugs are used for less serious conditions where treatment without NSAIDs may represent an acceptable alternative to both the patient and physician.

Laboratory Tests

Because serious GI tract ulceration and bleeding can occur without warning symptoms, physicians should follow chronically treated patients for the signs and symptoms of ulcer-

ation and bleeding and should inform them of the importance of this follow-up (see WARNINGS, *Risk of GI Ulcerations, Bleeding and Perforation with NSAID Therapy).*

Use in Pregnancy

CLINORIL is not recommended for use in pregnant women, since safety for use has not been established. The known effects of drugs of this class on the human fetus during the third trimester of pregnancy include: constriction of the ductus arteriosus prenatally, tricuspid incompetence, and pulmonary hypertension; non-closure of the ductus arteriosus postnatally which may be resistant to medical management; myocardial degenerative changes, platelet dysfunction with resultant bleeding, intracranial bleeding, renal dysfunction or failure, renal injury/dysgenesis which may result in prolonged or permanent renal failure, oligohydramnios, gastrointestinal bleeding or perforation, and increased risk of necrotizing enterocolitis.

In reproduction studies in the rat, a decrease in average fetal weight and an increase in numbers of dead pups were observed on the first day of the postpartum period at dosage levels of 20 and 40 mg/kg/day ($2^1/_2$ and 5 times the usual maximum daily dose in humans), although there was no adverse effect on the survival and growth during the remainder of the postpartum period. CLINORIL prolongs the duration of gestation in rats, as do other compounds of this class which also may cause dystocia and delayed parturition in pregnant animals. Visceral and skeletal malformations observed in low incidence among rabbits in some teratology studies did not occur at the same dosage levels in repeat studies, nor at a higher dosage level in the same species.

Nursing Mothers

Nursing should not be undertaken while a patient is on CLINORIL. It is not known whether sulindac is secreted in human milk; however, it is secreted in the milk of lactating rats.

Pediatric Use

Safety and effectiveness in pediatric patients have not been established.

Drug Interactions

DMSO should not be used with sulindac. Concomitant administration has been reported to reduce the plasma levels of the active sulfide metabolite and potentially reduce efficacy. In addition, this combination has been reported to cause peripheral neuropathy.

Although sulindac and its sulfide metabolite are highly bound to protein, studies, in which CLINORIL was given at a dose of 400 mg daily, have shown no clinically significant interaction with oral anticoagulants or oral hypoglycemic agents. However, patients should be monitored carefully until it is certain that no change in their anticoagulant or hypoglycemic dosage is required. Special attention should be paid to patients taking higher doses than those recommended and to patients with renal impairment or other metabolic defects that might increase sulindac blood levels.

The concomitant administration of aspirin with sulindac significantly depressed the plasma levels of the active sulfide metabolite. A double-blind study compared the safety and efficacy of CLINORIL 300 or 400 mg daily given alone or with aspirin 2.4 g/day for the treatment of osteoarthritis. The addition of aspirin did not alter the types of clinical or laboratory adverse experiences for CLINORIL; however, the combination showed an increase in the incidence of gastrointestinal adverse experiences. Since the addition of aspirin did not have a favorable effect on the therapeutic response to CLINORIL, the combination is not recommended.

The concomitant use of CLINORIL with other NSAIDs is not recommended due to the increased possibility of gastrointestinal toxicity, with little or no increase in efficacy.

Caution should be used if CLINORIL is administered concomitantly with methotrexate. Nonsteroidal anti-inflammatory drugs have been reported to decrease the tubular secretion of methotrexate and to potentiate its toxicity.

Administration of non-steroidal anti-inflammatory drugs concomitantly with cyclosporine has been associated with an increase in cyclosporine-induced toxicity, possibly due to decreased synthesis of renal prostacyclin. NSAIDs should be used with caution in patients taking cyclosporine, and renal function should be carefully monitored.

The concomitant administration of CLINORIL and diflunisal in normal volunteers resulted in lowering of the plasma levels of the active sulindac sulfide metabolite by approximately one-third.

Probenecid given concomitantly with sulindac had only a slight effect on plasma sulfide levels, while plasma levels of sulindac and sulfone were increased. Sulindac was shown to produce a modest reduction in the uricosuric action of probenecid, which probably is not significant under most circumstances.

Neither propoxyphene hydrochloride nor acetaminophen had any effect on the plasma levels of sulindac or its sulfide metabolite.

ADVERSE REACTIONS

The following adverse reactions were reported in clinical trials or have been reported since the drug was marketed. The probability exists of a causal relationship between CLINORIL and these adverse reactions. The adverse reactions which have been observed in clinical trials encompass observations in 1,865 patients, including 232 observed for at least 48 weeks.

Incidence Greater Than 1%

Gastrointestinal

The most frequent types of adverse reactions occurring with CLINORIL are gastrointestinal; these include gastrointestinal pain (10%), dyspepsia*, nausea* with or without vomiting, diarrhea*, constipation*, flatulence, anorexia and gastrointestinal cramps.

Dermatologic

Rash*, pruritus.

Central Nervous System

Dizziness*, headache*, nervousness.

Special Senses

Tinnitus.

Miscellaneous

Edema (see PRECAUTIONS).

*Incidence between 3% and 9%. Those reactions occurring in 1% to 3% of patients are not marked with an asterisk.

Incidence Less Than 1 in 100

Gastrointestinal

Gastritis, gastroenteritis or colitis. Peptic ulcer and gastrointestinal bleeding have been reported. GI perforation and intestinal strictures (diaphragms) have been reported rarely.

Liver function abnormalities; jaundice, sometimes with fever; cholestasis; hepatitis; hepatic failure.

There have been rare reports of sulindac metabolites in common bile duct "sludge" and in biliary calculi in patients with symptoms of cholecystitis who underwent a cholecystectomy.

Pancreatitis (see PRECAUTIONS).

Ageusia; glossitis.

Dermatologic

Stomatitis, sore or dry mucous membranes, alopecia, photosensitivity.

Erythema multiforme, toxic epidermal necrolysis, Stevens-Johnson syndrome, and exfoliative dermatitis have been reported.

Cardiovascular

Congestive heart failure, especially in patients with marginal cardiac function; palpitation; hypertension.

Hematologic

Thrombocytopenia; ecchymosis; purpura; leukopenia; agranulocytosis; neutropenia; bone marrow depression, including aplastic anemia; hemolytic anemia; increased prothrombin time in patients on oral anticoagulants (see PRECAUTIONS).

Genitourinary

Urine discoloration; dysuria; vaginal bleeding; hematuria; proteinuria; crystalluria; renal impairment, including renal failure; interstitial nephritis; nephrotic syndrome.

Renal calculi containing sulindac metabolites have been observed rarely.

Metabolic

Hyperkalemia.

Musculoskeletal

Muscle weakness.

Psychiatric

Depression; psychic disturbances including acute psychosis.

Nervous System

Vertigo; insomnia; somnolence; paresthesia; convulsions; syncope; aseptic meningitis.

Special Senses

Blurred vision; visual disturbances; decreased hearing; metallic or bitter taste.

Respiratory

Epistaxis.

Hypersensitivity Reactions

Anaphylaxis; angioneurotic edema; bronchial spasm; dyspnea.

Hypersensitivity vasculitis.

A potentially fatal apparent hypersensitivity syndrome has been reported. This syndrome may include constitutional symptoms (fever, chills, diaphoresis, flushing), cutaneous findings (rash or other dermatologic reactions—see above), conjunctivitis, involvement of major organs (changes in liver function including hepatic failure, jaundice, pancreatitis, pneumonitis with or without pleural effusion, leukopenia, leukocytosis, eosinophilia, disseminated intravascular coagulation, anemia, renal impairment, including renal failure), and other less specific findings (adenitis, arthralgia, arthritis, myalgia, fatigue, malaise, hypotension, chest pain, tachycardia).

Causal Relationship Unknown

A rare occurrence of fulminant necrotizing fasciitis, particularly in association with Group A β-hemolytic streptococcus, has been described in persons treated with non-steroidal anti-inflammatory agents, sometimes with fatal outcome (see also PRECAUTIONS, *General*).

Other reactions have been reported in clinical trials or since the drug was marketed, but occurred under circumstances where a causal relationship could not be established. However, in these rarely reported events, that possibility cannot be excluded. Therefore, these observations are listed to serve as alerting information to physicians.

Cardiovascular

Arrhythmia.

Metabolic

Hyperglycemia.

Nervous System

Neuritis.

Special Senses

Disturbances of the retina and its vasculature.

Miscellaneous

Gynecomastia.

MANAGEMENT OF OVERDOSAGE

Cases of overdosage have been reported and rarely, deaths have occurred. The following signs and symptoms may be observed following overdosage: stupor, coma, diminished urine output and hypotension.

In the event of overdosage, the stomach should be emptied by inducing vomiting or by gastric lavage, and the patient carefully observed and given symptomatic and supportive treatment.

Animal studies show that absorption is decreased by the prompt administration of activated charcoal and excretion is enhanced by alkalinization of the urine.

DOSAGE AND ADMINISTRATION

CLINORIL should be administered orally twice a day with food. The maximum dosage is 400 mg per day. Dosages above 400 mg per day are not recommended.

In osteoarthritis, rheumatoid arthritis, and ankylosing spondylitis, the recommended starting dosage is 150 mg twice a day. The dosage may be lowered or raised depending on the response.

A prompt response (within one week) can be expected in about one-half of patients with osteoarthritis, ankylosing spondylitis, and rheumatoid arthritis. Others may require longer to respond.

In acute painful shoulder (acute subacromial bursitis/supraspinatus tendinitis) and acute gouty arthritis, the recommended dosage is 200 mg twice a day. After a satisfactory response has been achieved, the dosage may be reduced according to the response. In acute painful shoulder, therapy for 7–14 days is usually adequate. In acute gouty arthritis, therapy for 7 days is usually adequate.

HOW SUPPLIED

No. 3360—Tablets CLINORIL 150 mg are yellow, hexagon-shaped, compressed tablets, coded MSD 941 on one side and CLINORIL on the other. They are supplied as follows:

NDC 0006-0941-68 in bottles of 100

(6505-01-071-5559, 150 mg 100's).

Shown in Product Identification Guide, page 322

No. 3353—Tablets CLINORIL 200 mg are yellow, hexagon-shaped, scored, compressed tablets, coded MSD 942 on one side and CLINORIL on the other. They are supplied as follows:

NDC 0006-0942-68 in bottles of 100

(6505-01-072-3426, 200 mg 100's).

Shown in Product Identification Guide, page 322

7858636 Issued June 1997

COGENTIN® Tablets ℞
(Benztropine Mesylate), U.S.P.
COGENTIN® Injection ℞
(Benztropine Mesylate), U.S.P.

DESCRIPTION

Benztropine mesylate is a synthetic compound containing structural features found in atropine and diphenhydramine. It is designated chemically as 8-azabicyclo[3.2.1] octane, 3-(diphenylmethoxy)-,*endo*, methanesulfonate. Its empirical formula is $C_{21}H_{25}NO{\cdot}CH_4O_3S$, and its structural formula is:

[See chemical structure at top of next column]

Benztropine mesylate is a crystalline white powder, very soluble in water, and has a molecular weight of 403.54.

Continued on next page

Information on the Merck & Co., Inc. products listed on these pages is the full prescribing information from product circulars in use August 31, 1998. For information, please call 1-800-NSC MERCK [1-800-672-6372].

Cogentin—Cont.

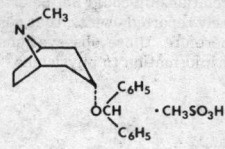

COGENTIN* (Benztropine Mesylate) is supplied as tablets in three strengths (0.5 mg, 1 mg, and 2 mg per tablet), and as a sterile injection for intravenous and intramuscular use. Tablets COGENTIN contain 0.5, 1 or 2 mg of benztropine mesylate. Each tablet contains the following inactive ingredients: calcium phosphate, cellulose, lactose, magnesium stearate and starch.

Each milliliter of the injection contains:

Benztropine mesylate .... 1 mg
Sodium chloride .... 9 mg
Water for Injection q.s. .... 1 mL

*Registered trademark of MERCK & CO., INC.

ACTIONS

COGENTIN possesses both anticholinergic and antihistaminic effects, although only the former have been established as therapeutically significant in the management of parkinsonism.

In the isolated guinea pig ileum, the anticholinergic activity of this drug is about equal to that of atropine; however, when administered orally to unanesthetized cats, it is only about half as active as atropine.

In laboratory animals, its antihistaminic activity and duration of action approach those of pyrilamine maleate.

INDICATIONS

For use as an adjunct in the therapy of all forms of parkinsonism.

Useful also in the control of extrapyramidal disorders (except tardive dyskinesia—see PRECAUTIONS) due to neuroleptic drugs (e.g., phenothiazines).

CONTRAINDICATIONS

Hypersensitivity to COGENTIN tablets or to any component of COGENTIN injection.

Because of its atropine-like side effects, this drug is contraindicated in pediatric patients under three years of age, and should be used with caution in older pediatric patients.

WARNINGS

Safe use in pregnancy has not been established.

COGENTIN may impair mental and/or physical abilities required for performance of hazardous tasks, such as operating machinery or driving a motor vehicle.

When COGENTIN is given concomitantly with phenothiazines, haloperidol, or other drugs with anticholinergic or antidopaminergic activity, patients should be advised to report gastrointestinal complaints, fever or heat intolerance promptly. Paralytic ileus, hyperthermia and heat stroke, all of which have sometimes been fatal, have occurred in patients taking anticholinergic-type antiparkinsonism drugs, including COGENTIN, in combination with phenothiazines and/or tricyclic antidepressants.

Since COGENTIN contains structural features of atropine, it may produce anhidrosis. For this reason, it should be administered with caution during hot weather, especially when given concomitantly with other atropine-like drugs to the chronically ill, the alcoholic, those who have central nervous system disease, and those who do manual labor in a hot environment. Anhidrosis may occur more readily when some disturbance of sweating already exists. If there is evidence of anhidrosis, the possibility of hyperthermia should be considered. Dosage should be decreased at the discretion of the physician so that the ability to maintain body heat equilibrium by perspiration is not impaired. Severe anhidrosis and fatal hyperthermia have occurred.

PRECAUTIONS

General

Since COGENTIN has cumulative action, continued supervision is advisable. Patients with a tendency to tachycardia and patients with prostatic hypertrophy should be observed closely during treatment.

Dysuria may occur, but rarely becomes a problem. Urinary retention has been reported with COGENTIN.

The drug may cause complaints of weakness and inability to move particular muscle groups, especially in large doses. For example, if the neck has been rigid and suddenly relaxes, it may feel weak, causing some concern. In this event, dosage adjustment is required.

Mental confusion and excitement may occur with large doses, or in susceptible patients. Visual hallucinations have been reported occasionally. Furthermore, in the treatment of extrapyramidal disorders due to neuroleptic drugs (e.g., phenothiazines), in patients with mental disorders, occasionally there may be intensification of mental symptoms. In such cases, antiparkinsonian drugs can precipitate a toxic psychosis. Patients with mental disorders should be kept under careful observation, especially at the beginning of treatment or if dosage is increased.

Tardive dyskinesia may appear in some patients on long-term therapy with phenothiazines and related agents, or may occur after therapy with these drugs has been discontinued. Antiparkinsonism agents do not alleviate the symptoms of tardive dyskinesia, and in some instances may aggravate them. COGENTIN is not recommended for use in patients with tardive dyskinesia.

The physician should be aware of the possible occurrence of glaucoma. Although the drug does not appear to have any adverse effect on simple glaucoma, it probably should not be used in angle-closure glaucoma.

Drug Interactions

Antipsychotic drugs such as phenothiazines or haloperidol; tricyclic antidepressants (see WARNINGS).

Pediatric use

Because of the atropine-like side effects, COGENTIN should be used with caution in pediatric patients over three years of age (see CONTRAINDICATIONS).

ADVERSE REACTIONS

The adverse reactions below, most of which are anticholinergic in nature, have been reported and within each category are listed in order of decreasing severity.

Cardiovascular

Tachycardia.

Digestive

Paralytic ileus, constipation, vomiting, nausea, dry mouth. If dry mouth is so severe that there is difficulty in swallowing or speaking, or loss of appetite and weight, reduce dosage, or discontinue the drug temporarily.

Slight reduction in dosage may control nausea and still give sufficient relief of symptoms. Vomiting may be controlled by temporary discontinuation, followed by resumption at a lower dosage.

Nervous System

Toxic psychosis, including confusion, disorientation, memory impairment, visual hallucinations; exacerbation of pre-existing psychotic symptoms; nervousness; depression; listlessness; numbness of fingers.

Special Senses

Blurred vision, dilated pupils.

Urogenital

Urinary retention, dysuria.

Metabolic/Immune or Skin

Occasionally, an allergic reaction, e.g., skin rash, develops. If this can not be controlled by dosage reduction, the medication should be discontinued.

Other

Heat stroke, hyperthermia, fever.

DOSAGE AND ADMINISTRATION

COGENTIN tablets should be used when patients are able to take oral medication.

The injection is especially useful for psychotic patients with acute dystonic reactions or other reactions that make oral medication difficult or impossible. It is recommended also when a more rapid response is desired than can be obtained with the tablets.

Since there is no significant difference in onset of effect after intravenous or intramuscular injection, usually there is no need to use the intravenous route. The drug is quickly effective after either route, with improvement sometimes noticeable a few minutes after injection. In emergency situations, when the condition of the patient is alarming, 1 to 2 mL of the injection normally will provide quick relief. If the parkinsonian effect begins to return, the dose can be repeated.

Because of cumulative action, therapy should be initiated with a low dose which is increased gradually at five or six-day intervals to the smallest amount necessary for optimal relief. Increases should be made in increments of 0.5 mg, to a maximum of 6 mg, or until optimal results are obtained without excessive adverse reactions.

Postencephalitic and

Idiopathic Parkinsonism—

The usual daily dose is 1 to 2 mg, with a range of 0.5 to 6 mg orally or parenterally.

As with any agent used in parkinsonism, dosage must be individualized according to age and weight, and the type of parkinsonism being treated. Generally, older patients and thin patients cannot tolerate large doses. Most patients with postencephalitic parkinsonism need fairly large doses and tolerate them well. Patients with a poor mental outlook are usually poor candidates for therapy.

In idiopathic parkinsonism, therapy may be initiated with a single daily dose of 0.5 to 1 mg at bedtime. In some patients, this will be adequate; in others 4 to 6 mg a day may be required.

In postencephalitic parkinsonism, therapy may be initiated in most patients with 2 mg a day in one or more doses. In highly sensitive patients, therapy may be initiated with 0.5 mg at bedtime, and increased as necessary.

Some patients experience greatest relief by taking the entire dose at bedtime; others react more favorably to divided doses, two to four times a day. Frequently, one dose a day is sufficient, and divided doses may be unnecessary or undesirable.

The long duration of action of this drug makes it particularly suitable for bedtime medication when its effects may last throughout the night, enabling patients to turn in bed during the night more easily, and to rise in the morning.

When COGENTIN is started, do not terminate therapy with other antiparkinsonian agents abruptly. If the other agents are to be reduced or discontinued, it must be done gradually. Many patients obtain greatest relief with combination therapy.

COGENTIN may be used concomitantly with SINEMET* (Carbidopa-Levodopa), or with levodopa, in which case periodic dosage adjustment may be required in order to maintain optimum response.

Drug-Induced Extrapyramidal Disorders—In treating extrapyramidal disorders due to neuroleptic drugs (e.g., phenothiazines), the recommended dosage is 1 to 4 mg once or twice a day orally or parenterally. Dosage must be individualized according to the need of the patient. Some patients require more than recommended; others do not need as much.

In acute dystonic reactions, 1 to 2 mL of the injection usually relieves the condition quickly. After that, the tablets, 1 to 2 mg twice a day, usually prevent recurrence.

When extrapyramidal disorders develop soon after initiation of treatment with neuroleptic drugs (e.g., phenothiazines), they are likely to be transient. One to 2 mg of COGENTIN tablets two or three times a day usually provides relief within one or two days. After one or two weeks, the drug should be withdrawn to determine the continued need for it. If such disorders recur, COGENTIN can be reinstituted.

Certain drug-induced extrapyramidal disorders that develop slowly may not respond to COGENTIN.

*Registered trademark of MERCK & CO., INC.

OVERDOSAGE

Manifestations—May be any of those seen in atropine poisoning or antihistamine overdosage: CNS depression, preceded or followed by stimulation; confusion; nervousness; listlessness; intensification of mental symptoms or toxic psychosis in patients with mental illness being treated with neuroleptic drugs (e.g., phenothiazines); hallucinations (especially visual); dizziness; muscle weakness; ataxia; dry mouth; mydriasis; blurred vision; palpitations; tachycardia; elevated blood pressure; nausea; vomiting; dysuria; numbness of fingers; dysphagia; allergic reactions, e.g., skin rash; headache; hot, dry, flushed skin; delirium; coma; shock; convulsions; respiratory arrest; anhidrosis; hyperthermia; glaucoma; constipation.

Treatment—Physostigmine salicylate, 1 to 2 mg, SC or IV, reportedly will reverse symptoms of anticholinergic intoxication.* A second injection may be given after 2 hours if required. Otherwise treatment is symptomatic and supportive. Induce emesis or perform gastric lavage (contraindicated in precomatose, convulsive, or psychotic states). Maintain respiration. A short-acting barbiturate may be used for CNS excitement, but with caution to avoid subsequent depression; supportive care for depression (avoid convulsant stimulants such as picrotoxin, pentylenetetrazol, or bemegride); artificial respiration for severe respiratory depression; a local miotic for mydriasis and cycloplegia; ice bags or other cold applications and alcohol sponges for hyperpyrexia, a vasopressor and fluids for circulatory collapse. Darken room for photophobia.

*Duvoisin, R.C.; Katz, R.J.; Amer. Med. Ass. 206:1963–1965, Nov. 25, 1968.

HOW SUPPLIED

No. 3297—Tablets COGENTIN, 0.5 mg, are white, round, scored, compressed tablets, coded MSD 21 on one side and COGENTIN on the other. They are supplied as follows:
NDC 0006-0021-68 in bottles of 100.
  Shown in Product Identification Guide, page 322
No. 3334—Tablets COGENTIN, 1 mg, are white, oval shaped, scored, compressed tablets, coded MSD 635 on one side and COGENTIN on the other. They are supplied as follows:
NDC 0006-0635-68 in bottles of 100.
  Shown in Product Identification Guide, page 322

No. 3172—Tablets COGENTIN, 2 mg, are white, round, scored, compressed tablets, coded MSD 60 on one side and COGENTIN on the other. They are supplied as follows:
NDC 0006-0060-68 in bottles of 100
(6505-01-230-8726, 2 mg 100's).
Shown in Product Identification Guide, page 322
No. 3275—Injection COGENTIN, 1 mg per mL, is a clear, colorless solution and is supplied as follows:
NDC 0006-3275-16 in boxes of 6×2 mL ampuls
(6505-00-785-0307, tray of 6×2 mL ampuls).
7924121 Issued July 1996

ColBENEMID® Tablets ℞
(Probenecid-Colchicine), U.S.P.

DESCRIPTION

ColBENEMID* (Probenecid-Colchicine) contains probenecid, which is a uricosuric agent, and colchicine, which has antigout activity, the mechanism of which is unknown.
Probenecid is the generic name for 4- [(dipropylamino) sulfonyl] benzoic acid (molecular weight 285.36). It has the following structural formula:

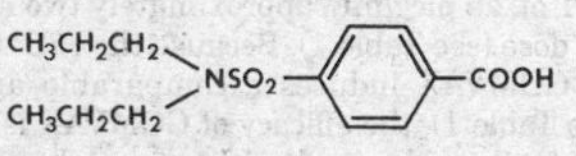

Probenecid is a white or nearly white, fine, crystalline powder. It is soluble in dilute alkali, in alcohol, in chloroform, and in acetone; it is practically insoluble in water and in dilute acids.
Colchicine is an alkaloid obtained from various species of Colchicum. The chemical name for colchicine is (*S*)-*N* -(5,6,7,9-tetrahydro-1,2,3,10-tetramethoxy-9-oxobenzo [*a*] heptalen-7-yl) acetamide (molecular weight 399.43). It has the following structural formula:

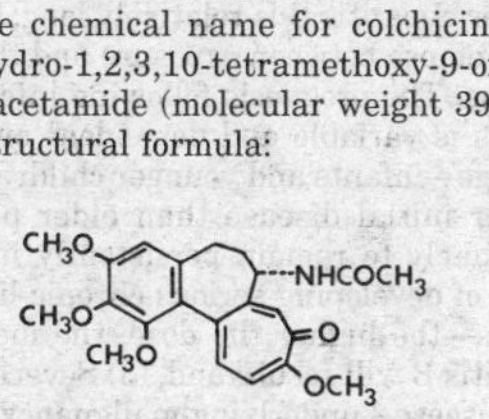

Colchicine consists of pale yellow scales or powder; it darkens on exposure to light. Colchicine is soluble in water, freely soluble in alcohol and in chloroform, and slightly soluble in ether.
Each tablet contains 0.5 g probenecid and 0.5 mg colchicine and the following inactive ingredients: calcium stearate, gelatin, magnesium carbonate, starch.

*Registered trademark of MERCK & CO., INC.

ACTIONS

Probenecid is a uricosuric and renal tubular blocking agent. It inhibits the tubular reabsorption of urate, thus increasing the urinary excretion of uric acid and decreasing serum urate levels. Effective uricosuria reduces the miscible urate pool, retards urate deposition, and promotes resorption of urate deposits.
Probenecid inhibits the tubular secretion of penicillin and usually increases penicillin plasma levels by any route the antibiotic is given. A 2-fold to 4-fold elevation has been demonstrated for various penicillins.
Probenecid also has been reported to inhibit the renal transport of many other compounds including aminohippuric acid (PAH), aminosalicylic acid (PAS), indomethacin, sodium iodomethamate and related iodinated organic acids, 17-ketosteroids, pantothenic acid, phenolsulfonphthalein (PSP), sulfonamides, and sulfonylureas. See also DRUG INTERACTIONS.
Probenecid decreases both hepatic and renal excretion of sulfobromophthalein (BSP). The tubular reabsorption of phosphorus is inhibited in hypoparathyroid but not in euparathyroid individuals.
Probenecid does not influence plasma concentrations of salicylates, nor the excretion of streptomycin, chloramphenicol, chlortetracycline, oxytetracycline, or neomycin.
The mode of action of colchicine in gout is unknown. It is not an analgesic, though it relieves pain in acute attacks of gout. It is not a uricosuric agent and will not prevent progression of gout to chronic gouty arthritis. It does have a prophylactic, suppressive effect that helps to reduce the incidence of acute attacks and to relieve the residual pain and mild discomfort that patients with gout occasionally feel.
In man and certain other animals, colchicine can produce a temporary leukopenia that is followed by leukocytosis.
Colchicine has other pharmacologic actions in animals: It alters neuromuscular function, intensifies gastrointestinal activity by neurogenic stimulation, increases sensitivity to central depressants, heightens response to sympathomimetic compounds, depresses the respiratory center, constricts blood vessels, causes hypertension by central vasomotor stimulation, and lowers body temperature.

INDICATIONS

For the treatment of chronic gouty arthritis when complicated by frequent, recurrent acute attacks of gout.

CONTRAINDICATIONS

Hypersensitivity to this product or to probenecid or colchicine.
Children under 2 years of age.
Not recommended in persons with known blood dyscrasias or uric acid kidney stones.
Therapy with ColBENEMID should not be started until an acute gouty attack has subsided.
Pregnancy: Probenecid crosses the placental barrier and appears in cord blood. Colchicine can arrest cell division in animals and plants. In certain species of animal under certain conditions, colchicine has produced teratogenic effects. The possibility of such effects in humans also has been reported. Because of the colchicine component, ColBENEMID is contraindicated in pregnant patients. The use of any drug in women of childbearing potential requires that the anticipated benefit be weighed against possible hazards.

WARNINGS

Exacerbation of gout following therapy with ColBENEMID may occur; in such cases additional colchicine or other appropriate therapy is advisable.
Probenecid increases plasma concentrations of methotrexate in both animals and humans. In animal studies, increased methotrexate toxicity has been reported. If ColBENEMID is given with methotrexate, the dosage of methotrexate should be reduced and serum levels may need to be monitored.
In patients on ColBENEMID the use of salicylates in either small or large doses is contraindicated because it antagonizes the uricosuric action of probenecid. The biphasic action of salicylates in the renal tubules accounts for the so-called "paradoxical effect" of uricosuric agents. In patients on ColBENEMID who require a mild analgesic agent the use of acetaminophen rather than small doses of salicylates would be preferred.
Rarely, severe allergic reactions and anaphylaxis have been reported with the use of ColBENEMID. Most of these have been reported to occur within several hours after readministration following prior usage of the drug.
The appearance of hypersensitivity reactions requires cessation of therapy with ColBENEMID.
Colchicine has been reported to adversely affect spermatogenesis in animals. Reversible azoospermia has been reported in one patient.

PRECAUTIONS

General
Hematuria, renal colic, costovertebral pain, and formation of uric acid stones associated with the use of ColBENEMID in gouty patients may be prevented by alkalization of the urine and a liberal fluid intake (*see* DOSAGE AND ADMINISTRATION). In these cases when alkali is administered, the acid-base balance of the patient should be watched.
Use with caution in patients with a history of peptic ulcer.
ColBENEMID has been used in patients with some renal impairment but dosage requirements may be increased. ColBENEMID may not be effective in chronic renal insufficiency particularly when the glomerular filtration rate is 30 mL/minute or less.
A reducing substance may appear in the urine of patients receiving probenecid. This disappears with discontinuance of therapy. Suspected glycosuria should be confirmed by using a test specific for glucose.
Adequate animal studies have not been conducted to determine the carcinogenicity potential of probenecid or this drug combination. Since colchicine is an established mutagen, its ability to act as a carcinogen must be suspected and administration of ColBENEMID should involve a weighing of the benefit-vs-risk when long-term administration is contemplated.
Drug Interactions
When probenecid is used to elevate plasma concentrations of penicillin, or other beta-lactams, or when such drugs are given to patients taking probenecid therapeutically, high plasma concentrations of the other drug may increase the incidence of adverse reactions associated with that drug. In the case of penicillin, or other beta-lactams, psychic disturbances have been reported.
The use of salicylates antagonizes the uricosuric action of probenecid (*see* WARNINGS). The uricosuric action of probenecid is also antagonized by pyrazinamide.
Probenecid produces an insignificant increase in free sulfonamide plasma concentrations but a significant increase in total sulfonamide plasma levels. Since probenecid decreases the renal excretion of conjugated sulfonamides, plasma concentrations of the latter should be determined from time to time when a sulfonamide and ColBENEMID are coadministered for prolonged periods. Probenecid may prolong or enhance the action of oral sulfonylureas and thereby increase the risk of hypoglycemia.
It has been reported that patients receiving probenecid require significantly less thiopental for induction of anesthesia. In addition, ketamine and thiopental anesthesia were significantly prolonged in rats receiving probenecid.
The concomitant administration of probenecid increases the mean plasma elimination half-life of a number of drugs which can lead to increased plasma concentrations. These include agents such as indomethacin, acetaminophen, naproxen, ketoprofen, meclofenamate, lorazepam, and rifampin. Although the clinical significance of this observation has not been established, a lower dosage of the drug may be required to produce a therapeutic effect, and increases in dosage of the drug in question should be made cautiously and in small increments when probenecid is being co-administrated. Although specific instances of toxicity due to this potential interaction have not been observed to date, physicians should be alert to this possibility.
Probenecid given concomitantly with sulindac had only a slight effect on plasma sulfide levels, while plasma levels of sulindac and sulfone were increased. Sulindac was shown to produce a modest reduction in the uricosuric action of probenecid, which probably is not significant under most circumstances.
In animals and in humans, probenecid has been reported to increase plasma concentrations of methotrexate (*see* WARNINGS).
Falsely high readings for theophylline have been reported in an *in vitro* study, using the Schack and Waxler technic, when therapeutic concentrations of theophylline and probenecid were added to human plasma.

ADVERSE REACTIONS

The following adverse reactions have been observed and within each category are listed in order of decreasing severity.
Probenecid
Central Nervous System: headache, dizziness.
Metabolic: precipitation of acute gouty arthritis.
Gastrointestinal: hepatic necrosis, vomiting, nausea, anorexia, sore gums.
Genitourinary: nephrotic syndrome, uric acid stones with or without hematuria, renal colic, costovertebral pain, urinary frequency.
Hypersensitivity: anaphylaxis, fever, urticaria, pruritus.
Hematologic: aplastic anemia, leukopenia, hemolytic anemia which in some patients could be related to genetic deficiency of glucose -6- phosphate dehydrogenase in red blood cells, anemia.
Integumentary: dermatitis, alopecia, flushing.
Colchicine
Side effects due to colchicine appear to be a function of dosage. The possibility of increased colchicine toxicity in the presence of hepatic dysfunction should be considered. The appearance of any of the following symptoms may require reduction of dosage or discontinuance of the drug.
Central Nervous System: peripheral neuritis.
Musculoskeletal: muscular weakness.
Gastrointestinal: nausea, vomiting, abdominal pain, or diarrhea may be particularly troublesome in the presence of peptic ulcer or spastic colon.
Hypersensitivity: urticaria.
Hematologic: aplastic anemia, agranulocytosis.
Integumentary: dermatitis, purpura, alopecia.
At toxic doses, colchicine may cause severe diarrhea, generalized vascular damage, and renal damage with hematuria and oliguria.

DOSAGE AND ADMINISTRATION

Therapy with ColBENEMID should not be *started* until an acute gouty attack has subsided. However, if an acute attack is precipitated *during* therapy, ColBENEMID may be continued without changing the dosage, and additional colchicine or other appropriate therapy should be given to control the acute attack.
The recommended adult dosage is 1 tablet of ColBENEMID daily for one week, followed by 1 tablet twice a day thereafter.

Continued on next page

Information on the Merck & Co., Inc. products listed on these pages is the full prescribing information from product circulars in use August 31, 1998. For information, please call 1-800-NSC MERCK [1-800-672-6372].

ColBenemid—Cont.

Some degree of renal impairment may be present in patients with gout. A daily dosage of 2 tablets may be adequate. However, if necessary, the daily dosage may be increased by 1 tablet every four weeks within tolerance (and usually not above 4 tablets per day) if symptoms of gouty arthritis are not controlled or the 24 hour uric acid excretion is not above 700 mg. As noted, probenecid may not be effective in chronic renal insufficiency particularly when the glomerular filtration rate is 30 mL/minute or less.

Gastric intolerance may be indicative of overdosage, and may be corrected by decreasing the dosage.

As uric acid tends to crystallize out of an acid urine, a liberal fluid intake is recommended, as well as sufficient sodium bicarbonate (3 to 7.5 g daily) or potassium citrate (7.5 g daily) to maintain an alkaline urine (see PRECAUTIONS). Alkalization of the urine is recommended until the serum urate level returns to normal limits and tophaceous deposits disappear, i.e., during the period when urinary excretion of uric acid is at a high level. Thereafter, alkalization of the urine and the usual restriction of purine-producing foods may be somewhat relaxed.

ColBENEMID (or probenecid) should be continued at the dosage that will maintain normal serum urate levels. When acute attacks have been absent for six months or more and serum urate levels remain within normal limits, the daily dosage of ColBENEMID may be decreased by 1 tablet every six months. The maintenance dosage should not be reduced to the point where serum urate levels tend to rise.

HOW SUPPLIED

No. 3283—Tablets ColBENEMID are white to off-white, capsule-shaped, scored tablets, coded MSD 614. Each tablet contains 0.5 g of probenecid and 0.5 mg of colchicine. They are supplied as follows:
NDC 0006-0614-68 bottles of 100.

Shown in Product Identification Guide, page 322
Storage
Protect from light.

7876427 Issued May 1989

COMVAX™   ℞
[Haemophilus b conjugate
(meningococcal protein conjugate) and
hepatitis B (recombinant) vaccine]

DESCRIPTION

COMVAX* [Haemophilus b Conjugate (Meningococcal Protein Conjugate) and Hepatitis B (Recombinant) Vaccine] is a sterile bivalent vaccine made of the antigenic components used in producing PedvaxHIB† [Haemophilus b Conjugate Vaccine (Meningococcal Protein Conjugate)] and RECOMBIVAX HB† [Hepatitis B Vaccine (Recombinant)]. These components are the *Haemophilus influenzae* type b capsular polysaccharide (PRP) that is covalently bound to an outer membrane protein complex (OMPC) of *Neisseria meningitidis* and hepatitis B surface antigen (HBsAg) from recombinant yeast cultures.

Haemophilus influenzae type b and *Neisseria meningitidis* serogroup B are grown in complex fermentation media. The PRP is purified from the culture broth by purification procedures which include ethanol fractionation, enzyme digestion, phenol extraction and diafiltration. The OMPC from *Neisseria meningitidis* is purified by detergent extraction, ultracentrifugation, diafiltration and sterile filtration.

The PRP-OMPC conjugate is prepared by the chemical coupling of the highly purified PRP (polyribosylribitol phosphate) of *Haemophilus influenzae* type b (Haemophilus b, Ross strain) to an OMPC of the B11 strain of *Neisseria meningitidis* serogroup B. The coupling of the PRP to the OMPC, which is necessary for enhanced immunogenicity of the PRP, is confirmed by analysis of the conjugate's components following chemical treatment which yields a unique amino acid. After conjugation, the aqueous bulk is then adsorbed onto an aluminum hydroxide adjuvant.

HBsAg is produced in recombinant yeast cells. A portion of the hepatitis B virus gene, coding for HBsAg, is cloned into yeast, and the vaccine for hepatitis B is produced from cultures of this recombinant yeast strain according to methods developed in the Merck Research Laboratories. The antigen is harvested and purified from fermentation cultures of a recombinant strain of the yeast *Saccharomyces cerevisiae* containing the gene for the *adw* subtype of HBsAg. The HBsAg protein is released from the yeast cells by cell disruption and purified by a series of physical and chemical methods. The vaccine contains no detectable yeast DNA but may contain not more than 1% yeast protein. The aqueous bulk is treated with formaldehyde and then adsorbed onto an aluminum hydroxide adjuvant.

After each PRP-OMPC and HBsAg aqueous bulk is adsorbed onto the aluminum hydroxide adjuvant, they are

then combined to produce COMVAX. Each 0.5 mL dose of COMVAX is formulated to contain 7.5 mcg of Haemophilus b PRP, 125 mcg of *Neisseria meningitidis* OMPC, 5 mcg of HBsAg, approximately 225 mcg of aluminum as aluminum hydroxide, and 35 mcg sodium borate (decahydrate) as a pH stabilizer, in 0.9% sodium chloride.

The product contains no preservative.

COMVAX is a sterile suspension for intramuscular injection.

---

*Trademark of MERCK & CO., Inc.
†Registered trademark of MERCK & CO., Inc.

CLINICAL PHARMACOLOGY

Haemophilus influenzae type b Disease

Prior to the introduction of *Haemophilus b* conjugate vaccines, *Haemophilus influenzae* type b (Hib) was the most frequent cause of bacterial meningitis and a leading cause of serious, systemic bacterial disease in young children worldwide.

Hib disease occurred primarily in children under 5 years of age, and in the United States prior to the initiation of a vaccine program was estimated to account for nearly 20,000 cases of invasive infections annually, approximately 12,000 of which were meningitis. The mortality rate from Hib meningitis is about 5%. In addition, up to 35% of survivors develop neurologic sequelae including seizures, deafness, and mental retardation. Other invasive diseases caused by this bacterium include cellulitis, epiglottitis, sepsis, pneumonia, septic arthritis, osteomyelitis, and pericarditis.

Prior to the introduction of the vaccine, it was estimated that 17% of all cases of Hib disease occurred in infants less than 6 months of age. The peak incidence of Hib meningitis occurred between 6 to 11 months of age. Forty-seven percent of all cases occurred by one year of age with the remaining 53% of cases occurring over the next four years.

Among children under 5 years of age, the risk of invasive Hib disease is increased in certain populations including the following

• Daycare attendees
• Lower socio-economic groups
• Blacks (especially those who lack the Km(1) immunoglobulin allotype)
• Caucasians who lack the G2m(23) immunoglobulin allotype)
• Native Americans
• Household contacts of cases
• Individuals with asplenia, sickle cell disease, or antibody deficiency syndromes.

An important virulence factor of the Hib bacterium is its polysaccharide capsule (PRP). Antibody to PRP (anti-PRP) has been shown to correlate with protection against Hib disease. While the anti-PRP level associated with protection using conjugated vaccines has not yet been determined, the level of anti-PRP associated with protection in studies using bacterial polysaccharide immune globulin or nonconjugated PRP vaccines ranged from ≥0.15 to ≥1.0 mcg/mL.

Nonconjugated PRP vaccines are capable of stimulating B-lymphocytes to produce antibody without the help of T-lymphocytes (T-independent). The responses to many other antigens are augmented by helper T-lymphocytes (T-dependent). PedvaxHIB is a PRP-conjugate vaccine in which the PRP is covalently bound to the OMPC carrier producing an antigen which is postulated to convert the T-independent antigen (PRP alone) into a T-dependent antigen resulting in both an enhanced antibody response and immunologic memory.

The protective efficacy of the PRP-OMPC component of COMVAX was demonstrated in a randomized, double-blind, placebo-controlled study involving 3486 Native American (Navajo) infants (The Protective Efficacy Study) who completed the primary two-dose regimen for lyophilized PedvaxHIB. This population has a much higher incidence of Hib disease than the United States population as a whole and also has a lower antibody response to Haemophilus b conjugate vaccines, including PedvaxHIB.

Each infant in this study received two doses of either placebo or lyophilized PedvaxHIB (15 mcg Haemophilus b PRP) with the first dose administered at a mean of 8 weeks of age and the second administered approximately two months later; DTP and OPV were administered concomitantly. In a subset of 416 subjects, lyophilized PedvaxHIB (15 mcg Haemophilus b PRP) induced anti-PRP levels >0.15 mcg/mL in 88% and >1.0 mcg/mL in 52% with a geometric mean titer (GMT) of 0.95 mcg/mL one to three months after the first dose; the corresponding anti-PRP levels one to three months following the second dose were 91% and 60%, respectively, with a GMT of 1.43 mcg/mL. These antibody responses were associated with a high level of protection.

Most subjects were initially followed until 15 to 18 months of age. During this time, 22 cases of invasive Haemophilus b disease occurred in the placebo group (8 cases after the first dose and 14 cases after the second dose) and only 1 case in the vaccine group (none after the first dose and 1 after the second dose). Following the primary two-dose regimen, the protective efficacy of lyophilized PedvaxHIB was calculated

to be 93% with a 95% confidence interval of 57-98%. In the two months between the first and second doses, the difference in number of cases of disease between placebo and vaccine recipients (8 vs 0 cases, respectively) was statistically significant (p=0.008). At termination of the study, placebo recipients were offered vaccine. All original participants were then followed two years and nine months from termination of the study. During this extended follow-up, invasive haemophilus b disease occurred in an additional 7 of the original placebo recipients prior to receiving vaccine and in 1 of the original vaccine recipients (who had received only 1 dose of vaccine). No cases of invasive haemophilus b disease were observed in placebo recipients after they received at least one dose of vaccine. Efficacy for this follow-up period, estimated from person-days at risk, was 96.6% (95 C.I., 72.2-99.9%) in children under 18 months of age and 100% (95 C.I., 23.5-100%) in children over 18 months of age.

Thus, in this study, a protective efficacy of 93% was achieved with an anti-PRP level of >1.0 mcg/mL in 60% of vaccinees and a GMT of 1.43 mcg/mL one to three months after the second dose. In a randomized, multicenter study comparing COMVAX (7.5 mcg Haemophilus b PRP; 5 mcg HBsAg) to concurrent administration of monovalent liquid PedvaxHIB and monovalent RECOMBIVAX HB, anti-PRP levels were measured in 576 of 645 infants who received two doses of COMVAX. In these infants, COMVAX induced anti-PRP levels >0.15 mcg/mL in 95% and >1.0 mcg/mL in 72% with a GMT of 2.5 mcg/mL, approximately two months after the second dose (see Table 1). Because the PRP-OMPC component of COMVAX induces a comparable anti-PRP response (see Table 1), the efficacy of COMVAX is expected to be similar to that obtained with monovalent lyophilized PedvaxHIB in the Protective Efficacy Trial in the prevention of invasive Hib disease.

Hepatitis B Disease

Hepatitis B virus is an important cause of viral hepatitis. There is no specific treatment for this disease. The incubation period for hepatitis B is relatively long; six weeks to six months may elapse between exposure and the onset of clinical symptoms. The prognosis following infection with hepatitis B virus is variable and dependent on at least three factors: (1) Age—infants and younger children usually experience milder initial disease than older persons but are much more likely to remain persistently infected and become at risk of developing serious chronic liver disease; (2) Dose of virus—the higher the dose, the more likely acute icteric hepatitis B will result; and, (3) Severity of associated underlying disease—underlying malignancy or pre-existing hepatic disease predisposes to increased mortality and morbidity.

Hepatitis B infection fails to resolve and progresses to a chronic carrier state in 5 to 10% of older children and adults and in up to 90% of infants; chronic infection also occurs more frequently after initial anicteric hepatitis B than after initial icteric disease. Consequently, carriers of HBsAg frequently give no history of having had recognized acute hepatitis. It has been estimated that more than 285 million people in the world today are persistently infected with hepatitis B virus. The Centers for Disease Control (CDC) estimates that there are approximately 0.75 to 1 million chronic carriers of hepatitis B virus in the USA. Chronic carriers represent the largest human reservoir of hepatitis B virus.

A serious complication of acute hepatitis B virus infection is massive hepatic necrosis while sequelae of chronic hepatitis B include cirrhosis of the liver, chronic active hepatitis, and hepatocellular carcinoma. Chronic carriers of HBsAg appear to be at increased risk of developing hepatocellular carcinoma. Although a number of etiologic factors are associated with development of hepatocellular carcinoma, the single most important etiologic factor appears to be chronic infection with hepatitis B virus.

The vehicles for transmission of the virus are most often blood and blood products but the viral antigen has also been found in tears, saliva, breast milk, urine, semen, and vaginal secretions. Hepatitis B virus is capable of surviving for days on environmental surfaces exposed to body fluids containing hepatitis B virus. Infection may occur when hepatitis B virus, transmitted by infected body fluids, is implanted via mucous surfaces or percutaneously introduced through accidental or deliberate breaks in the skin. Transmission of hepatitis B virus infection is often associated with close interpersonal contact with an infected individual and with crowded living conditions.

Hepatitis B is endemic throughout the world and is a serious medical problem in population groups at increased risk. Because vaccination limited to high-risk individuals has failed to substantially lower the overall incidence of hepatitis B infection, both the Advisory Committee on Immunization Practices (ACIP) and the Committee on Infectious Diseases of the American Academy of Pediatrics (AAP) have also endorsed universal infant immunization as part of a comprehensive strategy for the control of hepatitis B infection.

Multiple clinical studies have defined a protective antibody (anti-HBs) level as 1) 10 or more sample ratio units (SRU or

Table 1
Antibody Responses to COMVAX, liquid PedvaxHIB, and RECOMBIVAX HB

Vaccine	Age (months)	Time	N	Anti-PRP % Subjects with >0.15 mcg/mL	Anti-PRP % Subjects with >1.0 mcg/mL	Anti-PRP GMT (mcg/mL)	N	% Subjects ≥10 mIU/mL Anti-HBs	Anti-HBs GMT
COMVAX		Prevaccination	633	34.4	4.7	0.1	603	10.6	0.6
(7.5 mcg PRP,	2	Dose 1*	620	88.9	51.5	1.0	595	34.3	4.2
5 mcg HBsAg)	4	Dose 2*	576	94.8	72.4	2.5	571	92.1	113.9
	12/15	Dose 3**	570	99.3	92.6	9.5	571	98.4	4467.5
Liquid PedvaxHIB		Prevaccination	208	33.7	5.8	0.1	196	7.1	0.5
(7.5 mcg PRP)	2	Dose 1*	202	90.1	53.5	1.1	198	41.9	5.3
+	4	Dose 2*	186	95.2	76.3	2.8	185	98.4	255.7
RECOMBIVAX HB	12/15	Dose 3**	181	98.9	92.3	10.2	179	100.0	6943.9
(5 mcg HBsAg)									

*Postvaccination responses were determined approximately two months after doses 1 and 2.
**Postvaccination responses were determined approximately one month after administration of dose 3.

S/N) as determined by radioimmunoassay or 2) a positive result as determined by enzyme immunoassay. Note: 10 SRU is comparable to 10 mIU/mL of antibody. The ACIP and an international group of hepatitis B experts consider an anti-HBs titer ≥10 mIU/mL an adequate response to a complete course of hepatitis B vaccine and protective against clinically significant infection (antigenemia with or without clinical disease).

In clinical studies, 99% of 125 infants under 1 year of age born of non-carrier mothers developed a protective level of antibody (anti-HBs ≥10 mIU/mL) after receiving three 2.5-mcg doses of RECOMBIVAX HB at intervals of 0, 1, and 6 months.

In another clinical study, protective levels of antibody were achieved in 98% of 52 healthy infants after receiving 2.5 mcg of RECOMBIVAX HB at 2, 4, and 12 months of age. Protective anti-HBs levels were achieved in 100% of an additional 50 infants who also received three 2.5-mcg doses of RECOMBIVAX HB but at 2, 4, and 15 months of age.

The protective efficacy of three 5-mcg doses of RECOMBIVAX HB has been demonstrated in neonates born of mothers positive for both HBsAg and HBeAg (a core-associated antigenic complex which correlates with high infectivity). In a clinical study of infants who received one dose of Hepatitis B Immune Globulin at birth followed by the recommended three-dose regimen of RECOMBIVAX HB, chronic infection had not occurred in 96% of 130 infants after nine months of follow-up. The estimated efficacy in prevention of chronic hepatitis B infection was 95% as compared to the infection rate in untreated historical controls.

In a randomized, multicenter study comparing COMVAX to liquid PedvaxHIB and RECOMBIVAX HB, anti-HBs levels were measured in 571 of 598 infants who received 3 doses of COMVAX. In these infants, COMVAX induced protective anti-HBs levels (≥10 mIU/mL) in 98%. Because the HBs component of COMVAX induces a comparable anti-HBs response to that obtained with RECOMBIVAX HB, the efficacy of COMVAX is expected to be similar (Table 1).

COMVAX

The safety and immunogenicity of COMVAX (7.5 mcg Haemophilus b PRP, 5 mcg HBsAg) were compared with those of the component monovalent vaccines, liquid PedvaxHIB (7.5 mcg Haemophilus b PRP) and RECOMBIVAX HB (5 mcg HBsAg) given concurrently at separate sites, in combined clinical trials involving 1216 healthy infants. Each infant received a three-dose regimen of either COMVAX (n=856) or liquid PedvaxHIB and RECOMBIVAX HB administered either concomitantly (n=290) or one month apart (n=70) beginning at approximately 2 months of age; other standard pediatric vaccines (M-M-R†II [Measles, Mumps, and Rubella Virus Vaccine Live], DTP [diphtheria, tetanus, pertussis] or DTaP [diphtheria, tetanus, acellular pertussis] or OPV [oral poliovirus vaccine]) were administered concomitantly to most subjects. Antibody responses following the recommended three-dose regimen of COMVAX were similar to those following concurrent administration of the monovalent vaccines according to the same schedule. Table 1 summarizes antibody responses in a subset of infants from one multicenter, randomized, open-label study. These infants received a three-dose regimen of either COMVAX or liquid PedvaxHIB plus RECOMBIVAX HB at approximately 2, 4, and 12–15 months of age.

The anti-HBs GMT associated with the use of COMVAX was 4467.5 mIU/mL and the anti-HBs GMT associated with the concomitant use of monovalent PedvaxHIB plus monovalent RECOMBIVAX HB was 6943.9 mIU/mL. Although the difference is statistically significant (p=0.011), both values are much greater than the level of 10 mIU/mL previously established as marking a protective response to hepatitis B. These GMTs are also higher than those reported in a number of studies wherein healthy neonates or young infants received the currently licensed regimen of RECOMBIVAX HB consisting of 2.5 mcg doses administered on the standard 0, 1 and 6-month schedule. In those studies, the infants developed GMTs of 216–1269 mIU/mL. Another study has shown that infants given 2.5 mcg doses of RECOMBIVAX HB according to the schedule used for COMVAX (2, 4, and 12–15 months of age) developed GMTs of 1356–3424 mIU/mL. While a difference in the GMT between two vaccination regimens may result in differential retention of ≥10 mIU/mL of anti-HBs after a number of years, this is of no apparent clinical significance because of immunologic memory.

[See table 1 above]

Data are currently available for 38 infants in a study in which COMVAX was administered concomitantly with DTaP and IPV at 2 and 4 months of age. Two months after the second dose, 100% of the infants had ≥0.15 mcg/mL of anti-PRP, 84% had ≥1.0 mcg/mL of anti-PRP, 74% had ≥10 mIU/mL of anti-HBs (100% after 3 doses of COMVAX, n=19), and 100% possessed detectable antibody to all three types of poliovirus.

An additional 1756 infants were involved in clinical trials where COMVAX was administered concomitantly with either an investigational pneumococcal polysaccharide protein conjugate vaccine or an investigational preparation of diphtheria, tetanus, pertussis, and enhanced inactivated poliovirus vaccine. The serious adverse experience information for these subjects is provided in this circular (see ADVERSE REACTIONS).

Interchangeability of COMVAX and Licensed Haemophilus b Conjugate Vaccines or Recombinant Hepatitis B Vaccines

One multicenter study has shown similar safety profiles and similar anti-PRP and anti-HBs responses among children vaccinated with a three-dose course of COMVAX or a three-dose course of monovalent PedvaxHIB and monovalent RECOMBIVAX HB. Therefore, it is expected that responses would be comparable if COMVAX were used as a component of a mixed Haemophilus b conjugate vaccine series involving PedvaxHIB or a mixed hepatitis B vaccine series involving RECOMBIVAX HB. Published studies presenting limited clinical data have examined the interchangeability of other licensed Haemophilus b conjugate vaccines and PedvaxHIB. In addition, a clinical study has shown that in healthy neonates a regimen of hepatitis B vaccine can be initiated with another currently licensed hepatitis B vaccine and completed with RECOMBIVAX HB.

INDICATIONS AND USAGE

COMVAX is indicated for vaccination against invasive disease caused by *Haemophilus influenzae* type b and against infection caused by all known subtypes of hepatitis B virus in infants 6 weeks to 15 months of age born of HBsAg negative mothers. Infants born of HBsAg positive mothers should receive Hepatitis B Immune Globulin and Hepatitis B Vaccine (Recombinant) at birth and should complete the hepatitis B vaccination series given according to a particular schedule (see manufacturer's circular for Hepatitis B Vaccine [Recombinant]).

Infants born of mothers of unknown HBsAg status should receive Hepatitis B Vaccine (Recombinant) at birth and should complete the hepatitis B vaccination series given according to a particular schedule (see manufacturer's circular for Hepatitis B Vaccine [Recombinant]).

Vaccination with COMVAX should ideally begin at approximately 2 months of age or as soon thereafter as possible. In order to complete the three-dose regimen of COMVAX, vaccination should be initiated no later than 10 months of age. Infants in whom vaccination with a PRP-OMPC-containing product (i.e., PedvaxHIB, COMVAX) is not initiated until 11 months of age do not require three doses of PRP-OMPC; however, three doses of an HBsAg-containing product are required for complete vaccination against hepatitis B, regardless of age. For infants and children not vaccinated according to the recommended schedule see DOSAGE AND ADMINISTRATION.

Use With Other Vaccines

Results from clinical studies indicate that COMVAX can be administered concomitantly with DTP, OPV, eIPV (enhanced inactivated poliovirus vaccine), VARIVAX† [Varicella Virus Vaccine Live (Oka/Merck)], and M-M-R II, and with a booster dose of DTaP at approximately 15 months of age, using separate sites and syringes for injectable vaccines (see CLINICAL PHARMACOLOGY, *COMVAX*). No impairment of immune response to these individually tested vaccine antigens was demonstrated.

COMVAX has been administered concomitantly with the primary series of DTaP to a limited number of infants. No serious vaccine-related adverse events were reported. Immune response data are satisfactory for COMVAX but are currently unavailable for DTaP (see CLINICAL PHARMACOLOGY, *COMVAX*).

COMVAX SHOULD NOT BE USED IN INFANTS YOUNGER THAN 6 WEEKS OF AGE (see PRECAUTIONS).

CONTRAINDICATIONS

Hypersensitivity to any component of the vaccine.

WARNINGS

If COMVAX is used in persons with malignancies or those receiving immunosuppressive therapy or who are otherwise immunocompromised, the expected immune response may not be obtained.

Patients who develop symptoms suggestive of hypersensitivity after an injection should not receive further injections of the vaccine (see CONTRAINDICATIONS).

PRECAUTIONS

General

COMVAX will not protect against invasive disease caused by *Haemophilus influenzae* other than type b or against invasive disease (such as meningitis or sepsis) caused by other microorganisms. COMVAX will not prevent hepatitis by other viruses known to infect the liver. Because of the long incubation period for hepatitis B, it is possible for unrecognized infection to be present at the time the vaccine is given. The vaccine may not prevent hepatitis B in such patients.

As for any vaccine, adequate treatment provisions, including epinephrine, should be available for immediate use should an anaphylactic or anaphylactoid reaction occur.

As with other vaccines, COMVAX may not induce protective antibody levels immediately following vaccination and may not result in a protective antibody response in all individuals given the vaccine.

As reported with Haemophilus b Polysaccharide Vaccine and another Haemophilus b Conjugate Vaccine, cases of Haemophilus b disease may occur in the week after vaccination, prior to the onset of the protective effects of the vaccines.

The decision to administer or delay vaccination because of current or recent febrile illness depends on the severity of symptoms and on the etiology of the disease. The ACIP has recommended that immunization should be delayed during the course of an acute febrile illness. All vaccines can be administered to persons with minor illnesses such as diarrhea, mild upper-respiratory infection with or without low-grade fever, or other low-grade febrile illness. Persons with moderate or severe febrile illness should be vaccinated as soon as they have recovered from the acute phase of the illness.

Instructions to Health-care Provider

The health-care provider should determine the current health status and previous vaccination history of the vaccinee.

The health-care provider should question the patient, parent, or guardian about reactions to a previous dose of COMVAX, PedvaxHIB or other Haemophilus b conjugate vaccines or RECOMBIVAX HB or other hepatitis B vaccines.

Information for Patients

The health-care provider should provide the vaccine information required to be given with each vaccination to the patient, parent or guardian.

The health-care provider should inform the patient, parent or guardian of the benefits and risks associated with vaccination. For risks associated with vaccination, see WARNINGS, PRECAUTIONS, and ADVERSE REACTIONS.

Patients, parents and guardians should be instructed to report any serious adverse reactions to their health-care provider who in turn should report such events to the U.S. De-

Continued on next page

Information on the Merck & Co., Inc. products listed on these pages is the full prescribing information from product circulars in use August 31, 1998. For information, please call 1-800-NSC MERCK [1-800-672-6372].

Consult 1999 PDR® supplements and future editions for revisions

Comvax—Cont.

partment of Health and Human Services through the Vaccine Adverse Event Reporting System (VAERS), 1-800-822-7967.

Laboratory Test Interactions

Sensitive tests (e.g., Latex Agglutination Kits) may detect PRP derived from the vaccine in the urine of some vaccinees for at least 30 days following vaccination with lyophilized PedvaxHIB; in clinical studies with lyophilized PedvaxHIB, such children demonstrated a normal immune response to the vaccine. It is not known whether antigenuria will occur after vaccination with COMVAX.

Carcinogenesis, Mutagenesis, Impairment of Fertility

COMVAX has not been evaluated for its carcinogenic or mutagenic potential, or its potential to impair fertility.

Pregnancy

Pregnancy Category C: Animal reproduction studies have not been conducted with COMVAX. It is also not known whether COMVAX can cause fetal harm when administered to a pregnant woman or can affect reproduction capacity. COMVAX is not recommended for use in women of childbearing age.

Pediatric Use

COMVAX has been shown to be generally well tolerated and highly immunogenic in infants 6 weeks to 15 months of age. See DOSAGE AND ADMINISTRATION for recommended dosage schedules.

Safety and effectiveness of COMVAX in infants below the age of 6 weeks and above the age of 15 months have not been established. However, studies have demonstrated that PedvaxHIB is safe and immunogenic when administered to infants and children up to the age of 71 months and RECOMBIVAX HB is safe and immunogenic in persons of all ages.

COMVAX should not be used in infants younger than 6 weeks of age because this will lead to a reduced anti-PRP response and may lead to immune tolerance (impaired ability to respond to subsequent exposure to the PRP antigen). Infants born of HBsAg-positive mothers should not receive COMVAX but instead should receive Hepatitis B Immune Globulin and Hepatitis B Vaccine (Recombinant) at birth and should complete the hepatitis B vaccination series given according to a particular schedule (see manufacturer's circular for Hepatitis B Vaccine [Recombinant]). (See DOSAGE AND ADMINISTRATION.)

ADVERSE REACTIONS

In clinical trials involving the administration of 6705 doses of COMVAX to 2612 healthy infants 6 weeks to 15 months of age, COMVAX was generally well tolerated. Of these infants, 856 were involved in clinical trials (730 infants in controlled, randomized trials) in which most received COMVAX concomitantly with other licensed pediatric vaccines. These 856 infants were monitored for both serious and non-serious adverse experiences. The remaining 1756 infants were involved in trials where COMVAX was administered concomitantly with either an investigational pneumococcal polysaccharide protein conjugate vaccine or an investigational preparation of diphtheria, tetanus, pertussis, and inactivated poliovirus vaccine and were under surveillance for serious adverse experiences. The serious adverse experiences for these subjects are described following Table 2.

Adverse experiences observed within a five-day period following each dose of COMVAX were generally similar in type and frequency to those observed in infants who received concurrent injections of liquid PedvaxHIB and RECOMBIVAX HB at separate sites.

As judged by the investigators, no serious vaccine-related adverse experiences were observed during clinical trials.

Table 2 summarizes the local reactions and systemic complaints within five days of vaccination that were reported to occur among ≥1.0% of children given a three-dose course of COMVAX as well as the frequencies of these events among children in the study given concomitant injections of monovalent PedvaxHIB and RECOMBIVAX HB. In this randomized, multicenter study, 882 infants were assigned in a 3:1 ratio to receive either COMVAX or PedvaxHIB plus RECOMBIVAX HB at 2, 4, and 12–15 months of age, with the children monitored daily for five days after each injection for local reactions and systemic complaints.

[See table 2 below]

Among 856 infants from combined clinical trials who were monitored for both serious and non-serious adverse experiences, the following serious events were reported to occur in 13 infants during a 14-day period following vaccination with COMVAX (usually coadministered with other pediatric vaccines). These adverse experiences are grouped by case: viral infection; febrile seizure; asthma; diarrhea, vomiting, acidosis, dehydration, hypoglycemia, and seizure disorder; bacterial infection; bronchiolitis and reflux esophagitis; dehydration and fever; asthma, respiratory congestion, and tachypnea; asthma and upper respiratory infection; urinary tract infection and vomiting; pneumonia and asthma; apnea and reflux esophagitis; and vitreous hemorrhage. A causal relationship to the vaccine is unknown; however, these serious adverse events were judged not to be related to vaccination with COMVAX by the investigator.

Among 1756 infants who received COMVAX concomitantly with either an investigational pneumococcal polysaccharide protein conjugate vaccine or an investigational preparation of diphtheria, tetanus, pertussis, and inactivated poliovirus vaccine, the following serious events were reported to occur in 9 infants during a 14-day period following vaccination with COMVAX. These adverse experiences are grouped by case: respiratory syncytial virus; respiratory distress and otitis media; bronchiolitis in two vaccinees; viral gastroenteritis; skull fracture; bronchiolitis, respiratory syncytial virus, and pneumonia; respiratory syncytial virus and bronchiolitis; and upper respiratory infection, viral (see CLINICAL PHARMACOLOGY). A causal relationship to the vaccine is unknown; however, these serious events were judged not to be related to vaccination with COMVAX by the investigator.

In a group of infants (n=126) given a three-dose course of COMVAX after previously receiving a dose of Hepatitis B Vaccine (Recombinant) at or shortly after birth, the type, frequency, and severity of adverse experiences did not appear to be greater or different from those observed in infants given only COMVAX.

As with any vaccine, there is the possibility that broad use of COMVAX could reveal adverse experiences not observed in clinical trials.

Potential Adverse Effects

In addition, a variety of adverse effects have been reported with marketed use of either PedvaxHIB or RECOMBIVAX HB in infants and children through 71 months of age. These adverse effects are listed below.

PedvaxHIB
Hypersensitivity
Rarely, angioedema
Hematologic / Lymphatic
Lymphadenopathy
Nervous System
Febrile seizures
Skin
Sterile injection-site abscess; pain at the injection site
RECOMBIVAX HB
Hypersensitivity
Anaphylaxis and symptoms of hypersensitivity including reports of rash, pruritus, urticaria, edema, angioedema, arthralgia, dyspnea, hypotension, erythema multiforme, and ecchymoses
Cardiovascular System
Tachycardia; syncope
Digestive System
Elevation of liver enzymes
Hematologic
Increased erythrocyte sedimentation rate; thrombocytopenia
Musculoskeletal System
Arthritis
Nervous System
Bell's Palsy; Guillain-Barré Syndrome
Psychiatric / Behavioral
Agitation; somnolence; irritability
Skin
Stevens-Johnson Syndrome; alopecia.
Special Senses
Conjunctivitis; visual disturbances

DOSAGE AND ADMINISTRATION

FOR INTRAMUSCULAR ADMINISTRATION

Do not inject intravenously, intradermally, or subcutaneously.

Recommended Schedule

Infants born of HBsAg negative mothers should be vaccinated with three 0.5 mL doses of COMVAX, ideally at 2, 4, and 12-15 months of age. If the recommended schedule cannot be followed exactly, the interval between the first two doses should be at least two months and the interval between the second and third dose should be as close as possible to eight to eleven months.

Infants born of HBsAg-positive mothers should receive Hepatitis B Immune Globulin and Hepatitis B Vaccine (Recombinant) at birth and should complete the hepatitis B vaccination series given according to a particular schedule (see manufacturer's circular for Hepatitis B Vaccine [Recombinant]).

Infants born of mothers of unknown HBsAg status should receive Hepatitis B Vaccine (Recombinant) at birth and

Table 2
Local Reactions and Systemic Complaints Within 5 Days After Injection Reported to Occur in ≥1.0%† of Children Given a 3-Dose Course of COMVAX Compared to These Events in Children Given Concomitant Injections of PedvaxHIB and RECOMBIVAX HB

Event	Injection 1‡		Injection 2‡		Injection 3	
	COMVAX™ (N=660) %	PedvaxHIB and RECOMBIVAX HB*** (N=221) %	COMVAX™ (N=645) %	PedvaxHIB and RECOMBIVAX HB*** (N=213) %	COMVAX™ (N=593) %	PedvaxHIB and RECOMBIVAX HB*** (N=193) %
Injection Site Reactions						
Pain/Soreness*	34.5	37.6	24.3	25.8	23.9	21.2
Erythema (>1 in.)*	22.4 (2.7)	25.8 (2.7)	25.7 (1.4)	23.5 (3.3)	27.2 (3.0)	24.4 (1.6)
Swelling/Induration (>1 in.)*	27.6 (3.0)	33.5 (4.1)	30.4 (2.9)	31.0 (3.8)	27.2 (3.2)	29.5 (4.1)
Systemic Complaints						
Irritability*	57.0	46.6	50.7	44.1	32.2	29.0
Somnolence*	49.5	47.1	37.4	31.9	21.1	22.3
Crying—						
unusual, high pitched*	10.6	8.6	6.7	2.3	2.9	3.6
not otherwise specified	2.3	2.3	1.4	2.3	0.7	1.6
prolonged (>4 hrs.)*	2.4	2.3	0.8	1.4	0.2	0
Anorexia	3.9	2.3	2.0	0.9	0.8	0.5
Vomiting	2.1	1.8	2.5	0.9	1.0	1.6
Otitis media	0.5	0	2.0	1.4	2.7	1.6
Fever (°F, rectal equiv.)**						
101.0–102.9	14.2	11.9	13.8	12.2	10.5	6.4
≥103.0	0.8	0	1.6	1.4	2.7	4.3
Diarrhea	1.7	1.8	0.8	0.9	2.2	0.5
Upper respiratory infection	0.5	0.5	1.1	0.9	1.3	0.5
Rash	0.8	0	0.9	0	0.8	0.5
Rhinorrhea	0.2	0	1.1	0.9	1.3	2.1
Respiratory congestion	0.6	0.5	1.2	0.9	0.3	0.5
Cough	0.2	0	0.9	0.5	0.2	1.0
Candidiasis, oral	0.3	0.5	0.8	0	0.2	0
Rash, diaper	0.5	0.5	0.5	0.9	0.2	0

†Overall frequency of each event listed above is ≥1% even though the frequency after a given dose may be <1%.

‡Most children received DTP and OPV concomitantly with the first two doses of COMVAX or PedvaxHIB and RECOMBIVAX HB.

*Events prompted for on Vaccination Report Card given to parents/guardians of vaccinees.

**N for injections 1, 2, and 3 equals 655, 639, and 588, respectively, for COMVAX; N for injections 1, 2, and 3 equals 218, 213, and 187, respectively, for PedvaxHIB and RECOMBIVAX HB.

***Injection site reactions for PedvaxHIB and RECOMBIVAX HB based on occurrence with either of the monovalent components.

should complete the hepatitis B vaccination series given according to a particular schedule (see manufacturer's circular for Hepatitis B Vaccine [Recombinant]).

The subsequent administration of COMVAX for completion of the hepatitis B vaccination series in infants who were born of HBsAg positive mothers and received HBIG or infants born of mothers of unknown status has not been studied.

COMVAX should not be administered to any infant before the age of 6 weeks.

Modified Schedules

Children previously vaccinated with one or more doses of either hepatitis B vaccine or Haemophilus b conjugate vaccine

Children who receive one dose of hepatitis B vaccine at or shortly after birth may be administered COMVAX on the schedule of 2, 4, and 12–15 months of age. There are no data to support the use of a three-dose series of COMVAX in infants who have previously received more than one dose of hepatitis B vaccine. However, COMVAX may be administered to children otherwise scheduled to receive concurrent RECOMBIVAX HB and PedvaxHIB.

Children not vaccinated according to recommended schedule

Vaccination schedules for children not vaccinated according to the recommended schedule should be considered on an individual basis. The number of doses of a PRP-OMPC-containing product (i.e., COMVAX, PedvaxHIB) depends on the age that vaccination is begun. An infant 2 to 10 months of age should receive three doses of a product containing PRP-OMPC. An infant 11 to 14 months of age should receive two doses of a product containing PRP-OMPC. A child 15 to 71 months of age should receive one dose of a product containing PRP-OMPC. Infants and children, regardless of age, should receive three doses of an HBsAg-containing product. COMVAX is for intramuscular injection. The *anterolateral thigh* is the recommended site for intramuscular injection in infants. Data suggests that injections given in the buttocks frequently are given into fatty tissue instead of into muscle. Such injections have resulted in a lower seroconversion rate (for hepatitis B vaccine) than was expected.

Injection must be accomplished with a needle long enough to ensure intramuscular deposition of the vaccine. The ACIP has recommended that for intramuscular injections, the needle should be of sufficient length to reach the muscle mass itself. In a clinical trial with COMVAX (see CLINICAL PHARMACOLOGY, *COMVAX,* Table 1) vaccination was accomplished with a needle length of 5/8 inches in accordance with ACIP recommendations in effect at that time. ACIP currently recommends that needles of longer length (7/8 to 1 inch) be used.

The vaccine should be used as supplied; no reconstitution is necessary.

Shake well before withdrawal and use. Thorough agitation is necessary to maintain suspension of the vaccine.

Parenteral drug products should be inspected visually for extraneous particulate matter and discoloration prior to administration whenever solution and container permit. After thorough agitation, COMVAX is a slightly opaque, white suspension.

It is important to use a separate sterile syringe and needle for each patient to prevent transmission of infectious agents from one person to another.

HOW SUPPLIED

No. 4843—COMVAX is supplied as 7.5 mcg Haemophilus b PRP and 5 mcg HBsAg/0.5 mL in a 0.5 mL single dose vial. **NDC** 0006-4843-00.

No. 4898—COMVAX is supplied as 7.5 mcg Haemophilus b PRP and 5 mcg HBsAg/0.5 mL in a 0.5 mL single dose vial, in a box of 10 single dose vials. **NDC** 0006-4898-00.

Storage

Store vaccine at 2–8°C (36–46°F). Storage above or below the recommended temperature may reduce potency.

DO NOT FREEZE since freezing destroys potency.

9024701   Issued December 1996
COPYRIGHT © MERCK & CO., Inc., 1996
All rights reserved

CORTONE® Acetate Injectable Suspension   **R**
(Cortisone Acetate), U.S.P.
(Formerly called Sterile Suspension CORTONE®
Acetate)

For intramuscular injection only
NOT FOR INTRAVENOUS USE

DESCRIPTION

Cortisone acetate, a synthetic adrenocortical steroid, is a white or practically white, odorless, crystalline powder. It is stable in air. It is insoluble in water. The molecular weight is 402.49. It is designated chemically as 21-(acetyloxy)-17-hydroxypregn-4-ene-3,11,20-trione. The empirical formula is $C_{23}H_{30}O_6$ and the structural formula is:
[See chemical structure at top of next column]

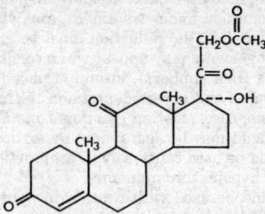

CORTONE* Acetate (Cortisone Acetate) Injectable Suspension is a sterile suspension containing 50 mg per milliliter of cortisone acetate in an aqueous medium (pH 5.0 to 7.0). Inactive ingredients per mL: sodium chloride, 9 mg; polysorbate 80, 4 mg; sodium carboxymethylcellulose, 5 mg; Water for Injection q.s. 1 mL. Benzyl alcohol, 9 mg, added as preservative.

No attempt should be made to alter CORTONE Acetate Injectable Suspension. Diluting it or mixing it with other substances may affect the state of suspension or change the rate of absorption and reduce its effectiveness.

---

*Registered trademark of MERCK & CO., Inc.

ACTIONS

CORTONE Acetate Injectable Suspension has a slow onset but long duration of action when compared with more soluble preparations. When daily corticosteroid therapy is required and oral therapy is not feasible, the required daily dosage may be given in a single intramuscular injection of this preparation.

Naturally occurring glucocorticoids (hydrocortisone and cortisone), which also have salt-retaining properties, are used as replacement therapy in adrenocortical deficiency states. They are also used for their potent anti-inflammatory effects in disorders of many organ systems.

Glucocorticoids cause profound and varied metabolic effects. In addition, they modify the body's immune responses to diverse stimuli.

INDICATIONS

When oral therapy is not feasible:
1. *Endocrine disorders*
Primary or secondary adrenocortical insufficiency (hydrocortisone or cortisone is the drug of choice; synthetic analogs may be used in conjunction with mineralocorticoids where applicable; in infancy, mineralocorticoid supplementation is of particular importance)
Acute adrenocortical insufficiency (hydrocortisone or cortisone is the drug of choice; mineralocorticoid supplementation may be necessary, particularly when synthetic analogs are used)
Preoperatively, and in the event of serious trauma or illness, in patients with known adrenal insufficiency or when adrenocortical reserve is doubtful
Shock unresponsive to conventional therapy if adrenocortical insufficiency exists or is suspected
    Congenital adrenal hyperplasia
    Nonsuppurative thyroiditis
    Hypercalcemia associated with cancer
2. *Rheumatic disorders*
As adjunctive therapy for short-term administration (to tide the patient over an acute episode or exacerbation) in:
    Post-traumatic osteoarthritis
    Synovitis of osteoarthritis
    Rheumatoid arthritis, including juvenile rheumatoid arthritis (selected cases may require low-dose maintenance therapy)
    Acute and subacute bursitis
    Epicondylitis
    Acute nonspecific tenosynovitis
    Acute gouty arthritis
    Psoriatic arthritis
    Ankylosing spondylitis
3. *Collagen diseases*
During an exacerbation or as maintenance therapy in selected cases of:
    Systemic lupus erythematosus
    Acute rheumatic carditis
    Systemic dermatomyositis (polymyositis)
4. *Dermatologic diseases*
    Pemphigus
    Severe erythema multiforme (Stevens-Johnson syndrome)
    Exfoliative dermatitis
    Bullous dermatitis herpetiformis
    Severe seborrheic dermatitis
    Severe psoriasis
    Mycosis fungoides
5. *Allergic states*
Control of severe or incapacitating allergic conditions intractable to adequate trials of conventional treatment in:

    Bronchial asthma
    Contact dermatitis
    Atopic dermatitis
    Serum sickness
    Seasonal or perennial allergic rhinitis
    Drug hypersensitivity reactions
    Urticarial transfusion reactions
    Acute noninfectious laryngeal edema (epinephrine is the drug of first choice)
6. *Ophthalmic diseases*
Severe acute and chronic allergic and inflammatory processes involving the eye, such as:
    Herpes zoster ophthalmicus
    Iritis, iridocyclitis
    Chorioretinitis
    Diffuse posterior uveitis and choroiditis
    Optic neuritis
    Sympathetic ophthalmia
    Anterior segment inflammation
    Allergic conjunctivitis
    Keratitis
    Allergic corneal marginal ulcers
7. *Gastrointestinal diseases*
To tide the patient over a critical period of the disease in:
    Ulcerative colitis (Systemic therapy)
    Regional enteritis (Systemic therapy)
8. *Respiratory diseases*
    Symptomatic sarcoidosis
    Berylliosis
    Fulminating or disseminated pulmonary tuberculosis when used concurrently with appropriate antituberculous chemotherapy
    Loeffler's syndrome not manageable by other means
    Aspiration pneumonitis
9. *Hematologic disorders*
    Acquired (autoimmune) hemolytic anemia
    Erythroblastopenia (RBC anemia)
    Congenital (erythroid) hypoplastic anemia
10. *Neoplastic diseases*
    For palliative management of:
    Leukemias and lymphomas in adults
    Acute leukemia of childhood
11. *Edematous states*
    To induce diuresis or remission of proteinuria in the nephrotic syndrome, without uremia, of the idiopathic type, or that due to lupus erythematosus
12. *Miscellaneous*
    Tuberculous meningitis with subarachnoid block or impending block when used concurrently with appropriate antituberculous chemotherapy
    Trichinosis with neurologic or myocardial involvement.

CONTRAINDICATIONS

Systemic fungal infections
Hypersensitivity to any component of this product

WARNINGS

Because rare instances of anaphylactoid reactions have occurred in patients receiving parenteral corticosteroid therapy, appropriate precautionary measures should be taken prior to administration, especially when the patient has a history of allergy to any drug. Anaphylactoid and hypersensitivity reactions have been reported for CORTONE Acetate Injectable Suspension (see ADVERSE REACTIONS).

In patients on corticosteroid therapy subjected to any unusual stress, increased dosage of rapidly acting corticosteroids before, during, and after the stressful situation is indicated.

Drug-induced secondary adrenocortical insufficiency may result from too rapid withdrawal of corticosteroids and may be minimized by gradual reduction of dosage. This type of relative insufficiency may persist for months after discontinuation of therapy; therefore, in any situation of stress occurring during that period, hormone therapy should be reinstituted. If the patient is receiving steroids already, dosage may have to be increased. Since mineralocorticoid secretion may be impaired, salt and/or a mineralocorticoid should be administered concurrently.

Corticosteroids may mask some signs of infection, and new infections may appear during their use. There may be decreased resistance and inability to localize infection when corticosteroids are used. Moreover, corticosteroids may affect the nitroblue-tetrazolium test for bacterial infection and produce false negative results.

Continued on next page

Cortone Acetate Injectable—Cont.

In cerebral malaria, a double-blind trial has shown that the use of corticosteroids is associated with prolongation of coma and a higher incidence of pneumonia and gastrointestinal bleeding.

Corticosteroids may activate latent amebiasis. Therefore, it is recommended that latent or active amebiasis be ruled out before initiating corticosteroid therapy in any patient who has spent time in the tropics or any patient with unexplained diarrhea.

Prolonged use of corticosteroids may produce posterior subcapsular cataracts, glaucoma with possible damage to the optic nerves, and may enhance the establishment of secondary ocular infections due to fungi or viruses.

Usage in pregnancy. Since adequate human reproduction studies have not been done with corticosteroids, use of these drugs in pregnancy or in women of childbearing potential requires that the anticipated benefits be weighed against the possible hazards to the mother and embryo or fetus. Infants born of mothers who have received substantial doses of corticosteroids during pregnancy should be carefully observed for signs of hypoadrenalism.

Corticosteroids appear in breast milk and could suppress growth, interfere with endogenous corticosteroid production, or cause other unwanted effects. Mothers taking pharmacologic doses of corticosteroids should be advised not to nurse.

Average and large doses of cortisone or hydrocortisone can cause elevation of blood pressure, salt and water retention, and increased excretion of potassium. These effects are less likely to occur with the synthetic derivatives except when used in large doses. Dietary salt restriction and potassium supplementation may be necessary. All corticosteroids increase calcium excretion.

Administration of live virus vaccines, including smallpox, is contraindicated in individuals receiving immunosuppressive doses of corticosteroids. If inactivated viral or bacterial vaccines are administered to individuals receiving immunosuppressive doses of corticosteroids, the expected serum antibody response may not be obtained.

Patients who are on drugs which suppress the immune system are more susceptible to infections than healthy individuals. Chickenpox and measles, for example, can have a more serious or even fatal course in non-immune patients on corticosteroids. In such patients who have not had these diseases, particular care should be taken to avoid exposure. The risk of developing a disseminated infection varies among individuals and can be related to the dose, route and duration of corticosteroid administration as well as to the underlying disease. If exposed to chickenpox, prophylaxis with varicella zoster immune globulin (VZIG) may be indicated. If chickenpox develops, treatment with antiviral agents may be considered. If exposed to measles, prophylaxis with immune globulin (IG) may be indicated. (See the respective package inserts for VZIG and IG for complete prescribing information.)

Similarly, corticosteroids should be used with great care in patients with known or suspected Strongyloides (threadworm) infestation. In such patients, corticosteroid-induced immunosuppression may lead to Strongyloides hyperinfection and dissemination with widespread larval migration, often accompanied by severe enterocolitis and potentially fatal gram-negative septicemia.

The use of CORTONE Acetate Injectable Suspension in active tuberculosis should be restricted to those cases of fulminating or disseminated tuberculosis in which the corticosteroid is used for the management of the disease in conjunction with an appropriate antituberculous regimen.

If corticosteroids are indicated in patients with latent tuberculosis or tuberculin reactivity, close observation is necessary as reactivation of the disease may occur. During prolonged corticosteroid therapy, these patients should receive chemoprophylaxis.

Literature reports suggest an apparent association between use of corticosteroids and left ventricular free wall rupture after a recent myocardial infarction; therefore, therapy with corticosteroids should be used with great caution in these patients.

PRECAUTIONS

CORTONE Acetate Injectable Suspension, like many other steroid formulations, is sensitive to heat. Therefore, it should not be autoclaved when it is desirable to sterilize the exterior of the vial.

Following prolonged therapy, withdrawal of corticosteroids may result in symptoms of the corticosteroid withdrawal syndrome including fever, myalgia, arthralgia, and malaise. This may occur in patients even without evidence of adrenal insufficiency.

There is an enhanced effect of corticosteroids in patients with hypothyroidism and in those with cirrhosis.

Corticosteroids should be used cautiously in patients with ocular herpes simplex for fear of corneal perforation.

The lowest possible dose of corticosteroid should be used to control the condition under treatment, and when reduction in dosage is possible, the reduction must be gradual.

Psychic derangements may appear when corticosteroids are used, ranging from euphoria, insomnia, mood swings, personality changes, and severe depression to frank psychotic manifestations. Also, existing emotional instability or psychotic tendencies may be aggravated by corticosteroids.

Aspirin should be used cautiously in conjunction with corticosteroids in hypoprothrombinemia.

Steroids should be used with caution in nonspecific ulcerative colitis, if there is a probability of impending perforation, abscess, or other pyogenic infection, also in diverticulitis, fresh intestinal anastomoses, active or latent peptic ulcer, renal insufficiency, hypertension, osteoporosis, and myasthenia gravis. Signs of peritoneal irritation following gastrointestinal perforation in patients receiving large doses of corticosteroids may be minimal or absent. Fat embolism has been reported as a possible complication of hypercortisonism.

When large doses are given, some authorities advise that antacids be administered between meals to help to prevent peptic ulcer.

Steroids may increase or decrease motility and number of spermatozoa in some patients.

Phenytoin, phenobarbital, ephedrine, and rifampin may enhance the metabolic clearance of corticosteroids, resulting in decreased blood levels and lessened physiologic activity, thus requiring adjustment in corticosteroid dosage.

The prothrombin time should be checked frequently in patients who are receiving corticosteroids and coumarin anticoagulants at the same time because of reports that corticosteroids have altered the response to the anticoagulants. Studies have shown that the usual effect produced by adding corticosteroids is inhibition of response to coumarins, although there have been some conflicting reports of potentiation not substantiated by studies.

When corticosteroids are administered concomitantly with potassium-depleting diuretics, patients should be observed closely for development of hypokalemia.

Injection of a steroid into an infected site is to be avoided.

Information for Patients

Susceptible patients who are on immunosuppressant doses of corticosteroids should be warned to avoid exposure to chickenpox or measles. Patients should also be advised that if they are exposed, medical advice should be sought without delay.

Pediatric Use

Growth and development of pediatric patients on prolonged corticosteroid therapy should be carefully followed.

ADVERSE REACTIONS

Fluid and electrolyte disturbances
 Sodium retention
 Fluid retention
 Congestive heart failure in susceptible patients
 Potassium loss
 Hypokalemic alkalosis
 Hypertension
Musculoskeletal
 Muscle weakness
 Steroid myopathy
 Loss of muscle mass
 Osteoporosis
 Vertebral compression fractures
 Aseptic necrosis of femoral and humeral heads
 Pathologic fracture of long bones
 Tendon rupture
Gastrointestinal
 Peptic ulcer with possible subsequent perforation and hemorrhage
 Perforation of the small and large bowel, particularly in patients with inflammatory bowel disease
 Pancreatitis
 Abdominal distention
 Ulcerative esophagitis
Dermatologic
 Impaired wound healing
 Thin fragile skin
 Petechiae and ecchymoses
 Erythema
 Increased sweating
 May suppress reactions to skin tests
 Other cutaneous reactions, such as allergic dermatitis, urticaria, angioneurotic edema
Neurologic
 Convulsions
 Increased intracranial pressure with papilledema (pseudotumor cerebri) usually after treatment
 Vertigo
 Headache
 Psychic disturbances
Endocrine
 Menstrual irregularities
 Development of cushingoid state

 Suppression of growth in children
 Secondary adrenocortical and pituitary unresponsiveness, particularly in times of stress, as in trauma, surgery, or illness
 Decreased carbohydrate tolerance
 Manifestations of latent diabetes mellitus
 Increased requirements for insulin or oral hypoglycemic agents in diabetics
 Hirsutism
Ophthalmic
 Posterior subcapsular cataracts
 Increased intraocular pressure
 Glaucoma
 Exophthalmos
Metabolic
 Negative nitrogen balance due to protein catabolism
Cardiovascular
 Myocardial rupture following recent myocardial infarction (see WARNINGS)
Other
 Anaphylactoid or hypersensitivity reactions
 Thromboembolism
 Weight gain
 Increased appetite
 Nausea
 Malaise

The following *additional* adverse reactions are related to parenteral corticosteroid therapy:
 Rare instances of blindness associated with intralesional therapy around the face and head
 Hyperpigmentation or hypopigmentation
 Subcutaneous and cutaneous atrophy
 Sterile abscess

OVERDOSAGE

Reports of acute toxicity and/or death following overdosage of glucocorticoids are rare. In the event of overdosage, no specific antidote is available; treatment is supportive and symptomatic.

The intraperitoneal LD_{50} of cortisone acetate in female mice was 1405 mg/kg.

DOSAGE AND ADMINISTRATION

NOT FOR INTRAVENOUS USE

For intramuscular injection only

DOSAGE REQUIREMENTS ARE VARIABLE AND MUST BE INDIVIDUALIZED ON THE BASIS OF THE DISEASE AND THE RESPONSE OF THE PATIENT.

The initial dosage varies from 20 to 300 mg a day depending on the disease being treated. In less severe diseases doses lower than 20 mg may suffice, while in severe diseases doses higher than 300 mg may be required. The initial dosage should be maintained or adjusted until the patient's response is satisfactory. If a satisfactory clinical response does not occur after a reasonable period of time, discontinue CORTONE Acetate Injectable Suspension and transfer the patient to other therapy.

After a favorable initial response, the proper maintenance dosage should be determined by decreasing the initial dosage in small amounts to the lowest dosage that maintains an adequate clinical response.

Patients should be observed closely for signs that might require dosage adjustment, including changes in clinical status resulting from remissions or exacerbations of the disease, individual drug responsiveness, and the effect of stress (e.g., surgery, infection, trauma). During stress it may be necessary to increase dosage temporarily.

If the drug is to be stopped after more than a few days of treatment, it usually should be withdrawn gradually.

HOW SUPPLIED

No. 7069—CORTONE Acetate Injectable Suspension is a white, mobile suspension, each mL containing 50 mg cortisone acetate, and is supplied as follows:
NDC 0006-7069-10 in 10 mL vials.
Storage
Sensitive to heat. Do not autoclave.
Protect from freezing.
      7411918   Issued February 1997

CORTONE® Acetate Tablets
(Cortisone Acetate), U.S.P.

℞

DESCRIPTION

Glucocorticoids are adrenocortical steroids, both naturally occurring and synthetic, which are readily absorbed from the gastrointestinal tract.

Cortisone acetate is a white or practically white, odorless, crystalline powder. It is stable in air. It is insoluble in water. The molecular weight is 402.49. It is designated chemically

as 21-(acetyloxy)-17-hydroxypregn-4-ene-3,11,20-trione. The empirical formula is $C_{23}H_{30}O_6$ and the structural formula is:

CORTONE* Acetate (Cortisone Acetate) tablets contain 25 mg of cortisone acetate in each tablet.
Inactive ingredients are lactose, magnesium stearate, and starch.

*Registered trademark of MERCK & CO., INC.

ACTIONS

Naturally occurring glucocorticoids (hydrocortisone and cortisone), which also have salt-retaining properties, are used as replacement therapy in adrenocortical deficiency states. They are also used for their potent anti-inflammatory effects in disorders of many organ systems.
Glucocorticoids cause profound and varied metabolic effects. In addition, they modify the body's immune responses to diverse stimuli.

INDICATIONS

1. *Endocrine Disorders*
Primary or secondary adrenocortical insufficiency (hydrocortisone or cortisone is the first choice; synthetic analogs may be used in conjunction with mineralocorticoids where applicable; in infancy mineralocorticoid supplementation is of particular importance).
  Congenital adrenal hyperplasia
  Nonsuppurative thyroiditis
  Hypercalcemia associated with cancer

2. *Rheumatic Disorders*
As adjunctive therapy for short-term administration (to tide the patient over an acute episode or exacerbation) in:
  Psoriatic arthritis
  Rheumatoid arthritis, including juvenile rheumatoid arthritis (selected cases may require low-dose maintenance therapy)
  Ankylosing spondylitis
  Acute and subacute bursitis
  Acute nonspecific tenosynovitis
  Acute gouty arthritis
  Post-traumatic osteoarthritis
  Synovitis of osteoarthritis
  Epicondylitis

3. *Collagen Diseases*
During an exacerbation or as maintenance therapy in selected cases of—
  Systemic lupus erythematosus
  Acute rheumatic carditis
  Systemic dermatomyositis (polymyositis)

4. *Dermatologic Diseases*
  Pemphigus
  Bullous dermatitis herpetiformis
  Severe erythema multiforme (Stevens-Johnson syndrome)
  Exfoliative dermatitis
  Mycosis fungoides
  Severe psoriasis
  Severe seborrheic dermatitis

5. *Allergic States*
Control of severe or incapacitating allergic conditions intractable to adequate trials of conventional treatment:
  Seasonal or perennial allergic rhinitis
  Bronchial asthma
  Contact dermatitis
  Atopic dermatitis
  Serum sickness
  Drug hypersensitivity reactions

6. *Ophthalmic Diseases*
Severe acute and chronic allergic and inflammatory processes involving the eye and its adnexa, such as—
  Allergic conjunctivitis
  Keratitis
  Allergic corneal marginal ulcers
  Herpes zoster ophthalmicus
  Iritis and iridocyclitis
  Chorioretinitis
  Anterior segment inflammation
  Diffuse posterior uveitis and choroiditis
  Optic neuritis
  Sympathetic ophthalmia

7. *Respiratory Diseases*
  Symptomatic sarcoidosis
  Loeffler's syndrome not manageable by other means
  Berylliosis
  Fulminating or disseminated pulmonary tuberculosis when used concurrently with appropriate antituberculous chemotherapy
  Aspiration pneumonitis

8. *Hematologic Disorders*
  Idiopathic thrombocytopenic purpura in adults
  Secondary thrombocytopenia in adults
  Acquired (autoimmune) hemolytic anemia
  Erythroblastopenia (RBC anemia)
  Congenital (erythroid) hypoplastic anemia

9. *Neoplastic Diseases*
For palliative management of:
  Leukemias and lymphomas in adults
  Acute leukemia of childhood

10. *Edematous States*
To induce a diuresis or remission of proteinuria in the nephrotic syndrome, without uremia, of the idiopathic type or that due to lupus erythematosus

11. *Gastrointestinal Diseases*
To tide the patient over a critical period of the disease in:
  Ulcerative colitis
  Regional enteritis

12. *Miscellaneous*
Tuberculous meningitis with subarachnoid block or impending block when used concurrently with appropriate antituberculous chemotherapy
Trichinosis with neurologic or myocardial involvement

CONTRAINDICATIONS

Systemic fungal infections
Hypersensitivity to this product

WARNINGS

In patients on corticosteroid therapy subjected to unusual stress, increased dosage of rapidly acting corticosteroids before, during, and after the stressful situation is indicated.
Drug-induced secondary adrenocortical insufficiency may result from too rapid withdrawal of corticosteroids and may be minimized by gradual reduction of dosage. This type of relative insufficiency may persist for months after discontinuation of therapy; therefore, in any situation of stress occurring during that period, hormone therapy should be reinstituted. If the patient is receiving steroids already, dosage may have to be increased. Since mineralocorticoid secretion may be impaired, salt and/or a mineralocorticoid should be administered concurrently.
Corticosteroids may mask some signs of infection, and new infections may appear during their use. There may be decreased resistance and inability to localize infection when corticosteroids are used. Moreover, corticosteroids may affect the nitroblue-tetrazolium test for bacterial infection and produce false negative results.
In cerebral malaria, a double-blind trial has shown that the use of corticosteroids is associated with prolongation of coma and a higher incidence of pneumonia and gastrointestinal bleeding.
Corticosteroids may activate latent amebiasis. Therefore, it is recommended that latent or active amebiasis be ruled out before initiating corticosteroid therapy in any patient who has spent time in the tropics or any patient with unexplained diarrhea.
Prolonged use of corticosteroids may produce posterior subcapsular cataracts, glaucoma with possible damage to the optic nerves, and may enhance the establishment of secondary ocular infections due to fungi or viruses.
Usage in pregnancy: Since adequate human reproduction studies have not been done with corticosteroids, use of these drugs in pregnancy or in women of childbearing potential requires that the anticipated benefits be weighed against the possible hazards to the mother and embryo or fetus. Infants born of mothers who have received substantial doses of corticosteroids during pregnancy should be carefully observed for signs of hypoadrenalism.
Corticosteroids appear in breast milk and could suppress growth, interfere with endogenous corticosteroid production, or cause other unwanted effects. Mothers taking pharmacologic doses of corticosteroids should be advised not to nurse.
Average and large doses of hydrocortisone or cortisone can cause elevation of blood pressure, salt and water retention, and increased excretion of potassium. These effects are less likely to occur with the synthetic derivatives except when used in large doses. Dietary salt restriction and potassium supplementation may be necessary. All corticosteroids increase calcium excretion.
Administration of live virus vaccines, including smallpox, is contraindicated in individuals receiving immunosuppressive doses of corticosteroids. If inactivated viral or bacterial vaccines are administered to individuals receiving immunosuppressive doses of corticosteroids, the expected serum antibody response may not be obtained. However, immunization procedures may be undertaken in patients who are receiving corticosteroids as replacement therapy, e.g., for Addison's disease.
Patients who are on drugs which suppress the immune system are more susceptible to infections than healthy individuals. Chickenpox and measles, for example, can have a more serious or even fatal course in non-immune patients on corticosteroids. In such patients who have not had these diseases, particular care should be taken to avoid exposure. The risk of developing a disseminated infection varies among individuals and can be related to the dose, route and duration of corticosteroid administration as well as to the underlying disease. If exposed to chickenpox, prophylaxis with varicella zoster immune globulin (VZIG) may be indicated. If chickenpox develops, treatment with antiviral agents may be considered. If exposed to measles, prophylaxis with immune globulin (IG) may be indicated. (See the respective package inserts for VZIG and IG for complete prescribing information.)
Similarly, corticosteroids should be used with great care in patients with known or suspected Strongyloides (threadworm) infestation. In such patients, corticosteroid-induced immunosuppression may lead to Strongyloides hyperinfection and dissemination with widespread larval migration, often accompanied by severe enterocolitis and potentially fatal gram-negative septicemia.
The use of CORTONE Acetate tablets in active tuberculosis should be restricted to those cases of fulminating or disseminated tuberculosis in which the corticosteroid is used for the management of the disease in conjunction with an appropriate antituberculous regimen.
If corticosteroids are indicated in patients with latent tuberculosis or tuberculin reactivity, close observation is necessary as reactivation of the disease may occur. During prolonged corticosteroid therapy, these patients should receive chemoprophylaxis.
Literature reports suggest an apparent association between use of corticosteroids and left ventricular free wall rupture after a recent myocardial infarction; therefore, therapy with corticosteroids should be used with great caution in these patients.

PRECAUTIONS

Following prolonged therapy, withdrawal of corticosteroids may result in symptoms of the corticosteroid withdrawal syndrome including fever, myalgia, arthralgia, and malaise. This may occur in patients even without evidence of adrenal insufficiency.
There is an enhanced effect of corticosteroids in patients with hypothyroidism and in those with cirrhosis.
Corticosteroids should be used cautiously in patients with ocular herpes simplex because of possible corneal perforation.
The lowest possible dose of corticosteroid should be used to control the condition under treatment, and when reduction in dosage is possible, the reduction should be gradual.
Psychic derangements may appear when corticosteroids are used, ranging from euphoria, insomnia, mood swings, personality changes, and severe depression, to frank psychotic manifestations. Also, existing emotional instability or psychotic tendencies may be aggravated by corticosteroids.
Aspirin should be used cautiously in conjunction with corticosteroids in hypoprothrombinemia.
Steroids should be used with caution in nonspecific ulcerative colitis, if there is a probability of impending perforation, abscess, or other pyogenic infection, diverticulitis, fresh intestinal anastomoses, active or latent peptic ulcer, renal insufficiency, hypertension, osteoporosis, and myasthenia gravis. Signs of peritoneal irritation following gastrointestinal perforation in patients receiving large doses of corticosteroids may be minimal or absent. Fat embolism has been reported as a possible complication of hypercortisonism.
When large doses are given, some authorities advise that corticosteroids be taken with meals and antacids taken between meals to help to prevent peptic ulcer.
Steroids may increase or decrease motility and number of spermatozoa in some patients.
Phenytoin, phenobarbital, ephedrine, and rifampin may enhance the metabolic clearance of corticosteroids, resulting in decreased blood levels and lessened physiologic activity, thus requiring adjustment in corticosteroid dosage.
The prothrombin time should be checked frequently in patients who are receiving corticosteroids and coumarin anticoagulants at the same time because of reports that corticosteroids have altered the response to these anticoagu-

Continued on next page

Cortone Acetate Tablets—Cont.

lants. Studies have shown that the usual effect produced by adding corticosteroids is inhibition of response to coumarins, although there have been some conflicting reports of potentiation not substantiated by studies.

When corticosteroids are administered concomitantly with potassium-depleting diuretics, patients should be observed closely for development of hypokalemia.

Information for Patients

Susceptible patients who are on immunosuppressant doses of corticosteroids should be warned to avoid exposure to chickenpox or measles. Patients should also be advised that if they are exposed, medical advice should be sought without delay.

Pediatric Use

Growth and development of pediatric patients on prolonged corticosteroid therapy should be carefully followed.

ADVERSE REACTIONS

Fluid and Electrolyte Disturbances
    Sodium retention
    Fluid retention
    Congestive heart failure in susceptible patients
    Potassium loss
    Hypokalemic alkalosis
    Hypertension
Musculoskeletal
    Muscle weakness
    Steroid myopathy
    Loss of muscle mass
    Osteoporosis
    Vertebral compression fractures
    Aseptic necrosis of femoral and humeral heads
    Pathologic fracture of long bones
    Tendon rupture
Gastrointestinal
    Peptic ulcer with possible perforation and hemorrhage
    Perforation of the small and large bowel, particularly in
    patients with inflammatory bowel disease
    Pancreatitis
    Abdominal distention
    Ulcerative esophagitis
Dermatologic
    Impaired wound healing
    Thin fragile skin
    Petechiae and ecchymoses
    Erythema
    Increased sweating
    May suppress reactions to skin tests
    Other cutaneous reactions, such as allergic dermatitis,
urticaria, angioneurotic edema
Neurologic
    Convulsions
    Increased intracranial pressure with papilledema (pseudotumor cerebri), usually after treatment
    Vertigo
    Headache
    Psychic disturbances
Endocrine
    Menstrual irregularities
    Development of cushingoid state
    Suppression of growth in children
    Secondary adrenocortical and pituitary unresponsiveness, particularly in times of stress, as in trauma, surgery, or illness
    Decreased carbohydrate tolerance
    Manifestations of latent diabetes mellitus
    Increased requirements for insulin or oral hypoglycemic
    agents in diabetics
    Hirsutism
Ophthalmic
    Posterior subcapsular cataracts
    Increased intraocular pressure
    Glaucoma
    Exophthalmos
Metabolic
    Negative nitrogen balance due to protein catabolism
Cardiovascular
    Myocardial rupture following recent myocardial infarction (see WARNINGS)
Other
    Hypersensitivity
    Thromboembolism
    Weight gain
    Increased appetite
    Nausea
    Malaise

OVERDOSAGE

Reports of acute toxicity and/or death following overdosage of glucocorticoids are rare. In the event of overdosage, no specific antidote is available; treatment is supportive and symptomatic.

The intraperitoneal LD_{50} of cortisone acetate in female mice was 1405 mg/kg.

DOSAGE AND ADMINISTRATION

For oral administration
DOSAGE REQUIREMENTS ARE VARIABLE AND MUST BE INDIVIDUALIZED ON THE BASIS OF THE DISEASE AND THE RESPONSE OF THE PATIENT.

The initial dosage varies from 25 to 300 mg a day depending on the disease being treated. In less severe diseases doses lower than 25 mg may suffice, while in severe diseases doses higher than 300 mg may be required. The initial dosage should be maintained or adjusted until the patient's response is satisfactory. If satisfactory clinical response does not occur after a reasonable period of time, discontinue CORTONE Acetate tablets and transfer the patient to other therapy.

After a favorable initial response, the proper maintenance dosage should be determined by decreasing the initial dosage in small amounts to the lowest dosage that maintains an adequate clinical response.

Patients should be observed closely for signs that might require dosage adjustment, including changes in clinical status resulting from remissions or exacerbations of the disease, individual drug responsiveness, and the effect of stress (e.g., surgery, infection, trauma). During stress it may be necessary to increase dosage temporarily.

If the drug is to be stopped after more than a few days of treatment, it usually should be withdrawn gradually.

HOW SUPPLIED

No. 7063—Tablets Cortone Acetate, 25 mg each, are white, round, scored, compressed tablets, coded MSD 219 on one side and CORTONE on the other. They are supplied as follows:

NDC 0006-0219-68 in bottles of 100.

Shown in Product Identification Guide, page 322
7930632   Issued February 1997

COSMEGEN® for Injection   ℞
(Dactinomycin for Injection), U.S.P.
(Actinomycin D)

WARNING

Dactinomycin is extremely corrosive to soft tissue. If extravasation occurs during intravenous use, severe damage to soft tissues will occur. In at least one instance, this has led to contracture of the arms.

DOSAGE

The dosage of COSMEGEN* (Dactinomycin for Injection) is calculated in micrograms (mcg). The usual adult dosage is 500 micrograms (0.5 mg) daily intravenously for a maximum of five days. The dosage for adults or children should not exceed 15 mcg/kg or 400–600 mcg/square meter of body surface daily intravenously for five days. Calculation of the dosage for obese or edematous patients should be on the basis of surface area in an effort to relate dosage to lean body mass.

---

*Registered trademark of MERCK & CO., INC.

DESCRIPTION

Dactinomycin is one of the actinomycins, a group of antibiotics produced by various species of *Streptomyces*. Dactinomycin is the principal component of the mixture of actinomycins produced by *Streptomyces parvullus*. Unlike other species of *Streptomyces*, this organism yields an essentially pure substance that contains only traces of similar compounds differing in the amino acid content of the peptide side chains. The empirical formula is $C_{62}H_{86}N_{12}O_{16}$ and the structural formula is:

[See chemical structure at top of next column]

COSMEGEN is a sterile, yellow lyophilized powder for injection by the intravenous route or by regional perfusion after reconstitution. Each vial contains 0.5 mg (500 mcg) of dactinomycin and 20.0 mg of mannitol.

CLINICAL PHARMACOLOGY

Action
Generally, the actinomycins exert an inhibitory effect on gram-positive and gram-negative bacteria and on some fungi. However, the toxic properties of the actinomycins (including dactinomycin) in relation to antibacterial activity are such as to preclude their use as antibiotics in the treatment of infectious diseases.

Because the actinomycins are cytotoxic, they have an antineoplastic effect which has been demonstrated in experimental animals with various types of tumor implant. This cytotoxic action is the basis for their use in the palliative treatment of certain types of cancer.

Pharmacokinetics and Metabolism
Results of a study in patients with malignant melanoma indicate that dactinomycin (^{3}H actinomycin D) is minimally metabolized, is concentrated in nucleated cells, and does not penetrate the blood-brain barrier. Approximately 30% of the dose was recovered in urine and feces in one week. The terminal plasma half-life for radioactivity was approximately 36 hours.

INDICATIONS AND USAGE

Wilms' Tumor
The neoplasm responding most frequently to COSMEGEN is Wilms' tumor. With low doses of both dactinomycin and radiotherapy, temporary objective improvement may be as good as and may last longer than with higher doses of each given alone. In the National Wilms' Tumor study, combination therapy with dactinomycin and vincristine together with surgery and radiotherapy, was shown to have significantly improved the prognosis of patients in groups II and III. Dactinomycin and vincristine were given for a total of seven cycles, so that maintenance therapy continued for approximately 15 months.

Postoperative radiotherapy in group I patients and optimal combination chemotherapy for those in group IV are unsettled issues. About 70 percent of lung metastases have disappeared with an appropriate combination of radiation, dactinomycin and vincristine.

Rhabdomyosarcoma
Temporary regression of the tumor and beneficial subjective results have occurred with dactinomycin in rhabdomyosarcoma which, like most soft tissue sarcomas, is comparatively radio-resistant.

Several groups have reported successful use of cyclophosphamide, vincristine, dactinomycin and doxorubicin hydrochloride in various combinations. Effective combinations have included vincristine and dactinomycin; vincristine, dactinomycin and cyclophosphamide (VAC therapy) and all four drugs in sequence. At present, the most effective treatment for children with inoperable or metastatic rhabdomyosarcoma has been VAC chemotherapy. Two-thirds of these children were doing well without evidence of disease at a median time of three years after diagnosis.

Carcinoma of Testis and Uterus
The sequential use of dactinomycin and methotrexate, along with meticulous monitoring of human chorionic gonadotropin levels until normal, has resulted in survival in the majority of women with metastatic choriocarcinoma. Sequential therapy is used if there is:

1. Stability in gonadotropin titers following two successive courses of an agent.
2. Rising gonadotropin titers during treatment.
3. Severe toxicity preventing adequate therapy.

In patients with nonmetastatic choriocarcinoma, dactinomycin or methotrexate or both, have been used successfully, with or without surgery.

Dactinomycin has been beneficial as a single agent in the treatment of metastatic nonseminomatour testicular carcinoma when used in cycles of 500 mcg/day for five consecutive days, every 6–8 weeks for periods of four months or longer.

Other Neoplasms
Dactinomycin has been given intravenously or by regional perfusion, either alone or with other antineoplastic compounds or x-ray therapy, in the palliative treatment of Ewing's sarcoma and sarcoma botryoides. For nonmetastatic Ewing's sarcoma, promising results were obtained when dactinomycin (45 mcg/m^2) and cyclophosphamide (1200 mg/m^2) were given sequentially and with radiotherapy, over an 18 month period. Those with metastatic disease remain the subject of continued investigation with a more aggressive chemotherapeutic regimen employed initially.

Temporary objective improvement and relief of pain and discomfort have followed the use of dactinomycin usually in

conjunction with radiotherapy for sarcoma botryoides. This palliative effect ranges from transitory inhibition of tumor growth to a considerable but temporary regression in tumor size.

COSMEGEN (Dactinomycin for Injection) and Radiation Therapy

Much evidence suggests that dactinomycin potentiates the effects of x-ray therapy. The converse also appears likely; i.e., dactinomycin may be more effective when radiation therapy also is given.

With combined dactinomycin-radiation therapy, the normal skin, as well as the buccal and pharyngeal mucosa, show early erythema. A smaller than usual x-ray dose when given with dactinomycin causes erythema and vesiculation, which progress more rapidly through the stages of tanning and desquamation. Healing may occur in four to six weeks rather than two to three months. Erythema from previous x-ray therapy may be reactivated by dactinomycin alone, even when irradiation occurred many months earlier, and especially when the interval between the two forms of therapy is brief. This potentiation of radiation effect represents a special problem when the irradiation treatment area includes the mucous membrane. When irradiation is directed toward the nasopharynx, the combination may produce severe oropharyngeal mucositis. *Severe reactions may ensue if high doses of both dactinomycin and radiation therapy are used or if the patient is particularly sensitive to such combined therapy.*

Because of this potentiating effect, dactinomycin may be tried in radio-sensitive tumors not responding to doses of x-ray therapy that can be tolerated. Objective improvement in tumor size and activity may be observed when lower, better tolerated doses of both types of therapy are employed.

COSMEGEN (Dactinomycin for Injection) and Perfusion Technic

Dactinomycin alone or with other antineoplastic agents has also been given by the isolation-perfusion technic, either as palliative treatment or as an adjunct to resection of a tumor. Some tumors considered resistant to chemotherapy and radiation therapy may respond when the drug is given by the perfusion technic. Neoplasms in which dactinomycin has been tried by this technic include various types of sarcoma, carcinoma, and adenocarcinoma.

In some instances tumors regressed, pain was relieved for variable periods, and surgery made possible. On other occasions, however, the outcome has been less favorable. Nevertheless, in selected cases, the drug by perfusion may provide more effective palliation than when given systemically.

Dactinomycin by the isolation-perfusion technic offers certain advantages, provided leakage of the drug through the general circulation into other areas of the body is minimal. By this technic the drug is in continuous contact with the tumor for the duration of treatment. The dose may be increased well over that used by the systemic route, usually without adding to the danger of toxic effects. If the agent is confined to an isolated part, it should not interfere with the patient's defense mechanism. Systemic absorption of toxic products from neoplastic tissue can be minimized by removing the perfusate when the procedure is finished.

CONTRAINDICATIONS

If dactinomycin is given at or about the time of infection with chicken pox or herpes zoster, a severe generalized disease, which may result in death, may occur.

PRECAUTIONS

General

COSMEGEN should be administered only under the supervision of a physician who is experienced in the use of cancer chemotherapeutic agents.

This drug is highly toxic and both powder and solution must be handled and administered with care. Inhalation of dust or vapors and contact with skin or mucous membranes, especially those of the eyes, must be avoided. Should accidental eye contact occur, copious irrigation with water should be instituted immediately, followed by prompt ophthalmologic consultation. Should accidental skin contact occur, the affected part must be irrigated immediately with copious amounts of water for at least 15 minutes.

As with all antineoplastic agents, dactinomycin is a toxic drug and very careful and frequent observation of the patient for adverse reactions is necessary. These reactions may involve any tissue of the body. The possibility of an anaphylactoid reaction should be borne in mind.

Increased incidence of gastrointestinal toxicity and marrow suppression has been reported when dactinomycin was given with x-ray therapy.

Particular caution is necessary when administering dactinomycin within two months of irradiation for the treatment of right-sided Wilms' tumor, since hepatomegaly and elevated SGOT levels have been noted.

Nausea and vomiting due to dactinomycin make it necessary to give this drug intermittently. It is extremely important to observe the patient daily for toxic side effects when multiple chemotherapy is employed, since a full course of therapy occasionally is not tolerated. If stomatitis, diarrhea, or severe hemopoietic depression appear during therapy, these drugs should be discontinued until the patient has recovered.

Recent reports indicate an increased incidence of second primary tumors following treatment with radiation and antineoplastic agents, such as dactinomycin. Multi-modal therapy creates the need for careful, long-term observation of cancer survivors.

Laboratory Tests

Many abnormalities of renal, hepatic, and bone marrow function have been reported in patients with neoplastic disease and receiving dactinomycin. It is advisable to check renal, hepatic, and bone marrow functions frequently.

Drug/Laboratory Test Interactions

It has been reported that dactinomycin may interfere with bioassay procedures for the determination of antibacterial drug levels.

Carcinogenesis, Mutagenesis, Impairment of Fertility

The International Agency on Research on Cancer has judged that dactinomycin is a positive carcinogen in animals. Local sarcomas were produced in mice and rats after repeated subcutaneous or intraperitoneal injection. Mesenchymal tumors occurred in male F344 rats given intraperitoneal injections of 0.05 mg/kg, 2 to 5 times per week for 18 weeks. The first tumor appeared at 23 weeks.

Dactinomycin has been shown to be mutagenic in a number of test systems *in vitro* and *in vivo* including human fibroblasts and leucocytes, and HELA cells. DNA damage and cytogenetic effects have been demonstrated in the mouse and the rat.

Adequate fertility studies have not been reported.

Pregnancy

Pregnancy Category C.

COSMEGEN has been shown to cause malformations and embryotoxicity in the rat, rabbit and hamster when given in doses of 50–100 mcg/kg intravenously (3–7 times the maximum recommended human dose). There are no adequate and well-controlled studies in pregnant women. COSMEGEN should be used during pregnancy only if the potential benefit justifies the potential risk to the fetus.

Nursing Mothers

It is not known whether this drug is excreted in human milk. Because many drugs are excreted in human milk and because of the potential for serious adverse reactions in nursing infants from COSMEGEN, a decision should be made whether to discontinue nursing or to discontinue the drug, taking into account the importance of the drug to the mother.

Pediatric Use

The greater frequency of toxic effects of dactinomycin in infants suggest that this drug should be given to infants only over the age of 6 to 12 months.

ADVERSE REACTIONS

Toxic effects (excepting nausea and vomiting) usually do not become apparent until two to four days after a course of therapy is stopped, and may not be maximal before one to two weeks have elapsed. Deaths have been reported. However, adverse reactions are usually reversible on discontinuance of therapy. They include the following:

Miscellaneous: malaise, fatigue, lethargy, fever, myalgia, proctitis, hypocalcemia.

Oral: cheilitis, dysphagia, esophagitis, ulcerative stomatitis, pharyngitis.

Gastrointestinal: anorexia, nausea, vomiting, abdominal pain, diarrhea, gastrointestinal ulceration, liver toxicity including ascites, hepatomegaly, hepatitis, and liver function test abnormalities. Nausea and vomiting, which occur early during the first few hours after administration, may be alleviated by giving antiemetics.

Hematologic: anemia, even to the point of aplastic anemia, agranulocytosis, leukopenia, thrombopenia, pancytopenia, reticulopenia. Platelet and white cell counts should be done *daily* to detect severe hemopoietic depression. If either count markedly decreases, the drug should be withheld to allow marrow recovery. This often takes up to three weeks.

Dermatologic: alopecia, skin eruptions, acne, flare-up of erythema or increased pigmentation of previously irradiated skin.

Soft tissues. Dactinomycin is extremely corrosive. If extravasation occurs during intravenous use, severe damage to soft tissues will occur. In at least one instance, this has led to contracture of the arms.

OVERDOSAGE

The intravenous LD_{50} of COSMEGEN in the rat is 460 mcg/kg.

DOSAGE AND ADMINISTRATION

Toxic reactions due to dactinomycin are frequent and may be severe (see ADVERSE REACTIONS), thus limiting in many instances the amount that may be given. However, the severity of toxicity varies markedly and is only partly dependent on the dose employed. The drug must be given in short courses.

Intravenous Use

The dosage of dactinomycin varies depending on the tolerance of the patient, the size and location of the neoplasm, and the use of other forms of therapy. It may be necessary to decrease the usual dosages suggested below when other chemotherapy or x-ray therapy is used concomitantly or has been used previously.

The dosage for adults or children should not exceed 15 mcg/kg or 400–600 mcg/square meter of body surface daily intravenously for five days. Calculation of the dosage for obese or edematous patients should be on the basis of surface area in an effort to relate dosage to lean body mass.

Adults: The usual adult dosage is 500 mcg (0.5 mg) daily intravenously for a maximum of five days.

Children: In children 15 mcg (0.015 mg) per kilogram of body weight is given intravenously daily for five days. An alternative schedule is a total dosage of 2500 mcg (2.5 mg) per square meter of body surface given intravenously over a one week period.

In both adults and children, a second course may be given after at least three weeks have elapsed, provided all signs of toxicity have disappeared.

Reconstitute COSMEGEN by adding 1.1 ml of **Sterile Water for Injection (without preservative)** using aseptic precautions. The resulting solution of dactinomycin will contain approximately 500 mcg (0.5 mg) per mL.

Parenteral drug products should be inspected visually for particulate matter and discoloration prior to administration, whenever solution and container permit. When reconstituted, COSMEGEN is a clear, gold-colored solution.

Once reconstituted, the solution of dactinomycin can be added to infusion solutions of Dextrose Injection 5 percent or Sodium Chloride Injection either directly or to the tubing of a running intravenous infusion.

Although reconstituted COSMEGEN is chemically stable, the product does not contain a preservative and accidental microbial contamination might result. Any unused portion should be discarded. Use of water containing preservatives (benzyl alcohol or parabens) to reconstitute COSMEGEN for Injection, results in the formation of a precipitate.

Partial removal of dactinomycin from intravenous solutions by cellulose ester membrane filters used in some intravenous in-line filters has been reported.

Since dactinomycin is extremely corrosive to soft tissue, precautions for materials of this nature should be observed.

If the drug is given directly into the vein without the use of an infusion, the "two-needle technic" should be used. Reconstitute and withdraw the calculated dose from the vial with one sterile needle. Use another sterile needle for direct injection into the vein.

Discard any unused portion of the dactinomycin solution.

Isolation-Perfusion Technic

The dosage schedules and the technic itself vary from one investigator to another; the published literature, therefore, should be consulted for details. In general, the following doses are suggested:

50 mcg (0.05 mg) per kilogram of body weight for lower extremity or pelvis.

35 mcg (0.035 mg) per kilogram of body weight for upper extremity.

It may be advisable to use lower doses in obese patients, or when previous chemotherapy or radiation therapy has been employed.

Complications of the perfusion technic are related mainly to the amount of drug that escapes into the systemic circulation and may consist of hemopoietic depression, absorption of toxic products from massive destruction of neoplastic tissue, increased susceptibility to infection, impaired wound healing, and superficial ulceration of the gastric mucosa. Other side effects may include edema of the extremity involved, damage to soft tissues of the perfused area, and (potentially) venous thrombosis.

HOW SUPPLIED

No. 3298—COSMEGEN for Injection is a lyophilized powder. In the dry form the compound is an amorphous yellow powder. The solution is clear and gold-colored. COSMEGEN for Injection is supplied as follows:

NDC 0006-3298-22 in vials containing 0.5 mg (500 micrograms) of dactinomycin and 20.0 mg of mannitol

(6505-00-902-1222, 0.5 mg).

Continued on next page

Information on the Merck & Co., Inc. products listed on these pages is the full prescribing information from product circulars in use August 31, 1998. For information, please call 1-800-NSC MERCK [1-800-672-6372].

Cosmegen—Cont.

Storage
Store at controlled room temperature, 15–30°C (59–86°F). Protect from light, humidity, and excessive heat.
Special Handling
Due to the drug's toxic and mutagenic properties, appropriate precautions including the use of appropriate safety equipment are recommended for the preparation of COSMEGEN for parenteral administration. The National Institutes of Health presently recommends that the preparation of injectable antineoplastic drugs should be performed in a Class II laminar flow biological safety cabinet and that personnel preparing drugs of this class should wear surgical gloves and a closed front surgical-type gown with knit cuffs.
9000829 Issued February 1997
COPYRIGHT © MERCK & CO., INC., 1983
All rights reserved

COSOPT™ Sterile Ophthalmic Solution ℞
(dorzolamide hydrochloride-timolol maleate ophthalmic solution)

DESCRIPTION

COSOPT* (dorzolamide hydrochloride-timolol maleate ophthalmic solution) is the combination of a topical carbonic anhydrase inhibitor and a topical beta-adrenergic receptor blocking agent.
Dorzolamide hydrochloride is described chemically as: (4*S*-*trans*)-4-(ethylamino)-5,6-dihydro-6-methyl-4*H*-thieno[2,3-*b*]thiopyran-2-sulfonamide 7,7-dioxide monohydrochloride. Dorzolamide hydrochloride is optically active. The specific rotation is:

[α] 25°C (C=1, water)=~-17°.
405 nm

Its empirical formula is $C_{10}H_{16}N_2O_4S_3$•HCl and its structural formula is:

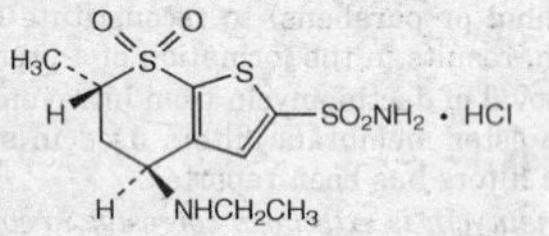

Dorzolamide hydrochloride has a molecular weight of 360.91. It is a white to off-white, crystalline powder, which is soluble in water and slightly soluble in methanol and ethanol.
Timolol maleate is described chemically as: (-)-1-(*tert*-butylamino)-3-[(4-morpholino-1,2,5-thiadiazol-3-yl)oxy]-2-propanol maleate (1:1) (salt). Timolol maleate possesses an asymmetric carbon atom in its structure and is provided as the levo-isomer. The nominal optical rotation of timolol maleate is:

[α] 25°C in 1N HCl (C=5)=-12.2°.
405 nm

Its molecular formula is $C_{13}H_{24}N_4O_3S$•$C_4H_4O_4$ and its structural formula is:

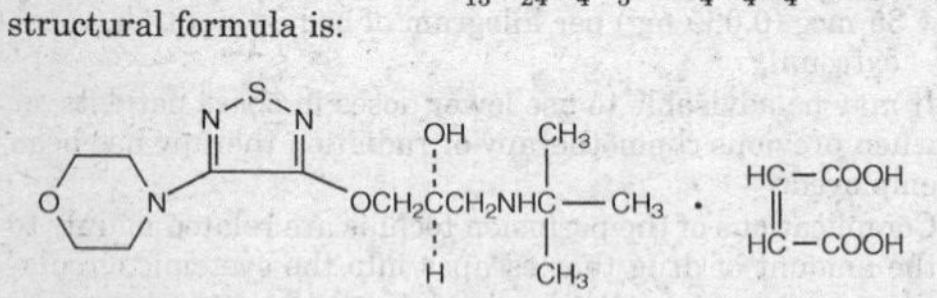

Timolol maleate has a molecular weight of 432.50. It is a white, odorless, crystalline powder which is soluble in water, methanol, and alcohol. Timolol maleate is stable at room temperature.
COSOPT is supplied as a sterile, isotonic, buffered, slightly viscous, aqueous solution. The pH of the solution is approximately 5.65, and the osmolarity is 242-323 mOsM. Each mL of COSOPT contains 20 mg dorzolamide (22.26 mg of dorzolamide hydrochloride) and 5 mg timolol (6.83 mg timolol maleate). Inactive ingredients are sodium citrate, hydroxyethyl cellulose, sodium hydroxide, mannitol, and water for injection. Benzalkonium chloride 0.0075% is added as a preservative.

*Trademark of MERCK & CO., Inc.

CLINICAL PHARMACOLOGY

Mechanism of Action
COSOPT is comprised of two components: dorzolamide hydrochloride and timolol maleate. Each of these two components decreases elevated intraocular pressure, whether or not associated with glaucoma, by reducing aqueous humor secretion. Elevated intraocular pressure is a major risk factor in the pathogenesis of optic nerve damage and glaucomatous visual field loss. The higher the level of intraocular pressure, the greater the likelihood of glaucomatous field loss and optic nerve damage.
Dorzolamide hydrochloride is an inhibitor of human carbonic anhydrase II. Inhibition of carbonic anhydrase in the ciliary processes of the eye decreases aqueous humor secretion, presumably by slowing the formation of bicarbonate ions with subsequent reduction in sodium and fluid transport. Timolol maleate is a $beta_1$ and $beta_2$ (non-selective) adrenergic receptor blocking agent that does not have significant intrinsic sympathomimetic, direct myocardial depressant, or local anesthetic (membrane-stabilizing) activity. The combined effect of these two agents administered as COSOPT b.i.d. results in additional intraocular pressure reduction compared to either component administered alone, but the reduction is not as much as when dorzolamide t.i.d. and timolol b.i.d. are administered concomitantly (see *Clinical Studies*).
Pharmacokinetics/Pharmacodynamics
Dorzolamide Hydrochloride
When topically applied, dorzolamide reaches the systemic circulation. To assess the potential for systemic carbonic anhydrase inhibition following topical administration, drug and metabolite concentrations in RBCs and plasma and carbonic anhydrase inhibition in RBCs were measured. Dorzolamide accumulates in RBCs during chronic dosing as a result of binding to CA-II. The parent drug forms a single N-desethyl metabolite, which inhibits CA-II less potently than the parent drug but also inhibits CA-I. The metabolite also accumulates in RBCs where it binds primarily to CA-I. Plasma concentrations of dorzolamide and metabolite are generally below the assay limit of quantitation (15nM). Dorzolamide binds moderately to plasma proteins (approximately 33%).
Dorzolamide is primarily excreted unchanged in the urine; the metabolite also is excreted in urine. After dosing is stopped, dorzolamide washes out of RBCs nonlinearly, resulting in a rapid decline of drug concentration initially, followed by a slower elimination phase with a half-life of about four months.
To simulate the systemic exposure after long-term topical ocular administration, dorzolamide was given orally to eight healthy subjects for up to 20 weeks. The oral dose of 2 mg b.i.d. closely approximates the amount of drug delivered by topical ocular administration of dorzolamide 2% t.i.d. Steady state was reached within 8 weeks. The inhibition of CA-II and total carbonic anhydrase activities was below the degree of inhibition anticipated to be necessary for a pharmacological effect on renal function and respiration in healthy individuals.
Timolol Maleate
In a study of plasma drug concentrations in six subjects, the systemic exposure to timolol was determined following twice daily topical administration of timolol maleate ophthalmic solution 0.5%. The mean peak plasma concentration following morning dosing was 0.46 ng/mL.
Clinical Studies
Clinical studies of 3 to 15 months duration were conducted to compare the IOP-lowering effect over the course of the day of COSOPT b.i.d. (dosed morning and bedtime) to individually- and concomitantly-administered 0.5% timolol (b.i.d.) and 2.0% dorzolamide (b.i.d. and t.i.d.). The IOP-lowering effect of COSOPT b.i.d. was greater (1-3 mmHg) than that of monotherapy with either 2.0% dorzolamide t.i.d. or 0.5% timolol b.i.d. The IOP-lowering effect of COSOPT b.i.d. was approximately 1 mmHg less than that of concomitant therapy with 2.0% dorzolamide t.i.d. and 0.5% timolol b.i.d.
Open-label extensions of two studies were conducted for up to 12 months. During this period, the IOP-lowering effect of COSOPT b.i.d. was consistent during the 12 month follow-up period.

INDICATIONS AND USAGE

COSOPT is indicated for the reduction of elevated intraocular pressure in patients with open-angle glaucoma or ocular hypertension who are insufficiently responsive to beta-blockers (failed to achieve target IOP determined after multiple measurements over time). The IOP-lowering of COSOPT b.i.d. was slightly less than that seen with the concomitant administration of 0.5% timolol b.i.d. and 2.0% dorzolamide t.i.d. (see CLINICAL PHARMACOLOGY, *Clinical Studies*).

CONTRAINDICATIONS

COSOPT is contraindicated in patients with (1) bronchial asthma; (2) a history of bronchial asthma; (3) severe chronic obstructive pulmonary disease (see WARNINGS); (4) sinus bradycardia; (5) second or third degree atrioventricular block; (6) overt cardiac failure (see WARNINGS); (7) cardiogenic shock; or (8) hypersensitivity to any component of this product.

WARNINGS

Systemic Exposure
COSOPT contains dorzolamine, a sulfonamide, and timolol maleate, a beta-adrenergic blocking agent; and although administered topically, is absorbed systemically. Therefore, the same types of adverse reactions that are attributable to sulfonamides and/or systemic administration of beta-adrenergic blocking agents may occur with topical administration. For example, severe respiratory reactions and cardiac reactions, including death due to bronchospasm in patients with asthma, and rarely death in association with cardiac failure, have been reported following systemic ophthalmic administration of timolol maleate (see CONTRAINDICATIONS). Fatalities have occurred, although rarely, due to severe reactions to sulfonamides including Stevens-Johnson syndrome, toxic epidermal necrolysis, fulminant hepatic necrosis, agranulocytosis, aplastic anemia, and other blood dyscrasias. Sensitization may recur when a sulfonamide is readministered irrespective of the route of administration. If signs of serious reactions or hypersensitivity occur, discontinue the use of this preparation.
Cardiac Failure
Sympathetic stimulation may be essential for support of the circulation in individuals with diminished myocardial contractility, and its inhibition by beta-adrenergic receptor blockade may precipitate more severe failure.
In Patients Without a History of Cardiac Failure continued depression of the myocardium with beta-blocking agents over a period of time can, in some cases, lead to cardiac failure. At the first sign or symptom of cardiac failure, COSOPT should be discontinued.
Obstructive Pulmonary Disease
Patients with chronic obstructive pulmonary disease (e.g., chronic bronchitis, emphysema) of mild or moderate severity, bronchospastic disease, or a history of bronchospastic disease (other than bronchial asthma or a history of bronchial asthma, in which COSOPT is contraindicated [see CONTRAINDICATIONS]) should, in general, not receive beta-blocking agents, including COSOPT.
Major Surgery
The necessity or desirability of withdrawal of beta-adrenergic blocking agents prior to major surgery is controversial. Beta-adrenergic receptor blockade impairs the ability of the heart to respond to beta-adrenergically mediated reflex stimuli. This may augment the risk of general anesthesia in surgical procedures. Some patients receiving beta-adrenergic receptor blocking agents have experienced protracted severe hypotension during anesthesia. Difficulty in restarting and maintaining the heartbeat has also been reported. For these reasons, in patients undergoing elective surgery, some authorities recommend gradual withdrawal of beta-adrenergic receptor blocking agents.
If necessary during surgery, the effects of beta-adrenergic blocking agents may be reversed by sufficient doses of adrenergic agonists.
Diabetes Mellitus
Beta-adrenergic blocking agents should be administered with caution in patients subject to spontaneous hypoglycemia or to diabetic patients (especially those with labile diabetes) who are receiving insulin or oral hypoglycemic agents. Beta-adrenergic receptor blocking agents may mask the signs and symptoms of acute hypoglycemia.
Thyrotoxicosis
Beta-adrenergic blocking agents may mask certain clinical signs (e.g., tachycardia) of hyperthyroidism. Patients suspected of developing thyrotoxicosis should be managed carefully to avoid abrupt withdrawal of beta-adrenergic blocking agents that might precipitate a thyroid storm.

PRECAUTIONS

General
Dorzolamide has not been studied in patients with severe renal impairment (CrCl < 30 mL/min). Because dorzolamide and its metabolite are excreted predominantly by the kidney, COSOPT is not recommended in such patients.
Dorzolamide has not been studied in patients with hepatic impairment and should therefore be used with caution in such patients.
While taking beta-blockers, patients with a history of atopy or a history of severe anaphylactic reactions to a variety of allergens may be more reactive to repeated accidental, diagnostic, or therapeutic challenge with such allergens. Such patients may be unresponsive to the usual doses of epinephrine used to treat anaphylactic reactions.
In clinical studies, local ocular adverse effects, primarily conjunctivitis and lid reactions, were reported with chronic administration of COSOPT. Many of these reactions had the clinical appearance and course of an allergic-type reaction that resolved upon discontinuation of drug therapy. If such reactions are observed, COSOPT should be discontinued and the patient evaluated before considering restarting the drug. (See ADVERSE REACTIONS.)

The management of patients with acute angle-closure glaucoma requires therapeutic interventions in addition to ocular hypotensive agents. COSOPT has not been studied in patients with acute angle-closure glaucoma.

Choroidal detachment after filtration procedures has been reported with the administration of aqueous suppressant therapy (e.g. timolol).

Beta-adrenergic blockade has been reported to potentiate muscle weakness consistent with certain myasthenic symptoms (e.g., diplopia, ptosis, and generalized weakness). Timolol has been reported rarely to increase muscle weakness in some patients with myasthenia gravis or myasthenic symptoms.

There have been reports of bacterial keratitis associated with the use of multiple dose containers of topical ophthalmic products. These containers had been inadvertently contaminated by patients who, in most cases, had a concurrent corneal disease or a disruption of the ocular epithelial surface. (See PRECAUTIONS, *Information for Patients*.)

Information for Patients

Patients with bronchial asthma, a history of bronchial asthma, severe chronic obstructive pulmonary disease, sinus bradycardia, second or third degree atrioventricular block, or cardiac failure should be advised not to take this product. (See CONTRAINDICATIONS.)

COSOPT contains dorzolamide (which is a sulfonamide) and although administered topically is absorbed systemically. Therefore the same types of adverse reactions that are attributable to sulfonamides may occur with topical administration. Patients should be advised that if serious or unusual reactions or signs of hypersensitivity occur, they should discontinue the use of the product (see WARNINGS).

Patients should be advised that if they develop any ocular reactions, particularly conjunctivitis and lid reactions, they should discontinue use and seek their physician's advice.

Patients should be instructed to avoid allowing the tip of the dispensing container to contact the eye or surrounding structures.

Patients should also be instructed that ocular solutions, if handled improperly or if the tip of the dispensing container contacts the eye or surrounding structures, can become contaminated by common bacteria known to cause ocular infections. Serious damage to the eye and subsequent loss of vision may result from using contaminated solutions. (See PRECAUTIONS, *General*.)

Patients also should be advised that if they have ocular surgery or develop an intercurrent ocular condition (e.g., trauma or infection), they should immediately seek their physician's advice concerning the continued use of the present multidose container.

If more than one topical ophthalmic drug is being used, the drugs should be administered at least ten minutes apart.

Patients should be advised that COSOPT contains benzalkonium chloride which may be absorbed by soft contact lenses. Contact lenses should be removed prior to administration of the solution. Lenses may be reinserted 15 minutes following administration of COSOPT.

Drug Interactions

Carbonic anhydrase inhibitors: There is a potential for an additive effect on the known systemic effects of carbonic anhydrase inhibition in patients receiving an oral carbonic anhydrase inhibitor and COSOPT. The concomitant administration of COSOPT and oral carbonic anhydrase inhibitors is not recommended.

Acid-base disturbances: Although acid-base and electrolyte disturbances were not reported in the clinical trials with dorzolamide hydrochloride ophthalmic solution, these disturbances have been reported with oral carbonic anhydrase inhibitors and have, in some instances, resulted in drug interactions (e.g., toxicity associated with high-dose salicylate therapy). Therefore, the potential for such drug interactions should be considered in patients receiving COSOPT.

Beta-adrenergic blocking agents: Patients who are receiving a beta-adrenergic blocking agent orally and COSOPT should be observed for potential additive effects of beta-blockade, both systemic and on intraocular pressure. The concomitant use of two topical beta-adrenergic blocking agents is not recommended.

Calcium antagonists: Caution should be used in the coadministration of beta-adrenergic blocking agents, such as COSOPT, and oral or intravenous calcium antagonists because of possible atrioventricular conduction disturbances, left ventricular failure, and hypotension. In patients with impaired cardiac function, coadministration should be avoided.

Catecholamine-depleting drugs: Close observation of the patient is recommended when a beta-blocker is administered to patients receiving catecholamine-depleting drugs such as reserpine, because of possible additive effects and the production of hypotension and/or marked bradycardia, which may result in vertigo, syncope, or postural hypotension.

Digitalis and calcium antagonists: The concomitant use of beta-adrenergic blocking agents with digitalis and calcium antagonists may have additive effects in prolonging atrioventricular conduction time.

Quinidine: Potentiated systemic beta-blockade (e.g., decreased heart rate) has been reported during combined treatment with quinidine and timolol, possibly because quinidine inhibits the metabolism of timolol via the P-450 enzyme, CYP2D6.

Injectable Epinephrine: (See PRECAUTIONS, General, Anaphylaxis.)

Carcinogenesis, Mutagenesis, Impairment of Fertility

In a two-year study of dorzolamide hydrochloride administered orally to male and female Sprague-Dawley rats, urinary bladder papillomas were seen in male rats in the highest dosage group of 20 mg/kg/day (250 times the recommended human ophthalmic dose). Papillomas were not seen in rats given oral doses equivalent to approximately 12 times the recommended human ophthalmic dose. No treatment-related tumors were seen in a 21-month study in female and male mice given oral doses up to 75 mg/kg/day (~900 times the recommended human ophthalmic dose).

The increased incidence of urinary bladder papillomas seen in the high-dose male rats is a class-effect of carbonic anhydrase inhibitors in rats. Rats are particularly prone to developing papillomas in response to foreign bodies, compounds causing crystalluria, and diverse sodium salts.

No changes in bladder urothelium were seen in dogs given oral dorzolamide hydrochloride for one year at 2 mg/kg/day (25 times the recommended human ophthalmic dose) or monkeys dosed topically to the eye at 0.4 mg/kg/day (~5 times the recommended human ophthalmic dose) for one year.

In a two-year study of timolol maleate administered orally to rats, there was a statistically significant increase in the incidence of adrenal pheochromocytomas in male rats administered 300 mg/kg/day (approximately 42,000 times the systemic exposure following the maximum recommended human ophthalmic dose). Similar differences were not observed in rats administered oral doses equivalent to approximately 14,000 times the maximum recommended human ophthalmic dose.

In a lifetime oral study of timolol maleate in mice, there were statistically significant increases in the incidence of benign and malignant pulmonary tumors, benign uterine polyps and mammary adenocarcinomas in female mice at 500 mg/kg/day, (approximately 71,000 times the systemic exposure following the maximum recommended human ophthalmic dose), but not at 5 or 50 mg/kg/day (approximately 700 or 7,000, respectively, times the systemic exposure following the maximum recommended human ophthalmic dose). In a subsequent study in female mice, in which post-mortem examinations were limited to the uterus and the lungs, a statistically significant increase in the incidence of pulmonary tumors was again observed at 500 mg/kg/day.

The increased occurrence of mammary adenocarcinomas was associated with elevations in serum prolactin which occurred in female mice administered oral timolol at 500 mg/kg/day, but not at doses of 5 or 50 mg/kg/day. An increased incidence of mammary adenocarcinomas in rodents has been associated with administration of several other therapeutic agents that elevate serum prolactin, but no correlation between serum prolactin levels and mammary tumors has been established in humans. Furthermore, in adult human female subjects who received oral dosages of up to 60 mg of timolol maleate (the maximum recommended human oral dosage), there were no clinically meaningful changes in serum prolactin.

The following tests for mutagenic potential were negative for dorzolamide: (1) *in vivo* (mouse) cytogenetic assay; (2) *in vitro* chromosomal aberration assay; (3) alkaline elution assay; (4) V-79 assay; and (5) Ames test.

Timolol maleate was devoid of mutagenic potential when tested *in vivo* (mouse) in the micronucleus test and cytogenetic assay (doses up to 800 mg/kg) and *in vitro* in a neoplastic cell transformation assay (up to 100 µg/mL). In Ames tests the highest concentrations of timolol employed, 5,000 or 10,000 µg/plate, were associated with statistically significant elevations of revertants observed with tester strain TA100 (in seven replicate assays), but not in the remaining three strains. In the assays with tester strain TA100, no consistent dose response relationship was observed, and the ratio of test to control revertants did not reach 2. A ratio of 2 is usually considered the criterion for a positive Ames test. Reproduction and fertility studies in rats with either timolol maleate or dorzolamide hydrochloride demonstrated no adverse effect on male or female fertility at doses up to approximately 100 times the systemic exposure following the maximum recommended human ophthalmic dose.

Pregnancy

Teratogenic Effects. Pregnancy Category C. Developmental toxicity studies with dorzolamide hydrochloride in rabbits at oral doses of ≥ 2.5 mg/kg/day (31 times the recommended human ophthalmic dose) revealed malformations of the vertebral bodies. These malformations occurred at doses that caused metabolic acidosis with decreased body weight gain in dams and decreased fetal weights. No treatment-related malformations were seen at 1.0 mg/kg/day (13 times the recommended human ophthalmic dose).

Teratogenicity studies with timolol in mice, rats, and rabbits at oral doses up to 50 mg/kg/day (7,000 times the systemic exposure following the maximum recommended human ophthalmic dose) demonstrated no evidence of fetal malformations. Although delayed fetal ossification was observed at this dose in rats, there were no adverse effects on postnatal development of offspring. Doses of 1000 mg/kg/day (142,000 times the systemic exposure following the maximum recommended human ophthalmic dose) were maternotoxic in mice and resulted in an increased number of fetal resorptions. Increased fetal resorptions were also seen in rabbits at doses of 14,000 times the systemic exposure following the maximum recommended human ophthalmic dose, in this case without apparent maternotoxicity.

There are no adequate and well-controlled studies in pregnant women. COSOPT should be used during pregnancy only if the potential benefit justifies the potential risk to the fetus.

Nursing Mothers

It is not known whether dorzolamide is excreted in human milk. Timolol maleate has been detected in human milk following oral and ophthalmic drug administration. Because of the potential for serious adverse reactions from COSOPT in nursing infants, a decision should be made whether to discontinue nursing or to discontinue the drug, taking into account the importance of the drug to the mother.

Pediatric Use

Safety and effectiveness in pediatric patients have not been established.

ADVERSE REACTIONS

COSOPT was evaluated for safety in 1035 patients with elevated intraocular pressure treated for open-angle-glaucoma or ocular hypertension. Approximately 5% of all patients discontinued therapy with COSOPT because of adverse reactions. The most frequently reported adverse events were taste perversion (bitter, sour, or unusual taste) or ocular burning and/or stinging in up to 30% of patients. Conjunctival hyperemia, blurred vision, superficial punctate keratitis or eye itching were reported between 5-15% of patients. The following adverse events were reported in 1-5% of patients: abdominal pain, back pain, blepharitis, bronchitis, cloudy vision, conjunctival discharge, conjunctival edema, conjunctival follicles, conjunctival injection, conjunctivitis, corneal erosion, corneal staining, cortical lens opacity, cough, dizziness, dryness of eyes, dyspepsia, eye debris, eye discharge, eye pain, eye tearing, eyelid edema, eyelid erythema, eyelid exudate/scales, eyelid pain or discomfort, foreign body sensation, glaucomatous cupping, headache, hypertension, influenza, lens nucleus coloration, lens opacity, nausea, nuclear lens opacity, pharyngitis, postsubcapsular cataract, sinusitis, upper respiratory infection, urinary tract infection, visual field defect, vitreous detachment.

The following adverse events have occurred either at low incidence (<1%) during clinical trials or have been reported during the use of COSOPT in clinical practice where these events were reported voluntarily from a population of unknown size and frequency of occurrence cannot be determined precisely. They have been chosen for inclusion based on factors such as seriousness, frequency of reporting, possible causal connection to COSOPT, or a combination of these factors: bradycardia, cardiac failure, chest pain, cerebral vascular accident, depression, diarrhea, dry mouth, dyspnea, hypotension, iridocyclitis, myocardial infarction, nasal congestion, skin rashes, paresthesia, photophobia, urolithiasis and vomiting.

Other adverse reactions that have been reported with the individual components are listed below:

Dorzolamide—Allergic/Hypersensitivity: Signs and symptoms of systemic allergic reactions including angioedema, bronchospasm, pruritus, urticaria; *Body as a Whole:* Asthenia/fatigue; *Skin:* Contact dermatitis; *Special Senses:* Signs and symptoms of ocular allergic reaction, and transient myopia.

Timolol (ocular administration)—Body as a Whole: Asthenia/fatigue; *Cardiovascular:* Arrhythmia, syncope, heart block, cerebral ischemia, worsening of angina pectoris, palpitation, cardiac arrest, pulmonary edema, claudication, Raynaud's phenomenon, and cold hands and feet; *Digestive:* Anorexia; *Immunologic:* Systemic lupus erythematosus; *Nervous System/Psychiatric:* Increase in signs and symptoms of myasthenia gravis, somnolence, insomnia, nightmares, behavioral changes and psychic disturbances including confusion, hallucinations, anxiety, disorientation,

Continued on next page

Information on the Merck & Co., Inc. products listed on these pages is the full prescribing information from product circulars in use August 31, 1998. For information, please call 1-800-NSC MERCK [1-800-672-6372].

Consult 1999 PDR® supplements and future editions for revisions

Cosopt—Cont.

nervousness, and memory loss; *Skin:* Alopecia, psoriasiform rash or exacerbation of psoriasis; *Hypersensitivity:* Signs and symptoms of systemic allergic reactions, including angioedema, urticaria, and localized and generalized rash; *Respiratory:* Bronchospasm (predominantly in patients with pre-existing bronchospastic disease), respiratory failure; *Endocrine:* Masked symptoms of hypoglycemia in diabetic patients (see WARNINGS); *Special Senses:* Ptosis; decreased corneal sensitivity; cystoid macular edema; visual disturbances including refractive changes and diplopia; pseudopemphigoid; choroidal detachment following filtration surgery (see PRECAUTIONS, *General*); and tinnitus; *Urogenital:* Retroperitoneal fibrosis, decreased libido, impotence, and Peyronie's disease.

The following additional adverse effects have been reported in clinical experience with ORAL timolol maleate or other ORAL beta-blocking agents and may be considered potential effects of ophthalmic timolol maleate: *Allergic:* Erythematous rash, fever combined with aching and sore throat, laryngospasm with respiratory distress; *Body as a Whole:* Extremity pain, decreased exercise tolerance, weight loss; *Cardiovascular:* Worsening of arterial insufficiency, vasodilatation; *Digestive:* Gastrointestinal pain, hepatomegaly, mesenteric arterial thrombosis, ischemic colitis; *Hematologic:* Nonthrombocytopenic purpura; thrombocytopenic purpura, agranulocytosis; *Endocrine:* Hyperglycemia, hypoglycemia; *Skin:* Pruritus, skin irritation, increased pigmentation, sweating; *Musculoskeletal:* Arthralgia; *Nervous System/Psychiatric:* Vertigo, local weakness, diminished concentration, reversible mental depression progressing to catatonia, an acute reversible syndrome characterized by disorientation for time and place, emotional lability, slightly clouded sensorium, and decreased performance on neuropsychometrics; *Respiratory:* Rales, bronchial obstruction; *Urogenital:* Urination difficulties.

OVERDOSAGE

There are no human data available on overdosage with COSOPT.

Symptoms consistent with systemic administration of beta-blockers or carbonic anhydrase inhibitors may occur, including electrolyte imbalance, development of an acidotic state, dizziness, headache, shortness of breath, bradycardia, bronchospasm, cardiac arrest and possible central nervous system effects. Serum electrolyte levels (particularly potassium) and blood pH levels should be monitored (see also ADVERSE REACTIONS).

A study of patients with renal failure showed that timolol did not dialyze readily.

DOSAGE AND ADMINISTRATION

The dose is one drop of COSOPT in the affected eye(s) two times daily.

If more than one topical ophthalmic drug is being used, the drugs should be administered at least ten minutes apart (see also PRECAUTIONS, *Drug Interactions*).

HOW SUPPLIED

COSOPT Ophthalmic Solution is a clear, colorless to nearly colorless, slightly viscous solution.

No. 3628 — COSOPT Ophthalmic Solution is supplied in an OCUMETER®*, a white, opaque, plastic ophthalmic dispenser with a controlled drop tip as follows:

NDC 0006-3628-03, 5 mL

NDC 0006-3628-10, 10 mL.

Storage

Store COSOPT between 15 and 25°C (59–77°F). Protect from light.

9098900 Issued April 1998

COPYRIGHT © MERCK & CO., Inc., 1998
All rights reserved

COZAAR® ℞
(Losartan Potassium Tablets)

USE IN PREGNANCY
When used in pregnancy during the second and third trimesters, drugs that act directly on the renin-angiotensin system can cause injury and even death to the developing fetus. When pregnancy is detected, COZAAR should be discontinued as soon as possible. See WARNINGS: *Fetal/Neonatal Morbidity and Mortality.*

DESCRIPTION

COZAAR* (losartan potassium), the first of a new class of antihypertensives, is an angiotensin II receptor (type AT_1) antagonist.

Losartan potassium, a non-peptide molecule, is chemically describedas2-butyl-4-chloro-1-[*p*-(*o*-1*H*-tetrazol-5-ylphenyl)-benzyl]imidazole-5-methanol monopotassium salt.

Its empirical formula is $C_{22}H_{22}ClKN_6O$, and its structural formula is:

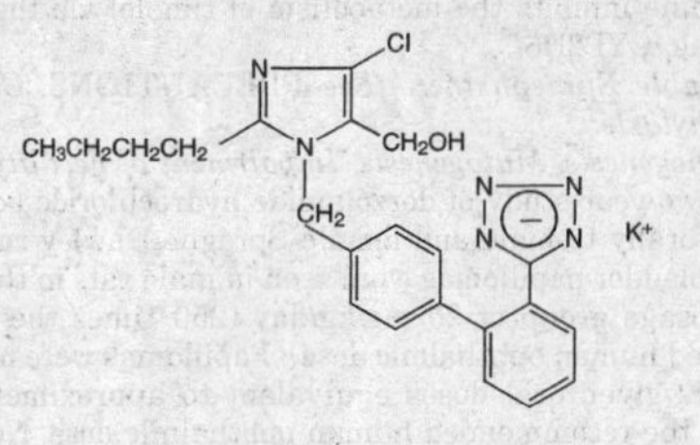

Losartan potassium is a white to off-white free-flowing crystalline powder with a molecular weight of 461.01. It is freely soluble in water, soluble in alcohols, and slightly soluble in common organic solvents, such as acetonitrile and methyl ethyl ketone. Oxidation of the 5-hydroxymethyl group on the imidazole ring results in the active metabolite of losartan.

COZAAR is available for oral administration containing either 25 mg or 50 mg of losartan potassium and the following inactive ingredients: microcrystalline cellulose, lactose hydrous, pregelatinized starch, magnesium stearate, hydroxypropyl cellulose, hydroxypropyl methylcellulose, titanium dioxide, D&C yellow No. 10 aluminum lake and FD&C blue No. 2 aluminum lake.

COZAAR 25 mg and 50 mg contain potassium in the following amounts: 2.12 mg (0.054 mEq) and 4.24 mg (0.108 mEq), respectively.

*Registered trademark of E. I. du Pont de Nemours and Company, Wilmington, Delaware, USA

CLINICAL PHARMACOLOGY

Mechanism of Action

Angiotensin II [formed from angiotensin I in a reaction catalyzed by angiotensin converting enzyme (ACE, kininase II)], is a potent vasoconstrictor, the primary vasoactive hormone of the renin-angiotensin system and an important component in the pathophysiology of hypertension. It also stimulates aldosterone secretion by the adrenal cortex. Losartan and its principal active metabolite block the vasoconstrictor and aldosterone-secreting effects of angiotensin II by selectively blocking the binding of angiotensin II to the AT_1 receptor found in many tissues, (e.g., vascular smooth muscle, adrenal gland). There is also an AT_2 receptor found in many tissues but it is not known to be associated with cardiovascular homeostatis. Both losartan and its principal active metabolite do not exhibit any partial agonist activity at the AT_1 receptor and have much greater affinity (about 1000-fold) for the AT_1 receptor than for the AT_2 receptor. *In vitro* binding studies indicate that losartan is a reversible, competitive inhibitor of the AT_1 receptor. The active metabolite is 10 to 40 times more potent by weight than losartan and appears to be a reversible, non-competitive inhibitor of the AT_1 receptor.

Neither losartan nor its active metabolite inhibits ACE (kininase II, the enzyme that converts angiotensin I to angiotensin II and degrades bradykinin); nor do they bind to or block other hormone receptors or ion channels known to be important in cardiovascular regulation.

Pharmacokinetics

General

Losartan is an orally active agent that undergoes substantial first-pass metabolism by cytochrome P450 enzymes. It is converted, in part, to an active carboxylic acid metabolite that is responsible for most of the angiotensin II receptor antagonism that follows losartan treatment. The terminal half-life of losartan is about 2 hours and of the metabolite is about 6–9 hours. The pharmacokinetics of losartan and its active metabolite are linear with oral losartan doses up to 200 mg and do not change over time. Neither losartan nor its metabolite accumulate in plasma upon repeated once-daily dosing.

Following oral administration, losartan is well absorbed (based on absorption of radiolabeled losartan) and undergoes substantial first-pass metabolism; the systemic bioavailability of losartan is approximately 33%. About 14% of an orally-administered dose of losartan is converted to the active metabolite. Mean peak concentrations of losartan and its active metabolite are reached in 1 hour and in 3–4 hours, respectively. While maximum plasma concentrations of losartan and its active metabolite are approximately equal, the AUC of the metabolite is about 4 times as great as that of losartan. A meal slows absorption of losartan and decreases its C_{max} but has only minor effects on losartan AUC or on the AUC of the metabolite (about 10% decreased).

Both losartan and its active metabolite are highly bound to plasma proteins, primarily albumin, with plasma free fractions of 1.3% and 0.2% respectively. Plasma protein binding is constant over the concentration range achieved with recommended doses. Studies in rats indicate that losartan crosses the blood-brain barrier poorly, if at all.

Losartan metabolites have been identified in human plasma and urine. In addition to the active carboxylic acid metabolite, several inactive metabolites are formed. Following oral and intravenous administration of ^{14}C-labeled losartan potassium, circulating plasma radioactivity is primarily attributed to losartan and its active metabolite. *In vitro* studies indicate that cytochrome P450 2C9 and 3A4 are involved in the biotransformation of losartan to its metabolites. Minimal conversion of losartan to the active metabolite (less than 1% of the dose compared to 14% of the dose in normal subjects) was seen in about one percent of individuals studied.

The volume of distribution of losartan is about 34 liters and of the active metabolite is about 12 liters. Total plasma clearance of losartan and the active metabolite is about 600 mL/min and 50 mL/min, respectively, with renal clearance of about 75 mL/min and 25 mL/min, respectively. When losartan is administered orally, about 4% of the dose is excreted unchanged in the urine and about 6% is excreted in urine as active metabolite. Biliary excretion contributes to the elimination of losartan and its metabolites. Following oral ^{14}C-labeled losartan, about 35% of radioactivity is recovered in the urine and about 60% in the feces. Following an intravenous dose of ^{14}C-labeled losartan, about 45% of radioactivity is recovered in the urine and 50% in the feces.

Special Populations

Pediatric: Losartan pharmacokinetics have not been investigated in patients <18 years of age.

Geriatric and Gender: Losartan pharmacokinetics have been investigated in the elderly (65–75 years) and in both genders. Plasma concentrations of losartan and its active metabolite are similar in elderly and young hypertensives. Plasma concentrations of losartan were about twice as high in female hypertensives as male hypertensives, but concentrations of the active metabolite were similar in males and females. No dosage adjustment is necessary (see DOSAGE AND ADMINISTRATION).

Race: Pharmacokinetic differences due to race have not been studied.

Renal Insufficiency: Plasma concentrations of losartan are not altered in patients with creatinine clearance above 30 mL/min. In patients with lower creatinine clearance, AUCs are about 50% greater and they are doubled in hemodialysis patients. Plasma concentrations of the active metabolite are not significantly altered in patients with renal impairment or in hemodialysis patients. Neither losartan nor its active metabolite can be removed by hemodialysis. No dosage adjustment is necessary for patients with renal impairment unless they are volume-depleted (see WARNINGS, *Hypotension—Volume-Depleted Patients* and DOSAGE AND ADMINISTRATION).

Hepatic Insufficiency: Following oral administration in patients with mild to moderate alcoholic cirrhosis of the liver, plasma concentrations of losartan and its active metabolite were, respectively, 5-times and about 1.7-times those in young male volunteers. Compared to normal subjects the total plasma clearance of losartan in patients with hepatic insufficiency was about 50% lower and the oral bioavailability was about 2-times higher. A lower starting dose is recommended for patients with a history of hepatic impairment (see DOSAGE AND ADMINISTRATION).

Drug Interactions

Losartan, administered for 12 days, did not affect the pharmacokinetics or pharmacodynamics of a single dose of warfarin. Losartan did not affect the pharmacokinetics of oral or intravenous digoxin. Coadministration of losartan and cimetidine led to an increase of about 18% in AUC of losartan but did not affect the pharmacokinetics of its active metabolite. Coadministration of losartan and phenobarbital led to a reduction of about 20% in the AUC of losartan and that of its active metabolite. Conversion of losartan to its active metabolite after intravenous administration is not affected by ketoconazole, an inhibitor of P450 3A4. There is no pharmacokinetic interaction between losartan and hydrochlorothiazide.

Pharmacodynamics and Clinical Effects

Losartan inhibits the pressor effect of angiotensin II (as well as angiotensin I) infusions. A dose of 100 mg inhibits the pressor effect by about 85% at peak with 25–40% inhibition persisting for 24 hours. Removal of the negative feedback of angiotensin II causes a 2–3 fold rise in plasma renin activity and consequent rise in angiotensin II plasma concentration in hypertensive patients. Losartan does not affect the response to bradykinin, whereas ACE inhibitors increase the response to bradykinin. Aldosterone plasma concentrations fall following losartan administration. In spite of the effect of losartan on aldosterone secretion, very little effect on serum potassium was observed.

In a single-dose study in normal volunteers, losartan had no effects on glomerular filtration rate, renal plasma flow or filtration fraction. In multiple dose studies in hypertensive patients, there were no notable effects on systemic or renal

prostaglandin concentrations, fasting triglycerides, total cholesterol or HDL-cholesterol or fasting glucose concentrations. There was a small uricosuric effect leading to a minimal decrease in serum uric acid (mean decrease <0.4 mg/dL) during chronic oral administration.

The antihypertensive effects of COZAAR were demonstrated principally in 4 placebo-controlled 6–12 week trials of dosages from 10 to 150 mg per day in patients with baseline diastolic blood pressures of 95–115. The studies allowed comparisons of two doses (50–100 mg/day) as once-daily or twice-daily regimens, comparisons of peak and trough effects, and comparisons of response by gender, age, and race. Three additional studies examined the antihypertensive effects of losartan and hydrochlorothiazide in combination.

The 4 studies of losartan monotherapy included a total of 1075 patients randomized to several doses of losartan and 334 to placebo. The 10 and 25 mg doses produced some effect at peak (6 hours after dosing) but small and inconsistent trough (24 hour) responses. Doses of 50, 100 and 150 mg once daily gave statistically significant systolic/diastolic mean decreases in blood pressure, compared to placebo in the range of 5.5–10.5/3.5–7.5 mmHg, with the 150 mg dose giving no greater effect than 50–100 mg. Twice-daily dosing at 50–100 mg/day gave consistently larger trough responses than once-daily dosing at the same total dose. Peak (6 hour) effects were uniformly, but moderately, larger than trough effects, with the trough-to-peak ratio for systolic and diastolic responses 50–95% and 60–90%, respectively.

Addition of a low dose of hydrochlorothiazide (12.5 mg) to losartan 50 mg once daily resulted in placebo-adjusted blood pressure reductions of 15.5/9.2 mmHg.

Analysis of age, gender, and race subgroups of patients showed that men and women, and patients over and under 65, had generally similar responses. Black patients, however, had notably smaller responses to losartan monotherapy.

The effect of losartan is substantially present within one week but in some studies the maximal effect occurred in 3–6 weeks. In long-term follow-up studies (without placebo control) the effect of losartan appeared to be maintained for up to a year. There is no apparent rebound effect after abrupt withdrawal of losartan. There was essentially no change in average heart rate in losartan-treated patients in controlled trials.

Persistent dry cough (with an incidence of a few percent) has been associated with ACE inhibitor use and in practice can be a cause of discontinuation of ACE inhibitor therapy. Two prospective, parallel-group, double-blind, randomized, controlled trials were conducted to assess the effects of losartan on the incidence of cough in hypertensive patients who had experienced cough while receiving ACE inhibitor therapy. Patients who had typical ACE inhibitor cough when challenged with lisinopril, whose cough disappeared on placebo, were randomized to losartan 50 mg, lisinopril 20 mg, or either placebo (one study, n=97) or 25 mg hydrochlorothiazide (n=135). The double-blind treatment period lasted up to 8 weeks. The incidence of cough is shown below.

Study 1†	HCTZ	Losartan	Lisinopril
Cough	25%	17%	69%
Study 2††	Placebo	Losartan	Lisinopril
Cough	35%	29%	62%

†Demographics = (89% caucasian, 64% female)
††Demographics = (90% caucasian, 51% female)

These studies demonstrate that the incidence of cough associated with losartan therapy, in a population that all had cough associated with ACE inhibitor therapy, is similar to that associated with hydrochlorothiazide or placebo therapy.

INDICATIONS AND USAGE

COZAAR is indicated for the treatment of hypertension. It may be used alone or in combination with other antihypertensive agents.

In considering the use of monotherapy with COZAAR, it should be noted that in controlled trials COZAAR had an effect on blood pressure that was notably less in black patients than in non-blacks, a finding similar to the small effect of angiotensin converting enzyme inhibitors in blacks.

CONTRAINDICATIONS

COZAAR is contraindicated in patients who are hypersensitive to any component of this product.

WARNINGS

Fetal/Neonatal Morbidity and Mortality

Drugs that act directly on the renin-angiotensin system can cause fetal and neonatal morbidity and death when administered to pregnant women. Several dozen cases have been reported in the world literature in patients who were taking angiotensin converting enzyme inhibitors. When pregnancy is detected, COZAAR should be discontinued as soon as possible.

The use of drugs that act directly on the renin-angiotensin system during the second and third trimesters of pregnancy has been associated with fetal and neonatal injury, including hypotension, neonatal skull hypoplasia, anuria, reversible or irreversible renal failure, and death. Oligohydramnios has also been reported, presumably resulting from decreased fetal renal function; oligohydramnios in this setting has been associated with fetal limb contractures, craniofacial deformation, and hypoplastic lung development. Prematurity, intrauterine growth retardation, and patent ductus arteriosus have also been reported, although it is not clear whether these occurrences were due to exposure to the drug.

These adverse effects do not appear to have resulted from intrauterine drug exposure that has been limited to the first trimester.

Mothers whose embryos and fetuses are exposed to an angiotensin II receptor antagonist only during the first trimester should be so informed. Nonetheless, when patients become pregnant, physicians should have the patient discontinue the use of COZAAR as soon as possible.

Rarely (probably less often than once in every thousand pregnancies), no alternative to an angiotensin II receptor antagonist will be found. In these rare cases, the mothers should be apprised of the potential hazards to their fetuses, and serial ultrasound examinations should be performed to assess the intraamniotic environment.

If oligohydramnios is observed, COZAAR should be discontinued unless it is considered life-saving for the mother. Contraction stress testing (CST), a non-stress test (NST), or biophysical profiling (BPP) may be appropriate, depending upon the week of pregnancy. Patients and physicians should be aware, however, that oligohydramnios may not appear until after the fetus has sustained irreversible injury.

Infants with histories of *in utero* exposure to an angiotensin II receptor antagonist should be closely observed for hypotension, oliguria, and hyperkalemia. If oliguria occurs, attention should be directed toward support of blood pressure and renal perfusion. Exchange transfusion or dialysis may be required as means of reversing hypotension and/or substituting for disordered renal function.

Losartan potassium has been shown to produce adverse effects in rat fetuses and neonates, including decreased body weight, delayed physical and behavioral development, mortality and renal toxicity. With the exception of neonatal weight gain (which was affected at doses as low as 10 mg/kg/day), doses associated with these effects exceeded 25 mg/kg/day (approximately three times the maximum recommended human dose of 100 mg on a mg/m^2 basis). These findings are attributed to drug exposure in late gestation and during lactation. Significant levels of losartan and its active metabolite were shown to be present in rat fetal plasma during late gestation and in rat milk.

Hypotension—Volume-Depleted Patients

In patients who are intravascularly volume-depleted (e.g., those treated with diuretics), symptomatic hypotension may occur after initiation of therapy with COZAAR. These conditions should be corrected prior to administration of COZAAR, or a lower starting dose should be used (see DOSAGE AND ADMINISTRATION).

PRECAUTIONS

General

Impaired Hepatic Function

Based on pharmacokinetic data which demonstrate significantly increased plasma concentrations of losartan in cirrhotic patients, a lower dose should be considered for patients with impaired liver function (see DOSAGE AND ADMINISTRATION and CLINICAL PHARMACOLOGY, *Pharmacokinetics*).

Hypersensitivity. See ADVERSE REACTIONS, *Post-Marketing Experience.*

Impaired Renal Function

As a consequence of inhibiting the renin-angiotensin-aldosterone system, changes in renal function have been reported in susceptible individuals treated with COZAAR; in some patients, these changes in renal function were reversible upon discontinuation of therapy.

In patients whose renal function may depend on the activity of the renin-angiotensin-aldosterone system (e.g., patients with severe congestive heart failure), treatment with angiotensin converting enzyme inhibitors has been associated with oliguria and/or progressive azotemia and (rarely) with acute renal failure and/or death. Similar outcomes have been reported with COZAAR.

In studies of ACE inhibitors in patients with unilateral or bilateral renal artery stenosis, increases in serum creatinine or BUN have been reported. Similar effects have been reported with COZAAR; in some patients, these effects were reversible upon discontinuation of therapy.

Information for Patients

Pregnancy: Female patients of childbearing age should be told about the consequences of second- and third-trimester exposure to drugs that act on the renin-angiotensin system, and they should also be told that these consequences do not appear to have resulted from intrauterine drug exposure that has been limited to the first trimester. These patients should be asked to report pregnancies to their physicians as soon as possible.

Drug Interactions

No significant drug-drug pharmacokinetic interactions have been found in interaction studies with hydrochlorothiazide, digoxin, warfarin, cimetidine and phenobarbital. (See CLINICAL PHARMACOLOGY, *Drug Interactions.*) Potent inhibitors of cytochrome P450 3A4 and 2C9 have not been studied clinically but *in vitro* studies show significant inhibition of the formation of the active metabolite by inhibitors of P450 3A4 (ketoconazole, troleandomycin, gestodene), or P450 2C9 (sulfaphenazole) and nearly complete inhibition by the combination of sulfaphenazole and ketoconazole. In humans, ketoconazole, an inhibitor of P450 3A4, did not affect the conversion of losartan to the active metabolite after intravenous administration of losartan. Inhibitors of cytochrome P450 2C9 have not been studied clinically. The pharmacodynamic consequences of concomitant use of losartan and inhibitors of P450 2C9 have not been examined.

As with other drugs that block angiotensin II or its effects, concomitant use of potassium-sparing diuretics (e.g., spironolactone, triamterene, amiloride), potassium supplements, or salt substitutes containing potassium may lead to increases in serum potassium.

Carcinogenesis, Mutagenesis, Impairment of Fertility

Losartan potassium was not carcinogenic when administered at maximally tolerated dosages to rats and mice for 105 and 92 weeks, respectively. Female rats given the highest dose (270 mg/kg/day) had a slightly higher incidence of pancreatic acinar adenoma. The maximally tolerated dosages (270 mg/kg/day in rats, 200 mg/kg/day in mice) provided systemic exposures for losartan and its pharmacologically active metabolite that were approximately 160- and 90-times (rats) and 30- and 15-times (mice) the exposure of a 50 kg human given 100 mg per day.

Losartan potassium was negative in the microbial mutagenesis and V-79 mammalian cell mutagenesis assays and in the *in vitro* alkaline elution and *in vitro* and *in vivo* chromosomal aberration assays. In addition, the active metabolite showed no evidence of genotoxicity in the microbial mutagenesis, *in vitro* alkaline elution, and *in vitro* chromosomal aberration assays.

Fertility and reproductive performance were not affected in studies with male rats given oral doses of losartan potassium up to approximately 150 mg/kg/day. The administration of toxic dosage levels in females (300/200 mg/kg/day) was associated with a significant ($p<0.05$) decrease in the number of corpora lutea/female, implants/female, and live fetuses/female at C-section. At 100 mg/kg/day only a decrease in the number of corpora lutea/female was observed. The relationship of these findings to drug-treatment is uncertain since there was no effect at these dosage levels on implants/pregnant female, percent post-implantation loss, or live animals/litter at parturition. In nonpregnant rats dosed at 135 mg/kg/day for 7 days, systemic exposure (AUCs) for losartan and its active metabolite were approximately 66 and 26 times the exposure achieved in man at the maximum recommended human daily dosage (100 mg).

Pregnancy

Pregnancy Categories C (first trimester) and D (second and third trimesters). See WARNINGS, *Fetal/Neonatal Morbidity and Mortality.*

Nursing Mothers

It is not known whether losartan is excreted in human milk, but significant levels of losartan and its active metabolite were shown to be present in rat milk. Because of the potential for adverse effects on the nursing infant, a decision should be made whether to discontinue nursing or discontinue the drug, taking into account the importance of the drug to the mother.

Pediatric Use

Safety and effectiveness in pediatric patients have not been established.

Use in the Elderly

Of the total number of patients receiving COZAAR in controlled clinical studies, 391 patients (19%) were 65 years and over, while 37 patients (2%) were 75 years and over. No overall differences in effectiveness or safety were observed between these patients and younger patients, but greater sensitivity of some older individuals cannot be ruled out.

Continued on next page

Information on the Merck & Co., Inc. products listed on these pages is the full prescribing information from product circulars in use August 31, 1998. For information, please call 1-800-NSC MERCK [1-800-672-6372].

Consult 1999 PDR® supplements and future editions for revisions

Cozaar—Cont.

ADVERSE REACTIONS

COZAAR has been evaluated for safety in more than 3300 patients treated for essential hypertension and 4058 patients/subjects overall. Over 1200 patients were treated for over 6 months and more than 800 for over one year. In general, treatment with COZAAR was well-tolerated. The overall incidence of adverse experiences reported with COZAAR was similar to placebo.
In controlled clinical trials, discontinuation of therapy due to clinical adverse experiences was required in 2.3 percent of patients treated with COZAAR and 3.7 percent of patients given placebo.
The following table of adverse events is based on four 6–12 week placebo controlled trials involving over 1000 patients on various doses (10–150 mg) of losartan and over 300 patients given placebo. All doses of losartan are grouped because none of the adverse events appeared to have a dose-related frequency. The table includes all adverse events, whether or not attributed to the treatment, occurring in at least 1% of patients treated with losartan and that were more frequent on losartan than placebo.

	Losartan (n=1075) Incidence	Placebo (n=334) Incidence
Digestive		
Diarrhea	2.4	2.1
Dyspepsia	1.3	1.2
Musculoskeletal		
Cramp, muscle	1.1	0.3
Myalgia	1.0	0.9
Pain, back	1.8	1.2
Pain, leg	1.0	0.0
Nervous System / Psychiatric		
Dizziness	3.5	2.1
Insomnia	1.4	0.6
Respiratory		
Congestion, nasal	2.0	1.2
Cough	3.4	3.3
Infection, upper respiratory	7.9	6.9
Sinus disorder	1.5	1.2
Sinusitis	1.0	0.3

The following adverse events were also reported at a rate of 1% or greater in patients treated with losartan, but were as, or more frequent, in the placebo group: asthenia/fatigue, edema/swelling, abdominal pain, chest pain, nausea, headache, pharyngitis.
Adverse events occurred at about the same rates in men and women, older and younger patients, and black and non-black patients.
A patient with known hypersensitivity to aspirin and penicillin, when treated with COZAAR, was withdrawn from study due to swelling of the lips and eyelids and facial rash, reported as angioedema, which returned to normal 5 days after therapy was discontinued.
Superficial peeling of palms and hemolysis was reported in one subject.
In addition to the adverse events above, potentially important events that occurred in at least two patients/subjects exposed to losartan or other adverse events that occurred in <1% of patients in clinical studies are listed below. It cannot be determined whether these events were causally related to losartan: *Body as a Whole:* facial edema, fever, orthostatic effects, syncope; *Cardiovascular:* angina pectoris, second degree AV block, CVA, hypotension, myocardial infarction, arrhythmias including atrial fibrillation, palpitation, sinus bradycardia, tachycardia, ventricular tachycardia, ventricular fibrillation; *Digestive:* anorexia, constipation, dental pain, dry mouth, flatulence, gastritis, vomiting; *Hematologic:* anemia; *Metabolic:* gout; *Musculoskeletal:* arm pain, hip pain, joint swelling, knee pain, musculoskeletal pain, shoulder pain, stiffness, arthralgia, arthritis, fibromyalgia, muscle weakness; *Nervous System / Psychiatric:* anxiety, anxiety disorder, ataxia, confusion, depression, dream abnormality, hypesthesia, decreased libido, memory impairment, migraine, nervousness, paresthesia, peripheral neuropathy, panic disorder, sleep disorder, somnolence, tremor, vertigo; *Respiratory:* dyspnea, bronchitis, pharyngeal discomfort, epistaxis, rhinitis, respiratory congestion; *Skin:* alopecia, dermatitis, dry skin, ecchymosis, erythema, flushing, photosensitivity, pruritus, rash, sweating, urticaria; *Special Senses:* blurred vision, burning/stinging in the eye, conjunctivitis, taste perversion, tinnitus, decrease in visual acuity; *Urogenital:* impotence, nocturia, urinary frequency, urinary tract infection.
Post-Marketing Experience
The following additional adverse reactions have been reported in post-marketing experience: *Hypersensitivity:* Angioedema (involving swelling of the face, lips, pharynx, and/or tongue) has been reported rarely in patients treated with losartan; some of these patients previously experienced angioedema with other drugs including ACE inhibitors; *Digestive:* Hepatitis (reported rarely).
Hyperkalemia has been reported.
Laboratory Test Findings
In controlled clinical trials, clinically important changes in standard laboratory parameters were rarely associated with administration of COZAAR.
Creatinine, Blood Urea Nitrogen: Minor increases in blood urea nitrogen (BUN) or serum creatinine were observed in less than 0.1 percent of patients with essential hypertension treated with COZAAR alone.
Hemoglobin and Hematocrit: Small decreases in hemoglobin and hematocrit (mean decreases of approximately 0.11 grams percent and 0.09 volume percent, respectively) occurred frequently in patients treated with COZAAR alone, but were rarely of clinical importance. No patients were discontinued due to anemia.
Liver Function Tests: Occasional elevations of liver enzymes and/or serum bilirubin have occurred. In patients with essential hypertension treated with COZAAR alone, one patient (<0.1%) was discontinued due to these laboratory adverse experiences.

OVERDOSAGE

Significant lethality was observed in mice and rats after oral administration of 1000 mg/kg and 2000 mg/kg, respectively, about 44 and 170 times the maximum recommended human dose on a mg/m^2 basis.
Limited data are available in regard to overdosage in humans. The most likely manifestation of overdosage would be hypotension and tachycardia; bradycardia could occur from parasympathetic (vagal) stimulation. If symptomatic hypotension should occur, supportive treatment should be instituted.
Neither losartan nor its active metabolite can be removed by hemodialysis.

DOSAGE AND ADMINISTRATION

The usual starting dose of COZAAR is 50 mg once daily, with 25 mg used in patients with possible depletion of intravascular volume (e.g., patients treated with diuretics) (see WARNINGS, *Hypotension—Volume-Depleted Patients*) and patients with a history of hepatic impairment (see PRECAUTIONS, *General*). COZAAR can be administered once or twice daily with total daily doses ranging from 25 mg to 100 mg.
If the antihypertensive effect measured at trough using once-a-day dosing is inadequate, a twice-a-day regimen at the same total daily dose or an increase in dose may give a more satisfactory response.
If blood pressure is not controlled by COZAAR alone, a low dose of a diuretic may be added. Hydrochlorothiazide has been shown to have an additive effect (see CLINICAL PHARMACOLOGY, *Pharmacodynamics and Clinical Effects*).
No initial dosage adjustment is necessary for elderly patients or for patients with renal impairment, including patients on dialysis.
COZAAR may be administered with other antihypertensive agents.
COZAAR may be administered with or without food.

HOW SUPPLIED

No. 3612—Tablets COZAAR, 25 mg, are light green, teardrop-shaped, film-coated tablets with code MRK on one side and 951 on the other. They are supplied as follows:
NDC 0006-0951-54 unit of use bottles of 90
(6505-01-414-4064, 25 mg 90's)
NDC 0006-0951-58 unit of use bottles of 100
(6505-01-414-4059, 25 mg 100's)
NDC 0006-0951-28 unit dose packages of 100
(6505-01-414-4063, 25 mg individually sealed 100's).
Shown in Product Identification Guide, page 323
No. 3613—Tablets COZAAR, 50 mg, are green, teardrop-shaped, film-coated tablets with code MRK 952 on one side and COZAAR on the other. They are supplied as follows:
NDC 0006-0952-31 unit of use bottles of 30
(6505-01-414-4062, 50 mg 30's)
NDC 0006-0952-54 unit of use bottles of 90
(6505-01-414-4060, 50 mg 90's)
NDC 0006-0952-58 unit of use bottles of 100
(6505-01-414-4058, 50 mg 100's)
NDC 0006-0952-28 unit dose packages of 100
(6505-01-414-4061, 50 mg individually sealed 100's)
NDC 0006-0952-82 bottles of 1,000.
Shown in Product Identification Guide, page 323
Storage
Store at controlled room temperature, 15–30°C (59–86°F). Keep container tightly closed. Protect from light.
Manufactured for:
MERCK & CO., INC., West Point, PA 19486, USA
by:
Du Pont Pharmaceuticals, Wilmington, DE 19880 USA

7882907 Issued March 1998
COPYRIGHT © MERCK & CO., Inc., 1995
All rights reserved

CRIXIVAN® Capsules ℞
(indinavir sulfate), U.S.P.

DESCRIPTION

CRIXIVAN* (indinavir sulfate) is an inhibitor of the human immunodeficiency virus (HIV) protease. CRIXIVAN Capsules are formulated as a sulfate salt and are available for oral administration in strengths of 200 and 400 mg of indinavir (corresponding to 250 and 500 mg indinavir sulfate, respectively). Each capsule also contains the inactive ingredients anhydrous lactose and magnesium stearate. The capsule shell has the following inactive ingredients and dyes: gelatin, titanium dioxide, silicon dioxide and sodium lauryl sulfate.
The chemical name for indinavir sulfate is [1(1*S*,2*R*),5(*S*)]-2,3,5-trideoxy-*N*-(2,3-dihydro-2-hydroxy-1 *H*-inden-1-yl)-5-[2-[[(1,1-dimethylethyl)amino]carbonyl]-4-(3-pyridinylmethyl)-1-piperazinyl] -2 -(phenylmethyl)-D-*erythro*-pentonamide sulfate (1:1) salt. Indinavir sulfate has the following structural formula:

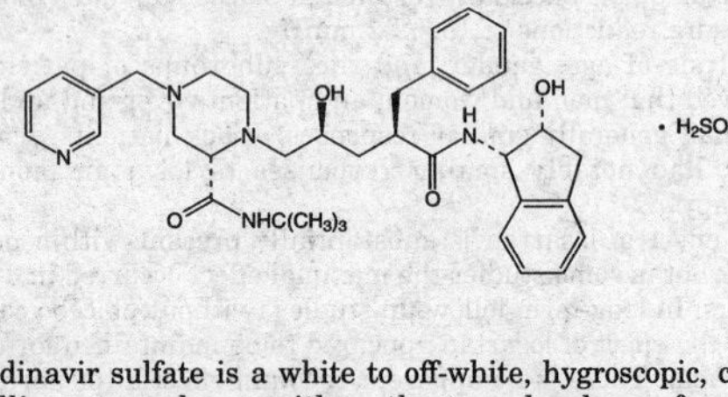

Indinavir sulfate is a white to off-white, hygroscopic, crystalline powder with the molecular formula $C_{36}H_{47}N_5O_4 \cdot H_2SO_4$ and a molecular weight of 711.88. It is very soluble in water and in methanol.

*Registered trademark of MERCK & CO., Inc.

MICROBIOLOGY

Mechanism of Action: HIV protease is an enzyme required for the proteolytic cleavage of the viral polyprotein precursors into the individual functional proteins found in infectious HIV. Indinavir binds to the protease active site and inhibits the activity of the enzyme. This inhibition prevents cleavage of the viral polyproteins resulting in the formation of immature noninfectious viral particles.
Antiretroviral Activity In Vitro: The relationship between *in vitro* susceptibility of HIV to indinavir and inhibition of HIV replication in humans has not been established. The *in vitro* activity of indinavir was assessed in cell lines of lymphoblastic and monocytic origin and in peripheral blood lymphocytes. HIV variants used to infect the different cell types include laboratory-adapted variants, primary clinical isolates and clinical isolates resistant to nucleoside analogue and nonnucleoside inhibitors of the HIV reverse transcriptase. The IC_{95} (95% inhibitory concentration) of indinavir in these test systems was in the range of 25 to 100 nM. In drug combination studies with the nucleoside analogues zidovudine and didanosine, as well as with an investigational nonnucleoside (L-697,661), indinavir showed synergistic activity in cell culture.
Drug Resistance: Isolates of HIV with reduced susceptibility to the drug have been recovered from some patients treated with indinavir. Viral resistance was correlated with the accumulation of mutations that resulted in the expression of amino acid substitutions in the viral protease. Eleven amino acid residue positions, at which substitutions are associated with resistance, have been identified. Resistance was mediated by the co-expression of multiple and variable substitutions at these positions. In general, higher levels of resistance were associated with the co-expression of greater numbers of substitutions.
Cross-Resistance to Other Antiviral Agents: Cross-resistance was noted between indinavir and the protease inhibitor ritonavir. Varying degrees of cross-resistance have been observed between indinavir and other HIV-protease inhibitors.

CLINICAL PHARMACOLOGY

Pharmacokinetics
Absorption: Indinavir was rapidly absorbed in the fasted state with a time to peak plasma concentration (T_{max}) of 0.8 ± 0.3 hours (mean ± S.D.) (n=11). A greater than dose-proportional increase in indinavir plasma concentrations was observed over the 200–1000 mg dose range. At a dosing

regimen of 800 mg every 8 hours, steady-state area under the plasma concentration time curve (AUC) was 30,691 ± 11,407 nM·hour (n=16), peak plasma concentration (C_{max}) was 12,617 ± 4037 nM (n=16), and plasma concentration eight hours post dose (trough) was 251 ± 178 nM (n=16).

Effect of Food on Oral Absorption: Administration of indinavir with a meal high in calories, fat, and protein (784 kcal, 48.6 g fat, 31.3 g protein) resulted in a 77% ± 8% reduction in AUC and an 84% ± 7% reduction in C_{max} (n=10). Administration with lighter meals (e.g., a meal of dry toast with jelly, apple juice, and coffee with skim milk and sugar or a meal of corn flakes, skim milk and sugar) resulted in little or no change in AUC, C_{max} or trough concentration.

Distribution: Indinavir was approximately 60% bound to human plasma proteins over a concentration range of 81 nM to 16,300 nM.

Metabolism: Following a 400-mg dose of ^{14}C-indinavir, 83 ± 1% (n=4) and 19 ± 3% (n=6) of the total radioactivity was recovered in feces and urine, respectively; radioactivity due to parent drug in feces and urine was 19.1% and 9.4%, respectively. Seven metabolites have been identified, one glucuronide conjugate and six oxidative metabolites. *In vitro* studies indicate that cytochrome P-450 3A4 (CYP3A4) is the major enzyme responsible for formation of the oxidative metabolites.

Elimination: Less than 20% of indinavir is excreted unchanged in the urine. Mean urinary excretion of unchanged drug was 10.4 ± 4.9% (n=10) and 12.0 ± 4.9% (n=10) following a single 700-mg and 1000-mg dose, respectively. Indinavir was rapidly eliminated with a half-life of 1.8 ± 0.4 hours (n=10). Significant accumulation was not observed after multiple dosing at 800 mg every 8 hours.

Special Populations
Hepatic Insufficiency: Patients with mild to moderate hepatic insufficiency and clinical evidence of cirrhosis had evidence of decreased metabolism of indinavir resulting in approximately 60% higher mean AUC following a single 400-mg dose (n=12). The half-life of indinavir increased to 2.8 ± 0.5 hours. Indinavir pharmacokinetics have not been studied in patients with severe hepatic insufficiency (see DOSAGE AND ADMINISTRATION, *Hepatic Insufficiency*).

Renal Insufficiency: The pharmacokinetics of indinavir have not been studied in patients with renal insufficiency.

Gender: Pharmacokinetics of indinavir appear to be comparable in men and women based on pharmacokinetic studies including 32 women (15 HIV-positive).

Race: Pharmacokinetics of indinavir appear to be comparable in Caucasians and Blacks based on pharmacokinetic studies including 42 Caucasians (26 HIV-positive) and 16 Blacks (4 HIV-positive).

Drug Interactions (also see PRECAUTIONS, *Drug Interactions*)
Specific drug interaction studies were performed with indinavir and a number of drugs.

Drugs That Should Not Be Coadministered With CRIXIVAN
Administration of indinavir (800 mg every 8 hours) with rifampin (600 mg once daily) for one week resulted in an 89% ± 9% decrease in indinavir AUC.

Drugs Requiring Dose Modification
Rifabutin: The coadministration of indinavir 800 mg every 8 hours with rifabutin either 300 mg once daily or 150 mg once daily was evaluated in two separate clinical studies. The results of these studies showed a decrease in indinavir AUC (32% ± 19% and 31% ± 15%, respectively) vs. indinavir 800 mg every 8 hours alone and an increase in rifabutin AUC (204% ± 142% and 60% ± 47%, respectively) vs. rifabutin 300 mg once daily alone. (See DOSAGE AND ADMINISTRATION, *Concomitant Therapy, Rifabutin*.)

Ketoconazole: Administration of a 400-mg dose of ketoconazole with a 400-mg dose of indinavir resulted in a 68% ± 48% increase in indinavir AUC (see DOSAGE AND ADMINISTRATION, *Concomitant Therapy, Ketoconazole*). The effects of administering a 400- or 800-mg dose of ketoconazole with an 800-mg dose of indinavir are not known.

Drugs Not Requiring Dose Modification
Nucleoside analogue antiretroviral agents: Administration of indinavir (1000 mg every 8 hours) with zidovudine (200 mg every 8 hours) for one week resulted in a 13% ± 48% increase in indinavir AUC and a 17% ± 23% increase in zidovudine AUC. In another study, administration of indinavir (800 mg every 8 hours) with zidovudine (200 mg every 8 hours) in combination with lamivudine (150 mg twice daily) for one week resulted in no change in indinavir AUC, a 36% increase in zidovudine AUC, and a 6% decrease in lamivudine AUC. Administration of indinavir (800 mg every 8 hours) in combination with stavudine (40 mg every 12 hours) for one week resulted in no change in indinavir AUC and a 25% ± 26% increase in stavudine AUC.

ORTHO-NOVUM 1/35:** Administration of indinavir (800 mg every 8 hours) with ORTHO-NOVUM 1/35 for one week resulted in a 24% ± 17% increase in ethinyl estradiol AUC and a 26% ± 14% increase in norethindrone AUC.

Cimetidine, Quinidine, Grapefruit Juice: Administration of a single 400-mg dose of indinavir following six days of cimetidine (600 mg every 12 hours) did not affect indinavir AUC. Administration of a single 400-mg dose of indinavir

with 8 oz. of grapefruit juice resulted in a <u>decrease</u> in indinavir AUC (26% ± 18%). Administration of a single 400-mg dose of indinavir with 200 mg of quinidine sulfate resulted in a 10% ± 26% increase in indinavir AUC.

Trimethoprim/Sulfamethoxazole, Fluconazole, Isoniazid, Clarithromycin: Administration of indinavir (400 mg every 6 hours) with trimethroprim/sulfamethoxazole (one double strength tablet every 12 hours) for one week resulted in no change in indinavir AUC, a 19% ± 31% increase in trimethoprim AUC, and no change in sulfamethoxazole AUC. Administration of indinavir (1000 mg every 8 hours) with fluconazole (400 mg once daily) for one week resulted in a 19% ± 33% decrease in indinavir AUC and no change in fluconazole AUC. Administration of indinavir (800 mg every 8 hours) with isoniazid (300 mg once daily) for one week resulted in no change in indinavir AUC and a 13% ± 15% increase in isoniazid AUC. Administration of indinavir (800 mg every 8 hours) with clarithromycin (500 mg every 12 hours) for one week resulted in a 29% ± 42% increase in indinavir AUC and a 53% ± 36% increase in clarithromycin AUC.

** Registered trademark of Ortho Pharmaceutical Corporation

INDICATIONS AND USAGE

CRIXIVAN in combination with antiretroviral agents is indicated for the treatment of HIV infection.
This indication is based on two clinical trials of approximately 1 year duration that demonstrated: 1) a reduction in the risk of AIDS defining illnesses or death; 2) a prolonged suppression of HIV RNA.

Description of Studies
In all clinical studies, with the exception of ACTG 320, the AMPLICOR HIV MONITOR assay was used to determine the level of circulating HIV RNA in serum. This is an experimental use of the assay. HIV RNA results should not be directly compared to results from other trials using different HIV RNA assays or using other sample sources.

Study ACTG 320 was a multicenter, randomized, double-blind clinical endpoint trial to compare the effect of CRIXIVAN in combination with zidovudine and lamivudine with that of zidovudine plus lamivudine on the progression to an AIDS-defining illness (ADI) or death. Patients were protease inhibitor and lamivudine naive and zidovudine experienced, with CD4 cell counts of ≤200 cells/mm³. The study enrolled 1156 HIV-infected patients (17% female, 28% Black, 18% Hispanic, mean age 39 years). The mean baseline CD4 cell count was 87 cells/mm³. The mean baseline HIV RNA for a subset of 190 patients was 4.98 $\log_{10}$ copies/mL (95,432 copies/mL). The study was terminated after a planned interim analysis, resulting in a median follow-up of 38 weeks and a maximum follow-up of 52 weeks. Results are shown in Table 1 and Figures 1 & 2.

Table 1
ACTG 320

Endpoint	Number (%) of Patients with AIDS-defining Illness or Death	
	IDV+ZDV+L (n=577)	ZDV+L (n=579)
HIV Progression or Death	35 (6.1)	63 (10.9)
Death*	10 (1.7)	19 (3.3)

*The number of deaths is inadequate to assess the impact of Indinavir on survival.
IDV = Indinavir, ZDV = Zidovudine, L = Lamivudine

Study ACTG 320: Figure 1
Indinavir Protocol ACTG 320 Zidovudine Experienced Plasma Viral RNA - Proportions Below 500 Copies/mL

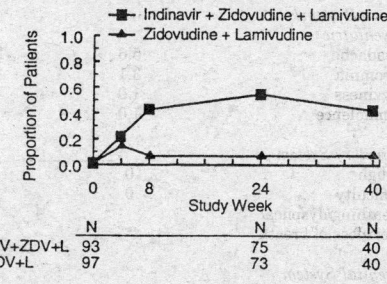

	N	N	N
IDV+ZDV+L	93	75	40
ZDV+L	97	73	40

[See figure 2 at top of next column]

Study 028, a double-blind, multicenter, randomized, clinical endpoint trial conducted in Brazil, compared the effects of CRIXIVAN plus zidovudine with those of CRIXIVAN alone or zidovudine alone on the progression to an ADI or death,

Study ACTG 320: Figure 2
ACTG 320 Zidovudine Experienced CD4 Cell Counts - Mean Change from Baseline

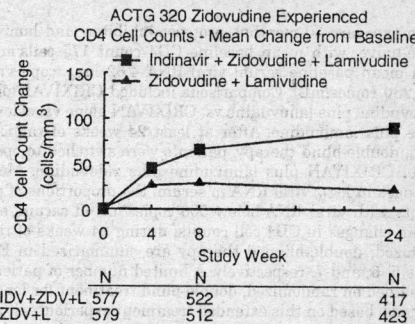

	N	N	N
IDV+ZDV+L	577	522	417
ZDV+L	579	512	423

and on surrogate marker responses. All patients were antiretroviral naive with CD4 cell counts of 50 to 250 cells/mm³. The study enrolled 996 HIV-1 seropositive patients [28% female, 11% Black, 1% Asian/Other, median age 33 years, mean baseline CD4 cell count of 152 cells/mm³, mean serum viral RNA of 4.44 $\log_{10}$ copies/mL (27,824 copies/mL)]. Treatment regimens containing zidovudine were modified in a blinded manner with the optional addition of lamivudine (median time: week 40). The median length of follow-up was 56 weeks with a maximum of 97 weeks. The study was terminated after a planned interim analysis, resulting in a median follow-up of 56 weeks and a maximum follow-up of 97 weeks. Results are shown in Table 2 and Figures 3 and 4.

Table 2
Protocol 028

Endpoint	Number (%) of Patients with AIDS-defining Illness or Death		
	IDV+ZDV (n=332)	IDV (n=332)	ZDV (n=332)
HIV Progression or Death	21 (6.3)	27 (8.1)	62 (18.7)
Death*	8 (2.4)	5 (1.5)	11 (3.3)

*The number of deaths is inadequate to assess the impact of Indinavir on survival.

Study 028: Figure 3
Indinavir Protocol 028 Zidovudine Naive Viral RNA - Proportions Below 500 Copies/mL in Serum

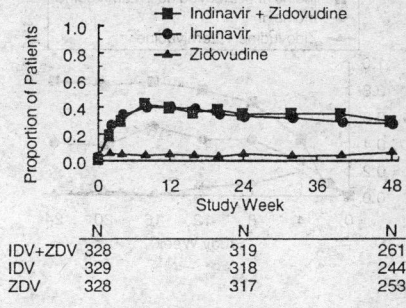

	N	N	N
IDV+ZDV	328	319	261
IDV	329	318	244
ZDV	328	317	253

Study 028: Figure 4
Indinavir Protocol 028 Zidovudine Naive CD4 Cell Counts - Mean Change from Baseline

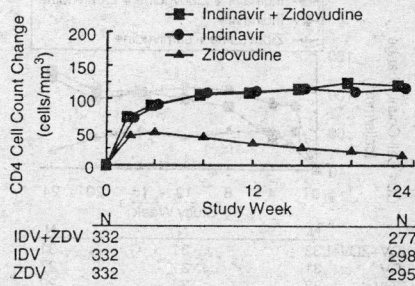

	N		N
IDV+ZDV	332		277
IDV	332		298
ZDV	332		295

Study 035 was a multicenter randomized trial in 97 HIV-1 seropositive patients who were zidovudine-experienced (me-

Continued on next page

Information on the Merck & Co., Inc. products listed on these pages is the full prescribing information from product circulars in use August 31, 1998. For information, please call 1-800-NSC MERCK [1-800-672-6372].

Consult 1999 PDR® supplements and future editions for revisions

Crixivan—Cont.

dian exposure 30 months), protease-inhibitor- and lamivudine-naive, with mean baseline CD4 count 175 cells/mm[3] and mean baseline serum viral RNA 4.62 $\log_{10}$ copies/mL (41,230 copies/mL). Comparisons included CRIXIVAN plus zidovudine plus lamivudine vs. CRIXIVAN alone vs. zidovudine plus lamivudine. After at least 24 weeks of randomized, double-blind therapy, patients were switched to open-label CRIXIVAN plus lamivudine plus zidovudine. Mean changes in $\log_{10}$ viral RNA in serum, the proportions of patients with viral RNA below 500 copies/mL in serum, and mean changes in CD4 cell counts, during 24 weeks of randomized, double-blinded therapy are summarized in Figures 5, 6, and 7, respectively. A limited number of patients remained on randomized, double-blind treatment for longer periods; based on this extended treatment experience, it appears that a greater number of subjects randomized to CRIXIVAN plus zidovudine plus lamivudine demonstrated HIV RNA levels below 500 copies/mL during one year of therapy as compared to those in other treatment groups.

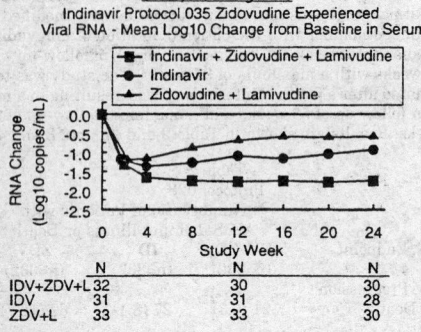

Study 035: Figure 5
Indinavir Protocol 035 Zidovudine Experienced
Viral RNA - Mean Log10 Change from Baseline in Serum

	N	N	N
IDV+ZDV+L	32	30	30
IDV	31	31	28
ZDV+L	33	33	30

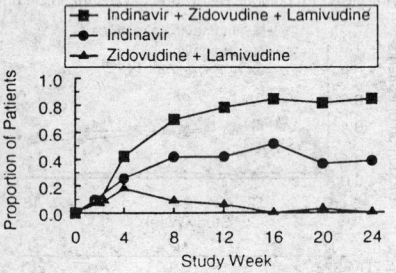

Study 035: Figure 6
Indinavir Protocol 035 Zidovudine Experienced
Viral RNA - Proportions Below 500 Copies/mL in Serum

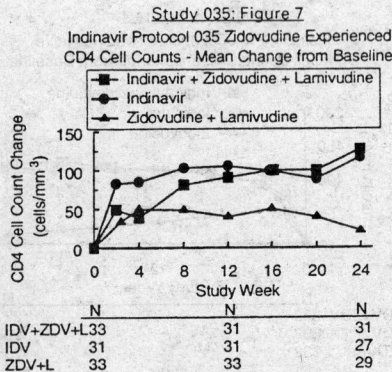

Study 035: Figure 7
Indinavir Protocol 035 Zidovudine Experienced
CD4 Cell Counts - Mean Change from Baseline

	N	N	N
IDV+ZDV+L	33	31	31
IDV	31	31	27
ZDV+L	33	33	29

Genotypic Resistance in Clinical Studies

Study 006 (10/15/93–10/12/94) was a dose-ranging study in which patients were initially treated with CRIXIVAN at a dose of <2.4 g/day followed by 2.4 g/day. Study 019 (6/23/94–4/10/95) was a randomized comparison of CRIXIVAN 600 mg every 6 hours, CRIXIVAN plus zidovudine, and zidovudine alone. Table 3 shows the incidence of genotypic resistance at 24 weeks in these studies.

Table 3
Genotypic Resistance at 24 Weeks

Treatment Group	Resistance to IDV n/N*	Resistance to ZDV n/N*
IDV	—	—
<2.4 g/day	31/37 (84%)	—
2.4 g/day	9/21 (43%)	1/17 (6%)
IDV/ZDV	4/22 (18%)	1/22 (5%)
ZDV	1/18 (6%)	11/17 (65%)

*N – includes patients with non-amplifiable virus at 24 weeks who had amplifiable virus at week 0.

CONTRAINDICATIONS

CRIXIVAN is contraindicated in patients with clinically significant hypersensitivity to any of its components.
CRIXIVAN should not be administered concurrently with terfenadine, cisapride, astemizole, triazolam, midazolam, or ergot derivatives. Inhibition of CYP3A4 by CRIXIVAN could result in elevated plasma concentrations of these drugs, potentially causing serious or life-threatening reactions.

WARNINGS

Nephrolithiasis

Nephrolithiasis has occurred with CRIXIVAN therapy. In some cases, nephrolithiasis has been associated with renal insufficiency or acute renal failure. If signs or symptoms of nephrolithiasis occur, (including flank pain, with or without hematuria or microscopic hematuria), temporary interruption (e.g., 1–3 days) or discontinuation of therapy may be considered. **Adequate hydration is recommended in all patients treated with CRIXIVAN. (See ADVERSE REACTIONS, *Post-Marketing Experience* and DOSAGE AND ADMINISTRATION, *Nephrolithiasis*.)**

Hemolytic Anemia

Acute hemolytic anemia, including cases resulting in death, has been reported in patients treated with CRIXIVAN. Once a diagnosis is apparent, appropriate measures for the treatment of hemolytic anemia should be instituted, including discontinuation of CRIXIVAN.

Hepatitis

Hepatitis including cases resulting in hepatic failure and death has been reported in patients treated with CRIXIVAN. Because the majority of these patients had confounding medical conditions and/or were receiving concomitant therapy(ies), a causal relationship between CRIXIVAN and these events has not been established.

Hyperglycemia

New onset diabetes mellitus, exacerbation of pre-existing diabetes mellitus and hyperglycemia have been reported during post-marketing surveillance in HIV-infected patients receiving protease inhibitor therapy. Some patients required either initiation or dose adjustments of insulin or oral hypoglycemic agents for treatment of these events. In some cases, diabetic ketoacidosis has occurred. In those patients who discontinued protease inhibitor therapy, hyperglycemia persisted in some cases. Because these events have been reported voluntarily during clinical practice, estimates of frequency cannot be made and a causal relationship between protease inhibitor therapy and these events has not been established.

PRECAUTIONS

General

Indirect hyperbilirubinemia has occurred frequently during treatment with CRIXIVAN and has infrequently been associated with increases in serum transaminases (see also ADVERSE REACTIONS, *Clinical Trials* and *Post-Marketing Experience*). It is not known whether CRIXIVAN will exacerbate the physiologic hyperbilirubinemia seen in neonates. (See *Pregnancy*)

Table 4
Clinical Adverse Experiences Reported in ≥2% of Patients

Adverse Experience	Studies 028 and 033* Considered Drug-Related and of Moderate or Severe Intensity			Study ACTG 320 of Unknown Drug Relationship and of Severe or Life-threatening Intensity	
	CRIXIVAN Percent (n=196)	CRIXIVAN plus Zidovudine Percent (n=196)	Zidovudine Percent (n=195)	CRIXIVAN plus Zidovudine plus Lamivudine Percent (n=571)	Zidovudine plus Lamivudine Percent (n=575)
Body as a Whole					
Abdominal pain	8.7	8.2	5.1	1.9	0.7
Asthenia/fatigue	3.6	9.2	7.7	2.4	4.5
Fever	0.5	0.5	0	3.8	3.0
Malaise	0.5	2.0	1.5	0	0
Digestive System					
Nausea	11.7	32.1	14.4	2.8	1.4
Diarrhea	4.6	4.1	2.1	0.9	1.2
Vomiting	4.1	12.2	4.6	1.4	1.4
Acid regurgitation	2.0	2.0	0.5	0.4	0
Anorexia	0.5	2.0	3.1	0.5	0.2
Dry mouth	0.5	0	2.1	0	0
Musculoskeletal System					
Back pain	2.0	1.0	1.5	0.9	0.7
Nervous System / Psychiatric					
Headache	5.6	11.7	5.1	2.4	2.8
Insomnia	3.1	1.5	0	0.2	0
Dizziness	1.0	3.6	0.5	0.5	0.7
Somnolence	1.0	1.5	3.6	0	0
Respiratory System					
Cough	0	0	0	1.6	1.0
Difficulty breathing/dyspnea/ shortness of breath	0	0.5	0.5	1.8	1.0
Urogenital System					
Nephrolithiasis**	3.1	1.5	0	2.6	0.3
Special Senses					
Taste perversion	2.6	3.6	2.1	0.2	0

*Includes, from Protocol 028, 224 patients with 12-week data and, from Protocol 033, 263 patients with a minimum of 12-week data as well as 100 patients with less than 12-week data.
**Including renal colic, and flank pain with and without hematuria

Table 5
Selected Laboratory Abnormalities of Severe or Life-threatening Intensity
Reported in Studies 028 and ACTG 320

	Study 028			Study ACTG 320	
	CRIXIVAN	CRIXIVAN plus Zidovudine	Zidovudine	CRIXIVAN plus Zidovudine plus Lamivudine	Zidovudine plus Lamivudine
	Percent (n=329)	Percent (n=321)	Percent (n=330)	Percent (n=571)	Percent (n=575)
Hematology					
Decreased hemoglobin <7.0 g/dL	0.6	0.9	3.0	2.4	3.5
Decreased platelet count <50 THS/mm^3	0.9	1.2	2.4	0.2	0.9
Decreased neutrophils <0.75 THS/mm^3	2.1	2.5	7.9	5.1	14.6
Blood chemistry					
Increased ALT >500% ULN*	5.5	5.9	5.2	2.6	2.6
Increased AST >500% ULN	4.0	2.8	3.6	3.3	2.8
Total serum bilirubin >250% ULN	12.5	10.6	1.5	6.1	1.4
Increased serum amylase >200% ULN	2.1	2.8	2.1	0.9	0.3
Increased glucose >250 mg/dL	0.9	1.2	0.6	1.6	1.9
Increased creatinine >300% ULN	0	0	0.6	0.2	0

* Upper limit of the normal range.

Coexisting Conditions
Patients with hemophilia: There have been reports of spontaneous bleeding in patients with hemophilia A and B treated with protease inhibitors. In some patients, additional factor VIII was required. In many of the reported cases, treatment with protease inhibitors was continued or restarted. A causal relationship between protease inhibitor therapy and these episodes has not been established. (See ADVERSE REACTIONS, *Post-Marketing Experience*.)
Patients with hepatic insufficiency due to cirrhosis: In these patients, the dosage of CRIXIVAN should be lowered because of decreased metabolism of CRIXIVAN (see DOSAGE AND ADMINISTRATION).
Patients with renal insufficiency: Patients with renal insufficiency have not been studied.
Information for Patients
CRIXIVAN is not a cure for HIV infection and patients may continue to develop opportunistic infections and other complications associated with HIV disease. The long-term effects of CRIXIVAN unknown at this time. CRIXIVAN has not been shown to reduce the risk of transmission of HIV to others through sexual contact or blood contamination.
Patients should be advised to remain under the care of a physician when using CRIXIVAN and should not modify or discontinue treatment without first consulting the physician. Therefore, if a dose is missed, patients should take the next dose at the regularly scheduled time and should not double this dose. Therapy with CRIXIVAN should be initiated and maintained at the recommended dosage.
For optimal absorption, CRIXIVAN should be administered without food but with water 1 hour before or 2 hours after a meal. Alternatively, CRIXIVAN may be administered with other liquids such as skim milk, juice, coffee, or tea, or with a light meal, e.g., dry toast with jelly, juice, and coffee with skim milk and sugar; or corn flakes, skim milk and sugar (see CLINICAL PHARMACOLOGY, *Effect of Food on Oral Absorption* and DOSAGE AND ADMINISTRATION). Ingestion of CRIXIVAN with a meal high in calories, fat, and protein reduces the absorption of indinavir.
CRIXIVAN Capsules are sensitive to moisture. Patients should be informed that CRIXIVAN should be stored and used in the original container and the desiccant should remain in the bottle.
Drug Interactions
Rifampin
Rifampin is a potent inducer of P-450 3A4 that markedly diminishes plasma concentrations of indinavir. Therefore, CRIXIVAN and rifampin should not be coadministered (see CLINICAL PHARMACOLOGY, *Drugs That Should Not Be Coadministered With CRIXIVAN*).
Rifabutin
When rifabutin and CRIXIVAN are coadministered, there is an increase in the plasma concentrations of rifabutin and a decrease in the plasma concentrations of indinavir. A dosage reduction of rifabutin and a dosage increase of CRIXIVAN

are necessary when rifabutin is coadministered with CRIXIVAN. The suggested dose adjustments are expected to result in rifabutin concentrations at least 50% higher than typically observed when rifabutin is administered alone at its usual dose (300 mg/day) and indinavir concentrations which may be slightly less than typically observed when indinavir is administered alone at its usual dose (800 mg every 8 hours). (See DOSAGE AND ADMINISTRATION, *Concomitant Therapy, Rifabutin;* CLINICAL PHARMACOLOGY, *Drug Interactions, Drugs Requiring Dose Modification, Rifabutin.*)
Ketoconazole
Due to an increase in the plasma concentrations of indinavir, a dosage reduction of indinavir should be considered when CRIXIVAN and ketoconazole are coadministered (see DOSAGE AND ADMINISTRATION, *Concomitant Therapy, Ketoconazole;* CLINICAL PHARMACOLOGY, *Drug Interactions, Drugs Requiring Dose Modification, Ketoconazole*).
Other
If CRIXIVAN and didanosine are administered concomitantly, they should be administered at least one hour apart on an empty stomach; a normal (acidic) gastric pH may be necessary for optimum absorption of indinavir, whereas acid rapidly degrades didanosine which is formulated with buffering agents to increase pH (consult the manufacturer's product circular for didanosine).
Interactions between indinavir and less potent CYP3A4 inducers than rifampin, such as phenobarbital, phenytoin, carbamazepine, and dexamethasone have not been studied. These agents should be used with caution if administered concomitantly with indinavir because decreased indinavir plasma concentrations may result.
Carcinogenesis, Mutagenesis, Impairment of Fertility
Carcinogenicity studies were conducted in mice and rats. In mice, no increased incidence of any tumor type was observed. The highest dose tested in rats was 640 mg/kg/day; at this dose a statistically significant increased incidence of thyroid adenomas was seen only in male rats. At that dose, daily systemic exposure in rats was approximately 1.3 times higher than daily systemic exposure in humans. No evidence of mutagenicity or genotoxicity was observed in *in vitro* microbial mutagenesis (Ames) tests, *in vitro* alkaline elution assays for DNA breakage, *in vitro* and *in vivo* chromosomal aberration studies, and *in vitro* mammalian cell mutagenesis assays. No treatment-related effects on mating, fertility, or embryo survival were seen in female rats and no treatment-related effects on mating performance were seen in male rats at doses providing systemic exposure comparable to or slightly higher than that with the clinical dose. In addition, no treatment-related effects were observed in fecundity or fertility of untreated females mated to treated males.
Pregnancy
Pregnancy Category C: Developmental toxicity studies were performed in rabbits (at doses up to 240 mg/kg/day), dogs

(at doses up to 80 mg/kg/day), and rats (at doses up to 640 mg/kg/day). The highest doses in these studies produced systemic exposures in these species comparable to or slightly greater than human exposure. No treatment-related external, visceral, or skeletal changes were observed in rabbits or dogs. No treatment-related external or visceral changes were observed in rats. Treatment-related increases over controls in the incidence of supernumerary ribs (at exposures at or below those in humans) and of cervical ribs (at exposures comparable to or slightly greater than those in humans) were seen in rats. In all three species, no treatment-related effects on embryonic/fetal survival or fetal weights were observed.
In rabbits, at a maternal dose of 240 mg/kg/day, no drug was detected in fetal plasma 1 hour after dosing. Fetal plasma drug levels 2 hours after dosing were approximately 3% of maternal plasma drug levels. In dogs, at a maternal dose of 80 mg/kg/day, fetal plasma drug levels were approximately 50% of maternal plasma drug levels both 1 and 2 hours after dosing. In rats, at maternal doses of 40 and 640 mg/kg/day, fetal plasma drug levels were approximately 10 to 15% and 10 to 20% of maternal plasma drug levels 1 and 2 hours after dosing, respectively.
Indinavir was administered to Rhesus monkeys during the third trimester of pregnancy (at doses up to 160 mg/kg twice daily) and to neonatal Rhesus monkeys (at doses up to 160 mg/kg twice daily). When administered to neonates, indinavir caused an exacerbation of the transient physiologic hyperbilirubinemia seen in this species after birth; serum bilirubin values were approximately fourfold above controls at 160 mg/kg twice daily. A similar exacerbation did not occur in neonates after *in utero* exposure to indinavir during the third trimester of pregnancy. In Rhesus monkeys, fetal plasma drug levels were approximately 1 to 2% of maternal plasma drug levels approximately 1 hour after maternal dosing at 40, 80, or 160 mg/kg twice daily.
Hyperbilirubinemia has occurred during treatment with CRIXIVAN (see PRECAUTIONS and ADVERSE REACTIONS). It is unknown whether CRIXIVAN administered to the mother in the perinatal period will exacerbate physiologic hyperbilirubinemia in neonates.
There are no adequate and well-controlled studies in pregnant women. CRIXIVAN should be used during pregnancy only if the potential benefit justifies the potential risk to the fetus.
Nursing Mothers
Studies in lactating rats have demonstrated that indinavir is excreted in milk. Although it is not known whether CRIXIVAN is excreted in human milk, there exists the potential for adverse effects from indinavir in nursing infants. Mothers should be instructed to discontinue nursing if they are receiving CRIXIVAN. This is consistent with the recommendation by the U.S. Public Health Service Centers for Disease Control and Prevention that HIV-infected mothers not breast-feed their infants to avoid risking postnatal transmission of HIV.
Pediatric Use
Safety and effectiveness in pediatric patients have not been established.

ADVERSE REACTIONS

Clinical Trials
Nephrolithiasis, including flank pain with or without hematuria (including microscopic hematuria), has been reported in approximately 9.3% (193/2071) of patients receiving CRIXIVAN in clinical trials at the recommended dose, compared to 2.1% in the control arms. Of the patients treated with CRIXIVAN who developed nephrolithiasis, 3.1% (6/193) were reported to develop hydronephrosis and 3.1% (6/193) underwent stent placement. Following the acute episode, 3.6% (7/193) of patients discontinued therapy. (See WARNINGS and DOSAGE AND ADMINISTRATION, *Nephrolithiasis.*)
Asymptomatic hyperbilirubinemia (total bilirubin ≥2.5 mg/dL), reported predominantly as elevated indirect bilirubin, has occurred in approximately 10% of patients treated with CRIXIVAN. In <1% this was associated with elevations in ALT or AST.
Hyperbilirubinemia and nephrolithiasis occurred more frequently at doses exceeding 2.4 g/day compared to doses ≤2.4 g/day.
Clinical adverse experiences reported in ≥2% of patients treated with CRIXIVAN alone, CRIXIVAN in combination with zidovudine or zidovudine plus lamivudine, zidovudine alone, or zidovudine plus lamivudine are presented in Table 4.
[See table 4 at bottom of previous page]

Continued on next page

Information on the Merck & Co., Inc. products listed on these pages is the full prescribing information from product circulars in use August 31, 1998. For information, please call 1-800-NSC MERCK [1-800-672-6372].

Crixivan—Cont.

In Phase I and II controlled trials, the following adverse events were reported significantly more frequently by those randomized to the arms containing CRIXIVAN than by those randomized to nucleoside analogues: rash, upper respiratory infection, dry skin, pharyngitis, taste perversion. Selected laboratory abnormalities of severe or life-threatening intensity reported in patients treated with CRIXIVAN alone, CRIXIVAN in combination with zidovudine or zidovudine plus lamivudine, zidovudine alone, or zidovudine plus lamivudine are presented in Table 5.

[See table 5 at top of previous page]

Post-Marketing Experience

Body As A Whole: redistribution/accumulation of body fat in areas such as the back of the neck, abdomen, and retroperitoneum.

Digestive System: liver function abnormalities; hepatitis including reports of hepatic failure (see WARNINGS).

Hematologic: increased spontaneous bleeding in patients with hemophilia (see PRECAUTIONS); acute hemolytic anemia (see WARNINGS).

Endocrine/Metabolic: new onset diabetes mellitus, exacerbation of pre-existing diabetes mellitus, hyperglycemia (see WARNINGS).

Hypersensitivity: anaphylactoid reactions.

Skin and Skin Appendage: rash including erythema multiforme and Stevens-Johnson Syndrome; hyperpigmentation; alopecia.

Urogenital System: nephrolithiasis; in some cases resulting in renal insufficiency or acute renal failure (see WARNINGS); crystalluria; interstitial nephritis.

Laboratory Abnormalities
Increased serum triglycerides.

OVERDOSAGE

It is not known whether CRIXIVAN is dialyzable by peritoneal or hemodialysis. Single oral or intraperitoneal doses of indinavir up to 20 times the related human dose in rats and 10 times the related human dose in mice caused no lethality.

DOSAGE AND ADMINISTRATION

The recommended dosage of CRIXIVAN is 800 mg (**two** 400-mg capsules) orally every 8 hours. The dosage is the same whether CRIXIVAN is used alone or in combination with other antiretroviral agents.

CRIXIVAN must be taken at intervals of 8 hours. For optimal absorption, CRIXIVAN should be administered without food but with water 1 hour before or 2 hours after a meal. Alternatively, CRIXIVAN may be administered with other liquids such as skim milk, juice, coffee, or tea, or with a light meal, e.g., dry toast with jelly, juice, and coffee with skim milk and sugar; or corn flakes, skim milk and sugar. (See CLINICAL PHARMACOLOGY, *Effect of Food on Oral Absorption*.)

To ensure adequate hydration, it is recommended that the patient drink at least 1.5 liters (approximately 48 ounces) of liquids during the course of 24 hours.

Concomitant Therapy

Rifabutin
Dose reduction of rifabutin to half the standard dose (consult the manufacturer's product circular for rifabutin) and a dose increase of CRIXIVAN to 1000 mg every 8 hours are recommended when rifabutin and CRIXIVAN are coadministered (see PRECAUTIONS, *Drug Interactions*).

Ketoconazole
Dose reduction of CRIXIVAN to 600 mg every 8 hours should be considered when administering ketoconazole concurrently.

Didanosine
If indinavir and didanosine are administered concomitantly, they should be administered at least one hour apart on an empty stomach (consult the manufacturer's product circular for didanosine).

Hepatic Insufficiency
The dosage of CRIXIVAN should be reduced to 600 mg every 8 hours in patients with mild-to-moderate hepatic insufficiency due to cirrhosis.

Nephrolithiasis
In addition to adequate hydration, medical management in patients who experience nephrolithiasis may include temporary interruption (e.g., 1–3 days) or discontinuation of therapy.

HOW SUPPLIED

CRIXIVAN Capsules are supplied as follows:

No. 3756—200 mg capsules: semi-translucent white capsules coded "**CRIXIVAN™ 200 mg**" in blue. Available as:
NDC 0006-0571-42 unit-of-use bottles of 270 (with desiccant)
NDC 0006-0571-43 unit-of-use bottles of 360 (with desiccant).

Shown in Product Identification Section, page 323

No. 3758—400 mg capsules: semi-translucent white capsules coded "**CRIXIVAN™ 400 mg**" in green. Available as:
NDC 0006-0573-62 unit-of-use bottles of 180 (with desiccant)
NDC 0006-0573-54 unit-of-use bottles of 90 (with desiccant).

Shown in Product Identification Guide, page 323

Storage
Store in a tightly-closed container at room temperature, 15–30°C (59–86°F). Protect from moisture.
CRIXIVAN Capsules are sensitive to moisture. CRIXIVAN should be dispensed and stored in the original container. The desiccant should remain in the original bottle.

7979807   Issued February 1998

COPYRIGHT © MERCK & CO., Inc., 1996, 1997
All rights reserved

CUPRIMINE® Capsules   ℞
(Penicillamine), U.S.P.

Physicians planning to use penicillamine should thoroughly familiarize themselves with its toxicity, special dosage considerations, and therapeutic benefits. Penicillamine should never be used casually. Each patient should remain constantly under the close supervision of the physician. Patients should be warned to report promptly any symptoms suggesting toxicity.

DESCRIPTION

Penicillamine is a chelating agent used in the treatment of Wilson's disease. It is also used to reduce cystine excretion in cystinuria and to treat patients with severe, active rheumatoid arthritis unresponsive to conventional therapy (see INDICATIONS). It is 3-mercapto-D-valine. It is a white or practically white, crystalline powder, freely soluble in water, slightly soluble in alcohol, and insoluble in ether, acetone, benzene, and carbon tetrachloride. Although its configuration is D, it is levorotatory as usually measured:

$$[\alpha]25° = -62.5° \pm 2° \ (c = 1, \ 1N \ NaOH),$$
D

calculated on a dried basis.
The empirical formula is $C_5H_{11}NO_2S$, giving it a molecular weight of 149.21. The structural formula is:

$$\begin{array}{c} SH \ \ NH_2 \\ | \ \ \ \ \ \ | \\ (CH_3)_2C{-}CHCOOH \end{array}$$

It reacts readily with formaldehyde or acetone to form a thiazolidine-carboxylic acid.
Capsules CUPRIMINE* (Penicillamine) for oral administration contain either 125 mg or 250 mg of penicillamine. Each capsule contains the following inactive ingredients: D & C Yellow 10, gelatin, lactose, magnesium stearate, and titanium dioxide. The 125 mg capsule also contains iron oxide.

---

*Registered trademark of MERCK & CO., INC.

CLINICAL PHARMACOLOGY

Penicillamine is a chelating agent recommended for the removal of excess copper in patients with Wilson's disease. From *in vitro* studies which indicate that one atom of copper combines with two molecules of penicillamine, it would appear that one gram of penicillamine should be followed by the excretion of about 200 milligrams of copper; however, the actual amount excreted is about one percent of this.
Penicillamine also reduces excess cystine excretion in cystinuria. This is done, at least in part, by disulfide interchange between penicillamine and cystine, resulting in formation of penicillamine-cysteine disulfide, a substance that is much more soluble than cystine and is excreted readily.
Penicillamine interferes with the formation of cross-links between tropocollagen molecules and cleaves them when newly formed.
The mechanism of action of penicillamine in rheumatoid arthritis is unknown although it appears to suppress disease activity. Unlike cytotoxic immunosuppressants, penicillamine markedly lowers IgM rheumatoid factor but produces no significant depression in absolute levels of serum immunoglobulins. Also unlike cytotoxic immunosuppressants which act on both, penicillamine *in vitro* depresses T-cell activity but not B-cell activity.
In vitro, penicillamine dissociates macroglobulins (rheumatoid factor) although the relationship of the activity to its effect in rheumatoid arthritis is not known.
In rheumatoid arthritis, the onset of therapeutic response to CUPRIMINE may not be seen for two or three months. In those patients who respond, however, the first evidence of suppression of symptoms such as pain, tenderness, and

swelling is generally apparent within three months. The optimum duration of therapy has not been determined. If remissions occur, they may last from months to years, but usually require continued treatment (see DOSAGE AND ADMINISTRATION).
In all patients receiving penicillamine, it is important that CUPRIMINE be given on an empty stomach, at least one hour before meals or two hours after meals, and at least one hour apart from any other drug, food, or milk. This permits maximum absorption and reduces the likelihood of inactivation by metal binding in the gastrointestinal tract.
Methodology for determining the bioavailability of penicillamine is not available; however, penicillamine is known to be a very soluble substance.

INDICATIONS

CUPRIMINE is indicated in the treatment of Wilson's disease, cystinuria, and in patients with severe, active rheumatoid arthritis who have failed to respond to an adequate trial of conventional therapy. Available evidence suggests that CUPRIMINE is not of value in ankylosing spondylitis.
Wilson's Disease—Wilson's disease (hepatolenticular degeneration) results from the interaction of an inherited defect and an abnormality in copper metabolism. The metabolic defect, which is the consequence of the autosomal inheritance of one abnormal gene from each parent, manifests itself in a greater positive copper balance than normal. As a result, copper is deposited in several organs and appears eventually to produce pathologic effects most prominently seen in the brain, where degeneration is widespread; in the liver, where fatty infiltration, inflammation, and hepatocellular damage progress to postnecrotic cirrhosis; in the kidney, where tubular and glomerular dysfunction results; and in the eye, where characteristic corneal copper deposits are known as Kayser-Fleischer rings.
Two types of patients require treatment for Wilson's disease: (1) the symptomatic, and (2) the asymptomatic in whom it can be assumed the disease will develop in the future if the patient is not treated.
Diagnosis, suspected on the basis of family or individual history, physical examination, or a low serum concentration of ceruloplasmin*, is confirmed by the demonstration of Kayser-Fleischer rings or, particularly in the asymptomatic patient, by the quantitative demonstration in a liver biopsy specimen of a concentration of copper in excess of 250 mcg/g dry weight.
Treatment has two objectives:
(1) to minimize dietary intake and absorption of copper.
(2) to promote excretion of copper deposited in tissues.
The first objective is attained by a daily diet that contains no more than one or two milligrams of copper. Such a diet should exclude, most importantly, chocolate, nuts, shellfish, mushrooms, liver, molasses, broccoli, and cereals enriched with copper, and be composed to as great an extent as possible of foods with a low copper content. Distilled or demineralized water should be used if the patient's drinking water contains more than 0.1 mg of copper per liter.
For the second objective, a copper chelating agent is used. In symptomatic patients this treatment usually produces marked neurologic improvement, fading of Kayser-Fleischer rings, and gradual amelioration of hepatic dysfunction and psychic disturbances.
Clinical experience to date suggests that life is prolonged with the above regimen.
Noticeable improvement may not occur for one to three months. Occasionally, neurologic symptoms become worse during initiation of therapy with CUPRIMINE. Despite this, the drug should not be discontinued permanently, although temporary interruption may result in clinical improvement of the neurological symptoms but it carries an increased risk of developing a sensitivity reaction upon resumption of therapy (see WARNINGS).
Treatment of asymptomatic patients has been carried out for over ten years. Symptoms and signs of the disease appear to be prevented indefinitely if daily treatment with CUPRIMINE can be continued.
Cystinuria—Cystinuria is characterized by excessive urinary excretion of the dibasic amino acids, arginine, lysine, ornithine, and cystine, and the mixed disulfide of cysteine and homocysteine. The metabolic defect that leads to cystinuria is inherited as an autosomal, recessive trait. Metabolism of the affected amino acids is influenced by at least two abnormal factors: (1) defective gastrointestinal absorption and (2) renal tubular dysfunction.
Arginine, lysine, ornithine, and cysteine are soluble substances, readily excreted. There is no apparent pathology connected with their excretion in excessive quantities.
Cystine, however, is so slightly soluble at the usual range of urinary pH that it is not excreted readily, and so crystallizes and forms stones in the urinary tract. Stone formation is the only known pathology in cystinuria.
Normal daily output of cystine is 40 to 80 mg. In cystinuria, output is greatly increased and may exceed 1 g/day. At 500 to 600 mg/day, stone formation is almost certain. When it is more than 300 mg/day, treatment is indicated.

Conventional treatment is directed at keeping urinary cystine diluted enough to prevent stone formation, keeping the urine alkaline enough to dissolve as much cystine as possible, and minimizing cystine production by a diet low in methionine (the major dietary precursor of cystine). Patients must drink enough fluid to keep urine specific gravity below 1.010, take enough alkali to keep urinary pH at 7.5 to 8, and maintain a diet low in methionine. This diet is not recommended in growing children and probably is contraindicated in pregnancy because of its low protein content (see PRECAUTIONS).

When these measures are inadequate to control recurrent stone formation, CUPRIMINE may be used as additional therapy. When patients refuse to adhere to conventional treatment, CUPRIMINE may be a useful substitute. It is capable of keeping cystine excretion to near normal values, thereby hindering stone formation and the serious consequences of pyelonephritis and impaired renal function that develop in some patients.

Bartter and colleagues depict the process by which penicillamine interacts with cystine to form penicillamine-cysteine mixed disulfide as:

$$CSSC + PS' \rightleftarrows CS' + CSSP$$
$$PSSP + CS' \rightleftarrows PS' + CSSP$$
$$CSSC + PSSP \rightleftarrows 2\ CSSP$$

CSSC = cystine
CS' = deprotonated cysteine
PSSP = penicillamine
PS' = deprotonated penicillamine sulfhydryl
CSSP = penicillamine-cysteine mixed disulfide

In this process, it is assumed that the deprotonated form of penicillamine, PS', is the active factor in bringing about the disulfide interchange.

Rheumatoid Arthritis —Because CUPRIMINE can cause severe adverse reactions, its use in rheumatoid arthritis should be restricted to patients who have severe, active disease and who have failed to respond to an adequate trial of conventional therapy. Even then, benefit-to-risk ratio should be carefully considered. Other measures, such as rest, physiotherapy, salicylates, and corticosteroids should be used, when indicated, in conjunction with CUPRIMINE (see PRECAUTIONS).

---

*For quantitative test for serum ceruloplasmin see: Morell, A.G.; Windsor, J.; Sternlieb, I.; Scheinberg, I.H.: Measurement of the concentration of ceruloplasmin in serum by determination of its oxidase activity, in "Laboratory Diagnosis of Liver Disease", F.W. Sunderman; F.W. Sunderman, Jr. (eds.), St. Louis, Warren H. Green, Inc., 1968, pp. 193-195.

CONTRAINDICATIONS

Except for the treatment of Wilson's disease or certain cases of cystinuria, use of penicillamine during pregnancy is contraindicated (see WARNINGS).

Although breast milk studies have not been reported in animals or humans, mothers on therapy with penicillamine should not nurse their infants.

Patients with a history of penicillamine-related aplastic anemia or agranulocytosis should not be restarted on penicillamine (see WARNINGS and ADVERSE REACTIONS).

Because of its potential for causing renal damage, penicillamine should not be administered to rheumatoid arthritis patients with a history or other evidence of renal insufficiency.

WARNINGS

The use of penicillamine has been associated with fatalities due to certain diseases such as aplastic anemia, agranulocytosis, thrombocytopenia, Goodpasture's syndrome, and myasthenia gravis.

Because of the potential for serious hematological and renal adverse reactions to occur at any time, routine urinalysis, white and differential blood cell count, hemoglobin determination, and direct platelet count must be done every two weeks for at least the first six months of penicillamine therapy and monthly thereafter. Patients should be instructed to report promptly the development of signs and symptoms of granulocytopenia and/or thrombocytopenia such as fever, sore throat, chills, bruising or bleeding. The above laboratory studies should then be promptly repeated.

Leukopenia and thrombocytopenia have been reported to occur in up to five percent of patients during penicillamine therapy. Leukopenia is of the granulocytic series and may or may not be associated with an increase in eosinophils. A confirmed reduction in WBC below 3500/mm³ mandates discontinuance of penicillamine therapy. Thrombocytopenia may be on an idiosyncratic basis, with decreased or absent megakaryocytes in the marrow, when it is part of an aplastic anemia. In other cases the thrombocytopenia is presumably on an immune basis since the number of megakaryocytes in the marrow has been reported to be normal or sometimes increased. The development of a platelet count below 100,000/mm³, even in the absence of clinical bleeding,

requires at least temporary cessation of penicillamine therapy. A progressive fall in either platelet count or WBC in three successive determinations, even though values are still within the normal range, likewise requires at least temporary cessation.

Proteinuria and/or hematuria may develop during therapy and may be warning signs of membranous glomerulopathy which can progress to a nephrotic syndrome. Close observation of these patients is essential. In some patients the proteinuria disappears with continued therapy; in others, penicillamine must be discontinued. When a patient develops proteinuria or hematuria the physician must ascertain whether it is a sign of drug-induced glomerulopathy or is unrelated to penicillamine.

Rheumatoid arthritis patients who develop moderate degrees of proteinuria may be continued cautiously on penicillamine therapy, provided that quantitative 24-hour urinary protein determinations are obtained at intervals of one to two weeks. Penicillamine dosage should not be increased under these circumstances. Proteinuria which exceeds 1 g/24 hours, or proteinuria which is progressively increasing, requires either discontinuance of the drug or a reduction in the dosage. In some patients, proteinuria has been reported to clear following reduction in dosage.

In rheumatoid arthritis patients, penicillamine should be discontinued if unexplained gross hematuria or persistent microscopic hematuria develops.

In patients with Wilson's disease or cystinuria the risks of continued penicillamine therapy in patients manifesting potentially serious urinary abnormalities must be weighed against the expected therapeutic benefits.

When penicillamine is used in cystinuria, an annual x-ray for renal stones is advised. Cystine stones form rapidly, sometimes in six months.

Up to one year or more may be required for any urinary abnormalities to disappear after penicillamine has been discontinued.

Because of rare reports of intrahepatic cholestasis and toxic hepatitis, liver function tests are recommended every six months for the duration of therapy.

Goodpasture's syndrome has occurred rarely. The development of abnormal urinary findings associated with hemoptysis and pulmonary infiltrates on x-ray requires immediate cessation of penicillamine.

Obliterative bronchiolitis has been reported rarely. The patient should be cautioned to report immediately pulmonary symptoms such as exertional dyspnea, unexplained cough or wheezing. Pulmonary function studies should be considered at that time.

Myasthenic syndrome sometimes progressing to myasthenia gravis has been reported. Ptosis and diplopia, with weakness of the extraocular muscles, are often early signs of myasthenia. In the majority of cases, symptoms of myasthenia have receded after withdrawal of penicillamine.

Most of the various forms of pemphigus have occurred during treatment with penicillamine. Pemphigus vulgaris and pemphigus foliaceus are reported most frequently, usually as a late complication of therapy. The seborrhea-like characteristics of pemphigus foliaceus may obscure an early diagnosis. When pemphigus is suspected, CUPRIMINE should be discontinued. Treatment has consisted of high doses of corticosteroids alone or, in some cases, concomitantly with an immunosuppressant. Treatment may be required for only a few weeks or months, but may need to be continued for more than a year.

Once instituted for Wilson's disease or cystinuria, treatment with penicillamine should, as a rule, be continued on a daily basis. Interruptions for even a few days have been followed by sensitivity reactions after reinstitution of therapy.

Pregnancy

Penicillamine has been shown to be teratogenic in rats when given in doses 6 times higher than the highest dose recommended for human use. Skeletal defects, cleft palates and fetal toxicity (resorptions) have been reported.

There are no controlled studies on the use of penicillamine in pregnant women. Although normal outcomes have been reported, characteristic congenital cutis laxa and associated birth defects have been reported in infants born of mothers who received therapy with penicillamine during pregnancy. Penicillamine should be used in women of childbearing potential only when the expected benefits outweigh the possible hazards. Women on therapy with penicillamine who are of childbearing potential should be apprised of this risk, advised to report promptly any missed menstrual periods or other indications of possible pregnancy, and followed closely for early recognition of pregnancy.

Wilson's Disease—Reported experience* shows that continued treatment with penicillamine throughout pregnancy protects the mother against relapse of the Wilson's disease, and that discontinuation of penicillamine has deleterious effects on the mother.

If penicillamine is administered during pregnancy to patients with Wilson's disease, it is recommended that the daily dosage be limited to 1 g. If cesarean section is planned,

the daily dosage should be limited to 250 mg during the last six weeks of pregnancy and postoperatively until wound healing is complete.

Cystinuria—If possible, penicillamine should not be given during pregnancy to women with cystinuria (see CONTRAINDICATIONS). There are reports of women with cystinuria on therapy with penicillamine who gave birth to infants with generalized connective tissue defects who died following abdominal surgery. If stones continue to form in these patients, the benefits of therapy to the mother must be evaluated against the risk to the fetus.

Rheumatoid Arthritis—Penicillamine should not be administered to rheumatoid arthritis patients who are pregnant (see CONTRAINDICATIONS) and should be discontinued promptly in patients in whom pregnancy is suspected or diagnosed.

There is a report that a woman with rheumatoid arthritis treated with less than one gram a day of penicillamine during pregnancy gave birth (cesarean delivery) to an infant with growth retardation, flattened face with broad nasal bridge, low set ears, short neck with loose skin folds, and unusually lax body skin.

---

*Scheinberg, I.H., Sternlieb, I.: N. Engl. J. Med. *293* : 1300-1302, Dec. 18, 1975.

PRECAUTIONS

Some patients may experience drug fever, a marked febrile response to penicillamine, usually in the second to third week following initiation of therapy. Drug fever may sometimes be accompanied by a macular cutaneous eruption.

In the case of drug fever in patients with Wilson's disease or cystinuria, penicillamine should be temporarily discontinued until the reaction subsides. Then penicillamine should be reinstituted with a small dose that is gradually increased until the desired dosage is attained. Systemic steroid therapy may be necessary, and is usually helpful, in such patients in whom toxic reactions develop a second or third time.

In the case of drug fever in rheumatoid arthritis patients, because other treatments are available, penicillamine should be discontinued and another therapeutic alternative tried since experience indicates that the febrile reaction will recur in a very high percentage of patients upon readministration of penicillamine.

The skin and mucous membranes should be observed for allergic reactions. Early and late rashes have occurred. Early rash occurs during the first few months of treatment and is more common. It is usually a generalized pruritic, erythematous, maculopapular or morbilliform rash and resembles the allergic rash seen with other drugs. Early rash usually disappears within days after stopping penicillamine and seldom recurs when the drug is restarted at a lower dosage. Pruritus and early rash may often be controlled by the concomitant administration of antihistamines. Less commonly, a late rash may be seen, usually after six months or more of treatment, and requires discontinuation of penicillamine. It is usually on the trunk, is accompanied by intense pruritus, and is usually unresponsive to topical corticosteroid therapy. Late rash may take weeks to disappear after penicillamine is stopped and usually recurs if the drug is restarted.

The appearance of a drug eruption accompanied by fever, arthralgia, lymphadenopathy or other allergic manifestations usually requires discontinuation of penicillamine.

Certain patients will develop a positive antinuclear antibody (ANA) test and some of these may show a lupus erythematosus-like syndrome similar to drug-induced lupus associated with other drugs. The lupus erythematosus-like syndrome is not associated with hypocomplementemia and may be present without nephropathy. The development of a positive ANA test does not mandate discontinuance of the drug; however, the physician should be alerted to the possibility that a lupus erythematosus-like syndrome may develop in the future.

Some patients may develop oral ulcerations which in some cases have the appearance of aphthous stomatitis. The stomatitis usually recurs on rechallenge but often clears on a lower dosage. Although rare, cheilosis, glossitis and gingivostomatitis have also been reported. These oral lesions are frequently dose-related and may preclude further increase in penicillamine dosage or require discontinuation of the drug.

Continued on next page

Information on the Merck & Co., Inc. products listed on these pages is the full prescribing information from product circulars in use August 31, 1998. For information, please call 1-800-NSC MERCK [1-800-672-6372].

Cuprimine—Cont.

Hypogeusia (a blunting or diminution in taste perception) has occurred in some patients. This may last two to three months or more and may develop into a total loss of taste; however, it is usually self-limited despite continued penicillamine treatment. Such taste impairment is rare in patients with Wilson's disease.

Penicillamine should not be used in patients who are receiving concurrently gold therapy, antimalarial or cytotoxic drugs, oxyphenbutazone or phenylbutazone because these drugs are also associated with similar serious hematologic and renal adverse reactions. Patients who have had gold salt therapy discontinued due to a major toxic reaction may be at greater risk of serious adverse reactions with penicillamine but not necessarily of the same type.

Patients who are allergic to penicillin may theoretically have cross-sensitivity to penicillamine. The possibility of reactions from contamination of penicillamine by trace amounts of penicillin has been eliminated now that penicillamine is being produced synthetically rather than as a degradation product of penicillin.

Because of their dietary restrictions, patients with Wilson's disease and cystinuria should be given 25 mg/day of pyridoxine during therapy, since penicillamine increases the requirement for this vitamin. Patients also may receive benefit from a multivitamin preparation, although there is no evidence that deficiency of any vitamin other than pyridoxine is associated with penicillamine. In Wilson's disease, multivitamin preparations must be copper-free.

Rheumatoid arthritis patients whose nutrition is impaired should also be given a daily supplement of pyridoxine. Mineral supplements should not be given, since they may block the response to penicillamine.

Iron deficiency may develop, especially in pediatric patients and in menstruating women. In Wilson's disease, this may be a result of adding the effects of the low copper diet, which is probably also low in iron, and the penicillamine to the effects of blood loss or growth. In cystinuria, a low methionine diet may contribute to iron deficiency, since it is necessarily low in protein. If necessary, iron may be given in short courses, but a period of two hours should elapse between administration of penicillamine and iron, since orally administered iron has been shown to reduce the effects of penicillamine.

Penicillamine causes an increase in the amount of soluble collagen. In the rat this results in inhibition of normal healing and also a decrease in tensile strength of intact skin. In man this may be the cause of increased skin friability at sites especially subject to pressure or trauma, such as shoulders, elbows, knees, toes, and buttocks. Extravasations of blood may occur and may appear as purpuric areas, with external bleeding if the skin is broken, or as vesicles containing dark blood. Neither type is progressive. There is no apparent association with bleeding elsewhere in the body and no associated coagulation defect has been found. Therapy with penicillamine may be continued in the presence of these lesions. They may not recur if dosage is reduced. Other reported effects probably due to the action of penicillamine on collagen are excessive wrinkling of the skin and development of small, white papules at venipuncture and surgical sites.

The effects of penicillamine on collagen and elastin make it advisable to consider a reduction in dosage to 250 mg/day, when surgery is contemplated. Reinstitution of full therapy should be delayed until wound healing is complete.

Carcinogenesis

Long-term animal carcinogenicity studies have not been done with penicillamine. There is a report that five of ten autoimmune disease-prone NZB hybrid mice developed lymphocytic leukemia after 6 months' intraperitoneal treatment with a dose of 400 mg/kg penicillamine 5 days per week.

Nursing Mothers

See CONTRAINDICATIONS.

Pediatric Use

The efficacy of CUPRIMINE in juvenile rheumatoid arthritis has not been established.

ADVERSE REACTIONS

Penicillamine is a drug with a high incidence of untoward reactions, some of which are potentially fatal. Therefore, it is mandatory that patients receiving penicillamine therapy remain under close medical supervision throughout the period of drug administration (see WARNINGS and PRECAUTIONS).

Reported incidences (%) for the most commonly occurring adverse reactions in rheumatoid arthritis patients are noted, based on 17 representative clinical trials reported in the literature (1270 patients).

Allergic—Generalized pruritus, early and late rashes (5%), pemphigus (see WARNINGS), and drug eruptions which may be accompanied by fever, arthralgia, or lymphadenopathy have occurred (see WARNINGS and PRECAUTIONS).

Some patients may show a lupus erythematosus-like syndrome similar to drug-induced lupus produced by other pharmacological agents (see PRECAUTIONS).

Urticaria and exfoliative dermatitis have occurred.

Thyroiditis has been reported; hypoglycemia in association with anti-insulin antibodies has been reported. These reactions are extremely rare.

Some patients may develop a migratory polyarthralgia, often with objective synovitis (see DOSAGE AND ADMINISTRATION).

Gastrointestinal—Anorexia, epigastric pain, nausea, vomiting, or occasional diarrhea may occur (17%).

Isolated cases of reactivated peptic ulcer have occurred, as have hepatic dysfunction and pancreatitis. Intrahepatic cholestasis and toxic hepatitis have been reported rarely. There have been a few reports of increased serum alkaline phosphatase, lactic dehydrogenase, and positive cephalin flocculation and thymol turbidity tests.

Some patients may report a blunting, diminution, or total loss of taste perception (12%); or may develop oral ulcerations. Although rare, cheilosis, glossitis, and gingivostomatitis have been reported (see PRECAUTIONS).

Gastrointestinal side effects are usually reversible following cessation of therapy.

Hematological—Penicillamine can cause bone marrow depression (see WARNINGS). Leukopenia (2%) and thrombocytopenia (4%) have occurred. Fatalities have been reported as a result of thrombocytopenia, agranulocytosis, aplastic anemia, and sideroblastic anemia.

Thrombotic thrombocytopenic purpura, hemolytic anemia, red cell aplasia, monocytosis, leukocytosis, eosinophilia, and thrombocytosis have also been reported.

Renal—Patients on penicillamine therapy may develop proteinuria (6%) and/or hematuria which, in some, may progress to the development of the nephrotic syndrome as a result of an immune complex membranous glomerulopathy (see WARNINGS).

Central Nervous System—Tinnitus, optic neuritis and peripheral sensory and motor neuropathies (including polyradiculoneuropathy, i.e., Guillain-Barre syndrome) have been reported. Muscular weakness may or may not occur with the peripheral neuropathies. Visual and psychic disturbances have been reported.

Neuromuscular—Myasthenia gravis (see WARNINGS).

Other—Adverse reactions that have been reported rarely include thrombophlebitis; hyperpyrexia (see PRECAUTIONS); falling hair or alopecia; lichen planus; polymyositis; dermatomyositis; mammary hyperplasia; elastosis perforans serpiginosa; toxic epidermal necrolysis; anetoderma (cutaneous macular atrophy); and Goodpasture's syndrome, a severe and ultimately fatal glomerulonephritis associated with intra-alveolar hemorrhage (see WARNINGS). Fatal renal vasculitis has also been reported. Allergic alveolitis, obliterative bronchiolitis, interstitial pneumonitis and pulmonary fibrosis have been reported in patients with severe rheumatoid arthritis, some of whom were receiving penicillamine. Bronchial asthma also has been reported.

Increased skin friability, excessive wrinkling of skin, and development of small white papules at venipuncture and surgical sites have been reported (see PRECAUTIONS).

The chelating action of the drug may cause increased excretion of other heavy metals such as zinc, mercury and lead. There have been reports associating penicillamine with leukemia. However, circumstances involved in these reports are such that a cause and effect relationship to the drug has not been established.

DOSAGE AND ADMINISTRATION

In all patients receiving penicillamine, it is important that CUPRIMINE be given on an empty stomach, at least one hour before meals or two hours after meals, and at least one hour apart from any other drug, food, or milk. Because penicillamine increases the requirement for pyridoxine, patients may require a daily supplement of pyridoxine (see PRECAUTIONS).

Wilson's Disease — Optimal dosage can be determined by measurement of urinary copper excretion and the determination of free copper in the serum. The urine must be collected in copper-free glassware, and should be quantitatively analyzed for copper before and soon after initiation of therapy with CUPRIMINE.

Determination of 24-hour urinary copper excretion is of greatest value in the first week of therapy with penicillamine. In the absence of any drug reaction, a dose between 0.75 and 1.5 g that results in an initial 24-hour cupriuresis of over 2 mg should be continued for about three months, by which time the most reliable method of monitoring maintenance treatment is the determination of free copper in the serum. This equals the difference between quantitatively determined total copper and ceruloplasmin-copper. Adequately treated patients will usually have less than 10 mcg free copper/dL of serum. It is seldom necessary to exceed a dosage of 2 g/day. If the patient is intolerant to therapy with CUPRIMINE, alternative treatment is trientine hydrochloride.

In patients who cannot tolerate as much as 1 g/day initially, initiating dosage with 250 mg/day, and increasing gradually to the requisite amount, gives closer control of the effects of the drug and may help to reduce the incidence of adverse reactions.

Cystinuria —It is recommended that CUPRIMINE be used along with conventional therapy. By reducing urinary cystine, it decreases crystalluria and stone formation. In some instances, it has been reported to decrease the size of, and even to dissolve, stones already formed.

The usual dosage of CUPRIMINE in the treatment of cystinuria is 2 g/day for adults, with a range of 1 to 4 g/day. For pediatric patients, dosage can be based on 30 mg/kg/day. The total daily amount should be divided into four doses. If four equal doses are not feasible, give the larger portion at bedtime. If adverse reactions necessitate a reduction in dosage, it is important to retain the bedtime dose.

Initiating dosage with 250 mg/day, and increasing gradually to the requisite amount, gives closer control of the effects of the drug and may help to reduce the incidence of adverse reactions.

In addition to taking CUPRIMINE, patients should drink copiously. It is especially important to drink about a pint of fluid at bedtime and another pint once during the night when urine is more concentrated and more acid than during the day. The greater the fluid intake, the lower the required dosage of CUPRIMINE.

Dosage must be individualized to an amount that limits cystine excretion to 100–200 mg/day in those with no history of stones, and below 100 mg/day in those who have had stone formation and/or pain. Thus, in determining dosage, the inherent tubular defect, the patient's size, age, and rate of growth, and his diet and water intake all must be taken into consideration.

The standard nitroprusside cyanide test has been reported useful as a qualitative measure of the effective dose[*]: Add 2 mL of freshly prepared 5 percent sodium cyanide to 5 mL of a 24-hour aliquot of protein-free urine and let stand ten minutes. Add 5 drops of freshly prepared 5 percent sodium nitroprusside and mix. Cystine will turn the mixture magenta. If the result is negative, it can be assumed that cystine excretion is less than 100 mg/g creatinine.

Although penicillamine is rarely excreted unchanged, it also will turn the mixture magenta. If there is any question as to which substance is causing the reaction, a ferric chloride test can be done to eliminate doubt: Add 3 percent ferric chloride dropwise to the urine. Penicillamine will turn the urine an immediate and quickly fading blue. Cystine will not produce any change in appearance.

[*]Lotz, M., Potts, J.T. and Bartter, F.C.: Brit. Med. J. *2* :521, Aug. 28, 1965 (in Medical Memoranda).

Rheumatoid Arthritis —The principal rule of treatment with CUPRIMINE in rheumatoid arthritis is patience. The onset of therapeutic response is typically delayed. Two or three months may be required before the first evidence of a clinical response is noted (see CLINICAL PHARMACOLOGY).

When treatment with CUPRIMINE has been interrupted because of adverse reactions or other reasons, the drug should be reintroduced cautiously by starting with a lower dosage and increasing slowly.

Initial Therapy—The currently recommended dosage regimen in rheumatoid arthritis begins with a single daily dose of 125 mg or 250 mg which is thereafter increased at one to three month intervals, by 125 mg or 250 mg/day, as patient response and tolerance indicate. If a satisfactory remission of symptoms is achieved, the dose associated with the remission should be continued (see *Maintenance Therapy*). If there is no improvement and there are no signs of potentially serious toxicity after two to three months of treatment with doses of 500–750 mg/day, increases of 250 mg/day at two to three month intervals may be continued until a satisfactory remission occurs (see *Maintenance Therapy*) or signs of toxicity develop (see WARNINGS and PRECAUTIONS). If there is no discernible improvement after three to four months of treatment with 1000 to 1500 mg of penicillamine/day, it may be assumed the patient will not respond and CUPRIMINE should be discontinued.

Maintenance Therapy—The maintenance dosage of CUPRIMINE must be individualized, and may require adjustment during the course of treatment. Many patients respond satisfactorily to a dosage within the 500–750 mg/day range. Some need less.

Changes in maintenance dosage levels may not be reflected clinically or in the erythrocyte sedimentation rate for two to three months after each dosage adjustment.

Some patients will subsequently require an increase in the maintenance dosage to achieve maximal disease suppression. In those patients who do respond, but who evidence incomplete suppression of their disease after the first six to nine months of treatment, the daily dosage of CUPRIMINE may be increased by 125 mg or 250 mg/day at three-month intervals. It is unusual in current practice to employ a dosage in excess of 1 g/day, but up to 1.5 g/day has sometimes been required.

Management of Exacerbations—During the course of treatment some patients may experience an exacerbation of disease activity following an initial good response. These may be self-limited and can subside within twelve weeks. They are usually controlled by the addition of non-steroidal anti-inflammatory drugs, and only if the patient has demonstrated a true "escape" phenomenon (as evidenced by failure of the flare to subside within this time period) should an increase in the maintenance dose ordinarily be considered. In the rheumatoid patient, migratory polyarthralgia due to penicillamine is extremely difficult to differentiate from an exacerbation of the rheumatoid arthritis. Discontinuance or a substantial reduction in dosage of CUPRIMINE for up to several weeks will usually determine which of these processes is responsible for the arthralgia.

Duration of Therapy—The optimum duration of therapy with CUPRIMINE in rheumatoid arthritis has not been determined. If the patient has been in remission for six months or more, a gradual, stepwise dosage reduction in decrements of 125 mg or 250 mg/day at approximately three month intervals may be attempted.

Concomitant Drug Therapy—CUPRIMINE should not be used in patients who are receiving gold therapy, antimalarial or cytotoxic drugs, oxyphenbutazone, or phenylbutazone (see PRECAUTIONS). Other measures, such as salicylates, other non-steroidal anti-inflammatory drugs, or systemic corticosteroids, may be continued when penicillamine is initiated. After improvement commences, analgesic and anti-inflammatory drugs may be slowly discontinued as symptoms permit. Steroid withdrawal must be done gradually, and many months of treatment with CUPRIMINE may be required before steroids can be completely eliminated.

Dosage Frequency—Based on clinical experience dosages up to 500 mg/day can be given as a single daily dose. Dosages in excess of 500 mg/day should be administered in divided doses.

HOW SUPPLIED

No. 3299—Capsules CUPRIMINE, 250 mg, are ivory-colored capsules containing a white or nearly white powder, and are coded CUPRIMINE and MSD 602. They are supplied as follows:
NDC 0006-0602-68 in bottles of 100
(6505-01-049-9494, 250 mg 100's).

Shown in Product Identification Guide, page 323
No. 3350—Capsules CUPRIMINE, 125 mg, are opaque ivory and gray capsules containing a white or nearly white powder, and are coded CUPRIMINE and MSD 672. They are supplied as follows:
NDC 0006-0672-68 in bottles of 100
(6505-01-097-1232, 125 mg 100's).

Shown in Product Identification Guide, page 323
Storage
Keep container tightly closed.
7873240   Issued February 1997
COPYRIGHT © MERCK & CO., INC., 1985, 1989
All rights reserved

DARANIDE® Tablets
(Dichlorphenamide), U.S.P.
℞

DESCRIPTION

DARANIDE* (Dichlorphenamide) is an oral carbonic anhydrase inhibitor. Dichlorphenamide, a dichlorinated benzenedisulfonamide, is known chemically as 4,5-dichloro-1,3-benzenedisulfonamide. Its empirical formula is $C_6H_6Cl_2N_2O_4S_2$ and its structural formula is:

Dichlorphenamide is a white or practically white, crystalline compound with a molecular weight of 305.16. It is very slightly soluble in water but soluble in dilute solutions of sodium carbonate and sodium hydroxide. Dilute alkaline solutions of dichlorphenamide are stable at room temperature.
DARANIDE is supplied as tablets, for oral administration, each containing 50 mg dichlorphenamide. Inactive ingredients are D&C Yellow 10, lactose, magnesium stearate, and starch.

*Registered trademark of MERCK & CO., INC.

CLINICAL PHARMACOLOGY

Carbonic anhydrase inhibitors reduce intraocular pressure by partially suppressing the secretion of aqueous humor (inflow), although the mechanism by which they do this is not fully understood. Evidence suggests that HCO_3^- ions are produced in the ciliary body by hydration of carbon dioxide under the influence of carbonic anhydrase and diffuse into the posterior chamber with Na^+ ions. The aqueous fluid contains more Na^+ and HCO_3^- ions than does plasma and consequently is hypertonic. Water is attracted to the posterior chamber by osmosis. Systemic administration of a carbonic anhydrase inhibitor has been shown to inactivate carbonic anhydrase in the ciliary body of the rabbit's eye and to reduce the high concentration of HCO_3^- ions in ocular fluids. As is the case with all carbonic anhydrase inhibitors, DARANIDE in high doses causes some decrease in renal blood flow and glomerular filtration rate.

In man, DARANIDE begins to act within an hour and maximal effect is observed in two to four hours. The lowered intraocular tension may be maintained for approximately 6 to 12 hours.

INDICATIONS AND USAGE

For adjunctive treatment of: chronic simple (open-angle) glaucoma, secondary glaucoma, and preoperatively in acute angle-closure glaucoma where delay of surgery is desired in order to lower intraocular pressure.

CONTRAINDICATIONS

DARANIDE is contraindicated in hepatic insufficiency, renal failure, adrenocortical insufficiency, hyperchloremic acidosis, or in conditions in which serum levels of sodium or potassium are depressed. DARANIDE should not be used in patients with severe pulmonary obstruction who are unable to increase their alveolar ventilation since their acidosis may be increased.
DARANIDE is contraindicated in patients who are hypersensitive to this product.

PRECAUTIONS

General
Potassium excretion is increased by DARANIDE and hypokalemia may develop with brisk diuresis, when severe cirrhosis is present, or during concomitant use of steroids or ACTH.
Interference with adequate oral electrolyte intake will also contribute to hypokalemia. Hypokalemia can sensitize or exaggerate the response of the heart to the toxic effects of digitalis (e.g., increased ventricular irritability). Hypokalemia may be avoided or treated by use of potassium supplements such as foods with a high potassium content. DARANIDE should be used with caution in patients with respiratory acidosis.

Drug Interactions
Caution is advised in patients receiving concomitant high-dose aspirin and carbonic anhydrase inhibitors, as anorexia, tachypnea, lethargy and coma have been rarely reported due to a possible drug interaction.

Carcinogenesis, Mutagenesis, Impairment of Fertility
Long-term studies in animals have not been performed to evaluate the effects upon fertility or carcinogenic potential of DARANIDE.

Pregnancy
Pregnancy Category C. Dichlorphenamide has been shown to be teratogenic in the rat (skeletal anomalies) when given in doses 100 times the human dose. There are no adequate and well-controlled studies in pregnant women. DARANIDE should not be used in women of childbearing age or in pregnancy, especially during the first trimester, unless the potential benefits outweigh the potential risks.

Nursing Mothers
It is not known whether dichlorphenamide is excreted in human milk. Because many drugs are excreted in human milk, caution should be exercised when dichlorphenamide is administered to a nursing woman.

Pediatric Use
Safety and effectiveness in pediatric patients have not been established.

ADVERSE REACTIONS

Certain side effects characteristic of carbonic anhydrase inhibitors may occur with DARANIDE, particularly with increasing doses. The most common effects include gastrointestinal disturbances (anorexia, nausea, and vomiting), drowsiness and paresthesias.
Included in the listing which follows are some adverse reactions which have not been reported with DARANIDE. However, pharmacological similarities among the carbonic anhydrase inhibitors make it advisable to consider the following reactions when dichlorphenamide is administered. *Central Nervous System/Psychiatric:* ataxia, tremor, tinnitus, headache, weakness, nervousness, globus hystericus, lassitude, depression, confusion, disorientation, dizziness; *Gastrointestinal:* constipation, hepatic insufficiency; *Metabolic:* loss of weight, metabolic acidosis, electrolyte imbalance (hypokalemia, hyperchloremia), hyperuricemia; *Hypersensitivity:* skin eruptions, pruritus, fever; *Hematologic:* leukopenia, agranulocytosis, thrombocytopenia; *Genitourinary:* urinary frequency, renal colic, renal calculi, phosphaturia.

OVERDOSAGE

The oral LD_{50} of DARANIDE is 1710 and 2600 mg/kg in the mouse and rat respectively.
Symptoms of overdosage or toxicity may include drowsiness, anorexia, nausea, vomiting, dizziness, paresthesias, ataxia, tremor and tinnitus.
In the event of overdosage, induce emesis or perform gastric lavage. The electrolyte disturbance most likely to be encountered from overdosage is hyperchloremic acidosis that may respond to bicarbonate administration. Potassium supplementation may be required. The patient should be carefully observed and given supportive treatment.

DOSAGE AND ADMINISTRATION

DARANIDE is usually given in conjunction with topical ocular hypotensive agents. In acute angle-closure glaucoma, it may be used together with miotics and osmotic agents in an attempt to reduce intraocular tension rapidly. If this is not quickly relieved, surgery may be mandatory.
Dosage must be adjusted carefully to meet the requirements of the individual patient. A priming dose of 100 to 200 mg of DARANIDE (2 to 4 tablets) is suggested for adults, followed by 100 mg (2 tablets) every 12 hours until the desired response has been obtained. The recommended maintenance dosage for adults is 25 to 50 mg ($^1/_2$ to 1 tablet) once to three times daily.

HOW SUPPLIED

No. 3256—Tablets DARANIDE, 50 mg each, are yellow, round, scored, compressed tablets, coded MSD 49 on one side and DARANIDE on the other. They are supplied as follows:
NDC 0006-0049-68 bottles of 100.
7870319   Issued October 1996
COPYRIGHT © MERCK & CO., INC., 1985
All rights reserved

DECADRON® Elixir
(Dexamethasone), U.S.P.
℞

DESCRIPTION

Glucocorticoids are adrenocortical steroids, both naturally occurring and synthetic, which are readily absorbed from the gastrointestinal tract.
Dexamethasone, a synthetic adrenocortical steroid, is a white to practically white, odorless, crystalline powder. It is stable in air. It is practically insoluble in water. The molecular weight is 392.47. It is designated chemically as 9-fluoro-11β,17,21-trihydroxy-16α-methylpregna -1, 4- diene-3,20-dione. The empirical formula is $C_{22}H_{29}FO_5$ and the structural formula is:

DECADRON* (Dexamethasone) elixir contains 0.5 mg of dexamethasone in each 5 mL. Benzoic acid, 0.1%, is added as a preservative. It also contains alcohol 5%. Inactive ingredients are FD&C Red 40, flavors, glycerin, purified water, and sodium saccharin.

*Registered trademark of MERCK & CO., INC.

ACTIONS

Naturally occurring glucocorticoids (hydrocortisone and cortisone), which also have salt-retaining properties, are used as replacement therapy in adrenocortical deficiency states.

Continued on next page

Decadron Elixir—Cont.

Their synthetic analogs, including dexamethasone, are primarily used for their potent anti-inflammatory effects in disorders of many organ systems.

Glucocorticoids cause profound and varied metabolic effects. In addition, they modify the body's immune responses to diverse stimuli.

At equipotent anti-inflammatory doses, dexamethasone almost completely lacks the sodium-retaining property of hydrocortisone and closely related derivatives of hydrocortisone.

INDICATIONS

1. *Endocrine Disorders*
   Primary or secondary adrenocortical insufficiency (hydrocortisone or cortisone is the first choice; synthetic analogs may be used in conjunction with mineralocorticoids where applicable; in infancy mineralocorticoid supplementation is of particular importance)
   Congenital adrenal hyperplasia
   Nonsuppurative thyroiditis
   Hypercalcemia associated with cancer
2. *Rheumatic Disorders*
   As adjunctive therapy for short-term administration (to tide the patient over an acute episode or exacerbation) in:
   Psoriatic arthritis
   Rheumatoid arthritis, including juvenile rheumatoid arthritis (selected cases may require low-dose maintenance therapy)
   Ankylosing spondylitis
   Acute and subacute bursitis
   Acute nonspecific tenosynovitis
   Acute gouty arthritis
   Post-traumatic osteoarthritis
   Synovitis of osteoarthritis
   Epicondylitis
3. *Collagen Diseases*
   During an exacerbation or as maintenance therapy in selected cases of—
   Systemic lupus erythematosus
   Acute rheumatic carditis
4. *Dermatologic Diseases*
   Pemphigus
   Bullous dermatitis herpetiformis
   Severe erythema multiforme (Stevens-Johnson syndrome)
   Exfoliative dermatitis
   Mycosis fungoides
   Severe psoriasis
   Severe seborrheic dermatitis
5. *Allergic States*
   Control of severe or incapacitating allergic conditions intractable to adequate trials of conventional treatment:
   Seasonal or perennial allergic rhinitis
   Bronchial asthma
   Contact dermatitis
   Atopic dermatitis
   Serum sickness
   Drug hypersensitivity reactions
6. *Ophthalmic Diseases*
   Severe acute and chronic allergic and inflammatory processes involving the eye and its adnexa, such as—
   Allergic conjunctivitis
   Keratitis
   Allergic corneal marginal ulcers
   Herpes zoster ophthalmicus
   Iritis and iridocyclitis
   Chorioretinitis
   Anterior segment inflammation
   Diffuse posterior uveitis and choroiditis
   Optic neuritis
   Sympathetic ophthalmia
7. *Respiratory Diseases*
   Symptomatic sarcoidosis
   Loeffler's syndrome not manageable by other means
   Berylliosis
   Fulminating or disseminated pulmonary tuberculosis when used concurrently with appropriate antituberculous chemotherapy
   Aspiration pneumonitis
8. *Hematologic Disorders*
   Idiopathic thrombocytopenic purpura in adults
   Secondary thrombocytopenia in adults
   Acquired (autoimmune) hemolytic anemia
   Erythroblastopenia (RBC anemia)
   Congenital (erythroid) hypoplastic anemia
9. *Neoplastic Diseases*
   For palliative management of:
   Leukemias and lymphomas in adults
   Acute leukemia of childhood
10. *Edematous States*
    To induce a diuresis or remission of proteinuria in the nephrotic syndrome, without uremia, of the idiopathic type or that due to lupus erythematosus

11. *Gastrointestinal Diseases*
    To tide the patient over a critical period of the disease in:
    Ulcerative colitis
    Regional enteritis
12. *Miscellaneous*
    Tuberculous meningitis with subarachnoid block or impending block when used concurrently with appropriate antituberculous chemotherapy
    Trichinosis with neurologic or myocardial involvement
13. *Diagnostic testing of adrenocortical hyperfunction.*

CONTRAINDICATIONS

Systemic fungal infections
Hypersensitivity to this product

WARNINGS

In patients on corticosteroid therapy subjected to unusual stress, increased dosage of rapidly acting corticosteroids before, during, and after the stressful situation is indicated.

Drug-induced secondary adrenocortical insufficiency may result from too rapid withdrawal of corticosteroids and may be minimized by gradual reduction of dosage. This type of relative insufficiency may persist for months after discontinuation of therapy; therefore, in any situation of stress occurring during that period, hormone therapy should be reinstituted. If the patient is receiving steroids already, dosage may have to be increased. Since mineralocorticoid secretion may be impaired, salt and/or a mineralocorticoid should be administered concurrently.

Corticosteroids may mask some signs of infection, and new infections may appear during their use. There may be decreased resistance and inability to localize infection when corticosteroids are used. Moreover, corticosteroids may affect the nitroblue-tetrazolium test for bacterial infection and produce false negative results.

In cerebral malaria, a double-blind trial has shown that the use of corticosteroids is associated with prolongation of coma and a higher incidence of pneumonia and gastrointestinal bleeding.

Corticosteroids may activate latent amebiasis. Therefore, it is recommended that latent or active amebiasis be ruled out before initiating corticosteroid therapy in any patient who has spent time in the tropics or any patient with unexplained diarrhea.

Prolonged use of corticosteroids may produce posterior subcapsular cataracts, glaucoma with possible damage to the optic nerves, and may enhance the establishment of secondary ocular infections due to fungi or viruses.

Usage in pregnancy: Since adequate human reproduction studies have not been done with corticosteroids, use of these drugs in pregnancy or in women of childbearing potential requires that the anticipated benefits be weighed against the possible hazards to the mother and embryo or fetus. Infants born of mothers who have received substantial doses of corticosteroids during pregnancy should be carefully observed for signs of hypoadrenalism.

Corticosteroids appear in breast milk and could suppress growth, interfere with endogenous corticosteroid production, or cause other unwanted effects. Mothers taking pharmacologic doses of corticosteroids should be advised not to nurse.

Average and large doses of hydrocortisone or cortisone can cause elevation of blood pressure, salt and water retention, and increased excretion of potassium. These effects are less likely to occur with the synthetic derivatives except when used in large doses. Dietary salt restriction and potassium supplementation may be necessary. All corticosteroids increase calcium excretion.

Administration of live virus vaccines, including smallpox, is contraindicated in individuals receiving immunosuppressive doses of corticosteroids. If inactivated viral or bacterial vaccines are administered to individuals receiving immunosuppressive doses of corticosteroids, the expected serum antibody response may not be obtained. However, immunization procedures may be undertaken in patients who are receiving corticosteroids as replacement therapy, e.g., for Addison's disease.

Patients who are on drugs which suppress the immune system are more susceptible to infections than healthy individuals. Chickenpox and measles, for example, can have a more serious or even fatal course in non-immune patients on corticosteroids. In such patients who have not had these diseases, particular care should be taken to avoid exposure. The risk of developing a disseminated infection varies among individuals and can be related to the dose, route and duration of corticosteroid administration as well as to the underlying disease. If exposed to chickenpox, prophylaxis with varicella zoster immune globulin (VZIG) may be indicated. If chickenpox develops, treatment with antiviral agents may be considered. If exposed to measles, prophylaxis with immune globulin (IG) may be indicated. (See the respective package inserts for VZIG and IG for complete prescribing information.)

Similarly, corticosteroids should be used with great care in patients with known or suspected Strongyloides (thread-

worm) infestation. In such patients, corticosteroid-induced immunosuppression may lead to Strongyloides hyperinfection and dissemination with widespread larval migration, often accompanied by severe enterocolitis and potentially fatal gram-negative septicemia.

The use of DECADRON elixir in active tuberculosis should be restricted to those cases of fulminating or disseminated tuberculosis in which the corticosteroid is used for the management of the disease in conjunction with an appropriate antituberculous regimen.

If corticosteroids are indicated in patients with latent tuberculosis or tuberculin reactivity, close observation is necessary as reactivation of the disease may occur. During prolonged corticosteroid therapy, these patients should receive chemoprophylaxis.

Literature reports suggest an apparent association between use of corticosteroids and left ventricular free wall rupture after a recent myocardial infarction; therefore, therapy with corticosteroids should be used with great caution in these patients.

PRECAUTIONS

Following prolonged therapy, withdrawal of corticosteroids may result in symptoms of the corticosteroid withdrawal syndrome including fever, myalgia, arthralgia, and malaise. This may occur in patients even without evidence of adrenal insufficiency.

There is an enhanced effect of corticosteroids in patients with hypothyroidism and in those with cirrhosis.

Corticosteroids should be used cautiously in patients with ocular herpes simplex because of possible corneal perforation.

The lowest possible dose of corticosteroid should be used to control the condition under treatment, and when reduction in dosage is possible, the reduction should be gradual.

Psychic derangements may appear when corticosteroids are used, ranging from euphoria, insomnia, mood swings, personality changes, and severe depression, to frank psychotic manifestations. Also, existing emotional instability or psychotic tendencies may be aggravated by corticosteroids.

Aspirin should be used cautiously in conjunction with corticosteroids in hypoprothrombinemia.

Steroids should be used with caution in nonspecific ulcerative colitis, if there is a probability of impending perforation, abscess, or other pyogenic infection, diverticulitis, fresh intestinal anastomoses, active or latent peptic ulcer, renal insufficiency, hypertension, osteoporosis, and myasthenia gravis. Signs of peritoneal irritation following gastrointestinal perforation in patients receiving large doses of corticosteroids may be minimal or absent. Fat embolism has been reported as a possible complication of hypercortisonism.

When large doses are given, some authorities advise that corticosteroids be taken with meals and antacids taken between meals to help to prevent peptic ulcer.

Steroids may increase or decrease motility and number of spermatozoa in some patients.

Phenytoin, phenobarbital, ephedrine, and rifampin may enhance the metabolic clearance of corticosteroids, resulting in decreased blood levels and lessened physiologic activity, thus requiring adjustment in corticosteroid dosage. These interactions may interfere with dexamethasone suppression tests which should be interpreted with caution during administration of these drugs.

False-negative results in the dexamethasone suppression test (DST) in patients being treated with indomethacin have been reported. Thus, results of the DST should be interpreted with caution in these patients.

The prothrombin time should be checked frequently in patients who are receiving corticosteroids and coumarin anticoagulants at the same time because of reports that corticosteroids have altered the response to these anticoagulants. Studies have shown that the usual effect produced by adding corticosteroids is inhibition of response to coumarins, although there have been some conflicting reports of potentiation not substantiated by studies.

When corticosteroids are administered concomitantly with potassium-depleting diuretics, patients should be observed closely for development of hypokalemia.

Information for Patients
Susceptible patients who are on immunosuppressant doses of corticosteroids should be warned to avoid exposure to chickenpox or measles. Patients should also be advised that if they are exposed, medical advice should be sought without delay.

Pediatric Use
Growth and development of pediatric patients on prolonged corticosteroid therapy should be carefully followed.

ADVERSE REACTIONS

Fluid and Electrolyte Disturbances
   Sodium retention
   Fluid retention
   Congestive heart failure in susceptible patients

Potassium loss
Hypokalemic alkalosis
Hypertension
Musculoskeletal
Muscle weakness
Steroid myopathy
Loss of muscle mass
Osteoporosis
Vertebral compression fractures
Aseptic necrosis of femoral and humeral heads
Pathologic fracture of long bones
Tendon rupture
Gastrointestinal
Peptic ulcer with possible perforation and hemorrhage
Perforation of the small and large bowel, particularly in patients with inflammatory bowel disease
Pancreatitis
Abdominal distention
Ulcerative esophagitis
Dermatologic
Impaired wound healing
Thin fragile skin
Petechiae and ecchymoses
Erythema
Increased sweating
May suppress reactions to skin tests
Other cutaneous reactions, such as allergic dermatitis, urticaria, angioneurotic edema
Neurologic
Convulsions
Increased intracranial pressure with papilledema (pseudotumor cerebri) usually after treatment
Vertigo
Headache
Psychic disturbances
Endocrine
Menstrual irregularities
Development of cushingoid state
Suppression of growth in children
Secondary adrenocortical and pituitary unresponsiveness, particularly in times of stress, as in trauma, surgery, or illness
Decreased carbohydrate tolerance
Manifestations of latent diabetes mellitus
Increased requirements for insulin or oral hypoglycemic agents in diabetics
Hirsutism
Ophthalmic
Posterior subcapsular cataracts
Increased intraocular pressure
Glaucoma
Exophthalmos
Metabolic
Negative nitrogen balance due to protein catabolism
Cardiovascular
Myocardial rupture following recent myocardial infarction (see WARNINGS)
Other
Hypersensitivity
Thromboembolism
Weight gain
Increased appetite
Nausea
Malaise
Hiccups

OVERDOSAGE

Reports of acute toxicity and/or death following overdosage of glucocorticoids are rare. In the event of overdosage, no specific antidote is available; treatment is supportive and symptomatic.
The oral LD_{50} of dexamethasone in female mice was 6.5 g/kg.

DOSAGE AND ADMINISTRATION

For oral administration
DOSAGE REQUIREMENTS ARE VARIABLE AND MUST BE INDIVIDUALIZED ON THE BASIS OF THE DISEASE AND THE RESPONSE OF THE PATIENT.
The initial dosage varies from 0.75 to 9 mg a day depending on the disease being treated. In less severe diseases doses lower than 0.75 mg may suffice, while in severe diseases doses higher than 9 mg may be required. The initial dosage should be maintained or adjusted until the patient's response is satisfactory. If satisfactory clinical response does not occur after a reasonable period of time, discontinue DECADRON elixir and transfer the patient to other therapy.
After a favorable initial response, the proper maintenance dosage should be determined by decreasing the initial dosage in small amounts to the lowest dosage that maintains an adequate clinical response.
Patients should be observed closely for signs that might require dosage adjustment, including changes in clinical sta-

tus resulting from remissions or exacerbations of the disease, individual drug responsiveness, and the effect of stress (e.g., surgery, infection, trauma). During stress it may be necessary to increase dosage temporarily.
If the drug is to be stopped after more than a few days of treatment, it usually should be withdrawn gradually.
The following milligram equivalents facilitate changing to DECADRON from other glucocorticoids:

DECADRON	Methylprednisolone and Triamcinolone	Prednisolone and Prednisone	Hydrocortisone	Cortisone
0.75 mg =	4 mg =	5 mg =	20 mg =	25 mg

Dexamethasone suppression tests
1. Tests for Cushing's syndrome
Give 1.0 mg of DECADRON orally at 11:00 p.m. Blood is drawn for plasma cortisol determination at 8:00 a.m. the following morning.
For greater accuracy, give 0.5 mg of DECADRON orally every 6 hours for 48 hours. Twenty-four hour urine collections are made for determination of 17-hydroxycorticosteroid excretion.
2. Test to distinguish Cushing's syndrome due to pituitary ACTH excess from Cushing's syndrome due to other causes
Give 2.0 mg of DECADRON orally every 6 hours for 48 hours. Twenty-four hour urine collections are made for determination of 17-hydroxycorticosteroid excretion.

HOW SUPPLIED

No. 7622—Elixir DECADRON, 0.5 mg dexamethasone per 5 mL, is a clear, red liquid and is supplied as follows:
NDC 0006-7622-55 bottles of 100 mL with calibrated dropper assembly.
NDC 0006-7622-66 bottles of 237 mL without dropper assembly.
(6505-01-137-8465, 237 mL).
Storage
Keep container tightly closed.
7412730 Issued February 1997

DECADRON® Tablets
(Dexamethasone), U.S.P. ℞

DESCRIPTION

Glucocorticoids are adrenocortical steroids, both naturally occurring and synthetic, which are readily absorbed from the gastrointestinal tract.
Dexamethasone, a synthetic adrenocortical steroid, is a white to practically white, odorless, crystalline powder. It is stable in air. It is practically insoluble in water. The molecular weight is 392.47. It is designated chemically as 9-fluoro-11β, 17, 21-trihydroxy-16α-methylpregna-1, 4-diene-3,20-dione. The empirical formula is $C_{22}H_{29}FO_5$ and the structural formula is:

DECADRON* (Dexamethasone) tablets are supplied in three potencies, 0.5 mg, 0.75 mg, and 4 mg. Inactive ingredients are calcium phosphate, lactose, magnesium stearate, and starch. Tablets DECADRON 0.5 mg also contain D&C Yellow 10 and FD&C Yellow 6. Tablets DECADRON 0.75 mg also contain FD&C Blue 1.

*Registered trademark of MERCK & CO., INC.

ACTIONS

Naturally occurring glucocorticoids (hydrocortisone and cortisone), which also have salt-retaining properties, are used as replacement therapy in adrenocortical deficiency states.

Their synthetic analogs including dexamethasone are primarily used for their potent anti-inflammatory effects in disorders of many organ systems.
Glucocorticoids cause profound and varied metabolic effects. In addition, they modify the body's immune responses to diverse stimuli.
At equipotent anti-inflammatory doses, dexamethasone almost completely lacks the sodium-retaining property of hydrocortisone and closely related derivatives of hydrocortisone.

INDICATIONS

1. *Endocrine Disorders*
Primary or secondary adrenocortical insufficiency (hydrocortisone or cortisone is the first choice; synthetic analogs may be used in conjunction with mineralocorticoids where applicable; in infancy mineralocorticoid supplementation is of particular importance)
Congenital adrenal hyperplasia
Nonsuppurative thyroiditis
Hypercalcemia associated with cancer
2. *Rheumatic Disorders*
As adjunctive therapy for short-term administration (to tide the patient over an acute episode or exacerbation) in:
Psoriatic arthritis
Rheumatoid arthritis, including juvenile rheumatoid arthritis (selected cases may require low-dose maintenance therapy)
Ankylosing spondylitis
Acute and subacute bursitis
Acute nonspecific tenosynovitis
Acute gouty arthritis
Post-traumatic osteoarthritis
Synovitis of osteoarthritis
Epicondylitis
3. *Collagen Diseases*
During an exacerbation or as maintenance therapy in selected cases of—
Systemic lupus erythematosus
Acute rheumatic carditis
4. *Dermatologic Diseases*
Pemphigus
Bullous dermatitis herpetiformis
Severe erythema multiforme (Stevens-Johnson syndrome)
Exfoliative dermatitis
Mycosis fungoides
Severe psoriasis
Severe seborrheic dermatitis
5. *Allergic States*
Control of severe or incapacitating allergic conditions intractable to adequate trials of conventional treatment:
Seasonal or perennial allergic rhinitis
Bronchial asthma
Contact dermatitis
Atopic dermatitis
Serum sickness
Drug hypersensitivity reactions
6. *Ophthalmic Diseases*
Severe acute and chronic allergic and inflammatory processes involving the eye and its adnexa, such as—
Allergic conjunctivitis
Keratitis
Allergic corneal marginal ulcers
Herpes zoster ophthalmicus
Iritis and iridocyclitis
Chorioretinitis
Anterior segment inflammation
Diffuse posterior uveitis and choroiditis
Optic neuritis
Sympathetic ophthalmia
7. *Respiratory Diseases*
Symptomatic sarcoidosis
Loeffler's syndrome not manageable by other means
Berylliosis
Fulminating or disseminated pulmonary tuberculosis when used concurrently with appropriate antituberculous chemotherapy
Aspiration pneumonitis
8. *Hematologic Disorders*
Idiopathic thrombocytopenic purpura in adults
Secondary thrombocytopenia in adults
Acquired (autoimmune) hemolytic anemia
Erythroblastopenia (RBC anemia)
Congenital (erythroid) hypoplastic anemia
9. *Neoplastic Diseases*
For palliative management of:

Continued on next page

Decadron Tablets—Cont.

Leukemias and lymphomas in adults
Acute leukemia of childhood
10. *Edematous States*
To induce a diuresis or remission of proteinuria in the nephrotic syndrome, without uremia, of the idiopathic type or that due to lupus erythematosus
11. *Gastrointestinal Diseases*
To tide the patient over a critical period of the disease in:
Ulcerative colitis
Regional enteritis
12. *Cerebral Edema* associated with primary or metastatic brain tumor, craniotomy, or head injury. Use in cerebral edema is not a substitute for careful neurosurgical evaluation and definitive management such as neurosurgery or other specific therapy.
13. *Miscellaneous*
Tuberculous meningitis with subarachnoid block or impending block when used concurrently with appropriate antituberculous chemotherapy
Trichinosis with neurologic or myocardial involvement
14. *Diagnostic testing of adrenocortical hyperfunction.*

CONTRAINDICATIONS

Systemic fungal infections
Hypersensitivity to this drug

WARNINGS

In patients on corticosteroid therapy subjected to unusual stress, increased dosage of rapidly acting corticosteroids before, during, and after the stressful situation is indicated. Drug-induced secondary adrenocortical insufficiency may result from too rapid withdrawal of corticosteroids and may be minimized by gradual reduction of dosage. This type of relative insufficiency may persist for months after discontinuation of therapy; therefore, in any situation of stress occurring during that period, hormone therapy should be reinstituted. If the patient is receiving steroids already, dosage may have to be increased. Since mineralocorticoid secretion may be impaired, salt and/or a mineralocorticoid should be administered concurrently.
Corticosteroids may mask some signs of infection, and new infections may appear during their use. There may be decreased resistance and inability to localize infection when corticosteroids are used. Moreover, corticosteroids may affect the nitroblue-tetrazolium test for bacterial infection and produce false negative results.
In cerebral malaria, a double-blind trial has shown that the use of corticosteroids is associated with prolongation of coma and a higher incidence of pneumonia and gastrointestinal bleeding.
Corticosteroids may activate latent amebiasis. Therefore, it is recommended that latent or active amebiasis be ruled out before initiating corticosteroid therapy in any patient who has spent time in the tropics or any patient with unexplained diarrhea.
Prolonged use of corticosteroids may produce posterior subcapsular cataracts, glaucoma with possible damage to the optic nerves, and may enhance the establishment of secondary ocular infections due to fungi or viruses.
Usage in pregnancy: Since adequate human reproduction studies have not been done with corticosteroids, use of these drugs in pregnancy or in women of childbearing potential requires that the anticipated benefits be weighed against the possible hazards to the mother and embryo or fetus. Infants born of mothers who have received substantial doses of corticosteroids during pregnancy should be carefully observed for signs of hypoadrenalism.
Corticosteroids appear in breast milk and could suppress growth, interfere with endogenous corticosteroid production, or cause other unwanted effects. Mothers taking pharmacologic doses of corticosteroids should be advised not to nurse.
Average and large doses of hydrocortisone or cortisone can cause elevation of blood pressure, salt and water retention, and increased excretion of potassium. These effects are less likely to occur with the synthetic derivatives except when used in large doses. Dietary salt restriction and potassium supplementation may be necessary. All corticosteroids increase calcium excretion.
Administration of live virus vaccines, including smallpox, is contraindicated in individuals receiving immunosuppressive doses of corticosteroids. If inactivated viral or bacterial vaccines are administered to individuals receiving immunosuppressive doses of corticosteroid the expected serum antibody response may not be obtained. However, immunization procedures may be undertaken in patients who are receiving corticosteroids as replacement therapy, e.g., for Addison's disease.
Patients who are on drugs which suppress the immune system are more susceptible to infections than healthy individuals. Chickenpox and measles, for example, can have a

more serious or even fatal course in non-immune patients on corticosteroids. In such patients who have not had these diseases, particular care should be taken to avoid exposure. The risk of developing a disseminated infection varies among individuals and can be related to the dose, route and duration of corticosteroid administration as well as to the underlying disease. If exposed to chickenpox, prophylaxis with varicella zoster immune globulin (VZIG) may be indicated. If chickenpox develops, treatment with antiviral agents may be considered. If exposed to measles, prophylaxis with immune globulin (IG) may be indicated. (See the respective package inserts for VZIG and IG for complete prescribing information.)
Similarly, corticosteroids should be used with great care in patients with known or suspected Strongyloides (threadworm) infestation. In such patients, corticosteroid-induced immunosuppression may lead to Strongyloides hyperinfection and dissemination with widespread larval migration, often accompanied by severe enterocolitis and potentially fatal gram-negative septicemia.
The use of DECADRON tablets in active tuberculosis should be restricted to those cases of fulminating or disseminated tuberculosis in which the corticosteroid is used for the management of the disease in conjunction with an appropriate antituberculous regimen.
If corticosteroids are indicated in patients with latent tuberculosis or tuberculin reactivity, close observation is necessary as reactivation of the disease may occur. During prolonged corticosteroid therapy, these patients should receive chemoprophylaxis.
Literature reports suggest an apparent association between use of corticosteroids and left ventricular free wall rupture after a recent myocardial infarction; therefore, therapy with corticosteroids should be used with great caution in these patients.

PRECAUTIONS

Following prolonged therapy, withdrawal of corticosteroids may result in symptoms of the corticosteroid withdrawal syndrome including fever, myalgia, arthralgia, and malaise. This may occur in patients even without evidence of adrenal insufficiency.
There is an enhanced effect of corticosteroids in patients with hypothyroidism and in those with cirrhosis.
Corticosteroids should be used cautiously in patients with ocular herpes simplex because of possible corneal perforation.
The lowest possible dose of corticosteroids should be used to control the condition under treatment, and when reduction in dosage is possible, the reduction should be gradual.
Psychic derangements may appear when corticosteroids are used, ranging from euphoria, insomnia, mood swings, personality changes, and severe depression, to frank psychotic manifestations. Also, existing emotional instability or psychotic tendencies may be aggravated by corticosteroids.
Aspirin should be used cautiously in conjunction with corticosteroids in hypoprothrombinemia.
Steroids should be used with caution in nonspecific ulcerative colitis, if there is a probability of impending perforation, abscess, or other pyogenic infection, diverticulitis, fresh intestinal anastomoses, active or latent peptic ulcer, renal insufficiency, hypertension, osteoporosis, and myasthenia gravis. Signs of peritoneal irritation following gastrointestinal perforation in patients receiving large doses of corticosteroids may be minimal or absent. Fat embolism has been reported as a possible complication of hypercortisonism.
When large doses are given, some authorities advise that corticosteroids be taken with meals and antacids taken between meals to help to prevent peptic ulcer.
Steroids may increase or decrease motility and number of spermatozoa in some patients.
Phenytoin, phenobarbital, ephedrine, and rifampin may enhance the metabolic clearance of corticosteroids, resulting in decreased blood levels and lessened physiologic activity, thus requiring adjustment in corticosteroid dosage. These interactions may interfere with dexamethasone suppression tests which should be interpreted with caution during administration of these drugs.
False-negative results in the dexamethasone suppression test (DST) in patients being treated with indomethacin have been reported. Thus, results of the DST should be interpreted with caution in these patients.
The prothrombin time should be checked frequently in patients who are receiving corticosteroids and coumarin anticoagulants at the same time because of reports that corticosteroids have altered the response to these anticoagulants. Studies have shown that the usual effect produced by adding corticosteroids is inhibition of response to coumarins, although there have been some conflicting reports of potentiation not substantiated by studies.
When corticosteroids are administered concomitantly with potassium-depleting diuretics, patients should be observed closely for development of hypokalemia.

Information for Patients
Susceptible patients who are on immunosuppressant doses of corticosteroids should be warned to avoid exposure to chickenpox or measles. Patients should also be advised that if they are exposed, medical advice should be sought without delay.
Pediatric Use
Growth and development of pediatric patients on prolonged corticosteroid therapy should be carefully followed.

ADVERSE REACTIONS

Fluid and Electrolyte Disturbances
Sodium retention
Fluid retention
Congestive heart failure in susceptible patients
Potassium loss
Hypokalemic alkalosis
Hypertension
Musculoskeletal
Muscle weakness
Steroid myopathy
Loss of muscle mass
Osteoporosis
Vertebral compression fractures
Aseptic necrosis of femoral and humeral heads
Pathologic fracture of long bones
Tendon rupture
Gastrointestinal
Peptic ulcer with possible perforation and hemorrhage
Perforation of the small and large bowel, particularly in patients with inflammatory bowel disease
Pancreatitis
Abdominal distention
Ulcerative esophagitis
Dermatologic
Impaired wound healing
Thin fragile skin
Petechiae and ecchymoses
Erythema
Increased sweating
May suppress reactions to skin tests
Other cutaneous reactions, such as allergic dermatitis, urticaria, angioneurotic edema
Neurologic
Convulsions
Increased intracranial pressure with papilledema (pseudotumor cerebri) usually after treatment
Vertigo
Headache
Psychic disturbances
Endocrine
Menstrual irregularities
Development of cushingoid state
Suppression of growth in children
Secondary adrenocortical and pituitary unresponsiveness, particularly in times of stress, as in trauma, surgery, or illness
Decreased carbohydrate tolerance
Manifestations of latent diabetes mellitus
Increased requirements for insulin or oral hypoglycemic agents in diabetics
Hirsutism
Ophthalmic
Posterior subcapsular cataracts
Increased intraocular pressure
Glaucoma
Exophthalmos
Metabolic
Negative nitrogen balance due to protein catabolism
Cardiovascular
Myocardial rupture following recent myocardial infarction (see WARNINGS)
Other
Hypersensitivity
Thromboembolism
Weight gain
Increased appetite
Nausea
Malaise
Hiccups

OVERDOSAGE

Reports of acute toxicity and/or death following overdosage of glucocorticoids are rare. In the event of overdosage, no specific antidote is available; treatment is supportive and symptomatic.
The oral LD$_{50}$ of dexamethasone in female mice was 6.5 g/kg.

DOSAGE AND ADMINISTRATION

For oral administration
DOSAGE REQUIREMENTS ARE VARIABLE AND MUST BE INDIVIDUALIZED ON THE BASIS OF THE DISEASE AND THE RESPONSE OF THE PATIENT.

The initial dosage varies from 0.75 to 9 mg a day depending on the disease being treated. In less severe diseases doses lower than 0.75 mg may suffice, while in severe diseases doses higher than 9 mg may be required. The initial dosage should be maintained or adjusted until the patient's response is satisfactory. If satisfactory clinical response does not occur after a reasonable period of time, discontinue DECADRON tablets and transfer the patient to other therapy.

After a favorable initial response, the proper maintenance dosage should be determined by decreasing the initial dosage in small amounts to the lowest dosage that maintains an adequate clinical response.

Patients should be observed closely for signs that might require dosage adjustment, including changes in clinical status resulting from remissions or exacerbations of the disease, individual drug responsiveness, and the effect of stress (e.g., surgery, infection, trauma). During stress it may be necessary to increase dosage temporarily.

If the drug is to be stopped after more than a few days of treatment, it usually should be withdrawn gradually.

The following milligram equivalents facilitate changing to DECADRON from other glucocorticoids:

DECADRON	Methylpred-nisolone and Triamcinolone	Prednisolone and Prednisone Hydrocortisone		Cortisone
0.75 mg =	4 mg =	5 mg =	20 mg =	25 =

In *acute, self-limited allergic disorders or acute exacerbations of chronic allergic disorders,* the following dosage schedule combining parenteral and oral therapy is suggested:

DECADRON* Phosphate (Dexamethasone Sodium Phosphate) injection, 4 mg per mL:

First Day
  1 or 2 mL, intramuscularly
DECADRON tablets, 0.75 mg:
Second Day
  4 tablets in two divided doses
Third Day
  4 tablets in two divided doses
Fourth Day
  2 tablets in two divided doses
Fifth Day
  1 tablet
Sixth Day
  1 tablet
Seventh Day
  No treatment
Eighth Day
  Follow-up visit

This schedule is designed to ensure adequate therapy during acute episodes, while minimizing the risk of overdosage in chronic cases.

In *cerebral edema,* DECADRON Phosphate (Dexamethasone Sodium Phosphate) injection is generally administered initially in a dosage of 10 mg intravenously followed by 4 mg every six hours intramuscularly until the symptoms of cerebral edema subside. Response is usually noted within 12 to 24 hours and dosage may be reduced after two to four days and gradually discontinued over a period of five to seven days. For palliative management of patients with recurrent or inoperable brain tumors, maintenance therapy with either DECADRON Phosphate (Dexamethasone Sodium Phosphate) injection or DECADRON tablets in a dosage of two mg two or three times daily may be effective.

Dexamethasone suppression tests
1. Tests for Cushing's syndrome
   Give 1.0 mg of DECADRON orally at 11:00 p.m. Blood is drawn for plasma cortisol determination at 8:00 a.m. the following morning.
   For greater accuracy, give 0.5 mg of DECADRON orally every 6 hours for 48 hours. Twenty-four hour urine collections are made for determination of 17-hydroxycorticosteroid excretion.
2. Test to distinguish Cushing's syndrome due to pituitary ACTH excess from Cushing's syndrome due to other causes
   Give 2.0 mg of DECADRON orally every 6 hours for 48 hours. Twenty-four hour urine collections are made for determination of 17-hydroxycorticosteroid excretion.

*Registered trademark of MERCK & CO., INC.

HOW SUPPLIED

Tablets DECADRON are compressed, pentagonal-shaped tablets, colored to distinguish potency. They are scored and coded on one side and embossed with DECADRON on the other. They are available as follows:
No. 7645—4 mg, white in color and coded MSD 97.
NDC 0006-0097-50 bottles of 50
  Shown in Product Identification Guide, page 323
No. 7601—0.75 mg, bluish-green in color and coded MSD 63.
NDC 0006-0063-12 5-12 PAK* (package of 12)
NDC 0006-0063-68 bottles of 100.
  Shown in Product Identification Guide, page 323
No. 7598—0.5 mg, yellow in color and coded MSD 41.
NDC 0006-0041-68 bottles of 100.
  Shown in Product Identification Guide, page 323

*Registered trademark of MERCK & CO., INC.
  7921148 Issued February 1997

DECADRON® Phosphate Injection ℞
(Dexamethasone Sodium Phosphate), U.S.P.

DESCRIPTION

Dexamethasone sodium phosphate, a synthetic adrenocortical steroid, is a white or slightly yellow, crystalline powder. It is freely soluble in water and is exceedingly hygroscopic. The molecular weight is 516.41. It is designated chemically as 9-fluoro-11β, 17-dihydroxy-16α-methyl-21-(phosphonooxy)pregna-1, 4-diene-3, 20-dione disodium salt. The empirical formula is $C_{22}H_{28}FNa_2O_8P$ and the structural formula is:

DECADRON* Phosphate (Dexamethasone Sodium Phosphate) injection is a sterile solution (pH 7.0 to 8.5) of dexamethasone sodium phosphate, sealed under nitrogen, and is supplied in two concentrations: 4 mg/mL and 24 mg/mL. The 24 mg/mL concentration offers the advantage of less volume in indications where high doses of corticosteroids by the intravenous route are needed.

Each milliliter of DECADRON Phosphate injection, 4 mg/mL, contains dexamethasone sodium phosphate equivalent to 4 mg dexamethasone phosphate or 3.33 mg dexamethasone. Inactive ingredients per mL: 8 mg creatinine, 10 mg sodium citrate, sodium hydroxide to adjust pH, and Water for Injection q.s., with 1 mg sodium bisulfite, 1.5 mg methylparaben, and 0.2 mg propylparaben added as preservatives.

Each milliliter of DECADRON Phosphate injection, 24 mg/mL, contains dexamethasone sodium phosphate equivalent to 24 mg dexamethasone phosphate or 20 mg dexamethasone. Inactive ingredients per mL: 8 mg creatinine, 10 mg sodium citrate, 0.5 mg disodium edetate, sodium hydroxide to adjust pH, and Water for Injection q.s., with 1 mg sodium bisulfite, 1.5 mg methylparaben, and 0.2 mg propylparaben added as preservatives.

---

*Registered trademark of MERCK & CO., INC.

ACTIONS

DECADRON Phosphate injection has a rapid onset but short duration of action when compared with less soluble preparations. Because of this, it is suitable for the treatment of acute disorders responsive to adrenocortical steroid therapy.

Naturally occurring glucocorticoids (hydrocortisone and cortisone), which also have salt-retaining properties, are used as replacement therapy in adrenocortical deficiency states. Their synthetic analogs, including dexamethasone, are primarily used for their potent anti-inflammatory effects in disorders of many organ systems.

Glucocorticoids cause profound and varied metabolic effects. In addition, they modify the body's immune responses to diverse stimuli.

At equipotent anti-inflammatory doses, dexamethasone almost completely lacks the sodium-retaining property of hydrocortisone and closely related derivatives of hydrocortisone.

INDICATIONS

  A. By intravenous or intramuscular injection when oral therapy is not feasible:

1. *Endocrine disorders*
Primary or secondary adrenocortical insufficiency (hydrocortisone or cortisone is the drug of choice; synthetic analogs may be used in conjunction with mineralocorticoids where applicable; in infancy, mineralocorticoid supplementation is of particular importance)
Acute adrenocortical insufficiency (hydrocortisone or cortisone is the drug of choice; mineralocorticoid supplementation may be necessary, particularly when synthetic analogs are used)
Preoperatively, and in the event of serious trauma or illness, in patients with known adrenal insufficiency or when adrenocortical reserve is doubtful
Shock unresponsive to conventional therapy if adrenocortical insufficiency exists or is suspected
Congenital adrenal hyperplasia
Nonsuppurative thyroiditis
Hypercalcemia associated with cancer
2. *Rheumatic disorders*
As adjunctive therapy for short-term administration (to tide the patient over an acute episode or exacerbation) in:
Post-traumatic osteoarthritis
Synovitis of osteoarthritis
Rheumatoid arthritis, including juvenile rheumatoid arthritis (selected cases may require low-dose maintenance therapy)
Acute and subacute bursitis
Epicondylitis
Acute nonspecific tenosynovitis
Acute gouty arthritis
Psoriatic arthritis
Ankylosing spondylitis
3. *Collagen diseases*
During an exacerbation or as maintenance therapy in selected cases of:
Systemic lupus erythematosus
Acute rheumatic carditis
4. *Dermatologic diseases*
Pemphigus
Severe erythema multiforme (Stevens-Johnson syndrome)
Exfoliative dermatitis
Bullous dermatitis herpetiformis
Severe seborrheic dermatitis
Severe psoriasis
Mycosis fungoides
5. *Allergic states*
Control of severe or incapacitating allergic conditions intractable to adequate trials of conventional treatment in:
Bronchial asthma
Contact dermatitis
Atopic dermatitis
Serum sickness
Seasonal or perennial allergic rhinitis
Drug hypersensitivity reactions
Urticarial transfusion reactions
Acute noninfectious laryngeal edema (epinephrine is the drug of first choice)
6. *Ophthalmic diseases*
Severe acute and chronic allergic and inflammatory processes involving the eye, such as:
Herpes zoster ophthalmicus
Iritis, iridocyclitis
Chorioretinitis
Diffuse posterior uveitis and choroiditis
Optic neuritis
Sympathetic ophthalmia
Anterior segment inflammation
Allergic conjunctivitis
Keratitis
Allergic corneal marginal ulcers
7. *Gastrointestinal diseases*
To tide the patient over a critical period of the disease in:
Ulcerative colitis (Systemic therapy)
Regional enteritis (Systemic therapy)
8. *Respiratory diseases*
Symptomatic sarcoidosis
Berylliosis
Fulminating or disseminated pulmonary tuberculosis when used concurrently with appropriate antituberculous chemotherapy
Loeffler's syndrome not manageable by other means
Aspiration pneumonitis
9. *Hematologic disorders*
Acquired (autoimmune) hemolytic anemia
Idiopathic thrombocytopenic purpura in adults (I.V. only; I.M. administration is contraindicated)
Secondary thrombocytopenia in adults
Erythroblastopenia (RBC anemia)

Continued on next page

Decadron Phosphate Inj.—Cont.

Congenital (erythroid) hypoplastic anemia
10. *Neoplastic diseases*
For palliative management of:
Leukemias and lymphomas in adults
Acute leukemia of childhood
11. *Edematous states*
To induce diuresis or remission of proteinuria in the nephrotic syndrome, without uremia, of the idiopathic type, or that due to lupus erythematosus
12. *Miscellaneous*
Tuberculous meningitis with subarachnoid block or impending block when used concurrently with appropriate antituberculous chemotherapy
Trichinosis with neurologic or myocardial involvement
13. *Diagnostic testing of adrenocortical hyperfunction*
14. *Cerebral Edema* associated with primary or metastatic brain tumor, craniotomy, or head injury. Use in cerebral edema is not a substitute for careful neurosurgical evaluation and definitive management such as neurosurgery or other specific therapy.
B. By intra-articular or soft tissue injection:
As adjunctive therapy for short-term administration (to tide the patient over an acute episode or exacerbation) in:
Synovitis of osteoarthritis
Rheumatoid arthritis
Acute and subacute bursitis
Acute gouty arthritis
Epicondylitis
Acute nonspecific tenosynovitis
Post-traumatic osteoarthritis.
C. By intralesional injection:
Keloids
Localized hypertrophic, infiltrated, inflammatory lesions of: lichen planus, psoriatic plaques, granuloma annulare, and lichen simplex chronicus (neurodermatitis)
Discoid lupus erythematosus
Necrobiosis lipoidica diabeticorum
Alopecia areata
May also be useful in cystic tumors of an aponeurosis or tendon (ganglia).

CONTRAINDICATIONS

Systemic fungal infections. (See WARNINGS regarding amphotericin B).
Hypersensitivity to any component of this product, including sulfites (see WARNINGS).

WARNINGS

Because rare instances of anaphylactoid reactions have occurred in patients receiving parenteral corticosteroid therapy, appropriate precautionary measures should be taken prior to administration, especially when the patient has a history of allergy to any drug. Anaphylactoid and hypersensitivity reactions have been reported for Injection DECADRON Phosphate (see ADVERSE REACTIONS).
Injection DECADRON Phosphate contains sodium bisulfite, a sulfite that may cause allergic-type reactions including anaphylactic symptoms and life-threatening or less severe asthmatic episodes in certain susceptible people. The overall prevalence of sulfite sensitivity in the general population is unknown and probably low. Sulfite sensitivity is seen more frequently in asthmatic than in nonasthmatic people.
Corticosteroids may exacerbate systemic fungal infections and therefore should not be used in the presence of such infections unless they are needed to control drug reactions due to amphotericin B. Moreover, there have been cases reported in which concomitant use of amphotericin B and hydrocortisone was followed by cardiac enlargement and congestive failure.
In patients on corticosteroid therapy subjected to any unusual stress, increased dosage of rapidly acting corticosteroids before, during, and after the stressful situation is indicated.
Drug-induced secondary adrenocortical insufficiency may result from too rapid withdrawal of corticosteroids and may be minimized by gradual reduction of dosage. This type of relative insufficiency may persist for months after discontinuation of therapy; therefore, in any situation of stress occurring during that period, hormone therapy should be reinstituted. If the patient is receiving steroids already, dosage may have to be increased. Since mineralocorticoid secretion may be impaired, salt and/or a mineralocorticoid should be administered concurrently.
Corticosteroids may mask some signs of infection, and new infections may appear during their use. There may be decreased resistance and inability to localize infection when corticosteroids are used. Moreover, corticosteroids may affect the nitroblue-tetrazolium test for bacterial infection and produce false negative results.

In cerebral malaria, a double-blind trial has shown that the use of corticosteroids is associated with prolongation of coma and a higher incidence of pneumonia and gastrointestinal bleeding.
Corticosteroids may activate latent amebiasis. Therefore, it is recommended that latent or active amebiasis be ruled out before initiating corticosteroid therapy in any patient who has spent time in the tropics or any patient with unexplained diarrhea.
Prolonged use of corticosteroids may produce posterior subcapsular cataracts, glaucoma with possible damage to the optic nerves, and may enhance the establishment of secondary ocular infections due to fungi or viruses.
Usage in pregnancy. Since adequate human reproduction studies have not been done with corticosteroids, use of these drugs in pregnancy or in women of childbearing potential requires that the anticipated benefits be weighed against the possible hazards to the mother and embryo or fetus. Infants born of mothers who have received substantial doses of corticosteroids during pregnancy should be carefully observed for signs of hypoadrenalism.
Corticosteroids appear in breast milk and could suppress growth, interfere with endogenous corticosteroid production, or cause other unwanted effects. Mothers taking pharmacologic doses of corticosteroids should be advised not to nurse.
Average and large doses of cortisone or hydrocortisone can cause elevation of blood pressure, salt and water retention, and increased excretion of potassium. These effects are less likely to occur with the synthetic derivatives except when used in large doses. Dietary salt restriction and potassium supplementation may be necessary. All corticosteroids increase calcium excretion.
Administration of live virus vaccines, including smallpox, is contraindicated in individuals receiving immunosuppressive doses of corticosteroids. If inactivated viral or bacterial vaccines are administered to individuals receiving immunosuppressive doses of corticosteroids, the expected serum antibody response may not be obtained. However, immunization procedures may be undertaken in patients who are receiving corticosteroids as replacement therapy, e.g., for Addison's disease.
Patients who are on drugs which suppress the immune system are more susceptible to infections than healthy individuals. Chickenpox and measles, for example, can have a more serious or even fatal course in non-immune patients on corticosteroids. In such patients who have not had these diseases, particular care should be taken to avoid exposure. The risk of developing a disseminated infection varies among individuals and can be related to the dose, route and duration of corticosteroid administration as well as to the underlying disease. If exposed to chickenpox, prophylaxis with varicella zoster immune globulin (VZIG) may be indicated. If chickenpox develops, treatment with antiviral agents may be considered. If exposed to measles, prophylaxis with immune globulin (IG) may be indicated. (See the respective package inserts for VZIG and IG for complete prescribing information.)
Similarly, corticosteroids should be used with great care in patients with known or suspected Strongyloides (threadworm) infestation. In such patients, corticosteroid-induced immunosuppression may lead to Strongyloides hyperinfection and dissemination with widespread larval migration, often accompanied by severe enterocolitis and potentially fatal gram-negative septicemia.
The use of DECADRON Phosphate injection in active tuberculosis should be restricted to those cases of fulminating or disseminated tuberculosis in which the corticosteroid is used for the management of the disease in conjunction with an appropriate antituberculous regimen.
If corticosteroids are indicated in patients with latent tuberculosis or tuberculin reactivity, close observation is necessary as reactivation of the disease may occur. During prolonged corticosteroid therapy, these patients should receive chemoprophylaxis.
Literature reports suggest an apparent association between use of corticosteroids and left ventricular free wall rupture after a recent myocardial infarction; therefore, therapy with corticosteroids should be used with great caution in these patients.

PRECAUTIONS

This product, like many other steroid formulations, is sensitive to heat. Therefore, it should not be autoclaved when it is desirable to sterilize the exterior of the vial.
Following prolonged therapy, withdrawal of corticosteroids may result in symptoms of the corticosteroid withdrawal syndrome including fever, myalgia, arthralgia, and malaise. This may occur in patients even without evidence of adrenal insufficiency.
There is an enhanced effect of corticosteroids in patients with hypothyroidism and in those with cirrhosis.
Corticosteroids should be used cautiously in patients with ocular herpes simplex for fear of corneal perforation.

The lowest possible dose of corticosteroid should be used to control the condition under treatment, and when reduction in dosage is possible, the reduction must be gradual.
Psychic derangements may appear when corticosteroids are used, ranging from euphoria, insomnia, mood swings, personality changes, and severe depression to frank psychotic manifestations. Also, existing emotional instability or psychotic tendencies may be aggravated by corticosteroids.
Aspirin should be used cautiously in conjunction with corticosteroids in hypoprothrombinemia.
Steroids should be used with caution in nonspecific ulcerative colitis, if there is a probability of impending perforation, abscess, or other pyogenic infection, also in diverticulitis, fresh intestinal anastomoses, active or latent peptic ulcer, renal insufficiency, hypertension, osteoporosis, and myasthenia gravis. Signs of peritoneal irritation following gastrointestinal perforation in patients receiving large doses of corticosteroids may be minimal or absent. Fat embolism has been reported as a possible complication of hypercortisonism.
When large doses are given, some authorities advise that antacids be administered between meals to help to prevent peptic ulcer.
Steroids may increase or decrease motility and number of spermatozoa in some patients.
Phenytoin, phenobarbital, ephedrine, and rifampin may enhance the metabolic clearance of corticosteroids resulting in decreased blood levels and lessened physiologic activity, thus requiring adjustment in corticosteroid dosage. These interactions may interfere with dexamethasone suppression tests which should be interpreted with caution during administration of these drugs.
False negative results in the dexamethasone suppression test (DST) in patients being treated with indomethacin have been reported. Thus, results of the DST should be interpreted with caution in these patients.
The prothrombin time should be checked frequently in patients who are receiving corticosteroids and coumarin anticoagulants at the same time because of reports that corticosteroids have altered the response to these anticoagulants. Studies have shown that the usual effect produced by adding corticosteroids is inhibition of response to coumarins, although there have been some conflicting reports of potentiation not substantiated by studies.
When corticosteroids are administered concomitantly with potassium-depleting diuretics, patients should be observed closely for development of hypokalemia.
Intra-articular injection of a corticosteroid may produce systemic as well as local effects.
Appropriate examination of any joint fluid present is necessary to exclude a septic process.
A marked increase in pain accompanied by local swelling, further restriction of joint motion, fever, and malaise is suggestive of septic arthritis. If this complication occurs and the diagnosis of sepsis is confirmed, appropriate antimicrobial therapy should be instituted.
Injection of a steroid into an infected site is to be avoided.
Corticosteroids should not be injected into unstable joints.
Patients should be impressed strongly with the importance of not overusing joints in which symptomatic benefit has been obtained as long as the inflammatory process remains active.
Frequent intra-articular injection may result in damage to joint tissues.
The slower rate of absorption by intramuscular administration should be recognized.
Information for Patients
Susceptible patients who are on immunosuppressant doses of corticosteroids should be warned to avoid exposure to chickenpox or measles. Patients should also be advised that if they are exposed, medical advice should be sought without delay.
Pediatric Use
Growth and development of pediatric patients on prolonged corticosteroid therapy should be carefully followed.

ADVERSE REACTIONS

Fluid and electrolyte disturbances
Sodium retention
Fluid retention
Congestive heart failure in susceptible patients
Potassium loss
Hypokalemic alkalosis
Hypertension
Musculoskeletal
Muscle weakness
Steroid myopathy
Loss of muscle mass
Osteoporosis
Vertebral compression fractures
Aseptic necrosis of femoral and humeral heads
Pathologic fracture of long bones
Tendon rupture
Gastrointestinal
Peptic ulcer with possible subsequent perforation and hemorrhage

Perforation of the small and large bowel, particularly in patients with inflammatory bowel disease
Pancreatitis
Abdominal distention
Ulcerative esophagitis
Dermatologic
Impaired wound healing
Thin fragile skin
Petechiae and ecchymoses
Erythema
Increased sweating
May suppress reactions to skin tests
Burning or tingling, especially in the perineal area (after I.V. injection)
Other cutaneous reactions, such as allergic dermatitis, urticaria, angioneurotic edema
Neurologic
Convulsions
Increased intracranial pressure with papilledema (pseudotumor cerebri) usually after treatment
Vertigo
Headache
Psychic disturbances
Endocrine
Menstrual irregularities
Development of cushingoid state
Suppression of growth in pediatric patients
Secondary adrenocortical and pituitary unresponsiveness, particularly in times of stress, as in trauma, surgery, or illness
Decreased carbohydrate tolerance
Manifestations of latent diabetes mellitus
Increased requirements for insulin or oral hypoglycemic agents in diabetics
Hirsutism
Ophthalmic
Posterior subcapsular cataracts
Increased intraocular pressure
Glaucoma
Exophthalmos
Retinopathy of prematurity
Metabolic
Negative nitrogen balance due to protein catabolism
Cardiovascular
Myocardial rupture following recent myocardial infarction (see WARNINGS)
Hypertrophic cardiomyopathy in low birth weight infants
Other
Anaphylactoid or hypersensitivity reactions
Thromboembolism
Weight gain
Increased appetite
Nausea
Malaise
Hiccups
The following *additional* adverse reactions are related to parenteral corticosteroid therapy:
Rare instances of blindness associated with intralesional therapy around the face and head
Hyperpigmentation or hypopigmentation
Subcutaneous and cutaneous atrophy
Sterile abscess
Postinjection flare (following intra-articular use)
Charcot-like arthropathy

OVERDOSAGE

Reports of acute toxicity and/or death following overdosage of glucocorticoids are rare. In the event of overdosage, no specific antidote is available; treatment is supportive and symptomatic.
Significant lethality was observed in female mice at single oral doses of 3630 mg/m^2 (1210 mg/kg) and single intravenous doses of 2382 mg/m^2 (794 mg/kg).

DOSAGE AND ADMINISTRATION

DECADRON Phosphate injection, 4 mg/mL—*For intravenous, intramuscular, intra-articular, intralesional, and soft tissue injection.*
DECADRON Phosphate injection, 24 mg/mL—*For intravenous injection only.*
DECADRON Phosphate injection can be given directly from the vial, or it can be added to Sodium Chloride Injection or Dextrose Injection and administered by intravenous drip.
Solutions used for intravenous administration or further dilution of this product should be preservative-free when used in the neonate, especially the premature infant.
When it is mixed with an infusion solution, sterile precautions should be observed. Since infusion solutions generally do not contain preservatives, mixtures should be used within 24 hours.

DOSAGE REQUIREMENTS ARE VARIABLE AND MUST BE INDIVIDUALIZED ON THE BASIS OF THE DISEASE AND THE RESPONSE OF THE PATIENT.
Intravenous and Intramuscular Injection
The initial dosage of DECADRON Phosphate injection varies from 0.5 to 9 mg a day depending on the disease being treated. In less severe diseases doses lower than 0.5 mg may suffice, while in severe diseases doses higher than 9 mg may be required.
The initial dosage should be maintained or adjusted until the patient's response is satisfactory. If a satisfactory clinical response does not occur after a reasonable period of time, discontinue DECADRON Phosphate injection and transfer the patient to other therapy.
After a favorable initial response, the proper maintenance dosage should be determined by decreasing the initial dosage in small amounts to the lowest dosage that maintains an adequate clinical response.
Patients should be observed closely for signs that might require dosage adjustment, including changes in clinical status resulting from remissions or exacerbations of the disease, individual drug responsiveness, and the effect of stress (e.g., surgery, infection, trauma). During stress it may be necessary to increase dosage temporarily.
If the drug is to be stopped after more than a few days of treatment, it usually should be withdrawn gradually.
When the intravenous route of administration is used, dosage usually should be the same as the oral dosage. In certain overwhelming, acute, life-threatening situations, however, administration in dosages exceeding the usual dosages may be justified and may be in multiples of the oral dosages. The slower rate of absorption by intramuscular administration should be recognized.
Shock
There is a tendency in current medical practice to use high (pharmacologic) doses of corticosteroids for the treatment of unresponsive shock. The following dosages of DECADRON phosphate injection have been suggested by various authors:

Author*	Dosage
Cavanagh[1]	3 mg/kg of body weight per 24 hours by constant intravenous infusion after an initial intravenous injection of 20 mg
Dietzman[2]	2 to 6 mg/kg of body weight as a single intravenous injection
Frank[3]	40 mg initially followed by repeat intravenous injection every 4 to 6 hours while shock persists
Oaks[4]	40 mg initially followed by repeat intravenous injection every 2 to 6 hours while shock persists
Schumer[5]	1 mg/kg of body weight as a single intravenous injection

Administration of high dose corticosteroid therapy should be continued only until the patient's condition has stabilized and usually not longer than 48 to 72 hours.
Although adverse reactions associated with high dose, short term corticosteroid therapy are uncommon, peptic ulceration may occur.

1. *Cavanagh, D.; Singh, K. B.: Endotoxin shock in pregnancy and abortion, in "Corticosteroids in the Treatment of Shock", Schumer, W.; Nyhus, L. M., Editors, Urbana, University of Illinois Press, 1970, pp. 86-96.
2. Dietzman, R. H.; Ersek, R. A.; Bloch, J. M.; Lillehei, R. C.: High-output, low-resistance gram-negative septic shock in man, Angiology 20: 691-700, Dec. 1969.
3. Frank, E.: Clinical observations in shock and management (In: Shields, T. F., ed.: Symposium on current concepts and management of shock), J. Maine Med. Ass. 59: 195-200, Oct. 1968.
4. Oaks, W. W.; Cohen, H. E.: Endotoxin shock in the geriatric patient, Geriat. 22: 120-130, Mar. 1967.
5. Schumer, W.; Nyhus, L. M.: Corticosteroid effect on biochemical parameters of human oligemic shock, Arch. Surg. 100: 405-408, Apr. 1970.

Cerebral Edema
DECADRON Phosphate injection is generally administered initially in a dosage of 10 mg intravenously followed by 4 mg every six hours intramuscularly until the symptoms of cerebral edema subside. Response is usually noted within 12 to 24 hours and dosage may be reduced after two to four days and gradually discontinued over a period of five to seven days. For palliative management of patients with recurrent or inoperable brain tumors, maintenance therapy with two mg two or three times a day may be effective.
Acute Allergic Disorders
In acute, self-limited allergic disorders or acute exacerbations of chronic allergic disorders, the following dosage schedule combining parenteral and oral therapy is suggested:
DECADRON Phosphate injection, 4 mg/mL: *first day*, 1 or 2 mL (4 or 8 mg), intramuscularly.
DECADRON* (Dexamethasone) tablets, 0.75 mg: *second and third days*, 4 tablets in two divided doses each day;

fourth day, 2 tablets in two divided doses; *fifth and sixth days*, 1 tablet each day; *seventh day*, no treatment; *eighth day*, follow-up visit.
This schedule is designed to ensure adequate therapy during acute episodes, while minimizing the risk of overdosage in chronic cases.

* Registered trademark of MERCK & CO., INC.

Intra-articular, Intralesional, and Soft Tissue Injection
Intra-articular, intralesional, and soft tissue injections are generally employed when the affected joints or areas are limited to one or two sites. Dosage and frequency of injection varies depending on the condition and the site of injection. The usual dose is from 0.2 to 6 mg. The frequency usually ranges from once every three to five days to once every two to three weeks. Frequent intra-articular injection may result in damage to joint tissues.
Some of the usual single doses are:

Site of Injection	Amount of Dexamethasone Phosphate (mg)
Large Joints (e.g., Knee)	2 to 4
Small Joints (e.g., Interphalangeal, Temporomandibular)	0.8 to 1
Bursae	2 to 3
Tendon Sheaths	0.4 to 1
Soft Tissue Infiltration	2 to 6
Ganglia	1 to 2

DECADRON Phosphate injection is particularly recommended for use in conjunction with one of the less soluble, longer-acting steroids for intra-articular and soft tissue injection.

HOW SUPPLIED

No 7628X—Injection DECADRON Phosphate, 4 mg per mL, is a clear, colorless solution, and is available in 1 mL, 5 mL, and 25 mL vials as follows:
NDC 0006-7628-66, boxes of 25 × 1 mL vials.
NDC 0006-7628-03, 5 mL vial
(6505-00-963-5355, 5 mL vial)
NDC 0006-7628-25, 25 mL vial.
FOR INTRAVENOUS USE ONLY:
No. 7646—Injection DECADRON Phosphate, 24 mg per mL, is a clear, colorless to light yellow solution and is available in 5 mL vials as follows:
NDC 0006-7646-03, 5 mL vial
(6505-01-153-3524, 5 mL vial).
Storage
Sensitive to heat. Do not autoclave.
Protect from freezing.
Protect from light. Store container in carton until contents have been used.
7347231   Issued July 1997

DECADRON® Phosphate with XYLOCAINE® ℞
Injection, Sterile
(Dexamethasone Sodium Phosphate-Lidocaine Hydrochloride)

For local injection only

NOT FOR INTRAVENOUS USE

DESCRIPTION

Dexamethasone sodium phosphate is a white or slightly yellow, crystalline powder. It is freely soluble in water and is exceedingly hygroscopic. The molecular weight is 516.41. It

Continued on next page

Decadron Phosphate w/Xylo.—Cont.

is designated chemically as 9-fluoro-11β,17-dihydroxy-16α-methyl-21-(phosphonooxy)pregna-1,4-diene-3,20-dione disodium salt. The empirical formula is $C_{22}H_{28}FNa_2O_8P$ and the structural formula is:

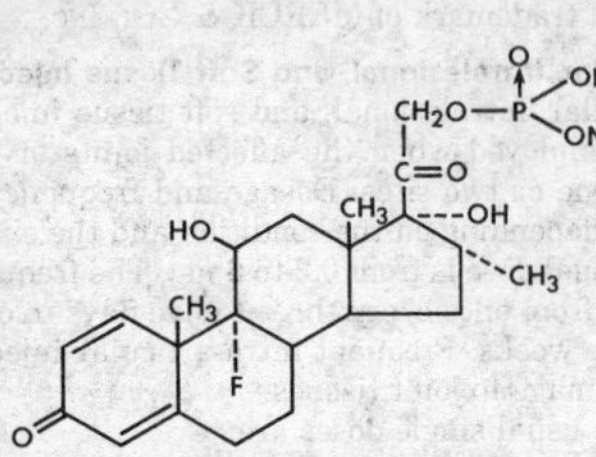

Lidocaine hydrochloride is a white, crystalline powder that is very soluble in water and alcohol, soluble in chloroform, and insoluble in ether. The molecular weight is 288.82. It is designated chemically as 2-(diethylamino)-*N* -(2,6- dimethylphenyl)acetamide, monohydrochloride, monohydrate. The empirical formula is $C_{14}H_{22}N_2O{\cdot}HCl{\cdot}H_2O$ and the structural formula is:

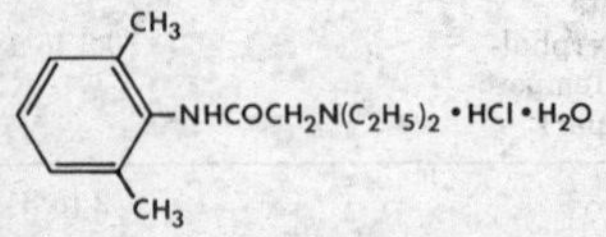

DECADRON* Phosphate with XYLOCAINE** (Dexamethasone Sodium Phosphate-Lidocaine Hydrochloride) injection is provided as a sterile solution (pH 6.5 to 6.9), sealed under nitrogen, for the convenience of physicians who prefer to treat patients with simultaneous administration of a corticosteroid and a local anesthetic.
Each milliliter contains dexamethasone sodium phosphate equivalent to dexamethasone phosphate, 4 mg; and lidocaine hydrochloride, 10 mg. Inactive ingredients per mL: citric acid anhydrous, 10 mg; creatinine, 8 mg; sodium bisulfite, 0.5 mg; disodium edetate, 0.5 mg; sodium hydroxide to adjust pH; and Water for Injection, q.s., 1 mL.
Methylparaben, 1.5 mg, and propylparaben, 0.2 mg, added as preservatives.

*Registered trademark of MERCK & CO., Inc.
**Registered trademark of Astra Pharmaceutical Products, Inc.

ACTIONS

DECADRON Phosphate (Dexamethasone Sodium Phosphate) is a synthetic glucocorticoid used primarily for its potent anti-inflammatory effects in disorders of many organ systems. Glucocorticoids cause profound and varied metabolic effects. In addition, they modify the body's immune responses to diverse stimuli.
XYLOCAINE (Lidocaine Hydrochloride) is a local anesthetic with a rapid onset and moderate duration of action. Local anesthesia appears within a few minutes after injection of DECADRON Phosphate with XYLOCAINE and lasts 45 minutes to one hour. By the time the anesthesia wears off, steroid activity usually has begun. If the anesthesia wears off before full steroid effect appears, there may be some discomfort beginning about an hour after injection and relief of pain may be delayed for a short time.

INDICATIONS

Acute and subacute bursitis
Acute and subacute nonspecific tenosynovitis

CONTRAINDICATIONS

Hypersensitivity to any component of this product, including sulfites (see WARNINGS).

Dexamethasone Sodium Phosphate
Systemic fungal infections
Lidocaine Hydrochloride
Patients with known history of hypersensitivity to local anesthetics of the amide type (e.g., mepivacaine, prilocaine)
Severe shock
Heart block

WARNINGS

Because rare instances of anaphylactoid reactions have occurred in patients receiving parenteral corticosteroid therapy, appropriate precautionary measures should be taken prior to administration, especially when the patient has a history of allergy to any drug. Anaphylactoid and hypersensitivity reactions have been reported for Injection DECADRON Phosphate with XYLOCAINE (see ADVERSE REACTIONS).
Injection DECADRON Phosphate with XYLOCAINE contains sodium bisulfite, a sulfite that may cause allergic-type reactions including anaphylactic symptoms and life-threatening or less severe asthmatic episodes in certain susceptible people. The overall prevalence of sulfite sensitivity in the general population is unknown and probably low. Sulfite sensitivity is seen more frequently in asthmatic than in nonasthmatic people.
Lidocaine Hydrochloride
RESUSCITATIVE EQUIPMENT AND DRUGS SHOULD BE IMMEDIATELY AVAILABLE WHEN ANY LOCAL ANESTHETIC IS USED.
Usage in pregnancy: The safe use of lidocaine hydrochloride has not been established with respect to adverse effects upon fetal development. Careful consideration should be given to this fact before administering this drug to women of childbearing potential, particularly during early pregnancy.
Dexamethasone Sodium Phosphate
In patients on corticosteroid therapy subjected to unusual stress, increased dosage of rapidly acting corticosteroids before, during, and after the stressful situation is indicated.
Drug-induced secondary adrenocortical insufficiency may result from too rapid withdrawal of corticosteroids and may be minimized by gradual reduction of dosage. This type of relative insufficiency may persist for months after discontinuation of therapy: therefore, in any situation of stress occurring during that period, hormone therapy should be reinstituted. If the patient is receiving steroids already, dosage may have to be increased. Since mineralocorticoid secretion may be impaired, salt and/or a mineralocorticoid should be administered concurrently.
Corticosteroids may mask some signs of infection, and new infections may appear during their use. There may be decreased resistance and inability to localize infection when corticosteroids are used. Moreover, corticosteroids may affect the nitroblue-tetrazolium test for bacterial infection and produce false negative results.
Corticosteroids may activate latent amebiasis. Therefore, it is recommended that latent or active amebiasis be ruled out before initiating corticosteroid therapy in any patient who has spent time in the tropics or any patient with unexplained diarrhea.
Prolonged use of corticosteroids may produce posterior subcapsular cataracts, glaucoma with possible damage to the optic nerves, and may enhance the establishment of secondary ocular infections due to fungi or viruses.
Usage in pregnancy: Since adequate human reproduction studies have not been done with corticosteroids, use of these drugs in pregnancy or in women of childbearing potential requires that the anticipated benefits be weighed against the possible hazards to the mother and embryo or fetus. Infants born of mothers who have received substantial doses of corticosteroids during pregnancy should be carefully observed for signs of hypoadrenalism.
Corticosteroids appear in breast milk and could suppress growth, interfere with endogenous corticosteroid production, or cause other unwanted effects. Mothers taking pharmacologic doses of corticosteroids should be advised not to nurse.
Average and large doses of cortisone or hydrocortisone can cause elevation of blood pressure, salt and water retention, and increased excretion of potassium. These effects are less likely to occur with the synthetic derivatives except when used in large doses. Dietary salt restriction and potassium supplementation may be necessary. All corticosteroids increase calcium excretion.
Administration of live virus vaccines, including smallpox, is contraindicated in individuals receiving immunosuppressive doses of corticosteroids. If inactivated viral or bacterial vaccines are administered to individuals receiving immunosuppressive doses of corticosteroids, the expected serum antibody response may not be obtained.
Patients who are on drugs which suppress the immune system are more susceptible to infections than healthy individuals. Chickenpox and measles, for example, can have a more serious or even fatal course in non-immune patients on corticosteroids. In such patients who have not had these diseases, particular care should be taken to avoid exposure. The risk of developing a disseminated infection varies among individuals and can be related to the dose, route and duration of corticosteroid administration as well as to the underlying disease. If exposed to chickenpox, prophylaxis with varicella zoster immune globulin (VZIG) may be indicated. If chickenpox develops, treatment with antiviral agents may be considered. If exposed to measles, prophylaxis with immune globulin (IG) may be indicated. (See the respective package inserts for VZIG and IG for complete prescribing information.)
Similarly, corticosteroids should be used with great care in patients with known or suspected Strongyloides (threadworm) infestation. In such patients, corticosteroid-induced immunosuppression may lead to Strongyloides hyperinfection and dissemination with widespread larval migration, often accompanied by severe enterocolitis and potentially fatal gram-negative septicemia.
If corticosteroids are indicated in patients with latent tuberculosis or tuberculin reactivity, close observation is necessary as reactivation of the disease may occur. During prolonged corticosteroid therapy, these patients should receive chemoprophylaxis.
Literature reports suggest an apparent association between use of corticosteroids and left ventricular free wall rupture after a recent myocardial infarction; therefore, therapy with corticosteroids should be used with great caution in these patients.

PRECAUTIONS

This product, like many other steroid formulations, is sensitive to heat. Therefore, it should not be autoclaved when it is desirable to sterilize the exterior of the vial.
Therapy with this preparation does not eliminate the need for conventional supportive measures. Although capable of ameliorating symptoms, and even suppressing them completely in some patients, it is not a cure. Neither the hormone nor the anesthetic has any effect on the basic cause of inflammation.
Supportive measures, such as analgesics, pertinent orthopedic procedures, heat or cold, rest, rehabilitation, and physiotherapy must be used as applicable. If physiotherapy is applied immediately following injection, it may cause severe pain.
In some patients, a single injection fully restores mobility. Patients should be strongly impressed with the importance of not overusing the affected part as long as the inflammatory process remains active.
Injection into an infected site is to be avoided.
Dexamethasone Sodium Phosphate
Following prolonged therapy, withdrawal of corticosteroids may result in symptoms of the corticosteroid withdrawal syndrome including fever, myalgia, arthralgia, and malaise. This may occur in patients even without evidence of adrenal insufficiency.
There is an enhanced effect of corticosteroids in patients with hypothyroidism and in those with cirrhosis.
Corticosteroids should be used cautiously in patients with ocular herpes simplex for fear of corneal perforation.
Psychic derangements may appear when corticosteroids are used, ranging from euphoria, insomnia, mood swings, personality changes, and severe depression to frank psychotic manifestations. Also, existing emotional instability or psychotic tendencies may be aggravated by corticosteroids.
Aspirin should be used cautiously in conjunction with corticosteroids in hypoprothrombinemia.
Steroids should be used with caution in non-specific ulcerative colitis, if there is a probability of impending perforation, abscess, or other pyogenic infection, also in diverticulitis, fresh intestinal anastomoses, active or latent peptic ulcer, renal insufficiency, hypertension, osteoporosis, and myasthenia gravis. Signs of peritoneal irritation following gastrointestinal perforation in patients receiving large doses of corticosteroids may be minimal or absent. Fat embolism has been reported as a possible complication of hypercortisonism.
When large doses are given, some authorities advise that antacids be administered between meals to help to prevent peptic ulcer.
Steroids may increase or decrease motility and number of spermatozoa in some patients.
Phenytoin, phenobarbital, ephedrine, and rifampin may enhance the metabolic clearance of corticosteroids, resulting in decreased blood levels and lessened physiologic activity, thus requiring adjustment in corticosteroid dosage.
The prothrombin time should be checked frequently in patients who are receiving corticosteroids and coumarin anticoagulants at the same time because of reports that corticosteroids have altered the response to these anticoagulants. Studies have shown that the usual effect produced by adding corticosteroids is inhibition of response to coumarins, although there have been some conflicting reports of potentiation not substantiated by studies.
When corticosteroids are administered concomitantly with potassium-depleting diuretics, patients should be observed closely for development of hypokalemia.
Lidocaine Hydrochloride
The safety and effectiveness of lidocaine hydrochloride depend on proper dosage, correct technique, adequate precautions, and readiness for emergencies.
Injection of repeated doses may cause significant increases in blood levels with each repeated dose due to slow accumulation of the drug or its metabolites. Tolerance varies with the status of the patient. Debilitated, elderly patients, acutely ill patients, and children should be given reduced doses commensurate with their age and physical status. INJECTIONS SHOULD ALWAYS BE MADE SLOWLY AND WITH FREQUENT ASPIRATIONS. Aspiration is advisable since it reduces the possibility of intravascular injection,

thereby keeping the incidence of side effects and anesthetic failures to a minimum. Consult standard textbooks for specific techniques and precautions for various local anesthetic procedures.

Lidocaine hydrochloride should be used with caution in persons with known drug sensitivities. Patients allergic to para-aminobenzoic acid derivatives (procaine, tetracaine, benzocaine, etc.) have not shown cross sensitivity to lidocaine hydrochloride.

Local anesthetics react with certain metals and cause the release of their respective ions which, if injected, may cause severe local irritation. Adequate precaution should be taken to avoid this type of interaction.

Information for Patients

Susceptible patients who are on immunosuppressant doses of corticosteroids should be warned to avoid exposure to chickenpox or measles. Patients should also be advised that if they are exposed, medical advice should be sought without delay.

Pediatric Use

Growth and development of pediatric patients on prolonged corticosteroid therapy should be carefully followed.

ADVERSE REACTIONS

Dexamethasone Sodium Phosphate
Fluid and electrolyte disturbances
   Sodium retention
   Fluid retention
   Congestive heart failure in susceptible patients
   Potassium loss
   Hypokalemic alkalosis
   Hypertension
Musculoskeletal
   Muscle weakness
   Steroid myopathy
   Loss of muscle mass
   Osteoporosis
   Vertebral compression fractures
   Aseptic necrosis of femoral and humeral heads
   Pathologic fracture of long bones
   Tendon rupture
Gastrointestinal
   Peptic ulcer with possible subsequent perforation and hemorrhage
   Perforation of the small and large bowel, particularly in patients with inflammatory bowel disease
   Pancreatitis
   Abdominal distention
   Ulcerative esophagitis
Dermatologic
   Impaired wound healing
   Thin fragile skin
   Petechiae and ecchymoses
   Erythema
   Increased sweating
   May suppress reactions to skin tests
   Other cutaneous reactions, such as allergic dermatitis, urticaria, angioneurotic edema
Neurologic
   Convulsions
   Increased intracranial pressure with papilledema (pseudotumor cerebri) usually after treatment
   Vertigo
   Headache
   Psychic disturbances
Endocrine
   Menstrual irregularities
   Development of cushingoid state
   Suppression of growth in children
   Secondary adrenocortical and pituitary unresponsiveness, particularly in times of stress, as in trauma, surgery, or illness
   Decreased carbohydrate tolerance
   Manifestations of latent diabetes mellitus
   Increased requirements for insulin or oral hypoglycemic agents in diabetics
   Hirsutism
Ophthalmic
   Posterior subcapsular cataracts
   Increased intraocular pressure
   Glaucoma
   Exophthalmos
Metabolic
   Negative nitrogen balance due to protein catabolism
Cardiovascular
   Myocardial rupture following recent myocardial infarction (see WARNINGS)
Other
   Anaphylactoid or hypersensitivity reactions
   Thromboembolism
   Weight gain
   Increased appetite
   Nausea
   Malaise
   Hiccups

The following *additional* adverse reactions are related to parenteral corticosteroid therapy:
   Rare instances of blindness associated with intralesional therapy around the face and head
   Hyperpigmentation or hypopigmentation
   Subcutaneous and cutaneous atrophy
   Sterile abscess
   Charcot-like arthropathy
Lidocaine Hydrochloride

Adverse reactions may result from high plasma levels due to excessive dosage, rapid absorption or inadvertent intravascular injection, or may result from a hypersensitivity, idiosyncrasy or diminished tolerance on the part of the patient. Such reactions are systemic in nature and involve the central nervous system and/or the cardiovascular system. CNS reactions are excitatory and/or depressant, and may be characterized by nervousness, dizziness, blurred vision, and tremors followed by drowsiness, convulsions, unconsciousness, and possibly respiratory arrest. The excitatory reactions may be very brief or may not occur at all, in which case the first manifestations of toxicity may be drowsiness merging into unconsciousness and respiratory arrest.

Cardiovascular reactions are depressant, and may be characterized by hypotension, myocardial depression, bradycardia and possibly cardiac arrest.

Treatment of a patient with toxic manifestations consists of assuring and maintaining a patent airway and supporting ventilation using oxygen and assisted or controlled respiration as required. This usually will be sufficient in the management of most reactions. Should circulatory depression occur, vasopressors, such as ephedrine or metaraminol, and intravenous fluids may be used. Should a convulsion persist despite oxygen therapy, small increments of an ultra-short acting barbiturate (thiopental or thiamylal) or a short acting barbiturate (pentobarbital or secobarbital) may be given intravenously.

Allergic reactions are characterized by cutaneous lesions, urticaria, edema or anaphylactoid reactions. The detection of sensitivity by skin testing is of doubtful value.

DOSAGE AND ADMINISTRATION

> **For local injection only**

NOT FOR INTRAVENOUS USE

DOSAGE AND FREQUENCY OF INJECTION ARE VARIABLE AND MUST BE INDIVIDUALIZED ON THE BASIS OF THE DISEASE AND THE RESPONSE OF THE PATIENT.

Injections should always be made slowly and with frequent aspiration.

The initial dose ranges from 0.1 to 0.75 mL depending on the disease being treated and the size of the area to be injected. Frequency of injection depends on symptomatic response. In some patients, acute conditions are controlled adequately by a single injection. In others, additional injections are required, usually at intervals of four to seven days. If satisfactory clinical response does not occur after a reasonable period of time, discontinue DECADRON Phosphate with XYLOCAINE Injection and transfer the patient to other therapy.

Patients should be observed closely for signs that might require dosage adjustment, including changes in clinical status resulting from remissions or exacerbations of the disease, and individual drug responsiveness.

The usual doses are:

	Acute and Subacute Bursitis	Acute and Subacute Nonspecific Tenosynovitis
Amount of injection (mL)	0.5 to 0.75	0.1 to 0.25
Amount of dexamethasone sodium phosphate (mg)	2 to 3	0.4 to 1
Amount of lidocaine hydrochloride (mg)	5 to 7.5	1 to 2.5

DECADRON Phosphate with XYLOCAINE may be given undiluted directly from the vial, or it may be diluted with Sterile Water for Injection or Sodium Chloride Injection, using up to five parts of diluent to each part of injection. Dilutions should be used within one hour, since there is a possibility of change in pH, and this may adversely affect the stability or activity of the components.

HOW SUPPLIED

No. 7625X—Injection DECADRON Phosphate with XYLOCAINE, containing 4 mg dexamethasone phosphate equivalent and 10 mg lidocaine hydrochloride per mL, is a clear, colorless solution, and is available as follows:
NDC 0006-7625-03 in 5 mL vials.
Storage
Sensitive to heat. Do not autoclave.
Protect from freezing.
        7349322   Issued February 1997

DECADRON® Phosphate   ℞
(Dexamethasone Sodium Phosphate), U.S.P.
0.05% Dexamethasone Phosphate Equivalent
Sterile Ophthalmic Ointment

DESCRIPTION

Dexamethasone sodium phosphate is 9-fluoro-11β,17-dihydroxy-16α-methyl-21-(phosphonooxy)pregna-1,4-diene-3,20-dione disodium salt. Its empirical formula is $C_{22}H_{28}FNa_2O_8P$ and its structural formula is:

Glucocorticoids are adrenocortical steroids, both naturally occurring and synthetic. Dexamethasone is a synthetic analog of naturally occurring glucocorticoids (hydrocortisone and cortisone). Dexamethasone sodium phosphate is a water soluble, inorganic ester of dexamethasone. Its molecular weight is 516.41.

Sterile Ophthalmic Ointment DECADRON* Phosphate (Dexamethasone Sodium Phosphate) is a topical steroid ointment containing dexamethasone sodium phosphate equivalent to 0.5 mg (0.05%) dexamethasone phosphate in each gram. Inactive ingredients: white petrolatum and mineral oil.

Dexamethasone sodium phosphate is an inorganic ester of dexamethasone.

---

*Registered trademark of MERCK & CO., Inc.

CLINICAL PHARMACOLOGY

Dexamethasone sodium phosphate suppresses the inflammatory response to a variety of agents and it probably delays or slows healing. No generally accepted explanation of these steroid properties have been advanced.

INDICATIONS AND USAGE

For the treatment of the following conditions:
Steroid responsive inflammatory conditions of the palpebral and bulbar conjunctiva, cornea, and anterior segment of the globe, such as allergic conjunctivitis, acne rosacea, superficial punctate keratitis, herpes zoster keratitis, iritis, cyclitis, selected infective conjunctivitis when the inherent hazard of steroid use is accepted to obtain an advisable diminution in edema and inflammation; corneal injury from chemical or thermal burns, or penetration of foreign bodies.

CONTRAINDICATIONS

Epithelial herpes simplex keratitis (dendritic keratitis).
Acute infectious stages of vaccinia, varicella, and many other viral diseases of the cornea and conjunctiva.
Mycobacterial infection of the eye.
Fungal diseases of ocular structures.
Hypersensitivity to a component of the medication.

WARNINGS

Prolonged use may result in ocular hypertension and/or glaucoma, with damage to the optic nerve, defects in visual

Continued on next page

Information on the Merck & Co., Inc. products listed on these pages is the full prescribing information from product circulars in use August 31, 1998. For information, please call 1-800-NSC MERCK [1-800-672-6372].

Decadron Phosphate Oint.—Cont.

acuity and fields of vision, and posterior subcapsular cataract formation. Prolonged use may suppress the host response and thus increase the hazard of secondary ocular infections. In those diseases causing thinning of the cornea or sclera, perforations have been known to occur with the use of topical corticosteroids. In acute purulent conditions of the eye, corticosteroids may mask infection or enhance existing infection. If these products are used for 10 days or longer, intraocular pressure should be routinely monitored even though it may be difficult in children and uncooperative patients.
Employment of corticosteroid medication in the treatment of herpes simplex other than epithelial herpes simplex keratitis, in which it is contraindicated, requires great caution; periodic slit-lamp microscopy is essential.

PRECAUTIONS

General
The possibility of persistent fungal infections of the cornea should be considered after prolonged corticosteroid dosing. There have been reports of bacterial keratitis associated with the use of multiple dose containers of topical ophthalmic products. These containers had been inadvertently contaminated by patients who, in most cases, had a concurrent corneal disease or a disruption of the ocular epithelial surface. (See PRECAUTIONS, *Information for Patients.*)
Information for Patients
Patients should be instructed to avoid allowing the tip of the dispensing container to contact the eye or surrounding structures.
Patients should also be instructed that ocular preparations, if handled improperly, can become contaminated by common bacteria known to cause ocular infections. Serious damage to the eye and subsequent loss of vision may result from using contaminated preparations. (See PRECAUTIONS, *General.*)
Patients should also be advised that if they develop an intercurrent ocular condition (e.g., trauma, ocular surgery or infection), they should immediately seek their physician's advice concerning the continued use of the present multidose container.
Carcinogenesis, Mutagenesis, Impairment of Fertility
Long-term animal studies have not been performed to evaluate the carcinogenic potential or the effect on fertility of Ophthalmic Ointment DECADRON Phosphate.
Pregnancy
Pregnancy Category C. Dexamethasone has been shown to be teratogenic in mice and rabbits following topical ophthalmic application in multiples of the therapeutic dose.
In the mouse, corticosteroids produce fetal resorptions and a specific abnormality, cleft palate. In the rabbit, corticosteroids have produced fetal resorptions and multiple abnormalities involving the head, ears, limbs, palate, etc.
There are no adequate or well-controlled studies in pregnant women. Ophthalmic Ointment DECADRON Phosphate should be used during pregnancy only if the potential benefit to the mother justifies the potential risk to the embryo or fetus. Infants born of mothers who have received substantial doses of corticosteroids during pregnancy should be observed carefully for signs of hypoadrenalism.
Nursing Mothers
Topically applied steroids are absorbed systemically. Therefore, because of the potential for serious adverse reactions in nursing infants from dexamethasone sodium phosphate, a decision should be made whether to discontinue nursing or discontinue the drug, taking into account the importance of the drug to the mother.
Pediatric Use
Safety and effectiveness in children have not been established.

ADVERSE REACTIONS

Glaucoma with optic nerve damage, visual acuity and field defects, posterior subcapsular cataract formation, secondary ocular infection from pathogens including herpes simplex, perforation of the globe.
Rarely, filtering blebs have been reported when topical steroids have been used following cataract surgery.
Rarely, stinging or burning may occur.

DOSAGE AND ADMINISTRATION

The duration of treatment will vary with the type of lesion and may extend from a few days to several weeks, according to therapeutic response. Relapses, more common in chronic active lesions than in self-limited conditions, usually respond to retreatment.
Apply a thin coating of ointment three or four times a day. When a favorable response is observed, reduce the number of daily applications to two, and later to one a day as a maintenance dose if this is sufficient to control symptoms.
Ophthalmic Ointment DECADRON Phosphate is particularly convenient when an eye pad is used. It may also be the preparation of choice for patients in whom therapeutic benefit depends on prolonged contact of the active ingredients with ocular tissues.

HOW SUPPLIED

No. 7615—0.05% Sterile Ophthalmic Ointment DECADRON Phosphate is a clear unctuous ointment and is supplied as follows:
NDC 0006-7615-04 in 3.5 g tubes
(6505-00-961-5508 0.05% 3.5 g).
7612331 Issued October 1993

DECADRON® Phosphate ℞
(Dexamethasone Sodium Phosphate), U.S.P.
0.1% Dexamethasone Phosphate Equivalent
Sterile Ophthalmic Solution

DESCRIPTION

Dexamethasone sodium phosphate is 9-fluoro-11β,17-dihydroxy-16α-methyl-21-(phosphonooxy)pregna-1,4-diene-3,20-dione disodium salt. Its empirical formula is $C_{22}H_{28}FNa_2O_8P$ and its structural formula is:

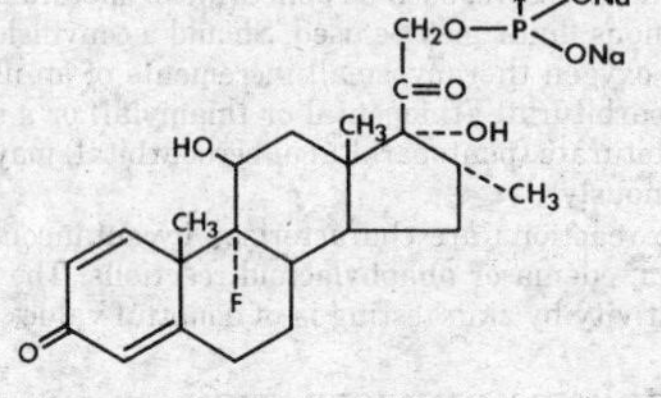

Glucocorticoids are adrenocortical steroids, both naturally occurring and synthetic. Dexamethasone is a synthetic analog of naturally occurring glucocorticoids (hydrocortisone and cortisone). Dexamethasone sodium phosphate is a water soluble, inorganic ester of dexamethasone. It is approximately three thousand times more soluble in water at 25°C than hydrocortisone. Its molecular weight is 516.41.
Ophthalmic Solution DECADRON* Phosphate (Dexamethasone Sodium Phosphate) in the 5 mL OCUMETER* ophthalmic dispenser is a topical steroid solution containing dexamethasone sodium phosphate equivalent to 1 mg (0.1%) dexamethasone phosphate in each milliliter of buffered solution. Inactive ingredients: creatinine, sodium citrate, sodium borate, polysorbate 80, disodium edetate, hydrochloric acid to adjust pH, and water for injection. Sodium bisulfite 0.1%, phenylethanol 0.25% and benzalkonium chloride 0.02% added as preservatives.

*Registered trademark of MERCK & CO., INC.

CLINICAL PHARMACOLOGY

Dexamethasone sodium phosphate suppresses the inflammatory response to a variety of agents and it probably delays or slows healing. No generally accepted explanation of these steroid properties have been advanced.

INDICATIONS AND USAGE

For the treatment of the following conditions:
Ophthalmic:
Steroid responsive inflammatory conditions of the palpebral and bulbar conjunctiva, cornea, and anterior segment of the globe, such as allergic conjunctivitis, acne rosacea, superficial punctate keratitis, herpes zoster keratitis, iritis, cyclitis, selected infective conjunctivitis when the inherent hazard of steroid use is accepted to obtain an advisable diminution in edema and inflammation; corneal injury from chemical or thermal burns, or penetration of foreign bodies.
Otic:
Steroid responsive inflammatory conditions of the external auditory meatus, such as allergic otitis externa, selected purulent and nonpurulent infective otitis externa when the hazard of steroid use is accepted to obtain an advisable diminution in edema and inflammation.

CONTRAINDICATIONS

Epithelial herpes simplex keratitis (dendritic keratitis).
Acute infectious stages of vaccinia, varicella, and many other viral diseases of the cornea and conjunctiva.
Mycobacterial infection of the eye.
Fungal diseases of ocular or auricular structures.
Hypersensitivity to any component of this product, including sulfites (see WARNINGS).
Perforation of a drum membrane.

WARNINGS

Prolonged use may result in ocular hypertension and/or glaucoma, with damage to the optic nerve, defects in visual acuity and fields of vision, and posterior subcapsular cataract formation. Prolonged use may suppress the host response and thus increase the hazard of secondary ocular infections. In those diseases causing thinning of the cornea or sclera, perforations have been known to occur with the use of topical corticosteroids. In acute purulent conditions of the eye or ear, corticosteroids may mask infection or enhance existing infection. If these products are used for 10 days or longer, intraocular pressure should be routinely monitored even though it may be difficult in children and uncooperative patients.
Employment of corticosteroid medication in the treatment of herpes simplex other than epithelial herpes simplex keratitis, in which it is contraindicated, requires great caution; periodic slit-lamp microscopy is essential.
Ophthalmic Solution DECADRON Phosphate contains sodium bisulfite, a sulfite that may cause allergic-type reactions including anaphylactic symptoms and life-threatening or less severe asthmatic episodes in certain susceptible people. The overall prevalence of sulfite sensitivity in the general population is unknown and probably low. Sulfite sensitivity is seen more frequently in asthmatic than in nonasthmatic people.

PRECAUTIONS

General
The possibility of persistent fungal infections of the cornea should be considered after prolonged corticosteroid dosing. There have been reports of bacterial keratitis associated with the use of multiple dose containers of topical ophthalmic products. These containers had been inadvertently contaminated by patients who, in most cases, had a concurrent corneal disease or a disruption of the ocular epithelial surface. (See PRECAUTIONS, *Information for Patients.*)
Information for Patients
Patients should be instructed to avoid allowing the tip of the dispensing container to contact the eye or surrounding structures.
Patients should also be instructed that ocular solutions, if handled improperly, can become contaminated by common bacteria known to cause ocular infections. Serious damage to the eye and subsequent loss of vision may result from using contaminated solutions. (See PRECAUTIONS, *General.*)
Patients should also be advised that if they develop an intercurrent ocular condition (e.g., trauma, ocular surgery or infection), they should immediately seek their physician's advice concerning the continued use of the present multidose container.
One of the preservatives in Ophthalmic Solution DECADRON Phosphate, benzalkonium chloride, may be absorbed by soft contact lenses. Patients wearing soft contact lenses should be instructed to wait at least 15 minutes after instilling Ophthalmic Solution DECADRON Phosphate before they insert their lenses.
Carcinogenesis, Mutagenesis, Impairment of Fertility
Long-term animal studies have not been performed to evaluate the carcinogenic potential or the effect on fertility of Ophthalmic Solution DECADRON Phosphate.
Pregnancy
Pregnancy Category C. Dexamethasone has been shown to be teratogenic in mice and rabbits following topical ophthalmic application in multiples of the therapeutic dose.
In the mouse, corticosteroids produce fetal resorptions and a specific abnormality, cleft palate. In the rabbit, corticosteroids have produced fetal resorptions and multiple abnormalities involving the head, ears, limbs, palate, etc.
There are no adequate or well-controlled studies in pregnant women. Ophthalmic Solution DECADRON Phosphate should be used during pregnancy only if the potential benefit to the mother justifies the potential risk to the embryo or fetus. Infants born of mothers who have received substantial doses of corticosteroids during pregnancy should be observed carefully for signs of hypoadrenalism.
Nursing Mothers
Topically applied steroids are absorbed systemically. Therefore, because of the potential for serious adverse reactions in nursing infants from dexamethasone sodium phosphate, a decision should be made whether to discontinue nursing or discontinue the drug, taking into account the importance of the drug to the mother.
Pediatric Use
Safety and effectiveness in pediatric patients have not been established.

ADVERSE REACTIONS

Glaucoma with optic nerve damage, visual acuity and field defects, posterior subcapsular cataract formation, secondary ocular infection from pathogens including herpes simplex, perforation of the globe.

Rarely, filtering blebs have been reported when topical steroids have been used following cataract surgery.

Rarely, stinging or burning may occur.

DOSAGE AND ADMINISTRATION

The duration of treatment will vary with the type of lesion and may extend from a few days to several weeks, according to therapeutic response. Relapses, more common in chronic active lesions than in self-limited conditions, usually respond to retreatment.

Eye—Instill one or two drops of solution into the conjunctival sac every hour during the day and every two hours during the night as initial therapy. When a favorable response is observed, reduce dosage to one drop every four hours. Later, further reduction in dosage to one drop three or four times daily may suffice to control symptoms.

Ear—Clean the aural canal thoroughly and sponge dry. Instill the solution directly into the aural canal. A suggested initial dosage is three or four drops two or three times a day. When a favorable response is obtained, reduce dosage gradually and eventually discontinue.

If preferred, the aural canal may be packed with a gauze wick saturated with solution. Keep the wick moist with the preparation and remove from the ear after 12 to 24 hours. Treatment may be repeated as often as necessary at the discretion of the physician.

HOW SUPPLIED

Sterile Ophthalmic Solution DECADRON Phosphate is a clear, colorless to pale yellow solution.

No. 7643—Ophthalmic Solution DECADRON Phosphate is supplied as follows:

NDC 0006-7643-03 in 5 mL white, opaque, plastic OCUMETER ophthalmic dispenser with a controlled drop tip. (6505-00-007-4536 0.1% 5 mL).

7261522 Issued September 1996

DECADRON-LA® Sterile Suspension
(Dexamethasone Acetate), U.S.P.   ℞

NOT FOR INTRAVENOUS USE

DESCRIPTION

Dexamethasone acetate, a synthetic adrenocortical steroid, is a white to practically white, odorless powder. It is a practically insoluble ester of dexamethasone. The structural formula is:

Dexamethasone acetate is present in DECADRON-LA* (Dexamethasone Acetate) sterile suspension as the monohydrate, with the empirical formula, $C_{24}H_{31}FO_6 \cdot H_2O$, and molecular weight, 452.52. Dexamethasone acetate is designated chemically as 21-(acetyloxy)-9-fluoro-11β,17-dihydroxy-16α-methylpregna-1,4-diene-3,20-dione.

DECADRON-LA sterile suspension is a sterile white suspension (pH 5.0 to 7.5) that settles on standing, but is easily resuspended by mild shaking.

Each milliliter contains dexamethasone acetate equivalent to 8 mg dexamethasone. Inactive ingredients per mL: 6.67 mg sodium chloride; 5 mg creatinine; 0.5 mg disodium edetate; 5 mg sodium carboxymethylcellulose; 0.75 mg polysorbate 80; sodium hydroxide to adjust pH; and Water for Injection, q.s. 1 mL, with 9 mg benzyl alcohol, and 1 mg sodium bisulfite added as preservatives.

*Registered trademark of MERCK & CO., Inc.

ACTIONS

DECADRON-LA sterile suspension is a long-acting, repository adrenocorticosteroid preparation with a prompt onset of action. It is suitable for intramuscular or local injection, but not when an immediate effect of short duration is desired.

Naturally occurring glucocorticoids (hydrocortisone and cortisone), which also have salt-retaining properties, are used as replacement therapy in adrenocortical deficiency states. Their synthetic analogs, including dexamethasone, are primarily used for their potent anti-inflammatory effects in disorders of many organ systems.

Glucocorticoids cause profound and varied metabolic effects. In addition, they modify the body's immune responses to diverse stimuli.

At equipotent anti-inflammatory doses, dexamethasone almost completely lacks the sodium-retaining property of hydrocortisone.

INDICATIONS

A.   By intramuscular injection when oral therapy is not feasible:

1.   *Endocrine disorders*
Congenital adrenal hyperplasia
Nonsuppurative thyroiditis
Hypercalcemia associated with cancer

2.   *Rheumatic disorders*
As adjunctive therapy for short-term administration (to tide the patient over an acute episode or exacerbation) in:
Post-traumatic osteoarthritis
Synovitis of osteoarthritis
Rheumatoid arthritis, including juvenile rheumatoid arthritis (selected cases may require low-dose maintenance therapy)
Acute and subacute bursitis
Epicondylitis
Acute nonspecific tenosynovitis
Acute gouty arthritis
Psoriatic arthritis
Ankylosing spondylitis

3.   *Collagen diseases*
During an exacerbation or as maintenance therapy in selected cases of:
Systemic lupus erythematosus
Acute rheumatic carditis

4.   *Dermatologic diseases*
Pemphigus
Severe erythema multiforme (Stevens-Johnson syndrome)
Exfoliative dermatitis
Bullous dermatitis herpetiformis
Severe seborrheic dermatitis
Severe psoriasis
Mycosis fungoides

5.   *Allergic states*
Control of severe or incapacitating allergic conditions intractable to adequate trials of conventional treatment in:
Bronchial asthma
Contact dermatitis
Atopic dermatitis
Serum sickness
Seasonal or perennial allergic rhinitis
Drug hypersensitivity reactions
Urticarial transfusion reactions

6.   *Ophthalmic diseases*
Severe acute and chronic allergic and inflammatory processes involving the eye, such as:
Herpes zoster ophthalmicus
Iritis, Iridocyclitis
Chorioretinitis
Diffuse posterior uveitis and choroiditis
Optic neuritis
Sympathetic ophthalmia
Anterior segment inflammation
Allergic conjunctivitis
Keratitis
Allergic corneal marginal ulcers

7.   *Gastrointestinal diseases*
To tide the patient over a critical period of the disease in:
Ulcerative colitis (Systemic therapy)
Regional enteritis (Systemic therapy)

8.   *Respiratory diseases*
Symptomatic sarcoidosis
Berylliosis
Loeffler's syndrome not manageable by other means
Aspiration pneumonitis

9.   *Hematologic disorders*
Acquired (autoimmune) hemolytic anemia
Secondary thrombocytopenia in adults
Erythroblastopenia (RBC anemia)
Congenital (erythroid) hypoplastic anemia

10.   *Neoplastic diseases*
For palliative management of:
Leukemias and lymphomas in adults
Acute leukemia of childhood

11.   *Edematous states*
To induce diuresis or remission of proteinuria in the nephrotic syndrome, without uremia, of the idiopathic type, or that due to lupus erythematosus

12.   *Miscellaneous*
Trichinosis with neurologic or myocardial involvement.

B.   By intra-articular or soft tissue injection as adjunctive therapy for short-term administration (to tide the patient over an acute episode or exacerbation) in:
Synovitis of osteoarthritis
Rheumatoid arthritis
Acute and subacute bursitis
Acute gouty arthritis
Epicondylitis
Acute nonspecific tenosynovitis
Post-traumatic osteoarthritis

C.   By intralesional injection in:
Keloids
Localized hypertrophic, infiltrated, inflammatory lesions of: lichen planus, psoriatic plaques, granuloma annulare, and lichen simplex chronicus (neurodermatitis)
Discoid lupus erythematosus
Necrobiosis lipoidica diabeticorum
Alopecia areata
May also be useful in cystic tumors of an aponeurosis or tendon (ganglia).

CONTRAINDICATIONS

Systemic fungal infections
Hypersensitivity to any component of this product, including sulfites (see WARNINGS).

WARNINGS

DO NOT INJECT INTRAVENOUSLY

Because rare instances of anaphylactoid reactions have occurred in patients receiving parenteral corticosteroid therapy, appropriate precautionary measures should be taken prior to administration, especially when the patient has a history of allergy to any drug. Anaphylactoid and hypersensitivity reactions have been reported for Sterile Suspension DECADRON-LA (see ADVERSE REACTIONS).

Sterile Suspension DECADRON-LA contains sodium bisulfite, a sulfite that may cause allergic-type reactions including anaphylactic symptoms and life-threatening or less severe asthmatic episodes in certain susceptible people. The overall prevalence of sulfite sensitivity in the general population is unknown and probably low. Sulfite sensitivity is seen more frequently in asthmatic than in nonasthmatic people.

In patients on corticosteroid therapy subjected to any unusual stress, increased dosage of rapidly acting corticosteroids before, during, and after the stressful situation is indicated.

Drug-induced secondary adrenocortical insufficiency may result from too rapid withdrawal of corticosteroids and may be minimized by gradual reduction of dosage. This type of relative insufficiency may persist for months after discontinuation of therapy; therefore, in any situation of stress occurring during that period, hormone therapy should be reinstituted. If the patient is receiving steroids already, dosage may have to be increased. Since mineralocorticoid secretion may be impaired, salt and/or a mineralocorticoid should be administered concurrently.

Corticosteroids may mask some signs of infection, and new infections may appear during their use. There may be decreased resistance and inability to localize infection when corticosteroids are used. Moreover, corticosteroids may affect the nitroblue-tetrazolium test for bacterial infection and produce false negative results.

In cerebral malaria, a double-blind trial has shown that the use of corticosteroids is associated with prolongation of coma and a higher incidence of pneumonia and gastrointestinal bleeding.

Corticosteroids may activate latent amebiasis. Therefore, it is recommended that latent or active amebiasis be ruled out before initiating corticosteroid therapy in any patient who has spent time in the tropics or any patient with unexplained diarrhea.

Prolonged use of corticosteroids may produce posterior subcapsular cataracts, glaucoma with possible damage to the optic nerves, and may enhance the establishment of secondary ocular infections due to fungi or viruses.

Usage in pregnancy.   Since adequate human reproduction studies have not been done with corticosteroids, use of these drugs in pregnancy or in women of childbearing potential requires that the anticipated benefits be weighed against the possible hazards to the mother and embryo or fetus. Infants born of mothers who have received substantial doses of corticosteroids during pregnancy should be carefully observed for signs of hypoadrenalism.

Corticosteroids appear in breast milk and could suppress growth, interfere with endogenous corticosteroid production, or cause other unwanted effects. Mothers taking pharmacologic doses of corticosteroids should be advised not to nurse.

Average and large doses of cortisone or hydrocortisone can cause elevation of blood pressure, salt and water retention, and increased excretion of potassium. These effects are less likely to occur with the synthetic derivatives except when used in large doses. Dietary salt restriction and potassium supplementation may be necessary. All corticosteroids increase calcium excretion.

Administration of live virus vaccines, including smallpox, is contraindicated in individuals receiving immunosuppres-

Continued on next page

Decadron-LA—Cont.

sive doses of corticosteroids. If inactivated viral or bacterial vaccines are administered to individuals receiving immunosuppressive doses of corticosteroids, the expected serum antibody response may not be obtained.

Patients who are on drugs which suppress the immune system are more susceptible to infections than healthy individuals. Chickenpox and measles, for example, can have a more serious or even fatal course in non-immune children or adults on corticosteroids. In such children or adults who have not had these diseases, particular care should be taken to avoid exposure. The risk of developing a disseminated infection varies among individuals and can be related to the dose, route and duration of corticosteroid administration as well as to the underlying disease. If exposed to chickenpox, prophylaxis with varicella zoster immune globulin (VZIG) may be indicated. If chickenpox develops, treatment with antiviral agents may be considered. If exposed to measles, prophylaxis with immune globulin (IG) may be indicated. (See the respective package inserts for VZIG and IG for complete prescribing information.)

Similarly, corticosteroids should be used with great care in patients with known or suspected Strongyloides (threadworm) infestation. In such patients, corticosteroid-induced immunosuppression may lead to Strongyloides hyperinfection and dissemination with widespread larval migration, often accompanied by severe enterocolitis and potentially fatal gram-negative septicemia.

If corticosteroids are indicated in patients with latent tuberculosis or tuberculin reactivity, close observation is necessary as reactivation of the disease may occur. During prolonged corticosteroid therapy, these patients should receive chemoprophylaxis.

Repository adrenocorticosteroid preparations may cause atrophy at the site of injection. To minimize the likelihood and/or severity of atrophy, do not inject subcutaneously, avoid injection into the deltoid muscle, and avoid repeated intramuscular injections into the same site if possible.

Dosage in children under 12 has not been established.

Literature reports suggest an apparent association between use of corticosteroids and left ventricular free wall rupture after a recent myocardial infarction; therefore, therapy with corticosteroids should be used with great caution in these patients.

PRECAUTIONS

DECADRON-LA sterile suspension is not recommended as initial therapy in acute, life-threatening situations.

This product, like many other steroid formulations, is sensitive to heat. Therefore, it should not be autoclaved when it is desirable to sterilize the exterior of the vial.

Following prolonged therapy, withdrawal of corticosteroids may result in symptoms of the corticosteroid withdrawal syndrome including fever, myalgia, arthralgia, and malaise. This may occur in patients even without evidence of adrenal insufficiency.

There is an enhanced effect of corticosteroids in patients with hypothyroidism and in those with cirrhosis.

Corticosteroids should be used cautiously in patients with ocular herpes simplex for fear of corneal perforation.

Psychic derangements may appear when corticosteroids are used, ranging from euphoria, insomnia, mood swings, personality changes, and severe depression to frank psychotic manifestations. Also, existing emotional instability or psychotic tendencies may be aggravated by corticosteroids.

Aspirin should be used cautiously in conjunction with corticosteroids in hypoprothrombinemia.

Steroids should be used with caution in nonspecific ulcerative colitis, if there is a probability of impending perforation, abscess, or other pyogenic infection, also in diverticulitis, fresh intestinal anastomoses, active or latent peptic ulcer, renal insufficiency, hypertension, osteoporosis, and myasthenia gravis. Signs of peritoneal irritation following gastrointestinal perforation in patients receiving large doses of corticosteroids may be minimal or absent. Fat embolism has been reported as a possible complication of hypercortisonism.

When large doses are given, some authorities advise that antacids be administered between meals to help to prevent peptic ulcer.

Growth and development of infants and children on prolonged corticosteroid therapy should be carefully followed. Steroids may increase or decrease motility and number of spermatozoa in some patients.

Phenytoin, phenobarbital, ephedrine, and rifampin may enhance the metabolic clearance of corticosteroids, resulting in decreased blood levels and lessened physiologic activity, thus requiring adjustment in corticosteroid dosage.

The prothrombin time should be checked frequently in patients who are receiving corticosteroids and coumarin anticoagulants at the same time because of reports that corticosteroids have altered the response to these anticoagulants. Studies have shown that the usual effect produced by

adding corticosteroids is inhibition of response to coumarins, although there have been some conflicting reports of potentiation not substantiated by studies.

When corticosteroids are administered concomitantly with potassium-depleting diuretics, patients should be observed closely for development of hypokalemia.

Intra-articular injection of a corticosteroid may produce systemic as well as local effects.

Appropriate examination of any joint fluid present is necessary to exclude a septic process.

A marked increase in pain accompanied by local swelling, further restriction of joint motion, fever, and malaise is suggestive of septic arthritis. If this complication occurs and the diagnosis of sepsis is confirmed, appropriate antimicrobial therapy should be instituted.

Injection of a steroid into an infected site is to be avoided. Corticosteroids should not be injected into unstable joints. Patients should be impressed strongly with the importance of not overusing joints in which symptomatic benefit has been obtained as long as the inflammatory process remains active.

Frequent intra-articular injection may result in damage to joint tissues.

Information for Patients

Susceptible patients who are on immunosuppressant doses of corticosteroids should be warned to avoid exposure to chickenpox or measles. Patients should also be advised that if they are exposed, medical advice should be sought without delay.

ADVERSE REACTIONS

Fluid and electrolyte disturbances
Sodium retention
Fluid retention
Congestive heart failure in susceptible patients
Potassium loss
Hypokalemic alkalosis
Hypertension
Musculoskeletal
Muscle weakness
Steroid myopathy
Loss of muscle mass
Osteoporosis
Vertebral compression fractures
Aseptic necrosis of femoral and humeral heads
Pathologic fracture of long bones
Tendon rupture
Gastrointestinal
Peptic ulcer with possible subsequent perforation and hemorrhage
Perforation of the small and large bowel, particularly in patients with inflammatory bowel disease
Pancreatitis
Abdominal distention
Ulcerative esophagitis
Dermatologic
Impaired wound healing
Thin fragile skin
Petechiae and ecchymoses
Erythema
Increased sweating
May suppress reactions to skin tests
Other cutaneous reactions, such as allergic dermatitis, urticaria, angioneurotic edema
Neurologic
Convulsions
Increased intracranial pressure with papilledema (pseudotumor cerebri) usually after treatment
Vertigo
Headache
Psychic disturbances
Endocrine
Menstrual irregularities
Development of cushingoid state
Suppression of growth in children
Secondary adrenocortical and pituitary unresponsiveness, particularly in times of stress, as in trauma, surgery, or illness
Decreased carbohydrate tolerance
Manifestations of latent diabetes mellitus
Increased requirements for insulin or oral hypoglycemic agents in diabetics
Hirsutism
Ophthalmic
Posterior subcapsular cataracts
Increased intraocular pressure
Glaucoma
Exophthalmos
Metabolic
Negative nitrogen balance due to protein catabolism
Cardiovascular
Myocardial rupture following recent myocardial infarction (see WARNINGS).
Other
Anaphylactoid or hypersensitivity reactions
Thromboembolism

Weight gain
Increased appetite
Nausea
Malaise
The following *additional* adverse reactions are related to parenteral corticosteroid therapy:
Rare instances of blindness associated with intralesional therapy around the face and head
Hyperpigmentation or hypopigmentation
Subcutaneous and cutaneous atrophy
Sterile abscess
Postinjection flare (following intra-articular use)
Charcot-like arthropathy
Scarring
Induration
Inflammation
Paresthesia
Delayed pain or soreness
Muscle twitching, ataxia, hiccups, and nystagmus have been reported in low incidence after injection of DECADRON-LA sterile suspension.

OVERDOSAGE

Reports of acute toxicity and/or death following overdosage of glucocorticoids are rare. In the event of overdosage, no specific antidote is available; treatment is supportive and symptomatic.

The intraperitoneal LD_{50} of dexamethasone acetate in female mice was 424 mg/kg.

DOSAGE AND ADMINISTRATION

For intramuscular, intralesional, intra-articular, and soft tissue injection.

Dosage Requirements Are Variable and Must Be Individualized on the Basis of the Disease and the Response of the Patient.

Dosage in children under 12 has not been established.
Intramuscular Injection
Dosage ranges from 1 to 2 mL, equivalent to 8 to 16 mg of dexamethasone. If further treatment is needed, dosage may be repeated at intervals of 1 to 3 weeks.
Intralesional Injection
The usual dose is 0.1 to 0.2 mL, equivalent to 0.8 to 1.6 mg of dexamethasone, per injection site.
Intra-articular and Soft Tissue Injection
The dose varies, depending on the location and the severity of inflammation. The usual dose is 0.5 to 2 mL, equivalent to 4 to 16 mg of dexamethasone. If further treatment is needed, dosage may be repeated at intervals of 1 to 3 weeks. Frequent intra-articular injection may result in damage to joint tissues.

HOW SUPPLIED

No. 7644—Sterile Suspension DECADRON-LA, 8 mg dexamethasone equivalent per mL, is a sterile white suspension, and is supplied as follows:
NDC 0006-7644-01 in 1 mL vials.
NDC 0006-7644-03 in 5 mL vials.
Storage
Sensitive to heat. Do not autoclave.
Protect from freezing.
     7498419 Issued October 1995

DECASPRAY® Topical Aerosol
(Dexamethasone), U.S.P.   ℞

DESCRIPTION

Topical Aerosol DECASPRAY* (Dexamethasone) is a topical steroid preparation, each 25 g of which contains 10 mg of dexamethasone. The topical corticosteroids constitute a class of primarily synthetic steroids used as anti-inflammatory and anti-pruritic agents.

Dexamethasone is 9-fluoro-11β,17,21-trihydroxy-16α-methylpregna-1, 4-diene-3, 20 dione. Its empirical formula is $C_{22}H_{29}FO_5$ and its structural formula is:

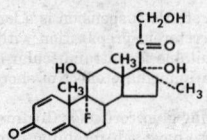

Dexamethasone has a molecular weight of 392.47.
The inactive ingredients are isopropyl myristate, and isobutane. Each second of spray dispenses approximately 0.075 mg of dexamethasone.

*Registered trademark of MERCK & CO., INC.

CLINICAL PHARMACOLOGY

Topical corticosteroids share anti-inflammatory, anti-pruritic, and vasoconstrictive actions.

The mechanism of anti-inflammatory activity of the topical corticosteroids is unclear. Various laboratory methods, including vasoconstrictor assays, are used to compare and predict potencies and/or clinical efficacies of the topical corticosteroids. There is some evidence to suggest that a recognizable correlation exists between vasoconstrictor potency and therapeutic efficacy in man.

Pharmacokinetics

The extent of percutaneous absorption of topical corticosteroids is determined by many factors including the vehicle, the integrity of the epidermal barrier, and the use of occlusive dressings.

Topical corticosteroids can be absorbed from normal intact skin. Inflammation and/or other disease processes in the skin increase percutaneous absorption. Occlusive dressings substantially increase the percutaneous absorption of topical corticosteroids. Thus, occlusive dressings may be a valuable therapeutic adjunct for treatment of resistant dermatoses. (See DOSAGE AND ADMINISTRATION.)

Once absorbed through the skin, topical corticosteroids are handled through pharmacokinetic pathways similar to systemically administered corticosteroids. Corticosteroids are bound to plasma proteins in varying degrees. Corticosteroids are metabolized primarily in the liver and are then excreted by the kidneys. Some of the topical corticosteroids and their metabolites are also excreted into the bile.

INDICATIONS AND USAGE

DECASPRAY Topical Aerosol is indicated for relief of the inflammatory and pruritic manifestations of corticosteroid-responsive dermatoses.

CONTRAINDICATIONS

Topical corticosteroids are contraindicated in those patients with a history of hypersensitivity to any of the components of the preparation.

WARNINGS

Avoid spraying in eyes or nose. Contents under pressure. Do not puncture or burn. Keep out of reach of children. Use only as directed. Intentional misuse by deliberately concentrating and inhaling the contents can be harmful or fatal.

Topically applied steroids are absorbed systemically. There may be rare instances in which this absorption results in immunosuppression. Patients who are on drugs which suppress the immune system are more susceptible to infections than healthy individuals. Chickenpox and measles, for example, can have a more serious or even fatal course in non-immune children or adults on corticosteroids. In such children or adults who have not had these diseases, particular care should be taken to avoid exposure. The risk of developing a disseminated infection varies among individuals and can be related to the dose, route and duration of corticosteroid administration as well as to the underlying disease. If exposed to chickenpox, prophylaxis with varicella zoster immune globulin (VZIG) may be indicated. If chickenpox develops, treatment with antiviral agents may be considered. If exposed to measles, prophylaxis with immune globulin (IG) may be indicated. (See the respective package inserts for VZIG and IG for complete prescribing information.)

PRECAUTIONS

General

Systemic absorption of topical corticosteroids has produced reversible hypothalamic-pituitary-adrenal (HPA) axis suppression, manifestations of Cushing's syndrome, hyperglycemia, and glycosuria in some patients.

Conditions which augment systemic absorption include the application of the more potent corticosteroids, use over large surface areas, prolonged use, and the addition of occlusive dressings.

Therefore, patients receiving a large dose of a potent topical corticosteroid applied to a large surface area or under an occlusive dressing should be evaluated periodically for evidence of HPA axis suppression by using urinary free cortisol and ACTH stimulation tests. If HPA axis suppression is noted, an attempt should be made to withdraw the drug, to reduce the frequency of application, or to substitute a less potent corticosteroid.

Recovery of HPA axis function is generally prompt and complete upon discontinuation of the drug. Infrequently, signs and symptoms of corticosteroid withdrawal may occur, requiring supplemental systemic corticosteroids.

Children may absorb proportionally larger amounts of topical corticosteroids and thus be more susceptible to systemic toxicity (See PRECAUTIONS, *Pediatric Use*).

If irritation develops, topical corticosteroids should be discontinued and appropriate therapy instituted.

In the presence of dermatological infections, the use of an appropriate antifungal or antibacterial agent should be instituted. If a favorable response does not occur promptly, the corticosteroid should be discontinued until the infection has been adequately controlled.

The product is not for ophthalmic use. However, if applied to the eyelids or skin near the eyes, the drug may enter the eyes. In patients with a history of herpes simplex keratitis ocular exposure to corticosteroids may lead to a recurrence. Prolonged ocular exposure may cause steroid glaucoma.

A few individuals may be sensitive to one or more of the components of this product. If any reaction indicating sensitivity is observed, discontinue use.

Generally, occlusive dressings should not be used on weeping or exudative lesions.

If occlusive dressing therapy is used, inspect lesions between dressings for development of infection. If infection develops, the technique should be discontinued and appropriate antimicrobial therapy instituted.

When large areas of the body are covered with an occlusive dressing, thermal homeostasis may be impaired. If elevation of body temperature occurs, use of the occlusive dressing should be discontinued.

CAUTION: Flammable. Do not use around open flame or while smoking.

Information for the Patient

Patients using topical corticosteroids should receive the following information and instructions:

1. This medication is to be used as directed by the physician. It is for external use only. Avoid contact with the eyes.
2. Patients should be advised not to use this medication for any disorder other than that for which it was prescribed.
3. The treated skin area should not be bandaged or otherwise covered or wrapped so as to be occlusive unless directed by the physician.
4. Patients should report any signs of local adverse reactions, especially under occlusive dressing.
5. Parents of pediatric patients should be advised not to use tight-fitting diapers or plastic pants on a child being treated in the diaper area, as these garments may constitute occlusive dressings.
6. Susceptible patients who are on immunosuppressant doses of corticosteroids should be warned to avoid exposure to chickenpox or measles. Patients should also be advised that if they are exposed, medical advice should be sought without delay.

Laboratory Tests

The following tests may be helpful in evaluating the HPA axis suppression:

• Urinary free cortisol test
• ACTH stimulation test

Carcinogenesis, Mutagenesis, and Impairment of Fertility

Long-term animal studies have not been performed to evaluate the carcinogenic potential or the effect on fertility of topical corticosteroids.

Studies to determine mutagenicity with prednisolone and hydrocortisone have revealed negative results.

Pregnancy

Pregnancy Category C: Corticosteroids are generally teratogenic in laboratory animals when administered systemically at relatively low dosage levels. The more potent corticosteroids have been shown to be teratogenic after dermal application in laboratory animals. There are no adequate and well-controlled studies in pregnant women on teratogenic effects from topically applied corticosteroids. Therefore, topical corticosteroids should be used during pregnancy only if the potential benefit justifies the potential risk to the fetus. Drugs of this class should not be used extensively on pregnant patients, in large amounts, or for prolonged periods of time.

Nursing Mothers

It is not known whether topical administration of corticosteroids could result in sufficient systemic absorption to produce detectable quantities in breast milk. Systemically administered corticosteroids are secreted into breast milk in quantities *not* likely to have a deleterious effect on the infant. Nevertheless, caution should be exercised when topical corticosteroids are administered to a nursing woman.

Pediatric Use

Pediatric patients may demonstrate greater susceptibility to topical corticosteroid-induced HPA axis suppression and Cushing's syndrome than mature patients because of a larger skin surface area to body weight ratio.

Hypothalamic-pituitary-adrenal (HPA) axis suppression, Cushing's syndrome, and intracranial hypertension have been reported in children receiving topical corticosteroids. Manifestations of adrenal suppression in children include linear growth retardation, delayed weight gain, low plasma cortisol levels, and absence of response to ACTH stimulation. Manifestations of intracranial hypertension include bulging fontanelles, headaches, and bilateral papilledema.

Administration of topical corticosteroids to children should be limited to the least amount compatible with an effective therapeutic regimen. Chronic corticosteroid therapy may interfere with the growth and development of children.

ADVERSE REACTIONS

The following adverse reactions are reported infrequently with topical corticosteroids, but may occur more frequently with the use of occlusive dressings. These reactions are listed in an approximate decreasing order of occurrence:

Burning
Itching
Irritation
Dryness
Folliculitis
Hypertrichosis
Acneiform eruptions
Hypopigmentation
Perioral dermatitis
Allergic contact dermatitis
Maceration of the skin
Secondary infection
Skin atrophy
Striae
Miliaria

OVERDOSAGE

Topically applied corticosteroids can be absorbed in sufficient amounts to produce systemic effects (See PRECAUTIONS).

DOSAGE AND ADMINISTRATION

Patients should be instructed in the correct way to use DECASPRAY. The preparation is readily applied, even on hairy areas. It does not have to be rubbed into the skin.

Optimal effects will be obtained with DECASPRAY when these directions are followed:

1. Keep the affected area clean to reduce the possibility of infection.
2. Shake the container *gently* once or twice each time before using. Hold it about six inches from the area to be treated. Effective medication may be obtained with the container held either upright or inverted, since it is fitted with a special valve that dispenses approximately the same dosage in either position.
3. Spray each four inch square of affected area for one or two seconds three or four times a day, depending on the nature of the condition and the response to therapy.
4. When a favorable response is obtained, reduce dosage gradually and eventually discontinue.
5. Occlusive dressings may be used for the management of psoriasis or recalcitrant conditions.

HOW SUPPLIED

No. 7623X—DECASPRAY is supplied as follows:
NDC 0006-7623-25 in a 25 g pressurized container.
DC 7413319 Issued April 1993
COPYRIGHT © MERCK & CO., INC., 1983
All rights reserved

DEMSER® Capsules   ℞
(Metyrosine), U.S.P.

DESCRIPTION

DEMSER* (Metyrosine) is (−)-α-methyl-*L* -tyrosine or (α-MPT). It has the following structural formula:

$$HO\!\!-\!\!\bigcirc\!\!-\!\!CH_2\!\!-\!\!\overset{\overset{\displaystyle CH_3}{|}}{\underset{\underset{\displaystyle NH_2}{|}}{C}}\!\!-\!\!COOH$$

Metyrosine is a white, crystalline compound of molecular weight 195. It is very slightly soluble in water, acetone, and methanol, and insoluble in chloroform and benzene. It is soluble in acidic aqueous solutions. It is also soluble in alkaline aqueous solutions, but is subject to oxidative degradation under these conditions.

Continued on next page

Demser—Cont.

DEMSER is supplied as capsules, for oral administration. Each capsule contains 250 mg metyrosine. Inactive ingredients are colloidal silicon dioxide, gelatin, hydroxypropyl cellulose, magnesium stearate, and titanium dioxide. The capsules may also contain any combination of D&C Red 33, D&C Yellow 10, FD&C Blue 1, and FD&C Blue 2.

*Registered trademark of MERCK & CO., INC.

CLINICAL PHARMACOLOGY

DEMSER inhibits tyrosine hydroxylase, which catalyzes the first transformation in catecholamine biosynthesis, i.e., the conversion of tyrosine to dihydroxyphenylalanine (DOPA). Because the first step is also the rate-limiting step, blockade of tyrosine hydroxylase activity results in decreased endogenous levels of catecholamines, usually measured as decreased urinary excretion of catecholamines and their metabolites.

In patients with pheochromocytoma, who produce excessive amounts of norepinephrine and epinephrine, administration of one to four grams of DEMSER per day has reduced catecholamine biosynthesis from about 35 to 80 percent as measured by the total excretion of catecholamines and their metabolites (metanephrine and vanillylmandelic acid). The maximum biochemical effect usually occurs within two to three days, and the urinary concentration of catecholamines and their metabolites usually returns to pretreatment levels within three to four days after DEMSER is discontinued. In some patients the total excretion of catecholamines and catecholamine metabolites may be lowered to normal or near normal levels (less than 10 mg/24 hours). In most patients the duration of treatment has been two to eight weeks, but several patients have received DEMSER for periods of one to 10 years.

Most patients with pheochromocytoma treated with DEMSER experience decreased frequency and severity of hypertensive attacks with their associated headache, nausea, sweating, and tachycardia. In patients who respond, blood pressure decreases progressively during the first two days of therapy with DEMSER; after withdrawal, blood pressure usually increases gradually to pretreatment values within two to three days.

Metyrosine is well absorbed from the gastrointestinal tract. From 53 to 88 percent (mean 69 percent) was recovered in the urine as unchanged drug following maintenance oral doses of 600 to 4000 mg/24 hours in patients with pheochromocytoma or essential hypertension. Less than 1% of the dose was recovered as catechol metabolites. These metabolites are probably not present in sufficient amounts to contribute to the biochemical effects of metyrosine. The quantities excreted, however, are sufficient to interfere with accurate determination of urinary catecholamines determined by routine techniques.

Plasma half-life of metyrosine determined over an 8-hour period after single oral doses was 3.4–3.7 hours in three patients.

For further information, refer to: Sjoerdsma, A.; Engelman, K.; Waldman, T. A.; Cooperman, L. H.; Hammond, W. G.: Pheochromocytoma: Current concepts of diagnosis and treatment, Ann. Intern. Med. 65: 1302–1326, Dec. 1966.

INDICATIONS AND USAGE

DEMSER is indicated in the treatment of patients with pheochromocytoma for:
1. Preoperative preparation of patients for surgery
2. Management of patients when surgery is contraindicated
3. Chronic treatment of patients with malignant pheochromocytoma.

DEMSER is not recommended for the control of essential hypertension.

CONTRAINDICATIONS

DEMSER is contraindicated in persons known to be hypersensitive to this compound.

WARNINGS

Maintain Fluid Volume During and After Surgery
When DEMSER is used preoperatively, alone or especially in combination with alpha-adrenergic blocking drugs, adequate intravascular volume must be maintained intraoperatively (especially after tumor removal) and postoperatively to avoid hypotension and decreased perfusion of vital organs resulting from vasodilatation and expanded volume capacity. Following tumor removal, large volumes of plasma may be needed to maintain blood pressure and central venous pressure within the normal range.

In addition, life-threatening arrhythmias may occur during anesthesia and surgery, and may require treatment with a beta blocker or lidocaine. During surgery, patients should have continuous monitoring of blood pressure and electrocardiogram.

Intraoperative Effects
While the preoperative use of DEMSER in patients with pheochromocytoma is thought to decrease intraoperative problems with blood pressure control, DEMSER does not eliminate the danger of hypertensive crises or arrhythmias during manipulation of the tumor, and the alpha-adrenergic blocking drug, phentolamine, may be needed.

Interaction with Alcohol
DEMSER may add to the sedative effects of alcohol and other CNS depressants, e.g., hypnotics, sedatives, and tranquilizers. (See PRECAUTIONS, *Information for Patients and Drug Interactions.*)

PRECAUTIONS

General
Metyrosine Crystalluria: **Crystalluria and urolithiasis have been found in dogs treated with DEMSER (Metyrosine) at doses similar to those used in humans, and crystalluria has also been observed in a few patients. To minimize the risk of crystalluria, patients should be urged to maintain water intake sufficient to achieve a daily urine volume of 2000 mL or more, particularly when doses greater than 2 g per day are given. Routine examination of the urine should be carried out. Metyrosine will crystallize as needles or rods. If metyrosine crystalluria occurs, fluid intake should be increased further. If crystalluria persists, the dosage should be reduced or the drug discontinued.**

Relatively Little Data Regarding Long-term Use: The total human experience with the drug is quite limited and few patients have been studied long-term. Chronic animal studies have not been carried out. Therefore, suitable laboratory tests should be carried out periodically in patients requiring prolonged use of DEMSER and caution should be observed in patients with impaired hepatic or renal function.

Information for Patients
When receiving DEMSER, patients should be warned about engaging in activities requiring mental alertness and motor coordination, such as driving a motor vehicle or operating machinery. DEMSER may have additive sedative effects with alcohol and other CNS depressants, e.g., hypnotics, sedatives, and tranquilizers.
Patients should be advised to maintain a liberal fluid intake. (See PRECAUTIONS, *General.*)

Drug Interactions
Caution should be observed in administering DEMSER to patients receiving phenothiazines or haloperidol because the extrapyramidal effects of these drugs can be expected to be potentiated by inhibition of catecholamine synthesis.
Concurrent use of DEMSER with alcohol or other CNS depressants can increase their sedative effects. (See WARNINGS and PRECAUTIONS, *Information for Patients.*)

Laboratory Test Interference
Spurious increases in urinary catecholamines may be observed in patients receiving DEMSER due to the presence of metabolites of the drug.

Carcinogenesis, Mutagenesis, Impairment of Fertility
Long-term carcinogenic studies in animals and studies on mutagenesis and impairment of fertility have not been performed with metyrosine.

Pregnancy
Pregnancy Category C. Animal reproduction studies have not been conducted with DEMSER. It is also not known whether DEMSER can cause fetal harm when administered to a pregnant woman or can affect reproduction capacity. DEMSER should be given to a pregnant woman only if clearly needed.

Nursing Mothers
It is not known whether DEMSER is excreted in human milk. Because many drugs are excreted in human milk, caution should be exercised when DEMSER is administered to a nursing woman.

Pediatric Use
Safety and effectiveness in pediatric patients below the age of 12 years have not been established.

ADVERSE REACTIONS

Central Nervous System
Sedation: The most common adverse reaction to DEMSER is moderate to severe sedation, which has been observed in almost all patients. It occurs at both low and high dosages. Sedative effects begin within the first 24 hours of therapy, are maximal after two to three days, and tend to wane during the next few days. Sedation usually is not obvious after one week unless the dosage is increased, but at dosages greater than 2000 mg/day some degree of sedation or fatigue may persist.

In most patients who experience sedation, temporary changes in sleep pattern occur following withdrawal of the drug. Changes consist of insomnia that may last for two or three days and feelings of increased alertness and ambition. Even patients who do not experience sedation while on DEMSER may report symptoms of psychic stimulation when the drug is discontinued.

Extrapyramidal Signs: Extrapyramidal signs such as drooling, speech difficulty, and tremor have been reported in

approximately 10 percent of patients. These occasionally have been accompanied by trismus and frank parkinsonism.
Anxiety and Psychic Disturbances: Anxiety and psychic disturbances such as depression, hallucinations, disorientation, and confusion may occur. These effects seem to be dose-dependent and may disappear with reduction of dosage.
Diarrhea
Diarrhea occurs in about 10 percent of patients and may be severe. Anti-diarrheal agents may be required if continuation of DEMSER is necessary.
Miscellaneous
Infrequently, slight swelling of the breast, galactorrhea, nasal stuffiness, decreased salivation, dry mouth, headache, nausea, vomiting, abdominal pain, and impotence or failure of ejaculation may occur. Crystalluria (see PRECAUTIONS) and transient dysuria and hematuria have been observed in a few patients. Hematologic disorders (including eosinophilia, anemia, thrombocytopenia, and thrombocytosis), increased SGOT levels, peripheral edema, and hypersensitivity reactions such as urticaria and pharyngeal edema have been reported rarely.

OVERDOSAGE

Signs of metyrosine overdosage include those central nervous system effects observed in some patients even at low dosages.
At doses exceeding 2000 mg/day, some degree of sedation or feeling of fatigue may persist. Doses of 2000–4000 mg/day can result in anxiety or agitated depression, neuromuscular effects (including fine tremor of the hands, gross tremor of the trunk, tightening of the jaw with trismus, diarrhea, and decreased salivation with dry mouth).
Reduction of drug dose or cessation of treatment results in the disappearance of these symptoms.
The acute toxicity of metyrosine was 442 mg/kg and 752 mg/kg in the female mouse and rat respectively.

DOSAGE AND ADMINISTRATION

The recommended initial dosage of DEMSER for adults and children 12 years of age and older is 250 mg orally four times daily. This may be increased by 250 mg to 500 mg every day to a maximum of 4.0 g/day in divided doses. When used for preoperative preparation, the optimally effective dosage of DEMSER should be given for at least five to seven days.
Optimally effective dosages of DEMSER usually are between 2.0 and 3.0 g/day, and the dose should be titrated by monitoring clinical symptoms and catecholamine excretion. In patients who are hypertensive, dosage should be titrated to achieve normalization of blood pressure and control of clinical symptoms. In patients who are usually normotensive, dosage should be titrated to the amount that will reduce urinary metanephrines and/or vanillylmandelic acid by 50 percent or more.
If patients are not adequately controlled by the use of DEMSER, an alpha-adrenergic blocking agent (phenoxybenzamine) should be added.
Use of DEMSER in children under 12 years of age has been limited and a dosage schedule for this age group cannot be given.

HOW SUPPLIED

No. 3355—Capsules DEMSER, 250 mg, are opaque, two-toned blue capsules coded MSD 690 on one side and DEMSER on the other. They are supplied as follows:
NDC 0006-0690-68 bottles of 100.

Shown in Product Identification Guide, page 323
7900807 Issued July 1996
COPYRIGHT© MERCK & CO., INC., 1985
All rights reserved

DIUPRES® Tablets   ℞
(Reserpine-Chlorothiazide), U.S.P.

WARNING

This fixed combination drug is not indicated for initial therapy of hypertension. Hypertension requires therapy titrated to the individual patient. If the fixed combination represents the dosage so determined, its use may be more convenient in patient management. The treatment of hypertension is not static, but must be re-evaluated as conditions in each patient warrant.

DESCRIPTION

DIUPRES* (Reserpine-Chlorothiazide) combines two antihypertensives: DIURIL* (Chlorothiazide) and reserpine.

Chlorothiazide

Chlorothiazide is a diuretic and antihypertensive. Its chemical name is 6-chloro-2*H* -1,2,4-benzothiadiazine- 7-sulfonamide 1,1-dioxide. Its empirical formula is $C_7H_6ClN_3O_4S_2$ and its structural formula is:

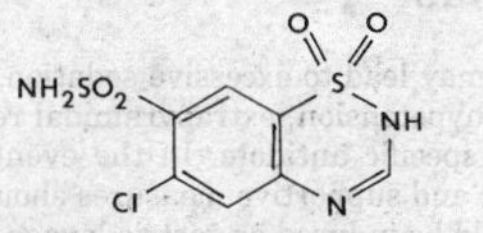

Chlorothiazide is a white, or practically white, crystalline powder with a molecular weight of 295.73, which is very slightly soluble in water, but readily soluble in dilute aqueous sodium hydroxide. It is soluble in urine to the extent of about 150 mg per 100 mL at pH 7.

Reserpine

The chemical name of reserpine is 11,17α-dimethoxy-18β-[(3, 4, 5-trimethoxybenzoyl)oxy] -3β,20α-yohimban- 16 β-carboxylic acid methylester. It is a crystalline alkaloid derived from Rauwolfia serpentina. Its empirical formula is $C_{33}H_{40}N_2O_9$ and its structural formula is:

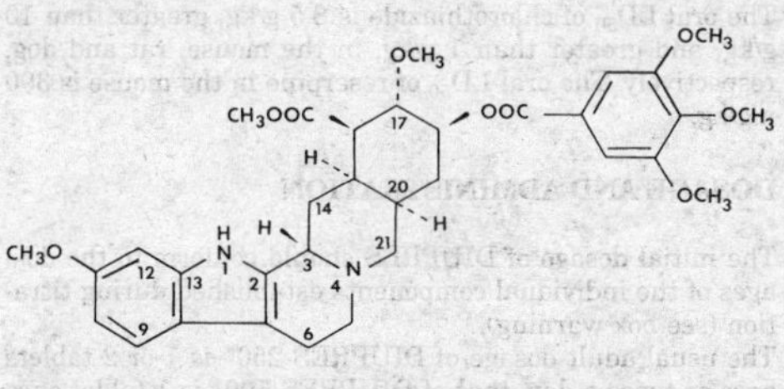

Reserpine is a white or pale buff to slightly yellowish, odorless, crystalline powder with a molecular weight of 608.69, is insoluble in water and freely soluble in glacial acetic acid.

DIUPRES is supplied as tablets in two strengths for oral use:

DIUPRES-250*, contains 250 mg of chlorothiazide and 0.125 mg of reserpine.

DIUPRES-500*, contains 500 mg of chlorothiazide and 0.125 mg of reserpine.

Each tablet contains the following inactive ingredients: FD&C Red 3, gelatin, lactose, magnesium stearate, starch and talc.

*Registered trademark of MERCK & CO., INC.

CLINICAL PHARMACOLOGY

Chlorothiazide

The mechanism of the antihypertensive effect of thiazides is unknown. Chlorothiazide does not usually affect normal blood pressure.

Chlorothiazide affects the distal renal tubular mechanism of electrolyte reabsorption. At maximal therapeutic dosage all thiazides are approximately equal in their diuretic efficacy.

Chlorothiazide increases excretion of sodium and chloride in approximately equivalent amounts. Natriuresis may be accompanied by some loss of potassium and bicarbonate.

After oral use diuresis begins within 2 hours, peaks in about 4 hours and lasts about 6 to 12 hours.

Reserpine

Reserpine has antihypertensive, bradycardic, and tranquilizing properties. It lowers arterial blood pressure by depletion of catecholamines. Reserpine is beneficial in relieving anxiety, tension, and headache in the hypertensive patient. It acts at the hypothalamic level of the central nervous system to promote relaxation without hypnosis or analgesia. The sleep pattern shown by the electroencephalogram following barbiturates does not occur with this drug. In laboratory animals spontaneous activity and response to external stimuli are decreased, but confusion or difficulty of movement is not evident.

The bradycardic action of reserpine promotes relaxation and may eliminate sinus tachycardia. It is most pronounced in subjects with sinus tachycardia and usually is not prominent in persons with a normal pulse rate.

Miosis, relaxation of the nictitating membrane, ptosis, hypothermia, and increased gastrointestinal activity are noted in animals given reserpine, sometimes in subclinical doses. None of these effects, except increased gastrointestinal activity, has been found to be clinically significant in man with therapeutic doses.

Pharmacokinetics and Metabolism

Chlorothiazide

Chlorothiazide is not metabolized but is eliminated rapidly by the kidney. The plasma half-life of chlorothiazide is 45–120 minutes. After oral doses, 10–15 percent is excreted unchanged in the urine. Chlorothiazide crosses the placental but not the blood-brain barrier and is excreted in breast milk.

Reserpine

Oral reserpine is rapidly absorbed from the gastrointestinal tract. Methylreserpate and trimethoxybenzoic acid are the primary metabolites which result from the hydrolytic cleavage of reserpine. Maximal blood levels are achieved approximately 2 hours after the oral dosage of ^3H-reserpine to six normal volunteers; within 96 hours approximately 8 percent was excreted in urine and 62 percent in feces. Reserpine appears in human breast milk. Reserpine crosses the placental barrier in guinea pigs.

INDICATIONS AND USAGE

Hypertension (see box warning).

CONTRAINDICATIONS

Chlorothiazide is contraindicated in anuria.

DIUPRES is contraindicated in hypersensitivity to chlorothiazide or other sulfonamide-derived drugs or to reserpine.

Electroshock therapy should not be given to patients while on reserpine, as severe and even fatal reactions have been reported with minimal convulsive electroshock dosage. After discontinuing reserpine, allow at least seven days before starting electroshock therapy.

Reserpine is contraindicated in patients:

— with active peptic ulcer
— with ulcerative colitis
— with a history of mental depression, especially suicidal tendencies.
— on therapy with monoamine oxidase (MAO) inhibitors.

WARNINGS

Chlorothiazide

Use with caution in severe renal disease. In patients with renal disease, thiazides may precipitate azotemia. Cumulative effects of the drug may develop in patients with impaired renal function.

Thiazides should be used with caution in patients with impaired hepatic function or progressive liver disease, since minor alterations of fluid and electrolyte balance may precipitate hepatic coma.

Thiazides may add to or potentiate the action of other antihypertensive drugs.

Sensitivity reactions may occur in patients with or without a history of allergy or bronchial asthma.

The possibility of exacerbation or activation of systemic lupus erythematosus has been reported.

Lithium generally should not be given with diuretics (see PRECAUTIONS, *Drug Interactions*).

Reserpine

Reserpine may cause mental depression. Recognition of depression may be difficult because this condition may often be disguised by somatic complaints (masked depression). The drug should be discontinued at first signs of depression such as despondency, early morning insomnia, loss of appetite, impotence or self-deprecation. Drug-induced depression may persist for several months after drug withdrawal and may be severe enough to result in suicide.

The occurrence of mental depression due to reserpine in doses of 0.25 mg daily or less is unusual. In any event, DIUPRES should be discontinued at the first sign of depression.

PRECAUTIONS

General

Chlorothiazide

All patients receiving diuretic therapy should be observed for evidence of fluid or electrolyte imbalance: namely, hyponatremia, hypochloremic alkalosis, and hypokalemia. Serum and urine electrolyte determinations are particularly important when the patient is vomiting excessively or receiving parenteral fluids. Warning signs or symptoms of fluid and electrolyte imbalance, irrespective of cause, include dryness of mouth, thirst, weakness, lethargy, drowsiness, restlessness, confusion, seizures, muscle pains or cramps, muscular fatigue, hypotension, oliguria, tachycardia, and gastrointestinal disturbances such as nausea and vomiting.

Hypokalemia may develop, especially with brisk diuresis, when severe cirrhosis is present or after prolonged therapy. Interference with adequate oral electrolyte intake will contribute to hypokalemia. Hypokalemia may cause cardiac arrhythmia and may also sensitize or exaggerate the response of the heart to the toxic effects of digitalis (e.g., increased ventricular irritability). Hypokalemia may be avoided or treated by use of potassium sparing diuretics or potassium supplements such as foods with a high potassium content.

Although any chloride deficit is generally mild and usually does not require specific treatment except under extraordinary circumstances (as in liver disease or renal disease), chloride replacement may be required in the treatment of metabolic alkalosis.

Dilutional hyponatremia may occur in edematous patients in hot weather. Appropriate therapy is water restriction, rather than administration of salt, except in rare instances when the hyponatremia is life threatening. In actual salt depletion, appropriate replacement is the therapy of choice.

Hyperuricemia may occur or acute gout may be precipitated in certain patients receiving thiazides.

In diabetic patients dosage adjustments of insulin or oral hypoglycemic agents may be required. Hyperglycemia may occur with thiazide diuretics. Thus latent diabetes mellitus may become manifest during thiazide therapy.

The antihypertensive effect of the drug may be enhanced in the postsympathectomy patient.

If progressive renal impairment becomes evident, consider withholding or discontinuing diuretic therapy.

Thiazides have been shown to increase the urinary excretion of magnesium; this may result in hypomagnesemia.

Thiazides may decrease urinary calcium excretion. Thiazides may cause intermittent and slight elevation of serum calcium in the absence of known disorders of calcium metabolism. Marked hypercalcemia may be evidence of hidden hyperparathyroidism. Thiazides should be discontinued before carrying out tests for parathyroid function.

Increases in cholesterol and triglyceride levels may be associated with thiazide diuretic therapy.

Reserpine

Since reserpine may increase gastric secretion and motility, it should be used cautiously in patients with a history of peptic ulcer, ulcerative colitis, or other gastrointestinal disorder. This compound may precipitate biliary colic in patients with gallstones, or bronchial asthma in susceptible persons.

Reserpine may cause hypotension including orthostatic hypotension.

Anxiety or depression, as well as psychosis, may develop during reserpine therapy. If depression is present when therapy is begun, it may be aggravated. Mental depression is unusual with reserpine doses of 0.25 mg daily or less. In any case, DIUPRES should be discontinued at the first sign of depression. Extreme caution should be used in treating patients with a history of mental depression, and the possibility of suicide should be kept in mind.

As with most antihypertensive therapy, caution should be exercised when treating hypertensive patients with renal insufficiency, since they adjust poorly to lowered blood pressure.

When two or more antihypertensives are given, the individual dosages may have to be reduced to prevent excessive drop in blood pressure. In hypertensive patients with coronary artery disease, it is important to avoid a precipitous drop in blood pressure.

Laboratory Tests

Periodic determination of serum electrolytes to detect possible electrolyte imbalance should be done at appropriate intervals.

Drug Interactions

Chlorothiazide

When given concurrently the following drugs may interact with thiazide diuretics.

Alcohol, barbiturates, or narcotics —potentiation of orthostatic hypotension may occur.

Antidiabetic drugs (oral agents and insulin)—dosage adjustment of the antidiabetic drug may be required.

Other antihypertensive drugs —additive effect or potentiation.

Cholestyramine and colestipol resins—Both cholestyramine and colestipol resins have the potential of binding thiazide diuretics and reducing diuretic absorption from the gastrointestinal tract.

Corticosteroids, ACTH —intensified electrolyte depletion, particularly hypokalemia.

Pressor amines (e.g., norepinephrine) —possible decreased response to pressor amines but not sufficient to preclude their use.

Skeletal muscle relaxants, nondepolarizing (e.g., tubocurarine) —possible increased responsiveness to the muscle relaxant.

Lithium —generally should not be given with diuretics. Diuretic agents reduce the renal clearance of lithium and add a high risk of lithium toxicity. Refer to the package insert for lithium preparations before use of such preparations with DIUPRES.

Non-steroidal Anti-inflammatory Drugs —In some patients, the administration of a non-steroidal anti-inflammatory agent can reduce the diuretic, natriuretic, and antihypertensive effects of loop, potassium-sparing and thiazide diuretics. Therefore, when DIUPRES and non-steroidal anti-inflammatory agents are used concomitantly, the patient should be observed closely to determine if the desired effect of the diuretic is obtained.

Continued on next page

Information on the Merck & Co., Inc. products listed on these pages is the full prescribing information from product circulars in use August 31, 1998. For information, please call 1-800-NSC MERCK [1-800-672-6372].

Diupres—Cont.

Reserpine

In hypertensive patients on reserpine therapy significant hypotension and bradycardia may develop during surgical anesthesia. The anesthesiologist should be aware that reserpine has been taken, since it may be necessary to give vagal blocking agents parenterally to prevent or reverse hypotension and/or bradycardia.

Use reserpine cautiously with digitalis and quinidine; cardiac arrhythmias have occurred with reserpine preparations.

Barbiturates enhance the central nervous system depressant effects of reserpine.

Monoamine oxidase (MAO) inhibitors: see CONTRAINDICATIONS.

Drug/Laboratory Test Interactions

Thiazides should be discontinued before carrying out tests for parathyroid function (see PRECAUTIONS, *General*).

Carcinogenesis, Mutagenesis, Impairment of Fertility

Carcinogenicity and mutagenicity studies have not been conducted with combinations of reserpine/chlorothiazide.

In a two-litter study in the rat at an oral dose of 50.0/0.025 mg/kg, the combination of chlorothiazide/reserpine did not impair fertility or produce abnormalities in the fetus.

Chlorothiazide

Carcinogenicity studies have not been done with chlorothiazide.

Chlorothiazide was not mutagenic *in vitro* in the Ames microbial mutagen test (using a maximum concentration of 5 mg/plate and *Salmonella typhimurium* strains TA 98 and TA 100) and was not mutagenic and did not induce mitotic nondisjunction in diploid strains of *Aspergillus nidulans*.

Chlorothiazide had no adverse effects on fertility in female rats at doses up to 60 mg/kg/day and no adverse effects on fertility in male rats at doses up to 40 mg/kg/day.

Reserpine

Reserpine at a concentration of 1 to 5000 mcg/plate had no mutagenic activity against four strains of *S. typhimurium* in vitro in the Ames microbial mutagen test with or without metabolic activation. Reserpine did not induce malignant transformation of mouse fibroblasts *in vitro* at concentrations of 0.3 to 10 mcg/mL.

A few chromosomal aberrations were induced by reserpine *in vitro* in cultured mouse mammary carcinoma cells but were considered negative in this study. The drug did not produce chromosomal aberrations in human peripheral leucocyte cultures although an increase in mitotic figures occurred. One study reported chromosomal aberrations and dominant lethal mutations in mice at doses up to 10 mg/kg of reserpine in the form of a pharmaceutical preparation. Another study did not show dominant lethal mutations in mice at IP doses of 0.92 and 4.6 mg/kg of reserpine.

Reserpine did not impair fertility in a two-litter study in the rat at an oral dose of 0.025 mg/kg.

Rodent studies have shown that reserpine is an animal tumorigen, causing an increased incidence of mammary fibroadenomas in female mice, malignant tumors of the seminal vesicle in male mice, and malignant adrenal medullary tumors in male rats. These findings arose in two year studies in which the drug was administered in the feed at concentrations of 5 and 10 ppm—about 100 to 300 times the usual human dose. The breast neoplasms are thought to be related to reserpine's prolactin-elevating effect. Several other prolactin-elevating drugs have also been associated with an increased incidence of mammary neoplasia in rodents.

The extent to which these findings indicate a risk to humans is uncertain. Tissue culture experiments show that about one-third of human breast tumors are prolactin-dependent *in vitro*, a factor of considerable importance if the use of the drug is contemplated in a patient with previously detected breast cancer. The possibility of an increased risk of breast cancer in reserpine users has been studied extensively; however, no firm conclusion has emerged. Although a few epidemiologic studies have suggested a slightly increased risk (less than twofold in all studies except one) in women who have used reserpine, other studies of generally similar design have not confirmed this. Epidemiologic studies conducted using other drugs (neuroleptic agents) that, like reserpine, increase prolactin levels and therefore would be considered rodent mammary carcinogens, have not shown an association between chronic administration of the drug and human mammary tumorigenesis. While long-term clinical observation has not suggested such an association, the available evidence is considered too limited to be conclusive at this time. An association of reserpine intake with pheochromocytoma or tumors of the seminal vesicles has not been explored.

Pregnancy

Use of diuretics during normal pregnancy is inappropriate and exposes mother and fetus to unnecessary hazard. Diuretics do not prevent development of toxemia of pregnancy and there is no satisfactory evidence that they are useful in the treatment of toxemia.

Teratogenic Effects—Pregnancy Category C: There are no adequate and well-controlled studies with DIUPRES or other combinations of reserpine/chlorothiazide in animals or pregnant women. DIUPRES may cause fetal harm when given to a pregnant woman. DIUPRES should be used during pregnancy only if the potential benefit justifies the potential risk to the fetus.

Reserpine: Reproduction studies in rats have shown that reserpine is teratogenic at doses of 1-2 mg/kg (125–250 times the maximum recommended human dose) IM or IP given early in pregnancy. A variety of abnormalities was produced including anophthalmia, absence of the axial skeleton, hydronephrosis, etc. Pregnancy in rabbits was interrupted when doses as low as 0.04 mg/kg (10 times the maximum recommended human dose) were given early or late in pregnancy.

Chlorothiazide: Thiazides cross the placental barrier and appear in cord blood.

Although reproduction studies performed with chlorothiazide doses of 50 mg/kg/day in rabbits, 60 mg/kg/day in rats and 500 mg/kg/day in mice revealed no external abnormalities of the fetus or impairment of growth and survival of the fetus due to chlorothiazide, such studies did not include complete examinations for visceral and skeletal abnormalities.

Nonteratogenic Effects

Reserpine: Reserpine has been demonstrated to cross the placental barrier in guinea pigs with depression of adrenal catecholamine stores in the newborn. There is some evidence that side effects such as nasal congestion, lethargy, depressed Moro reflex, and bradycardia may appear in infants born of reserpine-treated mothers.

Chlorothiazide: Chlorothiazide may cause fetal or neonatal jaundice, thrombocytopenia, and possibly other adverse reactions which have occurred in the adult.

Nursing Mothers

Thiazides and reserpine appear in breast milk. Because of the potential for serious adverse reactions in nursing infants from DIUPRES, a decision should be made whether to discontinue nursing or to discontinue the drug, taking into account the importance of the drug to the mother.

Pediatric Use

Safety and effectiveness of DIUPRES in pediatric patients have not been established.

ADVERSE REACTIONS

The following adverse reactions have been reported and, within each category, are listed in order of decreasing severity.

Chlorothiazide

Body as a Whole: Weakness.

Cardiovascular: Hypotension including orthostatic hypotension (may be aggravated by alcohol, barbiturates, narcotics or antihypertensive drugs).

Digestive: Pancreatitis, jaundice (intrahepatic cholestatic jaundice), diarrhea, vomiting, sialadenitis, cramping, constipation, gastric irritation, nausea, anorexia.

Hematologic: Aplastic anemia, agranulocytosis, leukopenia, hemolytic anemia, thrombocytopenia.

Hypersensitivity: Anaphylactic reactions, necrotizing angiitis (vasculitis and cutaneous vasculitis), respiratory distress including pneumonitis and pulmonary edema, photosensitivity, fever, urticaria, rash, purpura.

Metabolic: Electrolyte imbalance (see PRECAUTIONS), hyperglycemia, glycosuria, hyperuricemia.

Musculoskeletal: Muscle spasm.

Nervous System/Psychiatric: Vertigo, paresthesias, dizziness, headache, restlessness.

Renal: Renal failure, renal dysfunction, interstitial nephritis. (See WARNINGS.)

Skin: Erythema multiforme including Stevens-Johnson syndrome, exfoliative dermatitis including toxic epidermal necrolysis, alopecia.

Special Senses: Transient blurred vision, xanthopsia.

Urogenital: Impotence.

Reserpine

Cardiovascular: Angina pectoris, arrhythmia, premature ventricular contractions, other direct cardiac effects (e.g., fluid retention, congestive heart failure), bradycardia.

Digestive: Vomiting, diarrhea, nausea, hypersecretion and increased motility, anorexia, dryness of mouth, increased salivation.

Hematologic: Thrombocytopenic purpura, excessive bleeding following prostatic surgery.

Hypersensitivity: Pruritus, rash, flushing of skin.

Metabolic: Weight gain.

Musculoskeletal: Muscular aches.

Nervous System/Psychiatric: Mental depression, dull sensorium, syncope, paradoxical anxiety, excessive sedation, nightmares, headache, dizziness, nervousness, parkinsonism (usually reversible with decreased dosage or discontinuance of therapy).

Respiratory: Dyspnea, epistaxis, nasal congestion, enhanced susceptibility to colds.

Special Senses: Optic atrophy, uveitis, deafness, glaucoma, conjunctival injection, blurred vision.

Urogenital: Dysuria, impotence, decreased libido, nonpuerperal lactation.

OVERDOSAGE

Overdosage may lead to excessive sedation, mental depression, severe hypotension, extrapyramidal reactions.

There is no specific antidote. In the event of overdosage, symptomatic and supportive measures should be employed. Emesis should be induced or gastric lavage performed. Correct dehydration, electrolyte imbalance, hepatic coma and hypotension by established procedures. If required, give oxygen or artificial respiration for respiratory impairment. In the event of severe hypotension from the reserpine component, intravenous use of a vasopressor is indicated [e.g., ARAMINE* (Metaraminol Bitartrate), levarterenol, phenylephrine]. Anticholinergics may be needed to relieve gastrointestinal distress from reserpine. Because the effects of the rauwolfia alkaloids are prolonged, the patient should be closely observed for at least 72 hours.

Reserpine is not dialyzable. The degree to which chlorothiazide is removed by hemodialysis has not been established. The oral LD$_{50}$ of chlorothiazide is 8.5 g/kg, greater than 10 g/kg, and greater than 1 g/kg, in the mouse, rat and dog, respectively. The oral LD$_{50}$ of reserpine in the mouse is 390 mg/kg.

DOSAGE AND ADMINISTRATION

The initial dosage of DIUPRES should conform to the dosages of the individual components established during titration (see box warning).

The usual adult dosage of DIUPRES-250* is 1 or 2 tablets once or twice a day; that of DIUPRES-500* is 1 tablet once or twice a day.

Dosage may require adjustment according to the blood pressure response of the patient. For maintenance, dosage should be adjusted to the lowest requirement of the individual patient. Doses higher than 0.25 mg daily of reserpine should be used cautiously, because occurrence of serious mental depression and other side effects may increase considerably (see WARNINGS).

*Registered trademark of MERCK & CO., INC.

HOW SUPPLIED

No. 3261—Tablets DIUPRES-250 are pink, round, scored, compressed tablets, coded MSD 230 on one side and DIUPRES on the other. Each tablet contains 250 mg of chlorothiazide and 0.125 mg of reserpine. They are supplied as follows:

NDC 0006-0230-68 in bottles of 100
NDC 0006-0230-82 in bottles of 1000
Shown in Product Identification Guide, page 323

No. 3262—Tablets DIUPRES-500 are pink, round, scored, compressed tablets, coded MSD 405 on one side and DIUPRES on the other. Each tablet contains 500 mg of chlorothiazide and 0.125 mg of reserpine. They are supplied as follows:

NDC 0006-0405-68 in bottles of 100
NDC 0006-0405-82 in bottles of 1000
Shown in Product Identification Guide, page 323

Storage

Keep container tightly closed. Protect from light, moisture, freezing, –20°C (–4°F) and store at room temperature, 15–30°C (59–86°F).

7900347 Issued March 1995
COPYRIGHT © MERCK & CO., INC., 1986
All rights reserved

DIURIL® Sodium Intravenous
(Chlorothiazide Sodium), U.S.P.

℞

DESCRIPTION

Intravenous Sodium DIURIL* (Chlorothiazide Sodium) is a diuretic and antihypertensive. It is 6-chloro-2*H* -1,2,4-benzothiadiazine-7-sulfonamide 1,1-dioxide monosodium salt and its molecular weight is 317.71. Its empirical formula is $C_7H_5ClN_3NaO_4S_2$ and its structural formula is:

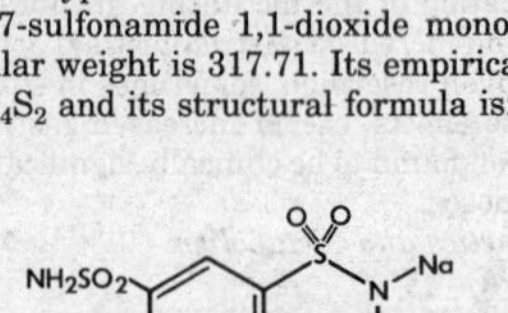

Intravenous Sodium DIURIL is a sterile lyophilized white powder and is supplied in a vial containing:

Chlorothiazide sodium equivalent
to chlorothiazide .... 0.5 g
Inactive ingredients:
Mannitol .... 0.25 g
Sodium hydroxide to adjust pH, with 0.4 mg thimerosal (mercury derivative) added as preservative.

DIURIL* (Chlorothiazide) is a diuretic and antihypertensive. It is 6-chloro-2*H* -1,2,4-benzothiadiazine-7-sulfonamide 1,1-dioxide. Its empirical formula is $C_7H_6ClN_3O_4S_2$ and its structural formula is:

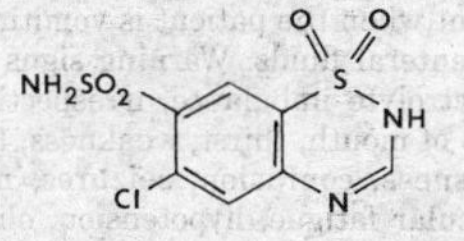

It is a white, or practically white, crystalline powder with a molecular weight of 295.72, which is very slightly soluble in water, but readily soluble in dilute aqueous sodium hydroxide. It is soluble in urine to the extent of about 150 mg per 100 mL at pH 7.

*Registered trademark of MERCK & CO., INC.

CLINICAL PHARMACOLOGY

The mechanism of the antihypertensive effect of thiazides is unknown. DIURIL (Chlorothiazide) does not usually affect normal blood pressure.
DIURIL (Chlorothiazide) affects the distal renal tubular mechanism of electrolyte reabsorption. At maximal therapeutic dosage all thiazides are approximately equal in their diuretic efficacy.
DIURIL (Chlorothiazide) increases excretion of sodium and chloride in approximately equivalent amounts. Natriuresis may be accompanied by some loss of potassium and bicarbonate.
After oral use diuresis begins within 2 hours, peaks in about 4 hours and lasts about 6 to 12 hours. Following intravenous use of Sodium DIURIL, onset of the diuretic action occurs in 15 minutes and the maximal action in 30 minutes.
Pharmacokinetics and Metabolism
DIURIL is not metabolized but is eliminated rapidly by the kidney; 96 percent of an intravenous dose is excreted unchanged in the urine within 23 hours. The plasma half-life of chlorothiazide is 45–120 minutes. Chlorothiazide crosses the placental but not the blood-brain barrier and is excreted in breast milk.

INDICATIONS AND USAGE

Intravenous Sodium DIURIL is indicated as adjunctive therapy in edema associated with congestive heart failure, hepatic cirrhosis, and corticosteroid and estrogen therapy.
Intravenous Sodium DIURIL has also been found useful in edema due to various forms of renal dysfunction such as nephrotic syndrome, acute glomerulonephritis, and chronic renal failure.
Use in Pregnancy. Routine use of diuretics during normal pregnancy is inappropriate and exposes mother and fetus to unnecessary hazard. Diuretics do not prevent development of toxemia of pregnancy and there is no satisfactory evidence that they are useful in the treatment of toxemia.
Edema during pregnancy may arise from pathologic causes or from the physiologic and mechanical consequences of pregnancy. Thiazides are indicated in pregnancy when edema is due to pathologic causes, just as they are in the absence of pregnancy (see PRECAUTIONS, *Pregnancy*). Dependent edema in pregnancy, resulting from restriction of venous return by the gravid uterus, is properly treated through elevation of the lower extremities and use of support stockings. Use of diuretics to lower intravascular volume in this instance is illogical and unnecessary. During normal pregnancy there is hypervolemia which is not harmful to the fetus or the mother in the absence of cardiovascular disease. However, it may be associated with edema, rarely generalized edema. If such edema causes discomfort, increased recumbency will often provide relief. Rarely this edema may cause extreme discomfort which is not relieved by rest. In these instances, a short course of diuretic therapy may provide relief and be appropriate.

CONTRAINDICATIONS

Anuria.
Hypersensitivity to any component of this product or to other sulfonamide-derived drugs.

WARNINGS

Intravenous use in infants and children has been limited and is not generally recommended.
Use with caution in severe renal disease. In patients with renal disease, thiazides may precipitate azotemia. Cumulative effects of the drug may develop in patients with impaired renal function.
Thiazides should be used with caution in patients with impaired hepatic function or progressive liver disease, since minor alterations of fluid and electrolyte balance may precipitate hepatic coma.
Thiazides may add to or potentiate the action of other antihypertensive drugs.
Sensitivity reactions may occur in patients with or without a history of allergy or bronchial asthma.
The possibility of exacerbation or activation of systemic lupus erythematosus has been reported.
Lithium generally should not be given with diuretics (see PRECAUTIONS, *Drug Interactions*).

PRECAUTIONS

General
All patients receiving diuretic therapy should be observed for evidence of fluid or electrolyte imbalance: namely, hyponatremia, hypochloremic alkalosis, and hypokalemia. Serum and urine electrolyte determinations are particularly important when the patient is vomiting excessively or receiving parenteral fluids. Warning signs or symptoms of fluid and electrolyte imbalance, irrespective of cause, include dryness of mouth, thirst, weakness, lethargy, drowsiness, restlessness, confusion, seizures, muscle pains or cramps, muscular fatigue, hypotension, oliguria, tachycardia, and gastrointestinal disturbances such as nausea and vomiting.
Hypokalemia may develop especially with brisk diuresis, when severe cirrhosis is present or after prolonged therapy. Interference with adequate oral electrolyte intake will also contribute to hypokalemia. Hypokalemia may cause cardiac arrhythmias and may also sensitize or exaggerate the response of the heart to the toxic effects of digitalis (e.g., increased ventricular irritability). Hypokalemia may be avoided or treated by use of potassium sparing diuretics or potassium supplements such as foods with a high potassium content.
Although any chloride deficit is generally mild and usually does not require specific treatment except under extraordinary circumstances (as in liver disease or renal disease), chloride replacement may be required in the treatment of metabolic alkalosis.
Dilutional hyponatremia may occur in edematous patients in hot weather; appropriate therapy is water restriction, rather than administration of salt, except in rare instances when the hyponatremia is life threatening. In actual salt depletion, appropriate replacement is the therapy of choice.
Hyperuricemia may occur or acute gout may be precipitated in certain patients receiving thiazides.
In diabetic patients dosage adjustments of insulin or oral hypoglycemic agents may be required. Hyperglycemia may occur with thiazide diuretics. Thus latent diabetes mellitus may become manifest during thiazide therapy.
The antihypertensive effects of the drug may be enhanced in the postsympathectomy patient.
If progressive renal impairment becomes evident, consider withholding or discontinuing diuretic therapy.
Thiazides have been shown to increase the urinary excretion of magnesium; this may result in hypomagnesemia.
Thiazides may decrease urinary calcium excretion. Thiazides may cause intermittent and slight elevation of serum calcium in the absence of known disorders of calcium metabolism. Marked hypercalcemia may be evidence of hidden hyperparathyroidism. Thiazides should be discontinued before carrying out tests for parathyroid function.
Increases in cholesterol and triglyceride levels may be associated with thiazide diuretic therapy.
Laboratory Tests
Periodic determination of serum electrolytes to detect possible electrolyte imbalance should be done at appropriate intervals.
Drug Interactions
When given concurrently the following drugs may interact with thiazide diuretics.
Alcohol, barbiturates, or narcotics —potentiation of orthostatic hypotension may occur.
Antidiabetic drugs —(oral agents and insulin)—dosage adjustment of the antidiabetic drug may be required.
Other antihypertensive drugs —additive effect or potentiation.
Corticosteroids, ACTH —intensified electrolyte depletion, particularly hypokalemia.
Pressor amines (e.g., norepinephrine) —possible decreased response to pressor amines but not sufficient to preclude their use.
Skeletal muscle relaxants, nondepolarizing (e.g., tubocurarine) —possible increased responsiveness to the muscle relaxant.
Lithium —generally should not be given with diuretics. Diuretic agents reduce the renal clearance of lithium and add a high risk of lithium toxicity. Refer to the package insert for lithium preparations before use of such preparations with Sodium DIURIL.
Non-steroidal Anti-inflammatory Drugs —In some patients, the administration of a non-steroidal anti-inflammatory agent can reduce the diuretic, natriuretic, and antihypertensive effects of loop, potassium-sparing and thiazide diuretics. Therefore, when Sodium DIURIL and non-steroidal anti-inflammatory agents are used concomitantly, the patient should be observed closely to determine if the desired effect of the diuretic is obtained.
Drug/Laboratory Test Interactions
Thiazides should be discontinued before carrying out tests for parathyroid function (see PRECAUTIONS, *General*).
Carcinogenesis, Mutagenesis, Impairment of Fertility
Carcinogenicity studies have not been conducted with chlorothiazide.
Chlorothiazide was not mutagenic *in vitro* in the Ames microbial mutagen test (using a maximum concentration of 5 mg/plate and *Salmonella typhimurium* strains TA98 and TA100) and was not mutagenic and did not induce mitotic nondisjunction in diploid-strains of *Aspergillus nidulans.*
Chlorothiazide had no adverse effects on fertility in female rats at doses up to 60 mg/kg/day and no adverse effects on fertility in male rats at doses up to 40 mg/kg/day. These doses are 1.5 and 1.0 times* the recommended maximum human dose, respectively, when compared on a body weight basis.

*Calculations based on a human body weight of 50 kg

Pregnancy
Teratogenic Effects —Pregnancy Category C: Although reproduction studies performed with chlorothiazide doses of 50 mg/kg/day in rabbits, 60 mg/kg/day in rats and 500 mg/kg/day in mice revealed no external abnormalities of the fetus or impairment of growth and survival of the fetus due to chlorothiazide, such studies did not include complete examinations for visceral and skeletal abnormalities. It is not known whether chlorothiazide can cause fetal harm when administered to a pregnant woman; however, thiazides cross the placental barrier and appear in cord blood. DIURIL should be used during pregnancy only if clearly needed (see INDICATIONS AND USAGE).
Nonteratogenic Effects: Chlorothiazide may cause fetal or neonatal jaundice, thrombocytopenia, and possibly other adverse reactions which have occurred in the adult.
Nursing Mothers
Because of the potential for serious adverse reactions in nursing infants from Intravenous Sodium DIURIL, a decision should be made whether to discontinue nursing or to discontinue the drug, taking into account the importance of the drug to the mother.
Pediatric Use
Safety and effectiveness of Intravenous Sodium DIURIL in pediatric patients have not been established.

ADVERSE REACTIONS

The following adverse reactions have been reported and, within each category, are listed in order of decreasing severity.
Body as a Whole: Weakness.
Cardiovascular: Hypotension including orthostatic hypotension (may be aggravated by alcohol, barbiturates, narcotics or antihypertensive drugs).
Digestive: Pancreatitis, jaundice (intrahepatic cholestatic jaundice), diarrhea, vomiting, sialadenitis, cramping, constipation, gastric irritation, nausea, anorexia.
Hematologic: Aplastic anemia, agranulocytosis, leukopenia, hemolytic anemia, thrombocytopenia.
Hypersensitivity: Anaphylactic reactions, necrotizing angiitis (vasculitis and cutaneous vasculitis), respiratory distress including pneumonitis and pulmonary edema, photosensitivity, fever, urticaria, rash, purpura.
Metabolic: Electrolyte imbalance (see PRECAUTIONS), hyperglycemia, glycosuria, hyperuricemia.
Musculoskeletal: Muscle spasm.
Nervous System/Psychiatric: Vertigo, paresthesias, dizziness, headache, restlessness.
Skin: Erythema multiforme including Stevens-Johnson syndrome, exfoliative dermatitis including toxic epidermal necrolysis, alopecia.
Special Senses: Transient blurred vision, xanthopsia.
Renal: Renal failure, renal dysfunction, interstitial nephritis (see WARNINGS); hematuria (following intravenous use).
Urogenital: Impotence.

Continued on next page

Information on the Merck & Co., Inc. products listed on these pages is the full prescribing information from product circulars in use August 31, 1998. For information, please call 1-800-NSC MERCK [1-800-672-6372].

Diuril Sodium —Cont.

Whenever adverse reactions are moderate or severe, thiazide dosage should be reduced or therapy withdrawn.

OVERDOSAGE

The most common signs and symptoms observed are those caused by electrolyte depletion (hypokalemia, hypochloremia, hyponatremia) and dehydration resulting from excessive diuresis. If digitalis has also been administered, hypokalemia may accentuate cardiac arrhythmias.
In the event of overdosage, symptomatic and supportive measures should be employed. Correct dehydration, electrolyte imbalance, hepatic coma and hypotension by established procedures. If required, give oxygen or artificial respiration for respiratory impairment.
The degree to which chlorothiazide sodium is removed by hemodialysis has not been established.
The intravenous LD_{50} of chlorothiazide in the mouse is 1.1 g/kg.

DOSAGE AND ADMINISTRATION

Intravenous Sodium DIURIL should be reserved for patients unable to take oral medication or for emergency situations.
Therapy should be individualized according to patient response. Use the smallest dosage necessary to achieve the required response.
Intravenous use in infants and children has been limited and is not generally recommended.
When medication can be taken orally, therapy with DIURIL tablets or oral suspension may be substituted for intravenous therapy, using the same dosage schedule as for the parenteral route.
Intravenous Sodium DIURIL may be given slowly by direct intravenous injection or by intravenous infusion.
Add 18 mL of Sterile Water for Injection to the vial to form an isotonic solution for intravenous injection. Never add less than 18 mL. When reconstituted with 18 mL of Sterile Water, the final concentration of Intravenous Sodium DIURIL is 28 mg/mL. Unused solution may be stored at room temperature for 24 hours, after which it must be discarded.
Parenteral drug products should be inspected visually for particulate matter and discoloration prior to use whenever solution and container permit. The solution is compatible with dextrose or sodium chloride solutions for intravenous infusion. Avoid simultaneous administration of solutions of chlorothiazide with whole blood or its derivatives.
Extravasation must be rigidly avoided. Do not give subcutaneously or intramuscularly.
The usual adult dosage is 0.5 to 1.0 g once or twice a day. Many patients with edema respond to intermittent therapy, i.e., administration on alternate days or on three to five days each week. With an intermittent schedule, excessive response and the resulting undesirable electrolyte imbalance are less likely to occur.

HOW SUPPLIED

No. 3250—Intravenous Sodium DIURIL is a dry, sterile lyophilized white powder usually in plug form, supplied in vials containing chlorothiazide sodium equivalent to 0.5 g of chlorothiazide.
NDC 0006-3250-32.
Storage
Store lyophilized powder between 2–25°C (36–77°F).
Store reconstituted solution at room temperature, 15–30°C (59–86°F), and discard unused portion after 24 hours.
7413535 Issued June 1995
COPYRIGHT © MERCK & CO., INC., 1986
All rights reserved

DIURIL® Tablets ℞
(Chlorothiazide), U.S.P.
DIURIL® Oral Suspension ℞
(Chlorothiazide), U.S.P.

DESCRIPTION

DIURIL* (Chlorothiazide) is a diuretic and antihypertensive. It is 6-chloro-2*H* -1,2,4 -benzothiadiazine-7-sulfonamide 1,1-dioxide. Its empirical formula is $C_7H_6ClN_3O_4S_2$ and its structural formula is:

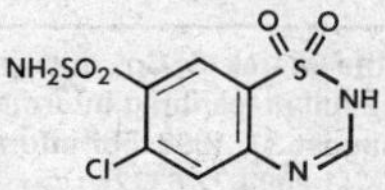

It is a white, or practically white, crystalline powder with a molecular weight of 295.73, which is very slightly soluble in water, but readily soluble in dilute aqueous sodium hydroxide. It is soluble in urine to the extent of about 150 mg per 100 mL at pH 7.
DIURIL is supplied as 250 mg and 500 mg tablets, for oral use. Each tablet contains the following inactive ingredients: gelatin, magnesium stearate, starch and talc. The 250 mg tablet also contains lactose.
Oral Suspension DIURIL contains 250 mg of chlorothiazide per 5 mL, alcohol 0.5 percent, with methylparaben 0.12 percent, propylparaben 0.02 percent, and benzoic acid 0.1 percent added as preservatives. The inactive ingredients are D&C Yellow 10, flavors, glycerin, purified water, sodium saccharin, sucrose and tragacanth.

*Registered trademark of MERCK & CO., INC.

CLINICAL PHARMACOLOGY

The mechanism of the antihypertensive effect of thiazides is unknown. DIURIL does not usually affect normal blood pressure.
DIURIL affects the distal renal tubular mechanism of electrolyte reabsorption. At maximal therapeutic dosage all thiazides are approximately equal in their diuretic efficacy.
DIURIL increases excretion of sodium and chloride in approximately equivalent amounts. Natriuresis may be accompanied by some loss of potassium and bicarbonate.
After oral use diuresis begins within 2 hours, peaks in about 4 hours and lasts about 6 to 12 hours.
Pharmacokinetics and Metabolism
DIURIL is not metabolized but is eliminated rapidly by the kidney. The plasma half-life of chlorothiazide is 45–120 minutes. After oral doses, 10–15 percent of the dose is excreted unchanged in the urine. Chlorothiazide crosses the placental but not the blood-brain barrier and is excreted in breast milk.

INDICATIONS AND USAGE

DIURIL is indicated as adjunctive therapy in edema associated with congestive heart failure, hepatic cirrhosis, and corticosteroid and estrogen therapy.
DIURIL has also been found useful in edema due to various forms of renal dysfunction such as nephrotic syndrome, acute glomerulonephritis, and chronic renal failure.
DIURIL is indicated in the management of hypertension either as the sole therapeutic agent or to enhance the effectiveness of other antihypertensive drugs in the more severe forms of hypertension.
Use in Pregnancy. Routine use of diuretics during normal pregnancy is inappropriate and exposes mother and fetus to unnecessary hazard. Diuretics do not prevent development of toxemia of pregnancy and there is no satisfactory evidence that they are useful in the treatment of toxemia.
Edema during pregnancy may arise from pathologic causes or from the physiologic and mechanical consequences of pregnancy. Thiazides are indicated in pregnancy when edema is due to pathologic causes, just as they are in the absence of pregnancy (see PRECAUTIONS, *Pregnancy*). Dependent edema in pregnancy, resulting from restriction of venous return by the gravid uterus, is properly treated through elevation of the lower extremities and use of support stockings. Use of diuretics to lower intravascular volume in this instance is illogical and unnecessary. During normal pregnancy there is hypervolemia which is not harmful to the fetus or the mother in the absence of cardiovascular disease. However, it may be associated with edema, rarely generalized edema. If such edema causes discomfort, increased recumbency will often provide relief. Rarely this edema may cause extreme discomfort which is not relieved by rest. In these instances, a short course of diuretic therapy may provide relief and be appropriate.

CONTRAINDICATIONS

Anuria.
Hypersensitivity to this product or to other sulfonamide-derived drugs.

WARNINGS

Use with caution in severe renal disease. In patients with renal disease, thiazides may precipitate azotemia. Cumulative effects of the drug may develop in patients with impaired renal function.
Thiazides should be used with caution in patients with impaired hepatic function or progressive liver disease, since minor alterations of fluid and electrolyte balance may precipitate hepatic coma.
Thiazides may add to or potentiate the action of other antihypertensive drugs.
Sensitivity reactions may occur in patients with or without a history of allergy or bronchial asthma.
The possibility of exacerbation or activation of systemic lupus erythematosus has been reported.
Lithium generally should not be given with diuretics (see PRECAUTIONS, *Drug Interactions).*

PRECAUTIONS

General
All patients receiving diuretic therapy should be observed for evidence of fluid or electrolyte imbalance: namely, hyponatremia, hypochloremic alkalosis, and hypokalemia. Serum and urine electrolyte determinations are particularly important when the patient is vomiting excessively or receiving parenteral fluids. Warning signs or symptoms of fluid and electrolyte imbalance, irrespective of cause, include dryness of mouth, thirst, weakness, lethargy, drowsiness, restlessness, confusion, seizures, muscle pains or cramps, muscular fatigue, hypotension, oliguria, tachycardia, and gastrointestinal disturbances such as nausea and vomiting.
Hypokalemia may develop, especially with brisk diuresis, when severe cirrhosis is present or after prolonged therapy. Interference with adequate oral electrolyte intake will also contribute to hypokalemia. Hypokalemia may cause cardiac arrhythmias and may also sensitize or exaggerate the response of the heart to the toxic effects of digitalis (e.g., increased ventricular irritability). Hypokalemia may be avoided or treated by use of potassium sparing diuretics or potassium supplements such as foods with a high potassium content.
Although any chloride deficit is generally mild and usually does not require specific treatment except under extraordinary circumstances (as in liver disease or renal disease), chloride replacement may be required in the treatment of metabolic alkalosis.
Dilutional hyponatremia may occur in edematous patients in hot weather; appropriate therapy is water restriction, rather than administration of salt, except in rare instances when the hyponatremia is life-threatening. In actual salt depletion, appropriate replacement is the therapy of choice.
Hyperuricemia may occur or acute gout may be precipitated in certain patients receiving thiazides.
In diabetic patients dosage adjustments of insulin or oral hypoglycemic agents may be required. Hyperglycemia may occur with thiazide diuretics. Thus latent diabetes mellitus may become manifest during thiazide therapy.
The antihypertensive effects of the drug may be enhanced in the post-sympathectomy patient.
If progressive renal impairment becomes evident, consider withholding or discontinuing diuretic therapy.
Thiazides have been shown to increase the urinary excretion of magnesium; this may result in hypomagnesemia.
Thiazides may decrease urinary calcium excretion. Thiazides may cause intermittent and slight elevation of serum calcium in the absence of known disorders of calcium metabolism. Marked hypercalcemia may be evidence of hidden hyperparathyroidism. Thiazides should be discontinued before carrying out tests for parathyroid function.
Increases in cholesterol and triglyceride levels may be associated with thiazide diuretic therapy.
Laboratory Tests
Periodic determination of serum electrolytes to detect possible electrolyte imbalance should be done at appropriate intervals.
Drug Interactions
When given concurrently the following drugs may interact with thiazide diuretics.
Alcohol, barbiturates, or narcotics —potentiation of orthostatic hypotension may occur.
Antidiabetic drugs (oral agents and insulin)—dosage adjustment of the antidiabetic drug may be required.
Other antihypertensive drugs —additive effect or potentiation.
Cholestyramine and colestipol resins—Both cholestyramine and colestipol resins have the potential of binding thiazide diuretics and reducing diuretic absorption from the gastrointestinal tract.
Corticosteroids, ACTH —intensified electrolyte depletion, particularly hypokalemia.
Pressor amines (e.g., norepinephrine) —possible decreased response to pressor amines but not sufficient to preclude their use.
Skeletal muscle relaxants, nondepolarizing (e.g., tubocurarine) —possible increased responsiveness to the muscle relaxant.
Lithium —generally should not be given with diuretics. Diuretic agents reduce the renal clearance of lithium and add a high risk of lithium toxicity. Refer to the package insert for lithium preparations before use of such preparations with DIURIL.
Non-steroidal Anti-inflammatory Drugs —In some patients, the administration of a non-steroidal anti-inflammatory agent can reduce the diuretic, natriuretic, and antihypertensive effects of loop, potassium-sparing and thiazide diuretics. Therefore, when DIURIL and non-steroidal anti-

inflammatory agents are used concomitantly, the patient should be observed closely to determine if the desired effect of the diuretic is obtained.

Drug/Laboratory Test Interactions

Thiazides should be discontinued before carrying out tests for parathyroid function (see PRECAUTIONS, *General*).

Carcinogenesis, Mutagenesis,
Impairment of Fertility

Carcinogenicity studies have not been conducted with chlorothiazide.

Chlorothiazide was not mutagenic *in vitro* in the Ames microbial mutagen test (using a maximum concentration of 5 mg/plate and *Salmonella typhimurium* strains TA98 and TA100) and was not mutagenic and did not induce mitotic nondisjunction in diploid-strains of *Aspergillus nidulans.*

Chlorothiazide had no adverse effects on fertility in female rats at doses up to 60 mg/kg/day and no adverse effects on fertility in male rats at doses up to 40 mg/kg/day. These doses are 1.5 and 1.0 times* the recommended maximum human dose, respectively, when compared on a body weight basis.

---

*Calculations based on a human body weight of 50 kg

Pregnancy

Teratogenic Effects —Pregnancy Category C: Although reproduction studies performed with chlorothiazide doses of 50 mg/kg/day in rabbits, 60 mg/kg/day in rats and 500 mg/kg/day in mice revealed no external abnormalities of the fetus or impairment of growth and survival of the fetus due to chlorothiazide, such studies did not include complete examinations for visceral and skeletal abnormalities. It is not known whether chlorothiazide can cause fetal harm when administered to a pregnant woman; however, thiazides cross the placental barrier and appear in cord blood. DIURIL should be used during pregnancy only if clearly needed (see INDICATIONS AND USAGE).

Nonteratogenic Effects: Chlorothiazide may cause fetal or neonatal jaundice, thrombocytopenia, and possibly other adverse reactions which have occurred in the adult.

Nursing Mothers

Because of the potential for serious adverse reactions in nursing infants from DIURIL, a decision should be made whether to discontinue nursing or to discontinue the drug, taking into account the importance of the drug to the mother.

ADVERSE REACTIONS

The following adverse reactions have been reported and, within each category, are listed in order of decreasing severity.

Body as a Whole: Weakness.

Cardiovascular: Hypotension including orthostatic hypotension (may be aggravated by alcohol, barbiturates, narcotics or antihypertensive drugs).

Digestive: Pancreatitis, jaundice (intrahepatic cholestatic jaundice), diarrhea, vomiting, sialadenitis, cramping, constipation, gastric irritation, nausea, anorexia.

Hematologic: Aplastic anemia, agranulocytosis, leukopenia, hemolytic anemia, thrombocytopenia.

Hypersensitivity: Anaphylactic reactions, necrotizing angiitis (vasculitis and cutaneous vasculitis), respiratory distress including pneumonitis and pulmonary edema, photosensitivity, fever, urticaria, rash, purpura.

Metabolic: Electrolyte imbalance (see PRECAUTIONS), hyperglycemia, glycosuria, hyperuricemia.

Musculoskeletal: Muscle spasm.

Nervous System/Psychiatric: Vertigo, paresthesias, dizziness, headache, restlessness.

Renal: Renal failure, renal dysfunction, interstitial nephritis. (See WARNINGS.)

Skin: Erythema multiforme including Stevens-Johnson syndrome, exfoliative dermatitis including toxic epidermal necrolysis, alopecia.

Special Senses: Transient blurred vision, xanthopsia.

Urogenital: Impotence.

Whenever adverse reactions are moderate or severe, thiazide dosage should be reduced or therapy withdrawn.

OVERDOSAGE

The most common signs and symptoms observed are those caused by electrolyte depletion (hypokalemia, hypochloremia, hyponatremia) and dehydration resulting from excessive diuresis. If digitalis has also been administered, hypokalemia may accentuate cardiac arrhythmias.

In the event of overdosage, symptomatic and supportive measures should be employed. Emesis should be induced or gastric lavage performed. Correct dehydration, electrolyte imbalance, hepatic coma and hypotension by established procedures. If required, give oxygen or artificial respiration for respiratory impairment.

The degree to which chlorothiazide sodium is removed by hemodialysis has not been established.

The oral LD_{50} of chlorothiazide is 8.5 g/kg, greater than 10 g/kg, and greater than 1 g/kg, in the mouse, rat and dog respectively.

DOSAGE AND ADMINISTRATION

Therapy should be individualized according to patient response. Use the smallest dosage necessary to achieve the required response.

Adults

For Edema

The usual adult dosage is 0.5 to 1.0 g once or twice a day. Many patients with edema respond to intermittent therapy, i.e., administration on alternate days or on three to five days each week. With an intermittent schedule, excessive response and the resulting undesirable electrolyte imbalance are less likely to occur.

For Control of Hypertension

The usual adult starting dosage is 0.5 or 1.0 g a day as a single or divided dose. Dosage is increased or decreased according to blood pressure response. Rarely some patients may require up to 2.0 g a day in divided doses.

Pediatric Patients

For Diuresis and For Control of Hypertension

The usual pediatric dosage is 5 to 10 mg per pound (10 to 20 mg/kg) per day in single or two divided doses, not to exceed 375 mg per day (2.5 to 7.5 mL or 1/2 to 1 1/2 teaspoonfuls of the oral suspension daily) in infants up to 2 years of age or 1 g per day in pediatric patients 2 to 12 years of age. In infants less than 6 months of age, doses up to 15 mg per pound (30 mg/kg) per day in two divided doses may be required.

HOW SUPPLIED

No. 3244—Tablets DIURIL, 250 mg, are white, round, scored, compressed tablets, coded MSD 214 on one side and DIURIL on the other. They are supplied as follows:

NDC 0006-0214-68 bottles of 100
NDC 0006-0214-82 bottles of 1000.

Shown in Product Identification Guide, page 323

No. 3245—Tablets DIURIL, 500 mg, are white, round, scored, compressed tablets, coded MSD 432 on one side and DIURIL on the other. They are supplied as follows:

NDC 0006-0432-68 bottles of 100
NDC 0006-0432-82 bottles of 1000
NDC 0006-0432-86 bottles of 5000.

Shown in Product Identification Guide, page 323

No. 3239—Oral Suspension DIURIL, 250 mg of chlorothiazide per 5 mL, is a yellow, creamy suspension, and is supplied as follows:

NDC 0006-3239-66 bottles of 237 mL
(6505-01-156-1600, 250 mg/5 mL, 237 mL).

Storage

Tablets DIURIL: Keep container tightly closed. Protect from moisture, freezing, -20°C (-4°F) and store at room temperature, 15–30°C (59–86°F).

Oral Suspension DIURIL: Keep container tightly closed. Protect from freezing, -20°C (-4°F) and store at room temperature, 15–30°C (59–86°F).

7897958 Issued June 1995

COPYRIGHT © MERCK & CO., INC., 1986
All rights reserved

DOLOBID® Tablets ℞
(Diflunisal), U.S.P.

DESCRIPTION

Diflunisal is 2′, 4′-difluoro-4-hydroxy-3-biphenylcarboxylic acid. Its empirical formula is $C_{13}H_8F_2O_3$ and its structural formula is:

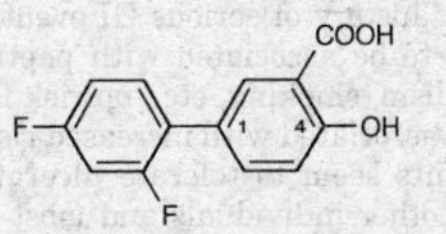

Diflunisal has a molecular weight of 250.20. It is a stable, white, crystalline compound with a melting point of 211–213°C. It is practically insoluble in water at neutral or acidic pH. Because it is an organic acid, it dissolves readily in dilute alkali to give a moderately stable solution at room temperature. It is soluble in most organic solvents including ethanol, methanol, and acetone.

DOLOBID* (Diflunisal) is available in 250 and 500 mg tablets for oral administration. Tablets DOLOBID contain the following inactive ingredients: cellulose, FD&C Yellow 6 hydroxypropyl cellulose, hydroxypropyl methylcellulose, magnesium stearate, starch, talc, and titanium dioxide.

---

*Registered trademark of MERCK & CO., INC.

CLINICAL PHARMACOLOGY

Action

DOLOBID is a non-steroidal drug with analgesic, anti-inflammatory and antipyretic properties. It is a peripherally-acting non-narcotic analgesic drug. Habituation, tolerance and addiction have not been reported.

Diflunisal is a difluorophenyl derivative of salicylic acid. Chemically, diflunisal differs from aspirin (acetylsalicylic acid) in two respects. The first of these two is the presence of a difluorophenyl substituent at carbon 1. The second difference is the removal of the 0-acetyl group from the carbon 4 position. Diflunisal is not metabolized to salicylic acid, and the fluorine atoms are not displaced from the difluorophenyl ring structure.

The precise mechanism of the analgesic and anti-inflammatory actions of diflunisal is not known. Diflunisal is a prostaglandin synthetase inhibitor. In animals, prostaglandins sensitize afferent nerves and potentiate the action of bradykinin in inducing pain. Since prostaglandins are known to be among the mediators of pain and inflammation, the mode of action of diflunisal may be due to a decrease of prostaglandins in peripheral tissues.

Pharmacokinetics and Metabolism

DOLOBID is rapidly and completely absorbed following oral administration with peak plasma concentrations occurring between 2 to 3 hours. The drug is excreted in the urine as two soluble glucuronide conjugates accounting for about 90% of the administered dose. Little or no diflunisal is excreted in the feces. Diflunisal appears in human milk in concentrations of 2–7% of those in plasma. More than 99% of diflunisal in plasma is bound to proteins.

As is the case with salicylic acid, concentration-dependent pharmacokinetics prevail when DOLOBID is administered; a doubling of dosage produces a greater than doubling of drug accumulation. The effect becomes more apparent with repetitive doses. Following single doses, peak plasma concentrations of 41 ± 11 μg/mL (mean ± S.D.) were observed following 250 mg doses, 87 ± 17 μg/mL were observed following 500 mg and 124 ± 11 μg/mL following single 1000 mg doses. However, following administration of 250 mg b.i.d., a mean peak level of 56 ± 14 μg/mL was observed on day 8, while the mean peak level after 500 mg b.i.d. for 11 days was 190 ± 33 μg/mL. In contrast to salicylic acid which has a plasma half-life of 2 1/2 hours, the plasma half-life of diflunisal is 3 to 4 times longer (8 to 12 hours), because of a difluorophenyl substituent at carbon 1. Because of its long half-life and nonlinear pharmacokinetics, several days are required for diflunisal plasma levels to reach steady state following multiple doses. For this reason, an initial loading dose is necessary to shorten the time to reach steady state levels, and 2 to 3 days of observation are necessary for evaluating changes in treatment regimens if a loading dose is not used.

Studies in baboons to determine passage across the blood-brain barrier have shown that only small quantities of diflunisal, under normal or acidotic conditions are transported into the cerebrospinal fluid (CSF). The ratio of blood/CSF concentrations after intravenous doses of 50 mg/kg or oral doses of 100 mg/kg of diflunisal was 100:1. In contrast, oral doses of 500 mg/kg of aspirin resulted in a blood/CSF ratio of 5:1.

Mild to Moderate Pain

DOLOBID is a peripherally-acting analgesic agent with a long duration of action. DOLOBID produces significant analgesia within 1 hour and maximum analgesia within 2 to 3 hours.

Consistent with its long half-life, clinical effects of DOLOBID mirror its pharmacokinetic behavior, which is the basis for recommending a loading dose when instituting therapy. Patients treated with DOLOBID, on the first dose, tend to have a slower onset of pain relief when compared with drugs achieving comparable peak effects. However, DOLOBID produces longer-lasting responses than the comparative agents.

Comparative single dose clinical studies have established the analgesic efficacy of DOLOBID at various dose levels relative to other analgesics. Analgesic effect measurements were derived from hourly evaluations by patients during eight and twelve-hour postdosing observation periods. The following information may serve as a guide for prescribing DOLOBID.

DOLOBID 500 mg was comparable in analgesic efficacy to aspirin 650 mg, acetaminophen 600 mg or 650 mg, and acetaminophen 650 mg with propoxyphene napsylate 100 mg. Patients treated with DOLOBID had longer lasting responses than the patients treated with the comparative analgesics.

DOLOBID 1000 mg was comparable in analgesic efficacy to acetaminophen 600 mg with codeine 60 mg. Patients treated with DOLOBID had longer lasting responses than the patients who received acetaminophen with codeine.

A loading dose of 1000 mg provides faster onset of pain relief, shorter time to peak analgesic effect, and greater peak analgesic effect than an initial 500 mg dose.

Continued on next page

Information on the Merck & Co., Inc. products listed on these pages is the full prescribing information from product circulars in use August 31, 1998. For information, please call 1-800-NSC MERCK [1-800-672-6372].

Dolobid—Cont.

In contrast to the comparative analgesics, a significantly greater proportion of patients treated with DOLOBID did not remedicate and continued to have a good analgesic effect eight to twelve hours after dosing. Seventy-five percent (75%) of patients treated with DOLOBID continued to have a good analgesic response at four hours. When patients having a good analgesic response at four hours were followed, 78% of these patients continued to have a good analgesic response at eight hours and 64% at twelve hours.

Chronic Anti-inflammatory Therapy in Osteoarthritis and Rheumatoid Arthritis

In the controlled, double-blind clinical trials in which DOLOBID (500 mg to 1000 mg a day) was compared with anti-inflammatory doses of aspirin (2–4 grams a day), patients treated with DOLOBID had a significantly lower incidence of tinnitus and of adverse effects involving the gastrointestinal system than patients treated with aspirin. (See also *Effect on Fecal Blood Loss*).

Osteoarthritis

The effectiveness of DOLOBID for the treatment of osteoarthritis was studied in patients with osteoarthritis of the hip and/or knee. The activity of DOLOBID was demonstrated by clinical improvement in the signs and symptoms of disease activity.

In a double-blind multicenter study of 12 weeks' duration in which dosages were adjusted according to patient response, DOLOBID, 500 or 750 mg daily, was shown to be comparable in effectiveness to aspirin, 2000 or 3000 mg daily. In open-label extensions of this study to 24 or 48 weeks, DOLOBID continued to show similar effectiveness and generally was well tolerated.

Rheumatoid Arthritis

In controlled clinical trials, the effectiveness of DOLOBID was established for both acute exacerbations and long-term management of rheumatoid arthritis. The activity of DOLOBID was demonstrated by clinical improvement in the signs and symptoms of disease activity.

In a double-blind multicenter study of 12 weeks' duration in which dosages were adjusted according to patient response, DOLOBID 500 or 750 mg daily was comparable in effectiveness to aspirin 2,600 or 3,900 mg daily. In open-label extensions of this study to 52 weeks, DOLOBID continued to be effective and was generally well tolerated.

DOLOBID 500, 750, or 1000 mg daily was compared with aspirin 2000, 3000, or 4000 mg daily in a multicenter study of 8 weeks' duration in which dosages were adjusted according to patient response. In this study, DOLOBID was comparable in efficacy to aspirin.

In a double-blind multicenter study of 12 weeks' duration in which dosages were adjusted according to patient needs, DOLOBID 500 or 750 mg daily and ibuprofen 1600 or 2400 mg daily were comparable in effectiveness and tolerability.

In a double-blind multicenter study of 12 weeks' duration, DOLOBID 750 mg daily was comparable in efficacy to naproxen 750 mg daily. The incidence of gastrointestinal adverse effects and tinnitus was comparable for both drugs. This study was extended to 48 weeks on an open-label basis. DOLOBID continued to be effective and generally well tolerated.

In patients with rheumatoid arthritis, DOLOBID and gold salts may be used in combination at their usual dosage levels. In clinical studies, DOLOBID added to the regimen of gold salts usually resulted in additional symptomatic relief but did not alter the course of the underlying disease.

Antipyretic Activity

DOLOBID is not recommended for use as an antipyretic agent. In single 250 mg, 500 mg, or 750 mg doses, DOLOBID produced measurable but not clinically useful decreases in temperature in patients with fever; however, the possibility that it may mask fever in some patients, particularly with chronic or high doses, should be considered.

Uricosuric Effect

In normal volunteers, an increase in the renal clearance of uric acid and a decrease in serum uric acid was observed when DOLOBID was administered at 500 mg or 750 mg daily in divided doses. Patients on long-term therapy taking DOLOBID at 500 mg to 1000 mg daily in divided doses showed a prompt and consistent reduction across studies in mean serum uric acid levels, which were lowered as much as 1.4 mg%. It is not known whether DOLOBID interferes with the activity of other uricosuric agents.

Effect on Platelet Function

As an inhibitor of prostaglandin synthetase, DOLOBID has a dose-related effect on platelet function and bleeding time. In normal volunteers, 250 mg b.i.d. for 8 days had no effect on platelet function, and 500 mg b.i.d., the usual recommended dose, had a slight effect. At 1000 mg b.i.d., which exceeds the maximum recommended dosage, however, DOLOBID inhibited platelet function. In contrast to aspirin, these effects of DOLOBID were reversible, because of the absence of the chemically labile and biologically reactive 0-acetyl group at the carbon 4 position. Bleeding time was not altered by a dose of 250 mg b.i.d., and was only slightly

increased at 500 mg b.i.d. At 1000 mg b.i.d., a greater increase occurred, but was not statistically significantly different from the change in the placebo group.

Effect on Fecal Blood Loss

When DOLOBID was given to normal volunteers at the usual recommended dose of 500 mg twice daily, fecal blood loss was not significantly different from placebo. Aspirin at 1000 mg four times daily produced the expected increase in fecal blood loss. DOLOBID at 1000 mg twice daily (NOTE: exceeds the recommended dosage) caused a statistically significant increase in fecal blood loss, but this increase was only one-half as large as that associated with aspirin 1300 mg twice daily.

Effect on Blood Glucose

DOLOBID did not affect fasting blood sugar in diabetic patients who were receiving tolbutamide or placebo.

INDICATIONS AND USAGE

DOLOBID is indicated for acute or long-term use for symptomatic treatment of the following:
1. Mild to moderate pain
2. Osteoarthritis
3. Rheumatoid arthritis

CONTRAINDICATIONS

Patients who are hypersensitive to this product.
Patients in whom acute asthmatic attacks, urticaria, or rhinitis are precipitated by aspirin or other non-steroidal anti-inflammatory drugs.

WARNINGS

Peptic ulceration and gastrointestinal bleeding have been reported in patients receiving DOLOBID. Fatalities have occurred rarely. Gastrointestinal bleeding is associated with higher morbidity and mortality in patients acutely ill with other conditions, the elderly and patients with hemorrhagic disorders. In patients with active gastrointestinal bleeding or an active peptic ulcer, the physician must weigh the benefits of therapy with DOLOBID against possible hazards, institute an appropriate ulcer regimen, and carefully monitor the patient's progress. When DOLOBID is given to patients with a history of either upper or lower gastrointestinal tract disease, it should be given only after consulting the ADVERSE REACTIONS section and under close supervision.

Risk of GI Ulcerations, Bleeding and Perforation with NSAID Therapy

Serious gastrointestinal toxicity such as bleeding, ulceration, and perforation, can occur at any time, with or without warning symptoms, in patients treated chronically with NSAID therapy. Although minor upper gastrointestinal problems, such as dyspepsia, are common, usually developing early in therapy, physicians should remain alert for ulceration and bleeding in patients treated chronically with NSAIDs even in the absence of previous GI tract symptoms. In patients observed in clinical trials of several months to two years duration, symptomatic upper GI ulcers, gross bleeding or perforation appear to occur in approximately 1% of patients treated for 3–6 months, and in about 2–4% of patients treated for one year. Physicians should inform patients about the signs and/or symptoms of serious GI toxicity and what steps to take if they occur.

Studies to date have not identified any subset of patients not at risk of developing peptic ulceration and bleeding. Except for a prior history of serious GI events and other risk factors known to be associated with peptic ulcer disease, such as alcoholism, smoking, etc., no risk factors (e.g., age, sex) have been associated with increased risk. Elderly or debilitated patients seem to tolerate ulceration or bleeding less well than other individuals and most spontaneous reports of fatal GI events are in this population. Studies to date are inconclusive concerning the relative risk of various NSAIDs in causing such reactions. High doses of any NSAID probably carry a greater risk of these reactions, although controlled clinical trials showing this do not exist in most cases. In considering the use of relatively large doses (within the recommended dosage range), sufficient benefit should be anticipated to offset the potential increased risk of GI toxicity.

PRECAUTIONS

General

Non-steroidal anti-inflammatory drugs, including DOLOBID, may mask the usual signs and symptoms of infection. Therefore, the physician must be continually on the alert for this and should use the drug with extra care in the presence of existing infection.

Although DOLOBID has less effect on platelet function and bleeding time than aspirin, at higher doses it is an inhibitor of platelet function; therefore, patients who may be adversely affected should be carefully observed when DOLOBID is administered (see CLINICAL PHARMACOLOGY).

Because of reports of adverse eye findings with agents of this class, it is recommended that patients who develop eye complaints during treatment with DOLOBID have ophthalmologic studies.

Peripheral edema has been observed in some patients taking DOLOBID. Therefore, as with other drugs in this class, DOLOBID should be used with caution in patients with compromised cardiac function, hypertension, or other conditions predisposing to fluid retention.

Acetylsalicylic acid has been associated with Reye syndrome. Because diflunisal is a derivative of salicylic acid, the possibility of its association with Reye syndrome cannot be excluded.

Hypersensitivity Syndrome

A potentially life-threatening, apparent hypersensitivity syndrome has been reported. This multisystem syndrome includes constitutional symptoms (fever, chills), and cutaneous findings (see ADVERSE REACTIONS, *Dermatologic*). It may also include involvement of major organs (changes in liver function, jaundice, leukopenia, thrombocytopenia, eosinophilia, disseminated intravascular coagulation, renal impairment, including renal failure), and less specific findings (adenitis, arthralgia, myalgia, arthritis, malaise, anorexia, disorientation). If evidence of hypersensitivity occurs, therapy with DOLOBID should be discontinued.

Renal Effects

As with other non-steroidal anti-inflammatory drugs, long term administration of diflunisal to animals has resulted in renal papillary necrosis and other abnormal renal pathology. In humans, there have been reports of acute interstitial nephritis with hematuria and proteinuria and occasionally nephrotic syndrome.

A second form of renal toxicity has been seen in patients with prerenal and renal conditions leading to a reduction in renal blood flow or blood volume, where the renal prostaglandins have a supportive role in the maintenance of renal perfusion. In these patients administration of an NSAID may cause a dose dependent reduction in prostaglandin formation and may precipitate overt renal decompensation. Patients at greatest risk of this reaction are those with conditions such as renal or hepatic dysfunction, diabetes mellitus, advanced age, extracellular volume depletion from any cause, congestive heart failure, septicemia, pyelonephritis, or concomitant use of any nephrotoxic drug. DOLOBID or other NSAIDs should be given with caution and renal function should be monitored in any patient who may have reduced renal reserve. Discontinuation of NSAID therapy is typically followed by recovery to the pretreatment state.

Since DOLOBID is eliminated primarily by the kidneys, patients with significantly impaired renal function should be closely monitored; a lower daily dosage should be anticipated to avoid excessive drug accumulation.

Information for Patients

DOLOBID, like other drugs of its class, is not free of side effects. The side effects of these drugs can cause discomfort and, rarely, there are more serious side effects such as gastrointestinal bleeding, which may result in hospitalization and even fatal outcomes.

NSAIDs (Non-steroidal Anti-inflammatory Drugs) are often essential agents in the management of arthritis and have a major role in the treatment of pain, but they also may be commonly employed for conditions which are less serious. Physicians may wish to discuss with their patients the potential risks (see WARNINGS, PRECAUTIONS and ADVERSE REACTIONS) and likely benefits of NSAID treatment, particularly when the drugs are used for less serious conditions where treatment without NSAIDs may represent an acceptable alternative to both the patient and physician.

Laboratory Tests

Liver Function Tests: As with other non-steroidal anti-inflammatory drugs, borderline elevations of one or more liver tests may occur in up to 15% of patients. These abnormalities may progress, may remain essentially unchanged, or may be transient with continued therapy. The SGPT (ALT) test is probably the most sensitive indicator of liver dysfunction. Meaningful (3 times the upper limit of normal) elevations of SGPT or SGOT (AST) occurred in controlled clinical trials in less than 1% of patients. A patient with symptoms and/or signs suggesting liver dysfunction, or in whom an abnormal liver test has occurred, should be evaluated for evidence of the development of more severe hepatic reactions while on therapy with DOLOBID. Severe hepatic reactions, including jaundice, have been reported with DOLOBID as well as with other non-steroidal anti-inflammatory drugs. Although such reactions are rare, if abnormal liver tests persist or worsen, if clinical signs and symptoms consistent with liver disease develop, or if systemic manifestations occur (e.g., eosinophilia, rash, etc.), DOLOBID should be discontinued, since liver reactions can be fatal.

Gastrointestinal: Because serious GI tract ulceration and bleeding can occur without warning symptoms, physicians should follow chronically treated patients for the signs and symptoms of ulceration and bleeding and should inform them of the importance of this follow-up (see WARNINGS, *Risk of GI Ulcerations, Bleeding and Perforation with NSAID Therapy*).

Drug Interactions

Oral Anticoagulants: In some normal volunteers, the concomitant administration of DOLOBID and warfarin, acenocoumarol, or phenprocoumon resulted in prolongation of prothrombin time. This may occur because diflunisal competitively displaces coumarins from protein binding sites. Accordingly, when DOLOBID is administered with oral anticoagulants, the prothrombin time should be closely monitored during and for several days after concomitant drug administration. Adjustment of dosage of oral anticoagulants may be required.

Tolbutamide: In diabetic patients receiving DOLOBID and tolbutamide, no significant effects were seen on tolbutamide plasma levels or fasting blood glucose.

Hydrochlorothiazide: In normal volunteers, concomitant administration of DOLOBID and hydrochlorothiazide resulted in significantly increased plasma levels of hydrochlorothiazide. DOLOBID decreased the hyperuricemic effect of hydrochlorothiazide.

Furosemide: In normal volunteers, the concomitant administration of DOLOBID and furosemide had no effect on the diuretic activity of furosemide. DOLOBID decreased the hyperuricemic effect of furosemide.

Antacids: Concomitant administration of antacids may reduce plasma levels of DOLOBID. This effect is small with occasional doses of antacids, but may be clinically significant when antacids are used on a continuous schedule.

Acetaminophen: In normal volunteers, concomitant administration of DOLOBID and acetaminophen resulted in an approximate 50% increase in plasma levels of acetaminophen. Acetaminophen had no effect on plasma levels of DOLOBID. Since acetaminophen in high doses has been associated with hepatotoxicity, concomitant administration of DOLOBID and acetaminophen should be used cautiously, with careful monitoring of patients.

Concomitant administration of DOLOBID and acetaminophen in dogs, but not in rats, at approximately 2 times the recommended maximum human therapeutic dose of each (40-52 mg/kg/day of DOLOBID/acetaminophen), resulted in greater gastrointestinal toxicity than when either drug was administered alone. The clinical significance of these findings has not been established.

Methotrexate: Caution should be used if DOLOBID is administered concomitantly with methotrexate. Non-steroidal anti-inflammatory drugs have been reported to decrease the tubular secretion of methotrexate and to potentiate its toxicity.

Cyclosporine: Administration of non-steroidal anti-inflammatory drugs concomitantly with cyclosporine has been associated with an increase in cyclosporine-induced toxicity, possibly due to decreased synthesis of renal prostacyclin. NSAIDs should be used with caution in patients taking cyclosporine, and renal function should be carefully monitored.

Drug Interactions: Non-steroidal Anti-inflammatory Drugs

The administration of diflunisal to normal volunteers receiving indomethacin decreased the renal clearance and significantly increased the plasma levels of indomethacin. In some patients the combined use of indomethacin and DOLOBID has been associated with fatal gastrointestinal hemorrhage. Therefore, indomethacin and DOLOBID should not be used concomitantly.

The concomitant use of DOLOBID and other NSAIDs is not recommended due to the increased possibility of gastrointestinal toxicity, with little or no increase in efficacy. The following information was obtained from studies in normal volunteers.

Aspirin: In normal volunteers, a small decrease in diflunisal levels was observed when multiple doses of DOLOBID and aspirin were administered concomitantly.

Sulindac: The concomitant administration of DOLOBID and sulindac in normal volunteers resulted in lowering of the plasma levels of the active sulindac sulfide metabolite by approximately one-third.

Naproxen: The concomitant administration of DOLOBID and naproxen in normal volunteers had no effect on the plasma levels of naproxen, but significantly decreased the urinary excretion of naproxen and its glucuronide metabolite. Naproxen had no effect on plasma levels of DOLOBID.

Drug/Laboratory Test Interactions

Serum Salicylate Assays: Caution should be used in interpreting the results of serum salicylate assays when diflunisal is present. Salicylate levels have been found to be falsely elevated with some assay methods.

Carcinogenesis, Mutagenesis, Impairment of Fertility

Diflunisal did not affect the type or incidence of neoplasia in a 105-week study in the rat given doses up to 40 mg/kg/day (equivalent to approximately 1.3 times the maximum recommended human dose), or in long-term carcinogenic studies in mice given diflunisal at doses up to 80 mg/kg/day (equivalent to approximately 2.7 times the maximum recommended human dose). It was concluded that there was no carcinogenic potential for DOLOBID.

Diflunisal passes the placental barrier to a minor degree in the rat. Diflunisal had no mutagenic activity after oral administration in the dominant lethal assay, in the Ames microbial mutagen test or in the V-79 Chinese hamster lung cell assay.

No evidence of impaired fertility was found in reproduction studies in rats at doses up to 50 mg/kg/day.

Pregnancy

Pregnancy Category C. A dose of 60 mg/kg/day of diflunisal (equivalent to two times the maximum human dose) was maternotoxic, embryotoxic, and teratogenic in rabbits. In three of six studies in rabbits, evidence of teratogenicity was observed at doses ranging from 40 to 50 mg/kg/day. Teratology studies in mice, at doses up to 45 mg/kg/day, and in rats at doses up to 100 mg/kg/day, revealed no harm to the fetus due to diflunisal. Aspirin and other salicylates have been shown to be teratogenic in a wide variety of species, including the rat and rabbit, at doses ranging from 50 to 400 mg/kg/day (approximately one to eight times the human dose). There are no adequate and well controlled studies with diflunisal in pregnant women. DOLOBID should be used during the first two trimesters of pregnancy only if the potential benefit justifies the potential risk to the fetus. The known effects of drugs of this class on the human fetus during the third trimester of pregnancy include: constriction of the ductus arteriosus prenatally, tricuspid incompetence, and pulmonary hypertension; non-closure of the ductus arteriosus postnatally which may be resistant to medical management; myocardial degenerative changes, platelet dysfunction with resultant bleeding, intracranial bleeding, renal dysfunction or failure, renal injury/dysgenesis which may result in prolonged or permanent renal failure, oligohydramnios, gastrointestinal bleeding or perforation, and increased risk of necrotizing enterocolitis. Use during the third trimester of pregnancy is not recommended.

In rats at a dose of one and one-half times the maximum human dose, there was an increase in the average length of gestation. Similar increases in the length of gestation have been observed with aspirin, indomethacin, and phenylbutazone, and may be related to inhibition of prostaglandin synthetase. Drugs of this class may cause dystocia and delayed parturition in pregnant animals.

Nursing Mothers

Diflunisal is excreted in human milk in concentrations of 2–7% of those in plasma. Because of the potential for serious adverse reactions in nursing infants from DOLOBID, a decision should be made whether to discontinue nursing or to discontinue the drug, taking into account the importance of the drug to the mother.

Pediatric Use

Safety and effectiveness of DOLOBID in pediatric patients have not been established. Use of DOLOBID in pediatric patients below the age of 12 years is not recommended.

The adverse effects observed following diflunisal administration to neonatal animals appear to be species, age, and dose-dependent. At dose levels approximately 3 times the usual human therapeutic dose, both aspirin (200 to 400 mg/kg/ day) and diflunisal (80 mg/kg/day) resulted in death, leukocytosis, weight loss, and bilateral cataracts in neonatal (4 to 5-day-old) beagle puppies after 2 to 10 doses. Administration of an 80 mg/kg/day dose of diflunisal to 25-day-old puppies resulted in lower mortality, and did not produce cataracts. In newborn rats, a 400 mg/kg/day dose of aspirin resulted in increased mortality and some cataracts, whereas the effects of diflunisal administration at doses up to 140 mg/kg/day were limited to a decrease in average body weight gain.

ADVERSE REACTIONS

The adverse reactions observed in controlled clinical trials encompass observations in 2,427 patients.

Listed below are the adverse reactions reported in the 1,314 of these patients who received treatment in studies of two weeks or longer. Five hundred thirteen patients were treated for at least 24 weeks, 255 patients were treated for at least 48 weeks, and 46 patients were treated for 96 weeks. In general, the adverse reactions listed below were 2 to 14 times less frequent in the 1,113 patients who received short-term treatment for mild to moderate pain.

Incidence Greater Than 1%

Gastrointestinal

The most frequent types of adverse reactions occurring with DOLOBID are gastrointestinal: these include nausea*, vomiting, dyspepsia*, gastrointestinal pain*, diarrhea*, constipation, and flatulence.

Psychiatric

Somnolence, insomnia.

Central Nervous System

Dizziness.

Special Senses

Tinnitus.

Dermatologic

Rash*.

Miscellaneous

Headache*, fatigue/tiredness.

Incidence Less Than 1 in 100

The following adverse reactions, occurring less frequently than 1 in 100, were reported in clinical trials or since the drug was marketed. The probability exists of a causal relationship between DOLOBID and these adverse reactions.

Dermatologic

Erythema multiforme, exfoliative dermatitis, Stevens-Johnson syndrome, toxic epidermal necrolysis, urticaria, pruritus, sweating, dry mucous membranes, stomatitis, photosensitivity.

Gastrointestinal

Peptic ulcer, gastrointestinal bleeding, anorexia, eructation, gastrointestinal perforation, gastritis.

Liver function abnormalities; jaundice, sometimes with fever; cholestasis; hepatitis.

Hematologic

Thrombocytopenia; agranulocytosis; hemolytic anemia.

Genitourinary

Dysuria; renal impairment, including renal failure; interstitial nephritis; hematuria; proteinuria.

Psychiatric

Nervousness, depression, hallucinations, confusion, disorientation.

Central Nervous System

Vertigo; light-headedness; paresthesias.

Special Senses

Transient visual disturbances including blurred vision.

Hypersensitivity Reactions

Acute anaphylactic reaction with bronchospasm; angioedema; flushing.

Hypersensitivity vasculitis.

Hypersensitivity syndrome (see PRECAUTIONS).

Miscellaneous

Asthenia, edema.

Causal Relationship Unknown

Other reactions have been reported in clinical trials or since the drug was marketed, but occurred under circumstances where a causal relationship could not be established. However, in these rarely reported events, that possibility cannot be excluded. Therefore, these observations are listed to serve as alerting information to physicians.

Respiratory

Dyspnea.

Cardiovascular

Palpitation, syncope.

Musculoskeletal

Muscle cramps.

Genitourinary

Nephrotic syndrome.

Special Senses

Hearing loss.

Miscellaneous

Chest pain.

A rare occurrence of fulminant necrotizing fasciitis, particularly in association with Group A β-hemolytic streptococcus, has been described in persons treated with non-steroidal anti-inflammatory agents, including diflunisal, sometimes with fatal outcome (see also PRECAUTIONS, *General*).

Potential Adverse Effects

In addition, a variety of adverse effects not observed with DOLOBID in clinical trials or in marketing experience, but reported with other non-steroidal analgesic/anti-inflammatory agents, should be considered potential adverse effects of DOLOBID.

*Incidence between 3% and 9%. Those reactions occurring in 1% to 3% are not marked with an asterisk.

OVERDOSAGE

Cases of overdosage have occurred and deaths have been reported. Most patients recovered without evidence of permanent sequelae. The most common signs and symptoms observed with overdosage were drowsiness, vomiting, nausea, diarrhea, hyperventilation, tachycardia, sweating, tinnitus, disorientation, stupor and coma. Diminished urine output and cardiorespiratory arrest have also been reported. The lowest dosage of DOLOBID at which a death has been reported was 15 grams without the presence of other drugs. In a mixed drug overdose, ingestion of 7.5 grams of DOLOBID resulted in death.

In the event of overdosage, the stomach should be emptied by inducing vomiting or by gastric lavage, and the patient carefully observed and given symptomatic and supportive treatment. Because of the high degree of protein binding, hemodialysis may not be effective.

Continued on next page

Information on the Merck & Co., Inc. products listed on these pages is the full prescribing information from product circulars in use August 31, 1998. For information, please call 1-800-NSC MERCK [1-800-672-6372].

Dolobid—Cont.

The oral LD_{50} of the drug is 500 mg/kg and 826 mg/kg in female mice and female rats respectively.

DOSAGE AND ADMINISTRATION

Concentration-dependent pharmacokinetics prevail when DOLOBID is administered; a doubling of dosage produces a greater than doubling of drug accumulation. The effect becomes more apparent with repetitive doses.
For mild to moderate pain, an initial dose of 1000 mg followed by 500 mg every 12 hours is recommended for most patients. Following the initial dose, some patients may require 500 mg every 8 hours.
A lower dosage may be appropriate depending on such factors as pain severity, patient response, weight, or advanced age; for example, 500 mg initially, followed by 250 mg every 8–12 hours.
For osteoarthritis and rheumatoid arthritis, the suggested dosage range is 500 mg to 1000 mg daily in two divided doses. The dosage of DOLOBID may be increased or decreased according to patient response.
Maintenance doses higher than 1500 mg a day are not recommended.
DOLOBID may be administered with water, milk or meals. Tablets should be swallowed whole, not crushed or chewed.

HOW SUPPLIED

Tablets DOLOBID are capsule-shaped, film-coated tablets supplied as follows:
No. 3390—250 mg peach colored, coded DOLOBID on one side and MSD 675 on the other.
NDC 0006-0675-61 unit of use bottles of 60
(6505-01-164-0501, 250 mg 60's).
Shown in Product Identification Guide, page 323
No. 3392—500 mg orange colored, coded DOLOBID on one side and MSD 697 on the other.
NDC 0006-0697-61 unit of use bottles of 60
(6505-01-144-9724, 500 mg 60's).
Shown in Product Identification Guide, page 323
7928832 Issued February 1997
COPYRIGHT © MERCK & CO., INC., 1988
All rights reserved

EDECRIN® Tablets ℞
(Ethacrynic Acid), U.S.P.

Intravenous
SODIUM EDECRIN® ℞
(Ethacrynate Sodium), U.S.P.

EDECRIN* (Ethacrynic Acid) is a potent diuretic which, if given in excessive amounts, may lead to profound diuresis with water and electrolyte depletion. Therefore, careful medical supervision is required, and dose and dose schedule must be adjusted to the individual patient's needs (see DOSAGE AND ADMINISTRATION).

DESCRIPTION

Ethacrynic acid is an unsaturated ketone derivative of an aryloxyacetic acid. It is designated chemically as [2,3-dichloro-4-(2-methylene-1-oxobutyl)phenoxy] acetic acid, and has a molecular weight of 303.14. Ethacrynic acid is a white, or practically white, crystalline powder, very slightly soluble in water, but soluble in most organic solvents such as alcohols, chloroform, and benzene. Its empirical formula is $C_{13}H_{12}Cl_2O_4$ and its structural formula is:

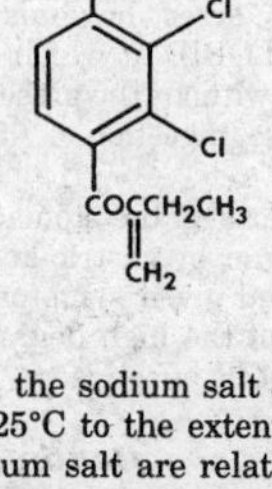

Ethacrynate sodium, the sodium salt of ethacrynic acid, is soluble in water at 25°C to the extent of about 7 percent. Solutions of the sodium salt are relatively stable at about pH 7 at room temperature for short periods, but as the pH or temperature increases the solutions are less stable. The molecular weight of ethacrynate sodium is 325.12. Its empirical formula is $C_{13}H_{11}Cl_2NaO_4$ and its structural formula is:
[See chemical structure at top of next column]

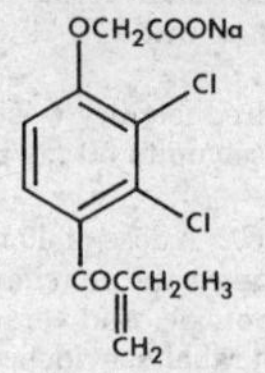

EDECRIN is supplied as 25 mg and 50 mg tablets for oral use. Each tablet contains the following inactive ingredients: colloidal silicon dioxide, lactose, magnesium stearate, starch and talc. The 50 mg tablet also contains D&C Yellow 10, FD&C Blue 1 and FD&C Yellow 6. Intravenous SODIUM EDECRIN* (Ethacrynate Sodium) is a sterile freeze-dried powder and is supplied in a vial containing:
Ethacrynate sodium equivalent to ethacrynic acid .... 50.0 mg
Inactive ingredients:
Mannitol .... 62.5 mg

*Registered trademark of MERCK & CO., INC.

CLINICAL PHARMACOLOGY

Pharmacokinetics and Metabolism
EDECRIN acts on the ascending limb of the loop of Henle and on the proximal and distal tubules. Urinary output is usually dose dependent and related to the magnitude of fluid accumulation. Water and electrolyte excretion may be increased several times over that observed with thiazide diuretics, since EDECRIN inhibits reabsorption of a much greater proportion of filtered sodium than most other diuretic agents. Therefore, EDECRIN is effective in many patients who have significant degrees of renal insufficiency (see WARNINGS concerning deafness). EDECRIN has little or no effect on glomerular filtration or on renal blood flow, except following pronounced reductions in plasma volume when associated with rapid diuresis.
The electrolyte excretion pattern of ethacrynic acid varies from that of the thiazides and mercurial diuretics. Initial sodium and chloride excretion is usually substantial and chloride loss exceeds that of sodium. With prolonged administration, chloride excretion declines, and potassium and hydrogen ion excretion may increase. EDECRIN is effective whether or not there is clinical acidosis or alkalosis.
Although EDECRIN, in carefully controlled studies in animals and experimental subjects, produces a more favorable sodium/potassium excretion ratio than the thiazides, in patients with increased diuresis excessive amounts of potassium may be excreted.
Onset of action is rapid, usually within 30 minutes after an oral dose of EDECRIN or within 5 minutes after an intravenous injection of SODIUM EDECRIN. After oral use, diuresis peaks in about 2 hours and lasts about 6 to 8 hours.
The sulfhydryl binding propensity of ethacrynic acid differs somewhat from that of the organomercurials. Its mode of action is not by carbonic anhydrase inhibition.
Ethacrynic acid does not cross the blood-brain barrier.

INDICATIONS AND USAGE

EDECRIN is indicated for treatment of edema when an agent with greater diuretic potential than those commonly employed is required.
1. Treatment of the edema associated with congestive heart failure, cirrhosis of the liver, and renal disease, including the nephrotic syndrome.
2. Short-term management of ascites due to malignancy, idiopathic edema, and lymphedema.
3. Short-term management of hospitalized pediatric patients, other than infants, with congenital heart disease or the nephrotic syndrome.
4. Intravenous SODIUM EDECRIN is indicated when a rapid onset of diuresis is desired, e.g., in acute pulmonary edema, or when gastrointestinal absorption is impaired or oral medication is not practicable.

CONTRAINDICATIONS

All diuretics, including ethacrynic acid, are contraindicated in anuria. If increasing electrolyte imbalance, azotemia, and/or oliguria occur during treatment of severe, progressive renal disease, the diuretic should be discontinued.
In a few patients this diuretic has produced severe, watery diarrhea. If this occurs, it should be discontinued and not used again.
Until further experience in infants is accumulated, therapy with oral and parenteral EDECRIN is contraindicated.
Hypersensitivity to any component of this product.

WARNINGS

The effects of EDECRIN on electrolytes are related to its renal pharmacologic activity and are dose dependent. The possibility of profound electrolyte and water loss may be avoided by weighing the patient throughout the treatment period, by careful adjustment of dosage, by initiating treatment with small doses, and by using the drug on an intermittent schedule when possible. When excessive diuresis occurs, the drug should be withdrawn until homeostasis is restored. When excessive electrolyte loss occurs, the dosage should be reduced or the drug temporarily withdrawn.
Initiation of diuretic therapy with EDECRIN in the cirrhotic patient with ascites is best carried out in the hospital. When maintenance therapy has been established, the individual can be satisfactorily followed as an outpatient.
EDECRIN should be given with caution to patients with advanced cirrhosis of the liver, particularly those with a history of previous episodes of electrolyte imbalance or hepatic encephalopathy. Like other diuretics it may precipitate hepatic coma and death.
Too vigorous a diuresis, as evidenced by rapid and excessive weight loss, may induce an acute hypotensive episode. In elderly cardiac patients, rapid contraction of plasma volume and the resultant hemoconcentration should be avoided to prevent the development of thromboembolic episodes, such as cerebral vascular thromboses and pulmonary emboli which may be fatal. Excessive loss of potassium in patients receiving digitalis glycosides may precipitate digitalis toxicity. Care should also be exercised in patients receiving potassium-depleting steroids.
A number of possibly drug-related deaths have occurred in critically ill patients refractory to other diuretics. These generally have fallen into two categories: (1) patients with severe myocardial disease who have been receiving digitalis and presumably developed acute hypokalemia with fatal arrhythmia; (2) patients with severely decompensated hepatic cirrhosis with ascites, with or without accompanying encephalopathy, who were in electrolyte imbalance and died because of intensification of the electrolyte defect.
Deafness, tinnitus, and vertigo with a sense of fullness in the ears have occurred, most frequently in patients with severe impairment of renal function. These symptoms have been associated most often with intravenous administration and with doses in excess of those recommended. The deafness has usually been reversible and of short duration (one to 24 hours). However, in some patients the hearing loss has been permanent. A number of these patients were also receiving drugs known to be ototoxic. EDECRIN may increase the ototoxic potential of other drugs (see PRECAUTIONS, subsection *Drug Interactions*).
Lithium generally should not be given with diuretics (see PRECAUTIONS, subsection *Drug Interactions*).

PRECAUTIONS

General
Weakness, muscle cramps, paresthesias, thirst, anorexia, and signs of hyponatremia, hypokalemia, and/or hypochloremic alkalosis may occur following vigorous or excessive diuresis and these may be accentuated by rigid salt restriction. Rarely tetany has been reported following vigorous diuresis. *During therapy with ethacrynic acid, liberalization of salt intake and supplementary potassium chloride are often necessary.*
When a metabolic alkalosis may be anticipated, e.g., in cirrhosis with ascites, the use of potassium chloride or a potassium-sparing agent before and during therapy with EDECRIN may mitigate or prevent the hypokalemia.
Loop diuretics have been shown to increase the urinary excretion of magnesium; this may result in hypomagnesemia.
The safety and efficacy of ethacrynic acid in hypertension have not been established. However, the dosage of coadministered antihypertensive agents may require adjustment.
Orthostatic hypotension may occur in patients receiving other antihypertensive agents when given ethacrynic acid.
EDECRIN has little or no effect on glomerular filtration or on renal blood flow, except following pronounced reductions in plasma volume when associated with rapid diuresis. A transient increase in serum urea nitrogen may occur. Usually, this is readily reversible when the drug is discontinued.
As with other diuretics used in the treatment of renal edema, hypoproteinemia may reduce responsiveness to ethacrynic acid and the use of salt-poor albumin should be considered.
A number of drugs, including ethacrynic acid, have been shown to displace warfarin from plasma protein; a reduction in the usual anticoagulant dosage may be required in patients receiving both drugs.
EDECRIN may increase the risk of gastric hemorrhage associated with corticosteroid treatment.
Laboratory Tests
Frequent serum electrolyte, CO_2 and BUN determinations should be performed early in therapy and periodically thereafter during active diuresis. Any electrolyte abnormalities should be corrected or the drug temporarily withdrawn.
Increases in blood glucose and alterations in glucose tolerance tests have been observed in patients receiving EDECRIN.

Drug Interactions
Lithium generally should not be given with diuretics because they reduce its renal clearance and add a high risk of lithium toxicity. Read circulars for lithium preparations before use of such concomitant therapy.
EDECRIN may increase the ototoxic potential of other drugs such as aminoglycoside and some cephalosporin antibiotics. Their concurrent use should be avoided.
A number of drugs, including ethacrynic acid, have been shown to displace warfarin from plasma protein; a reduction in the usual anticoagulant dosage may be required in patients receiving both drugs.
In some patients, the administration of a non-steroidal anti-inflammatory agent can reduce the diuretic, natriuretic, and antihypertensive effects of loop, potassium-sparing and thiazide diuretics. Therefore, when EDECRIN and non-steroidal anti-inflammatory agents are used concomitantly, the patient should be observed closely to determine if the desired effect of the diuretic is obtained.
Carcinogenesis, Mutagenesis, Impairment of Fertility
There was no evidence of a tumorigenic effect in a 79-week oral chronic toxicity study in rats at doses up to 45 times the human dose.
Ethacrynic acid had no effect on fertility in a two-litter study in rats or a two-generation study in mice at 10 times the human dose.
Pregnancy
Pregnancy Category B: Reproduction studies in the mouse and rabbit at doses up to 50 times the human dose showed no evidence of external abnormalities of the fetus due to EDECRIN.
In a two-litter study in the dog and rat, oral doses of 5 or 20 mg/kg/day ($2^1/_2$ or 10 times the human dose), respectively, did not interfere with pregnancy or with growth and development of the pups. Although there was reduction in the mean body weights of the fetuses in a teratogenic study in the rat at a dose level of 100 mg/kg (50 times the human dose), there was no effect on mortality or postnatal development. Functional and morphologic abnormalities were not observed.
There are, however, no adequate and well-controlled studies in pregnant women. Since animal reproduction studies are not always predictive of human response, EDECRIN should be used during pregnancy only if clearly needed.
Nursing Mothers
It is not known whether this drug is excreted in human milk. Because many drugs are excreted in human milk and because of the potential for serious adverse reactions in nursing infants from EDECRIN, a decision should be made whether to discontinue nursing or to discontinue the drug, taking into account the importance of the drug to the mother.
Pediatric Use
There are no well-controlled clinical trials in pediatric patients. The information on oral dosing in pediatric patients, other than infants, is supported by evidence from empiric use in this age group.
For information on oral use in pediatric patients, other than infants, see INDICATIONS AND USAGE and DOSAGE AND ADMINISTRATION.
Safety and effectiveness of oral and parenteral use in infants have not been established (see CONTRAINDICATIONS).
Safety and effectiveness of intravenous use in pediatric patients have not been established (see DOSAGE AND ADMINISTRATION, *Intravenous Use).*

ADVERSE REACTIONS

Gastrointestinal
Anorexia, malaise, abdominal discomfort or pain, dysphagia, nausea, vomiting, and diarrhea have occurred. These are more frequent with large doses or after one to three months of continuous therapy. A few patients have had sudden onset of profuse, watery diarrhea. Discontinue EDECRIN if diarrhea is severe and do not give it again. Gastrointestinal bleeding has occurred in some patients. Rarely, acute pancreatitis has been reported.
Metabolic
Reversible hyperuricemia and acute gout have been reported. Acute symptomatic hypoglycemia with convulsions occurred in two uremic patients who received doses above those recommended. Hyperglycemia has been reported. Rarely, jaundice and abnormal liver function tests have been reported in seriously ill patients receiving multiple drug therapy, including EDECRIN.
Hematologic
Agranulocytosis or severe neutropenia has been reported in a few critically ill patients also receiving agents known to produce this effect. Thrombocytopenia has been reported rarely. Henoch-Schönlein purpura has been reported rarely in patients with rheumatic heart disease receiving multiple drug therapy, including EDECRIN.
Special Senses (See WARNINGS)
Deafness, tinnitus and vertigo with a sense of fullness in the ears, and blurred vision have occurred.
Central Nervous System
Headache, fatigue, apprehension, confusion.
Miscellaneous
Skin rash, fever, chills, hematuria.
SODIUM EDECRIN occasionally has caused local irritation and pain after intravenous use.

OVERDOSAGE

Overdosage may lead to excessive diuresis with electrolyte depletion and dehydration.
In the event of overdosage, symptomatic and supportive measures should be employed. Emesis should be induced or gastric lavage performed. Correct dehydration, electrolyte imbalance, hepatic coma, and hypotension by established procedures. If required, give oxygen or artificial respiration for respiratory impairment.
In the mouse, the oral LD_{50} of ethacrynic acid is 627 mg/kg and the intravenous LD_{50} of ethacrynate sodium is 175 mg/kg.

DOSAGE AND ADMINISTRATION

Dosage must be regulated carefully to prevent a more rapid or substantial loss of fluid or electrolyte than is indicated or necessary. The magnitude of diuresis and natriuresis is largely dependent on the degree of fluid accumulation present in the patient. Similarly, the extent of potassium excretion is determined in large measure by the presence and magnitude of aldosteronism.
Oral Use
EDECRIN is available for oral use as 25 mg and 50 mg tablets.
Dosage: To Initiate Diuresis
In Adults: The smallest dose required to produce gradual weight loss (about 1 to 2 pounds per day) is recommended. Onset of diuresis usually occurs at 50 to 100 mg for adults. After diuresis has been achieved, the minimally effective dose (usually from 50 to 200 mg daily) may be given on a continuous or intermittent dosage schedule. Dosage adjustments are usually in 25 to 50 mg increments to avoid derangement of water and electrolyte excretion.
The patient should be weighed under standard conditions before and during the institution of diuretic therapy with this compound. Small alterations in dose should effectively prevent a massive diuretic response. The following schedule may be helpful in determining the smallest effective dose.

Day 1— 50 mg (single dose) after a meal
Day 2— 50 mg twice daily after meals, if necessary
Day 3— 100 mg in the morning and 50 to 100 mg following the afternoon or evening meal, depending upon response to the morning dose

A few patients may require initial and maintenance doses as high as 200 mg twice daily. These higher doses, which should be achieved gradually, are most often required in patients with severe, refractory edema.
In Pediatric Patients (excluding infants, see CONTRAINDICATIONS): The initial dose should be 25 mg. Careful stepwise increments in dosage of 25 mg should be made to achieve effective maintenance.
Maintenance Therapy
It is usually possible to reduce the dosage and frequency of administration once dry weight has been achieved.
EDECRIN (Ethacrynic Acid) may be given intermittently after an effective diuresis is obtained with the regimen outlined above. Dosage may be on an alternate daily schedule or more prolonged periods of diuretic therapy may be interspersed with rest periods. Such an intermittent dosage schedule allows time for correction of any electrolyte imbalance and may provide a more efficient diuretic response.
The chloruretic effect of this agent may give rise to retention of bicarbonate and a metabolic alkalosis. This may be corrected by giving chloride (ammonium chloride or arginine chloride). Ammonium chloride should not be given to cirrhotic patients.
EDECRIN has additive effects when used with other diuretics. For example, a patient who is on maintenance dosage of an oral diuretic may require additional intermittent diuretic therapy, such as an organomercurial, for the maintenance of basal weight. The intermittent use of EDECRIN orally may eliminate the need for injections of organomercurials. Small doses of EDECRIN may be added to existing diuretic regimens to maintain basal weight. This drug may potentiate the action of carbonic anhydrase inhibitors, with augmentation of natriuresis and kaliuresis. Therefore, when adding EDECRIN the initial dose and changes of dose should be in 25 mg increments, to avoid electrolyte depletion. Rarely, patients who failed to respond to ethacrynic acid have responded to older established agents.
While many patients do not require supplemental potassium, the use of potassium chloride or potassium-sparing agents, or both, during treatment with EDECRIN is advisable, especially in cirrhotic or nephrotic patients and in patients receiving digitalis.
Salt liberalization usually prevents the development of hyponatremia and hypochloremia. During treatment with EDECRIN, salt may be liberalized to a greater extent than with other diuretics. Cirrhotic patients, however, usually require at least moderate salt restriction concomitant with diuretic therapy.
Intravenous Use
Intravenous SODIUM EDECRIN is for intravenous use when oral intake is impractical or in urgent conditions, such as acute pulmonary edema.
The usual intravenous dose for the average sized adult is 50 mg, or 0.5 to 1.0 mg per kg of body weight. Usually only one dose has been necessary; occasionally a second dose at a new injection site, to avoid possible thrombophlebitis, may be required. A single intravenous dose not exceeding 100 mg has been used in critical situations.
Insufficient pediatric experience precludes recommendation for this age group.
To reconstitute the dry material, add 50 mL of 5 percent Dextrose Injection, or Sodium Chloride Injection to the vial. Occasionally, some 5 percent Dextrose Injection solutions may have a low pH (below 5). The resulting solution with such a diluent may be hazy or opalescent. Intravenous use of such a solution is not recommended. Inspect the vial containing Intravenous SODIUM EDECRIN for particulate matter and discoloration before use.
The solution may be given slowly through the tubing of a running infusion or by direct intravenous injection over a period of several minutes. Do not mix this solution with whole blood or its derivatives. Discard unused reconstituted solution after 24 hours.
SODIUM EDECRIN should not be given subcutaneously or intramuscularly because of local pain and irritation.

HOW SUPPLIED

No. 3321—Tablets EDECRIN, 25 mg, are white, capsule shaped, scored tablets, coded MSD 65 on one side and EDECRIN on the other. They are supplied as follows:
NDC 0006-0065-68 in bottles of 100.
Shown in Product Identification Guide, page 323
No. 3322—Tablets EDECRIN, 50 mg, are green, capsule shaped, scored tablets, coded MSD 90 on one side and EDECRIN on the other. They are supplied as follows:
NDC 0006-0090-68 in bottles of 100
(6505-00-834-0473, 50 mg bottles of 100).
Shown in Product Identification Guide, page 323
No. 3620—Intravenous SODIUM EDECRIN is a dry white material either in a plug form or as a powder. It is supplied in vials containing ethacrynate sodium equivalent to 50 mg of ethacrynic acid, **NDC** 0006-3620-50.
7901427 Issued June 1997
COPYRIGHT © MERCK & CO., INC., 1984
All rights reserved

ELSPAR® ℞
(Asparaginase)

WARNING

IT IS RECOMMENDED THAT ASPARAGINASE BE ADMINISTERED TO PATIENTS ONLY IN A HOSPITAL SETTING UNDER THE SUPERVISION OF A PHYSICIAN WHO IS QUALIFIED BY TRAINING AND EXPERIENCE TO ADMINISTER CANCER CHEMOTHERAPEUTIC AGENTS, BECAUSE OF THE POSSIBILITY OF SEVERE REACTIONS, INCLUDING ANAPHYLAXIS AND SUDDEN DEATH. THE PHYSICIAN MUST BE PREPARED TO TREAT ANAPHYLAXIS AT EACH ADMINISTRATION OF THE DRUG.
IN THE TREATMENT OF EACH PATIENT THE PHYSICIAN MUST WEIGH CAREFULLY THE POSSIBILITY OF ACHIEVING THERAPEUTIC BENEFIT VERSUS THE RISK OF TOXICITY. THE FOLLOWING DATA SHOULD BE THOROUGHLY REVIEWED BEFORE ADMINISTERING THE COMPOUND.

DESCRIPTION

ELSPAR* (Asparaginase) contains the enzyme L-asparagine amidohydrolase, type EC-2, derived from *Escherichia coli.* It is a white crystalline powder that is freely soluble in water and practically insoluble in methanol, acetone and chloroform. Its activity is expressed in terms of International Units (I.U.) according to the recommendation of the International Union of Biochemistry. The specific activity of ELSPAR is at least 225 I.U. per milligram of protein and each vial contains 10,000 I.U. of asparaginase and 80 mg of mannitol, an inactive ingredient, as a sterile, white lyophilized plug or powder for intravenous or intramuscular injection after reconstitution.

*Registered trademark of MERCK & CO., INC.

Continued on next page

Information on the Merck & Co., Inc. products listed on these pages is the full prescribing information from product circulars in use August 31, 1998. For information, please call 1-800-NSC MERCK [1-800-672-6372].

Elspar—Cont.

CLINICAL PHARMACOLOGY

Action

In a significant number of patients with acute leukemia, particularly lymphocytic, the malignant cells are dependent on an exogenous source of asparagine for survival. Normal cells, however, are able to synthesize asparagine and thus are affected less by the rapid depletion produced by treatment with the enzyme asparaginase. This is a unique approach to therapy based on a metabolic defect in asparagine synthesis of some malignant cells. ELSPAR, derived from *Escherichia coli*, is effective in inducing remissions in some patients with acute lymphocytic leukemia.

Asparagine Dependence Test

An asparagine dependence test has been utilized during the investigational studies. In this test leukemic cells obtained from some marrow cultures could be shown to require asparagine in *vitro,* suggesting sensitivity to asparaginase therapy in *vivo.* However, present data indicate that the correlation between asparagine dependence in such tests and the final response to therapy is sufficiently poor that the test is not recommended as a basis for selection of patients for treatment.

Pharmacokinetics and Metabolism

In a study in patients with metastatic cancer and leukemia, initial plasma levels of L-asparaginase following intravenous administration were correlated to dose. Daily administration resulted in a cumulative increase in plasma levels. Plasma half-life varied from 8 to 30 hours; it did not appear to be influenced by dosage, either single or repetitive, and could not be correlated with age, sex, surface area, renal or hepatic function, diagnosis or extent of disease. Apparent volume of distribution was approximately 70–80% of estimated plasma volume. There was some slow movement of asparaginase from vascular to extravascular, extracellular space. L-asparaginase was detected in the lymph. Cerebrospinal fluid levels were less than 1% of concurrent plasma levels. Only trace amounts appeared in the urine.

In a study in which patients with leukemia and metastatic cancer received intramuscular L-asparaginase, peak plasma levels of asparaginase were reached 14 to 24 hours after dosing. Plasma half-life was 39 to 49 hours. No asparaginase was detected in the urine.

INDICATIONS AND USAGE

ELSPAR is indicated in the therapy of patients with acute lymphocytic leukemia. This agent is useful primarily in combination with other chemotherapeutic agents in the induction of remissions of the disease in pediatric patients. ELSPAR should not be used as the sole induction agent unless combination therapy is deemed inappropriate. ELSPAR is not recommended for maintenance therapy.

CONTRAINDICATIONS

ELSPAR is contraindicated in patients with pancreatitis or a history of pancreatitis. Acute hemorrhagic pancreatitis, in some instances fatal, has been reported following asparaginase administration. Asparaginase is also contraindicated in patients who have had previous anaphylactic reactions to it.

WARNINGS

Allergic reactions to asparaginase are frequent and may occur during the primary course of therapy. They are not completely predictable on the basis of the intradermal skin test. Anaphylaxis and death have occurred even in a hospital setting with experienced observers.

Once a patient has received ELSPAR as part of a treatment regimen, retreatment with this agent at a later time is associated with increased risk of hypersensitivity reactions. In patients found by skin testing to be hypersensitive to asparaginase, and in any patient who has received a previous course of therapy with asparaginase, therapy with this agent should be instituted or reinstituted only after successful desensitization, and then only if in the judgement of the physician the possible benefit is greater than the increased risk. Desensitization itself may be hazardous. (See DOSAGE AND ADMINISTRATION, *Intradermal Skin Test.*)

In view of the unpredictability of the adverse reactions to asparaginase, it is recommended that this product be used in a hospital setting. Asparaginase has an adverse effect on liver function in the majority of patients. Therapy with asparaginase may increase pre-existing liver impairment caused by prior therapy or the underlying disease. Because of this there is a possibility that asparaginase may increase the toxicity of other medications.

The administration of ELSPAR *intravenously concurrently with or immediately before* a course of vincristine and prednisone may be associated with increased toxicity. (See DOSAGE AND ADMINISTRATION, *Recommended Induction Regimens.*)

PRECAUTIONS

General

This drug may be a contact irritant and both powder and solution must be handled and administered with care. Inhalation of dust or vapors and contact with skin or mucous membranes, especially those of the eyes, must be avoided. In case of contact, wash with copious amounts of water for at least 15 minutes.

Asparaginase has been reported to have immunosuppressive activity in animal experiments. Accordingly, the possibility that use of the drug in man may predispose to infection should be considered.

Asparaginase toxicity is reported to be greater in adults than in pediatric patients.

Laboratory Tests

The fall in circulating lymphoblasts often is quite marked; normal or below normal leukocyte counts are noted frequently within the first several days after initiating therapy. This may be accompanied by a marked rise in serum uric acid. The possible development of uric acid nephropathy should be borne in mind. Appropriate preventive measures should be taken, e.g., allopurinol, increased fluid intake, alkalization of urine. As a guide to the effects of therapy, the patient's peripheral blood count and bone marrow should be monitored frequently.

Frequent serum amylase determinations should be obtained to detect early evidence of pancreatitis. If pancreatitis occurs, therapy should be stopped and not reinstituted. Blood sugar should be monitored during therapy with ELSPAR because hyperglycemia may occur.

Drug Interactions

Tissue culture and animal studies indicate that ELSPAR can diminish or abolish the effect of methotrexate on malignant cells. This effect on methotrexate activity persists as long as plasma asparagine levels are suppressed. These results would seem to dictate against the clinical use of methotrexate with ELSPAR, or during the period following ELSPAR therapy when plasma asparagine levels are below normal.

Drug / Laboratory Test Interactions

L-asparaginase has been reported to interfere with the interpretation of thyroid function tests by producing a rapid and marked reduction in serum concentrations of thyroxine-binding globulin within two days after the first dose. Serum concentrations of thyroxine-binding globulin returned to pretreatment values within four weeks of the last dose of L-asparaginase.

Animal Toxicology

A one-month intravenous toxicity study of ELSPAR in dogs at doses of 250, 1000, and 2000 I.U./kg/day revealed reduced serum total protein and albumin with loss of body weight at the highest dose level and anorexia, emesis, and diarrhea at all dosage levels. A similar study in monkeys at doses of 100, 300, and 1000 I.U./kg/day also revealed reduction of serum total protein and albumin and body weight loss at all dosage levels. Bromsulfalein retention and fatty changes in the liver were noted in monkeys that were given 300 and 1000 I.U./kg/day. The rabbit was unusually sensitive to ELSPAR since a single intravenous dose of 1000 I.U./kg caused hypocalcemia associated with necrosis of the parathyroid cells, convulsions, and death in about one third of the animals. Some rabbits that died showed small thymic and lymph node hemorrhages and necrosis of the germinal centers in the lymph nodes and spleen. The intravenous administration of calcium gluconate alleviated or prevented the adverse effects.

Changes in the pancreatic islets (not pancreatitis) ranging from edema to necrosis were observed in the rabbits in the acute intravenous toxicity studies (doses of 12,500 to 50,000 I.U./kg) but not in rabbits that received 1000 I.U./kg. The anatomical changes and the hypocalcemia found in the rabbits were not observed in the subacute intravenous studies in the dogs and monkeys.

Carcinogenesis, Mutagenesis, Impairment of Fertility

The intraperitoneal injection of 2500 I.U./kg/ day for 4 days in newborn Swiss mice resulted in a small increase in pulmonary adenomas; lymphatic leukemia was not increased. L-asparaginase at concentrations of 152-909 I.U./plate was not mutagenic in the Ames microbial mutagen test with or without metabolic activation.

There are no adequate studies on the effects of asparaginase on fertility.

Pregnancy

Pregnancy Category C. In mice and rats ELSPAR has been shown to retard the weight gain of mothers and fetuses when given in doses of more than 1000 I.U./kg (the recommended human dose). Resorptions, gross abnormalities and skeletal abnormalities were observed. The intravenous administration of 50 or 100 I.U./kg (one-twentieth or one-tenth of the human dose) to pregnant rabbits on Day 8 and 9 of gestation resulted in dose dependent embryotoxicity and gross abnormalities. There are no adequate and well-controlled studies in pregnant women. ELSPAR should be used during pregnancy only if the potential benefit justifies the potential risk to the fetus.

Nursing Mothers

It is not known whether this drug is secreted in human milk. Because many drugs are secreted in human milk and because of the potential for serious adverse reactions in nursing infants from ELSPAR, a decision should be made whether to discontinue nursing or to discontinue the drug, taking into account the importance of the drug to the mother.

Pediatric Use

Asparaginase toxicity is reported to be greater in adults than in pediatric patients.

ADVERSE REACTIONS

Allergic reactions, including skin rashes, urticaria, arthralgia, respiratory distress, and acute anaphylaxis have been reported. (See WARNINGS.) Acute reactions have occurred in the absence of a positive skin test and during continued maintenance of therapeutic serum levels of ELSPAR.

In pediatric patients with advanced leukemia, a lower incidence of anaphylaxis has been reported with intramuscular administration, although there was a higher incidence of milder hypersensitivity reactions than with intravenous administration.

Fatal hyperthermia has been reported.

Pancreatitis, sometimes fulminant and fatal, has occurred during or following therapy with ELSPAR.

Hyperglycemia with glucosuria and polyuria has been reported in low incidence. Serum and urine acetone usually have been absent or negligible in these patients; this syndrome thus resembles hyperosmolar, nonketotic, hyperglycemia induced by a variety of other agents. This complication usually responds to discontinuance of ELSPAR, judicious use of intravenous fluid, and insulin, but may be fatal on occasion.

In addition to hypofibrinogenemia, depression of various other clotting factors has been reported. Most marked has been a decrease in plasma levels of factors V and VIII with a variable decrease in factors VII and IX. A decrease in circulating platelets has occurred in low incidence which, together with the increased levels of fibrin degradation products in the serum, may indicate development of a consumption coagulopathy. Bleeding has been a problem in only a minority of patients with demonstrable coagulopathy. However, intracranial hemorrhage and fatal bleeding associated with low fibrinogen levels have been reported. Increased fibrinolytic activity, apparently compensatory in nature, also has occurred.

Some patients have shown central nervous system effects consisting of depression, somnolence, fatigue, coma, confusion, agitation, and hallucinations varying from mild to severe. Rarely, a Parkinson-like syndrome has occurred, with tremor and a progressive increase in muscular tone. These side effects usually have reversed spontaneously after treatment was stopped. Therapy with ELSPAR is associated with an increase in blood ammonia during the conversion of asparagine to aspartic acid by the enzyme. No clear correlation exists between the degree of elevation of blood ammonia levels and the appearance of CNS changes. Chills, fever, nausea, vomiting, anorexia, abdominal cramps, weight loss, headache, and irritability may occur and usually are mild. Azotemia, usually pre-renal, occurs frequently. Acute renal shut down and fatal renal insufficiency have been reported during treatment. Proteinuria has occurred infrequently.

A variety of liver function abnormalities have been reported, including elevations of SGOT, SGPT, alkaline phosphatase, bilirubin (direct and indirect), and depression of serum albumin, cholesterol (total and esters), and plasma fibrinogen. Increases and decreases of total lipids have occurred. Marked hypoalbuminemia associated with peripheral edema has been reported. However, these abnormalities usually are reversible on discontinuance of therapy and some reversal may occur during the course of therapy. Fatty changes in the liver have been documented by biopsy. Malabsorption syndrome has been reported.

Rarely, transient bone marrow depression has been observed, as evidenced by a delay in return of hemoglobin or hematocrit levels to normal in patients undergoing hematologic remission of leukemia. Marked leukopenia has been reported.

OVERDOSAGE

The acute intravenous LD$_{50}$ of ELSPAR for mice was about 500,000 I.U./kg and for rabbits about 22,000 I.U./kg.

DOSAGE AND ADMINISTRATION

As a component of selected multiple agent induction regimens, ELSPAR may be administered by either the intravenous or the intramuscular route. When administered intravenously this enzyme should be given over a period of not

less than thirty minutes through the side arm of an already running infusion of Sodium Chloride Injection or Dextrose Injection 5% (D_5W). ELSPAR has little tendency to cause phlebitis when given intravenously. Anaphylactic reactions require the immediate use of epinephrine, oxygen, and intravenous steroids.
When administering ELSPAR intramuscularly, the volume at a single injection site should be limited to 2 ml. If a volume greater than 2 ml is to be administered, two injection sites should be used.
Unfavorable interactions of ELSPAR with some antitumor agents have been demonstrated. It is recommended therefore, that ELSPAR be used in combination regimens only by physicians familiar with the benefits and risks of a given regimen. During the period of its inhibition of protein synthesis and cell replication ELSPAR may interfere with the action of drugs such as methotrexate which require cell replication for their lethal effect. ELSPAR may interfere with the enzymatic detoxification of other drugs, particularly in the liver.
Recommended Induction Regimens:
When using chemotherapeutic agents in combination for the induction of remissions in patients with acute lymphocytic leukemia, regimens are sought which provide maximum chance of success while avoiding excessive cumulative toxicity or negative drug interactions.
One of the following combination regimens incorporating ELSPAR is recommended for acute lymphocytic leukemia in pediatric patients:
In the regimens below, Day 1 is considered to be the first day of therapy.
Regimen I
Prednisone 40 mg/square meter of body surface area per day orally in three divided doses for 15 days, followed by tapering of the dosage as follows:
20 mg/square meter for 2 days, 10 mg/square meter for 2 days, 5 mg/square meter for 2 days, 2.5 mg/square meter for 2 days and then discontinue.
Vincristine sulfate 2 mg/square meter of body surface area intravenously once weekly on Days 1, 8, and 15 of the treatment period. The maximum single dose should not exceed 2.0 mg.
Asparaginase 1,000 I.U./kg/day intravenously for ten successive days beginning on Day 22 of the treatment period.
Regimen II
Prednisone 40 mg/square meter of body surface area per day orally in three divided doses for 28 days (the total daily dose should be to the nearest 2.5 mg), following which the dosage of prednisone should be discontinued gradually over a 14 day period.
Vincristine sulfate 1.5 mg/square meter of body surface area intravenously weekly for four doses, on Days 1, 8, 15, and 22 of the treatment period. The maximum single dose should not exceed 2.0 mg.
Asparaginase 6,000 I.U./square meter of body surface area intramuscularly on Days 4, 7, 10, 13, 16, 19, 22, 25, and 28 of the treatment period. When a remission is obtained with either of the above regimens, appropriate maintenance therapy must be instituted. ELSPAR should not be used as part of a maintenance regimen. The above regimens do not preclude a need for special therapy directed toward the prevention of central nervous system leukemia.
It should be noted that ELSPAR has been used in combination regimens other than those recommended above. It is important to keep in mind that ELSPAR administered intravenously concurrently with or immediately before a course of vincristine and prednisone may be associated with increased toxicity. Physicians using a given regimen should be thoroughly familiar with its benefits and risks. Clinical data are insufficient for a recommendation concerning the use of combination regimens in adults. Asparaginase toxicity is reported to be greater in adults than in pediatric patients.
Use of ELSPAR as the sole induction agent should be undertaken only in an unusual situation when a combined regimen is inappropriate because of toxicity or other specific patient-related factors, or in cases refractory to other therapy. When ELSPAR is to be used as the sole induction agent for pediatric patients or adults the recommended dosage regimen is 200 I.U./kg/ day intravenously for 28 days. When complete remissions were obtained with this regimen, they were of short duration, 1 to 3 months. ELSPAR has been used as the sole induction agent in other regimens. Physicians using a given regimen should be thoroughly familiar with its benefits and risks.
Patients undergoing induction therapy must be carefully monitored and the therapeutic regimen adjusted according to response and toxicity.
Such adjustments should always involve decreasing dosages of one or more agents or discontinuation depending on the degree of toxicity. Patients who have received a course of ELSPAR, if retreated, have an increased risk of hypersensitivity reactions. Therefore, retreatment should be undertaken only when the benefit of such therapy is weighed against the increased risk.

Intradermal Skin Test:
Because of the occurrence of allergic reactions, an intradermal skin test should be performed prior to the initial administration of ELSPAR and when ELSPAR is given after an interval of a week or more has elapsed between doses. The skin test solution may be prepared as follows: Reconstitute the contents of a 10,000 I.U. vial with 5.0 ml of diluent. From this solution (2,000 I.U./ml) withdraw 0.1 ml and inject it into another vial containing 9.9 ml of diluent, yielding a skin test solution of approximately 20.0 I.U./ml. Use 0.1 ml of this solution (about 2.0 I.U.) for the intradermal skin test. The skin test site should be observed for at least one hour for the appearance of a wheal or erythema either of which indicates a positive reaction. An allergic reaction even to the skin test dose in certain sensitized individuals may rarely occur. A negative skin test reaction does not preclude the possibility of the development of an allergic reaction.

Desensitization:
Desensitization should be performed before administering the first dose of ELSPAR on initiation of therapy in positive reactors, and on retreatment of any patient in whom such therapy is deemed necessary after carefully weighing the increased risk of hypersensitivity reactions. Rapid desensitization of the patient may be attempted with progressively increasing amounts of intravenously administered ELSPAR provided adequate precautions are taken to treat an acute allergic reaction should it occur. One reported schedule begins with a total of 1 I.U. given intravenously and doubles the dose every 10 minutes, provided no reaction has occurred, until the accumulated total amount given equals the planned doses for that day.
For convenience the following table is included to calculate the number of doses necessary to reach the patient's total dose for that day:

Injection Number	ELSPAR Dose in I.U.	Accumulated Total Dose
1	1	1
2	2	3
3	4	7
4	8	15
5	16	31
6	32	63
7	64	127
8	128	255
9	256	511
10	512	1023
11	1024	2047
12	2048	4095
13	4096	8191
14	8192	16383
15	16384	32767
16	32768	65535
17	65536	131071
18	131072	262143

For example: A patient weighing 20 kg who is to receive 200 I.U./kg (total dose 4000 I.U.) would receive injections 1 through 12 during desensitization.

DIRECTIONS FOR RECONSTITUTION

Parenteral drug products should be inspected visually for particulate matter and discoloration prior to administration whenever solution and container permit. When reconstituted, ELSPAR should be a clear, colorless solution. If the solution becomes cloudy, discard.
For Intravenous Use
Reconstitute with Sterile Water for Injection or with Sodium Chloride Injection. The volume recommended for reconstitution is 5 ml for the 10,000 unit vials. Ordinary shaking during reconstitution does not inactivate the enzyme. This solution may be used for direct intravenous administration within an eight hour period following restoration. For administration by infusion, solutions should be diluted with the isotonic solutions, Sodium Chloride Injection or Dextrose Injection 5%. These solutions should be infused within eight hours and only if clear.
Occasionally, a very small number of gelatinous fiber-like particles may develop on standing. Filtration through a 5.0 micron filter during administration will remove the particles with no resultant loss in potency. Some loss of potency has been observed with the use of a 0.2 micron filter.
For Intramuscular Use
When ELSPAR is administered intramuscularly according to the schedule cited in the induction regimen, reconstitution is carried out by adding 2 ml Sodium Chloride Injection to the 10,000 unit vial. The resulting solution should be used within eight hours and only if clear.

HOW SUPPLIED

No. 4612 — ELSPAR is a white lyophilized plug or powder supplied as follows:
NDC 0006-4612-00 in a sterile 10 ml vial containing 10,000 I.U. of asparaginase and 80 mg mannitol, an inactive ingredient.
(6505-01-153-9650 10 mL vial)
Personnel preparing ELSPAR should avoid drug contact with skin, mucous membranes, or eyes and avoid inhaling the dust or vapor.
Store at 2–8°C (36–46°F). ELSPAR does not contain a preservative. Unused, reconstituted solution should be stored at 2 to 8°C (36 to 46°F) and discarded after eight hours, or sooner if it becomes cloudy.
7407112 Issued January 1997

FLEXERIL® Tablets ℞
(Cyclobenzaprine HCl), U.S.P.

DESCRIPTION

Cyclobenzaprine hydrochloride is a white, crystalline tricyclic amine salt with the empirical formula $C_{20}H_{21}N{\cdot}HCl$ and a molecular weight of 311.9. It has a melting point of 217°C, and a pK_a of 8.47 at 25°C. It is freely soluble in water and alcohol, sparingly soluble in isopropanol, and insoluble in hydrocarbon solvents. If aqueous solutions are made alkaline, the free base separates. Cyclobenzaprine HCl is designated chemically as 3-(5*H* -dibenzo[*a,d*]cyclohepten-5-ylidene)-*N, N* -dimethyl-1-propanamine hydrochloride, and has the following structural formula:

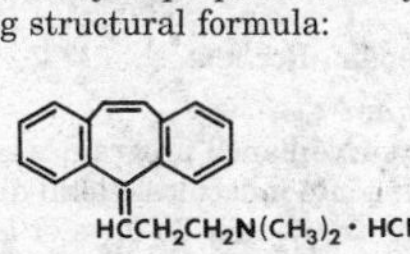

FLEXERIL* (Cyclobenzaprine HCl) is supplied as 10 mg tablets for oral administration.
Tablets FLEXERIL contain the following inactive ingredients: hydroxypropyl cellulose, hydroxypropyl methylcellulose, iron oxide, lactose, magnesium stearate, starch, and titanium dioxide.

*Registered trademark of MERCK & CO., INC.

CLINICAL PHARMACOLOGY

Cyclobenzaprine HCl relieves skeletal muscle spasm of local origin without interfering with muscle function. It is ineffective in muscle spasm due to central nervous system disease.
Cyclobenzaprine reduced or abolished skeletal muscle hyperactivity in several animal models. Animal studies indicate that cyclobenzaprine does not act at the neuromuscular junction or directly on skeletal muscle. Such studies show that cyclobenzaprine acts primarily within the central nervous system at brain stem as opposed to spinal cord levels, although its action on the latter may contribute to its overall skeletal muscle relaxant activity. Evidence suggests that the net effect of cyclobenzaprine is a reduction of tonic somatic motor activity, influencing both gamma (γ) and alpha (α) motor systems.
Pharmacological studies in animals showed a similarity between the effects of cyclobenzaprine and the structurally related tricyclic antidepressants, including reserpine antagonism, norepinephrine potentiation, potent peripheral and central anticholinergic effects, and sedation. Cyclobenzaprine caused slight to moderate increase in heart rate in animals.
Cyclobenzaprine is well absorbed after oral administration, but there is a large intersubject variation in plasma levels. Cyclobenzaprine is eliminated quite slowly with a half-life as long as one to three days. It is highly bound to plasma proteins, is extensively metabolized primarily to glucuronide-like conjugates, and is excreted primarily via the kidneys.
No significant effect on plasma levels or bioavailability of FLEXERIL or aspirin was noted when single or multiple doses of the two drugs were administered concomitantly. Concomitant administration of FLEXERIL and aspirin is usually well tolerated and no unexpected or serious clinical or laboratory adverse effects have been observed. No studies have been performed to indicate whether FLEXERIL enhances the clinical effect of aspirin or other analgesics, or whether analgesics enhance the clinical effect of FLEXERIL in acute musculoskeletal conditions.

Continued on next page

Information on the Merck & Co., Inc. products listed on these pages is the full prescribing information from product circulars in use August 31, 1998. For information, please call 1-800-NSC MERCK [1-800-672-6372].

Flexeril—Cont.

Clinical Studies
Controlled clinical studies show that FLEXERIL significantly improves the signs and symptoms of skeletal muscle spasm as compared with placebo. The clinical responses include improvement in muscle spasm as determined by palpation, reduction in local pain and tenderness, increased range of motion, and less restriction in activities of daily living. When daily observations were made, clinical improvement was observed as early as the first day of therapy.
Eight double-blind controlled clinical studies were performed in 642 patients comparing FLEXERIL, diazepam*, and placebo. Muscle spasm, local pain and tenderness, limitation of motion, and restriction in activities of daily living were evaluated. In three of these studies there was a significantly greater improvement with FLEXERIL than with diazepam, while in the other studies the improvement following both treatments was comparable.
Although the frequency and severity of adverse reactions observed in patients treated with FLEXERIL were comparable to those observed in patients treated with diazepam, dry mouth was observed more frequently in patients treated with FLEXERIL and dizziness more frequently in those treated with diazepam. The incidence of drowsiness, the most frequent adverse reaction, was similar with both drugs.
Analysis of the data from controlled studies shows that FLEXERIL produces clinical improvement whether or not sedation occurs.

*VALIUM® (diazepam, Roche)

Surveillance Program
A post-marketing surveillance program was carried out in 7607 patients with acute musculoskeletal disorders, and included 297 patients treated for 30 days or longer. The overall effectiveness of FLEXERIL was similar to that observed in the double-blind controlled studies; the overall incidence of adverse effects was less (see ADVERSE REACTIONS).

INDICATIONS AND USAGE

FLEXERIL is indicated as an adjunct to rest and physical therapy for relief of muscle spasm associated with acute, painful musculoskeletal conditions.
Improvement is manifested by relief of muscle spasm and its associated signs and symptoms, namely, pain, tenderness, limitation of motion, and restriction in activities of daily living.
FLEXERIL (Cyclobenzaprine HCl) should be used only for short periods (up to two or three weeks) because adequate evidence of effectiveness for more prolonged use is not available and because muscle spasm associated with acute, painful musculoskeletal conditions is generally of short duration and specific therapy for longer periods is seldom warranted.
FLEXERIL has not been found effective in the treatment of spasticity associated with cerebral or spinal cord disease, or in children with cerebral palsy.

CONTRAINDICATIONS

Hypersensitivity to the drug.
Concomitant use of monoamine oxidase inhibitors or within 14 days after their discontinuation.
Acute recovery phase of myocardial infarction, and patients with arrhythmias, heart block or conduction disturbances, or congestive heart failure.
Hyperthyroidism.

WARNINGS

Cyclobenzaprine is closely related to the tricyclic antidepressants, e.g., amitriptyline and imipramine. In short term studies for indications other than muscle spasm associated with acute musculoskeletal conditions, and usually at doses somewhat greater than those recommended for skeletal muscle spasm, some of the more serious central nervous system reactions noted with the tricyclic antidepressants have occurred (see WARNINGS, below, and ADVERSE REACTIONS).
FLEXERIL may interact with monoamine oxidase (MAO) inhibitors. Hyperpyretic crisis, severe convulsions, and deaths have occurred in patients receiving tricyclic antidepressants and MAO inhibitor drugs.
Tricyclic antidepressants have been reported to produce arrhythmias, sinus tachycardia, prolongation of the conduction time leading to myocardial infarction and stroke.
FLEXERIL may enhance the effects of alcohol, barbiturates, and other CNS depressants.

PRECAUTIONS

General
Because of its atropine-like action, FLEXERIL should be used with caution in patients with a history of urinary retention, angle-closure glaucoma, increased intraocular pressure, and in patients taking anticholinergic medication.
Information for Patients
FLEXERIL may impair mental and/or physical abilities required for performance of hazardous tasks, such as operating machinery or driving a motor vehicle.
Drug Interactions
FLEXERIL may enhance the effects of alcohol, barbiturates, and other CNS depressants.
Tricyclic antidepressants may block the antihypertensive action of guanethidine and similarly acting compounds.
Carcinogenesis, Mutagenesis, Impairment of Fertility
In rats treated with FLEXERIL for up to 67 weeks at doses of approximately 5 to 40 times the maximum recommended human dose, pale, sometimes enlarged, livers were noted and there was a dose-related hepatocyte vacuolation with lipidosis. In the higher dose groups this microscopic change was seen after 26 weeks and even earlier in rats which died prior to 26 weeks; at lower doses, the change was not seen until after 26 weeks.
Cyclobenzaprine did not affect the onset, incidence or distribution of neoplasia in an 81-week study in the mouse or in a 105-week study in the rat.
At oral doses of up to 10 times the human dose, cyclobenzaprine did not adversely affect the reproductive performance or fertility of male or female rats. Cyclobenzaprine did not demonstrate mutagenic activity in the male mouse at dose levels of up to 20 times the human dose.
Pregnancy
Pregnancy Category B: Reproduction studies have been performed in rats, mice and rabbits at doses up to 20 times the human dose, and have revealed no evidence of impaired fertility or harm to the fetus due to FLEXERIL. There are, however, no adequate and well-controlled studies in pregnant women. Because animal reproduction studies are not always predictive of human response, this drug should be used during pregnancy only if clearly needed.
Nursing Mothers
It is not known whether this drug is excreted in human milk. Because cyclobenzaprine is closely related to the tricyclic antidepressants, some of which are known to be excreted in human milk, caution should be exercised when FLEXERIL is administered to a nursing woman.
Pediatric Use
Safety and effectiveness of FLEXERIL in pediatric patients below 15 years of age have not been established.

ADVERSE REACTIONS

The following list of adverse reactions is based on the experience in 473 patients treated with FLEXERIL in controlled clinical studies, 7607 patients in the post-marketing surveillance program, and reports received since the drug was marketed. The overall incidence of adverse reactions among patients in the surveillance program was less than the incidence in the controlled clinical studies.
The adverse reactions reported most frequently with FLEXERIL were drowsiness, dry mouth and dizziness. The incidence of these common adverse reactions was lower in the surveillance program than in the controlled clinical studies:

	Clinical Studies	*Surveillance Program*
drowsiness	39%	16%
dry mouth	27%	7%
dizziness	11%	3%

Among the less frequent adverse reactions, there was no appreciable difference in incidence in controlled clinical studies or in the surveillance program. Adverse reactions which were reported in 1% to 3% of the patients were: fatigue/tiredness, asthenia, nausea, constipation, dyspepsia, unpleasant taste, blurred vision, headache, nervousness, and confusion.

Incidence Less Than 1 in 100

The following adverse reactions have been reported at an incidence of less than 1 in 100:
Body as a Whole: Syncope; malaise.
Cardiovascular: Tachycardia; arrhythmia; vasodilatation; palpitation; hypotension.
Digestive: Vomiting; anorexia; diarrhea; gastrointestinal pain; gastritis; thirst; flatulence; edema of the tongue; abnormal liver function and rare reports of hepatitis, jaundice and cholestasis.
Hypersensitivity: Anaphylaxis; angioedema; pruritus; facial edema; urticaria; rash.
Musculoskeletal: Local weakness.
Nervous System and Psychiatric: Ataxia; vertigo; dysarthria; tremors; hypertonia; convulsions; muscle twitching; disorientation; insomnia; depressed mood; abnormal sensations; anxiety; agitation; abnormal thinking and dreaming; hallucinations; excitement; paresthesia; diplopia.
Skin: Sweating.
Special Senses: Ageusia; tinnitus.
Urogenital: Urinary frequency and/or retention.

Causal Relationship Unknown

Other reactions, reported rarely for FLEXERIL under circumstances where a causal relationship could not be established or reported for other tricyclic drugs, are listed to serve as alerting information to physicians:
Body as a Whole: Chest pain; edema.
Cardiovascular: Hypertension; myocardial infarction; heart block; stroke.
Digestive: Paralytic ileus; tongue discoloration; stomatitis; parotid swelling.
Endocrine: Inappropriate ADH syndrome.
Hematic and Lymphatic: Purpura; bone marrow depression; leukopenia; eosinophilia; thrombocytopenia.
Metabolic, Nutritional and Immune: Elevation and lowering of blood sugar levels; weight gain or loss.
Musculoskeletal: Myalgia.
Nervous System and Psychiatric: Decreased or increased libido; abnormal gait; delusions; peripheral neuropathy; Bell's palsy; alteration in EEG patterns; extrapyramidal symptoms.
Respiratory: Dyspnea.
Skin: Photosensitization; alopecia.
Urogenital: Impaired urination; dilatation of urinary tract; impotence; testicular swelling; gynecomastia; breast enlargement; galactorrhea.

DRUG ABUSE AND DEPENDENCE

Pharmacologic similarities among the tricyclic drugs require that certain withdrawal symptoms be considered when FLEXERIL is administered, even though they have not been reported to occur with this drug. Abrupt cessation of treatment after prolonged administration may produce nausea, headache, and malaise. These are not indicative of addiction.

OVERDOSAGE

Manifestations: High doses may cause temporary confusion, disturbed concentration, transient visual hallucinations, agitation, hyperactive reflexes, muscle rigidity, vomiting, or hyperpyrexia, in addition to anything listed under ADVERSE REACTIONS. Based on the known pharmacologic actions of the drug, overdosage may cause drowsiness, hypothermia, tachycardia and other cardiac rhythm abnormalities such as bundle branch block, ECG evidence of impaired conduction, and congestive heart failure. Other manifestations may be dilated pupils, convulsions, severe hypotension, stupor, and coma.
The acute oral LD_{50} of FLEXERIL is approximately 338 and 425 mg/kg in mice and rats, respectively.
Treatment: Treatment is symptomatic and supportive. Empty the stomach as quickly as possible by emesis, followed by gastric lavage. After gastric lavage, activated charcoal may be administered. Twenty to 30 g of activated charcoal may be given every four to six hours during the first 24 to 48 hours after ingestion. An ECG should be taken and close monitoring of cardiac function must be instituted if there is any evidence of dysrhythmia. Maintenance of an open airway, adequate fluid intake, and regulation of body temperature are necessary.
The intravenous administration of 1-3 mg of physostigmine salicylate is reported to reverse symptoms of poisoning by atropine and other drugs with anticholinergic activity. Physostigmine may be helpful in the treatment of cyclobenzaprine overdose. Because physostigmine is rapidly metabolized, the dosage of physostigmine should be repeated as required, particularly if life-threatening signs such as arrhythmias, convulsions, and deep coma recur or persist after the initial dosage of physostigmine. Because physostigmine itself may be toxic, it is not recommended for routine use.
Standard medical measures should be used to manage circulatory shock and metabolic acidosis. Cardiac arrhythmias may be treated with neostigmine, pyridostigmine, or propranolol. When signs of cardiac failure occur, the use of a short-acting digitalis preparation should be considered. Close monitoring of cardiac function for not less than five days is advisable.
Anticonvulsants may be given to control seizures.
Dialysis is probably of no value because of low plasma concentrations of the drug.
Since overdosage is often deliberate, patients may attempt suicide by other means during the recovery phase. Deaths by deliberate or accidental overdosage have occurred with this class of drugs.

DOSAGE AND ADMINISTRATION

The usual dosage of FLEXERIL is 10 mg three times a day, with a range of 20 to 40 mg a day in divided doses. Dosage should not exceed 60 mg a day. Use of FLEXERIL for periods longer than two or three weeks is not recommended. (See INDICATIONS AND USAGE.)

HOW SUPPLIED

No. 3358—Tablets FLEXERIL, 10 mg, are butterscotch yellow, D-shaped, film coated tablets, coded MSD 931. They are supplied as follows:
NDC 0006-0931-68 in bottles of 100
(6505-01-062-8010, 10 mg 100's)
NDC 0006-0931-28 unit dose packages of 100
(6505-01-110-9926, 10 mg individually sealed 100's)
Shown in Product Identification Guide, page 323
7897214   Issued September 1996
COPYRIGHT © MERCK & CO., INC., 1985
All rights reserved

FOSAMAX® Tablets ℞
(alendronate sodium tablets)

DESCRIPTION

FOSAMAX* (alendronate sodium) is an aminobisphosphonate that acts as a specific inhibitor of osteoclast-mediated bone resorption. Bisphosphonates are synthetic analogs of pyrophosphate that bind to the hydroxyapatite found in bone.

Alendronate sodium is chemically described as (4-amino-1-hydroxybutylidene) bisphosphonic acid monosodium salt trihydrate.

The empirical formula of alendronate sodium is $C_4H_{12}NNaO_7P_2 \cdot 3H_2O$ and its formula weight is 325.12. The structural formula is:

$$\begin{array}{c} NH_2 \\ | \\ CH_2 \\ | \\ CH_2 \\ | \\ O \quad CH_2 \quad O \\ \| \quad | \quad \| \\ HO-P-C-P-ONa \cdot 3H_2O \\ | \quad | \quad | \\ OH \quad OH \quad OH \end{array}$$

Alendronate sodium is a white, crystalline, nonhygroscopic powder. It is soluble in water, very slightly soluble in alcohol, and practically insoluble in chloroform.

Tablets FOSAMAX for oral administration contain 6.53, 13.05 or 52.21 mg of alendronate monosodium salt trihydrate, which is the molar equivalent of 5.0, 10.0 and 40.0 mg, respectively, of free acid, and the following inactive ingredients: microcrystalline cellulose, anhydrous lactose, croscarmellose sodium, and magnesium stearate.

---

*Registered trademark of MERCK & CO., Inc.

CLINICAL PHARMACOLOGY

Mechanism of Action
Animal studies have indicated the following mode of action. At the cellular level, alendronate shows preferential localization to sites of bone resorption, specifically under osteoclasts. The osteoclasts adhere normally to the bone surface but lack the ruffled border that is indicative of active resorption. Alendronate does not interfere with osteoclast recruitment or attachment, but it does inhibit osteoclast activity. Studies in mice on the localization of radioactive [³H]alendronate in bone showed about 10-fold higher uptake on osteoclast surfaces than on osteoblast surfaces. Bones examined 6 and 49 days after [³H]alendronate administration in rats and mice, respectively, showed that normal bone was formed on top of the alendronate, which was incorporated inside the matrix. While incorporated in bone matrix, alendronate is not pharmacologically active. Thus, alendronate must be continuously administered to suppress osteoclasts on newly formed resorption surfaces. Histomorphometry in baboons and rats showed that alendronate treatment reduces bone turnover (i.e., the number of sites at which bone is remodeled). In addition, bone formation exceeds bone resorption at these remodeling sites, leading to progressive gains in bone mass.
Pharmacokinetics
Absorption
Relative to an intravenous (IV) reference dose, the mean oral bioavailability of alendronate in women was 0.7% for doses ranging from 5 to 40 mg when administered after an overnight fast and two hours before a standardized breakfast. Oral bioavailability of the 10 mg tablet in men (0.59%) was similar to that in women (0.78%) when administered after an overnight fast and 2 hours before breakfast.
A study examining the effect of timing of a meal on the bioavailability of alendronate was performed in 49 postmenopausal women. Bioavailability was decreased (by approximately 40%) when 10 mg alendronate was administered either 0.5 or 1 hour before a standardized breakfast, when

compared to dosing 2 hours before eating. In studies of treatment and prevention of osteoporosis, alendronate was effective when administered at least 30 minutes before breakfast.
Bioavailability was negligible whether alendronate was administered with or up to two hours after a standardized breakfast. Concomitant administration of alendronate with coffee or orange juice reduced bioavailability by approximately 60%.
Distribution
Preclinical studies (in male rats) show that alendronate transiently distributes to soft tissues following 1 mg/kg IV administration but is then rapidly redistributed to bone or excreted in the urine. The mean steady-state volume of distribution, exclusive of bone, is at least 28 L in humans. Concentrations of drug in plasma following therapeutic oral doses are too low (less than 5 ng/mL) for analytical detection. Protein binding in human plasma is approximately 78%.
Metabolism
There is no evidence that alendronate is metabolized in animals or humans.
Excretion
Following a single IV dose of [¹⁴C]alendronate, approximately 50% of the radioactivity was excreted in the urine within 72 hours and little or no radioactivity was recovered in the feces. Following a single 10 mg IV dose, the renal clearance of alendronate was 71 mL/min, and systemic clearance did not exceed 200 mL/min. Plasma concentrations fell by more than 95% within 6 hours following IV administration. The terminal half-life in humans is estimated to exceed 10 years, probably reflecting release of alendronate from the skeleton. Based on the above, it is estimated that after 10 years of oral treatment with FOSAMAX (10 mg daily) the amount of alendronate released daily from the skeleton is approximately 25% of that absorbed from the gastrointestinal tract.
Special Populations
Pediatric: Alendronate pharmacokinetics have not been investigated in patients <18 years of age.
Gender: Bioavailability and the fraction of an IV dose excreted in urine were similar in men and women.
Geriatric: Bioavailability and disposition (urinary excretion) were similar in elderly (≥ 65 years of age) and younger patients. No dosage adjustment is necessary (see DOSAGE AND ADMINISTRATION).
Race: Pharmacokinetic differences due to race have not been studied.
Renal Insufficiency: Preclinical studies show that, in rats with kidney failure, increasing amounts of drug are present in plasma, kidney, spleen, and tibia. In healthy controls, drug that is not deposited in bone is rapidly excreted in the urine. No evidence of saturation of bone uptake was found after 3 weeks dosing with cumulative IV doses of 35 mg/kg in young male rats. Although no clinical information is available, it is likely that, as in animals, elimination of alendronate via the kidney will be reduced in patients with impaired renal function. Therefore, somewhat greater accumulation of alendronate in bone might be expected in patients with impaired renal function.
No dosage adjustment is necessary for patients with mild-to-moderate renal insufficiency (creatinine clearance 35 to 60 mL/min). **FOSAMAX is not recommended for patients with more severe renal insufficiency (creatinine clearance <35 mL/min) due to lack of experience.**
Hepatic Insufficiency: As there is evidence that alendronate is not metabolized or excreted in the bile, no studies were conducted in patients with hepatic insufficiency. No dosage adjustment is necessary.
Drug Interactions (also see PRECAUTIONS, *Drug Interactions*)
Intravenous ranitidine was shown to double the bioavailability of oral alendronate. The clinical significance of this

increased bioavailability and whether similar increases will occur in patients given oral H_2-antagonists is unknown; no other specific drug interaction studies were performed. Products containing calcium and other multivalent cations are likely to interfere with absorption of alendronate.
[See table above]
Pharmacodynamics
Osteoporosis in postmenopausal women
Osteoporosis is characterized by low bone mass that leads to an increased risk of fracture. The diagnosis can be confirmed by the finding of low bone mass, evidence of fracture on x-ray, a history of osteoporotic fracture, or height loss or kyphosis, indicative of vertebral (spinal) fracture. Osteoporosis occurs in both males and females but is most common among women following the menopause, when bone turnover increases and the rate of bone resorption exceeds that of bone formation. These changes result in progressive bone loss and lead to osteoporosis in a significant proportion of women over age 50. Fractures, usually of the spine, hip, and wrist, are the common consequences. From age 50 to age 90, the risk of hip fracture in white women increases 50-fold and the risk of vertebral fracture 15- to 30-fold. It is estimated that approximately 40% of 50-year-old women will sustain one or more osteoporosis-related fractures of the spine, hip, or wrist during their remaining lifetimes. Hip fractures, in particular, are associated with substantial morbidity, disability, and mortality.
Alendronate is an aminobisphosphonate that binds to bone hydroxyapatite and specifically inhibits the activity of osteoclasts, the bone-resorbing cells. Alendronate reduces bone resorption with no direct effect on bone formation, although the latter process is ultimately reduced because bone resorption and formation are coupled during bone turnover. Alendronate thus reduces the elevated rate of bone turnover observed in postmenopausal women to approximate more closely that in premenopausal women. Alendronate is not an estrogen and does not have the benefits and risks of estrogen replacement therapy.
Daily oral doses of alendronate (5, 20, and 40 mg for six weeks) in postmenopausal women produced biochemical changes indicative of dose-dependent inhibition of bone resorption, including decreases in urinary calcium and urinary markers of bone collagen degradation (such as deoxypyridinoline and cross-linked N-telopeptides of type I collagen). These biochemical changes tended to return toward baseline values as early as 3 weeks following the discontinuation of therapy with alendronate and did not differ from placebo after 7 months.
In long-term (two- or three-year) osteoporosis treatment studies, FOSAMAX 10 mg/day reduced urinary excretion of markers of bone resorption, including deoxypyridinoline and cross-linked N-telopeptides of type I collagen, by approximately 50–60% to reach levels similar to those seen in healthy premenopausal women. Similar decreases were seen in patients in osteoporosis prevention studies who received FOSAMAX 5 mg/day. The decrease in the rate of bone resorption indicated by these markers was evident as early as one month and at three to six months reached a plateau that was maintained for the entire duration of treatment with FOSAMAX. In osteoporosis treatment studies FOSAMAX 10 mg/day decreased the markers of bone formation, osteocalcin and total serum alkaline phosphatase, by approximately 50% and 25–30%, respectively, to reach a plateau after 6 to 12 months. In osteoporosis prevention studies FOSAMAX 5 mg/day decreased these markers by approximately 40% and 15%, respectively. These data

Summary of Pharmacokinetic Parameters in the Normal Population

	Mean	90% Confidence Interval
Absolute bioavailability of 5 mg tablet, taken 2 hours before first meal of the day	0.63% (females)	(0.48, 0.83)
Absolute bioavailability of 10 mg tablet, taken 2 hours before first meal of the day	0.78% (females)	(0.61, 1.04)
	0.59% (males)	(0.43, 0.81)
Absolute bioavailability of 40 mg tablet, taken 2 hours before first meal of the day	0.06% (females)	(0.46, 0.78)
Renal Clearance (mL/min) (n=6)	71	(64, 78)

Continued on next page

Information on the Merck & Co., Inc. products listed on these pages is the full prescribing information from product circulars in use August 31, 1998. For information, please call 1-800-NSC MERCK [1-800-672-6372].

Consult 1999 PDR® supplements and future editions for revisions

Fosamax—Cont.

indicate that the rate of bone turnover reached a new steady-state, despite the progressive increase in the total amount of alendronate deposited within bone.
As a result of inhibition of bone resorption, asymptomatic reductions in serum calcium and phosphate concentrations were also observed following treatment with FOSAMAX. In the long-term studies, reductions from baseline in serum calcium (approximately 2%) and phosphate (approximately 4 to 6%) were evident the first month after the initiation of FOSAMAX 10 mg, but no further decreases were observed for the three-year duration of the studies. Similar reductions were observed with FOSAMAX 5 mg/day. The reduction in serum phosphate may reflect not only the positive bone mineral balance due to FOSAMAX but also a decrease in renal phosphate reabsorption.

Paget's disease of bone

Paget's disease of bone is a chronic, focal skeletal disorder characterized by greatly increased and disorderly bone remodeling. Excessive osteoclastic bone resorption is followed by osteoblastic new bone formation, leading to the replacement of the normal bone architecture by disorganized, enlarged, and weakened bone structure.
Clinical manifestations of Paget's disease range from no symptoms to severe morbidity due to bone pain, bone deformity, pathological fractures, and neurological and other complications. Serum alkaline phosphatase, the most frequently used biochemical index of disease activity, provides an objective measure of disease severity and response to therapy.
FOSAMAX decreases the rate of bone resorption directly, which leads to an indirect decrease in bone formation. In clinical trials, FOSAMAX 40 mg once daily for six months produced highly significant decreases in serum alkaline phosphatase as well as in urinary markers of bone collagen degradation. As a result of the inhibition of bone resorption, FOSAMAX induced generally mild, transient, and asymptomatic decreases in serum calcium and phosphate.

Clinical Studies

Treatment of osteoporosis in postmenopausal women

Effect on bone mineral density

The efficacy of FOSAMAX 10 mg once daily in postmenopausal women, 44 to 84 years of age, with osteoporosis (lumbar spine bone mineral density [BMD] of at least 2 standard deviations below the premenopausal mean) was demonstrated in four double-blind, placebo-controlled clinical studies of two or three years' duration. These included two large three-year, multicenter studies of virtually identical design, one performed in the United States (U.S.) and the other in 15 different countries (Multinational), which enrolled 478 and 516 patients, respectively. The following graph shows the mean increases in BMD of the lumbar spine, femoral neck, and trochanter in patients receiving FOSAMAX 10 mg/day relative to placebo-treated patients at three years for each of these studies.

**Increase in BMD
FOSAMAX 10 mg/day in Two Studies at Three Years**

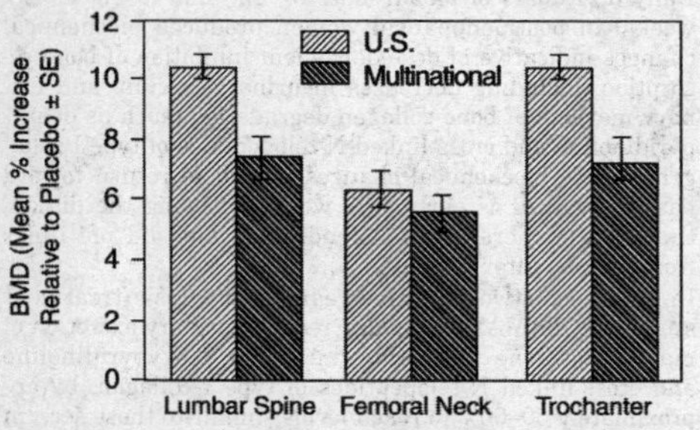

Highly significant increases in BMD, relative both to baseline and placebo, were seen at each measurement site in each study in patients who received FOSAMAX 10 mg/day. Total body BMD also increased significantly in each study, suggesting that the increases in bone mass of the spine and hip did not occur at the expense of other skeletal sites. Increases in BMD were evident as early as three months and continued throughout the three years of treatment. (See figures below for lumbar spine results.) Thus, FOSAMAX appears to reverse the progression of osteoporosis. FOSAMAX was similarly effective regardless of age, race, baseline rate of bone turnover, and baseline BMD in the range studied (at least 2 standard deviations below the premenopausal mean).
[See first graphic at top of next page]
In patients with postmenopausal osteoporosis treated with FOSAMAX for one or two years, the effects of treatment withdrawal were assessed. Following discontinuation, there were no further increases in bone mass and the rates of bone loss were similar to those of the placebo groups. These data indicate that continuous daily treatment with FOSAMAX is required to maintain the effect of the drug.

Effect on fracture incidence

To assess the effects of FOSAMAX on vertebral fracture incidence, the U.S. and Multinational studies were combined in an analysis that compared placebo to the pooled dosage groups of FOSAMAX (5 or 10 mg for three years or 20 mg for two years followed by 5 mg for one year). There was a significant 48% reduction in the proportion of patients treated with FOSAMAX experiencing one or more new vertebral fractures relative to those treated with placebo (3.2% vs. 6.2%). A reduction in the total number of new vertebral fractures (4.2 vs. 11.3 per 100 patients) was also observed. In the pooled analysis, patients who received FOSAMAX had a statistically significant smaller loss in stature than those who received placebo (−3.0 mm vs. −4.6 mm). Furthermore, of patients who sustained any vertebral fracture, those treated with FOSAMAX experienced less height loss (5.9 mm vs. 23.3 mm) due to a reduction in both the number and severity of fractures.
The Vertebral Fracture Study of the Fracture Intervention Trial (FIT) included results from 2027 patients who had at least one baseline vertebral (compression) fracture. The results of this study demonstrated the reduction in fracture incidence due to FOSAMAX. In this three-year, randomized, double-blind, placebo-controlled study, 1022 patients received FOSAMAX and 1005 patients received placebo. Treatment with FOSAMAX resulted in statistically significant and clinically meaningful reductions in the proportion of patients experiencing fractures as shown in the table below.
[See table at bottom of page]
Furthermore, treatment with FOSAMAX significantly reduced the incidence of total hospitalizations (24.9% vs. 30.4%).
The reduction in the incidence of vertebral fractures (FOSAMAX versus placebo) in the Vertebral Fracture Study of FIT (in which all women had at least one baseline vertebral fracture) was consistent with that in the combined U.S. and Multinational (U.S./Mult) treatment studies (see above), in which 80% of the women did not have a vertebral fracture at baseline. During these three-year studies, treatment with FOSAMAX reduced the proportion of women experiencing at least one new vertebral fracture in both study populations by approximately 50% (FIT: 47% reduction, $p<0.001$; U.S./Mult: 48% reduction, $p = 0.034$). Similarly, FOSAMAX reduced the proportion of women experiencing multiple (two or more) new vertebral fractures by approximately 90% in both studies ($p<0.001$). Thus, FOSAMAX reduces the incidence of fractures whether or not patients have experienced a previous vertebral fracture.
The two figures below display the cumulative incidence of patients with hip and wrist fractures over 3 years in the Vertebral Fracture Study of FIT. In both figures, the cumulative incidence of patients with these types of fracture is lower with FOSAMAX compared with placebo at all time points. FOSAMAX reduced the proportion of women experiencing hip fracture by 51% and wrist fracture by 48%. Proportionately similar reductions of hip and wrist fractures were seen in pooled earlier osteoporosis treatment studies.
[See second graphic on next page]
Overall, these results demonstrate the efficacy of FOSAMAX to reduce the incidence of fractures at the spine, hip and wrist, which are the three most common sites of osteoporotic fracture.

Bone histology

Bone histology in 270 postmenopausal patients with osteoporosis treated with FOSAMAX at doses ranging from 1 to 20 mg/day for one, two, or three years revealed normal mineralization and structure, as well as the expected decrease in bone turnover relative to placebo. These data, together with the normal bone histology and increased bone strength observed in rats and baboons exposed to long-term alendronate treatment, support the conclusion that bone formed during therapy with FOSAMAX is of normal quality.

Prevention of osteoporosis in postmenopausal women

Prevention of bone loss was demonstrated in two double-blind, placebo-controlled studies of postmenopausal women 40–60 years of age. One thousand six hundred nine patients (FOSAMAX 5 mg/day; n = 498) who were at least six months postmenopausal were entered into a two-year study without regard to their baseline BMD. In the other study, 447 patients (FOSAMAX 5 mg/day; n = 88), who were between six months and three years postmenopause, were treated for up to three years. In the placebo-treated patients BMD losses of approximately 1% per year were seen at the spine, hip (femoral neck and trochanter) and total body. In contrast, FOSAMAX 5 mg/day prevented bone loss in the majority of patients and induced significant increases in mean bone mass at each of these sites (see figures below). In addition, FOSAMAX 5 mg/day reduced the rate of bone loss at the forearm by approximately half relative to placebo. FOSAMAX 5 mg/day was similarly effective in this population regardless of age, time since menopause, race and baseline rate of bone turnover.
[See third graphic on next page]
Bone histology was normal in the 28 patients biopsied at the end of three years who received FOSAMAX at doses of up to 10 mg/day.

Paget's disease of bone

The efficacy of FOSAMAX 40 mg once daily for six months was demonstrated in two double-blind clinical studies of male and female patients with moderate to severe Paget's disease (alkaline phosphatase at least twice the upper limit of normal): a placebo-controlled multinational study and a U.S. comparative study with etidronate disodium 400 mg/day. The following figure shows the mean percent changes from baseline in serum alkaline phosphatase for up to six months of randomized treatment.

Effect on Serum Alkaline Phosphatase of FOSAMAX 40 mg/day Versus Placebo or Etidronate 400 mg/day

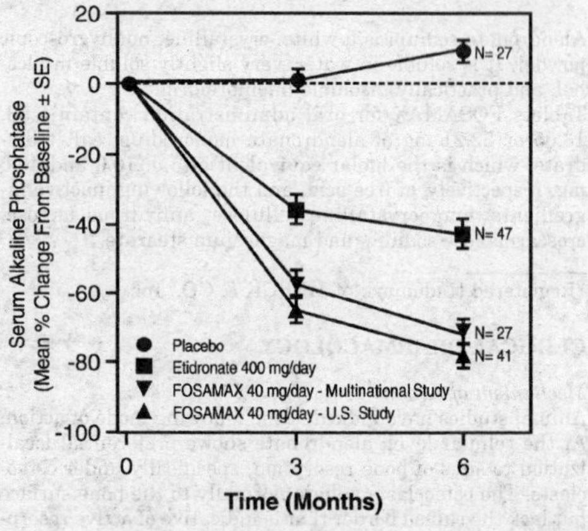

At six months the suppression in alkaline phosphatase in patients treated with FOSAMAX was significantly greater than that achieved with etidronate and contrasted with the complete lack of response in placebo-treated patients. Response (defined as either normalization of serum alkaline phosphatase or decrease from baseline ≥60%) occurred in approximately 85% of patients treated with FOSAMAX in the combined studies vs. 30% in the etidronate group and 0% in the placebo group. FOSAMAX was similarly effective irrespective of age, gender, race, prior use of other bisphosphonates, or baseline alkaline phosphatase within the range studied (at least twice the upper limit of normal).
Bone histology was evaluated in 33 patients with Paget's disease treated with FOSAMAX 40 mg/day for 6 months. As in patients treated for osteoporosis (see *Clinical Studies, Treatment of osteoporosis in postmenopausal women, Bone histology*), FOSAMAX did not impair mineralization, and the expected decrease in the rate of bone turnover was observed. Normal lamellar bone was produced during treatment with FOSAMAX, even where preexisting bone was woven and disorganized. Overall, bone histology data support the conclusion that bone formed during treatment with FOSAMAX is of normal quality.

ANIMAL PHARMACOLOGY

The relative inhibitory activities on bone resorption and mineralization of alendronate and etidronate were compared in the Schenk assay, which is based on histological examination of the epiphyses of growing rats. In this assay,

Effect of FOSAMAX on Fracture Incidence Over Three Years
in the Vertebral Fracture Study of FIT

	% of Patients FOSAMAX	Placebo	Reduction (%) in Fracture Incidence
Patients with:			
≥1 new vertebral fracture	8.0	15.0	47
≥2 new vertebral fractures	0.5	4.9	90
≥1 painful vertebral fracture	2.3	5.0	55
Hip fractures	1.1	2.2	51
Wrist (forearm) fractures	2.2	4.1	48

Time Course of Effect of FOSAMAX 10 mg/day Versus Placebo: Lumbar Spine BMD Percent Change From Baseline

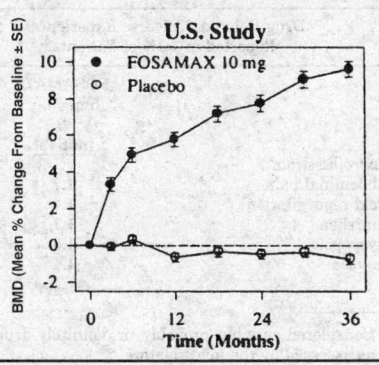

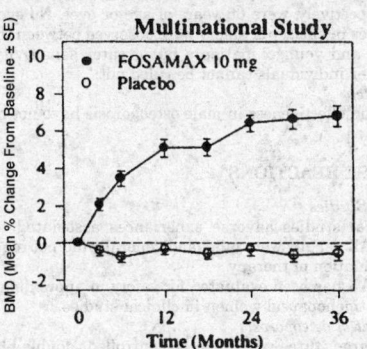

Cumulative Incidence of Patients with Hip and Wrist Fractures

FIT
(Vertebral Fracture Study)

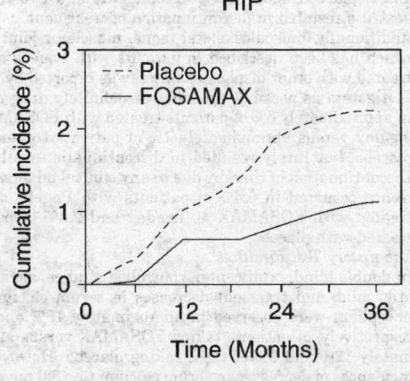

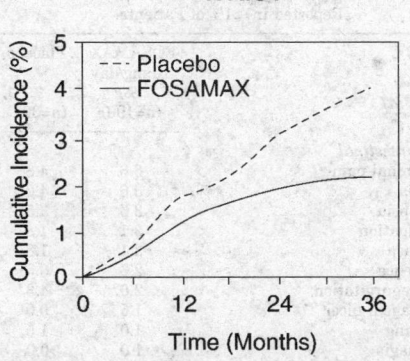

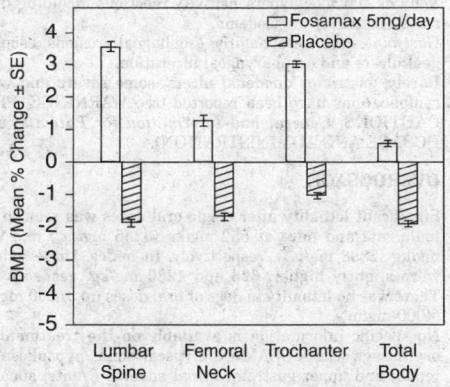

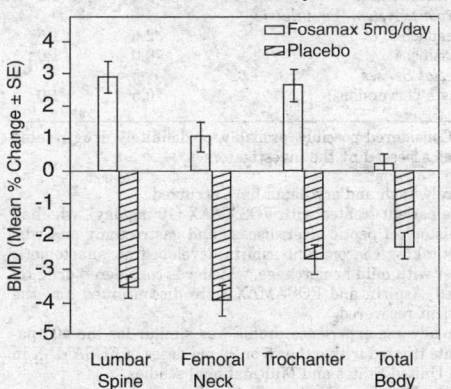

the lowest dose of alendronate that interfered with bone mineralization (leading to osteomalacia) was 6000-fold the antiresorptive dose. The corresponding ratio for etidronate was one to one. These data suggest that alendronate administered in therapeutic doses is highly unlikely to induce osteomalacia.

INDICATIONS AND USAGE

FOSAMAX is indicated for the treatment and prevention of osteoporosis in postmenopausal women.
- For the treatment of osteoporosis, FOSAMAX increases bone mass and prevents fractures, including those of the hip, wrist, and spine (vertebral compression fractures). Osteoporosis may be confirmed by the finding of low bone mass (for example, at least 2 standard deviations below the premenopausal mean) or by the presence or history of osteoporotic fracture. (See CLINICAL PHARMACOLOGY, *Pharmacodynamics*.)

- For the prevention of osteoporosis, FOSAMAX may be considered in postmenopausal women who are at risk of developing osteoporosis and for whom the desired clinical outcome is to maintain bone mass and to reduce the risk of future fracture.

Bone loss is particularly rapid in postmenopausal women younger than age 60. Risk factors often associated with the development of postmenopausal osteoporosis include early menopause; moderately low bone mass (for example, at least 1 standard deviation below the mean for healthy young adult women); thin body build; Caucasian or Asian race; and family history of osteoporosis. The presence of such risk factors may be important when considering the use of FOSAMAX for prevention of osteoporosis.

FOSAMAX is indicated for the treatment of Paget's disease of bone.
- Treatment is indicated in patients with Paget's disease of bone having alkaline phosphatase at least two times the

upper limit of normal, or those who are symptomatic, or those at risk for future complications from their disease.

CONTRAINDICATIONS
- Abnormalities of the esophagus which delay esophageal emptying such as stricture or achalasia
- Inability to stand or sit upright for at least 30 minutes
- Hypersensitivity to any component of this product
- Hypocalcemia (see PRECAUTIONS, *General*)

WARNINGS

FOSAMAX, like other bisphosphonates, may cause local irritation of the upper gastrointestinal mucosa.
Esophageal adverse experiences, such as esophagitis, esophageal ulcers and esophageal erosions, occasionally with bleeding, have been reported in patients receiving treatment with FOSAMAX. In some cases these have been severe and required hospitalization. Physicians should therefore be alert to any signs or symptoms signaling a possible esophageal reaction and patients should be instructed to discontinue FOSAMAX and seek medical attention if they develop dysphagia, odynophagia or retrosternal pain. The risk of severe esophageal adverse experiences appears to be greater in patients who lie down after taking FOSAMAX and/or who fail to swallow it with a full glass (6–8 oz) of water, and/or who continue to take FOSAMAX after developing symptoms suggestive of esophageal irritation. Therefore, it is very important that the full dosing instructions are provided to, and understood by, the patient (see DOSAGE AND ADMINISTRATION). In patients who cannot comply with dosing instructions due to mental disability, therapy with FOSAMAX should be used under appropriate supervision.
Because of possible irritant effects of FOSAMAX on the upper gastrointestinal mucosa and a potential for worsening of the underlying disease, caution should be used when FOSAMAX is given to patients with active upper gastrointestinal problems, (such as dysphagia, esophageal diseases, gastritis, duodenitis, or ulcers).

PRECAUTIONS

General
There have been rare (post-marketing) reports of gastric and duodenal ulcers, some severe and with complications, although no increased risk was observed in pre-marketing clinical trials.
FOSAMAX is not recommended for patients with renal insufficiency (creatinine clearance <35 mL/min). (See DOSAGE AND ADMINISTRATION.)
Causes of osteoporosis other than estrogen deficiency and aging should be considered.
Hypocalcemia must be corrected before initiating therapy with FOSAMAX (see CONTRAINDICATIONS). Other disturbances of mineral metabolism (such as vitamin D deficiency) should also be effectively treated. Presumably due to the effects of FOSAMAX on increasing bone mineral, small, asymptomatic decreases in serum calcium and phosphate may occur, especially in patients with Paget's disease, in whom the pretreatment rate of bone turnover may be greatly elevated. Adequate calcium and vitamin D intake should be ensured to provide for these enhanced needs.
Information for Patients
Patients should be instructed that the expected benefits of FOSAMAX may only be obtained when each tablet is swallowed with plain water the first thing upon arising for the day at least 30 minutes before the first food, beverage, or medication of the day. Even dosing with orange juice or coffee has been shown to markedly reduce the absorption of FOSAMAX (see CLINICAL PHARMACOLOGY, *Pharmacokinetics, Absorption*).
To facilitate delivery to the stomach and thus reduce the potential for esophageal irritation patients should be instructed to swallow FOSAMAX with a full glass of water (6–8 oz) and not to lie down for at least 30 minutes and until after their first food of the day. Patients should not chew or suck on the tablet because of a potential for oropharyngeal ulceration. Patients should be specifically instructed not to take FOSAMAX at bedtime or before arising for the day. Patients should be informed that failure to follow these instructions may increase their risk of esophageal problems. Patients should be instructed that if they develop symptoms of esophageal disease (such as difficulty or pain upon swallowing, retrosternal pain or new or worsening heartburn) they should stop taking FOSAMAX and consult their physician.
Patients should be instructed to take supplemental calcium and vitamin D, if daily dietary intake is inadequate. Weight-bearing exercise should be considered along with the modification of certain behavioral factors, such as excessive cigarette smoking, and/or alcohol consumption, if these factors exist.

Continued on next page

Fosamax—Cont.

Physicians should instruct their patients to read the patient package insert before starting therapy with FOSAMAX and to reread it each time the prescription is renewed.

Drug Interactions (also see CLINICAL PHARMACOLOGY, *Pharmacokinetics, Drug Interactions*)

Estrogen

The safety and effectiveness of the concomitant use of hormone replacement therapy and FOSAMAX in postmenopausal women has not been established.

Calcium Supplements/Antacids

It is likely that calcium supplements, antacids, and some oral medications will interfere with absorption of FOSAMAX. Therefore, patients must wait at least one-half hour after taking FOSAMAX before taking any other drug.

Aspirin

In clinical studies, the incidence of upper gastrointestinal adverse events was increased in patients receiving concomitant therapy with doses of FOSAMAX greater than 10 mg/day and aspirin-containing compounds.

Nonsteroidal Anti-inflammatory Drugs (NSAIDs)

FOSAMAX may be administered to patients taking NSAIDs. In a 3-year, controlled, clinical study (n = 2027) during which a majority of patients received concomitant NSAIDs, the incidence of upper gastrointestinal adverse events was similar in patients taking FOSAMAX 5 or 10 mg compared to those taking placebo. However, since NSAID use is associated with gastrointestinal irritation, caution should be used during concomitant use with FOSAMAX.

Carcinogenesis, Mutagenesis, Impairment of Fertility

Harderian gland (a retro-orbital gland not present in humans) adenomas were increased in high-dose female mice (p=0.003) in a 92-week carcinogenicity study at doses of alendronate of 1, 3, and 10 mg/kg/day (males) or 1, 2, and 5 mg/kg/day (females). These doses are equivalent to 0.5 to 4 times the 10 mg human dose based on surface area, mg/m^2.

Parafollicular cell (thyroid) adenomas were increased in high-dose male rats (p=0.003) in a 2-year carcinogenicity study at doses of 1 and 3.75 mg/kg body weight. These doses are equivalent to 1 and 3 times the 10 mg human dose based on surface area.

Alendronate was not genotoxic in the *in vitro* microbial mutagenesis assay with and without metabolic activation, in an *in vitro* mammalian cell mutagenesis assay, in an *in vitro* alkaline elution assay in rat hepatocytes, and in an *in vivo* chromosomal aberration assay in mice. In an *in vitro* chromosomal aberration assay in Chinese hamster ovary cells, however, alendronate was weakly positive at concentrations ≥5 mM in the presence of cytotoxicity.

Alendronate had no effect on fertility (male or female) in rats at oral doses up to 5 mg/kg/day (four times the 10 mg human dose based on surface area).

Pregnancy

Pregnancy Category C:

Reproduction studies in rats showed decreased postimplantation survival at 2 mg/kg/day and decreased body weight gain in normal pups at 1 mg/kg/day. Sites of incomplete fetal ossification were statistically significantly increased in rats beginning at 10 mg/kg/day in vertebral (cervical, thoracic, and lumbar), skull, and sternebral bones. The above doses ranged from 1 times (1 mg/kg) to 9 times (10 mg/kg) the 10 mg human dose based on surface area, mg/m^2. No similar fetal effects were seen when pregnant rabbits were treated at doses up to 35 mg/kg/day (50 times the 10 mg human dose based on surface area, mg/m^2).

Both total and ionized calcium decreased in pregnant rats at 15 mg/kg/day (13 times the 10 mg human dose based on surface area) resulting in delays and failures of delivery. Protracted parturition due to maternal hypocalcemia occurred in rats at doses as low as 0.5 mg/kg/day (0.5 times the recommended human dose) when rats were treated from before mating through gestation. Maternotoxicity (late pregnancy deaths) occurred in the female rats treated with 15 mg/kg/day for varying periods of time ranging from treatment only during pre-mating to treatment only during early, middle, or late gestation; these deaths were lessened but not eliminated by cessation of treatment. Calcium supplementation either in the drinking water or by minipump could not ameliorate the hypocalcemia or prevent maternal and neonatal deaths due to delays in delivery; calcium supplementation IV prevented maternal, but not fetal deaths.

There are no studies in pregnant women. FOSAMAX should be used during pregnancy only if the potential benefit justifies the potential risk to the mother and fetus.

Nursing Mothers

It is not known whether alendronate is excreted in human milk. Because many drugs are excreted in human milk, caution should be exercised when FOSAMAX is administered to nursing women.

Pediatric Use

Safety and effectiveness in pediatric patients have not been established.

Use in the Elderly

Of the patients receiving FOSAMAX in the two large osteoporosis treatment studies and Paget's disease studies (see CLINICAL PHARMACOLOGY, *Clinical Studies*), 45% and 70%, respectively, were 65 years of age or over. No overall differences in efficacy or safety were observed between these patients and younger patients but greater sensitivity of some older individuals cannot be ruled out.

Use in Men

Safety and effectiveness in male osteoporosis have not been established.

ADVERSE REACTIONS

Clinical Studies

In clinical studies adverse experiences associated with FOSAMAX usually were mild, and generally did not require discontinuation of therapy.

FOSAMAX has been evaluated for safety in approximately 3800 postmenopausal women in clinical studies.

Treatment of osteoporosis

In two large, three-year, placebo-controlled, double-blind, multicenter studies (United States and Multinational), discontinuation of therapy due to any clinical adverse experience occurred in 4.1% of 196 patients treated with FOSAMAX 10 mg/day and 6.0% of 397 patients treated with placebo. Adverse experiences reported by the investigators as possibly, probably, or definitely drug related in ≥1% of patients treated with either FOSAMAX 10 mg/day or placebo are presented in the following table.

Drug-Related**Adverse Experiences
Reported in ≥1% of Patients

	FOSAMAX 10 mg/day % (n=196)	Placebo % (n=397)
Gastrointestinal		
abdominal pain	6.6	4.8
nausea	3.6	4.0
dyspepsia	3.6	3.5
constipation	3.1	1.8
diarrhea	3.1	1.8
flatulence	2.6	0.5
acid regurgitation	2.0	4.3
esophageal ulcer	1.5	0.0
vomiting	1.0	1.5
dysphagia	1.0	0.0
abdominal distention	1.0	0.8
gastritis	0.5	1.3
Musculoskeletal		
musculoskeletal (bone, muscle or joint) pain	4.1	2.5
muscle cramp	0.0	1.0
Nervous System/Psychiatric		
headache	2.6	1.5
dizziness	0.0	1.0
Special Senses		
taste perversion	0.5	1.0

** Considered possibly, probably, or definitely drug related as assessed by the investigators

Rarely, rash and erythema have occurred.

One patient treated with FOSAMAX (10 mg/day), who had a history of peptic ulcer disease and gastrectomy and who was taking concomitant aspirin developed an anastomotic ulcer with mild hemorrhage, which was considered drug related. Aspirin and FOSAMAX were discontinued and the patient recovered.

The adverse experience profile was similar for the 401 patients treated with either 5 or 20 mg doses of FOSAMAX in the United States and Multinational studies.

In the Vertebral Fracture Study of the Fracture Intervention Trial, discontinuation of therapy due to any clinical adverse experience occurred in 7.6% of 1022 patients treated with FOSAMAX 5 mg/day for 2 years and 10 mg/day for the third year and 9.4% of 1005 patients treated with placebo. Similarly, discontinuations due to upper gastrointestinal adverse experiences were comparable: FOSAMAX, 2.6%; placebo, 2.6%. The overall adverse experience profile was similar to that seen in other studies with FOSAMAX 5 or 10 mg/day.

Prevention of osteoporosis

The safety of FOSAMAX in postmenopausal women 40–60 years of age has been evaluated in three double-blind, placebo-controlled studies involving over 1,400 patients randomized to receive FOSAMAX for either two or three years. In these studies the overall safety profiles of FOSAMAX 5 mg/day and placebo were similar. Discontinuation of therapy due to any clinical adverse experience occurred in 7.5% of 642 patients treated with FOSAMAX 5 mg/day and 5.7% of 648 patients treated with placebo. The adverse experiences reported by the investigators as possibly, probably or definitely drug related in ≥1% of patients treated with either FOSAMAX 5 mg/day or placebo are presented in the following table.

Drug-Related**Adverse Experiences
Reported in ≥1% of Patients

	FOSAMAX 5 mg/day % (n=642)	Placebo % (n=648)
Gastrointestinal		
abdominal pain	1.7	3.4
acid regurgitation	1.4	2.5
diarrhea	1.1	1.7
dyspepsia	1.9	1.7
nausea	1.4	1.4

** Considered possibly, probably, or definitely drug related as assessed by the investigators

Paget's disease of bone

In clinical studies (osteoporosis and Paget's disease), adverse experiences reported in 175 patients taking FOSAMAX 40 mg/day for 3–12 months were similar to those in postmenopausal women treated with FOSAMAX 10 mg/day. However, there was an apparent increased incidence of upper gastrointestinal adverse experiences in patients taking FOSAMAX 40 mg/day (17.7% FOSAMAX vs. 10.2% placebo). One case of esophagitis and two cases of gastritis resulted in discontinuation of treatment.

Additionally, musculoskeletal (bone, muscle or joint) pain, which has been described in patients with Paget's disease treated with other bisphosphonates, was reported by the investigators as possibly, probably, or definitely drug related in approximately 6% of patients treated with FOSAMAX 40 mg/day versus approximately 1% of patients treated with placebo, but rarely resulted in discontinuation of therapy.

Discontinuation of therapy due to any clinical adverse experience occurred in 6.4% of patients with Paget's disease treated with FOSAMAX 40 mg/day and 2.4% of patients treated with placebo.

Laboratory Test Findings

In double-blind, multicenter, controlled studies, asymptomatic, mild, and transient decreases in serum calcium and phosphate were observed in approximately 18% and 10%, respectively, of patients taking FOSAMAX versus approximately 12% and 3% of those taking placebo. However, the incidences of decreases in serum calcium to <8.0 mg/dL (2.0 mM) and serum phosphate to ≤2.0 mg/dL (0.65 mM) were similar in both treatment groups.

Post-Marketing Experience

The following adverse reactions have been reported in post-marketing use:

Body as a Whole: hypersensitivity reactions including urticaria and rarely angioedema.

Gastrointestinal: esophagitis, esophageal erosions, esophageal ulcers and oropharyngeal ulceration.

Rarely, gastric or duodenal ulcers, some severe and with complications have been reported (see WARNINGS, PRECAUTIONS, *General* and *Information for Patients*, and DOSAGE AND ADMINISTRATION).

OVERDOSAGE

Significant lethality after single oral doses was seen in female rats and mice at 552 mg/kg (3256 mg/m^2) and 966 mg/kg (2898 mg/m^2), respectively. In males, these values were slightly higher, 626 and 1280 mg/kg, respectively. There was no lethality in dogs at oral doses up to 200 mg/kg (4000 mg/m^2).

No specific information is available on the treatment of overdosage with FOSAMAX. Hypocalcemia, hypophosphatemia, and upper gastrointestinal adverse events, such as upset stomach, heartburn, esophagitis, gastritis, or ulcer, may result from oral overdosage. Milk or antacids should be given to bind alendronate. Due to the risk of esophageal irritation, vomiting should not be induced and the patient should remain fully upright.

Dialysis would not be beneficial.

DOSAGE AND ADMINISTRATION

FOSAMAX must be taken *at least* one-half hour before the first food, beverage, or medication of the day with plain water only (see PRECAUTIONS, *Information for Patients*). Other beverages (including mineral water), food, and some medications are likely to reduce the absorption of FOSAMAX (see PRECAUTIONS, *Drug Interactions*). Waiting less than 30 minutes, or taking FOSAMAX with food, beverages (other than plain water) or other medications will lessen the effect of FOSAMAX by decreasing its absorption into the body.

To facilitate delivery to the stomach and thus reduce the potential for esophageal irritation, FOSOMAX should only be

swallowed upon arising for the day with a full glass of water (6–8 oz) and patients should not lie down for at least 30 minutes and until after their first food of the day. FOSAMAX should not be taken at bedtime or before arising for the day. Failure to follow these instructions may increase the risk of esophageal adverse experiences (see WARNINGS).

Patients should receive supplemental calcium and vitamin D, if dietary intake is inadequate (see PRECAUTIONS, *General*).

No dosage adjustment is necessary for the elderly or for patients with mild-to-moderate renal insufficiency (creatinine clearance 35 to 60 mL/min). FOSAMAX is not recommended for patients with more severe renal insufficiency (creatinine clearance <35 mL/min) due to lack of experience.

Treatment of osteoporosis in postmenopausal women (see INDICATIONS AND USAGE)

The recommended dosage is 10 mg once a day.

Prevention of osteoporosis in postmenopausal women (see INDICATIONS AND USAGE)

The recommended dosage is 5 mg once a day.

Safety of treatment or prevention of osteoporosis with FOSAMAX for longer than four years has not been studied; extension studies are ongoing.

Paget's disease of bone

The recommended treatment regimen is 40 mg once a day for six months.

Retreatment of Paget's disease

In clinical studies in which patients were followed every six months, relapses during the 12 months following therapy occurred in 9% (3 out of 32) of patients who responded to treatment with FOSAMAX. Specific retreatment data are not available, although responses to FOSAMAX were similar in patients who had received prior bisphosphonate therapy and those who had not. Retreatment with FOSAMAX may be considered, following a six-month post-treatment evaluation period in patients who have relapsed, based on increases in serum alkaline phosphatase, which should be measured periodically. Retreatment may also be considered in those who failed to normalize their serum alkaline phosphatase.

HOW SUPPLIED

No. 3759—Tablets FOSAMAX, 5 mg, are white, round, uncoated tablets with an outline of a bone image on one side and code MRK 925 on the other. They are supplied as follows:

NDC 0006-0925-31 unit-of-use bottles of 30

NDC 0006-0925-58 unit-of-use bottles of 100.

Shown in Product Identification Guide, page 323

No. 3600—Tablets FOSAMAX, 10 mg, are white, round, uncoated tablets with a bone image and code MRK 936 on one side and a bone image and FOSAMAX on the other. They are supplied as follows:

NDC 0006-0936-31 unit-of-use bottles of 30 (6505-01-424-1106, 10 mg 30's)

NDC 0006-0936-58 unit-of-use bottles of 100

NDC 0006-0936-28 unit dose packages of 100 (6505-01-424-1113, 10 mg 100's)

NDC 0006-0936-82 bottles of 1000

NDC 0006-0936-72 carton of 25 UNIBLISTER™ cards of 31 tablets each.

Shown in Product Identification Guide, page 323

No. 3592—Tablets FOSAMAX, 40 mg, are white, triangular-shaped, uncoated tablets with code MRK 212 on one side and FOSAMAX on the other. They are supplied as follows:

NDC 0006-0212-31 unit-of-use bottles of 30 (6505-01-424-1111, 40 mg 30's).

Shown in Product Identification Guide, page 323

Storage

Store in a well-closed container at room temperature, 15–30°C (59–86°F).

7957007 Issued July 1997

COPYRIGHT © MERCK & CO., Inc., 1995
All rights reserved.

HUMORSOL® Sterile Ophthalmic Solution (Demecarium Bromide), U.S.P. For Topical Application into the Conjunctival Sac Only ℞

DESCRIPTION

Ophthalmic Solution HUMORSOL* (Demecarium Bromide) is a sterile solution supplied in two dosage strengths: 0.125 percent and 0.25 percent. The inactive ingredients are sodium chloride and water for injection; benzalkonium chloride 1:5000 is added as preservative. Demecarium bromide is a quaternary ammonium compound with a molecular weight of 716.60. Its chemical name is 3,3'-[1,10-decanediylbis [(methylimino)carbonyloxy]] bis [*N,N,N*-trimethylbenzenaminium] dibromide. Its empirical formula is $C_{32}H_{52}Br_2N_4O_4$ and its structural formula is:

[See chemical structure at top of next column]

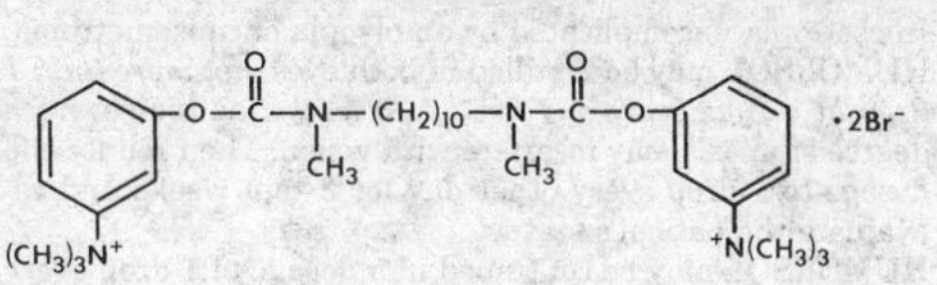

*Registered trademark of MERCK & CO., INC.

CLINICAL PHARMACOLOGY

HUMORSOL is a cholinesterase inhibitor with sustained activity. It acts mainly on true (erythrocyte) cholinesterase. Application of HUMORSOL to the eye produces intense miosis and ciliary muscle contraction due to inhibition of cholinesterase, allowing acetylcholine to accumulate at sites of cholinergic transmission. These effects are accompanied by increased capillary permeability of the ciliary body and iris, increased permeability of the blood-aqueous barrier, and vasodilation. Myopia may be induced or, if present, may be augmented by the increased refractive power of the lens that results from the accommodative effect of the drug. HUMORSOL indirectly produces some of the muscarinic and nicotinic effects of acetylcholine as quantities of the latter accumulate.

INDICATIONS AND USAGE

Open-angle glaucoma (HUMORSOL should be used in glaucoma only when shorter-acting miotics have proved inadequate.)

Conditions obstructing aqueous outflow, such as synechial formation, that are amenable to miotic therapy

Following iridectomy

Accommodative esotropia (accommodative convergent strabismus)

CONTRAINDICATIONS

Hypersensitivity to any component of this product.

Because of the toxicity of cholinesterase inhibitors in general, HUMORSOL is contraindicated in women who are or who may become pregnant. If this drug is used during pregnancy, or if the patient becomes pregnant while taking this drug, the patient should be apprised of the potential hazard to the fetus.

Because miotics may aggravate inflammation, HUMORSOL should not be used in active uveal inflammation and/or glaucoma associated with iridocyclitis.

WARNINGS

In patients receiving cholinesterase inhibitors such as HUMORSOL, succinylcholine should be administered with extreme caution before and during general anesthesia.

Because of possible adverse additive effects, HUMORSOL should be administered only with extreme caution to patients with myasthenia gravis who are receiving systemic anticholinesterase therapy; conversely, extreme caution should be exercised in the use of an anticholinesterase drug for the treatment of myasthenia gravis patients who are already undergoing topical therapy with cholinesterase inhibitors.

PRECAUTIONS

General

Gonioscopy is recommended prior to medication with HUMORSOL.

HUMORSOL should be used with caution in patients with chronic angle-closure (narrow-angle) glaucoma or in patients with narrow angles, because of the possibility of producing pupillary block and increasing angle blockage.

When an intraocular inflammatory process is present, the intensity and persistence of miosis and ciliary muscle contraction that result from anticholinesterase therapy require abstention from, or cautious use of, HUMORSOL.

Systemic effects are infrequent when HUMORSOL is instilled carefully. Compression of the lacrimal duct for several seconds immediately following instillation minimizes drainage into the nasal chamber with its extensive absorption surface. Wash the hands immediately after instillation.

Discontinue HUMORSOL if salivation, urinary incontinence, diarrhea, profuse sweating, muscle weakness, respiratory difficulties, shock, or cardiac irregularities occur.

Persons receiving cholinesterase inhibitors who are exposed to organophosphate-type insecticides and pesticides (gardeners, organophosphate plant or warehouse workers, farmers, residents of communities which are undergoing insecticide spraying or dusting, etc.) should be warned of the added systemic effects possible from absorption through the respiratory tract or skin. Wearing of respiratory masks, frequent washing, and clothing changes may be advisable.

Anticholinesterase drugs should be used with extreme caution, if at all, in patients with marked vagotonia, bronchial asthma, spastic gastrointesinal disturbances, peptic ulcer, pronounced bradycardia and hypotension, recent myocardial infarction, epilepsy, parkinsonism, and other disorders that may respond adversely to vagotonic effects.

After long-term use of HUMORSOL, dilation of blood vessels and resulting greater permeability increase the possibility of hyphema during ophthalmic surgery. Therefore, this drug should be discontinued before surgery.

Despite observance of all precautions and the use of only the recommended dose, there is some evidence that repeated administration may cause depression of the concentration of cholinesterase in the serum and erythrocytes, with resultant systemic effects.

There have been reports of bacterial keratitis associated with the use of multiple dose containers of topical ophthalmic products. These containers had been inadvertently contaminated by patients who, in most cases, had a concurrent corneal disease or a disruption of the ocular epithelial surface. (See PRECAUTIONS, *Information for Patients.*)

Information for Patients

Patients should be instructed to avoid allowing the tip of the dispensing container to contact the eye or surrounding structures.

Patients should also be instructed that ocular solutions, if handled improperly, can become contaminated by common bacteria known to cause ocular infections. Serious damage to the eye and subsequent loss of vision may result from using contaminated solutions. (See PRECAUTIONS, *General.*)

Patients should also be advised that if they develop an intercurrent ocular condition (e.g., trauma, ocular surgery or infection), they should immediately seek their physician's advice concerning the continued use of the present multidose container.

The preservative in HUMORSOL, benzalkonium chloride, may be absorbed by soft contact lenses. Patients wearing soft contact lenses should be instructed to wait at least 15 minutes after instilling HUMORSOL before they insert their lenses.

Drug Interactions

See WARNINGS regarding possible drug interactions of HUMORSOL with succinylcholine or with other anticholinesterase agents.

Carcinogenesis, Mutagenesis, Impairment of Fertility

Long-term studies in animals have not been performed to evaluate the effects of HUMORSOL on fertility or carcinogenic potential.

Pregnancy

Pregnancy Category X: See CONTRAINDICATIONS.

Nursing Mothers

It is not known whether this drug is excreted in human milk. Because of the potential for serious adverse reactions in nursing infants from HUMORSOL, a decision should be made whether to discontinue nursing or to discontinue the drug, taking into account the importance of the drug to the mother.

Pediatric Use

The occurrence of iris cysts is more frequent in pediatric patients. (See ADVERSE REACTIONS and DOSAGE AND ADMINISTRATION.)

Extreme caution should be exercised in pediatric patients receiving HUMORSOL who may require general anesthesia (see WARNINGS).

Since HUMORSOL is a potent cholinesterase inhibitor it should be kept out of the reach of children.

ADVERSE REACTIONS

Stinging, burning, lacrimation, lid muscle twitching, conjunctival and ciliary redness, brow ache, headache, and induced myopia with visual blurring may occur.

Activation of latent iritis or uveitis may occur.

As with all miotic therapy, retinal detachment has been reported occasionally.

Iris cysts may form, enlarge, and obscure vision. Occurrence is more frequent in children. The iris cyst usually shrinks upon discontinuance of the miotic. Rarely, the cyst may rupture or break free into the aqueous. Frequent examination for this occurrence is advised.

Lens opacities have been reported in patients on miotic therapy. Routine slit-lamp examinations, including the lens, should accompany prolonged use.

Paradoxical increase in intraocular pressure may follow anticholinesterase instillation. This may be alleviated by pupil-dilating medication.

Prolonged use may cause conjunctival thickening and obstruction of nasolacrimal canals.

Systemic effects, which occur rarely, are suggestive of increased cholinergic activity. Such effects may include nausea, vomiting, abdominal cramps, diarrhea, urinary incon-

Continued on next page

Information on the Merck & Co., Inc. products listed on these pages is the full prescribing information from product circulars in use August 31, 1998. For information, please call 1-800-NSC MERCK [1-800-672-6372].

Humorsol—Cont.

tinence, salivation, sweating, difficulty in breathing, bradycardia, or cardiac irregularities. Medical management of systemic effects may be indicated (see TREATMENT OF ADVERSE EFFECTS).

TREATMENT OF ADVERSE EFFECTS

If HUMORSOL is taken systemically by accident, or if systemic effects occur after topical application in the eye or from accidental skin contact, administer atropine sulfate parenterally (intravenously if necessary) in a dose (for adults) of 0.4 to 0.6 mg or more. The recommended dosage of atropine in infants and children up to 12 years of age is 0.01 mg/kg repeated every two hours as needed until the desired effect is obtained, or adverse effects of atropine preclude further usage. The maximum single dose should not exceed 0.4 mg.

The use of much larger doses of atropine in treating anticholinesterase intoxication in adults has been reported in the literature. Initially 2 to 6 mg may be given followed by 2 mg every hour or more often, as long as muscarinic effects continue. The greater possibility of atropinization with large doses, particularly in sensitive individuals, should be borne in mind.

Pralidoxime* chloride has been reported to be useful in treating systemic effects due to cholinesterase inhibitors. However, its use is recommended in addition to and not as substitute for atropine.

A short-acting barbiturate is indicated if convulsions occur that are not entirely relieved by atropine. Barbiturate dosage should be carefully adjusted to avoid central respiratory depression. Marked weakness or paralysis of muscles of respiration should be treated promptly by artificial respiration and maintenance of a clear airway.

The oral LD_{50} of HUMORSOL is 2.96 mg/kg in the mouse.

*PROTOPAM® Chloride (Pralidoxime Chloride). Ayerst Laboratories

DOSAGE AND ADMINISTRATION

HUMORSOL *is intended solely for topical use in the conjunctival sac.*

As HUMORSOL is an extremely potent drug, the physician should thoroughly familiarize himself with its use and the technic of instillation.

The required dose is applied in the conjunctival sac, with the patient supine, care being taken not to touch the cornea with the tip of the OCUMETER** ophthalmic dispenser. *The patient or person administering the medication should apply continuous gentle pressure on the lacrimal duct with the index finger for several seconds immediately following instillation of the drops. This is to prevent drainage overflow of solution into the nasal and pharyngeal spaces, which might cause systemic absorption. Wash the hands immediately after administration.*

HUMORSOL *should not be used more often than directed. Caution is necessary to avoid overdosage.*

Initial titration and dosage adjustments with HUMORSOL must be individualized to obtain maximal therapeutic effect. The patient must be closely observed during the initial period. If the response is not adequate within the first 24 hours, other measures should be considered.

Keep frequency of use to a minimum in all patients, but especially in children, to reduce the chance of iris cyst development (see ADVERSE REACTIONS).

Glaucoma

For initial therapy with HUMORSOL (0.125 percent or 0.25 percent) place 1 drop (children) or 1 or 2 drops (adults) in the glaucomatous eye. A decrease in intraocular pressure should occur within a few hours. During this period, keep the patient under supervision and make tonometric examinations at least hourly for 3 or 4 hours to be sure that no immediate rise in pressure occurs (see ADVERSE REACTIONS).

Duration of effect varies with the individual. The usual dosage can vary from as much as 1 or 2 drops twice a day to as little as 1 or 2 drops twice a week. The 0.125 percent strength used twice a day usually results in smooth control of the physiologic diurnal variation in intraocular pressure. This is probably the preferred dosage for most wide (open) angle glaucoma patients.

Strabismus

Essentially equal visual acuity of both eyes is a prerequisite to the successful treatment of esotropia with HUMORSOL. For initial evaluation it may be used as a diagnostic aid to determine if an accommodative factor exists. This is especially useful preoperatively in young children and in patients with normal hypermetropic refractive errors. One drop is given daily for 2 weeks, then 1 drop every 2 days for 2 to 3 weeks. If the eyes become straighter, an accommodative factor is demonstrated. This technic may supplement or complement standard testing with atropine and trial with glasses for the accommodative factor.

In esotropia uncomplicated by amblyopia or anisometropia, HUMORSOL may be instilled in both eyes, *not more than 1 drop at a time every day for 2 to 3 weeks,* as too severe a degree of miosis may interfere with vision. Then reduce the dosage to 1 drop every other day for 3 to 4 weeks and reevaluate the patient's status.

HUMORSOL may be continued in a dosage of 1 drop every 2 days to 1 drop twice a week. (The latter dosage may be maintained for several months.) Evaluate the patient's condition every 4 to 12 weeks. If improvement continues, change the schedule to 1 drop once a week and eventually to a trial without medication. However, if after 4 months, control of the condition still requires 1 drop every 2 days, therapy with HUMORSOL should be stopped.

**Registered trademark of MERCK & CO., INC.

HOW SUPPLIED

Sterile Ophthalmic Solution HUMORSOL is a clear, colorless, aqueous solution and is supplied in a 5 mL white, opaque, plastic OCUMETER ophthalmic dispenser with a controlled-drop tip:

No. 3255—0.125 percent solution.
NDC 0006-3255-03.

No. 3267—0.25 percent solution.
NDC 0006-3267-03.

Storage

Protect from freezing and excessive heat.

7414315 Issued September 1996

COPYRIGHT © MERCK & CO., INC., 1987
All rights reserved

HYDROCORTONE® ℞

Acetate Injectable Suspension
(Hydrocortisone Acetate), U.S.P.
(Formerly called Sterile Suspension HYDROCORTONE® Acetate)

For intra-articular, intralesional, and soft tissue injection only.

NOT FOR INTRAVENOUS USE

DESCRIPTION

Hydrocortisone acetate, a synthetic adrenocortical steroid, is a white to practically white, odorless, crystalline powder. It is insoluble in water and slightly soluble in alcohol and chloroform. The molecular weight is 404.50. It is designated chemically as 21-(acetyloxy)-11β,17-dihydroxypregn-4-ene-3,20-dione. The empirical formula is $C_{23}H_{32}O_6$ and the structural formula is:

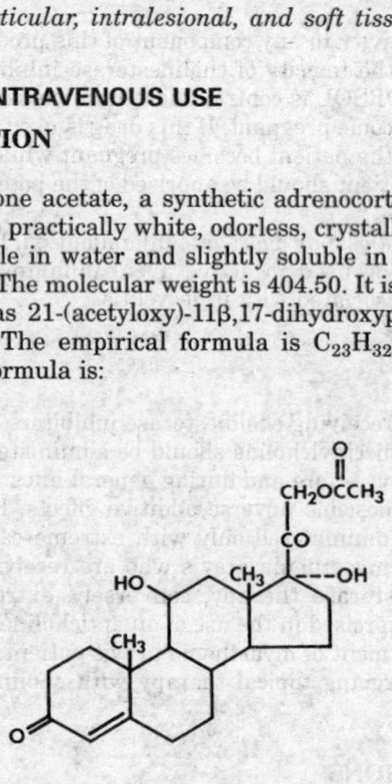

HYDROCORTONE* Acetate (Hydrocortisone Acetate) Injectable Suspension is a sterile suspension containing 50 mg per milliliter of hydrocortisone acetate in a suitable aqueous medium (pH -5.0 to 7.0). Inactive ingredients per mL: sodium chloride, 9 mg; polysorbate 80, 4 mg; sodium carboxymethylcellulose, 5 mg; and Water for Injection, q.s., 1 mL. Benzyl alcohol, 9 mg, added as preservative.

*Registered trademark of MERCK & CO., INC.

ACTIONS

HYDROCORTONE Acetate Injectable Suspension has a slow onset but long duration of action when compared with more soluble preparations. Because of its insolubility, it is suitable for intra-articular, intralesional, and soft tissue injection where its anti-inflammatory effects are confined mainly to the area in which it has been injected, although it is capable of producing systemic hormonal effects.

Naturally occurring glucocorticoids (hydrocortisone and cortisone), which also have salt-retaining properties, are used as replacement therapy in adrenocortical deficiency states. They are also used for their potent anti-inflammatory effect in disorders of many organ systems.

Glucocorticoids cause profound and varied metabolic effects. In addition, they modify the body's immune responses to diverse stimuli.

INDICATIONS

A. By intra-articular or soft tissue injection:

As adjunctive therapy for short-term administration (to tide the patient over an acute episode or exacerbation) in:

Synovitis of osteoarthritis
Rheumatoid arthritis
Acute and subacute bursitis
Acute gouty arthritis
Epicondylitis
Acute nonspecific tenosynovitis
Post-traumatic osteoarthritis

B. By intralesional injection:

Keloids

Localized hypertrophic, infiltrated, inflammatory lesions of: lichen planus, psoriatic plaques, granuloma annulare, and lichen simplex chronicus (neurodermatitis)

Discoid lupus erythematosus
Necrobiosis lipoidica diabeticorum
Alopecia areata

May also be useful in cystic tumors of an aponeurosis or tendon (ganglia).

CONTRAINDICATIONS

Systemic fungal infections
Hypersensitivity to any component of this product

WARNINGS

Because rare instances of anaphylactoid reactions have occurred in patients receiving parenteral corticosteroid therapy, appropriate precautionary measures should be taken prior to administration, especially when the patient has a history of allergy to any drug.

In patients on corticosteroid therapy subjected to any unusual stress, increased dosage of rapidly acting corticosteroids before, during, and after the stressful situation is indicated.

Drug-induced secondary adrenocortical insufficiency may result from too rapid withdrawal of corticosteroids and may be minimized by gradual reduction of dosage. This type of relative insufficiency may persist for months after discontinuation of therapy; therefore, in any situation of stress occurring during that period, hormone therapy should be reinstituted. If the patient is receiving steroids already, dosage may have to be increased. Since mineralocorticoid secretion may be impaired, salt and/or a mineralocorticoid should be administered concurrently.

Corticosteroids may mask some signs of infection, and new infections may appear during their use. There may be decreased resistance and inability to localize infection when corticosteroids are used. Moreover, corticosteroids may affect the nitroblue-tetrazolium test for bacterial infection and produce false negative results.

In cerebral malaria, a double-blind trial has shown that the use of corticosteroids is associated with prolongation of coma and a higher incidence of pneumonia and gastrointestinal bleeding.

Corticosteroids may activate latent amebiasis. Therefore, it is recommended that latent or active amebiasis be ruled out before initiating corticosteroid therapy in any patient who has spent time in the tropics or any patient with unexplained diarrhea.

Prolonged use of corticosteroids may produce posterior subcapsular cataracts, glaucoma with possible damage to the optic nerves, and may enhance the establishment of secondary ocular infections due to fungi or viruses.

Usage in pregnancy: Since adequate human reproduction studies have not been done with corticosteroids, use of these drugs in pregnancy or in women of childbearing potential requires that the anticipated benefits be weighed against the possible hazards to the mother and embryo or fetus. Infants born of mothers who have received substantial doses of corticosteroids during pregnancy should be carefully observed for signs of hypoadrenalism.

Corticosteroids appear in breast milk and could suppress growth, interfere with endogenous corticosteroid production, or cause other unwanted effects. Mothers taking pharmacologic doses of corticosteroids should be advised not to nurse.

Average and large doses of cortisone or hydrocortisone can cause elevation of blood pressure, salt and water retention, and increased excretion of potassium. These effects are less likely to occur with the synthetic derivatives except when used in large doses. Dietary salt restriction and potassium supplementation may be necessary. All corticosteroids increase calcium excretion.

Administration of live virus vaccines, including smallpox, is contraindicated in individuals receiving immunosuppressive doses of corticosteroids. If inactivated viral or bacterial vaccines are administered to individuals receiving immunosuppressive doses of corticosteroids, the expected serum antibody response may not be obtained.

Patients who are on drugs which suppress the immune system are more susceptible to infections than healthy individuals. Chickenpox and measles, for example, can have a

more serious or even fatal course in non-immune patients on corticosteroids. In such patients who have not had these diseases, particular care should be taken to avoid exposure. The risk of developing a disseminated infection varies among individuals and can be related to the dose, route and duration of corticosteroid administration as well as to the underlying disease. If exposed to chickenpox, prophylaxis with varicella zoster immune globulin (VZIG) may be indicated. If chickenpox develops, treatment with antiviral agents may be considered. If exposed to measles, prophylaxis with immune globulin (IG) may be indicated. (See the respective package inserts for VZIG and IG for complete prescribing information.)

Similarly, corticosteroids should be used with great care in patients with known or suspected Strongyloides (threadworm) infestation. In such patients, corticosteroid-induced immunosuppression may lead to Strongyloides hyperinfection and dissemination with widespread larval migration, often accompanied by severe enterocolitis and potentially fatal gram-negative septicemia.

If corticosteroids are indicated in patients with latent tuberculosis or tuberculin reactivity, close observation is necessary as reactivation of the disease may occur. During prolonged corticosteroid therapy, these patients should receive chemoprophylaxis.

Literature reports suggest an apparent association between use of corticosteroids and left ventricular free wall rupture after a recent myocardial infarction; therefore, therapy with corticosteroids should be used with great caution in these patients.

PRECAUTIONS

This product, like many other steroid formulations, is sensitive to heat. Therefore, it should not be autoclaved when it is desirable to sterilize the exterior of the vial.

Following prolonged therapy, withdrawal of corticosteroids may result in symptoms of the corticosteroid withdrawal syndrome including fever, myalgia, arthralgia, and malaise. This may occur in patients even without evidence of adrenal insufficiency.

There is an enhanced effect of corticosteroids in patients with hypothyroidism and in those with cirrhosis.

Corticosteroids should be used cautiously in patients with ocular herpes simplex for fear of corneal perforation.

Psychic derangements may appear when corticosteroids are used, ranging from euphoria, insomnia, mood swings, personality changes, and severe depression to frank psychotic manifestations. Also, existing emotional instability or psychotic tendencies may be aggravated by corticosteroids.

Aspirin should be used cautiously in conjunction with corticosteroids in hypoprothrombinemia.

Steroids should be used with caution in nonspecific ulcerative colitis, if there is a probability of impending perforation, abscess, or other pyogenic infection, also in diverticulitis, fresh intestinal anastomoses, active or latent peptic ulcer, renal insufficiency, hypertension, osteoporosis, and myasthenia gravis. Signs of peritoneal irritation following gastrointestinal perforation in patients receiving large doses of corticosteroids may be minimal or absent. Fat embolism has been reported as a possible complication of hypercortisonism.

When large doses are given, some authorities advise that antacids be administered between meals to help to prevent peptic ulcer.

Steroids may increase or decrease motility and number of spermatozoa in some patients.

Phenytoin, phenobarbital, ephedrine, and rifampin may enhance the metabolic clearance of corticosteroids resulting in decreased blood levels and lessened physiologic activity, thus requiring adjustment in corticosteroid dosage.

The prothrombin time should be checked frequently in patients who are receiving corticosteroids and coumarin anticoagulants at the same time because of reports that corticosteroids have altered the response to these anticoagulants. Studies have shown that the usual effect produced by adding corticosteroids is inhibition of response to coumarins, although there have been some conflicting reports of potentiation not substantiated by studies.

When corticosteroids are administered concomitantly with potassium-depleting diuretics, patients should be observed closely for development of hypokalemia.

Intra-articular injection of a corticosteroid may produce systemic as well as local effects.

Appropriate examination of any joint fluid present is necessary to exclude a septic process.

A marked increase in pain accompanied by local swelling, further restriction of joint motion, fever, and malaise is suggestive of septic arthritis. If this complication occurs and the diagnosis of sepsis is confirmed, appropriate antimicrobial therapy should be instituted.

Injection of a steroid into an infected site is to be avoided.

Corticosteroids should not be injected into unstable joints.

Patients should be impressed strongly with the importance of not overusing joints in which symptomatic benefit has been obtained as long as the inflammatory process remains active.

Frequent intra-articular injection may result in damage to joint tissues.

Information for Patients

Susceptible patients who are on immunosuppressant doses of corticosteroids should be warned to avoid exposure to chickenpox or measles. Patients should also be advised that if they are exposed, medical advice should be sought without delay.

Pediatric Use

Growth and development of pediatric patients on prolonged corticosteroid therapy should be carefully followed.

ADVERSE REACTIONS

Fluid and electrolyte disturbances
   Sodium retention
   Fluid retention
   Congestive heart failure in susceptible patients
   Potassium loss
   Hypokalemic alkalosis
   Hypertension
Musculoskeletal
   Muscle weakness
   Steroid myopathy
   Loss of muscle mass
   Osteoporosis
   Vertebral compression fractures
   Aseptic necrosis of femoral and humeral heads
   Pathologic fracture of long bones
   Tendon rupture
Gastrointestinal
   Peptic ulcer with possible subsequent perforation and hemorrhage
   Perforation of the small and large bowel, particularly in patients with inflammatory bowel disease
   Pancreatitis
   Abdominal distention
   Ulcerative esophagitis
Dermatologic
   Impaired wound healing
   Thin fragile skin
   Petechiae and ecchymoses
   Erythema
   Increased sweating
   May suppress reactions to skin tests
   Other cutaneous reactions, such as allergic dermatitis, urticaria, angioneurotic edema
Neurologic
   Convulsions
   Increased intracranial pressure with papilledema (pseudotumor cerebri) usually after treatment
   Vertigo
   Headache
   Psychic disturbances
Endocrine
   Menstrual irregularities
   Development of cushingoid state
   Suppression of growth in children
   Secondary adrenocortical and pituitary unresponsiveness, particularly in times of stress, as in trauma, surgery, or illness
   Decreased carbohydrate tolerance
   Manifestations of latent diabetes mellitus
   Increased requirements for insulin or oral hypoglycemic agents in diabetics
   Hirsutism
Ophthalmic
   Posterior subcapsular cataracts
   Increased intraocular pressure
   Glaucoma
   Exophthalmos
Metabolic
   Negative nitrogen balance due to protein catabolism
Cardiovascular
   Myocardial rupture following recent myocardial infarction (see WARNINGS)
Other
   Anaphylactoid or hypersensitivity reactions
   Thromboembolism
   Weight gain
   Increased appetite
   Nausea
   Malaise
The following *additional* adverse reactions are related to injection of corticosteroids:
   Rare instances of blindness associated with intralesional therapy around the face and head
   Hyperpigmentation or hypopigmentation
   Subcutaneous and cutaneous atrophy
   Sterile abscess
   Postinjection flare (following intra-articular use)
   Charcot-like arthropathy.

OVERDOSAGE

Reports of acute toxicity and/or death following overdosage of glucocorticoids are rare. In the event of overdosage, no specific antidote is available; treatment is supportive and symptomatic.

DOSAGE AND ADMINISTRATION
NOT FOR INTRAVENOUS USE

For intra-articular, intralesional, and soft tissue injection only

DOSAGE AND FREQUENCY OF INJECTION ARE VARIABLE AND MUST BE INDIVIDUALIZED ON THE BASIS OF THE DISEASE AND THE RESPONSE OF THE PATIENT.

The initial dose varies from 5 to 75 mg depending on the disease being treated and the size of the area to be injected. Frequency of injection depends on symptomatic response, and usually is once every two or three weeks. Severe conditions may require injection once a week. Frequent intra-articular injection may result in damage to joint tissues. If satisfactory clinical response does not occur after a reasonable period of time, discontinue HYDROCORTONE Acetate Injectable Suspension and transfer the patient to other therapy.

Patients should be observed closely for signs that might require dosage adjustment, including changes in clinical status resulting from remissions or exacerbations of the disease, and individual drug responsiveness.

Some of the usual single doses are:

Large Joints (e.g., Knee)	25 mg, occasionally 37.5 mg. Doses over 50 mg not recommended
Small Joints (e.g, Interphalangeal, Temporomandibular)	10 to 25 mg
Bursae	25 to 37.5 mg
Tendon Sheaths	5 to 12.5 mg
Soft Tissue Infiltration	25 to 50 mg, occasionally 75 mg
Ganglia	12.5 to 25 mg

For rapid onset of action, a soluble adrenocortical hormone preparation, such as DECADRON* Phosphate (Dexamethasone Sodium Phosphate) injection or HYDELTRASOL* (Prednisolone Sodium Phosphate) injection, may be given with HYDROCORTONE Acetate Injectable Suspension.

If desired, a local anesthetic may be used, and may be injected before HYDROCORTONE Acetate Injectable Suspension or mixed in a syringe with HYDROCORTONE Acetate Injectable Suspension and given simultaneously.

If used prior to intra-articular injection of the steroid, inject most of the anesthetic into the soft tissues of the surrounding area and instill a small amount into the joint.

If given together, mixing should be done in the injection syringe by drawing the steroid in *first* , then the anesthetic. In this way, the anesthetic will not be introduced inadvertently into the vial of steroid. *The mixture must be used immediately and any unused portion discarded.*

*Registered trademark of MERCK & CO., INC.

HOW SUPPLIED

No. 7519—HYDROCORTONE Acetate Injectable Suspension is a white, mobile suspension, containing 50 mg hydrocortisone acetate in each mL, and is supplied as follows: NDC 0006-7519-03 in 5 mL vials.
Storage
Sensitive to heat. Do not autoclave.
Protect from freezing.
         7348729   Issued February 1997

HYDROCORTONE® Phosphate Injection, Sterile   ℞
(Hydrocortisone Sodium Phosphate), U.S.P.

DESCRIPTION

Hydrocortisone sodium phosphate, a synthetic adrenocortical steroid, is a white to light yellow, odorless or practically

Continued on next page

Hydrocortone Phosphate—Cont.

odorless powder. It is freely soluble in water and is exceedingly hygroscopic. The molecular weight is 486.41. It is designated chemically as 11β,17-dihydroxy-21-(phosphonooxy)-pregn-4-ene-3,20-dione disodium salt. The empirical formula is $C_{21}H_{29}Na_2O_8P$ and the structural formula is:

HYDROCORTONE* Phosphate (Hydrocortisone Sodium Phosphate) injection is a sterile solution (pH 7.5 to 8.5), sealed under nitrogen, for intravenous, intramuscular, and subcutaneous administration.

Each milliliter contains hydrocortisone sodium phosphate equivalent to 50 mg hydrocortisone. Inactive ingredients per mL: 8 mg creatinine, 10 mg sodium citrate, sodium hydroxide to adjust pH, and Water for Injection, q.s. 1 mL, with 3.2 mg sodium bisulfite, 1.5 mg methylparaben, and 0.2 mg propylparaben added as preservatives.

---

* Registered trademark of MERCK & CO., INC.

ACTIONS

HYDROCORTONE Phosphate injection has a rapid onset but short duration of action when compared with less soluble preparations. Because of this, it is suitable for the treatment of acute disorders responsive to adrenocortical steroid therapy.

Naturally occurring glucocorticoids (hydrocortisone and cortisone), which also have salt-retaining properties, are used as replacement therapy in adrenocortical deficiency states. They are also used for their potent anti-inflammatory effects in disorders of many organ systems.

Glucocorticoids cause profound and varied metabolic effects. In addition, they modify the body's immune responses to diverse stimuli.

INDICATIONS

When oral therapy is not feasible:

1. *Endocrine disorders*
   Primary or secondary adrenocortical insufficiency (hydrocortisone or cortisone is the drug of choice; synthetic analogs may be used in conjunction with mineralocorticoids where applicable; in infancy, mineralocorticoid supplementation is of particular importance)
   Acute adrenocortical insufficiency (hydrocortisone or cortisone is the drug of choice; mineralocorticoid supplementation may be necessary, particularly when synthetic analogs are used)
   Preoperatively, and in the event of serious trauma or illness, in patients with known adrenal insufficiency or when adrenocortical reserve is doubtful
   Shock unresponsive to conventional therapy if adrenocortical insufficiency exists or is suspected
   Congenital adrenal hyperplasia
   Nonsuppurative thyroiditis
   Hypercalcemia associated with cancer

2. *Rheumatic disorders*
   As adjunctive therapy for short-term administration (to tide the patient over an acute episode or exacerbation) in:
   Post-traumatic osteoarthritis
   Synovitis of osteoarthritis
   Rheumatoid arthritis, including juvenile rheumatoid arthritis (selected cases may require low-dose maintenance therapy)
   Acute and subacute bursitis
   Epicondylitis
   Acute nonspecific tenosynovitis
   Acute gouty arthritis
   Psoriatic arthritis
   Ankylosing spondylitis

3. *Collagen diseases*
   During an exacerbation or as maintenance therapy in selected cases of:
   Systemic lupus erythematosus
   Acute rheumatic carditis
   Systemic dermatomyositis (polymyositis)

4. *Dermatologic diseases*
   Pemphigus
   Severe erythema multiforme (Stevens-Johnson syndrome)
   Exfoliative dermatitis
   Bullous dermatitis herpetiformis
   Severe seborrheic dermatitis
   Severe psoriasis
   Mycosis fungoides

5. *Allergic states*
   Control of severe or incapacitating allergic conditions intractable to adequate trials of conventional treatment in:
   Bronchial asthma
   Contact dermatitis
   Atopic dermatitis
   Serum sickness
   Seasonal or perennial allergic rhinitis
   Drug hypersensitivity reactions
   Urticarial transfusion reactions
   Acute noninfectious laryngeal edema (epinephrine is the drug of first choice)

6. *Ophthalmic diseases*
   Severe acute and chronic allergic and inflammatory processes involving the eye, such as:
   Herpes zoster ophthalmicus
   Iritis, iridocyclitis
   Chorioretinitis
   Diffuse posterior uveitis and choroiditis
   Optic neuritis
   Sympathetic ophthalmia
   Anterior segment inflammation
   Allergic conjunctivitis
   Keratitis
   Allergic corneal marginal ulcers

7. *Gastrointestinal diseases*
   To tide the patient over a critical period of the disease in:
   Ulcerative colitis (Systemic therapy)
   Regional enteritis (Systemic therapy)

8. *Respiratory diseases*
   Symptomatic sarcoidosis
   Berylliosis
   Fulminating or disseminated pulmonary tuberculosis when used concurrently with appropriate antituberculous chemotherapy
   Loeffler's syndrome not manageable by other means
   Aspiration pneumonitis

9. *Hematologic disorders*
   Acquired (autoimmune) hemolytic anemia
   Idiopathic thrombocytopenic purpura in adults (I.V. only; I.M. administration is contraindicated)
   Secondary thrombocytopenia in adults
   Erythroblastopenia (RBC anemia)
   Congenital (erythroid) hypoplastic anemia

10. *Neoplastic diseases*
    For palliative management of:
    Leukemias and lymphomas in adults
    Acute leukemia of childhood

11. *Edematous states*
    To induce diuresis or remission of proteinuria in the nephrotic syndrome, without uremia, of the idiopathic type, or that due to lupus erythematosus

12. *Miscellaneous*
    Tuberculous meningitis with subarachnoid block or impending block when used concurrently with appropriate antituberculous chemotherapy
    Trichinosis with neurologic or myocardial involvement

CONTRAINDICATIONS

Systemic fungal infections (see WARNINGS regarding amphotericin B)
Hypersensitivity to any component of this product, including sulfites (see WARNINGS).

WARNINGS

Because rare instances of anaphylactoid reactions have occurred in patients receiving parenteral corticosteroid therapy, appropriate precautionary measures should be taken prior to administration, especially when the patient has a history of allergy to any drug. Anaphylactoid and hypersensitivity reactions have been reported for Injection HYDROCORTONE Phosphate (see ADVERSE REACTIONS).

Injection HYDROCORTONE Phosphate contains sodium bisulfite, a sulfite that may cause allergic-type reactions including anaphylactic symptoms and life-threatening or less severe asthmatic episodes in certain susceptible people. The overall prevalence of sulfite sensitivity in the general population is unknown and probably low. Sulfite sensitivity is seen more frequently in asthmatic than in nonasthmatic people.

Corticosteroids may exacerbate systemic fungal infections and therefore should not be used in the presence of such infections unless they are needed to control drug reactions due to amphotericin B. Moreover, there have been cases reported in which concomitant use of amphotericin B and hydrocortisone was followed by cardiac enlargement and congestive failure.

In patients on corticosteroid therapy subjected to any unusual stress, increased dosage of rapidly acting corticosteroids before, during, and after the stressful situation is indicated.

Drug-induced secondary adrenocortical insufficiency may result from too rapid withdrawal of corticosteroids and may be minimized by gradual reduction of dosage. This type of relative insufficiency may persist for months after discontinuation of therapy; therefore, in any situation of stress occurring during that period, hormone therapy should be reinstituted. If the patient is receiving steroids already, dosage may have to be increased. Since mineralocorticoid secretion may be impaired, salt and/or a mineralocorticoid should be administered concurrently.

Corticosteroids may mask some signs of infection, and new infections may appear during their use. There may be decreased resistance and inability to localize infection when corticosteroids are used. Moreover, corticosteroids may affect the nitroblue-tetrazolium test for bacterial infection and produce false negative results.

In cerebral malaria, a double-blind trial has shown that the use of corticosteroids is associated with prolongation of coma and a higher incidence of pneumonia and gastrointestinal bleeding.

Corticosteroids may activate latent amebiasis. Therefore, it is recommended that latent or active amebiasis be ruled out before initiating corticosteroid therapy in any patient who has spent time in the tropics or any patient with unexplained diarrhea.

Prolonged use of corticosteroids may produce posterior subcapsular cataracts, glaucoma with possible damage to the optic nerves, and may enhance the establishment of secondary ocular infections due to fungi or viruses.

Usage in pregnancy. Since adequate human reproduction studies have not been done with corticosteroids, use of these drugs in pregnancy or in women of childbearing potential requires that the anticipated benefits be weighed against the possible hazards to the mother and embryo or fetus. Infants born of mothers who have received substantial doses of corticosteroids during pregnancy should be carefully observed for signs of hypoadrenalism.

Corticosteroids appear in breast milk and could suppress growth, interfere with endogenous corticosteroid production, or cause other unwanted effects. Mothers taking pharmacologic doses of corticosteroids should be advised not to nurse.

Average and large doses of cortisone or hydrocortisone can cause elevation of blood pressure, salt and water retention, and increased excretion of potassium. These effects are less likely to occur with the synthetic derivatives except when used in large doses. Dietary salt restriction and potassium supplementation may be necessary. All corticosteroids increase calcium excretion.

Administration of live virus vaccines, including smallpox, is contraindicated in individuals receiving immunosuppressive doses of corticosteroids. If inactivated viral or bacterial vaccines are administered to individuals receiving immunosuppressive doses of corticosteroids, the expected serum antibody response may not be obtained. However, immunization procedures may be undertaken in patients who are receiving corticosteroids as replacement therapy, e.g., for Addison's disease.

Patients who are on drugs which suppress the immune system are more susceptible to infections than healthy individuals. Chickenpox and measles, for example, can have a more serious or even fatal course in non-immune patients on corticosteroids. In such patients who have not had these diseases, particular care should be taken to avoid exposure. The risk of developing a disseminated infection varies among individuals and can be related to the dose, route and duration of corticosteroid administration as well as to the underlying disease. If exposed to chickenpox, prophylaxis with varicella zoster immune globulin (VZIG) may be indicated. If chickenpox develops, treatment with antiviral agents may be considered. If exposed to measles, prophylaxis with immune globulin (IG) may be indicated. (See the respective package inserts for VZIG and IG for complete prescribing information.)

Similarly, corticosteroids should be used with great care in patients with known or suspected Strongyloides (threadworm) infestation. In such patients, corticosteroid-induced immunosuppression may lead to Strongyloides hyperinfection and dissemination with widespread larval migration, often accompanied by severe enterocolitis and potentially fatal gram-negative septicemia.

The use of HYDROCORTONE Phosphate injection in active tuberculosis should be restricted to those cases of fulminating or disseminated tuberculosis in which the corticosteroid is used for the management of the disease in conjunction with an appropriate antituberculous regimen.

If corticosteroids are indicated in patients with latent tuberculosis or tuberculin reactivity, close observation is necessary as reactivation of the disease may occur. During prolonged corticosteroid therapy, these patients should receive chemoprophylaxis.

Literature reports suggest an apparent association between use of corticosteroids and left ventricular free wall rupture after a recent myocardial infarction; therefore, therapy with corticosteroids should be used with great caution in these patients.

PRECAUTIONS

This product, like many other steroid formulations, is sensitive to heat. Therefore, it should not be autoclaved when it is desirable to sterilize the exterior of the vial.

Following prolonged therapy, withdrawal of corticosteroids may result in symptoms of the corticosteroid withdrawal syndrome including fever, myalgia, arthralgia, and malaise. This may occur in patients even without evidence of adrenal insufficiency.

There is an enhanced effect of corticosteroids in patients with hypothyroidism and in those with cirrhosis.

Corticosteroids should be used cautiously in patients with ocular herpes simplex for fear of corneal perforation.

The lowest possible dose of corticosteroid should be used to control the condition under treatment, and when reduction in dosage is possible, the reduction must be gradual.

Psychic derangements may appear when corticosteroids are used, ranging from euphoria, insomnia, mood swings, personality changes, and severe depression to frank psychotic manifestations. Also, existing emotional instability or psychotic tendencies may be aggravated by corticosteroids.

Aspirin should be used cautiously in conjunction with corticosteroids in hypoprothrombinemia.

Steroids should be used with caution in nonspecific ulcerative colitis, if there is a probability of impending perforation, abscess, or other pyogenic infection, also in diverticulitis, fresh intestinal anastomoses, active or latent peptic ulcer, renal insufficiency, hypertension, osteoporosis, and myasthenia gravis. Signs of peritoneal irritation following gastrointestinal perforation in patients receiving large doses of corticosteroids may be minimal or absent. Fat embolism has been reported as a possible complication of hypercortisonism.

When large doses are given, some authorities advise that antacids be administered between meals to help to prevent peptic ulcer.

Steroids may increase or decrease motility and number of spermatozoa in some patients.

Phenytoin, phenobarbital, ephedrine, and rifampin may enhance the metabolic clearance of corticosteroids, resulting in decreased blood levels and lessened physiologic activity, thus requiring adjustment in corticosteroid dosage.

The prothrombin time should be checked frequently in patients who are receiving corticosteroids and coumarin anticoagulants at the same time because of reports that corticosteroids have altered the response to these anticoagulants. Studies have shown that the usual effect produced by adding corticosteroids is inhibition of response to coumarins, although there have been some conflicting reports of potentiation not substantiated by studies.

When corticosteroids are administered concomitantly with potassium-depleting diuretics, patients should be observed closely for development of hypokalemia.

Injection of a steroid into an infected site is to be avoided. The slower rate of absorption by intramuscular administration should be recognized.

Information for Patients

Susceptible patients who are on immunosuppressant doses of corticosteroids should be warned to avoid exposure to chickenpox or measles. Patients should also be advised that if they are exposed, medical advice should be sought without delay.

Pediatric Use

Growth and development of pediatric patients on prolonged corticosteroid therapy should be carefully followed.

ADVERSE REACTIONS

Fluid and electrolyte disturbances
  Sodium retention
  Fluid retention
  Congestive heart failure in susceptible patients
  Potassium loss
  Hypokalemic alkalosis
  Hypertension
Musculoskeletal
  Muscle weakness
  Steroid myopathy
  Loss of muscle mass
  Osteoporosis
  Vertebral compression fractures
  Aseptic necrosis of femoral and humeral heads
  Pathologic fracture of long bones
  Tendon rupture
Gastrointestinal
  Peptic ulcer with possible subsequent perforation and hemorrhage
  Perforation of the small and large bowel, particularly in patients with inflammatory bowel disease

  Pancreatitis
  Abdominal distention
  Ulcerative esophagitis
Dermatologic
  Impaired wound healing
  Thin fragile skin
  Petechiae and ecchymoses
  Erythema
  Increased sweating
  May suppress reactions to skin tests
  Burning or tingling, especially in the perineal area (after I.V. injection)
  Other cutaneous reactions, such as allergic dermatitis, urticaria, angioneurotic edema
Neurologic
  Convulsions
  Increased intracranial pressure with papilledema (pseudotumor cerebri) usually after treatment
  Vertigo
  Headache
  Psychic disturbances
Endocrine
  Menstrual irregularities
  Development of cushingoid state
  Suppression of growth in children
  Secondary adrenocortical and pituitary unresponsiveness, particularly in times of stress, as in trauma, surgery, or illness
  Decreased carbohydrate tolerance
  Manifestations of latent diabetes mellitus
  Increased requirements for insulin or oral hypoglycemic agents in diabetics
  Hirsutism
Ophthalmic
  Posterior subcapsular cataracts
  Increased intraocular pressure
  Glaucoma
  Exophthalmos
Metabolic
  Negative nitrogen balance due to protein catabolism
Cardiovascular
  Myocardial rupture following recent myocardial infarction (see WARNINGS)
Other
  Anaphylactoid or hypersensitivity reactions
  Thromboembolism
  Weight gain
  Increased appetite
  Nausea
  Malaise
The following *additional* adverse reactions are related to parenteral corticosteroid therapy:
  Rare instances of blindness associated with intralesional therapy around the face and head
  Hyperpigmentation or hypopigmentation
  Subcutaneous and cutaneous atrophy
  Sterile abscess

OVERDOSAGE

Reports of acute toxicity and/or death following overdosage of glucocorticoids are rare. In the event of overdosage, no specific antidote is available; treatment is supportive and symptomatic.

The intraperitoneal LD_{50} of hydrocortisone in female mice was 1740 mg/kg.

DOSAGE AND ADMINISTRATION

For intravenous, intramuscular, and subcutaneous injection. For single dose use only. Maintenance of sterility cannot be assured when used as a multiple dose vial.

HYDROCORTONE Phosphate injection can be given directly from the vial, or it can be added to Sodium Chloride Injection or Dextrose Injection and administered by intravenous drip.

Benzyl alcohol as a preservative has been associated with toxicity in premature infants. Solutions used for intravenous administration or further dilution of this product should be preservative-free when used in the neonate, especially the premature infant.

When it is mixed with an infusion solution, sterile precautions should be observed. Since infusion solutions generally do not contain preservatives, mixtures should be used within 24 hours.

DOSAGE REQUIREMENTS ARE VARIABLE AND MUST BE INDIVIDUALIZED ON THE BASIS OF THE DISEASE AND THE RESPONSE OF THE PATIENT.

The initial dosage varies from 15 to 240 mg a day depending on the disease being treated. In less severe diseases doses lower than 15 mg may suffice, while in severe diseases doses higher than 240 mg may be required. Usually the parenteral dosage ranges are one-third to one-half the oral dose given every 12 hours. However, in certain overwhelming, acute, life-threatening situations, administration in dosages exceeding the usual dosages may be justified and may be in multiples of the oral dosages.

The initial dosage should be maintained or adjusted until the patient's response is satisfactory. If a satisfactory clinical response does not occur after a reasonable period of time, discontinue HYDROCORTONE Phosphate injection and transfer the patient to other therapy.

After a favorable initial response, the proper maintenance dosage should be determined by decreasing the initial dosage in small amounts to the lowest dosage that maintains an adequate clinical response.

Patients should be observed closely for signs that might require dosage adjustment, including changes in clinical status resulting from remissions or exacerbations of the disease, individual drug responsiveness, and the effect of stress (e.g., surgery, infection, trauma). During stress it may be necessary to increase dosage temporarily.

If the drug is to be stopped after more than a few days of treatment, it usually should be withdrawn gradually.

HOW SUPPLIED

No. 7633—Injection HYDROCORTONE Phosphate, 50 mg hydrocortisone equivalent per mL, is a clear, light yellow solution, and is supplied as follows:
NDC 0006-7633-04 in 2 mL single dose vials.
Storage
Sensitive to heat. Do not autoclave.
    7498329   Issued February 1997

HYDROCORTONE® Tablets ℞
(Hydrocortisone), U.S.P.

DESCRIPTION

Glucocorticoids are adrenocortical steroids, both naturally occurring and synthetic, which are readily absorbed from the gastrointestinal tract.

Hydrocortisone is a white to practically white, odorless, crystalline powder, very slightly soluble in water. The molecular weight is 362.47. It is designated chemically as 11β,17,21-trihydroxypregn-4-ene-3,20-dione. The empirical formula is $C_{21}H_{30}O_5$ and the structural formula is:

Hydrocortisone is believed to be the principal hormone secreted by the adrenal cortex.

HYDROCORTONE* (Hydrocortisone) tablets contain 10 mg of hydrocortisone in each tablet.

Inactive ingredients are lactose, magnesium stearate, and starch.

*Registered trademark of MERCK & CO., INC.

ACTIONS

Naturally occurring glucocorticoids (hydrocortisone and cortisone), which also have salt-retaining properties, are used as replacement therapy in adrenocortical deficiency states. They are also used for their potent anti-inflammatory effects in disorders of many organ systems.

Glucocorticoids cause profound and varied metabolic effects. In addition, they modify the body's immune responses to diverse stimuli.

INDICATIONS

1. *Endocrine Disorders*
  Primary or secondary adrenocortical insufficiency (hydrocortisone or cortisone is the first choice; synthetic analogs may be used in conjunction with mineralocorticoids where applicable; in infancy mineralocorticoid supplementation is of particular importance)
    Congenital adrenal hyperplasia
    Nonsuppurative thyroiditis
    Hypercalcemia associated with cancer

Continued on next page

Hydrocortone Tablets—Cont.

2. *Rheumatic Disorders*
As adjunctive therapy for short-term administration (to tide the patient over an acute episode or exacerbation) in:
Psoriatic arthritis
Rheumatoid arthritis, including juvenile rheumatoid arthritis (selected cases may require low-dose maintenance therapy)
Ankylosing spondylitis
Acute and subacute bursitis
Acute nonspecific tenosynovitis
Acute gouty arthritis
Post-traumatic osteoarthritis
Synovitis of osteoarthritis
Epicondylitis
3. *Collagen Diseases*
During an exacerbation or as maintenance therapy in selected cases of—
Systemic lupus erythematosus
Acute rheumatic carditis
Systemic dermatomyositis (polymyositis)
4. *Dermatologic Diseases*
Pemphigus
Bullous dermatitis herpetiformis
Severe erythema multiforme (Stevens-Johnson syndrome)
Exfoliative dermatitis
Mycosis fungoides
Severe psoriasis
Severe seborrheic dermatitis
5. *Allergic States*
Control of severe or incapacitating allergic conditions intractable to adequate trials of conventional treatment:
Seasonal or perennial allergic rhinitis
Bronchial asthma
Contact dermatitis
Atopic dermatitis
Serum sickness
Drug hypersensitivity reactions
6. *Ophthalmic Diseases*
Severe acute and chronic allergic and inflammatory processes involving the eye and its adnexa, such as—
Allergic conjunctivitis
Keratitis
Allergic corneal marginal ulcers
Herpes zoster ophthalmicus
Iritis and iridocyclitis
Chorioretinitis
Anterior segment inflammation
Diffuse posterior uveitis and choroiditis
Optic neuritis
Sympathetic ophthalmia
7. *Respiratory Diseases*
Symptomatic sarcoidosis
Loeffler's syndrome not manageable by other means
Berylliosis
Fulminating or disseminated pulmonary tuberculosis when used concurrently with appropriate antituberculous chemotherapy
Aspiration pneumonitis
8. *Hematologic Disorders*
Idiopathic thrombocytopenic purpura in adults
Secondary thrombocytopenia in adults
Acquired (autoimmune) hemolytic anemia
Erythroblastopenia (RBC anemia)
Congenital (erythroid) hypoplastic anemia
9. *Neoplastic Diseases*
For palliative management of:
Leukemias and lymphomas in adults
Acute leukemia of childhood
10. *Edematous States*
To induce a diuresis or remission of proteinuria in the nephrotic syndrome, without uremia, of the idiopathic type or that due to lupus erythematosus
11. *Gastrointestinal Diseases*
To tide the patient over a critical period of the disease in:
Ulcerative colitis
Regional enteritis
12. *Miscellaneous*
Tuberculous meningitis with subarachnoid block or impending block when used concurrently with appropriate antituberculous chemotherapy
Trichinosis with neurologic or myocardial involvement

CONTRAINDICATIONS

Systemic fungal infections
Hypersensitivity to this product

WARNINGS

In patients on corticosteroid therapy subjected to unusual stress, increased dosage of rapidly acting corticosteroids before, during, and after the stressful situation is indicated.

Drug-induced secondary adrenocortical insufficiency may result from too rapid wthdrawal of corticosteroids and may be minimized by gradual reduction of dosage. This type of relative insufficiency may persist for months after discontinuation of therapy; therefore, in any situation of stress occurring during that period, hormone therapy should be reinstituted. If the patient is receiving steroids already, dosage may have to be increased. Since mineralocorticoid secretion may be impaired, salt and/or a mineralocorticoid should be administered concurrently.

Corticosteroids may mask some signs of infection, and new infections may appear during their use. There may be decreased resistance and inability to localize infection when corticosteroids are used. Moreover, corticosteroids may affect the nitroblue-tetrazolium test for bacterial infection and produce false negative results.

In cerebral malaria, a double-blind trial has shown that the use of corticosteroids is associated with prolongation of coma and a higher incidence of pneumonia and gastrointestinal bleeding.

Corticosteroids may activate latent amebiasis. Therefore, it is recommended that latent or active amebiasis be ruled out before initiating corticosteroid therapy in any patient who has spent time in the tropics or any patient with unexplained diarrhea.

Prolonged use of corticosteroids may produce posterior subcapsular cataracts, glaucoma with possible damage to the optic nerves, and may enhance the establishment of secondary ocular infections due to fungi or viruses.

Usage in pregnancy: Since adequate human reproduction studies have not been done with corticosteroids, use of these drugs in pregnancy or in women of childbearing potential requires that the anticipated benefits be weighed against the possible hazards to the mother and embryo or fetus. Infants born of mothers who have received substantial doses of corticosteroids during pregnancy should be carefully observed for signs of hypoadrenalism.

Corticosteroids appear in breast milk and could suppress growth, interfere with endogenous corticosteroid production, or cause other unwanted effects. Mothers taking pharmacologic doses of corticosteroids should be advised not to nurse.

Average and large doses of hydrocortisone or cortisone can cause elevation of blood pressure, salt and water retention, and increased excretion of potassium. These effects are less likely to occur with the synthetic derivatives except when used in large doses. Dietary salt restriction and potassium supplementation may be necessary. All corticosteroids increase calcium excretion.

Administration of live virus vaccines, including smallpox, is contraindicated in individuals receiving immunosuppressive doses of corticosteroids. If inactivated viral or bacterial vaccines are administered to individuals receiving immunosuppressive doses of corticosteroids, the expected serum antibody response may not be obtained. However, immunization procedures may be undertaken in patients who are receiving corticosteroids as replacement therapy, e.g., for Addison's disease.

Patients who are on drugs which suppress the immune system are more susceptible to infections than healthy individuals. Chickenpox and measles, for example, can have a more serious or even fatal course in non-immune patients on corticosteroids. In such patients who have not had these diseases, particular care should be taken to avoid exposure. The risk of developing a disseminated infection varies among individuals and can be related to the dose, route and duration of corticosteroid administration as well as to the underlying disease. If exposed to chickenpox, prophylaxis with varicella zoster immune globulin (VZIG) may be indicated. If chickenpox develops, treatment with antiviral agents may be considered. If exposed to measles, prophylaxis with immune globulin (IG) may be indicated. (See the respective package inserts for VZIG and IG for complete prescribing information.)

Similarly, corticosteroids should be used with great care in patients with known or suspected Strongyloides (threadworm) infestation. In such patients, corticosteroid-induced immunosuppression may lead to Strongyloides hyperinfection and dissemination with widespread larval migration, often accompanied by severe enterocolitis and potentially fatal gram-negative septicemia.

The use of HYDROCORTONE tablets in active tuberculosis should be restricted to those cases of fulminating or disseminated tuberculosis in which the corticosteroid is used for the management of the disease in conjunction with an appropriate antituberculous regimen.

If corticosteroids are indicated in patients with latent tuberculosis or tuberculin reactivity, close observation is necessary as reactivation of the disease may occur. During prolonged corticosteroid therapy, these patients should receive chemoprophylaxis.

Literature reports suggest an apparent association between use of corticosteroids and left ventricular free wall rupture after a recent myocardial infarction; therefore, therapy with corticosteroids should be used with great caution in these patients.

PRECAUTIONS

Following prolonged therapy, withdrawal of corticosteroids may result in symptoms of the corticosteroid withdrawal syndrome including fever, myalgia, arthralgia, and malaise. This may occur in patients even without evidence of adrenal insufficiency.

There is an enhanced effect of corticosteroids in patients with hypothyroidism and in those with cirrhosis.

Corticosteroids should be used cautiously in patients with ocular herpes simplex because of possible corneal perforation.

The lowest possible dose of corticosteroid should be used to control the condition under treatment, and when reduction in dosage is possible, the reduction should be gradual.

Psychic derangements may appear when corticosteroids are used, ranging from euphoria, insomnia, mood swings, personality changes, and severe depression, to frank psychotic manifestations. Also, existing emotional instability or psychotic tendencies may be aggravated by corticosteroids.

Aspirin should be used cautiously in conjunction with corticosteroids in hypoprothrombinemia.

Steroids should be used with caution in nonspecific ulcerative colitis, if there is a probability of impending perforation, abscess, or other pyogenic infection, diverticulitis, fresh intestinal anastomoses, active or latent peptic ulcer, renal insufficiency, hypertension, osteoporosis, and myasthenia gravis. Signs of peritoneal irritation following gastrointestinal perforation in patients receiving large doses of corticosteroids may be minimal or absent. Fat embolism has been reported as a possible complication of hypercortisonism.

When large doses are given, some authorities advise that corticosteroids be taken with meals and antacids taken between meals to help to prevent peptic ulcer.

Steroids may increase or decrease motility and number of spermatozoa in some patients.

Phenytoin, phenobarbital, ephedrine, and rifampin may enhance the metabolic clearance of corticosteroids, resulting in decreased blood levels and lessened physiologic activity, thus requiring adjustment in corticosteroid dosage.

The prothrombin time should be checked frequently in patients who are receiving corticosteroids and coumarin anticoagulants at the same time because of reports that corticosteroids have altered the response to these anticoagulants. Studies have shown that the usual effect produced by adding corticosteroids is inhibition of response to coumarins, although there have been some conflicting reports of potentiation not substantiated by studies.

When corticosteroids are administered concomitantly with potassium-depleting diuretics, patients should be observed closely for development of hypokalemia.

Information for Patients
Susceptible patients who are on immunosuppressant doses of corticosteroids should be warned to avoid exposure to chickenpox or measles. Patients should also be advised that if they are exposed, medical advice should be sought without delay.

Pediatric Use
Growth and development of pediatric patients on prolonged corticosteroid therapy should be carefully followed.

ADVERSE REACTIONS

Fluid and Electrolyte Disturbances
Sodium retention
Fluid retention
Congestive heart failure in susceptible patients
Potassium loss
Hypokalemic alkalosis
Hypertension
Musculoskeletal
Muscle weakness
Steroid myopathy
Loss of muscle mass
Osteoporosis
Vertebral compression fractures
Aseptic necrosis of femoral and humeral heads
Pathologic fracture of long bones
Tendon rupture
Gastrointestinal
Peptic ulcer with possible perforation and hemorrhage
Perforation of the small and large bowel, particularly in patients with inflammatory bowel disease
Pancreatitis
Abdominal distention
Ulcerative esophagitis
Dermatologic
Impaired wound healing
Thin fragile skin
Petechiae and ecchymoses
Erythema
Increased sweating
May suppress reactions to skin tests
Other cutaneous reactions, such as allergic dermatitis, urticaria, angioneurotic edema
Neurologic
Convulsions
Increased intracranial pressure with papilledema (pseudotumor cerebri) usually after treatment
Vertigo

Headache
Psychic disturbances
Endocrine
Menstrual irregularities
Development of cushingoid state
Suppression of growth in children
Secondary adrenocortical and pituitary unresponsiveness, particularly in times of stress, as in trauma, surgery, or illness
Decreased carbohydrate tolerance
Manifestations of latent diabetes mellitus
Increased requirements for insulin or oral hypoglycemic agents in diabetics
Hirsutism
Ophthalmic
Posterior subcapsular cataracts
Increased intraocular pressure
Glaucoma
Exophthalmos
Metabolic
Negative nitrogen balance due to protein catabolism
Cardiovascular
Myocardial rupture following recent myocardial infarction (see WARNINGS)
Other
Hypersensitivity
Thromboembolism
Weight gain
Increased appetite
Nausea
Malaise

OVERDOSAGE

Reports of acute toxicity and/or death following overdosage of glucocorticoids are rare. In the event of overdosage, no specific antidote is available; treatment is supportive and symptomatic.
The intraperitoneal LD_{50} of hydrocortisone in female mice was 1740 mg/kg.

DOSAGE AND ADMINISTRATION

For oral administration
DOSAGE REQUIREMENTS ARE VARIABLE AND MUST BE INDIVIDUALIZED ON THE BASIS OF THE DISEASE AND THE RESPONSE OF THE PATIENT.
The initial dosage varies from 20 to 240 mg a day depending on the disease being treated. In less severe diseases doses lower than 20 mg may suffice, while in severe diseases doses higher than 240 mg may be required. The initial dosage should be maintained or adjusted until the patient's response is satisfactory. If satisfactory clinical response does not occur after a reasonable period of time, discontinue HYDROCORTONE tablets and transfer the patient to other therapy.
After a favorable initial response, the proper maintenance dosage should be determined by decreasing the initial dosage in small amounts to the lowest dosage that maintains an adequate clinical response.
Patients should be observed closely for signs that might require dosage adjustment, including changes in clinical status resulting from remissions or exacerbations of the disease, individual drug responsiveness, and the effect of stress (e.g, surgery, infection, trauma). During stress it may be necessary to increase dosage temporarily.
If the drug is to be stopped after more than a few days of treatment, it usually should be withdrawn gradually.

HOW SUPPLIED

No. 7604—Tablets HYDROCORTONE, 10 mg each, are white, oval shaped compressed tablets, scored on one side, coded MSD 619, and are supplied as follows:
NDC 0006-0619-68 in bottles of 100.
Shown in Product Identification Guide, page 323
7920528   Issued February 1997

HydroDIURIL® Tablets   ℞
(Hydrochlorothiazide), U.S.P.

DESCRIPTION

HydroDIURIL* (Hydrochlorothiazide) is a diuretic and antihypertensive. It is the 3,4-dihydro derivative of chlorothiazide. Its chemical name is 6-chloro-3,4-dihydro-2*H*-1,2,4-benzothiadiazine-7-sulfonamide 1,1-dioxide. Its empirical formula is $C_7H_8ClN_3O_4S_2$ and its structural formula is:
[See chemical structure at top of next column]
It is a white, or practically white, crystalline powder with a molecular weight of 297.72, which is slightly soluble in water, but freely soluble in sodium hydroxide solution.
HydroDIURIL is supplied as 25 mg, 50 mg and 100 mg tablets for oral use. Each tablet contains the following inactive ingredients: calcium phosphate, FD&C Yellow 6, gelatin, lactose, magnesium stearate, starch and talc.

*Registered trademark of MERCK & CO., INC.

CLINICAL PHARMACOLOGY

The mechanism of the antihypertensive effect of thiazides is unknown. HydroDIURIL does not usually affect normal blood pressure.
HydroDIURIL affects the distal renal tubular mechanism of electrolyte reabsorption. At maximal therapeutic dosage all thiazides are approximately equal in their diuretic efficacy. HydroDIURIL increases excretion of sodium and chloride in approximately equivalent amounts. Natriuresis may be accompanied by some loss of potassium and bicarbonate.
After oral use diuresis begins within 2 hours, peaks in about 4 hours and lasts about 6 to 12 hours.
Pharmacokinetics and Metabolism
HydroDIURIL is not metabolized but is eliminated rapidly by the kidney. When plasma levels have been followed for at least 24 hours, the plasma half-life has been observed to vary between 5.6 and 14.8 hours. At least 61 percent of the oral dose is eliminated unchanged within 24 hours. Hydrochlorothiazide crosses the placental but not the blood-brain barrier and is excreted in breast milk.

INDICATIONS AND USAGE

HydroDIURIL is indicated as adjunctive therapy in edema associated with congestive heart failure, hepatic cirrhosis, and corticosteroid and estrogen therapy.
HydroDIURIL has also been found useful in edema due to various forms of renal dysfunction such as nephrotic syndrome, acute glomerulonephritis, and chronic renal failure. HydroDIURIL is indicated in the management of hypertension either as the sole therapeutic agent or to enhance the effectiveness of other antihypertensive drugs in the more severe forms of hypertension.
Use in Pregnancy. Routine use of diuretics during normal pregnancy is inappropriate and exposes mother and fetus to unnecessary hazard. Diuretics do not prevent development of toxemia of pregnancy and there is no satisfactory evidence that they are useful in the treatment of toxemia. Edema during pregnancy may arise from pathologic causes or from the physiologic and mechanical consequences of pregnancy. Thiazides are indicated in pregnancy when edema is due to pathologic causes, just as they are in the absence of pregnancy (see PRECAUTIONS, *Pregnancy*). Dependent edema in pregnancy, resulting from restriction of venous return by the gravid uterus, is properly treated through elevation of the lower extremities and use of support stockings. Use of diuretics to lower intravascular volume in this instance is illogical and unnecessary. During normal pregnancy there is hypervolemia which is not harmful to the fetus or the mother in the absence of cardiovascular disease. However, it may be associated with edema, rarely generalized edema. If such edema causes discomfort, increased recumbency will often provide relief. Rarely this edema may cause extreme discomfort which is not relieved by rest. In these instances, a short course of diuretic therapy may provide relief and be appropriate.

CONTRAINDICATIONS

Anuria.
Hypersensitivity to this product or to other sulfonamide-derived drugs.

WARNINGS

Use with caution in severe renal disease. In patients with renal disease, thiazides may precipitate azotemia. Cumulative effects of the drug may develop in patients with impaired renal function.
Thiazides should be used with caution in patients with impaired hepatic function or progressive liver disease, since minor alterations of fluid and electrolyte balance may precipitate hepatic coma.
Thiazides may add to or potentiate the action of other antihypertensive drugs.
Sensitivity reactions may occur in patients with or without a history of allergy or bronchial asthma.
The possibility of exacerbation or activation of systemic lupus erythematosus has been reported.
Lithium generally should not be given with diuretics (see PRECAUTIONS, *Drug Interactions*).

PRECAUTIONS

General
All patients receiving diuretic therapy should be observed for evidence of fluid or electrolyte imbalance: namely, hypo-

natremia, hypochloremic alkalosis, and hypokalemia. Serum and urine electrolyte determinations are particularly important when the patient is vomiting excessively or receiving parenteral fluids. Warning signs or symptoms of fluid and electrolyte imbalance, irrespective of cause, include dryness of mouth, thirst, weakness, lethargy, drowsiness, restlessness, confusion, seizures, muscle pains or cramps, muscular fatigue, hypotension, oliguria, tachycardia, and gastrointestinal disturbances such as nausea and vomiting.
Hypokalemia may develop, especially with brisk diuresis, when severe cirrhosis is present or after prolonged therapy. Interference with adequate oral electrolyte intake will also contribute to hypokalemia. Hypokalemia may cause cardiac arrhythmia and may also sensitize or exaggerate the response of the heart to the toxic effects of digitalis (e.g., increased ventricular irritability). Hypokalemia may be avoided or treated by use of potassium sparing diuretics or potassium supplements such as foods with a high potassium content.
Although any chloride deficit is generally mild and usually does not require specific treatment except under extraordinary circumstances (as in liver disease or renal disease), chloride replacement may be required in the treatment of metabolic alkalosis.
Dilutional hyponatremia may occur in edematous patients in hot weather; appropriate therapy is water restriction, rather than administration of salt, except in rare instances when the hyponatremia is life threatening. In actual salt depletion, appropriate replacement is the therapy of choice.
Hyperuricemia may occur or acute gout may be precipitated in certain patients receiving thiazides.
In diabetic patients dosage adjustments of insulin or oral hypoglycemic agents may be required. Hyperglycemia may occur with thiazide diuretics. Thus latent diabetes mellitus may become manifest during thiazide therapy.
The antihypertensive effects of the drug may be enhanced in the post-sympathectomy patient.
If progressive renal impairment becomes evident, consider withholding or discontinuing diuretic therapy.
Thiazides have been shown to increase the urinary excretion of magnesium; this may result in hypomagnesemia.
Thiazides may decrease urinary calcium excretion. Thiazides may cause intermittent and slight elevation of serum calcium in the absence of known disorders of calcium metabolism. Marked hypercalcemia may be evidence of hidden hyperparathyroidism. Thiazides should be discontinued before carrying out tests for parathyroid function.
Increases in cholesterol and triglyceride levels may be associated with thiazide diuretic therapy.
Laboratory Tests
Periodic determination of serum electrolytes to detect possible electrolyte imbalance should be done at appropriate intervals.
Drug Interactions
When given concurrently the following drugs may interact with thiazide diuretics.
Alcohol, barbiturates, or narcotics —potentiation of orthostatic hypotension may occur.
Antidiabetic drugs —(oral agents and insulin)—dosage adjustment of the antidiabetic drug may be required.
Other antihypertensive drugs —additive effect or potentiation.
Cholestyramine and colestipol resins—Absorption of hydrochlorothiazide is impaired in the presence of anionic exchange resins. Single doses of either cholestyramine or colestipol resins bind the hydrochlorothiazide and reduce its absorption from the gastrointestinal tract by up to 85 and 43 percent, respectively.
Corticosteroids, ACTH —intensified electrolyte depletion, particularly hypokalemia.
Pressor amines (e.g., norepinephrine) —possible decreased response to pressor amines but not sufficient to preclude their use.
Skeletal muscle relaxants, nondepolarizing (e.g., tubocurarine) —possible increased responsiveness to the muscle relaxant.
Lithium —generally should not be given with diuretics. Diuretic agents reduce the renal clearance of lithium and add a high risk of lithium toxicity. Refer to the package insert for lithium preparations before use of such preparations with HydroDIURIL.
Non-steroidal Anti-inflammatory Drugs —In some patients, the administration of a non-steroidal anti-inflammatory agent can reduce the diuretic, natriuretic, and antihypertensive effects of loop, potassium-sparing and thiazide diuretics. Therefore, when HydroDIURIL and non-steroidal

Continued on next page

HydroDiuril—Cont.

anti-inflammatory agents are used concomitantly, the patient should be observed closely to determine if the desired effect of the diuretic is obtained.

Drug/Laboratory Test Interactions
Thiazides should be discontinued before carrying out tests for parathyroid function (see PRECAUTIONS, *General*).

Carcinogenesis, Mutagenesis, Impairment of Fertility
Two-year feeding studies in mice and rats conducted under the auspices of the National Toxicology Program (NTP) uncovered no evidence of a carcinogenic potential of hydrochlorothiazide in female mice (at doses of up to approximately 600 mg/kg/day) or in male and female rats (at doses of up to approximately 100 mg/kg/day). The NTP, however, found equivocal evidence for hepatocarcinogenicity in male mice. Hydrochlorothiazide was not genotoxic *in vitro* in the Ames mutagenicity assay of *Salmonella typhimurium* strains TA 98, TA 100, TA 1535, TA 1537, and TA 1538 and in the Chinese Hamster Ovary (CHO) test for chromosomal aberrations, or *in vivo* in assays using mouse germinal cell chromosomes, Chinese hamster bone marrow chromosomes, and the *Drosophila* sex-linked recessive lethal trait gene. Positive test results were obtained only in the *in vitro* CHO Sister Chromatid Exchange (clastogenicity) and in the Mouse Lymphoma Cell (mutagenicity) assays, using concentrations of hydrochlorothiazide from 43 to 1300 µg/mL, and in the *Aspergillus nidulans* non-disjunction assay at an unspecified concentration.

Hydrochlorothiazide had no adverse effects on the fertility of mice and rats of either sex in studies wherein these species were exposed, via their diet, to doses of up to 100 and 4 mg/kg, respectively, prior to conception and throughout gestation.

Pregnancy
Teratogenic Effects—Pregnancy Category B: Studies in which hydrochlorothiazide was orally administered to pregnant mice and rats during their respective periods of major organogenesis at doses up to 3000 and 1000 mg hydrochlorothiazide/kg, respectively, provided no evidence of harm to the fetus.

There are, however, no adequate and well-controlled studies in pregnant women. Because animal reproduction studies are not always predictice of human response, this drug should be used during pregnancy only if clearly needed.

Nonteratogenic Effects: Thiazides cross the placental barrier and appear in cord blood. There is a risk of fetal or neonatal jaundice, thrombocytopenia, and possibly other adverse reactions that have occurred in adults.

Nursing Mothers
Thiazides are excreted in breast milk. Because of the potential for serious adverse reactions in nursing infants, a decision should be made whether to discontinue nursing or to discontinue hydrochlorothiazide, taking into account the importance of the drug to the mother.

Pediatric Use
Safety and effectiveness in children have not been established.

ADVERSE REACTIONS

The following adverse reactions have been reported and, within each category, are listed in order of decreasing severity.

Body as a Whole: Weakness.
Cardiovascular: Hypotension including orthostatic hypotension (may be aggravated by alcohol, barbiturates, narcotics or antihypertensive drugs).
Digestive: Pancreatitis, jaundice (intrahepatic cholestatic jaundice), diarrhea, vomiting, sialadenitis, cramping, constipation, gastric irritation, nausea, anorexia.
Hematologic: Aplastic anemia, agranulocytosis, leukopenia, hemolytic anemia, thrombocytopenia.
Hypersensitivity: Anaphylactic reactions, necrotizing angiitis (vasculitis and cutaneous vasculitis), respiratory distress including pneumonitis and pulmonary edema, photosensitivity, fever, urticaria, rash, purpura.
Metabolic: Electrolyte imbalance (see PRECAUTIONS), hyperglycemia, glycosuria, hyperuricemia.
Musculoskeletal: Muscle spasm.
Nervous System/Psychiatric: Vertigo, paresthesias, dizziness, headache, restlessness.
Renal: Renal failure, renal dysfunction, interstitial nephritis. (See WARNINGS.)
Skin: Erythema multiforme including Stevens-Johnson syndrome, exfoliative dermatitis including toxic epidermal necrolysis, alopecia.
Special Senses: Transient blurred vision, xanthopsia.
Urogenital: Impotence.
Whenever adverse reactions are moderate or severe, thiazide dosage should be reduced or therapy withdrawn.

OVERDOSAGE

The most common signs and symptoms observed are those caused by electrolyte depletion (hypokalemia, hypochloremia, hyponatremia) and dehydration resulting from excessive diuresis. If digitalis has also been administered, hypokalemia may accentuate cardiac arrhythmias.

In the event of overdosage, symptomatic and supportive measures should be employed. Emesis should be induced or gastric lavage performed. Correct dehydration, electrolyte imbalance, hepatic coma and hypotension by established procedures. If required, give oxygen or artificial respiration for respiratory impairment. The degree to which hydrochlorothiazide is removed by hemodialysis has not been established.

The oral LD_{50} of hydrochlorothiazide is greater than 10 g/kg in the mouse and rat.

DOSAGE AND ADMINISTRATION

Therapy should be individualized according to patient response. Use the smallest dosage necessary to achieve the required response.

Adults
For Edema
The usual adult dosage is 25 to 100 mg daily as a single or divided dose. Many patients with edema respond to intermittent therapy, i.e., administration on alternate days or on three to five days each week. With an intermittent schedule, excessive response and the resulting undesirable electrolyte imbalance are less likely to occur.
For Control of Hypertension
The usual initial dose in adults is 25 mg daily given as a single dose. The dose may be increased to 50 mg daily, given as a single or two divided doses. Doses above 50 mg are often associated with marked reductions in serum potassium (see also PRECAUTIONS).
Patients usually do not require doses in excess of 50 mg of hydrochlorothiazide daily when used concomitantly with other antihypertensive agents.

Infants and Children
For Diuresis and For Control of Hypertension
The usual pediatric dosage is 0.5 to 1 mg per pound (1 to 2 mg/kg) per day in single or two divided doses, not to exceed 37.5 mg per day in infants up to 2 years of age or 100 mg per day in children 2 to 12 years of age. In infants less than 6 months of age, doses up to 1.5 mg per pound (3 mg/kg) per day in two divided doses may be required.

HOW SUPPLIED

No. 3263—Tablets HydroDIURIL, 25 mg, are peach-colored, round, scored, compressed tablets, coded MSD 42. They are supplied as follows:
NDC 0006-0042-68 bottles of 100
NDC 0006-0042-82 bottles of 1000.
Shown in Product Identification Guide, page 323
No. 3264—Tablets HydroDIURIL, 50 mg, are peach-colored, round, scored, compressed tablets, coded MSD 105. They are supplied as follows:
NDC 0006-0105-68 bottles of 100
NDC 0006-0105-82 bottles of 1000
NDC 0006-0105-86 bottles of 5000.
Shown in Product Identification Guide, page 323
No. 3340—Tablets HydroDIURIL, 100 mg, are peach-colored, round, scored, compressed tablets, coded MSD 410. They are supplied as follows:
NDC 0006-0410-68 bottles of 100.
Shown in Product Identification Guide, page 323
Storage
Keep container tightly closed. Protect from light, moisture, freezing. −20°C (−4°F) and store at room temperature, 15–30°C (59–86°F).

7897449   Issued February 1994
COPYRIGHT © MERCK & CO., INC., 1986
All rights reserved

HYDROPRES® Tablets ℞
(Reserpine-Hydrochlorothiazide), U.S.P.

WARNING

This fixed combination drug is not indicated for initial therapy of hypertension. Hypertension requires therapy titrated to the individual patient. If the fixed combination represents the dosage so determined, its use may be more convenient in patient management. The treatment of hypertension is not static, but must be re-evaluated as conditions in each patient warrant.

DESCRIPTION

HYDROPRES* (Reserpine-Hydrochlorothiazide) combines two antihypertensives: HydroDIURIL* (Hydrochlorothiazide) and reserpine.

Hydrochlorothiazide
Hydrochlorothiazide is a diuretic and antihypertensive. It is the 3,4-dihydro derivative of chlorothiazide. Its chemical name is 6-chloro-3,4-dihydro-2*H*-1,2,4-benzothiadiazine-7-sulfonamide 1,1-dioxide. Its empirical formula is $C_7H_8ClN_3O_4S_2$ and its structural formula is:

Hydrochlorothiazide is a white, or practically white, crystalline powder with a molecular weight of 297.72, which is slightly soluble in water, but freely soluble in sodium hydroxide solution.

Reserpine
The chemical name for reserpine is (11, 17α-dimethoxy-18β-[(3,4,5-trimethoxybenzoyl)oxy]-3β, 20α-yohimban-16β-carboxylic acid methyl ester). It is a crystalline alkaloid derived from Rauwolfia serpentina. Its empirical formula is $C_{33}H_{40}N_2O_9$ and its structural formula is:

Reserpine is a white or pale buff to slightly yellowish, odorless, crystalline powder with a molecular weight of 608.69, is insoluble in water, and freely soluble in glacial acetic acid.
HYDROPRES is supplied as tablets in two strengths for oral use:
HYDROPRES 25, contains 25 mg of hydrochlorothiazide and 0.125 mg of reserpine.
HYDROPRES 50, contains 50 mg of hydrochlorothiazide and 0.125 mg of reserpine.
Each tablet contains the following inactive ingredients: calcium phosphate, D&C Yellow 10, FD&C Blue 1, FD&C Yellow 6, lactose, magnesium stearate, starch and talc.

*Registered trademark of MERCK & CO., INC.

CLINICAL PHARMACOLOGY

Hydrochlorothiazide
The mechanism of the antihypertensive effect of thiazides is unknown. Hydrochlorothiazide does not usually affect normal blood pressure.
Hydrochlorothiazide affects the distal renal tubular mechanism of electrolyte reabsorption. At maximal therapeutic dosage all thiazides are approximately equal in their diuretic efficacy.
Hydrochlorothiazide increases excretion of sodium and chloride in approximately equivalent amounts. Natriuresis may be accompanied by some loss of potassium and bicarbonate. After oral use, diuresis begins within 2 hours, peaks in about 4 hours and lasts about 6 to 12 hours.
Reserpine
Reserpine has antihypertensive, bradycardic, and tranquilizing properties. It lowers arterial blood pressure by depletion of catecholamines. Reserpine is beneficial in relieving anxiety, tension, and headache in the hypertensive patient. It acts at the hypothalamic level of the central nervous system to promote relaxation without hypnosis or analgesia. The sleep pattern shown by the electroencephalogram following barbiturates does not occur with this drug. In laboratory animals spontaneous activity and response to external stimuli are decreased, but confusion or difficulty of movement is not evident.
The bradycardic action of reserpine promotes relaxation and may eliminate sinus tachycardia. It is most pronounced in subjects with sinus tachycardia and usually is not prominent in persons with a normal pulse rate.
Miosis, relaxation of the nictitating membrane, ptosis, hypothermia, and increased gastrointestinal activity are noted in animals given reserpine, sometimes in subclinical doses. None of these effects, except increased gastrointestinal activity, has been found to be clinically significant in man with therapeutic doses.
Pharmacokinetics and Metabolism
Hydrochlorothiazide
Hydrochlorothiazide is not metabolized but is eliminated rapidly by the kidney. When plasma levels have been followed for at least 24 hours, the plasma half-life has been observed to vary between 5.6 and 14.8 hours. At least 61

percent of the oral dose is eliminated unchanged within 24 hours. Hydrochlorothiazide crosses the placental but not the blood-brain barrier and is excreted in breast milk.

Reserpine

Oral reserpine is rapidly absorbed from the gastrointestinal tract. Methylreserpate and trimethoxybenzoic acid are the primary metabolites which result from the hydrolytic cleavage of reserpine. Maximal blood levels were achieved approximately 2 hours after the oral dosage of ^{3}H-reserpine to six normal volunteers; within 96 hours approximately 8 percent was excreted in urine and 62 percent in feces. Reserpine appears in human breast milk. Reserpine crosses the placental barrier in guinea pigs.

INDICATION AND USAGE

Hypertension (see box warning).

CONTRAINDICATIONS

Hydrochlorothiazide is contraindicated in anuria.

HYDROPRES is contraindicated in hypersensitivity to hydrochlorothiazide or other sulfonamide-derived drugs or to reserpine.

Electroshock therapy should not be given to patients while on reserpine, as severe and even fatal reactions have been reported with minimal convulsive electroshock dosage. After discontinuing reserpine, allow at least seven days before starting electroshock therapy.

Reserpine is contraindicated in patients:

— with active peptic ulcer
— with ulcerative colitis
— with active or a history of mental depression, especially suicidal tendencies
— on therapy with monoamine oxidase (MAO) inhibitors.

WARNINGS

Hydrochlorothiazide

Use with caution in severe renal disease. In patients with renal disease, thiazides may precipitate azotemia. Cumulative effects of the drug may develop in patients with impaired renal function.

Thiazides should be used with caution in patients with impaired hepatic function or progressive liver disease, since minor alterations of fluid and electrolyte balance may precipitate hepatic coma.

Thiazides may add to or potentiate the action of other antihypertensive drugs.

Sensitivity reactions may occur in patients with or without a history of allergy or bronchial asthma.

The possibility of exacerbation or activation of systemic lupus erythematosus has been reported.

Lithium generally should not be given with diuretics (see PRECAUTIONS, *Drug Interactions*).

Reserpine

Reserpine may cause mental depression. Recognition of depression may be difficult because this condition may often be disguised by somatic complaints (masked depression). The drug should be discontinued at first signs of depression such as despondency, early morning insomnia, loss of appetite, impotence or self deprecation. Drug induced depression may persist for several months after drug withdrawal and may be severe enough to result in suicide.

The occurrence of mental depression due to reserpine in doses of 0.25 mg daily or less is unusual. In any event, HYDROPRES should be discontinued at the first sign of depression.

PRECAUTIONS

General

Hydrochlorothiazide

All patients receiving diuretic therapy should be observed for evidence of fluid or electrolyte imbalance: namely, hyponatremia, hypochloremic alkalosis, and hypokalemia. Serum and urine electrolyte determinations are particularly important when the patient is vomiting excessively or receiving parenteral fluids. Warning signs or symptoms of fluid and electrolyte imbalance irrespective of cause, include dryness of mouth, thirst, weakness, lethargy, drowsiness, restlessness, confusion, seizures, muscle pains or cramps, muscular fatigue, hypotension, oliguria, tachycardia, and gastrointestinal disturbances such as nausea and vomiting.

Hypokalemia may develop, especially with brisk diuresis, when severe cirrhosis is present or after prolonged therapy. Interference with adequate oral electrolyte intake will contribute to hypokalemia. Hypokalemia may cause cardiac arrhythmia and may also sensitize or exaggerate the response of the heart to the toxic effects of digitalis (e.g., increased ventricular irritability). Hypokalemia may be avoided or treated by use of potassium sparing diuretic or potassium supplements such as foods with a high potassium content.

Although any chloride deficit is generally mild and usually does not require specific treatment except under extraordinary circumstances (as in liver disease or renal disease), chloride replacement may be required in the treatment of metabolic alkalosis.

Dilutional hyponatremia may occur in edematous patients in hot weather. Appropriate therapy is water restriction, rather than administration of salt, except in rare instances when the hyponatremia is life threatening. In actual salt depletion, appropriate replacement is the therapy of choice.

Hyperuricemia may occur or acute gout may be precipitated in certain patients receiving thiazides.

In diabetic patients dosage adjustment of insulin or oral hypoglycemic agents may be required. Hyperglycemia may occur with thiazide diuretics. Thus latent diabetes mellitus may become manifest during thiazide therapy.

The antihypertensive effect of the drug may be enhanced in the postsympathectomy patient.

If progressive renal impairment becomes evident, consider withholding or discontinuing diuretic therapy.

Thiazides have been shown to increase the urinary excretion of magnesium; this may result in hypomagnesemia.

Thiazides may decrease urinary calcium excretion. Thiazides may cause intermittent and slight elevation of serum calcium in the absence of known disorders of calcium metabolism. Marked hypercalcemia may be evidence of hidden hyperparathyroidism. Thiazides should be discontinued before carrying out tests for parathyroid function.

Increases in cholesterol and triglyceride levels may be associated with thiazide diuretic therapy.

Reserpine

Since reserpine may increase gastric secretion and motility, it should be used cautiously in patients with a history of peptic ulcer, ulcerative colitis, or other gastrointestinal disorder. This compound may precipitate biliary colic in patients with gallstones, or bronchial asthma in susceptible persons.

Reserpine may cause hypotension including orthostatic hypotension.

Anxiety or depression, as well as psychosis, may develop during reserpine therapy. If depression is present when therapy is begun, it may be aggravated. Mental depression is unusual with reserpine doses of 0.25 mg daily or less. In any case, HYDROPRES should be discontinued at the first sign of depression. Extreme caution should be used in treating patients with a history of mental depression, and the possibility of suicide should be kept in mind.

As with most antihypertensive therapy, caution should be exercised when treating hypertensive patients with renal insufficiency, since they adjust poorly to lowered blood pressure.

When two or more antihypertensives are given, the individual dosages may have to be reduced to prevent excessive drop in blood pressure. In hypertensive patients with coronary artery disease, it is important to avoid a precipitous drop in blood pressure.

Laboratory Tests

Periodic determination of serum electrolytes to detect possible electrolyte imbalance should be done at appropriate intervals.

Drug Interactions

Hydrochlorothiazide

When given concurrently the following drugs may interact with thiazide diuretics.

Alcohol, barbiturates, or narcotics —potentiation of orthostatic hypotension may occur.

Antidiabetic drugs (oral agents and insulin) —dosage adjustment of the antidiabetic drug may be required.

Other antihypertensive drugs —additive effect or potentiation.

Cholestyramine and colestipol resins—Absorption of hydrochlorothiazide is impaired in the presence of anionic exchange resins. Single doses of either cholestyramine or colestipol resins bind the hydrochlorothiazide and reduce its absorption from the gastrointestinal tract by up to 85 and 43 percent, respectively.

Corticosteroids, ACTH —intensified electrolyte depletion, particularly hypokalemia.

Pressor amines (e.g., norepinephrine) —possible decreased response to pressor amines but not sufficient to preclude their use.

Skeletal muscle relaxants, nondepolarizing (e.g., tubocurarine) —possible increased responsiveness to the muscle relaxant.

Lithium —generally should not be given with diuretics. Diuretic agents reduce the renal clearance of lithium and add a high risk of lithium toxicity. Refer to the package insert for lithium preparations before use of such preparations with HYDROPRES.

Non-steroidal Anti-inflammatory Drugs —In some patients, the administration of a non-steroidal anti-inflammatory agent can reduce the diuretic, natriuretic, and antihypertensive effects of loop, potassium-sparing and thiazide diuretics. Therefore, when HYDROPRES and non-steroidal anti-inflammatory agents are used concomitantly, the patient should be observed closely to determine if the desired effect of the diuretic is obtained.

Reserpine

In hypertensive patients on reserpine therapy significant hypotension and bradycardia may develop during surgical anesthesia. The anesthesiologist should be aware that reserpine has been taken, since it may be necessary to give vagal blocking agents parenterally to prevent or reverse hypotension and/or bradycardia.

Use reserpine cautiously with digitalis and quinidine; cardiac arrhythmias have occurred with reserpine preparations.

Barbiturates enhance the central nervous system depressant effects of reserpine.

Monoamine oxidase (MAO) inhibitors: See CONTRAINDICATIONS.

Drug/Laboratory Test Interactions

Thiazides should be discontinued before carrying out tests for parathyroid function (see PRECAUTIONS, *General*).

Carcinogenesis, Mutagenesis, Impairment of Fertility

Carcinogenicity and mutagenicity studies have not been conducted with combinations of reserpine/hydrochlorothiazide.

In a two-litter study in the rat at an oral dose of 5.0/0.25 mg/kg, the combination of hydrochlorothiazide/reserpine did not impair fertility or produce abnormalities in the fetus.

Hydrochlorothiazide

Two-year feeding studies in mice and rats conducted under the auspices of the National Toxicology Program (NTP) uncovered no evidence of a carcinogenic potential of hydrochlorothiazide in female mice (at doses of up to approximately 600 mg/kg/day) or in male and female rats (at doses of up to approximately 100 mg/kg/day). The NTP, however, found equivocal evidence for hepatocarcinogenicity in male mice.

Hydrochlorothiazide was not genotoxic *in vitro* in the Ames mutagenicity assay of *Salmonella typhimurium* strains TA 98, TA 100, TA 1535, TA 1537, and TA 1538 and in the Chinese Hamster Ovary (CHO) test for chromosomal aberrations, or *in vivo* in assays using mouse germinal cell chromosomes, Chinese hamster bone marrow chromosomes, and the *Drosophila* sex-linked recessive lethal trait gene. Positive test results were obtained only in the *in vitro* CHO Sister Chromatid Exchange (clastogenicity) and in the Mouse Lymphoma Cell (mutagenicity) assays, using concentrations of hydrochlorothiazide from 43 to 1300 µg/mL, and in the *Aspergillus nidulans* non-disjunction assay at an unspecified concentration.

Hydrochlorothiazide had no adverse effects on the fertility of mice and rats of either sex in studies wherein these species were exposed, via their diet, to doses of up to 100 and 4 mg/kg, respectively, prior to conception and throughout gestation.

Reserpine

Reserpine at a concentration of 1 to 5000 mcg/plate had no mutagenic activity against four strains of *S. typhimurium in vitro* in the Ames microbial mutagen test with or without metabolic activation. Reserpine did not induce malignant transformation of mouse fibroblasts *in vitro* at concentrations of 0.3 to 10 mcg/mL.

A few chromosomal aberrations were induced by reserpine *in vitro* in cultured mouse mammary carcinoma cells but were considered negative in this study. The drug did not produce chromosomal aberrations in human peripheral leucocyte cultures although an increase in mitotic figures occurred. One study reported chromosomal aberrations and dominant lethal mutations in mice at doses up to 10 mg/kg of reserpine in the form of a pharmaceutical preparation. Another study did not show dominant lethal mutations in mice at IP doses of 0.92 and 4.6 mg/kg of reserpine.

Reserpine did not impair fertility in a two-litter study in the rat at an oral dose of 0.025 mg/kg.

Rodent studies have shown that reserpine is an animal tumorigen, causing an increased incidence of mammary fibroadenomas in female mice, malignant tumors of the seminal vesicles in male mice, and malignant adrenal medullary tumors in male rats. These findings arose in 2 year studies in which the drug was administered in the feed at concentrations of 5 and 10 ppm—about 100 to 300 times the usual human dose. The breast neoplasms are thought to be related to reserpine's prolactin-elevating effect. Several other prolactin-elevating drugs have also been associated with an increased incidence of mammary neoplasia in rodents.

The extent to which these findings indicate a risk to humans is uncertain. Tissue culture experiments show that about one-third of human breast tumors are prolactin-dependent *in vitro,* a factor of considerable importance if the use of the drug is contemplated in a patient with previously detected breast cancer. The possibility of an increased risk of breast cancer in reserpine users has been studied extensively; however, no firm conclusion has emerged. Although a few epidemiologic studies have suggested a slightly increased risk (less than twofold in all studies except one) in women who have used reserpine, other studies of generally

Continued on next page

Information on the Merck & Co., Inc. products listed on these pages is the full prescribing information from product circulars in use August 31, 1998. For information, please call 1-800-NSC MERCK [1-800-672-6372].

Hydropres—Cont.

similar design have not confirmed this. Epidemiologic studies conducted using other drugs (neuroleptic agents) that, like reserpine, increase prolactin levels and therefore would be considered rodent mammary carcinogens, have not shown an association between chronic administration of the drug and human mammary tumorigenesis. While long-term clinical observation has not suggested such an association, the available evidence is considered too limited to be conclusive at this time. An association of reserpine intake with pheochromocytoma or tumors of the seminal vesicles has not been explored.

Pregnancy
Use of diuretics during normal pregnancy is inappropriate and exposes mother and fetus to unnecessary hazard. Diuretics do not prevent development of toxemia of pregnancy and there is no satisfactory evidence that they are useful in the treatment of toxemia.

Teratogenic Effects —Pregnancy Category C: HYDROPRES may cause fetal harm when given to a pregnant woman. There are no adequate and well-controlled studies with HYDROPRES or other combinations of reserpine/hydrochlorothiazide in animals or pregnant women. HYDROPRES should be used during pregnancy only if the potential benefit justifies the potential risk to the fetus.

Reserpine: Reproduction studies in rats have shown that reserpine is teratogenic at doses of 1–2 mg/kg (125 to 250 times the maximum recommended human dose) IM or IP given early in pregnancy. A variety of abnormalities was produced including anophthalmia, absence of the axial skeleton, hydronephrosis, etc. Pregnancy in rabbits was interrupted when doses as low as 0.04 mg/kg (10 times the maximum recommended human dose) were given early or late in pregnancy.

Hydrochlorothiazide: Studies in which hydrochlorothiazide was orally administered to pregnant mice and rats during their respective periods of major organogenesis at doses up to 3000 and 1000 mg hydrochlorothiazide/kg, respectively, provided no evidence of harm to the fetus.

Nonteratogenic Effects

Reserpine: Reserpine has been demonstrated to cross the placental barrier in guinea pigs with depression of adrenal catecholamine stores in the newborn. There is some evidence that side effects such as nasal congestion, lethargy, depressed Moro reflex, and bradycardia may appear in infants born of reserpine-treated mothers.

Hydrochlorothiazide: Thiazides cross the placental barrier and appear in cord blood. There is a risk of fetal or neonatal jaundice, thrombocytopenia, and possibly other adverse reactions that have occurred in adults.

Nursing Mothers
Thiazides and reserpine appear in breast milk. Because of the potential for serious adverse reactions in nursing infants from HYDROPRES, a decision should be made whether to discontinue nursing or to discontinue the drug, taking into account the importance of the drug to the mother.

Pediatric Use
Safety and effectiveness of HYDROPRES in children has not been established.

ADVERSE REACTIONS

The following adverse reactions have been reported and, within each category, are listed in order of decreasing severity.

Hydrochlorothiazide
Body as a Whole: Weakness.
Cardiovascular: Hypotension including orthostatic hypotension (may be aggravated by alcohol, barbiturates, narcotics or antihypertensive drugs).
Digestive: Pancreatitis, jaundice (intrahepatic cholestatic jaundice), diarrhea, vomiting, sialadenitis, cramping, constipation, gastric irritation, nausea, anorexia.
Hematologic: Aplastic anemia, agranulocytosis, leukopenia, hemolytic anemia, thrombocytopenia.
Hypersensitivity: Anaphylactic reactions, necrotizing angiitis (vasculitis and cutaneous vasculitis), respiratory distress including pneumonitis and pulmonary edema, photosensitivity, fever, urticaria, rash, purpura.
Metabolic: Electrolyte imbalance (see PRECAUTIONS), hyperglycemia, glycosuria, hyperuricemia.
Musculoskeletal: Muscle spasm.
Nervous System/Psychiatric: Vertigo, paresthesias, dizziness, headache, restlessness.
Renal: Renal failure, renal dysfunction, interstitial nephritis. (See WARNINGS.)
Skin: Erythema multiforme including Stevens-Johnson syndrome, exfoliative dermatitis including toxic epidermal necrolysis, alopecia.
Special Senses: Transient blurred vision, xanthopsia.
Urogenital: Impotence.

Reserpine
Cardiovascular: Angina pectoris, arrhythmia, premature ventricular contractions, other direct cardiac effects (e.g., fluid retention, congestive heart failure), bradycardia.
Digestive: Vomiting, diarrhea, nausea, hypersecretion and increased motility, anorexia, dryness of mouth, increased salivation.
Hematologic: Thrombocytopenic purpura, excessive bleeding following prostatic surgery.
Hypersensitivity: Pruritus, rash, flushing of skin.
Metabolic: Weight gain.
Musculoskeletal: Muscular aches.
Nervous System/Psychiatric: Mental depression, dull sensorium, syncope, paradoxical anxiety, excessive sedation, nightmares, headache, dizziness, nervousness, parkinsonism (usually reversible with decreased dosage or discontinuance of therapy).
Respiratory: Dyspnea, epistaxis, nasal congestion, enhanced susceptibility to colds.
Special Senses: Optic atrophy, uveitis, deafness, glaucoma, conjunctival injection, blurred vision.
Urogenital: Dysuria, impotence, decreased libido, nonpuerperal lactation.

OVERDOSAGE

Overdosage may lead to excessive sedation, mental depression, severe hypotension, extrapyramidal reactions.

There is no specific antidote. In the event of overdosage, symptomatic and supportive measures should be employed. Emesis should be induced or gastric lavage performed. Correct dehydration, electrolyte imbalance, hepatic coma and hypotension by established procedures. If required, give oxygen or artificial respiration for respiratory impairment. In the event of severe hypotension from the reserpine component, intravenous use of a vasopressor is indicated [e.g., ARAMINE* (Metaraminol Bitartrate), levarterenol, phenylephrine]. Anticholinergics may be needed to relieve gastrointestinal distress from reserpine. Because the effects of the rauwolfia alkaloids are prolonged, the patient should be closely observed for at least 72 hours.

Reserpine is not dialyzable. The degree to which hydrochlorothiazide is removed by hemodialysis has not been established.

The oral LD$_{50}$ of hydrochlorothiazide is greater than 10 g/kg in the mouse and rat. The oral LD$_{50}$ of reserpine in the mouse is 390 mg/kg.

———

* Registered trademark of MERCK & CO., INC.

DOSAGE AND ADMINISTRATION

The initial dosage of HYDROPRES should conform to the dosages of the individual components established during titration (see box warning).

The usual adult dosage of HYDROPRES 25 is 1 or 2 tablets once a day; that of HYDROPRES 50 is 1 tablet once a day. Patients usually do not require doses in excess of 50 mg of hydrochlorothiazide daily when combined with other antihypertensive agents. Dosage may require adjustment according to the blood pressure response of the patient. For maintenance, dosage should be adjusted to the lowest requirements of the individual patient. Doses higher than 0.25 mg daily of reserpine should be used cautiously, because occurrence of serious mental depression and other side effects may increase considerably (see WARNINGS).

HOW SUPPLIED

No. 3265—Tablets HYDROPRES 25 are green, round, scored, compressed tablets, coded MSD 53. Each tablet contains 25 mg of hydrochlorothiazide and 0.125 mg of reserpine. They are supplied as follows:
NDC 0006-0053-68 in bottles of 100.
NDC 0006-0053-82 in bottles of 1000.
Shown in Product Identification Guide, page 323
No. 3266—Tablets HYDROPRES 50 are green, round, scored, compressed tablets, coded MSD 127. Each tablet contains 50 mg of hydrochlorothiazide and 0.125 mg of reserpine. They are supplied as follows:
NDC 0006-0127-68 in bottles of 100.
NDC 0006-0127-82 in bottles of 1000.
Shown in Product Identification Guide, page 323
Storage
Keep container tightly closed. Protect from light, moisture, freezing. −20°C (−4°F) and store at room temperature, 15–30°C (59–86°F).
7899046 Issued February 1995
COPYRIGHT © MERCK & CO., INC., 1986
All rights reserved

HYZAAR®   ℞
(Losartan Potassium-Hydrochlorothiazide Tablets)

> **USE IN PREGNANCY**
> **When used in pregnancy during the second and third trimesters, drugs that act directly on the renin-angiotensin system can cause injury and even death to the developing fetus.** When pregnancy is detected, HYZAAR should be discontinued as soon as possible. See WARNINGS: *Fetal/Neonatal Morbidity and Mortality.*

DESCRIPTION

HYZAAR* (losartan potassium-hydrochlorothiazide), combines an angiotensin II receptor (type AT$_1$) antagonist and a diuretic, hydrochlorothiazide.

Losartan potassium, a non-peptide molecule, is chemically described as 2-butyl-4-chloro-1-[p-(o-1H-tetrazol-5-ylphenyl)benzyl]imidazole-5-methanol monopotassium salt. Its empirical formula is $C_{22}H_{22}ClKN_6O$, and its structural formula is:

Losartan potassium is a white to off-white free-flowing crystalline powder with a molecular weight of 461.01. It is freely soluble in water, soluble in alcohols, and slightly soluble in common organic solvents, such as acetonitrile and methyl ethyl ketone.

Oxidation of the 5-hydroxymethyl group on the imidazole ring results in the active metabolite of losartan.

Hydrochlorothiazide is 6-chloro-3,4-dihydro-2H-1,2,4-benzothiadiazine-7-sulfonamide 1,1-dioxide. Its empirical formula is $C_7H_8ClN_3O_4S_2$ and its structural formula is:

Hydrochlorothiazide is a white, or practically white, crystalline powder with a molecular weight of 297.74, which is slightly soluble in water, but freely soluble in sodium hydroxide solution.

HYZAAR is available for oral administration containing 50 mg of losartan potassium, 12.5 mg of hydrochlorothiazide and the following inactive ingredients: microcrystalline cellulose, lactose hydrous, pregelatinized starch, magnesium stearate, hydroxypropyl cellulose, hydroxypropyl methylcellulose, titanium dioxide and D&C yellow No. 10 aluminum lake.

HYZAAR contains 4.24 mg (0.108 mEq) of potassium.

———

* Registered trademark of E.I. du Pont de Nemours and Company, Wilmington, Delaware, USA

CLINICAL PHARMACOLOGY

Mechanism of Action
Angiotensin II [formed from angiotensin I in a reaction catalyzed by angiotensin converting enzyme (ACE, kininase II)], is a potent vasoconstrictor, the primary vasoactive hormone of the renin-angiotensin system and an important component in the pathophysiology of hypertension. It also stimulates aldosterone secretion by the adrenal cortex. Losartan and its principal active metabolite block the vasoconstrictor and aldosterone-secreting effects of angiotensin II by selectively blocking the binding of angiotensin II to the AT$_1$ receptor found in many tissues, (e.g., vascular smooth muscle, adrenal gland). There is also an AT$_2$ receptor found in many tissues but it is not known to be associated with cardiovascular homeostasis. Both losartan and its principal active metabolite do not exhibit any partial agonist activity at the AT$_1$ receptor and have much greater affinity (about 1000-fold) for the AT$_1$ receptor than for the AT$_2$ receptor. *In vitro* binding studies indicate that losartan is a reversible, competitive inhibitor of the AT$_1$ receptor. The active metabolite is 10 to 40 times more potent by weight than losartan and appears to be a reversible, non-competitive inhibitor of the AT$_1$ receptor.

Neither losartan nor its active metabolite inhibits ACE (kininase II, the enzyme that converts angiotensin I to an-

giotensin II and degrades bradykinin); nor do they bind to or block other hormone receptors or ion channels known to be important in cardiovascular regulation.

Hydrochlorothiazide is a thiazide diuretic. Thiazides affect the renal tubular mechanisms of electrolyte reabsorption, directly increasing excretion of sodium and chloride in approximately equivalent amounts. Indirectly, the diuretic action of hydrochlorothiazide reduces plasma volume, with consequent increases in plasma renin activity, increases in aldosterone secretion, increases in urinary potassium loss, and decreases in serum potassium. The renin-aldosterone link is mediated by angiotensin II, so coadministration of an angiotensin II receptor antagonist tends to reverse the potassium loss associated with these diuretics.

The mechanism of the antihypertensive effect of thiazides is unknown.

Pharmacokinetics

General

Losartan Potassium

Losartan is an orally active agent that undergoes substantial first-pass metabolism by cytochrome P450 enzymes. It is converted, in part, to an active carboxylic acid metabolite that is responsible for most of the angiotensin II receptor antagonism that follows losartan treatment. The terminal half-life of losartan is about 2 hours and of the metabolite is about 6–9 hours. The pharmacokinetics of losartan and its active metabolite are linear with oral losartan doses up to 200 mg and do not change over time. Neither losartan nor its metabolite accumulate in plasma upon repeated once-daily dosing.

Following oral administration, losartan is well absorbed (based on absorption of radiolabeled losartan) and undergoes substantial first-pass metabolism; the systemic bioavailability of losartan is approximately 33%. About 14% of an orally-administered dose of losartan is converted to the active metabolite. Mean peak concentrations of losartan and its active metabolite are reached in 1 hour and in 3–4 hours, respectively. While maximum plasma concentrations of losartan and its active metabolite are approximately equal, the AUC of the metabolite is about 4 times as great as that of losartan. A meal slows absorption of losartan and decreases its C_{max} but has only minor effects on losartan AUC or on the AUC of the metabolite (about 10% decreased).

Both losartan and its active metabolite are highly bound to plasma proteins, primarily albumin, with plasma free fractions of 1.3% and 0.2% respectively. Plasma protein binding is constant over the concentration range achieved with recommended doses. Studies in rats indicate that losartan crosses the blood-brain barrier poorly, if at all.

Losartan metabolites have been identified in human plasma and urine. In addition to the active carboxylic acid metabolite, several inactive metabolites are formed. Following oral and intravenous administration of ^{14}C-labeled losartan potassium, circulating plasma radioactivity is primarily attributed to losartan and its active metabolite. *In vitro* studies indicate that cytochrome P450 2C9 and 3A4 are involved in the biotransformation of losartan to its metabolites. Minimal conversion of losartan to the active metabolite (less than 1% of the dose compared to 14% of the dose in normal subjects) was seen in about one percent of individuals studied.

The volume of distribution of losartan is about 34 liters and of the active metabolite is about 12 liters. Total plasma clearance of losartan and the active metabolite is about 600 mL/min and 50 mL/min, respectively, with renal clearance of about 75 mL/min and 25 mL/min, respectively. When losartan is administered orally, about 4% of the dose is excreted unchanged in the urine and about 6% is excreted in urine as active metabolite. Biliary excretion contributes to the elimination of losartan and its metabolites. Following oral ^{14}C-labeled losartan, about 35% of radioactivity is recovered in the urine and about 60% in the feces. Following an intravenous dose of ^{14}C-labeled losartan, about 45% of radioactivity is recovered in the urine and 50% in the feces.

Special Populations

Pediatric: Losartan pharmacokinetics have not been investigated in patients <18 years of age.

Geriatric and Gender: Losartan pharmacokinetics have been investigated in the elderly (65–75 years) and in both genders. Plasma concentrations of losartan and its active metabolite are similar in elderly and young hypertensives. Plasma concentrations of losartan were about twice as high in female hypertensives as male hypertensives, but concentrations of the active metabolite were similar in males and females.

Race: Pharmacokinetic differences due to race have not been studied.

Renal Insufficiency: Plasma concentrations of losartan are not altered in patients with creatinine clearance above 30 mL/min. In patients with lower creatinine clearance, AUCs are about 50% greater and are doubled in hemodialysis patients. Plasma concentrations of the active metabolite are not significantly altered in patients with renal impairment or in hemodialysis patients. Neither losartan nor its active metabolite can be removed by hemodialysis.

Hepatic Insufficiency: Following oral administration in patients with mild to moderate alcoholic cirrhosis of the liver, plasma concentrations of losartan and its active metabolite were, respectively, 5 times and about 1.7 times those in young male volunteers. Compared to normal subjects the total plasma clearance of losartan in patients with hepatic insufficiency was about 50% lower and the oral bioavailability was about 2-times higher. The lower starting dose of losartan recommended for use in patients with hepatic impairment cannot be given using HYZAAR. Its use in such patients as a means of losartan titration is, therefore, not recommended (see DOSAGE AND ADMINISTRATION).

Drug Interactions

Losartan Potassium

Losartan, administered for 12 days, did not affect the pharmacokinetics or pharmacodynamics of a single dose of warfarin. Losartan did not affect the pharmacokinetics of oral or intravenous digoxin. Coadministration of losartan and cimetidine led to an increase of about 18% in AUC of losartan but did not affect the pharmacokinetics of its active metabolite. Coadministration of losartan and phenobarbital led to a reduction of about 20% in the AUC of losartan and that of its active metabolite. Conversion of losartan to its active metabolite after intravenous administration is not affected by ketoconazole, an inhibitor of P450 3A4. There is no pharmacokinetic interaction between losartan and hydrochlorothiazide.

Hydrochlorothiazide

After oral administration of hydrochlorothiazide, diuresis begins within 2 hours, peaks in about 4 hours and lasts about 6 to 12 hours.

Hydrochlorothiazide is not metabolized but is eliminated rapidly by the kidney. When plasma levels have been followed for at least 24 hours, the plasma half-life has been observed to vary between 5.6 and 14.8 hours. At least 61 percent of the oral dose is eliminated unchanged within 24 hours. Hydrochlorothiazide crosses the placental but not the blood-brain barrier and is excreted in breast milk.

Pharmacodynamics and Clinical Effects

Losartan Potassium

Losartan inhibits the pressor effect of angiotensin II (as well as angiotensin I) infusions. A dose of 100 mg inhibits the pressor effect by about 85% at peak with 25–40% inhibition persisting for 24 hours. Removal of the negative feedback of angiotensin II causes a 2–3 fold rise in plasma renin activity and consequent rise in angiotensin II plasma concentration in hypertensive patients. Losartan does not affect the response to bradykinin, whereas ACE inhibitors increase the response to bradykinin. Aldosterone plasma concentrations fall following losartan administration. In spite of the effect of losartan on aldosterone secretion, very little effect on serum potassium was observed.

In a single-dose study in normal volunteers, losartan had no effects on glomerular filtration rate, renal plasma flow or filtration fraction. In multiple dose studies in hypertensive patients, there were no notable effects on systemic or renal prostaglandin concentrations, fasting triglycerides, total cholesterol or HDL-cholesterol or fasting glucose concentrations. There was a small uricosuric effect leading to a minimal decrease in serum uric acid (mean decrease <0.4 mg/dL) during chronic oral administration.

The antihypertensive effects of losartan were demonstrated principally in 4 placebo-controlled 6–12 week trials of dosages from 10 to 150 mg per day in patients with baseline diastolic blood pressures of 95–115. The studies allowed comparisons of two doses (50–100 mg/day) as once-daily or twice-daily regimens, comparisons of peak and trough effects, and comparisons of response by gender, age, and race. Three additional studies examined the antihypertensive effects of losartan and hydrochlorothiazide in combination.

The 4 studies of losartan monotherapy included a total of 1075 patients randomized to several doses of losartan and 334 to placebo. The 10 and 25 mg doses produced some effect at peak (6 hours after dosing) but small and inconsistent trough (24 hour) responses. Doses of 50, 100, and 150 mg once daily gave statistically significant systolic/diastolic mean decreases in blood pressure, compared to placebo in the range of 5.5–10.5/3.5–7.5 mmHg, with the 150 mg dose giving no greater effect than 50–100 mg. Twice-daily dosing at 50–100 mg/day gave consistently larger trough responses than once daily dosing at the same total dose. Peak (6 hour) effects were uniformly, but moderately larger than trough effects, with the trough to peak ratio for systolic and diastolic responses 50–95% and 60–90% respectively.

Analysis of age, gender, and race subgroups of patients showed that men and women, and patients over and under 65, had generally similar responses. Black patients, however, had notably smaller responses to losartan monotherapy.

The effect of losartan is substantially present within one week but in some studies the maximal effect occurred in 3–6 weeks. In long-term follow-up studies (without placebo control) the effect of losartan appeared to be maintained for up to a year. There is no apparent rebound effect after abrupt withdrawal of losartan. There was essentially no change in average heart rate in losartan-treated patients in controlled trials.

Persistent dry cough (with an incidence of a few percent) has been associated with ACE inhibitor use and in practice can be a cause of discontinuation of ACE inhibitor therapy. Two prospective, parallel-group, double-blind, randomized, controlled trials were conducted to assess the effects of losartan on the incidence of cough in hypertensive patients who had experienced cough while receiving ACE inhibitor therapy. Patients who had typical ACE inhibitor cough when challenged with lisinopril, whose cough disappeared on placebo, were randomized to losartan 50 mg, lisinopril 20 mg, or either placebo (one study, n=97) or 25 mg hydrochlorothiazide (n=135). The double-blind treatment period lasted up to 8 weeks. The incidence of cough is shown below.

Study 1†	HCTZ	Losartan	Lisinopril
Cough	25%	17%	69%
Study 2††	Placebo	Losartan	Lisinopril
Cough	35%	29%	62%

†Demographics = (89% caucasian, 64% female)
††Demographics = (90% caucasian, 51% female)

These studies demonstrate that the incidence of cough associated with losartan therapy, in a population that all had cough associated with ACE inhibitor therapy, is similar to that associated with hydrochlorothiazide or placebo therapy.

Losartan Potassium-Hydrochlorothiazide

The 3 controlled studies of losartan and hydrochlorothiazide included over 1300 patients assessing the antihypertensive efficacy of various doses of losartan (25, 50 and 100 mg) and concomitant hydrochlorothiazide (6.25, 12.5 and 25 mg). A factorial study compared the combination of losartan/hydrochlorothiazide 50/12.5 mg with its components and placebo. The combination of losartan/hydrochlorothiazide 50/12.5 mg resulted in an approximately additive placebo-adjusted systolic/diastolic response (15.5/9.0 mmHg for the combination compared to 8.5/5.0 mmHg for losartan alone and 7.0/3.0 mmHg for hydrochlorothiazide alone). Another study investigated the dose-response relationship of various doses of hydrochlorothiazide (6.25, 12.5 and 25 mg) or placebo on a background of losartan (50 mg) in patients not adequately controlled (SiDBP 93–120 mmHg) on losartan (50 mg) alone. The third study investigated the dose-response relationship of various doses of losartan (25, 50 and 100 mg) or placebo on a background of hydrochlorothiazide (25 mg) in patients not adequately controlled (SiDBP 93–120 mmHg) on hydrochlorothiazide (25 mg) alone. These studies showed an added antihypertensive response at trough (24 hours post-dosing) of hydrochlorothiazide 12.5 or 25 mg added to losartan 50 mg of 5.5/3.5 and 10.0/6.0 mmHg, respectively. Similarly, there was an added antihypertensive response at trough when losartan 50 or 100 mg was added to hydrochlorothiazide 25 mg of 9.0/5.5 and 12.5/6.5 mmHg, respectively. There was no significant effect on heart rate.

There was no difference in response for men and women or in patients over or under 65 years of age.

Black patients had a larger response to hydrochlorothiazide than non-black patients and a smaller response to losartan. The overall response to the combination was similar for black and non-black patients.

INDICATIONS AND USAGE

HYZAAR is indicated for the treatment of hypertension. This fixed dose combination is not indicated for initial therapy (see DOSAGE AND ADMINISTRATION).

CONTRAINDICATIONS

HYZAAR is contraindicated in patients who are hypersensitive to any component of this product.

Because of the hydrochlorothiazide component, this product is contraindicated in patients with anuria or hypersensitivity to other sulfonamide-derived drugs.

WARNINGS

Fetal/Neonatal Morbidity and Mortality

Drugs that act directly on the renin-angiotensin system can cause fetal and neonatal morbidity and death when administered to pregnant women. Several dozen cases have been reported in the world literature in patients who were taking angiotensin converting enzyme inhibitors. When pregnancy is detected, HYZAAR should be discontinued as soon as possible.

Continued on next page

Information on the Merck & Co., Inc. products listed on these pages is the full prescribing information from product circulars in use August 31, 1998. For information, please call 1-800-NSC MERCK [1-800-672-6372].

Hyzaar—Cont.

The use of drugs that act directly on the renin-angiotensin system during the second and third trimesters of pregnancy has been associated with fetal and neonatal injury, including hypotension, neonatal skull hypoplasia, anuria, reversible or irreversible renal failure, and death. Oligohydramnios has also been reported, presumably resulting from decreased fetal renal function; oligohydramnios in this setting has been associated with fetal limb contractures, craniofacial deformation, and hypoplastic lung development. Prematurity, intrauterine growth retardation, and patent ductus arteriosus have also been reported, although it is not clear whether these occurrences were due to exposure to the drug.

These adverse effects do not appear to have resulted from intrauterine drug exposure that has been limited to the first trimester.

Mothers whose embryos and fetuses are exposed to an angiotensin II receptor antagonist only during the first trimester should be so informed. Nonetheless, when patients become pregnant, physicians should have the patient discontinue the use of HYZAAR as soon as possible.

Rarely (probably less often than once in every thousand pregnancies), no alternative to an angiotensin II receptor antagonist will be found. In these rare cases, the mothers should be apprised of the potential hazards to their fetuses, and serial ultrasound examinations should be performed to assess the intra-amniotic environment.

If oligohydramnios is observed, HYZAAR should be discontinued unless it is considered life-saving for the mother. Contraction stress testing (CST), a non-stress test (NST), or biophysical profiling (BPP) may be appropriate, depending upon the week of pregnancy. Patients and physicians should be aware, however, that oligohydramnios may not appear until after the fetus has sustained irreversible injury.

Infants with histories of *in utero* exposure to an angiotensin II receptor antagonist should be closely observed for hypotension, oliguria, and hyperkalemia. If oliguria occurs, attention should be directed toward support of blood pressure and renal perfusion. Exchange transfusion or dialysis may be required as means of reversing hypotension and/or substituting for disordered renal function.

There was no evidence of teratogenicity in rats or rabbits treated with a maximum losartan potassium dose of 10 mg/kg/day in combination with 2.5 mg/kg/day of hydrochlorothiazide. At these dosages, respective exposures (AUCs) of losartan, its active metabolite, and hydrochlorothiazide in rabbits were approximately 5-, 1.5-, and 1.0-times those achieved in humans with 100 mg losartan in combination with 25 mg hydrochlorothiazide. AUC values for losartan, its active metabolite and hydrochlorothiazide, extrapolated from data obtained with losartan administered to rats at a dose of 50 mg/kg/day in combination with 12.5 mg/kg/day of hydrochlorothiazide, were approximately 6, 2, and 2 times greater than those achieved in humans with 100 mg of losartan in combination with 25 mg of hydrochlorothiazide. Fetal toxicity in rats, as evidenced by a slight increase in supernumerary ribs, was observed when females were treated prior to and throughout gestation with 10 mg/kg/day losartan in combination with 2.5 mg/kg/day hydrochlorothiazide. As also observed in studies with losartan alone, adverse fetal and neonatal effects, including decreased body weight, renal toxicity, and mortality, occurred when pregnant rats were treated during late gestation and/or lactation with 50 mg/kg/day losartan in combination with 12.5 mg/kg/day hydrochlorothiazide. Respective AUCs for losartan, its active metabolite and hydrochlorothiazide at these dosages in rats were approximately 35, 10 and 10 times greater than those achieved in humans with the administration of 100 mg of losartan in combination with 25 mg hydrochlorothiazide. When hydrochlorothiazide was administered without losartan to pregnant mice and rats during their respective periods of major organogenesis, at doses up to 3000 and 1000 mg/kg/day, respectively, there was no evidence of harm to the fetus.

Thiazides cross the placental barrier and appear in cord blood. There is a risk of fetal or neonatal jaundice, thrombocytopenia, and possibly other adverse reactions that have occurred in adults.

Hypotension—Volume-Depleted Patients
In patients who are intravascularly volume-depleted (e.g., those treated with diuretics), symptomatic hypotension may occur after initiation of therapy with HYZAAR. This condition should be corrected prior to administration of HYZAAR (see DOSAGE AND ADMINISTRATION).

Impaired Hepatic Function
Losartan Potassium-Hydrochlorothiazide
HYZAAR is not recommended for patients with hepatic impairment who require titration with losartan. The lower starting dose of losartan recommended for use in patients with hepatic impairment cannot be given using HYZAAR.
Hydrochlorothiazide
Thiazides should be used with caution in patients with impaired hepatic function or progressive liver disease, since minor alterations of fluid and electrolyte balance may precipitate hepatic coma.

Hypersensitivity Reaction
Hypersensitivity reactions to hydrochlorothiazide may occur in patients with or without a history of allergy or bronchial asthma, but are more likely in patients with such a history.
Systemic Lupus Erythematosus
Thiazide diuretics have been reported to cause exacerbation or activation of systemic lupus erythematosus.
Lithium Interaction
Lithium generally should not be given with thiazides (see PRECAUTIONS, *Drug Interactions, Hydrocholorothiazide, Lithium*).

PRECAUTIONS

General
Losartan Potassium-Hydrochlorothiazide
In double-blind clinical trials of various doses of losartan potassium and hydrochlorothiazide, the incidence of hypertensive patients who developed hypokalemia (serum potassium <3.5 mEq/L) was 6.7% versus 3.5% for placebo; the incidence of hyperkalemia (serum potassium >5.7 mEq/L) was 0.4%. No patient discontinued due to increases or decreases in serum potassium. The mean decrease in serum potassium in patients treated with various doses of losartan and hydrochlorothiazide was 0.123 mEq/L. In patients treated with various doses of losartan and hydrochlorothiazide, there was also a dose-related decrease in the hypokalemic response to hydrochlorothiazide as the dose of losartan was increased, as well as a dose-related decrease in serum uric acid with increasing doses of losartan.
Hydrochlorothiazide
Periodic determination of serum electrolytes to detect possible electrolyte imbalance should be performed at appropriate intervals.
All patients receiving thiazide therapy should be observed for clinical signs of fluid or electrolyte imbalance: hyponatremia, hypochloremic alkalosis, and hypokalemia. Serum and urine electrolyte determinations are particularly important when the patient is vomiting excessively or receiving parenteral fluids. Warning signs or symptoms of fluid and electrolyte imbalance, irrespective of cause, include dryness of mouth, thirst, weakness, lethargy, drowsiness, restlessness, confusion, seizures, muscle pains or cramps, muscular fatigue, hypotension, oliguria, tachycardia, and gastrointestinal disturbances such as nausea and vomiting.
Hypokalemia may develop, especially with brisk diuresis, when severe cirrhosis is present, or after prolonged therapy. Interference with adequate oral electrolyte intake will also contribute to hypokalemia. Hypokalemia may cause cardiac arrhythmia and may also sensitize or exaggerate the response of the heart to the toxic effects of digitalis (e.g., increased ventricular irritability).
Although any chloride deficit is generally mild and usually does not require specific treatment except under extraordinary circumstances (as in liver disease or renal disease), chloride replacement may be required in the treatment of metabolic alkalosis.
Dilutional hyponatremia may occur in edematous patients in hot weather; appropriate therapy is water restriction, rather than administration of salt except in rare instances when the hyponatremia is life-threatening. In actual salt depletion, appropriate replacement is the therapy of choice.
Hyperuricemia may occur or frank gout may be precipitated in certain patients receiving thiazide therapy. Because losartan decreases uric acid, losartan in combination with hydrochlorothiazide attenuates the diuretic-induced hyperuricemia.
In diabetic patients dosage adjustments of insulin or oral hypoglycemic agents may be required. Hyperglycemia may occur with thiazide diuretics. Thus latent diabetes mellitus may become manifest during thiazide therapy.
The antihypertensive effects of the drug may be enhanced in the postsympathectomy patient.
If progressive renal impairment becomes evident consider withholding or discontinuing diuretic therapy.
Thiazides have been shown to increase the urinary excretion of magnesium; this may result in hypomagnesemia.
Thiazides may decrease urinary calcium excretion. Thiazides may cause intermittent and slight elevation of serum calcium in the absence of known disorders of calcium metabolism. Marked hypercalcemia may be evidence of hidden hyperparathyroidism. Thiazides should be discontinued before carrying out tests for parathyroid function.
Increases in cholesterol and triglyceride levels may be associated with thiazide diuretic therapy.
Hypersensitivity. See ADVERSE REACTIONS, *Post-Marketing Experience*.
Impaired Renal Function
As a consequence of inhibiting the renin-angiotensin-aldosterone system, changes in renal function have been reported in susceptible individuals treated with losartan; in some patients, these changes in renal function were reversible upon discontinuation of therapy.
In patients whose renal function may depend on the activity of the renin-angiotensin-aldosterone system (e.g., patients

with severe congestive heart failure), treatment with angiotensin converting enzyme inhibitors has been associated with oliguria and/or progressive azotemia and (rarely) with acute renal failure and/or death. Similar outcomes have been reported with losartan.
In studies of ACE inhibitors in patients with unilateral or bilateral renal artery stenosis, increases in serum creatinine or BUN have been reported. Similar effects have been reported with losartan; in some patients, these effects were reversible upon discontinuation of therapy.
Thiazides should be used with caution in severe renal disease. In patients with renal disease, thiazides may precipitate azotemia. Cumulative effects of the drug may develop in patients with impaired renal function.
Information for Patients
Pregnancy: Female patients of childbearing age should be told about the consequences of second- and third-trimester exposure to drugs that act on the renin-angiotensin system, and they should also be told that these consequences do not appear to have resulted from intrauterine drug exposure that has been limited to the first trimester. These patients should be asked to report pregnancies to their physicians as soon as possible.
Symptomatic Hypotension: A patient receiving HYZAAR should be cautioned that lightheadedness can occur, especially during the first days of therapy, and that it should be reported to the prescribing physician. The patients should be told that if syncope occurs, HYZAAR should be discontinued until the physician has been consulted.
All patients should be cautioned that inadequate fluid intake, excessive perspiration, diarrhea, or vomiting can lead to an excessive fall in blood pressure, with the same consequences of lightheadedness and possible syncope.
Potassium Supplements: A patient receiving HYZAAR should be told not to use potassium supplements or salt substitutes containing potassium without consulting the prescribing physician (see PRECAUTIONS, *Drug Interactions, Losartan Potassium*).
Drug Interactions
Losartan Potassium
No significant drug-drug pharmacokinetic interactions have been found in interaction studies with hydrochlorothiazide, digoxin, warfarin, cimetidine and phenobarbital. (See CLINICAL PHARMACOLOGY, *Drug Interactions*.) Potent inhibitors of cytochrome P450 3A4 and 2C9 have not been studied clinically but *in vitro* studies show significant inhibition of the formation of the active metabolite by inhibitors of P450 3A4 (ketoconazole, troleandomycin, gestodene), or P450 2C9 (sulfaphenazole) and nearly complete inhibition by the combination of sulfaphenazole and ketoconazole. In humans, ketoconazole, an inhibitor of P450 3A4, did not affect the conversion of losartan to the active metabolite after intravenous administration of losartan. Inhibitors of cytochrome P450 2C9 have not been studied clinically. The pharmacodynamic consequences of concomitant use of losartan and inhibitors of P450 2C9 have not been examined.
As with other drugs that block angiotensin II or its effects, concomitant use of potassium-sparing diuretics (e.g., spironolactone, triamterene, amiloride), potassium supplements, or salt substitutes containing potassium may lead to increases in serum potassium (see PRECAUTIONS, *Information for Patients, Potassium Supplements*).
Hydrochlorothiazide
When administered concurrently the following drugs may interact with thiazide diuretics:
Alcohol, barbiturates, or narcotics—potentiation of orthostatic hypotension may occur.
Antidiabetic drugs (oral agents and insulin)—dosage adjustment of the antidiabetic drug may be required.
Other antihypertensive drugs—additive effect or potentiation.
Cholestyramine and colestipol resins—Absorption of hydrochlorothiazide is impaired in the presence of anionic exchange resins. Single doses of either cholestyramine or colestipol resins bind the hydrochlorothiazide and reduce its absorption from the gastrointestinal tract by up to 85 and 43 percent, respectively.
Corticosteroids, ACTH—intensified electrolyte depletion, particularly hypokalemia.
Pressor amines (e.g., norepinephrine)—possible decreased response to pressor amines but not sufficient to preclude their use.
Skeletal muscle relaxants, nondepolarizing (e.g., tubocurarine)—possible increased responsiveness to the muscle relaxant.
Lithium—should not generally be given with diuretics. Diuretic agents reduce the renal clearance of lithium and add a high risk of lithium toxicity. Refer to the package insert for lithium preparations before use of such preparations with HYZAAR.
Non-steroidal Anti-inflammatory Drugs—In some patients, the administration of a non-steroidal anti-inflammatory agent can reduce the diuretic, natriuretic, and antihypertensive effects of loop, potassium-sparing and thiazide diuretics. Therefore, when HYZAAR and non-steroidal anti-

inflammatory agents are used concomitantly, the patient should be observed closely to determine if the desired effect of the diuretic is obtained.

Carcinogenesis, Mutagenesis, Impairment of Fertility
Losartan Potassium-Hydrochlorothiazide
No carcinogenicity studies have been conducted with the losartan potassium-hydrochlorothiazide combination.
Losartan potassium-hydrochlorothiazide when tested at a weight ratio of 4:1, was negative in the Ames microbial mutagenesis assay and the V-79 Chinese hamster lung cell mutagenesis assay. In addition, there was no evidence of direct genotoxicity in the *in vitro* alkaline elution assay in rat hepatocytes and *in vitro* chromosomal aberration assay in Chinese hamster ovary cells at noncytotoxic concentrations.
Losartan potassium, coadministered with hydrochlorothiazide, had no effect on the fertility or mating behavior of male rats of dosages up to 135 mg/kg/day of losartan and 33.75 mg/kg/day of hydrochlorothiazide. These dosages have been shown to provide respective systemic exposures (AUCs) for losartan, its active metabolite and hydrochlorothiazide that are approximately 60, 60 and 30 times greater than those achieved in humans with 100 mg of losartan potassium in combination with 25 mg of hydrochlorothiazide. In female rats, however, the coadministration of doses as low as 10 mg/kg/day of losartan and 2.5 mg/kg/day of hydrochlorothiazide was associated with slight but statistically significant decreases in fecundity and fertility indices. AUC values for losartan, its active metabolite and hydrochlorothiazide, extrapolated from data obtained with losartan administered to rats at a dose of 50 mg/kg/day in combination with 12.5 mg/kg/day of hydrochlorothiazide, were approximately 6, 2, and 2 times greater than those achieved in humans with 100 mg of losartan in combination with 25 mg of hydrochlorothiazide.

Losartan Potassium
Losartan potassium was not carcinogenic when administered at maximally tolerated dosages to rats and mice for 105 and 92 weeks, respectively. Female rats given the highest dose (270 mg/kg/day) had a slightly higher incidence of pancreatic acinar adenoma. The maximally tolerated dosages (270 mg/kg/day in rats, 200 mg/kg/day in mice) provided systemic exposures for losartan and its pharmacologically active metabolite that were approximately 160 and 90 times (rats) and 30 and 15 times (mice) the exposure of a 50 kg human given 100 mg per day.
Losartan potassium was negative in the microbial mutagenesis and V-79 mammalian cell mutagenesis assays and in the *in vitro* alkaline elution and *in vitro* and *in vivo* chromosomal aberration assays. In addition, the active metabolite showed no evidence of genotoxicity in the microbial mutagenesis, *in vitro* alkaline elution, and *in vitro* chromosomal aberration assays.
Fertility and reproductive performance were not affected in studies with male rats given oral doses of losartan potassium up to approximately 150 mg/kg/day. The administration of toxic dosage levels in females (300/200 mg/kg/day) was associated with a significant (p<0.05) decrease in the number of corpora lutea/female, implants/female, and live fetuses/female at C-section. At 100 mg/kg/day only a decrease in the number of corpora lutea/female was observed. The relationship of these findings to drug-treatment is uncertain since there was no effect at these dosage levels on implants/pregnant female, percent post-implantation loss, or live animals/litter at parturition. In nonpregnant rats dosed at 135 mg/kg/day for 7 days, systemic exposure (AUCs) for losartan and its active metabolite were approximately 66 and 26 times the exposure achieved in man at the maximum recommended human daily dosage (100 mg).

Hydrochlorothiazide
Two-year feeding studies in mice and rats conducted under the auspices of the National Toxicology Program (NTP) uncovered no evidence of a carcinogenic potential of hydrochlorothiazide in female mice (at doses of up to approximately 600 mg/kg/day) or in male and female rats (at doses of up to approximately 100 mg/kg/day). The NTP, however, found equivocal evidence for hepatocarcinogenicity in male mice.
Hydrochlorothiazide was not genotoxic *in vitro* in the Ames mutagenicity assay of *Salmonella typhimurium* strains TA 98, TA 100, TA 1535, TA 1537, and TA 1538 and in the Chinese Hamster Ovary (CHO) test for chromosomal aberrations, or *in vivo* in assays using mouse germinal cell chromosomes, Chinese hamster bone marrow chromosomes, and the *Drosophila* sex-linked recessive lethal trait gene. Positive test results were obtained only in the *in vitro* CHO Sister Chromatid Exchange (clastogenicity) and in the Mouse Lymphoma Cell (mutagenicity) assays, using concentrations of hydrochlorothiazide from 43 to 1300 µg/mL, and in the *Aspergillus nidulans* non-disjunction assay at an unspecified concentration.
Hydrochlorothiazide had no adverse effects on the fertility of mice and rats of either sex in studies wherein these species were exposed, via their diet, to doses of up to 100 and 4 mg/kg, respectively, prior to mating and throughout gestation.

Pregnancy
Pregnancy Categories C (first trimester) and D (second and third trimesters). See WARNINGS, *Fetal/Neonatal Morbidity and Mortality*.

Nursing Mothers
It is not known whether losartan is excreted in human milk, but significant levels of losartan and its active metabolite were shown to be present in rat milk. Thiazides appear in human milk. Because of the potential for adverse effects on the nursing infant, a decision should be made whether to discontinue nursing or discontinue the drug, taking into account the importance of the drug to the mother.

Pediatric Use
Safety and effectiveness in pediatric patients have not been established.

Use in the Elderly
Of the total number of patients in controlled clinical studies of hypertension with HYZAAR, 107 patients (12.5%) were 65 years and over, while 9 patients (1.0%) were 75 years and over. No overall differences in effectiveness or safety were observed between these patients and younger patients, but greater sensitivity of some older individuals cannot be ruled out.

ADVERSE REACTIONS

Losartan potassium-hydrochlorothiazide has been evaluated for safety in 858 patients treated for essential hypertension. In clinical trials with losartan potassium-hydrochlorothiazide, no adverse experiences peculiar to this combination drug have been observed. Adverse experiences have been limited to those that were reported previously with losartan potassium and/or hydrochlorothiazide. The overall incidence of adverse experiences reported with the combination was comparable to placebo.
In general, treatment with losartan potassium-hydrochlorothiazide was well tolerated. For the most part, adverse experiences have been mild and transient in nature and have not required discontinuation of therapy. In controlled clinical trials, discontinuation of therapy due to clinical adverse experiences was required in only 2.8% and 2.3% of patients treated with the combination and placebo, respectively.
In these double-blind controlled clinical trials, the following adverse experiences reported with HYZAAR occurred in ≥1 percent of patients, and more often on drug than placebo, regardless of drug relationship:

	Losartan Potassium-Hydrochloro-thiazide (n=858)	Placebo (n=173)
Body as a Whole		
Abdominal pain	1.2	0.6
Edema/swelling	1.3	1.2
Cardiovascular		
Palpitation	1.4	0.0
Musculoskeletal		
Back pain	2.1	0.6
Nervous/Psychiatric		
Dizziness	5.7	2.9
Respiratory		
Cough	2.6	2.3
Sinusitis	1.2	0.6
Upper respiratory infection	6.1	4.6
Skin		
Rash	1.4	0.0

The following adverse events were also reported at a rate of 1% or greater, but were as, or more, common in the placebo group: asthenia/fatigue, diarrhea, nausea, headache, bronchitis, pharyngitis.
Adverse events occurred at about the same rates in men and women, older and younger patients, and black and non-black patients.
A patient with known hypersensitivity to aspirin and penicillin, when treated with losartan potassium, was withdrawn from study due to swelling of the lips and eyelids and facial rash, reported as angioedema, which returned to normal 5 days after therapy was discontinued.
Superficial peeling of palms and hemolysis was reported in one subject treated with losartan potassium.

Losartan Potassium
Other adverse experiences that have been reported with losartan, without regard to causality, are listed below:
Body as a Whole: chest pain, facial edema, fever, orthostatic effects, syncope; *Cardiovascular:* angina pectoris, arrhythmias including atrial fibrillation, sinus bradycardia, tachycardia, ventricular tachycardia and ventricular fibrillation, CVA, hypotension, myocardial infarction, second degree AV block; *Digestive:* anorexia, constipation, dental pain, dry mouth, dyspepsia, flatulence, gastritis, vomiting; *Hematologic:* anemia; *Metabolic:* gout; *Musculoskeletal:* arm pain, arthralgia, arthritis, fibromyalgia, hip pain, joint swelling, knee pain, leg pain, muscle cramps, muscle weakness, musculoskeletal pain, myalgia, shoulder pain, stiffness; *Nervous System/Psychiatric:* anxiety, anxiety disorder, ataxia, confusion, depression, dream abnormality, hypesthesia, insomnia, libido decreased, memory impairment, migraine, nervousness, panic disorder, paresthesia, peripheral neuropathy, sleep disorder, somnolence, tremor, vertigo; *Respiratory:* dyspnea, epistaxis, nasal congestion, pharyngeal discomfort, respiratory congestion, rhinitis, sinus disorder; *Skin:* alopecia, dermatitis, dry skin, ecchymosis, erythema, flushing, photosensitivity, pruritus, sweating, urticaria; *Special Senses:* blurred vision, burning/stinging in the eye, conjunctivitis, decrease in visual acuity, taste perversion, tinnitus; *Urogenital:* impotence, nocturia, urinary frequency, urinary tract infection.

Hydrochlorothiazide
Other adverse experiences that have been reported with hydrochlorothiazide, without regard to causality, are listed below:
Body as a Whole: weakness; *Digestive:* pancreatitis, jaundice (intrahepatic cholestatic jaundice), sialadenitis, cramping, gastric irritation; *Hematologic:* aplastic anemia, agranulocytosis, leukopenia, hemolytic anemia, thrombocytopenia; *Hypersensitivity:* purpura, photosensitivity, urticaria, necrotizing angiitis (vasculitis and cutaneous vasculitis), fever, respiratory distress including pneumonitis and pulmonary edema, anaphylactic reactions; *Metabolic:* hyperglycemia, glycosuria, hyperuricemia; *Musculoskeletal:* muscle spasm; *Nervous System/Psychiatric:* restlessness; *Renal:* renal failure, renal dysfunction, interstitial nephritis; *Skin:* erythema multiforme including Stevens-Johnson syndrome, exfoliative dermatitis including toxic epidermal necrolysis; *Special Senses:* transient blurred vision, xanthopsia.

Post-Marketing Experience
The following additional adverse reactions have been reported in post-marketing experience: *Hypersensitivity:* Angioedema (involving swelling of the face, lips, pharynx, and/or tongue) has been reported rarely in patients treated with losartan; some of these patients previously experienced angioedema with other drugs including ACE inhibitors; *Digestive:* Hepatitis has been reported rarely in patients treated with losartan.
Hyperkalemia has been reported with losartan.

Laboratory Test Findings
In controlled clinical trials, clinically important changes in standard laboratory parameters were rarely associated with administration of HYZAAR.

Creatinine, Blood Urea Nitrogen: Minor increases in blood urea nitrogen (BUN) or serum creatinine were observed in 0.6 and 0.8 percent, respectively, of patients with essential hypertension treated with HYZAAR alone. No patient discontinued taking HYZAAR due to increased BUN. One patient discontinued taking HYZAAR due to a minor increase in serum creatinine.

Hemoglobin and Hematocrit: Small decreases in hemoglobin and hematocrit (mean decreases of approximately 0.14 grams percent and 0.72 volume percent, respectively) occurred frequently in patients treated with HYZAAR alone, but were rarely of clinical importance. No patients were discontinued due to anemia.

Liver Function Tests: Occasional elevations of liver enzymes and/or serum bilirubin have occurred. In patients with essential hypertension treated with HYZAAR alone, no patients were discontinued due to these laboratory adverse experiences.

Serum Electrolytes: See PRECAUTIONS.

OVERDOSAGE

Losartan Potassium
Significant lethality was observed in mice and rats after oral administration of 1000 mg/kg and 2000 mg/kg, respectively, about 44 and 170 times the maximum recommended human dose on a mg/m² basis.
Limited data are available in regard to overdosage in humans. The most likely manifestation of overdosage would be hypotension and tachycardia; bradycardia could occur from parasympathetic (vagal) stimulation. If symptomatic hypotension should occur, supportive treatment should be instituted.
Neither losartan nor its active metabolite can be removed by hemodialysis.

Hydrochlorothiazide
The oral LD₅₀ of hydrochlorothiazide is greater than 10 g/kg in both mice and rats. The most common signs and symptoms observed are those caused by electrolyte depletion (hypokalemia, hypochloremia, hyponatremia) and dehydration resulting from excessive diuresis. If digitalis has also been administered, hypokalemia may accentuate cardiac arrhythmias. The degree to which hydrochlorothiazide is removed by hemodialysis has not been established.

Continued on next page

Information on the Merck & Co., Inc. products listed on these pages is the full prescribing information from product circulars in use August 31, 1998. For information, please call 1-800-NSC MERCK [1-800-672-6372].

Hyzaar—Cont.

DOSAGE AND ADMINISTRATION

The usual starting dose of losartan is 50 mg once daily, with 25 mg recommended for patients with intravascular volume depletion (e.g., patients treated with diuretics) (see WARNINGS, *Hypotension—Volume-Depleted Patients*) and patients with a history of hepatic impairment (see WARNINGS, *Impaired Hepatic Function*). Losartan can be administered once or twice daily at total daily doses of 25 to 100 mg. If the antihypertensive effect measured at trough using once-a-day dosing is inadequate, a twice-a-day regimen at the same total daily dose or an increase in dose may give a more satisfactory response.

Hydrochlorothiazide is effective in doses of 12.5 to 100 mg once daily and can be given at doses of 12.5 to 25 mg as HYZAAR.

To minimize dose-independent side effects, it is usually appropriate to begin combination therapy only after a patient has failed to achieve the desired effect with monotherapy.

The side effects (see WARNINGS) of losartan are generally rare and apparently independent of dose; those of hydrochlorothiazide are a mixture of dose-dependent (primarily hypokalemia) and dose-independent phenomena (e.g., pancreatitis), the former much more common than the latter. Therapy with any combination of losartan and hydrochlorothiazide will be associated with both sets of dose-independent side effects.

Replacement Therapy: The combination may be substituted for the titrated components.

Dose Titration by Clinical Effect: A patient whose blood pressure is not adequately controlled with losartan monotherapy (see above) may be switched to HYZAAR (losartan 50 mg/hydrochlorothiazide 12.5 mg) once daily. If blood pressure remains uncontrolled after about 3 weeks of therapy, the dose may be increased to two tablets once daily.

A patient whose blood pressure is inadequately controlled by 25 mg once daily of hydrochlorothiazide, or is controlled but who experiences hypokalemia with this regimen, may be switched to HYZAAR (losartan 50 mg/hydrochlorothiazide 12.5 mg) once daily, reducing the dose of hydrochlorothiazide without reducing the overall expected antihypertensive response. The clinical response to HYZAAR should be subsequently evaluated and if blood pressure remains uncontrolled after about 3 weeks of therapy, the dose may be increased to two tablets once daily.

The usual dose of HYZAAR is one tablet once daily. More than two tablets once daily is not recommended. The maximal antihypertensive effect is attained about 3 weeks after initiation of therapy.

Use in Patients with Renal Impairment: The usual regimens of therapy with HYZAAR may be followed as long as the patient's creatinine clearance is >30 mL/min. In patients with more severe renal impairment, loop diuretics are preferred to thiazides, so HYZAAR is not recommended.

Patients with Hepatic Impairment: HYZAAR is not recommended for titration in patients with hepatic impairment (see WARNINGS, *Impaired Hepatic Function*) because the appropriate 25 mg starting dose of losartan cannot be given.

HYZAAR may be administered with other antihypertensive agents.

HYZAAR may be administered with or without food.

HOW SUPPLIED

No. 3502—Tablets HYZAAR, 50-12.5 are yellow, teardrop shaped, film-coated tablets, coded MRK 717 on one side and HYZAAR on the other. Each tablet contains 50 mg of losartan potassium and 12.5 mg of hydrochlorothiazide. They are supplied as follows:

NDC 0006-0717-31 unit of use bottles of 30
NDC 0006-0717-54 unit of use bottles of 90
NDC 0006-0717-58 unit of use bottles of 100
(6505-01-416-4329, 50-12.5 100's).
NDC 0006-0717-28 unit dose packages of 100.

Shown in Product Identification Guide, page 323

Storage

Store at controlled room temperature, 15–30°C (59–86°F). Keep container tightly closed. Protect from light.

Manufactured for:
MERCK & CO., INC., West Point, PA 19486, USA
by:
Du Pont Pharmaceuticals, Wilmington, DE 19880 USA
7892805 Issued March 1998

COPYRIGHT © MERCK & CO., Inc., 1995
All rights reserved.

INDOCIN® Capsules, Oral Suspension and Suppositories (Indomethacin), U.S.P. ℞
INDOCIN® SR Capsules (Indomethacin), U.S.P. ℞

DESCRIPTION

INDOCIN* (Indomethacin) cannot be considered a simple analgesic and should not be used in conditions other than those recommended under INDICATIONS.

INDOCIN is supplied in four dosage forms. Capsules INDOCIN for oral administration contain either 25 mg or 50 mg of indomethacin and the following inactive ingredients: colloidal silicon dioxide, FD & C Blue 1, FD & C Red 3, gelatin, lactose, lecithin, magnesium stearate, and titanium dioxide. Capsules INDOCIN SR for sustained release oral administration contain 75 mg of indomethacin and the following inactive ingredients: cellulose, confectioner's sugar, FD & C Blue 1, FD & C Blue 2, FD & C Red 3, gelatin, hydroxypropyl methylcellulose, magnesium stearate, polyvinyl acetate-crotonic acid copolymer, starch, and titanium dioxide. Capsules INDOCIN SR conform to the requirements of the USP Drug Release Test 1 for Indomethacin Extended-release Capsules. Suspension INDOCIN for oral use contains 25 mg of indomethacin per 5 mL, alcohol 1%, and sorbic acid 0.1% added as a preservative and the following inactive ingredients: antifoam AF emulsion, flavors, purified water, sodium hydroxide or hydrochloric acid to adjust pH, sorbitol solution, tragacanth. Suppositories INDOCIN for rectal use contain 50 mg of indomethacin and the following inactive ingredients: butylated hydroxyanisole, butylated hydroxytoluene, edetic acid, glycerin, polyethylene glycol 3350, polyethylene glycol 8000 and sodium chloride. Indomethacin is a non-steroidal anti-inflammatory indole derivative designated chemically as 1-(4-chlorobenzoyl)-5-methoxy-2-methyl-*1H*-indole-3-acetic acid. Indomethacin is practically insoluble in water and sparingly soluble in alcohol. It has a pKa of 4.5 and is stable in neutral or slightly acidic media and decomposes in strong alkali. The suspension has a pH of 4.0–5.0. The structural formula is:

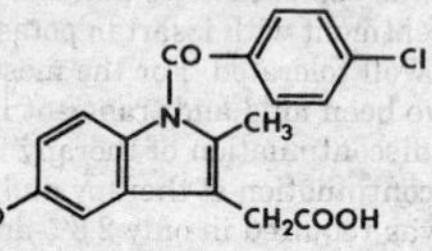

*Registered trademark of MERCK & CO., INC.

CLINICAL PHARMACOLOGY

INDOCIN is a non-steroidal drug with anti-inflammatory, antipyretic and analgesic properties. Its mode of action, like that of other anti-inflammatory drugs, is not known. However, its therapeutic action is not due to pituitary-adrenal stimulation.

INDOCIN is a potent inhibitor of prostaglandin synthesis *in vitro*. Concentrations are reached during therapy which have been demonstrated to have an effect *in vivo* as well. Prostaglandins sensitize afferent nerves and potentiate the action of bradykinin in inducing pain in animal models. Moreover, prostaglandins are known to be among the mediators of inflammation. Since indomethacin is an inhibitor of prostaglandin synthesis, its mode of action may be due to a decrease of prostaglandins in peripheral tissues.

INDOCIN has been shown to be an effective anti-inflammatory agent, appropriate for long-term use in rheumatoid arthritis, ankylosing spondylitis, and osteoarthritis.

INDOCIN affords relief of symptoms; it does not alter the progressive course of the underlying disease.

INDOCIN suppresses inflammation in rheumatoid arthritis as demonstrated by relief of pain, and reduction of fever, swelling and tenderness. Improvement in patients treated with INDOCIN for rheumatoid arthritis has been demonstrated by a reduction in joint swelling, average number of joints involved, and morning stiffness; by increased mobility as demonstrated by a decrease in walking time; and by improved functional capability as demonstrated by an increase in grip strength.

Indomethacin has been reported to diminish basal and CO_2 stimulated cerebral blood flow in healthy volunteers following acute oral and intravenous administration. In one study after one week of treatment with orally administered indomethacin, this effect on basal cerebral blood flow had disappeared. The clinical significance of this effect has not been established.

Capsules INDOCIN have been found effective in relieving the pain, reducing the fever, swelling, redness, and tenderness of acute gouty arthritis. Capsules INDOCIN rather than Capsules INDOCIN SR are recommended for treatment of acute gouty arthritis—see INDICATIONS.

Following single oral doses of Capsules INDOCIN 25 mg or 50 mg, indomethacin is readily absorbed, attaining peak plasma concentrations of about 1 and 2 mcg/mL, respectively, at about 2 hours. Orally administered Capsules INDOCIN are virtually 100% bioavailable, with 90% of the dose absorbed within 4 hours. A single 50 mg dose of Oral Suspension INDOCIN was found to be bioequivalent to a 50 mg INDOCIN capsule when each was administered with food.

Capsules INDOCIN SR 75 mg are designed to release 25 mg of the drug initially and the remaining 50 mg over approximately 12 hours (90% of dose absorbed by 12 hours). When measured over a 24-hour period, the cumulative amount and time-course of indomethacin absorption from a single Capsule INDOCIN SR are comparable to those of 3 doses of 25 mg Capsules INDOCIN given at 4–6 hour intervals.

Plasma concentrations of indomethacin fluctuate less and are more sustained following administration of Capsules INDOCIN SR than following administration of 25 mg Capsules INDOCIN given at 4–6 hour intervals. In multiple-dose comparisons, the mean daily steady-state plasma level of indomethacin attained with daily administration of Capsules INDOCIN SR 75 mg was indistinguishable from that following Capsules INDOCIN 25 mg given at 0, 6 and 12 hours daily. However, there was a significant difference in indomethacin plasma levels between the two dosage regimens especially after 12 hours.

Controlled clinical studies of safety and efficacy in patients with osteoarthritis have shown that one Capsule INDOCIN SR was clinically comparable to one 25 mg Capsule INDOCIN t.i.d.; and in controlled clinical studies in patients with rheumatoid arthritis, one Capsule INDOCIN SR taken in the morning and one in the evening were clinically indistinguishable from one 50 mg Capsule INDOCIN t.i.d.

Indomethacin is eliminated via renal excretion, metabolism, and biliary excretion. Indomethacin undergoes appreciable enterohepatic circulation. The mean half-life of indomethacin is estimated to be about 4.5 hours. With a typical therapeutic regimen of 25 or 50 mg t.i.d., the steady-state plasma concentrations of indomethacin are an average 1.4 times those following the first dose.

The rate of absorption is more rapid from the rectal suppository than from Capsules INDOCIN. Ordinarily, therefore, the total amount absorbed from the suppository would be expected to be at least equivalent to the capsule. In controlled clinical trials, however, the amount of indomethacin absorbed was found to be somewhat less (80–90%) than that absorbed from Capsules INDOCIN. This is probably because some subjects did not retain the material from the suppository for the one hour necessary to assure complete absorption. Since the suppository dissolves rather quickly rather than melting slowly, it is seldom recovered in recognizable form if the patient retains the suppository for more than a few minutes.

Indomethacin exists in the plasma as the parent drug and its desmethyl, desbenzoyl, and desmethyl-desbenzoyl metabolites, all in the unconjugated form. About 60 percent of an oral dosage is recovered in urine as drug and metabolites (26 percent as indomethacin and its glucuronide), and 33 percent is recovered in feces (1.5 percent as indomethacin).

About 99% of indomethacin is bound to protein in plasma over the expected range of therapeutic plasma concentrations. Indomethacin has been found to cross the blood-brain barrier and the placenta.

In a gastroscopic study in 45 healthy subjects, the number of gastric mucosal abnormalities was significantly higher in the group receiving Capsules INDOCIN than in the group taking Suppositories INDOCIN or placebo.

In a double-blind comparative clinical study involving 175 patients with rheumatoid arthritis, however, the incidence of upper gastrointestinal adverse effects with Suppositories or Capsules INDOCIN was comparable. The incidence of lower gastrointestinal adverse effects was greater in the suppository group.

INDICATIONS

Indomethacin has been found effective in active stages of the following:

1. Moderate to severe rheumatoid arthritis including acute flares of chronic disease.
2. Moderate to severe ankylosing spondylitis.
3. Moderate to severe osteoarthritis.
4. Acute painful shoulder (bursitis and/or tendinitis).
5. Acute gouty arthritis.

Capsules INDOCIN SR are recommended for all of the indications for Capsules INDOCIN except acute gouty arthritis.

INDOCIN may enable the reduction of steroid dosage in patients receiving steroids for the more severe forms of rheumatoid arthritis. In such instances the steroid dosage should be reduced slowly and the patients followed very closely for any possible adverse effects.

The use of INDOCIN in conjunction with aspirin or other salicylates is not recommended. Controlled clinical studies have shown that the combined use of INDOCIN and aspirin does not produce any greater therapeutic effect than the use of INDOCIN alone. Furthermore, in one of these clinical studies, the incidence of gastrointestinal side effects was significantly increased with combined therapy (see DRUG INTERACTIONS).

CONTRAINDICATIONS

INDOCIN should not be used in:

Patients who are hypersensitive to this product.

Patients in whom acute asthmatic attacks, urticaria, or rhinitis are precipitated by aspirin or other non-steroidal anti-inflammatory agents.

Suppositories INDOCIN are contraindicated in patients with a history of proctitis or recent rectal bleeding.

WARNINGS

General:

Because of the variability of the potential of INDOCIN to cause adverse reactions in the individual patient, the following are strongly recommended:

1. The lowest possible effective dose for the individual patient should be prescribed. Increased dosage tends to increase adverse effects, particularly in doses over 150–200 mg/day, without corresponding increase in clinical benefits.

2. Careful instructions to, and observations of, the individual patient are essential to the prevention of serious adverse reactions. As advancing years appear to increase the possibility of adverse reactions, INDOCIN should be used with greater care in the aged.

3. Effectiveness of INDOCIN in pediatric patients has not been established. INDOCIN should not be prescribed for pediatric patients 14 years of age and younger unless toxicity or lack of efficacy associated with other drugs warrants the risk.

   In experience with more than 900 pediatric patients reported in the literature or to the manufacturer who were treated with Capsules INDOCIN, side effects in pediatric patients were comparable to those reported in adults. Experience in pediatric patients has been confined to the use of Capsules INDOCIN.

   If a decision is made to use indomethacin for pediatric patients two years of age or older, such patients should be monitored closely and periodic assessment of liver function is recommended. There have been cases of hepatotoxicity reported in pediatric patients with juvenile rheumatoid arthritis, including fatalities. If indomethacin treatment is instituted, a suggested starting dose is 2 mg/kg/day given in divided doses. Maximum daily dosage should not exceed 4 mg/kg/day or 150–200 mg/day, whichever is less. As symptoms subside, the total daily dosage should be reduced to the lowest level required to control symptoms, or the drug should be discontinued.

4. If Capsules INDOCIN SR are used for initial therapy or during dosage adjustment, observe the patient closely (see DOSAGE AND ADMINISTRATION).

Gastrointestinal Effects:

Single or multiple ulcerations, including perforation and hemorrhage of the esophagus, stomach, duodenum or small and large intestine, have been reported to occur with INDOCIN. Fatalities have been reported in some instances. Rarely, intestinal ulceration has been associated with stenosis and obstruction.

Gastrointestinal bleeding without obvious ulcer formation and perforation of pre-existing sigmoid lesions (diverticulum, carcinoma, etc.) have occurred. Increased abdominal pain in ulcerative colitis patients or the development of ulcerative colitis and regional ileitis have been reported to occur rarely.

Because of the occurrence, and at times severity, of gastrointestinal reactions to INDOCIN, the prescribing physician must be continuously alert for any sign or symptom signaling a possible gastrointestinal reaction. The risks of continuing therapy with INDOCIN in the face of such symptoms must be weighed against the possible benefits to the individual patient.

INDOCIN should not be given to patients with active gastrointestinal lesions or with a history of recurrent gastrointestinal lesions except under circumstances which warrant the very high risk and where patients can be monitored very closely.

The gastrointestinal effects may be reduced by giving Capsules INDOCIN or Capsules INDOCIN SR immediately after meals, with food, or with antacids.

Risk of GI Ulcerations, Bleeding and Perforation with NSAID Therapy

Serious gastrointestinal toxicity such as bleeding, ulceration, and perforation, can occur at any time, with or without warning symptoms, in patients treated chronically with NSAID therapy. Although minor upper gastrointestinal problems, such as dyspepsia, are common, usually developing early in therapy, physicians should remain alert for ulceration and bleeding in patients treated chronically with NSAIDs even in the absence of previous GI tract symptoms. In patients observed in clinical trials of several months to two years duration, symptomatic upper GI ulcers, gross bleeding or perforation appear to occur in approximately 1% of patients treated for 3–6 months, and in about 2–4% of patients treated for one year. Physicians should inform patients about the signs and/or symptoms of serious GI toxicity and what steps to take if they occur.

Studies to date have not identified any subset of patients not at risk of developing peptic ulceration and bleeding. Except for a prior history of serious GI events and other risk factors known to be associated with peptic ulcer disease, such as alcoholism, smoking, etc., no risk factors (e.g., age, sex) have been associated with increased risk. Elderly or de-

bilitated patients seem to tolerate ulceration or bleeding less well than other individuals and most spontaneous reports of fatal GI events are in this population. Studies to date are inconclusive concerning the relative risk of various NSAIDs in causing such reactions. High doses of any NSAID probably carry a greater risk of these reactions, although controlled clinical trials showing this do not exist in most cases. In considering the use of relatively large doses (within the recommended dosage range), sufficient benefit should be anticipated to offset the potential increased risk of GI toxicity.

Renal Effects:

As with other non-steroidal anti-inflammatory drugs, long term administration of indomethacin to animals has resulted in renal papillary necrosis and other abnormal renal pathology. In humans, there have been reports of acute interstitial nephritis with hematuria, proteinuria, and occasionally nephrotic syndrome.

A second form of renal toxicity has been seen in patients with prerenal and renal conditions leading to a reduction in renal blood flow or blood volume, where the renal prostaglandins have a supportive role in the maintenance of renal perfusion. In these patients administration of an NSAID may cause a dose dependent reduction in prostaglandin formation and may precipitate overt renal decompensation. Patients at greatest risk of this reaction are those with conditions such as renal or hepatic dysfunction, diabetes mellitus, advanced age, extracellular volume depletion from any cause, congestive heart failure, septicemia, pyelonephritis, or concomitant use of any nephrotoxic drug. INDOCIN or other NSAIDs should be given with caution and renal function should be monitored in any patient who may have reduced renal reserve. Discontinuation of NSAID therapy is typically followed by recovery to the pretreatment state.

Increases in serum potassium concentration, including hyperkalemia, have been reported, even in some patients without renal impairment. In patients with normal renal function, these effects have been attributed to a hyporeninemic-hypoaldosteronism state (see PRECAUTIONS, *Drug Interactions*).

Since INDOCIN is eliminated primarily by the kidneys, patients with significantly impaired renal function should be closely monitored; a lower daily dosage should be anticipated to avoid excessive drug accumulation.

Ocular Effects:

Corneal deposits and retinal disturbances, including those of the macula, have been observed in some patients who had received prolonged therapy with INDOCIN. The prescribing physician should be alert to the possible association between the changes noted and INDOCIN. It is advisable to discontinue therapy if such changes are observed. Blurred vision may be a significant symptom and warrants a thorough ophthalmological examination. Since these changes may be asymptomatic, ophthalmologic examination at periodic intervals is desirable in patients where therapy is prolonged.

Central Nervous System Effects:

INDOCIN may aggravate depression or other psychiatric disturbances, epilepsy, and parkinsonism, and should be used with considerable caution in patients with these conditions. If severe CNS adverse reactions develop, INDOCIN should be discontinued.

INDOCIN may cause drowsiness; therefore, patients should be cautioned about engaging in activities requiring mental alertness and motor coordination, such as driving a car. INDOCIN may also cause headache. Headache which persists despite dosage reduction requires cessation of therapy with INDOCIN.

Use in Pregnancy and the Neonatal Period

INDOCIN is not recommended for use in pregnant women, since safety for use has not been established. The known effects of indomethacin and other drugs of this class on the human fetus during the third trimester of pregnancy include: constriction of the ductus arteriosus prenatally, tricuspid incompetence, and pulmonary hypertension; nonclosure of the ductus arteriosus postnatally which may be resistant to medical management; myocardial degenerative changes, platelet dysfunction with resultant bleeding, intracranial bleeding, renal dysfunction or failure, renal injury/dysgenesis which may result in prolonged or permanent renal failure, oligohydramnios, gastrointestinal bleeding or perforation, and increased risk of necrotizing enterocolitis. Teratogenic studies were conducted in mice and rats at dosages of 0.5, 1.0, 2.0, and 4.0 mg/kg/day. Except for retarded fetal ossification at 4 mg/kg/day considered secondary to the decreased average fetal weights, no increase in fetal malformations was observed as compared with control groups. Other studies in mice reported in the literature using higher doses (5 to 15 mg/kg/day) have described maternal toxicity and death, increased fetal resorptions, and fetal malformations. Comparable studies in rodents using high doses of aspirin have shown similar maternal and fetal effects.

As with other non-steroidal anti-inflammatory agents which inhibit prostaglandin synthesis, indomethacin has been found to delay parturition in rats.

In rats and mice, 4.0 mg/kg/day given during the last three days of gestation caused a decrease in maternal weight gain and some maternal and fetal deaths. An increased incidence of neuronal necrosis in the diencephalon in the live-born fetuses was observed. At 2.0 mg/kg/day, no increase in neuronal necrosis was observed as compared to the control groups. Administration of 0.5 or 4.0 mg/kg/day during the first three days of life did not cause an increase in neuronal necrosis at either dose level.

Use in Nursing Mothers

INDOCIN is excreted in the milk of lactating mothers. INDOCIN is not recommended for use in nursing mothers.

PRECAUTIONS

General

Non-steroidal anti-inflammatory drugs, including INDOCIN, may mask the usual signs and symptoms of infection. Therefore, the physician must be continually on the alert for this and should use the drug with extra care in the presence of existing infection.

Fluid retention and peripheral edema have been observed in some patients taking INDOCIN. Therefore, as with other non-steroidal anti-inflammatory drugs, INDOCIN should be used with caution in patients with cardiac dysfunction, hypertension, or other conditions predisposing to fluid retention.

In a study of patients with severe heart failure and hyponatremia, INDOCIN was associated with significant deterioration of circulatory hemodynamics, presumably due to inhibition of prostaglandin dependent compensatory mechanisms.

INDOCIN, like other non-steroidal anti-inflammatory agents, can inhibit platelet aggregation. This effect is of shorter duration than that seen with aspirin and usually disappears within 24 hours after discontinuation of INDOCIN. INDOCIN has been shown to prolong bleeding time (but within the normal range) in normal subjects. Because this effect may be exaggerated in patients with underlying hemostatic defects, INDOCIN should be used with caution in persons with coagulation defects.

As with other non-steroidal anti-inflammatory drugs, borderline elevations of one or more liver tests may occur in up to 15% of patients. These abnormalities may progress, may remain essentially unchanged, or may be transient with continued therapy. The SGPT (ALT) test is probably the most sensitive indicator of liver dysfunction. Meaningful (3 times the upper limit of normal) elevations of SGPT or SGOT (AST) occurred in controlled clinical trials in less than 1% of patients. A patient with symptoms and/or signs suggesting liver dysfunction, or in whom an abnormal liver test has occurred, should be evaluated for evidence of the development of more severe hepatic reaction while on therapy with INDOCIN. Severe hepatic reactions, including jaundice and cases of fatal hepatitis, have been reported with INDOCIN as with other non-steroidal anti-inflammatory drugs. Although such reactions are rare, if abnormal liver tests persist or worsen, if clinical signs and symptoms consistent with liver disease develop, or if systemic manifestations occur (e.g., eosinophilia, rash, etc.), INDOCIN should be discontinued.

Information for Patients

INDOCIN, like other drugs of its class, is not free of side effects. The side effects of these drugs can cause discomfort and, rarely, there are more serious side effects such as gastrointestinal bleeding, which may result in hospitalization and even fatal outcomes.

NSAIDs (Non-steroidal Anti-inflammatory Drugs) are often essential agents in the management of arthritis; but they also may be commonly employed for conditions which are less serious.

Physicians may wish to discuss with their patients the potential risks (see WARNINGS, PRECAUTIONS, and ADVERSE REACTIONS) and likely benefits of NSAID treatment, particularly when the drugs are used for less serious conditions where treatment without NSAIDs may represent an acceptable alternative to both the patient and physician.

Laboratory Tests

Because serious GI tract ulceration and bleeding can occur without warning symptoms, physicians should follow chronically treated patients for the signs and symptoms of ulceration and bleeding and should inform them of the importance of this follow-up (see WARNINGS, *Risk of GI Ulcerations, Bleeding and Perforation with NSAID Therapy*).

Carcinogenesis, Mutagenesis, Impairment of Fertility

In an 81-week chronic oral toxicity study in the rat at doses up to 1 mg/kg/day, indomethacin had no tumorigenic effect.

Continued on next page

Information on the Merck & Co., Inc. products listed on these pages is the full prescribing information from product circulars in use August 31, 1998. For information, please call 1-800-NSC MERCK [1-800-672-6372].

Indocin/Indocin SR—Cont.

Indomethacin produced no neoplastic or hyperplastic changes related to treatment in carcinogenic studies in the rat (dosing period 73–110 weeks) and the mouse (dosing period 62–88 weeks) at doses up to 1.5 mg/kg/day.

Indomethacin did not have any mutagenic effect in *in vitro* bacterial tests (Ames test and *E. coli* with or without metabolic activation) and a series of *in vivo* tests including the host-mediated assay, sex-linked recessive lethals in *Drosophila*, and the micronucleus test in mice.

Indomethacin at dosage levels up to 0.5 mg/kg/day had no effect on fertility in mice in a two generation reproduction study or a two litter reproduction study in rats.

Drug Interactions

In normal volunteers receiving indomethacin, the administration of diflunisal decreased the renal clearance and significantly increased the plasma levels of indomethacin. In some patients, combined use of INDOCIN and diflunisal has been associated with fatal gastrointestinal hemorrhage. Therefore, diflunisal and INDOCIN should not be used concomitantly.

In a study in normal volunteers, it was found that chronic concurrent administration of 3.6 g of aspirin per day decreases indomethacin blood levels approximately 20%.

The concomitant use of INDOCIN with other NSAIDs is not recommended due to the increased possibility of gastrointestinal toxicity, with little or no increase in efficacy.

Clinical studies have shown that INDOCIN does not influence the hypoprothrombinemia produced by anticoagulants. However, when any additional drug, including INDOCIN, is added to the treatment of patients on anticoagulant therapy, the patients should be observed for alterations of the prothrombin time.

When INDOCIN is given to patients receiving probenecid, the plasma levels of indomethacin are likely to be increased. Therefore, a lower total daily dosage of INDOCIN may produce a satisfactory therapeutic effect. When increases in the dose of INDOCIN are made, they should be made carefully and in small increments.

Caution should be used if INDOCIN is administered simultaneously with methotrexate. INDOCIN has been reported to decrease the tubular secretion of methotrexate and to potentiate its toxicity.

Administration of non-steroidal anti-inflammatory drugs concomitantly with cyclosporine has been associated with an increase in cyclosporine-induced toxicity, possibly due to decreased synthesis of renal prostacyclin. NSAIDs should be used with caution in patients taking cyclosporine, and renal function should be monitored.

Capsules INDOCIN 50 mg t.i.d. produced a clinically relevant elevation of plasma lithium and reduction in renal lithium clearance in psychiatric patients and normal subjects with steady state plasma lithium concentrations. This effect has been attributed to inhibition of prostaglandin synthesis. As a consequence, when INDOCIN and lithium are given concomitantly, the patient should be carefully observed for signs of lithium toxicity. (Read circulars for lithium preparations before use of such concomitant therapy.) In addition, the frequency of monitoring serum lithium concentration should be increased at the outset of such combination drug treatment.

INDOCIN given concomitantly with digoxin has been reported to increase the serum concentration and prolong the half-life of digoxin. Therefore, when INDOCIN and digoxin are used concomitantly, serum digoxin levels should be closely monitored.

In some patients, the administration of INDOCIN can reduce the diuretic, natriuretic, and, antihypertensive effects of loop, potassium-sparing, and thiazide diuretics. Therefore, when INDOCIN and diuretics are used concomitantly, the patient should be observed closely to determine if the desired effect of the diuretic is obtained.

INDOCIN reduces basal plasma renin activity (PRA), as well as those elevations of PRA induced by furosemide administration, or salt or volume depletion. These facts should be considered when evaluating plasma renin activity in hypertensive patients.

It has been reported that the addition of triamterene to a maintenance schedule of INDOCIN resulted in reversible acute renal failure in two of four healthy volunteers. INDOCIN and triamterene should not be administered together. INDOCIN and potassium-sparing diuretics each may be associated with increased serum potassium levels. The potential effects of INDOCIN and potassium-sparing diuretics on potassium kinetics and renal function should be considered when these agents are administered concurrently.

Most of the above effects concerning diuretics have been attributed, at least in part, to mechanisms involving inhibition of prostaglandin synthesis by INDOCIN.

Blunting of the antihypertensive effect of beta-adrenoceptor blocking agents by non-steroidal anti-inflammatory drugs including INDOCIN has been reported. Therefore, when using these blocking agents to treat hypertension, patients should be observed carefully in order to confirm that the desired therapeutic effect has been obtained. There are reports that INDOCIN can reduce the antihypertensive effect of captopril in some patients.

False-negative results in the dexamethasone suppression test (DST) in patients being treated with INDOCIN have been reported. Thus, results of the DST should be interpreted with caution in these patients.

Pediatric Use

Effectiveness in pediatric patients 14 years of age and younger has not been established (see WARNINGS).

ADVERSE REACTIONS

The adverse reactions for Capsules INDOCIN listed in the following table have been arranged into two groups: (1) incidence greater than 1%; and (2) incidence less than 1%. The incidence for group (1) was obtained from 33 double-blind controlled clinical trials reported in the literature (1,092 patients). The incidence for group (2) was based on reports in clinical trials, in the literature, and on voluntary reports since marketing. The probability of a causal relationship exists between INDOCIN and these adverse reactions, some of which have been reported only rarely.

In controlled clinical trials, the incidence of adverse reactions to Capsules INDOCIN SR and equal 24-hour doses of Capsules INDOCIN were similar.

The adverse reactions reported with Capsules INDOCIN may occur with use of the suppositories. In addition, rectal irritation and tenesmus have been reported in patients who have received the suppositories.

The adverse reactions reported with Capsules INDOCIN may also occur with use of the suspension.

[See table below]

[See table at bottom of next page]

Causal relationship unknown: Other reactions have been reported but occurred under circumstances where a causal relationship could not be established. However, in these rarely reported events, the possibility cannot be excluded. Therefore, these observations are being listed to serve as alerting information to physicians:

Cardiovascular: Thrombophlebitis

Hematologic: Although there have been several reports of leukemia, the supporting information is weak.

Genitourinary: Urinary frequency.

A rare occurrence of fulminant necrotizing fasciitis, particularly in association with Group A β-hemolytic streptococcus, has been described in persons treated with non-steroidal anti-inflammatory agents, including indomethacin, sometimes with fatal outcome (see also PRECAUTIONS, General).

OVERDOSAGE

The following symptoms may be observed following overdosage: nausea, vomiting, intense headache, dizziness, mental confusion, disorientation, or lethargy. There have been reports of paresthesias, numbness, and convulsions.

Treatment is symptomatic and supportive. The stomach should be emptied as quickly as possible if the ingestion is recent. If vomiting has not occurred spontaneously, the patient should be induced to vomit with syrup of ipecac. If the patient is unable to vomit, gastric lavage should be performed. Once the stomach has been emptied, 25 or 50 g of activated charcoal may be given. Depending on the condition of the patient, close medical observation and nursing care may be required. The patient should be followed for several days because gastrointestinal ulceration and hemorrhage have been reported as adverse reactions of indomethacin. Use of antacids may be helpful.

The oral LD_{50} of indomethacin in mice and rats (based on 14 day mortality response) was 50 and 12 mg/kg, respectively.

DOSAGE AND ADMINISTRATION

INDOCIN is available as 25 and 50 mg Capsules INDOCIN, 75 mg Capsules INDOCIN SR for oral use, Oral Suspension INDOCIN, containing 25 mg of indomethacin per 5 mL, and 50 mg Suppositories INDOCIN for rectal use. Capsules INDOCIN SR 75 mg once a day can be substituted for Capsules INDOCIN 25 mg t.i.d. However, there will be significant differences between the two dosage regimens in indomethacin blood levels, especially after 12 hours (see CLINICAL PHARMACOLOGY). In addition, Capsules INDOCIN SR 75 mg b.i.d. can be substituted for Capsules INDOCIN 50 mg t.i.d. Capsules INDOCIN SR may be substituted for all the indications for Capsules INDOCIN except acute gouty arthritis.

Adverse reactions appear to correlate with the size of the dose of INDOCIN in most patients but not all. Therefore, every effort should be made to determine the smallest effective dosage for the individual patient.

Incidence greater than 1%	Incidence less than 1%	
GASTROINTESTINAL		
nausea* with or without vomiting	anorexia	gastrointestinal bleeding without
dyspepsia* (including indigestion, heartburn and epigastric pain)	bloating (includes distention) flatulence peptic ulcer gastroenteritis	obvious ulcer formation and perforation of pre-existing sigmoid lesions
diarrhea	rectal bleeding	(diverticulum,
abdominal distress or pain	proctitis single or	carcinoma, etc.) development of
constipation	multiple ulcerations, including perforation and hemorrhage of the esophagus, stomach, duodenum or small and large intestines intestinal ulceration associated with stenosis and obstruction	ulcerative colitis and regional ileitis ulcerative stomatitis toxic hepatitis and jaundice (some fatal cases have been reported) intestinal strictures (diaphragms)
CENTRAL NERVOUS SYSTEM		
headache (11.7%)	anxiety (includes nervousness)	light-headedness syncope
dizziness*	muscle weakness	paresthesia
vertigo	involuntary muscle	aggravation of epilepsy
somnolence	movements	and parkinsonism
depression and fatigue (including malaise and listlessness)	insomnia muzziness psychic disturbances including psychotic episodes mental confusion drowsiness	depersonalization coma peripheral neuropathy convulsions dysarthria
SPECIAL SENSES		
tinnitus	ocular—corneal deposits and retinal disturbances, including those of the macula, have been reported in some patients on prolonged therapy with INDOCIN	blurred vision diplopia hearing disturbances, deafness

Always give Capsules INDOCIN, Capsules INDOCIN SR, or Oral Suspension INDOCIN with food, immediately after meals, or with antacids to reduce gastric irritation.

Pediatric Use

INDOCIN ordinarily should not be prescribed for pediatric patients 14 years of age and under (see WARNINGS).

Adult Use

Dosage Recommendations for Active Stages of the Following:

1. Moderate to severe rheumatoid arthritis including acute flares of chronic disease; moderate to severe ankylosing spondylitis; and moderate to severe osteoarthritis.

   Suggested Dosage:

   Capsules INDOCIN 25 mg b.i.d. or t.i.d. If this is well tolerated, increase the daily dosage by 25 or by 50 mg, if required by continuing symptoms, at weekly intervals until a satisfactory response is obtained or until a total daily dose of 150–200 mg is reached. DOSES ABOVE THIS AMOUNT GENERALLY DO NOT INCREASE THE EFFECTIVENESS OF THE DRUG.

In patients who have persistent night pain and/or morning stiffness, the giving of a large portion, up to a maximum of 100 mg, of the total daily dose at bedtime, either orally or by rectal suppositories, may be helpful in affording relief. The total daily dose should not exceed 200 mg. In acute flares of chronic rheumatoid arthritis, it may be necessary to increase the dosage by 25 mg or, if required, by 50 mg daily.

If Capsules INDOCIN SR 75 mg are used for initiating indomethacin treatment, one capsule daily should be the usual starting dose in order to observe patient tolerance since 75 mg per day is the maximum recommended starting dose for indomethacin (see above). If Capsules INDOCIN SR are used to increase the daily dose, patients should be observed for possible signs and symptoms of intolerance since the daily increment will exceed the daily increment recommended for the other dosage forms. For patients who require 150 mg of INDOCIN per day and have demonstrated acceptable tolerance, INDOCIN SR may be prescribed as one capsule twice daily.

If minor adverse effects develop as the dosage is increased, reduce the dosage rapidly to a tolerated dose and OBSERVE THE PATIENT CLOSELY.

If severe adverse reactions occur, STOP THE DRUG. After the acute phase of the disease is under control, an attempt to reduce the daily dose should be made repeatedly until the patient is receiving the smallest effective dose or the drug is discontinued.

Careful instructions to, and observations of, the individual patient are essential to the prevention of serious, irreversible, including fatal, adverse reactions.

As advancing years appear to increase the possibility of adverse reactions, INDOCIN should be used with greater care in the aged.

2. Acute painful shoulder (bursitis and/or tendinitis).

   Initial Dose:

   75–150 mg daily in 3 or 4 divided doses.

   The drug should be discontinued after the signs and symptoms of inflammation have been controlled for several days. The usual course of therapy is 7–14 days.

3. Acute gouty arthritis.

   Suggested Dosage:

   Capsules INDOCIN 50 mg t.i.d. until pain is tolerable. The dose should then be rapidly reduced to complete cessation of the drug. Definite relief of pain has been reported within 2 to 4 hours. Tenderness and heat usually subside in 24 to 36 hours, and swelling gradually disappears in 3 to 5 days.

HOW SUPPLIED

No. 3316—Capsules INDOCIN, 25 mg are opaque blue and white capsules, coded INDOCIN and MSD 25. They are supplied as follows:

NDC 0006-0025-68 bottles of 100
(6505-00-926-2154, 25 mg 100's).
NDC 0006-0025-82 bottles of 1000
(6505-00-931-0680, 25 mg 1000's).

Shown in Product Identification Guide, page 323

No. 3317—Capsules INDOCIN, 50 mg are opaque blue and white capsules, coded INDOCIN and MSD 50. They are supplied as follows:

NDC 0006-0050-68 bottles of 100.

Shown in Product Identification Guide, page 323

No. 3376—Oral Suspension INDOCIN, 25 mg per 5 mL, is an off-white suspension with a pineapple coconut mint flavor. It is supplied as follows:

NDC 0006-3376-66 in bottles of 237 mL.

No. 3370—Capsules INDOCIN SR, 75 mg each, are capsules with an opaque blue cap and clear body containing a mixture of blue and white pellets, coded INDOCIN SR and MSD 693. They are supplied as follows:

NDC 0006-0693-31 unit of use bottles of 30
(6505-01-135-7391, 75 mg 30's)
NDC 0006-0693-61 unit of use bottles of 60
(6505-01-137-4629, 75 mg 60's).

Shown in Product Identification Guide, page 323

No. 3354—Suppositories INDOCIN, 50 mg each, are white, opaque, rectal suppositories and are supplied as follows:

NDC 0006-0150-30, boxes of 30
(6505-01-231-7284, 50 mg 30's).

Shown in Product Identification Guide, page 323

Storage

Store Oral Suspension INDOCIN below 30°C (86°F). Avoid temperatures above 50°C (122°F). Protect from freezing. Store Suppositories INDOCIN below 30°C (86°F). Avoid transient temperatures above 40°C (104°F).

Suppositories INDOCIN are distributed by:
MERCK SHARP & DOHME, Division of Merck & Co., Inc. West Point, Pa. 19486
Manufactured by:
MERCK SHARP & DOHME
(Italia) S.p.A.
27100—Pavia, Italy
Capsules and Oral Suspension INDOCIN® and Capsules INDOCIN® SR are distributed and manufactured by:
MERCK SHARP & DOHME, Division of Merck & Co., Inc. West Point, Pa. 19486
7873325   Issued February 1997
COPYRIGHT © MERCK & CO., INC., 1988
All rights reserved

INDOCIN® I.V.   ℞
(Indomethacin Sodium Trihydrate)

DESCRIPTION

Sterile INDOCIN* I.V. (Indomethacin Sodium Trihydrate) for intravenous administration is lyophilized indomethacin sodium trihydrate. Each vial contains indomethacin sodium trihydrate equivalent to 1 mg indomethacin as a white to yellow lyophilized powder or plug. Variations in the size of the lyophilized plug and the intensity of color have no relationship to the quality or amount of indomethacin present in the vial.

Indomethacin sodium trihydrate is designated chemically as 1-(4-chlorobenzoyl)-5-methoxy-2-methyl-1H-indole-3-acetic acid, sodium salt, trihydrate. Its molecular weight is 433.82. Its empirical formula is $C_{19}H_{15}ClNNaO_4 \cdot 3H_2O$ and its structural formula is:

*Registered trademark of MERCK & CO., INC.

CLINICAL PHARMACOLOGY

Although the exact mechanism of action through which indomethacin causes closure of a patent ductus arteriosus is not known, it is believed to be through inhibition of prostaglandin synthesis. Indomethacin has been shown to be a potent inhibitor of prostaglandin synthesis, both *in vitro* and *in vivo*. In human newborns with certain congenital heart malformations, PGE 1 dilates the ductus arteriosus. In fetal

Continued on next page

Incidence greater than 1%	Incidence less than 1%	
CARDIOVASCULAR		
none	hypertension	congestive heart failure
	hypotension	arrhythmia;
	tachycardia	palpitations
	chest pain	
METABOLIC		
none	edema	hyperglycemia
	weight gain	glycosuria
	fluid retention	hyperkalemia
	flushing or sweating	
INTEGUMENTARY		
none	pruritus	exfoliative dermatitis
	rash; urticaria	erythema nodosum
	petechiae or	loss of hair
	ecchymosis	Stevens-Johnson
		syndrome
		erythema multiforme
		toxic epidermal
		necrolysis
HEMATOLOGIC		
none	leukopenia	aplastic anemia
	bone marrow	hemolytic anemia
	depression	agranulocytosis
	anemia secondary	thrombocytopenic
	to obvious or	purpura
	occult	disseminated intravascular
	gastrointestinal	coagulation
	bleeding	
HYPERSENSITIVITY		
none	acute anaphylaxis	dyspnea
	acute respiratory	asthma
	distress	purpura
	rapid fall in blood	angiitis
	pressure	pulmonary edema
	resembling a	fever
	shock-like state	
	angioedema	
GENITOURINARY		
none	hematuria	BUN elevation
	vaginal bleeding	renal insufficiency,
	proteinuria	including renal
	nephrotic syndrome	failure
	interstitial nephritis	
MISCELLANEOUS		
none	epistaxis	
	breast changes,	
	including	
	enlargement and	
	tenderness, or	
	gynecomastia	

* Reactions occurring in 3% to 9% of patients treated with INDOCIN. (Those reactions occurring in less than 3% of patients are unmarked.)

Information on the Merck & Co., Inc. products listed on these pages is the full prescribing information from product circulars in use August 31, 1998. For information, please call 1-800-NSC MERCK [1-800-672-6372].

Indocin I.V.—Cont.

and newborn lambs, E type prostaglandins have also been shown to maintain the patency of the ductus, and as in human newborns, indomethacin causes its constriction.

Studies in healthy young animals and in premature infants with patent ductus arteriosus indicated that, after the first dose of intravenous indomethacin, there was a transient reduction in cerebral blood flow velocity and cerebral blood flow. The clinical significance of this effect has not been established.

In double-blind placebo-controlled studies of INDOCIN I.V. in 460 small pre-term infants, weighing 1750 g or less, the infants treated with placebo had a ductus closure rate after 48 hours of 25 to 30 percent, whereas those treated with INDOCIN I.V. had a 75 to 80 percent closure rate. In one of these studies, a multicenter study, involving 405 pre-term infants, later re-opening of the ductus arteriosus occurred in 26 percent of infants treated with INDOCIN I.V., however, 70 percent of these closed subsequently without the need for surgery or additional indomethacin.

Pharmacokinetics and Metabolism

The disposition of indomethacin following intravenous administration (0.2 mg/kg) in pre-term neonates with patent ductus arteriosus has not been extensively evaluated. Even though the plasma half-life of indomethacin was variable among premature infants, it was shown to vary inversely with postnatal age and weight. In one study, of 28 infants who could be evaluated, the plasma half-life in those infants less than 7 days old averaged 20 hours (range: 3–60 hours, n = 18). In infants older than 7 days, the mean plasma half-life of indomethacin was 12 hours (range: 4–38 hours, n = 10). Grouping the infants by weight, mean plasma half-life in those weighing less than 1000 g was 21 hours (range: 9–60 hours, n = 10); in those infants weighing more than 1000 g, the mean plasma half-life was 15 hours (range: 3–52 hours, n = 18).

Following intravenous administration in adults, indomethacin is eliminated via renal excretion, metabolism, and biliary excretion. Indomethacin undergoes appreciable enterohepatic circulation. The mean plasma half-life of indomethacin is 4.5 hours. In the absence of enterohepatic circulation, it is 90 minutes. Indomethacin has been found to cross the blood-brain barrier and the placenta.

In adults, about 99 percent of indomethacin is bound to protein in plasma over the expected range of therapeutic plasma concentrations. The percent bound in neonates has not been studied. In controlled trials in premature infants, however, no evidence of bilirubin displacement has been observed as evidenced by increased incidence of bilirubin encephalopathy (kernicterus).

INDICATIONS AND USAGE

INDOCIN I.V. is indicated to close a hemodynamically significant patent ductus arteriosus in premature infants weighing between 500 and 1750 g when after 48 hours usual medical management (e.g., fluid restriction, diuretics, digitalis, respiratory support, etc.) is ineffective. Clear-cut clinical evidence of a hemodynamically significant patent ductus arteriosus should be present, such as respiratory distress, a continuous murmur, a hyperactive precordium, cardiomegaly and pulmonary plethora on chest x-ray.

CONTRAINDICATIONS

INDOCIN I.V. is contraindicated in: infants with proven or suspected infection that is untreated; infants who are bleeding, especially those with active intracranial hemorrhage or gastrointestinal bleeding; infants with thrombocytopenia; infants with coagulation defects; infants with or who are suspected of having necrotizing enterocolitis; infants with significant impairment of renal function; infants with congenital heart disease in whom patency of the ductus arteriosus is necessary for satisfactory pulmonary or systemic blood flow (e.g., pulmonary atresia, severe tetralogy of Fallot, severe coarctation of the aorta).

WARNINGS

Gastrointestinal Effects:

In the collaborative study, major gastrointestinal bleeding was no more common in those infants receiving indomethacin than in those infants on placebo. However, minor gastrointestinal bleeding (i.e., chemical detection of blood in the stool) was more commonly noted in those infants treated with indomethacin. Severe gastrointestinal effects have been reported in adults with various arthritic disorders treated chronically with oral indomethacin. [For further information, see package circular for Capsules INDOCIN* (Indomethacin).]

Central Nervous System Effects:

Prematurity per se, is associated with an increased incidence of spontaneous intraventricular hemorrhage. Because indomethacin may inhibit platelet aggregation, the poten-

tial for intraventricular bleeding may be increased. However, in the large multi-center study of INDOCIN I.V. (see CLINICAL PHARMACOLOGY), the incidence of intraventricular hemorrhage in babies treated with INDOCIN I.V. was not significantly higher than in the control infants.

Renal Effects:

INDOCIN I.V. may cause significant reduction in urine output (50 percent or more) with concomitant elevations of blood urea nitrogen and creatinine, and reductions in glomerular filtration rate and creatinine clearance. These effects in most infants are transient, disappearing with cessation of therapy with INDOCIN I.V. However, because adequate renal function can depend upon renal prostaglandin synthesis, INDOCIN I.V. may precipitate renal insufficiency, including acute renal failure, especially in infants with other conditions that may adversely affect renal function (e.g., extracellular volume depletion from any cause, congestive heart failure, sepsis, concomitant use of any nephrotoxic drug, hepatic dysfunction). When significant suppression of urine volume occurs after a dose of INDOCIN I.V., no additional dose should be given until the urine output returns to normal levels.

INDOCIN I.V. in pre-term infants may suppress water excretion to a greater extent than sodium excretion. When this occurs, a significant reduction in serum sodium values (i.e., hyponatremia) may result. Infants should have serum electrolyte determinations done during therapy with INDOCIN I.V. Renal function and serum electrolytes should be monitored (see PRECAUTIONS, *Drug Interactions* and DOSAGE AND ADMINISTRATION).

---

* Registered trademark of MERCK & CO., INC.

PRECAUTIONS

General

INDOCIN (Indomethacin) may mask the usual signs and symptoms of infection. Therefore, the physician must be continually on the alert for this and should use the drug with extra care in the presence of existing controlled infection.

Severe hepatic reactions have been reported in adults treated chronically with oral indomethacin for arthritic disorders. [For further information, see package circular for Capsules INDOCIN (Indomethacin)]. If clinical signs and symptoms consistent with liver disease develop in the neonate, or if systemic manifestations occur, INDOCIN I.V. should be discontinued.

INDOCIN I.V. may inhibit platelet aggregation. In one small study, platelet aggregation was grossly abnormal after indomethacin therapy (given orally to premature infants to close the ductus arteriosus). Platelet aggregation returned to normal by the tenth day. Premature infants should be observed for signs of bleeding.

The drug should be administered carefully to avoid extravascular injection or leakage as the solution may be irritating to tissue.

Drug Interactions

Since renal function may be reduced by INDOCIN I.V., consideration should be given to reduction in dosage of those medications that rely on adequate renal function for their elimination. Because the half-life of digitalis (given frequently to pre-term infants with patent ductus arteriosus and associated cardiac failure) may be prolonged when given concomitantly with indomethacin, the infant should be observed closely; frequent ECGs and serum digitalis levels may be required to prevent or detect digitalis toxicity early. Furthermore, in one study of premature infants treated with INDOCIN I.V. and also receiving either gentamicin or amikacin, both peak and trough levels of these aminoglycosides were significantly elevated.

Therapy with indomethacin may blunt the natriuretic effect of furosemide. This response has been attributed to inhibition of prostaglandin synthesis by non-steroidal anti-inflammatory drugs. In a study of 19 premature infants with patent ductus arteriosus treated with either INDOCIN I.V. alone or a combination of INDOCIN I.V. and furosemide, results showed that infants receiving both INDOCIN I.V. and furosemide had significantly higher urinary output, higher levels of sodium and chloride excretion, and higher glomerular filtration rates than did those infants receiving INDOCIN I.V. alone. In this study, the data suggested that therapy with furosemide helped to maintain renal function in the premature infant when INDOCIN I.V. was added to the treatment of patent ductus arteriosus.

Neonatal Effects

In rats and mice, oral indomethacin 4.0 mg/kg/day given during the last three days of gestation caused a decrease in maternal weight gain and some maternal and fetal deaths. An increased incidence of neuronal necrosis in the diencephalon in the live-born fetuses was observed. At 2.0 mg/kg/day, no increase in neuronal necrosis was observed as compared to the control groups. Administration of 0.5 or 4.0 mg/kg/day during the first three days of life did not cause an increase in neuronal necrosis at either dose level.

Pregnant rats, given 2.0 mg/kg/day and 4.0 mg/kg/day during the last trimester of gestation, delivered offspring whose

pulmonary blood vessels were both reduced in number and excessively muscularized. These findings are similar to those observed in the syndrome of persistent pulmonary hypertension of the newborn.

ADVERSE REACTIONS

In a double-blind placebo-controlled trial of 405 premature infants weighing less than or equal to 1750 g with evidence of large ductal shunting, in those infants treated with indomethacin (n = 206), there was a statistically significantly greater incidence of bleeding problems, including gross or microscopic bleeding into the gastrointestinal tract, oozing from the skin after needle stick, pulmonary hemorrhage, and disseminated intravascular coagulopathy. There was no statistically significant difference between treatment groups with reference to intracranial hemorrhage.

The infants treated with indomethacin sodium trihydrate also had a significantly higher incidence of transient oliguria and elevations of serum creatinine (greater than or equal to 1.8 mg/dL) than did the infants treated with placebo.

The incidences of retrolental fibroplasia (grades III and IV) and pneumothorax in infants treated with INDOCIN I.V. were no greater than in placebo controls and were statistically significantly lower than in surgically-treated infants. The following additional adverse reactions in infants have been reported from the collaborative study, anecdotal case reports, from other studies using rectal, oral, or intravenous indomethacin for treatment of patent ductus arteriosus or in marketed use. The rates are calculated from a database which contains experience of 849 indomethacin-treated infants reported in the medical literature, regardless of the route of administration. One year follow-up is available on 175 infants and shows no long-term sequelae which could be attributed to indomethacin. In controlled clinical studies, only electrolyte imbalance and renal dysfunction (of the reactions listed below) occurred statistically significantly more frequently after INDOCIN I.V. than after placebo. Reactions marked with a single asterick (*) occurred in 3–9 percent of indomethacin-treated infants: those marked with a double asterisk (**) occurred in 3–9 percent of both indomethacin- and placebo-treated infants. Unmarked reactions occurred in less than 3 percent of infants.

Renal: renal dysfunction in 41 percent of infants, including one or more of the following: reduced urinary output; reduced urine sodium, chloride, or potassium urine osmolality, free water clearance, or glomerular filtration, rate; elevated serum creatinine or BUN; uremia.

Cardiovascular: intracranial bleeding**, pulmonary hypertension.

Gastrointestinal: gastrointestinal bleeding*, vomiting, abdominal distention, transient ileus, localized perforation(s) of the small and/or large intestine.

Metabolic: hyponatremia*, elevated serum potassium*, reduction in blood sugar, including hypoglycemia, increased weight gain (fluid retention).

Coagulation: decreased platelet aggregation (see PRECAUTIONS).

The following adverse reactions have also been reported in infants treated with indomethacin, however, a causal relationship to therapy with INDOCIN I.V. has not been established:

Cardiovascular: bradycardia.

Respiratory: apnea, exacerbation of pre-existing pulmonary infection.

Metabolic: acidosis/alkalosis.

Hematologic: disseminated intravascular coagulation.

Gastrointestinal: necrotizing enterocolitis.

Ophthalmic: retrolental fibroplasia.**

A variety of additional adverse experiences have been reported in adults treated with oral indomethacin for moderate to severe rheumatoid arthritis, osteoarthritis, ankylosing spondylitis, acute painful shoulder and acute gouty arthritis (see section ADDITIONAL ADVERSE REACTIONS—ADULTS). Their relevance to the pre-term neonate receiving indomethacin for patent ductus arteriosus is unknown, however, the possibility exists that these experiences may be associated with the use of INDOCIN I.V. in pre-term neonates.

DOSAGE AND ADMINISTRATION

FOR INTRAVENOUS ADMINISTRATION ONLY.

Dosage recommendations for closure of the ductus arteriosus depends on the age of the infant at the time of therapy. A course of therapy is defined as three intravenous doses of INDOCIN I.V. given at 12–24 hour intervals, with careful attention to urinary output. If anuria or marked oliguria (urinary output < 0.6 mL/kg/hr) is evident at the scheduled time of the second or third dose of INDOCIN I.V., no additional doses should be given until laboratory studies indicate that renal function has returned to normal (see WARNINGS, *Renal Effects*).

Dosage according to age is as follows:

AGE at 1st dose	DOSAGE (mg/kg)		
	1st	2nd	3rd
Less than 48 hours	0.2	0.1	0.1
2–7 days	0.2	0.2	0.2
over 7 days	0.2	0.25	0.25

If the ductus arteriosus closes or is significantly reduced in size after an interval of 48 hours or more from completion of the first course of INDOCIN I.V., no further doses are necessary. If the ductus arteriosus re-opens, a second course of 1–3 doses may be given, each dose separated by a 12–24 hour interval as described above.

If the infant remains unresponsive to therapy with INDOCIN I.V. after 2 courses, surgery may be necessary for closure of the ductus arteriosus. If severe adverse reactions occur, STOP THE DRUG.

Directions for Use

Parenteral drug products should be inspected visually for particulate matter and discoloration prior to administration whenever solution and container permit.

The solution should be prepared only with 1 to 2 mL of preservative-free sterile Sodium Chloride Injection, 0.9 percent or preservative-free Sterile Water for Injection. Benzyl alcohol as a preservative has been associated with toxicity in newborns. Therefore, all diluents should be preservative-free. If 1 mL of diluent is used, the concentration of indomethacin in the solution will equal approximately 0.1 mg/ 0.1 mL; if 2 mL of diluent are used, the concentration of the solution will equal approximately 0.05 mg/0.1 mL. Any unused portion of the solution should be discarded because there is no preservative contained in the vial. A fresh solution should be prepared just prior to each administration. Once reconstituted, the indomethacin solution may be injected intravenously over 5–10 seconds.

Further dilution with intravenous infusion solutions is not recommended. INDOCIN I.V. is not buffered, and reconstitution with solutions at pH values below 6.0 may result in precipitation of the insoluble indomethacin free acid moiety.

HOW SUPPLIED

No. 3406—Sterile INDOCIN I.V. is a lyophilized white to yellow powder or plug supplied as single dose vials containing indomethacin sodium trihydrate, equivalent to 1 mg indomethacin.

NDC 0006-3406-17

(6505-01-209-1192, 3 single dose vials).

Storage

Store below 30°C (86°F). *Protect from light.* Store container in carton until contents have been used.

ADDITIONAL ADVERSE REACTIONS—ADULTS

The following adverse reactions have been reported in adults treated with oral indomethacin for moderate to severe rheumatoid arthritis, osteoarthritis, ankylosing spondylitis, acute painful shoulder and acute gouty arthritis. Complaints not of relevance in the treatment of the premature infant, such as anorexia, psychic disturbances, and blurred vision, are not listed.

Incidence 1% to 3%	Incidence less than 1%	

GASTROINTESTINAL

diarrhea	bloating (includes	gastrointestinal
constipation	distention)	bleeding without
	flatulence	obvious ulcer
	peptic ulcer	formation and
	gastroenteritis	perforation of
	rectal bleeding	pre-existing sigmoid
	proctitis	lesions
	single or multiple	development of
	ulcerations, includ-	ulcerative stomatitis
	ing perforation and	toxic hepatitis and
	hemorrhage of the	jaundice (some fatal
	esophagus, stomach,	cases have been
	duodenum or small	reported)
	and large intestines	intestinal strictures
	intestinal ulceration	(diaphragms)
	associated with	
	stenosis and	
	obstruction	

CENTRAL NERVOUS SYSTEM

none	involuntary muscle	aggravation of
	movements	epilepsy coma
		peripheral neuropathy
		convulsions

SPECIAL SENSES

none	hearing disturbances,	
	deafness	

CARDIOVASCULAR

none	hypertension	arrhythmia
	hypotension	congestive heart
	tachycardia	failure
		thrombophlebitis

METABOLIC

none	edema	hyperglycemia
	weight gain	glycosuria
	flushing	hyperkalemia

INTEGUMENTARY

none	rash; urticaria	exfoliative dermatitis
	petechiae or	erythema nodosum
	ecchymosis	loss of hair
		Stevens-Johnson
		syndrome
		erythema multiforme
		toxic epidermal
		necrolysis

HEMATOLOGIC

none	leukopenia	aplastic anemia
	bone marrow	hemolytic anemia
	depression	agranulocytosis
	anemia secondary to	thrombocytopenic
	obvious or occult	purpura
	gastrointestinal	
	bleeding	

HYPERSENSITIVITY

none	acute anaphylaxis	dyspnea
	acute respiratory	asthma
	distress	purpura
	rapid fall in blood	angiitis
	pressure resembling	pulmonary edema
	a shock-like state	

GENITOURINARY

none	hematuria	renal insufficiency,
	vaginal bleeding	including renal
		failure

MISCELLANEOUS

none	epistaxis	
	breast changes,	
	including en-	
	largement and	
	tenderness, or	
	gynecomastia	

See package circular for Capsules INDOCIN (Indomethacin) for additional information concerning adverse reactions and other cautionary statements.

7414814 Issued August 1995
COPYRIGHT © MERCK & CO., INC., 1985

INVERSINE® Tablets
(Mecamylamine HCl), U.S.P.   ℞

DESCRIPTION

INVERSINE* (Mecamylamine HCl) is a potent, oral antihypertensive agent and ganglion blocker, and is a secondary amine. It is N, 2,3,3-tetramethylbicyclo[2.2.1] heptan-2-amine hydrochloride. Its empirical formula is $C_{11}H_{21}N \cdot HCl$ and its structural formula is:

$$NHCH_3 \cdot HCl$$

It is a white, odorless, or practically odorless, crystalline powder, is highly stable, soluble in water and has a molecular weight of 203.75.

INVERSINE is supplied as tablets for oral use, each containing 2.5 mg mecamylamine HCl. Inactive ingredients are acacia, calcium phosphate, D&C Yellow 10, FD&C Yellow 6, lactose, magnesium stearate, starch, and talc.

*Registered trademark of MERCK & CO., INC.

CLINICAL PHARMACOLOGY

Mecamylamine reduces blood pressure in both normotensive and hypertensive individuals. It has a gradual onset of action ($^{1}/_{2}$ to 2 hours) and a long-lasting effect (usually 6 to 12 hours or more). A small oral dosage often produces a smooth and predictable reduction of blood pressure. Although this antihypertensive effect is predominantly orthostatic, the supine blood pressure is also significantly reduced.

Pharmacokinetics and Metabolism

Mecamylamine is almost completely absorbed from the gastrointestinal tract, resulting in consistent lowering of blood pressure in most patients with hypertensive cardiovascular disease. Mecamylamine is excreted slowly in the urine in the unchanged form. The rate of its renal elimination is influenced markedly by urinary pH. Alkalinization of the urine reduces, and acidification promotes, renal excretion of mecamylamine.

Mecamylamine crosses the blood-brain and placental barriers.

INDICATIONS AND USAGE

For the management of moderately severe to severe essential hypertension and in uncomplicated cases of malignant hypertension.

CONTRAINDICATIONS

INVERSINE should not be used in mild, moderate, labile hypertension and may prove unsuitable in uncooperative patients. It is contraindicated in coronary insufficiency or recent myocardial infarction.

INVERSINE should be given with great discretion, if at all, when renal insufficiency is manifested by a rising or elevated BUN. The drug is contraindicated in uremia. Patients receiving antibiotics and sulfonamides should generally not be treated with ganglion blockers. Other contraindications are glaucoma, organic pyloric stenosis or hypersensitivity to the product.

WARNINGS

Mecamylamine, a secondary amine, readily penetrates into the brain and thus may produce central nervous sytem effects. Tremor, choreiform movements, mental aberrations, and convulsions may occur rarely. These have occurred most often when large doses of INVERSINE were used, especially in patients with cerebral or renal insufficiency.

When ganglion blockers or other potent antihypertensive drugs are discontinued suddenly, hypertensive levels return. In patients with malignant hypertension and others, this may occur abruptly and may cause fatal cerebral vascular accidents or acute congestive heart failure. When INVERSINE is withdrawn, this should be done gradually and other antihypertensive therapy usually must be substituted. On the other hand, the effects of INVERSINE sometimes may last from hours to days after therapy is discontinued.

PRECAUTIONS

General

The patient's condition should be evaluated carefully, particularly as to renal and cardiovascular function. When renal, cerebral, or coronary blood flow is deficient, any additional impairment, which might result from added hypotension, must be avoided. The use of INVERSINE in patients with marked cerebral and coronary arteriosclerosis or after a recent cerebral accident requires caution.

The action of INVERSINE may be potentiated by excessive heat, fever, infection, hemorrhage, pregnancy, anesthesia, surgery, vigorous exercise, other antihypertensive drugs, alcohol, and salt depletion as a result of diminished intake or increased excretion due to diarrhea, vomiting, excessive sweating, or diuretics.

During therapy with INVERSINE, sodium intake should not be restricted but, if necessary, the dosage of the ganglion blocker must be adjusted.

Since urinary retention may occur in patients on ganglion blockers, caution is required in patients with prostatic hypertrophy, bladder neck obstruction, and urethral stricture. Frequent loose bowel movements with abdominal distention and decreased borborygmi may be the first signs of paralytic ileus. If these are present, INVERSINE should be discontinued immediately and remedial steps taken.

Information for Patients

INVERSINE may cause dizziness, lightheadedness, or fainting, especially when rising from a lying or sitting position. This effect may be increased by alcoholic beverages, exercise, or during hot weather. Getting up slowly may help alleviate such a reaction.

Drug Interactions

Patients receiving antibiotics and sulfonamides generally should not be treated with ganglion blockers.

The action of INVERSINE may be potentiated by anesthesia, other antihypertensive drugs and alcohol.

Carcinogenesis, Mutagenesis, Impairment of Fertility

Long-term studies in animals have not been performed to evaluate the effects upon fertility, mutagenic or carcinogenic potential of INVERSINE.

Continued on next page

Inversine—Cont.

Pregnancy

Pregnancy Category C. Animal reproduction studies have not been conducted with INVERSINE. It is not known whether INVERSINE can cause fetal harm when given to a pregnant woman or can affect reproductive capacity. INVERSINE should be given to a pregnant woman only if clearly needed.

Nursing Mothers

Because of the potential for serious adverse reactions in nursing infants from INVERSINE, a decision should be made whether to discontinue nursing or to discontinue the drug, taking into account the importance of the drug to the mother.

Pediatric Use

Safety and effectiveness in pediatric patients have not been established.

ADVERSE REACTIONS

The following adverse reactions have been reported and within each category are listed in order of decreasing severity.

Gastrointestinal: Ileus, constipation (sometimes preceded by small, frequent liquid stools), vomiting, nausea, anorexia, glossitis and dryness of mouth.

Cardiovascular: Orthostatic dizziness and syncope, postural hypotension.

Nervous System/Psychiatric: Convulsions, choreiform movements, mental aberrations, tremor, and paresthesias (see WARNINGS).

Respiratory: Interstitial pulmonary edema and fibrosis.

Urogenital: Urinary retention, impotence, decreased libido.

Special Senses: Blurred vision, dilated pupils.

Miscellaneous: Weakness, fatigue, sedation.

OVERDOSAGE

Signs of overdosage include: hypotension (which may progress to peripheral vascular collapse), postural hypotension, nausea, vomiting, diarrhea, constipation, paralytic ileus, urinary retention, dizziness, anxiety, dry mouth, mydriasis, blurred vision, or palpitations. A rise in intraocular pressure may occur.

Pressor amines may be used to counteract excessive hypotension. Since patients being treated with ganglion blockers are more than normally reactive to pressor amines, small doses of the latter are recommended to avoid excessive response.

The oral LD_{50} of mecamylamine in the mouse is 92 mg/kg.

DOSAGE AND ADMINISTRATION

Therapy is usually started with one 2.5 mg tablet of INVERSINE twice a day. This initial dosage should be modified by increments of one 2.5 mg tablet at intervals of not less than 2 days until the desired blood pressure response occurs (the criterion being a dosage just under that which causes signs of mild postural hypotension).

The average total daily dosage of INVERSINE is 25 mg, usually in three divided doses. However, as little as 2.5 mg daily may be sufficient to control hypertension in some patients. A range of two to four or even more doses may be required in severe cases when smooth control is difficult to obtain. In severe or urgent cases, larger increments at smaller intervals may be needed. Partial tolerance may develop in certain patients, requiring an increase in the daily dosage of INVERSINE.

Administration of INVERSINE after meals may cause a more gradual absorption and smoother control of excessively high blood pressure. The timing of doses in relation to meals should be consistent. Since the blood pressure response to antihypertensive drugs is increased in the early morning, the larger dose should be given at noontime and perhaps in the evening. The morning dose, as a rule, should be relatively small and in some instances may even be omitted.

The *initial regulation of dosage* should be determined by blood pressure readings in the erect position at the time of maximal effect of the drug, as well as by other signs and symptoms of orthostatic hypotension.

The *effective maintenance dosage* should be regulated by blood pressure readings in the erect position and by limitation of dosage to that which causes slight faintness or dizziness in this position. If the patient or a relative can use a sphygmomanometer, instructions may be given to reduce or omit a dose if faintness below a designated level or if faintness or lightheadedness occurs. *However, no change should be instituted without the knowledge of the physician.* Close supervision and education of the patient, as well as critical adjustment of dosage, are essential to successful therapy.

Other Antihypertensive Agents

When INVERSINE is given with other antihypertensive drugs, the dosage of these other agents, as well as that of INVERSINE, should be reduced to avoid excessive hypotension. However, thiazides should be continued in their usual dosage, while that of INVERSINE is decreased by at least 50 percent.

HOW SUPPLIED

No. 3219—Tablets INVERSINE, 2.5 mg, are yellow, round, scored, compressed tablets, coded MSD 52 on one side and INVERSINE on the other. They are supplied as follows:
NDC 0006-0052-68 in bottles of 100.

Shown in Product Identification Guide, page 323
7898723   Issued September 1996
COPYRIGHT © MERCK & CO., INC., 1985

LACRISERT® Sterile Ophthalmic Insert ℞
(hydroxypropyl cellulose ophthalmic insert), U.S.P.

DESCRIPTION

LACRISERT* (hydroxypropyl cellulose ophthalmic insert) is a sterile, translucent, rod-shaped, water soluble, ophthalmic insert made of hydroxypropyl cellulose, for administration into the inferior cul-de-sac of the eye.

The chemical name for hydroxypropyl cellulose is cellulose, 2-hydroxypropyl ether. It is an ether of cellulose in which hydroxypropyl groups ($-CH_2CHOHCH_3$) are attached to the hydroxyls present in the anhydroglucose rings of cellulose by ether linkages. A representative structure of the monomer is:

$$R=CH_2CHCH_3$$
$$OH$$

The molecular weight is typically 1×10^6.

Hydroxypropyl cellulose is an off-white, odorless, tasteless powder. It is soluble in water below 38°C, and in many polar organic solvents such as ethanol, propylene glycol, dioxane, methanol, isopropyl alcohol (95%), dimethyl sulfoxide, and dimethyl formamide.

Each LACRISERT is 5 mg of hydroxypropyl cellulose. LACRISERT contains no preservatives or other ingredients. It is about 1.27 mm in diameter by about 3.5 mm long.

LACRISERT is supplied in packages of 60 units, together with illustrated instructions and a special applicator for removing LACRISERT from the unit dose blister and inserting it into the eye. A spare applicator is included in each package.

*Registered trademark of MERCK & CO., INC.

CLINICAL PHARMACOLOGY

Pharmacodynamics

LACRISERT acts to stabilize and thicken the precorneal tear film and prolong the tear film breakup time which is usually accelerated in patients with dry eye states. LACRISERT also acts to lubricate and protect the eye.

LACRISERT usually reduces the signs and symptoms resulting from moderate to severe dry eye syndromes, such as conjunctival hyperemia, corneal and conjunctival staining with rose bengal, exudation, itching, burning, foreign body sensation, smarting, photophobia, dryness and blurred or cloudy vision. Progressive visual deterioration which occurs in some patients may be retarded, halted, or sometimes reversed.

In a multicenter crossover study the 5 mg LACRISERT administered once a day during the waking hours was compared to artificial tears used four or more times daily. There was a prolongation of tear film breakup time and a decrease in foreign body sensation associated with dry eye syndrome in patients during treatment with inserts as compared to artificial tears; these findings were statistically significantly different between the treatment groups. Improvement, as measured by amelioration of symptoms, by slit-lamp examination and by rose bengal staining of the cornea and conjunctiva, was greater in most patients with moderate to severe symptoms during treatment with LACRISERT. Patient comfort was usually better with LACRISERT than with artificial tears solution, and most patients preferred LACRISERT.

In most patients treated with LACRISERT for over one year, improvement was observed as evidenced by ameliora-tion of symptoms generally associated with keratoconjunctivitis sicca such as burning, tearing, foreign body sensation, itching, photophobia and blurred or cloudy vision. During studies in healthy volunteers, a thickened precorneal tear film was usually observed through the slit-lamp while LACRISERT was present in the conjunctival sac.

Pharmacokinetics and Metabolism

Hydroxypropyl cellulose is a physiologically inert substance. In a study of rats fed hydroxypropyl cellulose or unmodified cellulose at levels up to 5% of their diet, it was found that the two were biologically equivalent in that neither was metabolized.

Studies conducted in rats fed ^{14}C-labeled hydroxypropyl cellulose demonstrated that when orally administered, hydroxypropyl cellulose is not absorbed from the gastrointestinal tract and is quantitatively excreted in the feces.

Dissolution studies in rabbits showed that hydroxypropyl cellulose inserts became softer within 1 hour after they were placed in the conjunctival sac. Most of the inserts dissolved completely in 14 to 18 hours; with a single exception, all had disappeared by 24 hours after insertion. Similar dissolution of the inserts was observed during prolonged administration (up to 54 weeks).

INDICATIONS AND USAGE

LACRISERT is indicated in patients with moderate to severe dry eye syndromes, including keratoconjunctivitis sicca. LACRISERT is indicated especially in patients who remain symptomatic after an adequate trial of therapy with artificial tear solutions.

LACRISERT is also indicated for patients with:
Exposure keratitis
Decreased corneal sensitivity
Recurrent corneal erosions

CONTRAINDICATIONS

LACRISERT is contraindicated in patients who are hypersensitive to hydroxypropyl cellulose.

WARNINGS

Instructions for inserting and removing LACRISERT should be carefully followed.

PRECAUTIONS

General

If improperly placed, LACRISERT may result in corneal abrasion (see DOSAGE AND ADMINISTRATION).

Information for Patients

Patients should be advised to follow the instructions for using LACRISERT which accompany the package.

Because this product may produce transient blurring of vision, patients should be instructed to exercise caution when operating hazardous machinery or driving a motor vehicle.

Drug Interactions

Application of hydroxypropyl cellulose ophthalmic inserts to the eyes of unanesthetized rabbits immediately prior to or two hours before instilling pilocarpine, proparacaine HCl (0.5%), or phenylephrine (5%) did not markedly alter the magnitude and/or duration of the miotic, local corneal anesthetic, or mydriatic activity, respectively, of these agents.

Under various treatment schedules, the anti-inflammatory effect of ocularly instilled dexamethasone (0.1%) in unanesthetized rabbits with primary uveitis was not affected by the presence of hydroxypropyl cellulose inserts.

Carcinogenesis, Mutagenesis,
Impairment of Fertility

Feeding of hydroxypropyl cellulose to rats at levels up to 5% of their diet produced no gross or histopathologic changes or other deleterious effects.

Pediatric Use

Safety and effectiveness in pediatric patients have not been established.

ADVERSE REACTIONS

The following adverse reactions have been reported in patients treated with LACRISERT, but were in most instances mild and transient:
Transient blurring of vision (See PRECAUTIONS)
Ocular discomfort or irritation
Matting or stickiness of eyelashes
Photophobia
Hypersensitivity
Edema of the eyelids
Hyperemia

DOSAGE AND ADMINISTRATION

One LACRISERT ophthalmic insert in each eye once daily is usually sufficient to relieve the symptoms associated with moderate to severe dry eye syndromes. Individual patients

may require more flexibility in the use of LACRISERT; some patients may require twice daily use for optimal results.

Clinical experience with LACRISERT indicates that in some patients several weeks may be required before satisfactory improvement of symptoms is achieved.

LACRISERT is inserted into the inferior cul-de-sac of the eye beneath the base of the tarsus, not in apposition to the cornea, nor beneath the eyelid at the level of the tarsal plate. If not properly positioned, it will be expelled into the interpalpebral fissure, and may cause symptoms of a foreign body. Illustrated instructions are included in each package. While in the licensed practitioner's office, the patient should read the instructions, then practice insertion and removal of LACRISERT until proficiency is achieved.

NOTE: Occasionally LACRISERT is inadvertently expelled from the eye, especially in patients with shallow conjunctival fornices. The patient should be cautioned against rubbing the eye(s) containing LACRISERT, especially upon awakening, so as not to dislodge or expel the insert. If required, another LACRISERT ophthalmic insert may be inserted. If experience indicates that transient blurred vision develops in an individual patient, the patient may want to remove LACRISERT a few hours after insertion to avoid this. Another LACRISERT ophthalmic insert may be inserted if needed.

If LACRISERT causes worsening of symptoms, the patient should be instructed to inspect the conjunctival sac to make certain LACRISERT is in the proper location, deep in the inferior cul-de-sac of the eye beneath the base of the tarsus. If these symptoms persist, LACRISERT should be removed and the patient should contact the practitioner.

HOW SUPPLIED

No. 3380—LACRISERT, a sterile, translucent, rod-shaped, water soluble, ophthalmic insert made of hydroxypropyl cellulose, 5 mg, is supplied as follows:

NDC 0006-3380-60 in packages containing 60 unit doses, two reusable applicators and a storage container.
(6505-01-153-4360, 5 mg 60's).

Storage

Store below 30°C (86°F).

7415111 Issued October 1997
COPYRIGHT © MERCK & CO., INC., 1988
All rights reserved

M–M–R®ᵢᵢ   ℞
(Measles, Mumps, and Rubella Virus Vaccine Live), U.S.P.

DESCRIPTION

M-M-R* II (Measles, Mumps, and Rubella Virus Vaccine Live) is a live virus vaccine for immunization against measles (rubeola), mumps and rubella (German measles).

M-M-R II is a sterile lyophilized preparation of (1) ATTENUVAX* (Measles Virus Vaccine Live), a more attenuated line of measles virus, derived from Enders' attenuated Edmonston strain and grown in cell cultures of chick embryo; (2) MUMPSVAX* (Mumps Virus Vaccine Live), the Jeryl Lynn (B level) strain of mumps virus grown in cell cultures of chick embryo; and (3) MERUVAX* II (Rubella Virus Vaccine Live), the Wistar RA 27/3 strain of live attenuated rubella virus grown in human diploid cell (WI-38) culture. The vaccine viruses are the same as those used in the manufacture of ATTENUVAX (Measles Virus Vaccine Live), MUMPSVAX (Mumps Virus Vaccine Live) and MERUVAX II (Rubella Virus Vaccine Live). The three viruses are mixed before being lyophilized. The product contains no preservative.

The reconstituted vaccine is for subcutaneous administration. When reconstituted as directed, the dose for injection is 0.5 mL and contains not less than the equivalent of 1,000 $TCID_{50}$ (tissue culture infectious doses) of the U.S. Reference Measles Virus; 20,000 $TCID_{50}$ of the U.S. Reference Mumps Virus; and 1,000 $TCID_{50}$ of the U.S. Reference Rubella Virus. Each dose contains approximately 25 mcg of neomycin. The product contains no preservative. Sorbitol and hydrolyzed gelatin are added as stabilizers.

*Registered trademark of MERCK & CO., INC.

CLINICAL PHARMACOLOGY

Clinical studies of 279 triple seronegative children, 11 months to 7 years of age, demonstrated that M-M-R II is highly immunogenic and generally well tolerated. In these studies, a single injection of the vaccine induced measles hemagglutination-inhibition (HI) antibodies in 95 percent, mumps neutralizing antibodies in 96 percent, and rubella HI antibodies in 99 percent of susceptible persons.

The RA 27/3 rubella strain in M-M-R II elicits higher immediate post-vaccination HI, complement-fixing and neutraliz-

ing antibody levels than other strains of rubella vaccine and has been shown to induce a broader profile of circulating antibodies including anti-theta and anti-iota precipitating antibodies. The RA 27/3 rubella strain immunologically simulates natural infection more closely than other rubella vaccine viruses. The increased levels and broader profile of antibodies produced by RA 27/3 strain rubella virus vaccine appear to correlate with greater resistance to subclinical reinfection with the wild virus, and provide greater confidence for lasting immunity.

Vaccine induced antibody levels following administration of M-M-R II have been shown to persist up to 11 years without substantial decline. Continued surveillance will be necessary to determine further duration of antibody persistence.

INDICATIONS AND USAGE

M-M-R II is indicated for simultaneous immunization against measles, mumps, and rubella in persons 15 months of age or older. A second dose of M-M-R II or monovalent measles vaccine is recommended (see *Revaccination*).

Infants who are less than 15 months of age may fail to respond to the measles component of the vaccine due to presence in the circulation of residual measles antibody of maternal origin, the younger the infant, the lower the likelihood of seroconversion. In geographically isolated or other relatively inaccessible populations for whom immunization programs are logistically difficult, and in population groups in which natural measles infection may occur in a significant proportion of infants before 15 months of age, it may be desirable to give the vaccine to infants at an earlier age. Infants vaccinated under these conditions at less than 12 months of age should be revaccinated after reaching 15 months of age. There is some evidence to suggest that infants immunized at less than one year of age may not develop sustained antibody levels when later reimmunized. The advantage of early protection must be weighed against the chance for failure to respond adequately on reimmunization.

Previously unimmunized children of susceptible pregnant women should receive live attenuated rubella vaccine, because an immunized child will be less likely to acquire natural rubella and introduce the virus into the household.

Individuals planning travel outside the United States, if not immune, can acquire measles, mumps or rubella and import these diseases to the United States. Therefore, prior to International travel, individuals known to be susceptible to one or more of these diseases can receive either a single antigen vaccine (measles, mumps or rubella), or a combined antigen vaccine as appropriate. However, M-M-R II is preferred for persons likely to be susceptible to mumps and rubella; and if single-antigen measles vaccine is not readily available, travelers should receive M-M-R II regardless of their immune status to mumps or rubella.

Non-Pregnant Adolescent and Adult Females
Immunization of susceptible non-pregnant adolescent and adult females of childbearing age with live attenuated rubella virus vaccine is indicated if certain precautions are observed (see below and PRECAUTIONS). Vaccinating susceptible postpubertal females confers individual protection against subsequently acquiring rubella infection during pregnancy, which in turn prevents infection of the fetus and consequent congenital rubella injury.

Women of childbearing age should be advised not to become pregnant for three months after vaccination and should be informed of the reasons for this precaution.*

It is recommended that rubella susceptibility be determined by serologic testing prior to immunization.** If immune, as evidenced by a specific rubella antibody titer of 1:8 or greater (hemagglutination-inhibition test), vaccination is unnecessary. Congenital malformations do occur in up to seven percent of all live births. Their chance appearance after vaccination could lead to misinterpretation of the cause, particularly if the prior rubella-immune status of vaccinees is unknown.

Postpubertal females should be informed of the frequent occurrence of generally self-limited arthralgia and/or arthritis beginning 2 to 4 weeks after vaccination (see ADVERSE REACTIONS).

Postpartum Women
It has been found convenient in many instances to vaccinate rubella-susceptible women in the immediate postpartum period. (See *Nursing Mothers*).

Revaccination: Children first vaccinated when younger than 12 months of age should be revaccinated at 15 months of age.

The American Academy of Pediatrics (AAP), the Immunization Practices Advisory Committee (ACIP), and some state and local health agencies have recommended guidelines for routine measles revaccination and to help control measles outbreaks.†

Vaccines available for revaccination include monovalent measles vaccine [ATTENUVAX (Measles Virus Vaccine Live)] and polyvalent vaccines containing measles [e.g., M-M-R II, M-R-VAX‡ II (Measles and Rubella Virus Vaccine Live)]. If the prevention of sporadic measles outbreaks is

the sole objective, revaccination with a monovalent measles vaccine should be considered (see appropriate product circular). If concern also exists about immune status regarding mumps or rubella, revaccination with appropriate monovalent or polyvalent vaccine should be considered after consulting the appropriate product circulars. Unnecessary doses of a vaccine are best avoided by ensuring that written documentation of vaccination is preserved and a copy given to each vaccinee's parent or guardian.

Use with other Vaccines
Routine administration of DTP (diphtheria, tetanus, pertussis) and/or OPV (oral poliovirus vaccine) concomitantly with measles, mumps, and rubella vaccines is not recommended because there are limited data relating to the simultaneous administration of these antigens. M-M-R II should be given one month before or after administration of other vaccines. However, other schedules have been used. For example, the American Academy of Pediatrics has noted that when the patient may not return, some practitioners prefer to administer DTP, OPV, and M-M-R II on a single day. If done, separate sites and syringes should be used for DTP and M-M-R II. The Immunization Practices Advisory Committee (ACIP) recommends routine simultaneous administration of M-M-R II, DTP and OPV or inactivated polio vaccine (IPV) to all children $\geq$ 15 months who are eligible to receive these vaccines on the basis that there are equivalent antibody responses and no clinically significant increases in the frequency of adverse events when DTP, M-M-R II and OPV or IPV are administered either simultaneously at different sites or separately.†† Administration of M-M-R II at 15 months followed by DTP and OPV (or IPV) at 18 months remains an acceptable alternative, especially for children with caregivers known to be generally compliant with other health-care recommendations.

---

*NOTE: The Immunization Practices Advisory Committee (ACIP) has recommended "In view of the importance of protecting this age group against rubella, reasonable precautions in a rubella immunization program include asking females if they are pregnant, excluding those who say they are, and explaining the theoretical risks to the others."

**NOTE: The Immunization Practices Advisory Committee (ACIP) has stated "When practical, and when reliable laboratory services are available, potential vaccinees of childbearing age can have serologic tests to determine susceptibility to rubella. . . . However, routinely performing serologic tests for all females of childbearing age to determine susceptibility so that vaccine is given only to proven susceptibles is expensive and has been ineffective in some areas. Accordingly, the ACIP believes that rubella vaccination of a woman who is not known to be pregnant and has no history of vaccination is justifiable without serologic testing."

†NOTE: A primary difference among these recommendations is the timing of revaccination: the ACIP recommends routine revaccination at entry into kindergarten or first grade, whereas the AAP recommends routine revaccination at entrance to middle school or junior high school. In addition, some public health jurisdictions mandate the age for revaccination. The complete text of applicable guidelines should be consulted.

††NOTE: The Immunization Practices Advisory Committee (ACIP) recommends administering M-M-R II concomitantly with the fourth dose of DTP and the third dose of OPV to children 15 months of age or older providing that 6 months have elapsed since DTP-3; or, if fewer than three DTPs have been received, at least 6 weeks have elapsed since the last dose of DTP and OPV.

‡Registered trademark of MERCK & CO., INC.

CONTRAINDICATIONS

Do not give M-M-R II to pregnant females; the possible effects of the vaccine on fetal development are unknown at this time. If vaccination of postpubertal females is undertaken, pregnancy should be avoided for three months following vaccination. (See PRECAUTIONS, *Pregnancy*).

Anaphylactic or anaphylactoid reactions to neomycin (each dose of reconstituted vaccine contains approximately 25 mcg of neomycin).

History of anaphylactic or anaphylactoid reactions to eggs (see HYPERSENSITIVITY TO EGGS below).

Any febrile respiratory illness or other active febrile infection.

Active untreated tuberculosis.

Continued on next page

Information on the Merck & Co., Inc. products listed on these pages is the full prescribing information from product circulars in use August 31, 1998. For information, please call 1-800-NSC MERCK [1-800-672-6372].

M-M-R II—Cont.

Patients receiving immunosuppressive therapy. This contraindication does not apply to patients who are receiving corticosteroids as replacement therapy, e.g., for Addison's disease.

Individuals with blood dyscrasias, leukemia, lymphomas of any type, or other malignant neoplasms affecting the bone marrow or lymphatic systems.

Primary and acquired immunodeficiency states, including patients who are immunosuppressed in association with AIDS or other clinical manifestations of infection with human immunodeficiency viruses; cellular immune deficiencies; and hypogammaglobulinemic and dysgammaglobulinemic states.

Individuals with a family history of congenital or hereditary immunodeficiency, until the immune competence of the potential vaccine recipient is demonstrated.

HYPERSENSITIVITY TO EGGS

Live measles vaccine and live mumps vaccine are produced in chick embryo cell culture. Persons with a history of anaphylactic, anaphylactoid, or other immediate reactions (e.g., hives, swelling of the mouth and throat, difficulty breathing, hypotension, or shock) subsequent to egg ingestion should not be vaccinated. Evidence indicates that persons are not at increased risk if they have egg allergies that are not anaphylactic or anaphylactoid in nature. Such persons may be vaccinated in the usual manner. There is no evidence to indicate that persons with allergies to chickens or feathers are at increased risk of reaction to the vaccine.

PRECAUTIONS

General

Adequate treatment provisions including epinephrine, should be available for immediate use should an anaphylactic or anaphylactoid reaction occur.

Due caution should be employed in administration of M-M-R II to persons with a history of cerebral injury, individual or family histories of convulsions, or any other condition in which stress due to fever should be avoided. The physician should be alert to the temperature elevation which may occur following vaccination. (See ADVERSE REACTIONS).

Children and young adults who are known to be infected with human immunodeficiency viruses but without overt clinical manifestations of immunosuppression may be vaccinated; however, the vaccinees should be monitored closely for vaccine-preventable diseases because immunization may be less effective than for uninfected persons.

Vaccination should be deferred for at least 3 months following blood or plasma transfusions, or administration of human immune serum globulin.

Excretion of small amounts of the live attenuated rubella virus from the nose or throat has occurred in the majority of susceptible individuals 7–28 days after vaccination. There is no confirmed evidence to indicate that such virus is transmitted to susceptible persons who are in contact with the vaccinated individuals. Consequently, transmission through close personal contact, while accepted as a theoretical possibility, is not regarded as a significant risk. However, transmission of the rubella vaccine virus to infants via breast milk has been documented (see *Nursing Mothers*).

There are no reports of transmission of live attenuated measles or mumps viruses from vaccinees to susceptible contacts.

It has been reported that live attenuated measles, mumps and rubella virus vaccines given individually may result in a temporary depression of tuberculin skin sensitivity. Therefore, if a tuberculin test is to be done, it should be administered either before or simultaneously with M-M-R II. Children under treatment for tuberculosis have not experienced exacerbation of the disease when immunized with live measles virus vaccine; no studies have been reported to date of the effect of measles virus vaccines on untreated tuberculous children.

As for any vaccine, vaccination with M-M-R II may not result in seroconversion in 100% of susceptible persons given the vaccine.

Pregnancy

Pregnancy Category C

Animal reproduction studies have not been conducted with M-M-R II. It is also not known whether M-M-R II can cause fetal harm when administered to a pregnant woman or can affect reproduction capacity. Therefore, the vaccine should not be administered to pregnant females; furthermore, pregnancy should be avoided for three months following vaccination (see CONTRAINDICATIONS).

In counseling women who are inadvertently vaccinated when pregnant or who become pregnant within 3 months of vaccination, the physician should be aware of the following: (1) In a 10 year survey involving over 700 pregnant women who received rubella vaccine within 3 months before or after conception (of whom 189 received the Wistar RA 27/3 strain), none of the newborns had abnormalities compatible

with congenital rubella syndrome; (2) Although mumps virus is capable of infecting the placenta and fetus, there is no good evidence that it causes congenital malformations in humans. Mumps vaccine virus also has been shown to infect the placenta, but the virus has not been isolated from the fetal tissues from susceptible women who were vaccinated and underwent elective abortions; and (3) Reports have indicated that contracting of natural measles during pregnancy enhances fetal risk. Increased rates of spontaneous abortion, stillbirth, congenital defects and prematurity have been observed subsequent to natural measles during pregnancy. There are no adequate studies of the attenuated (vaccine) strain of measles virus in pregnancy. However, it would be prudent to assume that the vaccine strain of virus is also capable of inducing adverse fetal effects.

Nursing Mothers

It is not known whether measles or mumps vaccine virus is secreted in human milk. Recent studies have shown that lactating postpartum women immunized with live attenuated rubella vaccine may secrete the virus in breast milk and transmit it to breast-fed infants. In the infants with serological evidence of rubella infection, none exhibited severe disease; however, one exhibited mild clinical illness typical of acquired rubella. Caution should be exercised when M-M-R II is administered to a nursing woman.

ADVERSE REACTIONS

Burning and/or stinging of short duration at the injection site have been reported.

The adverse clinical reactions associated with the use of M-M-R II are those expected to follow administration of the monovalent vaccines given separately. These may include malaise, sore throat, cough, rhinitis, headache, dizziness, fever, rash, nausea, vomiting or diarrhea; mild local reactions such as erythema, induration, tenderness and regional lymphadenopathy; parotitis, orchitis, nerve deafness, thrombocytopenia and purpura; allergic reactions such as wheal and flare at the injection site or urticaria; polyneuritis; and arthralgia and/or arthritis (usually transient and rarely chronic).

Anaphylaxis and anaphylactoid reactions have been reported.

Vasculitis has been reported rarely.

Otitis media and conjunctivitis have been reported.

Moderate fever [101-102.9°F (38.3-39.4°C)] occurs occasionally, and high fever [above 103°F (39.4°C)] occurs less commonly. On rare occasions, children developing fever may exhibit febrile convulsions. Afebrile convulsions or seizures have occurred rarely following vaccination with live attenuated measles vaccine. Syncope, particularly at the time of mass vaccination, has been reported. Rash occurs infrequently and is usually minimal, but rarely may be generalized. Erythema multiforme has also been reported rarely.

Forms of optic neuritis, including retrobulbar neuritis, papillitis, and retinitis may infrequently follow viral infections, and have been reported to occur 1 to 3 weeks following inoculation with some live virus vaccines.

Clinical experience with live attenuated measles, mumps and rubella virus vaccines given individually indicates that encephalitis and other nervous system reactions have occurred very rarely. These might occur also with M-M-R II. Experience from more than 80 million doses of all live measles vaccines given in the U.S. through 1975 indicates that significant central nervous system reactions such as encephalitis and encephalopathy, occurring within 30 days after vaccination, have been temporally associated with measles vaccine very rarely. In no case has it been shown that reactions were actually caused by vaccine. The Center for Disease Control has pointed out that "a certain number of cases of encephalitis may be expected to occur in a large childhood population in a defined period of time even when no vaccines are administered". However, the data suggest the possibility that some of these cases may have been caused by measles vaccines. The risk of such serious neurological disorders following live measles virus vaccine administration remains far less than that for encephalitis and encephalopathy with natural measles (one per two thousand reported cases).

There have been rare reports of ocular palsies, Guillain-Barré syndrome, or ataxia occurring after immunization with vaccines containing live attenuated measles virus. The ocular palsies have occurred approximately 3–24 days following vaccination. No definite causal relationship has been established between these events and vaccination. Isolated reports of polyneuropathy including Guillain-Barré syndrome have also been reported after immunization with rubella-containing vaccines.

There have been reports of subacute sclerosing panencephalitis (SSPE) in children who did not have a history of natural measles but did receive measles vaccine. Some of these cases may have resulted from unrecognized measles in the first year of life or possibly from the measles vaccination. Based on estimated nationwide measles vaccine distribution, the association of SSPE cases to measles vaccination is about one case per million vaccine doses distributed. This is

far less than the association with natural measles, 6–22 cases of SSPE per million cases of measles. The results of a retrospective case-controlled study conducted by the Center for Disease Control suggest that the overall effect of measles vaccine has been to protect against SSPE by preventing measles with its inherent higher risk of SSPE.

Local reactions characterized by marked swelling, redness and vesiculation at the injection site of attenuated live measles virus vaccines, and systemic reactions including atypical measles, have occurred in persons who received killed measles vaccine previously. M-M-R II was not given under this condition in clinical trials. Rarely, more severe reactions that require hospitalization, including prolonged high fevers and extensive local reactions, have been reported. Panniculitis has been reported rarely following administration of measles vaccine.

Arthralgia and/or arthritis (usually transient and rarely chronic), and polyneuritis are features of natural rubella and vary in frequency and severity with age and sex, being greatest in adult females and least in prepubertal children. This type of involvement as well as myalgia and paresthesia, have also been reported following administration of MERUVAX II (Rubella Virus Vaccine Live).

Chronic arthritis has been associated with natural rubella infection and has been related to persistent virus and/or viral antigen isolated from body tissues. Only rarely have vaccine recipients developed chronic joint symptoms.

Following vaccination in children, reactions in joints are uncommon and generally of brief duration. In women, incidence rates for arthritis and arthralgia are generally higher than those seen in children (children: 0–3%; women: 12–20%), and the reactions tend to be more marked and of longer duration. Symptoms may persist for a matter of months or on rare occasions for years. In adolescent girls, the reactions appear to be intermediate in incidence between those seen in children and in adult women. Even in older women (35–45 years), these reactions are generally well tolerated and rarely interfere with normal activities.

DOSAGE AND ADMINISTRATION

FOR SUBCUTANEOUS ADMINISTRATION

Do not inject intravenously.

The dosage of vaccine is the same for all persons. Inject the total volume of the single dose vial (about 0.5 mL) or 0.5 mL of the 10 dose vial of reconstituted vaccine subcutaneously, preferably into the outer aspect of upper arm. *Do not give immune globulin (IG) concurrently with M-M-R II.*

During shipment, to insure that there is no loss of potency, the vaccine must be maintained at a temperature of 10°C (50°F) or less.

Before reconstitution, store M-M-R II at 2–8°C (36–46°F). *Protect from light.*

CAUTION: A sterile syringe free of preservatives, antiseptics, and detergents should be used for each injection and/or reconstitution of the vaccine because these substances may inactivate the live virus vaccine. A 25 gauge, $^5/_8''$ needle is recommended.

To reconstitute, use only the diluent supplied, since it is free of preservatives or other antiviral substances which might inactivate the vaccine.

Single Dose Vial —First withdraw the entire volume of diluent into the syringe to be used for reconstitution. Inject all the diluent in the syringe into the vial of lyophilized vaccine, and agitate to mix thoroughly. Withdraw the entire contents into a syringe and inject the total volume of restored vaccine subcutaneously.

It is important to use a separate sterile syringe and needle for each individual patient to prevent transmission of hepatitis B and other infectious agents from one person to another.

10 Dose Vial (available only to government agencies/institutions)

Withdraw the entire contents (7 mL) of the diluent vial into the sterile syringe to be used for reconstitution, and introduce into the 10 dose vial of lyophilized vaccine. Agitate to ensure thorough mixing. The outer labeling suggests "For Jet Injector or Syringe Use". Use with separate sterile syringes is permitted for containers of 10 doses or less. The vaccine and diluent do not contain preservatives; therefore, the user must recognize the potential contamination hazards and exercise special precautions to protect the sterility and potency of the product. The use of aseptic techniques and proper storage prior to and after restoration of the vaccine and subsequent withdrawal of the individual doses is essential. Use 0.5 mL of the reconstituted vaccine for subcutaneous injection.

It is important to use a separate sterile syringe and needle for each individual patient to prevent transmission of hepatitis B and other infectious agents from one person to another.

Each dose contains not less than the equivalent of 1,000 TCID$_{50}$ of the U.S. Reference Measles Virus, 20,000 TCID$_{50}$ of the U.S. Reference Mumps Virus and 1,000 TCID$_{50}$ of the U.S. Reference Rubella Virus.

Parenteral drug products should be inspected visually for particulate matter and discoloration prior to administration. M-M-R II, when reconstituted, is clear yellow.

HOW SUPPLIED

No. 4749—M-M-R II is supplied as a single-dose vial of lyophilized vaccine, **NDC** 0006-4749-00, and a vial of diluent.
No. 4681/4309—M-M-R II is supplied as follows: (1) a box of 10 single-dose vials of lyophilized vaccine (package A), **NDC** 0006-4681-00; and (2) a box of 10 vials of diluent (package B). To conserve refrigerator space, the diluent may be stored separately at room temperature (6505-00-165-6519, Ten Pack).
Available only to government agencies/institutions
No. 4682X—M-M-R II is supplied as one 10 dose vial of lyophilized vaccine, **NDC** 0006-4682-00, and one 7 mL vial of diluent.
Storage
It is recommended that the vaccine be used as soon as possible after reconstitution. Protect vaccine from light at all times, since such exposure may inactivate the virus. Store reconstituted vaccine in the vaccine vial in a dark place at 2–8°C (36–46°F) and discard if not used within 8 hours.

A.H.F.S. Category: 80:12
7678915 Issued March 1995

Copyright © MERCK & CO., INC., 1990
All rights reserved

M–R–VAX®$_{II}$ ℞
(Measles and Rubella Virus Vaccine Live), U.S.P.

DESCRIPTION

M-R-VAX* II (Measles and Rubella Virus Vaccine Live), is a live virus vaccine for immunization against measles (rubeola) and rubella (German measles).
M-R-VAX II is a sterile lyophilized preparation of (1) ATTENUVAX* (Measles Virus Vaccine Live), a more attenuated line of measles virus, derived from Enders' attenuated Edmonston strain and grown in cell cultures of chick embryo; and (2) MERUVAX* II (Rubella Virus Vaccine Live), the Wistar RA 27/3 strain of live attenuated rubella virus grown in human diploid cell (WI-38) culture. The vaccine viruses are the same as those used in the manufacture of ATTENUVAX (Measles Virus Vaccine Live) and MERUVAX II (Rubella Virus Vaccine Live). The two viruses are mixed before being lyophilized. The product contains no preservative.
The reconstituted vaccine is for subcutaneous administration. When reconstituted as directed, the dose for injection is 0.5 mL and contains not less than the equivalent of 1,000 $TCID_{50}$ (tissue culture infectious doses) of the U.S. Reference Measles Virus; and 1,000 $TCID_{50}$ of the U.S. Reference Rubella Virus. Each dose contains approximately 25 mcg of neomycin. The product contains no preservative. Sorbitol and hydrolized gelatin are added as stabilizers.

*Registered trademark of MERCK & CO., INC.

CLINICAL PHARMACOLOGY

Clinical studies of 237 double seronegative children, 10 months to 10 years of age, demonstrated that M-R-VAX II is highly immunogenic and generally well tolerated. In these studies, a single injection of the vaccine induced measles hemagglutination-inhibition (HI) antibodies in 95 percent and rubella HI antibodies in 99 percent of susceptible persons.
The RA 27/3 rubella strain in M-R-VAX II elicits higher immediate post-vaccination HI, complement-fixing and neutralizing antibody levels than other strains of rubella vaccine and has been shown to induce a broader profile of circulating antibodies including anti-theta and anti-iota precipitating antibodies. The RA 27/3 rubella strain immunologically simulates natural infection more closely than other rubella vaccine viruses. The increased levels and broader profile of antibodies produced by RA 27/3 strain rubella virus vaccine appear to correlate with greater resistance to subclinical reinfection with the wild virus, and provide greater confidence for lasting immunity.
Vaccine induced antibody levels following administration of M-R-VAX II have been shown to persist up to 11 years without substantial decline. Continued surveillance will be necessary to determine further duration of antibody persistence.

INDICATIONS AND USAGE

M-R-VAX II is indicated for simultaneous immunization against measles and rubella in persons 15 months of age or older. A second dose of M-R-VAX II or monovalent measles vaccine is recommended (see *Revaccination*).
Infants who are less than 15 months of age may fail to respond to the measles component of the vaccine due to presence in the circulation of residual measles antibody of maternal origin; the younger the infant, the lower the likelihood of seroconversion. In geographically isolated or other relatively inaccessible populations for whom immunization programs are logistically difficult, and in population groups in which natural measles infection may occur in a significant proportion of infants before 15 months of age, it may be desirable to give the vaccine to infants at an earlier age. Infants vaccinated under these conditions at less than 12 months of age should be revaccinated after reaching 15 months of age. There is some evidence to suggest that infants immunized at less than one year of age may not develop sustained antibody levels when later reimmunized. The advantage of early protection must be weighed against the chance for failure to respond adequately on reimmunization.
Previously unimmunized children of susceptible pregnant women should receive live attenuated rubella vaccine, because an immunized child will be less likely to acquire natural rubella and introduce the virus into the household.
Individuals planning travel outside the United States, if not immune, can acquire measles, mumps or rubella and import these diseases to the United States. Therefore, prior to International travel, individuals known to be susceptible to one or more of these diseases can receive either a single antigen vaccine (measles, mumps, or rubella), or a combined antigen vaccine as appropriate. However, M-M-R† II (Measles, Mumps, and Rubella Virus Vaccine Live) is preferred for persons likely to be susceptible to mumps and rubella; and if a single-antigen measles vaccine is not readily available, travelers should receive M-M-R II (Measles, Mumps, and Rubella Virus Vaccine Live) regardless of their immune status to mumps or rubella.
Non-Pregnant Adolescent and Adult Females
Immunization of susceptible non-pregnant adolescent and adult females of childbearing age with live attenuated rubella virus vaccine is indicated if certain precautions are observed (see below and PRECAUTIONS). Vaccinating susceptible postpubertal females confers individual protection against subsequently acquiring rubella infection during pregnancy, which in turn prevents infection of the fetus and consequent congenital rubella injury.
Women of childbearing age should be advised not to become pregnant for three months after vaccination and should be informed of the reason for this precaution.*
It is recommended that rubella susceptibility be determined by serologic testing prior to immunization.** If immune, as evidenced by a specific rubella antibody titer of 1:8 or greater (hemagglutination-inhibition test), vaccination is unnecessary. Congenital malformations do occur in up to seven percent of all live births. Their chance appearance after vaccination could lead to misinterpretation of the cause, particularly if the prior rubella-immune status of vaccinees is unknown.
Postpubertal females should be informed of the frequent occurrence of generally self-limited arthralgia and/or arthritis beginning 2 to 4 weeks after vaccination (see ADVERSE REACTIONS).
Postpartum Women
It has been found convenient in many instances to vaccinate rubella-susceptible women in the immediate postpartum period. (See *Nursing Mothers*).
Revaccination: Children first vaccinated when younger than 12 months of age should be revaccinated at 15 months of age.
The American Academy of Pediatrics (AAP), the Immunization Practices Advisory Committee (ACIP), and some state and local health agencies have recommended guidelines for routine measles revaccination and to help control measles outbreaks.***
Vaccines available for revaccination include monovalent measles vaccine [ATTENUVAX (Measles Virus Vaccine Live)] and polyvalent vaccines containing measles [e.g., M-M-R II (Measles, Mumps, and Rubella Virus Vaccine Live), M-R-VAX II]. If the prevention of sporadic measles outbreaks is the sole objective, revaccination with a monovalent measles vaccine should be considered (see appropriate product circular). If concern also exists about immune status regarding mumps or rubella, revaccination with appropriate monovalent or polyvalent vaccines should be considered after consulting the appropriate product circulars. Unnecessary doses of a vaccine are best avoided by ensuring that written documentation of vaccination is preserved and a copy given to each vaccinee's parent or guardian.
Use with other Vaccines
Routine administration of DTP (diphtheria, tetanus, pertussis) and/or OPV (oral poliovirus vaccine) concomitantly with measles, mumps and rubella vaccines is not recommended because there are insufficient data relating to the simultaneous administration of these antigens. However, the American Academy of Pediatrics has noted that in some circumstances, particularly when the patient may not return, some practitioners prefer to administer all these antigens on a single day. If done, separate sites and syringes should be used for DTP and M-R-VAX II.
M-R-VAX II should not be given less than one month before or after administration of other virus vaccines.

† Registered trademark of MERCK & CO., INC.
*NOTE: The Immunization Practices Advisory Committee (ACIP) has recommended "In view of the importance of protecting this age group against rubella, reasonable precautions in a rubella immunization program include asking females if they are pregnant, excluding those who say they are, and explaining the theoretical risks to the others."
**NOTE: The Immunization Practices Advisory Committee (ACIP) has stated "When practical, and when reliable laboratory services are available, potential vaccinees of childbearing age can have serologic tests to determine susceptibility to rubella. . . . However, routinely performing serologic tests for all females of childbearing age to determine susceptibility so that vaccine is given only to proven susceptibles is expensive and has been ineffective in some areas. Accordingly, the ACIP believes that rubella vaccination of a woman who is not known to be pregnant and has no history of vaccination is justifiable without serologic testing."
***NOTE: A primary difference among these recommendations is the timing of revaccination: the ACIP recommends routine revaccination at entry into Kindergarten or first grade, whereas the AAP recommends routine revaccination at entrance to middle school or junior high school. In addition, some public health jurisdictions mandate the age for revaccination. The complete text of applicable guidelines should be consulted.

CONTRAINDICATIONS

Do not give M-R-VAX II to pregnant females; the possible effects of the vaccine on fetal development are unknown at this time. If vaccination of postpubertal females is undertaken, pregnancy should be avoided for three months following vaccination. (See PRECAUTIONS, *Pregnancy*).
Anaphylactic or anaphylactoid reactions to neomycin (each dose of reconstituted vaccine contains approximately 25 mcg of neomycin).
History of anaphylactic or anaphylactoid reactions to eggs (see HYPERSENSITIVITY TO EGGS below).
Any febrile respiratory illness or other active febrile infection.
Active untreated tuberculosis.
Patients receiving immunosuppressive therapy. This contraindication does not apply to patients who are receiving corticosteroids as replacement therapy, e.g., for Addison's disease.
Individuals with blood dyscrasias, leukemia, lymphomas of any type, or other malignant neoplasms affecting the bone marrow or lymphatic systems.
Primary and acquired immunodeficiency states, including patients who are immunosuppressed in association with AIDS or other clinical manifestations of infection with human immunodeficiency viruses; cellular immune deficiencies; and hypogammaglobulinemic and dysgammaglobulinemic states.
Individuals with a family history of congenital or hereditary immunodeficiency, until the immune competence of the potential vaccine recipient is demonstrated.

HYPERSENSITIVITY TO EGGS

Live measles vaccine is produced in chick embryo cell culture. Persons with a history of anaphylactic, anaphylactoid, or other immediate reactions (e.g., hives, swelling of the mouth and throat, difficulty breathing, hypotension, or shock) subsequent to egg ingestion should not be vaccinated. Evidence indicates that persons are not at increased risk if they have egg allergies that are not anaphylactic or anaphylactoid in nature. Such persons may be vaccinated in the usual manner. There is no evidence to indicate that persons with allergies to chickens or feathers are at increased risk of reaction to the vaccine.

PRECAUTIONS

General
Adequate treatment provisions including epinephrine, should be available for immediate use should an anaphylactic or anaphylactoid reaction occur.
Due caution should be employed in administration of M-R-VAX II to persons with a history of cerebral injury, individual or family histories of convulsions, or any other condition in which stress due to fever should be avoided. The physi-

Continued on next page

Information on the Merck & Co., Inc. products listed on these pages is the full prescribing information from product circulars in use August 31, 1998. For information, please call 1-800-NSC MERCK [1-800-672-6372].

M-R-Vax II—Cont.

cian should be alert to the temperature elevation which may occur following vaccination. (See ADVERSE REACTIONS.)
Children and young adults who are known to be infected with human immunodeficiency viruses but without overt clinical manifestations of immunosuppression may be vaccinated; however, the vaccinees should be monitored closely for vaccine-preventable diseases because immunization may be less effective than for uninfected persons.
Vaccination should be deferred for at least 3 months following blood or plasma transfusions, or administration of human immune serum globulin.
Excretion of small amounts of the live attenuated rubella virus from the nose or throat has occurred in the majority of susceptible individuals 7–28 days after vaccination. There is no confirmed evidence to indicate that such virus is transmitted to susceptible persons who are in contact with the vaccinated individuals. Consequently, transmission through close personal contact, while accepted as a theoretical possibility, is not regarded as a significant risk. However, transmission of the rubella vaccine virus to infants via breast milk has been documented (see *Nursing Mothers*).
There are no reports of transmission of live attenuated measles virus from vaccinees to susceptible contacts.
It has been reported that live attenuated measles and rubella virus vaccines given individually may result in a temporary depression of tuberculin skin sensitivity. Therefore, if a tuberculin test is to be done, it should be administered either before or simultaneously with M-R-VAX II.
Children under treatment for tuberculosis have not experienced exacerbation of the disease when immunized with live measles virus vaccine; no studies have been reported to date of the effect of measles virus vaccines on untreated tuberculous children.
As for any vaccine, vaccination with M-R-VAX II may not result in seroconversion in 100% of susceptible persons given the vaccine.

Pregnancy

Pregnancy Category C

Animal reproduction studies have not been conducted with M-R-VAX II. It is also not known whether M-R-VAX II can cause fetal harm when administered to a pregnant woman or can affect reproduction capacity. Therefore, the vaccine should not be administered to pregnant females; futhermore, pregnancy should be avoided for three months following vaccination (see CONTRAINDICATIONS).
In counseling women who are inadvertently vaccinated when pregnant or who become pregnant within 3 months of vaccination, the physician should be aware of the following: (1) In a 10 year survey involving over 700 pregnant women who received rubella vaccine within 3 months before or after conception, (of whom 189 received the Wistar RA 27/3 strain), none of the newborns had abnormalities compatible with congenital rubella syndrome; (2) Reports have indicated that contracting of natural measles during pregnancy enhances fetal risk. Increased rates of spontaneous abortion, stillbirth, congenital defects and prematurity have been observed subsequent to natural measles during pregnancy. There are no adequate studies of the attenuated (vaccine) strain of measles virus in pregnancy. However, it would be prudent to assume that the vaccine strain of virus is also capable of inducing adverse fetal effects.

Nursing Mothers

It is not known whether measles vaccine virus is secreted in human milk. Recent studies have shown that lactating postpartum women immunized with live attenuated rubella vaccine may secrete the virus in breast milk and transmit it to breast-fed infants. In the infants with serological evidence of rubella infection, none exhibited severe disease; however, one exhibited mild clinical illness typical of acquired rubella. Caution should be exercised when M-R-VAX II is administered to a nursing woman.

ADVERSE REACTIONS

Burning and/or stinging of short duration at the injection site have been reported.
The adverse clinical reactions associated with the use of M-R-VAX II are those expected to follow administration of the monovalent vaccines given separately. These may include malaise, sore throat, cough, rhinitis, headache, dizziness, fever, rash, nausea, vomiting or diarrhea; mild local reactions such as erythema, induration, tenderness and regional lymphadenopathy; thrombocytopenia and purpura; allergic reactions such as wheal and flare at the injection site or urticaria; polyneuritis, and arthralgia and/or arthritis (usually transient and rarely chronic).
Anaphylaxis and anaphylactoid reactions have been reported.
Vasculitis has been reported rarely.
Moderate fever [101–102.9°F (38.3–39.4°C)] occurs occasionally, and high fever [above 103°F (39.4°C)] occurs less commonly. On rare occasions, children developing fever may exhibit febrile convulsions. Afebrile convulsions or seizures have occurred rarely following vaccination with live attenuated measles vaccine. Syncope, particularly at the time of mass vaccination, has been reported. Rash occurs infrequently and is usually minimal, but rarely may be generalized. Erythema multiforme has also been reported rarely.
Forms of optic neuritis, including retrobulbar neuritis, papillitis, and retinitis may infrequently follow viral infections, and have been reported to occur 1 to 3 weeks following inoculation with some live virus vaccines.
Clinical experience with live attenuated measles and rubella virus vaccines given individually indicates that encephalitis and other nervous system reactions have occurred very rarely. These might occur also with M-R-VAX II. Experience from more than 80 million doses of all live measles vaccines given in the U.S. through 1975 indicates that significant central nervous system reactions such as encephalitis and encephalopathy, occurring within 30 days after vaccination, have been temporally associated with measles vaccine very rarely. In no case has it been shown that reactions were actually caused by vaccine. The Center for Disease Control has pointed out that "a certain number of cases of encephalitis may be expected to occur in a large childhood population in a defined period of time even when no vaccines are administered". However, the data suggest the possibility that some of these cases may have been caused by measles vaccines. The risk of such serious neurological disorders following live measles virus vaccine administration remains far less than that for encephalitis and encephalopathy with natural measles (one per two thousand reported cases).
There have been rare reports of ocular palsies, Guillain-Barré syndrome, or ataxia occurring after immunization with vaccines containing live attenuated measles virus. The ocular palsies have occurred approximately 3–24 days following vaccination. No definite causal relationship has been established between these events and vaccination. Isolated reports of polyneuropathy including Guillain-Barré syndrome have also been reported after immunization with rubella-containing vaccines.
There have been reports of subacute sclerosing panencephalitis (SSPE) in children who did not have a history of natural measles but did receive measles vaccine. Some of these cases may have resulted from unrecognized measles in the first year of life or possibly from the measles vaccination. Based on estimated nationwide measles vaccine distribution, the association of SSPE cases to measles vaccination is about one case per million vaccine doses distributed. This is far less than the association with natural measles, 6–22 cases of SSPE per million cases of measles. The results of a retrospective case-controlled study conducted by the Center for Disease Control suggest that the overall effect of measles vaccine has been to protect against SSPE by preventing measles with its inherent higher risk of SSPE.
Local reactions characterized by marked swelling, redness and vesiculation at the injection site of attenuated live measles virus vaccines, and systemic reactions including atypical measles, have occurred in persons who received killed measles vaccine previously. M-R-VAX II was not given under this condition in clinical trials. Rarely, more severe reactions that require hospitalization, including prolonged high fevers and extensive local reactions, have been reported. Panniculitis has been reported rarely following administration of measles vaccine.
Arthralgia and/or arthritis (usually transient and rarely chronic), and polyneuritis are features of natural rubella and vary in frequency and severity with age and sex, being greatest in adult females and least in prepubertal children. This type of involvement as well as myalgia and paresthesia have also been reported following administration of MERUVAX II (Rubella Virus Vaccine Live).
Chronic arthritis has been associated with natural rubella infection and has been related to persistent virus and/or viral antigen isolated from body tissues. Only rarely have vaccine recipients developed chronic joint symptoms.
Following vaccination in children, reactions in joints are uncommon and generally of brief duration. In women, incidence rates for arthritis and arthralgia are generally higher than those seen in children (children: 0–3%; women: 12–20%), and the reactions tend to be more marked and of longer duration. Symptoms may persist for a matter of months or on rare occasions for years. In adolescent girls, the reactions appear to be intermediate in incidence between those seen in children and in adult women. Even in older women (35–45 years), these reactions are generally well tolerated and rarely interfere with normal activities.

DOSAGE AND ADMINISTRATION

FOR SUBCUTANEOUS ADMINISTRATION

Do not inject intravenously

The dosage of vaccine is the same for all persons. Inject the total volume of the single dose vial (about 0.5 mL) or 0.5 mL of the multiple dose vial of reconstituted vaccine subcutaneously, preferably into the outer aspect of upper arm. *Do not give immune globulin (IG) concurrently with* M-R-VAX II.
During shipment, to insure that there is no loss of potency, the vaccine must be maintained at a temperature of 10°C (50°F) or less.
Before reconstitution, store M-R-VAX II at 2–8°C (36–46°F).
Protect from light.
CAUTION: A sterile syringe free of preservatives, antiseptics, and detergents should be used for each injection and/or reconstitution of the vaccine because these substances may inactivate the live virus vaccine. A 25 gauge, 5/8" needle is recommended.
To reconstitute, use only the diluent supplied, since it is free of preservatives or other antiviral substances which might inactivate the vaccine.

Single Dose Vial —First withdraw the entire volume of diluent into the syringe to be used for reconstitution. Inject all the diluent in the syringe into the vial of lyophilized vaccine, and agitate to mix thoroughly. Withdraw the entire contents into a syringe and inject the total volume of restored vaccine subcutaneously.

It is important to use a separate sterile syringe and needle for each individual patient to prevent transmission of hepatitis B and other infectious agents from one person to another.

10 Dose Vial (available only to government agencies/institutions) —Withdraw the entire contents (7 mL) of the diluent vial into the sterile syringe to be used for reconstitution, and introduce into the 10 dose vial of lyophilized vaccine. Agitate to ensure thorough mixing. The outer labeling suggests "For Jet Injector or Syringe Use". Use with separate sterile syringes is permitted for containers of 10 doses or less. The vaccine and diluent do not contain preservatives; therefore, the user must recognize the potential contamination hazards and exercise special precautions to protect the sterility and potency of the product. The use of aseptic techniques and proper storage prior to and after restoration of the vaccine and subsequent withdrawal of the individual doses is essential. Use 0.5 mL of the reconstituted vaccine for subcutaneous injection.

It is important to use a separate sterile syringe and needle for each individual patient to prevent transmission of hepatitis B and other infectious agents from one person to another.

50 Dose Vial (available only to government agencies/institutions) —Withdraw the entire contents (30 mL) of diluent vial into the sterile syringe to be used for reconstitution and introduce into the 50 dose vial of lyophilized vaccine. Agitate to ensure thorough mixing. With full aseptic precautions, attach the vial to the sterilized multidose jet injector apparatus. Use 0.5 mL of the reconstituted vaccine for subcutaneous injection.

Each dose contains not less than the equivalent of 1,000 $TCID_{50}$ of the U.S. Reference Measles Virus and 1,000 $TCID_{50}$ of the U.S. Reference Rubella Virus.
Parenteral drug products should be inspected visually for particulate matter and discoloration prior to administration. M-R-VAX II, when reconstituted, is clear yellow.

HOW SUPPLIED

No. 4751—M-R-VAX II is supplied as a single-dose vial of lyophilized vaccine, **NDC** 0006-4751-00, and a vial of diluent.
No. 4677/4309—M-R-VAX II is supplied as follows: (1) a box of 10 single-dose vials of lyophilized vaccine (package A), **NDC** 0006-4677-00; and (2) a box of 10 vials of diluent (package B). To conserve refrigerator space, the diluent may be stored separately at room temperature (6505-01-098-8004, Ten Pack).
Available only to government agencies/institutions:
No. 4678—M-R-VAX II is supplied as one 10 dose vial of lyophilized vaccine, **NDC** 0006-4678-00, and one 7 mL vial of diluent.
No. 4679—M-R-VAX II is supplied as one 50 dose vial of lyophilized vaccine, **NDC** 0006-4679-00, and one 30 mL vial of diluent (6505-01-098-8005, 50 dose).

Storage

It is recommended that the vaccine be used as soon as possible after reconstitution. Protect vaccine from light at all times, since such exposure may inactivate the virus. Store reconstituted vaccine in the vaccine vial in a dark place at 2–8°C (36–46°F) and discard if not used within 8 hours.

A.H.F.S. Category: 80:12

7680217 Issued March 1995

COPYRIGHT © MERCK & CO., INC., 1990
All rights reserved

MAXALT® ℞
(RIZATRIPTAN BENZOATE)
TABLETS
MAXALT-MLT™ ℞
(RIZATRIPTAN BENZOATE)
ORALLY DISINTEGRATING TABLETS

DESCRIPTION

MAXALT* contains rizatriptan benzoate, a selective 5-hydroxytryptamine$_{1B/1D}$ (5-$HT_{1B/1D}$) receptor agonist.

Rizatriptan benzoate is described chemically as: *N,N*-dimethyl-5-(1*H*-1,2,4-triazol-1-ylmethyl)-1*H*-indole-3-ethanamine monobenzoate and its structural formula is:

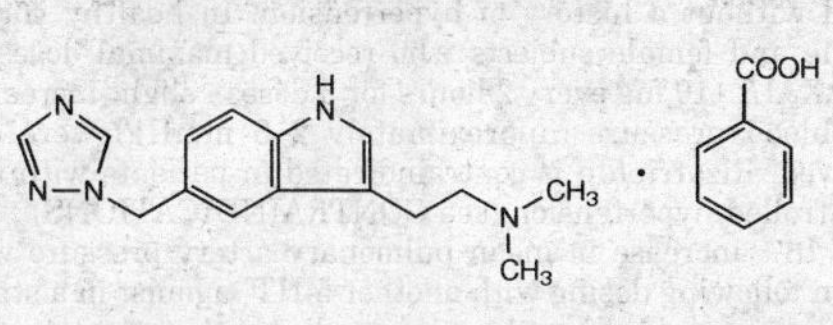

Its empirical formula is $C_{15}H_{19}N_5 \bullet C_7H_6O_2$, representing a molecular weight of the free base of 269.4. Rizatriptan benzoate is a white to off-white, crystalline solid that is soluble in water at about 42 mg per mL (expressed as free base) at 25°C.

MAXALT Tablets and MAXALT-MLT** Orally Disintegrating Tablets are available for oral administration in strengths of 5 and 10 mg (corresponding to 7.265 mg or 14.53 mg of the benzoate salt, respectively). Each compressed tablet contains the following inactive ingredients: lactose monohydrate, microcrystalline cellulose, pregelatinized starch, ferric oxide (red), and magnesium stearate.

Each lyophilized orally disintegrating tablet contains the following inactive ingredients: gelatin, mannitol, glycine, aspartame, and peppermint flavor.

* Registered trademark of MERCK & CO., Inc.
**Trademark of MERCK & CO., Inc.

CLINICAL PHARMACOLOGY

Mechanism of Action

Rizatriptan binds with high affinity to human cloned $5\text{-}HT_{1B}$ and $5\text{-}HT_{1D}$ receptors. Rizatriptan has weak affinity for other $5\text{-}HT_1$ receptor subtypes ($5\text{-}HT_{1A}$, $5\text{-}HT_{1E}$, $5\text{-}HT_{1F}$) and the $5\text{-}HT_7$ receptor, but has no significant activity at $5\text{-}HT_2$, $5\text{-}HT_3$, alpha- and beta-adrenergic, dopaminergic, histaminergic, muscarinic or benzodiazepine receptors.

Current theories on the etiology of migraine headache suggest that symptoms are due to local cranial vasodilatation and/or to the release of vasoactive and pro-inflammatory peptides from sensory nerve endings in an activated trigeminal system. The therapeutic activity of rizatriptan in migraine can most likely be attributed to agonist effects at $5\text{-}HT_{1B/1D}$ receptors on the extracerebral, intracranial blood vessels that become dilated during a migraine attack and on nerve terminals in the trigeminal system. Activation of these receptors results in cranial vessel constriction, inhibition of neuropeptide release and reduced transmission in trigeminal pain pathways.

Pharmacokinetics

Rizatriptan is completely absorbed following oral administration. The mean oral absolute bioavailability of the MAXALT Tablet is about 45%, and mean peak plasma concentrations (C_{max}) are reached in approximately 1–1.5 hours (T_{max}). The presence of a migraine headache did not appear to affect the absorption or pharmacokinetics of rizatriptan. Food has no significant effect on the bioavailability of rizatriptan but delays the time to reach peak concentration by an hour. In clinical trials, MAXALT was administered without regard to food. The plasma half-life of rizatriptan in males and females averages 2–3 hours.

The bioavailability and C_{max} of rizatriptan were similar following administration of MAXALT Tablets and MAXALT-MLT Orally Disintegrating Tablets, but the rate of absorption is somewhat slower with MAXALT-MLT, with T_{max} averaging 1.6–2.5 hours. AUC of rizatriptan is approximately 30% higher in females than in males. No accumulation occurred on multiple dosing.

The mean volume of distribution is approximately 140 liters in male subjects and 110 liters in female subjects. Rizatriptan is minimally bound (14%) to plasma proteins.

The primary route of rizatriptan metabolism is via oxidative deamination by monoamine oxidase-A (MAO-A) to the indole acetic acid metabolite, which is not active at the $5\text{-}HT_{1B/1D}$ receptor. N-monodesmethyl-rizatriptan, a metabolite with activity similar to that of parent compound at the $5\text{-}HT_{1B/1D}$ receptor, is formed to a minor degree. Plasma concentrations of N-monodesmethyl-rizatriptan are approximately 14% of those of parent compound, and it is eliminated at a similar rate. Other minor metabolites the N-oxide, the 6-hydroxy compound, and the sulfate conjugate of the 6-hydroxy metabolite are not active at the $5\text{-}HT_{1B/1D}$ receptor.

The total radioactivity of the administered dose recovered over 120 hours in urine and feces was 82% and 12%, respectively, following a single 10 mg oral administration of ^{14}C-rizatriptan. Following oral administration of ^{14}C-rizatriptan, rizatriptan accounted for about 17% of circulating plasma radioactivity. Approximately 14% of an oral dose is excreted in urine as unchanged rizatriptan while 51% is excreted as indole acetic acid metabolite, indicating substantial first pass metabolism.

Cytochrome P450 Isoforms: Rizatriptan is not an inhibitor of the activities of human liver cytochrome P450 isoforms 3A4/5, 1A2, 2C9, 2C19, or 2E1; rizatriptan is a competitive inhibitor (Ki=1400 nM) of cytochrome P450 2D6, but only at high, clinically irrelevant concentrations.

Special Populations

Age: Rizatriptan pharmacokinetics in healthy elderly non-migraineur volunteers (age 65–77 years) were similar to those in younger non-migraineur volunteers (age 18–45 years).

Gender: The mean $AUC_{0-\infty}$ and C_{max} of rizatriptan (10 mg orally) were about 30% and 11% higher in females as compared to males, respectively, while T_{max} occurred at approximately the same time.

Hepatic impairment: Following oral administration in patients with hepatic impairment caused by mild to moderate alcoholic cirrhosis of the liver, plasma concentrations of rizatriptan were similar in patients with mild hepatic insufficiency compared to a control group of healthy subjects; plasma concentrations of rizatriptan were approximately 30% greater in patients with moderate hepatic insufficiency. (See PRECAUTIONS.)

Renal impairment: In patients with renal impairment (creatinine clearance 10–60 mL/min/1.73 m^2), the $AUC_{0-\infty}$ of rizatriptan was not significantly different from that in healthy subjects. In hemodialysis patients, (creatinine clearance < 2 mL/min/1.73 m^2), however, the AUC for rizatriptan was approximately 44% greater than that in patients with normal renal function. (See PRECAUTIONS.)

Race: Pharmacokinetic data revealed no significant differences between African American and Caucasian subjects.

Drug Interactions (See also PRECAUTIONS, *Drug Interactions.*)

Monoamine oxidase inhibitors: Rizatriptan is principally metabolized via monoamine oxidase, 'A' subtype (MAO-A). Plasma concentrations of rizatriptan may be increased by drugs that are selective MAO-A inhibitors (e.g., moclobemide) or nonselective MAO inhibitors [type A and B] (e.g., isocarboxazid, phenelzine, tranylcypromine, and pargyline). In a drug interaction study, when MAXALT 10 mg was administered to subjects (n=12) receiving concomitant therapy with the selective, reversible MAO-A inhibitor, moclobemide 150 mg t.i.d., there were mean increases in rizatriptan AUC and C_{max} of 119% and 41% respectively; and the AUC of the active N-monodesmethyl metabolite of rizatriptan was increased more than 400%. The interaction would be expected to be greater with irreversible MAO inhibitors. No pharmacokinetic interaction is anticipated in patients receiving selective MAO-B inhibitors. (See CONTRAINDICATIONS; PRECAUTIONS, *Drug Interactions.*)

Propranolol: In a study of concurrent administration of propranolol 240 mg/day and a single dose of rizatriptan 10 mg in healthy subjects (n=11), mean plasma AUC for rizatriptan was increased by 70% during propranolol administration, and a fourfold increase was observed in one subject. The AUC of the active N-monodesmethyl metabolite of rizatriptan was not affected by propranolol. (See PRECAUTIONS; DOSAGE AND ADMINISTRATION.)

Nadolol/Metoprolol: In a drug interactions study, effects of multiple doses of nadolol 80 mg or metoprolol 100 mg every 12 hours on the pharmacokinetics of a single dose of 10 mg rizatriptan were evaluated in healthy subjects (n=12). No pharmacokinetic interactions were observed.

Paroxetine: In a study of the interaction between the selective serotonin reuptake inhibitor (SSRI) paroxetine 20 mg/day for two weeks and a single dose of MAXALT 10 mg in healthy subjects (n=12), neither the plasma concentrations of rizatriptan nor its safety profile were affected by paroxetine.

Oral contraceptives: In a study of concurrent administration of an oral contraceptive during 6 days of administration of MAXALT (10–30 mg/day) in healthy female volunteers (n=18), rizatriptan did not affect plasma concentrations of ethinyl estradiol or norethindrone.

Clinical Studies

The efficacy of MAXALT Tablets was established in four multicenter, randomized, placebo-controlled trials. Patients enrolled in these studies were primarily female (84%) and Caucasian (88%), with a mean age of 40 years (range of 18 to 71). Patients were instructed to treat a moderate to severe headache. Headache response, defined as a reduction of moderate or severe headache pain to no or mild headache pain, was assessed for up to 2 hours (Study 1) or up to 4 hours after dosing (Studies 2, 3 and 4). Associated symptoms of nausea, photophobia, and phonophobia and maintenance of response up to 24 hours postdose were evaluated. A second dose of MAXALT Tablets was allowed 2 to 24 hours after dosing for treatment of recurrent headache in Studies 1 and 2. Additional analgesics and/or antiemetics were allowed 2 hours after initial treatment for rescue in all four studies.

In all studies, the percentage of patients achieving headache response 2 hours after treatment was significantly greater in patients who received either MAXALT 5 or 10 mg compared to those who received placebo. In a separate study, doses of 2.5 mg were not different from placebo. Doses greater than 10 mg were associated with an increased incidence of adverse effects. The results from the 4 controlled studies using the marketed formulation are summarized in Table 1.

Table 1
Response Rates 2 Hours Following Treatment of Initial Headache

Study	Placebo	MAXALT Tablets 5 mg	MAXALT Tablets 10 mg
1	35% (n=304)	62%* (n=458)	71%*,** (n=456)
2†	37% (n=82)	—	77%* (n=320)
3	23% (n=80)	63%* (n=352)	—
4	40% (n=159)	60%* (n=164)	67%* (n=385)

*p value <0.05 in comparison with placebo
**p value <0.05 in comparison with 5 mg
†Results for initial headache only.

Comparisons of drug performance based upon results obtained in different clinical trials are never reliable. Because studies are conducted at different times, with different samples of patients, by different investigators, employing different criteria and/or different interpretations of the same criteria, under different conditions (dose, dosing regimen, etc.), quantitative estimates of treatment response and the timing of response may be expected to vary considerably from study to study.

The estimated probability of achieving an initial headache response within 2 hours following treatment is depicted in Figure 1.

Figure 1: Estimated Probability of Achieving an Initial Headache Response by 2 Hours††

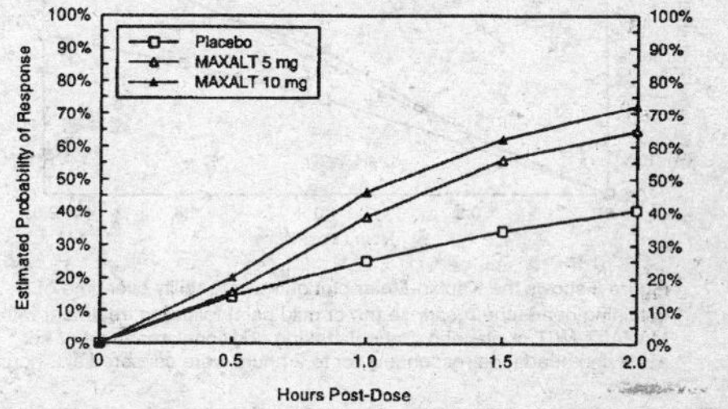

†† Figure 1 shows the Kaplan-Meier plot of the probability over time of obtaining headache response (no or mild pain) following treatment with rizatriptan or placebo. The averages displayed are based on pooled data from 4 placebo-controlled, outpatient trials providing evidence of efficacy (Studies 1, 2, 3, and 4). Patients taking additional treatment or not achieving headache response prior to 2 hours were censored at 2 hours.

For patients with migraine-associated photophobia, phonophobia, and nausea at baseline, there was a decreased incidence of these symptoms following administration of MAXALT compared to placebo.

Two to 24 hours following the initial dose of study treatment, patients were allowed to use additional treatment for pain response in the form of a second dose of study treatment or other medication. The estimated probability of patients taking a second dose or other medication for migraine over the 24 hours following the initial dose of study treatment is summarized in Figure 2.

Figure 2: Estimated Probability of Patients Taking a Second Dose of MAXALT Tablets or Other Medication for Migraines Over the 24 Hours Following the Initial Dose of Study Treatment†††

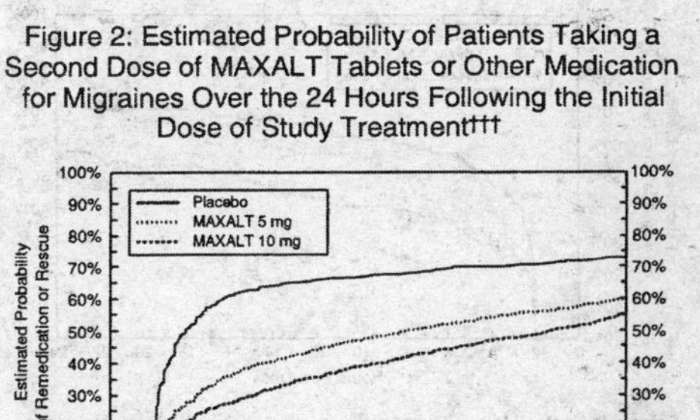

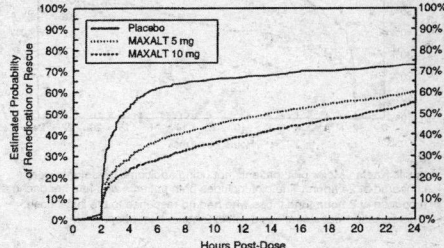

††† This Kaplan-Meier plot is based on data obtained in 4 placebo-controlled outpatient clinical trials (Studies 1, 2, 3, and 4). Patients not using additional treatments were censored at 24 hours. The plot includes both patients who had headache response at 2 hours and those who had no response to the initial dose. Remedication was not allowed within 2 hours post-dose.

Continued on next page

Information on the Merck & Co., Inc. products listed on these pages is the full prescribing information from product circulars in use August 31, 1998. For information, please call 1-800-NSC MERCK [1-800-672-6372].

Maxalt—Cont.

Efficacy was unaffected by the presence of aura; by the gender, or age of the patient; or by concomitant use of common migraine prophylactic drugs (e.g., beta-blockers, calcium channel blockers, tricyclic antidepressants) or oral contraceptives. There were insufficient data to assess the impact of race on efficacy.

MAXALT-MLT Orally Disintegrating Tablets

The efficacy of MAXALT-MLT 5 mg and 10 mg was demonstrated in a randomized, placebo-controlled trial that was similar in design to the trials of MAXALT Tablets. Patients were instructed to treat a moderate to severe headache. Of the 312 patients treated in the study, 88% were female and 91% were Caucasian, with a mean age of 40 years (range 18–65).

By 2 hours post-dosing, response rates in patients treated with MAXALT-MLT were approximately 66% in either the MAXALT-MLT 5 mg and 10 mg groups, compared to 47% in the placebo group. This difference was statistically significant.

The estimated probability of achieving an initial headache response by 2 hours following treatment with MAXALT-MLT is depicted in Figure 3.

Figure 3: Estimated Probability of Achieving an Initial Headache Response with MAXALT-MLT by 2 Hours‡

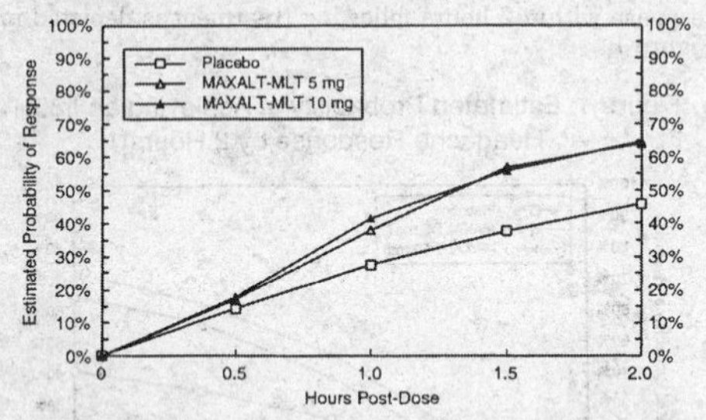

‡ Figure 3 shows the Kaplan-Meier plot of the probability over time of obtaining headache response (no or mild pain) following treatment with MAXALT-MLT or placebo. Patients taking additional treatment or not achieving headache response prior to 2 hours were censored at 2 hours.

For patients with migraine-associated photophobia and phonophobia at baseline, there was a decreased incidence of these symptoms following administration of MAXALT-MLT as compared to placebo.

Two to 24 hours following the initial dose of study treatment, patients were allowed to use additional treatment for pain response in the form of a second dose of study treatment or other medication. The estimated probability of patients taking a second dose or other medication for migraine over the 24 hours following the initial dose of study treatment is summarized in Figure 4.

Figure 4: Estimated Probability of Patients Taking a Second Dose of MAXALT-MLT or Other Medication for Migraines Over the 24 Hours Following the Initial Dose of Study Treatment‡‡

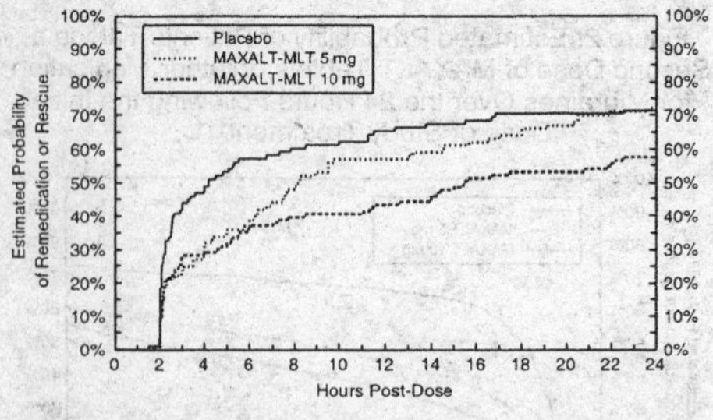

‡‡ In this Kaplan-Meier plot, patients not using additional treatments were censored at 24 hours. The plot includes both patients who had headache response at 2 hours and those who had no response to the initial dose. Remedication was not allowed within 2 hours post-dose.

INDICATIONS AND USAGE

MAXALT is indicated for the acute treatment of migraine attacks with or without aura in adults.

MAXALT is not intended for the prophylactic therapy of migraine or for use in the management of hemiplegic or basilar migraine (see CONTRAINDICATIONS). Safety and effectiveness of MAXALT has not been established for cluster headache, which is present in an older, predominantly male population.

CONTRAINDICATIONS

MAXALT should not be given to patients with ischemic heart disease (e.g., angina pectoris, history of myocardial infarction, or documented silent ischemia) or to patients who have symptoms or findings consistent with ischemic heart disease, coronary artery vasospasm, including Prinzmetal's variant angina, or other significant underlying cardiovascular disease (see WARNINGS).

Because MAXALT may increase blood pressure, it should not be given to patients with uncontrolled hypertension (see WARNINGS).

MAXALT should not be used within 24 hours of treatment with another 5-HT$_1$ agonist, or an ergotamine-containing or ergot-type medication like dihydroergotamine or methysergide.

MAXALT should not be administered to patients with hemiplegic or basilar migraine.

Concurrent administration of MAO inhibitors or use of rizatriptan within 2 weeks of discontinuation of MAO inhibitor therapy is contraindicated (see CLINICAL PHARMACOLOGY, *Drug Interactions* and PRECAUTIONS, *Drug Interactions*).

MAXALT is contraindicated in patients who are hypersensitive to rizatriptan or any of its inactive ingredients.

WARNINGS

MAXALT should only be used where a clear diagnosis of migraine has been established.

***Risk of Myocardial Ischemia and/or Infarction and Other Adverse Cardiac Events:* Because of the potential of this class of compounds (5-HT$_{1B/1D}$ agonists) to cause coronary vasospasm, MAXALT should not be given to patients with documented ischemic or vasospastic coronary artery disease (see CONTRAINDICATIONS). It is strongly recommended that rizatriptan not be given to patients in whom unrecognized coronary artery disease (CAD) is predicted by the presence of risk factors (e.g., hypertension, hypercholesterolemia, smoker, obesity, diabetes, strong family history of CAD, female with surgical or physiological menopause, or male over 40 years of age) unless a cardiovascular evaluation provides satisfactory clinical evidence that the patient is reasonably free of coronary artery and ischemic myocardial disease or other significant underlying cardiovascular disease. The sensitivity of cardiac diagnostic procedures to detect cardiovascular disease or predisposition to coronary artery vasospasm is modest, at best. If, during the cardiovascular evaluation, the patient's medical history, electrocardiographic or other investigations reveal findings indicative of, or consistent with, coronary artery vasospasm or myocardial ischemia, rizatriptan should not be administered (see CONTRAINDICATIONS).**

For patients with risk factors predictive of CAD, who are determined to have a satisfactory cardiovascular evaluation, it is strongly recommended that administration of the first dose of rizatriptan take place in the setting of a physician's office or similar medically staffed and equipped facility unless the patient has previously received rizatriptan. Because cardiac ischemia can occur in the absence of clinical symptoms, consideration should be given to obtaining on the first occasion of use an electrocardiogram (ECG) during the interval immediately following MAXALT, in these patients with risk factors.

It is recommended that patients who are intermittent long-term users of MAXALT and who have or acquire risk factors predictive of CAD, as described above, undergo periodic interval cardiovascular evaluation as they continue to use MAXALT.

The systematic approach described above is intended to reduce the likelihood that patients with unrecognized cardiovascular disease will be inadvertently exposed to rizatriptan.

Cardiac Events and Fatalities Associated with 5-HT$_1$ Agonists: Serious adverse cardiac events, including acute myocardial infarction, life-threatening disturbances of cardiac rhythm, and death have been reported within a few hours following the administration of other 5-HT$_1$ agonists. Considering the extent of use of 5-HT$_1$ agonists in patients with migraine, the incidence of these events is extremely low. Among the 3700 patients with migraine who participated in premarketing clinical trials of MAXALT, one patient was reported to have chest pain with possible ischemic ECG changes following a single dose of 10 mg.

Cerebrovascular Events and Fatalities Associated with 5-HT$_1$ Agonists: Cerebral hemorrhage, subarachnoid hemorrhage, stroke, and other cerebrovascular events have been reported in patients treated with other 5-HT$_1$ agonists; and some have resulted in fatalities. In a number of cases, it appears possible that the cerebrovascular events were primary, the agonist having been administered in the incorrect belief that the symptoms experienced were a consequence of migraine, when they were not. It should be noted that patients with migraine may be at increased risk of certain cerebrovascular events (e.g., stroke, hemorrhage, transient ischemic attack).

Other Vasospasm-Related Events: 5-HT$_1$ agonists may cause vasospastic reactions other than coronary artery vasospasm. Both peripheral vascular ischemia and colonic ischemia with abdominal pain and bloody diarrhea have been reported with 5-HT$_1$ agonists.

Increase in Blood Pressure: Significant elevation in blood pressure, including hypertensive crisis, has been reported on rare occasions in patients receiving 5-HT$_1$ agonists with and without a history of hypertension. In healthy young male and female subjects who received maximal doses of MAXALT (10 mg every 2 hours for 3 doses), slight increases in blood pressure (approximately 2–3 mmHg) were observed. Rizatriptan is contraindicated in patients with uncontrolled hypertension (see CONTRAINDICATIONS).

An 18% increase in mean pulmonary artery pressure was seen following dosing with another 5-HT$_1$ agonist in a study evaluating subjects undergoing cardiac catheterization.

PRECAUTIONS

General

As with other 5-HT$_{1B/1D}$ agonists, sensations of tightness, pain, pressure, and heaviness have been reported after treatment with MAXALT in the precordium, throat, neck and jaw. These events have not been associated with arrhythmias or definite ischemic ECG changes in clinical trials (one patient experienced chest pain with possible ischemic ECG changes). Because drugs in this class may cause coronary artery vasospasm, patients who experience signs or symptoms suggestive of angina following dosing should be evaluated for the presence of CAD or a predisposition to Prinzmetal's variant angina before receiving additional doses of medication, and should be monitored electrocardiographically if dosing is resumed and similar symptoms recur. Similarly, patients who experience other symptoms or signs suggestive of decreased arterial flow, such as ischemic bowel syndrome or Raynaud's syndrome following the use of any 5-HT$_1$ agonist are candidates for further evaluation (see WARNINGS).

Rizatriptan should also be administered with caution to patients with diseases that may alter the absorption, metabolism, or excretion of drugs (see CLINICAL PHARMACOLOGY, *Special Populations*).

Renally Impaired Patients: Rizatriptan should be used with caution in dialysis patients due to a decrease in the clearance of rizatriptan (see CLINICAL PHARMACOLOGY, *Special Populations*).

Hepatically Impaired Patients: Rizatriptan should be used with caution in patients with moderate hepatic insufficiency due to an increase in plasma concentrations of approximately 30% (see CLINICAL PHARMACOLOGY, *Special Populations*).

For a given attack, if a patient has no response to the first dose of rizatriptan, the diagnosis of migraine should be reconsidered before administration of a second dose.

Binding to Melanin-Containing Tissues

The propensity for rizatriptan to bind melanin has not been investigated. Based on its chemical properties, rizatriptan may bind to melanin and accumulate in melanin rich tissue (e.g., eye) over time. This raises the possibility that rizatriptan could cause toxicity in these tissues after extended use. There were, however, no adverse ophthalmologic changes related to treatment with rizatriptan in the one year dog toxicity study. Although no systematic monitoring of ophthalmologic function was undertaken in clinical trials, and no specific recommendations for ophthalmologic monitoring are offered, prescribers should be aware of the possibility of long-term ophthalmologic effects.

Phenylketonurics

Phenylketonuric patients should be informed that MAXALT-MLT Orally Disintegrating Tablets contain phenylalanine (a component of aspartame). Each 5-mg orally disintegrating tablet contains 1.05 mg phenylalanine, and each 10-mg orally disintegrating tablet contains 2.10 mg phenylalanine.

Information for Patients

Migraine or treatment with MAXALT may cause somnolence in some patients. Dizziness has also been reported in some patients receiving MAXALT. Patients should, therefore, evaluate their ability to perform complex tasks during migraine attacks and after administration of MAXALT.

Physicians should instruct their patients to read the patient package insert before taking MAXALT. See the accompanying PATIENT INFORMATION leaflet.

MAXALT-MLT Orally Disintegrating Tablets

Patients should be instructed not to remove the blister from the outer pouch until just prior to dosing. The blister pack should then be peeled open with dry hands and the orally disintegrating tablet placed on the tongue, where it will dissolve and be swallowed with the saliva.

Laboratory Tests

No specific laboratory tests are recommended for monitoring patients prior to and/or after treatment with MAXALT.

Drug Interactions (See also CLINICAL PHARMACOLOGY, *Drug Interactions*.)

Propranolol: Rizatriptan 5 mg should be used in patients taking propranolol, as propranolol has been shown to increase the plasma concentrations of rizatriptan by 70% (see CLINICAL PHARMACOLOGY, *Drug Interactions*; DOSAGE AND ADMINISTRATION).

Ergot-containing drugs: Ergot-containing drugs have been reported to cause prolonged vasospastic reactions. Because

there is a theoretical basis that these effects may be additive, use of ergotamine-containing or ergot-type medications (like dihydroergotamine or methysergide) and rizatriptan within 24 hours is contraindicated (see CONTRAINDICATIONS).

Other 5-HT₁ agonists: The administration of rizatriptan with other 5-HT₁ agonists has not been evaluated in migraine patients. Because their vasospastic effects may be additive, coadministration of rizatriptan and other 5-HT₁ agonists within 24 hours of each other is not recommended (see CONTRAINDICATIONS).

Selective serotonin reuptake inhibitors (SSRIs): SSRIs (e.g., fluoxetine, fluvoxamine, paroxetine, sertraline) have been reported, rarely, to cause weakness, hyperreflexia, and incoordination when coadministered with 5-HT₁ agonists. If concomitant treatment with rizatriptan and an SSRI is clinically warranted, appropriate observation of the patient is advised. No clinical or pharmacokinetic interactions were observed when MAXALT 10 mg was administered with paroxetine.

Monoamine oxidase inhibitors: Rizatriptan should not be administered to patients taking MAO-A inhibitors and nonselective MAO inhibitors; it has been shown that moclobemide (a specific MAO-A inhibitor) increased the systemic exposure of rizatriptan and its metabolite (see CLINICAL PHARMACOLOGY, *Drug Interactions*; CONTRAINDICATIONS).

Drug/Laboratory Test Interactions
MAXALT is not known to interfere with commonly employed clinical laboratory tests.

Carcinogenesis, Mutagenesis, Impairment of Fertility
Carcinogenesis: The lifetime carcinogenic potential of rizatriptan was evaluated in a 100-week study in mice and a 106-week study in rats at oral gavage doses of up to 125 mg/kg/day. Exposure data were not obtained in those studies, but plasma AUC's of parent drug measured in other studies after 5 and 21 weeks of oral dosing in mice and rats, respectively, indicate that the exposures to parent drug at the highest dose level in the carcinogenicity studies would have been approximately 150 times (mice) and 240 times (rats) average AUC's measured in humans after three 10 mg doses, the maximum recommended total daily dose. There was no evidence of an increase in tumor incidence related to rizatriptan in either species.

Mutagenesis: Rizatriptan, with and without metabolic activation, was neither mutagenic, nor clastogenic in a battery of *in vitro* and *in vivo* genetic toxicity studies, including: the microbial mutagenesis (Ames) assay, the *in vitro* mammalian cell mutagenesis assay in V-79 Chinese hamster lung cells, the *in vitro* alkaline elution assay in rat hepatocytes, the *in vitro* chromosomal aberration assay in Chinese hamster ovary cells and the *in vivo* chromosomal aberration assay in mouse bone marrow.

Impairment of Fertility: In a fertility study in rats, altered estrus cyclicity and delays in time to mating were observed in females treated orally with 100 mg/kg/day rizatriptan. Plasma drug exposure (AUC) at this dose was approximately 225 times the exposure in humans receiving the maximum recommended daily dose (MRDD) of 30 mg. The no-effect dose was 10 mg/kg/day (approximately 15 times the human exposure at the MRDD). There were no other fertility-related effects in the female rats. There was no impairment of fertility or reproductive performance in male rats treated with up to 250 mg/kg/day (approximately 550 times the human exposure at the MRDD).

Pregnancy: Pregnancy Category C
In a reproduction study in rats, birth weights and pre- and post-weaning weight gain were reduced in the offspring of females treated prior to and during mating and throughout gestation and lactation with doses of 10 and 100 mg/kg/day. Maternal plasma drug exposures (AUC) at these doses were approximately 15 and 225 times, respectively, the exposure in humans receiving the maximum recommended daily dose (MRDD) of 30 mg. The effects on offspring growth occurred in the absence of any apparent maternal toxicity in this study. The developmental no-effect dose was 2 mg/kg/day (maternal exposure approximately 1.5 times human exposure at the MRDD). The full spectrum of developmental toxicity is not known because adequately high doses, i.e., those producing some maternal toxicity, were not evaluated in the reproduction study. When higher, maternally toxic doses (250 mg/kg/day or greater) were evaluated over the same period of development in a rat dose range-finding study, pup mortality was increased.

In embryofetal development studies, no teratogenic effects were observed when pregnant rats and rabbits were administered doses of 100 and 50 mg/kg/day, respectively, during organogenesis. Fetal weights were decreased in conjunction with decreased maternal weight gain at the highest doses (maternal exposures approximately 225 and 115 times the human exposure at the MRDD in rats and rabbits, respectively). The developmental no-effect dose in these studies was 10 mg/kg/day in both rats and rabbits (maternal exposures approximately 15 times human exposure at the MRDD). Toxicokinetic studies demonstrated placental transfer of drug in both species.

There are no adequate and well-controlled studies in pregnant women; therefore, rizatriptan should be used during pregnancy only if the potential benefit justifies the potential risk to the fetus.

Nursing Mothers
It is not known whether this drug is excreted in human milk. Because many drugs are excreted in human milk, caution should be exercised when MAXALT is administered to women who are breast-feeding. Rizatriptan is extensively excreted in rat milk, at a level of 5-fold or greater than maternal plasma levels.

Pediatric Use
Safety and effectiveness of rizatriptan in pediatric patients have not been established; therefore, MAXALT is not recommended for use in patients under 18 years of age.

Use in the Elderly
The pharmacokinetics of rizatriptan were similar in elderly (aged ≥ 65 years) and in younger adults. Because migraine occurs infrequently in the elderly, clinical experience with MAXALT is limited in such patients. In clinical trials, there were no apparent differences in efficacy or in overall adverse experience rates between patients under 65 years of age and those 65 and above (n=17).

ADVERSE REACTIONS

Serious cardiac events, including some that have been fatal, have occurred following use of 5-HT₁ agonists. These events are extremely rare and most have been reported in patients with risk factors predictive of CAD. Events reported have included coronary artery vasospasm, transient myocardial ischemia, myocardial infarction, ventricular tachycardia, and ventricular fibrillation (see CONTRAINDICATIONS, WARNINGS, and PRECAUTIONS).

Incidence in Controlled Clinical Trials: Adverse experiences to rizatriptan were assessed in controlled clinical trials that included over 3700 patients who received single or multiple doses of MAXALT Tablets. The most common adverse events during treatment with MAXALT were asthenia/fatigue, somnolence, pain/pressure sensation and dizziness. These events appeared to be dose related. In long term extension studies where patients were allowed to treat multiple attacks for up to 1 year, 4% (59 out of 1525 patients) withdrew because of adverse experiences.

Table 2 lists the adverse events regardless of drug relationship (incidence ≥2% and greater than placebo) after a single dose of MAXALT. The events cited reflect experience gained under closely monitored conditions of clinical trials in a highly selected patient population. In actual clinical practice or in other clinical trials, these frequency estimates may not apply, as the conditions of use, reporting behavior, and the kinds of patients treated may differ.

Table 2
Incidence (≥ 2% and Greater than Placebo) of
Adverse Experiences After a Single Dose of MAXALT
Tablets or Placebo

	% of Patients		
Adverse Experiences	MAXALT 5 mg (N=977)	MAXALT 10 mg (N=1167)	Placebo (N=627)
Atypical Sensations	4	5	4
Paresthesia	3	4	<2
Pain and other Pressure Sensations	6	9	3
Chest Pain: tightness/pressure and/or heaviness	<2	3	1
Neck/throat/jaw: pain/tightness/pressure	<2	2	1
Regional Pain: tightness/pressure/ heaviness	<1	2	0
Pain, location unspecified	3	3	<2
Digestive	9	13	8
Dry Mouth	3	3	1
Nausea	4	6	4
Neurological	14	20	11
Dizziness	4	9	5
Headache	<2	2	<1
Somnolence	4	8	4
Other			
Asthenia/fatigue	4	7	2

MAXALT was generally well-tolerated. Adverse experiences were typically mild in intensity and were transient. The frequencies of adverse experiences in clinical trials did not increase when up to three doses were taken within 24 hours. Adverse event frequencies were also unchanged by concomitant use of drugs commonly taken for migraine prophylaxis (including propranolol), oral contraceptives, or analgesics. The incidences of adverse experiences were not affected by age or gender. There were insufficient data to assess the impact of race on the incidence of adverse events.

Other Events Observed in Association with the Administration of MAXALT: In the section that follows, the frequencies of less commonly reported adverse clinical events are presented. Because the reports include events observed in open studies, the role of MAXALT in their causation cannot be reliably determined. Furthermore, variability associated with adverse event reporting, the terminology used to describe adverse events, etc. limit the value of the quantitative frequency estimates provided. Event frequencies are calculated as the number of patients who used MAXALT (N=3716) and reported an event divided by the total number of patients exposed to MAXALT. All reported events are included, except those already listed in the previous table, those too general to be informative, and those not reasonably associated with the use of the drug. Events are further classified within body system categories and enumerated in order of decreasing frequency using the following definitions: frequent adverse events are those defined as those occurring in at least (>)1/100 patients; infrequent adverse experiences are those occurring in 1/100 to 1/1000 patients; and rare adverse experiences are those occurring in fewer than 1/1,000 patients.

General: Infrequent were chills, heat sensitivity, facial edema, hangover effect, and abdominal distention. Rare were fever, orthostatic effects, syncope and edema/swelling.
Atypical Sensations: Frequent were warm/cold sensations.
Cardiovascular: Frequent was palpitation. Infrequent were tachycardia, cold extremities, hypertension, arrhythmia, and bradycardia. Rare was angina pectoris.
Digestive: Frequent were diarrhea and vomiting. Infrequent were dyspepsia, thirst, acid regurgitation, dysphagia, constipation, flatulence, and tongue edema. Rare were anorexia, appetite increase, gastritis, paralysis (tongue), and eructation.
Metabolic: Infrequent was dehydration.
Musculoskeletal: Infrequent were muscle weakness, stiffness, myalgia, muscle cramp, musculoskeletal pain, arthralgia, and muscle spasm.
Neurological/Psychiatric: Frequent were hypesthesia, mental acuity decreased, euphoria and tremor. Infrequent were nervousness, vertigo, insomnia, anxiety, depression, disorientation, ataxia, dysarthria, confusion, dream abnormality, gait abnormality, irritability, memory impairment, agitation and hyperesthesia. Rare were: dysesthesia, depersonalization, akinesia/bradykinesia, apprehension, hyperkinesia, hypersomnia, and hyporeflexia.
Respiratory: Frequent was dyspnea. Infrequent were pharyngitis, irritation (nasal), congestion (nasal), dry throat, upper respiratory infection, yawning, respiratory congestion (nasal), dry nose, epistaxis, and sinus disorder. Rare were cough, hiccups, hoarseness, rhinorrhea, sneezing, tachypnea, and pharyngeal edema.
Special Senses: Infrequent were blurred vision, tinnitus, dry eyes, burning eye, eye pain, eye irritation, ear pain, and tearing. Rare were hyperacusis, smell perversion, photophobia, photopsia, itching eye, and eye swelling.
Skin and Skin Appendage: Frequent was flushing. Infrequent were sweating, pruritus, rash, and urticaria. Rare were erythema, acne, and photosensitivity.
Urogenital system: Frequent was hot flashes. Infrequent were urinary frequency, polyuria, and menstruation disorder. Rare was dysuria.

The adverse experience profile seen with MAXALT-MLT Orally Disintegrating Tablets was similar to that seen with MAXALT Tablets.

DRUG ABUSE AND DEPENDENCE

Although the abuse potential of MAXALT has not been specifically assessed, no abuse of, tolerance to, withdrawal from, or drug-seeking behavior was observed in patients who received MAXALT in clinical trials or their extensions. The 5-HT₁B/₁D agonists, as a class, have not been associated with drug abuse.

OVERDOSAGE

No overdoses of MAXALT were reported during clinical trials.

Rizatriptan 40 mg (administered as either a single dose or as two doses with a 2-hour interdose interval) was generally well tolerated in over 300 patients; dizziness and somnolence were the most common drug-related adverse effects.
In a clinical pharmacology study in which 12 subjects received rizatriptan, at total cumulative doses of 80 mg (given within four hours), two subjects experienced syncope and/or bradycardia. One subject, a female aged 29 years, developed vomiting, bradycardia, and dizziness beginning three hours

Continued on next page

Information on the Merck & Co., Inc. products listed on these pages is the full prescribing information from product circulars in use August 31, 1998. For information, please call 1-800-NSC MERCK [1-800-672-6372].

Consult 1999 PDR® supplements and future editions for revisions

Maxalt—Cont.

after receiving a total of 80 mg rizatriptan (administered over two hours); a third degree AV block, responsive to atropine, was observed an hour after the onset of the other symptoms. The second subject, a 25 year old male, experienced transient dizziness, syncope, incontinence, and a 5-second systolic pause (on ECG monitor) immediately after a painful venipuncture. The venipuncture occurred two hours after the subject had received a total of 80 mg rizatriptan (administered over four hours).

In addition, based on the pharmacology of rizatriptan, hypertension or other more serious cardiovascular symptoms could occur after overdosage. Gastrointestinal decontamination, (i.e., gastric lavage followed by activated charcoal) should be considered in patients suspected of an overdose with MAXALT. Clinical and electrocardiographic monitoring should be continued for at least 12 hours, even if clinical symptoms are not observed.

The effects of hemo- or peritoneal dialysis on serum concentrations of rizatriptan are unknown.

DOSAGE AND ADMINISTRATION

In controlled clinical trials, single doses of 5 and 10 mg of MAXALT Tablets or MAXALT-MLT were effective for the acute treatment of migraines in adults. There is evidence that the 10-mg dose may provide a greater effect than the 5-mg dose (see *Clinical Studies*). Individuals may vary in response to doses of MAXALT Tablets. The choice of dose should therefore be made on an individual basis, weighing the possible benefit of the 10-mg dose with the potential risk for increased adverse events.

Redosing: Doses should be separated by at least 2 hours; no more than 30 mg should be taken in any 24-hour period. The safety of treating, on average, more than four headaches in a 30-day period has not been established.

Patients receiving propranolol: In patients receiving propranolol, the 5-mg dose of MAXALT should be used, up to a maximum of 3 doses in any 24-hour period. (See CLINICAL PHARMACOLOGY, *Drug Interactions*.)

For MAXALT-MLT Orally Disintegrating Tablets, administration with liquid is not necessary. The orally disintegrating tablet is packaged in a blister within an outer aluminum pouch. Patients should be instructed not to remove the blister from the outer pouch until just prior to dosing. The blister pack should then be peeled open with dry hands and the orally disintegrating tablet placed on the tongue, where it will dissolve and be swallowed with the saliva.

HOW SUPPLIED

No. 3732—MAXALT Tablets, 5 mg, are pale pink, capsule-shaped, compressed tablets coded MRK on one side and 266 on the other. They are supplied as follows:
NDC 0006-0266-74, bottles of 500
　　Shown in Product Identification Guide, page 323
NDC 0006-0266-06, unit of use carrying case of 6 tablets.
No. 3733—MAXALT Tablets, 10 mg, are pale pink, capsule-shaped, compressed tablets coded MRK on one side and MRK 267 on the other. They are supplied as follows:
NDC 0006-0267-74, bottles of 500
NDC 0006-0267-06, unit of use carrying case of 6 tablets.
　　Shown in Product Identification Guide, page 323
No. 3800—MAXALT-MLT Orally Disintegrating Tablets, 5 mg, are white to off-white, round lyophilized orally disintegrating tablets debossed with a modified triangle on one side, and measuring 10.0–11.5 mm (side-to-side) with a peppermint flavor. Each orally disintegrating tablet is individually packaged in a blister inside an aluminum pouch (sachet). They are supplied as follows:
NDC 0006-3800-06, 2 × unit of use carrying case of 3 orally disintegrating tablets (6 tablets total).
　　Shown in Product Identification Guide, page 323
No. 3801—MAXALT-MLT Orally Disintegrating Tablets, 10 mg, are white to off-white, round lyophilized orally disintegrating tablets debossed with a modified square on one side, and measuring 12.0–13.8 mm (side-to-side) with a peppermint flavor. Each orally disintegrating tablet is individually packaged in a blister inside an aluminum pouch (sachet). They are supplied as follows:
NDC 0006-3801-06, 2 × unit of use carrying case of 3 orally disintegrating tablets (6 tablets total).
　　Shown in Product Identification Guide, page 323
Storage
Store MAXALT Tablets at room temperature, 15–30°C (59–86°F). Dispense in a tight container, if product is subdivided.
Store MAXALT-MLT Orally Disintegrating Tablets at room temperature, 15–30°C (59–86°F). The patient should be instructed not to remove the blister from the outer aluminum pouch until the patient is ready to consume the orally disintegrating tablet inside.
　　9122100　　　Issued June 1998
COPYRIGHT © MERCK & CO., Inc., 1998
All rights reserved

Patient Information about
MAXALT® (max-awlt) and MAXALT-MLT™
for Migraine
Generic name: rizatriptan benzoate

Please read this information before you start taking MAXALT*. Also, read the leaflet each time you renew your prescription, just in case anything has changed. Remember, this leaflet does not take the place of careful discussions with your doctor. You and your doctor should discuss MAXALT when you start taking your medication and at regular checkups.

What is MAXALT and what is it used for?

MAXALT is a medication used for the treatment of migraine attacks in adults. MAXALT is a member of a class of drugs called selective 5-HT$_{1B/1D}$ receptor agonists.

It is available as a traditional tablet (MAXALT) and as an orally disintegrating tablet (MAXALT-MLT**). Unless otherwise stated, the information contained in this leaflet applies both to MAXALT Tablets and to MAXALT-MLT orally disintegrating tablets.

Tell your doctor about your symptoms. Your doctor will decide if you have migraine. Use MAXALT only for a migraine attack. MAXALT should not be used to treat headaches that might be caused by other, more serious conditions.

You will find more information about migraine at the end of this leaflet.

---

*　Registered trademark of MERCK & CO., Inc.
**Trademark of MERCK & CO., Inc.

How should I take MAXALT?

Your doctor has prescribed either a 5 mg or 10 mg dosage of MAXALT or MAXALT-MLT for your migraine attack. When you have a migraine headache, take your medication as directed by your doctor.

MAXALT Tablets

If you are using MAXALT Tablets, swallow the tablet whole with liquid.

MAXALT-MLT Orally Disintegrating Tablets

If you are using MAXALT-MLT, leave the orally disintegrating tablet in its package until you are ready to take it. Remove the blister from the foil pouch. Do not push the tablet through the blister; rather, peel open the blister pack with dry hands and place the tablet on your tongue. The tablet will dissolve rapidly and be swallowed with your saliva. No liquid is needed to take the orally disintegrating tablet.

If your headache comes back after your initial dose, a second dose may be taken anytime after 2 hours of administering the first dose. For any attack where you have no response to the first dose, do not take a second dose without first consulting with your doctor. Do not take more than 30 mg of MAXALT in a 24-hour period, (for example, do not take more than three 10-mg tablets in a 24-hour period).

If you are receiving propranolol, you should use the 5-mg dose of MAXALT or MAXALT-MLT, up to a maximum of 3 doses (15 mg total) in a 24-hour period.

If your condition worsens, seek medical attention.

Who should not take MAXALT?

Do not take MAXALT if you:
- have had a serious allergic reaction to MAXALT or any of its ingredients
- have uncontrolled high blood pressure
- have heart disease or history of heart disease
- are currently taking monoamine oxidase (MAO) inhibitors*** such as phenelzine sulfate (NARDIL®) or tranylcypromine sulfate (PARNATE®) for mental depression, or have taken MAO inhibitors within the last two weeks.

MAXALT should not be used within 24 hours of treatment with another 5-HT$_1$ agonist*** such as sumatriptan (IMITREX®), naratriptan (AMERGE™) or zolmitriptan (ZOMIG™); or ergotamine-type medications such as ergotamine (BELLERGAL-S®, CAFERGOT®, ERGOMAR®, WIGRAINE®), dihydro-ergotamine (D.H.E. 45®), or methysergide (SANSERT®).

*** The brands listed are the trademarks of their respective owners and are not trademarks of Merck & Co., Inc.

What should I tell my doctor before and during treatment with MAXALT?

Tell your doctor:
- about any past or present medical problems
- about any history of high blood pressure, chest pain, shortness of breath or heart disease
- about any risk factors for heart disease
  - high blood pressure or diabetes
  - high cholesterol
  - obesity
  - smoking
  - family history of heart disease
  - post menopausal
  - male over 40
- about any allergies you have or have had
- if you are pregnant or plan to become pregnant
- if you are breast-feeding or plan to breast-feed

- about all drugs you are taking or plan to take, including those obtained without a prescription, and those you normally take for a migraine.

What if I am pregnant?

Do not use MAXALT if you are pregnant, think you might be pregnant, are trying to become pregnant, or are not using adequate contraception, unless you have discussed this with your doctor.

Can I take MAXALT with other medications?

Do not take MAXALT with any other drug in the same class within 24 hours, such as sumatriptan (IMITREX®), naratriptan (AMERGE™) or zolmitriptan (ZOMIG™).

Do not take MAXALT within 24 hours of taking ergotamine-type medications such as ergotamine (BELLERGAL-S®, CAFERGOT®, ERGOMAR®, WIGRAINE®), dihydro-ergotamine (D.H.E. 45®) or methysergide (SANSERT®) to treat your migraine.

Do not take MAXALT when you are taking monoamine oxidase (MAO) inhibitors, such as phenelzine sulfate (NARDIL®) or tranylcypromine sulfate (PARNATE®) for mental depression, or if it has been less than two weeks since you stopped taking an MAO inhibitor.

Ask your doctor for instructions about taking MAXALT if you are now taking propranolol (INDERAL®). (See **How should I take MAXALT?** section.)

What are the possible side effects of MAXALT?

Like all prescription drugs, MAXALT can cause side effects. In studies, MAXALT was generally well-tolerated. The side effects were usually mild and temporary. The following is **not** a complete list of side effects reported with MAXALT. Do not rely on this leaflet alone for information about side effects. Ask your doctor to discuss with you the more complete list of side effects.

In studies, the **most common** side effects reported were:
- **dizziness**
- **sleepiness, tiredness, fatigue**
- **pain or pressure sensation (e.g., in the chest or throat)**

If you experience dizziness, sleepiness, tiredness or fatigue, you should evaluate your ability to perform complex tasks such as driving or operating heavy machinery.

Other, **less common** side effects were related to the:

Heart and blood vessels – Alterations in heartbeat, increased blood pressure and cold extremities.

Muscles – Muscle weakness, stiffness, and spasm; and muscle and bone pain.

Nervous system – Nervousness, decreased mental sharpness, tremor, headache, abnormal sensation, vertigo, sleep disturbance, mood and personality changes, alterations in speech and movement, memory impairment, confusion and dream abnormality.

Digestive system – Stomach upset, diarrhea, dry mouth, constipation, gas, thirst, acid reflux, difficulty swallowing, tongue swelling, changes in appetite, burping and inability of the tongue to move.

Skin – Flushing (redness of the face lasting a short time), hot flashes, sweating, itching, rash, hives, acne and skin reaction to sunlight.

Respiratory – Difficult or rapid breathing, dryness or discomfort of the throat or nose, nose bleed, yawning and sinus disorder, cold-like symptoms, cough, hiccups and swelling of the throat.

Special Senses – Visual disturbances, ringing in the ears, ear pain, eye discomfort, swelling or tearing; alterations in hearing and smelling and visual intolerance to light.

Miscellaneous – Chills, heat sensitivity, swelling, bloating, hangover effect, fever, fainting, dizziness on standing up, warm/cold sensations, dehydration and changes in urination and menstruation.

Tell your doctor about these or any other symptoms. If the symptoms persist or worsen, seek medical attention promptly. In addition, tell your doctor if you experience any symptoms that suggest an allergic reaction (such as a rash or itching) after taking MAXALT.

There have been rare reports of serious heart-related side effects with this class of drugs.

What should I do if I take an overdose?

If you take more medication than you have been told to take, you should contact your doctor, hospital emergency department, or nearest poison control center immediately.

What is migraine and how does it differ from other headaches?

Migraine is an intense, throbbing, typically one-sided headache that often includes nausea, vomiting, sensitivity to light, and sensitivity to sound. According to many migraine sufferers, the pain and symptoms from a migraine headache are more intense than the pain and symptoms of a common headache.

Some people may have visual symptoms before the headache, such as flashing lights or wavy lines, called an aura. Migraine attacks typically last for hours or, rarely, for more than a day, and they can return frequently. The severity and frequency of migraine attacks may vary.

Based on your symptoms, your doctor will decide whether you have migraine.

Who gets migraine?
Migraine headaches tend to occur in members of the same family. Both men and women get migraine, but it is more common in women.
What may trigger a migraine attack?
Certain things are thought to trigger migraine attacks in some people. Some of these triggers are:
- certain foods or beverages (e.g., cheese, chocolate, citrus fruit, caffeine, alcohol)
- stress
- change in a behavior (e.g., under/oversleeping; missing a meal; change in diet)
- hormonal changes in women (e.g., menstruation)

You may be able to prevent migraine attacks or diminish their frequency if you understand what specifically triggers your attacks. Keeping a headache diary may help you identify and monitor the possible migraine triggers you encounter. Once the triggers are identified, you and your doctor can modify your treatment and lifestyle appropriately.
How does MAXALT work during a migraine attack?
Treatment with MAXALT:
1. Reduces swelling of blood vessels surrounding the brain. This swelling results in the headache pain of a migraine attack.
2. Blocks the release of substances from nerve endings that cause more pain and other symptoms of migraine.
3. Interrupts the sending of specific pain signals to your brain.

It is thought that each of these actions contributes to relief of your symptoms by MAXALT.
How should I store MAXALT?
Keep your medicine in a safe place where children cannot reach it. It may be harmful to children. Store your medication away from heat, light, moisture, and at a controlled room temperature 59°–86°F (15°–30°C). If your medication has expired, throw it away as instructed. If your doctor decides to stop your treatment, do not keep any leftover medicine unless your doctor tells you to do so. Throw away your medicine as instructed. Be sure that the discarded tablets are out of the reach of children.
If you are storing MAXALT-MLT, do not remove the blister from the outer aluminum pouch until you are ready to take the medication inside.
This leaflet provides a summary of information about MAXALT. If you have any questions or concerns about either MAXALT or migraine, talk to your doctor. In addition, talk to your pharmacist or other health care provider.
9122200 Issued June 1998
COPYRIGHT © MERCK & CO., Inc., 1998
All rights reserved

MEFOXIN® ℞
(Cefoxitin for Injection), U.S.P.

DESCRIPTION

MEFOXIN* (Cefoxitin for Injection) is a semi-synthetic, broad-spectrum cepha antibiotic sealed under nitrogen for intravenous administration. It is derived from cephamycin C, which is produced by *Streptomyces lactamdurans.* Its chemical name is sodium (6*R*, 7*S*)-3-(hydroxymethyl)-7-methoxy-8-oxo-7-[2-(2-thienyl)acetamido]-5-thia-1-azabicyclo[4.2.0]oct-2-ene-2-carboxylate carbamate (ester). The empirical formula is $C_{16}H_{16}N_3NaO_7S_2$, and the structural formula is:

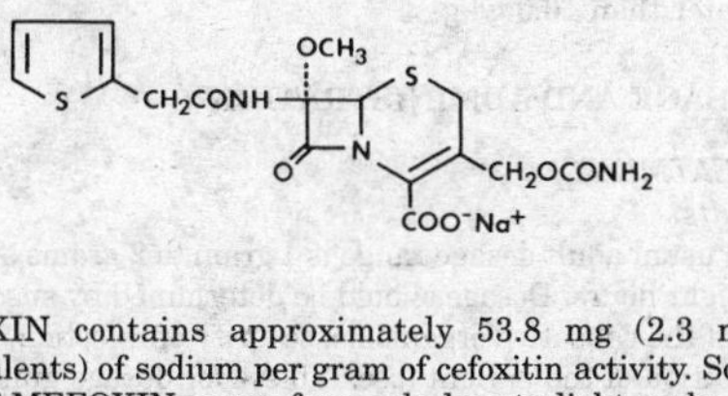

MEFOXIN contains approximately 53.8 mg (2.3 milliequivalents) of sodium per gram of cefoxitin activity. Solutions of MEFOXIN range from colorless to light amber in color. The pH of freshly constituted solutions usually ranges from 4.2 to 7.0.

*Registered trademark of MERCK & CO., INC.

CLINICAL PHARMACOLOGY

Clinical Pharmacology
Following an intravenous dose of 1 gram, serum concentrations were 110 mcg/mL at 5 minutes, declining to less than 1 mcg/mL at 4 hours. The half-life after an intravenous dose is 41 to 59 minutes. Approximately 85 percent of cefoxitin is excreted unchanged by the kidneys over a 6-hour period, resulting in high urinary concentrations. Probenecid slows tubular excretion and produces higher serum levels and increases the duration of measurable serum concentrations.
Cefoxitin passes into pleural and joint fluids and is detectable in antibacterial concentrations in bile.
Microbiology
The bactericidal action of cefoxitin results from inhibition of cell wall synthesis. Cefoxitin has *in vitro* activity against a wide range of gram-positive and gram-negative organisms. The methoxy group in the 7α position provides MEFOXIN with a high degree of stability in the presence of beta-lactamases, both penicillinases and cephalosporinases, of gram-negative bacteria. While *in vitro* studies have demonstrated the susceptibility of most strains of the following organisms, clinical efficacy for infections other than those included in the INDICATIONS AND USAGE section is unknown.
Gram-positive
Staphylococcus aureus, including penicillinase and non-penicillinase producing strains.
Staphylococcus epidermidis
Beta-hemolytic and other streptococci (most strains of enterococci, e.g., *Enterococcus faecalis* [formerly *Streptococcus faecalis*], are resistant)
Streptococcus pneumoniae
Gram-negative
Eikenella corrodens (beta-lactamase negative strains)
Escherichia coli
Klebsiella species (including *K. pneumoniae*)
Haemophilus influenzae
Neisseria gonorrhoeae, including penicillinase and non-penicillinase producing strains
Proteus mirabilis
Morganella morganii
Proteus vulgaris
Providencia species, including *Providencia rettgeri*
Anaerobic organisms
Peptococcus niger
Peptostreptococcus species
Clostridium species
Bacteroides species, including the *B. fragilis* group (includes *B. fragilis, B. distasonis, B. ovatus, B. thetaiotaomicron*).
MEFOXIN is inactive *in vitro* against most strains of *Pseudomonas aeruginosa* and enterococci and many strains of *Enterobacter cloacae.*
Methicillin-resistant staphylococci are almost uniformly resistant to MEFOXIN.

Susceptibility Tests
For fast-growing aerobic organisms, quantitative methods that require measurements of zone diameters give the most precise estimates of antibiotic susceptibility. One such procedure* has been recommended for use with discs to test susceptibility to cefoxitin. Interpretation involves correlation of the diameters obtained in the disc test with minimal inhibitory concentration (MIC) values for cefoxitin.
Reports from the laboratory giving results of the standardized single disc susceptibility test* using a 30 mcg cefoxitin disc should be interpreted according to the following criteria:
Organisms producing zones of 18 mm or greater are considered susceptible, indicating that the tested organism is likely to respond to therapy.
Organisms of intermediate susceptibility produce zones of 15 to 17 mm, indicating that the tested organism would be susceptible if high dosage is used or if the infection is confined to tissues and fluids (e.g., urine) in which high antibiotic levels are attained.
Resistant organisms produce zones of 14 mm or less, indicating that other therapy should be selected.
The cefoxitin disc should be used for testing cefoxitin susceptibility.
Cefoxitin has been shown by *in vitro* tests to have activity against certain strains of *Enterobacteriaceae* found resistant when tested with the cephalosporin class disc. For this reason, the cefoxitin disc should not be used for testing susceptibility to cephalosporins, and cephalosporin discs should not be used for testing susceptibility to cefoxitin.
Dilution methods, preferably the agar plate dilution procedure, are most accurate for susceptibility testing of obligate anaerobes.
A bacterial isolate may be considered susceptible if the MIC value for cefoxitin† is not more than 16 mcg/mL. Organisms are considered resistant if the MIC is greater than 32 mcg/mL.

* Bauer, A. W.; Kirby, W. M. M.; Sherris, J. C.; Turck, M.: Antibiotic susceptibility testing by a standardized single disc method, Amer. J. Clin. Path. *45* : 493–496, Apr. 1966. Standardized disc susceptibility test, Federal Register *37* : 20527–20529, 1972. National Committee for Clinical Laboratory Standards: Performance Standards for Antimicrobial Disc Susceptibility Tests–Fifth Edition; Approved Standard, NCCLS Document M2-A5, Vol 13, No. 24, NCCLS, Villanova, PA, December 1993.
† Determined by the ICS agar dilution method (Ericsson and Sherris, Acta Path. Microbiol. Scand. (B) Suppl. No. 217, 1971) or any other method that has been shown to give equivalent results.

INDICATIONS AND USAGE

Treatment
MEFOXIN is indicated for the treatment of serious infections caused by susceptible strains of the designated microorganisms in the diseases listed below.
(1) Lower respiratory tract infections, including pneumonia and lung abscess, caused by *Streptococcus pneumoniae,* other streptococci (excluding enterococci, e.g., *Enterococcus faecalis* [formerly *Streptococcus faecalis*]), *Staphylococcus aureus* (penicillinase and non-penicillinase producing), *Escherichia coli, Klebsiella* species, *Haemophilus influenzae,* and *Bacteroides* species.
(2) Urinary tract infections caused by *Escherichia coli, Klebsiella* species, *Proteus mirabilis, Morganella morganii, Proteus vulgaris* and *Providencia* species (including *P. rettgeri*).
(3) Intra-abdominal infections, including peritonitis and intra-abdominal abscess, caused by *Escherichia coli, Klebsiella* species, *Bacteroides* species including the *Bacteroides fragilis* group**, and *Clostridium* species.
(4) Gynecological infections, including endometritis, pelvic cellulitis, and pelvic inflammatory disease caused by *Escherichia coli, Neisseria gonorrhoeae* (penicillinase and non-penicillinase producing), *Bacteroides* species including *B. fragilis*, *Clostridium* species, *Peptococcus niger, Peptostreptococcus* species, and Group B streptococci. MEFOXIN, like cephalosporins, has no activity against *Chlamydia trachomatis.* Therefore, when MEFOXIN is used in the treatment of patients with pelvic inflammatory disease and *C. trachomatis* is one of the suspected pathogens, appropriate anti-chlamydial coverage should be added.
(5) Septicemia caused by *Streptococcus pneumoniae, Staphylococcus aureus* (penicillinase and non-penicillinase producing), *Escherichia coli, Klebsiella* species, and *Bacteroides* species including *B. fragilis.*
(6) Bone and joint infections caused by *Staphylococcus aureus* (penicillinase and non-penicillinase producing).
(7) Skin and skin structure infections caused by *Staphylococcus aureus* (penicillinase and non-penicillinase producing), *Staphylococcus epidermidis,* streptococci (excluding enterococci, e.g., *Enterococcus faecalis* [formerly *Streptococcus faecalis*]), *Escherichia coli, Proteus mirabilis, Klebsiella* species, *Bacteroides* species including *B. fragilis, Clostridium* species, *Peptococcus niger,* and *Peptostreptococcus* species.
Appropriate culture and susceptibility studies should be performed to determine the susceptibility of the causative organisms to MEFOXIN. Therapy may be started while awaiting the results of these studies.
In randomized comparative studies, MEFOXIN and cephalothin were comparably safe and effective in the management of infections caused by gram-positive cocci and gram-negative rods susceptible to the cephalosporins. MEFOXIN has a high degree of stability in the presence of bacterial beta-lactamases, both penicillinases and cephalosporinases. Many infections caused by aerobic and anaerobic gram-negative bacteria resistant to some cephalosporins respond to MEFOXIN. Similarly, many infections caused by aerobic and anaerobic bacteria resistant to some penicillin antibiotics (ampicillin, carbenicillin, penicillin G) respond to treatment with MEFOXIN. Many infections caused by mixtures of susceptible aerobic and anaerobic bacteria respond to treatment with MEFOXIN.
Prevention
MEFOXIN is indicated for the prophylaxis of infection in patients undergoing uncontaminated gastrointestinal surgery, vaginal hysterectomy, abdominal hysterectomy, or cesarean section.
If there are signs of infection, specimens for culture should be obtained for identification of the causative organism so that appropriate treatment may be instituted.

*******B. fragilis, B. distasonis, B. ovatus, B. thetaiotaomicron.*

CONTRAINDICATIONS

MEFOXIN is contraindicated in patients who have shown hypersensitivity to cefoxitin and the cephalosporin group of antibiotics.

WARNINGS

BEFORE THERAPY WITH 'MEFOXIN' IS INSTITUTED, CAREFUL INQUIRY SHOULD BE MADE TO DETER-

Continued on next page

Information on the Merck & Co., Inc. products listed on these pages is the full prescribing information from product circulars in use August 31, 1998. For information, please call 1-800-NSC MERCK [1-800-672-6372].

Mefoxin—Cont.

MINE WHETHER THE PATIENT HAS HAD PREVIOUS HYPERSENSITIVITY REACTIONS TO CEFOXITIN, CEPHALOSPORINS, PENICILLINS, OR OTHER DRUGS. THIS PRODUCT SHOULD BE GIVEN WITH CAUTION TO PENICILLIN-SENSITIVE PATIENTS. ANTIBIOTICS SHOULD BE ADMINISTERED WITH CAUTION TO ANY PATIENT WHO HAS DEMONSTRATED SOME FORM OF ALLERGY, PARTICULARLY TO DRUGS. IF AN ALLERGIC REACTION TO 'MEFOXIN' OCCURS, DISCONTINUE THE DRUG. SERIOUS HYPERSENSITIVITY REACTIONS MAY REQUIRE EPINEPHRINE AND OTHER EMERGENCY MEASURES.

Pseudomembranous colitis has been reported with nearly all antibacterial agents, including cefoxitin, and may range in severity from mild to life threatening. Therefore, it is important to consider this diagnosis in patients who present with diarrhea subsequent to the administration of antibacterial agents.

Treatment with antibacterial agents alters the normal flora of the colon and my permit overgrowth of clostridia. Studies indicate that a toxin produced by *Clostridium difficile* is one primary cause of "antibiotic-associated colitis."

After the diagnosis of pseudomembranous colitis has been established, appropriate therapeutic measures should be initiated. Mild cases of pseudomembranous colitis usually respond to drug discontinuation alone. In moderate to severe cases, consideration should be given to management with fluids and electrolytes, protein supplementation, and treatment with an antibacterial drug clinically effective against *Clostridium difficile* colitis.

PRECAUTIONS

General
The total daily dose should be reduced when MEFOXIN is administered to patients with transient or persistent reduction of urinary output due to renal insufficiency (see DOSAGE AND ADMINISTRATION), because high and prolonged serum antibiotic concentrations can occur in such individuals from usual doses.

Antibiotics (including cephalosporins) should be prescribed with caution in individuals with a history of gastrointestinal disease, particularly colitis.

As with other antibiotics, prolonged use of MEFOXIN may result in overgrowth of nonsusceptible organisms. Repeated evaluation of the patient's condition is essential. If superinfection occurs during therapy, appropriate measures should be taken.

Laboratory Tests
As with any potent antibacterial agent, periodic assessment of organ system functions, including renal, hepatic, and hematopoietic, is advisable during prolonged therapy.

Drug Interactions
Increased nephrotoxicity has been reported following concomitant administration of cephalosporins and aminoglycoside antibiotics.

Drug/Laboratory Test Interactions
As with cephalothin, high concentrations of cefoxitin (>100 micrograms/mL) may interfere with measurement of serum and urine creatinine levels by the Jaffé reaction, and produce false increases of modest degree in the levels of creatinine reported. Serum samples from patients treated with cefoxitin should not be analyzed for creatinine if withdrawn within 2 hours of drug administration.

High concentrations of cefoxitin in the urine may interfere with measurement of urinary 17-hydroxy-corticosteroids by the Porter-Silber reaction, and produce false increases of modest degree in the levels reported.

A false-positive reaction for glucose in the urine may occur. This has been observed with CLINITEST* reagent tablets.

Carcinogenesis, Mutagenesis, Impairment of Fertility
Long-term studies in animals have not been performed with cefoxitin to evaluate carcinogenic or mutagenic potential. Studies in rats treated intravenously with 400 mg/kg of cefoxitin (approximately three times the maximum recommended human dose) revealed no effects on fertility or mating ability.

Pregnancy
Pregnancy Category B. Reproduction studies performed in rats and mice at parenteral doses of approximately one to seven and one-half times the maximum recommended human dose did not reveal teratogenic or fetal toxic effects, although a slight decrease in fetal weight was observed.

There are, however, no adequate and well-controlled studies in pregnant women. Because animal reproduction studies are not always predictive of human response, this drug should be used during pregnancy only if clearly needed.

In the rabbit, cefoxitin was associated with a high incidence of abortion and maternal death. This was not considered to be a teratogenic effect but an expected consequence of the rabbit's unusual sensitivity to antibiotic-induced changes in the population of the microflora of the intestine.

Nursing Mothers
MEFOXIN is excreted in human milk in low concentrations. Caution should be exercised when MEFOXIN is administered to a nursing woman.

Pediatric Use
Safety and efficacy in pediatric patients from birth to three months of age have not yet been established. In pediatric patients three months of age and older, higher doses of MEFOXIN have been associated with an increased incidence of eosinophilia and elevated SGOT.

* Registered trademark of Ames Company, Division of Miles Laboratories, Inc.

ADVERSE REACTIONS

MEFOXIN is generally well tolerated. The most common adverse reactions have been local reactions following intravenous injection. Other adverse reactions have been encountered infrequently.

Local Reactions
Thrombophlebitis has occurred with intravenous administration.

Allergic Reactions
Rash (including exfoliative dermatitis and toxic epidermal necrolysis), pruritus, eosinophilia, fever, dyspnea, and other allergic reactions including anaphylaxis, interstitial nephritis and angioedema have been noted.

Cardiovascular
Hypotension

Gastrointestinal
Diarrhea, including documented pseudomembranous colitis which can appear during or after antibiotic treatment. Nausea and vomiting have been reported rarely.

Neuromuscular
Possible exacerbation of myasthenia gravis

Blood
Eosinophilia, leukopenia, including granulocytopenia, neutropenia, anemia, including hemolytic anemia, thrombocytopenia, and bone marrow depression. A positive direct Coombs test may develop in some individuals, especially those with azotemia.

Liver Function
Transient elevations in SGOT, SGPT, serum LDH, serum alkaline phosphatase; and jaundice have been reported.

Renal Function
Elevations in serum creatinine and/or blood urea nitrogen levels have been observed. As with the cephalosporins, acute renal failure has been reported rarely. The role of MEFOXIN in changes in renal function tests is difficult to assess, since factors predisposing to prerenal azotemia or to impaired renal function usually have been present.

In addition to the adverse reactions listed above which have been observed in patients treated with MEFOXIN, the following adverse reactions and altered laboratory test results have been reported for cephalosporin class antibiotics:
Urticaria, erythema multiforme, Stevens-Johnson syndrome, serum sickness-like reactions, abdominal pain, colitis, renal dysfunction, toxic nephropathy, false-positive test for urinary glucose, hepatic dysfunction including cholestasis, elevated bilirubin, aplastic anemia, hemorrhage, prolonged prothrombin time, pancytopenia, agranulocytosis, superinfection, vaginitis including vaginal candidiasis.

Several cephalosporins have been implicated in triggering seizures, particularly in patients with renal impairment when the dosage was not reduced. (See DOSAGE AND ADMINISTRATION.) If seizures associated with drug therapy occur, the drug should be discontinued. Anticonvulsant therapy can be given if clinically indicated.

OVERDOSAGE

The acute intravenous LD_{50} in the adult female mouse and rabbit was about 8.0 g/kg and greater than 1.0 g/kg respectively. The acute intraperitoneal LD_{50} in the adult rat was greater than 10.0 g/kg.

DOSAGE AND ADMINISTRATION

TREATMENT
Adults
The usual adult dosage range is 1 gram to 2 grams every six to eight hours. Dosage should be determined by susceptibility of the causative organisms, severity of infection, and the condition of the patient (see Table 1 for dosage guidelines). If *C. trachomatis* is a suspected pathogen, appropriate antichlamydial coverage should be added, because cefoxitin sodium has no activity against this organism.
[See table 1 above]
MEFOXIN may be used in patients with reduced renal function with the following dosage adjustments:
In adults with renal insufficiency, an initial loading dose of 1 gram to 2 grams may be given. After a loading dose, the recommendations for *maintenance dosage* (Table 2) may be used as a guide.
[See table 2 above]
When only the serum creatinine level is available, the following formula (based on sex, weight, and age of the patient) may be used to convert this value into creatinine clearance. The serum creatinine should represent a steady state of renal function.

Table 1—Guidelines for Dosage of MEFOXIN

Type of Infection	Daily Dosage	Frequency and Route
Uncomplicated forms* of infections such as pneumonia, urinary tract infection, cutaneous infection	3–4 grams	1 gram every 6–8 hours IV
Moderately severe or severe infections	6–8 grams	1 gram every 4 hours *or* 2 grams every 6–8 hours IV
Infections commonly needing antibiotics in higher dosage (e.g., gas gangrene)	12 grams	2 grams every 4 hours *or* 3 grams every 6 hours IV

*Including patients in whom bacteremia is absent or unlikely

Table 2—Maintenance Dosage of MEFOXIN in Adults with Reduced Renal Function

Renal Function	Creatinine Clearance (mL/min)	Dose (grams)	Frequency
Mild impairment	50–30	1–2	every 8–12 hours
Moderate impairment	29–10	1–2	every 12–24 hours
Severe impairment	9–5	0.5–1	every 12–24 hours
Essentially no function	<5	0.5–1	every 24–48 hours

Table 3—Preparation of Solution

MEFOXIN

Strength	Amount of Diluent to be Added (mL)*	Approximate Withdrawable Volume (mL)	Approximate Average Concentration (mg/mL)
1 gram Vial	10	10.5	95
2 gram Vial	10 or 20	11.1 or 21.0	180 or 95
1 gram Infusion Bottle	50 or 100	50 or 100	20 or 10
2 gram Infusion Bottle	50 or 100	50 or 100	40 or 20
10 gram Bulk	43 or 93	49 or 98.5	200 or 100

*Shake to dissolve and let stand until clear.

Males: $\frac{\text{Weight (kg)} \times (140 - \text{age})}{72 \times \text{serum creatinine (mg/100 mL)}}$

Females: $0.85 \times$ above value

In patients undergoing hemodialysis, the loading dose of 1 to 2 grams should be given after each hemodialysis, and the maintenance dose should be given as indicated in Table 2.

Antibiotic therapy for group A beta-hemolytic streptococcal infections should be maintained for at least 10 days to guard against the risk of rheumatic fever or glomerulonephritis. In staphylococcal and other infections involving a collection of pus, surgical drainage should be carried out where indicated.

Pediatric Patients

The recommended dosage in pediatric patients three months of age and older is 80 to 160 mg/kg of body weight per day divided into four to six equal doses. The higher dosages should be used for more severe or serious infections. The total daily dosage should not exceed 12 grams.

At this time no recommendation is made for pediatric patients from birth to three months of age (see PRECAUTIONS).

In pediatric patients with renal insufficiency, the dosage and frequency of dosage should be modified consistent with the recommendations for adults (see Table 2).

PREVENTION

Effective prophylactic use depends on the time of administration. MEFOXIN usually should be given one-half to one hour before the operation, which is sufficient time to achieve effective levels in the wound during the procedure. Prophylactic administration should usually be stopped within 24 hours since continuing administration of any antibiotic increases the possibility of adverse reactions but, in the majority of surgical procedures, does not reduce the incidence of subsequent infection.

For prophylactic use in uncontaminated gastrointestinal surgery, vaginal hysterectomy, or abdominal hysterectomy, the following doses are recommended:

Adults:

2 grams administered intravenously just prior to surgery (approximately one-half to one hour before the initial incision) followed by 2 grams every 6 hours after the first dose for no more than 24 hours.

Pediatric Patients (3 months and older):

30 to 40 mg/kg doses may be given at the times designated above.

Cesarean section patients:

For patients undergoing cesarean section, either a single 2 gram dose administered intravenously as soon as the umbilical cord is clamped OR a 3-dose regimen consisting of 2 grams given intravenously as soon as the umbilical cord is clamped followed by 2 grams 4 and 8 hours after the initial dose is recommended. (See CLINICAL STUDIES.)

* Registered trademark of MERCK & CO., INC.

PREPARATION OF SOLUTION

Table 3 is provided for convenience in constituting MEFOXIN for intravenous administration.

For Vials

One gram should be constituted with at least 10 mL, and 2 grams with 10 or 20 mL, of Sterile Water for Injection, Bacteriostatic Water for Injection, 0.9 percent Sodium Chloride Injection, or 5 percent Dextrose Injection. These primary solutions may be further diluted in 50 to 1000 mL of the diluents listed under the *Vials and Bulk Packages* portion of the *COMPATIBILITY AND STABILITY* section.

For Bulk Packages

The 10 gram bulk packages should be constituted with 43 or 93 mL of Sterile Water for Injection, Bacteriostatic Water for Injection, 0.9 percent Sodium Chloride Injection, or 5 percent Dextrose Injection. CAUTION: THE 10 GRAM BULK STOCK SOLUTION IS NOT FOR DIRECT INFUSION. These primary solutions may be further diluted in 50 to 1000 mL of the diluents listed under the *Vials and Bulk Packages* portion of the *COMPATIBILITY AND STABILITY* section.

Benzyl alcohol as a preservative has been associated with toxicity in neonates. While toxicity has not been demonstrated in pediatric patients greater than three months of age, in whom use of MEFOXIN may be indicated, small pediatric patients in this age range may also be at risk for benzyl alcohol toxicity. Therefore, diluent containing benzyl alcohol should not be used when MEFOXIN is constituted for administration to pediatric patients in this age range.

For Infusion Bottles

One or 2 grams of MEFOXIN for infusion may be constituted with 50 or 100 mL of 0.9 percent Sodium Chloride Injection, or 5 percent or 10 percent Dextrose Injection.

For ADD-Vantage®† Vials

See separate INSTRUCTIONS FOR USE OF MEFOXIN IN ADD-Vantage® VIALS. MEFOXIN in ADD-Vantage® vials should be constituted with ADD-Vantage® diluent containers containing 50 mL or 100 mL of either 0.9 percent Sodium Chloride Injection or 5 percent Dextrose Injection. MEFOXIN in ADD-Vantage® vials is for IV use only.

[See table three at top of previous page]

†Registered trademark of Abbott Laboratories.

ADMINISTRATION

MEFOXIN may be administered intravenously after constitution.

Parenteral drug products should be inspected visually for particulate matter and discoloration prior to administration whenever solution and container permit.

Intravenous Administration

The intravenous route is preferable for patients with bacteremia, bacterial septicemia, or other severe or life-threatening infections, or for patients who may be poor risks because of lowered resistance resulting from such debilitating conditions as malnutrition, trauma, surgery, diabetes, heart failure, or malignancy, particularly if shock is present or impending.

For intermittent intravenous administration, a solution containing 1 gram or 2 grams in 10 mL of Sterile Water for Injection can be injected over a period of three to five minutes. Using an infusion system, it may also be given over a longer period of time through the tubing system by which the patient may be receiving other intravenous solutions. However, during infusion of the solution containing MEFOXIN, it is advisable to temporarily discontinue administration of any other solutions at the same site.

For the administration of higher doses by continuous intravenous infusion, a solution of MEFOXIN may be added to an intravenous bottle containing 5 percent Dextrose Injection, 0.9 percent Sodium Chloride Injection, or 5 percent Dextrose and 0.9 percent Sodium Chloride Injection. BUTTERFLY† or scalp vein-type needles are preferred for this type of infusion.

Solutions of MEFOXIN, like those of most beta-lactam antibiotics, should not be added to aminoglycoside solutions (e.g., gentamicin sulfate, tobramycin sulfate, amikacin sulfate) because of potential interaction. However, MEFOXIN and aminoglycosides may be administered separately to the same patient.

† Registered trademark of Abbott Laboratories.

COMPATIBILITY AND STABILITY

Vials and Bulk Packages

MEFOXIN, as supplied in vials or the bulk package and constituted to 1 gram/10 mL with Sterile Water for Injection, Bacteriostatic Water for Injection (see *PREPARATION OF SOLUTION*), 0.9 percent Sodium Chloride Injection, or 5 percent Dextrose Injection, maintains satisfactory potency for 6 hours at room temperature or for one week under refrigeration (below 5°C).

These primary solutions may be further diluted in 50 to 1000 mL of the following diluents and maintain potency for an additional 18 hours at room temperature or an additional 48 hours under refrigeration:

- 0.9 percent Sodium Chloride Injection
- 5 percent or 10 percent Dextrose Injection
- 5 percent Dextrose and 0.9 percent Sodium Chloride Injection
- 5 percent Dextrose Injection with 0.2 percent or 0.45 percent saline solution
- Lactated Ringer's Injection
- 5 percent Dextrose in Lactated Ringer's Injection
- 10 percent invert sugar in water
- 10 percent invert sugar in saline solution
- 5 percent Sodium Bicarbonate Injection
- M/6 sodium lactate solution
- Mannitol 5% and 10%

Infusion Bottles

MEFOXIN, as supplied in infusion bottles and constituted with 50 to 100 mL of 0.9 percent Sodium Chloride Injection, or 5 percent or 10 percent Dextrose Injection, maintains satisfactory potency for 24 hours at room temperature or for 1 week under refrigeration (below 5°C).

ADD-Vantage® Vials

MEFOXIN is supplied in single dose ADD-Vantage® vials and should be prepared as directed in the accompanying INSTRUCTIONS FOR USE OF MEFOXIN IN ADD-Vantage® VIALS using ADD-Vantage® diluent containers containing 50 mL or 100 mL of either 0.9 percent Sodium Chloride Injection or 5 percent Dextrose Injection. When prepared with either of these diluents, MEFOXIN maintains satisfactory potency for 24 hours at room temperature.

After the periods mentioned above, any unused solutions should be discarded.

HOW SUPPLIED

Sterile MEFOXIN is a dry white to off-white powder supplied in vials and infusion bottles containing cefoxitin sodium as follows:

No. 3356—1 gram cefoxitin equivalent
NDC 0006-3356-45 in trays of 25 vials
(6505-01-119-6005, 1 g 25's).

No. 3368—1 gram cefoxitin equivalent
NDC 0006-3368-71 in trays of 10 infusion bottles
(6505-01-195-0649, 1 g infusion bottle 10's).

No. 3357—2 gram cefoxitin equivalent
NDC 0006-3357-53 in trays of 25 vials
(6505-01-104-6393, 2 g 25's).

No. 3369—2 gram cefoxitin equivalent
NDC 0006-3369-73 in trays of 10 infusion bottles
(6505-01-185-2624, 2 g infusion bottle 10's).

No. 3388—10 gram cefoxitin equivalent
NDC 0006-3388-67 in trays of 6 bulk bottles
(6505-01-263-0730, 10 g 6's).

No. 3548—1 gram cefoxitin equivalent
NDC 0006-3548-45 in trays of 25 ADD-Vantage® vials.
(6505-01-262-9509, 1 g ADD-Vantage® 25's).

No. 3549—2 gram cefoxitin equivalent
NDC 0006-3549-53 in trays of 25 ADD-Vantage® vials.
(6505-01-263-4531, 2 g ADD-Vantage® 25's).

Special storage instructions

MEFOXIN in the dry state should be stored between 2–25°C (36–77°F). Avoid exposure to temperatures above 50°C. The dry material as well as solutions tend to darken, depending on storage conditions; product potency, however, is not adversely affected.

CLINICAL STUDIES

A prospective, randomized, double-blind, placebo-controlled clinical trial was conducted to determine the efficacy of short-term prophylaxis with MEFOXIN in patients undergoing cesarean section who were at high risk for subsequent endometritis because of ruptured membranes. Patients were randomized to receive either three doses of placebo (n=58), a single dose of MEFOXIN (2 g) followed by two doses of placebo (n=64), or a three-dose regimen of MEFOXIN (each dose consisting of 2 g) (n=60), given intravenously, usually beginning at the time of clamping of the umbilical cord, with the second and third doses given 4 and 8 hours post-operatively. Endometritis occurred in 16/58 (27.6%) patients given placebo, 5/63 (7.9%) patients given a single dose of MEFOXIN, and 3/58 (5.2%) patients given three doses of MEFOXIN. The differences between the two groups treated with MEFOXIN and placebo with respect to endometritis were statistically significant ($p<0.01$) in favor of MEFOXIN. The differences between the one-dose and three-dose regimens of MEFOXIN were not statistically significant.

Two double-blind, randomized studies compared the efficacy of a single 2 gram intravenous dose of MEFOXIN to a single 2 gram dose of cefotetan in the prevention of surgical site-related infection (major morbidity) and non-site-related infections (minor morbidity) in patients following cesarean section. In the first study, 82/98 (83.7%) patients treated with MEFOXIN and 71/95 (74.7%) patients treated with cefotetan experienced no major or minor morbidity. The difference in the outcomes in this study (95% CI: −0.03, +0.21) was not statistically significant. In the second study, 65/75 (86.7%) patients treated with MEFOXIN and 62/76 (81.6%) patients treated with cefotetan experienced no major or minor morbidity. The difference in the outcomes in this study (95% CI: −0.08, +0.18) was not statistically significant.

In clinical trials of patients with intra-abdominal infections due to *Bacteroides fragilis* group microorganisms, eradication rates at 1 to 2 weeks posttreatment for isolates were in the range of 70% to 80%. Eradication rates for individual species are listed below:

Bacteroides distasonis	7/10	(70%)
Bacteroides fragilis	26/33	(79%)
Bacteroides ovatus	10/13	(77%)
B. thetaiotaomicron	13/18	(72%)

7882337 Issued October 1996

MEFOXIN®
Premixed Intravenous Solution
(Cefoxitin Injection) ℞

DESCRIPTION

Cefoxitin sodium is a semi-synthetic, broad-spectrum cepha antibiotic for intravenous administration. It is derived from cephamycin C, which is produced by *Streptomyces lactamdurans.* Its chemical name is sodium (6*R*,7*S*)-3-(hydroxymethyl)-7-methoxy-8-oxo-7-[2- (2-thienyl)acetamido]-5-thia-1-azabicyclo [4.2.0]oct-2-ene-2-carboxylate carbamate (ester). The empirical formula is $C_{16}H_{16}N_3NaO_7S_2$, and the molecular weight is 449.44. The structural formula is:

[See chemical structure at top of next column]

Cefoxitin sodium contains approximately 53.8 mg (2.3 milliequivalents) of sodium per gram of cefoxitin activity.

Continued on next page

Information on the Merck & Co., Inc. products listed on these pages is the full prescribing information from product circulars in use August 31, 1998. For information, please call 1-800-NSC MERCK [1-800-672-6372].

Mefoxin Premixed—Cont.

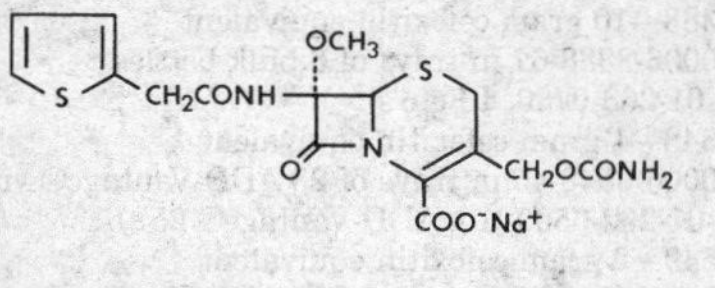

Premixed Intravenous Solution MEFOXIN* (Cefoxitin Sodium Injection) is supplied as a sterile, nonpyrogenic, frozen, iso-osmotic solution of cefoxitin sodium. Each 50 mL contains cefoxitin sodium equivalent to either 1 gram or 2 grams cefoxitin. Dextrose hydrous USP has been added to the above dosages to adjust osmolality (approximately 2 grams and 1.1 grams to 1 gram and 2 gram dosages, respectively). The pH is adjusted with sodium bicarbonate and may have been adjusted with hydrochloric acid. The pH is approximately 6.5. After thawing, the solution is intended for intravenous use only. Solutions of MEFOXIN range from colorless to light amber.

The plastic container is fabricated from a specially designed multilayer plastic (PL 2040). Solutions are in contact with the polyethylene layer of this container and can leach out certain chemical components of the plastic in very small amounts within the expiration period. The suitability and safety of the plastic have been confirmed in tests in animals according to the USP biological tests for plastic containers, as well as by tissue culture toxicity studies.

*Registered trademark of MERCK & CO., INC.

CLINICAL PHARMACOLOGY

Clinical Pharmacology

Following an intravenous dose of 1 gram of cefoxitin, serum concentrations were 110 mcg/mL at 5 minutes, declining to less than 1 mcg/mL at 4 hours. The half-life after an intravenous dose is 41 to 59 minutes. Approximately 85 percent of cefoxitin is excreted unchanged by the kidneys over a 6-hour period, resulting in high urinary concentrations. Probenecid slows tubular excretion and produces higher serum levels and increases the duration of measurable serum concentrations.

Cefoxitin passes into pleural and joint fluids and is detectable in antibacterial concentrations in bile.

Microbiology

The bactericidal action of cefoxitin results from inhibition of cell wall synthesis. Cefoxitin has *in vitro* activity against a wide range of gram-positive and gram-negative organisms. The methoxy group in the 7α position provides MEFOXIN with a high degree of stability in the presence of beta-lactamases, both penicillinases and cephalosporinases, of gram-negative bacteria. While *in vitro* studies have demonstrated the susceptibility of most strains of the following organisms, clinical efficacy for infections other than those included in the INDICATIONS AND USAGE section is unknown.

Gram-positive

- *Staphylococcus aureus,* including penicillinase and non-penicillinase producing strains
- *Staphylococcus epidermidis*
- Beta-hemolytic and other streptococci (most strains of enterococci, e.g., *Enterococcus faecalis* [formerly *Streptococcus faecalis*], are resistant)
- *Streptococcus pneumoniae*

Gram-negative

- *Eikenella corrodens* (beta-lactamase negative strains)
- *Escherichia coli*
- *Klebsiella* species (including *K. pneumoniae)*
- *Haemophilus influenzae*
- *Neisseria gonorrhoeae,* including penicillinase and non-penicillinase producing strains
- *Proteus mirabilis*
- *Morganella morganii*
- *Proteus vulgaris*
- *Providencia* species, including *Providencia rettgeri*

Anaerobic organisms

- *Peptococcus niger*
- *Peptostreptococcus* species
- *Clostridium* species
- *Bacteroides* species, including the *B. fragilis* group (includes *B. fragilis, B. distasonis, B. ovatus, B. thetaiotaomicron)*

MEFOXIN is inactive *in vitro* against most strains of *Pseudomonas aeruginosa* and enterococci and many strains of *Enterobacter cloacae.*

Methicillin-resistant staphylococci are almost uniformly resistant to MEFOXIN.

Susceptibility Tests

For fast-growing aerobic organisms, quantitative methods that require measurements of zone diameters give the most precise estimates of antibiotic susceptibility. One such procedure* has been recommended for use with discs to test susceptibility to cefoxitin. Interpretation involves correlation of the diameters obtained in the disc test with minimal inhibitory concentration (MIC) values for cefoxitin.

Reports from the laboratory giving results of the standardized single disc susceptibility test* using a 30 mcg cefoxitin disc should be interpreted according to the following criteria:

Organisms producing zones of 18 mm or greater are considered susceptible, indicating that the tested organism is likely to respond to therapy.

Organisms of intermediate susceptibility produce zones of 15 to 17 mm, indicating that the tested organism would be susceptible if high dosage is used or if the infection is confined to tissues and fluids (e.g., urine) in which high antibiotic levels are attained.

Resistant organisms produce zones of 14 mm or less, indicating that other therapy should be selected.

The cefoxitin disc should be used for testing cefoxitin susceptibility.

Cefoxitin has been shown by *in vitro* tests to have activity against certain strains of *Enterobacteriaceae* found resistant when tested with the cephalosporin class disc. For this reason, the cefoxitin disc should not be used for testing susceptibility to cephalosporins, and cephalosporin discs should not be used for testing susceptibility to cefoxitin.

Dilution methods, preferably the agar plate dilution procedure, are most accurate for susceptibility testing of obligate anaerobes.

A bacterial isolate may be considered susceptible if the MIC value for cefoxitin** is not more than 16 mcg/mL. Organisms are considered resistant if the MIC is greater than 32 mcg/mL.

* Bauer, A. W.; Kirby, W. M. M.; Sherris, J. C.; Turck, M.: Antibiotic susceptibility testing by a standardized single disc method, Amer. J. Clin. Path. *45* : 493–496, Apr. 1966. Standardized disc susceptibility test, Federal Register *37* : 20527–20529, 1972. National Committee for Clinical Laboratory Standards: Performance Standards for Antimicrobial Disc Susceptibility Tests—Fifth Edition; Approved Standard, NCCLS Document M2-A5, Vol 13, No. 24, NCCLS, Villanova, PA, December 1993.

** Determined by the ICS agar dilution method (Ericsson and Sherris, Acta Path. Microbiol. Scand. [B] Suppl. No. 217, 1971) or any other method that has been shown to give equivalent results.

INDICATIONS AND USAGE

MEFOXIN, supplied as a premixed solution in plastic containers, is intended for intravenous use only.

Treatment

MEFOXIN is indicated for the treatment of serious infections caused by susceptible strains of the designated microorganisms in the diseases listed below.

(1) **Lower respiratory tract infections,** including pneumonia and lung abscess, caused by *Streptococcus pneumoniae,* other streptococci (excluding enterococci, e.g., *Enterococcus faecalis* [formerly *Streptococcus faecalis*]), *Staphylococcus aureus* (penicillinase and non-penicillinase producing), *Escherichia coli, Klebsiella* species, *Haemophilus influenzae,* and *Bacteroides* species.

(2) **Urinary tract infections** caused by *Escherichia coli, Klebsiella* species, *Proteus mirabilis, Morganella morganii, Proteus vulgaris* and *Providencia* species (including *P. rettgeri*).

(3) **Intra-abdominal infections,** including peritonitis and intra-abdominal abscess, caused by *Escherichia coli, Klebsiella* species, *Bacteroides* species including the *Bacteroides fragilis* group***, and *Clostridium* species.

(4) **Gynecological infections,** including endometritis, pelvic cellulitis, and pelvic inflammatory disease caused by *Escherichia coli, Neisseria gonorrhoeae* (penicillinase and non-penicillinase producing), *Bacteroides* species including *B. fragilis, Clostridium* species, *Peptococcus niger, Peptostreptococcus* species, and Group B streptococci. MEFOXIN, like cephalosporins, has no activity against *Chlamydia trachomatis.* Therefore, when MEFOXIN is used in the treatment of patients with pelvic inflammatory disease and *C. trachomatis* is one of the suspected pathogens, appropriate antichlamydial coverage should be added.

(5) **Septicemia** caused by *Streptococcus pneumoniae, Staphylococcus aureus* (penicillinase and non-penicillinase producing), *Escherichia coli, Klebsiella* species, and *Bacteroides* species including *B. fragilis.*

(6) **Bone and joint infections** caused by *Staphylococcus aureus* (penicillinase and non-penicillinase producing).

(7) **Skin and skin structure infections** caused by *Staphylococcus aureus* (penicillinase and non-penicillinase producing), *Staphylococcus epidermidis,* streptococci (excluding enterococci, e.g., *Enterococcus faecalis* [formerly *Streptococcus faecalis*]), *Escherichia coli, Proteus mirabilis, Klebsiella* species, *Bacteroides* species including *B. fragilis, Clostridium* species, *Peptococcus niger,* and *Peptostreptococcus* species.

Appropriate culture and susceptibility studies should be performed to determine the susceptibility of the causative organisms to MEFOXIN. Therapy may be started while awaiting the results of these studies.

In randomized comparative studies, cefoxitin and cephalothin were comparably safe and effective in the management of infections caused by gram-positive cocci and gram-negative rods susceptible to the cephalosporins. MEFOXIN has a high degree of stability in the presence of bacterial beta-lactamases, both penicillinases and cephalosporinases.

Many infections caused by aerobic and anaerobic gram-negative bacteria resistant to some cephalosporins respond to MEFOXIN. Similarly, many infections caused by aerobic and anaerobic bacteria resistant to some penicillin antibiotics (ampicillin, carbenicillin, penicillin G) respond to treatment with MEFOXIN. Many infections caused by mixtures of susceptible aerobic and anaerobic bacteria respond to treatment with MEFOXIN.

Prevention

MEFOXIN is indicated for the prophylaxis of infection in patients undergoing uncontaminated gastrointestinal surgery, vaginal hysterectomy, abdominal hysterectomy, or cesarean section.

If there are signs of infection, specimens for culture should be obtained for identification of the causative organism so that appropriate treatment may be instituted.

*** *B. fragilis, B. distasonis, B. ovatus, B. thetaiotaomicron.*

CONTRAINDICATIONS

MEFOXIN is contraindicated in patients who have shown hypersensitivity to cefoxitin and the cephalosporin group of antibiotics.

WARNINGS

BEFORE THERAPY WITH 'MEFOXIN' IS INSTITUTED, CAREFUL INQUIRY SHOULD BE MADE TO DETERMINE WHETHER THE PATIENT HAS HAD PREVIOUS HYPERSENSITIVITY REACTIONS TO CEFOXITIN, CEPHALOSPORINS, PENICILLINS, OR OTHER DRUGS. THIS PRODUCT SHOULD BE GIVEN WITH CAUTION TO PENICILLIN-SENSITIVE PATIENTS. ANTIBIOTICS SHOULD BE ADMINISTERED WITH CAUTION TO ANY PATIENT WHO HAS DEMONSTRATED SOME FORM OF ALLERGY, PARTICULARLY TO DRUGS. IF AN ALLERGIC REACTION TO 'MEFOXIN' OCCURS, DISCONTINUE THE DRUG. SERIOUS HYPERSENSITIVITY REACTIONS MAY REQUIRE EPINEPHRINE AND OTHER EMERGENCY MEASURES.

Pseudomembranous colitis has been reported with nearly all antibacterial agents, including cefoxitin, and may range in severity from mild to life threatening. Therefore, it is important to consider this diagnosis in patients who present with diarrhea subsequent to the administration of antibacterial agents.

Treatment with antibacterial agents alters the normal flora of the colon and may permit overgrowth of clostridia. Studies indicate that a toxin produced by *Clostridium difficile* is one primary cause of "antibiotic-associated colitis."

After the diagnosis of pseudomembranous colitis has been established, appropriate therapeutic measures should be initiated. Mild cases of pseudomembranous colitis usually respond to drug discontinuation alone. In moderate to severe cases, consideration should be given to management with fluids and electrolytes, protein supplementation, and treatment with an antibacterial drug clinically effective against *Clostridium difficile* colitis.

PRECAUTIONS

General

The total daily dose should be reduced when MEFOXIN is administered to patients with transient or persistent reduction of urinary output due to renal insufficiency (see DOSAGE AND ADMINISTRATION, *TREATMENT*), because high and prolonged serum antibiotic concentrations can occur in such individuals from usual doses.

Antibiotics (including cephalosporins) should be prescribed with caution in individuals with a history of gastrointestinal disease, particularly colitis.

As with other antibiotics, prolonged use of MEFOXIN may result in overgrowth of nonsusceptible organisms. Repeated evaluation of the patient's condition is essential. If superinfection occurs during therapy, appropriate measures should be taken.

Do not use unless solution is clear and seal is intact.

Laboratory Tests

As with any potent antibacterial agent, periodic assessment of organ system functions, including renal, hepatic, and hematopoietic, is advisable during prolonged therapy.

Drug Interactions

Increased nephrotoxicity has been reported following concomitant administration of cephalosporins and aminoglycoside antibiotics.

Drug/Laboratory Test Interactions
As with cephalothin, high concentrations of cefoxitin (>100 micrograms/mL) may interfere with measurement of serum and urine creatinine levels by the Jaffé reaction, and produce false increases of modest degree in the levels of creatinine reported. Serum samples from patients treated with cefoxitin should not be analyzed for creatinine if withdrawn within 2 hours of drug administration.

High concentrations of cefoxitin in the urine may interfere with measurement of urinary 17-hydroxy-corticosteroids by the Porter-Silber reaction, and produce false increases of modest degree in the levels reported.

A false-positive reaction for glucose in the urine may occur. This has been observed with CLINITEST* reagent tablets.

---

* Registered trademark of Ames Company, Division of Miles Laboratories, Inc.

Carcinogenesis, Mutagenesis, Impairment of Fertility
Long term studies in animals have not been performed with cefoxitin to evaluate carcinogenic or mutagenic potential. Studies in rats treated intravenously with 400 mg/kg of cefoxitin (approximately three times the maximum recommended human dose) revealed no effects on fertility or mating ability.

Pregnancy
Pregnancy Category B. Reproduction studies performed in rats and mice at parenteral doses of approximately one to seven and one-half times the maximum recommended human dose did not reveal teratogenic or fetal toxic effects, although a slight decrease in fetal weight was observed.

There are, however, no adequate and well-controlled studies in pregnant women. Because animal reproduction studies are not always predictive of human response, this drug should be used during pregnancy only if clearly needed.

In the rabbit, cefoxitin was associated with a high incidence of abortion and maternal death. This was not considered to be a teratogenic effect but an expected consequence of the rabbit's unusual sensitivity to antibiotic-induced changes in the population of the microflora of the intestine.

Nursing Mothers
Cefoxitin is excreted in human milk in low concentrations. Caution should be exercised when MEFOXIN is administered to a nursing woman.

Pediatric Use
Safety and efficacy in pediatric patients from birth to three months of age have not yet been established. In pediatric patients three months of age and older, higher doses of cefoxitin have been associated with an increased incidence of eosinophilia and elevated SGOT.

The potential for toxic effects in pediatric patients from chemicals that may leach from the single-dose I.V. preparation in plastic has not been determined.

ADVERSE REACTIONS

Cefoxitin is generally well tolerated. The most common adverse reactions have been local reactions following intravenous injection. Other adverse reactions have been encountered infrequently.

Local Reactions
Thrombophlebitis has occurred with intravenous administration.

Allergic Reactions
Rash (including exfoliative dermatitis and toxic epidermal necrolysis), pruritus, eosinophilia, fever, dyspnea, and other allergic reactions including anaphylaxis, interstitial nephritis and angioedema have been noted.

Cardiovascular
Hypotension

Gastrointestinal
Diarrhea, including documented pseudomembranous colitis which can appear during or after antibiotic treatment. Nausea and vomiting have been reported rarely.

Neuromuscular
Possible exacerbation of myasthenia gravis.

Blood
Eosinophilia, leukopenia including granulocytopenia, neutropenia, anemia, including hemolytic anemia, thrombocytopenia, and bone marrow depression. A positive direct Coombs test may develop in some individuals, especially those with azotemia.

Liver Function
Transient elevations in SGOT, SGPT, serum LDH, and serum alkaline phosphatase; and jaundice have been reported.

Renal Function
Elevations in serum creatinine and/or blood urea nitrogen levels have been observed. As with the cephalosporins, acute renal failure has been reported rarely. The role of MEFOXIN in changes in renal function tests is difficult to assess, since factors predisposing to prerenal azotemia or to impaired renal function usually have been present.

In addition to the adverse reactions listed above which have been observed in patients treated with MEFOXIN, the following adverse reactions and altered laboratory test results have been reported for cephalosporin class antibiotics:

Urticaria, erythema multiforme, Stevens-Johnson syndrome, serum sickness-like reactions, abdominal pain, colitis, renal dysfunction, toxic nephropathy, false-positive test for urinary glucose, hepatic dysfunction including cholestasis, elevated bilirubin, aplastic anemia, hemorrhage, prolonged prothrombin time, pancytopenia, agranulocytosis, superinfection, vaginitis including vaginal candidiasis.

Several cephalosporins have been implicated in triggering seizures, particularly in patients with renal impairment when the dosage was not reduced. (See DOSAGE AND ADMINISTRATION.) If seizures associated with drug therapy occur, the drug should be discontinued. Anticonvulsant therapy can be given if clinically indicated.

OVERDOSAGE

The acute intravenous LD_{50} in the adult female mouse and rabbit was about 8.0 g/kg and greater than 1.0 g/kg respectively. The acute intraperitoneal LD_{50} in the adult rat was greater than 10.0 g/kg.

DOSAGE AND ADMINISTRATION

NOTE: MEFOXIN® in Galaxy† container is for intravenous infusion only.
TREATMENT
Adults
The usual adult dosage range is 1 gram to 2 grams every six to eight hours. Dosage should be determined by susceptibility of the causative organisms, severity of infection, and the condition of the patient (see Table 1 for dosage guidelines). If *C. trachomatis* is a suspected pathogen, appropriate antichlamydial coverage should be added, because cefoxitin sodium has no activity against this organism.

MEFOXIN may be used in patients with reduced renal function with the following dosage adjustments:
In adults with renal insufficiency, an initial loading dose of 1 gram to 2 grams may be given. After a loading dose, the recommendations for *maintenance dosage* (Table 2) may be used as a guide.

When only the serum creatinine level is available, the following formula (based on sex, weight, and age of the patient) may be used to convert this value into creatinine clearance. The serum creatinine should represent a steady state of renal function.

Males:

$$\frac{\text{Weight (kg)} \times (140 - \text{age})}{72 \times \text{serum creatinine (mg/100 mL)}}$$

Females: $0.85 \times$ male value

In patients undergoing hemodialysis, the loading dose of 1 to 2 grams should be given after each hemodialysis, and the maintenance dose should be given as indicated in Table 2. Antibiotic therapy for group A beta-hemolytic streptococcal infections should be maintained for at least 10 days to guard against the risk of rheumatic fever or glomerulonephritis. In staphylococcal and other infections involving a collection of pus, surgical drainage should be carried out where indicated.

Pediatric Patients
The recommended dosage in pediatric patients three months of age and older is 80 to 160 mg/kg of body weight per day divided into four to six equal doses. The higher dosages should be used for more severe or serious infections. The total daily dosage should not exceed 12 grams.

At this time no recommendation is made for pediatric patients from birth to three months of age (see PRECAUTIONS).

In pediatric patients with renal insufficiency, the dosage and frequency of dosage should be modified consistent with the recommendations for adults (see Table 2).

Table 1—Guidelines for Dosage of MEFOXIN

Type of Infection	Daily Dosage	Frequency and Route
Uncomplicated forms* of infections such as pneumonia, urinary tract infection, cutaneous infection	3–4 grams	1 gram every 6–8 hours IV
Moderately severe or severe infections	6–8 grams	1 gram every 4 hours *or* 2 grams every 6–8 hours IV
Infections commonly needing antibiotics in higher dosage (e.g., gas gangrene)	12 grams	2 grams every 4 hours *or* 3 grams every 6 hours IV

* Including patients in whom bacteremia is absent or unlikely.

Table 2—Maintenance Dosage of MEFOXIN in Adults with Reduced Renal Function

Renal Function	Creatinine Clearance (mL/min)	Dose (grams)	Frequency
Mild impairment	50–30	1–2	every 8–12 hours
Moderate impairment	29–10	1–2	every 12–24 hours
Severe impairment	9–5	0.5–1	every 12–24 hours
Essentially no function	<5	0.5–1	every 24–48 hours

PREVENTION
Effective prophylactic use depends on the time of administration. MEFOXIN usually should be given one-half to one hour before the operation, which is sufficient time to achieve effective levels in the wound during the procedure. Prophylactic administration should usually be stopped within 24 hours since continuing administration of any antibiotic increases the possibility of adverse reactions but, in the majority of surgical procedures, does not reduce the incidence of subsequent infection.

For prophylactic use in uncontaminated gastrointestinal surgery, vaginal hysterectomy, or abdominal hysterectomy, the following doses are recommended:
Adults:
2 grams administered intravenously just prior to surgery (approximately one-half to one hour before the initial incision) followed by 2 grams every 6 hours after the first dose for no more than 24 hours.
Pediatric Patients (3 months and older):
30 to 40 mg/kg doses may be given at the times designated above.
Cesarean section patients:
For patients undergoing cesarean section, either a single 2 gram dose administered intravenously as soon as the umbilical cord is clamped OR a 3-dose regimen consisting of 2 grams given intravenously as soon as the umbilical cord is clamped followed by 2 grams 4 and 8 hours after the initial dose is recommended. (See CLINICAL STUDIES.)
[See table 1 above]
[See table 2 above]

ADMINISTRATION
This premixed solution is for intravenous use only. Premixed Intravenous Solution MEFOXIN in Galaxy® containers (PL 2040 Plastic) is to be administered either as a continuous or intermittent infusion using sterile equipment. Scalp vein-type needles are preferred for this type of infusion. It is recommended that the intravenous administration apparatus be replaced at least once every 48 hours.

The intravenous route is preferred for patients with bacteremia, bacterial septicemia, or other severe or life-threatening infections, or for patients who may be poor risks because of lowered resistance resulting from such debilitating conditions as malnutrition, trauma, surgery, diabetes, heart failure, or malignancy, particularly if shock is present or impending.

Directions for Use of Galaxy® Containers (PL 2040 Plastic)
Thaw frozen container at room temperature, 25°C (77°F), or under refrigeration, 2–8°C (36–46°F). DO NOT FORCE THAW BY IMMERSION IN WATER BATHS OR BY MICROWAVE IRRADIATION.

After thawing, check for minute leaks by squeezing container firmly. If leaks are detected, discard solution as sterility may be impaired.

The container should be visually inspected for particulate matter and discoloration prior to administration. Components of the solution may precipitate in the frozen state and will dissolve upon reaching room temperature with little or no agitation. Agitate after solution has reached room temperature.

Do not use if the solution is cloudy or a precipitate has formed. If any seals or outlet ports are not intact, the con-

Continued on next page

Information on the Merck & Co., Inc. products listed on these pages is the full prescribing information from product circulars in use August 31, 1998. For information, please call 1-800-NSC MERCK [1-800-672-6372].

Mefoxin Premixed—Cont.

tainer should be discarded. Solutions of MEFOXIN tend to darken depending on storage conditions; product potency, however, is not adversely affected.

Additives should not be introduced into this solution.

CAUTION: Do not use plastic containers in series connections. Such use would result in air embolism due to residual air being drawn from the primary container before administration of the fluid from the secondary container is complete.

Preparation for Intravenous Administration:
1. Suspend container from eyelet support.
2. Remove plastic protector from outlet port at bottom of container.
3. Attach administration set. Refer to complete directions accompanying set.

MEFOXIN may be administered through the tubing system by which the patient may be receiving other intravenous solutions. However, during infusion of the solution containing MEFOXIN, it is advisable to temporarily discontinue administration of any other solutions at the same site.

Solutions of MEFOXIN, like those of most beta-lactam antibiotics, should not be added to aminoglycoside solutions (e.g., gentamicin sulfate, tobramycin sulfate, amikacin sulfate) because of potential interaction. However, MEFOXIN and aminoglycosides may be administered separately to the same patient.

---

†Galaxy® is a registered trademark of Baxter International Inc.

STABILITY

MEFOXIN, supplied as frozen, premixed, iso-osmotic solution in Galaxy® containers (PL 2040 Plastic), maintains satisfactory potency after thawing for 24 hours at a room temperature of 25°C (77°F) or 21 days under refrigeration, 2–8°C (36–46°F). After these periods, any unused solutions should be discarded.
DO NOT REFREEZE.

HOW SUPPLIED

Premixed Intravenous Solution MEFOXIN is supplied in single dose Galaxy® containers (PL 2040 Plastic) containing cefoxitin sodium as follows:

No. 2G3506—1 gram cefoxitin equivalent, iso-osmotic in 50 mL diluent containing approximately 2 grams dextrose hydrous USP

NDC 0006-3545-24 in boxes of 24
(6505-01-380-3410, 1 g 24's).

No. 2G3507—2 gram cefoxitin equivalent, iso-osmotic in 50 mL diluent containing approximately 1.1 grams dextrose hydrous USP

NDC 0006-3547-25 in boxes of 24
(6505-01-379-9245, 2 g 24's).

Special storage instructions

Store at or below −20°C (−4°F). [See Directions for Use of Galaxy® container (PL 2040 Plastic)].

MEFOXIN is also available in dry powder form in vials and infusion bottles containing sterile cefoxitin sodium equivalent to either 1 gram or 2 grams of cefoxitin, and in vials for pharmacy bulk use containing sterile cefoxitin sodium equivalent to 10 grams of cefoxitin, for constitution and intravenous administration (see appropriate product circular).

CLINICAL STUDIES

A prospective, randomized, double-blind, placebo-controlled clinical trial was conducted to determine the efficacy of short-term prophylaxis with MEFOXIN in patients undergoing cesarean section who were at high risk for subsequent endometritis because of ruptured membranes. Patients were randomized to receive either three doses of placebo (n=58), a single dose of MEFOXIN (2 g) followed by two doses of placebo (n=64), or a three-dose regimen of ME-FOXIN (each dose consisting of 2 g) (n=60), given intravenously, usually beginning at the time of clamping of the umbilical cord, with the second and third doses given 4 and 8 hours post-operatively. Endometritis occurred in 16/58 (27.6%) patients given placebo, 5/63 (7.9%) patients given a single dose of MEFOXIN, and 3/58 (5.2%) patients given three doses of MEFOXIN. The differences between the two groups treated with MEFOXIN and placebo with respect to endometritis were statistically significant (p<0.01) in favor of MEFOXIN. The differences between the one-dose and three-dose regimens of MEFOXIN were not statistically significant.

Two double-blind, randomized studies compared the efficacy of a single 2 gram intravenous dose of MEFOXIN to a single 2 gram dose of cefotetan in the prevention of surgical site-related infection (major morbidity) and non-site-related infections (minor morbidity) in patients following cesarean section. In the first study, 82/98 (83.7%) patients treated with MEFOXIN and 71/95 (74.7%) patients treated with ce-

fotetan experienced no major or minor morbidity. The difference in the outcomes in this study (95% CI: −0.03, +0.21) was not statistically significant. In the second study, 65/75 (86.7%) patients treated with MEFOXIN and 62/76 (81.6%) patients treated with cefotetan experienced no major or minor morbidity. The difference in the outcomes in this study (95% CI: −0.08, +0.18) was not statistically significant.

In clinical trials of patients with intra-abdominal infections due to *Bacteroides fragilis* group microorganisms, eradication rates at 1 to 2 weeks posttreatment for isolates were in the range of 70% to 80%. Eradication rates for individual species are listed below:

Bacteroides distasonis	7/10	(70%)
Bacteroides fragilis	26/33	(79%)
Bacteroides ovatus	10/13	(77%)
B. thetaiotaomicron	13/18	(72%)

Manufactured for:
MERCK & CO., INC., WEST POINT, PA 19486, USA
By:
BAXTER HEALTHCARE CORPORATION
Deerfield, Illinois 60015, USA
7948521 Issued October 1996
COPYRIGHT © MERCK & CO., INC., 1985, 1996
All rights reserved

MEPHYTON® Tablets ℞
(Phytonadione), U.S.P.
Vitamin K₁

DESCRIPTION

Phytonadione is a vitamin which is a clear, yellow to amber, viscous, and nearly odorless liquid. It is insoluble in water, soluble in chloroform and slightly soluble in ethanol. It has a molecular weight of 450.70.

Phytonadione is 2-methyl-3-phytyl-1, 4-naphthoquinone. Its empirical formula is $C_{31}H_{46}O_2$ and its structural formula is:

MEPHYTON* (Phytonadione) tablets containing 5 mg of phytonadione are yellow, compressed tablets, scored on one side. Inactive ingredients are acacia, calcium phosphate, colloidal silicon dioxide, lactose, magnesium stearate, starch, and talc.

*Registered trademark of MERCK & CO., INC.

CLINICAL PHARMACOLOGY

MEPHYTON tablets possess the same type and degree of activity as does naturally-occurring vitamin K, which is necessary for the production via the liver of active prothrombin (factor II), proconvertin (factor VII), plasma thromboplastin component (factor IX), and Stuart factor (factor X). The prothrombin test is sensitive to the levels of three of these four factors—II, VII, and X. Vitamin K is an essential cofactor for a microsomal enzyme that catalyzes the post-translational carboxylation of multiple, specific, peptide-bound glutamic acid residues in inactive hepatic precursors of factors II, VII, IX, and X. The resulting gamma-carboxyglutamic acid residues convert the precursors into active coagulation factors that are subsequently secreted by liver cells into the blood.

Oral phytonadione is adequately absorbed from the gastrointestinal tract only if bile salts are present. After absorption, phytonadione is initially concentrated in the liver, but the concentration declines rapidly. Very little vitamin K accumulates in tissues. Little is known about the metabolic fate of vitamin K. Almost no free unmetabolized vitamin K appears in bile or urine.

In normal animals and humans, phytonadione is virtually devoid of pharmacodynamic activity. However, in animals and humans deficient in vitamin K, the pharmacological action of vitamin K is related to its normal physiological function; that is, to promote the hepatic biosynthesis of vitamin K-dependent clotting factors.

MEPHYTON tablets generally exert their effect within 6 to 10 hours.

INDICATIONS AND USAGE

MEPHYTON is indicated in the following coagulation disorders which are due to faulty formation of factors II, VII, IX and X when caused by vitamin K deficiency or interference with vitamin K activity.

MEPHYTON tablets are indicated in:
— anticoagulant-induced prothrombin deficiency caused by coumarin or indanedione derivatives;
— hypoprothrombinemia secondary to antibacterial therapy;
— hypoprothrombinemia secondary to administration of salicylates;
— hypoprothrombinemia secondary to obstructive jaundice or biliary fistulas but only if bile salts are administered concurrently, since otherwise the oral vitamin K will not be absorbed.

CONTRAINDICATION

Hypersensitivity to any component of this medication.

WARNINGS

An immediate coagulant effect should not be expected after administration of phytonadione.

Phytonadione will not counteract the anticoagulant action of heparin.

When vitamin K₁ is used to correct excessive anticoagulant-induced hypoprothrombinemia, anticoagulant therapy still being indicated, the patient is again faced with the clotting hazards existing prior to starting the anticoagulant therapy. Phytonadione is not a clotting agent, but overzealous therapy with vitamin K₁ may restore conditions which originally permitted thromboembolic phenomena. Dosage should be kept as low as possible, and prothrombin time should be checked regularly as clinical conditions indicate.

Repeated large doses of vitamin K are not warranted in liver disease if the response to initial use of the vitamin is unsatisfactory. Failure to respond to vitamin K may indicate a congenital coagulation defect or that the condition being treated is unresponsive to vitamin K.

PRECAUTIONS

General

Temporary resistance to prothrombin-depressing anticoagulants may result, especially when larger doses of phytonadione are used. If relatively large doses have been employed, it may be necessary when reinstituting anticoagulant therapy to use somewhat larger doses of the prothrombin-depressing anticoagulant, or to use one which acts on a different principle, such as heparin sodium.

Laboratory Tests

Prothrombin time should be checked regularly as clinical conditions indicate.

Carcinogenesis, Mutagenesis, Impairment of Fertility

Studies of carcinogenicity or impairment of fertility have not been performed with MEPHYTON. MEPHYTON at concentrations up to 2000 mcg/plate with or without metabolic activation, was negative in the Ames microbial mutagen test.

Pregnancy

Pregnancy Category C: Animal reproduction studies have not been conducted with MEPHYTON. It is also not known whether MEPHYTON can cause fetal harm when administered to a pregnant woman or can affect reproduction capacity. MEPHYTON should be given to a pregnant woman only if clearly needed.

Pediatric Use

Safety and effectiveness in pediatric patients have not been established with MEPHYTON. Hemolysis, jaundice, and hyperbilirubinemia in newborns, particularly in premature infants, have been reported with vitamin K.

Nursing Mothers

It is not known whether this drug is excreted in human milk. Because many drugs are excreted in human milk, caution should be exercised when MEPHYTON is administered to a nursing woman.

ADVERSE REACTIONS

Transient "flushing sensations" and "peculiar" sensations of taste have been observed with parenteral phytonadione, as well as rare instances of dizziness, rapid and weak pulse, profuse sweating, brief hypotension, dyspnea, and cyanosis. Hyperbilirubinemia has been observed in the newborn following administration of parenteral phytonadione. This has occurred rarely and primarily with doses above those recommended.

OVERDOSAGE

The intravenous and oral LD₅₀s in the mouse are approximately 1.17 g/kg and greater than 24.18 g/kg, respectively.

DOSAGE AND ADMINISTRATION

MEPHYTON
Summary of Dosage Guidelines
(See circular text for details)

Adults	Initial Dosage
Anticoagulant-Induced Prothrombin Deficiency (caused by coumarin or indanedione derivatives)	2.5 mg–10 mg or up to 25 mg (rarely 50 mg)
Hypoprothrombinemia due to other causes (Antibiotics; Salicylates or other drugs; Factors limiting absorption or synthesis)	2.5 mg–25 mg or more (rarely up to 50 mg)

Anticoagulant-Induced Prothrombin Deficiency in Adults
To correct excessively prolonged prothrombin times caused by oral anticoagulant therapy—2.5 to 10 mg or up to 25 mg initially is recommended. In rare instances 50 mg may be required. Frequency and amount of subsequent doses should be determined by prothrombin time response or clinical condition. (See WARNINGS.) If, in 12 to 48 hours after oral administration, the prothrombin time has not been shortened satisfactorily, the dose should be repeated.
Hypoprothrombinemia Due to Other Causes in Adults
If possible, discontinuation or reduction of the dosage of drugs interfering with coagulation mechanisms (such as salicylates, antibiotics) is suggested as an alternative to administering concurrent MEPHYTON. The severity of the coagulation disorder should determine whether the immediate administration of MEPHYTON is required in addition to discontinuation or reduction of interfering drugs.
A dosage of 2.5 to 25 mg or more (rarely up to 50 mg) is recommended, the amount and route of administration depending upon the severity of the condition and response obtained.
The oral route should be avoided when the clinical disorder would prevent proper absorption. Bile salts must be given with the tablets when the endogenous supply of bile to the gastrointestinal tract is deficient.

HOW SUPPLIED

No. 7776—Tablets MEPHYTON, 5 mg vitamin K_1, are yellow, round, scored, compressed tablets, coded MSD 43 on one side and MEPHYTON on the other. They are supplied as follows:
NDC 0006-0043-68 bottles of 100
(6505-00-660-0460, 5 mg 100's).
Shown in Product Identification Guide, page 323
Storage:
Protect from light.
7918715 Issued August 1995
COPYRIGHT © MERCK & CO., INC., 1986, 1991
All rights reserved

MERUVAX®II ℞
(Rubella Virus Vaccine Live), U.S.P.
Wistar RA 27/3 Strain

DESCRIPTION

MERUVAX* II (Rubella Virus Vaccine Live) is a live virus vaccine for immunization against rubella (German measles).
MERUVAX II is a sterile lyophilized preparation of the Wistar Institute RA 27/3 strain of live attenuated rubella virus. The virus was adapted to and propagated in human diploid cell (WI-38) culture.
The reconstituted vaccine is for subcutaneous administration. When reconstituted as directed, the dose for injection is 0.5 mL and contains not less than the equivalent of 1,000 $TCID_{50}$ (tissue culture infectious doses) of the U.S. Reference Rubella Virus. Each dose also contains approximately 25 mcg of neomycin. The product contains no preservative. Sorbitol and hydrolyzed gelatin are added as stabilizers.

*Registered trademark of MERCK & CO., INC.

CLINICAL PHARMACOLOGY

MERUVAX II produces a modified, non-communicable rubella infection in susceptible persons.
Extensive clinical trials of rubella virus vaccines, prepared using RA 27/3 strain rubella virus, have been carried out in more than 28,000 human subjects (approximately 11,000 with MERUVAX II) in the U.S.A. and more than 20 additional countries. A single injection of the vaccine has been shown to induce rubella hemagglutination-inhibiting (HI) antibodies in 97% or more of susceptible persons. The RA 27/3 rubella strain elicits higher immediate post-vaccination HI, complement-fixing and neutralizing antibody levels than other strains of rubella vaccine and has been shown to induce a broader profile of circulating antibodies including anti-theta and anti-iota precipitating antibodies. The RA 27/3 rubella strain immunologically simulates natural infection more closely than other rubella vaccine viruses. The increased levels and broader profile of antibodies produced by RA 27/3 strain rubella virus vaccine appear to correlate with greater resistance to subclinical reinfection with the wild virus, and provide greater confidence for lasting immunity.
Vaccine-induced antibody levels have been shown to persist for at least 10 years without substantial decline. If the present pattern continues, it will provide a basis for the expectation that immunity following vaccination will be permanent. However, continued surveillance will be required to demonstrate this point.

INDICATIONS AND USAGE†

1. *Children Between 12 Months of Age and Puberty*
MERUVAX II is indicated for immunization against rubella (German measles) in persons from 12 months of age to puberty. A booster is not needed. It is not recommended for infants younger than 12 months because they may retain maternal rubella neutralizing antibodies that may interfere with the immune response. Children in kindergarten and the first grades of elementary school deserve priority for vaccination because often they are epidemiologically the major source of virus dissemination in the community. A history of rubella illness is usually not reliable enough to exclude children from immunization.
Previously unimmunized children of susceptible pregnant women should receive live attenuated rubella vaccine, because an immunized child will be less likely to acquire natural rubella and introduce the virus into the household.
2. *Adolescent and Adult Males*
Vaccination of adolescent or adult males may be a useful procedure in preventing or controlling outbreaks of rubella in circumscribed population groups (e.g., military bases and schools).
3. *Non-Pregnant Adolescent and Adult Females*
Immunization of susceptible non-pregnant adolescent and adult females of childbearing age with live attenuated rubella virus vaccine is indicated if certain precautions are observed (see below and PRECAUTIONS). Vaccinating susceptible postpubertal females confers individual protection against subsequently acquiring rubella infection during pregnancy, which in turn prevents infection of the fetus and consequent congenital rubella injury.
Women of childbearing age should be advised not to become pregnant for three months after vaccination and should be informed of the reason for this precaution.*
It is recommended that rubella susceptibility be determined by serologic testing prior to immunization.** If immune, as evidenced by a specific rubella antibody titer of 1:8 or greater (hemagglutination-inhibition test), vaccination is unnecessary. Congenital malformations do occur in up to seven percent of all live births. Their chance appearance after vaccination could lead to misinterpretation of the cause, particularly if the prior rubella-immune status of vaccinees is unknown.
Postpubertal females should be informed of the frequent occurrence of generally self-limited arthralgia and/or arthritis beginning 2 to 4 weeks after vaccination (see ADVERSE REACTIONS).
4. *Postpartum Women*
It has been found convenient in many instances to vaccinate rubella-susceptible women in the immediate postpartum period (see *Nursing Mothers*).
5. *International Travelers*
Individuals planning travel outside the United States, if not immune, can acquire measles, mumps or rubella and import these diseases to the United States. Therefore, prior to International travel, individuals known to be susceptible to one or more of these diseases can receive either a single antigen vaccine (measles, mumps or rubella), or a combined antigen vaccine as appropriate. However, M-M-R‡ II (Measles, Mumps, and Rubella Virus Vaccine Live) is preferred for persons likely to be susceptible to mumps and rubella; and if single-antigen measles vaccine is not readily available, travelers should receive M-M-R II (Measles, Mumps, and Rubella Virus Vaccine Live) regardless of their immune status to mumps or rubella.
Revaccination:
Children vaccinated when younger than 12 months of age should be revaccinated. Based on available evidence, there is no reason to routinely revaccinate persons who were vaccinated originally when 12 months of age or older. However, persons should be revaccinated if there is evidence to suggest that initial immunization was ineffective.
Use with Other Vaccines
Routine administration of DTP (diphtheria, tetanus, pertussis) and/or OPV (oral poliovirus vaccine) concomitantly with measles, mumps and rubella vaccines is not recommended because there are insufficient data relating to the simultaneous administration of these antigens. However, the American Academy of Pediatrics has noted that in some circumstances, particularly when the patient may not return, some practitioners prefer to administer all these antigens on a single day. If done, separate sites and syringes should be used for DTP and MERUVAX II.
MERUVAX II should not be given less than one month before or after administration of other virus vaccines.

†Based in part on the recommendation for rubella vaccine use of the Immunization Practices Advisory Committee (ACIP), Morbidity and Mortality Weekly Report: *33* (22): 301–310, 315–318, June 8, 1984.
*NOTE: The Immunization Practices Advisory Committee (ACIP) has recommended "In view of the importance of protecting this age group against rubella, reasonable precautions in a rubella immunization program include asking females if they are pregnant, excluding those who say they are, and explaining the theoretical risks to the others."
**NOTE: The Immunization Practices Advisory Committee (ACIP) has stated "When practical, and when reliable laboratory services are available, potential vaccinees of childbearing age can have serologic tests to determine susceptibility to rubella. . . . However, routinely performing serologic tests for all females of childbearing age to determine susceptibility so that vaccine is given only to proven susceptibles is expensive and has been ineffective in some areas. Accordingly, the ACIP believes that rubella vaccination of a woman who is not known to be pregnant and has no history of vaccination is justifiable without serologic testing."
‡Registered trademark of MERCK & CO., INC.

CONTRAINDICATIONS

Do not give MERUVAX II to pregnant females; the possible effects of the vaccine on fetal development are unknown at this time. If vaccination of postpubertal females is undertaken, pregnancy should be avoided for three months following vaccination. (See PRECAUTIONS, *Pregnancy*).
Anaphylactic or anaphylactoid reactions to neomycin (each dose of reconstituted vaccine contains approximately 25 mcg of neomycin).
Any febrile respiratory illness or other active febrile infection.
Active untreated tuberculosis.
Patients receiving immunosuppressive therapy. This contraindication does not apply to patients who are receiving corticosteroids as replacement therapy, e.g., for Addison's disease.
Individuals with blood dyscrasias, leukemia, lymphomas of any type, or other malignant neoplasms affecting the bone marrow or lymphatic systems.
Primary and acquired immunodeficiency states, including patients who are immunosuppressed in association with AIDS or other clinical manifestations of infection with human immunodeficiency viruses; cellular immune deficiencies; and hypogammaglobulinemic and dysgammaglobulinemic states.
Individuals with a family history of congenital or hereditary immunodeficiency, until the immune competence of the potential vaccine recipient is demonstrated.

PRECAUTIONS

General
Adequate treatment provisions including epinephrine, should be available for immediate use should an anaphylactic or anaphylactoid reaction occur.
Excretion of small amounts of the live attenuated rubella virus from the nose or throat has occurred in the majority of susceptible individuals 7–28 days after vaccination. There is no confirmed evidence to indicate that such virus is transmitted to susceptible persons who are in contact with the vaccinated individuals. Consequently, transmission through close personal contact, while accepted as a theoretical possibility, is not regarded as a significant risk. However, transmission of the vaccine virus to infants via breast milk has been documented (see *Nursing Mothers*).
There is no evidence that live rubella virus vaccine given after exposure to natural rubella virus will prevent illness. There is, however, no contraindication to vaccinating children already exposed to natural rubella.
Children and young adults who are known to be infected with human immunodeficiency viruses but without overt clinical manifestations of immunosuppression may be vac-

Continued on next page

Information on the Merck & Co., Inc. products listed on these pages is the full prescribing information from product circulars in use August 31, 1998. For information, please call 1-800-NSC MERCK [1-800-672-6372].

Meruvax II—Cont.

cinated; however, the vaccinees should be monitored closely for vaccine-preventable diseases because immunization may be less effective than for uninfected persons.
Vaccination should be deferred for at least three months following blood or plasma transfusions, or administration of human immune serum globulin. However, susceptible postpartum patients who received blood products may receive MERUVAX II prior to discharge provided that a repeat HI titer is drawn 6–8 weeks after vaccination to insure seroconversion. Similarly, although studies with other live rubella virus vaccines suggest that MERUVAX II may be given in the immediate postpartum period to those non-immune women who have received anti-Rho (D) globulin (human) without interfering with vaccine effectiveness, a follow-up post-vaccination HI titer should also be determined.
It has been reported that attenuated rubella virus vaccine, live, may result in a temporary depression of tuberculin skin sensitivity. Therefore, if a tuberculin test is to be done, it should be administered either before or simultaneously with MERUVAX II.
As for any vaccine, vaccination with MERUVAX II may not result in seroconversion in 100% of susceptible persons given the vaccine.
Pregnancy
Pregnancy Category C
Animal reproduction studies have not been conducted with MERUVAX II. It is also not known whether MERUVAX II can cause fetal harm when administered to a pregnant woman or can affect reproduction capacity. There is evidence suggesting transmission of rubella vaccine viruses to products of conception. Therefore, rubella vaccine should not be administered to pregnant females (see CONTRAINDICATIONS).
In counseling women who are inadvertently vaccinated when pregnant or who become pregnant within 3 months of vaccination, the physician should be aware of the following: In a 10 year survey involving over 700 pregnant women who received rubella vaccine within 3 months before or after conception, (of whom 189 received the Wistar RA 27/3 strain) none of the newborns had abnormalities compatible with congenital rubella syndrome.
Nursing Mothers
Recent studies have shown that lactating postpartum women immunized with live attenuated rubella vaccine may secrete the virus in breast milk and transmit it to breast-fed infants. In the infants with serological evidence of rubella infection, none exhibited severe disease; however, one exhibited mild clinical illness typical of acquired rubella. Caution should be exercised when MERUVAX II is administered to a nursing woman.

ADVERSE REACTIONS

Burning and/or stinging of short duration at the injection site have been reported.
Symptoms of the same kind as those seen following natural rubella may occur after vaccination. These include mild regional lymphadenopathy, urticaria, rash, malaise, sore throat, fever, headache, dizziness, nausea, vomiting, diarrhea, polyneuritis, and arthralgia and/or arthritis (usually transient and rarely chronic). Local pain, wheal and flare, induration, and erythema may occur at the site of injection. Reactions are usually mild and transient. Erythema multiforme has also been reported rarely.
Cough and rhinitis have also been reported.
Vasculitis has been reported rarely.
Anaphylaxis and anaphylactoid reactions have been reported.
Moderate fever [101–102.9°F (38.3–39.4°C)] occurs occasionally, and high fever [over 103°F (39.4°C)] occurs less commonly.
Syncope, particularly at the time of mass vaccination, has been reported.
Chronic arthritis has been associated with natural rubella infection and has been related to persistent virus and/or viral antigen isolated from body tissues. Only rarely have vaccine recipients developed chronic joint symptoms.
Following vaccination in children, reactions in joints are uncommon and generally of brief duration. In women, incidence rates for arthritis and arthralgia are generally higher than those seen in children (children: 0–3%; women: 12–20%) and the reactions tend to be more marked and of longer duration. Symptoms may persist for a matter of months or on rare occasions for years. In adolescent girls, the reactions appear to be intermediate in incidence between those seen in children and in adult women. Even in older women (35–45 years), these reactions are generally well tolerated and rarely interfere with normal activities.
Myalgia and paresthesia have been reported rarely after administration of MERUVAX II.
Forms of optic neuritis, including retrobulbar neuritis and papillitis may infrequently follow viral infections, and have been reported to occur 1 to 3 weeks following inoculation with some live virus vaccines.
Isolated reports of polyneuropathy including Guillain-Barré syndrome have been reported after immunization with rubella-containing vaccines.
Clinical experience with live rubella vaccines thus far indicates that encephalitis and other nervous system reactions have occurred very rarely in subjects who were given the vaccines, but a cause and effect relationship has not been established.
Thrombocytopenia with or without purpura has been reported.

DOSAGE AND ADMINISTRATION

FOR SUBCUTANEOUS ADMINISTRATION
Do not inject intravenously
The dosage of vaccine is the same for all persons. Inject the total volume of the single dose vial (about 0.5 mL) or 0.5 mL of the multiple dose vial of reconstituted vaccine subcutaneously, preferably into the outer aspect of upper arm. *Do not give immune globulin (IG) concurrently with* MERUVAX II.
To insure that there is no loss of potency during shipment, the vaccine must be maintained at a temperature of 10°C (50°F) or less.
Before reconstitution, store MERUVAX II at 2–8°C (36–46°F). *Protect from light.*
CAUTION: A sterile syringe free of preservatives, antiseptics, and detergents should be used for each injection and/or reconstitution of the vaccine because these substances may inactivate the live virus vaccine. A 25 gauge, $^5/_8$" needle is recommended.
To reconstitute, use only the diluent supplied, since it is free of preservatives or other antiviral substances which might inactivate the vaccine.
Single Dose Vial —First withdraw the entire volume of diluent into the syringe to be used for reconstitution. Inject all the diluent in the syringe into the vial of lyophilized vaccine, and agitate to mix thoroughly. Withdraw the entire contents into a syringe and inject the total volume of restored vaccine subcutaneously.
It is important to use a separate sterile syringe and needle for each individual patient to prevent transmission of hepatitis B and other infectious agents from one person to another.
10 Dose Vial (available only to government agencies / institutions) — Withdraw the entire contents (7 mL) of the diluent vial into the sterile syringe to be used for reconstitution, and introduce into the 10 dose vial of lyophilized vaccine. Agitate to ensure thorough mixing. The outer labeling suggests "For Jet Injector or Syringe Use". Use with separate sterile syringes is permitted for containers of 10 doses or less. The vaccine and diluent do not contain preservatives; therefore, the user must recognize the potential contamination hazards and exercise special precautions to protect the sterility and potency of the product. The use of aseptic techniques and proper storage prior to and after restoration of the vaccine and subsequent withdrawal of the individual doses is essential. Use 0.5 mL of the reconstituted vaccine for subcutaneous injection.
It is important to use a separate sterile syringe and needle for each individual patient to prevent transmission of hepatitis B and other infectious agents from one person to another.
50 Dose Vial (available only to government agencies / institutions) — Withdraw the entire contents (30 mL) of diluent vial into the sterile syringe to be used for reconstitution and introduce into the 50 dose vial of lyophilized vaccine. Agitate to ensure thorough mixing. With full aseptic precautions, attach the vial to the sterilized multidose jet injector apparatus. Use 0.5 mL of the reconstituted vaccine for subcutaneous injection.
Each dose contains not less than the equivalent of 1,000 $TCID_{50}$ of the U.S. Reference Rubella Virus.
Parenteral drug products should be inspected visually for particulate matter and discoloration prior to administration. MERUVAX II, when reconstituted, is clear yellow.

HOW SUPPLIED

No. 4747—MERUVAX II is supplied as a single-dose vial of lyophilized vaccine,
NDC 0006-4747-00, and a vial of diluent.
No. 4673/4309—MERUVAX II is supplied as follows: (1) a box of 10 single-dose vials of lyophilized vaccine (package A), **NDC** 0006-4673-00; and (2) a box of 10 vials of diluent (package B). To conserve refrigerator space, the diluent may be stored separately at room temperature.
(6505-00-145-0180, Ten Pack).
Available only to government agencies / institutions:
No. 4674—MERUVAX II is supplied as one 10 dose vial of lyophilized vaccine,
NDC 0006-4674-00, and one 7 mL vial of diluent.
No. 4675—MERUVAX II is supplied as one 50 dose vial of lyophilized vaccine,
NDC 0006-4675-00, and one 30 mL vial of diluent.
(6505-01-222-6468, 50 Dose).
Storage
It is recommended that the vaccine be used as soon as possible after reconstitution. Protect vaccine from light at all times, since such exposure may inactivate the virus. Store reconstituted vaccine in the vaccine vial in a dark place at 2–8°C (36–46°F) and discard if not used within 8 hours.

A.H.F.S. Category: 80:12
7680317 Issued March 1995
COPYRIGHT © MERCK & CO., INC., 1990
All rights reserved

MEVACOR® Tablets ℞
(Lovastatin)

DESCRIPTION

MEVACOR* (Lovastatin), is a cholesterol lowering agent isolated from a strain of *Aspergillus terreus.* After oral ingestion, lovastatin, which is an inactive lactone, is hydrolyzed to the corresponding β-hydroxyacid form. This is a principal metabolite and an inhibitor of 3-hydroxy-3-methylglutaryl-coenzyme A (HMG-CoA) reductase. This enzyme catalyzes the conversion of HMG-CoA to mevalonate, which is an early and rate limiting step in the biosynthesis of cholesterol.
Lovastatin is [1*S* -[1α(*R* *),3α,7β,8β(2*S* *,4*S* *),8aβ]]-1,2,3,7,8,8a-hexahydro-3,7-dimethyl-8-[2-(tetrahydro-4-hydroxy-6-oxo-2*H*-pyran-2-yl)ethyl]-1-naphthalenyl 2-methylbutanoate. The empirical formula of lovastatin is $C_{24}H_{36}O_5$ and its molecular weight is 404.55. Its structural formula is:

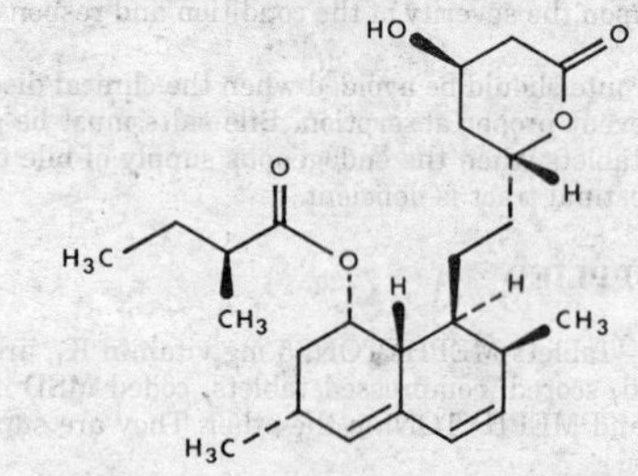

Lovastatin is a white, nonhygroscopic crystalline powder that is insoluble in water and sparingly soluble in ethanol, methanol, and acetonitrile.
Tablets MEVACOR are supplied as 10 mg, 20 mg and 40 mg tablets for oral administration. In addition to the active ingredient lovastatin, each tablet contains the following inactive ingredients: cellulose, lactose, magnesium stearate, and starch. Butylated hydroxyanisole (BHA) is added as a preservative. Tablets MEVACOR 10 mg also contain red ferric oxide and yellow ferric oxide. Tablets MEVACOR 20 mg also contain FD&C Blue 2. Tablets MEVACOR 40 mg also contain D&C Yellow 10 and FD&C Blue 2.

*Registered trademark of MERCK & CO., INC.

CLINICAL PHARMACOLOGY

The involvement of low-density lipoprotein (LDL) cholesterol in atherogenesis has been well-documented in clinical and pathological studies, as well as in many animal experiments.
Epidemiological studies have established that high LDL (low-density lipoprotein) cholesterol and low HDL (high-density lipoprotein) cholesterol are both risk factors for coronary heart disease. The Lipid Research Clinics Coronary Primary Prevention Trial (LRC-CPPT), coordinated by the National Institutes of Health (NIH) studied men aged 35–59 with total cholesterol levels 265 mg/dL (6.8 mmol/L) or greater, LDL cholesterol values 175 mg/dL (4.5 mmol/L) or greater and triglyceride levels not more than 300 mg/dL (3.4 mmol/L). This seven-year, double-blind, placebo-controlled study demonstrated that lowering LDL cholesterol with diet and cholestyramine decreased the combined rate of coronary heart disease death plus non-fatal myocardial infarction.
MEVACOR has been shown to reduce both normal and elevated LDL cholesterol concentrations. LDL is formed from VLDL and is catabolized predominantly by the high affinity LDL receptor. The mechanism of the LDL-lowering effect of MEVACOR may involve both reduction of VLDL cholesterol concentration, and induction of the LDL receptor, leading to reduced production and/or increased catabolism of LDL cholesterol. Apolipoprotein B also falls substantially during treatment with MEVACOR. Since each LDL particle con-

tains one molecule of apolipoprotein B, and since little apolipoprotein B is found in other lipoproteins, this strongly suggests that MEVACOR does not merely cause cholesterol to be lost from LDL, but also reduces the concentration of circulating LDL particles. In addition, MEVACOR can produce increases of variable magnitude in HDL cholesterol, and modestly reduces VLDL cholesterol and plasma triglycerides (see Tables I–III under *Clinical Studies*). The effects of MEVACOR on Lp(a), fibrinogen, and certain other independent biochemical risk markers for coronary heart disease are unknown.

MEVACOR is a specific inhibitor of HMG-CoA reductase, the enzyme which catalyzes the conversion of HMG-CoA to mevalonate. The conversion of HMG-CoA to mevalonate is an early step in the biosynthetic pathway for cholesterol.

Pharmacokinetics

Lovastatin is a lactone which is readily hydrolyzed *in vivo* to the corresponding β-hydroxyacid, a potent inhibitor of HMG-CoA reductase. Inhibition of HMG-CoA reductase is the basis for an assay in pharmacokinetic studies of the β-hydroxyacid metabolites (active inhibitors) and, following base hydrolysis, active plus latent inhibitors (total inhibitors) in plasma following administration of lovastatin.

Following an oral dose of ^{14}C-labeled lovastatin in man, 10% of the dose was excreted in urine and 83% in feces. The latter represents absorbed drug equivalents excreted in bile, as well as any unabsorbed drug. Plasma concentrations of total radioactivity (lovastatin plus ^{14}C-metabolites) peaked at 2 hours and declined rapidly to about 10% of peak by 24 hours postdose. Absorption of lovastatin, estimated relative to an intravenous reference dose, in each of four animal species tested, averaged about 30% of an oral dose. In animal studies, after oral dosing, lovastatin had high selectivity for the liver, where it achieved substantially higher concentrations than in non-target tissues. Lovastatin undergoes extensive first-pass extraction in the liver, its primary site of action, with subsequent excretion of drug equivalents in the bile. As a consequence of extensive hepatic extraction of lovastatin, the availability of drug to the general circulation is low and variable. In a single dose study in four hypercholesterolemic patients, it was estimated that less than 5% of an oral dose of lovastatin reaches the general circulation as active inhibitors. Following administration of lovastatin tablets the coefficient of variation, based on between-subject variability, was approximately 40% for the area under the curve (AUC) of total inhibitory activity in the general circulation.

Both lovastatin and its β-hydroxyacid metabolite are highly bound (>95%) to human plasma proteins. Animal studies demonstrated that lovastatin crosses the blood-brain and placental barriers.

The major active metabolites present in [illegible] human plasma are the β-hydroxyacid of lovastatin, its 6′-hydr[illegible]oxy derivative, and two additional metabolites. Peak plasma co[illegible]entrations of both active and total inhibitors were attained within 2 to 4 hours of dose administration. While the recommended therapeutic dose range is 10 to 80 mg/day, linearity of inhibitory activity in the general circulation was established by a single dose study employing lovastatin tablet dosages from 60 to as high as 120 mg. With a once-a-day dosing regimen, plasma concentrations of total inhibitors over a dosing interval achieved a steady state between the second and third days of therapy and were about 1.5 times those following a single dose. When lovastatin was given under fasting conditions, plasma concentrations of total inhibitors were on average about two-thirds those found when lovastatin was administered immediately after a standard test meal.

In a study of patients with severe renal insufficiency (creatinine clearance 10–30 mL/min), the plasma concentrations of total inhibitors after a single dose of lovastatin were approximately two-fold higher than those in healthy volunteers.

Clinical Studies

MEVACOR has been shown to be highly effective in reducing total and LDL cholesterol in heterozygous familial and non-familial forms of primary hypercholesterolemia and in mixed hyperlipidemia. A marked response was seen within 2 weeks, and the maximum therapeutic response occurred within 4–6 weeks. The response was maintained during continuation of therapy. Single daily doses given in the evening were more effective than the same dose given in the morning, perhaps because cholesterol is synthesized mainly at night.

In multicenter, double-blind studies in patients with familial or non-familial hypercholesterolemia, MEVACOR, administered in doses ranging from 10 mg q.p.m. to 40 mg b.i.d., was compared to placebo. MEVACOR consistently and significantly decreased total plasma cholesterol (TOTAL-C), LDL cholesterol (LDL-C), total cholesterol/HDL cholesterol (TOTAL-C/HDL-C) ratio and LDL cholesterol/HDL cholesterol (LDL-C/HDL-C) ratio. In addition, MEVACOR produced increases of variable magnitude in HDL cholesterol (HDL-C), and modestly decreased VLDL cholesterol (VLDL-C) and plasma triglycerides (TRIG.) (see Tables I through III for dose response results).

TABLE I
MEVACOR vs Placebo
(Mean Percent Change from Baseline After 6 Weeks)

DOSAGE	N	TOTAL-C	LDL-C	HDL-C	LDL-C/ HDL-C	TOTAL-C/ HDL/C	TRIG.
Placebo	33	−2	−1	−1	0	+1	+9
MEVACOR							
10 mg q.p.m.	33	−16	−21	+5	−24	−19	−10
20 mg q.p.m.	33	−19	−27	+6	−30	−23	+9
10 mg b.i.d.	32	−19	−28	+8	−33	−25	−7
40 mg q.p.m.	33	−22	−31	+5	−33	−25	−8
20 mg b.i.d.	36	−24	−32	+2	−32	−24	−6

TABLE II
MEVACOR vs. Cholestyramine
(Percent Change from Baseline After 12 Weeks)

TREATMENT	N	TOTAL-C (mean)	LDL-C (mean)	HDL-C (mean)	LDL-C/ HDL-C (mean)	TOTAL-C/ HDL-C (mean)	VLDL-C (median)	TRIG. (median)
MEVACOR								
20 mg b.i.d.	85	−27	−32	+9	−36	−31	−34	−21
40 mg b.i.d.	88	−34	−42	+8	−44	−37	−31	−27
Cholestyramine								
12 g b.i.d.	88	−17	−23	+8	−27	−21	+2	+11

TABLE III
MEVACOR vs. Placebo
(Percent Change from Baseline—
Average Values Between Weeks 12 and 48)

DOSAGE	N**	TOTAL-C (mean)	LDL-C (mean)	HDL-C (mean)	LDL-C/ HDL-C (mean)	TOTAL-C/ HDL-C (mean)	TRIG. (median)
Placebo	1663	+0.7	+0.4	+2.0	+0.2	+0.6	+4
MEVACOR							
20 mg q.p.m.	1642	−17	−24	+6.6	−27	−21	−10
40 mg q.p.m.	1645	−22	−30	+7.2	−34	−26	−14
20 mg b.i.d.	1646	−24	−34	+8.6	−38	−29	−16
40 mg b.i.d.	1649	−29	−40	+9.5	−44	−34	−19

**Patients enrolled

The results of a study in patients with primary hypercholesterolemia are presented in Table I.

[See table I above]

MEVACOR was compared to cholestyramine in a randomized openparallel study. The study was performed with patients with hypercholesterolemia who were at high risk of myocardial infarction. Summary results are presented in Table II.

[See table II above]

MEVACOR was studied in controlled trials in hypercholes-
[illegible] patients with well-controlled non-insulin depen-
terolem[illegible] mellitus with normal renal function. The ef-
dent diabetes [illegible] on lipids and lipoproteins and the safety
fect of MEVACOR [illegible] were similar tothat demonstrated in
profile of MEVACOR [illegible]EVACOR had no clinically impor-
studies in nondiabetics. M[illegible] the dose requirement of
tant effect on glycemic control or on [illegible]
oral hypoglycemic agents.

Expanded Clinical Evaluation of Lovastatin (EXCEL) Study

MEVACOR was compared to placebo in 8,245 patients with hypercholesterolemia (total cholesterol 240–300 mg/dL [6.2 mmol/L–7.6 mmol/L], LDL cholesterol >160 mg/dL [4.1 mmol/L]) in the randomized, double-blind, parallel, 48-week EXCEL study. All changes in the lipid measurements (Table III) in MEVACOR treated patients were dose-related and significantly different from placebo (p ≤0.001). These results were sustained throughout the study.

[See table III above]

Atherosclerosis

In the Canadian Coronary Atherosclerosis Intervention Trial (CCAIT), the effect of therapy with lovastatin on coronary atherosclerosis was assessed by coronary angiography in hyperlipidemic patients. In this randomized, double-blind, controlled clinical trial, patients were treated with conventional measures (usually diet and 325 mg of aspirin every other day) and either lovastatin 20–80 mg daily or placebo. Angiograms were evaluated at baseline and at two years by computerized quantitative coronary angiography (QCA). Lovastatin significantly slowed the progression of lesions as measured by the mean change per-patient in minimum lumen diameter (the primary endpoint) and percent diameter stenosis, and decreased the proportions of patients categorized with disease progression (33% vs. 50%) and with new lesions (16% vs. 32%).

In a similarly designed trial, the Monitored Atherosclerosis Regression Study (MARS), patients were treated with diet and either lovastatin 80 mg daily or placebo. No statistically significant difference between lovastatin and placebo was seen for the primary endpoint (mean change per patient in percent diameter stenosis of all lesions), or for most secondary QCA endpoints. Visual assessment by angiographers who formed a consensus opinion of overall angiographic change (Global Change Score) was also a secondary endpoint. By this endpoint, significant slowing of disease was seen, with regression in 23% of patients treated with lovastatin compared to 11% of placebo patients.

In the Familial Atherosclerosis Treatment Study (FATS), either lovastatin or niacin in combination with a bile acid sequestrant for 2.5 years in hyperlipidemic subjects significantly reduced the frequency of progression and increased the frequency of regression of coronary atherosclerotic lesions by QCA compared to diet and, in some cases, low-dose resin.

The effect of lovastatin on the progression of atherosclerosis in the coronary arteries has been corroborated by similar findings in another vasculature. In the Asymptomatic Carotid Artery Progression Study (ACAPS), the effect of therapy with lovastatin on carotid atherosclerosis was assessed by B-mode ultrasonography in hyperlipidemic patients with early carotid lesions and without known coronary heart disease at baseline. In this double-blind, controlled clinical trial, 919 patients were randomized in a 2 x 2 factorial design to placebo, lovastatin 10–40 mg daily and/or warfarin. Ultrasonograms of the carotid walls were used to determine the change per patient from baseline to three years in mean maximum intimal-medial thickness (IMT) of 12 measured segments. There was a significant regression of carotid lesions in patients receiving lovastatin alone compared to those receiving placebo alone (p=0.001). The predictive value of changes in IMT for stroke has not yet been established. In the lovastatin group there was a significant reduction in the number of patients with major cardiovascular events relative to the placebo group (5 vs. 14) and a significant reduction in all-cause mortality (1 vs. 8).

Eye

There was a high prevalence of baseline lenticular opacities in the patient population included in the early clinical trials with lovastatin. During these trials the appearance of new opacities was noted in both the lovastatin and placebo groups. There was no clinically significant change in visual acuity in the patients who had new opacities reported nor was any patient, including those with opacities noted at baseline, discontinued from therapy because of a decrease in visual acuity.

Continued on next page

Information on the Merck & Co., Inc. products listed on these pages is the full prescribing information from product circulars in use August 31, 1998. For information, please call 1-800-NSC MERCK [1-800-672-6372].

Mevacor—Cont.

A three-year, double-blind, placebo-controlled study in hypercholesterolemic patients to assess the effect of lovastatin on the human lens demonstrated that there were no clinically or statistically significant differences between the lovastatin and placebo groups in the incidence, type or progression of lenticular opacities. There are no controlled clinical data assessing the lens available for treatment beyond three years.

INDICATIONS AND USAGE

Therapy with lipid-altering agents should be a component of multiple risk factor intervention in those individuals at significantly increased risk for artherosclerotic vascular disease due to hypercholesterolemia. MEVACOR is indicated as an adjunct to diet for the reduction of elevated total and LDL cholesterol levels in patients with primary hypercholesterolemia (Types IIa and IIb***), when the response to diet restricted in saturated fat and cholesterol and to other nonpharmacological measures alone has been inadequate. MEVACOR is also indicated to slow the progression of coronary atherosclerosis in patients with coronary heart disease as part of a treatment strategy to lower total and LDL cholesterol to target levels.

Prior to initiating therapy with lovastatin, secondary causes for hypercholesterolemia (e.g., poorly controlled diabetes mellitus, hypothyroidism, nephrotic syndrome, dysproteinemias, obstructive liver disease, other drug therapy, alcoholism) should be excluded, and a lipid profile performed to measure TOTAL-C, HDL-C, and triglycerides (TG). For patients with TG less than 400 mg/dL (<4.5 mmol/L), LDL-C can be estimated using the following equation:

LDL-C = Total cholesterol − [0.2 × (triglycerides) + HDL-C]

For TG levels >400 mg/dL (>4.5 mmol/L), this equation is less accurate and LDL-C concentrations should be determined by ultracentrifugation. In hypertriglyceridemic patients, LDL-C may be low or normal despite elevated TOTAL-C. In such cases, MEVACOR is not indicated.

The National Cholesterol Education Program (NCEP) Treatment Guidelines are summarized below:

Definite Atherosclerotic Disease[†]	Two or More Other Risk Factors[††]	LDL-Cholesterol mg/dL (mmol/L)	
		Initiation Level	Goal
NO	NO	≥190 (≥4.9)	<160 (<4.1)
NO	YES	≥160 (≥4.1)	<130 (<3.4)
YES	YES or NO	≥130[†††] (≥3.4)	≤100 (≤2.6)

[†] Coronary heart disease or peripheral vascular disease (including symptomatic carotid artery disease).

[††] Other risk factors for coronary heart disease (CHD) include: age (males: ≥45 years; females: ≥55 years of premature menopause without estrogen replacement therapy); family history of premature CHD; current cigarette smoking; hypertension; confirmed HDL-C <35 mg/dL (<0.91 mmol/L); and diabetes mellitus. Subtract one risk factor if HDL-C is ≥60 mg/dL (≥1.6 mmol/L).

[†††] In CHD patients with LDL-C levels 100–129 mg/dL, the physician should exercise clinical judgment in deciding whether to initiate drug treatment.

At the time of hospitalization for an acute coronary event, consideration can be given to initiating drug therapy at discharge if the LDL-C is >130 mg/dL (see NCEP Guidelines above).

Since the goal of treatment is to lower LDL-C, the NCEP recommends that LDL-C levels be used to initiate and assess treatment response. Only if LDL-C levels are not available, should the TOTAL-C be used to monitor therapy.

Although MEVACOR may be useful to reduce elevated LDL cholesterol in patients with combined hypercholesterolemia and hypertriglyceridemia where hypercholesterolemia is the major abnormality (Type IIb hyperlipoproteinemia), it has not been studied in conditions where the major abnormality is elevation of chylomicrons, VLDL or IDL (i.e., hyperlipoproteinemia types I, III, IV, or V).***

***Classification of Hyperlipoproteinemias

Type	Lipoproteins elevated	Lipid Elevations	
		major	minor
I	(rare) chylomicrons	TG	→C
IIa	LDL	C	
IIb	LDL, VLDL	C	TG
III	(rare) IDL	C/TG	—
IV	VLDL	TG	→C
V	(rare) chylomicrons, VLDL	TG	→C

C = cholesterol, TG = triglycerides,
LDL = low-density lipoprotein,
VLDL = very low-density lipoprotein,
IDL = intermediate-density lipoprotein.

CONTRAINDICATIONS

Hypersensitivity to any component of this medication.
Active liver disease or unexplained persistent elevations of serum transaminases (see WARNINGS).
Concomitant therapy with the tetralol-class calcium channel blocker mibefradil (see WARNINGS, *Skeletal Muscle* and PRECAUTIONS, *Drug Interactions*).
Pregnancy and lactation. Atherosclerosis is a chronic process and the discontinuation of lipid-lowering drugs during pregnancy should have little impact on the outcome of long-term therapy of primary hypercholesterolemia. Moreoever, cholesterol and other products of the cholesterol biosynthesis pathway are essential components for fetal development, including synthesis of steroids and cell membranes. Because of the ability of inhibitors of HMG-CoA reductase such as MEVACOR to decrease the synthesis of cholesterol and possibly other products of the cholesterol biosynthesis pathway, MEVACOR is contraindicated during pregnancy and in nursing mothers. **MEVACOR should be administered to women of childbearing age only when such patients are highly unlikely to conceive.** If the patient becomes pregnant while taking this drug, MEVACOR should be discontinued immediately and the patient should be apprised of the potential hazard to the fetus (see PRECAUTIONS, *Pregnancy*).

WARNINGS

Liver Dysfunction

Marked persistent increases (to more than 3 times the upper limit of normal) in serum transaminases occurred in 1.9% of adult patients who received lovastatin for at least one year in early clinical trials (see ADVERSE REACTIONS). When the drug was interrupted or discontinued in these patients, the transaminase levels usually fell slowly to pretreatment levels. The increases usually appeared 3 to 12 months after the start of therapy with lovastatin, and were not associated with jaundice or other clinical signs or symptoms. There was no evidence of hypersensitivity. In the EXCEL study (see CLINICAL PHARMACOLOGY, *Clinical Studies*), the incidence of marked persistent increases in serum transaminases over 48 weeks was 0.1% for placebo, 0.1% at 20 mg/day, 0.9% at 40 mg/day, and 1.5% at 80 mg/day in patients on lovastatin. However, in postmarketing experience with MEVACOR, symptomatic liver disease has been reported rarely at all dosages (see ADVERSE REACTIONS).

It is recommended that liver function tests be performed before the initiation of treatment, at 6 and 12 weeks after initiation of therapy or elevation of dose, and periodically thereafter (e.g. seniannually). Patients who develop increased transaminase levels should be monitored with a second liver function evaluation to confirm the finding and be followed thereafter with frequent liver function tests until the abnormality(ies) return to normal. Should an increase in AST or ALT of three times the upper limit of normal or greater persist, withdrawal of therapy with MEVACOR is recommended.

The drug should be used with caution in patients who consume substantial quantities of alcohol and/or have a past history of liver disease. Active liver disease or unexplained transaminase elevations are contraindications to the use of lovastatin.

As with other lipid-lowering agents, moderate (less than three times the upper limit of normal) elevations of serum transaminases have been reported following therapy with MEVACOR (see ADVERSE REACTIONS). These changes appeared soon after initiation of therapy with MEVACOR, were often transient, were not accompanied by any symptoms and interruption of treatment was not required.

Skeletal Muscle

Rhabdomyolysis has been associated with lovastatin therapy alone, when combined with immunosuppressive therapy including cyclosporine in transplant patients, and when combined in non-transplant patients with either gemfibrozil or lipid-lowering doses (≥1 g/day) of nicotinic acid. Some of the affected patients had pre-existing renal insufficiency, usually as a consequence of long-standing diabetes. Acute renal failure from rhabdomyolysis has been seen more commonly with the lovastatin-gemfibrozil combination, and has also been reported in transplant patients receiving lovastatin plus cyclosporine.

Rhabdomyolysis has been reported during concomitant therapy with a related HMG-CoA reductase inhibitor and the tetralol-class calcium channel blocker mibefradil which is a potent cytochrome P-450 3A4 inhibitor (see CONTRAINDICATIONS).

Myopathy or rhabdomyolysis has occurred in transplant and non-transplant patients receiving MEVACOR or another HMG-CoA reductase inhibitor following the initiation of treatment with the antifungal agents itraconazole and ketoconazole. In a study in normal volunteers, plasma levels of lovastatin were increased about 20-fold when administered concomitantly with itraconazole. This is probably related to metabolism of both drugs by the same P-450 isoform. Based on this data, therapy with MEVACOR should be temporarily interrupted if systemic azole derivative antifungal therapy is required.

Rhabdomyolysis with or without renal impairment has been reported in patients receiving the macrolide antibiotics erythromycin and clarithromycin concomitantly with lovastatin. Rhabdomyolysis has also been reported with the concomitant use of the antidepressant nefazodone and another HMG-CoA reductase inhibitor. Therefore, patients receiving concomitant lovastatin and macrolide antibiotics or nefazodone should be carefully monitored.

Fulminant rhabdomyolysis has been seen as early as three weeks after initiation of combined therapy with gemfibrozil and lovastatin, but may be seen after several months. For these reasons, it is felt that, in most subjects who have had an unsatisfactory lipid response to either drug alone, the possible benefits of combined therapy with lovastatin and gemfibrozil do not outweigh the risks of severe myopathy, rhabdomyolysis, and acute renal failure. While it is not known whether this interaction occurs with fibrates other than gemfibrozil, myopathy and rhabdomyolysis have occasionally been associated with the use of other fibrates alone, including clofibrate. Therefore, the combined use of lovastatin with other fibrates should generally be avoided.

Physicians contemplating combined therapy with lovastatin and lipid-lowering doses of nicotinic acid or with immunosuppressive drugs should carefully weigh the potential benefits and risks and should carefully monitor patients for any signs and symptoms of muscle pain, tenderness, or weakness, particularly during the initial months of therapy and during any periods of upward dosage titration of either drug. Periodic CPK determinations may be considered in such situations, but there is no assurance that such monitoring will prevent the occurrence of severe myopathy. The monitoring of lovastatin drug and metabolite levels may be considered in transplant patients who are treated with immunosuppressives and lovastatin.

Lovastatin therapy should be temporarily withheld or discontinued in any patient with an acute, serious condition suggestive of a myopathy or having a risk factor predisposing to the development of renal failure secondary to rhabdomyolysis, including: severe acute infection, hypotension, major surgery, trauma, severe metabolic, endocrine and electrolyte disorders, and uncontrolled seizures. Also, as there are no known adverse consequences of brief interruption of therapy, treatment with lovastatin should be stopped a few days before elective major surgery.

Myalgia has been associated with lovastatin therapy. Transient, mildly elevated creatine phosphokinase levels are commonly seen in lovastatin-treated patients. However, in early clinical trials, approximately 0.5% of patients developed a myopathy, i.e., myalgia or muscle weakness associated with markedly elevated CPK levels. In the EXCEL study (see CLINICAL PHARMACOLOGY, *Clinical Studies*), five (0.1%) patients taking lovastatin alone (one at 40 mg q.p.m., and four at 40 mg b.i.d.) developed myopathy (muscle symptoms and CPK levels >10 times the upper limit of normal). Myopathy should be considered in any patient with diffuse myalgias, muscle tenderness or weakness, and/or marked elevation of CPK. Patients should be advised to report promptly unexplained muscle pain, tenderness or weakness, particularly if accompanied by malaise or fever. Lovastatin therapy should be discontinued if markedly elevated CPK levels occur or myopathy is diagnosed or suspected.

Most of the patients who have developed myopathy (including rhabdomyolysis) were taking lovastatin concomitantly with immunosuppressive drugs, gemfibrozil, or lipid-lowering doses of nicotinic acid. In initial clinical trials, about 30 percent of patients on concomitant immunosuppressive therapy including cyclosporine developed myopathy. Most of these patients were receiving lovastatin at doses of 40 to 80 mg/day. In reports from 7 subsequent studies, 148 cyclosporine-treated patients (105 cardiac and 43 renal) received concurrent lovastatin doses of 10 to 60 mg/day (the majority receiving 20 mg/day) for mean periods of 3 to 15 months. There was one case of rhabdomyolysis (0.6%) and one case of significant CPK elevation. In earlier studies of patients taking lovastatin in combination with gemfibrozil or niacin, the incidences of myopathy were approximately 5% and 2%, respectively.

In six patients with cardiac transplants taking immunosuppressive therapy including cyclosporine concomitantly with lovastatin 20 mg/day, the average plasma level of active metabolites derived from lovastatin was elevated to approximately four times the expected levels. Because of an apparent relationship between increased plasma levels of active

metabolites derived from lovastatin and myopathy, the daily dosage in patients taking immunosuppressants should not exceed 20 mg/day (see DOSAGE AND ADMINISTRATION). Even at this dosage, the benefits and risks of using lovastatin in patients taking immunosuppressants should be carefully considered.

PRECAUTIONS

General

Lovastatin may elevate creatine phosphokinase and transaminase levels (see WARNINGS and ADVERSE REACTIONS). This should be considered in the differential diagnosis of chest pain in a patient on therapy with lovastatin.

Homozygous Familial Hypercholesterolemia

MEVACOR is less effective in patients with the rare homozygous familial hypercholesterolemia, possibly because these patients have no functional LDL receptors. MEVACOR appears to be more likely to raise serum transaminases (see ADVERSE REACTIONS) in these homozygous patients.

Information for Patients

Patients should be advised to report promptly unexplained muscle pain, tenderness or weakness, particularly if accompanied by malaise or fever (see WARNINGS, Skeletal Muscle).

Drug Interactions

Mibefradil (see CONTRAINDICATIONS), Immunosuppressive Drugs, Itraconazole, Ketoconazole, Gemfibrozil, Niacin (Nicotinic Acid), Erythromycin, Clarithromycin, Nefazodone: See WARNINGS, Skeletal Muscle.

Coumarin Anticoagulants: In a small clinical trial in which lovastatin was administered to warfarin treated patients, no effect on prothrombin time was detected. However, another HMG-CoA reductase inhibitor has been found to produce a less than two seconds increase in prothrombin time in healthy volunteers receiving low doses of warfarin. Also, bleeding and/or increased prothrombin time have been reported in a few patients taking coumarin anticoagulants concomitantly with lovastatin. It is recommended that in patients taking anticoagulants, prothrombin time be determined before starting lovastatin and frequently enough during early therapy to insure that no significant alteration of prothrombin time occurs. Once a stable prothrombin time has been documented, prothrombin times can be monitored at the intervals usually recommended for patients on coumarin anticoagulants. If the dose of lovastatin is changed, the same procedure should be repeated. Lovastatin therapy has not been associated with bleeding or with changes in prothrombin time in patients not taking anticoagulants.

Antipyrine: Lovastatin had no effect on the pharmacokinetics of antipyrine or its metabolites. However, since lovastatin is metabolized by the cytochrome P-450 isoform 3A4, this does not preclude an interaction with other drugs metabolized by the same isoform.

Propranolol: In normal volunteers, there was no clinically significant pharmacokinetic or pharmacodynamic interaction with concomitant administration of single doses of lovastatin and propranolol.

Digoxin: In patients with hypercholesterolemia, concomitant administration of lovastatin and digoxin resulted in no effect on digoxin plasma concentrations.

Oral Hypoglycemic Agents: In pharmacokinetic studies of MEVACOR in hypercholesterolemic non-insulin dependent diabetic patients, there was no drug interaction with glipizide or with chlorpropamide (see CLINICAL PHARMACOLOGY, Clinical Studies).

Endocrine Function

HMG-CoA reductase inhibitors interfere with cholesterol synthesis and as such might theoretically blunt adrenal and/or gonadal steroid production. Results of clinical trials with drugs in this class have been inconsistent with regard to drug effects on basal and reserve steroid levels. However, clinical studies have shown that lovastatin does not reduce basal plasma cortisol concentration or impair adrenal reserve, and does not reduce basal plasma testosterone concentration. Another HMG-CoA reductase inhibitor has been shown to reduce the plasma testosterone response to HCG. In the same study, the mean testosterone response to HCG was slightly but not significantly reduced after treatment with lovastatin 40 mg daily for 16 weeks in 21 men. The effects of HMG-CoA reductase inhibitors on male fertility have not been studied in adequate numbers of male patients. The effects, if any, on the pituitary-gonadal axis in premenopausal women are unknown. Patients treated with lovastatin who develop clinical evidence of endocrine dysfunction should be evaluated appropriately. Caution should also be exercised if an HMG-CoA reductase inhibitor or other agent used to lower cholesterol levels is administered to patients also receiving other drugs (e.g., ketoconazole, spironolactone, cimetidine) that may decrease the levels or activity of endogenous steroid hormones.

CNS Toxicity

Lovastatin produced optic nerve degeneration (Wallerian degeneration of retinogeniculate fibers) in clinically normal dogs in a dose-dependent fashion starting at 60 mg/kg/day, a

	MEVACOR (N=613) %	Placebo (N=82) %	Cholestyramine (N=88) %
Gastrointestinal			
Constipation	4.9	—	34.1
Diarrhea	5.5	4.9	8.0
Dyspepsia	3.9	—	13.6
Flatus	6.4	2.4	21.6
Abdominal pain/cramps	5.7	2.4	5.7
Heartburn	1.6	—	8.0
Nausea	4.7	3.7	9.1
Musculoskeletal			
Muscle cramps	1.1	—	1.1
Myalgia	2.4	1.2	—
Nervous System / Psychiatric			
Dizziness	2.0	1.2	—
Headache	9.3	4.9	4.5
Skin			
Rash/pruritus	5.2	—	4.5
Special Senses			
Blurred vision	1.5	—	1.1
Dysgeusia	0.8	—	1.1

	Placebo (N=1663) %	MEVACOR 20 mg q.p.m. (N=1642) %	MEVACOR 40 mg q.p.m. (N=1645) %	MEVACOR 20 mg b.i.d. (N=1646) %	MEVACOR 40 mg b.i.d. (N=1649) %
Body As a Whole					
Asthenia	1.4	1.7	1.4	1.5	1.2
Gastrointestinal					
Abdominal pain	1.6	2.0	2.0	2.2	2.5
Constipation	1.9	2.0	3.2	3.2	3.5
Diarrhea	2.3	2.6	2.4	2.2	2.6
Dyspepsia	1.9	1.3	1.3	1.0	1.6
Flatulence	4.2	3.7	4.3	3.9	4.5
Nausea	2.5	1.9	2.5	2.2	2.2
Musculoskeletal					
Muscle cramps	0.5	0.6	0.8	1.1	1.0
Myalgia	1.7	2.6	1.8	2.2	3.0
Nervous System / Psychiatric					
Dizziness	0.7	0.7	1.2	0.5	0.5
Headache	2.7	2.6	2.8	2.1	3.2
Skin					
Rash	0.7	0.8	1.0	1.2	1.3
Special Senses					
Blurred vision	0.8	1.1	0.9	0.9	1.2

dose that produced mean plasma drug levels about 30 times higher than the mean drug level in humans taking the highest recommended dose (as measured by total enzyme inhibitory activity). Vestibulocochlear Wallerian-like degeneration and retinal ganglion cell chromatolysis were also seen in dogs treated for 14 weeks at 180 mg/kg/day, a dose which resulted in a mean plasma drug level (C_{max}) similar to that seen with the 60 mg/kg/day dose.

CNS vascular lesions, characterized by perivascular hemorrhage and edema, mononuclear cell infiltration of perivascular spaces, perivascular fibrin deposits and necrosis of small vessels, were seen in dogs treated with lovastatin at a dose of 180 mg/kg/day, a dose which produced plasma drug levels (C_{max}) which were about 30 times higher than the mean value in humans taking 80 mg/day.

Similar optic nerve and CNS vascular lesions have been observed with other drugs of this class.

Cataracts were seen in dogs treated for 11 and 28 weeks at 180 mg/kg/day and 1 year at 60 mg/kg/day.

Carcinogenesis, Mutagenesis, Impairment of Fertility

In a 21-month carcinogenic study in mice, there was a statistically significant increase in the incidence of hepatocellular carcinomas and adenomas in both males and females at 500 mg/kg/day. This dose produced a total plasma drug exposure 3 to 4 times that of humans given the highest recommended dose of lovastatin (drug exposure was measured as total HMG-CoA reductase inhibitory activity in extracted plasma). Tumor increases were not seen at 20 and 100 mg/kg/day, doses that produced drug exposures of 0.3 to 2 times that of humans at the 80 mg/day dose. A statistically significant increase in pulmonary adenomas was seen in female mice at approximately 4 times the human drug exposure. (Although mice were given 300 times the human dose [HD] on a mg/kg body weight basis, plasma levels of total inhibitory activity were only 4 times higher in mice than in humans given 80 mg of MEVACOR.)

There was an increase in incidence of papilloma in the nonglandular mucosa of the stomach of mice beginning at exposures of 1 to 2 times that of humans. The glandular mucosa was not affected. The human stomach contains only glandular mucosa.

In a 24-month carcinogenicity study in rats, there was a positive dose response relationship for hepatocellular carcinogenicity in males at drug exposures between 2–7 times that of human exposure at 80 mg/day (doses in rats were 5, 30 and 180 mg/kg/day).

An increased incidence of thyroid neoplasms in rats appears to be a response that has been seen with other HMG-CoA reductase inhibitors.

A chemically similar drug in this class was administered to mice for 72 weeks at 25, 100, and 400 mg/kg body weight, which resulted in mean serum drug levels approximately 3, 15, and 33 times higher than the mean human serum drug concentration (as total inhibitory activity) after a 40 mg oral dose. Liver carcinomas were significantly increased in high dose females and mid- and high dose males, with a maximum incidence of 90 percent in males. The incidence of adenomas of the liver was significantly increased in mid- and high dose females. Drug treatment also significantly increased the incidence of lung adenomas in mid- and high dose males and females. Adenomas of the Harderian gland (a gland of the eye of rodents) were significantly higher in high dose mice than in controls.

No evidence of mutagenicity was observed in a microbial mutagen test using mutant strains of *Salmonella typhimurium* with or without rat or mouse liver metabolic activation. In addition, no evidence of damage to genetic material was noted in an *in vitro* alkaline elution assay using rat or mouse hepatocytes, a V-79 mammalian cell forward mutation study, an *in vitro* chromosome aberration study in CHO cells, or an *in vivo* chromosomal aberration assay in mouse bone marrow.

Drug-related testicular atrophy, decreased spermatogenesis, spermatocytic degeneration and giant cell formation were seen in dogs starting at 20 mg/kg/day. Similar findings were seen with another drug in this class. No drug-related effects on fertility were found in studies with lovastatin in rats. However, in studies with a similar drug in this class, there was decreased fertility in male rats treated for 34 weeks at 25 mg/kg body weight, although this effect was not observed in a subsequent fertility study when this same

Continued on next page

Mevacor—Cont.

dose was administered for 11 weeks (the entire cycle of spermatogenesis, including epididymal maturation). In rats treated with this same reductase inhibitor at 180 mg/kg/day, seminiferous tubule degeneration (necrosis and loss of spermatogenic epithelium) was observed. No microscopic changes were observed in the testes from rats of either study. The clinical significance of these findings is unclear.

Pregnancy

Pregnancy Category X

See CONTRAINDICATIONS.

Safety in pregnant women has not been established.

Lovastatin has been shown to produce skeletal malformations at plasma levels 40 times the human exposure (for mouse fetus) and 80 times the human exposure (for rat fetus) based on mg/m^2 surface area (doses were 800 mg/kg/day). No drug-induced changes were seen in either species at multiples of 8 times (rat) or 4 times (mouse) based on surface area. No evidence of malformations was noted in rabbits at exposures up to 3 times the human exposure (dose of 15 mg/kg/day, highest tolerated dose).

Rare reports of congenital anomalies have been received following intrauterine exposure to HMG-CoA reductase inhibitors. In a review[†] of approximately 100 prospectively followed pregnancies in women exposed to MEVACOR or another structurally related HMG-CoA reductase inhibitor, the incidences of congenital anomalies, spontaneous abortions and fetal deaths/stillbirths did not exceed what would be expected in the general population. The number of cases is adequate only to exclude a 3 to 4-fold increase in congenital anomalies over the background incidence. In 89% of the prospectively followed pregnancies, drug treatment was initiated prior to pregnancy and was discontinued at some point in the first trimester when pregnancy was identified. As safety in pregnant women has not been established and there is no apparent benefit to therapy with MEVACOR during pregnancy (see CONTRAINDICATIONS), treatment should be immediately discontinued as soon as pregnancy is recognized. MEVACOR should be administered to women of child-bearing potential only when such patients are highly unlikely to conceive and have been informed of the potential hazard.

Nursing Mothers

It is not known whether lovastatin is excreted in human milk. Because a small amount of another drug in this class is excreted in human breast milk and because of the potential for serious adverse reactions in nursing infants, women taking MEVACOR should not nurse their infants (see CONTRAINDICATIONS).

Pediatric Use

Safety and effectiveness in pediatric patients have not been established. Because pediatric patients are not likely to benefit from cholesterol lowering for at least a decade and because experience with this drug is limited (no studies in subjects below the age of 20 years), treatment of pediatric patients with lovastatin is not recommended at this time.

[†]Manson, J.M., Freyssinges, C., Ducrocq, M.B., Stephenson, W.P., Postmarketing Surveillance of Lovastatin and Simvastatin Exposure During Pregnancy. *Reproductive Toxicology.* 10(6):439-446. 1996.

ADVERSE REACTIONS

MEVACOR is generally well tolerated; adverse reactions usually have been mild and transient. Less than 1% of patients were discontinued from controlled clinical studies of up to 14 weeks due to adverse experiences attributable to MEVACOR. About 3% of patients were discontinued from extensions of these studies due to adverse experiences attributable to MEVACOR; about half of these patients were discontinued due to increases in serum transaminases. The median duration of therapy in these extensions was 5.2 years.

In the EXCEL study (see CLINICAL PHARMACOLOGY, *Clinical Studies*), 4.6% of the patients treated up to 48 weeks were discontinued due to clinical or laboratory adverse experiences which were rated by the investigator as possibly, probably or definitely related to therapy with MEVACOR. The value for the placebo group was 2.5%.

Clinical Adverse Experiences

Adverse experiences reported in patients treated with MEVACOR in controlled clinical studies are shown in the table below:

[See first table at top of previous page]

Laboratory Tests

Marked persistent increases of serum transaminases have been noted (see WARNINGS).

About 11% of patients had elevations of creatine phosphokinase (CPK) levels of at least twice the normal value on one or more occasions. The corresponding values for the control agent cholestyramine was 9 percent. This was attributable to the noncardiac fraction of CPK. Large increases in CPK have sometimes been reported (see WARNINGS, *Skeletal Muscle*).

Expanded Clinical Evaluation of Lovastatin (EXCEL) Study

Clinical Adverse Experiences

MEVACOR was compared to placebo in 8,245 patients with hypercholesterolemia (total cholesterol 240–300 mg/dL [6.2–7.8 mmol/L]) in the randomized, double-blind, parallel, 48-week EXCEL study. Clinical adverse experiences reported as possibly, probably or definitely drug-related in ≥1% in any treatment group are shown in the table below. For no event was the incidence on drug and placebo statistically different.

[See second table at top of previous page]

Other clinical adverse experiences reported as possibly, probably or definitely drug-related in 0.5 to 1.0 percent of patients in any drug-related group are listed below. In all these cases the incidence on drug and placebo was not statistically different. *Body as a Whole:* chest pain; *Gastrointestinal:* acid regurgitation, dry mouth, vomiting; *Musculoskeletal:* leg pain, shoulder pain, arthralgia; *Nervous System/Psychiatric:* insomnia, paresthesia; *Skin:* alopecia, pruritus; *Special Senses:* eye irritation.

Concomitant Therapy

In controlled clinical studies in which lovastatin was administered concomitantly with cholestyramine, no adverse reactions peculiar to this concomitant treatment were observed. The adverse reactions that occurred were limited to those reported previously with lovastatin or cholestyramine. Other lipid-lowering agents were not administered concomitantly with lovastatin during controlled clinical studies. Preliminary data suggests that the addition of gemfibrozil to therapy with lovastatin is not associated with greater reduction in LDL cholesterol than that achieved with lovastatin alone. In uncontrolled clinical studies, most of the patients who have developed myopathy were receiving concomitant therapy with immunosuppressive drugs, gemfibrozil or niacin (nicotinic acid) (see WARNINGS, *Skeletal Muscle*).

The following effects have been reported with drugs in this class. Not all the effects listed below have necessarily been associated with lovastatin therapy.

Skeletal: muscle cramps, myalgia, myopathy, rhabdomyolysis, arthralgias.

Neurological: dysfunction of certain cranial nerves (including alteration of taste, impairment of extra-ocular movement, facial paresis), tremor, dizziness, vertigo, memory loss, paresthesia, peripheral neuropathy, peripheral nerve palsy, psychic disturbances, anxiety, insomnia, depression.

Hypersensitivity Reactions: An apparent hypersensitivity syndrome has been reported rarely which has included one or more of the following features: anaphylaxis, angioedema, lupus erythematous-like syndrome, polymyalgia rheumatica, vasculitis, purpura, thrombocytopenia, leukopenia, hemolytic anemia, positive ANA, ESR increase, eosinophilia, arthritis, arthralgia, urticaria, asthenia, photosensitivity, fever, chills, flushing, malaise, dyspnea, toxic epidermal necrolysis, erythema multiforme, including Stevens-Johnson syndrome.

Gastrointestinal: pancreatitis, hepatitis, including chronic active hepatitis, cholestatic jaundice, fatty change in liver; and rarely, cirrhosis, fulminant hepatic necrosis, and hepatoma; anorexia, vomiting.

Skin: alopecia, pruritus. A variety of skin changes (e.g., nodules, discoloration, dryness of skin/mucous membranes, changes to hair/nails) have been reported.

Reproductive: gynecomastia, loss of libido, erectile dysfunction.

Eye: progression of cataracts (lens opacities), ophthalmoplegia.

Laboratory Abnormalities: elevated transaminases, alkaline phosphatase, γ-glutamyl transpeptidase, and bilirubin; thyroid function abnormalities.

OVERDOSAGE

After oral administration of MEVACOR to mice the median lethal dose observed was >15 g/m^2.

Five healthy human volunteers have received up to 200 mg of lovastatin as a single dose without clinically significant adverse experiences. A few cases of accidental overdosage have been reported; no patients had any specific symptoms, and all patients recovered without sequelae. The maximum dose taken was 5–6 g.

Until further experience is obtained, no specific treatment of overdosage with MEVACOR can be recommended.

The dialyzability of lovastatin and its metabolites in man is not known at present.

DOSAGE AND ADMINISTRATION

The patient should be placed on a standard cholesterol-lowering diet before receiving MEVACOR and should continue on this diet during treatment with MEVACOR (see NCEP Treatment Guidelines for details on dietary therapy). MEVACOR should be given with meals.

The usual recommended starting dose is 20 mg once a day given with the evening meal. The recommended dosing range is 10–80 mg/day in single or two divided doses; the maximum recommended dose is 80 mg/day. Doses should be individualized according to the recommended goal of therapy (see NCEP Guidelines) and the patient's response (see Tables I to III under CLINICAL PHARMACOLOGY, *Clinical Studies* for dose response results). Patients requiring reductions in LDL cholesterol of 20% or more to achieve their goal (see INDICATIONS AND USAGE) should be started on 20 mg/day of MEVACOR. A starting dose of 10 mg may be considered for patients requiring smaller reductions. Adjustments should be made at intervals of 4 weeks or more. In patients taking immunosuppressive drugs concomitantly with lovastatin (see WARNINGS, *Skeletal Muscle*), therapy should begin with 10 mg of MEVACOR and should not exceed 20 mg/day.

Cholesterol levels should be monitored periodically and consideration should be given to reducing the dosage of MEVACOR if cholesterol levels fall significantly below the targeted range.

Concomitant Therapy

Preliminary evidence suggests that the cholesterol-lowering effects of lovastatin and the bile acid sequestrant, cholestyramine, are additive.

Dosage in Patients with Renal Insufficiency

In patients with severe renal insufficiency (creatinine clearance <30 mL/min), dosage increases above 20 mg/day should be carefully considered and, if deemed necessary, implemented cautiously (see CLINICAL PHARMACOLOGY and WARNINGS, *Skeletal Muscle*).

HOW SUPPLIED

No. 3560—Tablets MEVACOR 10 mg are peach, octagonal tablets, coded MSD 730 on one side and MEVACOR on the other. They are supplied as follows:

NDC 0006-0730-61 unit of use bottles of 60.

Shown in Product Identification Guide, page 323

No. 3561—Tablets MEVACOR 20 mg are light blue, octagonal tablets, coded MSD 731 on one side and MEVACOR on the other. They are supplied as follows:

NDC 0006-0731-61 unit of use bottles of 60 (6505-01-267-2497, 20 mg 60's)

NDC 0006-0731-94 unit of use bottles of 90

NDC 0006-0731-28 unit dose packages of 100 (6505-01-267-7925, 20 mg 100's)

NDC 0006-0731-82 bottles of 1000 (6505-01-359-1865, 20 mg 1000's)

NDC 0006-0731-87 bottles of 10,000 (6505-01-379-7905, 20 mg 10,000's).

Shown in Product Identification Guide, page 323

No. 3562—Tablets MEVACOR 40 mg are green, octagonal tablets, coded MSD 732 on one side and MEVACOR on the other. They are supplied as follows:

NDC 0006-0732-61 unit of use bottles of 60 (6505-01-310-0615, 40 mg 60's)

NDC 0006-0732-94 unit of use bottles of 90

NDC 0006-0732-82 bottles of 1000

NDC 0006-0732-87 bottles of 10,000 (6505-01-379-7903, 40 mg 10,000's).

Shown in Product Identification Guide, page 323

Storage

Store between 5–30°C (41–86°F). Tablets MEVACOR must be protected from light and stored in a well-closed, light-resistant container.

7825343 Issued April 1998

MIDAMOR® Tablets ℞
(Amiloride HCl), U.S.P.

DESCRIPTION

Amiloride HCl, an antikaliuretic-diuretic agent, is a pyrazine-carbonyl-guanidine that is unrelated chemically to other known antikaliuretic or diuretic agents. It is the salt of a moderately strong base (pKa 8.7). It is designated chemically as 3,5-diamino-6-chloro-*N*-(diaminomethylene) pyrazinecarboxamide monohydrochloride, dihydrate and has a molecular weight of 302.12. Its empirical formula is $C_6H_8ClN_7O \cdot HCl \cdot 2H_2O$ and its structural formula is:

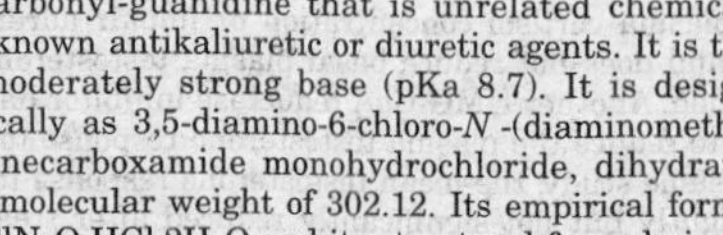

MIDAMOR* (Amiloride HCl) is available for oral use as tablets containing 5 mg of anhydrous amiloride HCl. Each tablet contains the following inactive ingredients: calcium phosphate, D&C Yellow 10, iron oxide, lactose, magnesium stearate and starch.

*Registered trademark of MERCK & CO., INC.

CLINICAL PHARMACOLOGY

MIDAMOR is a potassium-conserving (antikaliuretic) drug that possesses weak (compared with thiazide diuretics) natriuretic, diuretic, and antihypertensive activity. These effects have been partially additive to the effects of thiazide diuretics in some clinical studies. When administered with a thiazide or loop diuretic, MIDAMOR has been shown to decrease the enhanced urinary excretion of magnesium which occurs when a thiazide or loop diuretic is used alone. MIDAMOR has potassium-conserving activity in patients receiving kaliuretic-diuretic agents.

MIDAMOR is not an aldosterone antagonist and its effects are seen even in the absence of aldosterone.

MIDAMOR exerts its potassium sparing effect through the inhibition of sodium reabsorption at the distal convoluted tubule, cortical collecting tubule and collecting duct; this decreases the net negative potential of the tubular lumen and reduces both potassium and hydrogen secretion and their subsequent excretion. This mechanism accounts in large part for the potassium sparing action of amiloride.

MIDAMOR usually begins to act within 2 hours after an oral dose. Its effect on electrolyte excretion reaches a peak between 6 and 10 hours and lasts about 24 hours. Peak plasma levels are obtained in 3 to 4 hours and the plasma half-life varies from 6 to 9 hours. Effects on electrolytes increase with single doses of amiloride HCl up to approximately 15 mg.

Amiloride HCl is not metabolized by the liver but is excreted unchanged by the kidneys. About 50 percent of a 20 mg dose of MIDAMOR is excreted in the urine and 40 percent in the stool within 72 hours. MIDAMOR has little effect on glomerular filtration rate or renal blood flow. Because amiloride HCl is not metabolized by the liver, drug accumulation is not anticipated in patients with hepatic dysfunction, but accumulation can occur if the hepatorenal syndrome develops.

INDICATIONS AND USAGE

MIDAMOR is indicated as adjunctive treatment with thiazide diuretics or other kaliuretic-diuretic agents in congestive heart failure or hypertension to:

a. help restore normal serum potassium levels in patients who develop hypokalemia on the kaliuretic diuretic
b. prevent development of hypokalemia in patients who would be exposed to particular risk if hypokalemia were to develop, e.g., digitalized patients or patients with significant cardiac arrhythmias.

The use of potassium-conserving agents is often unnecessary in patients receiving diuretics for uncomplicated essential hypertension when such patients have a normal diet. MIDAMOR has little additive diuretic or antihypertensive effect when added to a thiazide diuretic.

MIDAMOR should rarely be used alone. It has weak (compared with thiazides) diuretic and antihypertensive effects. Used as single agents, potassium sparing diuretics, including MIDAMOR, result in an increased risk of hyperkalemia (approximately 10% with amiloride). MIDAMOR should be used alone only when persistent hypokalemia has been documented and only with careful titration of the dose and close monitoring of serum electrolytes.

CONTRAINDICATIONS

Hyperkalemia

MIDAMOR should not be used in the presence of elevated serum potassium levels (greater than 5.5 mEq per liter).

Antikaliuretic Therapy or Potassium Supplementation

MIDAMOR should not be given to patients receiving other potassium-conserving agents, such as spironolactone or triamterene. Potassium supplementation in the form of medication, potassium-containing salt substitutes or a potassium-rich diet should not be used with MIDAMOR except in severe and/or refractory cases of hypokalemia. Such concomitant therapy can be associated with rapid increases in serum potassium levels. If potassium supplementation is used, careful monitoring of the serum potassium level is necessary.

Impaired Renal Function

Anuria, acute or chronic renal insufficiency, and evidence of diabetic nephropathy are contraindications to the use of MIDAMOR. Patients with evidence of renal functional impairment (blood urea nitrogen [BUN] levels over 30 mg per 100 mL or serum creatinine levels over 1.5 mg per 100 mL) or diabetes mellitus should not receive the drug without careful, frequent and continuing monitoring of serum electrolytes, creatinine, and BUN levels. Potassium retention associated with the use of an antikaliuretic agent is accentuated in the presence of renal impairment and may result in the rapid development of hyperkalemia.

Hypersensitivity

MIDAMOR is contraindicated in patients who are hypersensitive to this product.

WARNINGS

Hyperkalemia

> Like other potassium-conserving agents, amiloride may cause hyperkalemia (serum potassium levels greater than 5.5 mEq per liter) which, if uncorrected, is potentially fatal. Hyperkalemia occurs commonly (about 10%) when amiloride is used without a kaliuretic diuretic. This incidence is greater in patients with renal impairment, diabetes mellitus (with or without recognized renal insufficiency), and in the elderly. When MIDAMOR is used concomitantly with a thiazide diuretic in patients without these complications, the risk of hyperkalemia is reduced to about 1–2 percent. It is thus essential to monitor serum potassium levels carefully in any patient receiving amiloride, particularly when it is first introduced, at the time of diuretic dosage adjustments, and during any illness that could affect renal function.

The risk of hyperkalemia may be increased when potassium-conserving agents, including MIDAMOR, are administered concomitantly with an angiotensin-converting enzyme inhibitor. (See PRECAUTIONS, *Drug Interactions.*) Warning signs or symptoms of hyperkalemia include paresthesias, muscular weakness, fatigue, flaccid paralysis of the extremities, bradycardia, shock, and ECG abnormalities. Monitoring of the serum potassium level is essential because mild hyperkalemia is not usually associated with an abnormal ECG.

When abnormal, the ECG in hyperkalemia is characterized primarily by tall, peaked T waves or elevations from previous tracings. There may also be lowering of the R wave and increased depth of the S wave, widening and even disappearance of the P wave, progressive widening of the QRS complex, prolongation of the PR interval, and ST depression.

Treatment of hyperkalemia: If hyperkalemia occurs in patients taking MIDAMOR, the drug should be discontinued immediately. If the serum potassium level exceeds 6.5 mEq per liter, active measures should be taken to reduce it. Such measures include the intravenous administration of sodium bicarbonate solution or oral or parenteral glucose with a rapid-acting insulin preparation. If needed, a cation exchange resin such as sodium polystyrene sulfonate may be given orally or by enema. Patients with persistent hyperkalemia may require dialysis.

Diabetes Mellitus

In diabetic patients, hyperkalemia has been reported with the use of all potassium-conserving diuretics, including MIDAMOR, even in patients without evidence of diabetic nephropathy. Therefore, MIDAMOR should be avoided, if possible, in diabetic patients and, if it is used, serum electrolytes and renal function must be monitored frequently. MIDAMOR should be discontinued at least three days before glucose tolerance testing.

Metabolic or Respiratory Acidosis

Antikaliuretic therapy should be instituted only with caution in severely ill patients in whom respiratory or metabolic acidosis may occur, such as patients with cardiopulmonary disease or poorly controlled diabetes. If MIDAMOR is given to these patients, frequent monitoring of acid-base balance is necessary. Shifts in acid-base balance alter the ratio of extracellular/intracellular potassium, and the development of acidosis may be associated with rapid increases in serum potassium levels.

PRECAUTIONS

General

Electrolyte Imbalance and BUN Increases

Hyponatremia and hypochloremia may occur when MIDAMOR is used with other diuretics and increases in BUN levels have been reported. These increases usually have accompanied vigorous fluid elimination, especially when diuretic therapy was used in seriously ill patients, such as those who had hepatic cirrhosis with ascites and metabolic alkalosis, or those with resistant edema. Therefore, when MIDAMOR is given with other diuretics to such patients, careful monitoring of serum electrolytes and BUN levels is important. In patients with pre-existing severe liver disease, hepatic encephalopathy, manifested by tremors, confusion, and coma, and increased jaundice, have been reported in association with diuretics, including amiloride HCl.

Drug Interactions

When amiloride HCl is administered concomitantly with an angiotensin-converting enzyme inhibitor, the risk of hyperkalemia may be increased. Therefore, if concomitant use of these agents is indicated because of demonstrated hypokalemia, they should be used with caution and with frequent monitoring of serum potassium. (See WARNINGS.)

Lithium generally should not be given with diuretics because they reduce its renal clearance and add a high risk of lithium toxicity. Read circulars for lithium preparations before use of such concomitant therapy.

In some patients, the administration of a non-steroidal anti-inflammatory agent can reduce the diuretic, natriuretic, and antihypertensive effects of loop, potassium-sparing and thiazide diuretics. Therefore, when MIDAMOR and non-steroidal anti-inflammatory agents are used concomitantly, the patient should be observed closely to determine if the desired effect of the diuretic is obtained. Since indomethacin and potassium-sparing diuretics, including MIDAMOR, may each be associated with increased serum potassium levels, the potential effects on potassium kinetics and renal function should be considered when these agents are administered concurrently.

Carcinogenicity, Mutagenicity, Impairment of Fertility

There was no evidence of a tumorigenic effect when amiloride HCl was administered for 92 weeks to mice at doses up to 10 mg/kg/day (25 times the maximum daily human dose). Amiloride HCl has also been administered for 104 weeks to male and female rats at doses up to 6 and 8 mg/kg/day (15 and 20 times the maximum daily dose for humans, respectively) and showed no evidence of carcinogenicity.

Amiloride HCl was devoid of mutagenic activity in various strains of *Salmonella typhimurium* with or without a mammalian liver microsomal activation system (Ames test).

Pregnancy

Pregnancy Category B. Teratogenicity studies with amiloride HCl in rabbits and mice given 20 and 25 times the maximum human dose, respectively, revealed no evidence of harm to the fetus, although studies showed that the drug crossed the placenta in modest amounts. Reproduction studies in rats at 20 times the expected maximum daily dose for humans showed no evidence of impaired fertility. At approximately 5 or more times the expected maximum daily dose for humans, some toxicity was seen in adult rats and rabbits and a decrease in rat pup growth and survival occurred.

There are, however, no adequate and well-controlled studies in pregnant women. Because animal reproduction studies are not always predictive of human response, this drug should be used during pregnancy only if clearly needed.

Nursing Mothers

Studies in rats have shown that amiloride is excreted in milk in concentrations higher than those found in blood, but it is not known whether MIDAMOR is excreted in human milk. Because many drugs are excreted in human milk and because of the potential for serious adverse reactions in nursing infants from MIDAMOR, a decision should be made whether to discontinue nursing or to discontinue the drug, taking into account the importance of the drug to the mother.

Pediatric Use

Safety and effectiveness in pediatric patients have not been established.

ADVERSE REACTIONS

MIDAMOR is usually well tolerated and, except for hyperkalemia (serum potassium levels greater than 5.5 mEq per liter—see WARNINGS), significant adverse effects have been reported infrequently. Minor adverse reactions were reported relatively frequently (about 20%) but the relationship of many of the reports to amiloride HCl is uncertain and the overall frequency was similar in hydrochlorothiazide treated groups. Nausea/anorexia, abdominal pain, flatulence, and mild skin rash have been reported and probably are related to amiloride. Other adverse experiences that have been reported with amiloride are generally those known to be associated with diuresis, or with the underlying disease being treated.

The adverse reactions for MIDAMOR listed in the following table have been arranged into two groups: (1) incidence greater than one percent; and (2) incidence one percent or less. The incidence for group (1) was determined from clinical studies conducted in the United States (837 patients treated with MIDAMOR). The adverse effects listed in group (2) include reports from the same clinical studies and voluntary reports since marketing. The probability of a causal relationship exists between MIDAMOR and these adverse reactions, some of which have been reported only rarely.

Incidence > 1%	Incidence ≤ 1%
Body as a Whole	
Headache*	Back pain
Weakness	Chest pain
Fatigability	Neck/shoulder ache
	Pain, extremeties
Cardiovascular	
None	Angina pectoris
	Orthostatic hypotension
	Arrhythmia
	Palpitation

Continued on next page

Information on the Merck & Co., Inc. products listed on these pages is the full prescribing information from product circulars in use August 31, 1998. For information, please call 1-800-NSC MERCK [1-800-672-6372].

Midamor—Cont.

Digestive
Nausea/anorexia*   Jaundice
Diarrhea*   GI bleeding
Vomiting*   Abdominal fullness
Abdominal pain   GI disturbance
Gas pain   Thirst
Appetite changes   Heartburn
Constipation   Flatulence
   Dyspepsia

Metabolic
Elevated serum   None
  potassium levels
  (> 5.5 mEq
  per liter)†

Skin
None   Skin rash
   Itching
   Dryness of mouth
   Pruritus
   Alopecia

Musculoskeletal
Muscle cramps   Joint pain
   Leg ache

Nervous
Dizziness   Paresthesia
Encephalopathy   Tremors
   Vertigo

Psychiatric
None   Nervousness
   Mental confusion
   Insomnia
   Decreased libido
   Depression
   Somnolence

Respiratory
Cough   Shortness of breath
Dyspnea

Special Senses
None   Visual disturbances
   Nasal congestion
   Tinnitus
   Increased intraocular
    pressure

Urogenital
Impotence   Polyuria
   Dysuria
   Urinary frequency
   Bladder spasms
   Gynecomastia

---

* Reactions occurring in 3% to 8% of patients treated with MIDAMOR. (Those reactions occurring in less than 3% of the patients are unmarked.)
† See WARNINGS.

Causal Relationship Unknown
Other reactions have been reported but occurred under circumstances where a causal relationship could not be established. However, in these rarely reported events, that possibility cannot be excluded. Therefore, these observations are listed to serve as alerting information to physicians.
   Activation of probable pre-existing peptic ulcer
   Aplastic anemia
   Neutropenia
   Abnormal liver function

OVERDOSAGE

No data are available in regard to overdosage in humans. The oral LD_{50} of amiloride hydrochloride (calculated as the base) is 56 mg/kg in mice and 36 to 85 mg/kg in rats, depending on the strain.
It is not known whether the drug is dialyzable.
The most likely signs and symptoms to be expected with overdosage are dehydration and electrolyte imbalance. These can be treated by established procedures. Therapy with MIDAMOR should be discontinued and the patient observed closely. There is no specific antidote. Emesis should be induced or gastric lavage performed. Treatment is symptomatic and supportive. If hyperkalemia occurs, active measures should be taken to reduce the serum potassium levels.

DOSAGE AND ADMINISTRATION

MIDAMOR should be administered with food.
MIDAMOR, one 5 mg tablet daily, should be added to the usual antihypertensive or diuretic dosage of a kaliuretic diuretic. The dosage may be increased to 10 mg per day, if necessary. More than two 5 mg tablets of MIDAMOR daily usually are not needed, and there is little controlled experi-

ence with such doses. If persistent hypokalemia is documented with 10 mg, the dose can be increased to 15 mg, then 20 mg, with careful monitoring of electrolytes.
In treating patients with congestive heart failure after an initial diuresis has been achieved, potassium loss may also decrease and the need for MIDAMOR should be reevaluated. Dosage adjustment may be necessary. Maintenance therapy may be on an intermittent basis.
If it is necessary to use MIDAMOR alone (see INDICATIONS), the starting dosage should be one 5 mg tablet daily. This dosage may be increased to 10 mg per day, if necessary. More than two 5 mg tablets usually are not needed, and there is little controlled experience with such doses. If persistent hypokalemia is documented with 10 mg, the dose can be increased to 15 mg, then 20 mg, with careful monitoring of electrolytes.

HOW SUPPLIED

No. 3381—Tablets MIDAMOR, 5 mg, are yellow, diamond-shaped, compressed tablets, coded MSD 92 on one side and MIDAMOR on the other. They are supplied as follows:
NDC 0006-0092-68 bottles of 100
(6505-01-127-8721 5 mg, 100's).
   Shown in Product Identification Guide, page 323
Storage
Protect from moisture, freezing and excessive heat.
      7905116   Issued August 1996
COPYRIGHT © MERCK & CO., INC., 1985
All rights reserved

MINTEZOL® Chewable Tablets   ℞
(Thiabendazole), U.S.P.

MINTEZOL® Suspension   ℞
(Thiabendazole), U.S.P.

DESCRIPTION

MINTEZOL* (Thiabendazole) is an anthelmintic provided as 500 mg chewable tablets, and as a suspension, containing 500 mg thiabendazole per 5 mL. The suspension also contains sorbic acid 0.1% added as a preservative. Inactive ingredients in the tablets are acacia, calcium phosphate, flavors, lactose, magnesium stearate, mannitol, methylcellulose, and sodium saccharin. Inactive ingredients in the suspension are an antifoam agent, flavors, polysorbate, purified water, sorbitol solution, and tragacanth.
Thiabendazole is a white to off-white odorless powder with a molecular weight of 201.26, which is practically insoluble in water but readily soluble in dilute acid and alkali. Its chemical name is 2-(4-thiazolyl)-1*H*-benzimidazole. The empirical formula is $C_{10}H_7N_3S$ and the structural formula is:

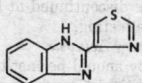

---

*Registered trademark of MERCK & CO., INC.

CLINICAL PHARMACOLOGY

In man, thiabendazole is rapidly absorbed and peak plasma concentration is reached within 1 to 2 hours after the oral administration of a suspension. It is metabolized almost completely to the 5-hydroxy form which appears in the urine as glucuronide or sulfate conjugates. In 48 hours, about 5% of the administered dose is recovered from the feces and about 90% from the urine. Most is excreted in the first 24 hours.
Mechanism of Action
The precise mode of action of thiabendazole on the parasite is unknown, but it may inhibit the helminth-specific enzyme fumarate reductase.
Thiabendazole is vermicidal and/or vermifugal against *Ascaris lumbricoides* ("common roundworm"), *Strongyloides stercoralis* (threadworm), *Necator americanus*, and *Ancylostoma duodenale* (hookworm), *Trichuris trichiura* (whipworm), *Ancylostoma braziliense* (dog and cat hookworm), *Toxocara canis* and *Toxocara cati* (ascarids), and *Enterobius vermicularis* (pinworm).
Its effect on larvae of *Trichinella spiralis* that have migrated to muscle is questionable.
Thiabendazole also suppresses egg and/or larval production and may inhibit the subsequent development of those eggs or larvae which are passed in the feces.

INDICATIONS AND USAGE

MINTEZOL is indicated for the treatment of:
   Strongyloidiasis (threadworm)
   Cutaneous larva migrans (creeping eruption)

   Visceral larva migrans
   Trichinosis: Relief of symptoms and fever and a reduction of eosinophilia have followed the use of MINTEZOL during the invasion stage of the disease.
Thiabendazole is usually inappropriate as first line therapy for enterobiasis (pinworm). However, when enterobiasis occurs with any of the conditions listed above, additional therapy is not required for most patients.
MINTEZOL should be used only in the following infestations when more specific therapy is not available or cannot be used or when further therapy with a second agent is desirable: Uncinariasis (hookworm: *Necator americanus* and *Ancylostoma duodenale*); Trichuriasis (whipworm); Ascariasis (large roundworm).

CONTRAINDICATION

Hypersensitivity to this product.
Thiabendazole is contraindicated as prophylactic treatment for pinworm infestation.

WARNINGS

If hypersensitivity reactions occur, the drug should be discontinued immediately and not be resumed. Erythema multiforme has been associated with thiabendazole therapy; in severe cases (Stevens-Johnson syndrome), fatalities have occurred.
Because CNS side effects may occur quite frequently, activities requiring mental alertness should be avoided.
Jaundice, cholestasis, and parenchymal liver damage have been reported in patients treated with MINTEZOL. In rare cases, liver damage has been severe and has led to irreversible hepatic failure. (See ADVERSE REACTIONS.)
Abnormal sensation in eyes, xanthopsia, blurred vision, drying of mucous membranes, and SICCA syndrome have been reported in patients treated with MINTEZOL. These adverse effects of the eye were in some cases persistent for prolonged intervals which have exceeded one year. (See ADVERSE REACTIONS.)
Thiabendazole should not usually be used as first line therapy for the treatment of enterobiasis. It should be reserved for use in patients who have experienced allergic reactions, or resistance to other treatments.

PRECAUTIONS

General
MINTEZOL is not suitable for the treatment of mixed infections with ascaris because it may cause these worms to migrate.
Ideally, supportive therapy is indicated for anemic, dehydrated or malnourished patients prior to initiation of the anthelmintic therapy.
In the presence of hepatic or renal dysfunction, patients should be carefully monitored.
MINTEZOL should be used only in patients in whom susceptible worm infestation has been diagnosed and should not be used prophylactically.
Information for Patients
Because CNS side effects may occur quite frequently, activities requiring mental alertness should be avoided.
Laboratory Tests
Rarely, a transient rise in liver function tests has occurred in patients receiving MINTEZOL.
Drug Interactions
Thiabendazole may compete with other drugs, such as theophylline, for sites of metabolism in the liver, thus elevating the serum levels of such compounds to potentially toxic levels. Therefore, when concomitant use of thiabendazole and xanthine derivatives is anticipated, it may be necessary to monitor blood levels and/or reduce the dosage of such compounds. Such concomitant use should be administered under careful medical supervision.
Carcinogenesis, Mutagenesis,
Impairment of Fertility
Thiabendazole has been used in numerous short- and long-term studies in animals at doses up to 15 times the usual human dose and was without carcinogenic effects. It did not adversely affect fertility in the mouse at $2^1/_2$ times the usual human dose or in the rat at a dose equivalent to the usual human dose. Thiabendazole had no mutagenic activity in *in vitro* microbial mutagen test, the micronucleus test and the host mediated assay *in vivo*.
Pregnancy
Pregnancy Category C: Reproduction and teratogenic studies done in the rabbit at a dose up to 15 times the usual human dose, in the rat at a dose equivalent to the human dose, and in the mouse at a dose up to $2^1/_2$ times the usual human dose, revealed no evidence of harm to the fetus. In an additional study in the mouse, no defects were observed when thiabendazole was given in an aqueous suspension, at a dose 10 times the usual human dose; however, cleft palate and axial skeletal defects were observed when thiabendazole was suspended in olive oil and given at the same dose. There are no adequate and well controlled studies in preg-

Therapeutic Regimens

Indication	Regimen	Comments
*STRONGYLOIDIASIS	2 doses per day for 2 successive days.	A single dose of 20 mg/lb or 50 mg/kg may be employed as an alternative schedule, but a higher incidence of side effects should be expected.
CUTANEOUS LARVA MIGRANS (Creeping Eruption)	2 doses per day for 2 successive days.	If active lesions are still present 2 days after completion of therapy, a second course is recommended.
VISCERAL LARVA MIGRANS	2 doses per day for 7 successive days.	Safety and efficacy data on the seven-day treatment course are limited.
*TRICHINOSIS	2 doses per day for 2–4 successive days according to the response of the patient.	The optimal dosage for the treatment of trichinosis has not been established.
Other Indications * Intestinal roundworms (including Ascariasis, Uncinariasis and Trichuriasis)	2 doses per day for 2 successive days.	A single dose of 20 mg/lb or 50 mg/kg may be employed as an alternative schedule, but a higher incidence of side effects should be expected.

* Clinical experience with thiabendazole for treatment of each of these conditions in pediatric patients weighing less than 30 lbs has been limited.

nant women. MINTEZOL should be used during pregnancy only if the potential benefit justifies the potential risk to the fetus.

Nursing Mothers
It is not known whether this drug is excreted in human milk. Because of the potential for serious adverse reactions in nursing infants from MINTEZOL, a decision should be made whether to discontinue nursing or to discontinue the drug, taking into account the importance of the drug to the mother.

Pediatric Use
The safety and effectiveness of thiabendazole for the treatment of Strongyloidiasis, Ascariasis, Uncinariasis, Trichuriasis and Trichinosis in pediatric patients weighing less than 30 lbs has been limited.

ADVERSE REACTIONS

Gastrointestinal: anorexia, nausea, vomiting, diarrhea, epigastric distress, abdominal pain, jaundice, cholestasis, parenchymal liver damage and hepatic failure. (See WARNINGS.)
Central Nervous System: dizziness, weariness, drowsiness, giddiness, headache, numbness, hyperirritability, convulsions, collapse, confusion, depression, floating sensation, weakness and lack of coordination.
Special Senses: tinnitus, abnormal sensation in eyes, xanthopsia, blurred vision, reduced vision, drying of mucous membranes (mouth, eyes, etc.), SICCA syndrome. (See WARNINGS.)
Cardiovascular: hypotension.
Metabolic: hyperglycemia.
Hematologic: transient leukopenia.
Genitourinary: hematuria, enuresis, malodor of the urine, crystalluria.
Hypersensitivity: pruritus, fever, facial flush, chills, conjunctival injection, angioedema, anaphylaxis, skin rashes (including perianal), erythema multiforme (including Stevens-Johnson syndrome), and lymphadenopathy.
Miscellaneous: appearance of live Ascaris in the mouth and nose.

OVERDOSAGE

Overdosage may be associated with transient disturbances of vision and psychic alterations.
There is no specific antidote in the event of overdosage. Therefore, symptomatic and supportive measures should be employed. Emesis should be induced or gastric lavage performed carefully.
The oral LD_{50} of MINTEZOL is 3.6 g/kg, 3.1 g/kg and 3.8 g/kg in the mouse, rat, and rabbit respectively.

DOSAGE AND ADMINISTRATION

The recommended maximum daily dose of MINTEZOL *is 3 grams.*
MINTEZOL should be given after meals if possible. Tablets MINTEZOL should be chewed before swallowing. Dietary restriction, complementary medications and cleansing enemas are not needed.
The usual dosage schedule for all conditions is two doses per day. The dosage is determined by the patient's weight.
A weight-dose chart follows:

Weight	Each Dose	
	g	mL
30 lb	0.25 (½ tablet)	2.5 (½ teaspoon)
50 lb	0.5 (1 tablet)	5.0 (1 teaspoon)
75 lb	0.75 (1½ tablets)	7.5 (1½ teaspoons)
100 lb	1.0 (2 tablets)	10.0 (2 teaspoons)
125 lb	1.25 (2½ tablets)	12.5 (2½ teaspoons)
150 lb & over	1.5 (3 tablets)	15.0 (3 teaspoons)

The regimen for each indication follows:
[See table at top of page]

HOW SUPPLIED

No. 3331 — MINTEZOL Suspension, 500 mg per 5 mL, is white to off-white and is supplied as follows:
NDC 0006-3331-60 in bottles of 120 mL
(6505-00-935-5835, 0.5 g/5 mL, 120 mL).
Storage
Store in a well-closed container at controlled room temperature [15–30°C (59–86°F)]. Protect from freezing.
No. 3332 — MINTEZOL Chewable Tablets, 500 mg, are white to off-white, orange-flavored, round, scored, compressed tablets, coded MSD 907 on one side and MINTEZOL on the other.
They are supplied as follows:
NDC 0006-0907-36 unit dose packages of 36
(6505-01-226-9909, 500 mg chewable, individually sealed 36's).
Shown in Product Identification Guide, page 323
Storage
Store in a well-closed container at controlled room temperature [15–30°C (59–86°F)].
7930814   Issued January 1998
COPYRIGHT © MERCK & CO., INC., 1983
All rights reserved

MODURETIC® Tablets
(Amiloride HCl-Hydrochlorothiazide), U.S.P.   ℞

DESCRIPTION

MODURETIC* (Amiloride HCl-Hydrochlorothiazide) combines the potassium-conserving action of amiloride HCl with the natriuretic action of hydrochlorothiazide.
Amiloride HCl is designated chemically as 3,5-diamino-6-chloro -*N*- (diaminomethylene) pyrazinecarboxamide monohydrochloride, dihydrate and has a molecular weight of 302.12. Its empirical formula is $C_6H_8ClN_7O \cdot HCl \cdot 2H_2O$ and its structural formula is:

Hydrochlorothiazide is designated chemically as 6-chloro-3,4-dihydro-2*H*-1,2,4-benzothiadiazine-7-sulfonamide 1,1-dioxide. Its empirical formula is $C_7H_8ClN_3O_4S_2$ and its structural formula is:

It is a white, or practically white, crystalline powder with a molecular weight of 297.74, which is slightly soluble in water, but freely soluble in sodium hydroxide solution.
MODURETIC is available for oral use as tablets containing 5 mg of anhydrous amiloride HCl and 50 mg of hydrochlorothiazide. Each tablet contains the following inactive ingredients: calcium phosphate, FD&C Yellow 6, guar gum, lactose, magnesium stearate and starch.

---

*Registered trademark of MERCK & CO., INC.

CLINICAL PHARMACOLOGY

MODURETIC provides diuretic and antihypertensive activity (principally due to the hydrochlorothiazide component), while acting through the amiloride component to prevent the excessive potassium loss that may occur in patients receiving a thiazide diuretic. Due to its amiloride component, the urinary excretion of magnesium is less with MODURETIC than with a thiazide or loop diuretic used alone (see PRECAUTIONS). The onset of the diuretic action of MODURETIC is within 1 to 2 hours and this action appears to be sustained for approximately 24 hours.
Amiloride HCl
Amiloride HCl is a potassium-conserving (antikaliuretic) drug that possesses weak (compared with thiazide diuretics) natriuretic, diuretic, and antihypertensive activity. These effects have been partially additive to the effects of thiazide diuretics in some clinical studies. Amiloride HCl has potassium-conserving activity in patients receiving kaliuretic-diuretic agents.
Amiloride HCl is not an aldosterone antagonist and its effects are seen even in the absence of aldosterone.
Amiloride HCl exerts its potassium sparing effect through the inhibition of sodium reabsorption at the distal convoluted tubule, cortical collecting tubule and collecting duct; this decreases the net negative potential of the tubular lumen and reduces both potassium and hydrogen secretion and their subsequent excretion. This mechanism accounts in large part for the potassium sparing action of amiloride. Amiloride HCl usually begins to act within 2 hours after an oral dose. Its effect on electrolyte excretion reaches a peak between 6 and 10 hours and lasts about 24 hours. Peak plasma levels are obtained in 3 to 4 hours and the plasma half-life varies from 6 to 9 hours. Effects on electrolytes increase with single doses of amiloride HCl up to approximately 15 mg.
Amiloride HCl is not metabolized by the liver but is excreted unchanged by the kidneys. About 50 percent of a 20 mg dose of amiloride HCl is excreted in the urine and 40 percent in the stool within 72 hours. Amiloride HCl has little effect on glomerular filtration rate or renal blood flow. Because amiloride HCl is not metabolized by the liver, drug accumulation is not anticipated in patients with hepatic dysfunction, but accumulation can occur if the hepatorenal syndrome develops.
Hydrochlorothiazide
The mechanism of the antihypertensive effect of thiazides is unknown. Thiazides do not usually affect normal blood pressure.
Hydrochlorothiazide is a diuretic and antihypertensive. It affects the distal renal tubular mechanism of electrolyte reabsorption. Hydrochlorothiazide increases excretion of sodium and chloride in approximately equivalent amounts. Natriuresis may be accompanied by some loss of potassium and bicarbonate.
After oral use diuresis begins within two hours, peaks in about four hours and lasts about 6 to 12 hours.
Hydrochlorothiazide is not metabolized but is eliminated rapidly by the kidney. When plasma levels have been followed for at least 24 hours, the plasma half-life has been observed to vary between 5.6 and 14.8 hours. At least 61

Continued on next page

Moduretic—Cont.

percent of the oral dose is eliminated unchanged within 24 hours. Hydrochlorothiazide crosses the placental but not the blood-brain barrier and is excreted in breast milk.

INDICATIONS AND USAGE

MODURETIC is indicated in those patients with hypertension or with congestive heart failure who develop hypokalemia when thiazides or other kaliuretic diuretics are used alone, or in whom maintenance of normal serum potassium levels is considered to be clinically important, e.g., digitalized patients, or patients with significant cardiac arrhythmias.

The use of potassium-conserving agents is often unnecessary in patients receiving diuretics for uncomplicated essential hypertension when such patients have a normal diet. MODURETIC may be used alone or as an adjunct to other antihypertensive drugs, such as methyldopa or beta blockers. Since MODURETIC enhances the action of these agents, dosage adjustments may be necessary to avoid an excessive fall in blood pressure and other unwanted side effects.

This fixed combination drug is not indicated for the initial therapy of edema or hypertension except in individuals in whom the development of hypokalemia cannot be risked.

CONTRAINDICATIONS

Hyperkalemia

MODURETIC should not be used in the presence of elevated serum potassium levels (greater than 5.5 mEq per liter).

Antikaliuretic Therapy or Potassium Supplementation

MODURETIC should not be given to patients receiving other potassium-conserving agents, such as spironolactone or triamterene. Potassium supplementation in the form of medication, potassium-containing salt substitutes or a potassium-rich diet should not be used with MODURETIC except in severe and/or refractory cases of hypokalemia. Such concomitant therapy can be associated with rapid increases in serum potassium levels. If potassium supplementation is used, careful monitoring of the serum potassium level is necessary.

Impaired Renal Function

Anuria, acute or chronic renal insufficiency, and evidence of diabetic nephropathy are contraindications to the use of MODURETIC. Patients with evidence of renal functional impairment (blood urea nitrogen [BUN] levels over 30 mg per 100 mL or serum creatinine levels over 1.5 mg per 100 mL) or diabetes mellitus should not receive the drug without careful, frequent and continuing monitoring of serum electrolytes, creatinine, and BUN levels. Potassium retention associated with the use of an antikaliuretic agent is accentuated in the presence of renal impairment and may result in the rapid development of hyperkalemia.

Hypersensitivity

MODURETIC is contraindicated in patients who are hypersensitive to this product, or to other sulfonamide-derived drugs.

WARNINGS

Hyperkalemia

Like other potassium-conserving diuretic combinations, MODURETIC may cause hyperkalemia (serum potassium levels greater than 5.5 mEq per liter). In patients without renal impairment or diabetes mellitus, the risk of hyperkalemia with MODURETIC is about 1-2 percent. This risk is higher in patients with renal impairment or diabetes mellitus (even without recognized diabetic nephropathy). Since hyperkalemia, if uncorrected, is potentially fatal, it is essential to monitor serum potassium levels carefully in any patient receiving MODURETIC, particularly when it is first introduced, at the time of dosage adjustments, and during any illness that could affect renal function.

The risk of hyperkalemia may be increased when potassium-conserving agents, including MODURETIC, are administered concomitantly with an angiotensin-converting enzyme inhibitor. (See PRECAUTIONS, *Drug Interactions*.) Warning signs or symptoms of hyperkalemia include paresthesias, muscular weakness, fatigue, flaccid paralysis of the extremities, bradycardia, shock, and ECG abnormalities. Monitoring of the serum potassium level is essential because mild hyperkalemia is not usually associated with an abnormal ECG.

When abnormal, the ECG in hyperkalemia is characterized primarily by tall, peaked T waves or elevations from previous tracings. There may also be lowering of the R wave and increased depth of the S wave, widening and even disap-

pearance of the P wave, progressive widening of the QRS complex, prolongation of the PR interval, and ST depression.

Treatment of hyperkalemia: If hyperkalemia occurs in patients taking MODURETIC, the drug should be discontinued immediately. If the serum potassium level exceeds 6.5 mEq per liter, active measures should be taken to reduce it. Such measures include the intravenous administration of sodium bicarbonate solution or oral or parenteral glucose with a rapid-acting insulin preparation. If needed, a cation exchange resin such as sodium polystyrene sulfonate may be given orally or by enema. Patients with persistent hyperkalemia may require dialysis.

Diabetes Mellitus

In diabetic patients, hyperkalemia has been reported with the use of all potassium-conserving diuretics, including amiloride HCl, even in patients without evidence of diabetic nephropathy. Therefore, MODURETIC should be avoided, if possible, in diabetic patients and, if it is used, serum electrolytes and renal function must be monitored frequently. MODURETIC should be discontinued at least three days before glucose tolerance testing.

Metabolic or Respiratory Acidosis

Antikaliuretic therapy should be instituted only with caution in severely ill patients in whom respiratory or metabolic acidosis may occur, such as patients with cardiopulmonary disease or poorly controlled diabetes. If MODURETIC is given to these patients, frequent monitoring of acid-base balance is necessary. Shifts in acid-base balance alter the ratio of extracellular/intracellular potassium, and the development of acidosis may be associated with rapid increases in serum potassium levels.

PRECAUTIONS

General

Electrolyte Imbalance and BUN Increases

Determination of serum electrolytes to detect possible electrolyte imbalance should be performed at appropriate intervals.

Patients should be observed for clinical signs of fluid or electrolyte imbalance: i.e., hyponatremia, hypochloremic alkalosis, and hypokalemia. Serum and urine electrolyte determinations are particularly important when the patient is vomiting excessively or receiving parenteral fluids. Warning signs or symptoms of fluid and electrolyte imbalance, irrespective of cause, include dryness of mouth, thirst, weakness, lethargy, drowsiness, restlessness, confusion, seizures, muscle pains or cramps, muscular fatigue, hypotension, oliguria, tachycardia, and gastrointestinal disturbances such as nausea and vomiting.

Hyponatremia and hypochloremia may occur during the use of thiazides and other diuretics. Any chloride deficit during thiazide therapy is generally mild and may be lessened by the amiloride HCl component of MODURETIC. Hypochloremia usually does not require specific treatment except under extraordinary circumstances (as in liver disease or renal disease). Dilutional hyponatremia may occur in edematous patients in hot weather; appropriate therapy is water restriction, rather than administration of salt, except in rare instances when the hyponatremia is life-threatening. In actual salt depletion, appropriate replacement is the therapy of choice.

Hypokalemia may develop during thiazide therapy, especially with brisk diuresis, when severe cirrhosis is present, during concomitant use of corticosteroids or ACTH, or after prolonged therapy. However, this usually is prevented by the amiloride HCl component of MODURETIC.

Interference with adequate oral electrolyte intake will also contribute to hypokalemia. Hypokalemia may cause cardiac arrhythmia and may also sensitize or exaggerate the response of the heart to the toxic effects of digitalis (e.g., increased ventricular irritability).

Thiazides have been shown to increase the urinary excretion of magnesium; this may result in hypomagnesemia. Amiloride HCl, a component of MODURETIC, has been shown to decrease the enhanced urinary excretion of magnesium which occurs when a thiazide or loop diuretic is used alone.

Increases in BUN levels have been reported with amiloride HCl and with hydrochlorothiazide. These increases usually have accompanied vigorous fluid elimination, especially when diuretic therapy was used in seriously ill patients, such as those who had hepatic cirrhosis with ascites and metabolic alkalosis, or those with resistant edema. Therefore, when MODURETIC is given to such patients, careful monitoring of serum electrolyte and BUN levels is important. In patients with pre-existing severe liver disease, hepatic encephalopathy, manifested by tremors, confusion, and coma, and increased jaundice, have been reported in association with diuretic therapy including amiloride HCl and hydrochlorothiazide.

In patients with renal disease, diuretics may precipitate azotemia. Cumulative effects of the components of MODURETIC may develop in patients with impaired renal

function. If renal impairment becomes evident, MODURETIC should be discontinued (see CONTRAINDICATIONS and WARNINGS).

Drug Interactions

In some patients, the administration of a non-steroidal anti-inflammatory agent can reduce the diuretic, natriuretic, and antihypertensive effects of loop, potassium-sparing and thiazide diuretics. Therefore, when MODURETIC and non-steroidal anti-inflammatory agents are used concomitantly, the patient should be observed closely to determine if the desired effect of the diuretic is obtained. Since indomethacin and potassium-sparing diuretics, including MODURETIC, may each be associated with increased serum potassium levels, the potential effects on potassium kinetics and renal function should be considered when these agents are administered concurrently.

Amiloride HCl

When amiloride HCl is administered concomitantly with an angiotensin-converting enzyme inhibitor, the risk of hyperkalemia may be increased. Therefore, if concomitant use of these agents in indicated because of demonstrated hypokalemia, they should be used with caution and with frequent monitoring of serum potassium. (See WARNINGS.)

Hydrochlorothiazide

When given concurrently the following drugs may interact with thiazide diuretics.

Alcohol, barbiturates, or narcotics —potentiation of orthostatic hypotension may occur.

Antidiabetic drugs (oral agents and insulin)—dosage adjustment of the antidiabetic drug may be required.

Other antihypertensive drugs —additive effect or potentiation.

Cholestyramine and colestipol resins—Absorption of hydrochlorothiazide is impaired in the presence of anionic exchange resins. Single doses of either cholestyramine or colestipol resins bind the hydrochlorothiazide and reduce its absorption from the gastrointestinal tract by up to 85 and 43 percent, respectively.

Corticosteroids, ACTH —intensified electrolyte depletion, particularly hypokalemia.

Pressor amines (e.g., norepinephrine) —possible decreased response to pressor amines but not sufficient to preclude their use.

Skeletal muscle relaxants, nondepolarizing (e.g., tubocurarine) —possible increased responsiveness to the muscle relaxant.

Lithium —generally should not be given with diuretics. Diuretic agents reduce the renal clearance of lithium and add a high risk of lithium toxicity. Refer to the package insert for lithium preparations before use of such preparations with MODURETIC.

Metabolic and Endocrine Effects

In diabetic patients, insulin requirements may be increased, decreased, or unchanged due to the hydrochlorothiazide component. Diabetes mellitus that has been latent may become manifest during administration of thiazide diuretics.

Because calcium excretion is decreased by thiazides, MODURETIC should be discontinued before carrying out tests for parathyroid function. Pathologic changes in the parathyroid glands, with hypercalcemia and hypophosphatemia have been observed in a few patients on prolonged thiazide therapy; however, the common complications of hyperparathyroidism such as renal lithiasis, bone resorption, and peptic ulceration have not been seen.

Hyperuricemia may occur or acute gout may be precipitated in certain patients receiving thiazide therapy.

Other Precautions

In patients receiving thiazides, sensitivity reactions may occur with or without a history of allergy or bronchial asthma. The possibility of exacerbation or activation of systemic lupus erythematosus has been reported with the use of thiazides.

Increases in cholesterol and triglyceride levels may be associated with thiazide diuretic therapy.

Carcinogenicity, Mutagenicity, Impairment of Fertility

Long-term studies in animals have not been performed to evaluate the effects upon fertility, mutagenicity or carcinogenic potential of MODURETIC.

Amiloride HCl

There was no evidence of a tumorigenic effect when amiloride HCl was administered for 92 weeks to mice at doses up to 10 mg/kg/day (25 times the maximum daily human dose). Amiloride HCl has also been administered for 104 weeks to male and female rats at doses up to 6 and 8 mg/kg/day (15 and 20 times the maximum daily dose for humans, respectively) and showed no evidence of carcinogenicity.

Amiloride HCl was devoid of mutagenic activity in various strains of *Salmonella typhimurium* with or without a mammalian liver microsomal activation system (Ames test).

Hydrochlorothiazide

Two-year feeding studies in mice and rats conducted under the auspices of the National Toxicology Program (NTP) uncovered no evidence of a carcinogenic potential of hydrochlorothiazide in female mice (at doses of up to approximately

600 mg/kg/day) or in male and female rats (at doses of up to approximately 100 mg/kg/day). The NTP, however, found equivocal evidence for hepatocarcinogenicity in male mice. Hydrochlorothiazide was not genotoxic *in vitro* in the Ames mutagenicity assay of *Salmonella typhimurium* strains TA 98, TA 100, TA 1535, TA 1537, and TA 1538 and in the Chinese Hamster Ovary (CHO) test for chromosomal aberrations, or *in vivo* in assays using mouse germinal cell chromosomes, Chinese hamster bone marrow chromosomes, and the *Drosophila* sex-linked recessive lethal trait gene. Positive test results were obtained only in the *in vitro* CHO Sister Chromatid Exchange (clastogenicity) and in the Mouse Lymphoma Cell (mutagenicity) assays, using concentrations of hydrochlorothiazide from 43 to 1300 μg/mL, and in the *Asperigillus nidulans* non-disjunction assay at an unspecified concentration.

Hydrochlorothiazide had no adverse effects on the fertility of mice and rats of either sex in studies wherein these species were exposed, via their diet, to doses of up to 100 and 4 mg/kg, respectively, prior to conception and throughout gestation.

Pregnancy

Pregnancy Category B. Teratogenicity studies have been performed with combinations of amiloride HCl and hydrochlorothiazide in rabbits and mice at doses up to 25 times the expected maximum daily dose for humans and have revealed no evidence of harm to the fetus. No evidence of impaired fertility in rats was apparent at dosage levels up to 25 times the expected maximum human daily dose. A perinatal and postnatal study in rats showed a reduction in maternal body weight gain during and after gestation at a daily dose of 25 times the expected maximum daily dose for humans. The body weights of alive pups at birth and at weaning were also reduced at this dose level. There are no adequate and well-controlled studies in pregnant women. Because animal reproduction studies are not always predictive of human responses, and because of the data listed below with the individual components, this drug should be used during pregnancy only if clearly needed.

Amiloride HCl

Teratogenicity studies with amiloride HCl in rabbits and mice given 20 and 25 times the maximum human dose, respectively, revealed no evidence of harm to the fetus, although studies showed that the drug crossed the placenta in modest amounts. Reproduction studies in rats at 20 times the expected maximum daily dose for humans showed no evidence of impaired fertility. At approximately 5 or more times the expected maximum daily dose for humans, some toxicity was seen in adult rats and rabbits and a decrease in rat pup growth and survival occurred.

Hydrochlorothiazide

Teratogenic Effects: Studies in which hydrochlorothiazide was orally administered to pregnant mice and rats during their respective periods of major organogenesis at doses up to 3000 and 1000 mg hydrochlorothiazide/kg, respectively, provided no evidence of harm to the fetus. There are, however, no adequate and well-controlled studies in pregnant women.

Nonteratogenic Effects: Thiazides cross the placental barrier and appear in cord blood. There is a risk of fetal or neonatal jaundice, thrombocytopenia, and possibly other adverse reactions that have occurred in adults.

Nursing Mothers

Studies in rats have shown that amiloride is excreted in milk in concentrations higher than those found in blood, but it is not known whether amiloride HCl is excreted in human milk. However, thiazides appear in breast milk. Because of the potential for serious adverse reactions in nursing infants, a decision should be made whether to discontinue nursing or to discontinue the drug, taking into account the importance of the drug to the mother.

Pediatric Use

Safety and effectiveness in pediatric patients have not been established.

ADVERSE REACTIONS

MODURETIC is usually well tolerated and significant clinical adverse effects have been reported infrequently. The risk of hyperkalemia (serum potassium levels greater than 5.5 mEq per liter) with MODURETIC is about 1–2 percent in patients without renal impairment or diabetes mellitus (see WARNINGS). Minor adverse reactions to amiloride HCl have been reported relatively frequently (about 20%) but the relationship of many of these reports to amiloride HCl is uncertain and the overall frequency was similar in hydrochlorothiazide treated groups. Nausea/anorexia, abdominal pain, flatulence, and mild skin rash have been reported and probably are related to amiloride. Other adverse experiences that have been reported with MODURETIC are generally those known to be associated with diuresis, thiazide therapy, or with the underlying disease being treated. Clinical trials have not demonstrated that combining amiloride and hydrochlorothiazide increases the risk of adverse reactions over those seen with the individual components.

The adverse reactions for MODURETIC listed in the following table have been arranged into two groups: (1) incidence greater than one percent; and (2) incidence one percent or less. The incidence for group (1) was determined from clinical studies conducted in the United States (607 patients treated with MODURETIC). The adverse effects listed in group (2) include reports from the same clinical studies and voluntary reports since marketing. The probability of a causal relationship exists between MODURETIC and these adverse reactions, some of which have been reported only rarely.

Incidence > 1%	Incidence > 1%
Body as a Whole	
Headache*	Malaise
Weakness*	Chest pain
Fatigue/tiredness	Back pain
	Syncope
Cardiovascular	
Arryhthmia	Tachycardia
	Digitalis toxicity
	Orthostatic hypotension
	Angina pectoris
Digestive	
Nausea/anorexia*	Constipation
Diarrhea	GI bleeding
Gastrointestinal	GI disturbance
pain	Appetite changes
Abdominal pain	Abdominal fullness
	Hiccups
	Thirst
	Vomiting
	Anorexia
	Flatulence
Metabolic	
Elevated serum	Gout
potassium levels	Dehydration
(>5.5 mEq)	Symptomatic
per liter)†	hyponatremia**
Musculoskeletal	
Leg ache	Muscle cramps/spasm
	Joint pain
Nervous	
Dizziness*	Paraesthesia/numbness
	Stupor
	Vertigo
Psychiatric	
None	Insomnia
	Nervousness
	Depression
	Sleepiness
	Mental confusion
Respiratory	
Dyspnea	None
Skin	
Rash*	Flushing
Pruritus	Diaphoresis
	Erythema multiforme including Stevens-Johnson syndrome
	Exfoliative dermatits including toxic epidermal necrolysis
	Alopecia
Special Senses	
None	Bad taste
	Visual disturbance
	Nasal congestion
Urogenital	
None	Impotence
	Nocturia
	Dysuria
	Incontinence
	Renal dysfunction including renal failure
	Gynecomastia

* Reactions occurring in 3% to 8% of patients treated with MODURETIC. (Those reactions occurring in less than 3% of the patients are unmarked.)

† See WARNINGS.

** See PRECAUTIONS.

Other adverse reactions that have been reported with the individual components and within each category are listed in order of decreasing severity:

Amiloride —Body as a Whole: Painful extremities, neck/shoulder ache, fatigability; *Cardiovascular:* Palpitation; *Digestive:* Activation of probable pre-existing peptic ulcer, abnormal liver function, jaundice, dyspepsia, heartburn; *Hematologic:* Aplastic anemia, neutropenia; *Integumentary:* Alopecia, itching, dry mouth; *Nervous System/Psychiatric:* Encephalopathy, tremors, decreased libido; *Respiratory:* Shortness of breath, cough; *Special Senses:* Increased intraocular pressure, tinnitus; *Urogenital:* Bladder spasms, polyuria, urinary frequency.

Hydrochlorothiazide —Digestive: Pancreatitis, jaundice (intrahepatic cholestatic jaundice), sialadenitis, cramping, gastric irritation; *Hematologic:* Aplastic anemia, agranulocytosis, leukopenia, hemolytic anemia, thrombocytopenia; *Hypersensitivity:* Anaphylactic reactions, necrotizing angiitis (vasculitis, cutaneous vasculitis), respiratory distress including pneumonitis and pulmonary edema, photosensitivity, fever, urticaria, purpura; *Metabolic:* Electrolyte imbalance (see PRECAUTIONS), hyperglycemia, glycosuria, hyperuricemia; *Nervous System/Psychiatric:* Restlessness; *Special Senses:* Transient blurred vision, xanthopsia; *Urogenital:* Interstitial nephritis (see WARNINGS).

OVERDOSAGE

No data are available in regard to overdosage in humans. The oral LD$_{50}$ of the combination drug is 189 and 422 mg/kg for female mice and female rats, respectively.

It is not known whether the drug is dialyzable.

No specific information is available on the treatment of overdosage with MODURETIC, and no specific antidote is available. Treatment is symptomatic and supportive. Therapy with MODURETIC should be discontinued and the patient observed closely. Suggested measures include induction of emesis and/or gastric lavage.

Amiloride HCl: No data are available in regard to overdosage in humans.

The oral LD$_{50}$ of amiloride HCl (calculated as the base) is 56 mg/kg in mice and 36 to 85 mg/kg in rats, depending on the strain.

The most common signs and symptoms to be expected with overdosage are dehydration and electrolyte imbalance. If hyperkalemia occurs, active measures should be taken to reduce the serum potassium levels.

Hydrochlorothiazide: The oral LD$_{50}$ of hydrochlorothiazide is greater than 10.0 g/kg in both mice and rats.

The most common signs and symptoms observed are those caused by electrolyte depletion (hypokalemia, hypochloremia, hyponatremia) and dehydration resulting from excessive diuresis. If digitalis has also been administered, hypokalemia may accentuate cardiac arrhythmias.

DOSAGE AND ADMINISTRATION

MODURETIC should be administered with food.

The usual starting dosage is 1 tablet a day. The dosage may be increased to 2 tablets a day, if necessary. More than 2 tablets of MODURETIC daily usually are not needed and there is no controlled experience with such doses. The daily dose is usually given as a single dose but may be given in divided doses. Once an initial diuresis has been achieved, dosage adjustment may be necessary. Maintenance therapy may be on an intermittent basis.

HOW SUPPLIED

No. 3385—Tablets MODURETIC are peach-colored, diamond-shaped, scored, compressed tablets, coded MSD 917 on one side and M on the other. Each tablet contains 5 mg of anhydrous amiloride HCl and 50 mg of hydrochlorothiazide. They are supplied as follows:

NDC 0006-0917-68 in bottles of 100 (6505-01-139-1498 100's)

NDC 0006-0917-28 unit dose packages of 100.

Shown in Product Identification Guide, page 323

Storage

Keep container tightly closed. Protect from light, moisture, freezing, –20°C (–4°F) and store at room temperature, 15–30°C (59–86°F).

7887325 Issued August 1996

MUMPSVAX®
(Mumps Virus Vaccine Live), U.S.P.
Jeryl Lynn Strain

℞

DESCRIPTION

MUMPSVAX* (Mumps Virus Vaccine Live) is a live virus vaccine for immunization against mumps.

MUMPSVAX is a sterile lyophilized preparation of the Jeryl Lynn (B level) strain of mumps virus. The virus was adapted to and propagated in cell cultures of chick embryo free of avian leukosis virus and other adventitious agents.

Continued on next page

Information on the Merck & Co., Inc. products listed on these pages is the full prescribing information from product circulars in use August 31, 1998. For information, please call 1-800-NSC MERCK [1-800-672-6372].

Mumpsvax—Cont.

The reconstituted vaccine is for subcutaneous administration. When reconstituted as directed, the dose for injection is 0.5 mL and contains not less than the equivalent of 20,000 TCID$_{50}$ (tissue culture infectious doses) of the U.S. Reference Mumps Virus. Each dose contains approximately 25 mcg of neomycin. The product contains no preservative. Sorbitol and hydrolized gelatin are added as stabilizers.

*Registered trademark of MERCK & CO., INC.

CLINICAL PHARMACOLOGY

MUMPSVAX produces a modified, non-communicable mumps infection in susceptible persons. Extensive clinical trials have demonstrated that MUMPSVAX is highly immunogenic and well tolerated. A single injection of the vaccine has been shown to induce mumps neutralizing antibodies in approximately 97 percent of susceptible children and approximately 93 percent of susceptible adults. The pattern of antibody response closely resembles that observed for natural mumps. Although the antibody level is significantly lower than that following natural infection, it is protective and long lasting. Vaccine-induced antibody levels have been shown to persist for at least 15 years with a rate of decline comparable to that seen in natural infection. If the present pattern continues, it will provide a basis for the expectation that immunity following vaccination will be permanent. However, continued surveillance will be required to demonstrate this point.

INDICATIONS AND USAGE

MUMPSVAX is indicated for immunization against mumps in persons 12 months of age or older. Most adults are likely to have been infected naturally and generally may be considered immune, even if they did not have clinically recognizable disease. A booster is not needed. It is not recommended for infants younger than 12 months because they may retain maternal mumps neutralizing antibodies which may interfere with the immune response.

Evidence indicates that the vaccine will not offer protection when given after exposure to natural mumps. Passively acquired antibody can interfere with the response to live, attenuated-virus vaccines. Therefore, administration of mumps virus vaccine should be deferred until approximately three months after passive immunization.

Individuals planning travel outside the United States, if not immune, can acquire measles, mumps or rubella and import these diseases to the United States. Therefore, prior to International travel, individuals known to be susceptible to one or more of these diseases can receive either a single antigen vaccine (measles, mumps or rubella), or a combined antigen vaccine as appropriate. However, M-M-R* II (Measles, Mumps, and Rubella Virus Vaccine Live) is preferred for persons likely to be susceptible to mumps and rubella; and if single-antigen measles vaccine is not readily available, travelers should receive M-M-R II (Measles, Mumps, and Rubella Virus Vaccine Live) regardless of their immune status to mumps or rubella.

Revaccination: Children vaccinated when younger than 12 months of age should be revaccinated. Based on available evidence, there is no reason to routinely revaccinate persons who were vaccinated originally when 12 months of age or older. However, persons should be revaccinated if there is evidence to suggest that initial immunization was ineffective.

Use with other Vaccines

Routine administration of DTP (diphtheria, tetanus, pertussis) and/or OPV (oral poliovirus vaccine) concomitantly with measles, mumps and rubella vaccines is not recommended because there are insufficient data relating to the simultaneous administration of these antigens. However, the American Academy of Pediatrics has noted that in some circumstances, particularly when the patient may not return, some practitioners prefer to administer all these antigens on a single day. If done, separate sites and syringes should be used for DTP and MUMPSVAX.

MUMPSVAX should not be given less than one month before or after administration of other virus vaccines.

*Registered trademark of MERCK & CO., INC.

CONTRAINDICATIONS

Do not give MUMPSVAX to pregnant females; the possible effects of the vaccine on fetal development are unknown at this time. If vaccination of postpubertal females is undertaken, pregnancy should be avoided for three months following vaccination (see PRECAUTIONS, *Pregnancy*).

Anaphylactic or anaphylactoid reactions to neomycin (each dose of reconstituted vaccine contains approximately 25 mcg of neomycin).

History of anaphylactic or anaphylactoid reactions to eggs (see HYPERSENSITIVITY TO EGGS below).

Any febrile respiratory illness or other active febrile infection.

Active untreated tuberculosis.

Patients receiving immunosuppressive therapy. This contraindication does not apply to patients who are receiving corticosteroids as replacement therapy, e.g., for Addison's disease.

Individuals with blood dyscrasias, leukemia, lymphomas of any type, or other malignant neoplasms affecting the bone marrow or lymphatic systems.

Primary and acquired immunodeficiency states, including patients who are immunosuppressed in association with AIDS or other clinical manifestations of infection with human immunodeficiency viruses; cellular immune deficiencies; and hypogammaglobulinemic and dysgammaglobulinemic states.

Individuals with a family history of congenital or hereditary immunodeficiency, until the immune competence of the potential vaccine recipient is demonstrated.

HYPERSENSITIVITY TO EGGS

Live mumps vaccine is produced in chick embryo cell culture. Persons with a history of anaphylactic, anaphylactoid, or other immediate reactions (e.g., hives, swelling of the mouth and throat, difficulty breathing, hypotension, or shock) subsequent to egg ingestion should be vaccinated only with extreme caution. Evidence indicates that persons are not at increased risk if they have egg allergies that are not anaphylactic or anaphylactoid in nature. Such persons may be vaccinated in the usual manner. There is no evidence to indicate that persons with allergies to chickens or feathers are at increased risk of reaction to the vaccine.

PRECAUTIONS

General

Adequate treatment provisions including epinephrine, should be available for immediate use should an anaphylactic or anaphylactoid reaction occur.

Children and young adults who are known to be infected with human immunodeficiency viruses but without overt clinical manifestations of immunosuppression may be vaccinated; however, the vaccinees should be monitored closely for vaccine-preventable diseases because immunization may be less effective than for uninfected persons.

Vaccination should be deferred for at least 3 months following blood or plasma transfusions, or administration of human immune serum globulin.

There are no reports of transmission of live mumps virus from vaccinees to susceptible contacts.

It has been reported that mumps virus vaccine, live, may result in a temporary depression of tuberculin skin sensitivity. Therefore, if a tuberculin test is to be done, it should be administered either before or simultaneously with MUMPSVAX.

As for any vaccine, vaccination with MUMPSVAX may not result in seroconversion in 100% of susceptible persons given the vaccine.

Pregnancy

Pregnancy Category C

Animal reproduction studies have not been conducted with MUMPSVAX. It is also not known whether MUMPSVAX can cause fetal harm when administered to a pregnant woman or can affect reproduction capacity. Therefore, mumps virus vaccine should not be given to persons known to be pregnant; furthermore, pregnancy should be avoided for three months following vaccination. Although mumps virus is capable of infecting the placenta and fetus, there is no good evidence that it causes congenital malformations in humans. Mumps vaccine virus also has been shown to infect the placenta, but the virus has not been isolated from the fetal tissues from susceptible women who were vaccinated and underwent elective abortions.

Nursing Mothers

It is not known whether mumps vaccine virus is secreted in human milk. Therefore, because many drugs are excreted in human milk, caution should be exercised when MUMPSVAX is administered to a nursing woman.

ADVERSE REACTIONS

Burning and/or stinging of short duration at the injection site have been reported.

Anaphylaxis and anaphylactoid reactions have been reported.

Mild fever occurs occasionally. Fever above 103°F (39.4°C) is uncommon.

Mild lymphadenopathy has been reported.

Cough and rhinitis have been reported after vaccination with other mumps-containing vaccines.

Diarrhea has been reported after vaccination with mumps-containing vaccines.

Vasculitis has been reported rarely after vaccination with other mumps-containing vaccines.

Parotitis has been reported to occur in very low incidence, and orchitis rarely, in persons who were vaccinated. In most instances investigated, prior exposure to natural mumps was established. In other instances, whether or not this was due to vaccine or to prior natural mumps exposure or to other causes has not been established.

Reports of purpura and allergic reactions such as wheal and flare at the injection site or urticaria have been extremely rare. Erythema multiforme has also been reported rarely.

Forms of optic neuritis, including retrobulbar neuritis and papillitis may infrequently follow viral infections, and have been reported to occur 1 to 3 weeks following inoculation with some live virus vaccines.

Syncope, particularly at the time of mass vaccination, has been reported.

Very rarely encephalitis, febrile seizures, nerve deafness and other nervous system reactions have occurred in vaccinees. A cause-effect relationship has not been established.

DOSAGE AND ADMINISTRATION

FOR SUBCUTANEOUS ADMINISTRATION

Do not inject intravenously

The dosage of vaccine is the same for all persons. Inject the total volume (about 0.5 mL) of reconstituted vaccine subcutaneously, preferably into the outer aspect of upper arm. *Do not give immune serum globulin (ISG) concurrently with* MUMPSVAX.

During shipment, to insure that there is no loss of potency, the vaccine must be maintained at a temperature of 10°C (50°F) or less.

Before reconstitution, store MUMPSVAX at 2–8°C (36–46°F). *Protect from light.*

CAUTION: A sterile syringe free of preservatives, antiseptics, and detergents should be used for each injection and/or reconstitution of the vaccine because these substances may inactivate the live virus vaccine. A 25 gauge, ⅝" needle is recommended.

To reconstitute, use only the diluent supplied, since it is free of preservatives or other antiviral substances which might inactivate the vaccine.

Single Dose Vial—First withdraw the entire volume of diluent into the syringe to be used for reconstitution. Inject all the diluent in the syringe into the vial of lyophilized vaccine, and agitate to mix thoroughly. Withdraw the entire contents into a syringe and inject the total volume of restored vaccine subcutaneously.

It is important to use a separate sterile syringe and needle for each individual patient to prevent transmission of hepatitis B and other infectious agents from one person to another.

10 Dose Vial (available only to government agencies/institutions)—Withdraw the entire contents (7 mL) of the diluent vial into the sterile syringe to be used for reconstitution, and introduce into the 10 dose vial of lyophilized vaccine. Agitate to ensure thorough mixing. The outer labeling suggests "For Jet Injector or Syringe Use". Use with separate sterile syringes is permitted for containers of 10 doses or less. The vaccine and diluent do not contain preservatives; therefore, the user must recognize the potential contamination hazards and exercise special precautions to protect the sterility and potency of the product. The use of aseptic techniques and proper storage prior to and after restoration of the vaccine and subsequent withdrawal of the individual doses is essential. Use 0.5 mL of the reconstituted vaccine for subcutaneous injection.

It is important to use a separate sterile syringe and needle for each individual patient to prevent transmission of hepatitis B and other infectious agents from one person to another.

50 Dose Vial (available only to government agencies/institutions)—Withdraw the entire contents (30 mL) of the diluent vial into the sterile syringe to be used for reconstitution and introduce into the 50 dose vial of lyophilized vaccine. Agitate to ensure thorough mixing. With full aseptic precautions, attach the vial to the sterilized multidose jet injector apparatus. Use 0.5 mL of the reconstituted vaccine for subcutaneous injection.

Each dose of MUMPSVAX contains not less than the equivalent of 20,000 TCID$_{50}$ of the U.S. Reference Mumps Virus. Parenteral drug products should be inspected visually for particulate matter and discoloration prior to administration. MUMPSVAX, when reconstituted, is clear yellow.

HOW SUPPLIED

No. 4753—MUMPSVAX is supplied as a single-dose vial of lyophilized vaccine, **NDC** 0006-4753-00, and a vial of diluent.

No. 4584X/4309—MUMPSVAX is supplied as follows: (1) a box of 10 single-dose vials of lyophilized vaccine (package A), **NDC** 0006-4584-00; and (2) a box of 10 vials of diluent (package B). To conserve refrigerator space, the diluent may be stored separately at room temperature (6505-01-037-6792, Ten Pack).

Available only to government agencies/institutions:
No. 4664X—MUMPSVAX is supplied as one 10 dose vial of lyophilized vaccine, **NDC** 0006-4664-00, and one 7 mL vial of diluent.
No. 4593X—MUMPSVAX is supplied as one 50 dose vial of lyophilized vaccine, **NDC** 0006-4593-00, and one 30 mL vial of diluent.
Storage
It is recommended that the vaccine be used as soon as possible after reconstitution. Protect vaccine from light at all times, since such exposure may inactivate the virus. Store reconstituted vaccine in the vaccine vial in a dark place at 2–8°C (36–46°F) and discard if not used within 8 hours.

A.H.F.S. Category: 80:12
DC 7680412 Issued March 1995

COPYRIGHT © MERCK & CO., INC., 1990
All rights reserved

MUSTARGEN®, Trituration of (Mechlorethamine HCl for Injection), U.S.P. ℞

DESCRIPTION

MUSTARGEN* (Mechlorethamine HCl), an antineoplastic nitrogen mustard also known as HN2 hydrochloride, is a nitrogen analog of sulfur mustard. It is a light yellow brown, crystalline, hygroscopic powder that is very soluble in water and also soluble in alcohol.
Mechlorethamine hydrochloride is designated chemically as 2-chloro-*N* -(2-chloroethyl)-*N* -methylethanamine hydrochloride. The molecular weight is 192.52 and the melting point is 108–111°C. The empirical formula is $C_5H_{11}Cl_2N{\cdot}HCl$, and the structural formula is:

$$CH_3N(CH_2CH_2Cl)_2{\cdot}HCl$$

Trituration of MUSTARGEN is a sterile, light yellow brown crystalline powder for injection by the intravenous or intracavitary routes after dissolution. Each vial of MUSTARGEN contains 10 mg of mechlorethamine hydrochloride triturated with sodium chloride q.s. 100 mg. When dissolved with 10 mL Sterile Water for Injection or 0.9% Sodium Chloride Injection, the resulting solution has a pH of 3–5 at a concentration of 1 mg mechlorethamine HCl per mL.

*Registered trademark of MERCK & CO., INC.

CLINICAL PHARMACOLOGY

Mechlorethamine, a biologic alkylating agent, has a cytotoxic action which inhibits rapidly proliferating cells.
Pharmacokinetics and Metabolism
In water or body fluids, mechlorethamine undergoes rapid chemical transformation and combines with water or reactive compounds of cells, so that the drug is no longer present in active form a few minutes after administration.

INDICATIONS AND USAGE

Before using MUSTARGEN *see CONTRAINDICATIONS, WARNINGS, PRECAUTIONS, ADVERSE REACTIONS, DOSAGE AND ADMINISTRATION, and HOW SUPPLIED, Special Handling.*
MUSTARGEN, administered intravenously, is indicated for the palliative treatment of Hodgkin's disease (Stages III and IV), lymphosarcoma, chronic myelocytic or chronic lymphocytic leukemia, polycythemia vera, mycosis fungoides, and bronchogenic carcinoma.
MUSTARGEN, administered intrapleurally, intraperitoneally, or intrapericardially, is indicated for the palliative treatment of metastatic carcinoma resulting in effusion.

CONTRAINDICATIONS

The use of MUSTARGEN is contraindicated in the presence of known infectious diseases and in patients who have had previous anaphylactic reactions to MUSTARGEN.

WARNINGS

> Extravasation of the drug into subcutaneous tissues results in a painful inflammation. The area usually becomes indurated and sloughing may occur. If leakage of drug is obvious, prompt infiltration of the area with sterile isotonic sodium thiosulfate ($^1/_6$ molar) and application of an ice compress for 6 to 12 hours may minimize the local reaction. For a $^1/_6$ molar solution of sodium thiosulfate, use 4.14 g of sodium thiosulfate per 100 mL of Sterile Water for Injection or 2.64 g of anhydrous sodium thiosulfate per 100 mL or dilute 4 mL of Sodium Thiosulfate Injection (10%) with 6 mL of Sterile Water for Injection.

Before using MUSTARGEN, *an accurate histologic diagnosis of the disease, a knowledge of its natural course, and an adequate clinical history are important. The hematologic status of the patient must first be determined. It is essential to understand the hazards and therapeutic effects to be expected. Careful clinical judgment must be exercised in selecting patients. If the indication for its use is not clear, the drug should not be used.*
As nitrogen mustard therapy may contribute to extensive and rapid development of amyloidosis, it should be used only if foci of acute and chronic suppurative inflammation are absent.
Usage in Pregnancy
Mechlorethamine hydrochloride can cause fetal harm when administered to a pregnant woman. MUSTARGEN has been shown to produce fetal malformations in the rat and ferret when given as single subcutaneous injections of 1 mg/kg (2–3 times the maximum recommended human dose). There are no adequate and well controlled studies in pregnant women. If this drug is used during pregnancy, or if the patient becomes pregnant while taking this drug, the patient should be apprised of the potential hazard to the fetus. Women of childbearing potential should be advised to avoid becoming pregnant.

PRECAUTIONS

General
This drug is highly toxic and both powder and solution must be handled and administered with care. Since MUSTARGEN is a powerful vesicant, it is intended primarily for intravenous use, and in most instances is given by this route. Inhalation of dust or vapors and contact with skin or mucous membranes, especially those of the eyes, must be avoided. Rubber gloves should be worn when handling MUSTARGEN. (See DOSAGE AND ADMINISTRATION and HOW SUPPLIED, *Special Handling.*)
Because of the toxicity of MUSTARGEN, and the unpleasant side effects following its use, the potential risk and discomfort from the use of this drug in patients with inoperable neoplasms or in the terminal stage of the disease must be balanced against the limited gain obtainable. These gains will vary with the nature and the status of the disease under treatment. The routine use of MUSTARGEN in all cases of widely disseminated neoplasms is to be discouraged.
The use of MUSTARGEN in patients with leukopenia, thrombocytopenia, and anemia, due to invasion of the bone marrow by tumor carries a greater risk. In such patients a good response to treatment with disappearance of the tumor from the bone marrow may be associated with improvement of bone marrow function. However, in the absence of a good response or in patients who have been previously treated with chemotherapeutic agents, hematopoiesis may be further compromised, and leukopenia, thrombocytopenia and anemia may become more severe and lead to the demise of the patient.
Tumors of bone and nervous tissue have responded poorly to therapy. Results are unpredictable in disseminated and malignant tumors of different types.
Precautions must be observed with the use of MUSTARGEN and x-ray therapy or other chemotherapy in alternating courses. Hematopoietic function is characteristically depressed by either form of therapy, and neither MUSTARGEN following x-ray therapy nor x-ray therapy subsequent to the drug should be given until bone marrow function has recovered. In particular, irradiation of such areas as sternum, ribs, and vertebrae shortly after a course of nitrogen mustard may lead to hematologic complications.
MUSTARGEN has been reported to have immunosuppressive activity. Therefore, it should be borne in mind that use of the drug may predispose the patient to bacterial, viral or fungal infection.
Hyperuricemia may develop during therapy with MUSTARGEN. The problem of urate precipitation should be anticipated, particularly in the treatment of the lymphomas, and adequate methods for control of hyperuricemia should be instituted and careful attention directed toward adequate fluid intake before treatment.
Since drug toxicity, especially sensitivity to bone marrow failure, seems to be more common in chronic lymphatic leukemia than in other conditions, the drug should be given in this condition with great caution, if at all.
Extreme caution must be used in exceeding the average recommended dose. (See OVERDOSAGE.)
Laboratory Tests
Many abnormalities of renal, hepatic, and bone marrow function have been reported in patients with neoplastic disease and receiving mechlorethamine. It is advisable to check renal, hepatic, and bone marrow functions frequently.
Carcinogenesis, Mutagenesis, Impairment of Fertility
Therapy with alkylating agents such as MUSTARGEN may be associated with an increased incidence of a second malignant tumor, especially when such therapy is combined with other antineoplastic agents or radiation therapy.
Young-adult female RF mice were injected intravenously with four doses of 2.4 mg/kg of mechlorethamine (0.1% solution) at 2-week intervals with observations for up to 2 years. An increased incidence of thymic lymphomas and pulmonary adenomas was observed. Painting mechlorethamine on the skin of mice for periods up to 33 weeks resulted in squamous cell tumors in 9 of 33 mice.
Mechlorethamine induced mutations in the Ames test, in *E. coli,* and *Neurospora crassa.* Mechlorethamine caused chromosome aberrations in a variety of plant and mammalian cells. Dominant lethal mutations were produced in ICR/Ha Swiss mice.
Mechlorethamine impaired fertility in the rat at a daily dose of 500 mg/kg intravenously for two weeks.
Pregnancy
Pregnancy Category D. See WARNINGS.
Nursing Mothers
It is not known whether this drug is excreted in human milk. Because many drugs are excreted in human milk and because of the potential for serious adverse reactions in nursing infants from MUSTARGEN, a decision should be made whether to discontinue nursing or to discontinue the drug, taking into account the importance of the drug to the mother.
Pediatric Use
Safety and effectiveness in pediatric patients have not been established by well-controlled studies. Use of MUSTARGEN in pediatric patients has been quite limited. MUSTARGEN has been used in Hodgkin's disease, stages III and IV, in combination with other oncolytic agents (MOPP schedule). The MOPP chemotherapy combination includes mechlorethamine, vincristine, procarbazine, and prednisone or prednisolone.

ADVERSE REACTIONS

Clinical use of MUSTARGEN *usually is accompanied by toxic manifestations.*
Local Toxicity
Thrombosis and thrombophlebitis may result from direct contact of the drug with the intima of the injected vein. Avoid high concentration and prolonged contact with the drug, especially in cases of elevated pressure in the antebrachial vein (e.g., in mediastinal tumor compression from severe vena cava syndrome).
Systemic Toxicity
General: Hypersensitivity reactions, including anaphylaxis, have been reported. Nausea, vomiting and depression of formed elements in the circulating blood are dose-limiting side effects and usually occur with the use of full doses of MUSTARGEN. Jaundice, alopecia, vertigo, tinnitus and diminished hearing may occur infrequently. Rarely, hemolytic anemia associated with such diseases as the lymphomas and chronic lymphocytic leukemia may be precipitated by treatment with alkylating agents including MUSTARGEN. Also, various chromosomal abnormalities have been reported in association with nitrogen mustard therapy.
MUSTARGEN is given preferably at night in case sedation for side effects is required. Nausea and vomiting usually occur 1 to 3 hours after use of the drug. Emesis may disappear in the first 8 hours, but nausea may persist for 24 hours. Nausea and vomiting may be so severe as to precipitate vascular accidents in patients with a hemorrhagic tendency. Premedication with antiemetics, in addition to sedatives, may help control severe nausea and vomiting. Anorexia, weakness and diarrhea may also occur.
Hematologic: The usual course of MUSTARGEN (total dose of 0.4 mg/kg either given as a single intravenous dose or divided into two or four daily doses of 0.2 or 0.1 mg/kg respectively) generally produces a lymphocytopenia within 24 hours after the first injection; significant granulocytopenia occurs within 6 to 8 days and lasts for 10 days to 3 weeks. Agranulocytosis appears to be relatively infrequent and recovery from leukopenia in most cases is complete within two weeks of the maximum reduction. Thrombocytopenia is variable but the time course of the appearance and recovery from reduced platelet counts generally parallels the sequence of granulocyte levels. In some cases severe thrombocytopenia may lead to bleeding from the gums and gastrointestinal tract, petechiae, and small subcutaneous hemorrhages; these symptoms appear to be transient and in most cases disappear with return to a normal platelet count. However, a severe and even uncontrollable depression of the hematopoietic system occasionally may follow the usual dose of MUSTARGEN, particularly in patients with widespread disease and debility and in patients previously treated with other antineoplastic agents or x-ray. Persistent pancytopenia has been reported. In rare instances, hemorrhagic complications may be due to hyperheparinemia. Erythrocyte and hemoglobin levels may decline during

Continued on next page

Information on the Merck & Co., Inc. products listed on these pages is the full prescribing information from product circulars in use August 31, 1998. For information, please call 1-800-NSC MERCK [1-800-672-6372].

Mustargen—Cont.

the first 2 weeks after therapy but rarely significantly. Depression of the hematopoietic system may be found up to 50 days or more after starting therapy.

Integumentary: Occasionally, a maculopapular skin eruption occurs, but this may be idiosyncratic and does not necessarily recur with subsequent courses of the drug. Erythema multiforme has been observed. Herpes zoster, a common complicating infection in patients with lymphomas, may first appear after therapy is instituted and on occasion may be precipitated by treatment. Further treatment should be discontinued during the acute phase of this illness to avoid progression to generalized herpes zoster.

Reproductive: Since the gonads are susceptible to MUSTARGEN, treatment may be followed by delayed catamenia, oligomenorrhea, or temporary or permanent amenorrhea. Impaired spermatogenesis, azoospermia, and total germinal aplasia have been reported in male patients treated with alkylating agents, especially in combination with other drugs. In some instances spermatogenesis may return in patients in remission, but this may occur only several years after intensive chemotherapy has been discontinued. Patients should be warned of the potential risk to their reproductive capacity.

OVERDOSAGE

With total doses exceeding 0.4 mg/kg of body weight for a single course, severe leukopenia, anemia, thrombocytopenia and a hemorrhagic diathesis with subsequent delayed bleeding may develop. Death may follow. The only treatment in instances of excessive dosage appears to be repeated blood product transfusions, antibiotic treatment of complicating infections and general supportive measures. The intravenous LD$_{50}$ of MUSTARGEN is 2 mg/kg and 1.6 mg/kg in the mouse and rat, respectively.

DOSAGE AND ADMINISTRATION

Intravenous Administration
The dosage of MUSTARGEN varies with the clinical situation, the therapeutic response and the magnitude of hematologic depression. A total dose of 0.4 mg/kg of body weight for each course usually is given either as a single dose or in divided doses of 0.1 to 0.2 mg/kg per day. Dosage should be based on ideal dry body weight. The presence of edema or ascites must be considered so that dosage will be based on actual weight unaugmented by these conditions.
The margin of safety in therapy with MUSTARGEN is narrow and considerable care must be exercised in the matter of dosage. Repeated examinations of blood are *mandatory* as a guide to subsequent therapy. (See OVERDOSAGE.)
Within a few minutes after intravenous injection, MUSTARGEN undergoes chemical transformation, combines with reactive compounds, and is no longer present in its active form in the blood stream. Subsequent courses should not be given until the patient has recovered hematologically from the previous course; this is best determined by repeated studies of the peripheral blood elements awaiting their return to normal levels. It is often possible to give repeated courses of MUSTARGEN as early as three weeks after treatment.
Preparation of Solution for Intravenous Administration
This drug is highly toxic and both powder and solution must be handled and administered with care. Since MUSTARGEN is a powerful vesicant, it is intended primarily for intravenous use, and in most instances is given by this route. Inhalation of dust or vapors and contact with skin or mucous membranes, especially those of the eyes, must be avoided. Rubber gloves should be worn when handling MUSTARGEN. Should accidental eye contact occur, copious irrigation with water, normal saline or a balanced salt ophthalmic irrigating solution should be instituted immediately, followed by prompt ophthalmologic consultation. Should accidental skin contact occur, the affected part must be irrigated immediately with copious amounts of water, for at least 15 minutes, followed by 2 percent sodium thiosulfate solution. (See also box warning and *Special Handling.*)
Each vial of MUSTARGEN contains 10 mg of mechlorethamine hydrochloride triturated with sodium chloride q.s. 100 mg. In neutral or alkaline aqueous solution it undergoes rapid chemical transformation and is highly unstable. Although solutions prepared according to instructions are acidic and do not decompose as rapidly, they should be prepared immediately before each injection since they will decompose on standing. When reconstituted, MUSTARGEN is a clear colorless solution. *Do not use if the solution is discolored or if droplets of water are visible within the vial prior to reconstitution.*
Using a sterile 10 mL syringe, inject 10 mL of Sterile Water for Injection or 10 mL Sodium Chloride Injection into a vial of MUSTARGEN. With the needle (syringe attached) still in the rubber stopper, shake the vial several times to dissolve the drug completely. The resultant solution contains 1 mg of mechlorethamine hydrochloride per mL.

Parenteral drug products should be inspected visually for particulate matter and discoloration prior to administration whenever solution and container permit.
Special Handling
Due to the drug's toxic and mutagenic properties, appropriate precautions including the use of appropriate safety equipment are recommended for the preparation of MUSTARGEN for parenteral administration. The National Institutes of Health presently recommends that the preparation of injectable anti-neoplastic drugs should be performed in a Class II laminar flow biological safety cabinet and that personnel preparing drugs of this class should wear surgical gloves and a closed front surgical-type gown with knit cuffs. Several other guidelines for proper handling and disposal of anti-cancer drugs have been published and should be considered. There is no general agreement that all of the procedures recommended in the guidelines are necessary or appropriate.
Accidental contact: Should accidental eye contact occur, copious irrigation with water, normal saline or a balanced salt ophthalmic irrigating solution should be instituted immediately, followed by prompt ophthalmologic consultation. Should accidental skin contact occur, the affected part must be irrigated immediately with copious amounts of water, for at least 15 minutes, followed by 2 percent sodium thiosulfate solution. (See also box warning.)
Technique for Intravenous Administration
Withdraw into the syringe the calculated volume of solution required for a single injection. *Dispose of any remaining solution after neutralization* (see below). Although the drug may be injected directly into any suitable vein, it is injected preferably into the rubber or plastic tubing of a flowing intravenous infusion set. This reduces the possibility of severe local reactions due to extravasation or high concentration of the drug. Injecting the drug into the tubing rather than adding it to the entire volume of the infusion fluid minimizes a chemical reaction between the drug and the solution. The rate of injection apparently is not critical provided it is completed within a few minutes.
Intracavitary Administration
Nitrogen mustard has been used by intracavitary administration with varying success in certain malignant conditions for the control of pleural, peritoneal, and pericardial effusions caused by malignant cells.
The technic and the dose used by any of these routes varies. Therefore, if MUSTARGEN is given by the intracavitary route, the published articles concerning such use should be consulted. *Because of the inherent risks involved, the physician should be experienced in the appropriate injection technics, and be thoroughly aware of the indications, dosages, hazards, and precautions as set forth in the published literature. When using MUSTARGEN by the intracavitary route, the general precautions concerning this agent should be borne in mind.*
As a general guide, reference is made especially to the technics of Weisberger et al. Intracavitary use is indicated in the presence of pleural, peritoneal, or pericardial effusion due to metastatic tumors. Local therapy with nitrogen mustard is used only when malignant cells are demonstrated in the effusion. Intracavitary injection is not recommended when the accumulated fluid is chylous in nature, since results are likely to be poor.
Paracentesis is first performed with most of the fluid being removed from the pleural or peritoneal cavity. The intracavitary use of MUSTARGEN may exert at least some of its effect through production of a chemical poudrage. Therefore, the removal of excess fluid allows the drug to more easily contact the peritoneal and pleural linings. For intrapleural or intrapericardial injection nitrogen mustard is introduced directly through the thoracentesis needle. For intraperitoneal injection it is given through a rubber catheter inserted into the trocar used for paracentesis or through a No. 18 gauge needle inserted at another site. This drug should be injected slowly, with frequent aspiration to ensure that a free flow of fluid is present. If fluid cannot be aspirated, pain and necrosis due to injection of solution outside the cavity may occur. Free flow of fluid also is necessary to prevent injection into a loculated pocket and to ensure adequate dissemination of nitrogen mustard.
The usual dose of nitrogen mustard for intracavitary injection is 0.4 mg/kg of body weight, though 0.2 mg/kg (or 10 to 20 mg) has been used by the intrapericardial route. The solution is prepared, as previously described for intravenous injection, by adding 10 mL of Sterile Water for Injection or 10 mL of Sodium Chloride Injection to the vial containing 10 mg of mechlorethamine hydrochloride. (Amounts of diluent of 50 to 100 mL of normal saline have also been used.) The position of the patient should be changed every 5 to 10 minutes for an hour after injection to obtain more uniform distribution of the drug throughout the serous cavity. The remaining fluid may be removed from the pleural or peritoneal cavity by paracentesis 24 to 36 hours later. The patient should be followed carefully by clinical and x-ray examination to detect reaccumulation of fluid.
Pain occurs rarely with intrapleural use; it is common with intraperitoneal injection and is often associated with nau-

sea, vomiting, and diarrhea of 2 to 3 days duration. Transient cardiac irregularities may occur with intrapericardial injection. Death, possibly accelerated by nitrogen mustard, has been reported following the use of this agent by the intracavitary route. Although absorption of MUSTARGEN when given by the intracavitary route is probably not complete because of its rapid deactivation by body fluids, the systemic effect is unpredictable. The acute side effects such as nausea and vomiting are usually mild. Bone marrow depression is generally milder than when the drug is given intravenously. Care should be taken to avoid use by the intracavitary route when other agents which may suppress bone marrow function are being used systemically.
Neutralization of Equipment and Unused Solution
To clean rubber gloves, tubing, glassware, etc., after giving MUSTARGEN, soak them in an aqueous solution containing equal volumes of sodium thiosulfate (5%) and sodium bicarbonate (5%) for 45 minutes. Excess reagents and reaction products are washed away easily with water. Any unused injection solution should be neutralized by mixing with an equal volume of sodium thiosulfate/sodium bicarbonate solution. Allow the mixture to stand for 45 minutes. Vials that have contained MUSTARGEN should be treated in the same way with thiosulfate/bicarbonate solution before disposal.

HOW SUPPLIED

No. 7753—Trituration of MUSTARGEN is a light yellow brown crystalline powder, each vial containing 10 mg mechlorethamine hydrochloride with sodium chloride q.s. 100 mg, and is supplied as follows:
NDC 0006-7753-31 in treatment sets of 4 vials.
Storage
Store at controlled room temperature 15–30°C (59–86°F). Protect from light and humidity. Solutions of mechlorethamine HCl decompose on standing; therefore, solutions of the drug should be prepared immediately before use.
7417931   Issued February 1997

MYOCHRYSINE® Injection (Gold Sodium Thiomalate), U.S.P.   ℞

Physicians planning to use MYOCHRYSINE (Gold Sodium Thiomalate) should thoroughly familiarize themselves with its toxicity and its benefits. The possibility of toxic reactions should always be explained to the patient before starting therapy. Patients should be warned to report promptly any symptoms suggesting toxicity. Before each injection of MYOCHRYSINE, the physician should review the results of laboratory work, and see the patient to determine the presence or absence of adverse reactions since some of these can be severe or even fatal.*

---

*Registered trademark of MERCK & CO., INC.

DESCRIPTION

MYOCHRYSINE is a sterile aqueous solution of gold sodium thiomalate. It contains 0.5 percent benzyl alcohol added as a preservative. The pH of the product is 5.8–6.5. Gold sodium thiomalate is a mixture of the mono- and disodium salts of gold thiomalic acid. The structural formula is:

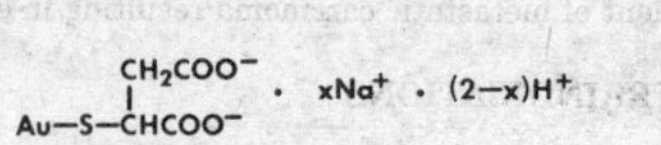

$$\begin{array}{c} CH_2COO^- \\ | \\ Au\!-\!S\!-\!CHCOO^- \end{array} \cdot\ xNa^+ \cdot (2\!-\!x)H^+$$

mercaptobutanedioic acid, monogold (1+) sodium salt

The molecular weight for $C_4H_3AuNa_2O_4S$ (the disodium salt) is 390.07 and for $C_4H_4AuNaO_4S$ (the monosodium salt) is 368.09.
MYOCHRYSINE is supplied as a solution for intramuscular injection containing 50 mg of gold sodium thiomalate per mL.

CLINICAL PHARMACOLOGY

The mode of action of gold sodium thiomalate is unknown. The predominant action appears to be a suppressive effect on the synovitis of active rheumatoid disease.

INDICATIONS AND USAGE

MYOCHRYSINE is indicated in the treatment of selected cases of active rheumatoid arthritis— both adult and juvenile type. The greatest benefit occurs in the early active

stage. In late stages of the illness when cartilage and bone damage have occurred, gold can only check the progression of rheumatoid arthritis and prevent further structural damage to joints. It cannot repair damage caused by previously active disease.

MYOCHRYSINE should be used only as *one part* of a complete program of therapy; alone it is not a complete treatment.

CONTRAINDICATIONS

Hypersensitivity to any component of this product.
Severe toxicity resulting from previous exposure to gold or other heavy metals.
Severe debilitation.
Systemic lupus erythematosus.

WARNINGS

Before treatment is started, the patient's hemoglobin, erythrocyte, white blood cell, differential and platelet counts should be determined, and urinalysis should be done to serve as basic reference. Urine should be analyzed for protein and sediment changes prior to each injection. Complete blood counts including platelet estimation should be made before every second injection throughout treatment. The occurrence of purpura or ecchymoses at any time always requires a platelet count.

Danger signals of possible gold toxicity include: rapid reduction of hemoglobin, leukopenia below 4000 WBC/mm^3, eosinophilia above 5 percent, platelet decrease below 100,000/mm^3, albuminuria, hematuria, pruritus, skin eruption, stomatitis, or persistent diarrhea. No additional injections of MYOCHRYSINE should be given unless further studies show these abnormalities to be caused by conditions other than gold toxicity.

PRECAUTIONS

General

Gold salts should not be used concomitantly with penicillamine.
The safety of coadministration with cytotoxic drugs has not been established.
Caution is indicated in the use of MYOCHRYSINE in patients with the following:
1. a history of blood dyscrasias such as granulocytopenia or anemia caused by drug sensitivity,
2. allergy or hypersensitivity to medications,
3. skin rash,
4. previous kidney or liver disease,
5. marked hypertension,
6. compromised cerebral or cardiovascular circulation.
Diabetes mellitus or congestive heart failure should be under control before gold therapy is instituted.

Carcinogenicity

Renal adenomas have been reported in long-term toxicity studies of rats receiving MYOCHRYSINE at high dose levels (2 mg/kg weekly for 45 weeks, followed by 6 mg/kg daily for 47 weeks), approximately 2 to 42 times the usual human dose. These adenomas are histologically similar to those produced in rats by chronic administration of experimental gold compounds and other heavy metals, such as lead. No reports have been received of renal adenomas in man in association with the use of MYOCHRYSINE.

Pregnancy

Pregnancy Category C.
MYOCHRYSINE has been shown to be teratogenic during the organogenetic period in rats and rabbits when given in doses, respectively, of 140 and 175 times the usual human dose. Hydrocephaly and microphthalmia were the malformations observed in rats when MYOCHRYSINE was administered subcutaneously at a dose of 25 mg/kg/day from day 6 through day 15 of gestation. In rabbits, limb malformations and gastroschisis were the malformations observed when MYOCHRYSINE was administered subcutaneously at doses of 20–45 mg/kg/day from day 6 through day 18 of gestation.
There are no adequate and well-controlled studies in pregnant women. MYOCHRYSINE should be used during pregnancy only if the potential benefit to the mother justifies the potential risk to the fetus.

Nursing Mothers

The presence of gold has been demonstrated in the milk of lactating mothers. In addition, gold has been found in the serum and red blood cells of a nursing infant. In view of the above findings and because of the potential for serious adverse reactions in nursing infants from MYOCHRYSINE, a decision should be made whether to discontinue nursing or to discontinue the drug, taking into account the importance of the drug to the mother. The slow excretion and persistence of gold in the mother, even after therapy is discontinued, must also be kept in mind.

ADVERSE REACTIONS

A variety of adverse reactions may develop during the initial phase (weekly injections) of therapy or during mainte-

nance treatment. Adverse reactions are observed most frequently when the cumulative dose of MYOCHRYSINE administered is between 400 and 800 mg. Very uncommonly, complications occur days to months after cessation of treatment.

Cutaneous reactions: Dermatitis is the most common reaction. *Any eruption, especially if pruritic, that develops during treatment with* MYOCHRYSINE *should be considered a reaction to gold until proven otherwise.* Pruritus often exists before dermatitis becomes apparent, and therefore should be considered a warning signal of impending cutaneous reaction. The most serious form of cutaneous reaction is generalized exfoliative dermatitis which may lead to alopecia and shedding of nails. Gold dermatitis may be aggravated by exposure to sunlight or an actinic rash may develop.

Mucous membrane reactions: Stomatitis is the second most common adverse reaction. Shallow ulcers on the buccal membranes, on the borders of the tongue, and on the palate or in the pharynx may occur as the only adverse reaction, or along with dermatitis. Sometimes diffuse glossitis or gingivitis develops. A metallic taste may precede these oral mucous membrane reactions and should be considered a warning signal.
Conjunctivitis is a rare reaction.

Renal reactions: Gold may be toxic to the kidney and produce a nephrotic syndrome or glomerulitis with hematuria. These renal reactions are usually relatively mild and subside completely if recognized early and treatment is discontinued. They may become severe and chronic if treatment is continued after onset of the reaction. Therefore, it is important to perform a *urinalysis before every injection*, and to discontinue treatment promptly if proteinuria or hematuria develops.

Hematologic reactions: Blood dyscrasia due to gold toxicity is rare, but because of the potential serious consequences it must be constantly watched for and recognized early by frequent blood examinations done throughout treatment. Granulocytopenia; thrombocytopenia, with or without purpura; hypoplastic and aplastic anemia; and eosinophilia have all been reported. These hematologic disorders may occur separately or in combinations.

Nitritoid and allergic reactions: Reactions of the "nitritoid type" which may resemble anaphylactoid effects have been reported. Flushing, fainting, dizziness and sweating are most frequently reported. Other symptoms that may occur include: nausea, vomiting, malaise, headache, and weakness.
More severe, but less common effects include: anaphylactic shock, syncope, bradycardia, thickening of the tongue, difficulty in swallowing and breathing, and angioneurotic edema. These effects may occur almost immediately after injection or as late as 10 minutes following injection. They may occur at any time during the course of therapy and if observed, treatment with MYOCHRYSINE should be discontinued.

Miscellaneous reactions: Gastrointestinal reactions have been reported, including nausea, vomiting, anorexia, abdominal cramps and diarrhea. Ulcerative enterocolitis, which can be severe or even fatal, has been reported rarely. There have been rare reports of reactions involving the eye such as iritis, corneal ulcers, and gold deposits in ocular tissues. Peripheral and central nervous system complications have been reported rarely. Peripheral neuropathy, with or without fasciculations, sensorimotor effects (including Guillain-Barré syndrome) and elevated spinal fluid protein have been reported. Central nervous system complications have included confusion, hallucinations and seizures. Usually these signs and symptoms cleared upon discontinuation of gold therapy.
Hepatitis, jaundice, with or without cholestasis, gold bronchitis, pulmonary injury manifested by interstitial pneumonitis and fibrosis, partial or complete hair loss and fever have also been reported.
Sometimes arthralgia occurs for a day or two after an injection of MYOCHRYSINE; this reaction usually subsides after the first few injections.

MANAGEMENT OF ADVERSE REACTIONS

Treatment with MYOCHRYSINE should be discontinued immediately when toxic reactions occur. Minor complications such as localized dermatitis, mild stomatitis, or slight proteinuria generally require no other therapy and resolve spontaneously with suspension of MYOCHRYSINE. Moderately severe skin and mucous membrane reactions often benefit from topical corticosteroids, oral antihistaminics, and soothing or anesthetic lotions.

If stomatitis or dermatitis becomes severe or more generalized, systemic corticosteroids (generally, prednisone 10 to 40 mg daily in divided doses) may provide symptomatic relief.
For serious renal, hematologic, pulmonary, and enterocolitic complications, high doses of systemic corticosteroids (prednisone 40 to 100 mg daily in divided doses) are recommended. The optimum duration of corticosteroid treatment

varies with the response of the individual patient. Therapy may be required for many months when adverse effects are unusually severe or progressive.
In patients whose complications do not improve with high-dose corticosteroid treatment, or who develop significant steroid-related adverse reactions, a chelating agent may be given to enhance gold excretion. Dimercaprol (BAL) has been used successfully, but patients must be monitored carefully as numerous untoward reactions may attend its use. Corticosteroids and a chelating agent may be used concomitantly.
MYOCHRYSINE *should not be reinstituted after severe or idiosyncratic reactions.*
MYOCHRYSINE may be readministered following resolution of mild reactions, using a reduced dosage schedule. If an initial test dose of 5 mg MYOCHRYSINE is well-tolerated, progressively larger doses (5 to 10 mg increments) may be given at weekly to monthly intervals until a dose of 25 to 50 mg is reached.

DOSAGE AND ADMINISTRATION

MYOCHRYSINE should be administered only by intramuscular injection, preferably intragluteally. It should be given with the patient lying down. He should remain recumbent for approximately 10 minutes after the injection.
Therapeutic effects from MYOCHRYSINE occur slowly. Early improvement, often limited to a reduction in morning stiffness, may begin after six to eight weeks of treatment, but beneficial effects may not be observed until after months of therapy.
Parenteral drug products should be inspected visually for particulate matter and discoloration prior to administration. Do not use if material has darkened. Color should not exceed pale yellow.
For the adult of average size the following dosage schedule is suggested:

Weekly Injections

1st injection	10 mg
2nd injection	25 mg

3rd and subsequent injections, 25 to 50 mg
until there is toxicity or major clinical improvement, or, in the absence of either of these, the cumulative dose of MYOCHRYSINE reaches one gram.
MYOCHRYSINE is continued until the cumulative dose reaches one gram unless toxicity or major clinical improvement occurs. If significant clinical improvement occurs before a cumulative dose of one gram has been administered, the dose may be decreased or the interval between injections increased as with maintenance therapy. Maintenance doses of 25 to 50 mg every other week for two to 20 weeks are recommended. If the clinical course remains stable, injections of 25 to 50 mg may be given every third and subsequently every fourth week indefinitely. Some patients may require maintenance treatment at intervals of one to three weeks. Should the arthritis exacerbate during maintenance therapy, weekly injections may be resumed temporarily until disease activity is suppressed.
Should a patient fail to improve during initial therapy (cumulative dose of one gram), several options are available:
1— the patient may be considered to be unresponsive and MYOCHRYSINE is discontinued
2— the same dose (25 to 50 mg) of MYOCHRYSINE may be continued for approximately ten additional weeks
3— the dose of MYOCHRYSINE may be increased by increments of 10 mg every one to four weeks, not to exceed 100 mg in a single injection.
If significant clinical improvement occurs using option 2 or 3, the maintenance schedule described above should be initiated. If there is no significant improvement or if toxicity occurs, therapy with MYOCHRYSINE should be stopped. The higher the individual dose of MYOCHRYSINE, the greater the risk of gold toxicity. Selection of one of these options for chrysotherapy should be based upon a number of factors, including the physician's experience with gold salt therapy, the course of the patient's condition, the choice of alternative treatments, and the availability of the patient for the close supervision required.

Juvenile Rheumatoid Arthritis

The pediatric dose of MYOCHRYSINE is proportional to the adult dose on a weight basis. After the initial test dose of 10 mg, the recommended dose for children is one mg per kilogram body weight, not to exceed 50 mg for a single injection. Otherwise, the guidelines given above for administration to adults also apply to children.

Concomitant Drug Therapy —Gold salts should not be used concomitantly with penicillamine.

Continued on next page

Information on the Merck & Co., Inc. products listed on these pages is the full prescribing information from product circulars in use August 31, 1998. For information, please call 1-800-NSC MERCK [1-800-672-6372].

Myochrysine—Cont.

The safety of coadministration with cytotoxic drugs has not been established. Other measures, such as salicylates, other non-steroidal anti-inflammatory drugs, or systemic corticosteroids, may be continued when MYOCHRYSINE is initiated. After improvement commences, analgesic and anti-inflammatory drugs may be discontinued slowly as symptoms permit.

HOW SUPPLIED

Injection MYOCHRYSINE is a light yellow to yellow solution which must be protected from light. It is supplied as follows:
No. 7762—50 mg of gold sodium thiomalate per mL as **NDC** 0006-7762-64 in boxes of 6 x 1 mL ampuls
NDC 0006-7762-10 in 10 mL vials
(6505-00-973-8579, 10 mL vial).
Storage
Protect from light.
Store container in carton until contents have been used.
      7594528   Issued April 1994
COPYRIGHT © MERCK & CO., INC., 1985
All rights reserved

NEODECADRON®
Sterile Ophthalmic Ointment
(Neomycin Sulfate-Dexamethasone
Sodium Phosphate), U.S.P.

℞

DESCRIPTION

Sterile Ophthalmic Ointment NEODECADRON* (Neomycin Sulfate-Dexamethasone Sodium Phosphate) is a topical corticosteroid-antibiotic ointment for ophthalmic use.
Dexamethasone sodium phosphate is 9-fluoro-11β, 17-dihydroxy-16α-methyl-21-(phosphonooxy)pregna-1, 4-diene-3, 20- dione disodium salt. Its empirical formula is $C_{22}H_{28}FNa_2O_8P$ and its structural formula is:

Dexamethasone is a synthetic analog of naturally occurring glucocorticoids (hydrocortisone and cortisone).
Dexamethasone sodium phosphate is a water soluble, inorganic ester of dexamethasone. Its molecular weight is 516.41.
Neomycin sulfate, an antibiotic of the aminoglycoside group, is a mixture of the sulfate salts of neomycin, produced by the growth of *Streptomyces fradiae* Waksman (Fam. Streptomycetaceae). Neomycin is a complex typically containing 8–13% neomycin C, less than 0.2% neomycin A, and the rest, neomycin B. The empirical formula for both neomycin B and neomycin C is $C_{23}H_{46}N_6O_{13}$, and the molecular weight for each is 614.65. Neomycin A (also referred to as neamine) has an empirical formula of $C_{12}H_{26}N_4O_6$ and a molecular weight of 322.36. The structural formulae for neomycin sulfate are:

Neomycin B $R_1=H, R_2=CH_2NH_2$
Neomycin C $R_1=CH_2NH_2, R_2=H$

Ophthalmic Ointment NEODECADRON contains in each gram: dexamethasone sodium phosphate equivalent to 0.5 mg (0.05%) dexamethasone phosphate and neomycin sulfate equivalent to 3.5 mg neomycin base. Inactive ingredients: white petrolatum and mineral oil.

---

*Registered trademark of MERCK & CO., INC.

CLINICAL PHARMACOLOGY

Corticosteroids suppress the inflammatory response to a variety of agents, and they probably delay or slow healing. Since corticosteroids may inhibit the body's defense mechanism against infection, a concomitant antimicrobial drug may be used when this inhibition is considered to be clinically significant in a particular case.
When a decision to administer both a corticosteroid and an antimicrobial is made, the administration of such drugs in combination has the advantage of greater patient compliance and convenience, with the added assurance that the appropriate dosage of both drugs is administered, plus assured compatibility of ingredients when both types of drug are in the same formulation and, particularly, that the correct volume of drug is delivered and retained.
The relative potency of corticosteroids depends on the molecular structure, concentration, and release from the vehicle.
Microbiology
The anti-infective component in Ophthalmic Ointment NEODECADRON is included to provide action against specific organisms susceptible to it. Neomycin sulfate is active *in vitro* against susceptible strains of the following microorganisms: *Staphylococcus aureus*, *Escherichia coli*, *Haemophilus influenzae*, *Klebsiella / Enterobacter* species, and *Neisseria* species. The product does not provide adequate coverage against: *Pseudomonas aeruginosa*, *Serratia marcescens*, and streptococci, including *Streptococcus pneumoniae*. (See INDICATIONS AND USAGE.)

INDICATIONS AND USAGE

For steroid-responsive inflammatory ocular conditions for which a corticosteroid is indicated and where bacterial infection or a risk of bacterial ocular infection exists.
Ocular steroids are indicated in inflammatory conditions of the palpebral and bulbar conjunctiva, cornea, and anterior segment of the globe where the inherent risk of steroid use in certain infective conjunctivitides is accepted to obtain a diminution in edema and inflammation. They are also indicated in chronic anterior uveitis and corneal injury from chemical, radiation, or thermal burns, or penetration of foreign bodies.
The use of a combination drug with an anti-infective component is indicated where the risk of infection is high or where there is an expectation that potentially dangerous numbers of bacteria will be present in the eye.
The particular anti-infective drug in this product is active against the following common bacterial eye pathogens:
   Staphylococcus aureus
   Escherichia coli
   Haemophilus influenzae
   Klebsiella / Enterobacter species
   Neisseria species
The product does not provide adequate coverage against:
   Pseudomonas aeruginosa
   Serratia marcescens
   Streptococci, including *Streptococcus pneumoniae*

CONTRAINDICATIONS

NEODECADRON is contraindicated in most viral diseases of the cornea and conjunctiva including epithelial herpes simplex keratitis (dendritic keratitis), vaccinia varicella, and also in mycobacterial infection of the eye and fungal diseases of ocular structures. NEODECADRON is also contraindicated in individuals with known or suspected hypersensitivity to any of the ingredients of this preparation and to other corticosteroids (see WARNINGS). Hypersensitivity to the antibiotic component occurs at a higher rate than for other components.

WARNINGS

NOT FOR INJECTION INTO THE EYE
Prolonged use of corticosteroids may result in ocular hypertension and/or glaucoma with damage to the optic nerve, defects in visual acuity and fields of vision, and in posterior subcapsular cataract formation.
Prolonged use of corticosteroids may suppress the host response and thus increase the hazard of secondary ocular infections. In those diseases causing thinning of the cornea or sclera, perforations have been known to occur with the use of topical corticosteroids. In acute purulent conditions of the eye, corticosteroids may mask infection or enhance existing infection.
If this product is used for 10 days or longer, intraocular pressure should be routinely monitored even though it may be difficult in children and uncooperative patients. Corticos-

steroids should be used with caution in the presence of ocular hypertension and/or glaucoma. Intraocular pressure should be checked frequently.
The use of corticosteroids after cataract surgery may delay healing and increase the incidence of filtering blebs.
Use of ocular corticosteroids may prolong the course and may exacerbate the severity of many viral infections of the eye (including herpes simplex). Employment of a corticosteroid medication in the treatment of patients with a history of herpes simplex requires great caution; periodic slit lamp microscopy is essential. (See CONTRAINDICATIONS.)
Neomycin sulfate may occasionally cause cutaneous sensitization. If any reaction indicating such sensitivity is observed, discontinue use.

PRECAUTIONS

General
The initial prescription and renewal of the medication order beyond 8 grams should be made by a physician only after examination of the patient with the aid of magnification, such as slit-lamp biomicroscopy and, where appropriate, fluorescein staining. If signs and symptoms fail to improve after two days, the patient should be re-evaluated.
The possibility of fungal infections of the cornea should be considered after prolonged corticosteroid dosing. Fungal cultures should be taken when appropriate.
If this product is used for 10 days or longer, intraocular pressure should be monitored (see WARNINGS).
There have been reports of bacterial keratitis associated with the use of multiple dose containers of topical ophthalmic products. These containers had been inadvertently contaminated by patients who, in most cases, had a concurrent corneal disease or a disruption of the ocular epithelial surface. (See PRECAUTIONS, *Information for Patients*.)
Information for Patients
Patients should be instructed to avoid allowing the tip of the dispensing container to contact the eye, eyelid, fingers, or any other surface. The use of this product by more than one person may spread infection. Keep tightly closed when not in use.
Patients should also be instructed that ocular preparations, if handled improperly, can become contaminated by common bacteria known to cause ocular infections. Serious damage to the eye and subsequent loss of vision may result from using contaminated preparations. (See PRECAUTIONS, *General*.)
If redness, irritation, swelling or pain persists or becomes aggravated, the patient should be advised to consult a physician. Patients should also be advised that if they have ocular surgery or develop an intercurrent ocular condition (e.g., trauma or infection), they should immediately seek their physician's advice.
Keep out of the reach of children.
Carcinogenesis, Mutagenesis, Impairment of Fertility
Long term animal studies have not been performed to evaluate the carcinogenic potential or the effect on fertility of Ophthalmic Ointment NEODECADRON. Treatment of human lymphocytes *in-vitro* with neomycin increased the frequency of chromosome aberrations at the highest concentration (80μg/mL) tested; however, the effects of neomycin on carcinogenesis and mutagenesis in humans are unknown.
Pregnancy
Teratogenic effects
Pregnancy Category C
Corticosteroids have been found to be teratogenic in animal studies. Ocular administration of 0.1% dexamethasone resulted in 15.6% and 32.3% incidence of fetal anomalies in two groups of pregnant rabbits. Fetal growth retardation and increased mortality rates have been observed in rats with chronic dexamethasone therapy. There are no adequate and well-controlled studies in pregnant women. Ophthalmic Ointment NEODECADRON should be used during pregnancy only if the potential benefit justifies the potential risk to the fetus. Infants born of mothers who have received substantial doses of corticosteroids during pregnancy should be observed carefully for signs of hypoadrenalism.
Nursing Mothers
It is not known whether topical administration of corticosteroids could result in sufficient systemic absorption to produce detectable quantities in human milk. Systemically-administered corticosteroids appear in human milk and could suppress growth, interfere with endogenous corticosteroid production, or cause other untoward effects. Because of the potential for serious adverse reactions in nursing infants from Ophthalmic Ointment NEODECADRON, a decision should be made whether to discontinue nursing or to discontinue the drug, taking into account the importance of the drug to the mother.
Pediatric Use
Safety and effectiveness in pediatric patients have not been established.

ADVERSE REACTIONS

Adverse reactions have occurred with corticosteroid/anti-infective combination drugs which can be attributed to the corticosteroid component, the anti-infective component, or the combination. Exact incidence figures are not available since no denominator of treated patients is available.

Reactions occurring most often from the presence of the anti-infective ingredient are allergic sensitizations. The reactions due to the corticosteroid component in decreasing order of frequency are: elevation of intraocular pressure (IOP) with possible development of glaucoma, and infrequent optic nerve damage; posterior subcapsular cataract formation; and delayed wound healing.

Secondary Infection: The development of secondary infection has occurred after use of combinations containing corticosteroids and antimicrobials. Fungal and viral infections of the cornea are particularly prone to develop coincidentally with long-term applications of a corticosteroid. The possibility of fungal invasion must be considered in any persistent corneal ulceration where corticosteroid treatment has been used.

DOSAGE AND ADMINISTRATION

NOT FOR INJECTION INTO THE EYE

The duration of treatment will vary with the type of lesion and may extend from a few days to several weeks, according to therapeutic response.

Apply a thin coating of Ophthalmic Ointment NEODECADRON three or four times a day. When a favorable response is observed, reduce the number of daily applications to two, and later to one a day as maintenance dose if this is sufficient to control symptoms.

Not more than 8 grams should be prescribed initially and the prescription should not be refilled without further evaluation as outlined in PRECAUTIONS above.

HOW SUPPLIED

No. 7617—Sterile Ophthalmic Ointment NEODECADRON is a clear, unctuous ointment, and is supplied as follows:
NDC 0006-7617-04 in 3.5 g tubes
(6505-00-982-0291 0.05% 3.5 g)
Storage
Store at controlled room temperature, 15°–30°C (59°–86°F).
7612628 Issued December 1995
COPYRIGHT © MERCK & CO., Inc., 1985, 1995
All rights reserved

NEODECADRON®
Sterile Ophthalmic Solution
(Neomycin Sulfate-Dexamethasone
Sodium Phosphate), U.S.P.

℞

DESCRIPTION

Ophthalmic Solution NEODECADRON* (Neomycin Sulfate-Dexamethasone Sodium Phosphate) is a topical corticosteroid-antibiotic solution for ophthalmic use.

Dexamethasone sodium phosphate is 9-fluoro-11β, 17-dihydroxy-16α-methyl-21-(phosphonooxy)pregna-1, 4-diene-3, 20-dione disodium salt. Its empirical formula is $C_{22}H_{28}FNa_2O_8P$ and its structural formula is:

Dexamethasone is a synthetic analog of naturally occurring glucocorticoids (hydrocortisone and cortisone).

Dexamethasone sodium phosphate is a water soluble, inorganic ester of dexamethasone. Its molecular weight is 516.41.

Neomycin sulfate, an antibiotic of the aminoglucoside group, is a mixture of the sulfate salts of neomycin, produced by the growth of *Streptomyces fradiae* Waksman (Fam. Stretomycetaceae). Neomycin is a complex typically containing 8–13% neomycin C, less than 0.2% neomycin A, and the rest, neomycin B. The empirical formula for both neomycin B and neomycin C is $C_{23}H_{46}N_6O_{13}$, and the molecular weight for each is 614.65. Neomycin A (also referred to as neamine) has an empirical formula of $C_{12}H_{26}N_4O_6$ and a molecular weight of 322.36. The structural formulae for neomycin sulfate are:

[See chemical structure at top of next column]

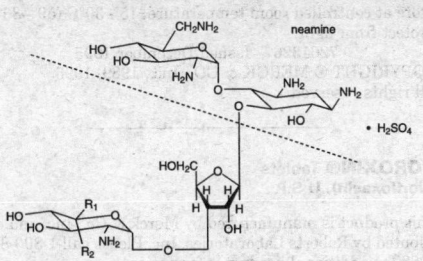

Neomycin B R₁=H, R₂=CH₂NH₂ → $R_1=H$, $R_2=CH_2NH_2$
Neomycin C $R_1=CH_2NH_2$, $R_2=H$

Each milliliter of buffered Ophthalmic Solution NEODECADRON in the OCUMETER* ophthalmic dispenser contains: dexamethasone sodium phosphate equivalent to 1 mg (0.1%) dexamethasone phosphate, and neomycin sulfate equivalent to 3.5 mg neomycin base. Inactive ingredients: creatinine, sodium citrate, sodium borate, polysorbate 80, disodium edetate, hydrochloric acid to adjust pH to 6.6–7.2, and water for injection. Benzalkonium chloride 0.02% and sodium bisulfite 0.1% added as preservatives.

* Registered trademark of MERCK & CO., Inc.

CLINICAL PHARMACOLOGY

Corticosteroids suppress the inflammatory response to a variety of agents, and they probably delay or slow healing. Since corticosteroids may inhibit the body's defense mechanism against infection, a concomitant antimicrobial drug may be used when this inhibition is considered to be clinically significant in a particular case.

When a decision to administer both a corticosteroid and an antimicrobial is made, the administration of such drugs in combination has the advantage of greater patient compliance and convenience, with the added assurance that the appropriate dosage of both drugs is administered, plus assured compatibility of ingredients when both types of drug are in the same formulation and, particularly, that the correct volume of drug is delivered and retained.

The relative potency of corticosteroids depends on the molecular structure, concentration, and release from the vehicle.

Microbiology

The anti-infective component in Ophthalmic Solution NEODECADRON is included to provide action against specific organisms susceptible to it. Neomycin sulfate is active *in vitro* against susceptible strains of the following microorganisms: *Staphylococcus aureus*, *Escherichia coli*, *Haemophilus influenzae*, *Klebsiella/Enterobacter* species, and *Neisseria* species. The product does not provide adequate coverage against: *Pseudomonas aeruginosa*, *Serratia marcescens*, and streptococci, including *Streptococcus pneumoniae*. (See INDICATIONS AND USAGE.)

INDICATIONS AND USAGE

For steroid-responsive inflammatory ocular conditions for which a corticosteroid is indicated and where bacterial infection or a risk of bacterial ocular infection exists.

Ocular steroids are indicated in inflammatory conditions of the palpebral and bulbar conjunctiva, cornea, and anterior segment of the globe where the inherent risk of steroid use in certain infective conjunctivitides is accepted to obtain a diminution in edema and inflammation. They are also indicated in chronic anterior uveitis and corneal injury from chemical, radiation, or thermal burns, or penetration of foreign bodies.

The use of a combination drug with an anti-infective component is indicated where the risk of infection is high or where there is an expectation that potentially dangerous numbers of bacteria will be present in the eye.

The particular anti-infective drug in this product is active against the following common bacterial eye pathogens:
Staphylococcus aureus
Escherichia coli
Haemophilus influenzae
Klebsiella/Enterobacter species
Neisseria species
The product does not provide adequate coverage against:
Pseudomonas aeruginosa
Serratia marcescens
Streptococci, including *Streptococcus pneumoniae*

CONTRAINDICATIONS

NEODECADRON is contraindicated in most viral diseases of the cornea and conjunctiva including epithelial herpes simplex keratitis (dendritic keratitis), vaccinia, varicella,

and also in mycobacterial infection of the eye and fungal diseases of ocular structures. NEODECADRON is also contraindicated in individuals with known or suspected hypersensitivity to any of the ingredients of this preparation, including sulfites, and to other corticosteroids (see WARNINGS). (Hypersensitivity to the antibiotic component occurs at a higher rate than for other components.)

WARNINGS

NOT FOR INJECTION INTO THE EYE

Prolonged use of corticosteroids may result in ocular hypertension and/or glaucoma with damage to the optic nerve, defects in visual acuity and fields of vision, and in posterior subcapsular cataract formation.

Prolonged use of corticosteroids may suppress the host response and thus increase the hazard of secondary ocular infections. In those diseases causing thinning of the cornea or sclera, perforations have been known to occur with the use of topical corticosteroids. In acute purulent conditions of the eye, corticosteroids may mask infection or enhance existing infection.

If this product is used for 10 days or longer, intraocular pressure should be routinely monitored even though it may be difficult in children and uncooperative patients. Corticosteroids should be used with caution in the presence of ocular hypertension and/or glaucoma. Intraocular pressure should be checked frequently.

The use of corticosteroids after cataract surgery may delay healing and increase the incidence of filtering blebs.

Use of ocular corticosteroids may prolong the course and may exacerbate the severity of many viral infections of the eye (including herpes simplex). Employment of a corticosteroid medication in the treatment of patients with a history of herpes simplex requires great caution; periodic slit lamp microscopy is essential. (See CONTRAINDICATIONS.)

Neomycin sulfate may occasionally cause cutaneous sensitization. If any reaction indicating such sensitivity is observed, discontinue use.

Ophthalmic Solution NEODECADRON contains sodium bisulfite, a sulfite that may cause allergic-type reactions including anaphylactic symptoms and life-threatening or less severe asthmatic episodes in certain susceptible people. The overall prevalence of sulfite sensitivity in the general population is unknown and probably low. Sulfite sensitivity is seen more frequently in asthmatic than in nonasthmatic people.

PRECAUTIONS

General

The initial prescription and renewal of the medication order beyond 20 milliliters should be made by a physician only after examination of the patient with the aid of magnification, such as slit lamp biomicroscopy and, where appropriate, fluorescein staining. If signs and symptoms fail to improve after two days, the patient should be re-evaluated.

The possibility of fungal infections of the cornea should be considered after prolonged corticosteroid dosing. Fungal cultures should be taken when appropriate.

If this product is used for 10 days or longer, intraocular pressure should be monitored (see WARNINGS).

There have been reports of bacterial keratitis associated with the use of multiple dose containers of topical ophthalmic products. These containers had been inadvertently contaminated by patients who, in most cases, had a concurrent corneal disease or a disruption of the ocular epithelial surface. (See PRECAUTIONS, *Information for Patients.*)

Information for Patients

Patients should be instructed to avoid allowing the tip of the dispensing container to contact the eye, eyelid, fingers, or any other surface. The use of this product by more than one person may spread infection. Keep tightly closed when not in use.

Patients should also be instructed that ocular preparations, if handled improperly, can become contaminated by common bacteria known to cause ocular infections. Serious damage to the eye and subsequent loss of vision may result from using contaminated preparations (see PRECAUTIONS, *General*).

If redness, irritation, swelling or pain persists or becomes aggravated, the patient should be advised to consult a physician. Patients should also be advised that if they have ocular surgery or develop an intercurrent ocular condition (e.g., trauma or infection), they should immediately seek their physician's advice.

One of the preservatives in Ophthalmic Solution NEODECADRON, benzalkonium chloride, may be absorbed by soft

Continued on next page

Neodecadron Solution—Cont.

contact lenses. Patients wearing soft contact lenses should be instructed to wait at least 15 minutes after instilling Ophthalmic Solution NEODECADRON before they insert their lenses.
Keep out of the reach of children.
Carcinogenesis, Mutagenesis, Impairment of Fertility
Long term animal studies have not been performed to evaluate the carcinogenic potential or the effect on fertility of Ophthalmic Solution NEODECADRON. Treatment of human lymphocytes *in-vitro* with neomycin increased the frequency of chromosome aberrations at the highest concentration (80 µg/mL) tested; however, the effects of neomycin on carcinogenesis and mutagenesis in humans are unknown.
Pregnancy
Teratogenic effects
Pregnancy Category C.
Corticosteroids have been found to be teratogenic in animal studies. Ocular administration of 0.1% dexamethasone resulted in 15.6% and 32.3% incidence of fetal anomalies in two groups of pregnant rabbits. Fetal growth retardation and increased mortality rates have been observed in rats with chronic dexamethasone therapy. There are no adequate and well-controlled studies in pregnant women. Ophthalmic Solution NEODECADRON should be used during pregnancy only if the potential benefit justifies the potential risk to the fetus. Infants born of mothers who have received substantial doses of corticosteroids during pregnancy should be observed carefully for signs of hypoadrenalism.
Nursing Mothers
It is not known whether topical administration of corticosteroids could result in sufficient systemic absorption to produce detectable quantities in human milk. Systemically-administered corticosteroids appear in human milk and could suppress growth, interfere with endogenous corticosteroid production, or cause other untoward effects. Because of the potential for serious adverse reactions in nursing infants from Ophthalmic Solution NEODECADRON, a decision should be made whether to discontinue nursing or to discontinue the drug, taking into account the importance of the drug to the mother.
Pediatric Use
Safety and effectiveness in pediatric patients have not been established.

ADVERSE REACTIONS

Adverse reactions have occurred with corticosteroid/anti-infective combination drugs which can be attributed to the corticosteroid component, the anti-infective component, the combination, or any other component of the product. Exact incidence figures are not available since no denominator of treated patients is available.
Reactions occurring most often from the presence of the anti-infective ingredient are allergic sensitizations. The reactions due to the corticosteroid component in decreasing order of frequency are: elevation of intraocular pressure (IOP) with possible development of glaucoma, and infrequent optic nerve damage; posterior subcapsular cataract formation; and delayed wound healing.
Secondary Infection: The development of secondary infection has occurred after use of combinations containing corticosteroids and antimicrobials. Fungal and viral infections of the cornea are particularly prone to develop coincidentally with long-term applications of a corticosteroid. The possibility of fungal invasion must be considered in any persistent corneal ulceration where corticosteroid treatment has been used.

DOSAGE AND ADMINISTRATION

The duration of treatment will vary with the type of lesion and may extend from a few days to several weeks, according to therapeutic response.
Instill one or two drops of Ophthalmic Solution NEODECADRON into the conjunctival sac every hour during the day and every two hours during the night as initial therapy. When a favorable response is observed, reduce dosage to one drop every four hours. Later, further reduction in dosage to one drop three or four times daily may suffice to control symptoms.
Not more than 20 milliliters should be prescribed initially and the prescription should not be refilled without further evaluation as outlined in PRECAUTIONS above.

HOW SUPPLIED

Sterile Ophthalmic Solution NEODECADRON is a clear, colorless to pale yellow solution.
No. 7639—Ophthalmic Solution NEODECADRON is supplied as follows:
NDC 0006-7639-03 in 5 mL white opaque, plastic OCUMETER ophthalmic dispenser with a controlled drop tip.
(6505-01-039-4352 0.1% 5 mL).
Storage
Store at controlled room temperature, 15°–30°C (59°–86°F).
Protect from light.
7261326 Issued December 1995

NOROXIN® Tablets (Norfloxacin), U.S.P. ℞

This product is manufactured by Merck & Co., Inc. and distributed by Roberts Laboratories, Inc. Please call 1-800-828-2088 for additional product information.

DESCRIPTION

NOROXIN+ (Norfloxacin) is a synthetic, broad-spectrum antibacterial agent for oral administration. Norfloxacin, a fluoroquinolone, is 1-ethyl-6-fluoro-1,4-dihydro-4-oxo-7-(1-piperazinyl)-3-quinolinecarboxylic acid. Its empirical formula is $C_{16}H_{18}FN_3O_3$ and the structural formula is:

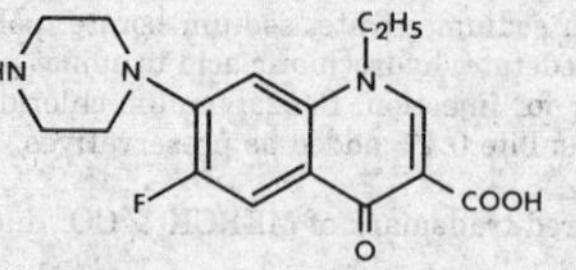

Norfloxacin is a white to pale yellow crystalline powder with a molecular weight of 319.34 and a melting point of about 221°C. It is freely soluble in glacial acetic acid, and very slightly soluble in ethanol, methanol and water.
NOROXIN is available in 400-mg tablets. Each tablet contains the following inactive ingredients: cellulose, croscarmellose sodium, hydroxypropyl cellulose, hydroxypropyl methylcellulose, iron oxide, magnesium stearate, and titanium dioxide.
Norfloxacin, a fluoroquinolone, differs from non-fluorinated quinolones by having a fluorine atom at the 6 position and a piperazine moiety at the 7 position.

+Registered trademark of MERCK & CO., INC.

CLINICAL PHARMACOLOGY

In fasting healthy volunteers, at least 30–40% of an oral dose of NOROXIN is absorbed. Absorption is rapid following single doses of 200 mg, 400 mg and 800 mg. At the respective doses, mean peak serum and plasma concentrations of 0.8, 1.5 and 2.4 µg/mL are attained approximately one hour after dosing. The presence of food and/or dairy products may decrease absorption. The effective half-life of norfloxacin in serum and plasma is 3–4 hours. Steady-state concentrations of norfloxacin will be attained within two days of dosing.
In healthy elderly volunteers (65–75 years of age with normal renal function for their age), norfloxacin is eliminated more slowly because of their slightly decreased renal function. Drug absorption appears unaffected. However, the effective half-life of norfloxacin in these elderly subjects is 4 hours.
The disposition of norfloxacin in patients with creatinine clearance rates greater than 30 mL/min/1.73m² is similar to that in healthy volunteers. In patients with creatinine clearance rates equal to or less than 30 mL/min/1.73m², the renal elimination of norfloxacin decreases so that the effective serum half-life is 6.5 hours. In these patients, alteration of dosage is necessary (see DOSAGE AND ADMINISTRATION). Drug absorption appears unaffected by decreasing renal function.
Norfloxacin is eliminated through metabolism, biliary excretion, and renal excretion. After a single 400-mg dose of NOROXIN, mean antimicrobial activities equivalent to 278, 773, and 82 µg of norfloxacin/g of feces were obtained at 12, 24, and 48 hours, respectively. Renal excretion occurs by both glomerular filtration and tubular secretion as evidenced by the high rate of renal clearance (approximately 275 mL/min). Within 24 hours of drug administration, 26 to 32% of the administered dose is recovered in the urine as norfloxacin with an additional 5–8% being recovered in the urine as six active metabolites of lesser antimicrobial potency. Only a small percentage (less than 1%) of the dose is recovered thereafter. Fecal recovery accounts for another 30% of the administered dose.
Two to three hours after a single 400-mg dose, urinary concentrations of 200 µg/mL or more are attained in the urine. In healthy volunteers, mean urinary concentrations of norfloxacin remain above 30 µg/mL for at least 12 hours following a 400-mg dose. The urinary pH may affect the solubility of norfloxacin. Norfloxacin is least soluble at urinary pH of 7.5 with greater solubility occurring at pHs above and below this value. The serum protein binding of norfloxacin is between 10 and 15%.
The following are mean concentrations of norfloxacin in various fluids and tissues measured 1 to 4 hours post-dose after two 400-mg doses, unless otherwise indicated:

Renal Parenchyma	7.3 µg/g
Prostate	2.5 µg/g
Seminal Fluid	2.7 µg/mL
Testicle	1.6 µg/g
Uterus/Cervix	3.0 µg/g
Vagina	4.3 µg/g
Fallopian Tube	1.9 µg/g
Bile	6.9 µg/mL (after two 200-mg doses)

Microbiology
Norfloxacin has *in vitro* activity against a broad range of gram-positive and gram-negative aerobic bacteria. The fluorine atom at the 6 position provides increased potency against gram-negative organisms, and the piperazine moiety at the 7 position is responsible for anti-pseudomonal activity.
Norfloxacin inhibits bacterial deoxyribonucleic acid synthesis and is bactericidal. At the molecular level, three specific events are attributed to norfloxacin in *E. coli* cells:
1) inhibition of the ATP-dependent DNA supercoiling reaction catalyzed by DNA gyrase,
2) inhibition of the relaxation of supercoiled DNA,
3) promotion of double-stranded DNA breakage.
Resistance to norfloxacin due to spontaneous mutation *in vitro* is a rare occurrence (range: 10^{-9} to 10^{-12} cells). Resistant organisms have emerged during therapy with norfloxacin in less than 1% of patients treated. Organisms in which development of resistance is greatest are the following:
Pseudomonas aeruginosa
Klebsiella pneumoniae
Acinetobacter spp.
Enterococcus spp.
For this reason, when there is a lack of satisfactory clinical response, repeat culture and susceptibility testing should be done. Nalidixic acid-resistant organisms are generally susceptible to norfloxacin *in vitro;* however, these organisms may have higher minimum inhibitory concentrations (MICs) to norfloxacin than nalidixic acid-susceptible strains. There is generally no cross-resistance between norfloxacin and other classes of antibacterial agents. Therefore, norfloxacin may demonstrate activity against indicated organisms resistant to some other antimicrobial agents including the aminoglycosides, penicillins, cephalosporins, tetracyclines, macrolides, and sulfonamides, including combinations of sulfamethoxazole and trimethoprim. Antagonism has been demonstrated *in vitro* between norfloxacin and nitrofurantoin.
Norfloxacin has been shown to be active against most strains of the following microorganisms both *in vitro* and in clinical infections as described in the **INDICATIONS AND USAGE** section.
Gram-positive aerobes:
Enterococcus faecalis
Staphylococcus aureus
Staphylococcus epidermidis
Staphylococcus saprophyticus
Streptococcus agalactiae
Gram-negative aerobes:
Citrobacter freundii
Enterobacter aerogenes
Enterobacter cloacae
Escherichia coli
Klebsiella pneumoniae
Neisseria gonorrhoeae
Proteus mirabilis
Proteus vulgaris
Pseudomonas aeruginosa
Serratia marcescens
The following *in vitro* data are available, **but their clinical significance is unknown.**
Norfloxacin exhibits *in vitro* minimal inhibitory concentrations (MIC's) of ≤4 µg/mL against most (≥90%) strains of the following microorganisms; however, the safety and effectiveness of norfloxacin in treating clinical infections due to these microorganisms have not been established in adequate and well-controlled clinical trials.
Gram-negative aerobes:
Citrobacter diversus
Edwardsiella tarda
Enterobacter agglomerans
Haemophilus ducreyi
Klebsiella oxytoca
Morganella morganii
Providencia alcalifaciens
Providencia rettgeri
Providencia stuartii
Pseudomonas fluorescens
Pseudomonas stutzeri
Other:
Ureaplasma urealyticum
NOROXIN is not generally active against obligate anaerobes.

Norfloxacin has not been shown to be active against *Treponema pallidum*. (See WARNINGS.)

Susceptibility Tests
Dilution Techniques:
Quantitative methods are used to determine antimicrobial minimal inhibitory concentrations (MIC's). These MIC's provide estimates of the susceptibility of bacteria to antimicrobial compounds. The MIC's should be determined using a standardized procedure. Standardized procedures are based on a dilution method[1] (broth, agar, or microdilution) or equivalent with standardized inoculum concentrations and standardized concentrations of norfloxacin powder. The MIC values should be interpreted according to the following criteria*:

MIC (µg/mL)	Interpretation
≤4	Susceptible (S)
8	Intermediate (I)
≥16	Resistant (R)

A report of "Susceptible" indicates that the pathogen is likely to be inhibited if the antimicrobial compound in the blood reaches the concentrations usually achievable. A report of "Intermediate" indicates that the result should be considered equivocal, and, if the microorganism is not fully susceptible to alternative, clinically feasible drugs, the test should be repeated. This category implies possible clinical applicability in body sites where the drug is physiologically concentrated or in situations where high dosage of drug can be used. This category also provides a buffer zone which prevents small uncontrolled technical factors from causing major discrepancies in interpretation. A report of "Resistant" indicates that the pathogen is not likely to be inhibited if the antimicrobial compound in the blood reaches the concentrations usually achievable; other therapy should be selected.

Standardized susceptibility test procedures require the use of laboratory control microorganisms to control the technical aspects of the laboratory procedures. Standard norfloxacin powder should provide the following MIC values:

Organism	MIC range (µg/mL)
E. coli ATCC 25922	0.03–0.12
E. faecalis ATCC 29212	2–8
P. aeruginosa ATCC 27853	1–4
S. aureus ATCC 29213	0.5–2

Diffusion Techniques:
Quantitative methods that require measurement of zone diameters also provide reproducible estimates of the susceptibility of bacteria to antimicrobial compounds. One such standardized procedure[2] requires the use of standardized inoculum concentrations. This procedure uses paper disks impregnated with 10-µg norfloxacin to test the susceptibility of microorganisms to norfloxacin. Reports from the laboratory providing results of the standard single-disk susceptibility test with a 10-µg norfloxacin disk should be interpreted according to the following criteria*:

Zone diameter (mm)	Interpretation
≥17	Susceptible (S)
13–16	Intermediate (I)
≤12	Resistant (R)

Interpretation should be as stated above for results using dilution techniques. Interpretation involves correlation of the diameter obtained in the disk test with the MIC for norfloxacin.

As with standard dilution techniques, diffusion methods require the use of laboratory control microorganisms that are used to control the technical aspects of the laboratory procedures. For the diffusion techniques, the 10-µg norfloxacin disk should provide the following zone diameters in these laboratory test quality control strains:

Organism	Zone Diameter (mm)
E. coli ATCC 25922	28–35
P. aeruginosa ATCC 27853	22–29
S. aureus ATCC 25923	17–28

*These interpretive criteria apply only to isolates from urinary tract infections. There are no established norfloxacin interpretive criteria for *Neisseria gonorrhoeae* or organisms isolated from other infection sites.

INDICATIONS AND USAGE

NOROXIN is indicated for the treatment of adults with the following infections caused by susceptible strains of the designated microorganisms:

Urinary tract infections:
Uncomplicated urinary tract infections (including cystitis) due to *Enterococcus faecalis, Escherichia coli, Klebsiella pneumoniae, Proteus mirabilis, Pseudomonas aeruginosa, Staphylococcus epidermidis, Staphylococcus saprophyticus, Citrobacter freundii**, Enterobacter aerogenes**, Enterobacter cloacae**, Proteus vulgaris**, Staphylococcus aureus**, or Streptococcus agalactiae**.

Complicated urinary tract infections due to *Enterococcus faecalis, Escherichia coli, Klebsiella pneumoniae, Proteus mirabilis, Pseudomonas aeruginosa*, or *Serratia marcescens**.

Sexually transmitted diseases (See WARNINGS.):
Uncomplicated urethral and cervical gonorrhea due to *Neisseria gonorrhoeae*.

Prostatitis:
Prostatitis due to *Escherichia coli*.
(See DOSAGE AND ADMINISTRATION for appropriate dosing instructions.)

Penicillinase production should have no effect on norfloxacin activity.

Appropriate culture and susceptibility tests should be performed before treatment in order to isolate and identify organisms causing the infection and to determine their susceptibility to norfloxacin. Therapy with norfloxacin may be initiated before results of these tests are known; once results become available, appropriate therapy should be given. Repeat culture and susceptibility testing performed periodically during therapy will provide information not only on the therapeutic effect of the antimicrobial agents but also on the possible emergence of bacterial resistance.

** Efficacy for this organism in this organ system was studied in fewer than 10 infections.

CONTRAINDICATIONS

NOROXIN (norfloxacin) is contraindicated in persons with a history of hypersensitivity, tendinitis, or tendon rupture associated with the use of norfloxacin or any member of the quinolone group of antimicrobial agents.

WARNINGS

THE SAFETY AND EFFICACY OF ORAL NORFLOXACIN IN CHILDREN, ADOLESCENTS (UNDER THE AGE OF 18), PREGNANT WOMEN, AND NURSING MOTHERS HAVE NOT BEEN ESTABLISHED. (See PRECAUTIONS—*Pregnancy, Nursing Mothers* and *Pediatric Use*.) The oral administration of single doses of norfloxacin, 6 times*** the recommended human clinical dose (on a mg/kg basis), caused lameness in immature dogs. Histologic examination of the weight-bearing joints of these dogs revealed permanent lesions of the cartilage. Other quinolones also produced erosions of the cartilage in weight-bearing joints and other signs of arthropathy in immature animals of various species. (See ANIMAL PHARMACOLOGY.)

Convulsions have been reported in patients receiving norfloxacin. Convulsions, increased intracranial pressure, and toxic psychoses have been reported in patients receiving drugs in this class. Quinolones may also cause central nervous system (CNS) stimulation which may lead to tremors, restlessness, lightheadedness, confusion, and hallucinations. If these reactions occur in patients receiving norfloxacin, the drug should be discontinued and appropriate measures instituted.

The effects of norfloxacin on brain function or on the electrical activity of the brain have not been tested. Therefore, until more information becomes available, norfloxacin, like all other quinolones, should be used with caution in patients with known or suspected CNS disorders, such as severe cerebral arteriosclerosis, epilepsy, and other factors which predispose to seizures. (See ADVERSE REACTIONS.)

Serious and occasionally fatal hypersensitivity (anaphylactoid or anaphylactic) reactions, some following the first dose, have been reported in patients receiving quinolone therapy. Some reactions were accompanied by cardiovascular collapse, loss of consciousness, tingling, pharyngeal or facial edema, dyspnea, urticaria and itching. Only a few patients had a history of hypersensitivity reactions. If an allergic reaction to norfloxacin occurs, discontinue the drug. Serious acute hypersensitivity reactions may require immediate emergency treatment with epinephrine. Oxygen, intravenous fluids, antihistamines, corticosteroids, pressor amines, and airway management, including intubation, should be administered as indicated.

Pseudomembranous colitis has been reported with nearly all antibacterial agents, including norfloxacin, and may range in severity from mild to life-threatening. Therefore, it is important to consider this diagnosis in patients who present with diarrhea subsequent to the administration of antibacterial agents.

Treatment with antibacterial agents alters the normal flora of the colon and may permit overgrowth of clostridia. Studies indicate that a toxin produced by *Clostridium difficile* is one primary cause of "antibiotic-associated colitis."

After the diagnosis of pseudomembranous colitis has been established, therapeutic measures should be initiated. Mild cases of pseudomembranous colitis usually respond to drug discontinuation alone. In moderate to severe cases, consideration should be given to management with fluids and electrolytes, protein supplementation, and treatment with an antibacterial drug clinically effective against *C. difficile* colitis.

Ruptures of the shoulder, hand, and Achilles tendons that required surgical repair or resulted in prolonged disability have been reported with norfloxacin. Norfloxacin should be discontinued if the patient experiences pain, inflammation, or rupture of a tendon. Patients should rest and refrain from exercise until the diagnosis of tendinitis or tendon rupture has been confidently excluded. Tendon rupture can occur at any time during or after therapy with norfloxacin.

Norfloxacin has not been shown to be effective in the treatment of syphilis. Antimicrobial agents used in high doses for short periods of time to treat gonorrhea may mask or delay the symptoms of incubating syphilis. All patients with gonorrhea should have a serologic test for syphilis at the time of diagnosis. Patients treated with norfloxacin should have a follow-up serologic test for syphilis after three months.

***Based on a patient weight of 50 kg.

PRECAUTIONS

General:
Needle-shaped crystals were found in the urine of some volunteers who received either placebo, 800 mg norfloxacin, or 1600 mg norfloxacin (at or twice the recommended daily dose, respectively) while participating in a double-blind, crossover study comparing single doses of norfloxacin with placebo. While crystalluria is not expected to occur under usual conditions with a dosage regimen of 400 mg b.i.d., as a precaution, the daily recommended dosage should not be exceeded and the patient should drink sufficient fluids to ensure a proper state of hydration and adequate urinary output.

Alteration in dosage regimen is necessary for patients with impaired renal function (see DOSAGE AND ADMINISTRATION).

Moderate to severe phototoxicity reactions have been observed in patients who are exposed to excessive sunlight while receiving some members of this drug class. Excessive sunlight should be avoided. Therapy should be discontinued if phototoxicity occurs.

Rarely, hemolytic reactions have been reported in patients with latent or actual defects in glucose-6-phosphate dehydrogenase activity who take quinolone antibacterial agents, including norfloxacin. (See ADVERSE REACTIONS.)

Information for Patients
Patients should be advised:
— to drink fluids liberally.
— that norfloxacin should be taken at least one hour before or at least two hours after a meal or ingestion of milk and/or other dairy products.
— that multivitamins or other products containing iron or zinc, or antacids should not be taken within the two-hour period before or within the two-hour period after taking norfloxacin. (See *Drug Interactions*.)
— that norfloxacin can cause dizziness and lightheadedness and, therefore, patients should know how they react to norfloxacin before they operate an automobile or machinery or engage in activities requiring mental alertness and coordination.
— to discontinue treatment and inform their physician if they experience pain, inflammation, or rupture of a tendon, and to rest and refrain from exercise until the diagnosis of tendinitis or tendon rupture has been confidently excluded.
— that norfloxacin may be associated with hypersensitivity reactions, even following the first dose, and to discontinue the drug at the first sign of a skin rash or other allergic reaction.
— to avoid undue exposure to excessive sunlight while receiving norfloxacin and to discontinue therapy if phototoxicity occurs.
— that some quinolones may increase the effects of theophylline and/or caffeine. (See *Drug Interactions*.)

Laboratory Tests
As with any potent antibacterial agent, periodic assessment of organ system functions, including renal, hepatic, and hematopoietic, is advisable during prolonged therapy.

Drug Interactions
Elevated plasma levels of theophylline have been reported with concomitant quinolone use. There have been reports of theophylline-related side effects in patients on concomitant therapy with norfloxacin and theophylline. Therefore, monitoring of theophylline plasma levels should be considered and dosage of theophylline adjusted as required.

Elevated serum levels of cyclosporine have been reported with concomitant use of cyclosporine with norfloxacin.

Continued on next page

Information on the Merck & Co., Inc. products listed on these pages is the full prescribing information from product circulars in use August 31, 1998. For information, please call 1-800-NSC MERCK [1-800-672-6372].

Noroxin—Cont.

Therefore cyclosporine serum levels should be monitored and appropriate cyclosporine dosage adjustments made when these drugs are used concomitantly.

Quinolones, including norfloxacin, may enhance the effects of the oral anticoagulant warfarin or its derivatives. When these products are administered concomitantly, prothrombin time or other suitable coagulation tests should be closely monitored.

Diminished urinary excretion of norfloxacin has been reported during the concomitant administration of probenecid and norfloxacin.

The concomitant use of nitrofurantoin is not recommended since nitrofurantoin may antagonize the antibacterial effect of NOROXIN in the urinary tract.

Multivitamins, or other products containing iron or zinc, antacids or sucralfate should not be administered concomitantly with, or within 2 hours of, the administration of norfloxacin, because they may interfere with absorption resulting in lower serum and urine levels of norfloxacin.

Some quinolones have also been shown to interfere with the metabolism of caffeine. This may lead to reduced clearance of caffeine and a prolongation of its plasma half-life.

Carcinogenesis, Mutagenesis, Impairment of Fertility
No increase in neoplastic changes was observed with norfloxacin as compared to controls in a study in rats, lasting up to 96 weeks at doses 8–9 times*** the usual human dose (on a mg/kg basis).

Norfloxacin was tested for mutagenic activity in a number of *in vivo* and *in vitro* tests. Norfloxacin had no mutagenic effect in the dominant lethal test in mice and did not cause chromosomal aberrations in hamsters or rats at doses 30–60 times*** the usual human dose (on a mg/kg basis). Norfloxacin had no mutagenic activity *in vitro* in the Ames microbial mutagen test, Chinese hamster fibroblasts and V-79 mammalian cell assay. Although norfloxacin was weakly positive in the Rec-assay for DNA repair, all other mutagenic assays were negative including a more sensitive test (V-79).

Norfloxacin did not adversely affect the fertility of male and female mice at oral doses up to 30 times*** the usual human dose (on a mg/kg basis).

Pregnancy
Teratogenic Effects. Pregnancy Category C. Norfloxacin has been shown to produce embryonic loss in monkeys when given in doses 10 times*** the maximum daily total human dose (on a mg/kg basis). At this dose, peak plasma levels obtained in monkeys were approximately 2 times those obtained in humans. There has been no evidence of a teratogenic effect in any of the animal species tested (rat, rabbit, mouse, monkey) at 6–50 times*** the maximum daily human dose (on a mg/kg basis). There are, however, no adequate and well controlled studies in pregnant women. Norfloxacin should be used during pregnancy only if the potential benefit justifies the potential risk to the fetus.

Nursing Mothers
It is not known whether norfloxacin is excreted in human milk.

When a 200-mg dose of NOROXIN was administered to nursing mothers, norfloxacin was not detected in human milk. However, because the dose studied was low, because other drugs in this class are secreted in human milk, and because of the potential for serious adverse reactions from norfloxacin in nursing infants, a decision should be made to discontinue nursing or to discontinue the drug, taking into account the importance of the drug to the mother.

Pediatric Use
The safety and effectiveness of oral norfloxacin in children and adolescents below the age of 18 years have not been established. Norfloxacin causes arthropathy in juvenile animals of several animal species. (See WARNINGS and ANIMAL PHARMACOLOGY.)

***Based on a patient weight of 50 kg.

ADVERSE REACTIONS

Single-Dose Studies
In clinical trials involving 82 healthy subjects and 228 patients with gonorrhea, treated with a single dose of norfloxacin, 6.5% reported drug-related adverse experiences. However, the following incidence figures were calculated without reference to drug relationship.

The most common adverse experiences (>1.0%) were: dizziness (2.6%), nausea (2.6%), headache (2.0%), and abdominal cramping (1.6%).

Additional reactions (0.3%–1.0%) were: anorexia, diarrhea, hyperhidrosis, asthenia, anal/rectal pain, constipation, dyspepsia, flatulence, tingling of the fingers, and vomiting.

Laboratory adverse changes considered drug-related were reported in 4.5% of patients/subjects. These laboratory changes were: increased AST (SGOT) (1.6%), decreased WBC (1.3%), decreased platelet count (1.0%), increased urine protein (1.0%), decreased hematocrit and hemoglobin (0.6%), and increased eosinophils (0.6%).

Multiple-Dose Studies
In clinical trials involving 52 healthy subjects and 1980 patients with urinary tract infections or prostatitis, treated with multiple doses of norfloxacin, 3.6% reported drug-related adverse experiences. However, the incidence figures below were calculated without reference to drug relationship.

The most common adverse experiences (>1.0%) were: nausea (4.2%), headache (2.8%), dizziness (1.7%), and asthenia (1.3%).

Additional reactions (0.3%–1.0%) were: abdominal pain, back pain, constipation, diarrhea, dry mouth, dyspepsia/heartburn, fever, flatulence, hyperhidrosis, loose stools, pruritus, rash, somnolence, and vomiting.

Less frequent reactions (0.1%–0.2%) included: abdominal swelling, allergies, anorexia, anxiety, bitter taste, blurred vision, bursitis, chest pain, chills, depression, dysmenorrhea, edema, erythema, foot or hand swelling, insomnia, mouth ulcer, myocardial infarction, palpitation, pruritus ani, renal colic, sleep disturbances, and urticaria.

Abnormal laboratory values observed in these patients/subjects were: eosinophilia (1.5%), elevation of ALT (SGPT) (1.4%), decreased WBC and/or neutrophil count (1.4%), elevation of AST (SGOT) (1.4%), and increased alkaline phosphatase (1.1%). Those occurring less frequently included increased BUN, increased LDH, increased serum creatinine, decreased hematocrit, and glycosuria.

Post Marketing
The most frequently reported adverse reaction in post-marketing experience is rash.

CNS effects characterized as generalized seizures and myoclonus have been reported with NOROXIN. A causal relationship to NOROXIN has not been established (see WARNINGS). Visual disturbances have been reported with drugs in this class.

The following additional adverse reactions have been reported since the drug was marketed:

Hypersensitivity Reactions
Hypersensitivity reactions have been reported including anaphylactoid reactions, angioedema, dyspnea, vasculitis, urticaria, arthritis, arthralgia and myalgia (see WARNINGS).

Skin
Toxic epidermal necrolysis, Stevens-Johnson syndrome and erythema multiforme, exfoliative dermatitis, photosensitivity

Gastrointestinal
Pseudomembranous colitis, hepatitis, jaundice including cholestatic jaundice, pancreatitis (rare), stomatitis. The onset of pseudomembranous colitis symptoms may occur during or after antibacterial treatment. (See WARNINGS.)

Renal
Interstitial nephritis, renal failure

Nervous System / Psychiatric
Peripheral neuropathy, Guillain-Barré syndrome, ataxia, paresthesia; psychic disturbances including psychotic reactions and confusion

Musculoskeletal
Tendinitis, tendon rupture, possible exacerbation of myasthenia gravis

Hematologic
Neutropenia, leukopenia, hemolytic anemia, sometimes associated with glucose-6-phosphate dehydrogenase deficiency; thrombocytopenia

Special Senses
Transient hearing loss (rare), tinnitus, diplopia

Other adverse events reported with quinolones include: agranulocytosis, albuminuria, candiduria, crystalluria, cylindruria, dysphagia, elevation of blood glucose, elevation of serum cholesterol, elevation of serum potassium, elevation of serum triglycerides, hematuria, hepatic necrosis, symptomatic hypoglycemia, nystagmus, postural hypotension, prolongation of prothrombin time, and vaginal candidiasis.

OVERDOSAGE

No significant lethality was observed in male and female mice and rats at single oral doses up to 4 g/kg.

In the event of acute overdosage, the stomach should be emptied by inducing vomiting or by gastric lavage, and the patient carefully observed and given symptomatic and supportive treatment. Adequate hydration must be maintained.

DOSAGE AND ADMINISTRATION

Tablets NOROXIN should be taken at least one hour before or at least two hours after a meal or ingestion of milk and/or other dairy products. Tablets NOROXIN should be taken with a glass of water. Patients receiving NOROXIN should be well hydrated (see PRECAUTIONS).

Normal Renal Function
The recommended daily dose of NOROXIN is as described in the following chart:
[See table below]

Renal Impairment
NOROXIN may be used for the treatment of urinary tract infections in patients with renal insufficiency. In patients with a creatinine clearance rate of 30 mL/min/1.73m² or less, the recommended dosage is one 400-mg tablet once daily for the duration given above. At this dosage, the urinary concentration exceeds the MICs for most urinary pathogens susceptible to norfloxacin, even when the creatinine clearance is less than 10 mL/min/1.73m².

When only the serum creatinine level is available, the following formula (based on sex, weight, and age of the patient) may be used to convert this value into creatinine clearance. The serum creatinine should represent a steady state of renal function.

Males: $\dfrac{(\text{weight in kg}) \times (140 - \text{age})}{(72) \times \text{serum creatinine (mg/100 mL)}}$

Females: $(0.85) \times (\text{above value})$

Elderly
Elderly patients being treated for urinary tract infections who have a creatinine clearance of greater than 30 mL/min/1.73m² should receive the dosages recommended under *Normal Renal Function.*

Elderly patients being treated for urinary tract infections who have a creatinine clearance of 30 mL/min/1.73m² or less should receive 400 mg once daily as recommended under *Renal Impairment.*

HOW SUPPLIED

No. 3522—Tablets NOROXIN 400 mg are dark pink, oval shaped, film-coated tablets, coded MSD 705 on one side and NOROXIN on the other. They are supplied as follows:
NDC 54092-097-01 bottles of 100
NDC 54092-097-20 unit of use bottles of 20
NDC 54092-097-52 unit dose packages of 100.
Shown in Product Identification Guide, page 323

Storage
Tablets NOROXIN should be stored in a tightly-closed container. Avoid storage at temperatures above 40°C (104°F).

ANIMAL PHARMACOLOGY

Norfloxacin and related drugs have been shown to cause arthropathy in immature animals of most species tested (see WARNINGS).

Crystalluria has occurred in laboratory animals tested with norfloxacin. In dogs, needle-shaped drug crystals were seen in the urine at doses of 50 mg/kg/day. In rats, crystals were reported following doses of 200 mg/kg/day.

Embryo lethality and slight maternotoxicity (vomiting and anorexia) were observed in cynomolgus monkeys at doses of 150 mg/kg/day or higher.

Ocular toxicity, seen with some related drugs, was not observed in any norfloxacin-treated animals.

REFERENCES

1. National Committee for Clinical Laboratory Standards, Methods for dilution antimicrobial susceptibility tests for

Infection	Description	Unit Dose	Frequency	Duration	Daily Dose
Urinary Tract	Uncomplicated UTI's (crystitis) due to *E. coli, K. pneumoniae,* or *P. mirabilis*	400 mg	q12h	3 days	800 mg
	Uncomplicated UTI's due to other indicated organisms	400 mg	q12h	7–10 days	800 mg
	Complicated UTI's	400 mg	q12h	10–21 days	800 mg
Sexually Transmitted Diseases	Uncomplicated Gonorrhea	800 mg	single dose	1 day	800 mg
Prostatitis	Acute or Chronic	400 mg	q12h	28 days	800 mg

bacteria that grow aerobically – 3rd ed., Approved Standard NCCLS Document M7–A3, Vol. 13, No. 25, NCCLS, Villanova, PA, 1993.
2. National Committee for Clinical Laboratory Standards, Performance standards for antimicrobial disk susceptibility tests – 5th ed., Approved Standard NCCLS Document M2–A5, Vol. 13, No. 24, NCCLS, Villanova, PA, 1993.
7898526 Issued May 1997
COPYRIGHT © MERCK & CO., INC., 1986, 1989
All rights reserved

Liquid PedvaxHIB® ℞
[Haemophilus b Conjugate Vaccine (Meningococcal Protein Conjugate)]

DESCRIPTION

PedvaxHIB* [Haemophilus b Conjugate Vaccine (Meningococcal Protein Conjugate)] is a highly purified capsular polysaccharide (polyribosylribitol phosphate or PRP) of *Haemophilus influenzae* type b (Haemophilus b, Ross strain) that is covalently bound to an outer membrane protein complex (OMPC) of the B11 strain of *Neisseria meningitidis* serogroup B. The covalent bonding of the PRP to the OMPC which is necessary for enhanced immunogenicity of the PRP is confirmed by quantitative analysis of the conjugate's components following chemical treatment which yields a unique amino acid. The potency of PedvaxHIB is determined by assay of PRP.
Haemophilus influenzae type b and *Neisseria meningitidis* serogroup B are grown in complex fermentation media. The PRP is purified from the culture broth by purification procedures which include ethanol fractionation, enzyme digestion, phenol extraction and diafiltration. The OMPC from *Neisseria meningitidis* is purified by detergent extraction, ultracentrifugation, diafiltration and sterile filtration.
Liquid PedvaxHIB is ready to use and does not require a diluent. Each 0.5 mL dose of Liquid PedvaxHIB is a sterile product formulated to contain: 7.5 mcg of Haemophilus b PRP, 125 mcg of *Neisseria meningitidis* OMPC and 225 mcg of aluminum as aluminum hydroxide, in 0.9% sodium chloride, but does not contain lactose or thimerosal.
Liquid PedvaxHIB is a slightly opaque white suspension. This vaccine is for intramuscular administration and not for intravenous injection. (See DOSAGE AND ADMINISTRATION.)

* Registered trademark of MERCK & CO., Inc.

CLINICAL PHARMACOLOGY

Prior to the introduction of Haemophilus b Conjugate Vaccines, *Haemophilus influenzae* type b (Hib) was the most frequent cause of bacterial meningitis and a leading cause of serious, systemic bacterial disease in young children worldwide.
Hib disease occurred primarily in children under 5 years of age in the United States prior to the initiation of a vaccine program and was estimated to account for nearly 20,000 cases of invasive infections annually, approximately 12,000 of which were meningitis. The mortality rate from Hib meningitis is about 5%. In addition, up to 35% of survivors develop neurologic sequelae including seizures, deafness, and mental retardation. Other invasive diseases caused by this bacterium include cellulitis, epiglottitis, sepsis, pneumonia, septic arthritis, osteomyelitis and pericarditis.
Prior to the introduction of the vaccine, it was estimated that 17% of all cases of Hib disease occurred in infants less than 6 months of age. The peak incidence of Hib meningitis occurs between 6 to 11 months of age. Forty-seven percent of all cases occur by one year of age with the remaining 53% of cases occurring over the next four years.
Among children under 5 years of age, the risk of invasive Hib disease is increased in certain populations including the following:
- Daycare attendees
- Lower socio-economic groups
- Blacks (especially those who lack the Km(1) immunoglobulin allotype)
- Caucasians who lack the G2m (n or 23) immunoglobulin allotype
- Native Americans
- Household contacts of cases
- Individuals with asplenia, sickle cell disease, or antibody deficiency syndromes

An important virulence factor of the Hib bacterium is its polysaccharide capsule (PRP). Antibody to PRP (anti-PRP) has been shown to correlate with protection against Hib disease. While the anti-PRP level associated with protection using conjugated vaccines has not yet been determined, the level of anti-PRP associated with protection in studies using bacterial polysaccharide immune globulin or nonconjugated PRP vaccines ranged from >0.15 to >1.0 mcg/mL.

TABLE 1
Antibody Responses in Navajo Infants

Vaccine	No. of Subjects	Time	% Subjects with >0.15 mcg/mL	% Subjects with >1.0 mcg/mL	Anti-PRP GMT (mcg/mL)
Lyophilized PedvaxHIB*	416**	Pre-Vaccination	44	10	0.16
	416	Post-Dose 1	88	52	0.95
	416	Post-Dose 2	91	60	1.43
Placebo*	461**	Pre-Vaccination	44	9	0.16
	461	Post-Dose 1	21	2	0.09
	461	Post-Dose 2	14	1	0.08
Lyophilized PedvaxHIB	27†	Prebooster	70	33	0.51
	27	Postbooster††	100	89	8.39

*Post-Vaccination values obtained approximately 1–3 months after each dose.
**The Protective Efficacy Study
†Immunogenicity Trial[34]
††Booster given at 12 months of age; Post-Vaccination values obtained 1 month after administration of booster dose.

Nonconjugated PRP vaccines are capable of stimulating B-lymphocytes to produce antibody without the help of T-lymphocytes (T-independent). The responses to many other antigens are augmented by helper T-lymphocytes (T-dependent). PedvaxHIB is a PRP-conjugate vaccine in which the PRP is covalently bound to the OMPC carrier producing an antigen which is postulated to convert the T-independent antigen (PRP alone) into a T-dependent antigen resulting in both an enhanced antibody response and immunologic memory.
Clinical Evaluation of PedvaxHIB
PedvaxHIB, in a lyophilized formulation (lyophilized PedvaxHIB), was initially evaluated in 3,486 Native American (Navajo) infants, who completed the primary two-dose regimen in a randomized, double-blind, placebo-controlled study (The Protective Efficacy Study). At the time of the study, this population had a much higher incidence of Hib disease than the United States population as a whole and also had a lower antibody response to Haemophilus b Conjugate Vaccines, including PedvaxHIB.
Each infant in this study received two doses of either placebo or lyophilized PedvaxHIB with the first dose administered at a mean of 8 weeks of age and the second administered approximately two months later; DTP and OPV were administered concomitantly. Antibody levels were measured in a subset of each group (TABLE 1).
[See table 1 above]
Most subjects were initially followed until 15 to 18 months of age. During this time, 22 cases of invasive Hib disease occurred in the placebo group (8 cases after the first dose and 14 cases after the second dose) and only 1 case in the vaccine group (none after the first dose and 1 after the second dose). Following the primary two-dose regimen, the protective efficacy of lyophilized PedvaxHIB was calculated to be 93% with a 95% confidence interval of 57%–98% (p=0.001, two-tailed). In the two months between the first and second doses, the difference in number of cases of disease between placebo and vaccine recipients (8 vs. 0 cases, respectively) was statistically significant (p=0.008, two-tailed); however, a primary two-dose regimen is required for infants 2–14 months of age.
At termination of the study, placebo recipients were offered vaccine. All original participants were then followed two years and nine months from termination of the study. During this extended follow-up, invasive Hib disease occurred in an additional seven of the original placebo recipients prior to receiving vaccine and in one of the original vaccine recipients (who had received only one dose of vaccine). No cases of invasive Hib disease were observed in placebo recipients after they received at least one dose of vaccine. Efficacy for this follow-up period, estimated from person-days at risk, was 96.6% (95 C.I., 72.2–99.9%) in children under 18 months of age and 100% (95 C.I., 23.5–100%) in children over 18 months of age.
Since protective efficacy with lyophilized PedvaxHIB was demonstrated in such a high risk population, it would be expected to be predictive of efficacy in other populations.
The safety and immunogenicity of lyophilized PedvaxHIB were evaluated in infants and children in other clinical studies that were conducted in various locations throughout the United States. PedvaxHIB was highly immunogenic in all age groups studied.
Lyophilized PedvaxHIB induced antibody levels greater than 1.0 mcg/mL in children who were poor responders to nonconjugated PRP vaccines. In a study involving such a subpopulation, 34 children ranging in age from 27 to 61 months who developed invasive Hib disease despite previous vaccination with nonconjugated PRP vaccines were randomly assigned to 2 groups. One group (n=14) was vaccinated with lyophilized PedvaxHIB and the other group (n=20) with a nonconjugated PRP vaccine at a mean interval of approximately 12 months after recovery from disease. All 14 children vaccinated with lyophilized PedvaxHIB but only 6 of 20 children re-vaccinated with a nonconjugated PRP vaccine achieved an antibody level of >1.0 mcg/mL. The 14 children who had not responded to revaccination with the nonconjugated PRP vaccine were then vaccinated with a single dose of lyophilized PedvaxHIB; following this vaccination, all achieved antibody levels of >1.0 mcg/mL.
In addition, lyophilized PedvaxHIB has been studied in children at high risk of Hib disease because of genetically-related deficiencies [Blacks who were Km(1) allotype negative and Caucasians who were G2m(23) allotype negative] and are considered hyporesponsive to nonconjugated PRP vaccines on this basis. The hyporesponsive children had anti-PRP responses comparable to those of allotype positive children of similar age range when vaccinated with lyophilized PedvaxHIB. All children achieved anti-PRP levels of >1.0 mcg/mL.
The safety and immunogenicity of Liquid PedvaxHIB were compared with those of lyophilized PedvaxHIB is a randomized clinical study involving 903 infants 2 to 6 months of age from the general U.S. population. DTP and OPV were administered concomitantly to most subjects. The antibody responses induced by each formulation of PedvaxHIB were similar. TABLE 2 shows antibody responses from this clinical study in subjects who received their first dose at 2 to 3 months of age.
[See table 2 at top of next page]
A booster dose of PedvaxHIB is required in infants who complete the primary two-dose regimen before 12 months of age. This booster dose will help maintain antibody levels during the first two years of life when children are at highest risk for invasive Hib disease. (See TABLE 2 and DOSAGE AND ADMINISTRATION.)
In four United States studies, antibody responses to lyophilized PedvaxHIB were evaluated in several subpopulations of infants initially vaccinated between 2 to 3 months of age. (See TABLE 3.)
[See table 3 at top of next page]
In two United States studies, antibody responses to Liquid PedvaxHIB were evaluated in several subpopulations of infants initially vaccinated between 2 to 3 months of age. (See TABLE 4.)
[See table 4 at top of next page]
Antibodies to the OMPC of *N. meningitidis* have been demonstrated in vaccinee sera, but the clinical relevance of these antibodies has not been established.
Interchangeability of Licensed Haemophilus b Conjugate Vaccines and PedvaxHIB
Published studies have examined the interchangeability of other licensed Haemophilus b Conjugate Vaccines and PedvaxHIB. According to the American Academy of Pediatrics, excellent immune responses have been achieved when different vaccines have been interchanged in the primary series. If PedvaxHIB is given in a series with one of the other products licensed for infants, the recommended number of doses to complete the series is determined by the other product and not by PedvaxHIB. PedvaxHIB may be interchanged with other licensed Haemophilus b Conjugate Vaccines for the booster dose.
Use with Other Vaccines
Results from clinical studies indicate that Liquid PedvaxHIB can be administered concomitantly with DTP, OPV, eIPV (enhanced inactivated poliovirus vaccine), VARIVAX* [Varicella Virus Vaccine Live (Oka/Merck)], M-M-R* II (Measles, Mumps, and Rubella Virus Vaccine Live) or RECOMBIVAX HB* [Hepatitis B Vaccine (Recombinant)]. No impairment of immune response to individual tested vaccine antigens was demonstrated.
The type, frequency and severity of adverse experiences observed in these studies with PedvaxHIB were similar to those seen when the other vaccines were given alone.

Continued on next page

Information on the Merck & Co., Inc. products listed on these pages is the full prescribing information from product circulars in use August 31, 1998. For information, please call 1-800-NSC MERCK [1-800-672-6372].

PedvaxHIB—Cont.

In addition, a PRP-OMPC-containing product, COMVAX* [Haemophilus b Conjugate (Meningococcal Protein Conjugate) and Hepatitis B (Recombinant) Vaccine], was given concomitantly with a booster dose of DTaP [diphtheria, tetanus, acellular pertussis] at approximately 15 months of age, using separate sites and syringes for injectable vaccines. No impairment of immune response to these individually tested vaccine antigens was demonstrated. COMVAX has also been administered concomitantly with the primary series of DTaP to a limited number of infants. PRP antibody responses are satisfactory for COMVAX, but immune responses are currently unavailable for DTaP (see Manufacturer's Product Circular for COMVAX). No serious vaccine-related adverse events were reported.

INDICATIONS AND USAGE

Liquid PedvaxHIB is indicated for routine vaccination against invasive disease caused by *Haemophilus influenzae* type b in infants and children 2 to 71 months of age.
Liquid PedvaxHIB will not protect against disease caused by *Haemophilus influenzae* other than type b or against other microorganisms that cause invasive disease such as meningitis or sepsis. As with any vaccine, vaccination with Liquid PedvaxHIB may not result in a protective antibody response in all individuals given the vaccine.
BECAUSE OF THE POTENTIAL FOR IMMUNE TOLERANCE, Liquid PedvaxHIB IS NOT RECOMMENDED FOR USE IN INFANTS YOUNGER THAN 6 WEEKS OF AGE. (See PRECAUTIONS.)

Revaccination
Infants completing the primary two-dose regimen before 12 months of age should receive a booster dose (see DOSAGE AND ADMINISTRATION).

CONTRAINDICATIONS

Hypersensitivity to any component of the vaccine or the diluent.
Persons who develop symptoms suggestive of hypersensitivity after an injection should not receive further injections of the vaccine.

PRECAUTIONS

General
As for any vaccine, adequate treatment provisions, including epinephrine, should be available for immediate use should an anaphylactoid reaction occur.
Special care should be taken to ensure that the injection does not enter a blood vessel.
It is important to use a separate sterile syringe and needle for each patient to prevent transmission of hepatitis B or other infectious agents from one person to another.
As with other vaccines, Liquid PedvaxHIB may not induce protective antibody levels immediately following vaccination.
As reported with Haemophilus b Polysaccharide Vaccine and another Haemophilus b Conjugate Vaccine, cases of Hib disease may occur in the week after vaccination, prior to the onset of the protective effects of the vaccines.
There is insufficient evidence that Liquid PedvaxHIB given immediately after exposure to natural *Haemophilus influenzae* type b will prevent illness.
The decision to administer or delay vaccination because of current or recent febrile illness depends on the severity of symptoms and on the etiology of the disease. The Advisory Committee on Immunization Practices (ACIP) has recommended that vaccination should be delayed during the course of an acute febrile illness. All vaccines can be administered to persons with minor illnesses such as diarrhea, mild upper-respiratory infection with or without low-grade fever, or other low-grade febrile illness. Persons with moderate or severe illness should be vaccinated as soon as they have recovered from the acute phase of the illness.
If PedvaxHIB is used in persons with malignancies or those receiving immunosuppressive therapy or who are otherwise immunocompromised, the expected immune response may not be obtained.

Instructions to Healthcare Provider
The healthcare provider should determine the current health status and previous vaccination history of the vaccinee.
The healthcare provider should question the patient, parent, or guardian about reactions to a previous dose of PedvaxHIB or other Haemophilus b Conjugate Vaccines.

Information for Patients
The healthcare provider should provide the vaccine information required to be given with each vaccination to the patient, parent, or guardian.

The healthcare provider should inform the patient, parent, or guardian of the benefits and risks associated with vaccination. For risks associated with vaccination, see ADVERSE REACTIONS.
Patients, parents, and guardians should be instructed to report any serious adverse reactions to their healthcare provider who in turn should report such events to the U.S. Department of Health and Human Services through the Vaccine Adverse Event Reporting System (VAERS), 1-800-822-7967.

Laboratory Test Interactions
Sensitive tests (e.g., Latex Agglutination Kits) may detect PRP derived from the vaccine in urine of some vaccinees for at least 30 days following vaccination with lyophilized

TABLE 2
Antibody Responses to Liquid and Lyophilized PedvaxHIB in Infants From the General U.S. Population

Formulation	Age (Months)	Time	No. of Subjects	% Subjects with anti-PRP >0.15 mcg/mL	% Subjects with anti-PRP >1.0 mcg/mL	Anti-PRP GMT (mcg/mL)
Liquid PedvaxHIB (7.5 mcg PRP)	2–3	Pre-Vaccination	487	32	7	0.12
		Post-Dose 1*	480	94	64	1.55
		Post-Dose 2**	393	97	80	3.22
	12–15	Prebooster	284	80	30	0.49
		Postbooster**	284	99	95	10.23
	24†	Persistence	94	97	55	1.29
Lyophilized PedvaxHIB (15 mcg PRP)	2–3	Pre-Vaccination	171	37	6	0.13
		Post-Dose 1*	169	97	72	1.88
		Post-Dose 2**	133	99	81	2.69
	12–15	Prebooster	87	71	28	0.39
		Postbooster**	87	99	91	7.64
	24†	Persistence	37	97	54	1.10

*Approximately two months Post-Vaccination
**Approximately one month Post-Vaccination
†Approximately

TABLE 3
Antibody Responses*
After Two Doses of Lyophilized PedvaxHIB Among Infants Initially Vaccinated at 2–3 Months of Age By Racial/Ethnic Group

Racial/Ethnic Groups	No. of Subjects	LYOPHILIZED % Subjects With Anti-PRP >0.15 mcg/mL	LYOPHILIZED % Subjects With Anti-PRP >1.0 mcg/mL	Anti-PRP GMT (mcg/mL)
Native American†	54	96	70	2.47
Caucasian	201	99	82	3.52
Hispanic	76	99	88	3.54
Black	23	100	96	5.40

* One month after the second dose
† Apache and Navajo

TABLE 4
Antibody Responses*
After Two Doses of Liquid PedvaxHIB Among Infants Initially Vaccinated at 2–3 Months of Age By Racial/Ethnic Group

Racial/Ethnic Groups	No. of Subjects	LIQUID % Subjects with Anti-PRP >0.15 mcg/mL	LIQUID % Subjects with Anti-PRP >1.0 mcg/mL	Anti-PRP GMT (mcg/mL)
Native American**	90	97	78	2.76
Caucasian	143	94	72	2.16
Hispanic	184	98	85	4.34
Black	18	100	94	7.58

* One month after the second dose
**Apache and Navajo

TABLE 5
Fever or Local Reactions in Subjects First Vaccinated at 2 to 6 Months of Age with Liquid PedvaxHIB*

Reaction	No. of Subjects Evaluated	Post-Dose 1 (hr) 6	Post-Dose 1 (hr) 24	Post-Dose 1 (hr) 48	No. of Subjects Evaluated	Post-Dose 2 (hr) 6	Post-Dose 2 (hr) 24	Post-Dose 2 (hr) 48
		Percentage				Percentage		
Fever** >38.3°C (≥101°F) Rectal	222	18.1	4.4	0.5	206	14.1	9.4	2.8
Erythema >2.5 cm diameter	674	2.2	1.0	0.5	562	1.6	1.1	0.4
Swelling >2.5 cm diameter	674	2.5	1.9	0.9	562	0.9	0.9	1.3

*DTP and OPV were administered concomitantly to most subjects.
** Fever was also measured by another method or reported as normal for an additional 345 infants after dose 1 and for an additional 249 infants after dose 2; however, these data are not included in this table.

PedvaxHIB; in clinical studies with lyophilized PedvaxHIB, such children demonstrated normal immune response to the vaccine.

Carcinogenesis, Mutagenesis, Impairment of Fertility

Liquid PedvaxHIB has not been evaluated for carcinogenic or mutagenic potential, or potential to impair fertility.

Pregnancy

Pregnancy Category C: Animal reproduction studies have not been conducted with PedvaxHIB. Liquid PedvaxHIB is not recommended for use in individuals 6 years of age and older.

Pediatric Use

Safety and effectiveness in infants below the age of 2 months and in children 6 years of age and older have not been established. In addition, Liquid PedvaxHIB should not be used in infants younger than 6 weeks of age because this will lead to a reduced anti-PRP response and may lead to immune tolerance (impaired ability to respond to subsequent exposure to the PRP antigen). Liquid PedvaxHIB is not recommended for use in individuals 6 years of age and older because they are generally not a risk of Hib disease.

ADVERSE REACTIONS

Liquid PedvaxHIB

In a multicenter clinical study (n=903) comparing the effects of Liquid PedvaxHIB with those of lyophilized PedvaxHIB, 1,699 doses of Liquid PedvaxHIB were administered to 678 healthy infants 2 to 6 months of age from the general U.S. population. DTP and OPV were administered concomitantly to most subjects. Both formulations of PedvaxHIB were generally well tolerated and no serious vaccine-related adverse reactions were reported.

During a three-day period following primary vaccination with Liquid PedvaxHIB in these infants, the most frequently reported (>1%) adverse reactions, without regard to causality, excluding those shown in TABLE 5, in decreasing order of frequency, were: irritability, sleepiness, injection site pain/soreness, injection site erythema (≤2.5 cm diameter, see also TABLE 5), injection site swelling/induration (≤2.5 cm diameter, see also TABLE 5), unusual high-pitched crying, prolonged crying (>4 hr), diarrhea, vomiting, crying, pain, otitis media, rash, and upper respiratory infection.

Selected objective observations reported by parents over a 48-hour period in these infants following primary vaccination with Liquid PedvaxHIB are summarized in TABLE 5.

[See table 5 on previous page]

Adverse reactions during a three-day period following administration of the booster dose were generally similar in type and frequency to those seen following primary vaccination.

Lyophilized PedvaxHIB

In The Protective Efficacy Study (see CLINICAL PHARMACOLOGY), 4,459 healthy Navajo infants 6 to 12 weeks of age received lyophilized PedvaxHIB or placebo. Most of these infants received DTP/OPV concomitantly. No differences were seen in the type and frequency of serious health problems expected in this Navajo population or in serious adverse experiences reported among those who received lyophilized PedvaxHIB and those who received placebo, and none was reported to be related to lyophilized PedvaxHIB. Only one serious reaction (tracheitis) was reported as possibly related to lyophilized PedvaxHIB and only one (diarrhea) as possibly related to placebo. Seizures occurred infrequently in both groups (9 occurred in vaccine recipients, 8 of whom also received DTP; 8 occurred in placebo recipients, 7 of whom also received DTP) and were not reported to be related to lyophilized PedvaxHIB.

In early clinical studies involving the administration of 8,086 doses of lyophilized PedvaxHIB alone to 5,027 healthy infants and children 2 months to 71 months of age, lyophilized PedvaxHIB was generally well tolerated. No serious adverse reactions were reported. In a subset of these infants, urticaria was reported in two children, and thrombocytopenia was seen in one child. A cause and effect relationship between these side effects and the vaccination has not been established.

Potential Adverse Reactions

The use of Haemophilus b Polysaccharide Vaccines and another Haemophilus b Conjugate Vaccine has been associated with the following additional adverse effects: early onset Hib disease and Guillain-Barré syndrome. A cause and effect relationship between these side effects and the vaccination was not established.

Post-Marketing Adverse Reactions

The following additional adverse reactions have been reported with the use of the lyophilized and liquid formulations of PedvaxHIB:

Hemic and Lymphatic System

Lymphadenopathy

Hypersensitivity

Rarely, angioedema

Nervous System

Febrile seizures

Skin

Sterile injection site abscess

DOSAGE AND ADMINISTRATION

Liquid PedvaxHIB

FOR INTRAMUSCULAR ADMINISTRATION

DO NOT INJECT INTRAVENOUSLY

If there is an interruption or delay between doses in the primary series, there is no need to repeat the series, but dosing should be continued at the next clinic visit. (See CONTRAINDICATIONS and PRECAUTIONS.)

2 to 14 Months of Age

Infants 2 to 14 months of age should receive a 0.5 mL dose of vaccine ideally beginning at 2 months of age followed by a 0.5 mL dose 2 months later (or as soon as possible thereafter). When the primary two-dose regimen is completed before 12 months of age, a booster dose is required (see below and TABLE 6). Infants born prematurely, regardless of birth weight, should be vaccinated at the same chronological age and according to the same schedule and precautions as full-term infants and children.

15 Months of Age and Older

Children 15 months of age and older previously unvaccinated against Hib disease should receive a single 0.5 mL dose of vaccine.

Booster Dose

In infants completing the primary two-dose regimen before 12 months of age, a booster dose (0.5 mL) should be administered at 12 to 15 months of age, but not earlier than 2 months after the second dose.

Vaccination regimens for Liquid PedvaxHIB by age group are outlined in TABLE 6.

TABLE 6
Vaccination Regimens for Liquid PedvaxHIB
By Age Groups

Age (Months) at First Dose	Primary	Age (Months) at Booster Dose
2–10	2 doses, 2 mo. apart	12–15
11–14	2 doses, 2 mo. apart	—
15–71	1 dose	—

Interchangeability

PedvaxHIB may be interchanged with other licensed Haemophilus b Conjugate Vaccines for the primary and booster doses. (See CLINICAL PHARMACOLOGY.)

Use with Other Vaccines

Results from clinical studies indicate that Liquid PedvaxHIB can be administered concomitantly with DTP, OPV, eIPV (enhanced inactivated poliovirus vaccine), VARIVAX [Varicella Virus Vaccine Live (Oka/Merck)], M-M-R II (Measles, Mumps, and Rubella Virus Vaccine Live) or RECOMBIVAX HB [Hepatitis B Vaccine (Recombinant)]. No impairment of immune response to these individually tested vaccine antigens was demonstrated.

The type, frequency and severity of adverse experiences observed in these studies with PedvaxHIB were similar to those seen with other vaccines when given alone. (See CLINICAL PHARMACOLOGY.)

In addition, a PRP-OMPC-containing product, COMVAX [Haemophilus b Conjugate (Meningococcal Protein Conjugate) and Hepatitis B (Recombinant) Vaccine], was given concomitantly with a booster dose of DTaP [diphtheria, tetanus, acellular pertussis] at approximately 15 months of age, using separate sites and syringes for injectable vaccines. No impairment of immune response to these individually tested vaccine antigens was demonstrated. COMVAX has also been administered concomitantly with the primary series of DTaP to a limited number of infants. PRP antibody responses are satisfactory for COMVAX, but immune responses are currently unavailable for DTaP (see Manufacturer's Product Circular for COMVAX). No serious vaccine-related adverse events were reported.

Parenteral drug products should be inspected visually for extraneous particulate matter and discoloration prior to administration whenever solution and container permit.

Liquid PedvaxHIB is a slightly opaque white suspension. (See DESCRIPTION.)

The vaccine should be used as supplied; no reconstitution is necessary.

Shake well before withdrawal and use. Thorough agitation is necessary to maintain suspension of the vaccine.

Inject 0.5 mL intramuscularly, preferably into the anterolateral thigh or the outer aspect of the upper arm. The buttocks should not be used for active vaccination of infants and children, because of the potential risk of injury to the sciatic nerve.

HOW SUPPLIED

Liquid PedvaxHIB is supplied as follows:

No. 4877—A single-dose vial of liquid vaccine, **NDC** 0006-4877-00.

No. 4897—A box of 10 single-dose vials of liquid vaccine, **NDC** 0006-4897-00.

Storage

Store vaccine at 2–8°C (34–46°F).

DO NOT FREEZE.

9018901 Issued March 1998

PEPCID® Tablets ℞
(Famotidine), U.S.P.
PEPCID® ℞
(Famotidine) for Oral Suspension

DESCRIPTION

The active ingredient in PEPCID* (Famotidine), is a histamine H_2-receptor antagonist. Famotidine is *N*′-(aminosulfonyl) -3- [[[2-[(diaminomethylene)amino] -4- thiazolyl]methyl]thio]propanimidamide. The empirical formula of famotidine is $C_8H_{15}N_7O_2S_3$ and its molecular weight is 337.43. Its structural formula is:

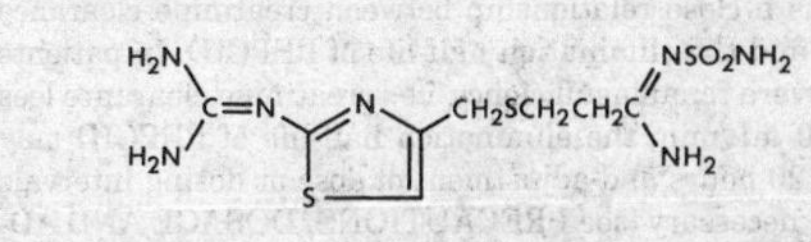

Famotidine is a white to pale yellow crystalline compound that is freely soluble in glacial acetic acid, slightly soluble in methanol, very slightly soluble in water, and practically insoluble in ethanol.

Each tablet for oral administration contains either 20 mg or 40 mg of famotidine and the following inactive ingredients: hydroxypropyl cellulose, hydroxypropyl methylcellulose, iron oxides, magnesium stearate, microcrystalline cellulose, corn starch, talc, titanium dioxide.

Each 5 mL of the oral suspension when prepared as directed contains 40 mg of famotidine and the following inactive ingredients: citric acid, flavors, microcrystalline cellulose and carboxymethylcellulose sodium, sucrose and xanthan gum. Added as preservatives are sodium benzoate 0.1%, sodium methylparaben 0.1%, and sodium propylparaben 0.02%.

*Registered trademark of MERCK & CO., INC.

CLINICAL PHARMACOLOGY

GI Effects

PEPCID is a competitive inhibitor of histamine H_2-receptors. The primary clinically important pharmacologic activity of PEPCID is inhibition of gastric secretion. Both the acid concentration and volume of gastric secretion are suppressed by PEPCID, while changes in pepsin secretion are proportional to volume output.

In normal volunteers and hypersecretors, PEPCID inhibited basal and nocturnal gastric secretion, as well as secretion stimulated by food and pentagastrin. After oral administration, the onset of the antisecretory effect occurred within one hour; the maximum effect was dose-dependent, occurring within one to three hours. Duration of inhibition of secretion by doses of 20 and 40 mg was 10 to 12 hours.

Single evening oral doses of 20 and 40 mg inhibited basal and nocturnal acid secretion in all subjects; mean nocturnal gastric acid secretion was inhibited by 86% and 94%, respectively, for a period of at least 10 hours. The same doses given in the morning suppressed food-stimulated acid secretion in all subjects. The mean suppression was 76% and 84% respectively 3 to 5 hours after administration, and 25% and 30% respectively 8 to 10 hours after administration. In some subjects who received the 20 mg dose, however, the antisecretory effect was dissipated within 6–8 hours. There was no cumulative effect with repeated doses. The nocturnal intragastric pH was raised by evening doses of 20 and 40 mg of PEPCID to mean values of 5.0 and 6.4, respectively. When PEPCID was given after breakfast, the basal daytime interdigestive pH at 3 and 8 hours after 20 or 40 mg of PEPCID was raised to about 5.

PEPCID had little or no effect on fasting or postprandial serum gastrin levels. Gastric emptying and exocrine pancreatic function were not affected by PEPCID.

Other Effects

Systemic effects of PEPCID in the CNS, cardiovascular, respiratory or endocrine systems were not noted in clinical pharmacology studies. Also, no antiandrogenic effects were

Continued on next page

Information on the Merck & Co., Inc. products listed on these pages is the full prescribing information from product circulars in use August 31, 1998. For information, please call 1-800-NSC MERCK [1-800-672-6372].

Pepcid—Cont.

noted. (See ADVERSE REACTIONS.) Serum hormone levels, including prolactin, cortisol, thyroxine (T_4), and testosterone, were not altered after treatment with PEPCID.

Pharmacokinetics

PEPCID is incompletely absorbed. The bioavailability of oral doses is 40–45%. PEPCID Tablets and PEPCID Oral Suspension are bioequivalent. Bioavailability may be slightly increased by food, or slightly decreased by antacids; however, these effects are of no clinical consequence. PEPCID undergoes minimal first-pass metabolism. After oral doses, peak plasma levels occur in 1–3 hours. Plasma levels after multiple doses are similar to those after single doses. Fifteen to 20% of PEPCID in plasma is protein bound. PEPCID has an elimination half-life of 2.5–3.5 hours. PEPCID is eliminated by renal (65–70%) and metabolic (30–35%) routes. Renal clearance is 250–450 mL/min, indicating some tubular excretion. Twenty-five to 30% of an oral dose and 65–70% of an intravenous dose are recovered in the urine as unchanged compound. The only metabolite identified in man is the S-oxide.

There is a close relationship between creatinine clearance values and the elimination half-life of PEPCID. In patients with severe renal insufficiency, i.e., creatinine clearance less than 10 mL/min, the elimination half-life of PEPCID may exceed 20 hours and adjustment of dose or dosing intervals may be necessary (see PRECAUTIONS, DOSAGE AND ADMINISTRATION).

In elderly patients, there are no clinically significant age-related changes in the pharmacokinetics of PEPCID.

Clinical Studies

Duodenal Ulcer

In a U.S. multicenter, double-blind study in outpatients with endoscopically confirmed duodenal ulcer, orally administered PEPCID was compared to placebo. As shown in Table 1, 70% of patients treated with PEPCID 40 mg h.s. were healed by week 4.

Table 1
Outpatients with Endoscopically
Confirmed Healed Duodenal Ulcers

	PEPCID 40 mg h.s. (N=89)	PEPCID 20 mg b.i.d. (N=84)	Placebo h.s. (N=97)
Week 2	*32%	*38%	17%
Week 4	*70%	*67%	31%

* Statistically significantly different than placebo (p< 0.001)

Patients not healed by week 4 were continued in the study. By week 8, 83% of patients treated with PEPCID had healed versus 45% of patients treated with placebo. The incidence of ulcer healing with PEPCID was significantly higher than with placebo at each time point based on proportion of endoscopically confirmed healed ulcers.

In this study, time to relief of daytime and nocturnal pain was significantly shorter for patients receiving PEPCID than for patients receiving placebo; patients receiving PEPCID also took less antacid than the patients receiving placebo.

Long-Term Maintenance

Treatment of Duodenal Ulcers

PEPCID, 20 mg p.o. h.s. was compared to placebo h.s. as maintenance therapy in two double-blind, multicenter studies of patients with endoscopically confirmed healed duodenal ulcers. In the U.S. study the observed ulcer incidence within 12 months in patients treated with placebo was 2.4 times greater than in the patients treated with PEPCID. The 89 patients treated with PEPCID had a cumulative observed ulcer incidence of 23.4% compared to an observed ulcer incidence of 56.6% in the 89 patients receiving placebo (p<0.01). These results were confirmed in an international study where the cumulative observed ulcer incidence within 12 months in the 307 patients treated with PEPCID was 35.7%, compared to an incidence of 75.5% in the 325 patients treated with placebo (p<0.01).

Gastric Ulcer

In both a U.S. and an international multicenter, double-blind study in patients with endoscopically confirmed active benign gastric ulcer, orally administered PEPCID, 40 mg h.s., was compared to placebo h.s. Antacids were permitted during the studies, but consumption was not significantly different between the PEPCID and placebo groups. As shown in Table 2, the incidence of ulcer healing (dropouts counted as unhealed) with PEPCID was statistically significantly better than placebo at weeks 6 and 8 in the U.S. study, and at weeks 4, 6 and 8 in the international study, based on the number of ulcers that healed, confirmed by endoscopy.

Table 2
Patients with Endoscopically
Confirmed Healed Gastric Ulcers

	U.S. Study		International Study	
	PEPCID 40 mg h.s. (N=74)	Placebo h.s. (N=75)	PEPCID 40 mg h.s. (N=149)	Placebo h.s. (N=145)
Week 4	45%	39%	**47%	31%
Week 6	**66%	44%	**65%	46%
Week 8	*78%	64%	**80%	54%

*,** Statistically significantly better than placebo (p≤0.05, p≤0.01 respectively)

Time to complete relief of daytime and nighttime pain was statistically significantly shorter for patients receiving PEPCID than for patients receiving placebo; however, in neither study was there a statistically significant difference in the proportion of patients whose pain was relieved by the end of the study (week 8).

Gastroesophageal Reflux Disease (GERD)

Orally administered PEPCID was compared to placebo in a U.S. study that enrolled patients with symptoms of GERD and without endoscopic evidence of erosion or ulceration of the esophagus. PEPCID 20 mg b.i.d. was statistically significantly superior to 40 mg h.s. and to placebo in providing a successful symptomatic outcome, defined as moderate or excellent improvement of symptoms (Table 3).

Table 3
% Successful Symptomatic Outcome

	PEPCID 20 mg b.i.d. (N=154)	PEPCID 40 mg h.s. (N=149)	Placebo (N=73)
Week 6	82**	69	62

** p≤0.01) vs Placebo

By two weeks of treatment, symptomatic success was observed in a greater percentage of patients taking PEPCID 20 mg b.i.d. compared to placebo (p≤0.01).

Symptomatic improvement and healing of endoscopically verified erosion and ulceration were studied in two additional trials. Healing was defined as complete resolution of all erosions or ulcerations visible with endoscopy. The U.S. study comparing PEPCID 40 mg p.o. b.i.d. to placebo and PEPCID 20 mg p.o. b.i.d. showed a significantly greater percentage of healing for PEPCID 40 mg b.i.d. at weeks 6 and 12 (Table 4).

Table 4
% Endoscopic Healing—U.S. Study

	PEPCID 40 mg b.i.d. (N=127)	PEPCID 20 mg b.i.d. (N=125)	Placebo (N=66)
Week 6	48**,++	32	18
Week 12	69**,+	54**	29

** p≤0.01 vs Placebo
+ p≤0.05 vs PEPCID 20 mg b.i.d.
++ p≤0.01 vs PEPCID 20 mg b.i.d.

As compared to placebo, patients who received PEPCID had faster relief of daytime and nighttime heartburn and a greater percentage of patients experienced complete relief of nighttime heartburn. These differences were statistically significant.

In the international study, when PEPCID 40 mg p.o. b.i.d. was compared to ranitidine 150 mg p.o. b.i.d., a statistically significantly greater percentage of healing was observed with PEPCID 40 mg b.i.d. at week 12 (Table 5). There was, however, no significant difference among treatments in symptom relief.

Table 5
% Endoscopic Healing—International Study

	PEPCID 40 mg b.i.d. (N=175)	PEPCID 20 mg b.i.d. (N=93)	Ranitidine 150 mg b.i.d. (N=172)
Week 6	48	52	42
Week 12	71*	68	60

* p≤0.05 vs Ranitidine 150 mg b.i.d.

Pathological Hypersecretory Conditions (e.g., Zollinger-Ellison Syndrome, Multiple Endocrine Adenomas)

In studies of patients with pathological hypersecretory conditions such as Zollinger-Ellison Syndrome with or without multiple endocrine adenomas, PEPCID significantly inhibited gastric acid secretion and controlled associated symptoms. Orally administered doses from 20 to 160 mg q 6 h maintained basal acid secretion below 10 mEq/hr; initial doses were titrated to the individual patient need and subsequent adjustments were necessary with time in some patients. PEPCID was well tolerated at these high dose levels for prolonged periods (greater than 12 months) in eight patients, and there were no cases reported of gynecomastia, increased prolactin levels, or impotence which were considered to be due to the drug.

INDICATIONS AND USAGE

PEPCID is indicated in:

1. *Short term treatment of active duodenal ulcer.* Most patients heal within 4 weeks; there is rarely reason to use PEPCID at full dosage for longer than 6 to 8 weeks. Studies have not assessed the safety of famotidine in uncomplicated active duodenal ulcer for periods of more than eight weeks.
2. *Maintenance therapy for duodenal ulcer patients at reduced dosage after healing of an active ulcer.* Controlled studies have not extended beyond one year.
3. *Short term treatment of active benign gastric ulcer.* Most patients heal within 6 weeks. Studies have not assessed the safety or efficacy of famotidine in uncomplicated active benign gastric ulcer for periods of more than 8 weeks.
4. *Short term treatment of gastroesophageal reflux disease (GERD).* PEPCID is indicated for short term treatment of patients with symptoms of GERD (see CLINICAL PHARMACOLOGY, *Clinical Studies*).
   PEPCID is also indicated for the short term treatment of esophagitis due to GERD including erosive or ulcerative disease diagnosed by endoscopy (see CLINICAL PHARMACOLOGY, *Clinical Studies*).
5. *Treatment of pathological hypersecretory conditions (e.g., Zollinger-Ellison Syndrome, multiple endocrine adenomas).*

CONTRAINDICATIONS

Hypersensitivity to any component of these products.

PRECAUTIONS

General

Symptomatic response to therapy with PEPCID does not preclude the presence of gastric malignancy.

Patients with Severe Renal Insufficiency

Longer intervals between doses or lower doses may need to be used in patients with severe renal insufficiency (creatinine clearance <10 mL/min) to adjust for the longer elimination half-life of famotidine. (See CLINICAL PHARMACOLOGY and DOSAGE AND ADMINISTRATION.) However, currently, no drug-related toxicity has been found with high plasma concentrations of famotidine.

Information for Patients

The patient should be instructed to shake the oral suspension vigorously for 5–10 seconds prior to each use. Unused constituted oral suspension should be discarded after 30 days.

Drug Interactions

No drug interactions have been identified. Studies with famotidine in man, in animal models, and *in vitro* have shown no significant interference with the disposition of compounds metabolized by the hepatic microsomal enzymes, e.g., cytochrome P450 system. Compounds tested in man include warfarin, theophylline, phenytoin, diazepam, aminopyrine and antipyrine. Indocyanine green as an index of hepatic drug extraction has been tested and no significant effects have been found.

Carcinogenesis, Mutagenesis, Impairment of Fertility

In a 106 week study in rats and a 92 week study in mice given oral doses of up to 2000 mg/kg/day (approximately 2500 times the recommended human dose for active duodenal ulcer), there was no evidence of carcinogenic potential for PEPCID.

Famotidine was negative in the microbial mutagen test (Ames test) using *Salmonella typhimurium* and *Escherichia coli* with or without rat liver enzyme activation at concentrations up to 10,000 mcg/plate. In *in vivo* studies in mice, with a micronucleus test and a chromosomal aberration test, no evidence of a mutagenic effect was observed.

In studies with rats given oral doses of up to 2000 mg/kg/day or intravenous doses of up to 200 mg/kg/day, fertility and reproductive performance were not affected.

Pregnancy

Pregnancy Category B

Reproductive studies have been performed in rats and rabbits at oral doses of up to 2000 and 500 mg/kg/day respectively and in both species at I.V. doses of up to 200 mg/kg/day, and have revealed no significant evidence of impaired fertility or harm to the fetus due to PEPCID. While no direct fetotoxic effects have been observed, sporadic abortions occurring only in mothers displaying marked decreased food intake were seen in some rabbits at oral doses of 200 mg/kg/day (250 times the usual human dose) or higher. There are, however, no adequate or well-controlled studies in pregnant women. Because animal reproductive studies are not always predictive of human response, this drug should be used during pregnancy only if clearly needed.

Nursing Mothers
Studies performed in lactating rats have shown that famotidine is secreted into breast milk. Transient growth depression was observed in young rats suckling from mothers treated with maternotoxic doses of at least 600 times the usual human dose. Famotidine is detectable in human milk. Because of the potential for serious adverse reactions in nursing infants from PEPCID, a decision should be made whether to discontinue nursing or discontinue the drug, taking into account the importance of the drug to the mother.

Pediatric Use
Safety and effectiveness in children have not been established.

Use in Elderly Patients
No dosage adjustment is required based on age (see CLINICAL PHARMACOLOGY, *Pharmacokinetics*). Dosage adjustment in the case of severe renal impairment may be necessary.

ADVERSE REACTIONS

The adverse reactions listed below have been reported during domestic and international clinical trials in approximately 2500 patients. In those controlled clinical trials in which PEPCID Tablets were compared to placebo, the incidence of adverse experiences in the group which received PEPCID Tablets, 40 mg at bedtime, was similar to that in the placebo group.

The following adverse reactions have been reported to occur in more than 1% of patients on therapy with PEPCID in controlled clinical trials, and may be causally related to the drug: headache (4.7%), dizziness (1.3%), constipation (1.2%) and diarrhea (1.7%).

The following other adverse reactions have been reported infrequently in clinical trials or since the drug was marketed. The relationship to therapy with PEPCID has been unclear in many cases. Within each category the adverse reactions are listed in order of decreasing severity:
Body as a Whole: fever, asthenia, fatigue
Cardiovascular: arrhythmia, AV block, palpitation
Gastrointestinal: cholestatic jaundice, liver enzyme abnormalities, vomiting, nausea, abdominal discomfort, anorexia, dry mouth
Hematologic: rare cases of agranulocytosis, pancytopenia, leukopenia, thrombocytopenia
Hypersensitivity: anaphylaxis, angioedema, orbital or facial edema, urticaria, rash, conjunctival injection
Musculoskeletal: musculoskeletal pain including muscle cramps, arthralgia
Nervous System/Psychiatric: grand mal seizure; psychic disturbances, which were reversible in cases for which follow-up was obtained, including hallucinations, confusion, agitation, depression, anxiety, decreased libido; paresthesia; insomnia; somnolence
Respiratory: bronchospasm
Skin: toxic epidermal necrolysis (very rare), alopecia, acne, pruritus, dry skin, flushing
Special Senses: tinnitus, taste disorder
Other: rare cases of impotence and rare cases of gynecomastia have been reported; however, in controlled clinical trials, the incidences were not greater than those seen with placebo.

The adverse reactions reported for PEPCID Tablets may also occur with PEPCID for Oral Suspension.

OVERDOSAGE

There is no experience to date with deliberate overdosage. Oral doses of up to 640 mg/day have been given to patients with pathological hypersecretory conditions with no serious adverse effects. In the event of overdosage, treatment should be symptomatic and supportive. Unabsorbed material should be removed from the gastrointestinal tract, the patient should be monitored, and supportive therapy should be employed.

The oral LD_{50} of famotidine in male and female rats and mice was greater than 3000 mg/kg and the minimum lethal acute oral dose in dogs exceeded 2000 mg/kg. Famotidine did not produce overt effects at high oral doses in mice, rats, cats and dogs, but induced significant anorexia and growth depression in rabbits starting with 200 mg/kg/day orally. The intravenous LD_{50} of famotidine for mice and rats ranged from 254–563 mg/kg and the minimum lethal single I.V. dose in dogs was approximately 300 mg/kg. Signs of acute intoxication in I.V. treated dogs were emesis, restlessness, pallor of mucous membranes or redness of mouth and ears, hypotension, tachycardia and collapse.

DOSAGE AND ADMINISTRATION

Duodenal Ulcer
Acute Therapy: The recommended adult oral dosage for active duodenal ulcer is 40 mg once a day at bedtime. Most patients heal within 4 weeks; there is rarely reason to use PEPCID at full dosage for longer than 6 to 8 weeks. A regimen of 20 mg b.i.d. is also effective.

Maintenance Therapy: The recommended oral dose is 20 mg once a day at bedtime.
Benign Gastric Ulcer
Acute Therapy: The recommended adult oral dosage for active benign gastric ulcer is 40 mg once a day at bedtime.
Gastroesophageal Reflux Disease (GERD)
The recommended oral dosage for treatment of patients with symptoms of GERD is 20 mg b.i.d. for up to 6 weeks. The recommended oral dosage for the treatment of patients with esophagitis including erosions and ulcerations and accompanying symptoms due to GERD is 20 or 40 mg b.i.d. for up to 12 weeks (see CLINICAL PHARMACOLOGY, *Clinical Studies*).
Pathological Hypersecretory Conditions (e.g., Zollinger-Ellison Syndrome, Multiple Endocrine Adenomas)
The dosage of PEPCID in patients with pathological hypersecretory conditions varies with the individual patient. The recommended adult oral starting dose for pathological hypersecretory conditions is 20 mg q 6 h. In some patients, a higher starting dose may be required. Doses should be adjusted to individual patient needs and should continue as long as clinically indicated. Doses up to 160 mg q 6 h have been administered to some patients with severe Zollinger-Ellison Syndrome.
Oral Suspension
PEPCID Oral Suspension may be substituted for PEPCID Tablets in any of the above indications. Each five mL contains 40 mg of famotidine after constitution of the powder with 46 mL of Purified Water as directed.
Directions for Preparing PEPCID Oral Suspension
Prepare suspension at time of dispensing. Slowly add 46 mL of Purified Water. Shake vigorously for 5–10 seconds immediately after adding the water and immediately before use.
Stability of PEPCID Oral Suspension
Unused constituted oral suspension should be discarded after 30 days.
Concomitant Use of Antacids
Antacids may be given concomitantly if needed.
Dosage Adjustment for Patients with Severe Renal Insufficiency
In patients with severe renal insufficiency, i.e., with a creatinine clearance less than 10 mL/min, the elimination half-life of PEPCID may exceed 20 hours, reaching approximately 24 hours in anuric patients. Although no relationship of adverse effects to high plasma levels has been established, to avoid excess accumulation of the drug, the dose of PEPCID may be reduced to 20 mg h.s. or the dosing interval may be prolonged to 36–48 hours as indicated by the patient's clinical response.

HOW SUPPLIED

No. 3535—PEPCID Tablets, 20 mg, are beige colored, U-shaped, film-coated tablets coded MSD 963 on one side and PEPCID on the other. They are supplied as follows:
NDC 0006-0963-31 unit of use bottles of 30
(6505-01-260-0902, 20 mg 30's)
NDC 0006-0963-94 unit of use bottles of 90
NDC 0006-0963-58 unit of use bottles of 100
NDC 0006-0963-28 unit dose package of 100
NDC 0006-0963-82 bottles of 1,000
NDC 0006-0963-87 bottles of 10,000
NDC 0006-0963-72 carton of 25
UNIBLISTER™ cards of 31 tablets each.
Shown in Product Identification Guide, page 323
No. 3536—PEPCID Tablets, 40 mg, are light brownish-orange, U-shaped, film-coated tablets coded MSD 964 on one side and PEPCID on the other. They are supplied as follows:
NDC 0006-0964-31 unit of use bottles of 30
(6505-01-257-3164, 40 mg 30's)
NDC 0006-0964-94 unit of use bottles of 90
NDC 0006-0964-58 unit of use bottles of 100
NDC 0006-0964-28 unit dose package of 100
(6505-01-318-0464, 40 mg individually sealed 100's)
NDC 0006-0964-82 bottles of 1,000
NDC 0006-0964-87 bottles of 10,000
NDC 0006-0964-72 carton of 25
UNIBLISTER™ cards of 31 tablets each.
Shown in Product Identification Guide, page 323
No. 3538—Oral Suspension PEPCID is a white to off-white powder containing 400 mg of famotidine for constitution. When constituted as directed, PEPCID Oral Suspension is a smooth, mobile, off-white, homogeneous suspension with a cherry-banana-mint flavor, containing 40 mg of famotidine per 5 mL.
NDC 0006-3538-92, bottles containing 400 mg famotidine.
Storage
Avoid storage of PEPCID Tablets at temperatures above 40°C (104°F).
Avoid storage of the powder for oral suspension at temperatures above 40°C (104°F). After constitution store the suspension below 30°C (86°F). Do not freeze. Discard unused suspension after 30 days.
7825028 Issued May 1996
COPYRIGHT © MERCK & CO., INC., 1986, 1988, 1991
All rights reserved

PEPCID® Injection Premixed ℞
(Famotidine)
PEPCID® Injection ℞
(Famotidine)

DESCRIPTION

The active ingredient in PEPCID* (Famotidine) Injection Premixed and PEPCID (famotidine) Injection is a histamine H_2-receptor antagonist. Famotidine is N'-(aminosulfonyl) - 3- [[[2-[(diaminomethylene)amino]-4-thiazolyl]methyl]thio]-propanimidamide. The empirical formula of famotidine is $C_8H_{15}N_7O_2S_3$ and its molecular weight is 337.43. Its structural formula is:

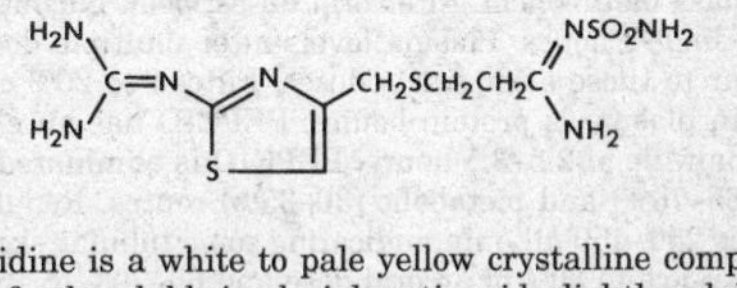

Famotidine is a white to pale yellow crystalline compound that is freely soluble in glacial acetic acid, slightly soluble in methanol, very slightly soluble in water, and practically insoluble in ethanol.
PEPCID Injection Premixed is supplied as a sterile solution, for intravenous use only, in plastic single dose containers. Each 50 mL of the premixed, iso-osmotic intravenous injection contains 20 mg famotidine, USP, and the following inactive ingredients: L-aspartic acid 6.8 mg, sodium chloride, USP, 450 mg, and Water for Injection. The pH ranges from 5.7 to 6.4 and may have been adjusted with additional L-aspartic acid or with sodium hydroxide.
The plastic container is fabricated from a specially designed multi-layer plastic (PL 2501). Solutions are in contact with the polyethylene layer of the container and can leach out certain chemical components of the plastic in very small amounts within the expiration period. The suitability and safety of the plastic have been confirmed in tests in animals according to the USP biological tests for plastic containers, as well as by tissue culture toxicity studies.
PEPCID (famotidine) Injection is supplied as a sterile concentrated solution for intravenous injection. Each mL of the solution contains 10 mg of famotidine and the following inactive ingredients: L-aspartic acid 4 mg, mannitol 20 mg, and Water for Injection q.s. 1 mL. The multidose injection also contains benzyl alcohol 0.9% added as preservative.

---

*Registered trademark of MERCK & CO., INC.

CLINICAL PHARMACOLOGY

GI Effects
PEPCID is a competitive inhibitor of histamine H_2-receptors. The primary clinically important pharmacologic activity of PEPCID is inhibition of gastric secretion. Both the acid concentration and volume of gastric secretion are suppressed by PEPCID, while changes in pepsin secretion are proportional to volume output.
In normal volunteers and hypersecretors, PEPCID inhibited basal and nocturnal gastric secretion, as well as secretion stimulated by food and pentagastrin. After oral administration, the onset of the antisecretory effect occurred within one hour; the maximum effect was dose-dependent, occurring within one to three hours. Duration of inhibition of secretion by doses of 20 and 40 mg was 10 to 12 hours. After intravenous administration, the maximum effect was achieved within 30 minutes. Single intravenous doses of 10 and 20 mg inhibited nocturnal secretion for a period of 10 to 12 hours. The 20 mg dose was associated with the longest duration of action in most subjects.
Single evening oral doses of 20 and 40 mg inhibited basal and nocturnal acid secretion in all subjects; mean nocturnal gastric acid secretion was inhibited by 86% and 94%, respectively, for a period of at least 10 hours. The same doses given in the morning suppressed food-stimulated acid secretion in all subjects. The mean suppression was 76% and 84% respectively, 3 to 5 hours after administration, and 25% and 30%, respectively, 8 to 10 hours after administration. In some subjects who received the 20 mg dose, however, the antisecretory effect was dissipated within 6–8 hours. There was no cumulative effect with repeated doses. The nocturnal intragastric pH was raised by evening doses of 20 and 40 mg of PEPCID to mean values of 5.0 and 6.4, respectively. When PEPCID was given after breakfast, the basal daytime interdigestive pH at 3 and 8 hours after 20 or 40 mg of PEPCID was raised to about 5.

Continued on next page

Information on the Merck & Co., Inc. products listed on these pages is the full prescribing information from product circulars in use August 31, 1998. For information, please call 1-800-NSC MERCK [1-800-672-6372].

Pepcid Injection—Cont.

PEPCID had little or no effect on fasting or postprandial serum gastrin levels. Gastric emptying and exocrine pancreatic function were not affected by PEPCID.

Other Effects

Systemic effects of PEPCID in the CNS, cardiovascular, respiratory or endocrine systems were not noted in clinical pharmacology studies. Also, no antiandrogenic effects were noted. (See ADVERSE REACTIONS.) Serum hormone levels, including prolactin, cortisol, thyroxine (T_4), and testosterone, were not altered after treatment with PEPCID.

Pharmacokinetics

Orally administered PEPCID is incompletely absorbed and its bioavailability is 40–45%. PEPCID undergoes minimal first-pass metabolism. After oral doses, peak plasma levels occur in 1–3 hours. Plasma levels after multiple doses are similar to those after single doses. Fifteen to 20% of PEPCID in plasma is protein bound. PEPCID has an elimination half-life of 2.5–3.5 hours. PEPCID is eliminated by renal (65–70%) and metabolic (30–35%) routes. Renal clearance is 250–450 mL/min, indicating some tubular excretion. Twenty-five to 30% of an oral dose and 65–70% of an intravenous dose are recovered in the urine as unchanged compound. The only metabolite identified in man is the S-oxide. There is a close relationship between creatinine clearance values and the elimination half-life of PEPCID. In patients with severe renal insufficiency, i.e., creatinine clearance less than 10 mL/min, the elimination half-life of PEPCID may exceed 20 hours and adjustment of dose or dosing intervals may be necessary (see PRECAUTIONS, DOSAGE AND ADMINISTRATION).

In elderly patients, there are no clinically significant age-related changes in the pharmacokinetics of PEPCID.

Clinical Studies

The majority of clinical study experience involved oral administration of PEPCID Tablets, and is provided herein for reference.

Duodenal Ulcer

In a U.S. multicenter, double-blind study in outpatients with endoscopically confirmed duodenal ulcer, orally administered PEPCID was compared to placebo. As shown in Table 1, 70% of patients treated with PEPCID 40 mg h.s. were healed by week 4.

Table 1
Outpatients with Endoscopically Confirmed Healed Duodenal Ulcers

	PEPCID 40 mg h.s. (N=89)	PEPCID 20 mg b.i.d. (N=84)	Placebo h.s. (N=97)
Week 2	*32%	*38%	17%
Week 4	*70%	*67%	31%

* Statistically significantly different than placebo (p< 0.001)

Patients not healed by week 4 were continued in the study. By week 8, 83% of patients treated with PEPCID had healed versus 45% of patients treated with placebo. The incidence of ulcer healing with PEPCID was significantly higher than with placebo at each time point based on proportion of endoscopically confirmed healed ulcers.

In this study, time to relief of daytime and nocturnal pain was significantly shorter for patients receiving PEPCID than for patients receiving placebo; patients receiving PEPCID also took less antacid than the patients receiving placebo.

Long-Term Maintenance
Treatment of Duodenal Ulcers

PEPCID, 20 mg p.o. h.s. was compared to placebo h.s. as maintenance therapy in two double-blind, multicenter studies of patients with endoscopically confirmed healed duodenal ulcers. In the U.S. study the observed ulcer incidence within 12 months in patients treated with placebo was 2.4 times greater than in the patients treated with PEPCID. The 89 patients treated with PEPCID had a cumulative observed ulcer incidence of 23.4% compared to an observed ulcer incidence of 56.6% in the 89 patients receiving placebo (p<0.01). These results were confirmed in an international study where the cumulative observed ulcer incidence within 12 months in the 307 patients treated with PEPCID was 35.7%, compared to an incidence of 75.5% in the 325 patients treated with placebo (p<0.01).

Gastric Ulcer

In both a U.S. and an international multicenter, double-blind study in patients with endoscopically confirmed active benign gastric ulcer, orally administered PEPCID, 40 mg h.s., was compared to placebo h.s. Antacids were permitted during the studies, but consumption was not significantly different between the PEPCID and placebo groups. As shown in Table 2, the incidence of ulcer healing (dropouts counted as unhealed) with PEPCID was statistically significantly better than placebo at weeks 6 and 8 in the U.S. study, and at weeks 4, 6 and 8 in the international study, based on the number of ulcers that healed, confirmed by endoscopy.

Table 2
Patients with Endoscopically Confirmed Healed Gastric Ulcers

	U.S. Study		International Study	
	PEPCID 40 mg h.s. (N=74)	Placebo h.s. (N=75)	PEPCID 40 mg h.s. (N=149)	Placebo h.s. (N=145)
Week 4	45%	39%	**47%	31%
Week 6	**66%	44%	**65%	46%
Week 8	*78%	64%	**80%	54%

*,** Statistically significantly better than placebo (p≤0.05, p≤0.01 respectively)

Time to complete relief of daytime and nighttime pain was statistically significantly shorter for patients receiving PEPCID than for patients receiving placebo; however, in neither study was there a statistically significant difference in the proportion of patients whose pain was relieved by the end of the study (week 8).

Gastroesophageal Reflux Disease (GERD)

Orally administered PEPCID was compared to placebo in a U.S. study that enrolled patients with symptoms of GERD and without endoscopic evidence of erosion or ulceration of the esophagus. PEPCID 20 mg b.i.d. was statistically significantly superior to 40 mg h.s. and to placebo in providing a successful symptomatic outcome, defined as moderate or excellent improvement of symptoms (Table 3).

Table 3
% Successful Symptomatic Outcome

	PEPCID 20 mg b.i.d. (N=154)	PEPCID 40 mg h.s. (N=49)	Placebo (N=73)
Week 6	82**	69	62

** p ≤0.01 vs Placebo

By two weeks of treatment, symptomatic success was observed in a greater percentage of patients taking PEPCID 20 mg b.i.d. compared to placebo (p ≤0.01).

Symptomatic improvement and healing of endoscopically verified erosion and ulceration were studied in two additional trials. Healing was defined as complete resolution of all erosions or ulcerations visible with endoscopy. The U.S. study comparing PEPCID 40 mg p.o. b.i.d. to placebo and PEPCID 20 mg p.o. b.i.d., showed a significantly greater percentage of healing for PEPCID 40 mg b.i.d. at weeks 6 and 12 (Table 4).

Table 4
% Endoscopic Healing—U.S. Study

	PEPCID 40 mg b.i.d. (N=127)	PEPCID 20 mg b.i.d. (N=125)	Placebo (N=66)
Week 6	48**,++	32	18
Week 12	69**,+	54**	29

** p ≤0.01 vs Placebo
+ p ≤0.05 vs PEPCID 20 mg b.i.d.
++ p ≤0.01 vs PEPCID 20 mg b.i.d.

As compared to placebo, patients who received PEPCID had faster relief of daytime and nighttime heartburn and a greater percentage of patients experienced complete relief of nighttime heartburn. These differences were statistically significant.

In the international study, when PEPCID 40 mg p.o. b.i.d. was compared to ranitidine 150 mg p.o. b.i.d., a statistically significantly greater percentage of healing was observed with PEPCID 40 mg b.i.d. at week 12 (Table 5). There was, however, no significant difference among treatments in symptom relief.

Table 5
% Endoscopic Healing—International Study

	PEPCID 40 mg b.i.d. (N=175)	PEPCID 20 mg b.i.d. (N=93)	Ranitidine 150 mg b.i.d. (N=172)
Week 6	48	52	42
Week 12	71*	68	60

* p ≤0.05 vs Ranitidine 150 mg b.i.d.

Pathological Hypersecretory Conditions
(e.g., Zollinger-Ellison Syndrome,
Multiple Endocrine Adenomas)

In studies of patients with pathological hypersecretory conditions such as Zollinger-Ellison Syndrome with or without multiple endocrine adenomas, PEPCID significantly inhibited gastric acid secretion and controlled associated symptoms. Orally administered doses from 20 to 160 mg q 6 h maintained basal acid secretion below 10 mEq/hr; initial doses were titrated to the individual patient need and subsequent adjustments were necessary with time in some patients. PEPCID was well tolerated at these high dose levels for prolonged periods (greater than 12 months) in eight patients, and there were no cases reported of gynecomastia, increased prolactin levels, or impotence which were considered to be due to the drug.

INDICATIONS AND USAGE

PEPCID Injection Premixed, supplied as a premixed solution in plastic containers (PL 2501 Plastic), and PEPCID Injection, supplied as a concentrated solution for intravenous injection, are intended for intravenous use only. PEPCID Injection Premixed and PEPCID Injection are indicated in some hospitalized patients with pathological hypersecretory conditions or intractable ulcers, or as an alternative to the oral dosage forms for short term use in patients who are unable to take oral medication for the following conditions:

1. *Short term treatment of active duodenal ulcer.* Most patients heal within 4 weeks; there is rarely reason to use PEPCID at full dosage for longer than 6 to 8 weeks. Studies have not assessed the safety of famotidine in uncomplicated active duodenal ulcer for periods of more than eight weeks.
2. *Maintenance therapy for duodenal ulcer patients at reduced dosage after healing of an active ulcer.* Controlled studies have not extended beyond one year.
3. *Short term treatment of active benign gastric ulcer.* Most patients heal within 6 weeks. Studies have not assessed the safety or efficacy of famotidine in uncomplicated active benign gastric ulcer for periods of more than 8 weeks.
4. *Short term treatment of gastroesophageal reflux disease (GERD).* PEPCID is indicated for short term treatment of patients with symptoms of GERD (see CLINICAL PHARMACOLOGY, *Clinical Studies*).
PEPCID is also indicated for the short term treatment of esophagitis due to GERD including erosive or ulcerative disease diagnosed by endoscopy (see CLINICAL PHARMACOLOGY, *Clinical Studies*).
5. *Treatment of pathological hypersecretory conditions (e.g., Zollinger-Ellison Syndrome, multiple endocrine adenomas).*

CONTRAINDICATIONS

Hypersensitivity to any component of these products.

PRECAUTIONS

General

Symptomatic response to therapy with PEPCID does not preclude the presence of gastric malignancy.

Patients with Severe Renal Insufficiency

Longer intervals between doses or lower doses may need to be used in patients with severe renal insufficiency (creatinine clearance <10 mL/min) to adjust for the longer elimination half-life of famotidine. (See CLINICAL PHARMACOLOGY, DOSAGE AND ADMINISTRATION.) However, currently, no drug-related toxicity has been found with high plasma concentrations of famotidine.

Drug Interactions

No drug interactions have been identified. Studies with famotidine in man, in animal models, and *in vitro* have shown no significant interference with the disposition of compounds metabolized by the hepatic microsomal enzymes, e.g., cytochrome P450 system. Compounds tested in man include warfarin, theophylline, phenytoin, diazepam, aminopyrine and antipyrine. Indocyanine green as an index of hepatic drug extraction has been tested and no significant effects have been found.

Carcinogenesis, Mutagenesis,
Impairment of Fertility

In a 106 week study in rats and a 92 week study in mice given oral doses of up to 2000 mg/kg/day (approximately 2500 times the recommended human dose for active duodenal ulcer), there was no evidence of carcinogenic potential for PEPCID.

Famotidine was negative in the microbial mutagen test (Ames test) using *Salmonella typhimurium* and *Escherichia coli* with or without rat liver enzyme activation at concentrations up to 10,000 mcg/plate. In *in vivo* studies in mice, with a micronucleus test and a chromosomal aberration test, no evidence of a mutagenic effect was observed.

In studies with rats given oral doses of up to 2000 mg/kg/day or intravenous doses of up to 200 mg/kg/day fertility and reproductive performance were not affected.

Pregnancy
Pregnancy Category B

Reproductive studies have been performed in rats and rabbits at oral doses of up to 2000 and 500 mg/kg/day, respectively, and in both species at I.V. doses of up to 200 mg/kg/day, and have revealed no significant evidence of impaired fertility or harm to the fetus due to PEPCID. While no di-

rect fetotoxic effects have been observed, sporadic abortions occurring only in mothers displaying marked decreased food intake were seen in some rabbits at oral doses of 200 mg/kg/day (250 times the usual human dose) or higher. There are, however, no adequate or well-controlled studies in pregnant women. Because animal reproductive studies are not always predictive of human response, this drug should be used during pregnancy only if clearly needed.

Nursing Mothers

Studies performed in lactating rats have shown that famotidine is secreted into breast milk. Transient growth depression was observed in young rats suckling from mothers treated with maternotoxic doses of at least 600 times the usual human dose. Famotidine is detectable in human milk. Because of the potential for serious adverse reactions in nursing infants from PEPCID, a decision should be made whether to discontinue nursing or discontinue the drug, taking into account the importance of the drug to the mother.

Pediatric Use

Safety and effectiveness in children have not been established.

Use in Elderly Patients

No dosage adjustment is required based on age (see CLINICAL PHARMACOLOGY, *Pharmacokinetics*). Dosage adjustment in the case of severe renal impairment may be necessary.

ADVERSE REACTIONS

The adverse reactions listed below have been reported during domestic and international clinical trials in approximately 2500 patients. In those controlled clinical trials in which PEPCID Tablets were compared to placebo, the incidence of adverse experiences in the group which received PEPCID Tablets, 40 mg at bedtime, was similar to that in the placebo group.

The following adverse reactions have been reported to occur in more than 1% of patients on therapy with PEPCID in controlled clinical trials, and may be causally related to the drug: headache (4.7%), dizziness (1.3%), constipation (1.2%) and diarrhea (1.7%).

The following other adverse reactions have been reported infrequently in clinical trials or since the drug was marketed. The relationship to therapy with PEPCID has been unclear in many cases. Within each category the adverse reactions are listed in order of decreasing severity:

Body as a Whole: fever, asthenia, fatigue

Cardiovascular: arrhythmia, AV block, palpitation

Gastrointestinal: cholestatic jaundice, liver enzyme abnormalities, vomiting, nausea, abdominal discomfort, anorexia, dry mouth

Hematologic: rare cases of agranulocytosis, pancytopenia, leukopenia, thrombocytopenia

Hypersensitivity: anaphylaxis, angioedema, orbital or facial edema, urticaria, rash, conjunctival injection

Musculoskeletal: musculoskeletal pain including muscle cramps, arthralgia

Nervous System/Psychiatric: grand mal seizure; psychic disturbances, which were reversible in cases for which follow-up was obtained, including hallucinations, confusion, agitation, depression, anxiety, decreased libido; paresthesia; insomnia; somnolence

Respiratory: bronchospasm

Skin: toxic epidermal necrolysis (very rare), alopecia, acne, pruritus, dry skin, flushing

Special Senses: tinnitus, taste disorder

Other: rare cases of impotence and rare cases of gynecomastia have been reported; however, in controlled clinical trials, the incidences were not greater than those seen with placebo.

The adverse reactions reported for PEPCID Tablets may also occur with PEPCID for Oral Suspension, PEPCID Injection Premixed or PEPCID Injection. In addition, transient irritation at the injection site has been observed with PEPCID Injection.

OVERDOSAGE

There is no experience to date with deliberate overdosage. Oral doses of up to 640 mg/day have been given to patients with pathological hypersecretory conditions with no serious adverse effects. In the event of overdosage, treatment should be symptomatic and supportive. Unabsorbed material should be removed from the gastrointestinal tract, the patient should be monitored, and supportive therapy should be employed.

The intravenous LD_{50} of famotidine for mice and rats ranged from 254–563 mg/kg and the minimum lethal single I.V. dose in dogs was approximately 300 mg/kg. Signs of acute intoxication in I.V. treated dogs were emesis, restlessness, pallor of mucous membranes or redness of mouth and ears, hypotension, tachycardia and collapse. The oral LD_{50} of famotidine in male and female rats and mice was greater than 3000 mg/kg and the minimum lethal acute oral dose in dogs exceeded 2000 mg/kg. Famotidine did not produce overt effects at high oral doses in mice, rats, cats and dogs, but induced significant anorexia and growth depression in rabbits starting with 200 mg/kg/day orally.

DOSAGE AND ADMINISTRATION

In some hospitalized patients with pathological hypersecretory conditions or intractable ulcers, or in patients who are unable to take oral medication, PEPCID Injection Premixed or PEPCID Injection may be administered until oral therapy can be instituted.

The recommended dosage for PEPCID Injection Premixed and PEPCID Injection is 20 mg q 12 h.

The doses and regimen for parenteral administration in patients with GERD have not been established.

Dosage Adjustments for Patients with Severe Renal Insufficiency

In patients with severe renal insufficiency, i.e., with a creatinine clearance less than 10 mL/min, the elimination half-life of PEPCID may exceed 20 hours, reaching approximately 24 hours in anuric patients. Although no relationship of adverse effects to high plasma levels has been established, to avoid excess accumulation of the drug, the dose of PEPCID Injection Premixed or PEPCID Injection may be reduced to 20 mg h.s. or the dosing interval may be prolonged to 36–48 hours as indicated by the patient's clinical response.

Pathological Hypersecretory Conditions (e.g., Zollinger-Ellison Syndrome, Multiple Endocrine Adenomas)

The dosage of PEPCID in patients with pathological hypersecretory conditions varies with the individual patient. The recommended adult intravenous dose is 20 mg q 12 h. Doses should be adjusted to individual patient needs and should continue as long as clinically indicated. In some patients, a higher starting dose may be required. Oral doses up to 160 mg q 6 h have been administered to some patients with severe Zollinger-Ellison Syndrome.

PEPCID Injection Premixed

PEPCID Injection Premixed, supplied in Galaxy** containers (PL 2501 Plastic), is a 50 mL iso-osmotic solution premixed with 0.9% sodium chloride for administration as an infusion over a 15–30 minute period. *This premixed solution is for intravenous use only using sterile equipment.*

Directions for Use of Galaxy® Containers

Check the container for minute leaks prior to use by squeezing the bag firmly. If leaks are found, discard solution as sterility may be impaired. Do not add supplementary medication. Do not use unless solution is clear and seal is intact.

CAUTION: Do not use plastic containers in series connections. Such use could result in air embolism due to residual air being drawn from the primary container before administration of the fluid from the secondary container is complete.

Preparation for administration:

1. Suspend container from eyelet support.
2. Remove plastic protector from outlet port at bottom of container.
3. Attach administration set. Refer to complete directions accompanying set.

To prepare PEPCID intravenous solutions, aseptically dilute 2 mL of PEPCID Injection (solution containing 10 mg/mL) with 0.9% Sodium Chloride Injection or other compatible intravenous solution (see *Stability, PEPCID Injection*) to a total volume of either 5 mL or 10 mL and inject over a period of not less than 2 minutes.

To prepare PEPCID intravenous infusion solutions, aseptically dilute 2 mL of PEPCID Injection with 100 mL of 5% dextrose or other compatible solution (see *Stability, PEPCID Injection*), and infuse over a 15–30 minute period.

Concomitant Use of Antacids

Antacids may be given concomitantly if needed.

Stability

Parenteral drug products should be inspected visually for particulate matter and discoloration prior to administration whenever solution and container permit.

PEPCID Injection Premixed

PEPCID Injection Premixed, as supplied premixed in 0.9% sodium chloride in Galaxy® containers (PL 2501 Plastic), is stable through the labeled expiration date when stored under the recommended conditions. (See HOW SUPPLIED, *Storage*).

PEPCID Injection

When added to or diluted with most commonly used intravenous solutions, e.g., Water for Injection, 0.9% Sodium Chloride Injection, 5% and 10% Dextrose Injection, or Lactated Ringer's Injection, diluted PEPCID Injection is physically and chemically stable (i.e., maintains at least 90% of initial potency) for 7 days at room temperature—see HOW SUPPLIED, *Storage.*

When added to or diluted with Sodium Bicarbonate Injection, 5%, PEPCID Injection at a concentration of 0.2 mg/mL (the recommended concentration of PEPCID intravenous infusion solutions) is physically and chemically stable (i.e., maintains at least 90% of initial potency) for 7 days at room temperature—see HOW SUPPLIED, *Storage.* However, a precipitate may form at higher concentrations of PEPCID Injection (>0.2 mg/mL) in Sodium Bicarbonate Injection, 5%.

** Galaxy® is a registered trademark of Baxter International Inc.

HOW SUPPLIED

FOR INTRAVENOUS USE ONLY

No. 3537—PEPCID (famotidine) Injection Premixed 20 mg per 50 mL is a clear, non-preserved, sterile solution premixed in a vehicle made iso-osmotic with Sodium Chloride, and is supplied as follows:

NDC 0006-3537-50, 50 mL single dose Galaxy® containers (PL 2501 Plastic).

No. 3539—PEPCID Injection 10 mg per 1 mL, is a non-preserved, clear, colorless solution and is supplied as follows:

NDC 0006-3539-04, 10 × 2 mL single dose vials (6505-01-281-1249, 10 mg per mL, 2 mL 10's).

No. 3541—PEPCID Injection 10 mg per 1 mL, is a clear, colorless solution and is supplied as follows:

NDC 0006-3541-14, 4 mL vials (6505-01-282-1180, 10 mg per mL, 4 mL)

NDC 0006–3541–20, 20 mL vials

NDC 0006–3541–49, 10 ×20 mL vials.

Storage

Store PEPCID Injection Premixed in Galaxy® containers (PL 2501 Plastic) at room temperature (25°C, 77°F). Exposure of the premixed product to excessive heat should be avoided. Brief exposure to temperatures up to 35°C (95°F) does not adversely affect the product.

Store PEPCID Injection at 2–8°C (36–46°F). If solution freezes, bring to room temperature; allow sufficient time to solubilize all the components.

Although diluted PEPCID Injection has been shown to be physically and chemically stable for 7 days at room temperature, there are no data on the maintenance of sterility after dilution. Therefore, it is recommended that if not used immediately after preparation, diluted solutions of PEPCID Injection should be refrigerated and used within 48 hours (see DOSAGE AND ADMINISTRATION).

PEPCID (famotidine) Injection Premixed is manufactured for:

MERCK & CO., INC., West Point, PA 19486, USA

By:

BAXTER HEALTHCARE CORPORATION

Deerfield, Illinois 60015 USA

PEPCID (famotidine) Injection is manufactured by:

MERCK & CO., INC., West Point, PA 19486, USA

9042506 Issued November 1997

COPYRIGHT © MERCK & CO., INC., 1993, 1995

All rights reserved

PERIACTIN® Tablets ℞

(Cyproheptadine HCl), U.S.P.

PERIACTIN® Syrup ℞

(Cyproheptadine HCl), U.S.P.

DESCRIPTION

PERIACTIN* (Cyproheptadine HCl) is an antihistaminic and antiserotonergic agent.

Cyproheptadine hydrochloride is a white to slightly yellowish, crystalline solid, with a molecular weight of 350.89, which is soluble in water, freely soluble in methanol, sparingly soluble in ethanol, soluble in chloroform, and practically insoluble in ether. It is the sesquihydrate of 4-(5*H*-dibenzo*[a,d]*cyclohepten-5-ylidene)-1-methylpiperidine hydrochloride. The empirical formula of the anhydrous salt is $C_{21}H_{21}N{\cdot}HCl$ and the structural formula of the anhydrous salt is:

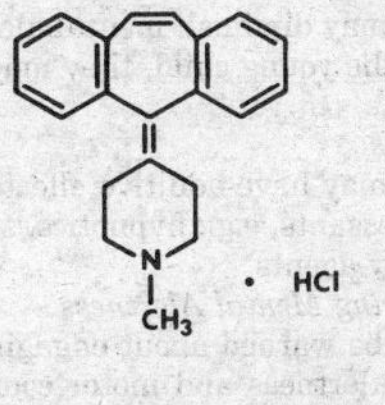

Continued on next page

Information on the Merck & Co., Inc. products listed on these pages is the full prescribing information from product circulars in use August 31, 1998. For information, please call 1-800-NSC MERCK [1-800-672-6372].

Periactin—Cont.

PERIACTIN is available in tablets, containing 4 mg of cyproheptadine hydrochloride, and as a syrup in which 5 mL contains 2 mg of cyproheptadine hydrochloride, with a pH range of 3.5 to 4.5.

The tablets also contain the following inactive ingredients: calcium phosphate, lactose, magnesium stearate, and starch. The syrup contains the following inactive ingredients: alcohol 5%, D & C Yellow 10, artificial flavors, glycerin, purified water, sodium saccharin, and sucrose, with sorbic acid 0.1% added as preservative.

* Registered trademark of MERCK & CO., INC.

CLINICAL PHARMACOLOGY

PERIACTIN is a serotonin and histamine antagonist with anticholinergic and sedative effects. Antiserotonin and antihistamine drugs appear to compete with serotonin and histamine, respectively, for receptor sites.

Pharmacokinetics and Metabolism

After a single 4 mg oral dose of ^{14}C-labelled cyproheptadine HCl in normal subjects, given as tablets or syrup, 2-20% of the radioactivity was excreted in the stools. Only about 34% of the stool radioactivity was unchanged drug, corresponding to less than 5.7% of the dose. At least 40% of the administered radioactivity was excreted in the urine. No significant difference in the mean urinary excretion exists between the tablet and syrup formulations. No detectable amounts of unchanged drug were present in the urine of patients on chronic 12-20 mg daily doses of PERIACTIN Syrup. The principal metabolite found in human urine has been identified as a quaternary ammonium glucuronide conjugate of cyproheptadine. Elimination is diminished in renal insufficiency.

INDICATIONS AND USAGE

Perennial and seasonal allergic rhinitis
Vasomotor rhinitis
Allergic conjunctivitis due to inhalant allergens and foods
Mild, uncomplicated allergic skin manifestations of urticaria and angioedema
Amelioration of allergic reactions to blood or plasma
Cold urticaria
Dermatographism
As therapy for anaphylactic reactions *adjunctive* to epinephrine and other standard measures after the acute manifestations have been controlled.

CONTRAINDICATIONS

Newborn or Premature Infants
This drug should *not* be used in newborn or premature infants.
Nursing Mothers
Because of the higher risk of antihistamines for infants generally and for newborns and prematures in particular, antihistamine therapy is contraindicated in nursing mothers.
Other Conditions
Hypersensitivity to cyproheptadine and other drugs of similar chemical structure:
  Monoamine oxidase inhibitor therapy
    (see DRUG INTERACTIONS)
  Angle-closure glaucoma
  Stenosing peptic ulcer
  Symptomatic prostatic hypertrophy
  Bladder neck obstruction
  Pyloroduodenal obstruction
  Elderly, debilitated patients

WARNINGS

Pediatric Patients
Overdosage of antihistamines, particularly in infants and young children, may produce hallucinations, central nervous system depression, convulsions, and death.
Antihistamines may diminish mental alertness; conversely, particularly, in the young child, they may occasionally produce excitation.
CNS Depressants
Antihistamines may have additive effects with alcohol and other CNS depressants, e.g., hypnotics, sedatives, tranquilizers, antianxiety agents.
Activities Requiring Mental Alertness
Patients should be warned about engaging in activities requiring mental alertness and motor coordination, such as driving a car or operating machinery.
Antihistamines are more likely to cause dizziness, sedation, and hypotension in elderly patients.

PRECAUTIONS

General
Cyproheptadine has an atropine-like action and, therefore, should be used with caution in patients with:

History of bronchial asthma
Increased intraocular pressure
Hyperthyroidism
Cardiovascular disease
Hypertension
Information for Patients
Antihistamines may diminish mental alertness; conversely, particularly, in the young child, they may occasionally produce excitation.
Patients should be warned about engaging in activities requiring mental alertness and motor coordination, such as driving a car or operating machinery.
Drug Interactions
MAO inhibitors prolong and intensify the anticholinergic effects of antihistamines.
Antihistamines may have additive effects with alcohol and other CNS depressants, e.g., hypnotics, sedatives, tranquilizers, antianxiety agents.
Carcinogenesis, Mutagenesis, Impairment of Fertility
Long-term carcinogenic studies have not been done with cyproheptadine.
Cyproheptadine had no effect on fertility in a two-litter study in rats or a two generation study in mice at about 10 times the human dose.
Cyproheptadine did not produce chromosome damage in human lymphocytes or fibroblasts *in vitro;* high doses (10^{-4} M) were cytotoxic. Cyproheptadine did not have any mutagenic effect in the Ames microbial mutagen test; concentrations of above 500 mcg/plate inhibited bacterial growth.
Pregnancy
Pregnancy Category B: Reproduction studies have been performed in rabbits, mice, and rats at oral or subcutaneous doses up to 32 times the maximum recommended human oral dose and have revealed no evidence of impaired fertility or harm to the fetus due to cyproheptadine. Cyproheptadine has been shown to be fetotoxic in rats when given by intraperitoneal injection in doses four times the maximum recommended human oral dose. Two studies in pregnant women, however, have not shown that cyproheptadine increases the risk of abnormalities when administered during the first, second and third trimesters of pregnancy. No teratogenic effects were observed in any of the newborns. Nevertheless, because the studies in humans cannot rule out the possibility of harm, cyproheptadine should be used during pregnancy only if clearly needed.
Nursing Mothers
It is not known whether this drug is excreted in human milk. Because many drugs are excreted in human milk, and because of the potential for serious adverse reactions in nursing infants from PERIACTIN, a decision should be made whether to discontinue nursing or to discontinue the drug, taking into account the importance of the drug to the mother (see CONTRAINDICATIONS).
Pediatric Use
Safety and effectiveness in pediatric patients below the age of two have not been established. See CONTRAINDICATIONS, *Newborn or Premature Infants*, and WARNINGS, *Children*.

ADVERSE REACTIONS

Adverse reactions which have been reported with the use of antihistamines are as follows:
Central Nervous System: Sedation and sleepiness (often transient), dizziness, disturbed coordination, confusion, restlessness, excitation, nervousness, tremor, irritability, insomnia, paresthesias, neuritis, convulsions, euphoria, hallucinations, hysteria, faintness.
Integumentary: Allergic manifestation of rash and edema, excessive perspiration, urticaria, photosensitivity.
Special Senses: Acute labyrinthitis, blurred vision, diplopia, vertigo, tinnitus.
Cardiovascular: Hypotension, palpitation, tachycardia, extrasystoles, anaphylactic shock.
Hematologic: Hemolytic anemia, leukopenia, agranulocytosis, thrombocytopenia.
Digestive System: Dryness of mouth, epigastric distress, anorexia, nausea, vomiting, diarrhea, constipation, jaundice.
Genitourinary: Urinary frequency, difficult urination, urinary retention, early menses.
Respiratory: Dryness of nose and throat, thickening of bronchial secretions, tightness of chest and wheezing, nasal stuffiness.
Miscellaneous: Fatigue, chills, headache, increased appetite/weight gain.

OVERDOSAGE

Antihistamine overdosage reactions may vary from central nervous system depression to stimulation especially in pediatric patients. Also, atropine-like signs and symptoms (dry mouth; fixed, dilated pupils; flushing, etc.) as well as gastrointestinal symptoms may occur.
If vomiting has not occurred spontaneously the patient should be induced to vomit with syrup of ipecac.

If the patient is unable to vomit, perform gastric lavage followed by activated charcoal. Isotonic or $^1/_2$ isotonic saline is the lavage of choice. Precautions against aspiration must be taken especially in infants and children.
When life threatening CNS signs and symptoms are present, intravenous physostigmine salicylate may be considered. Dosage and frequency of administration are dependent on age, clinical response, and recurrence after response. (See package circulars for physostigmine products.)
Saline cathartics, as milk of magnesia, by osmosis draw water into the bowel and, therefore, are valuable for their action in rapid dilution of bowel content.
Stimulants should *not* be used.
Vasopressors may be used to treat hypotension.
The oral LD_{50} of cyproheptadine is 123 mg/kg, and 295 mg/kg in the mouse and rat, respectively.

DOSAGE AND ADMINISTRATION

DOSAGE SHOULD BE INDIVIDUALIZED ACCORDING TO THE NEEDS AND THE RESPONSE OF THE PATIENT.
Each PERIACTIN tablet contains 4 mg of cyproheptadine hydrochloride. Each 5 mL of PERIACTIN syrup contains 2 mg of cyproheptadine hydrochloride.
Although intended primarily for administration to pediatric patients, the syrup is also useful for administration to adults who cannot swallow tablets.
Pediatric Patients
The total daily dosage for pediatric patients may be calculated on the basis of body weight or body area using approximately 0.25 mg/kg/day (0.11 mg/lb/day) or 8 mg per square meter of body surface (8 mg/m²). In small children for whom the calculation of dosage based upon body size is most important, it may be necessary to use PERIACTIN syrup to permit accurate dosage.
Age 2 to 6 years
The usual dose is 2 mg ($^1/_2$ tablet or 1 teaspoon) two or three times a day, adjusted as necessary to the size and response of the patient. The dose is not to exceed 12 mg a day.
Age 7 to 14 years
The usual dose is 4 mg (1 tablet or 2 teaspoons) two or three times a day, adjusted as necessary to the size and response of the patient. The dose is not to exceed 16 mg a day.
Adults
The total daily dose for adults should not exceed 0.5 mg/kg/day (0.23 mg/lb/day).
The therapeutic range is 4 to 20 mg a day, with the majority of patients requiring 12 to 16 mg a day. An occasional patient may require as much as 32 mg a day for adequate relief. It is suggested that dosage be initiated with 4 mg (1 tablet or 2 teaspoons) three times a day and adjusted according to the size and response of the patient.

HOW SUPPLIED

No. 3276—Tablets PERIACTIN, containing 4 mg of cyproheptadine hydrochloride each, are white, round, scored, compressed tablets, coded MSD 62 on one side and PERIACTIN on the other. They are supplied as follows:
NDC 0006-0062-68 bottles of 100
(6505-00-890-1884 4 mg 100's).
    Shown in Product Identification Guide, page 323
No. 3289X—Syrup PERIACTIN, 2 mg per 5 mL is a clear, yellow, syrupy liquid and is supplied as follows:
NDC 0006-3289-74 amber glass bottles of 473 mL.
Storage
Store Tablets PERIACTIN at controlled room temperature, 15–30°C (59–86°F), in a well-closed container.
Store Syrup PERIACTIN at controlled room temperature, 15–30°C (59–86°F), in a container which is kept tightly closed. Because of the risk of breakage, avoid freezing bottle.
        7926421   Issued March 1997
COPYRIGHT © MERCK & CO., INC., 1985
All rights reserved

PNEUMOVAX® 23
(PNEUMOCOCCAL VACCINE POLYVALENT)

℞

DESCRIPTION

PNEUMOVAX* 23 (Pneumococcal Vaccine Polyvalent), is a sterile, liquid vaccine for intramuscular or subcutaneous injection. It consists of a mixture of highly purified capsular polysaccharides from the 23 most prevalent or invasive pneumococcal types of *Streptococcus pneumoniae*, including the six serotypes that most frequently cause invasive drug-resistant pneumococcal infections among children and adults in the United States. (See Table 1.) The 23-valent vaccine accounts for at least 90% of pneumococcal blood isolates and at least 85% of all pneumococcal isolates from sites which are generally sterile as determined by ongoing surveillance of U.S. data.

Table 1
23 Pneumococcal Capsular Types Included in
PNEUMOVAX 23

Nomenclature	Pneumococcal Types
Danish	1 2 3 4 5 6B** 7F 8 9N 9V** 10A 11A 12F 14** 15B 17F 18C 19F** 19A** 20 22F 23F** 33F

**These serotypes most frequently cause drug-resistant pneumococcal infections

PNEUMOVAX 23 is manufactured according to methods developed by the MERCK Research Laboratories. Each 0.5 mL dose of vaccine contains 25 μg of each polysaccharide type dissolved in isotonic saline solution containing 0.25% phenol as preservative.
[See table 1 above]

---

*Registered trademark of MERCK & CO., Inc.

CLINICAL PHARMACOLOGY

Pneumococcal infection is a leading cause of death throughout the world and a major cause of pneumonia, bacteremia, meningitis, and otitis media.
Strains of drug-resistant *S. pneumoniae* have become increasingly common in the United States and in other parts of the world. In some areas as many as 35% of pneumococcal isolates have been reported to be resistant to penicillin. Many penicillin-resistant pneumococci are also resistant to other antimicrobial drugs (e.g., erythromycin, trimethoprim-sulfamethoxazole and extended-spectrum cephalosporins); therefore emphasizing the importance of vaccine prophylaxis against pneumococcal disease.

Epidemiology
Pneumococcal infection causes approximately 40,000 deaths annually in the United States.
At least 500,000 cases of pneumococcal pneumonia are estimated to occur annually in the United States; *S. pneumoniae* accounts for approximately 25–35% of cases of community-acquired bacterial pneumonia in persons who require hospitalization.
Pneumococcal disease accounts for an estimated 50,000 cases of pneumococcal bacteremia annually in the United States. Some studies suggest the overall annual incidence of bacteremia to be approximately 15 to 30 cases/100,000 population with 50 to 83 cases/100,000 for persons 65 years of age and older and 160 cases/100,000 for children less than two years of age.
The incidence of pneumococcal bacteremia is as high as 1% (940 cases/100,000 population) among persons with acquired immunodeficiency syndrome (AIDS).
In the United States, the risk of acquiring bacteremia is lower among whites than among persons in some other racial/ethnic groups (i.e., blacks, Alaskan Natives, and American Indians).
Despite appropriate antimicrobial therapy and intensive medical care, the overall case-fatality rate for pneumococcal bacteremia is 15–20% among adults, and among elderly patients this rate is approximately 30–40%. An overall case-fatality rate of 36% was documented for adult inner-city residents who were hospitalized for pneumococcal bacteremia.
In the United States, pneumococcal disease accounts for an estimated 3,000 cases of meningitis annually. The estimated overall annual incidence of pneumococcal meningitis is approximately 1 to 2 cases per 100,000 population. The incidence of pneumococcal meningitis is highest among children six to 24 months and persons aged ≥ 65 years; rates for blacks are twice as high as those for whites or Hispanics. Recurrent pneumococcal meningitis may occur in patients who have chronic cerebrospinal fluid leakage resulting from congenital lesions, skull fractures, or neurosurgical procedures.
Invasive pneumococcal disease (e.g., bacteremia or meningitis) and pneumonia cause high morbidity and mortality in spite of effective antimicrobial control by antibiotics. These effects of pneumococcal disease appear due to irreversible physiologic damage caused by the bacteria during the first 5 days following onset of illness, and occur irrespective of antimicrobial therapy. Vaccination offers an effective means of further reducing the mortality and morbidity of this disease.

Risk Factors
In addition to the very young and persons 65 years of age or older, patients with certain chronic conditions are at increased risk of developing pneumococcal infection and severe pneumococcal illness.
Patients with chronic cardiovascular diseases (e.g., congestive heart failure or cardiomyopathy), chronic pulmonary diseases (e.g., chronic obstructive pulmonary disease or emphysema), or chronic liver diseases (e.g., cirrhosis), diabetes mellitus, alcoholism or asthma (when it occurs with chronic bronchitis, emphysema, or long-term use of systemic corticosteroids) have an increased risk of pneumococcal disease. In adults, this population is generally immunocompetent.
Patients at high risk are those who have a decreased responsiveness to polysaccharide antigen or an increased rate of decline in serum antibody concentrations as a result of: immunosuppressive conditions (congenital immunodeficiency, human immunodeficiency virus [HIV] infection, leukemia, lymphoma, multiple myeloma, Hodgkin's disease, or generalized malignancy); organ or bone marrow transplantation; therapy with alkylating agents, antimetabolites, or systemic corticosteroids; chronic renal failure or nephrotic syndrome.
Patients at the highest risk of pneumococcal infection are those with functional or anatomic asplenia (e.g., sickle cell disease or splenectomy), because this condition leads to reduced clearance of encapsulated bacteria from the bloodstream. Children who have sickle cell disease or have had a splenectomy are at increased risk for fulminant pneumococcal sepsis associated with high mortality.

Immunogenicity
It has been established that the purified pneumococcal capsular polysaccharides induce antibody production and that such antibody is effective in preventing pneumococcal disease. Clinical studies have demonstrated the immunogenicity of each of the 23 capsular types when tested in polyvalent vaccines.
Studies with 12-, 14-, and 23-valent pneumococcal vaccines in children two years of age and older and in adults of all ages showed immunogenic responses. Protective capsular type-specific antibody levels generally develop by the third week following vaccination.
Bacterial capsular polysaccharides induce antibodies primarily by T-cell-independent mechanisms. Therefore, antibody response to most pneumococcal capsular types is generally poor or inconsistent in children aged < 2 years whose immune systems are immature.

Efficacy
The protective efficacy of pneumococcal vaccines containing 6 or 12 capsular polysaccharides was investigated in two controlled studies of young, healthy gold miners in South Africa, in whom there was a high attack rate for pneumococcal pneumonia and bacteremia. Capsular type-specific attack rates for pneumococcal pneumonia were observed for the period from 2 weeks through about 1 year after vaccination. Protective efficacy was 76% and 92%, respectively, in the two studies for the capsular types represented.
In similar studies carried out by Dr. R. Austrian and associates, using similar pneumococcal vaccines prepared for the National Institute of Allergy and Infectious Diseases, the reduction in pneumonia caused by the capsular types contained in the vaccines was 79%. Reduction in type-specific pneumococcal bacteremia was 82%.
A prospective study in France found pneumococcal vaccine to be 77% effective in reducing the incidence of pneumonia among nursing home residents.
In the United States, two postlicensure randomized controlled trials, in the elderly or patients with chronic medical conditions, who received a multivalent polysaccharide vaccine, did not support the efficacy of the vaccine for nonbacteremic pneumonia. However, these studies may have lacked sufficient statistical power to detect a difference in the incidence of laboratory-confirmed, nonbacteremic pneumococcal pneumonia between the vaccinated and nonvaccinated study groups.
A meta-analysis of nine randomized controlled trials of pneumococcal vaccine concluded that pneumococcal vaccine is efficacious in reducing the frequency of nonbacteremic pneumococcal pneumonia among adults in low risk groups but not in high-risk groups. These studies may have been limited because of the lack of specific and sensitive diagnostic tests for nonbacteremic pneumococcal pneumonia. The pneumococcal polysaccharide vaccine is not effective for the prevention of common upper respiratory disease in children. More recently, multiple, case-control studies have shown pneumococcal vaccine is effective in the prevention of serious pneumococcal disease, with point estimates of efficacy ranging from 56% to 81% in immunocompetent persons.
Only one case-control study did not document effectiveness against bacteremic disease possibly due to study limitations, including small sample size and incomplete ascertainment of vaccination status in patients. In addition, case-patients and persons who served as controls may not have been comparable regarding the severity of their underlying medical conditions, potentially creating a biased underestimate of vaccine effectiveness.
A serotype prevalence study, based on the Centers for Disease Control pneumococcal surveillance system, demonstrated 57% overall protective effectiveness against invasive infections caused by serotypes included in the vaccine in persons ≥ 6 years of age, 65–84% effectiveness among specific patient groups (e.g., persons with diabetes mellitus, coronary vascular disease, congestive heart failure, chronic pulmonary disease, and anatomic asplenia) and 75% effectiveness in immunocompetent persons aged ≥ 65 years of age. Vaccine effectiveness could not be confirmed for certain groups of immunocompromised patients; however, the study could not recruit sufficient numbers of unvaccinated patients from each disease group.
In an early study, vaccinated children and yound adults aged 2 to 25 years who had sickle cell disease, congenital asplenia, or undergone a splenectomy experienced significantly less bacteremic pneumococcal disease than patients who were not vaccinated.

Duration of Immunity
Following pneumococcal vaccination, serotype-specific antibody levels decline after 5–10 years. A more rapid decline in antibody levels may occur in some groups (e.g., children). Limited published data suggest that antibody levels may decline in the elderly > 60 years of age.
The Advisory Committee on Immunization Practices (ACIP) states that these findings indicate that revaccination may be needed to provide continued protection. (See INDICATIONS AND USAGE, *Revaccination*.)
The results from one epidemiologic study suggest that vaccination may provide protection for at least nine years after receipt of the initial dose. Decreasing estimates of effectiveness with increasing interval since vaccination, particularly among the very elderly (persons aged ≥ 85 years) have been reported.

INDICATIONS AND USAGE

PNEUMOVAX 23 is indicated for vaccination against pneumococcal disease caused by those pneumococcal types included in the vaccine. Effectiveness of the vaccine in the prevention of pneumococcal pneumonia and pneumococcal bacteremia has been demonstrated in controlled trials in South Africa, France and in case-control studies.
PNEUMOVAX 23 will not prevent disease caused by capsular types of pneumococcus other than those contained in the vaccine.
If it is known that a person has not received any pneumococcal vaccine or if earlier pneumococcal vaccination status is unknown, then persons in the categories listed below should be administered pneumococcal vaccine; however, if a person has received a primary dose of pneumococcal vaccine, before administering an additional dose of vaccine, please refer to the Revaccination section.
Vaccination with PNEUMOVAX 23 is recommended for selected individuals as follows:
Immunocompetent persons:
— routine vaccination for persons 50 years of age or older†
— persons aged ≥ 2 years with chronic cardiovascular disease (including congestive heart failure and cardiomyopathies), chronic pulmonary disease (including chronic obstructive pulmonary disease and emphysema), or diabetes mellitus
— persons aged ≥ 2 years with alcoholism, chronic liver disease (including cirrhosis) or cerebrospinal fluid leaks
— persons aged ≥ 2 years with functional or anatomic asplenia (including sickle cell disease and splenectomy)
— persons aged ≥ 2 years living in special environments or social settings (including Alaskan Natives and certain American Indian populations)
Immunocompromised persons:
— persons aged ≥ 2 years, including those with HIV infection, leukemia, lymphoma, Hodgkin's disease, multiple myeloma, generalized malignancy, chronic renal failure or nephrotic syndrome; those receiving immunosuppressive chemotherapy (including corticosteroids); and those who have received an organ or bone marrow transplant.

---

†NOTE: The ACIP recommends routine vaccination for immunocompetent persons 65 years of age and older.
Timing of Vaccination
Pneumococcal vaccine should be given at least two weeks before elective splenectomy, if possible.
For planning cancer chemotherapy or other immunosuppressive therapy (e.g., for patients with Hodgkin's disease or those who undergo organ or bone marrow transplantation), the interval between vaccination and initiation of immunosuppressive therapy should be at least two weeks. Vaccination during chemotherapy or radiation therapy should be avoided. Pneumococcal vaccine may be given several months following completion of chemotherapy or radiation therapy for neoplastic disease. In Hodgkin's disease, immune response to vaccination may be suboptimal for two years or longer after intensive chemotherapy (with or without radiation). For some patients, during the two years fol-

Continued on next page

Information on the Merck & Co., Inc. products listed on these pages is the full prescribing information from product circulars in use August 31, 1998. For information, please call 1-800-NSC MERCK [1-800-672-6372].

Pneumovax 23—Cont.

lowing the completion of chemotherapy or other immunosuppressive therapy (with or without radiation), significant improvement in antibody response has been observed, particularly as the interval between the end of treatment and pneumococcal vaccination increased.

Persons with asymptomatic or symptomatic HIV infection should be vaccinated as soon as possible after their diagnosis is confirmed.

Use With Other Vaccines

The ACIP states that pneumococcal vaccine may be administered at the same time as influenza vaccine (by separate injection in the other arm) without an increase in side effects or decreased antibody response to either vaccine. In contrast to pneumococcal vaccine, influenza vaccine is recommended annually, for appropriate populations.

Revaccination

Early studies have indicated that local reactions (i.e., arthus-type reactions) among adults receiving the second dose of 14–valent vaccine within 2 years after the first dose are more severe than those occurring after initial vaccination. However, subsequent studies have suggested that revaccination after intervals of ≥ 4 years is not associated with an increased incidence of adverse side effects.

Routine revaccination of immunocompetent persons previously vaccinated with 23–valent polysaccharide vaccine is not recommended. However, revaccination once is recommended for persons ≥ 2 years of age who are at highest risk of serious pneumococcal infection and those likely to have a rapid decline in pneumococcal antibody levels, provided that at least five years have passed since receipt of a first dose of pneumococcal vaccine.

The highest risk group includes persons with functional or anatomic asplenia (e.g., sickle cell disease or splenectomy), HIV infection, leukemia, lymphoma, Hodgkin's disease, multiple myeloma, generalized malignancy, chronic renal failure, nephrotic syndrome, or other conditions associated with immunosupression (e.g., organ or bone marrow transplantation), and those receiving immunosuppressive chemotherapy (including long-term systemic corticosteroids).

For children ≤ 10 years of age at revaccination and at highest risk of severe pneumococcal infection (e.g., children with functional or anatomic asplenia, including sickle cell disease or splenectomy or conditions associated with rapid antibody decline after initial vaccination including nephrotic syndrome, renal failure or renal transplantation), the ACIP recommends that revaccination may be considered three years after the previous dose.

If prior vaccination status is unknown for patients in the high risk group, patients should be given pneumococcal vaccine.

All persons ≥ 65 years of age who have not received vaccine within 5 years (and were < 65 years of age at the time of vaccination) should receive another dose of vaccine.

Because data are insufficient concerning the safety of pneumococcal vaccine when administered three or more times, revaccination following a second dose is not routinely recommended.

CONTRAINDICATIONS

Hypersensitivity to any component of the vaccine. Epinephrine injection (1:1000) must be immediately available should an acute anaphylactoid reaction occur due to any component of the vaccine.

WARNINGS

For planning cancer chemotherapy or other immunosuppressive therapy (e.g., for patients with Hodgkin's disease or those who undergo organ or bone marrow transplantation), the timing of the vaccination is critical. (See INDICATIONS AND USAGE, *Timing of Vaccination.*)

If the vaccine is used in persons receiving immunosuppressive therapy, the expected serum antibody response may not be obtained and potential impairment of future immune responses to pneumococcal antigens may occur. (See INDICATIONS AND USAGE, *Timing of Vaccination.*)

Intradermal administration may cause severe local reactions.

PRECAUTIONS

General

Caution and appropriate care should be exercised in administering PNEUMOVAX 23 to individuals with severely compromised cardiovascular and/or pulmonary function in whom a systemic reaction would pose a significant risk.

Any febrile respiratory illness or other active infection is reason for delaying use of PNEUMOVAX 23, except when, in the opinion of the physician, withholding the agent entails even greater risk.

In patients who require penicillin (or other antibiotic) prophylaxis against pneumococcal infection, such prophylaxis should not be discontinued after vaccination with PNEUMOVAX 23.

PNEUMOVAX 23 may not be effective in preventing infection resulting from basilar skull fracture or from external communication with cerebrospinal fluid.

Routine revaccination of immunocompetent persons previously vaccinated with a 23–valent vaccine is not recommended. However, revaccination once is recommended for persons aged ≥ 2 years who are at highest risk for serious pneumococcal infections and those likely to have a rapid decline in pneumococcal antibody levels. (See INDICATIONS AND USAGE, *Revaccination.*)

Instructions to Healthcare Provider

The healthcare provider should determine the current health status and previous vaccination history of the vaccinee. (See INDICATIONS AND USAGE, *Revaccination.*)

The healthcare provider should question the patient, parent or guardian about reactions to a previous dose of PNEUMOVAX 23 or other pneumococcal vaccine.

Information for Patients

The healthcare provider should inform the patient, parent or guardian of the benefits and risks associated with vaccination. For risks associated with vaccination, see WARNINGS, PRECAUTIONS, and ADVERSE REACTIONS.

Patients, parents, and guardians should be instructed to report any serious adverse reactions to their healthcare provider who in turn should report such events to the vaccine manufacturer or the U.S. Department of Health and Human Services through the Vaccine Adverse Event Reporting System (VAERS), 1-800-822-7967.

Pregnancy

Pregnancy Category C: Animal reproduction studies have not been conducted with PNEUMOVAX 23. It is also not known whether PNEUMOVAX 23 can cause fetal harm when administered to a pregnant woman or can affect reproduction capacity. PNEUMOVAX 23 should be given to a pregnant woman only if clearly needed.

Nursing Mothers

It is not known whether this drug is excreted in human milk. Because many drugs are excreted in human milk, caution should be excercised when PNEUMOVAX 23 is administered to a nursing woman.

Pediatric Use

In general, children less than 2 years of age respond poorly to the capsular types of PNEUMOVAX 23 that are most often the cause of pneumococcal disease in this age group. (See CLINICAL PHARMACOLOGY, *Immunogenicity.*) Safety and effectiveness in children below the age of 2 years have not been established. Accordingly, PNEUMOVAX 23 is not recommended in this age group.

ADVERSE REACTIONS

The following adverse experiences have been reported with PNEUMOVAX 23 in clinical trials and post-marketing experience:

The most common adverse experiences reported in clinical trials were:

Local reactions at injection site including soreness, warmth, erythema, swelling and induration

Fever ≤ 102°F.

Other adverse experiences reported in clinical trials and in post-marketing experience include:

Body as a Whole

Asthenia

Malaise

Fever (>102°F)

Digestive System

Nausea

Vomiting

Hematologic/Lymphatic

Lymphadenitis

Thrombocytopenia in patients with stabilized idiopathic thrombocytopenic purpura

Hemolytic anemia in patients who have had other hematologic disorders

Hypersensitivity

Anaphylactoid reactions

Serum Sickness

Musculoskeletal System

Arthralgia

Arthritis

Myalgia

Nervous System

Headache

Paresthesia

Radiculoneuropathy

Guillain-Barré Syndrome

Skin

Rash

Urticaria

DOSAGE AND ADMINISTRATION

Do not inject intravenously or intradermally.

Parenteral drug products should be inspected visually for particulate matter and discoloration prior to administration, whenever solution and container permit. PNEUMOVAX 23 is a clear, colorless solution.

Withdraw 0.5 mL from the vial using a sterile needle and syringe free of preservatives, antiseptics, and detergents.

Administer a single 0.5 mL dose of PNEUMOVAX 23 subcutaneously or intramuscularly (preferably in the deltoid muscle or lateral mid-thigh), with appropriate precautions to avoid intravascular administration.

It is important to use a separate sterile syringe and needle for each individual patient to prevent transmission of infectious agents from one person to another.

Store unopened and opened vials at 2–8°C (36–46°F). The vaccine is used directly as supplied. No dilution or reconstitution is necessary. Phenol 0.25% has been added as a preservative. All vaccine must be discarded after the expiration date.

Use With Other Vaccines

The ACIP states that pneumococcal vaccine may be administered at the same time as influenza vaccine (by separate injection in the other arm) without an increase in side effects or decreased antibody response to either vaccine. In contrast to pneumococcal vaccine, influenza vaccine is recommended annually, for appropriate populations.

HOW SUPPLIED

No. 4739 — PNEUMOVAX 23 is supplied as one 5-dose vial of liquid vaccine, **NDC** 0006-4739-00.

For use with syringe only (6505-01-092-0391).

No. 4943 — PNEUMOVAX 23 is supplied as a single-dose vial of liquid vaccine, in a box of 10 single-dose vials, **NDC** 0006-4943-00.

7999815   Issued April 1998

PRIMAXIN® I.M.   ℞
(Imipenem and Cilastatin for Injectable Suspension)
(Formerly called IMIPENEM-CILASTATIN SODIUM FOR SUSPENSION)

For Intramuscular Injection Only

DESCRIPTION

PRIMAXIN† I.M. (Imipenem and Cilastatin for Injectable Suspension) is a formulation of imipenem (a thienamycin antibiotic) and cilastatin sodium (the inhibitor of the renal dipeptidase, dehydropeptidase I). PRIMAXIN I.M. is a potent broad spectrum antibacterial agent for intramuscular administration.

Imipenem (N-formimidoylthienamycin monohydrate) is a crystalline derivative of thienamycin, which is produced by *Streptomyces cattleya.* Its chemical name is [5R-[5α, 6α (R*)]]-6-(1-hydroxyethyl)-3-[[2-[(iminomethyl)amino] ethyl]thio]-7-oxo-1-azabicyclo [3.2.0] hept-2-ene-2-carboxylic acid monohydrate. It is an off-white, nonhygroscopic crystalline compound with a molecular weight of 317.37. It is sparingly soluble in water, and slightly soluble in methanol. Its empirical formula is $C_{12}H_{17}N_3O_4S·H_2O$, and its structural formula is:

Cilastatin sodium is the sodium salt of a derivatized heptenoic acid. Its chemical name is [R- [R*,S*- (Z)]]-7-[(2-amino-2-carboxyethyl)thio]-2-[[(2, 2-dimethylcyclopropyl) carbonyl]amino]-2-heptenoic acid, monosodium salt. It is an off-white to yellowish-white, hygroscopic, amorphous compound with a molecular weight of 380.43. It is very soluble in water and in methanol. Its empirical formula is $C_{16}H_{25}N_2O_5SNa$, and its structural formula is:

PRIMAXIN I.M. 500 contains 32 mg of sodium (1.4 mEq) and PRIMAXIN I.M. 750 contains 48 mg of sodium (2.1 mEq). Prepared PRIMAXIN I.M. suspensions are white to light tan in color. Variations of color within this range do not affect the potency of the product.

† Registered trademark of MERCK & CO., Inc.

CLINICAL PHARMACOLOGY

Following intramuscular administrations of 500 or 750 mg doses of imipenem-cilastatin sodium in a 1:1 ratio with 1% lidocaine, peak plasma levels of imipenem antimicrobial ac-

tivity occur within 2 hours and average 10 and 12 mcg/mL, respectively. For cilastatin, peak plasma levels average 24 and 33 mcg/mL, respectively, and occur within 1 hour. When compared to intravenous administration of imipenem-cilastatin sodium, imipenem is approximately 75% bioavailable following intramuscular administration while cilastatin is approximately 95% bioavailable. The absorption of imipenem from the IM injection site continues for 6 to 8 hours while that for cilastatin is essentially complete within 4 hours. This prolonged absorption of imipenem following the administration of the intramuscular formulation of imipenem-cilastatin sodium results in an effective plasma half-life of imipenem of approximately 2 to 3 hours and plasma levels of the antibiotic which remain above 2 mcg/mL for at least 6 or 8 hours, following a 500 mg or 750 mg dose, respectively. This plasma profile for imipenem permits IM administration of the intramuscular formulation of imipenem-cilastatin sodium every 12 hours with no accumulation of cilastatin and only slight accumulation of imipenem.

A comparison of plasma levels of imipenem after a single dose of 500 mg or 750 mg of imipenem-cilastatin sodium (intravenous formulation) administered intravenously or of imipenem-cilastatin sodium (intramuscular formulation) diluted with 1% lidocaine and administered intramuscularly is as follows:

PLASMA CONCENTRATIONS OF IMIPENEM
(mcg/mL)

	500 MG		750 MG	
TIME	I.V.	I.M.	I.V.	I.M.
25 min	45.1	6.0	57.0	6.7
1 hr	21.6	9.4	28.1	10.0
2 hr	10.0	9.9	12.0	11.4
4 hr	2.6	5.6	3.4	7.3
6 hr	0.6	2.5	1.1	3.8
12 hr	ND†	0.5	ND†	0.8

† ND: Not Detectable (<0.3 mcg/mL)

Imipenem urine levels remain above 10 mcg/mL for the 12 hour dosing interval following the administration of 500 mg or 750 mg doses of the intramuscular formulation of imipenem-cilastatin sodium. Total urinary excretion of imipenem averages 50% while that for cilastatin averages 75% following either dose of the intramuscular formulation of imipenem-cilastatin sodium.

Imipenem, when administered alone, is metabolized in the kidneys by dehydropeptidase I resulting in relatively low levels in urine. Cilastatin sodium, an inhibitor of this enzyme, effectively prevents renal metabolism of imipenem so that when imipenem and cilastatin sodium are given concomitantly, increased levels of imipenem are achieved in the urine. The binding of imipenem to human serum proteins is approximately 20% and that of cilastatin is approximately 40%.

In a clinical study in which a 500 mg dose of the intramuscular formulation of imipenem-cilastatin sodium was administered to healthy subjects, the average peak level of imipenem in interstitial fluid (skin blister fluid) was approximately 5.0 mcg/mL within 3.5 hours after administration.

Imipenem-cilastatin sodium is hemodialyzable. However, usefulness of this procedure in the overdosage setting is questionable (see OVERDOSAGE).

Microbiology

The bactericidal activity of imipenem results from the inhibition of cell wall synthesis. Its greatest affinity is for penicillin-binding proteins (PBPs) 1A, 1B, 2, 4, 5 and 6 of *Escherichia coli,* and 1A, 1B, 2, 4 and 5 of *Pseudomonas aeruginosa.* The lethal effect is related to binding to PBP 2 and PBP 1B.

Imipenem has a high degree of stability in the presence of beta-lactamases, including penicillinases and cephalosporinases produced by gram-negative and gram-positive bacteria. It is a potent inhibitor of beta-lactamases from certain gram-negative bacteria which are inherently resistant to many beta-lactam antibiotics, e.g., *Pseudomonas aeruginosa, Serratia* spp. and *Enterobacter* spp.

Imipenem has *in vitro* activity against a wide range of gram-positive and gram-negative organisms. Imipenem is active against most strains of the following microorganisms *in vitro* and in clinical infections treated with the intramuscular formulation of imipenem-cilastatin sodium (see INDICATIONS AND USAGE).

Gram-positive aerobes:
- *Staphylococcus aureus* including penicillinase-producing strains
  - (NOTE: Methicillin-resistant staphylococci should be reported as resistant to imipenem.)
- Group D streptococcus including *Enterococcus faecalis* (formerly *S. faecalis*)
  - (NOTE: Imipenem is inactive *in vitro* against *Enterococcus faecium* [formerly *S. faecium*].)
- *Streptococcus pneumoniae*
- *Streptococcus pyogenes* (Group A streptococcus)
- *Streptococcus viridans* group

Gram-negative aerobes:
- *Acinetobacter* spp., including *A. calcoaceticus*
- *Citrobacter* spp.
- *Enterobacter cloacae*
- *Escherichia coli*
- *Haemophilus influenzae*
- *Klebsiella pneumoniae*
- *Pseudomonas aeruginosa*
  - (NOTE: Imipenem is inactive *in vitro* against *Xanthomonas (Pseudomonas) maltophilia* and *P. cepacia.*)

Gram-positive anaerobes:
- *Peptostreptococcus* spp.

Gram-negative anaerobes:
- *Bacteroides* spp., including
  - *Bacteroides distasonis*
  - *Bacteroides intermedius* (formerly *B. melaninogenicus intermedius*)
  - *Bacteroides fragilis*
  - *Bacteroides thetaiotaomicron*
- *Fusobacterium* spp.

Imipenem has been shown to be active *in vitro* against the following microorganisms; however, the clinical significance of these data is unknown.

Gram-positive aerobes:
- *Listeria monocytogenes*
- *Nocardia* spp.
- *Staphylococcus epidermidis* including penicillinase-producing strains.
  - (NOTE: Methicillin-resistant staphylococci should be reported as resistant to imipenem.)
- *Streptococcus agalactiae* (Group B streptococcus)
- Group C streptococcus
- Group G streptococcus

Gram-negative aerobes:
- *Achromobacter* spp.
- *Aeromonas hydrophila*
- *Alcaligenes* spp.
- *Bordetella bronchiseptica*
- *Campylobacter* spp.
- *Enterobacter* spp.
- *Gardnerella vaginalis*
- *Haemophilus parainfluenzae*
- *Hafnia* spp., including *H. alvei*
- *Klebsiella* spp., including *K. oxytoca*
- *Moraxella* spp.
- *Morganella morganii*
- *Neisseria gonorrhoeae* including penicillinase-producing strains
- *Pasteurella multocida*
- *Plesiomonas shigelloides*
- *Proteus mirabilis*
- *Proteus vulgaris*
- *Providencia rettgeri*
- *Providencia stuartii*
- *Salmonella* spp.
- *Serratia* spp., including *S. marcescens* and *S. proteamaculans* (formerly *S. liquefaciens*)
- *Shigella* spp.
- *Yersinia* spp., including *Y. enterocolitica* and *Y. pseudotuberculosis*

Gram-positive anaerobes:
- *Actinomyces* spp.
- *Clostridium* spp., including *C. perfringens*
- *Eubacterium* spp.
- *Peptococcus niger*
- *Propionibacterium* spp., including *P. acnes*

Gram-negative anaerobes:
- *Bacteroides bivius*
- *Bacteroides disiens*
- *Bacteroides ovatus*
- *Bacteroides vulgatus*
- *Porphyromonas asaccharolytica* (formerly *Bacteroides asaccharolyticus*)
- *Veillonella* spp.

In vitro tests show imipenem to act synergistically with aminoglycoside antibiotics against some isolates of *Pseudomonas aeruginosa.*

Susceptibility Tests:

Diffusion techniques:

Quantitative methods that require measurement of zone diameters give the most precise estimate of antibiotic susceptibility. One such standard procedure[1], which has been recommended for use with disks to test susceptibility of organisms to imipenem, uses the 10-mcg imipenem disk. Interpretation involves the correlation of the diameters obtained in the disk test with the minimum inhibitory concentration (MIC) for imipenem.

Reports from the laboratory giving results of the standard single-disk susceptibility test with a 10-mcg imipenem disk should be interpreted according to the following criteria:

Zone Diameter (mm)	Interpretation
≥16	Susceptible
14–15	Moderately Susceptible
≤13	Resistant

A report of "susceptible" indicates that the pathogen is likely to be inhibited by generally achievable blood levels. A report of "moderately susceptible" suggests that the organism would be susceptible if high dosage is used or if the infection is confined to tissues and fluids in which high antibiotic levels are attained. A report of "resistant" indicates that achievable concentrations are unlikely to be inhibitory and other therapy should be selected.

Standardized procedures require the use of laboratory control organisms. The 10-mcg imipenem disk should give the following zone diameters:

Organism	Zone Diameter (mm)
E. coli ATCC 25922	26–32
P. aeruginosa ATCC 27853	20–28

Dilution techniques:

Use a standardized dilution method[2] (broth, agar, microdilution) or equivalent with imipenem powder. The MIC values obtained should be interpreted according to the following criteria:

MIC (mcg/mL)	Interpretation
≤4	Susceptible
8	Moderately Susceptible
≥16	Resistant

As with standard diffusion techniques, dilution methods require the use of laboratory control organisms. Standard imipenem powder should provide the following MIC values:

Organism	MIC (mcg/mL)
E. coli ATCC 25922	0.06–0.25
S. aureus ATCC 29213	0.015–0.06
E. faecalis ATCC 29212	0.5–2.0
P. aeruginosa ATCC 27853	1.0–4.0

For anaerobic bacteria, the MIC of imipenem can be determined by agar or broth dilution (including microdilution) techniques.[3]

INDICATIONS AND USAGE

PRIMAXIN I.M. is indicated for the treatment of serious infections (listed below) of mild to moderate severity for which intramuscular therapy is appropriate. **PRIMAXIN I.M. is not intended for the therapy of severe or life-threatening infections, including bacterial sepsis or endocarditis, or in instances of major physiological impairments such as shock.**

PRIMAXIN I.M. is indicated for the treatment of infections caused by susceptible strains of the designated microorganisms in the conditions listed below:

(1) **Lower respiratory tract infections,** including pneumonia and bronchitis as an exacerbation of COPD, caused by *Streptococcus pneumoniae* and *Haemophilus influenzae.*

(2) **Intra-abdominal infections,** including acute gangrenous or perforated appendicitis and appendicitis with peritonitis, caused by Group D streptococcus including *Enterococcus faecalis**; *Streptococcus viridans* group*; *Escherichia coli; Klebsiella pneumoniae**; *Pseudomonas aeruginosa**; *Bacteroides* species including *B. fragilis, B. distasonis**, *B. intermedius** and *B. thetaiotaomicron**; *Fusobacterium* species and *Peptostreptococcus** species.

(3) **Skin and skin structure infections,** including abscesses, cellulitis, infected skin ulcers and wound infections caused by *Staphylococcus aureus* including penicillinase-producing strains; *Streptococcus pyogenes**; Group D streptococcus including *Enterococcus faecalis; Acinetobacter* species* including *A. calcoaceticus**; *Citrobacter* species*; *Escherichia coli; Enterobacter cloacae; Klebsiella pneumoniae**; *Pseudomonas aeruginosa** and *Bacteroides* species* including *B. fragilis**.

(4) **Gynecologic infections,** including postpartum endomyometritis, caused by Group D streptococcus including *Enterococcus faecalis**; *Escherichia coli; Klebsiella pneumoniae**; *Bacteroides intermedius**; and *Peptostreptococcus* species*.

As with other beta-lactam antibiotics, some strains of *Pseudomonas aeruginosa* may develop resistance fairly rapidly during treatment with PRIMAXIN I.M. During therapy of *Pseudomonas aeruginosa* infections, periodic susceptibility testing should be done when clinically appropriate.

*Efficacy for this organism in this organ system was studied in fewer than 10 infections.

CONTRAINDICATIONS

PRIMAXIN I.M. is contraindicated in patients who have shown hypersensitivity to any component of this product.

Continued on next page

Information on the Merck & Co., Inc. products listed on these pages is the full prescribing information from product circulars in use August 31, 1998. For information, please call 1-800-NSC MERCK [1-800-672-6372].

Consult 1999 PDR® supplements and future editions for revisions

Primaxin I.M.—Cont.

Due to the use of lidocaine hydrochloride diluent, this product is contraindicated in patients with a known hypersensitivity to local anesthetics of the amide type and in patients with severe shock or heart block. (Refer to the package circular for lidocaine hydrochloride).

WARNINGS

SERIOUS AND OCCASIONALLY FATAL HYPERSENSITIVITY (anaphylactic) REACTIONS HAVE BEEN REPORTED IN PATIENTS RECEIVING THERAPY WITH BETA-LACTAMS. THESE REACTIONS ARE MORE LIKELY TO OCCUR IN INDIVIDUALS WITH A HISTORY OF SENSITIVITY TO MULTIPLE ALLERGENS. THERE HAVE BEEN REPORTS OF INDIVIDUALS WITH A HISTORY OF PENICILLIN HYPERSENSITIVITY WHO HAVE EXPERIENCED SEVERE REACTIONS WHEN TREATED WITH ANOTHER BETA-LACTAM. BEFORE INITIATING THERAPY WITH PRIMAXIN® I.M., CAREFUL INQUIRY SHOULD BE MADE CONCERNING PREVIOUS HYPERSENSITIVITY REACTIONS TO PENICILLINS, CEPHALOSPORINS, OTHER BETA-LACTAMS, AND OTHER ALLERGENS. IF AN ALLERGIC REACTION OCCURS, PRIMAXIN® SHOULD BE DISCONTINUED. **SERIOUS ANAPHYLACTIC REACTIONS REQUIRE IMMEDIATE EMERGENCY TREATMENT WITH EPINEPHRINE. OXYGEN, INTRAVENOUS STEROIDS, AND AIRWAY MANAGEMENT, INCLUDING INTUBATION, MAY ALSO BE ADMINISTERED AS INDICATED.**

Pseudomembranous colitis has been reported with nearly all antibacterial agents, including PRIMAXIN, and may range in severity from mild to life-threatening. Therefore, it is important to consider this diagnosis in patients who present with diarrhea subsequent to the administration of antibacterial agents.

Treatment with antibacterial agents alters the normal flora of the colon and may permit overgrowth of clostridia. Studies indicate that a toxin produced by *Clostridium difficile* is one primary cause of "antibiotic-associated colitis".

After the diagnosis of pseudomembranous colitis has been established, therapeutic measures should be initiated. Mild cases of pseudomembranous colitis usually respond to drug discontinuation alone. In moderate to severe cases, consideration should be given to management with fluids and electrolytes, protein supplementation and treatment with an antibacterial drug effective against *C. difficile*.

Lidocaine HCl —Refer to the package circular for lidocaine HCl.

PRECAUTIONS

General

CNS adverse experiences such as myoclonic activity, confusional states, or seizures have been reported with PRIMAXIN I.V. (Imipenem and Cilastatin for Injection). These experiences have occurred most commonly in patients with CNS disorders (e.g., brain lesions or history of seizures) who also have compromised renal function. However, there were reports in which there was no recognized or documented underlying CNS disorder. These adverse CNS effects have not been seen with PRIMAXIN I.M.; however, should they occur during treatment, PRIMAXIN I.M. should be discontinued. Anticonvulsant therapy should be continued in patients with a known seizure disorder.

As with other antibiotics, prolonged use of PRIMAXIN I.M. may result in overgrowth of nonsusceptible organisms. Repeated evaluation of the patient's condition is essential. If superinfection occurs during therapy, appropriate measures should be taken.

Caution should be taken to avoid inadvertent injection into a blood vessel (see DOSAGE AND ADMINISTRATION). For additional precautions, refer to the package circular for lidocaine HCl.

Drug Interactions

Since concomitant administration of PRIMAXIN (Imipenem-Cilastatin Sodium) and probenecid results in only minimal increases in plasma levels of imipenem and plasma half-life, it is not recommended that probenecid be given with PRIMAXIN I.M.

PRIMAXIN I.M. should not be mixed with or physically added to other antibiotics. However, PRIMAXIN I.M. may be administered concomitantly with other antibiotics, such as aminoglycosides.

Carcinogenesis, Mutagenesis, Impairment of Fertility

Long term studies in animals have not been performed to evaluate carcinogenic potential of imipenem-cilastatin. Genetic toxicity studies were performed in a variety of bacterial and mammalian tests *in vivo* and *in vitro*. The tests used were: V79 mammalian cell mutagenesis assay (imipenem-cilastatin sodium alone and imipenem alone), Ames test (cilastatin sodium alone and imipenem alone), unscheduled DNA synthesis assay (imipenem-cilastatin sodium) and *in vivo* mouse cytogenetics test (imipenem-cilastatin sodium). None of these tests showed any evidence of genetic alterations.

Reproductive tests in male and female rats were performed with imipenem-cilastatin sodium at dosage levels up to 11 times† the maximum daily recommended human dose of the intramuscular formulation (on a mg/kg basis). Slight decreases in live fetal body weight were restricted to the highest dosage level. No other adverse effects were observed on fertility, reproductive performance, fetal viability, growth or postnatal development of pups. Similarly, no adverse effects on the fetus or on lactation were observed when imipenem-cilastatin sodium was administered to rats late in gestation.

Pregnancy: Teratogenic Effects

Pregnancy Category C: Teratology studies with cilastatin sodium in rabbits and rats at 10 and 33 times† the maximum recommended daily human dose of the intramuscular formulation (30 mg/kg/day) of PRIMAXIN, respectively, showed no evidence of adverse effects on the fetus. No evidence of teratogenicity was observed in rabbits and rats given imipenem at doses up to 2 and 30 times† the maximum recommended daily human dose of the intramuscular formulation of PRIMAXIN, respectively.

Teratology studies with imipenem-cilastatin sodium at doses up to 11 times† the maximum recommended human dose in pregnant mice and rats during the period of major organogenesis revealed no evidence of teratogenicity.

Imipenem-cilastatin sodium, when administered to pregnant rabbits at dosages above the usual human dose of the intramuscular formulation (1000–1500 mg/day), caused body weight loss, diarrhea, and maternal deaths. When comparable doses of imipenem-cilastatin sodium were given to nonpregnant rabbits, body weight loss, diarrhea, and deaths were also observed. This intolerance is not unlike that seen with other beta-lactam antibiotics in this species and is probably due to alteration of gut flora.

A teratology study in pregnant cynomolgus monkeys given imipenem-cilastatin sodium at doses of 40 mg/kg/day (bolus intravenous injection) or 160 mg/kg/day (subcutaneous injection) resulted in maternal toxicity including emesis, inappetence, body weight loss, diarrhea, abortion and death in some cases. In contrast, no significant toxicity was observed when nonpregnant cynomolgus monkeys were given doses of imipenem-cilastatin sodium up to 180 mg/kg/day (subcutaneous injection). When doses of imipenem-cilastatin sodium (approximately 100 mg/kg/day or approximately 3 times† the maximum daily recommended human dose of the intramuscular formulation) were administered to pregnant cynomolgus monkeys at an intraveous infusion rate which mimics human clinical use, there was minimal maternal intolerance (occasional emesis), no maternal deaths, no evidence of teratogenicity, but an increase in embryonic loss relative to the control groups.

There are, however, no adequate and well-controlled studies in pregnant women. PRIMAXIN I.M. should be used during pregnancy only if the potential benefit justifies the potential risk to the mother and fetus.

Nursing Mothers

It is not known whether imipenem-cilastatin sodium or lidocaine HCl (diluent) is excreted in human milk. Because many drugs are excreted in human milk, caution should be exercised when PRIMAXIN I.M. is administered to a nursing woman.

Pediatric Use

Safety and effectiveness in pediatric patients below the age of 12 years have not been established.

† Based on patient weight of 50 kg.

ADVERSE REACTIONS

PRIMAXIN I.M.

In 686 patients in multiple dose clinical trials of PRIMAXIN I.M., the following adverse reactions were reported:

Local Adverse Reactions

The most frequent adverse local clinical reaction that was reported as possibly, probably or definitely related to therapy with PRIMAXIN I.M. was pain at the injection site (1.2%).

Systemic Adverse Reactions

The most frequently reported systemic adverse clinical reactions that were reported as possibly, probably or definitely related to PRIMAXIN I.M. were nausea (0.6%), diarrhea (0.6%), vomiting (0.3%) and rash (0.4%).

Adverse Laboratory Changes

Adverse laboratory changes without regard to drug relationship that were reported during clinical trials were:

Hemic: decreased hemoglobin and hematocrit, eosinophilia, increased and decreased WBC, increased and decreased platelets, decreased erythrocytes, and increased prothrombin time.

Hepatic: increased AST, ALT, alkaline phosphatase, and bilirubin.

Renal: increased BUN and creatinine.

Urinalysis: presence of red blood cells, white blood cells, casts, and bacteria in the urine.

Potential ADVERSE EFFECTS:

In addition, a variety of adverse effects, not observed in clinical trials with PRIMAXIN I.M., have been reported with intravenous administration of PRIMAXIN I.V. (Imipenem and Cilastatin for Injection). Those listed below are to serve as alerting information to physicians.

Systemic Adverse Reactions

The most frequently reported systemic adverse clinical reactions that were reported as possibly, probably or definitely related to PRIMAXIN I.V. (Imipenem and Cilastatin for Injection) were fever, hypotension, seizures (see PRECAUTIONS), dizziness, pruritus, urticaria, and somnolence.

Additional adverse systemic clinical reactions reported possibly, probably or definitely drug related or reported since the drug was marketed are listed within each body system in order of decreasing severity: *Gastrointestinal:* pseudomembranous colitis (the onset of pseudomembranous colitis symptoms may occur during or after antibiotic treatment, see WARNINGS), hemorrhagic colitis, hepatitis, jaundice, gastroenteritis, abdominal pain, glossitis, tongue papillar hypertrophy, staining of the teeth and/or tongue, heartburn, pharyngeal pain, increased salivation; *Hematologic:* pancytopenia, bone marrow depression, thrombocytopenia, neutropenia, leukopenia, hemolytic anemia; *CNS:* encephalopathy, tremor, confusion, myoclonus, paresthesia, vertigo, headache, psychic disturbances including hallucinations; *Special Senses:* hearing loss, tinnitus, taste perversion; *Respiratory:* chest discomfort, dyspnea, hyperventilation, thoracic spine pain; *Cardiovascular:* palpitations, tachycardia; *Renal:* acute renal failure, oliguria/anuria, polyuria, urine discoloration; *Skin:* toxic epidermal necrolysis, Stevens-Johnson syndrome, erythema multiforme, angioneurotic edema, flushing, cyanosis, hyperhidrosis, skin texture changes, candidiasis, pruritus vulvae; *Body as a whole:* polyarthralgia, asthenia/weakness, drug fever.

Adverse Laboratory Changes

Adverse laboratory changes without regard to drug relationship that were reported during clinical trials or reported since the drug was marketed were:

Hepatic: increased LDH; *Hemic:* positive Coombs test, decreased neutrophils, agranulocytosis, increased monocytes, abnormal prothrombin time, increased lymphocytes, increased basophils; *Electrolytes:* decreased serum sodium, increased potassium, increased chloride; *Urinalysis:* presence of urine protein, urine bilirubin, and urine urobilinogen.

Lidocaine HCl —Refer to the package circular for lidocaine HCl.

OVERDOSAGE

The acute intravenous toxicity of imipenem-cilastatin sodium in a ratio of 1:1 was studied in mice at doses of 751 to 1359 mg/kg. Following drug administration, ataxia was rapidly produced and clonic convulsions were noted in about 45 minutes. Deaths occurred within 4–56 minutes at all doses.

The acute intravenous toxicity of imipenem-cilastatin sodium was produced within 5–10 minutes in rats at doses of 771 to 1583 mg/kg. In all dosage groups, females had decreased activity, bradypnea and ptosis with clonic convulsions preceding death; in males, ptosis was seen at all dose levels while tremors and clonic convulsions were seen at all but the lowest dose (771 mg/kg). In another rat study, female rats showed ataxia, bradypnea and decreased activity in all but the lowest dose (550 mg/kg); deaths were preceded by clonic convulsions. Male rats showed tremors at all doses and clonic convulsions and ptosis were seen at the two highest doses (1130 and 1734 mg/kg). Deaths occurred between 6 and 88 minutes with doses of 771 to 1734 mg/kg.

In the case of overdosage, discontinue PRIMAXIN I.M., treat symptomatically, and institute supportive measures as required. Imipenem-cilastatin sodium is hemodialyzable. However, usefulness of this procedure in the overdosage setting is questionable.

DOSAGE GUIDELINES

Type†/Location of Infection	Severity	Dosage Regimen
Lower respiratory tract Skin and skin structure Gynecologic	Mild/Moderate	500 or 750 mg q 12 h depending on the severity of infection
Intra-abdominal	Mild/Moderate	750 mg q 12 h

† See INDICATIONS AND USAGE section.

DOSAGE AND ADMINISTRATION

PRIMAXIN I.M. is for intramuscular use only.

The dosage recommendations for PRIMAXIN I.M. represent the quantity of imipenem to be administered. An equivalent amount of cilastatin is also present.

Patients with lower respiratory tract infections, skin and skin structure infections, and gynecologic infections of mild to moderate severity may be treated with 500 mg or 750 mg administered every 12 hours depending on the severity of the infection.

Intra-abdominal infection may be treated with 750 mg every 12 hours.

[See table at bottom of previous page]

Total daily IM dosages greater than 1500 mg per day are not recommended.

The dosage for any particular patient should be based on the location of and severity of the infection, the susceptibility of the infecting pathogen(s), and renal function.

The duration of therapy depends upon the type and severity of the infection. Generally, PRIMAXIN I.M. should be continued for at least two days after the signs and symptoms of infection have resolved. Safety and efficacy of treatment beyond fourteen days have not been established.

PRIMAXIN I.M. should be administered by deep intramuscular injection into a large muscle mass (such as the gluteal muscles or lateral part of the thigh) with a 21 gauge 2″ needle. Aspiration is necessary to avoid inadvertent injection into a blood vessel.

ADULTS WITH IMPAIRED RENAL FUNCTION

The safety and efficacy of PRIMAXIN I.M. have not been studied in patients with creatinine clearance of less than 20 mL/ min/1.73m². Serum creatinine alone may not be a sufficiently accurate measure of renal function. Creatinine clearance (T_{cc}) may be estimated from the following equation:

$$T_{cc} \text{ (Males)} = \frac{\text{(wt. in kg) } (140 - \text{age})}{(72) \text{ (creatinine in mg/dL)}}$$

$$T_{cc} \text{ (Females)} = 0.85 \times \text{above value}$$

PREPARATION FOR ADMINISTRATION

PRIMAXIN I.M. should be prepared for use with 1.0% lidocaine HCl solution† (without epinephrine). PRIMAXIN I.M. 500 should be prepared with 2 mL and PRIMAXIN I.M. 750 with 3 mL of lidocaine HCl. Agitate to form a suspension then withdraw and inject the entire contents of vial intramuscularly. The suspension of PRIMAXIN I.M. in lidocaine HCl should be used within one hour after preparation. **Note: The IM formulation is not for IV use.**

---

†Refer to the package circular for lidocaine HCl for detailed information concerning CONTRAINDICATIONS, WARNINGS, PRECAUTIONS, and ADVERSE REACTIONS.

COMPATIBILITY AND STABILITY

Before reconsitution:
The dry powder should be stored at a temperature below 25°C (77°F).

Suspensions for IM Administration
Suspensions of PRIMAXIN I.M. are white to light tan in color. Variations of color within this range do not affect the potency of the product.

The suspension of PRIMAXIN I.M. in lidocaine HCl should be used within one hour after preparation.

PRIMAXIN I.M. should not be mixed with or physically added to other antibiotics. However, PRIMAXIN I.M. may be administered concomitantly but at separate sites with other antibiotics, such as aminoglycosides.

HOW SUPPLIED

PRIMAXIN I.M. is supplied as a sterile powder mixture in vials for IM administration as follows:

No. 3582—500 mg imipenem equivalent and 500 mg cilastatin equivalent
NDC 0006-3582-75 in trays of 10 vials
(6505-01-337-3131 500 mg, 10's).

No. 3583—750 mg imipenem equivalent and 750 mg cilastatin equivalent
NDC 0006-3583-76 in trays of 10 vials
(6505-01-337-3130 750 mg, 10's).

REFERENCES

1. National Committee for Clinical Laboratory Standards, Performance Standards for Antimicrobial Disk Susceptibility Tests— Fourth Edition. Approved Standard NCCLS Document M2-A4, Vol. 10, No. 7 NCCLS, Villanova, PA, 1990.
2. National Committee for Clinical Laboratory Standards, Methods for Dilution Antimicrobial Susceptibility Tests for Bacteria that Grow Aerobically—Second Edition. Approved Standard NCCLS Document M7-A2, Vol. 10, No. 8 NCCLS, Villanova, PA, 1990.

3. National Committee for Clinical Laboratory Standards, Methods for Antimicrobial Susceptibility Testing of Anaerobic Bacteria—Second Edition. Tentative Standard NCCLS Document M11-T2, Villanova, PA, 1988.
    7632907   Issued August 1996
COPYRIGHT© MERCK & CO., INC., 1985, 1990
All rights reserved

PRIMAXIN® I.V.   ℞
(Imipenem and Cilastatin for Injection)
(Formerly called IMIPENEM-CILASTATIN SODIUM FOR INJECTION)

For Intravenous Injection Only

DESCRIPTION

PRIMAXIN† I.V. (Imipenem and Cilastatin for Injection) is a sterile formulation of imipenem (a thienamycin antibiotic) and cilastatin sodium (the inhibitor of the renal dipeptidase, dehydropeptidase I), with sodium bicarbonate added as a buffer. PRIMAXIN I.V. is a potent broad spectrum antibacterial agent for intravenous administration.

Imipenem (N-formimidoylthienamycin monohydrate) is a crystalline derivative of thienamycin, which is produced by *Streptomyces cattleya*. Its chemical name is (5R ,6S)-3-[[2-(formimidoylamino)ethyl]thio]-6-[(R)-1-hydroxyethyl]-7-oxo-1-azabicyclo[3.2.0]hept-2-ene-2-carboxylic acid monohydrate. It is an off-white, nonhygroscopic crystalline compound with a molecular weight of 317.37. It is sparingly soluble in water and slightly soluble in methanol. Its empirical formula is $C_{12}H_{17}N_3O_4S \cdot H_2O$, and its structural formula is:

Cilastatin sodium is the sodium salt of a derivatized heptenoic acid. Its chemical name is sodium (Z)-7-[[(R)-2-amino-2-carboxyethyl]thio] -2- [(S) - 2,2- dimethylcyclopropanecarboxamido]-2-heptenoate. It is an off-white to yellowish-white, hygroscopic, amorphous compound with a molecular weight of 380.43. It is very soluble in water and in methanol. Its empirical formula is $C_{16}H_{25}N_2O_5S$ Na, and its structural formula is:

PRIMAXIN I.V. is buffered to provide solutions in the pH range of 6.5 to 7.5. There is no significant change in pH when solutions are prepared and used as directed. (See **COMPATIBILITY AND STABILITY**.) PRIMAXIN I.V. 250 contains 18.8 mg of sodium (0.8 mEq) and PRIMAXIN I.V. 500 contains 37.5 mg of sodium (1.6 mEq). Solutions of PRIMAXIN I.V. range from colorless to yellow. Variations of color within this range do not affect the potency of the product.

---

†Registered trademark of MERCK & CO., INC.

CLINICAL PHARMACOLOGY

Adults
Intravenous Administration
Intravenous infusion of PRIMAXIN I.V. over 20 minutes results in peak plasma levels of imipenem antimicrobial activity that range from 14 to 24 µg/mL for the 250 mg dose, from 21 to 58 µg/mL for the 500 mg dose, and from 41 to 83 µg/mL for the 1000 mg dose. At these doses, plasma levels of imipenem antimicrobial activity decline to below 1 µg/mL or less in 4 to 6 hours. Peak plasma levels of cilastatin following a 20-minute intravenous infusion of PRIMAXIN I.V., range from 15 to 25 µg/mL for the 250 mg dose, from 31 to 49 µg/mL for the 500 mg dose, and from 56 to 88 µg/mL for the 1000 mg dose.

The plasma half-life of each component is approximately 1 hour. The binding of imipenem to human serum proteins is approximately 20% and that of cilastatin is approximately 40%. Approximately, 70% of the administered imipenem is recovered in the urine within 10 hours after which no further urinary excretion is detectable. Urine concentrations of imipenem in excess of 10 µg/mL can be maintained for up to 8 hours with PRIMAXIN I.V. at the 500-mg dose. Approximately, 70% of the cilastatin sodium dose is recovered in the urine within 10 hours of administration of PRIMAXIN I.V. No accumulation of imipenem/cilastatin in plasma or urine is observed with regimens administered as frequently as every 6 hours in patients with normal renal function.

Imipenem, when administered alone, is metabolized in the kidneys by dehydropeptidase I resulting in relatively low levels in urine. Cilastatin sodium, an inhibitor of this enzyme, effectively prevents renal metabolism of imipenem so that when imipenem and cilastatin sodium are given concomitantly, fully adequate antibacterial levels of imipenem are achieved in the urine.

After a 1 gram dose of PRIMAXIN I.V., the following average levels of imipenem were measured (usually at 1 hour post-dose except where indicated) in the tissues and fluids listed:

[See table at top of next page]

Imipenem-cilastatin sodium is hemodialyzable. However, usefulness of this procedure in the overdosage setting is questionable. (See **OVERDOSAGE**.)

Microbiology
The bactericidal activity of imipenem results from the inhibition of cell wall synthesis. Its greatest affinity is for penicillin binding proteins (PBPs) 1A, 1B, 2, 4, 5 and 6 of *Escherichia coli*, and 1A, 1B, 2, 4 and 5 of *Pseudomonas aeruginosa*. The lethal effect is related to binding to PBP 2 and PBP 1B.

Imipenem has a high degree of stability in the presence of beta-lactamases, both penicillinases and cephalosporinases produced by gram-negative and gram-positive bacteria. It is a potent inhibitor of beta-lactamases from certain gram-negative bacteria which are inherently resistant to most beta-lactam antibiotics, e.g., *Pseudomonas aeruginosa*, *Serratia* spp., and *Enterobacter* spp.

Imipenem has *in vitro* activity against a wide range of gram-positive and gram-negative organisms. Imipenem is active against most strains of the following microorganisms *in vitro* and in clinical infections treated with the intravenous formulation of imipenem-cilastatin sodium. (See **INDICATIONS AND USAGE.**)

Gram-positive aerobes:
    Enterococcus faecalis (formerly *S. faecalis*)
        (NOTE: Imipenem is inactive *in vitro* against *Enterococcus faecium* [formerly *S. faecium*].)
    Staphylococcus aureus including penicillinase-producing strains
    Staphylococcus epidermidis including penicillinase-producing strains
        (NOTE: Methicillin-resistant staphylococci should be reported as resistant to imipenem.)
    Streptococcus agalactiae (Group B streptococcus)
    Streptococcus pneumoniae
    Streptococcus pyogenes
Gram-negative aerobes:
    Acinetobacter spp.
    Citrobacter spp.
    Enterobacter spp.
    Escherichia coli
    Gardnerella vaginalis
    Haemophilus influenzae
    Haemophilus parainfluenzae
    Klebsiella spp.
    Morganella morganii
    Proteus vulgaris
    Providencia rettgeri
    Pseudomonas aeruginosa
        (NOTE: Imipenem is inactive *in vitro* against *Xanthomonas (Pseudomonas) maltophilia* and some strains of *P. cepacia*.)
    Serratia spp., including *S. marcescens*
Gram-positive anaerobes:
    Bifidobacterium spp.
    Clostridium spp.
    Eubacterium spp.
    Peptococcus spp.
    Peptostreptococcus spp.
    Propionibacterium spp.
Gram-negative anaerobes:
    Bacteroides spp., including *B. fragilis*
Fusobacterium spp.
The following *in vitro* data are available, **but their clinical significance is unknown.**

Imipenem exhibits *in vitro* minimum inhibitory concentrations (MIC's) of 4 µg/mL or less against most (≥90%) strains of the following microorganisms; however, the safety and effectiveness of imipenem in treating clinical infections due to these microorganisms have not been established in adequate and well-controlled clinical trials.

Continued on next page

Primaxin I.V.—Cont.

Gram-positive aerobes:
 Listeria monocytogenes
 Nocardia spp.
 Group C streptococcus
 Group G streptococcus
 Viridans group streptococci
Gram-negative aerobes:
 Achromobacter spp.
 Aeromonas hydrophila
 Alcaligenes spp.
 Bordetella bronchiseptica
 Campylobacter spp.
 Hafnia alvei
 Klebsiella oxytoca
 Klebsiella pneumoniae
 Moraxella spp.
 Neisseria gonorrhoeae including penicillinase-producing strains
 Pasteurella multocida
 Plesiomonas shigelloides
 Proteus mirabilis
 Providencia stuartii
 Salmonella spp.
 Serratia proteamaculans (formerly *S. liquefaciens*)
 Shigella spp.
 Yersinia spp., including *Y. enterocolitica* and *Y. pseudotuberculosis*
Gram-positive anaerobes:
 Actinomyces spp.
 Clostridium perfringens
 Propionibacterium acnes
Gram-negative anaerobes:
 Bacteroides spp., including *B. bivius, B. disiens, B. distasonis, B. intermedius* (formerly *B. melaninogenicus intermedius*), *B. ovatus, B. thetaiotaomicron,* and *B. vulgatus*
 Porphyromonas asaccharolytica (formerly *B. asaccharolyticus*)
 Veillonella spp.

In vitro tests show imipenem to act synergistically with aminoglycoside antibiotics against some isolates of *Pseudomonas aeruginosa.*

Susceptibility Tests:

Measurement of MIC or minimum bactericidal concentration (MBC) and achieved antimicrobial compound concentrations may be appropriate to guide therapy in some infections. (See **CLINICAL PHARMACOLOGY** section for further information on drug concentrations achieved in infected body sites and other pharmacokinetic properties of this antimicrobial drug product.)

Diffusion techniques:

Quantitative methods that require measurement of zone diameters provide reproducible estimates of the susceptibility of bacteria to antimicrobial compounds. One such standardized procedure[1] that has been recommended for use with disks to test the susceptibility of microorganisms to imipenem uses the 10-µg imipenem disk. Interpretation involves correlation of the diameter obtained in the disk test with the MIC for imipenem.

Reports from the laboratory providing results of the standard single-disk susceptibility test with a 10-µg imipenem disk should be interpreted according to the following criteria:

Zone Diameter (mm)	Interpretation
≥16	Susceptible (S)
14–15	Intermediate (I)
≤13	Resistant (R)

A report of "Susceptible" indicates that the pathogen is likely to be inhibited by usually achievable concentrations of the antimicrobial compound in blood. A report of "Intermediate" indicates that the result should be considered equivocal, and, if the microorganism is not fully susceptible to alternative, clinically feasible drugs, the test should be repeated. This category implies possible clinical applicability in body sites where the drug is physiologically concentrated or in situations where high dosage of drug can be used. This category also provides a buffer zone that prevents small uncontrolled technical factors from causing major discrepancies in interpretation. A report of "Resistant" indicates that usually achievable concentrations of the antimicrobial compound in the blood are unlikely to be inhibitory and that other therapy should be selected.

Standardized susceptibility test procedures require the use of laboratory control microorganisms. The 10-µg imipenem disk should provide the following diameters in these laboratory test quality control strains:

Microorganism	Zone Diameter (mm)
E. coli ATCC 25922	26–32
P. aeruginosa ATCC 27853	20–28

Dilution techniques:

Quantitative methods that are used to determine MIC's provide reproducible estimates of the susceptibility of bacteria

Tissue or Fluid	n	Imipenem Level µg/mL or µg/g	Range
Vitreous Humor	3	3.4 (3.5 hours post dose)	2.88–3.6
Aqueous Humor	5	2.99 (2 hours post dose)	2.4–3.9
Lung Tissue	8	5.6 (median)	3.5–15.5
Sputum	1	2.1	—
Pleural	1	22.0	—
Peritoneal	12	23.9 S.D. ±5.3 (2 hours post dose)	—
Bile	2	5.3 (2.25 hours post dose)	4.6 to 6.0
CSF (uninflamed)	5	1.0 (4 hours post dose)	0.26–2.0
CSF (inflamed)	7	2.6 (2 hours post dose)	0.5–5.5
Fallopian Tubes	1	13.6	—
Endometrium	1	11.1	—
Myometrium	1	5.0	—
Bone	10	2.6	0.4–5.4
Interstitial Fluid	12	16.4	10.0–22.6
Skin	12	4.4	NA
Fascia	12	4.4	NA

to antimicrobial compounds. One such procedure uses a standardized dilution method[2] (broth, agar, or microdilution) or equivalent with imipenem powder.

The MIC values obtained should be interpreted according to the following criteria:

MIC (µg/mL)	Interpretation
≤4	Susceptible (S)
8	Intermediate (I)
≥16	Resistant (R)

Interpretation should be as stated above for results using diffusion techniques.

As with standard diffusion techniques, dilution methods require the use of laboratory control microorganisms. Standard imipenem powder should provide the following MIC values:

Microorganism	MIC (µg/mL)
E. coli ATCC 25922	0.06–0.25
S. aureus ATCC 29213	0.015–0.06
E. faecalis ATCC 29212	0.5–2.0
P. aeruginosa ATCC 27853	1.0–4.0

Anaerobic techniques:

For anaerobic bacteria, the susceptibility to imipenem can be determined by the reference agar dilution method or by alternate standardized test methods.[3]

As with other susceptibility techniques, the use of laboratory control microorganisms is required. Standard imipenem powder should provide the following MIC values:
Reference Agar Dilution Testing:

Microorganism	MIC (µg/mL)
B. fragilis ATCC 25285	0.03–0.12
B. thetaiotaomicron ATCC 29741	0.06–0.25
E. lentum ATCC 43055	0.25–1.0

Broth Microdilution Testing:

Microorganism	MIC (µg/mL)
B. thetaiotaomicron ATCC 29741	0.06–0.25
E. lentum ATCC 43055	0.12–0.5

INDICATIONS AND USAGE

PRIMAXIN I.V. is indicated for the treatment of serious infections caused by susceptible strains of the designated microorganisms in the conditions listed below:

(1) **Lower respiratory tract infections.** *Staphylococcus aureus* (penicillinase-producing strains), *Acinetobacter* species, *Enterobacter* species, *Escherichia coli, Haemophilus influenzae, Haemophilus parainfluenzae*, Klebsiella* species, *Serratia marcescens*

(2) **Urinary tract infections** (complicated and uncomplicated). *Enterococcus faecalis, Staphylococcus aureus* (penicillinase-producing strains)*, *Enterobacter* species, *Escherichia coli, Klebsiella* species, *Morganella morganii*, Proteus vulgaris*, Providencia rettgeri*, Pseudomonas aeruginosa*

(3) **Intra-abdominal infections.** *Enterococcus faecalis, Staphylococcus aureus* (penicillinase-producing strains)*, *Staphylococcus epidermidis, Citrobacter* species, *Enterobacter* species, *Escherichia coli, Klebsiella* species, *Morganella morganii*, Proteus* species, *Pseudomonas aeruginosa, Bifidobacterium* species, *Clostridium* species, *Eubacterium* species, *Peptococcus* species, *Peptostreptococcus* species, *Propionibacterium* species*, *Bacteroides* species including *B. fragilis, Fusobacterium* species

(4) **Gynecologic infections.** *Enterococcus faecalis, Staphylococcus aureus* (penicillinase-producing strains)*, *Staphylococcus epidermidis, Streptococcus agalactiae* (Group B streptococcus), *Enterobacter* species*, *Escherichia coli, Gardnerella vaginalis, Klebsiella* species*, *Proteus* spe-

cies, *Bifidobacterium* species*, *Peptococcus* species*, *Peptostreptococcus* species, *Propionibacterium* species*, *Bacteroides* species including *B. fragilis**

(5) **Bacterial septicemia.** *Enterococcus faecalis, Staphylococcus aureus* (penicillinase-producing strains), *Enterobacter* species, *Escherichia coli, Klebsiella* species, *Pseudomonas aeruginosa, Serratia* species*, *Bacteroides* species including *B. fragilis**

(6) **Bone and joint infections.** *Enterococcus faecalis, Staphylococcus aureus* (penicillinase-producing strains), *Staphylococcus epidermidis, Enterobacter* species, *Pseudomonas aeruginosa*

(7) **Skin and skin structure infections.** *Enterococcus faecalis, Staphylococcus aureus* (penicillinase-producing strains), *Staphylococcus epidermidis, Acinetobacter* species, *Citrobacter* species, *Enterobacter* species, *Escherichia coli, Klebsiella* species, *Morganella morganii, Proteus vulgaris, Providencia rettgeri*, Pseudomonas aeruginosa, Serratia* species, *Peptococcus* species, *Peptostreptococcus* species, *Bacteroides* species including *B. fragilis, Fusobacterium* species*

(8) **Endocarditis.** *Staphylococcus aureus* (penicillinase-producing strains)

(9) **Polymicrobic infections.** PRIMAXIN I.V. is indicated for polymicrobic infections including those in which *S. pneumoniae* (pneumonia, septicemia), *S. pyogenes* (skin and skin structure), or nonpenicillinase-producing *S. aureus* is one of the causative organisms. However, monobacterial infections due to these organisms are usually treated with narrower spectrum antibiotics, such as penicillin G.

PRIMAXIN I.V. is not indicated in patients with meningitis because safety and efficacy have not been established.

For Pediatric Use information, See **PRECAUTIONS**, *Pediatric Use,* and **DOSAGE AND ADMINISTRATION** sections.

Because of its broad spectrum of bactericidal activity against gram-positive and gram-negative aerobic and anaerobic bacteria, PRIMAXIN I.V. is useful for the treatment of mixed infections and as presumptive therapy prior to the identification of the causative organisms.

Although clinical improvement has been observed in patients with cystic fibrosis, chronic pulmonary disease, and lower respiratory tract infections caused by *Pseudomonas aeruginosa,* bacterial eradication may not necessarily be achieved.

As with other beta-lactam antibiotics, some strains of *Pseudomonas aeruginosa* may develop resistance fairly rapidly during treatment with PRIMAXIN I.V. During therapy of *Pseudomonas aeruginosa* infections, periodic susceptibility testing should be done when clinically appropriate.

Infections resistant to other antibiotics, for example, cephalosporins, penicillin, and aminoglycosides, have been shown to respond to treatment with PRIMAXIN I.V.

---

*Efficacy for this organism in this organ system was studied in fewer than 10 infections.

CONTRAINDICATIONS

PRIMAXIN I.V. is contraindicated in patients who have shown hypersensitivity to any component of this product.

WARNINGS

SERIOUS AND OCCASIONALLY FATAL HYPERSENSITIVITY (ANAPHYLACTIC) REACTIONS HAVE BEEN REPORTED IN PATIENTS RECEIVING THERAPY WITH BETA-LACTAMS. THESE REACTIONS ARE MORE APT TO OCCUR IN PERSONS WITH A HISTORY OF SENSITIVITY TO MULTIPLE ALLERGENS.
THERE HAVE BEEN REPORTS OF PATIENTS WITH A HISTORY OF PENICILLIN HYPERSENSITIVITY WHO

HAVE EXPERIENCED SEVERE HYPERSENSITIVITY REACTIONS WHEN TREATED WITH ANOTHER BETA-LACTAM. BEFORE INITIATING THERAPY WITH PRIMAXIN I.V., CAREFUL INQUIRY SHOULD BE MADE CONCERNING PREVIOUS HYPERSENSITIVITY REACTIONS TO PENICILLINS, CEPHALOSPORINS, OTHER BETA-LACTAMS, AND OTHER ALLERGENS. IF AN ALLERGIC REACTION OCCURS, PRIMAXIN SHOULD BE DISCONTINUED.

SERIOUS ANAPHYLACTIC REACTIONS REQUIRE IMMEDIATE EMERGENCY TREATMENT WITH EPINEPHRINE. OXYGEN, INTRAVENOUS STEROIDS, AND AIRWAY MANAGEMENT, INCLUDING INTUBATION, MAY ALSO BE ADMINISTERED AS INDICATED.

Seizures and other CNS adverse experiences, such as confusional states and myoclonic activity, have been reported during treatment with PRIMAXIN I.V. (See **PRECAUTIONS**.)

Pseudomembranous colitis has been reported with nearly all antibacterial agents, including imipenem-cilastatin sodium, and may range in severity from mild to life threatening. Therefore, it is important to consider this diagnosis in patients who present with diarrhea subsequent to the administration of antibacterial agents.

Treatment with antibacterial agents alters the normal flora of the colon and may permit overgrowth of clostridia. Studies indicate that a toxin produced by *Clostridium difficile* is one primary cause of "antibiotic-associated colitis".

After the diagnosis of pseudomembranous colitis has been established, therapeutic measures should be initiated. Mild cases of pseudomembranous colitis usually respond to drug discontinuation alone. In moderate to severe cases, consideration should be given to management with fluids and electrolytes, protein supplementation and treatment with an antibacterial drug clinically effective against *C. difficile* colitis.

PRECAUTIONS

General

CNS adverse experiences such as confusional states, myoclonic activity, and seizures have been reported during treatment with PRIMAXIN I.V., especially when recommended dosages were exceeded. These experiences have occurred most commonly in patients with CNS disorders (e.g., brain lesions or history of seizures) and/or compromised renal function. However, there have been reports of CNS adverse experiences in patients who had no recognized or documented underlying CNS disorder or compromised renal function.

When recommended doses were exceeded, adult patients with creatinine clearances of ≤20 mL/min/1.73 m^2, whether or not undergoing hemodialysis, had a higher risk of seizure activity than those without impairment of renal function. Therefore, close adherence to the dosing guidelines for these patients is recommended. (See **DOSAGE AND ADMINISTRATION**.)

Patients with creatinine clearances of ≤5 mL/min/1.73 m^2 should not receive PRIMAXIN I.V. unless hemodialysis is instituted within 48 hours.

For patients on hemodialysis, PRIMAXIN I.V. is recommended only when the benefit outweighs the potential risk of seizures.

Close adherence to the recommended dosage and dosage schedules is urged, especially in patients with known factors that predispose to convulsive activity. Anticonvulsant therapy should be continued in patients with known seizure disorders. If focal tremors, myoclonus, or seizures occur, patients should be evaluated neurologically, placed on anticonvulsant therapy if not already instituted, and the dosage of PRIMAXIN I.V. re-examined to determine whether it should be decreased or the antibiotic discontinued.

As with other antibiotics, prolonged use of PRIMAXIN I.V. may result in overgrowth of nonsusceptible organisms. Repeated evaluation of the patient's condition is essential. If superinfection occurs during therapy, appropriate measures should be taken.

Laboratory Tests

While PRIMAXIN I.V. possesses the characteristic low toxicity of the beta-lactam group of antibiotics, periodic assessment of organ system functions, including renal, hepatic, and hematopoietic, is advisable during prolonged therapy.

Drug Interactions

Generalized seizures have been reported in patients who received ganciclovir and PRIMAXIN. These drugs should not be used concomitantly unless the potential benefits outweigh the risks.

Since concomitant administration of PRIMAXIN and probenecid results in only minimal increases in plasma levels of imipenem and plasma half-life, it is not recommended that probenecid be given with PRIMAXIN.

PRIMAXIN should not be mixed with or physically added to other antibiotics. However, PRIMAXIN may be administered concomitantly with other antibiotics, such as aminoglycosides.

Carcinogenesis, Mutagenesis, Impairment of Fertility

Long term studies in animals have not been performed to evaluate carcinogenic potential of imipenem-cilastatin. Genetic toxicity studies were performed in a variety of bacterial and mammalian tests in *in vivo* and *in vitro.* The tests used were: V79 mammalian cell mutagenesis assay (imipenem-cilastatin sodium alone and imipenem alone), Ames test (cilastatin sodium alone and imipenem alone), unscheduled DNA synthesis assay (imipenem-cilastatin sodium) and *in vivo* mouse cytogenetics test (imipenem-cilastatin sodium). None of these tests showed any evidence of genetic alterations.

Reproductive tests in male and female rats were performed with imipenem-cilastatin sodium at dosage levels up to 11 times† the usual human dose of the intravenous formulation (on a mg/kg basis). Slight decreases in live fetal body weight were restricted to the highest dosage level. No other adverse effects were observed on fertility, reproductive performance, fetal viability, growth or postnatal development of pups. Similarly, no adverse effects on the fetus or on lactation were observed when imipenem-cilastatin sodium was administered to rats late in gestation.

Pregnancy: Teratogenic Effects

Pregnancy Category C: Teratology studies with cilastatin sodium in rabbits and rats at 6 and 20 times† the maximum recommended human dose of the intravenous formulation of imipenem-cilastatin sodium (50 mg/kg/day†), respectively, showed no evidence of adverse effect on the fetus. No evidence of teratogenicity was observed in rabbits and rats given imipenem at doses up to 1 and 18 times† the maximum recommended daily human dose of the intravenous formulation of imipenem-cilastatin sodium, respectively.

Teratology studies with imipenem-cilastatin sodium at doses up to 11 times† the usual recommended human dose of the intravenous formulation (30 mg/kg/day†) in pregnant mice and rats during the period of major organogenesis revealed no evidence of teratogenicity.

Imipenem-cilastatin sodium, when administered to pregnant rabbits at dosages equivalent to the usual human dose of the intravenous formulation and higher, caused body weight loss, diarrhea, and maternal deaths. When comparable doses of imipenem-cilastatin sodium were given to non-pregnant rabbits, body weight loss, diarrhea, and deaths were also observed. This intolerance is not unlike that seen with other beta-lactam antibiotics in this species and is probably due to alteration of gut flora.

A teratology study in pregnant cynomolgus monkeys given imipenem-cilastatin sodium at doses of 40 mg/kg/day (bolus intravenous injection) or 160 mg/kg/day (subcutaneous injection) resulted in maternal toxicity including emesis, inappetence, body weight loss, diarrhea, abortion, and death in some cases. In contrast, no significant toxicity was observed when non-pregnant cynomolgus monkeys were given doses of imipenem-cilastatin sodium up to 180 mg/kg/day (subcutaneous injection). When doses of imipenem-cilastatin sodium (approximately 100 mg/kg/day or approximately 2 times† the maximum recommended daily human dose of the intravenous formulation) were administered to pregnant cynomolgus monkeys at an intravenous infusion rate which mimics human clinical use, there was minimal maternal intolerance (occasional emesis), no maternal deaths, no evidence of teratogenicity, but an increase in embryonic loss relative to control groups.

There are, however, no adequate and well-controlled studies in pregnant women. PRIMAXIN I.V. should be used during pregnancy only if the potential benefit justifies the potential risk to the mother and fetus.

Nursing Mothers

It is not known whether imipenem-cilastatin sodium is excreted in human milk. Because many drugs are excreted in human milk, caution should be exercised when PRIMAXIN I.V. is administered to a nursing woman.

Pediatric Use

Use of PRIMAXIN I.V. in pediatric patients, neonates to 16 years of age, is supported by evidence from adequate and well-controlled studies of PRIMAXIN I.V. in adults and by the following clinical studies and published literature in pediatric patients: Based on published studies of 178** pediatric patients ≥3 months of age (with non-CNS infections), the recommended dose of PRIMAXIN I.V. is 15–25 mg/kg/dose administered every six hours. Doses of 25 mg/kg/dose in patients 3 months to <3 years of age, and 15 mg/kg/dose in patients 3–12 years of age were associated with mean trough plasma concentrations of imipenem of 1.1±0.4 µg/mL and 0.6±0.2 µg/mL following multiple 60-minute infusions, respectively; trough urinary concentrations of imipenem were in excess of 10 µg/mL for both doses. These doses have provided adequate plasma and urine concentrations for the treatment of non-CNS infections. Based on studies in adults, the maximum daily dose for treatment of infections with fully susceptible organisms is 2.0 g per day, and of infections with moderately susceptible organisms (primarily some strains of *P. aeruginosa*) is 4.0 g/day. (See Table 1, **DOSAGE AND ADMINISTRATION**.) Higher doses (up to 90 mg/kg/day in older children) have been used in patients with cystic fibrosis. (See **DOSAGE AND ADMINISTRATION**.)

Based on studies of 135*** pediatric patients ≤3 months of age (weighing ≥1,500 gms), the following dosage schedule is recommended for non-CNS infections:

- <1 wk of age: 25 mg/kg every 12 hrs
- 1–4 wks of age: 25 mg/kg every 8 hrs
- 4 wks-3 mos. of age: 25 mg/kg every 6 hrs.

In a published dose-ranging study of smaller premature infants (670–1,890 gms) in the first week of life, a dose of 20 mg/kg q12h by 15–30 minutes infusion was associated with mean peak and trough plasma imipenem concentrations of 43 µg/mL and 1.7 µg/mL after multiple doses, respectively. However, moderate accumulation of cilastatin in neonates may occur following multiple doses of PRIMAXIN I.V. The safety of this accumulation is unknown.

PRIMAXIN I.V. is not recommended in pediatric patients with CNS infections because of the risk of seizures.

PRIMAXIN I.V. is not recommended in pediatric patients <30 kg with impaired renal function, as no data are available.

† Based on patient weight of 70 kg.
** Two patients were less than 3 months of age.
*** One patient was greater than 3 months of age.

ADVERSE REACTIONS

Adults

PRIMAXIN I.V. is generally well tolerated. Many of the 1,723 patients treated in clinical trials were severely ill and had multiple background diseases and physiological impairments, making it difficult to determine causal relationship of adverse experiences to therapy with PRIMAXIN I.V.

Local Adverse Reactions

Adverse local clinical reactions that were reported as possibly, probably or definitely related to therapy with PRIMAXIN I.V. were:

- Phlebitis/thrombophlebitis—3.1%
- Pain at the injection site—0.7%
- Erythema at the injection site—0.4%
- Vein induration—0.2%
- Infused vein infection—0.1%

Systemic Adverse Reactions

The most frequently reported systemic adverse clinical reactions that were reported as possibly, probably, or definitely related to PRIMAXIN I.V. were nausea (2.0%), diarrhea (1.8%), vomiting (1.5%), rash (0.9%), fever (0.5%), hypotension (0.4%), seizures (0.4%) (see **PRECAUTIONS**), dizziness (0.3%), pruritus (0.3%), urticaria (0.2%), somnolence (0.2%).

Additional adverse systemic clinical reactions reported as possibly, probably or definitely drug related occurring in less than 0.2% of the patients or reported since the drug was marketed are listed within each body system in order of decreasing severity: *Gastrointestinal* —pseudomembranous colitis (the onset of pseudomembranous colitis symptoms may occur during or after antibacterial treatment, see **WARNINGS**), hemorrhagic colitis, hepatitis, jaundice, gastroenteritis, abdominal pain, glossitis, tongue papillar hypertrophy, staining of the teeth and/or tongue, heartburn, pharyngeal pain, increased salivation; *Hematologic* —pancytopenia, bone marrow depression, thrombocytopenia, neutropenia, leukopenia, hemolytic anemia; *CNS* —encephalopathy, tremor, confusion, myoclonus, paresthesia, vertigo, headache, psychic disturbances including hallucinations; *Special Senses* —hearing loss, tinnitus, taste perversion; *Respiratory* —chest discomfort, dyspnea, hyperventilation, thoracic spine pain; *Cardiovascular* —palpitations, tachycardia; *Skin* —Stevens-Johnson syndrome, toxic epidermal necrolysis, erythema multiforme, angioneurotic edema, flushing, cyanosis, hyperhidrosis, skin texture changes, candidiasis, pruritus vulvae; *Body as a whole* —polyarthralgia, asthenia/weakness, drug fever; *Renal* —acute renal failure, oliguria/anuria, polyuria, urine discoloration. The role of PRIMAXIN I.V. in changes in renal function is difficult to assess, since factors predisposing to pre-renal azotemia or to impaired renal function usually have been present.

Adverse Laboratory Changes

Adverse laboratory changes without regard to drug relationship that were reported during clinical trials or reported since the drug was marketed were:

Hepatic: Increased ALT (SGPT), AST (SGOT), alkaline phosphatase, bilirubin and LDH

Hemic: Increased eosinophils, positive Coombs test, increased WBC, increased platelets, decreased hemoglobin and hematocrit, agranulocytosis, increased monocytes, abnormal prothrombin time, increased lymphocytes, increased basophils

Continued on next page

Information on the Merck & Co., Inc. products listed on these pages is the full prescribing information from product circulars in use August 31, 1998. For information, please call 1-800-NSC MERCK [1-800-672-6372].

Primaxin I.V.—Cont.

Electrolytes: Decreased serum sodium, increased potassium, increased chloride
Renal: Increased BUN, creatinine
Urinalysis: Presence of urine protein, urine red blood cells, urine white blood cells, urine casts, urine bilirubin, and urine urobilinogen
Pediatric Patients
In studies of 178 pediatric patients ≥3 months of age, the following adverse events were noted:

The Most Common Clinical Adverse Experiences Without Regard to Drug Relationship
(Patient Incidence >1%)

Adverse Experience	No. of Patients (%)
Digestive System	
Diarrhea	7* (3.9)
Gastroenteritis	2 (1.1)
Vomiting	2* (1.1)
Skin	
Rash	4 (2.2)
Irritation, I.V. site	2 (1.1)
Urogenital System	
Urine discoloration	2 (1.1)
Cardiovascular System	
Phlebitis	4 (2.2)

*One patient had both vomiting and diarrhea and is counted in each category.

In studies of 135 patients (newborn to 3 months of age), the following adverse events were noted:

The Most Common Clinical Adverse Experiences Without Regard to Drug Relationship
(Patient Incidence >1%)

Adverse Experience	No. of Patients (%)
Digestive System	
Diarrhea	4 (3.0%)
Oral Candidiasis	2 (1.5%)
Skin	
Rash	2 (1.5%)
Urogenital System	
Oliguria/anuria	3 (2.2%)
Cardiovascular System	
Tachycardia	2 (1.5%)
Nervous System	
Convulsions	8 (5.9%)

[See table at top right of page]

Patients (<3 Months of Age) With Normal Pretherapy but Abnormal During Therapy Laboratory Values

Laboratory Parameter	No. of Patients With Abnormalities* (%)
Eosinophil Count ↑	11 (9.0%)
Hematocrit ↓	3 (2.0%)
Hematocrit ↑	1 (1.0%)
Platelet Count ↑	5 (4.0%)
Platelet Count ↓	2 (2.0%)
Serum Creatinine ↑	5 (5.0%)
Bilirubin ↑	3 (3.0%)
Bilirubin ↓	1 (1.0%)
AST (SGOT) ↑	5 (6.0%)
ALT (SGPT) ↑	3 (3.0%)
Serum Alkaline Phosphate ↑	2 (3.0%)

*The denominator used for percentages was the number of patients for whom the test was performed during or post-treatment and, therefore, varies by test.

Examination of published literature and spontaneous adverse event reports suggested a similar spectrum of adverse events in adult and pediatric patients.

OVERDOSAGE

The acute intravenous toxicity of imipenem-cilastatin sodium in a ratio of 1:1 was studied in mice at doses of 751 to 1359 mg/kg. Following drug administration, ataxia was rapidly produced and clonic convulsions were noted in about 45 minutes. Deaths occurred within 4–56 minutes at all doses. The acute intravenous toxicity of imipenem-cilastatin sodium was produced within 5–10 minutes in rats at doses of 771 to 1583 mg/kg. In all dosage groups, females had decreased activity, bradypnea, and ptosis with clonic convulsions preceding death; in males, ptosis was seen at all dose levels while tremors and clonic convulsions were seen at all

Patients ≥3 Months of Age With Normal Pretherapy but Abnormal During Therapy Laboratory Values

Laboratory Parameter	Abnormality		No. of Patients With Abnormalities/ No. of Patients With Lab Done (%)	
Hemoglobin	Age	<5 mos.: <10 gm %	19/129	(14.7)
		6 mos.-12 yrs.: <11.5 gm%		
Hematocrit	Age	<5 mos.: <30 vol%	23/129	(17.8)
		6 mos.-12 yrs.: <34.5 vol %		
Neutrophils	≤1000/mm³ (absolute)		4/123	(3.3)
Eosinophils	≥7%		15/117	(12.8)
Platelet Count	≥500 ths/mm³		16/119	(13.4)
Urine Protein	≥1		8/97	(8.2)
Serum Creatinine	>1.2 mg/dl		0/105	(0)
BUN	>22 mg/dl		0/108	(0)
AST (SGOT)	>36 IU/L		14/78	(17.9)
ALT (SGPT)	>30 IU/L		10/93	(10.8)

but the lowest dose (771 mg/kg). In another rat study, female rats showed ataxia, bradypnea, and decreased activity in all but the lowest dose (550 mg/kg); deaths were preceded by clonic convulsions. Male rats showed tremors at all doses and clonic convulsions, and ptosis were seen at the two highest doses (1130 and 1734 mg/kg). Deaths occurred between 6 and 88 minutes with doses of 771 to 1734 mg/kg. In the case of overdosage, discontinue PRIMAXIN I.V., treat symptomatically, and institute supportive measures as required. Imipenem-cilastatin sodium is hemodialyzable. However, usefulness of this procedure in the overdosage setting is questionable.

DOSAGE AND ADMINISTRATION

Adults
The dosage recommendations for PRIMAXIN I.V. represent the quantity of imipenem to be administered. An equivalent amount of cilastatin is also present in the solution. Each 125 mg, 250 mg, or 500 mg dose should be given by intravenous administration over 20 to 30 minutes. Each 750 mg or 1000 mg dose should be infused over 40 to 60 minutes. In patients who develop nausea during the infusion, the rate of infusion may be slowed.
The total daily dosage for PRIMAXIN I.V. should be based on the type or severity of infection and given in equally divided doses based on consideration of degree of susceptibility of the pathogen(s), renal function, and body weight. Adult patients with impaired renal function, as judged by creatinine clearance ≤ 70 mL/min/1.73 m², require adjustment of dosage as described in the succeeding section of these guidelines.
Intravenous Dosage Schedule for Adults with Normal Renal Function and Body Weight ≥70 kg
Doses cited in Table I are based on a patient with normal renal function and a body weight of 70 kg. These doses should be used for a patient with a creatinine clearance of ≥71 mL/min/1.73 m² and a body weight of ≥70 kg. A reduction in dose must be made for a patient with a creatinine clearance ≤70 mL/min/1.73 m² and/or a body weight less than 70 kg. (See Tables II and III.)
Dosage regimens in column A of Table I are recommended for infections caused by fully susceptible organisms which represent the majority of pathogenic species. Dosage regimens in column B of Table I are recommended for infections caused by organisms with moderate susceptibility to imipenem, primarily some strains of *P. aeruginosa*.

TABLE I
INTRAVENOUS DOSAGE SCHEDULE FOR ADULTS WITH NORMAL RENAL FUNCTION AND BODY WEIGHT ≥ 70 kg

Type or Severity of Infection	A Fully susceptible organisms including gram-positive and gram-negative aerobes and anaerobes	B Moderately susceptible organisms, primarily some strains of *P. aeruginosa*
Mild	250 mg q6h (TOTAL DAILY DOSE=1.0g)	500 mg q6h (TOTAL DAILY DOSE=2.0g)
Moderate	500 mg q8h (TOTAL DAILY DOSE =1.5g) or 500 mg q6h (TOTAL DAILY DOSE=2.0g)	500 mg q6h (TOTAL DAILY DOSE=2.0g) or 1 g q8h (TOTAL DAILY DOSE=3.0g)
Severe, life threatening only	500 mg q6h (TOTAL DAILY DOSE=2.0g)	1 g q8h (TOTAL DAILY DOSE=3.0g) or 1 g q6h (TOTAL DAILY DOSE=4.0g)
Uncomplicated urinary tract infection	250 mg q6h (TOTAL DAILY DOSE=1.0g)	250 mg q6h (TOTAL DAILY DOSE=1.0g)
Complicated urinary tract infection	500 mg q6h (TOTAL DAILY DOSE=2.0g)	500 mg q6h (TOTAL DAILY DOSE=2.0g)

Due to the high antimicrobial activity of PRIMAXIN I.V., it is recommended that the maximum total daily dosage not exceed 50 mg/kg/day or 4.0 g/day, whichever is lower. There is no evidence that higher doses provide greater efficacy. However, patients over twelve years of age with cystic fibrosis and normal renal function have been treated with PRIMAXIN I.V. at doses up to 90 mg/kg/day in divided doses, not exceeding 4.0 g/day.

Reduced Intravenous Dosage Schedule for Adults with Impaired Renal Function and/or Body Weight <70 kg
Patients with creatinine clearance of ≤ 70 mL/min/1.73 m² and/or body weight less than 70 kg require dosage reduction of PRIMAXIN I.V. as indicated in the tables below. Creatinine clearance may be calculated from serum creatinine concentration by the following equation:

$$T_{cc} \text{ (Males)} = \frac{(\text{wt. in kg}) (140 - \text{age})}{(72) (\text{creatinine in mg/dL})}$$

$$T_{cc} \text{ (Females)} = 0.85 \times \text{above value}$$

To determine the dose for adults with impaired renal function and/or reduced body weight:

1. Choose a total daily dose from Table I based on infection characteristics.
2. a) If the total daily dose is 1.0 g, 1.5 g, or 2.0 g, use the appropriate subsection of Table II and continue with step 3.

   b) If the total daily dose is 3.0 g or 4.0 g, use the appropriate subsection of Table III and continue with step 3.
3. From Table II or III:

   a) Select the body weight on the far left which is closest to the patient's body weight (kg).

   b) Select the patient's creatinine clearance category.

   c) Where the row and column intersect is the reduced dosage regimen.

[See table II on next page]
[See table III on next page]

Patients with creatinine clearances of 6 to 20 mL/min/1.73 m² should be treated with PRIMAXIN I.V. 125 mg or 250 mg every 12 hours for most pathogens. There may be an increased risk of seizures when doses of 500 mg every 12 hours are administered to these patients.

Patients with creatinine clearance ≤5 mL/min/1.73 m² should not receive PRIMAXIN I.V. unless hemodialysis is instituted within 48 hours. There is inadequate information to recommend usage of PRIMAXIN I.V. for patients undergoing peritoneal dialysis.

Hemodialysis
When treating patients with creatinine clearances of ≤5 mL/min/1.73 m² who are undergoing hemodialysis, use the dosage recommendations for patients with creatinine clearances of 6–20 mL/min/1.73 m². (See *Reduced Intravenous*

Dosage Schedule for Adults with Impaired Renal Function and/or Body Weight <70 kg.) Both imipenem and cilastatin are cleared from the circulation during hemodialysis. The patient should receive PRIMAXIN I.V. after hemodialysis and at 12 hour intervals timed from the end of that hemodialysis session. Dialysis patients, especially those with background CNS disease, should be carefully monitored; for patients on hemodialysis, PRIMAXIN I.V. is recommended only when the benefit outweighs the potential risk of seizures. (See **PRECAUTIONS**.)

Pediatric Patients

See **PRECAUTIONS**, *Pediatric Patients*.

For pediatric patients ≥3 months of age, the recommended dose for non-CNS infections is 15–25 mg/kg/dose administered every six hours. Based on studies in adults, the maximum daily dose for treatment of infections with fully susceptible organisms is 2.0 g per day, and of infections with moderately susceptible organisms (primarily some strains of *P. aeruginosa*) is 4.0 g/day. Higher doses (up to 90 mg/kg/day in older children) have been used in patients with cystic fibrosis.

For pediatric patients ≤3 months of age (weighing ≥1,500 gms), the following dosage schedule is recommended for non-CNS infections:

   <1 wk of age: 25 mg/kg every 12 hrs
   1–4 wks of age: 25 mg/kg every 8 hrs
   4 wks–3 mos. of age: 25 mg/kg every 6 hrs.

Doses less than or equal to 500 mg should be given by intravenous infusion over 15 to 30 minutes. Doses greater than 500 mg should be given by intravenous infusion over 40 to 60 minutes.

PRIMAXIN I.V. is not recommended in pediatric patients with CNS infections because of the risk of seizures.

PRIMAXIN I.V. is not recommended in pediatric patients <30 kg with impaired renal function, as no data are available.

PREPARATION OF SOLUTION

Infusion Bottles

Contents of the infusion bottles of PRIMAXIN I.V. Powder should be restored with 100 mL of diluent (see list of diluents under **COMPATIBILITY AND STABILITY**) and shaken until a clear solution is obtained.

Vials

Contents of the vials must be suspended and transferred to 100 mL of an appropriate infusion solution.

A suggested procedure is to add approximately 10 mL from the appropriate infusion solution (see list of diluents under **COMPATIBILITY AND STABILITY**) to the vial. Shake well and transfer the resulting suspension to the infusion solution container.

Benzyl alcohol as a preservative has been associated with toxicity in neonates. While toxicity has not been demonstrated in pediatric patients greater than three months of age, small pediatric patients in this age range may also be at risk for benzyl alcohol toxicity. Therefore, diluents containing benzyl alcohol should not be used when PRIMAXIN I.V. is constituted for administration to pediatric patients in this age range.

CAUTION: THE SUSPENSION IS NOT FOR DIRECT INFUSION.

Repeat with an additional 10 mL of infusion solution to ensure complete transfer of vial contents to the infusion solution. **The resulting mixture should be agitated until clear.**

ADD-Vantage®† Vials

See separate INSTRUCTIONS FOR USE OF 'PRIMAXIN I.V.' IN ADD-Vantage® VIALS. PRIMAXIN I.V. in ADD-Vantage® vials should be reconstituted with ADD-Vantage® diluent containers containing 100 mL of either 0.9% Sodium Chloride Injection or 100 mL 5% Dextrose Injection.

---

† Registered trademark of Abbott Laboratories, Inc.

COMPATIBILITY AND STABILITY

Before reconstitution:

The dry powder should be stored at a temperature below 25°C (77°F).

Reconstituted solutions:

Solutions of PRIMAXIN I.V. range from colorless to yellow. Variations of color within this range do not affect the potency of the product.

PRIMAXIN I.V., as supplied in infusion bottles and vials and reconstituted as above with the following diluents, maintains satisfactory potency for four hours at room temperature or for 24 hours under refrigeration (5°C). Solutions of PRIMAXIN I.V. should not be frozen.

0.9% Sodium Chloride Injection
5% or 10% Dextrose Injection
5% Dextrose and 0.9% Sodium Chloride Injection
5% Dextrose Injection with 0.225% or 0.45% saline solution
5% Dextrose Injection with 0.15% potassium chloride solution
Mannitol 5% and 10%

PRIMAXIN I.V. is supplied in single dose ADD-Vantage® vials and should be prepared as directed in the accompanying INSTRUCTIONS FOR USE OF 'PRIMAXIN I.V.' IN ADD-Vantage® VIALS using ADD-Vantage® diluent containers containing 100 mL of either 0.9% Sodium Chloride Injection or 5% Dextrose Injection. When prepared with either of these diluents, PRIMAXIN I.V. maintains satisfactory potency for 4 hours at room temperature.

PRIMAXIN I.V. should not be mixed with or physically added to other antibiotics. However, PRIMAXIN I.V. may be administered concomitantly with other antibiotics, such as aminoglycosides.

HOW SUPPLIED

PRIMAXIN I.V. is supplied as a sterile powder mixture in vials and infusion bottles containing imipenem (anhydrous equivalent) and cilastatin sodium as follows:

No. 3514—250 mg imipenem equivalent and 250 mg cilastatin equivalent and 10 mg sodium bicarbonate as a buffer
NDC 0006-3514-58 in trays of 25 vials
(6505-01-332-4793 250 mg, 25's).
No. 3516—500 mg imipenem equivalent and 500 mg cilastatin equivalent and 20 mg sodium bicarbonate as a buffer
NDC 0006-3516-59 in trays of 25 vials
(6505-01-332-4794 500 mg, 25's).
No. 3515—250 mg imipenem equivalent and 250 mg cilastatin equivalent and 10 mg sodium bicarbonate as a buffer
NDC 0006-3515-74 in trays of 10 infusion bottles
(6505-01-246-4126 infusion bottle, 10's).
No. 3517—500 mg imipenem equivalent and 500 mg cilastatin equivalent and 20 mg sodium bicarbonate as a buffer
NDC 0006-3517-75 in trays of 10 infusion bottles
(6505-01-234-0240 infusion bottle, 10's).
No. 3551—250 mg imipenem equivalent and 250 mg cilastatin equivalent and 10 mg sodium bicarbonate as a buffer
NDC 0006-3551-58 in trays of 25 ADD-Vantage® vials.
No. 3552—500 mg imipenem equivalent and 500 mg cilastatin equivalent and 20 mg sodium bicarbonate as a buffer
NDC 0006-3552-59 in trays of 25 ADD-Vantage® vials.
(6505-01-279-9627 500 mg ADD-Vantage®, 25's).

REFERENCES

1. National Committee for Clinical Laboratory Standards, Performance Standards for Antimicrobial Disk Susceptibility Tests—Fifth Edition. Approved Standard NCCLS Document M2-A5, Vol. 13, No. 24 NCCLS, Villanova, PA, 1993.
2. National Committee for Clinical Laboratory Standards, Methods for Dilution Antimicrobial Susceptibility Tests for Bacteria that Grow Aerobically—Third Edition. Approved Standard NCCLS Document M7-A3, Vol. 13, No. 25 NCCLS, Villanova, PA, 1993.
3. National Committee for Clinical Laboratory Standards, Method for Antimicrobial Susceptibility Testing of Anaerobic Bacteria—Third Edition. Approved Standard NCCLS Document M11-A3, Vol. 13, No. 26 NCCLS, Villanova, PA, 1993.

7882123   Issued April 1998
COPYRIGHT© MERCK & CO., INC., 1987, 1994, 1998
All rights reserved

TABLE II
REDUCED INTRAVENOUS DOSAGE OF PRIMAXIN I.V. IN ADULT PATIENTS WITH IMPAIRED RENAL FUNCTION AND/OR BODY WEIGHT <70 kg

Body Weight (kg) is:	1.0 g/day and creatinine clearance (mL/min/1.73m²) is:				1.5 g/day and creatinine clearance (mL/min/1.73m²) is:				2.0 g/day and creatinine clearance (mL/min/1.73m²) is:			
	≥71	41–70	21–40	6–20	≥71	41–70	21–40	6–20	≥71	41–70	21–40	6–20
	then the reduced dosage regimen (mg) is:				then the reduced dosage regimen (mg) is:				then the reduced dosage regimen (mg) is:			
≥70	250 q6h	250 q8h	250 q12h	250 q12h	500 q8h	250 q6h	250 q8h	250 q12h	500 q6h	500 q8h	250 q6h	250 q12h
60	250 q8h	125 q6h	250 q12h	125 q12h	250 q6h	250 q8h	250 q8h	250 q12h	500 q6h	250 q8h	250 q8h	250 q12h
50	125 q6h	125 q6h	125 q8h	125 q12h	250 q6h	250 q8h	250 q12h	250 q12h	250 q6h	250 q8h	250 q8h	250 q12h
40	125 q6h	125 q8h	125 q12h	125 q12h	250 q8h	125 q6h	125 q8h	125 q12h	250 q6h	250 q8h	250 q12h	250 q12h
30	125 q8h	125 q8h	125 q12h	125 q12h	125 q6h	125 q8h	125 q8h	250 q12h	125 q8h	125 q6h	125 q8h	125 q12h

TABLE III
REDUCED INTRAVENOUS DOSAGE OF PRIMAXIN I.V. IN ADULT PATIENTS WITH IMPAIRED RENAL FUNCTION AND/OR BODY WEIGHT <70 kg

Body Weight (kg) is:	3.0 g/day and creatinine clearance (mL/min/1.73m²) is:				4.0 g/day and creatinine clearance (mL/min/1.73m²) is:			
	≥71	41–70	21–40	6–20	≥71	41–70	21–40	6–20
	then the reduced dosage regimen (mg) is:				then the reduced dosage regimen (mg) is:			
≥70	1000 q8h	500 q6h	500 q8h	500 q12h	1000 q6h	750 q8h	500 q8h	500 q12h
60	750 q8h	500 q8h	500 q8h	500 q12h	1000 q8h	750 q8h	500 q8h	500 q12h
50	500 q6h	500 q8h	250 q6h	250 q12h	750 q8h	500 q6h	500 q8h	500 q12h
40	500 q8h	250 q6h	250 q8h	250 q12h	500 q6h	500 q8h	250 q6h	250 q12h
30	250 q6h	250 q8h	250 q8h	250 q12h	500 q8h	250 q6h	250 q8h	250 q12h

PRINIVIL® Tablets   ℞
(Lisinopril)

USE IN PREGNANCY
When used in pregnancy during the second and third trimesters, ACE inhibitors can cause injury and even death to the developing fetus. When pregnancy is detected, PRINIVIL should be discontinued as soon as possible. See WARNINGS, *Fetal/Neonatal Morbidity and Mortality*.

DESCRIPTION

PRINIVIL* (Lisinopril), a synthetic peptide derivative, is an oral long-acting angiotensin converting enzyme inhibitor.

Continued on next page

Prinivil—Cont.

Lisinopril is chemically described as (*S*)-1-[N^2-(1-carboxy-3-phenylpropyl)-L-lysyl]-L-proline dihydrate. Its empirical formula is $C_{21}H_{31}N_3O_5 \cdot 2H_2O$ and its structural formula is:

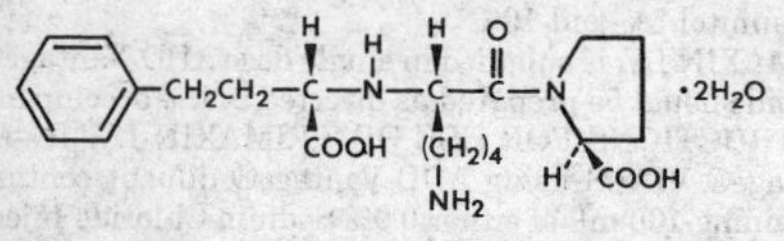

Lisinopril is a white to off-white, crystalline powder, with a molecular weight of 441.52. It is soluble in water and sparingly soluble in methanol and practically insoluble in ethanol.

PRINIVIL is supplied as 2.5 mg, 5 mg, 10 mg, 20 mg and 40 mg tablets for oral administration. In addition to the active ingredient lisinopril, each tablet contains the following inactive ingredients: calcium phosphate, mannitol, magnesium stearate, and starch. The 10 mg, 20 mg and 40 mg tablets also contain iron oxide.

*Registered trademark of MERCK & CO., INC.

CLINICAL PHARMACOLOGY

Mechanism of Action

Lisinopril inhibits angiotensin converting enzyme (ACE) in human subjects and animals. ACE is a peptidyl dipeptidase that catalyzes the conversion of angiotensin I to the vasoconstrictor substance, angiotensin II. Angiotensin II also stimulates aldosterone secretion by the adrenal cortex. The beneficial effects of lisinopril in hypertension and heart failure appear to result primarily from suppression of the renin-angiotensin-aldosterone system. Inhibition of ACE results in decreased plasma angiotensin II which leads to decreased vasopressor activity and to decreased aldosterone secretion. The latter decrease may result in a small increase of serum potassium. In hypertensive patients with normal renal function treated with PRINIVIL alone for up to 24 weeks, the mean increase in serum potassium was approximately 0.1 mEq/L; however, approximately 15 percent of patients had increases greater than 0.5 mEq/L and approximately six percent had a decrease greater than 0.5 mEq/L. In the same study, patients treated with PRINIVIL and hydrochlorothiazide for up to 24 weeks had a mean decrease in serum potassium of 0.1 mEq/L; approximately 4 percent of patients had increases greater than 0.5 mEq/L and approximately 12 percent had a decrease greater than 0.5 mEq/L. (See PRECAUTIONS.) Removal of angiotensin II negative feedback on renin secretion leads to increased plasma renin activity.

ACE is identical to kininase, an enzyme that degrades bradykinin. Whether increased levels of bradykinin, a potent vasodepressor peptide, play a role in the therapeutic effects of PRINIVIL remains to be elucidated.

While the mechanism through which PRINIVIL lowers blood pressure is believed to be primarily suppression of the renin-angiotensin-aldosterone system, PRINIVIL is antihypertensive even in patients with low-renin hypertension. Although PRINIVIL was antihypertensive in all races studied, black hypertensive patients (usually a low-renin hypertensive population) had a smaller average response to monotherapy than non-black patients.

Concomitant administration of PRINIVIL and hydrochlorothiazide further reduced blood pressure in black and non-black patients and any racial difference in blood pressure response was no longer evident.

Pharmacokinetics and Metabolism

Following oral administration of PRINIVIL, peak serum concentrations of lisinopril occur within about 7 hours, although there was a trend to a small delay in time taken to reach peak serum concentrations in acute myocardial infarction patients. Declining serum concentrations exhibit a prolonged terminal phase which does not contribute to drug accumulation. This terminal phase probably represents saturable binding to ACE and is not proportional to dose. Lisinopril does not appear to be bound to other serum proteins. Lisinopril does not undergo metabolism and is excreted unchanged entirely in the urine. Based on urinary recovery, the mean extent of absorption of lisinopril is approximately 25 percent, with large intersubject variability (6–60 percent) at all doses tested (5–80 mg). Lisinopril absorption is not influenced by the presence of food in the gastrointestinal tract. The absolute bioavailability of lisinopril is reduced to about 16% in patients with stable NYHA Class II-IV congestive heart failure, and the volume of distribution appears to be slightly smaller than that in normal subjects.

The oral bioavailability of lisinopril in patients with acute myocardial infarction is similar to that in healthy volunteers.

Upon multiple dosing, lisinopril exhibits an effective half-life of accumulation of 12 hours.

Impaired renal function decreases elimination of lisinopril, which is excreted principally through the kidneys, but this decrease becomes clinically important only when the glomerular filtration rate is below 30 mL/min. Above this glomerular filtration rate, the elimination half-life is little changed. With greater impairment, however, peak and trough lisinopril levels increase, time to peak concentration increases and time to attain steady state is prolonged. Older patients, on average, have (approximately doubled) higher blood levels and area under the plasma concentration time curve (AUC) than younger patients. (See DOSAGE AND ADMINISTRATION.) Lisinopril can be removed by hemodialysis.

Studies in rats indicate that lisinopril crosses the blood-brain barrier poorly. Multiple doses of lisinopril in rats do not result in accumulation in any tissues. Milk of lactating rats contains radioactivity following administration of ^{14}C lisinopril. By whole body autoradiography, radioactivity was found in the placenta following administration of labeled drug to pregnant rats, but none was found in the fetuses.

Pharmacodynamics and Clinical Effects

Hypertension: Administration of PRINIVIL to patients with hypertension results in a reduction of supine and standing blood pressure to about the same extent with no compensatory tachycardia. Symptomatic postural hypotension is usually not observed although it can occur and should be anticipated in volume and/or salt-depleted patients. (See WARNINGS.) When given together with thiazide-type diuretics, the blood pressure lowering effects of the two drugs are approximately additive.

In most patients studied, onset of antihypertensive activity was seen at one hour after oral administration of an individual dose of PRINIVIL, with peak reduction of blood pressure achieved by six hours. Although an antihypertensive effect was observed 24 hours after dosing with recommended single daily doses, the effect was more consistent and the mean effect was considerably larger in some studies with doses of 20 mg or more than with lower doses. However, at all doses studied, the mean antihypertensive effect was substantially smaller 24 hours after dosing than it was six hours after dosing.

In some patients achievement of optimal blood pressure reduction may require two to four weeks of therapy.

The antihypertensive effects of PRINIVIL are maintained during long-term therapy. Abrupt withdrawal of PRINIVIL has not been associated with a rapid increase in blood pressure or a significant increase in blood pressure compared to pretreatment levels.

Two dose-response studies utilizing a once daily regimen were conducted in 438 mild to moderate hypertensive patients not on a diuretic. Blood pressure was measured 24 hours after dosing. An antihypertensive effect of PRINIVIL was seen with 5 mg in some patients. However, in both studies blood pressure reduction occurred sooner and was greater in patients treated with 10, 20, or 80 mg of PRINIVIL. In controlled clinical studies, PRINIVIL 20–80 mg has been compared in patients with mild to moderate hypertension to hydrochlorothiazide 12.5–50 mg and with atenolol 50–200 mg; and in patients with moderate to severe hypertension to metoprolol 100–200 mg. It was superior to hydrochlorothiazide in effects on systolic and diastolic blood pressure in a population that was $^3/_4$ caucasian. PRINIVIL was approximately equivalent to atenolol and metoprolol in effects on diastolic blood pressure and had somewhat greater effects on systolic blood pressure.

PRINIVIL had similar effectiveness and adverse effects in younger and older (>65 years) patients. It was less effective in blacks than in caucasians.

In hemodynamic studies in patients with essential hypertension, blood pressure reduction was accompanied by a reduction in peripheral arterial resistance with little or no change in cardiac output and in heart rate. In a study in nine hypertensive patients, following administration of PRINIVIL, there was an increase in mean renal blood flow that was not significant. Data from several small studies are inconsistent with respect to the effect of PRINIVIL on glomerular filtration rate in hypertensive patients with normal renal function, but suggest that changes, if any, are not large.

In patients with renovascular hypertension PRINIVIL has been shown to be well tolerated and effective in controlling blood pressure (see PRECAUTIONS).

Heart Failure: During baseline-controlled clinical trials, in patients receiving digitalis and diuretics, single doses of PRINIVIL resulted in decreases in pulmonary capillary wedge pressure, systemic vascular resistance and blood pressure accompanied by an increase in cardiac output and no change in heart rate.

In two placebo controlled, 12-week clinical studies, PRINIVIL as adjunctive therapy to digitalis and diuretics improved the following signs and symptoms due to congestive heart failure: edema, rales, paroxysmal nocturnal dyspnea and jugular venous distention. In one of the studies beneficial response was also noted for: orthopnea, presence of third heart sound and the number of patients classified as NYHA Class III and IV. Exercise tolerance was also improved in this study. The effect of lisinopril on mortality in patients with heart failure has not been evaluated.

The once daily dosage for the treatment of congestive heart failure was the only dosage regimen used during clinical trial development and was determined by the measurement of hemodynamic responses.

Acute Myocardial Infarction: The Gruppo Italiano per lo Studio della Sopravvienza nell'Infarto Miocardico (GISSI-3) study was a multicenter, controlled, randomized, unblinded clinical trial conducted in 19,394 patients with acute myocardial infarction admitted to a coronary care unit. It was designed to examine the effects of short-term (6 week) treatment with lisinopril, nitrates, their combination, or no therapy on short-term (6 week) mortality and on long-term death and markedly impaired cardiac function. Patients presenting within 24 hours of the onset of symptoms who were hemodynamically stable were randomized, in a 2 × 2 factorial design, to six weeks of either

1) PRINIVIL alone (n = 4841),
2) nitrates alone (n = 4869),
3) PRINIVIL plus nitrates (n = 4841), or
4) open control (n = 4843).

All patients received routine therapies, including thrombolytics (72%), aspirin (84%), and a beta-blocker (31%), as appropriate, normally utilized in acute myocardial infarction (MI) patients.

The protocol excluded patients with hypotension (systolic blood pressure ≤100 mmHg), severe heart failure, cardiogenic shock and renal dysfunction (serum creatinine >2 mg/dL and/or proteinuria >500 mg/24 h). Doses of PRINIVIL were adjusted as necessary according to protocol. (See DOSAGE AND ADMINISTRATION.)

Study treatment was withdrawn at six weeks except where clinical conditions indicated continuation of treatment.

The primary outcomes of the trial were the overall mortality at six weeks and a combined endpoint at six months after the myocardial infarction, consisting of the number of patients who died, had late (day 4) clinical congestive heart failure, or had extensive left ventricular damage defined as ejection fraction ≤35%, or an akinetic-dyskinetic [A-D] score ≥45%. Patients receiving PRINIVIL (n = 9646) alone or with nitrates, had an 11 percent lower risk of death (2p [two-tailed] = 0.04) compared to patients receiving no PRINIVIL (n = 9672) (6.4 percent versus 7.2 percent, respectively) at six weeks. Although patients randomized to receive PRINIVIL for up to six weeks also fared numerically better on the combined endpoint at 6 months, the open nature of the assessment of heart failure, substantial loss of follow-up echocardiography, and substantial excess use of lisinopril between 6 weeks and 6 months in the group randomized to 6 weeks of lisinopril, preclude any conclusion about this endpoint.

Patients with acute myocardial infarction, treated with PRINIVIL had a higher (9.0 percent versus 3.7 percent, respectively) incidence of persistent hypotension (systolic blood pressure <90 mmHg for more than 1 hour) and renal dysfunction (2.4 percent versus 1.1 percent) in-hospital and at six weeks (increasing creatinine concentration to over 3 mg/dL or a doubling or more of the baseline serum creatinine concentration). See ADVERSE REACTIONS, *ACUTE MYOCARDIAL INFARCTION.*

INDICATIONS AND USAGE

Hypertension

PRINIVIL is indicated for the treatment of hypertension. It may be used alone as initial therapy or concomitantly with other classes of antihypertensive agents.

Heart Failure

PRINIVIL is indicated as adjunctive therapy in the management of heart failure in patients who are not responding adequately to diuretics and digitalis.

Acute Myocardial Infarction

PRINIVIL is indicated for the treatment of hemodynamically stable patients within 24 hours of acute myocardial infarction, to improve survival. Patients should receive, as appropriate, the standard recommended treatments such as thrombolytics, aspirin and beta-blockers.

In using PRINIVIL, consideration should be given to the fact that another angiotensin converting enzyme inhibitor, captopril, has caused agranulocytosis, particularly in patients with renal impairment or collagen vascular disease, and that available data are insufficient to show that PRINIVIL does not have a similar risk. (See WARNINGS.)

In considering use of PRINIVIL, it should be noted that in controlled clinical trials ACE inhibitors have an effect on blood pressure that is less in black patients than in non-blacks. In addition, it should be noted that black patients receiving ACE inhibitors have been reported to have a higher incidence of angioedema compared to non-blacks.

CONTRAINDICATIONS

PRINIVIL is contraindicated in patients who are hypersensitive to this product and in patients with a history of angioedema related to previous treatment with an angiotensin converting enzyme inhibitor.

WARNINGS

Anaphylactoid and Possibly Related Reactions

Presumably because angiotensin converting enzyme inhibitors affect the metabolism of eicosanoids and polypeptides, including endogenous bradykinin, patients receiving ACE inhibitors (including PRINIVIL) may be subject to a variety of adverse reactions, some of them serious.

Angioedema: Angioedema of the face, extremities, lips, tongue, glottis and/or larynx has been reported in patients treated with angiotensin converting enzyme inhibitors, including PRINIVIL. This may occur at any time during treatment. In such cases PRINIVIL should be promptly discontinued and appropriate therapy and monitoring should be provided until complete and sustained resolution of signs and symptoms has occurred. In instances where swelling has been confined to the face and lips the condition has generally resolved without treatment, although antihistamines have been useful in relieving symptoms. Angioedema associated with laryngeal edema may be fatal. **Where there is involvement of the tongue, glottis or larynx, likely to cause airway obstruction, appropriate therapy, e.g., subcutaneous epinephrine solution 1:1000 (0.3 mL to 0.5 mL) and/or measures necessary to ensure a patent airway, should be promptly provided.** (See ADVERSE REACTIONS.)

Patients with a history of angioedema unrelated to ACE inhibitor therapy may be at increased risk of angioedema while receiving an ACE inhibitor (see also INDICATIONS AND USAGE and CONTRAINDICATIONS).

Anaphylactoid reactions during desensitization: Two patients undergoing desensitizing treatment with hymenoptera venom while receiving ACE inhibitors sustained life-threatening anaphylactoid reactions. In the same patients, these reactions were avoided when ACE inhibitors were temporarily withheld, but they reappeared upon inadvertent rechallenge.

Anaphylactoid reactions during membrane exposure: Anaphylactoid reactions have been reported in patients dialyzed with high-flux membranes and treated concomitantly with an ACE inhibitor. Anaphylactoid reactions have also been reported in patients undergoing low-density lipoprotein apheresis with dextran sulfate absorption.

Hypotension

Excessive hypotension is rare in patients with uncomplicated hypertension treated with PRINIVIL alone.

Patients with heart failure given PRINIVIL commonly have some reduction in blood pressure with peak blood pressure reduction occurring 6 to 8 hours post dose, but discontinuation of therapy because of continuing symptomatic hypotension usually is not necessary when dosing instructions are followed; caution should be observed when initiating therapy. (See DOSAGE AND ADMINISTRATION.)

Patients at risk of excessive hypotension, sometimes associated with oliguria and/or progressive azotemia, and rarely with acute renal failure and/or death, include those with the following conditions or characteristics: heart failure with systolic blood pressure below 100 mmHg, hyponatremia, high dose diuretic therapy, recent intensive diuresis or increase in diuretic dose, renal dialysis, or severe volume and/or salt depletion of any etiology. It may be advisable to eliminate the diuretic (except in patients with heart failure), reduce the diuretic dose or increase salt intake cautiously before initiating therapy with PRINIVIL in patients at risk for excessive hypotension who are able to tolerate such adjustments. (See PRECAUTIONS, *Drug Interactions,* and ADVERSE REACTIONS.)

Patients with acute myocardial infarction in the GISSI-3 study had a higher (9.0 versus 3.7 percent) incidence of persistent hypotension (systolic blood pressure <90 mmHg for more than 1 hour) when treated with PRINIVIL. Treatment with PRINIVIL must not be initiated in acute myocardial infarction patients at risk of further serious hemodynamic deterioration after treatment with a vasodilator (e.g., systolic blood pressure of 100 mmHg or lower) or cardiogenic shock.

In patients at risk of excessive hypotension, therapy should be started under very close medical supervision and such patients should be followed closely for the first two weeks of treatment and whenever the dose of PRINIVIL and/or diuretic is increased. Similar considerations may apply to patients with ischemic heart or cerebrovascular disease, or in patients with acute myocardial infarction, in whom an excessive fall in blood pressure could result in a myocardial infarction or cerebrovascular accident.

If excessive hypotension occurs, the patient should be placed in the supine position and, if necessary, receive an intravenous infusion of normal saline. A transient hypotensive response is not a contraindication to further doses of PRINIVIL which usually can be given without difficulty once the blood pressure has stabilized. If symptomatic hypotension develops, a dose reduction or discontinuation of PRINIVIL or concomitant diuretic may be necessary.

Neutropenia/Agranulocytosis

Another angiotensin converting enzyme inhibitor, captopril, has been shown to cause agranulocytosis and bone marrow depression, rarely in uncomplicated patients but more frequently in patients with renal impairment especially if they also have a collagen vascular disease. Available data from clinical trials of PRINIVIL are insufficient to show that PRINIVIL does not cause agranulocytosis at similar rates. Marketing experience has revealed rare cases of neutropenia and bone marrow depression in which a causal relationship to lisinopril cannot be excluded. Periodic monitoring of white blood cell counts in patients with collagen vascular disease and renal disease should be considered.

Hepatic Failure: Rarely, ACE inhibitors have been associated with a syndrome that starts with cholestatic jaundice and progresses to fulminant hepatic necrosis, and (sometimes) death. The mechanism of this syndrome is not understood. Patients receiving ACE inhibitors who develop jaundice or marked elevations of hepatic enzymes should discontinue the ACE inhibitor and receive appropriate medical follow-up.

Fetal/Neonatal Morbidity and Mortality

ACE inhibitors can cause fetal and neonatal morbidity and death when administered to pregnant women. Several dozen cases have been reported in the world literature. When pregnancy is detected, ACE inhibitors should be discontinued as soon as possible.

The use of ACE inhibitors during the second and third trimesters of pregnancy has been associated with fetal and neonatal injury, including hypotension, neonatal skull hypoplasia, anuria, reversible or irreversible renal failure, and death. Oligohydramnios has also been reported, presumably resulting from decreased fetal renal function; oligohydramnios in this setting has been associated with fetal limb contractures, craniofacial deformation, and hypoplastic lung development. Prematurity, intrauterine growth retardation, and patent ductus arteriosus have also been reported, although it is not clear whether these occurrences were due to the ACE-inhibitor exposure.

These adverse effects do not appear to have resulted from intrauterine ACE-inhibitor exposure that has been limited to the first trimester. Mothers whose embryos and fetuses are exposed to ACE inhibitors only during the first trimester should be so informed. Nonetheless, when patients become pregnant, physicians should make every effort to discontinue the use of PRINIVIL as soon as possible.

Rarely (probably less often than once in every thousand pregnancies), no alternative to ACE inhibitors will be found. In these rare cases, the mothers should be apprised of the potential hazards to their fetuses, and serial ultrasound examinations should be performed to assess the intraamniotic environment.

If oligohydramnios is observed, PRINIVIL should be discontinued unless it is considered lifesaving for the mother. Contraction stress testing (CST), a non-stress test (NST), or biophysical profiling (BPP) may be appropriate, depending upon the week of pregnancy. Patients and physicians should be aware, however, that oligohydramnios may not appear until after the fetus has sustained irreversible injury.

Infants with histories of *in utero* exposure to ACE inhibitors should be closely observed for hypotension, oliguria, and hyperkalemia. If oliguria occurs, attention should be directed toward support of blood pressure and renal perfusion. Exchange transfusion or dialysis may be required as means of reversing hypotension and/or substituting for disordered renal function. Lisinopril, which crosses the placenta, has been removed from neonatal circulation by peritoneal dialysis with some clinical benefit, and theoretically may be removed by exchange transfusion, although there is no experience with the latter procedure.

No teratogenic effects of lisinopril were seen in studies of pregnant mice, rats, and rabbits. On a body surface area basis, the doses used were up to 55 times, 33 times, and 0.15 times, respectively, the maximum recommended human daily dose (MRHDD).

PRECAUTIONS

General

Impaired Renal Function: As a consequence of inhibiting the renin-angiotensin-aldosterone system, changes in renal function may be anticipated in susceptible individuals. In patients with severe congestive heart failure whose renal function may depend on the activity of the renin-angiotensin-aldosterone system, treatment with angiotensin converting enzyme inhibitors, including PRINIVIL, may be associated with oliguria and/or progressive azotemia and rarely with acute renal failure and/or death.

In hypertensive patients with unilateral or bilateral renal artery stenosis, increases in blood urea nitrogen and serum creatinine may occur. Experience with another angiotensin converting enzyme inhibitor suggests that these increases are usually reversible upon discontinuation of PRINIVIL and/or diuretic therapy. In such patients renal function should be monitored during the first few weeks of therapy.

Some patients with hypertension or heart failure with no apparent pre-existing renal vascular disease have developed increases in blood urea nitrogen and serum creatinine, usually minor and transient, especially when PRINIVIL has been given concomitantly with a diuretic. This is more likely to occur in patients with pre-existing renal impairment. Dosage reduction and/or discontinuation of the diuretic and/or PRINIVIL may be required.

Patients with acute myocardial infarction in the GISSI-3 study, treated with PRINIVIL, had a higher (2.4 percent versus 1.1 percent) incidence of renal dysfunction in-hospital and at six weeks (increasing creatinine concentration to over 3 mg/dL or a doubling or more of the baseline serum creatinine concentration). In acute myocardial infarction, treatment with PRINIVIL should be initiated with caution in patients with evidence of renal dysfunction, defined as serum creatinine concentration exceeding 2 mg/dL. If renal dysfunction develops during treatment with PRINIVIL (serum creatinine concentration exceeding 3 mg/dL or a doubling from the pre-treatment value) then the physician should consider withdrawal of PRINIVIL.

Evaluation of patients with hypertension, heart failure, or myocardial infarction should always include assessment of renal function. (See DOSAGE AND ADMINISTRATION.)

Hyperkalemia: In clinical trials hyperkalemia (serum potassium greater than 5.7 mEq/L) occurred in approximately 2.2 percent of hypertensive patients and 4.8 percent of patients with heart failure. In most cases these were isolated values which resolved despite continued therapy. Hyperkalemia was a cause of discontinuation of therapy in approximately 0.1 percent of hypertensive patients, 0.6 percent of patients with heart failure and 0.1 percent of patients with myocardial infarction. Risk factors for the development of hyperkalemia include renal insufficiency, diabetes mellitus, and the concomitant use of potassium-sparing diuretics, potassium supplements and/or potassium-containing salt substitutes, which should be used cautiously, if at all, with PRINIVIL. (See *Drug Interactions.*)

Cough: Presumably due to the inhibition of the degradation of endogenous bradykinin, persistent nonproductive cough has been reported with all ACE inhibitors, always resolving after discontinuation of therapy. ACE inhibitor-induced cough should be considered in the differential diagnosis of cough.

Surgery/Anesthesia: In patients undergoing major surgery or during anesthesia with agents that produce hypotension, PRINIVIL may block angiotensin II formation secondary to compensatory renin release. If hypotension occurs and is considered to be due to this mechanism, it can be corrected by volume expansion.

Information for Patients

Angioedema: Angioedema, including laryngeal edema, may occur at any time during treatment with angiotensin converting enzyme inhibitors, including lisinopril. Patients should be so advised and told to report immediately any signs or symptoms suggesting angioedema (swelling of face, extremities, eyes, lips, tongue, difficulty in swallowing or breathing) and to take no more drug until they have consulted with the prescribing physician.

Symptomatic Hypotension: Patients should be cautioned to report lightheadedness especially during the first few days of therapy. If actual syncope occurs, the patients should be told to discontinue the drug until they have consulted with the prescribing physician.

All patients should be cautioned that excessive perspiration and dehydration may lead to an excessive fall in blood pressure because of reduction in fluid volume. Other causes of volume depletion such as vomiting or diarrhea may also lead to a fall in blood pressure; patients should be advised to consult with their physician.

Hyperkalemia: Patients should be told not to use salt substitutes containing potassium without consulting their physician.

Neutropenia: Patients should be told to report promptly any indication of infection (e.g., sore throat, fever) which may be a sign of neutropenia.

Pregnancy: Female patients of childbearing age should be told about the consequences of second- and third-trimester exposure to ACE inhibitors, and they should also be told that these consequences do not appear to have resulted from intrauterine ACE-inhibitor exposure that has been limited to the first trimester. These patients should be asked to report pregnancies to their physicians as soon as possible.

NOTE: As with many other drugs, certain advice to patients being treated with PRINIVIL is warranted. This information is intended to aid in the safe and effective use of this medication. It is not a disclosure of all possible adverse or intended effects.

Drug Interactions

Hypotension—Patients on Diuretic Therapy: Patients on diuretics, and especially those in whom diuretic therapy was recently instituted, may occasionally experience an exces-

Continued on next page

Information on the Merck & Co., Inc. products listed on these pages is the full prescribing information from product circulars in use August 31, 1998. For information, please call 1-800-NSC MERCK [1-800-672-6372].

Prinivil—Cont.

sive reduction of blood pressure after initiation of therapy with PRINIVIL. The possibility of hypotensive effects with PRINIVIL can be minimized by either discontinuing the diuretic or increasing the salt intake prior to initiation of treatment with PRINIVIL. If it is necessary to continue the diuretic, initiate therapy with PRINIVIL at a dose of 5 mg daily, and provide close medical supervision after the initial dose until blood pressure has stabilized. (See WARNINGS, and DOSAGE AND ADMINISTRATION.) When a diuretic is added to the therapy of a patient receiving PRINIVIL, an additional antihypertensive effect is usually observed. Studies with ACE inhibitors in combination with diuretics indicate that the dose of the ACE inhibitor can be reduced when it is given with a diuretic. (See DOSAGE AND ADMINISTRATION.)

Indomethacin: In a study in 36 patients with mild to moderate hypertension where the antihypertensive effects of PRINIVIL alone were compared to PRINIVIL given concomitantly with indomethacin, the use of indomethacin was associated with a reduced effect, although the difference between the two regimens was not significant.

Other Agents: PRINIVIL has been used concomitantly with nitrates and/or digoxin without evidence of clinically significant adverse interactions. This included post myocardial infarction patients who were receiving intravenous or transdermal nitroglycerin. No clinically important pharmacokinetic interactions occurred when PRINIVIL was used concomitantly with propranolol or hydrochlorothiazide. The presence of food in the stomach does not alter the bioavailability of PRINIVIL.

Agents Increasing Serum Potassium: PRINIVIL attenuates potassium loss caused by thiazide-type diuretics. Use of PRINIVIL with potassium-sparing diuretics (e.g., spironolactone, triamterene, or amiloride), potassium supplements, or potassium-containing salt substitutes may lead to significant increases in serum potassium. Therefore, if concomitant use of these agents is indicated because of demonstrated hypokalemia, they should be used with caution and with frequent monitoring of serum potassium. Potassium sparing agents should generally not be used in patients with heart failure who are receiving PRINIVIL.

Lithium: Lithium toxicity has been reported in patients receiving lithium concomitantly with drugs which cause elimination of sodium, including ACE inhibitors. Lithium toxicity was usually reversible upon discontinuation of lithium and the ACE inhibitor. It is recommended that serum lithium levels be monitored frequently if PRINIVIL is administered concomitantly with lithium.

Carcinogenesis, Mutagenesis, Impairment of Fertility
There was no evidence of a tumorigenic effect when lisinopril was administered orally for 105 weeks to male and female rats at doses up to 90 mg/kg/day or for 92 weeks to male and female mice at doses up to 135 mg/kg/day. These

doses are 10 times and 7 times, respectively, the maximum recommended human daily dose (MRHDD) when compared on a body surface area basis.

Lisinopril was not mutagenic in the Ames microbial mutagen test with or without metabolic activation. It was also negative in a forward mutation assay using Chinese hamster lung cells. Lisinopril did not produce single strand DNA breaks in an *in vitro* alkaline elution rat hepatocyte assay. In addition, lisinopril did not produce increases in chromosomal aberrations in an *in vitro* test in Chinese hamster ovary cells or in an *in vivo* study in mouse bone marrow. There were no adverse effects on reproductive performance in male and female rats treated with up to 300 mg/kg/day of lisinopril (33 times the MRHDD when compared on a body surface area basis).

Pregnancy
Pregnancy Categories C (first trimester) *and D* (second and third trimesters). See WARNINGS, *Fetal/Neonatal Morbidity and Mortality.*

Nursing Mothers
Milk of lactating rats contains radioactivity following administration of ^{14}C lisinopril. It is not known whether this drug is secreted in human milk. Because many drugs are secreted in human milk, and because of the potential for serious adverse reactions in nursing infants from ACE inhibitors, a decision should be made whether to discontinue PRINIVIL, taking into account the importance of the drug to the mother.

Pediatric Use
Safety and effectiveness in pediatric patients have not been established.

ADVERSE REACTIONS

PRINIVIL has been found to be generally well tolerated in controlled clinical trials involving 1969 patients with hypertension or heart failure. For the most part, adverse experiences were mild and transient.

HYPERTENSION

In clinical trials in patients with hypertension treated with PRINIVIL, discontinuation of therapy due to clinical adverse experiences occurred in 5.7 percent of patients. The overall frequency of adverse experiences could not be related to total daily dosage within the recommended therapeutic dosage range.

For adverse experiences occurring in greater than one percent of patients with hypertension treated with PRINIVIL or PRINIVIL plus hydrochlorothiazide in controlled clinical trials and more frequently with PRINIVIL and/or PRINIVIL plus hydrochlorothiazide than placebo, comparative incidence data are listed in the table below:

[See table below]

Chest pain and back pain were also seen but were more common on placebo than PRINIVIL.

HEART FAILURE

In patients with heart failure treated with PRINIVIL for up to four years, discontinuation of therapy due to clinical adverse experiences occurred in 11.0 percent of patients. In controlled studies in patients with heart failure, therapy was discontinued in 8.1 percent of patients treated with PRINIVIL for up to 12 weeks, compared to 7.7 percent of patients treated with placebo for 12 weeks.

The following table lists those adverse experiences which occurred in greater than one percent of patients with heart failure treated with PRINIVIL or placebo for up to 12 weeks in controlled clinical trials and more frequently on PRINIVIL than placebo.

	Controlled Trials	
	PRINIVIL (n=407) Incidence (discontinuation) 12 weeks	Placebo (n=155) Incidence (discontinuation) 12 weeks
Body As A Whole		
Chest Pain	3.4 (0.2)	1.3 (0.0)
Abdominal Pain	2.2 (0.7)	1.9 (0.0)
Cardiovascular		
Hypotension	4.4 (1.7)	0.6 (0.6)
Digestive		
Diarrhea	3.7 (0.5)	1.9 (0.0)
Nervous/Psychiatric		
Dizziness	11.8 (1.2)	4.5 (1.3)
Headache	4.4 (0.2)	3.9 (0.0)
Respiratory		
Upper Respiratory Infection	1.5 (0.0)	1.3 (0.0)
Skin		
Rash	1.7 (0.5)	0.6 (0.6)

Also observed at >1% with PRINIVIL but more frequent or as frequent on placebo than PRINIVIL in controlled trials were asthenia, angina pectoris, nausea, dyspnea, cough and pruritus.

Worsening of heart failure, anorexia, increased salivation, muscle cramps, back pain, myalgia, depression, chest sound abnormalities and pulmonary edema were also seen in controlled clinical trials, but were more common on placebo than PRINIVIL.

ACUTE MYOCARDIAL INFARCTION

In the GISSI-3 trial, in patients treated with PRINIVIL for six weeks following acute myocardial infarction, discontinuation of therapy occurred in 17.6 percent of patients.

Patients treated with PRINIVIL had a significantly higher incidence of hypotension and renal dysfunction compared with patients not taking PRINIVIL.

In the GISSI-3 trial, hypotension (9.7 percent), renal dysfunction (2.0 percent), cough (0.5 percent), post-infarction angina (0.3 percent), skin rash and generalized edema (0.01 percent), and angioedema (0.01 percent) resulted in withdrawal of treatment. In elderly patients treated with PRINIVIL, discontinuation due to renal dysfunction was 4.2 percent.

Other clinical adverse experiences occurring in 0.3 to 1.0 percent of patients with hypertension or heart failure treated with PRINIVIL in controlled trials and rarer, serious, possibly drug-related events reported in uncontrolled studies or marketing experience are listed below, and within each category, are in order of decreasing severity:

Body as a Whole: Anaphylactoid reactions (see WARNINGS, *Anaphylactoid and Possible Related Reactions*), syncope, orthostatic effects, chest discomfort, pain, pelvic pain, flank pain, edema, facial edema, virus infection, fever, chills, malaise.

Cardiovascular: Cardiac arrest; myocardial infarction or cerebrovascular accident, possibly secondary to excessive hypotension in high risk patients (see WARNINGS, *Hypotension*); pulmonary embolism and infarction, arrhythmias (including ventricular tachycardia, atrial tachycardia, atrial fibrillation, bradycardia and premature ventricular contractions), palpitations, transient ischemic attacks, paroxysmal nocturnal dyspnea, orthostatic hypotension, decreased blood pressure, peripheral edema, vasculitis.

Digestive: Pancreatitis, hepatitis (hepatocellular or cholestatic jaundice) (see WARNINGS, *Hepatic Failure*), vomiting, gastritis, dyspepsia, heartburn, gastrointestinal cramps, constipation, flatulence, dry mouth.

Hematologic: Rare cases of bone marrow depression, neutropenia, and thrombocytopenia.

Endocrine: Diabetes mellitus.

Metabolic: Weight loss, dehydration, fluid overload, gout, weight gain.

Musculoskeletal: Arthritis, arthralgia, neck pain, hip pain, low back pain, joint pain, leg pain, knee pain, shoulder pain, arm pain, lumbago.

Nervous System/Psychiatric: Stroke, ataxia, memory impairment, tremor, peripheral neuropathy (e.g., dysesthesia) spasm, paresthesia, confusion, insomnia, somnolence, hypersomnia, irritability, and nervousness.

	Percent of Patients in Controlled Studies		
	PRINIVIL (n = 1349) Incidence (discontinuation)	PRINIVIL/ Hydrochlorothiazide (n = 629) Incidence (discontinuation)	Placebo (n =207) Incidence (discontinuation)
Body As A Whole			
Fatigue	2.5 (0.3)	4.0 (0.5)	1.0 (0.0)
Asthenia	1.3 (0.5)	2.1 (0.2)	1.0 (0.0)
Orthostatic Effects	1.2 (0.0)	3.5 (0.2)	1.0 (0.0)
Cardiovascular			
Hypotension	1.2 (0.5)	1.6 (0.5)	0.5 (0.5)
Digestive			
Diarrhea	2.7 (0.2)	2.7 (0.3)	2.4 (0.0)
Nausea	2.0 (0.4)	2.5 (0.2)	2.4 (0.0)
Vomiting	1.1 (0.2)	1.4 (0.1)	0.5 (0.0)
Dyspepsia	0.9 (0.0)	1.9 (0.0)	0.0 (0.0)
Musculoskeletal			
Muscle Cramps	0.5 (0.0)	2.9 (0.8)	0.5 (0.0)
Nervous/Psychiatric			
Headache	5.7 (0.2)	4.5 (0.5)	1.9 (0.0)
Dizziness	5.4 (0.4)	9.2 (1.0)	1.9 (0.0)
Paresthesia	0.8 (0.1)	2.1 (0.2)	0.0 (0.0)
Decreased Libido	0.4 (0.1)	1.3 (0.1)	0.0 (0.0)
Vertigo	0.2 (0.1)	1.1 (0.2)	0.0 (0.0)
Respiratory			
Cough	3.5 (0.7)	4.6 (0.8)	1.0 (0.0)
Upper Respiratory Infection	2.1 (0.1)	2.7 (0.1)	0.0 (0.0)
Common Cold	1.1 (0.1)	1.3 (0.1)	0.0 (0.0)
Nasal Congestion	0.4 (0.1)	1.3 (0.1)	0.0 (0.0)
Influenza	0.3 (0.1)	1.1 (0.1)	0.0 (0.0)
Skin			
Rash	1.3 (0.4)	1.6 (0.2)	0.5 (0.5)
Urogenital			
Impotence	1.0 (0.4)	1.6 (0.5)	0.0 (0.0)

Respiratory System: Malignant lung neoplasms, hemoptysis, pulmonary infiltrates, bronchospasm, asthma, pleural effusion, pneumonia, bronchitis, wheezing, orthopnea, painful respiration, epistaxis, laryngitis, sinusitis, pharyngeal pain, pharyngitis, rhinitis, rhinorrhea.

Skin: Urticaria, alopecia, herpes zoster, photosensitivity, skin lesions, skin infections, pemphigus, erythema, flushing, diaphoresis. Other severe skin reactions (including toxic epidermal necrolysis and Stevens-Johnson syndrome) have been reported rarely; causal relationship has not been established.

Special Senses: Visual loss, diplopia, blurred vision, tinnitus, photophobia.

Urogenital System: Acute renal failure, oliguria, anuria, uremia, progressive azotemia, renal dysfunction (see PRECAUTIONS and DOSAGE AND ADMINISTRATION), pyelonephritis, dysuria, urinary tract infection, breast pain.

Miscellaneous: A symptom complex has been reported which may include a positive ANA, an elevated erythrocyte sedimentation rate, arthralgia/arthritis, myalgia, fever, vasculitis, leukocytosis, eosinophilia, photosensitivity, rash, and other dermatological manifestations.

Angioedema: Angioedema has been reported in patients receiving PRINIVIL with an incidence higher in black than in non-black patients. Angioedema associated with laryngeal edema may be fatal. If angioedema of the face, extremities, lips, tongue, glottis and/or larynx occurs, treatment with PRINIVIL should be discontinued and appropriate therapy instituted immediately. (See WARNINGS.)

Hypotension: In hypertensive patients, hypotension occurred in 1.2 percent and syncope occurred in 0.1 percent of patients. Hypotension or syncope was a cause for discontinuation of therapy in 0.5 percent of hypertensive patients. In patients with heart failure, hypotension occurred in 5.3 percent and syncope occurred in 1.8 percent of patients. These adverse experiences were causes for discontinuation of therapy in 1.8 percent of these patients. In patients treated with PRINIVIL for six weeks after acute myocardial infarction, hypotension (systolic blood pressure 100 mmHg) resulted in discontinuation of therapy in 9.7 percent of the patients. (See WARNINGS.)

Fetal/Neonatal Morbidity and Mortality: See WARNINGS, *Fetal/Neonatal Morbidity and Mortality.*

Cough: See PRECAUTIONS, *Cough.*

Clinical Laboratory Test Findings

Serum Electrolytes: Hyperkalemia (see PRECAUTIONS), hyponatremia.

Creatinine, Blood Urea Nitrogen: Minor increases in blood urea nitrogen and serum creatinine, reversible upon discontinuation of therapy, were observed in about 2.0 percent of patients with essential hypertension treated with PRINIVIL alone. Increases were more common in patients receiving concomitant diuretics and in patients with renal artery stenosis. (See PRECAUTIONS.) Reversible minor increases in blood urea nitrogen and serum creatinine were observed in approximately 11.6 percent of patients with heart failure on concomitant diuretic therapy. Frequently, these abnormalities resolved when the dosage of the diuretic was decreased.

Hemoglobin and Hematocrit: Small decreases in hemoglobin and hematocrit (mean decreases of approximately 0.4 g percent and 1.3 vol percent, respectively) occurred frequently in patients treated with PRINIVIL but were rarely of clinical importance in patients without some other cause of anemia. In clinical trials, less than 0.1 percent of patients discontinued therapy due to anemia. Hemolytic anemia has been reported; a causal relationship to lisinopril cannot be excluded.

Liver Function Tests: Rarely, elevations of liver enzymes and/or serum bilirubin have occurred (see WARNINGS, *Hepatic Failure*).

In hypertensive patients, 2.0 percent discontinued therapy due to laboratory adverse experiences, principally elevations in blood urea nitrogen (0.6 percent), serum creatinine (0.5 percent) and serum potassium (0.4 percent). In the heart failure trials, 3.4 percent of patients discontinued therapy due to laboratory adverse experiences, 1.8 percent due to elevations in blood urea nitrogen and/or creatinine and 0.6 percent due to elevations in serum potassium. In the myocardial infarction trial, 2.0 percent of patients receiving PRINIVIL discontinued therapy due to renal dysfunction (increasing creatinine concentration to over 3 mg/dL or a doubling or more of the baseline serum creatinine concentration); less than 1.0 percent of patients discontinued therapy due to other laboratory adverse experiences: 0.1 percent with hyperkalemia and less than 0.1 percent with hepatic enzyme alterations.

OVERDOSAGE

Following a single oral dose of 20 g/kg, no lethality occurred in rats and death occurred in one of 20 mice receiving the same dose. The most likely manifestation of overdosage would be hypotension, for which the usual treatment would be intravenous infusion of normal saline solution. Lisinopril can be removed by hemodialysis.

DOSAGE AND ADMINISTRATION

Hypertension

Initial Therapy: In patients with uncomplicated essential hypertension not on diuretic therapy, the recommended initial dose is 10 mg once a day. Dosage should be adjusted according to blood pressure response. The usual dosage range is 20 to 40 mg per day administered in a single daily dose. The antihypertensive effect may diminish toward the end of the dosing interval regardless of the administered dose, but most commonly with a dose of 10 mg daily. This can be evaluated by measuring blood pressure just prior to dosing to determine whether satisfactory control is being maintained for 24 hours. If it is not, an increase in dose should be considered. Doses up to 80 mg have been used but do not appear to give a greater effect. If blood pressure is not controlled with PRINIVIL alone, a low dose of a diuretic may be added. Hydrochlorothiazide 12.5 mg has been shown to provide an additive effect. After the addition of a diuretic, it may be possible to reduce the dose of PRINIVIL.

Diuretic Treated Patients: In hypertensive patients who are currently being treated with a diuretic, symptomatic hypotension may occur occasionally following the initial dose of PRINIVIL. The diuretic should be discontinued, if possible, for two to three days before beginning therapy with PRINIVIL to reduce the likelihood of hypotension. (See WARNINGS.) The dosage of PRINIVIL should be adjusted according to blood pressure response. If the patient's blood pressure is not controlled with PRINIVIL alone, diuretic therapy may be resumed as described above.

If the diuretic cannot be discontinued, an initial dose of 5 mg should be used under medical supervision for at least two hours and until blood pressure has stabilized for at least an additional hour. (See WARNINGS and PRECAUTIONS, *Drug Interactions.*)

Concomitant administration of PRINIVIL with potassium supplements, potassium salt substitutes, or potassium-sparing diuretics may lead to increases of serum potassium (see PRECAUTIONS).

Dosage Adjustment in Renal Impairment: The usual dose of PRINIVIL (10 mg) is recommended for patients with a creatinine clearance > 30 mL/min (serum creatinine of up to approximately 3 mg/dL). For patients with creatinine clearance ≥ 10 mL/min ≤ 30 mL/min (serum creatinine ≥ 3 mg/dL), the first dose is 5 mg once daily. For patients with creatinine clearance < 10 mL/min (usually on hemodialysis) the recommended initial dose is 2.5 mg. The dosage may be titrated upward until blood pressure is controlled or to a maximum of 40 mg daily.

Renal Status	Creatinine-Clearance mL/min	Initial Dose mg/day
Normal Renal Function to Mild Impairment	> 30 mL/min	10 mg
Moderate to Severe Impairment	≥ 10 ≤ 30 mL/min	5 mg
Dialysis Patients*	< 10 mL/min	2.5 mg **

* See WARNINGS, *Anaphylactoid reactions during membrane exposure.*

** *Dosage or dosing interval should be adjusted depending on the blood pressure response.*

Heart Failure

PRINIVIL is indicated as adjunctive therapy with diuretics and digitalis. The recommended starting dose is 5 mg once a day.

When initiating treatment with lisinopril in patients with heart failure, the initial dose should be administered under medical observation, especially in those patients with low blood pressure (systolic blood pressure below 100 mmHg). The mean peak blood pressure lowering occurs six to eight hours after dosing. Observation should continue until blood pressure is stable. The concomitant diuretic dose should be reduced, if possible, to help minimize hypovolemia which may contribute to hypotension. (See WARNINGS and PRECAUTIONS, *Drug Interactions.*) The appearance of hypotension after the initial dose of PRINIVIL does not preclude subsequent careful dose titration with the drug, following effective management of the hypotension.

The usual effective dosage range is 5 to 20 mg per day administered as a single daily dose.

Dosage Adjustment in Patients with Heart Failure and Renal Impairment or Hyponatremia: In patients with heart failure who have hyponatremia (serum sodium <130 mEq/L) or moderate to severe renal impairment (creatinine clearance ≤30 mL/min or serum creatinine >3 mg/dL), therapy with PRINIVIL should be initiated at a dose of 2.5 mg once a day under close medical supervision. (See WARNINGS and PRECAUTIONS, *Drug Interactions.*)

Acute Myocardial Infarction

In hemodynamically stable patients within 24 hours of the onset of acute myocardial infarction, the first dose of PRINIVIL is 5 mg given orally, followed by 5 mg after 24 hours, 10 mg after 48 hours and then 10 mg of PRINIVIL once daily. Dosing should continue for six weeks. Patients should receive, as appropriate, the standard recommended treatments such as thrombolytics, aspirin and beta-blockers. Patients with a low systolic blood pressure (≤120 mmHg) when treatment is started or during the first 3 days after the infarct should be given a lower 2.5 mg oral dose of PRINIVIL (see WARNINGS). If hypotension occurs (systolic blood pressure ≤100 mmHg) a daily maintenance dose of 5 mg may be given with temporary reductions to 2.5 mg if needed. If prolonged hypotension occurs (systolic blood pressure <90 mmHg for more than 1 hour) PRINIVIL should be withdrawn. For patients who develop symptoms of heart failure, see DOSAGE AND ADMINISTRATION, *Heart Failure.*

Dosage Adjustment in Patients with Myocardial Infarction with Renal Impairment: In acute myocardial infarction, treatment with PRINIVIL should be initiated with caution in patients with evidence of renal dysfunction, defined as serum creatinine concentration exceeding 2 mg/dL. No evaluation of dosage adjustment in myocardial infarction patients with severe renal impairment has been performed.

Use in Elderly: In general, blood pressure response and adverse experiences were similar in younger and older patients given similar doses of PRINIVIL. Pharmacokinetic studies, however, indicate that maximum blood levels and area under the plasma concentration time curve (AUC) are doubled in older patients so that dosage adjustments should be made with particular caution.

HOW SUPPLIED

No. 3658—Tablets PRINIVIL, 2.5 mg, are white, round flat-faced beveled edged compressed tablets, coded MSD on one side and 15 on the other. They are supplied as follows:

NDC 0006-0015-28 unit dose packages of 100
NDC 0006-0015-31 unit of use bottles of 30
NDC 0006-0015-58 unit of use bottles of 100
NDC 0006-0015-72 carton of 25 UNIBLISTER™ cards of 31 tablets each.

Shown in Product Identification Guide, page 323

No. 3577—Tablets PRINIVIL, 5 mg, are white, shield shaped, scored, compressed tablets, with code MSD 19 on one side and PRINIVIL on the other. They are supplied as follows:

NDC 0006-0019-28 unit dose packages of 100
NDC 0006-0019-58 unit of use bottles of 100
(6505-01-281-2771, 5 mg 100's)
NDC 0006-0019-94 unit of use bottles of 90
NDC 0006-0019-82 bottles of 1,000
NDC 0006-0019-86 bottles of 5,000
(6505-01-367-8874, 5 mg 5,000's)
NDC 0006-0019-87 bottles of 10,000
(6505-01-377-8061, 5 mg 10,000's)
NDC 0006-0019-72 carton of 25 UNIBLISTER™ cards of 31 tablets each.

Shown in Product Identification Guide, page 323

No. 3578—Tablets PRINIVIL, 10 mg, are light yellow, shield shaped, compressed tablets, with code MSD 106 on one side and PRINIVIL on the other. They are supplied as follows:

NDC 0006-0106-28 unit dose packages of 100
(6505-01-342-4861, 10 mg individually sealed 100's)
NDC 0006-0106-31 unit of use bottles of 30
NDC 0006-0106-58 unit of use bottles of 100
(6505-01-275-0061, 10 mg 100's)
NDC 0006-0106-94 unit of use bottles of 90
NDC 0006-0106-82 bottles of 1,000
NDC 0006-0106-86 bottles of 5,000
(6505-01-368-6604, 10 mg 5,000's)
NDC 0006-0106-87 bottles of 10,000
(6505-01-377-8064, 10 mg 10,000's)
NDC 0006-0106-72 carton of 25 UNIBLISTER™ cards of 31 tablets each.

Shown in Product Identification Guide, page 323

No. 3579—Tablets PRINIVIL, 20 mg, are peach, shield shaped, compressed tablets, with code MSD 207 on one side and PRINIVIL on the other. They are supplied as follows:

NDC 0006-0207-28 unit dose packages of 100
NDC 0006-0207-31 unit of use bottles of 30
NDC 0006-0207-58 unit of use bottles of 100
(6505-01-282-6327, 20 mg 100's)
NDC 0006-0207-94 unit of use bottles of 90
NDC 0006-0207-82 bottles of 1,000
NDC 0006-0207-86 bottles of 5,000
(6505-01-368-2704)

Continued on next page

Information on the Merck & Co., Inc. products listed on these pages is the full prescribing information from product circulars in use August 31, 1998. For information, please call 1-800-NSC MERCK [1-800-672-6372].

Prinivil—Cont.

NDC 0006-0207-87 bottles of 10,000
(6505-01-8066, 20 mg 10,000's)
NDC 0006-0207-72 carton of 25 UNIBLISTER™ cards of 31 tablets each.

Shown in Product Identification Guide, page 323

No. 3580—Tablets PRINIVIL, 40 mg, are rose red, shield shaped, compressed tablets, with code MSD 237 on one side and PRINIVIL on the other. They are supplied as follows:
NDC 0006-0237-58 unit of use bottles of 100.

Shown in Product Identification Guide, page 323

Storage

Store at controlled room temperature, 15–30°C (59–86°F), and protect from moisture.

Dispense in a tight container, if product package is subdivided.

7825241 Issued March 1997

COPYRIGHT © MERCK & CO., Inc., 1988, 1989, 1992, 1993
All rights reserved

PRINZIDE® Tablets ℞
(Lisinopril-Hydrochlorothiazide)

USE IN PREGNANCY

When used in pregnancy during the second and third trimesters, ACE inhibitors can cause injury and even death to the developing fetus. When pregnancy is detected, PRINZIDE should be discontinued as soon as possible. See WARNINGS, *Pregnancy, Lisinopril, Fetal/Neonatal Morbidity and Mortality.*

DESCRIPTION

PRINZIDE* (Lisinopril-Hydrochlorothiazide) combines an angiotensin converting enzyme inhibitor, lisinopril, and a diuretic, hydrochlorothiazide.

Lisinopril, a synthetic peptide derivative, is an oral long-acting angiotensin converting enzyme inhibitor. It is chemically described as (*S*)-1-[N^2-(1-carboxy-3-phenylpropyl)-L-lysyl]-L-proline dihydrate. Its empirical formula is $C_{21}H_{31}N_3O_5{\cdot}2H_2O$ and its structural formula is:

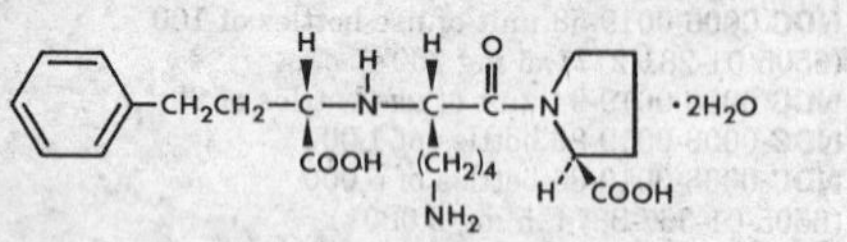

Lisinopril is a white to off-white, crystalline powder, with a molecular weight of 441.52. It is soluble in water, sparingly soluble in methanol, and practically insoluble in ethanol.

Hydrochlorothiazide is 6-chloro-3,4-dihydro-2*H*-1,2,4-benzothiadiazine-7-sulfonamide 1,1-dioxide. Its empirical formula is $C_7H_8ClN_3O_4S_2$ and its structural formula is:

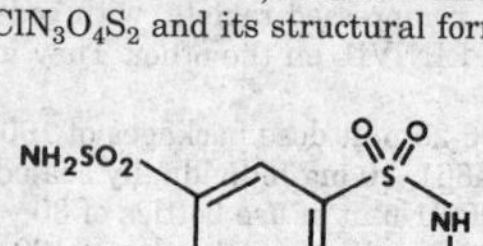

Hydrochlorothiazide is a white, or practically white, crystalline powder with a molecular weight of 297.73, which is slightly soluble in water, but freely soluble in sodium hydroxide solution.

PRINZIDE is available for oral use in three tablet combinations of lisinopril with hydrochlorothiazide: PRINZIDE 10-12.5, containing 10 mg lisinopril and 12.5 mg hydrochlorothiazide. PRINZIDE 20-12.5, containing 20 mg lisinopril and 12.5 mg hydrochlorothiazide and PRINZIDE 20-25, containing 20 mg lisinopril and 25 mg hydrochlorothiazide. Inactive ingredients are calcium phosphate, magnesium stearate, mannitol, and starch. PRINZIDE 10-12.5 also contains FD&C Blue #2 aluminum lake. PRINZIDE 20-12.5 and PRINZIDE 20-25 also contain iron oxide.

*Registered trademark of MERCK & CO., Inc.

CLINICAL PHARMACOLOGY

Lisinopril-Hydrochlorothiazide

As a result of its diuretic effects, hydrochlorothiazide increases plasma renin activity, increases aldosterone secretion, and decreases serum potassium. Administration of lisinopril blocks the renin-angiotensin-aldosterone axis and tends to reverse the potassium loss associated with the diuretic.

In clinical studies, the extent of blood pressure reduction seen with the combination of lisinopril and hydrochlorothiazide was approximately additive. The PRINZIDE 10-12.5 combination worked equally well in black and white patients. The PRINZIDE 20-12.5 and PRINZIDE 20-25 combinations appeared somewhat less effective in black patients, but relatively few black patients were studied. In most patients, the antihypertensive effect of PRINZIDE was sustained for at least 24 hours.

In a randomized, controlled comparison, the main antihypertensive effects of PRINZIDE 20-12.5 and PRINZIDE 20-25 were similar, suggesting that many patients who respond adequately to the latter combination may be controlled with PRINZIDE 20-12.5. (See DOSAGE AND ADMINISTRATION.)

Concomitant administration of lisinopril and hydrochlorothiazide has little or no effect on the bioavailability of either drug. The combination tablet is bioequivalent to concomitant administration of the separate entities.

Lisinopril

Mechanism of Action

Lisinopril inhibits angiotensin-converting enzyme (ACE) in human subjects and animals. ACE is a peptidyl dipeptidase that catalyzes the conversion of angiotensin I to the vasoconstrictor substance, angiotensin II. Angiotensin II also stimulates aldosterone secretion by the adrenal cortex. Inhibition of ACE results in decreased plasma angiotensin II which leads to decreased vasopressor activity and to decreased aldosterone secretion. The latter decrease may result in a small increase of serum potassium. Removal of angiotensin II negative feedback on renin secretion leads to increased plasma renin activity. In hypertensive patients with normal renal function treated with lisinopril alone for up to 24 weeks, the mean increase in serum potassium was less than 0.1 mEq/L; however, approximately 15 percent of patients had increases greater than 0.5 mEq/L and approximately six percent had a decrease greater than 0.5 mEq/L. In the same study, patients treated with lisinopril plus a thiazide diuretic showed essentially no change in serum potassium. (See PRECAUTIONS.)

ACE is identical to kininase, an enzyme that degrades bradykinin. Whether increased levels of bradykinin, a potent vasodepressor peptide, play a role in the therapeutic effects of lisinopril remains to be elucidated.

While the mechanism through which lisinopril lowers blood pressure is believed to be primarily suppression of the renin-angiotensin-aldosterone system, lisinopril is antihypertensive even in patients with low-renin hypertension. Although lisinopril was antihypertensive in all races studied, black hypertensive patients (usually a low-renin hypertensive population) had a smaller average response to lisinopril monotherapy than non-black patients.

Pharmacokinetics and Metabolism

Following oral administration of lisinopril, peak serum concentrations occur within about 7 hours. Declining serum concentrations exhibit a prolonged terminal phase which does not contribute to drug accumulation. This terminal phase probably represents saturable binding to ACE and is not proportional to dose. Lisinopril does not appear to be bound to other serum proteins.

Lisinopril does not undergo metabolism and is excreted unchanged entirely in the urine. Based on urinary recovery, the mean extent of absorption of lisinopril is approximately 25 percent, with large intersubject variability (6–60 percent) at all doses tested (5–80 mg). Lisinopril absorption is not influenced by the presence of food in the gastrointestinal tract.

Upon multiple dosing, lisinopril exhibits an effective half-life of accumulation of 12 hours.

Impaired renal function decreases elimination of lisinopril, which is excreted principally through the kidneys, but this decrease becomes clinically important only when the glomerular filtration rate is below 30 mL/min. Above this glomerular filtration rate, the elimination half-life is little changed. With greater impairment, however, peak and trough lisinopril levels increase, time to peak concentration increases and time to attain steady state is prolonged. Older patients, on average, have (approximately doubled) higher blood levels and area under the plasma concentration time curve (AUC) than younger patients. (See DOSAGE AND ADMINISTRATION.) Lisinopril can be removed by hemodialysis.

Studies in rats indicate that lisinopril crosses the blood-brain barrier poorly. Multiple doses of lisinopril in rats do not result in accumulation in any tissues. However, milk of lactating rats contains radioactivity following administration of ^{14}C lisinopril. By whole body autoradiography, radioactivity was found in the placenta following administration of labeled drug to pregnant rats, but none was found in the fetuses.

Pharmacodynamics

Administration of lisinopril to patients with hypertension results in a reduction of supine and standing blood pressure to about the same extent with no compensatory tachycardia. Symptomatic postural hypotension is usually not observed although it can occur and should be anticipated in volume and/or salt-depleted patients. (See WARNINGS.)

In most patients studied, onset of antihypertensive activity was seen at one hour after oral administration of an individual dose of lisinopril, with peak reduction of blood pressure achieved by six hours.

In some patients achievement of optimal blood pressure reduction may require two to four weeks of therapy.

At recommended single daily doses, antihypertensive effects have been maintained for at least 24 hours after dosing, although the effect at 24 hours was substantially smaller than the effect six hours after dosing.

The antihypertensive effects of lisinopril have continued during long-term therapy. Abrupt withdrawal of lisinopril has not been associated with a rapid increase in blood pressure; nor with a significant overshoot of pretreatment blood pressure.

In hemodynamic studies in patients with essential hypertension, blood pressure reduction was accompanied by a reduction in peripheral arterial resistance with little or no change in cardiac output and in heart rate. In a study in nine hypertensive patients, following administration of lisinopril, there was an increase in mean renal blood flow that was not significant. Data from several small studies are inconsistent with respect to the effect of lisinopril on glomerular filtration rate in hypertensive patients with normal renal function, but suggest that changes, if any, are not large.

In patients with renovascular hypertension lisinopril has been shown to be well tolerated and effective in controlling blood pressure (see PRECAUTIONS).

Hydrochlorothiazide

The mechanism of the antihypertensive effect of thiazides is unknown. Thiazides do not usually affect normal blood pressure.

Hydrochlorothiazide is a diuretic and antihypertensive. It affects the distal renal tubular mechanism of electrolyte reabsorption. Hydrochlorothiazide increases excretion of sodium and chloride in approximately equivalent amounts. Natriuresis may be accompanied by some loss of potassium and bicarbonate.

After oral use diuresis begins within two hours, peaks in about four hours and lasts about 6 to 12 hours.

Hydrochlorothiazide is not metabolized but is eliminated rapidly by the kidney. When plasma levels have been followed for at least 24 hours, the plasma half-life has been observed to vary between 5.6 and 14.8 hours. At least 61 percent of the oral dose is eliminated unchanged within 24 hours. Hydrochlorothiazide crosses the placental but not the blood-brain barrier.

INDICATIONS AND USAGE

PRINZIDE is indicated for the treatment of hypertension.

These fixed-dose combinations are not indicated for initial therapy (see DOSAGE AND ADMINISTRATION).

In using PRINZIDE, consideration should be given to the fact that an angiotensin converting enzyme inhibitor, captopril, has caused agranulocytosis, particularly in patients with renal impairment or collagen vascular disease, and that available data are insufficient to show that lisinopril does not have a similar risk. (See WARNINGS.)

In considering use of PRINZIDE, it should be noted that black patients receiving ACE inhibitors have been reported to have a higher incidence of angioedema compared to non-blacks. (See WARNINGS, *Angioedema.*)

CONTRAINDICATIONS

PRINZIDE is contraindicated in patients who are hypersensitive to any component of this product and in patients with a history of angioedema related to previous treatment with an angiotensin converting enzyme inhibitor. Because of the hydrochlorothiazide component, this product is contraindicated in patients with anuria or hypersensitivity to other sulfonamide-derived drugs.

WARNINGS

General

Lisinopril

Anaphylactoid and Possibly Related Reactions:

Presumably because angiotensin-converting enzyme inhibitors affect the metabolism of eicosanoids and polypeptides, including endogenous bradykinin, patients receiving ACE inhibitors (including PRINZIDE) may be subject to a variety of adverse reactions, some of them serious.

Angioedema: Angioedema of the face, extremities, lips, tongue, glottis and/or larynx has been reported rarely in patients treated with angiotensin converting enzyme inhibitors, including lisinopril. This may occur at any time during treatment. In such cases PRINZIDE should be promptly discontinued and appropriate therapy and monitoring should be provided until complete and sustained resolution of signs and symptoms has occurred. In instances where swelling has been confined to the face and lips the condition has generally resolved without treatment, although antihistamines have been useful in relieving symptoms. Angioedema associated with laryngeal edema may be fatal. **Where there is**

involvement of the tongue, glottis or larynx, likely to cause airway obstruction, subcutaneous epinephrine solution 1:1000 (0.3 mL to 0.5 mL) and/or measures necessary to ensure a patent airway, should be promptly provided. (See ADVERSE REACTIONS.)

Patients with a history of angioedema unrelated to ACE inhibitor therapy may be at increased risk of angioedema while receiving an ACE inhibitor (see also INDICATIONS AND USAGE and CONTRAINDICATIONS).

Anaphylactoid reactions during desensitization: Two patients undergoing desensitizing treatment with hymenoptera venom while receiving ACE inhibitors sustained life-threatening anaphylactoid reactions. In the same patients, these reactions were avoided when ACE inhibitors were temporarily withheld, but they reappeared upon inadvertent rechallenge.

Anaphylactoid reactions during membrane exposure: Anaphylactoid reactions have been reported in patients dialyzed with high-flux membranes and treated concomitantly with an ACE inhibitor. Anaphylactoid reactions have also been reported in patients undergoing low-density lipoprotein apheresis with dextran sulfate absorption.

Hypotension and Related Effects:
Excessive hypotension was rarely seen in uncomplicated hypertensive patients but is a possible consequence of lisinopril use in salt/volume-depleted persons, such as those treated vigorously with diuretics or patients on dialysis. (See PRECAUTIONS, *Drug Interactions* and ADVERSE REACTIONS.)

Syncope has been reported in 0.8 percent of patients receiving PRINZIDE. In patients with hypertension receiving lisinopril alone, the incidence of syncope was 0.1 percent. The overall incidence of syncope may be reduced by proper titration of the individual components. (See PRECAUTIONS, *Drug Interactions*, ADVERSE REACTIONS and DOSAGE AND ADMINISTRATION.)

In patients with severe congestive heart failure, with or without associated renal insufficiency, excessive hypotension has been observed and may be associated with oliguria and/or progressive azotemia, and rarely with acute renal failure and/or death. Because of the potential fall in blood pressure in these patients, therapy should be started under very close medical supervision. Such patients should be followed closely for the first two weeks of treatment and whenever the dose of lisinopril and/or diuretic is increased. Similar considerations apply to patients with ischemic heart or cerebrovascular disease in whom an excessive fall in blood pressure could result in a myocardial infarction or cerebrovascular accident.

If hypotension occurs, the patient should be placed in supine position and, if necessary, receive an intravenous infusion of normal saline. A transient hypotensive response is not a contraindication to further doses which usually can be given without difficulty once the blood pressure has increased after volume expansion.

Neutropenia/Agranulocytosis:
Another angiotensin converting enzyme inhibitor, captopril, has been shown to cause agranulocytosis and bone marrow depression, rarely in uncomplicated patients but more frequently in patients with renal impairment, especially if they also have a collagen vascular disease. Available data from clinical trials of lisinopril are insufficient to show that lisinopril does not cause agranulocytosis at similar rates. Marketing experience has revealed rare cases of neutropenia and bone marrow depression in which a causal relationship to lisinopril cannot be excluded. Periodic monitoring of white blood cell counts in patients with collagen vascular disease and renal disease should be considered.

Hepatic Failure:
Rarely, ACE inhibitors have been associated with a syndrome that starts with cholestatic jaundice and progresses to fulminant hepatic necrosis, and (sometimes) death. The mechanism of this syndrome is not understood. Patients receiving ACE inhibitors who develop jaundice or marked elevations of hepatic enzymes should discontinue the ACE inhibitor and receive appropriate medical follow-up.

Hydrochlorothiazide
Thiazides should be used with caution in severe renal disease. In patients with renal disease, thiazides may precipitate azotemia. Cumulative effects of the drug may develop in patients with impaired renal function.

Thiazides should be used with caution in patients with impaired hepatic function or progressive liver disease, since minor alterations of fluid and electrolyte balance may precipitate hepatic coma.

Sensitivity reactions may occur in patients with or without a history of allergy or bronchial asthma.

The possibility of exacerbation or activation of systemic lupus erythematosus has been reported.

Lithium generally should not be given with thiazides (see PRECAUTIONS, *Drug Interactions, Lisinopril* and *Hydrochlorothiazide*).

Pregnancy
Lisinopril-Hydrochlorothiazide
Teratogenicity studies were conducted in mice and rats with up to 90 mg/kg/day of lisinopril in combination with 10 mg/

kg/day of hydrochlorothiazide. This dose of lisinopril is 5 times (in mice) and 10 times (in rats) the maximum recommended human daily dose (MRHDD) when compared on a body surface area basis (mg/m²); the dose of hydrochlorothiazide is 0.9 times (in mice) and 1.8 times (in rats) the MRHDD. Maternal or fetotoxic effects were not seen in mice with the combination. In rats decreased maternal weight gain and decreased fetal weight occurred down to 3/10 mg/kg/day (the lowest dose tested). Associated with the decreased fetal weight was a delay in fetal ossification. The decreased fetal weight and delay in fetal ossification were not seen in saline-supplemented animals given 90/10 mg/kg/day.

When used in pregnancy during the second and third trimesters, ACE inhibitors can cause injury and even death to the developing fetus. When pregnancy is detected, PRINZIDE should be discontinued as soon as possible. (See *Lisinopril, Fetal/Neonatal Morbidity and Mortality*, below.)

Lisinopril
Fetal/Neonatal Morbidity and Mortality: ACE inhibitors can cause fetal and neonatal morbidity and death when administered to pregnant women. Several dozen cases have been reported in the world literature. When pregnancy is detected, ACE inhibitors should be discontinued as soon as possible.

The use of ACE inhibitors during the second and third trimesters of pregnancy has been associated with fetal and neonatal injury, including hypotension, neonatal skull hypoplasia, anuria, reversible or irreversible renal failure, and death. Oligohydramnios has also been reported, presumably resulting from decreased fetal renal function; oligohydramnios in this setting has been associated with fetal limb contractures, craniofacial deformation, and hypoplastic lung development. Prematurity, intrauterine growth retardation, and patent ductus arteriosus have also been reported, although it is not clear whether these occurrences were due to the ACE-inhibitor exposure.

These adverse effects do not appear to have resulted from intrauterine ACE-inhibitor exposure that has been limited to the first trimester. Mothers whose embryos and fetuses are exposed to ACE inhibitors only during the first trimester should be so informed. Nonetheless, when patients become pregnant, physicians should make every effort to discontinue the use of PRINZIDE as soon as possible.

Rarely (probably less often than once in every thousand pregnancies), no alternative to ACE inhibitors will be found. In these rare cases, the mothers should be apprised of the potential hazards to their fetuses, and serial ultrasound examinations should be performed to assess the intraamniotic environment.

If oligohydramnios is observed, PRINZIDE should be discontinued unless it is considered lifesaving for the mother. Contraction stress testing (CST), a non-stress test (NST), or biophysical profiling (BPP) may be appropriate, depending upon the week of pregnancy. Patients and physicians should be aware, however, that oligohydramnios may not appear until after the fetus has sustained irreversible injury.

Infants with histories of *in utero* exposure to ACE inhibitors should be closely observed for hypotension, oliguria, and hyperkalemia. If oliguria occurs, attention should be directed toward support of blood pressure and renal perfusion. Exchange transfusion or dialysis may be required as means of reversing hypotension and/or substituting for disordered renal function. Lisinopril, which crosses the placenta, has been removed from neonatal circulation by peritoneal dialysis with some clinical benefit, and theoretically may be removed by exchange transfusion, although there is no experience with the latter procedure.

No teratogenic effects of lisinopril were seen in studies of pregnant mice, rats, and rabbits. On a body surface area basis, the doses used were up to 55 times, 33 times, and 0.15 times, respectively, the MRHDD.

Hydrochlorothiazide
Studies in which hydrochlorothiazide was orally administered to pregnant mice and rats during their respective periods of major organogenesis at doses up to 3000 and 1000 mg/kg/day, respectively, provided no evidence of harm to the fetus. These doses are more than 150 times the MRHDD on a body surface area basis. Thiazides cross the placental barrier and appear in cord blood. There is a risk of fetal or neonatal jaundice, thrombocytopenia and possibly other adverse reactions that have occurred in adults.

PRECAUTIONS

General
Lisinopril
Impaired Renal Function: As a consequence of inhibiting the renin-angiotensin-aldosterone system, changes in renal function may be anticipated in susceptible individuals. In patients with severe congestive heart failure whose renal function may depend on the activity of the renin-angiotensin-aldosterone system, treatment with angiotensin converting enzyme inhibitors, including lisinopril, may be associated with oliguria and/or progressive azotemia and rarely with acute renal failure and/or death.

In hypertensive patients with unilateral or bilateral renal artery stenosis, increases in blood urea nitrogen and serum creatinine may occur. Experience with another angiotensin converting enzyme inhibitor suggests that these increases are usually reversible upon discontinuation of lisinopril and/or diuretic therapy. In such patients renal function should be monitored during the first few weeks of therapy. Some hypertensive patients with no apparent pre-existing renal vascular disease have developed increases in blood urea and serum creatinine, usually minor and transient, especially when lisinopril has been given concomitantly with a diuretic. This is more likely to occur in patients with pre-existing renal impairment. Dosage reduction of lisinopril and/or discontinuation of the diuretic may be required.

Evaluation of the hypertensive patient should always include assessment of renal function. (See DOSAGE AND ADMINISTRATION.)

Hyperkalemia: In clinical trials hyperkalemia (serum potassium greater than 5.7 mEq/L) occurred in approximately 1.4 percent of hypertensive patients treated with lisinopril plus hydrochlorothiazide. In most cases these were isolated values which resolved despite continued therapy. Hyperkalemia was not a cause of discontinuation of therapy. Risk factors for the development of hyperkalemia include renal insufficiency, diabetes mellitus, and the concomitant use of potassium-sparing diuretics, potassium supplements and/or potassium-containing salt substitutes, which should be used cautiously if at all with PRINZIDE. (See *Drug Interactions*.)

Cough: Presumably due to the inhibition of the degradation of endogenous bradykinin, persistent nonproductive cough has been reported with all ACE inhibitors, always resolving after discontinuation of therapy. ACE inhibitor-induced cough should be considered in the differential diagnosis of cough.

Surgery/Anesthesia: In patients undergoing major surgery or during anesthesia with agents that produce hypotension, lisinopril may block angiotensin II formation secondary to compensatory renin release. If hypotension occurs and is considered to be due to this mechanism, it can be corrected by volume expansion.

Hydrochlorothiazide
Periodic determination of serum electrolytes to detect possible electrolyte imbalance should be performed at appropriate intervals.

All patients receiving thiazide therapy should be observed for clinical signs of fluid or electrolyte imbalance: namely, hyponatremia, hypochloremic alkalosis, and hypokalemia. Serum and urine electrolyte determinations are particularly important when the patient is vomiting excessively or receiving parenteral fluids. Warning signs or symptoms of fluid and electrolyte imbalance, irrespective of cause, include dryness of mouth, thirst, weakness, lethargy, drowsiness, restlessness, confusion, seizures, muscle pains or cramps, muscular fatigue, hypotension, oliguria, tachycardia, and gastrointestinal disturbances such as nausea and vomiting.

Hypokalemia may develop, especially with brisk diuresis, when severe cirrhosis is present, or after prolonged therapy. Interference with adequate oral electrolyte intake will also contribute to hypokalemia. Hypokalemia may cause cardiac arrhythmia and may also sensitize or exaggerate the response of the heart to the toxic effects of digitalis (e.g., increased ventricular irritability). Because lisinopril reduces the production of aldosterone, concomitant therapy with lisinopril attenuates the diuretic-induced potassium loss (see *Drug Interactions, Agents Increasing Serum Potassium*).

Although any chloride deficit is generally mild and usually does not require specific treatment, except under extraordinary circumstances (as in liver disease or renal disease), chloride replacement may be required in the treatment of metabolic alkalosis.

Dilutional hyponatremia may occur in edematous patients in hot weather; appropriate therapy is water restriction, rather than administration of salt except in rare instances when the hyponatremia is life-threatening. In actual salt depletion, appropriate replacement is the therapy of choice.

Hyperuricemia may occur or frank gout may be precipitated in certain patients receiving thiazide therapy.

In diabetic patients dosage adjustments of insulin or oral hypoglycemic agents may be required. Hyperglycemia may occur with thiazide diuretics. Thus latent diabetes mellitus may become manifest during thiazide therapy.

The antihypertensive effects of the drug may be enhanced in the postsympathectomy patient.

If progressive renal impairment becomes evident consider withholding or discontinuing diuretic therapy.

Continued on next page

Information on the Merck & Co., Inc. products listed on these pages is the full prescribing information from product circulars in use August 31, 1998. For information, please call 1-800-NSC MERCK [1-800-672-6372].

Prinzide—Cont.

Thiazides have been shown to increase the urinary excretion of magnesium; this may result in hypomagnesemia.

Thiazides may decrease urinary calcium excretion. Thiazides may cause intermittent and slight elevation of serum calcium in the absence of known disorders of calcium metabolism. Marked hypercalcemia may be evidence of hidden hyperparathyroidism. Thiazides should be discontinued before carrying out tests for parathyroid function.

Increases in cholesterol and triglyceride levels may be associated with thiazide diuretic therapy.

Information for Patients

Angioedema: Angioedema, including laryngeal edema, may occur at any time during treatment with angiotensin converting enzyme inhibitors, including lisinopril. Patients should be so advised and told to report immediately any signs or symptoms suggesting angioedema (swelling of face, extremities, eyes, lips, tongue, difficulty in swallowing or breathing) and to take no more drug until they have consulted with the prescribing physician.

Symptomatic Hypotension: Patients should be cautioned to report lightheadedness especially during the first few days of therapy. If actual syncope occurs, the patients should be told to discontinue the drug until they have consulted with the prescribing physician.

All patients should be cautioned that excessive perspiration and dehydration may lead to an excessive fall in blood pressure because of reduction in fluid volume. Other causes of volume depletion such as vomiting or diarrhea may also lead to a fall in blood pressure; patients should be advised to consult with their physician.

Hyperkalemia: Patients should be told not to use salt substitutes containing potassium without consulting their physician.

Neutropenia: Patients should be told to report promptly any indication of infection (e.g., sore throat, fever) which may be a sign of neutropenia.

Pregnancy: Female patients of childbearing age should be told about the consequences of second- and third-trimester exposure to ACE inhibitors, and they should also be told that these consequences do not appear to have resulted from intrauterine ACE-inhibitor exposure that has been limited to the first trimester. These patients should be asked to report pregnancies to their physicians as soon as possible.

NOTE: As with many other drugs, certain advice to patients being treated with PRINZIDE is warranted. This information is intended to aid in the safe and effective use of this medication. It is not a disclosure of all possible adverse or intended effects.

Drug Interactions

Lisinopril

Hypotension—Patients on Diuretic Therapy: Patients on diuretics, and especially those in whom diuretic therapy was recently instituted, may occasionally experience an excessive reduction of blood pressure after initiation of therapy with lisinopril. The possibility of hypotensive effects with lisinopril can be minimized by either discontinuing the diuretic or increasing the salt intake prior to initiation of treatment with lisinopril. If it is necessary to continue the diuretic, initiate therapy with lisinopril at a dose of 5 mg daily, and provide close medical supervision after the initial dose for at least two hours and until blood pressure has stabilized for at least an additional hour. (See WARNINGS and DOSAGE AND ADMINISTRATION.) When a diuretic is added to the therapy of a patient receiving lisinopril, an additional antihypertensive effect is usually observed. (See DOSAGE AND ADMINISTRATION.)

Indomethacin: In a study in 36 patients with mild to moderate hypertension where the antihypertensive effects of lisinopril alone were compared to lisinopril given concomitantly with indomethacin, the use of indomethacin was associated with a reduced effect, although the difference between the two regimens was not significant.

Other Agents: Lisinopril has been used concomitantly with nitrates and/or digoxin without evidence of clinically significant adverse interactions. No meaningful clinically important pharmacokinetic interactions occurred when lisinopril was used concomitantly with propranolol, digoxin, or hydrochlorothiazide. The presence of food in the stomach does not alter the bioavailability of lisinopril.

Agents Increasing Serum Potassium: Lisinopril attenuates potassium loss caused by thiazide-type diuretics. Use of lisinopril with potassium-sparing diuretics (e.g., spironolactone, triamterene, or amiloride), potassium supplements, or potassium-containing salt substitutes may lead to significant increases in serum potassium. Therefore, if concomitant use of these agents is indicated, because of demonstrated hypokalemia, they should be used with caution and with frequent monitoring of serum potassium.

Lithium: Lithium toxicity has been reported in patients receiving lithium concomitantly with drugs which cause elimination of sodium, including ACE inhibitors. Lithium toxicity was usually reversible upon discontinuation of lithium and the ACE inhibitor. It is recommended that serum lithium levels be monitored frequently if lisinopril is administered concomitantly with lithium.

Hydrochlorothiazide

When administered concurrently the following drugs may interact with thiazide diuretics.

Alcohol, barbiturates, or narcotics —potentiation of orthostatic hypotension may occur.

Antidiabetic drugs (oral agents and insulin)—dosage adjustment of the antidiabetic drug may be required.

Other antihypertensive drugs —additive effect or potentiation.

Cholestyramine and colestipol resins —Absorption of hydrochlorothiazide is impaired in the presence of anionic exchange resins. Single doses of either cholestyramine or colestipol resins bind the hydrochlorothiazide and reduce its absorption from the gastrointestinal tract by up to 85 and 43 percent, respectively.

Corticosteroids, ACTH —intensified electrolyte depletion, particularly hypokalemia.

Pressor amines (e.g., norepinephrine) —possible decreased response to pressor amines but not sufficient to preclude their use.

Skeletal muscle relaxants, nondepolarizing (e.g., tubocurarine) —possible increased responsiveness to the muscle relaxant.

Lithium —should not generally be given with diuretics. Diuretic agents reduce the renal clearance of lithium and add a high risk of lithium toxicity. Refer to the package insert for lithium preparations before use of such preparations with PRINZIDE.

Non-steroidal Anti-inflammatory Drugs —In some patients, the administration of a non-steroidal anti-inflammatory agent can reduce the diuretic, natriuretic, and antihypertensive effects of loop, potassium-sparing and thiazide diuretics. Therefore, when PRINZIDE and non-steroidal anti-inflammatory agents are used concomitantly, the patient should be observed closely to determine if the desired effect of PRINZIDE is obtained.

Carcinogenesis, Mutagenesis, Impairment of Fertility

Lisinopril-Hydrochlorothiazide

Lisinopril in combination with hydrochlorothiazide was not mutagenic in a microbial mutagen test using *Salmonella typhimurium* (Ames test) or *Escherichia coli* with or without metabolic activation or in a forward mutation assay using Chinese hamster lung cells. Lisinopril-hydrochlorothiazide did not produce DNA single strand breaks in an *in vitro* alkaline elution rat hepatocyte assay. In addition, it did not produce increases in chromosomal aberrations in an *in vitro* test in Chinese hamster ovary cells or in an *in vivo* study in mouse bone marrow.

Lisinopril

There was no evidence of a tumorigenic effect when lisinopril was administered orally for 105 weeks to male and female rats at doses up to 90 mg/kg/day or for 92 weeks to male and female mice at doses up to 135 mg/kg/day. These doses are 10 times and 7 times, respectively, the maximum recommended human daily dose (MRHDD) when compared on a body surface area basis.

Lisinopril was not mutagenic in the Ames microbial mutagen test with or without metabolic activation. It was also negative in a forward mutation assay using Chinese hamster lung cells. Lisinopril did not produce single strand DNA breaks in an *in vitro* alkaline elution rat hepatocyte assay. In addition, lisinopril did not produce increases in chromosomal aberrations in an *in vitro* test in Chinese hamster ovary cells or in an *in vivo* study in mouse bone marrow.

There were no adverse effects on reproductive performance in male and female rats treated with up to 300 mg/kg/day of lisinopril (33 times the MRHDD when compared on a body surface area basis).

Hydrochlorothiazide

Two-year feeding studies in mice and rats conducted under the auspices of the National Toxicology Program (NTP) uncovered no evidence of a carcinogenic potential of hydrochlorothiazide in female mice at doses of up to approximately 600 mg/kg/day (53 times the MRHDD when compared on a body surface area basis) or in male and female rats at doses of up to approximately 100 mg/kg/day (18 times the MRHDD when compared on a body surface area basis). The NTP, however, found equivocal evidence for hepatocarcinogenicity in male mice.

Hydrochlorothiazide was not genotoxic *in vitro* in the Ames mutagenicity assay of *Salmonella typhimurium* strains TA 98, TA 100, TA 1535, TA 1537, and TA 1538 and in the Chinese Hamster Ovary (CHO) test for chromosomal aberrations, or *in vivo* in assays using mouse germinal cell chromosomes, Chinese hamster bone marrow chromosomes, and the *Drosophila* sex-linked recessive lethal trait gene. Positive test results were obtained only in the *in vitro* CHO Sister Chromatid Exchange (clastogenicity) and in the Mouse Lymphoma Cell (mutagenicity) assays, using concentrations of hydrochlorothiazide from 43 to 1300 µg/mL, and in the *Aspergillus nidulans* non-disjunction assay at an unspecified concentration.

Hydrochlorothiazide had no adverse effects on the fertility of mice and rats of either sex in studies wherein these species were exposed, via their diet, to doses of up to 100 and 4 mg/kg, respectively, prior to conception and throughout gestation. In mice and rats these doses are 9 times and 0.7 times, respectively, the MRHDD when compared on a body surface area basis.

Pregnancy

Pregnancy Categories C (first trimester) *and D* (second and third trimesters). See WARNINGS, *Pregnancy, Lisinopril, Fetal/Neonatal Morbidity and Mortality.*

Nursing Mothers

It is not known whether lisinopril is secreted in human milk. However, milk of lactating rats contains radioactivity following administration of ^{14}C lisinopril. In another study, lisinopril was present in rat milk at levels similar to plasma levels in the dams. Thiazides do appear in human milk. Because of the potential for serious reactions in nursing infants from ACE inhibitors and hydrochlorothiazide, a decision should be made whether to discontinue nursing or to discontinue PRINZIDE, taking into account the importance of the drug to the mother.

Pediatric Use

Safety and effectiveness in pediatric patients have not been established.

ADVERSE REACTIONS

PRINZIDE has been evaluated for safety in 930 patients, including 100 patients treated for 50 weeks or more.

In clinical trials with PRINZIDE no adverse experiences peculiar to this combination drug have been observed. Adverse experiences that have occurred have been limited to those that have been previously reported with lisinopril or hydrochlorothiazide.

The most frequent clinical adverse experiences in controlled trials (including open label extensions) with any combination of lisinopril and hydrochlorothiazide were: dizziness (7.5 percent), headache (5.2 percent), cough (3.9 percent), fatigue (3.7 percent) and orthostatic effects (3.2 percent), all of which were more common than in placebo-treated patients. Generally, adverse experiences were mild and transient in nature; but see WARNINGS regarding angioedema and excessive hypotension or syncope. Discontinuation of therapy due to adverse effects was required in 4.4 percent of patients, principally because of dizziness, cough, fatigue and muscle cramps.

	Percent of Patients in Controlled Studies	
	Lisinopril-Hydrochlorothiazide (n=930) Incidence (discontinuation)	Placebo (n=207) Incidence
Dizziness	7.5 (0.8)	1.9
Headache	5.2 (0.3)	1.9
Cough	3.9 (0.6)	1.0
Fatigue	3.7 (0.4)	1.0
Orthostatic Effects	3.2 (0.1)	1.0
Diarrhea	2.5 (0.2)	2.4
Nausea	2.2 (0.1)	2.4
Upper Respiratory Infection	2.2 (0.0)	0.0
Muscle Cramps	2.0 (0.4)	0.5
Asthenia	1.8 (0.2)	1.0
Paresthesia	1.5 (0.1)	0.0
Hypotension	1.4 (0.3)	0.5
Vomiting	1.4 (0.1)	0.5
Dyspepsia	1.3 (0.0)	0.0
Rash	1.2 (0.1)	0.5
Impotence	1.2 (0.3)	0.0

Adverse experiences occurring in greater than one percent of patients treated with lisinopril plus hydrochlorothiazide in controlled clinical trials are shown below.
[See table at bottom of previous page]
Clinical adverse experiences occurring in 0.3 to 1.0 percent of patients in controlled trials included: *Body as a Whole:* Chest pain, abdominal pain, syncope, chest discomfort, fever, trauma, virus infection. *Cardiovascular:* Palpitation, orthostatic hypotension. *Digestive:* Gastrointestinal cramps, dry mouth, constipation, heartburn. *Musculoskeletal:* Back pain, shoulder pain, knee pain, back strain, myalgia, foot pain. *Nervous/Psychiatric:* Decreased libido, vertigo, depression, somnolence. *Respiratory:* Common cold, nasal congestion, influenza, bronchitis, pharyngeal pain, dyspnea, pulmonary congestion, chronic sinusitis, allergic rhinitis, pharyngeal discomfort. *Skin:* Flushing, pruritus, skin inflammation, diaphoresis. *Special Senses:* Blurred vision, tinnitus, otalgia. *Urogenital:* Urinary tract infection.
Angioedema: Angioedema has been reported in patients receiving PRINZIDE, with an incidence higher in black than in non-black patients. Angioedema associated with laryngeal edema may be fatal. If angioedema of the face, extremities, lips, tongue, glottis and/or larynx occurs, treatment with PRINZIDE should be discontinued and appropriate therapy instituted immediately. (See WARNINGS.)
Hypotension: In clinical trials, adverse effects relating to hypotension occurred as follows: hypotension (1.4), orthostatic hypotension (0.5), other orthostatic effects (3.2). In addition syncope occurred in 0.8 percent of patients. (See WARNINGS.)
Cough: See PRECAUTIONS, *Cough.*
Clinical Laboratory Test Findings
Serum Electrolytes: See PRECAUTIONS.
Creatinine, Blood Urea Nitrogen: Minor reversible increases in blood urea nitrogen and serum creatinine were observed in patients with essential hypertension treated with PRINZIDE. More marked increases have also been reported and were more likely to occur in patients with renal artery stenosis. (See PRECAUTIONS.)
Serum Uric Acid, Glucose, Magnesium, Cholesterol, Triglycerides and Calcium: See PRECAUTIONS.
Hemoglobin and Hematocrit: Small decreases in hemoglobin and hematocrit (mean decreases of approximately 0.5 g percent and 1.5 vol percent, respectively) occurred frequently in hypertensive patients treated with PRINZIDE but were rarely of clinical importance unless another cause of anemia coexisted. In clinical trials, 0.4 percent of patients discontinued therapy due to anemia.
Liver Function Tests: Rarely, elevations of liver enzymes and/or serum bilirubin have occurred (see WARNINGS, *Hepatic Failure*).

Other adverse reactions that have been reported with the individual components are listed below:
Lisinopril —In clinical trials adverse reactions which occurred with lisinopril were also seen with PRINZIDE. In addition, and since lisinopril has been marketed, the following adverse reactions have been reported with lisinopril and should be considered potential adverse reactions for PRINZIDE: *Body as a Whole:* Anaphylactoid reactions (see WARNINGS, *Anaphylactoid and Possibly Related Reactions),* malaise, edema, facial edema, pain, pelvic pain, flank pain, chills; *Cardiovascular:* Cardiac arrest, myocardial infarction or cerebrovascular accident, possibly secondary to excessive hypotension in high risk patients (see WARNINGS, *Hypotension),* pulmonary embolism and infarction, worsening of heart failure, arrhythmias (including tachycardia, ventricular tachycardia, atrial tachycardia, atrial fibrillation, bradycardia, and premature ventricular contractions), angina pectoris, transient ischemic attacks, paroxysmal nocturnal dyspnea, decreased blood pressure, peripheral edema, vasculitis; *Digestive:* Pancreatitis, hepatitis (hepatocellular or cholestatic jaundice) (see WARNINGS, *Hepatic Failure*), gastritis, anorexia, flatulence, increased salivation; *Endocrine:* Diabetes mellitus; *Hematologic:* Rare cases of neutropenia, thrombocytopenia, and bone marrow depression have been reported. Hemolytic anemia has been reported; a causal relationship to lisinopril cannot be excluded; *Metabolic:* Gout, weight loss, dehydration, fluid overload, weight gain; *Musculoskeletal:* Arthritis, arthralgia, neck pain, hip pain, joint pain, leg pain, arm pain, lumbago; *Nervous System/Psychiatric:* Ataxia, memory impairment, tremor, insomnia, stroke, nervousness, confusion, peripheral neuropathy (e.g., paresthesia, dysesthesia), spasm, hypersomnia, irritability; *Respiratory:* Malignant lung neoplasms, hemoptysis, pulmonary edema, pulmonary infiltrates, bronchospasm, asthma, pleural effusion, pneumonia, wheezing, orthopnea, painful respiration, epistaxis, laryngitis, sinusitis, pharyngitis, rhinitis, rhinorrhea, chest sound abnormalities; *Skin:* Urticaria, alopecia, herpes zoster, photosensitivity, skin lesions, skin infections, pemphigus, erythema. Other severe skin reactions (including toxic epidermal necrolysis and Stevens-Johnson syndrome) have been reported rarely; causal relationship has not been established; *Speical Senses:* Visual loss, diplopia, photophobia; *Urogenital:* Acute renal failure, oliguria, anuria, uremia, progressive azotemia, renal dysfunction (see PRECAUTIONS and DOSAGE AND ADMINISTRATION), pyelonephritis, dysuria, breast pain.
Miscellaneous: A symptom complex has been reported which may include a positive ANA, an elevated erythrocyte sedimentation rate, arthralgia/arthritis, myalgia, fever, vasculitis, leukocytosis, eosinophilia, photosensitivity, rash, and other dermatological manifestations.
Fetal/Neonatal Morbidity and Mortality: See WARNINGS, *Pregnancy, Lisinopril, Fetal/Neonatal Morbidity and Mortality.*
Hydrochlorothiazide —Body as a Whole: Weakness; *Digestive:* Anorexia, gastric irritation, cramping, jaundice (intrahepatic cholestatic jaundice), pancreatitis, sialadenitis, constipation; *Hematologic:* Leukopenia, agranulocytosis, thrombocytopenia, aplastic anemia, hemolytic anemia; *Musculoskeletal:* Muscle spasm; *Nervous System/Psychiatric:* Restlessness; *Renal:* Renal failure, renal dysfunction, interstitial nephritis (see WARNINGS); *Skin:* Erythema multiforme including Stevens-Johnson syndrome, exfoliative dermatitis including toxic epidermal necrolysis, alopecia; *Special Senses:* Xanthopsia; *Hypersensitivity:* Purpura, photosensitivity, urticaria, necrotizing angiitis (vasculitis and cutaneous vasculitis), respiratory distress including pneumonitis and pulmonary edema, anaphylactic reactions.

OVERDOSAGE

No specific information is available on the treatment of overdosage with PRINZIDE. Treatment is symptomatic and supportive. Therapy with PRINZIDE should be discontinued and the patient observed closely. Suggested measures include induction of emesis and/or gastric lavage, and correction of dehydration, electrolyte imbalance and hypotension by established procedures.
Lisinopril
Following a single oral dose of 20 mg/kg, no lethality occurred in rats and death occurred in one of 20 mice receiving the same dose. The most likely manifestation of overdosage would be hypotension, for which the usual treatment would be intravenous infusion of normal saline solution. Lisinopril can be removed by hemodialysis.
Hydrochlorothiazide
Oral administration of a single oral dose of 10 mg/kg to mice and rats was not lethal. The most common signs and symptoms observed are those caused by electrolyte depletion (hypokalemia, hypochloremia, hyponatremia) and dehydration resulting from excessive diuresis. If digitalis has also been administered, hypokalemia may accentuate cardiac arrhythmias.

DOSAGE AND ADMINISTRATION

Lisinopril is an effective treatment of hypertension in once-daily doses of 10–80 mg, while hydrochlorothiazide is effective in doses of 25–100 mg. In clinical trials of lisinopril/hydrochlorothiazide combination therapy using lisinopril doses of 10–80 mg and hydrochlorothiazide doses of 6.25–50 mg, the antihypertensive response rates generally increased with increasing dose of either component.
The side effects (see WARNINGS) of lisinopril are generally rare and apparently independent of dose; those of hydrochlorothiazide are a mixture of dose-dependent phenomena (primarily hypokalemia) and dose-independent phenomena (e.g., pancreatitis), the former much more common than the latter. Therapy with any combination of lisinopril and hydrochlorothiazide will be associated with both sets of dose-independent side effects, but addition of lisinopril in clinical trials blunted the hypokalemia normally seen with diuretics.
To minimize dose-independent side effects, it is usually appropriate to begin combination therapy only after a patient has failed to achieve the desired effect with monotherapy.
Dose Titration Guided by Clinical Effect
A patient whose blood pressure is not adequately controlled with either lisinopril or hydrochlorothiazide monotherapy may be switched to PRINZIDE 10/12.5 or PRINZIDE 20/12.5. Further increases of either or both components could depend on clinical response. The hydrochlorothiazide dose should generally not be increased until 2–3 weeks have elapsed. Patients whose blood pressures are adequately controlled with 25 mg of daily hydrochlorothiazide, but who experience significant potassium loss with this regimen, may achieve similar or greater blood pressure control with less potassium loss if they are switched to PRINZIDE 10/12.5.
Replacement Therapy
The combination may be substituted for the titrated individual components.
Use in Renal Impairment
The usual regimens of therapy with PRINZIDE need not be adjusted as long as the patient's creatinine clearance is >30 mL /min/1.73 m^2 (serum creatinine approximately $\leq$3 mg/dL or 265 µmol/L. In patients with more severe renal impairment, loop diuretics are preferred to thiazides, so PRINZIDE is not recommended (see WARNINGS, *Anaphylactoid reactions during membrane exposure*).
Use in Elderly In general, blood pressure response and adverse experiences were similar in younger and older patients given PRINZIDE. However, in a multiple dose pharmacokinetic study in elderly versus young patients using the lisinopril/hydrochlorothiazide combination, area under the plasma concentration time curve (AUC) increased approximately 120% for lisinopril and approximately 80% for hydrochlorothiazide in older patients. Therefore, dosage adjustments in elderly patients should be made with particular caution.

HOW SUPPLIED

No. 3616—Tablets PRINZIDE 10-12.5 are blue hexagon-shaped tablets, coded MSD 145 on one side and PRINZIDE on the other. Each tablet contains 10 mg of lisinopril and 12.5 mg of hydrochlorothiazide. They are supplied as follows:
NDC 0006-0145-31 unit of use bottles of 30.
NDC 0006-0145-58 unit of use bottles of 100.
Shown in Product Identification Guide, page 323
No. 3594—Tablets PRINZIDE 20-12.5 are yellow, round, fluted-edge tablets, coded MSD 140 on one side and PRINZIDE on the other. Each tablet contains 20 mg of lisinopril and 12.5 mg of hydrochlorothiazide. They are supplied as follows:
NDC 0006-0140-31 unit of use bottles of 30
NDC 0006-0140-58 unit of use bottles of 100.
Shown in Product Identification Guide, page 323
No. 3595—Tablets PRINZIDE 20-25 are peach, round, fluted-edge tablets, coded MSD 142 on one side and PRINZIDE on the other. Each tablet contains 20 mg of lisinopril and 25 mg of hydrochlorothiazide. They are supplied as follows:
NDC 0006-0142-31 unit of use bottles of 30
NDC 0006-0142-58 unit of use bottles of 100.
Shown in Product Identification Guide, page 323
Storage
Store at controlled room temperature. 15–30°C (59–86°F).
Protect from excessive light and humidity.
Dispense in a well-closed container, if product package is subdivided.
7836328 Issued April 1996
COPYRIGHT © MERCK & CO., INC., 1989, 1992
All rights reserved

PROPECIA® ℞
(Finasteride)
Tablets, 1 mg

DESCRIPTION

PROPECIA* (finasteride), a synthetic 4-azasteroid compound, is a specific inhibitor of steroid Type II 5α-reductase, an intracellular enzyme that converts the androgen testosterone into 5α-dihydrotestosterone (DHT).
Finasteride is 4-azaandrost-1-ene-17-carboxamide,*N*-(1,1-dimethylethyl)-3-oxo-,(5α,17β)-. The empirical formula of finasteride is $C_{23}H_{36}N_2O_2$ and its molecular weight is 372.55. Its structural formula is:

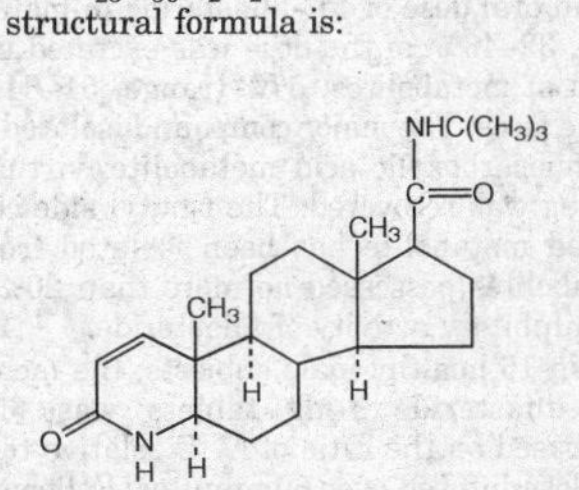

Finasteride is a white crystalline powder with a melting point near 250°C. It is freely soluble in chloroform and in lower alcohol solvents but is practically insoluble in water.
PROPECIA tablets for oral administration are film-coated tablets that contain 1 mg of finasteride and the following inactive ingredients: lactose monohydrate, microcrystalline cellulose, pregelatinized starch, sodium starch glycolate, docusate sodium, magnesium stearate, hydroxypropyl methylcellulose 2910, hydroxypropyl cellulose, titanium dioxide, talc, yellow ferric oxide, and red ferric oxide.

*Registered trademark of MERCK & CO., INC.

Continued on next page

Information on the Merck & Co., Inc. products listed on these pages is the full prescribing information from product circulars in use August 31, 1998. For information, please call 1-800-NSC MERCK [1-800-672-6372].

Propecia—Cont.

CLINICAL PHARMACOLOGY

Finasteride is a competitive and specific inhibitor of Type II 5α-reductase, an intracellular enzyme that converts the androgen testosterone into DHT. Two distinct isozymes are found in mice, rats, monkeys, and humans: Type I and II. Each of these isozymes is differentially expressed in tissues and developmental stages. In humans, Type I 5α-reductase is predominant in the sebaceous glands of most regions of skin, including scalp, and liver. Type I 5α-reductase is responsible for approximately one-third of circulating DHT. The Type II 5α-reductase isozyme is primarily found in prostate, seminal vesicles, epididymides, and hair follicles as well as liver, and is responsible for two-thirds of circulating DHT.

In humans, the mechanism of action of finasteride is based on its preferential inhibition of the Type II isozyme. Using native tissues (scalp and prostate), *in vitro* binding studies examining the potential of finasteride to inhibit either isozyme revealed a 100-fold selectivity for the human Type II 5α-reductase over Type I isozyme (IC_{50}=500 and 4.2 nM for Type I and II, respectively). For both isozymes, the inhibition by finasteride is accompanied by reduction of the inhibitor to dihydrofinasteride and adduct formation with NADP+. The turnover for the enzyme complex is slow ($t_{1/2}$ approximately 30 days for the Type II enzyme complex and 14 days for the Type I complex).

Finasteride has no affinity for the androgen receptor and has no androgenic, antiandrogenic, estrogenic, antiestrogenic, or progestational effects. Inhibition of Type II 5α-reductase blocks the peripheral conversion of testosterone to DHT, resulting in significant decreases in serum and tissue DHT concentrations. Finasteride produces a rapid reduction in serum DHT concentration, reaching 65% suppression within 24 hours of oral dosing with a 1-mg tablet. In men with male pattern hair loss (androgenetic alopecia), the balding scalp contains miniaturized hair follicles and increased amounts of DHT compared with hairy scalp. Administration of finasteride decreases scalp and serum DHT concentrations in these men. The relative contributions of these reductions to the treatment effect of finasteride have not been defined. By this mechanism, finasteride appears to interrupt a key factor in the development of androgenetic alopecia in those patients genetically predisposed.

Finasteride had no effect on circulating levels of cortisol, thyroid-stimulating hormone, or thyroxine, nor did it affect the plasma lipid profile (e.g., total cholesterol, low-density lipoproteins, high-density lipoproteins and triglycerides) or bone mineral density. In studies with finasteride, no clinically meaningful changes in luteinizing hormone (LH) or follicle-stimulating hormone (FSH) were detected. In healthy volunteers, treatment with finasteride did not alter the response of LH and FSH to gonadotropin-releasing hormone, indicating that the hypothalamic-pituitary-testicular axis was not affected. Mean circulating levels of testosterone and estradiol were increased by approximately 15% as compared to baseline, but these remained within the physiologic range.

Pharmacokinetics

Following an oral dose of ^{14}C-finasteride in man, a mean of 39% (range, 32–46%) of the dose was excreted in the urine in the form of metabolites; 57% (range, 51–64%) was excreted in the feces. The major compound isolated from urine was the monocarboxylic acid metabolite; virtually no unchanged drug was recovered. The t-butyl side chain monohydroxylated metabolite has been isolated from plasma. These metabolites possessed no more than 20% of the 5α-reductase inhibitory activity of finasteride.

In a study in 15 healthy male subjects, the mean bioavailability of finasteride 1-mg tablets was 65% (range 26–170%), based on the ratio of AUC relative to a 5-mg intravenous dose infused over 60 minutes. Following intravenous infusion, mean plasma clearance was 165 mL/min (range, 70–279 mL/min) and mean steady-state volume of distribution was 76 liters (range, 44–96 liters). In a separate study, the bioavailability of finasteride was not affected by food.

Approximately 90% of circulating finasteride is bound to plasma proteins. Finasteride has been found to cross the blood-brain barrier.

There is a slow accumulation phase for finasteride after multiple dosing. At steady state following dosing with 1 mg/day, maximum finasteride plasma concentration averaged 9.2 ng/mL (range, 4.9–13.7 ng/mL) and was reached 1 to 2 hours postdose; $AUC_{(0-24\ hr)}$ was 53 ng·hr/mL (range, 20–154 ng·hr/mL) and mean terminal half-life of elimination was 4.8 hours (range, 3.3–13.4 hours).

Semen levels have been measured in 35 men taking finasteride 1 mg daily for 6 weeks. In 60% (21 of 35) of the samples, finasteride levels were undetectable. The mean finasteride level was 0.26 ng/mL and the highest level measured was 1.52 ng/mL. Using this highest semen level measured and assuming 100% absorption from a 5-mL ejaculate

per day, human exposure through vaginal absorption would be up to 7.6 ng per day, which is 750 times lower than the exposure from the no-effect dose for developmental abnormalities in Rhesus monkeys (see PRECAUTIONS, *Pregnancy*).

The elimination rate of finasteride decreases somewhat with age. Mean terminal half-life is approximately 5–6 hours in men 18–60 years of age and 8 hours in men more than 70 years of age. These findings are of no clinical significance, and a reduction in dosage in the elderly is not warranted.

No dosage adjustment is necessary in patients with renal insufficiency. In patients with chronic renal impairment (creatinine clearance ranging from 9.0 to 55 mL/min), the values for AUC, maximum plasma concentration, half-life, and protein binding after a single dose of ^{14}C-finasteride were similar to those obtained in healthy volunteers. Urinary excretion of metabolites was decreased in patients with renal impairment. This decrease was associated with an increase in fecal excretion of metabolites. Plasma concentrations of metabolites were significantly higher in patients with renal impairment (based on a 60% increase in total radioactivity AUC). Furthermore, finasteride has been well tolerated in men with normal renal function receiving up to 80 mg/day for 12 weeks where exposure of these patients to metabolites would presumably be much greater.

Clinical Studies

The efficacy of PROPECIA was demonstrated in men (88% Caucasian) with mild to moderate androgenetic alopecia (male pattern hair loss) between 18 and 41 years of age. In order to prevent seborrheic dermatitis which might confound the assessment of hair growth in these studies (controlled phase and extensions), all men, whether treated with finasteride or placebo, were instructed to use a specified, medicated, tar-based shampoo (Neutrogena T/Gel®** Shampoo).

**Registered trademark of Johnson & Johnson

There were three double-blind, randomized, placebo-controlled studies of 12-month duration. The two primary endpoints were hair count and patient self-assessment; the two secondary endpoints were investigator assessment and ratings of photographs. The three studies were conducted in 1,879 men with mild to moderate, but not complete, hair loss. Two of the studies enrolled men with predominantly mild to moderate vertex hair loss (n=1,553). The third enrolled men having mild to moderate hair loss in the anterior midscalp area with or without vertex balding (n=326).

Two studies on Vertex Baldness

Of the men who completed the first 12 months of the two vertex baldness trials, 1,215 elected to continue in double-blind, placebo-controlled, 12-month extension studies. There were 547 men receiving PROPECIA for both the initial and extension periods (up to 24 months) and 60 men receiving placebo for the same periods. In addition, there were 65 men who received PROPECIA for the initial 12 months followed by placebo in the 12-month extension period, and 543 men who received placebo for the initial 12 months followed by PROPECIA in the 12-month extension period (See Figure below).

Hair counts were assessed by photographic enlargements of a representative area of active hair loss. In these two studies in men with vertex baldness, significant increases in hair count were demonstrated at 6 and 12 months in men treated with PROPECIA, while significant hair loss from

baseline was demonstrated in those treated with placebo. At 12 months there was a 107-hair difference from placebo (p<0.001, PROPECIA [n=679 evaluable men] vs placebo [n=672 evaluable men]) within a 1-inch diameter circle (5.1 cm²). Hair count was maintained in those men taking PROPECIA (n=433 evaluable men) for up to 24 months, while the placebo group (n=47 evaluable men) continued to show progressive hair loss. At 24 months, this resulted in a 138-hair difference between treatment groups (p<0.001) within the same area. Patients who switched from placebo to PROPECIA (n=426 evaluable men) at the end of the initial 12 months had an increase in hair count at 24 months. A change of treatment from PROPECIA to placebo (n=48 evaluable men) at the end of the initial 12 months resulted in reversal of the increase in hair count 12 months later, at 24 months. See figure below for combined study results.

At 12 months, 14% of men treated with PROPECIA had hair loss (defined as any decrease in hair count from baseline) compared with 58% of men in the placebo group. In men treated for up to 24 months, 17% of those treated with PROPECIA demonstrated hair loss compared with 72% of those in the placebo group.

[See figure below]

Patient self-assessment was obtained at each clinic visit from a self-administered questionnaire, which included questions on their perception of hair growth, hair loss, and appearance. This self-assessment demonstrated an increase in amount of hair, a decrease in hair loss, and improvement in appearance in men treated with PROPECIA. Overall improvement compared with placebo was seen as early as 3 months (p<0.05), with continued improvement over 24 months.

Investigator assessment was based on a 7-point scale evaluating increases or decreases in scalp hair at each patient visit. This assessment showed significantly greater increases in hair growth in men treated with PROPECIA compared with placebo as early as 3 months (p<0.001). At 12 months, the investigators rated 65% of men treated with PROPECIA as having increased hair growth compared with 37% in the placebo group. At 24 months, the investigators rated 80% of men treated with PROPECIA as having increased hair growth compared with 47% of men treated with placebo.

Standardized photographs of the head were assessed in a blinded fashion, at the beginning of the study and at 6, 12, 18 and 24 months. An independent panel rated increases or decreases in scalp hair on the same 7-point scale as the investigator assessment. At 12 months, 48% of men treated with PROPECIA had an increase as compared with 7% of men treated with placebo. At 24 months, an increase in hair growth was demonstrated in 66% of men treated with PROPECIA compared with 7% of men treated with placebo. Based on this assessment, continued treatment with PROPECIA resulted in further improvement. These results were observed in the context of no further increase in hair count between month 12 and month 24.

In one of the two vertex baldness studies, patients were questioned on non-scalp body hair growth. PROPECIA did not appear to affect non-scalp body hair.

Study on Hair Loss in the Anterior Mid-Scalp Area

A third study of 12-month duration, designed to assess the efficacy of PROPECIA in men with hair loss in the anterior mid-scalp area, also demonstrated significant increases in hair count compared with placebo. Increases in hair count were accompanied by improvements in patient self-assessment, investigator assessment, and ratings based on standardized photographs. Hair counts were obtained in the anterior mid-scalp area, and did not include the area of bitemporal recession or the anterior hairline.

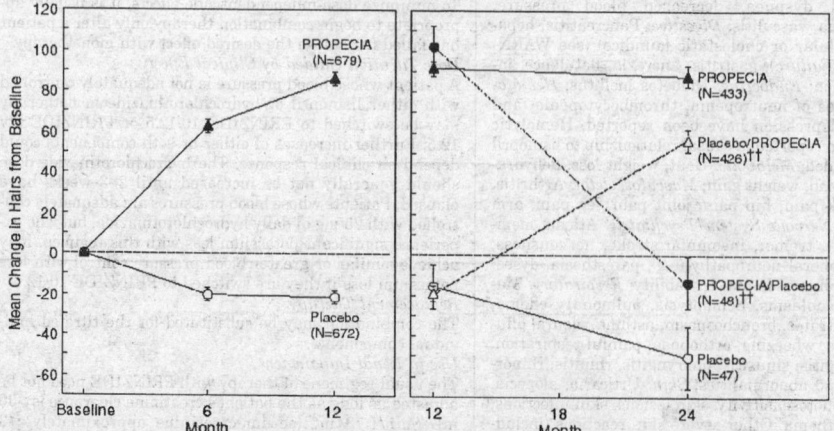

Effect on Hair Count†

Number of Hairs in a 1-Inch Diameter Circle
Mean Change ± 1 S.E.

PROPECIA (N=679)
Placebo (N=672)
PROPECIA (N=433)
Placebo/PROPECIA (N=426)††
PROPECIA/Placebo (N=48)††
Placebo (N=47)

† Pooled data from vertex hair loss studies (mean baseline hair count = 876)

†† At the end of initial 12-month period, treatment switched from PROPECIA to placebo (———PROPECIA/Placebo) or from placebo to PROPECIA (---------- Placebo/PROPECIA).

Summary of Clinical Studies
Clinical studies were conducted in men aged 18 to 41 with mild to moderate degrees of androgenetic alopecia. All men treated with PROPECIA or placebo received a tar-based shampoo (Neutrogena T/Gel®** Shampoo). Clinical improvement was seen as early as 3 months in the patients treated with PROPECIA and led to a net increase in scalp hair count and hair regrowth. In addition, clinical studies demonstrated slowing of hair loss with PROPECIA by patient self-assessment. These effects were maintained through the second year of treatment. Maintenance of or improvement in clinical efficacy has also been demonstrated in controlled and open-extension studies for up to 3 years.
Ethnic Analysis of Clinical Data
In a combined analysis of the two studies on vertex baldness, mean hair count changes from baseline were 91 vs −19 hairs (PROPECIA vs placebo) among Caucasians (n=1,185), 49 vs 27 hairs among Blacks (n=84), 53 vs −38 hairs among Asians (n=17), 67 vs 5 hairs among Hispanics (n=45) and 67 vs −15 hairs among other ethnic groups (n=20). Patient self-assessment showed improvement across racial groups with PROPECIA treatment, except for satisfaction of the frontal hairline and vertex in Black men, who were satisfied overall.
A sexual function questionnaire was self-administered by patients participating in the two vertex baldness trials to detect more subtle changes in sexual function. At Month 12, statistically significant differences in favor of placebo were found in 3 of 4 domains (sexual interest, erections, and perception of sexual problems). However, no significant difference was seen in the question on overall satisfaction with sex life.

INDICATIONS AND USAGE

PROPECIA is indicated for the treatment of male pattern hair loss (androgenetic alopecia) in **MEN ONLY**. Safety and efficacy were demonstrated in men between 18 to 41 years of age with mild to moderate hair loss of the vertex and anterior mid-scalp area (See CLINICAL PHARMACOLOGY, *Clinical Studies*).
Efficacy in bitemporal recession has not been established.
PROPECIA is not indicated in women (see CONTRAINDICATIONS).
PROPECIA is not indicated in children (see PRECAUTIONS, *Pediatric Use*).

CONTRAINDICATIONS

PROPECIA is contraindicated in the following:
Pregnancy. Finasteride use is contraindicated in women when they are or may potentially be pregnant. Because of the ability of 5α-reductase inhibitors to inhibit the conversion of testosterone to DHT, finasteride may cause abnormalities of the external genitalia of a male fetus of a pregnant woman who receives finasteride. If this drug is used during pregnancy, or if pregnancy occurs while taking this drug, the pregnant woman should be apprised of the potential hazard to the male fetus. (See also WARNINGS, EXPOSURE OF WOMEN - RISK TO MALE FETUS; and PRECAUTIONS, *Information for Patients* and *Pregnancy*.) In female rats, low doses of finasteride administered during pregnancy have produced abnormalities of the external genitalia in male offspring.
Hypersensitivity to any component of this medication.

WARNINGS

PROPECIA is not indicated for use in pediatric patients (See INDICATIONS AND USAGE; and PRECAUTIONS, *Pediatric Use*) or women (See also PRECAUTIONS, *Information for Patients* and *Pregnancy*; and HOW SUPPLIED, *Storage and Handling*.)
EXPOSURE OF WOMEN - RISK TO MALE FETUS
Women should not handle crushed or broken PROPECIA tablets when they are pregnant or may potentially be pregnant because of the possibility of absorption of finasteride and the subsequent potential risk to a male fetus. PROPECIA tablets are coated and will prevent contact with the active ingredient during normal handling, provided that the tablets have not been broken or crushed. (See also CONTRAINDICATIONS; PRECAUTIONS, *Information for Patients* and *Pregnancy*; and HOW SUPPLIED, *Storage and Handling*.)

PRECAUTIONS

General
Caution should be used in the administration of PROPECIA in patients with liver function abnormalities, as finasteride is metabolized extensively in the liver.
Information for Patients
Women should not handle crushed or broken PROPECIA tablets when they are pregnant or may potentially be pregnant because of the possibility of absorption of finasteride and the subsequent potential risk to a male fetus. PROPECIA tablets are coated and will prevent contact with the active ingredient during normal handling, provided that the tablets have not been broken or crushed. (See also CONTRAINDICATIONS; WARNINGS, EXPOSURE OF WOMEN - RISK TO MALE FETUS; PRECAUTIONS, *Pregnancy*; and HOW SUPPLIED, *Storage and Handling*.)
See also Patient Package Insert.
Drug/Laboratory Test Interactions
In clinical studies with PROPECIA in men 18–41 years of age, the mean value of serum prostate-specific antigen (PSA) decreased from 0.7 ng/mL at baseline to 0.5 ng/mL at Month 12. When finasteride is used in older men who have benign prostatic hyperplasia (BPH), PSA levels are decreased by approximately 50%. Until further information is gathered in men >41 years of age without BPH, consideration should be given to doubling the PSA level in men undergoing this test while taking PROPECIA.
Drug Interactions
No drug interactions of clinical importance have been identified. Finasteride does not appear to affect the cytochrome P450-linked drug metabolizing enzyme system. Compounds that have been tested in man include antipyrine, digoxin, propranolol, theophylline, and warfarin and no interactions were found.
Other concomitant therapy: Although specific interaction studies were not performed, finasteride doses of 1 mg or more were concomitantly used in clinical studies with acetaminophen, α-blockers, analgesics, angiotensin-converting enzyme (ACE) inhibitors, anticonvulsants, benzodiazepines, beta blockers, calcium-channel blockers, cardiac nitrates, diuretics, H_2 antagonists, HMG-CoA reductase inhibitors, prostaglandin synthetase inhibitors (NSAIDs), and quinolone anti-infectives without evidence of clinically significant adverse interactions.
Carcinogenesis, Mutagenesis, Impairment of Fertility
No evidence of a tumorigenic effect was observed in a 24-month study in Sprague-Dawley rats receiving doses of finasteride up to 160 mg/kg/day in males and 320 mg/kg/day in females. These doses produced respective systemic exposure in rats of 888 and 2,192 times those observed in man receiving the recommended human dose of 1 mg/day. All exposure calculations were based on calculated $AUC_{(0-24\ hr)}$ for animals and mean $AUC_{(0-24\ hr)}$ for man (0.05 μg·hr/mL).
In a 19-month carcinogenicity study in CD-1 mice, a statistically significant ($p \leq 0.05$) increase in the incidence of testicular Leydig cell adenomas was observed at a dose of 250 mg/kg/day (1,824 times the human exposure). In mice at a dose of 25 mg/kg/day (184 times the human exposure, estimated) and in rats at a dose of ≥40 mg/kg/day (312 times the human exposure) an increase in the incidence of Leydig cell hyperplasia was observed. A positive correlation between the proliferative changes in the Leydig cells and an increase in serum LH levels (2–3 fold above control) has been demonstrated in both rodent species treated with high doses of finasteride. No drug-related Leydig cell changes were seen in either rats or dogs treated with finasteride for 1 year at doses of 20 mg/kg/day and 45 mg/kg/day (240 and 2,800 times, respectively, the human exposure) or in mice treated for 19 months at a dose of 2.5 mg/kg/day (18.4 times the human exposure).
No evidence of mutagenicity was observed in an *in vitro* bacterial mutagenesis assay, a mammalian cell mutagenesis assay, or in an *in vitro* alkaline elution assay. In an *in vitro* chromosome aberration assay, when Chinese hamster ovary cells were treated with high concentrations (450–550 μmol) of finasteride, there was a slight increase in chromosome aberrations. These concentrations correspond to 18,000–22,000 times the peak plasma levels in man given a total dose of 1 mg. Further, the concentrations (450–550 μmol) used in *in vitro* studies are not achievable in a biological system. In an *in vivo* chromosome aberration assay in mice, no treatment-related increase in chromosome aberration was observed with finasteride at the maximum tolerated dose of 250 mg/kg/day (1,824 times the human exposure, estimated) as determined in the carcinogenicity studies.
In sexually mature male rabbits treated with finasteride at 80 mg/kg/day (4,344 times the estimated human exposure) for up to 12 weeks, no effect on fertility, sperm count, or ejaculate volume was seen. In sexually mature male rats treated with 80 mg/kg/day of finasteride (488 times the estimated human exposure), there were no significant effects on fertility after 6 or 12 weeks of treatment; however, when treatment was continued for up to 24 or 30 weeks, there was an apparent decrease in fertility, fecundity, and an associated significant decrease in the weights of the seminal vesicles and prostate. All these effects were reversible within 6 weeks of discontinuation of treatment. No drug-related effect on testes or on mating performance has been seen in rats or rabbits. This decrease in fertility in finasteride-treated rats is secondary to its effect on accessory sex organs (prostate and seminal vesicles) resulting in failure to form a seminal plug. The seminal plug is essential for normal fertility in rats but is not relevant in man.
Pregnancy
Teratogenic Effects: Pregnancy Category X
See CONTRAINDICATIONS.
PROPECIA is not indicated for use in women.
Administration of finasteride to pregnant rats at doses ranging from 100 μg/kg/day to 100 mg/kg/day (5–5,000 times the recommended human dose of 1 mg/day) resulted in dose-dependent development of hypospadias in 3.6 to 100% of male offspring. Pregnant rats produced male offspring with decreased prostatic and seminal vesicular weights, delayed preputial separation, and transient nipple development when given finasteride at ≥30 μg/kg/day (≥ 1.5 times the recommended human dose of 1 mg/day) and decreased anogenital distance when given finasteride at ≥3 μg/kg/day (one-fifth the recommended human dose of 1 mg/day). The critical period during which these effects can be induced in male rats has been defined to be days 16–17 of gestation. The changes described above are expected pharmacological effects of drugs belonging to the class of Type II 5α-reductase inhibitors and are similar to those reported in male infants with a genetic deficiency of Type II 5α-reductase. No abnormalities were observed in female offspring exposed to any dose of finasteride *in utero*.
No developmental abnormalities have been observed in first filial generation (F_1) male or female offspring resulting from mating finasteride-treated male rats (80 mg/kg/day; 488 times the human exposure) with untreated females. Administration of finasteride at 3 mg/kg/day (150 times the recommended human dose of 1 mg/day) during the late gestation and lactation period resulted in slightly decreased fertility in F_1 male offspring. No effects were seen in female offspring. No evidence of malformations has been observed in rabbit fetuses exposed to finasteride *in utero* from days 6–18 of gestation at doses up to 100 mg/kg/day (5000 times the recommended human dose of 1 mg/day). However, effects on male genitalia would not be expected since the rabbits were not exposed during the critical period of genital system development.
The *in utero* effects of finasteride exposure during the period of embryonic and fetal development were evaluated in the rhesus monkey (gestation days 20–100), a species more predictive of human development than rats or rabbits. Intravenous administration of finasteride to pregnant monkeys at doses as high as 800 ng/day (at least 750 times the highest estimated exposure of pregnant women to finasteride from semen of men taking 1 mg/day) resulted in no abnormalities in male fetuses. In confirmation of the relevance of the rhesus model for human fetal development, oral administration of a very high dose of finasteride (2 mg/kg/day; 100 times the recommended human dose of 1 mg/day or approximately 12 million times the highest estimated exposure to finasteride from semen of men taking 1 mg/day) to pregnant monkeys resulted in external genital abnormalities in male fetuses. No other abnormalities were observed in male fetuses and no finasteride-related abnormalities were observed in female fetuses at any dose.
Nursing Mothers
PROPECIA is not indicated for use in women.
It is not known whether finasteride is excreted in human milk.
Pediatric Use
PROPECIA is not indicated for use in pediatric patients.
Safety and effectiveness in pediatric patients have not been established.

ADVERSE REACTIONS

Clinical Studies for PROPECIA (finasteride 1 mg) in the Treatment of Male Pattern Hair Loss
In controlled clinical trials for PROPECIA of 12-month duration, 1.4% of the patients were discontinued due to adverse experiences that were considered to be possibly, probably or definitely drug-related (1.6% for placebo); 1.2% of patients on PROPECIA and 0.9% of patients on placebo discontinued therapy because of a drug-related sexual adverse experience. The following clinical adverse reactions were reported as possibly, probably or definitely drug-related in ≥1% of patients treated for 12 months with PROPECIA or placebo, respectively: decreased libido (1.8%, 1.3%), erectile dysfunction (1.3%, 0.7%) and ejaculation disorder (1.2%, 0.7%; primarily decreased volume of ejaculate:[0.8%, 0.4%]).
Integrated analysis of clinical adverse experiences showed that during treatment with PROPECIA, 36 (3.8%) of 945 men had reported one or more of these adverse experiences as compared to 20 (2.1%) of 934 men treated with placebo ($p=0.04$). Resolution occurred in all men who discontinued therapy with PROPECIA due to these side effects and in 58% of those who continued therapy.
In a study of finasteride 1 mg daily in healthy men, a median decrease in ejaculate volume of 0.3 mL (-11%) compared with 0.2 mL (−8%) for placebo was observed after 48

Continued on next page

Information on the Merck & Co., Inc. products listed on these pages is the full prescribing information from product circulars in use August 31, 1998. For information, please call 1-800-NSC MERCK [1-800-672-6372].

Propecia—Cont.

weeks of treatment. Two other studies showed that finasteride at 5 times the dosage of PROPECIA (5 mg daily) produced significant median decreases of approximately 0.5 mL (-25%) compared to placebo in ejaculate volume but this was reversible after discontinuation of treatment.

In the clinical studies with PROPECIA, the incidences for breast tenderness and enlargement, and for hypersensitivity reactions in finasteride-treated patients were not different from those in patients treated with placebo.

Controlled Clinical Trials and Long-Term Open Extension Studies for PROSCAR (finasteride 5 mg) in the Treatment of Benign Prostatic Hyperplasia*

In controlled clinical trials for PROSCAR of 12-month duration, 1.3% of the patients were discontinued due to adverse experiences that were considered to be possibly, probably or definitely drug-related (0.9% for placebo); only one patient on PROSCAR (0.2%) and one patient on placebo (0.2%) discontinued therapy because of a drug-related sexual adverse experience. The following clinical adverse reactions were reported as possibly, probably or definitely drug-related in ≥1% of patients treated for 12 months with PROSCAR or placebo, respectively: erectile dysfunction (3.7%, 1.1%), decreased libido (3.3%, 1.6%) and decreased volume of ejaculate (2.8%, 0.9%). The adverse experience profiles for patients treated with finasteride 1 mg/day for 12 months and those maintained on PROSCAR for 24 to 48 months were similar to that observed in the 12-month controlled studies with PROSCAR. Sexual adverse experiences resolved with continued treatment in over 60% of patients who reported them.

Adverse Effects Reported in Post-Marketing Experience for PROSCAR (finasteride 5 mg)

Breast tenderness and enlargement, as well as hypersensitivity reactions, including lip swelling and skin rash have been reported.

OVERDOSAGE

In clinical studies, single doses of finasteride up to 400 mg and multiple doses of finasteride up to 80 mg/day for three months did not result in adverse reactions. Until further experience is obtained, no specific treatment for an overdose with finasteride can be recommended.

Significant lethality was observed in male and female mice at single oral doses of 1,500 mg/m^2 (500 mg/kg) and in female and male rats at single oral doses of 2,360 mg/m^2 (400 mg/kg) and 5,900 mg/m^2 (1,000 mg/kg), respectively.

DOSAGE AND ADMINISTRATION

The recommended dosage is 1 mg once a day.

PROPECIA may be administered with or without meals.

In general, daily use for three months or more is necessary before benefit is observed. Continued use is recommended to sustain benefit. Withdrawal of treatment leads to reversal of effect within 12 months.

HOW SUPPLIED

No. 6550—PROPECIA tablets, 1 mg, are tan, octagonal, film-coated convex tablets with code MRK 71 on one side and PROPECIA 1 on the other. They are supplied as follows:

NDC 0006-0071-31 unit of use bottles of 30

NDC 0006-0071-61 ProPak™**- carton of 3 unit of use bottles of 30.

Shown in Product Identification Guide, page 323

Storage and Handling

Store at room temperature, 15–30°C (59–86°F). Keep container closed and protect from moisture.

Women should not handle crushed or broken PROPECIA tablets when they are pregnant or may potentially be pregnant because of the possibility of absorption of finasteride and the subsequent potential risk to a male fetus. PROPECIA tablets are coated and will prevent contact with the active ingredient during normal handling, provided that the tablets are not broken or crushed. (See WARNINGS, EXPOSURE OF WOMEN - RISK TO MALE FETUS; and PRECAUTIONS, *Information for Patients* and *Pregnancy*.)

**Trademark of MERCK & CO., Inc.

9090701 Issued December 1997

COPYRIGHT © MERCK & CO., Inc., 1997
All rights reserved.

PROSCAR®
(FINASTERIDE)
Tablets ℞

DESCRIPTION

PROSCAR* (finasteride), a synthetic 4-azasteroid compound, is a specific inhibitor of steroid Type II 5α-reductase, an intracellular enzyme that converts the androgen testosterone into 5α-dihydrotestosterone (DHT).

Mean (SD) Noncompartmental Pharmacokinetic Parameters After Multiple Doses of 5 mg/day in Older Men

	Mean (± SD)	
	45–60 years old (n=12)	≥70 years old (n=12)
AUC (ng•hr/mL)	389 (98)	463 (186)
Peak Concentration (ng/mL)	46.2 (8.7)	48.4 (14.7)
Time to Peak (hours)	1.8 (0.7)	1.8 (0.6)
Half-Life (hours)*	6.0 (1.5)	8.2 (2.5)

*First-dose values; all other parameters are last-dose values

Finasteride is 4-azaandrost-1-ene-17-carboxamide, *N*-(1,1-dimethylethyl)-3-oxo-,(5α,17β)-. The empirical formula of finasteride is $C_{23}H_{36}N_2O_2$ and its molecular weight is 372.55. Its structural formula is:

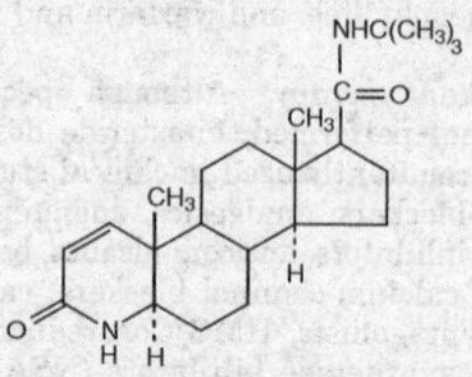

Finasteride is a white crystalline powder with a melting point near 250°C. It is freely soluble in chloroform and in lower alcohol solvents, but is practically insoluble in water. PROSCAR (finasteride) tablets for oral administration are film-coated tablets that contain 5 mg of finasteride and the following inactive ingredients: hydrous lactose, microcrystalline cellulose, pregelatinized starch, sodium starch glycolate, hydroxypropyl cellulose LF, hydroxypropylmethyl cellulose, titanium dioxide, magnesium stearate, talc, docusate sodium, FD&C Blue 2 aluminum lake and yellow iron oxide.

*Registered trademark of MERCK & CO., Inc.

CLINICAL PHARMACOLOGY

The development and enlargement of the prostate gland is dependent on the potent androgen, 5α-dihydrotestosterone (DHT). Type II 5α-reductase metabolizes testosterone to DHT in the prostate gland, liver and skin. DHT induces androgenic effects by binding to androgen receptors in the cell nuclei of these organs.

Finasteride is a competitive and specific inhibitor of Type II 5α-reductase with which it slowly forms a stable enzyme complex. Turnover from this complex is extremely slow ($t_{1/2}$ ~ 30 days). This has been demonstrated both *in vivo* and *in vitro*. Finasteride has no affinity for the androgen receptor. In man, the 5α-reduced steroid metabolites in blood and urine are decreased after administration of finasteride.

In man, a single 5-mg oral dose of PROSCAR produces a rapid reduction in serum DHT concentration, with the maximum effect observed 8 hours after the first dose. The suppression of DHT is maintained throughout the 24-hour dosing interval and with continued treatment. Daily dosing of PROSCAR at 5 mg/day for up to 4 years has been shown to reduce the serum DHT concentration by approximately 70%. The median circulating level of testosterone increased by approximately 10–20% but remained within the physiologic range.

Adult males with genetically inherited Type II 5α-reductase deficiency also have decreased levels of DHT. Except for the associated urogenital defects present at birth, no other clinical abnormalities related to Type II 5α-reductase deficiency have been observed in these individuals. These individuals have a small prostate gland throughout life and do not develop BPH.

In patients with BPH treated with finasteride (1–100 mg/day) for 7–10 days prior to prostatectomy, an approximate 80% lower DHT content was measured in prostatic tissue removed at surgery, compared to placebo; testosterone tissue concentration was increased up to 10 times over pretreatment levels, relative to placebo. Intraprostatic content of prostate-specific antigen (PSA) was also decreased.

In healthy male volunteers treated with PROSCAR for 14 days, discontinuation of therapy resulted in a return of DHT levels to pretreatment levels in approximately 2 weeks. In patients treated for three months, prostate volume, which declined by approximately 20%, returned to close to baseline value after approximately three months of discontinuation of therapy.

Pharmacokinetics

Absorption

In a study of 15 healthy young subjects, the mean bioavailability of finasteride 5-mg tablets was 63% (range 34–108%), based on the ratio of area under the curve (AUC) relative to an intravenous (IV) reference dose. Maximum finasteride plasma concentration averaged 37 ng/mL (range, 27–49 ng/mL) and was reached 1–2 hours postdose. Bioavailability of finasteride was not affected by food.

Distribution

Mean steady-state volume of distribution was 76 liters (range, 44–96 liters). Approximately 90% of circulating finasteride is bound to plasma proteins. There is a slow accumulation phase for finasteride after multiple dosing. After dosing with 5 mg/day of finasteride for 17 days, plasma concentrations of finasteride were 47 and 54% higher than after the first dose in men 45–60 years old (n=12) and ≥70 years old (n=12), respectively. Mean trough concentrations after 17 days of dosing were 6.2 ng/mL (range, 2.4–9.8 ng/mL) and 8.1 ng/mL (range, 1.8–19.7 ng/mL), respectively, in the two age groups. Although steady state was not reached in this study, mean trough plasma concentration in another study in patients with BPH (mean age, 65 years) receiving 5 mg/day was 9.4 ng/mL (range, 7.1–13.3 ng/mL; n=22) after over a year of dosing.

Finasteride has been shown to cross the blood brain barrier but does not appear to distribute preferentially to the CSF. In 2 studies of healthy subjects (n=69) receiving PROSCAR 5 mg/day for 6–24 weeks, finasteride concentrations in semen ranged from undetectable (<0.1 ng/mL) to 10.54 ng/mL. In an earlier study using a less sensitive assay, finasteride concentrations in the semen of 16 subjects receiving PROSCAR 5 mg/day ranged from undetectable (<1.0 ng/mL) to 21 ng/mL. Thus, based on a 5-mL ejaculate volume, the amount of finasteride in semen was estimated to be 50- to 100-fold less than the dose of finasteride (5 μg) that had no effect on circulating DHT levels in men (see also PRECAUTIONS, Pregnancy).

Metabolism

Finasteride is extensively metabolized in the liver, primarily via the cytochrome P450 3A4 enzyme subfamily. Two metabolites, the t-butyl side chain monohydroxylated and monocarboxylic acid metabolites, have been identified that possess no more than 20% of the 5α-reductase inhibitory activity of finasteride.

Excretion

In healthy young subjects (n=15), mean plasma clearance of finasteride was 165 mL/min (range, 70–279 mL/min) and mean elimination half-life in plasma was 6 hours (range, 3–16 hours). Following an oral dose of ^{14}C-finasteride in man (n=6), a mean of 39% (range, 32–46%) of the dose was excreted in the urine in the form of metabolites; 57% (range, 51–64%) was excreted in the feces.

The mean terminal half-life of finasteride in subjects ≥ 70 years of age was approximately 8 hours (range, 6–15 hours; n=12), compared with 6 hours (range, 4–12 hours; n=12) in subjects 45–60 years of age. As a result, mean AUC (0–24 hr) after 17 days of dosing was 15% higher in subjects ≥ 70 years of age than in subjects 45–60 years of age (p=0.02).

Special Populations

Pediatric: Finasteride pharmacokinetics have not been investigated in patients <18 years of age.

Gender: Finasteride pharmacokinetics in women are not available.

Geriatric: No dosage adjustment is necessary in the elderly. Although the elimination rate of finasteride is decreased in the elderly, these findings are of no clinical significance. See also *Pharmacokinetics*, *Excretion* and DOSAGE AND ADMINISTRATION.

Race: The effect of race on finasteride pharmacokinetics has not been studied.

Renal Insufficiency: No dosage adjustment is necessary in patients with renal insufficiency. In patients with chronic renal impairment, with creatinine clearances ranging from 9.0 to 55 mL/min, AUC, maximum plasma concentration, half-life, and protein binding after a single dose of ^{14}C-finasteride were similar to values obtained in healthy volunteers. Urinary excretion of metabolites was decreased in patients with renal impairment. This decrease was associated with an increase in fecal excretion of metabolites. Plasma concentrations of metabolites were significantly higher in patients with renal impairment (based on a 60%

Table 1
All Treatment Failures in PLESS

Event	Patients (%) *		Relative Risk**	95% CI	P Value**
	Placebo N=1503	Finasteride N=1513			
All Treatment Failures	37.1	26.2	0.68	(0.57 to 0.79)	<0.001
Surgical Interventions for BPH	10.1	4.6	0.45	(0.32 to 0.63)	<0.001
Acute Urinary Retention Requiring Catheterization	6.6	2.8	0.43	(0.28 to 0.66)	<0.001
Two consecutive symptoms scores ≥20	9.2	6.7			
Bladder Stone	0.4	0.5			
Incontinence	2.1	1.7			
Renal Failure	0.5	0.6			
UTI	5.7	4.9			
Discontinuation due to worsening of BPH, lack of improvement, or to receive other medical treatment	21.8	13.3			

*patients with multiple events may be counted more than once for each type of event
**Hazard ratio based on log rank test

increase in total radioactivity AUC). However, finasteride has been well tolerated in BPH patients with normal renal function receiving up to 80 mg/day for 12 weeks, where exposure of these patients to metabolites would presumably be much greater.

Hepatic Insufficiency: The effect of hepatic insufficiency on finasteride pharmacokinetics has not been studied. Caution should be used in the administration of PROSCAR in those patients with liver function abnormalities, as finasteride is metabolized extensively in the liver.

Drug Interactions (also see PRECAUTIONS, *Drug Interactions*)

No drug interactions of clinical importance have been identified. Finasteride does not appear to affect the cytochrome P450-linked drug metabolism enzyme system. Compounds that have been tested in man have included antipyrine, digoxin, propranolol, theophylline, and warfarin, and no clinically meaningful interactions were found.

Mean (SD) Pharmacokinetic Parameters in Healthy Young Subjects (n=15)

	Mean (± SD)
Bioavailability	63% (34–108%)*
Clearance (mL/min)	165 (55)
Volume of Distribution (L)	76 (14)
Half-Life (hours)	6.2 (2.1)

*Range

[See table at top of previous page]
Clinical Studies
PROSCAR 5 mg/day was initially evaluated in patients with symptoms of BPH and enlarged prostates by digital rectal examination in two 1-year, placebo-controlled, randomized, double-blind, studies and their 5-year open extensions.
PROSCAR was further evaluated in the PROSCAR Long-Term Efficacy and Safety Study (PLESS), a double-blind randomized, placebo-controlled, 4-year multicenter study. 3040 patients between the ages of 45 and 78, with moderate to severe symptoms of BPH and an enlarged prostate upon digital rectal examination, were randomized into the study (1524 to finasteride, 1516 to placebo) and 3016 patients were evaluable for efficacy. 1883 patients completed the 4-year study (1000 in the finasteride group, 883 in the placebo group).
Effect on Symptom Score
Symptoms were quantified using a score similar to the American Urological Association Symptom Score, which evaluated both obstructive symptoms (impairment of size and force of stream, sensation of incomplete bladder empty-

ing, delayed or interrupted urination) and irritative symptoms (nocturia, daytime frequency, need to strain or push the flow of urine) by rating on a 0 to 5 scale for six symptoms and a 0 to 4 scale for one symptom, for a total possible score of 34.
Patients in PLESS, had moderate to severe symptoms at baseline (mean of approximately 15 points on a 0–34 point scale). Patients randomized to PROSCAR who remained on therapy for 4 years had a mean (± 1 SD) decrease in symptom score of 3.3 (± 5.8) points compared with 1.3 (± 5.6) points in the placebo group. (See Figure 1.) A statistically significant improvement in symptom score was evident at 1 year in patients treated with PROSCAR vs placebo (−2.3 vs −1.6), and this improvement continued through Year 4.

Figure 1
Symptom Score in PLESS

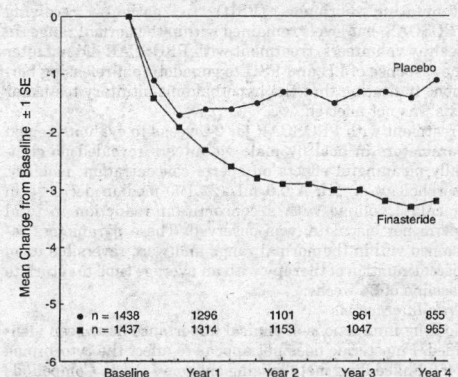

| ● n = 1438 | 1296 | 1101 | 961 | 855 |
| ■ n = 1437 | 1314 | 1153 | 1047 | 965 |

Results seen in earlier studies were comparable to those seen in PLESS. Although an early improvement in urinary symptoms was seen in some patients, a therapeutic trial of at least 6 months was generally necessary to assess whether a beneficial response in symptom relief had been achieved. The improvement in BPH symptoms was seen during the first year and maintained throughout an additional 5 years of open extension studies.
Effect on Acute Urinary Retention and the Need for Surgery
In PLESS, efficacy was also assessed by evaluating treatment failures. Treatment failure was prospectively defined as BPH-related urological events or clinical deterioration, lack of improvement and/or the need for alternative therapy. BPH-related urological events were defined as urological surgical intervention and acute urinary retention requiring catheterization. Complete event information was available for 92% of the patients. The following table (Table 1) summarizes the results.
[See table 1 above]

Compared with placebo, PROSCAR was associated with a significantly lower risk for acute urinary retention or the need for BPH-related surgery [13.2% for placebo vs 6.6% for PROSCAR; 51% reduction in risk, 95% CI: (34 to 63%)]. Compared with placebo, PROSCAR was associated with a significantly lower risk for surgery [10.1% for placebo vs 4.6% for PROSCAR; 55% reduction in risk, 95% CI: (37 to 68%)] and with a significantly lower risk of acute urinary retention [6.6% for placebo vs 2.8% for PROSCAR; 57% reduction in risk, 95% CI: (34 to 72%)]; See Figures 2 and 3.

Figure 2
Percent of Patients Having Surgery for BPH, Including TURP

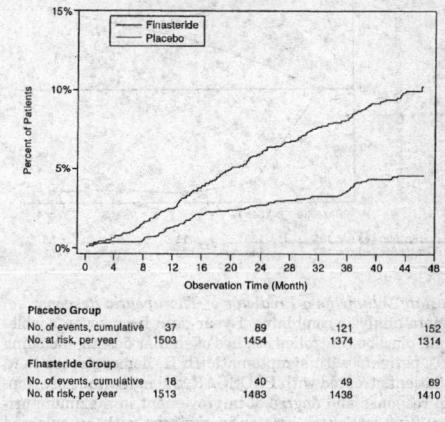

Placebo Group
No. of events, cumulative　37　89　121　152
No. at risk, per year　1503　1454　1374　1314

Finasteride Group
No. of events, cumulative　18　40　49　69
No. at risk, per year　1513　1483　1438　1410

Figure 3
Percent of Patients Developing Acute Urinary Retention (Spontaneous and Precipitated)

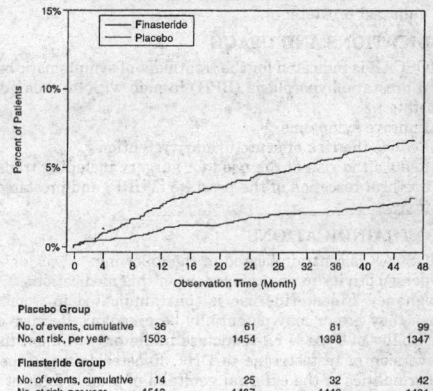

Placebo Group
No. of events, cumulative　36　61　81　99
No. at risk, per year　1503　1454　1398　1347

Finasteride Group
No. of events, cumulative　14　25　32　42
No. at risk, per year　1513　1487　1449　1421

Effect on Maximum Urinary Flow Rate
In the patients in PLESS who remained on therapy for the duration of the study and had evaluable urinary flow data, PROSCAR increased maximum urinary flow rate by 1.9 mL/sec compared with 0.2 mL/sec in the placebo group.
There was a clear difference between treatment groups in maximum urinary flow rate in favor of PROSCAR by month 4 (1.0 vs 0.3 mL/sec) which was maintained throughout the study. In the earlier 1-year studies, increase in maximum urinary flow rate was comparable to PLESS and was maintained through the first year and throughout an additional 5 years of open extension studies.
Effect on Prostate Volume
In PLESS, prostate volume was assessed yearly by magnetic resonance imaging (MRI) in a subset of patients. In patients treated with PROSCAR who remained on therapy, prostate volume was reduced compared with both baseline and placebo throughout the 4-year study. PROSCAR decreased prostate volume by 17.9% (from 55.9 cc at baseline to 45.8 cc at 4 years) compared with an increase of 14.1% (from 51.3 cc to 58.5 cc) in the placebo group (p<0.001). (See Figure 4.)

Continued on next page

Proscar—Cont.

Results seen in earlier studies were comparable to those seen in PLESS. Mean prostate volume at baseline ranged between 40-50 cc. The reduction in prostate volume was seen during the first year and maintained throughout an additional five years of open extension studies.

Figure 4
Prostate Volume in PLESS

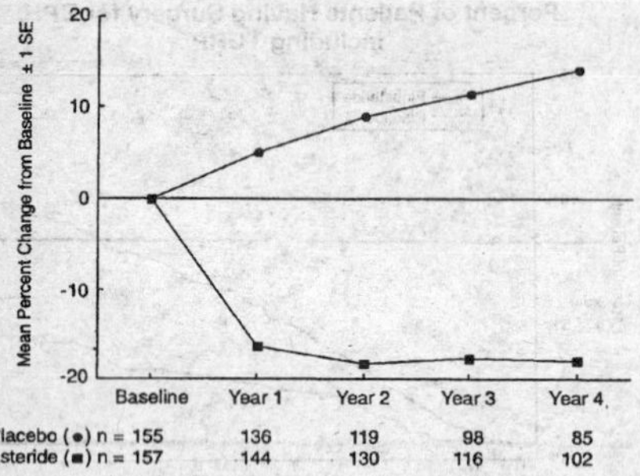
Mean Percent Change from Baseline ± 1 SE
20
10
0
-10
-20
Baseline
Year 1
Year 2
Year 3
Year 4
Placebo (●) n = 155 136 119 98 85
Finasteride (■) n = 157 144 130 116 102

Prostate Volume as a Predictor of Therapeutic Response
A meta-analysis combining 1-year data from seven double-blind, placebo-controlled studies of similar design, including 4491 patients with symptomatic BPH, demonstrated that, in patients treated with PROSCAR, the magnitude of symptom response and degree of improvement in maximum urinary flow rate were greater in patients with an enlarged prostate at baseline.

Summary of Clinical Studies
The data from these studies, showing improvement in BPH-related symptoms, reduction in treatment failure (BPH-related urological events), increased maximum urinary flow rates, and decreasing prostate volume, suggest that PROSCAR arrests the disease process of BPH in men with an enlarged prostate.

INDICATIONS AND USAGE

PROSCAR is indicated for the treatment of symptomatic benign prostatic hyperplasia (BPH) in men with an enlarged prostate to:

— Improve symptoms
— Reduce the risk of acute urinary retention
— Reduce the risk of the need for surgery including transurethral resection of the prostate (TURP) and prostatectomy.

CONTRAINDICATIONS

PROSCAR is contraindicated in the following:
Hypersensitivity to any component of this medication.
Pregnancy. Finasteride use is contraindicated in women when they are or may potentially be pregnant. Because of the ability of Type II 5α-reductase inhibitors to inhibit the conversion of testosterone to DHT, finasteride may cause abnormalities of the external genitalia of a male fetus of a pregnant woman who receives finasteride. If this drug is used during pregnancy, or if pregnancy occurs while taking this drug, the pregnant woman should be apprised of the potential hazard to the male fetus. (See also WARNINGS, EXPOSURE OF WOMEN—RISK TO MALE FETUS and PRECAUTIONS, *Information for Patients* and *Pregnancy*.)
In female rats, low doses of finasteride administered during pregnancy have produced abnormalities of the external genitalia in male offspring.

WARNINGS

PROSCAR is not indicated for use in pediatric patients (see PRECAUTIONS, *Pediatric Use*) or women (see also WARNINGS, EXPOSURE OF WOMEN—RISK TO MALE FETUS; PRECAUTIONS, *Information for Patients* and *Pregnancy*, and HOW SUPPLIED).
EXPOSURE OF WOMEN—RISK TO MALE FETUS
Women should not handle crushed or broken PROSCAR tablets when they are pregnant or may potentially be pregnant because of the possibility of absorption of finasteride and the subsequent potential risk to a male fetus. PROSCAR tablets are coated and will prevent contact with the active ingredient during normal handling, provided that the tablets have not been broken or crushed. (See CONTRAINDICATIONS; PRECAUTIONS, *Information for Patients* and *Pregnancy*, and HOW SUPPLIED).

PRECAUTIONS

General
Prior to initiating therapy with PROSCAR, appropriate evaluation should be performed to identify other conditions such as infection, prostate cancer, stricture disease, hypotonic bladder or other neurogenic disorders that might mimic BPH.
Patients with large residual urinary volume and/or severely diminished urinary flow should be carefully monitored for obstructive uropathy. These patients may not be candidates for finasteride therapy.
Caution should be used in the administration of PROSCAR in those patients with liver function abnormalities, as finasteride is metabolized extensively in the liver.

Effects on PSA and Prostate Cancer Detection
No clinical benefit has been demonstrated in patients with prostate cancer treated with PROSCAR. Patients with BPH and elevated PSA were monitored in controlled clinical studies with serial PSAs and prostate biopsies. In these studies, PROSCAR did not appear to alter the rate of prostate cancer detection. The overall incidence of prostate cancer was not significantly different in patients treated with PROSCAR or placebo.
PROSCAR causes a decrease in serum PSA levels by approximately 50% in patients with BPH, even in the presence of prostate cancer. This decrease is predictable over the entire range of PSA values, although it may vary in individual patients. Analysis of PSA data from over 3000 patients in PLESS confirmed that in typical patients treated with PROSCAR for six months or more, PSA values should be doubled for comparison with normal ranges in untreated men. This adjustment preserves the sensitivity and specificity of the PSA assay and maintains its ability to detect prostate cancer.
Any sustained increases in PSA levels while on PROSCAR should be carefully evaluated, including consideration of non-compliance to therapy with PROSCAR.

Information for Patients
Women should not handle crushed or broken PROSCAR tablets when they are pregnant or may potentially be pregnant because of the possibility of absorption of finasteride and the subsequent potential risk to the male fetus (see CONTRAINDICATIONS; WARNINGS, EXPOSURE OF WOMEN—RISK TO MALE FETUS; PRECAUTIONS, *Pregnancy* and HOW SUPPLIED).
Physicians should inform patients that the volume of ejaculate may be decreased in some patients during treatment with PROSCAR. This decrease does not appear to interfere with normal sexual function. However, impotence and decreased libido may occur in patients treated with PROSCAR (see ADVERSE REACTIONS).
Physicians should instruct their patients to read the patient package insert before starting therapy with PROSCAR and to reread it each time the prescription is renewed so that they are aware of current information for patients regarding PROSCAR.

Drug/Laboratory Test Interactions
In patients with BPH, PROSCAR has no effect on circulating levels of cortisol, estradiol, prolactin, thyroid-stimulating hormone, or thyroxine. No clinically meaningful effect was observed on the plasma lipid profile (i.e., total cholesterol, low density lipoproteins, high density lipoproteins and triglycerides) or bone mineral density. Increases of about 10% were observed in luteinizing hormone (LH) and follicle-stimulating hormone (FSH) in patients receiving PROSCAR, but levels remained within the normal range. In healthy volunteers, treatment with PROSCAR did not alter the response of LH and FSH to gonadotropin-releasing hormone indicating that the hypothalamic-pituitary-testicular axis was not affected.
Treatment with PROSCAR for 24 weeks to evaluate semen parameters in healthy male volunteers revealed no clinically meaningful effects on sperm concentration, mobility, morphology, or pH. A 0.6 mL (22.1%) median decrease in ejaculate volume with a concomitant reduction in total sperm per ejaculate, was observed. These parameters remained within the normal range and were reversible upon discontinuation of therapy with an average time to return to baseline of 84 weeks.

Drug Interactions
No drug interactions of clinical importance have been identified. Finasteride does not appear to affect the cytochrome P450-linked drug metabolizing enzyme system. Compounds that have been tested in man have included antipyrine, digoxin, propranolol, theophylline, and warfarin and no clinically meaningful interactions were found.
Other Concomitant Therapy: Although specific interaction studies were not performed, PROSCAR was concomitantly used in clinical studies with acetaminophen, acetylsalicylic acid, α-blockers, angiotensin-converting enzyme (ACE) inhibitors, analgesics, anti-convulsants, beta-adrenergic blocking agents, diuretics, calcium channel blockers, cardiac nitrates, HMG-CoA reductase inhibitors, nonsteroidal anti-inflammatory drugs (NSAIDSs), benzodiazepines, H_2 antagonists and quinolone anti-infectives without evidence of clinically significant adverse interactions.

Carcinogenesis, Mutagenesis, Impairment of Fertility
No evidence of a tumorigenic effect was observed in a 24-month study in Sprague-Dawley rats receiving doses of finasteride up to 160 mg/kg/day in males and 320 mg/kg/day in females. These doses produced respective systemic exposure in rats of 111 and 274 times those observed in man receiving the recommended human dose of 5 mg/day. All exposure calculations were based on calculated AUC (0–24hr) for animals and mean AUC (0–24 hr) for man (0.4 µg • hr/mL).
In a 19-month carcinogenicity study in CD-1 mice, a statistically significant (p≤0.05) increase in the incidence of testicular Leydig cell adenomas was observed at a dose of 250 mg/kg/day (228 times the human exposure). In mice at a dose of 25 mg/kg/day (23 times the human exposure, estimated) and in rats at a dose of ≥40 mg/kg/day (39 times the human exposure) an increase in the incidence of Leydig cell hyperplasia was observed. A positive correlation between the proliferative changes in the Leydig cells and an increase in serum LH levels (2–3 fold above control) has been demonstrated in both rodent species treated with high doses of finasteride. No drug-related Leydig cell changes were seen in either rats or dogs treated with finasteride for 1 year at doses of 20 mg/kg/day and 45 mg/kg/day (30 and 350 times, respectively, the human exposure) or in mice treated for 19 months at a dose of 2.5 mg/kg/day (2.3 times the human exposure, estimated).
No evidence of mutagenicity was observed in an *in vitro* bacterial mutagenesis assay, a mammalian cell mutagenesis assay, or in an *in vitro* alkaline elution assay. In an *in vitro* chromosome aberration assay, using Chinese hamster ovary cells, there was a slight increase in chromosome aberrations. These concentrations correspond to 3000–5000 times the peak plasma levels in man given a total dose of 5 mg. In an *in vivo* chromosome aberration assay in mice, no treatment-related increase in chromosome aberration was observed with finasteride at the maximum tolerated dose of 250 mg/kg/day (228 times the human exposure) as determined in the carcinogenicity studies.
In sexually mature male rabbits treated with finasteride at 80 mg/kg/day (543 times the human exposure) for up to 12 weeks, no effect on fertility, sperm count, or ejaculate volume was seen. In sexually mature male rats treated with 80 mg/kg/day of finasteride (61 times the human exposure), there were no significant effects on fertility after 6 or 12 weeks of treatment; however, when treatment was continued for up to 24 or 30 weeks, there was an apparent decrease in fertility, fecundity and an associated significant decrease in the weights of the seminal vesicles and prostate. All these effects were reversible within 6 weeks of discontinuation of treatment. No drug-related effect on testes or on mating performance has been seen in rats or rabbits. This decrease in fertility in finasteride-treated rats is secondary to its effect on accessory sex organs (prostate and seminal vesicles) resulting in failure to form a seminal plug. The seminal plug is essential for normal fertility in rats and is not relevant in man.

Pregnancy
Pregnancy Category X
See CONTRAINDICATIONS.
PROSCAR is not indicated for use in women.
Administration of finasteride to pregnant rats at doses ranging from 100 µg/kg/day to 100 mg/kg/day (1–1000 times the recommended human dose of 5 mg/day) resulted in dose-dependent development of hypospadias in 3.6 to 100% of male offspring. Pregnant rats produced male offspring with decreased prostatic and seminal vesicular weights, delayed preputial separation and transient nipple development when given finasteride at ≥30 µg/kg/day (≥3/10 of the recommended human dose of 5 mg/day) and decreased anogenital distance when given finasteride at ≥3 µg/kg/day (≥3/100 of the recommended human dose of 5 mg/day). The critical period during which these effects can be induced in male rats has been defined to be days 16–17 of gestation. The changes described above are expected pharmacological effects of drugs belonging to the class of Type II 5α-reductase inhibitors and are similar to those reported in male infants with a genetic deficiency of Type II 5α-reductase. No abnormalities were observed in female offspring exposed to any dose of finasteride *in utero*.
No developmental abnormalities have been observed in first filial generation (F_1) male or female offspring resulting from mating finasteride-treated male rats (80 mg/kg/day; 61 times the human exposure) with untreated females. Administration of finasteride at 3 mg/kg/day (30 times the recommended human dose of 5 mg/day) during the late gestation and lactation period resulted in slightly decreased fertility in F_1 male offspring. No effects were seen in female offspring. No evidence of malformations has been observed in rabbit fetuses exposed to finasteride *in utero* from days 6–18 of gestation at doses up to 100 mg/kg/day (1000 times the recommended human dose of 5 mg/day). However, effects on male genitalia would not be expected since the rabbits were not exposed during the critical period of genital system development.
The *in utero* effects of finasteride exposure during the period of embryonic and fetal development were evaluated in the rhesus monkey (gestation days 20–100), a species more predictive of human development than rats or rabbits. Intravenous administration of finasteride to pregnant monkeys at doses as high as 800 ng/day (at least 60 to 120 times the highest estimated exposure of pregnant women to finasteride from semen of men taking 5 mg/day) resulted in no abnormalities in male fetuses. In confirmation of the rele-

TABLE 2
Drug-Related Adverse Experiences

	Year 1 (%)		Years 2, 3 and 4* (%)	
	Finasteride	Placebo	Finasteride	Placebo
Impotence	8.1	3.7	5.1	5.1
Decreased Libido	6.4	3.4	2.6	2.6
Decreased Volume of Ejaculate	3.7	0.8	1.5	0.5
Ejaculation Disorder	0.8	0.1	0.2	0.1
Breast Enlargement	0.5	0.1	1.8	1.1
Breast Tenderness	0.4	0.1	0.7	0.3
Rash	0.5	0.2	0.5	0.1

*Combined Years 2–4
N = 1524 and 1516, finasteride vs placebo, respectively

vance of the rhesus model for human fetal development, oral administration of a dose of finasteride (2 mg/kg/day; 20 times the recommended human dose of 5 mg/day or approximately 1–2 million times the highest estimated exposure to finasteride from semen of men taking 5 mg/day) to pregnant monkeys resulted in external genital abnormalities in male fetuses. No other abnormalities were observed in male fetuses and no finasteride-related abnormalities were observed in female fetuses at any dose.

Nursing Mothers
PROSCAR is not indicated for use in women.
It is not known whether finasteride is excreted in human milk.

Pediatric Use
PROSCAR is not indicated for use in pediatric patients. Safety and effectiveness in pediatric patients have not been established.

ADVERSE REACTIONS

PROSCAR is generally well tolerated; adverse reactions usually have been mild and transient.

4-Year Placebo-Controlled Study
In PLESS, 1524 patients treated with PROSCAR and 1516 patients treated with placebo were evaluated for safety over a period of 4 years. The most frequently reported adverse reactions were related to sexual function. 3.7% (57 patients) treated with PROSCAR and 2.1% (32 patients) treated with placebo discontinued therapy as a result of adverse reactions related to sexual function, which are the most frequently reported adverse reactions.
Table 2 presents the only clinical adverse reactions considered possibly, probably or definitely drug related by the investigator, for which the incidence on PROSCAR was ≥1% and greater than placebo over the 4 years of the study. In years 2–4 of the study, there was no significant difference between treatment groups in the incidences of impotence, decreased libido and ejaculation disorder.
[See table 2 above]

Phase III Studies and 5-Year Open Extensions
The adverse experience profile in the 1–year, placebo-controlled, Phase III studies, the 5-year open extensions, and PLESS were similar.
There is no evidence of increased adverse experiences with increased duration of treatment with PROSCAR. New reports of drug-related sexual adverse experiences decreased with duration of therapy.
The following additional adverse effects have been reported in post-marketing experience:
—hypersensitivity reactions, including lip swelling.

OVERDOSAGE

Patients have received single doses of PROSCAR up to 400 mg and multiple doses of PROSCAR up to 80 mg/day for three months without adverse effects. Until further experience is obtained, no specific treatment for an overdose with PROSCAR can be recommended.
Significant lethality was observed in male and female mice at single oral doses of 1500 mg/m² (500 mg/kg) and in female and male rats at single oral doses of 2360 mg/m² (400 mg/kg) and 5900 mg/m² (1000 mg/kg), respectively.

DOSAGE AND ADMINISTRATION

The recommended dose is 5 mg orally once a day.
PROSCAR may be administered with or without meals.
No dosage adjustment is necessary for patients with renal impairment or for the elderly (see CLINICAL PHARMACOLOGY, *Pharmacokinetics*).

HOW SUPPLIED

No. 3094—PROSCAR tablets 5 mg are blue, modified apple-shaped, film-coated tablets, with the code MSD 72 on one side and PROSCAR on the other. They are supplied as follows:
NDC 0006-0072-31 unit of use bottles of 30 (6505-01-362-5331, 5 mg 30's)
NDC 0006-0072-58 unit of use bottles of 100 (6505-01-362-7422, 5 mg 100's)
NDC 0006-0072-28 unit dose packages of 100 (6505-01-362-5332, 5 mg individually sealed 100's).
Shown in Product Identification Guide, page 323
Storage and Handling
Store at room temperatures below 30°C (86°F). Protect from light and keep container tightly closed.
Women should not handle crushed or broken PROSCAR tablets when they are pregnant or may potentially be pregnant because of the possibility of absorption of finasteride and the subsequent potential risk to a male fetus (see WARNINGS, EXPOSURE OF WOMEN—RISK TO MALE FETUS, and PRECAUTIONS, *Information for Patients* and *Pregnancy*).
9132100 Issued March 1998
COPYRIGHT © MERCK & CO., INC., 1992, 1995, 1998
All rights reserved.

RECOMBIVAX HB®
Hepatitis B Vaccine (Recombinant)   ℞

DESCRIPTION

RECOMBIVAX HB* Hepatitis B Vaccine (Recombinant) is a non-infectious subunit viral vaccine derived from Hepatitis B surface antigen (HBsAg) produced in yeast cells. A portion of the hepatitis B virus gene, coding for HBsAg, is cloned into yeast, and the vaccine for hepatitis B is produced from cultures of this recombinant yeast strain according to methods developed in the Merck Research Laboratories.
The antigen is harvested and purified from fermentation cultures of a recombinant strain of the yeast *Saccharomyces cerevisiae* containing the gene for the *adw* subtype of HBsAg. The HBsAg protein is released from the yeast cells by cell disruption and purified by a series of physical and chemical methods. The vaccine contains no detectable yeast DNA but may contain not more than 1% yeast protein. The vaccine produced by the Merck method has been shown to be comparable to the plasma-derived vaccine in terms of animal potency (mouse, monkey, and chimpanzee) and protective efficacy (chimpanzee and human).
The vaccine against hepatitis B, prepared from recombinant yeast cultures, is free of association with human blood or blood products.
Each lot of hepatitis B vaccine is tested for safety, in mice and guinea pigs, and for sterility.
RECOMBIVAX HB is a sterile suspension for intramuscular injection. However, for persons at risk of hemorrhage following intramuscular injection, the vaccine may be administered subcutaneously. (See DOSAGE AND ADMINISTRATION).
RECOMBIVAX HB Hepatitis B Vaccine, (Recombinant) is supplied in four formulations.
Pediatric Formulation, 5 mcg/mL: each 0.5 mL dose contains 2.5 mcg of hepatitis B surface antigen.

Adolescent/High-Risk Infant, 10 mcg/mL: each 0.5 mL dose contains 5 mcg of hepatitis B surface antigen.
Adult Formulation, 10 mcg/mL: each 1 mL dose contains 10 mcg of hepatitis B surface antigen.
Dialysis Formulation, 40 mcg/mL: each 1 mL dose contains 40 mcg of hepatitis B surface antigen.
Each formulation contains thimerosal (mercury derivative) 1:20,000 added as a preservative and has been treated with formaldehyde prior to adsorption onto aluminum hydroxide. In each formulation, hepatitis B surface antigen is adsorbed onto approximately 0.5 mg of aluminum (provided as aluminum hydroxide) per mL of vaccine. The vaccine is of the *adw* subtype. RECOMBIVAX HB is indicated for vaccination of persons at risk of infection from hepatitis B virus including all known subtypes. RECOMBIVAX HB Dialysis Formulation is indicated for vaccination of adult predialysis and dialysis patients against infection caused by all known subtypes of hepatitis B virus.

* Registered trademark of MERCK & CO., INC.

CLINICAL PHARMACOLOGY

Hepatitis B virus is one of several hepatitis viruses that cause a systemic infection, with a major pathology in the liver. These include hepatitis A virus, hepatitis D virus, and C and E viruses, previously referred to as non-A, non-B hepatitis viruses.
Hepatitis B virus is an important cause of viral hepatitis. There is no specific treatment for this disease. The incubation period for hepatitis B is relatively long; six weeks to six months may elapse between exposure and the onset of clinical symptoms. The prognosis following infection with hepatitis B virus is variable and dependent on at least three factors: (1) Age—Infants and younger children usually experience milder initial disease than older persons; (2) Dose of virus—The higher the dose, the more likely acute icteric hepatitis B will result; and, (3) Severity of associated underlying disease —underlying malignancy or pre-existing hepatic disease predisposes to increased morbidity and mortality.
Persistence of viral infection (the chronic hepatitis B virus carrier state) occurs in 5–10% of persons following acute hepatitis B, and occurs more frequently after initial anicteric hepatitis B than after initial icteric disease. Consequently, carriers of hepatitis B surface antigen (HBsAg) frequently give no history of having had recognized acute hepatitis. The Centers for Disease Control and Prevention (CDC) estimates that there are approximately 200–300 million chronic carriers worldwide and 1.25 million chronic carriers of hepatitis B virus in the USA. Chronic carriers represent the largest human reservoir of hepatitis B.
The serious complications and sequelae of hepatitis B virus infection include massive hepatic necrosis, cirrhosis of the liver, chronic active hepatitis, and hepatocellular carcinoma. It is the cause of up to 80% of hepatocellular carcinomas. More than 250,000 people worldwide die each year of hepatitis B-associated acute and chronic liver disease. In the United States, hepatitis B-virus-related acute and chronic liver disease causes approximately 4-5000 deaths annually.
There is also evidence that several diseases other than hepatitis have been associated with hepatitis B virus infection through an immunologic mechanism involving antigen-antibody complexes. Such diseases include a syndrome with rash, urticaria, and arthralgia resembling serum sickness; periarteritis nodosa; membranous glomerulonephritis; and infantile papular acrodermatitis.
Although the vehicles for transmission of the virus are often blood and blood products, viral antigen has also been found in tears, saliva, breast milk, urine, semen and vaginal secretions. Hepatitis B virus is capable of surviving at least a month on environmental surfaces exposed to body fluids containing hepatitis B virus. Infection may occur when hepatitis B virus, transmitted by infected body fluids, is implanted via mucous surfaces or percutaneously introduced through accidental or deliberate breaks in the skin.
Transmission of hepatitis B virus infection is often associated with close interpersonal contact with an infected individual and with crowded living conditions. In such circumstances, transmission by inoculation via routes other than overt percutaneous ones may be quite common. Perinatal transmission of hepatitis B infection from infected mother to child, at or shortly after birth, can occur if the mother is a hepatitis B surface antigen (HBsAg) carrier or if the

Continued on next page

Recombivax HB—Cont.

mother has an acute hepatitis B infection in the third trimester. Infection in infancy by the hepatitis B virus usually leads to the chronic carrier state. Without prophylaxis, infants born to women whose sera are positive for both the hepatitis B surface antigen and the e antigen have an 85–90% likelihood of being infected and becoming a chronic carrier. Well-controlled studies have shown that administration of three 0.5 mL doses of Hepatitis B Immune Globulin (Human) starting at birth is 75% effective in preventing establishment of the chronic carrier state in these infants during the first year of life. However, the protective effect of Hepatitis B Immune Globulin (Human) is transient.

Hepatitis B is endemic throughout the world and is a serious medical problem in population groups at increased risk. Because vaccination limited to high-risk individuals has failed to substantially lower the overall incidence of hepatitis B infection, both the Advisory Committee on Immunization Practices (ACIP) and the Committee on Infectious Diseases of the American Academy of Pediatrics (AAP) have also endorsed universal infant immunization as part of a comprehensive strategy for the control of hepatitis B infection. In addition, the ACIP also recommends hepatitis B vaccination for all infants and children born after November 21, 1991 and catch-up vaccination of children at high risk of infection (children <11 years of age in households of Pacific Islander ethnicity or of first generation immigrants/refugees from countries with an intermediate or high endemicity of infection). These advisory groups further recommend broad-based vaccination of adolescents. The ACIP recommends that all individuals not previously vaccinated with hepatitis B vaccine be vaccinated at 11–12 years of age with the age-appropriate dose of vaccine and that the vaccination schedule take into account the feasibility of delivering three doses of vaccine to this age group. In addition, older unvaccinated adolescents with identified risk factors for hepatitis B virus infection should also be vaccinated. Similarly, the AAP recommends that universal immunization of all adolescents should be implemented when resources permit with emphasis on those individuals in high-risk settings. (Refer to INDICATIONS AND USAGE.)

Numerous epidemiological studies have shown that persons who develop anti-HBs following active infection with the hepatitis B virus are protected against the disease on reexposure to the virus.

Clinical studies have shown that RECOMBIVAX HB when injected into the deltoid muscle induced protective levels of antibody in 96% of 1213 healthy adults who received the recommended 3-dose regimen. Antibody responses varied with age; a protective level of antibody was induced in 98% of 787 young adults 20–29 years of age, 94% of 249 adults 30–39 years of age and in 89% of 177 adults ≥ 40 years of age. Studies with hepatitis B vaccine derived from plasma have shown that a lower response rate (81%) to vaccine may be obtained if the vaccine is administered as a buttock injection. Seroconversion rates and geometric mean antibody titers were measured 1 to 2 months after the 3rd dose. Multiple clinical studies have defined a protective antibody (anti-HBs) level as 1) 10 or more sample ratio units (SRU) as determined by radioimmunoassay or 2) a positive result as determined by enzyme immunoassay. Note: 10 SRU is comparable to 10 mIU/mL of antibody.

RECOMBIVAX HB is highly immunogenic in younger individuals. In clinical studies, 99% of 94 infants under 1 year of age born of non-carrier mothers, 96% of 48 children 1–10 years of age, and 99% of 112 children and adolescents 11–19 years of age developed a protective level of antibody following the recommended 3-dose regimen of vaccine (see DOSAGE AND ADMINISTRATION).

The protective efficacy of three 5 mcg doses of RECOMBIVAX HB has been demonstrated in neonates born of mothers positive for both HBsAg and HBeAg (a core-associated antigenic complex which correlates with high infectivity). In a clinical study of infants who received one dose of Hepatitis B Immune Globulin at birth followed by the recommended three dose regimen of RECOMBIVAX HB, chronic infection had not occurred in 96% of 130 infants after nine months of follow-up. The estimated efficacy in prevention of chronic hepatitis B infection was 95% as compared to the infection rate in untreated historical controls. Significantly fewer neonates became chronically infected when given one dose of Hepatitis B Immune Globulin at birth followed by the recommended three dose regimen of RECOMBIVAX HB when compared to historical controls who received only a single dose of Hepatitis B Immune Globulin. Testing for HBsAg and anti-HBs is recommended at 12–15 months of age. If HBsAg is not detectable, and anti-HBs is present, the child has been protected.

As demonstrated in the above study, Hepatitis B Immune Globulin, when administered simultaneously with RECOMBIVAX HB at separate body sites, did not interfere with the induction of protective antibodies against hepatitis B virus elicited by the vaccine.

The duration of the protective effect of RECOMBIVAX HB in healthy vaccinees is unknown at present and the need for booster doses is not yet defined. However, long-term follow-up (5 to 9 years) of approximately 3000 high-risk vaccinees (infants of carrier mothers, male homosexuals, Alaskan Natives) who developed an anti-HBs titer of ≥10 mIU/mL when given a similar plasma-derived vaccine of intervals of 0, 1, and 6 months showed that no subjects developed clinically apparent hepatitis B infection and that 5 subjects developed antigenemia, even though up to half of the subjects failed to maintain a titer at this level. Persistence of vaccine-induced immunologic memory among healthy vaccinees who responded to a primary course of plasma-derived or recombinant hepatitis B vaccine has been demonstrated by an anamnestic antibody response to a booster dose of RECOMBIVAX HB given 5–12 years later.

Predialysis and Dialysis Patients

Predialysis and dialysis adult patients respond less well to hepatitis B vaccines than do healthy individuals; however, vaccination of adult patients early in the course of their renal disease produces higher seroconversion rates than vaccination after dialysis has been initiated. In addition, the responses to these vaccines may be lower if the vaccine is administered as a buttock injection. When 40 mcg of Hepatitis B Vaccine (Recombinant) was administered in the deltoid muscle, 89% of 28 participants developed anti-HBs with 86% achieving levels ≥ 10 mIU/mL. However, when the same dosage of this vaccine was administered inappropriately either in the buttock or a combination of buttock and deltoid, 62% of 47 participants developed anti-HBs with 55% achieving levels of ≥ 10 mIU/mL.

A booster dose or revaccination with RECOMBIVAX HB Dialysis Formulation may be considered in predialysis/dialysis patients if the anti-HBs level is less than 10 mIU/mL.

Reports in the literature describe a more virulent form of hepatitis B associated with superinfections or coinfections by delta virus, an imcomplete RNA virus. Delta virus can only infect and cause illness in persons infected with hepatitis B virus since the delta agent requires a coat of HBsAg in order to become infectious. Therefore, persons immune to hepatitis B virus infection should also be immune to delta virus infection.

Interchangeability of Plasma-Derived and Recombinant Hepatitis B Vaccines

Although there have been no clinical studies in which a three-dose vaccine series was initiated with HEPTAVAX-B* (Hepatitis B Vaccine) and completed with RECOMBIVAX HB, or vice versa, extensive *in vitro* and *in vivo* studies have demonstrated that two vaccines are immunologically comparable.

*Registered trademark of MERCK & CO., INC.

INDICATIONS AND USAGE

RECOMBIVAX HB is indicated for vaccination against infection caused by all known subtypes of hepatitis B virus. **RECOMBIVAX HB Dialysis Formulation** is indicated for vaccination of adult predialysis and dialysis patients against infection caused by all known subtypes of hepatitis B virus.

Vaccination with RECOMBIVAX HB is recommended for:

1) Infants including those born to HBsAg positive mothers (high-risk infants).

2) Children born after November 21, 1991.

3) Adolescents (see CLINICAL PHARMACOLOGY).

4) Other persons of all ages in areas of high prevalence or those who are or may be at increased risk of infection with hepatitis B virus, such as:

- *Health Care Personnel*
  - Dentists and oral surgeons.
  - Physicians and surgeons.
  - Nurses.
  - Paramedical personnel and custodial staff who may be exposed to the virus via blood or other patient specimens.
  - Dental hygienists and dental nurses.
  - Laboratory personnel handling blood, blood products, and other patient specimens.
  - Dental, medical and nursing students.
- *Selected Patients and Patient Contacts*
  - Staff in hemodialysis units and hematology/oncology units.
  - Hemodialysis patients and patients with early renal failure before they require hemodialysis.
  - Patients requiring frequent and/or large volume blood transfusions or clotting factor concentrates (e.g., persons with hemophilia, thalassemia).
  - Clients (residents) and staff of institutions for the mentally handicapped.
  - Classroom contacts of deinstitutionalized mentally handicapped persons who have persistent hepatitis B surface antigenemia and who show aggressive behavior.
  - Household and other intimate contacts of persons with persistent hepatitis B surface antigenemia.
- *Sub-populations with a known high incidence of the disease,* such as:
  - Alaskan Natives.
  - Pacific Islanders.
  - Refugees from areas where hepatitis B virus infection is endemic.
  - Adoptees from countries where hepatitis B virus infection is endemic.
- *International Travelers*
- *Military Personnel identified as being at increased risk*
- *Morticians and Embalmers*
- *Blood bank and plasma fractionation workers*
- *Persons at Increased Risk of the Disease Due to Their Sexual Practices,* such as:
  - Persons who have heterosexual activity with multiple partners.
  - Persons who repeatedly contract sexually transmitted diseases.
  - Homosexual and bisexual adolescent and adult men.
  - Female prostitutes.
- *Prisoners*
- *Injection drug users*

Neither dosage strength will prevent hepatitis caused by other agents, such as hepatitis A virus, non-A, non-B hepatitis viruses, or other viruses known to infect the liver.

Revaccination

See CLINICAL PHARMACOLOGY

Use with Other Vaccines

Specific data are not yet available for the simultaneous administration of RECOMBIVAX HB with other vaccines. However, ACIP states that, in general, simultaneous administration of certain live and inactivated pediatric vaccines has not resulted in impaired antibody responses or increased rates of adverse reactions. Separate sites and syringes should be used for simultaneous administration of injectable vaccines.

CONTRAINDICATIONS

Hypersensitivity to yeast or any component of the vaccine.

WARNINGS

Patients who develop symptoms suggestive of hypersensitivity after an injection should not receive further injections of the vaccine (see CONTRAINDICATIONS).

Because of the long incubation period for hepatitis B, it is possible for unrecognized infection to be present at the time the vaccine is given. The vaccine may not prevent hepatitis B in such patients.

PRECAUTIONS

General

As with any percutaneous vaccine, epinephrine should be available for immediate use should an anaphylactoid reaction occur.

Any serious active infection is reason for delaying use of the vaccine except when in the opinion of the physician, withholding the vaccine entails a greater risk.

Caution and appropriate care should be exercised in administering the vaccine to individuals with severely compromised cardiopulmonary status or to others in whom a febrile or systemic reaction could pose a significant risk.

Pregnancy

Pregnancy Category C: Animal reproduction studies have not been conducted with the vaccine. It is also not known whether the vaccine can cause fetal harm when administered to a pregnant woman or can affect reproduction capacity. The vaccine should be given to a pregnant woman only if clearly needed.

Nursing Mothers

It is not known whether the vaccine is excreted in human milk. Because many drugs are excreted in human milk, cautions should be exercised when the vaccine is administered to a nursing woman.

Pediatric Use

RECOMBIVAX HB has been shown to be usually well-tolerated and highly immunogenic in infants and children of all ages. Newborns also respond well; maternally transferred antibodies do not interfere with the active immune response to the vaccine. See DOSAGE AND ADMINISTRATION for recommended pediatric dosage and for recommended dosage for infants born to HBsAg positive mothers. The safety and effectiveness of RECOMBIVAX HB Dialysis Formulation in children have not been established.

ADVERSE REACTIONS

RECOMBIVAX HB and RECOMBIVAX HB Dialysis Formulation are generally well-tolerated. No serious adverse reactions attributable to the vaccine have been reported during the course of clinical trials. No adverse experiences were reported during clinical trials which could be related to changes in the titers of antibodies to yeast. As with any vaccine, there is the possibility that broad use of the vaccine could reveal adverse reactions not observed in clinical trials. In a group of studies, 1636 doses of RECOMBIVAX HB were administered to 653 healthy infants and children (up to 10 years of age) who were monitored for 5 days after each dose.

Injection site reactions (including erythema and swelling) and systemic complaints were reported following 8% and 17% of the injections, respectively. The most frequently reported systemic adverse reactions (>1% injections), in decreasing order of frequency, were irritability, tiredness, fever (>101°F oral equivalent), crying, diarrhea, vomiting, diminished appetite, and insomnia.

In a group of studies, 3258 doses of RECOMBIVAX HB were administered to 1252 healthy adults who were monitored for 5 days after each dose. Injection site and systemic complaints were reported following 17% and 15% of the injections, respectively. The following adverse reactions were reported:

*Incidence Equal to or
Greater Than 1% of Injections*
LOCAL REACTION (INJECTION SITE)
Injection site reactions consisting principally of soreness, and including pain, tenderness, pruritus, erythema, ecchymosis, swelling, warmth, and nodule formation.
BODY AS A WHOLE
The most frequent systemic complaints include fatigue/weakness; headache; fever (≥100°F); and malaise.
DIGESTIVE SYSTEM
Nausea; and diarrhea
RESPIRATORY SYSTEM
Pharyngitis; and upper respiratory infection
Incidence Less than 1% of Injections
BODY AS A WHOLE
Sweating; achiness; sensation of warmth; lightheadedness; chills; and flushing
DIGESTIVE SYSTEM
Vomiting; abdominal pains/cramps; dyspepsia; and diminished appetite
RESPIRATORY SYSTEM
Rhinitis; influenza; and cough
NERVOUS SYSTEM
Vertigo/dizziness; and paresthesia
INTEGUMENTARY SYSTEM
Pruritus; rash (non-specified); angioedema; and urticaria
MUSCULOSKELETAL SYSTEM
Arthralgia including monoarticular; myalgia; back pain, neck pain; shoulder pain; and neck stiffness
HEMIC/LYMPHATIC SYSTEM
Lymphadenopathy
PSYCHIATRIC/BEHAVIORAL
Insomnia/Disturbed sleep
SPECIAL SENSES
Earache
UROGENITAL SYSTEM
Dysuria
CARDIOVASCULAR SYSTEM
Hypotension
Marketed Experience
The following additional adverse reactions have been reported with use of the marketed vaccine. In many instances, the relationship to the vaccine was unclear.
Hypersensitivity
Anaphylaxis and symptoms of immediate hypersensitivity reactions including rash, pruritus, urticaria, edema, angioedema, dyspnea, chest discomfort, bronchial spasm, palpitation, or symptoms consistent with a hypotensive episode have been reported within the first few hours after vaccination. An apparent hypersensitivity syndrome (serum-sickness-like) of delayed onset has been reported days to weeks after vaccination, including: arthralgia/arthritis (usually transient), fever, and dermatologic reactions such as urticaria, erythema multiforme, ecchymoses and erythema nodosum (See WARNINGS and PRECAUTIONS).
Digestive System
Elevation of liver enzymes; constipation.
Nervous System
Guillain-Barré Syndrome; multiple sclerosis; myelitis including transverse myelitis; peripheral neuropathy including Bell's Palsy; radiculopathy; herpes zoster; migraine; muscle weakness; hypesthesia.
Integumentary System
Stevens-Johnson Syndrome; petechiae.
Musculoskeletal System
Arthritis.
Hematologic
Increased erythrocyte sedimentation rate; thrombocytopenia.
Immune System
Systemic lupus erythematosus (SLE); lupus-like syndrome.
Psychiatric/Behavioral
Irritability; agitation; somnolence.
Special Senses
Optic neuritis; tinnitus; conjunctivitis; visual disturbances.
Cardiovascular System
Syncope; tachycardia.
The following adverse reaction has been reported with another Heaptitis B Vaccine (Recombinant) but not with RECOMBIVAX HB: keratitis.

DOSAGE AND ADMINISTRATION

Do not inject intravenously or intradermally.
RECOMBIVAX HB [Hepatitis B Vaccine (Recombinant)] DIALYSIS FORMULATION (40 mcg/mL) IS INTENDED ONLY FOR ADULT PREDIALYSIS/DIALYSIS PATIENTS.
RECOMBIVAX HB [Hepatitis B Vaccine (Recombinant)] PEDIATRIC, ADOLESCENT/HIGH-RISK INFANT, and ADULT FORMULATIONS (5 mcg/mL or 10 mcg/mL) ARE NOT INTENDED FOR USE IN PREDIALYSIS/DIALYSIS PATIENTS.
Table 1 summarizes the dose and formulation of RECOMBIVAX HB for specific populations. The vaccination regimen for each population EXCEPT Infants of HBsAg Positive Mothers (see Table 2) consists of 3 doses of vaccine given according to the following schedule:
1st dose: at elected date
2nd dose: 1 month later
3rd dose: 6 months after the first dose

Table 1

Group	Dose*	Formulation	Color Code
Infants born of:			
HBsAg Negative Mothers	2.5 mcg (0.5 mL)	Pediatric	Brown
HBsAg Positive Mothers†	5 mcg (0.5 mL)	Adolescent/High-Risk Infant	Yellow
1–10 years of age	2.5 mcg (0.5 mL)	Pediatric	Brown
11–19 years of age	5 mcg (0.5 mL)	Adolescent/High-Risk Infant	Yellow
≥20 years of age	10 mcg (1.0 mL)	Adult	Green
Predialysis and Dialysis Patients**	40 mcg/ 1.0 mL	Dialysis	Blue

† See Table 2
* If the suggested formulation is not available, the appropriate dosage can be achieved from another formulation provided that the total volume of vaccine administered does not exceed 1 mL. However, the Dialysis Formulation may be used only for adult predialysis/dialysis patients.
** See also recommendations for revaccination of Predialysis and Dialysis Patients under *Revaccination*, DOSAGE AND ADMINISTRATION.

RECOMBIVAX HB is for intramuscular injection. The *deltoid muscle* is the preferred site for intramuscular injection in adults. Data suggests that injections given in the buttocks frequently are given into fatty tissue instead of into muscle. Such injections have resulted in a lower seroconversion rate than was expected. The *anterolateral thigh* is the recommended site for intramuscular injection in infants and young children.
For persons at risk of hemorrhage following intramuscular injection, RECOMBIVAX HB may be administered subcutaneously. However, when other aluminum-adsorbed vaccines have been administered subcutaneously, an increased incidence of local reactions including subcutaneous nodules has been observed. Therefore, subcutaneous administration should be used only in persons (e.g., hemophiliacs) who are at risk of hemorrhage following intramuscular injections.
The vaccine should be used as supplied; no dilution or reconstitution is necessary. The full recommended dose of the vaccine should be used.
For Vial and Pre-filled Single Dose Syringe: Shake well before use. Thorough agitation at the time of administration is necessary to maintain suspension of the vaccine.
Parenteral drug products should be inspected visually for particulate matter and discoloration prior to administration. After thorough agitation, the vaccine is a slightly opaque, white suspension.
For Vial: Withdraw the recommended dose from the vial using a sterile needle and syringe free of preservatives, antiseptics, and detergents.
It is important to use a separate sterile syringe and needle for each individual patient to prevent transmission of hepatitis and other infectious agents from one person to another.
Injection must be accomplished with a needle long enough to ensure intramuscular deposition of the vaccine.
Dosage for Infants Born of HBsAg Positive Mothers (High-Risk Infants) or Mothers of Unknown HBsAg Status
The recommended regimen for infants born of HBsAg positive mothers is as follows:

Table 2

RECOMBIVAX HB	Birth	1 month	6 months
Adolescent/High-Risk Infant yellow color code	5 mcg** (0.5 mL)	5 mcg (0.5 mL)	5 mcg (0.5 mL)

HEPATITIS B IMMUNE GLOBULIN

| | 0.5 mL | — | — |

** The first 5 mcg/0.5 mL dose of RECOMBIVAX HB may be given at birth at the same time as Hepatitis B Immune Globulin, but should be administered in the opposite anterolateral thigh.

Dosage for Infants of Mothers of Unknown HBsAg Status
Recommendations from the ACIP for infants born of mothers of unknown HBsAg status are summarized as follows: In the event that a mother's HBsAg status is unknown, vaccination should be initiated as soon as possible with a 5 mcg/0.5 mL dose of vaccine (Adolescent/High-Risk Infant, yellow color code). If within 7 days of delivery the mother is determined to be HBsAg positive, the infant should also be given a dose of Hepatitis B Immune Globulin immediately; the vaccination series should then be completed with 5 mcg/0.5 mL dosages. If the mother's HBsAg antigen test is negative, then complete the vaccination series with 2.5 mcg/0.5 mL dosages (Pediatric Formulation, brown color code).
Revaccination
The duration of the protective effect of RECOMBIVAX HB in healthy vaccinees is unknown at present and the need for booster doses is not yet defined (see CLINICAL PHARMACOLOGY).
A booster dose or revaccination with RECOMBIVAX HB Dialysis Formulation (blue color code) may be considered in predialysis/dialysis patients if the anti-HBs level is less than 10 MIU/mL 1 to 2 months after the 3rd dose. The ACIP recommends that the need for booster doses of vaccine should be assessed by annual antibody testing and a booster dose given when antibody levels decline to <10 mIU/mL.
Known or Presumed Exposure to HBsAg
There are no prospective studies directly testing the efficacy of a combination of Hepatitis B Immune Globulin (Human) and RECOMBIVAX HB in preventing clinical hepatitis B following percutaneous, ocular or mucous membrane exposure to hepatitis B virus. However, since most persons with such exposures (e.g., health-care workers) are candidates for RECOMBIVAX HB and since combined Hepatitis B Immune Globulin (Human) plus vaccine is more efficacious than Hepatitis B Immune Globulin (Human) alone in perinatal exposures, the following guidelines are recommended for persons who have been exposed to hepatitis B virus such as through (1) percutaneous (needlestick), ocular, mucous membrane exposure to blood known or presumed to contain HBsAg, (2) human bites by known or presumed HBsAg carriers, that penetrate the skin, or (3) following intimate sexual contact with known or presumed HBsAg carriers:
Hepatitis B Immune Globulin (Human) (0.06 mL/kg) should be given intramuscularly as soon as possible after exposure and within 24 hours if possible. RECOMBIVAX HB (see dosage recommendation) should be given intramuscularly at a separate site within 7 days of exposure and second and third doses given one and six months, respectively, after the first dose.

HOW SUPPLIED

PEDIATRIC FORMULATION
No. 4799—RECOMBIVAX HB for pediatric use is supplied as 2.5 mcg/0.5 mL of HBsAg in a 0.5 mL single-dose vial, color coded with a brown cap and stripe on the vial labels and cartons, **NDC** 0006-4799-00.
No. 4761—RECOMBIVAX HB for pediatric use is supplied as 2.5 mcg/0.5 mL of HBsAg in a 3 mL multiple-dose vial, color coded with a brown cap and stripe on the vial labels and cartons, **NDC** 0006-4761-00 (6505-01-415-9815 2.5 mcg/0.5 mL, 3 mL).
No. 4874—RECOMBIVAX HB for pediatric use is supplied as 2.5 mcg/0.5 mL of HBsAg in a 0.5 mL single-dose vial, in a box of 10 single-dose vials, color coded with a brown cap and stripe on the vial labels and cartons, **NDC** 0006-4874-00.
No. 4875—RECOMBIVAX HB for pediatric use is supplied as 2.5 mcg/0.5 mL of HBsAg in a 3 mL multiple-dose vial, in a box of 10 multi-dose vials, color coded with a brown cap and stripe on the vial labels and cartons, **NDC** 0006-4875-00.
No. 4851—RECOMBIVAX HB for pediatric use is supplied as 2.5 mcg/0.5 mL of HBsAg in a 0.5 mL pre-filled single-dose glass syringe, in a box of 5 pre-filled single-dose syringes, color coded with a brown plunger rod and stripe on the syringe labels and cartons, **NDC** 0006-4851-00.

Continued on next page

Information on the Merck & Co., Inc. products listed on these pages is the full prescribing information from product circulars in use August 31, 1998. For information, please call 1-800-NSC MERCK [1-800-672-6372].

Recombivax HB—Cont.

ADOLESCENT/HIGH-RISK INFANT
No. 4769—RECOMBIVAX HB for adolescent use and for infants born of HBsAg+ mothers is supplied as 5 mcg/0.5 mL of HBsAg in a 0.5 mL single-dose vial, color coded with a yellow cap and stripe on the vial labels and cartons, **NDC** 0006-4769-00
(6505-01-415-9813 5 mcg/0.5 mL, 0.5 mL).
No. 4876—RECOMBIVAX HB for adolescent use and for infants born of HBsAg+ mothers is supplied as 5 mcg/0.5 mL of HBsAg in a 0.5 mL single-dose vial, in a box of 10 single-dose vials, color coded with a yellow cap and stripe on the vial labels and cartons, **NDC** 0006-4876-00.
No. 4849—RECOMBIVAX HB for adolescent use and for infants born of HBsAg+ mothers is supplied as 5 mcg/0.5 mL of HBsAg in a 0.5 mL pre-filled single-dose glass syringe, in a box of 5 pre-filled single-dose syringes, color coded with a yellow plunger rod and stripe on the syringe labels and cartons, **NDC** 0006-4849-00.
ADULT FORMULATION
No. 4775—RECOMBIVAX HB for adult use is supplied as 10 mcg/mL of HBsAg in a 1 mL single-dose vial, color coded with a green cap and stripe on the vial labels and cartons, **NDC** 0006-4775-00.
(6505-01-312-6410 10 mcg/mL, 1 mL).
No. 4773—RECOMBIVAX HB for adult use is supplied as 10 mcg/mL of HBsAg in a 3 mL multiple-dose vial, color coded with a green cap and stripe on the vial labels and cartons, **NDC** 0006-4773-00
(6505-01-266-3780 10 mcg/mL, 3 mL).
No. 4872—RECOMBIVAX HB for adult use is supplied as 10 mcg/mL of HBsAg in a 1 mL single-dose vial, in a box of 10 single-dose vials, color coded with a green cap and stripe on the vial labels and cartons, **NDC** 0006-4872-00.
No.4873—RECOMBIVAX HB for adult use is supplied as 10 mcg/mL of HBsAg in a 3 mL multiple-dose vial, in a box of 10 multi-dose vials, color coded with a green cap and stripe on the vial labels and cartons, **NDC** 0006-4873-00
(6505-10-415-9816 10 mcg/1.0 mL, 3 mL).
No. 4848—RECOMBIVAX HB for adult use is supplied as 10 mcg/mL of HBsAg in a 1 mL pre-filled single-dose glass syringe, in a box of 5 pre-filled single-dose syringes, color coded with a green plunger rod and stripe on the syringe labels and cartons, **NDC** 0006-4848-00.
DIALYSIS FORMULATION
No. 4776—RECOMBIVAX HB Dialysis Formulation is supplied as 40 mcg/mL of HBsAg in a 1 mL single-dose vial, color coded with a blue cap and stripe on the vial labels and cartons, **NDC** 0006-4776-00
(6505-01-317-1132 40 mcg/mL, 1 mL).
Storage
Store vials and syringes at 2–8°C (36°–46°F). Storage above or below the recommended temperature may reduce potency.
Do not freeze since freezing destroys potency.
7462215 Issued October 1997
COPYRIGHT © MERCK & CO., INC., 1986, 1989, 1993
All rights reserved

SINGULAIR® Tablets and Chewable Tablets ℞
(montelukast sodium)

DESCRIPTION

Montelukast sodium, the active ingredient in SINGULAIR*, is a selective and orally active leukotriene receptor antagonist that inhibits the cysteinyl leukotriene $CysLT_1$ receptor.
Montelukast sodium is described chemically as [R-(E)]-1-[[[1-[3-[2-(7-chloro-2-quinolinyl)ethenyl]phenyl]-3-[2-(1-hydroxy-1-methylethyl)phenyl]propyl]thio]methyl]cyclopropaneacetic acid, monosodium salt.
The empirical formula is $C_{35}H_{35}ClNNaO_3S$, and its molecular weight is 608.18. The structural formula is:

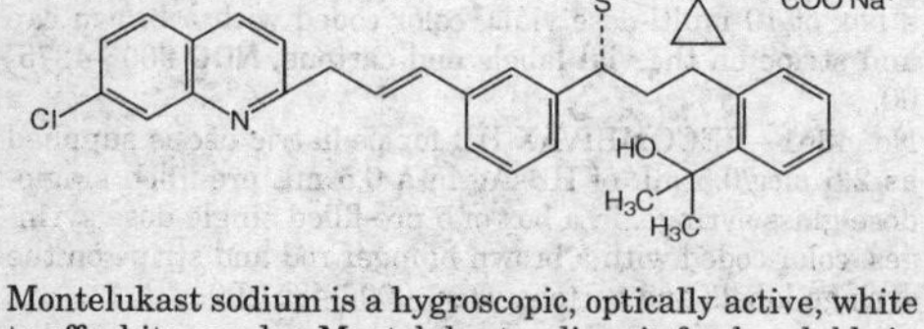

Montelukast sodium is a hygroscopic, optically active, white to off-white powder. Montelukast sodium is freely soluble in ethanol, methanol, and water and practically insoluble in acetonitrile.
Each 10-mg film-coated SINGULAIR tablet contains 10.4 mg montelukast sodium, which is the molar equivalent to 10.0 mg of free acid, and the following inactive ingredients: microcrystalline cellulose, lactose monohydrate, croscarmellose sodium, hydroxypropyl cellulose, and magnesium stearate. The film coating consists of: hydroxypropyl methylcellulose, hydroxypropyl cellulose, titanium dioxide, red iron oxide, yellow iron oxide, and carnauba wax.
Each 5-mg chewable SINGULAIR tablet contains 5.2 mg montelukast sodium, which is the molar equivalent to 5.0 mg of free acid, and the following inactive ingredients: mannitol, microcrystalline cellulose, hydroxypropyl cellulose, red ferric oxide, croscarmellose sodium, cherry flavor, aspartame, and magnesium stearate.

*Registered trademark of MERCK & CO., Inc.

CLINICAL PHARMACOLOGY

Mechanism of Action
The cysteinyl leukotrienes (LTC_4, LTD_4, LTE_4) are products of arachidonic acid metabolism and are released from various cells, including mast cells and eosinophils. These eicosanoids bind to cysteinyl leukotriene receptors (CysLT) found in the human airway. Cysteinyl leukotrienes and leukotriene receptor occupation have been correlated with the pathophysiology of asthma, including airway edema, smooth muscle contraction, and altered cellular activity associated with the inflammatory process, which contribute to the signs and symptoms of asthma.
Montelukast is an orally active compound that binds with high affinity and selectivity to the $CysLT_1$ receptor (in preference to other pharmacologically important airway receptors, such as the prostanoid, cholinergic, or β-adrenergic receptor). Montelukast inhibits physiologic actions of LTD_4 at the $CysLT_1$ receptor without any agonist activity.
Pharmacokinetics
Absorption
Montelukast is rapidly absorbed following oral administration. After administration of the 10-mg film-coated tablet to fasted adults, the mean peak montelukast plasma concentration (C_{max}) is achieved in 3 to 4 hours (T_{max}). The mean oral bioavailability is 64%. The oral bioavailability and C_{max} are not influenced by a standard meal in the morning.
For the 5-mg chewable tablet, the mean C_{max} is achieved in 2 to 2.5 hours after administration to adults in the fasted state. The mean oral bioavailability is 73% in the fasted state versus 63% when administered with a standard meal in the morning.
The safety and efficacy of SINGULAIR were demonstrated in clinical trials in which both formulations were administered in the evening without regard to the timing of food ingestion.
The comparative pharmacokinetics of montelukast when administered as two 5-mg chewable tablets versus one 10-mg film-coated tablet have not been evaluated.
Distribution
Montelukast is more than 99% bound to plasma proteins. The steady-state volume of distribution of montelukast averages 8 to 11 liters. Studies in rats with radiolabeled montelukast indicate minimal distribution across the blood-brain barrier. In addition, concentrations of radiolabeled material at 24 hours postdose were minimal in all other tissues.
Metabolism
Montelukast is extensively metabolized. In studies with therapeutic doses, plasma concentrations of metabolites of montelukast are undetectable at steady state in adults and pediatric patients.
In vitro studies using human liver microsomes indicate that cytochromes P450 3A4 and 2C9 are involved in the metabolism of montelukast. Clinical studies investigating the effect of known inhibitors of cytochromes P450 3A4 (e.g., ketoconazole, erythromycin) or 2C9 (e.g., fluconazole) on montelukast pharmacokinetics have not been conducted. Based on further *in vitro* results in human liver microsomes, therapeutic plasma concentrations of montelukast do not inhibit cytochromes P450 3A4, 2C9, 1A2, 2A6, 2C19, or 2D6 (see *Drug Interactions*).
Elimination
The plasma clearance of montelukast averages 45 mL/min in healthy adults. Following an oral dose of radiolabeled montelukast, 86% of the radioactivity was recovered in 5-day fecal collections and <0.2% was recovered in urine. Coupled with estimates of montelukast oral bioavailability, this indicates that montelukast and its metabolites are excreted almost exclusively via the bile.
In several studies, the mean plasma half-life of montelukast ranged from 2.7 to 5.5 hours in healthy young adults. The pharmacokinetics of montelukast are nearly linear for oral doses up to 50 mg. During once-daily dosing with 10-mg montelukast, there is little accumulation of the parent drug in plasma (~14%).
Special Populations
Gender: The pharmacokinetics of montelukast are similar in males and females.
Elderly: The pharmacokinetic profile and the oral bioavailability of a single 10-mg oral dose of montelukast are similar in elderly and younger adults. The plasma half-life of montelukast is slightly longer in the elderly. No dosage adjustment in the elderly is required.
Race: Pharmacokinetic differences due to race have not been studied.
Hepatic Insufficiency: Patients with mild-to-moderate hepatic insufficiency and clinical evidence of cirrhosis had evidence of decreased metabolism of montelukast resulting in 41% (90% CI=7%, 85%) higher mean montelukast area under the plasma concentration curve (AUC) following a single 10-mg dose. The elimination of montelukast was slightly prolonged compared with that in healthy subjects (mean half-life, 7.4 hours). No dosage adjustment is required in patients with mild-to-moderate hepatic insufficiency. The pharmacokinetics of SINGULAIR in patients with more severe hepatic impairment or with hepatitis have not been evaluated.
Renal Insufficiency: Since montelukast and its metabolites are not excreted in the urine, the pharmacokinetics of montelukast were not evaluated in patients with renal insufficiency. No dosage adjustment is recommended in these patients.
Adolescents and Pediatric Patients: The plasma concentration profile of montelukast following administration of the 10-mg film-coated tablet is similar in adolescents ≥15 years of age and young adults. The 10-mg film-coated tablet is recommended for use in patients ≥15 years of age.
Pharmacokinetic studies show that the plasma profile of the 5-mg chewable tablet in pediatric patients 6 to 14 years of age is similar to that of the 10-mg film-coated tablet in adults. The 5-mg chewable tablet should be used in pediatric patients 6 to 14 years of age.
Drug Interactions
Montelukast at a dose of 10 mg once daily dosed to pharmacokinetic steady state:
- did not cause clinically significant changes in the kinetics of a single intravenous dose of theophylline (predominantly a cytochrome P450 1A2 substrate).
- did not change the pharmacokinetic profile of warfarin (a substrate of cytochromes P450 2A6 and 2C9) or influence the effect of a single 30-mg oral dose of warfarin on prothrombin time or the INR (International Normalized Ratio).
- did not change the pharmacokinetic profile or urinary excretion of immunoreactive digoxin.
- did not change the plasma concentration profile of terfenadine (a substrate of cytochrome P450 3A4) or fexofenadine, its carboxylated metabolite, and did not prolong the QTc interval following coadministration with terfenadine 60 mg twice daily.

Montelukast at doses of ≥100 mg daily dosed to pharmacokinetic steady state:
- did not significantly alter the plasma concentrations of either component of an oral contraceptive containing norethindrone 1 mg/ethinyl estradiol 35 mcg.
- did not cause any clinically significant change in plasma profiles of prednisone or prednisolone following administration of either oral prednisone or intravenous prednisolone.

Phenobarbital, which induces hepatic metabolism, decreased the AUC of montelukast approximately 40% following a single 10-mg dose of montelukast. No dosage adjustment for SINGULAIR is recommended. It is reasonable to employ appropriate clinical monitoring when potent cytochrome P450 enzyme inducers, such as phenobarbital or rifampin, are co-administered with SINGULAIR.
Pharmacodynamics
Montelukast causes inhibition of airway cysteinyl leukotriene receptors as demonstrated by the ability to inhibit bronchoconstriction due to inhaled LTD_4 in asthmatics. Doses as low as 5 mg cause substantial blockage of LTD_4-induced bronchoconstriction. In a placebo-controlled, crossover study (n=12), SINGULAIR inhibited early- and late-phase bronchoconstriction due to antigen challenge by 75% and 57%, respectively.
The effect of SINGULAIR on eosinophils in the peripheral blood was examined in clinical trials in adults and pediatric asthmatic patients. SINGULAIR decreased mean peripheral blood eosinophils approximately 13 to 15% from baseline compared with placebo over the double-blind treatment periods. The relationship between this observation and the clinical benefits noted in the clinical trials is not known (see CLINICAL PHARMACOLOGY, *Clinical Studies*).
Clinical Studies
GENERAL
There have been no clinical trials evaluating the relative efficacy of morning versus evening dosing. Although the pharmacokinetics of montelukast are similar whether dosed in the morning or the evening, efficacy was demonstrated in clinical trials in adults and pediatric patients in which montelukast was administered in the evening without regard to the time of food ingestion.
ADOLESCENTS AND ADULTS 15 YEARS OF AGE AND OLDER
Clinical trials in adolescents and adults 15 years of age and older demonstrated there is no additional clinical benefit to montelukast doses above 10 mg once daily. This was shown in two chronic asthma trials using doses up to 200 mg once

daily and in one exercise challenge study using doses up to 50 mg, evaluated at the end of the once-daily dosing interval.

The efficacy of SINGULAIR for the chronic treatment of asthma in adolescents and adults 15 years of age and older was demonstrated in two (U.S. and Multinational) similarly designed, randomized, 12-week, double-blind, placebo-controlled trials in 1576 patients (795 treated with SINGULAIR, 530 treated with placebo, and 251 treated with active control). The patients studied were mild and moderate, non-smoking asthmatics who required approximately 5 puffs of inhaled β-agonist per day on an "as-needed" basis. The patients had a mean baseline percent of predicted forced expiratory volume in 1 second (FEV_1) of 66% (approximate range, 40 to 90%). The co-primary endpoints in these trials were FEV_1 and daytime asthma symptoms. Secondary endpoints included morning and evening peak expiratory flow rates (AM PEFR, PM PEFR), rescue β-agonist requirements, nocturnal awakening due to asthma, and other asthma-related outcomes. In both studies after 12 weeks, a random subset of patients receiving SINGULAIR was switched to placebo for an additional 3 weeks of double-blind treatment to evaluate for possible rebound effects. The results of the U.S. trial on the primary endpoint, FEV_1, expressed as mean percent change from baseline, are shown in FIGURE 1.

FIGURE 1
FEV_1 Mean Percent Change from Baseline
(U.S. Trial)

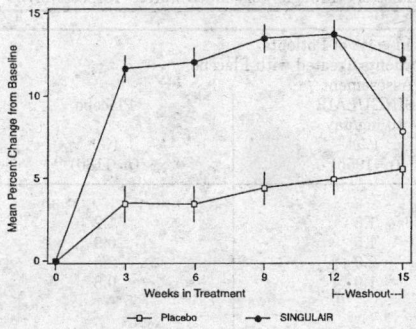

The effect of SINGULAIR on other primary and secondary endpoints is shown in TABLE 1 as combined analyses of the U.S. and Multinational trials.
[See table 1 below]
In adult patients, SINGULAIR reduced "as-needed" β-agonist use by 26.1% from baseline compared with 4.6% for placebo. In patients with nocturnal awakenings of at least 2 nights per week, SINGULAIR reduced the nocturnal awakenings by 34% from baseline, compared with 15% for placebo (combined analysis).

SINGULAIR, compared with placebo, significantly improved other protocol-defined, asthma-related outcome measurements (see TABLE 2).
[See table 2 at top of next page]
In one of these trials, a non-U.S. formulation of inhaled beclomethasone dipropionate dosed at 200 mcg (two puffs of 100 mcg ex-valve) twice daily with a spacer device was included as an active control. Over the 12-week treatment period, the mean percentage change in FEV_1 over baseline for SINGULAIR and beclomethasone were 7.49% vs 13.3% (p<0.001) respectively, see FIGURE 2; and the change in daytime symptom scores was -0.49 vs -0.70 on a 0 to 6 scale

(p<0.001) for SINGULAIR and beclomethasone, respectively. The percentages of individual patients treated with SINGULAIR or beclomethasone achieving any given percentage change in FEV_1 from baseline are shown in FIGURE 3.

FIGURE 2
FEV_1
Mean Percent Change From Baseline
(Multinational Trial)

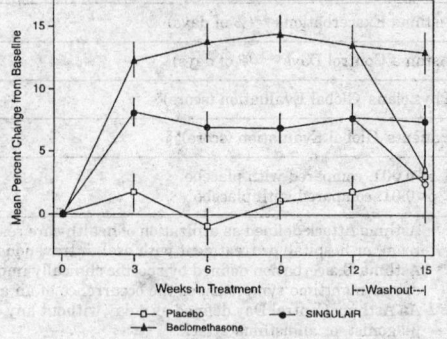

FIGURE 3
FEV_1
Distribution of Individual Patient Response
(Multinational Trial)

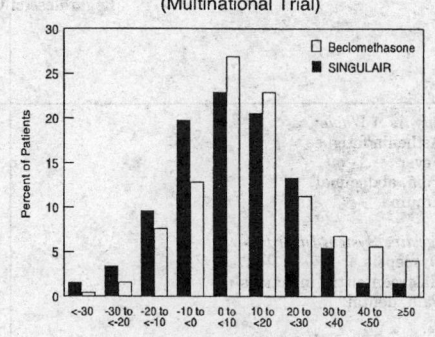

Onset of Action and Maintenance of Benefits
In each placebo-controlled trial in adults, the treatment effect of SINGULAIR, measured by daily diary card parameters, including symptom scores, "as-needed" β-agonist use, and PEFR measurements, was achieved after the first dose and was maintained throughout the dosing interval (24 hours). No significant change in treatment effect was observed during continuous once-daily evening administration in non-placebo-controlled extension trials for up to one year. Withdrawal of SINGULAIR in asthmatic patients after 12 weeks of continuous use did not cause rebound worsening of asthma.

PEDIATRIC PATIENTS 6 TO 14 YEARS OF AGE
The efficacy of SINGULAIR in pediatric patients 6 to 14 years of age was demonstrated in one 8-week double-blind, placebo-controlled trial in 336 patients (201 treated with

SINGULAIR and 135 treated with placebo) using an inhaled β-agonist on an "as-needed" basis. The patients had a mean baseline percent predicted FEV_1 of 72% (approximate range, 45 to 90%) and a mean daily inhaled β-agonist requirement of 3.4 puffs of albuterol. Approximately 36% of the patients were on inhaled corticosteroids.
Compared with placebo, treatment with one 5-mg SINGULAIR chewable tablet daily, resulted in a significant improvement in mean morning FEV_1 percent change from baseline (8.7% in the group treated with SINGULAIR vs 4.2% change from baseline in the placebo group, p<0.001). There was a significant decrease in the mean percentage change in daily "as-needed" inhaled β-agonist use (11.7% decrease from baseline in the group treated with SINGULAIR vs 8.2% increase from baseline in the placebo group, p<0.05). This effect represents a mean decrease from baseline of 0.56 and 0.23 puffs per day for the montelukast and placebo groups, respectively. Subgroup analyses indicated that younger pediatric patients aged 6 to 11 had efficacy results comparable to those of the older pediatric patients aged 12 to 14.
SINGULAIR, one 5-mg chewable tablet daily at bedtime, significantly decreased the percent of days asthma exacerbations occurred (SINGULAIR 20.6% vs placebo 25.7%, p≤0.05). (See TABLE 2 for definition of asthma exacerbation.) Parents' global asthma evaluations (parental evaluations of the patients' asthma, see TABLE 2 for definition of score) were significantly better with SINGULAIR compared with placebo (SINGULAIR 1.34 vs placebo 1.69, p≤0.05).
Similar to the adult studies, no significant change in the treatment effect was observed during continuous once-daily administration in one open-label extension trial without a concurrent placebo group for up to 6 months.

EFFECTS IN PATIENTS ON CONCOMITANT INHALED CORTICOSTEROIDS
Separate trials in adults evaluated the ability of SINGULAIR to add to the clinical effect of inhaled corticosteroids and to allow inhaled corticosteroid tapering when used concomitantly.
One randomized, placebo-controlled, parallel-group trial (n=226) enrolled stable asthmatic adults with a mean FEV_1 of approximately 84% of predicted who were previously maintained on various inhaled corticosteroids (delivered by metered-dose aerosol or dry powder inhalers). The types of inhaled corticosteroids and their mean baseline requirements included beclomethasone diproprionate (mean dose, 1203 mcg/day), triamcinolone acetonide (mean dose, 2004 mcg/day), flunisolide (mean dose, 1971 mcg/day), fluticasone propionate (mean dose, 1083 mcg/day), or budesonide (mean dose, 1192 mcg/day). Some of these inhaled corticosteroids were non-U.S.-approved formulations, and doses expressed may not be ex-actuator. The pre-study inhaled corticosteroid requirements were reduced by approximately 37% during a 5- to 7-week placebo run-in period designed to titrate patients toward their lowest effective inhaled corticosteroid dose. Treatment with SINGULAIR resulted in a further 47% reduction in mean inhaled corticosteroid dose compared with a mean reduction of 30% in the placebo group over the 12-week active treatment period (p≤0.05). Approximately 40% of the montelukast-treated patients and 29% of the placebo-treated patients could be tapered off inhaled corticosteroids and remained off inhaled corticosteroids at the conclusion of the study (p=NS). It is not known whether the results of this study are generalizable to asthmatics who require higher doses of inhaled corticosteroids or systemic corticosteroids.
In another randomized, placebo-controlled, parallel-group trial (n=642) in a similar population of adult patients previously maintained, but not adequately controlled, on inhaled corticosteroids (beclomethasone 336 mcg/day), the addition of SINGULAIR to beclomethasone resulted in statistically significant improvements in FEV_1 compared with those patients who were continued on beclomethasone alone or those patients who were withdrawn from beclomethasone and treated with montelukast or placebo alone over the last 10 weeks of the 16-week, blinded treatment period. Patients who were randomized to treatment arms containing beclomethasone had statistically significantly better asthma control than those patients randomized to SINGULAIR alone or placebo alone as indicated by FEV_1, daytime asthma symptoms, PEFR, nocturnal awakenings due to asthma, and "as-needed" β-agonist requirements.
In adult asthmatic patients with documented aspirin sensitivity, nearly all of whom were receiving concomitant inhaled and/or oral corticosteroids, a 4-week randomized, parallel-group trial (n=80) demonstrated that SINGULAIR, compared with placebo, resulted in significant improvement in parameters of asthma control. The magnitude of effect of SINGULAIR in aspirin-sensitive patients was similar to the

Continued on next page

TABLE 1
Effect of SINGULAIR on Primary and Secondary Endpoints
in Placebo-controlled Trials
(Combined Analyses - U.S. and Multinational Trials)

Endpoint	SINGULAIR		Placebo	
	Baseline	Mean Change from Baseline	Baseline	Mean Change from Baseline
Daytime Asthma Symptoms (0 to 6 scale)	2.43	-0.45*	2.45	-0.22
β-agonist (puffs per day)	5.38	-1.56*	5.55	-0.41
AM PEFR (L/min)	361.3	24.5*	364.9	3.3
PM PEFR (L/min)	385.2	17.9*	389.3	2.0
Nocturnal Awakenings (#/week)	5.37	-1.84*	5.44	-0.79

* p<0.001, compared with placebo

Information on the Merck & Co., Inc. products listed on these pages is the full prescribing information from product circulars in use August 31, 1998. For information, please call 1-800-NSC MERCK [1-800-672-6372].

Singulair—Cont.

effect observed in the general population of asthmatic patients studied. The effect of SINGULAIR on the bronchoconstrictor response to aspirin or other non-steroidal anti-inflammatory drugs in aspirin-sensitive asthmatic patients has not been evaluated (see PRECAUTIONS, *General*).

EFFECTS ON EXERCISE-INDUCED BRONCHOCONSTRICTION (ADULTS AND PEDIATRIC PATIENTS)

In a 12-week, randomized, double-blind, parallel group study of 110 adolescent and adult asthmatics 15 years of age and older, with a mean baseline FEV_1 percent of predicted of 83% and with documented exercise-induced exacerbation of asthma, treatment with SINGULAIR, 10 mg, once daily in the evening, resulted in a statistically significant reduction in mean maximal percent fall in FEV_1 and mean time to recovery to within 5% of the pre-exercise FEV_1. Exercise challenge was conducted at the end of the dosing interval (i.e., 20 to 24 hours after the preceding dose). This effect was maintained throughout the 12-week treatment period indicating that tolerance did not occur. SINGULAIR did not, however, prevent clinically significant deterioration in maximal percent fall in FEV_1 after exercise (i.e., ≥20% decrease from pre-exercise baseline) in 52% of patients studied. In a separate crossover study in adults, a similar effect was observed after two once-daily 10-mg doses of SINGULAIR.

In pediatric patients 6 to 14 years of age, using the 5-mg chewable tablet, a 2-day crossover study demonstrated effects similar to those observed in adults when exercise challenge was conducted at the end of the dosing interval (i.e., 20 to 24 hours after the preceding dose).

SINGULAIR should not be used as monotherapy for the treatment and management of exercise-induced bronchospasm. Patients who have exacerbations of asthma after exercise should continue to use their usual regimen of inhaled β-agonists as prophylaxis and have available for rescue a short-acting inhaled β-agonist (see PRECAUTIONS, *General* and *Information for Patients*).

INDICATIONS AND USAGE

SINGULAIR is indicated for the prophylaxis and chronic treatment of asthma in adults and pediatric patients 6 years of age and older.

CONTRAINDICATIONS

Hypersensitivity to any component of this product.

PRECAUTIONS

General

SINGULAIR is not indicated for use in the reversal of bronchospasm in acute asthma attacks, including status asthmaticus.

Patients should be advised to have appropriate rescue medication available. Therapy with SINGULAIR can be continued during acute exacerbations of asthma.

While the dose of inhaled corticosteroid may be reduced gradually under medical supervision, SINGULAIR should not be abruptly substituted for inhaled or oral corticosteroids.

SINGULAIR should not be used as monotherapy for the treatment and management of exercise-induced bronchospasm. Patients who have exacerbations of asthma after exercise should continue to use their usual regimen of inhaled β-agonists as prophylaxis and have available for rescue a short-acting inhaled β-agonist.

Patients with known aspirin sensitivity should continue avoidance of aspirin or non-steroidal anti-inflammatory agents while taking SINGULAIR. Although SINGULAIR is effective in improving airway function in asthmatics with documented aspirin sensitivity, it has not been shown to truncate bronchoconstrictor response to aspirin and other non-steroidal anti-inflammatory drugs in aspirin-sensitive asthmatic patients (see CLINICAL PHARMACOLOGY, *Clinical Studies*).

The reduction in systemic corticosteroid dose in patients receiving another leukotriene antagonist has been followed in rare cases by the occurrence of eosinophilia, vasculitic rash, worsening pulmonary symptoms, cardiac complications, and/or neuropathy sometimes presenting as Churg-Strauss syndrome, a systemic eosinophilic vasculitis. Although a causal relationship with leukotriene receptor antagonism has not been established and the phenomenon was not observed in clinical trials with montelukast, caution and appropriate clinical monitoring are recommended when systemic corticosteroid reduction is considered in patients receiving SINGULAIR.

Information for Patients

• Patients should be advised to take SINGULAIR daily as prescribed, even when they are asymptomatic, as well as during periods of worsening asthma, and to contact their physicians if their asthma is not well controlled.

• Patients should be advised that oral tablets of SINGULAIR are not for the treatment of acute asthma attacks. They should have appropriate short-acting inhaled β-agonist medication available to treat asthma exacerbations.

• Patients should be advised that, while using SINGULAIR, medical attention should be sought if short-acting inhaled bronchodilators are needed more often than usual, or if more than the maximum number of inhalations of short-acting bronchodilator treatment prescribed for 24-hour period are needed.

• Patients receiving SINGULAIR should be instructed not to decrease the dose or stop taking any other anti-asthma medications unless instructed by a physician.

• Patients who have exacerbations of asthma after exercise should be instructed to continue to use their usual regimen of inhaled β-agonists as prophylaxis unless otherwise instructed by their physician. All patients should have available for rescue a short-acting inhaled β-agonist.

• Patients with known aspirin sensitivity should be advised to continue avoidance of aspirin or non-steroidal anti-inflammatory agents while taking SINGULAIR.

Chewable Tablets

• *Phenylketonurics:* Phenylketonuric patients should be informed that the chewable tablet contains phenylalanine (a component of aspartame) 0.842 mg per 5-mg chewable tablet.

Drug Interactions

SINGULAIR has been administered with other therapies routinely used in the prophylaxis and chronic treatment of asthma with no apparent increase in adverse reactions. In drug-interaction studies, the recommended clinical dose of montelukast did not have clinically important effects on the pharmacokinetics of the following drugs: theophylline, prednisone, prednisolone, oral contraceptives (norethindrone 1 mg/ethinyl estradiol 35 mcg), terfenadine, digoxin, and warfarin.

Although additional specific interaction studies were not performed, SINGULAIR was used concomitantly with a wide range of commonly prescribed drugs in clinical studies without evidence of clinical adverse interactions. These medications included thyroid hormones, sedative hypnotics, non-steroidal anti-inflammatory agents, benzodiazepines, and decongestants.

Phenobarbital, which induces hepatic metabolism, decreased the AUC of montelukast approximately 40% following a single 10-mg dose of montelukast. No dosage adjustment for SINGULAIR is recommended. It is reasonable to

TABLE 2
Effect of SINGULAIR on Asthma-Related Outcome Measurements
(Combined Analyses - U.S. and Multinational Trials)

	SINGULAIR	Placebo
Asthma Attack* (% of patients)	11.6†	18.4
Oral Corticosteroid Rescue (% of patients)	10.7†	17.5
Discontinuation Due to Asthma (% of patients)	1.4‡	4.0
Asthma Exacerbations **(% of days)	12.8†	20.5
Asthma Control Days***(% of days)	38.5†	27.2
Physicians' Global Evaluation (score)§	1.77†	2.43
Patients' Global Evaluation (score)§§	1.60†	2.15

† p<0.001, compared with placebo
‡ p<0.01, compared with placebo

* Asthma Attack defined as utilization of health-care resources such as an unscheduled visit to a doctor's office, emergency room, or hospital; or treatment with oral, intravenous, or intramuscular corticosteroid.
** Asthma Exacerbation defined by specific clinically important decreases in PEFR, increase in β-agonist use, increases in day or nighttime symptoms, or the occurrence of an asthma attack.
*** An Asthma Control Day defined as a day without any of the following: nocturnal awakening, use of more than 2 puffs of β-agonist, or an asthma attack.
§ Physicians' evaluation of the patient's asthma, ranging from 0 to 6 ("very much better" through "very much worse," respectively).
§§ Patients' evaluation of asthma, ranging from 0 to 6 ("very much better" through "very much worse," respectively).

Adverse Experiences Occurring in ≥1% of Patients
with an Incidence Greater than that in Patients Treated with Placebo,
Regardless of Causality Assessment

	SINGULAIR 10 mg/day (%) (n=1955)	Placebo (%) (n=1180)
Body As A Whole		
Asthenia/fatigue	1.8	1.2
Fever	1.5	0.9
Pain, abdominal	2.9	2.5
Trauma	1.0	0.8
Digestive System Disorders		
Dyspepsia	2.1	1.1
Gastroenteritis, infectious	1.5	0.5
Pain, dental	1.7	1.0
Nervous System / Psychiatric		
Dizziness	1.9	1.4
Headache	18.4	18.1
Respiratory System Disorders		
Congestion, nasal	1.6	1.3
Cough	2.7	2.4
Influenza	4.2	3.9
Skin / Skin Appendages Disorder		
Rash	1.6	1.2
Laboratory Adverse Experiences*		
ALT increased	2.1	2.0
AST increased	1.6	1.2
Pyuria	1.0	0.9

*Number of patients tested (SINGULAIR and placebo, respectively): ALT and AST, 1935, 1170; pyuria, 1924, 1159.

employ appropriate clinical monitoring when potent cytochrome P450 enzyme inducers, such as phenobarbital or rifampin, are co-administered with SINGULAIR.

Carcinogenesis, Mutagenesis, and Impairment of Fertility

No evidence of tumorigenicity was seen in a 2-year carcinogenicity study in Sprague Dawley rats, at oral (gavage) doses up to 200 mg/kg/day (approximately 160 times the maximum recommended daily oral dose in adults and 190 times the maximum recommended daily oral dose in children, on a mg/m^2 basis) or in a 92-week carcinogenicity study in mice at oral doses up to 100 mg/kg/day (approximately 40 times the maximum recommended daily oral dose in adults and 50 times the maximum recommended daily oral dose in children, on a mg/m^2 basis).

Montelukast demonstrated no evidence of mutagenic or clastogenic activity in the following assays: the microbial mutagenesis assay, the V-79 mammalian cell mutagenesis assay, the alkaline elution assay in rat hepatocytes, the chromosomal aberration assay in Chinese hamster ovary cells, and in the *in vivo* mouse bone marrow chromosomal aberration assay.

In fertility studies in female rats, montelukast produced reductions in fertility and fecundity indices at an oral dose of 200 mg/kg (approximately 160 times the maximum recommended daily oral dose in adults, on a mg/m^2 basis). No effects on female fertility or fecundity were observed at an oral dose of 100 mg/kg (approximately 80 times the maximum recommended daily oral dose in adults, on a mg/m^2 basis).

Montelukast had no effects on fertility in male rats at oral doses up to 800 mg/kg (approximately 650 times the maximum recommended daily oral dose in adults, on a mg/m^2 basis).

Pregnancy, Teratogenic Effects

Pregnancy Category B:

No teratogenicity was observed in rats at oral doses up to 400 mg/kg/day (approximately 320 times the maximum recommended daily oral dose in adults, on a mg/m^2 basis) and in rabbits at oral doses up to 300 mg/kg/day (approximately 490 times the maximum recommended daily oral dose in adults, on a mg/m^2 basis). Montelukast crosses the placenta following oral dosing in rats and rabbits. There are, however, no adequate and well-controlled studies in pregnant women. Because animal reproduction studies are not always predictive of human response, SINGULAIR should be used during pregnancy only if clearly needed.

Nursing Mothers

Studies in rats have shown that montelukast is excreted in milk. It is not known if montelukast is excreted in human milk. Because many drugs are excreted in human milk, caution should be exercised when SINGULAIR is given to a nursing mother.

Pediatric Use

The safety and effectiveness in pediatric patients below the age of 6 years have not been established. Long-term trials evaluating the effect of chronic administration of SINGULAIR on linear growth in pediatric patients have not been conducted.

Geriatric Use

Of the total number of subjects in clinical studies of montelukast, 3.5% were 65 years of age and over and 0.4% were 75 years of age and over. No overall differences in safety or effectiveness were observed between these subjects and younger subjects, and other reported clinical experience has not identified differences in responses between the elderly and younger patients, but greater sensitivity of some older individuals cannot be ruled out.

ADVERSE REACTIONS

Adolescents and Adults 15 Years of Age and Older

SINGULAIR has been evaluated for safety in approximately 2600 adolescent and adult patients 15 years of age and older in clinical trials. In placebo-controlled clinical trials, the following adverse experiences reported with SINGULAIR occurred in greater than or equal to 1% of patients and at an incidence greater than that in patients treated with placebo, regardless of causality assessment:

[See second table at top of previous page]

The frequency of less common adverse events was comparable between SINGULAIR and placebo.

Cumulatively, 569 patients were treated with SINGULAIR for at least 6 months, 480 for one year, and 49 for two years in clinical trials. With prolonged treatment, the adverse experience profile did not significantly change.

Pediatric Patients 6 to 14 Years of Age

SINGULAIR has also been evaluated for safety in approximately 320 pediatric patients 6 to 14 years of age. Cumulatively, 169 pediatric patients were treated with SINGULAIR for at least 6 months, and 121 for one year or longer in clinical trials. The safety profile of SINGULAIR versus placebo in the double-blind, 8-week, pediatric efficacy trial was generally similar to the adult safety profile with the exception of the adverse events listed below. In pediatric patients receiving SINGULAIR, the following events occurred with a frequency ≥2% and more frequently than in pediatric patients who received placebo, regardless of causality assessment: diarrhea, laryngitis, pharyngitis, nausea, otitis, sinusitis, and viral infection. The frequency of less common adverse events was comparable between SINGULAIR and placebo. With prolonged treatment, the adverse experience profile did not significantly change.

OVERDOSAGE

No mortality occurred following single oral doses of montelukast up to 5000 mg/kg in mice (approximately 2000 times the maximum recommended daily oral dose in adults and 2400 times the maximum recommended daily oral dose in children, on a mg/m^2 basis) and rats (approximately 4100 times the maximum recommended daily oral dose in adults and 4800 times the maximum recommended daily oral dose in children, on a mg/m^2 basis).

No specific information is available on the treatment of overdosage with SINGULAIR. In chronic asthma studies, montelukast has been administered at doses up to 200 mg/day to patients for 22 weeks and, in short-term studies, up to 900 mg/day to patients for approximately a week without clinically important adverse experiences. In the event of overdose, it is reasonable to employ the usual supportive measures; e.g., remove unabsorbed material from the gastrointestinal tract, employ clinical monitoring, and institute supportive therapy, if required.

It is not known whether montelukast is removed by peritoneal dialysis or hemodialysis.

DOSAGE AND ADMINISTRATION

General Information:

Adolescents and Adults 15 Years of Age and Older

The dosage for adolescents and adults 15 years of age and older is one 10-mg tablet daily to be taken in the evening.

Pediatric Patients 6 to 14 Years of Age

The dosage for pediatric patients 6 to 14 years of age is one 5-mg chewable tablet daily to be taken in the evening. No dosage adjustment within this age group is necessary.

Safety and effectiveness in pediatric patients younger than 6 years of age have not been established.

The safety and efficacy of SINGULAIR was demonstrated in clinical trials where it was administered in the evening without regard to the time of food ingestion. There have been no clinical trials evaluating the relative efficacy of morning versus evening dosing.

HOW SUPPLIED

No. 3760—SINGULAIR Tablets, 5 mg, are pink, round, biconvex-shaped chewable tablets, with code MRK 275 on one side and SINGULAIR on the other. They are supplied as follows:

NDC 0006-0275-31 unit of use high-density polyethylene (HDPE) bottles of 30 with a polypropylene child-resistant cap, an aluminum foil induction seal, and a silica gel desiccant canister

NDC 0006-0275-54 unit of use high-density polyethylene (HDPE) bottles of 90 with a polypropylene child-resistant cap, an aluminum foil induction seal, and a silica gel desiccant canister

NDC 0006-0275-28 unit dose paper and aluminum foil-backed aluminum foil peelable blister packs of 100.

Shown in Product Identification Section, page 323

No. 3761—SINGULAIR Tablets, 10 mg, are beige, rounded square-shaped, film-coated tablets, with code MRK 117 on one side and SINGULAIR on the other. They are supplied as follows:

NDC 0006-0117-31 unit of use high-density polyethylene (HDPE) bottles of 30 with a polypropylene child-resistant cap, an aluminum foil induction seal, and a silica gel desiccant canister

NDC 0006-0117-54 unit of use high-density polyethylene (HDPE) bottles of 90 with a polypropylene child-resistant cap, an aluminum foil induction seal, and a silica gel desiccant canister

NDC 0006-0117-28 unit dose paper and aluminum foil-backed aluminum foil peelable blister pack of 100.

Shown in Product Identification Guide, page 323

Storage

Store the 5-mg chewable tablets and the 10-mg film-coated tablets at room temperature 15–30°C (59–86°F), protected from moisture and light.

9088800 Issued February 1998

COPYRIGHT © MERCK & CO., Inc., 1998
All rights reserved.

STROMECTOL® Tablets (ivermectin) ℞

DESCRIPTION

STROMECTOL® (Ivermectin) is a semisynthetic, anthelmintic agent for oral administration. Ivermectin is derived from the avermectins, a class of highly active broad-spectrum anti-parasitic agents isolated from the fermentation products of *Streptomyces avermitilis*. Ivermectin is a mixture containing at least 90% 5-*O*-demethyl-22,23-dihydroavermectin A_{1a} and less than 10% 5-*O*-demethyl-25-de(1-methylpropyl)-22,23-dihydro-25-(1-methylethyl)avermectin A_{1a}, generally referred to as 22,23-dihydroavermectin B_{1a} and B_{1b}, H_2B_{1a} and H_2B_{1b}, respectively. The respective empirical formulas are $C_{48}H_{74}O_{14}$ and $C_{47}H_{72}O_{14}$, with molecular weights of 875.10 and 861.07, respectively. The structural formulas are:

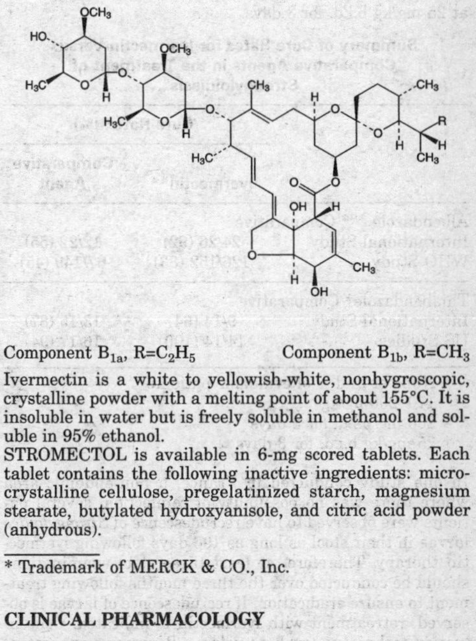

Component B_{1a}, R=C_2H_5 Component B_{1b}, R=CH_3

Ivermectin is a white to yellowish-white, nonhygroscopic, crystalline powder with a melting point of about 155°C. It is insoluble in water but is freely soluble in methanol and soluble in 95% ethanol.

STROMECTOL is available in 6-mg scored tablets. Each tablet contains the following inactive ingredients: microcrystalline cellulose, pregelatinized starch, magnesium stearate, butylated hydroxyanisole, and citric acid powder (anhydrous).

* Trademark of MERCK & CO., Inc.

CLINICAL PHARMACOLOGY

Pharmacokinetics

Following oral administration of ivermectin, plasma concentrations are approximately proportional to the dose. In two studies, after single 12-mg doses of STROMECTOL (2×6 mg) in fasting healthy volunteers (representing a mean dose of 165 μg/kg), the mean peak plasma concentrations of the major component (H_2B_{1a}) were 46.6 (±21.9) (range: 16.4–101.1) and 30.6 (±15.6) (range: 13.9–68.4) ng/mL respectively at approximately 4 hours after dosing. Ivermectin is metabolized in the liver, and ivermectin and/or its metabolites are excreted almost exclusively in the feces over an estimated 12 days, with less than 1% of the administered dose excreted in the urine. The apparent plasma half-life of ivermectin is approximately at least 16 hours following oral administration.

The effect(s) of food on the systemic availability of ivermectin has not been studied.

Microbiology

Ivermectin is a member of the avermectin class of broad-spectrum antiparasitic agents which have a unique mode of action. Compounds of the class bind selectively and with high affinity to glutamate-gated chloride ion channels which occur in invertebrate nerve and muscle cells. This leads to an increase in the permeability of the cell membrane to chloride ions with hyperpolarization of the nerve or muscle cell, resulting in paralysis and death of the parasite. Compounds of this class may also interact with other ligand-gated chloride channels, such as those gated by the neurotransmitter gamma-aminobutyric acid (GABA).

The selective activity of compounds of this class is attributable to the facts that some mammals do not have glutamate-gated chloride channels and that the avermectins have a low affinity for mammalian ligand-gated chloride channels. In addition, ivermectin does not readily cross the blood-brain barrier in humans.

Ivermectin is active against various life-cycle stages of many but not all nematodes. It is active against the tissue microfilariae of *Onchocerca volvulus* but not against the adult form. Its activity against *Strongyloides stercoralis* is limited to the intestinal stages.

Clinical Studies

Strongyloidiasis

Two controlled clinical studies using albendazole as the comparative agent were carried out in international sites where albendazole is approved for the treatment of strongy-

Continued on next page

Information on the Merck & Co., Inc. products listed on these pages is the full prescribing information from product circulars in use August 31, 1998. For information, please call 1-800-NSC MERCK [1-800-672-6372].

Consult 1999 PDR® supplements and future editions for revisions

Stromectol—Cont.

loidiasis of the gastrointestinal tract, and three controlled studies were carried out in the US and internationally using thiabendazole as the comparative agent. Efficacy, as measured by cure rate, was defined as the absence of larvae in at least two follow-up stool examinations 3 to 4 weeks post-therapy. Based on this criterion, efficacy was significantly greater for STROMECTOL (a single dose of 170 to 200 µg/kg) than for albendazole (200 mg b.i.d. for 3 days). STROMECTOL administered as a single dose of 200 µg/kg for 1 day was as efficacious as thiabendazole administered at 25 mg/kg b.i.d. for 3 days.

Summary of Cure Rates for Ivermectin Versus Comparative Agents in the Treatment of Strongyloidiasis

	Cure Rate* (%)	
	Ivermectin**	Comparative Agent
Albendazole *** Comparative		
International Study	24/26 (92)	12/22 (55)
WHO Study	126/152 (83)	67/149 (45)
Thiabendazole† Comparative		
International Study	9/14 (64)	13/15 (87)
US Studies	14/14 (100)	16/17 (94)

* Number and % of evaluable patients
** 170–200 µg/kg
*** 200 mg b.i.d. for 3 days
† 25 mg/kg b.i.d. for 3 days

In one study conducted in France, a non-endemic area where there was no possibility of reinfection, several patients were observed to have recrudescence of *Strongyloides* larvae in their stool as long as 106 days following ivermectin therapy. Therefore, at least three stool examinations should be conducted over the three months following treatment to ensure eradication. If recrudescence of larvae is observed, retreatment with ivermectin is indicated. Concentration techniques (such as using a Baermann apparatus) should be employed when performing these stool examinations, as the number of *Strongyloides* larvae per gram of feces may be very low.

Onchocerciasis

The evaluation of STROMECTOL in the treatment of onchocerciasis is based on the results of clinical studies involving 1278 patients. In a double-blind, placebo-controlled study involving adult patients with moderate to severe onchocercal infection, patients who received a single dose of 150 µg/kg STROMECTOL experienced an 83.2% and 99.5% decrease in skin microfilariae count (geometric mean) 3 days and 3 months after the dose, respectively. A marked reduction of > 90% was maintained for up to 12 months after the single dose. As with other microfilaricidal drugs, there was an increase in the microfilariae count in the anterior chamber of the eye at day 3 after treatment in some patients. However, at 3 and 6 months after the dose, a significantly greater percentage of patients treated with STROMECTOL had decreases in microfilariae count in the anterior chamber than patients treated with placebo.

In a separate open study involving pediatric patients ages 6 to 13 (n=103; weight range: 17–41 kg), similar decreases in skin microfilariae counts were observed for up to 12 months after dosing.

INDICATIONS AND USAGE

STROMECTOL is indicated for the treatment of the following infections:

Strongyloidiasis of the intestinal tract. STROMECTOL is indicated for the treatment of intestinal (i.e. nondisseminated) strongyloidiasis due to the nematode parasite *Strongyloides stercoralis.*

This indication is based on clinical studies of both comparative and open-label designs, in which from 64–100% of infected patients were cured following a single 200-µg/kg dose of ivermectin. (See *Clinical Studies.*)

Onchocerciasis. STROMECTOL is indicated for the treatment of onchocerciasis due to the nematode parasite *Onchocerca volvulus.*

This indication is based on randomized, double-blind, placebo-controlled and comparative studies conducted in 1427 patients in onchocerciasis-endemic areas of West Africa. The comparative studies used diethylcarbamazine citrate (DEC-C).

NOTE: STROMECTOL has no activity against adult *Onchocerca volvulus* parasites. The adult parasites reside in subcutaneous nodules which are infrequently palpable. Surgical excision of these nodules (nodulectomy) may be considered in the management of patients with onchocerciasis, since this procedure will eliminate the microfilariae-producing adult parasites.

CONTRAINDICATIONS

STROMECTOL is contraindicated in patients who are hypersensitive to any component of this product.

WARNINGS

Historical data have shown that microfilaricidal drugs, such as diethylcarbamazine citrate (DEC-C), might cause cutaneous and/or systemic reactions of varying severity (the Mazzotti reaction) and ophthalmological reactions in patients with onchocerciasis. These reactions are probably due to allergic and inflammatory responses to the death of microfilariae. Patients treated with STROMECTOL for onchocerciasis may experience these reactions in addition to clinical adverse reactions possibly, probably, or definitely related to the drug itself. (See ADVERSE REACTIONS, *Onchocerciasis.*)

The treatment of severe Mazzotti reactions has not been subjected to controlled clinical trials. Oral hydration, recumbency, intravenous normal saline, and/or parenteral corticosteroids have been used to treat postural hypotension. Antihistamines and/or aspirin have been used for most mild to moderate cases.

PRECAUTIONS

General

After treatment with microfilaricidal drugs, patients with hyperreactive onchodermatitis (sowda) may be more likely than others to experience severe advserse reactions, especially edema and aggravation of onchodermatitis.

Carcinogenesis, Mutagenesis, Impairment of Fertility

Long-term studies in animals have not been performed to evaluate the carcinogenic potential of ivermectin.

Ivermectin was not genotoxic *in vitro* in the Ames microbial mutagenicity assay of *Salmonella typhimurium* strains TA 1535, TA 1537, TA98, and TA100 with and without rat liver enzyme activation, the Mouse Lymphoma Cell Line L5178Y (cytotoxicity and mutagenicity) assays, or the unscheduled DNA synthesis assay in human fibroblasts.

Ivermectin had no adverse effects on the fertility in rats in studies at repeated doses of up to 3 times the maximum recommended human dose of 200 µg/kg (on a mg/m^2/day basis).

Information for Patients

STROMECTOL should be taken with water.

Strongyloidiasis: The patient should be reminded of the need for repeated stool examinations to document clearance of infection with *Strongyloides stercoralis.*

Onchocerciasis: The patient should be reminded that treatment with STROMECTOL does not kill the adult *Onchocerca* parasites, and therefore repeated follow-up and retreatment is usually required.

Pregnancy—Teratogenic Effects

Pregnancy Category C

Ivermectin has been shown to be teratogenic in mice, rats, and rabbits when given in repeated doses of 0.2, 8.1 and 4.5 times the maximum recommended human dose, respectively (on a mg/m^2/day basis). Teratogenicity was characterized in the three species tested by cleft palate; clubbed forepaws were additionally observed in rabbits. These development effects were found only at or near doses that were maternotoxic to the pregnant female. Therefore, ivermectin does not appear to be selectively fetotoxic to the developing fetus. There are, however, no adequate and well-controlled studies in pregnant women. Ivermectin should not be used during pregnancy since safety in pregnancy has not been established.

Nursing Mothers

STROMECTOL is excreted in human milk in low concentrations. Treatment of mothers who intend to breast feed should only be undertaken when the risk of delayed treatment to the mother outweighs the possible risk to the newborn.

Pediatric Use

Safety and effectiveness in pediatric patients weighing less than 15 kg have not been established.

Strongyloidiasis in Immunocompromised Hosts:

In immunocompromised (including HIV-infected) patients being treated for intestinal strongyloidiasis, repeated courses of therapy may be required. Adequate and well-controlled clinical studies have not been conducted in such patients to determine the optimal dosing regimen. Several treatments, i.e., at 2 week intervals, may be required, and cure may not be achievable. Control of extra-intestinal strongyloidiasis in these patients is difficult, and suppressive therapy, i.e., once per month may be helpful.

ADVERSE REACTIONS

Strongyloidiasis

In four clinical studies involving a total of 109 patients given either one or two doses of 170–200 µg/kg of STROMECTOL, the following adverse reactions were reported as possibly, probably, or definitely related to STROMECTOL:

Body as a whole: asthenia/fatigue (0.9%), abdominal pain (0.9%)

Gastrointestinal: anorexia (0.9%), constipation (0.9%), diarrhea (1.8%), nausea (1.8%), vomiting (0.9%)

Nervous System/Psychiatric: dizziness (2.8%), somnolence (0.9%), vertigo (0.9%), tremor (0.9%)

Skin: pruritus (2.8%), rash (0.9%), and urticaria (0.9%)

In comparative trials, patients treated with STROMECTOL experienced more abdominal distention and chest discomfort than patients treated with albendazole. However, STROMECTOL was better tolerated than thiabendazole in comparative studies involving 37 patients treated with thiabendazole.

The Mazzotti-type and ophthalmologic reactions associated with the treatment of onchocerciasis or the disease itself would not be expected to occur in strongyloidiasis patients treated with STROMECTOL. (See ADVERSE REACTIONS, *Onchocerciasis.*)

Laboratory Test Findings

In clinical trials involving 109 patients given either one or two doses of 170–200 µg/kg STROMECTOL, the following laboratory abnormalities were seen irrespective of drug relationship: elevation in ALT and/or AST (2%), decrease in leukocyte count (3%). Leukopenia and anemia were seen in one patient.

Onchocerciasis

In clinical trials involving 963 adult patients treated with 100 to 200 µg/kg STROMECTOL, worsening of the following Mazzotti reactions during the first 4 days post-treatment were reported: arthralgia/synovitis (9.3%), axillary lymph node enlargement and tenderness (11.0% and 4.4%, respectively), cervical lymph node enlargement and tenderness (5.3% and 1.2%, respectively), inguinal lymph node enlargement and tenderness (12.6% and 13.9%, respectively), other lymph node enlargement and tenderness (3.0% and 1.9%, respectively), pruritus (27.5%), skin involvement including edema, papular and pustular or frank urticarial rash (22.7%), and fever (22.6%). (See WARNINGS.)

In clinical trials, ophthalmological conditions were examined in 963 adult patients before treatment, at day 3, and months 3 and 6 after treatment with 100 to 200 µg/kg STROMECTOL. Changes observed were primarily deterioration from baseline 3 days post-treatment. Most changes either returned to baseline condition or improved over baseline severity at the month 3 and 6 visits. The percentages of patients with worsening of the following conditions at day 3, month 3 and 6, respectively, were: limbitis: 5.5%, 4.8%, and 3.5% and punctate opacity: 1.8%, 1.8%, and 1.4%. The corresponding percentages for patients treated with placebo were: limbitis: 6.2%, 9.9% and 9.4% and punctate opacity: 2.0%, 6.4% and 7.2%. (See WARNINGS.)

In clinical trials involving 963 adult patients who received 100 to 200 µg/kg STROMECTOL, the following clinical adverse reactions were reported as possibly, probably, or definitely related to the drug in ≥ 1% of the patients: facial edema (1.2%), peripheral edema (3.2%), orthostatic hypotension (1.1%), and tachycardia (3.5%). Drug-related headache and myalgia occurred in < 1% of patients (0.2%, and 0.4%, respectively). However, these were the most common adverse experiences reported overall during these trials regardless of causality (22.3% and 19.7%, respectively).

A similar safety profile was observed in an open study in pediatric patients ages 6 to 13.

Additionally, hypotension (mainly orthostatic hypotension) and worsening of bronchial asthma have been reported since the drug was registered overseas.

The following ophthalmological side effects do occur due to the disease itself but have also been reported after treatment with STROMECTOL: abnormal sensation in the eyes, eyelid edema, anterior uveitis, conjunctivitis, limbitis, keratitis, and chorioretinitis or choroiditis. These have rarely been severe or associated with loss of vision and have generally resolved without corticosteroid treatment.

Laboratory Test Findings

In controlled clinical trials, the following laboratory adverse experiences were reported as possibly, probably, or definitely related to the drug in ≥ 1% of the patients: eosinophilia (3%) and hemoglobin increase (1%).

OVERDOSAGE

Significant lethality was observed in mice and rats after single oral doses of 25 to 50 mg/kg and 40 to 50 mg/kg, respectively. No significant lethality was observed in dogs after single oral doses of up to 10 mg/kg. At these doses, the treatment related signs that were observed in these animals include ataxia, bradypnea, tremors, ptosis, decreased activity, emesis, and mydriasis.

In accidental intoxication with or significant exposure to unknown quantities of veterinary formulations of ivermectin in humans, either by ingestion, inhalation, injection, or exposure to body surfaces, the following adverse effects have been reported most frequently: rash, edema, headache, dizziness, asthenia, nausea, vomiting, and diarrhea. Other adverse effects that have been reported include: seizure, ataxia, dyspnea, abdominal pain, paresthesia, and urticaria.

In case of accidental poisoning, supportive therapy, if indicated, should include parenteral fluids and electrolytes, res-

piratory support (oxygen and mechanical ventilation if necessary) and pressor agents if clinically significant hypotension is present. Induction of emesis and/or gastric lavage as soon as possible, followed by purgatives and other routine anti-poison measures, may be indicated if needed to prevent absorption of ingested material.

DOSAGE AND ADMINISTRATION

Strongyloidiasis

The recommended dosage of STROMECTOL for the treatment of strongyloidiasis is a single oral dose designed to provide approximately 200 µg of ivermectin per kg of body weight. See Table 1 for dosage guidelines. Patients should take tablets with water. In general, additional doses are not necessary. However, follow-up stool examinations should be performed to verify eradication of infection (see *Clinical Studies*.)

Table 1
Dosage Guidelines for STROMECTOL for Strongyloidiasis

Body Weight (kg)	Single Oral Dose
15–24	1/2 tablet
25–35	1 tablet
36–50	1 1/2 tablets
51–65	2 tablets
66–79	2 1/2 tablets
≥80	200 µg/kg

Onchocerciasis

The recommended dosage of STROMECTOL for the treatment of onchocerciasis is a single oral dose designed to provide approximately 150 µg of ivermectin per kg of body weight. See Table 2 for dosage guidelines. Patients should take tablets with water. In mass distribution campaigns in international treatment programs, the most commonly used dose interval is 12 months. For the treatment of individual patients, retreatment may be considered at intervals as short as 3 months.

Table 2
Dosage Guidelines for STROMECTOL for Onchocerciasis

Body Weight (kg)	Single Oral Dose
15–25	1/2 tablet
26–44	1 tablet
45–64	1 1/2 tablets
65–84	2 tablets
≥85	150 µg/kg

HOW SUPPLIED

No. 8107—Tablets STROMECTOL 6 mg are white, scored, round, flat, beveled-edged tablets coded MSD 139 on one side and scored on the other. They are supplied as follows:
NDC 0006-0139-10 unit dose packages of 10.

Shown in Product Identification Guide, page 323

Storage

Store at temperatures below 30°C (86°F).

Dist. by:
MERCK & CO., INC.,
West Point, PA 19486, USA
Manufactured by:
MSD BV
Waarderweg 39
2031 BN Haarlem
Netherlands

9032300 Issued November 1996

COPYRIGHT MERCK & CO., Inc., 1996
All rights reserved.

SYPRINE® Capsules (Trientine Hydrochloride), U.S.P. ℞

DESCRIPTION

Trientine hydrochloride is *N,N'*-bis (2-aminoethyl)-1,2-ethanediamine dihydrochloride. It is a white to pale yellow crystalline hygroscopic powder. It is freely soluble in water, soluble in methanol, slightly soluble in ethanol, and insoluble in chloroform and ether.

The empirical formula is $C_6H_{18}N_4 \cdot 2HCl$ with a molecular weight of 219.2. The structural formula is:

$$NH_2(CH_2)_2NH(CH_2)_2NH(CH_2)_2NH_2 \cdot 2HCl$$

Trientine hydrochloride is a chelating compound for removal of excess copper from the body. SYPRINE* (Trientine Hydrochloride) is available as 250 mg capsules for oral administration. Capsules SYPRINE contain gelatin, iron oxides, stearic acid, and titanium dioxide as inactive ingredients.

*Registered trademark of MERCK & CO., INC.

CLINICAL PHARMACOLOGY

Introduction

Wilson's disease (hepatolenticular degeneration) is an autosomal inherited metabolic defect resulting in an inability to maintain a near-zero balance of copper. Excess copper accumulates possibly because the liver lacks the mechanism to excrete free copper into the bile. Hepatocytes store excess copper but when their capacity is exceeded copper is released into the blood and is taken up into extrahepatic sites. This condition is treated with a low copper diet and the use of chelating agents that bind copper to facilitate its excretion from the body.

Clinical Summary

Forty-one patients (18 male and 23 female) between the ages of 6 and 54 with a diagnosis of Wilson's disease and who were intolerant of d-penicillamine were treated in two separate studies with trientine hydrochloride. The dosage varied from 450 to 2400 mg per day. The average dosage required to achieve an optimal clinical response varied between 1000 mg and 2000 mg per day. The mean duration of trientine hydrochloride therapy was 48.7 months (range 2–164 months). Thirty-four of the 41 patients improved, 4 had no change in clinical global response, 2 were lost to follow-up and one showed deterioration in clinical condition. One of the patients who improved while on therapy with trientine hydrochloride experienced a recurrence of the symptoms of systemic lupus erythematosus which had appeared originally during therapy with penicillamine. Therapy with trientine hydrochloride was discontinued. No other adverse reactions, except iron deficiency, were noted among any of these 41 patients.

One investigator treated 13 patients with trientine hydrochloride following their development of intolerance to d-penicillamine. Retrospectively, he compared these patients to an additional group of 12 patients with Wilson's disease who were both tolerant of and controlled with d-penicillamine therapy, but who failed to continue any copper chelation therapy. The mean age at onset of disease of the latter group was 12 years as compared to 21 years for the former group. The trientine hydrochloride group received d-penicillamine for an average of 4 years as compared to an average of 10 years for the non-treated group.

Various laboratory parameters showed changes in favor of the patients treated with trientine hydrochloride. Free and total serum copper, SGOT, and serum bilirubin all showed mean increases over baseline in the untreated group which were significantly larger than with the patients treated with trientine hydrochloride. In the 13 patients treated with trientine hydrochloride, previous symptoms and signs relating to d-penicillamine intolerance disappeared in 8 patients, improved in 4 patients, and remained unchanged in one patient. The neurological status in the trientine hydrochloride group was unchanged or improved over baseline, whereas in the untreated group, 6 patients remained unchanged and 6 worsened. Kayser-Fleischer rings improved significantly during trientine hydrochloride treatment.

The clinical outcome of the two groups also differed markedly. Of the 13 patients on therapy with trientine hydrochloride (mean duration of therapy 4.1 years; range 1 to 13 years), all were alive at the data cutoff date, and in the non-treated group (mean years with no therapy 2.7 years; range 3 months to 9 years), 9 of the 12 died of hepatic disease.

Chelating Properties

Preclinical Studies

Studies in animals have shown that trientine hydrochloride has cupriuretic activities in both normal and copper-loaded rats. In general, the effects of trientine hydrochloride on urinary copper excretion are similar to those of equimolar doses of penicillamine, although in one study they were significantly smaller.

Human Studies

Renal clearance studies were carried out with penicillamine and trientine hydrochloride on separate occasions in selected patients treated with penicillamine for at least one year. Six-hour excretion rates of copper were determined off treatment and after a single dose of 500 mg of penicillamine or 1.2 g of trientine hydrochloride. The mean urinary excretion rates of copper were as follows:

No. of Patients	Single Dose Treatment	Basal Excretion Rate (µg Cu^{++}/6hr)	Test-dose Excretion Rate (µ Cu^{++}/6hr)
6	Trientine, 1.2 g	19	234
4	Penicillamine, 500 mg	17	320

In patients *not* previously treated with chelating agents, a similar comparison was made:

No. of Patients	Single Dose Treatment	Basal Excretion Rate (µ Cu^{++}/6hr)	Test-dose Excretion Rate (µ Cu++/6hr)
8	Trientine, 1.2 g	71	1326
7	Penicillamine, 500 mg	68	1074

These results demonstrate that SYPRINE is effective as a cupriuretic agent in patients with Wilson's disease although on a molar basis it appears to be less potent or less effective than penicillamine. Evidence from a radio-labelled copper study indicates that the different cupriuretic effect between these two drugs could be due to a difference in selectivity of the drugs for different copper pools within the body.

Pharmacokinetics

Data on the pharmacokinetics of trientine hydrochloride are not available. Dosage adjustment recommendations are based upon clinical use of the drug (see DOSAGE AND ADMINISTRATION).

INDICATIONS AND USAGE

SYPRINE is indicated in the treatment of patients with Wilson's disease who are intolerant of penicillamine. Clinical experience with SYPRINE is limited and alternate dosing regimens have not been well-characterized; all endpoints in determining an individual patient's dose have not been well defined. SYPRINE and penicillamine cannot be considered interchangeable. SYPRINE should be used when continued treatment with penicillamine is no longer possible because of intolerable or life endangering side effects.

Unlike penicillamine, SYPRINE is not recommended in cystinuria or rheumatoid arthritis. The absence of a sulfhydryl moiety renders it incapable of binding cystine and, therefore, it is of no use in cystinuria. In 15 patients with rheumatoid arthritis, SYPRINE was reported not to be effective in improving any clinical or biochemical parameter after 12 weeks of treatment.

SYPRINE is not indicated for treatment of biliary cirrhosis.

CONTRAINDICATIONS

Hypersensitivity to this product.

WARNINGS

Patient experience with trientine hydrochloride is limited (see CLINICAL PHARMACOLOGY). Patients receiving SYPRINE should remain under regular medical supervision throughout the period of drug administration. Patients (especially women) should be closely monitored for evidence of iron deficiency anemia.

PRECAUTIONS

General

There are no reports of hypersensitivity in patients who have been administered trientine hydrochloride for Wilson's disease. However, there have been reports of asthma, bronchitis and dermatitis occurring after prolonged environmental exposure in workers who use trientine hydrochloride as a hardener of epoxy resins. Patients should be observed closely for signs of possible hypersensitivity.

Information for Patients

Patients should be directed to take SYPRINE on an empty stomach, at least one hour before meals or two hours after meals and at least one hour apart from any other drug, food, or milk. The capsules should be swallowed whole with water and should not be opened or chewed. Because of the potential for contact dermatitis, any site of exposure to the capsule contents should be washed with water promptly. For the first month of treatment, the patient should have his temperature taken nightly, and he should be asked to report any symptom such as fever or skin eruption.

Laboratory Tests

The most reliable index for monitoring treatment is the determination of free copper in the serum, which equals the difference between quantitatively determined total copper and ceruloplasmin-copper. Adequately treated patients will usually have less than 10 mcg free copper/dL of serum.

Therapy may be monitored with a 24 hour urinary copper analysis periodically (i.e., every 6–12 months). Urine must be collected in copper-free glassware. Since a low copper diet should keep copper absorption down to less than one milligram a day, the patient probably will be in the desired state of negative copper balance if 0.5 to 1.0 milligram of copper is present in a 24-hour collection of urine.

Drug Interactions

In general, mineral supplements should not be given since they may block the absorption of SYPRINE. However, iron deficiency may develop, especially in children and menstruating or pregnant women, or as a result of the low copper diet recommended for Wilson's disease. If necessary, iron may be given in short courses, but since iron and SYPRINE each inhibit absorption of the other, two hours should elapse between administration of SYPRINE and iron.

Continued on next page

Information on the Merck & Co., Inc. products listed on these pages is the full prescribing information from product circulars in use August 31, 1998. For information, please call 1-800-NSC MERCK [1-800-672-6372].

Syprine—Cont.

It is important that SYPRINE be taken on an empty stomach, at least one hour before meals or two hours after meals and at least one hour apart from any other drug, food, or milk. This permits maximum absorption and reduces the likelihood of inactivation of the drug by metal binding in the gastrointestinal tract.

Carcinogenesis, Mutagenesis, Impairment of Fertility

Data on carcinogenesis, mutagenesis, and impairment of fertility are not available.

Pregnancy

Pregnancy Category C. Trientine hydrochloride was teratogenic in rats at doses similar to the human dose. The frequencies of both resorptions and fetal abnormalities, including hemorrhage and edema, increased while fetal copper levels decreased when trientine hydrochloride was given in the maternal diets of rats. There are no adequate and well-controlled studies in pregnant women. SYPRINE should be used during pregnancy only if the potential benefit justifies the potential risk to the fetus.

Nursing Mothers

It is not known whether this drug is excreted in human milk. Because many drugs are excreted in human milk, caution should be exercised when SYPRINE is administered to a nursing mother.

Pediatric Use

Controlled studies of the safety and effectiveness of SYPRINE in pediatric patients have not been conducted. It has been used clinically in pediatric patients as young as 6 years with no reported adverse experiences.

ADVERSE REACTIONS

Clinical experience with SYPRINE has been limited. The following adverse reactions have been reported in patients with Wilson's disease who were on therapy with trientine hydrochloride: iron deficiency, systemic lupus erythematosus (see CLINICAL PHARMACOLOGY).

SYPRINE is not indicated for treatment of biliary cirrhosis, but in one study of 4 patients treated with trientine hydrochloride for primary biliary cirrhosis, the following adverse reactions were reported: heartburn; epigastric pain and tenderness; thickening, fissuring and flaking of the skin; hypochromic microcytic anemia; acute gastritis; aphthoid ulcers; abdominal pain; melena; anorexia; malaise; cramps; muscle pain; weakness; rhabdomyolysis. A causal relationship of these reactions to drug therapy could not be rejected or established.

OVERDOSAGE

There is a report of an adult woman who ingested 30 grams of trientine hydrochloride without apparent ill effects. No other data on overdosage are available.

DOSAGE AND ADMINISTRATION

Systemic evaluation of dose and/or interval between dose has not been done. However, on limited clinical experience, the recommended initial dose of SYPRINE is 500–750 mg/day for pediatric patients and 750–1250 mg/day for adults given in divided doses two, three or four times daily. This may be increased to a maximum of 2000 mg/day for adults or 1500 mg/day for pediatric patients age 12 or under. The daily dose of SYPRINE should be increased only when the clinical response is not adequate or the concentration of free serum copper is persistently above 20 mcg/dL. Optimal long-term maintenance dosage should be determined at 6–12 month intervals (see PRECAUTIONS, *Laboratory Tests*).

It is important that SYPRINE be given on an empty stomach, at least one hour before meals or two hours after meals and at least one hour apart from any other drug, food, or milk. The capsules should be swallowed whole with water and should not be opened or chewed.

HOW SUPPLIED

No. 3408—Capsules SYPRINE, 250 mg, are light brown opaque capsules and are coded SYPRINE and MSD 661. They are supplied as follows:

NDC 0006-0661-68 in bottles of 100.

Shown in Product Identification Guide, page 323

Storage

Keep container tightly closed.

Store at 2°–8°C (36°–46°F).

7664602 Issued September 1996

COPYRIGHT © MERCK & CO., INC., 1985, 1989
All rights reserved

TIMOLIDE® Tablets ℞
(Timolol Maleate-Hydrochlorothiazide), U.S.P.

DESCRIPTION

TIMOLIDE* (Timolol Maleate-Hydrochlorothiazide) is for the treatment of hypertension. It combines the antihypertensive activity of two agents: a non-selective beta-adrenergic receptor blocking agent (timolol maleate) and a diuretic (hydrochlorothiazide).

Timolol maleate is (*S*)-1-[(1, 1-dimethylethyl) amino]-3-[[4-(4-morpholinyl)-1, 2, 5-thiadiazol -3- yl] oxy]-2-propanol (*Z*)-2-butenedioate (1:1) salt. Its empirical formula is $C_{13}H_{24}N_4O_3S \cdot C_4H_4O_4$ and its structural formula is:

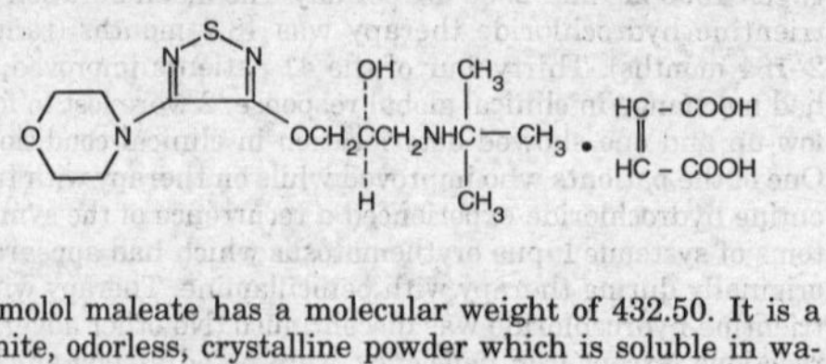

Timolol maleate has a molecular weight of 432.50. It is a white, odorless, crystalline powder which is soluble in water, methanol, and alcohol.

Hydrochlorothiazide is 6-chloro-3,4-dihydro-2*H*-1,2,4-benzothiadiazine-7-sulfonamide 1, 1- dioxide. Its empirical formula is $C_7H_8ClN_3O_4S_2$ and its structural formula is:

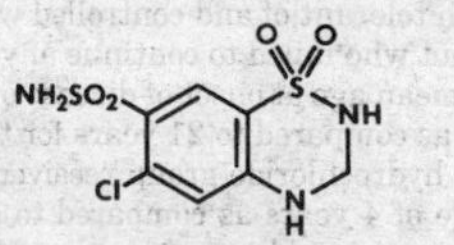

Hydrochlorothiazide has a molecular weight of 297.73. It is a white, or practically white, crystalline powder which is slightly soluble in water, but freely soluble in sodium hydroxide solution.

TIMOLIDE is supplied as tablets containing 10 mg of timolol maleate and 25 mg of hydrochlorothiazide for oral administration. Inactive ingredients are cellulose, FD&C Blue 2, magnesium stearate, and starch.

*Registered trademark of MERCK & CO., INC.

CLINICAL PHARMACOLOGY

TIMOLIDE

Timolol maleate and hydrochlorothiazide have been used singly and concomitantly for the treatment of hypertension. The antihypertensive effects of these agents are additive. The two components of TIMOLIDE have similar dosage schedules, and studies have shown that there is no interference with bioavailability when these agents are given together in the single combination tablet. Therefore, this combination provides a convenient formulation for the concomitant administration of these two entities.

In controlled clinical trials with TIMOLIDE in selected patients with mild to moderate essential hypertension, about 90 percent had a good to excellent response. In patients with more severe hypertension, TIMOLIDE may be administered with other antihypertensives such as ALDOMET* (Methyldopa) or a vasodilator.

Although the mechanisms of action of timolol maleate and hydrochlorothiazide in the treatment of hypertension have not been established, they are thought to be different; for example, hydrochlorothiazide increases plasma renin activity while timolol maleate reduces plasma renin activity.

Timolol Maleate

Timolol maleate is a $beta_1$ and $beta_2$ (non-selective) adrenergic receptor blocking agent that does not have significant intrinsic sympathomimetic, direct myocardial depressant, or local anesthetic activity.

Pharmacodynamics

Clinical pharmacology studies have confirmed the beta-adrenergic blocking activity as shown by (1) changes in resting heart rate and response of heart rate to changes in posture; (2) inhibition of isoproterenol-induced tachycardia; (3) alteration of the response to the Valsalva maneuver and amyl nitrite administration; and (4) reduction of heart rate and blood pressure changes on exercise.

Timolol maleate decreases the positive chronotropic, positive inotropic, bronchodilator, and vasodilator responses caused by beta-adrenergic receptor agonists. The magnitude of this decreased response is proportional to the existing sympathetic tone and the concentration of timolol maleate at receptor sites.

In normal volunteers, the reduction in heart rate response to a standard exercise was dose dependent over the test range of 0.5 to 20 mg, with a peak reduction at 2 hours of approximately 30% at higher doses.

Beta-adrenergic receptor blockade reduces cardiac output in both healthy subjects and patients with heart disease. In patients with severe impairment of myocardial function beta-adrenergic receptor blockade may inhibit the stimulatory effect of the sympathetic nervous system necessary to maintain adequate cardiac function.

Beta-adrenergic receptor blockade in the bronchi and bronchioles results in increased airway resistance from unopposed parasympathetic activity. Such an effect in patients with asthma or other bronchospastic conditions is potentially dangerous.

Clinical studies indicate that timolol maleate at a dosage of 20–60 mg/day reduces blood pressure without causing postural hypotension in most patients with essential hypertension. Administration of timolol maleate to patients with hypertension results initially in a decrease in cardiac output, little immediate change in blood pressure, and an increase in calculated peripheral resistance. With continued administration of timolol maleate blood pressure decreases within a few days, cardiac output usually remains reduced, and peripheral resistance falls toward pretreatment levels. Plasma volume may decrease or remain unchanged during therapy with timolol maleate. In the majority of patients with hypertension, timolol maleate also decreases plasma renin activity. Dosage adjustment to achieve optimal antihypertensive effect may require a few weeks. When therapy with timolol maleate is discontinued, the blood pressure tends to return to pretreatment levels gradually. In most patients the antihypertensive activity of timolol maleate is maintained with long-term therapy and is well tolerated.

The mechanism of the antihypertensive effects of beta-adrenergic receptor blocking agents is not established at this time. Possible mechanisms of action include reduction in cardiac output, reduction in plasma renin activity, and a central nervous system sympatholytic action.

Pharmacokinetics and Metabolism

Timolol maleate is rapidly and nearly completely absorbed (about 90%) following oral ingestion. Detectable plasma levels of timolol occur within one-half hour and peak plasma levels occur in about one to two hours. The drug half-life in plasma is approximately 4 hours and this is essentially unchanged in patients with moderate renal insufficiency. Timolol is partially metabolized by the liver and timolol and its metabolites are excreted by the kidney. Timolol is not extensively bound to plasma proteins; i.e., <10% by equilibrium dialysis and approximately 60% by ultrafiltration. An *in vitro* hemodialysis study, using ^{14}C timolol added to human plasma or whole blood, showed that timolol was readily dialyzed from these fluids; however, a study of patients with renal failure showed that timolol did not dialyze readily. Plasma levels following oral administration are about half those following intravenous administration indicating approximately 50% first pass metabolism. The level of beta sympathetic activity varies widely among individuals, and no simple correlation exists between the dose or plasma level of timolol maleate and its therapeutic activity. Therefore, objective clinical measurements such as reduction of heart rate and/or blood pressure should be used as guides in determining the optimal dosage for each patient.

Hydrochlorothiazide

Hydrochlorothiazide is a diuretic and antihypertensive agent. It affects the renal tubular mechanism of electrolyte reabsorption. Hydrochlorothiazide increases excretion of sodium and chloride in approximately equivalent amounts. Natriuresis may be accompanied by some loss of potassium and bicarbonate. The mechanism of the antihypertensive effect of thiazides may be related to the excretion and redistribution of body sodium. Hydrochlorothiazide usually does not cause clinically important changes in normal blood pressure.

*Registered trademark of MERCK & CO., INC.

INDICATIONS AND USAGE

TIMOLIDE is indicated for the treatment of hypertension. **This fixed combination drug is not indicated for initial therapy of hypertension. If the fixed combination represents the dose titrated to an individual patient's needs, it may be more convenient than the separate components.**

CONTRAINDICATIONS

TIMOLIDE is contraindicated in patients with bronchial asthma or with a history of bronchial asthma, or severe chronic obstructive pulmonary disease (see WARNINGS); sinus bradycardia; second and third degree atrioventricular block; overt cardiac failure (see WARNINGS); cardiogenic shock; anuria; hypersensitivity to this product or to sulfonamide-derived drugs.

WARNINGS

Cardiac Failure

Sympathetic stimulation may be essential for support of the circulation in individuals with diminished myocardial con-

tractility, and its inhibition by beta-adrenergic receptor blockade may precipitate more severe failure. Although beta blockers should be avoided in overt congestive heart failure, they can be used, if necessary, with caution in patients with a history of failure who are well-compensated, usually with digitalis and diuretics. Both digitalis and timolol maleate slow AV conduction. If cardiac failure persists, therapy with TIMOLIDE should be withdrawn.

In Patients Without a History of Cardiac Failure continued depression of the myocardium with beta-blocking agents over a period of time can, in some cases, lead to cardiac failure. At the first sign or symptom of cardiac failure, patients receiving TIMOLIDE should be digitalized and/or be given additional diuretic therapy. Observe the patient closely. If cardiac failure continues, despite adequate digitalization and diuretic therapy, TIMOLIDE should be withdrawn.

Renal and Hepatic Disease and Electrolyte Disturbances
Since timolol maleate is partially metabolized in the liver and excreted mainly by the kidneys, dosage reductions may be necessary when hepatic and/or renal insufficiency is present.

Although the pharmacokinetics of timolol maleate are not greatly altered by renal impairment, marked hypotensive responses have been seen in patients with marked renal impairment undergoing dialysis after 20 mg doses. Dosing in such patients should therefore be especially cautious.

In patients with renal disease, thiazides may precipitate azotemia, and cumulative effects may develop in the presence of impaired renal function. If progressive renal impairment becomes evident, TIMOLIDE should be discontinued. In patients with impaired hepatic function or progressive liver disease, even minor alterations in fluid and electrolyte balance may precipitate hepatic coma. Hepatic encephalopathy, manifested by tremors, confusion, and coma, has been reported in association with diuretic therapy including hydrochlorothiazide.

Exacerbation of Ischemic Heart Disease Following Abrupt Withdrawal —Hypersensitivity to catecholamines has been observed in patients withdrawn from beta blocker therapy; exacerbation of angina and, in some cases, myocardial infarction have occurred after *abrupt* discontinuation of such therapy. When discontinuing chronically administered timolol maleate, particularly in patients with ischemic heart disease, the dosage should be gradually reduced over a period of one to two weeks and the patient should be carefully monitored. If angina markedly worsens or acute coronary insufficiency develops, timolol maleate administration should be reinstituted promptly, at least temporarily, and other measures appropriate for the management of unstable angina should be taken. Patients should be warned against interruption or discontinuation of therapy without the physician's advice. Because coronary artery disease is common and may be unrecognized, it may be prudent not to discontinue timolol maleate therapy abruptly even in patients treated only for hypertension.

Obstructive Pulmonary Disease
PATIENTS WITH CHRONIC OBSTRUCTIVE PULMONARY DISEASE (e.g., CHRONIC BRONCHITIS, EMPHYSEMA) OF MILD OR MODERATE SEVERITY, BRONCHOSPASTIC DISEASE OR A HISTORY OF BRONCHOSPASTIC DISEASE (OTHER THAN BRONCHIAL ASTHMA OR A HISTORY OF BRONCHIAL ASTHMA, IN WHICH 'TIMOLIDE' IS CONTRAINDICATED, see CONTRAINDICATIONS), SHOULD IN GENERAL NOT RECEIVE BETA BLOCKERS, INCLUDING 'TIMOLIDE'. However, if TIMOLIDE is necessary in such patients, then the drug should be administered with caution since it may block bronchodilation produced by endogenous and exogenous catecholamine stimulation of beta$_2$ receptors.

Major Surgery
The necessity or desirability of withdrawal of beta-blocking therapy prior to major surgery is controversial. Beta-adrenergic receptor blockade impairs the ability of the heart to respond to beta-adrenergically mediated reflex stimuli. This may augment the risk of general anesthesia in surgical procedures. Some patients receiving beta-adrenergic receptor blocking agents have been subject to protracted severe hypotension during anesthesia. Difficulty in restarting and maintaining the heartbeat has also been reported. For these reasons, in patients undergoing elective surgery, some authorities recommend gradual withdrawal of beta-adrenergic receptor blocking agents.

If necessary during surgery, the effects of beta-adrenergic blocking agents may be reversed by sufficient doses of such agonists as isoproterenol, dopamine, dobutamine or levarterenol (see OVERDOSAGE).

Metabolic and Endocrine Effects
Beta-adrenergic blockade may mask certain clinical signs (e.g., tachycardia) of hyperthyroidism. Patients suspected of developing thyrotoxicosis should be managed carefully to avoid abrupt withdrawal of beta blockade which might precipitate a thyroid storm. Thiazides may decrease serum PBI levels without signs of thyroid disturbance.

Beta-adrenergic receptor blocking agents may mask the signs and symptoms of acute hypoglycemia. Therefore, TIMOLIDE should be administered with caution to patients subject to spontaneous hypoglycemia, or to diabetic patients (especially those with labile diabetes) who are receiving insulin or oral hypoglycemic agents. Insulin requirements in diabetic patients may be increased, decreased, or unchanged by thiazides. Diabetes mellitus which has been latent may become manifest during administration of thiazide diuretics.

Because calcium excretion is decreased by thiazides, TIMOLIDE should be discontinued before carrying out tests for parathyroid function. Pathologic changes in the parathyroid glands, with hypercalcemia and hypophosphatemia, have been observed in a few patients on prolonged thiazide therapy; however, the common complications of hyperparathyroidism such as renal lithiasis, bone resorption, and peptic ulceration have not been seen.

Hyperuricemia may occur or acute gout may be precipitated in certain patients receiving thiazide therapy.

PRECAUTIONS

General
Electrolyte and Fluid Balance Status: Periodic determination of serum electrolytes to detect possible electrolyte imbalance should be performed at appropriate intervals.

Patients should be observed for clinical signs of fluid or electrolyte imbalance, i.e., hyponatremia, hypochloremic alkalosis, and hypokalemia. Serum and urine electrolyte determinations are particularly important when the patient is vomiting excessively or receiving parenteral fluids. Warning signs or symptoms of fluid and electrolyte imbalance, irrespective of cause, include dryness of the mouth, thirst, weakness, lethargy, drowsiness, restlessness, confusion, seizures, muscle pains or cramps, muscular fatigue, hypotension, oliguria, tachycardia, and gastrointestinal disturbances such as nausea and vomiting.

Hypokalemia may develop, especially with brisk diuresis, when severe cirrhosis is present, or during concomitant use of corticosteroids or ACTH.

Interference with adequate oral electrolyte intake will also contribute to hypokalemia. Hypokalemia may cause cardiac arrhythmia and may also sensitize or exaggerate the response of the heart to the toxic effects of digitalis (e.g., increased ventricular irritability). Hypokalemia may be avoided or treated by use of potassium sparing diuretics or potassium supplements such as foods with a high potassium content.

Any chloride deficit during thiazide therapy is generally mild and usually does not require specific treatment except under extraordinary circumstances (as in liver disease or renal disease). Dilutional hyponatremia may occur in edematous patients in hot weather; appropriate therapy is water restriction rather than administration of salt except in rare instances when the hyponatremia is life threatening. In actual salt depletion, appropriate replacement is the therapy of choice.

Thiazides have been shown to increase urinary excretion of magnesium, which may result in hypomagnesemia.

Effects on Cholesterol and Triglyceride Levels:
Increases in cholesterol and triglyceride levels may be associated with thiazide diuretic therapy.

Muscle Weakness: Beta-adrenergic blockade has been reported to potentiate muscle weakness consistent with certain myasthenic symptoms (e.g., diplopia, ptosis, and generalized weakness). Timolol has been reported rarely to increase muscle weakness in some patients with myasthenia gravis or myasthenic symptoms.

Cerebrovascular Insufficiency: Because of potential effects of beta-adrenergic blocking agents relative to blood pressure and pulse, these agents should be used with caution in patients with cerebrovascular insufficiency. If signs or symptoms suggesting reduced cerebral blood flow are observed, consideration should be given to discontinuing these agents.

Drug Interactions
TIMOLIDE may potentiate the action of other antihypertensive agents used concomitantly. Close observation of the patient is recommended when TIMOLIDE is administered to patients receiving catecholamine-depleting drugs such as reserpine, because of possible additive effects and the production of hypotension and/or marked bradycardia, which may produce vertigo, syncope, or postural hypotension.

Blunting of the antihypertensive effect of beta-adrenoceptor blocking agents by non-steroidal anti-inflammatory drugs has been reported. In some patients, the administration of a non-steroidal anti-inflammatory agent can reduce the diuretic, natriuretic, and antihypertensive effects of loop, potassium-sparing and thiazide diuretics. Therefore, when TIMOLIDE and non-steroidal anti-inflammatory agents are used concomitantly, the patient should be observed closely to determine if the desired therapeutic effect has been obtained.

Literature reports suggest that oral calcium antagonists may be used in combination with beta-adrenergic blocking agents when heart function is normal, but should be

avoided in patients with impaired cardiac function. Hypotension, AV conduction disturbances, and left ventricular failure have been reported in some patients receiving beta-adrenergic blocking agents when an oral calcium antagonist was added to the treatment regimen. Hypotension was more likely to occur if the calcium antagonist were a dihydropyridine derivative, e.g., nifedipine, while left ventricular failure and AV conduction disturbances were more likely to occur with either verapamil or diltiazem.

Intravenous calcium antagonists should be used with caution in patients receiving beta-adrenergic blocking agents. The concomitant use of beta-adrenergic blocking agents with digitalis and either diltiazem or verapamil may have additive effects in prolonging AV conduction time.

Potentiated systemic beta-blockade (e.g., decreased heart rate) has been reported during combined treatment with quinidine and timolol, possibly because quinidine inhibits the metabolism of timolol via the P-450 enzyme, CYP2D6.

Beta adrenergic blocking agents may exacerbate the rebound hypertension which can follow the withdrawal of clonidine. If the two drugs are coadministered, the beta adrenergic blocking agent should be withdrawn several days before the gradual withdrawal of clonidine. If replacing clonidine by beta-blocker therapy, the introduction of beta adrenergic blocking agents should be delayed for several days after clonidine administration has stopped.

Risk from Anaphylactic Reaction: While taking beta-blockers, patients with a history of atopy or a history of severe anaphylactic reaction to a variety of allergens may be more reactive to repeated accidental, diagnostic, or therapeutic challenge with such allergens. Such patients may be unresponsive to the usual doses of epinephrine used to treat anaphylactic reactions.

In patients receiving thiazides, sensitivity reactions may occur with or without a history of allergy or bronchial asthma. The possible exacerbation or activation of systemic lupus erythematosus has been reported. The antihypertensive effects of thiazides may be enhanced in the post-sympathectomy patient.

Thiazides may decrease arterial responsiveness to norepinephrine. This diminution is not sufficient to preclude the therapeutic effectiveness of norepinephrine. Thiazides may increase the responsiveness to tubocurarine.

Lithium generally should not be given with diuretics because they reduce its renal clearance and add a high risk of lithium toxicity. Read circulars for lithium preparations before use of such preparations with TIMOLIDE.

Absorption of hydrochlorothiazide is impaired in the presence of anionic exchange resins. Single doses of either cholestyramine or colestipol resins bind the hydrochlorothiazide and reduce its absorption from the gastrointestinal tract by up to 85 and 43 percent, respectively.

Carcinogenesis, Mutagenesis, Impairment of Fertility
Carcinogenicity, mutagenicity, and fertility studies have not been conducted in animals with TIMOLIDE.

Timolol maleate: In a two-year study of timolol maleate in rats, there was a statistically significant increase in the incidence of adrenal pheochromocytomas in male rats administered 300 mg/kg/day (250 times* the maximum recommended daily human dose). Similar differences were not observed in rats administered doses equivalent to approximately 20 or 80 times* the maximum recommended daily human dose.

In a lifetime study in mice, there were statistically significant increases in the incidence of benign and malignant pulmonary tumors, benign uterine polyps and mammary adenocarcinoma in female mice at 500 mg/kg/day (approximately 400 times* the maximum recommended daily human dose), but not at 5 or 50 mg/kg/day. In a subsequent study in female mice, in which post-mortem examinations were limited to uterus and lungs, a statistically significant increase in the incidence of pulmonary tumors was again observed at 500 mg/kg/day.

The increased occurrence of mammary adenocarcinoma was associated with elevations of serum prolactin that occurred in female mice administered timolol at 500 mg/kg/day, but not at doses of 5 or 50 mg/kg/day. An increased incidence of mammary adenocarcinomas in rodents has been associated with administration of several other therapeutic agents which elevate serum prolactin, but no correlation between serum prolactin levels and mammary tumors has been established in man. Furthermore, in adult human female subjects who received oral dosages of up to 60 mg of timolol maleate, the maximum recommended daily human oral dosage, there were no clinically meaningful changes in serum prolactin.

Timolol maleate was devoid of mutagenic potential when evaluated *in vivo* (mouse) in the micronucleus test and cy-

Continued on next page

Information on the Merck & Co., Inc. products listed on these pages is the full prescribing information from product circulars in use August 31, 1998. For information, please call 1-800-NSC MERCK [1-800-672-6372].

Timolide—Cont.

togenetic assay (doses up to 800 mg/kg) and *in vitro* in a neoplastic cell transformation assay (up to 100 µg/mL). In Ames tests the highest concentrations of timolol employed, 5000 or 10,000 µg/plate, were associated with statistically significant elevations of revertants observed with tester strain TA100 (in seven replicate assays), but not in three additional strains. In the assays with tester strain TA100, no consistent dose response relationship was observed, nor did the ratio of test to control revertants reach 2. A ratio of 2 is usually considered the criterion for a positive Ames test. Reproduction and fertility studies in rats showed no adverse effect on male or female fertility at doses up to 125 times* the maximum recommended daily human dose.

Hydrochlorothiazide: Two-year feeding studies in mice and rats conducted under the auspices of the National Toxicology Program (NTP) uncovered no evidence of a carcinogenic potential of hydrochlorothiazide in female mice (at doses of up to approximately 600 mg/kg/day) or in male and female rats (at doses of up to approximately 100 mg/kg/day). The NTP, however, found equivocal evidence for hepatocarcinogenicity in male mice.

Hydrochlorothiazide was not genotoxic *in vitro* in the Ames mutagenicity assay of *Salmonella typhimurium* strains TA 98, TA 100, TA 1535, TA 1537, and TA 1538 and in the Chinese Hamster Ovary (CHO) test for chromosomal aberrations, or *in vivo* in assays using mouse germinal cell chromosomes, Chinese hamster bone marrow chromosomes, and the *Drosophila* sex-linked recessive lethal trait gene. Positive test results were obtained only in the *in vitro* CHO Sister Chromatid Exchange (clastogenicity) and in the Mouse Lymphoma Cell (mutagenicity) assay, using concentrations of hydrochlorothiazide from 43 to 1300 µg/mL, and in the *Aspergillus nidulans* nondisjunction assay at an unspecified concentration.

Hydrochlorothiazide had no adverse effects on the fertility of mice and rats of either sex in studies wherein these species were exposed, via their diet, to doses of up to 100 and 4 mg/kg, respectively, prior to conception and throughout gestation.

---

*Based on patient weight of 50 kg

Pregnancy

Teratogenic Effects—Pregnancy Category C. Combinations of timolol maleate and hydrochlorothiazide were studied for teratogenic potential in the mouse and rabbit. The timolol maleate/hydrochlorothiazide combinations were administered orally to pregnant mice and pregnant rabbits at dosage levels of 1/2.5, 4/10, or 8/10 mg/kg/day. No teratogenic, embryotoxic, fetotoxic, or maternotoxic effects attributable to treatment were observed in either species. There are no adequate and well-controlled studies in pregnant women with TIMOLIDE. Because of the data listed below with the individual components, TIMOLIDE should be used during pregnancy only if the potential benefit justifies the potential risk to the fetus.

Timolol Maleate: Teratogenicity studies with timolol maleate in mice, rats and rabbits at doses up to 50 mg/kg/day (approximately 40 times* the maximum recommended daily human dose) showed no evidence of fetal malformations. Although delayed fetal ossification was observed at this dose in rats, there were no adverse effects on postnatal development of offspring. Doses of 1000 mg/kg/day (approximately 830 times* the maximum recommended daily human dose) were maternotoxic in mice and resulted in an increased number of fetal resorptions. Increased fetal resorptions were also seen in rabbits at doses of approximately 40 times* the maximum recommended daily human dose, in this case without apparent maternotoxicity.

Hydrochlorothiazide: Studies in which hydrochlorothiazide was orally administered to pregnant mice and rats during their respecitve periods of major organogenesis at doses up to 3000 and 1000 mg hydrochlorothiazide/kg, respectively, provided no evidence of harm to the fetus.

Nonteratogenic Effects.

Hydrochlorothiazide: TIMOLIDE contains hydrochlorothiazide. Thiazides cross the placental barrier and appear in cord blood. The possible hazards to the fetus include fetal or neonatal jaundice, thrombocytopenia, and possibly other adverse reactions which have occurred in the adult.

---

* Based on patient weight of 50 kg

Nursing Mothers

Timolol maleate and thiazides have been detected in human milk. Because of the potential for serious adverse reactions from timolol and hydrochlorothiazide in nursing infants, a decision should be made whether to discontinue nursing or to discontinue the drug, taking into account the importance of the drug to the mother.

Pediatric Use

Safety and effectiveness in pediatric patients have not been established.

ADVERSE REACTIONS

TIMOLIDE is usually well tolerated in properly selected patients. Most adverse effects have been mild and transient.

The adverse reactions listed in the following table were spontaneously reported and have been arranged into two groups: (1) incidence greater than 1%; and (2) incidence less than 1%. The incidence was obtained from clinical studies conducted in the United States (257 patients treated with TIMOLIDE).

Incidence Greater Than 1%	*Incidence Less Than 1%*
BODY AS A WHOLE	
fatigue/tiredness (1.9%)	chest pain headache
asthenia (1.95)	
CARDIOVASCULAR	
hypotension (1.6%)	arrhythmia
bradycardia (1.2%)	syncope cardiac failure
DIGESTIVE SYSTEM	
none	diarrhea dyspepsia nausea gastrointestinal pain constipation
INTEGUMENTARY	
none	rash increased pigmentation dry mucous membranes
MUSCULOSKELETAL	
none	myalgia
NERVOUS SYSTEM	
dizziness (1.2%)	none
PSYCHIATRIC	
none	insomnia decreased libido nervousness confusion trouble concentrating somnolence
RESPIRATORY	
bronchial spasm (1.6%)	rales
dyspnea (1.2%)	
UROGENITAL	
none	renal colic

The following additional adverse effects have been reported in clinical experience with the drug: cerebral ischemia, cerebral vascular accident, gout, muscle cramps, oculogyric crisis, worsening of chronic obstructive pulmonary disease, earache, and impotence.

Other adverse reactions that have been reported with the individual components are listed below:

Timolol Maleate —Body as a Whole: extremity pain, decreased exercise tolerance, weight loss, fever; *Cardiovascular:* cardiac arrest, cerebral vascular accident, worsening of angina pectoris, sinoatrial block, AV block, worsening of arterial insufficiency, Raynaud's phenomenon, claudication, palpitations, vasodilatation, cold hands and feet, edema; *Digestive:* hepatomegaly, elevated liver function tests, vomiting; *Hematologic:* nonthrombocytopenic purpura; *Endocrine:* hyperglycemia, hypoglycemia; *Skin:* skin irritation, pruritus, sweating, alopecia; *Musculoskeletal:* arthralgia; *Nervous System:* local weakness, vertigo, paresthesia, increase in signs and symptoms of myasthenia gravis; *Psychiatric:* depression, nightmares, hallucinations; *Respiratory:* cough; *Special Senses:* visual disturbances, diplopia, ptosis, eye irritation, dry eyes, tinnitus; *Urogenital:* urination difficulties.

There have been reports of retroperitoneal fibrosis in patients receiving timolol maleate and in patients receiving other beta-adrenergic blocking agents. A causal relationship between this condition and therapy with beta-adrenergic blocking agents has not been established.

Hydrochlorothiazide —Body as a Whole: weakness; *Digestive:* anorexia, gastric irritation, vomiting, cramping, jaundice (intrahepatic cholestatic jaundice), pancreatitis, sialadenitis; *Nervous System/Psychiatric:* vertigo, paresthesias, restlessness; *Hematologic:* leukopenia, agranulocytosis, thrombocytopenia, aplastic anemia, hemolytic anemia; *Cardiovascular:* hypotension including orthostatic hypotension (may be aggravated by alcohol, barbiturates, narcotics or antihypertensive drugs); *Hypersensitivity:* purpura, photosensitivity, urticaria, necrotizing angiitis (vasculitis, cutaneous vasculitis), fever, respiratory distress including pneumonitis and pulmonary edema, anaphylactic reactions; *Metabolic:* hyperglycemia, glycosuria, hyperuricemia, electrolyte imbalance (see PRECAUTIONS); *Musculoskeletal:* muscle spasm; *Renal:* renal failure, renal dysfunction, interstitial nephritis (See WARNINGS); *Skin:* erythema multiforme including Stevens-Johnson syndrome, exfoliative dermatitis including toxic epidermal necrolysis, alopecia; *Special Senses:* transient blurred vision, xanthopsia.

Potential Adverse Effects: In addition, a variety of adverse effects not observed in clinical trials with timolol maleate, but reported with other beta-adrenergic blocking agents, should be considered potential adverse effects of timolol maleate: *Nervous System:* reversible mental depression progressing to catatonia; an acute reversible syndrome characterized by disorientation for time and place, short-term memory loss, emotional lability, slightly clouded sensorium, and decreased performance on neuropsychometrics; *Cardiovascular:* intensification of AV block (see CONTRAINDICATIONS); *Digestive:* mesenteric arterial thrombosis, ischemic colitis; *Hematologic:* agranulocytosis, thrombocytopenic purpura; *Allergic:* erythematous rash, fever combined with aching and sore throat, laryngospasm with respiratory distress; *Miscellaneous:* Peyronie's disease.

There have been reports of a syndrome comprising psoriasiform skin rash, conjunctivitis sicca, otitis, and sclerosing serositis attributed to the beta-adrenergic receptor blocking agent, practolol. This syndrome has not been reported with TIMOLIDE or BLOCADREN* (Timolol Maleate).

Clinical Laboratory Test Findings: Clinically important changes in standard laboratory parameters were rarely associated with the administration of TIMOLIDE. The changes in laboratory parameters were not progressive and usually were not associated with clinical manifestations. The most common changes were increases in serum triglycerides and uric acid and decreases in serum potassium and chloride. Decreases in HDL cholesterol have been reported.

---

*Registered trademark of MERCK & CO., INC.

OVERDOSAGE

No data are available with regard to overdosage with TIMOLIDE in humans.

Pretreatment of mice with hydrochlorothiazide (5 mg/kg) did not alter the LD_{50} of timolol (1320 mg/kg compared to 1300 mg/kg without pretreatment).

No specific information is available on the treatment of overdosage with TIMOLIDE, and no specific antidote is available. Treatment is symptomatic and supportive. Therapy with TIMOLIDE should be discontinued and the patient observed closely. Suggested measures include induction of emesis and/or gastric lavage, and correction of dehydration, electrolyte imbalance, and hypotension by established procedures.

Timolol Maleate

Overdosage has been reported with Tablets BLOCADREN* (timolol maleate). A 30-year-old female ingested 650 mg of BLOCADREN (maximum recommended daily dose—60 mg) and experienced second and third degree heart block. She recovered without treatment but approximately two months later developed irregular heartbeat, hypertension, dizziness, tinnitus, faintness, increased pulse rate and borderline first degree heart block.

The oral LD_{50} of the drug is 1190 and 900 mg/kg in female mice and female rats, respectively.

An *in vitro* hemodialysis study, using ^{14}C timolol added to human plasma or whole blood, showed that timolol was readily dialyzed from these fluids; however, a study of patients with renal failure showed that timolol did not dialyze readily.

The most common signs and symptoms to be expected with overdosage with a beta-adrenergic receptor blocking agent are symptomatic bradycardia, hypotension, bronchospasm, and acute cardiac failure. If overdosage occurs the following therapeutic measures should be considered:

(1) *Gastric lavage.*

(2) *Symptomatic bradycardia:* Use atropine sulfate intravenously in a dosage of 0.25 mg to 2 mg to induce vagal blockade. If bradycardia persists, intravenous isoproterenol hydrochloride should be administered cautiously. In refractory cases the use of a transvenous cardiac pacemaker may be considered.

(3) *Hypotension:* Use sympathomimetic pressor drug therapy, such as dopamine, dobutamine or levarterenol. In refractory cases the use of glucagon hydrochloride has been reported to be useful.

(4) *Bronchospasm:* Use isoproterenol hydrochloride. Additional therapy with aminophylline may be considered.

(5) *Acute cardiac failure:* Conventional therapy with digitalis, diuretics, and oxygen should be instituted immediately. In refractory cases the use of intravenous aminophylline is suggested. This may be followed, if necessary, by glucagon hydrochloride which has been reported to be useful.

(6) *Heart block (second or third degree):* Use isoproterenol hydrochloride or a transvenous cardiac pacemaker.

Hydrochlorothiazide

The most common signs and symptoms observed with hydrochlorothiazide overdosage are those caused by electrolyte depletion (hypokalemia, hypochloremia, hyponatremia) and dehydration resulting from excessive diuresis. If digitalis has also been administered, hypokalemia may accentuate cardiac arrhythmias.

---

*Registered trademark of MERCK & CO., INC.

DOSAGE AND ADMINISTRATION

The recommended starting and maintenance dosage is 1 tablet twice a day or 2 tablets once a day. Patients usually

do not require doses in excess of 50 mg of hydrochlorothiazide daily when combined with other antihypertensive agents. If the antihypertensive response is not satisfactory, another nondiuretic antihypertensive agent may be added.

HOW SUPPLIED

No. 3373—Tablets TIMOLIDE 10-25 are light blue, flat, hexagonal-shaped, compressed tablets, with code MSD 67 on one side and TIMOLIDE on the other. Each tablet contains 10 mg of timolol maleate and 25 mg of hydrochlorothiazide. They are supplied as follows:

NDC 0006-0067-68 bottles of 100.

Shown in Product Identification Guide, page 323

Storage

Store at controlled room temperature, 15–30°C (59–86°F). Keep container tightly closed. Protect from light.

7928432 Issued October 1997

COPYRIGHT © MERCK & CO., INC., 1985
All rights reserved

TIMOPTIC® Sterile Ophthalmic Solution 0.25% and 0.5% ℞
(Timolol Maleate Ophthalmic Solution), U.S.P.

DESCRIPTION

TIMOPTIC* (timolol maleate ophthalmic solution) is a non-selective beta-adrenergic receptor blocking agent. Its chemical name is (-)-1-(*tert*-butylamino)-3-[(4-morpholino-1,2,5-thiadiazol-3-yl)oxy]-2-propanol maleate (1:1) (salt). Timolol maleate possesses an asymmetric carbon atom in its structure and is provided as the levo-isomer. The nominal optical rotation of timolol maleate is:

$[\alpha]^{25°}_{405\ nm}$ in 0.1N HCl (C = 5%) = −12.2°.

Its molecular formula is $C_{13}H_{24}N_4O_3S{\cdot}C_4H_4O_4$ and its structural formula is:

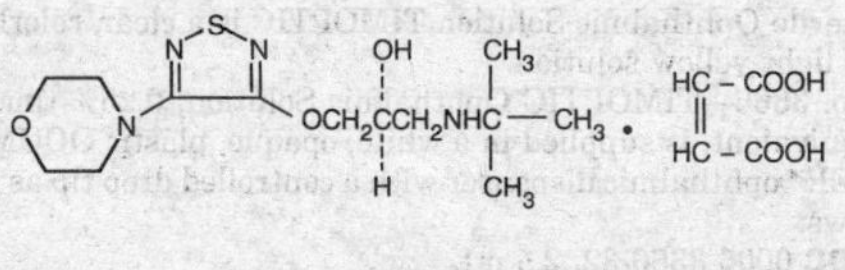

Timolol maleate has a molecular weight of 432.50. It is a white, odorless, crystalline powder which is soluble in water, methanol, and alcohol. TIMOPTIC is stable at room temperature.

TIMOPTIC Ophthalmic Solution is supplied as a sterile, isotonic, buffered, aqueous solution of timolol maleate in two dosage strengths: Each mL of TIMOPTIC 0.25% contains 2.5 mg of timolol (3.4 mg of timolol maleate). Each mL of TIMOPTIC 0.5% contains 5.0 mg of timolol (6.8 mg of timolol maleate). Inactive ingredients: monobasic and dibasic sodium phosphate, sodium hydroxide to adjust pH, and water for injection. Benzalkonium chloride 0.01% is added as preservative.

*Registered trademark of MERCK & CO., INC.

CLINICAL PHARMACOLOGY

Mechanism of Action

Timolol maleate is a $beta_1$ and $beta_2$ (non-selective) adrenergic receptor blocking agent that does not have significant intrinsic sympathomimetic, direct myocardial depressant, or local anesthetic (membrane-stabilizing) activity.

Beta-adrenergic receptor blockade reduces cardiac output in both healthy subjects and patients with heart disease. In patients with severe impairment of myocardial infarction, beta-adrenergic receptor blockade may inhibit the stimulatory effect of the sympathetic nervous system necessary to maintain adequate cardiac function.

Beta-adrenergic receptor blockade in the bronchi and bronchioles results in increased airway resistance from unopposed parasympathetic activity. Such an effect in patients with asthma or other bronchospastic conditions is potentially dangerous.

TIMOPTIC Ophthalmic Solution, when applied topically on the eye, has the action of reducing elevated as well as normal intraocular pressure, whether or not accompanied by glaucoma. Elevated intraocular pressure is a major risk factor in the pathogenesis of glaucomatous visual field loss. The higher the level of intraocular pressure, the greater the likelihood of glaucomatous visual field loss and optic nerve damage.

The onset of reduction in intraocular pressure following administration of TIMOPTIC can usually be detected within one-half hour after a single dose. The maximum effect usually occurs in one to two hours and significant lowering of intraocular pressure can be maintained for periods as long as 24 hours with a single dose. Repeated observations over a period of one year indicate that the intraocular pressure-lowering effect of TIMOPTIC is well maintained.

The precise mechanism of the ocular hypotensive action of TIMOPTIC is not clearly established at this time. Tonography and fluorophotometry studies in man suggest that its predominant action may be related to reduced aqueous formation. However, in some studies a slight increase in outflow facility was also observed.

Pharmacokinetics

In a study of plasma drug concentration in six subjects, the systemic exposure to timolol was determined following twice daily administration of TIMOPTIC 0.5%. The mean peak plasma concentration following morning dosing was 0.46 ng/mL and following afternoon dosing was 0.35 ng/mL.

Clinical Studies

In controlled multiclinic studies in patients with untreated intraocular pressures of 22 mmHg or greater, TIMOPTIC 0.25 percent or 0.5 percent administered twice a day produced a greater reduction in intraocular pressure than 1, 2, 3, or 4 percent pilocarpine solution administered four times a day or 0.5, 1, or 2 percent epinephrine hydrochloride solution administered twice a day.

In these studies, TIMOPTIC was generally well tolerated and produced fewer and less severe side effects than either pilocarpine or epinephrine. A slight reduction of resting heart rate in some patients receiving TIMOPTIC (mean reduction 2.9 beats/minute standard deviation 10.2) was observed.

INDICATIONS AND USAGE

TIMOPTIC Ophthalmic Solution is indicated in the treatment of elevated intraocular pressure in patients with ocular hypertension or open-angle glaucoma.

CONTRAINDICATIONS

TIMOPTIC is contraindicated in patients with (1) bronchial asthma; (2) a history of bronchial asthma; (3) severe chronic obstructive pulmonary disease (see **WARNINGS**); (4) sinus bradycardia; (5) second or third degree atrioventricular block; (6) overt cardiac failure (see **WARNINGS**); (7) cardiogenic shock; or (8) hypersensitivity to any component of this product.

WARNINGS

As with many topically applied ophthalmic drugs, this drug is absorbed systemically.

The same adverse reactions found with systemic administration of beta-adrenergic blocking agents may occur with topical administration. For example, severe respiratory reactions and cardiac reactions, including death due to bronchospasm in patients with asthma, and rarely death in association with cardiac failure, have been reported following systemic or ophthalmic administration of timolol maleate (see CONTRAINDICATIONS).

Cardiac Failure

Sympathetic stimulation may be essential for support of the circulation in individuals with diminished myocardial contractility, and its inhibition by beta-adrenergic receptor blockade may precipitate more severe failure.

In Patients Without a History of Cardiac Failure continued depression of the myocardium with beta-blocking agents over a period of time can, in some cases, lead to cardiac failure. At the first sign or symptom of cardiac failure TIMOPTIC should be discontinued.

Obstructive Pulmonary Disease

Patients with chronic obstructive pulmonary disease (e.g., chronic bronchitis, emphysema) of mild or moderate severity, bronchospastic disease, or a history of bronchospastic disease (other than bronchial asthma or a history of bronchial asthma, in which TIMOPTIC is contraindicated [see **CONTRAINDICATIONS**]) should, in general, not receive beta-blockers, including TIMOPTIC.

Major Surgery

The necessity or desirability of withdrawal of beta-adrenergic blocking agents prior to major surgery is controversial. Beta-adrenergic receptor blockade impairs the ability of the heart to respond to beta-adrenergically mediated reflex stimuli. This may augment the risk of general anesthesia in surgical procedures. Some patients receiving beta-adrenergic receptor blocking agents have experienced protracted severe hypotension during anesthesia. Difficulty in restarting and maintaining the heartbeat has also been reported. For these reasons, in patients undergoing elective surgery, some authorities recommend gradual withdrawal of beta-adrenergic receptor blocking agents.

If necessary during surgery, the effects of beta-adrenergic blocking agents may be reversed by sufficient doses of adrenergic agonists.

Diabetes Mellitus

Beta-adrenergic blocking agents should be administered with caution in patients subject to spontaneous hypoglycemia or to diabetic patients (especially those with labile diabetes) who are receiving insulin or oral hypoglycemic agents. Beta-adrenergic receptor blocking agents may mask the signs and symptoms of acute hypoglycemia.

Thyrotoxicosis

Beta-adrenergic blocking agents may mask certain clinical signs (e.g., tachycardia) of hyperthyroidism. Patients suspected of developing thyrotoxicosis should be managed carefully to avoid abrupt withdrawal of beta-adrenergic blocking agents that might precipitate a thyroid storm.

PRECAUTIONS

General

Because of potential effects of beta-adrenergic blocking agents on blood pressure and pulse, these agents should be used with caution in patients with cerebrovascular insufficiency. If signs or symptoms suggesting reduced cerebral blood flow develop following initiation of therapy with TIMOPTIC, alternative therapy should be considered.

There have been reports of bacterial keratitis associated with the use of multiple dose containers of topical ophthalmic products. These containers had been inadvertently contaminated by patients who, in most cases, had a concurrent corneal disease or a disruption of the ocular epithelial surface. (See **PRECAUTIONS**, *Information for Patients.*)

Choroidal detachment after filtration procedures has been reported with the administration of aqueous suppressant therapy (e.g. timolol).

Angle-closure glaucoma: In patients with angle-closure glaucoma, the immediate objective of treatment is to reopen the angle. This requires constricting the pupil. Timolol maleate has little or no effect on the pupil. TIMOPTIC should not be used alone in the treatment of angle-closure glaucoma.

Anaphylaxis: While taking beta-blockers, patients with a history of atopy or a history of severe anaphylactic reactions to a variety of allergens may be more reactive to repeated accidental, diagnostic, or therapeutic challenge with such allergens. Such patients may be unresponsive to the usual doses of epinephrine used to treat anaphylactic reactions.

Muscle Weakness: Beta-adrenergic blockade has been reported to potentiate muscle weakness consistent with certain myasthenic symptoms (e.g., diplopia, ptosis, and generalized weakness). Timolol has been reported rarely to increase muscle weakness in some patients with myasthenia gravis or myasthenic symptoms.

Information for Patients

Patients should be instructed to avoid allowing the tip of the dispensing container to contact the eye or surrounding structures.

Patients should also be instructed that ocular solutions, if handled improperly, can become contaminated by common bacteria known to cause ocular infections. Serious damage to the eye and subsequent loss of vision may result from using contaminated solutions. (See **PRECAUTIONS**, *General.*)

Patients should also be advised that if they have ocular surgery or develop an intercurrent ocular condition (e.g., trauma or infection), they should immediately seek their physician's advice concerning the use of the present multidose container.

Patients with bronchial asthma, a history of bronchial asthma, severe chronic obstructive pulmonary disease, sinus bradycardia, second or third degree atrioventricular block, or cardiac failure should be advised not to take this product. (See **CONTRAINDICATIONS.**)

Patients should be advised that TIMOPTIC contains benzalkonium chloride which may be absorbed by soft contact lenses. Contact lenses should be removed prior to administration of the solution. Lenses may be reinserted 15 minutes following TIMOPTIC administration.

Drug Interactions

Although TIMOPTIC used alone has little or no effect on pupil size, mydriasis resulting from concomitant therapy with TIMOPTIC and epinephrine has been reported occasionally.

Beta-adrenergic blocking agents: Patients who are receiving a beta-adrenergic blocking agent orally and TIMOPTIC should be observed for potential additive effects of beta-blockade, both systemic and on intraocular pressure. The concomitant use of two topical beta-adrenergic blocking agents is not recommended.

Calcium antagonists: Caution should be used in the coadministration of beta-adrenergic blocking agents, such as TIMOPTIC, and oral or intravenous calcium antagonists because of possible atrioventricular conduction disturbances,

Continued on next page

Information on the Merck & Co., Inc. products listed on these pages is the full prescribing information from product circulars in use August 31, 1998. For information, please call 1-800-NSC MERCK [1-800-672-6372].

Timoptic Sterile Ophthalmic—Cont.

left ventricular failure, and hypotension. In patients with impaired cardiac function, coadministration should be avoided.

Catecholamine-depleting drugs: Close observation of the patient is recommended when a beta blocker is administered to patients receiving catecholamine-depleting drugs such as reserpine, because of possible additive effects and the production of hypotension and/or marked bradycardia, which may result in vertigo, syncope, or postural hypotension.

Digitalis and calcium antagonists: The concomitant use of beta-adrenergic blocking agents with digitalis and calcium antagonists may have additive effects in prolonging atrioventricular conduction time.

Quinidine: Potentiated systemic beta-blockade (e.g., decreased heart rate) has been reported during combined treatment with quinidine and timolol, possibly because quinidine inhibits the metabolism of timolol via the P-450 enzyme, CYP2D6.

Injectable Epinephrine: (See **PRECAUTIONS**, *General, Anaphylaxis*)

Carcinogenesis, Mutagenesis, Impairment of Fertility

In a two-year oral study of timolol maleate administered orally to rats, there was a statistically significant increase in the incidence of adrenal pheochromocytomas in male rats administered 300 mg/kg/day (approximately 42,000 times the systemic exposure following the maximum recommended human ophthalmic dose). Similar differences were not observed in rats administered oral doses equivalent to approximately 14,000 times the maximum recommended human ophthalmic dose.

In a lifetime oral study in mice, there were statistically significant increases in the incidence of benign and malignant pulmonary tumors, benign uterine polyps and mammary adenocarcinomas in female mice at 500 mg/kg/day (approximately 71,000 times the systemic exposure following the maximum recommended human ophthalmic dose), but not at 5 or 50 mg/kg/day (approximately 700 or 7,000, respectively, times the systemic exposure following the maximum recommended human ophthalmic dose). In a subsequent study in female mice, in which post-mortem examinations were limited to the uterus and the lungs, a statistically significant increase in the incidence of pulmonary tumors was again observed at 500 mg/kg/day.

The increased occurrence of mammary adenocarcinomas was associated with elevations in serum prolactin which occurred in female mice administered oral timolol at 500 mg/kg/day, but not at doses of 5 or 50 mg/kg/day. An increased incidence of mammary adenocarcinomas in rodents has been associated with administration of several other therapeutic agents that elevate serum prolactin, but no correlation between serum prolactin levels and mammary tumors has been established in humans. Furthermore, in adult human female subjects who received oral dosages of up to 60 mg of timolol maleate (the maximum recommended human oral dosage), there were no clinically meaningful changes in serum prolactin.

Timolol maleate was devoid of mutagenic potential when tested *in vivo* (mouse) in the micronucleus test and cytogenetic assay (doses up to 800 mg/kg) and *in vitro* in a neoplastic cell transformation assay (up to 100 µg/mL). In Ames tests the highest concentrations of timolol employed, 5000 or 10,000 µg/plate, were associated with statistically significant elevations of revertants observed with tester strain TA100 (in seven replicate assays), but not in the remaining three strains. In the assays with tester strain TA100, no consistent dose response relationship was observed, and the ratio of test to control revertants did not reach 2. A ratio of 2 is usually considered the criterion for a positive Ames test.

Reproduction and fertility studies in rats demonstrated no adverse effect on male or female fertility at doses up to 21,000 times the systemic exposure following the maximum recommended human ophthalmic dose.

Pregnancy-Teratogenic effects:

Pregnancy Category C. Teratogenicity studies with timolol in mice, rats, and rabbits at oral doses up to 50 mg/kg/day (7,000 times the systemic exposure following the maximum recommended human ophthalmic dose) demonstrated no evidence of fetal malformations. Although delayed fetal ossification was observed at this dose in rats, there were no adverse effects on postnatal development of offspring. Doses of 1000 mg/kg/day (142,000 times the systemic exposure following the maximum recommended human ophthalmic dose) were maternotoxic in mice and resulted in an increased number of fetal resorptions. Increased fetal resorptions were also seen in rabbits at doses of 14,000 times the systemic exposure following the maximum recommended human ophthalmic dose, in this case without apparent maternotoxicity.

There are no adequate and well-controlled studies in pregnant women. TIMOPTIC should be used during pregnancy only if the potential benefit justifies the potential risk to the fetus.

Nursing Mothers

Timolol maleate has been detected in human milk following oral and ophthalmic drug administration. Because of the potential for serious adverse reactions from TIMOPTIC in nursing infants, a decision should be made whether to discontinue nursing or to discontinue the drug, taking into account the importance of the drug to the mother.

Pediatric Use

Safety and effectiveness in pediatric patients have not been established.

ADVERSE REACTIONS

The most frequently reported adverse experiences have been burning and stinging upon instillation (approximately one in eight patients).

The following additional adverse experiences have been reported less frequently with ocular administration of this or other timolol maleate formulations:

BODY AS A WHOLE

Headache, asthenia/fatigue, and chest pain.

CARDIOVASCULAR

Bradycardia, arrhythmia, hypotension, hypertension, syncope, heart block, cerebral vascular accident, cerebral ischemia, cardiac failure, worsening of angina pectoris, palpitation, cardiac arrest, pulmonary edema, edema, claudication, Raynaud's phenomenon, and cold hands and feet.

DIGESTIVE

Nausea, diarrhea, dyspepsia, anorexia, and dry mouth.

IMMUNOLOGIC

Systemic lupus erythematosus.

NERVOUS SYSTEM/PSYCHIATRIC

Dizziness, increase in signs and symptoms of myasthenia gravis, paresthesia, somnolence, insomnia, nightmares, behavioral changes and psychic disturbances including depression, confusion, hallucinations, anxiety, disorientation, nervousness, and memory loss.

SKIN

Alopecia and psoriasiform rash or exacerbation of psoriasis.

HYPERSENSITIVITY

Signs and symptoms of allergic reactions, including angioedema, urticaria, and localized and generalized rash.

RESPIRATORY

Bronchospasm (predominantly in patients with pre-existing bronchospastic disease), respiratory failure, dyspnea, nasal congestion, cough and upper respiratory infections.

ENDOCRINE

Masked symptoms of hypoglycemia in diabetic patients (see **WARNINGS**).

SPECIAL SENSES

Signs and symptoms of ocular irritation including conjunctivitis, blepharitis, keratitis, ocular pain, discharge (e.g., crusting), foreign body sensation, itching and tearing, and dry eyes; ptosis; decreased corneal sensitivity; cystoid macular edema; visual disturbances including refractive changes and diplopia; pseudopemphigoid; choroidal detachment following filtration surgery (see **PRECAUTIONS**, *General*), and tinnitus.

UROGENITAL

Retroperitoneal fibrosis, decreased libido, impotence, and Peyronie's disease.

The following additional adverse effects have been reported in clinical experience with ORAL timolol maleate or other ORAL beta-blocking agents and may be considered potential effects of ophthalmic timolol maleate: *Allergic:* Erythematous rash, fever combined with aching and sore throat, laryngospasm with respiratory distress; *Body as a Whole:* Extremity pain, decreased exercise tolerance, weight loss; *Cardiovascular:* Worsening of arterial insufficiency, vasodilatation; *Digestive:* Gastrointestinal pain, hepatomegaly, vomiting, mesenteric arterial thrombosis, ischemic colitis; *Hematologic:* Nonthrombocytopenic purpura; thrombocytopenic purpura, agranulocytosis; *Endocrine:* Hyperglycemia, hypoglycemia; *Skin:* Pruritus, skin irritation, increased pigmentation, sweating; *Musculoskeletal:* Arthralgia; *Nervous System/Psychiatric:* Vertigo, local weakness, diminished concentration, reversible mental depression progressing to catatonia, an acute reversible syndrome characterized by disorientation for time and place, emotional lability, slightly clouded sensorium, and decreased performance on neuropsychometrics; *Respiratory:* Rales, bronchial obstruction; *Urogenital:* Urination difficulties.

OVERDOSAGE

There have been reports of inadvertent overdosage with TIMOPTIC Ophthalmic Solution resulting in systemic effects similar to those seen with systemic beta-adrenergic blocking agents such as dizziness, headache, shortness of breath, bradycardia, bronchospasm, and cardiac arrest (see also **ADVERSE REACTIONS**).

Overdosage has been reported with Tablets BLOCADREN* (timolol maleate). A 30 year old female ingested 650 mg of BLOCADREN (maximum recommended oral daily dose is 60 mg) and experienced second and third degree heart block. She recovered without treatment but approximately two months later developed irregular heartbeat, hypertension, dizziness, tinnitus, faintness, increased pulse rate, and borderline first degree heart block.

Significant lethality was observed in female rats and female mice after a single dose of 900 and 1190 mg/kg (5310 and 3570 mg/m^2) of timolol, respectively.

An *in vitro* hemodialysis study, using ^{14}C timolol added to human plasma or whole blood, showed that timolol was readily dialyzed from these fluids; however, a study of patients with renal failure showed that timolol did not dialyze readily.

* Registered trademark of MERCK & CO., INC.

DOSAGE AND ADMINISTRATION

TIMOPTIC Ophthalmic Solution is available in concentrations of 0.25 and 0.5 percent. The usual starting dose is one drop of 0.25 percent TIMOPTIC in the affected eye(s) twice a day. If the clinical response is not adequate, the dosage may be changed to one drop of 0.5 percent solution in the affected eye(s) twice a day.

Since in some patients the pressure-lowering response to TIMOPTIC may require a few weeks to stabilize, evaluation should include a determination of intraocular pressure after approximately 4 weeks of treatment with TIMOPTIC.

If the intraocular pressure is maintained at satisfactory levels, the dosage schedule may be changed to one drop once a day in the affected eye(s). Because of diurnal variations in intraocular pressure, satisfactory response to the once-a-day dose is best determined by measuring the intraocular pressure at different times during the day.

Dosages above one drop of 0.5 percent TIMOPTIC twice a day generally have not been shown to produce further reduction in intraocular pressure. If the patient's intraocular pressure is still not at a satisfactory level on this regimen, concomitant therapy with other agent(s) for lowering intraocular pressure can be instituted. The concomitant use of two topical beta-adrenergic blocking agents is not recommended. (See PRECAUTIONS, *Drug Interactions, Beta-adrenergic blocking agents.*)

HOW SUPPLIED

Sterile Ophthalmic Solution TIMOPTIC is a clear, colorless to light yellow solution.

No. 3366—TIMOPTIC Ophthalmic Solution, 0.25% timolol equivalent, is supplied in a white, opaque, plastic OCUMETER* ophthalmic dispenser with a controlled drop tip as follows:

NDC 0006-3366-32, 2.5 mL
NDC 0006-3366-03, 5 mL
(6505-01-069-6518, 0.25% 5 mL)
NDC 0006-3366-10, 10 mL
(6505-01-093-5458, 0.25% 10 mL)
NDC 0006-3366-12, 15 mL.

No. 3367—TIMOPTIC Ophthalmic Solution, 0.5% timolol equivalent, is supplied in a white, opaque, plastic OCUMETER ophthalmic dispenser with a controlled drop tip as follows:

NDC 0006-3367-32, 2.5 mL
NDC 0006-3367-03, 5 mL
(6505-01-069-6519, 0.5% 5 mL)
NDC 0006-3367-10, 10 mL
(6505-01-092-0422, 0.5% 10 mL)
NDC 0006-3367-12, 15 mL.

Storage

Store at room temperature, 15–30°C (59–86°F). Protect from freezing. Protect from light.

*Registered trademark of MERCK & CO., INC.
9010840 Issued August 1997

TIMOPTIC® ℞

0.25% and 0.5%
(Timolol Maleate Ophthalmic Solution)
in OCUDOSE® (Dispenser), U.S.P.
Preservative-Free Sterile Ophthalmic Solution
in a Sterile Ophthalmic Unit Dose Dispenser

DESCRIPTION

Timolol maleate is a non-selective beta-adrenergic receptor blocking agent. Its chemical name is (-)-1-(*tert*-butylamino)-3-[(4-morpholino-1,2,5-thiadiazol-3-yl)oxy]-2-propanol maleate (1:1) (salt). Timolol maleate possesses an asymmetric carbon atom in its structure and is provided as the levo-isomer. The nominal optical rotation of timolol maleate is

$$[\alpha]^{25^\circ}_{405\ nm} \text{ in 0.1N HCl (C = 5\%) } = -12.2^\circ.$$

Its molecular formula is $C_{13}H_{24}N_4O_3S{\cdot}C_4H_4O_4$ and its structural formula is:

[See chemical structure at top of next column]

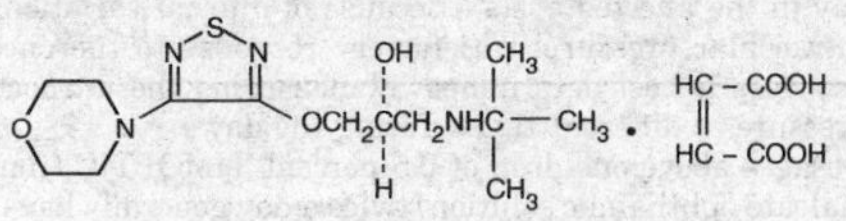

Timolol maleate has a molecular weight of 432.50. It is a white, odorless, crystalline powder which is soluble in water, methanol, and alcohol. Timolol maleate is stable at room temperature.

Timolol maleate ophthalmic solution is supplied in two formulations: Ophthalmic Solution TIMOPTIC* (timolol maleate ophthalmic solution), which contains the preservative benzalkonium chloride; and Ophthalmic Solution TIMOPTIC* (timolol maleate ophthalmic solution), the preservative-free formulation.

Preservative-free Ophthalmic Solution TIMOPTIC is supplied in OCUDOSE*, a unit dose container, as a sterile, isotonic, buffered, aqueous solution of timolol maleate in two dosage strengths: Each mL of Preservative-free TIMOPTIC in OCUDOSE 0.25% contains 2.5 mg of timolol (3.4 mg of timolol maleate). Each mL of Preservative-free TIMOPTIC in OCUDOSE 0.5% contains 5.0 mg of timolol (6.8 mg of timolol maleate). Inactive ingredients: monobasic and dibasic sodium phosphate, sodium hydroxide to adjust pH, and water for injection.

*Registered trademark of MERCK & CO., INC.

CLINICAL PHARMACOLOGY

Mechanism of Action

Timolol maleate is a $beta_1$ and $beta_2$ (non-selective) adrenergic receptor blocking agent that does not have significant intrinsic sympathomimetic, direct myocardial depressant, or local anesthetic (membrane-stabilizing) activity.

Beta-adrenergic receptor blockade reduces cardiac output in both healthy subjects and patients with heart disease. In patients with severe impairment of myocardial function beta-adrenergic receptor blockade may inhibit the stimulatory effect of the sympathetic nervous system necessary to maintain adequate cardiac function.

Beta-adrenergic receptor blockade in the bronchi and bronchioles results in increased airway resistance from unopposed parasympathetic activity. Such an effect in patients with asthma or other bronchospastic conditions is potentially dangerous.

TIMOPTIC (timolol maleate ophthalmic solution), when applied topically on the eye, has the action of reducing elevated as well as normal intraocular pressure, whether or not accompanied by glaucoma. Elevated intraocular pressure is a major risk factor in the pathogenesis of glaucomatous visual field loss. The higher the level of intraocular pressure, the greater the likelihood of glaucomatous visual field loss and optic nerve damage.

The onset of reduction in intraocular pressure following administration of TIMOPTIC (timolol maleate ophthalmic solution) can usually be detected within one-half hour after a single dose. The maximum effect usually occurs in one to two hours and significant lowering of intraocular pressure can be maintained for periods as long as 24 hours with a single dose. Repeated observations over a period of one year indicate that the intraocular pressure-lowering effect of TIMOPTIC (timolol maleate ophthalmic solution) is well maintained.

The precise mechanism of the ocular hypotensive action of TIMOPTIC (timolol maleate ophthalmic solution) is not clearly established at this time. Tonography and fluorophotometry studies in man suggest that its predominant action may be related to reduced aqueous formation. However, in some studies a slight increase in outflow facility was also observed.

Pharmacokinetics

In a study of plasma drug concentration in six subjects, the systemic exposure to timolol was determined following twice daily administration of TIMOPTIC 0.5%. The mean peak plasma concentration following morning dosing was 0.46 ng/mL and following afternoon dosing was 0.35 ng/mL.

Clinical Studies

In controlled multiclinic studies in patients with untreated intraocular pressures of 22 mmHg or greater, TIMOPTIC (timolol maleate ophthalmic solution) 0.25 percent or 0.5 percent administered twice a day produced a greater reduction in intraocular pressure than 1,2,3, or 4 percent pilocarpine solution administered four times a day or 0.5, 1, or 2 percent epinephrine hydrochloride solution administered twice a day.

In these studies, TIMOPTIC (timolol maleate ophthalmic solution) was generally well tolerated and produced fewer and less severe side effects than either pilocarpine or epinephrine. A slight reduction of resting heart rate in some patients receiving TIMOPTIC (timolol maleate ophthalmic solution) (mean reduction 2.9 beats/minute standard deviation 10.2) was observed.

INDICATIONS AND USAGE

Preservative-free TIMOPTIC in OCUDOSE is indicated in the treatment of elevated intraocular pressure in patients with ocular hypertension or open-angle glaucoma.

Preservative-free TIMOPTIC in OCUDOSE may be used when a patient is sensitive to the preservative in TIMOPTIC (timolol maleate ophthalmic solution), benzalkonium chloride, or when use of a preservative-free topical medication is advisable.

CONTRAINDICATIONS

Preservative-free TIMOPTIC in OCUDOSE is contraindicated in patients with (1) bronchial asthma; (2) a history of bronchial asthma; (3) severe chronic obstructive pulmonary disease (see **WARNINGS**); (4) sinus bradycardia; (5) second or third degree atrioventricular block; (6) overt cardiac failure (see **WARNINGS**); (7) cardiogenic shock; or (8) hypersensitivity to any component of this product.

WARNINGS

As with many topically applied ophthalmic drugs, this drug is absorbed systemically.

The same adverse reactions found with systemic administration of beta-adrenergic blocking agents may occur with topical administration. For example, severe respiratory reactions and cardiac reactions, including death due to bronchospasm in patients with asthma, and rarely death in association with cardiac failure, have been reported following systemic or ophthalmic administration of timolol maleate (see CONTRAINDICATIONS).

Cardiac Failure

Sympathetic stimulation may be essential for support of the circulation in individuals with diminished myocardial contractility, and its inhibition by beta-adrenergic receptor blockade may precipitate more severe failure.

In Patients Without a History of Cardiac Failure continued depression of the myocardium with beta-blocking agents over a period of time can, in some cases, lead to cardiac failure. At the first sign or symptom of cardiac failure Preservative-free TIMOPTIC in OCUDOSE should be discontinued.

Obstructive Pulmonary Disease

Patients with chronic obstructive pulmonary disease (e.g., chronic bronchitis, emphysema) of mild or moderate severity, bronchospastic disease, or a history of bronchospastic disease (other than bronchial asthma or a history of bronchial asthma, in which TIMOPTIC in OCUDOSE is contraindicated [see **CONTRAINDICATIONS**]) should, in general, not receive beta-blockers, including Preservative-free TIMOPTIC in OCUDOSE.

Major Surgery

The necessity or desirability of withdrawal of beta-adrenergic blocking agents prior to major surgery is controversial. Beta-adrenergic receptor blockade impairs the ability of the heart to respond to beta-adrenergically mediated reflex stimuli. This may augment the risk of general anesthesia in surgical procedures. Some patients receiving beta-adrenergic receptor blocking agents have experienced protracted severe hypotension during anesthesia. Difficulty in restarting and maintaining the heartbeat has also been reported. For these reasons, in patients undergoing elective surgery, some authorities recommend gradual withdrawal of beta-adrenergic receptor blocking agents.

If necessary during surgery, the effects of beta-adrenergic blocking agents may be reversed by sufficient doses of adrenergic agonists.

Diabetes Mellitus

Beta-adrenergic blocking agents should be administered with caution in patients subject to spontaneous hypoglycemia or to diabetic patients (especially those with labile diabetes) who are receiving insulin or oral hypoglycemic agents. Beta-adrenergic receptor blocking agents may mask the signs and symptoms of acute hypoglycemia.

Thyrotoxicosis

Beta-adrenergic blocking agents may mask certain clinical signs (e.g., tachycardia) of hyperthyroidism. Patients suspected of developing thyrotoxicosis should be managed carefully to avoid abrupt withdrawal of beta-adrenergic blocking agents that might precipitate a thyroid storm.

PRECAUTIONS

General

Because of potential effects of beta-adrenergic blocking agents on blood pressure and pulse, these agents should be used with caution in patients with cerebrovascular insufficiency. If signs or symptoms suggesting reduced cerebral blood flow develop following initiation of therapy with Preservative-free TIMOPTIC in OCUDOSE, alternative therapy should be considered.

Choroidal detachment after filtration procedures has been reported with the administration of aqueous suppressant therapy (e.g. timolol).

Angle-closure glaucoma: In patients with angle-closure glaucoma, the immediate objective of treatment is to reopen the angle. This requires constricting the pupil. Timolol maleate has little or no effect on the pupil. TIMOPTIC in OCUDOSE should not be used alone in the treatment of angle-closure glaucoma.

Anaphylaxis: While taking beta-blockers, patients with a history of atopy or a history of severe anaphylactic reactions to a variety of allergens may be more reactive to repeated accidental, diagnostic, or therapeutic challenge with such allergens. Such patients may be unresponsive to the usual doses of epinephrine used to treat anaphylactic reactions.

Muscle Weakness: Beta-adrenergic blockade has been reported to potentiate muscle weakness consistent with certain myasthenic symptoms (e.g., diplopia, ptosis, and generalized weakness). Timolol has been reported rarely to increase muscle weakness in some patients with myasthenia gravis or myasthenic symptoms.

Information for Patients

Patients should be instructed about the use of Preservative-free TIMOPTIC in OCUDOSE.

Since sterility cannot be maintained after the individual unit is opened, patients should be instructed to use the product immediately after opening, and to discard the individual unit and any remaining contents immediately after use.

Patients with bronchial asthma, a history of bronchial asthma, severe chronic obstructive pulmonary disease, sinus bradycardia, second or third degree atrioventricular block, or cardiac failure should be advised not to take this product. (See **CONTRAINDICATIONS**.)

Drug Interactions

Although TIMOPTIC (timolol maleate ophthalmic solution) used alone has little or no effect on pupil size, mydriasis resulting from concomitant therapy with TIMOPTIC (timolol maleate ophthalmic solution) and epinephrine has been reported occasionally.

Beta-adrenergic blocking agents: Patients who are receiving a beta-adrenergic blocking agent orally and Preservative-free TIMOPTIC in OCUDOSE should be observed for potential additive effects of beta-blockade, both systemic and on intraocular pressure. The concomitant use of two topical beta-adrenergic blocking agents is not recommended.

Calcium antagonists: Caution should be used in the coadministration of beta-adrenergic blocking agents, such as Preservative-free TIMOPTIC in OCUDOSE, and oral or intravenous calcium antagonists, because of possible atrioventricular conduction disturbances, left ventricular failure, and hypotension. In patients with impaired cardiac function, coadministration should be avoided.

Catecholamine-depleting drugs: Close observation of the patient is recommended when a beta blocker is administered to patients receiving catecholamine-depleting drugs such as reserpine, because of possible additive effects and the production of hyotension and/or marked bradycardia, which may result in vertigo, syncope, or postural hypotension.

Digitalis and calcium antagonists: The concomitant use of beta-adrenergic blocking agents with digitalis and calcium antagonists may have additive effects in prolonging atrioventricular conduction time.

Quinidine: Potentiated systemic beta-blockade (e.g., decreased heart rate) has been reported during combined treatment with quinidine and timolol, possibly because quinidine inhibits the metabolism of timolol via the P-450 enzyme, CYP2D6.

Injectable Epinephrine: (See **PRECAUTIONS**, *General, Anaphylaxis*)

Carcinogenesis, Mutagenesis, Impairment of Fertility

In a two-year oral study of timolol maleate administered orally to rats, there was a statistically significant increase in the incidence of adrenal pheochromocytomas in male rats administered 300 mg/kg/day (approximately 42,000 times the systemic exposure following the maximum recommended human ophthalmic dose). Similar differences were not observed in rats administered oral doses equivalent to approximately 14,000 times the maximum recommended human ophthalmic dose.

In a lifetime oral study in mice, there were statistically significant increases in the incidence of benign and malignant pulmonary tumors, benign uterine polyps and mammary adenocarcinomas in female mice at 500 mg/kg/day (approximately 71,000 times the systemic exposure following the maximum recommended human ophthalmic dose), but not at 5 or 50 mg/kg/day (approximately 700 or 7,000 times, respectively, the systemic exposure following the maximum recommended human ophthalmic dose). In a subsequent

Continued on next page

Information on the Merck & Co., Inc. products listed on these pages is the full prescribing information from product circulars in use August 31, 1998. For information, please call 1-800-NSC MERCK [1-800-672-6372].

Consult 1999 PDR® supplements and future editions for revisions

Timoptic in Ocudose—Cont.

study in female mice, in which post-mortem examinations were limited to the uterus and the lungs, a statistically significant increase in the incidence of pulmonary tumors was again observed at 500 mg/kg/day.

The increased occurrence of mammary adenocarcinomas was associated with elevations in serum prolactin which occurred in female mice administered oral timolol at 500 mg/kg/day, but not at doses of 5 or 50 mg/kg/day. An increased incidence of mammary adenocarcinomas in rodents has been associated with administration of several other therapeutic agents that elevate serum prolactin, but no correlation between serum prolactin levels and mammary tumors has been established in humans. Furthermore, in adult human female subjects who received oral dosages of up to 60 mg of timolol maleate (the maximum recommended human oral dosage), there were no clinically meaningful changes in serum prolactin.

Timolol maleate was devoid of mutagenic potential when tested *in vivo* (mouse) in the micronucleus test and cytogenetic assay (doses up to 800 mg/kg) and *in vitro* in a neoplastic cell transformation assay (up to 100 μg/mL). In Ames tests the highest concentrations of timolol employed, 5000 or 10,000 μg/plate, were associated with statistically significant elevations of revertants observed with tester strain TA 100 (in seven replicate assays), but not in the remaining three strains. In the assays with tester strain TA 100, no consistent dose response relationship was observed, and the ratio of test to control revertants did not reach 2. A ratio of 2 is usually considered the criterion for a positive Ames test.

Reproduction and fertility studies in rats demonstrated no adverse effect on male or female fertility at doses up to 21,000 times the systemic exposure following the maximum recommended human ophthalmic dose.

Pregnancy-Teratogenic effects:

Pregnancy Category C. Teratogenicity studies with timolol in mice, rats and rabbits at oral doses up to 50 mg/kg/day (7,000 times the systemic exposure following the maximum recommended human ophthalmic dose) demonstrated no evidence of fetal malformations. Although delayed fetal ossification was observed at this dose in rats, there were no adverse effects on postnatal development of offspring. Doses of 1000 mg/kg/day (142,000 times the systemic exposure following the maximum recommended human ophthalmic dose) were maternotoxic in mice and resulted in an increased number of fetal resorptions. Increased fetal resorptions were also seen in rabbits at doses of 14,000 times the systemic exposure following the maximum recommended human ophthalmic dose, in this case without apparent maternotoxicity.

There are no adequate and well-controlled studies in pregnant women. Preservative-free TIMOPTIC in OCUDOSE should be used during pregnancy only if the potential benefit justifies the potential risk to the fetus.

Nursing Mothers

Timolol maleate has been detected in human milk following oral and ophthalmic drug administration. Because of the potential for serious adverse reactions from timolol in nursing infants, a decision should be made whether to discontinue nursing or to discontinue the drug, taking into account the importance of the drug to the mother.

Pediatric Use

Safety and effectiveness in pediatric patients have not been established.

ADVERSE REACTIONS

The most frequently reported adverse experiences have been burning and stinging upon instillation (approximately one in eight patients).

The following additional adverse experiences have been reported less frequently with ocular administration of this or other timolol maleate formulations:

BODY AS A WHOLE

Headache, asthenia/fatigue, and chest pain.

CARDIOVASCULAR

Bradycardia, arrhythmia, hypotension, hypertension, syncope, heart block, cerebral vascular accident, cerebral ischemia, cardiac failure, worsening of angina pectoris, palpitation, cardiac arrest, pulmonary edema, edema, claudication, Raynaud's phenomenon, and cold hands and feet.

DIGESTIVE

Nausea, diarrhea, dyspepsia, anorexia, and dry mouth.

IMMUNOLOGIC

Systemic lupus erythematosus.

NERVOUS SYSTEM/PSYCHIATRIC

Dizziness, increase in signs and symptoms of myasthenia gravis, paresthesia, somnolence, insomnia, nightmares, behavioral changes and psychic disturbances including depression, confusion, hallucinations, anxiety, disorientation, nervousness, and memory loss.

SKIN

Alopecia and psoriasiform rash or exacerbation of psoriasis.

HYPERSENSITIVITY

Signs and symptoms of allergic reactions, including angioedema, urticaria, and localized and generalized rash.

RESPIRATORY

Bronchospasm (predominantly in patients with pre-existing bronchospastic disease), respiratory failure, dyspnea, nasal congestion, cough and upper respiratory infections.

ENDOCRINE

Masked symptoms of hypoglycemia in diabetic patients (see **WARNINGS**).

SPECIAL SENSES

Signs and symptoms of ocular irritation including conjunctivitis, blepharitis, keratitis, ocular pain, discharge (e.g., crusting), foreign body sensation, itching and tearing, and dry eyes; ptosis; decreased corneal sensitivity; cystoid macular edema; visual disturbances including refractive changes and diplopia; pseudopemphigoid; choroidal detachment following filtration surgery (see **PRECAUTIONS**, *General*), and tinnitus.

UROGENITAL

Retroperitoneal fibrosis, decreased libido, impotence, and Peyronie's disease.

The following additional adverse effects have been reported in clinical experience with ORAL timolol maleate or other ORAL beta blocking agents, and may be considered potential effects of ophthalmic timolol maleate: *Allergic:* Erythematous rash, fever combined with aching and sore throat, laryngospasm with respiratory distress; *Body as a Whole:* Extremity pain, decreased exercise tolerance, weight loss; *Cardiovascular:* Worsening of arterial insufficiency, vasodilatation; *Digestive:* Gastrointestinal pain, hepatomegaly, vomiting, mesenteric arterial thrombosis, ischemic colitis; *Hematologic:* Nonthrombocytopenic purpura; thrombocytopenic purpura; agranulocytosis; *Endocrine:* Hyperglycemia, hypoglycemia; *Skin:* Pruritus, skin irritation, increased pigmentation, sweating; *Musculoskeletal:* Arthralgia; *Nervous System/Psychiatric:* Vertigo, local weakness, diminished concentration, reversible mental depression progressing to catatonia; an acute reversible syndrome characterized by disorientation for time and place, emotional lability, slightly clouded sensorium, and decreased performance on neuropsychometrics; *Respiratory:* Rales, bronchial obstruction; *Urogenital:* Urination difficulties.

OVERDOSAGE

There have been reports of inadvertent overdosage with Ophthalmic Solution TIMOPTIC (timolol maleate ophthalmic solution) resulting in systemic effects similar to those seen with systemic beta-adrenergic blocking agents such as dizziness, headache, shortness of breath, bradycardia, bronchospasm, and cardiac arrest (see also **ADVERSE REACTIONS**).

Overdosage has been reported with Tablets BLOCADREN* (timolol maleate). A 30 year old female ingested 650 mg of BLOCADREN (maximum recommended oral daily dose is 60 mg) and experienced second and third degree heart block. She recovered without treatment but approximately two months later developed irregular heartbeat, hypertension, dizziness, tinnitus, faintness, increased pulse rate, and borderline first degree heart block.

Significant lethality was observed in female rats and female mice after a single dose of 900 and 1190 mg/kg (5310 and 3570 mg/m^2) of timolol, respectively.

An *in vitro* hemodialysis study, using ^{14}C timolol added to human plasma or whole blood, showed that timolol was readily dialyzed from these fluids; however, a study of patients with renal failure showed that timolol did not dialyze readily.

*Registered trademark of MERCK & CO., Inc.

DOSAGE AND ADMINISTRATION

Preservative-free TIMOPTIC in OCUDOSE is a sterile solution that does not contain a preservative. The solution from one individual unit is to be used immediately after opening for administration to one or both eyes. Since sterility cannot be guaranteed after the individual unit is opened, the remaining contents should be discarded immediately after administration.

Preservative-free TIMOPTIC in OCUDOSE is available in concentrations of 0.25 and 0.5 percent. The usual starting dose is one drop of 0.25 percent Preservative-free TIMOPTIC in OCUDOSE in the affected eye(s) administered twice a day. Apply enough gentle pressure on the individual container to obtain a single drop of solution. If the clinical response is not adequate, the dosage may be changed to one drop of 0.5 percent solution in the affected eye(s) administered twice a day.

Since in some patients the pressure-lowering response to Preservative-free TIMOPTIC in OCUDOSE may require a few weeks to stabilize, evaluation should include a determination of intraocular pressure after approximately 4 weeks of treatment with Preservative-free TIMOPTIC in OCUDOSE.

If the intraocular pressure is maintained at satisfactory levels, the dosage schedule may be changed to one drop once a day in the affected eye(s). Because of diurnal variations in intraocular pressure, satisfactory response to the once-a-day dose is best determined by measuring the intraocular pressure at different times during the day.

Dosages above one drop of 0.5 percent TIMOPTIC (timolol maleate ophthalmic solution) twice a day generally have not been shown to produce further reduction in intraocular pressure. If the patient's intraocular pressure is still not at a satisfactory level on this regimen, concomitant therapy with other agent(s) for lowering intraocular pressure can be instituted taking into consideration that the preparation(s) used concomitantly may contain one or more preservatives. The concomitant use of two topical beta-adrenergic blocking agents is not recommended. (See PRECAUTIONS, *Drug Interactions, Beta-adrenergic blocking agents.*)

HOW SUPPLIED

Preservative-free Sterile Ophthalmic Solution TIMOPTIC in OCUDOSE is a clear, colorless to light yellow solution.

No. 3542—Preservative-free TIMOPTIC, 0.25% timolol equivalent, is supplied in OCUDOSE, a clear polyethylene unit dose container. Each individual unit contains 0.3 mL of solution, and is available in a foil laminate overwrapped pouch as follows:

NDC 0006-3542-60; 60 Individual Unit Doses (6505-01-316-8791, 0.25% 60 Individual Unit Doses).

No. 3543—Preservative-free TIMOPTIC, 0.5% timolol equivalent, is supplied in OCUDOSE, a clear polyethylene unit dose container. Each individual unit contains 0.3 mL of solution, and is available in a foil laminate overwrapped pouch as follows:

NDC 0006-3543-60; 60 Individual Unit Doses (6505-01-284-5154, 0.5% 60 Individual Unit Doses).

Storage

Store at room temperature, 15-30°C (59-86°F). Protect from freezing. Protect from light.

Because evaporation can occur through the unprotected polyethylene unit dose container and prolonged exposure to direct light can modify the product, the unit dose container should be kept in the protective foil overwrap and used within one month after the foil package has been opened.

Mgf. by:
MERCK & CO, INC., West Point, PA 19486, USA
Filled by:
PACO
LAKEWOOD, NJ 08701, USA
7950515 Issued August 1997

TIMOPTIC-XE® ℞

0.25% and 0.5%
Sterile Ophthalmic Gel Forming Solution
(Timolol Maleate Ophthalmic Gel Forming Solution)

DESCRIPTION

TIMOPTIC-XE* (timolol maleate ophthalmic gel forming solution) is a non-selective beta-adrenergic receptor blocking agent. Its chemical name is (-)-1-(*tert*-butyl-amino)-3-[(4-morpholino-1,2,5-thiadiazol-3-yl)oxy]-2-propanol maleate (1:1) (salt). Timolol maleate possesses an asymmetric carbon atom in its structure and is provided as the levo-isomer. The nominal optical rotation of timolol maleate is:

$$[\alpha]^{25°}_{405\ nm} \text{ in 0.1N HCl (C=5\%)} = -12.2°.$$

Its molecular formula is $C_{13}H_{24}N_4O_3S \cdot C_4H_4O_4$ and its structural formula is:

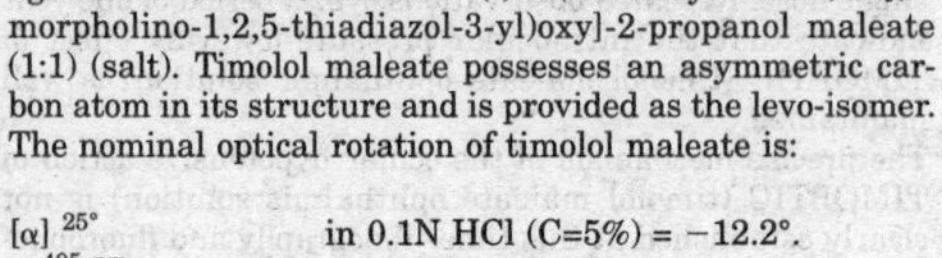

Timolol maleate has a molecular weight of 432.50. It is a white, odorless, crystalline powder which is soluble in water, methanol, and alcohol.

TIMOPTIC-XE Sterile Ophthalmic Gel Forming Solution is supplied as a sterile, isotonic, buffered, aqueous solution of timolol maleate in two dosage strengths. Each mL of TIMOPTIC-XE 0.25% contains 2.5 mg of timolol (3.4 mg of timolol maleate). Each mL of TIMOPTIC-XE 0.5% contains 5.0 mg of timolol (6.8 mg of timolol maleate). Inactive ingredients: GELRITE* gellan gum, tromethamine, mannitol, and water for injection. Preservative: benzododecinium bromide 0.012%.

GELRITE is a purified anionic heteropolysaccharide derived from gellan gum. An aqueous solution of GELRITE, in

the presence of a cation, has the ability to gel. Upon contact with the precorneal tear film, TIMOPTIC-XE forms a gel that is subsequently removed by the flow of tears.

* Registered trademark of Merck & Co., Inc.

CLINICAL PHARMACOLOGY

Mechanism of Action

Timolol maleate is a $beta_1$ and $beta_2$ (non-selective) adrenergic receptor blocking agent that does not have significant intrinsic sympathomimetic, direct myocardial depressant, or local anesthetic (membrane-stabilizing) activity.

TIMOPTIC-XE, when applied topically on the eye, has the action of reducing elevated, as well as normal intraocular pressure, whether or not accompanied by glaucoma. Elevated intraocular pressure is a major risk factor in the pathogenesis of glaucomatous visual field loss and optic nerve damage.

The precise mechanism of the ocular hypotensive action of TIMOPTIC-XE is not clearly established at this time. Tonography and fluorophotometry studies of TIMOPTIC* (timolol maleate ophthalmic solution) in man suggest that its predominant action may be related to reduced aqueous formation. However, in some studies, a slight increase in outflow facility was also observed.

Beta-adrenergic receptor blockade reduces cardiac output in both healthy subjects and patients with heart disease. In patients with severe impairment of myocardial function beta-adrenergic receptor blockade may inhibit the stimulatory effect of the sympathetic nervous system necessary to maintain adequate cardiac function.

Beta-adrenergic receptor blockade in the bronchi and bronchioles results in increased airway resistance from unopposed parasympathetic activity. Such an effect in patients with asthma or other bronchospastic conditions is potentially dangerous.

Pharmacokinetics

In a study of plasma drug concentration in six subjects, the systemic exposure to timolol was determined following once daily administration of TIMOPTIC-XE 0.5% in the morning. The mean peak plasma concentration following this morning dose was 0.28 ng/mL.

Clinical Studies

In controlled, double-masked, multicenter clinical studies, comparing TIMOPTIC-XE 0.25% to TIMOPTIC 0.25% and TIMOPTIC-XE 0.5% to TIMOPTIC 0.5%, TIMOPTIC-XE administered once a day was shown to be equally effective in lowering intraocular pressure as the equivalent concentration of TIMOPTIC administered twice a day. The effect of timolol in lowering intraocular pressure was evident for 24 hours with a single dose of TIMOPTIC-XE. Repeated observations over a period of six months indicate that the intraocular pressure-lowering effect of TIMOPTIC-XE was consistent. The results from the largest U.S. and international clinical trials comparing TIMOPTIC-XE 0.5% to TIMOPTIC 0.5% are shown in Figure 1.

Figure 1

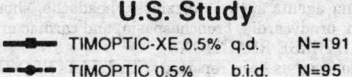

Mean IOP and Std Deviation (mm Hg) by Treatment Group

U.S. Study

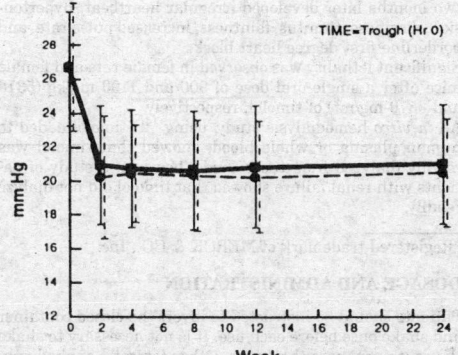

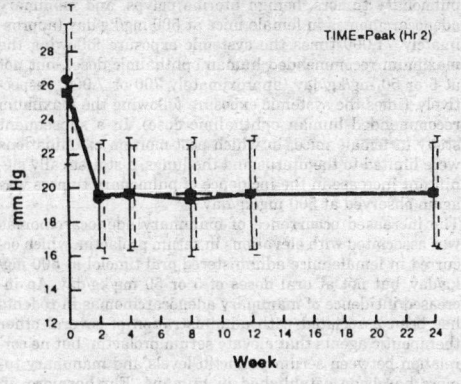

International Study

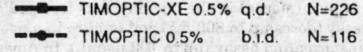

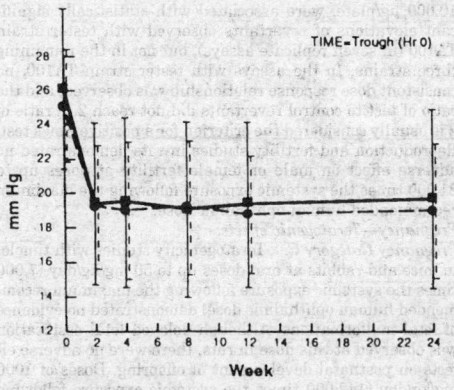

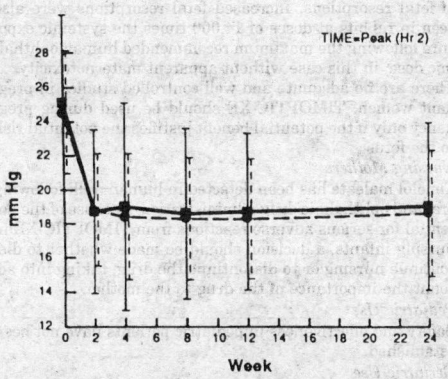

TIMOPTIC-XE administered once daily had a safety profile similar to that of an equivalent concentration of TIMOPTIC administered twice daily. Due to the physical characteristics of the formulation, there was a higher incidence of transient blurred vision in patients administered TIMOPTIC-XE. A slight reduction in resting heart rate was observed in some patients receiving TIMOPTIC-XE 0.5% (mean reduction 24 hours post-dose 0.8 beats/minute, mean reduction 2 hours post-dose 3.8 beats/minute). (See **ADVERSE REACTIONS**.)

TIMOPTIC-XE has not been studied in patients wearing contact lenses.

* Registered trademark of MERCK & CO., INC.

INDICATIONS AND USAGE

TIMOPTIC-XE Sterile Ophthalmic Gel Forming Solution is indicated in the treatment of elevated intraocular pressure in patients with ocular hypertension or open-angle glaucoma.

CONTRAINDICATIONS

TIMOPTIC-XE is contraindicated in patients with (1) bronchial asthma; (2) a history of bronchial asthma; (3) severe chronic obstructive pulmonary disease (see WARNINGS); (4) sinus bradycardia; (5) second or third degree atrioventricular block; (6) overt cardiac failure (see WARNINGS); (7) cardiogenic shock; or (8) hypersensitivity to any component of this product.

WARNINGS

As with many topically applied ophthalmic drugs, this drug is absorbed systemically.

The same adverse reactions found with systemic administration of beta-adrenergic blocking agents may occur with topical ophthalmic administration. For example, severe respiratory reactions and cardiac reactions, including death due to bronchospasm in patients with asthma, and rarely death in association with cardiac failure, have been reported following systemic or ophthalmic administration of timolol maleate. (See CONTRAINDICATIONS.)

Cardiac Failure

Sympathetic stimulation may be essential for support of the circulation in individuals with diminished myocardial contractility, and its inhibition by beta-adrenergic receptor blockade may precipitate more severe failure.

In Patients Without a History of Cardiac Failure, continued depression of the myocardium with beta-blocking agents over a period of time can, in some cases, lead to cardiac failure. At the first sign or symptom of cardiac failure, TIMOPTIC-XE should be discontinued.

Obstructive Pulmonary Disease

Patients with chronic obstructive pulmonary disease (e.g., chronic bronchitis, emphysema) of mild or moderate severity, bronchospastic disease, or a history of bronchospastic disease (other than bronchial asthma or a history of bronchial asthma, in which TIMOPTIC-XE is contraindicated [see **CONTRAINDICATIONS**]) should, in general, not receive beta-blockers, including TIMOPTIC-XE.

Major Surgery

The necessity or desirability of withdrawal of beta-adrenergic blocking agents prior to major surgery is controversial. Beta-adrenergic receptor blockade impairs the ability of the heart to respond to beta-adrenergically mediated reflex stimuli. This may augment the risk of general anesthesia in surgical procedures. Some patients receiving beta-adrenergic receptor blocking agents have experienced protracted, severe hypotension during anesthesia. Difficulty in restarting and maintaining the heartbeat has also been reported. For these reasons, in patients undergoing elective surgery, some authorities recommend gradual withdrawal of beta-adrenergic receptor blocking agents.

If necessary during surgery, the effects of beta-adrenergic blocking agents may be reversed by sufficient doses of adrenergic agonists.

Diabetes Mellitus

Beta-adrenergic blocking agents should be administered with caution in patients subject to spontaneous hypoglycemia or to diabetic patients (especially those with labile diabetes) who are receiving insulin or oral hypoglycemic agents. Beta-adrenergic receptor blocking agents may mask the signs and symptoms of acute hypoglycemia.

Thyrotoxicosis

Beta-adrenergic blocking agents may mask certain clinical signs (e.g., tachycardia) of hyperthyroidism. Patients suspected of developing thyrotoxicosis should be managed carefully to avoid abrupt withdrawal of beta-adrenergic blocking agents that might precipitate a thyroid storm.

PRECAUTIONS

General

Because of potential effects of beta-adrenergic blocking agents on blood pressure and pulse, these agents should be used with caution in patients with cerebrovascular insufficiency. If signs or symptoms suggesting reduced cerebral blood flow develop following initiation of therapy with TIMOPTIC-XE, alternative therapy should be considered. There have been reports of bacterial keratitis associated with the use of multiple dose containers of topical ophthalmic products. These containers had been inadvertently contaminated by patients who, in most cases, had a concurrent corneal disease or a disruption of the ocular epithelial surface. (See **PRECAUTIONS**, *Information for Patients*.) Choroidal detachment after filtration procedures has been reported with the administration of aqueous suppressant therapy (e.g. timolol).

Continued on next page

Timoptic-XE—Cont.

Angle-closure glaucoma: In patients with angle-closure glaucoma, the immediate objective of treatment is to reopen the angle. This may require constricting the pupil. Timolol maleate has little or no effect on the pupil. TIMOPTIC-XE should not be used alone in the treatment of angle-closure glaucoma.

Anaphylaxis: While taking beta-blockers, patients with a history of atopy or a history of severe anaphylactic reactions to a variety of allergens may be more reactive to repeated accidental, diagnostic, or therapeutic challenge with such allergens. Such patients may be unresponsive to the usual doses of epinephrine used to treat anaphylactic reactions.

Muscle Weakness: Beta-adrenergic blockade has been reported to potentiate muscle weakness consistent with certain myasthenic symptoms (e.g., diplopia, ptosis, and generalized weakness). Timolol has been reported rarely to increase muscle weakness in some patients with myasthenia gravis or myasthenic symptoms.

Information for Patients

Patients should be instructed to avoid allowing the tip of the dispensing container to contact the eye or surrounding structures.

Patients should also be instructed that ocular solutions, if handled improperly or if the tip of the dispensing container contacts the eye or surrounding structures, can become contaminated by common bacteria known to cause ocular infections. Serious damage to the eye and subsequent loss of vision may result from using contaminated solutions. (See **PRECAUTIONS,** *General.*)

Patients should also be advised that if they have ocular surgery or develop an intercurrent ocular condition (e.g., trauma or infection), they should immediately seek their physician's advice concerning the continued use of the present multidose container.

Patients should be instructed to invert the closed container and shake once before each use. It is not necessary to shake the container more than once.

Patients requiring concomitant topical ophthalmic medications should be instructed to administer these at least 10 minutes before instilling TIMOPTIC-XE.

Patients with bronchial asthma, a history of bronchial asthma, severe chronic obstructive pulmonary disease, sinus bradycardia, second or third degree atrioventricular block, or cardiac failure should be advised not to take this product. (See **CONTRAINDICATIONS.**)

Transient blurred vision, generally lasting from 30 seconds to 5 minutes, following instillation, and potential visual disturbances may impair the ability to perform hazardous tasks such as operating machinery or driving a motor vehicle.

Drug Interactions

Beta-adrenergic blocking agents: Patients who are receiving a beta-adrenergic blocking agent orally and TIMOPTIC-XE should be observed for potential additive effects of beta-blockade, both systemic and on intraocular pressure. The concomitant use of two topical beta-adrenergic blocking agents is not recommended.

Calcium antagonists: Caution should be used in the coadministration of beta-adrenergic blocking agents, such as TIMOPTIC-XE, and oral or intravenous calcium antagonists because of possible atrioventricular conduction disturbances, left ventricular failure, or hypotension. In patients with impaired cardiac function, coadministration should be avoided.

Catecholamine-depleting drugs: Close observation of the patient is recommended when a beta blocker is administered to patients receiving catecholamine-depleting drugs such as reserpine, because of possible additive effects and the production of hypotension and/or marked bradycardia, which may result in vertigo, syncope, or postural hypotension.

Digitalis and calcium antagonists: The concomitant use of beta-adrenergic blocking agents with digitalis and calcium antagonists may have additive effects in prolonging atrioventricular conduction time.

Quinidine: Potentiated systemic beta-blockade (e.g., decreased heart rate) has been reported during combined treatment with quinidine and timolol, possibly because quinidine inhibits the metabolism of timolol via the P-450 enzyme, CYP2D6.

Injectable Epinephrine: (See **PRECAUTIONS,** *General, Anaphylaxis:*)

Carcinogenesis, Mutagenesis, Impairment of Fertility

In a two-year study of timolol maleate administered orally to rats, there was a statistically significant increase in the incidence of adrenal pheochromocytomas in male rats administered 300 mg/kg/day (approximately 42,000 times the systemic exposure following the maximum recommended human ophthalmic dose). Similar differences were not observed in rats administered oral doses equivalent to approximately 14,000 times the maximum recommended human ophthalmic dose.

In a lifetime oral study in mice, there were statistically significant increases in the incidence of benign and malignant pulmonary tumors, benign uterine polyps, and mammary adenocarcinomas in female mice at 500 mg/kg/day (approximately 71,000 times the systemic exposure following the maximum recommended human ophthalmic dose), but not at 5 or 50 mg/kg/day (approximately 700 or 7,000, respectively, times the systemic exposure following the maximum recommended human ophthalmic dose). In a subsequent study in female mice, in which post-mortem examinations were limited to the uterus and the lungs, a statistically significant increase in the incidence of pulmonary tumors was again observed at 500 mg/kg/day.

The increased occurrence of mammary adenocarcinomas was associated with elevations in serum prolactin, which occurred in female mice administered oral timolol at 500 mg/kg/day, but not at oral doses of 5 or 50 mg/kg/day. An increased incidence of mammary adenocarcinomas in rodents has been associated with administration of several other therapeutic agents that elevate serum prolactin, but no correlation between serum prolactin levels and mammary tumors has been established in humans. Furthermore, in adult human female subjects who received oral dosages of up to 60 mg of timolol maleate (the maximum recommended human oral dosage), there were no clinically meaningful changes in serum prolactin.

Timolol maleate was devoid of mutagenic potential when tested *in vivo* (mouse) in the micronucleus test and cytogenetic assay (doses up to 800 mg) and *in vitro* in a neoplastic cell transformation assay (up to 100 µg/mL). In Ames tests, the highest concentrations of timolol employed, 5,000 or 10,000 µg/plate, were associated with statistically significant elevations of revertants observed with tester strain TA100 (in seven replicate assays), but not in the remaining three strains. In the assays with tester strain TA100, no consistent dose response relationship was observed, and the ratio of test to control revertants did not reach 2. A ratio of 2 is usually considered the criterion for a positive Ames test.

Reproduction and fertility studies in rats demonstrated no adverse effect on male or female fertility at doses up to 21,000 times the systemic exposure following the maximum recommended human ophthalmic dose.

Pregnancy—Teratogenic effects:

Pregnancy Category C. Teratogenicity studies with timolol in mice and rabbits at oral doses up to 50 mg/kg/day (7,000 times the systemic exposure following the maximum recommended human ophthalmic dose) demonstrated no evidence of fetal malformations. Although delayed fetal ossification was observed at this dose in rats, there were no adverse effects on postnatal development of offspring. Doses of 1000 mg/kg/day (142,000 times the systemic exposure following the maximum recommended human ophthalmic dose) were maternotoxic in mice and resulted in an increased number of fetal resorptions. Increased fetal resorptions were also seen in rabbits at doses of 14,000 times the systemic exposure following the maximum recommended human ophthalmic dose, in this case without apparent maternotoxicity.

There are no adequate and well-controlled studies in pregnant women. TIMOPTIC-XE should be used during pregnancy only if the potential benefit justifies the potential risk to the fetus.

Nursing Mothers

Timolol maleate has been detected in human milk following oral and ophthalmic drug administration. Because of the potential for serious adverse reactions from TIMOPTIC-XE in nursing infants, a decision should be made whether to discontinue nursing or to discontinue the drug, taking into account the importance of the drug to the mother.

Pediatric Use

Safety and effectiveness in pediatric patients have not been established.

Geriatric Use

Of the total number of patients in clinical studies of TIMOPTIC-XE, 46% were 65 years of age and over, while 14% were 75 years of age and over. No overall differences in effectiveness or safety were observed between these patients and younger patients, but greater sensitivity of some older individuals to the product cannot be ruled out.

ADVERSE REACTIONS

In clinical trials, transient blurred vision upon instillation of the drop was reported in approximately one in three patients (lasting from 30 seconds to 5 minutes). Less than 1% of patients discontinued from the studies due to blurred vision. The frequency of patients reporting burning and stinging upon instillation was comparable between TIMOPTIC-XE and TIMOPTIC (approximately one in eight patients).

Adverse experiences reported in 1–5% of patients were:

Ocular: Pain, conjunctivitis, discharge (e.g. crusting), foreign body sensation, itching and tearing;

Systemic: Headache, dizziness, and upper respiratory infections.

The following additional adverse experiences have been reported with the ocular administration of this or other timolol maleate formulations:

BODY AS A WHOLE
Asthenia/fatigue, and chest pain.

CARDIOVASCULAR
Bradycardia, arrhythmia, hypotension, hypertension, syncope, heart block, cerebral vascular accident, cerebral ischemia, cardiac failure, worsening of angina pectoris, palpitation, cardiac arrest, pulmonary edema, edema, claudication, Raynaud's phenomenon, and cold hands and feet.

DIGESTIVE
Nausea, diarrhea, dyspepsia, anorexia, and dry mouth.

IMMUNOLOGIC
Systemic lupus erythematosus.

NERVOUS SYSTEM/PSYCHIATRIC
Increase in signs and symptoms of myasthenia gravis, paresthesia, somnolence, insomnia, nightmares, behavioral changes and psychic disturbances including depression, confusion, hallucinations, anxiety, disorientation, nervousness, and memory loss.

SKIN
Alopecia and psoriasiform rash or exacerbation of psoriasis.

HYPERSENSITIVITY
Signs and symptoms of allergic reactions, including angioedema, urticaria, and localized and generalized rash.

RESPIRATORY
Bronchospasm (predominantly in patients with preexisting bronchospastic disease), respiratory failure, dyspnea, nasal congestion, and cough.

ENDOCRINE
Masked symptoms of hypoglycemia in diabetic patients (see **WARNINGS**).

SPECIAL SENSES
Signs and symptoms of ocular irritation including blepharitis, keratitis, and dry eyes; ptosis; decreased corneal sensitivity; cystoid macular edema; visual disturbances including refractive changes and diplopia; pseudopemphigoid; choroidal detachment following filtration surgery (see PRECAUTIONS, *General*); and tinnitus.

UROGENITAL
Retroperitoneal fibrosis, decreased libido, impotence, and Peyronie's disease.

The following additional adverse effects have been reported in clinical experience with ORAL timolol maleate or other ORAL beta-blocking agents and may be considered potential effects of ophthalmic timolol maleate: *Allergic:* Erythematous rash, fever combined with aching and sore throat, laryngospasm with respiratory distress; *Body as a Whole:* Extremity pain, decreased exercise tolerance, weight loss; *Cardiovascular:* Worsening of arterial insufficiency, vasodilatation; *Digestive:* Gastrointestinal pain, hepatomegaly, vomiting, mesenteric arterial thrombosis, ischemic colitis; *Hematologic:* Nonthrombocytopenic purpura, thrombocytopenic purpura, agranulocytosis; *Endocrine:* Hyperglycemia, hypoglycemia; *Skin:* Pruritus, skin irritation, increased pigmentation, sweating; *Musculoskeletal:* Arthralgia; *Nervous System/Psychiatric:* Vertigo, local weakness, diminished concentration, reversible mental depression progressing to catatonia, an acute reversible syndrome characterized by disorientation for time and place, emotional lability, slightly clouded sensorium, and decreased performance on neuropsychometrics; *Respiratory:* Rales, bronchial obstruction; *Urogenital:* Urination difficulties.

OVERDOSAGE

No data are available in regard to human overdosage with or accidental oral ingestion of TIMOPTIC-XE.

There have been reports of inadvertent overdosage with TIMOPTIC Ophthalmic Solution resulting in systemic effects similar to those seen with systemic beta-adrenergic blocking agents such as dizziness, headache, shortness of breath, bradycardia, bronchospasm, and cardiac arrest (see also ADVERSE REACTIONS).

Overdosage has been reported with Tablets BLOCADREN* (Timolol Maleate). A 30 year old female ingested 650 mg of BLOCADREN (maximum recommended oral daily dose is 60 mg) and experienced second and third degree heart block. She recovered without treatment but approximately two months later developed irregular heartbeat, hypertension, dizziness, tinnitus, faintness, increased pulse rate, and borderline first degree heart block.

Significant lethality was observed in female rats and female mice after a single oral dose of 900 and 1190 mg/kg (5310 and 3570 mg/m^2) of timolol, respectively.

An *in vitro* hemodialysis study, using ^{14}C timolol added to human plasma or whole blood, showed that timolol was readily dialyzed from these fluids; however, a study of patients with renal failure showed that timolol did not dialyze readily.

*Registered trademark of MERCK & CO., Inc.

DOSAGE AND ADMINISTRATION

Patients should be instructed to invert the closed container and shake once before each use. It is not necessary to shake the container more than once. Other topically applied ophthalmic medications should be administered at least 10

minutes before TIMOPTIC-XE. (See **PRECAUTIONS**, *Information for Patients* and accompanying INSTRUCTIONS FOR USE.)

TIMOPTIC-XE Sterile Ophthalmic Gel Forming Solution is available in concentrations of 0.25% and 0.5%. The dose is one drop of TIMOPTIC-XE (either 0.25% or 0.5%) in the affected eye(s) once a day.

Because in some patients the pressure-lowering response to TIMOPTIC-XE may require a few weeks to stabilize, evaluation should include a determination of intraocular pressure after approximately 4 weeks of treatment with TIMOPTIC-XE.

Dosages higher than one drop of 0.5% TIMOPTIC-XE once a day have not been studied. If the patient's intraocular pressure is still not at a satisfactory level on this regimen, concomitant therapy can be considered. The concomitant use of two topical beta-adrenergic blocking agents is not recommended. (See **PRECAUTIONS**, *Drug Interactions, Beta-adrenergic blocking agents*.)

When patients have been switched from therapy with TIMOPTIC administered twice daily to TIMOPTIC-XE administered once daily, the ocular hypotensive effect has remained consistent.

HOW SUPPLIED

TIMOPTIC-XE Sterile Ophthalmic Gel Forming Solution is a colorless to nearly colorless, slightly opalescent, and slightly viscous solution.

No. 3557—TIMOPTIC-XE Sterile Ophthalmic Gel Forming Solution, 0.25% timolol equivalent, is supplied in OCUMETER*, a white, opaque, plastic, ophthalmic dispenser with a controlled drop tip as follows:

NDC 0006-3557-32, 2.5 mL
(6505-01-388-0967, 0.25% 2.5 mL)
NDC 0006-3557-03, 5 mL
(6505-01-387-9495, 0.25% 5 mL).

No. 3558—TIMOPTIC-XE Sterile Ophthalmic Gel Forming Solution, 0.5% timolol equivalent, is supplied in OCUMETER, a white, opaque, plastic, ophthalmic dispenser with a controlled drop tip as follows:

NDC 0006-3558-32, 2.5 mL
(6505-01-388-0964, 0.5% 2.5 mL)
NDC 0006-3558-03, 5 mL
(6505-01-387-9482, 0.5% 5 mL).

Storage

Store between 15° and 25°C (59° and 77°F). **AVOID FREEZING.** Protect from light.

TIMOPTIC-XE®
0.25% and 0.5%
(Timolol Maleate Ophthalmic Gel Forming Solution)

INSTRUCTIONS FOR USE

Please follow these instructions carefully when using TIMOPTIC-XE*. Use TIMOPTIC-XE as prescribed by your doctor.

1. If you use other topically applied ophthalmic medications, they should be administered at least 10 minutes before TIMOPTIC-XE.
2. Wash hands before each use.
3. Invert the closed bottle and shake ONCE before each use. (It is not necessary to shake the bottle more than once.)

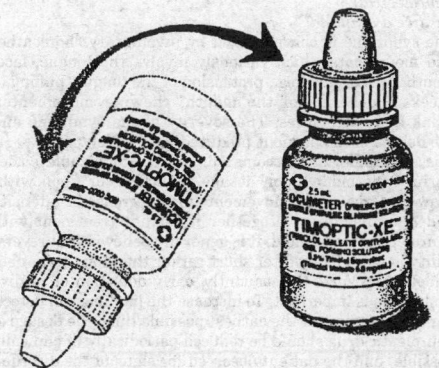

4. Remove the cap from the bottle carefully so that the dispenser tip does not touch anything. Place the cap in a clean, dry area.
5. Hold the bottle between the thumb and index finger. Use the index finger of the other hand to pull down the lower eyelid to form a pocket for the eye drop. Tilt your head back.
   [See figure at top of next column]
6. Place the dispenser tip close to your eye and gently squeeze the bottle to administer one drop. Remove pressure after a single drop has been released. If instructed, repeat steps 5 and 6 in the other eye.

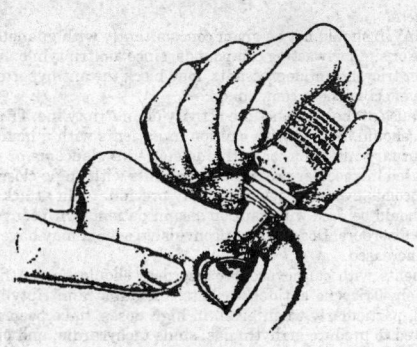

DO NOT ALLOW THE DISPENSER TIP TO TOUCH THE EYE OR SURROUNDING AREAS.

Ophthalmic medications, if handled improperly, can become contaminated by common bacteria known to cause eye infections. Serious damage to the eye and subsequent loss of vision may result from using contaminated ophthalmic medications. If you think your medication may be contaminated, or if you develop an eye infection, contact your doctor immediately concerning continued use of this bottle.

7. Replace the cap. Store the bottle at room temperature in an upright position in a clean area.
8. The dispenser tip is designed to provide a pre-measured drop; therefore, do NOT enlarge the hole of the dispenser.
9. Do NOT wash the tip of the dispenser with water, soap, or any other cleaner.

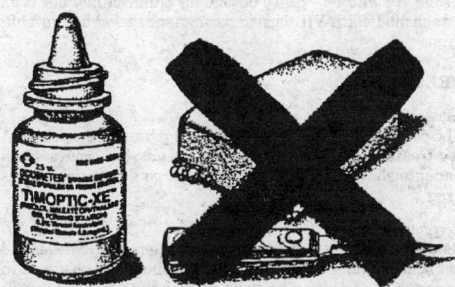

WARNING: Keep out of reach of children.
If you have any questions about the use of TIMOPTIC-XE, please consult your doctor.

TRIAVIL® Tablets   ℞
(Perphenazine-Amitriptyline HCl), U.S.P.

The following information was current at the time of publication in the 1995 edition of PDR. Effective December 1994, ownership and marketing responsibility for TRIAVIL was transferred to Lotus Biochemical. Please consult Lotus Biochemical for current prescribing information before prescribing this product.

DESCRIPTION

TRIAVIL* (Perphenazine-Amitriptyline HCl), a broad-spectrum psychotherapeutic agent for the management of outpatients and hospitalized patients with psychoses or neuroses characterized by mixtures of anxiety or agitation with symptoms of depression, is a combination of perphenazine and amitriptyline HCl. Since such mixed syndromes can occur in patients with various degrees of intensity of mental illness, TRIAVIL tablets are provided in multiple combinations to afford dosage flexibility for optimum management. TRIAVIL is a combination of perphenazine, a piperazine phenothiazine, and amitriptyline HCl, a dibenzocycloheptadiene.

Perphenazine

Perphenazine is 4-[3-(2-chloro-10*H*-phenothiazin-10-yl)propyl]-1-piperazineethanol. Its empirical formula is $C_{21}H_{26}ClN_3OS$ and its structural formula is:

[See chemical structure at top of next column]

Perphenazine has a molecular weight of 403.97. It is a white, odorless, bitter-tasting powder that is insoluble in water.

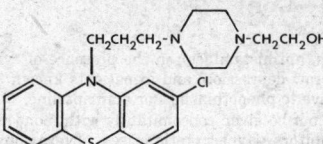

Amitriptyline HCl

Amitriptyline hydrochloride is 3-(10,11-dihydro-5*H*-dibenzo[*a, d*]cyclohepten-5-ylidene)-*N,N*-dimethyl-1-propanamine hydrochloride. Its empirical formula is $C_{20}H_{23}N \cdot HCl$ and its structural formula is:

Amitriptyline HCl, a dibenzocycloheptadiene derivative, has a molecular weight of 313.87. It is a white, odorless, crystalline compound which is freely soluble in water.

Tablets TRIAVIL are supplied in 5 potencies:
TRIAVIL 2-10, containing 2 mg of perphenazine
          and 10 mg of amitriptyline HCl.
TRIAVIL 2-25, containing 2 mg of perphenazine
          and 25 mg of amitriptyline HCl.
TRIAVIL 4-10, containing 4 mg of perphenazine
          and 10 mg of amitriptyline HCl.
TRIAVIL 4-25, containing 4 mg of perphenazine
          and 25 mg of amitriptyline HCl.
TRIAVIL 4-50, containing 4 mg of perphenazine
          and 50 mg of amitriptyline HCl.

Inactive ingredients are calcium phosphate, cellulose, hydroxypropyl cellulose, hydroxypropyl methylcellulose, lactose, magnesium stearate, starch, talc, and titanium dioxide. TRIAVIL 2-10 also contains FD&C Blue 1. TRIAVIL 2-25 and 4-50 also contain FD&C Yellow 6. TRIAVIL 4-10 also contains iron oxide. TRIAVIL 4-25 also contains D&C Yellow 10 and FD&C Yellow 6.

*Registered trademark of MERCK & CO., INC.

ACTIONS

Perphenazine—In common with all members of the piperazine group of phenothiazine derivatives, perphenazine has greater behavioral potency than phenothiazine derivatives of other groups without a corresponding increase in autonomic, hematologic, or hepatic side effects.

Extrapyramidal effects, however, may occur more frequently. These effects are interpreted as neuropharmacologic. They usually regress after discontinuation of the drug. Perphenazine is a potent tranquilizer and also a potent antiemetic. Orally, its milligram potency is about five or six times that of chlorpromazine with respect to behavioral effects. It is capable of alleviating symptoms of anxiety, tension, psychomotor excitement, and other manifestations of emotional stress without apparent dulling of mental acuity.

Amitriptyline HCl is an antidepressant with sedative effects. Its mechanism of action in man is not known. It is not a monoamine oxidase inhibitor and it does not act primarily by stimulation of the central nervous system.

INDICATIONS

TRIAVIL is recommended for treatment of (1) patients with *moderate to severe anxiety and/or agitation and depressed mood*, (2) patients with *depression in whom anxiety and/or agitation are severe*, and (3) patients with *depression and anxiety in association with chronic physical disease*. In many of these patients anxiety masks the depressive state so that, although therapy with a tranquilizer appears to be indicated, the administration of a tranquilizer alone will not be adequate.

Schizophrenic patients who have associated depressive symptoms should be considered for therapy with TRIAVIL. Many patients presenting symptoms such as agitation, anxiety, insomnia, psychomotor retardation, functional somatic complaints, a feeling of tiredness, loss of interest, and anorexia have responded well to therapy with TRIAVIL.

CONTRAINDICATIONS

TRIAVIL is contraindicated in depression of the central nervous system from drugs (barbiturates, alcohol, narcotics,

Continued on next page

Triavil—Cont.

analgesics, antihistamines); in the presence of evidence of bone marrow depression; and in patients known to be hypersensitive to phenothiazines or amitriptyline.
It should not be given concomitantly with monoamine oxidase inhibitors. Hyperpyretic crises, severe convulsions, and deaths have occurred in patients receiving tricyclic antidepressants and monoamine oxidase inhibitors simultaneously. When it is desired to replace a monoamine oxidase inhibitor with TRIAVIL, a minimum of 14 days should be allowed to elapse after the former is discontinued. TRIAVIL should then be initiated cautiously with gradual increase in dosage until optimum response is achieved.
Amitriptyline HCl is not recommended for use during the acute recovery phase following myocardial infarction.

WARNINGS

Tardive dyskinesia
Tardive dyskinesia, a syndrome consisting of potentially irreversible, involuntary dyskinetic movements may develop in patients treated with neuroleptic (antipsychotic) drugs. Although the prevalence of the syndrome appears to be highest among the elderly, especially elderly women, it is impossible to rely upon prevalence estimates to predict, at the inception of neuroleptic treatment, which patients are likely to develop the syndrome. Whether neuroleptic drug products differ in their potential to cause tardive dyskinesia is unknown.
Both the risk of developing the syndrome and the likelihood that it will become irreversible are believed to increase as the duration of treatment and the total cumulative dose of neuroleptic drugs administered to the patient increase. However, the syndrome can develop, although much less commonly, after relatively brief treatment periods at low doses.
There is no known treatment for established cases of tardive dyskinesia, although the syndome may remit, partially or completely, if neuroleptic treatment is withdrawn. Neuroleptic treatment, itself, however, may suppress (or partially suppress) the signs and symptoms of the syndrome and thereby may possibly mask the underlying disease process. The effect that symptomatic suppression has upon the long-term course of the syndrome is unknown.
Given these considerations, neuroleptics should be prescribed in a manner that is most likely to minimize the occurrence of tardive dyskinesia. Chronic neuroleptic treatment should generally be reserved for patients who suffer from a chronic mental illness that, 1) is known to respond to neuroleptic drugs, and, 2) for whom alternative, equally effective, but potentially less harmful treatments are *not* available or appropriate. In patients who do require chronic treatment, the smallest dose and the shortest duration of treatment producing a satisfactory clinical response should be sought. The need for continued treatment should be reassessed periodically.
If signs and symptoms of tardive dyskinesia appear in a patient on neuroleptics, drug discontinuation should be considered. However, some patients may require treatment despite the presence of the syndrome.
(For further information about the description of tardive dyskinesia and its clinical detection, please refer to the section on ADVERSE REACTIONS).
Neuroleptic Malignant Syndrome (NMS)
A potentially fatal symptom complex sometimes referred to as Neuroleptic Malignant Syndrome (NMS) has been reported in association with antipsychotic drugs. Clinical manifestations of NMS are hyperpyrexia, muscle rigidity, altered mental status and evidence of autonomic instability (irregular pulse or blood pressure, tachycardia, diaphoresis, and cardiac dysrhythmias).
The diagnostic evaluation of patients with this syndrome is complicated. In arriving at a diagnosis, it is important to identify cases where the clinical presentation includes both serious medical illness (e.g., pneumonia, systemic infection, etc.) and untreated or inadequately treated extrapyramidal signs and symptoms (EPS). Other important considerations in the differential diagnosis include central anticholinergic toxicity, heat stroke, drug fever and primary central nervous system (CNS) pathology.
The management of NMS should include 1) immediate discontinuation of antipsychotic drugs and other drugs not essential to concurrent therapy, 2) intensive symptomatic treatment and medical monitoring, and 3) treatment of any concomitant serious medical problems for which specific treatments are available. There is no general agreement about specific pharmacological treatment regimens for uncomplicated NMS.
If a patient requires antipsychotic drug treatment after recovery from NMS, the potential reintroduction of drug therapy should be carefully considered. The patient should be carefully monitored, since recurrences of NMS have been reported.

General
TRIAVIL should not be given concomitantly with guanethidine or similarly acting compounds, since amitriptyline, like other tricyclic antidepressants, may block the antihypertensive effect of these compounds.
Because of the atropine-like activity of amitriptyline, TRIAVIL should be used with caution in patients with a history of urinary retention, or with angle-closure glaucoma or increased intraocular pressure. In patients with angle-closure glaucoma, even average doses may precipitate an attack.
It should be used with caution also in patients with convulsive disorders. Dosage of anticonvulsive agents may have to be increased.
Patients with cardiovascular disorders should be watched closely. Tricyclic antidepressants, including amitriptyline HCl, particularly when given in high doses, have been reported to produce arrhythmias, sinus tachycardia, and prolongation of the conduction time. Myocardial infarction and stroke have been reported with drugs of this class.
Close supervision is required when amitriptyline HCl is given to hyperthyroid patients or those receiving thyroid medication.
TRIAVIL may enhance the response to alcohol and the effects of barbiturates and other CNS depressants. In patients who may use alcohol excessively, it should be borne in mind that the potentiation may increase the danger inherent in any suicide attempt or overdosage. Delirium has been reported with concurrent administration of amitriptyline and disulfiram.
Usage in Pregnancy—TRIAVIL is not recommended for use in pregnant patients or in nursing mothers at this time. Reproduction studies in rats have shown no fetal abnormalities; however, clinical experience and follow-up in pregnancy have been limited, and the possibility of adverse effects on fetal development must be considered.
Usage in Children—Since dosage for children has not been established, TRIAVIL is not recommended for use in children.

PRECAUTIONS

General
The possibility of suicide in depressed patients remains during treatment and until significant remission occurs. Such patients should not have access to large quantities of this drug.

Perphenazine
As with all phenothiazine compounds, perphenazine should not be used indiscriminately. Caution should be observed in giving it to patients who have previously exhibited severe adverse reactions to other phenothiazines.
Some of the untoward actions of perphenazine tend to appear more frequently when high doses are used. However, as with other phenothiazine compounds, patients receiving perphenazine in any dosage should be kept under close supervision.
The antiemetic effect of perphenazine may obscure signs of toxicity due to overdosage of other drugs, or render more difficult the diagnosis of disorders such as brain tumors or intestinal obstruction.
A significant, not otherwise explained, rise in body temperature may suggest individual intolerance to perphenazine, in which case TRIAVIL should be discontinued.
Neuroleptic drugs elevate prolactin levels; the elevation persists during chronic administration. Tissue culture experiments indicate that approximately one third of human breast cancers are prolactin dependent *in vitro,* a factor of potential importance if the prescription of these drugs is contemplated in a patient with a previously detected breast cancer. Although disturbances such as galactorrhea, amenorrhea, gynecomastia, and impotence have been reported, the clinical significance of elevated serum prolactin levels is unknown for most patients. An increase in mammary neoplasms has been found in rodents after chronic administration of neuroleptic drugs. Neither clinical studies nor epidemiologic studies conducted to date, however, have shown an association between chronic administration of these drugs and mammary tumorigenesis; the available evidence is considered too limited to be conclusive at this time.

Amitriptyline HCl
Depressed patients, particularly those with known manic depressive illness, may experience a shift to mania or hypomania. Patients with paranoid symptomatology may have an exaggeration of such symptoms. The tranquilizing effect of TRIAVIL seems to reduce the likelihood of these effects.
Concurrent administration of amitriptyline HCl and electroshock therapy may increase the hazards associated with such therapy. Such treatment should be limited to patients for whom it is essential.
Discontinue the drug several days before elective surgery if possible.
Both elevation and lowering of blood sugar levels have been reported.
Amitriptyline HCl should be used with caution in patients with impaired liver function.

Information for Patients
While on therapy with TRIAVIL, patients should be advised as to the possible impairment of mental and/or physical abilities required for performance of hazardous tasks, such as operating machinery or driving a motor vehicle.
Drug Interactions
Perphenazine
If hypotension develops, epinephrine should not be employed, as its action is blocked and partially reversed by perphenazine.
Phenothiazines may potentiate the action of central nervous system depressants (opiates, analgesics, antihistamines, barbiturates, alcohol) and atropine. In concurrent therapy with any of these, TRIAVIL should be given in reduced dosage. Phenothiazines also may potentiate the action of heat and phosphorous insecticides.
Amitriptyline HCl
When amitriptyline HCl is given with anticholinergic agents or sympathomimetic drugs, including epinephrine combined with local anesthetics, close supervision and careful adjustment of dosages are required.
Hyperpyrexia has been reported when amitriptyline HCl is administered with anticholinergic agents or with neuroleptic drugs, particularly during hot weather.
Paralytic ileus may occur in patients taking tricyclic antidepressants in combination with anticholinergic-type drugs.
Cimetidine is reported to reduce hepatic metabolism of certain tricyclic antidepressants, thereby delaying elimination and increasing steady-state concentrations of these drugs. Clinically significant effects have been reported with the tricyclic antidepressants when used concomitantly with cimetidine. Increases in plasma levels of tricyclic antidepressants, and in the frequency and severity of side effects, particularly anticholinergic, have been reported when cimetidine was added to the drug regimen. Discontinuation of cimetidine in well-controlled patients receiving tricyclic antidepressants and cimetidine may decrease the plasma levels and efficacy of the antidepressants.
Caution is advised if patients receive large doses of ethchlorvynol concurrently. Transient delirium has been reported in patients who were treated with 1 g of ethchlorvynol and 75-150 mg of amitriptyline HCl.

ADVERSE REACTIONS

To date, clinical evaluation of TRIAVIL has not revealed any adverse reactions peculiar to the combination. The adverse reactions that occurred were limited to those that have been reported previously for perphenazine and amitriptyline.
Treatment with TRIAVIL is commonly associated with sedation, hypotension, neurological impairments, and dry mouth.
Perphenazine
The common acute neurological effects of neuroleptic drugs, including perphenazine, consist of dystonia, akathisia or motor restlessness, and pseudoparkinsonism.
More chronic use of neuroleptics may be associated with the development of tardive dyskinesia. The salient features of this syndrome are described in the WARNINGS section and below.
The following adverse reactions have been reported and, within each category, are listed in order of decreasing severity.
Neurological:
Tardive dyskinesia:
The syndrome is characterized by involuntary choreoathetoid movements which variously involve the tongue, face, mouth, lips, or jaw (e.g., protrusion of the tongue, puffing of cheeks, puckering of the mouth, chewing movements), trunk and extremities. The severity of the syndrome and the degree of impairment produced vary widely.
The syndrome may become clinically recognizable either during treatment, upon dosage reduction, or upon withdrawal of treatment. Movements may decrease in intensity and may disappear altogether if further treatment with neuroleptics is withheld. It is generally believed that reversibility is more likely after short rather than long term neuroleptic exposure. Consequently, early detection of tardive dyskinesia is important. To increase the likelihood of detecting the syndrome at the earliest possible time, the dosage of neuroleptic drug should be reduced periodically (if clinically possible) and the patient observed for signs of the disorder.
It has been suggested that fine vermicular movements of the tongue may be an early sign of the syndrome, and that the full-blown syndrome may not develop if medication is stopped when lingual vermiculation appears.
1. Dystonia
This may present as acute, reversible torticollis, opisthotonos, carpopedal spasm, trismus, dysphagia, respiratory difficulty, oculogyric crisis, and protrusion of the tongue. Treatment consists of the parenteral administration of either an anticholinergic antiparkinsonian agent or diphenhydramine.
2. Akathisia
Akathisia presents as constant motor restlessness. The patient with akathisia often complains, *when asked,* about his/

her inability to stop moving. Akathisia should *not* be treated with an increased dose of neuroleptic; rather, the dose of antipsychotic may be lowered until the motor restlessness has subsided. The efficacy of anticholinergic treatment of this side effect is unestablished.
3. Pseudoparkinsonism
Pseudoparkinsonism refers to a drug-induced state similar to the classic syndrome. Generally, anticholinergic antiparksonian agents (i.e., benztropine, biperiden, procyclidine, or trihexphenidyl) and amantadine are helpful in alleviating symptoms that cannot be managed by neuroleptic dose reduction. The value of prophylactic antiparkinsonian drug therapy has not been established. The need for continued use of antiparkinsonian medication should be re-evaluated periodically.
Cardiovascular: Hypotension, hypertension, tachycardia, peripheral edema, occasional change in pulse rate, ECG abnormalities (quinidine-like effect), reversed epinephrine effect.
CNS and Neuromuscular: Neuroleptic malignant syndrome (see WARNINGS); extrapyramidal symptoms, including acute dyskinesia (see *Neurological*); reactivation of psychoses and production of catatonic-like states; paradoxical excitement; ataxia; muscle weakness; hypnotic effects; mild insomnia; lassitude; headache; hyperflexia; altered cerebrospinal fluid proteins.
Autonomic: Urinary frequency or incontinence, dry mouth or salivation, nasal congestion.
Allergic: Anaphylactoid reactions, laryngeal edema, asthma, angioneurotic edema.
Hematologic: Blood dyscrasias including pancytopenia, agranulocytosis, leukopenia, thrombocytopenic purpura, eosinophilia.
Gastrointestinal: Liver damage (jaundice, biliary stasis), obstipation, vomiting, nausea, constipation, anorexia.
Dermatologic: Eczema up to exfoliative dermatitis, urticaria, erythema, itching, photosensitivity.
Ophthalmic: Pigmentation of the cornea and lens, blurred vision.
Endocrine: Lactation, galactorrhea, hyperglycemia, gynecomastia, disturbances in menstrual cycle.
Other: False-positive pregnancy tests, including immunologic.
Other adverse reactions that should be considered because they have been reported with various phenothiazine compounds, but not with perphenazine, include:
CNS and Neuromuscular: Grand mal convulsions, cerebral edema.
Gastrointestinal: Polyphagia.
Dermatologic: Photophobia, pigmentation.
Ophthalmic: Pigmentary retinopathy.
Endocrine: Failure of ejaculation.
Amitriptyline HCl
Within each category the following adverse reactions are listed in order of decreasing severity. Included in the listing are a few adverse reactions which have not been reported with this specific drug. However, pharmacological similarities among the tricyclic antidepressant drugs require that each of the reactions be considered when amitriptyline is administered.
Cardiovascular: Myocardial infarction; stroke; heart block; arrhythmias; hypotension, particularly orthostatic hypotension; hypertension; tachycardia; palpitation.
CNS and Neuromuscular: Coma; seizures; hallucinations; delusions; confusional states; disorientation; incoordination; ataxia; tremors; peripheral neuropathy; numbness, tingling, and paresthesias of the extremities; extrapyramidal symptoms; dysarthria; disturbed concentration; excitement; anxiety; insomnia; restlessness; nightmares; drowsiness; dizziness; weakness; fatigue; headache; syndrome of inappropriate ADH (antidiuretic hormone) secretion; tinnitus; alteration in EEG patterns.
Anticholinergic: Paralytic ileus; hyperpyrexia; urinary retention, dilatation of the urinary tract; constipation; blurred vision, disturbance of accommodation, increased intraocular pressure, mydriasis; dry mouth.
Allergic: Skin rash; urticaria; photosensitization; edema of face and tongue.
Hematologic: Bone marrow depression including agranulocytosis, leukopenia, thrombocytopenia; purpura; eosinophilia.
Gastrointestinal: Rarely hepatitis (including altered liver function and jaundice); nausea; epigastric distress; vomiting; anorexia; stomatitis; peculiar taste; diarrhea; parotid swelling; black tongue.
Endocrine: Testicular swelling and gynecomastia in the male; breast enlargement and galactorrhea in the female; increased or decreased libido; elevation and lowering of blood sugar levels.
Other: Alopecia; edema; weight gain or loss; urinary frequency; increased perspiration.
Withdrawal Symptoms: After prolonged administration, abrupt cessation of treatment may produce nausea, headache, and malaise. Gradual dosage reduction has been reported to produce within two weeks, transient symptoms including irritability, restlessness, and dream and sleep disturbance. These symptoms are not indicative of addiction. Rare instances have been reported of mania or hypomania occurring within 2-7 days following cessation of chronic therapy with tricyclic antidepressants.

DOSAGE AND ADMINISTRATION

Since dosage for children has not been established, TRIAVIL is not recommended for use in children.
The total daily dose of TRIAVIL should not exceed four tablets of the 4-50 or eight tablets of any other dosage strength.
Initial Dosage
In psychoneurotic patients when anxiety and depression are of such a degree as to warrant combined therapy, one tablet of TRIAVIL 2-25 or TRIAVIL 4-25 three or four times a day or one tablet of TRIAVIL 4-50 twice a day is recommended.
In more severely ill patients with schizophrenia, TRIAVIL 4-25 is recommended in an initial dose of two tablets three times a day. If necessary, a fourth dose may be given at bedtime.
In elderly patients and adolescents, and some other patients in whom anxiety tends to predominate, TRIAVIL 4-10 may be administered three or four times a day initially, then adjusted as required for subsequent adequate therapy.

Maintenance Dosage
Depending on the condition being treated, therapeutic response may take from a few days to a few weeks or even longer. After a satisfactory response is noted, dosage should be reduced to the smallest amount necessary to obtain relief from the symptoms for which TRIAVIL is being administered. A useful maintenance dosage is one tablet of TRIAVIL 2-25 or 4-25 two to four times a day or one tablet of TRIAVIL 4-50 twice a day. TRIAVIL 2-10 and 4-10 can be used to increase flexibility in adjusting maintenance dosage to the lowest amount consistent with relief of symptoms. In some patients, maintenance dosage is required for many months.

OVERDOSAGE

Manifestations—High doses may cause temporary confusion, disturbed concentration, or transient visual hallucinations. Overdosage may cause drowsiness; hypothermia; tachycardia and other arrhythmic abnormalities, such as bundle branch block; ECG evidence of impaired conduction; congestive heart failure; dilated pupils; disorders of ocular motility; convulsions; severe hypotension; stupor; and coma. Other symptoms may be agitation, hyperactive reflexes, muscle rigidity, vomiting, hyperpyrexia, or any of the adverse reactions listed for perphenazine or amitriptyline.
Levarterenol (norepinephrine) may be used to treat hypotension, but not epinephrine.
All patients suspected of having taken an overdosage should be admitted to a hospital as soon as possible. *Treatment* is symptomatic and supportive. Empty the stomach as quickly as possible by emesis followed by gastric lavage upon arrival at the hospital. Saline emetics should not be used as the antiemetic effect of perphenazine may cause retention of the saline load and subsequent hypernatremia. Following gastric lavage, activated charcoal may be administered. Twenty to 30 g of activated charcoal may be given every four to six hours during the first 24 to 48 hours after ingestion. An ECG should be taken and close monitoring of cardiac function instituted if there is any sign of abnormality. Maintain an open airway and adequate fluid intake; regulate body temperature.
The intravenous administration of 1–3 mg of physostigmine salicylate is reported to reverse the symptoms of tricyclic antidepressant poisoning. Because physostigmine is rapidly metabolized, the dosage of physostigmine should be repeated as required particularly if life threatening signs such as arrhythmias, convulsions, and deep coma recur or persist after the initial dosage of physostigmine. On this basis, in severe overdosage with perphenazine-amitriptyline combinations, symptomatic treatment of central anticholinergic effects with physostigmine salicylate should be considered. Because physostigmine itself may be toxic, it is not recommended for routine use.
Standard measures should be used to manage circulatory shock and metabolic acidosis. Cardiac arrhythmias may be treated with neostigmine, pyridostigmine, or propranolol. Should cardiac failure occur, the use of digitalis should be considered. Close monitoring of cardiac function for not less than five days is advisable.
Anticonvulsants may be given to control convulsions. Amitriptyline and perphenazine increase the CNS depressant action but not the anticonvulsant action of barbiturates; therefore, an inhalation anesthetic, diazepam, or paraldehyde is recommended for control of convulsions. The management of acute symptoms of parkinsonism resulting from perphenazine intoxication may be treated with appropriate doses of COGENTIN* (Benztropine Mesylate) or diphenhydramine hydrochloride.**
Dialysis is of no value because of low plasma concentrations of the drug.
Since overdosage is often deliberate, patients may attempt suicide by other means during the recovery phase.
Deaths by deliberate or accidental overdosage have occurred with this class of drugs.

* Registered trademark of MERCK & CO., INC.
** BENADRYL® (Diphenhydramine Hydrochloride), Parke, Davis & Co.

HOW SUPPLIED

No. 3328—Tablets TRIAVIL 2–10 are blue, triangular, film coated tablets, coded MSD 914. They are supplied as follows:
NDC 0006-0914-68 bottles of 100
NDC 0006-0914-28 unit dose package of 100
NDC 0006-0914-74 bottles of 500.
Shown in Product Identification Guide, page 323
No. 3311—Tablets TRIAVIL 2–25 are orange, triangular, film coated tablets, coded MSD 921. They are supplied as follows:
NDC 0006-0921-68 bottles of 100
NDC 0006-0921-28 unit dose package of 100
NDC 0006-0921-74 bottles of 500.
(6505-01-210-4467 500's)
Shown in Product Identification Guide, page 323
No. 3310—Tablets TRIAVIL 4–10 are salmon, triangular, film coated tablets, coded MSD 934. They are supplied as follows:
NDC 0006-0934-68 bottles of 100
NDC 0006-0934-74 bottles of 500.
Shown in Product Identification Guide, page 323
No. 3312—Tablets TRIAVIL 4–25 are yellow, triangular, film coated tablets, coded MSD 946. They are supplied as follows:
NDC 0006-0946-68 bottles of 100
(6505-01-210-4468 100's)
NDC 0006-0946-28 unit dose package of 100
NDC 0006-0946-74 bottles of 500.
Shown in Product Identification Guide, page 323
No. 3364—Tablets TRIAVIL 4-50 are orange, diamond shaped, film coated tablets, coded MSD 517. They are supplied as follows:
NDC 0006-0517-60 bottles of 60
NDC 0006-0517-68 bottles of 100.
Shown in Product Identification Guide, page 323
Storage
Store Tablets TRIAVIL in a well-closed container. Avoid storage at temperatures above 40°C (104°F). In addition, Tablets TRIAVIL 2–10 must be protected from light and stored in a well-closed, light-resistant container.
A.H.F.S. Categories: 28:16:04, 28:16:08
DC 7398431 Issued September 1990

TRUSOPT® Sterile Ophthalmic Solution 2% ℞
(Dorzolamide Hydrochloride Ophthalmic Solution)

DESCRIPTION

TRUSOPT* (dorzolamide hydrochloride ophthalmic solution) is a carbonic anhydrase inhibitor formulated for topical ophthalmic use.
Dorzolamide hydrochloride is described chemically as: (4*S*-*trans*)-4-(ethylamino)-5,6-dihydro-6-methyl-4*H*-thieno [2,3-*b*]thiopyran-2-sulfonamide 7,7-dioxide monohydrochloride. Dorzolamide hydrochloride is optically active. The specific rotation is

$$\alpha^{25°}_{405} \text{ (C = 1, water) } = -17°.$$

Its empirical formula is $C_{10}H_{16}N_2O_4S_3 \cdot HCl$ and its structural formula is:

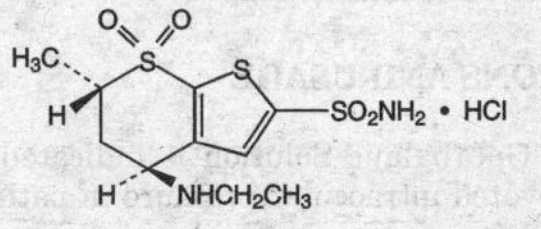

Dorzolamide hydrochloride has a molecular weight of 360.9 and a melting point of about 264°C. It is a white to off-white, crystalline powder, which is soluble in water and slightly soluble in methanol and ethanol.
TRUSOPT Sterile Ophthalmic Solution is supplied as a sterile, isotonic, buffered, slightly viscous, aqueous solution

Continued on next page

Information on the Merck & Co., Inc. products listed on these pages is the full prescribing information from product circulars in use August 31, 1998. For information, please call 1-800-NSC MERCK [1-800-672-6372].

Trusopt—Cont.

of dorzolamide hydrochloride. The pH of the solution is approximately 5.6. Each mL of TRUSOPT 2% contains 20 mg dorzolamide (22.3 mg of dorzolamide hydrochloride). Inactive ingredients are hydroxyethyl cellulose, mannitol, sodium citrate dihydrate, sodium hydroxide (to adjust pH) and water for injection. Benzalkonium chloride 0.0075% is added as a preservative.

* Registered trademark of MERCK & CO., Inc., Whitehouse Station, NJ, USA

CLINICAL PHARMACOLOGY

Mechanism of Action
Carbonic anhydrase (CA) is an enzyme found in many tissues of the body including the eye. It catalyzes the reversible reaction involving the hydration of carbon dioxide and the dehydration of carbonic acid. In humans, carbonic anhydrase exists as a number of isoenzymes, the most active being carbonic anhydrase II (CA-II), found primarily in red blood cells (RBCs), but also in other tissues. Inhibition of carbonic anhydrase in the ciliary processes of the eye decreases aqueous humor secretion, presumably by slowing the formation of bicarbonate ions with subsequent reduction in sodium and fluid transport. The result is a reduction in intraocular pressure (IOP).
TRUSOPT Ophthalmic Solution contains dorzolamide hydrochloride, an inhibitor of human carbonic anhydrase II. Following topical ocular administration, TRUSOPT reduces elevated intraocular pressure. Elevated intraocular pressure is a major risk factor in the pathogenesis of optic nerve damage and glaucomatous visual field loss.
Pharmacokinetics/Pharmacodynamics
When topically applied, dorzolamide reaches the systemic circulation. To assess the potential for systemic carbonic anhydrase inhibition following topical administration, drug and metabolite concentrations in RBCs and plasma and carbonic anhydrase inhibition in RBCs were measured. Dorzolamide accumulates in RBCs during chronic dosing as a result of binding to CA-II. The parent drug forms a single N-desethyl metabolite, which inhibits CA-II less potently than the parent drug but also inhibits CA-I. The metabolite also accumulates in RBCs where it binds primarily to CA-I. Plasma concentrations of dorzolamide and metabolite are generally below the assay limit of quantitation (15nM). Dorzolamide binds moderately to plasma proteins (approximately 33%). Dorzolamide is primarily excreted unchanged in the urine; the metabolite also is excreted in urine. After dosing is stopped, dorzolamide washes out of RBCs nonlinearly, resulting in a rapid decline of drug concentration initially, followed by a slower elimination phase with a half-life of about four months.
To simulate the systemic exposure after long-term topical ocular administration, dorzolamide was given orally to eight healthy subjects for up to 20 weeks. The oral dose of 2 mg b.i.d. closely approximates the amount of drug delivered by topical ocular administration of TRUSOPT 2% t.i.d. Steady state was reached within 8 weeks. The inhibition of CA-II and total carbonic anhydrase activities was below the degree of inhibition anticipated to be necessary for a pharmacological effect on renal function and respiration in healthy individuals.
Clinical Studies
The efficacy of TRUSOPT was demonstrated in clinical studies in the treatment of elevated intraocular pressure in patients with glaucoma or ocular hypertension (baseline IOP ≥23 mmHg). The IOP-lowering effect of TRUSOPT was approximately 3 to 5 mmHg throughout the day and this was consistent in clinical studies of up to one year duration. The efficacy of TRUSOPT when dosed less frequently than three times a day (alone or in combination with other products) has not been established.

INDICATIONS AND USAGE

TRUSOPT Ophthalmic Solution is indicated in the treatment of elevated intraocular pressure in patients with ocular hypertension or open-angle glaucoma.

CONTRAINDICATIONS

TRUSOPT is contraindicated in patients who are hypersensitive to any component of this product.

WARNINGS

TRUSOPT is a sulfonamide and although administered topically is absorbed systemically. Therefore, the same types of adverse reactions that are attributable to sulfonamides may occur with topical administration with TRUSOPT. Fatalities have occurred, although rarely, due to severe reactions to sulfonamides including Stevens-Johnson syndrome, toxic epidermal necrolysis, fulminant hepatic necrosis, agranulocytosis, aplastic anemia, and other blood dyscrasias. Sensitization may recur when a sulfonamide is readministered irrespective of the route of administration. If signs of serious reactions or hypersensitivity occur, discontinue the use of this preparation.

PRECAUTIONS

General
Carbonic anhydrase activity has been observed in both the cytoplasm and around the plasma membranes of the corneal endothelium. The effect of continued administration of TRUSOPT on the corneal endothelium has not been fully evaluated.
The management of patients with acute angle-closure glaucoma requires therapeutic interventions in addition to ocular hypotensive agents. TRUSOPT has not been studied in patients with acute angle-closure glaucoma.
TRUSOPT has not been studied in patients with severe renal impairment (CrCl < 30 mL/min). Because TRUSOPT and its metabolite are excreted predominantly by the kidney, TRUSOPT is not recommended in such patients.
TRUSOPT has not been studied in patients with hepatic impairment and should therefore be used with caution in such patients.
In clinical studies, local ocular adverse effects, primarily conjunctivitis and lid reactions, were reported with chronic administration of TRUSOPT. Many of these reactions had the clinical appearance and course of an allergic-type reaction that resolved upon discontinuation of drug therapy. If such reactions are observed, TRUSOPT should be discontinued and the patient evaluated before considering restarting the drug. (See **ADVERSE REACTIONS**.)
There is a potential for an additive effect on the known systemic effects of carbonic anhydrase inhibition in patients receiving an oral carbonic anhydrase inhibitor and TRUSOPT. The concomitant administration of TRUSOPT and oral carbonic anhydrase inhibitors is not recommended.
There have been reports of bacterial keratitis associated with the use of multiple dose containers of topical ophthalmic products. These containers had been inadvertently contaminated by patients who, in most cases, had a concurrent corneal disease or a disruption of the ocular epithelial surface.
Information for Patients
TRUSOPT is a sulfonamide and although administered topically is absorbed systemically. Therefore the same types of adverse reactions that are attributable to sulfonamides may occur with topical administration. Patients should be advised that if serious or unusual reactions or signs of hypersensitivity occur, they should discontinue the use of the product (see **WARNINGS**).
Patients should be advised that if they develop any ocular reactions, particularly conjunctivitis and lid reactions, they should discontinue use and seek their physician's advice.
Patients should be instructed to avoid allowing the tip of the dispensing container to contact the eye or surrounding structures.
Patients should also be instructed that ocular solutions, if handled improperly or if the tip of the dispensing container contacts the eye or surrounding structures, can become contaminated by common bacteria known to cause ocular infections. Serious damage to the eye and subsequent loss of vision may result from using contaminated solutions.
Patients also should be advised that if they have ocular surgery or develop an intercurrent ocular condition (e.g., trauma or infection), they should immediately seek their physician's advice concerning the continued use of the present multidose container.
If more than one topical ophthalmic drug is being used, the drugs should be administered at least ten minutes apart.
The preservative in TRUSOPT Ophthalmic Solution, benzalkonium chloride, may be absorbed by soft contact lenses. TRUSOPT should not be administered while wearing soft contact lenses.
Drug Interactions
Although acid-base and electrolyte disturbances were not reported in the clinical trials with TRUSOPT, these disturbances have been reported with oral carbonic anhydrase inhibitors and have, in some instances, resulted in drug interactions (e.g., toxicity associated with high-dose salicylate therapy). Therefore, the potential for such drug interactions should be considered in patients receiving TRUSOPT.
Carcinogenesis, Mutagenesis, Impairment of Fertility
In a two-year study of dorzolamide hydrochloride administered orally to male and female Sprague-Dawley rats, urinary bladder papillomas were seen in male rats in the highest dosage group of 20 mg/kg/day (250 times the recommended human ophthalmic dose). Papillomas were not seen in rats given oral doses equivalent to approximately 12 times the recommended human ophthalmic dose. No treatment-related tumors were seen in a 21-month study in female and male mice given oral doses up to 75 mg/kg/day (900 times the recommended human ophthalmic dose).
The increased incidence of urinary bladder papillomas seen in the high-dose male rats is a class-effect of carbonic anhydrase inhibitors in rats. Rats are particularly prone to developing papillomas in response to foreign bodies, compounds causing crystalluria, and diverse sodium salts.
No changes in bladder urothelium were seen in dogs given oral dorzolamide hydrochloride for one year at 2 mg/kg/day (25 times the recommended human ophthalmic dose) or monkeys dosed topically to the eye at 0.4 mg/kg/day (5 times the recommended human ophthalmic dose) for one year.
The following tests for mutagenic potential were negative: (1) *in vivo* (mouse) cytogenetic assay; (2) *in vitro* chromosomal aberration assay; (3) alkaline elution assay; (4) V-79 assay; and (5) Ames test.
In reproduction studies of dorzolamide hydrochloride in rats, there were no adverse effects on the reproductive capacity of males or females at doses up to 188 or 94 times, respectively, the recommended human ophthalmic dose.
Pregnancy
Teratogenic Effects. Pregnancy Category C. Developmental toxicity studies with dorzolamide hydrochloride in rabbits at oral doses of ≥2.5 mg/kg/day (31 times the recommended human ophthalmic dose) revealed malformations of the vertebral bodies. These malformations occurred at doses that caused metabolic acidosis with decreased body weight gain in dams and decreased fetal weights. No treatment-related malformations were seen at 1.0 mg/kg/day (13 times the recommended human ophthalmic dose). There were no treatment-related fetal malformations in developmental toxicity studies with dorzolamide hydrochloride in rats at oral doses up to 10 mg/kg/day (125 times the recommended human ophthalmic dose). There are no adequate and well-controlled studies in pregnant women. TRUSOPT should be used during pregnancy only if the potential benefit justifies the potential risk to the fetus.
Nursing Mothers
In a study of dorzolamide hydrochloride in lactating rats, decreases in body weight gain of 5 to 7% in offspring at an oral dose of 7.5 mg/kg/day (94 times the recommended human ophthalmic dose) were seen during lactation. A slight delay in postnatal development (incisor eruption, vaginal canalization and eye openings), secondary to lower fetal body weight, was noted.
It is not known whether this drug is excreted in human milk. Because many drugs are excreted in human milk and because of the potential for serious adverse reactions in nursing infants from TRUSOPT, a decision should be made whether to discontinue nursing or to discontinue the drug, taking into account the importance of the drug to the mother.
Pediatric Use
Safety and effectiveness in pediatric patients have not been established.
Geriatric Use
Of the total number of patients in clinical studies of TRUSOPT, 44% were 65 years of age and over, while 10% were 75 years of age and over. No overall differences in effectiveness or safety were observed between these patients and younger patients, but greater sensitivity of some older individuals to the product cannot be ruled out.

ADVERSE REACTIONS

In clinical studies, the most frequent adverse events associated with TRUSOPT were ocular burning, stinging, or discomfort immediately following ocular administration (approximately one-third of patients). Approximately one-quarter of patients noted a bitter taste following administration. Superficial punctate keratitis occurred in 10–15% of patients and signs and symptoms of ocular allergic reaction in approximately 10%. Events occurring in approximately 1–5% of patients were blurred vision, tearing, dryness, and photophobia. Other ocular events and systemic events were reported infrequently, including headache, nausea, asthenia/fatigue; and, rarely, skin rashes, urolithiasis, and iridocyclitis.
The following adverse reactions have been reported in postmarketing experience:
Hypersensitivity: signs and symptoms of systemic allergic reactions including angioedema, bronchospasm, pruritus, and urticaria;
Nervous System: dizziness, paresthesia;
Ocular: pain, redness, transient myopia (which resolved upon discontinuation of treatment);
Respiratory: dyspnea;
Skin: contact dermatitis.

OVERDOSAGE

Although no human data are available, electrolyte imbalance, development of an acidotic state, and possible central nervous system effects may occur. Serum electrolyte levels (particularly potassium) and blood pH levels should be monitored.
Significant lethality was observed in female rats and mice after single oral doses of dorzolamide hydrochloride 1927 mg/kg and 1320 mg/kg, respectively.

DOSAGE AND ADMINISTRATION

The dose is one drop of TRUSOPT Ophthalmic Solution in the affected eyes(s) three times daily.
TRUSOPT may be used concomitantly with other topical ophthalmic drug products to lower intraocular pressure. If more than one topical ophthalmic drug is being used, the drugs should be administered at least ten minutes apart.

HOW SUPPLIED

TRUSOPT Ophthalmic Solution is a slightly opalescent, nearly colorless, slightly viscous solution.
No. 3519—TRUSOPT Ophthalmic Solution 2% is supplied in OCUMETER®*, a white, opaque, plastic ophthalmic dispenser with a controlled drop tip as follows:
NDC 0006-3519-03, 5 mL
NDC 0006-3519-10, 10 mL
(6505-01-416-4328).
Storage
Store TRUSOPT Ophthalmic Solution at 15–30°C (59–86°F). Protect from light.

* Registered trademark of MERCK & CO., Inc.
9010004 Issued September 1997
COPYRIGHT© MERCK & CO., Inc., 1994
All rights reserved

URECHOLINE® Tablets ℞
(Bethanechol Chloride), U.S.P.
URECHOLINE® Injection ℞
(Bethanechol Chloride), U.S.P.

DESCRIPTION

URECHOLINE* (Bethanechol Chloride), a cholinergic agent, is a synthetic ester which is structurally and pharmacologically related to acetylcholine.
It is designated chemically as 2-[(aminocarbonyl)oxy]-*N, N, N*- trimethyl-1-propanaminium chloride. Its empirical formula is $C_7H_{17}ClN_2O_2$ and its structural formula is:

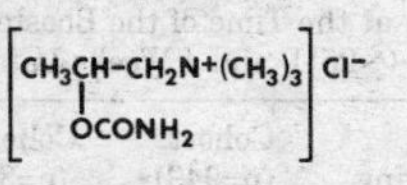
CH3CH–CH2N+(CH3)3 Cl−
OCONH2

It is a white, hygroscopic crystalline compound having a slight amine-like odor, freely soluble in water, and has a molecular weight of 196.68.
URECHOLINE is supplied as 5 mg, 10 mg, 25 mg, and 50 mg tablets for oral use. Inactive ingredients in the tablets are calcium phosphate, lactose, magnesium stearate, and starch. Tablets URECHOLINE 10 mg also contain FD&C Red 3 and FD&C Red 40. Tablets URECHOLINE 25 mg and 50 mg also contain D&C Yellow 10 and FD&C Yellow 6.
URECHOLINE is also supplied as a sterile solution **for subcutaneous use only.** The sterile solution is essentially neutral. Each milliliter contains bethanechol chloride, 5.15 mg, and Water for Injection, q.s., 1 mL. It may be autoclaved at 120° C for 20 minutes without discoloration or loss of potency.

*Registered trademark of MERCK & CO., Inc.

CLINICAL PHARMACOLOGY

Bethanechol chloride acts principally by producing the effects of stimulation of the parasympathetic nervous system. It increases the tone of the detrusor urinae muscle, usually producing a contraction sufficiently strong to initiate micturition and empty the bladder. It stimulates gastric motility, increases gastric tone, and often restores impaired rhythmic peristalsis.
Stimulation of the parasympathetic nervous system releases acetylcholine at the nerve endings. When spontaneous stimulation is reduced and therapeutic intervention is required, acetylcholine can be given, but it is rapidly hydrolyzed by cholinesterase, and its effects are transient. Bethanechol chloride is not destroyed by cholinesterase and its effects are more prolonged than those of acetylcholine.
Effects on the GI and urinary tracts sometimes appear within 30 minutes after oral administration of bethanechol chloride, but more often 60–90 minutes are required to reach maximum effectiveness. Following oral administration, the usual duration of action of bethanechol is one hour, although large doses (300–400 mg) have been reported to produce effects for up to six hours. Subcutaneous injection produces a more intense action on bladder muscle than does oral administration of the drug.
Because of the selective action of bethanechol, nicotinic symptoms of cholinergic stimulation are usually absent or minimal when orally or subcutaneously administered in therapeutic doses, while muscarinic effects are prominent. Muscarinic effects usually occur within 5–15 minutes after subcutaneous injection, reach a maximum in 15–30 minutes, and disappear within two hours. Doses that stimulate micturition and defecation and increase peristalsis do not ordinarily stimulate ganglia or voluntary muscles. Therapeutic test doses in normal human subjects have little effect on heart rate, blood pressure, or peripheral circulation.
Bethanechol chloride does not cross the blood-brain barrier because of its charged quaternary amine moiety. The metabolic fate and mode of excretion of the drug have not been elucidated.
A clinical study* was conducted on the relative effectiveness of oral and subcutaneous doses of bethanechol chloride on the stretch response of bladder muscle in patients with urinary retention. Results showed that 5 mg of the drug given subcutaneously stimulated a response that was more rapid in onset and of larger magnitude than an oral dose of 50 mg, 100 mg, or 200 mg. All the oral doses, however, had a longer duration of effect than the subcutaneous dose. Although the 50 mg oral dose caused little change in intravesical pressure in this study, this dose has been found in other studies to be clinically effective in the rehabilitation of patients with decompensated bladders.

*Diokno, A. C.; Lapides, J., Urol. *10:* 23–24, July 1977.

INDICATIONS AND USAGE

For the treatment of acute postoperative and postpartum nonobstructive (functional) urinary retention and for neurogenic atony of the urinary bladder with retention.

CONTRAINDICATIONS

Hypersensitivity to URECHOLINE tablets or to any component of URECHOLINE injection, hyperthyroidism, peptic ulcer, latent or active bronchial asthma, pronounced bradycardia or hypotension, vasomotor instability, coronary artery disease, epilepsy, and parkinsonism.
URECHOLINE should not be employed when the strength or integrity of the gastrointestinal or bladder wall is in question, or in the presence of mechanical obstruction; when increased muscular activity of the gastrointestinal tract or urinary bladder might prove harmful, as following recent urinary bladder surgery, gastrointestinal resection and anastomosis, or when there is possible gastrointestinal obstruction; in bladder neck obstruction, spastic gastrointestinal disturbances, acute inflammatory lesions of the gastrointestinal tract, or peritonitis; or in marked vagotonia.

WARNING

The sterile solution is for subcutaneous use only. It should never be given intramuscularly or intravenously. Violent symptoms of cholinergic over-stimulation, such as circulatory collapse, fall in blood pressure, abdominal cramps, bloody diarrhea, shock, or sudden cardiac arrest are likely to occur if the drug is given by either of these routes. Although rare, these same symptoms have occurred after subcutaneous injection, and may occur in cases of hypersensitivity or overdosage.

PRECAUTIONS

General
In urinary retention, if the sphincter fails to relax as URECHOLINE contracts the bladder, urine may be forced up the ureter into the kidney pelvis. If there is bacteriuria, this may cause reflux infection.
Information for Patients
URECHOLINE tablets should preferably be taken one hour before or two hours after meals to avoid nausea or vomiting. Dizziness, lightheadedness or fainting may occur, especially when getting up from a lying or sitting position.
Drug Interactions
Special care is required if this drug is given to patients receiving ganglion blocking compounds because a critical fall in blood pressure may occur. Usually, severe abdominal symptoms appear before there is such a fall in the blood pressure.
Carcinogenesis, Mutagenesis, Impairment of Fertility
Long-term studies in animals have not been performed to evaluate the effects upon fertility, mutagenic or carcinogenic potential of URECHOLINE.
Pregnancy
Pregnancy Category C. Animal reproduction studies have not been conducted with URECHOLINE. It is also not known whether URECHOLINE can cause fetal harm when administered to a pregnant woman or can affect reproduction capacity. URECHOLINE should be given to a pregnant woman only if clearly needed.
Nursing Mothers
It is not known whether this drug is secreted in human milk. Because many drugs are secreted in human milk and because of the potential for serious adverse reactions from URECHOLINE in nursing infants, a decision should be made whether to discontinue nursing or to discontinue the drug, taking into account the importance of the drug to the mother.
Pediatric Use
Safety and effectiveness in pediatric patients have not been established.

ADVERSE REACTIONS

Adverse reactions are rare following oral administration of bethanechol, but are more common following subcutaneous injection. Adverse reactions are more likely to occur when dosage is increased.
The following adverse reactions have been observed: *Body as a Whole:* malaise; *Digestive:* abdominal cramps or discomfort, colicky pain, nausea and belching, diarrhea, borborygmi, salivation; *Renal:* urinary urgency; *Nervous System:* headache; *Cardiovascular:* a fall in blood pressure with reflex tachycardia, vasomotor response; *Skin:* flushing producing a feeling of warmth, sensation of heat about the face, sweating; *Respiratory:* bronchial constriction, asthmatic attacks; *Special Senses:* lacrimation, miosis.
Causal Relationship Unknown: The following adverse reactions have been reported, and a causal relationship to therapy with URECHOLINE has not been established: *Body as a Whole:* hypothermia: *Nervous System:* seizures.

OVERDOSAGE

Early signs of overdosage are abdominal discomfort, salivation, flushing of the skin ("hot feeling"), sweating, nausea and vomiting.
Atropine is a specific antidote. The recommended dose for adults is 0.6 mg (1/100 grain). Repeat doses can be given every two hours, according to clinical response. The recommended dosage in infants and children up to 12 years of age is 0.01 mg/kg (to a maximum single dose of 0.4 mg) repeated every two hours as needed until the desired effect is obtained, or adverse effects of atropine preclude further usage. Subcutaneous injection of atropine is preferred except in emergencies when the intravenous route may be employed.
When URECHOLINE is administered subcutaneously, a syringe containing a dose of atropine sulfate should always be available to treat symptoms of toxicity.
The oral LD_{50} of bethanechol chloride is 1510 mg/kg in the mouse.

DOSAGE AND ADMINISTRATION

Dosage and route of administration must be individualized, depending on the type and severity of the condition to be treated.
Preferably give the drug when the stomach is empty. If taken soon after eating, nausea and vomiting may occur.
Oral—The usual adult dosage is 10 to 50 mg three or four times a day. The minimum effective dose is determined by giving 5 or 10 mg initially and repeating the same amount at hourly intervals until satisfactory response occurs or until a maximum of 50 mg has been given. The effects of the drug sometimes appear within 30 minutes and usually within 60 to 90 minutes. They persist for about an hour.
Subcutaneous—The usual dose is 1 mL (5.15 mg), although some patients respond satisfactorily to as little as 0.5 mL (2.575 mg). The minimum effective dose is determined by injecting 0.5 mL (2.575 mg) initially and repeating the same amount at 15 to 30 minute intervals to a maximum of four doses until satisfactory response is obtained, unless disturbing reactions appear. The minimum effective dose may be repeated thereafter three or four times a day as required.
Rarely, single doses up to 2 mL (10.30 mg) may be required. Such large doses may cause severe reactions and should be used only after adequate trial of single doses of 0.5 to 1 mL (2.575 to 5.15 mg) has established that smaller doses are not sufficient.
URECHOLINE is usually effective in 5 to 15 minutes after subcutaneous injection.
If necessary, the effects of the drug can be abolished promptly by atropine (see OVERDOSAGE).
Parenteral drug products should be inspected visually for particulate matter and discoloration prior to administration, whenever solution and container permit.

HOW SUPPLIED

Tablets URECHOLINE are round, compressed tablets, scored on one side. They are supplied as follows:

Continued on next page

Information on the Merck & Co., Inc. products listed on these pages is the full prescribing information from product circulars in use August 31, 1998. For information, please call 1-800-NSC MERCK [1-800-672-6372].

Urecholine—Cont.

No. 7785—5 mg, white in color, coded MSD 403 on one side and URECHOLINE on the other.
NDC 0006-0403-68 in bottles of 100.
   Shown in Product Identification Guide, page 323
No. 7787—10 mg, pink in color, coded MSD 412 on one side and URECHOLINE on the other.
NDC 0006-0412-68 in bottles of 100
(6505-00-616-7856 10 mg 100's).
   Shown in Product Identification Guide, page 323
No. 7788—25 mg, yellow in color, coded MSD 457 on one side and URECHOLINE on the other.
NDC 0006-0457-68 in bottles of 100
(6505-00-912-7440 25 mg, 100's).
   Shown in Product Identification Guide, page 323
No. 7790 — 50 mg, yellow in color, coded MSD 460 on one side and URECHOLINE on the other.
NDC 0006-0460-68 in bottles of 100.
   Shown in Product Identification Guide, page 323
No. 7786—Injection URECHOLINE, 5.15 mg per mL, is a clear, colorless solution, and is supplied as follows:
NDC 0006-7786-29 in box of 6 × 1 mL vials
(6505-00-616-8947 in box of 6 × 1 mL vials).
Storage
Store Tablets URECHOLINE in a tightly-closed container. Avoid storage at temperatures above 40°C (104°F).
Avoid storage of Injection URECHOLINE at temperatures below −20°C (−4°F) and above 40°C (104°F).
       7875834   Issued August 1997
COPYRIGHT © MERCK & CO., INC., 1984
All rights reserved

VAQTA®
(Hepatitis A Vaccine, Inactivated)   ℞

DESCRIPTION

VAQTA* [Hepatitis A Vaccine, Inactivated] is an inactivated whole virus vaccine derived from hepatitis A virus (HAV) grown in cell culture in human MRC-5 diploid fibroblasts. It contains inactivated virus of a strain which was originally derived by further serial passage of a proven attenuated strain. The virus is grown, harvested, purified by a combination of physical and high performance liquid chromatographic techniques developed at the Merck Research Laboratories, formalin inactivated, and then adsorbed onto aluminum hydroxide. One milliliter of the vaccine contains approximately 50 units (U) of hepatitis A virus antigen, which is purified and formulated without a preservative. Within the limits of current assay variability, the 50U dose of VAQTA contains less than 0.1 mcg of non-viral protein, less than 4×10^{-6} mcg of DNA, less than 10^{-4} mcg of bovine albumin, and less than 0.8 mcg of formaldehyde. Other process chemical residuals are less than 10 parts per billion (ppb).
VAQTA is a sterile suspension for intramuscular injection. VAQTA is supplied in two formulations:
Pediatric/Adolescent Formulation: each 0.5 mL dose contains approximately 25U of hepatitis A virus antigen adsorbed onto approximately 0.225 mg of aluminum provided as aluminum hydroxide, and 35 mcg of sodium borate as a pH stabilizer, in 0.9% sodium chloride.
Adult Formulation: each 1 mL dose contains approximately 50U of hepatitis A virus antigen adsorbed onto approximately 0.45 mg of aluminum provided as aluminum hydroxide, and 70 mcg of sodium borate as a pH stabilizer, in 0.9% sodium chloride.

*Registered trademark of MERCK & CO., Inc.

CLINICAL PHARMACOLOGY

Hepatitis A Disease
Hepatitis A virus is one of several hepatitis viruses that cause a systemic infection with pathology in the liver. The incubation period ranges from approximately 20 to 50 days. While the course of the disease is generally benign and does not result in chronic hepatitis, infection with hepatitis A virus remains an important cause of morbidity and occasional fulminant hepatitis and death.
Hepatitis A is transmitted most often by the fecal-oral route, with infection occurring primarily within private households. Common-source outbreaks due to contaminated food and water supplies have occurred following consumption of certain foods such as raw shellfish, and uncooked foods prepared by an infected food-handler or otherwise contaminated prior to ingestion (salads, sandwiches, frozen raspberries, etc.) Bloodborne transmission, while uncommon, is possible via blood transfusion, contaminated blood products, or from needles shared with an infected viremic individual. Sexual transmission has also been reported.
The disease burden due to hepatitis A in the United States has been estimated to be approximately 143,000 infections per year, of which 75,800 result in clinical hepatitis A disease, 11,400 hospitalizations, and 80 deaths due to fulminant hepatitis. Worldwide, it has been estimated that 1.4

million cases are reported annually. The clinical manifestations of hepatitis A infection often pass unrecognized in children ≤2 years of age whereas overt hepatitis A develops in the majority of infected older children and adults. Symptoms and signs of hepatitis A infection are similar to those associated with other types of viral hepatitis and include anorexia, nausea, fever/chills, jaundice, dark urine, light-colored stools, abdominal pain, malaise, and fatigue.
Clinical Trials
Clinical trials conducted worldwide with several formulations of the vaccine in 9181 healthy individuals ranging from 2 to 85 years of age have demonstrated that VAQTA is highly immunogenic and generally well tolerated.
Protection from hepatitis A disease has been shown to be related to the presence of antibody; an anamnestic antibody response occurs in healthy individuals with a history of infection who are subsequently re-exposed to hepatitis A virus. Similarly, protection after vaccination with VAQTA has been associated with the onset of seroconversion (≥10 mIU/mL of hepatitis A antibody, measured by a modification of the HAVAB** radioimmunoassay [RIA]) and with an anamnestic antibody response following booster vaccination with VAQTA.
Immunology
In combined clinical studies, 97% of 1214 healthy children and adolescents 2 through 17 years of age seroconverted with a geometric mean titer (GMT) of 43 mIU/mL within 4 weeks after a single ∼25U/0.5 mL intramuscular dose of VAQTA. Similarly, 95% of 1428 adults ≥18 years of age seroconverted with a GMT of 37 mIU/mL within 4 weeks after a single ∼50U/1.0 mL intramuscular dose of VAQTA. Furthermore, at 2 weeks post-vaccination, 69% (n=744) of adults seroconverted with a GMT of 16 mIU/mL after a single dose of VAQTA. Immune memory was demonstrated by an anamnestic antibody response in individuals who received a booster dose (see *Persistence*).
While a study evaluating VAQTA alone in a post-exposure setting has not been conducted, the concurrent use of VAQTA (∼50U) and immune globulin (IG, 0.06 mL/kg) was evaluated in a clinical study involving healthy adults 18 to 39 years of age. Table 1 provides seroconversion rates and GMT at 4 and 24 weeks after the first dose in each treatment group and at one month after a booster dose of VAQTA (administered at 24 weeks).

Table 1
Seroconversion Rates (%) and Geometric Mean Titers (GMT) after Vaccination with VAQTA plus IG, VAQTA Alone, and IG Alone

Weeks	VAQTA plus IG	VAQTA	IG
	Seroconversion Rate GMT (mIU/mL)		
4	100% 42 (n=129)	96% 38 (n=135)	87% 19 (n=30)
24	92% 83 (n=125)	97% 137 (n=132)	0% 5 (n=28)
28	100% 4872 (n=114)	100% 6498 (n=128)	N/A

* The seroconversion rate and the GMT in the group receiving VAQTA alone were significantly higher than in the group receiving VAQTA plus IG (p=0.05, p<0.001, respectively).
N/A=Not Applicable

Efficacy
A very high degree of protection has been demonstrated after a single dose of VAQTA in children and adolescents. The protective efficacy, immunogenicity and safety of VAQTA were evaluated in a randomized, double-blind, placebo-controlled study involving 1037 susceptible healthy children and adolescents 2 through 16 years of age in a U.S. community with recurrent outbreaks of hepatitis A (The Monroe Efficacy Study). Each child received an intramuscular dose of VAQTA (∼25U) or placebo. Among those individuals who were initially seronegative (by modified HAVAB), seroconversion was achieved in >99% of vaccine recipients within 4 weeks after vaccination. The onset of seroconversion following a single dose of VAQTA was shown to parallel the onset of protection against clinical hepatitis A disease.
Because of the long incubation period of the disease (approximately 20 to 50 days, or longer in children), the primary endpoint was based on clinically confirmed cases*** of hepatitis A occurring ≥50 days after vaccination to exclude any children incubating the infection before vaccination. In subjects who were initially seronegative, the protective efficacy of a single dose of VAQTA was observed to be

100% with 21 cases of clinically confirmed hepatitis A occurring in the placebo group and none in the vaccine group (p<0.001). A secondary endpoint was pre-defined as the number of clinically confirmed cases of hepatitis A ≥30 days. With this secondary endpoint, 28 cases of clinically confirmed hepatitis A occurred in the placebo group while none occurred in the vaccine group ≥30 days after vaccination. In addition, it was observed in this trial that no cases of clinically confirmed hepatitis A occurred in the vaccine group after day 16.† Following demonstration of protection with a single dose and termination of the study, a booster dose was administered to a subset of vaccinees 6, 12, or 18 months after the primary dose.
Persistence
The total duration of the protective effect of VAQTA in healthy vaccinees is unknown at present. However, seropositivity was shown to persist up to 18 months after a single ∼25U dose in a cohort of 35 out of 39 children and adolescents who participated in the Monroe Efficacy Study; 95% of this cohort responded anamnestically following a booster at 18 months. To date, no cases of clinically confirmed hepatitis A disease ≥50 days after vaccination have occurred in those vaccinees from The Monroe Efficacy Study monitored for up to 4 years.
The effectiveness of VAQTA for use in community outbreak control has been demonstrated by the fact that, although cases of imported infection have occurred, the study community has remained free of outbreaks. In contrast, three nearby sister communities to Monroe have continued to experience outbreaks.
In adults, seropositivity has been shown to persist up to 6 months after a single ∼50U dose. Studies are ongoing to evaluate longer-term persistence and the need, if any, for additional booster doses. Persistence of immunologic memory was demonstrated with an anamnestic antibody response to a booster dose of ∼25U given 6 to 18 months after the primary dose in children and adolescents (Table 2), and to a booster dose of ∼50U given 6 months after the primary dose to adults (Table 3).

Table 2
Children/Adolescents
Seroconversion Rates (%) and Geometric Mean Titers (GMT) for Cohorts of Initially Seronegative Vaccinees at the Time of the Booster (∼25U) and 4 Weeks Later

Weeks Following Initial ∼25U Dose	Cohort* (n=949) 0 and 6 Months	Cohort* (n=35) 0 and 12 Months	Cohort* (n=39) 0 and 18 Months
	Seroconversion Rate GMT (mIU/mL)		
24	97% 109	—	—
28	100% 10609	—	—
52	—	91% 48	—
56	—	100% 12308	—
78	—	—	90% 50
82	—	—	100% 9591

*Blood samples taken at both time points.

Table 3
Adults
Seroconversion Rates (%) and Geometric Mean Titers (GMT) for a Cohort of Vaccinees After a Booster Dose (∼50U) of VAQTA Administered at 6 Months

Weeks Following Initial ∼50U Dose	Cohort (n=1152) 0 and 6 Months
	Seroconversion Rate GMT (mIU/mL)
24	98% 134
28	100% 6010

** Trademark of Abbott Laboratories
*** The clinical case definition included all of the following occurring at the same time: 1) one or more typical clinical signs or symptoms of hepatitis A (e.g., jaundice, malaise, fever ≥ 38.3°C), 2) elevation of hepatitis A IgM antibody (HAVAB-M), 3) elevation of alanine transferase (ALT) ≥2 times the upper limit of normal.
† One vaccinee did not meet the pre-defined criteria for clinically confirmed hepatitis A but did have positive hepatitis A IgM and borderline liver enzyme (ALT) elevations on days 34, 50, and 58 after vaccination with mild clinical symptoms observed on days 49 and 50.

INDICATIONS AND USAGE

VAQTA is indicated for active pre-exposure prophylaxis against disease caused by hepatitis A virus in persons 2 years of age and older. Primary immunization should be given at least 2 weeks prior to expected exposure to HAV. Individuals who are or will be at increased risk of infection by HAV include:
TRAVELERS
Persons traveling to areas of higher endemicity for hepatitis A. These areas include, but are not limited to, Africa, Asia (except Japan), the Mediterranean basin, Eastern Europe, the Middle East, Central and South America, Mexico, and parts of the Caribbean. Current CDC (Centers for Disease Control and Prevention) advisories should be consulted with regard to specific locales.
MILITARY PERSONNEL
PEOPLE LIVING IN, OR RELOCATING TO, AREAS OF HIGH ENDEMICITY
CERTAIN ETHNIC AND GEOGRAPHIC POPULATIONS THAT EXPERIENCE CYCLIC HEPATITIS A EPIDEMICS SUCH AS:
Native peoples of Alaska and the Americas.
OTHERS
Persons engaging in high-risk sexual activity (such as homosexually active males); users of illicit injectable drugs; residents of a community experiencing an outbreak of hepatitis A.
Hemophiliacs and other recipients of therapeutic blood products (see PRECAUTIONS and DOSAGE AND ADMINISTRATION).
Although the epidemiology of hepatitis A does not permit the identification of other specific populations at high risk of disease, outbreaks of hepatitis A or exposure to hepatitis A virus have been described in a variety of populations in which VAQTA may be useful:
— Certain institutional workers (e.g., caretakers for the developmentally challenged)
— Employees of child day-care centers
— Laboratory workers who handle live hepatitis A virus
— Handlers of primate animals that may be harboring HAV
PEOPLE EXPOSED TO HEPATITIS A
For those requiring both immediate and long-term protection, VAQTA may be administered concomitantly with IG.
Revaccination
See DOSAGE AND ADMINISTRATION, *DOSAGE*.
Use With Other Vaccines
Data to recommend concurrent use with other vaccines are limited.
Use With Immune Globulin
For individuals requiring either post-exposure prophylaxis or combined immediate and longer-term protection (e.g., travelers departing on short notice to endemic areas), VAQTA may be administered concomitantly with IG using separate sites and syringes (see CLINICAL PHARMACOLOGY and DOSAGE AND ADMINISTRATION).
VAQTA IS NOT RECOMMENDED FOR USE IN INFANTS YOUNGER THAN 2 YEARS OF AGE SINCE DATA ON USE IN THIS AGE GROUP ARE NOT CURRENTLY AVAILABLE.

CONTRAINDICATIONS

Hypersensitivity to any component of the vaccine.

WARNINGS

Individuals who develop symptoms suggestive of hypersensitivity after an injection of VAQTA should not receive further injections of the vaccine (see CONTRAINDICATIONS). If VAQTA is used in individuals with malignancies or those receiving immunosuppressive therapy or who are otherwise immunocompromised, the expected immune response may not be obtained.

PRECAUTIONS

General
VAQTA will not prevent hepatitis caused by infectious agents other than hepatitis A virus. Because of the long incubation period (approximately 20 to 50 days) for hepatitis

Table 4
Local and Systemic Complaints (≥1%) in Healthy Children and Adolescents from The Monroe Efficacy Study

| | VAQTA | | |
Reaction	Dose 1*	Booster	Placebo*†
Injection-Site Complaints			
Pain	6.4% (33/515)	3.4% (16/475)	6.3% (32/510)
Tenderness	4.9% (25/515)	1.7% (8/475)	6.1% (31/510)
Erythema	1.9% (10/515)	0.8% (4/475)	1.8% (9/510)
Swelling	1.7% (9/515)	1.5% (7/475)	1.6% (8/510)
Warmth	1.7% (9/515)	0.6% (3/475)	1.6% (8/510)
Systemic Complaints			
Abdominal Pain	1.2% (6/519)	1.1% (5/475)	1.0% (5/518)
Pharyngitis	1.2% (6/519)	0% (0/475)	0.8% (4/518)
Headache	0.4% (2/519)	0.8% (4/475)	1.0% (5/518)

* No statistically significant differences between the two groups.
† Second injection of placebo not administered because code for the trial was broken.

A, it is possible for unrecognized hepatitis A infection to be present at the time the vaccine is given. The vaccine may not prevent hepatitis A in such individuals.
As with any vaccine, adequate treatment provisions, including epinephrine, should be available for immediate use should an anaphylactic or anaphylactoid reaction occur.
VAQTA should be administered with caution to people with bleeding disorders who are at risk of hemorrhage following intramuscular injection (see DOSAGE AND ADMINISTRATION).
As with any vaccine, vaccination with VAQTA may not result in a protective response in all susceptible vaccinees.
An acute infection or febrile illness may be reason for delaying use of VAQTA except when, in the opinion of the physician, withholding the vaccine entails a greater risk.
Carcinogenesis, Mutagenesis, Impairment of Fertility
VAQTA has not been evaluated for its carcinogenic or mutagenic potential, or its potential to impair fertility.
Pregnancy
Pregnancy Category C: Animal reproduction studies have not been conducted with VAQTA. It is also not known whether VAQTA can cause fetal harm when administered to a pregnant woman or can affect reproduction capacity. VAQTA should be given to a pregnant woman only if clearly needed.
Nursing Mothers
It is not known whether VAQTA is excreted in human milk. Because many drugs are excreted in human milk, caution should be exercised when VAQTA is administered to a woman who is breast feeding.
Pediatric Use
VAQTA has been shown to be generally well tolerated and highly immunogenic in individuals 2 through 17 years of age. See DOSAGE AND ADMINISTRATION for the recommended dosage schedule.
Safety and effectiveness in infants below 2 years of age have not been established.

ADVERSE REACTIONS

In combined clinical trials, 16,252 doses of VAQTA were administered to 9181 healthy children, adolescents, and adults. VAQTA was generally well tolerated.
No serious vaccine-related adverse experiences were observed during clinical trials.
The Monroe Efficacy Study
In this study, 1037 healthy children and adolescents, 2 through 16 years of age, received a primary dose of ∼25U of hepatitis A vaccine and a booster 6, 12, or 18 months later, or placebo. Subjects were observed during a 5-day period for fever and local complaints and during a 14-day period for systemic complaints. Injection-site complaints, generally mild and transient, were the most frequently reported complaints. Table 4 summarizes the local and systemic complaints (≥1%) reported in this study, without regard to causality. There were no significant differences in the rates of any complaints between vaccine and placebo recipients after Dose 1.
[See table 4 above]
Children/Adolescents — 2 through 17 Years of Age
In combined clinical trials (including Monroe Efficacy Study participants) involving 2595 healthy children and adolescents who received one or more ∼25U doses of hepatitis A vaccine, fever and local complaints were observed during a 5-day period following vaccination and systemic complaints during a 14-day period following vaccination. Injection-site complaints, generally mild and transient, were the most frequently reported complaints. Listed below are the complaints (≥1%) reported, without regard to causality, in decreasing order of frequency within each body system.
LOCALIZED INJECTION-SITE REACTIONS (generally mild and transient)
Pain (18.7%); tenderness (16.8%); warmth (8.6%); erythema (7.5%); swelling (7.3%); ecchymosis (1.3%).
BODY AS A WHOLE
Fever (≥102°F, Oral) (3.1%); abdominal pain (1.6%).

DIGESTIVE SYSTEM
Diarrhea (1.0%); vomiting (1.0%).
NERVOUS SYSTEM/PSYCHIATRIC
Headache (2.3%).
RESPIRATORY SYSTEM
Pharyngitis (1.5%); upper respiratory infection (1.1%); cough (1.0%).
LABORATORY FINDINGS
Very few laboratory abnormalities were reported and included isolated reports of elevated liver function tests, eosinophilia, and increased urine protein.
Adults—18 Years of Age and Older
In combined clinical trials involving 1529 healthy adults who received one or more ∼50U doses of hepatitis A vaccine, fever and local complaints were observed during a 5-day period following vaccination and systemic complaints during a 14-day period following vaccination. Injection-site complaints, generally mild and transient, were the most frequently reported complaints. Listed below are the complaints (≥1%) reported, without regard to causality, in decreasing order of frequency within each body system.
LOCALIZED INJECTION-SITE REACTIONS (generally mild and transient)
Tenderness (52.6%); pain (51.1%); warmth (17.3%); swelling (13.6%); erythema (12.9%); ecchymosis (1.5%); pain/soreness (1.2%).
BODY AS A WHOLE
Asthenia/fatigue (3.9%); fever (≥101°F, Oral) (2.6%); abdominal pain (1.3%).
DIGESTIVE SYSTEM
Diarrhea (2.4%); nausea (2.3%).
MUSCULOSKELETAL SYSTEM
Myalgia (2.0%); arm pain (1.3%); back pain (1.1%); stiffness (1.0%).
NERVOUS SYSTEM/PSYCHIATRIC
Headache (16.1%).
RESPIRATORY SYSTEM
Pharyngitis (2.7%); upper respiratory infection (2.8%); nasal congestion (1.1%).
UROGENITAL SYSTEM
Menstruation disorder (1.1%).
Allergic Reactions
Local and/or systemic allergic reactions that occurred in <1% of children/adolescents or adults in clinical trials regardless of causality included:
LOCAL
Injection site pruritus and/or rash.
SYSTEMIC
Bronchial constriction; asthma; wheezing; edema/swelling; rash; generalized erythema; urticaria; pruritus; eye irritation/itching; dermatitis. (See CONTRAINDICATIONS and WARNINGS.)
As with any vaccine, there is the possibility that use of VAQTA in very large populations might reveal adverse experiences not observed in clinical trials.

DOSAGE AND ADMINISTRATION

Do not inject intravenously, intradermally, or subcutaneously.
VAQTA is for intramuscular injection. The *deltoid muscle* is the preferred site for intramuscular injection.
DOSAGE
The vaccination regimen consists of one primary dose and one booster dose for healthy children, adolescents, and adults, as follows:

Continued on next page

Information on the Merck & Co., Inc. products listed on these pages is the full prescribing information from product circulars in use August 31, 1998. For information, please call 1-800-NSC MERCK [1-800-672-6372].

Vaqta—Cont.

Pediatric/Adolescent

Individuals 2 through 17 years of age should receive a single 0.5 mL (~25U) dose of vaccine at elected date and a booster dose of 0.5 mL (~25U) 6 to 18 months later.

Adult

Adults 18 years of age and older should receive a single 1.0 mL (~50U) dose of vaccine at elected date and a booster dose of 1.0 mL (~50U) 6 months later.

Use With Immune Globulin

VAQTA may be administered concomitantly with IG using separate sites and syringes. The vaccination regimen for VAQTA should be followed as stated above. Consult the manufacturer's product circular for the appropriate dosage of IG. A booster dose of VAQTA should be administered at the appropriate time as outlined above.

ADMINISTRATION

Known or Presumed Exposure to HAV/Travel to Endemic Areas

For individuals requiring either post-exposure prophylaxis or combined immediate and longer term protection (e.g., travelers departing on short notice to endemic areas), VAQTA may be administered concomitantly with IG using separate sites and syringes (see CLINICAL PHARMACOLOGY and DOSAGE AND ADMINISTRATION, *Use With Immune Globulin*).

Injection must be accomplished with a needle long enough to ensure intramuscular deposition of the vaccine. The Advisory Committee on Immunization Practices (ACIP) has recommended that "For all intramuscular injections, the needle should be long enough to reach the muscle mass and prevent vaccine from seeping into subcutaneous tissue, but not so long as to endanger underlying neurovascular structures or bone." For toddlers and older children they further state that "...the deltoid may be used if the muscle mass is adequate. The needle size can range from 22 to 25 gauge and from 5/8 to $1^1/_4$ inches, based on the size of the muscle...the anterolateral thigh may be used, but the needle should be longer—generally ranging from 7/8 to $1^1/_4$ inches." For adults they state that "...the deltoid is recommended for routine intramuscular vaccination among adults...The suggested needle size is 1 to $1^1/_2$ inches and 20 to 25 gauge."

For individuals with bleeding disorders who are at risk of hemorrhage following intramuscular injection, the ACIP recommends that when any intramuscular vaccine is indicated for such patients, "...it should be administered intramuscularly if, in the opinion of a physician familiar with the patient's bleeding risk, the vaccine can be administered with reasonable safety by this route. If the patient receives antihemophilia or other similar therapy, intramuscular vaccination can be scheduled shortly after such therapy is administered. A fine needle (≤23 gauge) can be used for the vaccination and firm pressure applied to the site (without rubbing) for at least two minutes. The patient or family should be instructed concerning the risk of hematoma from the injection."

The vaccine should be used as supplied; no reconstitution is necessary.

Shake well before withdrawal and use. Thorough agitation is necessary to maintain suspension of the vaccine. Discard if the suspension does not appear homogenous.

Parenteral drug products should be inspected visually for extraneous particulate matter and discoloration prior to administration whenever solution and container permit. After thorough agitation, VAQTA is a slightly opaque, white suspension.

It is important to use a separate sterile syringe and needle for each individual to prevent transmission of infectious agents from one person to another.

HOW SUPPLIED

PEDIATRIC/ADOLESCENT FORMULATION

Vials

No. 4831—VAQTA for pediatric/adolescent use is supplied as 25U/0.5 mL of hepatitis A virus protein in a 0.5 mL single-dose vial, NDC 0006-4831-00.

No. 4831—VAQTA for pediatric/adolescent use is supplied as 25U/0.5 mL of hepatitis A virus protein in a 0.5 mL single-dose vial, in a box of 5 single-dose vials, NDC 0006-4831-38.

Syringes

No. 4845—VAQTA for pediatric/adolescent use is supplied as 25U/0.5 mL of hepatitis A virus protein in a 0.5 mL single-dose prefilled syringe, NDC 0006-4845-00.

No. 4845—VAQTA for pediatric/adolescent use is supplied as 25U/0.5 mL of hepatitis A virus protein in a 0.5 mL single-dose prefilled syringe, in a box of 5 single-dose prefilled syringes, NDC 0006-4845-38.

ADULT FORMULATION

Vials

No. 4841—VAQTA for adult use is supplied as 50U/1 mL of hepatitis A virus protein in a 1 mL single-dose vial, NDC 0006-4841-00.

No. 4841—VAQTA for adult use is supplied as 50U/1 mL of hepatitis A virus protein in a 1 mL single-dose vial, in a box of 5 single-dose vials, NDC 0006-4841-38.

Syringes

No. 4844—VAQTA for adult use is supplied as 50U/1 mL of hepatitis A virus protein in a 1 mL single-dose prefilled syringe, NDC 0006-4844-00.

No. 4844—VAQTA for adult use is supplied as 50U/1 mL of hepatitis A virus protein in a 1 mL single-dose prefilled syringe, in a box of 5 single-dose, prefilled syringes, NDC 0006-4844-38.

Storage

Store vaccine at 2–8°C (36–46°F).

DO NOT FREEZE since freezing destroys potency.

Syringes of VAQTA are also filled by:

Evans Medical Ltd.

Gaskill Road, Speke, Liverpool L24 9GR, England
7977500   Issued March 1996

COPYRIGHT © MERCK & CO., Inc., 1996

All rights reserved

VARIVAX®   ℞
[Varicella Virus Vaccine Live (Oka/Merck)]

DESCRIPTION

VARIVAX* [Varicella Virus Vaccine Live (Oka/Merck)] is a preparation of the Oka/Merck strain of live, attenuated varicella virus. The virus was initially obtained from a child with natural varicella, then introduced into human embryonic lung cell cultures, adapted to and propagated in embryonic guinea pig cell cultures and finally propagated in human diploid cell cultures (WI-38). Further passage of the virus for varicella vaccine was performed at Merck Research Laboratories (MRL) in human diploid cell cultures (MRC-5) that were free of adventitious agents. This live, attenuated varicella vaccine is a lyophilized preparation containing sucrose, phosphate, glutamate, and processed gelatin as stabilizers.

VARIVAX, when reconstituted as directed, is a sterile preparation for subcutaneous administration. Each 0.5 mL dose contains the following: a minimum of 1350 PFU (plaque forming units) of Oka/Merck varicella virus when reconstituted and stored at room temperature for 30 minutes, approximately 25 mg of sucrose, 12.5 mg hydrolyzed gelatin, 3.2 mg sodium chloride, 0.5 mg monosodium L-glutamate, 0.45 mg of sodium phosphate dibasic, 0.08 mg of potassium phosphate monobasic, 0.08 mg of potassium chloride; residual components of MRC-5 cells including DNA and protein; and trace quantities of sodium phosphate monobasic, EDTA, neomycin, and fetal bovine serum. The product contains no preservative.

To maintain potency, the lyophilized vaccine must be kept frozen at an average temperature of −15°C (+5°F) or colder and must be used before the expiration date (see HOW SUPPLIED, *Stability* and *Storage*). Storage in any freezer (e.g., chest, frost-free) that reliably maintains an average temperature of −15°C (+5°F) or colder and has a separate sealed freezer door is acceptable.

*Registered trademark of MERCK & CO., Inc.

CLINICAL PHARMACOLOGY

Varicella is a highly communicable disease in children, adolescents, and adults caused by the varicella-zoster virus. The disease usually consists of 300 to 500 maculopapular and/or vesicular lesions accompanied by a fever (oral temperature ≥100°F) in up to 70% of individuals. Approximately 3.5 million cases of varicella occurred annually from 1980–1994 in the United States with the peak incidence occurring in children five to nine years of age. The incidence rate of chickenpox is 8.3–9.1% per year in children 1–9 years of age. The attack rate of natural varicella following household exposure among healthy susceptible children was shown to be 87%. Although it is generally a benign, self-limiting disease, varicella may be associated with serious complications (e.g., bacterial superinfection, pneumonia, encephalitis, Reye's Syndrome), and/or death.

Evaluation of Clinical Efficacy Afforded by VARIVAX

Clinical Data in Children

In combined clinical trials of VARIVAX at doses ranging from 1,000–17,000 PFU, the majority of subjects who received VARIVAX and were exposed to wild-type virus were either completely protected from chickenpox or developed a milder form (for clinical description see below) of the disease. The protective efficacy of VARIVAX was evaluated in three different ways: 1) by comparing chickenpox rates in vaccinees versus historical controls, 2) by assessment of protection from disease following household exposure, and 3) by a placebo-controlled, double-blind clinical trial.

In early clinical trials, a total of 4142 children received 1000–1625 PFU of attenuated virus per dose of VARIVAX

and have been followed for up to six years post single-dose vaccination. In this group there was considerable variation in chickenpox rates among studies and study sites, and much of the reported data were acquired by passive follow-up. It was observed that 2.1%–3.6% of vaccinees per year reported chickenpox (called breakthrough cases). This represents an approximate 67% (57–77%) decrease from the total number of cases expected based on attack rates in children aged 1–9 over this same period (8.3–9.1%). In those who developed breakthrough chickenpox postvaccination, the majority experienced mild disease (median number of lesions <50). In one study, a total of 47% (27/58) of breakthrough cases had <50 lesions compared with 8% (7/92) in unvaccinated individuals, and 7% (4/58) of breakthrough cases had >300 lesions compared with 50% (46/92) in unvaccinated individuals. In studies of vaccinated children who contracted chickenpox after a household exposure, 57% (31/54) of the cases reported <50 lesions, while 1.9% (1/54) reported >300 lesions with an oral temperature above 100°F. In later clinical trials with the current vaccine, a total of 1164 children received 2900–9000 PFU of attenuated virus per dose of VARIVAX and have been followed for up to three years post single-dose vaccination. It was observed that 0.2%–1.0% of vaccinees per year reported breakthrough chickenpox for up to three years post single-dose vaccination. This represents an approximate 93% decrease from the total number of cases expected based on attack rates in children aged 1–9 over this same period (8.3%–9.1%). In those who developed breakthrough chickenpox postvaccination, the majority experienced mild disease.

Among a subset of vaccinees who were actively followed, 259 were exposed to an individual with chickenpox in a household setting. There were no reports of breakthrough chickenpox in 80% of exposed children; 20% reported a mild form of chickenpox. This represents a 77% reduction in the expected number of cases when compared to the historical attack rate of varicella following household exposure to chickenpox of 87% in unvaccinated individuals.

Although no placebo-controlled trial was carried out with VARIVAX using the current vaccine, a placebo-controlled trial was conducted using a formulation containing 17,000 PFU per dose. In this trial, a single dose of VARIVAX protected 96–100% of children against chickenpox over a two-year period. The study enrolled healthy individuals 1 to 14 years of age (n=491 vaccine, n=465 placebo). In the first year, 8.5% of placebo recipients contracted chickenpox, while no vaccine recipient did, for a calculated protection rate of 100% during the first varicella season. In the second year, when only a subset of individuals agreed to remain in the blinded study (n=163 vaccine, n=161 placebo), 96% protective efficacy was calculated for the vaccine group as compared to placebo.

There are insufficient data to assess the rate of protection against the complications of chickenpox (e.g., encephalitis, hepatitis, pneumonia) in children.

Clinical Data in Adolescents and Adults

Although no placebo-controlled trial was carried out in adolescents and adults, efficacy was determined by evaluation of protection when vaccinees received 2 doses of VARIVAX 4 or 8 weeks apart and were subsequently exposed to chickenpox in a household setting. In up to two years of active follow-up, 17 of 64 (27%) vaccinees reported breakthrough chickenpox following household exposure; of the 17 cases, 12 (71%) reported <50 lesions, 5 reported 50–300 lesions, and none reported >300 lesions with an oral temperature above 100°F. In combined clinical studies of adolescents and adults (n=1019) who received two doses of VARIVAX and later developed breakthrough chickenpox and reported numbers of lesions (42 of 1019), 25 of 42 (60%) reported <50 lesions, 16 of 42 (38%) reported 50–300 lesions, and 1 of 42 (2%) reported >300 lesions and an oral temperature above 100°F.

The attack rate of unvaccinated adults exposed to a single contact in a household has not been previously studied. When compared to the previously reported attack rate of natural varicella of 87% following household exposure among unvaccinated children, this represents an approximate 70% reduction in the expected number of cases in the household setting.

There are insufficient data to assess the rate of protection of VARIVAX against the serious complications of chickenpox in adults (e.g., encephalitis, hepatitis, pneumonitis) and during pregnancy (congenital varicella syndrome).

Immunogenicity of VARIVAX

Clinical trials with several formulations of the vaccine containing attenuated virus ranging from 1000 to 17,000 PFU per dose have demonstrated that VARIVAX induces detectable immune responses in a high proportion of individuals and is generally well tolerated in healthy individuals ranging from 12 months to 55 years of age.

Seroconversion as defined by the acquisition of any detectable varicella antibodies (gpELISA >0.3, a highly sensitive assay which is not commercially available) was observed in 97% of vaccinees at approximately 4–6 weeks postvaccination in 6889 susceptible children 12 months to 12 years of age. Rates of breakthrough disease were significantly lower

among children with varicella antibody titers ≥5 compared to children with titers <5. Titers ≥5 were induced in approximately 76% of children vaccinated with a single dose of vaccine at 1000–17,000 PFU per dose. In a multicenter study involving susceptible adolescents and adults 13 years of age and older, two doses of VARIVAX administered four to eight weeks apart induced a seroconversion rate (gpELISA >0.3) of approximately 75% in 539 individuals four weeks after the first dose and of 99% in 479 individuals four weeks after the second dose. The average antibody response in vaccinees who received the second dose eight weeks after the first dose was higher than that in those, who received the second dose four weeks after the first dose. In another multicenter study involving adolescents and adults, two doses of VARIVAX administered eight weeks apart induced a seroconversion rate (gpELISA >0.3) of 94% in 142 individuals six weeks after the first dose and 99% in 122 individuals six weeks after the second dose.

VARIVAX also induces cell-mediated immune responses in vaccinees. The relative contributions of humoral immunity and cell-mediated immunity to protection from chickenpox are unknown.

Persistence of Immune Response
Studies in vaccinees examining chickenpox breakthrough rates over 5 years showed the lowest rates (0.2–2.9%) in the first two years postvaccination, with somewhat higher but stable rates in the third through fifth year. The severity of reported breakthrough chickenpox, as measured by number of lesions and maximum temperature, appeared not to increase with time since vaccination.

In clinical studies involving healthy children who received 1 dose of vaccine, detectable varicella antibodies (gpELISA >0.3) were present in 98.8% (3775/3822) at 1 year, 98.9% (1057/1069) at 2 years, 97.5% (548/562) at 3 years, and 99.5% (220/221) at 4 years postvaccination. Antibody levels were present at least one year in 97.2% (423/435) of healthy adolescents and adults who received two doses of live varicella vaccine separated by 4 to 8 weeks. A boost in antibody levels has been observed in vaccinees following exposure to natural varicella which could account for the apparent long-term persistence of antibody levels after vaccination in these studies. The duration of protection from varicella obtained using VARIVAX in the absence of wild-type boosting is unknown. VARIVAX also induces cell-mediated immune responses in vaccinees. The relative contributions of humoral immunity and cell-mediated immunity to protection from chickenpox are unknown.

Transmission
In the placebo-controlled trial, transmission of vaccine virus was assessed in household settings (during the 8-week postvaccination period) in 416 susceptible placebo recipients who were household contacts of 445 vaccine recipients. Of the 416 placebo recipients, three developed chickenpox and seroconverted, nine reported a varicella-like rash and did not seroconvert, and six had no rash but seroconverted. If vaccine virus transmission occurred, it did so at a very low rate and possibly without recognizable clinical disease in contacts. These cases may represent either natural varicella from community contacts or a low incidence of transmission of vaccine virus from vaccinated contacts (see PRECAUTIONS, *Transmission*). Post-marketing experience suggests that transmission of vaccine virus may occur rarely between healthy vaccinees who develop a varicella-like rash and healthy susceptible contacts. Transmission of vaccine virus from vaccinees without a varicella-like rash has been reported but has not been confirmed.

Herpes Zoster
Overall, 9454 healthy children (12 months to 12 years of age) and 1648 adolescents and adults (13 years of age and older) have been vaccinated with Oka/Merck live attenuated varicella vaccine in clinical trials. Eight cases of herpes zoster have been reported in children during 42,556 person years of follow-up in clinical trials, resulting in a calculated incidence of at least 18.8 cases per 100,000 person years. The completeness of this reporting has not been determined. One case of herpes zoster has been reported in the adolescent and adult age group during 5410 person years of follow-up in clinical trials resulting in a calculated incidence of 18.5 cases per 100,000 person years.

All nine cases were mild and without sequelae. Two cultures (one child and one adult) obtained from vesicles were positive for wild-type varicella zoster virus as confirmed by restriction endonuclease analysis. The long-term effect of VARIVAX on the incidence of herpes zoster, particularly in those vaccinees exposed to natural varicella, is unknown at present.

In children, the reported rate of zoster in vaccine recipients appears not to exceed that previously determined in a population-based study of healthy children who had experienced natural varicella. The incidence of zoster in adults who have had natural varicella infection is higher than that in children.

Reye's Syndrome
Reye's Syndrome has occurred in children and adolescents following natural varicella infection, the majority of whom had received salicylates. In clinical studies in healthy chil-

dren and adolescents in the United States, physicians advised varicella vaccine recipients not to use salicylates for six weeks after vaccination. There were no reports of Reye's Syndrome in varicella vaccine recipients during these studies.

Studies with Other Vaccines
In combined clinical studies involving 1080 children 12 to 36 months of age, 653 received VARIVAX and M-M-R*II (Measles, Mumps, and Rubella Virus Vaccine Live) concomitantly at separate sites and 427 received the vaccines six weeks apart. Seroconversion rates and antibody levels were comparable between the two groups at approximately six weeks postvaccination to each of the virus vaccine components. No differences were noted in adverse reactions reported in those who received VARIVAX concomitantly with M-M-R II (Measles, Mumps, and Rubella Virus Vaccine Live) at separate sites and those who received VARIVAX and M-M-R II (Measles, Mumps, and Rubella Virus Vaccine Live) at different times (see PRECAUTIONS, *Drug Interactions, Use with Other Vaccines*).

In a clinical study involving 318 children 12 months to 42 months of age, 160 received an investigational vaccine (a formulation combining measles, mumps, rubella, and varicella in one syringe) concomitantly with booster doses of DTaP (diphtheria, tetanus, acellular pertussis) and OPV (oral poliovirus vaccine) while 144 received M-M-R II (Measles, Mumps, and Rubella Virus Vaccine Live) concomitantly with booster doses of DTaP and OPV followed by VARIVAX 6 weeks later. At six weeks postvaccination, seroconversion rates for measles, mumps, rubella, and varicella and the percentage of vaccinees whose titers were boosted for diphtheria, tetanus, pertussis, and polio were comparable between the two groups, but anti-varicella levels were decreased when the investigational vaccine containing varicella was administered concomitantly with DTaP. No clinically significant differences were noted in adverse reactions between the two groups.

In another clinical study involving 307 children 12 to 18 months of age, 150 received an investigational vaccine (a formulation combining measles, mumps, rubella, and varicella in one syringe) concomitantly with a booster dose of PedvaxHIB* [Haemophilus b Conjugate Vaccine (Meningococcal Protein Conjugate)] while 130 received M-M-R II (Measles, Mumps, and Rubella Virus Vaccine Live) concomitantly with a booster dose of PedvaxHIB followed by VARIVAX 6 weeks later. At six weeks postvaccination, seroconversion rates for measles, mumps, rubella, and varicella, and geometric mean titers for PedvaxHIB were comparable between the two groups, but anti-varicella levels were decreased when the investigational vaccine containing varicella was administered concomitantly with PedvaxHIB. No clinically significant differences in adverse reactions were seen between the two groups.

VARIVAX is recommended for subcutaneous administration. However, during clinical trials, some children received VARIVAX intramuscularly resulting in seroconversion rates similar to those in children who received the vaccine by the subcutaneous route. Persistence of antibody and efficacy in those receiving intramuscular injections have not been defined.

---

* Registered trademark of MERCK & Co., Inc.

INDICATIONS AND USAGE

VARIVAX is indicated for vaccination against varicella in individuals 12 months of age and older.

Revaccination
The duration of protection of VARIVAX is unknown at present and the need for booster doses is not defined. However, a boost in antibody levels has been observed in vaccinees following exposure to natural varicella as well as following a booster dose of VARIVAX administered four to six years postvaccination.

In a highly vaccinated population, immunity for some individuals may wane due to lack of exposure to natural varicella as a result of shifting epidemiology. Post-marketing surveillance studies are ongoing to evaluate the need and timing for booster vaccination.

Vaccination with VARIVAX may not result in protection of all healthy, susceptible children, adolescents, and adults (see CLINICAL PHARMACOLOGY).

CONTRAINDICATIONS

A history of hypersensitivity to any component of the vaccine, including gelatin.

A history of anaphylactoid reaction to neomycin (each dose of reconstituted vaccine contains trace quantities of neomycin).

Individuals with blood dyscrasias, leukemia, lymphomas of any type, or other malignant neoplasms affecting the bone marrow or lymphatic systems.

Individuals receiving immunosuppressive therapy. Individuals who are on immunosuppressant drugs are more susceptible to infections than healthy individuals. Vaccination

with live attenuated varicella vaccine can result in a more extensive vaccine-associated rash or disseminated disease in individuals on immunosuppressant doses of corticosteroids.

Individuals with primary and acquired immunodeficiency states, including those who are immunosuppressed in association with AIDS or other clinical manifestations of infection with human immunodeficiency virus; cellular immune deficiencies; and hypogammaglobulinemic and dysgammaglobulinemic states.

A family history of congenital or hereditary immunodeficiency, unless the immune competence of the potential vaccine recipient is demonstrated.

Active untreated tuberculosis.

Any febrile respiratory illness or other active febrile infection.

Pregnancy; the possible effects of the vaccine on fetal development are unknown at this time. However, natural varicella is known to sometimes cause fetal harm. If vaccination of postpubertal females is undertaken, pregnancy should be avoided for three months following vaccination. (See PRECAUTIONS, *Pregnancy*).

WARNINGS

Children and adolescents with acute lymphoblastic leukemia (ALL) in remission can receive the vaccine under an investigational protocol. More information is available by contacting the VARIVAX coordinating center, Bio-Pharm Clinical Services, Inc., 4 Valley Square, Blue Bell, PA 19422 (215) 283-0897.

PRECAUTIONS

General
Adequate treatment provisions, including epinephrine injection (1:1000), should be available for immediate use should an anaphylactoid reaction occur.

The duration of protection from varicella infection after vaccination with VARIVAX is unknown.

It is not known whether VARIVAX given immediately after exposure to natural varicella virus will prevent illness.

Vaccination should be deferred for at least 5 months following blood or plasma transfusions, or administration of immune globulin or varicella zoster immune globulin (VZIG). Following administration of VARIVAX, any immune globulin including VZIG should not be given for 2 months thereafter unless its use outweighs the benefits of vaccination.

Vaccine recipients should avoid use of salicylates for 6 weeks after vaccination with VARIVAX as Reye's Syndrome has been reported following the use of salicylates during natural varicella infection (see CLINICAL PHARMACOLOGY, *Reye's Syndrome*).

The safety and efficacy of VARIVAX have not been established in children and young adults who are known to be infected with human immunodeficiency viruses with and without evidence of immunosuppression (see also CONTRAINDICATIONS).

Care is to be taken by the health care provider for safe and effective use of VARIVAX.

The health care provider should question the patient, parent, or guardian about reactions to a previous dose of VARIVAX or a similar product.

The health care provider should obtain the previous immunization history of the vaccinee.

VARIVAX should not be injected into a blood vessel.

Vaccination should be deferred in patients with a family history of congenital or hereditary immunodeficiency until the patient's own immune system has been evaluated.

A separate sterile needle and syringe should be used for administration of each dose of VARIVAX to prevent transfer of infectious diseases.

Needles should be disposed of properly and should not be recapped.

Transmission
Post-marketing experience suggests that transmission of vaccine virus may occur rarely between healthy vaccinees who develop a varicella-like rash and healthy susceptible contacts. Transmission of vaccine virus from vaccinees without a varicella-like rash has been reported but has not been confirmed.

Therefore, vaccine recipients should attempt to avoid, whenever possible, close association with susceptible high-risk individuals for up to six weeks. In circumstances where contact with high-risk individuals is unavoidable, the potential risk of transmission of vaccine virus should be weighed against the risk of acquiring and transmitting natural varicella virus. Susceptible high-risk individuals include:

Continued on next page

Information on the Merck & Co., Inc. products listed on these pages is the full prescribing information from product circulars in use August 31, 1998. For information, please call 1-800-NSC MERCK [1-800-672-6372].

Consult 1999 PDR® supplements and future editions for revisions

Varivax—Cont.

- immunocompromised individuals
- pregnant women without documented history of chickenpox or laboratory evidence of prior infection
- newborn infants of mothers without documented history of chickenpox or laboratory evidence of prior infection

Information for Patients
The health care provider should inform the patient, parent or guardian of the benefits and risks of VARIVAX.
Patients, parents, or guardians should be instructed to report any adverse reactions to the health care provider.
The U.S. Department of Health and Human Services has established a Vaccine Adverse Event Reporting System (VAERS) to accept all reports of suspected adverse events after the administration of any vaccine, including but not limited to the reporting of events required by the National Childhood Vaccine Injury Act of 1986. The VAERS toll-free number for VAERS forms and information is 1-800-822-7967.
Pregnancy should be avoided for three months following vaccination.

Drug Interactions
See PRECAUTIONS, *General,* regarding the administration of immune globulins, salicylates, and transfusions.
Drug Interactions, Use with Other Vaccines
Results from clinical studies indicate that VARIVAX can be administered concomitantly with M-M-R II (Measles, Mumps, and Rubella Virus Vaccine Live).
Limited data from an experimental product containing varicella vaccine suggest that VARIVAX can be administered concomitantly with DTaP (diphtheria, tetanus, acellular pertussis) and PedvaxHIB using separate sites and syringes (see CLINICAL PHARMACOLOGY, *Studies with Other Vaccines*). However, there are no data relating to simultaneous administration of VARIVAX with DTP or OPV.
Carcinogenesis, Mutagenesis, Impairment of Fertility
VARIVAX has not been evaluated for its carcinogenic or mutagenic potential, or its potential to impair fertility.
Pregnancy
Pregnancy Category C: Animal reproduction studies have not been conducted with VARIVAX. It is also not known whether VARIVAX can cause fetal harm when administered to a pregnant woman or can affect reproduction capacity. Therefore, VARIVAX should not be administered to pregnant females; furthermore, pregnancy should be avoided for three months following vaccination (see CONTRAINDICATIONS).
Nursing Mothers
It is not known whether varicella vaccine virus is secreted in human milk. Therefore, because some viruses are secreted in human milk, caution should be exercised if VARIVAX is administered to a nursing woman.
Pediatric Use
No clinical data are available on safety or efficacy of VARIVAX in children less than one year of age and administration to infants under twelve months of age is not recommended.

ADVERSE REACTIONS

In clinical trials, VARIVAX was administered to 11,102 healthy children, adolescents, and adults. VARIVAX was generally well tolerated.
In a double-blind placebo controlled study among 914 healthy children and adolescents who were serologically confirmed to be susceptible to varicella, the only adverse reactions that occurred at a significantly (p<0.05) greater rate in vaccine recipients than in placebo recipients were pain and redness at the injection site.
Children 1 to 12 Years of Age
In clinical trials involving healthy children monitored for up to 42 days after a single dose of VARIVAX, the frequency of fever, injection-site complaints, or rashes were reported as follows:
[See table 1 above]
In addition, the most frequently (≥1%) reported adverse experiences, without regard to causality, are listed in decreasing order of frequency: upper respiratory illness, cough, irritability/nervousness, fatigue, disturbed sleep, diarrhea, loss of appetite, vomiting, otitis, diaper rash/contact rash, headache, teething, malaise, abdominal pain, other rash, nausea, eye complaints, chills, lymphadenopathy, myalgia, lower respiratory illness, allergic reactions (including allergic rash, hives), stiff neck, heat rash/prickly heat, arthralgia, eczema/dry skin/dermatitis, constipation, itching.
Pneumonitis has been reported rarely (<1%) in children vaccinated with VARIVAX; a causal relationship has not been established.
Febrile seizures have occurred rarely (<0.1%) in children vaccinated with VARIVAX; a causal relationship has not been established.
Adolescents and Adults 13 Years of Age and Older
In clinical trials involving healthy adolescents and adults, the majority of whom received two doses of VARIVAX and

Table 1
Fever, Local Reactions, or Rashes (%) in Children
0 to 42 Days Postvaccination

Reaction	N	Post dose 1	Peak Occurrence in Postvaccination Days
Fever ≥102°F (39°C) Oral	8827	14.7%	0–42
Injection-site complaints (pain/soreness, swelling and/or erythema, rash, pruritus, hematoma, induration, stiffness)	8916	19.3%	0–2
Varicella-like rash (injection site) Median number of lesions	8916	3.4% 2	8–19
Varicella-like rash (generalized) Median number of lesions	8916	3.8% 5	5–26

Table 2
Fever, Local Reactions, or Rashes (%) in Adolescents and Adults
0 to 42 Days Postvaccination

Reaction	N	Post Dose 1	Peak Occurrence in Postvaccination Days	N	Post Dose 2	Peak Occurrence in Postvaccination Days
Fever ≥100°F (37.7°C) Oral	1584	10.2%	14-27	956	9.5%	0–42
Injection-site complaints (soreness, erythema, swelling, rash, pruritus, pyrexia, hematoma, induration, numbness)	1606	24.4%	0–2	955	32.5%	0–2
Varicella-like rash (injection site) Median number of lesions	1606	3% 2	6–20	955	1% 2	0–6
Varicella-like rash (generalized) Median number of lesions	1606	5.5% 5	7–21	955	0.9% 5.5	0–23

were monitored for up to 42 days after any dose, the frequency of fever, injection-site complaints, or rashes were reported as follows:
[See table 2 above]
In addition, the most frequently (≥1%) reported adverse experiences, without regard to causality, are listed in decreasing order of frequency: upper respiratory illness, headache, fatigue, cough, myalgia, disturbed sleep, nausea, malaise, diarrhea, stiff neck, irritability/nervousness, lymphadenopathy, chills, eye complaints, abdominal pain, loss of appetite, arthralgia, otitis, itching, vomiting, other rashes, constipation, lower respiratory illness, allergic reactions (including allergic rash, hives), contact rash, cold/canker sore.
As with any vaccine, there is the possibility that broad use of the vaccine could reveal adverse reactions not observed in clinical trials.
The following additional adverse reactions have been reported since the vaccine has been marketed:
Body As A Whole
Anaphylaxis.
Hemic and Lymphatic System
Thrombocytopenia.
Nervous/Psychiatric
Encephalitis; Guillain-Barré syndrome; transverse myelitis; Bell's palsy; ataxia; paresthesia.
Respiratory
Pharyngitis.
Skin
Stevens-Johnson syndrome; erythema multiforme; Henoch-Schönlein purpura; secondary bacterial infections of skin and soft tissue, including impetigo and cellulitis; herpes zoster.

DOSAGE AND ADMINISTRATION

FOR SUBCUTANEOUS ADMINISTRATION
Do not inject intravenously
Children 12 months to 12 years of age should receive a single 0.5 mL dose administered subcutaneously.
Adolescents and adults 13 years of age and older should receive a 0.5 mL dose administered subcutaneously at elected date and a second 0.5 mL dose 4 to 8 weeks later.
VARIVAX is for subcutaneous administration. The outer aspect of the upper arm (deltoid) is the preferred site of injection.
VARIVAX **SHOULD BE STORED FROZEN** at an average temperature of −15°C (+5°F) or colder until it is reconstituted for injection (see HOW SUPPLIED, *Storage*). Any freezer (e.g. chest, frost-free) that reliably maintains an average temperature of −15°C and has a separate sealed freezer door is acceptable for storing VARIVAX. The diluent should

be stored separately at room temperature or in the refrigerator. To reconstitute the vaccine, first withdraw 0.7 mL of diluent into the syringe to be used for reconstitution. Inject all the diluent in the syringe into the vial of lyophilized vaccine and gently agitate to mix thoroughly. Withdraw the entire contents into a syringe and inject the total volume (about 0.5 mL) of reconstituted vaccine subcutaneously, preferably into the outer aspect of the upper arm (deltoid) or the anterolateral thigh. **IT IS RECOMMENDED THAT THE VACCINE BE ADMINISTERED IMMEDIATELY AFTER RECONSTITUTION, TO MINIMIZE LOSS OF POTENCY. DISCARD IF RECONSTITUTED VACCINE IS NOT USED WITHIN 30 MINUTES.**
CAUTION: A sterile syringe free of preservatives, antiseptics, and detergents should be used for each injection and/or reconstitution of VARIVAX because these substances may inactivate the vaccine virus.
It is important to use a separate sterile syringe and needle for each patient to prevent transmission of infectious agents from one individual to another.
To reconstitute the vaccine, use only the Merck sterile diluent supplied with VARIVAX, M-M-R II, or the component vaccines of M-M-R II, since it is free of preservatives and other anti-viral substances which might inactivate the vaccine virus.
Do not freeze reconstituted vaccine.
Do not give immune globulin including Varicella Zoster Immune Globulin concurrently with VARIVAX (see also PRECAUTIONS).
Parenteral drug products should be inspected visually for particulate matter and discoloration prior to administration, whenever solution and container permit. VARIVAX when reconstituted is a clear, colorless to pale yellow liquid.

HOW SUPPLIED

No. 4826/4309—VARIVAX is supplied as follows: (1) a single-dose vial of lyophilized vaccine, **NDC** 0006-4826-00 (package A); and (2) a box of 10 vials of diluent (package B).
No. 4827/4309—VARIVAX is supplied as follows: (1) a box of 10 single-dose vials of lyophilized vaccine (package A), **NDC** 0006-4827-00; and (2) a box of 10 vials of diluent (package B)
(6505-01-413-1331, Ten Pack).
Stability
VARIVAX retains a potency level of 1500 PFU or higher per dose for at least 18 months in a frost-free freezer with an average temperature of −15°C (+5°F) or colder.
VARIVAX has a minimum potency level of approximately 1350 PFU 30 minutes after reconstitution at room temperature (20-25°C, 68-77°F).

Prior to reconstitution, VARIVAX retains potency when stored for up to 72 continuous hours at refrigerator temperature (2-8°C, 36-46°F).
For information regarding stability under other conditions other than those recommended, call 1-800-9-VARIVAX.
Storage
During shipment, to ensure that there is no loss of potency, the vaccine must be maintained at a temperature of −20°C (−4°F) or colder.
Before reconstitution, store the lyophilized vaccine in a freezer at an average temperature of −15°C (+5°F) or colder. Any freezer (e.g. chest, frost-free) that reliably maintains an average temperature of −15°C and has a separate sealed freezer door is acceptable for storing VARIVAX.
VARIVAX may be stored at refrigerator temperature (2-8°C, 36-46°F) for up to 72 continuous hours prior to reconstitution. Vaccine stored at 2-8°C which is not used within 72 hours of removal from −15°C storage should be discarded.
Before reconstitution, protect from light.
The diluent should be stored separately at room temperature (20-25°C, 68-77°F), or in the refrigerator.
7999907 Issued March 1998
Copyright © MERCK & CO., Inc., 1995
All rights reserved

VASERETIC® Tablets ℞
(Enalapril Maleate-Hydrochlorothiazide), U.S.P.

USE IN PREGNANCY
When used in pregnancy during the second and third trimesters, ACE inhibitors can cause injury and even death to the developing fetus. When pregnancy is detected, VASERETIC should be discontinued as soon as possible. See WARNINGS, *Pregnancy, Enalapril Maleate, Fetal/Neonatal Morbidity and Mortality.*

DESCRIPTION

VASERETIC* (Enalapril Maleate-Hydrochlorothiazide) combines an angiotensin converting enzyme inhibitor, enalapril maleate, and a diuretic, hydrochlorothiazide.
Enalapril maleate is the maleate salt of enalapril, the ethyl ester of a long-acting angiotensin converting enzyme inhibitor, enalaprilat. Enalapril maleate is chemically described as (*S*)-1-[*N*-[1-(ethoxycarbonyl)-3-phenylpropyl]-L-alanyl]-L-proline, (*Z*)-2-butenedioate salt (1:1). Its empirical formula is $C_{20}H_{28}N_2O_5 \cdot C_4H_4O_4$, and its structural formula is:

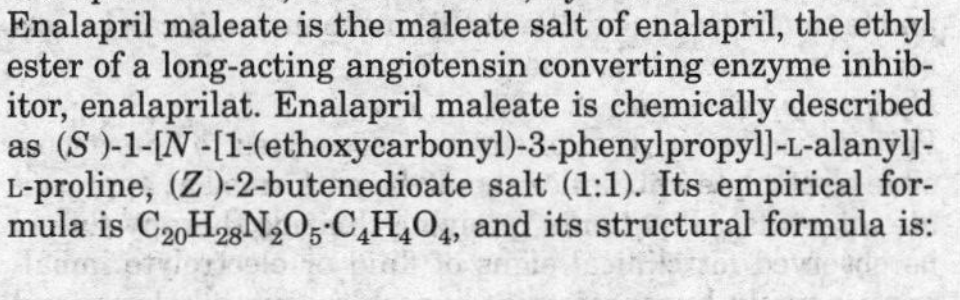

Enalapril maleate is a white to off-white crystalline powder with a molecular weight of 492.53. It is sparingly soluble in water, soluble in ethanol, and freely soluble in methanol.
Enalapril is a pro-drug; following oral administration, it is bioactivated by hydrolysis of the ethyl ester to enalaprilat, which is the active angiotensin converting enzyme inhibitor.
Hydrochlorothiazide is 6-chloro-3,4-dihydro-2*H*-1,2,4-benzothiadiazine-7-sulfonamide 1,1-dioxide. Its empirical formula is $C_7H_8ClN_3O_4S_2$ and its structural formula is:

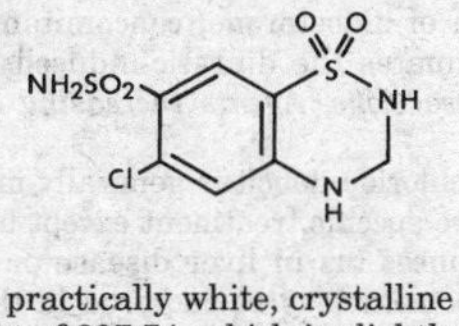

It is a white, or practically white, crystalline powder with a molecular weight of 297.74, which is slightly soluble in water, but freely soluble in sodium hydroxide solution.
VASERETIC is available in two tablet combinations of enalapril maleate with hydrochlorothiazide: VASERETIC 5–12.5, containing 5 mg enalapril maleate and 12.5 mg hydrochlorothiazide and VASERETIC 10–25, containing 10 mg enalapril maleate and 25 mg hydrochlorothiazide. Inactive ingredients are: iron oxides, lactose, magnesium stearate, starch and other ingredients.

*Registered trademark of MERCK & CO., Inc.

CLINICAL PHARMACOLOGY

As a result of its diuretic effects, hydrochlorothiazide increases plasma renin activity, increases aldosterone secretion, and decreases serum potassium. Administration of enalapril maleate blocks the renin-angiotensin-aldosterone axis and tends to reverse the potassium loss associated with the diuretic.
In clinical studies, the extent of blood pressure reduction seen with the combination of enalapril maleate and hydrochlorothiazide was approximately additive. The antihypertensive effect of VASERETIC was usually sustained for at least 24 hours.
Concomitant administration of enalapril maleate and hydrochlorothiazide has little, or no effect on the bioavailability of either drug. The combination tablet is bioequivalent to concomitant administration of the separate entities.
Enalapril Maleate
Mechanism of Action: Enalapril, after hydrolysis to enalaprilat, inhibits angiotensin-converting enzyme (ACE) in human subjects and animals. ACE is a peptidyl dipeptidase that catalyzes the conversion of angiotensin I to the vasoconstrictor substance, angiotensin II. Angiotensin II also stimulates aldosterone secretion by the adrenal cortex. Inhibition of ACE results in decreased plasma angiotensin II, which leads to decreased vasopressor activity and to decreased aldosterone secretion. Although the latter decrease is small, it results in small increases of serum potassium. In hypertensive patients treated with enalapril maleate alone for up to 48 weeks, mean increases in serum potassium of approximately 0.2 mEq/L were observed. In patients treated with enalapril maleate plus a thiazide diuretic, there was essentially no change in serum potassium. (See PRECAUTIONS.) Removal of angiotensin II negative feedback on renin secretion leads to increased plasma renin activity.
ACE is identical to kininase, an enzyme that degrades bradykinin. Whether increased levels of bradykinin, a potent vasodepressor peptide, play a role in the therapeutic effects of enalapril remains to be elucidated.
While the mechanism through which enalapril lowers blood pressure is believed to be primarily suppression of the renin-angiotensin-aldosterone system, enalapril is antihypertensive even in patients with low-renin hypertension. Although enalapril was antihypertensive in all races studied, black hypertensive patients (usually a low-renin hypertensive population) had a smaller average response to enalapril maleate monotherapy than non-black patients. In contrast, hydrochlorothiazide was more effective in black patients than enalapril. Concomitant administration of enalapril maleate and hydrochlorothiazide was equally effective in black and non-black patients.
Pharmacokinetics and Metabolism: Following oral administration of enalapril maleate, peak serum concentrations of enalapril occur within about one hour. Based on urinary recovery, the extent of absorption of enalapril is approximately 60 percent. Enalapril absorption is not influenced by the presence of food in the gastrointestinal tract. Following absorption, enalapril is hydrolyzed to enalaprilat, which is a more potent angiotensin converting enzyme inhibitor than enalapril; enalaprilat is poorly absorbed when administered orally. Peak serum concentrations of enalaprilat occur three to four hours after an oral dose of enalapril maleate. Excretion of enalaprilat and enalapril is primarily renal. Approximately 94 percent of the dose is recovered in the urine and feces as enalaprilat or enalapril. The principal components in urine are enalaprilat, accounting for about 40 percent of the dose, and intact enalapril. There is no evidence of metabolites of enalapril, other than enalaprilat.
The serum concentration profile of enalaprilat exhibits a prolonged terminal phase, apparently representing a small fraction of the administered dose that has been bound to ACE. The amount bound does not increase with dose, indicating a saturable site of binding. The effective half-life for accumulation of enalaprilat following multiple doses of enalapril maleate is 11 hours.
The disposition of enalapril and enalaprilat in patients with renal insufficiency is similar to that in patients with normal renal function until the glomerular filtration rate is 30 mL/min or less. With glomerular filtration rate ≤30 mL/min, peak and trough enalaprilat levels increase, time to peak concentration increases and time to steady state may be delayed. The effective half-life of enalaprilat following multiple doses of enalapril maleate is prolonged at this level of renal insufficiency. Enalaprilat is dialyzable at the rate of 62 mL/min.
Studies in dogs indicate that enalapril crosses the blood-brain barrier poorly, if at all; enalaprilat does not enter the brain. Multiple doses of enalapril maleate in rats do not result in accumulation in any tissues. Milk of lactating rats contains radioactivity following administration of ^{14}C enalapril maleate. Radioactivity was found to cross the placenta following administration of labeled drug to pregnant hamsters.
Pharmacodynamics: Administration of enalapril maleate to patients with hypertension of severity ranging from mild to severe results in a reduction of both supine and standing blood pressure usually with no orthostatic component. Symptomatic postural hypotension is infrequent with enalapril alone but it can be anticipated in volume-depleted patients, such as patients treated with diuretics. In clinical trials with enalapril and hydrochlorothiazide administered concurrently, syncope occurred in 1.3 percent of patients. (See WARNINGS and DOSAGE AND ADMINISTRATION.)
In most patients studied, after oral administration of a single dose of enalapril maleate, onset of antihypertensive activity was seen at one hour with peak reduction of blood pressure achieved by four to six hours.
At recommended doses, antihypertensive effects of enalapril maleate monotherapy have been maintained for at least 24 hours. In some patients the effects may diminish toward the end of the dosing interval; this was less frequently observed with concomitant administration of enalapril maleate and hydrochlorothiazide.
Achievement of optimal blood pressure reduction may require several weeks of enalapril therapy in some patients.
The antihypertensive effects of enalapril have continued during long term therapy. Abrupt withdrawal of enalapril has not been associated with a rapid increase in blood pressure.
In hemodynamic studies in patients with essential hypertension, blood pressure reduction produced by enalapril was accompanied by a reduction in peripheral arterial resistance with an increase in cardiac output and little or no change in heart rate. Following administration of enalapril maleate, there is an increase in renal blood flow; glomerular filtration rate is usually unchanged. The effects appear to be similar in patients with renovascular hypertension.
In a clinical pharmacology study, indomethacin or sulindac was administered to hypertensive patients receiving enalapril maleate. In this study there was no evidence of a blunting of the antihypertensive action of enalapril maleate.
Hydrochlorothiazide
The mechanism of the antihypertensive effect of thiazides is unknown. Thiazides do not usually affect normal blood pressure. Hydrochlorothiazide is a diuretic and antihypertensive. It affects the distal renal tubular mechanism of electrolyte reabsorption. Hydrochlorothiazide increases excretion of sodium and chloride in approximately equivalent amounts. Natriuresis may be accompanied by some loss of potassium and bicarbonate. After oral use diuresis begins within two hours, peaks in about four hours and lasts about 6 to 12 hours. Hydrochlorothiazide is not metabolized but is eliminated rapidly by the kidney. When plasma levels have been followed for at least 24 hours, the plasma half-life has been observed to vary between 5.6 and 14.8 hours. At least 61 percent of the oral dose is eliminated unchanged within 24 hours. Hydrochlorothiazide crosses the placental but not the blood-brain barrier.

INDICATIONS AND USAGE

VASERETIC is indicated for the treatment of hypertension.
These fixed dose combinations are not indicated for initial treatment (see DOSAGE AND ADMINISTRATION).
In using VASERETIC, consideration should be given to the fact that another angiotensin converting enzyme inhibitor, captopril, has caused agranulocytosis, particularly in patients with renal impairment or collagen vascular disease, and that available data are insufficient to show that enalapril does not have a similar risk. (See WARNINGS.)
In considering use of VASERETIC, it should be noted that black patients receiving ACE inhibitors have been reported to have a higher incidence of angioedema compared to non-blacks. (See WARNINGS, *Angioedema.*)

CONTRAINDICATIONS

VASERETIC is contraindicated in patients who are hypersensitive to any component of this product and in patients with a history of angioedema related to previous treatment with an angiotensin converting enzyme inhibitor. Because of the hydrochlorothiazide component, this product is contraindicated in patients with anuria or hypersensitivity to other sulfonamide-derived drugs.

WARNINGS

General
Enalapril Maleate
Hypotension: Excessive hypotension was rarely seen in uncomplicated hypertensive patients but is a possible consequence of enalapril use in severely salt/volume depleted persons such as those treated vigorously with diuretics or patients on dialysis.
Syncope has been reported in 1.3 percent of patients receiving VASERETIC. In patients receiving enalapril alone, the incidence of syncope is 0.5 percent. The overall incidence of syncope may be reduced by proper titration of the individual components. (See PRECAUTIONS, *Drug Interactions,* ADVERSE REACTIONS and DOSAGE AND ADMINISTRATION.)
In patients with severe congestive heart failure, with or without associated renal insufficiency, excessive hypotension has been observed and may be associated with oliguria and/or progressive azotemia, and rarely with acute renal

Continued on next page

Information on the Merck & Co., Inc. products listed on these pages is the full prescribing information from product circulars in use August 31, 1998. For information, please call 1-800-NSC MERCK [1-800-672-6372].

Vaseretic—Cont.

failure and/or death. Because of the potential fall in blood pressure in these patients, therapy should be started under very close medical supervision. Such patients should be followed closely for the first two weeks of treatment and whenever the dose of enalapril and/or diuretic is increased. Similar considerations may apply to patients with ischemic heart or cerebrovascular disease, in whom an excessive fall in blood pressure could result in a myocardial infarction or cerebrovascular accident.

If hypotension occurs, the patient should be placed in the supine position and, if necessary, receive an intravenous infusion of normal saline. A transient hypotensive response is not a contraindication to further doses, which usually can be given without difficulty once the blood pressure has increased after volume expansion.

Anaphylactoid and Possibly Related Reactions:

Presumably because angiotensin-converting enzyme inhibitors affect the metabolism of eicosanoids and polypeptides, including endogenous bradykinin, patients receiving ACE inhibitors (including VASERETIC) may be subject to a variety of adverse reactions, some of them serious.

Angioedema: Angioedema of the face, extremities, lips, tongue, glottis and/or larynx has been reported in patients treated with angiotensin converting enzyme inhibitors, including enalapril. This may occur at any time during treatment. In such cases VASERETIC should be promptly discontinued and appropriate therapy and monitoring should be provided until complete and sustained resolution of signs and symptoms has occurred. In instances where swelling has been confined to the face and lips the condition has generally resolved without treatment, although antihistamines have been useful in relieving symptoms. Angioedema associated with laryngeal edema may be fatal. **Where there is involvement of the tongue, glottis or larynx, likely to cause airway obstruction, appropriate therapy, e.g., subcutaneous epinephrine solution 1:1000 (0.3 mL to 0.5 mL) and/or measures necessary to ensure a patent airway, should be promptly provided.** (See ADVERSE REACTIONS.)

Patients with a history of angioedema unrelated to ACE inhibitor therapy may be at increased risk of angioedema while receiving an ACE inhibitor (see also INDICATIONS AND USAGE and CONTRAINDICATIONS).

Anaphylactoid reactions during desensitization: Two patients undergoing desensitizing treatment with hymenoptera venom while receiving ACE inhibitors sustained life-threatening anaphylactoid reactions. In the same patients, these reactions were avoided when ACE inhibitors were temporarily withheld, but they reappeared upon inadvertent rechallenge.

Anaphylactoid reactions during membrane exposure: Anaphylactoid reactions have been reported in patients dialyzed with high-flux membranes and treated concomitantly with an ACE inhibitor. Anaphylactoid reactions have also been reported in patients undergoing low-density lipoprotein apheresis with dextran sulfate absorption.

Neutropenia/Agranulocytosis: Another angiotensin converting enzyme inhibitor, captopril, has been shown to cause agranulocytosis and bone marrow depression, rarely in uncomplicated patients but more frequently in patients with renal impairment especially if they also have a collagen vascular disease. Available data from clinical trials of enalapril are insufficient to show that enalapril does not cause agranulocytosis at similar rates. Marketing experience has revealed several cases of neutropenia or agranulocytosis in which a causal relationship to enalapril cannot be excluded. Periodic monitoring of white blood cell counts in patients with collagen vascular disease and renal disease should be considered.

Hepatic Failure: Rarely, ACE inhibitors have been associated with a syndrome that starts with cholestatic jaundice and progresses to fulminant hepatic necrosis, and (sometimes) death. The mechanism of this syndrome is not understood. Patients receiving ACE inhibitors who develop jaundice or marked elevations of hepatic enzymes should discontinue the ACE inhibitor and receive appropriate medical follow-up.

Hydrochlorothiazide

Thiazides should be used with caution in severe renal disease. In patients with renal disease, thiazides may precipitate azotemia. Cumulative effects of the drug may develop in patients with impaired renal function.

Thiazides should be used with caution in patients with impaired hepatic function or progressive liver disease, since minor alterations of fluid and electrolyte balance may precipitate hepatic coma.

Sensitivity reactions may occur in patients with or without a history of allergy or bronchial asthma.

The possibility of exacerbation or activation of systemic lupus erythematosus has been reported.

Lithium generally should not be given with thiazides (see PRECAUTIONS, *Drug Interactions, Enalapril Maleate* and *Hydrochlorothiazide*).

Pregnancy

Enalapril-Hydrochlorothiazide

There was no teratogenicity in mice given up to 30 mg/kg/day or in rats given up to 90 mg/kg/day of enalapril in combination with 10 mg/kg/day of hydrochlorothiazide. These doses of enalapril are 4.3 and 26 times (mice and rats, respectively) the maximum recommended human daily dose (MRHDD) when compared on a body surface area basis (mg/m^2); the dose of hydrochlorothiazide is 0.8 times (in mice) and 1.6 times (in rats) the MRHDD. At these doses, fetotoxicity expressed as a decrease in average fetal weight occurred in both species. No fetotoxicity occurred at lower doses; 30/10 mg/kg/day of enalapril-hydrochlorothiazide in rats and 10/10 mg/kg/day of enalapril-hydrochlorothiazide in mice.

When used in pregnancy during the second and third trimesters, ACE inhibitors can cause injury and even death to the developng fetus. When pregnancy is detected, VASERETIC should be discontinued as soon as possible. (See *Enalapril Maleate, Fetal/Neonatal Morbidity and Mortality,* below.)

Enalapril Maleate

Fetal/Neonatal Morbidity and Mortality: ACE inhibitors can cause fetal and neonatal morbidity and death when administered to pregnant women. Several dozen cases have been reported in the world literature. When pregnancy is detected, ACE inhibitors should be discontinued as soon as possible.

The use of ACE inhibitors during the second and third trimesters of pregnancy has been associated with fetal and neonatal injury, including hypotension, neonatal skull hypoplasia, anuria, reversible or irreversible renal failure, and death. Oligohydramnios has also been reported, presumably resulting from decreased fetal renal function; oligohydramnios in this setting has been associated with fetal limb contractures, craniofacial deformation, and hypoplastic lung development. Prematurity, intrauterine growth retardation, and patent ductus arteriosus have also been reported, although it is not clear whether these occurrences were due to the ACE-inhibitor exposure.

These adverse effects do not appear to have resulted from intrauterine ACE-inhibitor exposure that has been limited to the first trimester. Mothers whose embryos and fetuses are exposed to ACE inhibitors only during the first trimester should be so informed. Nonetheless, when patients become pregnant, physicians should make every effort to discontinue the use of VASERETIC as soon as possible.

Rarely (probably less often than once in every thousand pregnancies), no alternative to ACE inhibitors will be found. In these rare cases, the mothers should be apprised of the potential hazards to their fetuses, and serial ultrasound examinations should be performed to assess the intraamniotic environment.

If oligohydramnios is observed, VASERETIC should be discontinued unless it is considered lifesaving for the mother. Contraction stress testing (CST), a non-stress test (NST), or biophysical profiling (BPP) may be appropriate, depending upon the week of pregnancy. Patients and physicians should be aware, however, that oligohydramnios may not appear until after the fetus has sustained irreversible injury.

Infants with histories of *in utero* exposure to ACE inhibitors should be closely observed for hypotension, oliguria, and hyperkalemia. If oliguria occurs, attention should be directed toward support of blood pressure and renal perfusion. Exchange transfusion or dialysis may be required as means of reversing hypotension and/or substituting for disordered renal functon. Enalapril, which crosses the placenta, has been removed from neonatal circulation by peritoneal dialysis with some clinical benefit, and theoretically may be removed by exchange transfusion, although there is no experience with the latter procedure.

No teratogenic effects of enalapril were seen in studies of pregnant rats and rabbits. On a body surface area basis, the doses were 57 times and 12 times, respectively, the MRHDD.

Hydrochlorothiazide

Studies in which hydrochlorothiazide was orally administered to pregnant mice and rats during their respective periods of major organogenesis at doses up to 3000 and 1000 mg/kg/day, respectively, provided no evidence of harm to the fetus. These doses are more than 150 times the MRHDD on a body surface area basis. Thiazides cross the placental barrier and appear in cord blood. There is a risk of fetal or neonatal jaundice, thrombocytopenia, and possibly other adverse reactions that have occurred in adults.

PRECAUTIONS

General

Enalapril Maleate

Impaired Renal Function: As a consequence of inhibiting the renin-angiotensin-aldosterone system, changes in renal function may be anticipated in susceptible individuals. In patients with severe congestive heart failure whose renal function may depend on the activity of the renin-angiotensin-aldosterone system, treatment with angiotensin converting enzyme inhibitors, including enalapril, may be associated with oliguria and/or progressive azotemia and rarely with acute renal failure and/or death.

In clinical studies in hypertensive patients with unilateral or bilateral renal artery stenosis, increases in blood urea nitrogen and serum creatinine were observed in 20 percent of patients. These increases were almost always reversible upon discontinuation of enalapril and/or diuretic therapy. In such patients renal function should be monitored during the first few weeks of therapy.

Some patients with hypertension or heart failure with no apparent pre-existing renal vascular disease have developed increases in blood urea and serum creatinine, usually minor and transient, especially when enalapril has been given concomitantly with a diuretic. This is more likely to occur in patients with pre-existing renal impairment. Dosage reduction of enalapril and/or discontinuation of the diuretic may be required.

Evaluation of the hypertensive patient should always include assessment of renal function.

Hyperkalemia: Elevated serum potassium (greater than 5.7 mEq/L) was observed in approximately one percent of hypertensive patients in clinical trials treated with enalapril alone. In most cases these were isolated values which resolved despite continued therapy, although hyperkalemia was a cause of discontinuation of therapy in 0.28 percent of hypertensive patients. Hyperkalemia was less frequent (approximately 0.1 percent) in patients treated with enalapril plus hydrochlorothiazide. Risk factors for the development of hyperkalemia include renal insufficiency, diabetes mellitus, and the concomitant use of potassium-sparing diuretics, potassium supplements and/or potassium-containing salt substitutes, which should be used cautiously, if at all, with enalapril. (See *Drug Interactions.*)

Cough: Presumably due to the inhibition of the degradation of endogenous bradykinin, persistent nonproductive cough has been reported with all ACE inhibitors, always resolving after discontinuation of therapy. ACE inhibitor-induced cough should be considered in the differential diagnosis of cough.

Surgery/Anesthesia: In patients undergoing major surgery or during anesthesia with agents that produce hypotension, enalapril may block angiotensin II formation secondary to compensatory renin release. If hypotension occurs and is considered to be due to this mechanism, it can be corrected by volume expansion.

Hydrochlorothiazide

Periodic determination of serum electrolytes to detect possible electrolyte imbalance should be performed at appropriate intervals. All patients receiving thiazide therapy should be observed for clinical signs of fluid or electrolyte imbalance: namely hyponatremia, hypochloremic alkalosis, and hypokalemia. Serum and urine electrolyte determinations are particularly important when the patient is vomiting excessively or receiving parenteral fluids. Warning signs or symptoms of fluid and electrolyte imbalance, irrespective of cause, include dryness of mouth, thirst, weakness, lethargy, drowsiness, restlessness, confusion, seizures, muscle pains or cramps, muscular fatigue, hypotension, oliguria, tachycardia, and gastrointestinal disturbances such as nausea and vomiting.

Hypokalemia may develop, especially with brisk diuresis, when severe cirrhosis is present, or after prolonged therapy. Interference with adequate oral electrolyte intake will also contribute to hypokalemia. Hypokalemia may cause cardiac arrhythmia and may also sensitize or exaggerate the response of the heart to the toxic effects of digitalis (e.g., increased ventricular irritability). Because enalapril reduces the production of aldosterone, concomitant therapy with enalapril attenuates the diuretic-induced potassium loss (see *Drug Interactions, Agents Increasing Serum Potassium*).

Although any chloride deficit is generally mild and usually does not require specific treatment except under extraordinary circumstances (as in liver disease or renal disease), chloride replacement may be required in the treatment of metabolic alkalosis.

Dilutional hyponatremia may occur in edematous patients in hot weather; appropriate therapy is water restriction, rather than administration of salt except in rare instances when the hyponatremia is life-threatening. In actual salt depletion, appropriate replacement is the therapy of choice.

Hyperuricemia may occur or frank gout may be precipitated in certain patients receiving thiazide therapy.

In diabetic patients dosage adjustments of insulin or oral hypoglycemic agents may be required. Hyperglycemia may occur with thiazide diuretics. Thus latent diabetes mellitus may become manifest during thiazide therapy.

The antihypertensive effects of the drug may be enhanced in the postsympathectomy patient.

If progressive renal impairment becomes evident consider withholding or discontinuing diuretic therapy.

Thiazides have been shown to increase the urinary excretion of magnesium; this may result in hypomagnesemia.

Thiazides may decrease urinary calcium excretion. Thiazides may cause intermittent and slight elevation of serum

calcium in the absence of known disorders of calcium metabolism. Marked hypercalcemia may be evidence of hidden hyperparathyroidism. Thiazides should be discontinued before carrying out tests for parathyroid function.
Increases in cholesterol and triglyceride levels may be associated with thiazide diuretic therapy.
Information for Patients
Angioedema: Angioedema, including laryngeal edema, may occur at any time during treatment with angiotensin converting enzyme inhibitors, including enalapril. Patients should be so advised and told to report immediately any signs or symptoms suggesting angioedema (swelling of face, extremities, eyes, lips, tongue, difficulty in swallowing or breathing) and to take no more drug until they have consulted with the prescribing physician.
Hypotension: Patients should be cautioned to report lightheadedness especially during the first few days of therapy. If actual syncope occurs, the patients should be told to discontinue the drug until they have consulted with the prescribing physician.
All patients should be cautioned that excessive perspiration and dehydration may lead to an excessive fall in blood pressure because of reduction in fluid volume. Other causes of volume depletion such as vomiting or diarrhea may also lead to a fall in blood pressure; patients should be advised to consult with the physician.
Hyperkalemia: Patients should be told not to use salt substitutes containing potassium without consulting their physician.
Neutropenia: Patients should be told to report promptly any indication of infection (e.g., sore throat, fever) which may be a sign of neutropenia.
Pregnancy: Female patients of childbearing age should be told about the consequences of second- and third-trimester exposure to ACE inhibitors, and they should also be told that these consequences do not appear to have resulted from intrauterine ACE-inhibitor exposure that has been limited to the first trimester. These patients should be asked to report pregnancies to their physicians as soon as possible.
NOTE: As with many other drugs, certain advice to patients being treated with VASERETIC is warranted. This information is intended to aid in the safe and effective use of this medication. It is not a disclosure of all possible adverse or intended effects.
Drug Interactions
Enalapril Maleate
Hypotension —Patients on Diuretic Therapy: Patients on diuretics and especially those in whom diuretic therapy was recently instituted, may occasionally experience an excessive reduction of blood pressure after initiation of therapy with enalapril. The possibility of hypotensive effects with enalapril can be minimized by either discontinuing the diuretic or increasing the salt intake prior to initiation of treatment with enalapril. If it is necessary to continue the diuretic, provide medical supervision for at least two hours and until blood pressure has stabilized for at least an additional hour. (See WARNINGS, and DOSAGE AND ADMINISTRATION.)
Agents Causing Renin Release: The antihypertensive effect of enalapril is augmented by antihypertensive agents that cause renin release (e.g., diuretics).
Other Cardiovascular Agents: Enalapril has been used concomitantly with beta adrenergic-blocking agents, methyldopa, nitrates, calcium-blocking agents, hydralazine and prazosin without evidence of clinically significant adverse interactions.
Agents Increasing Serum Potassium: Enalapril attenuates diuretic-induced potassium loss. Potassium-sparing diuretics (e.g., spironolactone, triamterene, or amiloride), potassium supplements, or potassium-containing salt substitutes may lead to significant increases in serum potassium. Therefore, if concomitant use of these agents is indicated because of demonstrated hypokalemia they should be used with caution and with frequent monitoring of serum potassium.
Lithium: Lithium toxicity has been reported in patients receiving lithium concomitantly with drugs which cause elimination of sodium, including ACE inhibitors. A few cases of lithium toxicity have been reported in patients receiving concomitant enalapril and lithium and were reversible upon discontinuation of both drugs. It is recommended that serum lithium levels be monitored frequently if enalapril is administered concomitantly with lithium.
Hydrochlorothiazide
When administered concurrently the following drugs may interact with thiazide diuretics:
Alcohol, barbiturates, or narcotics —potentiation of orthostatic hypotension may occur.
Antidiabetic drugs (oral agents and insulin)—dosage adjustment of the antidiabetic drug may be required.
Other antihypertensive drugs —additive effect or potentiation.
Cholestyramine and colestipol resins —Absorption of hydrochlorothiazide is impaired in the presence of anionic exchange resins. Single doses of either cholestyramine or colestipol resins bind the hydrochlorothiazide and reduce its absorption from the gastrointestinal tract by up to 85 and 43 percent, respectively.
Corticosteroids, ACTH —intensified electrolyte depletion, particularly hypokalemia.
Pressor amines (e.g., norepinephrine) —possible decreased response to pressor amines but not sufficient to preclude their use.
Skeletal muscle relaxants, nondepolarizing (e.g., tubocurarine) —possible increased responsiveness to the muscle relaxant.
Lithium —should not generally be given with diuretics. Diuretic agents reduce the renal clearance of lithium and add a high risk of lithium toxicity. Refer to the package insert for lithium preparations before use of such preparations with VASERETIC.
Non-steroidal Anti-inflammatory Drugs —In some patients, the administration of a non-steroidal anti-inflammatory agent can reduce the diuretic, natriuretic, and antihypertensive effects of loop, potassium-sparing and thiazide diuretics. Therefore, when VASERETIC and non-steroidal anti-inflammatory agents are used concomitantly, the patient should be observed closely to determine if the desired effect of the diuretic is obtained.
Carcinogenesis, Mutagenesis, Impairment of Fertility
Enalapril in combination with hydrochlorothiazide was not mutagenic in the Ames microbial mutagen test with or without metabolic activation. Enalapril-hydrochlorothiazide did not produce DNA single strand breaks in an *in vitro* alkaline elution assay in rat hepatocytes or chromosomal aberrations in an *in vivo* mouse bone marrow assay.
Enalapril Maleate
There was no evidence of a tumorigenic effect when enalapril was administered for 106 weeks to male and female rats at doses up to 90 mg/kg/day or for 94 weeks to male and female mice at doses up to 90 and 180 mg/kg/day, respectively. These doses are 26 times (in rats and female mice) and 13 times (in male mice) the maximum recommended human daily dose (MRHDD) when compared on a body surface area basis.
Neither enalapril maleate nor the active diacid was mutagenic in the Ames microbial mutagen test with or without metabolic activation. Enalapril was also negative in the following genotoxicity studies: rec-assay, reverse mutation assay with *E. coli*, sister chromatid exchange with cultured mammalian cells, and the micronucleus test with mice, as well as in an *in vivo* cytogenic study using mouse bone marrow.
There were no adverse effects on reproductive performance of male and female rats treated with up to 90 mg/kg/day of enalapril (26 times the MRHDD when compared on a body surface area basis).
Hydrochlorothiazide
Two year feeding studies in mice and rats conducted under the auspices of the National Toxicology Program (NTP) uncovered no evidence of a carcinogenic potential of hydrochlorothiazide in female mice at doses up to approximately 600 mg/kg/day (53 times the MRHDD when compared on a body surface area basis) or in male and female rats at doses up to approximately 100 mg/kg/day (18 times the MRHDD when compared on a body surface area basis). The NTP, however, found equivocal evidence for hepatocarcinogenicity in male mice.
Hydrochlorothiazide was not genotoxic *in vitro* in the Ames mutagenicity assay of *Salmonella typhimurium* strains TA 98, TA 100, TA 1535, TA 1537, and TA 1538 and in the Chinese Hamster Ovary (CHO) test for chromosomal aberrations, or *in vivo* in assays using mouse germinal cell chromosomes, Chinese hamster bone marrow chromosomes, and the *Drosophila* sex-linked recessive lethal trait gene. Positive test results were obtained only in the *in vitro* CHO Sister Chromatid Exchange (clastogenicity) and in the Mouse Lymphoma Cell (mutagenicity) assays, using concentrations of hydrochlorothiazide from 43 to 1300 μg/mL, and in the *Aspergillus nidulans* non-disjunction assay at an unspecified concentration.
Hydrochlorothiazide had no adverse effects on the fertility of mice and rats of either sex in studies wherein these species were exposed, via their diet, to doses of up to 100 and 4 mg/kg, respectively, prior to mating and throughout gestation. In mice and rats these doses are 9 times and 0.7 times, respectively, the MRHDD when compared on a body surface area basis.
Pregnancy
Pregnancy Categories C (first trimester) *and D* (second and third trimesters). See WARNINGS, *Pregnancy, Enalapril Maleate, Fetal/Neonatal Morbidity and Mortality.*
Nursing Mothers
Enalapril, enalaprilat, and hydrochlorothiazide have been detected in human breast milk. Because of the potential for serious reactions in nursing infants from either drug, a decision should be made whether to discontinue nursing or to discontinue VASERETIC, taking into account the importance of the drug to the mother.
Pediatric Use
Safety and effectiveness in pediatric patients have not been established.

ADVERSE REACTIONS

VASERETIC has been evaluated for safety in more than 1500 patients, including over 300 patients treated for one year or more. In clinical trials with VASERETIC no adverse experiences peculiar to this combination drug have been observed. Adverse experiences that have occurred, have been limited to those that have been previously reported with enalapril or hydrochlorothiazide.
The most frequent clinical adverse experiences in controlled trials were: dizziness (8.6 percent), headache (5.5 percent), fatigue (3.9 percent) and cough (3.5 percent). Generally, adverse experiences were mild and transient in nature. Adverse experiences occurring in greater than two percent of patients treated with VASERETIC in controlled clinical trials are shown below.

	Percent of Patients in Controlled Studies	
	VASERETIC (n=1580) Incidence (discontinuation)	Placebo (n=230) Incidence
Dizziness	8.6 (0.7)	4.3
Headache	5.5 (0.4)	9.1
Fatigue	3.9 (0.8)	2.6
Cough	3.5 (0.4)	0.9
Muscle Cramps	2.7 (0.2)	0.9
Nausea	2.5 (0.4)	1.7
Asthenia	2.4 (0.3)	0.9
Orthostatic Effects	2.3 (<0.1)	0.0
Impotence	2.2 (0.5)	0.5
Diarrhea	2.1 (<0.1)	1.7

Clinical adverse experiences occurring in 0.5 to 2.0 percent of patients in controlled trials included: *Body As A Whole:* Syncope, chest pain, abdominal pain; *Cardiovascular:* Orthostatic hypotension, palpitation, tachycardia; *Digestive:* Vomiting, dyspepsia, constipation, flatulence, dry mouth; *Nervous/Psychiatric:* Insomnia, nervousness, paresthesia, somnolence, vertigo; *Skin:* Pruritus, rash; *Other:* Dyspnea, gout, back pain, arthralgia, diaphoresis, decreased libido, tinnitus, urinary tract infection.
Angioedema: Angioedema has been reported in patients receiving VASERETIC, with an incidence higher in black than in non-black patients. Angioedema associated with laryngeal edema may be fatal. If angioedema of the face, extremities, lips, tongue, glottis and/or larynx occurs, treatment with VASERETIC should be discontinued and appropriate therapy instituted immediately. (See WARNINGS.)
Hypotension: In clinical trials, adverse effects relating to hypotension occurred as follows: hypotension (0.9 percent), orthostatic hypotension (1.5 percent), other orthostatic effects (2.3 percent). In addition syncope occurred in 1.3 percent of patients. (See WARNINGS.)
Cough: See PRECAUTIONS, *Cough.*
Clinical Laboratory Test Findings
Serum Electrolytes: See PRECAUTIONS.
Creatinine, Blood Urea Nitrogen: In controlled clinical trials minor increases in blood urea nitrogen and serum creatinine, reversible upon discontinuation of therapy, were observed in about 0.6 percent of patients with essential hypertension treated with VASERETIC. More marked increases have been reported in other enalapril experience. Increases are more likely to occur in patients with renal artery stenosis. (See PRECAUTIONS.)
Serum Uric Acid, Glucose, Magnesium, and Calcium: See PRECAUTIONS.
Hemoglobin and Hematocrit: Small decreases in hemoglobin and hematocrit (mean decreases of approximately 0.3 g percent and 1.0 vol percent, respectively) occur frequently in hypertensive patients treated with VASERETIC but are rarely of clinical importance unless another cause of anemia coexists. In clinical trials, less than 0.1 percent of patients discontinued therapy due to anemia.
Liver Function Tests: Rarely, elevations of liver enzymes and/or serum bilirubin have occurred (see WARNINGS, *Hepatic Failure*).
Other adverse reactions that have been reported with the individual components are listed below and, within each category, are in order of decreasing severity.
Enalapril Maleate —Enalapril has been evaluated for safety in more than 10,000 patients. In clinical trials ad-

Continued on next page

Information on the Merck & Co., Inc. products listed on these pages is the full prescribing information from product circulars in use August 31, 1998. For information, please call 1-800-NSC MERCK [1-800-672-6372].

Vaseretic—Cont.

verse reactions which occurred with enalapril were also seen with VASERETIC. However, since enalapril has been marketed, the following adverse reactions have been reported: *Body As A Whole:* Anaphylactoid reactions (see WARNINGS, *Anaphylactoid reactions during membrane exposure*); *Cardiovascular:* Cardiac arrest; myocardial infarction or cerebrovascular accident, possibly secondary to excessive hypotension in high risk patients (see WARNINGS, *Hypotension*); pulmonary embolism and infarction; pulmonary edema; rhythm disturbances including atrial tachycardia and bradycardia, atrial fibrillation; hypotension; angina pectoris, Raynaud's phenomenon; *Digestive:* Ileus, pancreatitis, hepatic failure, hepatitis (hepatocellular [proven on rechallenge] or cholestatic jaundice) (see WARNINGS, *Hepatic Failure*), melena, anorexia, glossitis, stomatitis, dry mouth; *Hematologic:* Rare cases of neutropenia, thrombocytopenia and bone marrow depression. Hemolytic anemia, including cases of hemolysis in patients with G-6-PD deficiency, has been reported; a causal relationship to enalapril cannot be excluded. *Nervous System/Psychiatric:* Depression, confusion, ataxia, peripheral neuropathy (e.g., paresthesia, dysesthesia), dream abnormality; *Urogenital:* Renal failure, oliguria, renal dysfunction, (see PRECAUTIONSand DOSAGE AND ADMINISTRATION), flank pain, gynecomastia; *Respiratory:* Pulmonary infiltrates, bronchospasm, pneumonia, bronchitis, rhinorrhea, sore throat and hoarseness, asthma, upper respiratory infection; *Skin:* Exfoliative dermatitis, toxic epidermal necrolysis, Stevens-Johnson syndrome, herpes zoster, erythema multiforme, urticaria, pemphigus, alopecia, flushing, photosensitivity; *Special Senses:* Blurred vision, taste alteration, anosmia, conjunctivitis, dry eyes, tearing.

Miscellaneous: A symptom complex has been reported which may include some or all of the following: a positive ANA, an elevated erythrocyte sedimentation rate, arthralgia/arthritis, myalgia/myositis, fever, serositis, vasculitis, leukocytosis, eosinophilia, photosensitivity, rash and other dermatologic manifestations.

Fetal/Neonatal Morbidity and Mortality: See WARNINGS, *Pregnancy, Enalapril Maleate, Fetal/Neonatal Morbidity and Mortality.*

Hydrochlorothiazide—Body as a Whole: Weakness; *Digestive:* Pancreatitis, jaundice (intrahepatic cholestatic jaundice), sialadenitis, cramping, gastric irritation, anorexia; *Hematologic:* Aplastic anemia, agranulocytosis, leukopenia, hemolytic anemia, thrombocytopenia; *Hypersensitivity:* Purpura, photosensitivity, urticaria, necrotizing angiitis (vasculitis and cutaneous vasculitis), fever, respiratory distress including pneumonitis and pulmonary edema, anaphylactic reactions; *Musculoskeletal:* Muscle spasm; *Nervous system/Psychiatric:* Restlessness; *Renal:* Renal failure, renal dysfunction, interstitial nephritis (see WARNINGS); *Skin:* Erythema multiforme including Stevens-Johnson syndrome, exfoliative dermatitis including toxic epidermal necrolysis, alopecia; *Special Senses:* Transient blurred vision, xanthopsia.

OVERDOSAGE

No specific information is available on the treatment of overdosage with VASERETIC. Treatment is symptomatic and supportive. Therapy with VASERETIC should be discontinued and the patient observed closely. Suggested measures include induction of emesis and/or gastric lavage, and correction of dehydration, electrolyte imbalance and hypotension by established procedures.

Enalapril Maleate —Single oral doses of enalapril above 1,000 mg/kg and ≥1,775 mg/kg were associated with lethality in mice and rats, respectively. The most likely manifestation of overdosage would be hypotension, for which the usual treatment would be intravenous infusion of normal saline solution. Enalaprilat may be removed from general circulation by hemodialysis and has been removed from neonatal circulation by peritoneal dialysis.

Hydrochlorothiazide —Lethality was not observed after administration of an oral dose of 10 g/kg to mice and rats. The most common signs and symptoms observed are those caused by electrolyte depletion (hypokalemia, hypochloremia, hyponatremia) and dehydration resulting from excessive diuresis. If digitalis has also been administered, hypokalemia may accentuate cardiac arrhythmias.

DOSAGE AND ADMINISTRATION

Enalapril and hydrochlorothiazide are effective treatments for hypertension. The usual dosage range of enalapril is 10 to 40 mg per day administered in a single or two divided doses; hydrochlorothiazide is effective in doses of 25 to 100 mg daily. The side effects (see WARNINGS) of enalapril are generally rare and apparently independent of dose; those of hydrochlorothiazide are a mixture of dose-dependent phenomena (primarily hypokalemia) and dose-independent phenomena (e.g., pancreatitis), the former much more common than the latter. Therapy with any combination of enalapril and hydrochlorothiazide will be associated with both sets of dose-independent side effects but the addition of enalapril in clinicial trials blunted the hypokalemia normally seen with diuretics. To minimize dose-independent side effects, it is usually appropriate to begin combination therapy only after a patient has failed to achieve the desired effect with monotherapy.

Dose Titration Guided by Clinical Effect: A patient whose blood pressure is not adequately controlled with either enalapril or hydrochlorothiazide monotherapy may be given VASERETIC 5–12.5 or VASERETIC 10–25. Further increases of enalapril, hydrochlorothiazide or both depend on clinical response. The hydrochlorothiazide dose should generally not be increased until 2–3 weeks have elapsed. In general, patients do not require doses in excess of 20 mg of enalapril or 50 mg of hydrochlorothiazide. The daily dosage should not exceed four tablets of VASERETIC 5–12.5 or two tablets of VASERETIC 10–25.

Replacement Therapy: The combination may be substituted for the titrated components.

Use in Renal Impairment: The usual regimens of therapy with VASERETIC need not be adjusted as long as the patient's creatinine clearance is >30 mL/min/1.73 m^2 (serum creatinine approximately ≤3 mg/dL or 265 μmol/L). In patients with more severe renal impairment, loop diuretics are preferred to thiazides, so enalapril maleate-hydrochlorothiazide is not recommended (see WARNINGS, *Anaphylactoid reactions during membrane exposure*).

Use in Elderly: Clinical studies in VASERETIC did not include sufficient numbers of patients aged 65 and over to determine whether they respond differently from younger patients. In general, dose selection for an elderly patient should be cautious, usually starting at the low end of the dosing range.

HOW SUPPLIED

No. 3644—Tablets VASERETIC 5-12.5 are green, squared capsule-shaped compressed tablets, coded MSD on one side and 173 on the other. Each tablet contains 5 mg of enalapril maleate and 12.5 mg of hydrochlorothiazide. They are supplied as follows:

NDC 0006-0173-68 bottles of 100 (with desiccant).

Shown in Product Identification Guide, page 323

No. 3418—Tablets VASERETIC 10-25, are rust, squared capsule-shaped, compressed tablets, coded MSD 720 on one side and VASERETIC on the other. Each tablet contains 10 mg of enalapril maleate and 25 mg of hydrochlorothiazide. They are supplied as follows:

NDC 0006-0720-68 bottles of 100 (with desiccant).

Shown in Product Identification Guide, page 323

Storage

Store below 30°C (86°F) and avoid transient temperatures above 50°C (122°F). Keep container tightly closed. Protect from moisture.

Dispense in a tight container, if product package is subdivided.

7843631 Issued February 1997

COPYRIGHT © MERCK & CO., INC., 1989, 1992
All rights reserved

VASOTEC® I.V. Injection ℞
(Enalaprilat)

USE IN PREGNANCY

When used in pregnancy during the second and third trimesters, ACE inhibitors can cause injury and even death to the developing fetus. When pregnancy is detected, VASOTEC I.V. should be discontinued as soon as possible. See WARNINGS, *Fetal/Neonatal Morbidity and Mortality.*

DESCRIPTION

VASOTEC* I.V. (Enalaprilat) is a sterile aqueous solution for intravenous administration. Enalaprilat is an angiotensin converting enzyme inhibitor. It is chemically described as (*S*)-1-[*N*-(1-carboxy-3-phenylpropyl)-L-alanyl]-L-proline dihydrate. Its empirical formula is $C_{18}H_{24}N_2O_5 \cdot 2H_2O$ and its structural formula is:

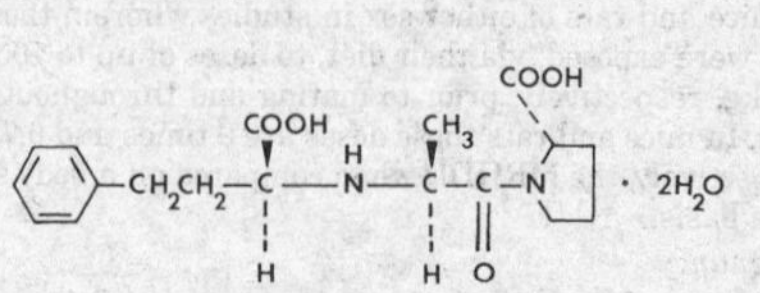

Enalaprilat is a white to off-white, crystalline powder with a molecular weight of 384.43. It is sparingly soluble in methanol and slightly soluble in water.

Each milliliter of VASOTEC I.V. contains 1.25 mg enalaprilat (anhydrous equivalent); sodium chloride to adjust tonicity; sodium hydroxide to adjust pH; water for injection, q.s.; with benzyl alcohol, 9 mg, added as a preservative.

*Registered trademark of MERCK & CO., INC.

CLINICAL PHARMACOLOGY

Enalaprilat, an angiotensin-converting enzyme (ACE) inhibitor when administered intravenously, is the active metabolite of the orally administered pro-drug, enalapril maleate. Enalaprilat is poorly absorbed orally.

Mechanism of Action

Intravenous enalaprilat, or oral enalapril, after hydrolysis to enalaprilat, inhibits ACE in human subjects and animals. ACE is a peptidyl dipeptidase that catalyzes the conversion of angiotensin I to the vasoconstrictor substance, angiotensin II. Angiotensin II also stimulates aldosterone secretion by the adrenal cortex. Inhibition of ACE results in decreased plasma angiotensin II, which leads to decreased vasopressor activity and to decreased aldosterone secretion. Although the latter decrease is small, it results in small increases of serum potassium. In hypertensive patients treated with enalapril alone for up to 48 weeks, mean increases in serum potassium of approximately 0.2 mEq/L were observed. In patients treated with enalapril plus a thiazide diuretic, there was essentially no change in serum potassium. (See PRECAUTIONS.) Removal of angiotensin II negative feedback on renin secretion leads to increased plasma renin activity.

ACE is identical to kininase, an enzyme that degrades bradykinin. Whether increased levels of bradykinin, a potent vasodepressor peptide, play a role in the therapeutic effects of enalaprilat remains to be elucidated.

While the mechanism through which enalaprilat lowers blood pressure is believed to be primarily suppression of the renin-angiotensin-aldosterone system, enalaprilat has antihypertensive activity even in patients with low-renin hypertension. In clinical studies, black hypertensive patients (usually a low-renin hypertensive population) had a smaller average response to enalaprilat monotherapy than non-black patients.

Pharmacokinetics and Metabolism

Following intravenous administration of a single dose, the serum concentration profile of enalaprilat is polyexponential with a prolonged terminal phase, apparently representing a small fraction of the administered dose that has been bound to ACE. The amount bound does not increase with dose, indicating a saturable site of binding. The effective half-life for accumulation of enalaprilat, as determined from oral administration of multiple doses of enalapril maleate, is approximately 11 hours. Excretion of enalaprilat is primarily renal with more than 90 percent of an administered dose recovered in the urine as unchanged drug within 24 hours. Enalaprilat is poorly absorbed following oral administration.

The disposition of enalaprilat in patients with renal insufficiency is similar to that in patients with normal renal function until the glomerular filtration rate is 30 mL/min or less. With glomerular filtration rate ≤30 mL/min, peak and trough enalaprilat levels increase, time to peak concentration increases and time to steady state may be delayed. The effective half-life of enalaprilat is prolonged at this level of renal insufficiency. (See DOSAGE AND ADMINISTRATION.) Enalaprilat is dialyzable at the rate of 62 mL/min. Studies in dogs indicate that enalaprilat does not enter the brain, and that enalaprilat crosses the blood-brain barrier poorly, if at all. Multiple doses of enalapril maleate in rats do not result in accumulation in any tissues. Milk in lactating rats contains radioactivity following administration of ^{14}C enalapril maleate. Radioactivity was found to cross the placenta following administration of labeled drug to pregnant hamsters.

Pharmacodynamics

VASOTEC I.V. results in the reduction of both supine and standing systolic and diastolic blood pressure, usually with no orthostatic component. Symptomatic postural hypotension is therefore infrequent, although it might be anticipated in volume-depleted patients (see WARNINGS). The onset of action usually occurs within fifteen minutes of administration with the maximum effect occurring within one to four hours. The abrupt withdrawal of enalaprilat has not been associated with a rapid increase in blood pressure.

The duration of hemodynamic effects appears to be dose-related. However, for the recommended dose, the duration of action in most patients is approximately six hours.

Following administration of enalapril, there is an increase in renal blood flow; glomerular filtration rate is usually unchanged. The effects appear to be similar in patients with renovascular hypertension.

INDICATIONS AND USAGE

VASOTEC I.V. is indicated for the treatment of hypertension when oral therapy is not practical.

VASOTEC I.V. has been studied with only one other antihypertensive agent, furosemide, which showed approximately additive effects on blood pressure. Enalapril, the pro-drug of

enalaprilat, has been used extensively with a variety of other antihypertensive agents, without apparent difficulty except for occasional hypotension.
In using VASOTEC I.V., consideration should be given to the fact that another angiotensin converting enzyme inhibitor, captopril, has caused agranulocytosis, particularly in patients with renal impairment or collagen vascular disease, and that available data are insufficient to show that VASOTEC I.V. does not have a similar risk. (See WARNINGS.)
In considering use of VASOTEC I.V., it should be noted that in controlled clinical trials ACE inhibitors have an effect on blood pressure that is less in black patients than in non-blacks. In addition, it should be noted that black patients receiving ACE inhibitors have been reported to have a higher incidence of angioedema compared to non-blacks. (See WARNINGS, *Angioedema.*)

CONTRAINDICATIONS

VASOTEC I.V. is contraindicated in patients who are hypersensitive to any component of this product and in patients with a history of angioedema related to previous treatment with an angiotensin converting enzyme inhibitor.

WARNINGS

Hypotension
Excessive hypotension is rare in uncomplicated hypertensive patients but is a possible consequence of the use of enalaprilat especially in severely salt/volume depleted persons such as those treated vigorously with diuretics or patients on dialysis. Patients at risk for excessive hypotension, sometimes associated with oliguria and/or progressive azotemia, and rarely with acute renal failure and/or death, include those with the following conditions or characteristics: heart failure, hyponatremia, high dose diuretic therapy, recent intensive diuresis or increase in diuretic dose, renal dialysis, or severe volume and/or salt depletion of any etiology. It may be advisable to eliminate the diuretic, reduce the diuretic dose or increase salt intake cautiously before initiating therapy with VASOTEC I.V. in patients at risk for excessive hypotension who are able to tolerate such adjustment. (See PRECAUTIONS, *Drug Interactions,* ADVERSE REACTIONS, and DOSAGE AND ADMINISTRATION.) In patients with heart failure, with or without associated renal insufficiency, excessive hypotension has been observed and may be associated with oliguria and/or progressive azotemia, and rarely with acute renal failure and/or death. Because of the potential for an excessive fall in blood pressure especially in these patients, therapy should be followed closely whenever the dose of enalaprilat is adjusted and/or diuretic is increased. Similar consideration may apply to patients with ischemic heart or cerebrovascular disease, in whom an excessive fall in blood pressure could result in a myocardial infarction or cerebrovascular accident.
If hypotension occurs, the patient should be placed in the supine position and, if necessary, receive an intravenous infusion of normal saline. A transient hypotensive response is not a contraindication to further doses, which usually can be given without difficulty once the blood pressure has increased after volume expansion.
Anaphylactoid and Possibly Related Reactions
Presumably because angiotensin-converting enzyme inhibitors affect the metabolism of eicosanoids and polypeptides, including endogenous bradykinin, patients receiving ACE inhibitors (including VASOTEC I.V.) may be subject to a variety of adverse reactions, some of them serious.
Angioedema: Angioedema of the face, extremities, lips, tongue, glottis and/or larynx has been reported in patients treated with angiotensin converting enzyme inhibitors, including enalaprilat. This may occur at any time during treatment. In such cases VASOTEC I.V. should be promptly discontinued and appropriate therapy and monitoring should be provided until complete and sustained resolution of signs and symptoms has occurred. In instances where swelling has been confined to the face and lips the condition has generally resolved without treatment, although antihistamines have been useful in relieving symptoms. Angioedema associated with laryngeal edema may be fatal. **Where there is involvement of the tongue, glottis or larynx, likely to cause airway obstruction, appropriate therapy, e.g., subcutaneous epinephrine solution 1:1000 (0.3 mL to 0.5 mL) and/or measures necessary to ensure a patent airway, should be promptly provided.** (See ADVERSE REACTIONS.)
Patients with a history of angioedema unrelated to ACE inhibitor therapy may be at increased risk of angioedema while receiving an ACE inhibitor (see also INDICATIONS AND USAGE and CONTRAINDICATIONS).
Anaphylactoid reactions during desensitization: Two patients undergoing desensitizing treatment with hymenoptera venom while receiving ACE inhibitors sustained life-threatening anaphylactoid reactions. In the same patients, these reactions were avoided when ACE inhibitors were temporarily withheld, but they reappeared upon inadvertent rechallenge.
Anaphylactoid reactions during membrane exposure: Anaphylactoid reactions have been reported in patients dialyzed with high-flux membranes and treated concomitantly with an ACE inhibitor. Anaphylactoid reactions have also been reported in patients undergoing low-density lipoprotein apheresis with dextran sulfate absorption.
Neutropenia/Agranulocytosis
Another angiotensin converting enzyme inhibitor, captopril, has been shown to cause agranulocytosis and bone marrow depression, rarely in uncomplicated patients but more frequently in patients with renal impairment especially if they also have a collagen vascular disease. Available data from clinical trials of enalapril are insufficient to show that enalapril does not cause agranulocytosis in similar rates. Marketing experience has revealed several cases of neutropenia, or agranulocytosis in which a causal relationship to enalapril cannot be excluded. Periodic monitoring of white blood cell counts in patients with collagen vascular disease and renal disease should be considered.
Hepatic Failure
Rarely, ACE inhibitors have been associated with a syndrome that starts with cholestatic jaundice and progresses to fulminant hepatic necrosis, and (sometimes) death. The mechanism of this syndrome is not understood. Patients receiving ACE inhibitors who develop jaundice or marked elevations of hepatic enzymes should discontinue the ACE inhibitor and receive appropriate medical follow-up.
Fetal/Neonatal Morbidity and Mortality
ACE inhibitors can cause fetal and neonatal morbidity and death when administered to pregnant women. Several dozen cases have been reported in the world literature. When pregnancy is detected, ACE inhibitors should be discontinued as soon as possible.
The use of ACE inhibitors during the second and third trimesters of pregnancy has been associated with fetal and neonatal injury, including hypotension, neonatal skull hypoplasia, anuria, reversible or irreversible renal failure, and death. Oligohydramnios has also bee reported, presumably resulting from decreased fetal renal function: oligohydramnois in this setting has been associated with fetal limb contractures, craniofacial deformation, and hypoplastic lung development. Prematurity, intrauterine growth retardation, and patent ductus arteriosus have also been reported, although it is not clear whether these occurrences were due to the ACE-inhibitor exposure.
These adverse effects do not appear to have resulted from intrauterine ACE-inhibitor exposure that has been limited to the first trimester. Mothers whose embryos and fetuses are exposed to ACE inhibitors only during the first trimester should be so informed. Nonetheless, when patients become pregnant, physicians should make every effort to discontinue the use of VASOTEC I.V. as soon as possible.
Rarely (probably less often than once in every thousand pregnancies), no alternative to ACE inhibitors will be found. In these rare cases, the mothers should be apprised of the potential hazards to their fetuses, and serial ultrasound examinations should be performed to assess the intraamniotic environment.
If oligohydramnois is observed, VASOTEC I.V. should be discontinued unless it is considered lifesaving for the mother. Contraction stress testing (CST), a non-stress test (NST), or biophysical profiling (BPP) may be appropriate, depending upon the week of pregnancy. Patients and physicians should be aware, however, that oligohydramnois may not appear until after the fetus has sustained irreversible injury.
Infants with histories of *in utero* exposure to ACE inhibitors should be closely observed for hypotension, oliguria, and hyperkalemia. If oliguria occurs, attention should be directed toward support of blood pressure and renal perfusion. Exchange transfusion or dialysis may be required as means of reversing hypotension and/or substituting for disordered renal function. Enalapril, which crosses the placenta, has been removed from neonatal circulation by peritoneal dialysis with some clinical benefit, and theoretically may be removed by exchange transfusion, although there is no experience with the latter procedure.
No teratogenic effects of oral enalapril were seen in studies of pregnant rats and rabbits. On a body surface area basis, the doses used were 57 times and 12 times, respectively, the maximum recommended human daily dose (MRHDD).

PRECAUTIONS

General
Impaired Renal Function: As a consequence of inhibiting the renin-angiotensin-aldosterone system, changes in renal function may be anticipated in susceptible individuals. In patients with severe heart failure whose renal function may depend on the activity of the renin-angiotensin-aldosterone system, treatment with angiotensin converting enzyme inhibitors, including enalapril or enalaprilat, may be associated with oliguria and/or progressive azotemia and rarely with acute renal failure and/or death.
In clinical studies in hypertensive patients with unilateral or bilateral renal artery stenosis, increases in blood urea nitrogen and serum creatinine were observed in 20 percent of patients receiving enalapril. These increases were almost always reversible upon discontinuation of enalapril or enalapril and/or diuretic therapy. In such patients renal function should be monitored during the first few weeks of therapy.
Some hypertensive patients with no apparent pre-existing renal vascular disease have developed increases in blood urea and serum creatinine, usually minor and transient, especially when enalaprilat has been given concomitantly with a diuretic. This is more likely to occur in patients with pre-existing renal impairment. Dosage reduction of enalaprilat and/or discontinuation of the diuretic may be required.
Evaluation of the hypertensive patient should always include assessment of renal function. (See DOSAGE AND ADMINISTRATION.)
Hyperkalemia: Elevated serum potassium (greater than 5.7 mEq/L) was observed in approximately one percent of hypertensive patients in clinical trials receiving enalapril. In most cases these were isolated values which resolved despite continued therapy. Hyperkalemia was a cause of discontinuation of therapy in 0.28 percent of hypertensive patients. Risk factors for the development of hyperkalemia include renal insufficiency, diabetes mellitus, and the concomitant use of potassium-sparing agents or potassium supplements, which should be used cautiously, if at all, with VASOTEC I.V. (See *Drug Interactions.*)
Cough: Presumably due to the inhibition of the degradation of endogenous bradykinin, persistent nonproductive cough has been reported with all ACE inhibitors, always resolving after discontinuation of therapy. ACE inhibitor-induced cough should be considered in the differential diagnosis of cough.
Surgery/Anesthesia: In patients undergoing major surgery or during anesthesia with agents that produce hypotension, enalaprilat may block angiotensin II formation secondary to compensatory renin release. If hypotension occurs and is considered to be due to this mechanism, it can be corrected by volume expansion.
Drug Interactions
Hypotension—Patients on Diuretic Therapy: Patients on diuretics and especially those in whom diuretic therapy was recently instituted, may occasionally experience an excessive reduction of blood pressure after initiation of therapy with enalaprilat. The possibility of hypotensive effects with enalaprilat can be minimized by administration of an intravenous infusion of normal saline, discontinuing the diuretic or increasing the salt intake prior to initiation of treatment with enalaprilat. If it is necessary to continue the diuretic, provide close medical supervision for at least one hour after the initial dose of enalaprilat. (See WARNINGS.)
Agents Causing Renin Release: The antihypertensive effect of VASOTEC I.V. appears to be augmented by antihypertensive agents that cause renin release (e.g., diuretics.)
Other Cardiovascular Agents: VASOTEC I.V. has been used concomitantly with digitalis, beta adrenergic-blocking agents, methyldopa, nitrates, calcium-blocking agents, hydralazine and prazosin without evidence of clinically significant adverse interactions.
Agents Increasing Serum Potassium: VASOTEC I.V. attenuates potassium loss caused by thiazide-type diuretics. Potassium-sparing diuretics (e.g., spironolactone, triamterene, or amiloride), potassium supplements, or potassium-containing salt substitutes may lead to significant increases in serum potassium. Therefore, if concomitant use of these agents is indicated because of demonstrated hypokalemia, they should be used with caution and with frequent monitoring of serum potassium.
Lithium: Lithium toxicity has been reported in patients receiving lithium concomitantly with drugs which cause elimination of sodium, including ACE inhibitors. A few cases of lithium toxicity have been reported in patients receiving concomitant enalapril and lithium and were reversible upon discontinuation of both drugs. It is recommended that serum lithium levels be monitored frequently if enalapril is administered concomitantly with lithium.
Carcinogenesis, Mutagenesis, Impairment of Fertility
Carcinogenicity studies have not been done with VASOTEC I.V.
VASOTEC I.V. is the bioactive form of its ethyl ester, enalapril maleate. There was no evidence of a tumorigenic effect when enalapril was administered for 106 weeks to male and female rats at doses up to 90 mg/kg/day or for 94 weeks to male and female mice at doses up to 90 and 180 mg/kg/day, respectively. These doses are 26 times (in rats and female mice) and 13 times (in male mice) the maximum recommended human daily dose (MRHDD) when compared on a body surface area basis.

Continued on next page

Information on the Merck & Co., Inc. products listed on these pages is the full prescribing information from product circulars in use August 31, 1998. For information, please call 1-800-NSC MERCK [1-800-672-6372].

Vasotec I.V.—Cont.

VASOTEC I.V. was not mutagenic in the Ames microbial mutagen test with or without metabolic activation. Enalapril showed no drug-related changes in the following genotoxicity studies: rec-assay, reverse mutation assay with *E. coli*, sister chromatid exchange with cultured mammalian cells, the micronucleus test with mice, and in an *in vivo* cytogenic study using mouse bone marrow. There were no adverse effects on reproductive performance of male and female rats treated with up to 90 mg/kg/day of enalapril (26 times the MRHDD when compared on a body surface area basis).

Pregnancy
Pregnancy Categories C (first trimester) and *D* (second and third trimesters). See WARNINGS, *Fetal/Neonatal Morbidity and Mortality.*
Nursing Mothers
Enalapril and enalaprilat have been detected in human breast milk. Because of the potential for serious adverse reactions in nursing infants from enalapril, a decision should be made whether to discontinue nursing or to discontinue VASOTEC I.V., taking into account the importance of the drug to the mother.
Pediatric Use
Safety and effectiveness in pediatric patients have not been established.

ADVERSE REACTIONS

VASOTEC I.V. has been found to be generally well tolerated in controlled clinical trials involving 349 patients (168 with hypertension, 153 with congestive heart failure and 28 with coronary artery disease). The most frequent clinically significant adverse experience was hypotension (3.4 percent), occurring in eight patients (5.2 percent) with congestive heart failure, three (1.8 percent) with hypertension and one with coronary artery disease. Other adverse experiences occurring in greater than one percent of patients were: headache (2.9 percent) and nausea (1.1 percent).
Adverse experiences occurring in 0.5 to 1.0 percent of patients in controlled clinical trials included: myocardial infarction, fatigue, dizziness, fever, rash and constipation.
Angioedema: Angioedema has been reported in patients receiving enalaprilat, with an incidence higher in black than in non-black patients. Angioedema associated with laryngeal edema may be fatal. If angioedema of the face, extremities, lips, tongue, glottis and/or larynx occurs, treatment with enalaprilat should be discontinued and appropriate therapy instituted immediately. (See WARNINGS.)
Cough: See PRECAUTIONS, *Cough.*
Enalapril Maleate
Since enalapril is converted to enalaprilat, those adverse experiences associated with enalapril might also be expected to occur with VASOTEC I.V.
The following adverse experiences have been reported with enalapril and, within each category, are listed in order of decreasing severity.
Body As A Whole: Syncope, orthostatic effects, anaphylactoid reactions (see WARNINGS, *Anaphylactoid reactions during membrane exposure*), chest pain, abdominal pain, asthenia.
Cardiovascular: Cardiac arrest; myocardial infarction or cerebrovascular accident, possibly secondary to excessive hypotension in high risk patients (see WARNINGS, *Hypotension*); pulmonary embolism and infarction; pulmonary edema; rhythm disturbances including atrial tachycardia and bradycardia; atrial fibrillation; orthostatic hypotension; angina pectoris; palpitation, Raynaud's phenomenon.
Digestive: Ileus, pancreatitis, hepatic failure, hepatitis (hepatocellular [proven on rechallenge] or cholestatic jaundice) (see WARNINGS, *Hepatic Failure*), melena, diarrhea, vomiting, dyspepsia, anorexia, glossitis, stomatitis, dry mouth.
Hematologic: Rare cases of neutropenia, thrombocytopenia and bone marrow depression.
Musculoskeletal: Muscle cramps.
Nervous/Psychiatric: Depression, vertigo, confusion, ataxia, somnolence, insomnia, nervousness, peripheral neuropathy (e.g. paresthesia, dysesthesia), dream abnormality.
Respiratory: Bronchospasm, dyspnea, pneumonia, bronchitis, cough, rhinorrhea, sore throat and hoarseness, asthma, upper respiratory infection, pulmonary infiltrates.
Skin: Exfoliative dermatitis, toxic epidermal necrolysis, Stevens-Johnson syndrome, pemphigus, herpes zoster, erythema multiforme, urticaria, pruritus, alopecia, flushing, diaphoresis, photosensitivity.
Special Senses: Blurred vision, taste alteration, anosmia, tinnitus, conjunctivitis, dry eyes, tearing.
Urogenital: Renal failure, oliguria, renal dysfunction (see PRECAUTIONS and DOSAGE AND ADMINISTRATION), urinary tract infection, flank pain, gynecomastia, impotence.
Miscellaneous: A symptom complex has been reported which may include some or all of the following: a positive ANA, an elevated erythrocyte sedimentation rate, arthral-

gia/arthritis, myalgia/myositis, fever, serositis, vasculitis, leukocytosis, eosinophilia, photosensitivity, rash and other dermatologic manifestations.
Hypotension: Combining the results of clinical trials in patients with hypertension or congestive heart failure, hypotension (including postural hypotension, and other orthostatic effects) was reported in 2.3 percent of patients following the initial dose of enalapril or during extended therapy. In the hypertensive patients, hypotension occurred in 0.9 percent and syncope occurred in 0.5 percent of patients. Hypotension or syncope was a cause for discontinuation of therapy in 0.1 percent of hypertensive patients. (See WARNINGS.)
Fetal/Neonatal Morbidity and Mortality: See WARNINGS, *Fetal/Neonatal Morbidity and Mortality.*
Clinical Laboratory Test Findings
Serum Electrolytes: Hyperkalemia (see PRECAUTIONS), hyponatremia.
Creatinine, Blood Urea Nitrogen: In controlled clinical trials minor increases in blood urea nitrogen and serum creatinine, reversible upon discontinuation of therapy, were observed in about 0.2 percent of patients with essential hypertension treated with enalapril alone. Increases are more likely to occur in patients receiving concomitant diuretics or in patients with renal artery stenosis. (See PRECAUTIONS.)
Hematology: Small decreases in hemoglobin and hematocrit (mean decreases of approximately 0.3 g percent and 1.0 vol percent, respectively) occur frequently in hypertensive patients treated with enalapril but are rarely of clinical importance unless another cause of anemia coexists. In clinical trials, less than 0.1 percent of patients discontinued therapy due to anemia. Hemolytic anemia, including cases of hemolysis in patients with G-6-PD deficiency, has been reported; a causal relationship to enalapril cannot be excluded.
Liver Function Tests: Elevations of liver enzymes and/or serum bilirubin have occurred (see WARNINGS, *Hepatic Failure*).

OVERDOSAGE

In clinical studies, some hypertensive patients received a maximum dose of 80 mg of enalaprilat intravenously over a fifteen minute period. At this high dose, no adverse effects beyond those as associated with the recommended dosages were observed.
A single intravenous dose of ≤ 4167 mg/kg of enalaprilat was associated with lethality in female mice. No lethality occurred after an intravenous dose of 3472 mg/kg.
The most likely manifestation of overdosage would be hypotension, for which the usual treatment would be intravenous infusion of normal saline solution.
Enalaprilat may be removed from general circulation by hemodialysis and has been removed from neonatal circulation by peritoneal dialysis.

DOSAGE AND ADMINISTRATION

FOR INTRAVENOUS ADMINISTRATION ONLY
The dose in hypertension is 1.25 mg every six hours administered intravenously over a five minute period. A clinical response is usually seen within 15 minutes. Peak effects after the first dose may not occur for up to four hours after dosing. The peak effects of the second and subsequent doses may exceed those of the first.
No dosage regimen for VASOTEC I.V. has been clearly demonstrated to be more effective in treating hypertension than 1.25 mg every six hours. However, in controlled clinical studies in hypertension, doses as high as 5 mg every six hours were well tolerated for up to 36 hours. There has been inadequate experience with doses greater than 20 mg per day.
In studies of patients with hypertension, VASOTEC I.V. has not been administered for periods longer than 48 hours. In other studies, patients have received VASOTEC I.V. for as long as seven days.
The dose for patients being converted to VASOTEC I.V. from oral therapy for hypertension with enalapril maleate is 1.25 mg every six hours. For conversion from intravenous to oral therapy, the recommended initial dose of Tablets VASOTEC (Enalapril Maleate) is 5 mg once a day with subsequent dosage adjustments as necessary.
Patients on Diuretic Therapy
For patients on diuretic therapy the recommended starting dose for hypertension is 0.625 mg administered intravenously over a five minute period. A clinical response is usually seen within 15 minutes. Peak effects after the first dose may not occur for up to four hours after dosing, although most of the effect is usually apparent within the first hour. If after one hour there is an inadequate clinical response, the 0.625 mg dose may be repeated. Additional doses of 1.25 mg may be administered at six hour intervals.
For conversion from intravenous to oral therapy, the recommended initial dose of Tablets VASOTEC (Enalapril Maleate) for patients who have responded to 0.625 mg of enalaprilat every six hours is 2.5 mg once a day with subsequent dosage adjustment as necessary.

Dosage Adjustment in Renal Impairment
The usual dose of 1.25 mg of enalaprilat every six hours is recommended for patients with a creatinine clearance >30 mL/min (serum creatinine of up to approximately 3 mg/dL). For patients with creatinine clearance ≤30 mL/min (serum creatinine ≥3 mg/dL), the initial dose is 0.625 mg. (See WARNINGS.)
If after one hour there is an inadequate clinical response, the 0.625 mg dose may be repeated. Additional doses of 1.25 mg may be administered at six hour intervals.
For dialysis patients, see below, *Patients at Risk of Excessive Hypotension.*
For conversion from intravenous to oral therapy, the recommended initial dose of Tablets VASOTEC (Enalapril Maleate) is 5 mg once a day for patients with creatinine clearance >30 mL/min and 2.5 mg once daily for patients with creatinine clearance ≤30 mL/min. Dosage should then be adjusted according to blood pressure response.
Patients at Risk of Excessive Hypotension
Hypertensive patients at risk of excessive hypotension include those with the following concurrent conditions or characteristics: heart failure, hyponatremia, high dose diuretic therapy, recent intensive diuresis or increase in diuretic dose, renal dialysis, or severe volume and/or salt depletion of any etiology (see WARNINGS). Single doses of enalaprilat as low as 0.2 mg have produced excessive hypotension in normotensive patients with these diagnoses. Because of the potential for an extreme hypotensive response in these patients, therapy should be started under very close medical supervision. The starting dose should be no greater than 0.625 mg administered intravenously over a period of no less than five minutes and preferably longer (up to one hour).
Patients should be followed closely whenever the dose of enalaprilat is adjusted and/or diuretic is increased.
Administration
VASOTEC I.V. should be administered as a slow intravenous infusion, as indicated above, over at least five minutes. It may be administered as provided or diluted with up to 50 mL of a compatible diluent.
Parenteral drug products should be inspected visually for particulate matter and discoloration prior to use whenever solution and container permit.
Compatibility and Stability
VASOTEC I.V. as supplied and mixed with the following intravenous diluents has been found to maintain full activity for 24 hours at room temperature:
5 percent Dextrose Injection
0.9 percent Sodium Chloride Injection
0.9 percent Sodium Chloride Injection in 5 percent Dextrose
5 percent Dextrose in Lactated Ringer's Injection
McGaw ISOLYTE* E.

* Registered trademark of American Hospital Supply Corporation.

HOW SUPPLIED

No. 3508—VASOTEC I.V., 1.25 mg per mL, is a clear, colorless solution and is supplied in vials containing 1 mL and 2 mL.
NDC 0006-3508-01, 1 mL vials
(6505-01-356-8505, 1 mL vial)
NDC 0006-3508-04, 2 mL vials
(6505-01-305-6988, 2 mL vial).
Storage
Store below 30°C (86°F).

7875728   Issued February 1997
COPYRIGHT © MERCK & CO., INC., 1989, 1991, 1992
All rights reserved

VASOTEC® Tablets   ℞
(Enalapril Maleate), U.S.P.

USE IN PREGNANCY
When used in pregnancy during the second and third trimesters, ACE inhibitors can cause injury and even death to the developing fetus. When pregnancy is detected, VASOTEC should be discontinued as soon as possible. See WARNINGS, *Fetal/Neonatal Morbidity and Mortality.*

DESCRIPTION

VASOTEC* (Enalapril Maleate) is the maleate salt of enalapril, the ethyl ester of a long-acting angiotensin converting enzyme inhibitor, enalaprilat. Enalapril maleate is chemically described as (*S*)-1-[*N*-[1-(ethoxycarbonyl)-3- phenylpropyl]-L-alanyl]-L-proline, (*Z*)-2-butenedioate salt (1:1). Its empirical formula is $C_{20}H_{28}N_2O_5 \cdot C_4H_4O_4$, and its structural formula is:
[See chemical structure at top of next column]

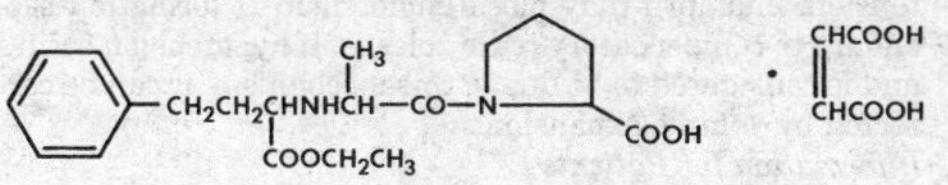

Enalapril maleate is a white to off-white, crystalline powder with a molecular weight of 492.53. It is sparingly soluble in water, soluble in ethanol, and freely soluble in methanol.
Enalapril is a pro-drug; following oral administration, it is bioactivated by hydrolysis of the ethyl ester to enalaprilat, which is the active angiotensin converting enzyme inhibitor.
Enalapril maleate is supplied as 2.5 mg, 5 mg, 10 mg, and 20 mg tablets for oral administration. In addition to the active ingredient enalapril maleate, each tablet contains the following inactive ingredients: lactose, magnesium stearate, starch, and other ingredients. The 2.5 mg, 10 mg and 20 mg tablets also contain iron oxides.

*Registered trademark of MERCK & CO., INC.

CLINICAL PHARMACOLOGY

Mechanism of Action
Enalapril, after hydrolysis to enalaprilat, inhibits angiotensin-converting enzyme (ACE) in human subjects and animals. ACE is a peptidyl dipeptidase that catalyzes the conversion of angiotensin I to the vasoconstrictor substance, angiotensin II. Angiotensin II also stimulates aldosterone secretion by the adrenal cortex. The beneficial effects of enalapril in hypertension and heart failure appear to result primarily from suppression of the renin-angiotensin-aldosterone system. Inhibition of ACE results in decreased plasma angiotensin II, which leads to decreased vasopressor activity and to decreased aldosterone secretion. Although the latter decrease is small, it results in small increases of serum potassium. In hypertensive patients treated with VASOTEC alone for up to 48 weeks, mean increases in serum potassium of approximately 0.2 mEq/L were observed. In patients treated with VASOTEC plus a thiazide diuretic, there was essentially no change in serum potassium. (See PRECAUTIONS.) Removal of angiotensin II negative feedback on renin secretion leads to increased plasma renin activity.
ACE is identical to kininase, an enzyme that degrades bradykinin. Whether increased levels of bradykinin, a potent vasodepressor peptide, play a role in the therapeutic effects of VASOTEC remains to be elucidated.
While the mechanism through which VASOTEC lowers blood pressure is believed to be primarily suppression of the renin-angiotensin-aldosterone system, VASOTEC is antihypertensive even in patients with low-renin hypertension. Although VASOTEC was antihypertensive in all races studied, black hypertensive patients (usually a low-renin hypertensive population) had a smaller average response to enalapril monotherapy than non-black patients.
Pharmacokinetics and Metabolism
Following oral administration of VASOTEC, peak serum concentrations of enalapril occur within about one hour. Based on urinary recovery, the extent of absorption of enalapril is approximately 60 percent. Enalapril absorption is not influenced by the presence of food in the gastrointestinal tract. Following absorption, enalapril is hydrolyzed to enalaprilat, which is a more potent angiotensin converting enzyme inhibitor than enalapril; enalaprilat is poorly absorbed when administered orally. Peak serum concentrations of enalaprilat occur three to four hours after an oral dose of enalapril maleate. Excretion of VASOTEC is primarily renal. Approximately 94 percent of the dose is recovered in the urine and feces as enalaprilat or enalapril. The principal components in urine are enalaprilat, accounting for about 40 percent of the dose, and intact enalapril. There is no evidence of metabolites of enalapril, other than enalaprilat.
The serum concentration profile of enalaprilat exhibits a prolonged terminal phase, apparently representing a small fraction of the administered dose that has been bound to ACE. The amount bound does not increase with dose, indicating a saturable site of binding. The effective half-life for accumulation of enalaprilat following multiple doses of enalapril maleate is 11 hours.
The disposition of enalapril and enalaprilat in patients with renal insufficiency is similar to that in patients with normal renal function until the glomerular filtration rate is 30 mL/min or less. With glomerular filtration rate ≤30 mL/min, peak and trough enalaprilat levels increase, time to peak concentration increases and time to steady state may be delayed. The effective half-life of enalaprilat following multiple doses of enalapril maleate is prolonged at this level of renal insufficiency. (See DOSAGE AND ADMINISTRATION.) Enalaprilat is dialyzable at the rate of 62 mL/min.
Studies in dogs indicate that enalapril crosses the blood-brain barrier poorly, if at all; enalaprilat does not enter the brain. Multiple doses of enalapril maleate in rats do not result in accumulation in any tissues. Milk of lactating rats contains radioactivity following administration of ^{14}C enalapril maleate. Radioactivity was found to cross the placenta following administration of labeled drug to pregnant hamsters.
Pharmacodynamics and Clinical Effects
Hypertension: Administration of VASOTEC to patients with hypertension of severity ranging from mild to severe results in a reduction of both supine and standing blood pressure usually with no orthostatic component. Symptomatic postural hypotension is therefore infrequent, although it might be anticipated in volume-depleted patients. (See WARNINGS.)
In most patients studied, after oral administration of a single dose of enalapril, onset of antihypertensive activity was seen at one hour with peak reduction of blood pressure achieved by four to six hours.
At recommended doses, antihypertensive effects have been maintained for at least 24 hours. In some patients the effects may diminish toward the end of the dosing interval (see DOSAGE AND ADMINISTRATION).
In some patients achievement of optimal blood pressure reduction may require several weeks of therapy.
The antihypertensive effects of VASOTEC have continued during long term therapy. Abrupt withdrawal of VASOTEC has not been associated with a rapid increase in blood pressure.
In hemodynamic studies in patients with essential hypertension, blood pressure reduction was accompanied by a reduction in peripheral arterial resistance with an increase in cardiac output and little or no change in heart rate. Following administration of VASOTEC, there is an increase in renal blood flow; glomerular filtration rate is usually unchanged. The effects appear to be similar in patients with renovascular hypertension.
When given together with thiazide-type diuretics, the blood pressure lowering effects of VASOTEC are approximately additive.
In a clinical pharmacology study, indomethacin or sulindac was administered to hypertensive patients receiving VASOTEC. In this study there was no evidence of a blunting of the antihypertensive action of VASOTEC.
Heart Failure: In trials in patients treated with digitalis and diuretics, treatment with enalapril resulted in decreased systemic vascular resistance, blood pressure, pulmonary capillary wedge pressure and heart size, and increased cardiac output and exercise tolerance. Heart rate was unchanged or slightly reduced, and mean ejection fraction was unchanged or increased. There was a beneficial effect on severity of heart failure as measured by the New York Heart Association (NYHA) classification and on symptoms of dyspnea and fatigue. Hemodynamic effects were observed after the first dose, and appeared to be maintained in uncontrolled studies lasting as long as four months. Effects on exercise tolerance, heart size, and severity and symptoms of heart failure were observed in placebo-controlled studies lasting from eight weeks to over one year.
Heart Failure, Mortality Trials: In a multicenter, placebo-controlled clinical trial, 2,569 patients with all degrees of symptomatic heart failure and ejection fraction ≤35 percent were randomized to placebo or enalapril and followed for up to 55 months (SOLVD-Treatment). Use of enalapril was associated with an 11 percent reduction in all-cause mortality and a 30 percent reduction in hospitalization for heart failure. Diseases that excluded patients from enrollment in the study included severe stable angina (>2 attacks/day), hemodynamically significant valvular or outflow tract obstruction, renal failure (creatinine >2.5 mg/dL), cerebral vascular disease (e.g., significant carotid artery disease), advanced pulmonary disease, malignancies, active myocarditis and constrictive pericarditis. The mortality benefit associated with enalapril does not appear to depend upon digitalis being present.
A second multicenter trial used the SOLVD protocol for study of asymptomatic or minimally symptomatic patients. SOLVD-Prevention patients, who had left ventricular ejection fraction ≤35% and no history of symptomatic heart failure, were randomized to placebo (n=2117) or enalapril (n=2111) and followed for up to 5 years. The majority of patients in the SOLVD-Prevention trial had a history of ischemic heart disease. A history of myocardial infarction was present in 80 percent of patients, current angina pectoris in 34 percent, and a history of hypertension in 37 percent. No statistically significant mortality effect was demonstrated in this population. Enalapril-treated subjects had 32% fewer first hospitalizations for heart failure, and 32% fewer total heart failure hospitalizations. Compared to placebo, 32 percent fewer patients receiving enalapril developed symptoms of overt heart failure. Hospitalizations for cardiovascular reasons were also reduced. There was an insignificant reduction in hospitalizations for any cause in the enalapril treatment group (for enalapril vs. placebo, respectively, 1166 vs. 1201 first hospitalizations, 2649 vs. 2840 total hospitalizations), although the study was not powered to look for such an effect.
The SOLVD-Prevention trial was not designed to determine whether treatment of asymptomatic patients with low ejection fraction would be superior, with respect to preventing hospitalization, to closer follow-up and use of enalapril at the earliest sign of heart failure. However, under the conditions of follow-up in the SOLVD-Prevention trial (every 4 months at the study clinic; personal physician as needed), 68% of patients on placebo who were hospitalized for heart failure had no prior symptoms recorded which would have signaled initiation of treatment.
The SOLVD-Prevention trial was also not designed to show whether enalapril modified the progression of underlying heart disease.
In another multicenter, placebo-controlled trial (CONSENSUS) limited to patients with NYHA class IV congestive heart failure and radiographic evidence of cardiomegaly, use of enalapril was associated with improved survival. The results are shown in the following table.

	SURVIVAL (%)	
	Six Months	One Year
VASOTEC (n=127)	74	64
Placebo (n=126)	56	48

In both CONSENSUS and SOLVD-Treatment trials, patients were also usually receiving digitalis, diuretics or both.

INDICATIONS AND USAGE

Hypertension
VASOTEC is indicated for the treatment of hypertension.
VASOTEC is effective alone or in combination with other antihypertensive agents, especially thiazide-type diuretics. The blood pressure lowering effects of VASOTEC and thiazides are approximately additive.
Heart Failure
VASOTEC is indicated for the treatment of symptomatic congestive heart failure, usually in combination with diuretics and digitalis. In these patients VASOTEC improves symptoms, increases survival, and decreases the frequency of hospitalization (see CLINICAL PHARMACOLOGY, *Heart Failure, Mortality Trials* for details and limitations of survival trials).
Asymptomatic Left Ventricular Dysfunction
In clinically stable asymptomatic patients with left ventricular dysfunction (ejection fraction ≤35 percent), VASOTEC decreases the rate of development of overt heart failure and decreases the incidence of hospitalization for heart failure. (See CLINICAL PHARMACOLOGY, *Heart Failure, Mortality Trials* for details and limitations of survival trials.)
In using VASOTEC consideration should be given to the fact that another angiotensin converting enzyme inhibitor, captopril, has caused agranulocytosis, particularly in patients with renal impairment or collagen vascular disease, and that available data are insufficient to show that VASOTEC does not have a similar risk. (See WARNINGS.)
In considering use of VASOTEC, it should be noted that in controlled clinical trials ACE inhibitors have an effect on blood pressure that is less in black patients than in non-blacks. In addition, it should be noted that black patients receiving ACE inhibitors have been reported to have a higher incidence of angioedema compared to non-blacks. (See WARNINGS, *Angioedema*.)

CONTRAINDICATIONS

VASOTEC is contraindicated in patients who are hypersensitive to this product and in patients with a history of angioedema related to previous treatment with an angiotensin converting enzyme inhibitor.

WARNINGS

Anaphylactoid and Possibly Related Reactions
Presumably because angiotensin-converting enzyme inhibitors affect the metabolism of eicosanoids and polypeptides, including endogenous bradykinin, patients receiving ACE inhibitors (including VASOTEC) may be subject to a variety of adverse reactions, some of them serious.
Angioedema: Angioedema of the face, extremities, lips, tongue, glottis and/or larynx has been reported in patients treated with angiotensin converting enzyme inhibitors, including VASOTEC. This may occur at any time during treatment. In such cases VASOTEC should be promptly discontinued and appropriate therapy and monitoring should be provided until complete and sustained resolution of signs and symptoms has occurred. In instances where swelling has been confined to the face and lips the condition has generally resolved without treatment, although antihistamines

Continued on next page

Information on the Merck & Co., Inc. products listed on these pages is the full prescribing information from product circulars in use August 31, 1998. For information, please call 1-800-NSC MERCK [1-800-672-6372].

Vasotec Tablets—Cont.

have been useful in relieving symptoms. Angioedema associated with laryngeal edema may be fatal. **Where there is involvement of the tongue, glottis or larynx, likely to cause airway obstruction, appropriate therapy, e.g., subcutaneous epinephrine solution 1:1000 (0.3 mL to 0.5 mL) and/or measures necessary to ensure a patent airway, should be promptly provided.** (See ADVERSE REACTIONS.)

Patients with a history of angioedema unrelated to ACE inhibitor therapy may be at increased risk of angioedema while receiving an ACE inhibitor (see also INDICATIONS AND USAGE and CONTRAINDICATIONS).

Anaphylactoid reactions during desensitization: Two patients undergoing desensitizing treatment with hymenoptera venom while receiving ACE inhibitors sustained life-threatening anaphylactoid reactions. In the same patients, these reactions were avoided when ACE inhibitors were temporarily withheld, but they reappeared upon inadvertent rechallenge.

Anaphylactoid reactions during membrane exposure: Anaphylactoid reactions have been reported in patients dialyzed with high-flux membranes and treated concomitantly with an ACE inhibitor. Anaphylactoid reactions have also been reported in patients undergoing low-density lipoprotein apheresis with dextran sulfate absorption.

Hypotension

Excessive hypotension is rare in uncomplicated hypertensive patients treated with VASOTEC alone. Patients with heart failure given VASOTEC commonly have some reduction in blood pressure, especially with the first dose, but discontinuation of therapy for continuing symptomatic hypotension usually is not necessary when dosing instructions are followed; caution should be observed when initiating therapy. (See DOSAGE AND ADMINISTRATION.) Patients at risk for excessive hypotension, sometimes associated with oliguria and/or progressive azotemia, and rarely with acute renal failure and/or death, include those with the following conditions or characteristics: heart failure, hyponatremia, high dose diuretic therapy, recent intensive diuresis or increase in diuretic dose, renal dialysis, or severe volume and/or salt depletion of any etiology. It may be advisable to eliminate the diuretic (except in patients with heart failure), reduce the diuretic dose or increase salt intake cautiously before initiating therapy with VASOTEC in patients at risk for excessive hypotension who are able to tolerate such adjustments. (See PRECAUTIONS, *Drug Interactions* and ADVERSE REACTIONS.) In patients at risk for excessive hypotension, therapy should be started under very close medical supervision and such patients should be followed closely for the first two weeks of treatment and whenever the dose of enalapril and/or diuretic is increased. Similar considerations may apply to patients with ischemic heart or cerebrovascular disease, in whom an excessive fall in blood pressure could result in a myocardial infarction or cerebrovascular accident.

If excessive hypotension occurs, the patient should be placed in the supine position and, if necessary, receive an intravenous infusion of normal saline. A transient hypotensive response is not a contraindication to further doses of VASOTEC, which usually can be given without difficulty once the blood pressure has stabilized. If symptomatic hypotension develops, a dose reduction or discontinuation of VASOTEC or concomitant diuretic may be necessary.

Neutropenia/Agranulocytosis

Another angiotensin converting enzyme inhibitor, captopril, has been shown to cause agranulocytosis and bone marrow depression, rarely in uncomplicated patients but more frequently in patients with renal impairment especially if they also have a collagen vascular disease. Available data from clinical trials of enalapril are insufficient to show that enalapril does not cause agranulocytosis at similar rates. Marketing experience has revealed several cases of neutropenia or agranulocytosis in which a causal relationship to enalapril cannot be excluded. Periodic monitoring of white blood cell counts in patients with collagen vascular disease and renal disease should be considered.

Hepatic Failure

Rarely, ACE inhibitors have been associated with a syndrome that starts with cholestatic jaundice and progresses to fulminant hepatic necrosis, and (sometimes) death. The mechanism of this syndrome is not understood. Patients receiving ACE inhibitors who develop jaundice or marked elevations of hepatic enzymes should discontinue the ACE inhibitor and receive appropriate medical follow-up.

Fetal/Neonatal Morbidity and Mortality

ACE inhibitors can cause fetal and neonatal morbidity and death when administered to pregnant women. Several dozen cases have been reported in the world literature. When pregnancy is detected, ACE inhibitors should be discontinued as soon as possible.

The use of ACE inhibitors during the second and third trimesters of pregnancy has been associated with fetal and neonatal injury, including hypotension, neonatal skull hypoplasia, anuria, reversible or irreversible renal failure, and death. Oligohydramnios has also been reported, presumably resulting from decreased fetal renal function: oligohydramnios in this setting has been associated with fetal limb contractures, craniofacial deformation, and hypoplastic lung development. Prematurity, intrauterine growth retardation, and patent ductus arteriosus have also been reported, although it is not clear whether these occurrences were due to the ACE-inhibitor exposure.

These adverse effects do not appear to have resulted from intrauterine ACE-inhibitor exposure that has been limited to the first trimester. Mothers whose embryos and fetuses are exposed to ACE inhibitors only during the first trimester should be so informed. Nonetheless, when patients become pregnant, physicians should make every effort to discontinue the use of VASOTEC as soon as possible.

Rarely (probably less often than once in every thousand pregnancies), no alternative to ACE inhibitors will be found. In these rare cases, the mothers should be apprised of the potential hazards to their fetuses, and serial ultrasound examinations should be performed to assess the intraamniotic environment.

If oligohydramnios is observed, VASOTEC should be discontinued unless it is considered lifesaving for the mother. Contraction stress testing (CST), a non-stress test (NST), or biophysical profiling (BPP) may be appropriate, depending upon the week of pregnancy. Patients and physicians should be aware, however, that oligohydramnois may not appear until after the fetus has sustained irreversible injury.

Infants with histories of *in utero* exposure to ACE inhibitors should be closely observed for hypotension, oliguria, and hyperkalemia. If oliguria occurs, attention should be directed toward support of blood pressure and renal perfusion. Exchange transfusion or dialysis may be required as means of reversing hypotension and/or substituting for disordered renal function. Enalapril, which crosses the placenta, has been removed from neonatal circulation by peritoneal dialysis with some clinical benefit, and theoretically may be removed by exchange transfusion, although there is no experience with the latter procedure.

No teratogenic effects of enalapril were seen in studies of pregnant rats and rabbits. On a body surface area basis, the doses used were 57 times and 12 times, respectively, the maximum recommended human daily dose (MRHDD).

PRECAUTIONS

General

Impaired Renal Function: As a consequence of inhibiting the renin-angiotensin-aldosterone system, changes in renal function may be anticipated in susceptible individuals. In patients with severe heart failure whose renal function may depend on the activity of the renin-angiotensin-aldosterone system, treatment with angiotensin converting enzyme inhibitors, including VASOTEC, may be associated with oliguria and/or progressive azotemia and rarely with acute renal failure and/or death.

In clinical studies in hypertensive patients with unilateral or bilateral renal artery stenosis, increases in blood urea nitrogen and serum creatinine were observed in 20 percent of patients. These increases were almost always reversible upon discontinuation of enalapril and/or diuretic therapy. In such patients renal function should be monitored during the first few weeks of therapy.

Some patients with hypertension or heart failure with no apparent pre-existing renal vascular disease have developed increases in blood urea and serum creatinine, usually minor and transient, especially when VASOTEC has been given concomitantly with a diuretic. This is more likely to occur in patients with pre-existing renal impairment. Dosage reduction and/or discontinuation of the diuretic and/or VASOTEC may be required.

Evaluation of patients with hypertension or heart failure should always include assessment of renal function. (See DOSAGE AND ADMINISTRATION.)

Hyperkalemia: Elevated serum potassium (greater than 5.7 mEq/L) was observed in approximately one percent of hypertensive patients in clinical trials. In most cases these were isolated values which resolved despite continued therapy. Hyperkalemia was a cause of discontinuation of therapy in 0.28 percent of hypertensive patients. In clinical trials in heart failure, hyperkalemia was observed in 3.8 percent of patients but was not a cause for discontinuation.

Risk factors for the development of hyperkalemia include renal insufficiency, diabetes mellitus, and the concomitant use of potassium-sparing diuretics, potassium supplements and/or potassium-containing salt substitutes, which should be used cautiously, if at all, with VASOTEC. (See *Drug Interactions.*)

Cough: Presumably due to the inhibition of the degradation of endogenous bradykinin, persistent nonproductive cough has been reported with all ACE inhibitors, always resolving after discontinuation of therapy. ACE inhibitor-induced cough should be considered in the differential diagnosis of cough.

Surgery/Anesthesia: In patients undergoing major surgery or during anesthesia with agents that produce hypotension, enalapril may block angiotensin II formation secondary to compensatory renin release. If hypotension occurs and is considered to be due to this mechanism, it can be corrected by volume expansion.

Information for Patients

Angioedema: Angioedema, including laryngeal edema, may occur at any time during treatment with angiotensin converting enzyme inhibitors, including enalapril. Patients should be so advised and told to report immediately any signs or symptoms suggesting angioedema (swelling of face, extremities, eyes, lips, tongue, difficulty in swallowing or breathing) and to take no more drug until they have consulted with the prescribing physician.

Hypotension: Patients should be cautioned to report lightheadedness, especially during the first few days of therapy. If actual syncope occurs, the patients should be told to discontinue the drug until they have consulted with the prescribing physician.

All patients should be cautioned that excessive perspiration and dehydration may lead to an excessive fall in blood pressure because of reduction in fluid volume. Other causes of volume depletion such as vomiting or diarrhea may also lead to a fall in blood pressure; patients should be advised to consult with the physician.

Hyperkalemia: Patients should be told not to use salt substitutes containing potassium without consulting their physician.

Neutropenia: Patients should be told to report promptly any indication of infection (e.g., sore throat, fever) which may be a sign of neutropenia.

Pregnancy: Female patients of childbearing age should be told about the consequences of second- and third-trimester exposure to ACE inhibitors, and they should also be told that these consequences do not appear to have resulted from intrauterine ACE-inhibitor exposure that has been limited to the first trimester. These patients should be asked to report pregnancies to their physicians as soon as possible.

NOTE: As with many other drugs, certain advice to patients being treated with enalapril is warranted. This information is intended to aid in the safe and effective use of this medication. It is not a disclosure of all possible adverse or intended effects.

Drug Interactions

Hypotension—Patients on Diuretic Therapy: Patients on diuretics and especially those in whom diuretic therapy was recently instituted, may occasionally experience an excessive reduction of blood pressure after initiation of therapy with enalapril. The possibility of hypotensive effects with enalapril can be minimized by either discontinuing the diuretic or increasing the salt intake prior to initiation of treatment with enalapril. If it is necessary to continue the diuretic, provide close medical supervision after the initial dose for at least two hours and until blood pressure has stabilized for at least an additional hour. (See WARNINGS and DOSAGE AND ADMINISTRATION.)

Agents Causing Renin Release: The antihypertensive effect of VASOTEC is augmented by antihypertensive agents that cause renin release (e.g., diuretics).

Other Cardiovascular Agents: VASOTEC has been used concomitantly with beta adrenergic-blocking agents, methyldopa, nitrates, calcium-blocking agents, hydralazine, prazosin and digoxin without evidence of clinically significant adverse interactions.

Agents Increasing Serum Potassium: VASOTEC attenuates potassium loss caused by thiazide-type diuretics. Potassium-sparing diuretics (e.g., spironolactone, triamterene, or amiloride), potassium supplements, or potassium-containing salt substitutes may lead to significant increases in serum potassium. Therefore, if concomitant use of these agents is indicated because of demonstrated hypokalemia, they should be used with caution and with frequent monitoring of serum potassium. Potassium sparing agents should generally not be used in patients with heart failure receiving VASOTEC.

Lithium: Lithium toxicity has been reported in patients receiving lithium concomitantly with drugs which cause elimination of sodium, including ACE inhibitors. A few cases of lithium toxicity have been reported in patients receiving concomitant VASOTEC and lithium and were reversible upon discontinuation of both drugs. It is recommended that serum lithium levels be monitored frequently if enalapril is administered concomitantly with lithium.

Carcinogenesis, Mutagenesis, Impairment of Fertility

There was no evidence of a tumorigenic effect when enalapril was administered for 106 weeks to male and female rats at doses up to 90 mg/kg/day or for 94 weeks to male and female mice at doses up to 90 and 180 mg/kg/day, respectively. These doses are 26 times (in rats and female mice) and 13 times (in male mice) the maximum recommended human daily dose (MRHDD) when compared on a body surface area basis.

Neither enalapril maleate nor the active diacid was mutagenic in the Ames microbial mutagen test with or without metabolic activation. Enalapril was also negative in the following genotoxicity studies: rec-assay, reverse mutation as-

say with *E. coli*, sister chromatid exchange with cultured mammalian cells, and the micronucleus test with mice, as well as in an *in vivo* cytogenic study using mouse bone marrow.

There were no adverse effects on reproductive performance of male and female rats treated with up to 90 mg/kg/day of enalapril (26 times the MRHDD when compared on a body surface area basis).

Pregnancy
Pregnancy Categories C (first trimester) and *D* (second and third trimesters). See WARNINGS, *Fetal/Neonatal Morbidity and Mortality.*
Nursing Mothers
Enalapril and enalaprilat have been detected in human breast milk. Because of the potential for serious adverse reactions in nursing infants from enalapril, a decision should be made whether to discontinue nursing or to discontinue VASOTEC, taking into account the importance of the drug to the mother.
Pediatric Use
Safety and effectiveness in pediatric patients have not been established.

ADVERSE REACTIONS

VASOTEC has been evaluated for safety in more than 10,000 patients, including over 1000 patients treated for one year or more. VASOTEC has been found to be generally well tolerated in controlled clinical trials involving 2987 patients.

For the most part, adverse experiences were mild and transient in nature. In clinical trials, discontinuation of therapy due to clinical adverse experiences was required in 3.3 percent of patients with hypertension and in 5.7 percent of patients with heart failure. The frequency of adverse experiences was not related to total daily dosage within the usual dosage ranges. In patients with hypertension the overall percentage of patients treated with VASOTEC reporting adverse experiences was comparable to placebo.

HYPERTENSION
Adverse experiences occurring in greater than one percent of patients with hypertension treated with VASOTEC in controlled clinical trials are shown below. In patients treated with VASOTEC, the maximum duration of therapy was three years; in placebo treated patients the maximum duration of therapy was 12 weeks.

	VASOTEC (n = 2314) Incidence (discontinuation)	Placebo (n = 230) Incidence
Body As A Whole		
Fatigue	3.0 (<0.1)	2.6
Orthostatic Effects	1.2 (<0.1)	0.0
Asthenia	1.1 (0.1)	0.9
Digestive		
Diarrhea	1.4 (<0.1)	1.7
Nausea	1.4 (0.2)	1.7
Nervous/Psychiatric		
Headache	5.2 (0.3)	9.1
Dizziness	4.3 (0.4)	4.3
Respiratory		
Cough	1.3 (0.1)	0.9
Skin		
Rash	1.4 (0.4)	0.4

HEART FAILURE
Adverse experiences occurring in greater than one percent of patients with heart failure treated with VASOTEC are shown below. The incidences represent the experiences from both controlled and uncontrolled clinical trials (maximum duration of therapy was approximately one year). In the placebo treated patients, the incidences reported are from the controlled trials (maximum duration of therapy is 12 weeks). The percentage of patients with severe heart failure (NYHA Class IV) was 29 percent and 43 percent for patients treated with VASOTEC and placebo, respectively.

	VASOTEC (n = 673) Incidence (discontinuation)	Placebo (n = 339) Incidence
Body As A Whole		
Orthostatic Effects	2.2 (0.1)	0.3
Syncope	2.2 (0.1)	0.9
Chest Pain	2.1 (0.0)	2.1
Fatigue	1.8 (0.0)	1.8
Abdominal Pain	1.6 (0.4)	2.1
Asthenia	1.6 (0.1)	0.3
Cardiovascular		
Hypotension	6.7 (1.9)	0.6
Orthostatic Hypotension	1.6 (0.1)	0.3
Angina Pectoris	1.5 (0.1)	1.8
Myocardial Infarction	1.2 (0.3)	1.8

Digestive		
Diarrhea	2.1 (0.1)	1.2
Nausea	1.3 (0.1)	0.6
Vomiting	1.3 (0.0)	0.9
Nervous/Psychiatric		
Dizziness	7.9 (0.6)	0.6
Headache	1.8 (0.1)	0.9
Vertigo	1.6 (0.1)	1.2
Respiratory		
Cough	2.2 (0.0)	0.6
Bronchitis	1.3 (0.0)	0.9
Dyspnea	1.3 (0.1)	0.4
Pneumonia	1.0 (0.0)	2.4
Skin		
Rash	1.3 (0.0)	2.4
Urogenital		
Urinary Tract Infection	1.3 (0.0)	2.4

Other serious clinical adverse experiences occurring since the drug was marketed or adverse experiences occurring in 0.5 to 1.0 percent of patients with hypertension or heart failure in clinical trials are listed below and, within each category, are in order of decreasing severity.
Body As A Whole: Anaphylactoid reactions (see WARNINGS, *Anaphylactoid and Possibly Related Reactions*).
Cardiovascular: Cardiac arrest; myocardial infarction or cerebrovascular accident, possibly secondary to excessive hypotension in high risk patients (see WARNINGS, *Hypotension*); pulmonary embolism and infarction; pulmonary edema; rhythm disturbances including atrial tachycardia and bradycardia; atrial fibrillation; palpitation, Raynaud's phenomenon.
Digestive: Ileus, pancreatitis, hepatic failure, hepatitis (hepatocellular [proven on rechallenge] or cholestatic jaundice) (see WARNINGS, *Hepatic Failure*), melena, anorexia, dyspepsia, constipation, glossitis, stomatitis, dry mouth.
Hematologic: Rare cases of neutropenia, thrombocytopenia and bone marrow depression.
Musculoskeletal: Muscle cramps.
Nervous/Psychiatric: Depression, confusion, ataxia, somnolence, insomnia, nervousness, peripheral neuropathy (e.g., paresthesia, dysesthesia), dream abnormality.
Respiratory: Bronchospasm, rhinorrhea, sore throat and hoarseness, asthma, upper respiratory infection, pulmonary infiltrates.
Skin: Exfoliative dermatitis, toxic epidermal necrolysis, Stevens-Johnson syndrome, pemphigus, herpes zoster, erythema multiforme, urticaria, pruritus, alopecia, flushing, diaphoresis, photosensitivity.
Special Senses: Blurred vision, taste alteration, anosmia, tinnitus, conjunctivitis, dry eyes, tearing.
Urogenital: Renal failure, oliguria, renal dysfunction (see PRECAUTIONS and DOSAGE AND ADMINISTRATION), flank pain, gynecomastia, impotence.
Miscellaneous: A symptom complex has been reported which may include some or all of the following: a positive ANA, an elevated erythrocyte sedimentation rate, arthralgia/arthritis, myalgia/myositis, fever, serositis, vasculitis, leukocytosis, eosinophilia, photosensitivity, rash and other dermatologic manifestations.
Angioedema: Angioedema has been reported in patients receiving VASOTEC, with an incidence higher in black than in non-black patients. Angioedema associated with laryngeal edema may be fatal. If angioedema of the face, extremities, lips, tongue, glottis and/or larynx occurs, treatment with VASOTEC should be discontinued and appropriate therapy instituted immediately. (See WARNINGS.)
Hypotension: In the hypertensive patients, hypotension occurred in 0.9 percent and syncope occurred in 0.5 percent of patients following the initial dose or during extended therapy. Hypotension or syncope was a cause for discontinuation of therapy in 0.1 percent of hypertensive patients. In heart failure patients, hypotension occurred in 6.7 percent and syncope occurred in 2.2 percent of patients. Hypotension or syncope was a cause for discontinuation of therapy in 1.9 percent of patients with heart failure. (See WARNINGS.)
Fetal/Neonatal Morbidity and Mortality: See WARNINGS, *Fetal/Neonatal Morbidity and Mortality.*
Cough: See PRECAUTIONS, *Cough.*
Clinical Laboratory Test Findings
Serum Electrolytes: Hyperkalemia (see PRECAUTIONS), hyponatremia.
Creatinine, Blood Urea Nitrogen: In controlled clinical trials minor increases in blood urea nitrogen and serum creatinine, reversible upon discontinuation of therapy, were observed in about 0.2 percent of patients with essential hypertension treated with VASOTEC alone. Increases are more likely to occur in patients receiving concomitant diuretics or in patients with renal artery stenosis. (See PRECAUTIONS.) In patients with heart failure who were also receiving diuretics with or without digitalis increases in blood urea nitrogen or serum creatinine, usually reversible upon discontinuation of VASOTEC and/or other concomitant di-

uretic therapy, were observed in about 11 percent of patients. Increases in blood urea nitrogen or creatinine were a cause for discontinuation in 1.2 percent of patients.
Hematology: Small decreases in hemoglobin and hematocrit (mean decreases of approximately 0.3 g percent and 1.0 vol percent, respectively) occur frequently in either hypertension or congestive heart failure patients treated with VASOTEC but are rarely of clinical importance unless another cause of anemia coexists. In clinical trials, less than 0.1 percent of patients discontinued therapy due to anemia. Hemolytic anemia, including cases of hemolysis in patients with G-6-PD deficiency, has been reported; a causal relationship to enalapril cannot be excluded.
Liver Function Tests: Elevations of liver enzymes and/or serum bilirubin have occurred (see WARNINGS, *Hepatic Failure*).

OVERDOSAGE

Limited data are available in regard to overdosage in humans.
Single oral doses of enalapril above 1,000 mg/kg and ≥1,775 mg/kg were associated with lethality in mice and rats, respectively.
The most likely manifestation of overdosage would be hypotension, for which the usual treatment would be intravenous infusion of normal saline solution.
Enalaprilat may be removed from general circulation by hemodialysis and has been removed from neonatal circulation by peritoneal dialysis.

DOSAGE AND ADMINISTRATION

Hypertension
In patients who are currently being treated with a diuretic, symptomatic hypotension occasionally may occur following the initial dose of VASOTEC. The diuretic should, if possible, be discontinued for two to three days before beginning therapy with VASOTEC to reduce the likelihood of hypotension. (See WARNINGS.) If the patient's blood pressure is not controlled with VASOTEC alone, diuretic therapy may be resumed.
If the diuretic cannot be discontinued an initial dose of 2.5 mg should be used under medical supervision for at least two hours and until blood pressure has stabilized for at least an additional hour. (See WARNINGS and PRECAUTIONS, *Drug Interactions.*)
The recommended initial dose in patients not on diuretics is 5 mg once a day. Dosage should be adjusted according to blood pressure response. The usual dosage range is 10 to 40 mg per day administered in a single dose or two divided doses. In some patients treated once daily, the antihypertensive effect may diminish toward the end of the dosing interval. In such patients, an increase in dosage or twice daily administration should be considered. If blood pressure is not controlled with VASOTEC alone, a diuretic may be added.
Concomitant administration of VASOTEC with potassium supplements, potassium salt substitutes, or potassium-sparing diuretics may lead to increases of serum potassium (see PRECAUTIONS).
Dosage Adjustment in Hypertensive Patients with Renal Impairment
The usual dose of enalapril is recommended for patients with a creatinine clearance >30 mL/min (serum creatinine of up to approximately 3 mg/dL). For patients with creatinine clearance ≤30 mL/min (serum creatinine ≥3 mg/dL), the first dose is 2.5 mg once daily. The dosage may be titrated upward until blood pressure is controlled or to a maximum of 40 mg daily.

Renal Status	Creatinine-Clearance mL/min	Initial Dose mg/day
Normal Renal Function	>80 mL/min	5 mg
Mild Impairment	≤80 >30 mL/min	5 mg
Moderate to Severe Impairment	≤30 mL/min	2.5 mg
Dialysis Patients*	—	2.5 mg on dialysis days**

Continued on next page

Vasotec Tablets—Cont.

* See WARNINGS, *Anaphylactoid reactions during membrane exposure.*
** Dosage on nondialysis days should be adjusted depending on the blood pressure response.

Heart Failure
VASOTEC is indicated for the treatment of symptomatic heart failure, usually in combination with diuretics and digitalis. In the placebo-controlled studies that demonstrated improved survival, patients were titrated as tolerated up to 40 mg, administered in two divided doses.
The recommended initial dose is 2.5 mg. The recommended dosing range is 2.5 to 20 mg given twice a day. Doses should be titrated upward, as tolerated, over a period of a few days or weeks. The maximum daily dose administered in clinical trials was 40 mg in divided doses.
After the initial dose of VASOTEC, the patient should be observed under medical supervision for at least two hours and until blood pressure has stabilized for at least an additional hour. (See WARNINGS and PRECAUTIONS, *Drug Interactions.*) If possible, the dose of any concomitant diuretic should be reduced which may diminish the likelihood of hypotension. The appearance of hypotension after the initial dose of VASOTEC does not preclude subsequent careful dose titration with the drug, following effective management of the hypotension.
Asymptomatic Left Ventricular Dysfunction
In the trial that demonstrated efficacy, patients were started on 2.5 mg twice daily and were titrated as tolerated to the targeted daily dose of 20 mg (in divided doses).
After the initial dose of VASOTEC, the patient should be observed under medical supervision for at least two hours and until blood pressure has stabilized for at least an additional hour. (See WARNINGS and PRECAUTIONS, *Drug Interactions.*) If possible, the dose of any concomitant diuretic should be reduced which may diminish the likelihood of hypotension. The appearance of hypotension after the initial dose of VASOTEC does not preclude subsequent careful dose titration with the drug, following effective management of the hypotension.
Dosage Adjustment in Patients with Heart Failure and Renal Impairment or Hyponatremia
In patients with heart failure who have hyponatremia (serum sodium less than 130 mEq/L) or with serum creatinine greater than 1.6 mg/dL, therapy should be initiated at 2.5 mg daily under close medical supervision. (See DOSAGE AND ADMINISTRATION, *Heart Failure,* WARNINGS and PRECAUTIONS, *Drug Interactions.*) The dose may be increased to 2.5 mg b.i.d., then 5 mg b.i.d. and higher as needed, usually at intervals of four days or more if at the time of dosage adjustment there is not excessive hypotension or significant deterioration of renal function. The maximum daily dose is 40 mg.

HOW SUPPLIED

No. 3411—Tablets VASOTEC, 2.5 mg, are yellow, biconvex barrel shaped, scored, compressed tablets with code MSD 14 on one side and VASOTEC on the other. They are supplied as follows:
NDC 0006-0014-94 unit of use bottles of 90 (with desiccant)
NDC 0006-0014-68 bottles of 100 (with desiccant)
NDC 0006-0014-28 unit dose packages of 100
NDC 0006-0014-98 unit of use bottles of 180 (with desiccant)
NDC 0006-0014-82 bottles of 1,000 (with desiccant)
NDC 0006-0014-87 bottles of 10,000 (with desiccant) (6505-01-379-5607, 2.5 mg 10,000's).
Shown in Product Identification Guide, page 323
No. 3412—Tablets VASOTEC, 5 mg, are white, barrel shaped, scored, compressed tablets, with code MSD 712 on one side and VASOTEC on the other. They are supplied as follows:
NDC 0006-0712-94 unit of use bottles of 90 (with desiccant)
NDC 0006-0712-68 bottles of 100 (with desiccant) (6505-01-236-8880, 5 mg 100's)
NDC 0006-0712-28 unit dose packages of 100 (6505-01-244-4811, 5 mg individually sealed 100's)
NDC 0006-0712-98 unit of use bottles of 180 (with desiccant)
NDC 0006-0712-82 bottles of 1,000 (with desiccant)
NDC 0006-0712-81 bottles of 4,000 (with desiccant)
NDC 0006-0712-87 bottles of 10,000 (with desiccant) (6505-01-379-5575, 5 mg 10,000's).
Shown in Product Identification Guide, page 323
No. 3413—Tablets VASOTEC, 10 mg, are salmon, barrel shaped, compressed tablets, with code MSD 713 on one side and VASOTEC on the other. They are supplied as follows:
NDC 0006-0713-94 unit of use bottles of 90 (with desiccant)
NDC 0006-0713-68 bottles of 100 (with desiccant) (6505-01-236-8881, 10 mg 100's)
NDC 0006-0713-28 unit dose packages of 100 (6505-01-314-6028, 10 mg individually sealed 100's)
NDC 0006-0713-98 unit of use bottles of 180 (with desiccant)
NDC 0006-0713-82 bottles of 1,000 (with desiccant)
NDC 0006-0713-81 bottles of 4,000 (with desiccant)
NDC 0006-0713-87 bottles of 10,000 (with desiccant) (6505-01-378-8022, 10 mg 10,000's).
Shown in Product Identification Guide, page 323
No. 3414—Tablets VASOTEC, 20 mg, are peach, barrel shaped, compressed tablets, with code MSD 714 on one side and VASOTEC on the other. They are supplied as follows:
NDC 0006-0714-94 unit of use bottles of 90 (with desiccant)
NDC 0006-0714-68 bottles of 100 (with desiccant) (6505-01-237-0545, 20 mg 100's)
NDC 0006-0714-28 unit dose packages of 100 (6505-01-318-0465, 20 mg individually sealed 100's)
NDC 0006-0714-82 bottles of 1,000 (with desiccant)
NDC 0006-0714-87 bottles of 10,000 (with desiccant) (6505-01-378-8780, 20 mg 10,000's).
Shown in Product Identification Guide, page 323
Storage
Store below 30°C (86°F) and avoid transient temperatures above 50°C (122°F). Keep container tightly closed. Protect from moisture.
Dispense in a tight container, if product package is subdivided.

7825155 Issued February 1997
COPYRIGHT © MERCK & CO., INC., 1988, 1989, 1992, 1993
All rights reserved

VIVACTIL® Tablets (Protriptyline HCl), U.S.P. ℞

DESCRIPTION

Protriptyline HCl is *N*- methyl-5*H* -dibenzo[*a,d*]-cycloheptene-5-propanamine hydrochloride. Its empirical formula is $C_{19}H_{21}N \cdot HCl$ and its structural formula is:

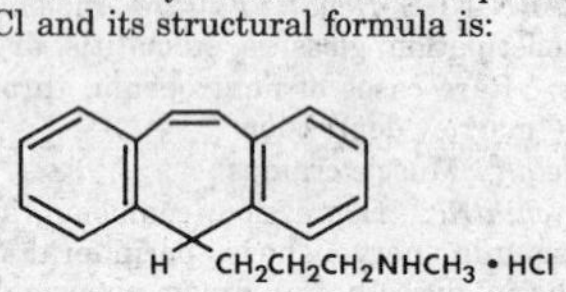

Protriptyline HCl, a dibenzocycloheptene derivative, has a molecular weight of 299.84. It is a white to yellowish powder that is freely soluble in water and soluble in dilute HCl.
VIVACTIL* (Protriptyline HCl) is supplied as 5 mg and 10 mg film coated tablets. Inactive ingredients are calcium phosphate, cellulose, guar gum, hydroxypropyl cellulose, hydroxypropyl methylcellulose, lactose, magnesium stearate, starch, talc, and titanium dioxide. Tablets VIVACTIL 5 mg and 10 mg also contain FD&C Yellow 6. Tablets VIVACTIL 10 mg also contain D&C Yellow 10.

*Registered trademark of MERCK & CO., INC.

ACTIONS

VIVACTIL is an antidepressant agent. The mechanism of its antidepressant action in man is not known. It is not a monoamine oxidase inhibitor, and it does not act primarily by stimulation of the central nervous system.
VIVACTIL has been found in some studies to have a more rapid onset of action than imipramine or amitriptyline. The initial clinical effect may occur within one week. Sedative and tranquilizing properties are lacking. The rate of excretion is slow.

INDICATIONS

VIVACTIL is indicated for the treatment of symptoms of mental depression in patients who are under close medical supervision. Its activating properties make it particularly suitable for withdrawn and anergic patients.

CONTRAINDICATIONS

VIVACTIL is contraindicated in patients who have shown prior hypersensitivity to it.
It should not be given concomitantly with a monoamine oxidase inhibiting compound. Hyperpyretic crises, severe convulsions, and deaths have occurred in patients receiving tricyclic antidepressant and monoamine oxidase inhibiting drugs simultaneously. When it is desired to substitute VIVACTIL for a monoamine oxidase inhibitor, a minimum of 14 days should be allowed to elapse after the latter is discontinued. VIVACTIL should then be initiated cautiously with gradual increase in dosage until optimum response is achieved.
This drug should not be used during the acute recovery phase following myocardial infarction.

WARNINGS

VIVACTIL may block the antihypertensive effect of guanethidine or similarly acting compounds.
VIVACTIL should be used with caution in patients with a history of seizures, and, because of its autonomic activity, in patients with a tendency to urinary retention, or increased intraocular tension.
Tachycardia and postural hypotension may occur more frequently with VIVACTIL than with other antidepressant drugs. VIVACTIL should be used with caution in elderly patients and patients with cardiovascular disorders; such patients should be observed closely because of the tendency of the drug to produce tachycardia, hypotension, arrhythmias, and prolongation of the conduction time. Myocardial infarction and stroke have occurred with drugs of this class.
On rare occasions, hyperthyroid patients or those receiving thyroid medication may develop arrhythmias when this drug is given.
In patients who may use alcohol excessively, it should be borne in mind that the potentiation may increase the danger inherent in any suicide attempt or overdosage.
Pediatric Usage
The safety and effectiveness of VIVACTIL in pediatric patients have not been established.
Usage in Pregnancy
Safe use in pregnancy and lactation has not been established; therefore, use in pregnant women, nursing mothers or women who may become pregnant requires that possible benefits be weighed against possible hazards to mother and child.
In mice, rats, and rabbits, doses about ten times greater than the recommended human doses had no apparent adverse effects on reproduction.

PRECAUTIONS

General
When protriptyline HCl is used to treat the depressive component of schizophrenia, psychotic symptoms may be aggravated. Likewise, in manic-depressive psychosis, depressed patients may experience a shift toward the manic phase if they are treated with an antidepressant drug. Paranoid delusions, with or without hostility, may be exaggerated. In any of these circumstances, it may be advisable to reduce the dose of VIVACTIL or to use a major tranquilizing drug concurrently.
Symptoms, such as anxiety or agitation, may be aggravated in overactive or agitated patients.
The possibility of suicide in depressed patients remains during treatment and until significant remission occurs. This type of patient should not have access to large quantities of the drug.
Concurrent administration of VIVACTIL and electroshock therapy may increase the hazards of therapy. Such treatment should be limited to patients for whom it is essential.
Discontinue the drug several days before elective surgery, if possible.
Both elevation and lowering of blood sugar levels have been reported.
Information for Patients
While on therapy with VIVACTIL, patients should be advised as to the possible impairment of mental and/or physical abilities required for performance of hazardous tasks, such as operating machinery or driving a motor vehicle.
Drug Interactions
When VIVACTIL is given with anticholinergic agents or sympathomimetic drugs, including epinephrine combined with local anesthetics, close supervision and careful adjustment of dosages are required.
Hyperpyrexia has been reported when tricyclic antidepressants are administered with anticholinergic agents or with neuroleptic drugs, particularly during hot weather.
Cimetidine is reported to reduce hepatic metabolism of certain tricyclic antidepressants, thereby delaying elimination and increasing steady-state concentrations of these drugs. Clinically significant effects have been reported with the tricyclic antidepressants when used concomitantly with cimetidine. Increases in plasma levels of tricyclic antidepressants, and in the frequency and severity of side effects, particularly anticholinergic, have been reported when cimetidine was added to the drug regimen. Discontinuation of cimetidine in well-controlled patients receiving tricyclic antidepressants and cimetidine may decrease the plasma levels and efficacy of the antidepressants.
It may enhance the response to alcohol and the effects of barbiturates and other CNS depressants.
Drugs Metabolized by Cytochrome P450 2D6: The biochemical activity of the drug-metabolizing isozyme, cytochrome P450 2D6 (debrisoquine hydroxylase), is reduced in a subset of the Caucasian population (about 7–10% of Caucasians are so called "poor metabolizers"); reliable estimates of the prevalence of reduced P450 2D6 isozyme activity among Asian, African, and other populations are not yet available. Poor metabolizers have higher than expected plasma concentrations of tricyclic antidepressants (TCAs) when given usual doses. Depending on the fraction of drug metabolized by P450 2D6, the increase in plasma concentration may be small or quite large (8-fold increase in plasma AUC of the TAC).

In addition, certain drugs inhibit the activity of this isozyme and make normal metabolizers resemble poor metabolizers. An individual who is stable on a given dose of TCA may become abruptly toxic when given one of these inhibiting drugs as concomitant therapy. The drugs that inhibit cytochrome P450 2D6 include some that are not metabolized by the enzyme (quinidine; cimetidine) and many that are substrates for P450 2D6 (many other antidepressants, phenothiazines, and the Type 1C antiarrhythmics, propafenone and flecainide). While all the selective serotonin reuptake inhibitors (SSRIs), e.g., fluoxetine, sertraline, and paroxetine, inhibit P450 2D6, they may vary in the extent of inhibition. The extent to which SSRI-TCA interactions may pose clinical problems will depend on the degree of inhibition and the pharmacokinetics of the SSRI involved. Nevertheless, caution is indicated in the coadministration of TCAs with any of the SSRIs, and also in switching from one class to the other. Of particular importance, sufficient time must elapse before initiating TCA treatment in a patient being withdrawn from fluoxetine, given the long half-life of the parent and active metabolite (at least 5 weeks may be necessary). Concomitant use of tricyclic antidepressants with drugs that can inhibit cytochrome P450 2D6 may require lower doses than usually prescribed for either the tricyclic antidepressant or the other drug. Furthermore, whenever one of these other drugs is withdrawn from co-therapy, an increased dose of tricyclic antidepressant may be required. It is desirable to monitor TCA plasma levels whenever a TCA is going to be coadministered with another drug known to be an inhibitor of P450 2D6.

Pediatric Use

The safety and effectiveness of VIVACTIL in pediatric patients have not been established.

ADVERSE REACTIONS

Within each category the following adverse reactions are listed in order of decreasing severity. Included in the listing are a few adverse reactions which have not been reported with this specific drug. However, the pharmacological similarities among the tricyclic antidepressant drugs require that each of the reactions be considered when protriptyline is administered. VIVACTIL is more likely to aggravate agitation and anxiety and produce cardiovascular reactions such as tachycardia and hypotension.

Cardiovascular: Myocardial infarction; stroke; heart block; arrhythmias; hypotension, particularly orthostatic hypotension; hypertension; tachycardia; palpitation.

Psychiatric: Confusional states (especially in the elderly) with hallucinations, disorientation, delusions, anxiety, restlessness, agitation; hypomania; exacerbation of psychosis; insomnia, panic, and nightmares.

Neurological: Seizures; incoordination; ataxia; tremors; peripheral neuropathy; numbness, tingling, and paresthesias of extremities; extrapyramidal symptoms; drowsiness; dizziness; weakness and fatigue; headache; syndrome of inappropriate ADH (antidiuretic hormone) secretion; tinnitus; alteration in EEG patterns.

Anticholinergic: Paralytic ileus; hyperpyrexia; urinary retention, delayed micturition, dilatation of the urinary tract; constipation; blurred vision, disturbance of accommodation, increased intraocular pressure, mydriasis; dry mouth and rarely associated sublingual adenitis.

Allergic: Drug fever; petechiae, skin rash, urticaria, itching, photosensitization (avoid excessive exposure to sunlight); edema (general, or of face and tongue).

Hematologic: Agranulocytosis; bone marrow depression; leukopenia; thrombocytopenia; purpura; eosinophilia.

Gastrointestinal: Nausea and vomiting; anorexia; epigastric distress; diarrhea; peculiar taste; stomatitis; abdominal cramps; black tongue.

Endocrine: Impotence, increased or decreased libido; gynecomastia in the male; breast enlargement and galactorrhea in the female; testicular swelling; elevation or depression of blood sugar levels.

Other: Jaundice (simulating obstructive); altered liver function; parotid swelling; alopecia; flushing; weight gain or loss, urinary frequency, nocturia; perspiration.

Withdrawal Symptoms: Though not indicative of addiction, abrupt cessation of treatment after prolonged therapy may produce nausea, headache, and malaise.

DOSAGE AND ADMINISTRATION

Dosage should be initiated at a low level and increased gradually, noting carefully the clinical response and any evidence of intolerance.

Usual Adult Dosage—Fifteen to 40 mg a day divided into 3 or 4 doses. If necessary, dosage may be increased to 60 mg a day. Dosages above this amount are not recommended. Increases should be made in the morning dose.

Adolescent and Elderly Patients—In general, lower dosages are recommended for these patients. Five mg 3 times a day may be given initially, and increased gradually if necessary. In elderly patients, the cardiovascular system must be monitored closely if the daily dose exceeds 20 mg.

When satisfactory improvement has been reached, dosage should be reduced to the smallest amount that will maintain relief of symptoms.

Minor adverse reactions require reduction in dosage. Major adverse reactions or evidence of hypersensitivity require prompt discontinuation of the drug.

The safety and effectiveness of VIVACTIL in pediatric patients have not been established.

OVERDOSAGE

Deaths may occur from overdosage with this class of drugs. Multiple drug ingestion (including alcohol) is common in deliberate tricyclic antidepressant overdose. As management of overdose is complex and changing, it is recommended that the physician contact a poison control center for current information on treatment. Signs and symptoms of toxicity develop rapidly after tricyclic antidepressant overdose, therefore, hospital monitoring is required as soon as possible.

MANIFESTATIONS

Critical manifestations of overdosage include: cardiac dysrhythmias, severe hypotension, convulsions, and CNS depression, including coma. Changes in the electrocardiogram, particularly in QRS axis or width, are clinically significant indicators of tricyclic antidepressant toxicity.

Other signs of overdose may include: confusion, disturbed concentration, transient visual hallucinations, dilated pupils, agitation, hyperactive reflexes, stupor, drowsiness, muscle rigidity, vomiting, hypothermia, hyperpyrexia, or any of the symptoms listed under ADVERSE REACTIONS.

MANAGEMENT

General

Obtain an ECG and immediately initiate cardiac monitoring. Protect the patient's airway, establish an intravenous line and initiate gastric decontamination. A minimum of six hours of observation with cardiac monitoring and observation for signs of CNS or respiratory depression, hypotension, cardiac dysrhythmias and/or conduction blocks, and seizures is necessary. If signs of toxicity occur at any time during this period, extended monitoring is required. There are case reports of patients succumbing to fatal dysrhythmias late after overdose. These patients had clinical evidence of significant poisoning prior to death and most received inadequate gastrointestinal decontamination. Monitoring of plasma drug levels should not guide management of the patient.

Gastrointestinal Decontamination

All patients suspected of a tricyclic antidepressant overdose should receive gastrointestinal decontamination. This should include large volume gastric lavage followed by activated charcoal. If consciousness is impaired, the airway should be secured prior to lavage. Emesis is contraindicated.

Cardiovascular

A maximal limb-lead QRS duration of ≥ 0.10 seconds may be the best indication of the severity of the overdose. Intravenous sodium bicarbonate should be used to maintain the serum pH in the range of 7.45 to 7.55. If the pH response is inadequate, hyperventilation may also be used. Concomitant use of hyperventilation and sodium bicarbonate should be done with extreme caution, with frequent pH monitoring. A pH >7.60 or a pCO_2 <20 mmHg is undesirable. Dysrhythmias unresponsive to sodium bicarbonate therapy/hyperventilation may respond to lidocaine, bretylium or phenytoin. Type 1A and 1C antiarrhythmics are generally contraindicated (e.g., quinidine, disopyramide, and procainamide).

In rare instances, hemoperfusion may be beneficial in acute refractory cardiovascular instability in patients with acute toxicity. However, hemodialysis, peritoneal dialysis, exchange transfusions, and forced diuresis generally have been reported as ineffective in tricyclic antidepressant poisoning.

CNS

In patients with CNS depression, early intubation is advised because of the potential for abrupt deterioration. Seizures should be controlled with benzodiazepines or, if these are ineffective, other anticonvulsants (e.g., phenobarbital, phenytoin). Physostigmine is not recommended except to treat life-threatening symptoms that have been unresponsive to other therapies, and then only in close consultation with a poison control center.

PSYCHIATRIC FOLLOW-UP

Since overdosage is often deliberate, patients may attempt suicide by other means during the recovery phase. Psychiatric referral may be appropriate.

PEDIATRIC MANAGEMENT

The principles of management of child and adult overdosages are similar. It is strongly recommended that the physician contact the local poison control center for specific pediatric treatment.

HOW SUPPLIED

No. 3313—Tablets VIVACTIL, 5 mg, are orange, oval, film coated tablets, coded MSD 26. They are supplied as follows:

NDC 0006-0026-68 bottles of 100
(6505-00-369-7297, 5 mg 100).

Shown in Product Identification Guide, page 323

No. 3314—Tablets VIVACTIL, 10 mg, are yellow, oval, film coated tablets, coded MSD 47. They are supplied as follows:

NDC 0006-0047-68 bottles of 100
(6505-00-462-7353, 10 mg 100's)

NDC 0006-0047-28 unit dose packages of 100.

Shown in Product Identification Guide, page 323

Storage

Store Tablets VIVACTIL in a tightly closed container. Avoid storage at temperatures above 40°C (104°F).

METABOLISM

Metabolic studies indicate that protriptyline is well absorbed from the gastrointestinal tract and is rapidly sequestered in tissues. Relatively low plasma levels are found after administration, and only a small amount of unchanged drug is excreted in the urine of dogs and rabbits. Preliminary studies indicate that demethylation of the secondary amine moiety occurs to a significant extent, and that metabolic transformation probably takes place in the liver. It penetrates the brain rapidly in mice and rats, and moreover that which is present in the brain is almost all unchanged drug.

Studies on the disposition of radioactive protriptyline in human test subjects showed significant plasma levels within 2 hours, peaking at 8 to 12 hours, then declining gradually.

Urinary excretion studies in the same subjects showed significant amounts of radioactivity in 2 hours. The rate of excretion was slow. Cumulative urinary excretion during 16 days accounted for approximately 50% of the drug. The fecal route of excretion did not seem to be important.

7904023 Issued July 1996

ZOCOR® Tablets ℞
(Simvastatin)

DESCRIPTION

ZOCOR* (simvastatin) is a lipid-lowering agent that is derived synthetically from a fermentation product of *Aspergillus terreus.* After oral ingestion, simvastatin, which is an inactive lactone, is hydrolyzed to the corresponding β-hydroxyacid form. This is an inhibitor of 3-hydroxy-3-methylglutaryl-coenzyme A (HMG-CoA) reductase. This enzyme catalyzes the conversion of HMG-CoA to mevalonate, which is an early and rate-limiting step in the biosynthesis of cholesterol.

Simvastatin is butanoic acid, 2,2-dimethyl-,1,2,3,7,8,8a-hexahydro-3,7-dimethyl-8-[2-(tetrahydro-4-hydroxy-6-oxo-2*H*-pyran-2-yl)-ethyl]-1-naphthalenyl ester, [1*S*-[1α,3α,7β,8β(2*S**,4*S**),-8aβ]]. The empirical formula of simvastatin is $C_{25}H_{38}O_5$ and its molecular weight is 418.57. Its structural formula is:

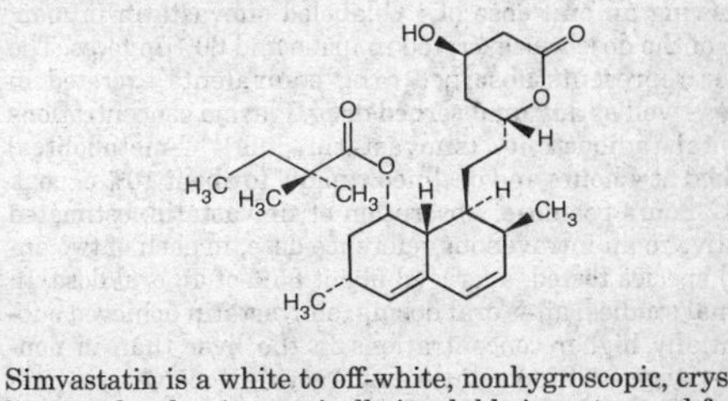

Simvastatin is a white to off-white, nonhygroscopic, crystalline powder that is practically insoluble in water, and freely soluble in chloroform, methanol and ethanol.

Tablets ZOCOR for oral administration contain either 5 mg, 10 mg, 20 mg, 40 mg or 80 mg of simvastatin and the following inactive ingredients: cellulose, hydroxypropyl cellulose, hydroxypropyl methylcellulose, iron oxides, lactose, magnesium stearate, starch, talc, titanium dioxide and other ingredients. Butylated hydroxyanisole is added as a preservative.

*Registered trademark of MERCK & CO., Inc.

CLINICAL PHARMACOLOGY

The involvement of low-density lipoprotein (LDL) cholesterol in atherogenesis has been well-documented in clinical and pathological studies, as well as in many animal experiments. Epidemiological studies have established that high LDL (low-density lipoprotein) cholesterol and low HDL

Continued on next page

Information on the Merck & Co., Inc. products listed on these pages is the full prescribing information from product circulars in use August 31, 1998. For information, please call 1-800-NSC MERCK [1-800-672-6372].

Zocor—Cont.

(high-density lipoprotein) cholesterol are both risk factors for coronary heart disease. Though frequently found in association with low HDL, elevated plasma triglycerides (TG) has not been established as an independent risk factor for coronary heart disease. The independent effect of raising HDL or lowering TG on the risk of coronary and cardiovascular morbidity and mortality has not been determined.

In the Scandinavian Simvastatin Survival Study (4S), the effect of improving lipoprotein levels with ZOCOR on total mortality was assessed in 4444 patients with coronary heart disease (CHD) and baseline total cholesterol (TOTAL-C) 212–309 mg/dL (5.5–8.0 mmol/L). The patients were followed for a median of 5.4 years. In this multicenter, randomized, double-blind, placebo-controlled study, ZOCOR significantly reduced the risk of mortality by 30% (11.5% vs 8.2%, placebo vs ZOCOR); of CHD mortality by 42% (8.5% vs 5.0%); and of having a hospital-verified non-fatal myocardial infarction by 37% (19.6% vs 12.9%). Furthermore, ZOCOR significantly reduced the risk for undergoing myocardial revascularization procedures (coronary artery bypass grafting or percutaneous transluminal coronary angioplasty) by 37% (17.2% vs 11.4%) [see CLINICAL PHARMACOLOGY, *Clinical Studies*].

ZOCOR has been shown to reduce both normal and elevated LDL cholesterol concentrations. LDL is formed from very-low-density lipoprotein (VLDL) and is catabolized predominantly by the high affinity LDL receptor. The mechanism of the LDL-lowering effect of ZOCOR may involve both reduction of VLDL cholesterol concentration, and induction of the LDL receptor, leading to reduced production and/or increased catabolism of LDL cholesterol. Apolipoprotein B (Apo B) also falls substantially during treatment with ZOCOR. As each LDL particle contains one molecule of apolipoprotein B, and since in patients with predominant elevations in LDL-C (without accompanying elevation in VLDL) little apolipoprotein B is found in other lipoproteins, this strongly suggests that ZOCOR does not merely cause cholesterol to be lost from LDL, but also reduces the concentration of circulating LDL particles. In addition, ZOCOR reduces VLDL cholesterol and plasma triglycerides (TG) and increases HDL cholesterol. The effects of ZOCOR on Lp(a), fibrinogen, and certain other independent biochemical risk markers for coronary heart disease are unknown.

ZOCOR is a specific inhibitor of HMG-CoA reductase, the enzyme that catalyzes the conversion of HMG-CoA to mevalonate. The conversion of HMG-CoA to mevalonate is an early step in the biosynthetic pathway for cholesterol.

Pharmacokinetics

Simvastatin is a lactone that is readily hydrolyzed *in vivo* to the corresponding β-hydroxyacid, a potent inhibitor of HMG-CoA reductase. Inhibition of HMG-CoA reductase is the basis for an assay in pharmacokinetic studies of the β-hydroxyacid metabolites (active inhibitors) and, following base hydrolysis, active plus latent inhibitors (total inhibitors) in plasma following administration of simvastatin.

Following an oral dose of ^{14}C-labeled simvastatin in man, 13% of the dose was excreted in urine and 60% in feces. The latter represents absorbed drug equivalents excreted in bile, as well as any unabsorbed drug. Plasma concentrations of total radioactivity (simvastatin plus ^{14}C-metabolites) peaked at 4 hours and declined rapidly to about 10% of peak by 12 hours postdose. Absorption of simvastatin, estimated relative to an intravenous reference dose, in each of two animal species tested, averaged about 85% of an oral dose. In animal studies, after oral dosing, simvastatin achieved substantially higher concentrations in the liver than in non-target tissues. Simvastatin undergoes extensive first-pass extraction in the liver, its primary site of action, with subsequent excretion of drug equivalents in the bile. As a consequence of extensive hepatic extraction of simvastatin (estimated to be >60% in man), the availability of drug to the general circulation is low. In a single-dose study in nine healthy subjects, it was estimated that less than 5% of an oral dose of simvastatin reaches the general circulation as active inhibitors. Following administration of simvastatin tablets, the coefficient of variation, based on between-subject variability, was approximately 48% for the area under the concentration-time curve (AUC) for total inhibitory activity in the general circulation.

Both simvastatin and its β-hydroxyacid metabolite are highly bound (approximately 95%) to human plasma proteins. Animal studies have not been performed to determine whether simvastatin crosses the blood-brain and placental barriers. However, when radiolabeled simvastatin was administered to rats, simvastatin-derived radioactivity crossed the blood-brain barrier.

The major active metabolites of simvastatin present in human plasma are the β-hydroxyacid of simvastatin and its 6′-hydroxy, 6′-hydroxymethyl, and 6′-exomethylene derivatives. Peak plasma concentrations of both active and total inhibitors were attained within 1.3 to 2.4 hours postdose. While the recommended therapeutic dose range is 5 to 80 mg/day, there was no substantial deviation from linearity of AUC of inhibitors in the general circulation with an increase in dose to as high as 120 mg. Relative to the fasting state, the plasma profile of inhibitors was not affected when simvastatin was administered immediately before an A.H.A. recommended low-fat meal.

Kinetic studies with another reductase inhibitor, having a similar principal route of elimination, have suggested that for a given dose level higher systemic exposure may be achieved in patients with severe renal insufficiency (as measured by creatinine clearance).

Clinical Studies

ZOCOR has been shown to be highly effective in reducing total and LDL cholesterol in heterozygous familial and non-familial forms of hypercholesterolemia and in mixed hyperlipidemia. A marked response was seen within 2 weeks, and the maximum therapeutic response occurred within 4–6 weeks. The response was maintained during chronic therapy. Furthermore, improving lipoprotein levels with ZOCOR improved survival in patients with CHD and hypercholesterolemia treated with 20–40 mg per day for a median of 5.4 years.

In a multicenter, double-blind, placebo-controlled, dose-response study in patients with familial or non-familial hypercholesterolemia, ZOCOR given as a single-dose in the evening (the recommended dosing) was similarly effective as when given on a twice-daily basis. ZOCOR consistently and significantly decreased total plasma cholesterol (TOTAL-C), LDL cholesterol (LDL-C), total cholesterol/HDL cholesterol (TOTAL-C/HDL-C) ratio, and LDL cholesterol/HDL cholesterol (LDL-C/HDL-C) ratio. ZOCOR also decreased triglycerides (TG) and increased HDL cholesterol (HDL-C).

The results of 3 separate studies depicting the dose response to simvastatin in patients with primary hypercholesterolemia are presented in TABLE I.

[See table I below]

The mean reduction in LDL cholesterol was 47% at the 80-mg dose. Of the 664 patients randomized to 80 mg, 475 patients with plasma triglycerides ≤ 200 mg/dL had a median reduction in triglycerides of 21%, while in 189 patients with triglycerides > 200 mg/dL, the median reduction in triglycerides was 36%. In these studies, patients with triglycerides > 350 mg/dL were excluded.

In a controlled clinical study, 12 patients 15–39 years of age with homozygous familial hypercholesterolemia received simvastatin 40 mg/day in a single dose or in 3 divided doses, or 80 mg/day in 3 divided doses. Eleven of the 12 patients had reductions in LDL cholesterol. In those patients with reductions, the mean LDL cholesterol changes for the 40- and 80-mg doses were 14% (range 8% to 23%, median 12%) and 30% (range 14% to 46%, median 29%), respectively. One patient had an increase of 15% in LDL cholesterol. Another patient with absent LDL cholesterol receptor function had an LDL cholesterol reduction of 41% with the 80-mg dose.

In the Scandinavian Simvastatin Survival Study (4S), the effect of therapy with ZOCOR on total mortality was assessed in 4444 patients with coronary heart disease (CHD) and baseline total cholesterol 212–309 mg/dL (5.5–8.0 mmol/L). In this multicenter, randomized, double-blind, placebo-controlled study, patients were treated with standard care, including diet, and either ZOCOR 20–40 mg daily (n=2221) or placebo (n=2223) for a median duration of 5.4 years. Over the course of the study, treatment with ZOCOR led to mean reductions in total cholesterol, LDL cholesterol and triglycerides of 25%, 35%, and 10%, respectively, and a mean increase in HDL cholesterol of 8%. ZOCOR significantly reduced the risk of mortality (Figure 1) by 30%, (p=0.0003, 182 deaths in the ZOCOR group vs 256 deaths in the placebo group). The risk of CHD mortality was significantly reduced by 42%, (p=0.00001, 111 vs 189). There was no statistically significant difference between groups in non-cardiovascular mortality. ZOCOR also significantly decreased the risk of having major coronary events (CHD mortality plus hospital-verified and silent non-fatal myocardial infarction [MI]) (Figure 2) by 34%, (p<0.00001, 431 patients vs 622 patients with one or more events). The risk of having a hospital-verified non-fatal MI was reduced by 37%. ZOCOR significantly reduced the risk for undergoing myocardial revascularization procedures (coronary artery bypass grafting or percutaneous transluminal coronary angioplasty) by 37%, (p<0.00001, 252 patients vs 383 patients). Furthermore, ZOCOR significantly reduced the risk of fatal plus non-fatal cerebrovascular events (combined stroke and transient ischemic attacks) by 28% (p=0.033, 75 patients vs 102 patients). ZOCOR reduced the risk of major coronary events to a similar extent across the range of baseline total and LDL cholesterol levels. The risk of mortality was significantly decreased in patients ≥60 years of age by 27% and in patients <60 years of age by 37%. Because there were only 53 female deaths, the effect of ZOCOR on mortality in women could not be adequately assessed. However, ZOCOR significantly lessened the risk of having major coronary events by 34% (60 women vs 91 women with one or more event). The randomization was stratified by angina alone (21% of each treatment group) or a previous MI. Because there were only 57 deaths among the patients with angina alone at baseline, the effect of ZOCOR on mortality in this subgroup could not be adequately assessed. However, trends in reduced coronary mortality, major coronary events and revascularization procedures were consistent between this group and the total study cohort.

Figure 1

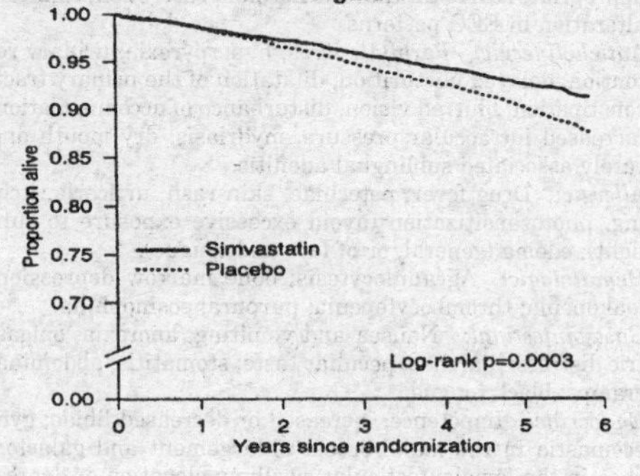
Proportion alive
Simvastatin
Placebo
Log-rank p=0.0003
Years since randomization

Figure 2

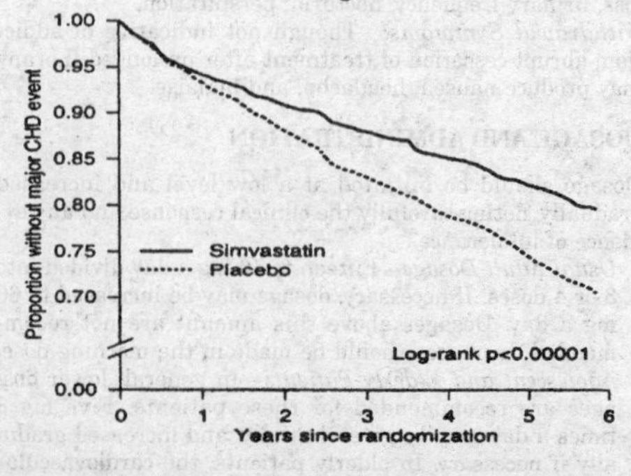
Proportion without major CHD event
Simvastatin
Placebo
Log-rank p<0.00001
Years since randomization

In the Multicenter Anti-Atheroma Study, the effect of therapy with simvastatin on atherosclerosis was assessed by

Table I
Dose Response in Patients with Primary Hypercholesterolemia
(Mean Percent Change from Baseline After 6 to 24 Weeks)

TREATMENT	N	TOTAL-C	LDL-C	HDL-C	TG*
Lower Dose Comparative Study (Mean % Change at Week 6)					
ZOCOR					
5 mg q.p.m.	109	−19	−26	10	−12
10 mg q.p.m.	110	−23	−30	12	−15
Scandinavian Simvastatin Survival Study (Mean % Change at Week 6)					
Placebo	2223	−1	−1	0	3
ZOCOR					
20 mg q.p.m.	2221	−28	−38	8	−15
Upper Dose Comparative Study (Mean % Change averaged at Weeks 18 and 24)					
ZOCOR					
40 mg q.p.m.	433	−31	−41	9	−18
80 mg q.p.m.	664	−36	−47	8	−24

* median percent change

		LDL-Cholesterol mg/dL (mmol/L)	
Definite Atherosclerotic Disease†	Two or More Other Risk Factors††	Initiation Level	Goal
NO	NO	≥190 (≥4.9)	<160 (<4.1)
NO	YES	≥160 (≥4.1)	<130 (<3.4)
YES	YES OR NO	≥130††† (≥3.4)	≤100 (≤2.6)

---

† Coronary heart disease or peripheral vascular disease (including symptomatic carotid artery disease).

†† Other risk factors for coronary heart disease (CHD) include: age (males: ≥45 years; females: ≥55 years or premature menopause without estrogen replacement therapy); family history of premature CHD; current cigarette smoking; hypertension; confirmed HDL-C <35 mg/dL (<0.91 mmol/L); and diabetes mellitus. Subtract one risk factor if HDL-C is ≥60 mg/dL (≥1.6 mmol/L).

††† In CHD patients with LDL-C levels 100–129 mg/dL, the physician should exercise clinical judgment in deciding whether to initiate drug treatment.

quantitative coronary angiography in hypercholesterolemic men and women with coronary heart disease. In this randomized, double-blind, controlled trial, patients with a mean baseline total cholesterol value of 245 mg/dL (6.4 mmol/L) and a mean baseline LDL value of 170 mg/dL (4.4 mmol/L) were treated with conventional measures and with simvastatin 20 mg/day or placebo. Angiograms were evaluated at baseline, two and four years. A total of 347 patients had a baseline angiogram and at least one follow-up angiogram. The co-primary endpoints of the trial were mean change per-patient in minimum and mean lumen diameters, indicating focal and diffuse disease, respectively. Simvastatin significantly slowed the progression of lesions as measured in the final angiogram by both these parameters (mean changes in minimum lumen diameter: −0.04 mm with simvastatin vs −0.12 mm with placebo; mean changes in mean lumen diameter: −0.03 mm with simvastatin vs −0.08 mm with placebo), as well as by change from baseline in percent diameter stenosis (0.9% simvastatin vs 3.6% placebo). After four years, the groups also differed significantly in the proportions of patients categorized with disease progression (23% simvastatin vs 33% placebo) and disease regression (18% simvastatin vs 12% placebo). In addition, simvastatin significantly decreased the proportion of patients with new lesions (13% simvastatin vs 24% placebo) and with new total occlusions (5% vs 11%). The mean change per-patient in mean and minimum lumen diameters calculated by comparing angiograms in the subset of 274 patients who had matched angiographic projections at baseline, two and four years is presented below (Figures 3 and 4).

Figure 3

Mean Lumen Diameter
(Mean and Standard Error)

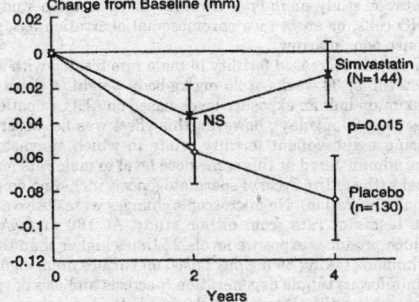

[See figure 4 at top of next column]

Endocrine Function

In clinical studies, simvastatin did not impair adrenal reserve or significantly reduce basal plasma cortisol concentration. Small reductions from baseline in basal plasma testosterone in men were observed in clinical studies with simvastatin, an effect also observed with other inhibitors of HMG-CoA reductase and the bile acid sequestrant cholestyramine. There was no effect on plasma gonadotropin levels. In a placebo-controlled 12-week study there was no significant effect of simvastatin 80 mg on the plasma testosterone response to hCG. In another 24-week study simvastatin 20–40 mg had no detectable effect on spermatogenesis. In 4S, in which 4444 patients were randomized to simvastatin 20–40 mg or placebo daily for a median duration of 5.4 years, the incidence of male sexual adverse events in the two treatment groups was not significantly different. Be-

Figure 4

Minimum Lumen Diameter
(Mean and Standard Error)

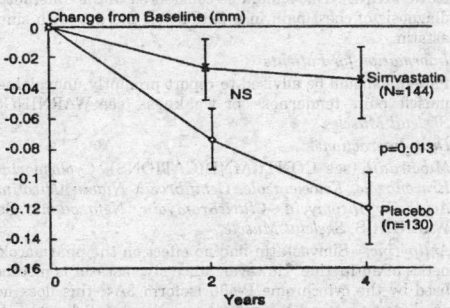

cause of these factors, the small changes in plasma testosterone are unlikely to be clinically significant. The effects, if any, on the pituitary-gonadal axis in pre-menopausal women are unknown.

INDICATIONS AND USAGE

Therapy with lipid-altering agents should be considered in those individuals at increased risk for atherosclerosis-related clinical events as a function of cholesterol level, the presence of coronary heart disease, or other risk factors. Lipid-altering agents should be used in addition to a diet restricted in saturated fat and cholesterol when the response to diet and other nonpharmacological measures alone has been inadequate (see NCEP Guidelines, below).

Coronary Heart Disease

In patients with coronary heart disease and hypercholesterolemia, ZOCOR is indicated to:

• Reduce the risk of total mortality by reducing coronary death;

• Reduce the risk of non-fatal myocardial infarction;

• Reduce the risk for undergoing myocardial revascularization procedures.

• Reduce the risk of stroke or transient ischemic attack.

(For a discussion of efficacy results by gender and other predefined subgroups, see CLINICAL PHARMACOLOGY, *Clinical Studies*.)

Hyperlipidemia

ZOCOR is indicated as an adjunct to diet to reduce elevated TOTAL-C LDL-C, Apo B, and TG levels in patients with primary hypercholesterolemia (heterozygous familial and non-familial) and mixed dyslipidemia (Fredrickson Types IIa and IIb**).

ZOCOR is also indicated to reduce TOTAL-C and LDL-C in patients with homozygous familial hypercholesterolemia as an adjunct to other lipid-lowering treatments (e.g., LDL apheresis) or if such treatments are unavailable.

General Recommendations

Prior to initiating therapy with simvastatin, secondary causes for hypercholesterolemia (e.g., poorly controlled diabetes mellitus, hypothyroidism, nephrotic syndrome, dysproteinemias, obstructive liver disease, other drug therapy, alcoholism) should be excluded, and a lipid profile performed to measure TOTAL-C, HDL-C, and triglycerides. For patients with TG less than 400 mg/dL (<4.5 mmol/L), LDL-C can be estimated using the following equation:

LDL-C = Total cholesterol − [0.20 × (triglycerides) + HDL-C]

For TG levels >400 mg/dL (>4.5 mmol/L), this equation is less accurate and LDL-C concentration should be deter-

mined by ultracentrifugation. In many hypertriglyceridemic patients, LDL-C may be low or normal despite elevated TOTAL-C. In such cases, ZOCOR is not indicated.

Lipid determinations should be performed at intervals of no less than four weeks and dosage adjusted according to the patient's response to therapy.

The National Cholesterol Education Program (NCEP) Treatment Guidelines are summarized below:

[See table at left]

At the time of hospitalization for an acute coronary event, consideration can be given to initiating drug therapy at discharge if the LDL-C is ≥ 130 mg/dL (see NCEP Guidelines, above).

Since the goal of treatment is to lower LDL-C, the NCEP recommends that LDL-C levels be used to initiate and assess treatment response. Only if LDL-C levels are not available, should the TOTAL-C be used to monitor therapy.

ZOCOR is indicated to reduce elevated LDL cholesterol and triglyceride levels in patients with Type IIb hyperlipoproteinemia (where hypercholesterolemia is the major abnormality). However, it has not been studied in conditions where the major abnormality is elevation of chylomicrons, VLDL or IDL (i.e., hyperlipoproteinemia types I, III, IV, or V).**

**Classification of Hyperlipoproteinemias

		Lipid Elevations	
Type	Lipoproteins elevated	major	minor
I (rare)	chylomicrons	TG	↑→C
IIa	LDL	C	—
IIb	LDL, VLDL	C	TG
III (rare)	IDL	C/TG	—
IV	VLDL	TG	↑→C
V (rare)	chylomicrons, VLDL	TG	↑→C

C = cholesterol, TG = triglycerides,
LDL = low-density lipoprotein,
VLDL = very-low-density lipoprotein,
IDL = intermediate-density lipoprotein.

CONTRAINDICATIONS

Hypersensitivity to any component of this medication.

Active liver disease or unexplained persistent elevations of serum transaminases (see WARNINGS).

Concomitant therapy with the tetralol-class calcium channel blocker mibefradil (see PRECAUTIONS, *Drug Interactions*).

Pregnancy and lactation. Atherosclerosis is a chronic process and the discontinuation of lipid-lowering drugs during pregnancy should have little impact on the outcome of long-term therapy of primary hypercholesterolemia. Moreover, cholesterol and other products of the cholesterol biosynthesis pathway are essential components for fetal development, including synthesis of steroids and cell membranes. Because of the ability of inhibitors of HMG-CoA reductase such as ZOCOR to decrease the synthesis of cholesterol and possibly other products of the cholesterol biosynthesis pathway, ZOCOR is contraindicated during pregnancy and in nursing mothers. **ZOCOR should be administered to women of childbearing age only when such patients are highly unlikely to conceive.** If the patient becomes pregnant while taking this drug, ZOCOR should be discontinued immediately and the patient should be apprised of the potential hazard to the fetus (see PRECAUTIONS, *Pregnancy*).

WARNINGS

Skeletal Muscle

Simvastatin and other inhibitors of HMG-CoA reductase occasionally cause myopathy, which is manifested as muscle pain or weakness associated with grossly elevated creatine kinase (> 10X the upper limit of normal [ULN]). **Rhabdomyolysis, with or without acute renal failure secondary to myoglobinuria, has been reported rarely.** In the Scandinavian Simvastatin Survival Study, there was one case of myopathy among 1399 patients taking simvastatin 20 mg and no cases among 822 patients taking 40 mg daily for a median duration of 5.4 years. In two 6-month controlled clinical studies, there was one case of myopathy among 436 patients taking 40 mg and 5 cases among 669 patients taking 80 mg. The risk of myopathy is increased by concomitant therapy with certain drugs, some of which were excluded by the designs of these studies (see below).

Myopathy caused by drug interactions.

The incidence and severity of myopathy are increased by concomitant administration of HMG-CoA reductase inhibi-

Continued on next page

Information on the Merck & Co., Inc. products listed on these pages is the full prescribing information from product circulars in use August 31, 1998. For information, please call 1-800-NSC MERCK [1-800-672-6372].

Zocor—Cont.

tors with drugs that can cause myopathy when given alone, such as gemfibrozil and other fibrates, and lipid-lowering doses (≥ 1 g/day) of niacin (nicotinic acid).
In addition, the risk of myopathy appears to be increased by high levels of HMG-CoA reductase inhibitory activity in plasma. Simvastatin is metabolized by the cytochrome P450 isoform 3A4. Certain drugs which share this metabolic pathway can raise the plasma levels of simvastatin and may increase the risk of myopathy. These include cyclosporine, itraconazole, ketoconazole and other antifungal azoles, the macrolide antibiotics erythromycin and clarithromycin, and the antidepressant nefazodone.
Reducing the risk of myopathy.
1. General measures. Patients starting therapy with simvastatin should be advised of the risk of myopathy, and told to report promptly unexplained muscle pain, tenderness or weakness. A creatine kinase (CK) level above 10X ULN in a patient with unexplained muscle symptoms indicates myopathy. **Simvastatin therapy should be discontinued if myopathy is diagnosed or suspected.** In most cases, when patients were promptly discontinued from treatment, muscle symptoms and CK increases resolved.
Of the patients with rhabdomyolysis, many had complicated medical histories. Some had preexisting renal insufficiency, usually as a consequence of long-standing diabetes. In such patients, dose escalation requires caution. Also, as there are no known adverse consequences of brief interruption of therapy, treatment with simvastatin should be stopped a few days before elective major surgery and when any major acute medical or surgical condition supervenes.
2. Measures to reduce the risk of myopathy caused by drug interactions (see above and PRECAUTIONS, *Drug Interactions*). Physicians contemplating combined therapy with simvastatin and any of the interacting drugs should weigh the potential benefits and risks, and should carefully monitor patients for any signs and symptoms of muscle pain, tenderness, or weakness, particularly during the initial months of therapy and during any periods of upward dosage titration of either drug. Periodic CK determinations may be considered in such situations, but there is no assurance that such monitoring will prevent myopathy.
The combined use of simvastatin with fibrates or niacin should be avoided unless the benefit of further alteration in lipid levels is likely to outweigh the increased risk of this drug combination. Combinations of fibrates or niacin with low doses of simvastatin have been used without myopathy in small, short-term clinical trials with careful monitoring. Addition of these drugs to simvastatin typically provides little additional reduction in LDL cholesterol, but further reductions of triglycerides and further increases in HDL cholesterol may be obtained. If one of these drugs must be used with simvastatin, clinical experience suggests that the risk of myopathy is less with niacin than with the fibrates.
In patients taking concomitant cyclosporine, fibrates or niacin, the dose of simvastatin should generally not exceed 10 mg (see DOSAGE AND ADMINISTRATION, *General Recommendations* and *Concomitant Lipid-Lowering Therapy*), as the risk of myopathy increases substantially at higher doses. Interruption of simvastatin therapy during a course of treatment with a systemic antifungal azole or a macrolide antibiotic should be considered.
Liver Dysfunction
Persistent increases (to more than 3 times the upper limit of normal) in serum transaminases have occurred in approximately 1% of patients who received simvastatin in clinical trials. When drug treatment was interrupted or discontinued in these patients, the transaminase levels usually fell slowly to pretreatment levels. The increases were not associated with jaundice or other clinical signs or symptoms. There was no evidence of hypersensitivity.
In the Scandinavian Simvastatin Survival Study (see CLINICAL PHARMACOLOGY, *Clinical Studies*), the number of patients with more than one transaminase elevation to >3 times the upper limit of normal, over the course of the study, was not significantly different between the simvastatin and placebo groups (14 [0.7%] vs. 12 [0.6%]). Elevated transaminases resulted in the discontinuation of 8 patients from therapy in the simvastatin group (n=2,221) and 5 in the placebo group (n=2,223). Of the 1986 simvastatin treated patients in 4S with normal liver function tests (LFTs) at baseline, only 8 (0.4%) developed consecutive LFT elevations to >3 times the upper limit of normal and/or were discontinued due to transaminase elevations during the 5.4 years (median follow-up) of the study. Among these 8 patients, 5 initially developed these abnormalities within the first year. All of the patients in this study received a starting dose of 20 mg of simvastatin; 37% were titrated to 40 mg.
In 2 controlled clinical studies in 1105 patients, the 12-month incidence of persistent hepatic transaminase elevation without regard to drug relationship was 0.9% and 2.1% at the 40- and 80-mg dose, respectively. No patients developed persistent liver function abnormalities following the initial 6 months of treatment at a given dose.
It is recommended that liver function tests be performed before the initiation of treatment, and periodically thereafter (e.g., semiannually) for the first year of treatment or until one year after the last elevation in dose. Patients titrated to the 80 mg dose should receive an additional test at 3 months. Patients who develop increased transaminase levels should be monitored with a second liver function evaluation to confirm the finding and be followed thereafter with frequent liver function tests until the abnormality(ies) return to normal. Should an increase in AST or ALT of three times the upper limit of normal or greater persist, withdrawal of therapy with ZOCOR is recommended.
The drug should be used with caution in patients who consume substantial quantities of alcohol and/or have a past history of liver disease. Active liver diseases or unexplained transaminase elevations are contraindications to the use of simvastatin.
As with other lipid-lowering agents, moderate (less than three times the upper limit of normal) elevations of serum transaminases have been reported following therapy with simvastatin. These changes appeared soon after initiation of therapy with simvastatin, were often transient, were not accompanied by any symptoms and did not require interruption of treatment.

PRECAUTIONS

General
Simvastatin may cause elevation of creatine kinase and transaminase levels (see WARNINGS and ADVERSE REACTIONS). This should be considered in the differential diagnosis of chest pain in a patient on therapy with simvastatin.
Information for Patients
Patients should be advised to report promptly unexplained muscle pain, tenderness, or weakness (see WARNINGS, *Skeletal Muscle*).
Drug Interactions
Mibefradil (see CONTRAINDICATIONS), *Cyclosporine, Itraconazole, Ketoconazole, Gemfibrozil, Niacin (Nicotinic Acid), Erythromycin, Clarithromycin, Nefazodone:* See WARNINGS, *Skeletal Muscle*.
Antipyrine: Simvastatin had no effect on the pharmacokinetics of antipyrine. However, since simvastatin is metabolized by the cytochrome P-450 isoform 3A4, this does not preclude an interaction with other drugs metabolized by the same isoform (see WARNINGS, *Skeletal Muscle*).
Propranolol: In healthy male volunteers there was a significant decrease in mean C_{max}, but no change in AUC, for simvastatin total and active inhibitors with concomitant administration of single doses of ZOCOR and propranolol. The clinical relevance of this finding is unclear. The pharmacokinetics of the enantiomers of propranolol were not affected.
Digoxin: Concomitant administration of a single dose of digoxin in healthy male volunteers receiving simvastatin resulted in a slight elevation (less than 0.3 ng/mL) in digoxin concentrations in plasma (as measured by a radioimmunoassay) compared to concomitant administration of placebo and digoxin. Patients taking digoxin should be monitored appropriately when simvastatin is initiated.
Warfarin: In two clinical studies, one in normal volunteers and the other in hypercholesterolemic patients, simvastatin 20–40 mg/day modestly potentiated the effect of coumarin anticoagulants: the prothrombin time, reported as International Normalized Ratio (INR), increased from a baseline of 1.7 to 1.8 and from 2.6 to 3.4 in the volunteer and patient studies, respectively. With other reductase inhibitors, clinically evident bleeding and/or increased prothrombin time has been reported in a few patients taking coumarin anticoagulants concomitantly. In such patients, prothrombin time should be determined before starting simvastatin and frequently enough during early therapy to insure that no significant alteration of prothrombin time occurs. Once a stable prothrombin time has been documented, prothrombin times can be monitored at the intervals usually recommended for patients on coumarin anticoagulants. If the dose of simvastatin is changed or discontinued, the same procedure should be repeated. Simvastatin therapy has not been associated with bleeding or with changes in prothrombin time in patients not taking anticoagulants.
CNS Toxicity
Optic nerve degeneration was seen in clinically normal dogs treated with simvastatin for 14 weeks at 180 mg/kg/day, a dose that produced mean plasma drug levels about 12 times higher than the mean drug level in humans taking 80 mg/day.
A chemically similar drug in this class also produced optic nerve degeneration (Wallerian degeneration of retinogeniculate fibers) in clinically normal dogs in a dose-dependent fashion starting at 60 mg/kg/day, a dose that produced mean plasma drug levels about 30 times higher than the mean drug level in humans taking the highest recommended dose (as measured by total enzyme inhibitory activity). This same drug also produced vestibulocochlear Wallerian-like degeneration and retinal ganglion cell chromatolysis in dogs treated for 14 weeks at 180 mg/kg/day, a dose that resulted in a mean plasma drug level similar to that seen with the 60 mg/kg/day dose.
CNS vascular lesions, characterized by perivascular hemorrhage and edema, mononuclear cell infiltration of perivascular spaces, perivascular fibrin deposits and necrosis of small vessels were seen in dogs treated with simvastatin at a dose of 360 mg/kg/day, a dose that produced mean plasma drug levels that were about 14 times higher than the mean drug levels in humans taking 80 mg/day. Similar CNS vascular lesions have been observed with several other drugs of this class.
There were cataracts in female rats after two years of treatment with 50 and 100 mg/kg/day (22 and 25 times the human AUC at 80 mg/day, respectively) and in dogs after three months at 90 mg/kg/day (19 times) and at two years at 50 mg/kg/day (5 times).
Carcinogenesis, Mutagenesis, Impairment of Fertility
In a 72-week carcinogenicity study, mice were administered daily doses of simvastatin of 25, 100, and 400 mg/kg body weight, which resulted in mean plasma drug levels approximately 1, 4, and 8 times higher than the mean human plasma drug level, respectively (as total inhibitory activity based on AUC) after an 80-mg oral dose. Liver carcinomas were significantly increased in high-dose females and mid- and high-dose males with a maximum incidence of 90 percent in males. The incidence of adenomas of the liver was significantly increased in mid- and high-dose females. Drug treatment also significantly increased the incidence of lung adenomas in mid- and high-dose males and females. Adenomas of the Harderian gland (a gland of the eye of rodents) were significantly higher in high-dose mice than in controls. No evidence of a tumorigenic effect was observed at 25 mg/kg/day.
In a separate 92-week carcinogenicity study in mice at doses up to 25 mg/kg/day, no evidence of a tumorigenic effect was observed (mean plasma drug levels were 1 times higher than humans given 80 mg simvastatin as measured by AUC).
In a two-year study in rats at 25 mg/kg/day, there was a statistically significant increase in the incidence of thyroid follicular adenomas in female rats exposed to approximately 11 times higher levels of simvastatin than in humans given 80 mg simvastatin (as measured by AUC).
A second two-year rat carcinogenicity study with doses of 50 and 100 mg/kg/day produced hepatocellular adenomas and carcinomas (in female rats at both doses and in males at 100 mg/kg/day). Thyroid follicular cell adenomas were increased in males and females at both doses; thyroid follicular cell carcinomas were increased in females at 100 mg/kg/day. The increased incidence of thyroid neoplasms appears to be consistent with findings from other HMG-CoA reductase inhibitors. These treatment levels represented plasma drug levels (AUC) of approximately 7 and 15 times (males) and 22 and 25 times (females) the mean human plasma drug exposure after an 80 milligram daily dose.
No evidence of mutagenicity was observed in a microbial mutagenicity (Ames) test with or without rat or mouse liver metabolic activation. In addition, no evidence of damage to genetic material was noted in an *in vitro* alkaline elution assay using rat hepatocytes, a V-79 mammalian cell forward mutation study, an *in vitro* chromosome aberration study in CHO cells, or an *in vivo* chromosomal aberration assay in mouse bone marrow.
There was decreased fertility in male rats treated with simvastatin for 34 weeks at 25 mg/kg body weight (4 times the maximum human exposure level, based on AUC, in patients receiving 80 mg/day); however, this effect was not observed during a subsequent fertility study in which simvastatin was administered at this same dose level to male rats for 11 weeks (the entire cycle of spermatogenesis including epididymal maturation). No microscopic changes were observed in the testes of rats from either study. At 180 mg/kg/day, (which produces exposure levels 22 times higher than those in humans taking 80 mg/day based on surface area, mg/m^2), seminiferous tubule degeneration (necrosis and loss of spermatogenic epithelium) was observed. In dogs, there was drug-related testicular atrophy, decreased spermatogenesis, spermatocytic degeneration and giant cell formation at 10 mg/kg/day, (approximately 2 times the human exposure, based on AUC, at 80 mg/day). The clinical significance of these findings is unclear.
Pregnancy
Pregnancy Category X
See CONTRAINDICATIONS.
Safety in pregnant women has not been established.
Simvastatin was not teratogenic in rats at doses of 25 mg/kg/day or in rabbits at doses up to 10 mg/kg daily. These doses resulted in 3 times (rat) or 3 times (rabbit) the human exposure based on mg/m^2 surface area. However, in studies with another structurally-related HMG-CoA reductase inhibitor, skeletal malformations were observed in rats and mice.
Rare reports of congenital anomalies have been received following intrauterine exposure to HMG-CoA reductase inhibitors. In a review*** of approximately 100 prospectively fol-

lowed pregnancies in women exposed to ZOCOR or another structurally related HMG-CoA reductase inhibitor, the incidences of congenital anomalies, spontaneous abortions and fetal deaths/stillbirths did not exceed what would be expected in the general population. The number of cases is adequate only to exclude a 3- to 4-fold increase in congenital anomalies over the background incidence. In 89% of the prospectively followed pregnancies, drug treatment was initiated prior to pregnancy and was discontinued at some point in the first trimester when pregnancy was identified. As safety in pregnant women has not been established and there is no apparent benefit to therapy with ZOCOR during pregnancy (see CONTRAINDICATIONS), treatment should be immediately discontinued as soon as pregnancy is recognized. ZOCOR should be administered to women of childbearing potential only when such patients are highly unlikely to conceive and have been informed of the potential hazards.

Nursing Mothers

It is not known whether simvastatin is excreted in human milk. Because a small amount of another drug in this class is excreted in human milk and because of the potential for serious adverse reactions in nursing infants, women taking simvastatin should not nurse their infants (see CONTRAINDICATIONS).

Pediatric Use

Safety and effectiveness in pediatric patients have not been established. Because pediatric patients are not likely to benefit from cholesterol lowering for at least a decade and because experience with this drug is limited (no studies in subjects below the age of 20 years), treatment of pediatric patients with simvastatin is not recommended at this time.

*** Manson, J.M., Freyssinges, C., Ducrocq, M.B., Stephenson, W.P., Postmarketing Surveillance of Lovastatin and Simvastatin Exposure During Pregnancy, *Reproductive Toxicology*, 10(6):439–446, 1996.

ADVERSE REACTIONS

In the pre-marketing controlled clinical studies and their open extensions (2423 patients with mean duration of follow-up of approximately 18 months), 1.4% of patients were discontinued due to adverse experiences attributable to ZOCOR. Adverse reactions have usually been mild and transient. ZOCOR has been evaluated for serious adverse reactions in more than 21,000 patients and is generally well-tolerated.

Clinical Adverse Experiences

Adverse experiences occurring at an incidence of 1 percent or greater in patients treated with ZOCOR, regardless of causality, in controlled clinical studies are shown in the table below:

	ZOCOR (N = 1583) %	Placebo (N = 157) %	Cholestyramine (N = 179) %
Body as a Whole			
Abdominal pain	3.2	3.2	8.9
Asthenia	1.6	2.5	1.1
Gastrointestinal			
Constipation	2.3	1.3	29.1
Diarrhea	1.9	2.5	7.8
Dyspepsia	1.1	—	4.5
Flatulence	1.9	1.3	14.5
Nausea	1.3	1.9	10.1
Nervous System / Psychiatric			
Headache	3.5	5.1	4.5
Respiratory			
Upper respiratory infection	2.1	1.9	3.4

Scandinavian Simvastatin Survival Study Clinical Adverse Experiences

In the Scandinavian Simvastatin Survival Study (4S) (see CLINICAL PHARMACOLOGY, *Clinical Studies*) involving 4444 patients treated with 20–40 mg/day of ZOCOR (n=2221) or placebo (n=2223), the safety and tolerability profiles were comparable between groups over the median 5.4 years of the study. The clinical adverse experiences reported as possibly, probably, or definitely drug-related in ≥0.5% in either treatment group are shown in the table below:

	ZOCOR (N = 2,221) %	Placebo (N = 2,223) %
Body as a Whole		
Abdominal pain	0.9	0.9
Gastrointestinal		
Diarrhea	0.5	0.3
Dyspepsia	0.6	0.5
Flatulence	0.9	0.7
Nausea	0.4	0.6
Musculoskeletal		
Myalgia	1.2	1.3
Skin		
Eczema	0.8	0.8
Pruritus	0.5	0.4
Rash	0.6	0.6
Special Senses		
Cataract	0.5	0.8

The following effects have been reported with drugs in this class. Not all the effects listed below have necessarily been associated with simvastatin therapy.

Skeletal: muscle cramps, myalgia, myopathy, rhabdomyolysis, arthralgias.

Neurological: dysfunction of certain cranial nerves (including alteration of taste, impairment of extra-ocular movement, facial paresis), tremor, dizziness, vertigo, memory loss, paresthesia, peripheral neuropathy, peripheral nerve palsy, psychic disturbances, anxiety, insomnia, depression.

Hypersensitivity Reactions: An apparent hypersensitivity syndrome has been reported rarely which has included one or more of the following features: anaphylaxis, angioedema, lupus erythematous-like syndrome, polymyalgia rheumatica, vasculitis, purpura, thrombocytopenia, leukopenia, hemolytic anemia, positive ANA, ESR increase, eosinophilia, arthritis, arthralgia, urticaria, asthenia, photosensitivity, fever, chills, flushing, malaise, dyspnea, toxic epidermal necrolyis, erythema multiforme, including Stevens-Johnson syndrome.

Gastrointestinal: Pancreatitis, hepatitis, including chronic active hepatitis, cholestatic jaundice, fatty change in liver, and, rarely, cirrhosis, fulminant hepatic necrosis, and hepatoma; anorexia, vomiting.

Skin: alopecia, pruritus. A variety of skin changes (e.g., nodules, discoloration, dryness of skin/mucous membranes, changes to hair/nails) have been reported.

Reproductive: gynecomastia, loss of libido, erectile dysfunction.

Eye: progression of cataracts (lens opacities), ophthalmoplegia.

Laboratory Abnormalities: elevated transaminases, alkaline phosphatase, γ-glutamyl transpeptidase, and bilurubin; thyroid function abnormalities.

Laboratory Tests

Marked persistent increases of serum transaminases have been noted (see WARNINGS, *Liver Dysfunction*). About 5% of patients had elevations of creatine kinase (CK) levels of 3 or more times the normal value on one or more occasions. This was attributable to the noncardiac fraction of CK. Muscle pain or dysfunction usually was not reported (see WARNINGS, *Skeletal Muscle*).

Concomitant Therapy

In controlled clinical studies in which simvastatin was administered concomitantly with cholestyramine, no adverse reactions peculiar to this concomitant treatment were observed. The adverse reactions that occurred were limited to those reported previously with simvastatin or cholestyramine. The combined use of simvastatin with fibrates should generally be avoided (see WARNINGS, *Skeletal Muscle*).

OVERDOSAGE

Significant lethality was observed in mice after a single oral dose of 9 g/m^2. No evidence of lethality was observed in rats or dogs treated with doses of 30 and 100 g/m^2, respectively. No specific diagnostic signs were observed in rodents. At these doses the only signs seen in dogs were emesis and mucoid stools.

A few cases of overdosage with ZOCOR have been reported; no patients had any specific symptoms, and all patients recovered without sequelae. The maximum dose taken was 450 mg. Until further experience is obtained, no specific treatment of overdosage with ZOCOR can be recommended. The dialyzability of simvastatin and its metabolites in man is not known at present.

DOSAGE AND ADMINISTRATION

The patient should be placed on a standard cholesterol-lowering diet before receiving ZOCOR and should continue on this diet during treatment with ZOCOR (see NCEP Treatment Guidelines for details on dietary therapy).

The recommended usual starting dose is 20 mg once a day in the evening. Patients who require only a moderate reduction of LDL cholesterol may be started at 10 mg. See below for dosage recommendations for patients receiving concomitant therapy with cyclosporine, fibrates or niacin, and for those with severe renal insufficiency.

The recommended dosing range is 5–80 mg/day as a single dose in the evening. Doses should be individualized according to baseline LDL-C levels, the recommended goal of therapy (see NCEP Guidelines) and the patient's response. Adjustments of dosage should be made at intervals of 4 weeks or more.

Cholesterol levels should be monitored periodically and consideration should be given to reducing the dosage of ZOCOR if cholesterol falls significantly below the targeted range.

Dosage in Patients with Homozygous Familial Hypercholesterolemia

Based on the results of a controlled clinical study, the recommended dosage for patients with homozygous familial hypercholesterolemia is ZOCOR 40 mg/day in the evening or 80 mg/day in 3 divided doses of 20 mg, 20 mg, and an evening dose of 40 mg. ZOCOR should be used as an adjunct to other lipid-lowering treatments (e.g., LDL apheresis) in these patients or if such treatments are unavailable.

General Recommendations

In the elderly, maximum reductions in LDL cholesterol may be achieved with daily doses of 20 mg of ZOCOR or less.

In patients taking cyclosporine concomitantly with simvastatin (see WARNINGS, *Skeletal Muscle*), therapy should begin with 5 mg of ZOCOR and should not exceed 10 mg/day.

Concomitant Lipid-Lowering Therapy

ZOCOR is effective alone or when used concomitantly with bile-acid sequestrants. Use of ZOCOR with fibrates or niacin should generally be avoided. However, if ZOCOR is used in combination with fibrates or niacin, the dose of ZOCOR should not exceed 10 mg (see WARNINGS, *Skeletal Muscle*).

Dosage in Patients with Renal Insufficiency

Because ZOCOR does not undergo significant renal excretion, modification of dosage should not be necessary in patients with mild to moderate renal insufficiency. However, caution should be exercised when ZOCOR is administered to patients with severe renal insufficiency; such patients should be started at 5 mg/day and be closely monitored (see CLINICAL PHARMACOLOGY, *Pharmacokinetics* and WARNINGS, *Skeletal Muscle*).

HOW SUPPLIED

No. 3588 — Tablets ZOCOR 5 mg are buff, shield-shaped, film-coated tablets, coded MSD 726 on one side and ZOCOR on the other. They are supplied as follows:

NDC 0006-0726-61 unit of use bottles of 60
(6505-01-354-4549, 5 mg 60's)
NDC 0006-0726-54 unit of use bottles of 90
(6505-01-354-4548, 5 mg 90's)
NDC 0006-0726-28 unit dose packages of 100.

Shown in Product Identification Guide, page 324

No. 3589 — Tablets ZOCOR 10 mg are peach, shield-shaped, film-coated tablets, coded MSD 735 on one side and ZOCOR on the other. They are supplied as follows:

NDC 0006-0735-61 unit of use bottles of 60
(6505-01-354-4545, 10 mg 60's)
NDC 0006-0735-54 unit of use bottles of 90
(6505-01-354-4544, 10 mg 90's)
NDC 0006-0735-28 unit dose packages of 100
(6505-01-354-4543, 10 mg individually sealed 100's)
NDC 0006-0735-82 bottles of 1000
(6505-01-373-7290, 10 mg 1000's)
NDC 0006-0735-87 bottles of 10,000
(6505-01-378-8058, 10 mg 10,000's).

Shown in Product Identification Guide, page 324

No. 3590 — Tablets ZOCOR 20 mg are tan, shield-shaped, film-coated tablets, coded MSD 740 on one side and ZOCOR on the other. They are supplied as follows:

NDC 0006-0740-61 unit of use bottles of 60
(6505-01-354-4547, 20 mg 60's)
NDC 0006-0740-28 unit dose packages of 100
NDC 0006-0740-82 bottles of 1000
NDC 0006-0740-87 bottles of 10,000
(6505-01-378-8771, 20 mg 10,000's).

Shown in Product Identification Guide, page 324

No. 3591 — Tablets ZOCOR 40 mg are brick red, shield-shaped, film-coated tablets, coded MSD 749 on one side and ZOCOR on the other. They are supplied as follows:

NDC 0006-0749-61 unit of use bottles of 60
(6505-01-354-4546, 40 mg 60's).

Shown in Product Identification Guide, page 324

No. 6577 — Tablets ZOCOR 80 mg are brick red, capsule-shaped, film-coated tablets, coded MSD 543 on one side and 80 on the other. They are supplied as follows:

NDC 0006-0543-61 unit of use bottles of 60.

Shown in Product Identification Guide, page 324

Storage

Store between 5–30°C (41–86°F).

7825430 Issued July 1998

COPYRIGHT © MERCK & CO., Inc., 1991, 1995
All rights reserved.

Information on the Merck & Co., Inc. products listed on these pages is the full prescribing information from product circulars in use August 31, 1998. For information, please call 1-800-NSC MERCK [1-800-672-6372].

Mericon Industries, Inc.
8819 N. PIONEER ROAD
PEORIA, IL 61615

Direct Inquiries to:
William R. Connelly
(309) 693-2150
FAX: (309) 693-2158

BIOTIN OTC
['bī-ō-tĭn]
biotin supplement–high potency

ACTIVE INGREDIENTS
Biotin 5 mg
DIRECTIONS
Take one capsule daily or as directed by your physician.
HOW SUPPLIED
Biotin is supplied as capsules in bottles of 120.
NDC 00394-0130-12

FLORICAL® OTC
[flor ĭ cal]
(fluoride and calcium supplement)

ACTIVE INGREDIENTS
Florical® contains 3.75 mg fluoride (as sodium fluoride), 145 mg calcium (as calcium carbonate)
DIRECTIONS
Take one tablet or capsule daily, or as recommended by physician.
HOW SUPPLIED
Florical® is supplied as tablets or capsules in bottles of 100 or 500.
NDC 00394-0102-02 (Capsules 100's)
NDC 00394-0102-05 (Capsules 500's)
NDC 00394-0100-02 (Tablets 100's)
NDC 00394-0100-05 (Tablets 500's)

MONOCAL® OTC
[mon ō cal]
(fluoride and calcium supplement)

ACTIVE INGREDIENTS
Monocal® contains 3 mg fluoride (as monofluorophosphate) and 250 mg calcium (as calcium carbonate)
DIRECTIONS
Take one tablet daily, or as recommended by physician.
HOW SUPPLIED
Monocal® is supplied as tablets in bottles of 100.
NDC 00394-0105-02

Merz Pharmaceuticals
DIVISION OF MERZ, INC.
4215 TUDOR LANE (27410)
P.O. Box 18806
GREENSBORO, NC 27419

Direct Inquiries to:
Director of Regulatory Affairs
(910) 856-2003

FAX: (910) 856-0107

For Medical Information Contact:
In Emergencies:
Director of Regulatory Affairs
(910) 856-2003
FAX: (910) 856-0107

ANATUSS® DM SYRUP OTC

DESCRIPTION
Each 5 ml of ANATUSS DM SYRUP for oral administration contains:
Guaifenesin	100 mg
Pseudoephedrine Hydrochloride	30 mg
Dextromethorphan Hydrobromide	10 mg
In a good tasting cherry flavored vehicle.

HOW SUPPLIED
ANATUSS DM SYRUP is supplied in pints NDC #0259-0383-16, 4 oz bottles NDC #0259-0383-04.

ANATUSS® DM TABLETS OTC

DESCRIPTION
Each orange, oval European scored ANATUSS DM TABLET for oral administration contains:
Guaifenesin	400 mg
Pseudoephedrine Hydrochloride	60 mg
Dextromethorphan Hydrobromide	20 mg

HOW SUPPLIED
ANATUSS DM TABLETS are available as orange, oval shaped tablets, deep-scored on one side with an "M" appearing on the left of the score and a "P" appearing on the right of the score and 0382 appearing on the reverse side of the tablet.
In bottles of 100: NDC #0259-0382-01, in bottles of 20: NDC #0259-0382-21.

ANATUSS® LA TABLETS ℞

DESCRIPTION
Each off-white European scored Anatuss LA Tablet for oral administration contains:
Guaifenesin	400 mg
Pseudoephedrine Hydrochloride	120 mg
Guaifenesin, 3-(2-methoxyphenoxy)-1,2-Propanediol, a white odorless, crystalline material with a slightly bitter aromatic taste. Pseudoephedrine Hydrochloride, [1-(methylamino)ethyl]benzenemethanol, a white crystalline, almost odorless powder with a bitter taste.

HOW SUPPLIED
Anatuss LA Tablets are available as off-white oval-shaped tablets, deep-scored on one side with an "M" appearing on the left of the score and an "R" appearing on the right of the score and 0379 appearing on the bottom side of the tablet.
In bottles of 100: NDC #0259-0379-01.

ELDERCAPS® ℞

DESCRIPTION
Each capsule contains: Vitamin A Acetate, 4000 I.U.; Vitamin D_3, 400 I.U.; Vitamin E, 25 I.U.; Ascorbic Acid, 200 mg.; Thiamine Mononitrate, 10 mg.; Riboflavin, 5 mg.; Pyridoxine HCl, 2 mg.; Niacinamide, 25 mg.; d-Calcium Pantothenate, 10 mg.; Zinc 25 mg (as 69 mg of Zinc Sulfate monohydrate); Magnesium 6.95 mg (as 35 mg of Magnesium Sulfate Dry Powder); Manganese 1.63 mg (as 5 mg of Manganese Sulfate Monohydrate); Folic Acid, 1 mg.

HOW SUPPLIED
ELDERCAPS are supplied in bottles of 100: NDC #0259-0393-01.

ELDERTONIC® OTC

DESCRIPTION
Each 45 ml. contains: Thiamine HCl, 1.5 mg.; Riboflavin, 1.7 mg. (as Riboflavin 5'-Phosphate Sodium); Pyridoxine HCl, 2.0 mg.; Cyanocobalamin, 6.0 mcg.; Dexpanthenol, 10.0 mg.; Niacinamide, 20.0 mg.; Zinc, 15 mg. (as zinc sulfate); Manganese, 2.0 mg. (as manganese sulfate); Magnesium (minimum content as added magnesium), 2.0 mg. (as magnesium sulfate); Alcohol, 13.5%.
In a special sherry wine base.

INDICATIONS
B-complex vitamins with minerals for nutritional supplementation.

DOSAGE
Adults: one tablespoonful three times a day with meals.

WARNING
Do not exceed recommended dosage unless directed by a physician.

USAGE IN PREGNANCY
Safe use of this product in pregnancy has not been established.

CAUTION
Keep out of the reach of children.

HOW SUPPLIED
ELDERTONIC available in 8 oz. bottles: NDC #0259-0351-08, Pint bottles: NDC #0259-0351-16, Quart bottles: NDC #0259-0351-32, Gallons: NDC #0259-0351-28.

MAY–VITA® ELIXIR ℞

DESCRIPTION
Each 45 ml. contains: Dexpanthenol, 10 mg; Niacinamide, 40 mg.; Pyridoxine HCl (B-6), 4 mg.; Cyanocobalamin (B-12), 12 mcg.; Folic Acid, 1 mg.; Iron, 36 mg. (as polysaccharide iron complex); Zinc, 15 mg. (as zinc sulfate); Manganese, 4 mg. (as manganese sulfate); Alcohol, 13%.

INDICATIONS
For vitamin and mineral replacement therapy in deficiency states and for treatment of iron deficiency anemia and/or nutritional megaloblastic anemias due to inadequate diet.

WARNINGS
Folic acid alone is improper therapy in the treatment of pernicious anemia and other megaloblastic anemias where vitamin B_{12} is deficient.

PRECAUTIONS
Folic acid, especially in doses above 0.1 mg. daily, may obscure pernicious anemia, in that hematologic remission may occur while neurological manifestations remain progressive.

ADVERSE REACTIONS
Allergic sensitization has been reported following both oral and parenteral administration of folic acid.

USE IN PREGNANCY
Safe use of this product in pregnancy has not been established.

DOSAGE
Usual adult dosage is one tablespoonful (15 ml.) three times daily with meals. Do not exceed recommended dosage unless directed by a physician.

HOW SUPPLIED
MAY-VITA ELIXIR is supplied in Pint bottles: NDC #0259-0366-16.

NU-IRON® 150 CAPSULES OTC
(polysaccharide-iron complex)

NU-IRON® ELIXIR (polysaccharide-iron complex)
Sugar Free Dye Free

DESCRIPTION
NU-IRON is a highly water soluble complex of iron and a low molecular weight polysaccharide.
Each NU-IRON 150 Capsule contains:
Iron (elemental) .... 150 mg.
(as Polysaccharide Iron Complex)
Each 5 ml. of NU-IRON Elixir contains:
Iron (elemental) .... 100 mg.
(as Polysaccharide Iron Complex)
Alcohol 10%

ACTION AND USES
NU-IRON is a non-ionic, easily assimilated, relatively non-toxic form of iron. Full therapeutic doses may be achieved with virtually no gastrointestinal side effects. There is no metallic aftertaste and no staining of teeth.

INDICATIONS
For treatment of uncomplicated iron deficiency anemia.

CONTRAINDICATIONS
Hemochromatosis, hemosiderosis or a known hypersensitivity to any of the ingredients.

DOSAGE
ADULTS: One or two NU-IRON 150 Capsules daily, or one or two teaspoonsful NU-IRON Elixir daily. CHILDREN; 6 to 12 years old; one teaspoonful NU-IRON Elixir daily. For younger children consult physician.

HOW SUPPLIED
NU-IRON 150 CAPSULES in blister paks of 100 (10 × 10): NDC #0259-0291-01, NDC #0259-0291-50.
NU-IRON ELIXIR in 8 oz bottles: NDC #0259-0292-08.

NU–IRON® PLUS ELIXIR ℞
(polysaccharide-iron complex)
Sugar Free Dye Free

DESCRIPTION

Each 5 ml of NU-IRON
PLUS ELIXIR contains:

Iron (elemental)	100 mg
(as Polysaccharide Iron Complex)	
Folic Acid	1 mg
Vitamin B12	25 mcg
Alcohol	10%

HOW SUPPLIED

NU-IRON PLUS ELIXIR is supplied in 8 oz bottles: NDC #0259-0342-08.

NU–IRON® V TABLETS ℞
(polysaccharide-iron complex with vitamins)

DESCRIPTION

Each maroon film-coated tablet contains:
IRON, ELEMENTAL (As a polysaccharide-iron complex) 60 mg; Folic Acid 1 mg; Ascorbic Acid 50 mg. (as sodium ascorbate); Cyanocobalamin (Vitamin B-12) 3 mcg.; Vitamin A 4000 I.U.; Vitamin D-2 400 I.U.; Thiamine Mononitrate 3 mg.; Riboflavin 3 mg.; Pyridoxine Hydrochloride 2 mg.; Niacinamide 10 mg.; Calcium Carbonate 312 mg.

HOW SUPPLIED

NU-IRON V TABLETS are available as maroon film-coated capsule-shaped tablets. In bottles of 100: NDC #0259-0331-01.

SEDAPAP® TABLETS ℞
(Butalbital and Acetaminophen Tablets)
50 mg/650 mg

DESCRIPTION

Butalbital and acetaminophen is supplied in tablet form for oral administration.
Butalbital (5-allyl-5-isobutylbarbituric acid), a slightly bitter, white, odorless, crystalline powder, is a short to intermediate-acting barbiturate. It has the following structural formula:

$C_{11}H_{16}N_2O_3$ MW = 224.26

Acetaminophen (4'-hydroxyacetanalide), a slightly bitter, white, odorless, crystalline powder, is a non-opiate, non-salicylate analgesic and antipyretic. It has the following structural formula:

$C_8H_9NO_2$ MW = 151.16

Each Sedapap Tablet contains:

Butalbital	50 mg
(Warning: May be habit forming)	
Acetaminophen	650 mg

In addition, each tablet contains the following inactive ingredients: colloidal silicon dioxide, croscarmellose sodium, crospovidone, microcrystalline cellulose, povidone, pregelatinized starch and stearic acid.

CLINICAL PHARMACOLOGY

This combination drug product is intended as a treatment for tension headache.
It consists of a fixed combination of butalbital, and acetaminophen. The role each component plays in the relief of the complex of symptoms known as tension headache is incompletely understood.
Pharmacokinetics: The behavior of the individual components is described below.
Butalbital: Butalbital is well absorbed from the gastrointestinal tract and is expected to distribute to most tissues in the body. Barbiturates in general may appear in breast milk and readily cross the placental barrier. They are bound to plasma and tissue proteins to a varying degree and binding increases directly as a function of lipid solubility.

Elimination of butalbital is primarily via the kidney (59% to 88% of the dose) as unchanged drug or metabolites. The plasma half-life is about 35 hours. Urinary excretion products include parent drug (about 3.6% of the dose), 5-isobutyl-5-(2,3-dihydroxypropyl) barbituric acid (about 24% of the dose), 5-allyl-5(3-hydroxy-2-methyl-1-propyl) barbituric acid (about 4.8% of the dose), products with the barbituric acid ring hydrolyzed with excretion of urea (about 14% of the dose), as well as unidentified materials. Of the material excreted in the urine, 32% is conjugated.
See OVERDOSAGE for toxicity information.
Acetaminophen: Acetaminophen is rapidly absorbed from the gastrointestinal tract and is distributed throughout most body tissues. The plasma half-life is 1.25 to 3 hours, but may be increased by liver damage and following overdosage. Elimination of acetaminophen is principally by liver metabolism (conjugation) and subsequent renal excretion of metabolites. Approximately 85% of an oral dose appears in the urine within 24 hours of administration, most as the glucuronide conjugate, with small amounts of other conjugates and unchanged drug.
See OVERDOSAGE for toxicity information.

INDICATIONS AND USAGE

Butalbital and Acetaminophen Tablets are indicated for the relief of the symptom complex of tension (or muscle contraction) headache.
Evidence supporting the efficacy and safety of this combination product in the treatment of multiple recurrent headaches is unavailable. Caution in this regard is required because butalbital is habit-forming and potentially abusable.

CONTRAINDICATIONS

This product is contraindicated under the following conditions:
• Hypersensitivity or intolerance to any component of this product.
• Patients with porphyria.

WARNINGS

Butalbital is habit-forming and potentially abusable. Consequently, the extended use of this product is not recommended.

PRECAUTIONS

General: Butalbital and Acetaminophen Tablets should be prescribed with caution in certain special-risk patients, such as the elderly or debilitated, and those with severe impairment of renal or hepatic function, or acute abdominal conditions.
Information for Patients: This product may impair mental and/or physical abilities required for the performance of potentially hazardous tasks such as driving a car or operating machinery. Such tasks should be avoided while taking this product.
Alcohol and other CNS depressants may produce an additive CNS depression, when taken with this combination product, and should be avoided.
Butalbital may be habit-forming. Patients should take the drug only for as long as it is prescribed, in the amounts prescribed, and no more frequently than prescribed.
Laboratory Tests: In patients with severe hepatic or renal disease, effects of therapy should be monitored with serial liver and/or renal function tests.
Drug Interactions: The CNS effects of butalbital may be enhanced by monoamine oxidase (MAO) inhibitors.
Butalbital and acetaminophen may enhance the effects of: other narcotic analgesics, alcohol, general anesthetics, tranquilizers such as chlordiazepoxide, sedative-hypnotics, or other CNS depressants, causing increased CNS depression.
Drug/Laboratory Test Interactions: Acetaminophen may produce false-positive test results for urinary 5-hydroxyindoleacetic acid.
Carcinogenesis, Mutagenesis, Impairment of Fertility: No adequate studies have been conducted in animals to determine whether acetaminophen or butalbital have a potential for carcinogenesis, mutagenesis or impairment of fertility.
Pregnancy: Teratogenic Effects: Pregnancy Category C: Animal reproduction studies have not been conducted with this combination product. It is also not known whether butalbital and acetaminophen can cause fetal harm when administered to a pregnant woman or can affect reproduction capacity. This product should be given to a pregnant woman only when clearly needed.
Nonteratogenic Effects: Withdrawal seizures were reported in a two-day-old male infant whose mother had taken butalbital-containing drug during the last two months of pregnancy. Butalbital was found in the infant's serum. The infant was given phenobarbital 5 mg/kg, which was tapered without further seizure or other withdrawal symptoms.
Nursing Mothers: Barbiturates and acetaminophen are excreted in breast milk in small amounts, but the significance of their effects on nursing infants is not known. Because of potential for serious adverse reactions in nursing infants from butalbital and acetaminophen, a decision

should be made whether to discontinue nursing or to discontinue the drug, taking into account the importance of the drug to the mother.
Pediatric Use: Safety and effectiveness in pediatric patients below the age of 12 have not been established.

ADVERSE REACTIONS

Frequently Observed: The most frequently reported adverse reactions are drowsiness, lightheadedness, dizziness, sedation, shortness of breath, nausea, vomiting, abdominal pain, and intoxicated feeling.
Infrequently Observed: All adverse events tabulated below are classified as infrequent.
Central Nervous: headache, shaky feeling, tingling, agitation, fainting, fatigue, heavy eyelids, high energy, hot spells, numbness, sluggishness, seizure. Mental confusion, excitement or depression can also occur due to intolerance, particularly in elderly or debilitated patients, or due to overdosage of butalbital.
Autonomic Nervous: dry mouth, hyperhidrosis.
Gastrointestinal: difficulty swallowing, heartburn, flatulence, constipation.
Cardiovascular: tachycardia.
Musculoskeletal: leg pain, muscle fatigue.
Genitourinary: diuresis.
Miscellaneous: pruritus, fever, earache, nasal congestion, tinnitus, euphoria, allergic reactions.
Several cases of dermatological reactions, including toxic epidermal necrolysis and erythema multiforme, have been reported.
The following adverse drug events may be borne in mind as a potential effect of the components of this product. Potential effects of high dosage are listed in the OVERDOSAGE section.
Acetaminophen: allergic reactions, rash, thrombocytopenia, agranulocytosis.

DRUG ABUSE AND DEPENDENCE

Abuse and Dependence: Butalbital: Barbiturates may be habit-forming: Tolerance, psychological dependence, and physical dependence may occur especially following prolonged use of high doses of barbiturates. The average daily dose for the barbiturate addict is usually about 1500 mg. As tolerance to barbiturates develops, the amount needed to maintain the same level of intoxication increases; tolerance to a fatal dosage, however, does not increase more than twofold. As this occurs, the margin between an intoxication dosage and fatal dosage becomes smaller. The lethal dose of a barbiturate is far less if alcohol is also ingested. Major withdrawal symptoms (convulsions and delirium) may occur within 16 hours and last up to 5 days after abrupt cessation of these drugs. Intensity of withdrawal symptoms gradually declines over a period of approximately 15 days. Treatment of barbiturate dependence consists of cautious and gradual withdrawal of the drug. Barbiturate-dependent patients can be withdrawn by using a number of different withdrawal regimens. One method involves initiating treatment at the patient's regular dosage level and gradually decreasing the daily dosage as tolerated by the patient.

OVERDOSAGE

Following an acute overdosage of butalbital and acetaminophen, toxicity may result from the barbiturate or the acetaminophen.
Signs and Symptoms: Toxicity from barbiturate poisoning include drowsiness, confusion, and coma; respiratory depression; hypotension; and hypovolemic shock.
In acetaminophen overdosage: dose-dependent, potentially fatal hepatic necrosis is the most serious adverse effect. Renal tubular necrosis, hypoglycemic coma and thrombocytopenia may also occur. Early symptoms following a potentially hepatotoxic overdose may include: nausea, vomiting, diaphoresis and general malaise. Clinical and laboratory evidence of hepatic toxicity may not be apparent until 48 to 72 hours post-ingestion. In adults hepatic toxicity has rarely been reported with acute overdoses of less than 10 grams, or fatalities with less than 15 grams.
Treatment: A single or multiple overdose with this combination product is a potentially lethal polydrug overdose, and consultation with a regional poison control center is recommended.
Immediate treatment includes support of cardiorespiratory function and measures to reduce drug absorption. Vomiting should be induced mechanically, or with syrup of ipecac, if the patient is alert (adequate pharyngeal and laryngeal reflexes). Oral activated charcoal (1 g/kg) should follow gastric emptying. The first dose should be accompanied by an appropriate cathartic. If repeated doses are used, the cathartic might be included with alternate doses as required. Hypotension is usually hypovolemic and should respond to fluids. Pressors should be avoided. A cuffed endotracheal tube should be inserted before gastric lavage of the unconscious patient and, when necessary, to provide assisted respiration. If renal function is normal, forced diuresis may aid in

Continued on next page

Sedapap—Cont.

the elimination of the barbiturate. Alkalinization of the urine increases renal excretion of some barbiturates, especially phenobarbital.

Meticulous attention should be given to maintaining adequate pulmonary ventilation. In severe cases of intoxication, peritoneal dialysis, or preferably hemodialysis may be considered. If hypoprothrombinemia occurs due to acetaminophen overdose, vitamin K should be administered intravenously.

If the dose of acetaminophen may have exceeded 140 mg/kg, acetylcysteine should be administered as early as possible. Serum acetaminophen levels should be obtained, since levels four or more hours following ingestion help predict acetaminophen toxicity. Do not await acetaminophen assay results before initiating treatment. Hepatic enzymes should be obtained initially, and repeated at 24-hour intervals. Methemoglobinemia over 30% should be treated with methylene blue by slow intravenous administration.

Toxic Doses (for adults):

Butalbital: toxic dose 1 g	(20 tablets)
Acetaminophen: toxic dose 10 g	(15 tablets)

DOSAGE AND ADMINISTRATION

Oral: One table every four hours as needed. Total daily dosage should not exceed 6 tablets.

Extended and repeated use of this product is not recommended because of the potential for physical dependence.

HOW SUPPLIED

SEDAPAP® TABLETS (Butalbital and Acetaminophen Tablets) 50 mg/650 mg are supplied in bottles of 100 tablets, NDC 0259-0392-01. Each tablet contains butalbital 50 mg (Warning: May be habit forming) and acetaminophen 650 mg. Tablets are uncoated, white, capsule-shaped and are debossed "MP" score "392" on one side.

Storage: Protect from light and moisture. Store at controlled room temperature, 15° - 30°C (59° - 86°F).

Dispense in a tight, light-resistant container with a child-resistant closure.

CAUTION: Federal law prohibits dispensing without prescription.

MFG. FOR:

MERZ PHARMACEUTICALS™
Greensboro, NC 27407

BY:

MIKART, INC.
Atlanta, GA 30318

Rev. 4/97	Code 805A00
30-1168-00	

STERAPRED® 5 mg UNIPAK   ℞
STERAPRED® 5 mg 12 Day UNIPAK

DESCRIPTION

Each white tablet contains:
Prednisone .... 5 mg.

HOW SUPPLIED

STERAPRED 5 mg UNIPAK available in 21 tablet tapered dose dispensing pack. NDC #0259-0390-21.
STERAPRED 5 mg 12 DAY UNIPAK available in 48 tablet tapered dose dispensing pack. NDC #0259-0391-48.

STERAPRED® DS UNIPAK   ℞
STERAPRED® DS 12 DAY UNIPAK

DESCRIPTION

Each white tablet contains:
Prednisone .... 10 mg.

HOW SUPPLIED

STERAPRED DS UNIPAK available in 21 tablet tapered dose dispensing pack: NDC #0259-0364-21.
STERAPRED DS 12 DAY UNIPAK available in 48 tablet tapered dose dispensing pack: NDC #0259-0389-48.

Milex Products, Inc.
**4311 N. NORMANDY
CHICAGO, IL 60634-1403**

Direct Inquiries to:
1-800-621-1278

AMINO-CERV™   ℞
[ah-me 'no-serv]
pH 5.5 Cervical Creme

ACTIVE INGREDIENTS

Urea 8.34%, Sodium Propionate 0.50%, Methionine 0.83%, Cystine 0.35%, Inositol 0.83%, Benzalkonium Chloride 0.000004%. Buffered to pH of 5.5 in a water-miscible creme base.

DESCRIPTION

An AMINO-ACID and UREA creme specifically formulated for cervical treatment: Cervicitis (mild), postpartum cervicitis, postpartum cervical tears, post surgical cervical procedures.

ADVANTAGES

METHIONINE and CYSTINE are amino-acids necessary for wound healing and forming of epithelial tissue. INOSITOL acts as an essential growth factor and promotes epithelialization.

UREA aids in debridement, dissolves the coagulum and promotes epithelialization. Its solvent action on fibroblasts prevents the formation of excessive tissue—thus preventing stenosis when used as directed.

BENZALKONIUM CHLORIDE serves to lower surface tension and thus aids in spreading the medication. Along with SODIUM PROPIONATE it also exerts a bacteriostatic effect.

AMINO-CERV is geared to the higher pH of the healthy cervix in contrast with pH 4 vaginal preparations. With its pH factor of 5.5 Amino-Cerv promotes faster healing of the cervix, yet will not adversely affect a healthy vagina.

DIRECTIONS

When immediate postpartum bleeding has subsided (usually from 24 to 48 hours after delivery), one Milex Jector full of AMINO-CERV creme should be applied nightly for four weeks. In mild cervicitis (not requiring cautery or cryosurgery) one applicatorful of AMINO-CERV should be injected in the vagina nightly upon retiring for 2 weeks. A small amount of AMINO-CERV should be applied immediately following a surgical cervical procedure with the exception of a cold coning procedure. One applicatorful should be injected nightly upon retiring for 2 to 4 weeks (the duration of treatment depends on extent of the surgical procedure). In each of the post surgical visits, the physician should again apply a small amount of AMINO-CERV with a probe or applicator. The canal is to be completely probed on the last visit.

After COLD CONING, one applicatorful should be injected upon retiring about 24 hours after surgery and nightly thereafter for four weeks. During the four weekly office visits following cold coning, a small amount of AMINO-CERV should be applied with a probe or applicator into the canal by the physician. The canal is to be completely probed on the last visit.

Reasons For Variation of Directions
(1) After most surgical procedures, cauterization, cryosurgery and laser surgery, immediate use of AMINO-CERV is indicated to aid in dissolving dead or burned tissue.
(2) After cold coning, there is no dead tissue to slough off. Therefore, a wait of 24 hours or longer is desirable for normal healing to take place and for some fibroblasts to be laid down before applying the AMINO-CERV (which has a solvent action on both the fibroblasts and the absorbable sutures). When NONABSORBABLE sutures are used, AMINO-CERV can be used immediately.

CONTRAINDICATIONS

Deleterious side effects have not been a problem at the doses recommended. The usual precautions against allergic reactions should be observed.

STORAGE

Store at room temperature.

PACKAGING

2³/₄ oz. tube with MILEX-JECTOR (2 weeks supply, 14 applications).

Mission Pharmacal
Company
**10999 IH 10 WEST
SUITE 1000
SAN ANTONIO, TX 78230-1355**

Direct Inquiries to:
PO Box 786099
San Antonio, TX 78278–6099
TOLL FREE: (800) 292-7364
(210) 696-8400
FAX: (210) 696-6010
For Medical Information Contact:
In Emergencies:
George Alexandrides
(830) 249-9822
FAX: (830) 816-2545

CITRACAL® Ⓤ
[sit 'ra-cal]
ultradense calcium citrate dietary supplement

INGREDIENTS

Calcium (as Ultradense™ calcium citrate) 200 mg., polyethylene glycol, croscarmellose sodium, HPMC, color added, magnesium silicate, magnesium stearate.

SENSITIVE PATIENTS

CITRACAL® contains no wheat, barley, yeast or rye; is sugar, dairy and gluten free and contains no artificial colors.

ONE TABLET PROVIDES

200 mg. calcium (elemental), equaling 20% of the U.S. recommended daily allowance for adults and children 4 or more years of age.

FOUR TABLETS PROVIDE

800 mg. calcium (elemental), equaling 80% of the U.S. recommended daily allowance for adults and children 4 or more years of age.

DIRECTIONS

Take 1 to 2 tablets twice daily or as recommended by a physician, pharmacist or health professional.

HOW SUPPLIED

CITRACAL® is supplied as white, nearly oval shaped, coated tablets in bottles of 100 NDC 0178-0800-01, and bottles of 200 NDC 0178-0800-20.
Ⓤ = Kosher Parvae approved by Orthodox Union.

CITRACAL® Caplets + D Ⓤ
[sit 'ra-cal]
ultradense calcium citrate dietary supplement

INGREDIENTS

CITRACAL® Caplets + D are supplied in an ultra-dense caplet formulation, each containing calcium (as Ultradense™ calcium citrate) 315 mg., polyethylene glycol, croscarmellose sodium, HPMC, color added, magnesium silicate, magnesium stearate, vitamin D₃ (200IU).

HOW SUPPLIED

CITRACAL® Caplets + D are available in bottles of 60 NDC 0178-0815-60; bottles of 120 NDC 0178-0815-12, and bottles of 180 NDC 0178-0815-18.
Ⓤ= Kosher Parvae approved by Orthodox Union.

CITRACAL® LIQUITAB® Ⓤ
[sit 'ra-cal]
calcium citrate dietary supplement

INGREDIENTS: CITRACAL® LIQUITAB® is supplied as effervescent tablets each containing calcium (as calcium citrate) 500 mg., citric acid, adipic acid, saccharin sodium, orange flavor, cellulose gum, aspartame.

This product contains NutraSweet®.
Phenylketonurics: Contains 6 mg. phenylalanine per tablet.

HOW SUPPLIED

CITRACAL® LIQUITAB® is available in bottles of 30 tablets. **NDC** 0178-0811-30.
Ⓤ = Kosher Parvae Approved by Orthodox Union

CALCET®ⓤ
[kăl 'cet]
Calcium Dietary Supplement
NDC-0178-0251-01

HOW SUPPLIED
CALCET® tablets are supplied as yellow, rectangular shaped, coated tablets in bottles of 100 tablets.
ⓤ = Kosher Parvae approved by Orthodox Union

CALCET PLUS®
[kăl 'cet]
Calcium-Iron-Zinc-Multivitamin
NDC 0178-0252-60

> **WARNING:** Accidental overdose of **iron-containing** products is a leading cause of fatal poisoning in children under 6. Keep this product out of reach of children. In case of accidental overdose, call a doctor or poison control center immediately. If you are pregnant or nursing a baby, seek the advice of a health professional before using this product.

HOW SUPPLIED
CALCET PLUS tablets are supplied as white, elliptical shaped, coated tablets in bottles of 60's.

FOSFREE®
[fos 'frē]
Calcium—Iron—Multivitamin
NDC 0178-0031-60
NDC 0178-0031-12

> **WARNING:** Accidental overdose of **iron-containing** products is a leading cause of fatal poisoning in children under 6. Keep this product out of reach of children. In case of accidental overdose, call a doctor or poison control center immediately. If you are pregnant or nursing a baby, seek the advice of a health professional before using this product.

HOW SUPPLIED
FOSFREE® is supplied as yellow, elliptical shaped, coated tablets in bottles of either 60 or 120 tablets.

IROMIN–G®
[i 'rō-min]
Hematinic Dietary Supplement
NDC-0178-0081-01

> **WARNING:** Accidental overdose of **iron-containing** products is a leading cause of fatal poisoning in children under 6. Keep this product out of reach of children. In case of accidental overdose, call a doctor or poison control center immediately.

HOW SUPPLIED
IROMIN-G® is supplied as red bolus shaped coated tablets in bottles of 100 tablets.

MISSION PRENATAL DIETARY SUPPLEMENT SERIES

MISSION PRENATAL®
Vitamins—Iron—Calcium—.4 mg. Folic Acid
NDC 0178-0132-01

MISSION PRENATAL® F.A
Vitamins—Iron—Calcium—Zinc—.8mg Folic Acid
NDC 0178-0153-01

MISSION PRENATAL® H.P.
Vitamins—Iron—Calcium—0.8 mg. Folic Acid
NDC 0178-0161-01

> **WARNING:** Accidental overdose of **iron-containing** products is a leading cause of fatal poisoning in children under 6. Keep this product out of reach of children. In case of accidental overdose, call a doctor or poison control center immediately.

HOW SUPPLIED
MISSION® PRENATAL is supplied as pink, rectangular-shaped, sugar-coated tablets in bottles of 100.

MISSION® PRENATAL F.A. is supplied as blue, rectangular-shaped, sugar coated tablets in bottles of 100.
MISSION® PRENATAL H.P. is supplied as green, rectangular-shaped, sugar-coated tablets in bottles of 100.

MISSION PRENATAL® Rx
Prenatal Supplement with Vitamins and Minerals
NDC 0178-0007-01
℞

> **WARNING:** Accidental overdose of **iron-containing** products is a leading cause of fatal poisoning in children under 6. KEEP THIS PRODUCT OUT OF THE REACH OF CHILDREN. In case of accidental overdose, call a doctor or poison control center immediately.

HOW SUPPLIED
MISSION PRENATAL Rx is supplied as pink, elliptical shape, film-coated tablets in bottles of 100.

MISSION PHARMACAL UROLOGICALS

UROCIT®–K
[yu 'ro-cĭt kay]
Potassium Citrate
℞

DESCRIPTION
Urocit-K is a citrate salt of potassium. Its empirical formula is $K_3C_6H_5O_7 \cdot H_2O$, and its structural formula is:

$$\begin{array}{l} CH_2\!-\!\!-\!\!-COOK \\ \mid \\ HO\!-\!\!-\!\!-C\!-\!\!-\!\!-COOK \cdot H_2O \\ \mid \\ CH_2\!-\!\!-\!\!-COOK \end{array}$$

Potassium citrate is a white granular powder that is soluble in water at 154 g/100 ml, almost insoluble in alcohol, and insoluble in organic solvents.
Urocit-K is supplied as wax matrix tablets, containing 5 meq (540 mg) potassium citrate and 10 meq (1080 mg) potassium citrate each, for oral administration.

CLINICAL PHARMACOLOGY
When Urocit-K is given orally, the metabolism of absorbed citrate produces an alkaline load. The induced alkaline load in turn increases urinary pH and raises urinary citrate by augmenting citrate clearance without measurably altering ultrafilterable serum citrate. Thus, Urocit-K therapy appears to increase urinary citrate principally by modifying the renal handling of citrate, rather than by increasing the filtered load of citrate. The increased filtered load of citrate may play some role, however, as in small comparisons of oral citrate and oral bicarbonate, citrate had a greater effect on urinary citrate.
In addition to raising urinary pH and citrate, Urocit-K increases urinary potassium by approximately the amount contained in the medication. In some patients, Urocit-K causes a transient reduction in urinary calcium.
The changes induced by Urocit-K produce a urine that is less conducive to the crystallization of stone-forming salts (calcium oxalate, calcium phosphate and uric acid). Increased citrate in the urine, by complexing with calcium, decreases calcium ion activity and thus the saturation of calcium oxalate. Citrate also inhibits the spontaneous nucleation of calcium oxalate and calcium phosphate (brushite). The increase in urinary pH also decreases calcium ion activity by increasing calcium complexation to dissociated anions. The rise in urinary pH also increases the ionization of uric acid to more soluble urate ion.
Urocit-K therapy does not alter the urinary saturation of calcium phosphate, since the effect of increased citrate complexation of calcium is opposed by the rise in pH-dependent dissociation of phosphate. Calcium phosphate stones are more stable in alkaline urine.
In the setting of normal renal function, the rise in urinary citrate following a single dose begins by the first hour and lasts for 12 hours. With multiple doses the rise in citrate excretion reaches its peak by the third day and averts the normally wide circadian fluctuation in urinary citrate, thus maintaining urinary citrate at a higher, more constant level throughout the day. When the treatment is withdrawn, urinary citrate begins to decline toward the pre-treatment level on the first day.
The rise in citrate excretion is directly dependent on the Urocit-K dosage. Following long-term treatment, Urocit-K at a dosage of 60 meq/day raises urinary citrate by approximately 400 mg/day and increases urinary pH by approximately 0.7 units.

In patients with severe renal tubular acidosis or chronic diarrheal syndrome where urinary citrate may be very low (<100 mg/day), Urocit®-K may be relatively ineffective in raising urinary citrate. A higher dose of Urocit®-K may therefore be required to produce a satisfactory citraturic response. In patients with renal tubular acidosis in whom urinary pH may be high, Urocit®-K produces a relatively small rise in urinary pH.

INDICATIONS AND USAGE
Potassium citrate is indicated for the management of renal tubular acidosis (RTA) with calcium stones, hypocitraturic calcium oxalate nephrolithiasis of any etiology, and uric acid lithiasis with or without calcium stones.

CONTRAINDICATIONS
Urocit®-K is contraindicated in patients with hyperkalemia (or who have conditions predisposing them to hyperkalemia), as a further rise in serum potassium concentration may produce cardiac arrest. Such conditions include: chronic renal failure, uncontrolled diabetes mellitus, acute dehydration, strenuous physical exercise in unconditioned individuals, adrenal insufficiency, extensive tissue breakdown, or the administration of a potassium-sparing agent (such as triamterene, spironolactone or amiloride).
Urocit®-K is contraindicated in patients in whom there is cause for arrest or delay in tablet passage through the gastrointestinal tract, such as those suffering from delayed gastric emptying, esophageal compression, intestinal obstruction or stricture or those taking anticholinergic medication. Because of its ulcerogenic potential, Urocit®-K should not be given to patients with peptic ulcer disease.
Urocit®-K is contraindicated in patients with active urinary tract infection (with either urea-splitting or other organisms, in association with either calcium or struvite stones). The ability of Urocit®-K to increase urinary citrate may be attenuated by bacterial enzymatic degradation of citrate. Moreover, the rise in urinary pH resulting from Urocit®-K therapy might promote further bacterial growth.
Urocit®-K is contraindicated in patients with renal insufficiency (glomerular filtration rate of less than 0.7 ml/kg/min), because of the danger of soft tissue calcification and increased risk for the development of hyperkalemia.

WARNINGS
HYPERKALEMIA: In patients with impaired mechanisms for excreting potassium, Urocit®-K administration can produce hyperkalemia and cardiac arrest. Potentially fatal hyperkalemia can develop rapidly and be asymptomatic. The use of Urocit®-K in patients with chronic renal failure, or any other condition which impairs potassium excretion such as severe myocardial damage or heart failure, should be avoided.

INTERACTION WITH POTASSIUM-SPARING DIURETICS
Concomitant administration of Urocit®-K and a potassium-sparing diuretic (such as triamterene, spironolactone or amiloride) should be avoided, since the simultaneous administration of these agents can produce severe hyperkalemia.

GASTROINTESTINAL LESIONS
Because of reports of upper gastrointestinal mucosal lesions following administration of potassium chloride (wax-matrix), and endoscopic examination of the upper gastrointestinal mucosa was performed in 30 normal volunteers after they had taken glycopyrrolate 2 mg. p.o. t.i.d., Urocit®-K 95 meq/day, wax-matrix potassium chloride 96 meq/day or wax matrix placebo, in thrice daily schedule in the fasting state for one week. Urocit®-K and the wax-matrix formulation of potassium chloride were indistinguishable but both were significantly more irritating than the wax-matrix placebo. In a subsequent similar study, lesions were less severe when glycopyrrolate was omitted.
Solid dosage forms of potassium chloride have produced stenotic and/or ulcerative lesions of the small bowel and deaths. These lesions are caused by a high local concentration of potassium ions in the region of the dissolving tablets, which injured the bowel. In addition, perhaps because wax-matrix preparations are not enteric-coated and release some of their potassium content in the stomach, there have been reports of upper gastrointestinal bleeding associated with these products. The frequency of gastrointestinal lesions with wax-matrix potassium chloride products is estimated at one per 100,000 patient-years. Experience with Urocit®-K is limited, but a similar frequency of gastrointestinal lesions should be anticipated.
If there is severe vomiting, abdominal pain or gastro-intestinal bleeding, Urocit®-K should be discontinued immediately and the possibility of bowel perforation or obstruction investigated.

PRECAUTIONS
Information For Patients:
Physicians should consider reminding the patient of the following:

Continued on next page

Urocit-K—Cont.

To take each dose without crushing, chewing or sucking the tablet.

To take this medicine only as directed. This is especially important if the patient is also taking both diuretics and digitalis preparations.

To check with physician if there is trouble swallowing tablets or if the tablet seems to stick in the throat.

To check with the doctor at once if tarry stools or other evidence of gastrointestinal bleeding is noticed.

Laboratory Tests: Regular serum potassium determinations are recommended. Careful attention should be paid to acid-base balance, other serum electrolyte levels, the electrocardiogram, and the clinical status of the patient, particularly in the presence of cardiac disease, renal disease or acidosis.

Drug Interactions: POTASSIUM-SPARING DIURETICS: See WARNINGS section.

DRUGS THAT SLOW GASTROINTESTINAL TRANSIT TIME (such as anticholinergics) can be expected to increase the gastrointestinal irritation produced by potassium salts. (See CONTRAINDICATIONS section).

Carcinogenesis, Mutagenesis, Impairment Of Fertility: Long-term carcinogenicity studies in animals have not been performed.

Pregnancy Category C: Animal reproduction studies have not been conducted with Urocit®-K. It is also not known whether Urocit®-K can cause fetal harm when administered to a pregnant woman or can affect reproduction capacity. Urocit®-K should be given to a pregnant woman only if clearly needed.

Nursing Mothers: The normal potassium ion content of human milk is about 13 meq/l. It is not known if Urocit®-K has an effect on this content. Caution should be exercised when Urocit®-K is administered to a nursing woman.

Pediatric Use: Safety and effectiveness in children have not been established.

ADVERSE REACTIONS

Some patients may develop minor gastrointestinal complaints during Urocit®-K therapy, such as abdominal discomfort, vomiting, diarrhea, loose bowel movements or nausea. These symptoms are due to the irritation of the gastrointestinal tract, and may be alleviated by taking the dose with meals or snack, or by reducing the dosage. Patients may find intact matrices in feces. (See also CONTRAINDICATIONS, WARNINGS)

OVERDOSAGE

The administration of potassium salts to persons without predisposing conditions for hyperkalemia (see CONTRAINDICATIONS) rarely causes serious hyperkalemia at recommended dosages. It is important to recognize that hyperkalemia is usually asymptomatic and may be manifested only by an increased serum potassium concentration and characteristic electrocardiographic changes (peaking of T-wave, loss of P-wave, depression of S-T segment and prolongation of the QT interval). Late manifestations include muscle paralysis and cardiovascular collapse from cardiac arrest.

Treatment measures for hyperkalemia include the following: (1) elimination of potassium-rich foods, medications containing potassium, and of potassium-sparing diuretics, (2) intravenous administration of 300–500 ml/hr of 10% dextrose solution containing 10–20 units of insulin/1000 ml, (3) correction of acidosis, if present, with intravenous sodium bicarbonate, and (4) use of exchange resins, hemodialysis or peritoneal dialysis.

In treating hyperkalemia, it should be recalled that in patients who have been stabilized on digitalis, too rapid a lowering of the serum potassium concentration can produce digitalis toxicity.

DOSAGE AND ADMINISTRATION

Treatment with Urocit®-K should be added to a regimen that limits salt intake (avoidance of foods with high salt content and of added salt at the table) and encourages high fluid intake (urine volume should be at least two liters per day). The objective of treatment with Urocit®-K is to provide Urocit®-K in sufficient dosage to restore normal urinary citrate (greater than 320 mg/day and as close to the normal mean of 640 mg/day as possible), and to increase urinary pH to a level of 6.0 to 7.0.

In patients with severe hypocitraturia (urinary citrate of less than 150 mg/day), therapy should be initiated at a dosage of 60 meq/day (20 meq three times/day or 15 meq four times/day with meals or within 30 minutes after meals or bedtime snack). In patients with mild-moderate hypocitraturia (>150 mg/day), therapy should be initiated at a dosage of 30 meq/day (10 meq three times/day with meals). Twenty-four hour urinary citrate and/or urinary pH measurements should be used to determine the adequacy of the initial dosage and to evaluate the effectiveness of any dosage change. In addition, urinary citrate and/or pH should be measured every four months.

Doses of Urocit®-K greater than 100 meq/day have not been studied and should be avoided.

Serum electrolytes (sodium, potassium, chloride and carbon dioxide), serum creatinine, and complete blood count should be monitored every four months. Treatment should be discontinued if there is hyperkalemia, a significant rise in serum creatinine, or a significant fall in blood hematocrit or hemoglobin.

HOW SUPPLIED

Urocit®-K is available for oral administration in tablet form in the following sizes: (NDC 0178-0600-01) 5 meq potassium citrate and (NDC 0178-0610-01) 10 meq potassium citrate, packaged in bottles of 100 each.

Store in a cool, dry place.

CAUTION: Federal law prohibits dispensing without a prescription.

Rev. 02890

Mission
PHARMACAL COMPANY
San Antonio, TX 78296-1676

LITHOSTAT®
[lith 'o-stat]
Acetohydroxamic Acid (AHA)

℞

DESCRIPTION

Acetohydroxamic acid (AHA) is a stable, synthetic compound derived from hydroxylamine and ethyl acetate. Its molecular structure is similar to urea:

$$H-\underset{\underset{H}{|}}{\overset{\overset{H}{|}}{C}}-\underset{}{\overset{\overset{O}{\|}}{C}}-\underset{\underset{H}{|}}{N}-OH$$

ACETOHYDROXAMIC ACID (AHA)

AHA is weakly acidic, highly soluble in water, and chelates metals - notably iron. The molecular weight is 75.068. AHA has a pKa of 9.32 and a melting point of 89–91°C. Available as 250 mg tablets.

HOW SUPPLIED

LITHOSTAT®, NDC 0178-0500-01, is available for oral administration as 250 mg white colored, round tablets, in unit of use packages of 100 tablets.

THIOLA™
[thi-ól-a]
Tiopronin Tablets

℞

DESCRIPTION

THIOLA™ (Tiopronin) is a reducing and complexing thiol compound. Tiopronin is N-(2-Mercaptopropionyl) glycine and has the following structure:

$$CH_3-\underset{\underset{SH}{|}}{\overset{\overset{\bullet}{}}{CH}}-CONHCH_2-COOH$$

Tiopronin has the empirical formula $C_5H_9NO_3S$ and a molecular weight of 163.20. It has one asymmetric center and therefore exists as dl (racemic) mixture.

Tiopronin is a white crystalline powder which is freely soluble in water.

THIOLA™ tablets are white sugar coated tablets, each containing 100 mg. of Tiopronin and are taken orally.

HOW SUPPLIED

THIOLA™ (NDC 0178-0900-01), is available for oral administration as 100 mg. round, white, sugar coated tablets in bottles of 100 tablets each.

CALCIBIND®
[kal 'sĕ-bīnd]
Cellulose Sodium Phosphate
Oral Powder

℞

DESCRIPTION

Cellulose Sodium Phosphate (CSP), the active ingredient in CALCIBIND®, is a synthetic compound made by phosphorylation of cellulose and has the following structural formula:

[See chemical structure at top of next column]

Where n indicates the degree of polymerization and has an average value of approximately 3000. The molecular weight of CSP monomer is 286.1 and the average molecular weight of the polymer is 858,000.

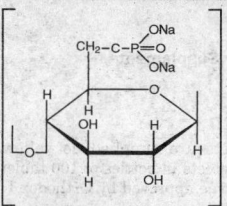

It has an inorganic bound phosphate of 31–36%, free phosphate of 3.5%, sodium content of approximately 11% and a calcium binding capacity of 1.8 mmol of Ca per gram of the oral powder. It has excellent ion exchange properties, the sodium ion exchanging for calcium. When taken orally, CSP binds calcium, the complex of calcium and cellulose phosphate being excreted in feces. The dosage of CALCIBIND® is powder for oral administration.

HOW SUPPLIED

CALCIBIND® NDC 0178-0255-30 is available for oral administration in bottles of 300 grams of CSP bulk powder.

THERA-GESIC®
[thĕr 'ə-jĕ-zik]
(Methyl Salicylate 15%, Menthol 1%)
TOPICAL THERAPEUTIC ANALGESIC CREME

OTC

DESCRIPTION

THERA-GESIC® contains methyl salicylate and menthol in a rapidly absorbed greaseless base containing carbomer 934, dimethicone, glycerine, methylparaben, propylparaben, sodium laurel sulfate, trolamine, water.

INDICATION

Effective temporary relief of arthritis pain and muscle soreness.

WARNINGS

FOR EXTERNAL USE ONLY. Use only as directed. Keep away from children to avoid accidental poisoning. Keep away from eyes, mucous membranes, broken or irritated skin. Do not use THERA-GESIC® if you have skin sensitive to oil of wintergreen (methyl salicylate). If skin irritation develops, if pain lasts 7 days or more, or if redness is present, discontinue use and consult a physician immediately. DO NOT SWALLOW. If swallowed induce vomiting, call a physician. Contact a physician before applying this medicine to children, including teenagers with chicken pox or flu.

DIRECTIONS

ADULTS AND CHILDREN 12 OR MORE YEARS OF AGE: An application of THERA-GESIC® is the gentle massaging of several thin layers of creme into and around the sore or painful area. The number of thin layers controls the intensity of the action. One thin layer provides a mild effect, two thin layers provide a strong effect and three thin layers provide a very strong effect. Do not apply more than 3 to 4 times daily. Once THERA-GESIC® has penetrated the skin, the area may be washed, leaving it dry, clean and fragrance-free without decreasing the effectiveness of the product. IF YOU INTEND TO WRAP, BANDAGE OR COVER THE AREA WHERE YOU HAVE APPLIED THERA-GESIC®, IT MUST BE WASHED THOROUGHLY TO AVOID EXCESSIVE IRRITATION. DO NOT USE A HEATING PAD AFTER APPLICATION OF THERA-GESIC®.

HOW SUPPLIED

NDC 0178-0320-03	3 oz. tube
NDC 0178-0320-05	5 oz. tube

Store in a cool place.

IDENTIFICATION PROBLEM?
Turn to the **Product Identification Guide,**
where you'll find more than
1600 products pictured in actual
size and full color.

Monarch Pharmaceuticals
355 BEECHAM STREET
BRISTOL, TN 37620

Direct Inquiries to:
800-776-3637
FAX: 423-989-6279

Medical Emergency Contact:
Dr. Henry Richards, M.D.
800-546-4906
FAX: 423-989-6137

ANUSOL–HC® 2.5%
(Hydrocortisone Cream, USP)   ℞

Rx only

DESCRIPTION

The topical corticosteroids constitute a class of primarily synthetic steroids used as antiinflammatory and antipruritic agents. Anusol-HC 2.5% (Hydrocortisone Cream, USP) is a topical corticosteroid with hydrocortisone 2.5% (active ingredient) in a water-washable cream containing the following inactive ingredients: benzyl alcohol. petrolatum, stearyl alcohol, propylene glycol. isopropyl myristate, polyoxyl 40 stearate, carbomer 934, sodium lauryl sulfate, edetate disodium, sodium hydroxide to adjust the pH, and purified water.

Hydrocortisone has the chemical name Pregn-4-ene-3,20-dione, 11,17,21, trihydroxy-,(11β) and the following chemical structure:

MOLECULAR FORMULA $C_{21}H_{30}O_5$
MOLECULAR WEIGHT 362.47
CAS REGISTRY NUMBER 50-23-7

CLINICAL PHARMACOLOGY

Topical corticosteroids share antiinflammatory, antipruritic and vasoconstrictive actions.

The mechanism of antiinflammatory activity of the topical corticosteroids is unclear. Various laboratory methods, including vasoconstrictor assays, are used to compare and predict potencies and/or clinical efficacies of the topical corticosteroids. There is some evidence to suggest that a recognizable correlation exists between vasoconstrictor potency and therapeutic efficacy in man.

Pharmacokinetics: The extent of percutaneous absorption of topical corticosteroids is determined by many factors including the vehicle, the integrity of the epidermal barrier, and the use of occlusive dressings.

Topical corticosteroids can be absorbed from normal intact skin. Inflammation and/or other disease processes in the skin increase percutaneous absorption. Occlusive dressings substantially increase the percutaneous absorption of topical corticosteroids. Thus, occlusive dressings may be a valuable therapeutic adjunct for treatment of resistant dermatoses (see DOSAGE AND ADMINISTRATION).

Once absorbed through the skin, topical corticosteroids are handled through pharmacokinetic pathways similar to systemically administered corticosteroids. Corticosteroids are bound to plasma proteins in varying degrees. Corticosteroids are metabolized primarily in the liver and are then excreted by the kidneys. Some of the topical corticosteroids and their metabolites are also excreted into the bile.

INDICATIONS AND USAGE

Topical corticosteroids are indicated for the relief of the inflammatory and pruritic manifestations of corticosteroid-responsive dermatoses.

CONTRAINDICATIONS

Topical corticosteroids are contraindicated in those patients with a history of hypersensitivity to any of the components of the preparation.

PRECAUTIONS

General: Systemic absorption of topical corticosteroids has produced reversible hypothalamic-pituitary-adrenal (HPA) axis suppression, manifestations of Cushing's syndrome, hyperglycemia, and glucosuria in some patients.

Conditions which augment systemic absorption include the application of the more potent steroids, use over large surface areas, prolonged use, and the addition of occlusive dressings.

If HPA axis suppression is noted (by using the urinary free cortisol and ACTH stimulation tests) an attempt should be made to withdraw the drug or to reduce the frequency of application.

Recovery of HPA axis function is generally prompt and complete upon discontinuation of the drug. Infrequently, signs and symptoms of steroid withdrawal may occur, requiring supplemental systemic corticosteroids.

Pediatric patients may absorb proportionally larger amounts of topical corticosteroids and thus be more susceptible to systemic toxicity (see PRECAUTIONS—Use in Pediatric Patients).

If irritation develops, topical corticosteroids should be discontinued and appropriate therapy instituted. In the presence of dermatological infections, the use of an appropriate antifungal or antibacterial agent should be instituted. If a favorable response does not occur promptly, the corticosteroid should be discontinued until the infection has been adequately controlled.

Information for the Patient: Patients using topical corticosteroids should receive the following information and instructions:
1. This medication is to be used as directed by the physician. It is for external use only. Avoid contact with the eyes.
2. Patients should be advised not to use this medication for any disorder other than for which it has been prescribed.
3. The treated skin area should not be bandaged or otherwise covered or wrapped as to be occlusive unless directed by the physician.
4. Patients should report any signs of local adverse reactions especially under occlusive dressing.
5. Parents of pediatric patients should be advised not to use tight-fitting diapers or plastic pants on a child being treated in the diaper area, as these garments may constitute occlusive dressings.

Laboratory Tests: The urinary free cortisol test and the ACTH stimulation test may be helpful in evaluating the HPA axis suppression.

Carcinogenesis, Mutagenesis, and Impairment of Fertility: Long-term animal studies have not been performed to evaluate the carcinogenic potential or the effect on fertility of topical corticosteroids. Studies to determine mutagenicity with hydrocortisone have revealed negative results.

Pregnancy Category C: Corticosteroids are generally teratogenic in laboratory animals when administered systemically at relatively low dosage levels. The more potent corticosteroids have been shown to be teratogenic after dermal application in laboratory animals. There are no adequate and well-controlled studies in pregnant women on teratogenic effects from topically applied corticosteroids.

Therefore, topical corticosteroids should be used during pregnancy only if the potential benefit justifies the potential risk to the fetus. Drugs of this class should not be used extensively on pregnant patients, in large amounts, or for prolonged periods of time.

Nursing Mothers: It is not known whether topical administration of corticosteroids could result in sufficient systemic absorption to produce detectable quantities in breast milk. Systemically administered corticosteroids are secreted into breast milk in quantities not likely to have a deleterious effect on the infant. Nevertheless, caution should be exercised when topical corticosteroids are administered to a nursing woman.

Use in Pediatric Patients: PEDIATRIC PATIENTS MAY DEMONSTRATE GREATER SUSCEPTIBILITY TO TOPICAL CORTICOSTEROID-INDUCED HPA AXIS SUPPRESSION AND CUSHING'S SYNDROME THAN MATURE PATIENTS BECAUSE OF A LARGER SKIN SURFACE AREA TO BODY WEIGHT RATIO.

Hypothalamic-pituitary-adrenal (HPA) axis suppression, Cushing's syndrome, and intracranial hypertension have been reported in pediatric patients receiving topical corticosteroids. Manifestations of adrenal suppression in pediatric patients include linear growth retardation, delayed weight gain, low plasma cortisol levels, and absence of response to ACTH stimulation. Manifestations of intracranial hypertension include bulging fontanelles, headaches, and bilateral papilledema.

Administration of topical corticosteroids to pediatric patients should be limited to the least amount compatible with an effective therapeutic regimen. Chronic corticosteroid therapy may interfere with the growth and development of pediatric patients.

ADVERSE REACTIONS

The following local adverse reactions are reported infrequently with topical corticosteroids, but may occur more frequently with the use of occlusive dressings. These reactions are listed in an approximate decreasing order of occurrence:
Burning
Itching
Irritation
Dryness
Folliculitis
Hypertrichosis
Acneiform eruptions
Hypopigmentation
Perioral dermatitis
Allergic contact dermatitis
Maceration of the skin
Secondary infection
Skin atrophy
Striae
Miliaria

OVERDOSAGE

Topically applied corticosteroids can be absorbed in sufficient amounts to produce systemic effects. (See PRECAUTIONS).

DOSAGE AND ADMINISTRATION

Anusol-HC 2.5% (Hydrocortisone Cream, USP) should be applied to the affected area two to four times daily depending on the severity of the condition.

Occlusive dressings may be used for the management of psoriasis or recalcitrant conditions. If an infection develops, the use of occlusive dressings should be discontinued and appropriate antimicrobial therapy instituted.

HOW SUPPLIED

Anusol-HC 2.5% (Hydrocortisone Cream, USP) is supplied in 30 gram tubes NDC 61570-313-11.

Store at controlled room temperature 15°–30°C (59°–86°F). Store away from heat. Protect from freezing.
Revised September 1996
Manufactured by
Allergan Herbert
Skin Care Division of Allergan, Inc.
Irvine, CA 92713 USA
Distributed by: Monarch Pharmaceuticals, Inc.
Bristol, TN 37620
Shown in Product Identification Guide, page 324

ANUSOL–HC® 25–mg SUPPOSITORIES   ℞
[ăn ′ū-sōl ″]
(Hydrocortisone Acetate)

DESCRIPTION

Each Anusol-HC 25-mg Suppository contains 25 mg hydrocortisone acetate in a hydrogenated cocoglyceride base. Hydrocortisone acetate is a corticosteroid. Chemically, hydrocortisone acetate is pregn-4-ene-3,20-dione, 21-(acetyloxy)-11,17-dihydroxy-,(11β) with the following structural formula:

CLINICAL PHARMACOLOGY

In normal subjects, about 26 percent of hydrocortisone acetate is absorbed when the hydrocortisone acetate suppository is applied to the rectum. Absorption of hydrocortisone acetate may vary across abraded or inflamed surfaces.

Topical steroids are primarily effective because of their antiinflammatory, antipruritic and vasoconstrictive action.

INDICATIONS AND USAGE

For use in inflamed hemorrhoids, post irradiation (factitial) proctitis, as an adjunct in the treatment of chronic ulcerative colitis, cryptitis, other inflammatory conditions of the anorectum, and pruritus ani.

CONTRAINDICATION

Anusol-HC suppositories are contraindicated in those patients with a history of hypersensitivity to any of the components.

PRECAUTIONS

Do not use unless adequate proctologic examination is made.

If irritation develops, the product should be discontinued and appropriate therapy instituted.

In the presence of an infection, the use of an appropriate antifungal or antibacterial agent should be instituted. If a favorable response does not occur promptly, the corticosteroid should be discontinued until the infection has been adequately controlled.

No long-term studies in animals have been performed to evaluate the carcinogenic potential of corticosteroid suppositories.

Information for Patients

Staining of fabric may occur with use of the suppository. Precautionary measures are recommended.

Continued on next page

Anusol-HC Suppositories—Cont.

Pregnancy Category C
In laboratory animals, topical steroids have been associated with an increase in the incidence of fetal abnormalities when gestating females have been exposed to rather low dosage levels. There are no adequate and well-controlled studies in pregnant women. Anusol-HC suppositories should only be used during pregnancy if the potential benefit justifies the risk to the fetus. Drugs of this class should not be used extensively on pregnant patients, in large amounts, or for prolonged periods of time.

It is not known whether this drug is excreted in human milk, and because many drugs are excreted in human milk and because of the potential for serious adverse reactions in nursing infants from Anusol-HC suppositories, a decision should be made whether to discontinue nursing or to discontinue the drug, taking into account the importance of the drug to the mother.

ADVERSE REACTIONS
The following local adverse reactions have been reported with corticosteroid suppositories:
1. Burning
2. Itching
3. Irritation
4. Dryness
5. Folliculitis
6. Hypopigmentation
7. Allergic Contact Dermatitis
8. Secondary infection

DRUG ABUSE AND DEPENDENCE
Drug abuse and dependence have not been reported in patients treated with Anusol-HC suppositories.

OVERDOSAGE
If signs and symptoms of systemic overdosage occur discontinue use.

DOSAGE AND ADMINISTRATION
Usual dosage: One suppository in the rectum morning and night for two weeks in nonspecific proctitis. In more severe cases, one suppository three times daily; or two suppositories twice daily. In factitial proctitis, recommended therapy is six to eight weeks or less, according to response.

OPENING INSTRUCTIONS

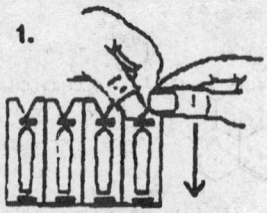
1.

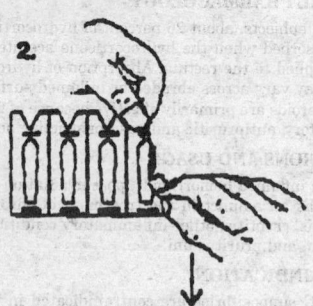
2.

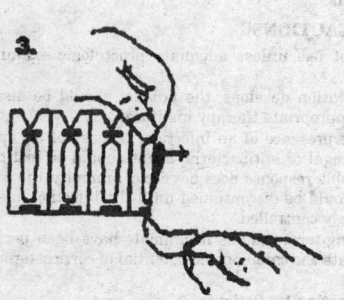
3.

Avoid excessive handling of the suppository. It is designed to melt at body temperature.

1. Tear at the "V" cut and peel the foil in a downward motion.
2. Continue tearing downward to almost the full length of the suppository.
3. Gently remove the suppository from the foil packet.

HOW SUPPLIED
Anusol-HC 25-mg Suppositories are off-white, smooth surfaced, rod shaped with one rounded end. Package of 12 suppositories NDC 61570-172-61 and package of 24 suppositories NDC 61570-172-62.

Store below 30° C (86° F). Protect from freezing.
Revised September 1993
Rx only
Manufactured by: Alpharma USPD Inc.
Baltimore, MD 21244
Shown in Product Identification Guide, page 324
Distributed by: Monarch Pharmaceuticals, Inc.
Bristol, TN 37620

CHLOROMYCETIN® OPHTHALMIC ℞
[chlōrō ' mycētin]
(Chloramphenicol for Ophthalmic Solution, USP)

> **WARNING**
> Bone marrow hypoplasia including aplastic anemia and death has been reported following local application of chloramphenicol. Chloramphenicol should not be used when less potentially dangerous agents would be expected to provide effective treatment

DESCRIPTION
Each vial of Chloromycetin Ophthalmic contains 25 mg of Chloromycetin (chloramphenicol) with boric acid-sodium borate buffer. Sodium hydroxide may have been added for adjustment of pH. A 15 mL bottle of Sterile Distilled Water is included in each package for use as a diluent in the preparation of a solution of Chloromycetin suitable for ophthalmic use. By varying the quantity of diluent used, solutions ranging in strength from 0.16% to 0.5% may be prepared. Both the powder for solution and the diluent contain no preservatives. Sterile powder.
The chemical names for chloramphenicol are
(1) Acetamide, 2,2-dichloro-*N*-[2-hydroxy-1-(hydroxymethyl)-2-(4-nitrophenyl) ethyl]-, and
(2) D-*tbreo*(—)-2,2-Dichloro-*N*-[β-hydroxy-α-(hydroxymethyl)-*p*-nitrophenethyl] acetamide.
Chloramphenicol has the following empirical and structural formulas:

$$O_2N-C_6H_4-\underset{H}{\overset{OH}{C}}-\underset{NHCOCHCl_2}{\overset{H}{C}}-CH_2OH$$

$C_{11}H_{12}Cl_2N_2O_3$ Mol. Wt. 323.13

CLINICAL PHARMACOLOGY
Chloramphenicol is a broad-spectrum antibiotic originally isolated from *Streptomyces venezuelae*. It is primarily bacteriostatic and acts by inhibition of protein synthesis by interfering with the transfer or activated amino acids from soluble RNA to ribosomes. It has been noted that chloramphenicol is found in measurable amounts in the aqueous humor following local application to the eye. Development of resistance to chloramphenicol can be regarded as minimal for staphylococci and many other species of bacteria.

INDICATIONS AND USAGE
Chloramphenicol should be used only in those serious infections for which less potentially dangerous drugs are ineffective or contraindicated. Bacteriological studies should be performed to determine the causative organisms and their sensitivity to chloramphenicol (see Boxed Warning).
Chloromycetin Ophthalmic (Chloramphenicol for Ophthalmic Solution, USP) is indicated for the treatment of surface ocular infections involving the conjunctiva and/or cornea caused by chloramphenicol-susceptible organisms.
The particular antiinfective drug in this product is active against the following common bacterial eye pathogens:
Staphylococcus aureus
Streptococci, including *Streptococcus pneumoniae*
Escherichia coli
Haemophilus influenzae
Klebsiella / Enterobacter species
Moraxella lacunata
(Morax-Axenfeld bacillus)
Neisseria species

The product does not provide adequate coverage against:
Pseudomonas aeruginosa
Serratia marcescens

CONTRAINDICATIONS
This product is contraindicated in persons sensitive to any of its components.

WARNINGS
SEE BOXED WARNING

PRECAUTIONS
The prolonged use of antibiotics may occasionally result in overgrowth of nonsusceptible organisms, including fungi. If new infections appear during medication, the drug should be discontinued and appropriate measures should be taken. In all serious infections the topical use of chloramphenicol should be supplemented by appropriate systemic medication.

ADVERSE REACTIONS
Blood dyscrasias have been reported in association with the use of chloramphenicol (see WARNINGS).
Transient burning or stinging sensations may occur with use of Chloromycetin Ophthalmic Solution.

DOSAGE AND ADMINISTRATION
Two drops applied to the affected eye every three hours, or more frequently if deemed advisable by the prescribing physician. Administration should be continued day and night for the first 48 hours, after which the interval between applications may be increased. Treatment should be continued for at least 48 hours after the eye appears normal.

Directions for dispensing—Prepare solution by adding sterile distilled water to the vial as follows:

Strength of solution desired	Add sterile distilled water
0.5%	5 mL
0.25%	10 mL
0.16%	15 mL

Solutions remain stable at room temperature for ten days.

HOW SUPPLIED
NDC 61570-321-31 Chloromycetin Ophthalmic (Chloramphenicol for Ophthalmic Solution, USP) is supplied in a package containing dry ingredients in a 15 mL vial and also a vial containing 15 mL of Sterile Distilled Water for use as a diluent in preparing the solution for ophthalmic use. A sterilized dropper-cap assembly for use on the vial of solution is included in the package.
Store below 30°C (86°F).
Chloromycetin, brand of chloramphenicol. Reg US Pat Off
Rx only
Distributed by: Monarch Pharmaceuticals, Inc.
Bristol, TN 37620

CHLOROMYCETIN® ℞
Ophthalmic Ointment, 1%
[chlorō mycētin]
(Chloramphenicol Ophthalmic Ointment, USP)

> **WARNING**
> Bone marrow hypoplasia including aplastic anemia and death has been reported following local application of chloramphenicol. Chloramphenicol should not be used when less potentially dangerous agents would be expected to provide effective treatment.

DESCRIPTION
Each gram of Chloromycetin Ophthalmic Ointment, 1% contains 10 mg chloramphenicol in a special base of liquid petrolatum and polyethylene. It contains no preservatives. Sterile ointment.
The chemical names for chloramphenicol are:
(1) Acetamide, 2,2-dichloro-*N*-[2-hydroxy-1-(hydroxymethyl)-2-(4-nitrophenyl) ethyl]-, and
(2) D-*threo*-(—)-2,2-Dichloro-*N*-[β-hydroxy-α-(hydroxymethyl)-*p*-nitrophenethyl] acetamide.
Chloramphenicol has the following empirical and structural formulas:

$$O_2N-C_6H_4-\underset{H}{\overset{OH}{C}}-\underset{NHCOCHCl_2}{\overset{H}{C}}-CH_2OH$$

$C_{11}H_{12}Cl_2N_2O_5$ Mol Wt 323.13

CLINICAL PHARMACOLOGY
Chloramphenicol is a broad-spectrum antibiotic originally isolated from *Streptomyces venezuelae*. It is primarily bacteriostatic and acts by inhibition of protein synthesis by interfering with the transfer of activated amino acids from soluble RNA to ribosomes. It has been noted that chloramphenicol is found in measurable amounts in the aqueous humor following local application to the eye. Development of resistance to chloramphenicol can be regarded as minimal for staphylococci and many other species of bacteria.

INDICATIONS AND USAGE

Chloramphenicol should be used only in those serious infections for which less potentially dangerous drugs are ineffective or contraindicated. Bacteriological studies should be performed to determine the causative organisms and their sensitivity to chloramphenicol (see Boxed Warning). Chloromycetin Ophthalmic Ointment, 1% (Chloramphenicol Ophthalmic Ointment, USP) is indicated for the treatment of surface ocular infections involving the conjunctiva and/or cornea caused by chloramphenicol-susceptible organisms. The particular antiinfective drug in this product is active against the following common bacterial eye pathogens:

Staphylococcus aureus
Streptococci, including *Streptococcus pneumoniae*
Escherichia coli
Haemophilus influenzae
Klebsiella / Enterobacter species
Moraxella lacunata
  (Morax-Axenfeld bacillus)
Neisseria species
The product does not provide adequate coverage against:
Pseudomonas aeruginosa
Serratia marcescens

CONTRAINDICATIONS

This product is contraindicated in persons sensitive to any of its components.

WARNINGS

SEE BOXED WARNING
Ophthalmic ointments may retard corneal wound healing.

PRECAUTIONS

The prolonged use of antibiotics may occasionally result in overgrowth of nonsusceptible organisms, including fungi. If new infections appear during medication, the drug should be discontinued and appropriate measures should be taken. In all serious infections the topical use of chloramphenicol should be supplemented by appropriate systemic medication.

ADVERSE REACTIONS

Blood dyscrasias have been reported in association with the use of chloramphenicol (see WARNINGS).
Allergic or inflammatory reactions due to individual hypersensitivity and occasional burning or stinging may occur with the use of Chloromycetin Ophthalmic Ointment.

DOSAGE AND ADMINISTRATION

A small amount of ointment placed in the lower conjunctival sac every three hours, or more frequently if deemed advisable by the prescribing physician. Administration should be continued day and night for the first 48 hours, after which the interval between applications may be increased. Treatment should be continued for at least 48 hours after the eye appears normal.

HOW SUPPLIED

N DC 61570-307-01
Chloromycetin Ophthalmic Ointment, 1% (Chloramphenicol Ophthalmic Ointment, USP) is supplied, sterile, in ophthalmic ointment tubes of 3.5 grams.
Chloromycetin, brand of chloramphenicol. Reg US Pat Off
Rx only.
Distributed by: Monarch Pharmaceuticals, Inc., Bristol, TN 37620

COLY-MYCIN® M PARENTERAL   ℞

[cŏly-mycĭn]
(Sterile Colistimethate Sodium, USP)

FOR INTRAMUSCULAR AND INTRAVENOUS USE

DESCRIPTION

Coly-Mycin® M Parenteral (Sterile Colistimethate Sodium, USP) is a sterile parenteral antibiotic product which, when reconstituted (see Reconstitution), is suitable for intramuscular or intravenous administration.
Each vial contains colistimethate sodium or pentasodium colistinmethanesulfonate (150 mg colistin base activity). Colistimethate sodium is a polypeptide antibiotic with an approximate molecular weight of 1750. The empirical formula is $C_{58}H_{105}N_{16}Na_5O_{28}S_5$ and the structural formula is represented below:

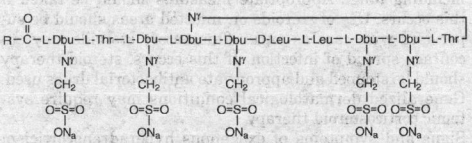

Dbu is 2, 4-diaminobutanoic acid, R is 5-methylheptyl in colistin A and
5-methylhexyl in colistin B

TABLE 1. Suggested Modification of Dosage Schedules of Coly-Mycin M Parenteral for Adults with Impaired Renal Function

Renal Function		Degree of Impairment		
	Normal	Mild	Moderate	Considerable
Plasma creatinine, mg/100 mL	0.7–1.2	1.3–1.5	1.6–2.5	2.6–4.0
Urea clearance, % of normal	80–100	40–70	25–40	10–25
Dosage				
Unit dose of Coly-Mycin M, mg	100–150	75–115	66–150	100–150
Frequency, times/day	4 to 2	2	2 or 1	every 36 hr
Total daily dose, mg	300	150–230	133–150	100
Approximate daily dose, mg/kg/day	5.0	2.5–3.8	2.5	1.5

CLINICAL PHARMACOLOGY

Typical serum and urine levels following a single 150 mg dose of Coly-Mycin M Parenteral IM or IV in normal adult subjects are shown in Figure 1.

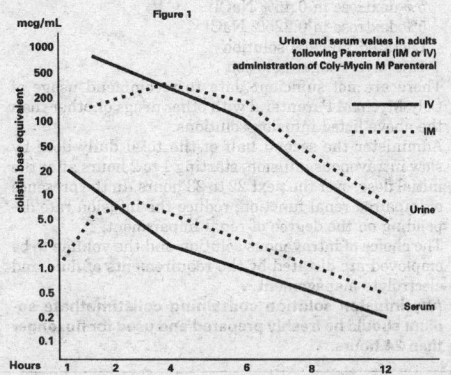

Higher serum levels were obtained at 10 minutes following IV administration. Serum concentration declined with a half-life of 2–3 hours following either intravenous or intramuscular administration in adults and in the pediatric population, including premature infants.
Average urine levels ranged from about 270 mcg/mL at 2 hours to about 15 mcg/mL at 8 hours after intravenous administration and from 200 to about 25 mcg/mL during a similar period following intramuscular administration.
Microbiology: Colistimethate sodium is a surface active agent which penetrates into and disrupts the bacterial cell membrane. It has been shown to have bactericidal activity against most strains of the following microorganisms, both *in vitro* and in clinical infections as described in the INDICATIONS AND USAGE section:
Aerobic gram-negative microorganisms:
Enterobacter aerogenes, Escherichia coli, Klebsiella pneumoniae, and *Pseudomonas aeruginosa*
Susceptibility Tests: Colistimethate sodium is no longer listed as an antimicrobial for routine testing and reporting by clinical microbiology laboratories.

INDICATIONS AND USAGE

Coly-Mycin M Parenteral is indicated for the treatment of acute or chronic infections due to sensitive strains of certain gram-negative bacilli. It is particularly indicated when the infection is caused by sensitive strains of *Pseudomonas aeruginosa*. This antibiotic is not indicated for infections due to *Proteus* or *Neisseria.* Coly-Mycin M Parenteral has proven clinically effective in treatment of infections due to the following gram-negative organisms: *Enterobacter aerogenes, Escherichia coli, Klebsiella pneumoniae,* and *Pseudomonas aeruginosa.*
Coly-Mycin M Parenteral may be used to initiate therapy in serious infections that are suspected to be due to gram-negative organisms and in the treatment of infections due to susceptible gram-negative pathogenic bacilli.

CONTRAINDICATIONS

The use of Coly-Mycin M Parenteral is contraindicated for patients with a history of sensitivity to the drug or any of its components.

WARNINGS

Maximum daily dose should not exceed 5 mg/kg/day (2.3 mg/lb) with normal renal function.

Transient neurological disturbances may occur. These include circumoral paresthesia or numbness, tingling or formication of the extremities, generalized pruritus, vertigo, dizziness, and slurring of speech. For these reasons, patients should be warned not to drive vehicles or use hazardous machinery while on therapy. Reduction of dosage may alleviate symptoms. Therapy need not be discontinued, but such patients should be observed with particular care.
Nephrotoxicity can occur and is probably a dose-dependent effect of colistimethate sodium. These manifestations of nephrotoxicity are reversible following discontinuation of the antibiotic.
Overdosage can result in renal insufficiency, muscle weakness, and apnea (see OVERDOSAGE section). See PRECAUTIONS, Drug Interactions subsection for use concomitantly with other antibiotics and curariform drugs.
Respiratory arrest has been reported following intramuscular administration of colistimethate sodium. Impaired renal function increases the possibility of apnea and neuromuscular blockade following administration of colistimethate sodium. Therefore, it is important to follow recommended dosing guidelines. See DOSAGE AND ADMINISTRATION section for use in renal impairment.
Pseudomembranous colitis has been reported with nearly all antimicrobial agents, and may range in severity from mild to life-threatening. Therefore, it is important to consider this diagnosis in patients who present with diarrhea subsequent to the administration of antibacterial agents
Treatment with antibacterial agents alters the normal flora of the colon and may permit overgrowth of clostridia. Studies indicate that a toxin produced by *Clostridium difficile* is a primary cause of "antibiotic-associated colitis."
After the diagnosis of pseudomembranous colitis has been established, appropriate therapeutic measures should be initiated. Mild cases of pseudomembranous colitis usually respond to drug discontinuation alone. In moderate-to-severe cases, consideration should be given to management with fluids and electrolytes, protein supplementation, and treatment with an antibacterial drug clinically effective against *Clostridium difficile* colitis.

PRECAUTIONS

General
Since Coly-Mycin M Parenteral is eliminated mainly by renal excretion, it should be used with caution when the possibility of impaired renal function exists. The decline in renal function with advanced age should be considered.
When actual renal impairment is present, Coly-Mycin M Parenteral may be used, but the greatest caution should be exercised and the dosage should be reduced in proportion to the extent of the impairment. Administration of amounts of Coly-Mycin M Parenteral in excess of renal excretory capacity will lead to high serum levels and can result in further impairment of renal function, initiating a cycle which, if not recognized, can lead to acute renal insufficiency, renal shutdown, and further concentration of the antibiotic to toxic levels in the body. At this point, interference of nerve transmission at neuromuscular junctions may occur and result in muscle weakness and apnea (see OVERDOSAGE section). Signs indicating the development of impaired renal function include: diminishing urine output, rising BUN and serum creatinine and decreased creatinine clearance. Therapy

Continued on next page

Coly-Mycin M—Cont.

with Coly-Mycin M Parenteral should be discontinued immediately if signs of impaired renal function occur. However, if it is necessary to reinstate the drug, dosing should be adjusted accordingly after drug plasma levels have fallen (see DOSAGE AND ADMINISTRATION section).

Drug Interactions

Certain other antibiotics (aminoglycosides and polymyxin) have also been reported to interfere with the nerve transmission at the neuromuscular junction. Based on this reported activity, they should not be given concomitantly with Coly-Mycin M Parenteral except with the greatest caution. Curariform muscle relaxants (eg, tubocurarine) and other drugs, including ether, succinylcholine, gallamine, decamethonium and sodium citrate, potentiate the neuromuscular blocking effect and should be used with extreme caution in patients being treated with Coly-Mycin M Parenteral. Sodium cephalothin may enhance the nephrotoxicity of Coly-Mycin M Parenteral. The concomitant use of sodium cephalothin and Coly-Mycin M Parenteral should be avoided.

Carcinogenesis, Mutagenesis, Impairment of Fertility

Long-term animal carcinogenicity studies and genetic toxicology studies have not been performed with colistimethate sodium. There were no adverse effects on fertility or reproduction in rats at doses of 9.3 mg/kg/day (0.30 times the maximum daily human dose when based on mg/mm²).

Pregnancy - Teratogenic Effects

Pregnancy Category C: Colistimethate sodium given intramuscularly during organogenesis to rabbits at 4.15 and 9.3 mg/kg resulted in talipes varus in 2.6% and 2.9% of fetuses, respectively. These doses are 0.25 and 0.55 times the maximum daily human dose based on mg/mm². In addition, increased resorption occurred at 9.3 mg/kg. Colistimethate sodium was not teratogenic in rats at 4.15 or 9.3 mg/kg. These doses are 0.13 and 0.30 times the maximum daily human dose based on mg/mm². There are no adequate and well-controlled studies in pregnant women. Since colistimethate sodium is transferred across the placental barrier in humans, it should be used during pregnancy only if the potential benefit justifies the potential risk to the fetus.

Nursing Mothers

It is not known whether colistimethate sodium is excreted in human breast milk. However, colistin sulphate is excreted in human breast milk. Therefore, caution should be exercised when colistimethate sodium is administered to nursing women.

Pediatric Use

In clinical studies, colistimethate sodium was administered to the pediatric population (neonates, infants, children and adolescents). Although adverse reactions appear to be similar in the adult and pediatric populations, subjective symptoms of toxicity may not be reported by pediatric patients. Close clinical monitoring of pediatric patients is recommended.

ADVERSE REACTIONS

The following adverse reactions have been reported:
Gastrointestinal: gastrointestinal upset
Nervous System: tingling of extremities and tongue, slurred speech, dizziness, vertigo and paresthesia
Integumentary: generalized itching, urticaria and rash
Body as a Whole: fever
Laboratory Deviations: increased blood urea nitrogen (BUN), elevated creatinine and decreased creatinine clearance
Respiratory System: respiratory distress and apnea
Renal System: nephrotoxicity and decreased urine output

OVERDOSAGE

Overdosage with colistimethate sodium can cause neuromuscular blockade characterized by paresthesia, lethargy, confusion, dizziness, ataxia, nystagmus, disorders of speech and apnea. Respiratory muscle paralysis may lead to apnea, respiratory arrest and death.

Overdosage with the drug can also cause acute renal failure, manifested as decreased urine output and increases in serum concentrations of BUN and creatinine.

As in any case of overdose, colistimethate sodium therapy should be discontinued and general supportive measures should be utilized.

It is unknown whether colistimethate sodium can be removed by hemodialysis or peritoneal dialysis in overdose cases.

DOSAGE AND ADMINISTRATION

Important: Coly-Mycin M Parenteral is supplied in vials containing colistimethate sodium equivalent to 150 mg colistin base activity per vial.

Reconstitution: The **150 mg** vial should be reconstituted with **2.0 mL** Sterile Water for Injection, USP. The reconstituted solution provides colistimethate sodium at a concentration equivalent to 75 mg/mL colistin base activity. During reconstitution swirl **gently** to avoid frothing.

Parenteral drug products should be inspected visually for particulate matter and discoloration prior to administration, whenever solution and container permit. If these conditions are observed, the product should not be used.

Dosage

Adults and pediatric patients—Intravenous or Intramuscular Administration: Coly-Mycin M Parenteral should be given in 2 to 4 divided doses at dose levels of 2.5 to 5 mg/kg per day for patients with normal renal function, depending on the severity of the infection.

In obese individuals, dosage should be based on ideal body weight.

The daily dose should be reduced in the presence of renal impairment. Modifications of dosage in the presence of renal impairment are presented in Table 1.

[See table 1 on previous page]

Note: The suggested unit dose is 2.5–5 mg/kg; however, the time INTERVAL between injections should be increased in the presence of impaired renal function.

INTRAVENOUS ADMINISTRATION

1. Direct Intermittent Administration—Slowly inject one-half of the total daily dose over a period of 3 to 5 minutes every 12 hours.

2. Continuous Infusion—Slowly inject one-half of the total daily dose over 3 to 5 minutes. Add the remaining half of the total daily dose of Coly-Mycin M Parenteral to one of the following:

   0.9% NaCl
   5% dextrose in 0.9% NaCl
   5% dextrose in water
   5% dextrose in 0.45% NaCl
   5% dextrose in 0.225% NaCl
   Lactated Ringer's solution
   10% invert sugar solution

There are not sufficient data to recommend usage of Coly-Mycin M Parenteral with other drugs or other than the above listed infusion solutions.

Administer the second half of the total daily dose by slow intravenous infusion, starting 1 to 2 hours after the initial dose, over the next 22 to 23 hours. In the presence of impaired renal function, reduce the infusion rate depending on the degree of renal impairment.

The choice of intravenous solution and the volume to be employed are dictated by the requirements of fluid and electrolyte management.

Any infusion solution containing colistimethate sodium should be freshly prepared and used for no longer than 24 hours.

HOW SUPPLIED

Coly-Mycin M Parenteral is supplied in vials containing colistimethate sodium (equivalent to 150 mg colistin base activity per vial) as a white to slightly yellow lyophilized cake and is available as one vial per carton NDC 61570-414-51

Store between 15°–30°C (59°–86°F).

Store reconstituted solution in refrigerator 2°–8°C (36°–46°F) or between 15°–30°C (59°–86°F) and use within 7 days.

Rx only.

Distributed by: Monarch Pharmaceuticals, Inc,. Bristol, TN 37620

Shown in Product Identification Guide, page 324

CORTISPORIN® Cream ℞

[cŏr 'tĭ-spŏrin']

(neomycin and polymyxin B sulfates and hydrocortisone acetate cream, USP)

DESCRIPTION

CORTISPORIN Cream (neomycin and polymyxin B sulfates and hydrocortisone acetate cream, USP) is a topical antibacterial cream. Each gram contains: neomycin sulfate equivalent to 3.5 mg neomycin base, polymyxin B sulfate equivalent to 10,000 polymyxin B units, and hydrocortisone acetate 5 mg (0.5%). The inactive ingredients are liquid petrolatum, white petrolatum, propylene glycol, polyoxyethylene polyoxypropylene compound, emulsifying wax, purified water, and 0.25% methylparaben added as a preservative. Sodium hydroxide or sulfuric acid may be added to adjust pH.

Neomycin sulfate is the sulfate salt of neomycin B and C, which are produced by the growth of *Streptomyces fradiae* Waksman (Fam. Streptomycetaceae). It has a potency equivalent of not less than 600 µg of neomycin standard per mg, calculated on an anhydrous basis. The structural formulae are:

[See chemical structure at top of next column]

Polymyxin B sulfate is the sulfate salt of polymyxin B_1 and B_2, which are produced by the growth of *Bacillus polymyxa* (Prazmowski) Migula (Fam. Bacillaceae). It has a potency of

Neomycin B (R_1=H, R_2=CH$_2$NH$_2$)
Neomycin C (R_1=CH$_2$NH$_2$, R_2=H)

not less than 6,000 polymyxin B units per mg, calculated on an anhydrous basis. The structural formulae are:

Polymyxin B_1 (R=CH$_3$)
Polymyxin B_2 (R=H)
DAB=α,γ-diaminobutyric acid

Hydrocortisone acetate is the acetate ester of hydrocortisone, an anti-inflammatory hormone. Its chemical name is 21-(acetyloxy)-11β,17-dihydroxypregn-4-ene-3,20-dione. Its structural formula is:

The base is a smooth vanishing cream with a pH of approximately 5.0.

CLINICAL PHARMACOLOGY

Corticoids suppress the inflammatory response to a variety of agents and they may delay healing. Since corticoids may inhibit the body's defense mechanism against infection, a concomitant antimicrobial drug may be used when this inhibition is considered to be clinically significant in a particular case.

The anti-infective components in the combination are included to provide action against specific organisms susceptible to them. Polymyxin B sulfate and neomycin sulfate together are considered active against the following microorganisms:

Staphylococcus aureus, Escherichia coli, Haemophilus influenzae, Klebsiella-Enterobacter species, *Neisseria* species, and *Pseudomonas aeruginosa*. The product does not provide adequate coverage against *Serratia marcescens* and streptococci, including *Streptococcus pneumoniae*.

The relative potency of corticosteroids depends on the molecular structure, concentration, and release from the vehicle.

The acid pH helps restore normal cutaneous acidity. Owing to its excellent spreading and penetrating properties, the cream facilitates treatment of hairy and intertriginous areas. It may also be of value in selective cases where the lesions are moist.

INDICATIONS AND USAGE

For the treatment of corticosteroid-responsive dermatoses with secondary infection. It has not been demonstrated that this steroid-antibiotic combination provides greater benefit than the steroid component alone after 7 days of treatment (see WARNINGS).

CONTRAINDICATIONS

Not for use in the eyes or in the external ear canal if the eardrum is perforated. This product is contraindicated in tuberculous, fungal, or viral lesions of the skin (herpes simplex, vaccinia, and varicella). This product is contraindicated in those individuals who have shown hypersensitivity to any of its components.

WARNINGS

Because of the concern of nephrotoxicity and ototoxicity associated with neomycin, this combination should not be used over a wide area or for extended periods of time.

PRECAUTIONS

General: As with any antibacterial preparation, prolonged use may result in overgrowth of nonsusceptible organisms, including fungi. Appropriate measures should be taken if this occurs. Use of steroids on infected areas should be supervised with care as anti-inflammatory steroids may encourage spread of infection. If this occurs, steroid therapy should be stopped and appropriate antibacterial drugs used. Generalized dermatological conditions may require systemic corticosteroid therapy.

Signs and symptoms of exogenous hyperadrenocorticism can occur with the use of topical corticosteroids, including adrenal suppression. Systemic absorption of topically ap-

plied steroids will be increased if extensive body surface areas are treated or if occlusive dressings are used. Under these circumstances, suitable precautions should be taken when long-term use is anticipated.

Specifically, sufficient percutaneous absorption of hydrocortisone can occur in pediatric patients during prolonged use to cause cessation of growth, as well as other systemic signs and symptoms of hyperadrenocorticism.

Information for Patients: If redness, irritation, swelling or pain persists or increases, discontinue use and notify physician. Do not use in the eyes.

Laboratory Tests: Systemic effects of excessive levels of hydrocortisone may include a reduction in the number of circulating eosinophils and a decrease in urinary excretion of 17-hydroxycorticosteroids.

Carcinogenesis, Mutagenesis, Impairment of Fertility: Long-term studies in animals (rats, rabbits, mice) showed no evidence of carcinogenicity attributable to oral administration of corticosteroids.

Pregnancy: *Teratogenic Effects:* Pregnancy Category C. Corticosteroids have been shown to be teratogenic in rabbits when applied topically at concentrations of 0.5% on days 6 to 18 of gestation and in mice when applied topically at a concentration of 15% on days 10 to 13 of gestation. There are no adequate and well-controlled studies in pregnant women. Corticosteroids should be used during pregnancy only if the potential benefit justifies the potential risk to the fetus.

Nursing Mothers: Hydrocortisone acetate appears in human milk following oral administration of the drug. Since systemic absorption of hydrocortisone may occur when applied topically, caution should be exercised when CORTISPORIN Cream is used by a nursing woman.

Pediatric Use: Safety and effectiveness in pediatric patients have not been established (see PRECAUTIONS: General).

ADVERSE REACTIONS

Neomycin occasionally causes skin sensitization. Ototoxicity and nephrotoxicity have also been reported (see WARNINGS). Adverse reactions have occurred with topical use of antibiotic combinations including neomycin and polymyxin B. Exact incidence figures are not available since no denominator of treated patients is available. The reaction occurring most often is allergic sensitization. In one clinical study, using a 20% neomycin patch, neomycin-induced allergic skin reactions occurred in two of 2,175 (0.09%) individuals in the general population.[1] In another study, the incidence was found to be approximately 1%.[2]

The following local adverse reactions have been reported with topical corticosteroids, especially under occlusive dressings: burning, itching, irritation, dryness, folliculitis, hypertrichosis, acneiform eruptions, hypopigmentation, perioral dermatitis, allergic contact dermatitis, maceration of the skin, secondary infection, skin atrophy, striae, and miliaria.

When steroid preparations are used for long periods of time in intertriginous areas or over extensive body areas, with or without occlusive non-permeable dressings, striae may occur; also there exists the possibility of systemic side effects when steroid preparations are used over large areas or for a long period of time.

DOSAGE AND ADMINISTRATION

A small quantity of the cream should be applied 2 to 4 times daily, as required. The cream should, if conditions permit, be gently rubbed into the affected areas.

HOW SUPPLIED

Tube of 7.5 g (NDC 61570-032-75).

Store at 15° to 25°C (59° to 77°F).

Rx only

REFERENCES

1. Leyden JJ, Kligman AM. Contact dermatitis to neomycin sulfate. *JAMA.* 1979;242:1276-1278.
2. Prystowsky SD, Allen AM, Smith RW, et al. Allergic contact hypersensitivity to nickel, neomycin, ethylenediamine, and benzocaine. *Arch Dermatol.* 1979;115:959-962.

Distributed by: Monarch Pharmaceuticals, Inc., Bristol, TN 37620

Manufactured by: Catalytica Pharmaceuticals, Inc., Greenville, NC 27834

Rev. 1/98

CORTISPORIN® Ointment   ℞

[cŏr′tĭ-spōrin]

(neomycin and polymyxin B sulfates, bacitracin zinc, and hydrocortisone ointment, USP)

DESCRIPTION

CORTISPORIN Ointment (neomycin and polymyxin B sulfates, bacitracin zinc, and hydrocortisone ointment, USP) is a topical antibacterial ointment. Each gram contains: neomycin sulfate equivalent to 3.5 mg neomycin base, polymyxin B sulfate equivalent to 5,000 polymyxin B units, bacitracin zinc equivalent to 400 bacitracin units, hydrocortisone 10 mg (1%), and white petrolatum, qs.

Neomycin sulfate is the sulfate salt of neomycin B and C, which are produced by the growth of *Streptomyces fradiae* Waksman (Fam. Streptomycetaceae). It has a potency equivalent of not less than 600 µg of neomycin standard per mg, calculated on an anhydrous basis. The structural formulae are:

Neomycin B (R_1=H, R_2=CH_2NH_2)
Neomycin C (R_1=CH_2NH_2, R_2=H)

Polymyxin B sulfate is the sulfate salt of polymyxin B_1 and B_2, which are produced by the growth of *Bacillus polymyxa* (Prazmowski) Migula (Fam. Bacillaceae). It has a potency of not less than 6,000 polymyxin B units per mg, calculated on an anhydrous basis. The structural formulae are:

Polymyxin B_1 (R=CH_3)
Polymyxin B_2 (R=H)
DAB=α,γ-diaminobutyric acid

Bacitracin zinc is the zinc salt of bacitracin, a mixture of related cyclic polypeptides (mainly bacitracin A) produced by the growth of an organism of the *licheniformis* group of *Bacillus subtilis* (Fam. Bacillaceae). It has a potency of not less than 40 bacitracin units per mg. The structural formula is:

Hydrocortisone, 11β,17,21-trihydroxypregn-4-ene-3, 20-dione, is an anti-inflammatory hormone. Its structural formula is:

CLINICAL PHARMACOLOGY

Corticoids suppress the inflammatory response to a variety of agents and they may delay healing. Since corticoids may inhibit the body's defense mechanism against infection, a concomitant antimicrobial drug may be used when this inhibition is considered to be clinically significant in a particular case.

The anti-infective components in the combination are included to provide action against specific organisms susceptible to them. Polymyxin B sulfate, bacitracin zinc, and neomycin sulfate are considered active against the following microorganisms: *Staphylococcus aureus,* streptococci, including *Streptococcus pneumoniae, Escherichia coli, Haemophilus influenzae, Klebsiella-Enterobacter* species, *Neisseria* species, and *Pseudomonas aeruginosa.*

The product does not provide adequate coverage against *Serratia marcescens.*

The relative potency of corticosteroids depends on the molecular structure, concentration, and release from the vehicle.

INDICATIONS AND USAGE

For the treatment of corticosteroid-responsive dermatoses with secondary infection. It has not been demonstrated that this steroid-antibiotic combination provides greater benefit than the steroid component alone after 7 days of treatment (see WARNINGS).

CONTRAINDICATIONS

Not for use in the eyes or in the external ear canal if the eardrum is perforated. This product is contraindicated in tuberculous, fungal, or viral lesions of the skin (herpes simplex, vaccinia, and varicella). This product is contraindicated in those individuals who have shown hypersensitivity to any of its components.

WARNINGS

Because of the concern of nephrotoxicity and ototoxicity associated with neomycin, this combination should not be used over a wide area or for extended periods of time.

PRECAUTIONS

General: As with any antibiotic preparation, prolonged use may result in the overgrowth of nonsusceptible organisms, including fungi. Appropriate measures should be taken if this occurs. Use of steroids on infected areas should be supervised with care as anti-inflammatory steroids may encourage spread of infection. If this occurs, steroid therapy should be stopped and appropriate antibacterial drugs used. Generalized dermatological conditions may require systemic corticosteroid therapy.

Signs and symptoms of exogenous hyperadrenocorticism can occur with the use of topical corticosteroids, including adrenal suppression. Systemic absorption of topically applied steroids will be increased if extensive body surface areas are treated or if occlusive dressings are used. Under these circumstances, suitable precautions should be taken when long-term use is anticipated.

Specifically, sufficient percutaneous absorption of hydrocortisone can occur in pediatric patients during prolonged use to cause cessation of growth, as well as other systemic signs and symptoms of hyperadrenocorticism.

Information for Patients: If redness, irritation, swelling, or pain persists or increases, discontinue use and notify physician. Do not use in the eyes.

Laboratory Tests: Systemic effects of excessive levels of hydrocortisone may include a reduction in the number of circulating eosinophils and a decrease in urinary excretion of 17-hydroxycorticosteroids.

Carcinogenesis, Mutagenesis, Impairment of Fertility: Long-term studies in animals (rats, rabbits, mice) showed no evidence of carcinogenicity attributable to oral administration of corticosteroids.

Pregnancy: *Teratogenic Effects:* Pregnancy Category C. Corticosteroids have been shown to be teratogenic in rabbits when applied topically at concentrations of 0.5% on days 6 to 18 of gestation and in mice when applied topically at a concentration of 15% on days 10 to 13 of gestation. There are no adequate and well-controlled studies in pregnant women. Corticosteroids should be used during pregnancy only if the potential benefit justifies the potential risk to the fetus.

Nursing Mothers: Hydrocortisone appears in human milk following oral administration of the drug. Since systemic absorption of hydrocortisone may occur when applied topically, caution should be exercised when CORTISPORIN Ointment is used by a nursing woman.

Pediatric Use: Safety and effectiveness in pediatric patients have not been established (see PRECAUTIONS: General).

ADVERSE REACTIONS

Neomycin occasionally causes skin sensitization. Ototoxicity and nephrotoxicity have also been reported (see WARNINGS). Adverse reactions have occurred with topical use of antibiotic combinations including neomycin, bacitracin, and polymyxin B. Exact incidence figures are not available since no denominator of treated patients is available. The reaction occurring most often is allergic sensitization. In one clinical study, using a 20% neomycin patch, neomycin-induced allergic skin reactions occurred in two of 2,175 (0.09%) individuals in the general population.[1] In another study, the incidence was found to be approximately 1%.[2]

The following local adverse reactions have been reported with topical corticosteroids, especially under occlusive dressings: burning, itching, irritation, dryness, folliculitis, hypertrichosis, acneiform eruptions, hypopigmentation, perioral dermatitis, allergic contact dermatitis, maceration of the skin, secondary infection, skin atrophy, striae, and miliaria.

When steroid preparations are used for long periods of time in intertriginous areas or over extensive body areas, with or without occlusive non-permeable dressings, striae may occur; also there exists the possibility of systemic side effects when steroid preparations are used over large areas or for a long period of time.

DOSAGE AND ADMINISTRATION

A thin film is applied 2 to 4 times daily to the affected area.

HOW SUPPLIED

Tube of ½ oz with applicator tip (NDC 61570-031-50).

Store at 15° to 25°C (59° to 77°F).

Rx only

REFERENCES

1. Leyden JJ, Kligman AM. Contact dermatitis to neomycin sulfate. *JAMA.* 1979;242:1276–1278.

Continued on next page

Cortisporin Ointment—Cont.

2. Prystowsky SD, Allen AM, Smith RW, et al. Allergic contact hypersensitivity to nickel, neomycin, ethylenediamine, and benzocaine. *Arch Dermatol.* 1979;115:959–962.

Distributed by: Monarch Pharmaceuticals, Inc., Bristol, TN 37620
Manufactured by: Catalytica Pharmaceuticals, Inc., Greenville, NC 27834

Rev. 1/98

CORTISPORIN® ℞
Ophthalmic Ointment Sterile
[*cŏr 'tĭ-spŏrin*]
(neomycin and polymyxin B sulfates, bacitracin zinc, and hydrocortisone ophthalmic ointment, USP)

DESCRIPTION

CORTISPORIN® Ophthalmic Ointment (neomycin and polymyxin B sulfates, bacitracin zinc, and hydrocortisone ophthalmic ointment) is a sterile antimicrobial and anti-inflammatory ointment for ophthalmic use. Each gram contains: neomycin sulfate equivalent to 3.5 mg neomycin base, polymyxin B sulfate equivalent to 10,000 polymyxin B units, bacitracin zinc equivalent to 400 bacitracin units, hydrocortisone 10 mg (1%), and white petrolatum, q.s.
Neomycin sulfate is the sulfate salt of neomycin B and C, which are produced by the growth of *Streptomyces fradiae* Waksman (Fam. Streptomycetaceae). It has a potency equivalent of not less than 600 µg of neomycin standard per mg, calculated on an anhydrous basis. The structural formulae are:

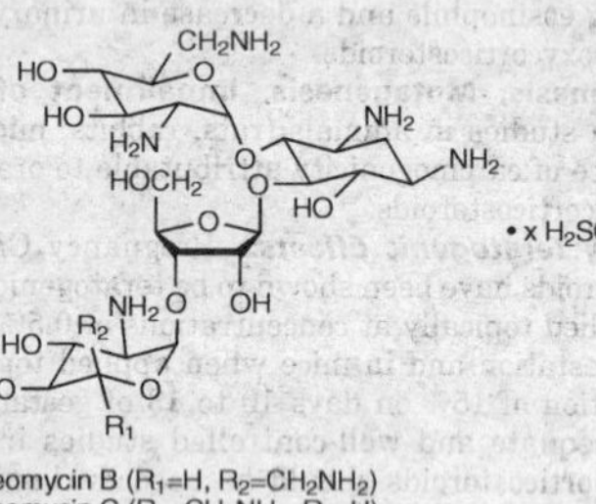

Neomycin B (R_1=H, R_2=CH_2NH_2)
Neomycin C (R_1=CH_2NH_2, R_2=H)

Polymyxin B sulfate is the sulfate salt of polymyxin B_1 and B_2, which are produced by the growth of *Bacillus polymyxa* (Prazmowski) Migula (Fam. Bacillaceae). It has a potency of not less than 6,000 polymyxin B units per mg, calculated on an anhydrous basis. The structural formulae are:

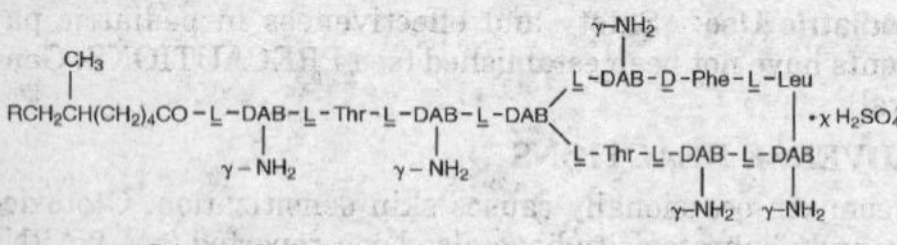

Polymyxin B_1 (R=CH_3)
Polymyxin B_2 (R=H)
DAB=α,γ-diaminobutyric acid

Bacitracin zinc is the zinc salt of bacitracin, a mixture of related cyclic polypeptides (mainly bacitracin A) produced by the growth of an organism of the *licheniformis* group of *Bacillus subtilis* var Tracy. It has a potency of not less than 40 bacitracin units per mg. The structural formula is:

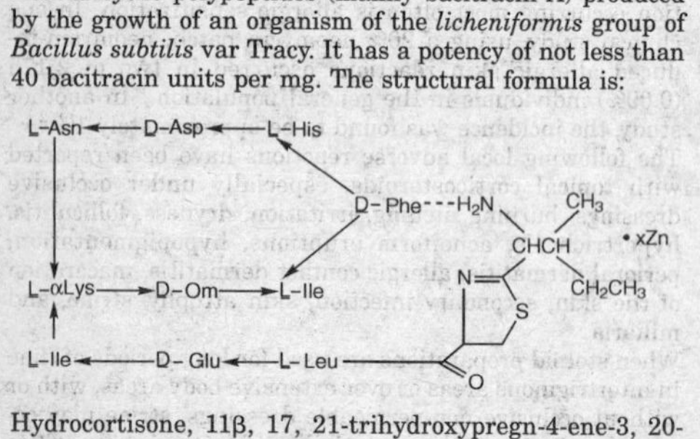

Hydrocortisone, 11β, 17, 21-trihydroxypregn-4-ene-3, 20-dione, is an anti-inflammatory hormone. Its structural formula is:

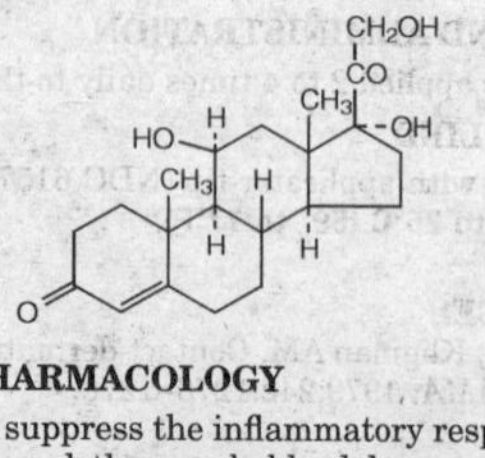

CLINICAL PHARMACOLOGY

Corticosteroids suppress the inflammatory response to a variety of agents and they probably delay or slow healing. Since corticosteroids may inhibit the body's defense mechanism against infection, concomitant antimicrobial drugs may be used when this inhibition is considered to be clinically significant in a particular case.
When a decision to administer both a corticosteroid and antimicrobials is made, the administration of such drugs in combination has the advantage of greater patient compliance and convenience, with the added assurance that the appropriate dosage of all drugs is administered. When each type of drug is in the same formulation, compatibility of ingredients is assured and the correct volume of drug is delivered and retained.
The relative potency of corticosteroids depends on the molecular structure, concentration, and release from the vehicle.
Microbiology: The anti-infective components in CORTISPORIN Ophthalmic Ointment are included to provide action against specific organisms susceptible to it. Neomycin sulfate and polymyxin B sulfate are active in vitro against susceptible strains of the following microorganisms: *Staphylococcus aureus*, streptococci including *Streptococcus pneumoniae, Escherichia coli, Haemophilus influenzae, Klebsiella/Enterobacter* species, *Neisseria* species, and *Pseudomonas aeruginosa*. The product does not provide adequate coverage against *Serratia marcescens* (see INDICATIONS AND USAGE).

INDICATIONS AND USAGE

CORTISPORIN Ophthalmic Ointment is indicated for steroid-responsive inflammatory ocular conditions for which a corticosteroid is indicated and where bacterial infection or a risk of bacterial infection exists.
Ocular corticosteroids are indicated in inflammatory conditions of the palpebral and bulbar conjunctiva, cornea, and anterior segment of the globe where the inherent risk of corticosteroid use in certain infective conjunctivitides is accepted to obtain a diminution in edema and inflammation. They are also indicated in chronic anterior uveitis and corneal injury from chemical, radiation, or thermal burns, or penetration of foreign bodies.
The use of a combination drug with an anti-infective component is indicated where the risk of infection is high or where there is an expectation that potentially dangerous numbers of bacteria will be present in the eye (see CLINICAL PHARMACOLOGY: Microbiology).
The particular anti-infective drugs in this product are active against the following common bacterial eye pathogens: *Staphylococcus aureus*, streptococci, including *Streptococcus pneumoniae, Escherichia coli, Haemophilus influenzae, Klebsiella/Enterobacter* species, *Neisseria* species, and *Pseudomonas aeruginosa.*
The product does not provide adequate coverage against *Serratia marcescens.*

CONTRAINDICATIONS

CORTISPORIN Ophthalmic Ointment is contraindicated in most viral diseases of the cornea and conjunctiva including: epithelial herpes simplex keratitis (dendritic keratitis), vaccinia and varicella, and also in mycobacterial infection of the eye and fungal diseases of ocular structures.
CORTISPORIN Ophthalmic Ointment is also contraindicated in individuals who have shown hypersensitivity to any of its components. Hypersensitivity to the antibiotic component occurs at a higher rate than for other components.

WARNINGS

NOT FOR INJECTION INTO THE EYE. CORTISPORIN Ophthalmic Ointment should never be directly introduced into the anterior chamber of the eye. Ophthalmic ointments may retard corneal wound healing.
Prolonged use of corticosteroids may result in ocular hypertension and/or glaucoma, with damage to the optic nerve, defects in visual acuity and fields of vision, and in posterior subcapsular cataract formation.
Prolonged use may suppress the host response and thus increase the hazard of secondary ocular infections. In those diseases causing thinning of the cornea or sclera, perforations have been known to occur with the use of topical corticosteroids. In acute purulent conditions of the eye, corticosteroids may mask infection or enhance existing infection.
If these products are used for 10 days or longer, intraocular pressure should be routinely monitored even though it may be difficult in uncooperative patients. Corticosteroids should be used with caution in the presence of glaucoma.
The use of corticosteroids after cataract surgery may delay healing and increase the incidence of filtering blebs.
Use of the ocular corticosteroids may prolong the course and may exacerbate the severity of many viral infections of the eye (including herpes simplex). Employment of corticosteroid medication in the treatment of herpes simplex requires great caution.
Topical antibiotics, particularly neomycin sulfate, may cause cutaneous sensitization. A precise incidence of hypersensitivity reactions (primarily skin rash) due to topical antibiotics is not known. The manifestations of sensitization to topical antibiotics are usually itching, reddening, and edema of the conjunctiva and eyelid. A sensitization reaction may manifest simply as a failure to heal. During long-term use of topical antibiotic products, periodic examination for such signs is advisable, and the patient should be told to discontinue the product if they are observed. Symptoms usually subside quickly on withdrawing the medication. Applications of products containing these ingredients should be avoided for the patient thereafter (see PRECAUTIONS: General).

PRECAUTIONS

General: The initial prescription and renewal of the medication order beyond 8 grams should be made by a physician only after examination of the patient with the aid of magnification, such as slit lamp biomicroscopy and, where appropriate, fluorescein staining. If signs and symptoms fail to improve after two days, the patient should be re-evaluated.
The possibility of fungal infections of the cornea should be considered after prolonged corticosteroid dosing. Fungal cultures should be taken when appropriate.
If this product is used for 10 days or longer, intraocular pressure should be monitored (see WARNINGS).
There have been reports of bacterial keratitis associated with the use of topical ophthalmic products in multiple-dose containers which have been inadvertently contaminated by patients, most of whom had a concurrent corneal disease or a disruption of the ocular epithelial surface (see PRECAUTIONS: Information for Patients).
Allergic cross-reactions may occur which could prevent the use of any or all of the following antibiotics for the treatment of future infections: kanamycin, paromomycin, streptomycin, and possibly gentamicin.
Information for Patients: Patients should be instructed to avoid allowing the tip of the dispensing container to contact the eye, eyelid, fingers, or any other surface. The use of this product by more than one person may spread infection.
Patients should also be instructed that ocular products, if handled improperly, can become contaminated by common bacteria known to cause ocular infections. Serious damage to the eye and subsequent loss of vision may result from using contaminated products (see PRECAUTIONS: General).
If the condition persists or gets worse, or if a rash or allergic reaction develops, the patient should be advised to stop use and consult a physician. Do not use this product if you are allergic to any of the listed ingredients.
Keep tightly closed when not in use. Keep out of the reach of children.
Carcinogenesis, Mutagenesis, Impairment of Fertility: Long-term studies in animals to evaluate carcinogenic or mutagenic potential have not been conducted with polymyxin B sulfate or bacitracin. Treatment of cultured human lymphocytes in vitro with neomycin increased the frequency of chromosome aberrations at the highest concentrations (80 µg/mL) tested; however, the effects of neomycin on carcinogenesis and mutagenesis in humans are unknown.
Long-term studies in animals (rats, rabbits, mice) showed no evidence of carcinogenicity or mutagenicity attributable to oral administration of corticosteroids. Long-term animal studies have not been performed to evaluate the carcinogenic potential of topical corticosteroids. Studies to determine mutagenicity with hydrocortisone have revealed negative results.
Polymyxin B has been reported to impair the motility of equine sperm, but its effects on male or female fertility are unknown. No adverse effects on male or female fertility, litter size, or survival were observed in rabbits given bacitracin zinc 100 gm/ton of diet. Long-term animal studies have not been performed to evaluate the effect on fertility of topical corticosteroids.
Pregnancy: *Teratogenic Effects:* Pregnancy Category C. Corticosteroids have been found to be teratogenic in rabbits when applied topically at concentrations of 0.5% on days 6 to 18 of gestation and in mice when applied topically at a concentration of 15% on days 10 to 13 of gestation. There are no adequate and well-controlled studies in pregnant women. CORTISPORIN Ophthalmic Ointment should be used during pregnancy only if the potential benefit justifies the potential risk to the fetus.
Nursing Mothers: It is not known whether topical administration of corticosteroids could result in sufficient systemic absorption to produce detectable quantities in human milk. Systemically administered corticosteroids appear in human milk and could suppress growth, interfere with endogenous corticosteroid production, or cause other untoward effects. Because of the potential for serious adverse reactions in nursing infants from CORTISPORIN Ophthalmic Ointment, a decision should be made whether to discontinue nursing or to discontinue the drug, taking into account the importance of the drug to the mother.
Pediatric Use: Safety and effectiveness in children have not been established.

ADVERSE REACTIONS

Adverse reactions have occurred with corticosteroid/anti-infective combination drugs which can be attributed to the corticosteroid component, the anti-infective component, or the combination. The exact incidence is not known.

Reactions occurring most often from the presence of the anti-infective ingredient are allergic sensitization reactions including itching, swelling, and conjunctival erythema (see WARNINGS). More serious hypersensitivity reactions, including anaphylaxis, have been reported rarely.
The reactions due to the corticosteroid component in decreasing order of frequency are: elevation of intraocular pressure (IOP) with possible development of glaucoma, and infrequent optic nerve damage; posterior subcapsular cataract formation; and delayed wound healing.
Secondary Infection: The development of the secondary infection has occurred after use of combinations containing corticosteroids and antimicrobials. Fungal and viral infections of the cornea are particularly prone to develop coincidentally with long-term applications of a corticosteroid. The possibility of fungal invasion must be considered in any persistent corneal ulceration where corticosteroid treatment has been used.
Local irritation on installation has been reported.

DOSAGE AND ADMINISTRATION

Apply the ointment in the affected eye every 3 or 4 hours, depending on the severity of the condition.
Not more than 8 grams should be prescribed initially and the prescription should not be refilled without further evaluation as outlined in PRECAUTIONS above.

HOW SUPPLIED

Tube of 1/8 oz. (3.5 g) with ophthalmic tip (NDC 61570-035-35).
Rx only
Store at 15° to 25°C (59° to 77°F).
Distributed by: Monarch Pharmaceuticals, Inc., Bristol, TN 37620
Manufactured by: Catalytica Pharmaceuticals, Inc., Greenville, NC 27834

CORTISPORIN® ℞
OPHTHALMIC SUSPENSION STERILE
(neomycin and polymyxin B sulfates and hydrocortisone ophthalmic suspension, USP)

DESCRIPTION

CORTISPORIN Ophthalmic Suspension (neomycin and polymyxin B sulfates and hydrocortisone ophthalmic suspension) is a sterile antimicrobial and anti-inflammatory suspension for ophthalmic use. Each mL contains: neomycin sulfate equivalent to 3.5 mg neomycin base, polymyxin B sulfate equivalent to 10,000 polymyxin B units, and hydrocortisone 10 mg (1%). The vehicle contains thimerosal 0.001% (added as a preservative) and the inactive ingredients cetyl alcohol, glyceryl monostearate, mineral oil, polyoxyl 40 stearate, propylene glycol, and Water for Injection. Sulfuric acid may be added to adjust pH.
Neomycin sulfate is the sulfate salt of neomycin B and C, which are produced by the growth of *Streptomyces fradiae* Waksman (Fam. Streptomycetaceae). It has a potency equivalent of not less than 600 µg of neomycin standard per mg, calculated on an anhydrous basis. The structural formulae are:

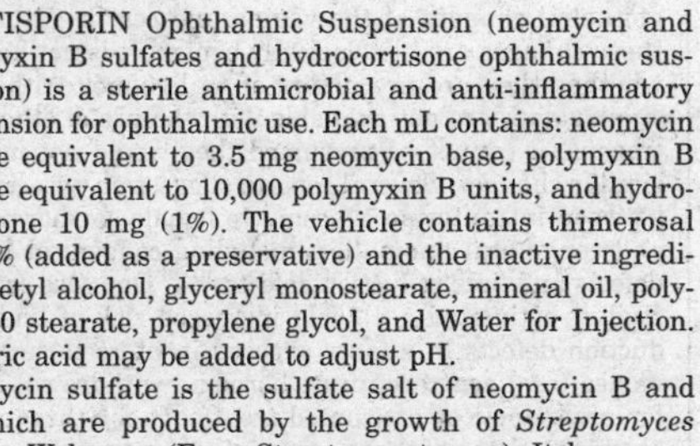

Neomycin B (R_1=H, R_2=CH_2NH_2)
Neomycin C (R_1=CH_2NH_2, R_2=H)

Polymyxin B sulfate is the sulfate salt of polymyxin B_1 and B_2, which are produced by the growth of *Bacillus polymyxa* (Prazmowski) Migula (Fam. Bacillaceae). It has a potency of not less than 6,000 polymyxin B units per mg, calculated on an anhydrous basis. The structural formulae are:

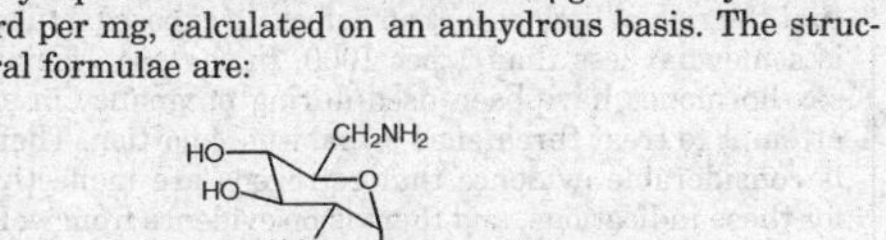

Polymyxin B_1 (R=CH_3)
Polymyxin B_2 (R=H)
DAB=α, γ-diaminobutyric acid

Hydrocortisone, 11β,17,21-trihydroxypregn-4-ene-3,20-dione, is an anti-inflammatory hormone. Its structural formula is:
[See chemical structure at top of next column]

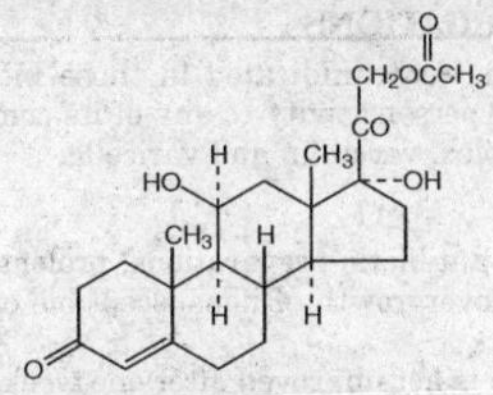

CLINICAL PHARMACOLOGY

Corticosteroids suppress the inflammatory response to a variety of agents, and they probably delay or slow healing. Since corticosteroids may inhibit the body's defense mechanism against infection, concomitant antimicrobial drugs may be used when this inhibition is considered to be clinically significant in a particular case.
When a decision to administer both a corticosteroid and antimicrobials is made, the administration of such drugs in combination has the advantage of greater patient compliance and convenience, with the added assurance that the appropriate dosage of all drugs is administered. When each type of drug is in the same formulation, compatibility of ingredients is assured and the correct volume of drug is delivered and retained.
The relative potency of corticosteroids depends on the molecular structure, concentration, and release from the vehicle.
Microbiology: The anti-infective components in CORTISPORIN Ophthalmic Suspension are included to provide action against specific organisms susceptible to it. Neomycin sulfate and polymyxin B sulfate are active in vitro against susceptible strains of the following microorganisms: *Staphylococcus aureus, Escherichia coli, Haemophilus influenzae, Klebsiella/Enterobacter species, Neisseria species,* and *Pseudomonas aeruginosa*. The product does not provide adequate coverage against Serratia marcescens and streptococci, including Streptococcus pneumoniae (see INDICATIONS AND USAGE).

INDICATIONS AND USAGE

CORTISPORIN Ophthalmic Suspension is indicated for steroid-responsive inflammatory ocular conditions for which a corticosteroid is indicated and where bacterial infection or a risk of bacterial infection exists.
Ocular corticosteroids are indicated in inflammatory conditions of the palpebral and bulbar conjunctiva, cornea, and anterior segment of the globe where the inherent risk of corticosteroid use in certain infective conjunctivitides is accepted to obtain a diminution in edema and inflammation. They are also indicated in chronic anterior uveitis and corneal injury from chemical, radiation, or thermal burns, or penetration of foreign bodies.
The use of a combination drug with an anti-infective component is indicated where the risk of infection is high or where there is an expectation that potentially dangerous numbers of bacteria will be present in the eye (see CLINICAL PHARMACOLOGY: Microbiology).
The particular anti-infective drugs in this product are active against the following common bacterial eye pathogens: *Staphylococcus aureus, Escherichia coli, Haemophilus influenzae, Klebsiella/Enterobacter species, Neisseria species,* and *Pseudomonas aeruginosa.*
The product does not provide adequate coverage against Serratia marcescens and streptococci, including *Streptococcus pneumoniae.*

CONTRAINDICATIONS

CORTISPORIN Ophthalmic Suspension is contraindicated in most viral diseases of the cornea and conjunctiva including: epithelial herpes simplex keratitis (dendritic keratitis), vaccinia and varicella, and also in mycobacterial infection of the eye and fungal diseases of ocular structures.
CORTISPORIN Ophthalmic Suspension is also contraindicated in individuals who have shown hypersensitivity to any of its components. Hypersensitivity to the antibiotic component occurs at a higher rate than for other components.

WARNINGS

NOT FOR INJECTION INTO THE EYE. CORTISPORIN Ophthalmic Suspension should never be directly introduced into the anterior chamber of the eye.
Prolonged use of corticosteroids may result in ocular hypertension and/or glaucoma, with damage to the optic nerve, defects in visual acuity and fields of vision, and in posterior subcapsular cataract formation.
Prolonged use may suppress the host response and thus increase the hazard of secondary ocular infections. In those diseases causing thinning of the cornea or sclera, perforations have been known to occur with the use of topical corticosteroids. In acute purulent conditions of the eye, corticosteroids may mask infection or enhance existing infection.
If these products are used for 10 days or longer, intraocular pressure should be routinely monitored even though it may be difficult in uncooperative patients. Corticosteroids should be used with caution in the presence of glaucoma.
The use of corticosteroids after cataract surgery may delay healing and increase the incidence of filtering blebs.
Use of ocular corticosteroids may prolong the course and may exacerbate the severity of many viral infections of the eye (including herpes simplex). Employment of corticosteroid medication in the treatment of herpes simplex requires great caution.
Topical antibiotics, particularly, neomycin sulfate, may cause cutaneous sensitization. A precise incidence of hypersensitivity reactions (primarily skin rash) due to topical antibiotics is not known. The manifestations of sensitization to topical antibiotics are usually itching, reddening, and edema of the conjunctiva and eyelid. A sensitization reaction may manifest simply as a failure to heal. During long-term use of topical antibiotic products, periodic examination for such signs is advisable, and the patient should be told to discontinue the product if they are observed. Symptoms usually subside quickly on withdrawing the medication. Application of products containing these ingredients should be avoided for the patient thereafter (see PRECAUTIONS: General).

PRECAUTIONS

General: The initial prescription and renewal of the medication order beyond 20 milliliters should be made by a physician only after examination of the patient with the aid of magnification, such as slit lamp biomicroscopy and, where appropriate, fluorescein staining. If signs and symptoms fail to improve after 2 days, the patient should be re-evaluated.
The possibility of fungal infections of the cornea should be considered after prolonged corticosteroid dosing. Fungal cultures should be taken when appropriate.
If this product is used for 10 days or longer, intraocular pressure should be monitored (see WARNINGS).
There have been reports of bacterial keratitis associated with the use of topical ophthalmic products in multiple-dose containers which have been inadvertently contaminated by patients, most of whom had a concurrent corneal disease or a disruption of the ocular epithelial surface (see PRECAUTIONS: Information for Patients).
Allergic cross-reactions may occur which could prevent the use of any or all of the following antibiotics for the treatment of future infections: kanamycin, paromomycin, streptomycin, and possibly gentamicin.
Information for Patients: Patients should be instructed to avoid allowing the tip of the dispensing container to contact the eye, eyelid, fingers, or any other surface. The use of this product by more than one person may spread infection.
Patients should also be instructed that ocular products, if handled improperly, can become contaminated by common bacteria known to cause ocular infections. Serious damage to the eye and subsequent loss of vision may result from using contaminated products (see PRECAUTIONS: General).
If the condition persists or gets worse, or if a rash or allergic reaction develops, the patient should be advised to stop use and consult a physician. Do not use this product if you are allergic to any of the listed ingredients.
Keep tightly closed when not in use. Keep out of reach of children.
Carcinogenesis, Mutagenesis, Impairment of Fertility: Long-term studies in animals to evaluate carcinogenic or mutagenic potential have not been conducted with polymyxin B sulfate. Treatment of cultured human lymphocytes in vitro with neomycin increased the frequency of chromosome aberrations at the highest concentrations (80 mg/mL) tested; however, the effects of neomycin on carcinogenesis and mutagenesis in humans are unknown.
Long-term studies in animals (rats, rabbits, mice) showed no evidence of carcinogenicity or mutagenicity attributable to oral administration of corticosteroids. Long-term animal studies have not been performed to evaluate the carcinogenic potential of topical corticosteroids. Studies to determine mutagenicity with hydrocortisone have revealed negative results.
Polymyxin B has been reported to impair the motility of equine sperm, but its effects on male or female fertility are unknown. Long-term animal studies have not been performed to evaluate the effect on fertility of topical corticosteroids.
Pregnancy: ***Teratogenic Effects:*** Pregnancy Category C. Corticosteroids have been found to be teratogenic in rabbits when applied topically at concentrations of 0.5% on days 6 to 18 of gestation and in mice when applied topically at a concentration of 15% on days 10 to 13 of gestation. There are no adequate and well-controlled studies in pregnant women. CORTISPORIN Ophthalmic Suspension should be used during pregnancy only if the potential benefit justifies the potential risk to the fetus.
Nursing Mothers: It is not known whether topical administration of corticosteroids could result in sufficient systemic absorption to produce detectable quantities in human milk. Systemically administered corticosteroids appear in human milk and could suppress growth, interfere with endogenous corticosteroid production, or cause other untoward effects.

Continued on next page

Cortisporin Ophthalmic Susp.—Cont.

Because of the potential for serious adverse reactions in nursing infants from CORTISPORIN Ophthalmic Suspension, a decision should be made whether to discontinue nursing or to discontinue the drug, taking into account the importance of the drug to the mother.

Pediatric Use: Safety and effectiveness in pediatric patients have not been established.

ADVERSE REACTIONS

Adverse reactions have occurred with corticosteroid/anti-infective combination drugs which can be attributed to the corticosteroid component, the anti-infective component, or the combination. The exact incidence is not known.

Reactions occurring most often from the presence of the anti-infective ingredient are allergic sensitization reactions including itching, swelling, and conjunctival erythema (see WARNINGS). More serious hypersensitivity reactions, including anaphylaxis, have been reported rarely.

The reactions due to the corticosteroid component in decreasing order of frequency are: elevation of intraocular pressure (IOP) with possible development of glaucoma, and infrequent optic nerve damage; posterior subcapsular cataract formation; and delayed wound healing.

Secondary Infection: The development of secondary infection has occurred after use of combinations containing corticosteroids and antimicrobials. Fungal and viral infections of the cornea are particularly prone to develop coincidentally with long-term applications of a corticosteroid. The possibility of fungal invasion must be considered in any persistent corneal ulceration where corticosteroid treatment has been used.

Local irritation on instillation has also been reported.

DOSAGE AND ADMINISTRATION

One or two drops in the affected eye every 3 or 4 hours, depending on the severity of the condition. The suspension may be used more frequently if necessary.

Not more than 20 milliliters should be prescribed initially and the prescription should not be refilled without further evaluation as outlined in PRECAUTIONS above.

SHAKE WELL BEFORE USING.

HOW SUPPLIED

Plastic DROP DOSE® dispenser bottle of 7.5 mL (NDC 61570-036-75).

Rx only

Store at 15° to 25°C (59° to 77°F).

Distributed by: Monarch Pharmaceuticals, Inc., Bristol, TN 37620

Manufactured By: Catalytica Pharmaceutical, Inc. Greenville, NC 27835

5/97

Shown in Product Identification Guide, page 324

CORTISPORIN®-TC Otic Suspension with Neomycin and Hydrocortisone ℞

[*cŏr 'tĭ -spŏrin*]

(colistin sulfate - neomycin sulfate - thonzonium bromide - hydrocortisone acetate otic suspension)

DESCRIPTION

Cortisporin®-TC Otic Suspension with Neomycin and Hydrocortisone (colistin sulfate—neomycin sulfate—thonzonium bromide—hydrocortisone acetate otic suspension) is a sterile aqueous suspension containing in each mL: Colistin base activity, 3mg (as the sulfate); Neomycin base activity, 3.3 mg (as the sulfate); Hydrocortisone acetate, 10 mg (1%); Thonzonium bromide, 0.5 mg (0.05%); Polysorbate 80, acetic acid, and sodium acetate in a buffered aqueous vehicle. Thimerosal (mercury derivative), 0.002%, added as a preservative. It is a nonviscous liquid, buffered at pH 5, for instillation into the canal of the external ear or direct application to the affected aural skin.

CLINICAL PHARMACOLOGY

1. Colistin sulfate - an antibiotic with bactericidal action against most gram-negative organisms, notably *Pseudomonas aeruginosa, E coli*, and *Klebsiella-Aerobacter*.
2. Neomycin sulfate - a broad-spectrum antibiotic bactericidal to many pathogens, notably *Staph aureus* and *Proteus sp*.
3. Hydrocortisone acetate - a corticosteroid that controls inflammation, edema, pruritus, and other dermal reactions.
4. Thonzonium bromide - a surface-active agent that promotes tissue contact by dispersion and penetration of the cellular debris and exudate.

INDICATIONS AND USAGE

For the treatment of superficial bacterial infections of the external auditory canal, caused by organisms susceptible to the action of the antibiotics; and for the treatment of infections of mastoidectomy and fenestration cavities, caused by organisms susceptible to the antibiotics.

CONTRAINDICATIONS

This product is contraindicated in those individuals who have shown hypersensitivity to any of its components, and in herpes simplex, vaccinia, and varicella.

WARNINGS

As with other antibiotic preparations, prolonged treatment may result in overgrowth of nonsusceptible organisms and fungi.

If the infection is not improved after one week, cultures and susceptibility tests should be repeated to verify the identity of the organism and to determine whether therapy should be changed.

Patients who prefer to warm the medication before using should be cautioned against heating the suspension above body temperature, in order to avoid loss of potency.

PRECAUTIONS

General

If sensitization or irritation occurs, medication should be discontinued promptly.

This drug should be used with care in cases of perforated eardrum and in longstanding cases of chronic otitis media because of the possibility of ototoxicity caused by neomycin.

Treatment should not be continued for longer than ten days.

Allergic cross-reactions may occur which could prevent the use of any or all of the following antibiotics for the treatment of future infections: kanamycin, paromomycin, streptomycin, and possibly gentamicin.

ADVERSE REACTIONS

Neomycin is a not uncommon cutaneous sensitizer. There are articles in the current literature that indicate an increase in the prevalence of persons sensitive to neomycin.

DOSAGE AND ADMINISTRATION

The external auditory canal should be thoroughly cleansed and dried with a sterile cotton applicator.

When using the calibrated dropper:

For adults, 5 drops of the suspension should be instilled into the affected ear 3 or 4 times daily. For pediatric patients, 4 drops are suggested because of the smaller capacity of the ear canal.

This dosage correlates to the 4 drops (for adults) and 3 drops (for pediatric patients) recommended when using the dropper-bottle container for this product.

The patient should lie with the affected ear upward and then the drops should be instilled. This position should be maintained for 5 minutes to facilitate penetration of the drops into the ear canal. Repeat, if necessary, for the opposite ear.

If preferred, a cotton wick may be inserted into the canal and then the cotton may be saturated with the suspension. This wick should be kept moist by adding further solution every 4 hours. The wick should be replaced at least once every 24 hours.

HOW SUPPLIED

Cortisporin®-TC Otic Suspension is supplied as:

NDC 61570-090-10 .... 10-mL bottle with dropper

Each mL contains: Colistin sulfate equivalent to 3 mg of colistin base activity, Neomycin sulfate equivalent to 3.3 mg neomycin base activity, Hydrocortisone acetate 10mg (1%), Thonzonium bromide 0.5 mg (0.05%), and Polysorbate 80 in an aqueous vehicle buffered with acetic acid and sodium acetate. Thimerosal (mercury derivative) 0.002% added as a preservative.

A sterilized dropper-cap assembly for use on the bottle of suspension is included in the package.

Shake well before using.

Store at controlled room temperature 15°–30° C (59°–86° F). Stable for 18 months at room temperature; prolonged exposure to higher temperatures should be avoided.

Rx only.

Distributed by:
Monarch Pharmaceuticals, Inc.
Bristol, TN 37620

Manufactured by:
Parkedale Pharmaceuticals, Inc.
Rochester, MI 48307

Rev. 3/98
090G030

Shown in Product Identification Guide, page 324

MENEST™ ℞

[*men-est '*]

brand of esterified estrogens tablets, USP

WARNINGS

1. ESTROGENS HAVE BEEN REPORTED TO INCREASE THE RISK OF ENDOMETRIAL CARCINOMA.

Three independent case control studies have shown an increased risk of endometrial cancer in postmenopausal women exposed to exogenous estrogens for prolonged periods.[1–3] This risk was independent of the other known risk factors for endometrial cancer. These studies are further supported by the finding that incidence rates of endometrial cancer have increased sharply since 1969 in eight different areas of the United States with population-based cancer reporting systems, an increase which may be related to the rapidly expanding use of estrogens during the last decade.[4]

The three case control studies reported that the risk of endometrial cancer in estrogen users was about 4.5 to 13.9 times greater than in nonusers. The risk appears to depend on both duration of treatment[1] and on estrogen dose.[3] In view of these findings, when estrogens are used for the treatment of menopausal symptoms, the lowest dose that will control symptoms should be utilized and medication should be discontinued as soon as possible. When prolonged treatment is medically indicated, the patient should be reassessed on at least a semiannual basis to determine the need for continued therapy. Although the evidence must be considered preliminary, one study suggests that cyclic administration of low doses of estrogen may carry less risk than continuous administration[3]; it therefore appears prudent to utilize such a regimen.

Close clinical surveillance of all women taking estrogens is important. In all cases of undiagnosed persistent or recurring abnormal vaginal bleeding, adequate diagnostic measures should be undertaken to rule out malignancy.

There is no evidence at present that "natural" estrogens are more or less hazardous than "synthetic" estrogens at equiestrogenic doses.

2. ESTROGENS SHOULD NOT BE USED DURING PREGNANCY.

The use of female sex hormones, both estrogens and progestagens, during early pregnancy may seriously damage the offspring. It has been shown that females exposed in utero to diethylstilbestrol, a nonsteroidal estrogen, have an increased risk of developing in later life a form of vaginal or cervical cancer that is ordinarily extremely rare.[5,6] The risk has been estimated as not greater than 4 per 1000 exposures.[7] Furthermore, a high percentage of such exposed women (from 30 to 90 percent) have been found to have vaginal adenosis,[8–12] epithelial changes of the vagina and cervix. Although these changes are histologically benign, it is not known whether they are precursors of malignancy. Although similar data are not available with the use of other estrogens, it cannot be presumed they would not induce similar changes. Several reports suggest an association between intrauterine exposure to female sex hormones and congenital anomalies, including congenital heart defects and limb reduction defects.[13–16] One case control study[16] estimated a 4.7-fold increased risk of limb reduction defects in infants exposed in utero to sex hormones (oral contraceptives, hormone withdrawal tests for pregnancy, or attempted treatment for threatened abortion). Some of these exposures were very short and involved only a few days of treatment. The data suggest that the risk of limb reduction defects in exposed fetuses is somewhat less than 1 per 1000. In the past, female sex hormones have been used during pregnancy in an attempt to treat threatened or habitual abortion. There is considerable evidence that estrogens are ineffective for these indications, and there is no evidence from well-controlled studies that progestagens are effective for these uses. If Menest (esterified estrogens tablets) is used during pregnancy, or if the patient becomes pregnant while taking this drug, she should be apprised of the potential risks to the fetus, and the advisability of pregnancy continuation.

DESCRIPTION

Esterified estrogens is a mixture of the sodium salts of the sulfate esters of the estrogenic substances, principally estrone, that are of the type excreted by pregnant mares. The content of total esterified estrogens is not less than 90 percent and not more than 110 percent of the labeled amount. Esterified estrogens contain not less than 75 percent and not more than 85 percent of sodium estrone sulfate, and not less than 6 percent and not more than 15 percent of sodium equilin sulfate, in such proportion that the total of these two components is not less than 90 percent, all percentages being calculated on the basis of the total esterified estrogens content.

Inactive Ingredients: Ethyl cellulose, fragrances, hydroxypropyl cellulose, hydroxypropyl methylcellulose 2910, lactose, magnesium stearate, methylcellulose, polyethylene glycol, sodium bicarbonate, shellac, starch, stearic acid, titanium dioxide, and vanillin. Dyes in the form of aluminum lakes are contained in each tablet strength as follows: **0.3 mg Tablet:** FD&C Yellow No. 6, D&C Yellow No. 10. **0.625 mg Tablet:** FD&C Yellow No. 6, D&C Yellow No. 10. **1.25 mg Tablet:** FD&C Yellow No. 6, D&C Yellow No. 10, FD&C Blue No. 1. **2.5 mg Tablet:** D&C Red No. 30.

CLINICAL PHARMACOLOGY

Estrogens are important in the development and maintenance of the female reproductive system and secondary sex characteristics. They promote growth and development of the vagina, uterus, and fallopian tubes, and enlargement of the breasts. Indirectly, they contribute to the shaping of the skeleton, maintenance of tone and elasticity of urogenital structures, changes in the epiphyses of the long bones that allow for the pubertal growth spurt and its termination, growth of axillary and pubic hair, and pigmentation of the nipples and genitals. Decline of estrogenic activity at the end of the menstrual cycle can bring on menstruation, although the cessation of progesterone secretion is the most important factor in the mature ovulatory cycle. However, in the preovulatory or nonovulatory cycle, estrogen is the primary determinant in the onset of menstruation. Estrogens also affect the release of pituitary gonadotropins. The pharmacologic effects of esterified estrogens are similar to those of endogenous estrogens. They are soluble in water and are well absorbed from the gastrointestinal tract.

In responsive tissues (female genital organs, breasts, hypothalamus, pituitary) estrogens enter the cell and are transported into the nucleus. As a result of estrogen action, specific RNA and protein synthesis occurs. Metabolism and inactivation occur primarily in the liver. Some estrogens are excreted into the bile; however, they are reabsorbed from the intestine and returned to the liver through the portal venous system. Water soluble estrogen conjugates are strongly acidic and are ionized in body fluids, which favor excretion through the kidneys since tubular reabsorption is minimal.

INDICATIONS AND USAGE

Menest (esterified estrogens tablets) is indicated in the treatment of:

1. Moderate to severe *vasomotor* symptoms associated with the menopause. (There is no evidence that estrogens are effective for nervous symptoms or depression which might occur during menopause, and they should not be used to treat these conditions.)
2. Atrophic vaginitis.
3. Kraurosis vulvae.
4. Female hypogonadism.
5. Female castration.
6. Primary ovarian failure.
7. Breast cancer (for palliation only) in appropriately selected women and men with metastatic disease.
8. Prostatic carcinoma—palliative therapy of advanced disease.

MENEST (esterified estrogens tablets) HAS NOT BEEN SHOWN TO BE EFFECTIVE FOR ANY PURPOSE DURING PREGNANCY AND ITS USE MAY CAUSE SEVERE HARM TO THE FETUS (SEE BOXED WARNING).

CONTRAINDICATIONS

Estrogens should not be used in women (or men) with any of the following conditions:

1. Known or suspected cancer of the breast except in appropriately selected patients being treated for metastatic disease.
2. Known or suspected estrogen-dependent neoplasia.
3. Known or suspected pregnancy (See Boxed Warning).
4. Undiagnosed abnormal genital bleeding.
5. Active thrombophlebitis or thromboembolic disorders.
6. A past history of thrombophlebitis, thrombosis or thromboembolic disorders associated with previous estrogen use (except when used in treatment of breast or prostatic malignancy).

WARNINGS

1. *Induction of malignant neoplasms.* Long-term continuous administration of natural and synthetic estrogens in certain animal species increases the frequency of carcinomas of the breast, cervix, vagina, and liver. There is now evidence that estrogens increase the risk of carcinoma of the endometrium in humans. (See Boxed Warning.) At the present time there is no satisfactory evidence that estrogens given to postmenopausal women increase the risk of cancer of the breast[18] although a recent long-term followup of a single physician's practice has raised this possibility.[18A] Because of the animal data, there is a need for caution in prescribing estrogens for women with a strong family history of breast cancer or who have breast nodules, fibrocystic disease, or abnormal mammograms.
2. *Gall bladder disease.* A recent study has reported a 2- to 3-fold increase in the risk of surgically confirmed gall bladder disease in women receiving postmenopausal estrogens,[18] similar to the 2-fold increase previously noted in users of oral contraceptives.[19–24] In the case of oral contraceptives the increased risk appeared after 2 years of use.[24]
3. *Effects similar to those caused by estrogen-progestagen oral contraceptives.* There are several serious adverse effects of oral contraceptives, most of which have not, up to now, been documented as consequences of postmenopausal estrogen therapy. This may reflect the comparatively low doses of estrogen used in post-menopausal women. It would be expected that the larger doses of estrogen used to treat prostatic or breast cancer or postpartum breast engorgement are more likely to result in these adverse effects and, in fact, it has been shown that there is an increased risk of thrombosis in men receiving estrogens for prostatic cancer and women for postpartum breast engorgement.[20–23]

   a. *Thromboembolic disease.* It is now well established that users of oral contraceptives have an increased risk of various thromboembolic and thrombotic vascular diseases, such as thrombophlebitis, pulmonary embolism, stroke, and myocardial infarction.[24–31] Cases of retinal thrombosis, mesenteric thrombosis, and optic neuritis have been reported in oral contraceptive users. There is evidence that the risk of several of these adverse reactions is related to the dose of the drug.[32, 33] An increased risk of post-surgery thromboembolic complications has also been reported in users of oral contraceptives.[34,35] If feasible, estrogen should be discontinued at least 4 weeks before surgery of the type associated with an increased risk of thromboembolism, or during periods of prolonged immobilization.

   While an increased rate of thromboembolic and thrombotic disease in postmenopausal users of estrogens has not been found,[18–36] this does not rule out the possibility that such an increase may be present or that subgroups of women who have underlying risk factors or who are receiving relatively large doses of estrogens may have increased risk.

   Therefore estrogens should not be used in persons with active thrombophlebitis or thromboembolic disorders, and they should not be used (except in treatment of malignancy) in persons with a history of such disorders in association with estrogen use. They should be used with caution in patients with cerebral vascular or coronary artery disease and only for those in whom estrogens are clearly needed.

   Large doses of estrogen (5 mg esterified estrogens per day), comparable to those used to treat cancer of the prostate and breast, have been shown in a large prospective clinical trial in men[37] to increase the risk of nonfatal myocardial infarction, pulmonary embolism and thrombophlebitis. When estrogen doses of this size are used, any of the thromboembolic and thrombotic adverse effects associated with oral contraceptive use should be considered a clear risk.

   b. *Hepatic adenoma.* Benign hepatic adenomas appear to be associated with the use of oral contraceptives.[38–40] Although benign, and rare, these may rupture and may cause death through intra-abdominal hemorrhage. Such lesions have not yet been reported in association with other estrogen or progestagen preparations but should be considered in estrogen users having abdominal pain and tenderness, abdominal mass, or hypovolemic shock. Hepatocellular carcinoma has also been reported in women taking estrogen-containing oral contraceptives.[39] The relationship of this malignancy to these drugs is not known at this time.

   c. *Elevated blood pressure.* Increased blood pressure is not uncommon in women using oral contraceptives. There is now a report that this may occur with use of estrogens in the menopause[41] and blood pressure should be monitored with estrogen use, especially if high doses are used.

   d. *Glucose tolerance.* A worsening of glucose tolerance has been observed in a significant percentage of patients on estrogen-containing oral contraceptives. For this reason, diabetic patients should be carefully observed while receiving estrogen.
4. *Hypercalcemia.* Administration of estrogens may lead to severe hypercalcemia in patients with breast cancer and bone metastases. If this occurs, the drug should be stopped and appropriate measures taken to reduce the serum calcium level.

See footnotes at end of article.

PRECAUTIONS

A. *General Precautions:*

1. A complete medical and family history should be taken prior to the initiation of any estrogen therapy. The pretreatment and periodic physical examinations should include special reference to blood pressure, breast, abdomen, and pelvic organs, and should include a Papanicolau smear. As a general rule, estrogen should not be prescribed for longer than 1 year without another physical examination being performed.
2. Fluid retention—Because estrogens may cause some degree of fluid retention, conditions which might be influenced by this factor, such as epilepsy, migraine, and cardiac or renal dysfunction, require careful observation.
3. Certain patients may develop undesirable manifestations of excessive estrogenic stimulation, such as abnormal or excessive uterine bleeding, mastodynia, etc.
4. Oral contraceptives appear to be associated with an increased incidence of mental depression.[24] Although it is not clear whether this is due to the estrogenic or progestagenic component of the contraceptive, patients with a history of depression should be carefully observed.
5. Pre-existing uterine leiomyomata may increase in size during estrogen use.
6. The pathologist should be advised of estrogen therapy when relevant specimens are submitted.
7. Patients with a past history of jaundice during pregnancy have an increased risk of recurrence of jaundice while receiving estrogen-containing oral contraceptive therapy. If jaundice develops in any patient receiving estrogen, the medication should be discontinued while the cause is investigated.
8. Estrogens may be poorly metabolized in patients with impaired liver function and they should be administered with caution in such patients.
9. Because estrogens influence the metabolism of calcium and phosphorus, they should be used with caution in patients with metabolic bone diseases that are associated with hypercalcemia or in patients with renal insufficiency.
10. Because of the effects of estrogens on epiphyseal closure, they should be used judiciously in young patients in whom bone growth is not complete.
11. The lowest effective dose appropriate for the specific indication should be utilized. Studies of the addition of a progestin for 7 or more days of a cycle of estrogen administration have reported a lowered incidence of endometrial hyperplasia. Morphological and biochemical studies of endometrium suggest that 10 to 13 days of progestin are needed to provide maximal maturation of the endometrium and to eliminate any hyperplastic changes. Whether this will provide protection from endometrial carcinoma has not been clearly established.
    There are possible additional risks which may be associated with the inclusion of progestin in estrogen replacement regimens. The potential risks include adverse effects on carbohydrate and lipid metabolism. The choice of progestin and dosage may be important in minimizing these adverse effects.
12. Certain endocrine and liver function tests may be affected by estrogen-containing oral contraceptives. The following similar changes may be expected with larger doses of estrogen:
    a. Increased sulfobromophthalein retention.
    b. Increased prothrombin and factors VII, VIII, IX, and X; decreased antithrombin 3; increased norepinephrine-induced platelet aggregability.
    c. Increased thyroid binding globulin (TBG) leading to increased circulating total thyroid hormone, as measured by PBI, T4 by column or T4 by radioimmunoassay. Free T3 resin uptake is decreased, reflecting the elevated TBG; free T4 concentration is unaltered.
    d. Impaired glucose tolerance.
    e. Decreased pregnanediol excretion.
    f. Reduced response to metyrapone test.
    g. Reduced serum folate concentration.
    h. Increased serum triglyceride and phospholipid concentration.

B. *Information for patients:* See text which appears after PHYSICIAN REFERENCES.

C. *Pregnancy Category X*—See Contraindications and Boxed Warning.

D. *Nursing Mothers.* As a general principle, the administration of any drug to nursing mothers should be done only when clearly necessary since many drugs are excreted in human milk.

ADVERSE REACTIONS

(See Warnings regarding induction of neoplasia, adverse effects on the fetus, increased incidence of gall bladder disease, and adverse effects similar to those of oral contraceptives, including thromboembolism.) The following additional adverse reactions have been reported with estrogenic therapy, including oral contraceptives:

1. *Genitourinary system.*
   Breakthrough bleeding, spotting, change in menstrual flow.
   Dysmenorrhea.
   Premenstrual-like syndrome.
   Amenorrhea during and after treatment.
   Increase in size of uterine fibromyomata.
   Vaginal candidiasis.
   Change in cervical eversion and in degree of cervical secretion.
   Cystitis-like syndrome.
2. *Breasts.*
   Tenderness, enlargement, secretion.
3. *Gastrointestinal.*
   Nausea, vomiting.
   Abdominal cramps, bloating.
   Cholestatic jaundice.

Continued on next page

Menest—Cont.

4. *Skin.*
Chloasma or melasma which may persist when drug is discontinued.
Erythema multiforme.
Erythema nodosum.
Hemorrhagic eruption.
Loss of scalp hair.
Hirsutism.
5. *Eyes.*
Steepening of corneal curvature.
Intolerance to contact lenses.
6. *CNS.*
Headache, migraine, dizziness.
Mental depression.
Chorea.
7. *Miscellaneous.*
Increase or decrease in weight.
Reduced carbohydrate tolerance.
Aggravation of porphyria.
Edema.
Changes in libido.

ACUTE OVERDOSAGE

Numerous reports of ingestion of large doses of estrogen-containing oral contraceptives by young children indicate that serious ill effects do not occur. Overdosage of estrogen may cause nausea, and withdrawal bleeding may occur in females.

DOSAGE AND ADMINISTRATION

1. *Given cyclically for short term use only:*
For treatment of moderate to severe *vasomotor symptoms, atrophic vaginitis* or *kraurosis vulvae* associated with the menopause.
The lowest dose that will control symptoms should be chosen and medication should be discontinued as promptly as possible.
Administration should be cyclic (e.g., 3 weeks on and 1 week off).
Attempts to discontinue or taper medication should be made at 3 to 6 month intervals.
USUAL DOSAGE RANGES:
Vasomotor symptoms—1.25 mg daily. If the patient has not menstruated within the last 2 months or more, cyclic administration is started arbitrarily. If the patient is menstruating, cyclic administration is started on day 5 of bleeding.
Atrophic vaginitis and kraurosis vulvae—0.3 mg to 1.25 mg or more daily, depending upon the tissue response of the individual patient. Administer cyclically.
2. *Given cyclically:* Female hypogonadism; female castration; primary ovarian failure.
USUAL DOSAGE RANGES:
Female hypogonadism—2.5 to 7.5 mg daily, in divided doses for 20 days, followed by a rest period of 10 days' duration. If bleeding does not occur by the end of this period, the same dosage schedule is repeated. The number of courses of estrogen therapy necessary to produce bleeding may vary depending on responsiveness of the endometrium. If bleeding occurs before the end of the 10 day period, begin a 20 day estrogen-progestin cyclic regimen with Menest (esterified estrogens tablets), 2.5 to 7.5 mg daily in divided doses, for 20 days. During the last 5 days of estrogen therapy, give an oral progestin. If bleeding occurs before this regimen is concluded, therapy is discontinued and may be resumed on the fifth day of bleeding.
Female castration and primary ovarian failure—1.25 mg daily, cyclically. Adjust dosage upward or downward according to severity of symptoms and response of the patient. For maintenance, adjust dosage to lowest level that will provide effective control.
3. *Given chronically:* Inoperable progressing prostatic cancer—1.25 to 2.5 mg three times daily. The effectiveness of therapy can be judged by phosphatase determinations as well as by symptomatic improvement of the patient.
Inoperable progressing breast cancer in appropriately selected men and postmenopausal women. (See INDICATIONS AND USAGE)—Suggested dosage is 10 mg three times daily for a period of at least 3 months.
Treated patients with an intact uterus should be monitored closely for signs of endometrial cancer and appropriate diagnostic measures should be taken to rule out malignancy in the event of persistent or recurring abnormal vaginal bleeding.

HOW SUPPLIED

Tablets:

0.3 mg yellow, film-coated oblong tablet imprinted with BMP 125 100's: NDC 61570-072-01

0.625 mg orange, film-coated oblong tablet imprinted with BMP 126 100's: NDC 61570-073-01

1.25 mg green, film-coated oblong tablet imprinted with BMP 127 100's: NDC 61570-074-01

2.5 mg pink, film-coated oblong tablet imprinted with BMP 128 50's: NDC 61570-075-50

PHYSICIAN REFERENCES

1. Ziel HK, Finkel WD: Increased Risk of Endometrial Carcinoma Among Users of Conjugated Estrogens, *New England Journal of Medicine* 293:1167–1170, 1975.
2. Smith DC, Prentic R, Thompson DJ, Hermann WL: Association of Exogenous Estrogen and Endometrial Carcinoma, *New England Journal of Medicine* 293:1164–1167, 1975.
3. Mack TM, Pike MC, Henderson BE, et al: Estrogens and Endometrial Cancer in a Retirement Community, *New England Journal of Medicine* 294:1262–1267, 1976.
4. Weiss NS, Szekely DR, Austin DF: Increasing Incidence of Endometrial Cancer in the United States, *New England Journal of Medicine* 294:1259–1262, 1976.
5. Herbst AL, Ulfelder H, Poskanzer DC: Adenocarcinoma of Vagina, *New England Journal of Medicine* 284:878–881, 1971.
6. Greenwald P, Barlow J, Nasca P, Burnett W: Vaginal Cancer After Maternal Treatment with Synthetic Estrogens, *New England Journal of Medicine* 285:390–392, 1971.
7. Lanier A, Noller K, Decker D, et al: Cancer and Stilbestrol. A Follow-up of 1719 Persons Exposed to Estrogens in Utero and Born 1943–1959, *Mayo Clinic Proceedings* 48:793–799, 1973.
8. Herbst A, Kurman R, Scully R: Vaginal and Cervical Abnormalities After Exposure to Stilbestrol In Utero, *Obstetrics and Gynecology* 40:287–298, 1972.
9. Herbst A, Robboy S, Macdonald G, Scully R: The Effects of Local Progesterone on Stilbestrol-Associated Vaginal Adenosis, *American Journal of Obstetrics and Gynecology* 118:607–615, 1974.
10. Herbst A, Poskanzer D, Robboy S, et al: Prenatal Exposure to Stilbestrol, A Prospective Comparison of Exposed Female Offspring with Unexposed Controls, *New England Journal of Medicine* 292:334–339, 1975.
11. Stafl A, Mattingly R, Foley D, Fetherston W: Clinical Diagnosis of Vaginal Adenosis, *Obstetrics and Gynecology* 43:118–128, 1974.
12. Sherman AI, Goldrath M, Berlin A, et al: Cervical-Vaginal Adenosis After *In Utero* Exposure to Synthetic Estrogens, *Obstetrics and Gynecology* 44:531–545, 1974.
13. Gal I, Kirman B, Stern J: Hormone Pregnancy Tests and Congenital Malformation, *Nature* 216:83, 1967.
14. Levy EP, Cohen A, Fraser FC: Hormone Treatment During Pregnancy and Congenital Heart Defects, *Lancet* 1:611, 1973.
15. Nora J, Nora A: Birth Defects and Oral Contraceptives, *Lancet* 1:941–942, 1973.
16. Janerich DT, Piper JM, Glebatis, DM: Oral Contraceptives and Congenital Limb-Reduction Defects, *New England Journal of Medicine* 291:697–700, 1974.
17. Estrogens for Oral or Parenteral Use, *Federal Register* 40:8212, 1975.
18. Boston Collaborative Drug Surveillance Program: Surgically Confirmed Gall Bladder Disease, Venous Thromboembolism and Breast Tumors in Relations to Post-Menopausal Estrogen Therapy, *New England Journal of Medicine* 290:15–19, 1974.
18a.Hoover R, Gray LA Sr, Cole P, MacMahon B: Menopausal Estrogens and Breast Cancer, *New England Journal of Medicine* 295:401–405, 1976.
19. Boston Collaborative Drug Surveillance Program: Oral Contraceptives and Venous Thromboembolic Disease, Surgically Confirmed Gall Bladder Disease, and Breast Tumors, *Lancet* 1:1399–1404, 1973.
20. Daniel DG, Campbell H, Turnbull AC: Puerperal Thromboembolism and Suppression of Lactation, *Lancet* 2:287–289, 1967.
21. The Veterans Administration Cooperative Urological Research Group: Carcinoma of the Prostate: Treatment Comparisons, *Journal of Urology* 98:516–522, 1967.
22. Bailar JC: Thromboembolism and Oestrogen Therapy, *Lancet* 2:560, 1967.
23. Blackard C, Doe R, Mellinger G, Byar D: Incidence of Cardiovascular Disease and Death in Patients Receiving Diethylstilbestrol for Carcinoma of the Prostate, *Cancer* 26:249–256, 1970.
24. Royal College of General Practitioners: Oral Contraception and Thromboembolic Disease, *Journal of the Royal College of General Practitioners* 13:267–279, 1967.
25. Inman WHW, Vessey MP: Investigation of Deaths from Pulmonary, Coronary and Cerebral Thrombosis and Embolism in Women of Child-Bearing Age, *British Medical Journal* 2:193–199, 1968.
26. Vessey MP, Doll R: Investigation of Relation Between Use of Oral Contraceptives and Thromboembolic Disease. A Further Report, *British Medical Journal* 2:651–657, 1969.
27. Sartwell PE, Masi AT, Arthes FG, et al: Thromboembolism and Oral Contraceptives: An Epidemiological Case Control Study, *American Journal of Epidemiology* 90:365–380, 1969.
28. Collaborative Group for the Study of Stroke in Young Women: Oral Contraception and Increased Risk of Cerebral Ischemia or Thrombosis, *New England Journal of Medicine* 288:871–878, 1973.
29. Collaborative Group for the Study of Stroke in Young Women: Oral Contraceptives and Stroke in Young Women: Associated Risk Factors, *Journal of the American Medical Association* 231:718–722, 1975.
30. Mann JI, Inman WHW: Oral Contraceptives and Death from Myocardial Infarction, *British Medical Journal* 2:245–248, 1975.
31. Mann JI, Vessey MP, Thorogood M, Doll R: Myocardial Infarction in Young Women with Special Reference to Oral Contraceptive Practice, *British Medical Journal* 2:241–245, 1975.
32. Inman WHW, Vessey VP, Westerholm B, Engelund A: Thromboembolic Disease and the Steroidal Content of Oral Contraceptives, *British Medical Journal* 2:203–209, 1970.
33. Stolley PD, Tonascia JA, Tockman MS, et al: Thrombosis with Low-Estrogen Oral Contraceptives, *American Journal of Epidemiology* 102:197–208, 1975.
34. Vessey MP, Doll R, Fairbairn AS, Glober G: Post-Operative Thromboembolism and the Use of the Oral Contraceptives, *British Medical Journal* 3:123–126, 1970.
35. Greene GR, Sartwell PE: Oral Contraceptive Use in Patients with Thromboembolism Following Surgery, Trauma or Infection, *American Journal of Public Health* 62:680–685, 1972.
36. Rosenberg L, Armstrong MB, Jick H: Myocardial Infarction and Estrogen Therapy in Postmenopausal Women, *New England Journal of Medicine* 294:1256–1259, 1976.
37. Coronary Drug Project Research Group: The Coronary Drug Project: Initial Findings Leading to Modification of Its Research Protocol, *Journal of the American Medical Association* 214:1303–1313, 1970.
38. Baum J, Holtz F, Bookstein JJ, Klein EW: Possible Association Between Benign Hepatomas and Oral Contraceptives, *Lancet* 2:926–928, 1973.
39. Mays ET, Christopherson WM, Mahr MM, Williams HC: Hepatic Changes in Young Women Ingesting Contraceptive Steroids, Hepatic Hemorrhage and Primary Hepatic Tumors, *Journal of the American Medical Association* 235:730–782, 1976.
40. Edmondson HA, Henderson B, Benton B: Liver Cell Adenomas Associated with the Use of Oral Contraceptives, *New England Journal of Medicine* 294:470–472, 1976.
41. Pfeffer RI, Van Den Noort S: Estrogen Use and Stroke Risk in Postmenopausal Women, *American Journal of Epidemiology* 103:445–456, 1976.

PATIENT INFORMATION

WHAT YOU SHOULD KNOW ABOUT ESTROGENS

Estrogens are female hormones produced by the ovaries. The ovaries make several different kinds of estrogens. In addition, scientists have been able to make a variety of synthetic estrogens. As far as we know, all these estrogens have similar properties and therefore much the same usefulness, side effects, and risks. This leaflet is intended to help you understand what estrogens are used for, the risks involved in their use, and how to use them as safely as possible.
This leaflet includes the most important information about estrogens, but not all the information. If you want to know more, you can ask your doctor or pharmacist to let you read the package insert prepared for the doctor.

USES OF ESTROGEN

Estrogens are prescribed by doctors for a number of purposes, including:
1. To provide estrogen during a period of adjustment when a woman's ovaries no longer produce it, in order to prevent certain uncomfortable symptoms of estrogen deficiency. (All women normally stop producing estrogens, generally between the ages of 45 and 55; this is called the menopause.)
2. To prevent symptoms of estrogen deficiency when a woman's ovaries have been removed surgically before the natural menopause.
3. To prevent pregnancy. (Estrogens are given along with a progestagen, another female hormone; these combinations are called oral contraceptives or birth control pills. Patient labeling is available to women taking oral contraceptives, and they will not be discussed in this leaflet.)
4. To treat certain cancers in women and men.
THERE IS NO PROPER USE OF ESTROGENS IN A PREGNANT WOMAN.

ESTROGENS IN THE MENOPAUSE

In the natural course of their lives, all women eventually experience a decrease in estrogen production. This usually occurs between ages 45 and 55, but may occur earlier or later. Sometimes the ovaries may need to be removed before natural menopause by an operation, producing a "surgical menopause."
When the amount of estrogen in the blood begins to decrease, many women may develop typical symptoms: Feelings of warmth in the face, neck, and chest or sudden in-

tense episodes of heat and sweating throughout the body (called "hot flashes" or "hot flushes"). These symptoms are sometimes very uncomfortable. A few women eventually develop changes in the vagina (called "atrophic vaginitis") which cause discomfort, especially during and after intercourse.

Estrogens can be prescribed to treat these symptoms of the menopause. It is estimated that considerably more than half of all women undergoing the menopause have only mild symptoms or no symptoms at all and therefore do not need estrogens. Other women may need estrogens for a few months, while their bodies adjust to lower estrogen levels. Sometimes the need will be for periods longer than 6 months. In an attempt to avoid overstimulation of the uterus (womb), estrogens are usually given cyclically during each month of use, that is 3 weeks of pills followed by 1 week without pills.

Sometimes women experience nervous symptoms or depression during menopause. There is no evidence that estrogens are effective for such symptoms and they should not be used to treat them, although other treatments may be needed.

You may have heard that taking estrogens for long periods (years) after menopause will keep your skin soft and supple and keep you feeling young. There is no evidence that this is so, however, and such long-term treatment carries important risks.

THE DANGERS OF ESTROGENS

1. *Cancer of the uterus.* If estrogens are used in the postmenopausal period for more than a year, there is an increased risk of *endometrial cancer* (cancer of the uterus). Women taking estrogens have roughly 5 to 10 times as great a chance of getting this cancer as women who take no estrogens. To put this another way, while a postmenopausal woman not taking estrogens has 1 chance in 1,000 each year of getting cancer of the uterus, a woman taking estrogens has 5 to 10 chances in 1,000 each year. For this reason *it is important to take estrogens only when you really need them.*

   The risk of this cancer is greater the longer estrogens are used and also seems to be greater when larger doses are taken. For this reason *it is important to take the lowest dose of estrogen that will control symptoms and to take it only as long as it is needed.* If estrogens are needed for longer periods of time, your doctor will want to re-evaluate your need for estrogens at least every 6 months.

   Women using estrogens should report any irregular vaginal bleeding to their doctors; such bleeding may be of no importance, but it can be an early warning of cancer of the uterus. If you have undiagnosed vaginal bleeding, you should not use estrogens until a diagnosis is made and you are certain there is no cancer of the uterus. If you have had your uterus completely removed (total hysterectomy) there is no danger of developing cancer of the uterus.
2. *Other possible cancers.* Estrogens can cause development of other tumors in animals, such as tumors of the breast, cervix, vagina, or liver, when given for a long time. At present there is no good evidence that women using estrogen in the menopause have an increased risk of such tumors, but there is no way yet to be sure they do not; and one study raises the possibility that use of estrogens in the menopause may increase risk of breast cancer many years later. This is a further reason to use estrogens only when clearly needed. While you are taking estrogens, it is important that you go to your doctor at least once a year for a physical examination. Also, if members of your family have had breast cancer or if you have breast nodules or abnormal mammograms (breast x-rays), your doctor may wish to carry out more frequent examinations of your breasts.
3. *Gall bladder disease.* Women who use estrogens after menopause are more likely to develop gall bladder disease needing surgery than women who do not use estrogens. Birth control pills have a similar effect.
4. *Abnormal blood clotting.* Oral contraceptives increase the risk of blood clotting in various parts of the body. This can result in a stroke (if the clot is in the brain), a heart attack (clot in a blood vessel of the heart), or a pulmonary embolus (a clot which forms in the legs or pelvis, then breaks off and travels to the lungs). Any of these can be fatal.

   At this time use of estrogens in the menopause is not known to cause such blood clotting, but this has not been fully studied and there could still prove to be such a risk. It is recommended that if you have had clotting in the legs or lungs or a heart attack or stroke while you were using estrogens or birth control pills, you should not use estrogens (unless they are being used to treat cancer of the breast or prostate). If you have had a stroke or heart attack or if you have angina pectoris, estrogens should be used with great caution and only if clearly needed (for example, if you have severe symptoms of the menopause).

SPECIAL WARNING ABOUT PREGNANCY

You should not receive estrogen if you are pregnant. If this should occur there is a greater than usual chance that the developing child will be born with a birth defect, although the possibility remains fairly small. A female child may have an increased risk of developing cancer of the vagina or cervix later in life (in the teens or twenties). Every possible effort should be made to avoid exposure to estrogens during pregnancy. If exposure occurs, see your doctor.

OTHER EFFECTS OF ESTROGENS

In addition to the serious known risks of estrogens described above, estrogens have the following side effects and potential risks:

1. *Nausea and vomiting.* The most common side effect of estrogen therapy is nausea. Vomiting is less common.
2. *Effects on breasts.* Estrogens may cause breast tenderness or enlargement and may cause the breasts to secrete a liquid. These effects are not dangerous.
3. *Effects on the uterus.* Estrogens may cause benign fibroid tumors of the uterus to get larger. Some women will have menstrual bleeding when estrogens are stopped. But if the bleeding occurs on days you are still taking estrogens you should report this to your doctor.
4. *Effects on liver.* Women taking oral contraceptives develop on rare occasions a tumor of the liver which can rupture and bleed into the abdomen. So far, these tumors have not been reported in women using estrogens in the menopause, but you should report any swelling or unusual pain or tenderness in the abdomen to your doctor immediately.

   Women with a past history of jaundice (yellowing of the skin and white parts of the eyes) may get jaundice again during estrogen use. If this occurs, stop taking estrogen and see your doctor.
5. *Other effects.* Estrogens may cause excess fluid to be retained in the body. This may make some conditions worse, such as epilepsy, migraine, heart disease, or kidney disease.

SUMMARY

Estrogens have important uses, but they have serious risks as well. You must decide, with your doctor, whether the risks are acceptable to you in view of the benefits of treatment. Except where your doctor has prescribed estrogens for use in special cases of cancer of the breast or prostate, you should not use estrogens if you have cancer of the breast or uterus, are pregnant, have undiagnosed abnormal vaginal bleeding, clotting in the legs or lungs, or have had a stroke, heart attack or angina, or clotting in the legs or lungs in the past while you were taking estrogens.

You can use estrogens as safely as possible by understanding that your doctor will require regular physical examinations while you are taking them and will try to discontinue the drug as soon as possible and use the smallest dose possible. Be alert for signs of trouble including:

1. Abnormal bleeding from the vagina.
2. Pains in the calves or chest or sudden shortness of breath, or coughing blood (indicating possible clots in the legs, heart, or lungs).
3. Severe headache, dizziness, faintness, or changes in vision (indicating possible developing clots in the brain or eye).
4. Breast lumps (you should ask your doctor how to examine your own breasts).
5. Jaundice (yellowing of the skin).
6. Mental depression.

Based on his or her assessment of your medical needs, your doctor has prescribed this drug for you. Do not give the drug to anyone else.

Rx Only

Manufactured by: King Pharmaceuticals, Inc.
Bristol, TN 37620
Distributed by: Monarch Pharmaceuticals, Inc.
Bristol, TN 37620

Shown in Product Identification Guide, page 324

PEDIOTIC® SUSPENSION STERILE ℞
(neomycin and polymyxin B sulfates and hydrocortisone otic suspension, USP)

DESCRIPTION

PEDIOTIC Suspension (neomycin and polymyxin B sulfates and hydrocortisone otic suspension) is a sterile antibacterial and anti-inflammatory suspension for otic use. Each mL contains: neomycin sulfate equivalent to 3.5 mg neomycin base, polymyxin B sulfate equivalent to 10,000 polymyxin B units, and hydrocortisone 10 mg (1%). The vehicle contains thimerosal 0.001% (added as a preservative) and the inactive ingredients cetyl alcohol, glyceryl monostearate, mineral oil, polyoxyl 40 stearate, propylene glycol, and Water for Injection. Sulfuric acid may be added to adjust pH. PEDIOTIC Suspension has a minimum pH of 4.1, which is less acidic than the minimum pH of 3.0 for CORTISPORIN® Otic Suspension.

Neomycin sulfate is the sulfate salt of neomycin B and C, which are produced by the growth of *Streptomyces fradiae* Waksman (Fam. Streptomycetaceae). It has a potency equivalent of not less than 600 µg of neomycin standard per mg, calculated on an anhydrous basis. The structural formulae are:

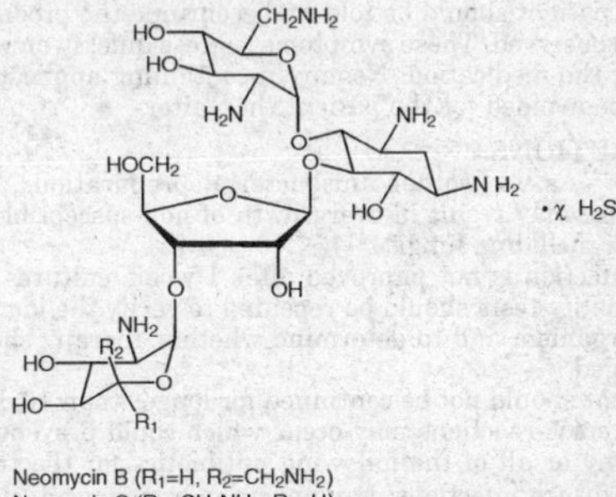

Neomycin B (R_1=H, R_2=CH_2NH_2)
Neomycin C (R_1=CH_2NH_2, R_2=H)

Polymyxin B sulfate is the sulfate salt of polymyxin B_1 and B_2, which are produced by the growth of *Bacillus polymyxa* (Prazmowski) Migula (Fam. Bacillaceae). It has a potency of not less than 6,000 polymyxin B units per mg, calculated on an anhydrous basis. The structural formulae are:

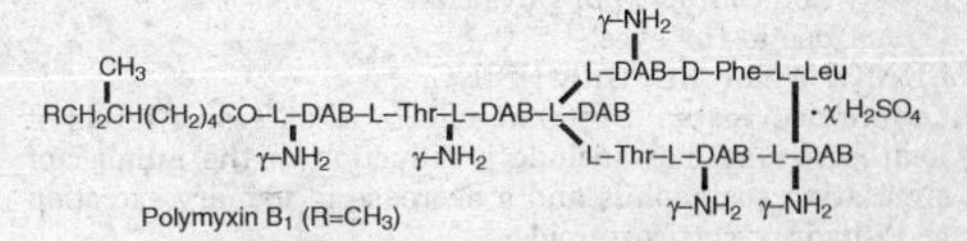

Polymyxin B_1 (R=CH_3)
Polymyxin B_2 (R=H)
DAB=α, γ-diaminobutyric acid

Hydrocortisone, 11β, 17, 21-trihydroxypregn-4-ene-3,20-dione, is an anti-inflammatory hormone. Its structural formula is:

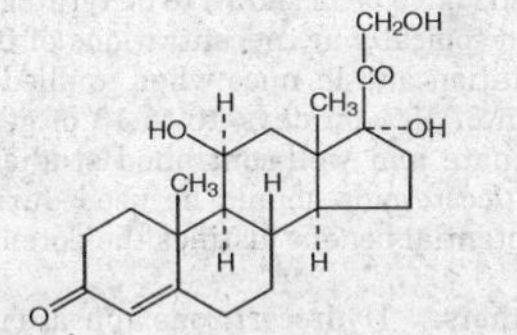

CLINICAL PHARMACOLOGY

Corticoids suppress the inflammatory response to a variety of agents and they may delay healing. Since corticoids may inhibit the body's defense mechanism against infection, a concomitant antimicrobial drug may be used when this inhibition is considered to be clinically significant in a particular case.

The anti-infective components in the combination are included to provide action against specific organisms susceptible to them. Neomycin sulfate and polymyxin B sulfate together are considered active against the following microorganisms: *Staphylococcus aureus, Escherichia coli, Haemophilus influenzae, Klebsiella-Enterobacter* species, *Neisseria* species, and *Pseudomonas aeruginosa.* This product does not provide adequate coverage against *Serratia marcescens* and streptococci, including *Streptococcus pneumoniae.*

The relative potency of corticosteroids depends on the molecular structure, concentration, and release from the vehicle.

INDICATIONS AND USAGE

For the treatment of superficial bacterial infections of the external auditory canal caused by organisms susceptible to the action of the antibiotics, and for the treatment of infections of mastoidectomy and fenestration cavities caused by organisms susceptible to the antibiotics.

CONTRAINDICATIONS

This product is contraindicated in those individuals who have shown hypersensitivity to any of its components, and in herpes simplex, vaccinia, and varicella infections.

WARNINGS

This product should be used with care in cases of perforated eardrum and in long-standing cases of chronic otitis media because of the possibility of ototoxicity. Neomycin sulfate may cause cutaneous sensitization. A precise incidence of hypersensitivity reactions (primarily skin rash) due to topical neomycin is not known.

When using neomycin-containing products to control secondary infection in the chronic dermatoses, such as chronic otitis externa or stasis dermatitis, it should be borne in mind that the skin in these conditions is more liable than is normal skin to become sensitized to many substances, including neomycin. The manifestation of sensitization to neomycin is usually a low-grade reddening with swelling, dry

Continued on next page

Pediotic—Cont.

scaling, and itching; it may be manifest simply as a failure to heal. Periodic examination for such signs is advisable, and the patient should be told to discontinue the product if they are observed. These symptoms regress quickly on withdrawing the medication. Neomycin-containing applications should be avoided for the patient thereafter.

PRECAUTIONS

General: As with other antibacterial preparations, prolonged use may result in overgrowth of non-susceptible organisms, including fungi.

If the infection is not improved after 1 week, cultures and susceptibility tests should be repeated to verify the identity of the organism and to determine whether therapy should be changed.

Treatment should not be continued for longer than 10 days.

Allergic cross-reactions may occur which could prevent the use of any or all of the following antibiotics for the treatment of future infections: kanamycin, paromomycin, streptomycin, and possibly gentamicin.

Information for Patients: Avoid contaminating the dropper with material from the ear, fingers, or other source. This caution is necessary if the sterility of the drops is to be preserved.

If sensitization or irritation occurs, discontinue use immediately and contact your physician.

Do not use in the eyes.

SHAKE WELL BEFORE USING.

Laboratory Tests: Systemic effects of excessive levels of hydrocortisone may include a reduction in the number of circulating eosinophils and a decrease in urinary excretion of 17-hydroxycorticosteroids.

Carcinogenesis, Mutagenesis, Impairment of Fertility: Long-term studies in animals (rats, rabbits, mice) showed no evidence of carcinogenicity attributable to oral administration of corticosteroids.

Pregnancy: ***Teratogenic Effects:*** Pregnancy Category C. Corticosteroids have been shown to be teratogenic in rabbits when applied topically at concentrations of 0.5% on days 6 to 18 of gestation and in mice when applied topically at a concentration of 15% on days 10 to 13 of gestation. There are no adequate and well-controlled studies in pregnant women. Corticosteroids should be used during pregnancy only if the potential benefit justifies the potential risk to the fetus.

Nursing Mothers: Hydrocortisone appears in human milk following oral administration of the drug. Since systemic absorption of hydrocortisone may occur when applied topically, caution should be exercised when PEDIOTIC is used by a nursing woman.

Pediatric Use: See DOSAGE AND ADMINISTRATION.

ADVERSE REACTIONS

Neomycin occasionally causes skin sensitization. Ototoxicity and nephrotoxicity have also been reported (see WARNINGS). Adverse reactions have occurred with topical use of antibiotic combinations including neomycin and polymyxin B. Exact incidence figures are not available since no denominator of treated patients is available. The reaction occurring most often is allergic sensitization. In one clinical study, using a 20% neomycin patch, neomycin-induced allergic skin reactions occurred in two of 2,175 (0.09%) individuals in the general population.[1] In another study, the incidence was found to be approximately 1%.[2]

The following local adverse reactions have been reported with topical corticosteroids, especially under occlusive dressings: burning, itching, irritation, dryness, folliculitis, hypertrichosis, acneiform eruptions, hypopigmentation, perioral dermatitis, allergic contact dermatitis, maceration of the skin, secondary infection, skin atrophy, striae, and miliaria. Stinging and burning have been reported rarely when this drug has gained access to the middle ear.

DOSAGE AND ADMINISTRATION

The external auditory canal should be thoroughly cleansed and dried with a sterile cotton applicator.

For adults, 4 drops of the suspension should be instilled into the affected ear 3 or 4 times daily. For infants and children, 3 drops are suggested because of the smaller capacity of the ear canal.

The patient should lie with the affected ear upward and then the drops should be instilled. This position should be maintained for 5 minutes to facilitate penetration of the drops into the ear canal. Repeat, if necessary, for the opposite ear.

If preferred, a cotton wick may be inserted into the canal and then the cotton may be saturated with the suspension. This wick should be kept moist by adding further suspension every 4 hours. The wick should be replaced at least once every 24 hours.

SHAKE WELL BEFORE USING.

HOW SUPPLIED

Bottle of 7.5 mL with sterilized dropper (NDC 61570-038-75). Store at 15° to 25°C (59° to 77°F).

Rx only

REFERENCES

1. Leyden JJ, Kligman AM. Contact dermatitis to neomycin sulfate. *JAMA*. 1979;242:1276-1278.
2. Prystowsky SD, Allen AM, Smith RW, Nonomura JH, Odom RB, Akers WA. Allergic contact hypersensitivity to nickel, neomycin, ethylenediamine, and benzocaine: relationships between age, sex, history of exposure, and reactivity to standard patch tests and use tests in a general population. *Arch Dermatol*. 1979;115:959-962.

Distributed by: Monarch Pharmaceuticals, Inc.
Bristol, TN 37620
Manufactured by: Catalytica Pharmaceutical, Inc.
Greenville, NC 27835

5/97
0932683

PROCANBID® ℞

[*prō căn 'bĭd*]
(Procainamide Hydrochloride Extended-Release Tablets*)
***Procanbid is not USP for dissolution.**

WARNINGS:
Positive ANA Titer: The prolonged administration of procainamide often leads to the development of a positive antinuclear antibody (ANA) test, with or without symptoms of a lupus erythematosus-like syndrome. If a positive ANA titer develops, the benefits versus risks of continued procainamide therapy should be assessed.

DESCRIPTION

Procanbid (Procainamide Hydrochloride Extended-Release Tablets), a Group 1A cardiac antiarrhythmic drug, is p-amino-N-[2-(diethylamino) ethyl]benzamide monohydrochloride, molecular weight 271.79. Its structural formula is:

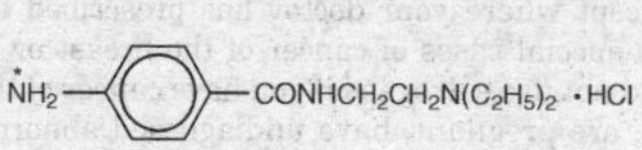

(*Site of acetylation to N-acetylprocainamide)

Procainamide hydrochloride differs from procaine which is the p-aminobenzoyl ester of 2-(diethylamino)-ethanol. Procainamide as the free base has a pK_a of 9.24; the monohydrochloride is very soluble in water.

Procanbid (Procainamide Hydrochloride Extended-Release Tablets) contains 500 mg or 1000 mg of procainamide hydrochloride for oral administration. The release of procainamide hydrochloride is controlled by 2 mechanisms using patented technology. The core of the tablet consists of a wax matrix which is then coated with a polymeric, control-release layer. Both strengths of Procanbid contain black iron oxide; candelilla wax, FCC; carnauba wax, NF; colloidal silicon dioxide, NF; hydroxypropyl cellulose, NF; hydroxypropylmethyl cellulose; magnesium stearate, NF; polyacrylate dispersion; polyethylene glycol 3350, NF; polyethylene glycol 8000, NF; propylene glycol; simethicone emulsion, USP; talc, USP; and titanium dioxide. The 1000-mg tablet additionally contains polysorbate 80.

CLINICAL PHARMACOLOGY

Mechanism of Action: Procainamide (PA) increases the effective refractory period of the atria, and to a lesser extent the bundle of His-Purkinje system and ventricles of the heart. It reduces impulse conduction velocity in the atria, His-Purkinje fibers, and ventricular muscle, but has variable effects on the atrioventricular (A-V) node, a direct slowing action and a weaker vagolytic effect that may speed A-V conduction slightly. Myocardial excitability is reduced in the atria, Purkinje fibers, papillary muscles, and ventricles by an increase in the threshold for excitation, combined with inhibition of ectopic pacemaker activity by retardation of the slow phase of diastolic depolarization, thus decreasing automaticity especially in ectopic sites. Contractility of the undamaged heart is usually not affected by therapeutic concentrations, although slight reduction of cardiac output may occur, and may be significant in the presence of myocardial damage. Therapeutic levels of PA may exert vagolytic effects and produce slight acceleration of heart rate, while high or toxic concentrations may prolong A-V conduction time or induce A-V block, or even cause abnormal automaticity and spontaneous firing, by unknown mechanisms.

The electrocardiogram may reflect these effects by showing slight sinus tachycardia (due to the anticholinergic action) and widened QRS complexes and, less regularly, prolonged Q-T and P-R intervals (due to longer systole and slower conduction), as well as some decrease in QRS and T wave amplitude. These direct effects of PA on electrical activity, conduction, responsiveness, excitability, and automaticity are characteristic of a Group 1A antiarrhythmic agent, the prototype for which is quinidine; PA effects are very similar. However, PA has weaker vagal blocking action than does quinidine, does not induce alpha-adrenergic blockade, and is less depressing to cardiac contractility.

Pharmacokinetics and Drug Metabolism

Absorption/Bioavailability: PA is well absorbed following oral administration. The absolute bioavailability from immediate-release PA HCl capsules is approximately 85% in patients and healthy subjects. Bioavailability of Procanbid is similar to that of PA HCl extended-release tablets, USP (Procan®SR) which have been shown to be similar to that of immediate-release PA.

The Procanbid patented delivery system is designed to control the rate of PA release such that absorption is sustained throughout a 12-hour dosing interval. After administration of Procanbid with a high-fat meal, the extent of PA absorption was increased by about 20%. Peak, trough, and average plasma PA concentrations following twice daily administration of Procanbid to healthy subjects are similar to those achieved when Procan SR is administered 4 times daily. In patients with frequent ventricular premature depolarizations (VPDs), peak and steady-state average PA concentrations following administration of Procanbid every 12 hours are bioequivalent to those following administration of an equivalent daily dose of Procan SR. While corresponding minimum concentrations are slightly lower than those for Procan SR, they remain within the acceptable therapeutic range of 3 to 10 mcg/mL.

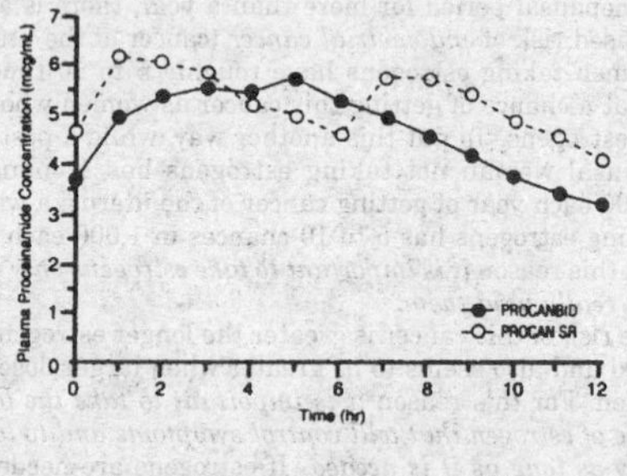

Figure 1. Mean Steady-State Plasma Concentrations Following Administration of Two 1000-mg Procanbid Tablets Every 12 Hours or One 1000-mg Procan SR Tablet Every 6 Hours to Patients with VPDs.

Twice-daily administration of two 1000-mg Procanbid tablets to patients with frequent VPDs produced a mean plasma PA concentration of 4.6 mcg/mL. Average peak and trough levels are within the generally accepted therapeutic range of 3 to 10 mcg/mL. Relative proportions of PA and N-acetylprocainamide (NAPA) during administration of Procanbid are similar to those following administration of immediate-release PA or Procan SR.

Distribution: Plasma protein binding of PA is insignificant, approximately 20%. The apparent volume of distribution is approximately 2 L/kg. It is not known if PA crosses the placenta.

Metabolism/Excretion: The elimination half-life of PA is 3 to 4 hours in patients with normal renal function, but reduced renal function prolongs the half-life (see Special Populations). PA is mainly eliminated intact by the kidneys. The only metabolite of any significance is N-acetylprocainamide (NAPA). Renal excretion accounts for >80% of the elimination of NAPA. Approximately 16 to 21% of PA is metabolized to NAPA in "slow acetylators"; in "rapid acetylators" the range is 24 to 33%. In white and black populations the numbers of rapid and slow acetylators are about 50%. The plasma concentration of NAPA is lower than the PA concentration in most individuals. The reverse may occur in individuals forming more of the metabolite while also having reduced kidney function. NAPA has significant antiarrhythmic activity.

An average of 65% of the dose was recovered as intact drug in the urine after intravenous administration of PA. The renal clearance of PA ranged from 400 to 600 mL/min. Active renal secretion ranged from 300 to 500 mL/min, and is thus the major elimination pathway for PA. The tubular secretion utilizes the base-secreting system also responsible for secretion of metformin, cimetidine, ranitidine, triamterene, and flecainide. Thus there is a potential for drug-drug interactions at this level.

Special Populations: *Patients with Renal Disease:* Decline in renal function, such as that occurring with advancing age or renal disease, increases the PA elimination half-life which can result in relatively high plasma concentrations of PA (see WARNINGS). Accumulation of NAPA due to impaired renal function can be more extensive than accumulation of PA.

Patients with Congestive Heart Failure: PA clearance is reduced in patients with severe heart failure, in part due to decreased renal perfusion (see WARNINGS).

Age, Gender, and Race: PA clearance decreases with increasing patient age, in part due to concurrent decreases in

renal function. However, the pharmacokinetics of PA and NAPA are similar in young healthy subjects (mean age 32 yr) and patients with frequent VPDs (mean age 60 yr) following administration of Procanbid every 12 hours. Steady state plasma procainamide concentrations in women receiving Procanbid are 30 percent higher than those seen in men receiving the same dosing regimen. When corrected for body surface area this difference is only 16 percent. Concentrations of N-acetylprocainamide are not significantly different among men and women whether corrected for body surface area or not. Procanbid tablets produce similar PA and NAPA concentrations in black and caucasian individuals.

Pharmacodynamics: While therapeutic plasma PA concentrations have been reported to be 3 to 10 mcg/mL, patients such as those with sustained ventricular tachycardia may need higher concentrations for adequate control. This may justify an increased risk of toxicity (see OVERDOSAGE). Where programmed ventricular stimulation has been used to evaluate efficacy of PA in preventing recurring ventricular tachyarrhythmias, an average plasma PA concentration of 13.6 mcg/mL was necessary for adequate control. Action of PA on the central nervous system is not prominent, but high concentrations may cause tremors.

A double-blind, placebo-controlled, dose-response, formulation-crossover study was conducted, comparing the suppression of VPDs by Procanbid administered every 12 hours and Procan SR administered every 6 hours. Similar VPD suppression was observed following administration of both formulations for 1 week each. Procanbid demonstrated significant pharmacologic activity (mean percent change from baseline in VPDs) compared with placebo, and a significant linear dose-response relationship was observed. VPD suppression was maintained throughout the dosing interval.

In this study, VPD rate tended to decrease with increasing concentration of PA and NAPA; however, PA concentration alone was a poor predictor of antiarrhythmic effect. The concentration-effect relationship for administration of Procanbid every 12 hours was indistinguishable from that for administration of Procan SR every 6 hours.

INDICATIONS AND USAGE

Procanbid tablets are indicated for the treatment of documented ventricular arrhythmias, such as sustained ventricular tachycardia, that in the judgment of the physician are life-threatening. Because of the proarrhythmic effects of procainamide, its use with lesser arrhythmias is generally not recommended. Treatment of patients with asymptomatic ventricular premature depolarizations should be avoided.

Initiation of procainamide treatment, as with other antiarrhythmic agents used to treat life-threatening arrhythmias, should be carried out in the hospital.

Antiarrhythmic drugs have not been shown to enhance survival in patients with ventricular arrhythmias.

Because procainamide has the potential to produce serious hematologic disorders (0.5%), particularly leukopenia or agranulocytosis (sometimes fatal), its use should be reserved for patients in whom, in the opinion of the physician, the benefits of treatment clearly outweigh the risks. (See WARNINGS and Boxed Warning.)

CONTRAINDICATIONS

Complete Heart Block: Procainamide should not be administered to patients with complete heart block because of its effects in suppressing nodal or ventricular pacemakers and the hazard of asystole. It may be difficult to recognize complete heart block in patients with ventricular tachycardia, but if significant slowing of ventricular rate occurs during PA treatment without evidence of A-V conduction appearing, PA should be stopped. In cases of second degree A-V block or various types of hemiblock, PA should be avoided or discontinued because of the possibility of increased severity of block unless the ventricular rate is controlled by an electrical pacemaker.

Idiosyncratic Hypersensitivity: In patients sensitive to procaine or other ester-type local anesthetics, cross sensitivity to PA is unlikely; however, it should be borne in mind, and PA should not be used if it produces acute allergic dermatitis, asthma, or anaphylactic symptoms.

Lupus Erythematosus: An established diagnosis of systemic lupus erythematosus is a contraindication to PA therapy, since aggravation of symptoms is highly likely.

Torsades De Pointes: In the unusual ventricular arrhythmia called "les torsades de pointes" (twisting of the points), characterized by alternation of 1 or more ventricular premature beats in the directions of the QRS complexes on ECG in persons with prolonged Q-T and often enhanced U waves, Group 1A antiarrhythmic drugs are contraindicated. Administration of PA in such cases may aggravate this special type of ventricular extrasystole or tachycardia instead of suppressing it.

WARNINGS

Mortality: In the National Heart, Lung, and Blood Institute's Cardiac Arrhythmia Suppresion Trial (CAST), a long-term, multi-centered, randomized, double-blind study in patients with asymptomatic non-life-threatening ventricular arrhythmias who had a myocardial infarction more than 6 days but less than 2 years previously, an excessive mortality or non-fatal cardiac arrest rate (7.7%) was seen in patients treated with encainide or flecainide compared with that seen in patients assigned to carefully matched placebo-treated groups (3.0%). The average duration of treatment with encainide or flecainide in this study was 10 months.

The applicability of the CAST results to other populations (eg, those without recent myocardial infarction) is uncertain. Considering the known proarrhythmic properties of procainamide and the lack of evidence of improved survival for any antiarrhythmic drug in patients without life-threatening arrhythmias, the use of Procanbid as well as other antiarrhythmic agents should be reserved for patients with life-threatening ventricular arrhythmias.

BLOOD DYSCRASIAS: Agranulocytosis, bone marrow depression, neutropenia, hypoplastic anemia, and thrombocytopenia have been reported in patients receiving procainamide hydrochloride at a rate of approximately 0.5%. Most of these patients received procainamide hydrochloride within the recommended dosage range. Fatalities have occurred (with approximately 20%–25% mortality in reported cases of agranulocytosis). Since most of these events have been noted during the first 12 weeks of therapy, it is recommended that complete blood counts including white cell, differential, and platelet counts be performed at weekly intervals for the first 3 months of therapy, and periodically thereafter. Complete blood counts should be performed promptly if the patient develops any signs of infection (such as fever, chills, sore throat, or stomatitis), bruising, or bleeding. If any of these hematologic disorders are identified, procainamide hydrochloride should be discontinued. Blood counts usually return to normal within 1 month of discontinuation. Caution should be used in patients with pre-existing marrow failure or cytopenia of any type (see ADVERSE REACTIONS).

Digitalis Intoxication: Caution should be exercised in the use of procainamide in arrhythmias associated with digitalis intoxication. Procainamide can suppress digitalis-induced arrhythmias; however, if there is concomitant marked disturbance of atrioventricular conduction, additional depression of conduction and ventricular asystole or fibrillation may result. Therefore, use of procainamide should be considered only if discontinuation of digitalis, and therapy with potassium lidocaine, or phenytoin are ineffective.

First Degree Heart Block: Caution should be exercised also if the patient exhibits or develops first degree heart block while taking PA, and dosage reduction is advised in such cases. If the block persists despite dosage reduction, continuation of PA administration must be evaluated on the basis of current benefit versus risk of increased heart block.

Predigitalization for Atrial Flutter or Fibrillation: Patients with atrial flutter or fibrillation should be cardioverted or digitalized prior to PA administration to avoid enhancement of A-V conduction which may result in ventricular rate acceleration beyond tolerable limits. Adequate digitalization reduces but does not eliminate the possibility of sudden increase in ventricular rate as the atrial rate is slowed by PA in these arrhythmias.

Congestive Heart Failure: For patients in congestive heart failure, and those with acute ischemic heart disease or cardiomyopathy, caution should be used in PA therapy, since even slight depression of myocardial contractility may further reduce the cardiac output of the damaged heart.

Concurrent Other Antiarrhythmic Agents: Concurrent use of PA with other Group 1A antiarrhythmic agents such as quinidine or disopyramide may produce enhanced prolongation of conduction or depression of contractility and hypotension, especially in patients with cardiac decompensation. Such use should be reserved for patients with serious arrhythmias unresponsive to a single drug and employed only if close observation is possible.

Renal Insufficiency: Renal insufficiency may lead to accumulation of high plasma concentrations of PA and/or NAPA from conventional oral doses of PA, with effects similar to those of overdosage (see OVERDOSAGE), unless dosage is adjusted for the individual patient.

Myasthenia Gravis: Patients with myasthenia gravis may show worsening of symptoms from PA due to its procaine-like effect on diminishing acetylcholine release at skeletal muscle motor nerve endings, so that PA administration may be hazardous without optimal adjustment of anticholinesterase medications and other precautions.

PRECAUTIONS

General: Immediately after initiation of PA therapy, patients should be closely observed for possible hypersensitivity reactions, especially if procaine or local anesthetic sensitivity is suspected, and for muscular weakness if myasthenia gravis is a possibility.

In conversion of atrial fibrillation to normal sinus rhythm by any means, dislodgment of mural thrombi may lead to embolization, which should be kept in mind.

Based upon the approximate half-life of 3 hours for PA, pharmacokinetic steady state would be reached within 1 day. After achieving and maintaining therapeutic plasma concentrations and satisfactory electrocardiographic and clinical responses, continued frequent periodic monitoring of vital signs and electrocardiograms is advised. If evidence of QRS widening of more than 25% or marked prolongation of the Q-T interval occurs, concern for overdosage is appropriate, and reduction in dosage is advisable if a 50% increase occurs. Elevated serum creatinine or urea nitrogen, reduced creatinine clearance, or history of renal insufficiency, as well ase use in older patients (over age 50), provide grounds to anticipate that less than the usual dosage may suffice, since the urinary elimination of PA and NAPA may be reduced, leading to gradual accumulation beyond normally predicted amounts. If facilities are available for measurement of plasma PA and NAPA, or acetylation capability, individual dose adjustment for optimal therapeutic concentrations may be easier, but close observation of clinical effectiveness is the most important criterion.

In the longer term, periodic complete blood counts are useful to detect possible idiosyncratic hematologic effects of PA on neutrophil, platelet, or red cell homeostatis; agranulocytosis has been reported to occur occasionally in patients on long-term PA therapy. A rising titer of serum ANA may precede clinical symptoms of the lupoid syndrome (see Boxed Warning and ADVERSE REACTIONS). If the lupus erythematosus-like syndrome develops in a patient with recurrent life-threatening arrhythmias not controlled by other agents, corticosteroid suppressive therapy may be used concomitantly with PA. Since the PA-induced lupoid syndrome rarely includes dangerous pathologic renal changes, PA therapy may not necessarily have to be stopped unless the symptoms of serositis and the possibility of further lupoid effects are of greater risk than the benefit of PA in controlling arrhythmias. Patients with rapid acetylation capability are less likely to develop the lupoid syndrome after prolonged PA therapy.

Information for Patients: The physician is advised to explain to the patient that close cooperation in adhering to the prescribed dosage schedule is of great importance in controlling the cardiac arrhythmia safely. The patient should understand clearly that more medication is not necessarily better and may be dangerous, that skipping doses or increasing intervals between doses to suit personal convenience may lead to loss of control of the heart problem, and that "making up" missed doses by doubling up later may be hazardous.

The patient should be encouraged to disclose any past history of drug sensitivity, especially to procaine or other local anesthetic agents, and to report any history of kidney disease, congestive heart failure, myasthenia gravis, liver disease, or lupus erythematosus.

The patient should be counseled to report promptly any symptoms of arthralgia, myalgia, fever, chills, skin rash, easy bruising, sore throat or sore mouth, infections, dark urine or icterus, wheezing, muscular weakness, chest or abdominal pain, palpitations, nausea, vomiting, anorexia, diarrhea, hallucinations, dizziness, or depression.

The patient should be advised not to break or chew the tablet as this would interfere with designed dissolution characteristics. The tablet matrix or Procanbid may be seen in the stool since it does not disintegrate following release of procainamide.

Laboratory Tests: Laboratory tests such as complete blood count (CBC), electrocardiogram, and serum creatinine or urea nitrogen may be indicated, depending on the clinical situation, and periodic rechecking of the CBC and ANA may be helpful in early detection of untoward reactions.

Drug Interactions: If other antiarrhythmic drugs are being used, additive effects on the heart may occur with PA administration, and dosage reduction may be necessary (see WARNINGS).

Anticholinergic drugs administered concurrently with PA may produce additive antivagal effects on A-V nodal conduction, although this is not as well documented for PA as for quinidine.

Coadministration of cimetidine decreases renal clearance of PA, potentially leading to clinically significant increases in plasma concentrations. Large (> 300 mg/day) doses of ranitidine possibly have this effect also. Plasma PA concentrations higher than those for administration of PA alone have been reported for coadministration with either amiodarone or trimethoprim. Alcohol (ethanol) consumption tends to decrease the half-life of PA in the blood through induction of its acetylation to NAPA.

Patients taking PA who require neuromuscular blocking agents such as succinylcholine may require less than usual doses of the latter, due to PA effects of reducing acetylcholine release.

Continued on next page

Procanbid—Cont.

Drug/Laboratory Test Interactions: Suprapharmacologic concentrations of lidocaine and meprobamate may inhibit fluorescence of PA and NAPA, and propranolol shows a native fluorescence close to the PA/NAPA peak wavelengths, so that tests which depend on fluorescence measurement may be affected.

Carcinogenesis, Mutagenesis, Impairment of Fertility: Long-term studies in animals have not been performed.

Pregnancy Category C: Animal reproduction studies have not been conducted with PA. It also is not known whether PA can cause fetal harm when administered to a pregnant woman or can affect reproduction capacity. PA should be given to a pregnant woman only if clearly needed.

Nursing Mothers: Both PA and NAPA are excreted in human milk, and absorbed by the nursing infant. Because of the potential for serious adverse reactions in nursing infants, a decision to discontinue nursing or the drug should be made, taking into account the importance of the drug to the mother.

Pediatric Use: Safety and effectiveness in pediatric patients have not been established.

ADVERSE REACTIONS

Cardiovascular System: Hypotension following oral PA administration is rare. Hypotension and serious disturbances of cardiac rhythm such as ventricular asystole or fibrillation are more common after intravenous administration (see OVERDOSAGE, WARNINGS). Second degree heart block has been reported in 2 of almost 500 patients taking PA orally.

Multisystem Effects: A lupus erythematosus-like syndrome of arthralgia, pleural or abdominal pain, and sometimes arthritis, pleural effusion, pericarditis, fever, chills, myalgia, and possibly related hematologic or skin lesions (see below) is fairly common after prolonged PA administration, perhaps more often in patients who are slow acetylators (see Boxed Warning and PRECAUTIONS). While some studies have reported less than 1 in 500, others have reported this syndrome in up to 30% of patients on long-term oral PA therapy. If discontinuation of PA does not reverse the lupoid symptoms, corticosteroid treatment may be effective.

Hematologic System: Neutropenia, thrombocytopenia, or hemolytic anemia may rarely be encountered. Agranulocytosis has occurred after repeated use of PA, and deaths have been reported (see WARNINGS and Boxed Warning).

Skin: Angioneurotic edema, urticaria, pruritus, flushing, and maculopapular rash have also occurred occasionally.

Gastrointestinal System: Anorexia, nausea, vomiting, abdominal pain, bitter taste, or diarrhea may occur in 3 to 4 percent of patients taking oral procainamide.

Elevated Liver Enzymes: Elevations of transaminase with and without elevations of alkaline phosphatase and bilirubin have been reported in patients taking oral procainamide. Some patients have had clinical symptoms (eg, malaise, right upper quadrant pain). Deaths from liver failure have been reported.

Nervous System: Dizziness or giddiness, weakness, mental depression, and psychosis with hallucinations have been reported occasionally.

OVERDOSAGE

Progressive widening of the QRS complex, prolonged Q-T and P-R intervals, lowering of the R and T waves, as well as increasing A-V block, may be seen with doses which are excessive for a given patient. Increased ventricular extrasystoles or even ventricular tachycardia or fibrillation may occur. After intravenous administration but seldom after oral therapy, transient high plasma concentrations of PA may induce hypotension, affecting systolic more than diastolic pressures, especially in hypertensive patients. Such high levels may also produce central nervous depression, tremor, and even respiratory depression.

Plasma levels above 10 mcg/mL are increasingly associated with toxic findings, which are seen occasionally in the 10 to 12 mcg/mL range, more often in the 12 to 15 mcg/mL range, and commonly in patients with plasma levels greater than 15 mcg/mL. A single oral dose of IR PA 2000 mg may produce overdosage symptoms, while 3000 mg of IR PA may be dangerous, especially if the patient is a slow acetylator, has decreased renal function, or underlying organic heart disease.

Treatment of overdosage or toxic manifestations includes general supportive measures, close observation, monitoring of vital signs and possibly intravenous pressor agents, and mechanical cardiorespiratory support. If available, PA and NAPA plasma levels may be helpful in assessing the potential degree of toxicity and response to therapy. Both PA and NAPA are removed from the circulation by hemodialysis but not peritoneal dialysis. No specific antidote for PA is known.

DOSAGE AND ADMINISTRATION

The dose should be adjusted for the individual patient, based on clinical assessment of the degree of underlying myocardial disease, the patient's age, and renal function. For patients who have been receiving another formulation of procainamide, the dose of the other formulation can function as a general guide, but re-titration with Procanbid is recommended.

As a general guide, for younger patients with normal renal function, an initial total daily oral dose of up to 50 mg/kg of body weight of Procanbid tablets may be used, given in 2 divided doses, every 12 hours, to maintain therapeutic blood concentrations. For older patients, especially those over 50 years of age, or for patients with renal, hepatic, or cardiac insufficiency, lesser amounts or longer intervals may produce adequate blood concentrations, and decrease the probability of occurrence of dose-related adverse reactions.

CARE SHOULD BE TAKEN WHEN DISPENSING PROCANBID TO ASSURE THE BID DOSAGE FORM HAS BEEN PRESCRIBED AND DISPENSED. Procanbid tablets should be swallowed whole and should not be bitten or cut.

To provide up to 50 mg/kg of body weight per day*

Patients Weighing	Dose
88-110 lb (40-50 kg)	1000 mg q12 hrs
132-154 lb (60-70 kg)	1500 mg q12 hrs
176-198 lb (80-90 kg)	2000 mg q12 hrs
>220 lb (>100 kg)	2500 mg q12 hrs

* Initial dosage schedule guide only, to be adjusted for each patient individually, based on age, cardiorenal function, blood concentration (if available), and clinical response.

HOW SUPPLIED

Procanbid tablets are supplied as follows:

500 mg: White, film-coated, elliptical tablets, coded "PROCANBID" on one side and "500" on the other.

N 61570-069-60 Bottles of 60

N 61570-069-70 Unit dose packages of 100 (10 strips of 10 tablets each).

1000 mg: Gray, film-coated, elliptical tablets, coded "PROCANBID" on one side and "1000" on the other.

N 61570-071-60 Bottles of 60

N 61570-071-70 Unit dose packages of 100 (10 strips of 10 tablets each).

Dispense in well-closed containers as defined in the USP.

Store at 20°–25°C (68°–77°F) [see USP].

Rx only.

Distributed by:
Monarch Pharmaceuticals, Inc.
Bristol, TN 37620
Manufactured by: Warner-Lambert Co Rev. 3/98
Morris Plains, NJ 07950 USA

Shown in Product Identification Guide, page 324

SEPTRA® I.V. Infusion ℞

[sĕp 'tra]

(trimethoprim and sulfamethoxazole)

DESCRIPTION

SEPTRA I.V. Infusion (trimethoprim and sulfamethoxazole), a sterile solution for intravenous infusion only, is a synthetic antibacterial combination product. Each mL contains 16 mg trimethoprim and 80 mg sulfamethoxazole compounded with 40% propylene glycol, 10% ethyl alcohol, and 0.3% diethanolamine; 1% benzyl alcohol and 0.1% sodium metabisulfite added as preservatives, Water for Injection, and pH adjusted to approximately 10 with sodium hydroxide.

Trimethoprim is 5-[(3,4,5-trimethoxyphenyl)methyl]-2,4-pyrimidinediamine. It is a white to light yellow, odorless, bitter compound with a molecular weight of 290.32 and the molecular formula $C_{14}H_{18}N_4O_3$. The structural formula is:

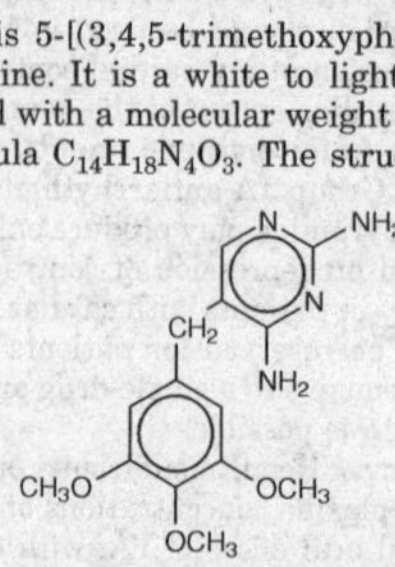

Sulfamethoxazole is 4-amino-*N*-(5-methyl-3-isoxazolyl)benzenesulfonamide. It is an almost white, odorless, tasteless compound with a molecular weight of 253.28 and the molecular formula $C_{10}H_{11}N_3O_3S$. The structural formula is:

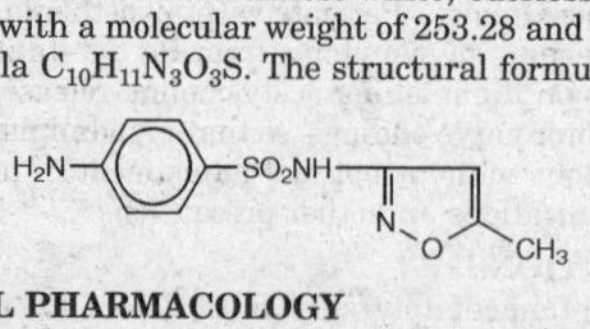

CLINICAL PHARMACOLOGY

Following a 1-hour intravenous infusion of a single dose of 160 mg trimethoprim and 800 mg sulfamethoxazole to 11 patients whose weight ranged from 105 lb to 165 lb (mean, 143 lb), the mean peak plasma concentrations of trimethoprim and sulfamethoxazole were 3.4 ± 0.3 mcg/mL and 46.3 ± 2.7 mcg/mL, respectively. Following repeated intravenous administration of the same dose at 8-hour intervals, the mean plasma concentrations just prior to and immediately after each infusion at steady-state were 5.6 ± 0.6 mcg/mL and 8.8 ± 0.9 mcg/mL for trimethoprim and 70.6 ± 7.3 mcg/mL and 105.6 ± 10.9 mcg/mL for sulfamethoxazole. The mean plasma half-life was 11.3 ± 0.7 hours for trimethoprim and 12.8 ± 1.8 hours for sulfamethoxazole. All of these 11 patients had normal renal function and their ages ranged from 17 to 78 years (median, 60 years).[1]

Pharmacokinetic studies in pediatric patients and adults suggest an age-dependent half-life of trimethoprim as indicated in the following table.[2]

Age (years)	No. of Patients	Mean TMP Half-life (hours)
<1	2	7.67
1-10	9	5.49
10-20	5	8.19
20-63	6	12.82

Patients with severely impaired renal function exhibit an increase in the half-lives of both components, requiring dosage regimen adjustment (see DOSAGE AND ADMINISTRATION).

Both trimethoprim and sulfamethoxazole exist in the blood as unbound, protein-bound, and metabolized forms; sulfamethoxazole also exists as the conjugated form. The metabolism of sulfamethoxazole occurs predominately by N_4-acetylation, although the glucuronide conjugate has been identified. The principal metabolites of trimethoprim are the 1- and 3-oxides and the 3′- and 4′-hydroxy derivatives. The free forms of trimethoprim and sulfamethoxazole are considered to be the therapeutically active forms. Approximately 44% of trimethoprim and 70% of sulfamethoxazole are bound to plasma proteins. The presence of 10 mg percent sulfamethoxazole in plasma decreases the protein binding of trimethoprim by an insignificant degree; trimethoprim does not influence the protein binding of sulfamethoxazole.

Excretion of trimethoprim and sulfamethoxazole is primarily by the kidneys through both glomerular filtration and tubular secretion. Urine concentrations of both trimethoprim and sulfamethoxazole are considerably higher than are the concentrations in the blood. The percent of dose excreted in urine over a 12-hour period following the intravenous administration of the first dose of 240 mg of trimethoprim and 1,200 mg of sulfamethoxazole on day 1 ranged from 17% to 42.4% as free trimethoprim; 7% to 12.7% as free sulfamethoxazole; and 36.7% to 56% as total (free plus the N_4-acetylated metabolite) sulfamethoxazole. When administered together as SEPTRA, neither trimethoprim nor sulfamethoxazole affects the urinary excretion pattern of the other.

Both trimethoprim and sulfamethoxazole distribute to sputum and vaginal fluid; trimethoprim also distributes to bronchial secretions, and both pass the placental barrier and are excreted in human milk.

Microbiology: Sulfamethoxazole inhibits bacterial synthesis of dihydrofolic acid by competing with *para*-aminobenzoic acid (PABA). Trimethoprim blocks the production of tetrahydrofolic acid from dihydrofolic acid by binding to and reversibly inhibiting the required enzyme, dihydrofolate reductase. Thus, SEPTRA blocks two consecutive steps in the biosynthesis of nucleic acids and proteins essential to many bacteria.

In vitro studies have shown that bacterial resistance develops more slowly with SEPTRA than with trimethoprim or sulfamethoxazole alone.

In vitro serial dilution tests have shown that the spectrum of antibacterial activity of SEPTRA includes common bacterial pathogens with the exception of *Pseudomonas aeruginosa*. The following organisms are usually susceptible: *Escherichia coli, Klebsiella* species, *Enterobacter* species, *Morganella morganii, Proteus mirabilis*, indole-positive *Proteus* species, including *Proteus vulgaris, Haemophilus influenzae* (including ampicillin-resistant strains), *Streptococcus pneumoniae, Shigella flexneri*, and *Shigella sonnei*. It should be noted, however, that there are little clinical data on the use of SEPTRA I.V. Infusion in serious systemic infections due to *Haemophilus influenzae* and *Streptococcus pneumoniae*.

[See table at top of next page]

Susceptibility Testing: The recommended quantitative disc susceptibility method may be used for estimating the susceptibility of bacteria to SEPTRA.[3,4] With this procedure, a report from the laboratory of "Susceptible to trimethoprim and sulfamethoxazole" indicates that the infection is likely to respond to therapy with SEPTRA. If the infection is confined to the urine, a report of "Intermediate susceptibility to trimethoprim and sulfamethoxazole" also indicates that the infection is likely to respond. A report of "Resistant to trimethoprim and sulfamethoxazole" indicates that the infection is unlikely to respond to therapy with SEPTRA.

Representative Minimum Inhibitory Concentration Values for Organisms Susceptible to SEPTRA (MIC-mcg/mL)

Bacteria	TMP Alone	SMX Alone	TMP/SMX (1:19) TMP	TMP/SMX (1:19) SMX
Escherichia coli	0.05-1.5	1.0-245	0.05-0.5	0.95-9.5
Proteus species (indole positive)	0.5-5.0	7.35-300	0.05-1.5	0.95-28.5
Morganella morganii	0.5-5.0	7.35-300	0.05-1.5	0.95-28.5
Proteus mirabilis	0.5-1.5	7.35-30	0.05-0.15	0.95-2.85
Klebsiella species	0.15-5.0	2.45-245	0.05-1.5	0.95-28.5
Enterobacter species	0.15-5.0	2.45-245	0.05-1.5	0.95-28.5
Haemophilus influenzae	0.15-1.5	2.85-95	0.015-0.15	0.285-2.85
Streptococcus pneumoniae	0.15-1.5	7.35-24.5	0.05-0.15	0.95-2.85
*Shigella flexneri**	<0.01-0.04	<0.16->320	<0.002-0.03	0.04-0.625
*Shigella sonnei**	0.02-0.08	0.625->320	0.004-0.06	0.08-1.25

TMP = trimethoprim   SMX = sulfamethoxazole
*Rudoy RC, Nelson JD, Haltalin KC. *Antimicrobial Agents and Chemotherapy.* 1974;5:439-443.

INDICATIONS AND USAGE

Pneumocystis Carinii Pneumonia: SEPTRA I.V. Infusion is indicated in the treatment of *Pneumocystis carinii* pneumonia in pediatric patients and adults.

Shigellosis: SEPTRA I.V. Infusion is indicated in the treatment of enteritis caused by susceptible strains of *Shigella flexneri* and *Shigella sonnei* in pediatric patients and adults.

Urinary Tract Infections: SEPTRA I.V. Infusion is indicated in the treatment of severe or complicated urinary tract infections due to susceptible strains of *Escherichia coli, Klebsiella* species, *Enterobacter* species, *Morganella morganii,* and *Proteus* species when oral administration of SEPTRA is not feasible and when the organism is not susceptible to single-agent antibacterials effective in the urinary tract.

Although appropriate culture and susceptibility studies should be performed, therapy may be started while awaiting the results of these studies.

CONTRAINDICATIONS

SEPTRA is contraindicated in patients with a known hypersensitivity to trimethoprim or sulfonamides and in patients with documented megaloblastic anemia due to folate deficiency. SEPTRA is also contraindicated in pregnant patients at term and in nursing mothers, because sulfonamides pass the placenta and are excreted in the milk and may cause kernicterus. SEPTRA is contraindicated in pediatric patients less than 2 months of age.

WARNINGS

FATALITIES ASSOCIATED WITH THE ADMINISTRATION OF SULFONAMIDES, ALTHOUGH RARE, HAVE OCCURRED DUE TO SEVERE REACTIONS, INCLUDING STEVENS-JOHNSON SYNDROME, TOXIC EPIDERMAL NECROLYSIS, FULMINANT HEPATIC NECROSIS, AGRANULOCYTOSIS, APLASTIC ANEMIA, AND OTHER BLOOD DYSCRASIAS. SULFONAMIDES, INCLUDING SULFONAMIDE-CONTAINING PRODUCTS SUCH AS TRIMETHOPRIM/SULFAMETHOXAZOLE, SHOULD BE DISCONTINUED AT THE FIRST APPEARANCE OF SKIN RASH OR ANY SIGN OF ADVERSE REACTION. In rare instances, a skin rash may be followed by a more severe reaction, such as Stevens-Johnson syndrome, toxic epidermal necrolysis, hepatic necrosis, and serious blood disorders (see PRECAUTIONS).

Clinical signs, such as rash, sore throat, fever, arthralgia, pallor, purpura, or jaundice may be early indications of serious reactions.

Cough, shortness of breath, and pulmonary infiltrates are hypersensitivity reactions of the respiratory tract that have been reported in association with sulfonamide treatment.

The sulfonamides should not be used for the treatment of group A beta-hemolytic streptococcal infections. In an established infection, they will not eradicate the streptococcus and, therefore, will not prevent sequelae such as rheumatic fever.

Pseudomembranous colitis has been reported with nearly all antibacterial agents, including trimethoprim/sulfamethoxazole, and may range in severity from mild to life-threatening. Therefore, it is important to consider this diagnosis in patients who present with diarrhea subsequent to the administration of antibacterial agents.

Treatment with antibacterial agents alters the normal flora of the colon and may permit overgrowth of clostridia. Studies indicate that a toxin produced by *Clostridium difficile* is one primary cause of "antibiotic-associated colitis."

After the diagnosis of pseudomembranous colitis has been established, therapeutic measures should be initiated. Mild cases of pseudomembranous colitis usually respond to drug discontinuation alone. In moderate to severe cases, consideration should be given to management with fluids and electrolytes, protein supplementation, and treatment with an antibacterial drug effective against *C. difficile.*

Contains sodium metabisulfite, a sulfite that may cause allergic-type reactions including anaphylactic symptoms and life-threatening or less severe asthmatic episodes in certain susceptible people. The overall prevalence of sulfite sensitivity in the general population is unknown and probably low. Sulfite sensitivity is seen more frequently in asthmatic than in nonasthmatic people.

Contains benzyl alcohol. In newborn infants, benzyl alcohol has been associated with an increased incidence of neurological and other complications which are sometimes fatal.

PRECAUTIONS

General: SEPTRA should be given with caution to patients with impaired renal or hepatic function, to those with possible folate deficiency (e.g., the elderly, chronic alcoholics, patients receiving anticonvulsant therapy, patients with malabsorption syndrome, and patients in malnutrition states), and to those with severe allergy or bronchial asthma. In glucose-6-phosphate dehydrogenase-deficient individuals, hemolysis may occur. This reaction is frequently dose-related. Adequate fluid intake must be maintained in order to prevent crystalluria and stone formation (see CLINICAL PHARMACOLOGY and DOSAGE AND ADMINISTRATION).

Local irritation and inflammation due to extravascular infiltration of the infusion has been observed with SEPTRA I.V. Infusion. If these occur, the infusion should be discontinued and restarted at another site.

Use in the Elderly: There may be an increased risk of severe adverse reactions in elderly patients, particularly when complicating conditions exist, e.g., impaired kidney and/or liver function, or concomitant use of other drugs. Severe skin reactions, or generalized bone marrow suppression (see WARNINGS and ADVERSE REACTIONS), or a specific decrease in platelets (with or without purpura) are the most frequently reported severe adverse reactions in elderly patients. In those concurrently receiving certain diuretics, primarily thiazides, an increased incidence of thrombocytopenia with purpura has been reported. Appropriate dosage adjustments should be made for patients with impaired kidney function (see DOSAGE AND ADMINISTRATION).

Use in the Treatment of *Pneumocystis carinii* Pneumonia in Patients with Acquired Immunodeficiency Syndrome (AIDS): The incidence of side effects, particularly rash, fever, leukopenia, and elevated aminotransferase (transaminase) values in AIDS patients who are being treated with SEPTRA for *Pneumocystis carinii* pneumonia has been reported to be greatly increased compared with the incidence normally associated with the use of SEPTRA in non-AIDS patients. The incidence of hyperkalemia and hyponatremia appears to be increased in AIDS patients receiving SEPTRA.

The concomitant use of leucovorin with trimethoprim-sulfamethoxazole for the acute treatment of *Pneumocystis carinii* pneumonia in patients with HIV infection was associated with increased rates of treatment failure and morbidity in a placebo-controlled study.

Laboratory Tests: Appropriate culture and susceptibility studies should be performed before and throughout treatment. Complete blood counts should be done frequently in patients receiving SEPTRA; if a significant reduction in the count of any formed blood element is noted, SEPTRA should be discontinued. Urinalyses with careful microscopic examination and renal function tests should be performed during therapy, particularly for those patients with impaired renal function.

Drug Interactions: In elderly patients concurrently receiving certain diuretics, primarily thiazides, an increased incidence of thrombocytopenia with purpura has been reported.

It has been reported that SEPTRA may prolong the prothrombin time in patients who are receiving the anticoagulant warfarin. This interaction should be kept in mind when SEPTRA is given to patients already on anticoagulant therapy, and the coagulation time should be reassessed.

SEPTRA may inhibit the hepatic metabolism of phenytoin. SEPTRA, given at a common clinical dosage, increased the phenytoin half-life by 39% and decreased the phenytoin metabolic clearance rate by 27%. When administering these drugs concurrently, one should be alert for possible excessive phenytoin effect.

Sulfonamides can also displace methotrexate from plasma protein binding sites, thus increasing free methotrexate concentrations.

Drug/Laboratory Test Interactions: SEPTRA, specifically the trimethoprim component, can interfere with a serum methotrexate assay as determined by the competitive binding protein technique (CBPA) when a bacterial dihydrofolate reductase is used as the binding protein. No interference occurs, however, if methotrexate is measured by a radioimmunoassay (RIA).

The presence of trimethoprim and sulfamethoxazole may also interfere with the Jaffé alkaline picrate reaction assay for creatinine, resulting in over-estimations of about 10% in the range of normal values.

Carcinogenesis, Mutagenesis, Impairment of Fertility: *Carcinogenesis:* Long-term studies in animals to evaluate carcinogenic potential have not been conducted with SEPTRA I.V. Infusion.

Mutagenesis: Bacterial mutagenic studies have not been performed with sulfamethoxazole and trimethoprim in combination. Trimethoprim was demonstrated to be non-mutagenic in the Ames assay. In studies at two laboratories, no chromosomal damage was detected in cultured Chinese hamster ovary cells at concentrations approximately 500 times human plasma levels; at concentrations approximately 1,000 times human plasma levels in these same cells, a low level of chromosomal damage was induced at one of the laboratories. No chromosomal abnormalities were observed in cultured human leukocytes at concentrations of trimethoprim up to 20 times human steady-state plasma levels. No chromosomal effects were detected in peripheral lymphocytes of human subjects receiving 320 mg of trimethoprim in combination with up to 1,600 mg of sulfamethoxazole per day for as long as 112 weeks.

Impairment of Fertility: SEPTRA I.V. Infusion has not been studied in animals for evidence of impairment of fertility. However, studies in rats at oral dosages as high as 70 mg/kg trimethoprim plus 350 mg/kg sulfamethoxazole daily showed no adverse effects on fertility or general reproductive performance.

Pregnancy: *Teratogenic Effects:* Pregnancy Category C. In rats, oral doses of 533 mg/kg sulfamethoxazole or 200 mg/kg trimethoprim produced teratological effects manifested mainly as cleft palates. The highest dose which did not cause cleft palates in rats was 512 mg/kg sulfamethoxazole or 192 mg/kg trimethoprim when administered separately. In two studies in rats, no teratogenicity was observed when 512 mg/kg of sulfamethoxazole was used in combination with 128 mg/kg of trimethoprim. In one study, however, cleft palates were observed in one litter out of nine when 355 mg/kg of sulfamethoxazole was used in combination with 88 mg/kg of trimethoprim.

In some rabbit studies, an overall increase in fetal loss (dead and resorbed and malformed conceptuses) was associated with doses of trimethoprim six times the human therapeutic dose.

While there are no large, well-controlled studies on the use of trimethoprim and sulfamethoxazole in pregnant women, Brumfitt and Pursell,[5] in a retrospective study, reported the outcome of 186 pregnancies during which the mother received either placebo or oral trimethoprim and sulfamethoxazole. The incidence of congenital abnormalities was 4.5% (3 of 66) in those who received placebo and 3.3% (4 of 120) in those receiving trimethoprim and sulfamethoxazole. There were no abnormalities in the 10 children whose mothers received the drug during the first trimester. In a separate survey, Brumfitt and Pursell also found no congenital abnormalities in 35 children whose mothers had received oral trimethoprim and sulfamethoxazole at the time of conception or shortly thereafter.

Because trimethoprim and sulfamethoxazole may interfere with folic acid metabolism, SEPTRA I.V. Infusion should be used during pregnancy only if the potential benefit justifies the potential risk to the fetus.

Nonteratogenic Effects: See CONTRAINDICATIONS section.

Nursing Mothers: See CONTRAINDICATIONS section.

Pediatric Use: SEPTRA I.V. Infusion is not recommended for pediatric patients younger than 2 months of age (see CONTRAINDICATIONS).

ADVERSE REACTIONS

The most common adverse effects are gastrointestinal disturbances (nausea, vomiting, anorexia) and allergic skin reactions (such as rash and urticaria). **FATALITIES ASSOCIATED WITH THE ADMINISTRATION OF SULFONAMIDES, ALTHOUGH RARE, HAVE OCCURRED DUE TO SEVERE REACTIONS, INCLUDING STEVENS-JOHNSON SYNDROME, TOXIC EPIDERMAL NECROLYSIS, FULMINANT HEPATIC NECROSIS, AGRANULOCYTOSIS, APLASTIC ANEMIA, OTHER BLOOD DYSCRASIAS, AND HYPERSENSITIVITY OF**

Continued on next page

Septra I.V. Infusion—Cont.

THE RESPIRATORY TRACT (SEE WARNINGS). Local reaction, pain, and slight irritation on I.V. administration are infrequent. Thrombophlebitis has rarely been observed.

Hematologic: Agranulocytosis, aplastic anemia, thrombocytopenia, leukopenia, neutropenia, hemolytic anemia, megaloblastic anemia, hypoprothrombinemia, methemoglobinemia, eosinophilia.

Allergic: Stevens-Johnson syndrome, toxic epidermal necrolysis, anaphylaxis, allergic myocarditis, erythema multiforme, exfoliative dermatitis, angioedema, drug fever, chills, Henoch-Schönlein purpura, serum sickness-like syndrome, generalized allergic reactions, generalized skin eruptions, conjunctival and scleral injection, photosensitivity, pruritus, urticaria, and rash. In addition, periarteritis nodosa and systemic lupus erythematosus have been reported.

Gastrointestinal: Hepatitis, including cholestatic jaundice and hepatic necrosis, elevation of serum transaminase and bilirubin, pseudomembranous enterocolitis, pancreatitis, stomatitis, glossitis, nausea, emesis, abdominal pain, diarrhea, anorexia.

Genitourinary: Renal failure, interstitial nephritis, BUN and serum creatinine elevation, toxic nephrosis with oliguria and anuria, and crystalluria.

Metabolic: Hyperkalemia, hyponatremia.

Neurologic: Aseptic meningitis, convulsions, peripheral neuritis, ataxia, vertigo, tinnitus, headache.

Psychiatric: Hallucinations, depression, apathy, nervousness.

Endocrine: The sulfonamides bear certain chemical similarities to some goitrogens, diuretics (acetazolamide and the thiazides), and oral hypoglycemic agents. Cross-sensitivity may exist with these agents. Diuresis and hypoglycemia have occurred rarely in patients receiving sulfonamides.

Musculoskeletal: Arthralgia and myalgia.

Respiratory System: Cough, shortness of breath, and pulmonary infiltrates (see WARNINGS).

Miscellaneous: Weakness, fatigue, insomnia.

OVERDOSAGE

Acute: Since there has been no extensive experience in humans with single doses of SEPTRA I.V. Infusion in excess of 25 mL (400 mg trimethoprim and 2,000 mg sulfamethoxazole), the maximum tolerated dose in humans is unknown. Signs and symptoms of overdosage reported with sulfonamides include anorexia, colic, nausea, vomiting, dizziness, headache, drowsiness, and unconsciousness. Pyrexia, hematuria, and crystalluria may be noted. Blood dyscrasias and jaundice are potential late manifestations of overdosage. Signs of acute overdosage with trimethoprim include nausea, vomiting, dizziness, headache, mental depression, confusion, and bone marrow depression.

General principles of treatment include the administration of intravenous fluids if urine output is low and renal function is normal. Acidification of the urine will increase renal elimination of trimethoprim.

The patient should be monitored with blood counts and appropriate blood chemistries, including electrolytes. If a significant blood dyscrasia or jaundice occurs, specific therapy should be instituted for these complications. Peritoneal dialysis is not effective and hemodialysis is only moderately effective in eliminating trimethoprim and sulfamethoxazole.

Chronic: Use of SEPTRA I.V. Infusion at high doses and/or for extended periods of time may cause bone marrow depression manifested as thrombocytopenia, leukopenia, and/or megaloblastic anemia. If signs of bone marrow depression occur, the patient should be given leucovorin; 5 to 15 mg leucovorin daily has been recommended by some investigators.

Animal Toxicity: The LD_{50} of SEPTRA I.V. Infusion in mice is 700 mg/kg or 7.3 mL/kg; in rats and rabbits the LD_{50} is >500 mg/kg or >5.2 mL/kg. The vehicle produced the same LD_{50} in each of these species as the active drug.

The signs and symptoms noted in mice, rats, and rabbits with SEPTRA I.V. Infusion or its vehicle at the high I.V. doses used in acute toxicity studies included ataxia, decreased motor activity, loss of righting reflex, tremors or convulsions, and/or respiratory depression.

DOSAGE AND ADMINISTRATION

CONTRAINDICATED IN PEDIATRIC PATIENTS LESS THAN 2 MONTHS OF AGE. CAUTION-SEPTRA I.V. INFUSION MUST BE DILUTED IN 5% DEXTROSE IN WATER SOLUTION PRIOR TO ADMINISTRATION. DO NOT MIX SEPTRA I.V. INFUSION WITH OTHER DRUGS OR SOLUTIONS. RAPID INFUSION OR BOLUS INJECTION MUST BE AVOIDED.

Dosage: ***Pediatric Patients and Adults:***

Pneumocystis Carinii Pneumonia: Total daily dose is 15 to 20 mg/kg (based on the trimethoprim component) given in three to four equally divided doses every 6 or 8 hours for up to 14 days. One investigator noted that a total daily dose of 10 to 15 mg/kg was sufficient in 10 adult patients with normal renal function.[6]

Severe Urinary Tract Infections and Shigellosis: Total daily dose is 8 to 10 mg/kg (based on the trimethoprim component) given in two to four equally divided doses every 6, 8, or 12 hours for up to 14 days for severe urinary tract infections and 5 days for shigellosis. The maximum recommended daily dose is 60 mL per day.

For Patients with Impaired Renal Function: When renal function is impaired, a reduced dosage should be employed using the following table:

Creatinine Clearance (mL/min)	Recommended Dosage Regimen
Above 30	Use Standard Regimen
15-30	½ the Usual Regimen
Below 15	Use Not Recommended

Method of Preparation: SEPTRA I.V. Infusion must be diluted. EACH 5 mL SHOULD BE ADDED TO 125 mL OF 5% DEXTROSE IN WATER. After diluting with 5% dextrose in water, the solution should not be refrigerated and should be used within 6 hours. If a dilution of 5 mL per 100 mL of 5% dextrose in water is desired, it should be used within 4 hours. If upon visual inspection there is cloudiness or evidence of crystallization after mixing, the solution should be discarded and a fresh solution prepared.

Multiple-Dose Vial: After initial entry into the vial, the remaining contents must be used within 48 hours.

The following infusion systems have been tested and found satisfactory: unit-dose glass containers; unit-dose polyvinyl chloride and polyolefin containers. No other systems have been tested and, therefore, no others can be recommended.

Dilution: EACH 5 mL OF SEPTRA I.V. INFUSION SHOULD BE ADDED TO 125 mL OF 5% DEXTROSE IN WATER.

NOTE: **In those instances where fluid restriction is desirable,** each 5 mL may be added to 75 mL of 5% dextrose in water. Under these circumstances the solution should be mixed just prior to use and should be administered within 2 hours. If upon visual inspection there is cloudiness or evidence of crystallization after mixing, the solution should be discarded and a fresh solution prepared.

DO NOT MIX SEPTRA I.V. INFUSION-5% DEXTROSE IN WATER WITH DRUGS OR SOLUTIONS IN THE SAME CONTAINER.

Administration: The solution should be given by intravenous infusion over a period of 60 to 90 minutes. Rapid infusion or bolus injections must be avoided. SEPTRA I.V. Infusion should not be given intramuscularly.

HOW SUPPLIED

5-mL vials, containing 80 mg trimethoprim (16 mg/mL) and 400 mg sulfamethoxazole (80 mg/mL) for infusion with 5% dextrose in water. Contains benzyl alcohol (see WARNINGS). Tray of 10 (NDC 61570-056-10).

10-mL multiple-dose vials, containing 160 mg trimethoprim (16 mg/mL) and 800 mg sulfamethoxazole (80 mg/mL) for infusion with 5% dextrose in water. Contains benzyl alcohol (see WARNINGS). Tray of 10 (NDC 61570-054-10).

20-mL multiple-dose vials, containing 320 mg trimethoprim (16 mg/mL) and 1,600 mg sulfamethoxazole (80 mg/mL) for infusion with 5% dextrose in water. Contains benzyl alcohol (see WARNINGS). Tray of 10 (NDC 61570-055-10).

Store at 15° to 25°C (59° to 77°F). DO NOT REFRIGERATE.

Also available in tablets containing 80 mg trimethoprim and 400 mg sulfamethoxazole (bottle of 100); DS (double strength) tablets containing 160 mg trimethoprim and 800 mg sulfamethoxazole (bottles of 100 and 250); and oral suspension containing 40 mg trimethoprim and 200 mg sulfamethoxazole in each 5 mL (pink, cherry-flavored: bottle of 1 pint [473 mL], 100 mL–package of 6; and purple, grape-flavored: bottle of 1 pint [473 mL]).

REFERENCES

1. Grose WE, Bodey GP, Loo TL. Clinical pharmacology of intravenously administered trimethoprim-sulfamethoxazole. *Antimicrob Agents Chemother*. 1979;15:447-451.
2. Siber GR, Gorham C, Durbin W, Lesko L, Levin MJ. Pharmacology of intravenous trimethoprim-sulfamethoxazole in children and adults. In: Nelson JD, Grassi C, eds. *Current Chemotherapy of Infectious Disease*. Washington, DC: American Society for Microbiology; 1980;1:691-692.
3. Bauer AW, Kirby WMM, Sherris JC, Turck M. Antibiotic susceptibility testing by a standardized single disk method. *Am J Clin Pathol*. 1966;45:493-496.
4. National Committee for Clinical Laboratory Standards. Performance standards for antimicrobial disk susceptibility tests, 2nd ed. Villanova, PA. 1979.
5. Brumfitt W, Pursell R. Trimethoprim-sulfamethoxazole in the treatment of bacteriuria in women. *J Infect Dis*. 1973;128(suppl):S657-S663.
6. Winston DJ, Lau WK, Gale RP, Young LS. Trimethoprim-sulfamethoxazole for the treatment of *Pneumocystis carinii* pneumonia. *Ann Int Med*. 1980;92:762-769.

Distributed by: Monarch Pharmaceuticals, Inc., Bristol, TN 37620

Manufactured by: Catalytica Pharmaceuticals, Inc., Greenville, NC 27834

Rev. 1/98

595716

SEPTRA®Tablets ℞

[sĕp 'tra]

SEPTRA® DS (Double Strength) Tablets ℞
SEPTRA® Suspension ℞
SEPTRA® Grape Suspension ℞

(trimethoprim and sulfamethoxazole)

DESCRIPTION

SEPTRA (trimethoprim and sulfamethoxazole) is a synthetic antibacterial combination product. Each SEPTRA Tablet contains 80 mg trimethoprim and 400 mg sulfamethoxazole and the inactive ingredients docusate sodium, FD&C Red No. 40, magnesium stearate, povidone, and sodium starch glycolate.

Each SEPTRA DS (double strength) Tablet contains 160 mg trimethoprim and 800 mg sulfamethoxazole and the inactive ingredients docusate sodium, FD&C Red No. 40, magnesium stearate, povidone, and sodium starch glycolate.

Each teaspoonful (5 mL) of SEPTRA Suspension contains 40 mg trimethoprim and 200 mg sulfamethoxazole and the inactive ingredients alcohol 0.26%, methylparaben 0.1% and sodium benzoate 0.1% (added as preservatives), carboxymethylcellulose sodium, citric acid, FD&C Red No. 40 and Yellow No. 6, flavor, glycerin, microcrystalline cellulose, polysorbate 80, saccharin sodium, and sorbitol. Each teaspoonful (5 mL) of SEPTRA Grape Suspension contains 40 mg trimethoprim and 200 mg sulfamethoxazole and the inactive ingredients alcohol 0.26%, methylparaben 0.1%, and sodium benzoate 0.1% (added as preservatives), carboxymethylcellulose sodium, citric acid, FD&C Red No. 40 and Blue No. 1, flavor, glycerin, microcrystalline cellulose, polysorbate 80, saccharin sodium, and sorbitol. Both tablet and suspension forms are for oral administration.

Trimethoprim is 5-[(3,4,5-trimethoxyphenyl)methyl]-2,4-pyrimidinediamine. It is a white to light yellow, odorless, bitter compound with a molecular weight of 290.32, and the molecular formula $C_{14}H_{18}N_4O_3$. The structural formula is:

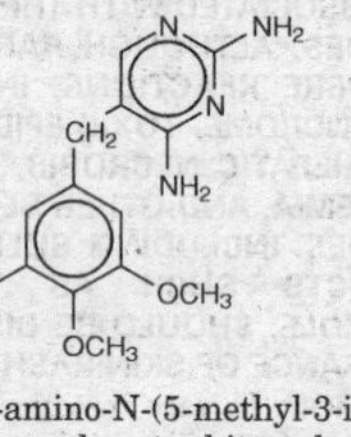

Sulfamethoxazole is 4-amino-N-(5-methyl-3-isoxazolyl)benzenesulfonamide. It is an almost white, odorless, tasteless compound with a molecular weight of 253.28, and the molecular formula $C_{10}H_{11}N_3O_3S$. The structural formula is:

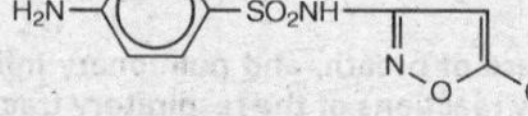

CLINICAL PHARMACOLOGY

SEPTRA is rapidly absorbed following oral administration. Both sulfamethoxazole and trimethoprim exist in the blood as unbound, protein-bound, and metabolized forms; sulfamethoxazole also exists as the conjugated form. The metabolism of sulfamethoxazole occurs predominately by N_4-acetylation, although the glucuronide conjugate has been identified. The principal metabolites of trimethoprim are the 1- and 3-oxides and the 3′- and 4′-hydroxy derivatives. The free forms of sulfamethoxazole and trimethoprim are considered to be the therapeutically active forms. Approximately 44% of trimethoprim and 70% of sulfamethoxazole are bound to plasma proteins. The presence of 10 mg percent sulfamethoxazole in plasma decreases the protein binding of trimethoprim by an insignificant degree; trimethoprim does not influence the protein binding of sulfamethoxazole.

Peak blood levels for the individual components occur 1 to 4 hours after oral administration. The mean serum half-lives of sulfamethoxazole and trimethoprim are 10 and 8 to 10 hours, respectively. However, patients with severely impaired renal function exhibit an increase in the half-lives of both components, requiring dosage regimen adjustment (see DOSAGE AND ADMINISTRATION). Detectable amounts of trimethoprim and sulfamethoxazole are present in the blood 24 hours after drug administration. During administration of 160 mg trimethoprim and 800 mg sulfamethox-

azole b.i.d., the mean steady-state plasma concentration of trimethoprim was 1.72 mcg/mL. The steady-state minimal plasma levels of free and total sulfamethoxazole were 57.4 mcg/mL and 68.0 mcg/mL, respectively. These steady-state levels were achieved after 3 days of drug administration.[1]

Excretion of sulfamethoxazole and trimethoprim is primarily by the kidneys through both glomerular filtration and tubular secretion. Urine concentrations of both sulfamethoxazole and trimethoprim are considerably higher than are the concentrations in the blood. The average percentage of the dose recovered in urine from 0 to 72 hours after a single oral dose is 84.5% for total sulfonamide and 66.8% for free trimethoprim. Thirty percent of the total sulfonamide is excreted as free sulfamethoxazole, with the remaining as N_4-acetylated metabolite.[2] When administered together as SEPTRA, neither sulfamethoxazole nor trimethoprim affects the urinary excretion pattern of the other. Both trimethoprim and sulfamethoxazole distribute to sputum, vaginal fluid, and middle ear fluid; trimethoprim also distributes to bronchial secretions, and both pass the placental barrier and are excreted in human milk.

Microbiology: Sulfamethoxazole inhibits bacterial synthesis of dihydrofolic acid by competing with *para*-aminobenzoic acid (PABA). Trimethoprim blocks the production of tetrahydrofolic acid from dihydrofolic acid by binding to and reversibly inhibiting the required enzyme, dihydrofolate reductase. Thus, SEPTRA blocks two consecutive steps in the biosynthesis of nucleic acids and proteins essential to many bacteria.

In vitro studies have shown that bacterial resistance develops more slowly with SEPTRA than with either trimethoprim or sulfamethoxazole alone.

In vitro serial dilution tests have shown that the spectrum of antibacterial activity of SEPTRA includes the common urinary tract pathogens with the exception of *Pseudomonas aeruginosa*. The following organisms are usually susceptible: *Escherichia coli, Klebsiella* species, *Enterobacter* species, *Morganella morganii, Proteus mirabilis*, and indole-positive *Proteus* species including *Proteus vulgaris*.

The usual spectrum of antimicrobial activity of SEPTRA includes bacterial pathogens isolated from middle ear exudate and from bronchial secretions (*Haemophilus influenzae*, including ampicillin-resistant strains, and *Streptococcus pneumoniae*), and enterotoxigenic strains of *Escherichia coli* (ETEC) causing bacterial gastroenteritis. *Shigella flexneri* and *Shigella sonnei* are also usually susceptible.

[See table above]

REPRESENTATIVE MINIMUM INHIBITORY CONCENTRATION VALUES FOR ORGANISMS SUSCEPTIBLE TO SEPTRA (MIC-µg/mL)

Bacteria	TMP Alone	SMX Alone	TMP/SMX (1:19) TMP	TMP/SMX (1:19) SMX
Escherichia coli	0.05–1.5	1.0–245	0.05–0.5	0.95–9.5
Escherichia coli (enterotoxigenic strains)	0.015–0.15	0.285–>950	0.005–0.15	0.095–2.85
Proteus species (indole positive)	0.5–5.0	7.35–300	0.05–1.5	0.95–28.5
Morganella morganii	0.5–5.0	7.35–300	0.05–1.5	0.95–28.5
Proteus mirabilis	0.5–1.5	7.35–30	0.05–0.15	0.95–2.85
Klebsiella species	0.15–5.0	2.45–245	0.05–1.5	0.95–28.5
Enterobacter species	0.15–5.0	2.45–245	0.05–1.5	0.95–28.5
Haemophilus influenzae	0.15–1.5	2.85–95	0.015–0.15	0.285–2.85
Streptococcus pneumoniae	0.15–1.5	7.35–24.5	0.05–0.15	0.95–2.85
*Shigella flexneri**	<0.01–0.04	<0.16–>320	<0.002–0.03	0.04–0.625
*Shigella sonnei**	0.02–0.08	0.625–>320	0.004–0.06	0.08–1.25

TMP=trimethoprimSMX=sulfamethoxazole

*Rudoy RC, Nelson JD, Haltalin KC. *Antimicrobial Agents and Chemotherapy* 1974;5:439–443.

Susceptibility Testing: The recommended quantitative disc susceptibility method may be used for estimating the susceptibility of bacteria to SEPTRA.[3,4] With this procedure, a report from the laboratory of "Susceptible to trimethoprim and sulfamethoxazole" indicates that the infection is likely to respond to therapy with SEPTRA. If the infection is confined to the urine, a report of "Intermediate susceptibility to trimethoprim and sulfamethoxazole" also indicates that the infection is likely to respond. A report of "Resistant to trimethoprim and sulfamethoxazole" indicates that the infection is unlikely to respond to therapy with SEPTRA.

INDICATIONS AND USAGE

Urinary Tract Infections: For the treatment of urinary tract infections due to susceptible strains of the following organisms: *Escherichia coli, Klebsiella* species, *Enterobacter* species, *Morganella morganii, Proteus mirabilis,* and *Proteus vulgaris*. It is recommended that initial episodes of uncomplicated urinary tract infections be treated with a single effective antibacterial agent rather than the combination.

Acute Otitis Media: For the treatment of acute otitis media in pediatric patients due to susceptible strains of *Streptococcus pneumoniae* or *Haemophilus influenzae* when, in the judgment of the physician, SEPTRA offers some advantage over the use of other antimicrobial agents. To date, there are limited data on the safety of repeated use of SEPTRA in pediatric patients under two years of age. SEPTRA is not indicated for prophylactic or prolonged administration in otitis media at any age.

Acute Exacerbations of Chronic Bronchitis in Adults: For the treatment of acute exacerbations of chronic bronchitis due to susceptible strains of *Streptococcus pneumoniae* or *Haemophilus influenzae* when, in the judgment of the physician, SEPTRA offers some advantage over the use of a single antimicrobial agent.

Travelers' Diarrhea in Adults: For the treatment of travelers' diarrhea due to susceptible strains of enterotoxigenic *E. coli*. Shigellosis: For the treatment of enteritis caused by susceptible strains of *Shigella flexneri* and *Shigella sonnei* when antibacterial therapy is indicated.

***Pneumocystis Carinii* Pneumonia:** For the treatment of documented *Pneumocystis carinii* pneumonia. For prophylaxis against *Pneumocystis carinii* pneumonia in individuals who are immunosuppressed and considered to be at an increased risk of developing *Pneumocystis carinii* pneumonia.

CONTRAINDICATIONS

SEPTRA is contraindicated in patients with a known hypersensitivity to trimethoprim or sulfonamides and in patients with documented megaloblastic anemia due to folate deficiency. SEPTRA is also contraindicated in pregnant patients at term and in nursing mothers, because sulfonamides pass the placenta and are excreted in the milk and may cause kernicterus. SEPTRA is contraindicated in pediatric patients less than 2 months of age.

WARNINGS

FATALITIES ASSOCIATED WITH THE ADMINISTRATION OF SULFONAMIDES, ALTHOUGH RARE, HAVE OCCURRED DUE TO SEVERE REACTIONS, INCLUDING STEVENS-JOHNSON SYNDROME, TOXIC EPIDERMAL NECROLYSIS, FULMINANT HEPATIC NECROSIS, AGRANULOCYTOSIS, APLASTIC ANEMIA, AND OTHER BLOOD DYSCRASIAS. SULFONAMIDES, INCLUDING SULFONAMIDE-CONTAINING PRODUCTS SUCH AS TRIMETHOPRIM/SULFAMETHOXAZOLE, SHOULD BE DISCONTINUED AT THE FIRST APPEARANCE OF SKIN RASH OR ANY SIGN OF ADVERSE REACTION. In rare instances, a skin rash may be followed by a more severe reaction, such as Stevens-Johnson syndrome, toxic epidermal necrolysis, hepatic necrosis, and serious blood disorder (see PRECAUTIONS).

Clinical signs, such as rash, sore throat, fever, arthralgia, pallor, purpura, or jaundice may be early indications of serious reactions.

Cough, shortness of breath, and pulmonary infiltrates are hypersensitivity reactions of the respiratory tract that have been reported in association with sulfonamide treatment.

The sulfonamides should not be used for the treatment of group A beta-hemolytic streptococcal infections. In an established infection, they will not eradicate the streptococcus and, therefore, will not prevent sequelae such as rheumatic fever.

Pseudomembranous colitis has been reported with nearly all antibacterial agents, including trimethoprim/sulfamethoxazole, and may range in severity from mild to life-threatening. Therefore, it is important to consider this diagnosis in patients who present with diarrhea subsequent to the administration of antibacterial agents.

Treatment with antibacterial agents alters the normal flora of the colon and may permit overgrowth of clostridia. Studies indicate that a toxin produced by Clostridium difficile is one primary cause of "antibiotic-associated colitis."

After the diagnosis of pseudomembranous colitis has been established, therapeutic measures should be initiated. Mild cases of pseudomembranous colitis usually respond to drug discontinuation alone. In moderate to severe cases, consideration should be given to management with fluids and electrolytes, protein supplementation, and treatment with an antibacterial drug effective against *C. difficile*.

PRECAUTIONS

General: SEPTRA should be given with caution to patients with impaired renal or hepatic function, to those with possible folate deficiency (e.g., the elderly, chronic alcoholics, patients receiving anticonvulsant therapy, patients with malabsorption syndrome, and patients in malnutrition states), and to those with severe allergy or bronchial asthma. In glucose-6-phosphate dehydrogenase-deficient individuals, hemolysis may occur. This reaction is frequently dose-related (see CLINICAL PHARMACOLOGY and DOSAGE AND ADMINISTRATION).

Use in the Elderly: There may be an increased risk of severe adverse reactions in elderly patients, particularly when complicating conditions exist, e.g., impaired kidney and/or liver function, or concomitant use of other drugs. Severe skin reactions, or generalized bone marrow suppression (see WARNINGS and ADVERSE REACTIONS), or a specific decrease in platelets (with or without purpura) are the most frequently reported severe adverse reactions in elderly patients. In those concurrently receiving certain diuretics, primarily thiazides, an increased incidence of thrombocytopenia with purpura has been reported. Appropriate dosage adjustments should be made for patients with impaired kidney function (see DOSAGE AND ADMINISTRATION).

Use in the Treatment of and Prophylaxis for *Pneumocystis carinii* Pneumonia in Patients with Acquired Immunodeficiency Syndrome (AIDS): The incidence of side effects, particularly rash, fever, leukopenia, and elevated aminotransferase (transaminase) values in AIDS patients who are being treated with SEPTRA for *Pneumocystis carinii* pneumonia has been reported to be greatly increased compared with the incidence normally associated with the use of SEPTRA in non-AIDS patients. The incidence of hyperkalemia and hyponatremia appears to be increased in AIDS patients receiving SEPTRA. Adverse effects are generally less severe in patients receiving SEPTRA for prophylaxis. A history of mild intolerance to SEPTRA in AIDS patients does not appear to predict intolerance of subsequent secondary prophylaxis. However, if a patient develops skin rash or any sign of adverse reaction, therapy with SEPTRA should be re-evaluated (see WARNINGS).

The concomitant use of leucovorin with trimethoprim-sulfamethoxazole for the acute treatment of *Pneumocystis carinii* pneumonia in patients with HIV infection was associated with increased rates of treatment failure and morbidity in a placebo-controlled study.

Information for Patients: Patients should be instructed to maintain an adequate fluid intake in order to prevent crystalluria and stone formation.

Laboratory Tests: Complete blood counts should be done frequently in patients receiving SEPTRA; if a significant reduction in the count of any formed blood element is noted, SEPTRA should be discontinued. Urinalyses with careful microscopic examination and renal function tests should be performed during therapy, particularly for those patients with impaired renal function.

Drug Interactions: In elderly patients concurrently receiving certain diuretics, primarily thiazides, an increased incidence of thrombocytopenia with purpura has been reported.

Continued on next page

Septra Tablets/Suspension—Cont.

It has been reported that SEPTRA may prolong the prothrombin time in patients who are receiving the anticoagulant warfarin. This interaction should be kept in mind when SEPTRA is given to patients already on anticoagulant therapy, and the coagulation time should be reassessed.
SEPTRA may inhibit the hepatic metabolism of phenytoin. SEPTRA, given at a common clinical dosage, increased the phenytoin half-life by 39% and decreased the phenytoin metabolic clearance rate by 27%. When administering these drugs concurrently, one should be alert for possible excessive phenytoin effect.
Sulfonamides can also displace methotrexate from plasma protein binding sites, thus increasing free methotrexate concentrations.
Drug/Laboratory Test Interactions: SEPTRA, specifically the trimethoprim component, can interfere with a serum methotrexate assay as determined by the competitive binding protein technique (CBPA) when a bacterial dihydrofolate reductase is used as the binding protein. No interference occurs, however, if methotrexate is measured by a radioimmunoassay (RIA).
The presence of trimethoprim and sulfamethoxazole may also interfere with the Jaffé alkaline picrate reaction assay for creatinine, resulting in overestimations of about 10% in the range of normal values.
Carcinogenesis, Mutagenesis, Impairment of Fertility: ***Carcinogenesis***: Long-term studies in animals to evaluate carcinogenic potential have not been conducted with SEPTRA.
Mutagenesis: Bacterial mutagenic studies have not been performed with sulfamethoxazole and trimethoprim in combination. Trimethoprim was demonstrated to be non-mutagenic in the Ames assay. In studies at two laboratories, no chromosomal damage was detected in cultured Chinese hamster ovary cells at concentrations approximately 500 times human plasma levels; at concentrations approximately 1,000 times human plasma levels in these same cells, a low level of chromosomal damage was induced at one of the laboratories. No chromosomal abnormalities were observed in cultured human leukocytes at concentrations of trimethoprim up to 20 times human steady-state plasma levels. No chromosomal effects were detected in peripheral lymphocytes of human subjects receiving 320 mg of trimethoprim in combination with up to 1,600 mg of sulfamethoxazole per day for as long as 112 weeks.
Impairment of Fertility: No adverse effects on fertility or general reproductive performance were observed in rats given oral dosages as high as 70 mg/kg/day trimethoprim plus 350 mg/kg/day sulfamethoxazole.
Pregnancy: *Teratogenic Effects:* Pregnancy Category C. In rats, oral doses of 533 mg/kg sulfamethoxazole or 200 mg/kg trimethoprim produced teratological effects manifested mainly as cleft palates. The highest dose which did not cause cleft palates in rats was 512 mg/kg sulfamethoxazole or 192 mg/kg trimethoprim when administered separately. In two studies in rats, no teratogenicity was observed when 512 mg/kg of sulfamethoxazole was used in combination with 128 mg/kg of trimethoprim. In one study, however, cleft palates were observed in one litter out of nine when 355 mg/kg of sulfamethoxazole was used in combination with 88 mg/kg of trimethoprim.
In some rabbit studies, an overall increase in fetal loss (dead and resorbed and malformed conceptuses) was associated with doses of trimethoprim six times the human therapeutic dose.
While there are no large, well-controlled studies on the use of trimethoprim and sulfamethoxazole in pregnant women, Brumfitt and Pursell,[5] in a retrospective study, reported the outcome of 186 pregnancies during which the mother received either placebo or trimethoprim and sulfamethoxazole. The incidence of congenital abnormalities was 4.5% (3 of 66) in those who received placebo and 3.3% (4 of 120) in those receiving trimethoprim and sulfamethoxazole. There were no abnormalities in the 10 children whose mothers received the drug during the first trimester. In a separate survey, Brumfitt and Pursell also found no congenital abnormalities in 35 children whose mothers had received oral trimethoprim and sulfamethoxazole at the time of conception or shortly thereafter.
Because trimethoprim and sulfamethoxazole may interfere with folic acid metabolism, SEPTRA should be used during pregnancy only if the potential benefit justifies the potential risk to the fetus.
Nonteratogenic Effects: See CONTRAINDICATIONS section.
Nursing Mothers: See CONTRAINDICATIONS section.
Pediatric Use: SEPTRA is not recommended for pediatric patients younger than 2 months of age (see INDICATIONS AND USAGE and CONTRAINDICATIONS).

ADVERSE REACTIONS

The most common adverse effects are gastrointestinal disturbances (nausea, vomiting, anorexia) and allergic skin reactions (such as rash and urticaria). **FATALITIES ASSOCIATED WITH THE ADMINISTRATION OF SULFONAMIDES, ALTHOUGH RARE, HAVE OCCURRED DUE TO SEVERE REACTIONS, INCLUDING STEVENS-JOHNSON SYNDROME, TOXIC EPIDERMAL NECROLYSIS, FULMINANT HEPATIC NECROSIS, AGRANULOCYTOSIS, APLASTIC ANEMIA, OTHER BLOOD DYSCRASIAS, AND HYPERSENSITIVITY OF THE RESPIRATORY TRACT (SEE WARNINGS).**
Hematologic: Agranulocytosis, aplastic anemia, thrombocytopenia, leukopenia, neutropenia, hemolytic anemia, megaloblastic anemia, hypoprothrombinemia, methemoglobinemia, eosinophilia.
Allergic: Stevens-Johnson syndrome, toxic epidermal necrolysis, anaphylaxis, allergic myocarditis, erythema multiforme, exfoliative dermatitis, angioedema, drug fever, chills, Henoch-Schönlein purpura, serum sickness-like syndrome, generalized allergic reactions, generalized skin eruptions, photosensitivity, conjunctival and scleral injection, pruritus, urticaria, and rash. In addition, periarteritis nodosa and systemic lupus erythematosus have been reported.
Gastrointestinal: Hepatitis, including cholestatic jaundice and hepatic necrosis, elevation of serum transaminase and bilirubin, pseudo membranous enterocolitis, pancreatitis, stomatitis, glossitis, nausea, emesis, abdominal pain, diarrhea, anorexia.
Genitourinary: Renal failure, interstitial nephritis, BUN and serum creatinine elevation, toxic nephrosis with oliguria and anuria, and crystalluria.
Metabolic: Hyperkalemia, hyponatremia.
Neurologic: Aseptic meningitis, convulsions, peripheral neuritis, ataxia, vertigo, tinnitus, headache.
Psychiatric: Hallucinations, depression, apathy, nervousness.
Endocrine: The sulfonamides bear certain chemical similarities to some goitrogens, diuretics (acetazolamide and the thiazides), and oral hypoglycemic agents. Cross-sensitivity may exist with these agents. Diuresis and hypoglycemia have occurred rarely in patients receiving sulfonamides.
Musculoskeletal: Arthralgia and myalgia.
Respiratory System: Cough, shortness of breath, and pulmonary infiltrates (see WARNINGS).
Miscellaneous: Weakness, fatigue, insomnia.

OVERDOSAGE

Acute: The amount of a single dose of SEPTRA that is either associated with symptoms of overdosage or is likely to be life-threatening has not been reported. Signs and symptoms of overdosage reported with sulfonamides include anorexia, colic, nausea, vomiting, dizziness, headache, drowsiness, and unconsciousness. Pyrexia, hematuria, and crystalluria may be noted. Blood dyscrasias and jaundice are potential late manifestations of overdosage. Signs of acute overdosage with trimethoprim include nausea, vomiting, dizziness, headache, mental depression, confusion, and bone marrow depression.
General principles of treatment include the institution of gastric lavage or emesis; forcing oral fluids; and the administration of intravenous fluids if urine output is low and renal function is normal. Acidification of the urine will increase renal elimination of trimethoprim. The patient should be monitored with blood counts and appropriate blood chemistries, including electrolytes. If a significant blood dyscrasia or jaundice occurs, specific therapy should be instituted for these complications. Peritoneal dialysis is not effective and hemodialysis is only moderately effective in eliminating trimethoprim and sulfamethoxazole.
Chronic: Use of SEPTRA at high doses and/or for extended periods of time may cause bone marrow depression manifested as throm bocytopenia, leukopenia, and/or megaloblastic anemia. If signs of bone marrow depression occur, the patient should be given leucovorin; 5 to 15 mg leucovorin daily has been recommended by some investigators.

DOSAGE AND ADMINISTRATION

Contraindicated in pediatric patients less than 2 months of age.
Urinary Tract Infections And Shigellosis In Adults And Pediatric Patients and Acute Otitis Media in Pediatric Patients: *Adults*: The usual adult dosage in the treatment of urinary tract infections is one SEPTRA DS (double strength) tablet, two SEPTRA tablets, or four teaspoonfuls (20 mL) SEPTRA Suspension every 12 hours for 10 to 14 days. An identical daily dosage is used for 5 days in the treatment of shigellosis.
Pediatric Patients: The recommended dose for pediatric patients with urinary tract infections or acute otitis media is 8 mg/kg trimethoprim and 40 mg/kg sulfamethoxazole per 24 hours, given in two divided doses every 12 hours for 10 days. An identical daily dosage is used for 5 days in the treatment of shigellosis. The following table is a guideline for the attainment of this dosage:
Pediatric Patients: Two Months of Age or Older

Weight		Dose-Every 12 Hours	
lb	kg	Teaspoonfuls	Tablets
22	10	1 (5 mL)	
44	20	2 (10 mL)	1
66	30	3 (15 mL)	1½
88	40	4 (20 mL)	2 (or 1 DS Tablet)

For Patients With Impaired Renal Function: When renal function is impaired a reduced dosage should be employed using the following table:

Creatinine Clearance (mL/min)	Recommended Dosage Regimen
Above 30	Use Standard Regimen
15-30	½ the Usual Regimen
Below 15	Use Not Recommended

Acute Exacerbations of Chronic Bronchitis in Adults: The usual adult dosage in the treatment of acute exacerbations of chronic bronchitis is one SEPTRA DS (double strength) tablet, two SEPTRA tablets, or four teaspoonfuls (20 mL) SEPTRA Suspension every 12 hours for 14 days.
Travelers' Diarrhea in Adults: For the treatment of travelers' diarrhea, the usual adult dosage is one SEPTRA DS (double strength) tablet, two SEPTRA tablets, or four teaspoonfuls (20 mL) of SEPTRA Suspension every 12 hours for 5 days.
Pneumocystis Carinii Pneumonia: Treatment: Adults and Pediatric Patients:
The recommended dosage for treatment of patients with documented *Pneumocystis carinii* pneumonia is 15 to 20 mg/kg trimethoprim and 75 to 100 mg/kg sulfamethoxazole per 24 hours given in equally divided doses every 6 hours for 14 to 21 days. The following table is a guideline for the upper limit of this dosage:

Weight		Dose-Every 6 Hours	
lb	kg	Teaspoonfuls	Tablets
18	8	1 (5 mL)	
35	16	2 (10 mL)	1
53	24	3 (15 mL)	1½
70	32	4 (20 mL)	2 (or 1 DS Tablet)
88	40	5 (25 mL)	2½
106	48	6 (30 mL)	3 (or 1½ DS Tablets)
141	64	8 (40 mL)	4 (or 2 DS Tablets)
176	80	10 (50 mL)	5 (or 2½ DS Tablets)

For the lower limit dose (15 mg/kg trimethoprim and 75 mg/kg sulfamethoxazole per 24 hours) administer 75% of the dose in the above table.
Prophylaxis: Adults:
The recommended dosage for prophylaxis in adults is one SEPTRA DS (double strength) tablet daily.
Pediatric Patients:
For pediatric patients, the recommended dose is 150 mg/m^2/day trimethoprim with 750 mg/m^2/day sulfamethoxazole given orally in equally divided doses twice a day, on 3 consecutive days per week. The total daily dose should not exceed 320 mg trimethoprim and 1,600 mg sulfamethoxazole. The following table is a guideline for the attainment of this dosage in pediatric patients:

Body Surface Area	Dose - every 12 hours	
(m^2)	Teaspoonfuls	Tablets
0.26	½ (2.5 mL)	
0.53	1 (5 mL)	½
1.06	2 (10 mL)	1

HOW SUPPLIED

TABLETS (pink, scored, round-shaped) containing 80 mg trimethoprim and 400 mg sulfamethoxazole: Bottles of 100 (NDC 61570-052-01). Imprint on tablets "SEPTRA" and "Y2B."
DS (DOUBLE STRENGTH) TABLETS (pink, scored, oval-shaped) containing 160 mg trimethoprim and 800 mg sulfamethoxazole: Bottles of 100 (NDC 61570-053-01) and 250 (NDC 61570-053-52). Imprint on tablets "SEPTRA DS" and "02C."
ORAL SUSPENSIONS (pink, cherry-flavored) containing 40 mg trimethoprim and 200 mg sulfamethoxazole in each teaspoonful (5 mL): Bottle of 1 pint (473 mL) (NDC 61570-050-16) and 100 mL-package of 6 (NDC 61570-050-11); and (purple, grape-flavored) containing 40 mg trimethoprim and 200 mg sulfamethoxazole in each teaspoonful (5 mL): Bottle of 1 pint (473 mL) (NDC 61570-051-16).
Tablets should be stored at 15° to 25°C (59° to 77°F) in a dry place and protected from light.
Suspensions should be stored at 15° to 25°C (59° to 77°F) and protected from light.
Also available:
SEPTRA I.V. Infusion: 5 mL vials, containing 80 mg trimethoprim (16 mg/mL) and 400 mg sulfamethoxazole (80 mg/mL), tray of 10;
10 mL multiple dose vials containing 160 mg trimethoprim (16 mg/mL) and 800 mg sulfamethoxazole (80 mg/mL), tray of 10;
20 mL multiple dose vials containing 320 mg trimethoprim (16 mg/mL) and 1600 mg sulfamethoxazole (80 mg/mL), tray of 10.
Rx only

REFERENCES

1. Kremers P, Duvivier J, Heusghem C. Pharmacokinetic studies of co-trimoxazole in man after single and repeated doses. *J Clin Pharmacol*. 1974;14:112–117.
2. Kaplan SA, Weinfeld RE, Abruzzo CW, McFaden K, Jack ML, Weissman L. Pharmacokinetic profile of trimethoprim-sulfamethoxazole in man. *J Infect Dis*. 1973;128(suppl):S547–S555.
3. Antibiotic susceptibility discs; certification procedure. *Federal Register*. 1972;37:20527–20529.
4. Bauer AW, Kirby WMM, Sherris JC, Turck M. Antibiotic susceptibility testing by standardized single disk method. *Am J Clin Pathol*. 1966;45:493–496.
5. Brumfitt W, Pursell R. Trimethoprim-sulfamethoxazole in the treatment of bacteriuria in women. *J Infect Dis*. 1973;128(suppl):S657–S663.

Distributed by: Monarch Pharmaceuticals, Inc., Bristol, TN 37620
Manufactured by: Catalytica Pharmaceuticals, Inc., Greenville, NC 27834

Rev. 1/98

THALITONE® ℞
(chlorthalidone tablets, USP)
15 & 25 mg

DESCRIPTION

Thalitone® (chlorthalidone USP) is an antihypertensive/diuretic supplied as 15 or 25 mg tablets for oral use. It is a monosulfamyl diuretic that differs chemically from thiazide diuretics in that a double ring system is incorporated in its structure. It is a racemic mixture of 2-chloro-5-(1-hydroxy-3-oxo-1-isoindolinyl) benzenesulfonamide, with the following structural formula:

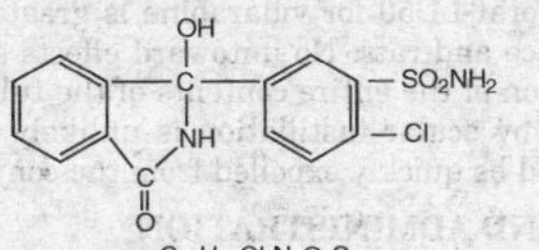

$C_{14}H_{11}Cl\,N_2O_4S$
Mol. Wt. 338.76

Chlorthalidone is practically insoluble in water, in ether and in chloroform; soluble in methanol; slightly soluble in alcohol.
The inactive ingredients are colloidal silicon dioxide, lactose, magnesium stearate, microcrystalline cellulose, povidone, sodium starch glycolate.

CLINICAL PHARMACOLOGY

Chlorthalidone is a long-acting oral diuretic with antihypertensive activity. Its diuretic action commences a mean of 2.6 hours after dosing and continues for up to 72 hours. The drug produces diuresis with increased excretion of sodium and chloride. The diuretic effects of chlorthalidone and the benzothiadiazine (thiazide) diuretics appear to arise from similar mechanisms and the maximal effect of chlorthalidone and the thiazides appear to be similar. The site of the action appears to be the distal convoluted tubule of the nephron. The diuretic effects of chlorthalidone lead to decreased extracellular fluid volume, plasma volume, cardiac output, total exchangeable sodium, glomerular filtration rate, and renal plasma flow. Although the mechanism of action of chlorthalidone and related drugs is not wholly clear, sodium and water depletion appear to provide a basis for its antihypertensive effect. Like the thiazide diuretics, chlorthalidone produces dose-related reductions in serum potassium levels, elevations in serum uric acid and blood glucose, and it can lead to decreased sodium and chloride levels.
The mean plasma half-life of chlorthalidone is about 40 to 60 hours. It is eliminated primarily as unchanged drug in the urine. Non-renal routes of elimination have yet to be clarified. In the blood, approximately 75% of the drug is bound to plasma proteins.
Thalitone® (chlorthalidone USP) has been formulated with PVP (povidone polyvinylpyrrolidone), a bioavailability enhancer that provides 104% to 116% bioavailability relative to an oral solution of chlorthalidone. Thalitone® cannot be substituted for other formulations of chlorthalidone and likewise, other formulations of chlorthalidone cannot be substituted for Thalitone®.

INDICATIONS AND USAGE

Thalitone® (chlorthalidone USP) is indicated in the management of hypertension either alone or in combination with other antihypertensive drugs.
Chlorthalidone is indicated as adjunctive therapy in edema associated with congestive heart failure, hepatic cirrhosis, and corticosteroid and estrogen therapy.
Chlorthalidone has also been found useful in edema due to various forms of renal dysfunction such as nephrotic syndrome, acute glomerulonephritis, and chronic renal failure.
Usage in Pregnancy The routine use of diuretics in an otherwise healthy woman is inappropriate and exposes mother and fetus to unnecessary hazard. Diuretics do not prevent development of toxemia of pregnancy and there is no satisfactory evidence that they are useful in the treatment of developed toxemia.
Edema during pregnancy may arise from pathological causes or from the physiologic and mechanical consequences of pregnancy. Chlorthalidone is indicated in pregnancy when edema is due to pathologic causes just as it is in the absence of pregnancy (however, see WARNINGS below). Dependent edema in pregnancy resulting from restriction of venous return by the expanded uterus is properly treated through elevation of the lower extremities and use of support hose; use of diuretics to lower intravascular volume in this case is illogical and unnecessary. There is hypervolemia during normal pregnancy that is harmful to neither the fetus nor the mother (in the absence of cardiovascular disease) but that is associated with edema, including generalized edema, in the majority of pregnancy women. If this edema produces discomfort, increased recumbency will often provide relief. In rare instances, this edema may cause extreme discomfort that is not relieved by rest. In these cases, a short course of diuretics may provide relief and may be appropriate.

CONTRAINDICATIONS

Anuria. Known hypersensitivity to chlorthalidone or other sulfonamide-derived drugs.

WARNINGS

Thalitone® (chlorthalidone USP) should be used with caution in severe renal disease. In patients with renal disease, chlorthalidone or related drugs may precipitate azotemia. Cumulative effects of the drug may develop in patients with impaired renal function.
Chlorthalidone should be used with caution in patients with impaired hepatic function or progressive liver disease, because minor alterations of fluid and electrolyte balance may precipitate hepatic coma.
Sensitivity reactions may occur in patients with a history of allergy or bronchial asthma.
The possibility of exacerbation or activation of systemic lupus erythematosus has been reported with thiazide diuretics which are structurally related to chlorthalidone. However, systemic lupus erythematosus has not been reported following chlorthalidone administration.

PRECAUTIONS

General Hypokalemia and other electrolyte abnormalities, including hyponatremia and hypochloremic alkalosis, are common in patients receiving chlorthalidone. These abnormalities are dose-related but may occur even at the lowest marketed doses of chlorthalidone. Serum electrolytes should be determined before initiating therapy and at periodic intervals during therapy. Serum and urine electrolyte determinations are particularly important when the patient is vomiting excessively or receiving parenteral fluids. All patients taking chlorthalidone should be observed for clinical signs of electrolyte imbalance, including dryness of mouth, thirst, weakness, lethargy, drowsiness, restlessness, muscle pains or cramps, muscular fatigue, hypotension, oliguria, tachycardia, palpitations and gastrointestinal disturbances, such as nausea and vomiting. Digitalis therapy may exaggerate metabolic effects of hypokalemia especially with reference to myocardial activity.
Any chloride deficit is generally mild and usually does not require specific treatment except under extraordinary circumstances (as in liver disease or renal disease). Dilutional hyponatremia may occur in edematous patients in hot weather; appropriate therapy is water restriction, rather than administration of salt, except in rare instances when the hyponatremia is life-threatening. In cases of actual salt depletion, appropriate replacement is the therapy of choice.
Thiazide-like diuretics have been shown to increase the urinary excretion of magnesium; this may result in hypomagnesemia.
Calcium excretion is decreased by thiazide-like drugs. Pathological changes in the parathyroid gland with hypercalcemia and hypophosphatemia have been observed in a few patients on thiazide therapy. The common complications of hyperparathyroidism such as renal lithiasis, bone resorption and peptic ulceration have not been seen.
Uric Acid Hyperuricemia may occur or frank gout may be precipitated in certain patients receiving chlorthalidone.
Other Increases in serum glucose may occur and latent diabetes mellitus may become manifest during chlorthalidone therapy (see PRECAUTIONS Drug Interactions). Chlorthalidone and related drugs may decrease serum PBI levels without signs of thyroid disturbance.
Information For Patients Patients should inform their doctor if they have: 1) had an allergic reaction to chlorthalidone or other diuretics or have asthma 2) kidney disease 3) liver disease 4) gout 5) systemic lupus erythematosus, or 6) been taking other drugs such as cortisone, digitalis, lithium carbonate, or drugs for diabetes.
Patients should be cautioned to contact their physician if they experience any of the following symptoms of potassium loss: excess thirst, tiredness, drowsiness, restlessness, muscle pains or cramps, nausea, vomiting or increased heart rate or pulse.
Patients should also be cautioned that taking alcohol can increase the chance of dizziness occurring.
Laboratory Tests Periodic determination of serum electrolytes to detect possible electrolyte imbalance should be performed at appropriate intervals.
All patients receiving chlorthalidone should be observed for clinical signs of fluid or electrolyte imbalance: namely, hyponatremia, hypochloremic alkalosis and hypokalemia. Serum and urine electrolyte determinations are particularly important when the patient is vomiting excessively or receiving parenteral fluids.
Drug Interactions Chlorthalidone may add to or potentiate the action of other antihypertensive drugs.
Insulin requirements in diabetic patients may be increased, decreased or unchanged. Higher dosage of oral hypoglycemic agents may be required.
Chlorthalidone and related drugs may increase the responsiveness to tubocurarine.
Chlorthalidone and related drugs may decrease arterial responsiveness to norepinephrine. This diminution is not sufficient to preclude effectiveness of the pressor agent for therapeutic use.
Lithium renal clearance is reduced by chlorthalidone, increasing the risk of lithium toxicity.
Drug/Laboratory Test Interactions Chlorthalidone and related drugs may decrease serum PBI levels without signs of thyroid disturbance.
Carcinogenesis, Mutagenesis, Impairment of Fertility No information is available.
Pregnancy/Teratogenic Effects PREGNANCY CATEGORY B: Reproduction studies have been performed in the rat and the rabbit at doses up to 420 times the human dose and have revealed no evidence of harm to the fetus due to chlorthalidone. There are, however, no adequate and well-controlled studies in pregnant women. Because animal reproduction studies are not always predictive of human response, this drug should be used during pregnancy only if clearly needed.
Pregnancy/Non-Teratogenic Effects Thiazides cross the placental barrier and appear in cord blood. The use of chlorthalidone and related drugs in pregnant women requires that the anticipated benefits of the drug be weighed against possible hazards to the fetus. These hazards include fetal or neonatal jaundice, thrombocytopenia, and possibly other adverse reactions that have occurred in the adult.
Nursing Mothers Thiazides are excreted in human milk. Because of the potential for serious adverse reactions in nursing infants from chlorthalidone, a decision should be made whether to discontinue nursing or to discontinue the drug, taking into account the importance of the drug to the mother.
Pediatric Use Safety and effectiveness in children have not been established.

ADVERSE REACTIONS

The following adverse reactions have been observed, but there is not enough systematic collection of data to support an estimate of their frequency.
Gastrointestinal System Reactions: anorexia, gastric irritation, nausea, vomiting, cramping, diarrhea, constipation, jaundice (intrahepatic cholestatic jaundice), pancreatitis.
Central Nervous System Reactions: dizziness, vertigo, paresthesias, headache, xanthopsia.
Hematologic Reactions: leukopenia, agranulocytosis, thrombocytopenia, aplastic anemia.
Dermatologic-Hypersensitivity Reactions: purpura, photosensitivity, rash, urticaria, necrotizing angiitis (vasculitis) (cutaneous vasculitis), Lyell's syndrome (toxic epidermal necrolysis).
Cardiovascular Reaction: Orthostatic hypotension may occur and may be aggravated by alcohol, barbiturates or narcotics.
Other Adverse Reactions: hyperglycemia, glycosuria, hyperuricemia, muscle spasm, weakness, restlessness, impotence.
Whenever adverse reactions are moderate or severe, chlorthalidone dosage should be reduced or therapy withdrawn.

OVERDOSAGE

Symptoms of acute overdosage include nausea, weakness, dizziness and disturbances of electrolyte balance. The oral LD_{50} of the drug in the mouse and the rat is more than 25,000 mg/kg body weight. The minimum lethal dose (MLD) in humans has not been established. There is no specific antidote but gastric lavage is recommended, followed by supportive treatment. Where necessary, this may include intravenous dextrose-saline with potassium, administered with caution.

DOSAGE AND ADMINISTRATION

Therapy should be initiated with the lowest possible dose, then titrated according to individual patient response. A single dose given in the morning with food is recommended; divided doses are unnecessary.

Continued on next page

Thalitone—Cont.

Hypertension Therapy in most patients should be initiated with a single daily dose of 15 mg. If the response is insufficient after a suitable trial, the dosage may be increased to 30 mg and then to a single daily dose of 45-50 mg. If additional control is required, the addition of a second antihypertensive drug is recommended. Increases in serum uric acid and decreases in serum potassium are dose-related over the 15-50 mg/day range and beyond.

Edema INITIATION: Adults, initially 30 to 60 mg daily or 60 mg on alternate days. Some patients may require 90 to 120 mg at these intervals or up to 120 mg daily. Dosages above this level, however, do not usually produce a greater response.

MAINTENANCE: Maintenance doses may often be lower than initial doses and should be adjusted according to the individual patient. Effectiveness is well sustained during continued use.

HOW SUPPLIED

White, kidney-shaped, compressed tablets coded HTI/77 containing 15 mg of chlorthalidone in bottles of 100 (NDC 61570-024-01) and white, kidney-shaped compressed scored tablets coded HTI/76 containing 25 mg of chlorthalidone in bottles of 100 (NDC 61570-023-01).

Storage: Store below 30°C (86°F).

Rx only

Distributed by: Monarch Pharmaceuticals, Inc.,
Bristol, TN 37620
Manufactured by:
King Pharmaceuticals, Inc
Bristol, TN 37620

1/97

Shown in Product Identification Guide, page 324

VIRA-A®

[vī 'ra-ā]

(Vidarabine Ophthalmic Ointment, USP) 3%

℞

DESCRIPTION

VIRA-A is the trade name for vidarabine (also known as adenine arabinoside and Ara-A), an antiviral drug for the topical treatment of epithelial keratitis caused by Herpes simplex virus. The chemical name is 9H-Purin-6-amine, 9-β-D-arabinofuranosyl-, monohydrate. Each gram of the ophthalmic ointment contains 30 mg of vidarabine monohydrate equivalent to 28.11 mg of vidarabine in a sterile, inert, petrolatum base.

The empirical and structural formulas are:

$C_{10}H_{13}H_5O_4 \cdot H_2O$ Mol. Wt. 285.26

CLINICAL PHARMACOLOGY

VIRA-A is rapidly deaminated to arabinosylhypoxanthine (Ara-Hx), the principal metabolite. Ara-Hx also possesses *in vitro* antiviral activity but this activity is less than that of VIRA-A. Because of the low solubility of VIRA-A, trace amounts of both VIRA-A and Ara-Hx can be detected in the aqueous humor only if there is an epithelial defect in the cornea. If the cornea is normal, only trace amounts of Ara-Hx can be recovered from the aqueous humor.

Systemic absorption of VIRA-A should not be expected to occur following ocular administration and swallowing lacrimal secretions. In laboratory animals, VIRA-A is rapidly deaminated in the gastrointestinal tract to Ara-Hx.

In contrast to topical idoxuridine, VIRA-A demonstrated less cellular toxicity in the regenerating corneal epithelium of the rabbit.

In controlled and uncontrolled clinical trials, an average of seven and nine days of continuous VIRA-A Ophthalmic Ointment, 3%, therapy was required to achieve corneal re-epithelialization. In the controlled trials, 70 of 81 subjects (86%) re-epithelialized at the end of three weeks of therapy. In the uncontrolled trials, 101 of 142 subjects (71%) re-epithelialized at the end of three weeks. Seventy-five percent of the subjects in these uncontrolled trials had either not healed previously or had developed hypersensitivity to topical idoxuridine therapy.

Microbiology

Vidarabine is a purine nucleoside obtained from fermentation cultures of *Streptomyces antibioticus*. The antiviral mechanism of action has not been established. Vidarabine appears to interfere with the early steps of viral DNA synthesis.

Vidarabine has been shown to possess antiviral activity against the following viruses *in vitro*:

Herpes simplex types 1 and 2
Vaccinia
Varicella-Zoster

Except for Rhabdovirus and Oncornavirus, vidarabine does not display *in vitro* antiviral activity against other RNA or DNA viruses, including Adenovirus.

Susceptibility Tests—No universal, standardized, quantitative *in vitro* procedures have as yet been developed to estimate the susceptibility of viruses to antiviral agents.

INDICATIONS AND USAGE

VIRA-A Ophthalmic Ointment, 3%, is indicated for the treatment of acute keratoconjunctivitis and recurrent epithelial keratitis due to Herpes simplex virus types 1 and 2. The clinical diagnosis of keratitis caused by Herpes simplex virus is usually established by the presence of typical dendritic or geographic lesions on slit-lamp examination. It is also effective in superficial keratitis caused by Herpes simplex virus which has not responded to topical idoxuridine or when toxic or hypersensitivity reactions due to idoxuridine have occurred. The effectiveness of VIRA-A Ophthalmic Ointment, 3%, against stromal keratitis and uveitis due to Herpes simplex virus has not been established.

CONTRAINDICATIONS

VIRA-A Ophthalmic Ointment, 3%, is contraindicated in patients who develop hypersensitivity reactions to it.

WARNINGS

Normally, corticosteroids alone are contraindicated in Herpes simplex virus infections of the eye. If VIRA-A Ophthalmic Ointment, 3%, is administered concurrently with topical corticosteroid therapy, corticosteroid-induced ocular side effects must be considered. These include corticosteroid-induced glaucoma or cataract formation and progression of a bacterial or viral infection.

VIRA-A is not effective against RNA virus or adenoviral ocular infections. It is also not effective against bacterial, fungal, or chlamydial infections of the cornea or nonviral trophic ulcers.

Although viral resistance to VIRA-A has not been observed, this possibility may exist.

PRECAUTIONS

General

The diagnosis of keratoconjunctivitis due to Herpes simplex virus should be established clinically prior to prescribing VIRA-A Ophthalmic Ointment, 3%.

Patients should be forewarned that VIRA-A Ophthalmic Ointment, 3%, like any ophthalmic ointment, may produce a temporary visual haze.

Carcinogenesis

Chronic parenteral (IM) studies of vidarabine have been conducted in mice and rats.

In the mouse study, there was a statistically significant increase in liver tumor incidence among the vidarabine-treated females. In the same study some vidarabine-treated male mice developed kidney neoplasia. No renal tumors were found in the vehicle-treated control mice or the vidarabine-treated female mice.

In the rat study, intestinal, testicular, and thyroid neoplasia occurred with greater frequency among the vidarabine-treated animals than in the vehicle-treated controls. The increases in thyroid adenoma incidence in the high-dose (50 mg/kg) males and the low-dose (30 mg/kg) females were statistically significant.

Hepatic megalocytosis, associated with vidarabine treatment, has been found in short and long-term rodent (rat and mouse) studies. It is not clear whether or not this represents a preneoplastic change.

The recommended frequency and duration of administration should not be exceeded (see DOSAGE AND ADMINISTRATION).

Mutagenesis

Results of *in vitro* experiments indicate that vidarabine can be incorporated into mammalian DNA and can induce mutation in mammalian cells (mouse L5178Y cell line). Thus far, *in vivo* studies have not been as conclusive, but there is some evidence (dominant lethal assay in mice) that vidarabine may be capable of producing mutagenic effects in male germ cells.

It has also been reported that vidarabine causes chromosome breaks and gaps when added to human leukocytes *in vitro*. While the significance of these effects in terms of mutagenicity is not fully understood, there is a well-known correlation between the ability of various agents to produce such effects and their ability to produce heritable genetic damage.

Pregnancy Category C

VIRA-A parenterally is teratogenic in rats and rabbits. Ten percent VIRA-A ointment applied to 10% of the body surface during organogenesis induced fetal abnormalities in rabbits. When 10% VIRA-A ointment was applied to 2% to 3% of the body surface of rabbits, no fetal abnormalities were found. This dose greatly exceeds the total recommended ophthalmic dose in humans. The possibility of embryonic or fetal damage in pregnant women receiving VIRA-A Ophthalmic Ointment, 3%, is remote. The topical ophthalmic dose is small, and the drug relatively insoluble. Its ocular penetration is very low. However, a safe dose for a human embryo or fetus has not been established. There are no adequate and well-controlled studies in pregnant women. VIRA-A should be used during pregnancy only if the potential benefit justifies the potential risk to the fetus.

Nursing Mothers

It is not known whether VIRA-A is secreted in human milk. Because many drugs are excreted in human milk and because of the potential for tumorigenicity shown for VIRA-A in animal studies, a decision should be made whether to discontinue nursing or to discontinue the drug, taking into account the importance of the drug to the mother. However, breast milk excretion is unlikely because VIRA-A is rapidly deaminated in the gastrointestinal tract.

Pediatric Use

The safety and effectiveness in pediatric patients below the age of 2 years have not been established.

ADVERSE REACTIONS

Lacrimation, foreign body sensation, conjunctival injection, burning, irritation, superficial punctate keratitis, pain, photophobia, punctal occlusion, and sensitivity have been reported with VIRA-A Ophthalmic Ointment, 3%. The following have also been reported but appear disease-related: uveitis, stromal edema, secondary glaucoma, trophic defects, corneal vascularization, and hyphema.

OVERDOSAGE

Acute massive overdosage by oral ingestion of the ophthalmic ointment has not occurred. However, the rapid deamination to arabinosylhypoxanthine should preclude any difficulty. The oral LD50 for vidarabine is greater than 5020 mg/kg in mice and rats. No untoward effects should result from ingestion of the entire contents of the tube.

Overdosage by ocular instillation is unlikely because any excess should be quickly expelled from the conjunctival sac.

DOSAGE AND ADMINISTRATION

Administer approximately one-half inch of VIRA-A Ophthalmic Ointment, 3%, into the lower conjunctival sac five times daily at three-hour intervals.

If there are no signs of improvement after 7 days, or complete re-epithelialization has not occurred in 21 days, other forms of therapy should be considered. Some severe cases may require longer treatment.

Too frequent administration should be avoided.

After re-epithelialization has occurred, treatment for an additional 7 days at a reduced dosage (such as twice daily) is recommended in order to prevent recurrence.

The following topical antibiotics: gentamicin, erythromycin, chloramphenicol; or topical steroids: prednisolone or dexamethasone have been administered concurrently with VIRA-A Ophthalmic Ointment, 3%.

HOW SUPPLIED

NDC 61570-367-71

VIRA-A Ophthalmic Ointment, 3%, is supplied sterile in ophthalmic ointment tubes of 3.5 g. The base is a 60:40 mixture of solid and liquid petrolatum.

Store at room temperature 15°-30°C (59°F-86°F).

Rx only.

Distributed by: Monarch Pharmaceuticals, Inc.
Bristol, TN 37620
Manufactured by: Parkedale Pharmaceuticals, Inc., Rochester, MI 48307

Rev. 4/98

Muro Pharmaceutical, Inc.
an ASTA Medica company
890 EAST STREET
TEWKSBURY, MA 01876-1496

Direct Inquiries to:
Professional Service Department
(800) 225-0974
(978) 851-5981

BROMFED® CAPSULES ℞
[brōm 'fĕd]

A light green and clear capsule containing white beads
Extended-Release.
Each capsule contains:
Brompheniramine maleate .... 12 mg
Pseudoephedrine hydrochloride .... 120 mg
in a specially prepared base to provide prolonged action.

BROMFED-PD® CAPSULES ℞
A dark green and clear capsule containing white beads.
Extended-Release.
Each capsule contains:
Brompheniramine maleate .... 6 mg
Pseudoephedrine hydrochloride .... 60 mg
in a specially prepared base to provide prolonged action.

BROMFED® AND BROMFED-PD® CAPSULES also contain as inactive ingredients: Benzyl Alcohol, Butyl Paraben, Carboxymethylcellulose Sodium, D & C Yellow #10, Edetate Calcium Disodium, FD&C Blue #1, FD&C Yellow #6, Gelatin, Methyl Paraben, Pharmaceutical Glaze, Propyl Paraben, Sodium Lauryl Sulfate, Sodium Propionate, Starch, Sucrose and other ingredients.

BROMFED® TABLETS ℞
A white scored tablet.
Each tablet contains:
Brompheniramine maleate .... 4 mg
Pseudoephedrine hydrochloride .... 60 mg
Also contains as inactive ingredients colloidal silicon dioxide, lactose, magnesium stearate, microcrystalline cellulose and sodium starch glycolate.

BROMFED® contains ingredients of the following therapeutic classes: antihistamine and decongestant.

CLINICAL PHARMACOLOGY
Brompheniramine maleate is an alkylamine type antihistamine. This group of antihistamines are among the most active histamine antagonists and are generally effective in relatively low doses. The drugs are not so prone to produce drowsiness and are among the most suitable agents for daytime use; but again, a significant proportion of patients do experience this effect. Pseudoephedrine hydrochloride is a sympathomimetic which acts predominantly on alpha receptors and has little action on beta receptors. It therefore functions as an oral nasal decongestant with minimal CNS stimulation.

INDICATIONS
For the treatment of the symptoms of seasonal and perennial allergic rhinitis, and vasomotor rhinitis, including nasal obstruction (congestion).

CONTRAINDICATIONS
Hypersensitivity to any of the ingredients. Also contraindicated in patients with severe hypertension, severe coronary artery disease, patients on MAO inhibitor therapy, patients with narrow-angle glaucoma, urinary retention, peptic ulcer and during an asthmatic attack.

WARNINGS
Considerable caution should be exercised in patients with hypertension, diabetes mellitus, ischemic heart disease, hyperthyroidism, increased intraocular pressure and prostatic hypertrophy. The elderly (60 years and older) are more likely to exhibit adverse reactions.
Antihistamines may cause excitability, especially in pediatric patients. At dosages higher than the recommended dose, nervousness, dizziness or sleeplessness may occur.

PRECAUTIONS
General: Caution should be exercised in patients with high blood pressure, heart disease, diabetes or thyroid disease. The antihistamine in this product may exhibit additive effects with other CNS depressants, including alcohol.
Information for Patients: Antihistamines may cause drowsiness. Ambulatory patients who operate machinery or motor vehicles should be cautioned accordingly.
Drug Interactions: MAO inhibitors and beta adrenergic blockers increase the effects of sympathomimetics. Sympathomimetics may reduce the antihypertensive effects of methyldopa, mecamylamine, reserpine and veratrum alkaloids. Concomitant use of antihistamines with alcohol and other CNS depressants may have an additive effect.

Pregnancy
The safety or use of this product in pregnancy has not been established.

ADVERSE REACTIONS
Adverse reactions include drowsiness, lassitude, nausea, giddiness, dryness of the mouth, blurred vision, cardiac palpitations, flushing, increased irritability or excitement (especially in pediatric patients).
Pediatric Use: Antihistamines may cause excitability especially in the pediatric population. Safety and effectiveness of Bromfed® Capsules has not been established in pediatric patients less than 12 years of age, and safety and effectiveness of Bromfed-PD® Capsules has not been established in pediatric patients less than 6 years of age. See Contraindications, Warnings, and Precautions for complete information.

OVERDOSAGE
KEEP THIS AND ALL DRUGS OUT OF THE REACH OF CHILDREN. IN CASE OF SUSPECTED OVERDOSE, IMMEDIATELY CALL YOUR REGIONAL POISON CONTROL CENTER AND/OR SEEK PROFESSIONAL ASSISTANCE.
Symptoms of overdosage may be caused by pseudoephedrine. Symptoms of overdosage with pseudoephedrine include anxiety, tenseness, respiratory difficulty, headache and awareness of the slow forceful heartbeat.
Treatment of Overdose: The stomach should be emptied promptly by emetics and/or gastric lavage. The installation of activated charcoal also should be considered. Cardiac function and serum electrolytes should be monitored and treatment instigated if indicated. If convulsions or marked CNS excitement occurs, diazepam may be used.

DOSAGE AND ADMINISTRATION:
BROMFED® CAPSULES
Adults and pediatric patients 12 years of age and over: 1 capsule every 12 hours.
BROMFED-PD® CAPSULES
Pediatric patients 6 to under 12 years of age: 1 capsule every 12 hours. Adults and pediatric patients 12 years of age and over: 1-2 capsules every 12 hours.
BROMFED® TABLETS
Adults and pediatric patients 12 years of age and over: One tablet every 4 hours not to exceed 6 doses in 24 hours. Pediatric patients 6 to under 12 years of age: One-half tablet every 4 hours not to exceed 6 doses in 24 hours. Do not give to pediatric patients under 6 years except under the advice and supervision of a physician.

HOW SUPPLIED:
BROMFED® CAPSULES
Bottle of 100 (NDC 0451-4000-50) and 500 (NDC 0451-4000-60). Each capsule is coded "BROMFED" "MURO 12-120."
BROMFED-PD® CAPSULES
Bottle of 100 (NDC 0451-4001-50) and 500 (NDC 0451-4001-60). Each capsule is coded "BROMFED-PD" "MURO 6-60."
BROMFED® TABLETS
Bottle of 100 (NDC 0451-4060-50). Each tablet is coded "MURO 4060" on one side and scored on the reverse side. Dispense in tight child-resistant containers as defined in USP/NF. Store at controlled room temperature between 15°-30°C (59°-86°F).
Rx only
I-4000-17   5/98
Dist. by:
Muro Pharmaceutical, Inc.
an ASTA Medica company
Tewksbury, MA 01876–1496
Mfd. by:
SCHWARZ PHARMA MANUFACTURING, INC.
Seymour, IN 47274

GUAIFED® CAPSULES ℞

A white opaque and clear capsule containing white beads.
Each capsule contains:
Pseudoephedrine hydrochloride .... 120 mg
in a specially prepared base to provide prolonged action.
Guaifenesin .... 250 mg
designed for immediate release to provide rapid action.

GUAIFED-PD® CAPSULES ℞

A blue and clear capsule containing white beads.
Each capsule contains:
Pseudoephedrine hydrochloride .... 60 mg
in a specially prepared base to provide prolonged action.
Guaifenesin .... 300 mg
designed for immediate release to provide rapid action.

GUAIFED® AND GUAIFED-PD® CAPSULES also contain as inactive ingredients: Benzyl Alcohol, Butyl Paraben, Edetate Calcium Disodium, Gelatin, Methyl Paraben, Pharma-

ceutical Glaze, Propyl Paraben, Sodium Lauryl Sulfate, Sodium Propionate, Starch, Sucrose, Titanium Dioxide, FD&C Blue #1 (Guaifed-PD® only) and other ingredients.

GUAIFED® and **GUAIFED-PD®** contains ingredients of the following therapeutic classes: nasal decongestant and expectorant.

CLINICAL PHARMACOLOGY
Pseudoephedrine hydrochloride is a sympathomimetic which acts predominantly on alpha adrenergic receptors in the mucosa of the respiratory tract, producing vasoconstriction and has little action on beta receptors. It therefore functions as an oral nasal decongestant with minimal CNS stimulation. Pseudoephedrine hydrochloride also increases sinus drainage and secretions. Guaifenesin is an expectorant which increases the output of phlegm (sputum) and bronchial secretions by reducing adhesiveness and surface tension. The increased flow of less viscid secretions promotes ciliary action and changes a dry, unproductive cough to one that is more productive and less frequent.

INDICATIONS
For temporary relief of nasal congestion and dry non-productive cough associated with the common cold and other respiratory allergies. Helps drainage of the bronchial tubes by thinning the mucus.

CONTRAINDICATIONS
This product is contraindicated in patients with known hypersensitivity to any of its ingredients. Also contraindicated in patients with severe hypertension, severe coronary artery disease and patients on MAO inhibitor therapy. Should not be used during pregnancy or in nursing mothers. Considerable caution should be exercised in patients with hypertension, diabetes mellitus, ischemic heart disease, hyperthyroidism, increased intraocular pressure and prostatic hypertrophy. The elderly (60 years or older) are more likely to exhibit adverse reactions. At dosages higher than the recommended dose, nervousness, dizziness or sleeplessness may occur.

WARNINGS
Do not take this product for persistent or chronic cough such as occurs with smoking, asthma, or emphysema, or where cough is accompanied by excessive secretions except under the advice and supervision of a physician. This medication should be taken a few hours prior to bedtime to minimize the possibility of sleeplessness. Take this medication with a glass of water after each dose, to help loosen mucus in the lungs.

PRECAUTIONS
General: Caution should be exercised in patients with high blood pressure, heart disease, diabetes or thyroid disease and in patients who exhibit difficulty in urination due to enlargement of the prostate gland. Check with a physician if symptoms do not improve within 7 days or if accompanied by high fever, rash or persistent headache.
Drug Interactions: Do not take this product if you are presently taking a prescription drug for high blood pressure or depression, without first consulting a physician. MAO inhibitors and beta adrenergic blockers may increase the effect of sympathomimetics. Sympathomimetics may reduce the antihypertensive effects of methyldopa, mecamylamine, reserpine and veratrum alkaloids. Pseudoephedrine hydrochloride may increase the possibility of cardiac arrhythmias in patients taking digitalis glycosides.
Pregnancy
Pregnancy Category B
It has been shown that pseudophedrine hydrochloride can cause reduced average weight, length, and rate of skeletal ossification in the animal fetus.
Nursing Mothers: Pseudoephedrine is excreted in breast milk; use by nursing mother is not recommended because of the higher than usual risk of side effects from sympathomimetic amines for infants, especially newborn and premature infants.
Geriatrics: Pseudoephedrine should be used with caution in the elderly because they may be more sensitive to the effects of the sympathomimetics.

ADVERSE REACTIONS
Adverse reactions include nausea, cardiac palpitations, increased irritability or excitement, headache, dizziness, tachycardia, diarrhea, drowsiness, stomach pain, seizures, slowed heart rate, shortness of breath and/or troubled breathing.
Pediatric Use: Safety and effectiveness in pediatric patients less than 6 years of age has not been established for **GUAIFED-PD®**, and safety and effectiveness in pediatric patients less than 12 years of age has not been established for **GUAIFED®**. See Contraindications, Warnings, and Precautions for complete information.

OVERDOSAGE
KEEP THIS AND ALL DRUGS OUT OF THE REACH OF CHILDREN. IN CASE OF SUSPECTED OVERDOSE, IM-

Continued on next page

Guaifed—Cont.

MEDIATELY CALL YOUR REGIONAL POISON CONTROL CENTER and/or SEEK PROFESSIONAL ASSISTANCE.

Symptoms of overdosage may be caused by pseudoephedrine. Symptoms of overdosage with pseudoephedrine include anxiety, tenseness, respiratory difficulty, headache and awareness of the slow forceful heartbeat.

Treatment of Overdose: The stomach should be emptied promptly by emetics and/or gastric lavage. The instillation of activated charcoal also should be considered. Cardiac function and serum electrolytes should be monitored and treatment instigated if indicated. If convulsions or marked CNS excitement occurs, diazepam may be used.

DOSAGE AND ADMINISTRATION

GUAIFED® CAPSULES

Adults and pediatric patients 12 years of age and over: 1 capsules every 12 hours.

GUAIFED-PD® CAPSULES

Pediatric patients 6 to under 12 years of age: 1 capsule every 12 hours.

Adults and pediatric patients 12 years of age and over: 1–2 capsules every 12 hours.

HOW SUPPLIED

GUAIFED® CAPSULES

Bottles of 100 (NDC 0451-4002-50). Bottle of 500 (NDC 0451-4002-60).

Each capsule is coded "GUAIFED" "MURO 120–250."

GUAIFED-PD® CAPSULES

Bottles of 100 (NDC 0451-4003-50). Bottle of 500 (NDC 0451-4003-60).

Each capsule is coded "GUAIFED-PD" "MURO 60–300."

Dispense in tight, child-resistant containers as defined in USP/NF.

Store at controlled room temperature.

Keep this and all drugs out of reach of children.

Rx only

I-4003-9   5/98

Dist. by:

MURO Pharmaceutical, Inc.

an ASTA Medica company

Tewksbury, MA 01876-1496

Mfd. by:

SCHWARZ PHARMA MANUFACTURING, INC.

Seymour, IN 47274

PRELONE® SYRUP   ℞

[prē-lōnĕ]

(Prednisolone Syrup, USP 15 mg per 5 mL)

DESCRIPTION

Prednisolone syrup contains prednisolone which is a glucocorticoid. Glucocorticoids are adrenocortical steroids, both naturally occurring and synthetic, which are readily absorbed from the gastrointestinal tract. Prednisolone is a white to practically white, odorless, crystalline powder. It is very slightly soluble in water, slightly soluble in alcohol, in chloroform, in dioxane, and in methanol.

The chemical name for Prednisolone is pregna-1,4-diene-3, 20-dione, 11, 17, 21-tridihydroxy. Its molecular weight is 360.45. The molecular formula is $C_{21}H_{28}O_5$, and the structural formula is:

PRELONE® Syrup contains 15 mg of prednisolone in each 5 mL. Benzoic acid, 0.1% is added as a preservative. It also contains alcohol 5%, citric acid, edetate disodium, glycerine, propylene glycol, purified water, sodium saccharin, sucrose, artificial wild cherry flavor, FD&C blue #1 and red #40.

CLINICAL PHARMACOLOGY

Naturally occurring glucocorticoids (hydrocortisone and cortisone), which also have salt-retaining properties, are used as replacement therapy in adrenocortical deficiency states. Their synthetic analogs such as prednisolone are primarily used for their potent anti-inflammatory effects in disorders of many organ systems.

Glucocorticoids such as prednisolone cause profound and varied metabolic effects. In addition, they modify the body's immune responses to diverse stimuli.

INDICATIONS AND USAGE

PRELONE® Syrup is indicated in the following conditions:

1. **Endocrine Disorders**

   Primary or secondary adrenocortical insufficiency (hydrocortisone or cortisone is the first choice: synthetic analogs may be used in conjunction with mineralocorticoids where applicable; in infancy mineralocorticoid supplementation is of particular importance).

   Congenital adrenal hyperplasia

   Nonsuppurative thyroiditis

   Hypercalcemia associated with cancer

2. **Rheumatic Disorders**

   As adjunctive therapy for short-term administration (to tide the patient over an acute episode or exacerbation) in:

   Psoriatic arthritis

   Rheumatoid arthritis, including juvenile rheumatoid arthritis (selected cases may require low-dose maintenance therapy)

   Ankylosing spondylitis

   Acute and subacute bursitis

   Acute nonspecific tenosynovitis

   Acute gouty arthritis

   Post-traumatic osteoarthritis

   Synovitis of osteoarthritis

   Epicondylitis

3. **Collagen Diseases**

   During an exacerbation or as maintenance therapy in selected cases of:

   Systemic lupus erythematosus

   Acute rheumatic carditis

4. **Dermatologic Diseases**

   Pemphigus

   Bullous dermatitis herpetiformis

   Severe erythema multiforme (Stevens-Johnson syndrome)

   Exfoliative dermatitis

   Mycosis fungoides

   Severe psoriasis

   Severe seborrheic dermatitis

5. **Allergic States**

   Control of severe or incapacitating allergic conditions intractable to adequate trials of conventional treatment:

   Seasonal or perennial allergic rhinitis

   Bronchial asthma

   Contact dermatitis

   Atopic dermatitis

   Serum sickness

   Drug hypersensitivity reactions

6. **Ophthalmic diseases**

   Severe acute and chronic allergic and inflammatory processes involving the eye and its adnexa such as:

   Allergic corneal marginal ulcers

   Herpes zoster ophthalmicus

   Anterior segment inflammation

   Diffuse posterior uveitis and choroiditis

   Sympathetic ophthalmia

   Allergic conjunctivitis

   Keratitis

   Chorioretinitis

   Optic neuritis

   Iritis and iridocyclitis

7. **Respiratory Diseases**

   Symptomatic sarcoidosis

   Loeffler's syndrome not manageable by other means

   Berylliosis

   Fulminating or disseminated pulmonary tuberculosis when used concurrently with appropriate antituberculous chemotherapy

   Aspiration pneumonitis

8. **Hematologic Disorders**

   Idiopathic thrombocytopenic purpura in adults

   Secondary thrombocytopenia in adults

   Acquired (autoimmune) hemolytic anemia

   Erythroblastopenia (RBC anemia)

   Congenital (erythroid) hypoplastic anemia

9. **Neoplastic Diseases**

   For palliative management of:

   Acute leukemia of childhood

   Leukemias and lymphomas in adults

10. **Edematous States**

    To induce a diuresis or remission of proteinuria in the nephrotic syndrome, without uremia, of the idiopathic type or that due to lupus erythematosus.

11. **Gastrointestinal Diseases**

    To tide the patient over a critical period of the disease in:

    Ulcerative colitis

    Regional enteritis

12. **Miscellaneous**

    Tuberculous meningitis with subarachnoid block or impending block used concurrently with appropriate antituberculous chemotherapy. Trichinosis with neurologic or myocardial involvement.

In addition to the above indications *PRELONE® Syrup* is indicated for systemic dermatomyositis (polymyositis).

CONTRAINDICATIONS

Systemic fungal infections.

WARNINGS

In patients on corticosteroid therapy subjected to unusual stress, increased dosage of rapidly acting corticosteroids before, during, and after the stressful situation is indicated. Corticosteroids may mask some signs of infection, and new infections may appear during their use. There may be decreased resistance and inability to localize infection when corticosteroids are used.

Prolonged use of corticosteroids may produce posterior subcapsular cataracts, glaucoma with possible damage to the optic nerves, and may enhance the establishment of secondary ocular infections due to fungi or viruses.

Use in pregnancy: Since adequate human reproduction studies have not been done with corticosteroids, the use of these drugs in pregnancies, nursing mothers or women of childbearing potential requires that the possible benefits of the drug be weighed against the potential hazards to the mother and embryo or fetus. Infants born of mothers who have received substantial doses of corticosteroids during pregnancy should be carefully observed for signs of hypoadrenalism.

Average and large doses of hydrocortisone or cortisone can cause elevation of blood pressure, salt and water retention, and increased excretion of potassium. These effects are less likely to occur with the synthetic derivatives except when used in large doses. Dietary salt restriction and potassium supplementation may be necessary. All corticosteroids increase calcium excretion.

While on corticosteroid therapy, patients should not be vaccinated against smallpox. Other immunization procedures should not be undertaken in patients who are on corticosteroids, especially on high dose, because of possible hazards of neurological complications and a lack of antibody response.

Children who are on drugs which suppress the immune system are more susceptible to infections than healthy children. Chickenpox and measles, for example, can have a more serious or even fatal course in non-immune children or adults on corticosteroids. In such children or adults who have not had these diseases, particular care should be taken to avoid exposure. How the dose, route and duration of corticosteroid administration affects the risk of developing a disseminated infection is not known. The contribution of the underlying disease and/or prior corticosteroid treatment to the risk is also not known. If exposed to chickenpox, prophylaxis with varicella zoster immune globulin (VZIG) may be indicated. If exposed to measles, prophylaxis with pooled intravenous immunoglobulin (IVIG) may be indicated. (See the respective package inserts for complete VZIG and IVIG prescribing information.) If chickenpox develops, treatment with antiviral agents may be considered.

The use of *PRELONE® Syrup* in active tuberculosis should be restricted to those cases of fulminating or disseminated tuberculosis in which the corticosteroid is used for the management of the disease in conjunction with an appropriate antituberculous regimen.

If corticosteroids are indicated in patients with latent tuberculosis or tuberculin reactivity, close observation is necessary as reactivation of the disease may occur. During prolonged corticosteroid therapy, these patients should receive chemoprophylaxis.

PRECAUTIONS

Information for patients: Patients who are on immunosuppressant doses of corticosteroids should be warned to avoid exposure to chickenpox or measles. Patients should also be advised that if they are exposed, medical advice should be sought without delay.

General: Drug-induced secondary adrenocortical insufficiency may be minimized by gradual reduction of dosage. This type of relative insufficiency may persist for months after discontinuation of therapy; therefore, in any situation of stress occurring during that period hormone therapy should be reinstituted. Since mineralocorticoid secretion may be impaired, salt and/or a mineralocorticoid should be administered concurrently.

There is an enhanced effect of corticosteroids on patients with hypothyroidism and in those with cirrhosis.

Corticosteroids should be used cautiously in patients with ocular herpes simplex because of possible corneal perforation.

The lowest possible dose of corticosteroid should be used to control the condition under treatment, and when reduction in dosage is possible, the reduction should be gradual.

Psychic derangements may appear when corticosteroids are used, ranging from euphoria, insomnia, mood swings, personality changes, and severe depression, to frank psychotic manifestations. Also, existing emotional instability or psychotic tendencies may be aggravated by corticosteroids.

Aspirin should be used cautiously in conjunction with corticosteroids in hypoprothrombinemia.

Steroids should be used with caution in nonspecific ulcerative colitis, if there is a probability of impending perforation, abscess or other pyogenic infections; diverticulitis; fresh intestinal anastomoses; active or latent peptic ulcer; renal insufficiency; hypertension; osteoporosis; and myasthenia gravis.
Growth and development of infants and children on prolonged corticosteroid therapy should be carefully observed.

ADVERSE REACTIONS

Fluid and Electrolyte Disturbances
- Sodium retention
- Fluid retention
- Congestive heart failure in susceptible patients
- Potassium loss
- Hypokalemic alkalosis
- Hypertension

Musculoskeletal
- Muscle weakness
- Steroid myopathy
- Loss of muscle mass
- Osteoporosis
- Vertebral compression fractures
- Aseptic necrosis of femoral and humeral heads
- Pathologic fracture of long bones

Gastrointestinal
- Peptic ulcer with possible perforation and hemorrhage
- Pancreatitis
- Abdominal distention
- Ulcerative esophagitis

Dermatologic
- Impaired wound healing
- Thin fragile skin
- Petechiae and ecchymoses
- Facial erythema
- Increased sweating
- May suppress reactions to skin tests

Neurological
- Convulsions
- Increased intracranial pressure with papilledema (pseudo-tumor cerebri) usually after treatment
- Vertigo
- Headache

Endocrine
- Menstrual irregularities
- Development of Cushingoid state
- Suppression of growth in children
- Secondary adrenocortical and pituitary unresponsiveness, particularly in times of stress, as in trauma, surgery or illness
- Decreased carbohydrate tolerance
- Manifestations of latent diabetes mellitus
- Increased requirements for insulin or oral hypoglycemic agents in diabetics

Ophthalmic
- Posterior subcapsular cataracts
- Increased intraocular pressure
- Glaucoma
- Exophthalmos

Metabolic
- Negative nitrogen balance due to protein catabolism

DOSAGE AND ADMINISTRATION

Dosage of ***PRELONE® Syrup*** should be individualized according to the severity of the disease and the response of the patient. For infants and children, the recommended dosage should be governed by the same considerations rather than strict adherence to the ratio indicated by age or body weight.
Hormone therapy is an adjunct to and not a replacement for conventional therapy.
Dosage should be decreased or discontinued gradually when the drug has been administered for more than a few days.
The severity, prognosis, expected duration of the disease, and the reaction of the patient to medication are primary factors in determining dosage.
If a period of spontaneous remission occurs in a chronic condition, treatment should be discontinued.
Blood pressure, body weight, routine laboratory studies, including two-hour postprandial blood glucose and serum potassium, and a chest X-ray should be obtained at regular intervals during prolonged therapy. Upper GI X-rays are desirable in patients with known or suspected peptic ulcer disease.
The initial dosage of ***PRELONE® Syrup*** may vary from 5 mg to 60 mg per day depending on the specific disease entity being treated. In situations of less severity lower doses will generally suffice while in selected patients higher initial doses may be required. The initial dosage should be maintained or adjusted until a satisfactory response is noted. If after a reasonable period of time there is a lack of satisfactory clinical response, ***PRELONE® Syrup*** should be discontinued and the patient transferred to other appropriate therapy. **IT SHOULD BE EMPHASIZED THAT DOSAGE REQUIREMENTS ARE VARIABLE AND MUST BE INDIVIDUALIZED ON THE BASIS OF THE DISEASE UNDER TREATMENT AND THE RESPONSE OF THE PATIENT.**
After a favorable response is noted, the proper maintenance dosage should be determined by decreasing the initial drug dosage in small decrements at appropriate time intervals until the lowest dosage which will maintain an adequate clinical response is reached. It should be kept in mind that constant monitoring is needed in regard to drug dosage. Included in the situations which may make dosage adjustments necessary are changes in clinical status secondary to remissions or exacerbations in the disease process, the patient's individual drug responsiveness, and the effect of patient exposure to stressful situations not directly related to the disease entity under treatment. In this latter situation it may be necessary to increase the dosage of ***PRELONE® Syrup*** for a period of time consistent with the patient's condition. If after long-term therapy the drug is to be stopped, it is recommended that it be withdrawn gradually rather than abruptly.

HOW SUPPLIED

PRELONE® Syrup is a cherry flavored red liquid containing 15mg of Prednisolone in each 5 mL (teaspoonful) and is supplied in 240 mL bottles (NDC 0451-1500-08) and 480 mL bottles (0451-1500-16).
Pharmacist: Dispense with suitable calibrated measuring device to assure proper measuring of dose.

Dose/Volume Chart

15 mg prednisolone = 1 teaspoon
10 mg prednisolone = 2/3 teaspoon
7.5 mg prednisolone = 1/2 teaspoon
5 mg prednisolone = 1/3 teaspoon

Dispense in tight, light-resistant and child-resistant containers as defined in USP/NF.
Store at room temperature. Do Not Refrigerate.
Rx only
Muro Pharmaceutical, Inc.
an ASTA Medica company
890 East Street • Tewksbury, Massachusetts 01876-1496
I-1500-13 3/98

VOLMAX® ℞
(albuterol sulfate)
Extended-Release Tablets

DESCRIPTION

Volmax® (albuterol sulfate) Extended-Release Tablets contain albuterol sulfate, the racemic form of albuterol and a relatively selective beta$_2$-adrenergic bronchodilator, in an extended-release formulation. Albuterol sulfate has the chemical name (±), α_1-[(*tert*-butylamino)methyl]-4-hydroxy-*m*-xylene-α, α′-diol sulfate (2:1) (salt), and the following chemical structure:

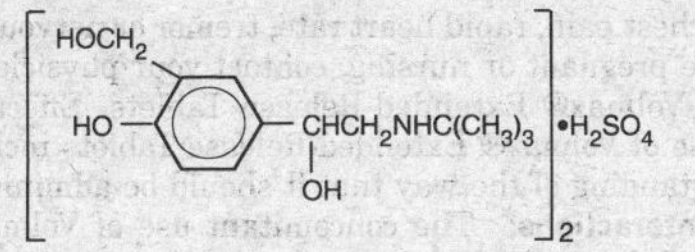

HOCH2
HO
CHCH2NHC(CH3)3
•H2SO4
OH
2

Albuterol sulfate has a molecular weight of 576.7, and the molecular formula is $(C_{13}H_{21}NO_3)_2 \bullet H_2SO_4$. Albuterol sulfate is a white crystalline powder, soluble in water and slightly soluble in ethanol.
The World Health Organization recommended name for albuterol base is salbutamol.
Each Volmax® Extended-Release Tablet for oral administration contains 4 mg or 8 mg of albuterol as 4.8 mg or 9.6 mg, respectively, of albuterol sulfate in a nondeformable cellulosic material that serves as the rate-controlling membrane. Each tablet also contains the inactive ingredients cellulose acetate, croscarmellose sodium, FD&C Blue No. 1 (4 mg tablet only), hydroxypropyl cellulose (8 mg tablet only), hydroxypropyl methylcellulose, magnesium stearate, povidone, silica, sodium chloride, and titanium dioxide.

CLINICAL PHARMACOLOGY

In vitro studies and *in vivo* pharmacologic studies have demonstrated that albuterol has a preferential effect on beta$_2$-adrenergic receptors compared with isoproterenol. While it is recognized that beta$_2$-adrenergic receptors are the predominant receptors in bronchial smooth muscle, data indicate that there is a population of beta$_2$-receptors in the human heart existing in a concentration between 10% and 50%. The precise function of these receptors has not been established. (See Warnings).
The pharmacologic effects of beta-adrenergic agonist drugs, including albuterol, are at least in part attributable to stimulation through beta-adrenergic receptors on intracellular adenyl cyclase, the enzyme that catalyzes the conversion of adenosine triphosphate (ATP) to cyclic-3′, 5′-adenosine monophosphate (cyclic AMP). Increased cyclic AMP levels are associated with relaxation of bronchial smooth muscle and inhibition of release of mediators of immediate hypersensitivity from cells, especially from mast cells.
Albuterol has been shown in most controlled clinical trials to have more effect on the respiratory tract, in the form of bronchial smooth muscle relaxation, than isoproterenol at comparable doses while producing fewer cardiovascular effects.
Albuterol is longer acting than isoproterenol in most patients by any route of administration because it is not a substrate for the cellular uptake processes for catecholamines nor for catechol-*O*-methyl transferase.
Animal studies show that albuterol does not pass the blood-brain barrier.
Studies in laboratory animals (minipigs, rodents, and dogs) recorded the occurrence of cardiac arrhythmias and sudden death (with histologic evidence of myocardial necrosis) when beta-agonists and methylxanthines were administered concurrently. The significance of these findings when applied to humans is currently unknown.
Pharmacokinetics and Disposition: In a single-dose study comparing one 8 mg Volmax® Extended-Release Tablet with two 4 mg immediate-release Ventolin® (albuterol sulfate, USP) Tablets in 17 normal adult volunteers, the extent of availability of Volmax® Extended-Release Tablets was shown to be about 80% of Ventolin® Tablets with or without food. In addition, lower mean peak plasma concentration and longer time to reach the peak level were observed with Volmax® Extended-Release Tablets as compared to Ventolin® Tablets. The single-dose study results also showed that food decreases the rate of absorption of albuterol from Volmax® Extended-Release Tablets without altering the extent of bioavailability. In addition, the study indicated that food causes a more gradual increase in the fraction of the available dose absorbed from the extended-release formulation as compared with the fasting condition.
In another single-dose study in adults, 8 mg and 4 mg Volmax® Extended-Release Tablets were shown to deliver dose-proportional plasma concentrations in the fasting state. Definitive studies for the effect of food on 4 mg Volmax® Extended-Release Tablets have not been conducted. However, since food lowers the rate of absorption of 8 mg Volmax® Extended-Release Tablets, it is expected that food reduces the rate of absorption of 4 mg Volmax® Extended-Release Tablets also.
Volmax® Extended-Release Tablets have been formulated to provide duration of action of up to 12 hours. In an 8-day, multiple-dose, crossover study, 15 normal adult male volunteers were given 8 mg Volmax® Extended-Release Tablets every 12 ours or 4 mg Ventolin® (albuterol sulfate, USP) Tablets every 6 hours. Each dose of Volmax® Extended-Release Tablets and the corresponding doses of Ventolin® Tablets were administered in the postprandial state. Steady-state plasma concentrations were reached within 2 days for both formulations. Fluctuations (C_{max}-C_{min}/$C_{average}$) in plasma concentrations were similar for Volmax® Extended-Release Tablets administered at 12-hour intervals and Ventolin® Tablets administered every 6 hours. In addition, the relative bioavailability of Volmax® Extended-Release Tablets was approximately 100% of the immediate-release tablet at steady state. A summary of these results is shown in the following table:
[See table at top of next page]
The mean plasma albuterol concentration versus time data at steady state after the administration of Volmax® Extended-Release Tablets 8 mg q12h are displayed in the following graph:
[See figure at top of next column]
Pharmacokinetic studies of 4- and 8-mg Volmax® Extended-Release Tablets have not been conducted in pediatric patients. Bioavailability of 4- and 8-mg Volmax® Extended-Release Tablets in pediatric patients relative to 2- and 4-mg immediate release albuterol has been extrapolated from adult studies showing comparability at steady-state dosing and reduced bioavailability after single dose administration.

INDICATIONS AND USAGE

Volmax® Extended-Release Tablets are indicated for the relief of bronchospasm in adults and children 6 years of age and older with reversible obstructive airway disease.

CONTRAINDICATIONS

Volmax® Extended-Release Tablets are contraindicated in patients with a history of hypersensitivity to albuterol or any of its components.

WARNINGS

Immediate hypersensitivity reactions may occur after administration of albuterol, as demonstrated by rare cases of urticaria, angioedema, rash, bronchospasm, and oropharyngeal edema.
Cardiovascular Effects: Volmax® Extended-Release Tablets, like all other beta-adrenergic agonists, can produce a clinically significant cardiovascular effect in some patients, as measured by pulse rate, blood pressure, and/or symptoms. Although such effects are uncommon after administration of Volmax® Extended-Release Tablets at recom-

Continued on next page

Volmax—Cont.

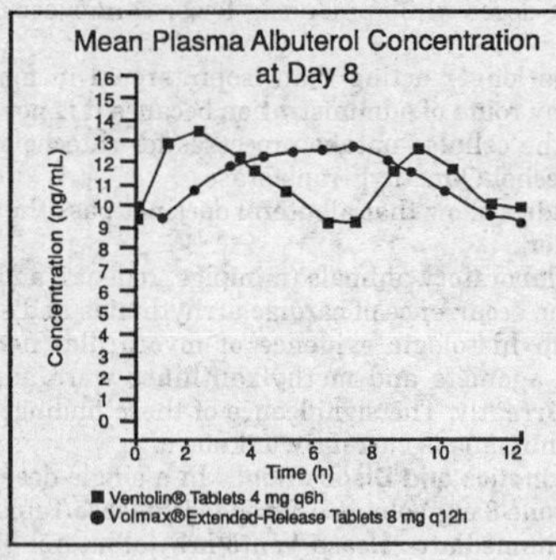
Mean Plasma Albuterol Concentration
at Day 8
Concentration (ng/mL)
Time (h)
■ Ventolin® Tablets 4 mg q6h
● Volmax® Extended-Release Tablets 8 mg q12h

mended doses, if they occur, the drug may need to be discontinued. In addition, beta-agonists have been reported to produce electrocardiogram (ECG) changes, such as flattening of the T wave, prolongation of the QTc interval, and ST segment depression. The clinical significance of these findings is unknown. Therefore, Volmax® Extended-Release Tablets, like all sympathomimetic amines, should be used with caution in patients with cardiovascular disorders, especially coronary insufficiency, cardiac arrhythmias, and hypertension.

Deterioration of Asthma: Asthma may deteriorate acutely over a period of hours or chronically over several days or longer. If the patient needs more doses of Volmax® Extended-Release Tablets than usual, this may be a marker of destabilization of asthma and requires reevaluation of the patient and the treatment regimen, giving special consideration to the possible need to anti-inflammatory treatment; e.g., corticosteroids.

Use of Anti-Inflammatory Agents: The use of beta adrenergic agonist bronchodilators alone may not be adequate to control asthma in many patients. Early consideration should be given to adding anti-inflammatory agents; e.g., corticosteroids.

Paradoxical Bronchospasm: Volmax® Extended-Release Tablets can produce paradoxical bronchospasm, which may be lifethreatening. If paradoxical bronchospasm occurs, Volmax® Extended-Release Tablet should be discontinued immediately and alternative therapy instituted.

Rarely, erythema multiforme and Steven-Johnson syndrome have been associated with the administration of oral albuterol in children.

PRECAUTIONS

General: Albuterol, as with all sympathomimetic amines, should be used with caution in patients with cardiovascular disorders, especially coronary insufficiency, cardiac arrhythmias, and hypertension; in patients with convulsive disorders, hyperthyroidism, or diabetes melllitus; and in patients who are unusually responsive to sympathomimetic amines.

In controlled clinical trials in adults, patients treated with Volmax® Extended-Release Tablets had increases in selected serum chemistry values and decreases in selected hematologic values. Increases in SGPT were more frequent among patients treated with Volmax® Extended-Release Tablets (12 of 247 patients, 4.9%) than among the theophylline (6 of 188 patients, 3.2%) and placebo (1 of 138 patients, 0.7%) groups. Increases in serum glucose concentration were also more frequent among patients treated with Volmax® Extended-Release Tablets (23 of 234 patients, 9.8%) than among theothephylline (11 of 173 patients, 6.45%) and placebo (3 of 129 patients, 2.3%) groups. Increases in SGOT were also more frequent among patient treated with Volmax® Extended-Release Tablets (10 of 248 patients, 4%) and theophylline (5 of 193, 2.6%) than among patients treated with placebo. Decreases in white blood cell counts were more frequent in patients treated with Volmax® Extended-Release Tablets (10 of 247 patients, 4%) compared with patients receiving theophylline (2 of 185 patients. 1.1%) and patients receiving placebo (1 of 141 patients, 0.7%). Decreases in hemoglobin and hematocrit were more frequent in patients receiving Volmax® Extended-Release Tablets (16 of 228 patients, 7.0%, and 17 of 230 patients, 7.4%, respectively) than in patients receiving theophylline (5 of 171 patients, 2.9%, and 9 of 173 patients, 5.2%, respectively) and patients receiving placebo (5 of 129 patients, 3.9%, and 3 of 132 patients, 2.3%, respectively). The clinical significance of these results is unknown.

Large doses of intravenous albuterol have been reported to aggravate pre-existing diabetes mellitus and ketoacidosis. As with other beta-agonists, albuterol may produce significant hypokalemia in some patients, possibly through intracellular shunting, which has the potential to produce adverse cardiovascular effects. The decrease is usually transient, not requiring supplementation.

Mean Values at Steady State

	C_{max} (ng/mL)	C_{max} (ng/mL)	T_{max} (h)	T_{12} (h)	AUC (ng•h/mL)
VOLMAX®	13.7	8.1	6.0	9.3	134
Ventolin®	13.9	8.1	2.6	7.2	132

Event	Volmax® (n=330)	Theophylline (n=197	Other β-Agonists (n=20)	Placebo (n=178)
Nervousness	8.5%	5.1%	10.0%	2.8%
Tremor	24.2%	6.1%	35.0%	1.1%
Headache	18.8%	26.9%	35.0%	20.8%
Tachycardia	2.7%	0.5%	5.0%	0%
Palpitations	2.4%	0.5%	0%	1.1%
Muscle Cramps	2.7%	0.5%	5.0%	0.6%
Insomnia	2.4%	6.1%	0%	1.7%
Nausea/Vomiting	4.2%	19.8%	5.0%	3.9%
Dizziness	1.5%	2.0%	0%	5.1%
Somnolence	0.3%	1.0%	0%	0.6%

As with other nondeformable material, caution should be used when administering Volmax® Extended-Release Tablets to patients with pre-existing gastrointestinal narrowing from any cause. There have been rare reports of gastrointestinal obstruction in such patients occurring in association with ingestion of products containing delivery systems similar to that contained in Volmax® Extended-Release Tablets.

Information for Patients:

Each Volmax® Extended-Release Table contains a small hole that is part of the unique extended-release system. Volmax® Extended-Release Tablets must be swallowed whole with the aid of liquids. DO NOT CHEW OR CRUSH THESE TABLETS.

The outer coating of the tablet is not absorbed and is excreted in the feces; in some instances the empty outer coating may be noticeable in the stool.

The action of Volmax® Extended-Release Tablets should last up to 12 hours or longer. Volmax® Extended-Release Tablets should not be used more frequently than recommended. Do not increase the dose or frequency of Volmax® Extended-Release Tablets without consulting your physician. If you find that treatment with Volmax® Extended-Release Tablets becomes less effective for symptomatic relief, your symptoms become worse, and/or you need to use the product more frequently than usual, you should seek medical attention immediately. While you are using Volmax® Extended-Release Tablets, other inhaled drugs and asthma medications should be taken only as directed by your physician. Common adverse effects include palpitations, chest pain, rapid heart rate, tremor or nervousness. If you are pregnant or nursing, contact your physician about use of Volmax® Extended-Release Tablets. Effective and safe use of Volmax® Extended-Release Tablets includes an understanding of the way that it should be administered.

Drug Interactions: The concomitant use of Volmax® Extended-Release Tablets and other oral sympathomimetic agents is not recommended since such combined use may lead to deleterious cardiovascular effects. This recommendation does not preclude the judicious use of an aerosol bronchodilator of the adrenergic stimulant type in patients receiving Volmax® Extended-Release Tablets. Such concomitant use, however, should be individualized and not given on a routine basis. If regular coadministration is required, then alternative therapy should be considered.

Monoamine Oxidase Inhibitors or Tricyclic Antidepressants: Albuterol should be administered with extreme caution to patients being treated with monoamine oxidase inhibitors or tricyclic antidepressants, or within 2 weeks of discontinuation of such agents, because the action of albuterol on the vascular system may be potentiated.

Beta Blockers: Beta-adrenergic receptor blocking agents not only block the pulmonary effect of beta agonists, such as Volmax® Extended-Release Tablets, but may produce severe bronchospasm in asthmatic patients. Therefore, patients with asthma should not normally be treated with beta-blockers. However, under certain circumstances, e.g., as prophylaxis after myocardial infarction, there may be no acceptable alternatives to the use of beta-adrenergic blocking agents in patients with asthma. In this setting, cardioselective beta-blockers could be considered, although they should be administered with caution.

Diuretics: The ECG changes and/or hypokalemia that may result from the administration of nonpotassium-sparing diuretics (such as loop or thiazide diuretics) can be acutely worsened by beta-agonists, especially when the recommended dose of the beta-agonist is exceeded. Although the clinical significance of these effects is not known, caution is advised in the coadministration of beta-agonists with non potassium-sparing diuretics.

Digoxin: Mean decreases of 16% to 22% in serum digoxin levels were demonstrated after single dose intravenous and oral administration of albuterol, respectively, to normal volunteers who had received digoxin for 10 days. The clinical significance of these findings for patients with obstructive airway disease who are receiving albuterol and digoxin on a chronic basis is unclear. Nevertheless, it would be prudent to carefully evaluate the serum digoxin levels in patients who are currently receiving digoxin and albuterol.

CARCINOGENESIS, MUTAGENESIS, IMPAIRMENT OF FERTILITY: In a 2-year study in Sprague-Dawley rats, albuterol sulfate caused a significant dose-related increase in the incidence of benign leiomyomas of the mesovarium at dietary doses of 2.0, 10, and 50 mg/kg, (approximately 1/2, 3, and 15 times, respectively, the maximum recommended daily oral dose for adults on a mg/m^2 basis, or, approximately 2/5, 2, and 10 times, respectively, the maximum recommended daily oral dose for children on a mg/m^2 basis). In another study this effect was blocked by the coadministration of propranolol, a non-selective beta-adrenergic antagonist. In a 18 month study in CD-1 mice, albuterol sulfate showed no evidence of tumorigenicity at dietary doses of up to 500 mg/kg (approximately 65 times the maximum recommended daily oral dose for adults on a mg/m^2 basis, or, approximately 50 times the maximum recommended daily oral dose for children on a mg/m^2 basis). In a 22 month study in the Golden hamster, albuterol sulfate showed no evidence of tumorigenicity at dietary doses of 50 mg/kg. (approximately 7 times the maximum recommended daily oral dose for adults and children on a mg/m^2 basis).

Albuterol sulfate was not mutagenic in the Ames test with or without metabolic activation using tester strains *S. typhimurium* TA 1537, TA 1538, and TA98 or *E. coli* WP2, WP2uvrA, and WP67. No forward mutation was seen in yeast strain *S. cerevisiae* S9 nor any mitotic gene conversion in yeast strain *S. cerevisiae* JD1 with or without metabolic activation. Fluctuation assays in *S. typhimurium* TA98 and *E. coli* WP2, both with metabolic activation, were negative. Albuterol sulfate was not clastogenic in a human peripheral lymphocyte assay or in an AH1 strain mouse micronucleus assay at intraperitoneal doses of up to 200 mg/kg.

Reproduction studies in rats demonstrated no evidence of impaired fertility at oral doses up to 50 mg/kg, (approximately 15 times the maximum recommended daily oral dose for adults on a mg/m^2 basis).

Pregnancy: Teratogenic Effects: Pregnancy Category C: Albuterol Sulfate has been shown to be teratogenic in mice. A study in CD-1 mice at subcutaneous (SC) doses of 0.025, 0.25, and 2.5 mg/kg, (approximately 3/1000, 3/100, and 3/10 times the maximum recommended daily oral dose for adults on a mg/m^2 basis), showed cleft palate formation in 5 of 111 (4.5%) fetuses at 0.25 mg/kg and in 10 of 108 (9.3%) fetuses at 2.5 mg/kg. The drug did not induce cleft palate formation at the lowest dose, 0.025 mg/kg. Cleft palate also occurred in 22 of 72 (30.5%) fetuses of females treated with 2.5 mg/kg, of isoproterenol (positive control) subcutaneously (approximately 3/10 times the maximum recommended daily oral dose for adults on a mg/m^2 basis). A reproduction study in Stride Dutch rabbits revealed cranioschisis in 7/19 fetuses (37%) when albuterol sulfate was administered orally at a 50 mg/kg dose, (approximately 25 times the maximum recommended daily oral dose for adults on a mg/m^2 basis).

There are no adequate and well-controlled studies in pregnant women. Albuterol should be used during pregnancy only if the potential benefit justifies the potential risk to the fetus.

During worldwide marketing experience, various congenital anomalies, including cleft palate and limb defects, have been rarely reported in the offspring of patients being treated with albuterol. Some of the mothers were taking multiple medications during their pregnancies. No consistent pattern of defects can be discerned, and a relationship between albuterol use and the congenital anomalies has not been established.

Labor and Delivery: Because of the potential for beta-agonist interference with uterine contractility, use of Volmax® Extended-Release Tablets for relief of bronchospasm during labor should be restricted to those patients in whom the benefits clearly outweigh the risks.

Tocolysis: Albuterol has not been approved for the management of pre-term labor. The benefit risk ratio when albuterol is administered for tocolysis has not been established. Serious adverse reactions, including pulmonary edema, have been reported during or following treatment of premature labor with beta$_2$-agonists, including albuterol.

Nursing Mothers: It is not known whether albuterol is excreted in human milk. Because of the potential for tumorigenicity shown for albuterol in animal studies, a decision should be made whether to discontinue nursing or to discontinue the drug, taking into account the importance of the drug to the mother.

Pediatric Use: The safety and effectiveness of Volmax® Extended-Release Tablets have been established in pediatric patients 6 years of age or older. Use of Volmax® Extended-Release Tablets in these age groups is supported by evidence from adequate and well-controlled studies of Volmax® Extended-Release Tablets in adults; the likelihood that the disease course, pathophysiology, and the drug's effect in pediatric and adult patients are substantially similar; the established safety and effectiveness of immediate release albuterol tablets in pediatric patients 6 years of age and older; and clinical trials that support the safety of Volmax ® Extended-Release Tablets in pediatric patients over 6 years of age. The recommended dose of Volmax® Extended-Release Tablets for the pediatric population is based upon the recommended pediatric dosing of immediate-release albuterol tablets and pharmacokinetic studies in adults showing comparable bioavailability at steadystate dosing and reduced bioavailability after single dose administration. Safety and effectiveness in pediatric patients below 6 years of age have not been established.

ADVERSE REACTIONS

The adverse reactions to albuterol are similar in nature to reactions to other sympathomimetic agents. The most frequent adverse reactions to albuterol are nervousness, tremor, headache, tachycardia, and palpitations. Less frequent adverse reactions are muscle cramps, insomnia, nausea, weakness, dizziness, drowsiness, flushing, restlessness, irritability, chest discomfort, and difficulty in micturition. Rare cases of urticaria, angioedema, rash bronchospasm, and oropharyngeal edema have been reported after the use of albuterol.

In addition, albuterol, like other sympathomimetic agents, can cause adverse reactions such as hypertension, angina, vomiting, vertigo, central nervous system stimulation, unusual taste, and drying or irritation of the oropharynx.

In controlled clinical trials of adult patients conducted in the United States, the following incidence of adverse events was reported:

[See second table at top of previous page]

A trend was observed among patients treated with Volmax® Extended-Release Tablets toward increasing frequency of muscle cramps with increasing patient age (12–20 years, 1.2%; 21–30 years, 2.6%; 31–40 years, 6.9%; 41–50 years, 6.9%), compared with no such events in the placebo group. Also observed was an increasing frequency of tremor with increasing patient age (12–20 years, 29.4%; 21–30 years, 29.9%; 31–40 years, 27.6%; 41–50 years, 37.9%), compared to 2.9% or less in the placebo group.

The reactions are generally transient in nature, and it is usually not necessary to discontinue treatment with Volmax® Extended-Release Tablets.

OVERDOSAGE

The expected symptoms with overdosage are those of excessive beta-adrenergic stimulation and/or occurrence or exaggeration of any of the symptoms listed under ADVERSE REACTIONS; e.g., seizures, angina, hypertension or hypotension, tachycardia with rates up to 200 beats per minute, arrhythmias, nervousness, headache, tremor, dry mouth, palpitation, nausea, dizziness, fatigue, malaise, and insomnia. Hypokalemia may also occur. As with all sympathomimetic aerosol medications, cardiac arrest and even death may be associated with abuse of Volmax® Extended-Release Tablets.

Treatment consists of discontinuation of Volmax® Extended-Release Tablets together with appropriate symptomatic therapy. The judicious use of a cardioselective beta-receptor blocker may be considered, bearing in mind that such medication can produce bronchospasm. There is insufficient evidence to determine if dialysis is beneficial for overdosage of Volmax® Extended-Release Tablets.

The oral median lethal dose of albuterol sulfate in mice is greater than 2000 mg/kg, (approximately 250 times the maximum recommended daily oral dose for adults on a mg/m^2 basis, or, approximately 200 times the maximum recommended daily oral dose for chidlren on a mg/m^2 basis). In mature rats, the subcutaneous median lethal dose of albuterol sulfate is approximately 450 mg/kg (approximately 110 times the maximum recommended daily oral dose for adults on a mg/m^2 basis, or approximately 90 times the maximum recommended daily oral dose for children on a mg/m^2 basis). In small young rats, the subcutaneous median lethal dose is approximately 2000 mg/kg, (approximately 500 times the maximum recommended daily oral dose for adults on a mg/m^2 basis, or, approximately 400 times the maximum recommended daily oral dose for children on a mg/m^2 basis).

DOSAGE AND ADMINISTRATION

The following dosages of VOLMAX® Extended-Release Tablets are expressed in terms of albuterol base:

Usual Dosage:

Adults and Pediatric Patients 12 years of age and older: The usual recommended dosage for adults and pediatric patients over 12 years of age is 8 mg every 12 hours. In some patients, 4 mg every 12 hours may be sufficient.

Pediatric Patients 6 to 12 years of age: The usual recommended dosage for children 6 through 12 years of age is 4 mg every 12 hours.

Dosage adjustment in Adults and Pediatric Patients 12 years of age and older: In unusual circumstances, such as adults of low body weight, it may be desirable to use a starting dosage of 4 mg every 12 hours and progress to 8 mg every 12 hours according to response.

If control of reversible airway obstruction is not achieved with the recommended doses in patients on otherwise optimized asthma therapy, the doses may be cautiously increased stepwise under the control of the supervising physician to a maximum dose of 32 mg per day in divided doses (i.e., q12h).

Dosage adjustment in Pediatric Patients 6 to 12 years of age: If control of reversible airway obstruction is not achieved with the recommended doses in patients on otherwise optimized asthma therapy, the doses may be cautiously increased stepwise under the control of the supervising physician to a maximum dose of 24 mg per day in divided doses (i.e., q12h).

Switching from oral Ventolin® products: Patients currently maintained on Ventolin® (albuterol sulfate, USP) Tablets or Ventolin® (albuterol sulfate) Syrup can be switched to Volmax® Extended-Release Tablets. For example, the administration of one 4 mg Volmax® Extended-Release Tablets every 12 hours is comparable to one 2 mg Ventolin® Tablet every 6 hours. Multiples of this regimen up to the maximum recommended daily dose also apply.

Each Volmax® Extended-Release Tablet contains a small hole that is part of the unique extended-release system. Volmax® Extended-Release Tablets must be swallowed whole with the aid of liquids. DO NOT CHEW OR CRUSH THESE TABLETS.

HOW SUPPLIED

Volmax® Extended-Release Tablets, 4 mg of albuterol as the sulfate, are light blue, hexagonal tablets printed with "Volmax" on one side and the number "4" on the other in dark blue ink. They are supplied in HDPE bottles with child-resistant closures of 100 tablets (NDC 0451-0398-50) and HDPE bottles of 500 tablets (NDC 0451-0398-60).

Volmax® Extended-Release Tablets, 8 mg of albuterol as the sulfate, are white, hexagonal tablets printed with "Volmax" on one side and the number "8" on the other in dark blue ink. They are supplied in HDPE bottles with child-resistant closures of 100 tablets (NDC 0451-0399-50) and HDPE bottles of 500 tablets (NDC 0451-0399-60).

Store between 2° and 30° C (36° and 86° F).

Muro Pharmaceutical, Inc.
An ASTA Medica company
Marketed by: Muro Pharmaceutical, Inc.
Tewksbury, MA 01876-1496
Manufactured by: Glaxo Operations UK Ltd. England
Muro® is a registered trademark of
Muro Pharmaceutical, Inc.
*Ventolin® is a registered trademark of Glaxo-Wellcome Operations, Inc.
1/98   I-0398-0399-8

Mylan Pharmaceuticals Inc.
781 CHESTNUT RIDGE ROAD
P.O. BOX 4310
MORGANTOWN, WV 26504-4310

Direct Inquiries to:
(304) 599-2595
For Medical Information Contact:
Pharmacy Affairs Department
(800) 82-MYLAN
Sales and Ordering:
Sales Department
(800) RX-MYLAN

The following list of Mylan products is provided to facilitate identification. It includes the color(s) and identification codes for all tablets and capsules.

PRODUCT	IDENTIFICATION CODE
GENERIC NAME	(Front/nicarBack*)
Description	
Color(s)	
ACEBUTOLOL HYDROCHLORIDE	MYLAN 1200
Capsules, 200 mg ℞	
Med. Orange & Med. Orange	
ACEBUTOLOL HYDROCHLORIDE	MYLAN 1400
Capsules, 400 mg ℞	
Med. Orange & Med. Orange	
ACYCLOVIR	MYLAN 2200
Capsules, 200 mg ℞	
Lavender & Lavender	
ACYCLOVIR	ACY 400/Blank
Tablets, 400 mg ℞	
White	
ACYCLOVIR	ACY 800/Blank
Tablets, 800 mg ℞	
White	
ALBUTEROL	M255/Blank
Tablets, USP, 2 mg ℞	
White	
ALBUTEROL	M572/Blank
Tablets, USP, 4 mg ℞	
White	
ALLOPURINOL	M31/Blank
Tablets, USP, 100 mg ℞	
White	
ALLOPURINOL	M71/Blank
Tablets, USP, 300 mg ℞	
White	
ALPRAZOLAM	MYLAN A/Scored
Tablets, USP, 0.25 mg Ⓒ/℞	
White	
ALPRAZOLAM	MYLAN A3/Scored
Tablets, USP, 0.5 mg Ⓒ/℞	
Peach	
ALPRAZOLAM	MYLAN A1/Scored
Tablets, USP, 1 mg Ⓒ/℞	
Blue	
ALPRAZOLAM	MYLAN A4/Scored
Tablets, USP, 2 mg Ⓒ/℞	
White	
AMILORIDE HYDROCHLORIDE and HYDROCHLOROTHIAZIDE	M577/Blank
Tablets, USP, 5 mg/50 mg ℞	
Lt. Orange	
AMITRIPTYLINE HYDROCHLORIDE	M77/Blank
Tablets, USP, 10 mg ℞	
White	
AMITRIPTYLINE HYDROCHLORIDE	M51/Blank
Tablets, USP, 25 mg ℞	
Lt. Green	
AMITRIPTYLINE HYDROCHLORIDE	M36/Blank
Tablets, USP, 50 mg ℞	
Brown	
AMITRIPTYLINE HYDROCHLORIDE	M37/Blank
Tablets, USP, 75 mg ℞	
Blue	
AMITRIPTYLINE HYDROCHLORIDE	M38/Blank
Tablets, USP, 100 mg ℞	
Orange	
AMITRIPTYLINE HYDROCHLORIDE	M39/Blank
Tablets, USP, 150 mg ℞	
Flesh	
ATENOLOL	M/231
Tablets, 50 mg ℞	
White	
ATENOLOL	M/757
Tablets, 100 mg ℞	
White	

Continued on next page

Product Listing—Cont.

ATENOLOL and CHLORTHALIDONE   M63/Blank
Tablets, 50 mg/25 mg ℞
White

ATENOLOL and CHLORTHALIDONE   M64/Blank
Tablets, 100 mg/25 mg ℞
White

BROMOCRIPTINE MESYLATE   BCT 2 1/2/Blank
Tablets, USP, 2.5 mg ℞
White

BUMETANIDE   MYLAN/245
Tablets, USP, 0.5 mg ℞
Lt. Green

BUMETANIDE   MYLAN/370
Tablets, USP, 1 mg ℞
Yellow

BUMETANIDE   MYLAN/417
Tablets, USP, 2 mg ℞
Peach

CAPTOPRIL   MC1/Scored
Tablets, USP, 12.5 mg ℞
White

CAPTOPRIL   MC2/Scored
Tablets, USP, 25 mg ℞
White

CAPTOPRIL   MC3/Blank
Tablets, USP, 50 mg ℞
White

CAPTOPRIL   MC4/Blank
Tablets, USP, 100 mg ℞
White

CAPTOPRIL and HYDROCHLOROTHIAZIDE M81/Scored
Tablets, USP, 25 mg/15 mg ℞
White

CAPTOPRIL and HYDROCHLOROTHIAZIDE M84/Scored
Tablets, USP, 50 mg/15 mg ℞
White

CAPTOPRIL and HYDROCHLOROTHIAZIDE M83/Scored
Tablets, USP, 25 mg/25 mg ℞
White

CAPTOPRIL and HYDROCHLOROTHIAZIDE M86/Scored
Tablets, USP, 50 mg/25 mg ℞
Peach

CEFACLOR   MYLAN 7250
Capsules, USP, 250 mg ℞
Pink & White

CEFACLOR   MYLAN 7500
Capsules, USP, 500 mg ℞
Pink & Gray

CEFACLOR   —
Powders for Oral Suspension, USP, 125 mg/5 mL ℞

CEFACLOR   —
Powders for Oral Suspension, USP, 187 mg/5 mL ℞

CEFACLOR   —
Powders for Oral Suspension, USP, 250 mg/5 mL ℞

CEFACLOR   —
Powders for Oral Suspension, USP, 375 mg/5 mL ℞

CEPHALEXIN   MYLAN 6025
Capsules, USP, 250 mg ℞
Dark Blue & White

CEPHALEXIN   MYLAN 6050
Capsules, USP, 500 mg ℞
Dark Blue & Lt. Blue

CEPHALEXIN   —
Powders for Oral Suspension, USP, 125 mg/5 mL ℞

CEPHALEXIN   —
Powders for Oral Suspension, USP, 250 mg/5 mL ℞

CHLORDIAZEPOXIDE and   MYLAN/211
AMITRIPTYLINE HYDROCHLORIDE
Tablets, USP, 5 mg/12.5 mg Ⓝ/℞
Green

CHLORDIAZEPOXIDE and   MYLAN/277
AMITRIPTYLINE HYDROCHLORIDE
Tablets, USP, 10 mg/25 mg Ⓝ/℞
White

CHLOROTHIAZIDE   M50/Blank
Tablets, USP, 250 mg ℞
White

CHLOROTHIAZIDE   MYLAN 162/Blank
Tablets, USP, 500 mg ℞
White

CHLORPROPAMIDE   MYLAN 197/100
Tablets, USP, 100 mg ℞
Green

CHLORPROPAMIDE   MYLAN 210/250
Tablets, USP, 250 mg ℞
Green

CHLORTHALIDONE   M35/Blank
Tablets, USP, 25 mg ℞
Lt. Yellow

CHLORTHALIDONE   M75/Blank
Tablets, USP, 50 mg ℞
Lt. Green

CIMETIDINE   M/53
Tablets, USP, 200 mg ℞
Green

CIMETIDINE   M/317
Tablets, USP, 300 mg ℞
Green

CIMETIDINE   M/372
Tablets, USP, 400 mg ℞
Green

CIMETIDINE   M541/Blank
Tablets, USP, 800 mg ℞
Green

CLOMIPRAMINE HYDROCHLORIDE   MYLAN 3025
Capsules, 25 mg ℞
Medium Orange & Flesh

CLOMIPRAMINE HYDROCHLORIDE   MYLAN 3050
Capsules, 50 mg ℞
Yellow & Flesh

CLOMIPRAMINE HYDROCHLORIDE   MYLAN 3075
Capsules, 75 mg ℞
Swedish Orange & Flesh

CLONIDINE HYDROCHLORIDE   MYLAN 152/Blank
Tablets, USP, 0.1 mg ℞
White

CLONIDINE HYDROCHLORIDE   MYLAN 186/Blank
Tablets, USP, 0.2 mg ℞
White

CLONIDINE HYDROCHLORIDE   MYLAN 199/Blank
Tablets, USP, 0.3 mg ℞
White

CLORAZEPATE DIPOTASSIUM   M30/Blank
Tablets, 3.75 mg Ⓝ/℞
Blue

CLORAZEPATE DIPOTASSIUM   M40/Blank
Tablets, 7.5 mg Ⓝ/℞
Peach

CLORAZEPATE DIPOTASSIUM   M70/Blank
Tablets, 15 mg Ⓝ/℞
White

CYCLOBENZAPRINE HYDROCHLORIDE   M/751
Tablets, USP, 10 mg ℞
Butterscotch-Yellow

DIAZEPAM   MYLAN 271/Scored
Tablets, USP, 2 mg Ⓝ/℞
White

DIAZEPAM   MYLAN 345/Scored
Tablets, USP, 5 mg Ⓝ/℞
Orange

DIAZEPAM   MYLAN 477/Scored
Tablets, USP, 10 mg Ⓝ/℞
Green

DILTIAZEM HYDROCHLORIDE   M23/Blank
Tablets, USP, 30 mg ℞
White

DILTIAZEM HYDROCHLORIDE   M45/Scored
Tablets, USP, 60 mg ℞
White

DILTIAZEM HYDROCHLORIDE   M135/Scored
Tablets, USP, 90 mg ℞
White

DILTIAZEM HYDROCHLORIDE   M525/Scored
Tablets, USP, 120 mg ℞
White

DILTIAZEM HYDROCHLORIDE   MYLAN 5220
Extended-release Capsules, USP, 120 mg ℞
Lt. Pink & Flesh

DILTIAZEM HYDROCHLORIDE   MYLAN 5280
Extended-release Capsules, USP, 180 mg ℞
Lavender / Flesh

DILTIAZEM HYDROCHLORIDE   MYLAN 5340
Extended-release Capsules, USP, 240 mg ℞
Lt Blue / Flesh

DILTIAZEM HYDROCHLORIDE   MYLAN 6060
Extended-release Capsules, USP, 60 mg ℞
Coral & White

DILTIAZEM HYDROCHLORIDE   MYLAN 6090
Extended-release Capsules, USP, 90 mg ℞
Coral & Ivory

DILTIAZEM HYDROCHLORIDE   MYLAN 6120
Extended-release Capsules, USP, 120 mg ℞
Coral & Coral

DIPHENOXYLATE HYDRO-   M15/Blank
CHLORIDE and ATROPINE SULFATE
Tablets, USP, 2.5 mg/0.025 mg Ⓝ/℞
White

DOXEPIN HYDROCHLORIDE   MYLAN 1049
Capsules, USP, 10 mg ℞
Buff & Buff

DOXEPIN HYDROCHLORIDE   MYLAN 3125
Capsules, USP, 25 mg ℞
Ivory & White

DOXEPIN HYDROCHLORIDE   MYLAN 4250
Capsules, USP, 50 mg ℞
Ivory & Ivory

DOXEPIN HYDROCHLORIDE   MYLAN 5375
Capsules, USP, 75 mg ℞
Lt. Green & Lt. Green

DOXEPIN HYDROCHLORIDE   MYLAN 6410
Capsules, USP, 100 mg ℞
Lt. Green & White

DOXYCYCLINE HYCLATE   MYLAN 145
Capsules, USP, 50 mg ℞
Aqua Blue & White

DOXYCYCLINE HYCLATE   MYLAN 148
Capsules, USP, 100 mg ℞
Aqua Blue & Aqua Blue

DOXYCYCLINE HYCLATE   MYLAN 167/100
Tablets, USP, 100 mg ℞
Beige

ERYTHROMYCIN ETHYLSUCCINATE   M400/Blank
Tablets, USP, 400 mg ℞
Beige

ERYTHROMYCIN STEARATE   MYLAN 106/250
Tablets, USP, 250 mg ℞
Yellow

ERYTHROMYCIN STEARATE   MYLAN 107/500
Tablets, USP, 500 mg ℞
Yellow

ETODOLAC   MYLAN 7200
Capsules, 200 mg ℞
Brown & Brown

ETODOLAC   MYLAN 7233
Capsules, 300 mg ℞
Lt. Brown & Lt. Brown

ETODOLAC   MYLAN/237
Tablets, 400 mg ℞
White

FENOPROFEN CALCIUM   M471/Scored
Tablets, USP, 600 mg ℞
Lt. Orange

FLUPHENAZINE HYDROCHLORIDE   M/4
Tablets, USP, 1 mg ℞
White

FLUPHENAZINE HYDROCHLORIDE   M/9
Tablets, USP, 2.5 mg ℞
Yellow

FLUPHENAZINE HYDROCHLORIDE   M/74
Tablets, USP, 5 mg ℞
Green

FLUPHENAZINE HYDROCHLORIDE   M/97
Tablets, USP, 10 mg ℞
Orange

FLURAZEPAM HYDROCHLORIDE   MYLAN 4415
Capsules, USP, 15 mg Ⓝ/℞
White & Powder Blue

FLURAZEPAM HYDROCHLORIDE   MYLAN 4430
Capsules, USP, 30 mg Ⓝ/℞
Powder Blue & Powder Blue

FLURBIPROFEN   M76/Blank
Tablets, USP, 50 mg ℞
Beige

FLURBIPROFEN   M93/Blank
Tablets, USP, 100 mg ℞
Beige

FUROSEMIDE   M2/Blank
Tablets, USP, 20 mg ℞
White

FUROSEMIDE   MYLAN 216/40
Tablets, USP, 40 mg ℞
White

FUROSEMIDE   MYLAN 232/80
Tablets, USP, 80 mg ℞
White

GEMFIBROZIL   MYLAN/517
Tablets, USP, 600 mg ℞
White

GLIPIZIDE   MYLAN G1/Blank
Tablets, 5 mg ℞
White

GLIPIZIDE   MYLAN G2/Blank
Tablets, 10 mg ℞
White

GUANFACINE   M/G4
Tablets, USP, 1 mg ℞
White

GUANFACINE   M/G5
Tablets, USP, 2 mg ℞
Blue

HALOPERIDOL   MYLAN 351/Scored
Tablets, USP, 0.5 mg ℞
Orange

HALOPERIDOL   MYLAN 257/Scored
Tablets, USP, 1 mg ℞
Orange

HALOPERIDOL   MYLAN 214/Scored
Tablets, USP, 2 mg ℞
Orange

HALOPERIDOL   MYLAN 327/Scored
Tablets, USP, 5 mg ℞
Orange

HYDROXYCHLOROQUINE SULFATE   M/373
Tablets, USP, 200 mg ℞
White

IBUPROFEN Tablets, USP, 400 mg ℞ *White*	MYLAN 1401/Blank
IBUPROFEN Tablets, USP, 600 mg ℞ *White*	MYLAN 1601/Blank
IBUPROFEN Tablets, USP, 800 mg ℞ *White*	MYLAN 1801/Blank
INDAPAMIDE Tablets, USP, 1.25 mg ℞ *Pink*	M/69
INDAPAMIDE Tablets, USP, 2.5 mg ℞ *White*	M/80
INDOMETHACIN Capsules, USP, 25 mg ℞ *Lt. Green & Lt. Green*	MYLAN 143
INDOMETHACIN Capsules, USP, 50 mg ℞ *Lt. Green & Lt. Green*	MYLAN 147
KETOPROFEN Capsules, 50 mg ℞ *Lt. Celery & Lt. Celery*	MYLAN 4070
KETOPROFEN Capsules, 75 mg ℞ *Lt. Aqua & Lt. Aqua*	MYLAN 5750
KETOROLAC TROMETHAMINE Tablets, USP, 10 mg ℞ *White*	M134
LACTULOSE Solution, USP, 10 g/15 mL ℞	—
LOPERAMIDE HYDROCHLORIDE Capsules, USP, 2 mg ℞ *Lt. Brown & Lt. Brown*	MYLAN 2100
LORAZEPAM Tablets, USP, 0.5 mg ℂⁿ/℞ *White*	M/321
LORAZEPAM Tablets, USP, 1 mg ℂⁿ/℞ *White*	MYLAN 457/Blank
LORAZEPAM Tablets, USP, 2 mg ℂⁿ/℞ *White*	MYLAN 777/Blank
MAPROTILINE HYDROCHLORIDE Tablets, USP, 25 mg ℞ *White*	M/60
MAPROTILINE HYDROCHLORIDE Tablets, USP, 50 mg ℞ *Blue*	M/87
MAPROTILINE HYDROCHLORIDE Tablets, USP, 75 mg ℞ *White*	M/92
MECLOFENAMATE SODIUM Capsules, USP, 50 mg ℞ *Coral & Coral*	MYLAN 2150
MECLOFENAMATE SODIUM Capsules, USP, 100 mg ℞ *Coral & White*	MYLAN 3000
METHOTREXATE Tablets, USP, 2.5 mg ℞ *Orange*	M14/Blank
METHYCLOTHIAZIDE Tablets, USP, 5 mg ℞ *Blue*	M29/Blank
METHYLDOPA Tablets, USP, 250 mg ℞ *Beige*	MYLAN/611
METHYLDOPA Tablets, USP, 500 mg ℞ *Beige*	MYLAN/421
METHYLDOPA and HYDROCHLOROTHIAZIDE Tablets, USP, 250 mg/15 mg ℞ *Green*	MYLAN/507
METHYLDOPA and HYDROCHLOROTHIAZIDE Tablets, USP, 250 mg/25 mg ℞ *Green*	MYLAN/711
METOPROLOL TARTRATE Tablets, USP, 50 mg ℞ *Pink*	M32/Scored
METOPROLOL TARTRATE Tablets, USP, 100 mg ℞ *Lt. Blue*	M47/Scored
NADOLOL Tablets, USP, 20 mg ℞ *Yellow*	M28/Blank
NADOLOL Tablets, USP, 40 mg ℞ *Yellow*	M171/Blank
NADOLOL Tablets, USP, 80 mg ℞ *Yellow*	M132/Blank
NAPROXEN Tablets, USP, 250 mg ℞ *White*	MYLAN/377
NAPROXEN Tablets, USP, 375 mg ℞ *White*	MYLAN/555
NAPROXEN Tablets, USP, 500 mg ℞ *White*	MYLAN/451
NAPROXEN SODIUM Tablets, USP, 275 mg ℞ *Lt. Blue*	M/537
NAPROXEN SODIUM Tablets, USP, 550 mg ℞ *Lt. Blue*	MYLAN/733
NICARDIPINE HYDROCHLORIDE Capsules, 20 mg ℞ *Ivory*	MYLAN 1020
NICARDIPINE HYDROCHLORIDE Capsules, 30 mg ℞ *Blue Green & Yellow*	MYLAN 1430
NITROFURANTOIN Capsules, USP, 50 mg ℞ *Lt. Brown & Lt. Brown*	MYLAN 1650
NITROFURANTOIN Capsules, USP, 100 mg ℞ *Gray & Gray*	MYLAN 1700
NITROGLYCERIN TRANSDERMAL SYSTEM Patches, 0.2 mg ℞	Nitroglycerin 0.2 mg/hr
NITROGLYCERIN TRANSDERMAL SYSTEM Patches, 0.4 mg ℞	Nitroglycerin 0.4 mg/hr
NITROGLYCERIN TRANSDERMAL SYSTEM Patches, 0.6 mg ℞	Nitroglycerin 0.6 mg/hr
NORTRIPTYLINE HYDROCHLORIDE Capsules, USP, 10 mg ℞ *Swedish Orange & Swedish Orange*	MYLAN 1410
NORTRIPTYLINE HYDROCHLORIDE Capsules, USP, 25 mg ℞ *Orange & Swedish Orange*	MYLAN 2325
NORTRIPTYLINE HYDROCHLORIDE Capsules, USP, 50 mg ℞ *Yellow & Swedish Orange*	MYLAN 3250
NORTRIPTYLINE HYDROCHLORIDE Capsules, USP, 75 mg ℞ *Brown & Swedish Orange*	MYLAN 4175
PENTOXIFYLLINE Extended-release Tablets, 400 mg ℞ *Lavender*	MYLAN/357
PERPHENAZINE and AMITRIPTYLINE HYDROCHLORIDE Tablets, USP, 2 mg/10 mg ℞ *White*	MYLAN/330
PERPHENAZINE and AMITRIPTYLINE HYDROCHLORIDE Tablets, USP, 2 mg/25 mg ℞ *Purple*	MYLAN/442
PERPHENAZINE and AMITRIPTYLINE HYDROCHLORIDE Tablets, USP, 4 mg/10 mg ℞ *Blue*	MYLAN/727
PERPHENAZINE and AMITRIPTYLINE HYDROCHLORIDE Tablets, USP, 4 mg/25 mg ℞ *Orange*	MYLAN/574
PERPHENAZINE and AMITRIPTYLINE HYDROCHLORIDE Tablets, USP, 4 mg/50 mg ℞ *Purple*	MYLAN/73
PINDOLOL Tablets, USP, 5 mg ℞ *White*	M52/Blank
PINDOLOL Tablets, USP, 10 mg ℞ *White*	M127/Blank
PIROXICAM Capsules, USP, 10 mg ℞ *Dark Green & Olive*	MYLAN 1010
PIROXICAM Capsules, USP, 20 mg ℞ *Medium Green & Medium Green*	MYLAN 2020
PRAZOSIN HYDROCHLORIDE Capsules, USP, 1 mg ℞ *Dk. Green & Lt. Brown*	MYLAN 1101
PRAZOSIN HYDROCHLORIDE Capsules, USP, 2 mg ℞ *Brown & Lt. Brown*	MYLAN 2302
PRAZOSIN HYDROCHLORIDE Capsules, USP, 5 mg ℞ *Lt. Blue & Lt. Brown*	MYLAN 3205
PROBENECID Tablets, USP, 500 mg ℞ *Yellow*	MYLAN 156/500
PROCHLORPERAZINE MALEATE Tablets, USP, 5 mg ℞ *Maroon*	M/P1
PROCHLORPERAZINE MALEATE Tablets, USP, 10 mg ℞ *Maroon*	M/P2
PROPOXYPHENE COMPOUND Capsules, USP, 65 mg ℂⁿ/℞ *Gray & Red*	MYLAN 131
PROPOXYPHENE HYDROCHLORIDE Capsules, USP, 65 mg ℂⁿ/℞ *Pink & Pink*	MYLAN 129
PROPOXYPHENE HYDROCHLORIDE and ACETAMINOPHEN Tablets, USP, 65 mg/650 mg ℂⁿ/℞ *Orange*	MYLAN/130
PROPOXYPHENE NAPSYLATE and ACETAMINOPHEN Tablets, USP, 100 mg/650 mg ℂⁿ/℞ *Pink*	MYLAN/155
PROPOXYPHENE NAPSYLATE and ACETAMINOPHEN Tablets, USP, 100 mg/650 mg ℂⁿ/℞ *White*	MYLAN/1155
PROPRANOLOL HYDROCHLORIDE Tablets, USP, 10 mg ℞ *Orange*	MYLAN 182/10
PROPRANOLOL HYDROCHLORIDE Tablets, USP, 20 mg ℞ *Blue*	MYLAN 183/20
PROPRANOLOL HYDROCHLORIDE Tablets, USP, 40 mg ℞ *Green*	MYLAN 184/40
PROPRANOLOL HYDROCHLORIDE Tablets, USP, 80 mg ℞ *Yellow*	MYLAN 185/80
PROPRANOLOL HYDROCHLO- RIDE and HYDROCHLOROTHIAZIDE Tablets, USP, 40 mg/25 mg ℞ *White*	MYLAN 731/Scored
PROPRANOLOL HYDROCHLO- RIDE and HYDROCHLOROTHIAZIDE Tablets, USP, 80 mg/25 mg ℞ *White*	MYLAN 347/Scored
RANITIDINE Tablets, USP, 150 mg ℞ *White*	G/00 30
RANITIDINE Tablets, USP, 300 mg ℞ *White*	G/00 31
SPIRONOLACTONE Tablets, USP, 25 mg ℞ *White*	MYLAN 146/25
SPIRONOLACTONE and HYDROCHLOROTHIAZIDE Tablets, USP, 25 mg/25 mg ℞ *Ivory*	M41/Blank
SULINDAC Tablets, USP, 150 mg ℞ *Yellow-Orange*	MYLAN/427
SULINDAC Tablets, USP, 200 mg ℞ *Yellow-Orange*	MYLAN 531/Blank
TEMAZEPAM Capsules, USP, 15 mg ℂⁿ/℞ *Peach & Peach*	MYLAN 4010
TEMAZEPAM Capsules, USP, 30 mg ℂⁿ/℞ *Yellow & Yellow*	MYLAN 5050
TETRACYCLINE HYDROCHLORIDE Capsules, USP, 250 mg ℞ *Orange & Yellow*	MYLAN 101
TETRACYCLINE HYDROCHLORIDE Capsules, USP, 500 mg ℞ *Black & Yellow*	MYLAN 102
THIORIDAZINE HYDROCHLORIDE Tablets, USP, 10 mg ℞ *Orange*	M54/10
THIORIDAZINE HYDROCHLORIDE Tablets, USP, 25 mg ℞ *Orange*	M58/25
THIORIDAZINE HYDROCHLORIDE Tablets, USP, 50 mg ℞ *Orange*	M59/50
THIORIDAZINE HYDROCHLORIDE Tablets, USP, 100 mg ℞ *Orange*	M61/100
THIOTHIXENE Capsules, USP, 1 mg ℞ *Caramel & Powder Blue*	MYLAN 1001
THIOTHIXENE Capsules, USP, 2 mg ℞ *Caramel & Yellow*	MYLAN 2002
THIOTHIXENE Capsules, USP, 5 mg ℞ *Caramel & White*	MYLAN 3005

Continued on next page

Product Listing—Cont.

THIOTHIXENE MYLAN 5010
Capsules, USP, 10 mg ℞
Caramel & Peach

TIMOLOL MALEATE M55/Blank
Tablets, USP, 5 mg ℞
Green

TIMOLOL MALEATE M221/Blank
Tablets, USP, 10 mg ℞
Green

TIMOLOL MALEATE M715/Blank
Tablets, USP, 20 mg ℞
Green

TOLAZAMIDE MYLAN 217/250
Tablets, USP, 250 mg ℞
White

TOLAZAMIDE MYLAN 551/Blank
Tablets, USP, 500 mg ℞
White

TOLBUTAMIDE M13/Blank
Tablets, USP, 500 mg ℞
White

TOLMETIN SODIUM MYLAN 5200
Capsules, USP, 400 mg ℞
Lt. Blue & Lt. Blue

TOLMETIN SODIUM M313/Blank
Tablets, USP, 600 mg ℞
Beige

TRIAMTERENE and HYDROCHLOROTHIAZIDE MYLAN 2537
Capsules, USP, 37.5 mg/25 mg ℞
Olive & Yellow

TRIAMTERENE and HYDROCHLOROTHIAZIDE MYLAN/TH1
Tablets, USP, 37.5 mg/25 mg ℞
Green

TRIAMTERENE and HYDROCHLOROTHIAZIDE MYLAN/TH2
Tablets, USP, 75 mg/50 mg ℞
Yellow

TRIFLUOPERAZINE HYDROCHLORIDE M/T3
Tablets, USP, 1 mg ℞
White

TRIFLUOPERAZINE HYDROCHLORIDE M/T4
Tablets, USP, 2 mg ℞
White

TRIFLUOPERAZINE HYDROCHLORIDE M/T5
Tablets, USP, 5 mg ℞
Lavender

TRIFLUOPERAZINE HYDROCHLORIDE M/T6
Tablets, USP, 10 mg ℞
Lavender

VERAPAMIL HYDROCHLORIDE MYLAN 512/Blank
Tablets, USP, 80 mg ℞
White

VERAPAMIL HYDROCHLORIDE MYLAN 772/Blank
Tablets, USP, 120 mg ℞
White

VERAPAMIL HYDROCHLORIDE MYLAN/244
Extended-release Tablets, 120 mg
Blue

VERAPAMIL HYDROCHLORIDE M312/Blank
Extended-release Tablets, 180 mg
Blue

VERAPAMIL HYDROCHLORIDE M411/Blank
Extended-release Tablets, 240 mg ℞
Blue

*Front/Back Side for Tablets or Both Cap and Body for Capsules.

CAPTOPRIL TABLETS, USP ℞

12.5 mg, 25 mg, 50 mg and 100 mg

USE IN PREGNANCY

When used in pregnancy during the second and third trimesters, ACE inhibitors can cause injury and even death to the developing fetus. When pregnancy is detected, captopril should be discontinued as soon as possible. See **WARNINGS: Fetal/Neonatal Morbidity and Mortality.**

DESCRIPTION

Captopril is a specific competitive inhibitor of angiotensin I-converting enzyme (ACE), the enzyme responsible for the conversion of angiotensin I to angiotensin II.

Captopril is designated chemically as 1-[(2S)-3-mercapto-2-methylpropionyl]-L-proline (MW 217.29).

Captopril is a white to off-white crystalline powder that may have a slight sulfurous odor; it is soluble in water (approx. 160 mg/mL), methanol, and ethanol and sparingly soluble in chloroform and ethyl acetate.

The structural formula is:

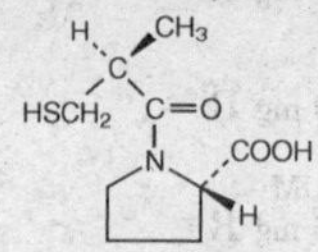

$C_9H_{15}NO_3S$

Each tablet for oral administration contains 12.5 mg, 25 mg, 50 mg or 100 mg of captopril and the following inactive ingredients: anhydrous lactose, colloidal silicon dioxide, crospovidone, microcrystalline cellulose and stearic acid.

CLINICAL PHARMACOLOGY

Mechanism of Action: The mechanism of action of captopril has not yet been fully elucidated. Its beneficial effects in hypertension and heart failure appear to result primarily from suppression of the renin-angiotensin-aldosterone system. However, there is no consistent correlation between renin levels and response to the drug. Renin, an enzyme synthesized by the kidneys, is released into the circulation where it acts on a plasma globulin substrate to produce angiotensin I, a relatively inactive decapeptide. Angiotensin I is then converted by angiotensin converting enzyme (ACE) to angiotensin II, a potent endogenous vasoconstrictor substance. Angiotensin II also stimulates aldosterone secretion from the adrenal cortex, thereby contributing to sodium and fluid retention.

Captopril prevents the conversion of angiotensin I to angiotensin II by inhibition of ACE, a peptidyldipeptide carboxy hydrolase. This inhibition has been demonstrated in both healthy human subjects and in animals by showing that the elevation of blood pressure caused by exogenously administered angiotensin I was attenuated or abolished by captopril. In animal studies, captopril did not alter the pressor responses to a number of other agents, including angiotensin II and norepinephrine, indicating specificity of action.

ACE is identical to "bradykininase", and captopril may also interfere with the degradation of the vasodepressor peptide, bradykinin. Increased concentrations of bradykinin or prostaglandin E_2 may also have a role in the therapeutic effect of captopril.

Inhibition of ACE results in decreased plasma angiotensin II and increased plasma renin activity (PRA), the latter resulting from loss of negative feedback on renin release caused by reduction in angiotensin II. The reduction of angiotensin II leads to decreased aldosterone secretion, and, as a result, small increases in serum potassium may occur along with sodium and fluid loss.

The antihypertensive effects persist for a longer period of time than does demonstrable inhibition of circulating ACE. It is not known whether the ACE present in vascular endothelium is inhibited longer than the ACE in circulating blood.

Pharmacokinetics: After oral administration of therapeutic doses of captopril, rapid absorption occurs with peak blood levels at about one hour. The presence of food in the gastrointestinal tract reduces absorption by about 30 to 40 percent; captopril therefore should be given one hour before meals. Based on carbon-14 labeling, average minimal absorption is approximately 75 percent. In a 24-hour period, over 95 percent of the absorbed dose is eliminated in the urine; 40 to 50 percent is unchanged drug; most of the remainder is the disulfide dimer of captopril and captopril-cysteine disulfide.

Approximately 25 to 30 percent of the circulating drug is bound to plasma proteins. The apparent elimination half-life for total radioactivity in blood is probably less than 3 hours. An accurate determination of half-life of unchanged captopril is not, at present, possible, but it is probably less than 2 hours. In patients with renal impairment, however, retention of captopril occurs (see DOSAGE AND ADMINISTRATION).

Pharmacodynamics: Administration of captopril results in a reduction of peripheral arterial resistance in hypertensive patients with either no change, or an increase, in cardiac output. There is an increase in renal blood flow following administration of captopril and glomerular filtration rate is usually unchanged.

Reductions of blood pressure are usually maximal 60 to 90 minutes after oral administration of an individual dose of captopril. The duration of effect is dose related. The reduction in blood pressure may be progressive, so to achieve maximal therapeutic effects, several weeks of therapy may be required. The blood pressure lowering effects of captopril and thiazide-type diuretics are additive. In contrast, captopril and beta-blockers have a less than additive effect.

Blood pressure is lowered to about the same extent in both standing and supine positions. Orthostatic effects and tachycardia are infrequent but may occur in volume-depleted patients. Abrupt withdrawal of captopril has not been associated with a rapid increase in blood pressure.

In patients with heart failure, significantly decreased peripheral (systemic vascular) resistance and blood pressure (afterload), reduced pulmonary capillary wedge pressure (preload) and pulmonary vascular resistance, increased cardiac output, and increased exercise tolerance time (ETT) have been demonstrated. These hemodynamic and clinical effects occur after the first dose and appear to persist for the duration of therapy. Placebo controlled studies of 12 weeks duration in patients who did not respond adequately to diuretics and digitalis show no tolerance to beneficial effects on ETT; open studies, with exposure up to 18 months in some cases, also indicate that ETT benefit is maintained. Clinical improvement has been observed in some patients where acute hemodynamic effects were minimal.

The Survival and Ventricular Enlargement (SAVE) study was a multicenter, randomized, double-blind, placebo-controlled trial conducted in 2,231 patients (age 21 to 79 years) who survived the acute phase of a myocardial infarction and did not have active ischemia. Patients had left ventricular dysfunction (LVD), defined as a resting left ventricular ejection fraction ≤40%, but at the time of randomization were not sufficiently symptomatic to require ACE inhibitor therapy for heart failure. About half of the patients had had symptoms of heart failure in the past. Patients were given a test dose of 6.25 mg oral captopril and were randomized within 3 to 16 days post-infarction to receive either captopril or placebo in addition to conventional therapy. Captopril was initiated at 6.25 mg or 12.5 mg tid and after two weeks titrated to a target maintenance dose of 50 mg tid. About 80% of patients were receiving the target dose at the end of the study. Patients were followed for a minimum of two years and for up to five years, with an average follow-up of 3.5 years.

Baseline blood pressure was 113/70 mm Hg and 112/70 mm Hg for the placebo and captopril groups, respectively. Blood pressure increased slightly in both treatment groups during the study and was somewhat lower in the captopril group (119/74 vs. 125/77 mm Hg at 1 yr).

Therapy with captopril improved long-term survival and clinical outcomes compared to placebo. The risk reduction for all cause mortality was 19% (P = 0.02) and for cardiovascular death was 21% (P = 0.014). Captopril treated subjects had 22% (P = 0.034) fewer first hospitalizations for heart failure. Compared to placebo, 22% fewer patients receiving captopril developed symptoms of overt heart failure. There was no significant difference between groups in total hospitalizations for all cause (2056 placebo; 2036 captopril).

In a multicenter study, a marketed brand of captopril tablets were well tolerated in the presence of other therapies such as aspirin, beta blockers, nitrates, vasodilators, calcium antagonists and diuretics.

Studies in rats and cats indicate that captopril does not cross the blood-brain barrier to any significant extent.

INDICATIONS AND USAGE

Hypertension: Captopril tablets are indicated for the treatment of hypertension.

In using captopril, consideration should be given to the risk of neutropenia/agranulocytosis (see WARNINGS).

Captopril may be used as initial therapy for patients with normal renal function, in whom the risk is relatively low. In patients with impaired renal function, particularly those with collagen vascular disease, captopril should be reserved for hypertensives who have either developed unacceptable side effects on other drugs, or have failed to respond satisfactorily to drug combinations.

Captopril is effective alone and in combination with other antihypertensive agents, especially thiazide-type diuretics. The blood pressure lowering effects of captopril and thiazides are approximately additive.

Heart Failure: Captopril tablets are indicated in the treatment of congestive heart failure usually in combination with diuretics and digitalis. The beneficial effect of captopril in heart failure does not require the presence of digitalis, however, most controlled clinical trial experience with captopril has been in patients receiving digitalis, as well as diuretic treatment.

Left Ventricular Dysfunction After Myocardial Infarction: Captopril tablets are indicated to improve survival following myocardial infarction in clinically stable patients with left ventricular dysfunction manifested as an ejection fraction ≤ 40% and to reduce the incidence of overt heart failure and subsequent hospitalizations for congestive heart failure in these patients.

In considering use of captopril tablets, it should be noted that in controlled trials ACE inhibitors have an effect on blood pressure that is less in black patients than in non-blacks. In addition, ACE inhibitors (for which adequate data are available) cause a higher rate of angioedema in black than in non-black patients (see WARNINGS: Angioedema).

CONTRAINDICATIONS

Captopril tablets are contraindicated in patients who are hypersensitive to this product or any other angiotensin-converting enzyme inhibitor (e.g., a patient who has experienced angioedema during therapy with any other ACE inhibitor).

WARNINGS

Anaphylactoid and Possibly Related Reactions: Presumably because angiotensin-converting enzyme inhibitors af-

fect the metabolism of eicosanoids and polypeptides, including endogenous bradykinin, patients receiving ACE inhibitors (including captopril) may be subject to a variety of adverse reactions, some of them serious.

Angioedema: Angioedema involving the extremities, face, lips, mucous membranes, tongue, glottis or larynx has been seen in patients treated with ACE inhibitors, including captopril. If angioedema involves the tongue, glottis or larynx, airway obstruction may occur and be fatal. Emergency therapy, including but not necessarily limited to, subcutaneous administration of a 1:1000 solution of epinephrine should be promptly instituted.

Swelling confined to the face, mucous membranes of the mouth, lips and extremities has usually resolved with discontinuation of captopril; some cases required medical therapy. (See PRECAUTIONS: Information for Patients and ADVERSE REACTIONS.)

Anaphylactoid Reactions During Desensitization: Two patients undergoing desensitizing treatment with hymenoptera venom while receiving ACE inhibitors sustained life-threatening anaphylactoid reactions. In the same patients, these reactions were avoided when ACE inhibitors were temporarily withheld, but they reappeared upon inadvertent rechallenge.

Anaphylactoid Reactions During Membrane Exposure: Anaphylactoid reactions have been reported in patients dialyzed with high-flux membranes and treated concomitantly with an ACE inhibitor. Anaphylactoid reactions have also been reported in patients undergoing low-density lipoprotein apheresis with dextran sulfate absorption.

Neutropenia/Agranulocytosis: Neutropenia (< 1000/mm³) with myeloid hypoplasia has resulted from use of captopril. About half of the neutropenic patients developed systemic or oral cavity infections or other features of the syndrome of agranulocytosis.

The risk of neutropenia is dependent on the clinical status of the patient:

In clinical trials in patients with hypertension who have normal renal function (serum creatinine less than 1.6 mg/dL and no collagen vascular disease), neutropenia has been seen in one patient out of over 8,600 exposed.

In patients with some degree of renal failure (serum creatinine at least 1.6 mg/dL) but no collagen vascular disease, the risk of neutropenia in clinical trials was about 1 per 500, a frequency over 15 times that for uncomplicated hypertension. Daily doses of captopril were relatively high in these patients, particularly in view of their diminished renal function. In foreign marketing experience in patients with renal failure, use of allopurinol concomitantly with captopril has been associated with neutropenia but this association has not appeared in U.S. reports.

In patients with collagen vascular diseases (e.g., systemic lupus erythematosus, scleroderma) and impaired renal function, neutropenia occurred in 3.7 percent of patients in clinical trials.

While none of the over 750 patients in formal clinical trials of heart failure developed neutropenia, it has occurred during the subsequent clinical experience. About half of the reported cases had serum creatinine ≥ 1.6 mg/dL and more than 75 percent were in patients also receiving procainamide. In heart failure, it appears that the same risk factors for neutropenia are present.

The neutropenia has usually been detected within three months after captopril was started. Bone marrow examinations in patients with neutropenia consistently showed myeloid hypoplasia, frequently accompanied by erythroid hypoplasia and decreased numbers of megakaryocytes (e.g., hypoplastic bone marrow and pancytopenia); anemia and thrombocytopenia were sometimes seen.

In general, neutrophils returned to normal in about two weeks after captopril was discontinued, and serious infections were limited to clinically complex patients. About 13 percent of the cases of neutropenia have ended fatally, but almost all fatalities were in patients with serious illness, having collagen vascular disease, renal failure, heart failure or immunosuppressant therapy, or a combination of these complicating factors.

Evaluation of the hypertensive or heart failure patient should always include assessment of renal function.

If captopril is used in patients with impaired renal function, white blood cell and differential counts should be evaluated prior to starting treatment and at approximately two-week intervals for about three months, then periodically.

In patients with collagen vascular disease or who are exposed to other drugs known to affect the white cells or immune response, particularly when there is impaired renal function, captopril should be used only after an assessment of benefit and risk, and then with caution.

All patients treated with captopril should be told to report any signs of infection (e.g., sore throat, fever). If infection is suspected, white cell counts should be performed without delay.

Since discontinuation of captopril and other drugs has generally led to prompt return of the white count to normal,

upon confirmation of neutropenia (neutrophil count < 1000/mm³) the physician should withdraw captopril and closely follow the patient's course.

Proteinuria: Total urinary proteins greater than 1 g per day were seen in about 0.7 percent of patients receiving captopril. About 90 percent of affected patients had evidence of prior renal disease or received relatively high doses of captopril (in excess of 150 mg/day), or both. The nephrotic syndrome occurred in about one-fifth of proteinuric patients. In most cases, proteinuria subsided or cleared within six months whether or not captopril was continued. Parameters of renal function, such as BUN and creatinine, were seldom altered in the patients with proteinuria.

Hypotension: Excessive hypotension was rarely seen in hypertensive patients but is a possible consequence of captopril use in salt/volume depleted persons (such as those treated vigorously with diuretics), patients with heart failure or those patients undergoing renal dialysis. (See PRECAUTIONS: Drug Interactions.)

In heart failure, where the blood pressure was either normal or low, transient decreases in mean blood pressure greater than 20 percent were recorded in about half of the patients. This transient hypotension is more likely to occur after any of the first several doses and is usually well tolerated, producing either no symptoms or brief mild light-headedness, although in rare instances it has been associated with arrhythmia or conduction defects. Hypotension was the reason for discontinuation of drug in 3.6 percent of patients with heart failure.

BECAUSE OF THE POTENTIAL FALL IN BLOOD PRESSURE IN THESE PATIENTS, THERAPY SHOULD BE STARTED UNDER VERY CLOSE MEDICAL SUPERVISION. A starting dose of 6.25 or 12.5 mg tid may minimize the hypotensive effect. Patients should be followed closely for the first two weeks of treatment and whenever the dose of captopril and/or diuretic is increased. In patients with heart failure, reducing the dose of diuretic, if feasible, may minimize the fall in blood pressure.

Hypotension is not *per se* a reason to discontinue captopril. Some decrease of systemic blood pressure is a common and desirable observation upon initiation of captopril treatment in heart failure. The magnitude of the decrease is greatest early in the course of treatment; this effect stabilizes within a week or two, and generally returns to pretreatment levels, without a decrease in therapeutic efficacy, within two months.

Fetal/Neonatal Morbidity and Mortality: ACE inhibitors can cause fetal and neonatal morbidity and death when administered to pregnant women. Several dozen cases have been reported in the world literature. When pregnancy is detected, ACE inhibitors should be discontinued as soon as possible.

The use of ACE inhibitors during the second and third trimesters of pregnancy has been associated with fetal and neonatal injury, including hypotension, neonatal skull hypoplasia, anuria, reversible or irreversible renal failure, and death. Oligohydramnios has also been reported, presumably resulting from decreased fetal renal function; oligohydramnios in this setting has been associated with fetal limb contractures, craniofacial deformation, and hypoplastic lung development. Prematurity, intrauterine growth retardation, and patent ductus arteriosus have also been reported, although it is not clear whether these occurrences were due to the ACE-inhibitor exposure.

These adverse effects do not appear to have resulted from intrauterine ACE-inhibitor exposure that has been limited to the first trimester. Mothers whose embryos and fetuses are exposed to ACE inhibitors only during the first trimester should be so informed. Nonetheless, when patients become pregnant, physicians should make every effort to discontinue the use of captopril as soon as possible.

Rarely (probably less often than once in every thousand pregnancies), no alternative to ACE inhibitors will be found. In these rare cases, the mothers should be apprised of the potential hazards to their fetuses, and serial ultrasound examinations should be performed to assess the intra-amniotic environment.

If oligohydramnios is observed, captopril should be discontinued unless it is considered life-saving for the mother. Contraction stress testing (CST), a non-stress test (NST), or biophysical profiling (BPP) may be appropriate, depending upon the week of pregnancy. Patients and physicians should be aware, however, that oligohydramnios may not appear until after the fetus has sustained irreversible injury.

Infants with histories of *in utero* exposure to ACE inhibitors should be closely observed for hypotension, oliguria, and hyperkalemia. If oliguria occurs, attention should be directed toward support of blood pressure and renal perfusion. Exchange transfusion or dialysis may be required as a means of reversing hypotension and/or substituting for disordered renal function. While captopril may be removed from the adult circulation by hemodialysis, there is inadequate data concerning the effectiveness of hemodialysis for removing it from the circulation of neonates or children. Peritoneal dialysis is not effective for removing captopril; there is no information concerning exchange transfusion for removing captopril from the general circulation.

When captopril was given to rabbits at doses about 0.8 to 70 times (on a mg/kg basis) the maximum recommended human dose, low incidences of craniofacial malformations were seen. No teratogenic effects of captopril were seen in studies of pregnant rats and hamsters. On a mg/kg basis, the doses used were up to 150 times (in hamsters) and 625 times (in rats) the maximum recommended human dose.

Hepatic Failure: Rarely, ACE inhibitors have been associated with a syndrome that starts with cholestatic jaundice and progresses to fulminant hepatic necrosis and (sometimes) death. The mechanism of this syndrome is not understood. Patients receiving ACE inhibitors who develop jaundice or marked elevations of hepatic enzymes should discontinue the ACE inhibitor and receive appropriate medical follow-up.

PRECAUTIONS

General: *Impaired Renal Function: Hypertension:* Some patients with renal disease, particularly those with severe renal artery stenosis have developed increases in BUN and serum creatinine after reduction of blood pressure with captopril. Captopril dosage reduction and/or discontinuation of diuretic may be required. For some of these patients, it may not be possible to normalize blood pressure and maintain adequate renal perfusion.

Heart Failure: About 20 percent of patients develop stable elevations of BUN and serum creatinine greater than 20 percent above normal or baseline upon long-term treatment with captopril. Less than 5 percent of patients, generally those with severe preexisting renal disease, required discontinuation of treatment due to progressively increasing creatinine; subsequent improvement probably depends upon the severity of the underlying renal disease.

See CLINICAL PHARMACOLOGY, DOSAGE AND ADMINISTRATION, ADVERSE REACTIONS: Altered Laboratory Findings.

Hyperkalemia: Elevations in serum potassium have been observed in some patients treated with ACE inhibitors, including captopril. When treated with ACE inhibitors, patients at risk for the development of hyperkalemia include those with: renal insufficiency; diabetes mellitus; and those using concomitant potassium-sparing diuretics, potassium supplements or potassium-containing salt substitutes; or other drugs associated with increases in serum potassium. (See PRECAUTIONS: Information for Patients and Drug Interactions; ADVERSE REACTIONS: Altered Laboratory Findings.)

Cough: Presumably due to the inhibition of the degradation of endogenous bradykinin, persistent nonproductive cough has been reported with all ACE inhibitors, always resolving after discontinuation of therapy. ACE inhibitor-induced cough should be considered in the differential diagnosis of cough.

Valvular Stenosis: There is concern, on theoretical grounds, that patients with aortic stenosis might be at particular risk of decreased coronary perfusion when treated with vasodilators because they do not develop as much afterload reduction as others.

Surgery/Anesthesia: In patients undergoing major surgery or during anesthesia with agents that produce hypotension, captopril will block angiotensin II formation secondary to compensatory renin release. If hypotension occurs and is considered to be due to this mechanism, it can be corrected by volume expansion.

Hemodialysis: Recent clinical observations have shown an association of hypersensitivity-like (anaphylactoid) reactions during hemodialysis with high-flux dialysis membranes (e.g., AN69) in patients receiving ACE inhibitors. In these patients, consideration should be given to using a different type of dialysis membrane or a different class of medication. (See WARNINGS: Anaphylactoid Reactions During Membrane Exposure.)

Information For Patients: Patients should be advised to immediately report to their physician any signs or symptoms suggesting angioedema (e.g., swelling of face, eyes, lips, tongue, larynx and extremities; difficulty in swallowing or breathing; hoarseness) and to discontinue therapy. (See WARNINGS: Angioedema.)

Patients should be told to report promptly any indication of infection (e.g., sore throat, fever), which may be a sign of neutropenia, or of progressive edema which might be related to proteinuria and nephrotic syndrome.

All patients should be cautioned that excessive perspiration and dehydration may lead to an excessive fall in blood pressure because of reduction in fluid volume. Other causes of volume depletion such as vomiting or diarrhea may also lead to a fall in blood pressure; patients should be advised to consult with the physician.

Patients should be advised not to use potassium-sparing diuretics, potassium supplements or potassium-containing salt substitutes without consulting their physician. (See PRECAUTIONS: General and Drug Interactions; ADVERSE REACTIONS.)

Continued on next page

Captopril—Cont.

Patients should be warned against interruption or discontinuation of medication unless instructed by the physician. Heart failure patients on captopril therapy should be cautioned against rapid increases in physical activity.

Patients should be informed that captopril should be taken one hour before meals (see DOSAGE AND ADMINISTRATION).

Pregnancy: Female patients of childbearing age should be told about the consequences of second- and third-trimester exposure to ACE inhibitors, and they should also be told that these consequences do not appear to have resulted from intrauterine ACE-inhibitor exposure that has been limited to the first trimester. These patients should be asked to report pregnancies to their physicians as soon as possible.

Drug Interactions: *Hypotension-Patients on Diuretic Therapy:* Patients on diuretics and especially those in whom diuretic therapy was recently instituted, as well as those on severe dietary salt restriction or dialysis, may occasionally experience a precipitous reduction of blood pressure usually within the first hour after receiving the initial dose of captopril.

The possibility of hypotensive effects with captopril can be minimized by either discontinuing the diuretic or increasing the salt intake approximately one week prior to initiation of treatment with captopril or initiating therapy with small doses (6.25 or 12.5 mg). Alternatively, provide medical supervision for at least one hour after the initial dose. If hypotension occurs, the patient should be placed in a supine position and, if necessary, receive an intravenous infusion of normal saline. This transient hypotensive response is not a contraindication to further doses which can be given without difficulty once the blood pressure has increased after volume expansion.

Agents Having Vasodilator Activity: Data on the effect of concomitant use of other vasodilators in patients receiving captopril for heart failure are not available; therefore, nitroglycerin or other nitrates (as used for management of angina) or other drugs having vasodilator activity should, if possible, be discontinued before starting captopril. If resumed during captopril therapy, such agents should be administered cautiously, and perhaps at lower dosage.

Agents Causing Renin Release: Captopril's effect will be augmented by antihypertensive agents that cause renin release. For example, diuretics (e.g., thiazides) may activate the renin-angiotensin-aldosterone system.

Agents Affecting Sympathetic Activity: The sympathetic nervous system may be especially important in supporting blood pressure in patients receiving captopril alone or with diuretics. Therefore, agents affecting sympathetic activity (e.g., ganglionic blocking agents or adrenergic neuron blocking agents) should be used with caution. Beta-adrenergic blocking drugs add some further antihypertensive effect to captopril, but the overall response is less than additive.

Agents Increasing Serum Potassium: Since captopril decreases aldosterone production, elevation of serum potassium may occur. Potassium-sparing diuretics such as spironolactone, triamterene, or amiloride, or potassium supplements should be given only for documented hypokalemia, and then with caution, since they may lead to a significant increase of serum potassium. Salt substitutes containing potassium should also be used with caution.

Inhibitors of Endogenous Prostaglandin Synthesis: It has been reported that indomethacin may reduce the antihypertensive effect of captopril, especially in cases of low renin hypertension. Other nonsteroidal anti-inflammatory agents (e.g., aspirin) may also have this effect.

Lithium: Increased serum lithium levels and symptoms of lithium toxicity have been reported in patients receiving concomitant lithium and ACE inhibitor therapy. These drugs should be co-administered with caution and frequent monitoring of serum lithium levels is recommended. If a diuretic is also used, it may increase the risk of lithium toxicity.

Drug/Laboratory Test Interactions: Captopril may cause a false-positive urine test for acetone.

Carcinogenesis, Mutagenesis and Impairment of Fertility: Two-year studies with doses of 50 to 1350 mg/kg/day in mice and rats failed to show any evidence of carcinogenic potential. The high dose in these studies is 150 times the maximum recommended human dose of 450 mg, assuming a 50 kg subject. On a body-surface-area basis, the high doses for mice and rats are 13 and 26 times the maximum recommended human dose, respectively.

Studies in rats have revealed no impairment of fertility.

Animal Toxicology: Chronic oral toxicity studies were conducted in rats (2 years), dogs (47 weeks; 1 year), mice (2 years), and monkeys (1 year). Significant drug-related toxicity included effects on hematopoiesis, renal toxicity, erosion/ulceration of the stomach, and variation of retinal blood vessels.

Reductions in hemoglobin and/or hematocrit values were seen in mice, rats, and monkeys at doses 50 to 150 times the maximum recommended human dose (MRHD) of 450 mg,

assuming a 50 kg subject. On a body-surface-area basis, these doses are 5 to 25 times maximum recommended human dose (MRHD). Anemia, leukopenia, thrombocytopenia, and bone marrow suppression occurred in dogs at doses 8 to 30 times MRHD on a body-weight basis (4 to 15 times MRHD on a surface-area basis). The reductions in hemoglobin and hematocrit values in rats and mice were only significant at 1 year and returned to normal with continued dosing by the end of the study. Marked anemia was seen at all dose levels (8 to 30 times MRHD) in dogs, whereas moderate to marked leukopenia was noted only at 15 and 30 times MRHD and thrombocytopenia at 30 times MRHD. The anemia could be reversed upon discontinuation of dosing. Bone marrow suppression occurred to a varying degree, being associated only with dogs that died or were sacrificed in a moribund condition in the 1 year study. However, in the 47-week study at a dose 30 times MRHD, bone marrow suppression was found to be reversible upon continued drug administration.

Captopril caused hyperplasia of the juxtaglomerular apparatus of the kidneys in mice and rats at doses 7 to 200 times MRHD on a body-weight basis (0.6 to 35 times MRHD on a surface-area basis); in monkeys at 20 to 60 times MRHD on a body-weight basis (7 to 20 times MRHD on a surface-area basis); and in dogs at 30 times MRHD on a body-weight basis (15 times MRHD on a surface-area basis).

Gastric erosions/ulcerations were increased in incidence in male rats at 20 to 200 times MRHD on a body-weight basis (3.5 and 35 times MRHD on a surface-area basis); in dogs at 30 times MRHD on a body-weight basis (15 times MRHD on a surface-area basis); and in monkeys at 65 times MRHD on a body-weight basis (20 times MRHD on a surface-area basis). Rabbits developed gastric and intestinal ulcers when given oral doses approximately 30 times MRHD on a body-weight basis (10 times MRHD on a surface-area basis) for only 5 to 7 days.

In the two-year rat study, irreversible and progressive variations in the caliber of retinal vessels (focal sacculations and constrictions) occurred at all dose levels (7 to 200 times MRHD) on a body-weight basis; 1 to 35 times MRHD on a surface-area basis in a dose-related fashion. The effect was first observed in the 88th week of dosing, with a progressively increased incidence thereafter, even after cessation of dosing.

Pregnancy Categories C (first trimester) and D (second and third trimesters): See WARNINGS: Fetal/Neonatal Morbidity and Mortality.

Nursing Mothers: Concentrations of captopril in human milk are approximately one percent of those in maternal blood. Because of the potential for serious adverse reactions in nursing infants from captopril, a decision should be made whether to discontinue nursing or to discontinue the drug, taking into account the importance of captopril to the mother. (See PRECAUTIONS: Pediatric Use.)

Pediatric Use: Safety and effectiveness in pediatric patients have not been established. There is limited experience reported in the literature with the use of captopril in the pediatric population; dosage, on a weight basis, was generally reported to be comparable to or less than that used in adults.

Infants, especially newborns, may be more susceptible to the adverse hemodynamic effects of captopril. Excessive, prolonged and unpredictable decreases in blood pressure and associated complications, including oliguria and seizures, have been reported.

Captopril should be used in pediatric patients only if other measures for controlling blood pressure have not been effective.

ADVERSE REACTIONS

Reported incidences are based on clinical trials involving approximately 7000 patients.

Renal: About one of 100 patients developed proteinuria (see WARNINGS).

Each of the following has been reported in approximately 1 to 2 of 1000 patients and are of uncertain relationship to drug use: renal insufficiency, renal failure, nephrotic syndrome, polyuria, oliguria, and urinary frequency.

Hematologic: Neutropenia/agranulocytosis has occurred (see WARNINGS). Cases of anemia, thrombocytopenia, and pancytopenia have been reported.

Dermatologic: Rash, often with pruritus, and sometimes with fever, arthralgia, and eosinophilia, occurred in about 4 to 7 (depending on renal status and dose) of 100 patients, usually during the first four weeks of therapy. It is usually maculopapular, and rarely urticarial. The rash is usually mild and disappears within a few days of dosage reduction, short-term treatment with an antihistaminic agent, and/or discontinuing therapy; remission may occur even if captopril is continued. Pruritus, without rash, occurs in about 2 of 100 patients. Between 7 and 10 percent of patients with skin rash have shown an eosinophilia and/or positive ANA titers. A reversible associated pemphigoid-like lesion, and photosensitivity, have also been reported.

Flushing or pallor has been reported in 2 to 5 of 1000 patients.

Cardiovascular: Hypotension may occur; see WARNINGS and PRECAUTIONS (Drug Interactions) for discussion of hypotension with captopril therapy.

Tachycardia, chest pain, and palpitations have each been observed in approximately 1 of 100 patients.

Angina pectoris, myocardial infarction, Raynaud's syndrome, and congestive heart failure have each occurred in 2 to 3 of 1000 patients.

Dysgeusia: Approximately 2 to 4 (depending on renal status and dose) of 100 patients developed a diminution or loss of taste perception. Taste impairment is reversible and usually self-limited (2 to 3 months) even with continued drug administration. Weight loss may be associated with the loss of taste.

Angioedema: Angioedema involving the extremities, face, lips, mucous membranes, tongue, glottis or larynx has been reported in approximately one in 1000 patients. Angioedema involving the upper airways has caused fatal airway obstruction. (See WARNINGS: Angioedema and PRECAUTIONS: Information for Patients.)

Cough: Cough has been reported in 0.5 to 2% of patients treated with captopril in clinical trials (see PRECAUTIONS: General: *Cough*).

The following have been reported in about 0.5 to 2 percent of patients but did not appear at increased frequency compared to placebo or other treatments used in controlled trials: gastric irritation, abdominal pain, nausea, vomiting, diarrhea, anorexia, constipation, aphthous ulcers, peptic ulcer, dizziness, headache, malaise, fatigue, insomnia, dry mouth, dyspnea, alopecia, paresthesias.

Other clinical adverse effects reported since the drug was marketed are listed below by body system. In this setting, an incidence or causal relationship cannot be accurately determined.

Body as a Whole: Anaphylactoid reactions (see WARNINGS: Anaphylactoid and Possible Related Reactions and PRECAUTIONS: Hemodialysis).

General: Asthenia, gynecomastia.

Cardiovascular: Cardiac arrest, cerebrovascular accident/insufficiency, rhythm disturbances, orthostatic hypotension, syncope.

Dermatologic: Bullous pemphigus, erythema multiforme (including Stevens-Johnson syndrome), exfoliative dermatitis.

Gastrointestinal: Pancreatitis, glossitis, dyspepsia.

Hematologic: Anemia, including aplastic and hemolytic.

Hepatobiliary: Jaundice, hepatitis, including rare cases of necrosis, cholestasis.

Metabolic: Symptomatic hyponatremia.

Musculoskeletal: Myalgia, myasthenia.

Nervous/Psychiatric: Ataxia, confusion, depression, nervousness, somnolence.

Respiratory: Bronchospasm, eosinophilic pneumonitis, rhinitis.

Special Senses: Blurred vision.

Urogenital: Impotence.

As with other ACE inhibitors, a syndrome has been reported which may include: fever, myalgia, arthralgia, interstitial nephritis, vasculitis, rash or other dermatologic manifestations, eosinophilia and an elevated ESR.

Fetal/Neonatal Morbidity and Mortality: See WARNINGS: Fetal/Neonatal Morbidity and Mortality.

Altered Laboratory Findings: *Serum Electrolytes: Hyperkalemia:* small increases in serum potassium, especially in patients with renal impairment (see PRECAUTIONS).

Hyponatremia: particularly in patients receiving a low sodium diet or concomitant diuretics.

BUN/Serum Creatinine: Transient elevations of BUN or serum creatinine especially in volume or salt depleted patients or those with renovascular hypertension may occur. Rapid reduction of longstanding or markedly elevated blood pressure can result in decreases in the glomerular filtration rate and, in turn, lead to increases in BUN or serum creatinine.

Hematologic: A positive ANA has been reported.

Liver Function Tests: Elevations of liver transaminases, alkaline phosphatase, and serum bilirubin have occurred.

OVERDOSAGE

Correction of hypotension would be of primary concern. Volume expansion with an intravenous infusion of normal saline is the treatment of choice for restoration of blood pressure.

While captopril may be removed from the adult circulation by hemodialysis, there is inadequate data concerning the effectiveness of hemodialysis for removing it from the circulation of neonates or children. Peritoneal dialysis is not effective for removing captopril; there is no information concerning exchange transfusion for removing captopril from the general circulation.

DOSAGE AND ADMINISTRATION

Captopril should be taken one hour before meals. Dosage must be individualized.

Hypertension: Initiation of therapy requires consideration of recent antihypertensive drug treatment, the extent of blood pressure elevation, salt restriction, and other clinical

circumstances. If possible, discontinue the patient's previous antihypertensive drug regimen for one week before starting captopril.
The initial dose of captopril is 25 mg bid or tid. If satisfactory reduction of blood pressure has not been achieved after one or two weeks, the dose may be increased to 50 mg bid or tid. Concomitant sodium restriction may be beneficial when captopril is used alone.
The dose of captopril in hypertension usually does not exceed 50 mg tid. Therefore, if the blood pressure has not been satisfactorily controlled after one to two weeks at this dose, (and the patient is not already receiving a diuretic), a modest dose of a thiazide-type diuretic (e.g., hydrochlorothiazide, 25 mg daily), should be added. The diuretic dose may be increased at one- to two-week intervals until its highest usual antihypertensive dose is reached.
If captopril is being started in a patient al ready receiving a diuretic, captopril therapy should be initiated under close medical supervision (see WARNINGS and PRECAUTIONS [Drug Interactions] regarding hypotension), with dosage and titration of captopril as noted above.
If further blood pressure reduction is required, the dose of captopril may be increased to 100 mg bid or tid and then, if necessary, to 150 mg bid or tid (while continuing the diuretic). The usual dose range is 25 to 150 mg bid or tid. A maximum daily dose of 450 mg captopril should not be exceeded.
For patients with severe hypertension (e.g., accelerated or malignant hypertension), when temporary discontinuation of current antihypertensive therapy is not practical or desirable, or when prompt titration to more normotensive blood pressure levels is indicated, diuretic should be continued but other current antihypertensive medication stopped and captopril dosage promptly initiated at 25 mg bid or tid, under close medical supervision.
When necessitated by the patient's clinical condition, the daily dose of captopril may be increased every 24 hours or less under continuous medical supervision until a satisfactory blood pressure response is obtained or the maximum dose of captopril is reached. In this regimen, addition of a more potent diuretic, e.g., furosemide, may also be indicated.
Beta-blockers may also be used in conjunction with captopril therapy (see PRECAUTIONS: Drug Interactions), but the effects of the two drugs are less than additive.
Heart Failure: Initiation of therapy requires consideration of recent diuretic therapy and the possibility of severe salt/volume depletion. In patients with either normal or low blood pressure, who have been vigorously treated with diuretics and who may be hyponatremic and/or hypovolemic, a starting dose of 6.25 or 12.5 mg tid may minimize the magnitude or duration of the hypotensive effect (see WARNINGS: Hypotension); for these patients, titration to the usual daily dosage can then occur within the next several days.
For most patients the usual initial daily dosage is 25 mg tid. After a dose of 50 mg tid is reached, further increases in dosage should be delayed, where possible, for at least two weeks to determine if a satisfactory response occurs. Most patients studied have had a satisfactory clinical improvement at 50 or 100 mg tid. A maximum daily dose of 450 mg of captopril should not be exceeded.
Captopril should generally be used in conjunction with a diuretic and digitalis. Captopril therapy must be initiated under very close medical supervision.
Left Ventricular Dysfunction After Myocardial Infarction: The recommended dose for long-term use in patients following a myocardial infarction is a target maintenance dose of 50 mg tid.
Therapy may be initiated as early as three days following a myocardial infarction. After a single dose of 6.25 mg, captopril therapy should be initiated at 12.5 mg tid. Captopril should then be increased to 25 mg tid during the next several days and to a target dose of 50 mg tid over the next several weeks as tolerated (see CLINICAL PHARMACOLOGY).
Captopril may be used in patients treated with other post-myocardial infarction therapies, e.g., thrombolytics, aspirin, beta-blockers.
Dosage Adjustment in Renal Impairment: Because captopril is excreted primarily by the kidneys, excretion rates are reduced in patients with impaired renal function. These patients will take longer to reach steady-state captopril levels and will reach higher steady-state levels for a given daily dose than patients with normal renal function. Therefore, these patients may respond to smaller or less frequent doses.
Accordingly, for patients with significant renal impairment, initial daily dosage of captopril should be reduced, and smaller increments utilized for titration, which should be quite slow (one- to two-week intervals). After the desired therapeutic effect has been achieved, the dose should be slowly back-titrated to determine the minimal effective dose. When concomitant diuretic therapy is required, a loop diuretic (e.g., furosemide), rather than a thiazide diuretic, is preferred in patients with severe renal impairment. (See WARNINGS: Anaphylactoid Reactions During Membrane Exposure and PRECAUTIONS: Hemodialysis.)

HOW SUPPLIED

Captopril tablets are available containing 12.5 mg, 25 mg, 50 mg or 100 mg of captopril.
The 12.5 mg tablets are white, partially scored (both sides), oval tablets marked with M to the left of the score and C1 to the right of the score on one side. They are available as follows:

NDC 0378-3007-01
bottles of 100 tablets
NDC 0378-3007-10
bottles of 1000 tablets

The 25 mg tablets are white, quadrisect scored, round tablets marked with M over C2 on the non-scored side. They are available as follows:

NDC 0378-3012-01
bottles of 100 tablets
NDC 0378-3012-10
bottles of 1000 tablets

The 50 mg tablets are white, scored, round tablets marked with M over C3 on the scored side. They are available as follows:

NDC 0378-3017-01
bottles of 100 tablets
NDC 0378-3017-10
bottles of 1000 tablets

The 100 mg tablets are white, scored, round tablets marked with M over C4 on the scored side. They are available as follows:

NDC 0378-3022-01
bottles of 100 tablets

Captopril tablets may exhibit a slight sulfurous odor.
Bottles contain a desiccant-charcoal canister.
STORE AT CONTROLLED ROOM TEMPERATURE 15°–30°C (59°–86°F).
PROTECT FROM MOISTURE.
Dispense in a tight container using a child-resistant closure.
Rx only
Mylan Pharmaceuticals Inc.
Morgantown, WV 26505

REVISED MARCH 1998
CAPT:R7

Nabi®

5800 PARK OF COMMERCE BLVD., N.W.
BOCA RATON, FL 33487

For Medical Information Contact:
Generally:
Immunotherapy Customer Service
(800) 458-HBIG (4244)
(305) 625-5303
800-4-WINRHO
800-327-7106 - AUTOPLEX
800-685-5579 - Medical
FAX: (305) 625-0925
In Emergencies:
Immunotherapy Customer Service
FAX: (305) 625-0925
(800) 458-HBIG (4244)
(800) 4WINRHO (494-6746)
(800) 327-7106 AUTOPLEX

AUTOPLEX® T ℞
Anti-Inhibitor Coagulant Complex
Heat Treated

Caution: This product is to be used only in patients with inhibitors to Factor VIII.

Warning: This is a potent drug with potential hazards. For maximal safety and efficacy, carefully read and follow directions below.

DESCRIPTION

Anti-Inhibitor Coagulant Complex, Heat Treated, Autoplex® T*, is a sterile product prepared from pooled human plasma with subsequent alcohol fractionation to Cohn Fraction IV_1. It contains, in concentrated form, variable amounts of activated and precursor vitamin K-dependent clotting factors. Factors of the kinin generating system are also present. The product is standardized by its ability to correct the clotting time of Factor VIII deficient plasma or Factor VIII deficient plasma which contains inhibitors to Factor VIII.
When reconstituted, this product contains a maximum of 2 units per mL of heparin and a residual amount of polyethylene glycol (2 mg per mL, maximum). It also contains 0.02 M sodium citrate and the sodium content is 177 ±15 milliequivalents per liter.
Laboratory testing of several lots of Anti-Inhibitor Coagulant Complex, Heat Treated, Autoplex® T, has shown the presence of Factor VIII coagulant antigen (VIII:CAg). Although anamnestic response to this antigen following administration of the product was not observed during the clinical trials, the possibility of such a response does exist.
Each lot of Anti-Inhibitor Coagulant Complex, Heat Treated, Autoplex® T, is assayed and labeled for units of Hyland Factor VIII correctional activity. Factor VIII correctional activity may not be exclusively related to the efficacious components(s). (See **Clinical Pharmacology**.)
During the manufacturing process, this product was heated for 6 days at 60°C. This heating step is designed to reduce the risk of transmission of hepatitis and other viral diseases. However, no procedure has been shown to be totally effective in removing hepatitis infectivity from Anti-Inhibitor Coagulant Complex.
Anti-Inhibitor Coagulant Complex, Heat Treated, Autoplex® T, **must** be administered intravenously.

*This product and/or its manufacture covered by U.S. Patent Nos. 4,286,056, 4,287,180, 4,357,321, 4,382,083, 4,459,288, and 4,495,278.

CLINICAL PHARMACOLOGY

The Factor VIII correctional activity of Anti-Inhibitor Coagulant Complex, Heat Treated, Autoplex® T, is thought to be, in part, related to the Factor Xa content of the product. It is additionally hypothesized that the elevated Factor VII-VIIa content of this product is also a contributing factor in the *in vivo* reestablishment of normal hemostasis by way of Factor X activation in conjunction with tissue factor, phospholipid and ionic calcium.
Control of thrombin formation is regulated by (1) the presence of antithrombin III and other serine protease inhibitors which neutralize Factors IXa and Xa, (2) the short biological half-lives of Factors VII and VIIa and (3) the presence of the circulating Factor VIII inhibitor which additionally controls overactivation of the intrinsic coagulation system.
In work with human immunodeficiency virus (HIV), substantial reduction in viral content has been reported in a recent study of the effects of ethanol fractionation, the process by which Anti-Inhibitor Coagulant Complex, Heat Treated, Autoplex® T, is manufactured. Wells, *et al*, report 1 to 4 log reduction in each fractionation step they examined.[1]
The effectiveness of the 6-day heating step in reducing viral infectivity was assessed by *in vitro* viral inactivation studies, using as markers, viruses not commonly found in plasma. When known quantities of these viruses were added to the product, the heat treatment employed inactivated the following quantities of virus:

Sindbis	10.0 Log_{10}
Vesicular stomatitis	5.0 Log_{10}
Herpes simplex	1.6 Log_{10}
HIV	4.5 Log_{10}

In separate experiments, HIV was also studied and these data are reported in the table above.
A retrospective study conducted with patients receiving unheated Anti-Inhibitor Coagulant Complex, Autoplex®, supports the effectiveness of the purification process in reducing viral burden in the product. In the study, none of the patients who received that product exclusively seroconverted for HIV antibodies, while 56% of those patients who received other treatment modalities seroconverted during the three year study.[2]

INDICATIONS AND USAGE

Anti-Inhibitor Coagulant Complex, Heat Treated, Autoplex® T, is indicated for use in patients with Factor VIII inhibitors who are bleeding or are to undergo surgery.[3-6] The intravenous administration of this preparation is intended to control bleeding episodes in such patients.
Approximately 10% of individuals with hemophilia A (classical hemophilia) have laboratory-measurable inhibitors to Factor VIII.[7] For these patients, the treatment of choice depends upon the following factors: the severity of the bleeding episode, the existing level of inhibitor and whether the patient responds to infusion of Factor VIII with increasing antibody titers (anamnestic rise of Factor VIII antibody).
The following table is presented as a guide in determining the preferred therapy with respect to the use of Anti-Inhibitor Coagulant Complex or Antihemophilic Factor (Human) in patients with Factor VIII inhibitors. Inhibitor level categories are given in the shaded areas of the table and the corresponding recommended product or products are given in the unshaded areas. Other regimens have been proposed.[8]
[See table at top of next page]
Patients whose present Factor VIII inhibitor levels are greater than 10 Bethesda Units, as well as patients whose inhibitor levels are historically known to rise to greater than 10 Bethesda Units following treatment with Antihemophilic Factor (Human), should be treated with Anti-Inhibitor Coagulant Complex.

Continued on next page

Autoplex T—Cont.

Patients whose present Factor VIII inhibitor levels are between 2 and 10 Bethesda Units and whose inhibitor levels are historically known to remain in this range following treatment with Antihemophilic Factor (Human) may be treated with either Antihemophilic Factor (Human) or Anti-Inhibitor Coagulant Complex, depending on the patient's clinical history and the severity of the bleeding episode. Patients with Factor VIII inhibitor levels of less than 2 Bethesda Units whose inhibitor levels are historically known to remain at 2 Bethesda Units or less following treatment with Antihemophilic Factor (Human) may be treated with appropriate doses of Antihemophilic Factor (Human).

For patients who have low levels of Factor VIII inhibitor and whose history does not include adequate laboratory indications of an anamnestic response to Antihemophilic Factor (Human), the treatment of choice should be based on clinical judgement. In such patients who are having noncritical or minor bleeding episodes, the use of Anti-Inhibitor Coagulant Complex, Heat Treated, Autoplex® T, will maintain the inhibitor at a low level and allow the use of other coagulant therapeutic agents in subsequent major emergencies.

CONTRAINDICATIONS

The use of Anti-Inhibitor Coagulant Complex, Heat Treated, Autoplex® T, is contraindicated in patients with signs of fibrinolysis and in patients with disseminated intravascular coagulation (DIC).

WARNINGS

Anti-Inhibitor Coagulant Complex, Heat Treated, Autoplex® T, is made from human plasma. Products made from human plasma may contain infectious agents, such as viruses, that can cause disease. The risk that such products will transmit an infectious agent has been reduced by screening plasma donors for prior exposure to certain viruses, by testing for the presence of certain current virus infections, and by inactivating and/or removing certain viruses (See Clinical Pharmacology). Despite these measures, such products can still potentially transmit disease. There is also the possibility that unknown infectious agents may be present in such products. ALL infections thought by a physician possibly to have been transmitted by this product should be reported by the physician or other healthcare provider to the U.S. distributor, Nabi®, at 1-800-327-7106. The physician should discuss the risks and benefits of this product with the patient. Physicians should also report adverse reactions or any disease condition which may occur concomitantly with the administration of this product to the U.S. distributor, Nabi®.

If the infusion of the concentrate occurs more than 1 hour following reconstitution, there may be increased prekallikrein activator (PKA) with consequent hypotension.

PRECAUTIONS

General

Some viruses, such as parvovirus B19 or hepatitis A, are particularly difficult to remove or inactivate at this time. Parvovirus B19 most seriously affects pregnant women, or immune-compromised individuals. Symptoms of parvovirus B19 infection include fever, drowsiness, chills, and runny nose followed about two weeks later by a rash, and joint pain. Evidence of hepatitis A may include several days to weeks of poor appetite, tiredness, and low-grade fever followed by nausea, vomiting, and pain in the belly. Dark urine and a yellowed complexion are also common symptoms. Patients should be encouraged to consult their physician if such symptoms appear.

Certain components used in the packaging of this product contain natural rubber latex.

Identification of the clotting deficiency as that caused by the presence of Factor VIII inhibitors is essential before the administration of Anti-Inhibitor Coagulant Complex, Heat Treated, Autoplex® T, is initiated.

Signs and/or symptoms of hypotension may occur with this product. In these cases, stopping the infusion allows the symptoms to disappear. With all but the most reactive individuals, the infusion may be resumed at a slower rate.

If clinical signs of intravascular coagulation occur, the infusion should be stopped promptly and the patient monitored for DIC by the appropriate laboratory tests. Symptoms of DIC include changes in blood pressure and pulse rate, respiratory distress, chest pain and cough. Laboratory indications of DIC include prolonged thrombin time, prothrombin time and partial thromboplastin time tests. Other indications of DIC are decreased fibrinogen concentration, decreased platelet count and/or the presence of fibrinogen/fibrin degradation products.

Special caution should be taken in the use of this concentrate in newborns, where a high morbidity and mortality may be associated with hepatitis, and in individuals with pre-existing liver disease.

Laboratory Tests

In some cases, laboratory tests such as the activated partial thromboplastin time test may not correlate with clinical response, in that the appearance of hemostatic improvement may occur without a reduction of partial thromboplastin time. However, the prothrombin time would be expected to be shortened.

HISTORICAL MAXIMUM LEVEL OF FACTOR VIII INHIBITOR	PRESENT LEVEL OF FACTOR VIII INHIBITOR <2 B.U.[a]	2-10 B.U.	>10 B.U.
<2 B.U.	AHF[b]	AICC[c] or AHF	AICC
2-10 B.U.	AICC or AHF	AICC or AHF	AICC
>10 B.U.	AICC	AICC	AICC

[a]B.U. designates Bethesda Units.
[b]AHF designates Antihemophilic Factor (Human).
[c]AICC designates Anti-Inhibitor Coagulant Complex.

In children, fibrinogen levels should be determined prior to the initial infusion and monitored during the course of the treatment.

Drug Interactions

Since only limited data are available on the administration of highly activated prothrombin complex products together with antifibrinolytic agents such as epsilon-aminocaproic acid (EACA) or tranexamic acid,[6] the concomitant use of Anti-Inhibitor Coagulant Complex, Heat Treated, Autoplex® T, with such agents is not recommended.

Pregnancy

Pregnancy Category C. Animal reproduction studies have not been conducted with Anti-Inhibitor Coagulant Complex, Heat Treated, Autoplex® T. It is also not known whether Anti-Inhibitor Coagulant Complex, Heat Treated, Autoplex® T, can cause fetal harm when administered to a pregnant woman or can affect reproduction capacity. Anti-Inhibitor Coagulant Complex, Heat Treated, Autoplex® T, should be given to a pregnant woman only if clearly needed.

ADVERSE REACTIONS

As with other plasma preparations, reactions manifested by fever, chills or indications of protein sensitivity may be observed with the administration of Anti-Inhibitor Coagulant Complex, Heat Treated, Autoplex® T. Signs and/or symptoms of high prekallikrein activity, such as changes in blood pressure or pulse rate may also be observed. It is advisable that appropriate medications be available for the treatment of acute allergic reactions or acute vasoactive reactions, should they occur.

A rate of infusion that is too rapid may cause headache, flushing, and changes in pulse rate and blood pressure. In such instances, stopping the infusion allows the symptoms to disappear promptly. With all but the most reactive individuals, infusion may be resumed at a slower rate.

DOSAGE AND ADMINISTRATION

Each bottle of Anti-Inhibitor Coagulant Complex, Heat Treated, Autoplex® T, is labeled with the number of Hyland Factor VIII Correctional Units that it contains. One Hyland Factor VIII Correctional Unit is that quantity of activated prothrombin complex which, upon addition to an equal volume of Factor VIII deficient or inhibitor plasma, will correct the clotting time (ellagic acid-activated partial thromboplastin time) to 35 seconds (normal).

The recommended dosage range is 25 to 100 Hyland Factor VIII Correctional Units per kg of body weight, depending upon the severity of hemorrhage. If no hemostatic improvement is observed approximately 6 hours following the initial administration, the dosage should be repeated.

Subsequent dosage and administration intervals should be adjusted according to the patient's clinical response. (See **Laboratory Tests.**)

Reconstitution: Use Aseptic Technique

1. Bring Anti-Inhibitor Coagulant Complex, Heat Treated, Autoplex® T (dry concentrate) and Sterile Water for Injection, USP, (diluent) to room temperature.
2. Remove caps from concentrate and diluent bottles to expose central portions of rubber stoppers.
3. Cleanse stoppers with germicidal solution.
4. Remove protective covering from one end of the double-ended needle and insert exposed needle through **diluent** stopper.
5. Remove protective covering from the other end of the double-ended needle. Invert diluent bottle over the upright concentrate bottle, then **rapidly** insert free end of the needle through the concentrate bottle stopper at its center. Vacuum in the concentrate bottle will draw in diluent.
6. Disconnect the two bottles by removing needle from the diluent bottle, then remove needle from concentrate bottle stopper. Swirl or rotate the concentrate bottle until all material is dissolved. Do not shake vigorously.

Parenteral drug products should be inspected visually for particulate matter and discoloration prior to administration, whenever solution and container permit.

Note: Do not refrigerate after reconstitution.

Rate of Administration

It is recommended that Anti-Inhibitor Coagulant Complex, Heat Treated, Autoplex® T, be infused initially at a rate of 2 mL/min. If infusion at this rate is well tolerated the administration rate may be gradually increased to 10 mL/min.

Administration: Use Aseptic Technique

When reconstitution of Anti-Inhibitor Coagulant Complex, Heat Treated, Autoplex® T, is complete, its infusion should commence as soon as practical; however, it must be completed within 1 hour.

The reconstituted solution should be at room temperature during infusion.

A. Intravenous Drip Infusion

When a Hyland administration set is used, follow directions for use printed on the administration set container. When an administration set from another source is used, follow directions accompanying that set where necessary. The use of a Hyland administration set is recommended as it contains a suitable filter.

B. Intravenous Syringe Injection

1. Attach filter needle to syringe and draw back plunger to admit air into the syringe.
2. Insert needle into the reconstituted Anti-Inhibitor Coagulant Complex, Heat Treated, Autoplex® T.
3. Inject air into bottle and then withdraw the reconstituted material into the syringe.
4. Remove and discard the filter needle from the syringe; attach a suitable needle and inject intravenously as instructed under **Rate of Administration**.
5. If patient is to receive more than one bottle of concentrate, the contents of two bottles may be drawn into the same syringe by drawing up each bottle through a separate used filter needle. This practice lessens the loss of concentrate. Please note: filter needles are intended to filter the contents of a single bottle of Anti-Inhibitor coagulant Complex, Heat Treated, Autoplex® T, only.

HOW SUPPLIED

Anti-Inhibitor Coagulant Complex, Heat Treated, Autoplex® T, is furnished with a suitable volume of Sterile Water for Injection, USP; a double-ended needle; a filter needle; and a package insert.

Storage

Anti-Inhibitor Coagulant Complex, Heat Treated, Autoplex® T, should be stored under ordinary refrigeration (2 – 8°C, 36 – 46°F). Avoid freezing to prevent damage to the diluent bottle.

REFERENCES

1. Wells MA, Wittek AE, Epstein JS, *et al*: Inactivation and partition of human T-cell lymphotropic virus, type III, during ethanol fractionation. **Transfusion 26**:210-213, 1986
2. Gazengel C, Larrieu MJ: Lack of seroconversion for LAV/HTLV-III in patients exclusively given unheated activated prothrombin complex prepared with ethanol step. **Lancet 2**:1189, 1985
3. Kurczynski EM, Penner JA: Activated prothrombin concentrate for patients with factor VIII inhibitors. **New Eng J Med 291**:164-167, 1974
4. Penner JA, Kelly PE: Management of patients with factor VIII or IX inhibitors. **Semin Thromb Hemostas 1**:386-399, 1975
5. Buchanan GR, Kevy SV: Use of prothrombin complex concentrates in hemophiliacs with inhibitors: Clinical and laboratory studies. **Pediatrics 62**:767-774, 1978
6. Mannucci PM, Federici F, Vigano S, *et al*: Multiple dental extractions with a new prothrombin complex concentrate in two patients with factor VIII inhibitors. **Thromb Res 15**:359-364, 1979
7. Shapiro SS: Antibodies to blood coagulation factors. **Clinics in Haematology 8**:207-214, 1979

8. Roberts HR: Hemophiliacs with inhibitors: Therapeutic options. **New Eng J. Med 305**:757-758, 1981

BIBLIOGRAPHY

Fekete LF, Holst SL, Peetoom F, *et al*: "Auto" Factor IX Concentrate: A new therapeutic approach to treatment of hemophilia A patients with inhibitors. **Proceedings, 14th International Congress of Haematology** . Sao Paulo, Brazil, 1972
Kelly P, Penner JA: Antihemophilic factor inhibitors: Management with prothrombin complex concentrates. **JAMA 236** :2061, 1976
Seligsohn U, Kasper CK, Østerud B, *et al*: Activated factor VII. Presence in factor IX concentrates and persistence in the circulation after infusion. **Blood 53**:828, 1979
Abildgaard CF, Penner JA, Watson-Williams EJ: Anti-Inhibitor Coagulant Complex (Autoplex) for treatment of factor VIII inhibitors in hemophilia. **Blood 56**:978, 1980

NDC 59730-6059-7
Distributed by:
Nabi®
Boca Raton, FL 33487 USA
Manufactured by:
Baxter Healthcare Corporation
Hyland Division
Glendale, CA 91203 USA
U.S. License No. 140
6849
Revised April 1998

H-BIG® ℞
HEPATITIS B IMMUNE GLOBULIN (HUMAN)

DESCRIPTION

Hepatitis B Immune Globulin (Human), H-BIG®, is a sterile solution of immunoglobulin (16.5 ± 1.5% protein) which is prepared from the pooled plasma of individuals with high titers of antibody to the hepatitis B surface antigen (anti-HBs), by the Cohn-Oncley cold alcohol fractionation process. **Hepatitis B Immune Globulin (Human) is intended only for intramuscular injection**. The product is stabilized with 0.3M glycine and contains 1:10,000 thimerosal (a mercury derivative) as a preservative. The solution has been adjusted to a pH of 6.8 ± 0.4 with sodium hydroxide or hydrochloric acid. Each vial of H-BIG® contains anti-HBs equivalent to or exceeding the potency of anti-HBs in a U.S. Reference hepatitis B immune globulin (Center for Biologics Evaluation and Research, FDA). The high titer plasma was fractionated by Centeon. The plasma used to make Fraction II powder for potency adjustment was fractionated by Centeon and/or Michigan Department of Public Health.

CLINICAL PHARMACOLOGY

Hepatitis B Immune Globulin (Human) provides passive immunization for individuals exposed to the hepatitis B virus as evidenced by a reduction in the attack rate of hepatitis B following its use.[1-7] Clinical studies[7,8] indicate the advantage of simultaneous administration of Hepatitis B Vaccine and Hepatitis B Immune Globulin (Human), H-BIG®. Neonatal studies[7,9] demonstrated the combined use of Hepatitis B Vaccine and Hepatitis B Immune Globulin (Human) to be more effective in the maintenance of protective antibody levels than prophylactic administration of Hepatitis B Vaccine or Hepatitis B Immune Globulin (Human) alone.

No prospective studies have been performed on the efficacy of concurrent Hepatitis B Vaccine and Hepatitis B Immune Globulin (Human) administration following parenteral exposure, mucous membrane contact or oral ingestion in adults; however, the Recommendation of the Immunization Practices Advisory Committee (ACIP) advises that the combination prophylaxis be provided based upon the increased efficacy found with that regimen in neonates.[6,7] In passive immunization with the administration of the recommended dose of Hepatitis B Immune Globulin (Human), a maximum serum level of circulating anti-HBs was seen in 2–4 days, the half-life was about 25 days and a detectable level persists for approximately two months or longer.[10] Cases of type B hepatitis are rarely seen following exposure to HBV in persons with preexisting anti-HBs. H-BIG® is produced by the Cohn-Oncley cold alcohol fractionation method.

INDICATIONS AND USAGE

H-BIG® is indicated for post-exposure to prophylaxis[4,6] following either parenteral exposure (accidental "needle-stick"), direct mucous membrane contact (accidental splash), sexual exposure[6], or oral ingestion (pipetting accident) involving HBsAg positive materials such as blood, plasma and serum. H-BIG® is also indicated in post-exposure prophylaxis in infants born to hepatitis B surface antigen positive (HBsAg positive) mothers.[4,6,7] Such infants are at risk of becoming chronic carriers.[11,12,13] The risk is especially great if the mother is also HBeAg positive.[14,15] The carrier state can be prevented in about 75% of such exposures if newborns are given Hepatitis B Immune Globulin (Human), immediately after birth and in the early months of life.[4] Concurrent H-BIG® and Hepatitis B Vaccine administration does not appear to interfere with antibody responses to Hepatitis B Vaccine and increases efficacy to about 94%.[6,7,9]

CONTRAINDICATIONS

There are no specific contraindications for H-BIG®. No adverse reactions have been seen in individuals with preexisting hepatitis B surface antigen (HBsAg) although data regarding this occurrence are limited. Some individuals may demonstrate hypersensitivity to the glycine and/or thimerosal components used to stabilize and preserve this product.

WARNINGS

H-BIG® should be given with caution to patients with a history of prior systemic allergic reactions following the administration of human immunoglobulin preparations. Persons with an isolated deficiency of Immunoglobulin A (IgA) have the potential for developing antibodies to such immunoglobulin, which could result in anaphylactic reactions to subsequent administration of any blood products containing IgA.[18] As with any other immune globulin preparation, H-BIG® should be given to such persons only if the expected benefits outweigh the potential risks. In patients who have severe thrombocytopenia or any coagulation disorder that would contraindicate intramuscular injections, H-BIG® should be given only if the expected benefits outweigh the potential risks.

PRECAUTIONS

General

H-BIG® should be administered with caution to patients with a history of prior systemic allergic reactions following the administration of human immune globulin preparations. Hypersensitivity reactions to injections of immune globulin occur rarely, however, the incidence of these reactions may be increased in patients receiving repeated injections of immune globulin.[19] Epinephrine should be available for treatment of acute allergic symptoms. **H-BIG® should not be administered intravenously because of the potential for serious reactions**. Injections should be made intramuscularly, and care should be taken to draw back on the plunger of the syringe before injections in order to be certain that the needle is not in a blood vessel or nerve. If blood or any unusual discoloration is present in the syringe, H-BIG® should not be injected. The needle should be withdrawn and syringe discarded. A new dose of Hepatitis B Immune Globulin (Human) should be prepared and the procedure for administration repeated at a different site, using a new syringe and needle.

There is no evidence that HIV-1, the causative virus of AIDS, is transmitted by H-BIG®, which is prepared by the Cohn-Oncley cold ethanol process.[20]

Drug Interactions

Although administration of Hepatitis B Immune Globulin (Human) did not interfere with measles vaccination[16] it is not known whether H-BIG® may interfere with the immune response to vaccination with other live virus vaccines, including mumps and rubella. Therefore, vaccination with live virus vaccines should be deferred until approximately three (3) months after administration of Hepatitis B Immune Globulin (Human). It may be necessary to revaccinate persons who received H-BIG® shortly after live virus vaccination. Hepatitis B Vaccine may be administered at the same time, but at a different injection site, without interference.[3] No interactions with other products are known.

Pregnancy Category C

Animal reproduction studies have not been conducted with Hepatitis B Immune Globulin (Human). It is also not known whether H-BIG® can cause fetal harm when administered to a pregnant woman or can affect reproduction capacity. H-BIG® should be given to a pregnant woman only if clearly needed.

Nursing Mothers

It is not known whether this drug is excreted in human milk. Since many drugs are excreted in human milk, caution should be exercised when Hepatitis B Immune Globulin (Human) is administered to a nursing woman.

ADVERSE REACTIONS

Local pain and tenderness at the injection site, and urticaria and angioedema may occur. Anaphylactic reactions, although rare, have been reported following the injection of human immunoglobulin preparations.[17] Anaphylaxis is more likely to occur if H-BIG® is administered intravenously, therefore, **H-BIG® must be administered ONLY intramuscularly**. In highly allergic individuals, repeated injections may lead to anaphylactic shock.[22,23] Persons with an isolated deficiency of Immunoglobulin A (IgA) have the potential for developing antibodies to such immunoglobulin, which could result in anaphylactic reactions to subsequent administration of any blood products containing IgA.[18]

OVERDOSAGE

Although no data are available, clinical experience with other immunoglobulin preparations suggests that the only manifestations would be pain and tenderness of the injection site.

DOSAGE AND ADMINISTRATION

Parenteral drug products should be inspected visually for particulate matter and discoloration prior to administration whenever solution and container permit. H-BIG® is a clear, very slightly amber, moderately viscous liquid. **H-BIG® should be administered intramuscularly, preferably in the gluteal or deltoid region**. H-BIG® should never be administered into or near blood vessels or nerves. DO NOT INJECT INTRAVENOUSLY.

If blood or any unusual discoloration is present in the syringe, H-BIG® should not be injected. The needle should be withdrawn and syringe discarded. A new dose of Hepatitis B Immune Globulin (Human) should be prepared and the procedure for administration repeated at a different site, using a new syringe and needle. It is important to use a separate sterile syringe and needle for each individual patient, in order to prevent transmission of hepatitis B and other infectious agents from one person to another. **Any vial that has been entered into should be used promptly. Partially used vials should be discarded and not saved for future use.**

Adults

The Immunization Practices Advisory Committee (ACIP) recommends that Hepatitis B Immune Globulin (Human) and Hepatitis B Vaccine be given concurrently.[6]

Recommendations for adults who have not been previously vaccinated against hepatitis B are the following: H-BIG® (0.06 mL/kg) should be administered intramuscularly as soon as possible after exposure and within 24 hours if possible. Hepatitis B Vaccine (see appropriate product circular for dosage recommendations), should be given intramuscularly, within seven (7) days of exposure. Second and third doses should be administered at one (1) and six (6) months, respectively, after the first dose.

Recommendations for adults who have been previously vaccinated against hepatitis B are the following: Persons should have their anti-HBs titers checked promptly. For those with known adequate antibody levels (10 mIU/mL anti-HBs are approximately equal to 10 SRU), no injection is required.[6] Those with inadequate or unknown titers should receive a dose of Hepatitis B Immune Globulin (Human) and one of Hepatitis B Vaccine simultaneously at two (2) different sites. The recommended dose of H-BIG® is 0.06 mL/kg (usually 3–5 mL), administered as soon as possible after exposure (preferably within 24 hours). Doses over 5 mL should be administered in the multiple sites to minimize discomfort. Immunization with Hepatitis B Vaccine should begin as soon as possible, but within seven (7) days. For use of Hepatitis B Vaccine, see appropriate manufacturer's literature. If the individual refuses the Hepatitis B Vaccine, a second dose of H-BIG® (0.06 mL/kg) should be given one (1) month after the first dose.

Newborns

Infants born to HBsAg positive mothers are at high risk of becoming chronic carriers of hepatitis B virus and of developing the chronic sequelae of hepatitis B virus infection. Controlled studies have shown that administration of three (3) 0.5 mL doses of H-BIG® starting at birth is 75% effective in preventing establishment of the chronic carrier state in these infants during the first year of life.[24] Protection can be transient, whereupon the effectiveness of the Hepatitis B Immune Globulin (Human) would decline thereafter. Results from clinical studies indicate that the administration of one (1) 0.5 mL dose of H-BIG® at birth and the recommended three (3) doses of Hepatitis B Vaccine be given concurrently to infants born to HBsAg positive mothers (especially those mothers who are HBeAg positive).[4,6,7,9,25,26] The recommended dose of H-BIG® for at risk newborns is 0.5 mL as soon after birth as possible, preferably no later than twelve (12) hours. Immunization with Hepatitis B Vaccine should begin promptly within seven (7) days of birth. For information on Hepatitis B Vaccine, refer to the appropriate manufacturer's literature. If administration of the first dose of Hepatitis B Vaccine is delayed for as long as three (3) months, then a 0.5 mL dose of H-BIG® should be repeated at three (3) months. If the Hepatitis B Vaccine is refused, then the 0.5 mL dose of H-BIG® should be repeated at three (3) and six (6) months.

Testing for HBsAg and anti-HBs is recommended at 12–15 months of age. If HBsAg is not detectable and anti-HBs is present, the child has been protected.[6] The recommended dosage for infants born to HBsAg positive mothers is the following:

	BIRTH	WITHIN 7 DAYS	1 MONTH	6 MONTHS
Hepatitis B Vaccine**	—	0.5 mL*	0.5 mL	0.5 mL
H-BIG®	0.5 mL	—	—	—

*The first dose of Hepatitis B Vaccine may be given at birth at the same time as Hepatitis B Immune Globulin (Human), but should be administered in the anterolateral aspect of the opposite thigh.

**See DOSAGE AND ADMINISTRATION section on the circular for the Hepatitis B Vaccine that you are utilizing.

Continued on next page

H-Big—Cont.

HOW SUPPLIED

H-BIG® is supplied as follows:
NDC 59730-8399-2 in a 0.5 mL unit **single dose** syringe.
NDC 59730-8399-1 in a 1.0 mL **single dose** vial.
NDC 59730-8399-5 in a 5.0 mL **single dose** vial.

STORAGE

Store at 2–8°C, (35–46°F). DO NOT FREEZE. DO NOT USE AFTER EXPIRATION DATE.
Caution: Federal (USA) law prohibits dispensing without prescription.

REFERENCES

1. Grady GF, Lee VA: Hepatitis B immune globulin—prevention of hepatitis from accidental exposure among medical personnel. *N Engl J Med* 293(21); 1067–1070, 1975.
2. Seeff LB, Wright EC, et al: Type B hepatitis after needle stick exposure; prevention with Hepatitis B Immune Globulin. *Ann Int Med* 88(3): 285–293, 1978.
3. Krugman S, Giles JP: Viral hepatitis, type B (MS-2-strain). Further observations on natural history and prevention *N Engl J Med* 288(15): 755–760, 1973.
4. Beasley RP, et al: Hepatitis B immune globulin (H-BIG) efficacy in the interruptions of perinatal transmission of hepatitis B virus carrier state, *Lancet* 2(8243): 388–393, 1981.
5. Hoofnagle JH, Seeff LB, et al: Passive-active immunity from hepatitis B immune globulin. *Ann Int Med*91:813–818, 1979.
6. Centers for Disease Control: Recommendations for Protection Against Viral Hepatitis. *Morbid Mortal Wkly Rep*. 34(22): 313–335, June 1985.
7. Beasley RP, et al: Prevention of perinatally transmitted hepatitis B virus infections with Hepatitis B Immune Globulin and Hepatitis B Vaccine. *Lancet* 3(8359): 1099–1102, 1983.
8. Szmuness W, et al: Passive—active immunisation against hepatitis B: Immunogenicity studies in adult Americans. *Lancet* 1:575–577, 1981.
9. Mazel JA, et al: Passive—active immunisation of neonates of HBsAg positive carrier mothers: preliminary observations *British Medical Journal* 208;513–515, 1984.
10. Scheiermann N, Kuwert EK: Uptake and elimination of hepatitis B immunoglobulins after intramuscular application in man, *Develop Biol Standard* 54,347–355, 1983.
11. Jhaveri R, Rosenfeld W, Salazar JD, et al: High titer multiple dose therapy with HBIG newborn infants of HBsAg positive mothers. *J Pediatr* 97(2);305–308, 1980.
12. Stevens CE, Beasley RP, Tsui J, et al: Vertical transmission of hepatitis B antigen in Taiwan, *N Engl J Med* 292(15); 771–774, 1975.
13. Shiraki Y, Toshihara N, Kawana T, et al: Hepatitis B surface antigen and chronic hepatitis in infants born to asymptomatic carrier mothers, *Am J Dis Child* 131(6);644–647, 1977.
14. Okada K, Kamiyama M, et al: e antigen and anti-e antigen in the serum of asymptomatic carrier mothers as indicators of positive and negative transmission of hepatitis B virus to their infants, *N Engl J Med* 294(14); 746–749, 1976.
15. Beasley RP, Trepo C, Stevens CE, et al: The e antigen and vertical transmission of hepatitis B surface antigen. *Am J Epidemiol*105(2);94–98, 1977.
16. Beasley RP, Hwang LY: Measles vaccination not interfered with by Hepatitis B Immune Globulin, *Lancet* 1:161, 1982.
17. Ellis EF, Henney CS: Adverse reactions following administration of human gamma globulin. *J Allerg*43:45–54, 1969.
18. Fudenberg HH. Sensitization to immunoglobulins and hazards of gamma globulin therapy. *Immunoglobulins. Biologic Aspects and Clinical Uses* Edited by Ezlo Merler, National Academy of Sciences, Washington DC; 211–220, 1970.
19. Bruhl HH. Adverse reactions to large doses of Human Immune serum globulin (IsG). Clinical observations. *Minn Med*60 (9): 673–676, Sept. 1977.
20. Zuck TF, Preston MS, Tankersley DL, et al. *N England J Med* 314(22): 1454–1455, May 1986.
21. Owings WJ. Hypersensitivity to gamma globulin. A case report. *J. Med Ass Alabama* 23; 74, Sept. 1953.
22. Baybutt JE. Hypersensitivity to immune serum globulin Report of a case. *Amer. Med Ass* 171;415, Sept. 26 1959.
23. Beasley RP, Hwang L, Lee GC et al. Efficacy of Hepatitis B Immuno Globulin for prevention of perinatal transmission of the hepatitis B virus carrier state. Final report of a randomized double-blind, placebo-controlled trial. *Hepatology 3;* 135–141, 1983.
24. Stevens CE, Taylor PE, Tong MJ et al. Hepatitis B Vaccine: an overview. In *Viral Hepatitis and Liver Disease.* Vyas GN, Deinstag JL, Hoofnagle JH (eds.) Grune & Stratton Inc; 275–291, 1984.
25. Stevens CE, Toy PT, Long MJ et al. Perinatal hepatitis B transmission in the United States. *JAMA* 253(12); 1740–1745, 1985.

Hepatitis B Immune Globulin (Human), H-BIG®
U.S. License No. 43
Manufactured by Abbott Laboratories, North Chicago, IL 60064

Distributed by Nabi®, Miami, FL 33169, USA
H-BIG® is a registered trademark of Nabi®.
01230-30-HEP-140797

WinRho SDF™ ℞

[*win' rō s d f*]

Rh$_o$ (D) Immune Globuline Intravenous (Human)

DESCRIPTION

Rh$_o$ (D) Immune Globulin Intravenous (Human) (Rh$_o$ (D) IGIV) — WinRho SDF™ — is a sterile, freeze- dried gamma globulin (IgG) fraction containing antibodies to Rh$_o$ (D). WinRho SDF™ is prepared from human plasma by an anion-exchange column chromatography method.[1–3] The manufacturing process includes a solvent detergent treatment step (using tri-n-butyl phosphate and Triton X-100) that is effective in inactivating lipid enveloped viruses such as hepatitis B, hepatitis C, and HIV.[4] WinRho SDF™ is filtered using a Planova 35 nm Virus Filter which has been validated to be effective in the removal of some nonlipid enveloped viruses.[5–6] These two processes are designed to increase product safety by reducing the risk of transmission of enveloped and nonenveloped viruses, respectively.

The product potency is expressed in international units by comparison to the World Health Organization (WHO) standard. A 300 µg (1,500 International Unit [IU]*) vial contains sufficient anti-Rh$_o$ (D) to effectively suppress the immunizing potential of approximately 17 mL of Rh$_o$ (D) positive red blood cells. This product contains approximately 5 µg/mL IgA per 120 µg (600 IU) vial.

The product is stabilized with 0.1 M glycine, 0.04 M sodium chloride, and 0.01% polysorbate 80. It contains no preservative.

Treatment of ITP

For use in the treatment of immune thrombocytopenic purpura (ITP), WinRho SDF™ **must be administered intravenously.**

Suppression of Rh Isoimmunization

For use in the suppression of Rh isoimmunization, WinRho SDF™ may be administered either intramuscularly or intravenously.

**In the past, a full dose of Rh$_o$ (D) Immune Globulin (Human) has traditionally been referred to as a "300 µg" dose. Potency and dosing recommendations are now expressed in IU by comparison to the WHO anti-D standard. The conversion of "µg" to "IU" is 1 µg = 5 IU.*

CLINICAL PHARMACOLOGY

Treatment of ITP

WinRho SDF™, Rh$_o$ (D) Immune Globulin Intravenous (Human), has been shown to increase platelet counts in non-splenectomized, Rh$_o$ (D) positive patients with ITP. Platelet counts usually rise within one to two days and peak within seven to 14 days after initiation of therapy. The duration of response is variable; however, the average duration is approximately 30 days. The mechanism of action is not completely understood, but is thought to be due to the formation of anti-Rh$_o$ (D)-coated red blood cell complexes resulting in Fc receptor blockade, thus sparing antibody-coated platelets.[7–8]

Suppression of Rh Isoimmunization

WinRho SDF™ is used to suppress the immune response of non-sensitized Rh$_o$ (D) negative individuals following exposure to Rh$_o$ (D) positive red blood cells by fetomaternal hemorrhage during delivery of an Rh$_o$ (D) positive infant, abortion (spontaneous or induced), amniocentesis, abdominal trauma, or mismatched transfusion.[9–11] The mechanism of action is not completely understood.

WinRho SDF™, when administered within 72 hours of a full-term delivery of an Rh$_o$ (D) positive infant by an Rh$_o$ (D) negative mother, will reduce the incidence of Rh isoimmunization from 12 – 13% to 1 – 2%. The 1 – 2% is, for the most part, due to isoimmunization during the last trimester of pregnancy. When treatment is given both antenatally at 28 weeks gestation and postpartum, the Rh immunization rate drops to about 0.1%.[12–15]

When 120 µg (600 IU) of Rh$_o$ (D) IGIV is administered to pregnant women, passive anti-Rh$_o$ (D) antibodies are not detectable in the circulation for more than six weeks and therefore a dose of 300 µg (1,500 IU) should be used for antenatal administration.

In a clinical study with Rh$_o$ (D) negative volunteers (nine males and one female), Rh$_o$ (D) positive red cells were completely cleared from the circulation within eight hours of intravenous administration of Rh$_o$ (D) IGIV. There was no indication of Rh isoimmunization of these subjects at six months after the clearance of the Rh$_o$ (D) positive red cells.

Pharmacokinetics — IM versus IV Administration

In a clinical study involving Rh$_o$ (D) negative volunteers, two subjects received 120 µg (600 IU) Rh$_o$ (D) IGIV by intravenous (IV) administration and two subjects received this dose by intramuscular (IM) administration. Peak levels (36 to 48 ng/mL) were reached within two hours of IV administration and peak levels (18 to 19 ng/mL) were reached at five to 10 days after IM administration. The calculated areas under the curve were the same for both routes of administration. The $t_{1/2}$ for anti-Rh$_o$ (D) was about 24 days following IV administration and about 30 days following IM administration.

INDICATIONS AND CLINICAL USE

Treatment of ITP

WinRho SDF™, Rh$_o$ (D) Immune Globulin Intravenous (Human), is recommended for the treatment of non-splenectomized, Rh$_o$ (D) positive

- children with chronic or acute ITP,
- adults with chronic ITP, or
- children and adults with ITP secondary to HIV infection

in clinical situations requiring an increase in platelet count to prevent excessive hemorrhage.

Suppression of Rh Isoimmunization

Pregnancy and Other Obstetric Conditions

WinRho SDF™ is recommended for the suppression of Rh isoimmunization in non-sensitized, Rh$_o$ (D) negative women within 72 hours after spontaneous or induced abortions, amniocentesis, chorionic villus sampling, ruptured tubal pregnancy, abdominal trauma or transplacental hemorrhage or in the normal course of pregnancy unless the blood type of the fetus or father is known to be Rh$_o$ (D) negative.

In the case of maternal bleeding due to threatened abortion, WinRho SDF™ should be administered as soon as possible. Suppression of Rh isoimmunization reduces the likelihood of hemolytic disease in an Rh$_o$ (D) positive fetus in present and future pregnancies.

The criteria for an Rh-incompatible pregnancy requiring administration of WinRho SDF™ at 28 weeks gestation and within 72 hours after delivery are:

- the mother must be Rh$_o$ (D) negative,
- the mother is carrying a child whose father is either Rh$_o$ (D) positive or Rh$_o$ (D) unknown,
- the baby is either Rh$_o$ (D) positive or Rh$_o$ (D) unknown, and
- the mother must not be previously sensitized to the Rh$_o$ (D) factor.

Transfusion

WinRho SDF™, Rh$_o$ (D) Immune Globulin Intravenous (Human), is recommended for the suppression of Rh isoimmunization in Rh$_o$ (D) negative female children and female adults in their childbearing years transfused with Rh$_o$ (D) positive red blood cells or blood components containing Rh$_o$ (D) positive red blood cells. Treatment should be initiated within 72 hours of exposure. Treatment should be given (without preceding exchange transfusion) only if the transfused Rh$_o$ (D) positive blood represents less than 20% of the total circulating red cells. A 300 µg (1,500 IU) dose will suppress the immunizing potential of approximately 17 mL of Rh$_o$ (D) positive red blood cells.

CLINICAL TRIALS

Treatment of ITP

Efficacy was documented in four subgroups of patients with ITP:

Childhood Chronic ITP

In an open-label, single arm, multicenter study, 24 non-splenectomized, Rh$_o$ (D) positive children with ITP of greater than six months duration were treated initially with 50 µg/kg (250 IU/kg) Rh$_o$ (D) Immune Globulin Intravenous (Human) (25 µg/kg [125 IU/kg] on days 1 and 2), with subsequent doses ranging from 25 to 55 µg/kg (125 to 275 IU/kg). Response was defined as a platelet increase to at least 50,000/mm^3 and a doubling of the baseline. Nineteen of 24 patients responded for an overall response rate of 79%, an overall mean peak platelet count of 229,400/mm^3 (range 43,300 to 456,000), and a mean duration of response of 36.5 days (range 6 to 84).[16–17]

Childhood Acute ITP

A multicenter, randomized, controlled trial comparing Rh$_o$ (D) IGIV to high dose and low dose Immune Globulin Intravenous (Human) and prednisone was conducted in 146 non-splenectomized, Rh$_o$ (D) positive children with acute ITP and platelet counts less than 20,000/mm^3. Of 38 patients receiving Rh$_o$ (D) IGIV (25 µg/kg [125 IU/kg] on days 1 and 2), 32 patients (84%) responded (platelet count ≥ 50,000/mm^3) with a mean peak platelet count of 319,500/mm^3 (range 61,000 to 892,000), with no statistically significant differences compared to other treatment arms. The mean times to achieving ≥ 20,000/mm^3 or ≥ 50,000/mm^3 platelets for patients receiving Rh$_o$ (D) IGIV were 1.9 and 2.8 days, respectively. When comparing the different therapies for time to

platelet count ≥ 20,000/mm^3 or ≥ 50,000/mm^3, no statistically significant differences among treatment groups were detected, with a range of 1.3 to 1.9 days and 2.0 to 3.2 days, respectively.[18–19]

Adult Chronic ITP

Twenty-four non-splenectomized, Rh_o (D) positive adults with ITP of greater than six months duration and platelet counts < 30,000/mm^3 or requiring therapy were enrolled in a single-arm, open-label trial and treated with 20 to 75 µg/kg (100 to 375 IU/kg) Rh_o (D) IGIV (mean dose 46.2 µg/kg [231 IU/kg]). Twenty-one of 24 patients responded (increase ≥ 20,000/mm^3) during the first two courses of therapy for an overall response rate of 88% with a mean peak platelet count of 92,300/mm^3 (range 8,000 to 229,000).[20–21]

ITP Secondary to HIV Infection

Eleven children and 52 adults, who were non-splenectomized and Rh_o (D) positive, with all Walter Reed classes of HIV infection and ITP, with initial platelet counts of ≤ 30,000/mm^3 or requiring therapy, were treated with 20 to 75 µg/kg (100 to 375 IU/kg) Rh_o (D) IGIV in an open label trial. Rh_o (D) IGIV was administered for an average of 7.3 courses (range 1 to 57) over a mean period of 407 days (range 6 to 1,952). Fifty-seven of 63 patients responded (increase ≥ 20,000/mm^3) during the first six courses of therapy for an overall response rate of 90%. The overall mean change in platelet count for six courses was 60,900/mm^3 (range −2,000 to 565,000), and the mean peak platelet count was 81,700/mm^3 (range 16,000 to 593,000).[21–23]

Suppression of Rh Isoimmunization

The pivotal study[24] supporting this indication was conducted in 1,186 non-sensitized, Rh_o (D) negative pregnant women in cases in which the blood types of the fathers were either Rh_o (D) positive or unknown. Rh_o (D) IGIV was administered according to one of three regimens: 1) 93 women received 120 µg (600 IU) at 28 weeks; 2) 131 women received 240 µg (1200 IU) each at 28 and 34 weeks; 3) 962 women received 240 µg (1200 IU) at 28 weeks. All women received a postnatal administration of 120 µg (600 IU) if the newborn was found to be Rh_o (D) positive. Of 1,186 women who received antenatal Rh_o (D)IGIV, 806 were given Rh_o (D) IGIV postnatally following the delivery of an Rh_o (D) positive infant, of which 325 women underwent testing at six months after delivery for evidence of Rh isoimmunization. Of these 325 women, 23 would have been expected to display signs of Rh isoimmunization; however, none was observed ($p < 0.001$ in a Chi-square test of significance of difference between observed and expected isoimmunization in the absence of Rh_o (D) IGIV).

CONTRAINDICATIONS

Treatment of ITP **and**
Suppression of Rh Isoimmunization

Individuals known to have had an anaphylactic or severe systemic reaction to human globulin should not receive WinRho SDF™, Rh_o (D) Immune Globulin Intravenous (Human), or any other Immune Globulin (Human). WinRho SDF™ contains trace amounts of IgA (approximately 5 µg/mL per 120 µg [600 IU] vial). Individuals who are deficient in IgA may have the potential for developing IgA antibodies and have anaphylactic reactions. The physician must weigh the potential benefit of treatment with WinRho SDF™ against the potential for hypersensitivity reactions.

WARNINGS

WinRho SDF™, Rh_o (D) Immune Globulin Intravenous (Human), is made from human plasma. Products made from human plasma may contain infectious agents, such as viruses, that can cause disease. The risk that such products will transmit an infectious agent has been reduced by screening plasma donors for prior exposure to certain viruses, by testing for the presence of certain current virus infections, and by inactivating and/or removing certain viruses. The WinRho SDF™ manufacturing process includes a solvent detergent treatment step (using tri-n-butyl phosphate and Triton X-100) that is effective in inactivating lipid enveloped viruses such as hepatitis B, hepatitis C, and HIV. WinRho SDF™ is filtered using a Planova 35 nm Virus Filter that is effective in reducing the level of some non-lipid enveloped viruses such as hepatitis A. These two processes are designed to increase product safety by reducing the risk of transmission of lipid enveloped and non-lipid enveloped viruses, respectively. Despite these measures, such products can still potentially transmit disease. There is also the possibility that unknown infectious agents may be present in such products. ALL infections thought by a physician possibly to have been transmitted by this product should be reported by the physician or other healthcare provider to the distributor, Nabi® at 1-800-4WINRHO (1-800- 494-6746). The physician should discuss the risks and benefits of this product with the patient.

Treatment of ITP

WinRho SDF™ must be administered via the intravenous route for the treatment of ITP as its efficacy has not been established by the intramuscular or subcutaneous routes.

WinRho SDF™ should not be administered to Rh_o (D) negative or splenectomized individuals as its efficacy in these patients has not been demonstrated.

Suppression of Rh Isoimmunization

For the suppression of Rh isoimmunization in the mother, do not administer to the infant.

PRECAUTIONS

WinRho SDF™, Rh_o (D) Immune Globulin Intravenous (Human), should not be administered as immunoglobulin replacement therapy for immune globulin deficiency syndromes.

Treatment of ITP

If the patient has a lower than normal hemoglobin level (less than 10 g/dL), a reduced dose of 25 to 40 µg/kg (125 to 200 IU/kg) should be given to minimize the risk of increasing the severity of anemia in the patient. WinRho SDF™, Rh_o (D) Immune Globulin Intravenous (Human), must be used with extreme caution in patients with a hemoglobin level that is less than 8 g/dL due to the risk of increasing the severity of the anemia.

Suppression of Rh Isoimmunization

WinRho SDF™ should not be administered to Rh_o (D) negative individuals who are Rh immunized as evidenced by standard manual Rh antibody screening tests.

A large fetomaternal hemorrhage late in pregnancy or following delivery may cause a weak mixed field positive D^u test result. Such an individual should be assessed for a large fetomaternal hemorrhage and the dose of WinRho SDF™ adjusted accordingly. WinRho SDF™ should be administered if there is any doubt about the mother's blood type.

Laboratory Tests

In addition to anti-D, WinRho SDF™ contains trace amounts of anti-C, E, A and B. These antibodies may be detected by laboratory screening tests.

Treatment of ITP

The presence of passively administered anti-Rh_o (D) can lead to a positive direct antiglobulin (Coomb's) test. Interpretation of this result must be made in the context of the patient's clinical condition and supporting laboratory data.

Suppression of Rh Isoimmunization

The presence of passively administered anti-Rh_o (D) in maternal or fetal blood can lead to a positive direct antiglobulin (Coomb's) test. If there is an uncertainty about the mother's Rh group or immune status, WinRho SDF™ should be administered to the mother.

Drug Interactions

Treatment of ITP **and**
Suppression of Rh Isoimmunization

Administration of WinRho SDF™ with other drugs has not been evaluated. Refer to Dosage and Administration section for information on drug compatibility.

Pregnancy Category C

Treatment of ITP **and**
Suppression of Rh Isoimmunization

Animal reproduction studies have not been conducted with WinRho SDF™. It is not known whether WinRho SDF™ can cause fetal harm when administered to a pregnant woman or can affect reproductive capacity. WinRho SDF™ should be given to a pregnant woman only if clearly needed.

ADVERSE REACTIONS

Treatment of ITP

WinRho SDF™, Rh_o (D) Immune Globulin Intravenous (Human), is administered to Rh_o (D) positive patients with ITP. Therefore, side effects related to the destruction of Rh_o (D) positive red cells, such as decreased hemoglobin, can be expected. At the recommended initial intravenous dose of 50 µg/kg (250 IU/kg), the mean maximum decrease in hemoglobin was 1.70 g/dL (range +0.40 to −6.1 g/dL). At a reduced dose, ranging from 25 to 40 µg/kg (125 to 200 IU/kg), the mean maximum decrease in hemoglobin was 0.81 g/dL (range +0.65 to −1.9 g/dL). Only 5/137 (3.7%) of patients had a maximum decrease in hemoglobin of greater than 4 g/dL (range 4.2 to 6.1 g/dL). In most cases, the red blood cell destruction is believed to occur in the spleen. However, there have been rare reports of acute onset of hemoglobinuria consistent with intravascular hemolysis and possibly accompanied by reversible acute renal impairment. Some cases occurred in patients receiving red blood cell transfusion concurrent with WinRho SDF™.

In trials in subjects (n=161) with childhood acute ITP, adults and children with chronic ITP, and adults and children with ITP secondary to HIV, 60/848 (7%) of infusions were associated with at least one adverse event that was considered to be related to the study medication. The most common adverse events were headache (19 infusions; 2%), chills (14 infusions; <2%), and fever (nine infusions; 1%). All are expected adverse events associated with infusions of immunoglobulins.

Suppression of Rh Isoimmunization

Adverse reactions to Rh_o (D) Immune Globulin Intravenous (Human) are infrequent in Rh_o (D) negative individuals. In the clinical trial[24] of 1,186 Rh_o (D) negative pregnant women, no adverse events were attributed to Rh_o (D) IGIV. Discomfort and slight swelling at the site of injection and slight elevation in temperature have been reported in a small number of cases. A post-marketing survey conducted since the Canadian licensure of Rh_o (D) IGIV in 1980 for this indication included data obtained from 31,059 injections (25,068 for routine Rh prophylaxis and 5,991 following abortions, amniocentesis, chorionic villus sampling and antepartum hemorrhage). There were 9,905 Rh_o (D) negative women who delivered Rh_o (D) positive infants, almost all of whom had received antenatal as well as postnatal prophylaxis. Of the patients followed in this survey, there were 26 reported treatment failures that resulted in the development of Rh_o (D) antibodies. There were no adverse experiences related to Rh_o (D) IGIV reported in this survey.

General Adverse Reactions

In addition to the adverse reactions described above, the following have been reported infrequently in clinical trials and/or postmarketing experience, in patients treated for ITP or the suppression of Rh isoimmunization, and are thought to be temporally associated with WinRho SDF™, Rh_o (D) Immune Globulin Intravenous (Human), use: asthenia, abdominal or back pain, hypotension, pallor, diarrhea, increased LDH, arthralgia, myalgia, dizziness, hyperkinesia, somnolence, vasodilation, pruritis, rash, and sweating. As is the case with all drugs of this nature, there is a remote chance of an idiosyncratic or anaphylactic reaction with WinRho SDF™ in individuals with hypersensitivity to blood products.

SYMPTOMS AND TREATMENT OF OVERDOSAGE

Treatment of ITP **and**
Suppression of Rh Isoimmunization

There are no reports of known overdoses in patients being treated for Rh isoimmunization or ITP. In clinical studies with nonpregnant Rh_o (D) positive patients with ITP (n=141) treated with 120 to 6,500 µg (600 to 32,500 IU) of Rh_o (D) IGIV, there were no signs or symptoms that warranted medical intervention. However, these same doses were associated with a mild, transient hemolytic anemia.

DOSAGE AND ADMINISTRATION

Treatment of ITP **and**
Suppression of Rh Isoimmunization

WinRho SDF™, Rh_o (D) Immune Globulin Intravenous (Human), should be reconstituted only with the accompanying vial of 0.9% Sodium Chloride Injection. It should not be administered with other products.

Reconstitution

Intravenous Administration

Aseptically reconstitute the product shortly before use with 2.5 mL of 0.9% Sodium Chloride Injection for 120 µg (600 IU) and 300 µg (1,500 IU) and 8.5 mL of 0.9% Sodium Chloride Injection for 1,000 µg (5,000 IU) (see the next table). Inject the diluent slowly onto the inside wall of the vial and gently swirl until dissolved. Do not shake.

Intramuscular Administration

Aseptically reconstitute the product shortly before use with 1.25 mL of 0.9% Sodium Chloride Injection for 120 µg (600 IU) and 300 µg (1,500 IU) and 8.5 mL of 0.9% Sodium Chloride Injection for 1,000 µg (5,000 IU) (see the next table). Inject the diluent slowly onto the inside wall of the vial and gently swirl until dissolved. Do not shake.

Reconstitution of WinRho SDF™

Vial Size	Volume of Diluent to be Added to Vial
Intravenous Injection	—
120 µg (600 IU)	2.5 mL
300 µg (1,500 IU)	2.5 mL
1,000 µg (5,000 IU)	8.5 mL
Intramuscular Injection	—
120 µg (600 IU)	1.25 mL
300 µg (1,500 IU)	1.25 mL
1,000 µg (5,000 IU)	8.5 mL*

*To be administered into several sites

Injection

Parenteral products such as WinRho SDF™ should be inspected for particulate matter and discoloration prior to administration. Use the product within 12 hours of reconstitution. Discard any unused portion.

Intravenous Administration

Infuse the entire dose into a suitable vein over three to five minutes. WinRho SDF™, Rh_o (D) Immune Globulin Intravenous (Human), should be administered separately from other drugs.

Intramuscular Administration

Administer into the deltoid muscle of the upper arm or the anterolateral aspects of the upper thigh. Due to the risk of

Continued on next page

WinRho SDF—Cont.

sciatic nerve injury, the gluteal region should not be used as a routine injection site. If the gluteal region is used, use only the upper, outer quadrant.

Treatment of ITP

WinRho SDF™ **must be given by intravenous administration** for the treatment of ITP.

Initial Dosing: After confirming that the patient is Rh_o (D) positive, an initial dose of 50 µg/kg (250 IU/kg) body weight, given as a single injection, is recommended for the treatment of ITP. The initial dose may be administered in two divided doses given on separate days, if desired. If the patient has a hemoglobin level that is less than 10 g/dL, a reduced dose of 25 to 40 µg/kg (125 to 200 IU/kg) should be given to minimize the risk of increasing the severity of anemia in the patient. All patients should be monitored to determine clinical response by assessing platelet counts, red cell counts, hemoglobin, and reticulocyte levels.

Subsequent Dosing: If subsequent therapy is required to elevate platelet counts, an intravenous dose of 25 to 60 µg/kg (125 to 300 IU/kg) body weight of WinRho SDF™ is recommended. The frequency and dose used in maintenance therapy should be determined by the patient's clinical response by assessing platelet counts, red cell counts, hemoglobin, and reticulocyte levels.

If patient responded to initial dose with a satisfactory increase in platelets:

Maintenance Therapy:
Dosing (25–60 µg/kg [125–300 IU/kg]) individualized based on platelet and Hgb levels.

If patient did not respond to initial dose, administer a subsequent dose based on Hgb:

If Hgb between 8–10 g/dL,
redose between 25–40 µg/kg
(125–200 IU/kg).
If Hgb >10 g/dL,
redose between 50–60 µg/kg
(250–300 IU/kg).
If Hgb <8 g/dL, use with caution.

The following equations are provided to determine the dosage and number of vials needed for the treatment of ITP:
• weight in lbs. + 2.2083 = weight in kg
• weight in kg X selected µg (IU) dosing level = dosage
• dosage + vial size = number of vials needed

Suppression of Rh Isoimmunization

WinRho SDF™ may be given by intravenous or intramuscular administration for the suppression of Rh isoimmunization.

Pregnancy

The same dosage, as described below, is to be administered by either the intramuscular or intravenous routes.

A 300 µg (1,500 IU) dose of WinRho SDF™, Rh_o (D) Immune Globulin Intravenous (Human), should be administered at 28 weeks gestation. If WinRho SDF™ is administered early in the pregnancy, it is recommended that WinRho SDF™ be administered at 12-week intervals in order to maintain an adequate level of passively acquired anti-Rh.

A 120 µg (600 IU) dose should be administered as soon as possible after delivery of a confirmed Rh_o (D) positive baby and normally no later than 72 hours after delivery. In the event that the Rh status of the baby is not known at 72 hours, WinRho SDF™ should be administered to the mother at 72 hours after delivery. If more than 72 hours have elapsed, WinRho SDF™ should not be withheld, but administered as soon as possible up to 28 days after delivery.

Other Obstetric Conditions

The same dosage, as described below, is to be administered by either the intramuscular or intravenous routes.

A 120 µg (600 IU) dose of WinRho SDF™ should be administered immediately after abortion, amniocentesis (after 34 weeks gestation) or any other manipulation late in pregnancy (after 34 weeks gestation) associated with increased risk of Rh isoimmunization. Administration should take place within 72 hours after the event.

A 300 µg (1,500 IU) dose of $WinRh_o$ SDF™ should be administered immediately after amniocentesis before 34 weeks gestation or after chorionic villus sampling. This dose should be repeated every 12 weeks while the woman is pregnant. In the case of threatened abortion, WinRho SDF™ should be administered as soon as possible.

Obstetric Indications and Recommended Dose

Indication	Dose (Administer IM or IV)
Pregnancy:	—
•28 weeks gestation	300 µg (1,500 IU)
•Postpartum (if newborn Rh positive)	120 µg (600 IU)
Obstetric Conditions:	—
•Threatened abortion at any time	300 µg (1,500 IU)
•Amniocentesis and chorionic villus sampling before 34 weeks gestation	300 µg (1,500 IU)
•Abortion, aminocentesis, or any other manipulation after 34 weeks gestation	120 µg (600 IU)

Transfusion

WinRho SDF™ should be administered within 72 hours after exposure for treatment of incompatible blood transfusions or massive fetal hemorrhage.

Transfusion Indication and Recommended Dose

Route of Administration	WinRho SDF™ Dose	
	If exposed to Rh_o(D) Positive Whole Blood:	If exposed to Rh_o(D) Positive Red Blood Cells:
Intravenous	9 µg (45 IU)/ mL Blood	18 µg (90 IU)/ mL Cells
Intramuscular	12 µg (60 IU)/ mL Blood	24 µg (120 IU)/ mL Cells

Administer 600 µg (3,000 IU) **every 8 hours via the intravenous route**, until the total dose, calculated from the above table, is administered.
Administer 1,200 µg (6,000 IU) **every 12 hours via the intramuscular route**, until the total dose, calculated from the above table, is administered.

HOW SUPPLIED

WinRho SDF™, Rh_o (D) Immune Globulin Intravenous (Human), is available in packages containing:

NDC Number	Contents
60492-0021-1	A box containing a single dose vial of 120 µg (600 IU) anti-Rh_o(D) IGIV, a single dose vial of 2.5 mL 0.9% Sodium Chloride Injection, and a package insert
60492-0023-1	A box containing a single dose vial of 300 µg (1,500 IU) anti-Rh_o (D) IGIV, a single dose vial of 2.5 mL 0.9% Sodium Chloride Injection, and a package insert
60492-0024-1	A box containing a vial of 1,000 µg (5,000 IU) anti-Rh_o (D) IGIV, a vial of 8.5 mL 0.9% Sodium Chloride Injection, and a package insert

STORAGE

Store at 2 to 8°C (35 to 46°F). Do not freeze. Do not use after expiration date.
If the reconstituted product is not used immediately, store it at room temperature for no longer than 12 hours. Do not freeze the reconstituted product. Discard the product if not administered within 12 hours.

CAUTION

U.S. federal law prohibits dispensing without prescription.

REFERENCES

1. Bowman, JM, et al.: Low protein Rh immune globulin (Rh IgG)-purity, stability, activity and prophylactic value. *Vox Sang* 1973; 24:301–316.
2. Bowman, JM, et al.: WinRho: Rh immune globulin prepared by ion exchange for intravenous use. *Can. Med. Assoc. J.* 1980; 123:1121–1125.
3. Friesen, AD, et al.: Column ion-exchange preparation and characterization of an Rh immune globulin (WinRho) for intravenous use. *J. Appl. Biochem.* 1981; 3:164–175.
4. Horowitz, B: Investigations into the application of tri(n-butyl)phosphate/detergent mixtures to blood derivatives. Morgenthaler J (ed): *Virus Inactivation in Plasma Products, Curr. Stud. Hematol. Blood. Transfus.* 1989; 56:83–96.
5. Information on file at Cangene Corporation.
6. Burnouf, T: Value of virus filtration as a method for improving the safety of plasma products. *Vox Sang.* 1996; 70:235-236.
7. Ballow, M: Mechanisms of action of intravenous immunoglobulin therapy and potential use in autoimmune connective tissue diseases. *Cancer.* 1991; 68:1430–1436.
8. Kniker, WT: Immunosuppressive agents, γ-globulin, immunomodulation, immunization, and apheresis. *J. Aller. Clin. Immunol.* 1989; 84:1104–1106.
9. Chown, B, et al.: The effect of anti-D IgG on D-positive recipients. *Can. Med. Assoc. J.* 1970; 102:1161–1164.
10. Bowman, JM and Chown, B: Prevention of Rh immunization after massive Rh-positive transfusion. *Can. Med. Assoc. J.* 1968; 99:385–388.
11. Bowman, JM: Suppression of Rh isoimmunization: a review. *Obstet. & Gynec.* 1978; 52:385–393.
12. Bowman, JM, et al.: Rh isoimmunization during pregnancy: antenatal prophylaxis. *Can. Med. Assoc. J.* 1978; 118:623–627.
13. Bowman, JM, and Pollock, JM: Antenatal prophylaxis of Rh isoimmunization: 28 weeks'- gestation service program. *Can. Med. Assoc. J.* 1978; 118:627–630.
14. Bowman, JM, and Pollock, JM: Failures of intravenous Rh immune globulin prophylaxis: An analysis of the reasons for such failures. *Trans. Med. Rev.* 1987; 1:101–11.
15. Bowman, JM: Antenatal suppression of Rh alloimmunization. *Clin Obstet. & Gynec.* 1991; 34:296–303.
16. Unpublished data on file, CITP Report, May 1993.
17. Andrew, M, et al.: A multicenter study of the treatment of childhood chronic idiopathic thrombocytopenic purpura with anti-D. *J Pediatrics* 120:522–527, 1992.
18. Unpublished data on file, AITP Report, May 1993.
19. Blanchette, V, et al.: Randomised trial of intravenous immunoglobulin G, intravenous anti-D, and oral prednisone in childhood acute immune thrombocytopenic purpura. *Lancet* 1994; 344: 703–707.
20. Unpublished data on file, BITP-2 Report, May 1993.
21. Bussel, JB, et al.: Intravenous anti-D treatment of immune thrombocytopenic purpura: Analysis of efficacy, toxicity, and mechanism of effect. *Blood* 1991; 77: 1884-1893.
22. Unpublished data on file, BITP-1 Report, May 1993.
23. Bussel, JB, et al.: IV anti-D treatment of ITP: Results in 210 cases. Abstract, *The American Society of Hematology,* Anaheim, CA, December, 1992.
24. Unpublished data on file, WR3 Report, May 1993.

Manufactured by:
Cangene Corporation
Winnipeg, Canada R3T 5Y3
U.S. License No. 1201
Distributed by:
Nabi®
Boca Raton, FL 33487
Part No. 07.0205.02

Neurex Corporation

**3760 HAVEN AVENUE
MENLO PARK, CA 94025**

Direct Inquiries to:
888-853-NXCO (6926)

CORLOPAM®
brand of (fenoldopam mesylate) Injection

Rx

DESCRIPTION

CORLOPAM (fenoldopam mesylate) is a dopamine D_1-like receptor agonist. The product is formulated as a solution to be diluted for intravenous infusion. Chemically it is 6-chloro-2,3,4,5-tetrahydro-1-(4-hydroxyphenyl)-[1H]-3-benzazepine-7,8-diol methanesulfonate with the following structure:

fenoldopam mesylate

Fenoldopam mesylate is a white to off-white powder with a molecular weight of 401.87 and a molecular formula of $C_{16}H_{16}ClNO_3 \cdot CH_3SO_3H$. It is sparingly soluble in water, ethanol and methanol, and is soluble in propylene glycol. Ampules: Each 1 mL contains, in sterile aqueous solution, citric acid 3.44 mg; fenoldopam mesylate equivalent to fenoldopam 10 mg; propylene glycol 518 mg; sodium citrate dihydrate 0.61 mg; sodium metabisulfite 1 mg.

CLINICAL PHARMACOLOGY
Mechanism of Action

Fenoldopam is a rapid-acting vasodilator. It is an agonist for D_1-like dopamine receptors and binds with moderate affinity to α_2-adrenoceptors. It has no significant affinity for D_2-like receptors, α_1 and β adrenoceptors, $5HT_1$ and $5HT_2$ receptors, or muscarinic receptors. Fenoldopam is a racemic mixture with the R-isomer responsible for the biological ac-

Table 1
CORLOPAM Plasma Concentrations in Normotensive, Mild to Moderate and Malignant Hypertensive Patients
CORLOPAM PLASMA CONCENTRATION (ng/mL)

CORLOPAM Infusion Rate (µg/kg/min)	Patient Populations		
	Normotensive Subjects n=10	Mild to Moderate Hypertensive Patients n=7	Malignant Hypertension Patients n=20
0.1	3.2	4.0	3.3

tivity. The R-isomer has approximately 250-fold higher affinity for D_1-like receptors than does the S-isomer. In nonclinical studies, fenoldopam had no agonist effect on presynaptic D_2-like dopamine receptors, or α- or β-adrenoceptors, nor did it affect angiotensin-converting enzyme activity. Fenoldopam may increase norepinephrine plasma concentration.

In animals, fenoldopam has vasodilating effects in coronary, renal, mesenteric and peripheral arteries. All vascular beds, however, do not respond uniformly to fenoldopam. Vasodilating effects have been demonstrated in renal efferent and afferent arterioles. In humans, increases in renal blood flow were demonstrated in hypertensive and normal subjects treated with intravenous fenoldopam in two small controlled trials. No beneficial clinical effect on renal function has been shown in patients with heart failure or hepatic or severe renal disease.

Pharmacokinetics

Administered as a constant infusion at rates of 0.01 to 1.6 µg/kg/min, fenoldopam produced steady-state plasma concentrations that were proportional to infusion rates. The elimination half-life was about 5 minutes in mild to moderate hypertensives, with little difference between the R (active) and S isomers. Steady state concentrations are attained in about 20 minutes (4 half-lives). The steady state plasma concentrations of fenoldopam, at comparable infusion rates, were similar in normotensive subjects and in patients with mild to moderate hypertension or hypertensive emergencies (Table 1).
[See table 1 above]

Clearance of parent (active) fenoldopam is not altered in patients with end-stage renal disease on continuous ambulatory peritoneal dialysis (CAPD) and is not affected on average, in severe hepatic failure. The effects of hemodialysis on the pharmacokinetics of fenoldopam have not been evaluated.

In radiolabelled studies in rats, no more than 0.005% of fenoldopam crossed the blood-brain barrier.

Excretion and Metabolism

Radiolabeled studies show that about 90% of infused fenoldopam is eliminated in urine, 10% in feces. Elimination is largely by conjugation, without participation of cytochrome P-450 enzymes. The principal routes of conjugation are methylation, glucuronidation, and sulfation. Only 4% of the administered dose is excreted unchanged. Animal data indicate that the metabolites are inactive.

Special Population: The pharmacokinetics of fenoldopam were not influenced by age, gender, or race in hypertensive emergency patients. Effects of renal and hepatic dysfunction are described above. There have been no formal drug-drug interaction studies using intravenous fenoldopam.

Pharmacodynamics and Clinical Studies

In a randomized double-blind, placebo-controlled, 5-group study in 32 patients with mild to moderate essential hypertension (diastolic blood pressure between 95 and 119 mmHg), and a mean baseline pressure of about 154/98 mmHg, and heart rate of about 75 bpm, fixed-rate IV infusions of CORLOPAM produced dose-related reductions in systolic and diastolic blood pressure. Infusions were maintained at a fixed rate for 48 hours. Table 2 shows the results of the study. The onset of response was rapid at all infusion rates, with the 15-minute response representing 50–100% of the one-hour response in all groups. There was some suggestion of partial tolerance at 48 hours in the two higher dose infusions, but a substantial effect persisted through 48 hours. When infusions were stopped, blood pressure gradually returned to pretreatment values with no evidence of rebound. This study suggests that there is no greater response to 0.8 µg/kg/min than to 0.4 µg/kg/min.
[See table 2 below]

In a multicenter, randomized, double-blind comparison of four infusion rates, CORLOPAM was administered as constant rate infusions of 0.01, 0.03, 0.1 and 0.3 µg/kg/min for up to 24 hours to 94 patients experiencing hypertensive emergencies (defined as diastolic blood pressure ≥ 120 mmHg with evidence of compromise of end-organ function involving the cardiovascular, renal, cerebral or retinal systems). Infusion rates could be doubled after one hour if clinically indicated. There were dose-related, rapid-onset, decreases in systolic and diastolic blood pressures and increases in heart rate (Table 3).
[See table 3 at bottom of next page]

Two hundred and thirty six severely hypertensive patients (DBP ≥ 120 mm Hg), with or without end-organ compromise, were randomized to receive in two open-label studies either fenoldopam or nitroprusside. The response rate was 79% (92/117) in the fenoldopam group and 77% (90/119) in the nitroprusside group. Response required a decline in supine diastolic blood pressure to less than 110 mm Hg if the baseline were between 120 and 150 mm Hg, inclusive, or by ≥ 40 mm Hg if the baseline were ≥ 150 mm Hg. Patients were titrated to the desired effect. For fenoldopam, the dose ranged from 0.1 to 1.5 µg/kg/min; for nitroprusside, the dose ranged from 1.0 to 8.0 µg/kg/min. As in the study in mild to moderate hypertensives, most of the effect seen at one hour is present at 15 minutes. The additional effect seen after 1 hour occurs in all groups and may not be drug-related (there was no placebo group to evaluate this).

INDICATIONS AND USAGE

CORLOPAM is indicated for the in-hospital, short-term (up to 48 hours) management of severe hypertension when rapid, but quickly reversible, emergency reduction of blood pressure is clinically indicated, including malignant hypertension with deteriorating end-organ function. Transition to oral therapy with another agent can begin at any time after blood pressure is stable during CORLOPAM infusion.

CONTRAINDICATIONS

None known.

WARNINGS

Contains sodium metabisulfite, a sulfite that may cause allergic-type reactions including anaphylactic symptoms and life-threatening or less severe asthmatic episodes in certain susceptible people. The overall prevalence of sulfite sensitivity in the general population is unknown and probably low. Sulfite sensitivity is seen more frequently is asthmatic than in nonasthmatic people.

PRECAUTIONS

Intraocular Pressure: In a clinical study of 12 patients with open-angle glaucoma or ocular hypertension (mean baseline intraocular pressure was 29.2 mmHg with a range of 22.0–33.0 mmHg), infusion of CORLOPAM at escalating doses ranging from 0.05–0.5 µg/kg/min over a 3.5 hour period caused a dose-dependent increase in intraocular pressure (IOP). At the peak effect, the intraocular pressure was raised by a mean of 6.5 mmHg (range −2.0 to +8.5 mmHg, corrected for placebo effect). Upon discontinuation of the CORLOPAM infusion, the IOP returned to baseline values within 2 hours. CORLOPAM administration to patients with glaucoma or intraocular hypertension should be undertaken with caution.

Tachycardia: CORLOPAM causes a dose-related tachycardia (Table 2 and Table 3), particularly with infusion rates above 0.1 µg/kg/min. Tachycardia diminishes over time but remains substantial at higher doses.

Hypotension: CORLOPAM may occasionally produce symptomatic hypotension and close monitoring of blood pressure during administration is essential. (See Adverse Reactions.) It is particularly important to avoid systemic hypotension when administering the drug to patients who have sustained an acute cerebral infarction or hemorrhage.

Hypokalemia: Decreases in serum potassium occasionally to values below 3.0 meq/L were observed after less than 6 hours of fenoldopam infusion. It is not clear if the hypokalemia reflects a pressure natriuresis with enhanced potassium-sodium exchange or a direct drug effect. During clinical trials, electrolytes were monitored at intervals of 6 hours. Hypokalemia was treated with either oral or intravenous potassium supplementation. Patient management should include appropriate attention to serum electrolytes.

Table 2
PHARMACODYNAMIC EFFECTS OF FENOLDOPAM IN MILD TO MODERATE HYPERTENSIVE PATIENTS

Time Point and Mean Change From Time Zero ± SE	Infusion Rate (µg/kg/min)				
	Placebo n = 7	0.04 n = 7	0.1 n = 7	0.4 n = 5	0.8 n = 6
15 Minutes of Infusion*					
Systolic BP	0 ± 6	−15 ± 6	−19 ± 8	−14 ± 4	−24 ± 6
Diastolic BP	0 ± 2	−5 ± 3	−12 ± 4	−15 ± 3	−20 ± 4
Heart Rate	+2 ± 2	+3 ± 2	+5 ± 1	+16 ± 3	+19 ± 3
30 Minutes of Infusion*					
Systolic BP	−6 ± 5	−17 ± 6	−18 ± 6	−14 ± 4	−26 ± 6
Diastolic BP	−6 ± 3	−7 ± 3	−16 ± 4	−14 ± 3	−20 ± 2
Heart Rate	+2 ± 2	+3 ± 2	+10 ± 2	+18 ± 3	+23 ± 3
1 Hour of Infusion*					
Systolic BP	−15 ± 4	−22 ± 7	−22 ± 7	−26 ± 9	−22 ± 9
Diastolic BP	−5 ± 3	−9 ± 2	−18 ± 4	−19 ± 4	−21 ± 1
Heart Rate	+1 ± 3	+5 ± 2	+12 ± 3	+19 ± 4	+25 ± 4
4 Hours of Infusion*					
Systolic BP	−14 ± 5	−16 ± 9	−31 ± 15	−22 ± 11	−25 ± 7
Diastolic BP	−14 ± 8	−8 ± 4	−19 ± 9	−25 ± 3	−20 ± 1
Heart Rate	+5 ± 3	+6 ± 3	+10 ± 4	+21 ± 2	+27 ± 7
24 Hours of Infusion*					
Systolic BP	−20 ± 6	−23 ± 8	−35 ± 7	−22 ± 6	−23 ± 11
Diastolic BP	−11 ± 6	−11 ± 5	−23 ± 10	−22 ± 5	−13 ± 3
Heart Rate	+6 ± 3	+5 ± 3	+13 ± 2	+17 ± 4	+15 ± 3
48 Hours of Infusion*					
Systolic BP	−12 ± 8	−31 ± 6	−22 ± 8	−9 ± 6	−14 ± 10
Diastolic BP	−9 ± 5	−10 ± 6	−9 ± 7	−9 ± 2	−9 ± 3
Heart Rate	+1 ± 2	0 ± 4	+1 ± 4	+12 ± 3	+8 ± 3

* Mean change from time zero ± S.E.

Continued on next page

Corlopam—Cont.

Drug Interactions: Although there have been no formal interaction studies, intravenous CORLOPAM has been administered safely with drugs such as digitalis and sublingual nitroglycerin. There is limited experience with concomitant antihypertensive agents such as beta-blockers, alpha-blockers, calcium channel-blockers, ACE inhibitors, and diuretics (both thiazide-like and loop).

Carcinogenesis, Mutagenesis, Impairment of Fertility: In a 24-month study, mice treated orally with fenoldopam at 12.5, 25, or 50 mg/kg/day, reduced to 25 mg/kg/day on day 209 of study, showed no increase above controls in the incidence of neoplasms. Female mice in the highest dose group had an increased incidence and degree of severity of a fibro osseous lesion of the sternum compared with control or low-dose animals. Compared to controls, female mice in the middle- and upper-dose groups had a higher incidence and degree of severity of chronic nephritis. These pathologic lesions were not seen in male mice treated with fenoldopam. In a 24-month study, rats treated orally with fenoldopam at 5, 10 or 20 mg/kg/day, with the mid- and high-dose groups increased to 15 or 25 mg/kg/day, respectively, on day 372 of the study, showed no increase above controls in the incidence or type of neoplasms. Compared with the controls, rats in the mid- and high-dose groups had a higher incidence of hyperplasia of collecting duct epithelium at the tip of the renal papilla.

In in vitro assays, fenoldopam did not induce bacterial gene mutation in the Ames test or mammalian gene mutation in the Chinese hamster ovary (CHO) cell assay. In the in vitro chromosomal aberration assay with CHO cells, fenoldopam was associated with statistically significant and dose-dependent increases in chromosomal aberrations, and in the proportion of aberrant metaphases. However, no chromosomal damage was seen in the in vivo mice micronucleus or bone marrow assays. The data support the conclusion that fenoldopam is not genotoxic or clastogenic.

Oral fertility and general reproduction performance studies in male and female rats at 12.5, 37.5 or 75 mg/kg/day revealed no impairment of fertility or reproduction performance due to fenoldopam.

Pregnancy: Pregnancy Category B. Oral reproduction studies have been performed in rats and rabbits at doses of 12.5 to 200 mg/kg/day and 6.25 to 25 mg/kg/day, respectively. Studies have revealed maternal toxicity at the highest doses tested but no evidence of impaired fertility or harm to the fetus due to fenoldopam. However, there are no adequate and well-controlled studies in pregnant women. Since animal reproduction studies are not always predictive of human response, fenoldopam should be used in pregnancy only if clearly needed.

Nursing Mothers: Fenoldopam is excreted in milk in rats. It is not known whether this drug is excreted in human milk. Because many drugs are excreted in human milk, caution should be exercised when CORLOPAM is administered to a nursing woman.

Pediatric Use: Safety and effectiveness in children have not been established.

ADVERSE REACTIONS

CORLOPAM causes a dose-related fall in blood pressure and increase in heart rate (see Precautions, Tachycardia, and Hypotension). In controlled clinical studies of severe hypertension in patients with end-organ damage, 3% (4/137) of patients withdrew because of excessive falls in blood pressure. Increased heart rate could, in theory, lead to ischemic cardiac events or worsened heart failure, although these events have not been observed. The most common events reported as associated with CORLOPAM use are headache, cutaneous dilation (flushing), nausea, and hypotension, each reported in more than 5% of patients.

Adverse reactions in controlled trials in hypertension
Adverse events occurring more than once in any dosing group (once if potentially important or plausibly drug-related) in the fixed-dose constant-infusion studies are presented in the following Table by infusion-rate group. There was no clear dose relationship, except possibly for headache, nausea, flushing.

[See table 4 on next page]

Adverse effects in overall data base
The adverse event incidences listed below are based on observations of over 1,000 CORLOPAM treated patients and not listed in the Table above.

Events reported with a frequency between 0.5–5% in patients treated with IV CORLOPAM
Cardiovascular: extrasystoles, palpitations, bradycardia, heart failure, ischemic heart disease, myocardial infarction, angina pectoris
Metabolic: elevated BUN, elevated serum glucose, elevated transaminase, elevated LDH
General Body: non-specific chest pain, pyrexia
Hematologic/Lymphatic: leukocytosis, bleeding
Respiratory: dyspnea, upper respiratory disorder
Genitourinary: oliguria
Musculoskeletal: limb cramp

ANIMAL TOXICOLOGY

Unusual toxicology findings (arterial lesions in the rat) with fenoldopam are summarized below. These findings have not been observed in mice or dogs. No evidence of a similar lesion in humans has been observed.

Arterial lesions characterized by medial necrosis and hemorrhage have been seen in renal and splanchnic arteries of rats given fenoldopam mesylate by continuous intravenous infusion at doses of 1 to 100 µg/kg/min for 24 hours. The incidence of these lesions is dose related. Arterial lesions morphologically identical to those observed with fenoldopam have been reported in rats infused with dopamine. Data suggest that the mechanism for this injury involves activation of D_1-like dopaminergic receptors. Such lesions have not been seen in dogs given doses up to 100 µg/kg/min by continuous intravenous infusion for 24 hours, nor were they seen in dogs infused at the same dose for 6 hours daily for 24 days. The clinical significance of this finding is not known.

Oral administration of fenoldopam doses of 10 to 15 mg/kg/day or 20 to 25 mg/kg/day to rats for 24 months induced a higher incidence of polyarteritis nodosa compared to controls. Such lesions were not seen in rats given 5 mg/kg/day of fenoldopam or in mice given the drug at doses up to 50 mg/kg/day for 24 months.

OVERDOSAGE

Intentional CORLOPAM overdosage has not been reported. The most likely reaction would be excessive hypotension which should be treated with drug discontinuation and appropriate supportive measures.

DOSAGE AND ADMINISTRATION

The optimal magnitude and rate of blood pressure reduction in acutely hypertensive patients have not been rigorously determined, but, in general, both delay and too rapid decreases appear undesirable in sick patients. An initial CORLOPAM dose may be chosen from Tables 2 and 3 in the Clinical Pharmacology Section that produces the desired magnitude and rate of blood pressure reduction in a given clinical situation. Doses below 0.1 µg/kg/min have very modest effects and appear only marginally useful in this population. In general, as the initial dose increases, there is a greater and more rapid blood pressure reduction. However, lower initial doses (0.03–0.1 µg/kg/min) titrated slowly have been associated with less reflex tachycardia than have higher initial doses (≥ 0.3 µg/kg/min). In clinical trials, doses from 0.01–1.6 µg/kg/min have been studied. Most of the effect of a given infusion rate is attained in 15 minutes.

CORLOPAM should be administered by continuous intravenous infusion. **A bolus dose should not be used.** Hypotension and rapid decreases of blood pressure should be avoided. The initial dose should be titrated upward or downward, no more frequently than every 15 minutes (and less frequently as goal pressure is approached) to achieve the desired therapeutic effect. The recommended increments for titration are 0.05–0.1 µg/kg/min.

Use of a calibrated, mechanical infusion pump is recommended for proper control of infusion rate during CORLOPAM infusion. In clinical trials, CORLOPAM treatment was safely performed **without** the need for intra-arterial blood pressure monitoring; blood pressure and heart rate were monitored at frequent intervals, typically every 15 minutes. Frequent blood pressure monitoring is recommended.

Use of beta-blockers in conjunction with CORLOPAM has not been studied in hypertensive patients and, if possible, concomitant use should be avoided. If the drugs are used together, caution should be exercised because unexpected hypotension could result from beta-blocker inhibition of the reflex response to fenoldopam.

The CORLOPAM infusion can be abruptly discontinued or gradually tapered prior to discontinuation. Oral antihypertensive agents can be added during CORLOPAM infusion or following its discontinuation. Patients in controlled clinical trials have received intravenous CORLOPAM for as long as 48 hours.

PREPARATION OF INFUSION SOLUTION
WARNING: CONTENTS OF AMPULES MUST BE DILUTED BEFORE INFUSION. EACH AMPULE IS FOR SINGLE USE ONLY.
Dilution:
The CORLOPAM Injection ampule concentrate must be diluted in 0.9% Sodium Chloride Injection USP or 5% Dextrose Injection USP using the following dilution schedule:

mL of Concentrate (mg of drug)	Added to	Final Concentration
4 mL (40 mg)	1000 mL	40 µg/mL
2 mL (20 mg)	500 mL	40 µg/mL
1 mL (10 mg)	250 mL	40 µg/mL

The drug dose rate must be individualized according to body weight and according to the desired rapidity and extent of pharmacodynamic effect. The following Table provides the calculated infusion volume in mL/min for a range of drug doses and body weights. The infusion should be administered using a calibrated mechanical infusion pump that can accurately and reliably deliver the desired infusion rate.

[See table 5 on next page]
The diluted solution is stable under normal ambient light and temperature conditions for at least 24 hours. Diluted solution that is not used within 24 hours of preparation

Table 3
PHARMACODYNAMIC EFFECTS OF FENOLDOPAM IN HYPERTENSIVE EMERGENCY PATIENTS

Time Point and Pharmacodynamic Parameters	Infusion Rate µg/kg/min			
	0.01 n = 25	0.03 n = 24	0.1 n = 22	0.3 n = 23
Pre-Infusion Baseline				
Systolic BP – mean ± SE	210 ± 21	208 ± 26	205 ± 24	211 ± 17
Diastolic BP – mean ± SE	136 ± 16	135 ± 11	133 ± 14	136 ± 15
Heart rate – mean ± SE	87 ± 20	84 ± 14	81 ± 19	80 ± 14
15 minutes of Infusion*				
Systolic BP	−5 ± 4	−7 ± 4	−16 ± 4	−19 ± 4
Diastolic BP	−5 ± 3	−8 ± 3	−12 ± 2	−21 ± 2
Heart rate	−2 ± 3	+1 ± 1	+2 ± 1	+11 ± 2
30 Minutes of Infusion*				
Systolic BP	−6 ± 4	−11 ± 4	−21 ± 3	−16 ± 4
Diastolic BP	−10 ± 3	−12 ± 3	−17 ± 3	−20 ± 2
Heart rate	−2 ± 3	−1 ± 1	+3 ± 2	+12 ± 3
1 Hour of Infusion*				
Systolic BP	−5 ± 3	−9 ± 4	−19 ± 4	−22 ± 4
Diastolic BP	−8 ± 3	−13 ± 3	−18 ± 2	−23 ± 2
Heart rate	−1 ± 3	0 ± 2	+3 ± 2	+11 ± 3
4 Hours of Infusion*				
Systolic BP	−14 ± 4	−20 ± 5	−23 ± 4	−37 ± 4
Diastolic BP	−12 ± 3	−18 ± 3	−21 ± 3	−29 ± 3
Heart rate	−2 ± 4	0 ± 2	+4 ± 2	+11 ± 2

* Mean change from baseline ± S.E.

Table 4
ADVERSE EVENTS* FROM FIXED-DOSE INFUSION STUDIES BY DOSE GROUP

Body System	Event	Placebo (n = 7)	0.01 (n = 26)	0.03-0.04 (n = 31)	0.1 (n = 28)	0.3-0.4 (n = 29)	0.6-0.8 (n = 11)
		CORLOPAM Doses (µg/kg/min)					
Body, General	Headache	1	5	4	7	8	6
	Injection site reaction	0	1	3	0	3	2
	ST-T abnormalities (primarily T-wave inversion)	0	2	4	0	1	0
	Flushing	0	0	0	0	1	3
Cardiovascular	Hypotension**	0	0	0	2	0	2
	Postural hypotension	0	2	0	0	0	0
	Tachycardia**	0	0	0	0	0	2
	Nausea	0	3	0	3	5	4
	Vomiting	0	2	0	2	1	2
Digestive	Abdominal pain/ fullness	0	2	0	0	2	1
	Constipation	0	0	0	0	0	2
	Diarrhea	0	0	0	0	2	0
Metabolic and Nutritional	Increased creatinine**	0	0	2	0	0	0
	Hypokalemia**	0	2	0	0	1	0
	Nervousness/ anxiety	0	0	1	0	0	2
Nervous	Insomnia	0	2	0	0	0	0
	Dizziness	0	1	1	2	2	0
Respiratory	Nasal congestion	0	0	0	0	0	2
Skin and Appendages	Sweating	0	0	0	1	1	2
Urogenital	Urinary tract infection	0	2	0	1	0	0
Musculoskeletal	Back pain	0	1	0	1	2	2

* Includes events reported by 2 or more patients receiving CORLOPAM treatment across all dose groups.
** Investigator defined; no protocol definition.

Table 5
INFUSION RATES (mL/min) TO ACHIEVE A GIVEN DRUG DOSE RATE (µg/kg/min)

Body Weight (kg)	0.025 µg/kg/min	0.05 µg/kg/min	0.1 µg/kg/min	0.2 µg/kg/min	0.3 µg/kg/min
	Drug Dose Rate				
	Infusion Rates (mL/min)				
40	0.025	0.05	0.10	0.20	0.30
50	0.031	0.06	0.13	0.25	0.38
60	0.038	0.08	0.15	0.30	0.45
70	0.044	0.09	0.18	0.35	0.53
80	0.050	0.10	0.20	0.40	0.60
90	0.056	0.11	0.23	0.45	0.68
100	0.063	0.13	0.25	0.50	0.75
110	0.069	0.14	0.28	0.55	0.83
120	0.075	0.15	0.30	0.60	0.90
130	0.081	0.16	0.33	0.65	0.98
140	0.088	0.18	0.35	0.70	1.05
150	0.094	0.19	0.38	0.75	1.13

should be discarded. Parenteral products should be inspected visually. If particulate matter or cloudiness is observed, the drug should be discarded.

HOW SUPPLIED

Ampules: 10 mg/mL in single-dose ampules of 5 mL, in packages of one. NDC 62860-0003-1

10 mg/mL in single-dose ampules of 2 mL, in packages of one. NDC 62860-0002-2
10 mg/mL in single-dose ampules of 1 mL, in packages of one. NDC 62860-0004-1

Store at 2–30° C.
© Neurex Corporation, December, 1997
Shown in Product Identification Guide, page 324

Neutrogena Dermatologics
5760 WEST 96th STREET
LOS ANGELES, CA 90045

Direct Inquiries to:
Diane Foster
(310) 642-1150
FAX: (310) 337-2156
For Medical Information Contact:
In Emergencies:
Kamran Mather, Ph.D.
(310) 642-1150
FAX: (310) 216-5399

MELANEX®   ℞
Topical Solution
(Hydroquinone USP, 3.0%)
FOR EXTERNAL USE ONLY

CAUTION: Federal law prohibits dispensing without prescription.

DESCRIPTION

Each milliliter of Melanex® Topical Solution contains 30 mg of hydroquinone in a hydroalcoholic base of purified water, SD Alcohol 40 (45%), Laureth-4, Isopropyl Alcohol (4%), Propylene Glycol, Ascorbic Acid.

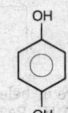

$C_6H_6O_2$ 110.11
1,4 DIHYDROXYBENZENE
Hydroquinone

CLINICAL PHARMACOLOGY

It has been suggested the primary action of hydroquinone is directed at tyrosinase.[1] The selective inhibition of the enzyme affects melanogenesis in the melanocytes resulting in cessation of melanin formation and subsequent reduction in pigmentation. Additional studies indicate hydroquinone acts on the essential subcellular metabolic processes of melanocytes with resultant cytolysis, i.e., non-enzyme-mediated depigmentation.[2]

INDICATIONS AND USAGE

Melanex® is indicated in the temporary depigmentation of hyperpigmented skin conditions such as chloasma, melasma, freckles, senile lentigines, and other forms of melanin hyperpigmentation.

DOSAGE AND ADMINISTRATION

Apply to affected areas twice daily, in the morning and before bedtime. During the day, an effective broad spectrum sunscreen like Neutrogena® Sunblock SPF 15 or SPF 30 should be used and unnecessary solar exposure avoided, or protective clothing should be worn to cover the treated area in order to prevent repigmentation from occurring.

CONTRAINDICATIONS

Melanex® is contraindicated in persons who have shown hypersensitivity to hydroquinone or any of the other ingredients. The safety of topical treatment with hydroquinone during pregnancy has not been established.

PRECAUTIONS

Concurrent use of Melanex® with peroxide products may result in transient dark staining of skin areas so treated. This is due to the oxidation of hydroquinone by the peroxide. This transient staining can be removed by discontinuing concurrent usage and normal soap cleansing.

FOR EXTERNAL USE ONLY

Hydroquinone preparations may produce skin irritation in susceptible individuals and have a slight potential to produce allergic response. Therefore, the physician should use appropriate caution. If rash or irritation develops, discontinue use and consult physician. Do not use on children under 12 years.

If no improvement is seen after two months of treatment, use of product should be discontinued. Avoid contact with eyes. In case of accidental contact, patient should rinse eyes thoroughly with water and contact physician. A bitter taste and anesthetic effect may occur if applied to lips. Keep out of reach of children. Use of Melanex® in paranasal and infraorbital areas increases the chance of irritation (see **ADVERSE REACTIONS**).

Continued on next page

Melanex—Cont.

ADVERSE REACTIONS

The following have been reported: dryness and fissuring of the paranasal and infraorbital areas, erythema, and stinging. Hydroquinone has been known to produce irritation and sensitization in susceptible individuals.

HOW SUPPLIED: 1 fl. oz. (30 ML) bottle with plastic rod and Appliderm® Applicator unit.

NOTE: Slight darkening of the Melanex® solution is normal and will not affect potency. See expiration date on bottle.

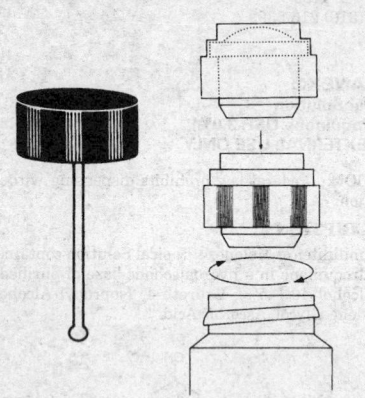

Store at room temperature or below. Avoid excessive heat.
(1) JIMBOW K., OBATHA H., PATHAK M., FITZPATRICK T.B. Mechanism and Depigmentation of Hydroquinone, Journal of Investigative Dermatology 1974, 62:436–449.
(2) op. cit.
For additional information please call:
Neutrogena Technical Department toll-free (800) 421-6857; in California call (800) 649-1150.
NDC 10812-930-01
Distributed by
Neutrogena Dermatologics
5760 W. 96th St.
Los Angeles, CA 90045
Shown in Product Identification Guide, page 324

NeXstar Pharmaceuticals, Inc.
**650 CLIFFSIDE DRIVE
SAN DIMAS, CA 91773 USA**

For Medical Inquiries:
800-403-3945
Customer Service
800-403-3945

DAUNOXOME®   ℞
(daunorubicin citrate liposome injection)

WARNINGS

1. Cardiac function should be monitored regularly in patients receiving DaunoXome because of the potential risk for cardiac toxicity and congestive heart failure. Cardiac monitoring is advised especially in those patients who have received prior anthracyclines or who have pre-existing cardiac disease.
1. Severe myelosuppression may occur.
2. DaunoXome should be administered only under the supervision of a physician who is experienced in the use of cancer chemotherapeutic agents.
3. Dosage should be reduced in patients with impaired hepatic function. **(See DOSAGE AND ADMINISTRATION)**
4. A triad of back pain, flushing, and chest tightness has been reported in 13.8% of the patients (16/116) treated with DaunoXome in the Phase III clinical trial, and in 2.7% of treatment cycles (27/994). This triad generally occurs during the first five minutes of the infusion, subsides with interruption of the infusion, and generally does not recur if the infusion is then resumed at a slower rate.

DESCRIPTION

DaunoXome is a sterile, pyrogen-free, preservative-free product in a single use vial for intravenous infusion.

DaunoXome contains an aqueous solution of the citrate salt of daunorubicin encapsulated within lipid vesicles (liposomes) composed of a lipid bilayer of distearoylphosphatidylcholine and cholesterol (2:1 molar ratio), with a mean diameter of about 45 nm. The lipid to drug weight ratio is 18.7:1 (total lipid:daunorubicin base), equivalent to a 10:5:1 molar ratio of distearoylphosphatidylcholine:cholesterol: daunorubicin. Daunorubicin is an anthracycline antibiotic with antineoplastic activity, originally obtained from *Streptomyces peucetius*. Daunorubicin has a 4-ring anthracycline moiety linked by a glycosidic bond to daunosamine, an amino sugar. Daunorubicin may also be isolated from *Streptomyces coeruleorubidus* and has the following chemical name: (8S-cis)-8-acetyl-10-[(3-amino-2,3,6-trideoxy-α-L-lyxo-hexopyranosyl)oxy]-7,8,9,10-tetrahydro-6,8,11-trihydroxy-1-methoxy-5,12-naphthacenedione hydrochloride. Daunorubicin citrate has the following chemical structure:

DSPC (distearoylphosphatidylcholine) has the following chemical structure:

The following represents the idealized, spherical morphology of a liposome:

This represents the aqueous core that contains daunorubicin citrate.

The diameter of the liposomes in DaunoXome is between 35 and 65 nm.

⊸ represents a molecule of DSPC.

Note: Liposomal encapsulation can substantially affect a drug's functional properties relative to those of the unencapsulated drug.

In addition, different liposomal drug products may vary from one another in the chemical composition and physical form of the liposomes. Such differences can substantially affect the functional properties of liposomal drug products. Each vial contains daunorubicin citrate equivalent to 50 mg of daunorubicin base, encapsulated in liposomes consisting of 701 mg distearoylphosphatidylcholine and 171 mg cholesterol. The liposomes encapsulating daunorubicin are dispersed in an aqueous medium containing 2, 125 mg sucrose, 94 mg glycine, and 7 mg calcium chloride dihydrate in a total volume of 25 mL/vial. The pH of the dispersion is between 4.9 and 6.0. The liposome dispersion should appear red and translucent.

CLINICAL PHARMACOLOGY

Mechanism of Action
DaunoXome is a liposomal preparation of daunorubicin formulated to maximize the selectivity of daunorubicin for solid tumors *in situ*. While in the circulation, the DaunoXome formulation helps to protect the entrapped daunorubicin from chemical and enzymatic degradation, minimizes protein binding, and generally decreases uptake by normal (non-reticuloendothelial system) tissues. The specific mechanism by which DaunoXome is able to deliver daunorubicin to solid tumors *in situ* is not known. However, it is believed to be a function of increased permeability of the tumor neovasculature to some particles in the size range of

DaunoXome. In animal studies, daunorubicin has been shown to accumulate in tumors to a greater extent when administered as DaunoXome than when administered as daunorubicin. Once within the tumor environment, daunorubicin is released over time enabling it to exert its antineoplastic activity.

Pharmacokinetics
Following intravenous injection of DaunoXome, plasma clearance of daunorubicin shows monoexponential decline. The pharmacokinetic parameter values for total daunorubicin following a single 40 mg/m^2 dose of DaunoXome administered over a 30–60 minute period to patients with AIDS-related Kaposi's sarcoma and following a single rapid intravenous, 80 mg/m^2 dose of conventional daunorubicin to patients with disseminated solid malignancies are shown in Table 1.

TABLE 1
PHARMACOKINETIC PARAMETERS OF DAUNOXOME IN AIDS PATIENTS WITH KAPOSI'S SARCOMA AND REPORTED PARAMETERS FOR CONVENTIONAL DAUNORUBICIN

Parameter (units)	[a]DaunoXome	[b]Conventional Daunorubicin
Plasma Clearance (mL/min)	17.3 ±6.1	[c]236 ±181
Volume of Distribution (L)	6.4 ±1.5	1006 ±622
Distribution Half-Life (h)	4.41 ±2.33	0.77 ±0.3
Elimination Half-Life (h)	—	55.4 ±13.7

[a]N=30, [b]N=4, [c] Calculated

The plasma pharmacokinetics of DaunoXome differ significantly from the results reported for conventional daunorubicin hydrochloride. DaunoXome has a small steady-state volume of distribution 6.4 L, (probably because it is confined to vascular fluid volume), and clearance of 17 mL/min. These differences in the volume of distribution and clearance result in a higher daunorubicin exposure (in terms of plasma AUC) from DaunoXome than with conventional daunorubicin hydrochloride. The apparent elimination half-life of DaunoXome is 4.4 hours, far shorter than that of daunorubicin, and probably represents a distribution half-life. Although preclinical biodistribution data in animals suggest that DaunoXome crosses the normal blood-brain barrier, it is unknown whether DaunoXome crosses the blood-brain barrier in humans.

Metabolism: Daunorubicinol, the major active metabolite of daunorubicin, was detected at low levels in the plasma following intravenous administration of DaunoXome.

No formal assessments of pharmacokinetic drug-drug interactions between DaunoXome and other agents have been conducted.

Special Populations: The pharmacokinetics of DaunoXome have not been evaluated in women, in different ethnic groups, or in subjects with renal and hepatic insufficiency.

Clinical Study
In an open-label, randomized, controlled clinical study conducted at 13 centers in the U.S.A. and Canada in advanced (25 or more mucocutaneous lesions; the development of 10 or more lesions in a one month period of time; symptomatic visceral involvement; or tumor-associated edema) HIV-related Kaposi's sarcoma, two treatment regimens were compared as first line cytotoxic therapy: DaunoXome 40 mg/m^2 and ABV (doxorubicin (Adriamycin®*) 10 mg/m^2, bleomycin 15 U, and vincristine 1.0 mg). All drugs were administered intravenously every 2 weeks. Responses were assessed using the AIDS Clinical Trials Group Oncology Committee of the National Institute of Allergy and Infectious Diseases (ACTG) criteria (a response required at least one of any of the following for at least 28 days; a. ≥50% reduction in the number; b. ≥50% reduction in the sums of the products of the largest perpendicular diameters of bidimensionally measurable marker lesions; or c. complete flattening of ≥50% of all previously raised lesions). Table II summarizes the efficacy results.
*Andriamycin is a registered trademark of Adria Laboratories, Columbus, OH.

TABLE II
EFFICACY DATA
FIRST LINE CYTOTOXIC THERAPY FOR ADVANCED KAPOSI'S SARCOMA

	DaunoXome n=116	ABV n=111
Response Rate	23%*	30%
Duration of Response, Median	110 days**	113 days

Time to Progression, Median	92 days***	105 days
Survival	342 days****	291 days

* The 95% confidence interval for difference in the response rates (ABV - DaunoXome) was [−5%, 18%]

** The hazard ratio (ABV/DaunoXome) for duration of response was 0.80, and the 95% confidence intervals were (0.44, 1.46)

*** The hazard ratio (ABV/DaunoXome) for time to progression was 0.78, and the 95% confidence intervals were (0.57, 1.07)

**** The hazard ratio for mortality (ABV/DaunoXome) was 1.29, and 95% confidence intervals were (0.92, 1.79)

Twenty of the 33 ABV responders responded to therapy by criteria more stringent than flattening of lesions (i.e., shrinkage of lesions and/or reduction in the number of lesions). Eleven of the 27 DaunoXome responders responded to therapy by criteria other than flattening of lesions. Photographic evidence of tumor response to DaunoXome and ABV was comparable across all anatomic sites (e.g., face, oral cavity, trunk, legs, and feet).

INDICATIONS AND USAGE

DaunoXome is indicated as a first line cytotoxic therapy for advanced HIV-associated Kaposi's sarcoma. DaunoXome is not recommended in patients with less than advanced HIV-related Kaposi's sarcoma.

CONTRAINDICATIONS

Therapy with DaunoXome is contraindicated in patients who have experienced a serious hypersensitivity reaction to previous doses of DaunoXome or to any of its constituents.

WARNINGS

DaunoXome is intended for administration under the supervision of a physician who is experienced in the use of cancer chemotherapeutic agents.

The primary toxicity of DaunoXome is myelosuppression, especially of the granulocytic series, which may be severe, with much less marked effects on the platelets and erythroid series. Careful hematologic monitoring is required and since patients with HIV infection are immunocompromised, patients must be observed carefully for evidence of intercurrent or opportunistic infections.

Special attention must be given to the potential cardiac toxicity of DaunoXome, particularly in patients who have received prior anthracyclines or who have pre-existing cardiac disease. Although there is no reliable means of predicting congestive heart failure, cardiomyopathy induced by anthracyclines is usually associated with a decrease of the left ventricular ejection fraction (LVEF). Cardiac function should be evaluated in each patient by means of a history and physical examination before each course of DaunoXome and determination of LVEF should be performed at total cumulative doses of DaunoXome of 320 mg/m^2, 480 mg/m^2 and every 240 mg/m^2 thereafter.

A triad of back pain, flushing, and chest tightness has been reported in 13.8% of the patients (16/116) treated with DaunoXome in the randomized clinical trial and in 2.7% of treatment cycles (27/994). This triad generally occurs during the first five minutes of the infusion, subsides with interruption of the infusion, and generally does not recur if the infusion is then resumed at a slower rate. This combination of symptoms appears to be related to the lipid component of DaunoXome, as a similar set of signs and symptoms has been observed with other liposomal products not containing daunorubicin.

Daunorubicin has been associated with local tissue necrosis at the site of drug extravasation. Although no such local tissue necrosis has been observed with DaunoXome, care should be taken to ensure that there is no extravasation of drug when DaunoXome is administered.

Dosage should be reduced in patients with impaired hepatic function. (See DOSAGE AND ADMINISTRATION)

Pregnancy Category D

DaunoXome can cause fetal harm when administered to a pregnant woman. DaunoXome was administered to rats on gestation days 6 through 15 at 0.3, 1.0 or 2.0 mg/kg/day, (about 1/20th, 1/6th, or 1/3rd the recommended human dose on a mg/m^2 basis). DaunoXome produced severe maternal toxicity and embryolethality at 2.0 mg/kg/day and was embryotoxic and caused fetal malformations (anophthalmia, microphthalmia, incomplete ossification) at 0.3 mg/kg/day. Embryotoxicity was characterized by increased embryofetal deaths, reduced number of litters, and reduced litter sizes.

There are no studies of DaunoXome in pregnant women. If DaunoXome is used during pregnancy, or if the patient becomes pregnant while taking DaunoXome, the patient must be warned of the potential hazard to the fetus. Patients should be advised to avoid becoming pregnant while taking DaunoXome.

PRECAUTIONS
Drug Interactions
In the patient population studied, DaunoXome has been administered to patients receiving a variety of concomitant medications (e.g., antiretroviral agents, antiviral agents, anti-infective agents). Although interactions of DaunoXome with other drugs have not been observed, no systematic studies of interactions have been conducted.

Carcinogenesis, Mutagenesis, and Impairment of Fertility
No carcinogenesis, mutagenesis, or impairment of fertility studies were conducted with DaunoXome.

Carcinogenesis: Carcinogenicity and mutagenicity studies have been conducted with daunorubicin, the active component of DaunoXome. A high incidence of mammary tumors was observed about 120 days after a single intravenous dose of 12.5 mg/kg daunorubicin in rats (about 2 times the human dose on a mg/m^2 basis). Mutagenesis: Daunorubicin was mutagenic in in vitro tests (Ames assay, V79 hamster cell assay), and clastogenic in in vitro (CCRFCEM human lymphoblasts) and in in vivo (SCE assay in mouse bone marrow) tests. Impairment of Fertility: Daunorubicin intravenous doses of 0.25 mg/kg/day (about 8 times the human dose on a mg/m^2 basis) in male dogs caused testicular atrophy and total aplasia of spermatocytes in the seminiferous tubules.

Pregnancy
Pregnancy "Category D". See WARNINGS Section.

Pediatric Use
Safety and effectiveness in pediatric patients have not been established.

Use in the Elderly
Safety and effectiveness in the elderly have not been established.

Special Populations
Safety has not been established in patients with pre-existing hepatic or renal dysfunction.

ADVERSE REACTIONS

DaunoXome contains daunorubicin, encapsulated within a liposome. Conventional daunorubicin has acute myelosuppression as its dose limiting side effect, with the greatest effect on the granulocytic series. In addition, daunorubicin causes alopecia, and nausea and vomiting in a significant number of patients treated. Extravasation of conventional daunorubicin can cause severe local tissue necrosis. Chronic therapy at total doses above 300 mg/m^2 causes a cumulative-dose-related cardiomyopathy with congestive heart failure.

Administered as DaunoXome, daunorubicin has substantially altered pharmacokinetics and some differences in toxicity. The most important acute toxicity of DaunoXome remains myelosuppression, principally of the granulocytic series, with much less marked effects on the platelets and erythroid series.

In an open-label, randomized, controlled clinical trial conducted in 13 centers in the U.S.A. and Canada in advanced HIV-related Kaposi's sarcoma, two treatment regimens were compared as first line cytotoxic therapy: DaunoXome and ABV (doxorubicin (Adriamycin®*), bleomycin, and vincristine). All drugs were administered intravenously every 2 weeks. The safety data presented below include all reported or observed adverse experiences, including those not considered to be drug related. Patients with advanced HIV-associated Kaposi's sarcoma are seriously ill due to their underlying infection and are receiving several concomitant medications including potentially toxic antiviral and antiretroviral agents. The contribution of the study drugs to the adverse experience profile is therefore difficult to establish.

Table III summarizes the important safety data.

TABLE III
SUMMARY OF IMPORTANT SAFETY DATA

	DaunoXome (N=116) % of patients	ABV (N=111) % of patients
Neutropenia (<1000 cells/mm^3)	36%	35%
Neutropenia (<500 cells/mm^3)	15%	5%
Opportunistic Infections/ Illnesses, % of patients	40%	27%
Median time to first Opportunistic Infections/ Illnesses	214 days	412 days**
Number of cases with absolute reduction in ejection fraction of 20–25%*	3	1
Number of cases removed from therapy due to cardiac causes*	2	0
Alopecia All grades % of patients	8%	36%***
Neuropathy All grades % of patients	13%	41%***

* The denominator is uncertain since there were several instances of missing repeat cardiac evaluations

** p=0.21

*** p<0.001

A triad of back pain, flushing and chest tightness was reported in 13.8% of the patients (16/116) treated with DaunoXome in the Phase III clinical trial and in 2.7% of treatment cycles (27/994). Most of the episodes were mild to moderate in severity (12% of patients and 2.5% of treatment cycles).

Mild alopecia was reported in 6% of patients treated with DaunoXome and moderate alopecia in 2% of patients. Mild nausea was reported in 35% of DaunoXome patients, moderate nausea in 16% of patients and severe nausea in 3% of patients. For patients treated with DaunoXome, mild vomiting was reported in 10%, moderate in 10%, and severe in 3% of patients. Although grade 3–4 injection site inflammation was reported in 2 patients treated with DaunoXome, no instances of local tissue necrosis were observed with extravasation.

Table IV is a listing of all the mild-moderate and severe adverse events reported on both treatment arms in Protocol 103-09 in ≥5% of DaunoXome patients.

TABLE IV
ADVERSE EXPERIENCES: PROTOCOL 103–09

	DaunoXome (N=116)		ABV (N=111)	
	Mild Moderate	Severe	Mild Moderate	Severe
Nausea	51%	3%	45%	5%
Fatigue	43%	6%	44%	7%
Fever	42%	5%	49%	5%
Diarrhea	34%	4%	29%	6%
Cough	26%	2%	19%	0%
Dyspnea	23%	3%	17%	3%
Headache	22%	3%	23%	2%
Allergic Reactions	21%	3%	19%	2%
Abdominal Pain	20%	3%	23%	4%
Anorexia	21%	2%	26%	2%
Vomiting	20%	3%	26%	2%
Rigors	19%	0%	23%	0%
Back Pain	16%	0%	8%	0%
Increased Sweating	12%	2%	12%	0%
Neuropathy	12%	1%	38%	3%
Rhinitis	12%	0%	6%	0%
Edema	9%	2%	8%	1%
Chest Pain	9%	1%	7%	0%
Depression	7%	3%	6%	0%
Malaise	9%	1%	11%	1%
Stomatitis	9%	1%	8%	0%
Alopecia	8%	0%	36%	0%
Dizziness	8%	0%	9%	0%
Sinusitis	8%	0%	5%	1%
Arthralgia	7%	0%	6%	0%
Constipation	7%	0%	18%	0%

DaunoXome—Cont.

Myalgia	7%	0%	12%	0%
Pruritus	7%	0%	14%	0%
Insomnia	6%	0%	14%	0%
Influenza-like symptoms	5%	0%	5%	0%
Tenesmus	4%	1%	1%	0%
Abnormal vision	3%	2%	3%	0%

The following adverse events were reported in ≤5% of patients treated with DaunoXome, tabulated by body system.
Body As A Whole: Infection site inflammation
Cardiovascular: Hot flushes, hypertension, palpitation, syncope, tachycardia
Digestive: Increased appetite, dysphagia, GI hemorrhage, gastritis, gingival bleeding, hemorrhoids, hepatomegaly, melena, dry mouth, tooth caries
Hemic and Lymphatic: Lymphadenopathy, splenomegaly
Metabolic and Nutritional: Dehydration, thirst
Nervous: Amnesia, anxiety, ataxia, confusion, convulsions, emotional liability, abnormal gait, hallucination, hyperkinesia, hypertonia, meningitis, somnolence, abnormal thinking, tremor
Respiratory: Hemoptysis, hiccups, pulmonary infiltration, increased sputum
Skin: Folliculitis, seborrhea, dry skin
Special Senses: Conjunctivitis, deafness, earache, eye pain, taste perversion, tinnitus
Urogenital: Dysuria, nocturia, polyuria

OVERDOSAGE
The symptoms of acute overdosage are increased severities of the observed dose-limiting toxicities of therapeutic doses of DaunoXome, myelosuppression (especially granulocytopenia), fatigue, and nausea and vomiting.

DOSAGE AND ADMINISTRATION
DaunoXome should be administered intravenously over a 60 minute period at a dose of 40 mg/m^2, with doses repeated every two weeks. Blood counts should be repeated prior to each dose, and therapy withheld if the absolute granulocyte count is less than 750 cells/mm^3. Treatment should be continued until there is evidence of progressive disease (e.g., based on best response achieved: new visceral sites of involvement, or progression of visceral disease; development of 10 or more new, cutaneous lesions or a 25% increase in the number of lesions compared to baseline; a change in the character of 25% or more of all previously counted flat lesions to raised; increase in surface area of the indicator lesions), or until other intercurrent complications of HIV disease preclude continuation of therapy.
Patients with Impaired Hepatic and Renal Function
Limited clinical experience exists in treating hepatically and renally impaired patients with DaunoXome.
Therefore, based on experience with daunorubicin HCl, it is recommended that the dosage of DaunoXome *be reduced* if the bilirubin or creatinine is elevated as follows: Serum bilirubin 1.2 to 3 mg/dL, give $^3/_4$ the normal dose; serum bilirubin or creatinine >3 mg/dL, give $^1/_2$ the normal dose. Do not mix DaunoXome with other drugs.
Preparation Of Solution
DaunoXome should be diluted 1:1 with 5% Dextrose Injection (D5W) before administration. Each vial of DaunoXome contains daunorubicin citrate equivalent to 50 mg daunorubicin base, at a concentration of 2 mg/mL. The recommended concentration after dilution is 1 mg daunorubicin/mL of solution.
Use aseptic technique.
Aseptic technique must be strictly observed in all handling, since no preservative or bacteriostatic agent is present in DaunoXome or in the materials recommended for dilution. Withdraw the calculated volume of DaunoXome from the vial into a sterile syringe, and transfer it into a sterile infusion bag containing an equivalent amount of D5W. Administer diluted DaunoXome immediately. If not used immediately, diluted DaunoXome should be stored refrigerated at 2°–8°C (36°–46°F) for a maximum of 6 hours
Caution: The only fluid which may be mixed with DaunoXome is D5W; DaunoXome must not be mixed with saline, bacteriostatic agents such as benzyl alcohol, or any other solution.
Do not use an in-line filter for the intravenous infusion of DaunoXome.
All parenteral drug products should be inspected visually for particulate matter and discoloration prior to administration, whenever solution and container permit. DaunoXome is a translucent dispersion of liposomes that scatters light to some degree. Do not use DaunoXome if it appears opaque, or has precipitate or foreign matter present.

Procedures for proper handling and disposal of anticancer drugs should be followed.[1–7]

HOW SUPPLIED
DaunoXome is a translucent, red, liposomal dispersion supplied in single use vials, each sealed with a synthetic rubber stopper and aluminum sealing ring with a plastic cap. DaunoXome provides daunorubicin citrate equivalent to 50 mg of daunorubicin base, at a concentration of 2 mg/mL. DaunoXome is supplied under NDC 56146-0301-1 for a single unit pack, NDC 56146-0301-4 for a 4-unit pack, and NDC 56146-0301-0 for a 10-unit pack.
Storage
Store DaunoXome in a refrigerator, 2°–8°C (36°–46°F). Do not freeze. Protect from light.
U.S. PATENT NUMBERS
The United States Patent Numbers applicable to DaunoXome are: 5,441,745; 5,435,989; 5,019,369; 4,946,683; 4,753,788; and additional patents pending.

REFERENCES
1. Recommendations for the Safe Handling of Parenteral Antineoplastic Drugs. NIH Publication No. 83-2621. For sale by the Superintendent of Documents, US Government Printing Office, Washington, DC 20402.
2. AMA Council Report, Guidelines for Handling Parenteral Antineoplastics. JAMA 1985; 253(11): 1590-1592.
3. National Study Commission on Cytotoxic Exposure–Recommendations for Handling Cytotoxic Agents. Available from Louis P. Jeffrey, Sc.D., Chairman, National Study Commission on Cytotoxic Exposure Massachusetts College of Pharmacy and Allied Health Sciences, 179 Longwood Avenue, Boston, Massachusetts 02115.
4. Clinical Oncological Society of Australia. Guidelines and Recommendations for Safe Handling of Antineoplastic Agents. Med. J. Australia 1983; 1: 426-428.
5. Jones RB, et al; Safe Handling of Chemotherapeutic Agents: A report from the Mount Sinai Medical Center. CA-A Cancer Journal for Clinicians 1983; (Sept/Oct) 258-263.
6. American Society of Hospital Pharmacists Technical Assistance Bulletin on Handling Cytotoxic and Hazardous Drugs. Am. J. Hosp. Pharm. 1990; 47: 1033-1049.
7. OSHA Work-Practice Guidelines for Personnel Dealing with Cytotoxic (Antineoplastic) Drugs. Am. J. Hosp. Pharm. 1986; 43: 1193-1204.

NEXSTAR   P0098
Pharmaceuticals, Inc.   rev. 4/96
NeXstar Pharmaceuticals, Inc.
650 Cliffside Drive • San Dimas, CA 91773 USA
DaunoXome is a registered trademark of NeXstar Pharmaceuticals, Inc.
Copyright 1996, NeXstar Pharmaceuticals, Inc.
All rights reserved.

Niche Pharmaceuticals, Inc.
P.O. BOX 449
200 N. OAK STREET
ROANOKE, TX 76262

Direct Inquiries to:
Steve F. Brandon
(817) 491-2770
FAX: (817) 491-3533

For Medical Information Contact:
In Emergencies:
Gerald L. Beckloff, M.D.
(817) 491-2770
FAX: (817) 491-3533

MAGTAB®SR   OTC
[măg-tăb]
(Magnesium L-lactate dihydrate)
Sustained release Magnesium Supplement

DESCRIPTION
MagTab®SR is a sustained release oral magnesium supplement. Each pale yellow caplets contain 7mEq (84 Mg) magnesium as magnesium L-lactate dihydrate *835 Mg in a sustained release wax matrix formulation).

INDICATIONS/USES
As a dietary supplement, MagTab®SR, is indicated for patients with, or at risk for, magnesium deficiency. Hypomagnesemia and/or magnesium deficiency can result from inadequate nutritional intake or absorption, magnesium depleting drugs such as diuretics, or alcoholism.

WARNINGS
Patients with renal disease should not take magnesium supplements without the advice and direct supervision of a physician. Excessive dosage of magnesium can cause loose stools or diarrhea.

DOSAGE
As a dietary supplement, take 1 or 2 caplets b.i.d. or as directed by a physician.

HOW SUPPLIED
MagTab®SR is available for oral administration as uncoated yellow caplets, in bottles of 60 and 100.
U.S. Patent Number: 5,002,774

UNIFIBER®   OTC
[uni fi' ber]
(Powdered Cellulose)
3 grams Fiber per tablespoon

DESCRIPTION
Unifiber is an all natural insoluble bulk fiber supplement that promotes normal bowel function by adding needed bulk to the diet. Unifiber contains powdered cellulose 75%, water 5%, corn syrup 19%, and xanthan gum 1%. Unifiber mixes easily with liquids or soft foods, and is tasteless, non-gelling, and pleasant to take. One tablespoon of Unifiber provides 3 grams of concentrated dietary fiber.
NUTRITION INFORMATION
Each 4 gram (1T) serving of Unifiber contains 3 grams of fiber, 4 calories, 0% fat, 0% cholesterol, 0% protein, and is free of all electrolytes.

INDICATION/USES
As a dietary supplement, Unifiber is indicated for patients needing a concentrated source of fiber to help maintain and promote normal bowel function. Because Unifiber is electrolyte free and contains no excitoxins, it is an ideal fiber supplement for patients on a restricted diet, such as the OB patient, kidney patients on dialysis, diabetic patients, and the elderly.

CONTRAINDICATIONS
Intestinal obstruction or fecal impaction.

DOSAGE
Adults: Stir one tablespoon into a glass with 3 or 4 ounces of fruit juice, milk, or water; or mix with soft foods such as applesauce, mashed potatoes, or pudding. Can be taken up to 3 times daily if needed, or as recommended by a doctor. Generally produces effect in 12–72 hours.
Tube Feedings: Mix one tablespoon in 30–60 cc of water.
Children (6 to 12 years): ½ dose 2 or 3 times daily.

HOW SUPPLIED
Unifiber is available over the counter in powder containers of 5 oz (35 servings), 9 oz (63 servings), or 16 oz (113 servings)

North American Vaccine, Inc.
10150 OLD COLUMBIA ROAD
COLUMBIA, MD 21046

Direct Inquiries to:
Ph: (301) 419-8400

CERTIVA™   ℞
Diphtheria and Tetanus Toxoids and Acellular Pertussis Vaccine Adsorbed

DESCRIPTION
Certiva™ (Diphtheria and Tetanus Toxoids and Acellular Pertussis Vaccine Adsorbed) is a sterile combination of diphtheria, tetanus, and pertussis toxoids (one pertussis antigen, inactivated pertussis toxin) adsorbed onto aluminum hydroxide.[1] It is intended for intramuscular injection only. After shaking, Certiva™ is a homogeneous white suspension.
The pertussis toxin (PT) is isolated from Phase 1 *Bordetella pertussis* grown in modified Stainer-Scholte medium. After purification by affinity chromatography, which includes the use of fetuin, a bovine serum protein, as an affinity ligand, PT is detoxified using hydrogen peroxide.
Diphtheria toxin is derived from *Corynebacterium diphtheriae* grown in Stainer's Diphtheria Culture Medium, containing casein hydrolysate, and is purified by fractional precipitation with ammonium sulfate. Tetanus toxin is derived from *Clostridium tetani* grown in modified Mueller and Miller Medium, containing casein hydrolysate, and is purified

by precipitation with ammonium sulfate.[2] The purified diphtheria and tetanus toxins are detoxified using formaldehyde.

Each antigen is individually adsorbed onto aluminum hydroxide.[2] Each 0.5 ml dose of vaccine is formulated to contain 15 Lf diphtheria toxoid, 6 Lf tetanus toxoid, 40 mcg pertussis toxoid, 0.5 mg aluminum as aluminum hydroxide, and is preserved with 0.01% thimerosal (mercury derivative). The product may contain residual fetuin. The residual free formaldehyde content by assay is less than or equal to 10 ppm. The diphtheria and tetanus toxoids each induce not less than 2 units of antitoxin per ml in the guinea pig potency test. The potency of the pertussis toxoid is evaluated by measurement of antibody titers to pertussis toxin in immunized mice using an ELISA.

Diphtheria and tetanus toxoid bulks for further manufacturing use are produced by Statens Seruminstitut, Copenhagen, Denmark. The pertussis toxoid is manufactured by North American Vaccine, Inc., Beltsville, Maryland. Final formulation and release of Certiva™ are conducted by North American Vaccine, Inc.

CLINICAL PHARMACOLOGY

Immunization against diphtheria, tetanus and pertussis, using a conventional whole-cell pertussis DTP vaccine (Diphtheria and Tetanus Toxoids and Pertussis Vaccine Adsorbed) has been routine practice during infancy and childhood in the United States since the late 1940s. Widespread immunization in the United States has played a major role in dramatically reducing the incidence of cases and deaths from each of these diseases.[3]

Diphtheria

Diphtheria is a disease resulting from infection of the respiratory tract or skin with *Corynebacterium diphtheriae*. The disease can be localized to the site of infection or can be associated with systemic toxicity, which may include myocarditis and neuritis and is caused by diphtheria exotoxin, an extracellular protein metabolite of toxigenic strains of *C. diphtheriae*. Humans are the only known reservoir for *C. diphtheriae*. More than 200,000 cases of diphtheria, primarily among children, were reported in the United States in 1921, before the general use of diphtheria toxoid vaccine.[3] Approximately 5–10% of cases were fatal; the highest case-fatality rates were in the very young and the elderly. Immunization programs with diphtheria toxoid introduced in the 1940's had a significant impact on the epidemiology of the disease. Only 24 cases of respiratory diphtheria were reported in the United States from 1980 to 1989, and 15 cases from 1990 to 1994; however, the case-fatality rate has remained constant at about 5–10%.[3,4] Although diphtheria is currently a rare disease in the United States, the disease has remained endemic in many developing countries and recent outbreaks have occurred in areas of the former Soviet Union.[5]

A complete vaccination series with diphtheria toxoid substantially reduces the risk and severity of disease, and protection is thought to last for at least 10 years.[3] Serum antitoxin concentrations of at least 0.01 antitoxin units per ml are generally regarded as protective.[6,7] Vaccination does not eliminate carriage of *C. diphtheriae* from the pharynx, nose, or skin.[3] Efficacy of the diphtheria toxoid used in Certiva™ was determined on the basis of immunogenicity studies, with a comparison to a serological correlate of protection (≥0.01 antitoxin units per ml) established by the Panel on Review of Bacterial Vaccines and Toxoids.[7] In a clinical study with Certiva™, 99.7% of 299 U.S. infants had protective titers to diphtheria toxin (≥0.01 antitoxin units per ml) in sera obtained one month after the third dose; vaccination at 2, 4, and 6 months of age.

Tetanus

Tetanus is a disease characterized by neuromuscular dysfunction resulting from the effects of a potent exotoxin elaborated by *Clostridium tetani*, a microorganism which is commonly found in the outdoor environment (usually soil). Persons with the disease exhibit muscular rigidity and spasms that can either be localized or generalized, depending on host factors and the site of inoculation. With the routine use of tetanus toxoid, the occurrence of tetanus in the United States has decreased markedly, from 560 reported cases in 1947 to an average of 57 cases reported annually from 1985-1994.[3,4] Tetanus in the United States is primarily a disease of older adults. Of 99 cases with complete information reported to the Centers for Disease Control and Prevention during 1987-1988, 68% were ≥50 years of age, only 6 were <20 years of age. No cases of neonatal tetanus were reported. Overall, the case fatality rate was 21%. The disease continues to occur almost exclusively among persons who are unvaccinated or inadequately vaccinated or whose vaccination histories are unknown or uncertain.[8]

Spores of *C. tetani* are ubiquitous. Serologic tests indicate that naturally acquired immunity to tetanus toxin does not occur in the United States. Thus, universal primary immunization with subsequent maintenance of adequate antitoxin levels by means of timed boosters is needed to protect all age groups.[3] Tetanus toxoid is a highly effective antigen, and a completed primary series generally induces protective levels of at least 0.01 antitoxin units per ml, a level which has been reported to be protective.[7] It is thought that protection persists for at least 10 years.[3,9] Efficacy of the tetanus toxoid in Certiva™ was determined on the basis of immunogenicity studies with a comparison to a serological correlate of protection (≥0.01 antitoxin units per ml) established by the Panel on Review of Bacterial Vaccines and Toxoids.[7] In a clinical study with Certiva™, 100% of 299 U.S. infants had a protective level of tetanus toxoid (≥0.01 antitoxin units per ml) in sera obtained one month after the third dose; vaccination at 2, 4, and 6 months of age.

TABLE 1

POSITIVE PERTUSSIS CULTURES IN THE GÖTEBORG REGION OF SWEDEN (1989–1997)

	Before Pertussis Immunization*						Period of Mass Immunization with Certiva™-EU and Pertussis Toxoid		
Month / *Year*	*1989–1990*	*1990–1991*	*1991–1992*	*1992–1993*	*1993–1994*	*1994–1995*	*1995–1996*	*1996–1997*	*1997–*
July	61	78	55	52	90	67	104	14	3
August	44	92	55	72	100	96	100	37	6
September	54	70	56	73	86	70	75	18	11
October	84	130	60	82	99	78	93	8	7
November	97	105	61	66	126	96	100	8	3
December	76	62	35	66	88	118	53	8	0
January	76	121	58	78	138	113	48	9	—
February	59	102	40	72	86	55	30	1	—
March	60	81	37	81	75	50	28	2	—
April	51	73	18	92	50	85	15	1	—
May	73	64	41	69	88	69	22	1	—
June	47	46	59	92	55	63	8	1	—
Total Positive	782	1024	575	895	1081	960	676	108	*30*
Total Cultures	3150	3801	2934	3608	4272	4105	2809	784	*299*

*National recommendation for routine pediatric pertussis vaccination reinstituted January 1996

Pertussis

Pertussis (whooping cough) is a disease of the respiratory tract caused by *Bordetella pertussis*. Pertussis is highly communicable (attack rates in unimmunized household contacts of up to 90% have been reported) and can cause severe disease, particularly among the very young.[3] Since immunization against pertussis became widespread, the number of reported cases and associated mortality in the United States have declined from an average annual incidence and mortality of 150 cases and 6 deaths per 100,000, respectively, in the early 1940's, to annual reported incidences of 1.6, 2.6, and 1.8 cases per 100,000 population in 1992, 1993, and 1994, respectively, and estimated annual incidences of 2.0 and 2.4 cases per 100,000 population for 1995 and 1996, respectively.[10,11] Precise epidemiologic data do not exist because bacteriological confirmation of pertussis can be obtained in less than half of the suspected cases. Most reported illness from *B. pertussis* occurs in infants and young children in whom complications can be severe. From 1980 to 1989, of 10,749 pertussis cases reported nationally in infants less than 1 year of age, 69% were hospitalized, 22% had pneumonia, 3% had seizures, 0.9% had encephalopathy, and 0.6% died.[12] Older children and adults, in whom classic signs are often absent, may go undiagnosed and may serve as reservoirs of disease.[13]

Routine vaccination with whole-cell DTP vaccine has significantly reduced pertussis-related morbidity and mortality. However, concerns regarding reactogenicity of whole-cell DTP vaccine have spurred development of safer pertussis vaccines. The role of different components produced by *B. pertussis* in either the pathogenesis of, or the immunity to, pertussis is not well understood. Certiva™-EU, which contains one pertussis antigen, pertussis toxoid, has been shown to be effective in preventing World Health Organization (WHO)-defined pertussis after three doses of vaccine administered at 3, 5, and 12 months of age.

Efficacy

Between 1991–1994, a double-blind, randomized, placebo-controlled efficacy trial of Certiva™-EU was conducted in Göteborg, Sweden, where pertussis is endemic and pertussis immunization had been stopped in 1979. Certiva™-EU contains the same amount of pertussis toxoid (40 mcg) per dose as Certiva™, but contains more diphtheria toxoid (25 Lf vs. 15 Lf) and more tetanus toxoid (7 Lf vs. 6 Lf) per dose than Certiva™. A total of 3,450 healthy infants from 96 Child Health Centers were randomized to receive Certiva™-EU (n=1,724) or Statens Seruminstitut Diphtheria and Tetanus Toxoids Adsorbed Vaccine (DT) (n=1,726) at 3, 5, and 12 months of age.[14,15] Cases of pertussis were identified by obtaining nasopharyngeal cultures for *B. pertussis* and acute and convalescent serum samples in all subjects and family members with coughing episodes lasting ≥ 7 days. Duration of cough and severity of symptoms were determined by telephone interview and/or office visit at approximately 4 weeks and again at 60 days after report of cough lasting ≥ 7 days.

The main observation period started 30 days after the third dose of vaccine and lasted a mean of 17 months. During this period, WHO-defined pertussis (paroxysmal cough for ≥ 21 days with one or more of the following: positive culture, positive culture in a family member, or a significant rise in serum PT-IgG or FHA-IgG) was identified in 72 (4.3%) of 1,682 Certiva™-EU recipients and 240 (14.3%) of 1,676 DT recipients.[14,15,16] Case rates per 100 person-years of follow-up were 2.89 in the Certiva™-EU group and 10.17 in the DT group. Starting one month after the third dose, the protective efficacy of Certiva™-EU against WHO-defined pertussis was 72% (95% CI: 62% to 78%). Protective efficacy against WHO-defined pertussis for the period starting 30 days after the second dose of vaccine up until administration of the third dose was 60% (95% CI: 13% to 83%) (10 cases in 1,708 Certiva™-EU recipients, 25 cases in 1,717 DT recipients).[15]

When the definition of pertussis was expanded to include clinically milder disease with respect to type and duration of cough, with infection confirmed by culture and/or serologic testing, the efficacy of Certiva™-EU during the main observation period was 63% (95% CI: 52% to 71%) against ≥ 21 days of any cough and 54% (95% CI: 43% to 64%) against ≥ 7 days of any cough.[14] After the main observation period, follow-up was continued for an additional 6 month period during which the study was unblinded. During this period the efficacy of Certiva™-EU remained high against WHO-defined pertussis at 77% (95% CI: 65% to 85%) in children whose median age was then 36.5 months.[15,17]

Protective efficacy was also estimated in vaccine recipients who had household exposure to WHO-defined pertussis during the main observation period. Nineteen (19) of 88 Certiva™-EU recipients and 50 of 63 DT recipients were identified with a secondary case of pertussis (defined as paroxysmal cough for ≥ 21 days with infection confirmed by culture and/or serologic testing and with an onset between 6–60 days after onset in the primary case). The protective efficacy of Certiva™-EU in preventing WHO-defined pertussis after household exposure was 73% (95% CI: 57% to 86%) based on comparing the proportion of exposed subjects who were identified with pertussis in each vaccine group.[15,18]

Effectiveness

An epidemiologic, open-label, Mass Vaccination Project was initiated in June 1995 in the Göteborg region of Sweden to study the safety and effectiveness of Certiva™-EU and pertussis toxoid vaccines in infants and children. Effectiveness was determined by regional surveillance of pertussis cultures. Nasopharyngeal cultures were obtained from coughing individuals of all ages with suspected pertussis at the discretion of their treating physician. Cultures were analyzed by the single regional reference laboratory (Department of Clinical Bacteriology, Sahlgrenska Hospital, Göteborg, Sweden) as part of an established surveillance system from which pertussis culture data have been generated and reported since 1976. Table 1 depicts the monthly positive pertussis cultures collected from July 1989 through December 1997 (two and one half years into the project). Between 1989 and 1994 (the period before initiation of the Mass Vaccination Project), the yearly number of positive pertussis cultures varied, ranging from 575 out of 2,934 total cultures to 1,081 out of 4,272 total cultures. By the second year of the Mass Vaccination Project (July 1996 - June 1997), a total of 108 out of 784 cultures were positive for pertussis, the majority from children not participating in the Project with the remainder from children having received at least 1 dose of

Continued on next page

Certiva—Cont.

vaccine. During the next 6 months (July 1997 - December 1997), 30 cultures out of a total of 299 were pertussis positive, the majority from children not participating in the Project.

[See table 1 at top of previous page]

Immune Response to Certiva™

In a study of Swedish infants comparing Certiva™ to Certiva™-EU, serum antibody levels to PT after three doses of Certiva™ administered at 2, 4, and 6 months of age (n=116) were significantly higher than those after two doses of Certiva™-EU administered at 3 and 5 months of age (n=103), but were significantly lower than those observed after three doses of Certiva™-EU administered at 3, 5, and 12 months of age (n=101).[15] The antibody response to PT after a fourth dose of Certiva™ administered at 15 months of age (n=114) was similar to that after the third dose of Certiva™-EU at 12 months of age (n=101).[15] In a study of U.S. infants, serum antibody titers to PT following four doses of Certiva™ administered at 2, 4, 6, and 15-21 months of age (n=89) were similar to those achieved following three doses of Certiva™-EU administered at 3, 5, and 12 months of age [subset of Swedish children from the efficacy trial (n=232)].[15] While a serologic correlate of protection for pertussis has not been established, the antibody response to PT in U.S. infants after doses of Certiva™ at 2, 4, 6, and 15-21 months of age was comparable to that achieved in Swedish infants in whom efficacy was demonstrated after three doses of Certiva™-EU at 3, 5, and 12 months of age.

Immune Response To Simultaneously Administered Vaccines

In a clinical study conducted in the United States, infants received Certiva™ at 2, 4, and 6 months of age, and at each time point, the majority were simultaneously immunized with *Haemophilus influenzae* type b conjugate vaccine (HibTITER, 96–99%), polio vaccine live oral (OPV) (83–97%), and hepatitis B vaccine (18–80%). Immune responses to these simultaneously administered vaccines were evaluated in a subset. After a third dose of OPV, 95–96% of infants had protective neutralizing antibody to poliovirus types 1 and 3 (n=219).[15] After the third dose of HibTITER, 61% of infants achieved anti-PRP antibody levels ≥ 1 mcg/ml (n=249), compared to 73% of infants (n=77) who received HibTITER simultaneously with whole-cell DTP in the same study; these rates (61% vs. 73%) are not significantly different (p=0.078), but the study design lacked statistical power (80%) to rule out a difference of 15% (α=5%). After two doses of hepatitis B vaccine administered concurrently with Certiva™, 99% had anti-HBsAg titers ≥ 10 mIU/ml (n=101)[15]; the total number of hepatitis B vaccine doses received by these infants is unknown, because the number of doses received prior to entry into the study at 2 months of age was not recorded.

One-hundred thirty-three (133) infants who received 3 doses of Certiva™ in the above study received a fourth dose of Certiva™ at 15-21 months of age and were simultaneously immunized with measles, mumps, and rubella (MMR) vaccine and HibTITER. Anti-PRP antibody levels ≥ 1.0 mcg/ml were achieved in 100% of subjects (n=84); antibodies to measles, mumps, and rubella were detected in 91-95% of subjects (n=55).[15]

In another study of 221 children who received Certiva™ at 4 to 6 years of age, 89% and 16% simultaneously received polio, and measles, mumps, and rubella vaccination, respectively. Antibodies to measles, mumps and rubella were detected in 100% of tested subjects (n=32) and neutralization titers to polio types 1, 2, and 3 were achieved in 99% of tested subjects (n=105; 102 with OPV and 3 with inactivated polio vaccine).[15]

INDICATIONS AND USAGE

Certiva™ is indicated for active immunization against diphtheria, tetanus, and pertussis (whooping cough) in infants and children 6 weeks to 7 years of age (prior to seventh birthday). Completion of a primary series of pertussis vaccination early in life is strongly recommended because of the substantial risks of complications of pertussis in infancy.[3]

This product is not recommended for immunizing persons on or after their seventh birthday (See **DOSAGE AND ADMINISTRATION**).

In instances where the pertussis vaccine component is contraindicated, Diphtheria and Tetanus Toxoids Adsorbed (For Pediatric Use) (DT) should be used for each of the remaining doses (See **CONTRAINDICATIONS**).

Tetanus Immune Globulin (Human TIG) and/or equine Diphtheria Antitoxin should be used if passive immunization is required.[3]

Individuals who have recovered from culture-confirmed pertussis do not need additional doses of Certiva™ but should receive additional doses of DT to complete the recommended immunization series.

Certiva™ is not to be used for treatment of actual infection with diphtheria, tetanus or pertussis.

As with any vaccine, vaccination with Certiva™ may not protect 100% of recipients.

CONTRAINDICATIONS

Hypersensitivity to any component of the vaccine, including thimerosal (a mercury derivative), is a contraindication (See **DESCRIPTION**).

It is a contraindication to use this vaccine after an immediate anaphylactic reaction temporally associated with a previous dose. Because of uncertainty as to which component of the vaccine might be responsible, no further vaccination with any diphtheria, tetanus or pertussis component should be carried out. Alternatively, because of the importance of tetanus vaccinations, such individuals may be referred for evaluation by an allergist.[3]

The decision to administer or delay vaccination because of a current or recent febrile illness depends largely on the severity of the symptoms and their etiology. Although a moderate or severe febrile illness is sufficient reason to postpone vaccinations, minor illnesses such as mild upper-respiratory infections with or without low-grade fever are not contraindications.[3,19,20,21,22]

Elective immunization procedures should be deferred during an outbreak of poliomyelitis.[23]

Data on the use of Certiva™ in children for whom whole-cell pertussis vaccine is contraindicated are not available. Until such data are available, it would be prudent to consider CDC Advisory Committee on Immunization Practices (ACIP) and American Academy of Pediatrics (AAP) contraindications to pertussis-containing vaccines as contraindications to Certiva™.[3,20,21]

The ACIP states that "if either of the following events occurs after administration of DTaP or whole-cell DTP, subsequent vaccination with DTaP or whole-cell DTP is contraindicated"[22]:

- An immediate anaphylactic reaction.
- Encephalopathy not attributable to another identifiable cause (e.g., an acute, severe central nervous system disorder occurring within 7 days after vaccination and generally consisting of major alterations in consciousness, unresponsiveness, or generalized or focal seizures that persist more than a few hours, without recovery within 24 hours.) In such cases, DT vaccine should be administered for the remaining doses in the vaccination schedule to ensure protection against diphtheria and tetanus.

WARNINGS

The ACIP and AAP state that if any of the following events occur in temporal relation to receipt of DTP or DTaP, the decision to give subsequent doses of vaccine containing the pertussis component should be carefully considered. There may be circumstances, such as a high incidence of pertussis, in which the potential benefits outweigh possible risks, particularly because these events have not been proven to cause permanent sequelae. The following events were previously considered contraindications and are now considered precautions by the ACIP[22]:

- Temperature of ≥105°F (≥40.5°C) within 48 hours, not attributable to another identifiable cause.
- Collapse or shock-like state (hypotonic hyporesponsive episode) within 48 hours.
- Persistent crying lasting ≥3 hours, occurring within 48 hours.
- Convulsions with or without fever, occurring within 3 days.

Data on the use of Certiva™ in children with a personal history of convulsion or an evolving or changing disorder of the central nervous system are not available. In the opinion of the manufacturer, the presence of a personal history of convulsion or an evolving or changing disorder of the central nervous system is considered a warning against further immunization with this vaccine.

The ACIP and AAP recommend considering deferral of immunization against pertussis in children with progressive neurologic disorder, personal history of convulsion, and known or suspected neurologic conditions which predispose to seizures or neurologic deterioration until the child's health status has been fully assessed, a treatment regimen established and the condition stabilized.[3,20,21,22]

Children with a personal or family history of convulsion may have an increased risk of seizure following DTP vaccination compared with children without such histories.[24,25] However, the ACIP recognizes in certain instances that infants and children with stable neurologic conditions, including well-controlled seizures, may be vaccinated and that the occurrence of single seizures (temporally unassociated with DTP) does not contraindicate DTP vaccination if the seizures can be satisfactorily explained. In addition, the ACIP does not consider a family history of convulsions or other central nervous system disorders to be a contraindication to pertussis vaccination.[20,22,25] Data on the use of Certiva™ in these infants and children are not available.

The decision to administer a pertussis-containing vaccine to children with stable central nervous system disorders, such as well-controlled seizures or satisfactorily explained single seizures, must be made by the attending physician on a case-by-case basis, taking into account all relevant factors and an assessment of the potential risks and benefits for each child. The physician should review the full text of the ACIP and AAP guidelines prior to considering vaccination for such children. In addition, the parent or guardian should be advised of the potential increased risk involved (See **INFORMATION FOR VACCINE RECIPIENTS AND PARENTS**).

For children at higher risk of seizures than the general population, the ACIP recommends that acetaminophen or ibuprofen may be administered at the time of DTaP vaccination and for 24 hours thereafter (using an age-appropriate dose and dosing interval) to reduce the possibility of post-vaccination fever.[22]

A committee from the Institute of Medicine (IOM) has concluded that evidence is consistent with a causal relationship between whole-cell DTP and acute neurologic illness, and under special circumstances, between whole-cell DTP and chronic neurologic disease in the context of the National Childhood Encephalopathy Study (NCES) report.[26,27] However, the IOM committee concluded that evidence was insufficient to indicate whether or not whole-cell DTP vaccine increased the overall risk of chronic neurological disease.[27] The ACIP indicated that the results of the NCES were insufficient to determine whether DTP administration before the acute neurological event influenced the potential for neurologic dysfunction 10 years later.[20] Acute encephalopathy or permanent neurological injury have not been reported in clinical trials after administration of Certiva™, but experience with this vaccine is insufficient to rule this out (See **ADVERSE REACTIONS**).

Certiva™ should not be given to infants or children with thrombocytopenia or any coagulation disorder that would contraindicate intramuscular injection unless the potential benefit clearly outweighs the risk of administration. If the decision is made to administer Certiva™ to children with coagulation disorders, it should be given with caution (See **DRUG INTERACTIONS**).[19]

PRECAUTIONS

Care is to be taken by the physician for the safe and effective use of this vaccine.

1. Prior to administration of any dose of Certiva™, the physician should review the child's medical history. The physician should also review the child's previous immunization history for possible vaccine sensitivity and occurrence of any symptoms or signs of an adverse event after immunization, in order to determine the existence of any contraindication to immunization with Certiva™ and to allow an assessment of benefits and risks (See **CONTRAINDICATIONS** and **ADVERSE REACTIONS**).
2. Before the injection of any biological, the physician should take all precautions known for the prevention of allergic or any other side reactions, including understanding the use of the biological concerned and the nature of the side effects and adverse reactions that may follow its use. Epinephrine injection (1:1,000) and other appropriate agents used for the control of immediate allergic reactions must be immediately available should an acute anaphylactic reaction occur.
3. Children with impaired immune responsiveness, whether due to the use of immunosuppressive therapy (including irradiation, corticosteroids, antimetabolites, alkylating agents, and cytotoxic agents), a genetic defect, human immunodeficiency virus (HIV) infection, or other causes, may have reduced immune response to active immunization procedures. Deferral of immunization may be considered in individuals receiving immunosuppressive therapy. Other groups should receive this vaccine according to the usual recommended schedule (See **DRUG INTERACTIONS**).[28]
4. Certiva™ is not contraindicated based on the presence of HIV infection.[3]
5. Special care should be taken to ensure that the injection does not enter a blood vessel.
6. A separate, sterile syringe and needle or a sterile disposable unit should be used for each subject to prevent transmission of hepatitis or other infectious agents from person to person. Needles should not be recapped but should be disposed of properly.

Caution: The packaging stopper of this product contains natural rubber latex which may cause allergic reactions.

INFORMATION FOR VACCINE RECIPIENTS AND PARENTS

Parents or guardians of infants and children to be vaccinated should be fully informed of the benefits and risks of vaccination with Certiva™ and the importance of completing the immunization series, unless contraindicated.

The physician should inform the parents or guardians about the potential for adverse reactions that have been temporally associated with Certiva™ and other pertussis vaccine administrations. The parents or guardians of infants and children with family history of convulsions or other central nervous system disorders should be advised of the potential increased risk of seizures following DTP vaccinations.

Prior to each immunization, the parent or guardian should be provided with the Vaccine Information Materials (VIMs), as required by the National Childhood Vaccine Injury Act of

1986.[29] Parents or guardians should be instructed to report any severe or unusual reactions to their health-care provider.

The U.S. Department of Health and Human Services has established a Vaccine Adverse Event Reporting System (VAERS) to accept all reports of suspected adverse events after the administration of any vaccine, including, but not limited to, the reporting of events required by the National Childhood Vaccine Injury Act of 1986.[29,30] The toll-free number for VAERS forms and information is 1-800-822-7967.

DRUG INTERACTIONS

For information regarding simultaneous administration with other vaccines, refer to **DOSAGE AND ADMINISTRATION** and **CLINICAL PHARMACOLOGY**.

As with other intramuscular injections, the vaccine should not be given to infants or children on anticoagulant therapy, unless the potential benefit clearly outweighs the risk of administration (see **WARNINGS**).

Immunosuppressive therapies, including irradiation, antimetabolites, alkylating agents, cytotoxic drugs, and corticosteroids (administered in greater than physiologic doses), may reduce the immune response to vaccines. Although no specific studies with pertussis-containing vaccines under these circumstances are available, if immunosuppressive therapy will be discontinued shortly, it would be reasonable to defer immunization until the patient has been off therapy for at least one month; otherwise, the patient should be vaccinated while still on therapy.[3,28] If Certiva™ has been administered to persons receiving immunosuppressive therapy, receiving a recent injection of immune globulin or having an immunodeficiency disorder, an adequate immunologic response may not be obtained.

Tetanus Immune Globulin, or Diphtheria Antitoxin, if used, should be given in a separate site, with a separate needle and syringe.

CARCINOGENESIS, MUTAGENESIS, IMPAIRMENT OF FERTILITY

Certiva™ has not been evaluated for its carcinogenic or mutagenic potentials or impairment of fertility.

PREGNANCY

REPRODUCTIVE STUDIES - PREGNANCY CATEGORY C

Animal reproduction studies have not been conducted with Certiva™. It is not known whether Certiva™ can cause fetal harm when administered to a pregnant woman or can affect reproductive capacity. Certiva™ is NOT recommended for use in a pregnant woman. This vaccine is not recommended for persons 7 years of age or older (See **PEDIATRIC USE**).

PEDIATRIC USE

SAFETY AND EFFECTIVENESS OF Certiva™ IN INFANTS BELOW 6 WEEKS OF AGE HAVE NOT BEEN ESTABLISHED (SEE **DOSAGE AND ADMINISTRATION SECTION**).

THIS VACCINE IS NOT RECOMMENDED FOR PERSONS 7 YEARS OF AGE AND OLDER.

Tetanus and Diphtheria Toxoids Adsorbed for adult use (Td) is to be used in individuals 7 years of age or older.

ADVERSE REACTIONS

In clinical studies in the United States and Sweden, 11,560 doses of Certiva™ (10,608 intramuscular, 952 subcutaneous) and 30,951 doses of Certiva™-EU (5,574 with thimerosal; 25,377 without thimerosal; all subcutaneous) have been administered.[15] In these studies, 3,698 infants received 10,615 doses of Certiva™ as a 3-dose series at 2, 4, and 6 months of age; 682 of these infants received a 4th consecutive dose of Certiva™ at 15–24 months of age; no children have received 5 consecutive doses of Certiva™. Forty-two (42) children received Certiva™ as a 4th dose at 15–22 months of age, following 3 doses of whole-cell DTP vaccine; 221 children received Certiva™ as a 5th dose at 4–6 years of age, following 3 doses of whole-cell DTP and a 4th dose of whole-cell DTP or acellular DTaP vaccine. In addition, 1,875 infants received 5,574 doses of Certiva™-EU as a 3-dose series at 3, 5 and 12 months of age.[14,15] In an ongoing study, 11,859 infants are completing a 3-dose series at 3, 5, and 12 months of age and have been evaluated after 25,377 doses to date.[15] In a comparative study, local and systemic adverse reactions commonly associated with whole-cell DTP vaccination occurred less frequently after vaccination with Certiva™.[15] Studies have shown, however, that the rate of erythema, swelling, and fever increased with successive doses of Certiva™ (Tables 2, 3, and 6).

In a double-blind safety and immunogenicity study in the United States, 1,303 infants were randomized to receive Certiva™ (n=977) or U.S. licensed whole-cell DTP vaccine manufactured by Lederle Laboratories (n=326) at 2, 4, and 6 months of age. At each time point, 96–99% of subjects also received *Haemophilus influenzae* type b conjugate vaccine, 83–97% received polio vaccine live oral, and 18–80% received hepatitis B vaccine. Safety data were actively collected using standardized diary cards and follow-up telephone calls at 1, 3, and 7 days after each vaccination, and are available for 972 and 323 infants, respectively, who received at least one dose of Certiva™ or whole-cell DTP. Local injection site reactions and systemic reactions such as fever (≥ 38°C), irritability, decreased appetite, and drowsiness were significantly less frequent after Certiva™ than after whole-cell DTP (Table 2). Within 7 days after vaccination, there were no deaths and five hospitalizations (3 Certiva™ recipients: 1 with cold/high fever on day 6, 1 with ear infection on day 6, 1 with febrile seizure and respiratory infection on day 4; 2 whole-cell DTP recipients: 1 with diarrhea on day 4, 1 with hives/allergic reaction on day 4), none judged to be vaccine-related by the investigators.[15]

TABLE 2

ADVERSE EVENTS (%) OCCURRING WITHIN 72 HOURS AFTER INTRAMUSCULAR VACCINATION OF U.S. INFANTS WITH CERTIVA™ OR WHOLE-CELL DTP AT 2, 4, AND 6 MONTHS OF AGE

	Certiva™ Reaction %			Whole-Cell Pertussis DTP Reaction %			p-values*
	Dose 1 2 Mos.	Dose 2 4 Mos.	Dose 3 6 Mos.	Dose 1 2 Mos.	Dose 2 4 Mos.	Dose 3 6 Mos.	Combined Doses DTaP:DTP
Local *n=*	*972*	*898*	*868*	*323*	*295*	*279*	*2,738 : 897*
Redness (any)	5.2	8.5	13.0	22.1	29.9	27.2	<0.0001
Redness ≥ 3 cm	0.2	0.6	1.3	5.6	1.4	2.2	<0.0001
Swelling (any)	8.0	8.6	8.6	29.9	23.4	20.4	<0.0001
Swelling ≥ 3 cm	1.9	1.2	1.3	14.0	9.2	5.0	<0.0001
Tenderness/pain	8.4	6.8	5.4	28.6	15.9	18.0	<0.0001
Systemic‡							
Fever ≥ 38°C†	3.2	7.2	11.4	15.7	19.7	25.5	<0.0001
Fever ≥ 39°C†	0.2	1.7	2.1	0	2.5	7.1	NS (p=0.052)
Irritability	34.2	30.3	27.0	55.4	38.6	34.8	<0.0001
Drowsiness	38.3	21.2	12.4	45.2	25.1	20.4	<0.001
Decreased appetite	14.5	11.7	9.2	22.0	10.5	14.3	<0.01
Vomiting	14.3	8.2	7.3	13.3	7.5	6.5	NS
High-pitched/unusual crying	0.3	0	0.1	0.6	0	0	NS#
Persistent crying ≥ 3 hours	0.1	0.1	0	0.6	0	0	NS#
Hypotonic-hyporesponsive episode	0.1**	0	0	0	0	0.7	NS#
Seizures/convulsions	0	0	0	0	0	0.4	NS#

* Two-tailed Fisher's exact test/Certiva™:whole-cell DTP across all doses

‡ Other age-appropriate vaccines concomitantly administered with Certiva™

† Rectal temperatures only, denominators for Certiva™ at doses 1, 2 and 3 are 524, 363 and 282, respectively, and for whole-cell DTP 172, 122 and 98, respectively, for a total of 1,169 Certiva™ doses and 392 whole-cell DTP doses

\# NS = no significant (p>0.05); study not powered to detect significant differences for the predicted event rates

** Database record represents one subject after dose 1; no medical attention sought, child received doses two, three and four without incident

[See table 2 above]

In an open-label study in the United States, safety results are available from 2,480 infants who received at least one dose of a three-dose series of Certiva™ administered at 2, 4, and 6 months of age. At each time point, 95–98% of subjects also received *Haemophilus influenzae* type b conjugate vaccine, 71–94% received polio vaccine live oral, and 7–50% received hepatitis B vaccine. Safety data were actively collected using standardized diary cards and follow-up telephone calls at 1, 2, 3, and 7 days after each vaccination (Table 3). Within 7 days after vaccination, there were no reports of seizures, hypotonic-hyporesponsive episodes (HHE), or deaths; seven hospitalizations occurred (bronchiolitis, RSV pneumonia, pyelonephrosis, urinary tract infection, breath-holding episode, stridor, otitis media/fever), none of which were judged to be vaccine-related by the investigators.[15] Of the 2,283 infants who completed the 3-dose series, 316 received a 4th dose at 15–24 months of age. Standardized diary cards and telephone follow-up at 2 and 7 days post-vaccination were used to actively collect safety data. There were no reports of serious adverse events during the first 7 days after vaccination. The most common complaints were irritability, injection site redness (of any size) and pain (Table 3).[15]

[See table 3 at top of next page]

In an open-label study, 175 children who had previously received either whole-cell DTP (n=42) or Certiva™ (n=133) at 2, 4, and 6 months of age were immunized with Certiva™ at 15–21 months of age. Standardized diary cards and telephone follow-up at 2 and 7 days post-vaccination were used to actively collect safety data (Table 4).

[See table 4 on next page]

Table 5 lists the frequency of adverse reactions in 221 U.S. children who received Certiva™ at 4–6 years of age. These children had previously received 3 doses of a whole-cell DTP vaccine at 2, 4, and 6 months of age and either a whole-cell DTP or DTaP vaccine at 12–24 months of age.

[See table 5 on next page]

In the randomized, double-blinded, placebo-controlled efficacy trial in Göteborg, Sweden, a total of 3,450 infants were vaccinated with either DT (1,726 infants) or Certiva™-EU (1,724 infants) at 3, 5, and 12 months of age; no other vaccines were administered concurrently. Safety data were actively collected using standardized diary cards and telephone follow-up 7 days after each vaccination and monthly for general health and disease surveillance. Within 7 days after vaccination, there were no reports of hypotonic-hyporesponsive episodes or deaths; 28 hospitalizations (12 Certiva™-EU, 16 DT) occurred, none judged to be vaccine-related by the investigators. Rates of both fever and local injection site reactions increased with the number of vaccinations in both groups. Rates for fever were similar between the two groups within the first seven days following a vaccination. Injection site redness and swelling were more common among Certiva™-EU-vaccinated than among DT-vaccinated children after the second injection (Table 6).[14,15]

[See table 6 at top of page 1977]

Other adverse events (irritability, crying, feeding problems, vomiting, sleeping problems, respiratory infections, diarrhea and physician visits) were seen with similar frequency in the two groups after each vaccination.

When the total U.S. clinical trial experience with Certiva™ is considered (10,587 doses administered to 3,715 infants and children), adverse event rates per 1,000 doses meeting AAP and ACIP criteria as absolute contraindications or precautions to further pertussis immunization and occurring within 72 hours after immunization were: persistent, inconsolable crying for ≥ 3 hours, 0.57; fever ≥ 40.5°C, 0; seizures (febrile and afebrile), 0; hypotonic-hyporesponsive episode, 0.09 (database record represents one subject after dose 1; no medical attention sought; child received doses 2, 3, and 4 without incident).

For Certiva™-EU (5,574 doses containing thimerosal administered to 1,875 Swedish infants with active follow-up) rates per 1,000 doses for similar adverse events occurring within 7 days of vaccination were the following: persistent crying for ≥ 3 hours, 1.44; fever ≥ 40.5°C, 1.79; seizures (febrile) within 48 hours of vaccination, 0.36; hypotonic-hyporesponsive episode, 0. Rates of serious adverse events that are less common than those reported in these actively monitored trials are not known at this time.

In an open-label study in Sweden, 11,859 infants have received 25,377 doses of Certiva™-EU (without thimerosal) at 3, 5, and 12 months of age, and serious adverse events were ascertained through evaluation of hospitalization databases and spontaneous reporting. Within 7 days after vaccination, there were three hospitalizations for seizures (2 within 48 hours after vaccination); no hospitalizations for diagnoses judged by the investigators to be consistent with hypotonic-hyporesponsive episodes; and two deaths attributed to Sudden Infant Death Syndrome (SIDS), neither judged to be vaccine-related.[15] In this study, 32,799 children 1–5 years of age have received 81,613 doses of a vaccine containing pertussis toxoid (but not the tetanus and diphtheria toxoids; 6,764 doses were administered as Certiva™-EU as the first dose at 1 year of age) on a 0, 2, and 8 month schedule, and were monitored the same way as the infants. Within 7 days after vaccination, there were seven hospitalizations for seizures (none within 48 hours after vaccination); no hospitalizations for diagnoses judged by the investigators to be consistent with hypotonic-hyporesponsive episodes; and no deaths.

Continued on next page

Certiva—Cont.

In the overall clinical trial experience involving 17,690 infants and children who received 42,490 doses of Certiva™ or Certiva™-EU, there were no occurrences of anaphylaxis or encephalopathy. Nine deaths were reported, two occurring within 7 days after vaccination; none of these events was determined to be related to vaccination. Causes of death included four cases of Sudden Infant Death Syndrome (SIDS), 1 accidental suffocation, 1 invasive bacterial infection, 1 cerebral edema (unknown cause), 2 unknown (history of cardiac malformation or myelomeningocele).[15] The rate of SIDS was 0.6 per thousand infants vaccinated with Certiva™ in the U.S. studies, and 0.1 per thousand infants vaccinated with Certiva™-EU in Swedish studies.[15] The incidence of SIDS in Sweden from 1985 – 1992 was between 0.7 and 1.1 cases per thousand live births with a decline from 0.7 to 0.4 cases per thousand live births between 1992 and 1995.[31,32] From 1979 to 1996, the incidence of SIDS in the U.S. has declined from 1.5 to 0.74 cases per thousand live births.[33] By chance alone, some cases of SIDS can be expected to follow receipt of whole-cell DTP or DTaP.[21] In the clinical trial experience of 32,799 children who received 81,613 doses of pertussis toxoid vaccine, there were no reports of anaphylaxis or encephalopathy.[15] Of five reported deaths, none occurred within 7 days after vaccination and none was determined to be related to vaccination. Causes of death included 1 invasive bacterial infection, 1 unexpected sudden death, 1 murder, 1 hepatoblastoma, and 1 unknown (history of cardiac malformation).[15] Rarely, an anaphylactic reaction (i.e., hives, swelling of the mouth, difficulty breathing, hypotension or shock) has been reported after receiving preparations containing diphtheria, tetanus, and/or pertussis antigens.[3]

Arthus-type hypersensitivity reactions, characterized by severe local reactions (generally starting 2 to 8 hours after an injection) may follow receipt of tetanus toxoid. A few cases of peripheral neuropathy have been reported following tetanus toxoid administration, although the IOM concluded that the evidence is inadequate to accept or reject a causal relation.[34] A review by the IOM found a causal relation between tetanus toxoid and brachial neuritis and Guillain-Barré Syndrome.[34] The following illnesses have been reported as temporally associated with the administration of tetanus toxoid containing vaccines: neurological complications[35,36] including cochlear lesion[37], brachial plexus neuropathies[38], paralysis of the radial nerve[39], paralysis of the recurrent laryngeal nerve, accommodation paresis, and EEG disturbances with encephalopathy.[40,41] In the differential diagnosis of polyradiculoneuropathies following administration of a vaccine containing tetanus toxoid, tetanus toxoid should be considered as a possible etiology.[41]

Additional Adverse Reactions Evaluated in Conjunction with Whole-cell DTP Vaccination

Whole-cell DTP has been associated with acute encephalopathy.[27] In the National Childhood Encephalopathy Study (NCES), a large, case-control study in England, children 2 to 35 months of age with serious acute neurologic disorders (cases), such as encephalopathy or complicated convulsion(s), were compared to children without acute neurologic disorders who were matched for age, sex, and residence (controls).[42] Cases were more likely to have received whole-cell DTP vaccine within 7 days before onset of illness than were controls within 7 days before being the exact age as their matched case child at the time of onset of illness (relative risk, 3.3). The attributable risk for all neurologic events was estimated to be 1:140,000 doses of whole-cell DTP vaccine administered.[42]

A detailed follow-up to the NCES indicated that cases were significantly more likely than controls to have chronic nervous system dysfunction 10 years later.[43] These cases who developed chronic nervous system dysfunction were more likely to have received whole-cell DTP vaccine within 7 days before onset of acute illness than were controls within 7 days before being the exact age as their matched case child at the time of onset of acute illness (relative risk, 5.5). A committee of the IOM has concluded that the evidence is consistent with a causal relation between whole-cell DTP and acute neurologic illness, and that the balance of the evidence is consistent with a causal relation between whole-cell DTP and the forms of nervous system dysfunction described in the NCES in those children who experience a serious acute neurologic illness within 7 days after receiving whole-cell DTP vaccine. However, the IOM committee also concluded that the evidence is insufficient to indicate whether or not whole-cell DTP increases the overall risk in children for chronic nervous system dysfunction.[27] The ACIP indicated that the results of the NCES were insufficient to determine whether whole-cell DTP administration before the acute neurological event influenced the potential for neurologic dysfunction 10 years later.[20] Subsequent studies have failed to provide evidence in support of a causal relationship between whole-cell DTP vaccination and either serious acute neurologic illness or permanent neurologic injury.[36,44,45,46]

TABLE 3
ADVERSE EVENTS (%) OCCURRING WITHIN 72 HOURS AFTER INTRAMUSCULAR VACCINATION OF U.S. INFANTS WITH CERTIVA™ AT 2, 4, AND 6, AND 15–24 MONTHS OF AGE

	Certiva™			
	Dose 1 2 Mos.	Dose 2 4 Mos.	Dose 3 6 Mos.	Dose 4 15 Mos.
Local n*=	2480	2374	2283	316
Redness (any)	4.4	7.7	10.9	21.0
Redness ≥ 3 cm	0.2	0.3	0.5	5.7
Swelling (any)	3.6	5.4	7.9	12.7
Swelling ≥ 3 cm	0.6	0.4	1.1	4.5
Tenderness/pain (any)**	5.9	4.0	3.9	19.0
Systemic‡				
Fever ≥ 38°C†	1.5	3.5	5.0	10.5
Fever ≥ 39°C†#	0.1	0.4	1.0	2.6
Irritability	33.4	27.9	26.4	22.5
Drowsiness	33.5	17.1	11.1	11.4
Decreased appetite	15.4	10.5	10.0	8.9
Vomiting/spitting up	7.3	4.9	4.5	3.8
High-pitched, unusual crying	0.2	0.1	0	0
Persistent crying ≥ 3 hours#	0.1	0.04	0	0

* Denominators vary less than 1.2% from the column totals
**85% of events reported were mild in intensity
‡ Other age-appropriate vaccines concomitantly administered with Certiva™
† Rectal temperatures only, fever rates based on 6,447 total Certiva™ doses at 2, 4 and 6 months of age, and 266 at 15 months of age
# Within 48 hours of vaccination, there were no fevers ≥40.3°C (rectal) and no persistent, inconsolable crying ≥ 3 hours

TABLE 4
ADVERSE EVENTS (%) OCCURRING WITHIN 72 HOURS FOLLOWING AN INTRAMUSCULAR DOSE OF CERTIVA™ AT 15–21 MONTHS OF AGE IN CHILDREN WHO RECEIVED THREE DOSES OF CERTIVA™ OR WHOLE-CELL DTP VACCINE AT 2, 4, AND 6 MONTHS OF AGE[15]

	Vaccine received at 2, 4, and 6 mo. of age	
	Certiva™	Whole-cell DTP
EVENTS n=	133	42
Local (any)		
Redness	15.3	7.1
Swelling	9.9	9.5
Pain	9.0	7.1
Systemic*		
Fever ≥ 38°C‡	2.1	15.4
Decreased appetite	9.8	14.3
Vomiting	3.8	0
Drowsiness	7.5	14.3
Irritability	19.6	21.4
High-pitched/unusual crying	0	0
Persistent crying ≥ 3 hours	0.8†	0

* Other age-appropriate vaccines concomitantly administered with Certiva™
‡ Denominatin for rectal temperatures for Certiva™ primed and whole-cell DTP primed subjects are 48 and 13, respectively; 38°C =100.4°F
† Represents one subject who was bitten by ants

TABLE 5
ADVERSE EVENTS (%) OCCURRING WITHIN 7 DAYS FOLLOWING AN INTRAMUSCULAR DOSE OF CERTIVA™ AT 4–6 YEARS OF AGE (5TH DOSE IN THE SERIES) IN 221 CHILDREN HAVING RECEIVED ALL OF THEIR PREVIOUS AGE-APPROPRIATE PERTUSSIS VACCINATIONS[15]

Local Events (any)			Systemic Events**				
Redness	Swelling	Pain*	Fever >38°C	Decreased Appetite	Vomiting	Drowsiness	Irritability
19.5	18.1	36.2	4.5	6.8	5.0	10.0	8.1

* 83% of subjects reported pain of mild intensity; the remaining 17% were of moderate intensity as judged by the caregiver
**Other age-appropriate concomitantly administered with Certiva™

Onset of infantile spasms has occurred in infants who have recently received whole-cell DTP vaccines or DT. Analysis of data from the NCES on children with infantile spasms showed that receipt of DT or whole-cell DTP vaccines was not causally related to infantile spasms.[26,47] The incidence of onset of infantile spasms increases at 3 to 9 months of age, the time period in which the second and third doses of vaccine are generally given. Therefore, some cases of infantile spasms can be expected to be related by chance alone to recent receipt of whole-cell DTP vaccine.[26,47]

Sudden Infant Death Syndrome (SIDS) has been reported in infants following administration of whole-cell DTP or DTaP vaccine. Large case-control studies of SIDS in the U.S. have shown that receipt of whole-cell DTP vaccine was not causally related to SIDS.[26,48,49] It should be recognized that the first three immunizing doses of whole-cell DTP vaccine or DTaP vaccine are usually administered to infants 2 to 6 months old and that approximately 85% of SIDS cases occur at ages 1 to 6 months, with the peak incidence occurring at 6 weeks to 4 months of age. By chance alone, some cases of SIDS can be expected to follow receipt of whole-cell DTP or DTaP vaccine.[48] A review by a committee of the IOM concluded that available evidence did not indicate a causal relation between whole-cell DTP vaccines and SIDS.[26]

A bulging fontanel associated with increased intracranial pressure which occurred within 24 hours following whole-cell DTP immunization has been reported, although a causal relationship has not been established.[26,35]

The above findings regarding possible association of unusual neurologic events and SIDS relate only to DTP vaccines containing whole-cell pertussis. At this time there are insufficient data to determine their relevance to Certiva™ immunization.

ADVERSE EVENT REPORTING

Adverse events occurring after vaccine administration should be reported by the health-care provider to the U.S. Department of Health and Human Services through the Vaccine Adverse Event Reporting System (VAERS).[30] The toll-free number for VAERS forms and information is 1-800-822-7967. The National Vaccine Injury Compensation Pro-

TABLE 6
ADVERSE EVENTS (%) OCCURRING AFTER SUBCUTANEOUS* VACCINATION OF SWEDISH INFANTS WITH CERTIVA™-EU AT 3, 5, AND 12 MONTHS OF AGE

	Dose 1 3 Mos.		Dose 2 5 Mos.		Dose 3 12 Mos.	
	Certiva™-EU	DT	Certiva™-EU	DT	Certiva™-EU	DT
n=	1724	1726	1708	1717	1692	1687
Within 7 days of vaccination						
Redness (any)	22.2	18.8	50.9	39.5	57.6	49.3
Redness ≥ 4 cm	0.1	0.2	2.0	0.8	10.0	7.9
Swelling (any)	10.8	10.5	34.7	28.7	45.9	38.9
Swelling ≥ 4 cm	0.2	0.2	1.9	0.9	9.1	6.7
Seizures**	0	0	0	0	0.2	0
Within 48 hours of vaccination						
Fever ≥ 38°C†	6.4	6.5	10.9	11.4	16.8	16.6
Fever ≥ 39°C†	0.5	0	1.4	0.8	2.5	2.3
Persistent crying ≥ 3 hrs	0.1	0.2	0.2	0.1	0	0

* Subcutaneous administration may result in an increased frequency of local injection site complaints when compared to intramuscular administration.[14] Certiva™ is for *intramsucular* injection only (see DESCRIPTION and DOSAGE AND ADMINISTRATION)

**Three febrile events: two with concomitant respiratory tract infection and one with concomitant gastroenteritis; no afebrile seizures were reported

† Rectal temperatures

gram, established by the National Childhood Vaccine Injury Act of 1986, requires physicians and other health-care providers who administer vaccines to maintain permanent vaccination records (including a record of the name of the vaccine manufacturer, lot number of the vaccine administered, date of administration and the name, address and title of the person administering the vaccine) and to report occurrences of certain adverse events to the U.S. Department of Health and Human Services. Reportable events include those listed in the Act (*i.e.*, those listed in the Vaccine Injury Table) for each vaccine and events specified in the package insert as contraindications to further doses of the vaccine.[29,30]

The health-care provider also should report these events to the Director of Medical Affairs, North American Vaccine, Inc., 10150 Old Columbia Road, Columbia MD 21046, or call toll-free 1-888-628-2829.

DOSAGE AND ADMINISTRATION
General
The vaccine should be inspected visually for extraneous particulate matter and/or discoloration prior to administration. If these conditions exist, the vaccine should not be used. Shake vial well to obtain a homogeneous suspension before withdrawing each dose. Inject 0.5 ml of Certiva™ intramuscularly only. The preferred injection sites are the anterolateral aspect of the thigh and the deltoid muscle of the upper arm. The vaccine should not be injected into the gluteal area or areas where there may be a major nerve trunk. Before injection, the skin over the injection site should be cleansed with suitable germicide. After insertion of the needle, aspirate to ensure that the needle has not entered a blood vessel.
Fractional doses (doses < 0.5 ml) should not be given since the safety and efficacy of fractional doses have not been determined.

IMMUNIZATION SERIES
A 0.5 ml intramuscular injection of Certiva™ is recommended for administration at 2, 4, and 6 months of age, at intervals of six to eight weeks, with a fourth dose given at 15–20 months of age (see CLINICAL PHARMACOLOGY). The interval between the third and fourth doses should be at least 6 months. The customary age for the first dose is two months of age, but the vaccine may be given starting at six weeks of age. It is recommended that Certiva™ be given for all doses in the series because no interchangeability data on DTaP vaccines exist.
Certiva™ may be used to complete the immunization series in infants who have received one or two doses of whole-cell DTP vaccine. However, the safety and efficacy of Certiva™ in such infants have not been evaluated.
Certiva™ as a fourth dose is recommended at 15–20 months of age in children who have received three doses of whole-cell DTP vaccine. The interval between the third and fourth dose should be at least 6 months.
Certiva™ as a fifth dose is recommended at 4–6 years of age (prior to the seventh birthday) in children who have received 4 doses of a whole-cell DTP vaccine or 3 doses of a whole-cell DTP vaccine followed by one dose of a DTaP vaccine. A fifth dose is not needed if the fourth dose was given on or after the fourth birthday. At this time, there are no data to establish the frequency of adverse events following a fifth dose of Certiva™ in children who previously received 4 doses of Certiva™.

ADDITIONAL DOSING INFORMATION
If any recommended dose of pertussis vaccine cannot be given, DT (For Pediatric Use) should be given as needed to complete the series.

Interruption of the recommended schedule with a delay between doses should not interfere with the final immunity achieved with Certiva™. There is no need to start the series over again, regardless of the time elapsed between doses. A reduced or fractional dose (dose < 0.5 ml) should not be given, because the safety and efficacy of reduced doses have not been determined.[19]
Pre-term infants should be vaccinated according to their chronological age from birth.[19]
Persons 7 years of age or older should not be immunized with Certiva™. They should receive Tetanus and Diphtheria Toxoids (Td) for adult use for routine booster immunization against tetanus and diphtheria.

SIMULTANEOUS VACCINE ADMINISTRATION
In clinical trials, Certiva™ was routinely administered, at separate sites, concomitantly with one or more of the following vaccines: polio vaccine live oral (OPV), hepatitis B vaccine, *Haemophilus influenzae* type b conjugate vaccine (Hib), and measles, mumps and rubella vaccine (MMR) (see CLINICAL PHARMACOLOGY).
No data are available on the simultaneous administration of inactivated polio vaccine (IPV) as a primary series or varicella vaccine with Certiva™.
When concomitant administration of other vaccines is required, they should be given with different syringes and at different injection sites.
The ACIP encourages routine simultaneous administration of acellular DTaP, Hib, IPV or OPV, hepatitis B, MMR and varicella vaccines for children who are at the recommended age to receive these vaccines and for whom no specific contraindications exist at the time of the visit, unless, in the judgment of the provider, complete vaccination of the child will not be compromised by administering vaccines at different visits.[19,22] Simultaneous administration is particularly important if the child might not return for subsequent vaccinations.

HOW SUPPLIED
Vial, 15 Dose (7.5 ml)
NDC 62448-4012-1
STORAGE
Store between 2–8°C (35–46°F). DO NOT FREEZE.

REFERENCES
1. Sekura R, *et al.* Clinical, metabolic and antibody responses of adult volunteers to an investigational vaccine composed of pertussis toxin inactivated by hydrogen peroxide. J Pediatrics 1988;113:806–813.
2. Aggerbeck H, Fenger C, and Heron I. Booster vaccination against diphtheria, tetanus in man. Comparison of calcium phosphate and aluminum hydroxide as adjuvants—II. Vaccine 1995;13:1366–1374.
3. Diphtheria, Tetanus and Pertussis: Recommendations for Vaccine Use and Other Preventive Measures, Recommendations of the Immunization Practices Advisory Committee (ACIP). MMWR 1991;40(RR-10): 1–28.
4. CDC, Summary of notifiable diseases, United States, 1994. MMWR 1995;43(53):70–71.
5. CDC. Diphtheria Epidemic - New Independent States of the Former Soviet Union, 1990-1994. MMWR 1995;44(10):177–181.
6. Ipsen J. Immunization of adults against diphtheria and tetanus. N Engl J Med 1954 Sep 16;251(12):459–466.
7. DHHS, FDA, Biological products; bacterial vaccines and toxoids: implementation of efficacy review; proposed rule. Federal Register 1985;50(240):51002–51117.
8. CDC. Tetanus - United States, 1987 and 1988. MMWR 1990;39(3):37–44.
9. Diphtheria, Tetanus and Pertussis: Guidelines for Vaccine Prophylaxis and Other Preventive Measures, Recommendation of the Immunization Practices Advisory Committee (ACIP). MMWR 1985 July 12;34(27):405–426.
10. Pertussis—United States, January 1992-June 1995. MMWR 1995 Jul 21;44(28):525–527.
11. Atkinson W, ed.; Epidemiology and Prevention of Vaccine-Preventable Diseases ("The Pink Book"); 4th Edition; Atlanta, Centers for Disease Control and Prevention; September 1997.
12. Farizo KM *et al.* Epidemiologic features of pertussis in the United States 1980-1989. Clin Infect Dis 1992;14: 708–719.
13. Nennig MF, *et al.* Prevalence and incidence of adult pertussis in an urban population. JAMA 1996; 275:1672–1674.
14. Trollfors B, *et al.* A placebo-controlled trial of a pertussis-toxoid vaccine. N Engl J Med 1995;333:1045–1050.
15. Data on file Certiva™ at North American Vaccine, Inc.
16. Case Definition of Pertussis. (citation) World Health Organization (WHO) Meeting 1991 Jan 10–11. Technical Report No. 01-A1-1S12S.
17. Taranger J, *et al.* Unchanged efficacy of a pertussis toxoid vaccine throughout the two years after the third vaccination of infants. Pediatr. Infect. Dis. J. 1997;16:180–184.
18. Trollfors B., *et al.* Efficacy of a monocomponent pertussis toxoid vaccine after household exposure to pertussis. J Pediatr. 1997; 130:532–536.
19. ACIP. General recommendations on immunization. MMWR 1994;43(RR-1).
20. CDC. Update: Vaccine side effects, adverse reactions, contraindications, and precautions. Recommendations of the Advisory Committee on Immunization Practices. MMWR 1996;45(RR-12):1–35.
21. American Academy of Pediatrics. Report of the Committee on Infectious Diseases (Red Book). American Academy of Pediatrics, Evanston (IL); 24th edition; 1997: pg. 404.
22. CDC. Pertussis vaccination: Use of acellular pertussis vaccines among infants and young children. Recommendations of the Advisory Committee on Immunization Practices (ACIP). MMWR 1997;46(RR-7):1–25.
23. Sutter, R.W., *et al.* Attributable risk of DTP (Diphtheria and Tetanus Toxoids and Pertussis Vaccine) injection in provoking paralytic poliomyelitis during a large outbreak in Oman. J Infect Dis 1992; 165:444–449.
24. Livengood, J.R., *et al.* Family history of convulsions and use of pertussis vaccine. J Pediatr 1989; 115:527–531.
25. Stetler, H.C., *et al.* History of convulsions and use of pertussis vaccine. J Pediatr 1985; 107:175–179.
26. Howson CP, *et al.* Adverse effects of pertussis and rubella vaccines: Pertussis vaccines and CNS disorders. Institute of Medicine (IOM); Washington (DC): National Academy Press; 1991.
27. Stratton KR, *et al.* DPT vaccine and chronic nervous system dysfunction: A New Analysis. Institute of Medicine (IOM). Washington, DC: National Academy Press, 1994 (Supplement).
28. CDC. Use of vaccines and immune globulins for persons with altered immunocompetence. Recommendations of the Advisory Committee on Immunization Practices (ACIP). MMWR 1993; Vol. 42 (No. RR-4):1–3.
29. National Childhood Vaccine Injury Act: Requirements for Permanent Vaccination Records and for Reporting of Selected Events after Vaccination. MMWR 1988 Apr 8;37(13):197–200.
30. CDC. Vaccine Adverse Event Reporting System-United States. MMWR 1990;39:730–733.
31. Willinger M., *et al.* Infant sleep position and risk for sudden infant death syndrome: Report of meeting held January 13 and 14, 1994. National Institutes of Health, Bethesda, MD. Pediatrics 1994; 93:814–819.
32. Epidemiological Center, National Board of Health and Welfare, Sweden. 1997. Causes of death in Sweden, 1995.
33. Guyer B, et al. Annual summary of vital statistics-1996. Pediatrics 1997; 100(6):905–918.
34. Stratton KR, *et al.* Adverse events associated with childhood vaccines—evidence bearing on causality. Institute of Medicine (IOM). Washington (DC): National Academy Press;1994.
35. Jacob J, *et al.* Increased intracranial pressure after diphtheria, tetanus and pertussis immunization. Am J Dis Child 1979; 133:217–218.
36. Walker AM, *et al.* Neurologic events following diphtheria-tetanus-pertussis immunization. Pediatrics 1988;81: 345–349.
37. Wilson GS. Allergic manifestations— Post-vaccinal neuritis. In: The hazards of immunization. London, England. The Athlone Press; 1967. p. 153–156.
38. Tsairis P, *et al.* Natural history of brachial plexus neuropathy. Arch Neurol 1972;27:109–117.

Continued on next page

Certiva—Cont.

39. Blumstein GI, *et al*. Peripheral neuropathy following tetanus toxoid administration. JAMA 1966;198:1030-1031.
40. CDC. Adverse events following immunization. MMWR Surveillance Report 1985-86; No. 3; issued Feb 1989.
41. Schlenska GK. Unusual neurological complications following tetanus-toxoid administration. J Neurol 1977;215:299–302.
42. Miller, D.L., *et al*. Pertussis immunisation and serious acute neurological illness in children. Br Med J 1981; 282:1595–1599.
43. Miller, D.L., *et al*. Pertussis immunisation and serious acute neurological illnesses in children. Br Med J 1993; 307:1171–1176.
44. Pollock TM, *et al*. A 7-year survey of disorders attributed to vaccination in North West Thames region. Lancet 1983; 1:753–757.
45. Griffin MR, *et al*. Risk of seizures and encephalopathy after immunization with the diphtheria-tetanus-pertussis vaccine. JAMA 1990; 263(12):1641–1645.
46. Shields WD, *et al*. Relationship of pertussis immunization to the onset of neurologic disorders: a retrospective epidemiologic study. J Pediatr 1988; 113:801–805.
47. Bellman MH, *et al*. Infantile spasms and pertussis immunization. Lancet 1983 7 May:1031–1034.
48. Walker AM, *et al*. Diphtheria-tetanus-pertussis immunization and sudden infant death syndrome. Am J Public Health 1987;77:945–971.
49. Griffin, M.R., *et al*. Risk of sudden infant death syndrome after immunization with the diphtheria-tetanus-pertussis vaccine. N Engl J Med 1988; 319:618–623.

May 1, 1998

Manufactured by:
North American Vaccine, Inc.
Beltsville, MD 20705
Marketed by:
North American Vaccine, Inc.
and
Ross Products Division
Abbott Laboratories, Inc.
Columbus, OH 43215

Northampton Medical, Inc.
(See UCB Pharma, Inc.)

Novartis Consumer Health, Inc.
560 MORRIS AVENUE
SUMMIT, NJ 07901-1312

Direct Inquiries to:
Consumer & Professional Affairs
(800) 452-0051
FAX: (800) 635-2801
or write to the above address.

DULCOLAX®   OTC
brand of bisacodyl USP

DESCRIPTION AND CLINICAL PHARMACOLOGY
Dulcolax is a contact stimulant laxative, administered either orally or rectally, which acts directly on the colonic mucosa to produce normal peristalsis throughout the large intestine. The active ingredient in Dulcolax, bisacodyl, is a colorless, tasteless compound that is practically insoluble in water or alkaline solution. Its chemical name is: bis(p-acetoxyphenyl)-2-pyridylmethane. Bisacodyl is very poorly absorbed, if at all, in the small intestine following oral administration, or in the large intestine following rectal administration. On contact with the mucosa or submucosal plexi of the large intestine, bisacodyl stimulates sensory nerve endings to produce parasympathetic reflexes resulting in increased peristaltic contractions of the colon. It has also been shown to promote fluid and ion accumulation in the colon, which increases the laxative effect. A bowel movement is usually produced approximately 6 hours after oral administration (8–12 hours if taken at bedtime), and approximately 15 minutes to 1 hour after rectal administration, providing satisfactory cleansing of the bowel which may, under certain circumstances, obviate the need for colonic irrigation.
Dulcolax (brand of bisacodyl USP) is available as enteric coated tablets of 5 mg each or as suppositories of 10 mg each. Each tablet also contains: acacia, acetylated monoglyceride, carnauba wax, cellulose acetate phthalate, corn starch, D&C Red No. 30 aluminum lake, D&C Yellow No. 10 aluminum lake, dibutyl phthalate, docusate sodium, gelatin, glycerin, iron oxides, kaolin, lactose, magnesium stearate, methylparaben, pharmaceutical glaze, polyethylene glycol, povidone, propylparaben, sodium benzoate, sorbitan monooleate, sucrose, talc, titanium dioxide, and white wax. Each suppository also contains hydrogenated vegetable oil. Tablets and suppositories contain less than 0.2 mg sodium per dosage unit and are thus dietetically sodium-free.

INDICATIONS AND USAGE
For the relief of occasional constipation and irregularity. For use as part of a bowel cleansing regimen in preparing the patient for surgery or for preparing the colon for x-ray endoscopic examination. Dulcolax will not replace the colonic irrigations usually given patients before intracolonic surgery, but is useful in the preliminary emptying of the colon prior to those procedures. Dulcolax may also be used in postoperative care (i.e., restoration of normal bowel hygiene), antepartum care, postpartum care, and in preparation for delivery.

CONTRAINDICATIONS
Stimulant laxatives, such as Dulcolax, are contraindicated for patients with acute surgical abdomen, appendicitis, rectal bleeding, gastroenteritis, or intestinal obstruction.

WARNINGS AND PRECAUTIONS
Use of Dulcolax is not recommended when abdominal pain, nausea, or vomiting are present. Long term administration of Dulcolax is not recommended in the treatment of chronic constipation. This product should not be used beyond 7 days unless deemed necessary. Rectal bleeding or failure to have a bowel movement after Dulcolax use may indicate a serious condition. If this occurs, the patient should discontinue use of the product.
This and all medication should be kept out of the reach of children.
Pregnancy Category B
Teratology
Reproduction studies of oral doses of Dulcolax (bisacodyl) have been performed in rats administered up to 70 times the human dose, and have revealed no evidence of impaired fertility or damage to the fetus. At the dose which equated to 70 times the human dose, there was some evidence of lower litter survival at weaning. There are, however, no adequate and well-controlled studies in pregnant women, hence Dulcolax should be used during pregnancy only at the discretion of the physician.
Extent of Drug Absorption
In a pharmacokinetic (crossover) study involving 12 patients (Roth, 1988), plasma levels of bisacodyl were measured following oral administration of a 10 mg reference solution and two 5 mg Dulcolax tablets, and following rectal administration of one 10 mg Dulcolax suppository. With the solution dose, the average Cmax was 237 ng/ml; with the tablet dose, the average Cmax was 26 ng/ml (11% of the solution Cmax); with the suppository dose, in six patients the plasma level was below the limit of detection, and in the remaining six patients, the average Cmax was 31 ng/ml (13% of the solution Cmax in those particular patients). These data demonstrate the low level of systemic absorption of bisacodyl resulting from Dulcolax use.

ADVERSE DRUG REACTIONS
The process of restoring normal bowel function by use of a laxative may result in some abdominal discomfort.

OVERDOSAGE
There are no specific antidotes that are required to be administered in the event of overdosage; however, supportive care may be required in order to prevent dehydration and/or electrolyte imbalance.

DOSAGE AND ADMINISTRATION
Tablets
Adults and children 12 years of age and over: Take 2 or 3 tablets (usually 2) in a single dose once daily.
Children 6 to under 12 years of age: Take 1 tablet once daily. Expect results in 8–12 hours if taken at bedtime or within 6 hours if taken before breakfast. Do not chew or crush tablets. Do not administer tablets within 1 hour after taking an antacid or milk.
Children under 6 years of age: Oral administration is not recommended due to the requirement to swallow tablets whole.
Suppositories
Adults and children 12 years of age and over: Use 1 suppository once daily. Remove foil wrapper. Lie on your side and, with pointed end first, push suppository high into the rectum so it will not slip out. Retain it for 15 to 20 minutes. If you feel the suppository must come out immediately, it was not inserted high enough and should be pushed higher.
Children under 12 years of age: One half of one 10 mg suppository once daily.
If the suppository seems soft, hold in foil wrapper under cold water for one or two minutes. In the presence of anal fissures or hemorrhoids, suppository may be coated at the tip with petroleum jelly before insertion.
Preparation for x-ray endoscopy: For barium enemas, no food should be given following oral administration to prevent reaccumulation of material in the rectum, and a suppository should be administered one to two hours prior to examination.

HOW SUPPLIED
Dulcolax, brand of bisacodyl, is supplied as either light orange enteric coated tablets of 5 mg each in boxes of 10, 25, 50, and 100, or as suppositories of 10 mg each in boxes of 4, 8, 16, and 50.
NDC 0067-6200 (tablets)
NDC 0067-6100 (suppositories)
Store Dulcolax tablets and suppositories at temperatures below 77°F (25°C). Avoid excessive humidity.
Dulcolax is also supplied in a Bowel Prep Kit. Each kit contains one Dulcolax suppository (10 mg), four Dulcolax tablets (5 mg each), and complete patient instructions.

BIBLIOGRAPHY
Roth, V.W. et al: "Pharmacokinetics and Laxative Effect of Bisacodyl after Administration of Various Dosage Forms"; Arzneim.-Forsch. 38 (I), No. 4, pp. 570–4 (1988).
Additional literature references available upon request.
Shown in Product Identification Guide, page 324

EX-LAX® LAXATIVE Pills   OTC
Regular Strength Ex-Lax,
Maximum Strength Ex-Lax
Ex-Lax Stool Softener Caplets

(See PDR For Nonprescription Drugs)

EX-LAX® Regular Strength CHOCOLATED LAXATIVE
Pieces   OTC

(See PDR For Nonprescription Drugs)

GAS–X®   OTC
ANTIGAS CHEWABLE TABLETS
EXTRA STRENGTH GAS–X®
ANTIGAS CHEWABLE TABLETS
EXTRA STRENGTH GAS–X®
ANTIGAS SOFTGELS
EXTRA STRENGTH GAS-X ANTIGAS LIQUIDS
SIMETHICONE - ANTIGAS

(See PDR For Nonprescription Drugs)

HABITROL®   ℞
(nicotine transdermal system)
Systemic delivery of 21, 14, or 7 mg/day over 24 hours
Prescribing Information

DESCRIPTION
Habitrol is a transdermal system that provides systemic delivery of nicotine following its application to intact skin for 24 hours.
Nicotine is a tertiary amine composed of a pyridine and a pyrrolidine ring. It is a colorless-to-pale yellow, freely water-soluble, strongly alkaline, oily, volatile, hygroscopic liquid obtained from the tobacco plant. Nicotine has a characteristic pungent odor and turns brown on exposure to air or light. Of its two stereoisomers, S(-)-nicotine is the more active and is the more prevalent form in tobacco. The free alkaloid is absorbed rapidly through the skin and respiratory tract.
Structural Formula

Chemical Name: S-3(1-methyl-2-pyrrolidinyl) pyridine
Molecular Formula: $C_{10}H_{14}N_2$
Molecular Weight: 162.23
Ionization Constants: pK_{a1}=7.84, pK_{a2}=3.04
Octanol-Water Partition Coefficient: 15:1 at pH 7

Habitrol systems are round, flat, 0.6-mm-thick multi-layer units containing nicotine as the active agent. Proceeding from the visible surface toward the surface attached to the skin are: (1) a tan-colored aluminized backing film; (2) a pressure-sensitive acrylate adhesive; (3) a layer containing a methacrylic acid copolymer solution of nicotine dispersed in a pad of nonwoven viscose and cotton; (4) an adhesive

layer similar in composition to (2) above; (5) a protective aluminized release liner which overlays the adhesive layer and must be removed prior to use.

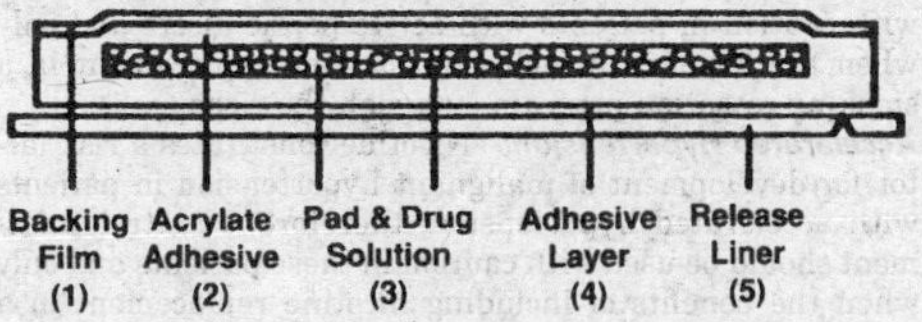
Backing Film (1)
Acrylate Adhesive (2)
Pad & Drug Solution (3)
Adhesive Layer (4)
Release Liner (5)

Nicotine is the active ingredient; other components of the system are pharmacologically inactive.
The amount of nicotine delivered to the patient from each system (29 mcg/cm^2-h) is nearly proportional to the surface area. About 60% of the total amount of nicotine remains in the system 24 hours after application. Habitrol systems are labeled as to the dose actually absorbed by the patient. The dose of nicotine absorbed from a Habitrol system represents 98% of the amount released from the system in 24 hours.

Dose Absorbed in 24 hours (mg/day)	System Surface Area (cm^2)	Total Nicotine Content (mg)
21	30	52.5
14	20	35.0
7	10	17.5

CLINICAL PHARMACOLOGY

Pharmacologic Action

Nicotine, the chief alkaloid in tobacco products, binds stereoselectively to acetylcholine receptors at the autonomic ganglia, in the adrenal medulla, at neuromuscular junctions, and in the brain. Two types of central nervous system effects are believed to be the basis of nicotine's positively reinforcing properties. A stimulating effect, exerted mainly in the cortex via the locus ceruleus, produces increased alertness and cognitive performance. A "reward" effect via the "pleasure system" in the brain is exerted in the limbic system. At low doses the stimulant effects predominate while at high doses the reward effects predominate. Intermittent intravenous administration of nicotine activates neurohormonal pathways, releasing acetylcholine, norepinephrine, dopamine, serotonin, vasopressin, beta-endorphin, growth hormone, and ACTH.

Pharmacodynamics

The cardiovascular effects of nicotine include peripheral vasoconstriction, tachycardia, and elevated blood pressure. Acute and chronic tolerance to nicotine develops from smoking tobacco or ingesting nicotine preparations. Acute tolerance (a reduction in response for a given dose) develops rapidly (less than 1 hour), however, not at the same rate for different physiologic effects (skin temperature, heart rate, subjective effects). Withdrawal symptoms such as cigarette craving can be reduced in some individuals by plasma nicotine levels lower than those from smoking.
Withdrawal from nicotine in addicted individuals is characterized by craving, nervousness, restlessness, irritability, mood lability, anxiety, drowsiness, sleep disturbances, impaired concentration, increased appetite, minor somatic complaints (headache, myalgia, constipation, fatigue), and weight gain. Nicotine toxicity is characterized by nausea, abdominal pain, vomiting, diarrhea, diaphoresis, flushing, dizziness, disturbed hearing and vision, confusion, weakness, palpitations, altered respiration, and hypotension.
The cardiovascular effects of Habitrol 14 mg/day systems used continuously for 24 hours were compared with smoking every hour during waking hours, for 10 days. A small increase in blood pressure was detectable on the first day but not after 10 days. Heart rate was increased by 3%–7% and stroke volume decreased by 5%–12% on the 10th day of application. Habitrol treatment had no significant influence on cutaneous blood flow or skin temperature.
Both smoking and nicotine can increase circulating cortisol and catecholamines, and tolerance does not develop to the catecholamine-releasing effects of nicotine. Changes in the response to a concomitantly administered adrenergic agonist or antagonist should be watched for when nicotine intake is altered during Habitrol therapy and/or smoking cessation (see PRECAUTIONS, Drug Interactions).

Pharmacokinetics

The volume of distribution following IV administration of nicotine is approximately 2 to 3 L/kg and the half-life ranges from 1 to 2 hours. The major eliminating organ is the liver, and average plasma clearance is about 1.2 L/min; the kidney and lung also metabolize nicotine. There is no significant skin metabolism of nicotine. More than 20 metabolites of nicotine have been identified, all of which are believed to be less active than the parent compound. The primary metabolite of nicotine in plasma, cotinine, has a half-life of 15 to 20 hours and concentrations that exceed nicotine by 10-fold.

Quit Rates After Week 3 by Treatment

Concomitant Support	Treatment	Number of Patients	After 7 Weeks (range)	After Weaning (range)
Yes†	Habitrol	260	19–54%	8–43%
	Placebo*	256	9–30%	8–30%
No††	Habitrol	141	4–28%	4–20%
	Placebo*	135	0–24%	0–22%

* Sub Therapeutic (ST) Placebo systems contained 13% of the nicotine found in the respective-sized active system to allow blinding as to color and odor.
† Two trials with 9 clinics, number of patients per treatment ranged from 22 to 39.
†† One trial with 5 clinics, number of patients per treatment ranged from 24 to 40.

Plasma-protein binding of nicotine is <5%. Therefore, changes in nicotine binding from use of concomitant drugs or alterations of plasma proteins by disease states would not be expected to have significant consequences.
The primary urinary metabolites are cotinine (15% of the dose) and trans-3-hydroxycotinine (45% of the dose). About 10% of nicotine is excreted unchanged in the urine. As much as 30% may be excreted in the urine with high urine flow rates and urine acidification below pH 5.
The pharmacokinetic model which best fits the plasma nicotine concentrations from Habitrol systems is an open, two-compartment disposition model with a skin depot through which nicotine enters the central circulation compartment. The nicotine from the drug matrix is released slowly from the system. Therefore, the decline of plasma nicotine concentrations during the last 12 hours is determined primarily by release of nicotine from the system through the skin.

Steady-State Plasma Nicotine Concentrations for Two Consecutive Applications of Habitrol 21 mg/day (Mean ± 2SD, N=9)

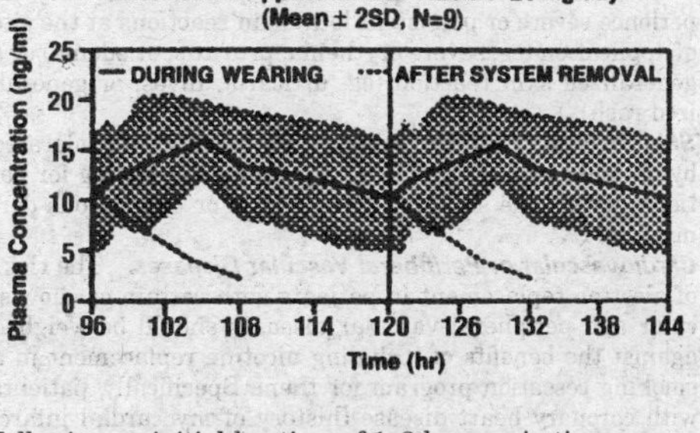
Plasma Concentration (ng/ml)
25
20
15
10
5
0
DURING WEARING
AFTER SYSTEM REMOVAL
96
102
108
114
120
126
132
138
144
Time (hr)

Following an initial lag time of 1–2 hours, nicotine concentrations increase to a broad peak between 6 and 12 hours and then decrease gradually. Steady state for nicotine is attained within 2 days of initiating Habitrol treatment and average plasma nicotine concentrations are, on average, 25% higher compared to single dose applications. Upon application of a new system and removal of the old system there is, in some patients, a slight and transient (30–60 min.) increase in nicotine plasma concentration and its variability. Plasma nicotine concentrations are proportional to dose (ie, linear kinetics are observed) for the three dosages of Habitrol systems. Nicotine kinetics are similar for all sites of application on the back, abdomen, or side.
Following removal of Habitrol systems, plasma nicotine concentrations decline in an exponential fashion with an apparent mean half-life of 3–4 hours (see dotted line in graph) compared with 1–2 hours for IV administration, due to continued absorption from the skin depot. Most nonsmoking patients will have nondetectable nicotine concentrations in 10 to 12 hours.

Steady-State Nicotine Pharmacokinetic Parameters for Habitrol Systems
(mean, standard deviation, range)

Parameter (units)	14 mg/day (N=9) Mean	SD	Range	21 mg/day (N=9) Mean	SD	Range
C_{max} (ng/mL)	12	4	6–16	17	2	13–19
C_{avg} (ng/mL)	9	3	5–12	13	2	9–17
C_{min} (ng/mL)	6	2	3–10	9	2	7–14
T_{max} (hrs)	5	3	0– 8	6	3	2– 9

C_{max}: maximum observed plasma concentration
C_{avg}: average plasma concentration
C_{min}: minimum observed plasma concentration
T_{max}: time of maximum plasma concentration

Clinical Studies

The efficacy of Habitrol treatment as an aid to smoking cessation was demonstrated in three placebo-controlled, double-blind trials in otherwise healthy patients smoking at least one pack per day (N=792). In two of the trials Habitrol therapy was combined with concomitant support and in one trial Habitrol was used without concomitant support. In all three trials, patients were treated for 7 weeks (3 weeks of titration and 4 weeks of maintenance) followed by 3 weeks of weaning. Quitting was defined as total abstinence from smoking as measured by patient diary and verified by expired carbon monoxide. The "quit rates" are the proportions of all persons initially enrolled who abstained after week 3. The two trials in otherwise healthy smokers with concomitant support showed that Habitrol therapy was more effective than placebo after 7 weeks. Quit rates were still significantly different after the additional 3-week weaning period. The quit rates varied approximately 3-fold among clinics for each treatment when Habitrol therapy was used with a concomitant support program. Data from these two studies (N=516) are combined in the Quit Rate table. Greater variability and decreased quit rates were demonstrated in both placebo and Habitrol treatment groups when concomitant support was not employed (N=276, see table).
[See table above]
Patients who used Habitrol treatment in clinical trials had a significant reduction in craving for cigarettes, a major nicotine withdrawal symptom, as compared to placebo-treated patients (see graph). Reduction in craving, as with quit rate, is quite variable. This variability is presumed to be due to inherent differences in patient populations, eg, patient motivation, concomitant illnesses, number of cigarettes smoked per day, number of years smoking, exposure to other smokers, socioeconomic status, etc, as well as differences among the clinics.

Severity of Craving by Treatment in the Two Clinical Trials with Concurrent Group Therapy (N=427)

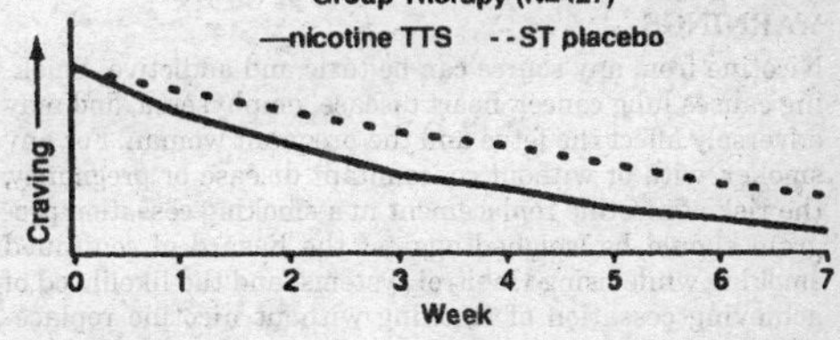
—nicotine TTS
- - ST placebo
Craving
0
1
2
3
4
5
6
7
Week

Patients using Habitrol systems dropped out of the trials less frequently than did patients receiving placebo. Quit rates for the 32 patients over age 60 were comparable to the quit rates for the 369 patients aged 60 and under.

Individualization of Dosage

It is important to make sure that patients read the instructions made available to them and have their questions answered. They should clearly understand the directions for applying and disposing of Habitrol systems. They should be instructed to stop smoking completely when the first system is applied.
The success or failure of smoking cessation depends heavily on the quality, intensity, and frequency of supportive care. Patients are more likely to quit smoking if they are seen frequently and participate in formal smoking cessation programs.
The goal of Habitrol therapy is complete abstinence. Significant health benefits have not been demonstrated for reduction of smoking. If a patient is unable to stop smoking by the fourth week of therapy, treatment should probably be discontinued. Patients who have not stopped smoking after 4 weeks of Habitrol therapy are unlikely to quit on that attempt.
Patients who fail to quit on any attempt may benefit from interventions to improve their chances for success on subsequent attempts. Patients who were unsuccessful should be counseled to determine why they failed. Patients should then probably be given a "therapy holiday" before the next attempt. A new quit attempt should be encouraged when the factors that contributed to failure can be eliminated or reduced, and conditions are more favorable.
Based on the clinical trials, a reasonable approach to assisting patients in their attempt to quit smoking is to assign their initial Habitrol dosage using the recommended dosing schedule (see Dosing Schedule). The need for dose adjustment should be assessed during the first 2 weeks. Patients should continue the dose selected with counseling and support over the following month. Those who have successfully stopped smoking during that time should be supported during 4 to 8 weeks of weaning, after which treatment should be terminated.

Continued on next page

Habitrol—Cont.

Therapy should generally begin with the Habitrol 21 mg/day dose (see Dosing Schedule below) except if the patient is small (less than 100 lbs), is a light smoker (less than $\frac{1}{2}$ pack of cigarettes per day) or has cardiovascular disease.

Dosing Schedule

	Otherwise Healthy Patients	Other Patients*
Initial/Starting Dose	21 mg/day	14 mg/day
Duration of Treatment	4–8 weeks	4–8 weeks
First Weaning Doseg	14 mg/day	7 mg/day
Duration of Treatment	2–4 weeks	2–4 weeks
Second Weaning Dose	7 mg/day	
Duration of Treatment	2–4 weeks	

* small patient (less than 100 lbs)
  or light smoker (less than 10 cigarettes/day)
  or patient with cardiovascular disease

The symptoms of nicotine withdrawal and excess overlap (see Pharmacodynamics and ADVERSE REACTIONS). Since patients using Habitrol treatment may also smoke intermittently, it may be difficult to determine if patients are experiencing nicotine withdrawal or nicotine excess.

The controlled clinical trials using Habitrol therapy suggest that abnormal dreams are more often symptoms of nicotine excess while flatulence, anxiety, and depression are more often symptoms of nicotine withdrawal.

INDICATIONS AND USAGE

Habitrol treatment is indicated as an aid to smoking cessation for the relief of nicotine withdrawal symptoms. Habitrol treatment should be used as a part of a comprehensive behavioral smoking cessation program.

The use of Habitrol systems for longer than 3 months has not been studied.

CONTRAINDICATIONS

Use of Habitrol systems is contraindicated in patients with hypersensitivity or allergy to nicotine or to any of the components of the therapeutic system.

WARNINGS

Nicotine from any source can be toxic and addictive. Smoking causes lung cancer, heart disease, emphysema, and may adversely affect the fetus and the pregnant woman. For any smoker, with or without concomitant disease or pregnancy, the risk of nicotine replacement in a smoking cessation program should be weighed against the hazard of continued smoking while using Habitrol systems, and the likelihood of achieving cessation of smoking without nicotine replacement.

Pregnancy Warning

Tobacco smoke, which has been shown to be harmful to the fetus, contains nicotine, hydrogen cyanide, and carbon monoxide. Nicotine has been shown in animal studies to cause fetal harm. It is therefore presumed that Habitrol treatment can cause fetal harm when administered to a pregnant woman. The effect of nicotine delivery by Habitrol systems has not been examined in pregnancy (see PRECAUTIONS, Other Effects). Therefore, pregnant smokers should be encouraged to attempt cessation using educational and behavioral interventions before using pharmacological approaches. If Habitrol therapy is used during pregnancy, or if the patient becomes pregnant while using Habitrol treatment, the patient should be apprised of the potential hazard to the fetus.

Safety Note Concerning Children

The amounts of nicotine that are tolerated by adult smokers can produce symptoms of poisoning and could prove fatal if Habitrol systems are applied or ingested by children or pets. Used 21 mg/day systems contain about 60% (32 mg) of their initial drug content. Therefore, patients should be cautioned to keep both used and unused Habitrol systems out of the reach of children and pets.

PRECAUTIONS

General

The patient should be urged to stop smoking completely when initiating Habitrol therapy (see DOSAGE AND ADMINISTRATION). Patients should be informed that if they continue to smoke while using Habitrol systems, they may experience adverse effects due to peak nicotine levels higher than those experienced from smoking alone. If there is a clinically significant increase in cardiovascular or other effects attributable to nicotine, the Habitrol dose should be reduced or Habitrol treatment discontinued (see WARNINGS). Physicians should anticipate that concomitant medications may need dosage adjustment (see Drug Interactions).

The use of Habitrol systems beyond 3 months by patients who stop smoking should be discouraged because the chronic consumption of nicotine by any route can be harmful and addicting.

Allergic Reactions: In a 12-week, open-label dermal irritation and sensitization study of Habitrol systems, 22 of 223 patients exhibited definite erythema at 24 hours after application. Upon rechallenge, 3 patients exhibited mild-to-moderate contact allergy. Patients with contact sensitization should be cautioned that a serious reaction could occur from exposure to other nicotine-containing products or smoking. In the efficacy trials, erythema following system removal was typically seen in about 17% of patients, some edema in 4%, and dropouts due to skin reactions occurred in 6% of patients.

Patients should be instructed to promptly discontinue the Habitrol treatment and contact their physicians if they experience severe or persistent local skin reactions at the site of application (eg, severe erythema, pruritus, or edema) or a generalized skin reaction (eg, urticaria, hives, or generalized rash).

Skin Disease: Habitrol systems are usually well tolerated by patients with normal skin, but may be irritating for patients with some skin disorders (atopic or eczematous dermatitis).

Cardiovascular or Peripheral Vascular Diseases: The risks of nicotine replacement in patients with certain cardiovascular and peripheral vascular diseases should be weighed against the benefits of including nicotine replacement in a smoking cessation program for them. Specifically, patients with coronary heart disease (history of myocardial infarction and/or angina pectoris), serious cardiac arrhythmias, or vasospastic diseases (Buerger's disease, Prinzmetal's variant angina) should be carefully screened and evaluated before nicotine replacement is prescribed.

Tachycardia occurring in association with the use of Habitrol treatment was reported occasionally. If serious cardiovascular symptoms occur with Habitrol treatment, it should be discontinued.

Habitrol treatment should generally not be used in patients during the immediate post-myocardial infarction period, patients with serious arrhythmias, and patients with severe or worsening angina pectoris.

Renal or Hepatic Insufficiency: The pharmacokinetics of nicotine have not been studied in the elderly or in patients with renal or hepatic impairment. However, given that nicotine is extensively metabolized and that its total system clearance is dependent on liver blood flow, some influence of hepatic impairment on drug kinetics (reduced clearance) should be anticipated. Only severe renal impairment would be expected to affect the clearance of nicotine or its metabolites from the circulation (see CLINICAL PHARMACOLOGY, Pharmacokinetics).

Endocrine Diseases: Habitrol treatment should be used with caution in patients with hyperthyroidism, pheochromocytoma, or insulin-dependent diabetes since nicotine causes the release of catecholamines by the adrenal medulla.

Peptic Ulcer Disease: Nicotine delays healing in peptic ulcer disease; therefore, Habitrol treatment should be used with caution in patients with active peptic ulcers and only when the benefits of including nicotine replacement in a smoking cessation program outweigh the risks.

Accelerated Hypertension: Nicotine constitutes a risk factor for development of malignant hypertension in patients with accelerated hypertension; therefore, Habitrol treatment should be used with caution in these patients and only when the benefits of including nicotine replacement in a smoking cessation program outweigh the risks.

Information for Patients: A patient instruction sheet is included in the package of Habitrol systems dispensed to the patient. It contains important information and instructions on how to use and dispose of Habitrol systems properly. Patients should be encouraged to ask questions of the physician and pharmacist.

Patients must be advised to keep both used and unused systems out of the reach of children and pets.

Drug Interactions

Smoking cessation, with or without nicotine replacement, may alter the pharmacokinetics of certain concomitant medications.

[See table below]

Carcinogenesis, Mutagenesis, Impairment of Fertility

Nicotine itself does not appear to be a carcinogen in laboratory animals. However, nicotine and its metabolites increased the incidence of tumors in the cheek pouches of hamsters and forestomach of F344 rats, respectively, when given in combination with tumor-initiators. One study, which could not be replicated, suggested that cotinine, the primary metabolite of nicotine, may cause lymphoreticular sarcoma in the large intestine in rats.

Nicotine and cotinine were not mutagenic in the Ames *Salmonella* test. Nicotine induced repairable DNA damage in an *E. coli* test system. Nicotine was shown to be genotoxic in a test system using Chinese hamster ovary cells. In rats and rabbits, implantation can be delayed or inhibited by a reduction in DNA synthesis that appears to be caused by nicotine. Studies have shown a decrease in litter size in rats treated with nicotine during gestation.

Pregnancy Category D (see WARNINGS)

The harmful effects of cigarette smoking on maternal and fetal health are clearly established. These include low birth weight, an increased risk of spontaneous abortion, and increased perinatal mortality. The specific effects of Habitrol treatment on fetal development are unknown. Therefore, pregnant smokers should be encouraged to attempt cessation using educational and behavioral interventions before using pharmacological approaches.

Spontaneous abortion during nicotine replacement therapy has been reported; as with smoking, nicotine as a contributing factor cannot be excluded.

Habitrol treatment should be used during pregnancy only if the likelihood of smoking cessation justifies the potential risk of use of nicotine replacement by the patient, who may continue to smoke.

Teratogenicity

Animal Studies: Nicotine was shown to produce skeletal abnormalities in the offspring of mice when given doses toxic to the dams (25 mg/kg/day IP or SC).

Human Studies: Nicotine teratogenicity has not been studied in humans except as a component of cigarette smoke (each cigarette smoked delivers about 1 mg of nicotine). It has not been possible to conclude whether cigarette smoking is teratogenic to humans.

Other Effects

Animal Studies: A nicotine bolus (up to 2 mg/kg) to pregnant rhesus monkeys caused acidosis, hypercarbia, and hypotension (fetal and maternal concentrations were about 20 times those achieved after smoking 1 cigarette in 5 minutes). Fetal breathing movements were reduced in the fetal lamb after intravenous injection of 0.25 mg/kg nicotine to the ewe (equivalent to smoking 1 cigarette every 20 seconds for 5 minutes). Uterine blood flow was reduced about 30% after infusion of 0.1 mg/kg/min nicotine for 20 minutes to pregnant rhesus monkeys (equivalent to smoking about six cigarettes every minute for 20 minutes).

Human Experience: Cigarette smoking during pregnancy is associated with an increased risk of spontaneous abortion, low-birth-weight infants and perinatal mortality. Nicotine and carbon monoxide are considered the most likely mediators of these outcomes. The effects of cigarette smoking on fetal cardiovascular parameters have been studied near term. Cigarettes increased fetal aortic blood flow and heart rate and decreased uterine blood flow and fetal breathing movements. Habitrol treatment has not been studied in pregnant humans.

Labor and Delivery

Habitrol systems are not recommended to be left on during labor and delivery. The effects of nicotine on the mother or the fetus during labor are unknown.

May Require a Decrease in Dose at Cessation of Smoking	Possible Mechanism
Acetaminophen, caffeine, imipramine, oxazepam, pentazocine, propranolol, theophylline	Deinduction of hepatic enzymes on smoking cessation
Insulin	Increase of subcutaneous insulin absorption with smoking cessation
Adrenergic antagonists (eg, prazosin, labetalol)	Decrease in circulating catecholamines with smoking cessation

May Require an Increase in Dose at Cessation of Smoking	Possible Mechanism
Adrenergic agonists (eg, isoproterenol, phenylephrine)	Decrease in circulating catecholamines with smoking cessation

Nursing Mothers
Caution should be exercised when Habitrol therapy is administered to nursing women. The safety of Habitrol treatment in nursing infants has not been examined. Nicotine passes freely into breast milk; the milk-to-plasma ratio averages 2.9. Nicotine is absorbed orally. An infant has the ability to clear nicotine by hepatic first-pass clearance; however, the efficiency of removal is probably lowest at birth. The nicotine concentrations in milk can be expected to be lower with Habitrol treatment when used as directed than with cigarette smoking, as maternal plasma nicotine concentrations are generally reduced with nicotine replacement. The risk of exposure of the infant to nicotine from Habitrol systems should be weighed against the risks associated with the infant's exposure to nicotine from continued smoking by the mother (passive smoke exposure and contamination of breast milk with other components of tobacco smoke) and from Habitrol systems alone or in combination with continued smoking.

Pediatric Use
Habitrol systems are not recommended for use in children because the safety and effectiveness of Habitrol treatment in children and adolescents who smoke have not been evaluated.

Geriatric Use
Forty-eight patients over the age of 60 participated in clinical trials of Habitrol therapy. Habitrol therapy appeared to be as effective in this age group as in younger smokers.

ADVERSE REACTIONS

Assessment of adverse events in the 792 patients who participated in controlled clinical trials is complicated by the occurrence of GI and CNS effects of nicotine withdrawal as well as nicotine excess. The actual incidences of both are confounded by concurrent smoking by many of the patients. In the trials, when reporting adverse events, the investigators did not attempt to identify the cause of the symptom.

Topical Adverse Events
The most common adverse event associated with topical nicotine is a short-lived erythema, pruritus, or burning at the application site, which was seen at least once in 35% of patients on Habitrol treatment in the clinical trials. Local erythema after system removal was noted at least once in 17% of patients and local edema in 4%. Erythema generally resolved within 24 hours. Cutaneous hypersensitivity (contact sensitization) occurred in 2% of patients on Habitrol treatment (see PRECAUTIONS, Allergic Reactions).

Probably Causally Related
The following adverse events were reported more frequently in Habitrol-treated patients than in placebo-treated patients or exhibited a dose response in clinical trials.

Digestive system—Diarrhea*, dyspepsia*.
Mouth/Tooth disorders—Dry mouth.
Musculoskeletal system—Arthralgia*, myalgia*.
Nervous system—Abnormal dreams†, somnolence†.

Frequencies for 21 mg/day system.
* Reported in 3% to 9% of patients.
† Reported in 1% to 3% of patients.
Unmarked if reported in <1% of patients.

Causal Relationship Unknown
Adverse events reported in Habitrol- and placebo-treated patients at about the same frequency in clinical trials are listed below. The clinical significance of the association between Habitrol treatment and these events is unknown, but they are reported as alerting information for the clinician.
Body as a whole—Allergy†, back pain†.
Cardiovascular system—Hypertension*.
Digestive system—Abdominal pain†, constipation†, nausea*, vomiting.
Nervous system—Dizziness*, concentration impaired†, headache (17%), insomnia*.
Respiratory system—Cough increased†, pharyngitis†, sinus itis†.
Urogenital system—Dysmenorrhea*.

Frequencies for 21 mg/day system
* Reported in 3% to 9% of patients.
† Reported in 1% to 3% of patients.
Unmarked if reported in <1% of patients.

DRUG ABUSE AND DEPENDENCE

Habitrol systems are likely to have a low abuse potential based on differences between it and cigarettes in four characteristics commonly considered important in contributing to abuse: much slower absorption, much smaller fluctuations in blood levels, lower blood levels of nicotine, and less frequent use (ie, once daily).
Dependence on nicotine polacrilex chewing gum replacement therapy has been reported. Such dependence might also occur from transference to Habitrol systems of tobacco-based nicotine dependence. The use of the system beyond 3 months has not been evaluated and should be discouraged. To minimize the risk of dependence, patients should be encouraged to withdraw gradually from Habitrol treatment after 4 to 8 weeks of usage. Recommended dose reduction is to progressively decrease the dose every 2 to 4 weeks (see DOSAGE AND ADMINISTRATION).

OVERDOSAGE

The effects of applying several Habitrol systems simultaneously or of swallowing Habitrol systems are unknown (see WARNINGS, Safety Note Concerning Children).
The oral LD_{50} for nicotine in rodents varies with species but is in excess of 24 mg/kg; death is due to respiratory paralysis. The oral minimum lethal dose of nicotine in dogs is greater than 5 mg/kg. The oral minimum acute lethal dose for nicotine in human adults is reported to be 40 to 60 mg (<1 mg/kg).
Two or three Habitrol 30 cm^2 systems in capsules fed to dogs weighing 8–17 kg were emetic, but did not produce any other significant clinical signs. The administration of these patches corresponds to about 6–17 mg/kg of nicotine.
Signs and symptoms of an overdose of Habitrol systems would be expected to be the same as those of acute nicotine poisoning including: pallor, cold sweat, nausea, salivation, vomiting, abdominal pain, diarrhea, headache, dizziness, disturbed hearing and vision, tremor, mental confusion, and weakness. Prostration, hypotension, and respiratory failure may ensue with large overdoses. Lethal doses produce convulsions quickly and death follows as a result of peripheral or central respiratory paralysis or, less frequently, cardiac failure.

Overdose From Topical Exposure
The Habitrol system should be removed immediately if the patient shows signs of overdosage and the patient should seek immediate medical care. The skin surface may be flushed with water and dried. No soap should be used since it may increase nicotine absorption. Nicotine will continue to be delivered into the bloodstream for several hours (see CLINICAL PHARMACOLOGY, Pharmacokinetics) after removal of the system because of a depot of nicotine in the skin.

Overdose From Ingestion
Persons ingesting Habitrol systems should be referred to a health care facility for management. Due to the possibility of nicotine-induced seizures, activated charcoal should be administered. In unconscious patients with a secure airway, instill activated charcoal via nasogastric tube. A saline cathartic or sorbitol added to the first dose of activated charcoal may speed gastrointestinal passage of the system. Repeated doses of activated charcoal should be administered as long as the system remains in the gastrointestinal tract since it will continue to release nicotine for many hours.

Management of Nicotine Poisoning
Other supportive measures include diazepam or barbiturates for seizures, atropine for excessive bronchial secretions or diarrhea, respiratory support for respiratory failure, and vigorous fluid support for hypotension and cardiovascular collapse.

DOSAGE AND ADMINISTRATION

Patients must desire to stop smoking and should be instructed to *stop smoking immediately* as they begin using Habitrol therapy. The patient should read the patient instruction sheet on Habitrol treatment and be encouraged to ask any questions. Treatment should be initiated with Habitrol 21 mg/day or 14 mg/day systems (see CLINICAL PHARMACOLOGY, Individualization of Dosage). Dosage cannot be adjusted by cutting a Habitrol system.
Once the appropriate dosage is selected the patient should begin 4–6 weeks of therapy at that dosage. The patient should stop smoking cigarettes completely during this period. If the patient is unable to stop cigarette smoking within 4 weeks, Habitrol therapy should probably be stopped, since few additional patients in clinical trials were able to quit after this time.

Recommended Dosing Schedule for Healthy Patients[a]
(see Individualization of Dosage)

Dose	Duration
Habitrol 21 mg/day	First 6 Weeks
Habitrol 14 mg/day	Next 2 Weeks[b]
Habitrol 7 mg/day	Last 2 Weeks[c]

[a] Start with Habitrol 14 mg/day for 6 weeks for patients who:
—have cardiovascular disease
—weigh less than 100 pounds
—smoke less than 1/2 a pack of cigarettes/day
Decrease dose to Habitrol 7 mg/day for the final 2–4 weeks.

[b] Patients who have successfully abstained from smoking should have their dose of Habitrol reduced after each 2–4 weeks of treatment until the 7 mg/day dose has been used for 2–4 weeks (see Individualization of Dosage).

[c] The entire course of nicotine substitution and gradual withdrawal should take 8–12 weeks, depending on the size of the initial dose. The use of Habitrol beyond 3 months has not been studied.

The Habitrol system should be applied promptly upon its removal from the protective pouch to prevent evaporative loss of nicotine from the system. Habitrol systems should be used only when the pouch is intact to assure that the product has not been tampered with.
Habitrol systems should be applied only once a day to a non-hairy, clean, and dry skin site on the trunk or upper, outer arm. After 24 hours, the used Habitrol system should be removed and a new system applied to an alternate skin site. Skin sites should not be reused for at least a week. Patients should be cautioned not to continue to use the same system for more than 24 hours.

Safety and Handling
Habitrol systems can be a dermal irritant and can cause contact sensitization. Although exposure of health care workers to nicotine from Habitrol systems should be minimal, care should be taken to avoid unnecessary contact with active systems. If active systems are handled, wash hands with water alone, since soap may increase nicotine absorption. Do not touch eyes. KEEP OUT OF THE REACH OF CHILDREN.

Disposal
When the used system is removed from the skin, it should be folded over and placed in the protective pouch which contained the new system. The used system should be immediately disposed of in such a way to prevent its access by children or pets. See patient information for further directions for handling and disposal.

HOW SUPPLIED

Habitrol systems are individually packaged in child-resistant pouches and should not be used if individual pouches are unsealed.
[See table above]

Nicotine Delivery Rate *(in vivo)*	Nicotine in System	System Size	Package Size	NDC Number
21 mg/day	52.5 mg	30 cm^2	30 systems	0067-0810-21
14 mg/day	35.0 mg	20 cm^2	30 systems	0067-0820-14
7 mg/day	17.5 mg	10 cm^2	30 systems	0067-0830-07

How to Store
Do not store above 86°F (30°C) because Habitrol systems are sensitive to heat. A slight discoloration of the system is not significant.
Do not store unpouched. Once removed from the protective pouch, Habitrol systems should be applied promptly since nicotine is volatile and the system may lose strength.
The use of this product is covered by U.S. Patent No. 4,597,961.

CAUTION: Federal law prohibits dispensing without prescription.

Novartis Consumer Health, Inc.
Dist. by:
Novartis Consumer Health, Inc.
Summit, NJ 07901-1312

HABITROL®
(nicotine transdermal system)
Patient Instructions

IMPORTANT

YOUR DOCTOR HAS PRESCRIBED THIS DRUG FOR YOUR USE ONLY. DO NOT LET ANYONE ELSE USE IT. KEEP THIS MEDICINE OUT OF THE REACH OF CHILDREN AND PETS. Nicotine can be very toxic and harmful. Small amounts of nicotine can cause serious illness in children. Even used Habitrol patches contain enough nicotine to poison children and pets. Be sure to throw Habitrol patches away out of the reach of children and pets. If a child puts on Habitrol patches or plays with a Habitrol patch that is out of the sealed pouch, take it away from the child and contact a poison control center, or contact a doctor immediately.
Women: Nicotine in any form may cause harm to your unborn baby if you use nicotine while you are pregnant. Do not use Habitrol patches if you are pregnant or nursing unless advised by your doctor. If you become pregnant while using Habitrol patches or if you think you might be pregnant, stop smoking and don't use Habitrol patches until you have talked to your doctor.
This leaflet will provide you with general information about nicotine and specific instructions about how to use Habitrol patches. It is important that you read it carefully and completely before you start using Habitrol patches. Be sure to read the PRECAUTIONS section before using Habitrol patches, because, as with all drugs, Habitrol treatment has

Continued on next page

Habitrol—Cont.

side effects. Since this leaflet is only a summary of information, be sure to ask your doctor if you have any questions or want to know more.

INTRODUCTION

IT IS IMPORTANT THAT YOU ARE FIRMLY COMMITTED TO GIVING UP SMOKING.

Habitrol is a skin patch containing nicotine designed to help you quit smoking cigarettes. When you wear a Habitrol patch, it releases nicotine through the skin into your bloodstream while you're wearing it. The nicotine which is in your skin will still be entering your bloodstream for several hours after you take the patch off.

It is the nicotine in cigarettes that causes addiction to smoking. Habitrol therapy replaces some of the nicotine you crave when you are stopping smoking. Habitrol patches may also help relieve other symptoms of nicotine withdrawal that may occur when you stop smoking such as irritability, frustration, anger, anxiety, difficulty in concentration, and restlessness.

There are three doses of Habitrol. Your doctor has chosen the Habitrol patch with the correct dose for you and may adjust it during the first week or two. After about 6 weeks, your doctor will give you smaller Habitrol patches approximately every two weeks. The smaller patches give you less nicotine. In time, you will be completely off nicotine. You cannot adjust the nicotine dose by cutting a Habitrol patch.

INFORMATION ABOUT HABITROL PATCHES

How Habitrol Patches Work

Habitrol patches contain nicotine. When you put a Habitrol patch on your skin, nicotine passes from the patch through the skin and into your blood.

How to Apply a Habitrol Patch

Step 1. Choose a non-hairy, clean, dry area on your trunk or upper, outer part of your arm. Do not put a Habitrol patch on skin that is very oily, burned, broken out, cut, or irritated in any way.

Step 2. Do not remove the Habitrol patch from its sealed, child-resistant, protective pouch until you are ready to use it. Carefully cut open the child-resistant pouch. Discard the used patch you take off by folding it in half and putting it into the opened pouch. Throw it away in the trash out of the reach of children and pets (see Step 7).

Step 3. A shiny protective liner covers the sticky side of the Habitrol patch—the side that will be put on your skin. The liner has a precut slit to help you remove it from the patch. With the silver side facing you, pull the liner away from the Habitrol patch starting at the precut slit. Hold the Habitrol patch at the edge (touch the sticky side as little as possible) and pull off the other piece of the protective liner. Throw away this liner.

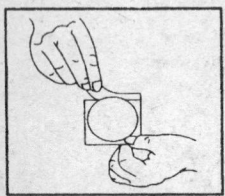 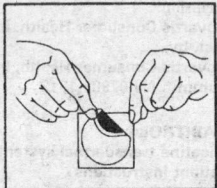

Step 4. Immediately apply the sticky side of the Habitrol patch to your skin. Press the Habitrol patch firmly on your skin with the palm of your hand for about 10 seconds. Make sure it sticks well to your skin, expecially around the edges.

Step 5. Wash your hands when you have finished applying the Habitrol patch. Nicotine on your hands could get into your eyes and nose and could cause stinging, redness, or more serious problems.

Step 6. After approximately 24 hours, remove the patch you have been wearing. Choose a *different* place on your skin to apply the next Habitrol patch and repeat Steps 1 to 5. Do not return to a previously used skin site for at least one week. Do not leave the Habitrol patch on for more than 24 hours because it may irritate your skin and because it loses strength after 24 hours.

Step 7. Fold the used Habitrol patch in half with the sticky side together. After you have put on a new Habitrol patch, take its pouch and place the used, folded Habitrol patch inside of it. Throw the pouch in the trash away from children and pets.

When to Apply a Habitrol Patch

If you apply the Habitrol patch at about the same time each day, it will help you to remember when to put on a new Habitrol patch. If you want to change the time when you put

on your patch, you can do so. Just remove the Habitrol patch you are wearing and put on a new one. After that, apply the Habitrol patch at the new time each day.

If Your Habitrol Patch Gets Wet

Water will not harm the Habitrol patch you are wearing. You can bathe, swim, use a hot tub, or shower while you are wearing a Habitrol patch.

If Your Habitrol Patch Comes Off

If your Habitrol patch falls off, put on a new one. Remove the Habitrol patch at your regular time to keep your schedule the same, or 24 hours after applying the replacement patch if you wish to change the time each day that you apply a new patch. Before putting on a new patch, make sure you select a non-hairy area which is not irritated and is clean and dry.

Disposing of a Habitrol Patch

Fold the used Habitrol patch in half with the sticky side together. After you put on a new Habitrol patch, take its opened pouch or aluminum foil and place the used, folded Habitrol patch inside of it. THROW THE POUCH IN THE TRASH AWAY FROM CHILDREN AND PETS.

Storage Instructions

Keep the Habitrol patch in its protective pouch until you are ready to use it. Do not store your Habitrol patches above 86°F (30°C) because the patch is sensitive to heat. Remember, the inside of your car can reach temperatures much higher than this in the summer.

PRECAUTIONS

What to Ask Your Doctor

Ask your doctor about possible problems with Habitrol therapy. Be sure to tell your doctor if you have had any of the following:
- a recent heart attack (myocardial infarction)
- irregular heart beat (arrhythmia)
- severe or worsening heart pain (angina pectoris)
- allergies to drugs
- rashes from adhesive tape or bandages
- skin diseases
- very high blood pressure
- stomach ulcers
- overactive thyroid
- diabetes requiring insulin
- kidney or liver disease

If You Are Taking Medicines

Habitrol patch use, together with stopping smoking, may change the effect of other medicines. It is important to tell your doctor about all the medicines you are taking.

What to Watch For (Adverse Effects)

You should not smoke while using the Habitrol patch. It is possible to get too much nicotine (an overdose), especially if you use a Habitrol patch and smoke at the same time. Signs of an overdose would include bad headaches, dizziness, upset stomach, drooling, vomiting, diarrhea, cold sweat, blurred vision, difficulty with hearing, mental confusion, and weakness. An overdose might cause you to faint.

If Your Skin Reacts to the Habitrol Patch

When you first put on a Habitrol patch, mild itching, burning, or tingling is normal and should go away within an hour. After you remove a Habitrol patch, the skin under the patch might be somewhat red. Your skin should not stay red for more than a day. If you get a skin rash after using a Habitrol patch, or if the skin under the patch becomes swollen or very red, call your doctor. Do not put on a new patch. You may be allergic to one of the components of the Habitrol patch.

If you do become allergic to the nicotine in the Habitrol patch, you could get sick from using cigarettes or other nicotine-containing products.

What to Do When Problems Occur

IF YOU NOTICE ANY WORRISOME SYMPTOMS OR PROBLEMS, TAKE OFF THE HABITROL PATCH AND CALL YOUR DOCTOR AT ONCE.

CHILD-RESISTANT POUCH. DO NOT USE IF INDIVIDUAL POUCHES ARE UNSEALED.

Dist. by:
Novartis Consumer Health, Inc.
Summit, NJ 07901-1312

Shown in Product Identification Guide, page 324

MAALOX®   OTC

Magnesia and Alumina
Oral Suspension
Antacid

Liquids
Cooling Mint
Smooth Cherry
Refreshing Lemon

DESCRIPTION

Maalox® Antacid is used for the relief of acid indigestion, heartburn, sour stomach and upset stomach associated with these symptoms.

Active Ingredients	Maalox Suspension 5 mL teaspoon
Magnesium Hydroxide	200 mg
Aluminum Hydroxide (equivalent to dried gel, USP)	225 mg

INACTIVE INGREDIENTS

Cooling Mint
Calcium saccharin, flavor, guar gum, methylparaben, propylparaben, purified water, sorbitol.
Smooth Cherry and Refreshing Lemon
Calcium saccharin, flavors, methylparaben, propylparaben, purified water, sorbitol and xanthan gum.

Minimum Recommended Dosage: Maalox Suspension	
	Per 2 Tsp. (10 mL)
Acid neutralizing capacity	NLT 26.6 mEq
Sodium content	NMT 2.5 mg

DIRECTIONS FOR USE

Two to four teaspoonfuls, four times a day or as directed by a physician.

PATIENT WARNINGS

Do not take more than 16 teaspoonfuls in a 24-hour period or use the maximum dosage for more than 2 weeks or use if you have kidney disease except under the advice and supervision of a physician. Keep this and all drugs out of the reach of children.

DRUG INTERACTION PRECAUTION

Antacids may interact with certain prescription drugs. If you are presently taking a prescription drug, do not take this product without checking with your physician or other health professional.

Professional Labeling

INDICATIONS

As an antacid for symptomatic relief of hyperacidity associated with the diagnosis of peptic ulcer, gastritis, peptic esophagitis, gastric hyperacidity, heartburn, or hiatal hernia.

WARNINGS

Prolonged use of aluminum-containing antacids in patients with renal failure may result in or worsen dialysis osteomalacia. Elevated tissue aluminum levels contribute to the development of the dialysis encephalopathy and osteomalacia syndromes. Small amounts of aluminum are absorbed from the gastrointestinal tract and renal excretion of aluminum is impaired in renal failure. Aluminum is not well removed by dialysis because it is bound to albumin and transferrin, which do not cross dialysis membranes. As a result, aluminum is deposited in bone, and dialysis osteomalacia may develop when large amounts of aluminum are ingested orally by patients with impaired renal function.

Aluminum forms insoluble complexes with phosphate in the gastrointestinal tract, thus decreasing phosphate absorption. Prolonged use of aluminum-containing antacids by normophosphatemic patients may result in hypophosphatemia if phosphate intake is not adequate. In its more severe forms, hypophosphatemia can lead to anorexia, malaise, muscle weakness, and osteomalacia.

HOW SUPPLIED

Maalox® Cooling Mint Suspension is available in plastic bottles of 5 oz (0067-0330-62), 12 oz (0067-0330-71) and 26 oz (0067-0330-44).

Maalox® Smooth Cherry Suspension is available in plastic bottles of 12 oz (0067-0331-71) and 26 oz (0067-0331-44).

Maalox® Refreshing Lemon Suspension is available in plastic bottles of 12 oz (0067-0222-71) and 26 oz (0067-0222-44).

MAALOX® ANTACID/ANTI-GAS   OTC
Alumina, Magnesia and Simethicone Tablets
Antacid/Anti-Gas

Tablets
Lemon, Cherry, and Mint Flavors
☐ **Physician-proven Maalox® formula for antacid effectiveness.**
☐ **Simethicone, at a recognized clinical dose, for antiflatulent action.**

DESCRIPTION
Maalox® Antacid/Anti-Gas, a balanced combination of magnesium and aluminum hydroxides plus simethicone, is a non-constipating antacid/anti-gas product which comes in pleasant tasting flavors.

COMPOSITION
To provide symptomatic relief of hyperacidity plus alleviation of gas symptoms, each tablet contains:

Active Ingredients	Maalox® Antacid/Anti-Gas Per Tablet
Magnesium Hydroxide	200 mg
Aluminum Hydroxide (equivalent to dried gel, USP)	200 mg
Simethicone	25 mg

INACTIVE INGREDIENTS
Maalox® Antacid/Anti-Gas Tablets: D&C Red No. 30, D&C Yellow No. 10, dextrose, flavors, magnesium stearate, mannitol, saccharin sodium, sorbitol, starch, sucrose, talc.
To aid in establishing proper dosage schedules, the following information is provided:

Minimum Recommended Dosage:	Per Tablet
Acid neutralizing capacity	NLT 12.6 mEq
Sodium content*	NMT 1 mg
Sugar content	0.54 g
Lactose content	None

*Dietetically insignificant.

DIRECTIONS FOR USE
Chew 1 to 4 tablets 4 times a day or as directed by a physician.

PATIENT WARNINGS
Do not take more than 16 tablets in a 24-hour period or use the maximum dosage for more than 2 weeks or use if you have kidney disease except under the advice and supervision of a physician. Keep this and all drugs out of the reach of children.

DRUG INTERACTION PRECAUTION
Antacids may interact with certain prescription drugs. If you are presently taking a prescription drug, do not take this product without checking with your physician or other health professional.

Professional Labeling
INDICATIONS
As an antacid for symptomatic relief of hyperacidity associated with the diagnosis of peptic ulcer, gastritis, peptic esophagitis, gastric hyperacidity, heartburn, or hiatal hernia. As an antiflatulent to alleviate the symptoms of gas, including postoperative gas pain.

WARNINGS
Prolonged use of aluminum-containing antacids in patients with renal failure may result in or worsen dialysis osteomalacia. Elevated tissue aluminum levels contribute to the development of the dialysis encephalopathy and osteomalacia syndromes. Small amounts of aluminum are absorbed from the gastrointestinal tract and renal excretion of aluminum is impaired in renal failure. Aluminum is not well removed by dialysis because it is bound to albumin and transferrin, which do not cross dialysis membranes. As a result, aluminum is deposited in bone, and dialysis osteomalacia may develop when large amounts of aluminum are ingested orally by patients with impaired renal function.
Aluminum forms insoluble complexes with phosphate in the gastrointestinal tract, thus decreasing phosphate absorption. Prolonged use of aluminum-containing antacids by normophosphatemic patients may result in hypophosphatemia if phosphate intake is not adequate. In its more severe forms, hypophosphatemia can lead to anorexia, malaise, muscle weakness, and osteomalacia.

ADVANTAGES
Maalox® Antacid/Anti-Gas Tablets are uniquely palatable—an important feature which encourages patients to follow your dosage directions. Maalox® Antacid/Anti-Gas Tablets have the time-proven, nonconstipating, sodium-free* Maalox® formula—useful for those patients suffering from the problems associated with hyperacidity. Additionally, Maalox® Antacid/Anti-Gas Tablets contain simethicone to alleviate discomfort associated with entrapped gas.
*Dietetically insignificant.

HOW SUPPLIED
Maalox® Antacid/Anti-Gas Refreshing Lemon Tablets are available in plastic bottles of 50 tablets (0067-0339-50) and 100 tablets (0067-0339-67), tray of 12 rolls (0067-0339-23), and 3 roll packs of 36 tablets (0067-0339-33).
Maalox® Antacid/Anti-Gas Smooth Cherry Tablets are available in plastic bottles of 50 tablets (0067-0341-50) and 100 tablets (0067-0341-68).
Maalox® Antacid/Anti-Gas Tablets are also available in **assorted flavor** bottles of 50 tablets (0067-7346-50) and 100 tablets (0067-7346-68), tray of 12 rolls (0067-7346-23) and 3 roll packs of 36 tablets (0067-7346-33).

EXTRA STRENGTH   OTC
MAALOX® ANTACID/ANTI-GAS
Alumina, Magnesia and Simethicone Oral Suspensions and Tablets, Antacid/Anti-Gas

Suspensions and Tablets
☐ **Refreshing Lemon**
  Smooth Cherry
  Cooling Mint
☐ **Physician-proven Maalox® formula for antacid effectiveness.**
☐ **Simethicone, at a recognized clinical dose, for antiflatulent action.**

DESCRIPTION
Extra Strength Maalox® Antacid/Anti-Gas, a balanced combination of magnesium and aluminum hydroxides plus simethicone, is a non-constipating antacid/anti-gas product to provide symptomatic relief of acid indigestion, heartburn, symptoms referred to as gas and sour stomach associated with these suspensions. Available in suspensions in Refreshing Lemon, Smooth Cherry, and Cooling Mint flavors and in tablets in Cooling Mint and assorted (Refreshing Lemon/Smooth Cherry/Cooling Mint) flavors.

COMPOSITION
To provide symptomatic relief of hyperacidity plus alleviation of gas symptoms, each teaspoonful/tablet contains:

Active Ingredients	Extra Strength Maalox® Antacid/Anti-Gas Per Tsp. (5 mL)	Per Tablet
Magnesium Hydroxide	450 mg	350 mg
Aluminum Hydroxide (equivalent to dried gel, USP)	500 mg	350 mg
Simethicone	40 mg	30 mg

INACTIVE INGREDIENTS
Suspensions: Calcium Saccharin, FD&C Red No. 40 (Smooth Cherry only), Guar Gum, Flavors, Methylparaben, Propylparaben, Purified Water, and Sorbitol.
Tablets: D&C Red No. 30, D&C Yellow No. 10, Dextrose, FD&C Blue No. 1, Flavors, Magnesium Stearate, Mannitol, Saccharin Sodium, Sorbitol, Starch, Sucrose.

DIRECTIONS FOR USE
Suspensions; 2 to 4 teaspoonfuls, 4 times per day, or as directed by a physician. Tablets; chew 1 to 3 tablets, 4 times per day, or as directed by a physician.

PATIENT WARNINGS
Do not take more than 12 teaspoonfuls or 12 tablets in a 24-hour period or use the maximum dosage for more than 2 weeks or use if you have kidney disease except under the advice and supervision of a physician. Keep this and all drugs out of the reach of children.

DRUG INTERACTION PRECAUTION
Antacids may interact with certain prescription drugs. If you are presently taking a prescription drug, do not take this product without checking with your physician or other health professional.
To aid in establishing proper dosage schedules, the following information is provided:

	Minimum Recommended Dosage: Extra Strength Maalox® Antacid/Anti-Gas	
	Per 2 Tsp. (10 mL)	Per Tablet
Acid neutralizing capacity	59.6 mEq	NLT 22.1 mEq
Sodium content*	<2.5 mg	<1.7 mg

*Dietetically insignificant.

Professional Labeling
INDICATIONS
As an antacid for symptomatic relief of hyperacidity associated with the diagnosis of peptic ulcer, gastritis, peptic esophagitis, gastric hyperacidity, heartburn, or hiatal hernia. As an antiflatulent to alleviate the symptoms of gas, including postoperative gas pain.

ADVANTAGES
Among antacids, Extra Strength Maalox® Antacid/Anti-Gas Suspension and Extra Strength Maalox® Antacid/Anti-Gas Tablets are uniquely palatable—an important feature which encourages patients to follow your dosage directions. Extra Strength Maalox® Antacid/Anti-Gas Suspension and Extra Strength Maalox® Antacid/Anti-Gas Tablets have the time-proven, nonconstipating, sodium-free* Maalox® formula—useful for those patients suffering from the problems associated with hyperacidity. Additionally, Extra Strength Maalox® Antacid/Anti-Gas Suspension and Extra Strength Maalox® Antacid/Anti-Gas Tablets contain simethicone to relieve symptoms referred to as gas.
*Dietetically insignificant.

WARNINGS
Prolonged use of aluminum-containing antacids in patients with renal failure may result in or worsen dialysis osteomalacia. Elevated tissue aluminum levels contribute to the development of the dialysis encephalopathy and osteomalacia syndromes. Small amounts of aluminum are absorbed from the gastrointestinal tract and renal excretion of aluminum is impaired in renal failure. Aluminum is not well removed by dialysis because it is bound to albumin and transferrin, which do not cross dialysis membranes. As a result, aluminum is deposited in bone, and dialysis osteomalacia may develop when large amounts of aluminum are ingested orally by patients with impaired renal function.
Aluminum forms insoluble complexes with phosphate in the gastrointestinal tract, thus decreasing phosphate absorption. Prolonged use of aluminum-containing antacids by normophosphatemic patients may result in hypophosphatemia if phosphate intake is not adequate. In its more severe forms, hypophosphatemia can lead to anorexia, malaise, muscle weakness, and osteomalacia.

HOW SUPPLIED
Extra Strength Maalox® Antacid/Anti-Gas Suspensions Available in Refreshing Lemon in the following sizes: 5 fl. oz. (148 mL) (0067-0333-62), 12 fl. oz. (355 mL) (0067-0333-71) and 26 fl. oz. (769 mL) (0067-0333-44).
Smooth Cherry is available in plastic bottles of 12 fl. oz. (355 mL) (0067-0336-71) and 26 fl. oz. (769 mL) (0067-0336-44).
Cooling Mint is available in plastic bottles of 12 fl. oz. (355 mL) (0067-0338-71) and 26 fl. oz. (769 mL) (0067-0338-44).
Extra Strength Maalox® Antacid/Anti-Gas Cooling Mint Tablets are available in bottles of 38 tablets (0067-0345-38) and 75 tablets (0067-0345-75).
Extra Strength Maalox® Antacid/Anti-Gas assorted flavors tablets are available in bottles of 38 tablets (0067-7214-38) and 75 tablets (0067-7214-75).

Fiber Therapy
PERDIEM®   OTC
Psyllium Fiber

DESCRIPTION
Fiber Therapy Perdiem contains a 100% natural bulk-forming fiber that gently helps relieve occasional constipation

Continued on next page

Perdiem Fiber—Cont.

(irregularity). Fiber Therapy Perdiem contains no synthetic stimulants. Perdiem's unique form, is easy to swallow and requires no mixing. Fiber Therapy Perdiem generally takes effect within 12 to 72 hours.

INDICATIONS

For relief of occasional constipation. This product generally produces bowel movement in 12 to 72 hours.

ACTIVE INGREDIENTS

100% psyllium (Plantago hydrocolloid).
Each rounded (6 gm) teaspoon contains:
4.03 gm psyllium, 36.1 mg potassium and 1.80 mg sodium.
Only 4 Calories

INACTIVE INGREDIENTS

Acacia, iron oxides, natural flavors, paraffin, sucrose, talc, titanium dioxide.

DIRECTIONS FOR USE

Perdiem requires no mixing in liquids for use.
THIS PRODUCT (CHILD OR ADULT DOSE) MUST BE FOLLOWED WITH AT LEAST 8 OUNCES (A FULL GLASS) OF COOL WATER OR OTHER FLUID. TAKING THIS PRODUCT WITHOUT ENOUGH LIQUID MAY CAUSE CHOKING (SEE WARNINGS)
Adults and Children 12 Years and Older: In the evening and/or before breakfast, 1 to 2 rounded teaspoonfuls placed in the mouth and swallowed with at least 8 oz. of cool liquid.
Children 7 to 11 Years Old: One rounded teaspoonful one to two times daily with at least 8 oz. of cool liquid. Perdiem is not intended for use in children under the age of 7 years.
For Severe Cases of Constipation: Perdiem may be taken more frequently, up to 2 rounded teaspoonfuls every 6 hours not to exceed 5 teaspoonfuls in a 24-hour period.
PERDIEM SHOULD NOT BE CHEWED.

WARNINGS

TAKING THIS PRODUCT WITHOUT ADEQUATE FLUID MAY CAUSE IT TO SWELL AND BLOCK THE THROAT OR ESOPHAGUS AND MAY CAUSE CHOKING. DO NOT TAKE THIS PRODUCT IF YOU HAVE DIFFICULTY IN SWALLOWING. IF YOU EXPERIENCE CHEST PAIN, VOMITING OR DIFFICULTY IN SWALLOWING OR BREATHING AFTER TAKING THIS PRODUCT, SEEK IMMEDIATE MEDICAL ATTENTION.
People with esophageal narrowing should not use bulk-forming agents.
If you have noticed a sudden change in bowel habits that persists over a two-week period, consult a doctor before using any laxative product.
If use of this product for constipation has produced no effect within one week or if rectal bleeding occurs after use of any bulk fiber or laxative, discontinue use and consult a doctor. Do not use if you have a history of psyllium allergy or experience abdominal pain, nausea or vomiting unless directed by a doctor.

HOW SUPPLIED

250 gm (8.8 oz.) canisters (NDC 0067-0795-70)

Overnight Relief
PERDIEM®   OTC
100% Natural Bulk Fiber Plus Vegetable Laxative

DESCRIPTION

Overnight Relief Perdiem is a unique combination of natural bulk-forming psyllium fiber plus a natural senna laxative. Perdiem's unique combination of ingredients provides gentle, predictable overnight relief of constipation without synthetic laxative ingredients. Perdiem's unique form is easy to swallow, has a great mint taste and requires no mixing. Overnight Relief Perdiem generally takes effect within 12 hours, so you can depend on it to work overnight.

INDICATIONS

For relief of occasional constipation. This product generally produces bowel movement within 12 hours.

ACTIVE INGREDIENTS

82% psyllium (Plantago hydrocolloid) and 18% senna (Cassia Pod Concentrate).
Each rounded (6 gm) teaspoonful contains:
3.25 gm psyllium, 0.74 gm senna, 35.5 mg potassium and 1.8 mg sodium.
Only 4 Calories

INACTIVE INGREDIENTS

Acacia, iron oxides, natural flavors, paraffin, sucrose, talc.

DIRECTIONS FOR USE

Perdiem requires no mixing in liquids for use.
THIS PRODUCT (CHILD OR ADULT DOSE) MUST BE FOLLOWED WITH AT LEAST 8 OUNCES (A FULL GLASS) OF COOL WATER OR OTHER FLUID.

TAKING THIS PRODUCT WITHOUT ENOUGH LIQUID MAY CAUSE CHOKING (SEE WARNINGS).
Adults and Children 12 Years and Older: In the evening and/or before breakfast, 1 to 2 rounded teaspoonfuls placed in the mouth and swallowed with at least 8 oz. of cool liquid.
Children 7 to 11 Years Old: One rounded teaspoonful one to two times daily with at least 8 oz. of cool liquid.
Perdiem is not intended for use in children under the age of 7 years.
For Severe Cases of Constipation: Perdiem may be taken more frequently, up to 2 rounded teaspoonfuls every 6 hours not to exceed 5 teaspoonfuls in a 24-hour period.
PERDIEM SHOULD NOT BE CHEWED.

PRECAUTIONS

Pregnancy category B. Results from limited animal reproduction studies have not demonstrated a risk to the fetus. However, because there are not adequate and well-controlled studies in pregnant women, this product should be used during pregnancy only if clearly needed.

WARNINGS

TAKING THIS PRODUCT WITHOUT ADEQUATE FLUID MAY CAUSE IT TO SWELL AND BLOCK THE THROAT OR ESOPHAGUS AND MAY CAUSE CHOKING. DO NOT TAKE THIS PRODUCT IF YOU HAVE DIFFICULTY IN SWALLOWING. IF YOU EXPERIENCE CHEST PAIN, VOMITING OR DIFFICULTY IN SWALLOWING OR BREATHING AFTER TAKING THIS PRODUCT, SEEK IMMEDIATE MEDICAL ATTENTION.
People with esophageal narrowing should not use bulk-forming agents.
If you have noticed a sudden change in bowel habits that persists over a two-week period, consult a doctor before using any laxative product.
If use of this product for constipation has produced no effect within one week or if rectal bleeding occurs after use of any bulk fiber or laxative, discontinue use and consult a doctor. Do not use if you have a history of psyllium allergy or experience abdominal pain, nausea or vomiting unless directed by a doctor.

HOW SUPPLIED

400 gm (14 oz.) canisters (NDC 0067-0690-39)
250 gm (8.8 oz.) canisters (NDC 0067-0690-70)
6×6 gm Individual packets (NDC 0067-0690-16)

SLOW FE®   OTC
Slow Release Iron Tablets

DESCRIPTION

SLOW FE supplies ferrous sulfate, for the treatment of iron deficiency and iron deficiency anemia with a significant reduction in the incidence of the common side effects associated with taking oral iron preparations. The wax matrix delivery system of SLOW FE is designed to maximize the release of ferrous sulfate in the duodenum and the jejunum where it is best tolerated and absorbed. SLOW FE has been clinically shown to be associated with a lower incidence of constipation, diarrhea and abdominal discomfort when compared to an immediate release iron tablet[1] and a leading sustained release iron capsule.[2]

FORMULA

Each tablet contains: Active Ingredient: 160 mg dried ferrous sulfate USP, equivalent to 50 mg elemental iron. Inactive Ingredients: cetostearyl alcohol, hydroxypropyl methylcellulose, lactose, magnesium stearate, polysorbate 80, talc, titanium dioxide, yellow iron oxide, FD&C blue #2 aluminum lake.

DOSAGE

ADULTS—one or two tablets daily or as recommended by a physician. A maximum of four tablets daily may be taken. CHILDREN—one tablet daily. Tablets must be swallowed whole.

WARNING

The treatment of any anemic condition should be under the advice and supervision of a physician. As oral iron products interfere with absorption of oral tetracycline antibiotics, these products should not be taken within two hours of each other. As with any drug, if you are pregnant or nursing a baby, seek the advice of a health professional before using this product.
Accidental overdose of iron-containing products is a leading cause of fatal poisonings in children under 6. KEEP THIS PRODUCT OUT OF REACH OF CHILDREN. In case of accidental overdose, call a doctor or poison control center immediately.
Tamper-Evident Packaging.

HOW SUPPLIED

Blister Packages of 30, 60, and 90 ct supplied in Child-Resistant packaging.
Do not store above 30°C (86°F). Protect from moisture.

REFERENCES

1. Brock C et al. Adverse effects of iron supplementation: A comparative trial of a wax-matrix iron preparation and conventional ferrous sulfate tablets. *Clin Ther.* 1985; 7:568–573.
2. Brock C, Curry H. Comparative incidence of side effects of a wax-matrix and a sustained-release iron preparation. *Clin Ther.* 1985;7:492–496.
Shown in Product Identification Guide, page 324

SLOW FE® WITH FOLIC ACID   OTC
(Slow Release Iron + Folic Acid)

DESCRIPTION

Slow Fe + Folic Acid delivers 50 mg. elemental iron (160 mg. dried ferrous sulfate) plus 400 mcg. folic acid using the unique wax matrix delivery system described above (for SLOW FE® Slow Release Iron Tablets) .
Provides women of childbearing potential with the daily target level of folic acid to reduce the risk of neural tube birth defects. These birth defects are rare, but serious, and occur within 28 days of conception, often before a woman knows she's pregnant.

FORMULA

Each tablet contains: Active Ingredients: 160 mg. dried ferrous sulfate, USP (equivalent to 50 mg. elemental iron) and 400 mcg. folic acid. Inactive Ingredients: cetostearyl alcohol, hydroxypropyl methylcellulose, lactose, magnesium stearate, polysorbate 80, talc, titanium dioxide, yellow iron oxide.

DOSAGE

ADULTS—One or two tablets once a day or as recommended by a physician. A maximum of two tablets daily may be taken. CHILDREN UNDER 12—Consult a physician. Tablets must be swallowed whole.

WARNING

The treatment of any anemic condition should be under the advice and supervision of a physician. As oral iron products interfere with absorption of oral tetracycline antibiotics, these products should not be taken within two hours of each other. Intake of folic acid from all sources should be limited to 1000 mcg. per day to prevent the masking of Vitamin B_{12} deficiencies. Should you become pregnant while using this product, consult a physician as soon as possible about good prenatal care and the continued use of this product. If you are already pregnant or nursing a baby, seek the advice of a health care professional before using this product. Accidental overdose of iron-containing products is a leading cause of fatal poisonings in children under 6. KEEP THIS PRODUCT OUT OF REACH OF CHILDREN. In case of accidental overdose, call a doctor or poison control center immediately.

HOW SUPPLIED

Blister packages of 20 supplied in Child-Resistant packaging.
Do not store above 30°C (86°F). Protect from moisture.
CHILD-RESISTANT
Blister packaged for your protection. Do not use if individual seals are broken.
NOVARTIS CONSUMER HEALTH, INC.
560 Morris Ave.
Summit, N.J. 07901-1312
Shown in Product Identification Guide, page 324

TAVIST•D® Tablets and Caplets   OTC
12 Hour Relief
Antihistamine/Nasal Decongestant

(See PDR For Nonprescription Drugs)

TAVIST® Allergy (Formerly Tavist•1®) Tablets   OTC
12 Hour Relief
Antihistamine

(See PDR For Nonprescription Drugs)

TAVIST® Sinus Caplets   OTC
Relief of Sinus Symptoms
Analgesic (Pain Reliever)/Nasal Decongestant

(See PDR for Nonprescription Drugs)

THERAFLU® OTC

Flu and Cold Hot Liquid Medicine
Flu, Cold & Cough Lemon Flavored Hot
Liquid Medicine
Maximum Strength NightTime Flu, Cold &
Cough Lemon Flavored Hot Liquid Medicine
Maximum Strength No Drowsiness
Flu, Cold & Cough Lemon Flavored
Hot Liquid Medicine
Maximum Strength Sore Throat & Cold
Apple Cinnamon Flavored Hot Liquid Medicine
Maximum Strength Non-Drowsy
Flu, Cold & Cough Caplets
Maximum Strength NightTime Flu, Cold & Cough
Caplets
Maximum Strength Sore Throat & Cough
Cherry Flavored Hot Liquid Medicine

(See PDR For Nonprescription Drugs)

TRIAMINIC® AM COUGH AND OTC
DECONGESTANT FORMULA

(See PDR for Nonprescription Drugs)

TRIAMINIC® AM DECONGESTANT OTC
FORMULA

(See PDR For Nonprescription Drugs)

TRIAMINIC® EXPECTORANT OTC

(See PDR For Nonprescription Drugs)

TRIAMINIC® EXPECTORANT DH ©

DESCRIPTION

Each teaspoonful (5 mL) of TRIAMINIC® Expectorant DH contains:
hydrocodone bitartrate 1.67 mg (Warning: May be habit forming), phenylpropanolamine hydrochloride, USP, 12.5 mg, pheniramine maleate, USP, 6.25 mg, pyrilamine maleate, USP, 6.25 mg, and guaifenesin 100 mg.
Inactive ingredients:
alcohol (5%), benzoic acid, D&C Yellow 10, FD&C Blue 1, FD&C Yellow 6, ethyl vanillin, flavors, menthol, purified water, sorbitol, spearmint oil, sucrose.

HOW SUPPLIED

TRIAMINIC® Expectorant DH (green) is available in pint bottles. Store at room temperature; tight, light-resistant container. TRIAMINIC® Expectorant DH is a Schedule III controlled substance.

TRIAMINIC TRIAMINICOL® OTC

(See PDR For Nonprescription Drugs)

TRIAMINIC® NightTime OTC

(See PDR For Nonprescription Drugs)

TRIAMINIC® Rx PEDIATRIC ORAL SOLUTION

DESCRIPTION

Each mL of TRIAMINIC® Rx Pediatric Oral Solution contains:
phenylpropanolamine hydrochloride, USP, 20 mg, pheniramine maleate, USP, 10 mg, and pyrilamine maleate, USP, 10 mg.
Inactive ingredients:
benzoic acid, flavor, glycerin, purified water, D&C Red 33, sorbitol, sucrose, FD&C Yellow 6.

HOW SUPPLIED

TRIAMINIC Rx Pediatric Oral Solution is available in a 15 ml plastic squeeze bottle that delivers approximately 24 drops per ml. Store at room temperature.

TRIAMINIC® Severe Cold & Fever OTC

(See PDR For Nonprescription Drugs)

TRIAMINIC® SORE THROAT FORMULA OTC

(See PDR For Nonprescription Drugs)

TRIAMINIC® SYRUP OTC

(See PDR For Nonprescription Drugs)

TRIAMINIC® DM OTC

(See PDR For Nonprescription Drugs)

TRANSDERM SCŌP® R
[trans-derm scōpe]
scopolamine 1.5 mg

Transdermal Therapeutic System

Programmed to deliver *in vivo* approximately 1.0 mg of scopolamine over 3 days

DESCRIPTION

The Transderm Scōp system is a circular flat patch designed for continuous release of scopolamine following application to an area of intact skin on the head, behind the ear. Clinical evaluation has demonstrated that the system provides effective antiemetic and antinauseant actions when tested against motion-sickness stimuli in adults. The Transderm Scōp system is a film 0.2 mm thick and 2.5 cm^2, with four layers. Proceeding from the visible surface towards the surface attached to the skin, these layers are: (1) a backing layer of tan-colored , aluminized, polyester film; (2) a drug reservoir of scopolamine, light mineral oil, and polyisobutylene; (3) a microporous polypropylene membrane that controls the rate of delivery of scopolamine from the system to the skin surface; and (4) an adhesive formulation of light mineral oil, polyisobutylene, and scopolamine. A protective peel strip of siliconized polyester, which covers the adhesive layer, is removed before the system is used. The inactive components, light mineral oil (12.4 mg) and polyisobutylene (11.4 mg), are not released from the system.

Cross section of the system:

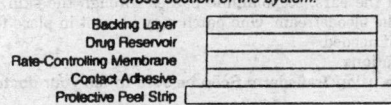

Backing Layer
Drug Reservoir
Rate-Controlling Membrane
Contact Adhesive
Protective Peel Strip

CLINICAL PHARMACOLOGY

The sole active agent of Transderm Scōp is scopolamine, a belladonna alkaloid with well-known pharmacological properties. The drug has a long history of oral and parenteral use for central anticholinergic activity, including prophylaxis of motion sickness. The mechanism of action of scopolamine in the central nervous system (CNS) is not definitely known but may include anticholinergic effects. The ability of scopolamine to prevent motion-induced nausea is believed to be associated with inhibition of vestibular input to the CNS, which results in inhibition of the vomiting reflex. In addition, scopolamine may have a direct action on the vomiting center within the reticular formation of the brain stem. Applied to the postauricular skin, Transderm Scōp provides for a gradual release of scopolamine from an adhesive matrix of light mineral oil and polyisobutylene.
Scopolamine is well-absorbed percutaneously following topical application of the Transderm Scōp patch behind the ear. The Transderm Scōp system contains 1.5 mg of scopolamine. The system is programmed to deliver approximately 1.0 mg of scopolamine at an approximately constant rate to the systemic circulation over the 3–day lifetime of the system. An initial priming dose of scopolamine, released from the adhesive layer of the system, saturates the skin binding sites and rapidly brings the plasma concentration of scopolamine to the required steady-state level. A continuous controlled release of scopolamine, which flows from the drug reservoir through the rate-controlling membrane, maintains the plasma concentration at a constant level. The distribution of scopolamine is not well characterized. It crosses the placenta as well as the blood-brain barrier and may be reversibly bound to plasma proteins. Similarly, the metabolic and excretory disposition of scopolamine has not been fully determined. It appears to be highly metabolized to a conjugated form and a very small amount of unchanged scopolamine is excreted in the urine. Average peak plasma concentrations of 87 pg/ml for free scopolamine and 354 pg/ml for total (i.e., free + conjugated) scopolamine were attained on average within 24 hours following administration of a single Transderm Scōp patch to human volunteers. Following the administration of a single patch, the average half-life of elimination for total scopolamine was approximately 10 hours. The urinary excretion rate after 24 hours was 0.7 µg/hr. for free scopolamine and 3.8 µg/hr. for total sco-

polamine. After patch removal, depletion of scopolamine bound to skin receptors at the site of application results in a gradual decrease in scopolamine plasma concentration.

INDICATIONS AND USAGE

Transderm Scōp is indicated for prevention of nausea and vomiting associated with motion sickness in adults. The patch should be applied only to skin in the postauricular area.
Clinical Results: Transderm Scōp provides antiemetic protection within several hours following application of the patch behind the ear. In 195 adult subjects of different racial origins who participated in clinical efficacy studies at sea or in a controlled motion environment, there was a 75% reduction in the incidence of motion-induced nausea and vomiting. Transderm Scōp provided significantly greater protection than that obtained with oral dimenhydrinate.

CONTRAINDICATIONS

Transderm Scōp is specifically contraindicated in persons who are hypersensitive to the drug scopolamine or to other belladonna alkaloids, or to any ingredient or component in the formulation or delivery system, or in patients with angle-closure (narrow angle) glaucoma.

WARNINGS

Transderm Scōp should not be used in children and should be used with special caution in the elderly. See PRECAUTIONS.
Since drowsiness, disorientation, and confusion may occur with the use of scopolamine, patients should be warned of the possibility and cautioned against engaging in activities that require mental alertness, such as driving a motor vehicle or operating dangerous machinery.
Potentially alarming idiosyncratic reactions may occur with ordinary therapeutic doses of scopolamine.

PRECAUTIONS
General
Scopolamine should be used with caution in patients with pyloric obstruction, or urinary bladder neck obstruction. Caution should be exercised when administering an antiemetic or antimuscarinic drug to patients suspected of having intestinal obstruction.
Transderm Scōp should be used with special caution in the elderly or in individuals with impaired metabolic, liver, or kidney functions, because of the increased likelihood of CNS effects.
Caution should be exercised in patients with a history of seizure or psychosis, since scopolamine can potentially aggravate both disorders.
Information for Patients
Since scopolamine can cause temporary dilation of the pupils and blurred vision if it comes in contact with the eyes, patients should be strongly advised to wash their hands thoroughly with soap and water immediately after handling the patch. In addition, it is important that used patches be disposed of properly to avoid contact with children or pets. Patients should be advised to remove the patch immediately and contact a physician in the unlikely event that they experience symptoms of acute narrow-angle glaucoma (pain in and reddening of the eyes accompanied by dilated pupils). Patients should also be instructed to remove the patch if they develop any difficulties in urinating.
Patients should be warned against driving a motor vehicle or operating dangerous machinery while wearing the patch. Patients who engage in these activities should also be aware of the possibility of withdrawal symptoms when the patch is removed. Patients who expect to participate in underwater sports should be cautioned regarding the potentially disorienting effects of scopolamine. A patient brochure is available.
Drug Interactions
Scopolamine should be used with care in patients taking drugs, including alcohol, capable of causing CNS effects. Special attention should be given to drugs having anticholinergic properties, e.g., belladonna alkaloids, antihistamines (including meclizine), and antidepressants.
Carcinogenesis, Mutagenesis, Impairment of Fertility
No long-term studies in animals have been performed to evaluate carcinogenic potential. Fertility studies were performed in female rats and revealed no evidence of impaired fertility or harm to the fetus due to scopolamine hydrobromide administered by daily subcutaneous injection. In the highest-dose group (plasma level approximately 500 times the level achieved in humans using a transdermal system), reduced maternal body weights were observed.
Pregnancy Category C
Teratogenic studies were performed in pregnant rats and rabbits with scopolamine hydrobromide administered by daily intravenous injection. No adverse effects were recorded in the rats. In the rabbits, the highest dose (plasma level approximately 100 times the level achieved in humans using a transdermal system) of drug administered had a

Continued on next page

Transderm Scōp—Cont.

marginal embryotoxic effect. Transderm Scōp should be used during pregnancy only if the anticipated benefit justifies the potential risk to the fetus.

Nursing Mothers

It is not known whether scopolamine is excreted in human milk. Because many drugs are excreted in human milk, caution should be exercised when Transderm Scōp is administered to a nursing woman.

Pediatric Use

Children are particularly susceptible to the side effects of belladonna alkaloids. Transderm Scōp should not be used in children because it is not known whether this system will release an amount of scopolamine that could produce serious adverse effects in children.

ADVERSE REACTIONS

The most frequent adverse reaction to Transderm Scōp is dryness of the mouth. This occurs in about two thirds of the people. A less frequent adverse reaction is drowsiness, which occurs in less than one sixth of the people. Transient impairment of eye accommodation, including blurred vision and dilation of the pupils, is also observed.

The following adverse reactions have also been reported on infrequent occasions during the use of Transderm Scōp: disorientation; memory disturbances; dizziness; restlessness; hallucinations; confusion; difficulty urinating; rashes and erythema; acute narrow-angle glaucoma; and dry, itchy, or red eyes.

Drug Withdrawal: Symptoms including dizziness, nausea, vomiting, headache, and disturbances of equilibrium have been reported in a few patients following discontinuation of the use of the Transderm Scōp system. These symptoms have occurred most often in patients who have used the systems for more than three days.

OVERDOSAGE

Overdosage with scopolamine may cause disorientation, memory disturbances, dizziness, restlessness, hallucinations, confusion, psychosis and convulsions, bronchospasm and respiratory depression, and muscular weakness. Should these symptoms occur, the Transderm Scōp patch should be removed immediately, adequate hydration should be maintained, and appropriate symptomatic treatment initiated.

Current recommendations for the treatment of severe, life-threatening antimuscarinic symptoms are as follows; the prescriber is urged, however, to contact his or her local Poison Control Center for additional recommendations.

Physostigmine salicylate:

In Adults: Administered intravenously in doses of 0.5 to 2 mg at a rate not to exceed 1 mg per minute. If symptoms recur, doses of 0.5 to 2 mg may be repeated up to a total dose of 5 mg.

In Children: 0.02 mg/kg administered intramuscularly or intravenously every 5 to 10 minutes, until a therapeutic effect is seen or a total dose of 2 mg is achieved. Infusion rate should not exceed 0.5 mg per minute.

OR

Neostigmine methylsulfate:

In Adults: Administered intramuscularly in doses of 0.5 to 1 mg, repeated every 2 to 3 hours; OR intravenously in doses of 0.5 to 2 mg, repeated as needed.

Small doses of a short-acting barbiturate (e.g., 100 mg thiopental sodium) or benzodiazepine, or a rectal infusion of 2% solution of chloral hydrate may control agitation or delirium. Intravenous norepinephrine bitartrate or metaraminol bitartrate may be given cautiously to restore blood pressure. To treat respiratory depression, administer artificial respiration with oxygen.

DOSAGE AND ADMINISTRATION

Initiation of Therapy: One Transderm Scōp patch (programmed to deliver approximately 1.0 mg of scopolamine over 3 days) should be applied to the hairless area behind one ear at least 4 hours before the antiemetic effect is required. Only one patch should be worn at any time.

Handling: After the patch is applied on dry skin behind the ear, the hands should be washed thoroughly with soap and water and dried. Upon removal, the patch should be discarded, and the hands and application site washed thoroughly with soap and water and dried, to prevent any traces of scopolamine from coming into direct contact with the eyes. (A patient brochure is available.)

Continuation of Therapy: Should the patch become displaced, it should be discarded and a fresh one placed on the hairless area behind the other ear. If therapy is required for longer than 3 days, the first patch should be discarded, and a fresh one placed on the hairless area behind the other ear.

HOW SUPPLIED

The Transderm Scōp system is a tan-colored circular patch, 2.5 cm^2, on a clear, oversized, hexagonal peel strip, which is removed prior to use.

Each Transderm Scōp system contains 1.5 mg of scopolamine and is programmed to deliver *in vivo* approximately 1.0 mg of scopolamine over 3 days. Transderm Scōp is available in packages of four patches. Each patch is foil wrapped. Patient instructions are included.

1 Package (4 patches) .... NDC 0067-4345-04

The system should be stored between 15° and 30°C (59° and 86°F).

CAUTION

Federal law prohibits dispensing without prescription.

Distributed by:

Novartis Consumer Health, Inc.

Summit, New Jersey 07901-1312

Please read this instruction sheet carefully before opening the system package.

Information for the Patient

TRANSDERM SCŌP®

Generic Name: scopolamine, pronounced skoe-POL-a-meen

Transdermal Therapeutic System

The Transderm Scōp system helps to prevent the nausea and vomiting of motion sickness for up to 3 days. It is a round adhesive patch that you place behind your ear several hours before you travel. Wear only one patch at any time.

Be sure to wash your hands thoroughly with soap and water immediately after handling the patch, so that any drug that might get on your hands will not come into contact with your eyes.

Avoid drinking alcohol while using Transderm Scōp. Also, be careful about driving or operating any machinery while using the system because the drug might make you drowsy.

DO NOT USE TRANSDERM SCŌP IF YOU ARE ALLERGIC TO SCOPOLAMINE OR HAVE GLAUCOMA.

TRANSDERM SCŌP SHOULD NOT BE USED IN CHILDREN AND SHOULD BE USED WITH CAUTION IN THE ELDERLY.

How The Transderm Scōp System Works

A group of nerve fibers deep inside the ear helps people keep their balance. For some people, the motion of ships, airplanes, trains, automobiles, and buses increases the activity of these nerve fibers. This increased activity causes the *dizziness, nausea, and vomiting* of motion sickness. People may have one, some, or all of these symptoms.

Transderm Scōp contains the drug scopolamine, which helps reduce the activity of the nerve fibers in the inner ear. When a Transderm Scōp patch is placed on the skin behind one of the ears, scopolamine passes through the skin and into the bloodstream. One patch may be kept in place for 3 days if needed.

Precautions

Before using Transderm Scōp be sure to tell your doctor if you

- Are pregnant or nursing (or planning to become pregnant)
- Have (or have had) glaucoma (increased pressure in the eyeball)
- Have (or have had) any metabolic, liver, or kidney disease
- Have any obstructions of the stomach or intestine
- Have any trouble urinating or any bladder obstruction
- Have any skin allergy or have had a skin reaction such as a rash or redness to any drug, especially scopolamine, or chemical or food substance.

Any of these conditions could make Transderm Scōp unsuitable for you. Also tell your doctor if you are taking any other medicines.

In the unlikely event that you experience pain in the eye and reddened whites of the eye, which may be accompanied by widening of the pupil and blurred vision, remove the patch immediately and consult your doctor. As indicated below under Side Effects, widening of the pupils and blurred vision without pain or reddened whites of the eye is usually temporary and not serious.

Transderm Scōp should not be used in children. The safety of its use in children has not been determined. Children and the elderly may be particularly sensitive to the effects of scopolamine.

Side Effects

The most common side effect experienced by people using Transderm Scōp is dryness of the mouth. This occurs in about two thirds of the people. A less frequent side effect is drowsiness, which occurs in less than one sixth of the people. Temporary blurring of vision and dilation (widening) of the pupils may occur, especially if the drug is on your hands and comes in contact with the eyes. On infrequent occasions, disorientation, memory disturbances, dizziness, restlessness, hallucinations, confusion, difficulty urinating, skin rashes or redness, dry, itchy, or red eyes and eye pain have been reported. If these effects do occur, remove the patch and call your doctor. Since drowsiness, disorientation, and confusion may occur with the use of scopolamine, be careful driving or operating any dangerous machinery, especially when you first start using the drug system.

In addition, if you plan to participate in underwater sports while wearing the patch, you should discuss with your doctor the potentially disorienting effects of scopolamine.

Drug Withdrawal: Symptoms including dizziness, nausea, vomiting, headache, and disturbances of equilibrium have been reported in a few people following discontinuation of the Transderm Scōp system. These symptoms have occurred most often in people who have used the systems for more than three days. We recommend that you consult your doctor if these symptoms occur.

Eye Effects: Temporary blurring of vision and dilation (widening) of the pupils may occur, especially if the drug is on your fingers or hands and comes into contact with the eyes. Dry, itchy, or reddened whites of the eye and eye pain have been reported infrequently. In the unlikely event that you experience pain in the eye and reddened whites of the eye, which may be accompanied by widening of the pupil and blurred vision, remove the patch and consult your doctor promptly. Widening of the pupils and blurred vision without pain, or reddened whites of the eye, are usually temporary and not serious.

How to Use Transderm Scōp

Transderm Scōp should be stored between 15-30°C (59-86°F) until you are ready to use it.

1. Plan to apply one Transderm Scōp patch at least 4 hours before you need it. **Wear only one patch at any time.**
2. Select a hairless area of skin behind one ear, taking care to avoid any cuts or irritations. Wipe the area with a clean, dry tissue.
3. Peel the package open and remove the patch (Figure 1).

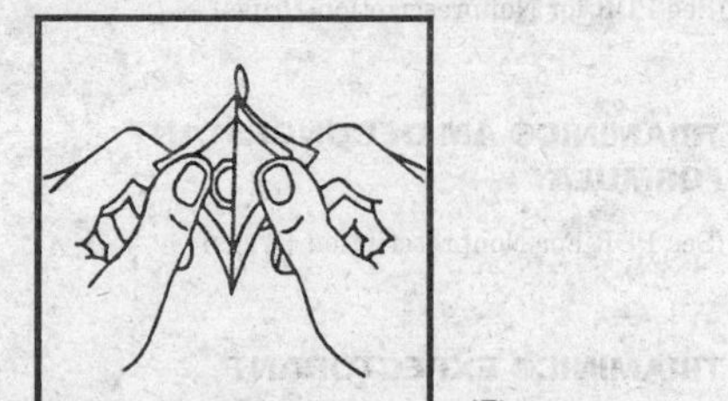

(Figure 1)

4. Remove the clear plastic six-sided backing from the round patch. Try not to touch the adhesive surface on the patch with your hands (Figure 2).

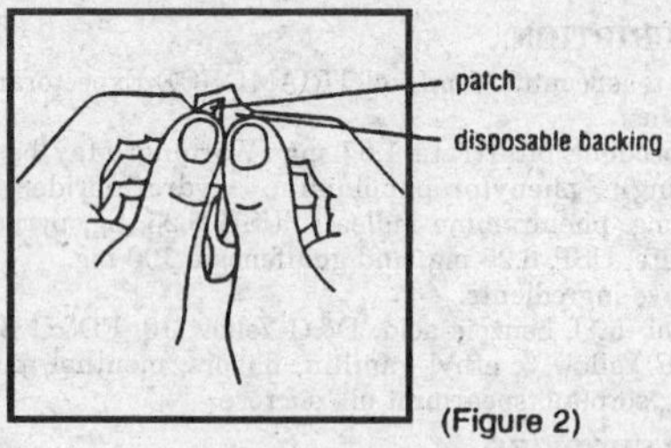

(Figure 2)

5. Firmly apply the adhesive surface (metallic side) to the dry area of skin behind the ear so that the tan-colored side is showing (Figure 3). Make good contact, especially around the edge. Once you have placed the patch behind your ear, do not move it for as long as you want to use it (up to 3 days).

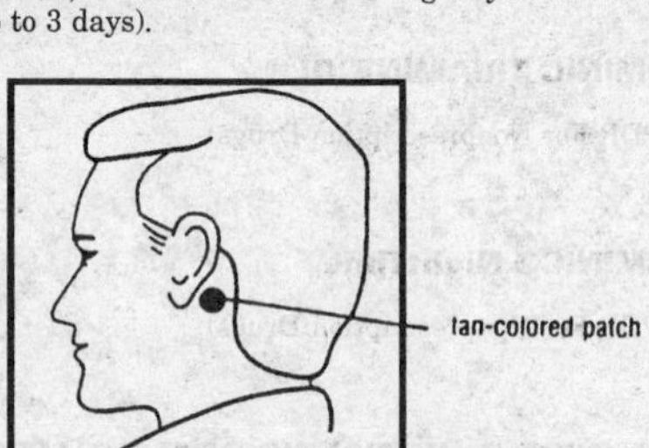

(Figure 3)

6. ***Important:* After the patch is in place, be sure to wash your hands thoroughly with soap and water to remove any scopolamine. If this drug were to contact your eyes, it could cause temporary blurring of vision and dilation (widening) of the pupils (the dark circles in the center of your eyes). Unless accompanied by eye pain and redness (see Precautions), this is not serious and your pupils should return to normal.**
7. Remove the patch after 3 days and throw it away. (You may remove it sooner if you are no longer concerned about motion sickness.) After removing the patch, be sure to wash your hands and the area behind your ear thoroughly with soap and water. The patch will still contain some active ingredient after use. Therefore, to avoid accidental contact or ingestion by children or pets, fold the used patch in half with the sticky side together and dispose in the trash out of the reach of children and pets.
8. If you wish to control nausea for longer than 3 days, *remove* the first patch after 3 days and place a new one *behind the other ear*, repeating instruction 2 to 7.

9. Keep the patch dry, if possible, to prevent it from falling off. Limited contact with water, however, as in bathing or swimming, will not affect the system. In the unlikely event that the patch falls off, throw it away and put a new one behind the other ear.

This leaflet presents a summary of information about Transderm Scōp. If you would like more information or if you have any questions, ask your doctor or pharmacist. A more technical leaflet is available, written for your doctor. If you would like to read the leaflet, ask your pharmacist to show you a copy. You may need the help of your doctor or pharmacist to understand some of the information.

Distributed by:
Novartis Consumer Health, Inc.
Summit, N.J. 07901-1312

Shown in Product Identification Guide, page 324

Novartis Pharmaceuticals Corporation

NOVARTIS PHARMACEUTICALS CORPORATION
59 Route 10
East Hanover, NJ 07936
(for branded products)

GENEVA PHARMACEUTICALS, INC.
A NOVARTIS COMPANY
2655 West Midway Boulevard
PO Box 446
Broomfield, CO 80038-0446
(for branded generic product listing refer to Geneva Pharmaceuticals, Inc.)

For Information Contact (*branded products*):

Customer Response Department
(888) NOW-NOVARTIS [888-669-6682]

Global Internet Address:
http: //www.novartis.com

For Information Contact (*branded generic products*):

Customer Support Department
(800) 525-8747
(303) 466-2400
FAX: (303) 469-6467

ACTIGALL® ℞

[*ăct-ĭ-găll*]
ursodiol USP
Capsules

Caution: Federal law prohibits dispensing without prescription.

The following prescribing information is based on official labeling in effect on August 1, 1998.

SPECIAL NOTE

Gallbladder stone dissolution with Actigall treatment requires months of therapy. Complete dissolution does not occur in all patients and recurrence of stones within 5 years has been observed in up to 50% of patients who do dissolve their stones on bile acid therapy. Patients should be carefully selected for therapy with ursodiol, and alternative therapies should be considered.

DESCRIPTION

Actigall is a bile acid available as 300-mg capsules suitable for oral administration.

Actigall is ursodiol USP (ursodeoxycholic acid), a naturally occurring bile acid found in small quantities in normal human bile and in larger quantities in the biles of certain species of bears. It is a bitter-tasting, white powder freely soluble in ethanol, methanol, and glacial acetic acid; sparingly soluble in chloroform; slightly soluble in ether; and insoluble in water. The chemical name for ursodiol is 3α, 7β-dihydroxy-5β-cholan-24-oic acid ($C_{24}H_{40}O_4$). Ursodiol USP has a molecular weight of 392.58. Its structure is shown below:

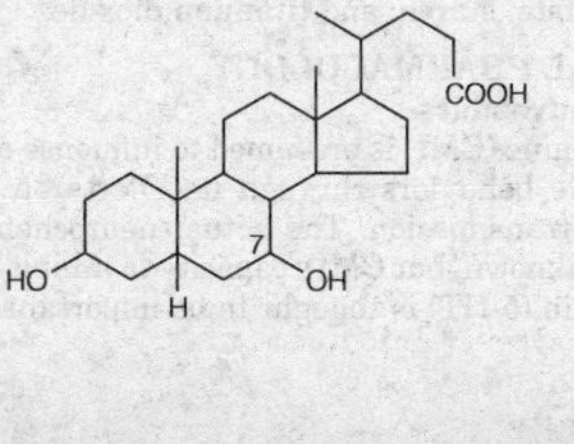

Inactive Ingredients. Colloidal silicon dioxide, ferric oxide, gelatin, magnesium stearate, starch (corn), and titanium dioxide.

CLINICAL PHARMACOLOGY

About 90% of a therapeutic dose of Actigall is absorbed in the small bowel after oral administration. After absorption, ursodiol enters the portal vein and undergoes efficient extraction from portal blood by the liver (i.e., there is a large "first-pass" effect) where it is conjugated with either glycine or taurine and is then secreted into the hepatic bile ducts. Ursodiol in bile is concentrated in the gallbladder and expelled into the duodenum in gallbladder bile via the cystic and common ducts by gallbladder contractions provoked by physiologic responses to eating. Only small quantities of ursodiol appear in the systemic circulation and very small amounts are excreted into urine. The sites of the drug's therapeutic actions are in the liver, bile, and gut lumen.

Beyond conjugation, ursodiol is not altered or catabolized appreciably by the liver or intestinal mucosa. A small proportion of orally administered drug undergoes bacterial degradation with each cycle of enterohepatic circulation. Ursodiol can be both oxidized and reduced at the 7-carbon, yielding either 7-keto-lithocholic acid or lithocholic acid, respectively. Further, there is some bacterially catalyzed deconjugation of glyco- and tauro- ursodeoxycholic acid in the small bowel. Free ursodiol, 7-keto-lithocholic acid, and lithocholic acid are relatively insoluble in aqueous media and larger proportions of these compounds are lost from the distal gut into the feces. Reabsorbed free ursodiol is reconjugated by the liver. Eighty percent of lithocholic acid formed in the small bowel is excreted in the feces, but the 20% that is absorbed is sulfated at the 3-hydroxyl group in the liver to relatively insoluble lithocholyl conjugates which are excreted into bile and lost in feces. Absorbed 7-keto-lithocholic acid is stereospecifically reduced in the liver to chenodiol.

Lithocholic acid causes cholestatic liver injury and can cause death from liver failure in certain species unable to form sulfate conjugates. Lithocholic acid is formed by 7-dehydroxylation of the dihydroxy bile acids (ursodiol and chenodiol) in the gut lumen. The 7-dehydroxylation reaction appears to be alpha-specific, i.e., chenodiol is more efficiently 7-dehydroxylated than ursodiol and, for equimolar doses of ursodiol and chenodiol, levels of lithocholic acid appearing in bile are lower with the former. Man has the capacity to sulfate lithocholic acid. Although liver injury has not been associated with ursodiol therapy, a reduced capacity to sulfate may exist in some individuals, but such a deficiency has not yet been clearly demonstrated.

Pharmacodynamics

Ursodiol suppresses hepatic synthesis and secretion of cholesterol, and also inhibits intestinal absorption of cholesterol. It appears to have little inhibitory effect on synthesis and secretion into bile of endogenous bile acids, and does not appear to affect secretion of phospholipids into bile.

With repeated dosing, bile ursodeoxycholic acid concentrations reach a steady state in about 3 weeks. Although insoluble in aqueous media, cholesterol can be solubilized in at least two different ways in the presence of dihydroxy bile acids. In addition to solubilizing cholesterol in micelles, ursodiol acts by an apparently unique mechanism to cause dispersion of cholesterol as liquid crystals in aqueous media. Thus, even though administration of high doses (e.g., 15-18 mg/kg/day) does not result in a concentration of ursodiol higher than 60% of the total bile acid pool, ursodiol-rich bile effectively solubilizes cholesterol. The overall effect of ursodiol is to increase the concentration level at which saturation of cholesterol occurs.

The various actions of ursodiol combine to change the bile of patients with gallstones from cholesterol-precipitating to cholesterol-solubilizing, thus resulting in bile conducive to cholesterol stone dissolution.

After ursodiol dosing is stopped, the concentration of the bile acid in bile falls exponentially, declining to about 5%-10% of its steady-state level in about 1 week.

Clinical Results

Gallstone Dissolution

On the basis of clinical trial results in a total of 868 patients with radiolucent gallstones treated in 8 studies (three in the U.S. involving 282 patients, one in the U.K. involving 130 patients, and four in Italy involving 456 patients) for periods ranging from 6-78 months with Actigall doses ranging from about 5 to 20 mg/kg/day, an Actigall dose of about 8-10 mg/kg/day appeared to be the best dose. With an Actigall dose of about 10 mg/kg/day, complete stone dissolution can be anticipated in about 30% of unselected patients with uncalcified gallstones <20 mm in maximal diameter treated for up to 2 years. Patients with calcified gallstones prior to treatment, or patients who develop stone calcification or gallbladder nonvisualization on treatment, and patients with stones >20 mm in maximal diameter rarely dissolve their stones. The chance of gallstone dissolution is increased up to 50% in patients with floating or floatable stones (i.e., those with high cholesterol content), and is inversely related to stone size for those <20 mm in maximal diameter. Complete dissolution was observed in 81% of patients with stones up to 5 mm in diameter. Age, sex, weight, degree of obesity, and serum cholesterol level are not related to the chance of stone dissolution with Actigall.

A nonvisualizing gallbladder by oral cholecystogram prior to the initiation of therapy is not a contraindication to Actigall therapy (the group of patients with nonvisualizing gallbladders in the Actigall studies had complete stone dissolution rates similar to the group of patients with visualizing gallbladders). However, gallbladder nonvisualization developing during ursodiol treatment predicts failure of complete stone dissolution and in such cases therapy should be discontinued.

Partial stone dissolution occurring within 6 months of beginning therapy with Actigall appears to be associated with a >70% chance of eventual complete stone dissolution with further treatment; partial dissolution observed within 1 year of starting therapy indicates a 40% probability of complete dissolution.

Stone recurrence after dissolution with Actigall therapy was seen within 2 years in 8/27 (30%) of patients in the U.K. studies. Of 16 patients in the U.K. study whose stones had previously dissolved on chenodiol but later recurred, 11 had complete dissolution on Actigall. Stone recurrence has been observed in up to 50% of patients within 5 years of complete stone dissolution on ursodiol therapy. Serial ultrasonographic examinations should be obtained to monitor for recurrence of stones, bearing in mind that radiolucency of the stones should be established before another course of Actigall is instituted. A prophylactic dose of Actigall has not been established.

Gallstone Prevention

Two placebo-controlled, multicenter, double-blind, randomized, parallel group trials in a total of 1316 obese patients were undertaken to evaluate Actigall in the prevention of gallstone formation in obese patients undergoing rapid weight loss. The first trial consisted of 1004 obese patients with a body mass index (BMI) ≥38 who underwent weight loss induced by means of a very low calorie diet for a period of 16 weeks. An intent-to-treat analysis of this trial showed that gallstone formation occurred in 23% of the placebo group, while those patients on 300, 600, or 1200 mg/day of Actigall experienced a 6%, 3%, and 2% incidence of gallstone formation, respectively. The mean weight loss for this 16-week trial was 47 lb for the placebo group, and 47, 48, and 50 lb for the 300, 600, and 1200 mg/day Actigall groups, respectively.

The second trial consisted of 312 obese patients (BMI ≥40) who underwent rapid weight loss through gastric bypass surgery. The trial drug treatment period was for 6 months following this surgery. Results of this trial showed that gallstone formation occurred in 23% of the placebo group, while those patients on 300, 600, or 1200 mg/day of Actigall experienced a 9%, 1%, and 5% incidence of gallstone formation, respectively. The mean weight loss for this 6-month trial was 64 lb for the placebo group, and 67, 74, and 72 lb for the 300, 600, and 1200 mg/day Actigall groups, respectively.

ALTERNATIVE THERAPIES

Watchful Waiting

Watchful waiting has the advantage that no therapy may ever be required. For patients with silent or minimally symptomatic stones, the rate of development of moderate-to-severe symptoms or gallstone complications is estimated to be between 2% and 6% per year, leading to a cumulative rate of 7% to 27% in 5 years. Presumably the rate is higher for patients already having symptoms.

Cholecystectomy

For patients with symptomatic gallstones, surgery offers the advantage of immediate and permanent stone removal, but carries a high risk in some patients. About 5% of cholecystectomized patients have residual symptoms or retained common duct stones. The spectrum of surgical risk varies as a function of age and the presence of disease other than cholelithiasis.

Mortality Rates for Cholecystectomy in the U.S.
(National Halothane Study, JAMA 1966; 197:775-8)
27,600 Cholecystectomies (Smoothed Rates)
Deaths/1000 Operations***

Low Risk Patients*	Age (Yrs)	Cholecystectomy	Cholecystectomy + Common Duct Exploration
Women	0-49	.54	2.13
	50-69	2.80	10.10
Men	0-49	1.04	4.12
	50-69	5.41	19.23
High Risk Patients**			
Women	0-49	12.66	47.62
	50-69	17.24	58.82

Continued on next page

Actigall—Cont.

Men	0-49	24.39	90.91
	50-69	33.33	111.11

* In good health or with moderate systemic disease.
** With severe or extreme systemic disease.
*** Includes both elective and emergency surgery.

Women in good health or who have only moderate systemic disease and are under 49 years of age have the lowest surgical mortality rate (0.054); men in all categories have a surgical mortality rate twice that of women. Common duct exploration quadruples the rates in all categories. The rates rise with each decade of life and increase tenfold or more in all categories with severe or extreme systemic disease.

INDICATIONS AND USAGE
1. Actigall is indicated for patients with radiolucent, noncalcified gallbladder stones <20 mm in greatest diameter in whom elective cholecystectomy would be undertaken except for the presence of increased surgical risk due to systemic disease, advanced age, idiosyncratic reaction to general anesthesia, or for those patients who refuse surgery. Safety of use of Actigall beyond 24 months is not established.
2. Actigall is indicated for the prevention of gallstone formation in obese patients experiencing rapid weight loss.

CONTRAINDICATIONS
1. Actigall will not dissolve calcified cholesterol stones, radiopaque stones, or radiolucent bile pigment stones. Hence, patients with such stones are not candidates for Actigall therapy.
2. Patients with compelling reasons for cholecystectomy including unremitting acute cholecystitis, cholangitis, biliary obstruction, gallstone pancreatitis, or biliary-gastrointestinal fistula are not candidates for Actigall therapy.
3. Allergy to bile acids.

PRECAUTIONS
Liver Tests
Ursodiol therapy has not been associated with liver damage. Lithocholic acid, a naturally occurring bile acid, is known to be a liver-toxic metabolite. This bile acid is formed in the gut from ursodiol less efficiently and in smaller amounts than that seen from chenodiol. Lithocholic acid is detoxified in the liver by sulfation and, although man appears to be an efficient sulfater, it is possible that some patients may have a congenital or acquired deficiency in sulfation, thereby predisposing them to lithocholate-induced liver damage.
Abnormalities in liver enzymes have not been associated with Actigall therapy and, in fact, Actigall has been shown to decrease liver enzyme levels in liver disease. However, patients given Actigall should have SGOT (AST) and SGPT (ALT) measured at the initiation of therapy and thereafter as indicated by the particular clinical circumstances.
Drug Interactions
Bile acid sequestering agents such as cholestyramine and colestipol may interfere with the action of Actigall by reducing its absorption. Aluminum-based antacids have been shown to adsorb bile acids in vitro and may be expected to interfere with Actigall in the same manner as the bile acid sequestering agents. Estrogens, oral contraceptives, and clofibrate (and perhaps other lipid-lowering drugs) increase hepatic cholesterol secretion, and encourage cholesterol gallstone formation and hence may counteract the effectiveness of Actigall.
Carcinogenesis, Mutagenesis, Impairment of Fertility
Ursodeoxycholic acid was tested in 2-year oral carcinogenicity studies in CD-1 mice and Sprague-Dawley rats at daily doses of 50, 250, and 1000 mg/kg/day. It was not tumorigenic in mice. In the rat study, it produced statistically significant dose-related increased incidences of pheochromocytomas of adrenal medulla in males (p=0.014, Peto trend test) and females (p=0.004, Peto trend test). A 78-week rat study employing intrarectal instillation of lithocholic acid and tauro-deoxycholic acid, metabolites of ursodiol and chenodiol, has been conducted. These bile acids alone did not produce any tumors. A tumor-promoting effect of both metabolites was observed when they were co-administered with a carcinogenic agent. Results of epidemiologic studies suggest that bile acids might be involved in the pathogenesis of human colon cancer in patients who had undergone a cholecystectomy, but direct evidence is lacking. Ursodiol is not mutagenic in the Ames test. Dietary administration of lithocholic acid to chickens is reported to cause hepatic adenomatous hyperplasia.
Pregnancy Category B
Reproduction studies have been performed in rats and rabbits with ursodiol doses up to 200-fold the therapeutic dose and have revealed no evidence of impaired fertility or harm to the fetus at doses of 20- to 100-fold the human dose in rats and at 5-fold the human dose (highest dose tested) in rabbits. Studies employing 100- to 200-fold the human dose in rats have shown some reduction in fertility rate and litter size. There have been no adequate and well-controlled studies of the use of ursodiol in pregnant women; but inadvertent exposure of 4 women to therapeutic doses of the drug in the first trimester of pregnancy during the Actigall trials led to no evidence of effects on the fetus or newborn baby. Although it seems unlikely, the possibility that ursodiol can cause fetal harm cannot be ruled out; hence, the drug is not recommended for use during pregnancy.

Nursing Mothers
It is not known whether ursodiol is excreted in human milk. Because many drugs are excreted in human milk, caution should be exercised when Actigall is administered to a nursing mother.
Pediatric Use
The safety and effectiveness of Actigall in pediatric patients have not been established.

ADVERSE REACTIONS
The nature and frequency of adverse experiences were similar across all groups.
The following tables provide comprehensive listings of the adverse experiences reported that occurred with a 5% incidence level:

GALLSTONE DISSOLUTION

	Ursodiol 8-10 mg/kg/day (N=155)		Placebo (N=159)	
	N	(%)	N	(%)
Body as a Whole				
Allergy	8	(5.2)	7	(4.4)
Chest Pain	5	(3.2)	10	(6.3)
Fatigue	7	(4.5)	8	(5.0)
Infection Viral	30	(19.4)	41	(25.8)
Digestive System				
Abdominal Pain	67	(43.2)	70	(44.0)
Cholecystitis	8	(5.2)	7	(4.4)
Constipation	15	(9.7)	14	(8.8)
Diarrhea	42	(27.1)	34	(21.4)
Dyspepsia	26	(16.8)	18	(11.3)
Flatulence	12	(7.7)	12	(7.5)
Gastrointestinal Disorder	6	(3.9)	8	(5.0)
Nausea	22	(14.2)	27	(17.0)
Vomiting	15	(9.7)	11	(6.9)
Musculoskeletal System				
Arthralgia	12	(7.7)	24	(15.1)
Arthritis	9	(5.8)	4	(2.5)
Back Pain	11	(7.1)	18	(11.3)
Myalgia	9	(5.8)	9	(5.7)
Nervous System				
Headache	28	(18.1)	34	(21.4)
Insomnia	3	(1.9)	8	(5.0)
Respiratory System				
Bronchitis	10	(6.5)	6	(3.8)
Coughing	11	(7.1)	7	(4.4)
Pharyngitis	13	(8.4)	5	(3.1)
Rhinitis	8	(5.2)	11	(6.9)
Sinusitis	17	(11.0)	18	(11.3)
Upper Respiratory Tract Infection	24	(15.5)	21	(13.2)
Urogenital System				
Urinary Tract Infection	10	(6.5)	7	(4.4)

GALLSTONE PREVENTION

	Actigall 600 mg (N=322)		Placebo (N=325)	
	N	(%)	N	(%)
Body as a Whole				
Fatigue	25	(7.8)	33	(10.2)
Infection Viral	29	(9.0)	29	(8.9)
Influenza-like Symptoms	21	(6.5)	19	(5.8)
Digestive System				
Abdominal Pain	20	(6.2)	39	(12.0)
Constipation	85	(26.4)	72	(22.2)
Diarrhea	81	(25.2)	68	(20.9)
Flatulence	15	(4.7)	24	(7.4)
Nausea	56	(17.4)	43	(13.2)
Vomiting	44	(13.7)	44	(13.5)
Musculoskeletal System				
Back Pain	38	(11.8)	21	(6.5)
Musculoskeletal Pain	19	(5.9)	15	(4.6)
Nervous System				
Dizziness	53	(16.5)	42	(12.9)
Headache	80	(24.8)	78	(24.0)
Respiratory System				
Pharyngitis	10	(3.1)	19	(5.8)
Sinusitis	17	(5.3)	18	(5.5)
Upper Respiratory Tract Infection	40	(12.4)	35	(10.8)
Skin and Appendages				
Alopecia	17	(5.3)	8	(2.5)
Urogenital System				
Dysmenorrhea	18	(5.6)	19	(5.8)

OVERDOSAGE
Neither accidental nor intentional overdosing with Actigall has been reported. Doses of Actigall in the range of 16-20 mg/kg/day have been tolerated for 6-37 months without symptoms by 7 patients. The LD_{50} for ursodiol in rats is over 5000 mg/kg given over 7-10 days and over 7500 mg/kg for mice. The most likely manifestation of severe overdose with Actigall would probably be diarrhea, which should be treated symptomatically.

DOSAGE AND ADMINISTRATION
Gallstone Dissolution
The recommended dose for Actigall treatment of radiolucent gallbladder stones is 8-10 mg/kg/day given in 2 or 3 divided doses.
Ultrasound images of the gallbladder should be obtained at 6-month intervals for the first year of Actigall therapy to monitor gallstone response. If gallstones appear to have dissolved, Actigall therapy should be continued and dissolution confirmed on a repeat ultrasound examination within 1 to 3 months. Most patients who eventually achieve complete stone dissolution will show partial or complete dissolution at the first on-treatment reevaluation. If partial stone dissolution is not seen by 12 months of Actigall therapy, the likelihood of success is greatly reduced.
Gallstone Prevention
The recommended dosage of Actigall for gallstone prevention in patients undergoing rapid weight loss is 600 mg/day (300 mg b.i.d.).

HOW SUPPLIED
Capsules 300 mg — opaque, white, pink (imprinted Actigall 300 mg)
Bottles of 100 .... NDC 0078-0319-05
Do not store above 86°F (30°C).
Dispense in tight container (USP).

C97-12 (Rev. 12/97)

Distributed by
Novartis Pharmaceuticals Corporation
East Hanover, New Jersey 07936
Shown in Product Identification Guide, page 324

ANAFRANIL®   ℞
[aña fränill]
clomipramine hydrochloride
Capsules

Caution: Federal law prohibits dispensing without prescription.
The following prescribing information is based on official labeling in effect on August 1, 1998.

DESCRIPTION
Anafranil, clomipramine hydrochloride, is an antiobsessional drug that belongs to the class (dibenzazepine) of pharmacologic agents known as tricyclic antidepressants. Anafranil is available as capsules of 25, 50, and 75 mg for oral administration.
Clomipramine hydrochloride is 3-chloro-5-[3-(dimethylamino)propyl]-10,11-dihydro-5H-dibenz[b,f]azepine monohydrochloride and its structural formula is

Clomipramine hydrochloride is a white to off-white crystalline powder. It is freely soluble in water, in methanol, and in methylene chloride, and insoluble in ethyl ether and in hexane. Its molecular weight is 351.3.
Inactive Ingredients. D&C Red No. 33 (25-mg capsules only), D&C Yellow No. 10, FD&C Blue No. 1 (50-mg capsules only), FD&C Yellow No. 6, gelatin, magnesium stearate, methylparaben, propylparaben, silicon dioxide, sodium lauryl sulfate, starch, and titanium dioxide.

CLINICAL PHARMACOLOGY
Pharmacodynamics
Clomipramine (CMI) is presumed to influence obsessive and compulsive behaviors through its effects on serotonergic neuronal transmission. The actual neurochemical mechanism is unknown, but CMI's capacity to inhibit the reuptake of serotonin (5-HT) is thought to be important.

Pharmacokinetics

Absorption/Bioavailability: CMI from Anafranil capsules is as bioavailable as CMI from a solution. The bioavailability of CMI from capsules is not significantly affected by food. In a dose proportionality study involving multiple CMI doses, steady-state plasma concentrations (C_{SS}) and area-under-plasma-concentration-time curves (AUC) of CMI and CMI's major active metabolite, desmethylclomipramine (DMI), were not proportional to dose over the ranges evaluated, i.e., between 25-100 mg/day and between 25-150 mg/day, although C_{SS} and AUC are approximately linearly related to dose between 100-150 mg/day. The relationship between dose and CMI/DMI concentrations at higher daily doses has not been systematically assessed, but if there is significant dose dependency at doses above 150 mg/day, there is the potential for dramatically higher C_{SS} and AUC even for patients dosed within the recommended range. This may pose a potential risk to some patients (see WARNINGS and PRECAUTIONS, Drug Interactions).

After a single 50-mg oral dose, maximum plasma concentrations of CMI occur within 2-6 hours (mean, 4.7 hr) and range from 56 ng/mL to 154 ng/mL (mean, 92 ng/mL). After multiple daily doses of 150 mg of Anafranil, steady-state maximum plasma concentrations range from 94 ng/mL to 339 ng/mL (mean, 218 ng/mL) for CMI and from 134 ng/mL to 532 ng/mL (mean, 274 ng/mL) for DMI. No pharmacokinetic information is available for doses ranging from 150 mg/day to 250 mg/day, the maximum recommended daily dose.

Distribution: CMI distributes into cerebrospinal fluid (CSF) and brain and into breast milk. DMI also distributes into CSF, with a mean CSF/plasma ratio of 2.6. The protein binding of CMI is approximately 97%, principally to albumin, and is independent of CMI concentration. The interaction between CMI and other highly protein-bound drugs has not been fully evaluated, but may be important *(see* PRECAUTIONS, Drug Interactions).

Metabolism: CMI is extensively biotransformed to DMI and other metabolites and their glucuronide conjugates. DMI is pharmacologically active, but its effects on OCD behaviors are unknown. These metabolites are excreted in urine and feces, following biliary elimination. After a 25-mg radiolabeled dose of CMI in two subjects, 60% and 51%, respectively, of the dose were recovered in the urine and 32% and 24%, respectively, in feces. In the same study, the combined urinary recoveries of CMI and DMI were only about 0.8-1.3% of the dose administered. CMI does not induce drug-metabolizing enzymes, as measured by antipyrine half-life.

Elimination: Evidence that the C_{SS} and AUC for CMI and DMI may increase disproportionately with increasing oral doses suggests that the metabolism of CMI and DMI may be capacity limited. This fact must be considered in assessing the estimates of the pharmacokinetic parameters presented below, as these were obtained in individuals exposed to doses of 150 mg. If the pharmacokinetics of CMI and DMI are nonlinear at doses above 150 mg, their elimination half-lives may be considerably lengthened at doses near the upper end of the recommended dosing range (i.e., 200 mg/day to 250 mg/day). Consequently, CMI and DMI may accumulate, and this accumulation may increase the incidence of any dose- or plasma-concentration-dependent adverse reactions, in particular seizures (see WARNINGS).

After a 150-mg dose, the half-life of CMI ranges from 19 hours to 37 hours (mean, 32 hr) and that of DMI ranges from 54 hours to 77 hours (mean, 69 hr). Steady-state levels after multiple dosing are typically reached within 7-14 days for CMI. Plasma concentrations of the metabolite exceed the parent drug on multiple dosing. After multiple dosing with 150 mg/day, the accumulation factor for CMI is approximately 2.5 and for DMI is 4.6. Importantly, it may take two weeks or longer to achieve this extent of accumulation at constant dosing because of the relatively long elimination half-lives of CMI and DMI (see DOSAGE AND ADMINISTRATION). The effects of hepatic and renal impairment on the disposition of Anafranil have not been determined.

Interactions: Coadministration of haloperidol with CMI increases plasma concentrations of CMI. Coadministration of CMI with phenobarbital increases plasma concentrations of phenobarbital (see PRECAUTIONS, Drug Interactions). Younger subjects (18-40 years of age) tolerated CMI better and had significantly lower steady-state plasma concentrations, compared with subjects over 65 years of age. Children under 15 years of age had significantly lower plasma concentration/dose ratios, compared with adults. Plasma concentrations of CMI were significantly lower in smokers than in nonsmokers.

INDICATIONS AND USAGE

Anafranil is indicated for the treatment of obsessions and compulsions in patients with Obsessive-Compulsive Disorder (OCD). The obsessions or compulsions must cause marked distress, be time-consuming, or significantly interfere with social or occupational functioning, in order to meet the DSM-III-R (circa 1989) diagnosis of OCD.

Obsessions are recurrent, persistent ideas, thoughts, images, or impulses that are ego-dystonic. Compulsions are repetitive, purposeful, and intentional behaviors performed in response to an obsession or in a stereotyped fashion, and are recognized by the person as excessive or unreasonable.

The effectiveness of Anafranil for the treatment of OCD was demonstrated in multicenter, placebo-controlled, parallel-group studies, including two 10-week studies in adults and one 8-week study in children and adolescents 10-17 years of age. Patients in all studies had moderate-to-severe OCD (DSM-III), with mean baseline ratings on the Yale-Brown Obsessive Compulsive Scale (YBOCS) ranging from 26 to 28 and a mean baseline rating of 10 on the NIMH Clinical Global Obsessive Compulsive Scale (NIMH-OC). Patients taking CMI experienced a mean reduction of approximately 10 on the YBOCS, representing an average improvement on this scale of 35% to 42% among adults and 37% among children and adolescents. CMI-treated patients experienced a 3.5 unit decrement on the NIMH-OC. Patients on placebo showed no important clinical response on either scale. The maximum dose was 250 mg/day for most adults and 3 mg/kg/day (up to 200 mg) for all children and adolescents.

The effectiveness of Anafranil for long-term use (i.e., for more than 10 weeks) has not been systematically evaluated in placebo-controlled trials. The physician who elects to use Anafranil for extended periods should periodically reevaluate the long-term usefulness of the drug for the individual patient (see DOSAGE AND ADMINISTRATION).

CONTRAINDICATIONS

Anafranil is contraindicated in patients with a history of hypersensitivity to Anafranil or other tricyclic antidepressants.

Anafranil should not be given in combination, or within 14 days before or after treatment, with a monoamine oxidase (MAO) inhibitor. Hyperpyretic crisis, seizures, coma, and death have been reported in patients receiving such combinations.

Anafranil is contraindicated during the acute recovery period after a myocardial infarction.

WARNINGS

Seizures

During premarket evaluation, seizure was identified as the most significant risk of Anafranil use.

The observed cumulative incidence of seizures among patients exposed to Anafranil at doses up to 300 mg/day was 0.64% at 90 days, 1.12% at 180 days, and 1.45% at 365 days. The cumulative rates correct the crude rate of 0.7% (25 of 3519 patients) for the variable duration of exposure in clinical trials.

Although dose appears to be a predictor of seizure, there is a confounding of dose and duration of exposure, making it difficult to assess independently the effect of either factor alone. The ability to predict the occurrence of seizures in subjects exposed to doses of CMI greater than 250 mg is limited, given that the plasma concentration of CMI may be dose-dependent and may vary among subjects given the same dose. Nevertheless, prescribers are advised to limit the daily dose to a maximum of 250 mg in adults and 3 mg/kg (or 200 mg) in children and adolescents (see DOSAGE AND ADMINISTRATION).

Caution should be used in administering Anafranil to patients with a history of seizures or other predisposing factors, e.g., brain damage of varying etiology, alcoholism, and concomitant use with other drugs that lower the seizure threshold.

Rare reports of fatalities in association with seizures have been reported by foreign postmarketing surveillance, but not in U.S. clinical trials. In some of these cases, Anafranil had been administered with other epileptogenic agents; in others, the patients involved had possibly predisposing medical conditions. Thus a causal association between Anafranil treatment and these fatalities has not been established.

Physicians should discuss with patients the risk of taking Anafranil while engaging in activities in which sudden loss of consciousness could result in serious injury to the patient or others, e.g., the operation of complex machinery, driving, swimming, climbing.

PRECAUTIONS

General

Suicide: Since depression is a commonly associated feature of OCD, the risk of suicide must be considered. Prescriptions for Anafranil should be written for the smallest quantity of capsules consistent with good patient management, in order to reduce the risk of overdose.

Cardiovascular Effects: Modest orthostatic decreases in blood pressure and modest tachycardia were each seen in approximately 20% of patients taking Anafranil in clinical trials; but patients were frequently asymptomatic. Among approximately 1400 patients treated with CMI in the premarketing experience who had ECGs, 1.5% developed abnormalities during treatment, compared with 3.1% of patients receiving active control drugs and 0.7% of patients receiving placebo. The most common ECG changes were PVCs, ST-T wave changes, and intraventricular conduction abnormalities. These changes were rarely associated with significant clinical symptoms. Nevertheless, caution is necessary in treating patients with known cardiovascular disease, and gradual dose titration is recommended.

Psychosis, Confusion, and Other Neuropsychiatric Phenomena: Patients treated with Anafranil have been reported to show a variety of neuropsychiatric signs and symptoms including delusions, hallucinations, psychotic episodes, confusion, and paranoia. Because of the uncontrolled nature of many of the studies, it is impossible to provide a precise estimate of the extent of risk imposed by treatment with Anafranil. As with tricyclic antidepressants to which it is closely related, Anafranil may precipitate an acute psychotic episode in patients with unrecognized schizophrenia.

Mania/Hypomania: During premarketing testing of Anafranil in patients with affective disorder, hypomania or mania was precipitated in several patients. Activation of mania or hypomania has also been reported in a small proportion of patients with affective disorder treated with marketed tricyclic antidepressants, which are closely related to Anafranil.

Hepatic Changes: During premarketing testing, Anafranil was occasionally associated with elevations in SGOT and SGPT (pooled incidence of approximately 1% and 3%, respectively) of potential clinical importance (i.e., values greater than 3 times the upper limit of normal). In the vast majority of instances, these enzyme increases were not associated with other clinical findings suggestive of hepatic injury; moreover, none were jaundiced. Rare reports of more severe liver injury, some fatal, have been recorded in foreign postmarketing experience. Caution is indicated in treating patients with known liver disease, and periodic monitoring of hepatic enzyme levels is recommended in such patients.

Hematologic Changes: Although no instances of severe hematologic toxicity were seen in the premarketing experience with Anafranil, there have been postmarketing reports of leukopenia, agranulocytosis, thrombocytopenia, anemia, and pancytopenia in association with Anafranil use. As is the case with tricyclic antidepressants to which Anafranil is closely related, leukocyte and differential blood counts should be obtained in patients who develop fever and sore throat during treatment with Anafranil.

Central Nervous System: More than 30 cases of hyperthermia have been recorded by nondomestic postmarketing surveillance systems. Most cases occurred when Anafranil was used in combination with other drugs. When Anafranil and a neuroleptic were used concomitantly, the cases were sometimes considered to be examples of a neuroleptic malignant syndrome.

Sexual Dysfunction: The rate of sexual dysfunction in male patients with OCD who were treated with Anafranil in the premarketing experience was markedly increased compared with placebo controls (i.e., 42% experienced ejaculatory failure and 20% experienced impotence, compared with 2.0% and 2.6%, respectively, in the placebo group). Approximately 85% of males with sexual dysfunction chose to continue treatment.

Weight Changes: In controlled studies of OCD, weight gain was reported in 18% of patients receiving Anafranil, compared with 1% of patients receiving placebo. In these studies, 28% of patients receiving Anafranil had a weight gain of at least 7% of their initial body weight, compared with 4% of patients receiving placebo. Several patients had weight gains in excess of 25% of their initial body weight. Conversely, 5% of patients receiving Anafranil and 1% receiving placebo had weight losses of at least 7% of their initial body weight.

Electroconvulsive Therapy: As with closely related tricyclic antidepressants, concurrent administration of Anafranil with electroconvulsive therapy may increase the risks; such treatment should be limited to those patients for whom it is essential, since there is limited clinical experience.

Surgery: Prior to elective surgery with general anesthetics, therapy with Anafranil should be discontinued for as long as is clinically feasible, and the anesthetist should be advised.

Use in Concomitant Illness: As with closely related tricyclic antidepressants, Anafranil should be used with caution in the following:

(1)Hyperthyroid patients or patients receiving thyroid medication, because of the possibility of cardiac toxicity;

(2)Patients with increased intraocular pressure, a history of narrow-angle glaucoma, or urinary retention, because of the anticholinergic properties of the drug;

(3)Patients with tumors of the adrenal medulla (e.g., pheochromocytoma, neuroblastoma) in whom the drug may provoke hypertensive crises;

(4)Patients with significantly impaired renal function.

Withdrawal Symptoms: A variety of withdrawal symptoms have been reported in association with abrupt discontinuation of Anafranil, including dizziness, nausea, vomiting, headache, malaise, sleep disturbance, hyperthermia, and irritability. In addition, such patients may experi-

Continued on next page

Anafranil—Cont.

ence a worsening of psychiatric status. While the withdrawal effects of Anafranil have not been systematically evaluated in controlled trials, they are well known with closely related tricyclic antidepressants, and it is recommended that the dosage be tapered gradually and the patient monitored carefully during discontinuation (see DRUG ABUSE AND DEPENDENCE).

Information for Patients

Physicians are advised to discuss the following issues with patients for whom they prescribe Anafranil:

(1) The risk of seizure (see WARNINGS);

(2) The relatively high incidence of sexual dysfunction among males (see Sexual Dysfunction);

(3) Since Anafranil may impair the mental and/or physical abilities required for the performance of complex tasks, and since Anafranil is associated with a risk of seizures, patients should be cautioned about the performance of complex and hazardous tasks (see WARNINGS);

(4) Patients should be cautioned about using alcohol, barbiturates, or other CNS depressants concurrently, since Anafranil may exaggerate their response to these drugs;

(5) Patients should notify their physician if they become pregnant or intend to become pregnant during therapy;

(6) Patients should notify their physician if they are breastfeeding.

Drug Interactions

The risks of using Anafranil in combination with other drugs have not been systematically evaluated. Given the primary CNS effects of Anafranil, caution is advised in using it concomitantly with other CNS-active drugs (see Information for Patients). Anafranil should *not* be used with MAO inhibitors (see CONTRAINDICATIONS).

Close supervision and careful adjustment of dosage are required when Anafranil is administered with anticholinergic or sympathomimetic drugs.

Several tricyclic antidepressants have been reported to block the pharmacologic effects of guanethidine, clonidine, or similar agents, and such an effect may be anticipated with CMI because of its structural similarity to other tricyclic antidepressants.

The plasma concentration of CMI has been reported to be increased by the concomitant administration of haloperidol; plasma levels of several closely related tricyclic antidepressants have been reported to be increased by the concomitant administration of methylphenidate or hepatic enzyme inhibitors (e.g., cimetidine, fluoxetine) and decreased by the concomitant administration of hepatic enzyme inducers (e.g., barbiturates, phenytoin), and such an effect may be anticipated with CMI as well. Administration of CMI has been reported to increase the plasma levels of phenobarbital, if given concomitantly (see CLINICAL PHARMACOLOGY, Interactions).

Drugs Metabolized by P450 2D6: The biochemical activity of the drug metabolizing isozyme cytochrome P450 2D6 (debrisoquin hydroxylase) is reduced in a subset of the Caucasian population (about 7%-10% of Caucasians are so-called "poor metabolizers"); reliable estimates of the prevalence of reduced P450 2D6 isozyme activity among Asian, African and other populations are not yet available. Poor metabolizers have higher than expected plasma concentrations of tricyclic antidepressants (TCAs) when given usual doses. Depending on the fraction of drug metabolized by P450 2D6, the increase in plasma concentration may be small, or quite large (8 fold increase in plasma AUC of the TCA). In addition, certain drugs inhibit the activity of this isozyme and make normal metabolizers resemble poor metabolizers. An individual who is stable on a given dose of TCA may become abruptly toxic when given one of these inhibiting drugs as concomitant therapy. The drugs that inhibit cytochrome P450 2D6 include some that are not metabolized by the enzyme (quinidine; cimetidine) and many that are substrates for P450 2D6 (many other antidepressants, phenothiazines, and the Type 1C antiarrhythmics propafenone and flecainide). While all the selective serotonin reuptake inhibitors (SSRIs), e.g., fluoxetine, sertraline, and paroxetine, inhibit P450 2D6, they may vary in the extent of inhibition. The extent to which SSRI-TCA interactions may pose clinical problems will depend on the degree of inhibition and the pharmacokinetics of the SSRI involved. Nevertheless, caution is indicated in the co-administration of TCAs with any of the SSRIs and also in switching from one class to the other. Of particular importance, sufficient time must elapse before initiating TCA treatment in a patient being withdrawn from fluoxetine, given the long half-life of the parent and active metabolite (at least 5 weeks may be necessary). Concomitant use of tricyclic antidepressants with drugs that can inhibit cytochrome P450 2D6 may require lower doses than usually prescribed for either the tricyclic antidepressant or the other drug. Furthermore, whenever one of these drugs is withdrawn from co-therapy, an increased dose of tricyclic antidepressant may be required. It is desirable to monitor

TCA plasma levels whenever a TCA is going to be co-administered with another drug known to be an inhibitor of P450 2D6.

Because Anafranil is highly bound to serum protein, the administration of Anafranil to patients taking other drugs that are highly bound to protein (e.g., warfarin, digoxin) may cause an increase in plasma concentrations of these drugs, potentially resulting in adverse effects. Conversely, adverse effects may result from displacement of protein-bound Anafranil by other highly bound drugs (see CLINICAL PHARMACOLOGY, Distribution).

Carcinogenesis, Mutagenesis, Impairment of Fertility

In a 2-year bioassay, no clear evidence of carcinogenicity was found in rats given doses 20 times the maximum daily human dose. Three out of 235 treated rats had a rare tumor (hemangioendothelioma); it is unknown if these neoplasms are compound related.

In reproduction studies, no effects on fertility were found in rats given doses approximately 5 times the maximum daily human dose.

Pregnancy Category C

No teratogenic effects were observed in studies performed in rats and mice at doses up to 20 times the maximum daily human dose. Slight nonspecific fetotoxic effects were seen in the offspring of pregnant mice given doses 10 times the maximum daily human dose. Slight nonspecific embryotoxicity was observed in rats given doses 5-10 times the maximum daily human dose.

There are no adequate or well-controlled studies in pregnant women. Withdrawal symptoms, including jitteriness, tremor, and seizures, have been reported in neonates whose mothers had taken Anafranil until delivery. Anafranil should be used during pregnancy only if the potential benefit justifies the potential risk to the fetus.

Nursing Mothers

Anafranil has been found in human milk. Because of the potential for adverse reactions, a decision should be made whether to discontinue nursing or to discontinue the drug, taking into account the importance of the drug to the mother.

Pediatric Use

In a controlled clinical trial in children and adolescents (10-17 years of age), 46 outpatients received Anafranil for up to 8 weeks. In addition, 150 adolescent patients have received Anafranil in open-label protocols for periods of

several months to several years. Of the 196 adolescents studied, 50 were 13 years of age or less and 146 were 14-17 years of age. The adverse reaction profile in this age group (see ADVERSE REACTIONS) is similar to that in adults.

The risks, if any, that may be associated with Anafranil's extended use in children and adolescents with OCD have not been systematically assessed. The evidence supporting the conclusion that Anafranil is safe for use in children and adolescents is derived from relatively short term clinical studies and from extrapolation of experience gained with adult patients. In particular, there are no studies that directly evaluate the effects of long term Anafranil use on the growth, development, and maturation of children and adolescents. Although there is no evidence to suggest that Anafranil adversely affects growth, development or maturation, the absence of such findings is not adequate to rule out a potential for such effects in chronic use.

The safety and effectiveness in pediatric patients below the age of 10 have not been established. Therefore, specific recommendations cannot be made for the use of Anafranil in pediatric patients under the age of 10.

Use in Elderly

Anafranil has not been systematically studied in older patients; but 152 patients at least 60 years of age participating in U.S. clinical trials received Anafranil for periods of several months to several years. No unusual age-related adverse events have been identified in this elderly population, but these data are insufficient to rule out possible age-related differences, particularly in elderly patients who have concomitant systemic illnesses or who are receiving other drugs concomitantly.

ADVERSE REACTIONS

Commonly Observed

The most commonly observed adverse events associated with the use of Anafranil and not seen at an equivalent incidence among placebo-treated patients were gastrointestinal complaints, including dry mouth, constipation, nausea, dyspepsia, and anorexia; nervous system complaints, including somnolence, tremor, dizziness, nervousness, and myoclonus; genitourinary complaints, including changed libido, ejaculatory failure, impotence, and micturition disorder; and other miscellaneous complaints, including fatigue, sweating, increased appetite, weight gain, and visual changes.

Incidence of Treatment-Emergent Adverse Experience in Placebo-Controlled Clinical Trials
(Percentage of Patients Reporting Event)

Body System/ Adverse Event*	Adults Anafranil (N=322)	Adults Placebo (N=319)	Children and Adolescents Anafranil (N=46)	Children and Adolescents Placebo (N=44)
Nervous System				
Somnolence	54	16	46	11
Tremor	54	2	33	2
Dizziness	54	14	41	14
Headache	52	41	28	34
Insomnia	25	15	11	7
Libido change	21	3	-	-
Nervousness	18	2	4	2
Myoclonus	13	-	2	-
Increased appetite	11	2	-	2
Paresthesia	9	3	2	2
Memory impairment	9	1	7	2
Anxiety	9	4	2	-
Twitching	7	1	4	5
Impaired concentration	5	2	-	-
Depression	5	1	-	-
Hypertonia	4	1	2	-
Sleep disorder	4	-	9	5
Psychosomatic disorder	3	-	-	-
Yawning	3	-	-	-
Confusion	3	-	2	-
Speech disorder	3	-	-	-
Abnormal dreaming	3	-	-	2
Agitation	3	-	-	-
Migraine	3	-	-	-
Depersonalization	2	-	2	-
Irritability	2	2	-	-
Emotional lability	2	-	-	2
Panic reaction	1	-	2	-
Aggressive reaction	-	-	2	-
Paresis	-	-	2	-
Skin and Appendages				
Increased sweating	29	3	9	-
Rash	8	1	4	2
Pruritus	6	-	2	2
Dermatitis	2	-	-	-
Acne	2	2	-	5
Dry skin	2	-	-	5
Urticaria	1	-	-	-
Abnormal skin odor	-	-	2	-

* Events reported by at least 1% of Anafranil patients are included.

Incidence of Treatment-Emergent Adverse Experience in Placebo-Controlled Clinical Trials (Percentage of Patients Reporting Event)

Body System/ Adverse Event*	Adults		Children and Adolescents	
	Anafranil (N=322)	Placebo (N=319)	Anafranil (N=46)	Placebo (N=44)
Digestive System				
Dry mouth	84	17	63	16
Constipation	47	11	22	9
Nausea	33	14	9	11
Dyspepsia	22	10	13	2
Diarrhea	13	9	7	5
Anorexia	12	-	22	2
Abdominal pain	11	9	13	16
Vomiting	7	2	7	-
Flatulence	6	3	-	2
Tooth disorder	5	-	-	-
Gastrointestinal disorder	2	-	-	2
Dysphagia	2	-	-	-
Esophagitis	1	-	-	-
Eructation	-	-	2	2
Ulcerative stomatitis	-	-	2	-
Body as a Whole				
Fatigue	39	18	35	9
Weight increase	18	1	2	-
Flushing	8	-	7	-
Hot flushes	5	-	2	-
Chest pain	4	4	7	-
Fever	4	-	2	7
Allergy	3	3	7	5
Pain	3	2	4	2
Local edema	2	4	-	-
Chills	2	1	-	-
Weight decrease	-	-	2	-
Otitis media	-	-	4	5
Asthenia	-	-	2	-
Halitosis	-	-	2	-
Cardiovascular System				
Postural hypotension	6	-	4	-
Palpitation	4	2	4	-
Tachycardia	4	-	2	-
Syncope	-	-	2	-
Respiratory System				
Pharyngitis	14	9	-	5
Rhinitis	12	10	7	9
Sinusitis	6	4	2	5
Coughing	6	6	4	5
Bronchospasm	2	-	7	2
Epistaxis	2	-	-	2
Dyspnea	-	-	2	-
Laryngitis	-	1	2	-

* Events reported by at least 1% of Anafranil patients are included.

Leading to Discontinuation of Treatment

Approximately 20% of 3616 patients who received Anafranil in U.S. premarketing clinical trials discontinued treatment because of an adverse event. Approximately one-half of the patients who discontinued (9% of the total) had multiple complaints, none of which could be classified as primary. Where a primary reason for discontinuation could be identified, most patients discontinued because of nervous system complaints (5.4%), primarily somnolence. The second-most-frequent reason for discontinuation was digestive system complaints (1.3%), primarily vomiting and nausea.

Incidence in Controlled Clinical Trials

The following table enumerates adverse events that occurred at an incidence of 1% or greater among patients with OCD who received Anafranil in adult or pediatric placebo-controlled clinical trials. The frequencies were obtained from pooled data of clinical trials involving either adults receiving Anafranil (N=322) or placebo (N=319) or children treated with Anafranil (N=46) or placebo (N=44). The prescriber should be aware that these figures cannot be used to predict the incidence of side effects in the course of usual medical practice, in which patient characteristics and other factors differ from those that prevailed in the clinical trials. Similarly, the cited frequencies cannot be compared with figures obtained from other clinical investigations involving different treatments, uses, and investigators. The cited figures, however, provide the physician with a basis for estimating the relative contribution of drug and nondrug factors to the incidence of side effects in the populations studied.

[See table at bottom of previous page]
[See table above]
[See table at bottom of next page]

Other Events Observed During the Premarketing Evaluation of Anafranil

During clinical testing in the U.S., multiple doses of Anafranil were administered to approximately 3600 subjects. Untoward events associated with this exposure were recorded by clinical investigators using terminology of their own choosing. Consequently, it is not possible to provide a meaningful estimate of the proportion of individuals experiencing adverse events without first grouping similar types of untoward events into a smaller number of standardized event categories.

In the tabulations that follow, a modified World Health Organization dictionary of terminology has been used to classify reported adverse events. The frequencies presented, therefore, represent the proportion of the 3525 individuals exposed to Anafranil who experienced an event of the type cited on at least one occasion while receiving Anafranil. All events are included except those already listed in the previous table, those reported in terms so general as to be uninformative, and those in which an association with the drug was remote. It is important to emphasize that although the events reported occurred during treatment with Anafranil, they were not necessarily caused by it.

Events are further categorized by body system and listed in order of decreasing frequency according to the following definitions: frequent adverse events are those occurring on one or more occasions in at least 1/100 patients; infrequent adverse events are those occurring in 1/100 to 1/1000 patients; rare events are those occurring in less than 1/1000 patients.

Body as a Whole: Infrequent-general edema, increased susceptibility to infection, malaise. *Rare*-dependent edema, withdrawal syndrome.

Cardiovascular System: Infrequent-abnormal ECG, arrhythmia, bradycardia, cardiac arrest, extrasystoles, pallor. *Rare*-aneurysm, atrial flutter, bundle branch block, cardiac failure, cerebral hemorrhage, heart block, myocardial infarction, myocardial ischemia, peripheral ischemia, thrombophlebitis, vasospasm, ventricular tachycardia.

Digestive System: Infrequent-abnormal hepatic function, blood in stool, colitis, duodenitis, gastric ulcer, gastritis, gastroesophageal reflux, gingivitis, glossitis, hemorrhoids, hepatitis, increased saliva, irritable bowel syndrome, peptic ulcer, rectal hemorrhage, tongue ulceration, tooth caries. *Rare*-cheilitis, chronic enteritis, discolored feces, gastric dilatation, gingival bleeding, hiccup, intestinal obstruction, oral/pharyngeal edema, paralytic ileus, salivary gland enlargement.

Endocrine System: Infrequent-hypothyroidism. *Rare*-goiter, gynecomastia, hyperthyroidism.

Hemic and Lymphatic System: Infrequent-lymphadenopathy. *Rare*-leukemoid reaction, lymphoma-like disorder, marrow depression.

Metabolic and Nutritional Disorder: Infrequent-dehydration, diabetes mellitus, gout, hypercholesterolemia, hyperglycemia, hyperuricemia, hypokalemia. *Rare*-fat intolerance, glycosuria.

Musculoskeletal System: Infrequent-arthrosis. *Rare*-dystonia, exostosis, lupus erythematosus rash, bruising, myopathy, myositis, polyarteritis nodosa, torticollis.

Nervous System: Frequent-abnormal thinking, vertigo. *Infrequent*-abnormal coordination, abnormal EEG, abnormal gait, apathy, ataxia, coma, convulsions, delirium, delusion, dyskinesia, dysphonia, encephalopathy, euphoria, extrapyramidal disorder, hallucinations, hostility, hyperkinesia, hypnagogic hallucinations, hypokinesia, leg cramps, manic reaction, neuralgia, paranoia, phobic disorder, psychosis, sensory disturbance, somnambulism, stimulation, suicidal ideation, suicide attempt, teeth-grinding. *Rare*-anticholinergic syndrome, aphasia, apraxia, catalepsy, cholinergic syndrome, choreoathetosis, generalized spasm, hemiparesis, hyperesthesia, hyperreflexia, hypoesthesia, illusion, impaired impulse control, indecisiveness, mutism, neuropathy, nystagmus, oculogyric crisis, oculomotor nerve paralysis, schizophrenic reaction, stupor, suicide.

Respiratory System: Infrequent-bronchitis, hyperventilation, increased sputum, pneumonia. *Rare*-cyanosis, hemoptysis, hypoventilation, laryngismus.

Skin and Appendages: Infrequent-alopecia, cellulitis, cyst, eczema, erythematous rash, genital pruritus, maculopapular rash, photosensitivity reaction, psoriasis, pustular rash, skin discoloration. *Rare*-chloasma, folliculitis, hypertrichosis, piloerection, seborrhea, skin hypertrophy, skin ulceration.

Special Senses: Infrequent-abnormal accommodation, deafness, diplopia, earache, eye pain, foreign body sensation, hyperacusis, parosmia, photophobia, scleritis, taste loss. *Rare*-blepharitis, chromatopsia, conjunctival hemorrhage, exophthalmos, glaucoma, keratitis, labyrinth disorder, night blindness, retinal disorder, strabismus, visual field defect.

Urogenital System: Infrequent-endometriosis, epididymitis, hematuria, nocturia, oliguria, ovarian cyst, perineal pain, polyuria, prostatic disorder, renal calculus, renal pain, urethral disorder, urinary incontinence, uterine hemorrhage, vaginal hemorrhage. *Rare*-albuminuria, anorgasmy, breast engorgement, breast fibroadenosis, cervical dysplasia, endometrial hyperplasia, premature ejaculation, pyelonephritis, pyuria, renal cyst, uterine inflammation, vulvar disorder.

DRUG ABUSE AND DEPENDENCE

Anafranil has not been systematically studied in animals or humans for its potential for abuse, tolerance, or physical dependence. While a variety of withdrawal symptoms have been described in association with Anafranil discontinuation (see PRECAUTIONS, Withdrawal Symptoms), there is no evidence for drug-seeking behavior, except for a single report of potential Anafranil abuse by a patient with a history of dependence on codeine, benzodiazepines, and multiple psychoactive drugs. The patient received Anafranil for depression and panic attacks and appeared to become dependent after hospital discharge.

Despite the lack of evidence suggesting an abuse liability for Anafranil in foreign marketing, it is not possible to predict the extent to which Anafranil might be misused or abused once marketed in the U.S. Consequently, physicians should carefully evaluate patients for a history of drug abuse and follow such patients closely.

OVERDOSAGE

Deaths may occur from overdosage with this class of drugs. Multiple drug ingestion (including alcohol) is common in deliberate tricyclic overdose. As the management is complex and changing, it is recommended that the physician contact a poison control center for current information on treatment. Signs and symptoms of toxicity develop rapidly after tricyclic overdose. Therefore, hospital monitoring is required as soon as possible.

Human Experience

In U.S. clinical trials, 2 deaths occurred in 12 reported cases of acute overdosage with Anafranil either alone or in combination with other drugs. One death involved a patient suspected of ingesting a dose of 7000 mg. The second death involved a patient suspected of ingesting a dose of 5750 mg. The 10 nonfatal cases involved doses of up to 5000 mg, accompanied by plasma levels of up to 1010 ng/mL. All 10 patients completely recovered. Among reports from other countries of Anafranil overdose, the lowest dose associated with a fatality was 750 mg. Based upon postmarketing reports in the United Kingdom, CMI's lethality in overdose

Continued on next page

Anafranil—Cont.

is considered to be similar to that reported for closely related tricyclic compounds marketed as antidepressants.

Manifestations

Signs and symptoms vary in severity depending upon factors such as the amount of drug absorbed, the age of the patient, and the time elapsed since drug ingestion. Critical manifestations of overdose include cardiac dysrhythmias, severe hypotension, convulsions, and CNS depression including coma. Changes in the electrocardiogram, particularly in QRS axis or width, are clinically significant indicators of tricyclic toxicity. Other CNS manifestations may include drowsiness, stupor, ataxia, restlessness, agitation, delirium, severe perspiration, hyperactive reflexes, muscle rigidity, and athetoid and choreiform movements. Cardiac abnormalities may include tachycardia, signs of congestive heart failure, and in very rare cases, cardiac arrest. Respiratory depression, cyanosis, shock, vomiting, hyperpyrexia, mydriasis, and oliguria or anuria may also be present.

Management

Obtain an ECG and immediately initiate cardiac monitoring. Protect the patient's airway, establish an intravenous line, and initiate gastric decontamination. A minimum of 6 hours of observation with cardiac monitoring and observation for signs of CNS or respiratory depression, hypotension, cardiac dysrhythmias and/or conduction blocks, and seizures is necessary.

If signs of toxicity occur at any time during this period, extended monitoring is required. There are case reports of patients succumbing to fatal dysrhythmias late after overdose; these patients had clinical evidence of significant poisoning prior to death and most received inadequate gastrointestinal decontamination. Monitoring of plasma drug levels should not guide management of the patient.

Gastrointestinal Decontamination: All patients suspected of tricyclic overdose should receive gastrointestinal decontamination. This should include large volume gastric lavage followed by activated charcoal. If consciousness is impaired, the airway should be secured prior to lavage. Emesis is contraindicated.

Cardiovascular: A maximal limb-lead QRS duration of ≥ 0.10 seconds may be the best indication of the severity of the overdose. Intravenous sodium bicarbonate should be used to maintain the serum pH in the range of 7.45 to 7.55. If the pH response is inadequate, hyperventilation may also be used. Concomitant use of hyperventilation and sodium bicarbonate should be done with extreme caution, with frequent pH monitoring. A pH >7.60 or a Pco_2 <20 mmHg is undesirable. Dysrhythmias unresponsive to sodium bicarbonate therapy/hyperventilation may respond to lidocaine, bretylium, or phenytoin. Type 1A and 1C antiarrhythmics are generally contraindicated (e.g., quinidine, disopyramide, and procainamide).

In rare instances, hemoperfusion may be beneficial in acute refractory cardiovascular instability in patients with acute toxicity. However, hemodialysis, peritoneal dialysis, exchange transfusions, and forced diuresis generally have been reported as ineffective in tricyclic poisoning.

CNS: In patients with CNS depression, early intubation is advised because of the potential for abrupt deterioration. Seizures should be controlled with benzodiazepines, or if these are ineffective, other anticonvulsants (e.g., phenobarbital, phenytoin). Physostigmine is not recommended except to treat life-threatening symptoms that have been unresponsive to other therapies, and then only in consultation with a poison control center.

Psychiatric Follow-up: Since overdosage is often deliberate, patients may attempt suicide by other means during the recovery phase. Psychiatric referral may be appropriate.

Pediatric Management: The principles of management of child and adult overdosages are similar. It is strongly recommended that the physician contact the local poison control center for specific pediatric treatment.

DOSAGE AND ADMINISTRATION

The treatment regimens described below are based on those used in controlled clinical trials of Anafranil in 520 adults, and 91 children and adolescents with OCD. During initial titration, Anafranil should be given in divided doses with meals to reduce gastrointestinal side effects. The goal of this initial titration phase is to minimize side effects by permitting tolerance to side effects to develop or allowing the patient time to adapt if tolerance does not develop.

Because both CMI and its active metabolite, DMI, have long elimination half-lives, the prescriber should take into consideration the fact that steady-state plasma levels may not be achieved until 2-3 weeks after dosage change (see CLINICAL PHARMACOLOGY). Therefore, after initial titration, it may be appropriate to wait 2-3 weeks between further dosage adjustments.

Initial Treatment/Dose Adjustment (Adults)

Treatment with Anafranil should be initiated at a dosage of 25 mg daily and gradually increased, as tolerated, to approximately 100 mg during the first 2 weeks. During initial titration, Anafranil should be given in divided doses with meals to reduce gastrointestinal side effects. Thereafter, the dosage may be increased gradually over the next several weeks, up to a maximum of 250 mg daily. After titration, the total daily dose may be given once daily at bedtime to minimize daytime sedation.

Initial Treatment/Dose Adjustment (Children and Adolescents)

As with adults, the starting dose is 25 mg daily and should be gradually increased (also given in divided doses with meals to reduce gastrointestinal side effects) during the first 2 weeks, as tolerated, up to a daily maximum of 3 mg/kg or 100 mg, whichever is smaller. Thereafter, the dosage may be increased gradually over the next several weeks up to a daily maximum of 3 mg/kg or 200 mg, whichever is smaller (see PRECAUTIONS, Pediatric Use). As with adults, after titration, the total daily dose may be given once daily at bedtime to minimize daytime sedation.

Maintenance/Continuation Treatment (Adults, Children, and Adolescents)

While there are no systematic studies that answer the question of how long to continue Anafranil, OCD is a chronic condition and it is reasonable to consider continuation for a responding patient. Although the efficacy of Anafranil after 10 weeks has not been documented in controlled trials, patients have been continued in therapy under double-blind conditions for up to 1 year without loss of benefit. However, dosage adjustments should be made to maintain the patient on the lowest effective dosage, and patients should be periodically reassessed to determine the need for treatment. During maintenance, the total daily dose may be given once daily at bedtime.

HOW SUPPLIED

Capsules 25 mg-ivory/melon yellow (imprinted ANAFRANIL 25 mg)
    Bottles of 100 .... NDC 0078-0316-05
    Unit Dose (blister pack)
    Box of 100 (strips of 10) .... NDC 0078-0316-06
Capsules 50 mg-ivory/aqua blue (imprinted ANAFRANIL 50 mg)
    Bottles of 100 .... NDC 0078-0317-05
    Unit Dose (blister pack)
    Box of 100 (strips of 10) .... NDC 0078-0317-06
Capsules 75 mg-ivory/yellow (imprinted ANAFRANIL 75 mg)
    Bottles of 100 .... NDC 0078-0318-05
    Unit Dose (blister pack)
    Box of 100 (strips of 10) .... NDC 0078-0318-06
Do not store above 30°C (86°F). Protect from moisture.
Dispense in tight container (USP).

ANIMAL TOXICOLOGY

Testicular and lung changes commonly associated with tricyclic compounds have been observed with Anafranil. In 1- and 2-year studies in rats, changes in the testes (atrophy, aspermatogenesis, and calcification) and drug-induced phospholipidosis in the lungs were observed at doses 4 times the maximum daily human dose. Testicular atrophy was also observed in a 1-year oral toxicity study in dogs at 10 times the maximum daily human dose.

C98-13 (Rev. 4/98)

Shown in Product Identification Guide, page 324

Incidence of Treatment-Emergent Adverse Experience in Placebo-Controlled Clinical Trials (Percentage of Patients Reporting Event)

Body System/ Adverse Event*	Adults		Children and Adolescents	
	Anafranil (N=322)	Placebo (N=319)	Anafranil (N=46)	Placebo (N=44)
Urogenital System				
Male and Female Patients Combined				
Micturition disorder	14	2	4	2
Urinary tract infection	6	1	-	-
Micturition frequency	5	3	-	-
Urinary retention	2	-	7	-
Dysuria	2	2	-	-
Cystitis	2	-	-	-
Female Patients Only	(N=182)	(N=167)	(N=10)	(N=21)
Dysmenorrhea	12	14	10	10
Lactation (nonpuerperal)	4	-	-	-
Menstrual disorder	4	2	-	-
Vaginitis	2	-	-	-
Leukorrhea	2	-	-	-
Breast enlargement	2	-	-	-
Breast pain	1	-	-	-
Amenorrhea	1	-	-	-
Male Patients Only	(N=140)	(N=152)	(N=36)	(N=23)
Ejaculation failure	42	2	6	-
Impotence	20	3	-	-
Special Senses				
Abnormal vision	18	4	7	2
Taste perversion	8	-	4	-
Tinnitus	6	-	4	-
Abnormal lacrimation	3	2	-	-
Mydriasis	2	-	-	-
Conjunctivitis	1	-	2	-
Anisocoria	-	-	2	-
Blepharospasm	-	-	2	-
Ocular allergy	-	-	2	-
Vestibular disorder	-	-	2	2
Musculoskeletal				
Myalgia	13	9	-	-
Back pain	6	6	-	-
Arthralgia	3	5	-	-
Muscle weakness	1	-	2	-
Hemic and Lymphatic				
Purpura	3	-	-	-
Anemia	-	-	2	2
Metabolic and Nutritional				
Thirst	2	2	-	2

* Events reported by at least 1% of Anafranil patients are included.

APLIGRAF™   ℞
[*ă-plĭ-grăf*]
(Graftskin)

Caution: Federal law restricts this device to sale by or on the order of a physician (or properly licensed practitioner).

The following prescribing information is based on official labeling in effect on August 1, 1998.

1. DEVICE DESCRIPTION

Apligraf is a viable, bi-layered, skin construct: the epidermal layer is formed by human keratinocytes and has a well-differentiated stratum corneum; the dermal layer is composed of human fibroblasts in a bovine Type I collagen lattice. While matrix proteins and cytokines found in human skin are present in Apligraf, Apligraf does not contain Langerhans cells, melanocytes, macrophages, lymphocytes, blood vessels or hair follicles. Apligraf is manufactured under aseptic conditions from human neonatal male foreskin tissue. The fibroblast and ke-

ratinocyte cell banks which are the source of the cells from which Apligraf is derived are tested for human and animal viruses, retroviruses, bacteria, fungi, yeast, mycoplasma, karyology, isoenzymes, and tumorigenicity. The final product is tested for morphology, cell viability, epidermal coverage, sterility, mycoplasma, and physical container integrity. Product manufacture also includes reagents derived from animal materials including bovine pituitary extract. All animal derived reagents are tested for viruses, retroviruses, bacteria, fungi, yeast, and mycoplasma before use, and all bovine material is obtained from countries free from bovine spongiform encephalopathy (BSE).

2. INTENDED USE/INDICATIONS

Apligraf is indicated for use with standard therapeutic compression for the treatment of non-infected partial and full-thickness skin ulcers due to venous insufficiency of greater than 1 month duration and which have not adequately responded to conventional ulcer therapy.

3. CONTRAINDICATIONS

- Apligraf is contraindicated for use on clinically infected wounds.
- Apligraf is contraindicated in patients with known allergies to bovine collagen.
- Apligraf is contraindicated in patients with a known hypersensitivity to the components of the Apligraf agarose shipping medium (Section 8).

4. WARNINGS

Warning: DO NOT OPEN AND DO NOT USE Apligraf after the expiration date or if the pH is not within the acceptable range (6.8-7.7) as determined by the provided color chart (Section 9).

Warning: Allergic reactions to the components in the Apligraf agarose shipping medium (Section 8) and bovine collagen, (a component of Apligraf), have been reported. Discontinue product use if a patient shows evidence of an immunologic reaction. Patients should notify their physician of any symptoms of an allergic reaction. In studies with 361 patients, no allergic reactions to Apligraf were reported.

5. PRECAUTIONS

Caution: Do not use Apligraf if there is evidence of container damage or product contamination.

Caution: Apligraf should not be reused, frozen or sterilized after opening.

Caution: Apligraf should be kept in its tray on the shipping medium in the sealed bag under controlled temperature (20°C-31°C) until ready for use.

Caution: Apligraf should be handled using sterile technique and placed on a prepared wound bed within 5 minutes of opening the package.

Caution: Do not use cytotoxic agents, including Dakin's solution, Mafenide Acetate, Scarlet Red Dressing, Tincoban, Zinc Sulfate, Povidone-iodine solution, or Chlorhexidine with Apligraf. In *in vitro* and *in vivo* histology studies, exposure to these agents degraded Apligraf. Device exposure to Mafenide Acetate, Polymyxin/Nystatin or Dakin's Solution also reduced Apligraf cell viability.

Caution: Diagnosis of wound infection may be complicated by the white or yellow appearance of Apligraf after it becomes hydrated with wound fluid. Apligraf-treated wounds with respect to signs of suspected infection, including a change from baseline at the ulcer site for pain, edema, erythema, drainage, odor, warmth and/or unexplained fever, should be evaluated and treated according to standard practice for infection.

Caution: The persistence of Apligraf cells on the wound and the safety of this device in venous ulcer patients beyond one year has not been evaluated. In clinical studies with Apligraf there have been no reports of long term sequelae associated with Apligraf use.

Caution: The safety and the effectiveness of Apligraf have not been established for patients receiving greater than 5 device applications.

6. ADVERSE EVENTS

All reported adverse events which occurred in the Apligraf cohort in the pivotal clinical study at an incidence of 1% or greater are listed in Table 1. The adverse events are listed in descending order according to frequency. This table lists all adverse events reported in the study including those attributed and not attributed to treatment.
[See table 1 above]
Adverse events were recorded as mild, moderate, severe or life-threatening. There were 1 life-threatening and 3 severe infections reported in the Apligraf group and none in the control arm. Of the four events, two severe infections were considered related to treatment, however, one occurred one month after the last application of Apligraf and the other occurred following application on a pre-existing *Pseudomonas* infection.

Table 1
Adverse Events Reported in Greater than 1.0% of Apligraf Patients

	Apligraf (n=161)	Control (n=136)
	Total	Total
Suspected Wound Infection[1] (study site)	47 (29.2%)	19 (14.0%)
Suspected Wound Infection[1] (non-study site)	16 (9.9%)	15 (11.0%)
Cellulitis[2] (study site)	13 (8.1%)	11 (8.1%)
Cellulitis[2] (non-study site)	12 (7.5%)	7 (5.1%)
Dermatitis (non-study site)	10 (6.2%)	10 (7.4%)
Exudate (study site)	9 (5.6%)	0 (0.0%)
Peripheral Edema	8 (5.0%)	7 (5.1%)
Pain (study site)	7 (4.3%)	7 (5.1%)
Death	6 (3.7%)	6 (4.4%)
Skin Ulcer (non-study site)	6 (3.7%)	5 (3.7%)
Pain (non-study site)	5 (3.1%)	4 (2.9%)
Pruritus (non-study site)	5 (3.1%)	2 (1.5%)
Skin Ulcer (study site)	5 (3.1%)	3 (2.2%)
Infection (non-wound)	4 (2.5%)	1 (0.7%)
Positive Wound Culture[3] (study site)	4 (2.5%)	3 (2.2%)
Rhinitis	4 (2.5%)	1 (0.7%)
Dermatitis (study site)	4 (2.5%)	2 (1.5%)
Pain (overall body)	3 (1.8%)	2 (1.5%)
Congestive Heart Failure	3 (1.8%)	0 (0.0%)
Accidental Injury (musculoskeletal)	3 (1.8%)	0 (0.0%)
Dyspnea	3 (1.8%)	1 (0.7%)
Pharyngitis	3 (1.8%)	0 (0.0%)
Rash (study site)	3 (1.8%)	2 (1.5%)
Accidental Injury (overall body)	2 (1.3%)	1 (0.7%)
Asthenia	2 (1.3%)	0 (0.0%)
Arrhythmia	2 (1.3%)	0 (0.0%)
Abscess (non-study site)	2 (1.3%)	0 (0.0%)
Arthralgia	2 (1.3%)	2 (1.5%)
Cough Increased	2 (1.3%)	0 (0.0%)
Rash (non-study site)	2 (1.3%)	5 (3.7%)
Erythema (study site)	2 (1.3%)	1 (0.7%)
Kidney Failure	2 (1.3%)	0 (0.0%)
Urinary Tract Infection	2 (1.3%)	5 (3.7%)

In the clinical trial the following definitions were used:
[1] *Suspected wound infection:* a wound with at least some clinical signs and symptoms of infection such as increased exudate, odor, redness, swelling, heat, pain, tenderness to the touch, and purulent discharge; quantitative culture was not required.
[2] *Cellulitis:* a non-suppurative inflammation of the subcutaneous tissues extending along connective tissue planes and across intercellular spaces; widespread swelling, redness, and pain without definite localization.
[3] *Positive wound culture:* reported as an adverse event, but not reported as a wound infection.

7. CLINICAL STUDIES

Study Design
A prospective, randomized, controlled, multi-center, multi-specialty, unmasked study was conducted to evaluate the safety and effectiveness of Apligraf and compression therapy in comparison to an active treatment concurrent control of zinc paste gauze and compression therapy. The study population included consenting patients who were 18-89 years old, available for one year follow-up, with venous insufficiency confirmed by plethysmography (venous reflux <20 sec.); associated with non-infected partial and/or full thickness skin loss ulcer (IAET Stage 2 or 3) of greater than one month duration and which had not adequately responded to conventional ulcer therapy. Patients were excluded for ankle brachial index <0.65, severe rheumatoid arthritis, collagen vascular disease, pregnancy/lactation, cellulitis, osteomyelitis, ulcer with necrotic, avascular or bone/tendon/fascia exposed-bed, clinically significant wound healing impairment due to uncontrolled diabetes, or renal, hepatic, hematologic, neurologic or immune insufficiency or due to immunosuppressive agents such as corticosteroids (>15 mg/day), radiation therapy or chemotherapy; or enrollment in studies within the past 30 days for investigational devices or within the past three months for investigational drugs related to wound healing.
Extremities with multiple ulcers were enrolled; however, only one ulcer per extremity was studied. Non-study ulcer care was not specifically defined. Study ulcer care was defined for the treatment (Apligraf and compression therapy) and control (zinc paste gauze and compression therapy), treatment groups in two phases:
1) Active Phase (0-8 weeks): All patients received: i) a non-adherent, ii) a non-occlusive, and iii) a therapeutic compression dressing on day 0, mid-week during the first week (day 3-5) and at weeks 1-8. Control treated patients also received zinc impregnated gauze at each visit. All Apligraf patients received Apligraf on day 0. At the day 3-5 and weeks 1, 2, and 3 visits, if less than 50% Apligraf take was observed, then patients received an additional application of Apligraf. Patients were not allowed to receive more than 5 Apligraf applications total.
2) Maintenance Phase (8-52 weeks): Closed-ulcer extremities received non-specified elastic compression stockings. Open-ulcer extremities continued with dressing changes.
Wound closure was defined as 100% epithelialization without drainage and assessed by clinical observation at visits on day 0, day 3-5, weekly from weeks 1-8, months 3 and 6 after initial treatment application or until wound closure was achieved. Additional follow-up visits were 9 and 12 months after initial treatment.

Study Results
The incidence of wound closure at set visits up to 6 months is presented below as the raw data results (Figure 1) and the results after adjustment for pooled center, baseline ulcer duration, and baseline area (Figure 2).

Figure 1
Efficacy Cohort (n=240)
Raw Frequency of Complete Wound Closure as a Function of Time

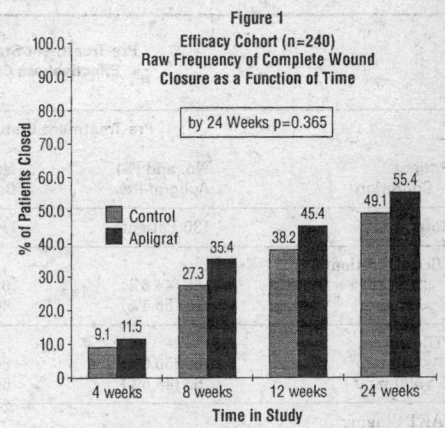

by 24 Weeks p=0.365

[See figure 2 at top of next column]

Ulcer recurrence
At six months, the incidence of ulcer recurrence was 8.3% (6/72) for Apligraf- and 7.4% (4/54) for control-treated patients. The incidence of ulcer recurrence by 12 months was 18.1% (13/72) in the Apligraf group and 22.2% (12/54) in the control group.

Suspected wound infection
In the effectiveness cohort, there were 33/130 (25.4%) Apligraf-treated and 15/110 (13.6%) control-treated ulcers with suspected wound infection. While the overall incidence

Continued on next page

Apligraf—Cont.

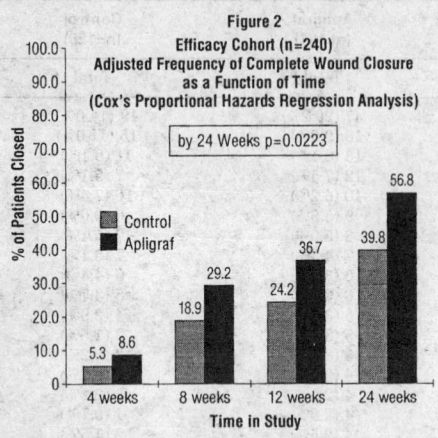

Figure 2
Efficacy Cohort (n=240)
Adjusted Frequency of Complete Wound Closure
as a Function of Time
(Cox's Proportional Hazards Regression Analysis)

by 24 Weeks p=0.0223

of wound infection was higher in the Apligraf arm, the incidence of wound closure (Figures 1 and 2) was also higher for Apligraf-treated patients.

Baseline status impact on wound closure

The impact of patient baseline status on wound closure was evaluated for the patient populations above and below the median values for ulcer duration and ulcer size as well as for baseline IAET Ulcer Stage, the presence of diabetes, and a patient's Ankle Brachial Index. The results of these analyses are displayed in Table 2.

[See table 2 below]

Secondary endpoints

Clinical assessment (scale 1-4) of wound depth (IAET staging), erythema, edema, wound pain, fibrin, exudate, granulation tissue, and overall assessment by changes in mean score and analysis of variance from baseline to the 6 month visit indicated no differences between treatment groups at 6 months.

Immune response

In tests of patients' sera there were no observations of antibody responses against bovine Type I collagen, bovine serum proteins or the Class I HLA antigens on human dermal fibroblasts, and human epidermal cells. T-cell specific responses were also not observed against bovine Type I collagen, human fibroblasts or human keratinocytes. There was also no clinical evidence of Apligraf rejection by any patient.

8. HOW SUPPLIED

Apligraf is supplied sealed in a heavy gauge polyethylene bag with a 10% CO_2/air atmosphere and agarose nutrient medium, ready for single use. To maintain cell viability, Apligraf should be kept in the sealed bag at 20°C-31°C until use. Apligraf is supplied as a circular disk approximately 75 mm in diameter and 0.75 mm thick. The agarose shipping medium contains agarose, L-glutamine, hydrocortisone/bovine serum albumin, bovine insulin, human transferrin, triiodothyronine, ethanolamine, O-phosphorylethanolamine, adenine, selenious acid, DMEM powder, HAM's F-12 powder, sodium bicarbonate, calcium chloride, and water for injection.

To maintain cell viability, the product is aseptically manufactured, but not terminally sterilized. Apligraf is shipped following a preliminary sterility test with a 48 hour incubation to determine the absence of microbial growth. Final (14 day incubation) sterility tests results are not available at the time of application.

9. DIRECTIONS FOR USE

Apligraf is indicated for use with standard therapeutic compression for the treatment of non-infected partial and full-thickness skin ulcers due to venous insufficiency of greater than 1 month duration and which have not adequately responded to conventional ulcer therapy. Apligraf consists of living cells which must be kept sealed in its nutrient medium and 10% CO_2/air atmosphere under controlled temperature (20°C–31°C) and used within 5 minutes of opening.

Preparation of the Venous Ulcer Wound Bed Prior to Apligraf Application

1. Wound Infection:
Apligraf should not be applied over infected or deteriorating wounds until the underlying condition has been resolved.

2. Bacterial Containment:
Antimicrobial agents may be used during the week prior to Apligraf application to reduce the risk of infection. Dakin's solution, Mafenide Acetate, Scarlet Red Dressing, Tincoban, Zinc Sulfate, Povidone-iodine solution, and Chlorhexidine have been determined to be cytotoxic to Apligraf.

3. Wound Bed Preparation:
Apligraf should be applied to a clean, debrided wound after thoroughly irrigating the wound with a non-cytotoxic solution. Oozing or bleeding resulting from debridement should be stopped through the use of gentle pressure. Previous ulcer treatments other than standard therapeutic compression should be discontinued.

4. Control of Heavy Exudation:
Heavy exudation may displace Apligraf and reduce adherence. Exudation should be minimized by appropriate clinical treatment. If exudation persists, Apligraf should be made permeable to exudate by perforating the Apligraf to allow for drainage.

Suggested Technique for the Application of Apligraf to the Wound

1. Check expiration date. If expired, do not open or use.
2. Check product pH. If not 6.8-7.7 by the provided color pH chart, do not open or use.
3. Prepare a sterile field and atraumatic instruments: forceps.
4. Cut open the sealed polyethylene bag and transfer the plastic tray to the sterile field with aseptic technique.

5. Lift off the tray lid and note epidermal and dermal layer orientation: Apligraf is packaged with the epidermal (dull, matte finish) layer facing up and the dermal (glossy) layer facing down.
6. Using the sterile atraumatic instrument, gently dislodge approximately 0.5 inch of Apligraf away from the wall of the tray.
7. With sterile gloved hands, insert one index finger under the released section of Apligraf. Use the other index finger to grasp the Apligraf in a second spot along the edge of the device. Holding the Apligraf in two places lift the entire Apligraf out of the tray using a smooth, even motion. This easy motion should prevent Apligraf from bending and folding over onto itself. To minimize Apligraf damage: avoid Apligraf contact with foreign bodies and minimize handling Apligraf except by its margins.
8. Do not allow Apligraf to fold or wrinkle on itself. If excessive folding occurs, Apligraf can be floated (epidermal surface up) onto warm sterile saline solution in a sterile tray.
9. Apligraf should be placed such that the dermal layer (the glossy layer closest to the medium) is in direct contact with the wound surface. Trim Apligraf so as to cover the wound bed with 1/8-1/4″ margins.
10. Secure Apligraf with a three-layer dressing so as to assure contact to wound bed:
    • Apply a non-adherent dressing over the ulcer and Apligraf, extending 0.5 inch beyond the ulcer perimeter and inflamed skin margins.
    • Apply a non-occlusive dressing such as fine mesh gauze. This may be folded or rolled as a bolster.
    • Apply a self adherent elastic wrap from metatarsals to tibial plateau so that therapeutic compression is applied to the ulcer site.

Frequency of Dressing Changes and Apligraf Applications

1. The wound should be inspected and the dressing changed at least once a week during the immediate post application period. More frequent changes may be required on highly exudative wounds.
2. Additional applications of Apligraf may be necessary. Prior to additional applications, non-adherent remnants of Apligraf should be gently removed. Healing tissue or adherent Apligraf should not be disrupted. The wound bed should be cleansed with a non-cytotoxic solution prior to additional applications of Apligraf. Additional applications of Apligraf should not be applied over areas where Apligraf is adherent.
3. The wound site should continue to be dressed with a non-adherent dressing, pressure bolster and elastic overwrap as described above.
4. Upon complete wound closure, patients should be continued with compression therapy such as support stockings.
5. The safety and the effectiveness of Apligraf have not been established for patients receiving greater than 5 device applications.

10. PATIENT'S MANUAL

A brochure will be made available to:
1. Provide basic information about chronic wounds.
2. Address standard patient care while receiving Apligraf treatment.
3. Educate patients on Apligraf-related healing process.

11. PEEL-OFF LABEL

Remove the peel-off label from the lower right corner of the Apligraf package label and place it in the patient's chart. This label bears a unique lot number and expiration date of the Apligraf.

Apligraf™ (Graftskin)
Essential Prescribing Information
Numbers in parentheses ( ) refer to sections in the main part of the product labeling.

Device Description
Apligraf is a bi-layered viable skin construct manufactured using neonatal foreskin keratinocytes and fibroblasts with bovine Type I collagen. **(1)**

Intended Use/Indications
Apligraf is indicated for use with standard therapeutic compression in the treatment of uninfected partial and/or full-thickness skin loss ulcers due to venous insufficiency of greater than 1 month duration and which have not adequately responded to conventional ulcer therapy. **(2)**

Contraindications
Apligraf is contraindicated for use on clinically infected wounds and in patients with known allergies to bovine collagen or hypersensitivity to the components of the shipping medium. **(3, 4, 5, 8)**

Warnings and Precautions
If expiration date or product pH (6.8-7.7) is not within the acceptable range DO NOT OPEN AND DO NOT USE the product. A clinical determination of wound infection should be made based on all of the signs and symptoms of infection. **(4, 5)**

Table 2
Pre-Treatment Status and Wound Closure
Effectiveness Cohort (n=240 patients)

Patient Condition	Pre-Treatment Status		Number and Percent of Wound Closure by 6 months	
	No. and (%) Apligraf Pts.	No. and (%) Control Pts.	Apligraf	Control
Total	130 Patients	110 Patients	72 (55.4%)	54 (49.1%)
Ulcer Duration				
≤1 year	58 (44.6%)	62 (56.3%)	38/58 (65.5%)	45/62 (72.6%)
>1 year	72 (55.4%)	48 (43.6%)	34/72 (47.2%)	9/48 (18.8%)
***Ulcer Area**				
<500 mm²	65 (50.0%)	60 (54.5%)	45/65 (69.2%)	35/60 (58.3%)
>500 mm²	63 (48.5%)	50 (45.5%)	26/63 (41.3%)	19/50 (38.0%)
IAET Staging				
Stage II	63 (48.5%)	56 (50.9%)	34/63 (54.0%)	32/56 (57.1%)
Stage III	67 (51.5%)	54 (49.1%)	38/67 (56.7%)	22/54 (40.7%)
Diabetes				
Yes[1]	25 (19.2%)	11 (10.0%)	12/25 (48.0%)	4/11 (36.4%)
No	105 (80.8%)	99 (90.0%)	60/105 (57.1%)	50/99 (50.5%)
****Ankle Brachial Index data (ABI)**				
>0.65 ≤0.8	9 (6.9%)	10 (9.1%)	4/9 (44.4%)	4/10 (40.0%)
>0.8 ≤1.0	43 (33.1%)	50 (45.5%)	26/43 (60.5%)	27/50 (54.0%)
>1.0	75 (57.7%)	49 (44.5%)	40/75 (53.3%)	22/49 (44.9%)

*Baseline ulcer area missing for two patients in the Apligraf™ group.
**ABI data are missing for 3 Apligraf and 1 control patient.
[1] This category includes both insulin-dependent and non-insulin dependent diabetes patients, because the insulin-dependence of patients was not determined in this clinical trial.

Adverse Events

In the controlled clinical study conducted in patients with ulcers due to venous insufficiency of greater than one month in duration, suspected infection was reported more frequently in Apligraf-treated (29.2%) than control patients (14.0%). There were 1 life-threatening and 3 severe infections in the Apligraf group and none in the control arm. Of these, two severe infections were considered related to treatment, however, one occurred one month after the last application of Apligraf and the other occurred following application on a pre-existing *Pseudomonas* infection.

While the overall incidence of wound infection was higher in the Apligraf arm, the incidence of wound closure was 72/130 (55.4%) and 54/110 (49.1%) for Apligraf and control treated patients, respectively. **(6, 7)**

Maintaining Device Effectiveness

Apligraf has been processed under aseptic conditions and should be handled observing sterile technique. It should be kept in its tray on the medium in the sealed bag under controlled temperature (20°C–31°C) until ready for use. Apligraf should be placed on the wound bed within 5 minutes of opening the package. Handling before application to the wound site should be minimal. If there is any question that Apligraf may be contaminated or compromised, it should not be used. Apligraf should not be used beyond the listed expiration date. **(9)**

Use in Specific Populations

The safety and effectiveness of Apligraf has not been established in pregnant women, acute wounds, burns, and ulcers caused by diabetic neuropathy or pressure.

Patient Counseling Information

Patients should be counseled regarding the importance of complying with compression therapy or other treatment which may be prescribed in conjunction with Apligraf.

How Supplied

Apligraf is supplied sealed in a heavy gauge polyethylene bag with a 10% CO_2/air atmosphere and agarose nutrient medium, ready for single use. To maintain cell viability, Apligraf should be kept in the sealed bag at 20°C-31°C until use. Apligraf is supplied as a circular disk approximately 75 mm in diameter and 0.75 mm thick. **(8)**

Manufactured by:
Organogenesis Inc.
Canton, MA 02021
Marketed and distributed by:
Novartis Pharmaceuticals Corporation
East Hanover, New Jersey 07936

                                    USA-Z01
MAY 1998   300-111-0

AREDIA®   ℞

[ă rē dē ă]
pamidronate disodium for injection
For Intravenous Infusion

Rx only
The following prescribing information is based on official labeling in effect on August 1, 1998.

Prescribing Information

DESCRIPTION

Aredia, pamidronate disodium (APD), is a bone-resorption inhibitor available in 30-mg, 60-mg, or 90-mg vials for intravenous administration. Each 30-mg, 60-mg, and 90-mg vial contains, respectively, 30 mg, 60 mg, and 90 mg of sterile, lyophilized pamidronate disodium and 470 mg, 400 mg, and 375 mg of mannitol, USP. The pH of a 1% solution of pamidronate disodium in distilled water is approximately 8.3. Aredia, a member of the group of chemical compounds known as bisphosphonates, is an analog of pyrophosphate. Pamidronate disodium is designated chemically as phosphonic acid (3-amino-1-hydroxypropylidene) bis-, disodium salt, pentahydrate, (APD), and its structural formula is

PO₃HNa

NH₂ – CH₂ – CH₂ – C – OH • 5H₂O

PO₃HNa

Pamidronate disodium is a white-to-practically-white powder. It is soluble in water and in 2N sodium hydroxide, sparingly soluble in 0.1N hydrochloric acid and in 0.1N acetic acid, and practically insoluble in organic solvents. Its molecular formula is $C_3H_9NO_7P_2Na_2\cdot5H_2O$ and its molecular weight is 369.1.

Inactive Ingredients. Mannitol, USP, and phosphoric acid (for adjustment to pH 6.5 prior to lyophilization).

CLINICAL PHARMACOLOGY

The principal pharmacologic action of Aredia is inhibition of bone resorption. Although the mechanism of antiresorptive

Table 1
Mean (SD, CV%) Pamidronate Pharmacokinetic Parameters in Cancer Patients
(n=6 for each group)

Dose (infusion rate)	Maximum Concentration (µg/mL)	Percent of dose excreted in urine	Total Clearance (mL/min)	Renal Clearance (mL/min)
30 mg (4 hrs)	0.73 (0.14, 19.1%)	43.9 (14.0, 31.9%)	136 (44, 32.4%)	58 (27, 46.5%)
60 mg (4 hrs)	1.44 (0.57, 39.6%)	47.4 (47.4, 54.4%)	88 (56, 63.6%)	42 (28, 66.7%)
90 mg (4 hrs)	2.61 (0.74, 28.3%)	45.3 (25.8, 56.9%)	103 (37, 35.9%)	44 (16, 36.4%)
90 mg (24 hrs)	1.38 (1.97, 142.7%)	47.5 (10.2, 21.5%)	101 (58, 57.4%)	52 (42, 80.8%)

action is not completely understood, several factors are thought to contribute to this action. Aredia adsorbs to calcium phosphate (hydroxyapatite) crystals in bone and may directly block dissolution of this mineral component of bone. *In vitro* studies also suggest that inhibition of osteoclast activity contributes to inhibition of bone resorption. In animal studies, at doses recommended for the treatment of hypercalcemia, Aredia inhibits bone resorption apparently without inhibiting bone formation and mineralization. Of relevance to the treatment of hypercalcemia of malignancy is the finding that Aredia inhibits the accelerated bone resorption that results from osteoclast hyperactivity induced by various tumors in animal studies.

Pharmacokinetics

Cancer patients (n=24) who had minimal or no bony involvement were given an intravenous infusion of 30, 60, or 90 mg of Aredia over 4 hours and 90 mg of Aredia over 24 hours (Table 1).

Distribution

The mean ± SD body retention of pamidronate was calculated to be 54 ± 16% of the dose over 120 hours.

Metabolism

Pamidronate is not metabolized and is exclusively eliminated by renal excretion.

Excretion

After administration of 30, 60, and 90 mg of Aredia over 4 hours, and 90 mg of Aredia over 24 hours, an overall mean ± SD of 46 ± 16% of the drug was excreted unchanged in the urine within 120 hours. Cumulative urinary excretion was linearly related to dose. The mean ± SD elimination half-life is 28 ± 7 hours. Mean ± SD total and renal clearances of pamidronate were 107 ± 50 mL/min and 49 ± 28 mL/min, respectively. The rate of elimination from bone has not been determined.

Special Populations

There are no data available on the effects of age, gender, or race on the pharmacokinetics of pamidronate.

Pediatric

Pamidronate is not labeled for use in the pediatric population.

Renal Insufficiency

The pharmacokinetics of pamidronate were studied in cancer patients (n=19) with normal and varying degrees of renal impairment. Each patient received a single 90-mg dose of Aredia infused over 4 hours. The renal clearance of pamidronate in patients was found to closely correlate with creatinine clearance (see Figure 1). A trend toward a lower percentage of drug excreted unchanged in urine was observed in renally impaired patients. Adverse experiences noted were not found to be related to changes in renal clearance of pamidronate. Given the recommended dose, 90 mg infused over 4 hours, excessive accumulation of pamidronate in renally impaired patients is not anticipated if Aredia is administered on a monthly basis.

Figure 1: Pamidronate renal clearance as a function of creatinine clearance in patients with normal and impaired renal function. The lines are the mean prediction line and 95% confidence intervals.

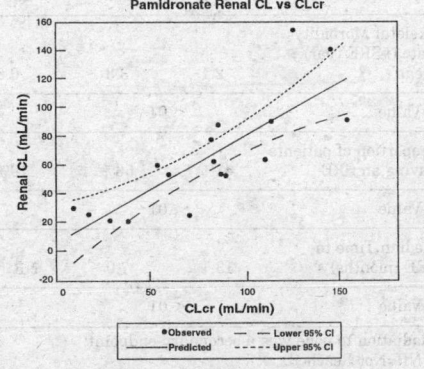

Pamidronate Renal CL vs CLcr

● Observed   —— Lower 95% CI
■ Predicted   - - - - Upper 95% CI

Hepatic Insufficiency

There are no human pharmacokinetic data for Aredia in patients who have hepatic insufficiency.

Drug-Drug Interactions

There are no human pharmacokinetic data for drug interactions with Aredia.

[See table 1 above]

After intravenous administration of radiolabeled pamidronate in rats, approximately 50%-60% of the compound was rapidly adsorbed by bone and slowly eliminated from the body by the kidneys. In rats given 10 mg/kg bolus injections of radiolabeled Aredia, approximately 30% of the compound was found in the liver shortly after administration and was then redistributed to bone or eliminated by the kidneys over 24-48 hours. Studies in rats injected with radiolabeled Aredia showed that the compound was rapidly cleared from the circulation and taken up mainly by bones, liver, spleen, teeth, and tracheal cartilage. Radioactivity was eliminated from most soft tissues within 1-4 days; was detectable in liver and spleen for 1 and 3 months, respectively; and remained high in bones, trachea, and teeth for 6 months after dosing. Bone uptake occurred preferentially in areas of high bone turnover. The terminal phase of elimination half-life in bone was estimated to be approximately 300 days.

Pharmacodynamics

Serum phosphate levels have been noted to decrease after administration of Aredia, presumably because of decreased release of phosphate from bone and increased renal excretion as parathyroid hormone levels, which are usually suppressed in hypercalcemia associated with malignancy, return toward normal. Phosphate therapy was administered in 30% of the patients in response to a decrease in serum phosphate levels. Phosphate levels usually returned toward normal within 7-10 days.

Urinary calcium/creatinine and urinary hydroxyproline/creatinine ratios decrease and usually return to within or below normal after treatment with Aredia. These changes occur within the first week after treatment, as do decreases in serum calcium levels, and are consistent with an antiresorptive pharmacologic action.

Hypercalcemia of Malignancy

Osteoclastic hyperactivity resulting in excessive bone resorption is the underlying pathophysiologic derangement in metastatic bone disease and hypercalcemia of malignancy. Excessive release of calcium into the blood as bone is resorbed results in polyuria and gastrointestinal disturbances, with progressive dehydration and decreasing glomerular filtration rate. This, in turn, results in increased renal resorption of calcium, setting up a cycle of worsening systemic hypercalcemia. Correction of excessive bone resorption and adequate fluid administration to correct volume deficits are therefore essential to the management of hypercalcemia.

Most cases of hypercalcemia associated with malignancy occur in patients who have breast cancer; squamous-cell tumors of the lung or head and neck; renal-cell carcinoma; and certain hematologic malignancies, such as multiple myeloma and some types of lymphomas. A few less-common malignancies, including vasoactive intestinal-peptide-producing tumors and cholangiocarcinoma, have a high incidence of hypercalcemia as a metabolic complication. Patients who have hypercalcemia of malignancy can generally be divided into two groups, according to the pathophysiologic mechanism involved.

In humoral hypercalcemia, osteoclasts are activated and bone resorption is stimulated by factors such as parathyroid-hormone-related protein, which are elaborated by the tumor and circulate systemically. Humoral hypercalcemia usually occurs in squamous-cell malignancies of the lung or head and neck or in genitourinary tumors such as renal-cell carcinoma or ovarian cancer. Skeletal metastases may be absent or minimal in these patients.

Continued on next page

Aredia—Cont.

Extensive invasion of bone by tumor cells can also result in hypercalcemia due to local tumor products that stimulate bone resorption by osteoclasts. Tumors commonly associated with locally mediated hypercalcemia include breast cancer and multiple myeloma.

Total serum calcium levels in patients who have hypercalcemia of malignancy may not reflect the severity of hypercalcemia, since concomitant hypoalbuminemia is commonly present. Ideally, ionized calcium levels should be used to diagnose and follow hypercalcemic conditions; however, these are not commonly or rapidly available in many clinical situations. Therefore, adjustment of the total serum calcium value for differences in albumin levels is often used in place of measurement of ionized calcium; several nomograms are in use for this type of calculation (see DOSAGE AND ADMINISTRATION).

Clinical Trials

In one double-blind clinical trial, 52 patients who had hypercalcemia of malignancy were enrolled to receive 30 mg, 60 mg, or 90 mg of Aredia as a single 24-hour intravenous infusion if their corrected serum calcium levels were ≥12.0 mg/dL after 48 hours of saline hydration.

The mean baseline-corrected serum calcium for the 30-mg, 60-mg, and 90-mg groups were 13.8 mg/dL, 13.8 mg/dL, and 13.3 mg/dL, respectively.

The majority of patients (64%) had decreases in albumin-corrected serum calcium levels by 24 hours after initiation of treatment. Mean-corrected serum calcium levels at days 2-7 after initiation of treatment with Aredia were significantly reduced from baseline in all three dosage groups. As a result, by 7 days after initiation of treatment with Aredia, 40%, 61%, and 100% of the patients receiving 30 mg, 60 mg, and 90 mg of Aredia, respectively, had normal-corrected serum calcium levels. Many patients (33%-53%) in the 60-mg and 90-mg dosage groups continued to have normal-corrected serum calcium levels, or a partial response (≥15% decrease of corrected serum calcium from baseline), at day 14.

In a second double-blind, controlled clinical trial, 65 cancer patients who had corrected serum calcium levels of ≥12.0 mg/dL after at least 24 hours of saline hydration were randomized to receive either 60 mg of Aredia as a single 24-hour intravenous infusion or 7.5 mg/kg of Didronel (etidronate disodium) as a 2-hour intravenous infusion daily for 3 days. Thirty patients were randomized to receive Aredia and 35 to receive Didronel.

The mean baseline-corrected serum calcium for the Aredia 60-mg and Didronel groups were 14.6 mg/dL and 13.8 mg/dL, respectively.

By day 7, 70% of the patients in the Aredia group and 41% of the patients in the Didronel group had normal-corrected serum calcium levels (P<0.05). When partial responders (≥15% decrease of serum calcium from baseline) were also included, the response rates were 97% for the Aredia group and 65% for the Didronel group (P<0.01). Mean-corrected serum calcium for the Aredia and Didronel groups decreased from baseline values to 10.4 and 11.2 mg/dL, respectively, on day 7. At day 14, 43% of patients in the Aredia group and 18% of patients in the Didronel group still had normal-corrected serum calcium levels, or maintenance of a partial response. For responders in the Aredia and Didronel groups, the median duration of response was similar (7 and 5 days, respectively). The time course of effect on corrected serum calcium is summarized in the following table.

Change in Corrected Serum Calcium by Time from Initiation of Treatment

Time (hr)	Mean Change from Baseline in Corrected Serum Calcium (mg/dL) Aredia	Didronel	P-Value[1]
Baseline	14.6	13.8	
24	−0.3	−0.5	
48	−1.5	−1.1	
72	−2.6	−2.0	
96	−3.5	−2.0	<0.01
168	−4.1	−2.5	<0.01

[1]Comparison between treatment groups

In a third multicenter, randomized, parallel double-blind trial, a group of 69 cancer patients with hypercalcemia was enrolled to receive 60 mg of Aredia as a 4- or 24-hour infusion, which was compared to a saline treatment group. Patients who had a corrected serum calcium level of ≥12.0 mg/dL after 24 hours of saline hydration were eligible for this trial.

The mean baseline-corrected serum calcium levels for Aredia 60-mg 4-hour infusion, Aredia 60-mg 24-hour infusion, and saline infusion were 14.2 mg/dL, 13.7 mg/dL, and 13.7 mg/dL, respectively.

By day 7 after initiation of treatment, 78%, 61%, and 22% of the patients had normal-corrected serum calcium levels for the 60-mg 4-hour infusion, 60-mg 24-hour infusion, and saline infusion, respectively. At day 14, 39% of the patients in the Aredia 60-mg 4-hour infusion group and 26% of the patients in the Aredia 60-mg 24-hour infusion group had normal-corrected serum calcium levels or maintenance of a partial response.

For responders, the median duration of complete responses was 4 days and 6.5 days for Aredia 60-mg 4-hour infusion and Aredia 60-mg 24-hour infusion, respectively.

In all three trials, patients treated with Aredia had similar response rates in the presence or absence of bone metastases. Concomitant administration of furosemide did not affect response rates.

Thirty-two patients who had recurrent or refractory hypercalcemia of malignancy were given a second course of 60 mg of Aredia over a 4- or 24-hour period. Of these, 41% showed a complete response and 16% showed a partial response to the retreatment, and these responders had about a 3-mg/dL fall in mean-corrected serum calcium levels 7 days after retreatment.

Unlike Aredia 60 mg, the drug has not been investigated in a controlled clinical trial employing a 90-mg dose infused over a 4-hour period.

Paget's Disease

Paget's disease of bone (osteitis deformans) is an idiopathic disease characterized by chronic, focal areas of bone destruction complicated by concurrent excessive bone repair, affecting one or more bones. These changes result in thickened but weakened bones that may fracture or bend under stress. Signs and symptoms may be bone pain, deformity, fractures, neurological disorders resulting from cranial and spinal nerve entrapment and from spinal cord and brain stem compression, increased cardiac output to the involved bone, increased serum alkaline phosphatase levels (reflecting increased bone formation) and/or urine hydroxyproline excretion (reflecting increased bone resorption).

Clinical Trials

In one double-blind clinical trial, 64 patients with moderate to severe Paget's disease of bone were enrolled to receive 5 mg, 15 mg, or 30 mg of Aredia as a single 4-hour infusion on 3 consecutive days, for total doses of 15 mg, 45 mg, and 90 mg of Aredia.

The mean baseline serum alkaline phosphatase levels were 1409 U/L, 983 U/L, and 1085 U/L, and the mean baseline urine hydroxyproline/creatinine ratios were 0.25, 0.19, and 0.19 for the 15-mg, 45-mg, and 90-mg groups, respectively.

The effects of Aredia on serum alkaline phosphatase (SAP) and urine hydroxyproline/creatinine ratios (UOHP/C) are summarized in the following table:

Percent of Patients With Significant % Decreases in SAP and UOHP/C

% Decrease	SAP 15 mg	SAP 45 mg	SAP 90 mg	UOHP/C 15 mg	UOHP/C 45 mg	UOHP/C 90 mg
≥50	26	33	60	15	47	72
≥30	40	65	83	35	57	85

The median maximum percent decreases from baseline in serum alkaline phosphatase and urine hydroxyproline/creatinine ratios were 25%, 41%, and 57%, and 25%, 47%, and 61% for the 15-mg, 45-mg, and 90-mg groups, respectively. The median time to response (≥50% decrease) for serum alkaline phosphatase was approximately 1 month for the 90-mg group, and the response duration ranged from 1 to 372 days.

No statistically significant differences between treatment groups, or statistically significant changes from baseline were observed for the bone pain response, mobility, and global evaluation in the 45-mg and 90-mg groups. Improvement in radiologic lesions occurred in some patients in the 90-mg group.

Twenty-five patients who had Paget's disease were retreated with 90 mg of Aredia. Of these, 44% had a ≥50% decrease in serum alkaline phosphatase from baseline after treatment, and 39% had a ≥50% decrease in urine hydroxyproline/creatinine ratio from baseline after treatment.

Osteolytic Bone Metastases of Breast Cancer and Osteolytic Lesions of Multiple Myeloma

Osteolytic bone metastases commonly occur in patients with multiple myeloma or breast cancer. These cancers demonstrate a phenomenon known as osteotropism, meaning they possess an extraordinary affinity for bone. The distribution of osteolytic bone metastases in these cancers is predominantly in the axial skeleton, particularly the spine, pelvis, and ribs, rather than the appendicular skeleton, although lesions in the proximal femur and humerus are not uncommon. This distribution is similar to the red bone marrow in which slow blood flow possibly assists attachment of metastatic cells. The surface-to-volume ratio of trabecular bone is much higher than cortical bone, and therefore disease processes tend to occur more floridly in trabecular bone than at sites of cortical tissue.

These bone changes can result in patients having evidence of osteolytic skeletal destruction leading to severe bone pain that requires either radiation therapy or narcotic analgesics (or both) for symptomatic relief. These changes also cause pathologic fractures of bone in both the axial and appendicular skeleton. Axial skeletal fractures of the vertebral bodies may lead to spinal cord compression or vertebral body collapse with significant neurologic complications. Also, patients may experience episode(s) of hypercalcemia.

Clinical Trials

In a double-blind, randomized, placebo-controlled trial, 392 patients with advanced multiple myeloma were enrolled to receive Aredia or placebo in addition to their underlying antimyeloma therapy to determine the effect of Aredia on the occurrence of skeletal-related events (SREs). SREs were defined as episodes of pathologic fractures, radiation therapy to bone, surgery to bone, and spinal cord compression. Patients received either 90 mg of Aredia or placebo as a monthly 4-hour intravenous infusion for 9 months. Of the 392 patients, 377 were evaluable for efficacy (196 Aredia, 181 placebo). The proportion of patients developing any SRE was significantly smaller in the Aredia group (24% vs 41%, P<0.001), and the mean skeletal morbidity rate (#SRE/year) was significantly smaller for Aredia patients than for placebo patients (mean: 1.1 vs 2.1, P<.02). The times to the first SRE occurrence, pathologic fracture, and radiation to bone were significantly longer in the Aredia group (P=.001, .006, and .046, respectively). Moreover, fewer Aredia patients suffered any pathologic fracture (17% vs 30%, P=.004) or needed radiation to bone (14% vs 22%, P=.049).

In addition, decreases in pain scores from baseline occurred at the last measurement for those Aredia patients with pain at baseline (P=.026) but not in the placebo group. At the last measurement, a worsening from baseline was observed in the placebo group for the Spitzer quality of life variable (P<.001) and ECOG performance status (P<.011) while there was no significant deterioration from baseline in these parameters observed in Aredia-treated patients.*

After 21 months, the proportion of patients experiencing any skeletal event remained significantly smaller in the Aredia group than the placebo group (P=.015). In addition, the mean skeletal morbidity rate (#SRE/year) was 1.3 vs 2.2 for Aredia patients vs placebo patients (P=.008), and time to first SRE was significantly longer in the Aredia group com-

	Breast Cancer Patients Receiving Chemotherapy: Any SRE A	Any SRE P	Radiation[†] A	Radiation[†] P	Breast Cancer Patients Receiving Hormonal Therapy: Any SRE A	Any SRE P	Radiation[†] A	Radiation[†] P
N	185	195	185	195	182	189	182	189
Skeletal Morbidity Rate (#SRE/year) Mean	2.1	3.3	0.6	1.1	2.4	3.5	0.6	1.1
P-Value	<.01		<.01		.05		<.01	
Proportion of patients having an SRE	43%	56%	19%	33%	47%	55%	21%	33%
P-Value	<.01		<.01		.11		.01	
Median Time to SRE (months)	13.1	7.0	NR**	NR**	10.9	7.4	NR**	NR**
P-Value	<.01		<.01		.16		<.01	

[†]Radiation to bone was a secondary endpoint.
**NR=Not Reached.

Mean Change (Δ) from Baseline‡ at Last Measurement

| | Breast Cancer Patients Receiving Chemotherapy | | | | | Breast Cancer Patients Receiving Hormonal Therapy | | | | |
| | Aredia | | Placebo | | A vs P | Aredia | | Placebo | | A vs P |
	N	Mean Δ	N	Mean Δ	P-Value*	N	Mean Δ	N	Mean Δ	P-Value*
Pain Score	175	+0.3	183	+1.1	<.05	173	−0.3	179	++0.8	<.01
Analgesic Score	175	+0.3	183	+0.9	.05	173	+0.4	179	++1.5	<.01
ECOG PS	178	+0.6	186	+0.8	.03	175	+0.5	182	++0.6	.23
Spitzer QOL	177	−1.2	185	−1.6	.11	173	−0.9	181	−1.4	.07

‡ Decreases in pain, analgesic scores and ECOG PS, and increases in Spitzer QOL indicate an improvement from baseline.
* The statistical significance of analyses of these secondary endpoints of pain, quality of life, and performance status in all three trials may be overestimated since numerous analyses were performed.

Treatment-Related Adverse Experiences Reported in Three U.S. Controlled Clinical Trials

Percent of Patients

| | Aredia | | | Didronel | Saline |
	60 mg over 4 hr n=23	60 mg over 24 hr n=73	90 mg over 24 hr n=17	7.5 mg/kg × 3 days n=35	n=23
General					
Edema	0	1	0	0	0
Fatigue	0	0	12	0	0
Fever	26	19	18	9	0
Fluid overload	0	0	0	6	0
Infusion-site reaction	0	4	18	0	0
Moniliasis	0	0	6	0	0
Rigors	0	0	0	0	4
Gastrointestinal					
Abdominal pain	0	1	0	0	0
Anorexia	4	1	12	0	0
Constipation	4	0	6	3	0
Diarrhea	0	1	0	0	0
Dyspepsia	4	0	0	0	0
Gastrointestinal hemorrhage	0	0	6	0	0
Nausea	4	0	18	6	0
Stomatitis	0	1	0	3	0
Vomiting	4	0	0	0	0
Respiratory					
Dyspnea	0	0	0	3	0
Rales	0	0	6	0	0
Rhinitis	0	0	6	0	0
Upper respiratory infection	0	3	0	0	0
CNS					
Anxiety	0	0	0	0	4
Convulsions	0	0	0	3	0
Insomnia	0	1	0	0	0
Nervousness	0	0	0	0	4
Psychosis	4	0	0	0	0
Somnolence	0	1	6	0	0
Taste perversion	0	0	0	3	0
Cardiovascular					
Atrial fibrillation	0	0	6	0	4
Atrial flutter	0	1	0	0	0
Cardiac failure	0	1	0	0	0
Hypertension	0	0	6	0	4
Syncope	0	0	6	0	0
Tachycardia	0	0	6	0	4
Endocrine					
Hypothyroidism	0	0	6	0	0
Hemic and Lymphatic					
Anemia	0	0	6	0	0
Leukopenia	4	0	0	0	0
Neutropenia	0	1	0	0	0
Thrombocytopenia	0	1	0	0	0
Musculoskeletal					
Myalgia	0	1	0	0	0
Urogenital					
Uremia	4	0	0	0	0
Laboratory Abnormalities					
Hypocalcemia	0	1	12	0	0
Hypokalemia	4	4	18	0	0
Hypomagnesemia	4	10	12	3	4
Hypophosphatemia	0	9	18	3	0
Abnormal liver function	0	0	0	3	0

pared to placebo (P=.016). Fewer Aredia patients suffered vertebral pathologic fractures (16% vs 27%, P=.005). Survival of all patients was not different between treatment groups.

Two double-blind, randomized, placebo-controlled trials compared the safety and efficacy of 90 mg of Aredia infused over 2 hours every 3 to 4 weeks for 12 months to that of placebo in preventing SREs in breast cancer patients with osteolytic bone metastases who had one or more predominantly lytic metastases of at least 1 cm in diameter: one in patients being treated with antineoplastic chemotherapy and the second in patients being treated with hormonal antineoplastic therapy at trial entry.

382 patients receiving chemotherapy were randomized, 185 to Aredia and 197 to placebo. 372 patients receiving hormonal therapy were randomized, 182 to Aredia and 190 to placebo. All but three patients were evaluable for efficacy. The efficacy results on SREs are shown in the table below: [See table at bottom of previous page]

Bone lesion response was radiographically assessed at baseline and at 3, 6, and 12 months. The complete + partial response rate was 33% in Aredia patients and 18% in placebo patients treated with chemotherapy (P=.001). No difference was seen between Aredia and placebo in hormonally-treated patients.

Pain and analgesic scores, ECOG performance status and Spitzer quality of life index were measured at baseline and periodically during the trials. The changes from baseline to the last measurement carried forward are shown in the table below:
[See first table above]

INDICATIONS AND USAGE

Hypercalcemia of Malignancy

Aredia, in conjunction with adequate hydration, is indicated for the treatment of moderate or severe hypercalcemia associated with malignancy, with or without bone metastases. Patients who have either epidermoid or non-epidermoid tumors respond to treatment with Aredia. Vigorous saline hydration, an integral part of hypercalcemia therapy, should be initiated promptly and an attempt should be made to restore the urine output to about 2 L/day throughout treatment. Mild or asymptomatic hypercalcemia may be treated with conservative measures (i.e., saline hydration, with or without loop diuretics). Patients should be hydrated adequately throughout the treatment, but overhydration, especially in those patients who have cardiac failure, must be avoided. Diuretic therapy should not be employed prior to correction of hypovolemia. The safety and efficacy of Aredia in the treatment of hypercalcemia associated with hyperparathyroidism or with other non-tumor-related conditions has not been established.

Paget's Disease

Aredia is indicated for the treatment of patients with moderate to severe Paget's disease of bone. The effectiveness of Aredia was demonstrated primarily in patients with serum alkaline phosphatase ≥3 times the upper limit of normal. Aredia therapy in patients with Paget's disease has been effective in reducing serum alkaline phosphatase and urinary hydroxyproline levels by ≥50% in at least 50% of patients, and by ≥30% in at least 80% of patients. Aredia therapy has also been effective in reducing these biochemical markers in patients with Paget's disease who failed to respond, or no longer responded to other treatments.

Osteolytic Bone Metastases of Breast Cancer and Osteolytic Lesions of Multiple Myeloma

Aredia is indicated, in conjunction with standard antineoplastic therapy, for the treatment of osteolytic bone metastases of breast cancer and osteolytic lesions of multiple myeloma. The Aredia treatment effect appeared to be smaller in the study of breast cancer patients receiving hormonal therapy than in the study of those receiving chemotherapy (see CLINICAL PHARMACOLOGY, Osteolytic Bone Metastases of Breast Cancer and Osteolytic Lesions of Multiple Myeloma, Clinical Trials section).

CONTRAINDICATIONS

Aredia is contraindicated in patients with clinically significant hypersensitivity to Aredia or other bisphosphonates.

WARNINGS

In both rats and dogs, nephropathy has been associated with intravenous (bolus and infusion) administration of Aredia.

Two 7-day intravenous infusion studies were conducted in the dog wherein Aredia was given for 1, 4, or 24 hours at doses of 1-20 mg/kg for up to 7 days. In the first study, the compound was well tolerated at 3 mg/kg (1.7 × highest recommended human dose [HRHD] for a single intravenous infusion) when administered for 4 or 24 hours, but renal findings such as elevated BUN and creatinine levels and renal tubular necrosis occurred when 3 mg/kg was infused for 1 hour and at doses of ≥10 mg/kg. In the second study, slight renal tubular necrosis was observed in 1 male at 1 mg/kg when infused for 4 hours. Additional findings included elevated BUN levels in several treated animals and renal tubular dilation and/or inflammation at ≥1 mg/kg after each infusion time.

Aredia was given to rats at doses of 2, 6, and 20 mg/kg and to dogs at doses of 2, 4, 6, and 20 mg/kg as a 1-hour infusion, once a week, for 3 months followed by a 1-month recovery period. In rats, nephrotoxicity was observed at ≥6 mg/kg and included increased BUN and creatinine levels and tubular degeneration and necrosis. These findings were still present at 20 mg/kg at the end of the recovery period. In dogs, moribundity/death and renal toxicity occurred at 20 mg/kg as did kidney findings of elevated BUN and creatinine levels at ≥6 mg/kg and renal tubular degeneration at ≥4 mg/kg. The kidney changes were partially reversible at 6 mg/kg. In both studies, the dose level that produced no adverse renal effects was considered to be 2 mg/kg (1.1 × HRHD for a single intravenous infusion).

Continued on next page

Aredia—Cont.

Patients who receive an intravenous infusion of Aredia should have periodic evaluations of standard laboratory and clinical parameters of renal function.

Studies conducted in young rats have reported the disruption of dental dentine formation following single- and multi-dose administration of bisphosphonates. The clinical significance of these findings is unknown.

PRECAUTIONS

General

Standard hypercalcemia-related metabolic parameters, such as serum levels of calcium, phosphate, magnesium, and potassium, should be carefully monitored following initiation of therapy with Aredia. Cases of asymptomatic hypophosphatemia (12%), hypokalemia (7%), hypomagnesemia (11%), and hypocalcemia (5%-12%), were reported in Aredia-treated patients. Rare cases of symptomatic hypocalcemia (including tetany) have been reported in association with Aredia therapy. If hypocalcemia occurs, short-term calcium therapy may be necessary. In Paget's disease of bone, 17% of patients treated with 90 mg of Aredia showed serum calcium levels below 8 mg/dL.

Aredia has not been tested in patients who have class Dc renal impairment (creatinine >5.0 mg/dL), and in few multiple myeloma patients with serum creatinine ≥3.0 mg/dL. (See also CLINICAL PHARMACOLOGY, Pharmacokinetics.) Clinical judgment should determine whether the potential benefit outweighs the potential risk in such patients.

Laboratory Tests

Serum calcium, electrolytes, phosphate, magnesium and creatinine, and CBC, differential, and hematocrit/hemoglobin must be closely monitored in patients treated with Aredia. Patients who have preexisting anemia, leukopenia, or thrombocytopenia should be monitored carefully in the first 2 weeks following treatment.

Drug Interactions

Concomitant administration of a loop diuretic had no effect on the calcium-lowering action of Aredia.

Carcinogenesis, Mutagenesis, Impairment of Fertility

In a 104-week carcinogenicity study (daily oral administration) in rats, there was a positive dose response relationship for benign adrenal pheochromocytoma in males (P <0.00001). Although this condition was also observed in females, the incidence was not statistically significant. When the dose calculations were adjusted to account for the limited oral bioavailability of Aredia in rats, the lowest daily dose associated with adrenal pheochromocytoma was similar to the intended clinical dose. Adrenal pheochromocytoma was also observed in low numbers in the control animals and is considered a relatively common spontaneous neoplasm in the rat. Aredia (daily oral administration) was not carcinogenic in an 80-week study in mice.

Aredia was nonmutagenic in six mutagenicity assays: Ames test, *Salmonella* and *Escherichia*/liver-microsome test, nucleus-anomaly test, sister-chromatid-exchange study, point-mutation test, and micronucleus test in the rat.

In rats, decreased fertility occurred in first-generation offspring of parents who had received 150 mg/kg of Aredia orally; however, this occurred only when animals were mated with members of the same dose group. Aredia has not been administered intravenously in such a study.

Pregnancy Category C

There are no adequate and well-controlled studies in pregnant women.

Bolus intravenous studies conducted in rats and rabbits determined that Aredia produces maternal toxicity and embryo/fetal effects when given during organogenesis at doses of 0.6 to 8.3 times the highest recommended human dose for a single intravenous infusion. As it has been shown that Aredia can cross the placenta in rats and has produced marked maternal and nonteratogenic embryo/fetal effects in rats and rabbits, it should not be given to women during pregnancy.

Nursing Mothers

It is not known whether Aredia is excreted in human milk. Because many drugs are excreted in human milk, caution should be exercised when Aredia is administered to a nursing woman.

Pediatric Use

Safety and effectiveness of Aredia in pediatric patients have not been established.

ADVERSE REACTIONS

Clinical Studies

Hypercalcemia of Malignancy

Transient mild elevation of temperature by at least 1°C was noted 24 to 48 hours after administration of Aredia in 34% of patients in clinical trials. In the saline trial, 18% of patients had a temperature elevation of at least 1°C 24 to 48 hours after treatment.

Drug-related local soft-tissue symptoms (redness, swelling or induration and pain on palpation) at the site of catheter insertion were most common (18%) in patients treated with 90 mg of Aredia. When all on-therapy events are considered, that rate rises to 41%. Symptomatic treatment resulted in rapid resolution in all patients.

Rare cases of uveitis, iritis, scleritis, and episcleritis have been reported, including one case of scleritis, and one case of uveitis upon separate rechallenges.

Four of 128 patients (3%) who received Aredia during the three U.S. controlled hypercalcemia clinical studies were reported to have had seizures, 2 of whom had preexisting seizure disorders. None of the seizures were considered to be drug-related by the investigators. However, a possible relationship between the drug and the occurrence of seizures cannot be ruled out. It should be noted that in the saline arm 1 patient (4%) had a seizure.

At least 15% of patients treated with Aredia for hypercalcemia of malignancy also experienced the following adverse events during a clinical trial:

General: Fluid overload, generalized pain

Cardiovascular: Hypertension

Gastrointestinal: Abdominal pain, anorexia, constipation, nausea, vomiting

Genitourinary: Urinary tract infection

Musculoskeletal: Bone pain

Laboratory abnormality: Anemia, hypokalemia, hypomagnesemia, hypophosphatemia

Many of these adverse experiences may have been related to the underlying disease state.

The following table lists the adverse experiences considered to be treatment-related during comparative, controlled U.S. trials.

[See second table on previous page]

Paget's Disease

Transient mild elevation of temperature >1°C above-pretreatment baseline was noted within 48 hours after completion of treatment in 21% of the patients treated with 90 mg of Aredia in clinical trials.

Drug-related musculoskeletal pain and nervous system symptoms (dizziness, headache, paresthesia, increased sweating) were more common in patients with Paget's disease treated with 90 mg of Aredia than in patients with hypercalcemia of malignancy treated with the same dose.

Adverse experiences considered to be related to trial drug, which occurred in at least 5% of patients with Paget's disease treated with 90 mg of Aredia in two U.S. clinical trials, were fever, nausea, back pain, and bone pain.

At least 10% of all Aredia-treated patients with Paget's disease also experienced the following adverse experiences during clinical trials:

Cardiovascular: Hypertension

Musculoskeletal: Arthrosis, bone pain

Nervous system: Headache

Most of these adverse experiences may have been related to the underlying disease state.

Osteolytic Bone Metastases of Breast Cancer and Osteolytic Lesions of Multiple Myeloma

The most commonly reported (>15%) adverse experiences occurred with similar frequencies in the Aredia and placebo treatment groups, and most of these adverse experiences may have been related to the underlying disease state or cancer therapy.

[See table below]

Toxicities commonly associated with chemotherapy, including cytopenia, infection, nausea and vomiting, and cachexia, were not more frequent or severe in Aredia patients than in placebo patients, although viral infection, herpes zoster, and anorexia all occurred more frequently in the Aredia arm of the study. Mineral and electrolyte disturbances, including hypocalcemia, were reported rarely and in similar percentages of Aredia-treated patients compared with those in the placebo group. The reported frequencies of hypocalcemia, hypokalemia, hypophosphatemia, and hypomagnesemia for Aredia-treated patients were 3.0%, 8.7%, 1.6%, and 3.8%, respectively, and for placebo-treated patients were 1.2%, 10.6%, 1.7%, and 4.2%, respectively. In previous hypercalcemia of malignancy trials, patients treated with Aredia (60 or 90 mg over 24 hours) developed electrolyte abnormalities more frequently (see ADVERSE REACTIONS, Hypercalcemia of Malignancy).

Arthralgias and myalgias were reported slightly more frequently in the Aredia group than in the placebo group (11.5% and 22.6% vs 8.0% and 16.9%, respectively).

In multiple myeloma patients, there were five Aredia-related serious and unexpected adverse experiences. Four of these were reported during the 12-month extension of the multiple myeloma trial. Three of the reports were of worsening renal function developing in patients with progressive multiple myeloma or multiple myeloma-associated amyloidosis. The fourth report was the adult respiratory distress syndrome developing in a patient recovering from pneumonia and acute gangrenous cholecystitis. One Aredia-treated patient experienced an allergic reaction characterized by swollen and itchy eyes, runny nose, and scratchy throat within 24 hours after the sixth infusion.

In the breast cancer trials, there were four Aredia-related adverse experiences, all moderate in severity, that caused a patient to discontinue participation in the trial. One was due to interstitial pneumonitis, another to malaise and dyspnea. One Aredia patient discontinued the trial due to a symptomatic hypocalcemia. Another Aredia patient discontinued therapy due to severe bone pain after each infusion, which the investigator felt was trial-drug-related.

Post-Marketing Experience

Rare instances of allergic manifestations have been reported, including hypotension, dyspnea, or angioedema, and very rarely, anaphylactic shock. Aredia is contraindicated in patients with clinically significant hyper sensitivity to Aredia or other bisphosphonates (See CONTRAINDICATIONS).

Commonly Reported Adverse Experiences in Three U.S. Controlled Clinical Trials

	Aredia 90 mg over 2 hr N=367 %	Aredia 90 mg over 4 hr N=205 %	All Aredia 90 mg N=572 %	Placebo N=573 %
General				
Asthenia	16.6	16.1	16.4	15.4
Fatigue	29.7	31.7	30.4	35.5
Fever	33.5	39.0	35.5	30.5
Metastases	21.3	1.0	14.0	13.6
Digestive System				
Anorexia	22.9	17.1	20.8	18.0
Constipation	27.2	28.3	27.6	30.9
Diarrhea	22.9	26.8	24.3	26.2
Dyspepsia	11.4	17.6	13.6	12.4
Nausea	55.6	35.6	48.4	46.4
Pain, Abdominal	16.1	19.5	17.3	14.0
Vomiting	39.0	16.6	30.9	28.1
Hemic and Lymphatic				
Anemia	28.1	47.8	35.1	32.6
Granulocytopenia	14.7	20.5	16.8	17.3
Thrombocytopenia	7.9	16.6	11.0	13.1
Musculoskeletal System				
Myalgia	21.0	25.4	22.6	16.9
Skeletal Pain	58.6	61.0	59.4	69.1
CNS				
Headache	23.7	24.4	24.0	19.7
Insomnia	18.8	17.1	18.2	17.3
Respiratory System				
Coughing	18.3	26.3	21.2	18.8
Dyspnea	24.0	22.0	23.3	18.7
Upper Respiratory Infection	12.8	32.2	19.8	20.9
Urogenital System				
Urinary Tract Infection	13.9	15.6	14.5	10.8

OVERDOSAGE

There have been several cases of drug maladministration of intravenous Aredia in hypercalcemia patients with total doses of 225 mg to 300 mg given over $2^1/_2$ to 4 days. All of these patients survived, but they experienced hypocalcemia that required intravenous and/or oral administration of calcium.

In addition, one obese woman (95 kg) who was treated with 285 mg of Aredia/day for 3 days experienced high fever (39.5°C), hypotension (from 170/90 mmHg to 90/60 mmHg), and transient taste perversion, noted about 6 hours after the first infusion. The fever and hypotension were rapidly corrected with steroids.

If overdosage occurs, symptomatic hypocalcemia could also result; such patients should be treated with short-term intravenous calcium.

DOSAGE AND ADMINISTRATION

Hypercalcemia of Malignancy

Consideration should be given to the severity of as well as the symptoms of hypercalcemia. Vigorous saline hydration alone may be sufficient for treating mild, asymptomatic hypercalcemia. Overhydration should be avoided in patients who have potential for cardiac failure. In hypercalcemia associated with hematologic malignancies, the use of glucocorticoid therapy may be helpful.

Moderate Hypercalcemia

The recommended dose of Aredia in moderate hypercalcemia (corrected serum calcium* of approximately 12-13.5 mg/dL) is 60 to 90 mg. The 60-mg dose is given as an initial, SINGLE-DOSE, intravenous infusion over at least 4 hours. The 90-mg dose must be given by an initial, SINGLE-DOSE, intravenous infusion over 24 hours.

Severe Hypercalcemia

The recommended dose of Aredia in severe hypercalcemia (corrected serum calcium* >13.5 mg/dL) is 90 mg. The 90-mg dose must be given by an initial, SINGLE-DOSE, intravenous infusion over 24 hours.

*Albumin-corrected serum calcium (CCa, mg/dL) = serum calcium, mg/dL + 0.8 (4.0-serum albumin, g/dL).

Retreatment

A limited number of patients have received more than one treatment with Aredia for hypercalcemia. Retreatment with Aredia, in patients who show complete or partial response initially, may be carried out if serum calcium does not return to normal or remain normal after initial treatment. **It is recommended that a minimum of 7 days elapse before retreatment, to allow for full response to the initial dose.** The dose and manner of retreatment is identical to that of the initial therapy.

Paget's Disease

The recommended dose of Aredia in patients with moderate to severe Paget's disease of bone is 30 mg daily, administered as a 4-hour infusion on 3 consecutive days for a total dose of 90 mg.

Retreatment

A limited number of patients with Paget's disease have received more than one treatment of Aredia in clinical trials. When clinically indicated, patients should be retreated at the dose of initial therapy.

Osteolytic Bone Lesions of Multiple Myeloma

The recommended dose of Aredia in patients with osteolytic bone lesions of multiple myeloma is 90 mg administered as a 4-hour infusion given on a monthly basis.

Patients with marked Bence-Jones proteinuria and dehydration should receive adequate hydration prior to Aredia infusion.

Limited information is available on the use of Aredia in multiple myeloma patients with a serum creatinine ≥3.0 mg/dL.

The optimal duration of therapy is not yet known (see CLINICAL TRIALS section).

Osteolytic Bone Metastases of Breast Cancer

The recommended dose of Aredia in patients with osteolytic bone metastases is 90 mg administered over a 2-hour infusion given every 3-4 weeks.

Aredia has been frequently used with doxorubicin, fluorouracil, cyclophosphamide, methotrexate, mitoxantrone, vinblastine, dexamethasone, prednisone, melphalan, vincristine, megesterol, and tamoxifen. It has been given less frequently with etoposide, cisplatin, cytabrine, paclitaxel, and aminoglutethimide.

Preparation of Solution

Reconstitution

Aredia is reconstituted by adding 10 mL of Sterile Water for Injection, USP, to each vial, resulting in a solution of 30 mg/10 mL, 60 mg/10 mL, or 90 mg/10 mL. The pH of the reconstituted solution is 6.0-7.4. The drug should be completely dissolved before the solution is withdrawn.

Hypercalcemia of Malignancy

The daily dose must be administered as an intravenous infusion over at least 4 hours for the 60-mg dose, and over 24 hours for the 90-mg dose. The recommended dose should be diluted in 1000 mL of sterile 0.45% or 0.9% Sodium Chloride, USP, or 5% Dextrose Injection, USP. This infusion solution is stable for up to 24 hours at room temperature.

Paget's Disease

The recommended daily dose of 30 mg should be diluted in 500 mL of sterile 0.45% or 0.9% Sodium Chloride, USP, or 5% Dextrose Injection, USP, and administered over a 4-hour period for 3 consecutive days.

Osteolytic Bone Metastases of Breast Cancer

The recommended dose of 90 mg should be diluted in 250 mL of sterile 0.45% or 0.9% Sodium Chloride, USP, or 5% Dextrose Injection, USP, and administered over a 2-hour period every 3-4 weeks.

Osteolytic Bone Lesions of Multiple Myeloma

The recommended dose of 90 mg should be diluted in 500 mL of sterile 0.45% or 0.9% Sodium Chloride, USP, or 5% Dextrose Injection, USP, and administered over a 4-hour period on a monthly basis.

Aredia must not be mixed with calcium-containing infusion solutions, such as Ringer's solution, and should be given in a single intravenous solution and line separate from all other drugs.

Note: **Parenteral drug products should be inspected visually for particulate matter and discoloration prior to administration, whenever solution and container permit.**

Aredia reconstituted with Sterile Water for Injection may be stored under refrigeration at 36°-46°F (2°-8°C) for up to 24 hours.

HOW SUPPLIED

Vials–30 mg–each contains 30 mg of sterile, lyophilized pamidronate disodium and 470 mg of mannitol, USP.
Carton of 4 vials .... NDC 0083-2601-04

Vials–60 mg–each contains 60 mg of sterile, lyophilized pamidronate disodium and 400 mg of mannitol, USP.
Carton of 1 vial .... NDC 0083-2606-01

Vials–90 mg–each contains 90 mg of sterile, lyophilized pamidronate disodium and 375 mg of mannitol, USP.
Carton of 1 vial .... NDC 0083-2609-01

Do not store above 86°F (30°C).

C98-23 (Rev. 5/98)

Shown in Product Identification Guide, page 324

BRETHINE® ℞

[*breth-een '*]

terbutaline sulfate tablets USP

Tablets of 5 mg

Tablets of 2.5 mg

The following prescribing information is based on official labeling in effect on August 1, 1998.

DESCRIPTION

Brethine, terbutaline sulfate USP, is a bronchodilator available as tablets of 2.5 mg (2.05 mg of the free base) and 5 mg (4.1 mg of the free base) for oral administration. Terbutaline sulfate is ±-α-[(*tert*-Butylamino)methyl]-3,5-dihydroxybenzyl alcohol sulfate (2:1) (salt).

Terbutaline sulfate USP is a white to gray-white crystalline powder. It is odorless or has a faint odor of acetic acid. It is soluble in water and in 0.1N hydrochloric acid, slightly soluble in methanol, and insoluble in chloroform. Its molecular weight is 548.65.

Inactive Ingredients. Cellulose compounds, lactose, magnesium stearate, povidone, and starch.

ACTIONS

Brethine is a β-adrenergic receptor agonist which has been shown by *in vitro* and *in vivo* pharmacological studies in animals to exert a preferential effect on β_2-adrenergic receptors such as those located in bronchial smooth muscle. Controlled clinical studies in patients who were administered the drug orally have revealed proportionally greater changes in pulmonary function parameters than in heart rate or blood pressure. While this *suggests* a relative preference for the β_2 receptor in man, the usual cardiovascular effects commonly associated with sympathomimetic agents were also observed with Brethine.

Brethine has been shown in controlled clinical studies to relieve bronchospasm in chronic obstructive pulmonary disease.

This action is manifested by a clinically significant increase in pulmonary function as demonstrated by an increase of 15% or more in FEV_1 and in $FEF_{25-75\%}$. Following administration of Brethine tablets, a measurable change in flow rate is usually observed in 30 minutes, and a clinically significant improvement in pulmonary function occurs at 60–120 minutes. The maximum effect usually occurs within 120-180 minutes. Brethine also produces a clinically significant decrease in airway and pulmonary resistance which persists for at least four hours or longer. Significant bronchodilator action, as measured by various pulmonary function determinations (airway resistance, $FEF_{25-75\%}$, or PEFR), has been demonstrated in some studies for periods up to eight hours.

Clinical studies were conducted in which the effectiveness of Brethine was evaluated in comparison with ephedrine over periods up to three months. Both drugs continued to produce significant improvement in pulmonary function throughout this period of treatment.

INDICATIONS

Brethine is indicated as a bronchodilator for bronchial asthma and for reversible bronchospasm which may occur in association with bronchitis and emphysema.

CONTRAINDICATIONS

Brethine is contraindicated when there is known hypersensitivity to sympathomimetic amines.

WARNINGS

There have been rare reports of seizures in patients receiving terbutaline; seizures did not recur in these patients after the drug was discontinued.

Controlled clinical studies and other clinical experience have shown that Brethine, like other β-adrenergic agonists, can produce a significant cardiovascular effect in some patients, as measured by pulse rate, blood pressure, symptoms, and/or ECG changes.

Usage in Pregnancy: Animal reproductive studies have been negative with respect to adverse effects on fetal development. The safe use of Brethine has not, however, been established in human pregnancy. As with any medication, the use of the drug in pregnancy, lactation, or women of childbearing potential requires that the expected therapeutic benefit of the drug be weighed against its possible hazards to the mother or child.

Usage in Pediatrics: Brethine tablets are not presently recommended for children below the age of 12 years due to insufficient clinical data in this pediatric group.

PRECAUTIONS

Brethine should be used with caution in patients with diabetes, hypertension, hyperthyroidism, and a history of seizures. Large doses of intravenous terbutaline sulfate have been reported to aggravate preexisting diabetes and ketoacidosis.

As with other sympathomimetic bronchodilator agents, Brethine should be administered cautiously to cardiac patients, especially those with associated arrhythmias. The concomitant use of Brethine with other sympathomimetic agents is not recommended, since their combined effect on the cardiovascular system may be deleterious to the patient. However, this does not preclude the use of an aerosol bronchodilator of the adrenergic stimulant type for the relief of an acute bronchospasm in patients receiving chronic oral Brethine therapy.

Terbutaline sulfate should not be used for tocolysis. Serious adverse reactions may occur after administration of terbutaline sulfate to women in labor. In the mother, these include increased heart rate, transient hyperglycemia, hypokalemia, cardiac arrhythmias, pulmonary edema, and myocardial ischemia. Increased fetal heart rate and neonatal hypoglycemia may occur as a result of maternal administration.

Immediate hypersensitivity reactions and exacerbation of bronchospasm have been reported after terbutaline administration.

PEDIATRIC USE

Safety and effectiveness in pediatric patients below the age of 12 years have not been established.

ADVERSE REACTIONS

Commonly observed side effects include nervousness and tremor. Other reported reactions include headache, increased heart rate, palpitations, drowsiness, nausea, vomiting, sweating, and muscle cramps. These reactions are generally transient in nature and usually do not require treatment. The frequency of these side effects appears to diminish with continued therapy. In general, all the side effects observed are characteristic of those commonly seen with sympathomimetic amines.

There have been rare reports of elevations in liver enzymes and of hypersensitivity vasculitis.

DOSAGE AND ADMINISTRATION

The usual oral dose of Brethine for adults is 5 mg administered at approximately six-hour intervals, three times daily, during the hours the patient is usually awake. If side effects are particularly disturbing, the dose may be reduced to 2.5 mg three times daily, and still provide a clinically significant improvement in pulmonary function. A dose of 2.5 mg, three times daily, also is recommended for children in the 12- to 15-year group. Brethine is not recommended at present for use in children below the age of 12 years. In adults, a total dose of 15 mg should not be exceeded in a 24-hour period. In children, a total dose of 7.5 mg should not be exceeded in a 24-hour period.

OVERDOSAGE

Overdosage experience is limited. Excessive beta-adrenergic receptor stimulation may augment the signs or symptoms listed under **ADVERSE REACTIONS** and they may be accompanied by other adrenergic effects. Treat the alert patient who has taken excessive oral medication by emptying the stomach by means of induced emesis, followed by gastric lavage. In the unconscious patient, secure the airway with a cuffed endotracheal tube before beginning lavage (do not induce emesis). Instillation of activated charcoal slurry may help reduce absorption of terbutaline sulfate. Maintain adequate respiratory exchange. Provide cardiac and respiratory support as needed. Continue observation until symptom-free.

Continued on next page

Brethine Tablets—Cont.

HOW SUPPLIED

Tablets 2.5 mg—oval, white, scored (imprinted Geigy 72)
Bottles of 100 .... NDC 0028-0072-01
Bottles of 1000 .... NDC 0028-0072-10
Gy-Pak®—One Unit
12 bottles—100 tablets each .... NDC 0028-0072-65
Unit Dose (blister pack)
Box of 100 (strips of 10) .... NDC 0028-0072-61
Tablets 5 mg—round, white, scored (imprinted Geigy 105)
Bottles of 100 .... NDC 0028-0105-01
Bottles of 1000 .... NDC 0028-0105-10
Gy-Pak®—One Unit
12 bottles—100 tablets each .... NDC 0028-0105-65
Unit Dose (blister pack)
Box of 100 (strips of 10) .... NDC 0028-0105-61
Store at controlled room temperature 59°-86°F (15°-30°C).
Dispense in tight, light-resistant container (USP).

C95-48 (Rev. 11/95)

Shown in Product Identification Guide, page 324

BRETHINE®
[*breth-een '*]
terbutaline sulfate Injection USP
Ampuls
A sterile aqueous solution for subcutaneous injection

℞

The following prescribing information is based on official labeling in effect on August 1, 1998.

DESCRIPTION

Brethine, terbutaline sulfate injection USP, is a β-adrenergic agonist bronchodilator available as a sterile, non-pyrogenic, aqueous solution in ampuls, for subcutaneous administration. Each milliliter of solution contains 1 mg of terbutaline sulfate USP (0.82 mg of the free base); sodium chloride ACS, for isotonicity; and hydrochloric acid ACS, for adjustment to a target pH of 4. Terbutaline sulfate is $(\pm)$-α-[(*tert*-butylamino)methyl]-3,5-dihydroxybenzyl alcohol sulfate (2:1) (salt). The empirical formula is $(C_{12}H_{19}NO_3)_2 \cdot H_2SO_4$ and the structural formula is:

$$\left[\text{HO} \underset{\text{HO}}{\bigcirc} \text{-CHCH}_2\text{NHC(CH}_3)_3 \atop \text{OH} \right]_2 \cdot H_2SO_4$$

Terbutaline sulfate USP is a white to gray-white crystalline powder. It is odorless or has a faint odor of acetic acid. It is soluble in water and in 0.1N hydrochloric acid, slightly soluble in methanol, and insoluble in chloroform. Its molecular weight is 548.65.

CLINICAL PHARMACOLOGY

Brethine is a β-adrenergic receptor agonist. In vitro and in vivo studies in animals have shown that Brethine exerts a preferential effect on β_2-adrenergic receptors. While it is recognized that β_2-adrenergic receptors are the predominant receptors in bronchial smooth muscle, recent data indicate that there is a population of β_2-receptors in the human heart, existing in a concentration between 10%–50%. The precise function of these, however, is not yet established (see WARNINGS). Controlled clinical studies in patients given Brethine subcutaneously have not revealed a preferential β_2-adrenergic effect.

The pharmacologic effects of β-adrenergic agonists, including Brethine, are at least in part attributable to stimulation through β-adrenergic receptors of intracellular adenylcyclase, the enzyme which catalyzes the conversion of adenosine triphosphate (ATP) to cyclic 3', 5'-adenosine monophosphate (cAMP). Increased cAMP levels are associated with relaxation of bronchial smooth muscle and inhibition of release of mediators of immediate hypersensitivity from cells, especially from mast cells.

Controlled clinical studies have shown that Brethine relieves bronchospasm in acute and chronic obstructive pulmonary disease by significantly increasing pulmonary flow rates (e.g., an increase of 15% or more in FEV_1). After subcutaneous administration of 0.25 mg of Brethine, a measurable change in flow rate usually occurs within 5 minutes, and a clinically significant increase in FEV_1 occurs within 15 minutes. The maximum effect usually occurs within 30–60 minutes, and clinically significant bronchodilator activity may continue for 1.5 to 4 hours. The duration of clinically significant improvement is comparable to that observed with equimilligram doses of epinephrine.

Recent studies in laboratory animals (minipigs, rodents, and dogs) recorded the occurrence of cardiac arrhythmias and sudden death (with histological evidence of necrosis) when β-agonists and methylxanthines were administered concurrently. The significance of these findings when applied to humans is currently unknown.

Pharmacokinetics

After subcutaneous administration of 0.25 mg of terbutaline sulfate to two male subjects, peak terbutaline serum concentrations of 5.2 and 5.3 ng/mL were observed at about 20 minutes after dosing. Further studies are needed to confirm these results.

Elimination half-life of the drug in 10 of 14 patients was approximately 2.9 hr after subcutaneous administration, but longer elimination half-lives (between 6-14 hr) were found in the other 4 patients. About 90% of the drug was excreted in the urine at 96 hr after subcutaneous administration, with about 60% of this being unchanged drug. It appears that the sulfate conjugate is a major metabolite of terbutaline and urinary excretion is the primary route of elimination.

INDICATIONS AND USAGE

Brethine is indicated for the prevention and reversal of bronchospasm in patients with bronchial asthma and reversible bronchospasm associated with bronchitis and emphysema.

CONTRAINDICATIONS

Brethine is contraindicated in patients known to be hypersensitive to sympathomimetic amines or any component of this drug product.

WARNINGS

There have been rare reports of seizures in patients receiving terbutaline; seizures did not recur in these patients after the drug was discontinued.

Controlled clinical studies and other clinical experience have shown that Brethine, like other β-adrenergic agonists, can produce a significant cardiovascular effect in some patients, as measured by pulse rate, blood pressure, symptoms, and/or ECG changes.

PRECAUTIONS

General

Since Brethine is a sympathomimetic amine, it should be used with caution in patients with cardiovascular disorders, including ischemic heart disease, hypertension, and cardiac arrhythmias; in patients with hyperthyroidism or diabetes mellitus; and in patients who are unusually responsive to sympathomimetic amines or who have convulsive disorders. Significant changes in systolic and diastolic blood pressure can be expected to occur in some patients after use of any β-adrenergic bronchodilator.

Immediate hypersensitivity reactions and exacerbations of bronchospasm have been reported after terbutaline administration.

Terbutaline sulfate should not be used for tocolysis.

Drug Interactions

The concomitant use of Brethine with other sympathomimetic agents is not recommended, since the combined effect on the cardiovascular system may be deleterious to the patient.

β-adrenergic agonists should be administered with caution to patients being treated with monoamine oxidase inhibitors or tricyclic antidepressants, since the action of β-adrenergic agonists on the vascular system may be potentiated.

Carcinogenesis, Mutagenesis, Impairment of Fertility

In a 2-year oral study in the rat, terbutaline sulfate caused a significant dose-related increase in the incidence of benign leiomyomas of the mesovarium at doses corresponding to 5000, 50,000, 100,000, and 200,000 times the maximum recommended human subcutaneous dose (0.01 mg/kg). The rel-

evance of these findings to humans is not known. An 18-month oral study in mice revealed no evidence of tumorigenicity at doses up to 200 mg/kg (20,000 times the maximum recommended human subcutaneous dose). Mutagenicity studies have not been performed. A reproduction study in rats at oral doses up to 5000 times the maximum subcutaneous dose (0.01 mg/kg) revealed no evidence of impaired fertility.

Pregnancy Category B

Reproduction studies performed in mice, rats, or rabbits at doses up to 1500 times the subcutaneous maximum daily human dose of 0.01 mg/kg have revealed no evidence of impaired fertility or harm to the fetus due to Brethine. Increased levels of maternal and fetal blood glucose have been observed after intravenous administration of terbutaline to near-term pregnant baboons at doses up to 4 times the maximum recommended human subcutaneous dose.

There are, however, no adequate and well-controlled studies in pregnant women. Because animal reproduction studies are not always predictive of human response, this drug should be used during pregnancy only if clearly needed. Administration of the drug under these conditions requires careful benefit-to-risk determination.

Labor and Delivery

Terbutaline sulfate should not be used for tocolysis. Serious adverse reactions may occur after administration of terbutaline sulfate to women in labor. In the mother, these include increased heart rate, transient hyperglycemia, hypokalemia, cardiac arrhythmias, pulmonary edema, and myocardial ischemia. Increased fetal heart rate and neonatal hypoglycemia may occur as a result of maternal administration.

Nursing Mothers

It is not known whether this drug is excreted in human milk. Therefore, Brethine should be used during nursing only if the potential benefit justifies the possible risk to the newborn.

Pediatric Use

Brethine is not recommended for pediatric patients under the age of 12 years because of insufficient clinical data to establish safety and effectiveness.

ADVERSE REACTIONS

Adverse reactions observed with Brethine are similar to those commonly seen with other sympathomimetic agents. All these reactions are transient in nature and usually do not require treatment.

The following table compares adverse reactions seen in patients treated with terbutaline sulfate injection (0.25 mg and 0.5 mg) with those seen in patients treated with epinephrine injection (0.25 mg and 0.5 mg), during eight double-blind crossover studies involving a total of 214 patients.
[See table below]

There have been rare reports of elevations in liver enzymes and of hypersensitivity vasculitis with terbutaline administration.

OVERDOSAGE

Acute Toxicity

Intravenous LD_{50}'s (mg/kg): rats, 61.5; mice, 48.4. Oral LD_{50} in rats is > 5000 mg/kg.

Incidence (%) of Adverse Reactions

Reaction	Terbutaline (%) 0.25 mg N=77	Terbutaline (%) 0.5 mg N=205	Epinephrine (%) 0.25 mg N=153	Epinephrine (%) 0.5 mg N=61
Central Nervous System				
Tremors	7.8	38.0	16.3	18.0
Nervousness	16.9	30.7	8.5	31.1
Dizziness	1.3	10.2	7.8	3.3
Headache	7.8	8.8	3.3	9.8
Drowsiness	11.7	9.8	14.4	8.2
Cardiovascular				
Palpitations	7.8	22.9	7.8	29.5
Tachycardia	1.3	1.5	2.6	0.0
Respiratory				
Dyspnea	0.0	2.0	2.0	0.0
Chest discomfort	1.3	1.5	2.6	0.0
Gastrointestinal				
Nausea/vomiting	1.3	3.9	1.3	11.5
Systemic				
Weakness	1.3	0.5	2.6	1.6
Flushed feeling	0.0	2.4	1.3	0.0
Sweating	0.0	2.4	0.0	0.0
Pain at injection site	2.6	0.5	2.6	1.6

Note: Some patients received more than one dosage strength of terbutaline sulfate and epinephrine. In addition, there were reports of anxiety, muscle cramps, and dry mouth (<0.5%).

Signs and Symptoms
Excessive β-adrenergic receptor stimulation may augment the signs and symptoms listed under ADVERSE REACTIONS.
Treatment
There is no specific antidote. Treatment consists of discontinuation of Brethine along with the institution of appropriate symptomatic therapy.

DOSAGE AND ADMINISTRATION

Ampuls should be used only for subcutaneous administration and not intravenous infusion. Sterility and accurate dosing cannot be assured if the ampuls are not used in accordance with DOSAGE AND ADMINISTRATION.
The usual subcutaneous dose of Brethine is 0.25 mg injected into the lateral deltoid area. If significant clinical improvement does not occur within 15-30 minutes, a second dose of 0.25 mg may be administered. If the patient then fails to respond within another 15-30 minutes, other therapeutic measures should be considered. The total dose within 4 hours should not exceed 0.5 mg.
Note: Parenteral drug products should be inspected visually for particulate matter and discoloration prior to administration, whenever solution and container permit.

HOW SUPPLIED

Ampuls 1 mg/mL—The drug is supplied at a volume of 1 mL contained in a 2 mL clear glass ampul. Each ampul contains 1 mg of Brethine per 1 mL of solution; 0.25 ml of solution will provide the usual clinical dose of 0.25 mg. Ampuls are expiration-dated.
Box of 10 ampuls .... NDC 0028-7507-23
Box of 100 ampuls .... NDC 0028-7507-01
Keep at controlled room temperature 59°-86°F (15°-30°C).
Protect from light by storing ampuls in original carton until dispensed. Do not use if solution is discolored.
C95-51 (Rev. 12/95)
Shown in Product Identification Guide, page 324

CATAFLAM® ℞
diclofenac potassium
Immediate-Release Tablets

VOLTAREN® ℞
diclofenac sodium
Delayed-Release (enteric-coated) Tablets

VOLTAREN®-XR ℞
diclofenac sodium
Extended-Release Tablets

The following prescribing information is based on official labeling in effect on August 1, 1998.
Prescribing Information

DESCRIPTION

Diclofenac, as the sodium or potassium salt, is a benzeneacetic acid derivative, designated chemically as 2-[(2,6-dichlorophenyl)amino] benzeneacetic acid, monosodium or monopotassium salt. The structural formula is shown in Figure 1.

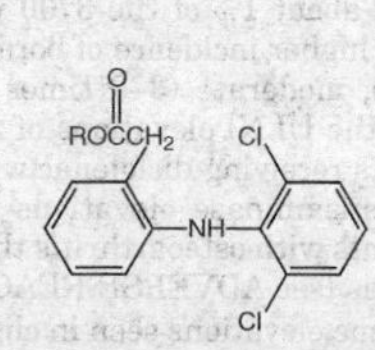

R = K: Cataflam®, diclofenac potassium
R = Na: Voltaren® or Voltaren®-XR, diclofenac sodium
Diclofenac, as the sodium or potassium salt, is a faintly yellowish white to light beige, virtually odorless, slightly hygroscopic crystalline powder. Molecular weights of the sodium and potassium salts are 318.14 and 334.25, respectively. It is freely soluble in methanol, soluble in ethanol, and practically insoluble in chloroform and in dilute acid. Diclofenac sodium is sparingly soluble in water while diclofenac potassium is soluble in water. The n-octanol/water partition coefficient is, for both diclofenac salts, 13.4 at pH 7.4 and 1545 at pH 5.2. Both salts have a single dissociation constant (pKa) of 4.0 ± 0.2 at 25° C in water.
Diclofenac potassium is available as **Cataflam Immediate-Release Tablets** of 50 mg for oral administration.
CATAFLAM Inactive Ingredients: Calcium phosphate, colloidal silicon dioxide, iron oxides, magnesium stearate, microcrystalline cellulose, polyethylene glycol, povidone, sodium starch glycolate, starch, sucrose, talc, titanium dioxide.
Diclofenac sodium is available as **VOLTAREN Delayed-Release (enteric-coated) Tablets** of 25 mg, 50 mg, and 75 mg for oral administration, and **VOLTAREN-XR Extended-Release Tablets** of 100 mg.
VOLTAREN Inactive Ingredients: Hydroxypropyl methylcellulose, iron oxide, lactose, magnesium stearate, methacrylic acid copolymer, microcrystalline cellulose, polyethylene glycol, povidone, propylene glycol, sodium hydroxide, sodium starch glycolate, talc, titanium dioxide, D&C Yellow No. 10 Aluminum Lake (25-mg tablet only), FD&C Blue No. 1 Aluminum Lake (50-mg tablet only).
VOLTAREN-XR Inactive Ingredients: Cetyl alcohol, hydroxypropyl methylcellulose, iron oxide, magnesium stearate, polyethylene glycol, polysorbate, povidone, silicon dioxide, sucrose, talc, titanium dioxide.

CLINICAL PHARMACOLOGY

Pharmacodynamics
Diclofenac, the anion in Cataflam, Voltaren, and Voltaren-XR, is a nonsteroidal anti-inflammatory drug (NSAID). In pharmacologic studies, diclofenac has shown anti-inflammatory, analgesic, and antipyretic activity. As with other NSAIDs, its mode of action is not known; its ability to inhibit prostaglandin synthesis, however, may be involved in its anti-inflammatory activity, as well as contribute to its efficacy in relieving pain related to inflammation and primary dysmenorrhea. With regard to its analgesic effect, diclofenac is not a narcotic.
Pharmacokinetics
Cataflam Immediate-Release Tablets, Voltaren Delayed-Release Tablets, and Voltaren-XR Extended-Release Tablets, contain the same therapeutic moiety, diclofenac. They differ in the cationic portion of the salt (see DESCRIPTION), as well as in their release characteristics. Cataflam Immediate-Release Tablets are formulated to release diclofenac in the stomach. Voltaren Delayed-Release (enteric-coated) Tablets are in a pharmaceutical formulation that resists dissolution in the low pH of gastric fluid but allows a rapid release of drug in the higher pH-environment of the duodenum. Conversely, Voltaren-XR Extended-Release Tablets are formulated to release drug over a prolonged period. The primary pharmacokinetic difference between the three products is in the pattern of drug release and absorption, as described below and shown in Table 1.

Table 1
Mean (% CV) Pharmacokinetics of Diclofenac Following Single Oral Doses of CATAFLAM, VOLTAREN Delayed-Release, and VOLTAREN-XR

Drug	Dose (mg)	AUC (ng·hr/mL)	C_{max} (ng/mL)	T_{max} (hr)
Cataflam	50	1309 (21.7%)	1312 (44.1%)	1.00 (74.6%)
Voltaren	50	1429 (38.4%)	1417 (22.4%)	2.22 (49.8%)
Voltaren-XR	100	2079 (33.7%)	417 (40.7%)	5.25 (28.3%)

For this reason, separate sections are provided below to describe the different absorption profiles of Cataflam Immediate-Release Tablets, Voltaren Delayed-Release Tablets, and Voltaren-XR Extended-Release Tablets.
Absorption
Under fasting condition, diclofenac is completely absorbed from the gastrointestinal tract. However, due to first-pass metabolism, only about 50% of the absorbed dose is systemically available.
Cataflam Immediate-Release Tablets: In some fasting volunteers, measurable plasma levels are observed within 10 minutes of dosing with Cataflam. Peak plasma levels are achieved in approximately 1 hour in fasting normal volunteers, with a range from 0.33 to 2 hours.
The extent of diclofenac absorption is not significantly affected when Cataflam is taken with food. However, the rate of absorption is reduced by food, as indicated by a delay in T_{max} and decrease in C_{max} values by approximately 30%. After repeated oral administration of Cataflam 50 mg t.i.d. no accumulation of diclofenac in plasma occurred.
Voltaren Delayed-Release Tablets: Peak plasma levels are achieved in 2 hours in fasting normal volunteers, with a range from 1 to 4 hours. The area-under-the-plasma-concentration curve (AUC) is dose-proportional within the range of 25 mg to 150 mg. Peak plasma levels are less than dose-proportional and are approximately 1.0, 1.5, and 2.0 μg/mL for 25-mg, 50-mg, and 75-mg doses, respectively. It should be noted that the administration of several individual Voltaren tablets may not yield equivalent results in peak concentration as the administration of one tablet of a higher strength. This is probably due to the staggered gastric emptying of tablets into the duodenum. After repeated oral administration of Voltaren 50 mg b.i.d., diclofenac did not accumulate in plasma.
When Voltaren is taken with food, there is usually a delay in the onset of absorption of 1 to 4.5 hours, with delays as long as 10 hours in some patients, and a reduction in peak plasma levels of approximately 40%. The extent of absorption of diclofenac, however, is not significantly affected by food intake.
Voltaren-XR Extended-Release Tablets: The extent of diclofenac absorption from the extended-release tablet is not significantly affected when the drug is taken with food, however, food significantly altered the absorption pattern as indicated by a delay of 1 to 2 hours in T_{max} and a two-fold increase in C_{max} values. The plasma profile of the extended-release tablet, under fasting conditions, was characterized by multiple peaks and high intersubject variability in blood profiles. In contrast, the plasma profile for the extended-release tablets under fed conditions showed a more consistent absorption pattern with a single peak usually occurring between 5 and 6 hours after the meal.
Distribution
Plasma concentrations of diclofenac decline from peak levels in a biexponential fashion, with the terminal phase having a half-life of approximately 2 hours. Clearance and volume of distribution are about 350 mL/min and 550 mL/kg, respectively. More than 99% of diclofenac is reversibly bound to human plasma albumin.
As with other NSAIDs, diclofenac diffuses into and out of the synovial fluid. Diffusion into the joint occurs when plasma levels are higher than those in the synovial fluid, after which the process reverses and synovial fluid levels are higher than plasma levels. It is not known whether diffusion into the joint plays a role in the effectiveness of diclofenac.
Metabolism and Elimination
Diclofenac is eliminated through metabolism and subsequent urinary and biliary excretion of the glucuronide and the sulfate conjugates of the metabolites. Approximately 65% of the dose is excreted in the urine, and approximately 35% in the bile.
Conjugates of unchanged diclofenac account for 5%–10% of the dose excreted in the urine and for less than 5% excreted in the bile. Little or no unchanged unconjugated drug is excreted. Conjugates of the principal metabolite account for 20%–30% of the dose excreted in the urine and for 10%–20% of the dose excreted in the bile. Conjugates of three other metabolites together account for 10%–20% of the dose excreted in the urine and for small amounts excreted in the bile. The elimination half-life values for these metabolites are shorter than those for the parent drug. Urinary excretion of an additional metabolite (half-life 80 hours) accounts for only 1.4% of the oral dose. The degree of accumulation of diclofenac metabolites is unknown. Some of the metabolites may have activity.
Special Populations
A 4-week study, comparing plasma level profiles of diclofenac (Voltaren 50 mg b.i.d.) in younger (26–46 years) versus older (66–81 years) adults, did not show differences between age groups (10 patients per age group).
Geriatric Population: An 8-day study, comparing the kinetics of diclofenac (100 mg Voltaren-XR q.d.) in osteoarthritis patients older than 65 years versus younger than 65 years showed no significant differences between the two groups with respect to peak plasma levels, time to peak levels, or AUC.
Patients with Renal and/or Hepatic Impairment: To date, no differences in the pharmacokinetics of diclofenac have been detected in studies of patients with renal (50 mg intravenously) or hepatic impairment (100-mg oral solution). In patients with renal impairment (N=5, creatinine clearance 3 to 42 mL/min), AUC values and elimination rates were comparable to those in healthy subjects. In patients with biopsy-confirmed cirrhosis or chronic active hepatitis (variably elevated transaminases and mildly elevated bilirubins, N=10), diclofenac concentrations and urinary elimination values were comparable to those in healthy subjects.
Clinical Studies
Cataflam Immediate-Release Tablets in Analgesia/Primary Dysmenorrhea: The analgesic efficacy of Cataflam was demonstrated in trials of patients with postoperative pain (following gynecologic, oral, and orthopedic surgery), osteoarthritis of the knee, and primary dysmenorrhea. The effectiveness of Cataflam in studies of pain or primary dysmenorrhea showed that onset of analgesia began, in some patients, as soon as 30 minutes, and relief of pain lasted as long as 8 hours, following single 50-mg or 100-mg doses. Duration of pain relief was judged by the time at which approximately half of the patients need remedication. The onset and duration of pain relief for either the 50-mg or 100-mg dose was essentially the same, whether patients had moderate or severe pain at baseline.
Cataflam was studied in single-dose and multiple-dose pain trials. The pain models in single-dose studies were post-dental extraction and post-gynecologic surgery: the efficacy of the 50-mg dose (N=258) and the 100-mg dose (N=255) was comparable to aspirin 650 mg in onset of pain relief, but generally provided a longer duration of analgesia than aspirin. The pain models for multiple-dose trials were post-orthopedic surgery pain as well as pain associated with primary dysmenorrhea: the efficacy of the 50-mg dose (N=101) and the 100-mg dose (N=442), followed by 50 mg every 8 hours, was comparable to naproxen sodium 550 mg followed by 275 mg every 8 hours. In one study of chronic pain, in patients with osteoarthritis (N=196), Cataflam 50 mg t.i.d. was comparable in efficacy to ibuprofen 800 mg t.i.d. and Voltaren Delayed-Release Tablets 50 mg t.i.d.

Continued on next page

Cataflam/Voltaren—Cont.

Voltaren Delayed-Release Tablets in Osteoarthritis: Voltaren was evaluated for the management of the signs and symptoms of osteoarthritis of the hip or knee in a total of 633 patients treated for up to 3 months in placebo- and active-controlled clinical trials against aspirin (N=449), and naproxen (N=92). Voltaren was given both in variable (100–150 mg/day) and fixed (150 mg/day) dosing schedules in either b.i.d. or t.i.d. dosing regimens. In these trials, Voltaren was found to be comparable to 2400 to 3600 mg/day of aspirin or 500 mg/day of naproxen. Voltaren was effective when administered as either b.i.d. or t.i.d. dosing regimens.

Voltaren Delayed-Release Tablets in Rheumatoid Arthritis: Voltaren was evaluated for managing the signs and symptoms of rheumatoid arthritis in a total of 468 patients treated for up to 3 months in placebo- and active-controlled clinical trials against aspirin (N=290), and ibuprofen (N=74). Voltaren was given in a fixed (150 or 200 mg/day) dosing schedule as either b.i.d. or t.i.d. dosing regimens. Voltaren was found to be comparable to 3600 to 4800 mg/day of aspirin, and 2400 mg/day of ibuprofen. Voltaren was used b.i.d. or t.i.d., administering 150 mg/day in most trials, but 50 mg q.i.d. (200 mg/day) was also studied.

Voltaren Delayed-Release Tablets in Ankylosing Spondylitis: Voltaren was evaluated for the management of the signs and symptoms of ankylosing spondylitis in a total of 132 patients in one active-controlled clinical trial against indomethacin (N=130). Both Voltaren and indomethacin patients were started on 25 mg t.i.d. and were permitted to increase the dose 25 mg/day each week to a maximum dose of 125 mg/day. Voltaren 75–125 mg/day was found to be comparable to indomethacin 75–125 mg/day.

Voltaren-XR Extended-Release Tablets in Osteoarthritis: The use of Voltaren-XR Tablets in controlling the signs and symptoms of osteoarthritis was assessed in two double-blind, controlled trials in which 742 patients participated and 517 patients were treated for 3 months. In one active- and placebo-controlled study, Voltaren-XR Tablets at doses of 100 mg q.d. were comparable to Voltaren Delayed-Release Tablets 50 mg b.i.d. in patients whose osteoarthritis symptoms were stabilized after 2 weeks of treatment with Voltaren Delayed-Release Tablets 75 mg b.i.d. In another study, Voltaren-XR Tablets at doses of 100 mg q.d. and 100 mg b.i.d. were compared to Voltaren Delayed-Release Tablets 50 mg q.i.d. Voltaren-XR Tablets 100 mg b.i.d. were comparable to Voltaren Delayed-Release Tablets 50 mg q.i.d. With the Voltaren-XR Tablet formulation, although there was a trend toward greater efficacy at doses of 200 mg daily than 100 mg daily, there was also an increase in side effects when 200 mg of Voltaren-XR Tablets were administered to patients with osteoarthritis.

Voltaren-XR Extended-Release Tablets in Rheumatoid Arthritis: The use of Voltaren-XR Tablets in controlling the signs and symptoms of rheumatoid arthritis was assessed in two double-blind, controlled trials in which 704 patients participated and 441 patients were treated for 3 months. In one active- and placebo-controlled study, Voltaren-XR Tablets 100 mg q.d. were comparable to Voltaren Delayed-Release Tablets 50 mg b.i.d. in patients whose rheumatoid arthritis symptoms were stabilized after 2 weeks' treatment of Voltaren Delayed-Release Tablets 75 mg b.i.d. In another study, Voltaren-XR Tablets at doses of 100 mg q.d. and 100 mg b.i.d. were compared to Voltaren Delayed-Release Tablets 50 mg q.i.d.; Voltaren-XR Tablets 100 mg b.i.d. were comparable to Voltaren Delayed-Release Tablets 50 mg q.i.d. There was a trend toward greater efficacy with doses of 200 mg daily as compared to 100 mg daily of Voltaren-XR Tablets. There was also an increase in side effects when 200 mg of Voltaren-XR Tablets were administered to patients with rheumatoid arthritis.

Special Studies *(The clinical significance of the findings outlined below is unknown.)*

G.I. Blood Loss/Endoscopy Data: G.I. blood loss and endoscopy studies were performed with Voltaren Delayed-Release (enteric-coated) Tablets that, unlike Immediate-Release Tablets, do not dissolve in the stomach where the endoscopic lesions are primarily seen; Cataflam Immediate-Release Tablets have not been similarly studied. A repeat-dose endoscopy study, in patients with rheumatoid arthritis or osteoarthritis treated with Voltaren Delayed-Release Tablets 75 mg b.i.d. (N=101), or naproxen (immediate-release tablets) 500 mg b.i.d. (N=103) for 3 months, resulted in a significantly smaller number of patients with an increase in endoscopy score from baseline and a significantly lower mean endoscopy score after treatment in the Voltaren-treated patients. Two repeat-dose endoscopic studies, in normal volunteers showed that daily doses of Voltaren Delayed-Release Tablets 75 or 100 mg (N=6 and N=14, respectively) for 1 week caused fewer gastric lesions, and those that did occur had lower scores than those observed following daily 500-mg doses of naproxen (immediate-release tablets). In healthy subjects, the daily administration of 150 mg of Voltaren (N=8) for 3 weeks resulted in a mean fecal blood loss less than that observed with 3.0 g of aspirin daily (N=8). In four repeat-dose studies, mean fecal blood loss with 150 mg of Voltaren was also less than that observed with 750 mg of naproxen (N=8 and N=6) or 150 mg of indomethacin (N=8 and N=6).

INDIVIDUALIZATION OF DOSAGE

Diclofenac, like other NSAIDs, shows interindividual differences in both pharmacokinetics and clinical response (pharmacodynamics). Consequently, the recommended strategy for initiating therapy is to use a starting dose likely to be effective for the majority of patients and to adjust dosage thereafter based on observation of diclofenac's beneficial and adverse effects.

In patients weighing less than 60 kg (132 lb), or where the severity of the disease, concomitant medication, or other diseases warrant, the maximum recommended total daily dose of Cataflam, Voltaren, or Voltaren-XR should be reduced. Experience with other NSAIDs has shown that starting therapy with maximum doses in patients at increased risk due to renal or hepatic disease, low body weight (<60 kg), advanced age, a known ulcer diathesis, or known sensitivity to NSAID effects, is likely to increase frequency of adverse reactions and is not recommended (see PRECAUTIONS).

Osteoarthritis/Rheumatoid Arthritis/Ankylosing Spondylitis: The usual starting dose of Cataflam Immediate-Release Tablets or Voltaren Delayed-Release for patients with osteoarthritis, is 100 to 150 mg/day, using a b.i.d. or t.i.d. dosing regimen. For patients with osteoarthritis, the ususal starting dose of Voltaren-XR Extended-Release Tablets is 100 mg q.d. In two variable-dose clinical trials in osteoarthritis using Voltaren Delayed-Release Tablets, of 266 patients started on 100 mg/day, 176 chose to increase the dose to 150 mg/day. Dosages above 200 mg/day have not been studied in patients with osteoarthritis.

For most patients with rheumatoid arthritis, the usual starting dose of Cataflam Immediate-Release Tablets or Voltaren Delayed-Release Tablets is 150 mg/day, using a b.i.d. or t.i.d. dosing regimen. The usual starting dose of Voltaren-XR Extended-Release Tablets is 100 mg q.d. Patients requiring more relief of pain and inflammation may increase the dose to 200 mg/day. In clinical trials, patients receiving 200 mg/day were less likely to drop from the trial due to lack of efficacy than patients receiving 150 mg/day as Voltaren Delayed-Release Tablets or 100 mg/day as Voltaren-XR Extended-Release Tablets. Dosages above 225 mg/day are not recommended in patients with rheumatoid arthritis because of increased risk of adverse events.

The recommended dose of Voltaren Delayed-Release Tablets for patients with ankylosing spondylitis is 100 to 125 mg/day, using a q.i.d. dosing regimen (see DOSAGE AND ADMINISTRATION regarding the 125 mg/day dosing regimen). In a variable-dose clinical trial, of 132 patients started on 75 mg/day, 122 chose to increase the dose to 125 mg/day. Dosages above 125 mg/day have not been studied in patients with ankylosing spondylitis.

Analgesia/Primary Dysmenorrhea: Because of earlier absorption of diclofenac from Cataflam Immediate-Release Tablets, it is the formulation indicated for management of pain and primary dysmenorrhea when prompt onset of pain relief is desired. The results of clinical trials suggest an initial Cataflam dose of 50 mg for pain or for primary dysmenorrhea, followed by doses of 50 mg every 8 hours, as needed. With experience, some patients with recurring pain, such as dysmenorrhea, may find that an initial dose of 100 mg of Cataflam, followed by 50-mg doses, will provide better relief. After the first day, when the maximum recommended dose may be 200 mg, the total daily dose should generally not exceed 150 mg.

INDICATIONS AND USAGE

Cataflam Immediate-Release Tablets and Voltaren Delayed-Release Tablets are indicated for the acute and chronic treatment of signs and symptoms of osteoarthritis and rheumatoid arthritis. Voltaren-XR Extended-Release Tablets are indicated for chronic therapy of osteoarthritis and rheumatoid arthritis. In addition, Cataflam Immediate-Release Tablets and Voltaren Delayed-Release Tablets are indicated for the treatment of ankylosing spondylitis. Only Cataflam is indicated for the management of pain and primary dysmenorrhea, when prompt pain relief is desired, because it is formulated to provide earlier plasma concentrations of diclofenac (see CLINICAL PHARMACOLOGY, Pharmacokinetics and Clinical Studies).

CONTRAINDICATIONS

Diclofenac in all formulations, Cataflam, Voltaren, and Voltaren-XR, is contraindicated in patients with known hypersensitivity to diclofenac and diclofenac-containing products. Diclofenac should not be given to patients who have experienced asthma, urticaria, or other allergic-type reactions after taking aspirin or other NSAIDs. Severe, rarely fatal, anaphylactic-like reactions to diclofenac have been reported in such patients (see WARNINGS—Anaphylactoid Reactions, and PRECAUTIONS—Preexisting Asthma).

WARNINGS

Gastrointestinal Effects

Peptic ulceration and gastrointestinal bleeding have been reported in patients receiving diclofenac. Physicians and patients should therefore remain alert for ulceration and bleeding in patients treated chronically with diclofenac even in the absence of previous G.I. tract symptoms. It is recommended that patients be maintained on the lowest dose of diclofenac possible, consistent with achieving a satisfactory therapeutic response.

Risk of G.I. Ulcerations, Bleeding, and Perforation with NSAID Therapy: Serious gastrointestinal toxicity such as bleeding, ulceration, and perforation can occur at any time, with or without warning symptoms, in patients treated chronically with NSAID therapy. Although minor upper gastrointestinal problems, such as dyspepsia, are common, usually developing early in therapy, physicians should remain alert for ulceration and bleeding in patients treated chronically with NSAIDs even in the absence of previous G.I. tract symptoms. In patients observed in clinical trials of several months to 2 years' duration, symptomatic upper G.I. ulcers, gross bleeding, or perforation appear to occur in approximately 1% of patients for 3–6 months, and in about 2%–4% of patients treated for 1 year. Physicians should inform patients about the signs and/or symptoms of serious G.I. toxicity and what steps to take if they occur.

Studies to date have not identified any subset of patients not at risk of developing peptic ulceration and bleeding. Except for a prior history of serious G.I. events and other risk factors known to be associated with peptic ulcer disease, such as alcoholism, smoking, etc., no risk factors (e.g., age, sex) have been associated with increased risk. Elderly or debilitated patients seem to tolerate ulceration or bleeding less well than other individuals, and most spontaneous reports of fatal G.I. events are in this population. Studies to date are inconclusive concerning the relative risk of various NSAIDs in causing such reactions. High doses of any NSAID probably carry a greater risk of these reactions, although controlled clinical trials showing this do not exist in most cases. In considering the use of relatively large doses (within the recommended dosage range), sufficient benefit should be anticipated to offset the potential increased risk of G.I. toxicity.

Hepatic Effects

Elevations of one or more liver tests may occur during diclofenac therapy. These laboratory abnormalities may progress, may remain unchanged, or may be transient with continued therapy. Borderline elevations (i.e., less than 3 times the ULN [=the Upper Limit of the Normal range]), or greater elevations of transaminases occurred in about 15% of diclofenac-treated patients. Of the hepatic enzymes, ALT (SGPT) is the one recommended for the monitoring of liver injury.

In clinical trials, meaningful elevations (i.e., more than 3 times the ULN) of AST (SGOT) (ALT was not measured in all studies) occurred in about 2% of approximately 5700 patients at some time during Voltaren treatment. In a large, open, controlled trial, meaningful elevations of ALT and/or AST occurred in about 4% of 3700 patients treated for 2–6 months, including marked elevations (i.e., more than 8 times the ULN) in about 1% of the 3700 patients. In that open-label study, a higher incidence of borderline (less than 3 times the ULN), moderate (3–8 times the ULN), and marked (>8 times the ULN) elevations of ALT or AST was observed in patients receiving diclofenac when compared to other NSAIDs. Transaminase elevations were seen more frequently in patients with osteoarthritis than in those with rheumatoid arthritis (see ADVERSE REACTIONS).

In addition to enzyme elevations seen in clinical trials, postmarketing surveillance has found rare cases of severe hepatic reactions, including liver necrosis, jaundice, and fulminant fatal hepatitis with and without jaundice. Some of these rare reported cases underwent liver transplantation.

Physicians should measure transaminases periodically in patients receiving long-term therapy with diclofenac, because severe hepatotoxicity may develop without a prodrome of distinguishing symptoms. The optimum times for making the first and subsequent transaminase measurements are not known. In the largest U.S. trial (open-label) that involved 3700 patients monitored first at 8 weeks and 1200 patients monitored again at 24 weeks, almost all meaningful elevations in transaminases were detected before patients became symptomatic. In 42 of the 51 patients in all trials who developed marked transaminase elevations, abnormal tests occurred during the first 2 months of therapy with diclofenac. Postmarketing experience has shown severe hepatic reactions can occur at any time during treatment with diclofenac. Cases of drug-induced hepatotoxicity have been reported in the first month, and in some cases, the first two months of therapy. Based on these experiences, transaminases should be monitored within 4 to 8 weeks after initiating treatment with diclofenac (see PRECAUTIONS—Laboratory Tests). As with other NSAIDs, if abnormal liver tests persist or worsen, if clinical signs and/or symptoms consistent with liver disease de-

velop, or if systemic manifestations occur (e.g., eosinophilia, rash, etc.), diclofenac should be discontinued immediately. To minimize the possibility that hepatic injury will become severe between transaminase measurements, physicians should inform patients of the warning signs and symptoms of hepatotoxicity (e.g., nausea, fatigue, lethargy, pruritus, jaundice, right upper quadrant tenderness, and "flu-like" symptoms), and the appropriate action patients should take if these signs and symptoms appear.

Anaphylactoid Reactions

As with other NSAIDs, anaphylactoid reactions may occur in patients without prior exposure to diclofenac. Diclofenac should not be given to patients with the aspirin triad. The triad typically occurs in asthmatic patients who experience rhinitis with or without nasal polyps, or who exhibit severe, potentially fatal bronchospasm after taking aspirin or other nonsteroidal anti-inflammatory drugs. Fatal reactions have been reported in such patients (see CONTRAINDICATIONS, and PRECAUTIONS—Preexisting Asthma). Emergency help should be sought in cases where an anaphylactoid reaction occurs.

Advanced Renal Disease

In cases with advanced kidney disease, treatment with diclofenac, as with other NSAIDs, should only be initiated with close monitoring of the patient's kidney functions (see PRECAUTIONS—Renal Effects).

Pregnancy

In late pregnancy, diclofenac should, as with other NSAIDs, be avoided because it will cause premature closure of the ductus arteriosus (see PRECAUTIONS—Pregnancy, *Teratogenic Effects, Pregnancy Category B,* and Labor and Delivery).

PRECAUTIONS

General

Cataflam Immediate-Release Tablets, Voltaren Delayed-Release Tablets, and Voltaren-XR Extended-Release Tablets should not be used concomitantly with other diclofenac-containing products since they also circulate in plasma as the diclofenac anion.

Fluid Retention and Edema: Fluid retention and edema have been observed in some patients taking diclofenac. Therefore, as with other NSAIDs, diclofenac should be used with caution in patients with a history of cardiac decompensation, hypertension, or other conditions predisposing to fluid retention.

Hematologic Effects: Anemia is sometimes seen in patients receiving diclofenac or other NSAIDs. This may be due to fluid retention, G.I. blood loss, or an incompletely described effect upon erythropoiesis.

Renal Effects: As a class, NSAIDs have been associated with renal papillary necrosis and other abnormal renal pathology in long-term administration to animals. In oral diclofenac studies in animals, some evidence of renal toxicity was noted. Isolated incidents of papillary necrosis were observed in a few animals at high doses (20–120 mg/kg) in several baboon subacute studies. In patients treated with diclofenac, rare cases of interstitial nephritis and papillary necrosis have been reported (see ADVERSE REACTIONS).

A second form of renal toxicity, generally associated with NSAIDs, is seen in patients with conditions leading to a reduction in renal blood flow or blood volume, where renal prostaglandins have a supportive role in the maintenance of renal perfusion. In these patients, administration of an NSAID results in a dose-dependent decrease in prostaglandin synthesis and, secondarily, in a reduction of renal blood flow, which may precipitate overt renal failure. Patients at greatest risk of this reaction are those with impaired renal function, heart failure, liver dysfunction, those taking diuretics, and the elderly. Discontinuation of NSAID therapy is typically followed by recovery to the pretreatment state.

Cases of significant renal failure in patients receiving diclofenac have been reported from marketing experience, but were not observed in over 4000 patients in clinical trials during which serum creatinine and BUN values were followed serially. There were only 11 patients (0.3%) whose serum creatinine and concurrent serum BUN values were greater than 2.0 mg/dL and 40 mg/dL, respectively, while on diclofenac (mean rise in the 11 patients: creatinine 2.3 mg/dL and BUN 28.4 mg/dL).

Since diclofenac metabolites are eliminated primarily by the kidneys, patients with significantly impaired renal function should be more closely monitored than subjects with normal renal function.

Porphyria: The use of diclofenac in patients with hepatic porphyria should be avoided. To date, 1 patient has been described in whom diclofenac probably triggered a clinical attack of porphyria. The postulated mechanism, demonstrated in rats, for causing such attacks by diclofenac, as well as some other NSAIDs, is through stimulation of the porphyrin precursor delta-aminolevulinic acid (ALA).

Aseptic Meningitis: As with other NSAIDs, aseptic meningitis with fever and coma has been observed on rare occasions in patients on diclofenac therapy. Although it is probably more likely to occur in patients with systemic lupus erythematosus and related connective tissue diseases, it has been reported in patients who do not have an underlying chronic disease. If signs or symptoms of meningitis develop in a patient on diclofenac, the possibility of its being related to diclofenac should be considered.

Preexisting Asthma: About 10% of patients with asthma may have aspirin-sensitive asthma. The use of aspirin in patients with aspirin-sensitive asthma has been associated with severe bronchospasm which can be fatal. Since cross-reactivity, including bronchospasm, between aspirin and other nonsteroidal anti-inflammatory drugs has been reported in such aspirin-sensitive patients, diclofenac should not be administered to patients with this form of aspirin sensitivity and should be used with caution in all patients with preexisting asthma.

Other Precautions: The pharmacologic activity of diclofenac may reduce fever and inflammation, thus diminishing their utility as diagnostic signs in detecting underlying conditions.

In order to avoid exacerbation of manifestations of adrenal insufficiency, patients who have been on prolonged corticosteroid treatment should have their therapy tapered slowly rather than discontinued abruptly when diclofenac is added to the treatment program.

Blurred and/or diminished vision, scotomata, and/or changes in color vision have been reported. If a patient develops such complaints while receiving diclofenac, the drug should be discontinued and the patient should have an ophthalmologic examination which includes central visual fields and color vision testing.

Information for Patients

Diclofenac, like other drugs of its class, is not free of side effects. The side effects of these drugs can cause discomfort and, rarely, more serious side effects, such as gastrointestinal bleeding, and more rarely, liver toxicity (see WARNINGS, Hepatic Effects), which may result in hospitalization and even fatal outcomes.

NSAIDs are often essential agents in the management of arthritis and have a major role in the management of pain, but they also may be commonly employed for conditions that are less serious.

Physicians may wish to discuss with their patients the potential risks (see WARNINGS, PRECAUTIONS, and ADVERSE REACTIONS) and likely benefits of NSAID treatment, particularly when the drugs are used for less serious conditions where treatment without NSAIDs may represent an acceptable alternative to both the patient and physician.

Because serious G.I. tract ulceration and bleeding can occur without warning symptoms, physicians should follow chronically treated patients for the signs and symptoms of ulceration and bleeding and should inform them of the importance of this follow-up (see WARNINGS, Gastrointestinal Effects, *Risk of G.I. Ulcerations, Bleeding, and Perforation with NSAID Therapy*). If diclofenac is used chronically, patients should also be instructed to report any signs and symptoms that might be due to hepatotoxicity of diclofenac; these symptoms may become evident between visits when periodic liver laboratory tests are performed (see WARNINGS, Hepatic Effects, and PRECAUTIONS—Laboratory Tests).

Laboratory Tests

Hepatic Effects: Transaminases and other hepatic enzymes should be monitored in patients treated with NSAIDs. For patients on diclofenac therapy, it is recommended that a determination be made within 4 weeks of initiating therapy and at intervals thereafter. If clinical signs and symptoms consistent with liver disease develop, or if systemic manifestations occur (e.g., eosinophilia, rash, etc.) and abnormal liver tests are detected, persist or worsen, diclofenac should be discontinued immediately.

Hematologic Effects: Patients on long-term treatment with NSAIDs, including diclofenac, should have their hemoglobin or hematocrit checked periodically for signs or symptoms of anemia. Appropriate measures should be taken in case such signs of anemia occur.

Drug Interactions

Aspirin: Concomitant administration of diclofenac and aspirin is not recommended because diclofenac is displaced from its binding sites during the concomitant administration of aspirin, resulting in lower plasma concentrations, peak plasma levels, and AUC values.

Anticoagulants: While studies have not shown diclofenac to interact with anticoagulants of the warfarin type, caution should be exercised, nonetheless, since interactions have been seen with other NSAIDs. Because prostaglandins play an important role in hemostasis, and NSAIDs affect platelet function as well, concurrent therapy with all NSAIDs, including diclofenac, and warfarin requires close monitoring of patients to be certain that no change in their anticoagulant dosage is required.

Digoxin, Methotrexate, Cyclosporine: Diclofenac, like other NSAIDs, may affect renal prostaglandins and increase the toxicity of certain drugs. Ingestion of diclofenac may increase serum concentrations of digoxin and methotrexate and increase cyclosporine's nephrotoxicity. Patients who begin taking diclofenac or who increase their diclofenac dose or any other NSAID while taking digoxin, methotrexate, or cyclosporine may develop toxicity characteristics for these drugs. They should be observed closely, particularly if renal function is impaired. In the case of digoxin, serum levels should be monitored.

Lithium: Diclofenac decreases lithium renal clearance and increases lithium plasma levels. In patients taking diclofenac and lithium concomitantly, lithium toxicity may develop.

Oral Hypoglycemics: Diclofenac does not alter glucose metabolism in normal subjects nor does it alter the effects of oral hypoglycemic agents. There are rare reports, however, from marketing experiences, of changes in effects of insulin or oral hypoglycemic agents in the presence of diclofenac that necessitated changes in the doses of such agents. Both hypo- and hyperglycemic effects have been reported. A direct causal relationship has not been established, but physicians should consider the possibility that diclofenac may alter a diabetic patient's response to insulin or oral hypoglycemic agents.

Diuretics: Diclofenac and other NSAIDs can inhibit the activity of diuretics. Concomitant treatment with potassium-sparing diuretics may be associated with increased serum potassium levels.

Other Drugs: In small groups of patients (7–10/interaction study), the concomitant administration of azathioprine, gold, chloroquine, D-penicillamine, prednisolone, doxycycline, or digitoxin did not significantly affect the peak levels and AUC values of diclofenac. Phenobarbital toxicity has been reported to have occurred in a patient on chronic phenobarbital treatment following the initiation of diclofenac therapy.

Protein Binding

In vitro, diclofenac interferes minimally or not at all with the protein binding of salicylic acid (20% decrease in binding), tolbutamide, prednisolone (10% decrease in binding), or warfarin. Benzylpenicillin, ampicillin, oxacillin, chlortetracycline, doxycycline, cephalothin, erythromycin, and sulfamethoxazole have no influence *in vitro* on the protein binding of diclofenac in human serum.

Drug/Laboratory Test Interactions

Effect on Blood Coagulation: Diclofenac increases platelet aggregaton time but does not affect bleeding time, plasma thrombin clotting time, plasma fibrinogen, or factors V and VII to XII. Statistically significant changes in prothrombin and partial thromboplastin times have been reported in normal volunteers. The mean changes were observed to be less than 1 second in both instances, however, and are unlikely to be clinically important. Diclofenac is a prostaglandin synthetase inhibitor, however, and all drugs that inhibit prostaglandin synthesis interfere with platelet function to some degree; therefore, patients who may be adversely affected by such an action should be carefully observed.

Carcinogenesis, Mutagenesis, Impairment of Fertility

Long-term carcinogenicity studies in rats given diclofenac sodium up to 2 mg/kg/day (or 12 mg/m^2/day, approximately the human dose) have revealed no significant increases in tumor incidence. There was a slight increase in benign mammary fibroadenomas in mid-dose-treated (0.5 mg/kg/day or 3 mg/m^2/day) female rats (high-dose females had excessive mortality), but the increase was not significant for this common rat tumor. A 2-year carcinogenicity study conducted in mice employing diclofenac sodium at doses up to 0.3 mg/kg/day (0.9 mg/m^2/day) in males and 1 mg/kg/day (3 mg/m^2/day) in females did not reveal any oncogenic potential. Diclofenac sodium did not show mutagenic activity in *in vitro* point mutation assays in mammalian (mouse lymphoma) and microbial (yeast, Ames) test systems and was nonmutagenic in several mammalian *in vitro* and *in vivo* tests, including dominant lethal and male germinal epithelial chromosomal studies in mice, and nucleus anomaly and chromosomal aberration studies in Chinese hamsters. Diclofenac sodium administered to male and female rats at 4 mg/kg/day (24 mg/m^2/day) did not affect fertility.

Pregnancy, *Teratogenic Effects, Pregnancy Category B*

Reproduction studies have been performed in mice given diclofenac sodium (up to 20 mg/kg/day or 60 mg/m^2/day) and in rats and rabbits given diclofenac sodium (up to 10 mg/kg/day or 60 mg/m^2/day for rats, and 80 mg/m^2/day for rabbits), and have revealed no evidence of teratogenicity despite the induction of maternal toxicity and fetal toxicity. In rats, maternally toxic doses were associated with dystocia, prolonged gestation, reduced fetal weights and growth, and reduced fetal survival. Diclofenac has been shown to cross the placental barrier in mice and rats. There are, however, no adequate and well-controlled studies in pregnant women. Because animal reproduction studies are not always predictive of human response, this drug should not be used during pregnancy unless the benefits to the mother justify the potential risk to the fetus. Because of the risk to the fetus resulting in premature closure of the ductus arteriosus, diclofenac should be avoided in late pregnancy.

Continued on next page

Cataflam/Voltaren—Cont.

Labor and Delivery
The effects of diclofenac on labor and delivery in pregnant women are unknown. Because of the known effects of prostaglandin-inhibiting drugs on the fetal cardiovascular system (closure of ductus arteriosus), use of diclofenac during late pregnancy should be avoided and, as with other nonsteroidal anti-inflammatory drugs, it is possible that diclofenac may inhibit uterine contractions and delay parturition.

Nursing Mothers
Because of the potential for serious adverse reactions in nursing infants from diclofenac, a decision should be made whether to discontinue nursing or to discontinue the drug, taking into account the importance of the drug to the mother.

Pediatric Use
Safety and effectiveness of diclofenac in pediatric patients have not been established.

Geriatric Use
Of the more than 6000 patients treated with diclofenac in U.S. trials, 31% were older than 65 years of age. No overall difference was observed between efficacy, adverse event, or pharmacokinetic profiles of older and younger patients. As with any NSAID, the elderly are likely to tolerate adverse reactions less well than younger patients.

ADVERSE REACTIONS

Adverse reaction information is derived from blinded, controlled, and open-label clinical trials, as well as worldwide marketing experience. In the description below, rates of more common events represent clinical study results; rarer events are derived principally from marketing experience and publications, and accurate rate estimates are generally not possible.

In 718 patients treated for shorter periods, i.e., 2 weeks or less, with Cataflam Immediate-Release Tablets, adverse reactions were reported one-half to one-tenth as frequently as by patients treated for longer periods. In a 6-month, double-blind trial comparing Cataflam Immediate-Release Tablets (N=196) versus Voltaren Delayed-Release Tablets (N=197) versus ibuprofen (N=197), adverse reactions were similar in nature and frequency. In controlled clinical trials, the incidence of adverse reactions for Voltaren Delayed-Release Tablets and Voltaren-XR Extended-Release Tablets at comparable doses were similar.

The incidence of common adverse reactions (greater than 1%) is based upon controlled clinical trials in 1543 patients treated up to 13 weeks with Voltaren Delayed-Release Tablets. By far the most common adverse effects were gastrointestinal symptoms, most of them minor, occurring in about 20%, and leading to discontinuation in about 3%, of patients. Peptic ulcer or G.I. bleeding occurred in clinical trials in 0.6% (95% confidence interval: 0.2% to 1%) of approximately 1800 patients during their first 3 months of diclofenac treatment and in 1.6% (95% confidence interval: 0.8% to 2.4%) of approximately 800 patients followed for 1 year.

Gastrointestinal symptoms were followed in frequency by central nervous system side effects such as headache (7%) and dizziness (3%).

Meaningful (exceeding 3 times the Upper Limit of Normal) elevations of ALT (SGPT) or AST (SGOT) occurred at an overall rate of approximately 2% during the first 2 months of Voltaren treatment. Unlike aspirin-related elevations, which occur more frequently in patients with rheumatoid arthritis, these elevations were more frequently observed in patients with osteoarthritis (2.6%) than in patients with rheumatoid arthritis (0.7%). Marked elevations (exceeding 8 times the ULN) were seen in 1% of patients treated for 2–6 months (see WARNINGS, Hepatic Effects).

The following adverse reactions were reported in patients treated with diclofenac:

Incidence Greater Than 1%—Causal Relationship Probable:
(All derived from clinical trials.)

*Incidence, 3% to 9% (incidence of unmarked reactions is 1%–3%).

Body as a Whole: Abdominal pain or cramps,* headache,* fluid retention, abdominal distention.

Digestive: Diarrhea,* indigestion,* nausea,* constipation,* flatulence, liver test abnormalities,* PUB, i.e., peptic ulcer, with or without bleeding and/or perforation, or bleeding without ulcer (see above and also WARNINGS).

Nervous System: Dizziness.

Skin and Appendages: Rash, pruritus.

Special Senses: Tinnitus.

Incidence Less Than 1%—Causal Relationship Probable:
(Adverse reactions reported only in worldwide marketing experience or in the literature, not seen in clinical trials, are considered rare and are *italicized*.)

Body as a Whole: Malaise, swelling of lips and tongue, photosensitivity, *anaphylaxis*, anaphylactoid reactions.

Cardiovascular: Hypertension, congestive heart failure.

Digestive: Vomiting, jaundice, melena, *esophageal lesions*, aphthous stomatitis, dry mouth and mucous membranes, bloody diarrhea, hepatitis, *hepatic necrosis, cirrhosis, hepatorenal syndrome*, appetite change, pancreatitis with or without concomitant hepatitis, *colitis*.

Hemic and Lymphatic: Hemoglobin decrease, leukopenia, thrombocytopenia, *eosinophilia, hemolytic anemia, aplastic anemia, agranulocytosis*, purpura, *allergic purpura*.

Metabolic and Nutritional Disorders: Azotemia.

Nervous System: Insomnia, drowsiness, depression, diplopia, anxiety, irritability, *aseptic meningitis, convulsions*.

Respiratory: Epistaxis, asthma, laryngeal edema.

Skin and Appendages: Alopecia, urticaria, eczema, dermatitis, *bullous eruption, erythema multiforme major*, angioedema, *Stevens-Johnson syndrome*.

Special Senses: Blurred vision, taste disorder, reversible and irreversible hearing loss, scotoma.

Urogenital: *Nephrotic syndrome*, proteinuria, *oliguria, interstitial nephritis, papillary necrosis, acute renal failure*.

Incidence Less Than 1%—Causal Relationship Unknown:
(The following reactions have been reported in patients taking diclofenac under circumstances that do not permit a clear attribution of the reaction to diclofenac. These reactions are being included as alerting information to physicians. Adverse reactions reported only in worldwide marketing experience or in the literature, not seen in clinical trials, are considered rare and are *italicized*.)

Body as a Whole: Chest pain.

Cardiovascular: Palpitations, *flushing*, tachycardia, premature ventricular contractions, myocardial infarction, *hypotension*.

Digestive: *Intestinal perforation*.

Hemic and Lymphatic: *Bruising*.

Metabolic and Nutritional Disorders: Hypoglycemia, *weight loss*.

Nervous System: Paresthesia, memory disturbance, nightmares, tremor, tic, *abnormal coordination, disorientation, psychotic reaction*.

Respiratory: Dyspnea, hyperventilation, edema of pharynx.

Skin and Appendages: Excess perspiration, *exfoliative dermatitis*.

Special Senses: Vitreous floaters, night blindness, amblyopia.

Urogenital: Urinary frequency, nocturia, hematuria, impotence, vaginal bleeding.

OVERDOSAGE

Worldwide reports of overdosage with diclofenac cover 66 cases. In approximately one-half of these reports of overdosage, concomitant medications were also taken. The highest dose of diclofenac was 5.0 g in a 17-year-old male who suffered loss of consciousness, increased intracranial pressure, aspiration pneumonitis, and died 2 days after overdose. The next highest doses of diclofenac were 4.0 g and 3.75 g. The 24-year-old female who took 4.0 g and the 28- and 42-year-old females, each of whom took 3.75 g, did not develop any clinically significant signs or symptoms. However, there was a report of a 17-year-old female who experienced vomiting and drowsiness after an overdose of 2.37 g of diclofenac.

Animal LD_{50} values show a wide range of susceptibilities to acute overdosage, with primates being more resistant to acute toxicity than rodents (LD_{50} in mg/kg—rats, 55; dogs, 500; monkeys, 3200).

In case of acute overdosage, it is recommended that the stomach be emptied by vomiting or lavage. Forced diuresis may theoretically be beneficial because the drug is excreted in the urine. The effect of dialysis or hemoperfusion in the elimination of diclofenac (99% protein-bound: see CLINICAL PHARMACOLOGY) remains unproven. In addition to supportive measures, the use of oral activated charcoal may help to reduce the absorption of diclofenac.

DOSAGE AND ADMINISTRATION

Diclofenac may be administered as 50-mg Cataflam Immediate-Release Tablets, as 25-mg, 50-mg, and 75-mg Voltaren Delayed-Release Tablets, or as 100-mg Voltaren-XR Extended-Release Tablets. Cataflam Immediate-Release Tablets is the formulation indicated for management of acute pain and primary dysmenorrhea when prompt onset of pain relief is desired because of earlier absorption of diclofenac. For the same reason, Voltaren-XR is not indicated for the management of acute painful conditions and should be used as chronic therapy in patients with osteoarthritis and rheumatoid arthritis.

The dosage of diclofenac should be individualized to the lowest effective dose to minimize adverse effects (see INDIVIDUALIZATION OF DOSAGE).

Osteoarthritis: The recommended dosage is 100 to 150 mg/day: Cataflam or Voltaren Delayed-Release 50 mg b.i.d. or t.i.d; or Voltaren Delayed-Release 75 mg b.i.d. The recommended dosage for chronic therapy with Voltaren-XR is 100 mg q.d. Dosages of Voltaren-XR Extended Release Tablets of 200 mg daily are not recommended for patients with osteoarthritis. Dosages above 200 mg/day have not been studied in patients with osteoarthritis.

Rheumatoid Arthritis: The recommended dosage is 100 to 200 mg/day: Cataflam or Voltaren Delayed-Release 50 mg t.i.d. or q.i.d.; or Voltaren Delayed-Release 75 mg b.i.d. The recommended dosage for chronic therapy with Voltaren-XR is 100 mg q.d. In the rare patient where Voltaren-XR 100 mg/day is unsatisfactory, the dose may be increased to 100 mg b.i.d. if the benefits outweigh the clinical risks. Dosages above 225 mg/day are not recommended in patients with rheumatoid arthritis.

Ankylosing Spondylitis: The recommended dosage is 100 to 125 mg/day: Voltaren 25 mg q.i.d. with an extra 25-mg dose at bedtime if necessary. Dosages above 125 mg/day have not been studied in patients with ankylosing spondylitis.

Analgesia and Primary Dysmenorrhea: The recommended starting dose of Cataflam Immediate-Release Tablets is 50 mg t.i.d. With experience, physicians may find that in some patients an initial dose of 100 mg of Cataflam, followed by 50-mg doses, will provide better relief. After the first day, when the maximum recommended dose may be 200 mg, the total daily dose should generally not exceed 150 mg.

HOW SUPPLIED

Cataflam Tablets

50 mg–light brown, round, biconvex (imprinted CATAFLAM on one side and 50 on the other side)
Bottles of 100 .... NDC 0028-0151-01
Unit Dose (blister pack)
Box of 100 (strips of 10) .... NDC 0028-0151-61

Voltaren *Delayed-Release* Tablets

25 mg–yellow, biconvex, triangular-shaped (imprinted VOLTAREN 25 on one side)
Bottles of 60 .... NDC 0028-0258-60
Bottles of 100 .... NDC 0028-0258-01
Unit Dose (blister pack)
Box of 100 (strips of 10) .... NDC 0028-0258-61

50 mg–light brown, biconvex, triangular-shaped (imprinted VOLTAREN 50 on one side)
Bottles of 60 .... NDC 0028-0262-60
Bottles of 100 .... NDC 0028-0262-01
Bottles of 1000 .... NDC 0028-0262-10
Unit Dose (blister pack)
Box of 100 (strips of 10) .... NDC 0028-0262-61

75 mg–light pink, biconvex, triangular-shaped (imprinted VOLTAREN 75 on one side)
Bottles of 60 .... NDC 0028-0264-60
Bottles of 100 .... NDC 0028-0264-01
Bottles of 1000 .... NDC 0028-0264-10
Unit Dose (blister pack)
Box of 100 (strips of 10) .... NDC 0028-0264-61

Voltaren-XR *Extended-Release* Tablets

100 mg–light pink, coated, round, biconvex, with beveled edges (imprinted Voltaren-XR on one side and 100 on the other side)
Bottles of 100 .... NDC 0028-0205-01
Unit Dose (blister pack)
Box of 100 (strips of 10) .... NDC 0028-0205-61

Do not store above 86°F (30°C). Protect from moisture. Dispense in ***tight*** container (USP).

C96-10 (Rev. 2/96)

Dist. by:
Ciba-Geigy Corporation
Pharmaceuticals Division
Ardsley, New York 10502
Shown in Product Identification Guide, pages 324 and 326

CLOZARIL® ℞

[*klō 'ză-ril*]
(clozapine) Tablets

Caution: Federal law prohibits dispensing without prescription.

The following prescribing information is based on official labeling in effect on August 1, 1998.

DESCRIPTION

CLOZARIL® (clozapine), an atypical antipsychotic drug, is a tricyclic dibenzodiazepine derivative, 8-chloro-11-(4-methyl-1-piperazinyl)-5*H*-dibenzo [*b,e*] [1,4] diazepine.
The structural formula is:

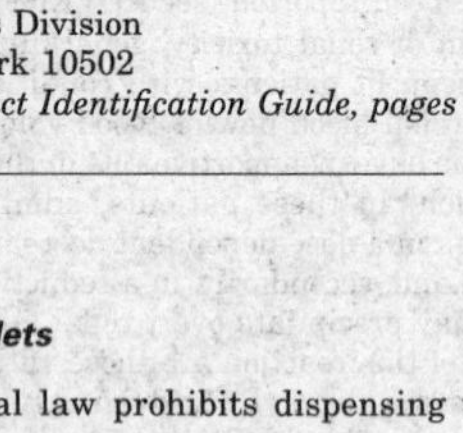

$C_{18}H_{19}ClN_4$ Mol. wt. 326.83

CLOZARIL® (clozapine) is available in pale yellow tablets of 25 mg and 100 mg for oral administration.

25 mg and 100 mg Tablets

Active Ingredient: clozapine is a yellow, crystalline powder, very slightly soluble in water.

Inactive Ingredients: colloidal silicon dioxide, NF; lactose, NF; magnesium stearate, NF; povidone, USP; starch, NF; and talc, USP.

CLINICAL PHARMACOLOGY

Pharmacodynamics

CLOZARIL® (clozapine) is classified as an 'atypical' antipsychotic drug because its profile of binding to dopamine receptors and its effects on various dopamine mediated behaviors differ from those exhibited by more typical antipsychotic drug products. In particular, although CLOZARIL® (clozapine) does interfere with the binding of dopamine at D_1, D_2, D_3 and D_5 receptors, and has a high affinity for the D_4 receptor, it does not induce catalepsy nor inhibit apomorphine-induced stereotypy. This evidence, consistent with the view that CLOZARIL® (clozapine) is preferentially more active at limbic than at striatal dopamine receptors, may explain the relative freedom of CLOZARIL® (clozapine) from extrapyramidal side effects.

CLOZARIL® (clozapine) also acts as an antagonist at adrenergic, cholinergic, histaminergic and serotonergic receptors.

Absorption, Distribution, Metabolism and Excretion

In man, CLOZARIL® (clozapine) tablets (25 mg and 100 mg) are equally bioavailable relative to a clozapine solution. Following a dosage of 100 mg b.i.d., the average steady state peak plasma concentration was 319 ng/mL (range: 102-771 ng/mL), occurring at the average of 2.5 hours (range: 1-6 hours) after dosing. The average minimum concentration at steady state was 122 ng/mL (range: 41-343 ng/mL), after 100 mg b.i.d. dosing. Food does not appear to affect the systemic bioavailability of CLOZARIL® (clozapine). Thus, CLOZARIL® (clozapine) may be administered with or without food.

Clozapine is approximately 97% bound to serum proteins. The interaction between CLOZARIL® (clozapine) and other highly protein-bound drugs has not been fully evaluated but may be important. *(See PRECAUTIONS)*

Clozapine is almost completely metabolized prior to excretion and only trace amounts of unchanged drug are detected in the urine and feces. Approximately 50% of the administered dose is excreted in the urine and 30% in the feces. The demethylated, hydroxylated and N-oxide derivatives are components in both urine and feces. Pharmacological testing has shown the desmethyl metabolite to have only limited activity, while the hydroxylated and N-oxide derivatives were inactive.

The mean elimination half-life of clozapine after a single 75 mg dose was 8 hours (range: 4-12 hours), compared to a mean elimination half-life, after achieving steady state with 100 mg b.i.d. dosing, of 12 hours (range: 4-66 hours). A comparison of single-dose and multiple-dose administration of clozapine showed that the elimination half-life increased significantly after multiple dosing relative to that after single-dose administration, suggesting the possibility of concentration dependent pharmacokinetics. However, at steady state, linearly dose-proportional changes with respect to AUC (area under the curve), peak and minimum clozapine plasma concentrations were observed after administration of 37.5 mg, 75 mg, and 150 mg b.i.d.

Human Pharmacology

In contrast to more typical antipsychotic drugs, CLOZARIL® (clozapine) therapy produces little or no prolactin elevation.

As is true of more typical antipsychotic drugs, clinical EEG studies have shown that CLOZARIL® (clozapine) increases delta and theta activity and slows dominant alpha frequencies. Enhanced synchronization occurs, and sharp wave activity and spike and wave complexes may also develop. Patients, on rare occasions, may report an intensification of dream activity during CLOZARIL® (clozapine) therapy. REM sleep was found to be increased to 85% of the total sleep time. In these patients, the onset of REM sleep occurred almost immediately after falling asleep.

INDICATIONS AND USAGE

CLOZARIL® (clozapine) is indicated for the management of severely ill schizophrenic patients who fail to respond adequately to standard antipsychotic drug treatment. Because of the significant risk of agranulocytosis and seizure associated with its use, CLOZARIL® (clozapine) should be used only in patients who have failed to respond adequately to treatment with appropriate courses of standard antipsychotic drugs, either because of insufficient effectiveness or the inability to achieve an effective dose due to intolerable adverse effects from those drugs. *(See WARNINGS)*

The effectiveness of CLOZARIL® (clozapine) in a treatment resistant schizophrenic population was demonstrated in a 6-week study comparing CLOZARIL® (clozapine) and chlorpromazine. Patients meeting DSM-III criteria for schizophrenia and having a mean BPRS total score of 61 were demonstrated to be treatment resistant by history and by open, prospective treatment with haloperidol before entering into the double-blind phase of the study. The superiority of CLOZARIL® (clozapine) to chlorpromazine was documented in statistical analyses employing both categorical and continuous measures of treatment effect.

Because of the significant risk of agranulocytosis and seizure, events which both present a continuing risk over time, the extended treatment of patients failing to show an acceptable level of clinical response should ordinarily be avoided. In addition, the need for continuing treatment in patients exhibiting beneficial clinical responses should be periodically re-evaluated.

CONTRAINDICATIONS

CLOZARIL® (clozapine) is contraindicated in patients with a previous hypersensitivity to clozapine or any other component of this drug, in patients with myeloproliferative disorders, uncontrolled epilepsy, or a history of CLOZARIL® (clozapine) induced agranulocytosis or severe granulocytopenia. As with more typical antipsychotic drugs, CLOZARIL® (clozapine) is contraindicated in severe central nervous system depression or comatose states from any cause.

CLOZARIL® (clozapine) should not be used simultaneously with other agents having a well-known potential to cause agranulocytosis or otherwise suppress bone marrow function. The mechanism of CLOZARIL® (clozapine) induced agranulocytosis is unknown; nonetheless, it is possible that causative factors may interact synergistically to increase the risk and/or severity of bone marrow suppression.

WARNINGS

General

BECAUSE OF THE SIGNIFICANT RISK OF AGRANULOCYTOSIS, A POTENTIALLY LIFE-THREATENING ADVERSE EVENT *(SEE FOLLOWING)*, CLOZARIL® (clozapine) SHOULD BE RESERVED FOR USE IN THE TREATMENT OF SEVERELY ILL SCHIZOPHRENIC PATIENTS WHO FAIL TO SHOW AN ACCEPTABLE RESPONSE TO ADEQUATE COURSES OF STANDARD ANTIPSYCHOTIC DRUG TREATMENT, EITHER BECAUSE OF INSUFFICIENT EFFECTIVENESS OR THE INABILITY TO ACHIEVE AN EFFECTIVE DOSE DUE TO INTOLERABLE ADVERSE EFFECTS FROM THOSE DRUGS. CONSEQUENTLY, BEFORE INITIATING TREATMENT WITH CLOZARIL® (clozapine), IT IS STRONGLY RECOMMENDED THAT A PATIENT BE GIVEN AT LEAST 2 TRIALS, EACH WITH A DIFFERENT STANDARD ANTIPSYCHOTIC DRUG PRODUCT, AT AN ADEQUATE DOSE, AND FOR AN ADEQUATE DURATION.

PATIENTS WHO ARE BEING TREATED WITH CLOZARIL® (clozapine) MUST HAVE A BASELINE WHITE BLOOD CELL (WBC) AND DIFFERENTIAL COUNT BEFORE INITIATION OF TREATMENT, AND A WBC COUNT EVERY WEEK FOR THE FIRST SIX MONTHS. THEREAFTER, IF ACCEPTABLE WBC COUNTS (WBC greater than or equal to 3,000/mm^3, ANC ≥1500/mm^3) HAVE BEEN MAINTAINED DURING THE FIRST 6 MONTHS OF CONTINUOUS THERAPY, WBC COUNTS CAN BE MONITORED EVERY OTHER WEEK. WBC COUNTS MUST BE MONITORED WEEKLY FOR AT LEAST 4 WEEKS AFTER THE DISCONTINUATION OF CLOZARIL® (clozapine).

CLOZARIL® (clozapine) IS AVAILABLE ONLY THROUGH A DISTRIBUTION SYSTEM THAT ENSURES MONITORING OF WBC COUNTS ACCORDING TO THE SCHEDULE DESCRIBED BELOW PRIOR TO DELIVERY OF THE NEXT SUPPLY OF MEDICATION.

Agranulocytosis

Agranulocytosis, defined as an absolute neutrophil count (ANC) of less than 500/mm^3, has been estimated to occur in association with CLOZARIL® (clozapine) use at a cumulative incidence at 1 year of approximately 1.3%, based on the occurrence of 15 US cases out of 1743 patients exposed to CLOZARIL® (clozapine) during its clinical testing prior to domestic marketing. All of these cases occurred at a time when the need for close monitoring of WBC counts was already recognized. This reaction could prove fatal if not detected early and therapy interrupted. Of the 149 cases of agranulocytosis reported worldwide in association with CLOZARIL® (clozapine) use as of December 31, 1989, 32% were fatal. However, few of these deaths occurred since 1977, at which time the knowledge of CLOZARIL® (clozapine) induced agranulocytosis became more widespread, and close monitoring of WBC counts more widely practiced. Nevertheless, it is unknown at present what the case fatality rate will be for CLOZARIL® (clozapine) induced agranulocytosis, despite strict adherence to the required frequency of monitoring. In the U.S., under a weekly WBC monitoring system with CLOZARIL® (clozapine), there have been 585 cases of agranulocytosis as of August 21, 1997; 19 were fatal. During this period 150, 409 patients received CLOZARIL® (clozapine). A hematologic risk analysis was conducted based upon the available information in the Clozaril® National Registry (CNR) for U.S. patients. Based upon a cut-off date of April 30, 1995, the incidence rates of agranulocytosis based upon a weekly monitoring schedule, rose steeply during the first two months of therapy, peaking in the third month. Among Clozaril® (clozapine) patients who continued the drug beyond the third month, the weekly incidence of agranulocytosis fell to a substantial degree, so that by the sixth month the weekly incidence of agranulocytosis was reduced to 3 per 1000 person-years. After six months, the weekly incidence of agranulocytosis declines still further, however, never reaches zero. It should be noted that any type of reduction in the frequency of monitoring WBC counts may result in an increase incidence of agranulocytosis.

Because of the substantial risk for developing agranulocytosis in association with CLOZARIL® (clozapine) use, which may persist over an extended period of time, patients must have a blood sample drawn for a WBC count before initiation of treatment with CLOZARIL® (clozapine), and must have subsequent WBC counts done at least weekly for the first 6 months of continuous treatment. If WBC counts remain acceptable (WBC greater than or equal to 3000/mm^3, ANC ≥1500/mm^3) during this period, WBC counts may be monitored every other week thereafter. After discontinuation of CLOZARIL® (clozapine), weekly WBC counts should be continued for an additional 4 weeks. If a patient is on CLOZARIL® (clozapine) therapy for less than 6 months with no abnormal blood events and there is a break on therapy which is less than or equal to 1 month, then patients can continue where they left off with weekly WBC testing for 6 months. When this 6 month period has been completed, the frequency of WBC count monitoring can be reduced to every other week. If a patient is on CLOZARIL® (clozapine) therapy for less than 6 months with no abnormal blood events and there is a break on therapy which is greater than 1 month, then patients should be tested weekly for an additional 6 month period before biweekly testing is initiated. If a patient is on CLOZARIL® (clozapine) therapy for less than 6 months and experiences an abnormal blood event as described below but remains a rechallengeable patient [patients cannot be reinitiated on CLOZARIL® (clozapine) therapy if WBC counts fall below 2000/mm^3 or the ANC falls below 1000/mm^3 during CLOZARIL® (clozapine) therapy], the patient must re-start the 6 month period of weekly WBC monitoring at day 0.

If a patient is on CLOZARIL® (clozapine) therapy for 6 months or longer with no abnormal blood events and there is a break on therapy which is 1 year or less, then the patient can continue WBC count monitoring every other week if CLOZARIL® (clozapine) therapy is reinitiated. If a patient is on CLOZARIL® (clozapine) therapy for 6 months or longer with no abnormal blood events and there is a break on therapy which is greater than 1 year, then, if CLOZARIL® (clozapine) therapy is reinitiated, the patient must have WBC counts monitored weekly for an additional 6 months. If a patient on CLOZARIL® (clozapine) therapy for 6 months or longer and subsequently has an abnormal blood event, but remains a rechallengeable patient, then the patient must re-start weekly WBC count monitoring until an additional 6 months of CLOZARIL® (clozapine) therapy has been received. The distribution of CLOZARIL® (clozapine) is contingent upon performance of the required blood tests.

Treatment should not be initiated if the WBC count is less than 3500/mm^3, or if the patient has a history of a myeloproliferative disorder, or previous CLOZARIL® (clozapine) induced agranulocytosis or granulocytopenia. Patients should be advised to report immediately the appearance of lethargy, weakness, fever, sore throat or any other signs of infection. If, after the initiation of treatment, the total WBC count has dropped below 3500/mm^3 or it has dropped by a substantial amount from baseline, even if the count is above 3500/mm^3, or if immature forms are present, a repeat WBC count and a differential count should be done. A substantial drop is defined as a single drop of 3,000 or more in the WBC count or a cumulative drop of 3,000 or more within 3 weeks. If subsequent WBC counts and the differential count reveal a total WBC count between 3000 and 3500/mm^3 and an ANC above 1500/mm^3, twice weekly WBC counts and differential counts should be performed.

If the total WBC count falls below 3000/mm^3 or the ANC below 1500/mm^3, CLOZARIL® (clozapine) therapy should be interrupted, WBC count and differential should be performed daily, and patients should be carefully monitored for flu-like symptoms or other symptoms suggestive of infection. CLOZARIL® (clozapine) therapy may be resumed if no symptoms of infection develop, and if the total WBC count returns to levels above 3000/mm^3 and the ANC returns to levels above 1500/mm^3. However, in this event, twice-weekly WBC counts and differential counts should continue until total WBC counts return to levels above 3500/mm^3.

Continued on next page

Clozaril—Cont.

If the total WBC count falls below 2000/mm³ or the ANC falls below 1000/mm³, bone marrow aspiration should be considered to ascertain granulopoietic status. Protective isolation with close observation may be indicated if granulopoiesis is determined to be deficient. Should evidence of infection develop, the patient should have appropriate cultures performed and an appropriate antibiotic regimen instituted.

Patients whose total WBC counts fall below 2000/mm³, or ANCs below 1000/mm³ during CLOZARIL® (clozapine) therapy should have daily WBC count and differential. These patients should not be re-challenged with CLOZARIL® (clozapine). Patients discontinued from CLOZARIL® (clozapine) therapy due to significant WBC suppression have been found to develop agranulocytosis upon rechallenge, often with a shorter latency on re-exposure. To reduce the chances of rechallenge occurring in patients who have experienced significant bone marrow suppression during CLOZARIL® (clozapine) therapy, a single, national master file will be maintained confidentially.

Except for evidence of significant bone marrow suppression during initial CLOZARIL® (clozapine) therapy, there are no established risk factors, based on worldwide experience, for the development of agranulocytosis in association with CLOZARIL® (clozapine) use. However, a disproportionate number of the US cases of agranulocytosis occurred in patients of Jewish background compared to the overall proportion of such patients exposed during domestic development of CLOZARIL® (clozapine). Most of the US cases occurred within 4-10 weeks of exposure, but neither dose nor duration is a reliable predictor of this problem. No patient characteristics have been clearly linked to the development of agranulocytosis in association with CLOZARIL® (clozapine) use, but agranulocytosis associated with other antipsychotic drugs has been reported to occur with a greater frequency in women, the elderly and in patients who are cachectic or have serious underlying medical illness; such patients may also be at particular risk with CLOZARIL® (clozapine). To reduce the risk of agranulocytosis developing undetected, CLOZARIL® (clozapine) is available only through a distribution system that ensures monitoring of WBC counts according to the schedule described above prior to delivery of the next supply of medication.

Interrupted Therapy (WBC <3000/mm³ ANC <1500/mm³) for Bi-Weekly Monitoring

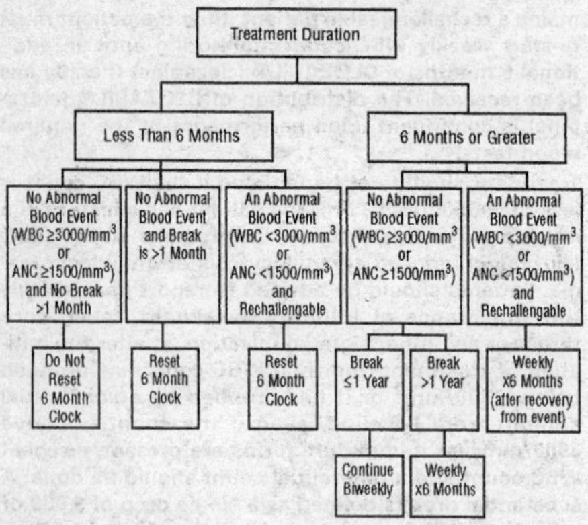

Eosinophilia

In clinical trials, 1% of patients developed eosinophilia, which, in rare cases, can be substantial. If a differential count reveals a total eosinophil count above 4,000/mm³, CLOZARIL® (clozapine) therapy should be interrupted until the eosinophil count falls below 3,000/mm³.

Seizures

Seizure has been estimated to occur in association with CLOZARIL® (clozapine) use at a cumulative incidence at one year of approximately 5%, based on the occurrence of one or more seizures in 61 of 1743 patients exposed to CLOZARIL® (clozapine) during its clinical testing prior to domestic marketing (i.e., crude rate of 3.5%). Dose appears to be an important predictor of seizure, with a greater likelihood of seizure at the higher CLOZARIL® (clozapine) doses used.

Caution should be used in administering CLOZARIL® (clozapine) to patients having a history of seizures or other predisposing factors. Because of the substantial risk of seizure associated with CLOZARIL® (clozapine) use, patients should be advised not to engage in any activity where sudden loss of consciousness could cause serious risk to themselves or others, e.g., the operation of complex machinery, driving an automobile, swimming, climbing, etc.

Adverse Cardiovascular and Respiratory Effects

Orthostatic hypotension with or without syncope can occur with CLOZARIL® (clozapine) treatment and may represent a continuing risk in some patients. Rarely (approximately 1 case per 3,000 patients), collapse can be profound and be accompanied by respiratory and/or cardiac arrest. Orthostatic hypotension is more likely to occur during initial titration in association with rapid dose escalation and may even occur on first dose. In one report, initial doses as low as 12.5 mg were associated with collapse and respiratory arrest. When restarting patients who have had even a brief interval off CLOZARIL® (clozapine), i.e., 2 days or more since the last dose, it is recommended that treatment be reinitiated with one-half of a 25 mg tablet (12.5 mg) once or twice daily *(see DOSAGE AND ADMINISTRATION)*.

Some of the cases of collapse/respiratory arrest/cardiac arrest during initial treatment occurred in patients who were being administered benzodiazepines; similar events have been reported in patients taking other psychotropic drugs or even CLOZARIL® (clozapine) by itself. Although it has not been established that there is an interaction between CLOZARIL® (clozapine) and benzodiazepines or other psychotropics, caution is advised when clozapine is initiated in patients taking a benzodiazepine or any other psychotropic drug.

Tachycardia, which may be sustained, has also been observed in approximately 25% of patients taking CLOZARIL® (clozapine), with patients having an average increase in pulse rate of 10-15 bpm. The sustained tachycardia is not simply a reflex response to hypotension, and is present in all positions monitored. Either tachycardia or hypotension may pose a serious risk for an individual with compromised cardiovascular function.

A minority of CLOZARIL® (clozapine) treated patients experience ECG repolarization changes similar to those seen with other antipsychotic drugs, including S-T segment depression and flattening or inversion of T waves, which all normalize after discontinuation of CLOZARIL® (clozapine). The clinical significance of these changes is unclear. However, in clinical trials with CLOZARIL® (clozapine), several patients experienced significant cardiac events, including ischemic changes, myocardial infarction, arrhythmias and sudden death. In addition there have been postmarketing reports of congestive heart failure, myocarditis, with or without eosinophilia, and pericarditis/pericardial effusions in association with CLOZARIL® (clozapine) use. Causality assessment was difficult in many of these cases because of serious preexisting cardiac disease and plausible alternative causes. Rare instances of sudden death have been reported in psychiatric patients, with or without associated antipsychotic drug treatment, and the relationship of these events to antipsychotic drug use is unknown.

CLOZARIL® (clozapine) should be used with caution in patients with known cardiovascular and/or pulmonary disease, and the recommendation for gradual titration of dose should be carefully observed.

Neuroleptic Malignant Syndrome (NMS)

A potentially fatal symptom complex sometimes referred to as Neuroleptic Malignant Syndrome (NMS) has been reported in association with antipsychotic drugs. Clinical manifestations of NMS are hyperpyrexia, muscle rigidity, altered mental status and evidence of autonomic instability (irregular pulse or blood pressure, tachycardia, diaphoresis, and cardiac dysrhythmias).

The diagnostic evaluation of patients with this syndrome is complicated. In arriving at a diagnosis, it is important to identify cases where the clinical presentation includes both serious medical illness (e.g., pneumonia, systemic infection, etc.) and untreated or inadequately treated extrapyramidal signs and symptoms (EPS). Other important considerations in the differential diagnosis include central anticholinergic toxicity, heat stroke, drug fever and primary central nervous system (CNS) pathology.

The management of NMS should include 1) immediate discontinuation of antipsychotic drugs and other drugs not essential to concurrent therapy, 2) intensive symptomatic treatment and medical monitoring, and 3) treatment of any concomitant serious medical problems for which specific treatments are available. There is no general agreement about specific pharmacological treatment regimens for uncomplicated NMS.

If a patient requires antipsychotic drug treatment after recovery from NMS, the potential reintroduction of drug therapy should be carefully considered. The patient should be carefully monitored, since recurrences of NMS have been reported.

There have been several reported cases of NMS in patients receiving CLOZARIL® (clozapine) alone or in combination with lithium or other CNS-active agents.

Tardive Dyskinesia

A syndrome consisting of potentially irreversible, involuntary, dyskinetic movements may develop in patients treated with antipsychotic drugs. Although the prevalence of the syndrome appears to be highest among the elderly, especially elderly women, it is impossible to rely upon prevalence estimates to predict, at the inception of treatment, which patients are likely to develop the syndrome.

There are several reasons for predicting that CLOZARIL® (clozapine) may be different from other antipsychotic drugs in its potential for inducing tardive dyskinesia, including the preclinical finding that it has a relatively weak dopamine blocking effect and the clinical finding of a virtual absence of certain acute extrapyramidal symptoms, e.g., dystonia. A few cases of tardive dyskinesia have been reported in patients on CLOZARIL® (clozapine) who had been previously treated with other antipsychotic agents, so that a causal relationship cannot be established. There have been no reports of tardive dyskinesia directly attributable to CLOZARIL® (clozapine) alone. Nevertheless, it cannot be concluded, without more extended experience, that CLOZARIL® (clozapine) is incapable of inducing this syndrome.

Both the risk of developing the syndrome and the likelihood that it will become irreversible are believed to increase as the duration of treatment and the total cumulative dose of antipsychotic drugs administered to the patient increase. However, the syndrome can develop, although much less commonly, after relatively brief treatment periods at low doses. There is no known treatment for established cases of tardive dyskinesia, although the syndrome may remit, partially or completely, if antipsychotic drug treatment is withdrawn. Antipsychotic drug treatment, itself, however, may suppress (or partially suppress) the signs and symptoms of the syndrome and thereby may possibly mask the underlying process. The effect that symptom suppression has upon the long-term course of the syndrome is unknown.

Given these considerations, CLOZARIL® (clozapine) should be prescribed in a manner that is most likely to minimize the occurrence of tardive dyskinesia. As with any antipsychotic drug, chronic CLOZARIL® (clozapine) use should be reserved for patients who appear to be obtaining substantial benefit from the drug. In such patients, the smallest dose and the shortest duration of treatment should be sought. The need for continued treatment should be reassessed periodically.

If signs and symptoms of tardive dyskinesia appear in a patient on CLOZARIL® (clozapine), drug discontinuation should be considered. However, some patients may require treatment with CLOZARIL® (clozapine) despite the presence of the syndrome.

PRECAUTIONS

General

Because of the significant risk of agranulocytosis and seizure, both of which present a continuing risk over time, the extended treatment of patients failing to show an acceptable level of clinical response should ordinarily be avoided. In addition, the need for continuing treatment in patients exhibiting beneficial clinical responses should be periodically re-evaluated. Although it is not known whether the risk would be increased, it is prudent either to avoid CLOZARIL® (clozapine) or use it cautiously in patients with a previous history of agranulocytosis induced by other drugs.

Fever

During CLOZARIL® (clozapine) therapy, patients may experience transient temperature elevations above 100.4°F (38°C), with the peak incidence within the first 3 weeks of treatment. While this fever is generally benign and self limiting, it may necessitate discontinuing patients from treatment. On occasion, there may be an associated increase or decrease in WBC count. Patients with fever should be carefully evaluated to rule out the possibility of an underlying infectious process or the development of agranulocytosis. In the presence of high fever, the possibility of Neuroleptic Malignant Syndrome (NMS) must be considered. There have been several reports of NMS in patients receiving CLOZARIL® (clozapine), usually in combination with lithium or other CNS-active drugs. *[See Neuroleptic Malignant Syndrome (NMS), under WARNINGS]*

Pulmonary Embolism

The possibility of pulmonary embolism should be considered in patients receiving CLOZARIL® (clozapine) who present with deep vein thrombosis, acute dyspnea, chest pain or with other respiratory signs and symptoms. As of December 31, 1993 there were 18 cases of fatal pulmonary embolism in association with CLOZARIL® (clozapine) therapy in users

10-54 years of age. Based upon the extent of use observed in the Clozaril National Registry, the mortality rate associated with pulmonary embolus was 1 death per 3450 person-years of use. This rate was about 27.5 times higher than that in the general population of a similar age and gender (95% Confidence Interval; 17.1,42.2). Deep vein thrombosis has also been observed in association with CLOZARIL® (clozapine) therapy. Whether pulmonary embolus can be attributed to CLOZARIL® (clozapine) or some characteristic(s) of its users is not clear, but the occurrence of deep vein thrombosis or respiratory symptomatology should suggest its presence.

Hyperglycemia

Severe hyperglycemia, sometimes leading to ketoacidosis, has been reported during CLOZARIL® (clozapine) treatment in patients with no prior history of hyperglycemia. While a causal relationship to CLOZARIL® (clozapine) use has not been definitively established, glucose levels normalized in most patients after discontinuation of CLOZARIL® (clozapine), and a rechallenge in one patient produced a recurrence of hyperglycemia. The effect of CLOZARIL® (clozapine) on glucose metabolism in patients with diabetes mellitus has not been studied. The possibility of impaired glucose tolerance should be considered in patients receiving CLOZARIL® (clozapine) who develop symptoms of hyperglycemia, such as polydipsia, polyuria, polyphagia, and weakness. In patients with significant treatment-emergent hyperglycemia, the discontinuation of CLOZARIL® (clozapine) should be considered.

Hepatitis

Caution is advised in patients using CLOZARIL® (clozapine) who have concurrent hepatic disease. Hepatitis has been reported in both patients with normal and pre-existing liver function abnormalities. In patients who develop nausea, vomiting, and/or anorexia during CLOZARIL® (clozapine) treatment, liver function tests should be performed immediately. If the elevation of these values is clinically relevant or if symptoms of jaundice occur, treatment with CLOZARIL® (clozapine) should be discontinued.

Anticholinergic Toxicity

CLOZARIL® (clozapine) has very potent anticholinergic effects and great care should be exercised in using this drug in the presence of prostatic enlargement or narrow angle glaucoma. In addition, CLOZARIL® (clozapine) use has been associated with varying degrees of impairment of intestinal peristalsis, ranging from constipation to intestinal obstruction, fecal impaction and paralytic ileus *(see ADVERSE REACTIONS)*. On rare occasions, these cases have been fatal. Constipation should be initially treated by ensuring adequate hydration, and use of ancillary therapy such as bulk laxatives. Consultation with a gastroenterologist is advisable in more serious cases.

Interference with Cognitive and Motor Performance

Because of initial sedation, CLOZARIL® (clozapine) may impair mental and/or physical abilities, especially during the first few days of therapy. The recommendations for gradual dose escalation should be carefully adhered to, and patients cautioned about activities requiring alertness.

Use in Patients with Concomitant Illness

Clinical experience with CLOZARIL® (clozapine) in patients with concomitant systemic diseases is limited. Nevertheless, caution is advisable in using CLOZARIL® (clozapine) in patients with renal or cardiac disease.

Use in Patients Undergoing General Anesthesia

Caution is advised in patients being administered general anesthesia because of the CNS effects of CLOZARIL® (clozapine). Check with the anesthesiologist regarding continuation of CLOZARIL® (clozapine) therapy in a patient scheduled for surgery.

Information for Patients

Physicians are advised to discuss the following issues with patients for whom they prescribe CLOZARIL® (clozapine):

— Patients who are to receive CLOZARIL® (clozapine) should be warned about the significant risk of developing agranulocytosis. They should be informed that weekly blood tests are required for the first 6 months, if acceptable WBC counts (WBC greater than or equal to 3000/mm^3, ANC $\geq$ 1500/mm^3) have been maintained during the first 6 months of continuous therapy, then WBC counts can be monitored every other week in order to monitor for the occurrence of agranulocytosis, and that CLOZARIL® (clozapine) tablets will be made available only through a special program designed to ensure the required blood monitoring. Patients should be advised to report immediately the appearance of lethargy, weakness, fever, sore throat, malaise, mucous membrane ulceration or other possible signs of infection. Particular attention should be paid to any flu-like complaints or other symptoms that might suggest infection.

— Patients should be informed of the significant risk of seizure during CLOZARIL® (clozapine) treatment, and they should be advised to avoid driving and any other potentially hazardous activity while taking CLOZARIL® (clozapine).

— Patients should be advised of the risk of orthostatic hypotension, especially during the period of initial dose titration.

— Patients should be informed that if they stop taking CLOZARIL® (clozapine) for more than 2 days, they should not restart their medication at the same dosage, but should contact their physician for dosing instructions.

— Patients should notify their physician if they are taking, or plan to take, any prescription or over-the-counter drugs or alcohol.

— Patients should notify their physician if they become pregnant or intend to become pregnant during therapy.

— Patients should not breast feed an infant if they are taking CLOZARIL® (clozapine).

Drug Interactions

The risks of using CLOZARIL® (clozapine) in combination with other drugs have not been systematically evaluated. The mechanism of CLOZARIL® (clozapine) induced agranulocytosis is unknown; nonetheless, the possibility that causative factors may interact synergistically to increase the risk and/or severity of bone marrow suppression warrants consideration. Therefore, CLOZARIL® (clozapine) should not be used with other agents having a well-known potential to suppress bone marrow function.

Given the primary CNS effects of CLOZARIL® (clozapine), caution is advised in using it concomitantly with other CNS-active drugs or alcohol.

Orthostatic hypotension in patients taking clozapine can, in rare cases (approximately 1 case per 3,000 patients), be accompanied by profound collapse and respiratory and/or cardiac arrest. Some of the cases of collapse/respiratory arrest/cardiac arrest during initial treatment occurred in patients who were being administered benzodiazepines; similar events have been reported in patients taking other psychotropic drugs or even CLOZARIL® (clozapine) by itself. Although it has not been established that there is an interaction between CLOZARIL® (clozapine) and benzodiazepines or other psychotropics, caution is advised when clozapine is initiated in patients taking a benzodiazepine or any other psychotropic drug.

Because CLOZARIL® (clozapine) is highly bound to serum protein, the administration of CLOZARIL® (clozapine) to a patient taking another drug which is highly bound to protein (e.g., warfarin, digitoxin) may cause an increase in plasma concentrations of these drugs, potentially resulting in adverse effects. Conversely, adverse effects may result from displacement of protein-bound CLOZARIL® (clozapine) by other highly bound drugs.

Cimetidine and erythromycin may both increase plasma levels of CLOZARIL® (clozapine), potentially resulting in adverse effects. Although concomitant use of CLOZARIL® (clozapine) and carbamazepine is not recommended, it should be noted that discontinuation of concomitant carbamazepine administration may result in an increase in CLOZARIL® (clozapine) plasma levels. Phenytoin may decrease CLOZARIL® (clozapine) plasma levels, resulting in a decrease in effectiveness of a previously effective CLOZARIL® (clozapine) dose.

Elevated serum levels of clozapine have been observed when CLOZARIL® (clozapine) is administered with selective serotonin reuptake inhibitors (SSRI's), e.g. fluoxetine and fluvoxamine. Therefore, such combined treatment should be approached with caution and patients should be monitored closely when CLOZARIL® (clozapine) is combined with an SSRI. A reduced CLOZARIL® (clozapine) dose should be considered.

A subset (3%-10%) of the population has reduced activity of certain drug metabolizing enzymes such as the cytochrome P450 isozyme P450 2D6. Such individuals are referred to as "poor metabolizers" of drugs such as debrisoquin, dextromethorphan, the tricyclic antidepressants, and clozapine. These individuals may develop higher than expected plasma concentrations of clozapine when given usual doses. In addition, certain drugs that are metabolized by this isozyme, including many antidepressants (clozapine, selective serotonin reuptake inhibitors, and others), may inhibit the activity of this isozyme, and thus may make normal metabolizers resemble poor metabolizers with regard to concomitant therapy with other drugs metabolized by this enzyme system, leading to drug interaction.

Concomitant use of clozapine with other drugs metabolized by cytochrome P450 2D6 may require lower doses than usually prescribed for either clozapine or the other drug. Therefore, co-administration of clozapine with other drugs that are metabolized by this isozyme, including antidepressants, phenothiazines, carbamazepine, and Type 1C antiarrhythmics (e.g., propafenone, flecainide and encainide), or that inhibit this enzyme (e.g., quinidine), should be approached with caution.

CLOZARIL® (clozapine) may also potentiate the hypotensive effects of antihypertensive drugs and the anticholinergic effects of atropine-type drugs. The administration of epinephrine should be avoided in the treatment of drug induced hypotension because of a possible reverse epinephrine effect.

Carcinogenesis, Mutagenesis, Impairment of Fertility

No carcinogenic potential was demonstrated in long-term studies in mice and rats at doses approximately 7 times the typical human dose on a mg/kg basis. Fertility in male and female rats was not adversely affected by clozapine. Clozapine did not produce genotoxic or mutagenic effects when assayed in appropriate bacterial and mammalian tests.

Pregnancy Category B

Reproduction studies have been performed in rats and rabbits at doses of approximately 2-4 times the human dose and have revealed no evidence of impaired fertility or harm to the fetus due to clozapine. There are, however, no adequate and well-controlled studies in pregnant women. Because animal reproduction studies are not always predictive of human response, and in view of the desirability of keeping the administration of all drugs to a minimum during pregnancy, this drug should be used only if clearly needed.

Nursing Mothers

Animal studies suggest that clozapine may be excreted in breast milk and have an effect on the nursing infant. Therefore, women receiving CLOZARIL® (clozapine) should not breast feed.

Pediatric Use

Safety and effectiveness in pediatric patients have not been established.

ADVERSE REACTIONS

Associated with Discontinuation of Treatment

Sixteen percent of 1080 patients who received CLOZARIL® (clozapine) in premarketing clinical trials discontinued treatment due to an adverse event, including both those that could be reasonably attributed to CLOZARIL® (clozapine) treatment and those that might more appropriately be considered intercurrent illness. The more common events considered to be causes of discontinuation included: CNS, primarily drowsiness/sedation, seizures, dizziness/syncope; cardiovascular, primarily tachycardia, hypotension and ECG changes; gastrointestinal, primarily nausea/vomiting; hematologic, primarily leukopenia/granulocytopenia/agranulocytosis; and fever. None of the events enumerated accounts for more than 1.7% of all discontinuations attributed to adverse clinical events.

Commonly Observed

Adverse events observed in association with the use of CLOZARIL® (clozapine) in clinical trials at an incidence of greater than 5% were: central nervous system complaints, including drowsiness/sedation, dizziness/vertigo, headache and tremor; autonomic nervous system complaints, including salivation, sweating, dry mouth and visual disturbances; cardiovascular findings, including tachycardia, hypotension and syncope; and gastrointestinal complaints, including constipation and nausea; and fever. Complaints of drowsiness/sedation tend to subside with continued therapy or dose reduction. Salivation may be profuse, especially during sleep, but may be diminished with dose reduction.

Incidence in Clinical Trials

The following table enumerates adverse events that occurred at a frequency of 1% or greater among CLOZARIL® (clozapine) patients who participated in clinical trials. These rates are not adjusted for duration of exposure.

Treatment-Emergent Adverse Experience Incidence Among Patients Taking CLOZARIL® (clozapine) in Clinical Trials (N = 842) (Percentage of Patients Reporting)

Body System Adverse Event[a]	Percent
Central Nervous System	
Drowsiness/Sedation	39
Dizziness/Vertigo	19
Headache	7
Tremor	6
Syncope	6
Disturbed sleep/Nightmares	4
Restlessness	4
Hypokinesia/Akinesia	4
Agitation	4
Seizures (convulsions)	3[b]
Rigidity	3
Akasthisia	3
Confusion	3
Fatigue	2
Insomnia	2
Hyperkinesia	1
Weakness	1
Lethargy	1
Ataxia	1
Slurred speech	1
Depression	1
Epileptiform movements/Myoclonic jerks	1
Anxiety	1

Continued on next page

Clozaril—Cont.

Cardiovascular

Tachycardia	25[b]
Hypotension	9
Hypertension	4
Chest pain/Angina	1
ECG change/Cardiac abnormality	1

Gastrointestinal

Constipation	14
Nausea	5
Abdomnial discomfort/Heartburn	4
Nausea/Vomiting	3
Vomiting	3
Diarrhea	2
Liver test abnormality	1
Anorexia	1

Urogenital

Urinary abnormalities	2
Incontinence	1
Abnormal ejaculation	1
Urinary urgency/frequency	1
Urinary retention	1

Autonomic Nervous System

Salivation	31
Sweating	6
Dry mouth	6
Visual disturbances	5

Integumentary (Skin)

Rash	2

Musculoskeletal

Muscle weakness	1
Pain (back, neck, legs)	1
Muscle spasm	1
Muscle pain, ache	1

Respiratory

Throat discomfort	1
Dyspnea, shortness of breath	1
Nasal congestion	1

Hemic/Lymphatic

Leukopenia/Decreased WBC/Neutropenia	3
Agranulocytosis	1[b]
Eosinophilia	1

Miscellaneous

Fever	5
Weight gain	4
Tongue numb/sore	1

[a] Events reported by at least 1% of CLOZARIL® (clozapine) patients are included.

[b] Rate based on population of approximately 1700 exposed during premarket clinical evaluation of CLOZARIL® (clozapine).

Other Events Observed During the Premarketing Evaluation of CLOZARIL® (clozapine)

This section reports additional, less frequent adverse events which occurred among the patients taking CLOZARIL® (clozapine) in clinical trials. Various adverse events were reported as part of the total experience in these clinical studies; a causal relationship to CLOZARIL® (clozapine) treatment cannot be determined in the absence of appropriate controls in some of the studies. The table above enumerates adverse events that occurred at a frequency of at least 1% of patients treated with CLOZARIL® (clozapine). The list below includes all additional adverse experiences reported as being temporally associated with the use of the drug which occurred at a frequency less than 1%, enumerated by organ system.

Central Nervous System: loss of speech, amentia, tics, poor coordination, delusions/hallucinations, involuntary movement, stuttering, dysarthria, amnesia/memory loss, histrionic movements, libido increase or decrease, paranoia, shakiness, Parkinsonism, and irritability.

Cardiovascular System: edema, palpitations, phlebitis/thrombophlebitis, cyanosis, premature ventricular contraction, bradycardia, and nose bleed.

Gastrointestinal System: abdominal distention, gastroenteritis, rectal bleeding, nervous stomach, abnormal stools, hematemesis, gastric ulcer, bitter taste, and eructation.

Urogenital System: dysmenorrhea, impotence, breast pain/discomfort, and vaginal itch/infection.

Autonomic Nervous System: numbness, polydypsia, hot flashes, dry throat, and mydriasis.

Integumentary (Skin): pruritus, pallor, eczema, erythema, bruise, dermatitis, petechiae, and urticaria.

Musculoskeletal System: twitching and joint pain.

Respiratory System: coughing, pneumonia/pneumonia-like symptoms, rhinorrhea, hyperventilation, wheezing, bronchitis, laryngitis, and sneezing.

Hemic and Lymphatic System: anemia and leukocytosis.

Miscellaneous: chills/chills with fever, malaise, appetite increase, ear disorder, hypothermia, eyelid disorder, bloodshot eyes, and nystagmus.

Postmarketing Clinical Experience

Postmarketing experience has shown an adverse experience profile similar to that presented above. Voluntary reports of adverse events temporally associated with CLOZARIL® (clozapine) not mentioned above that have been received since market introduction and that may have no causal relationship with the drug include the following:

Central Nervous System: delirium; EEG abnormal; exacerbation of psychosis; myoclonus; overdose; paresthesia; possible mild cataplexy; and status epilepticus.

Cardiovascular System: atrial or ventricular fibrillation and periorbital edema.

Gastrointestinal System: acute pancreatitis; dysphagia; fecal impaction; intestinal obstruction/paralytic ileus; and salivary gland swelling.

Hepatobiliary System: cholestasis; hepatitis; jaundice.

Hepatic System: cholestasis.

Urogenital System: acute interstitial nephritis and priapism.

Integumentary (Skin): hypersensitivity reactions: photosensitivity, vasculitis, erythema multiforme, and Stevens-Johnson Syndrome.

Musculoskeletal System: myasthenic syndrome and rhabdomyolysis.

Respiratory System: aspiration and pleural effusion.

Hemic and Lymphatic System: deep vein thrombosis; elevated hemoglobin/hematocrit; ESR increased; pulmonary embolism; sepsis; thrombocytosis; and thrombocytopenia.

Miscellaneous: CPK elevation; hyperglycemia; hyperuricemia; hyponatremia; and weight loss.

DRUG ABUSE AND DEPENDENCE

Physical and psychological dependence have not been reported or observed in patients taking CLOZARIL® (clozapine).

OVERDOSAGE

Human Experience

The most commonly reported signs and symptoms associated with CLOZARIL® (clozapine) overdose are: altered states of consciousness, including drowsiness, delirium and coma; tachycardia; hypotension; respiratory depression or failure; hypersalivation. Aspiration pneumonia and cardiac arrhythmias have also been reported. Seizures have occurred in a minority of reported cases. Fatal overdoses have been reported with CLOZARIL® (clozapine), generally at doses above 2500 mg. There have also been reports of patients recovering from overdoses well in excess of 4 g.

Management of Overdose

Establish and maintain an airway; ensure adequate oxygenation and ventilation. Activated charcoal, which may be used with sorbitol, may be as or more effective than emesis or lavage, and should be considered in treating overdosage. Cardiac and vital signs monitoring is recommended along with general symptomatic and supportive measures. Additional surveillance should be continued for several days because of the risk of delayed effects. Avoid epinephrine and derivatives when treating hypotension, and quinidine and procainamide when treating cardiac arrhythmia.

There are no specific antidotes for CLOZARIL® (clozapine). Forced diuresis, dialysis, hemoperfusion and exchange transfusion are unlikely to be of benefit.

In managing overdosage, the physician should consider the possibility of multiple drug involvement.

Up-to-date information about the treatment of overdose can often be obtained from a certified Regional Poison Control Center. Telephone numbers of certified Poison Control Centers are listed in the Physicians' Desk Reference®.*

DOSAGE AND ADMINISTRATION

Upon initiation of CLOZARIL® (clozapine) therapy, up to a 1 week supply of additional CLOZARIL® (clozapine) tablets may be provided to the patient to be held for emergencies (e.g., weather, holidays).

Initial Treatment

It is recommended that treatment with CLOZARIL® (clozapine) begin with one-half of a 25 mg tablet (12.5 mg) once or twice daily and then be continued with daily dosage increments of 25-50 mg/day, if well-tolerated, to achieve a target dose of 300-450 mg/day by the end of 2 weeks. Subsequent dosage increments should be made no more than once or twice-weekly, in increments not to exceed 100 mg. Cautious titration and a divided dosage schedule are necessary to minimize the risks of hypotension, seizure, and sedation.

In the multicenter study that provides primary support for the effectiveness of CLOZARIL® (clozapine) in patients resistant to standard antipsychotic drug treatment, patients were titrated during the first 2 weeks up to a maximum dose of 500 mg/day, on a t.i.d. basis, and were then dosed in a total daily dose range of 100-900 mg/day, on a t.i.d. basis thereafter, with clinical response and adverse effects as guides to correct dosing.

Therapeutic Dose Adjustment

Daily dosing should continue on a divided basis as an effective and tolerable dose level is sought. While many patients may respond adequately at doses between 300-600 mg/day, it may be necessary to raise the dose to the 600-900 mg/day range to obtain an acceptable response. [Note: In the multicenter study providing the primary support for the superiority of CLOZARIL® (clozapine) in treatment resistant patients, the mean and median CLOZARIL® (clozapine) doses were both approximately 600 mg/day.]

Because of the possibility of increased adverse reactions at higher doses, particularly seizures, patients should ordinarily be given adequate time to respond to a given dose level before escalation to a higher dose is contemplated. Dosing should not exceed 900 mg/day.

Because of the significant risk of agranulocytosis and seizure, events which both present a continuing risk over time, the extended treatment of patients failing to show an acceptable level of clinical response should ordinarily be avoided.

Maintenance Treatment

While the maintenance effectiveness of CLOZARIL® (clozapine) in schizophrenia is still under study, the effectiveness of maintenance treatment is well established for many other antipsychotic drugs. It is recommended that responding patients be continued on CLOZARIL® (clozapine), but at the lowest level needed to maintain remission. Because of the significant risk associated with the use of CLOZARIL® (clozapine), patients should be periodically reassessed to determine the need for maintenance treatment.

Discontinuation of Treatment

In the event of planned termination of CLOZARIL® (clozapine) therapy, gradual reduction in dose is recommended over a 1-2 week period. However, should a patient's medical condition require abrupt discontinuation (e.g., leukopenia), the patient should be carefully observed for the recurrence of psychotic symptoms.

Reinitiation of Treatment in Patients Previously Discontinued

When restarting patients who have had even a brief interval off CLOZARIL® (clozapine), i.e., 2 days or more since the last dose, it is recommended that treatment be reinitiated with one-half of a 25 mg tablet (12.5 mg) once or twice daily (see WARNINGS). If that dose is well tolerated, it may be feasible to titrate patients back to a therapeutic dose more quickly than is recommended for initial treatment. However, any patient who has previously experienced respiratory or cardiac arrest with initial dosing, but was then able to be successfully titrated to a therapeutic dose, should be re-titrated with extreme caution after even 24 hours of discontinuation.

Certain additional precautions seem prudent when reinitiating treatment. The mechanisms underlying CLOZARIL® (clozapine) induced adverse reactions are unknown. It is conceivable, however, that re-exposure of a patient might enhance the risk of an untoward event's occurrence and increase its severity. Such phenomena, for example, occur when immune mediated mechanisms are responsible. Consequently, during the reinitiation of treatment, additional caution is advised. Patients discontinued for WBC counts below 2000/mm³ or an ANC below 1000/mm³ must *not* be restarted on CLOZARIL® (clozapine). (See WARNINGS)

HOW SUPPLIED

CLOZARIL® (clozapine) is available as 25 mg and 100 mg round, pale-yellow, uncoated tablets with a facilitated score.

CLOZARIL® (clozapine) Tablets

25 mg

Engraved with "CLOZARIL" once on the periphery of one side.
Engraved with a facilitated score and "25" once on the other side.
Bottle of 100 (NDC 0078-0126-05).
Unit dose packages of 100: 2 × 5 strips, 10 blisters per strip (NDC 0078-0126-06).

100 mg

Engraved with "CLOZARIL" once on the periphery of one side.
Engraved with a facilitated score and "100" once on the other side.
Bottle of 100 (NDC 0078-0127-05).
Unit dose packages of 100: 2 × 5 strips, 10 blisters per strip (NDC 0078-0127-06).

Store and Dispense

Storage temperature should not exceed 86°F (30°C). Drug dispensing should not ordinarily exceed a weekly supply. If a patient is eligible for WBC testing every other week, then a two week supply of CLOZARIL® (clozapine) can be dispensed. Dispensing should be contingent upon the results of a WBC count.

*Trademark of Medical Economics Company, Inc.

REV: MARCH 1998 30718909
Shown in Product Identification Guide, page 324

CYTADREN® TABLETS ℞
[*sight 'a-dren*]
aminoglutethimide tablets USP

Caution: Federal law prohibits dispensing without prescription.

The following prescribing information is based on official labeling in effect on August 1, 1998.

DESCRIPTION
Cytadren, aminoglutethimide tablets USP, is an inhibitor of adrenocortical steroid synthesis, available as 250-mg tablets for oral administration. Its chemical name is 3-(4-amino-phenyl)-3-ethyl-2,6-piperidinedione, and its structural formula is

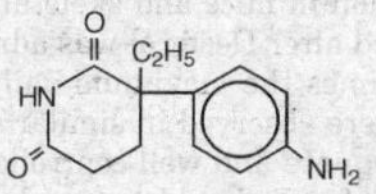

Aminoglutethimide USP is a fine, white or creamy white, crystalline powder. It is very slightly soluble in water, and readily soluble in most organic solvents. It forms water-soluble salts with strong acids. Its molecular weight is 232.28.
Inactive Ingredients. Cellulose compounds, colloidal silicon dioxide, starch, stearic acid, and talc.

CLINICAL PHARMACOLOGY
Cytadren inhibits the enzymatic conversion of cholesterol to Δ^5-pregnenolone, resulting in a decrease in the production of adrenal glucocorticoids, mineralocorticoids, estrogens, and androgens.
Cytadren blocks several other steps in steroid synthesis, including the C-11, C-18, and C-21 hydroxylations and the hydroxylations required for the aromatization of androgens to estrogens, mediated through the binding of Cytadren to cytochrome P-450 complexes.
A decrease in adrenal secretion of cortisol is followed by an increased secretion of pituitary adrenocorticotropic hormone (ACTH), which will overcome the blockade of adrenocortical steroid synthesis by Cytadren. The compensatory increase in ACTH secretion can be suppressed by the simultaneous administration of hydrocortisone. Since Cytadren increases the rate of metabolism of dexamethasone but not that of hydrocortisone, the latter is preferred as the adrenal glucocorticoid replacement.
Although Cytadren inhibits the synthesis of thyroxine by the thyroid gland, the compensatory increase in thyroid-stimulating hormone (TSH) is frequently of sufficient magnitude to overcome the inhibition of thyroid synthesis due to Cytadren. In spite of an increase in TSH, Cytadren has not been associated with increased prolactin secretion.
Note: Cytadren was marketed previously as an anticonvulsant but was withdrawn from marketing for that indication in 1966 because of the effects on the adrenal gland.

Pharmacokinetics
Cytadren is rapidly and completely absorbed after oral administration. In 6 healthy male volunteers, maximum plasma levels of Cytadren averaged 5.9 µg/mL at a median of 1.5 hours after ingestion of two 250-mg tablets. The bioavailability of tablets is equivalent to equal doses given as a solution. After ingestion of a single oral dose, 34%-54% is excreted in the urine as unchanged drug during the first 48 hours, and an additional fraction as the N-acetyl derivative.
The half-life of Cytadren in normal volunteers given single oral doses averaged 12.5 ± 1.6 hours.
Upon withdrawal of therapy with Cytadren, the ability of the adrenal glands to synthesize steroid returns, usually within 72 hours.

INDICATIONS AND USAGE
Cytadren is indicated for the suppression of adrenal function in selected patients with Cushing's syndrome. Morning levels of plasma cortisol in patients with adrenal carcinoma and ectopic ACTH-producing tumors were reduced on the average to about one half of the pretreatment levels, and in patients with adrenal hyperplasia to about two thirds of the pretreatment levels, during 1-3 months of therapy with Cytadren. Data available from the few patients with adrenal adenoma suggest similar reductions in plasma cortisol levels. Measurements of plasma cortisol showed reductions to at least 50% of baseline or to normal levels in one third or more of the patients studied, depending on diagnostic groups and time of measurement.
Because Cytadren does not affect the underlying disease process, it is used primarily as an interim measure until more definitive therapy such as surgery can be undertaken or in cases where such therapy is not appropriate. Only small numbers of patients have been treated for longer than 3 months. A decreased effect or "escape phenomenon" seems to occur more frequently in patients with pituitary-dependent Cushing's syndrome, probably because of increasing ACTH levels in response to decreasing glucocorticoid levels.
Cytadren should be used only in those patients who are responsive to treatment.

CONTRAINDICATIONS
Cytadren is contraindicated in those patients with serious forms, and/or more severe manifestations, of hypersensitivity to glutethimide or aminoglutethimide.

WARNINGS
Cytadren may cause adrenocortical hypofunction, especially under conditions of stress, such as surgery, trauma, or acute illness. Patients should be carefully monitored and given hydrocortisone and mineralocorticoid supplements as indicated. Dexamethasone should not be used. (See PRECAUTIONS, Drug Interactions.)
Cytadren also may suppress aldosterone production by the adrenal cortex and may cause orthostatic or persistent hypotension. The blood pressure should be monitored in all patients at appropriate intervals. Patients should be advised of the possible occurrence of weakness and dizziness as symptoms of hypotension, and of measures to be taken should they occur.
The effects of Cytadren may be potentiated if it is taken in combination with alcohol.
Cytadren can cause fetal harm when administered to a pregnant woman. In the earlier experience with the drug in about 5000 patients, two cases of pseudohermaphroditism were reported in female infants whose mothers were treated with Cytadren and concomitant anticonvulsants. Normal pregnancies have also occurred in patients treated with Cytadren.
When administered to rats at doses $^1/_2$ and $1^1/_4$ times the maximum daily human dose, Cytadren caused a decrease in fetal implantation, an increase in fetal deaths, and a variety of teratogenic effects. The compound also caused pseudohermaphroditism in rats treated with approximately 3 times the maximum daily human dose. If this drug must be used during pregnancy, or if the patient becomes pregnant while taking the drug, the patient should be apprised of the potential hazard to the fetus.

PRECAUTIONS
General
This drug should be administered only by physicians familiar with its use and hazards. Therapy should be initiated in a hospital. (See DOSAGE AND ADMINISTRATION.)

Information for Patients
Patients should be warned that drowsiness may occur and that they should not drive, operate potentially dangerous machinery, or engage in other activities that may become hazardous because of decreased alertness.
Patients should also be warned of the possibility of hypotension and its symptoms (see WARNINGS).

Laboratory Tests
Hypothyroidism may occur in association with Cytadren; hence, appropriate clinical observations should be made and laboratory studies of thyroid function performed as indicated. Supplementary thyroid hormone may be required.
Hematologic abnormalities in patients receiving Cytadren have been reported (see ADVERSE REACTIONS). Therefore, baseline hematologic studies should be performed, followed by periodic hematologic evaluation.
Since elevations in SGOT, alkaline phosphatase, and bilirubin have been reported, appropriate clinical observations and regular laboratory studies should be performed before and during therapy.
Serum electrolyte levels should be determined periodically.

Drug Interactions
Cytadren accelerates the metabolism of dexamethasone; therefore, if glucocorticoid replacement is needed, hydrocortisone should be prescribed.
Aminoglutethimide diminishes the effect of coumarin and warfarin.

Carcinogenesis, Mutagenesis, Impairment of Fertility
A 2-year carcinogenicity study of Cytadren conducted in rats at doses of 10-60 mg/kg/day (approximately 0.04 to 0.2 times the maximum daily therapeutic dose based on surface area, mg/m^2) revealed a highly statistically significant dose-related trend in the incidence of benign and malignant neoplasms of the adrenal cortex and thyroid follicular cells in both sexes. A borderline statistically significant increase (0.05 level) in ovarian tubular adenomas was observed at 60 mg/kg/day. Urinary bladder papillomas also showed a statistically significant dose-related trend in males.
Cytadren affects fertility in female rats (see WARNINGS). The relevance of these findings to humans is not known.

Pregnancy Category D
See WARNINGS.

Nursing Mothers
It is not known whether this drug is excreted in human milk. Because many drugs are excreted in human milk and because of the potential for serious adverse reactions in nursing infants from Cytadren, a decision should be made whether to discontinue nursing or to discontinue the drug, taking into account the importance of the drug to the mother.

Pediatric Use
Safety and effectiveness in pediatric patients have not been established (see CLINICAL STUDIES IN CHILDREN).

ADVERSE REACTIONS
Untoward effects have been reported in about 2 out of 3 patients with Cushing's syndrome who were treated for 4 or more weeks with Cytadren as the only adrenocortical suppressant.
The most frequent and reversible side effects were drowsiness (approximately 1 in 3 patients), morbilliform skin rash (1 in 6 patients), nausea and anorexia (each approximately 1 in 8 patients), and dizziness (about 1 in 20 patients). The dizziness was possibly caused by lowered vascular resistance or orthostasis. These reactions often disappear spontaneously with continued therapy.

Other Effects Observed
Hematologic: Single instances of neutropenia, leukopenia (patient received concomitant *o,p '* -DDD), pancytopenia (patient received concomitant 5-fluorouracil), and agranulocytosis occurred in 4 of 27 patients with Cushing's syndrome caused by adrenal carcinoma who were treated for at least 4 weeks. In 1 patient with adrenal hyperplasia, hemoglobin levels and hematocrit decreased during the course of treatment with Cytadren. From the earlier experience with the drug used as an anticonvulsant in 1,214 patients, transient leukopenia was the only hematologic effect and was reported once; Coombs'-negative hemolytic anemia also occurred once. In approximately 300 patients with non-adrenal malignancy, 1 in 25 showed some degree of anemia, and 1 in 150 developed pancytopenia during treatment with Cytadren.
Endocrine: Adrenal insufficiency occurred in about 1 in 30 patients with Cushing's syndrome who were treated with Cytadren for 4 or more weeks. This insufficiency tended to involve glucocorticoids as well as mineralocorticoids. Hypothyroidism is occasionally associated with thyroid enlargement and may be detected or confirmed by measuring plasma levels of the thyroid hormone. Masculinization and hirsutism have occasionally occurred in females, as has precocious sexual development in males.
Central Nervous System: Headache was reported in about 1 in 20 patients.
Cardiovascular: Hypotension, occasionally orthostatic, occurred in 1 in 30 patients receiving Cytadren. Tachycardia occurred in 1 in 40 patients.
Gastrointestinal and Liver: Vomiting occurred in 1 in 30 patients. Isolated instances of abnormal findings on liver function tests were reported. Suspected hepatotoxicity occurred in less than 1 in 1000 patients.
Skin: In addition to rash (1 in 6 patients, and often reversible with continued therapy), pruritus was reported in 1 in 20 patients. These may be allergic or hypersensitive reactions. Urticaria has occurred rarely.
Miscellaneous: Fever was reported in several patients who were treated with Cytadren for less than 4 weeks; some of these patients also received other drugs. Myalgia occurred in 1 in 30 patients.
Pulmonary hypersensitivity, including allergic alveolitis and interstitial alveolar infiltrates, has occurred rarely.

OVERDOSAGE
Acute Toxicity
No deaths due to overdosage with Cytadren have been reported.
The highest known doses that have been survived are 7 g (33-year-old woman), 7.5-10 g (16-year-old girl), and 10 g (10-year-old boy).
Oral LD_{50}'s (mg/kg): rats, 1800; dogs, >100. Intravenous LD_{50}'s (mg/kg): rats, 156; dogs, >100.

Signs and Symptoms
An acute overdose with Cytadren may reduce the production of steroids in the adrenal cortex to a degree that is clinically relevant. The following manifestations may be expected:
Respiratory Function: Respiratory depression, hypoventilation.
Cardiovascular System: Hypotension, hypovolemic shock due to dehydration.
Central Nervous System/Muscles: Somnolence, lethargy, coma, ataxia, dizziness, fatigue. (Extreme weakness has been reported with divided doses of 3 g daily.)
Gastrointestinal System: Nausea, vomiting.
Renal Function: Loss of sodium and water.
Laboratory Findings: Hyponatremia, hypochloremia, hyperkalemia, hypoglycemia.
The signs and symptoms of acute overdosage with Cytadren may be aggravated or modified if alcohol, hypnotics, tranquilizers, or tricyclic antidepressants have been taken at the same time.

Continued on next page

Cytadren—Cont.

Treatment
Symptomatic treatment of overdosage is recommended.
Since aminoglutethimide and glutethimide are chemically related, measures that have been used in successfully removing glutethimide from the body might be useful in removing aminoglutethimide.
Gastric lavage and unspecified supportive treatment have been employed. Full consciousness following deep coma was regained 40 hours or less after ingestion of 3 or 4 g without lavage. No evidence of hematologic, renal, or hepatic effects was subsequently found.
Close monitoring should be provided, and appropriate measures taken to support vital functions, if necessary.
If deficiency of circulating glucocorticoid develops, an intravenous infusion of a soluble hydrocortisone preparation (100 mg of hydrocortisone sodium succinate in 500 mL of isotonic sodium chloride solution) and 50 mL of 40% glucose solution should be given within 3 hours. After the initial infusion is completed, an intravenous administration of hydrocortisone, 10 mg per hour, should be continued until the patient is able to take oral cortisone.
If hypovolemia or hypotension occurs, an intravenous administration of norepinephrine, 10 mg, in 500 mL of isotonic sodium chloride should be administered according to the patient's needs and response. After rehydration, 500 mL of plasma or blood should be given for maintenance of sufficient circulatory volume.
Dialysis may be considered in severe intoxication.

DOSAGE AND ADMINISTRATION
Adults
Treatment should be instituted in a hospital until a stable dosage regimen is achieved. Therapy should be initiated with 250 mg orally four times daily, preferably at 6-hour intervals. Adrenocortical response should be followed by careful monitoring of plasma cortisol levels until the desired level of suppression is achieved. If the level of cortisol suppression is inadequate, the dosage may be increased in increments of 250 mg daily at intervals of 1-2 weeks to a total daily dose of 2 g. Dose reduction or temporary discontinuation of therapy may be required in the event of adverse effects, including extreme drowsiness, severe skin rash, or excessively low cortisol levels. If a skin rash persists for longer than 5-8 days or becomes severe, the drug should be discontinued. It may be possible to reinstate therapy at a lower dosage following the disappearance of a mild or moderate rash. Mineralocorticoid replacement (e.g., fludrocortisone) may be necessary. If glucocorticoid replacement therapy is needed, 20–30 mg of hydrocortisone orally in the morning will replace endogenous secretion.

HOW SUPPLIED
Tablets 250 mg — white, round, scored into quarters (imprinted CIBA 24)
Bottles of 100 .... NDC 0083-0024-30
Protect from light.
Do not store above 30°F (86°C).
Dispense in tight, light-resistant container (USP).

CLINICAL STUDIES IN CHILDREN
Clinical investigations included 9 patients aged $2^1/_2$ to 16 years; 4 of these were aged 10 or less. Seven of the patients received other therapies (drugs or irradiation) either with Cytadren or within a short period before initiation of therapy with Cytadren. Diagnoses included 5 patients with adrenal carcinoma, 3 with adrenal hyperplasia, and 1 with ectopic ACTH-producing tumor. Duration of treatment ranged from 3 days to $6^1/_2$ months. Dosages ranged from 0.375 g to 1.5 g daily. In general, smaller doses were used for younger patients; for example, a $2^1/_2$-year-old received 0.5-0.75 g daily, a $3^1/_2$-year-old received 0.5 g daily, and all others over 10 years of age received 0.75-1.5 g daily. Results are difficult to evaluate because of the concomitant therapy, duration of therapy, or inadequate laboratory documentation. Most patients did show decreases in plasma or urinary steroids at some time during treatment, but these may have been due to other therapeutic modalities or their combinations.

C97-37 (Rev. 1/98)

DESFERAL® ℞
[*des 'fer-all*]
deferoxamine mesylate for injection USP
Vials

Caution: Federal law prohibits dispensing without a prescription.

The following prescribing information is based on official labeling in effect on August 1, 1998.

DESCRIPTION
Desferal, deferoxamine mesylate USP, is an iron-chelating agent, available in vials for intramuscular, subcutaneous, and intravenous administration. Each vial contains 500 mg of deferoxamine mesylate USP in sterile, lyophilized form. Deferoxamine mesylate is *N*-[5-[3-[(5-aminopentyl) hydroxycarbamoyl]propionamido]-pentyl]-3-[[5-(*N*-hydroxyacetamido)pentyl]carbamoyl] propionohydroxamic acid monomethanesulfonate (salt), and it structural formula is

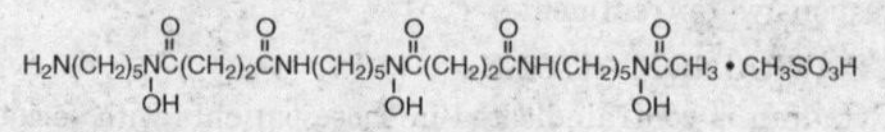

Deferoxamine mesylate USP is a white to off-white powder. It is freely soluble in water and slightly soluble in methanol. Its molecular weight is 656.79.

CLINICAL PHARMACOLOGY
Desferal chelates iron by forming a stable complex that prevents the iron from entering into further chemical reactions. It readily chelates iron from ferritin and hemosiderin but not readily from transferrin; it does not combine with the iron from cytochromes and hemoglobin. Desferal does not cause any demonstrable increase in the excretion of electrolytes or trace metals. Theoretically, 100 parts by weight of Desferal is capable of binding approximately 8.5 parts by weight of ferric iron.
Desferal is metabolized principally by plasma enzymes, but the pathways have not yet been defined. The chelate is readily soluble in water and passes easily through the kidney, giving the urine a characteristic reddish color. Some is also excreted in the feces via the bile.

INDICATIONS AND USAGE
Desferal is indicated for the treatment of acute iron intoxication and of chronic iron overload due to transfusion-dependent anemias.
Acute Iron Intoxication
Desferal is an adjunct to, and not a substitute for, standard measures used in treating acute iron intoxication, which may include the following: induction of emesis with syrup of ipecac; gastric lavage; suction and maintenance of a clear airway; control of shock with intravenous fluids, blood, oxygen, and vasopressors; and correction of acidosis.
Chronic Iron Overload
Desferal can promote iron excretion in patients with secondary iron overload from multiple transfusions (as may occur in the treatment of some chronic anemias, including thalassemia). Long-term therapy with Desferal slows accumulation of hepatic iron and retards or eliminates progression of hepatic fibrosis.
Iron mobilization with Desferal is relatively poor in patients under the age of 3 years with relatively little iron overload. The drug should ordinarily not be given to such patients unless significant iron mobilization (e.g., 1 mg or more of iron per day) can be demonstrated.
Desferal is not indicated for the treatment of primary hemochromatosis, since phlebotomy is the method of choice for removing excess iron in this disorder.

CONTRAINDICATIONS
Desferal is contraindicated in patients with severe renal disease or anuria, since the drug and the iron chelate are excreted primarily by the kidney.

WARNINGS
Ocular and auditory disturbances have been reported when Desferal was administered over prolonged periods of time, at high doses, or in patients with low ferritin levels. The ocular disturbances observed have been blurring of vision; cataracts after prolonged administration in chronic iron overload; decreased visual acuity including visual loss; impaired peripheral, color, and night vision; and retinal pigmentary abnormalities. The auditory abnormalities reported have been tinnitus and hearing loss including high frequency sensorineural hearing loss. In most cases, both ocular and auditory disturbances were reversible upon immediate cessation of treatment. Slit-lamp examinations performed in patients treated with Desferal for acute iron intoxication have not revealed cataracts.
Visual acuity tests, slit-lamp examinations, funduscopy and audiometry are recommended periodically in patients treated for prolonged periods of time. Toxicity is more likely to be reversed if symptoms or test abnormalities are detected early.
High doses of Desferal and concomitant low ferritin levels have also been associated with growth retardation. After reduction of Desferal dose, growth velocity may partially resume to pretreatment rates.
Adult respiratory distress syndrome, also reported in children, has been described following treatment with excessively high intravenous doses of Desferal in patients with acute iron intoxication or thalassemia.

PRECAUTIONS
General
Flushing of the skin, urticaria, hypotension, and shock have occurred in a few patients when Desferal was administered by rapid intravenous injection. THEREFORE, DESFERAL SHOULD BE GIVEN INTRAMUSCULARLY OR BY SLOW SUBCUTANEOUS OR INTRAVENOUS INFUSION.
Iron overload increases susceptibility of patients to Yersinia enterocolitica infections. In some rare cases, treatment with Desferal has enhanced this susceptibility, resulting in generalized infections by providing this bacteria with a siderophore otherwise missing. In such cases, Desferal treatment should be discontinued until the infection is resolved.
In patients undergoing hemodialysis while receiving Desferal, there have been rare reports of fungal infections (i.e., mucormycosis) that have sometimes been fatal; however, a causal relationship to the drug has not been established.
Information for Patients
Patients should be informed that occasionally their urine may show a reddish discoloration.
Carcinogenesis, Mutagenesis, Impairment of Fertility
Long-term carcinogenicity studies in animals have not been performed with Desferal.
Cytotoxicity may occur, since Desferal has been shown to inhibit DNA synthesis *in vitro*.
Pregnancy Category C
Delayed ossification in mice and skeletal anomalies in rabbits were observed after Desferal was administered in daily doses up to 4.5 times the maximum daily human dose. No adverse effects were observed in similar studies in rats.
There are no adequate and well-controlled studies in pregnant women. Desferal should be used during pregnancy only if the potential benefit justifies the potential risk to the fetus.
Nursing Mothers
It is not known whether this drug is excreted in human milk. Because many drugs are excreted in human milk, caution should be exercised when Desferal is administered to a nursing woman.
Pediatric Use
Safety and effectiveness in pediatric patients under the age of 3 years have not been established (see INDICATIONS AND USAGE).

ADVERSE REACTIONS
The following adverse reactions have been observed, but there are not enough data to support an estimate of their frequency.
Skin: Localized irritation and pain, swelling and induration, pruritus, erythema, wheal formation.
Hypersensitive Reactions: Generalized erythema (rash), urticaria, anaphylactic reaction.
Cardiovascular: Tachycardia, hypotension, shock.
Digestive: Abdominal discomfort, diarrhea, nausea, vomiting.
Special Senses: Ocular and auditory disturbances (see WARNINGS).
Other: Dysuria, leg cramps, fever.

OVERDOSAGE
Acute Toxicity
Intravenous LD_{50}'s (mg/kg): mice, 287; rats, 329.
Signs and Symptoms
Since Desferal is available only for parenteral administration, acute poisoning is unlikely to occur. However, tachycardia, hypotension, and gastrointestinal symptoms have occasionally developed in patients who received overdoses of Desferal.
Treatment
There is no specific antidote.
Signs and symptoms of overdosage may be eliminated by reducing the dosage.
Desferal is readily dialyzable.

DOSAGE AND ADMINISTRATION
Acute Iron Intoxication
Intramuscular Administration
This route is preferred and should be used for ALL PATIENTS NOT IN SHOCK.
Dosage. A dose of 1000 mg (2 vials) should be administered initially. This may be followed by 500 mg (1 vial) every 4 hours for two doses. Depending upon the clinical response, subsequent doses of 500 mg may be administered every 4-12 hours. The total amount administered should not exceed 6000 mg in 24 hours.
Preparation of Solution. Desferal is dissolved by adding 2 mL of Sterile Water for Injection to each vial, resulting in a solution of 250 mg/mL. The drug should be completely dissolved before the solution is withdrawn. Desferal is then administered intramuscularly. See *Note* below.
Intravenous Administration
THIS ROUTE SHOULD BE USED ONLY FOR PATIENTS IN A STATE OF CARDIOVASCULAR COLLAPSE AND THEN ONLY BY SLOW INFUSION. THE RATE OF INFUSION SHOULD NOT EXCEED 15 MG/KG/HR.
Dosage. An initial dose of 1000 mg (2 vials) should be administered at a rate NOT TO EXCEED 15 mg/kg/hr. This may be followed by 500 mg every 4 hours for two doses. Depending upon the clinical response, subsequent doses of 500 mg may be administered every 4-12 hours. The total amount administered should not exceed 6000 mg in 24 hours.

As soon as the clinical condition of the patient permits, intravenous administration should be discontinued and the drug should be administered intramuscularly.

Preparation of Solution. Desferal is dissolved by adding 2 mL of Sterile Water for Injection to each vial, resulting in a solution of 250 mg/mL. The drug should be completely dissolved before the solution is withdrawn. The solution is then added to physiologic saline, glucose in water, or Ringer's lactate solution and administered at a rate NOT TO EXCEED 15 mg/kg/hr. See *Note* below.

Chronic Iron Overload

The more effective of the following routes of administration must be chosen on an individual basis for each patient.

Intramuscular Administration

A daily dose of 500-1000 mg (1-2 vials) should be administered intramuscularly. In addition, 2000 mg should be administered intravenously with each unit of blood transfused; however, Desferal should be administered separately from the blood. The rate of intravenous infusion must not exceed 15 mg/kg/hr.

Subcutaneous Administration

A daily dose of 1000-2000 mg (2-4 vials) (20-40 mg/kg/day) should be administered over 8-24 hours, utilizing a small portable pump capable of providing continuous mini-infusion. The duration of infusion must be individualized. In some patients, as much iron will be excreted after a short infusion of 8-12 hours as with the same dose given over 24 hours.

Preparation of Solution for Subcutaneous or Intramuscular Administration. Desferal is dissolved by adding 2 mL of Sterile Water for Injection to each vial, resulting in a solution of 250 mg/mL. The drug should be completely dissolved before the solution is withdrawn into the syringe to be used for administration. See *Note* below.

***Note:* Parenteral drug products should be inspected visually for particulate matter and discoloration prior to administration, whenever solution and container permit.**

Desferal reconstituted with Sterile Water for Injection may be stored under sterile conditions and protected from light at room temperature for not longer than 1 week. Do not refrigerate reconstituted solution.

Reconstituting Desferal in solvents or under conditions other than indicated may result in precipitation. Turbid solutions should not be used.

HOW SUPPLIED

Vials – each containing 500 mg of sterile, lyophilized deferoxamine mesylate

Cartons of 4 vials .... NDC 0083-3801-04

Do not store above 77°F (25°C).

Distributed by C97-13 (Rev. 10/97)
Novartis Pharmaceuticals Corporation
East Hanover, New Jersey 07936

D.H.E. 45® ℞

(dihydroergotamine mesylate)
Injection, USP

Rx only

The following prescribing information is based on official labeling in effect on August 1, 1998.

DESCRIPTION

D.H.E. 45® is ergotamine hydrogenated in the 9, 10 position as the mesylate salt. D.H.E. 45® is known chemically as ergotaman-3′,6′,18-trione,9,-10-dihydro-12′-hydroxy-2′-methyl-5′- (phenylmethyl)-,(5′α)-, monomethanesulfonate. Its molecular weight is 679.80 and its empirical formula is $C_{33}H_{37}N_5O_5 \bullet CH_4O_3S$).

The chemical structure is:

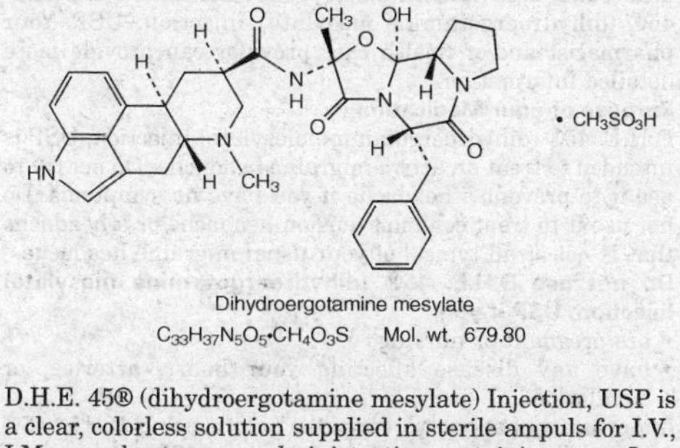

Dihydroergotamine mesylate
$C_{33}H_{37}N_5O_5 \cdot CH_4O_3S$ Mol. wt. 679.80

D.H.E. 45® (dihydroergotamine mesylate) Injection, USP is a clear, colorless solution supplied in sterile ampuls for I.V., I.M., or subcutaneous administration containing per mL:

dihydroergotamine mesylate, USP .... 1 mg
methanesulfonic acid/sodium hydroxide, qs to
.... pH 3.6 ± 0.4
alcohol, USP .... 6.1% by vol.
glycerin, USP .... 15% by wt.
water for injection, USP, qs to .... 1 mL

CLINICAL PHARMACOLOGY

Mechanism of Action

Dihydroergotamine binds with high affinity to $5\text{-}HT_{1D\alpha}$ and $5\text{-}HT_{1D\beta}$ receptors. It also binds with high affinity to serotonin $5\text{-}HT_{1A}$, $5\text{-}HT_{2A}$, and $5\text{-}HT_{2C}$ receptors, noradrenaline α_{2A}, α_{2B} and α, receptors, and dopamine D_{2L} and D_3 receptors.

The therapeutic activity of dihydroergotamine in migraine is generally attributed to the agonist effect at $5\text{-}HT_{1D}$ receptors. Two current theories have been proposed to explain the efficacy of $5\text{-}HT_{1D}$ receptor agonists in migraine. One theory suggests that activation of $5\text{-}HT_{1D}$ receptors located on intracranial blood vessels, including those on arterio-venous anastomoses, leads to vasoconstriction, which correlates with the relief of migraine headache. The alternative hypothesis suggests that activation of $5\text{-}HT_{1D}$ receptors on sensory nerve endings of the trigeminal system results in the inhibition of pro-inflammatory neuropeptide release.

In addition, dihydroergotamine possesses oxytocic properties. *(See CONTRAINDICATIONS)*

Pharmacokinetics

Absorption

Absolute bioavailability for the subcutaneous and intramuscular route have not been determined, however, no difference was observed in dihydroergotamine bioavailability from intramuscular and subcutaneous doses. Dihydroergotamine mesylate is poorly bioavailable following oral administration.

Distribution

Dihydroergotamine mesylate is 93% plasma protein bound. The apparent steady-state volume of distribution is approximately 800 liters.

Metabolism

Four dihydroergotamine mesylate metabolites have been identified in human plasma following oral administration. The major metabolite, 8′-β-hydroxydihydroergotamine, exhibits affinity equivalent to its parent for adrenergic and 5-HT receptors and demonstrates equivalent potency in several venoconstrictor activity models, *in vivo* and *in vitro*. The other metabolites, i.e., dihydrolysergic acid, dihydrolysergic amide, and a metabolite formed by oxidative opening of the proline ring are of minor importance. Following nasal administration, total metabolites represent only 20%-30% of plasma AUC. Quantitative pharmacokinetic characterization of the four metabolites has not been performed.

Excretion

The major excretory route of dihydroergotamine is via the bile in the feces. The total body clearance is 1.5 L/min which reflects mainly hepatic clearance. Only 6%-7% of unchanged dihydroergotamine is excreted in the urine after intramuscular injection. The renal clearance (0.1 L/min) is unaffected by the route of dihydroergotamine administration. The decline of plasma dihydroergotamine after intramuscular or intravenous administration is multi-exponential with a terminal half-life of about 9 hours.

Subpopulations

No studies have been conducted on the effect of renal or hepatic impairment, gender, race, or ethnicity on dihydroergotamine pharmacokinetics. D.H.E. 45® (dihydroergotamine mesylate) Injection, USP is contraindicated in patients with severely impaired hepatic or renal function. *(See CONTRAINDICATIONS)*

Interactions

Pharmacokinetic interactions (increased blood levels) have been reported in patients treated orally with dihydroergotamine and macrolide antibiotics, principally troleandomycin, presumably due to inhibition of cytochrome P450 3A metabolism of dihydroergotamine by troleandomycin. Dihydroergotamine has also been shown to be an inhibitor of cytochrome P450 3A catalyzed reactions. No pharmacokinetic interactions involving other cytochrome P450 isoenzymes are known.

INDICATIONS AND USAGE

D.H.E. 45® (dihydroergotamine mesylate) Injection, USP is indicated for the acute treatment of migraine headaches with or without aura and the acute treatment of cluster headache episodes.

CONTRAINDICATIONS

D.H.E. 45® (dihydroergotamine mesylate) Injection, USP should not be given to patients with ischemic heart disease (angina pectoris, history of myocardial infarction, or documented silent ischemia) or to patients who have clinical symptoms or findings consistent with coronary artery vasospasm including Prinzmetal's variant angina. *(See WARNINGS)*

Because D.H.E. 45® (dihydroergotamine mesylate) Injection, USP may increase blood pressure, it should not be given to patients with uncontrolled hypertension.

D.H.E. 45® (dihydroergotamine mesylate) Injection, USP, $5\text{-}HT_1$ agonists (e.g., sumatriptan), ergotamine-containing or ergot-type medications or methysergide should not be used within 24 hours of each other.

D.H.E. 45® (dihydroergotamine mesylate) Injection, USP should not be administered to patients with hemiplegic or basilar migraine.

In addition to those conditions mentioned above, D.H.E. 45® (dihydroergotamine mesylate) Injection, USP is also contraindicated in patients with known peripheral arterial disease, sepsis, following vascular surgery and severely impaired hepatic or renal function.

D.H.E. 45® (dihydroergotamine mesylate) Injection, USP may cause fetal harm when administered to a pregnant woman. Dihydroergotamine possesses oxytocic properties and, therefore, should not be administered during pregnancy. If this drug is used during pregnancy, or if the patient becomes pregnant while taking this drug, the patient should be apprised of the potential hazard to the fetus.

There are no adequate studies of dihydroergotamine in human pregnancy, but developmental toxicity has been demonstrated in experimental animals. In embryo-fetal development studies of dihydroergotamine mesylate nasal spray, intranasal administration to pregnant rats throughout the period of organogenesis resulted in decreased fetal body weights and/or skeletal ossification at doses of 0.16 mg/day (associated with maternal plasma dihydroergotamine exposures [AUC] approximately 0.4-1.2 times the exposures in humans receiving the MRDD of 4 mg) or greater. A no effect level for embryo-fetal toxicity was not established in rats. Delayed skeletal ossification was also noted in rabbit fetuses following intranasal administration of 3.6 mg/day (maternal exposures approximately 7 times human exposures at the MRDD) during organogenesis. A no effect level was seen at 1.2 mg/day (maternal exposures approximately 2.5 times human exposures at the MRDD). When dihydroergotamine mesylate nasal spray was administered intranasally to female rats during pregnancy and lactation, decreased body weights and impaired reproductive function (decreased mating indices) were observed in the offspring at doses of 0.16 mg/day or greater. A no effect level was not established. Effects on development occurred at doses below those that produced evidence of significant maternal toxicity in these studies. Dihydroergotamine-induced intrauterine growth retardation has been attributed to reduced uteroplacental blood flow resulting from prolonged vasoconstriction of the uterine vessels and/or increased myometrial tone.

D.H.E. 45® (dihydroergotamine mesylate) Injection, USP is contraindicated in patients who have previously shown hypersensitivity to ergot alkaloids.

Dihydroergotamine mesylate should not be used by nursing mothers. *(See PRECAUTIONS)*

Dihydroergotamine mesylate should not be used with peripheral and central vasoconstrictors because the combination may result in additive or synergistic elevation of blood pressure.

WARNINGS

D.H.E. 45® (dihydroergotamine mesylate) Injection, USP should only be used where a clear diagnosis of migraine headache has been established.

Risk of Myocardial Ischemia and/or Infarction and Other Adverse Cardiac Events

D.H.E. 45® (dihydroergotamine mesylate) Injection, USP should not be used by patients with documented ischemic or vasospastic coronary artery disease. *(See CONTRAINDICATIONS.)* It is strongly recommended that D.H.E. 45® (dihydroergotamine mesylate) Injection, USP not be given to patients in whom unrecognized coronary artery disease (CAD) is predicted by the presence of risk factors (e.g., hypertension, hypercholesterolemia, smoker, obesity, diabetes, strong family history of CAD, females who are surgically or physiologically postmenopausal, or males who are over 40 years of age) unless a cardiovascular evaluation provides satisfactory clinical evidence that the patient is reasonably free of coronary artery and ischemic myocardial disease or other significant underlying cardiovascular disease. The sensitivity of cardiac diagnostic procedures to detect cardiovascular disease or predisposition to coronary artery vasospasm is modest, at best. If, during the cardiovascular evaluation, the patient's medical history or electrocardiographic investigations reveal findings indicative of or consistent with coronary artery vasospasm or myocardial ischemia, D.H.E. 45® (dihydroergotamine mesylate) Injection, USP should not be administered. *(See CONTRAINDICATIONS)*

For patients with risk factors predictive of CAD who are determined to have a satisfactory cardiovascular evaluation, it is strongly recommended that administration of the first dose of D.H.E. 45® (dihydroergotamine mesylate) Injection, USP take place in the setting of a physician's office or similar medically staffed and equipped facility unless the patient has previously received dihydroergotamine mesylate. Because cardiac ischemia can occur in the absence of clinical symptoms, consideration should be given to obtaining on the first occasion of use an electrocardiogram (ECG) during the interval immediately following D.H.E. 45® (dihydroergotamine mesylate) Injection, USP, in those patients with risk factors.

Continued on next page

D.H.E. 45—Cont.

It is recommended that patients who are intermittent long-term users of D.H.E. 45® (dihydroergotamine mesylate) Injection, USP and who have or acquire risk factors predictive of CAD, as described above, undergo periodic interval cardiovascular evaluation as they continue to use D.H.E. 45® (dihydroergotamine mesylate) Injection, USP.
The systematic approach described above is currently recommended as a method to identify patients in whom D.H.E. 45® (dihydroergotamine mesylate) Injection, USP may be used to treat migraine headaches with an acceptable margin of cardiovascular safety.

Cardiac Events and Fatalities
The potential for adverse cardiac events exists. Serious adverse cardiac events, including acute myocardial infarction, life-threatening disturbances of cardiac rhythm, and death have been reported to have occurred following the administration of dihydroergotamine mesylate injection. Considering the extent of use of dihydroergotamine mesylate in patients with migraine, the incidence of these events is extremely low.

Drug-Associated Cerebrovascular Events and Fatalities
Cerebral hemorrhage, subarachnoid hemorrhage, stroke, and other cerebrovascular events have been reported in patients treated with D.H.E. 45® (dihydroergotamine mesylate) Injection, USP; and some have resulted in fatalities. In a number of cases, it appears possible that the cerebrovascular events were primary, the D.H.E. 45® (dihydroergotamine mesylate) Injection, USP having been administered in the incorrect belief that the symptoms experienced were a consequence of migraine, when they were not. It should be noted that patients with migraine may be at increased risk of certain cerebrovascular events (e.g., stroke, hemorrhage, transient ischemic attack).

Other Vasospasm Related Events
D.H.E. 45® (dihydroergotamine mesylate) Injection, USP, like other ergot alkaloids, may cause vasospastic reactions other than coronary artery vasospasm. Myocardial, peripheral vascular, and colonic ischemia have been reported with D.H.E. 45® (dihydroergotamine mesylate) Injection, USP.
D.H.E. 45® (dihydroergotamine mesylate) Injection, USP associated vasospastic phenomena may also cause muscle pains, numbness, coldness, pallor, and cyanosis of the digits. In patients with compromised circulation, persistent vasospasm may result in gangrene or death. D.H.E. 45® (dihydroergotamine mesylate) Injection, USP should be discontinued immediately if signs or symptoms of vasoconstriction develop.

Increase In Blood Pressure
Significant elevation in blood pressure has been reported on rare occasions in patients with and without a history of hypertension treated with dihydroergotamine mesylate injection. D.H.E. 45® (dihydroergotamine mesylate) Injection, USP is contraindicated in patients with uncontrolled hypertension. *(See CONTRAINDICATIONS)*
An 18% increase in mean pulmonary artery pressure was seen following dosing with another 5-HT$_1$ agonist in a study evaluating subjects undergoing cardiac catheterization.

PRECAUTIONS

General
D.H.E. 45® (dihydroergotamine mesylate) Injection, USP may cause coronary artery vasospasm; patients who experience signs or symptoms suggestive of angina following its administration should, therefore, be evaluated for the presence of CAD or a predisposition to variant angina before receiving additional doses. Similarly, patients who experience other symptoms or signs suggestive of decreased arterial flow, such as ischemic bowel syndrome or Raynaud's syndrome following the use of any 5-HT agonist are candidates for further evaluation. *(See WARNINGS)*

Information for Patients
The text of a patient information sheet is printed at the end of this insert. To assure safe and effective use of D.H.E. 45® (dihydroergotamine mesylate) Injection, USP, the information and instructions provided in the patient information sheet should be discussed with patients.
Patients should be advised to report to the physician immediately any of the following: numbness or tingling in the fingers and toes, muscle pain in the arms and legs, weakness in the legs, pain in the chest, temporary speeding or slowing of the heart rate, swelling, or itching.
Prior to the initial use of the product by a patient, the prescriber should take steps to ensure that the patient understands how to use the product as provided. *(See Patient Information Sheet and product packaging)*

Drug Interactions

Vasoconstrictors
D.H.E. 45® (dihydroergotamine mesylate) Injection, USP should not be used with peripheral vasoconstrictors because the combination may cause synergistic elevation of blood pressure.

Sumatriptan
Sumatriptan has been reported to cause coronary artery vasospasm, and its effect could be additive with D.H.E. 45® (dihydroergotamine mesylate) Injection, USP. Sumatriptan and D.H.E. 45® (dihydroergotamine mesylate) Injection, USP should not be taken within 24 hours of each other. *(See CONTRAINDICATIONS)*

Beta Blockers
Although the results of a clinical study did not indicate a safety problem associated with the administration of D.H.E. 45® (dihydroergotamine mesylate) Injection, USP to subjects already receiving propranolol, there have been reports that propranolol may potentiate the vasoconstrictive action of ergotamine by blocking the vasodilating property of epinephrine.

Nicotine
Nicotine may provoke vasoconstriction in some patients, predisposing to a greater ischemic response to ergot therapy.

Macrolide Antibiotics
(e.g., erythromycin and troleandomycin)
Agents of the ergot alkaloid class, of which D.H.E. 45® (dihydroergotamine mesylate) Injection, USP is a member, have been shown to interact with antibiotics of the macrolide class, resulting in increased plasma levels of unchanged alkaloids and peripheral vasoconstriction. Vasospastic reactions have been reported with therapeutic doses of ergotamine-containing drugs when co-administered with these antibiotics.

SSRI's
Weakness, hyperreflexia, and incoordination have been reported rarely when 5-HT$_1$ agonists have been co-administered with SSRI's (e.g., fluoxetine, fluvoxamine, paroxetine, sertraline). There have been no reported cases from spontaneous reports of drug interaction between SSRI's and D.H.E. 45® (dihydroergotamine mesylate) Injection, USP.

Oral Contraceptives
The effect of oral contraceptives on the pharmacokinetics of D.H.E. 45® (dihydroergotamine mesylate) Injection, USP has not been studied.

Carcinogenesis, Mutagenesis, Impairment of Fertility

Carcinogenesis
Assessment of the carcinogenic potential of dihydroergotamine mesylate in mice and rats is ongoing.

Mutagenesis
Dihydroergotamine mesylate was clastogenic in two *in vitro* chromosomal aberration assays, the V79 Chinese hamster cell assay with metabolic activation and the cultured human peripheral blood lymphocyte assay. There was no evidence of mutagenic potential when dihydroergotamine mesylate was tested in the presence or absence of metabolic activation in two gene mutation assays (the Ames test and the *in vitro* mammalian Chinese hamster V79/HGPRT assay) and in an assay for DNA damage (the rat hepatocyte unscheduled DNA synthesis test). Dihydroergotamine was not clastogenic in the *in vivo* mouse and hamster micronucleus tests.

Impairment of Fertility
Impairment of fertility was not evaluated for D.H.E. 45® (dihydroergotamine mesylate) Injection, USP. There was no evidence of impairment of fertility in rats given intranasal doses of Migranal® Nasal Spray up to 1.6 mg/day (associated with mean plasma dihydroergotamine mesylate exposures [AUC] approximately 9 to 11 times those in humans receiving the MRDD of 4 mg).

Pregnancy

Pregnancy Category X. See CONTRAINDICATIONS.

Nursing Mothers
Ergot drugs are known to inhibit prolactin. It is likely that D.H.E. 45® (dihydroergotamine mesylate) Injection, USP is excreted in human milk, but there are no data on the concentration of dihydroergotamine in human milk. It is known that ergotamine is excreted in breast milk and may cause vomiting, diarrhea, weak pulse, and unstable blood pressure in nursing infants. Because of the potential for these serious adverse events in nursing infants exposed to D.H.E. 45® (dihydroergotamine mesylate) Injection, USP, nursing should not be undertaken with the use of D.H.E. 45® (dihydroergotamine mesylate) Injection, USP. *(See CONTRAINDICATIONS)*

Pediatric Use
Safety and effectiveness in pediatric patients have not been established.

ADVERSE REACTIONS

Serious cardiac events, including some that have been fatal, have occurred following use of D.H.E. 45® (dihydroergotamine mesylate) Injection, USP, but are extremely rare. Events reported have included coronary artery vasospasm, transient myocardial ischemia, myocardial infarction, ventricular tachycardia, and ventricular fibrillation. *(See CONTRAINDICATIONS, WARNINGS, and PRECAUTIONS)*

Post-introduction Reports
The following events derived from postmarketing experience have been occasionally reported in patients receiving D.H.E. 45® (dihydroergotamine mesylate) Injection, USP: vasospasm, paraesthesia, hypertension, dizziness, anxiety, dyspnea, headache, flushing, diarrhea, rash, increased sweating, and pleural and retroperitoneal fibrosis after long-term use of dihydroergotamine. Extremely rare cases of myocardial infarction and stroke have been reported. A causal relationship has not been established.
D.H.E. 45® (dihydroergotamine mesylate) Injection, USP is not recommended for prolonged daily use. *(See DOSAGE AND ADMINISTRATION)*

DRUG ABUSE AND DEPENDENCE

Currently available data have not demonstrated drug abuse or psychological dependence with dihydroergotamine. However, cases of drug abuse and psychological dependence in patients on other forms of ergot therapy have been reported. Thus, due to the chronicity of vascular headaches, it is imperative that patients be advised not to exceed recommended dosages.

OVERDOSAGE

To date, there have been no reports of acute overdosage with this drug. Due to the risk of vascular spasm, exceeding the recommended dosages of D.H.E. 45® (dihydroergotamine mesylate) Injection, USP is to be avoided. Excessive doses of dihydroergotamine may result in peripheral signs and symptoms of ergotism. Treatment includes discontinuance of the drug, local application of warmth to the affected area, the administration of vasodilators, and nursing care to prevent tissue damage.
In general, the symptoms of an acute D.H.E. 45® (dihydroergotamine mesylate) Injection, USP overdose are similar to those of an ergotamine overdose, although there is less pronounced nausea and vomiting with D.H.E. 45® (dihydroergotamine mesylate) Injection, USP. The symptoms of an ergotamine overdose include the following: numbness, tingling, pain, and cyanosis of the extremities associated with diminished or absent peripheral pulses; respiratory depression; an increase and/or decrease in blood pressure, usually in that order; confusion, delirium, convulsions, and coma; and/or some degree of nausea, vomiting, and abdominal pain.
In laboratory animals, significant lethality occurs when dihydroergotamine is given at I.V. doses of 44 mg/kg in mice, 130 mg/kg in rats, and 37 mg/kg in rabbits.
Up-to-date information about the treatment of overdosage can often be obtained from a certified Regional Poison Control Center. Telephone numbers of certified Poison Control Centers are listed in the Physician's Desk Reference® (PDR).*

DOSAGE AND ADMINISTRATION

D.H.E. 45® (dihydroergotamine mesylate) Injection, USP should be administered in a dose of 1 mL intravenously, intramuscularly or subcutaneously. The dose can be repeated, as needed, at 1 hour intervals to a total dose of 3 mL for intramuscular or subcutaneous delivery or 2 mL for intravenous delivery in a 24 hour period. The total weekly dosage should not exceed 6 mL.

HOW SUPPLIED

D.H.E. 45® (dihydroergotamine mesylate) Injection, USP
Available as a clear, colorless, sterile solution in single 1 mL sterile ampuls containing 1 mg of dihydroergotamine mesylate per mL, in packages of 10 (NDC 0078-0041-01).
Store below 77° F (25° C), in light-resistant containers. Do not refrigerate or freeze.
To assure constant potency, protect the ampuls from light and heat. Administer only if clear and colorless.

INSTRUCTION FOR PATIENTS ON SUBCUTANEOUS SELF-INJECTION

Information for the Patient

D.H.E. 45® (dihydroergotamine mesylate) Injection, USP
Before self-injecting D.H.E. 45® (dihydroergotamine mesylate) Injection, USP by subcutaneous administration, you will need to obtain professional instruction on how to properly administer your medication. Below are some of the steps you should follow carefully. Read this leaflet completely before using this medication.
This leaflet does not contain all of the information on D.H.E. 45® (dihydroergotamine mesylate) Injection, USP. Your pharmacist and/or health care provider can provide more detailed information.

Purpose of your Medication
D.H.E. 45® (dihydroergotamine mesylate) Injection, USP is intended to treat an active migraine headache. Do not try to use it to prevent a headache if you have no symptoms. Do not use it to treat common tension headache or a headache that is not at all typical of your usual migraine headache.

Do not use D.H.E. 45® (dihydroergotamine mesylate) Injection, USP if you:
- are pregnant or nursing.
- have any disease affecting your heart, arteries, or circulation.

Important questions to consider before using D.H.E. 45® (dihydroergotamine mesylate) Injection, USP
Please answer the following questions before you use your D.H.E. 45® (dihydroergotamine mesylate) Injection, USP. If you answer YES to any of these questions or are unsure of the answer, you should talk to your doctor before using D.H.E. 45® (dihydroergotamine mesylate) Injection, USP.
- Do you have high blood pressure?

- Do you have chest pain, shortness of breath, heart disease, or have you had any surgery on your heart arteries?
- Do you have risk factors for heart disease (such as high blood pressure, high cholesterol, obesity, diabetes, smoking, strong family history of heart disease, or you are postmenopausal or a male over 40)?
- Do you have any problems with blood circulation in your arms or legs, fingers, or toes?
- Are you pregnant? Do you think you might be pregnant? Are you trying to become pregnant? Are you sexually active and not using birth control? Are you breast feeding?
- Have you ever had to stop taking this or any other medication because of an allergy or bad reaction?
- Are you taking any other migraine medications, erythromycin or other antibiotics, or medications for blood pressure prescribed by your doctor, or other medicines obtained from your drugstore without a doctor's prescription?
- Do you smoke?
- Have you had, or do you have, any disease of the liver or kidney?
- Is this headache different from your usual migraine attacks?

REMEMBER TO TELL YOUR DOCTOR IF YOU HAVE ANSWERED YES TO ANY OF THESE QUESTIONS BEFORE YOU USE D.H.E. 45® (dihydroergotamine mesylate) Injection, USP

Side Effects To Watch Out For

Although the following reactions rarely occur, they can be serious and should be reported to your physician immediately:

- Numbness or tingling in your fingers and toes.
- Pain, tightness, or discomfort in your chest.
- Muscle pain or cramps in your arms and legs.
- Weakness in your legs.
- Temporary speeding or slowing of your heart rate.
- Swelling or itching.

Dosage

Your doctor will have told you what dose to use for each migraine attack. Should you get another migraine attack in the same day as the attack you treated, you must not treat it with D.H.E. 45® (dihydroergotamine mesylate) Injection, USP unless at least 6 hours have elapsed since your last injection. No more than 6 mL of D.H.E. 45® (dihydroergotamine mesylate) Injection, USP should be injected during a one-week period.

Learn what to do in case of an Overdose

If you have used more medication than you have been instructed, contact your doctor, hospital emergency department, or nearest poison control center immediately.

How to use the D.H.E. 45® (dihydroergotamine mesylate) Injection, USP

1. Use available training materials.
   - Read and follow the instructions in the patient instruction booklet which is provided with the D.H.E. 45® (dihydroergotamine mesylate) Injection, USP package before attempting to use the product.
   - If there are any questions concerning the use of your D.H.E. 45® (dihydroergotamine mesylate) Injection, USP, ask your Doctor or pharmacist.
2. Preparing for the Injection
   - Carefully examine the ampul (glass vial) of D.H.E. 45® (dihydroergotamine mesylate) Injection, USP for any cracks or breaks, and the liquid for discoloration, cloudiness, or particles. If any of these defects are present, use a new ampul, make certain it is intact, and return the defective ampul to your doctor or pharmacy. Once you open an ampul, if it is not used within an hour, it should be thrown away.
3. Locating an Injection Site
   - Administer your subcutaneous Injection in the middle of your thigh, well above the knee.
4. Drawing the Medication into the Syringe
   - Wash your hands thoroughly with soap and water.
   - Check the dose of your medication.
   - Look to see if there is any liquid at the top of the ampul. If there is, gently flick the ampul with your finger to get all the liquid into the bottom portion of the ampul.
   - Hold the bottom of the ampul in one hand. Clean the ampul neck with an alcohol wipe using your other hand. Then place the alcohol wipe around the neck of the ampul and break it open by pressing your thumb against the neck of the ampul.
   - Tilt the ampul down at a 45° angle. Insert the needle into the solution in the ampul.
   - Draw up the medication by pulling back the plunger slowly and steadily until you reach your dose.
   - Check the syringe for air bubbles. Hold it with the needle pointing upward. If there are air bubbles, tap your finger against the barrel of the syringe to get the bubbles to the top. Slowly and carefully push the plunger up so that the bubbles are pushed out through the needle and you see a drop of medication.
   - When there are no air bubbles, check the dose of the medication. If the dose is incorrect, repeat steps 6 through 8 until you draw up the right dose.
5. Preparing the Injection Site
   - With a new alcohol wipe, clean the selected injection site thoroughly with a firm, circular motion from inside to outside. Wait for the injection site to dry before injecting.
6. Administering the Injection
   - Hold the syringe/needle in your right hand.
   - With your left hand, firmly grasp about a 1-inch fold of skin at the injection site.
   - Push the needle shaft, bevel side up, all the way into the fold of skin at a 45° to 90° angle, then release the fold of skin.
   - While holding the syringe with your left hand, use your right hand to draw back slightly on the plunger.
   - If you do not see any blood coming back into the syringe, inject the medication by pushing down on the plunger. If you do see blood in the syringe, that means the needle has penetrated a vein. If this happens, pull the needle/syringe out of the skin slightly and draw back on the plunger again. If no blood is seen this time, inject the medication.
   - Use your right hand to pull the needle out of your skin quickly at the same angle you injected it. Immediately press the alcohol wipe on the injection site and rub.

Check the expiration date printed on the ampul containing medication. If the expiration date has passed, do not use it.

Answers to patients' questions about D.H.E. 45® (dihydroergotamine mesylate) Injection, USP

What if I need help in using my D.H.E. 45® (dihydroergotamine mesylate) Injection, USP?

If you have any questions or if you need help in opening, putting together, or using D.H.E. 45® (dihydroergotamine mesylate) Injection, USP, speak to your doctor or pharmacist.

How much medication should I use and how often?

Your doctor will have told you what dose to use for each migraine attack. Should you get another migraine attack in the same day as the attack you treated, you must not treat it with D.H.E. 45® (dihydroergotamine mesylate) Injection, USP unless at least 6 hours have elapsed since your last injection. No more than 6 mL of D.H.E. 45® (dihydroergotamine mesylate) Injection, USP should be injected during a one-week period. Do not use more than this amount unless instructed to do so by your doctor.

If you have any other unanswered question about D.H.E. 45® (dihydroergotamine mesylate) Injection, USP, consult your doctor or pharmacist.

*Trademark of Medical Economics Company, Inc.

REV: MAY 1998 30220906

DIOVAN™
valsartan
Capsules ℞

The following prescribing information is based on official labeling in effect on August 1, 1998.

Prescribing Information

> **USE IN PREGNANCY**
> **When used in pregnancy during the second and third trimesters, drugs that act directly on the renin-angiotensin system can cause injury and even death to the developing fetus.** When pregnancy is detected, Diovan should be discontinued as soon as possible. See **WARNINGS: Fetal/Neonatal Morbidity and Mortality.**

DESCRIPTION

Diovan (valsartan) is a nonpeptide, orally active, and specific angiotensin II antagonist acting on the AT_1 receptor subtype.

Valsartan is chemically described as *N*-(1-oxopentyl)-*N*-[[2'-(1*H*-tetrazol-5-yl)[1,1'-biphenyl]-4-yl]methyl]-L-valine. Its empirical formula is $C_{24}H_{29}N_5O_3$, its molecular weight is 435.5, and its structural formula is

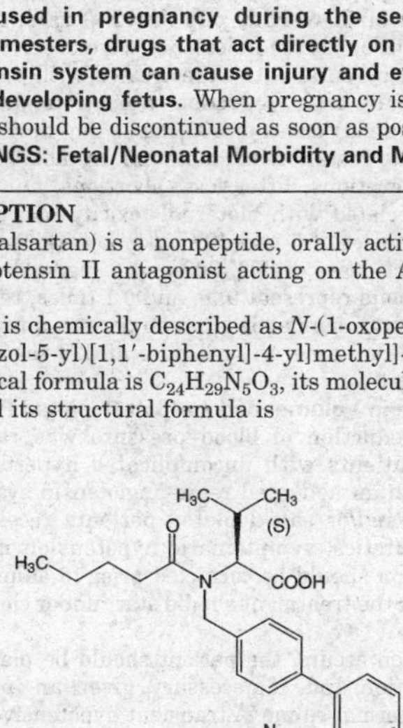

Valsartan is a white to practically white fine powder. It is soluble in ethanol and methanol and slightly soluble in water.

Diovan is available as capsules for oral administration, containing either 80 mg or 160 mg of valsartan. The inactive ingredients of the capsules are cellulose compounds, crospovidone, gelatin, iron oxides, magnesium stearate, povidone, sodium lauryl sulfate, and titanium dioxide.

CLINICAL PHARMACOLOGY

Mechanism of Action

Angiotensin II is formed from angiotensin I in a reaction catalyzed by angiotensin-converting enzyme (ACE, kininase II). Angiotensin II is the principal pressor agent of the renin-angiotensin system, with effects that include vasoconstriction, stimulation of synthesis and release of aldosterone, cardiac stimulation, and renal reabsorption of sodium. Valsartan blocks the vasoconstrictor and aldosterone-secreting effects of angiotensin II by selectively blocking the binding of angiotensin II to the AT_1 receptor in many tissues, such as vascular smooth muscle and the adrenal gland. Its action is therefore independent of the pathways for angiotensin II synthesis.

There is also an AT_2 receptor found in many tissues, but AT_2 is not known to be associated with cardiovascular homeostasis. Valsartan has much greater affinity (about 20,000-fold) for the AT_1 receptor than for the AT_2 receptor. The primary metabolite of valsartan is essentially inactive with an affinity for the AT_1 receptor about one 200th that of valsartan itself.

Blockade of the renin-angiotensin system with ACE inhibitors, which inhibit the biosynthesis of angiotensin II from angiotensin I, is widely used in the treatment of hypertension. ACE inhibitors also inhibit the degradation of bradykinin, a reaction also catalyzed by ACE. Because valsartan does not inhibit ACE (kininase II), it does not affect the response to bradykinin. Whether this difference has clinical relevance is not yet known. Valsartan does not bind to or block other hormone receptors or ion channels known to be important in cardiovascular regulation.

Blockade of the angiotensin II receptor inhibits the negative regulatory feedback of angiotensin II on renin secretion, but the resulting increased plasma renin activity and angiotensin II circulating levels do not overcome the effect of valsartan on blood pressure.

Pharmacokinetics

Valsartan peak plasma concentration is reached 2 to 4 hours after dosing. Valsartan shows bi-exponential decay kinetics following intravenous administration, with an average elimination half-life of about 6 hours. Absolute bioavailability for the capsule formulation is about 25% (range 10%–35%). Food decreases the exposure (as measured by AUC) to valsartan by about 40% and peak plasma concentration (C_{max}) by about 50%. AUC and C_{max} values of valsartan increase approximately linearly with increasing dose over the clinical dosing range. Valsartan does not accumulate appreciably in plasma following repeated administration.

Metabolism and Elimination

Valsartan, when administered as an oral solution, is primarily recovered in feces (about 83% of dose) and urine (about 13% of dose). The recovery is mainly as unchanged drug, with only about 20% of dose recovered as metabolites. The primary metabolite, accounting for about 9% of dose, is valeryl 4-hydroxy valsartan. The enzyme(s) responsible for valsartan metabolism have not been identified but do not seem to be CYP 450 isozymes.

Following intravenous administration, plasma clearance of valsartan is about 2 L/h and its renal clearance is 0.62 L/h (about 30% of total clearance).

Distribution

The steady state volume of distribution of valsartan after intravenous administration is small (17 L), indicating that valsartan does not distribute into tissues extensively. Valsartan is highly bound to serum proteins (95%), mainly serum albumin.

Special Populations

Pediatric: The pharmacokinetics of valsartan have not been investigated in patients <18 years of age.

Geriatric: Exposure (measured by AUC) to valsartan is higher by 70% and the half-life is longer by 35% in the elderly than in the young. No dosage adjustment is necessary (see DOSAGE AND ADMINISTRATION).

Gender: Pharmacokinetics of valsartan does not differ significantly between males and females.

Renal Insufficiency: There is no apparent correlation between renal function (measured by creatinine clearance) and exposure (measured by AUC) to valsartan in patients with different degrees of renal impairment. Consequently, dose adjustment is not required in patients with mild-to-moderate renal dysfunction. No studies have been performed in patients with severe impairment of renal function (creatinine clearance <10 mL/min). Valsartan is not removed from the plasma by hemodialysis. In the case of severe renal disease, exercise care with dosing of valsartan (see DOSAGE AND ADMINISTRATION).

Continued on next page

Diovan—Cont.

Hepatic Insufficiency: On average, patients with mild-to-moderate chronic liver disease have twice the exposure (measured by AUC values) to valsartan of healthy volunteers (matched by age, sex and weight). In general, no dosage adjustment is needed in patients with mild-to-moderate liver disease. Care should be exercised in patients with liver disease (see DOSAGE AND ADMINISTRATION).

Pharmacodynamics and Clinical Effects

Valsartan inhibits the pressor effect of angiotensin II infusions. An oral dose of 80 mg inhibits the pressor effect by about 80% at peak with approximately 30% inhibition persisting for 24 hours. No information on the effect of larger doses is available.

Removal of the negative feedback of angiotensin II causes a 2- to 3-fold rise in plasma renin and consequent rise in angiotensin II plasma concentration in hypertensive patients. Minimal decreases in plasma aldosterone were observed after administration of valsartan; very little effect on serum potassium was observed.

In multiple-dose studies in hypertensive patients with stable renal insufficiency and patients with renovascular hypertension, valsartan had no clinically significant effects on glomerular filtration rate, filtration fraction, creatinine clearance, or renal plasma flow.

In multiple-dose studies in hypertensive patients, valsartan had no notable effects on total cholesterol, fasting triglycerides, fasting serum glucose, or uric acid.

The antihypertensive effects of Diovan were demonstrated principally in 7 placebo-controlled, 4- to 12-week trials (one in patients over 65) of dosages from 10 to 320 mg/day in patients with baseline diastolic blood pressures of 95–115. The studies allowed comparison of once-daily and twice-daily regimens of 160 mg/day; comparison of peak and trough effects; comparison (in pooled data) of response by gender, age, and race; and evaluation of incremental effects of hydrochlorothiazide.

Administration of valsartan to patients with essential hypertension results in a significant reduction of sitting, supine, and standing systolic and diastolic blood pressure, usually with little or no orthostatic change.

In most patients, after administration of a single oral dose, onset of antihypertensive activity occurs at approximately 2 hours, and maximum reduction of blood pressure is achieved within 6 hours. The antihypertensive effect persists for 24 hours after dosing, but there is a decrease from peak effect at lower doses (40 mg) presumably reflecting loss of inhibition of angiotensin II. At higher doses, however, (160 mg) there is little difference in peak and trough effect. During repeated dosing, the reduction in blood pressure with any dose is substantially present within 2 weeks, and maximal reduction is generally attained after 4 weeks.

In long-term follow-up studies (without placebo control), the effect of valsartan appeared to be maintained for up to two years. The antihypertensive effect is independent of age, gender or race. The latter finding regarding race is based on pooled data and should be viewed with caution, because antihypertensive drugs that affect the renin-angiotensin system (that is, ACE inhibitors and angiotensin-II blockers) have generally been found to be less effective in low-renin hypertensives (frequently blacks) than in high-renin hypertensives (frequently whites). In pooled, randomized, controlled trials of Diovan that included a total of 140 blacks and 830 whites, valsartan and an ACE-inhibitor control were generally at least as effective in blacks as whites. The explanation for this difference from previous findings is unclear.

Abrupt withdrawal of valsartan has not been associated with a rapid increase in blood pressure.

The blood pressure lowering effect of valsartan and thiazide-type diuretics are approximately additive.

The 7 studies of valsartan monotherapy included over 2000 patients randomized to various doses of valsartan and about 800 patients randomized to placebo. Doses below 80 mg were not consistently distinguished from those of placebo at trough, but doses of 80, 160 and 320 mg produced dose-related decreases in systolic and diastolic blood pressure, with the difference from placebo of approximately 6–9/3–5 mmHg at 80–160 mg and 9/6 mmHg at 320 mg. In a controlled trial the addition of HCTZ to valsartan 80 mg resulted in additional lowering of systolic and diastolic blood pressure by approximately 6/3 and 12/5 mmHg for 12.5 and 25 mg of HCTZ, respectively, compared to valsartan 80 mg alone.

Patients with an inadequate response to 80 mg once daily were titrated to either 160 mg once daily or 80 mg twice daily, which resulted in a comparable response in both groups.

In controlled trials, the antihypertensive effect of once-daily valsartan 80 mg was similar to that of once-daily enalapril 20 mg or once-daily lisinopril 10 mg.

There was essentially no change in heart rate in valsartan-treated patients in controlled trials.

INDICATIONS AND USAGE

Diovan is indicated for the treatment of hypertension. It may be used alone or in combination with other antihypertensive agents.

CONTRAINDICATIONS

Diovan is contraindicated in patients who are hypersensitive to any component of this product.

WARNINGS

Fetal/Neonatal Morbidity and Mortality

Drugs that act directly on the renin-angiotensin system can cause fetal and neonatal morbidity and death when administered to pregnant women. Several dozen cases have been reported in the world literature in patients who were taking angiotensin-converting enzyme inhibitors. When pregnancy is detected, Diovan should be discontinued as soon as possible.

The use of drugs that act directly on the renin-angiotensin system during the second and third trimesters of pregnancy has been associated with fetal and neonatal injury, including hypotension, neonatal skull hypoplasia, anuria, reversible or irreversible renal failure, and death. Oligohydramnios has also been reported, presumably resulting from decreased fetal renal function; oligohydramnios in this setting has been associated with fetal limb contractures, craniofacial deformation, and hypoplastic lung development. Prematurity, intrauterine growth retardation, and patent ductus arteriosus have also been reported, although it is not clear whether these occurrences were due to exposure to the drug.

These adverse effects do not appear to have resulted from intrauterine drug exposure that has been limited to the first trimester. Mothers whose embryos and fetuses are exposed to an angiotensin II receptor antagonist only during the first trimester should be so informed. Nonetheless, when patients become pregnant, physicians should advise the patient to discontinue the use of valsartan as soon as possible.

Rarely (probably less often than once in every thousand pregnancies), no alternative to a drug acting on the renin-angiotensin system will be found. In these rare cases, the mothers should be apprised of the potential hazards to their fetuses, and serial ultrasound examinations should be performed to assess the intra-amniotic environment.

If oligohydramnios is observed, valsartan should be discontinued unless it is considered life-saving for the mother. Contraction stress testing (CST), a nonstress test (NST), or biophysical profiling (BPP) may be appropriate, depending upon the week of pregnancy. Patients and physicians should be aware, however, that oligohydramnios may not appear until after the fetus has sustained irreversible injury.

Infants with histories of in utero exposure to an angiotensin II receptor antagonist should be closely observed for hypotension, oliguria, and hyperkalemia. If oliguria occurs, attention should be directed toward support of blood pressure and renal perfusion. Exchange transfusion or dialysis may be required as means of reversing hypotension and/or substituting for disordered renal function.

No teratogenic effects were observed when valsartan was administered to pregnant mice and rats at oral doses up to 600 mg/kg/day and to pregnant rabbits at oral doses up to 10 mg/kg/day. However, significant decreases in fetal weight, pup birth weight, pup survival rate, and slight delays in developmental milestones were observed in studies in which parental rats were treated with valsartan at oral, maternally toxic (reduction in body weight gain and food consumption) doses of 600 mg/kg/day during organogenesis or late gestation and lactation. In rabbits, fetotoxicity (i.e., resorptions, litter loss, abortions, and low body weight) associated with maternal toxicity (mortality) was observed at doses of 5 and 10 mg/kg/day. The no observed adverse effect doses of 600, 200 and 2 mg/kg/day in mice, rats and rabbits represent 9, 6, and 0.1 times, respectively, the maximum recommended human dose on a mg/m² basis. (Calculations assume an oral dose of 320 mg/day and a 60-kg patient).

Hypotension in Volume- and /or Salt-Depleted Patients

Excessive reduction of blood pressure was rarely seen (0.1%) in patients with uncomplicated hypertension. In patients with an activated renin-angiotensin system, such as volume- and/or salt-depleted patients receiving high doses of diuretics, symptomatic hypotension may occur. This condition should be corrected prior to administration of Diovan, or the treatment should start under close medical supervision.

If hypotension occurs, the patient should be placed in the supine position and, if necessary, given an intravenous infusion of normal saline. A transient hypotensive response is not a contraindication to further treatment, which usually can be continued without difficulty once the blood pressure has stabilized.

PRECAUTIONS

General

Impaired Hepatic Function: As the majority of valsartan is eliminated in the bile, patients with mild-to-moderate hepatic impairment, including patients with biliary obstructive disorders, showed lower valsartan clearance (higher AUCs). Care should be exercised in administering Diovan to these patients.

Impaired Renal Function: As a consequence of inhibiting the renin-angiotensin-aldosterone system, changes in renal function may be anticipated in susceptible individuals. In patients whose renal function may depend on the activity of the renin-angiotensin-aldosterone system (e.g., patients with severe congestive heart failure), treatment with angiotensin-converting enzyme inhibitors and angiotensin receptor antagonists has been associated with oliguria and/or progressive azotemia and (rarely) with acute renal failure and/or death. Diovan would be expected to behave similarly.

In studies of ACE inhibitors in patients with unilateral or bilateral renal artery stenosis, increases in serum creatinine or blood urea nitrogen have been reported. In a 4-day trial of valsartan in 12 patients with unilateral renal artery stenosis, no significant increases in serum creatinine or blood urea nitrogen were observed. There has been no long-term use of Diovan in patients with unilateral or bilateral renal artery stenosis, but an effect similar to that seen with ACE inhibitors should be anticipated.

Information for Patients

Pregnancy: Female patients of childbearing age should be told about the consequences of second- and third-trimester exposure to drugs that act on the renin-angiotensin system, and they should also be told that these consequences do not appear to have resulted from intrauterine drug exposure that has been limited to the first trimester. These patients should be asked to report pregnancies to their physicians as soon as possible.

Drug Interactions

No clinically significant pharmacokinetic interactions were observed when valsartan was coadministered with amlodipine, atenolol, cimetidine, digoxin, furosemide, glyburide, hydrochlorothiazide, or indomethacin. The valsartan-atenolol combination was more antihypertensive than either component, but it did not lower the heart rate more than atenolol alone.

Coadministration of valsartan and warfarin did not change the pharmacokinetics of valsartan or the time-course of the anticoagulant properties of warfarin.

CYP 450 Interactions: The enzyme(s) responsible for valsartan metabolism have not been identified but do not seem to be CYP 450 isozymes. The inhibitory or induction potential of valsartan on CYP 450 is also unknown.

Carcinogenesis, Mutagenesis, Impairment of Fertility

There was no evidence of carcinogenicity when valsartan was administered in the diet to mice and rats for up to 2 years at doses up to 160 and 200 mg/kg/day, respectively. These doses in mice and rats are about 2.6 and 6 times, respectively, the maximum recommended human dose on a mg/m² basis. (Calculations assume an oral dose of 320 mg/day and a 60-kg patient.)

Mutagenicity assays did not reveal any valsartan-related effects at either the gene or chromosome level. These assays included bacterial mutagenicity tests with *Salmonella* (Ames) and *E coli;* a gene mutation test with Chinese hamster V79 cells; a cytogenetic test with Chinese hamster ovary cells; and a rat micronucleus test.

Valsartan had no adverse effects on the reproductive performance of male or female rats at oral doses up to 200 mg/kg/day. This dose is 6 times the maximum recommended human dose on a mg/m² basis. (Calculations assume an oral dose of 320 mg/day and a 60-kg patient.)

Pregnancy Categories C (first trimester) and D (second and third trimesters)

See WARNINGS, Fetal/Neonatal Morbidity and Mortality.

Nursing Mothers

It is not known whether valsartan is excreted in human milk, but valsartan was excreted in the milk of lactating rats. Because of the potential for adverse effects on the nursing infant, a decision should be made whether to discontinue nursing or discontinue the drug, taking into account the importance of the drug to the mother.

Pediatric Use

Safety and effectiveness in pediatric patients have not been established.

Geriatric Use

In the controlled clinical trials of valsartan, 1214 (36.2%) of patients treated with valsartan were ≥ 65 years and 265 (7.9%) were ≥ 75 years. No overall difference in the efficacy or safety of valsartan was observed in this patient population, but greater sensitivity of some older individuals cannot be ruled out.

ADVERSE REACTIONS

Diovan has been evaluated for safety in more than 4000 patients, including over 400 treated for over 6 months, and more than 160 for over 1 year. Adverse experiences have generally been mild and transient in nature and have only infrequently required discontinuation of therapy. The overall incidence of adverse experiences with Diovan was similar to placebo.

The overall frequency of adverse experiences was neither dose-related nor related to gender, age, race, or regimen. Discontinuation of therapy due to side effects was required in 2.3% of valsartan patients and 2.0% of placebo patients. The most common reasons for discontinuation of therapy with Diovan were headache and dizziness.

The adverse experiences that occurred in placebo-controlled clinical trials in at least 1% of patients treated with Diovan and at a higher incidence in valsartan (n=2316) than placebo (n=888) patients included viral infection (3% vs. 2%), fatigue (2% vs. 1%), and abdominal pain (2% vs. 1%).

Headache, dizziness, upper respiratory infection, cough, diarrhea, rhinitis, sinusitis, nausea, pharyngitis, edema, and arthralgia occurred at a more than 1% rate but at about the same incidence in placebo and valsartan patients.

In trials in which valsartan was compared to an ACE inhibitor with or without placebo, the incidence of dry cough was significantly greater in the ACE-inhibitor group (7.9%) than in the groups who received valsartan (2.6%) or placebo (1.5%). In a 129-patient trial limited to patients who had had dry cough when they had previously received ACE inhibitors, the incidences of cough in patients who received valsartan, HCTZ, or lisinopril were 20%, 19%, and 69% respectively ($p<0.001$).

Dose-related orthostatic effects were seen in less than 1% of patients. An increase in the incidence of dizziness was observed in patients treated with Diovan 320 mg (8%) compared to 10 to 160 mg (2% to 4%).

Diovan has been used concomitantly with hydrochlorothiazide without evidence of clinically important adverse interactions.

Other adverse experiences that occurred in controlled clinical trials of patients treated with Diovan (>0.2% of valsartan patients) are listed below. It cannot be determined whether these events were causally related to Diovan.

Body as a Whole: Allergic reaction and asthenia
Cardiovascular: Palpitations
Dermatologic: Pruritus and rash
Digestive: Constipation, dry mouth, dyspepsia, and flatulence
Musculoskeletal: Back pain, muscle cramps, and myalgia
Neurologic and Psychiatric: Anxiety, insomnia, paresthesia, and somnolence
Respiratory: Dyspnea
Special Senses: Vertigo
Urogenital: Impotence

Other reported events seen less frequently in clinical trials included chest pain, syncope, anorexia, vomiting, and angioedema.

Clinical Laboratory Test Findings

In controlled clinical trials, clinically important changes in standard laboratory parameters were rarely associated with administration of Diovan.

Creatinine: Minor elevations in creatinine occurred in 0.8% of patients taking Diovan and 0.6% given placebo in controlled clinical trials.

Hemoglobin and Hematocrit: Greater than 20% decreases in hemoglobin and hematocrit were observed in 0.4% and 0.8%, respectively, of Diovan patients, compared with 0.1% and 0.1% in placebo-treated patients. One valsartan patient discontinued treatment for microcytic anemia.

Liver function tests: Occasional elevations (greater than 150%) of liver chemistries occurred in Diovan-treated patients. Three patients (<0.1%) treated with valsartan discontinued treatment for elevated liver chemistries.

Neutropenia: Neutropenia was observed in 1.9% of patients treated with Diovan and 0.8% of patients treated with placebo.

Serum Potassium: Greater than 20% increases in serum potassium were observed in 4.4% of Diovan-treated patients compared to 2.9% of placebo-treated patients. No patient treated with valsartan discontinued therapy for hyperkalemia.

OVERDOSAGE

Limited data are available related to overdosage in humans. The most likely manifestations of overdosage would be hypotension and tachycardia; bradycardia could occur from parasympathetic (vagal) stimulation. If symptomatic hypotension should occur, supportive treatment should be instituted.

Valsartan is not removed from the plasma by hemodialysis. Valsartan was without grossly observable adverse effects at single oral doses up to 2000 mg/kg in rats and up to 1000 mg/kg in marmosets, except for salivation and diarrhea in the rat and vomiting in the marmoset at the highest dose (60 and 37 times, respectively, the maximum recommended human dose on a mg/m^2 basis). (Calculations assume an oral dose of 320 mg/day and a 60-kg patient.)

DOSAGE AND ADMINISTRATION

The recommended starting dose of Diovan is 80 mg once daily when used as monotherapy in patients who are not volume-depleted. Diovan may be used over a dose range of 80 mg to 320 mg daily, administered once-a-day.

The antihypertensive effect is substantially present within 2 weeks and maximal reduction is generally attained after 4 weeks. If additional antihypertensive effect is required, the dosage may be increased to 160 mg or 320 mg or a diuretic may be added. Addition of a diuretic has a greater effect than dose increases beyond 80 mg.

No initial dosage adjustment is required for elderly patients, for patients with mild or moderate renal impairment, or for patients with mild or moderate liver insufficiency. Care should be exercised with dosing of Diovan in patients with hepatic or severe renal impairment.

Diovan may be administered with other antihypertensive agents.

Diovan may be administered with or without food.

HOW SUPPLIED

Diovan is available as capsules containing valsartan 80 mg or 160 mg. Both strengths are packaged in bottles of 100 capsules and 4000 capsules and unit dose blister packages. Capsules are imprinted as follows:

80 mg Capsule - Light grey/light pink opaque, imprinted CG FZF

Bottles of 100	NDC 0083-4000-01
Bottles of 4000	NDC 0083-4000-41
Unit Dose (blister pack) Box of 100 (strips of 10)	NDC 0083-4000-61

160 mg Capsule - Dark grey/light pink opaque, imprinted CG GOG

Bottles of 100	NDC 0083-4001-01
Bottles of 4000	NDC 0083-4001-41
Unit Dose (blister pack) Box of 100 (strips of 10)	NDC 0083-4001-61

Store below 30°C (86°F). Protect from moisture.
Dispense in tight container (USP).

C97-6 (Rev. 4/97)

Dist. by:
Ciba-Geigy Corporation
Pharmaceuticals Division
Summit, New Jersey 07901

Shown in Product Identification Guide, page 324

DIOVAN HCT™ ℞

valsartan and hydrochlorothiazide
Combination Tablets
80 mg/12.5 mg
160 mg/12.5 mg

Rx only

The following prescribing information is based on official labeling in effect on November 1, 1998.

USE IN PREGNANCY
When used in pregnancy during the second and third trimesters, drugs that act directly on the renin-angiotensin system can cause injury and even death to the developing fetus. When pregnancy is detected, Diovan HCT should be discontinued as soon as possible. See **WARNINGS: Fetal/Neonatal Morbidity and Mortality.**

DESCRIPTION

Diovan HCT is a combination of valsartan, an orally active, specific angiotensin II antagonist acting on the AT$_1$ receptor subtype, and hydrochlorothiazide, a diuretic.

Valsartan, a nonpeptide molecule, is chemically described as *N*-(1-oxopentyl)-*N*-[[2'-(1*H*-tetrazol-5-yl)[1,1'-biphenyl]-4-yl]methyl]-L-Valine. Its empirical formula is $C_{24}H_{29}N_5O_3$, its molecular weight is 435.5, and its structural formula is

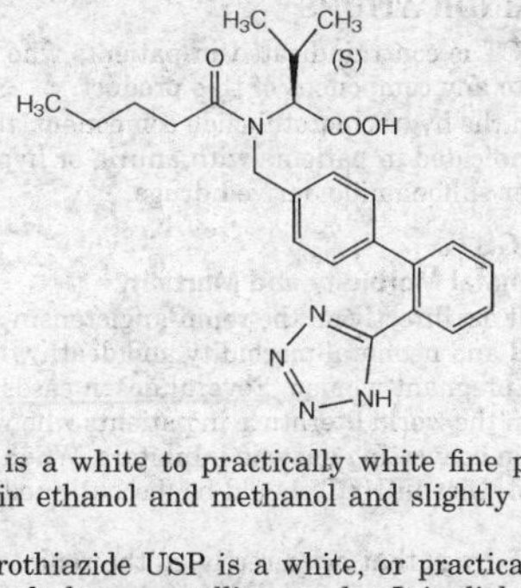

Valsartan is a white to practically white fine powder. It is soluble in ethanol and methanol and slightly soluble in water.

Hydrochlorothiazide USP is a white, or practically white, practically odorless, crystalline powder. It is slightly soluble in water; freely soluble in sodium hydroxide solution, in *n*-butylamine, and in dimethylformamide; sparingly soluble in methanol; and insoluble in ether, in chloroform, and in dilute mineral acids. Hydrochlorothiazide is chemically described as 6-chloro-3,4-dihydro-2*H*-1,2,4-benzothiadiazine-7-sulfonamide 1,1-dioxide. Hydrochlorothiazide is a thiazide diuretic. Its empirical formula is $C_7H_8ClN_3O_4S_2$, its molecular weight is 297.73, and its structural formula is

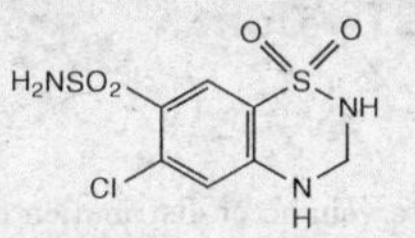

Diovan HCT tablets are formulated for oral administration with a combination of 80 mg or 160 mg of valsartan and 12.5 mg of hydrochlorothiazide USP. The inactive ingredients of the tablets are colloidal silicon dioxide, crospovidone, hydroxypropyl methylcellulose, iron oxides, magnesium stearate, microcrystalline cellulose, polyethylene glycol, talc, and titanium dioxide.

CLINICAL PHARMACOLOGY

Mechanism of Action

Angiotensin II is formed from angiotensin I in a reaction catalyzed by angiotensin-converting enzyme (ACE, kininase II). Angiotensin II is the principal pressor agent of the renin-angiotensin system, with effects that include vasoconstriction, stimulation of synthesis and release of aldosterone, cardiac stimulation, and renal reabsorption of sodium. Valsartan blocks the vasoconstrictor and aldosterone-secreting effects of angiotensin II by selectively blocking the binding of angiotensin II to the AT$_1$ receptor in many tissues, such as vascular smooth muscle and the adrenal gland. Its action is therefore independent of the pathways for angiotensin II synthesis.

There is also an AT$_2$ receptor found in many tissues, but AT$_2$ is not known to be associated with cardiovascular homeostasis. Valsartan has much greater affinity (about 20,000-fold) for the AT$_1$ receptor than for the AT$_2$ receptor. The primary metabolite of valsartan is essentially inactive with an affinity for the AT$_1$ receptor about one 200th that of valsartan itself.

Blockade of the renin-angiotensin system with ACE inhibitors, which inhibit the biosynthesis of angiotensin II from angiotensin I, is widely used in the treatment of hypertension. ACE inhibitors also inhibit the degradation of bradykinin, a reaction also catalyzed by ACE. Because valsartan does not inhibit ACE (kininase II) it does not affect the response to bradykinin. Whether this difference has clinical relevance is not yet known. Valsartan does not bind to or block other hormone receptors or ion channels known to be important in cardiovascular regulation.

Blockade of the angiotensin II receptor inhibits the negative regulatory feedback of angiotensin II on renin secretion, but the resulting increased plasma renin activity and angiotensin II circulating levels do not overcome the effect of valsartan on blood pressure.

Hydrochlorothiazide is a thiazide diuretic. Thiazides affect the renal tubular mechanisms of electrolyte reabsorption, directly increasing excretion of sodium and chloride in approximately equivalent amounts. Indirectly, the diuretic action of hydrochlorothiazide reduces plasma volume, with consequent increases in plasma renin activity, increases in aldosterone secretion, increases in urinary potassium loss, and decreases in serum potassium. The renin-aldosterone link is mediated by angiotensin II, so coadministration of an angiotensin II receptor antagonist tends to reverse the potassium loss associated with these diuretics.

The mechanism of the antihypertensive effect of thiazides is unknown.

Pharmacokinetics

Valsartan

Valsartan peak plasma concentration is reached 2 to 4 hours after dosing. Valsartan shows bi-exponential decay kinetics following intravenous administration, with an average elimination half-life of about 6 hours. Absolute bioavailability for the capsule formulation is about 25% (range 10%-35%). Food decreases the exposure (as measured by AUC) to valsartan by about 40% and peak plasma concentration (C_{max}) by about 50%. AUC and C_{max} values of valsartan increase approximately linearly with increasing dose over the clinical dosing range. Valsartan does not accumulate appreciably in plasma following repeated administration.

Metabolism and Elimination

Valsartan

Valsartan, when administered as an oral solution, is primarily recovered in feces (about 83% of dose) and urine (about 13% of dose). The recovery is mainly as unchanged drug, with only about 20% of dose recovered as metabolites. The primary metabolite, accounting for about 9% of dose, is valeryl 4-hydroxy valsartan. The enzyme(s) responsible for valsartan metabolism have not been identified but do not seem to be CYP 450 isozymes.

Following intravenous administration, plasma clearance of valsartan is about 2 L/h and its renal clearance is 0.62 L/h (about 30% of total clearance).

Hydrochlorothiazide

Hydrochlorothiazide is not metabolized but is eliminated rapidly by the kidney. At least 61% of the oral dose is eliminated as unchanged drug within 24 hours. The elimination half-life is between 5.8 and 18.9 hours.

Continued on next page

Diovan HCT—Cont.

Distribution

Valsartan

The steady state volume of distribution of valsartan after intravenous administration is small (17 L), indicating that valsartan does not distribute into tissues extensively. Valsartan is highly bound to serum proteins (95%), mainly serum albumin.

Hydrochlorothiazide

Hydrochlorothiazide crosses the placental but not the blood-brain barrier and is excreted in breast milk.

Special Populations

Pediatric: The pharmacokinetics of valsartan have not been investigated in patients <18 years of age.

Geriatric: Exposure (measured by AUC) to valsartan is higher by 70% and the half-life is longer by 35% in the elderly than in the young. No dosage adjustment is necessary *(see DOSAGE AND ADMINISTRATION)*.

Gender: Pharmacokinetics of valsartan does not differ significantly between males and females.

Race: Pharmacokinetic differences due to race have not been studied.

Renal Insufficiency: There is no apparent correlation between renal function (measured by creatinine clearance) and exposure (measured by AUC) to valsartan in patients with different degrees of renal impairment. Consequently, dose adjustment is not required in patients with mild-to-moderate renal dysfunction. No studies have been performed in patients with severe impairment of renal function (creatinine clearance <10 mL/min). Valsartan is not removed from the plasma by hemodialysis. In the case of severe renal disease, exercise care with dosing of valsartan *(see DOSAGE AND ADMINISTRATION)*.

Thiazide diuretics are eliminated by the kidney, with a terminal half-life of 5-15 hours. In a study of patients with impaired renal function (mean creatinine clearance of 19 mL/min), the half-life of hydrochlorothiazide elimination was lengthened to 21 hours.

Hepatic Insufficiency: On average, patients with mild-to-moderate chronic liver disease have twice the exposure (measured by AUC values) to valsartan of healthy volunteers (matched by age, sex and weight). In general, no dosage adjustment is needed in patients with mild-to-moderate liver disease. Care should be exercised in patients with liver disease *(see DOSAGE AND ADMINISTRATION)*.

Pharmacodynamics and Clinical Effects

Valsartan – Hydrochlorothiazide

In controlled clinical trials including over 1500 patients, 730 patients were exposed to valsartan (80 and 160 mg) and concomitant hydrochlorothiazide (12.5 and 25 mg). A factorial trial compared the combinations of 80/12.5 mg, 80/25 mg, 160/12.5 mg and 160/25 mg with their respective components and placebo. The combination of valsartan and hydrochlorothiazide resulted in additive placebo-adjusted decreases in systolic and diastolic blood pressure at trough of 15-21/8-11 mmHg at 80/12.5 mg to 160/25 mg, compared to 7-10/4-6 mmHg for valsartan 80 mg to 160 mg and 6-10/3-5 mmHg for hydrochlorothiazide 12.5 mg to 25 mg, alone.

In another controlled trial the addition of hydrochlorothiazide to valsartan 80 mg resulted in additional lowering of systolic and diastolic blood pressure by approximately 6/3 and 12/5 mmHg for 12.5 mg and 25 mg of hydrochlorothiazide, respectively, compared to valsartan 80 mg alone.

The maximal antihypertensive effect was attained 4 weeks after the initiation of therapy, the first time point at which blood pressure was measured in these trials.

In long-term follow-up studies (without placebo control) the effect of the combination of valsartan and hydrochlorothiazide appeared to be maintained for up to two years. The antihypertensive effect is independent of age or gender. The overall response to the combination was similar for black and non-black patients.

There was essentially no change in heart rate in patients treated with the combination of valsartan and hydrochlorothiazide in controlled trials.

Valsartan

Valsartan inhibits the pressor effect of angiotensin II infusions. An oral dose of 80 mg inhibits the pressor effect by about 80% at peak with approximately 30% inhibition persisting for 24 hours. No information on the effect of larger doses is available.

Removal of the negative feedback of angiotensin II causes a 2- to 3-fold rise in plasma renin and consequent rise in angiotensin II plasma concentration in hypertensive patients. Minimal decreases in plasma aldosterone were observed after administration of valsartan; very little effect on serum potassium was observed.

In multiple-dose studies in hypertensive patients with stable renal insufficiency and patients with renovascular hypertension, valsartan had no clinically significant effects on glomerular filtration rate, filtration fraction, creatinine clearance, or renal plasma flow.

In multiple-dose studies in hypertensive patients, valsartan had no notable effects on total cholesterol, fasting triglycerides, fasting serum glucose, or uric acid.

The antihypertensive effects of valsartan were demonstrated principally in 7 placebo-controlled, 4- to 12-week trials (one in patients over 65) of dosages from 10 to 320 mg/day in patients with baseline diastolic blood pressures of 95-115. The studies allowed comparison of once-daily and twice-daily regimens of 160 mg/day; comparison of peak and trough effects; comparison (in pooled data) of response by gender, age, and race; and evaluation of incremental effects of hydrochlorothiazide.

Administration of valsartan to patients with essential hypertension results in a significant reduction of sitting, supine, and standing systolic and diastolic blood pressure, usually with little or no orthostatic change.

In most patients, after administration of a single oral dose, onset of antihypertensive activity occurs at approximately 2 hours, and maximum reduction of blood pressure is achieved within 6 hours. The antihypertensive effect persists for 24 hours after dosing, but there is a decrease from peak effect at lower doses (40 mg) presumably reflecting loss of inhibition of angiotensin II. At higher doses, however (160 mg), there is little difference in peak and trough effect. During repeated dosing, the reduction in blood pressure with any dose is substantially present within 2 weeks, and maximal reduction is generally attained after 4 weeks. In long-term follow-up studies (without placebo control) the effect of valsartan appeared to be maintained for up to two years. The antihypertensive effect is independent of age, gender or race. The latter finding regarding race is based on pooled data and should be viewed with caution, because antihypertensive drugs that affect the renin-angiotensin system (that is, ACE inhibitors and angiotensin-II blockers) have generally been found to be less effective in low-renin hypertensives (frequently blacks) than in high-renin hypertensives (frequently whites). In pooled, randomized, controlled trials of Diovan that included a total of 140 blacks and 830 whites, valsartan and an ACE-inhibitor control were generally at least as effective in blacks as whites. The explanation for this difference from previous findings is unclear.

Abrupt withdrawal of valsartan has not been associated with a rapid increase in blood pressure.

The 7 studies of valsartan monotherapy included over 2000 patients randomized to various doses of valsartan and about 800 patients randomized to placebo. Doses below 80 mg were not consistently distinguished from those of placebo at trough, but doses of 80, 160 and 320 mg produced dose-related decreases in systolic and diastolic blood pressure, with the difference from placebo of approximately 6-9/3-5 mmHg at 80-160 mg and 9/6 mmHg at 320 mg.

Patients with an inadequate response to 80 mg once daily were titrated to either 160 mg once daily or 80 mg twice daily, which resulted in a comparable response in both groups.

In controlled trials, the antihypertensive effect of once daily valsartan 80 mg was similar to that of once daily enalapril 20 mg or once daily lisinopril 10 mg.

There was essentially no change in heart rate in valsartan-treated patients in controlled trials.

Hydrochlorothiazide

After oral administration of hydrochlorothiazide, diuresis begins within 2 hours, peaks in about 4 hours and lasts about 6 to 12 hours.

INDICATIONS AND USAGE

Diovan HCT is indicated for the treatment of hypertension. This fixed dose combination is not indicated for initial therapy *(see DOSAGE AND ADMINISTRATION)*.

CONTRAINDICATIONS

Diovan HCT is contraindicated in patients who are hypersensitive to any component of this product.

Because of the hydrochlorothiazide component, this product is contraindicated in patients with anuria or hypersensitivity to other sulfonamide-derived drugs.

WARNINGS

Fetal/Neonatal Morbidity and Mortality

Drugs that act directly on the renin-angiotensin system can cause fetal and neonatal morbidity and death when administered to pregnant women. Several dozen cases have been reported in the world literature in patients who were taking angiotensin-converting enzyme inhibitors. When pregnancy is detected, Diovan HCT should be discontinued as soon as possible.

The use of drugs that act directly on the renin-angiotensin system during the second and third trimesters of pregnancy has been associated with fetal and neonatal injury, including hypotension, neonatal skull hypoplasia, anuria, reversible or irreversible renal failure, and death. Oligohydramnios has also been reported, presumably resulting from decreased fetal renal function; oligohydramnios in this setting has been associated with fetal limb contractures, craniofacial deformation, and hypoplastic lung development. Prematurity, intrauterine growth retardation, and patent ductus arteriosus have also been reported, although it is not clear whether these occurrences were due to exposure to the drug.

These adverse effects do not appear to have resulted from intrauterine drug exposure that has been limited to the first trimester.

Mothers whose embryos and fetuses are exposed to an angiotensin II receptor antagonist only during the first trimester should be so informed. Nonetheless, when patients become pregnant, physicians should advise the patient to discontinue the use of Diovan HCT as soon as possible.

Rarely (probably less often than once in every thousand pregnancies), no alternative to a drug acting on the renin-angiotensin system will be found. In these rare cases, the mothers should be apprised of the potential hazards to their fetuses, and serial ultrasound examinations should be performed to assess the intraamniotic environment.

If oligohydramnios is observed, Diovan HCT should be discontinued unless it is considered life-saving for the mother. Contraction stress testing (CST), a nonstress test (NST), or biophysical profiling (BPP) may be appropriate, depending upon the week of pregnancy. Patients and physicians should be aware, however, that oligohydramnios may not appear until after the fetus has sustained irreversible injury.

Infants with histories of in utero exposure to an angiotensin II receptor antagonist should be closely observed for hypotension, oliguria, and hyperkalemia. If oliguria occurs, attention should be directed toward support of blood pressure and renal perfusion. Exchange transfusion or dialysis may be required as means of reversing hypotension and/or substituting for disordered renal function.

Valsartan – Hydrochlorothiazide in Animals

There was no evidence of teratogenicity in mice, rats, or rabbits treated orally with valsartan at doses up to 600, 100 and 10 mg/kg/day, respectively, in combination with hydrochlorothiazide at doses up to 188, 31 and 3 mg/kg/day. These non-teratogenic doses in mice, rats and rabbits, respectively, represent 18, 7 and 1 times the maximum recommended human dose (MRHD) of valsartan and 38, 13 and 2 times the MRHD of hydrochlorothiazide on a mg/m^2 basis. (Calculations assume an oral dose of 160 mg/day valsartan in combination with 25 mg/day hydrochlorothiazide and a 60-kg patient.)

Fetotoxicity was observed in association with maternal toxicity in rats and rabbits at valsartan doses of ≥200 and 10 mg/kg/day, respectively, in combination with hydrochlorothiazide doses of ≥63 and 3 mg/kg/day. Fetotoxicity in rats was considered to be related to decreased fetal weights and included fetal variations of sternebrae, vertebrae, ribs and/or renal papillae. Fetotoxicity in rabbits included increased numbers of late resorptions with resultant increases in total resorptions, postimplantation losses and decreased number of live fetuses. The no observed adverse effect doses in mice, rats and rabbits for valsartan were 600, 100 and 3 mg/kg/day, respectively, in combination with hydrochlorothiazide doses of 188, 31 and 1 mg/kg/day. These no adverse effect doses in mice, rats and rabbits, respectively, represent 5, 1.5 and 0.06 times the MRHD of valsartan and 38, 13 and 0.5 times the MRHD of hydrochlorothiazide on a mg/m^2 basis. (Calculations assume an oral dose of 160 mg/day valsartan in combination with 25 mg/day hydrochlorothiazide and a 60-kg patient.)

Valsartan in Animals

No teratogenic effects were observed when valsartan was administered to pregnant mice and rats at oral doses up to 600 mg/kg/day and to pregnant rabbits at oral doses up to 10 mg/kg/day. However, significant decreases in fetal weight, pup birth weight, pup survival rate, and slight delays in developmental milestones were observed in studies in which parental rats were treated with valsartan at oral, maternally toxic (reduction in body weight gain and food consumption) doses of 600 mg/kg/day during organogenesis or late gestation and lactation. In rabbits, fetotoxicity (i.e., resorptions, litter loss, abortions, and low body weight) associated with maternal toxicity (mortality) was observed at doses of 5 and 10 mg/kg/day. The no observed adverse effect doses of 600, 200 and 2 mg/kg/day in mice, rats and rabbits represent 18, 12 and 0.2 times, respectively, the maximum recommended human dose on a mg/m^2 basis. (Calculations assume an oral dose of 160 mg/day and a 60-kg patient.)

Hydrochlorothiazide in Animals

Under the auspices of the National Toxicology Program, pregnant mice and rats that received hydrochlorothiazide via gavage at doses up to 3000 and 1000 mg/kg/day, respectively, on gestation days 6 through 15 showed no evidence of teratogenicity. These doses of hydrochlorothiazide in mice and rats represent 608 and 405 times, respectively, the maximum recommended human dose on a mg/m^2 basis. (Calculations assume an oral dose of 25 mg/day and a 60-kg patient.)

Intrauterine exposure to thiazide diuretics is associated with fetal or neonatal jaundice, thrombocytopenia, and possibly other adverse reactions that have occurred in adults.

Hypotension in Volume- and/or Salt-Depleted Patients

Excessive reduction of blood pressure was rarely seen (0.5%) in patients with uncomplicated hypertension treated

with Diovan HCT. In patients with an activated renin-angiotensin system, such as volume- and/or salt-depleted patients receiving high doses of diuretics, symptomatic hypotension may occur. This condition should be corrected prior to administration of Diovan HCT, or the treatment should start under close medical supervision.

If hypotension occurs, the patient should be placed in the supine position and, if necessary, given an intravenous infusion of normal saline. A transient hypotensive response is not a contraindication to further treatment, which usually can be continued without difficulty once the blood pressure has stabilized.

Hydrochlorothiazide

Impaired Hepatic Function

Thiazide diuretics should be used with caution in patients with impaired hepatic function or progressive liver disease, since minor alterations of fluid and electrolyte balance may precipitate hepatic coma.

Hypersensitivity Reaction

Hypersensitivity reactions to hydrochlorothiazide may occur in patients with or without a history of allergy or bronchial asthma, but are more likely in patients with such a history.

Systemic Lupus Erythematosus

Thiazide diuretics have been reported to cause exacerbation or activation of systemic lupus erythematosus.

Lithium Interaction

Lithium generally should not be given with thiazides (see PRECAUTIONS, Drug Interactions, Hydrochlorothiazide, Lithium).

PRECAUTIONS

Serum Electrolytes

Valsartan – Hydrochlorothiazide

In the controlled trials of various doses of the combination of valsartan and hydrochlorothiazide the incidence of hypertensive patients who developed hypokalemia (serum potassium <3.5 mEq/L) was 4.5%; the incidence of hyperkalemia (serum potassium >5.7 mEq/L) was 0.3%. Two patients (0.3%) discontinued from a trial for decreases in serum potassium.

In controlled clinical trials of Diovan HCT, the average change in serum potassium was near zero in subjects who received Diovan HCT 160/12.5 mg, but the average subject who received Diovan HCT 80/12.5 mg, 80/25 mg or 160/25 mg experienced a mild reduction in serum potassium.

In clinical trials, the opposite effects of valsartan (80 or 160 mg) and hydrochlorothiazide (12.5 mg) on serum potassium approximately balanced each other in many patients. In other patients, one or the other effect may be dominant. Periodic determinations of serum electrolytes to detect possible electrolyte imbalance should be performed at appropriate intervals.

Hydrochlorothiazide

All patients receiving thiazide therapy should be observed for clinical signs of fluid or electrolyte imbalance: hyponatremia, hypochloremic alkalosis, and hypokalemia. Serum and urine electrolyte determinations are particularly important when the patient is vomiting excessively or receiving parenteral fluids. Warning signs or symptoms of fluid and electrolyte imbalance, irrespective of cause, include dryness of mouth, thirst, weakness, lethargy, drowsiness, restlessness, confusion, seizures, muscle pains or cramps, muscular fatigue, hypotension, oliguria, tachycardia, and gastrointestinal disturbances such as nausea and vomiting.

Hypokalemia may develop, especially with brisk diuresis, when severe cirrhosis is present, or after prolonged therapy. Interference with adequate oral electrolyte intake will also contribute to hypokalemia. Hypokalemia may cause cardiac arrhythmia and may also sensitize or exaggerate the response of the heart to the toxic effects of digitalis (e.g., increased ventricular irritability).

Although any chloride deficit is generally mild and usually does not require specific treatment except under extraordinary circumstances (as in liver disease or renal disease), chloride replacement may be required in the treatment of metabolic alkalosis.

Dilutional hyponatremia may occur in edematous patients in hot weather; appropriate therapy is water restriction, rather than administration of salt except in rare instances when the hyponatremia is life-threatening. In actual salt depletion, appropriate replacement is the therapy of choice. Hyperuricemia may occur or frank gout may be precipitated in certain patients receiving thiazide therapy.

In diabetic patients dosage adjustments of insulin or oral hypoglycemic agents may be required. Hyperglycemia may occur with thiazide diuretics. Thus latent diabetes mellitus may become manifest during thiazide therapy.

The antihypertensive effects of the drug may be enhanced in the postsympathectomy patient.

If progressive renal impairment becomes evident, consider withholding or discontinuing diuretic therapy.

Thiazides have been shown to increase the urinary excretion of magnesium; this may result in hypomagnesemia.

Thiazides may decrease urinary calcium excretion. Thiazides may cause intermittent and slight elevation of serum calcium in the absence of known disorders of calcium metabolism. Marked hypercalcemia may be evidence of hidden hyperparathyroidism. Thiazides should be discontinued before carrying out tests for parathyroid function. Increases in cholesterol and triglyceride levels may be associated with thiazide diuretic therapy.

Impaired Hepatic Function

Valsartan

As the majority of valsartan is eliminated in the bile, patients with mild-to-moderate hepatic impairment, including patients with biliary obstructive disorders, showed lower valsartan clearance (higher AUCs). Care should be exercised in administering valsartan to these patients.

Impaired Renal Function

Valsartan

As a consequence of inhibiting the renin-angiotensin-aldosterone system, changes in renal function may be anticipated in susceptible individuals. In patients whose renal function may depend on the activity of the renin-angiotensin-aldosterone system (e.g., patients with severe congestive heart failure), treatment with angiotensin-converting enzyme inhibitors and angiotensin receptor antagonists has been associated with oliguria and/or progressive azotemia and (rarely) with acute renal failure and/or death. Valsartan would be expected to behave similarly.

In studies of ACE inhibitors in patients with unilateral or bilateral renal artery stenosis, increases in serum creatinine or blood urea nitrogen have been reported. In a 4-day trial of valsartan in 12 patients with unilateral renal artery stenosis, no significant increases in serum creatinine or blood urea nitrogen were observed. There has been no long-term use of valsartan in patients with unilateral or bilateral renal artery stenosis, but an effect similar to that seen with ACE inhibitors should be anticipated.

Hydrochlorothiazide

Thiazides should be used with caution in severe renal disease. In patients with renal disease, thiazides may precipitate azotemia. Cumulative effects of the drug may develop in patients with impaired renal function.

Information for Patients

Pregnancy: Female patients of childbearing age should be told about the consequences of second- and third-trimester exposure to drugs that act on the renin-angiotensin system, and they should also be told that these consequences do not appear to have resulted from intrauterine drug exposure that has been limited to the first trimester. These patients should be asked to report pregnancies to their physicians as soon as possible.

Symptomatic Hypotension: A patient receiving Diovan HCT should be cautioned that lightheadedness can occur, especially during the first days of therapy, and that it should be reported to the prescribing physician. The patients should be told that if syncope occurs, Diovan HCT should be discontinued until the physician has been consulted.

All patients should be cautioned that inadequate fluid intake, excessive perspiration, diarrhea, or vomiting can lead to an excessive fall in blood pressure, with the same consequences of lightheadedness and possible syncope.

Potassium Supplements: A patient receiving Diovan HCT should be told not to use potassium supplements or salt substitutes containing potassium without consulting the prescribing physician.

Drug Interactions

Valsartan

No clinically significant pharmacokinetic interactions were observed when valsartan was coadministered with amlodipine, atenolol, cimetidine, digoxin, furosemide, glyburide, hydrochlorothiazide, or indomethacin. The valsartan-atenolol combination was more antihypertensive than either component, but it did not lower the heart rate more than atenolol alone.

Coadministration of valsartan and warfarin did not change the pharmacokinetics of valsartan or the time-course of the anticoagulant properties of warfarin.

CYP 450 Interactions: The enzyme(s) responsible for valsartan metabolism have not been identified but do not seem to be CYP 450 isozymes. The inhibitory or induction potential of valsartan on CYP 450 is also unknown.

Hydrochlorothiazide

When administered concurrently the following drugs may interact with thiazide diuretics:

Alcohol, barbiturates, or narcotics - Potentiation of orthostatic hypotension may occur.

Antidiabetic drugs (oral agents and insulin) - Dosage adjustment of the antidiabetic drug may be required.

Other antihypertensive drugs - Additive effect or potentiation.

Cholestyramine and colestipol resins - Absorption of hydrochlorothiazide is impaired in the presence of anionic exchange resins. Single doses of either cholestyramine or

colestipol resins bind the hydrochlorothiazide and reduce its absorption from the gastrointestinal tract by up to 85% and 43% respectively.

Corticosteroids, ACTH - Intensified electrolyte depletion, particularly hypokalemia.

Pressor amines (e.g., norepinephrine) - Possible decreased response to pressor amines but not sufficient to preclude their use.

Skeletal muscle relaxants, nondepolarizing (e.g., tubocurarine) - Possible increased responsiveness to the muscle relaxant.

Lithium - Should not generally be given with diuretics. Diuretic agents reduce the renal clearance of lithium and add a high risk of lithium toxicity. Refer to the package insert for lithium preparations before use of such preparations with Diovan HCT.

Non-steroidal anti-inflammatory Drugs - In some patients, the administration of a non-steroidal anti-inflammatory agent can reduce the diuretic, natriuretic, and antihypertensive effects of loop, potassium-sparing and thiazide diuretics. Therefore, when Diovan HCT and non-steroidal anti-inflammatory agents are used concomitantly, the patient should be observed closely to determine if the desired effect of the diuretic is obtained.

Carcinogenesis, Mutagenesis, Impairment of Fertility

Valsartan – Hydrochlorothiazide

No carcinogenicity, mutagenicity or fertility studies have been conducted with the combination of valsartan and hydrochlorothiazide. However, these studies have been conducted for valsartan as well as hydrochlorothiazide alone. Based on the preclinical safety and human pharmacokinetic studies, there is no indication of any adverse interaction between valsartan and hydrochlorothiazide.

Valsartan

There was no evidence of carcinogenicity when valsartan was administered in the diet to mice and rats for up to 2 years at doses up to 160 and 200 mg/kg/day, respectively. These doses in mice and rats are about 5 and 12 times, respectively, the maximum recommended human dose on a mg/m^2 basis. (Calculations assume an oral dose of 160 mg/day and a 60-kg patient.)

Mutagenicity assays did not reveal any valsartan-related effects at either the gene or chromosome level. These assays included bacterial mutagenicity tests with Salmonella (Ames) and E coli; a gene mutation test with Chinese hamster V79 cells; a cytogenetic test with Chinese hamster ovary cells; and a rat micronucleus test.

Valsartan had no adverse effects on the reproductive performance of male or female rats at oral doses up to 200 mg/kg/day. This dose is about 12 times the maximum recommended human dose on a mg/m^2 basis. (Calculations assume an oral dose of 160 mg/day and a 60-kg patient.)

Hydrochlorothiazide

Two-year feeding studies in mice and rats conducted under the auspices of the National Toxicology Program (NTP) uncovered no evidence of a carcinogenic potential of hydrochlorothiazide in female mice (at doses of up to approximately 600 mg/kg/day) or in male and female rats (at doses of up to approximately 100 mg/kg/day). The NTP, however, found equivocal evidence for hepatocarcinogenicity in male mice. Hydrochlorothiazide was not genotoxic In Vitro in the Ames mutagenicity assay of Salmonella Typhimurium strains TA 98, TA 100, TA 1535, TA 1537, and TA 1538 and in the Chinese Hamster Ovary (CHO) test for chromosomal aberrations, or In Vivo in assays using mouse germinal cell chromosomes, Chinese hamster bone marrow chromosomes, and the Drosophila sex-linked recessive lethal trait gene. Positive test results were obtained only in the In Vitro CHO Sister Chromatid Exchange (clastogenicity) and in the Mouse Lymphoma Cell (mutagenicity) assays, using concentrations of hydrochlorothiazide from 43 to 1300 mcgm/mL, and in the Aspergillus Nidulans non-disjunction assay at an unspecified concentration.

Hydrochlorothiazide had no adverse effects on the fertility of mice and rats of either sex in studies wherein these species were exposed, via their diet, to doses of up to 100 and 4 mg/kg, respectively, prior to mating and throughout gestation.

Pregnancy Categories C (first trimester) and D (second and third trimesters)

See WARNINGS, Fetal/Neonatal Morbidity and Mortality.

Nursing Mothers

It is not known whether valsartan is excreted in human milk, but valsartan was excreted in the milk of lactating rats. Thiazides appear in human milk. Because of the potential for adverse effects on the nursing infant, a decision should be made whether to discontinue nursing or discontinue the drug, taking into account the importance of the drug to the mother.

Pediatric Use

Safety and effectiveness in pediatric patients have not been established.

Continued on next page

Diovan HCT—Cont.

Geriatric Use
In the controlled clinical trials of Diovan HCT, 117 (16%) of patients treated with valsartan-hydrochlorothiazide were ≥65 years and 16 (2.2%) were ≥75 years. No overall difference in the efficacy or safety of valsartan-hydrochlorothiazide was observed between these patients and younger patients, but greater sensitivity of some older individuals cannot be ruled out.

ADVERSE REACTIONS

Diovan HCT has been evaluated for safety in more than 1,300 patients, including over 360 treated for over 6 months, and 170 for over 1 year. Adverse experiences have generally been mild and transient in nature and have only infrequently required discontinuation of therapy. The overall incidence of adverse experiences with Diovan HCT was comparable to placebo.

The overall frequency of adverse experiences was neither dose-related nor related to gender, age or race. In controlled clinical trials, discontinuation of therapy due to side effects was required in 3.6% of valsartan-hydrochlorothiazide patients and 4.3% of placebo patients. The most common reasons for discontinuation of therapy with Diovan HCT were headache, fatigue and dizziness.

The adverse experiences that occurred in controlled clinical trials in at least 2% of patients treated with Diovan HCT and at a higher incidence in valsartan-hydrochlorothiazide (n=730) than placebo (n=93) patients included dizziness (9% vs 7%), viral infection (3% vs 1%), fatigue (5% vs 1%), pharyngitis (3% vs 1%), coughing (3% vs 0%) and diarrhea (3% vs 0%).

Headache, upper respiratory infection, sinusitis, back pain and chest pain occurred at a more than 2% rate but at about the same incidence in placebo and valsartan-hydrochlorothiazide patients.

Dose-related orthostatic effects were seen in less than 1% of patients. A dose-related increase in the incidence of dizziness was observed in patients treated with Diovan HCT from 80/12.5 mg (6%) to 160/25 mg (16%).

Other adverse experiences that have been reported with valsartan-hydrochlorothiazide (>0.2% of valsartan-hydrochlorothiazide patients in controlled clinical trials) without regard to causality, are listed below:

Body as a Whole: Allergic reaction, anaphylaxis, asthenia, and dependent edema.
Cardiovascular: Palpitations, syncope, and tachycardia.
Dermatologic: Flushing, rash, sunburn, and increased sweating.
Digestive: Increased appetite, constipation, dyspepsia, flatulence, dry mouth, nausea, abdominal pain, and vomiting.
Metabolic: Dehydration and gout.
Musculoskeletal: Arthralgia, muscle cramps, muscle weakness, arm pain, and leg pain.
Neurologic and Psychiatric: Anxiety, depression, insomnia, decreased libido, paresthesia, and somnolence.
Respiratory: Bronchospasm, dyspnea, and epistaxis.
Special Senses: Tinnitus, vertigo, and abnormal vision.
Urogenital: Dysuria, impotence, micturition frequency, and urinary tract infection.

Valsartan
In trials in which valsartan was compared to an ACE inhibitor with or without placebo, the incidence of dry cough was significantly greater in the ACE inhibitor group (7.9%) than in the groups who received valsartan (2.6%) or placebo (1.5%). In a 129-patient trial limited to patients who had had dry cough when they had previously received ACE inhibitors, the incidences of cough in patients who received valsartan, hydrochlorothiazide, or lisinopril were 20%, 19%, 69% respectively ($p < 0.001$).

Other reported events seen less frequently in clinical trials included chest pain, syncope, anorexia, vomiting, and angioedema.

Hydrochlorothiazide
Other adverse experiences that have been reported with hydrochlorothiazide, without regard to causality, are listed below:

Body As A Whole: weakness;
Digestive: pancreatitis, jaundice (intrahepatic cholestatic jaundice), sialadenitis, cramping, gastric irritation;
Hematologic: aplastic anemia, agranulocytosis, leukopenia, hemolytic anemia, thrombocytopenia;
Hypersensitivity: purpura, photosensitivity, urticaria, necrotizing angiitis (vasculitis and cutaneous vasculitis), fever, respiratory distress including pneumonitis and pulmonary edema, anaphylactic reactions;
Metabolic: hyperglycemia, glycosuria, hyperuricemia;
Musculoskeletal: muscle spasm;
Nervous System/Psychiatric: restlessness;
Renal: renal failure, renal dysfunction, interstitial nephritis;
Skin: erythema multiforme including Stevens-Johnson syndrome, exfoliative dermatitis including toxic epidermal necrolysis;
Special Senses: transient blurred vision, xanthopsia.

Clinical Laboratory Test Findings
In controlled clinical trials, clinically important changes in standard laboratory parameters were rarely associated with administration of Diovan HCT.

Creatinine: Minor elevations in creatinine occurred in 1.4% of patients taking Diovan HCT and 1.1% given placebo in controlled clinical trials.

Hemoglobin and Hematocrit: Greater than 20% decreases in hemoglobin and hematocrit were observed in 0.1% and 1.0%, respectively, of Diovan HCT patients, compared with 0.0% in placebo-treated patients.

Liver function tests: Occasional elevations (greater than 150%) of liver chemistries occurred in Diovan HCT-treated patients.

Neutropenia: Neutropenia was observed in 0.6% of patients treated with Diovan HCT and 0.0% of patients treated with placebo.

Serum Electrolytes: *See PRECAUTIONS.*

OVERDOSAGE

Valsartan – Hydrochlorothiazide
Limited data are available related to overdosage in humans. The most likely manifestations of overdosage would be hypotension and tachycardia; bradycardia could occur from parasympathetic (vagal) stimulation. If symptomatic hypotension should occur, supportive treatment should be instituted.

Valsartan is not removed from the plasma by dialysis.

The degree to which hydrochlorothiazide is removed by hemodialysis has not been established. The most common signs and symptoms observed in patients are those caused by electrolyte depletion (hypokalemia, hypochloremia, hyponatremia) and dehydration resulting from excessive diuresis. If digitalis has also been administered, hypokalemia may accentuate cardiac arrhythmias.

In rats and marmosets, single oral doses of valsartan up to 1524 and 762 mg/kg in combination with hydrochlorothiazide at doses up to 476 and 238 mg/kg, respectively, were very well tolerated without any treatment-related effects. These no adverse effect doses in rats and marmosets, respectively, represent 93 and 56 times the maximum recommended human dose (MRHD) of valsartan and 188 and 113 times the MRHD of hydrochlorothiazide on a mg/m^2 basis. (Calculations assume an oral dose of 160 mg/day valsartan in combination with 25 mg/day hydrochlorothiazide and a 60-kg patient.)

Valsartan
Valsartan was without grossly observable adverse effects at single oral doses up to 2000 mg/kg in rats and up to 1000 mg/kg in marmosets, except for salivation and diarrhea in the rat and vomiting in the marmoset at the highest dose (31 and 18 times, respectively, the maximum recommended human dose on a mg/m^2 basis). (Calculations assume an oral dose of 160 mg/day and a 60-kg patient.)

Hydrochlorothiazide
The oral LD_{50} of hydrochlorothiazide is greater than 10 g/kg in both mice and rats, which represents 2027 and 4054 times, respectively, the maximum recommended human dose on a mg/m^2 basis. (Calculations assume an oral dose of 25 mg/day and a 60-kg patient.)

DOSAGE AND ADMINISTRATION

The recommended starting dose of valsartan is 80 mg once daily when used as monotherapy in patients who are not volume depleted. Valsartan may be used over a dose range of 80 mg to 320 mg daily, administered once-a-day. Hydrochlorothiazide is effective in doses of 12.5 to 50 mg once daily, and can be given at doses of 12.5 mg to 25 mg as Diovan HCT.

To minimize dose-independent side effects, it is usually appropriate to begin combination therapy only after a patient has failed to achieve the desired effect with monotherapy.

The side effects *(see WARNINGS)* of valsartan are generally rare and apparently independent of dose; those of hydrochlorothiazide are a mixture of dose-dependent phenomena (primarily hypokalemia) and dose-independent phenomena (e.g., pancreatitis), the former much more common than the latter. Therapy with any combination of valsartan and hydrochlorothiazide will be associated with both sets of dose-independent side effects.

Replacement Therapy: The combination may be substituted for the titrated components.

Dose titration by Clinical Effect: Diovan HCT is available as tablets containing either valsartan 80 mg or 160 mg and hydrochlorothiazide 12.5 mg. A patient whose blood pressure is not adequately controlled with valsartan monotherapy (see above) may be switched to Diovan HCT, valsartan 80 mg/hydrochlorothiazide 12.5 mg once daily. If blood pressure remains uncontrolled after about 3-4 weeks of therapy, either valsartan or both components may be increased depending on clinical response. There are no studies evaluating doses of valsartan greater than 160 mg in combination with hydrochlorothiazide 25 mg.

A patient whose blood pressure is inadequately controlled by 25 mg once daily of hydrochlorothiazide, or is controlled but who experiences hypokalemia with this regimen, may be switched to Diovan HCT (valsartan 80 mg/hydrochlorothiazide 12.5 mg) once daily, reducing the dose of hydrochlorothiazide without reducing the overall expected antihypertensive response. The clinical response to Diovan HCT should be subsequently evaluated and if blood pressure remains uncontrolled after 3-4 weeks of therapy, the dose may be titrated up to valsartan 160 mg/hydrochlorothiazide 25 mg.

The maximal antihypertensive effect is attained about 4 weeks after initiation of therapy.

Patients with Renal Impairment: The usual regimens of therapy with Diovan HCT may be followed as long as the patient's creatinine clearance is >30 mL/min. In patients with more severe renal impairment, loop diuretics are preferred to thiazides, so Diovan HCT is not recommended.

Patients with Hepatic Impairment: Care should be exercised with dosing of Diovan HCT in patients with hepatic impairment.

Other: No initial dosage adjustment is required for elderly patients.

Diovan HCT may be administered with other antihypertensive agents.

Diovan HCT may be administered with or without food.

HOW SUPPLIED

Diovan HCT is available as tablets containing either valsartan 80 mg or 160 mg and hydrochlorothiazide 12.5 mg. Both strengths are packaged in bottles of 100 tablets and 4000 tablets and unit dose blister packages. Tablets are imprinted as follows:

80/12.5 mg Tablet - Light orange, imprinted CG on one side HGH on the other

Bottles of 100	NDC 0078-0314-05
Bottles of 4000	NDC 0078-0314-97
Unit Dose (blister pack)	NDC 0078-0314-06
Box of 100 (strips of 10)	

160/12.5 mg Tablet - Dark red, imprinted CG on one side HHH on the other

Bottles of 100	NDC 0078-0315-05
Bottles of 4000	NDC 0078-0315-97
Unit Dose (blister pack)	NDC 0078-0315-06
Box of 100 (strips of 10)	

Storage: Store below 30°C (86°F). Protect from moisture. Dispense in tight container (USP).

666760 C98-20 (Rev. 4/98)

Distributed by
Novartis Pharmaceuticals Corporation
East Hanover, New Jersey 07936

Shown in Product Identification Guide, page 324

DYNACIRC® ℞
[*dī-nă serk*]
(isradipine) CAPSULES

CAUTION: Federal law prohibits dispensing without prescription.

The following prescribing information is based on official labeling in effect on August 1, 1998.

DESCRIPTION

DynaCirc® (isradipine) is a calcium antagonist available for oral administration in capsules containing 2.5 mg or 5 mg. The structural formula of isradipine is:

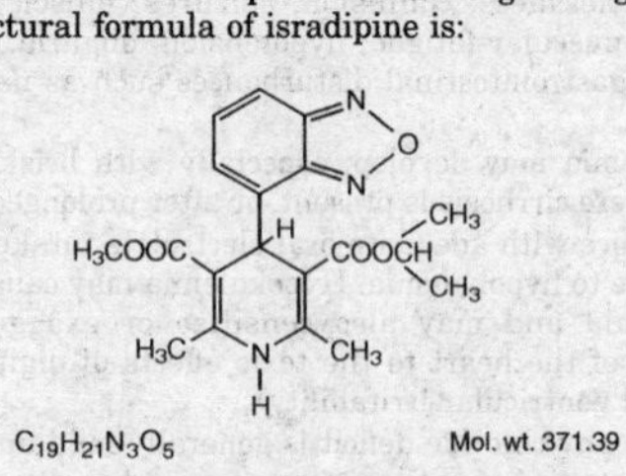

$C_{19}H_{21}N_3O_5$ Mol. wt. 371.39

Chemically, isradipine is 3,5-Pyridinedicarboxylic acid, 4-(4-benzofurazanyl)-1,4-dihydro-2,6-dimethyl-, methyl 1-methyl-ethyl ester. Isradipine is a yellow, fine crystalline powder which is odorless or has a faint characteristic odor. Isradipine is practically insoluble in water (<10 mg/L at 37°C), but is soluble in ethanol and freely soluble in acetone, chloroform and methylene chloride.

Active Ingredient: isradipine
Inactive Ingredients: colloidal silicon dioxide, D&C Red No. 7 Calcium Lake, FD&C Red No. 40 (5 mg capsule only), FD&C Yellow No. 6 Aluminum Lake, gelatin, lactose, starch, titanium dioxide and other ingredients.

The 2.5 mg and 5 mg capsules may also contain: benzyl alcohol, butylparaben, edetate calcium disodium, methylparaben, propylparaben, sodium propionate.

CLINICAL PHARMACOLOGY

Mechanism of Action
Isradipine is a dihydropyridine calcium channel blocker. It binds to calcium channels with high affinity and specificity and inhibits calcium flux into cardiac and smooth muscle.

The effects observed in mechanistic experiments *in vitro* and studied in intact animals and man are compatible with this mechanism of action and are typical of the class.

Except for diuretic activity, the mechanism of which is not clearly understood, the pharmacodynamic effects of isradipine observed in whole animals can also be explained by calcium channel blocking activity, especially dilating effects in arterioles which reduce systemic resistance and lower blood pressure, with a small increase in resting heart rate. Although like other dihydropyridine calcium channel blockers, isradipine has negative inotropic effects *in vitro*, studies conducted in intact anesthetized animals have shown that the vasodilating effect occurs at doses lower than those which affect contractility. In patients with normal ventricular function, isradipine's afterload reducing properties lead to some increase in cardiac output.

Effects in patients with impaired ventricular function have not been fully studied.

Clinical Effects

Dose-related reductions in supine and standing blood pressure are achieved within 2-3 hours following single oral doses of 2.5 mg, 5 mg, 10 mg, and 20 mg DynaCirc® (isradipine), with a duration of action (at least 50% of peak response) of more than 12 hours following administration of the highest dose.

DynaCirc® (isradipine) has been shown in controlled, double-blind clinical trials to be an effective antihypertensive agent when used as monotherapy, or when added to therapy with thiazide-type diuretics. During chronic administration, divided doses (b.i.d.) in the range of 5-20 mg daily have been shown to be effective, with response at trough (prior to next dose) over 50% of the peak blood pressure effect. The response is dose-related between 5-10 mg daily. DynaCirc® (isradipine) is equally effective in reducing supine, sitting, and standing blood pressure.

On chronic administration, increases in resting pulse rate averaged about 3-5 beats/min. These increases were not dose-related.

Hemodynamics

In man, peripheral vasodilation produced by DynaCirc® (isradipine) is reflected by decreased systemic vascular resistance and increased cardiac output. Hemodynamic studies conducted in patients with normal left ventricular function produced, following intravenous isradipine administration, increases in cardiac index, stroke volume index, coronary sinus blood flow, heart rate, and peak positive left ventricular dP/dt. Systemic, coronary, and pulmonary vascular resistance were decreased. These studies were conducted with doses of isradipine which produced clinically significant decreases in blood pressure. The clinical consequences of these hemodynamic effects, if any, have not been evaluated.

Effects on heart rate are variable, dependent upon rate of administration and presence of underlying cardiac condition. While increases in both peak positive dP/dt and LV ejection fraction are seen when intravenous isradipine is given, it is impossible to conclude that these represent a positive inotropic effect due to simultaneous changes in preload and afterload. In patients with coronary artery disease undergoing atrial pacing during cardiac catheterization, intravenous isradipine diminished abnormalities of systolic performance. In patients with moderate left ventricular dysfunction, oral and intravenous isradipine in doses which reduce blood pressure by 12%-30%, resulted in improvement in cardiac index without increase in heart rate, and with no change or reduction in pulmonary capillary wedge pressure. Combination of isradipine and propranolol did not significantly affect left ventricular dP/dt max. The clinical consequences of these effects have not been evaluated.

Electrophysiologic Effects

In general, no detrimental effects on the cardiac conduction system were seen with the use of DynaCirc® (isradipine). Electrophysiologic studies were conducted on patients with normal sinus and atrioventricular node function. Intravenous isradipine in doses which reduce systolic blood pressure did not affect PR, QRS, AH* or HV* intervals.

No changes were seen in Wenckebach cycle length, atrial, and ventricular refractory periods. Slight prolongation of QT$_c$ interval of 3% was seen in one study. Effects on sinus node recovery time (CSNRT) were mild or not seen.

In patients with sick sinus syndrome, at doses which significantly reduced blood pressure, intravenous isradipine resulted in no depressant effect on sinus and atrioventricular node function.

*AH = conduction time from low right atrium to His bundle deflection, or AV nodal conduction time; HV = conduction time through His bundle and the bundle branch-Purkinje system.

Pharmacokinetics and Metabolism

Isradipine is 90%-95% absorbed and is subject to extensive first-pass metabolism, resulting in a bioavailability of about 15%-24%. Isradipine is detectable in plasma within 20 minutes after administration of single oral doses of 2.5-20 mg, and peak concentrations of approximately 1 ng/mL/mg dosed occur about 1.5 hours after drug administration. Administration of DynaCirc® (isradipine) with food signifi-

cantly increases the time to peak by about an hour, but has no effect on the total bioavailability (area under the curve) of the drug. Isradipine is 95% bound to plasma proteins. Both peak plasma concentration and AUC exhibit a linear relationship to dose over the 0-20 mg dose range. The elimination of isradipine is biphasic with an early half-life of $1^1/_2$–2 hours, and a terminal half-life of about 8 hours. The total body clearance of isradipine is 1.4 L /min and the apparent volume of distribution is 3 L /kg.

Isradipine is completely metabolized prior to excretion, and no unchanged drug is detected in the urine. Six metabolites have been characterized in blood and urine, with the mono acids of the pyridine derivative and a cyclic lactone product accounting for >75% of the material identified. Approximately 60%-65% of an administered dose is excreted in the urine and 25%-30% in the feces. Mild renal impairment (creatinine clearance 30-80 mL /min) increases the bioavailability (AUC) of isradipine by 45%. Progressive deterioration reverses this trend, and patients with severe renal failure (creatinine clearance <10 mL /min) who have been on hemodialysis show a 20%-50% lower AUC than healthy volunteers. No pharmacokinetic information is available on drug therapy during hemodialysis. In elderly patients, C$_{max}$ and AUC are increased by 13% and 40%, respectively; in patients with hepatic impairment, C$_{max}$ and AUC are increased by 32% and 52%, respectively *(see DOSAGE AND ADMINISTRATION)*.

INDICATIONS AND USAGE

Hypertension

DynaCirc® (isradipine) is indicated in the management of hypertension. It may be used alone or concurrently with thiazide-type diuretics.

CONTRAINDICATIONS

DynaCirc® (isradipine) is contraindicated in individuals who have shown hypersensitivity to any of the ingredients in the formulation.

WARNINGS

None

PRECAUTIONS

General

Blood Pressure: Because DynaCirc® (isradipine) decreases peripheral resistance, like other calcium blockers DynaCirc® (isradipine) may occasionally produce symptomatic hypotension. However, symptoms like syncope and severe dizziness have rarely been reported in hypertensive patients administered DynaCirc® (isradipine), particularly at the initial recommended doses *(see DOSAGE AND ADMINISTRATION)*.

Use in Patients with Congestive Heart Failure: Although acute hemodynamic studies in patients with congestive heart failure have shown that DynaCirc® (isradipine) reduced afterload without impairing myocardial contractility, it has a negative inotropic effect at high doses *in vitro*, and possibly in some patients. Caution should be exercised when using the drug in congestive heart failure patients, particularly in combination with a beta-blocker.

Drug Interactions

Nitroglycerin: DynaCirc® (isradipine) has been safely coadministered with nitroglycerin.

Hydrochlorothiazide: A study in normal healthy volunteers has shown that concomitant administration of DynaCirc® (isradipine) and hydrochlorothiazide does not result in altered pharmacokinetics of either drug. In a study in hypertensive patients, addition of isradipine to existing hydrochlorothiazide therapy did not result in any unexpected adverse effects, and isradipine had an additional antihypertensive effect.

Propranolol: In a single dose study in normal volunteers, coadministration of propranolol had a small effect on the rate but no effect on the extent of isradipine bioavailability. Significant increases in AUC (27%) and C$_{max}$ (58%) and decreases in t$_{max}$ (23%) of propranolol were noted in this study. However, concomitant administration of 5 mg b.i.d. isradipine and 40 mg b.i.d. propranolol to healthy volunteers under steady-state conditions had no relevant effect on either drug's bioavailability. AUC and C$_{max}$ differences were <20% between isradipine given singly and in combination with propranolol, and between propranolol given singly and in combination with isradipine.

Cimetidine: In a study in healthy volunteers, a one-week course of cimetidine at 400 mg b.i.d. with a single 5 mg dose of isradipine on the sixth day showed an increase in isradipine mean peak plasma concentrations (36%) and significant increase in area under the curve (50%). If isradipine therapy is initiated in a patient currently receiving cimetidine, careful monitoring for adverse reactions is advised and downward dose adjustment may be required.

Rifampicin: In a study in healthy volunteers, a six-day course of rifampicin at 600 mg/day followed by a single 5 mg dose of isradipine resulted in a reduction in isradipine levels to below detectable limits. If rifampicin therapy is required, isradipine concentrations and therapeutic effects are likely to be markedly reduced or abolished as a consequence of increased metabolism and higher clearance of isradipine.

Warfarin: In a study in healthy volunteers, no clinically relevant pharmacokinetic or pharmacodynamic interaction between isradipine and racemic warfarin was seen when two single oral doses of warfarin (0.7 mg/kg body weight) were administered during 11 days of multiple-dose treatment with 5 mg b.i.d. isradipine. Neither racemic warfarin nor isradipine binding to plasma proteins *in vitro* was altered by the addition of the other drug.

Digoxin: The concomitant administration of DynaCirc® (isradipine) and digoxin in a single-dose pharmacokinetic study did not affect renal, non-renal, and total body clearance of digoxin.

Fentanyl Anesthesia: Severe hypotension has been reported during fentanyl anesthesia with concomitant use of a beta blocker and a calcium channel blocker. Even though such interactions have not been seen in clinical studies with DynaCirc® (isradipine), an increased volume of circulating fluids might be required if such an interaction were to occur.

Carcinogenesis, Mutagenesis, Impairment of Fertility

Treatment of male rats for 2 years with 2.5, 12.5, or 62.5 mg/kg/day isradipine admixed with the diet (approximately 6, 31, and 156 times the maximum recommended daily dose based on a 50 kg man) resulted in dose dependent increases in the incidence of benign Leydig cell tumors and testicular hyperplasia relative to untreated control animals. These findings, which were replicated in a subsequent experiment, may have been indirectly related to an effect of isradipine on circulating gonadotropin levels in the rats; a comparable endocrine effect was not evident in male patients receiving therapeutic doses of the drug on a chronic basis. Treatment of mice for two years with 2.5, 15, or 80 mg/kg/day isradipine in the diet (approximately 6, 38, and 200 times the maximum recommended daily dose based on a 50 kg man) showed no evidence of oncogenicity. There was no evidence of mutagenic potential based on the results of a battery of mutagenic tests. No effect on fertility was observed in male and female rats treated with up to 60 mg/kg/day isradipine.

Pregnancy

Pregnancy Category C: Isradipine was administered orally to rats and rabbits during organogenesis. Treatment of pregnant rats with doses of 6, 20, or 60 mg/kg/day produced a significant reduction in maternal weight gain during treatment with the highest dose (150 times the maximum recommended human daily dose) but with no lasting effects on the mother or the offspring. Treatment of pregnant rabbits with doses of 1, 3, or 10 mg/kg/day (2.5, 7.5, and 25 times the maximum recommended human daily dose) produced decrements in maternal body weight gain and increased fetal resorptions at the two higher doses. There was no evidence of embryotoxicity at doses which were not maternotoxic and no evidence of teratogenicity at any dose tested. In a peri /postnatal administration study in rats, reduced maternal body weight gain during late pregnancy at oral doses of 20 and 60 mg/kg/day isradipine was associated with reduced birth weights and decreased peri and postnatal pup survival.

There are no adequate and well controlled studies in pregnant women. The use of DynaCirc® (isradipine) during pregnancy should only be considered if the potential benefit outweighs potential risks.

Nursing Mothers

It is not known whether DynaCirc® (isradipine) is excreted in human milk. Because many drugs are excreted in human milk, and because of the potential for adverse effects of DynaCirc® (isradipine) on nursing infants, a decision should be made as to whether to discontinue nursing or discontinue the drug, taking into account the importance of the drug to the mother.

Pediatric Use

Safety and effectiveness in pediatric patients have not been established.

ADVERSE REACTIONS

In multiple dose U.S. studies in hypertension, 1228 patients received DynaCirc® (isradipine) alone or in combination with other agents, principally a thiazide diuretic, 934 of them in controlled comparisons with placebo or active agents. An additional 652 patients (which includes 374 normal volunteers) received DynaCirc® (isradipine) in U.S. studies of conditions other than hypertension, and 1321 patients received DynaCirc® (isradipine) in non-U.S. studies. About 500 patients received DynaCirc® (isradipine) in long-term hypertension studies, 410 of them for at least 6 months. The adverse reaction rates given below are principally based on controlled hypertension studies, but rarer serious events are derived from all exposures to DynaCirc® (isradipine), including foreign marketing experience.

Most adverse reactions were mild and related to the vasodilatory effects of DynaCirc® (dizziness, edema, palpitations, flushing, tachycardia), and many were transient. About 5% of isradipine patients left studies prematurely because of adverse reactions (vs. 3% of placebo patients and 6% of active control patients), principally due to headache, edema, dizziness, palpitations, and gastrointestinal disturbances.

Continued on next page

Dynacirc—Cont.

The following table shows the most common adverse reactions, volunteered or elicited, considered by the investigator to be at least possibly drug related. The results for the DynaCirc® (isradipine) treated patients are presented for all doses pooled together (reported by 1% or greater of patients receiving any dose of isradipine), and also for the two treatment regimens most applicable to the treatment of hypertension with DynaCirc® (isradipine): (1) initial and maintenance dose of 2.5 mg b.i.d., and (2) initial dose of 2.5 mg b.i.d. followed by maintenance dose of 5.0 mg b.i.d.
[See first table above]

Except for headache, which is not clearly drug-related (see previous table), the more frequent adverse reactions listed show little change, or increase slightly, in frequency over time, as shown in the following table:
[See second table above]

Edema, palpitations, fatigue, and flushing appear to be dose-related, especially at the higher doses of 15-20 mg/day. In open-label, long-term studies of up to two years in duration, the adverse events reported were generally the same as those reported in the short-term controlled trials. The overall frequencies of these adverse events were slightly higher in the long-term than in the controlled studies, but as in the controlled trials most adverse reactions were mild and transient.

The following adverse experiences were reported in 0.5%–1.0% of the isradipine-treated patients in hypertension studies, or are rare. More serious events from this and other data sources, including postmarketing exposure, are shown in italics. The relationship of these adverse events to isradipine administration is uncertain.

Skin: pruritus, *urticaria*
Musculoskeletal: cramps of legs /feet
Respiratory: cough
Cardiovascular: shortness of breath, hypotension, *atrial fibrillation, ventricular fibrillation, myocardial infarction, heart failure*
Gastrointestinal: abdominal discomfort, constipation, diarrhea
Urogenital: nocturia
Nervous System: drowsiness, insomnia, lethargy, nervousness, impotence, decreased libido, depression, *syncope, paresthesia* (which includes numbness and tingling), *transient ischemic attack, stroke*
Autonomic: hyperhidrosis, visual disturbance, dry mouth, numbness
Miscellaneous: throat discomfort, *leukopenia, elevated liver function tests*

OVERDOSAGE

Minimal empirical data are available on DynaCirc® (isradipine) overdosage. Three individual suicide attempts with dosages of isradipine reported to be from 20 mg up to 100 mg resulted in lethargy, sinus tachycardia and, in the case of the person ingesting 100 mg, transient hypotension which responded to fluid therapy. A foreign report of the ingestion of 200 mg of isradipine with ethanol resulted only in flushing, tachycardia with ST depression on ECG, and hypotension, all of which were reversible. The ingestion of 5 mg of isradipine by a 22-month old child and the accidental ingestion of 100 mg of isradipine by a 58-year old female did not result in any sequelae.

Available data suggest that, as with other dihydropyridines, overdosage with DynaCirc® (isradipine) might result in excessive peripheral vasodilatation with subsequent marked and probably prolonged systemic hypotension, and tachycardia. Emesis, gastric lavage, administration of activated charcoal followed in 30 minutes by a saline cathartic would be reasonable therapy. Isradipine is highly protein-bound and *not* removed by hemodialysis. Overdosage characterized by clinically significant hypotension should be treated with active cardiovascular support including monitoring of cardiac and respiratory function, elevation of lower extremities, and attention to circulating fluid volume and urine output. A vasoconstrictor (such as epinephrine, norepinephrine, or levarterenol) may be helpful in restoring a normotensive state, provided that there is no contraindication to its use.

Refractory hypotension or AV conduction disturbances may be treated with intravenous calcium salts, or glucagon. Cimetidine should be withheld in such instances due to the risk of further increasing plasma isradipine levels.

Significant lethality was observed in mice given oral doses of over 200 mg/kg and rabbits given about 50 mg/kg of isradipine. Rats tolerated doses of over 2000 mg/kg without effects on survival.

DOSAGE AND ADMINISTRATION

The dosage of DynaCirc® (isradipine) should be individualized. The recommended initial dose of DynaCirc® (isradipine) is 2.5 mg b.i.d. alone or in combination with a thiazide diuretic. An antihypertensive response usually occurs within 2-3 hours. Maximal response may require 2-4 weeks. If a satisfactory reduction in blood pressure does not occur

after this period, the dose may be adjusted in increments of 5 mg/day at 2-4 week intervals up to a maximum of 20 mg/day. Most patients, however, show no additional response to doses above 10 mg/day, and adverse effects are increased in frequency above 10 mg/day.

The bioavailability of DynaCirc® (increased AUC) is increased in elderly patients (above 65 years of age), patients with hepatic functional impairment, and patients with mild renal impairment. Ordinarily, the starting dose should still be 2.5 mg b.i.d. in these patients.

HOW SUPPLIED

DynaCirc® (isradipine) Capsules

2.5 mg

White, imprinted twice with the DynaCirc® (isradipine) logo and "DynaCirc" on one end, and "2.5" and "⟨S⟩" on the other.

Bottles of 100 capsules (NDC 0078-0226-05)

Bottles of 60 capsules (NDC 0078-0226-44)

5 mg

Light pink, imprinted twice with the DynaCirc® (isradipine) logo and "DynaCirc" on one end, and "5" and "⟨S⟩" on the other.

Bottles of 100 capsules (NDC 0078-0227-05)

Bottles of 60 capsules (NDC 0078-0227-44)

Store and Dispense

Below 86°F (30°C) in a tight container. Protect from light.
[REV: MARCH 1996   30119906]

Shown in Product Identification Guide, page 324

Adverse Experience	DynaCirc® (isradipine)					
	All Doses N = 934	2.5 mg b.i.d 199	5 mg b.i.d† 150	10 mg b.i.d†† 59	Placebo 297	Active Controls* 414
	%	%	%	%	%	%
Headache	13.7	12.6	10.7	22.0	14.1	9.4
Dizziness	7.3	8.0	5.3	3.4	4.4	8.2
Edema	7.2	3.5	8.7	8.5	3.0	2.9
Palpitations	4.0	1.0	4.7	5.1	1.4	1.5
Fatigue	3.9	2.5	2.0	8.5	0.3	6.3
Flushing	2.6	3.0	2.0	5.1	0.0	1.2
Chest Pain	2.4	2.5	2.7	1.7	2.4	2.9
Nausea	1.8	1.0	2.7	5.1	1.7	3.1
Dyspnea	1.8	0.5	2.7	3.4	1.0	2.2
Abdominal Discomfort	1.7	0.0	3.3	1.7	1.7	3.9
Tachycardia	1.5	1.0	1.3	3.4	0.3	0.5
Rash	1.5	1.5	2.0	1.7	0.3	0.7
Pollakiuria	1.5	2.0	1.3	3.4	0.0	<1.0
Weakness	1.2	0.0	0.7	0.0	0.0	1.2
Vomiting	1.1	1.0	1.3	0.0	0.3	0.2
Diarrhea	1.1	0.0	2.7	3.4	2.0	1.9

† Initial dose of 2.5 mg b.i.d. followed by maintenance dose of 5.0 mg b.i.d.
†† Initial dose of 2.5 mg b.i.d. followed by sequential titration to 5.0 mg b.i.d., 7.5 mg b.i.d., and maintenance dose of 10.0 mg b.i.d.
* Propranolol, prazosin, hydrochlorothiazide, enalapril, captopril.

Incidence Rates for DynaCirc® (isradipine) (All Doses) by Week (%)

Week	1	2	3	4	5	6
n	694	906	649	847	432	494
Adverse Reaction						
Headache	6.5	6.1	5.2	5.2	5.8	4.5
Dizziness	1.6	1.9	1.7	2.2	2.3	2.0
Edema	1.2	2.5	3.2	3.2	5.3	5.5
Palpitations	1.2	1.3	1.4	1.9	2.1	1.4
Fatigue	0.4	1.0	1.4	1.2	1.2	1.6
Flushing	1.2	1.3	2.0	1.4	2.1	1.4

Week	7	8	9	10	11	12
n	153	377	261	362	107	105
Adverse Reaction						
Headache	2.0	2.7	1.9	2.8	2.8	3.8
Dizziness	2.0	1.9	2.3	3.9	4.7	3.8
Edema	5.9	5.0	4.6	4.7	3.8	3.8
Palpitations	1.3	0.8	0.8	1.7	1.9	2.9
Fatigue	2.0	2.7	1.5	1.4	0.9	1.9
Flushing	3.3	1.3	1.1	0.8	0.0	0.0

DYNACIRC CR®   ℞
[dĭ-nă-serk]
(isradipine)
Controlled Release Tablets

Caution: Federal law prohibits dispensing without prescription.

The following prescribing information is based on official labeling in effect on August 1, 1998.

DESCRIPTION

DynaCirc CR® contains isradipine, a calcium antagonist. It is available for once-daily oral administration as a controlled release 5 mg and 10 mg tablet for DynaCirc CR® (isradipine). DynaCirc CR® is a registered trademark for isradipine GITS (Gastrointestinal Therapeutic System) tablets.

The structural formula of isradipine is:

$C_{19}H_{21}N_3O_5$ Mol. wt. 371.39

Chemically, isradipine is 3,5-Pyridinedicarboxylic acid, 4-(4-benzofurazanyl)-1,4-dihydro-2,6-dimethyl-, methyl 1-methylethyl ester. Isradipine is a yellow, fine crystalline powder which is odorless or has a faint characteristic odor. Isradipine is practically insoluble in water (<10 mg/L at 37°C), but is soluble in ethanol and freely soluble in acetone, chloroform and methylene chloride.

Active Ingredient: isradipine

Inactive Ingredients: butylated hydroxytoluene; cellulose acetate; hydroxypropyl methylcellulose; magnesium stearate; polyethylene glycol; polyethylene oxide; polysorbate 80; propylene glycol; red ferric oxide; silicon dioxide; sodium chloride; titanium dioxide; yellow ferric oxide.

System Components and Performance

Isradipine is delivered from the DynaCirc CR® (isradipine) Controlled Release Tablet as follows: a semipermeable membrane surrounds an osmotically active drug core. The core is composed of two layers: an "active" layer containing the drug, and a pharmacologically inert but osmotically active "push" layer. After ingestion, the tablet overcoating is quickly dissipated in the gastrointestinal tract, allowing water to enter the tablet through the semipermeable membrane. The polyethylene oxide polymer swells in the osmotic ("push") layer and exerts pressure against the "active" drug layer, releasing isradipine as a fine suspension through the laser-drilled tablet orifice which has been positioned on the "active" drug layer side. Drug delivery is essentially constant as long as the osmotic gradient remains constant and, after either 5 mg or 10 mg of isradipine is released, gradually falls to a negligible amount. The controlled rate of drug delivery into the gastrointestinal lumen is independent of pH or gastrointestinal motility. The delivery of isradipine in DynaCirc CR® (isradipine) Controlled Release Tablets depends on the existence of an osmotic gradient between the contents of the bilayer core and the fluid in the GI tract. The biologically inert core of the tablet remains intact and, unless it becomes trapped, is eliminated in the feces.

CLINICAL PHARMACOLOGY

Mechanism of Action

Isradipine is a dihydropyridine calcium channel blocker. It binds to calcium channels with high affinity and specificity and inhibits calcium flux into cardiac and smooth muscle. The effects observed in mechanistic experiments *in vitro* and studied in intact animals and man are compatible with this mechanism of action and are typical of the class.

Except for diuretic activity, the mechanism of which is not clearly understood, the pharmacodynamic effects of isradipine observed in whole animals can also be explained by calcium channel blocking activity, especially dilating effects in arterioles which reduce systemic resistance and lower blood pressure, with a small increase in resting heart rate. Although like other dihydropyridine calcium channel blockers, isradipine has negative inotropic effects *in vitro*, studies conducted in intact anesthetized animals have shown that the vasodilating effect occurs at doses lower than those which affect contractility. In patients with normal ventricular function, isradipine's afterload reducing properties lead to some increase in cardiac output.

Effects in patients with impaired ventricular function have not been fully studied.

Clinical Effects

In randomized, placebo-controlled, double-blind, clinical trials, DynaCirc CR® (isradipine) Controlled Release Tablets have been shown to have antihypertensive effects proportional to doses between 5 and 20 mg, administered once daily. DynaCirc CR® (isradipine) produced statistically significant reductions in supine and standing blood pressure, compared with placebo, 24 hours postdose. The endpoint results of one parallel group dose-ranging trial showed mean responses 24 hours after ingestion of DynaCirc CR® (isradipine) (systolic/diastolic) -5.2/-2.8, -13.4/-9.7, -15.6/-10.2 and -15.5/-11.8 mmHg, for 5, 10, 15 and 20 mg doses, respectively, change from baseline greater than concurrent placebo. The antihypertensive effect of any one dose begins in about 2 hours and reaches a peak at about 8–10 hours postdose. At the recommended starting dose (5 mg) the trough response (24 hours after dosing) was about 76% that of the peak. At doses of 10, 15 and 20 mg, the trough blood pressure response was about equal to that at peak effect. In association with the fall in blood pressure, resting heart rate is slightly increased, on average from 1–3 beats/minute. The antihypertensive response to DynaCirc CR® (isradipine) has not been detected to be influenced by gender or age.

Hemodynamics

In man, peripheral vasodilation produced by immediate-release DynaCirc® (isradipine) is reflected by decreased systemic vascular resistance and increased cardiac output. Hemodynamic studies conducted in patients with normal left ventricular function produced, following intravenous isradipine administration, increases in cardiac index, stroke volume index, coronary sinus blood flow, heart rate and peak positive left ventricular dP/dt. Systemic, coronary, and pulmonary vascular resistance was decreased. These studies were conducted with doses of isradipine which produced clinically significant decreases in blood pressure. The clinical consequences of these hemodynamic effects, if any, have not been evaluated.

Effects on heart rate are variable, dependent upon rate of administration and presence of underlying cardiac condition. While increases in both peak positive dP/dt and LV ejection fraction are seen when intravenous isradipine is given, it is impossible to conclude that these represent a positive inotropic effect due to simultaneous changes in preload and afterload. In patients with coronary artery disease undergoing atrial pacing during cardiac catheterization, intravenous isradipine diminished abnormalities of systolic performance. In patients with moderate left ventricular dysfunction, oral and intravenous isradipine in doses which reduce blood pressure by 12%–30%, resulted in improvement in cardiac index without increase in heart rate, and with no change or reduction in pulmonary capillary wedge pressure. Combination of isradipine and propranolol did not significantly affect left ventricular dP/dt max. The clinical consequences of these effects have not been evaluated.

Electrophysiologic Effects

In general, no detrimental effects on the cardiac conduction system were seen with the use of immediate-release DynaCirc® (isradipine). Electrophysiologic studies were conducted on patients with normal sinus and atrioventricular node function. Intravenous isradipine in doses which reduce systolic blood pressure did not affect PR, QRS, AH* or HV* intervals.

No changes were seen in Wenckebach cycle length, atrial, and ventricular refractory periods. Slight prolongation of QT_c interval of 3% was seen in one study. Effects on sinus node recovery time (CSNRT) were mild or not seen.

In patients with sick sinus syndrome, at doses which significantly reduced blood pressure, intravenous isradipine resulted in no depressant effect on sinus and atrioventricular node function.

*AH = conduction time from low right atrium to His bundle deflection, or AV nodal conduction time; HV = conduction time through His bundle and the bundle branch-Purkinje system.

Pharmacokinetics and Metabolism

With the immediate-release formulation DynaCirc® (isradipine) Capsules, 90%–95% of the orally administered dose is absorbed. Because of the biotransformation of isradipine during its first-pass through the portal circulation, the bioavailability of DynaCirc CR® (isradipine) ranges from 15%–24%. Isradipine is 95% bound to plasma proteins. Peak concentrations of approximately 1 ng/mL/mg dosed occur about 1.5 hours after DynaCirc® (isradipine) Capsules administration. The elimination of isradipine is biphasic with an early half-life of $1^1/_2$–2 hours, and a terminal half-life of about 8 hours, resulting in trough concentrations of about 0.1 ng/mL/mg dosed of immediate-release DynaCirc® (isradipine) Capsules.

In single dose studies of DynaCirc CR® (isradipine) Controlled Release Tablets, after a 2–3 hour lag time, concentrations of isradipine plateau between 7 and 18 hours post-dosing (reaching a C_{max} of 3–4 ng/mL with an AUC of 62–73 ng•h/mL for a 10 mg dose) and then a concentration >50% of the peak exists for 17–20 hours.

There is no evidence of dose dumping either in the presence or absence of food. Food has been shown to decrease the extent of bioavailability of DynaCirc CR® (isradipine) by up to 25%.

The pharmacokinetics of DynaCirc CR® (isradipine) Controlled Release Tablets are linear over the dose range of 5–20 mg, in that the plasma drug concentrations are proportional to the dose administered.

Isradipine is completely metabolized prior to excretion, and no unchanged drug is detected in the urine. The major routes of isradipine metabolism are ring oxidation of the dihydropyridine moiety to give the corresponding pyridine, and ester cleavage, with or without concomitant oxidation of the dihydropyridine moiety, giving the corresponding carboxylic acids. The cytochrome P-450 IIIA4 system is implicated in the formation of these metabolites, which are hemodynamically inactive. Approximately 60%–65% of an administered dose is excreted in the urine and 25%–30% in the feces. With immediate-release DynaCirc® (isradipine), mild renal impairment (creatinine clearance 30–80 mL/min) increases the AUC of isradipine by 45%. Progressive deterioration reverses this trend, and patients with severe renal failure (creatinine clearance <10 mL/min) who have been on hemodialysis show a 20%–50% lower AUC than healthy volunteers. In elderly patients administered DynaCirc® (isradipine) Capsules, C_{max} and AUC are increased by 13% and 40%, respectively; in patients with hepatic impairment, C_{max} and AUC are increased by 32% and 52%, respectively *(see DOSAGE AND ADMINISTRATION).*

INDICATIONS AND USAGE

Hypertension

DynaCirc CR® (isradipine) is indicated in the management of hypertension. It may be used alone or concurrently with thiazide-type diuretics.

CONTRAINDICATIONS

DynaCirc CR® (isradipine) is contraindicated in individuals who have shown hypersensitivity to any of the ingredients in the formulation.

WARNINGS

None

PRECAUTIONS

General

Blood Pressure: Because DynaCirc CR® (isradipine) decreases peripheral resistance, like other calcium blockers DynaCirc CR® (isradipine) may occasionally produce symptomatic hypotension. However, symptoms like syncope and severe dizziness have rarely been reported in hypertensive patients administered DynaCirc CR® (isradipine), particularly at the initial recommended doses *(see DOSAGE AND ADMINISTRATION).*

Use in Patients with Congestive Heart Failure: Although acute hemodynamic studies in patients with congestive heart failure have shown that immediate-release DynaCirc® (isradipine) reduced afterload without impairing myocardial contractility, it has a negative inotropic effect at high doses *in vitro* and possibly in some patients. Caution should be exercised when using DynaCirc CR® (isradipine) in congestive heart failure patients, particularly in combination with a beta-blocker.

Peripheral Edema: Peripheral edema, when it occurs, is usually mild to moderate in severity. It is a localized phenomenon thought to be associated with vasodilation of arterioles and other small blood vessels, and not due to left ventricular dysfunction or generalized fluid retention. Peripheral edema is dose-related with an incidence ranging from approximately 9% at 5 mg; 13% at 10 mg; 16% at 15 mg; and 36% at the highest dose studied (20 mg once-daily). With patients whose hypertension is complicated by congestive heart failure, care should be taken to differentiate this edema from the effects of decreasing left ventricular function. Although the frequency of edema is correlated with dose, no DynaCirc CR® (isradipine) treated patients discontinued the short-term (6 weeks or less), placebo-controlled hypertension studies as a result of edema. Less than 5% of DynaCirc CR® (isradipine) treated patients in long-term studies discontinued due to edema.

Other: As with any other non-deformable material, caution should be used when administering DynaCirc CR® (isradipine) in patients with pre-existing severe gastrointestinal narrowing (pathologic or iatrogenic). There have been reports of obstructive symptoms in patients with known strictures associated with ingestion of other GITS products.

Information for Patients: DynaCirc CR® (isradipine) Controlled Release Tablets should be swallowed whole. Do not chew, divide or crush tablets. Do not be concerned if you occasionally notice in your stool something resembling a tablet. In DynaCirc CR® (isradipine), the medication is contained within a nonabsorbable shell that has been specially designed to slowly release the drug for your body to absorb. When this process is completed, the empty tablet shell is eliminated in the stool.

Drug Interactions

Nitroglycerin: Immediate-release DynaCirc® (isradipine) has been safely coadministered with nitroglycerin.

Hydrochlorothiazide: A study in normal healthy volunteers has shown that concomitant administration of immediate-release DynaCirc® (isradipine) and hydrochlorothiazide does not result in altered pharmacokinetics of either drug. In a study in hypertensive patients, addition of isradipine to existing hydrochlorothiazide therapy did not result in any unexpected adverse effects, and isradipine had an additional antihypertensive effect.

Propranolol: In a single dose study in normal volunteers using immediate-release DynaCirc® (isradipine), coadministration of propranolol had a small effect on the rate but no effect on the extent of isradipine bioavailability. Significant increases in AUC (27%) and C_{max} (58%) and decreases in t_{max} (23%) of propranolol were noted in this study.

Digoxin: The concomitant administration of immediate-release DynaCirc® (isradipine) and digoxin in a single-dose pharmacokinetic study did not affect renal, non-renal and total body clearance of digoxin.

Fentanyl Anesthesia: Severe hypotension has been reported during fentanyl anesthesia with concomitant use of a beta blocker and a calcium channel blocker. An increased volume of circulating fluids might be required if such an interaction were to occur.

Carcinogenesis, Mutagenesis, Impairment of Fertility

Treatment of male rats for 2 years with 2.5, 12.5, or 62.5 mg/kg/day isradipine admixed with the diet (approximately 6, 31, and 156 times the maximum recommended daily dose based on a 50 kg man) resulted in dose dependent increases in the incidence of benign Leydig cell tumors and testicular hyperplasia relative to untreated control animals. These findings, which were replicated in a subsequent experiment, may have been indirectly related to an effect of isradipine on circulating gonadotropin levels in the rats;

Continued on next page

Dynacirc CR—Cont.

a comparable endocrine effect was not evident in male patients receiving therapeutic doses of the drug on a chronic basis. Treatment of mice for two years with 2.5, 15, or 80 mg/kg/day isradipine in the diet (approximately 6, 38, and 200 times the maximum recommended dose based on a 50 kg man) showed no evidence of oncogenicity. There was no evidence of mutagenic potential based on the results of a battery of mutagenic tests. No effect on fertility was observed in male and female rats treated with up to 60 mg/kg/day isradipine.

Pregnancy

Pregnancy Category C: Isradipine was administered orally to rats and rabbits during organogenesis. Treatment of pregnant rats with doses of 6, 20, or 60 mg/kg/day produced a significant reduction in maternal weight gain during treatment with the highest dose (150 times the maximum recommended human daily dose) but with no lasting effects on the mother or the offspring. Treatment of pregnant rabbits with doses of 1, 3, or 10 mg/kg/day (2.5, 7.5, and 25 times the maximum recommended human daily dose) produced decrements in maternal body weight gain and increased fetal resorption at the two higher doses. There was no evidence of embryotoxicity at doses which were not maternotoxic and no evidence of teratogenicity at any dose tested. In a peri/postnatal administration study in rats, reduced maternal body weight gain during late pregnancy at oral doses of 20 and 60 mg/kg/day isradipine was associated with reduced birth weights and decreased peri and postnatal pup survival.

There are no adequate and well controlled studies in pregnant women. The use of DynaCirc CR® (isradipine) during pregnancy should only be considered if the potential benefit outweighs potential risks.

Nursing Mothers

It is not known whether DynaCirc® (isradipine) is excreted in human milk. Because many drugs are excreted in human milk, and because of the potential for adverse effects of DynaCirc® (isradipine) on nursing infants, a decision should be made as to whether to discontinue nursing or discontinue the drug, taking into account the importance of the drug to the mother.

Pediatric Use

Safety and effectiveness have not been established in children.

ADVERSE REACTIONS

In a controlled clinical trial with DynaCirc CR® (isradipine), dose-related edema occurred at an incidence of approximately 9% at 5 mg; 13% at 10 mg; 16% at 15 mg; and 36% at the highest dose studied (20 mg), was mild to moderate in severity, and was not related to age or gender.

The incidences of elicited or volunteered adverse reactions (excluding non-drug related) in the following tables are based on 6-week multicenter, placebo-controlled, double-blind hypertension studies. Less than 1% of DynaCirc CR® (isradipine) or placebo-treated patients discontinued from these studies due to adverse reactions.

The most common adverse experiences (≥1.0%) reported with DynaCirc CR® (isradipine) in a dose-response study are shown in the following table. There were no discontinuations of patients treated with DynaCirc CR® (isradipine) in this study due to these common side effects.

Most Frequently Reported Newly-Occurring Adverse Reactions in Dose-Response Study

Adverse Reactions (Excluding Non-Drug Related)	DynaCirc CR® (isradipine)				
	5 mg (N=79)	10 mg (N=79)	15 mg (N=82)	20 mg (N=78)	Placebo Group (N=83)
Headache	13.9%	12.7%	18.3%	10.3%	15.7%
Edema	8.9%	12.7%	15.9%	35.9%	3.6%
Dizziness	5.1%	6.3%	3.7%	6.4%	2.4%
Constipation	3.8%	1.3%	1.2%	2.6%	0.0%
Fatigue	2.5%	7.6%	3.7%	3.8%	2.4%
Flushing	2.5%	3.8%	1.2%	1.3%	1.2%
Abdominal Discomfort	1.3%	5.1%	3.7%	5.1%	1.2%
Rash	1.3%	1.3%	0.0%	2.6%	0.0%

The table below shows elicited or volunteered adverse experiences for DynaCirc CR® (isradipine) treated patients in two 6-week, placebo-controlled, multicenter studies, at doses from 5–20 mg, and considered by the investigator to be at least possibly drug related. The results for DynaCirc CR® (isradipine) treated patients are presented for all doses pooled together (reported by at least 1.0% of active drug treated patients). The incidence of adverse reactions are listed below:

Adverse Reactions (Excluding Non-Drug Related)	Treatment Group	
	DynaCirc CR® (isradipine) (N=422)	Placebo (N=186)
Edema	15.2%	2.2%
Headache	13.0%	12.4%
Dizziness	4.7%	2.7%
Fatigue	4.3%	2.2%
Abdominal Discomfort	2.8%	0.5%
Flushing	1.9%	0.5%
Constipation	1.7%	0.0%
Palpitations	1.2%	0.0%
Nausea	1.2%	1.6%
Abdominal Distention	1.2%	0.0%

The following adverse experiences were reported in 0.5%–1.0% or less of DynaCirc CR® (isradipine) or immediate-release DynaCirc® (isradipine) treated patients in hypertensive studies, or were noted in postmarketing experience with immediate-release DynaCirc® (isradipine) Capsules. More serious events are shown in italics. The relationship of these adverse experiences to isradipine administration is uncertain.

Skin: pruritus, *urticaria*
Musculoskeletal: backache/pain, joint pain, neck pain/sore/stiff, legs ache/pain, cramps of legs/feet
Respiratory: dyspnea, nasal congestion, cough
Cardiovascular: epistaxis, tachycardia, chest pain, shortness of breath, hypotension, *syncope, atrial or ventricular fibrillation, myocardial infarction, heart failure*
Gastrointestinal: diarrhea, vomiting, appetite increased or decreased
Urogenital: pollakiuria, impotence, dysuria, nocturia

Central Nervous: drowsiness, insomnia, lethargy, nervousness, libido decrease/frigidity, impotence, depression, *paresthesia* (which includes numbness and tingling), *transient ischemic attack, stroke*
Autonomic: dry mouth, hyperhidrosis, visual disturbance
Miscellaneous: weight gain, throat discomfort, *drug fever, leukopenia, elevated liver function tests*

No gastrointestinal bleeding has been reported in clinical trials with DynaCirc CR® (isradipine) Controlled Release Tablets.

In a long-term (one-year) DynaCirc CR® (isradipine) open-label, hypertension trial, the adverse events reported were generally the same as those seen in the short-term placebo-controlled studies. About 6% of DynaCirc CR® (isradipine) treated patients discontinued the long-term trial due to adverse reactions.

With immediate-release DynaCirc® (isradipine) Capsules, most of the adverse experiences were transient, mild, and related to vasodilatory effects. The following table shows the most common adverse events reported in U.S. clinical trials for immediate-release DynaCirc® (isradipine) Capsules, volunteered or elicited, and considered by the investigator to be at least possibly drug related. [See table below]

In open-label, long-term studies of up to two years in duration with immediate-release DynaCirc® (isradipine) Capsules, the adverse experiences reported were generally the same as those reported in the short-term controlled trials. The overall frequencies of these adverse events were slightly higher in the long-term than in the controlled studies, but in the controlled studies most adverse reactions were mild and transient.

OVERDOSAGE

Although there is no well documented experience with DynaCirc® (isradipine) overdosage, available data suggest that, as with other dihydropyridines, gross overdosage would result in excessive peripheral vasodilation with subsequent marked and probably prolonged systemic hypotension. Clinically significant hypotension overdosage calls for active cardiovascular support including monitoring of cardiac and respiratory function, elevation of lower extremities and attention to circulating fluid volume and urine output. A vasoconstrictor (such as epinephrine, norepinephrine, or levarterenol) may be helpful in restoring vascular tone and blood pressure, provided that there is no contraindication to its use. Since isradipine is highly protein bound, dialysis is not likely to be of benefit.

Significant lethality was observed in mice given oral doses of over 200 mg/kg and rabbits given about 50 mg/kg of isradipine. Rats tolerated doses of over 2000 mg/kg without effects on survival.

DOSAGE AND ADMINISTRATION

The dosage of DynaCirc CR® (isradipine) Controlled Release Tablets should be individualized. The recommended initial dose of DynaCirc CR® (isradipine) is 5 mg once-daily as monotherapy or in combination with a thiazide diuretic. An antihypertensive response usually occurs within 2 hours, with the peak antihypertensive response occurring 8–10 hours post-dose; blood pressure reduction is maintained for at least 24 hours following drug administration. If necessary, the dose may be adjusted in increments of 5 mg at 2–4 week intervals up to a maximum dose of 20 mg/day. Adverse experiences are increased in frequency above 10 mg/day.

DynaCirc CR® (isradipine) Controlled Release Tablets should be swallowed whole and should not be bitten or divided.

The bioavailability (increased AUC) of immediate-release DynaCirc® (isradipine) is increased in elderly patients (above 65 years of age), patients with hepatic functional impairment, and patients with mild renal impairment. Ordinarily, a starting dose of DynaCirc CR® (isradipine) 5 mg once-daily should be used in these patients.

HOW SUPPLIED

DynaCirc CR® (isradipine) Controlled Release Tablets
5 mg
A light pink, round, standard biconvex and film coated tablet. Printing is in red with "Dynacirc CR" in a semicircle with "5" centered within the semicircle.
Bottles of 100 controlled release tablets (NDC 0078-0235-05)
Bottles of 30 controlled release tablets (NDC 0078-0235-15)
10 mg
A beige, round, standard biconvex and film coated tablet. Printing is in red with "DynaCirc CR" in a semicircle with "10" centered within the semicircle.
Bottles of 100 controlled release tablets (NDC 0078-0236-05)
Bottles of 30 controlled release tablets (NDC 0078-0236-15)
Store and Dispense
Below 86°F (30°C) in a tight container, protected from moisture and humidity.

[REV: AUGUST 1996   37022904]
Shown in Product Identification Guide, page 324

	DynaCirc® (isradipine)					
Adverse Experience	All Doses	2.5 mg b.i.d.	5 mg b.i.d.†	10 mg b.i.d.††	Placebo (N=297) %	Active Controls* (N=414) %
Headache	13.7	12.6	10.7	22.0	14.1	9.4
Dizziness	7.3	8.0	5.3	3.4	4.4	8.2
Edema	7.2	3.5	8.7	8.5	3.0	2.9
Palpitations	4.0	1.0	4.7	5.1	1.4	1.5
Fatigue	3.9	2.5	2.0	8.5	0.3	6.3
Flushing	2.6	3.0	2.0	5.1	0.0	1.2
Chest Pain	2.4	2.5	2.7	1.7	2.4	2.9
Nausea	1.8	1.0	2.7	5.1	1.7	3.1
Dyspnea	1.8	0.5	2.7	3.4	1.0	2.2
Abdominal Discomfort	1.7	0.0	3.3	1.7	1.7	3.9
Tachycardia	1.5	1.0	1.3	3.4	0.3	0.5
Rash	1.5	1.5	2.0	1.7	0.3	0.7
Pollakiuria	1.5	2.0	1.3	3.4	0.0	<1.0
Weakness	1.2	0.0	0.7	0.0	0.0	1.2
Vomiting	1.1	0.0	1.3	0.0	0.3	0.2
Diarrhea	1.1	0.0	2.7	3.4	2.0	1.9

†Initial dose of 2.5 mg b.i.d. followed by maintenance dose of 5.0 mg b.i.d.
††Initial dose of 2.5 mg b.i.d. followed by sequential titration to 5.0 mg b.i.d., 7.5 mg b.i.d., and maintenance dose of 10.0 mg b.i.d.
*Propranolol, prazosin, hydrochlorothiazide, enalapril, captopril.

ESTRADERM® ℞

[ĕs tră derm]

estradiol transdermal system

Continuous delivery for twice-weekly application

Caution: Federal law prohibits dispensing without a prescription.

The following prescribing information is based on official labeling in effect on August 1, 1998.

Prescribing Information

1. ESTROGENS HAVE BEEN REPORTED TO INCREASE THE RISK OF ENDOMETRIAL CARCINOMA IN POSTMENOPAUSAL WOMEN.

Close clinical surveillance of all women taking estrogens is important. Adequate diagnostic measures, including endometrial sampling when indicated, should be undertaken to rule out malignancy in all cases of undiagnosed persistent or recurring abnormal vaginal bleeding. There is no evidence that "natural" estrogens are more or less hazardous than "synthetic" estrogens at equiestrogenic doses.

2. ESTROGENS SHOULD NOT BE USED DURING PREGNANCY.

Estrogen therapy during pregnancy is associated with an increased risk of congenital defects in the reproductive organs of the fetus, and possibly other birth defects. Studies of women who received diethylstilbestrol (DES) during pregnancy have shown that female offspring have an increased risk of vaginal adenosis, squamous cell dysplasia of the uterine cervix, and clear cell vaginal cancer later in life; male offspring have an increased risk of urogenital abnormalities and possible testicular cancer later in life. The 1985 DES Task Force concluded that use of DES during pregnancy is associated with a subsequent increased risk of breast cancer in the mothers, although a causal relationship remains unproven and the observed level of excess risk is similar to that for a number of other breast cancer risk factors.

There is no indication for estrogen therapy during pregnancy. Estrogens are ineffective for the prevention or treatment of threatened or habitual abortion. Estrogens are not indicated for the prevention of postpartum breast engorgement.

DESCRIPTION

Estraderm, estradiol transdermal system, is designed to release 17β-estradiol through a rate-limiting membrane continuously upon application to intact skin.

Two systems are available to provide nominal in vivo delivery of 0.05 or 0.1 mg of estradiol per day via skin of average permeability (interindividual variation in skin permeability is approximately 20%). Each corresponding system having an active surface area of 10 or 20 cm^2 contains 4 or 8 mg of estradiol USP and 0.3 or 0.6 mL of alcohol USP, respectively. The composition of the systems per unit area is identical.

Estradiol USP (17β-estradiol) is a white, crystalline powder, chemically described as estra-1,3,5 (10)-triene-3,17β-diol. The structural formula is

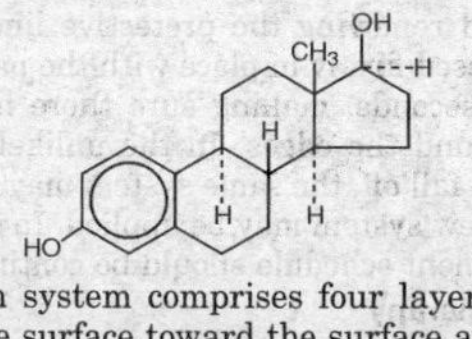

The Estraderm system comprises four layers. Proceeding from the visible surface toward the surface attached to the skin, these layers are (1) a transparent polyester film, (2) a drug reservoir of estradiol USP and alcohol USP gelled with hydroxypropyl cellulose, (3) an ethylene-vinyl acetate copolymer membrane, and (4) an adhesive formulation of light mineral oil and polyisobutylene. A protective liner (5) of siliconized polyethylene terephthalate film is attached to the adhesive surface and must be removed before the system can be used.

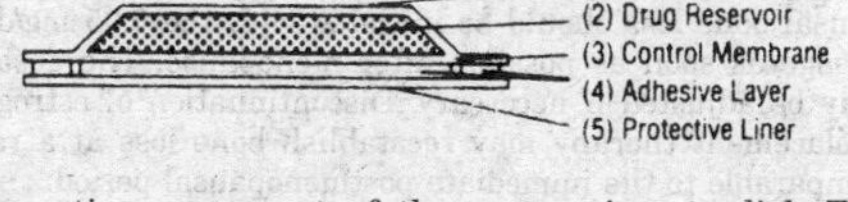

The active component of the system is estradiol. The remaining components of the system are pharmacologically inactive. Alcohol is also released from the system during use.

CLINICAL PHARMACOLOGY

The Estraderm system releases estradiol, the major estrogenic hormone secreted by the human ovary. Although circulating estrogens exist in a dynamic equilibrium of metabolic interconversions, estradiol is the principal intracellular human estrogen and is substantially more potent than estrone or estriol at the receptor level.

Estraderm provides systemic estrogen replacement therapy. Estrogen receptors have been identified in tissues of the reproductive tract, breast, pituitary, hypothalamus, liver, and in the bone of women. Among numerous effects, estradiol is largely responsible for the development and maintenance of the female reproductive system and of secondary sexual characteristics. By a direct action, it causes growth and development of the vagina, uterus, and fallopian tubes. With other hormones, such as pituitary hormones and progesterone, they cause enlargement of the breasts through promotion of ductal growth, stromal development, and the accretion of fat. Estrogens contribute to the shaping of the skeleton, to the maintenance of tone and elasticity of urogenital structures, to changes in the epiphyses of the long bones that allow for the pubertal growth spurt and its termination, to the growth of axillary and pubic hair, and to the pigmentation of the nipples and genitals. Estrogens are intricately involved with other hormones, especially progesterone, in the processes of the ovulatory menstrual cycle and pregnancy and affect the release of pituitary gonadotropins.

Loss of ovarian estradiol secretion after menopause can result in instability of thermoregulation, causing hot flushes associated with sleep disturbance and excessive sweating, and urogenital atrophy, causing dyspareunia and urinary incontinence. Estradiol replacement therapy alleviates many of these symptoms of estradiol deficiency in the menopausal woman.

Transdermal administration produces therapeutic serum levels of estradiol with lower circulating levels of estrone and estrone conjugates and requires smaller total doses than does oral therapy. Because estradiol has a short half-life (~1 hour), transdermal administration of estradiol allows a rapid decline in blood levels after an Estraderm system is removed, e.g., in a cycling regimen.

In a study using transdermally administered estradiol, 0.1 mg daily, plasma levels increased by 66 pg/mL, resulting in an average plasma level of 73 pg/mL. There were no significant increases in the concentration of renin substrate or other hepatic proteins (sex hormone-binding globulin, thyroxine-binding globulin, and corticosteroid-binding globulin).

Pharmacokinetics

Administration of Estraderm produces mean serum concentrations of estradiol comparable to those produced by daily oral administration of estradiol at about 20 times the daily transdermal dose. In single-application studies in 14 postmenopausal women using Estraderm systems that provided 0.05 and 0.1 mg of exogenous estradiol per day, these systems produced increased blood levels within 4 hours and maintained respective mean serum estradiol concentrations of 32 and 67 pg/mL above baseline over the application period. At the same time, increases in estrone serum concentration averaged only 9 and 27 pg/mL above baseline, respectively. Serum concentrations of estradiol and estrone returned to preapplication levels within 24 hours after removal of the system. The estimated daily urinary output of estradiol conjugates increased 5 to 10 times the baseline values and returned to near baseline within 2 days after removal of the system.

By comparison, estradiol (2 mg/day) administered orally to postmenopausal women resulted in increases in mean serum concentration of 59 pg/mL of estradiol and 302 pg/mL of estrone above baseline on the third consecutive day of dosing. Urinary output of estradiol conjugates after oral administration increased to about 100 times the baseline values and did not approach baseline until 7-8 days after the last dose.

In a 3-week multiple-application study of 14 postmenopausal women in which Estraderm 0.05 was applied twice weekly, the mean increments in steady-state serum concentration were 30 pg/mL for estradiol and 12 pg/mL for estrone. Urinary output of estradiol conjugates returned to baseline within 3 days after removal of the last (6th) system, indicating little or no estrogen accumulation in the body.

INDICATIONS AND USAGE

Estraderm® (estradiol transdermal system) is indicated in the following:

1. Treatment of moderate-to-severe vasomotor symptoms associated with menopause. There is no adequate evidence that estrogens are effective for nervous symptoms or depression that might occur during menopause, and they should not be used to treat these conditions.
2. Treatment of atrophic vaginitis and kraurosis vulvae.
3. Treatment of atrophic urethritis.
4. Treatment of hypoestrogenism due to hypogonadism, castration, or primary ovarian failure.
5. Prevention of osteoporosis (loss of bone mass). The mainstays of prevention and management of osteoporosis are estrogen, an adequate lifetime calcium intake, and exercise. Estrogen replacement therapy is the most effective single modality for the prevention of postmenopausal osteoporosis in women. Estrogen replacement therapy reduces bone resorption and retards or halts postmenopausal bone loss. Case-controlled studies have shown an approximately 60% reduction in hip and wrist fractures in women whose estrogen replacement was begun within a few years of menopause. Studies also suggest that estrogen reduces the rate of vertebral fractures. Even when started as late as 6 years after menopause, estrogen prevents further loss of bone mass for as long as treatment is continued. When estrogen therapy is discontinued, bone mass declines at a rate comparable to the immediate postmenopausal period. A well-controlled, double-blind, prospective trial conducted at the Mayo Clinic has demonstrated that treatment with Estraderm prevents bone loss in postmenopausal women at a dosage of 0.05 mg/day.

Treatment with Estraderm 0.05 mg showed full maintenance of bone density with a slight (0.8%), but not significant, increase. Placebo treatment resulted in a significant loss of more than 6% below baseline vertebral bone mass. Patients using either Estraderm 0.1 or 0.05 mg had significantly greater bone densities than those using placebo.

Women are at higher risk than men because they have less bone mass, and for several years following natural or induced menopause, the rate of bone mass decline is accelerated. Early menopause is one of the strongest predictors for the development of osteoporosis. In addition, other factors affecting the skeleton that are associated with osteoporosis include race (white and Asian women are at higher risk than black women); genetic factors (small build, family history); endocrine factors (nulliparity, thyrotoxicosis, hyperparathyroidism, Cushing's syndrome, hyperprolactinemia, Type I diabetes); life-style (cigarette smoking, alcohol abuse, sedentary habits); and nutrition (below-average body weight, dietary calcium intake). Calcium deficiency has been implicated in the pathogenesis of the disease. Therefore, when not contraindicated, it is recommended that postmenopausal women receive calcium supplementation.

Immobilization and prolonged bed rest produce rapid bone loss, while weight-bearing exercise has been shown both to reduce bone loss and to increase bone mass. The optimal type and amount of physical activity that would prevent osteoporosis have not been established.

CONTRAINDICATIONS

Patients with known hypersensitivity to any of the components of the therapeutic system should not use Estraderm. Estrogens should not be used in women with any of the following conditions:

1. Known or suspected pregnancy (see Boxed Warning). Estrogen may cause fetal harm when administered to a pregnant woman.
2. Known or suspected cancer of the breast.
3. Known or suspected estrogen-dependent neoplasia.
4. Undiagnosed abnormal genital bleeding.
5. Active thrombophlebitis or thromboembolic disorders, or a documented history of these conditions.

WARNINGS

1. *Induction of malignant neoplasms.* Some studies have suggested a possible increased incidence of breast cancer in those women taking estrogen therapy at higher doses or for prolonged periods of time. The majority of studies, however, have not shown an association with the usual doses used for estrogen replacement therapy. Women on this therapy should have regular breast examinations and should be instructed in breast self-examination. The reported endometrial cancer risk among unopposed estrogen users is about 2- to 12-fold greater than in nonusers and appears dependent on duration of treatment and on estrogen dose. Most studies show no significant increased risk associated with use of estrogens for less than 1 year. The greatest risk appears associated with prolonged use with increased risks of 15- to 24-fold for 5 to 10 years or more. In three studies, persistence of risk was demonstrated for 8 to over 15 years after cessation of estrogen treatment. In one study, a significant decrease in the incidence of endometrial cancer occurred 6 months after estrogen withdrawal. Concurrent progestin therapy may offset this risk, but the overall health impact in postmenopausal women is not known (see PRECAUTIONS).

Estrogen therapy during pregnancy is associated with an increased risk of fetal congenital reproductive tract disorders. In female offspring, there is an increased risk of vaginal adenosis, squamous cell dysplasia of the cervix, and clear cell vaginal cancer later in life; in males, urogenital and possibly testicular abnormalities. Although some of these changes are benign, it is not known whether they are precursors of malignancy.

2. *Gallbladder disease.* Two studies have reported a 2- to 4-fold increase in the risk of surgically confirmed gallbladder disease in postmenopausal women receiving

Continued on next page

Estraderm—Cont.

oral estrogen replacement therapy, similar to the 2-fold increase previously noted in users of oral contraceptives.

3. *Cardiovascular disease.* Large doses of oral estrogen (5 mg conjugated estrogens per day), comparable to those used to treat cancer of the prostate and breast, have been shown in a large prospective clinical trial in men to increase the risk of nonfatal myocardial infarction, pulmonary embolism, and thrombophlebitis. It cannot necessarily be extrapolated from men to women. However, to avoid the theoretical cardiovascular risk to women caused by high estrogen doses, the dose for estrogen replacement therapy should not exceed the lowest effective dose.

4. *Elevated blood pressure.* Occasional blood pressure increases during postmenopausal estrogen replacement therapy have been attributed to idiosyncratic reactions to estrogens. More often, blood pressure has remained the same or has dropped. Postmenopausal estrogen use does not increase the risk of stroke; nonetheless, blood pressure should be monitored at regular intervals with estrogen use, especially if high doses are used. Ethinyl estradiol and conjugated estrogens have been shown to increase renin substrate. In contrast to these oral estrogens, transdermally administered estradiol does not affect renin substrate.

5. *Hypercalcemia.* Administration of estrogen may lead to severe hypercalcemia in patients with breast cancer and bone metastases. If this occurs, the drug should be stopped and appropriate measures taken to reduce the serum calcium level.

PRECAUTIONS

General

1. *Addition of a progestin.* Studies of the addition of a progestin for 10 or more days of a cycle of estrogen administration have reported a lowered incidence of endometrial hyperplasia than would be induced by estrogen treatment alone. Morphologic and biochemical studies of endometria suggest that 10 to 14 days of progestin are needed to provide maximal maturation of the endometrium and to reduce the likelihood of hyperplastic changes. There are possible additional risks that may be associated with the use of progestins in estrogen replacement regimens. These include (1) adverse effects on lipoprotein metabolism (lowering HDL and raising LDL), which could diminish the purported cardioprotective effect of estrogen therapy (see PRECAUTIONS, below); (2) impairment of glucose tolerance; and (3) possible enhancement of mitotic activity in breast epithelial tissue, although few epidemiologic data are available to address this point (see PRECAUTIONS, below). The choice of progestin, its dose, and its regimen may be important in minimizing these adverse effects, but these issues will require further study before they are clarified.

2. *Cardiovascular risk.* A causal relationship between estrogen replacement therapy and reduction of cardiovascular disease in postmenopausal women has not been proven. Furthermore, the effect of added progestins on this putative benefit is not yet known.

In recent years, many published studies have suggested that there may be a cause-effect relationship between postmenopausal oral estrogen replacement therapy *without added progestins* and a decrease in cardiovascular disease in women. Although most of the observational studies that assessed this statistical association have reported a 20% to 50% reduction in coronary heart disease risk and associated mortality in estrogen takers, the following should be considered when interpreting these reports:

1. Because only one of these studies was randomized and it was too small to yield statistically significant results, all relevant studies were subject to selection bias. The apparently reduced risk of coronary artery disease cannot be attributed with certainty to estrogen replacement therapy. It may instead have been caused by lifestyle and medical characteristics of the women studied with the possibility that healthier women were selected for estrogen therapy. Thus, ongoing and future large-scale randomized trials may fail to confirm this apparent benefit.
2. Current medical practice often includes the use of concomitant progestin therapy in women with intact uteri (see PRECAUTIONS and WARNINGS). While the effects of added progestins on the risk of ischemic heart disease are not known, all available progestins reverse at least some of the favorable effects of estrogens on HDL and LDL levels.
3. While the effects of added progestins on the risk of breast cancer are also unknown, available epidemiological evidence suggests that progestins do not reduce, and may enhance, the moderately increased breast cancer incidence that has been reported with prolonged estrogen replacement therapy (see WARNINGS, above).

Because relatively long-term use of estrogens by women with uteri has been shown to induce endometrial cancer, physicians often recommend that women who are deemed candidates for hormone replacement should take progestins as well as estrogens. When considering prescribing concomitant estrogens and progestins for hormone replacement therapy, physicians and patients are advised to carefully weigh the potential benefits and risks of the added progestin. Large-scale, randomized, placebo-controlled, prospective clinical trials are required to clarify these issues.

3. *Physical examination.* A complete medical and family history should be taken prior to the initiation of any estrogen therapy. The pretreatment and periodic physical examinations should include special reference to blood pressure, breasts, abdomen, and pelvic organs and should include a Papanicolaou smear. As a general rule, estrogen should not be prescribed for longer than 1 year without another physical examination being performed.

4. *Hypercoagulability.* Some studies have shown that women taking estrogen replacement therapy have hypercoagulability, primarily related to decreased antithrombin activity. This effect appears dose- and duration-dependent and is less pronounced than that associated with oral contraceptive use. Also, postmenopausal women tend to have increased coagulation parameters at baseline compared to premenopausal women. Epidemiological studies, which employed primarily orally administered estrogen products, have suggested that hormone replacement therapy (HRT) may be associated with an increased relative risk of developing venous thromboembolism (VTE), i.e., deep venous thrombosis or pulmonary embolism. Risk/benefit should therefore be carefully weighed in consultation with the patient when prescribing either oral or transdermal HRT to women with a risk factor for VTE.

5. *Familial hyperlipoproteinemia.* Estrogen therapy may be associated with massive elevations of plasma triglycerides, leading to pancreatitis and other complications in patients with familial defects of lipoprotein metabolism.

6. *Fluid retention.* Because estrogens may cause some degree of fluid retention, conditions that might be influenced by this factor, such as asthma, epilepsy, migraine, and cardiac or renal dysfunction, require careful observation.

7. *Uterine bleeding and mastodynia.* Certain patients may develop undesirable manifestations of estrogenic stimulation, such as abnormal uterine bleeding and mastodynia.

8. *Impaired liver function.* Estrogens may be poorly metabolized in patients with impaired liver function and should be administered with caution.

Information for the Patient

See text of Patient Package Insert, which appears after the HOW SUPPLIED section.

Laboratory Tests

Estrogen administration should generally be guided by clinical response at the smallest dose, rather than laboratory monitoring, for relief of symptoms for those indications in which symptoms are observable. For prevention and treatment of osteoporosis, however, see DOSAGE AND ADMINISTRATION. Tests used to measure adequacy of estrogen replacement therapy include serum estrone and estradiol levels and suppression of serum gonadotropin levels.

Drug/Laboratory Test Interactions

Some of these drug/laboratory test interactions have been observed only with estrogen-progestin combinations (oral contraceptives):

1. Accelerated prothrombin time, partial thromboplastin time, and platelet aggregation time; increased platelet count; increased factors II, VII antigen, VIII antigen, VIII coagulant activity, IX, X, XII, VII-X complex, II-VII-X complex, and beta-thromboglobulin; decreased levels of antifactor Xa and antithrombin III; decreased antithrombin III activity; increased levels of fibrinogen and fibrinogen activity; increased plasminogen antigen and activity.
2. Increased thyroid-binding globulin (TBG) leading to increased circulating total thyroid hormone, as measured by T_4 levels determined either by column or by radioimmunoassay. Free T_3 resin uptake is decreased, reflecting the elevated TBG; free T_4 and free T_3 concentrations are unaltered.
3. Other binding proteins may be elevated in serum, i.e., corticosteroid-binding globulin (CBG), sex hormone-binding globulin (SHBG), leading to increased circulating corticosteroids and sex steroids respectively. Free or biologically active hormone concentrations are unchanged. Other plasma proteins may be increased (angiotensinogen/renin substrate, alpha-1–antitrypsin, ceruloplasmin).
4. Increased plasma HDL and HDL-2 subfraction concentrations, reduced LDL cholesterol concentration, increased triglyceride levels.
5. Impaired glucose tolerance.
6. Reduced response to metyrapone test.
7. Reduced serum folate concentration.

Carcinogenesis, Mutagenesis, Impairment of Fertility

Long-term, continuous administration of natural and synthetic estrogens in certain animal species increases the frequency of carcinomas of the breast, cervix, vagina, testis, and liver (see CONTRAINDICATIONS and WARNINGS).

Pregnancy Category X

Estrogens should not be used during pregnancy (see CONTRAINDICATIONS and Boxed Warning).

Nursing Mothers

As a general principle, the administration of any drug to nursing mothers should be done only when clearly necessary since many drugs are excreted in human milk.

Pediatric Use

The safety and effectiveness in pediatric patients have not been established.

ADVERSE REACTIONS

(See WARNINGS regarding induction of neoplasia, adverse effects on the fetus, gallbladder disease, cardiovascular disease, elevated blood pressure, and hypercalcemia.)

The most commonly reported adverse reaction to Estraderm in clinical trials was redness and irritation at the application site. This occurred in about 17% of the women treated and caused approximately 2% to discontinue therapy. Reports of rash have been rare. There have also been rare reports of severe systemic allergic reactions.

The following additional adverse reactions have been reported with estrogen therapy:

1. *Genitourinary system.* Changes in vaginal bleeding pattern and abnormal withdrawal bleeding or flow; breakthrough bleeding; spotting; increase in size of uterine leiomyomata; vaginal candidiasis; change in amount of cervical secretion.
2. *Breasts.* Tenderness, enlargement.
3. *Gastrointestinal.* Nausea, vomiting; abdominal cramps, bloating; cholestatic jaundice; gallbladder disease.
4. *Skin.* Chloasma or melasma that may persist when drug is discontinued; erythema multiforme; erythema nodosum; hemorrhagic eruption; loss of scalp hair; hirsutism.
5. *Eyes.* Steepening of corneal curvature; intolerance to contact lenses.
6. *CNS.* Headache, migraine, dizziness; mental depression; chorea.
7. *Miscellaneous.* Increase or decrease in weight; reduced carbohydrate tolerance; aggravation of porphyria; edema; changes in libido.

ACUTE OVERDOSAGE

Serious ill effects have not been reported following acute ingestion of large doses of estrogen-containing oral contraceptives by young children. Overdosage of estrogen may cause nausea and vomiting, and withdrawal beeding may occur in females.

DOSAGE AND ADMINISTRATION

The adhesive side of the Estraderm system should be placed on a clean, dry area of the skin on the trunk of the body (including the buttocks and abdomen). The site selected should be one that is not exposed to sunlight. *Estraderm should not be applied to the breasts.* The Estraderm system should be replaced twice weekly. The sites of application must be rotated, with an interval of at least 1 week allowed between applications to a particular site. The area selected should not be oily, damaged, or irritated. The waistline should be avoided, since tight clothing may rub the system off. The system should be applied immediately after opening the pouch and removing the protective liner. The system should be pressed firmly in place with the palm of the hand for about 10 seconds, making sure there is good contact, especially around the edges. In the unlikely event that a system should fall off, the same system may be reapplied. If necessary, a new system may be applied. In either case, the original treatment schedule should be continued.

Initiation of Therapy

Estraderm is currently available in two dosage forms—0.05 mg and 0.1 mg. For treatment of moderate-to-severe vasomotor symptoms, atrophic vaginitis, and atrophic urethritis associated with menopause, initiate therapy with Estraderm 0.05 applied to the skin twice weekly. The lowest dose that will control symptoms should be chosen, and medication should be discontinued as promptly as possible. Attempts to discontinue or taper medication given only for these menopausal symptoms should be made at 3-month to 6-month intervals.

Prophylactic therapy with Estraderm to prevent postmenopausal bone loss should be initiated with the 0.05 mg/day dosage as soon as possible after menopause. The dosage may be adjusted if necessary. Discontinuation of estrogen replacement therapy may reestablish bone loss at a rate comparable to the immediate postmenopausal period.

In women not currently taking oral estrogens, treatment with Estraderm may be initiated at once. In women who are currently taking oral estrogen, treatment with Estraderm should be initiated 1 week after withdrawal of oral hormone replacement therapy, or sooner if menopausal symptoms reappear in less than 1 week.

Therapeutic Regimen

Estraderm therapy may be given continuously in patients who do not have an intact uterus. In those patients with an intact uterus, Estraderm may be given on a cyclic schedule (e.g., 3 weeks on drug followed by 1 week off drug).

HOW SUPPLIED

Estraderm estradiol transdermal system 0.05 mg/day – each 10 cm^2 system contains 4 mg of estradiol USP for nominal* delivery of 0.05 mg of estradiol per day.

Patient Calendar Pack
of 8 Systems .... NDC 0083-2310-08
Carton of 6 Patient Calendar Packs
of 8 Systems .... NDC 0083-2310-62
Carton of 1 Patient Calendar Pack
of 24 Systems .... NDC 0083-2310-24

Estraderm estradiol transdermal system 0.1 mg/day – each 20 cm^2 system contains 8 mg of estradiol USP for nominal* delivery of 0.1 mg of estradiol per day.

Patient Calendar Pack
of 8 Systems .... NDC 0083-2320-08
Carton of 6 Patient Calendar Packs
of 8 Systems .... NDC 0083-2320-62
Carton of 1 Patient Calendar Pack
of 24 Systems .... NDC 0083-2320-24

*See DESCRIPTION.

Do not store above 86°F (30°C).

Do not store unpouched. Apply immediately upon removal from the protective pouch.

C97-35 (Rev. 5/98)

Information for the Patient

ESTRADERM® ℞

Generic name: estradiol transdermal system pronounced ess-tra-DYE-all

1. ESTROGENS INCREASE THE RISK OF CANCER OF THE UTERUS IN WOMEN WHO HAVE HAD THEIR MENOPAUSE ("CHANGE OF LIFE").

If you use any estrogen-containing drug, it is important to visit your doctor regularly and report any unusual vaginal bleeding right away. Vaginal bleeding after menopause may be a warning sign of uterine cancer. Your doctor should evaluate any unusual vaginal bleeding to find out the cause.

2. ESTROGENS SHOULD NOT BE USED DURING PREGNANCY.

Estrogens do not prevent miscarriage (spontaneous abortion) and are not needed in the days following childbirth. If you take estrogens during pregnancy, your unborn child has a greater than usual chance of having birth defects. The risk of developing these defects is small, but clearly larger than the risk in children whose mothers did not take estrogens during pregnancy. These birth defects may affect the baby's urinary system and sex organs. Daughters born to mothers who took DES (an estrogen drug) have a higher than usual chance of developing cancer of the vagina or cervix when they become teenagers or young adults. Sons may have a higher than usual chance of developing cancer of the testicles when they become teenagers or young adults.

INTRODUCTION

Your doctor has prescribed Estraderm for the treatment of your menopausal symptoms and/or to prevent osteoporosis. During menopause, production of estrogen hormones by your body decreases well below the amounts normally produced during your fertile years. In many women, this decrease in estrogen production causes uncomfortable symptoms, most noticeably, hot flushes and sleep disturbance. Estrogens can be given to reduce or eliminate these symptoms and/or to prevent osteoporosis.

The Estraderm system that your doctor has prescribed for you releases small amounts of estradiol through the skin in a continuous way. Estradiol is the same hormone that your ovaries produce abundantly before menopause. Your doctor will prescribe the lowest dose you require, depending upon your individual response. The dose is adjusted by the size of the Estraderm system used; the systems are available in two sizes. The length of treatment will depend on the reason for use.

INFORMATION ABOUT ESTRADERM

How Estraderm Works

Estraderm contains estradiol. When applied to the skin as directed below, the Estraderm system releases estradiol, which flows through the skin into the bloodstream.

How and Where to Apply Estraderm

Each Estraderm system is individually sealed in a protective pouch. Tear open this pouch at the indentation (do not use scissors) and remove the system. Bubbles in the system are normal.

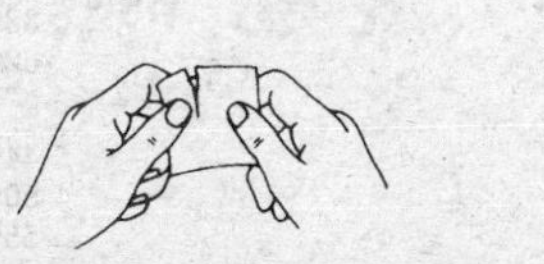

A stiff protective liner covers the adhesive side of the system – the side that will be placed against your skin. This liner must be removed before applying the system. Slide the protective liner sideways between your thumb and index finger. Then hold the system at one edge. Remove the protective liner and discard it. Try to avoid touching the adhesive.

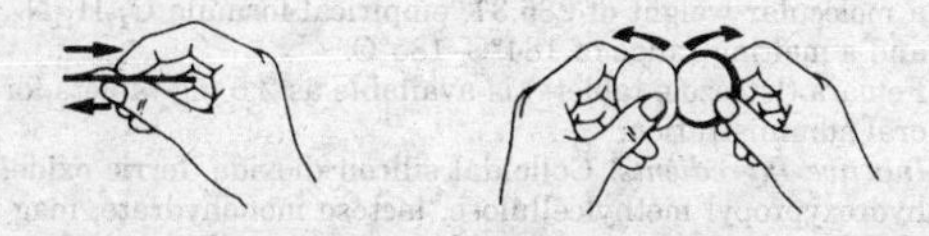

Apply the adhesive side of the system to a clean, dry area of the skin on the trunk of the body (including the buttocks and abdomen).

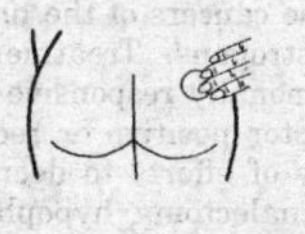

The site selected should be one that is not exposed to sunlight. Some women may find that it is more comfortable to wear Estraderm on the buttocks. *Do not apply Estraderm to your breasts.* The sites of application must be rotated, with an interval of at least 1 week allowed between applications to a particular site. The area selected should not be oily, damaged, or irritated. Avoid the waistline, since tight clothing may rub the system off. Apply the system immediately after opening the pouch and removing the protective liner. Press the system firmly in place with the palm of your hand for about 10 seconds, making sure there is good contact, especially around the edges.

The Estraderm system should be worn continuously until it is time to replace it with a new system. You may wish to experiment with different locations when applying a new system, to find ones that are most comfortable for you and where clothing will not rub on the system.

When to Apply Estraderm

The Estraderm system should be replaced twice weekly. Your Estraderm package contains a calendar checklist on the back to help you remember a schedule. Mark the 2-day schedule you plan to follow. Always change the system on the 2 days of the week you have marked.

When changing the system, remove the used Estraderm and discard it. Any adhesive that might remain on your skin can be easily rubbed off. Then place the new Estraderm on a different skin site. (The same skin site should not be used again for at least 1 week after removal of the system.)

Please note: Contact with water when you are bathing, swimming, or showering will not affect the system. In the unlikely event that a system should fall off, put this same system back on and continue to follow your original treatment schedule. If necessary, you may apply a new system but continue to follow your original schedule.

Benefits of Treatment With Estraderm

Regular use of Estraderm twice weekly offers relief of moderate-to-severe symptoms of menopause and has been shown to help prevent osteoporosis, which is a thinning of the bones that makes them more fragile. In the years following the menopause, unless estrogen therapy is taken regularly, your bones can rapidly lose strength, possibly leading to osteoporosis and bone fractures. Estraderm may prevent this bone loss and the development of osteoporosis and may help you to avoid fractures of your spine ("dowager's hump"), wrist, and hip later in life.

Small quantities of the naturally occurring hormone estradiol are absorbed through the skin from the Estraderm system, ensuring a continuous supply of circulating hormone in the body.

There is no medical evidence that the use of any estrogen during menopause will keep you feeling young, keep your skin soft, or relieve nervousness.

USES OF ESTROGEN

To reduce moderate-to-severe menopausal symptoms. Estrogens are hormones produced by the ovaries. The decrease in the amount of estrogen that occurs in all women, usually between ages 45 and 55, causes the menopause. Sometimes the ovaries are removed by an operation, causing "surgical menopause." When the amount of estrogen begins to decrease, some women develop very uncomfortable symptoms, such as feelings of warmth in the face, neck, and chest or sudden intense episodes of heat and sweating ("hot flashes"). The use of drugs containing estrogens can help the body adjust to lower estrogen levels.

Some women have only mild menopausal symptoms, or none at all, and do not need estrogen therapy for these particular symptoms. Other women may need estrogens for a few months while their bodies adjust to lower estrogen levels. For the treatment of menopausal symptoms only, most women need estrogen replacement therapy for no longer than 6 months. The prevention of osteoporosis may require longer-term therapy.

To prevent osteoporosis (brittle bones). After age 40, and especially after menopause, women begin to lose bone more rapidly, and some women develop osteoporosis. This thinning of the bones makes the bones weaker and more likely to break, often leading to fractures of the spine, hip, and wrist. Taking estrogens after the menopause slows down or halts bone loss and may prevent bones from breaking. Rapid loss of bone may begin soon after estrogen therapy is discontinued. Eating foods that are high in calcium (such as milk products) or taking calcium supplements and certain types of exercise may also help prevent osteoporosis. Before you change your calcium intake or exercise habits, it is important to discuss these life-style changes with your doctor to find out if they are safe for you. Since estrogen use is associated with some risk, its use in the prevention of osteoporosis should be confined to women who appear to be susceptible to this condition. The following characteristics are often present in women who are likely to develop osteoporosis: early menopause; white or Asian race; a family history of osteoporosis in a mother, sister, or aunt; slight build; cigarette smoking; alcohol abuse; or sedentary life-style.

Women who had their menopause by the surgical removal of their ovaries at a relatively young age may be good candidates for Estraderm therapy to help prevent osteoporosis.

To treat atrophic vaginitis (itching, burning, dryness in or around the vagina) *and atrophic urethritis* (which may cause difficulty or burning on urination).

WHEN ESTROGENS SHOULD NOT BE USED

During pregnancy. Although the possibility is fairly small, there is a greater risk of having a child born with a birth defect if you take estrogens during pregnancy. A male child may have an increased risk of developing abnormalities of the urinary system and sex organs. A female child may have an increased risk of developing cancer of the vagina or cervix in her teens or twenties. Estrogen is not effective in preventing miscarriage (abortion). In addition, estrogen should not be used after childbirth to prevent the breast from filling with milk, or while breast-feeding.

If you have undiagnosed vaginal bleeding. Unusual vaginal bleeding can be a warning sign of uterine cancer, especially if it happens after menopause. Your doctor must find out the proper treatment, if any. Taking estrogens without visiting your doctor can cause you serious harm if your vaginal bleeding is caused by cancer of the uterus.

If you have any circulation problems. Estrogen therapy should be used only after consultation with your doctor and only in recommended doses. Patients with a tendency for abnormal blood clotting should avoid estrogen use (see DANGERS OF ESTROGENS).

If you have had cancer. Since estrogens increase the risk of certain cancers, you should not take estrogens if you have ever had cancer of the breast or uterus.

When they are ineffective. Sometimes women experience nervous symptoms or depression during menopause. There is no evidence that estrogens are effective for such symptoms. You may have heard that taking estrogens for long periods (years) after menopause will keep your skin soft and supple and keep you feeling young. There is no evidence for these claims, and such long-term treatment may carry serious risks.

DANGERS OF ESTROGENS

Cancer of the uterus. The risk of cancer of the uterus increases the longer estrogens are used and when larger doses are taken. One study showed that when estrogens are discontinued, this increased risk of cancer seems to fall off quickly. Three other studies showed that the risk for uterine cancer stayed high for 8 to more than 15 years after stopping estrogen treatment. Because of this risk, *it is important to take the lowest dose of estrogen that will control your symptoms and to take it only as long as you need it.* Using progestin therapy together with estrogen therapy may reduce the higher risk of uterine cancer related to estrogen use (see OTHER INFORMATION).

If you have had your uterus removed (total hysterectomy), there is no danger of developing cancer of the uterus.

Cancer of the breast. The majority of studies have shown no association between the usual doses used for estrogen replacement therapy and breast cancer. Some studies have suggested a possible increased incidence of breast cancer in those women taking estrogens for prolonged periods of time and especially if higher doses are used.

Regular breast examinations by a health professional and monthly self-examination are recommended for women receiving estrogen therapy, as they are for all women.

Gallbladder disease. Women who use estrogens after menopause are more likely to develop gallbladder disease needing surgery than women who do not use estrogens.

Continued on next page

Estraderm—Cont.

Abnormal blood clotting. Taking estrogens may increase the risk of blood clots. These clots can cause a stroke, heart attack, or pulmonary embolus, any of which may be fatal.

SIDE EFFECTS

In addition to the risks listed above, the following side effects have been reported with estrogen use:
- Nausea and vomiting.
- Breast tenderness or enlargement.
- Enlargement of benign tumors of the uterus.
- Retention of excess fluid. This may make some conditions worsen, such as asthma, epilepsy, migraine, heart disease, or kidney disease.
- A spotty darkening of the skin, particularly on the face.
- Skin irritation, redness, or rash may occur at the site of Estraderm application.

REDUCING RISK OF ESTROGEN USE

If you decide to take estrogen replacement therapy, you can reduce your risks by carefully monitoring your treatment.
See your doctor regularly. While you are taking estrogens, it is important that you visit your doctor at least once a year for a physical examination. If members of your family have had breast cancer or if you have ever had breast nodules or an abnormal mammogram (breast x-ray), you may need to have more frequent breast examinations.
Reevaluate your need for estrogens. You and your doctor should reevaluate your need for estrogens at least every 6 months.
Be alert for signs of trouble. Report these or any other unusual side effects to your doctor immediately:
- Abnormal bleeding from the vagina.
- Pains in the calves or chest, a sudden shortness of breath, or coughing blood (indicating possible clots in the legs, heart, or lungs).
- Severe headache, dizziness, faintness, or changes in vision, indicating possible clots in the brain or eye.
- Breast lumps.
- Yellowing of the skin.
- Pain, swelling, or tenderness in the abdomen.
- Skin irritation, redness, or rash.

OTHER INFORMATION

If your uterus has not been removed, your doctor may choose to prescribe a progestin, a different hormonal drug, to be used in association with estrogen treatment. Progestins lower the risk of developing endometrial hyperplasia, a possible precancerous condition of the uterine lining, which may occur while using estrogens. There are possible additional risks that may be associated with the inclusion of a progestin in estrogen treatment. The possible risks include unfavorable effects on blood fats and sugars, as well as a possible further increase in breast cancer risk that may be associated with long-term estrogen use.
Some research has suggested that estrogens taken *without progestins* may protect women against developing heart disease. However, this effect of estrogens is not certain.
You are cautioned to discuss very carefully with your doctor or health care provider all the possible risks and benefits of long-term estrogen and progestin treatment, as they affect you personally.
Your doctor has prescribed this drug for you and you alone. Do not give the drug to anyone else.
If you will be taking calcium supplements as part of the treatment to help prevent osteoporosis, check with your doctor about the amounts recommended.
Keep this and all other drugs out of the reach of children. In case of overdose, remove the Estraderm system and call your doctor, hospital, or poison control center immediately.
This leaflet provides the most important information about estrogens. If you want to read more, ask your doctor or pharmacist to let you read the professional labeling.

C97-36 (Rev. 5/98)
C97-35/C97-36 (Rev. 5/98)

Shown in Product Identification Guide, page 324

FEMARA™ ℞

[fĕ 'mără]
(letrozole tablets)
2.5 mg Tablets

The following prescribing information is based on official labeling in effect on August 1, 1998.

Prescribing Information

DESCRIPTION

Femara (letrozole tablets) for oral administration contain 2.5 mg of letrozole, a nonsteroidal aromatase inhibitor (inhibitor of estrogen synthesis). It is chemically described as 4,4'-(1H-1,2,4-Triazol-1-ylmethylene)dibenzonitrile, and its structural formula is
[See chemical structure at top of next column]
Letrozole is a white to yellowish crystalline powder, practically odorless, freely soluble in dichloromethane, slightly

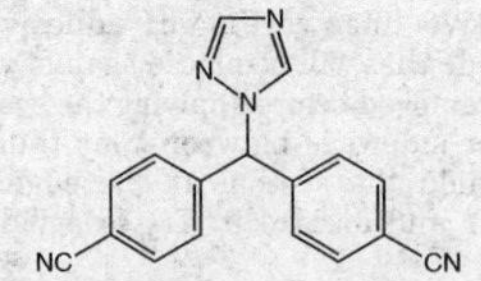

soluble in ethanol, and practically insoluble in water. It has a molecular weight of 285.31, empirical formula $C_{17}H_{11}N_5$, and a melting range of 184°C–185°C.
Femara (letrozole tablets) is available as 2.5 mg tablets for oral administration.
Inactive Ingredients. Colloidal silicon dioxide, ferric oxide, hydroxypropyl methylcellulose, lactose monohydrate, magnesium stearate, maize starch, microcrystalline cellulose, polyethylene glycol, sodium starch glycolate, talc, and titanium dioxide.

CLINICAL PHARMACOLOGY

Mechanism of Action

The growth of some cancers of the breast is stimulated or maintained by estrogens. Treatment of breast cancer thought to be hormonally responsive (i.e., estrogen and/or progesterone receptor positive or receptor unknown) has included a variety of efforts to decrease estrogen levels (ovariectomy, adrenalectomy, hypophysectomy) or inhibit estrogen effects (antiestrogens and progestational agents). These interventions lead to decreased tumor mass or delayed progression of tumor growth in some women.
In postmenopausal women, estrogens are mainly derived from the action of the aromatase enzyme, which converts adrenal androgens (primarily androstenedione and testosterone) to estrone and estradiol. The suppression of estrogen biosynthesis in peripheral tissues and in the cancer tissue itself can therefore be achieved by specifically inhibiting the aromatase enzyme.
Letrozole is a nonsteroidal competitive inhibitor of the aromatase enzyme system; it inhibits the conversion of androgens to estrogens. In adult nontumor- and tumor-bearing female animals, letrozole is as effective as ovariectomy in reducing uterine weight, elevating serum LH, and causing the regression of estrogen-dependent tumors. In contrast to ovariectomy, treatment with letrozole does not lead to an increase in serum FSH. Letrozole selectively inhibits gonadal steroidogenesis but has no significant effect on adrenal mineralocorticoid or glucocorticoid synthesis.
Letrozole inhibits the aromatase enzyme by competitively binding to the heme of the cytochrome P450 subunit of the enzyme, resulting in a reduction of estrogen biosynthesis in all tissues. Treatment of women with letrozole significantly lowers serum estrone, estradiol and estrone sulfate and has not been shown to significantly affect adrenal corticosteroid synthesis, aldosterone synthesis, or synthesis of thyroid hormones.

Pharmacokinetics

Letrozole is rapidly and completely absorbed from the gastrointestinal tract and absorption is not affected by food. It is metabolized slowly to an inactive metabolite whose glucuronide conjugate is excreted renally, representing the major clearance pathway. About 90% of radiolabeled letrozole is recovered in urine. Letrozole's terminal elimination half-life is about 2 days and steady-state plasma concentration after daily 2.5 mg dosing is reached in 2–6 weeks. Plasma concentrations at steady-state are 1.5 to 2 times higher than predicted from the concentrations measured after a single dose, indicating a slight non-linearity in the pharmacokinetics of letrozole upon daily administration of 2.5 mg. These steady-state levels are maintained over extended periods, however, and continuous accumulation of letrozole does not occur. Letrozole is weakly protein bound and has a large volume of distribution (approximately 1.9 L/kg).

Metabolism and Excretion

Metabolism to a pharmacologically-inactive carbinol metabolite (4,4'-methanolbisbenzonitrile) and renal excretion of the glucuronide conjugate of this metabolite is the major pathway of letrozole clearance. Of the radiolabel recovered in urine, at least 75% was the glucuronide of the carbinol metabolite, about 9% was two unidentified metabolites, and 6% was unchanged letrozole.
In human microsomes with specific CYP isozyme activity, CYP 3A4 metabolized letrozole to the carbinol metabolite while CYP 2A6 formed both this metabolite and its ketone analog. In human liver microsomes, letrozole strongly inhibited CYP 2A6 and moderately inhibited CYP 2C19.

Special Populations

Pediatric, Geriatric and Race:
In the study populations (adults ranging in age from 35 to >80 years), no change in pharmacokinetic parameters was observed with increasing age. Differences in letrozole pharmacokinetics between adult and pediatric populations have not been studied. Differences in letrozole pharmacokinetics due to race have not been studied.

Renal Insufficiency:
In a study of volunteers with varying renal function (24-hour creatinine clearance: 9–116 mL/min), no effect of renal function on the pharmacokinetics of single doses of 2.5 mg of Femara (letrozole tablets) was found. In addition, in a study of 347 patients with advanced breast cancer, about half of whom received 2.5 mg Femara and half 0.5 mg Femara, renal impairment (calculated creatinine clearance: 20–50 mL/min) did not affect steady-state plasma letrozole concentration.

Hepatic Insufficiency:
In a study of subjects with varying degrees of non-metastatic hepatic dysfunction (e.g., cirrhosis, Child-Pugh classification A and B), the mean AUC values of the volunteers with moderate hepatic impairment were 37% higher than in normal subjects, but still within the range seen in subjects without impaired function. Patients with severe hepatic impairment (Child-Pugh classification C) have not been studied (see DOSAGE & ADMINISTRATION Hepatic Impairment).

Drug/Drug Interactions:
A pharmacokinetic interaction study with cimetidine showed no clinically significant effect on letrozole pharmacokinetics. An interaction study with warfarin showed no clinically significant effect of letrozole on warfarin pharmacokinetics.
There is no clinical experience to date on the use of Femara in combination with other anti-cancer agents.

Pharmacodynamics

In postmenopausal patients with advanced breast cancer, daily doses of 0.1 mg to 5 mg Femara suppress plasma concentrations of estradiol, estrone, and estrone sulfate by 75%–95% from baseline with maximal suppression achieved within two–three days. Suppression is dose-related, with doses of 0.5 mg and higher giving many values of estrone and estrone sulfate that were below the limit of detection in the assays. Estrogen suppression was maintained throughout treatment in all patients treated at 0.5 mg or higher.
Letrozole is highly specific in inhibiting aromatase activity. There is no impairment of adrenal steroidogenesis. No clinically-relevant changes were found in the plasma concentrations of cortisol, aldosterone, 11-deoxycortisol, 17-hydroxy-progesterone, ACTH or in plasma renin activity among postmenopausal patients treated with a daily dose of Femara 0.1 mg to 5 mg. The ACTH stimulation test performed after 6 and 12 weeks of treatment with daily doses of 0.1, 0.25, 0.5, 1, 2.5, and 5 mg did not indicate any attenuation of aldosterone or cortisol production. Glucocorticoid or mineralocorticoid supplementation is, therefore, not necessary.
No changes were noted in plasma concentrations of androgens (androstenedione and testosterone) among healthy postmenopausal women after 0.1, 0.5, and 2.5 mg single doses of Femara or in plasma concentrations of androstenedione among postmenopausal patients treated with daily doses of 0.1 mg to 5 mg. This indicates that the blockade of estrogen biosynthesis does not lead to accumulation of androgenic precursors. Plasma levels of LH and FSH were not affected by letrozole in patients, nor was thyroid function as evaluated by TSH levels, T3 uptake, and T4 levels

Clinical Studies

Femara was initially studied at doses of 0.1 mg to 5.0 mg daily in six non-comparative phase I/II trials in 181 postmenopausal estrogen/progesterone receptor positive or unknown advanced breast cancer patients previously

Table I: Selected Study Population Demographics

Parameter	megestrol acetate study	aminoglutethimide study
No. of Participants	552	557
Receptor Status		
ER/PR Positive	57%	56%
ER/PR Unknown	43%	44%
Previous Therapy		
Adjuvant Only	33%	38%
Therapeutic +/− Adj.	66%	62%
Sites of Disease		
Visceral Metastases	40%	44%
Soft Tissue Metastases	56%	50%
Bony Metastases	50%	55%

treated with at least antiestrogen therapy. Patients had received other hormonal therapies and also may have received cytotoxic therapy. Eight (20%) of forty patients treated with Femara 2.5 mg daily in phase I/II trials achieved an objective tumor response (complete or partial response).

Two large randomized controlled multinational (predominantly European) trials were conducted in patients with advanced breast cancer who had progressed despite antiestrogen therapy. Patients were randomized to Femara 0.5 mg daily, Femara 2.5 mg daily, or a comparator (megestrol acetate 160 mg daily in one study; and aminoglutethimide 250 mg bid with corticosteroid supplementation in the other study). In each study over 60% of the patients had received therapeutic antiestrogens, and about one-fifth of these patients had had an objective response. The megestrol acetate controlled study was double-blind; the other study was open label. Selected baseline characteristics for each study are shown in the following table:

[See table 1 at bottom of previous page]

Confirmed objective tumor response (complete response plus partial response) was the primary endpoint of the trials. Responses were measured according to the Union Internationale Contre le Cancer (UICC) criteria and verified by independent, blinded review. All responses were confirmed by a second evaluation 4–12 weeks after the documentation of the initial response.

The following table shows the results for the first trial, with a minimum follow-up of 15 months, that compared Femara 0.5 mg, Femara 2.5 mg, and megestrol acetate 160 mg daily. (All analyses are unadjusted.)

[See table 2 below]

The Kaplan-Meier Curve for progression for the megestrol acetate study is shown below.

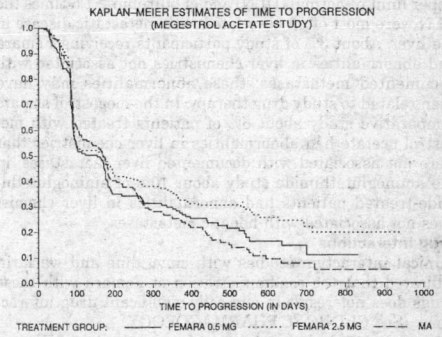

KAPLAN–MEIER ESTIMATES OF TIME TO PROGRESSION (MEGESTROL ACETATE STUDY)

TREATMENT GROUP: — FEMARA 0.5 MG — FEMARA 2.5 MG – – – MA

The results for the study comparing Femara to aminoglutethimide, with a minimum follow-up of nine months, are shown in the following table.
(Unadjusted analysis are used).

[See table 3 below]

The Kaplan-Meier Curve for progression for the aminoglutethimide study is shown below.

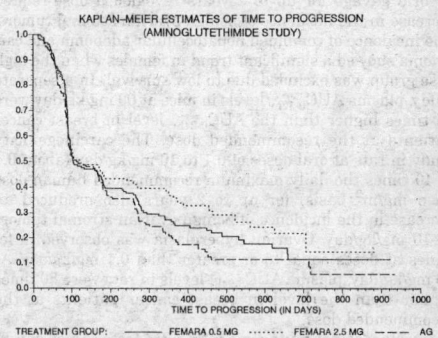

KAPLAN–MEIER ESTIMATES OF TIME TO PROGRESSION (AMINOGLUTETHIMIDE STUDY)

TREATMENT GROUP: — FEMARA 0.5 MG — FEMARA 2.5 MG – – – AG

Table 2: Megestrol Acetate Study Results

	Femara 0.5 mg N = 188	Femara 2.5 mg N = 174	Megestrol Acetate N = 190
Objective Response (CR + PR)	22 (11.7%)	41 (23.6%)	31 (16.3%)
Median Duration of Response	552 days	(Not reached)	561 days
Median Time to Progression	154 days	170 days	168 days
Median Survival	633 days	730 days	659 days
Odds Ratio for Response	Femara 2.5: Femara 0.5 = 2.33 (95% CI: 1.32, 4.17); p = 0.004*		Femara 2.5: Megestrol = 1.58 (95% CI: 0.94, 2.66); p = 0.08*
Relative Risk of Progression	Femara 2.5: Femara 0.5 = 0.81 (95% CI: 0.63, 1.03); p = 0.09*		Femara 2.5: Megestrol = 0.77 (95% CI: 0.60, 0.98), p = 0.03*

*two-sided p-value

Table 3: Aminoglutethimide Study Results

	Femara 0.5 N = 193	Femara 2.5 N = 185	Aminoglutethimide N = 179
Objective Response (CR + PR)	34 (17.6%)	34 (18.4%)	22 (12.3%)
Median Duration of Response	619 days	706 days	450 days
Median Time to Progression	103 days	123 days	112 days
Median Survival	636 days	792 days	592 days
Odds Ratio for Response	Femara 2.5: Femara 0.5 = 1.05 (95% CI: 0.62, 1.79); p = 0.85*		Femara 2.5: Aminoglutethimide = 1.61 (95% CI: 0.90, 2.87); p = 0.11*
Relative Risk of Progression	Femara 2.5: Femara 0.5 = .86 (95% CI: 0.68, 1.11); p = 0.25*		Femara 2.5: Aminoglutethimide = 0.74 (95% CI: 0.57, 0.94); p = 0.02*

*two-sided p-value

Adverse Experience	Percentage (%) of Patients with Adverse Events			
	Pooled Femara 2.5 mg (n=359) %	Pooled Femara 0.5 mg (n=380) %	Megestrol Acetate 160 mg (n=189) %	Aminoglutethimide 500 mg (n=178) %
Body as a Whole				
Fatigue	8	6	11	3
Chest pain	6	3	7	3
Peripheral edema[1]	5	5	8	3
Asthenia	4	5	4	5
Weight increase	2	2	9	3
Cardiovascular				
Hypertension	5	7	5	6
Digestive System				
Nausea	13	15	9	14
Vomiting	7	7	5	9
Constipation	6	7	9	7
Diarrhea	6	5	3	4
Pain-abdominal	6	5	9	8
Anorexia	5	3	5	5
Dyspepsia	3	4	6	5
Infections/Infestations				
Viral infection	6	5	6	3
Lab Abnormality				
Hypercholesterolemia	3	3	0	6
Musculoskeletal System				
Musculoskeletal[2]	21	22	30	14
Arthralgia	8	8	8	3
Nervous System				
Headache	9	12	9	7
Somnolence	3	2	2	9
Dizziness	3	5	7	3
Respiratory System				
Dyspnea	7	9	16	5
Coughing	6	5	7	5
Skin and Appendages				
Hot flushes	6	5	4	3
Rash[3]	5	4	3	12
Pruritus	1	2	5	3

[1] Includes peripheral edema, leg edema, dependent edema, edema
[2] Includes musculoskeletal pain, skeletal pain, back pain, arm pain, leg pain
[3] Includes rash, erythematous rash, maculopapular rash, psoriaform rash, vesicular rash

INDICATIONS AND USAGE

Femara (letrozole tablets) is indicated for the treatment of advanced breast cancer in postmenopausal women with disease progression following antiestrogen therapy.

CONTRAINDICATIONS

Femara is contraindicated in patients with known hypersensitivity to Femara or any of its excipients.

WARNINGS

Pregnancy

Letrozole may cause fetal harm when administered to pregnant women. Studies in rats at doses equal to or greater than 0.003 mg/kg (about 1/100 the daily maximum recommended human dose on a mg/m² basis) administered during the period of organogenesis, have shown that letrozole is embryotoxic and fetotoxic, as indicated by intrauterine mortality, increased resorption, increased postimplantation loss, decreased numbers of live fetuses and fetal anomalies including absence and shortening of renal papilla, dilation of ureter, edema and incomplete ossification of frontal skull and metatarsals. Letrozole was teratogenic in rats. A 0.03 mg/kg dose (about 1/10 the daily maximum recommended human dose on a mg/m² basis) caused fetal domed head and cervical/centrum vertebral fusion.

Letrozole is embryotoxic at doses equal to or greater than 0.002 mg/kg and fetotoxic when administered to rabbits at 0.02 mg/kg (about 1/100,000 and 1/10,000 the daily maximum recommended human dose on a mg/m² basis, respectively). Fetal anomalies included incomplete ossification of the skull, sternebrae, and fore- and hindlegs.

There are no studies in pregnant women. Femara is indicated for postmenopausal women. If there is exposure to letrozole during pregnancy, the patient should be apprised of the potential hazard to the fetus and potential risk for loss of the pregnancy.

PRECAUTIONS

Laboratory Tests

No dose-related effect of Femara on any hematologic or clinical chemistry parameter was evident. Moderate decreases in lymphocyte counts, of uncertain clinical significance, were observed in some patients receiving Femara (letrozole tablets) 2.5 mg. This depression was transient in about half

Continued on next page

Femara—Cont.

of those affected. Two patients on Femara developed thrombocytopenia; relationship to the study drug was unclear. Patient withdrawal due to laboratory abnormalities, whether related to study treatment or not, was infrequent. Increases in SGOT, SGPT, and gamma GT ≥5 times the upper limit of normal (ULN) and of bilirubin ≥1.5 times the ULN were most often associated with metastatic disease in the liver. About 3% of study participants receiving Femara had abnormalities in liver chemistries not associated with documented metastases; these abnormalities may have been related to study drug therapy. In the megestrol acetate comparative study about 8% of patients treated with megestrol acetate had abnormalities in liver chemistries that were not associated with documented liver metastases; in the aminoglutethimide study about 10% of aminoglutethimide-treated patients had abnormalities in liver chemistries not associated with hepatic metastases.

Drug Interactions

Clinical interaction studies with cimetidine and warfarin indicated that the coadministration of Femara with these drugs does not result in clinically-significant drug interactions. (See CLINICAL PHARMACOLOGY)

There is no clinical experience to date on the use of Femara in combination with other anti-cancer agents.

Drug/Laboratory Test-Interactions

None observed.

Carcinogenesis, Mutagenesis, Impairment of Fertility

A conventional carcinogenesis study in mice at doses of 0.6 to 60 mg/kg/day (about one to 100 times the daily maximum recommended human dose on a mg/m^2 basis) administered by oral gavage for up to 2 years revealed a dose-related increase in the incidence of benign ovarian stromal tumors. The incidence of combined hepatocellular adenoma and carcinoma showed a significant trend in females when the high dose group was excluded due to low survival. In a separate study, plasma $AUC_{0\text{-}12hr}$ levels in mice at 60 mg/kg/day were 55 times higher than the $AUC_{0\text{-}24hr}$ level in breast cancer patients at the recommended dose. The carcinogenicity study in rats at oral doses of 0.1 to 10 mg/kg/day (about 0.4 to 40 times the daily maximum recommended human dose on a mg/m^2 basis) for up to 2 years also produced an increase in the incidence of benign ovarian stromal tumors at 10 mg/kg/day. Ovarian hyperplasia was observed in females at doses equal to or greater than 0.1 mg/kg/day. At 10 mg/kg/day, plasma $AUC_{0\text{-}24hr}$ levels in rats were 80 times higher than the level in breast cancer patients at the recommended dose.

Letrozole was not mutagenic in *in vitro* tests (Ames and E. coli bacterial tests) but was observed to be a potential clastogen in *in vitro* assays (CHO K1 and CCL 61 Chinese hamster ovary cells). Letrozole was not clastogenic *in vivo* (micronucleus test in rats).

Studies to investigate the effect of letrozole on fertility have not been conducted; however, repeated dosing caused sexual inactivity in females and atrophy of the reproductive tract in males and females at doses of 0.6, 0.1 and 0.03 mg/kg in mice, rats and dogs, respectively (about one, 0.4 and 0.4 the daily maximum recommended human dose on a mg/m^2 basis, respectively).

Pregnancy: Pregnancy Category D (See WARNINGS).

Nursing Mothers

It is not known if letrozole is excreted in human milk. Because many drugs are excreted in human milk, caution should be exercised when letrozole is administered to a nursing woman (See WARNINGS AND PRECAUTIONS).

Pediatric Use

The safety and effectiveness in pediatric patients have not been established.

Geriatric Use

The mean age of patients in the two randomized trials, that compared Femara (0.5 mg and 2.5 mg) to megestrol acetate and to aminoglutethimide, was 64 years. Thirty percent of patients were ≥70 years old. The proportion of patients responding to each dose of Femara was similar for women ≥70 years old and <70 years old.

ADVERSE REACTIONS

Femara (letrozole tablets) was generally well tolerated in two controlled clinical trials.

Study discontinuations in the megestrol acetate comparison study for adverse events other than progression of tumor occurred in 5/188 (2.7%) of patients on Femara 0.5 mg, in 4/174 (2.3%) of the patients on Femara 2.5 mg, and in 15/190 (7.9%) of patients on megestrol acetate. There were fewer thromboembolic events at both Femara doses than on the megestrol acetate arm (2 of 362 patients or 0.6% vs. 9 of 190 patients or 4.7%). There was also less vaginal bleeding (1 of 362 patients or 0.3% vs. 6 of 190 patients or 3.2%) on letrozole than on megestrol acetate. In the aminoglutethimide comparison study, discontinuations for reasons other than progression occurred in 6/193 (3.1%) of patients on 0.5 mg Femara, 7/185 (3.8%) of patients on 2.5 mg Femara, and 7/178 (3.9%) of patients on aminoglutethimide.

Comparisons of the incidence of adverse events revealed no significant differences between the high and low dose Femara groups in either study. Most of the adverse events observed in all treatment groups were mild to moderate in severity and it was generally not possible to distinguish adverse reactions due to treatment from the consequences of the patient's metastatic breast cancer, the effects of estrogen deprivation, or intercurrent illness.

Adverse events, regardless of relationship to study drug, that were reported in at least 5% of the patients treated with Femara 0.5 mg, Femara 2.5 mg, megestrol acetate, or aminoglutethimide in the two controlled trials are shown in the following table:

[See table at bottom of previous page]

Other less frequent (<5%) adverse experiences considered consequential and reported in at least 3 patients treated with Femara, included hypercalcemia, fracture, depression, anxiety, pleural effusion, alopecia, increased sweating and vertigo.

OVERDOSAGE

No experience with Femara (letrozole tablets) overdose has been reported. In single dose studies the highest dose used was 30 mg, which was well tolerated; in multiple dose trials, the largest dose of 5 mg was well tolerated.

Lethality was observed in mice and rats following single oral doses that were equal to or greater than 2000 mg/kg (about 4000 to 8000 times the daily maximum recommended human dose on a mg/m^2 basis); death was associated with reduced motor activity, ataxia and dyspnea. Lethality was observed in cats following single IV doses that were equal to or greater than 10 mg/kg (about 50 times the daily maximum recommended human dose on a mg/m^2 basis); death was preceded by depressed blood pressure and arrhythmias.

There is no experience in humans with an overdose of Femara, so firm recommendations for treatment are not possible. Emesis could be induced if the patient is alert. In general, supportive care and frequent monitoring of vital signs is appropriate.

DOSAGE & ADMINISTRATION

Adult and Elderly Patients

The recommended dose of Femara (letrozole tablets) is one 2.5 mg tablet administered once a day, without regard to meals. Treatment with Femara should continue until tumor progression is evident. No dose adjustment is required for elderly patients. Patients treated with Femara do not require glucocorticoid or mineralocorticoid replacement therapy.

Renal Impairment

(See CLINICAL PHARMACOLOGY.) No dosage adjustment is required for patients with renal impairment if creatinine clearance is ≥10 mL/min.

Hepatic Impairment

(See CLINICAL PHARMACOLOGY.) Although letrozole blood concentrations were modestly increased in subjects with moderate hepatic impairment due to cirrhosis, no dosage adjustment is recommended for patients with mild-to-moderate hepatic impairment. Patients with severe impairment of liver function have not been studied. Because letrozole is eliminated almost exclusively by hepatic metabolism, patients with severe impairment of liver function should be dosed with caution.

HOW SUPPLIED

2.5 mg tablets – dark yellow, film-coated, round, slightly biconvex, with beveled edges (imprinted with the letters FV on one side and CG on the other side).

Packaged in HDPE bottles with a safety screw cap.

Bottles of 30 tablets .... NDC 0078-0249-15

Store at 25°C (77°F); excursions permitted to 15°C–30°C (59°F–86°F) [see USP Controlled Room Temperature].

C97-8 (Rev. 7/97)

Shown in Product Identification Guide, page 324

FIORICET® ℞

[fē-ōr 'ĭ-set]

(Butalbital, Acetaminophen, and Caffeine Tablets, USP)

Caution: Federal law prohibits dispensing without prescription.

The following prescribing information is based on official labeling in effect on August 1, 1998.

DESCRIPTION

Fioricet® (Butalbital, Acetaminophen, and Caffeine Tablets, USP) is supplied in tablet form for oral administration.

Each tablet contains the following active ingredients:

butalbital, USP .... 50 mg
acetaminophen, USP .... 325 mg
caffeine, USP .... 40 mg

Inactive Ingredients: crospovidone, FD&C Blue #1, magnesium stearate, microcrystalline cellulose, povidone, pregelatinized starch, and stearic acid.

Butalbital (5-allyl-5-isobutylbarbituric acid), is a short to intermediate-acting barbiturate. It has the following structural formula:

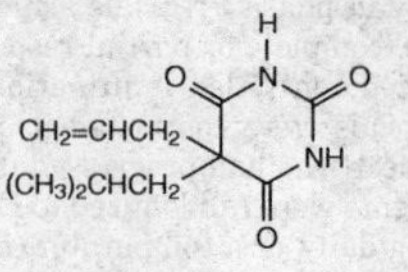

$C_{11}H_{16}N_2O_3$ Mol. wt. 224.26

Acetaminophen (4′-hydroxyacteanilide), is a non-opiate, non-salicylate analgesic and antipyretic. It has the following structural formula:

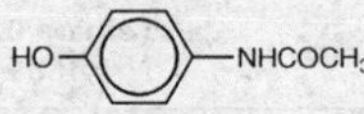

$C_8H_9NO_2$ Mol. wt. 151.17

Caffeine (1,3,7-trimethylxanthine), is a central nervous system stimulant. It has the following structural formula:

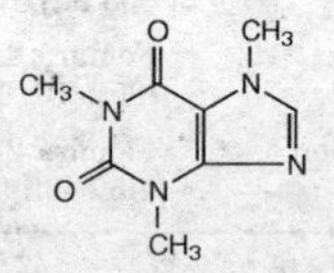

$C_8H_{10}N_4O_2$ Mol. wt. 194.19

CLINICAL PHARMACOLOGY

This combination drug product is intended as a treatment for tension headache.

It consists of a fixed combination of butalbital, acetaminophen, and caffeine. The role each component plays in the relief of the complex of symptoms known as tension headache is incompletely understood.

Pharmacokinetics

The behavior of the individual components is described below.

Butalbital

Butalbital is well absorbed from the gastrointestinal tract and is expected to distribute to most tissues in the body. Barbiturates in general may appear in breast milk and readily cross the placental barrier. They are bound to plasma and tissue proteins to a varying degree and binding increases directly as a function of lipid solubility.

Elimination of butalbital is primarily via the kidney (59% to 88% of the dose) as unchanged drug or metabolites. The plasma half-life is about 35 hours. Urinary excretion products include parent drug (about 3.6% of the dose), 5-isobutyl-5-(2,3-dihydroxypropyl) barbituric acid (about 24% of the dose), 5-allyl-5(3-hydroxy-2-methyl-1-propyl) barbituric acid (about 4.8% of the dose), products with the barbituric acid ring hydrolyzed with excretion of urea (about 14% of the dose), as well as unidentified materials. Of the material excreted in the urine, 32% is conjugated.

The *in vitro* plasma protein binding of butalbital is 45% over the concentration range of 0.5-20 mcg/mL. This falls within the range of plasma protein binding (20%-45%) reported with other barbiturates such as phenobarbital, pentobarbital, and secobarbital sodium. The plasma-to-blood concentration ratio was almost unity, indicating that there is no preferential distribution of butalbital into either plasma or blood cells.

See *OVERDOSAGE* for toxicity information.

Acetaminophen

Acetaminophen is rapidly absorbed from the gastrointestinal tract and is distributed throughout most body tissues. The plasma half-life is 1.25 to 3 hours, but may be increased by liver damage and following overdosage. Elimination of acetaminophen is principally by liver metabolism (conjugation) and subsequent renal excretion of metabolites. Approximately 85% of an oral dose appears in the urine within 24 hours of administration, most as the glucuronide conjugate, with small amounts of other conjugates and unchanged drug.

See *OVERDOSAGE* for toxicity information.

Caffeine

Like most xanthines, caffeine is rapidly absorbed and distributed in all body tissues and fluids, including the CNS, fetal tissues, and breast milk.

Caffeine is cleared through metabolism and excretion in the urine. The plasma half-life is about 3 hours. Hepatic biotransformation prior to excretion results in about equal amounts of 1-methyl-xanthine and 1-methyluric acid. Of the 70% of the dose that is recovered in the urine, only 3% is unchanged drug.

See *OVERDOSAGE* for toxicity information.

INDICATIONS AND USAGE

Fioricet® (Butalbital, Acetaminophen, and Caffeine Tablets) is indicated for the relief of the symptom complex of tension (or muscle contraction) headache.

Evidence supporting the efficacy and safety of this combination product in the treatment of multiple recurrent head-

aches is unavailable. Caution in this regard is required because butalbital is habit-forming and potentially abusable.

CONTRAINDICATIONS

This product is contraindicated under the following conditions:

–Hypersensitivity or intolerance to any component of this product

–Patients with porphyria.

WARNINGS

Butalbital is habit-forming and potentially abusable. Consequently, the extended use of this product is not recommended.

PRECAUTIONS

General

Butalbital, acetaminophen, and caffeine tablets should be prescribed with caution in certain special-risk patients, such as the elderly or debilitated, and those with severe impairment of renal or hepatic function, or acute abdominal conditions.

Information for Patients

This product may impair mental and/or physical abilities required for the performance of potentially hazardous tasks such as driving a car or operating machinery. Such tasks should be avoided while taking this product.

Alcohol and other CNS depressants may produce an additive CNS depression when taken with this combination product, and should be avoided.

Butalbital may be habit-forming. Patients should take the drug only for as long as it is prescribed, in the amounts prescribed, and no more frequently than prescribed.

Laboratory Tests

In patients with severe hepatic or renal disease, effects of therapy should be monitored with serial liver and/or renal function tests.

Drug Interactions

The CNS effects of butalbital may be enhanced by monoamine oxidase (MAO) inhibitors.

Butalbital, acetaminophen, and caffeine may enhance the effects of: other narcotic analgesics, alcohol, general anesthetics, tranquilizers such as chlordiazepoxide, sedative-hypnotics, or other CNS depressants, causing increased CNS depression.

Drug/Laboratory Test Interactions

Acetaminophen may produce false-positive test results for urinary 5-hydroxyindoleacetic acid.

Carcinogenesis, Mutagenesis, Impairment of Fertility

No adequate studies have been conducted in animals to determine whether acetaminophen or butalbital have a potential for carcinogenesis, mutagenesis or impairment of fertility.

Pregnancy

Teratogenic Effects

Pregnancy Category C: Animal reproduction studies have not been conducted with this combination product. It is also not known whether butalbital, acetaminophen, and caffeine can cause fetal harm when administered to a pregnant woman or can affect reproduction capacity. This product should be given to a pregnant woman only when clearly needed.

Nonteratogenic Effects

Withdrawal seizures were reported in a two-day-old male infant whose mother had taken a butalbital-containing drug during the last two months of pregnancy. Butalbital was found in the infant's serum. The infant was given phenobarbital 5 mg/kg, which was tapered without further seizure or other withdrawal symptoms.

Nursing Mothers

Caffeine, barbiturates, and acetaminophen are excreted in breast milk in small amounts, but the significance of their effects on nursing infants is not known. Because of potential for serious adverse reactions in nursing infants from butalbital, acetaminophen, and caffeine, a decision should be made whether to discontinue nursing or to discontinue the drug, taking into account the importance of the drug to the mother.

Pediatric Use

Safety and effectiveness in pediatric patients below the age of 12 have not been established.

ADVERSE REACTIONS

Frequently Observed

The most frequently reported adverse reactions are drowsiness, lightheadedness, dizziness, sedation, shortness of breath, nausea, vomiting, abdominal pain, and intoxicated feeling.

Infrequently Observed

All adverse events tabulated below are classified as infrequent.

Central Nervous System: headache, shaky feeling, tingling, agitation, fainting, fatigue, heavy eyelids, high energy, hot spells, numbness, sluggishness, seizure. Mental confusion, excitement, or depression can also occur due to intolerance, particularly in elderly or debilitated patients, or due to overdosage of butalbital.

Autonomic Nervous System: dry mouth, hyperhidrosis.

Gastrointestinal: difficulty swallowing, heartburn, flatulence, constipation.

Cardiovascular: tachycardia.

Musculoskeletal: leg pain, muscle fatigue.

Genitourinary: diuresis.

Miscellaneous: pruritus, fever, earache, nasal congestion, tinnitus, euphoria, allergic reactions.

Several cases of dermatological reactions, including toxic epidermal necrolysis and erythema multiforme, have been reported.

The following adverse drug events may be borne in mind as potential effects of the components of this product. Potential effects of high dosage are listed in the OVERDOSAGE section.

Acetaminophen: allergic reactions, rash, thrombocytopenia, agranulocytosis.

Caffeine: cardiac stimulation, irritability, tremor, dependence, nephrotoxicity, hyperglycemia.

DRUG ABUSE AND DEPENDENCE

Abuse and Dependence

Butalbital

Barbiturates may be habit-forming: Tolerance, psychological dependence, and physical dependence may occur especially following prolonged use of high doses of barbiturates. The average daily dose for the barbiturate addict is usually about 1500 mg. As tolerance to barbiturates develops, the amount needed to maintain the same level of intoxication increases; tolerance to a fatal dosage, however, does not increase more than two-fold. As this occurs, the margin between an intoxication dosage and fatal dosage becomes smaller. The lethal dose of a barbiturate is far less if alcohol is also ingested. Major withdrawal symptoms (convulsions and delirium) may occur within 16 hours and last up to 5 days after abrupt cessation of these drugs. Intensity of withdrawal symptoms gradually declines over a period of approximately 15 days. Treatment of barbiturate dependence consists of cautious and gradual withdrawal of the drug. Barbiturate-dependent patients can be withdrawn by using a number of different withdrawal regimens. One method involves initiating treatment at the patient's regular dosage level and gradually decreasing the daily dosage as tolerated by the patient.

OVERDOSAGE

Following an acute overdosage of butalbital, acetaminophen, and caffeine, toxicity may result from the barbiturate or the acetaminophen. Toxicity due to caffeine is less likely, due to the relatively small amounts in this formulation.

Signs and Symptoms

Toxicity from *barbiturate* poisoning include drowsiness, confusion, and coma; respiratory depression; hypotension; and hypovolemic shock.

In *acetaminophen* overdosage: dose-dependent, potentially fatal hepatic necrosis is the most serious adverse effect. Renal tubular necroses, hypoglycemic coma, and thrombocytopenia may also occur. Early symptoms following a potentially hepatotoxic overdose may include: nausea, vomiting, diaphoresis, and general malaise. Clinical and laboratory evidence of hepatic toxicity may not be apparent until 48 to 72 hours post-ingestion. In adults hepatic toxicity has rarely been reported with acute overdoses of less than 10 grams, or fatalities with less than 15 grams.

Acute *caffeine* poisoning may cause insomnia, restlessness, tremor, and delirium, tachycardia and extrasystoles.

Treatment

A single or mulitple overdose with this combination product is a potentially lethal polydrug overdose, and consultation with a regional poison control center is recommended.

Immediate treatment includes support of cardiorespiratory function and measures to reduce drug absorption. Vomiting should be induced mechanically, or with syrup of ipecac, if the patient is alert (adequate pharyngeal and laryngeal reflexes). Oral activated charcoal (1 g/kg) should follow gastric emptying. The first dose should be accompanied by an appropriate cathartic. If repeated doses are used, the cathartic might be included with alternate doses as required. Hypotension is usually hypovolemic and should respond to fluids. Pressors should be avoided. A cuffed endotracheal tube should be inserted before gastric lavage of the unconscious patient and when necessary, to provide assisted respiration. If renal function is normal, forced diuresis may aid in the elimination of the barbiturate. Alkalinization of the urine increases renal excretion of some barbiturates, especially phenobarbital.

Meticulous attention should be given to maintaining adequate pulmonary ventilation. In severe cases of intoxication, peritoneal dialysis, or preferably hemodialysis may be considered. If hypoprothrombinemia occurs due to acetaminophen overdose, vitamin K should be administered intravenously.

If the dose of acetaminophen may have exceeded 140 mg/kg, acetylcysteine should be administered as early as possible. Serum acetaminophen levels should be obtained, since levels four or more hours following ingestion help predict acet-

aminophen toxicity. Do not await acetaminophen assay results before initiating treatment. Hepatic enzymes should be obtained initially, and repeated at 24-hour intervals. Methemoglobinemia over 30% should be treated with methylene blue by slow intravenous administration.

Toxic Doses (for adults)

Butalbital:	toxic dose	1g	(20 tablets)
Acetaminophen:	toxic dose	10g	(30 tablets)
Caffeine:	toxic dose	1g	(25 tablets)

In all cases of suspected overdosage, call your Regional Poison Control Center to obtain the most up-to-date information about the treatment of overdosage. Telephone numbers of certified Regional Poison Control Centers are listed in the Physicians' Desk Reference®*.

DOSAGE AND ADMINISTRATION

One or 2 tablets every 4 hours as needed. Total daily dosage should not exceed 6 tablets.

Extended and repeated use of this product is not recommended because of the potential for physical dependence.

HOW SUPPLIED

Fioricet® (Butalbital, Acetaminophen, and Caffeine Tablets, USP)

Containing 50 mg butalbital, 325 mg acetaminophen, and 40 mg caffeine. Available as light-blue, unscored round compressed tablets, engraved "FIORICET" and "△," on one side, three-head profile "⟨⟨⟨" on other side. Bottles of 100 (NDC 0078-0084-05) and 500 (NDC 0078-0084-08).

Unit dose packages of 100, 10 blister strips of 10 tablets (NDC 0078-0084-06).

Store and Dispense

Store below 86°F (30°C); dispense in a tight container.

*Trademark of Medical Economics, Inc.

REV: MARCH 1998   30131904

Shown in Product Identification Guide, page 324

FIORICET® with CODEINE   Ⓒ Ⅲ ℞

[fē -ōr' ĭ-set]

(butalbital, acetaminophen, caffeine, and codeine phosphate) Capsules

Caution: Federal law prohibits dispensing without prescription.

The following prescribing information is based on official labeling in effect on August 1, 1998.

DESCRIPTION

Fioricet® with Codeine (butalbital, acetaminophen, caffeine, and codeine phosphate) is supplied in capsule form for oral administration.

Each capsule contains:

codeine phosphate, USP	30 mg ($^{1}/_{2}$ gr)

Warning: May be habit-forming.

butalbital, USP	50 mg

Warning: May be habit-forming.

caffeine, USP	40 mg
acetaminophen, USP	325 mg

Codeine phosphate [morphine-3-methyl ether phosphate (1:1) (salt) hemihydrate, $C_{18}H_{24}NO_7P$, anhydrous mw 397.37], is a narcotic analgesic and antitussive.

Butalbital (5-allyl-5-isobutylbarbituric acid, $C_{11}H_{16}N_2O_3$, mw 224.26), is a short- to intermediate-acting barbiturate.

Caffeine (1,3,7-trimethylxanthine, $C_8H_{10}N_4O_2$, mw 194.19), is a central nervous system stimulant.

Acetaminophen (4'-hydroxyacetanilide, $C_8H_9NO_2$, mw 151.16), is a non-opiate, non-salicylate analgesic and antipyretic.

Active Ingredients: codeine phosphate, USP, butalbital, USP, caffeine, USP, and acetaminophen, USP.

Inactive Ingredients: black iron oxide, colloidal silicon dioxide, D&C Red #7 (calcium lake), D&C Red #33, FD&C Blue #1, FD&C Blue #1 (aluminum lake), gelatin, magnesium stearate, pregelatinized starch, red iron oxide, sodium lauryl sulfate, and titanium dioxide.

May also include: benzyl alcohol, butylparaben, carboxymethylcellulose sodium, edetate calcium disodium, methylparaben, propylparaben, silicon dioxide, and sodium propionate.

CLINICAL PHARMACOLOGY

Fioricet® with Codeine (butalbital, acetaminophen, caffeine, and codeine phosphate) is a combination drug product intended as a treatment for tension headache.

Fioricet® consists of a fixed combination of butalbital 50 mg, acetaminophen 325 mg and caffeine 40 mg. The role each component plays in the relief of the complex of symptoms known as tension headache is incompletely understood.

Continued on next page

Fioricet with Codeine—Cont.

Pharmacokinetics

The behavior of the individual components is described below.

Codeine

Codeine is readily absorbed from the gastrointestinal tract. It is rapidly distributed from the intravascular spaces to the various body tissues, with preferential uptake by parenchymatous organs such as the liver, spleen and kidney. Codeine crosses the blood-brain barrier, and is found in fetal tissue and breast milk. The plasma concentration does not correlate with brain concentration or relief of pain; however, codeine is not bound to plasma proteins and does not accumulate in body tissues.

The plasma half-life is about 2.9 hours. The elimination of codeine is primarily via the kidneys, and about 90% of an oral dose is excreted by the kidneys within 24 hours of dosing. The urinary secretion products consist of free and glucuronide conjugated codeine (about 70%), free and conjugated norcodeine (about 10%), free and conjugated morphine (about 10%), normorphine (4%), and hydrocodone (1%). The remainder of the dose is excreted in the feces.

At therapeutic doses, the analgesic effect reaches a peak within 2 hours and persists between 4 and 6 hours.

See *OVERDOSAGE* for toxicity information.

Butalbital

Butalbital is well absorbed from the gastrointestinal tract and is expected to distribute to most tissues in the body. Barbiturates in general may appear in breast milk and readily cross the placental barrier. They are bound to plasma and tissue proteins to a varying degree and binding increases directly as a function of lipid solubility.

Elimination of butalbital is primarily via the kidney (59%–88% of the dose) as unchanged drug or metabolites. The plasma half-life is about 35 hours. Urinary excretion products include parent drug (about 3.6% of the dose), 5-isobutyl-5-(2,3-dihydroxypropyl) barbituric acid (about 24% of the dose), 5-allyl-5(3-hydroxy-2-methyl-1-propyl) barbituric acid (about 4.8% of the dose), products with the barbituric acid ring hydrolyzed with excretion of urea (about 14% of the dose), as well as unidentified materials. Of the material excreted in the urine, 32% is conjugated.

The *in vitro* plasma protein binding of butalbital is 45% over the concentration range of 0.5-20 μg/mL. This falls within the range of plasma protein binding (20%–45%) reported with other barbiturates such as phenobarbital, pentobarbital, and secobarbital sodium. The plasma-to-blood concentration ratio was almost unity indicating that there is no preferential distribution of butalbital into either plasma or blood cells.

See *OVERDOSAGE* for toxicity information.

Caffeine

Like most xanthines, caffeine is rapidly absorbed and distributed in all body tissues and fluids, including the CNS, fetal tissues, and breast milk.

Caffeine is cleared through metabolism and excretion in the urine. The plasma half-life is about 3 hours. Hepatic biotransformation prior to excretion results in about equal amounts of 1-methylxanthine and 1-methyluric acid. Of the 70% of the dose that is recovered in the urine, only 3% is unchanged drug.

See *OVERDOSAGE* for toxicity information.

Acetaminophen

Acetaminophen is rapidly absorbed from the gastrointestinal tract and is distributed throughout most body tissues. The plasma half-life is 1.25–3 hours, but may be increased by liver damage and following overdosage. Elimination of acetaminophen is principally by liver metabolism (conjugation) and subsequent renal excretion of metabolites. Approximately 85% of an oral dose appears in the urine within 24 hours of administration, most as the glucuronide conjugate, with small amounts of other conjugates and unchanged drug.

See *OVERDOSAGE* for toxicity information.

INDICATIONS

Fioricet® with Codeine (butalbital, acetaminophen, caffeine, and codeine phosphate) is indicated for the relief of the symptom complex of tension (or muscle contraction) headache.

Evidence supporting the efficacy and safety of Fioricet® with Codeine (butalbital, acetaminophen, caffeine, and codeine phosphate) in the treatment of multiple recurrent headaches is unavailable. Caution in this regard is required because codeine and butalbital are habit-forming and potentially abusable.

CONTRAINDICATIONS

Fioricet® with Codeine (butalbital, acetaminophen, caffeine, and codeine phosphate) is contraindicated under the following conditions:

— Hypersensitivity or intolerance to acetaminophen, caffeine, butalbital, or codeine.

— Patients with porphyria.

WARNINGS

In the presence of head injury or other intracranial lesions, the respiratory depressant effects of codeine and other narcotics may be markedly enhanced, as well as their capacity for elevating cerebrospinal fluid pressure. Narcotics also produce other CNS depressant effects, such as drowsiness, that may further obscure the clinical course of the patients with head injuries.

Codeine or other narcotics may obscure signs on which to judge the diagnosis or clinical course of patients with acute abdominal conditions.

Butalbital and codeine are both habit-forming and potentially abusable. Consequently, the extended use of Fioricet® with Codeine (butalbital, acetaminophen, caffeine, and codeine phosphate) is not recommended.

PRECAUTIONS

General

Fioricet® with Codeine (butalbital, acetaminophen, caffeine, and codeine phosphate) should be prescribed with caution in certain special-risk patients such as the elderly or debilitated, and those with severe impairment of renal or hepatic function, head injuries, elevated intracranial pressure, acute abdominal conditions, hypothyroidism, urethral stricture, Addison's disease, or prostatic hypertrophy.

Information for Patients

Fioricet® with Codeine (butalbital, acetaminophen, caffeine, and codeine phosphate) may impair mental and/or physical abilities required for the performance of potentially hazardous tasks such as driving a car or operating machinery. Such tasks should be avoided while taking Fioricet® with Codeine (butalbital, acetaminophen, caffeine, and codeine phosphate).

Alcohol and other CNS depressants may produce an additive CNS depression, when taken with Fioricet® with Codeine (butalbital, acetaminophen, caffeine, and codeine phosphate), and should be avoided.

Codeine and butalbital may be habit-forming. Patients should take the drug only for as long as it is prescribed, in the amounts prescribed, and no more frequently than prescribed.

Laboratory Tests

In patients with severe hepatic or renal disease, effects of therapy should be monitored with serial liver and/or renal function tests.

Drug Interactions

The CNS effects of butalbital may be enhanced by monoamine oxidase (MAO) inhibitors.

Fioricet® with Codeine (butalbital, acetaminophen, caffeine, and codeine phosphate) may enhance the effects of:

—Other narcotic analgesics, alcohol, general anesthetics, tranquilizers such as chlordiazepoxide, sedative-hypnotics, or other CNS depressants, causing increased CNS depression.

Drug/Laboratory Test Interactions

Codeine

Codeine may increase serum amylase levels.

Acetaminophen

Acetaminophen may produce false-positive test results for urinary 5-hydroxyindoleacetic acid.

Carcinogenesis, Mutagenesis, Impairment of Fertility

No adequate studies have been conducted in animals to determine whether acetaminophen, codeine and butalbital have a potential for carcinogenesis or mutagenesis. No adequate studies have been conducted in animals to determine whether acetaminophen and butalbital have a potential for impairment of fertility.

Pregnancy

Teratogenic Effects

Pregnancy Category C: Animal reproduction studies have not been conducted with Fioricet® with Codeine (butalbital, acetaminophen, caffeine, and codeine phosphate). It is also not known whether Fioricet® with Codeine (butalbital, acetaminophen, caffeine, and codeine phosphate) can cause fetal harm when administered to a pregnant woman or can affect reproduction capacity. Fioricet® with Codeine (butalbital, acetaminophen, caffeine, and codeine phosphate) should be given to a pregnant woman only when clearly needed.

Nonteratogenic Effects

Withdrawal seizures were reported in a two-day-old male infant whose mother had taken a butalbital-containing drug during the last 2 months of pregnancy. Butalbital was found in the infant's serum. The infant was given phenobarbital 5 mg/kg, which was tapered without further seizure or other withdrawal symptoms.

Labor and Delivery

Use of codeine during labor may lead to respiratory depression in the neonate.

Nursing Mothers

Caffeine, barbiturates, acetaminophen and codeine are excreted in breast milk in small amounts, but the significance of their effects on nursing infants is not known. Because of potential for serious adverse reactions in nursing infants from Fioricet® with Codeine (butalbital, acetaminophen, caffeine, and codeine phosphate), a decision should be made whether to discontinue nursing or to discontinue the drug, taking into account the importance of the drug to the mother.

Pediatric Use

Safety and effectiveness in pediatric patients have not been established.

ADVERSE REACTIONS

Frequently Observed

The most frequently reported adverse reactions are drowsiness, lightheadedness, dizziness, sedation, shortness of breath, nausea, vomiting, abdominal pain, and intoxicated feeling.

Infrequently Observed

All adverse events tabulated below are classified as infrequent.

Central Nervous: headache, shaky feeling, tingling, agitation, fainting, fatigue, heavy eyelids, high energy, hot spells, numbness, sluggishness, seizure. Mental confusion, excitement or depression can also occur due to intolerance, particularly in elderly or debilitated patients, or due to overdosage of butalbital.

Autonomic Nervous: dry mouth, hyperhidrosis.

Gastrointestinal: difficulty swallowing, heartburn, flatulence, constipation.

Cardiovascular: tachycardia.

Musculoskeletal: leg pain, muscle fatigue.

Genitourinary: diuresis.

Miscellaneous: pruritus, fever, earache, nasal congestion, tinnitus, euphoria, allergic reactions.

The following adverse reactions have been voluntarily reported as temporally associated with Fiorinal® with Codeine, a related product containing aspirin, butalbital, caffeine, and codeine.

Central Nervous: abuse, addiction, anxiety, disorientation, hallucination, hyperactivity, insomnia, libido decrease, nervousness, neuropathy, psychosis, sexual activity increase, slurred speech, twitching, unconsciousness, vertigo.

Autonomic Nervous: epistaxis, flushing, miosis, salivation.

Gastrointestinal: anorexia, appetite increased, diarrhea, esophagitis, gastroenteritis, gastrointestinal spasms, hiccup, mouth burning, pyloric ulcer.

Cardiovascular: chest pain, hypotensive reaction, palpitations, syncope.

Skin: erythema, erythema multiforme, exfoliative dermatitis, hives, rash, toxic epidermal necrolysis.

Urinary: kidney impairment, urinary difficulty.

Miscellaneous: allergic reaction, anaphylactic shock, cholangiocarcinoma, drug interaction with erythromycin (stomach upset), edema.

The following adverse drug events may be borne in mind as potential effects of the components of Fioricet® with Codeine (butalbital, acetaminophen, caffeine, and codeine phosphate). Potential effects of high dosage are listed in the *OVERDOSAGE* section.

Acetaminophen: allergic reactions, rash, thrombocytopenia, agranulocytosis.

Caffeine: cardiac stimulation, irritability, tremor, dependence, nephrotoxicity, hyperglycemia.

Codeine: nausea, vomiting, drowsiness, lightheadedness, constipation, pruritus.

Several cases of dermatological reactions, including toxic epidermal necrolysis and erythema multiforme, have been reported for Fioricet® (Butalbital, Acetaminophen, and Caffeine Tablets, USP).

DRUG ABUSE AND DEPENDENCE

Controlled Substance

Fioricet® with Codeine (butalbital, acetaminophen, caffeine, and codeine phosphate) is controlled by the Drug Enforcement Administration and is classified under Schedule III.

Abuse and Dependence

Codeine

Codeine can produce drug dependence of the morphine type and, therefore, has the potential for being abused. Psychological dependence, physical dependence, and tolerance may develop upon repeated administration and it should be prescribed and administered with the same degree of caution appropriate to the use of other oral narcotic medications.

Butalbital

Barbiturates may be habit-forming: Tolerance, psychological dependence, and physical dependence may occur especially following prolonged use of high doses of barbiturates. The average daily dose for the barbiturate addict is usually about 1,500 mg. As tolerance to barbiturates develops, the amount needed to maintain the same level of intoxication increases; tolerance to a fatal dosage, however, does not increase more than two fold. As this occurs, the margin between an intoxication dosage and fatal dosage becomes smaller. The lethal dose of a barbiturate is far less if alcohol is also ingested. Major withdrawal symptoms (convulsions and delirium) may occur within 16 hours and last up to 5 days after abrupt cessation of these drugs. Intensity of withdrawal symptoms gradually declines over a period of approximately 15 days. Treatment of barbiturate depend-

ence consists of cautious and gradual withdrawal of the drug. Barbiturate-dependent patients can be withdrawn by using a number of different withdrawal regimens. One method involves initiating treatment at the patient's regular dosage level and gradually decreasing the daily dosage as tolerated by the patient.

OVERDOSAGE

Following an acute overdosage of Fioricet® with Codeine (butalbital, acetaminophen, caffeine, and codeine phosphate), toxicity may result from the barbiturate, the codeine, or the acetaminophen. Toxicity due to the caffeine is less likely, due to the relatively small amounts in this formulation.

Signs and Symptoms

Toxicity from ***barbiturate*** poisoning includes drowsiness, confusion, and coma; respiratory depression; hypotension; and hypovolemic shock. Toxicity from ***codeine*** poisoning includes the opioid triad of: pinpoint pupils, depression of respiration, and loss of consciousness. Convulsions may occur. In ***acetaminophen*** overdosage: dose-dependent, potentially fatal hepatic necrosis is the most serious adverse effect. Renal tubular necroses, hypoglycemic coma, and thrombocytopenia may also occur. Early symptoms following a potentially hepatotoxic overdose may include: nausea, vomiting, diaphoresis, and general malaise. Clinical and laboratory evidence of hepatic toxicity may not be apparent until 48–72 hours post-ingestion. In adults hepatic toxicity has rarely been reported with acute overdoses of less than 10 grams, or fatalities with less than 15 grams. Acute ***caffeine*** poisoning may cause insomnia, restlessness, tremor, and delirium, tachycardia, and extrasystoles.

Treatment

A single or multiple overdose with Fioricet® with Codeine (butalbital, acetaminophen, caffeine and codeine phosphate) is a potentially lethal polydrug overdose, and consultation with a regional poison control center is recommended. Immediate treatment includes support of cardiorespiratory function and measures to reduce drug absorption. Vomiting should be induced mechanically, or with syrup of ipecac, if the patient is alert (adequate pharyngeal and laryngeal reflexes). Oral activated charcoal (1 g/kg) should follow gastric emptying. The first dose should be accompanied by an appropriate cathartic. If repeated doses are used, the cathartic might be included with alternate doses as required. Hypotension is usually hypovolemic and should respond to fluids. The value of vasopressor agents such as Norepinephrine or Phenylephrine Hydrochloride in treating hypotension is questionable since they increase vasoconstriction and decrease blood flow. However, if prolonged support of blood pressure is required, Norepinephrine Bitartrate (Levophed®)* may be given I.V. with the usual precautions and serial blood pressure monitoring. A cuffed endotracheal tube should be inserted before gastric lavage of the unconscious patient and, when necessary, to provide assisted respiration. If renal function is normal, forced diuresis may aid in the elimination of the barbiturate. Alkalinization of the urine increases renal excretion of some barbiturates, especially phenobarbital.

Meticulous attention should be given to maintaining adequate pulmonary ventilation. In severe cases of intoxication, peritoneal dialysis, or preferably hemodialysis may be considered. If hypoprothrombinemia occurs due to acetaminophen overdose, vitamin K should be administered intravenously.

Naloxone, a narcotic antagonist, can reverse respiratory depression and coma associated with opioid overdose. Naloxone 0.4–2 mg is given parenterally. Since the duration of action of codeine may exceed that of the naloxone, the patient should be kept under continuous surveillance and repeated doses of the antagonist should be administered as needed to maintain adequate respiration. A narcotic antagonist should not be administered in the absence of clinically significant respiratory or cardiovascular depression.

If the dose of acetaminophen may have exceeded 140 mg/kg, N-acetyl-cysteine should be administered as early as possible. Serum acetaminophen levels should be obtained, since levels 4 or more hours following ingestion help predict acetaminophen toxicity. Do not await acetaminophen assay results before initiating treatment. Hepatic enzymes should be obtained initially, and repeated at 24-hour intervals.

Methemoglobinemia over 30% should be treated with methylene blue by slow intravenous administration.

Toxic doses (for adults)

Butalbital:	toxic dose 1.0 g (20 capsules of Fioricet® with Codeine)
Acetaminophen:	toxic dose 10 g (30 capsules of Fioricet® with Codeine)
Caffeine:	toxic dose 1.0 g (25 capsules of Fioricet® with Codeine)
Codeine:	toxic dose 240 mg (8 capsules of Fioricet® with Codeine)

DOSAGE AND ADMINISTRATION

One or 2 capsules every 4 hours. Total daily dosage should not exceed 6 capsules.

Extended and repeated use of this product is not recommended because of the potential for physical dependence.

HOW SUPPLIED

Fioricet® with Codeine (butalbital, acetaminophen, caffeine, and codeine phosphate) Capsules

Dark blue, opaque cap with a grey, opaque body. Cap is imprinted twice in light-blue with "FIORICET" and "CODEINE". Body is imprinted twice with four-head profile "((((" in red.

Bottle of 100 (NDC 0078-0243-05)

Store and Dispense

Below 86°F (30°C); tight container.

*Levophed is a registered Trademark of Sanofi Winthrop Pharmaceuticals.

[REV: FEBRUARY 1996 30132902]

Shown in Product Identification Guide, page 324

FIORINAL® Ⓒ℞

[fē-or'ĭ-nol]

(butalbital, aspirin, and caffeine)

Capsules, USP

Caution: Federal law prohibits dispensing without prescription.

The following information is based on official labeling in effect on August 1, 1998.

DESCRIPTION

Each Fiorinal® (butalbital, aspirin, and caffeine) Capsule for oral administration contains: butalbital, USP, 50 mg; aspirin, USP, 325 mg; caffeine, USP, 40 mg.

Butalbital, 5-allyl-5-isobutyl-barbituric acid, has an empirical formula of $C_{11}H_{16}N_2O_3$ and a molecular weight of 224.26.

Aspirin, benzoic acid, 2-(acetyloxy)-, has an empirical formula of $C_9H_8O_4$ and a molecular weight of 180.16.

Caffeine, 1, 3, 7-trimethylxanthine, has an empirical formula of $C_8H_{10}N_4O_2$ and a molecular weight of 194.19.

Active Ingredients: aspirin, USP, butalbital, USP, and caffeine, USP.

Inactive Ingredients: D&C Yellow #10, gelatin, microcrystalline cellulose, sodium lauryl sulfate, starch, and talc.

May Also Include: benzyl alcohol, butylparaben, color additives including FD&C Blue #1, FD&C Green #3, FD&C Yellow #6, edetate calcium disodium, methylparaben, propylparaben, silicon dioxide, and sodium propionate.

CLINICAL PHARMACOLOGY

Pharmacologically, Fiorinal® (butalbital, aspirin, and caffeine) combines the analgesic properties of aspirin with the anxiolytic and muscle relaxant properties of butalbital.

The clinical effectiveness of Fiorinal® (butalbital, aspirin, and caffeine) in tension headache has been established in double-blind, placebo-controlled, multi-clinic trials. A factorial design study compared Fiorinal® (butalbital, aspirin, and caffeine) with each of its major components. This study demonstrated that each component contributes to the efficacy of Fiorinal® (butalbital, aspirin, and caffeine) in the treatment of the target symptoms of tension headache (headache pain, psychic tension, and muscle contraction in the head, neck, and shoulder region). For each symptom and the symptom complex as a whole, Fiorinal® (butalbital, aspirin, and caffeine) was shown to have significantly superior clinical effects to either component alone.

Pharmacokinetics

The behavior of the individual components is described below.

Aspirin

The systemic availability of aspirin after an oral dose is highly dependent on the dosage form, the presence of food, the gastric emptying time, gastric pH, antacids, buffering agents, and particle size. These factors affect not necessarily the extent of absorption of total salicylates but more the stability of aspirin prior to absorption.

During the absorption process and after absorption, aspirin is mainly hydrolyzed to salicylic acid and distributed to all body tissues and fluids, including fetal tissues, breast milk, and the central nervous system (CNS). Highest concentrations are found in plasma, liver, renal cortex, heart, and lung. In plasma, about 50%-80% of the salicylic acid and its metabolites are loosely bound to plasma proteins.

The clearance of total salicylates is subject to saturable kinetics; however, first-order elimination kinetics are still a good approximation for doses up to 650 mg. The plasma half-life for aspirin is about 12 minutes and for salicylic acid and/or total salicylates is about 3.0 hours.

The elimination of therapeutic doses is through the kidneys either as salicylic acid or other biotransformation products. The renal clearance is greatly augmented by an alkaline urine as is produced by concurrent administration of sodium bicarbonate or potassium citrate.

The biotransformation of aspirin occurs primarily in the hepatocytes. The major metabolites are salicyluric acid (75%), the phenolic and acyl glucuronides of salicylate (15%), and gentisic and gentisuric acid (1%). The bioavailability of the aspirin component of Fiorinal® (butalbital, aspirin, and caffeine) is equivalent to that of a solution except for a slower rate of absorption. A peak concentration of 8.80 µg/mL was obtained at 40 minutes after a 650 mg dose. See *OVERDOSAGE* for toxicity information.

Butalbital

Butalbital is well absorbed from the gastrointestinal tract and is expected to distribute to most of the tissues in the body. Barbiturates, in general, may appear in breast milk and readily cross the placental barrier. They are bound to plasma and tissue proteins to a varying degree and binding increases directly as a function of lipid solubility.

Elimination of butalbital is primarily via the kidney (59%-88% of the dose) as unchanged drug or metabolites. The plasma half-life is about 35 hours. Urinary excretion products included parent drug (about 3.6% of the dose), 5-isobutyl-5-(2,3-dihydroxypropyl) barbituric acid (about 24% of the dose), 5-allyl-5(3-hydroxy-2-methyl-1-propyl) barbituric acid (about 4.8% of the dose), products with the barbituric acid ring hydrolyzed with excretion of urea (about 14% of the dose), as well as unidentified materials. Of the material excreted in the urine, 32% was conjugated.

The bioavailability of the butalbital component of Fiorinal® (butalbital, aspirin, and caffeine) is equivalent to that of a solution except for a decrease in the rate of absorption. A peak concentration of 2020 ng/mL is obtained at about 1.5 hours after a 100 mg dose.

The *in vitro* plasma protein binding of butalbital is 45% over the concentration range of 0.5-20 µg/mL. This falls within the range of plasma protein binding (20%-45%) reported with other barbiturates such as phenobarbital, pentobarbital, and secobarbital sodium. The plasma-to-blood concentration ratio was almost unity indicating that there is no preferential distribution of butalbital into either plasma or blood cells.

See *OVERDOSAGE* for toxicity information.

Caffeine

Like most xanthines, caffeine is rapidly absorbed and distributed in all body tissues and fluids, including the CNS, fetal tissues, and breast milk.

Caffeine is cleared rapidly through metabolism and excretion in the urine. The plasma half-life is about 3.0 hours. Hepatic biotransformation prior to excretion results in about equal amounts of 1-methylxanthine and 1-methyluric acid. Of the 70% of the dose that has been recovered in the urine, only 3% was unchanged drug.

The bioavailability of the caffeine component for Fiorinal® (butalbital, aspirin, and caffeine) is equivalent to that of a solution except for a slightly longer time to peak. A peak concentration of 1660 ng/mL was obtained in less than an hour for an 80 mg dose.

See *OVERDOSAGE* for toxicity information.

INDICATIONS

Fiorinal® (butalbital, aspirin, and caffeine) is indicated for the relief of the symptom complex of tension (or muscle contraction) headache. Evidence supporting the efficacy and safety of Fiorinal® (butalbital, aspirin, and caffeine) in the treatment of multiple recurrent headaches is unavailable. Caution in this regard is required because butalbital is habit-forming and potentially abusable.

CONTRAINDICATIONS

Fiorinal® (butalbital, aspirin, and caffeine) is contraindicated under the following conditions:

1. Hypersensitivity or intolerance to aspirin, caffeine, or butalbital.
2. Patients with a hemorrhagic diathesis (e.g., hemophilia, hypoprothrombinemia, von Willebrand's disease, the thrombocytopenias, thrombasthenia and other ill-defined hereditary platelet dysfunctions, severe vitamin K deficiency and severe liver damage).
3. Patients with the syndrome of nasal polyps, angioedema and bronchospastic reactivity to aspirin or other nonsteroidal anti-inflammatory drugs. Anaphylactoid reactions have occurred in such patients.
4. Peptic ulcer or other serious gastrointestinal lesions.
5. Patients with porphyria.

WARNINGS

Therapeutic doses of aspirin can cause anaphylactic shock and other severe allergic reactions. It should be ascertained if the patient is allergic to aspirin, although a specific history of allergy may be lacking.

Significant bleeding can result from aspirin therapy in patients with peptic ulcer or other gastrointestinal lesions, and in patients with bleeding disorders. Aspirin administered preoperatively may prolong the bleeding time. Butalbital is habit-forming and potentially abusable. Consequently, the extended use of Fiorinal® (butalbital, aspirin, and caffeine) is not recommended. Results from epidemiologic studies indicate an association between aspirin and Reye's Syndrome. Caution should be used in administering this product to children, including teenagers, with chicken pox or flu.

Continued on next page

Fiorinal—Cont.

PRECAUTIONS

General

Fiorinal® (butalbital, aspirin, and caffeine) should be prescribed with caution for certain special-risk patients such as the elderly or debilitated, and those with severe impairment of renal or hepatic function, coagulation disorders, head injuries, elevated intracranial pressure, acute abdominal conditions, hypothyroidism, urethral stricture, Addison's disease, or prostatic hypertrophy.

Aspirin should be used with caution in patients on anticoagulant therapy and in patients with underlying hemostatic defects, and extreme caution in the presence of peptic ulcer. Precautions should be taken when administering salicylates to persons with known allergies. Hypersensitivity to aspirin is particularly likely in patients with nasal polyps, and relatively common in those with asthma.

Information for Patients

Patients should be informed that Fiorinal® (butalbital, aspirin, and caffeine) contains aspirin and should not be taken by patients with an aspirin allergy.

Fiorinal® (butalbital, aspirin, and caffeine) may impair the mental and /or physical abilities required for performance of potentially hazardous tasks such as driving a car or operating machinery. Such tasks should be avoided while taking Fiorinal® (butalbital, aspirin, and caffeine).

Alcohol and other CNS depressants may produce an additive CNS depression when taken with Fiorinal® (butalbital, aspirin, and caffeine) and should be avoided.

Butalbital may be habit-forming. Patients should take the drug only for as long as it is prescribed, in the amounts prescribed, and no more frequently than prescribed.

Laboratory Tests

In patients with severe hepatic or renal disease, effects of therapy should be monitored with serial liver and/or renal function tests.

Drug Interactions

The CNS effects of butalbital may be enhanced by monoamine oxidase (MAO) inhibitors.

In patients receiving concomitant corticosteroids and chronic use of aspirin, withdrawal of corticosteroids may result in salicylism because corticosteroids enhance renal clearance of salicylates and their withdrawal is followed by return to normal rates of renal clearance.

Fiorinal® (butalbital, aspirin, and caffeine) may enhance the effects of:

1. Oral anticoagulants, causing bleeding by inhibiting prothrombin formation in the liver and displacing anticoagulants from plasma protein binding sites.
2. Oral antidiabetic agents and insulin, causing hypoglycemia by contributing an additive effect, if dosage of Fiorinal® (butalbital, aspirin, and caffeine) exceeds maximum recommended daily dosage.
3. 6-mercaptopurine and methotrexate, causing bone marrow toxicity and blood dyscrasias by displacing these drugs from secondary binding sites, and, in the case of methotrexate, also reducing its excretion.
4. Non-steroidal anti-inflammatory agents, increasing the risk of peptic ulceration and bleeding by contributing additive effects.
5. Other narcotic analgesics, alcohol, general anesthetics, tranquilizers such as chlordiazepoxide, sedative-hypnotics, or other CNS depressants, causing increased CNS depression.

Fiorinal® (butalbital, aspirin, and caffeine) may diminish the effects of:

Uricosuric agents such as probenecid and sulfinpyrazone, reducing their effectiveness in the treatment of gout. Aspirin competes with these agents for protein binding sites.

Drug/Laboratory Test Interactions

Aspirin: Aspirin may interfere with the following laboratory determinations in blood: serum amylase, fasting blood glucose, cholesterol, protein, serum glutamic-oxaloacetic transaminase (SGOT), uric acid, prothrombin time and bleeding time. Aspirin may interfere with the following laboratory determinations in urine: glucose, 5-hydroxyindoleacetic acid, Gerhardt ketone, vanillylmandelic acid (VMA), uric acid, diacetic acid, and spectrophotometric detection of barbiturates.

Carcinogenesis, Mutagenesis, Impairment of Fertility

Adequate long-term studies have been conducted in mice and rats with aspirin, alone or in combination with other drugs, in which no evidence of carcinogenesis was seen. No adequate studies have been conducted in animals to determine whether aspirin has a potential for mutagenesis or impairment of fertility. No adequate studies have been conducted in animals to determine whether butalbital has a potential for carcinogenesis, mutagenesis, or impairment of fertility.

Usage in Pregnancy

Teratogenic Effects:

Pregnancy Category C. Animal reproduction studies have not been conducted with Fiorinal® (butalbital, aspirin, and caffeine). It is also not known whether Fiorinal® (butalbital, aspirin, and caffeine) can cause fetal harm when administered to a pregnant woman or can affect reproduction capacity. Fiorinal® (butalbital, aspirin, and caffeine) should be given to a pregnant woman only when clearly needed.

Nonteratogenic Effects:

Withdrawal seizures were reported in a two-day-old male infant whose mother had taken a butalbital-containing drug during the last 2 months of pregnancy. Butalbital was found in the infant's serum. The infant was given phenobarbital 5mg/kg, which was tapered without further seizure or other withdrawal symptoms.

Studies of aspirin use in pregnant women have not shown that aspirin increases the risk of abnormalities when administered during the first trimester of pregnancy. In controlled studies involving 41,337 pregnant women and their offspring, there was no evidence that aspirin taken during pregnancy caused stillbirth, neonatal death or reduced birth weight. In controlled studies of 50,282 pregnant women and their offspring, aspirin administration in moderate and heavy doses during the first four lunar months of pregnancy showed no teratogenic effect.

Therapeutic doses of aspirin in pregnant women close to term may cause bleeding in mother, fetus, or neonate. During the last 6 months of pregnancy, regular use of aspirin in high doses may prolong pregnancy and delivery.

Labor and Delivery

Ingestion of aspirin prior to delivery may prolong delivery or lead to bleeding in the mother or neonate.

Nursing Mothers

Aspirin, caffeine, and barbiturates are excreted in breast milk in small amounts, but the significance of their effects on nursing infants is not known. Because of potential for serious adverse reactions in nursing infants from Fiorinal® (butalbital, aspirin, and caffeine), a decision should be made whether to discontinue nursing or to discontinue the drug, taking into account the importance of the drug to the mother.

Pediatric Use

Safety and effectiveness in pediatric patients have not been established.

ADVERSE REACTIONS

The most frequent adverse reactions are drowsiness and dizziness. Less frequent adverse reactions are lightheadedness and gastrointestinal disturbances including nausea, vomiting, and flatulence. A single incidence of bone marrow suppression has been reported with the use of Fiorinal® (butalbital, aspirin, and caffeine). Several cases of dermatological reactions including toxic epidermal necrolysis and erythema multiforme have been reported.

DRUG ABUSE AND DEPENDENCE

Controlled Substance

Fiorinal® (butalbital, aspirin, and caffeine) is controlled by the Drug Enforcement Administration and is classified under Schedule III.

Abuse and Dependence

Butalbital

Barbiturates may be habit-forming: Tolerance, psychological dependence, and physical dependence may occur especially following prolonged use of high doses of barbiturates. The average daily dose for the barbiturate addict is usually about 1,500 mg. As tolerance to barbiturates develops, the amount needed to maintain the same level of intoxication increases; tolerance to a fatal dosage, however, does not increase more than twofold. As this occurs, the margin between an intoxication dosage and fatal dosage becomes smaller. The lethal dose of a barbiturate is far less if alcohol is also ingested. Major withdrawal symptoms (convulsions and delirium) may occur within 16 hours and last up to 5 days after abrupt cessation of these drugs. Intensity of withdrawal symptoms gradually declines over a period of approximately 15 days. Treatment of barbiturate dependence consists of cautious and gradual withdrawal of the drug. Barbiturate-dependent patients can be withdrawn by using a number of different withdrawal regimens. One method involves initiating treatment at the patient's regular dosage level and gradually decreasing the daily dosage as tolerated by the patient.

OVERDOSAGE

The toxic effects of acute overdosage of Fiorinal® (butalbital, aspirin, and caffeine) are attributable mainly to its barbiturate component, and, to a lesser extent, aspirin. Because toxic effects of caffeine occur in very high dosages only, the possibility of significant caffeine toxicity from Fiorinal® (butalbital, aspirin, and caffeine) overdosage is unlikely.

Signs and Symptoms

Symptoms attributable to ***acute barbiturate poisoning*** include drowsiness, confusion, and coma; respiratory depression; hypotension; hypovolemic shock. Symptoms attributable to ***acute aspirin poisoning*** include hyperpnea; acid-base disturbances with development of metabolic acidosis; vomiting and abdominal pain; tinnitus; hyperthermia; hypoprothrombinemia; restlessness; delirium; convulsions. ***Acute caffeine poisoning*** may cause insomnia, restlessness, tremor, and delirium; tachycardia and extrasystoles.

Treatment

Treatment consists primarily of management of barbiturate intoxication and the correction of the acid-base imbalance due to salicylism. Vomiting should be induced mechanically or with emetics in the conscious patient. Gastric lavage may be used if the pharyngeal and laryngeal reflexes are present and if less than 4 hours have elapsed since ingestion. A cuffed endotracheal tube should be inserted before gastric lavage of the unconscious patient and when necessary to provide assisted respiration. Diuresis, alkalinization of the urine, and correction of electrolyte disturbances should be accomplished through administration of intravenous fluids such as 1% sodium bicarbonate in 5% dextrose in water. Meticulous attention should be given to maintaining adequate pulmonary ventilation. The value of vasopressor agents such as Norepinephrine or Phenylephrine Hydrochloride in treating hypotension is questionable since they increase vasoconstriction and decrease blood flow. However, if prolonged support of blood pressure is required, Norepinephrine Bitartrate (Levophed®)* may be given I.V. with the usual precautions and serial blood pressure monitoring. In severe cases of intoxication, peritoneal dialysis, hemodialysis, or exchange transfusion may be lifesaving. Hypoprothrombinemia should be treated with Vitamin K, intravenously.

Up-to-date information about the treatment of overdose can often be obtained from a Certified Regional Poison Control Center. Telephone numbers of Certified Regional Poison Control Centers are listed in the Physicians' Desk Reference®.**

Toxic and Lethal Doses

Butalbital: toxic dose 1.0 g (20 capsules of Fiorinal®)

Aspirin: toxic blood level greater than 30 mg/100 mL; lethal dose 10-30 g

Caffeine: toxic dose 1.0 g (25 capsules of Fiorinal®)

DOSAGE AND ADMINISTRATION

One or 2 capsules every 4 hours. Total daily dose should not exceed 6 capsules.

Extended and repeated use of this product is not recommended because of the potential for physical dependence.

HOW SUPPLIED

Fiorinal® (butalbital, aspirin, and caffeine) Capsules, USP

Bright kelly green cap with a lime green body, imprinted "FIORINAL 78-103" on each half of capsule.

Packages of 100 (NDC 0078-0103-05).

Packages of 500 (NDC 0078-0103-08).

ControlPak® package, 25 capsules (continuous reverse-numbered roll of sealed blisters) (NDC 0078-0103-13).

Store and Dispense

Below 77°F (25°C), tight container.

*Levophed is a registered Trademark of Sanofi Winthrop Pharmaceuticals.

**Trademark of Medical Economics Company, Inc.

[REV: MARCH 1998 30130905]

Shown in Product Identification Guide, page 324

FIORINAL® with CODEINE Ⓒ℞

[fē-or 'ĭ-nol]

(butalbital, aspirin, caffeine, and codeine phosphate)

Capsules, USP

CAUTION: Federal law prohibits dispensing without prescription.

The following prescribing information is based on official labeling in effect on August 1, 1998.

DESCRIPTION

Fiorinal® with Codeine (butalbital, aspirin, caffeine, and codeine phosphate) is supplied in capsule form for oral administration.

Each capsule contains:

codeine phosphate, USP	30 mg ($^1/_2$ gr)
Warning: May be habit-forming.	
butalbital, USP	50 mg
Warning: May be habit-forming.	
caffeine, USP	40 mg
aspirin, USP	325 mg

Codeine phosphate [morphine-3-methyl ether phosphate (1:1) (salt) hemihydrate. $C_{18}H_{24}NO_7P$, anhydrous mw 397.37], is a narcotic analgesic and antitussive.

Butalbital (5-allyl-5-isobutylbarbituric acid, $C_{11}H_{16}N_2O_3$, mw 224.26), is a short- to intermediate-acting barbiturate.

Caffeine (1,3,7-trimethylxanthine, $C_8H_{10}N_4O_2$, mw 194.19), is a central nervous stimulant.

Aspirin is benzoic acid, 2-(acetyloxy)-, $C_9H_8O_4$, mw 180.16, is an analgesic, antipyretic, anti-inflammatory.

Inactive Ingredients: D&C Yellow #10, FD&C Blue #1, FD&C Red #3, FD&C Yellow #6, gelatin, microcrystalline cellulose, sodium lauryl sulfate, starch, talc, titanium dioxide.

May Also Include: benzyl alcohol, butylparaben, edetate calcium disodium, glycerin, methylparaben, propylparaben, silicon dioxide, sodium propionate.

CLINICAL PHARMACOLOGY

Fiorinal® with Codeine (butalbital, aspirin, caffeine, and codeine phosphate) is a combination drug product intended as a treatment for tension headache.

Fiorinal® (butalbital, aspirin, and caffeine) consists of a fixed combination of caffeine 40 mg, butalbital 50 mg, and aspirin 325 mg. The role each component plays in the relief of the complex of symptoms known as tension headache is incompletely understood.

Pharmacokinetics

Bioavailability: The bioavailability of the components of the fixed combination of Fiorinal® with Codeine (butalbital, aspirin, caffeine, and codeine phosphate) is identical to their bioavailability when Fiorinal® (butalbital, aspirin, and caffeine) and Codeine are administered separately in equivalent molar doses.

The behavior of the individual components is described below.

Aspirin

The systemic availability of aspirin after an oral dose is highly dependent on the dosage form, the presence of food, the gastric emptying time, gastric pH, antacids, buffering agents, and particle size. These factors affect not necessarily the extent of absorption of total salicylates but more the stability of aspirin prior to absorption.

During the absorption process and after absorption, aspirin is mainly hydrolyzed to salicylic acid and distributed to all body tissues and fluids, including fetal tissues, breast milk, and the central nervous system (CNS). Highest concentrations are found in plasma, liver, renal cortex, heart, and lung. In plasma, about 50%-80% of the salicylic acid and its metabolites are loosely bound to plasma proteins.

The clearance of total salicylates is subject to saturable kinetics; however, first-order elimination kinetics are still a good approximation for doses up to 650 mg. The plasma half-life for aspirin is about 12 minutes and for salicylic acid and/or total salicylates is about 3.0 hours.

The elimination of therapeutic doses is through the kidneys either as salicylic acid or other biotransformation products. The renal clearance is greatly augmented by an alkaline urine as is produced by concurrent administration of sodium bicarbonate or potassium citrate.

The biotransformation of aspirin occurs primarily in the hepatocytes. The major metabolites are salicyluric acid (75%), the phenolic and acyl glucuronides of salicylate (15%), and gentisic and gentisuric acid (1%). The bioavailability of the aspirin component of Fiorinal® with Codeine (butalbital, aspirin, caffeine, and codeine phosphate) capsules is equivalent to that of a solution except for a slower rate of absorption. A peak concentration of 8.80 µg/mL was obtained at 40 minutes after a 650 mg dose.

See *OVERDOSAGE* for toxicity information.

Codeine

Codeine is readily absorbed from the gastrointestinal tract. It is rapidly distributed from the intravascular spaces to the various body tissues, with preferential uptake by parenchymatous organs such as the liver, spleen, and kidney. Codeine crosses the blood-brain barrier, and is found in fetal tissue and breast milk. The plasma concentration does not correlate with brain concentration or relief of pain, however, codeine is not bound to plasma proteins and does not accumulate in body tissues.

The plasma half-life is about 2.9 hours. The elimination of codeine is primarily via the kidneys, and about 90% of an oral dose is excreted by the kidneys within 24 hours of dosing. The urinary secretion products consist of free and glucuronide-conjugated codeine (about 70%), free and conjugated norcodeine (about 10%), free and conjugated morphine (about 10%), normorphine (4%), and hydrocodone (1%). The remainder of the dose is excreted in the feces.

At therapeutic doses, the analgesic effect reaches a peak within 2 hours and persists between 4 and 6 hours.

The bioavailability of the codeine component of Fiorinal® with Codeine (butalbital, aspirin, caffeine, and codeine phosphate) capsules is equivalent to that of a solution. Peak concentrations of 198 ng/mL were obtained at 1 hour after a 60 mg dose.

See *OVERDOSAGE* for toxicity information.

Butalbital

Butalbital is well absorbed from the gastrointestinal tract and is expected to distribute to most of the tissues in the body. Barbiturates, in general, may appear in breast milk and readily cross the placental barrier. They are bound to plasma and tissue proteins to a varying degree and binding increases directly as a function of lipid solubility.

Elimination of butalbital is primarily via the kidney (59%-88% of the dose) as unchanged drug or metabolites. The plasma half-life is about 35 hours. Urinary excretion products included parent drug (about 3.6% of the dose), 5-isobutyl-5-(2,3-dihydroxypropyl) barbituric acid (about 24% of the dose), 5-allyl-5(3-hydroxy-2-methyl-1-propyl) barbituric acid (about 4.8% of the dose), products with the

barbituric acid ring hydrolyzed with excretion of urea (about 14% of the dose), as well as unidentified materials. Of the material excreted in the urine, 32% was conjugated. The bioavailability of the butalbital component of Fiorinal® with Codeine (butalbital, aspirin, caffeine, and codeine phosphate) capsules is equivalent to that of a solution except for a decrease in the rate of absorption. A peak concentration of 2020 ng/mL is obtained at about 1.5 hours after a 100 mg dose.

The *in vitro* plasma protein binding of butalbital is 45% over the concentration range of 0.5-20 µg/mL. This falls within the range of plasma protein binding (20%-45%) reported with other barbiturates such as phenobarbital, pentobarbital, and secobarbital sodium. The plasma-to-blood concentration ratio was almost unity indicating that there is no preferential distribution of butalbital into either plasma or blood cells.

See *OVERDOSAGE* for toxicity information.

Caffeine

Like most xanthines, caffeine is rapidly absorbed and distributed in all body tissues and fluids, including the CNS, fetal tissues, and breast milk.

Caffeine is cleared rapidly through metabolism and excretion in the urine. The plasma half-life is about 3 hours. Hepatic biotransformation prior to excretion results in about equal amounts of 1-methyl-xanthine and 1-methyluric acid. Of the 70% of the dose that has been recovered in the urine, only 3% was unchanged drug.

The bioavailability of the caffeine component for Fiorinal® with Codeine (butalbital, aspirin, caffeine, and codeine phosphate) capsules is equivalent to that of a solution except for a slightly longer time to peak. A peak concentration of 1660 ng/mL was obtained in less than an hour for an 80 mg dose.

See *OVERDOSAGE* for toxicity information.

INDICATIONS

Fiorinal® with Codeine (butalbital, aspirin, caffeine, and codeine phosphate) is indicated for the relief of the symptom complex of tension (or muscle contraction) headache.

Evidence supporting the efficacy of Fiorinal® with Codeine (butalbital, aspirin, caffeine, and codeine phosphate) is derived from 2 multi-clinic trials that compared patients with tension headache randomly assigned to 4 parallel treatments: Fiorinal® with Codeine (butalbital, aspirin, caffeine, and codeine phosphate), codeine, Fiorinal® (butalbital, aspirin, and caffeine), and placebo. Response was assessed over the course of the first 4 hours of each of 2 distinct headaches, separated by at least 24 hours. Fiorinal® with Codeine (butalbital, aspirin, caffeine, and codeine phosphate) proved statistically significantly superior to each of its components (Fiorinal®, codeine) and to placebo on measures of pain relief.

Evidence supporting the efficacy and safety of Fiorinal® with Codeine (butalbital, aspirin, caffeine, and codeine phosphate) in the treatment of multiple recurrent headaches is unavailable. Caution in this regard is required because codeine and butalbital are habit-forming and potentially abusable.

CONTRAINDICATIONS

Fiorinal® with Codeine (butalbital, aspirin, caffeine, and codeine phosphate) is contraindicated under the following conditions:

1. Hypersensitivity or intolerance to aspirin, caffeine, butalbital or codeine.
2. Patients with a hemorrhagic diathesis (e.g., hemophilia, hypoprothrombinemia, von Willebrand's disease, the thrombocytopenias, thrombasthenia and other ill-defined hereditary platelet dysfunctions, severe vitamin K deficiency and severe liver damage.)
3. Patients with the syndrome of nasal polyps, angioedema and bronchospastic reactivity to aspirin or other non-steroidal anti-inflammatory drugs. Anaphylactoid reactions have occurred in such patients.
4. Peptic ulcer or other serious gastrointestinal lesions.
5. Patients with porphyria.

WARNINGS

Therapeutic doses of aspirin can cause anaphylactic shock and other severe allergic reactions. It should be ascertained if the patient is allergic to aspirin, although a specific history of allergy may be lacking.

Significant bleeding can result from aspirin therapy in patients with peptic ulcer or other gastrointestinal lesions, and in patients with bleeding disorders.

Aspirin administered pre-operatively may prolong the bleeding time.

In the presence of head injury or other intracranial lesions, the respiratory depressant effects of codeine and other narcotics may be markedly enhanced, as well as their capacity for elevating cerebrospinal fluid pressure. Narcotics also produce other CNS depressant effects, such as drowsiness, that may further obscure the clinical course of patients with head injuries.

Codeine or other narcotics may obscure signs on which to judge the diagnosis or clinical course of patients with acute abdominal conditions.

Butalbital and codeine are both habit-forming and potentially abusable. Consequently, the extended use of Fiorinal® with Codeine (butalbital, aspirin, caffeine, and codeine phosphate) is not recommended.

Results from epidemiologic studies indicate an association between aspirin and Reye's Syndrome. Caution should be used in administering this product to children, including teenagers, with chicken pox or flu.

PRECAUTIONS

General

Fiorinal® with Codeine, (butalbital, aspirin, caffeine, and codeine phosphate) should be prescribed with caution for certain special-risk patients such as the elderly or debilitated, and those with severe impairment of renal or hepatic function, coagulation disorders, or head injuries, elevated intracranial pressure, acute abdominal conditions, hypothyroidism, urethral stricture, Addison's disease, prostatic hypertrophy, and peptic ulcer.

Aspirin should be used with caution in patients on anticoagulant therapy and in patients with underlying hemostatic defects.

Precautions should be taken when administering salicylates to persons with known allergies. Hypersensitivity to aspirin is particularly likely in patients with nasal polyps, and relatively common in those with asthma.

Information for Patients

Patients should be informed that Fiorinal® with Codeine (butalbital, aspirin, caffeine, and codeine phosphate) contains aspirin and should not be taken by patients with an aspirin allergy.

Fiorinal® with Codeine (butalbital, aspirin, caffeine, and codeine phosphate) may impair the mental and /or physical abilities required for performance of potentially hazardous tasks such as driving a car or operating machinery. Such tasks should be avoided while taking Fiorinal® with Codeine (butalbital, aspirin, caffeine, and codeine phosphate). Alcohol and other CNS depressants may produce an additive CNS depression when taken with Fiorinal® with Codeine (butalbital, aspirin, caffeine, and codeine phosphate), and should be avoided.

Codeine and butalbital may be habit-forming. Patients should take the drug only for as long as it is prescribed, in the amounts prescribed, and no more frequently than prescribed.

Laboratory Tests

In patients with severe hepatic or renal disease, effects of therapy should be monitored with serial liver and /or renal function tests.

Drug Interactions

The CNS effects of butalbital may be enhanced by monoamine oxidase (MAO) inhibitors.

In patients receiving concomitant corticosteroids and chronic use of aspirin, withdrawal of corticosteroids may result in salicylism because corticosteroids enhance renal clearance of salicylates and their withdrawal is followed by return to normal rates of renal clearance.

Fiorinal® with Codeine (butalbital, aspirin, caffeine, and codeine phosphate) may enhance the effects of:

1. Oral anticoagulants, causing bleeding by inhibiting prothrombin formation in the liver and displacing anticoagulants from plasma protein binding sites.
2. Oral antidiabetic agents and insulin, causing hypoglycemia by contributing an additive effect, if dosage of Fiorinal® with Codeine (butalbital, aspirin, caffeine, and codeine phosphate) exceeds maximum recommended daily dosage.
3. 6-mercaptopurine and methotrexate, causing bone marrow toxicity and blood dyscrasias by displacing these drugs from secondary binding sites, and, in the case of methotrexate, also reducing its excretion.
4. Non-steroidal anti-inflammatory agents, increasing the risk of peptic ulceration and bleeding by contributing additive effects.
5. Other narcotic analgesics, alcohol, general anesthetics, tranquilizers such as chlordiazepoxide, sedative-hypnotics, or other CNS depressants, causing increased CNS depression.

Fiorinal® with Codeine (butalbital, aspirin, caffeine, and codeine phosphate) may diminish the effects of:

Uricosuric agents such as probenecid and sulfinpyrazone, reducing their effectiveness in the treatment of gout. Aspirin competes with these agents for protein binding sites.

Drug/Laboratory Test Interactions

Aspirin: Aspirin may interfere with the following laboratory determinations in blood: serum amylase, fasting blood glucose, cholesterol, protein, serum glutamic-oxalacetic transaminase (SGOT), uric acid, prothrombin time and bleeding time. Aspirin may interfere with the following laboratory determinations in urine: glucose, 5-hydroxyindoleacetic

Continued on next page

Fiorinal with Codeine—Cont.

acid, Gerhardt ketone, vanillylmandelic acid (VMA), uric acid, diacetic acid, and spectrophotometric detection of barbiturates.

Codeine: Codeine may increase serum amylase levels.

Carcinogenesis, Mutagenesis, Impairment of Fertility

Adequate long-term studies have been conducted in mice and rats with aspirin, alone or in combination with other drugs, in which no evidence of carcinogenesis was seen. No adequate studies have been conducted in animals to determine whether aspirin has a potential for mutagenesis or impairment of fertility. No adequate studies have been conducted in animals to determine whether butalbital has a potential for carcinogenesis, mutagenesis, or impairment of fertility.

Usage in Pregnancy

Teratogenic Effects:

Pregnancy Category C. Animal reproduction studies have not been conducted with Fiorinal® with Codeine (butalbital, aspirin, caffeine, and codeine phosphate). It is also not known whether Fiorinal® with Codeine (butalbital, aspirin, caffeine, and codeine phosphate) can cause fetal harm when administered to a pregnant woman or can affect reproduction capacity. Fiorinal® with Codeine (butalbital, aspirin, caffeine, and codeine phosphate) should be given to a pregnant woman only when clearly needed.

Nonteratogenic Effects:

Although Fiorinal® with Codeine (butalbital, aspirin, caffeine, and codeine phosphate) was not implicated in the birth defect, a female infant was born with lissencephaly, pachygyria and heterotopic gray matter. The infant was born 8 weeks prematurely to a woman who had taken an average of 90 Fiorinal® with Codeine (butalbital, aspirin, caffeine, and codeine phosphate) capsules each month from the first few days of pregnancy. The child's development was mildly delayed and from one year of age she had partial simple motor seizures.

Withdrawal seizures were reported in a two-day-old male infant whose mother had taken a butalbital-containing drug during the last 2 months of pregnancy. Butalbital was found in the infant's serum. The infant was given phenobarbital 5mg/kg, which was tapered without further seizure or other withdrawal symptoms.

Studies of aspirin use in pregnant women have not shown that aspirin increases the risk of abnormalities when administered during the first trimester of pregnancy. In controlled studies involving 41,337 pregnant women and their offspring, there was no evidence that aspirin taken during pregnancy caused stillbirth, neonatal death or reduced birth weight. In controlled studies of 50,282 pregnant women and their offspring, aspirin administration in moderate and heavy doses during the first four lunar months of pregnancy showed no teratogenic effect.

Reproduction studies have been performed in rabbits and rats at doses up to 150 times the human dose and have revealed no evidence of impaired fertility or harm to the fetus due to codeine.

Therapeutic doses of aspirin in pregnant women close to term may cause bleeding in mother, fetus, or neonate. During the last 6 months of pregnancy, regular use of aspirin in high doses may prolong pregnancy and delivery.

Labor and Delivery

Ingestion of aspirin prior to delivery may prolong delivery or lead to bleeding in the mother or neonate. Use of codeine during labor may lead to respiratory depression in the neonate.

Nursing Mothers

Aspirin, caffeine, barbiturates and codeine are excreted in breast milk in small amounts, but the significance of their effects on nursing infants is not known. Because of potential for serious adverse reactions in nursing infants from Fiorinal® with Codeine (butalbital, aspirin, caffeine, and codeine phosphate), a decision should be made whether to discontinue nursing or to discontinue the drug, taking into account the importance of the drug to the mother.

Pediatric Use

Safety and effectiveness in pediatric patients have not been established.

ADVERSE REACTIONS

Commonly Observed

The most commonly reported adverse events associated with the use of Fiorinal® with Codeine (butalbital, aspirin, caffeine, and codeine phosphate) and not reported at an equivalent incidence by placebo-treated patients were nausea and/or abdominal pain, drowsiness, and dizziness.

Associated with Treatment Discontinuation

Of the 382 patients treated with Fiorinal® with Codeine (butalbital, aspirin, caffeine, and codeine phosphate) in controlled clinical trials, three (0.8%) discontinued treatment with Fiorinal® with Codeine (butalbital, aspirin, caffeine, and codeine phosphate) because of adverse events. One patient each discontinued treatment for the following reasons: gastrointestinal upset; lightheadedness and heavy eyelids; and drowsiness and generalized tingling.

Incidence in Controlled Clinical Trials

The following table summarizes the incidence rates of the adverse events reported by at least 1% of the Fiorinal® with Codeine (butalbital, aspirin, caffeine, and codeine phosphate) treated patients in controlled clinical trials comparing Fiorinal® with Codeine (butalbital, aspirin, caffeine, and codeine phosphate) to placebo, and provides a comparison to the incidence rates reported by the placebo-treated patients.

The prescriber should be aware that these figures cannot be used to predict the incidence of side effects in the course of usual medical practice where patient characteristics and other factors differ from those that prevailed in the clinical trials. Similarly, the cited frequencies cannot be compared with figures obtained from other clinical investigations involving different treatments, uses, and investigators.

Adverse Events Reported by at Least 1% of Fiorinal® with Codeine (butalbital, aspirin, caffeine, and codeine phosphate) Treated Patients During Placebo Controlled Clinical Trials

	Incidence Rate of Adverse Events	
Body System/ Adverse Event	Fiorinal®/Codeine (butalbital, aspirin, caffeine, and codeine phosphate) (N=382)	Placebo (N=377)
Central Nervous		
Drowsiness	2.4%	0.5%
Dizziness/ Lightheadedness	2.6%	0.5%
Intoxicated Feeling	1.0%	0%
Gastrointestinal		
Nausea/ Abdominal Pain	3.7%	0.8%

Other Adverse Events Reported During Controlled Clinical Trials

The listing that follows represents the proportion of the 382 patients exposed to Fiorinal® with Codeine (butalbital, aspirin, caffeine, and codeine phosphate) while participating in the controlled clinical trials who reported, on at least one occasion, an adverse event of the type cited. All reported adverse events, except those already presented in the previous table, are included. It is important to emphasize that, although the adverse events reported did occur while the patient was receiving Fiorinal® with Codeine (butalbital, aspirin, caffeine, and codeine phosphate), the adverse events were not necessarily caused by Fiorinal® with Codeine (butalbital, aspirin, caffeine, and codeine phosphate). Adverse events are classified by body system and frequency. "Frequent" is defined as an adverse event which occurred in at least 1/100 (1%) of the patients; all adverse events listed in the previous table are frequent. "Infrequent" is defined as an adverse event that occurred in less than 1/100 patients but at least 1/1000 patients. All adverse events tabulated below are classified as infrequent.

Central Nervous: headache, shaky feeling, tingling, agitation, fainting, fatigue, heavy eyelids, high energy, hot spells, numbness, and sluggishness.

Autonomic Nervous: dry mouth and hyperhidrosis.

Gastrointestinal: vomiting, difficulty swallowing, and heartburn.

Cardiovascular: tachycardia.

Musculoskeletal: leg pain and muscle fatigue.

Genitourinary: diuresis.

Miscellaneous: pruritus, fever, earache, nasal congestion, and tinnitus.

Voluntary reports of adverse drug events, temporally associated with Fiorinal® with Codeine (butalbital, aspirin, caffeine, and codeine phosphate), that have been received since market introduction and that were not reported in clinical trials by the patients treated with Fiorinal® with Codeine (butalbital, aspirin, caffeine, and codeine phosphate), are listed below. Many or most of these events may have no causal relationship with the drug and are listed according to body system.

Central Nervous: Abuse, addiction, anxiety, depression, disorientation, hallucination, hyperactivity, insomnia, libido decrease, nervousness, neuropathy, psychosis, sedation, sexual activity increase, slurred speech, twitching, unconsciousness, vertigo.

Autonomic Nervous: epistaxis, flushing, miosis, salivation.

Gastrointestinal: anorexia, appetite increased, constipation, diarrhea, esophagitis, gastroenteritis, gastrointestinal spasm, hiccup, mouth burning, pyloric ulcer.

Cardiovascular: chest pain, hypotensive reaction, palpitations, syncope.

Skin: erythema, erythema multiforme, exfoliative dermatitis, hives, rash, toxic epidermal necrolysis.

Urinary: kidney impairment, urinary difficulty.

Miscellaneous: allergic reaction, anaphylactic shock, cholangiocarcinoma, drug interaction with erythromycin (stomach upset), edema.

The following adverse drug events may be borne in mind as potential effects of the components of Fiorinal® with Codeine (butalbital, aspirin, caffeine, and codeine phosphate). Potential effects of high dosage are listed in the *OVERDOSAGE* section of this insert.

Aspirin: occult blood loss, hemolytic anemia, iron deficiency anemia, gastric distress, heartburn, nausea, peptic ulcer, prolonged bleeding time, acute airway obstruction, renal toxicity when taken in high doses for prolonged periods, impaired urate excretion, hepatitis.

Caffeine: cardiac stimulation, irritability, tremor, dependence, nephrotoxicity, hyperglycemia.

Codeine: nausea, vomiting, drowsiness, lightheadedness, constipation, pruritus.

DRUG ABUSE AND DEPENDENCE

Controlled Substance

Fiorinal® with Codeine (butalbital, aspirin, caffeine, and codeine phosphate) is controlled by the Drug Enforcement Administration and is classified under Schedule III.

Abuse and Dependence

Codeine

Codeine can produce drug dependence of the morphine type and, therefore, has the potential for being abused. Psychological dependence, physical dependence, and tolerance may develop upon repeated administration and it should be prescribed and administered with the same degree of caution appropriate to the use of other oral narcotic medications.

Butalbital

Barbiturates may be habit-forming: Tolerance, psychological dependence, and physical dependence may occur especially following prolonged use of high doses of barbiturates. The average daily dose for the barbiturate addict is usually about 1,500 mg. As tolerance to barbiturates develops, the amount needed to maintain the same level of intoxication increases; tolerance to a fatal dosage, however, does not increase more than twofold. As this occurs, the margin between an intoxication dosage and fatal dosage becomes smaller. The lethal dose of a barbiturate is far less if alcohol is also ingested. Major withdrawal symptoms (convulsions and delirium) may occur within 16 hours and last up to 5 days after abrupt cessation of these drugs. Intensity of withdrawal symptoms gradually declines over a period of approximately 15 days. Treatment of barbiturate dependence consists of cautious and gradual withdrawal of the drug. Barbiturate-dependent patients can be withdrawn by using a number of different withdrawal regimens. One method involves initiating treatment at the patient's regular dosage level and gradually decreasing the daily dosage as tolerated by the patient.

OVERDOSAGE

The toxic effects of acute overdosage of Fiorinal® with Codeine (butalbital, aspirin, caffeine, and codeine phosphate) capsules are attributable mainly to the barbiturate and codeine components, and, to a lesser extent, aspirin. Because toxic effects of caffeine occur in very high dosages only, the possibility of significant caffeine toxicity from Fiorinal® with Codeine (butalbital, aspirin, caffeine, and codeine phosphate) overdosage is unlikely.

Signs and Symptoms

Symptoms attributable to ***acute barbiturate poisoning*** include drowsiness, confusion, and coma; respiratory depression; hypotension; hypovolemic shock. Symptoms attributable to ***acute aspirin poisoning*** include hyperpnea; acid-base disturbances with development of metabolic acidosis; vomiting and abdominal pain; tinnitus, hyperthermia; hypoprothrombinemia; restlessness; delirium; convulsions. ***Acute caffeine poisoning*** may cause insomnia, restlessness, tremor, and delirium; tachycardia and extrasystoles. Symptoms of ***acute codeine poisoning*** include the opioid triad of: pinpoint pupils, marked depression of respiration, and loss of consciousness. Convulsions may occur.

Treatment

The following paragraphs describe one approach to the treatment of overdose with Fiorinal® with Codeine (butalbital, aspirin, caffeine, and codeine phosphate). However, because strategies for the management of an overdose continually evolve, consultation with a regional poison control center is strongly encouraged.

Treatment consists primarily of management of barbiturate intoxication, reversal of the effects of codeine, and the correction of the acid-base imbalance due to salicylism. Vomiting should be induced mechanically or with emetics in the conscious patient. Gastric lavage may be used if the pharyngeal and laryngeal reflexes are present and if less than 4 hours have elapsed since ingestion. A cuffed endotracheal tube should be inserted before gastric lavage of the unconscious patient and when necessary to provide assisted respiration. Diuresis, alkalinization of the urine, and correction of electrolyte disturbances should be accomplished through administration of intravenous fluids such as 1% sodium bicarbonate and 5% dextrose in water.

Meticulous attention should be given to maintaining adequate pulmonary ventilation. The value of vasopressor agents such as Norepinephrine or Phenylephrine Hydrochloride in treating hypotension is questionable since they increase vasoconstriction and decrease blood flow. However, if prolonged support of blood pressure is required, Norepinephrine Bitartrate (Levophed®)* may be given I.V. with the usual precautions and serial blood pressure monitoring. In severe cases of intoxication, peritoneal dialysis, hemodialysis, or exchange transfusion may be lifesaving. Hypoprothrombinemia should be treated with vitamin K, intravenously.

Methemoglobinemia over 30% should be treated with methylene blue by slow intravenous administration.

Naloxone, a narcotic antagonist, can reverse respiratory depression and coma associated with opioid overdose. Typically, a dose of 0.4-2.0 mg is given parenterally and may be repeated if an adequate response is not achieved. Since the duration of action of codeine may exceed that of the antagonist, the patient should be kept under continued surveillance and repeated doses of the antagonist should be administered as needed to maintain adequate respiration. A narcotic antagonist should not be administered in the absence of clinically significant respiratory or cardiovascular depression.

Up-to-date information about the treatment of overdose can be obtained from a Certified Regional Poison Control Center. Telephone numbers of Certified Regional Poison Control Centers are listed in the Physicians' Desk Reference®.**

Toxic and Lethal Doses
Butalbital: toxic dose 1.0 g (adult); lethal dose 2.0-5.0 g (20 capsules of Fiorinal® with Codeine)
Aspirin: toxic blood level greater than 30 mg/100 mL; lethal dose 10-30 g (adult)
Caffeine: toxic dose greater than 1.0 g; (25 capsules of Fiorinal® with Codeine); lethal dose unknown
Codeine: toxic dose 240 mg (8 capsules of Fiorinal® with Codeine); lethal dose 0.5-1.0 g (adult)

DOSAGE AND ADMINISTRATION

One or 2 capsules every 4 hours. Total daily dosage should not exceed 6 capsules.

Extended and repeated use of this product is not recommended because of the potential for physical dependence.

HOW SUPPLIED
Fiorinal® with Codeine
(butalbital, aspirin, caffeine, and codeine phosphate)
Capsules, USP
Imprinted " Ⓢ " F-C on one half, "SANDOZ 78-107" other half, color is blue and red.
Bottles of 100 (NDC 0078-0107-05)
ControlPak® package of 25: continuous reverse-numbered roll of sealed blisters (NDC 0078-0107-13)
Store and Dispense
Below 77°F (25°C); tight container.
* Levophed is a registered Trademark of Sanofi Winthrop Pharmaceuticals.
** Trademark of Medical Economics Company.
[REV: FEBRUARY 1996 30133903]
Shown in Product Identification Guide, page 325

LAMISIL®
[lä″ mə ′səl]   ℞
(terbinafine hydrochloride cream) Cream, 1%
FOR TOPICAL DERMATOLOGIC USE ONLY—NOT FOR OPHTHALMIC, ORAL, OR INTRAVAGINAL USE

Caution: Federal (USA) law prohibits dispensing without a prescription.
The following prescribing information is based on official labeling in effect on August 1, 1998.

DESCRIPTION
Lamisil® Cream, 1%, contains the synthetic antifungal compound, terbinafine hydrochloride. It is intended for topical dermatologic use only.
Chemically, terbinafine hydrochloride is (E)-N-(6,6-dimethyl-2-hepten-4-ynyl)-N-methyl-1-naphthalenemethanamine hydrochloride. The compound has the empirical formula $C_{21}H_{26}ClN$, a molecular weight of 327.90, and the following structural formula:
[See chemical structure at top of next column]

Successful Outcomes

Therapy	1 Week Therapy			4 Weeks Therapy	
	At 1 wk (end of Rx)	At 4 wks (3 wk f/up)	At 6 wks (5 wk f/up)	At 4 wks (end of Rx)	At 6 wks (2 wk f/up)
Lamisil®	14% 11/79	51% 40/78	65% 51/78	71% 94/133	73% 97/132
Vehicle	6% 5/79	13% 10/75	12% 8/69	NA	NA
Active Control	NA	NA	NA	63% 84/133	59% 79/134

Terbinafine hydrochloride is a white to off-white fine crystalline powder. It is freely soluble in methanol and methylene chloride, soluble in ethanol, and slightly soluble in water.

Each gram of Lamisil® Cream, 1%, contains 10 mg of terbinafine hydrochloride in a white cream base of benzyl alcohol NF, cetyl alcohol NF, cetyl palmitate, isopropyl myristate NF, polysorbate 60 NF, purified water USP, sodium hydroxide NF, sorbitan monostearate NF, and stearyl alcohol NF.

CLINICAL PHARMACOLOGY
Pharmacokinetics
Following a single application of 100 μL of Lamisil® (terbinafine hydrochloride cream) Cream, 1%, (containing 1 mg of ^{14}C-terbinafine) to a 30 cm² area of the ventral forearm of 6 healthy subjects, the recovery of radioactivity in urine and feces averaged 3.5% of the administered dose.

In a study of 16 healthy subjects, 8 of whose skin was artificially compromised by stripping the stratum corneum to the viable layer, single and multiple applications (average 0.1 mg/cm² B.I.D. for 5 days) of terbinafine as Lamisil® (terbinafine hydrochloride cream) Cream, 1%, were made to various sites. In this study, systemic absorption was highly variable. The maximum measured plasma concentration of terbinafine was 11.4 ng/mL, and the maximum measured plasma concentration of the de-methylated metabolite was 11.0 ng/mL. In many patients there were no detectable plasma levels of either parent compound or metabolite. Urinary excretion accounted for up to 9% of the topically applied dose; the majority excreted less than 4%. No measurement of fecal drug content was performed.

In a study of 10 patients with tinea cruris, once daily application of Lamisil® (terbinafine hydrochloride cream) Cream, 1%, for 7 days resulted in plasma concentrations of terbinafine of 0–11 ng/mL on day 7. Plasma concentrations of the metabolites of terbinafine ranged from 11–80 ng/mL in these patients.

Approximately 75% of cutaneously absorbed terbinafine is eliminated in the urine predominantly as metabolites.

Microbiology
Terbinafine hydrochloride is a synthetic allylamine derivative. Terbinafine hydrochloride exerts its antifungal effect by inhibiting squalene epoxidase, a key enzyme in sterol biosynthesis in fungi. This action results in a deficiency in ergosterol and a corresponding accumulation of squalene within the fungal cell. Depending on the concentration of the drug and the fungal species tested *in vitro*, terbinafine hydrochloride may be fungicidal; however, the clinical significance of these data is unknown. *In vitro*, mammalian squalene epoxidase is only inhibited at higher (4,000-fold) concentrations.

Terbinafine has been shown to be active against most strains of the following organisms both *in vitro* and in clinical infections at indicated body sites (See INDICATIONS AND USAGE):

Epidermophyton floccosum
Trichophyton mentagrophytes
Trichophyton rubrum

The following *in vitro* data are available; however, their clinical significance is unknown. Terbinafine exhibits satisfactory *in vitro* MIC's against most strains of the following organisms; however, the safety and efficacy of terbinafine in treating clinical infections due to these organisms have not been established in adequate and well-controlled clinical trials:

Microsporum canis
Microsporum gypseum
Microsporum nanum
Trichophyton verrucosum

CLINICAL STUDIES
In the following data presentations, the term "successful outcome" refers to those patients evaluated at a specific time point, who had both negative mycological results (culture and KOH preparation) and a total clinical score of less than or equal to 2. The clinical score is the sum of the scores of each sign and symptom graded on a scale of 0=absent, 1=mild, 2=moderate, and 3=severe. Mean clinical scores at entry ranged from 6–11 in the pivotal clinical trials.

All studies included as a minimum, clinical evaluation of erythema, desquamation/scaling, and pruritus (also fissuring in the moccasin studies).

A. Tinea Pedis (Interdigital Type)
In 3 studies of Lamisil® (terbinafine hydrochloride cream) Cream, 1%, used B.I.D. in the treatment of tinea pedis, 2 (combined in the table below) were vehicle-controlled (placebo) evaluations of 1 week treatment duration. The third study (see table below) was of 4 weeks therapy compared to another active drug.
[See table above]

B. Tinea Corporis/Cruris
Two studies (combined below) compared Lamisil® (terbinafine hydrochloride cream) Cream, 1%, to vehicle (placebo), applied once daily for 1 week in the treatment of tinea corporis/cruris.

In the table below, sites of infection are separated into 2 groups: (1) tinea corporis and (2) tinea cruris. Patients with mixed tinea corporis/cruris are included in both groups.

Successful Outcomes

Disease	Therapy	At 1 wk (end of Rx)	At 4 wks (3 wk f/up)
Corporis	Lamisil®	21% 7/33	83% 25/30
	Vehicle	0% 0/31	31% 4/13
Cruris	Lamisil®	43% 21/49	92% 45/49
	Vehicle	9% 5/58	25% 7/28

C. Plantar Tinea Pedis (Moccasin Type)
Two studies of Lamisil® (terbinafine hydrochloride cream) Cream, 1%, used in the treatment of plantar tinea pedis (moccasin type), were vehicle-controlled (placebo) evaluations of 2 weeks treatment duration (B.I.D.).
In the following table, patients are categorized according to whether or not they had associated toenail onychomycosis.

Successful Outcomes

Associated Disease	Therapy	At 2 wks (end of Rx)	At 8 wks (6 wks f/up)
Without Onychomycosis	Lamisil®	23% (3%)* 7/30	65% (29%) 20/31
	Vehicle	12% (4%) 3/25	15% (0%) 4/26
With Onychomycosis	Lamisil®	3% (2%) 2/64	48% (21%) 32/66
	Vehicle	1% (0%) 1/69	1% (0%) 1/70

*The % of patients with complete eradication of signs and symptoms is given in parentheses.

INDICATIONS AND USAGE
Lamisil® (terbinafine hydrochloride cream) Cream, 1%, is indicated for the topical treatment of the following dermatologic infections: interdigital tinea pedis (athlete's foot), tinea cruris (jock itch), or tinea corporis (ringworm) due to *Epidermophyton floccosum, Trichophyton mentagrophytes,* or *Trichophyton rubrum* and plantar tinea pedis (moccasin type) due to *Trichophyton mentagrophytes* or *Trichophyton rubrum.* (See DOSAGE AND ADMINISTRATION).

Continued on next page

Lamisil Cream—Cont.

Diagnosis of the disease should be confirmed either by direct microscopic examination of scrapings from infected tissue mounted in a solution of potassium hydroxide or by culture.

CONTRAINDICATIONS

Lamisil® (terbinafine hydrochloride cream) Cream, 1%, is contraindicated in individuals who have known or suspected hypersensitivity to terbinafine or any other of its components.

WARNINGS

Lamisil® (terbinafine hydrochloride cream) Cream, 1%, is not for ophthalmic, oral, or intravaginal use.

PRECAUTIONS

General

If irritation or sensitivity develops with the use of Lamisil® (terbinafine hydrochloride cream) Cream, 1%, treatment should be discontinued and appropriate therapy instituted.

Information for Patients

The patient should be told to:

1. Use Lamisil® (terbinafine hydrochloride cream) Cream, 1%, as directed by the physician and avoid contact with the eyes, nose, mouth, or other mucous membranes,
2. Use the medication for the treatment time recommended by the physician,
3. Inform the physician if the area of application shows signs of increased irritation or possible sensitization (redness, itching, burning, blistering, swelling, or oozing),
4. Avoid the use of occlusive dressings unless otherwise directed by the physician.

Drug Interactions

Potential interactions between Lamisil® (terbinafine hydrochloride cream) Cream, 1%, and other drugs have not been systematically evaluated.

Carcinogenesis, Mutagenesis, Impairment of Fertility

In a 2-year oral carcinogenicity study in mice, a 4% incidence of splenic hemangiosarcomas and a 6% incidence of leiomyosarcoma-like tumors of the seminal vesicles were observed in males at the highest dose level, 156 mg/kg/day (equivalent to at least 390 times the maximum potential exposure at the recommended human topical dose). In a carcinogenicity study in rats at the highest dose level, 69 mg/kg/day (equivalent to at least 173 times the maximum potential exposure at the recommended human topical dose), a 6% incidence of both liver tumors and skin lipomas were observed in males. In rats, the formation of liver tumors was associated with peroxisomal proliferation.

A battery of *in vitro* and *in vivo* genotoxicity tests, including Ames assay, mutagenicity evaluation in Chinese hamster ovarian cells, chromosome aberration test, sister chromatid exchanges, and mouse micronucleus test revealed no evidence for a mutagenic or clastogenic potential for the drug.

Reproductive studies in rats administered up to 300 mg/kg/day orally (equivalent to at least 750 times the maximum potential exposure at the recommended human topical dose) did not reveal any adverse effects on fertility or other reproductive parameters. Intravaginal mucosal application of terbinafine hydrochloride at 150 mg/day in pregnant rabbits did not increase the incidence of abortions or premature deliveries or affect fetal parameters.

Pregnancy

Pregnancy Category B: Oral doses of terbinafine hydrochloride, up to 300 mg/kg/day (equivalent to at least 750 times the maximum potential exposure at the recommended human topical dose), during organogenesis in rats and rabbits were not teratogenic. Similarly, a subcutaneous study in rats at doses up to 100 mg/kg/day (equivalent to at least 250 times the maximum potential exposure at the recommended human topical dose) and a percutaneous study in rabbits, including doses up to 150 mg/kg/day (equivalent to at least 350 times the maximum potential exposure at the recommended human topical dose) did not reveal any teratogenic potential.

There are, however, no adequate and well-controlled studies in pregnant women. Because animal reproduction studies are not always predictive of human response, this drug should be used only if clearly indicated during pregnancy.

The above comparisons between oral animal doses and maximum potential exposure at the recommended human topical doses are based upon the application to human skin of 0.1 mg of terbinafine/cm^2, the assumption of average human cutaneous exposure of 100 cm^2 [assuming the use of 1 gram of Lamisil® (terbinafine hydrochloride cream) Cream, 1%, per dose], and a maximum theoretical (100%) human cutaneous absorption. At present, comparative animal and human systemic exposure pharmacokinetic data are not available.

Nursing Mothers

After a single oral dose of 500 mg of terbinafine hydrochloride to 2 volunteers, the total dose of terbinafine hydrochloride secreted in human milk during the 72-hour post-dosing period was 0.65 mg in one person and 0.15 mg in the other. The total excretion of terbinafine in human milk was 0.13% and 0.03% of the administered dose, respectively. The concentrations of the de-methylated metabolite measured in the human milk of these 2 volunteers were below the detection limit of the assay used (150 ng/mL of milk).

Because of the small amount of data on human neonatal exposure, a decision should be made whether to discontinue nursing or to discontinue the drug, taking into account the importance of the drug to the mother, as well as the findings of tumors in male mice and rats following oral administration of terbinafine hydrochloride and the lack of data on carcinogenicity in neonatal animals.

Nursing mothers should avoid application of Lamisil® (terbinafine hydrochloride cream) Cream, 1%, to the breast.

Pediatric Use

Safety and efficacy in pediatric patients below the age of 12 years have not been established.

ADVERSE REACTIONS

In clinical trials, 6 (0.3%) of 2379 patients treated with Lamisil® (terbinafine hydrochloride cream) Cream, 1%, discontinued therapy due to adverse events and 56 (2.4%) reported adverse reactions thought to be possibly, probably, or, definitely related to drug therapy. These reactions included irritation (1%), burning/tingling (0.9%), itching (0.2%), and dryness (0.2%).

OVERDOSAGE

Overdosage of terbinafine hydrochloride in humans has not been reported to date. Acute overdosage with topical application of terbinafine hydrochloride is unlikely due to the limited absorption of topically applied drug and would not be expected to lead to a life threatening situation.

Overdosage in rats and mice by the oral and intravenous routes of drug administration has produced sedation, drowsiness, ataxia, dyspnea, exophthalmus, and piloerection. The majority of deaths in animals occurred following oral administration of doses exceeding 3 grams/kilogram or following 200 mg/kg administered intravenously. In rabbits, overdosage produced erythema, edema, and scale formation following topical administration of doses in excess of 1.5 grams/kilogram.

When terbinafine hydrochloride cream, 1%, was administered as a single oral dose at 10 and 25 mL/kg (100 and 250 mg/kg, respectively) to rats and mice, no deaths or other drug-related toxicities were observed.

DOSAGE AND ADMINISTRATION

In the treatment of **interdigital tinea pedis** (athlete's foot), Lamisil® (terbinafine hydrochloride cream) Cream, 1%, should be applied to cover the affected and immediately surrounding areas twice daily until clinical signs and symptoms are significantly improved. In many patients this occurs by day 7 of drug therapy. The duration of drug therapy should be for a minimum of 1 week and should not exceed 4 weeks. *(See CLINICAL STUDIES.)*

In the treatment of **tinea cruris** (jock itch) or **tinea corporis** (ringworm), Lamisil® (terbinafine hydrochloride cream) Cream, 1%, should be applied to cover the affected and immediately surrounding areas once or twice daily until clinical signs and symptoms are significantly improved. In many patients this occurs by day 7 of drug therapy. The duration of drug therapy should be for a minimum of 1 week and should not exceed 4 weeks. *(See CLINICAL STUDIES.)*

In the treatment of **plantar tinea pedis** (moccasin type), Lamisil® (terbinafine hydrochloride cream) Cream, 1%, should be applied to cover the affected area and immediately surrounding areas twice daily for 2 weeks. Treatment outcome may be influenced by the presence of onychomycosis, where patients who have an associated toenail infection may be less likely to have a favorable clinical and mycological response to therapy. *(See CLINICAL STUDIES.)*

Note:

Improvement is gradual. In many patients treated with shorter durations of therapy (1–2 weeks), improvement continues during the 2–6 weeks after drug therapy has been completed. As a consequence, patients should not be considered therapeutic failures until they have been observed for a period of 2–6 weeks off therapy. *(See CLINICAL STUDIES.)*

If successful outcome is not achieved during the post-treatment observation period, the diagnosis should be reviewed.

HOW SUPPLIED

Lamisil® (terbinafine hydrochloride cream) Cream, 1%

Tubes of 15 grams (NDC 0078-0170-40)
Tubes of 30 grams (NDC 0078-0170-46)
Store between 5° and 30°C (41° and 86°F)
REV: MARCH 1997 38052903

Shown in Product Identification Guide, page 325

LAMISIL® SOLUTION, 1% ℞

[la″ mə′ səl]
(terbinafine hydrochloride solution)

FOR TOPICAL DERMATOLOGIC USE ONLY– NOT FOR OPHTHALMIC, ORAL, OR INTRAVAGINAL USE.

Caution: Federal (USA) law prohibits dispensing without prescription.

The following prescribing information is based on official labeling in effect on August 1, 1998.

DESCRIPTION

Lamisil® Solution, 1% (terbinafine hydrochloride solution) contains the synthetic antifungal compound, terbinafine hydrochloride. It is intended for topical dermatologic use only. Chemically, terbinafine hydrochloride is (E)-N-(6,6-dimethyl-2-hepten-4-ynyl)-N-methyl-1-naphthalenemethanamine hydrochloride. The compound has the empirical formula $C_{21}H_{26}ClN$, a molecular weight of 327.90 and the following structural formula:

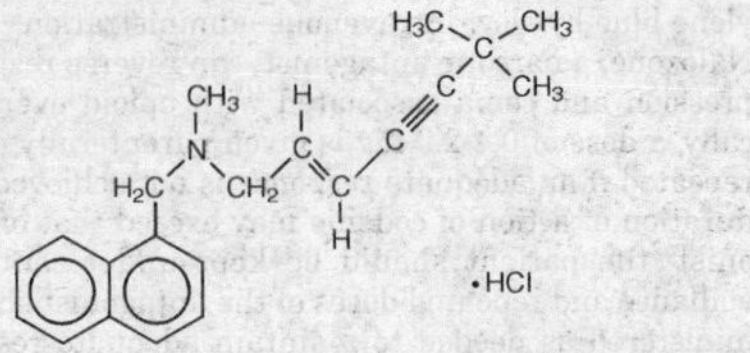

Terbinafine hydrochloride is a white to off-white fine crystalline powder. It is freely soluble in methanol and methylene chloride, soluble in ethanol, and slightly soluble in water.

Each gram of Lamisil® Solution, 1% (terbinafine hydrochloride solution) contains 10 mg of terbinafine hydrochloride in a solution of cetomacrogol 1000, ethanol (28.7%), propylene glycol, and purified water, USP.

CLINICAL PHARMACOLOGY

Pharmacokinetics

Absorption: In a study of 10 patients with tinea cruris, once daily application of Lamisil® Solution, 1% (terbinafine hydrochloride solution) for 7 days (total amount of terbinafine hydrochloride applied averaged 0.8 g) resulted in plasma concentrations of terbinafine of up to 21 ng/mL on day 7, representing approximately 2% of plasma concentrations achieved with a 250 mg terbinafine hydrochloride tablet. Plasma concentrations of the N-demethylated metabolite of terbinafine ranged up to 14 ng/mL in these patients. In subjects with healthy skin, neither the parent nor the N-demethylated metabolite were detected in the plasma following once daily dosing for seven days with 0.3 g of 1% terbinafine hydrochloride solution.

Distribution: The skin pharmacokinetics of Lamisil® Solution, 1% (terbinafine hydrochloride solution), delivered by spray was compared to the 1% Cream in 36 healthy subjects following both single and multiple applications (approximately 5 mg of terbinafine hydrochloride was applied to roughly a 190 cm^2 area on the back). Maximum mean total stratum corneum drug concentrations (C_{max}) averaged 720 and 810 ng/cm^2 on days 1 and 7, respectively. No significant differences in total stratum corneum AUC (area under the curve), C_{max} and half-life were seen between the 1% spray and the 1% cream after 1 or 7 days of treatment. Similar skin levels of terbinafine are achieved by delivery of Lamisil® Solution, 1% (terbinafine hydrochloride solution) from the spray bottle or from application of Lamisil® 1% Cream (terbinafine hydrochloride cream).

Metabolism: It is unknown whether or not there is any significant skin metabolism of topically applied terbinafine. Radiolabeled studies with oral dosage forms indicate that terbinafine is highly metabolized into a number of metabolites which undergo conjugation and excretion into the urine. The primary metabolite seen in the urine (10% of the oral dose) is N-demethyl terbinafine.

Elimination: The half-life of terbinafine when absorbed through the skin, regardless of the method of topical administration, is ~21 hours. Approximately 75% of cutaneously absorbed terbinafine is eliminated in the urine, predominately as metabolites.

Microbiology: Terbinafine hydrochloride is a synthetic allylamine derivative. Terbinafine hydrochloride is hypothesized to act by inhibiting the epoxidation of squalene, thus blocking the biosynthesis of ergosterol, an essential component of fungal cell membranes. The allylamine derivatives, like the benzylamines, act at an earlier step in the ergosterol biosynthesis pathway than the azole class of antifungal drugs. Depending on the concentration of the drug and the fungal species tested *in vitro*, terbinafine hydrochloride may be fungicidal. However, the clinical significance of *in vitro* data is unknown.

Terbinafine has been shown to be active against most strains of the following organisms both *in vitro* and in clinical infections as described in the *INDICATIONS AND USAGE* section:

Epidermophyton floccosum
Malassezia furfur (formerly *Pityrosporum ovale*)
Trichophyton mentagrophytes
Trichophyton rubrum

The following *in vitro* data are available, **but their clinical significance is unknown.** *In vitro*, terbinafine exhibits satisfactory MIC's against most strains of the following microorganisms; however, the safety and efficacy of terbinafine in

treating clinical infections due to these microorganisms have not been established in adequate and well-controlled clinical trials:

Microsporum canis
Microsporum gypseum
Microsporum nanum
Trichophyton verrucosum

INDICATIONS AND USAGE

Lamisil® Solution, 1% (terbinafine hydrochloride solution) is indicated for the topical treatment of the following dermatologic infections: tinea (pityriasis) versicolor due to *Malassezia furfur* (formerly *Pityrosporum ovale*), and tinea pedis (athlete's foot), tinea cruris (jock itch), or tinea corporis (ringworm), due to *Trichophyton rubrum*, *Trichophyton mentagrophytes*, or *Epidermophyton floccosum* (See DOSAGE AND ADMINISTRATION). Diagnosis of disease should be confirmed either by culture [except *Malassezia furfur* (formerly *Pityrosporum ovale*)] or direct microscopic examination of scrapings from infected tissue mounted in a solution of potassium hydroxide.

CONTRAINDICATIONS

Lamisil® Solution, 1% (terbinafine hydrochloride solution) is contraindicated in individuals who have known or suspected hypersensitivity to terbinafine or any other of its components.

WARNINGS

Lamisil® Solution, 1% (terbinafine hydrochloride solution) is not for ophthalmic, oral, or intravaginal use.

PRECAUTIONS

General: Lamisil® Solution, 1% (terbinafine hydrochloride solution) contains 28.7% alcohol. If irritation or sensitivity develops with the use of Lamisil® Solution, 1% (terbinafine hydrochloride solution) treatment should be discontinued and appropriate therapy instituted.

Lamisil® Solution, 1% (terbinafine hydrochloride solution) may be irritating to the eyes.

Information for Patients: *The patient should be told to:*

1. Use Lamisil® Solution, 1% (terbinafine hydrochloride solution) as directed by the physician and avoid contact with the eyes, nose, mouth, or other mucous membranes. The spray form should not be used on the face. In case of accidental contact with the eyes, rinse eyes thoroughly with running water and consult a physician if any symptoms persist.

2. Apply Lamisil® Solution, 1% (terbinafine hydrochloride solution) once daily for the indications of tinea corporis and tinea cruris, and twice daily for the indications of tinea pedis and tinea (pityriasis) versicolor.

3. Cleanse and dry the affected areas thoroughly before applying Lamisil® Solution. Sufficient solution should be applied to wet the treatment area(s) thoroughly, and to cover the affected skin and surrounding area.

4. Use the medication for the full treatment time (1 week) even though symptoms may have improved.

5. Inform the physician if the area of application shows signs of increased irritation or possible sensitization (redness, itching, burning, blistering, swelling, or oozing).

6. Notify the physician if there is no improvement after one week of treatment.

7. Avoid the use of occlusive dressings unless otherwise directed by the physician.

Drug Interactions: Potential interactions between Lamisil® Solution, 1% (terbinafine hydrochloride solution) and other drugs have not been systematically evaluated.

Carcinogenesis, Mutagenesis, Impairment of Fertility: In a 28-month oral carcinogenicity study in rats, a marginal increase in the incidence of liver tumors was observed in males at the highest dose level, 69 mg/kg/day (in terms of mg/m²/day equivalent to 34 times the maximum potential exposure at the recommended topical human dose*). There was no dose-related trend, and the mid-dose male rats, 20 mg/kg/day (in terms of mg/m²/day equivalent to 10 times the maximum potential exposure at the recommended topical human dose*), did not have any tumors. No increased incidence in liver tumors was noted in female rats at dose levels up to 97 mg/kg/day (in terms of mg/m²/day equivalent to 47 times the maximum potential exposure at the recommended topical human dose*) or in male or female mice treated orally for 23 months at doses up to 156 mg/kg/day (in terms of mg/m²/day equivalent to 38 times the maximum potential exposure at the recommended topical human dose*).

A wide range of oral *in vivo* studies in mice, rats, dogs, and monkeys, and *in vitro* studies using rat, monkey, and human hepatocytes suggest that the development of liver tumors in the high-dose male rats may be associated with peroxisome proliferation and support the conclusion that this is a rat-specific finding.

The results of a variety of *in vitro* (mutations in *E. coli* and *Salmonella*, DNA repair in rat hepatocytes, mutagenicity in Chinese hamster fibroblasts, chromosome aberration and sister chromatid exchanges in Chinese hamster lung cells) and *in vivo* (chromosome aberration in Chinese hamsters, micronucleus test in mice) genotoxicity tests gave no evi-

dence of a mutagenic or clastogenic potential and demonstrated the absence of tumor-initiating or cell-proliferating activity.

Oral reproduction studies in rats at doses up to 300 mg/kg/day (in terms of mg/m²/day equivalent to 146 times the maximum potential exposure at the recommended topical human dose*) did not reveal any specific effects on fertility or other reproductive parameters. Intravaginal application of terbinafine hydrochloride at 150 mg/day (in terms of mg/m²/day equivalent to 165 times the maximum potential exposure at the recommended topical human dose*) in pregnant rabbits did not increase the incidence of abortions, premature deliveries, or fetal abnormalities.

Pregnancy: *Pregnancy Category B:* Oral doses of terbinafine hydrochloride up to 300 mg/kg/day (in terms of mg/m²/day equivalent to 146 and 329 times the maximum potential exposure at the recommended topical human dose*) during organogenesis in rats and rabbits, respectively, were not teratogenic. Similarly, a subcutaneous study in rats at doses up to 100 mg/kg/day (in terms of mg/m²/day equivalent to 49 times the maximum potential exposure at the recommended topical human dose*) and a percutaneous study in rabbits, including doses up to 150 mg/kg/day (in terms of mg/m²/day equivalent to 329 times the maximum potential exposure at the recommended topical human dose*), did not reveal any teratogenic potential. There are, however, no adequate and well-controlled studies in pregnant women. Because animal reproduction studies are not always predictive of human response, Lamisil® Solution, 1% (terbinafine hydrochloride solution) should be used only if clearly indicated during pregnancy.

*The above comparisons between oral animal doses and the maximum potential exposure at the recommended topical human dose are based upon the application to human skin of 0.1 mg of terbinafine/cm² twice daily, the assumption of average human cutaneous exposure of 100 cm² (assuming the use of 1 gram of Lamisil® Solution/dose), and the theoretical maximum human cutaneous absorption of 100%.

Nursing Mothers: After a single oral dose of 500 mg of terbinafine hydrochloride to two volunteers, the total dose of terbinafine secreted in human milk during the 72-hour post-dosing period was 0.65 mg in one person and 0.15 mg in the other. The total excretion of terbinafine in human milk was 0.13% and 0.03% of the administered dose, respectively. This 500 mg dose represents about 50 times the percutaneous exposure as described in the previous paragraph. The concentrations of the N-demethylated metabolite measured in the human milk of these two volunteers were below the detection limit of the assay used (150 ng/mL of milk).

Because of the small amount of data on human neonatal exposure, a decision should be made whether to discontinue nursing or to discontinue the drug, taking into account the importance of the drug to the mother.

Nursing mothers should avoid application of Lamisil® Solution, 1% (terbinafine hydrochloride solution) to the breast.

Pediatric Use: The safety and efficacy of Lamisil® Solution, 1% (terbinafine hydrochloride solution) have not been established in pediatric patients.

ADVERSE REACTIONS

Clinical Trials: In clinical trials, 2 (0.2%) of 898 patients treated with Lamisil® Solution, 1% (terbinafine hydrochloride solution) and 2 (0.6%) of 306 patients treated with placebo (vehicle) discontinued therapy due to adverse events. For Lamisil® Solution-treated patients, adverse reactions thought to be possibly, probably, or definitely related to drug therapy included application site reactions (burning or irritation) (1.3%), itching (1.1%), skin exfoliation (1.0%), and erythematous rash (0.9%).

OVERDOSAGE

Present clinical experience regarding overdose with Lamisil® is limited. Up to 5 grams of terbinafine hydrochloride tablets [equivalent to approximately 17 bottles of Lamisil® Solution, 1% (terbinafine hydrochloride solution)] have been taken without inducing severe or life-threatening adverse reactions. The symptoms of overdose associated with oral terbinafine hydrochloride included nausea, vomiting, abdominal pain, dizziness, rash, urinary frequency, and headache. There has been no experience of overdose with topical formulations of terbinafine. However, the alcohol content (28.7% alcohol) of Lamisil® Solution, 1% (terbinafine hydrochloride solution) has to be taken into account. Terbinafine overdosage in rats and mice by the oral and intravenous routes of drug administration has produced sedation, drowsiness, ataxia, dyspnea, exophthalmus, and piloerection. The majority of deaths in animals occurred following oral administration of doses exceeding 3 g/kg or following 200 mg/kg administered intravenously. In rabbits, overdosage produced erythema, edema, and scale formation following topical administration of doses in excess of 1.5 g/kg.

When 1% terbinafine hydrochloride solution was administered as a single oral dose at 20 or 25 mL/kg (200 and 250 mg/kg, respectively) to rats and mice, no deaths or other drug-related toxicities were observed.

DOSAGE AND ADMINISTRATION

Lamisil® Solution, 1% (terbinafine hydrochloride solution) is applied once or twice daily, depending on the indication. The affected areas should be cleansed and dried thoroughly before applying Lamisil® Solution, 1% (terbinafine hydrochloride solution). Sufficient solution should be applied to wet the treatment area(s) thoroughly, and to cover the affected skin and surrounding area. (See CLINICAL STUDIES)

Duration and Frequency of Treatment:

Tinea (pityriasis) versicolor: 1 week, twice a day
Tinea corporis, cruris: 1 week, once a day
Tinea pedis: 1 week, twice a day

If successful outcome is not achieved during the post treatment period, the diagnosis should be reviewed.

CLINICAL STUDIES

In the majority of patients, relief of signs and symptoms begins within the one week treatment period with continued improvement occurring over a period of 2-7 weeks after treatment has concluded. In the following data presentations, the term "mycological cure" refers to those patients evaluated at a specific timepoint who had negative mycological results [*both* culture and microscopy – except in tinea (pityriasis) versicolor where only microscopy was used]. The term "effective treatment" refers to an outcome with both a mycological cure and a *total* clinical score representing minimal residual signs and symptoms [less than or equal to 1 for tinea (pityriasis) versicolor and less than or equal to 2 for tinea corporis, tinea cruris and tinea pedis with no more than a score of 1 in any sign or symptom]. The clinical score is the sum of the scores for each sign and symptom graded on a scale of 0 = absent, 1 = mild, 2 = moderate, and 3 = severe. All tinea (pityriasis) versicolor studies included clinical evaluation of erythema, desquamation, and pruritus. All tinea pedis, tinea corporis, and tinea cruris studies included clinical evaluation of erythema, desquamation, pruritus, vesicles, encrustation, and pustules. The term "complete cure" refers to a case with both a mycological cure and a total clinical score of 0.

Note: The following tables are extracted from the final reports for each study. The Intent-to-Treat Populations were used to generate these tables where EOT is End-of-Treatment (week 1) and EOS is End-of-Study (week 8 or last visit before leaving study).

A. Tinea (pityriasis) Versicolor: In two studies of Lamisil® Solution, 1% (terbinafine hydrochloride solution), applied twice daily for 1 week in the treatment of tinea (pityriasis) versicolor (Lamisil®: N=173, Vehicle: N=81), the combined efficacy results were as follows:

Response	Therapy	EOT	EOS
Mycological Cure	Lamisil®	50.6%	78.8%
	Vehicle	43.6%	35.8%
Effective Treatment	Lamisil®	39.3%	74.3%
	Vehicle	24.1%	29.6%
Complete Cure	Lamisil®	19.4%	57.6%
	Vehicle	11.4%	27.2%

B. Tinea Pedis: The results of one study of Lamisil® Solution, 1% (terbinafine hydrochloride solution) applied twice daily for 1 week in the treatment of tinea pedis (Lamisil®: N=58, Vehicle: N=28) are shown below. These results were supported by other clinical trials.

Response	Therapy	EOT	EOS
Mycological Cure	Lamisil®	42.9%	87.9%
	Vehicle	14.3%	14.3%
Effective Treatment	Lamisil®	17.9%	65.5%
	Vehicle	3.6%	3.6%
Complete Cure	Lamisil®	1.8%	20.7%
	Vehicle	3.6%	0%

C. Tinea Corporis/Cruris: The results of one study of Lamisil® Solution, 1% (terbinafine hydrochloride solution) applied once daily for 1 week in the treatment of tinea corporis or tinea cruris (Lamisil®: N=72, Vehicle: N=37) are shown below:

Response	Therapy	EOT	EOS
Mycological Cure	Lamisil®	78.3%	84.7%
	Vehicle	11.1%	27.8%
Effective Treatment	Lamisil®	37.7%	70.8%
	Vehicle	0%	11.1%

Lamisil Solution—Cont.

Complete Cure	Lamisil®	5.7%	52.8%
	Vehicle	0%	2.8%

HOW SUPPLIED

Lamisil® Solution, 1% (terbinafine hydrochloride solution) is supplied in a 30 mL pump spray bottle containing 290 mg of terbinafine hydrochloride (NDC 0078-0328-82) with a spray-pump assembly, which will also function upside-down, and protective cap.
Store at 5°C to 25°C (41°F to 77°F); do not refrigerate.

NOVEMBER 1997 30152801

Shown in Product Identification Guide, page 325

LAMISIL® ℞

[la″ mə 'səl]
(terbinafine hydrochloride tablets)
Tablets

Caution: Federal law prohibits dispensing without prescription.

The following prescribing information is based on official labeling in effect on August 1, 1998.

DESCRIPTION

Lamisil® (terbinafine hydrochloride tablets) Tablets contain the synthetic allylamine antifungal compound terbinafine hydrochloride.
Chemically, terbinafine hydrochloride is (E)-*N*-(6,6-dimethyl-2-hepten-4-ynyl)-*N*-methyl-1-naphthalenemethanamine hydrochloride. The empirical formula $C_{21}H_{26}ClN$ with a molecular weight of 327.90, and the following structural formula:

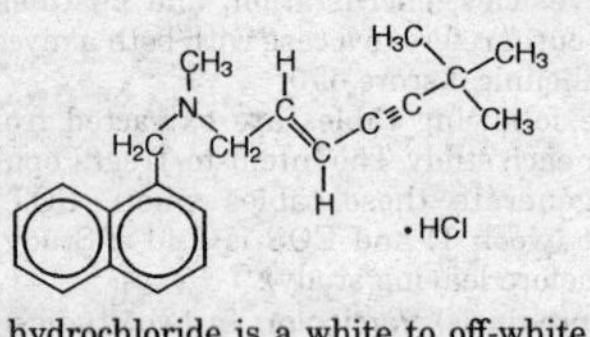

Terbinafine hydrochloride is a white to off-white fine crystalline powder. It is freely soluble in methanol and methylene chloride, soluble in ethanol, and slightly soluble in water.

Each tablet contains:
Active Ingredients: terbinafine hydrochloride (equivalent to 250 mg base)
Inactive Ingredients: colloidal silicon dioxide, NF; hydroxypropyl methylcellulose, USP; magnesium stearate, NF; microcrystalline cellulose, NF; sodium starch glycolate, NF

CLINICAL PHARMACOLOGY

Pharmacokinetics
Following oral administration, terbinafine is well absorbed (>70%) and the bioavailability of Lamisil® (terbinafine hydrochloride tablets) Tablets as a result of first-pass metabolism is approximately 40%. Peak plasma concentrations of 1 µg/mL appear within 2 h after a single 250 mg dose; the AUC (area under the curve) is approximately 4.56 µg·h/mL. An increase in the AUC of terbinafine of less than 20% is observed when Lamisil® is administered with food. No clinically relevant age-dependent changes in steady-state plasma concentrations of terbinafine have been reported. In patients with renal impairment (creatinine clearance ≤50 mL/min) or hepatic cirrhosis, the clearance of terbinafine is decreased by approximately 50% compared to normal volunteers. No effect of gender on the blood levels of terbinafine was detected in clinical trials. In plasma, terbinafine is >99% bound to plasma proteins and there are no specific binding sites. At steady-state, in comparison to a single dose, the peak concentration of terbinafine is 25% higher and plasma AUC increases by a factor of 2.5; the increase in plasma AUC is consistent with an effective half-life of ~36 hours. Terbinafine is distributed to the sebum and skin. A terminal half-life of 200–400 h may represent the slow elimination of terbinafine from tissues such as skin and adipose. Prior to excretion, terbinafine is extensively metabolized. No metabolites have been identified that have antifungal activity similar to terbinafine. Approximately 70% of the administered dose is eliminated in the urine.

Microbiology
Terbinafine hydrochloride is a synthetic allylamine derivative. Terbinafine hydrochloride exerts its antifungal effect by inhibiting squalene epoxidase, a key enzyme in sterol biosynthesis in fungi. This action results in a deficiency in ergosterol and a corresponding accumulation of sterol within the fungal cell. Depending on the concentration of the drug and the fungal species tested *in vitro*, terbinafine hydrochloride may be fungicidal; however, the clinical significance of these data is unknown. *In vitro*, mammalian squalene epoxidase is only inhibited at higher (4,000-fold) concentrations.
Terbinafine has been shown to be active against most strains of the following organisms both *in vitro* and in clinical infections of the nail.

Trichophyton rubrum
Trichophyton mentagrophytes

Blood and tissue levels of terbinafine following oral dosing with Lamisil® 250 mg QD exceed *in vitro* MIC's against most strains of the following organisms which can infect the nail; however, the efficacy of terbinafine in treating nail infections due to these organisms has not been studied in controlled clinical trials.

Epidermophyton floccosum
Microsporum gypseum
Microsporum nanum
Trichophyton verrucosum
Candida albicans
Scopulariopsis brevicaulis

CLINICAL STUDIES

The efficacy of Lamisil® (terbinafine hydrochloride tablets) Tablets in the treatment of onychomycosis is illustrated by the response of patients with toenail and/or fingernail infections who participated in two US/Canadian placebo-controlled clinical trials.
Results of the toenail study, as assessed at week 48 (12 weeks of treatment with 36 weeks follow-up after completion of therapy), demonstrated mycological cure, defined as simultaneous occurrence of negative KOH plus negative culture, in 70% of patients. Fifty-nine percent (59%) of patients experienced effective treatment (mycological cure plus 0% nail involvement or >5mm of new unaffected nail growth); 38% of patients demonstrated mycological cure plus clinical cure (0% nail involvement).
Results of the fingernail study, as assessed at week 24 (6 weeks of treatment with 18 weeks follow-up after completion of therapy), demonstrated mycological cure in 79% of patients, effective treatment in 75% of the patients, and mycological cure plus clinical cure in 59% of the patients.
The mean time to overall success was approximately 10 months for the toenail study and 4 months for the fingernail study. In the toenail study, for patients evaluated at least six months after achieving clinical cure and at least one year after completing Lamisil® therapy, the clinical relapse rate was approximately 15%.

INDICATIONS AND USAGE

Lamisil® (terbinafine hydrochloride tablets) Tablets are indicated for the treatment of onychomycosis of the toenail or fingernail due to dermatophytes (tinea unguium) *(see DOSAGE AND ADMINISTRATION).*

CONTRAINDICATIONS

Lamisil® (terbinafine hydrochloride tablets) Tablets are contraindicated in individuals with hypersensitivity to terbinafine.

WARNINGS

Rare cases of symptomatic hepatobiliary dysfunction including cholestatic hepatitis have been reported. Treatment with Lamisil® (terbinafine hydrochloride tablets) Tablets should be discontinued if hepatobiliary dysfunction develops *(see PRECAUTIONS).* There have been isolated reports of serious skin reactions (e.g., Stevens-Johnson Syndrome and toxic epidermal necrolysis). If progressive skin rash occurs, treatment with Lamisil® should be discontinued.

PRECAUTIONS

General
Changes in the ocular lens and retina have been reported following the use of Lamisil® (terbinafine hydrochloride tablets) Tablets in controlled trials. The clinical significance of these changes is unknown. Hepatic function (hepatic enzyme) tests are recommended in patients administered Lamisil® for more than six weeks or in those who develop unexplained nausea, anorexia, or fatigue *(see WARNINGS).*
In patients with either pre-existing liver disease or renal impairment (creatinine clearance ≤50 mL/min), the use of Lamisil® has not been adequately studied, and therefore, is not recommended *(see CLINICAL PHARMACOLOGY, Pharmacokinetics).*
Transient decreases in absolute lymphocyte counts (ALC) have been observed in controlled clinical trials. In placebo-controlled trials, 8/465 Lamisil®-treated patients (1.7%) and 3/137 placebo-treated patients (2.2%) had decreases in ALC to below 1000/mm^3 on two or more occasions. The clinical significance of this observation is unknown. However, in patients with known or suspected immunodeficiency, physicians should consider monitoring complete blood counts in individuals using Lamisil® therapy for greater than six weeks.
Isolated cases of severe neutropenia have been reported. These were reversible upon discontinuation of Lamisil®, with or without supportive therapy. If clinical signs and symptoms suggestive of secondary infection occur, a complete blood count should be obtained. If the neutrophil count is ≤1,000 cells/mm^3, Lamisil® should be discontinued and supportive management started.

Drug Interactions
In vitro studies with human liver microsomes showed that terbinafine does not inhibit the metabolism of tolbutamide, ethinylestradiol, ethoxycoumarin, and cyclosporine. *In vivo* drug-drug interaction studies conducted in normal volunteer subjects showed that terbinafine does not affect the clearance of antipyrine, digoxin, and the antihistamine terfenadine. Terbinafine does not affect the clearance of warfarin or warfarin's effect on prothrombin time. Terbinafine decreases the clearance of intravenously administered caffeine by 19%. Terbinafine increases the clearance of cyclosporine by 15%.
Terbinafine clearance is increased 100% by rifampin, a CyP450 enzyme inducer, and decreased 33% by cimetidine, a CyP450 enzyme inhibitor. Terbinafine clearance is decreased 16% by terfenadine. Terbinafine clearance is unaffected by cyclosporine.
There is no information available from prospectively conducted drug interaction studies with the following classes of drugs: oral contraceptives, hormone replacement therapies, hypoglycemics, theophyllines, phenytoins, thiazide diuretics, beta blockers, and calcium channel blockers.

Carcinogenesis, Mutagenesis, Impairment of Fertility
In a 28-month oral carcinogenicity study in rats, a marginal increase in the incidence of liver tumors was observed in males at the highest dose level, 69 mg/kg/day [13.8× the maximum recommended human dose (MRHD) based on body weight (BW) and 3.6× the MRHD based on body surface area (BSA)]. There was no dose-related trend and the mid-dose male rats (20 mg/kg/day; 4.0× the MRHD based on BW and 1.0× the MRHD based on BSA) did not have any tumors. No increased incidence in liver tumors was noted in female rats at dose levels up to 97 mg/kg/day (19.4× the MRHD based on BW and 4.5× the MRHD based on BSA) or in male or female mice treated orally for 23 months at doses up to 156 mg/kg/day (31.2× the MRHD based on BW and 3.9× the MRHD based on BSA).
A wide range of *in vivo* studies in mice, rats, dogs, and monkeys, and *in vitro* studies using rat, monkey, and human hepatocytes suggest that the development of liver tumors in the high-dose male rats may be associated with peroxisome proliferation, and support the conclusion that this is a rat-specific finding. *In vivo* investigations included evaluations of the effects of Lamisil® on liver weight, morphology, and ultrastructure; hepatic cytochrome P450; and peroxisome proliferation assessed morphologically and biochemically (peroxisomal enzymes) in mice, rats, dogs, and monkeys. The effects of Lamisil® and two known metabolites on hepatic morphology and peroxisomal and P450 enzyme activities were also evaluated *in vivo* in male rats and *in vitro* in primary hepatocyte cultures from male rats and humans and from monkeys. The results of the *in vivo* investigations indicated that oral administration of Lamisil® (500 mg/kg/day) resulted in peroxisome proliferation in rats, and that these effects did not occur in mice, dogs, or monkeys. Further, *in vitro* studies indicated that peroxisome proliferation occurred in rat hepatocytes, but not in monkey or human hepatocytes.
Systemic exposure to Lamisil®, assessed by the steady-state plasma unbound fraction area under the curve (AUC) for terbinafine and metabolites, was 7.7 and 9.7 µg·h/mL for male and female rats, respectively, and 11.2 and 13.1 µg·h/mL for male and female mice, respectively, at doses comparable to the high doses in the carcinogenicity studies. In human subjects at the MRHD (a daily dose of 250 mg of Lamisil®), the unbound AUC was 0.466 µg·h/mL. The resulting safety margins for humans, based on relative systemic exposure (AUC unbound), in rats and mice were 17 to 21 and 24 to 28, respectively.
The results of a variety of *in vitro* and *in vivo* genotoxicity tests gave no evidence of a mutagenic or clastogenic potential, and demonstrated the absence of tumor-initiating or cell-proliferating activity.
Oral reproduction studies in rats at doses up to 300 mg/kg/day (60× the MRHD based on BW and approximately 12× the MRHD based on BSA) did not reveal any specific effects on fertility or other reproductive parameters. Intravaginal application of terbinafine hydrochloride at 150 mg/day in pregnant rabbits did not increase the incidence of abortions or premature deliveries nor affect fetal parameters.

Pregnancy
Pregnancy Category B: Oral reproduction studies have been performed in rabbits and rats at doses up to 300 mg/kg/day (60× the MRHD based on BW and 9× to 12× the MRHD, in rabbits and rats, respectively, based on BSA) and have revealed no evidence of impaired fertility or harm to the fetus due to terbinafine. There are, however, no adequate and well-controlled studies in pregnant women. Because animal reproduction studies are not always predictive of human response, and because treatment of onychomycosis can be postponed until after pregnancy is completed, it is recommended that Lamisil® not be initiated during pregnancy.

Nursing Mothers
After oral administration, terbinafine is present in breast milk of nursing mothers. The ratio of terbinafine in milk to plasma is 7:1. Treatment with Lamisil® is not recommended in nursing mothers.

Pediatric Use

The safety and efficacy of Lamisil® have not been established in pediatric patients.

ADVERSE REACTIONS

The most frequently reported adverse events observed in the 3 US/Canadian placebo-controlled trials are listed in the table below. The adverse events reported encompass gastrointestinal symptoms (including diarrhea, dyspepsia, and abdominal pain), liver test abnormalities, rashes, urticaria, pruritus, and taste disturbances. In general, the adverse events were mild, transient, and did not lead to discontinuation from study participation.

	Adverse Event		Discontinuation	
	Lamisil® (%) n=465	Placebo (%) n=137	Lamisil® (%) n=465	Placebo (%) n=137
Headache	12.9	9.5	0.2	0.0
Gastrointestinal Symptoms:				
Diarrhea	5.6	2.9	0.6	0.0
Dyspepsia	4.3	2.9	0.4	0.0
Abdominal Pain	2.4	1.5	0.4	0.0
Nausea	2.6	2.9	0.2	0.0
Flatulence	2.2	2.2	0.0	0.0
Dermatological Symptoms:				
Rash	5.6	2.2	0.9	0.7
Pruritus	2.8	1.5	0.2	0.0
Urticaria	1.1	0.0	0.2	0.0
Liver Enzyme Abnormalities*	3.3	1.4	0.2	0.0
Taste Disturbance	2.8	0.7	0.2	0.0
Visual Disturbance	1.1	1.5	0.9	0.0

* Liver enzyme abnormalities $\geq 2\times$ the upper limit of the normal range.

Rare adverse events, based on worldwide experience with Lamisil® (terbinafine hydrochloride tablets) Tablets use, include: symptomatic idiosyncratic hepatobiliary dysfunction (including cholestatic hepatitis) *(see WARNINGS and PRECAUTIONS)*, serious skin reactions *(see WARNINGS)*, severe neutropenia *(see PRECAUTIONS)*, thrombocytopenia and allergic reactions (including anaphylaxis). Rarely, Lamisil® may cause taste disturbance (including taste loss) which usually recovers within several weeks after discontinuation of the drug.
Other adverse reactions which have been reported include malaise, fatigue, vomiting, arthralgia, myalgia, and hair loss.

OVERDOSAGE

Clinical experience regarding overdose with Lamisil® (terbinafine hydrochloride tablets) is limited. Doses up to 5 grams (20 times the therapeutic daily dose) have been taken without inducing serious adverse reactions. The symptoms of overdose included nausea, vomiting, abdominal pain, dizziness, rash, frequent urination, and headache.

DOSAGE AND ADMINISTRATION

Lamisil® (terbinafine hydrochloride tablets) Tablets, one 250 mg tablet, should be taken once daily for 6 weeks by patients with fingernail onychomycosis. Lamisil®, one 250 mg tablet, should be taken once daily for 12 weeks by patients with toenail onychomycosis. The optimal clinical effect is seen some months after mycological cure and cessation of treatment. This is related to the period required for outgrowth of healthy nail.

HOW SUPPLIED

Lamisil®
(terbinafine hydrochloride tablets)
Tablets
Supplied as white to yellow-tinged white circular, bi-convex, bevelled tablets containing 250 mg of terbinafine imprinted with "LAMISIL" in circular form on one side and code "250" on the other.
Bottles of 100 tablets
NDC 0078-0179-05
Bottles of 30 tablets
NDC 0078-0179-15
Store tablets below 25°C (77°F); in a tight container. Protect from light.

REV: OCTOBER 1997   37051904
Shown in Product Identification Guide, page 325

LESCOL®   ℞

[lĕs-cŏl]
(fluvastatin sodium)
Capsules

Caution: Federal law prohibits dispensing without prescription.
The following prescribing information is based on official labeling in effect on September 1, 1998.

DESCRIPTION

Lescol® (fluvastatin sodium) is a water soluble cholesterol lowering agent which acts through the inhibition of 3-hydroxy-3-methylglutaryl-coenzyme A (HMG-CoA) reductase. Fluvastatin sodium is $[R^*,S^*-(E)]-(\pm)$-7-[3-(4-fluorophenyl)-1-(1-methylethyl)-1H-indol-2-yl]-3,5-dihydroxy-6-heptenoic acid, monosodium salt. The structural formula is:

$C_{24}H_{25}FNO_4 \cdot Na$ Mol. wt. 433.46

This molecular entity is the first entirely synthetic HMG-CoA reductase inhibitor, and is in part structurally distinct from the fungal derivatives of this therapeutic class.
Fluvastatin sodium is a white to pale yellow, hygroscopic powder soluble in water, ethanol and methanol. Lescol® (fluvastatin sodium) is supplied as capsules containing fluvastatin sodium, equivalent to 20 mg or 40 mg of fluvastatin, for oral administration.
Active Ingredient: fluvastatin sodium
Inactive Ingredients: gelatin, magnesium stearate, microcrystalline cellulose, pregelatinized starch, red iron oxide, sodium lauryl sulfate, talc, titanium dioxide, yellow iron oxide, and other ingredients.
May Also Include: benzyl alcohol, black iron oxide, butylparaben, carboxymethylcellulose sodium, edetate calcium disodium, methylparaben, propylparaben, silicon dioxide and sodium propionate.

CLINICAL PHARMACOLOGY

A variety of clinical studies have demonstrated that elevated levels of total cholesterol (Total-C), low density lipoprotein cholesterol (LDL-C), and apolipoprotein B (a membrane transport complex for LDL-C) promote human atherosclerosis. Similarly, decreased levels of HDL-cholesterol (HDL-C) and its transport complex, apolipoprotein A, are associated with the development of atherosclerosis. Epidemiologic investigations have established that cardiovascular morbidity and mortality vary directly with the level of Total-C and LDL-C and inversely with the level of HDL-C. In patients with hypercholesterolemia, treatment with Lescol® (fluvastatin sodium) reduced Total-C, LDL-C, and apolipoprotein B. Lescol® (fluvastatin sodium) also moderately reduced triglycerides (TG) while producing an increase in HDL-C of variable magnitude. The agent had no consistent effect on either Lp(a) or fibrinogen. The effect of Lescol® (fluvastatin sodium)-induced changes in lipoprotein levels, including reduction of serum cholesterol, on cardiovascular morbidity or mortality has not been determined.

Mechanism of Action

Lescol® (fluvastatin sodium) is a competitive inhibitor of HMG-CoA reductase, which is responsible for the conversion of 3-hydroxy-3-methylglutaryl-coenzyme A (HMG-CoA) to mevalonate, a precursor of sterols, including cholesterol. The inhibition of cholesterol biosynthesis reduces the cholesterol in hepatic cells, which stimulates the synthesis of LDL receptors and thereby increases the uptake of LDL particles. The end result of these biochemical processes is a reduction of the plasma cholesterol concentration.

Pharmacokinetics/Metabolism

Oral Absorption
Fluvastatin is absorbed rapidly and completely following oral administration, with peak concentrations reached in less than 1 hour. Following administration of a 10 mg dose,

the absolute bioavailability is 24% (range 9%-50%). Administration with food reduces the rate but not the extent of absorption. At steady-state, administration of fluvastatin with the evening meal results in a two-fold decrease in C_{max} and more than two-fold increase in t_{max} as compared to administration 4 hours after the evening meal. No significant difference in extent of absorption or in the lipid-lowering effects were observed between the two administrations. After single or multiple doses above 20 mg, fluvastatin exhibits saturable first-pass metabolism resulting in higher-than-expected plasma fluvastatin concentrations. The inactive enantiomer accounts for about 60% of the increase.

Distribution
Fluvastatin is 98% bound to plasma proteins. The mean volume of distribution (VD_{ss}) is estimated at 34.4 liters. The parent drug is targeted to the liver and no active metabolites are present systemically.

Metabolism
Iuvastatin is metabolized in the liver, primarily via hydroxylation of the indole ring at the 5- and 6-positions. N-dealkylation and beta-oxidation of the side-chain also occurs. The hydroxy metabolites have some pharmacologic activity, but do not circulate in the blood. Both enantiomers of fluvastatin are metabolized in a similar manner.

Elimination
Fluvastatin is primarily (about 90%) eliminated in the feces as metabolites, with less than 2% present as unchanged drug.

Special Populations: Renal Insufficiency:
No significant (<6%) renal excretion of fluvastatin occurs in humans.

Hepatic Insufficiency:
Fluvastatin is subject to saturable first-pass metabolism/sequestration by the liver and is eliminated primarily via the biliary route. Therefore, the potential exists for drug accumulation in patients with hepatic insufficiency. Caution should therefore be exercised when fluvastatin sodium is administered to patients with a history of liver disease or heavy alcohol ingestion *(see WARNINGS)*.

Age: Plasma levels of fluvastatin are not affected by age.

Gender: Women tend to have slightly higher (but statistically insignificant) fluvastatin concentrations than men. This is most likely due to body weight differences, as adjusting for body weight decreases the magnitude of the differences seen.

Pediatric: No data are available. Fluvastatin is not indicated for use in the pediatric population.

Steady-state plasma concentrations show no evidence of accumulation of fluvastatin following administration of up to 80 mg daily, as evidenced by a beta-elimination half-life of less than 3 hours. However, under conditions of maximum rate of absorption (i.e., fasting) systemic exposure to fluvastatin is increased 33% to 53% compared to a single 20 mg or 40 mg dose.

Single-dose and steady-state pharmacokinetic parameters in 33 subjects with hypercholesterolemia are summarized below:
[See table below]

Clinical Studies

Lescol® (fluvastatin sodium) has been studied in 19 controlled studies worldwide for patients with Type IIa or IIb hyperlipoproteinemia. Lescol® (fluvastatin sodium) alone was administered to 2326 patients in daily dose regimens of 20 mg, 40 mg, and 80 mg (40 mg b.i.d.) in trials from 6-36 weeks in duration. In the largest single randomized study with Lescol® (fluvastatin sodium) (n=292), treatment at a dose of 20 mg QPM resulted in a highly significant decrease in LDL-C of 22% after nine weeks of study. In the largest single study (n=210) of patients randomized to 40 mg daily and limited to FH patients, a mean LDL-C reduction of 24% was observed. This effect was observed after 4 weeks of treatment and was maintained during the additional 8 weeks of fluvastatin administration. In the largest single controlled study (N=266) of patients randomized to 80 mg (40 mg b.i.d.) daily, a mean LDL-C reduction of 35% was observed during the initial evaluation period (average of 4 and 8 weeks exposure) and a mean LDL-C reduction of 32%

Continued on next page

	C_{max} (ng/mL) mean±SD (range)	AUC (ng·h/mL) mean±SD (range)	t_{max} (hr) mean±SD (range)	CL/F (L/hr) mean±SD (range)	$t_{1/2}$ (hr) mean±SD (range)
20 mg single dose (n=17)	166±106 (48.9-517)	207±65 (111-288)	0.9±0.4 (0.5-2.0)	107±38.1 (69.5-181)	2.5±1.7 (0.5-6.6)
20 mg b.i.d. (n=17)	200±86 (71.8-366)	275±111 (91.6-467)	1.2±0.9 (0.5-4.0)	87.8±45 (42.8-218)	2.8±1.7 (0.9-6.0)
40 mg single dose (n=16)	273±189 (72.8-812)	456±259 (207-1221)	1.2±0.7 (0.75-3.0)	108±44.7 (32.8-193)	2.7±1.3 (0.8-5.9)
40 mg b.i.d. (n=16)	432±236 (119-990)	697±275 (359-1559)	1.2±0.6 (0.5-2.5)	64.2±21.1 (25.7-111)	2.7±1.3 (0.7-5.0)

Lescol—Cont.

was observed at endpoint (28 weeks exposure). In a long term open-label free titration study, after 96 weeks LDL-C decreases of 25% (20 mg, N=68), 31% (40 mg, N=298), and 34% (80 mg, N=209) were observed. Reductions in Apo B were also seen as a result of treatment with Lescol® (fluvastatin sodium). Small but statistically significant increases in HDL-C and corresponding decreases in TG were also noted. No consistent effect on Lp(a) was found.

Atherosclerosis

In the Lipoprotein and Coronary Atherosclerosis Study (LCAS), the effect of Lescol® (fluvastatin sodium) therapy on coronary atherosclerosis was assessed by quantitative coronary angiography (QCA) in patients with coronary artery disease and mild to moderate hypercholesterolemia (baseline LDL-C range 115–190 mg/dL). In this randomized double-blind, placebo controlled trial, 429 patients were treated with conventional measures (Step 1 AHA Diet) and either Lescol® (fluvastatin sodium) 40 mg/day or placebo. In order to provide treatment to patients receiving placebo with LDL-C levels ≥160 mg/dL at baseline, adjunctive therapy with cholestyramine was added after week 12 to all patients in the study with baseline LDL-C values of ≥160 mg/dL. These baseline levels were present in 25% of the study population. Quantitative coronary angiograms were evaluated at baseline and 2.5 years in 340 (79%) angiographic evaluable patients.

Lescol® (fluvastatin sodium) significantly slowed the progression of coronary atheroclerosis. Compared to placebo, Lescol® (fluvastatin sodium) significantly slowed the progression of lesions as measured by within-patient per-lesion change in minimum lumen diameter (MLD), the primary endpoint (see Figure 1 below), percent diameter stenosis (Figure 2), and the formation of new lesions (13% of all fluvastatin patients versus 22% of all placebo patients). Additionally, a significant difference in favor of Lescol® (fluvastatin sodium) was found between all fluvastatin and all placebo patients in the distribution among the three categories of definite progression, definite regression, and mixed or no change. Beneficial angiographic results (change in MLD) were independent of patients' gender and consistent across a range of baseline LDL-C levels.

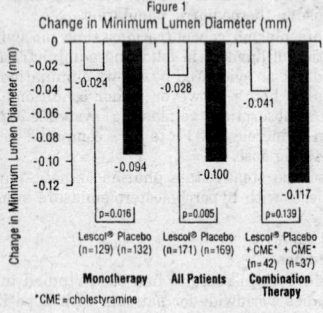

Figure 1
Change in Minimum Lumen Diameter (mm)

*CME = cholestyramine

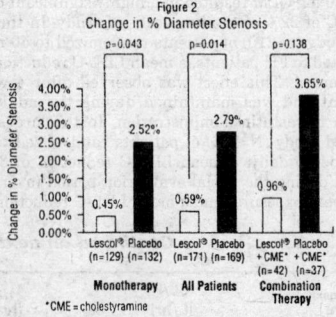

Figure 2
Change in % Diameter Stenosis

*CME = cholestyramine

INDICATIONS AND USAGE

Therapy with lipid-altering agents should be a component of multiple risk factor intervention in those individuals at significantly increased risk for atherosclerosis vascular disease due to hypercholesterolemia. Lescol® (fluvastatin sodium) is indicated as an adjunct to diet in the treatment of elevated total cholesterol (Total-C) and LDL-C levels in patients with primary hypercholesterolemia (Type IIa and IIb) whose response to dietary restriction of saturated fat and cholesterol and other nonpharmacological measures has not been adequate.

Definite Atherosclerotic Disease*	Two or More Other Risk Factors**	LDL-Cholesterol mg/dL (mmol/L) Initiation Level	Goal
NO	NO	≥190 (≥4.9)	<160 (<4.1)
NO	YES	≥160 (≥4.1)	<130 (<3.4)
YES	YES or NO	≥130 (≥3.4)	≤100 (≤2.6)

* Coronary heart disease or peripheral vascular disease (including symptomatic carotid artery disease).
** Other risk factors for coronary heart disease (CHD) include: age (males: ≥45 years; females ≥55 years or premature menopause without estrogen replacement therapy); family history of premature CHD; current cigarette smoking; hypertension; confirmed HDL-C <35 mg/dL (<0.91 mmol/L); and diabetes mellitus. Subtract one risk factor if HDL-C is ≥60 mg/dL (≥1.6 mmol/L).

Lescol® (fluvastatin sodium) is also indicated to slow the progression of coronary atherosclerosis in patients with coronary heart disease as part of a treatment strategy to lower total and LDL cholesterol to target levels.

Therapy with lipid-altering agents should be considered only after secondary causes for hyperlipidemia such as poorly controlled diabetes mellitus, hypothyroidism, nephrotic syndrome, dysproteinemias, obstructive liver disease, other medication, or alcoholism, have been excluded. Prior to initiation of fluvastatin sodium, a lipid profile should be performed to measure Total-C, HDL-C and TG. For patients with TG <400 mg/dL (<4.5 mmol/L). LDL-C can be estimated using the following equation:

$$LDL\text{-}C = Total\text{-}C - HDL\text{-}C - 1/5\ TG$$

For TG levels >400 mg/dL (>4.5 mmol/L), this equation is less accurate and LDL-C concentrations should be determined by ultracentrifugation. In many hypertriglyceridemic patients LDL-C may be low or normal despite elevated Total-C. In such cases, Lescol® (fluvastatin sodium) is not indicated.

Lipid determinations should be performed at intervals of no less than 4 weeks and dosage adjusted according to the patient's response to therapy.

The National Cholesterol Education Program (NCEP) Treatment Guidelines are summarized below:
[See table above]
Since the goal of treatment is to lower LDL-C, the NCEP recommends that the LDL-C levels be used to initiate and assess treatment response. Only if LDL-C levels are not available, should the Total-C be used to monitor therapy.
[See table below]
Lescol® (fluvastatin sodium) has not been studied in conditions where the major abnormality is elevation of chylomicrons, VLDL, or IDL (i.e., hyperlipoproteinemia Types I, III, IV, or V).

CONTRAINDICATIONS

Hypersensitivity to any component of this medication. Lescol® (fluvastatin sodium) is contraindicated in patients with active liver disease or unexplained, persistent elevations in serum transaminases (see WARNINGS).

Pregnancy and Lactation

Atherosclerosis is a chronic process and discontinuation of lipid-lowering drugs during pregnancy should have little impact on the outcome of long-term therapy of primary hypercholesterolemia. Cholesterol and other products of cholesterol biosynthesis are essential components for fetal development (including synthesis of steroids and cell membranes). Since HMG-CoA reductase inhibitors decrease cholesterol synthesis and possibly the synthesis of other biologically active substances derived from cholesterol, they may cause fetal harm when administered to pregnant women. Therefore, HMG-CoA reductase inhibitors are contraindicated during pregnancy and in nursing mothers. **Fluvastatin sodium should be administered to women of childbearing age only when such patients are highly unlikely to conceive and have been informed of the potential hazards.** If the patient becomes pregnant while taking this class of drug, therapy should be discontinued and the patient apprised of the potential hazard to the fetus.

WARNINGS

Liver Enzymes

Biochemical abnormalities of liver function have been associated with HMG-CoA reductase inhibitors and other lipid-lowering agents. A small number of patients treated with Lescol® (fluvastatin sodium) is worldwide controlled trials (N=25, 1.1%) developed dose-related, persistent elevations of transaminase levels to more than 3 times the upper limit of normal. Fourteen of these patients (0.6%) were discontinued from therapy. In all clinical trials, a total of 33/2969 patients (1.1%) had persistent transaminase elevations with an average fluvastatin exposure of approximately 71.2 weeks; 19 of these patients (0.6%) were discontinued. The majority of patients with these abnormal biochemical findings were asymptomatic.

It is recommended that liver function tests be performed before the initiation of treatment, at 6 and 12 weeks after initiation of therapy or elevation in dose, and periodically thereafter (e.g., semiannually). Liver enzyme changes generally occur in the first 3 months of treatment with Lescol® (fluvastatin sodium). Patients who develop increased transaminase levels should be monitored with a second liver function evaluation to confirm the finding and be followed thereafter with frequent liver function tests until the abnormality(ies) return to normal. Should an increase in AST or ALT of three times the upper limit of normal or greater persist, withdrawal of fluvastatin sodium therapy is recommended.

Active liver disease or unexplained transaminase elevations are contraindications to the use of Lescol® (fluvastatin sodium) (see CONTRAINDICATIONS). Caution should be exercised when fluvastatin sodium is administered to patients with a history of liver disease or heavy alcohol ingestion (see CLINICAL PHARMACOLOGY: Pharmacokinetics/Metabolism). Such patients should be closely monitored.

Skeletal Muscle: Rhabdomyolysis with renal dysfunction secondary to myoglobinuria has been reported with fluvastatin and with other drugs in this class. Myopathy, defined as muscle aching or muscle weakness in conjunction with increases in creatine phosphokinase (CPK) values to greater than 10 times the upper limit of normal, has been reported rarely.

Myopathy should be considered in any patients with diffuse myalgias, muscle tenderness or weakness, and/or marked elevation of CPK. Patients should be advised to report promptly unexplained muscle pain, tenderness or weakness, particularly if accompanied by malaise or fever. Fluvastatin sodium therapy should be discontinued if markedly elevated CPK levels occur or myopathy is diagnosed or suspected. Fluvastatin sodium therapy should also be temporarily withheld in any patient experiencing an acute or serious condition predisposing to the development of renal failure secondary to rhabdomyolysis, e.g., sepsis; hypotension; major surgery; trauma; severe metabolic, endocrine, or electrolyte disorders; or uncontrolled epilepsy.

The risk of myopathy and or rhabdomyolysis during treatment with HMG-CoA reductase inhibitors has been reported to be increased if therapy with either cyclosporine,

Classification of Hyperlipoproteinemias

Type	Lipoproteins Elevated	Lipid Elevations Major	Minor
I (rare)	Chylomicrons	TG	↑ → C
IIa	LDL	C	—
IIb	LDL, VLDL	C	TG
III (rare)	IDL	C/TG	—
IV	VLDL	TG	↑ → C
V (rare	Chylomicrons, VLDL	TG	↑ → C

C = cholesterol, TG = triglycerides, LDL = low density lipoprotein, VLDL = very low density lipoprotein, IDL = intermediate density lipoprotein

gemfibrozil, erythromycin, or niacin is administered concurrently. Myopathy was not observed in a clinical trial in 74 patients involving patients who were treated with fluvastatin sodium together with niacin.

Uncomplicated myalgia has been observed infrequently in patients treated with Lescol® (fluvastatin sodium) at rates indistinguishable from placebo.

The use of fibrates alone may occassionally be associated with myopathy. The combined use of HMG-CoA reductase inhibitors and fibrates should generally be avoided.

PRECAUTIONS

General

Before instituting therapy with Lescol® (fluvastatin sodium), an attempt should be made to control hypercholesterolemia with appropriate diet, exercise, and weight reduction in obese patients, and to treat other underlying medical problems *(see INDICATIONS AND USAGE)*.

The HMG-CoA reductase inhibitors may cause elevation of creatine phosphokinase and transaminase levels *(see WARNINGS and ADVERSE REACTIONS)*. This should be considered in the differential diagnosis of chest pain in a patient on therapy with fluvastatin sodium.

Homozygous Familial Hypercholesterolemia

HMG-CoA reductase inhibitors are reported to be less effective in patients with rare homozygous familial hypercholesterolemia, possibly because these patients have few functional LDL receptors.

Information for Patients

Patients should be advised to report promptly unexplained muscle pain, tenderness or weakness, particularly if accompanied by malaise or fever.

Women should be informed that if they become pregnant while receiving Lescol® (fluvastatin sodium) the drug should be discontinued immediately to avoid possible harmful effects on a developing fetus from a relative deficit of cholesterol and biological products derived from cholesterol. In addition, Lescol® (fluvastatin sodium) should not be taken during nursing. *(See CONTRAINDICATIONS)*

Drug Interactions

Immunosuppressive Drugs, Gemfibrozil, Niacin (Nicotinic Acid), Erythromycin: *See WARNINGS: Skeletal Muscle.*

Antipyrine: Administration of fluvastatin sodium does not influence the metabolism and excretion of antipyrine, either by induction or inhibition. Antipyrine is a model for drugs metabolized by the microsomal hepatic enzyme system; therefore, interactions with other drugs metabolized by this mechanism are not expected.

Niacin/Propranolol: Concomitant administration of fluvastatin sodium with niacin or propranolol has no effect on the bioavailability of fluvastatin sodium.

Cholestyramine: Administration of fluvastatin sodium concomitantly with, or up to 4 hours after cholestyramine, results in fluvastatin decreases of more than 50% for AUC and 50%-80% for C_{max}. However, administration of fluvastatin sodium 4 hours after cholestyramine resulted in a clinically significant additive effect compared with that achieved with either component drug.

Digoxin: In a crossover study involving 18 patients chronically receiving digoxin, a single 40 mg dose of fluvastatin had no effect on digoxin AUC, but had an 11% increase in digoxin C_{max} and small increase in digoxin urinary clearance. Patients taking digoxin should be monitored appropriately when fluvastatin therapy is initiated.

Cimetidine/Ranitidine/Omeprazole: Concomitant administration of fluvastatin sodium with cimetidine, ranitidine and omeprazole results in a significant increase in the fluvastatin C_{max} (43%, 70% and 50%, respectively) and AUC (24%-33%), with an 18%-23% decrease in plasma clearance.

Rifampicin: Administration of fluvastatin sodium to subjects pretreated with rifampicin results in significant reduction in C_{max} (59%) and AUC (51%), with a large increase (95%) in plasma clearance.

Warfarin: *In vitro* protein binding studies demonstrated no interaction at therapeutic concentrations. Concomitant administration of a single dose of warfarin (30 mg) in young healthy males receiving fluvastatin sodium (40 mg/day × 8 days) resulted in no elevation of racemic warfarin concentration. There was also no effect on prothrombin complex activity when compared to concomitant administration of placebo and warfarin. However, bleeding and/or increased prothrombin times have been reported in patients taking coumarin anticoagulants concomitantly with other HMG-CoA reductase inhibitors. Therefore, patients receiving warfarin-type anticoagulants should have their prothrombin times closely monitored when fluvastatin sodium is initiated or the dosage of fluvastatin sodium is changed.

Endocrine Function: HMG-CoA reductase inhibitors interfere with cholesterol synthesis and lower circulating cholesterol levels and, as such, might theoretically blunt adrenal or gonadal steroid hormone production.

Fluvastatin exhibited no effect upon non-stimulated cortisol levels and demonstrated no effect upon thyroid metabolism as assessed by TSH. Small declines in total testosterone have been noted in treated groups, but no commensurate elevation in LH occurred, suggesting that the observation was not due to a direct effect upon testosterone production. No effect upon FSH in males was noted. Due to the limited number of premenopausal females studied to date, no conclusions regarding the effect of fluvastatin upon female sex hormones may be made.

Two clinical studies in patients receiving fluvastatin at doses up to 80 mg daily for periods of 24 to 28 weeks demonstrated no effect of treatment upon the adrenal response to ACTH stimulation. A clinical study evaluated the effect of fluvastatin at doses up to 80 mg daily for 28 weeks upon the gonadal response to HCG stimulation. Although the mean total testosterone response was significantly reduced ($p<0.05$) relative to baseline in the 80 mg group, it was not significant in comparison to the changes noted in groups receiving either 40 mg of fluvastatin or placebo.

Patients treated with fluvastatin sodium who develop clinical evidence of endocrine dysfunction should be evaluated appropriately. Caution should be exercised if an HMG-CoA reductase inhibitor or other agent used to lower cholesterol levels is administered to patients receiving other drugs (e.g., ketoconazole, spironolactone, or cimetidine) that may decrease the levels of endogenous steroid hormones.

CNS Toxicity

CNS effects, as evidenced by decreased activity, ataxia, loss of righting reflex, and ptosis were seen in the following animal studies: the 18-month mouse carcinogenicity study at 50 mg/kg/day, the 6-month dog study at 36 mg/kg/day, the 6-month hamster study at 40 mg/kg/day, and in acute, high-dose studies in rats and hamsters (50 mg/kg), rabbits (300 mg/kg) and mice (1500 mg/kg). CNS toxicity in the acute high-dose studies was characterized (in mice) by conspicuous vacuolation in the ventral white columns of the spinal cord at a dose of 5000 mg/kg and (in rat) by edema with separation of myelinated fibers of the ventral spinal tracts and sciatic nerve at a dose of 1500 mg/kg. CNS toxicity, characterized by periaxonal vacuolation, was observed in the medulla of dogs that died after treatment for 5 weeks with 48 mg/kg/day; this finding was not observed in the remaining dogs when the dose level was lowered to 36 mg/kg/day. CNS vascular lesions, characterized by perivascular hemorrhages, edema, and mononuclear cell infiltration of perivascular spaces, have been observed in dogs treated with other members of this class. No CNS lesions have been observed after chronic treatment for up to 2 years with fluvastatin in the mouse (at doses up to 350 mg/kg/day), rat (up to 24 mg/kg/day), or dog (up to 16 mg/kg/day).

Prominent bilateral posterior Y suture lines in the ocular lens were seen in dogs after treatment with 1, 8, and 16 mg/kg/day for 2 years.

Carcinogenesis, Mutagenesis, Impairment of Fertility

A 2-year study was performed in rats at dose levels of 6, 9, and 18-24 (escalated after 1 year) mg/kg/day. These treatment levels represented plasma drug levels of approximately 9, 13, and 26-35 times the mean human plasma drug concentration after a 40 mg oral dose. A low incidence of forestomach squamous papillomas and 1 carcinoma of the forestomach at the 24 mg/kg/day dose level was considered to reflect the prolonged hyperplasia induced by direct contact exposure to fluvastatin sodium rather than to a systemic effect of the drug. In addition, an increased incidence of thyroid follicular cell adenomas and carcinomas was recorded for males treated with 18-24 mg/kg/day. The increased incidence of thyroid follicular cell neoplasm in male rats with fluvastatin sodium appears to be consistent with findings from other HMG-CoA reductase inhibitors. In contrast to other HMG-CoA reductase inhibitors, no hepatic adenomas or carcinomas were observed.

The carcinogenicity study conducted in mice at dose levels of 0.3, 15 and 30 mg/kg/day revealed, as in rats, a statistically significant increase in forestomach squamous cell papillomas in males and females at 30 mg/kg/day and in females at 15 mg/kg/day. These treatment levels represented plasma drug levels of approximately 0.05, 2, and 7 times the mean human plasma drug concentration after a 40 mg oral dose.

No evidence of mutagenicity was observed *in vitro*, with or without rat-liver metabolic activation, in the following studies: microbial mutagen tests using mutant strains of *Salmonella typhimurium* or *Escherichia coli;* malignant transformation assay in BALB/3T3 cells; unscheduled DNA synthesis in rat primary hepatocytes; chromosomal aberrations in V79 Chinese Hamster cells; HGPRT V79 Chinese Hamster cells. In addition, there was no evidence of mutagenicity *in vivo* in either a rat or mouse micronucleus test.

In a study in rats at dose levels for females of 0.6, 2 and 6 mg/kg/day and at dose levels for males of 2, 10 and 20 mg/kg/day, fluvastatin sodium had no adverse effects on the fertility or reproductive performance.

Seminal vesicles and testes were small in hamsters treated for 3 months at 20 mg/kg/day (approximately three times the 40 milligram human daily dose based on surface area, mg/m^2). There was tubular degeneration and aspermatogenesis in testes as well as vesiculitis of seminal vesicles. Vesiculitis of seminal vesicles and edema of the testes were also seen in rats treated for 2 years at 18 mg/kg/day (approximately 4 times the human C_{max} achieved with a 40 milligram daily dose).

Pregnancy

Pregnancy Category X

See CONTRAINDICATIONS.

Fluvastatin sodium produced delays in skeletal development in rats at doses of 12 mg/kg/day and in rabbits at doses of 10 mg/kg/day. Malaligned thoracic vertebrae were seen in rats at 36 mg/kg, a dose that produced maternal toxicity. These doses resulted in 2 times (rat at 12 mg/kg) or 5 times (rabbit at 10 mg/kg) the 40 mg human exposure based on mg/m^2 surface area. A study in which female rats were dosed during the third trimester at 12 and 24 mg/kg/day resulted in maternal mortality at or near term and postpartum. In addition, fetal and neonatal lethality were apparent. No effects on the dam or fetus occurred at 2 mg/kg/day. A second study at levels of 2, 6, 12 and 24 mg/kg/day confirmed the findings in the first study with neonatal mortality beginning at 6 mg/kg. A modified Segment III study was performed at dose levels of 12 or 24 mg/kg/day with or

Continued on next page

Adverse Event	Lescol® (fluvastatin sodium) (%) (N=2326)	Placebo (%) (N=960)
Integumentary		
Rash	2.3	2.4
Musculoskeletal		
Back Pain	5.7	6.6
Myalgia	5.0	4.5
Arthralgia	4.0	4.1
Arthritis	2.1	2.0
Respiratory		
Upper Respiratory Tract Infection	16.2	16.5
Pharyngitis	3.8	3.8
Rhinitis	4.7	4.9
Sinusitis	2.6	1.9
Coughing	2.4	2.9
Gastrointestinal		
Dyspepsia	7.9	3.2
Diarrhea	4.9	4.2
Abdominal Pain	4.9	3.8
Nausea	3.2	2.0
Constipation	3.1	3.3
Flatulence	2.6	2.5
Misc. Tooth Disorder	2.1	1.7
Central Nervous System		
Dizziness	2.2	2.5
Psychiatric Disorders		
Insomnia	2.7	1.4
Miscellaneous		
Headache	8.9	7.8
Influenza-Like Symptoms	5.1	5.7
Accidental Trauma	5.1	4.8
Fatigue	2.7	2.3
Allergy	2.3	2.2

Lescol—Cont.

without the presence of concurrent supplementation with mevalonic acid, a product of HMG-CoA reductase which is essential for cholesterol biosynthesis. The concurrent administration of mevalonic acid completely prevented the maternal and neonatal mortality but did not prevent low body weights in pups at 24 mg/kg on days 0 and 7 postpartum. Therefore, the maternal and neonatal lethality observed with fluvastatin sodium reflect its exaggerated pharmacologic effect during pregnancy. There are no data with fluvastatin sodium in pregnant women. However, rare reports of congenital anomalies have been received following intrauterine exposure to other HMG-CoA reductase inhibitors. There has been one report of severe congenital bony deformity, tracheo-esophageal fistula, and anal atresia (VATER association) in a baby born to a woman who took another HMG-CoA reductase inhibitor with dextroamphetamine sulfate during the first trimester of pregnancy. **Lescol® (fluvastatin sodium) should be administered to women of child-bearing potential only when such patients are highly unlikely to conceive and have been informed of the potential hazards.** If a woman becomes pregnant while taking Lescol® (fluvastatin sodium), the drug should be discontinued and the patient advised again as to the potential hazards to the fetus.

Nursing Mothers

Based on preclinical data, drug is present in breast milk in a 2:1 ratio (milk:plasma). Because of the potential for serious adverse reactions in nursing infants, nursing women should not take Lescol® (fluvastatin sodium) *(see CONTRAINDICATIONS).*

Pediatric Use

Safety and effectiveness in individuals less than 18 years old have not been established. Treatment in patients less than 18 years of age is not recommended at this time.

Geriatric Use

The effect of age on the pharmacokinetics of fluvastatin sodium was evaluated. Results indicate that for the general patient population plasma concentrations of fluvastatin sodium do not vary either as a function of age or gender. *(See also CLINICAL PHARMACOLOGY: Pharmacokinetics/Metabolism.)* Elderly patients (≥65 years of age) demonstrated a greater treatment response in respect to LDL-C, Total-C and LDL/HDL ratio than patients <65 years of age.

ADVERSE REACTIONS

In all clinical studies, 1.0% (32/2969) of fluvastatin treated patients were discontinued due to adverse experiences attributed to study drug (mean exposure approximately 16 months ranging in duration from 1 to >36 months). This results in controlled studies in an exposure adjusted rate of 0.8% (32/4051) per patient year in fluvastatin patients compared to an incidence of 1.1% (4/355) in placebo patients. Adverse reactions have usually been of mild to moderate severity.

Adverse experiences occurring in controlled studies with a frequency >2% regardless of causality include the following: [See table at bottom of previous page]

The following effects have been reported with drugs in this class. Not all the effects listed below have necessarily been associated with fluvastatin sodium therapy.

Skeletal: muscle cramps, myalgia, myopathy, rhabdomyolysis, arthralgias.

Neurological: dysfunction of certain cranial nerves (including alteration of taste, impairment of extra-ocular movement, facial paresis), tremor, dizziness vertigo, memory loss, paresthesia, peripheral neuropathy, peripheral nerve palsy, psychic disturbances, anxiety, insomnia, depression.

Hypersensitivity Reactions: An apparent hypersensitivity syndrome has been reported rarely which has included one or more of the following features: anaphylaxis, angioedema, lupus erythematosus-like syndrome, polymyalgia rheumatica, vasculitis, purpura, thrombocytopenia, leukopenia, hemolytic anemia, positive ANA, ESR increase, eosinophilia, arthritis, arthralgia, urticaria, asthenia, photosensitivity, fever, chills, flushing, malaise, dyspnea, toxic epidermal necrolysis, erythema multiforme, including Stevens-Johnson syndrome.

Gastrointestinal: pancreatitis, hepatitis, including chronic active hepatitis, cholestatic jaundice, fatty change in liver, and, rarely, cirrhosis, fulminant hepatic necrosis, and hepatoma; anorexia, vomiting.

Skin: alopecia, pruritus. A variety of skin changes (e.g., nodules, discoloration, dryness of skin/mucous membranes, changes to hair/nails) have been reported.

Reproductive: gynecomastia, loss of libido, erectile dysfunction.

Eye: progression of cataracts (lens opacities), ophthalmoplegia.

Laboratory Abnormalities: elevated transaminases, alkaline phosphatase, γ-glutamyl transpeptidase, and bilirubin; thyroid function abnormalities.

Concomitant Therapy

Fluvastatin sodium has been administered concurrently with cholestyramine and nicotinic acid. No adverse reactions unique to the combination or in addition to those previously reported for this class of drugs alone have been reported. Myopathy and rhabdomyolysis (with or without acute renal failure) have been reported when another HMG-CoA reductase inhibitor was used in combination with immunosuppressive drugs, gemfibrozil, erythromycin, or lipid-lowering doses of nicotinic acid. Concomitant therapy with HMG-CoA reductase inhibitors and these agents is generally not recommended. *(See WARNINGS: Skeletal Muscle.)*

OVERDOSAGE

The approximate oral LD_{50} is greater than 2 g/kg in mice and greater than 0.7 g/kg in rats.

The maximum single oral dose received by healthy volunteers was 60 mg. No clinically significant adverse experiences were seen at this dose. There has been a single report of 2 children, one 2 years old and the other 3 years of age, either of whom may have possibly ingested fluvastatin sodium. The maximum amount of fluvastatin sodium that could have been ingested was 80 mg (4 × 20 mg capsules). Vomiting was induced by ipecac in both children and no capsules were noted in their emesis. Neither child experienced any adverse symptoms and both recovered from the incident without problems.

Should an accidental overdose occur, treat symptomatically and institute supportive measures as required. The dialyzability of fluvastatin sodium and of its metabolites in humans is not known at present.

Information about the treatment of overdose can often be obtained from a certified Regional Poison Control Center. Telephone numbers of certified Regional Poison Control Centers are listed in the Physicians' Desk Reference®.*

DOSAGE AND ADMINISTRATION

The patient should be placed on a standard cholesterol-lowering diet before receiving Lescol® (fluvastatin sodium) and should continue on this diet during treatment with Lescol® (fluvastatin sodium). (See NCEP Treatment Guidelines for details on dietary therapy.)

The recommended starting dose for the majority of patients is 20-40 mg once daily at bedtime. The recommended dosing range is 20-80 mg/day. The daily regimen of 80 mg should be administered in divided doses, i.e., 40 mg b.i.d., and should be reserved for those whose LDL-cholesterol response is inadequate at 40 mg/day. Lescol® (fluvastatin sodium) may be taken without regard to meals, since there are no apparent differences in the lipid-lowering effects of fluvastatin sodium administered with the evening meal or 4 hours after the evening meal. Since the maximal reductions in LDL-C of a given dose are seen within 4 weeks, periodic lipid determinations should be performed and dosage adjustment made according to the patient's response to therapy and established treatment guidelines. The therapeutic effect of Lescol® (fluvastatin sodium) is maintained with prolonged administration.

Concomitant Therapy

Lipid-lowering effects on total cholesterol and LDL cholesterol are additive when Lescol® (fluvastatin sodium) is combined with a bile-acid binding resin or niacin. When administering a bile-acid resin (e.g., cholestyramine) and fluvastatin sodium, Lescol® (fluvastatin sodium) should be administered at bedtime, at least 2 hours following the resin to avoid a significant interaction due to drug binding to resin. *(See also ADVERSE REACTIONS: Concomitant Therapy.)*

Dosage in Patients with Renal Insufficiency

Since fluvastatin sodium is cleared hepatically with less than 6% of the administered dose excreted into the urine, dose adjustments for mild to moderate renal impairment are not necessary. Caution should be exercised with severe impairment.

HOW SUPPLIED

Lescol® (fluvastatin sodium) Capsules

20 mg

Brown and light brown imprinted twice with "S" and "20" on one half and "LESCOL" and the Lescol® (fluvastatin sodium) logo twice on the other half of the capsule.

Bottles of 30 capsules (NDC 0078-0176-15)

Bottles of 100 capsules (NDC 0078-0176-05)

40 mg

Brown and gold imprinted twice with "S" and "40" on one half and "LESCOL" and the Lescol® (fluvastatin sodium) logo twice on the other half of the capsule.

Bottles of 30 capsules (NDC 0078-0234-15)

Bottles of 100 capsules (NDC 0078-0234-05)

Store and Dispense

Below 86°F (30°C) in a tight container. Protect from light.

*Trademark of Medical Economics Company, Inc.

REV: SEPTEMBER 1998 30753908

Shown in Product Identification Guide, page 325

LOPRESSOR® ℞

[*lō-prēs-ōr*]

metoprolol tartrate tablets, USP

metoprolol tartrate injection, USP

Caution: Federal law prohibits dispensing without prescription.

The following prescribing information is based on official labeling in effect on October 1, 1998.

DESCRIPTION

Lopressor, metoprolol tartrate, is a selective $beta_1$-adrenoreceptor blocking agent, available as 50- and 100-mg tablets for oral administration and in 5-ml ampuls for intravenous administration. Each ampul contains a sterile solution of metoprolol tartrate USP, 5 mg, and sodium chloride USP, 45 mg. Metoprolol tartrate is (±)-1-(isopropylamino)-3-[*p*-(2-methoxyethyl)phenoxy]-2-propanol (2:1) *dextro*-tartrate salt, and its structural formula is

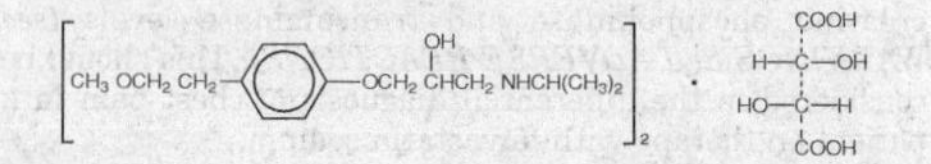
CH3 OCH2 CH2
OH
OCH2 CHCH2 NHCH(CH3)2
2
COOH
H—C—OH
HO—C—H
COOH

Metoprolol tartrate is a white, practically odorless, crystalline powder with a molecular weight of 684.82. It is very soluble in water; freely soluble in methylene chloride, in chloroform, and in alcohol; slightly soluble in acetone; and insoluble in ether.

Inactive Ingredients. Tablets contain cellulose compounds, colloidal silicon dioxide, D&C Red No. 30 aluminum lake (50-mg tablets), FD&C Blue No. 2 aluminum lake (100-mg tablets), lactose, magnesium stearate, polyethylene glycol, propylene glycol, povidone, sodium starch glycolate, talc, and titanium dioxide.

CLINICAL PHARMACOLOGY

Lopressor is a beta-adrenergic receptor blocking agent. In vitro and in vivo animal studies have shown that it has a preferential effect on $beta_1$ adrenoreceptors, chiefly located in cardiac muscle. This preferential effect is not absolute, however, and at higher doses, Lopressor also inhibits $beta_2$ adrenoreceptors, chiefly located in the bronchial and vascular musculature.

Clinical pharmacology studies have confirmed the beta-blocking activity of metoprolol in man, as shown by (1) reduction in heart rate and cardiac output at rest and upon exercise, (2) reduction of systolic blood pressure upon exercise, (3) inhibition of isoproterenol-induced tachycardia, and (4) reduction of reflex orthostatic tachycardia.

Relative $beta_1$ selectivity has been confirmed by the following: (1) In normal subjects, Lopressor is unable to reverse the $beta_2$ -mediated vasodilating effects of epinephrine. This contrasts with the effect of nonselective ($beta_1$ plus $beta_2$) beta blockers, which completely reverse the vasodilating effects of epinephrine. (2) In asthmatic patients, Lopressor reduces FEV_1 and FVC significantly less than a nonselective beta blocker, propranolol, at equivalent $beta_1$-receptor blocking doses.

Lopressor has no intrinsic sympathomimetic activity, and membrane-stabilizing activity is detectable only at doses much greater than required for beta blockade. Lopressor crosses the blood-brain barrier and has been reported in the CSF in a concentration 78% of the simultaneous plasma concentration. Animal and human experiments indicate that Lopressor slows the sinus rate and decreases AV nodal conduction.

In controlled clinical studies, Lopressor has been shown to be an effective antihypertensive agent when used alone or as concomitant therapy with thiazide-type diuretics, at dosages of 100-450 mg daily. In controlled, comparative, clinical studies, Lopressor has been shown to be as effective an antihypertensive agent as propranolol, methyldopa, and thiazide-type diuretics, and to be equally effective in supine and standing positions.

The mechanism of the antihypertensive effects of beta-blocking agents has not been elucidated. However, several possible mechanisms have been proposed: (1) competitive antagonism of catecholamines at peripheral (especially cardiac) adrenergic neuron sites, leading to decreased cardiac output; (2) a central effect leading to reduced sympathetic outflow to the periphery; and (3) suppression of renin activity.

By blocking catecholamine-induced increases in heart rate, in velocity and extent of myocardial contraction, and in blood pressure, Lopressor reduces the oxygen requirements of the heart at any given level of effort, thus making it useful in the long-term management of angina pectoris. However, in patients with heart failure, beta-adrenergic blockade may increase oxygen requirements by increasing left ventricular fiber length and end-diastolic pressure.

Although beta-adrenergic receptor blockade is useful in the treatment of angina and hypertension, there are situations in which sympathetic stimulation is vital. In patients with severely damaged hearts, adequate ventricular function may depend on sympathetic drive. In the presence of AV block, beta blockade may prevent the necessary facili-

tating effect of sympathetic activity on conduction. Beta$_2$-adrenergic blockade results in passive bronchial constriction by interfering with endogenous adrenergic bronchodilator activity in patients subject to bronchospasm and may also interfere with exogenous bronchodilators in such patients.

In controlled clinical trials, Lopressor, administered two or four times daily, has been shown to be an effective antianginal agent, reducing the number of angina attacks and increasing exercise tolerance. The dosage used in these studies ranged from 100-400 mg daily. A controlled, comparative, clinical trial showed that Lopressor was indistinguishable from propranolol in the treatment of angina pectoris.

In a large (1,395 patients randomized), double-blind, placebo-controlled clinical study, Lopressor was shown to reduce 3-month mortality by 36% in patients with suspected or definite myocardial infarction.

Patients were randomized and treated as soon as possible after their arrival in the hospital, once their clinical condition had stabilized and their hemodynamic status had been carefully evaluated. Subjects were ineligible if they had hypotension, bradycardia, peripheral signs of shock, and/or more than minimal basal rales as signs of congestive heart failure. Initial treatment consisted of intravenous followed by oral administration of Lopressor or placebo, given in a coronary care or comparable unit. Oral maintenance therapy with Lopressor or placebo was then continued for 3 months. After this double-blind period, all patients were given Lopressor and followed up to 1 year.

The median delay from the onset of symptoms to the initiation of therapy was 8 hours in both the Lopressor and placebo treatment groups. Among patients treated with Lopressor, there were comparable reductions in 3-month mortality for those treated early ($\leq$ 8 hours) and those in whom treatment was started later. Significant reductions in the incidence of ventricular fibrillation and in chest pain following initial intravenous therapy were also observed with Lopressor and were independent of the interval between onset of symptoms and initiation of therapy.

The precise mechanism of action of Lopressor in patients with suspected or definite myocardial infarction is not known.

In this study, patients treated with metoprolol received the drug both very early (intravenously) and during a subsequent 3-month period, while placebo patients received no beta-blocker treatment for this period. The study thus was able to show a benefit from the overall metoprolol regimen but cannot separate the benefit of very early intravenous treatment from the benefit of later beta-blocker therapy. Nonetheless, because the overall regimen showed a clear beneficial effect on survival without evidence of an early adverse effect on survival, one acceptable dosage regimen is the precise regimen used in the trial. Because the specific benefit of very early treatment remains to be defined however, it is also reasonable to administer the drug orally to patients at a later time as is recommended for certain other beta blockers.

Pharmacokinetics

In man, absorption of Lopressor is rapid and complete. Plasma levels following oral administration, however, approximate 50% of levels following intravenous administration, indicating about 50% first-pass metabolism.

Plasma levels achieved are highly variable after oral administration. Only a small fraction of the drug (about 12%) is bound to human serum albumin. Elimination is mainly by biotransformation in the liver, and the plasma half-life ranges from approximately 3-7 hours. Less than 5% of an oral dose of Lopressor is recovered unchanged in the urine; the rest is excreted by the kidneys as metabolites that appear to have no clinical significance. The systemic availability and half-life of Lopressor in patients with renal failure do not differ to a clinically significant degree from those in normal subjects. Consequently, no reduction in dosage is usually needed in patients with chronic renal failure.

Significant beta-blocking effect (as measured by reduction of exercise heart rate) occurs within 1 hour after oral administration, and its duration is dose-related. For example, a 50% reduction of the maximum registered effect after single oral doses of 20, 50, and 100 mg occurred at 3.3, 5.0, and 6.4 hours, respectively, in normal subjects. After repeated oral dosages of 100 mg twice daily, a significant reduction in exercise systolic blood pressure was evident at 12 hours. Following intravenous administration of Lopressor, the urinary recovery of unchanged drug is approximately 10%. When the drug was infused over a 10-minute period, in normal volunteers, maximum beta blockade was achieved at approximately 20 minutes. Doses of 5 mg and 15 mg yielded a maximal reduction in exercise-induced heart rate of approximately 10% and 15%, respectively. The effect on exercise heart rate decreased linearly with time at the same rate for both doses, and disappeared at approximately 5 hours and 8 hours for the 5-mg and 15-mg doses, respectively.

Equivalent maximal beta-blocking effect is achieved with oral and intravenous doses in the ratio of approximately 2.5:1.

There is a linear relationship between the log of plasma levels and reduction of exercise heart rate. However, antihypertensive activity does not appear to be related to plasma levels. Because of variable plasma levels attained with a given dose and lack of a consistent relationship of antihypertensive activity to dose, selection of proper dosage requires individual titration.

In several studies of patients with acute myocardial infarction, intravenous followed by oral administration of Lopressor caused a reduction in heart rate, systolic blood pressure, and cardiac output. Stroke volume, diastolic blood pressure, and pulmonary artery end diastolic pressure remained unchanged.

In patients with angina pectoris, plasma concentration measured at 1 hour is linearly related to the oral dose within the range of 50-400 mg. Exercise heart rate and systolic blood pressure are reduced in relation to the logarithm of the oral dose of metoprolol. The increase in exercise capacity and the reduction in left ventricular ischemia are also significantly related to the logarithm of the oral dose.

INDICATIONS AND USAGE

Hypertension

Lopressor tablets are indicated for the treatment of hypertension. They may be used alone or in combination with other antihypertensive agents.

Angina Pectoris

Lopressor is indicated in the long-term treatment of angina pectoris.

Myocardial Infarction

Lopressor ampuls and tablets are indicated in the treatment of hemodynamically stable patients with definite or suspected acute myocardial infarction to reduce cardiovascular mortality. Treatment with intravenous Lopressor can be initiated as soon as the patient's clinical condition allows (see DOSAGE AND ADMINISTRATION, CONTRAINDICATIONS, and WARNINGS). Alternatively, treatment can begin within 3 to 10 days of the acute event (see DOSAGE AND ADMINISTRATION).

CONTRAINDICATIONS

Hypertension and Angina

Lopressor is contraindicated in sinus bradycardia, heart block greater than first degree, cardiogenic shock, and overt cardiac failure (see WARNINGS).

Myocardial Infarction

Lopressor is contraindicated in patients with a heart rate <45 beats/min; second- and third-degree heart block; significant first-degree heart block (P-R interval $\geq$0.24 sec); systolic blood pressure <100 mmHg; or moderate-to-severe cardiac failure (see WARNINGS).

WARNINGS

Hypertension and Angina

Cardiac Failure: Sympathetic stimulation is a vital component supporting circulatory function in congestive heart failure, and beta blockade carries the potential hazard of further depressing myocardial contractility and precipitating more severe failure. In hypertensive and angina patients who have congestive heart failure controlled by digitalis and diuretics, Lopressor should be administered cautiously. Both digitalis and Lopressor slow AV conduction.

In Patients Without a History of Cardiac Failure: Continued depression of the myocardium with beta-blocking agents over a period of time can, in some cases, lead to cardiac failure. At the first sign or symptom of impending cardiac failure, patients should be fully digitalized and/or given a diuretic. The response should be observed closely. If cardiac failure continues, despite adequate digitalization and diuretic therapy, Lopressor should be withdrawn.

Ischemic Heart Disease: Following abrupt cessation of therapy with certain beta-blocking agents, exacerbations of angina pectoris and, in some cases, myocardial infarction have occurred. When discontinuing chronically administered Lopressor, particularly in patients with ischemic heart disease, the dosage should be gradually reduced over a period of 1-2 weeks and the patient should be carefully monitored. If angina markedly worsens or acute coronary insufficiency develops, Lopressor administration should be reinstated promptly, at least temporarily, and other measures appropriate for the management of unstable angina should be taken. Patients should be warned against interruption or discontinuation of therapy without the physician's advice. Because coronary artery disease is common and may be unrecognized, it may be prudent not to discontinue Lopressor therapy abruptly even in patients treated only for hypertension.

Bronchospastic Diseases: PATIENTS WITH BRONCHOSPASTIC DISEASES SHOULD, IN GENERAL, NOT RECEIVE BETA-BLOCKERS. Because of its relative beta$_1$ selectivity, however, Lopressor may be used with caution in patients with bronchospastic disease who do not respond to, or cannot tolerate, other antihypertensive treatment. Since beta$_1$ selectivity is not absolute, a beta$_2$-stimulating agent

should be administered concomitantly, and the lowest possible dose of Lopressor should be used. In these circumstances it would be prudent initially to administer Lopressor in smaller doses three times daily, instead of larger doses two times daily, to avoid the higher plasma levels associated with the longer dosing interval. (See DOSAGE AND ADMINISTRATION.)

Major Surgery: The necessity or desirability of withdrawing beta-blocking therapy prior to major surgery is controversial; the impaired ability of the heart to respond to reflex adrenergic stimuli may augment the risks of general anesthesia and surgical procedures.

Lopressor, like other beta blockers, is a competitive inhibitor of beta-receptor agonists, and its effects can be reversed by administration of such agents, e.g., dobutamine or isoproterenol. However, such patients may be subject to protracted severe hypotension. Difficulty in restarting and maintaining the heart beat has also been reported with beta blockers.

Diabetes and Hypoglycemia: Lopressor should be used with caution in diabetic patients if a beta-blocking agent is required. Beta blockers may mask tachycardia occurring with hypoglycemia, but other manifestations such as dizziness and sweating may not be significantly affected.

Thyrotoxicosis: Beta-adrenergic blockade may mask certain clinical signs (e.g., tachycardia) of hyperthyroidism. Patients suspected of developing thyrotoxicosis should be managed carefully to avoid abrupt withdrawal of beta blockade, which might precipitate a thyroid storm.

Myocardial Infarction

Cardiac Failure: Sympathetic stimulation is a vital component supporting circulatory function, and beta blockade carries the potential hazard of depressing myocardial contractility and precipitating or exacerbating minimal cardiac failure.

During treatment with Lopressor, the hemodynamic status of the patient should be carefully monitored. If heart failure occurs or persists despite appropriate treatment, Lopressor should be discontinued.

Bradycardia: Lopressor produces a decrease in sinus heart rate in most patients; this decrease is greatest among patients with high initial heart rates and least among patients with low initial heart rates. Acute myocardial infarction (particularly inferior infarction) may in itself produce significant lowering of the sinus rate. If the sinus rate decreases to <40 beats/min, particularly if associated with evidence of lowered cardiac output, atropine (0.25-0.5 mg) should be administered intravenously. If treatment with atropine is not successful, Lopressor should be discontinued, and cautious administration of isoproterenol or installation of a cardiac pacemaker should be considered.

AV Block: Lopressor slows AV conduction and may produce significant first- (P-R interval $\geq$ 0.26 sec), second-, or third-degree heart block. Acute myocardial infarction also produces heart block.

If heart block occurs, Lopressor should be discontinued and atropine (0.25-0.5 mg) should be administered intravenously. If treatment with atropine is not successful, cautious administration of isoproterenol or installation of a cardiac pacemaker should be considered.

Hypotension: If hypotension (systolic blood pressure $\leq$ 90 mmHg) occurs, Lopressor should be discontinued, and the hemodynamic status of the patient and the extent of myocardial damage carefully assessed. Invasive monitoring of central venous, pulmonary capillary wedge, and arterial pressures may be required. Appropriate therapy with fluids, positive inotropic agents, balloon counterpulsation, or other treatment modalities should be instituted. If hypotension is associated with sinus bradycardia or AV block, treatment should be directed at reversing these (see above).

Bronchospastic Diseases: PATIENTS WITH BRONCHOSPASTIC DISEASES SHOULD, IN GENERAL, NOT RECEIVE BETA BLOCKERS. Because of its relative beta$_1$ selectivity, Lopressor may be used with extreme caution in patients with bronchospastic disease. Because it is unknown to what extent beta$_2$-stimulating agents may exacerbate myocardial ischemia and the extent of infarction, these agents should *not* be used prophylactically. If bronchospasm not related to congestive heart failure occurs, Lopressor should be discontinued. A theophylline derivative or a beta$_2$ agonist may be administered cautiously, depending on the clinical condition of the patient. Both theophylline derivatives and beta$_2$ agonists may produce serious cardiac arrhythmias.

PRECAUTIONS

General

Lopressor should be used with caution in patients with impaired hepatic function.

Information for Patients

Patients should be advised to take Lopressor regularly and continuously, as directed, with or immediately following meals. If a dose should be missed, the patient should take

Continued on next page

Lopressor—Cont.

only the next scheduled dose (without doubling it). Patients should not discontinue Lopressor without consulting the physician.

Patients should be advised (1) to avoid operating automobiles and machinery or engaging in other tasks requiring alertness until the patient's response to therapy with Lopressor has been determined; (2) to contact the physician if any difficulty in breathing occurs; (3) to inform the physician or dentist before any type of surgery that he or she is taking Lopressor.

Laboratory Tests

Clinical laboratory findings may include elevated levels of serum transaminase, alkaline phosphatase, and lactate dehydrogenase.

Drug Interactions

Catecholamine-depleting drugs (e.g., reserpine) may have an additive effect when given with beta-blocking agents. Patients treated with Lopressor plus a catecholamine depletor should therefore be closely observed for evidence of hypotension or marked bradycardia, which may produce vertigo, syncope, or postural hypotension.

Risk of Anaphylactic Reaction. While taking beta-blockers, patients with a history of severe anaphylactic reaction to a variety of allergens may be more reactive to repeated challenge, either accidental, diagnostic, or therapeutic. Such patients may be unresponsive to the usual doses of epinephrine used to treat allergic reactions.

Carcinogenesis, Mutagenesis, Impairment of Fertility

Long-term studies in animals have been conducted to evaluate carcinogenic potential. In a 2-year study in rats at three oral dosage levels of up to 800 mg/kg per day, there was no increase in the development of spontaneously occurring benign or malignant neoplasms of any type. The only histologic changes that appeared to be drug related were an increased incidence of generally mild focal accumulation of foamy macrophages in pulmonary alveoli and a slight increase in biliary hyperplasia. In a 21-month study in Swiss albino mice at three oral dosage levels of up to 750 mg/kg per day, benign lung tumors (small adenomas) occurred more frequently in female mice receiving the highest dose than in untreated control animals. There was no increase in malignant or total (benign plus malignant) lung tumors, nor in the overall incidence of tumors or malignant tumors. This 21-month study was repeated in CD-1 mice, and no statistically or biologically significant differences were observed between treated and control mice of either sex for any type of tumor.

All mutagenicity tests performed (a dominant lethal study in mice, chromosome studies in somatic cells, a Salmonella/mammalian-microsome mutagenicity test, and a nucleus anomaly test in somatic interphase nuclei) were negative.

No evidence of impaired fertility due to Lopressor was observed in a study performed in rats at doses up to 55.5 times the maximum daily human dose of 450 mg.

Pregnancy Category C

Lopressor has been shown to increase postimplantation loss and decrease neonatal survival in rats at doses up to 55.5 times the maximum daily human dose of 450 mg. Distribution studies in mice confirm exposure of the fetus when Lopressor is administered to the pregnant animal. These studies have revealed no evidence of impaired fertility or teratogenicity. There are no adequate and well-controlled studies in pregnant women. Because animal reproduction studies are not always predictive of human response, this drug should be used during pregnancy only if clearly needed.

Nursing Mothers

Lopressor is excreted in breast milk in very small quantity. An infant consuming 1 liter of breast milk daily would receive a dose of less than 1 mg of the drug. Caution should be exercised when Lopressor is administered to a nursing woman.

Pediatric Use

Safety and effectiveness in pediatric patients have not been established.

ADVERSE REACTIONS

Hypertension and Angina

Most adverse effects have been mild and transient.

Central Nervous System: Tiredness and dizziness have occurred in about 10 of 100 patients. Depression has been reported in about 5 of 100 patients. Mental confusion and short-term memory loss have been reported. Headache, nightmares, and insomnia have also been reported.

Cardiovascular: Shortness of breath and bradycardia have occurred in approximately 3 of 100 patients. Cold extremities; arterial insufficiency, usually of the Raynaud type; palpitations; congestive heart failure; peripheral edema; and hypotension have been reported in about 1 of 100 patients. (See CONTRAINDICATIONS, WARNINGS, and PRECAUTIONS.)

Respiratory: Wheezing (bronchospasm) and dyspnea have been reported in about 1 of 100 patients (see WARNINGS).

Gastrointestinal: Diarrhea has occurred in about 5 of 100 patients. Nausea, dry mouth, gastric pain, constipation, flatulence, and heartburn have been reported in about 1 of 100 patients.

Hypersensitive Reactions: Pruritus or rash have occurred in about 5 of 100 patients. Worsening of psoriasis has also been reported.

Miscellaneous: Peyronie's disease has been reported in fewer than 1 of 100,000 patients. Musculoskeletal pain, blurred vision, and tinnitus have also been reported.

There have been rare reports of reversible alopecia, agranulocytosis, and dry eyes. Discontinuation of the drug should be considered if any such reaction is not otherwise explicable.

The oculomucocutaneous syndrome associated with the beta blocker practolol has not been reported with Lopressor.

Myocardial Infarction

Central Nervous System: Tiredness has been reported in about 1 of 100 patients. Vertigo, sleep disturbances, hallucinations, headache, dizziness, visual disturbances, confusion, and reduced libido have also been reported, but a drug relationship is not clear.

Cardiovascular: In the randomized comparison of Lopressor and placebo described in the CLINICAL PHARMACOLOGY section, the following adverse reactions were reported:

	Lopressor	*Placebo*
Hypotension (systolic BP < 90 mmHg)	27.4%	23.2%
Bradycardia (heart rate < 40 beats/min)	15.9%	6.7%
Second- or third-degree heart block	4.7%	4.7%
First-degree heart block (P-R ≥ 0.26 sec)	5.3%	1.9%
Heart failure	27.5%	29.6%

Respiratory: Dyspnea of pulmonary origin has been reported in fewer than 1 of 100 patients.

Gastrointestinal: Nausea and abdominal pain have been reported in fewer than 1 of 100 patients.

Dermatologic: Rash and worsened psoriasis have been reported, but a drug relationship is not clear.

Miscellaneous: Unstable diabetes and claudication have been reported, but a drug relationship is not clear.

Potential Adverse Reactions

A variety of adverse reactions not listed above have been reported with other beta-adrenergic blocking agents and should be considered potential adverse reactions to Lopressor.

Central Nervous System: Reversible mental depression progressing to catatonia; an acute reversible syndrome characterized by disorientation for time and place, short-term memory loss, emotional lability, slightly clouded sensorium, and decreased performance on neuropsychometrics.

Cardiovascular: Intensification of AV block (See CONTRAINDICATIONS).

Hematologic: Agranulocytosis, nonthrombocytopenic purpura, thrombocytopenic purpura.

Hypersensitive Reactions: Fever combined with aching and sore throat, laryngospasm, and respiratory distress.

OVERDOSAGE

Acute Toxicity

Several cases of overdosage have been reported, some leading to death.

Oral LD_{50}'s (mg/kg): mice, 1158-2460; rats, 3090-4670.

Signs and Symptoms

Potential signs and symptoms associated with overdosage with Lopressor are bradycardia, hypotension, bronchospasm, and cardiac failure.

Treatment

There is no specific antidote.

In general, patients with acute or recent myocardial infarction may be more hemodynamically unstable than other patients and should be treated accordingly (see WARNINGS, Myocardial Infarction).

On the basis of the pharmacologic actions of Lopressor, the following general measures should be employed:

Elimination of the Drug: Gastric lavage should be performed.

Bradycardia: Atropine should be administered. If there is no response to vagal blockade, isoproterenol should be administered cautiously.

Hypotension: A vasopressor should be administered, e.g., levarterenol or dopamine.

Bronchospasm: A $beta_2$-stimulating agent and/or a theophylline derivative should be administered.

Cardiac Failure: A digitalis glycoside and diuretic should be administered. In shock resulting from inadequate cardiac contractility, administration of dobutamine, isoproterenol, or glucagon may be considered.

DOSAGE AND ADMINISTRATION

Hypertension

The dosage of Lopressor should be individualized. Lopressor should be taken with or immediately following meals.

The usual initial dosage is 100 mg daily in single or divided doses, whether used alone or added to a diuretic. The dosage may be increased at weekly (or longer) intervals until optimum blood pressure reduction is achieved. In general, the maximum effect of any given dosage level will be apparent after 1 week of therapy. The effective dosage range is 100 to 450 mg per day. Dosages above 450 mg per day have not been studied. While once-daily dosing is effective and can maintain a reduction in blood pressure throughout the day, lower doses (especially 100 mg) may not maintain a full effect at the end of the 24-hour period, and larger or more frequent daily doses may be required. This can be evaluated by measuring blood pressure near the end of the dosing interval to determine whether satisfactory control is being maintained throughout the day. $Beta_1$ selectivity diminishes as the dose of Lopressor is increased.

Angina Pectoris

The dosage of Lopressor should be individualized. Lopressor should be taken with or immediately following meals.

The usual initial dosage is 100 mg daily, given in two divided doses. The dosage may be gradually increased at weekly intervals until optimum clinical response has been obtained or there is pronounced slowing of the heart rate. The effective dosage range is 100-400 mg per day. Dosages above 400 mg per day have not been studied. If treatment is to be discontinued, the dosage should be reduced gradually over a period of 1-2 weeks. (See WARNINGS.)

Myocardial Infarction

Early Treatment: During the early phase of definite or suspected acute myocardial infarction, treatment with Lopressor can be initiated as soon as possible after the patient's arrival in the hospital. Such treatment should be initiated in a coronary care or similar unit immediately after the patient's hemodynamic condition has stabilized.

Treatment in this early phase should begin with the intravenous administration of three bolus injections of 5 mg of Lopressor each; the injections should be given at approximately 2-minute intervals. During the intravenous administration of Lopressor, blood pressure, heart rate, and electrocardiogram should be carefully monitored.

In patients who tolerate the full intravenous dose (15 mg), Lopressor tablets, 50 mg every 6 hours, should be initiated 15 minutes after the last intravenous dose and continued for 48 hours. Thereafter, patients should receive a maintenance dosage of 100 mg twice daily (see *Late Treatment* below).

Patients who appear not to tolerate the full intravenous dose should be started on Lopressor tablets either 25 mg or 50 mg every 6 hours (depending on the degree of intolerance) 15 minutes after the last intravenous dose or as soon as their clinical condition allows. In patients with severe intolerance, treatment with Lopressor should be discontinued (see WARNINGS).

Late Treatment: Patients with contraindications to treatment during the early phase of suspected or definite myocardial infarction, patients who appear not to tolerate the full early treatment, and patients in whom the physician wishes to delay therapy for any other reason should be started on Lopressor tablets, 100 mg twice daily, as soon as their clinical condition allows. Therapy should be continued for at least 3 months. Although the efficacy of Lopressor beyond 3 months has not been conclusively established, data from studies with other beta blockers suggest that treatment should be continued for 1-3 years.

Note: **Parenteral drug products should be inspected visually for particulate matter and discoloration prior to administration, whenever solution and container permit.**

HOW SUPPLIED

Metoprolol tartrate tablets, USP

Tablets 50 mg — capsule-shaped, biconvex, pink, scored (imprinted GEIGY on one side and 51 twice on the scored side)

Bottles of 100 .... NDC 0028-0051-01
Bottles of 1000 .... NDC 0028-0051-10
Unit Dose (blister pack)
Box of 100 (strips of 10) .... NDC 0028-0051-61

Tablets 100 mg — capsule-shaped, biconvex, light blue, scored (imprinted GEIGY on one side and 71 twice on the scored side)

Bottles of 100 .... NDC 0028-0071-01
Bottles of 1000 .... NDC 0028-0071-10
Unit Dose (blister pack)
Box of 100 (strips of 10) .... NDC 0028-0071-61

Store between 15°C-30°C (59°F-86°F). Protect from moisture.

Dispense in tight, light-resistant container (USP).

Metoprolol tartrate injection, USP

Ampuls 5 mL —each containing 5 mg of metoprolol tartrate
Tray of 4 packs of 3 ampuls .... NDC 0028-4201-33

Do not store above 30°C (86°F). Protect from light.

C98-18 (Rev. 5/98)

Distributed by:
Novartis Pharmaceuticals Corporation
East Hanover, New Jersey 07936

Shown in Product Identification Guide, page 325

LOPRESSOR HCT® ℞

[lō-prĕs-ōr]

metoprolol tartrate USP and hydrochlorothiazide USP
50/25 Tablets
100/25 Tablets
100/50 Tablets
Beta Blocker/Diuretic Antihypertensive

Caution: Federal law prohibits dispensing without prescription.

The following prescribing information is based on official labeling in effect on August 1, 1998.

Prescribing Information

DESCRIPTION

Lopressor HCT has the antihypertensive effect of Lopressor®, metoprolol tartrate, a selective $beta_1$-adrenoreceptor blocking agent, and the antihypertensive and diuretic actions of hydrochlorothiazide. It is available as tablets for oral administration. The 50/25 tablets contain 50 mg of metoprolol tartrate USP and 25 mg of hydrochlorothiazide USP; the 100/25 tablets contain 100 mg of metoprolol tartrate USP and 25 mg of hydrochlorothiazide USP; and the 100/50 tablets contain 100 mg of metoprolol tartrate USP and 50 mg of hydrochlorothiazide USP.

Metoprolol tartrate USP is (±)-1-Isopropylamino-3-[*p*-(2-methoxyethyl)phenoxy]-2-propanol 2:1 *dextro*-tartrate salt, and its structural formula is

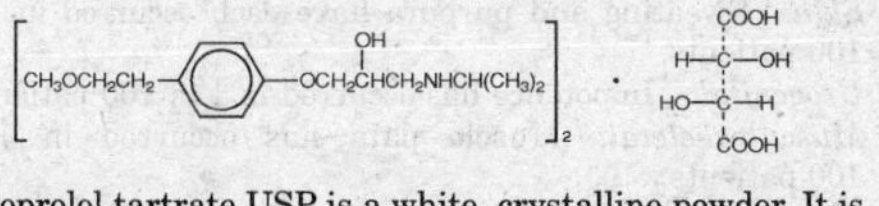

Metoprolol tartrate USP is a white, crystalline powder. It is very soluble in water; freely soluble in methylene chloride, in chloroform, and in alcohol; slightly soluble in acetone; and insoluble in ether. Its molecular weight is 684.82.

Hydrochlorothiazide is 6-chloro-3,4-dihydro-2*H*-1,2,4-benzothiadiazine-7-sulfonamide 1,1-dioxide and its structural formula is

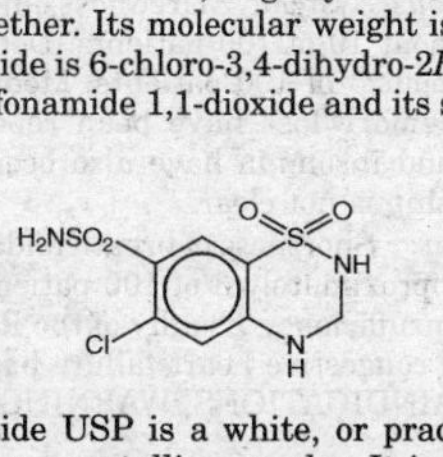

Hydrochlorothiazide USP is a white, or practically white, practically odorless, crystalline powder. It is freely soluble in sodium hydroxide solution, in *n*-butylamine, and in dimethylformamide; sparingly soluble in methanol; slightly soluble in water; and insoluble in ether, in chloroform, and in dilute mineral acids. Its molecular weight is 297.73.

Inactive Ingredients: Cellulose compounds, colloidal silicon dioxide, D&C Yellow No. 10 (100/50-mg tablets), FD&C Blue No. 1 (50/25-mg tablets), FD&C Red No. 40 and FD&C Yellow No. 6 (100/25-mg tablets), lactose, magnesium stearate, povidone, sodium starch glycolate, corn starch, stearic acid, and sucrose.

CLINICAL PHARMACOLOGY

Lopressor

Lopressor is a beta-adrenergic receptor blocking agent. *In vitro* and *in vivo* animal studies have shown that it has a preferential effect on $beta_1$ adrenoreceptors, chiefly located in cardiac muscle. This preferential effect is not absolute, however, and at higher doses, Lopressor also inhibits $beta_2$ adrenoreceptors, chiefly located in the bronchial and vascular musculature.

Clinical pharmacology studies have confirmed the beta-blocking activity of metoprolol in man, as shown by (1) reduction in heart rate and cardiac output at rest and upon exercise, (2) reduction of systolic blood pressure upon exercise, (3) inhibition of isoproterenol-induced tachycardia, and (4) reduction of reflex orthostatic tachycardia.

Relative $beta_1$ selectivity has been confirmed by the following: (1) In normal subjects, Lopressor is unable to reverse the $beta_2$-mediated vasodilating effects of epinephrine. This contrasts with the effect of nonselective ($beta_1$ plus $beta_2$) beta blockers, which completely reverse the vasodilating effects of epinephrine. (2) In asthmatic patients, Lopressor reduces FEV_1 and FVC significantly less than a nonselective beta blocker, propranolol at equivalent $beta_1$-receptor blocking doses.

Lopressor has no intrinsic sympathomimetic activity and only weak membrane-stabilizing activity. Lopressor crosses the blood-brain barrier and has been reported in the CSF in a concentration 78% of the simultaneous plasma concentration. Animal and human experiments indicate that Lopressor slows the sinus rate and decreases AV nodal conduction.

In controlled clinical studies, Lopressor has been shown to be an effective antihypertensive agent when used alone or as concomitant therapy with thiazide-type diuretics, at dosages of 100-450 mg daily. In controlled, comparative, clinical studies, Lopressor has been shown to be as effective an antihypertensive agent as propranolol, methyldopa, and thiazide-type diuretics, and to be equally effective in supine and standing positions.

The mechanism of the antihypertensive effects of beta-blocking agents has not been elucidated. However, several possible mechanisms have been proposed: (1) competitive antagonism of catecholamines at peripheral (especially cardiac) adrenergic neuron sites, leading to decreased cardiac output; (2) a central effect leading to reduced sympathetic outflow to the periphery; and (3) suppression of renin activity.

In man, absorption of Lopressor is rapid and complete. Plasma levels following oral administration, however, approximate 50% of levels following intravenous administration, indicating about 50% first-pass metabolism. Plasma levels achieved are highly variable after oral administration. Only a small fraction of the drug (about 12%) is bound to human serum albumin. Elimination is mainly by biotransformation in the liver, and the plasma half-life ranges from approximately 3 to 7 hours. Less than 5% of an oral dose of Lopressor is recovered unchanged in the urine; the rest is excreted by the kidneys as metabolites that appear to have no clinical significance. The systemic availability and half-life of Lopressor in patients with renal failure do not differ to a clinically significant degree from those in normal subjects. Consequently, no reduction in dosage is usually needed in patients with chronic renal failure.

Significant beta-blocking effect (as measured by reduction of exercise heart rate) occurs within 1 hour after oral administration, and its duration is dose-related. For example, a 50% reduction of the maximum registered effect after single oral doses of 20, 50, and 100 mg occurred at 3.3, 5.0, and 6.4 hours, respectively, in normal subjects. After repeated oral dosages of 100 mg twice daily, a significant reduction in exercise systolic blood pressure was evident at 12 hours. There is a linear relationship between the log of plasma levels and reduction of exercise heart rate. However, antihypertensive activity does not appear to be related to plasma levels. Because of variable plasma levels attained with a given dose and lack of a consistent relationship of antihypertensive activity to dose, selection of proper dosage requires individual titration.

Hydrochlorothiazide

Thiazides affect the renal tubular mechanism of electrolyte reabsorption. At maximal therapeutic dosage, all thiazides are approximately equal in their diuretic potency. Thiazides increase excretion of sodium and chloride in approximately equivalent amounts. Natriuresis causes a secondary loss of potassium.

The mechanism of the antihypertensive effect of thiazides is unknown. Thiazides do not affect normal blood pressure.

The onset of action of thiazides occurs in 2 hours and the peak effect at about 4 hours. The action persists for approximately 6-12 hours. Hydrochlorothiazide is rapidly absorbed, as indicated by peak plasma concentrations 1-2.5 hours after oral administration. Plasma levels of the drug are proportional to dose; the concentration in whole blood is 1.6-1.8 times higher than in plasma. Thiazides are eliminated rapidly by the kidney. After oral administration of 25- to 100-mg doses, 72-97% of the dose is excreted in the urine, indicating dose-independent absorption. Hydrochlorothiazide is eliminated from plasma in a biphasic fashion with a terminal half-life of 10–17 hours. Plasma protein binding is 67.9%. Plasma clearance is 15.9-30.0 L/hr; volume of distribution is 3.6-7.8 L/kg.

Gastrointestinal absorption of hydrochlorothiazide is enhanced when administered with food. Absorption is decreased in patients with congestive heart failure, and the pharmacokinetics are considerably different in these patients.

INDICATIONS AND USAGE

Lopressor HCT is indicated for the management of hypertension.

This fixed-combination drug is not indicated for initial therapy of hypertension. If the fixed combination represents the dose titrated to the individual patient's needs, therapy with the fixed combination may be more convenient than with the separate components.

CONTRAINDICATIONS

Lopressor

Lopressor is contraindicated in sinus bradycardia, heart block greater than first degree, cardiogenic shock, and overt cardiac failure (see WARNINGS).

Hydrochlorothiazide

Hydrochlorothiazide is contraindicated in patients with anuria or hypersensitivity to this or other sulfonamide-derived drugs (see WARNINGS).

WARNINGS

Lopressor

Cardiac Failure. Sympathetic stimulation is a vital component supporting circulatory function in congestive heart failure, and beta blockade carries the potential hazard of further depressing myocardial contractility and precipitating more severe failure. In hypertensive patients who have congestive heart failure controlled by digitalis and diuretics, Lopressor should be administered cautiously. Both digitalis and Lopressor slow AV conduction.

In Patients Without a History of Cardiac Failure. Continued depression of the myocardium with beta-blocking agents over a period of time can, in some cases, lead to cardiac failure. At the first sign or symptom of impending cardiac failure, patients should be fully digitalized and/or given a diuretic. The response should be observed closely. If cardiac failure continues, despite adequate digitalization and diuretic therapy, Lopressor should be withdrawn.

Ischemic Heart Disease. Following abrupt cessation of therapy with certain beta-blocking agents, exacerbations of angina pectoris and, in some cases, myocardial infarction have been reported. Even in the absence of overt angina pectoris, when discontinuing therapy, Lopressor should not be withdrawn abruptly, and patients should be cautioned against interruption of therapy without the physician's advice (see PRECAUTIONS, Information for Patients).

Bronchospastic Diseases. **PATIENTS WITH BRONCHOSPASTIC DISEASES SHOULD, IN GENERAL, NOT RECEIVE BETA BLOCKERS. Because of its relative $beta_1$ selectivity, however, Lopressor may be used with caution in patients with bronchospastic disease who do not respond to, or cannot tolerate, other antihypertensive treatment. Since $beta_1$ selectivity is not absolute, a $beta_2$-stimulating agent should be administered concomitantly, and the lowest possible dose of Lopressor should be used. In these circumstances it would be prudent initially to administer Lopressor in smaller doses three times daily, instead of larger doses two times daily, to avoid the higher plasma levels associated with the longer dosing interval. (See DOSAGE AND ADMINISTRATION.)**

Major Surgery. The necessity or desirability of withdrawing beta-blocking therapy prior to major surgery is controversial; the impaired ability of the heart to respond to reflex adrenergic stimuli may augment the risks of general anesthesia and surgical procedures.

Lopressor, like other beta blockers, is a competitive inhibitor of beta-receptor agonists, and its effects can be reversed by administration of such agents, e.g., dobutamine or isoproterenol. However, such patients may be subject to protracted severe hypotension. Difficulty in restarting and maintaining the heartbeat has also been reported with beta blockers.

Diabetes and Hypoglycemia. Lopressor should be used with caution in diabetic patients if a beta-blocking agent is required. Beta blockers may mask tachycardia occurring with hypoglycemia, but other manifestations such as dizziness and sweating may not be significantly affected. Selective beta blockers do not potentiate insulin-induced hypoglycemia and, unlike nonselective beta blockers, do not delay recovery of blood glucose to normal levels.

Thyrotoxicosis. Beta-adrenergic blockade may mask certain clinical signs (e.g., tachycardia) or hyperthyroidism. Patients suspected of developing thyrotoxicosis should be managed carefully to avoid abrupt withdrawal of beta blockade, which might precipitate a thyroid storm.

Hydrochlorothiazide

Thiazides should be used with caution in patients with severe renal disease. In patients with renal disease, thiazides may precipitate azotemia. Cumulative effects of the drug may develop in patients with impaired renal function.

Thiazides should be used with caution in patients with impaired hepatic function or progressive liver disease, since minor alterations of fluid and electrolyte imbalance may precipitate hepatic coma.

Thiazides may add to or potentiate the action of other antihypertensive drugs. Potentiation occurs with ganglionic or peripheral adrenergic blocking drugs.

Sensitivity reactions are more likely to occur in patients with a history of allergy or bronchial asthma.

The possibility of exacerbation or activation of systemic lupus erythematosus has been reported.

PRECAUTIONS

General

Lopressor. Lopressor should be used with caution in patients with impaired hepatic function.

Hydrochlorothiazide. All patients receiving thiazide therapy should be observed for clinical signs of fluid or electrolyte imbalance, namely hyponatremia, hypochloremic alkalosis, and hypokalemia (see Laboratory Tests and Drug/Drug Interactions). Warning signs are dryness of mouth, thirst, weakness, lethargy, drowsiness, restlessness, muscle pains or cramps, muscular fatigue, hypotension, oliguria, tachycardia, and gastrointestinal disturbance, such as nausea or vomiting.

Hypokalemia may develop, especially in cases of brisk diuresis or severe cirrhosis.

Interference with adequate oral intake of electrolytes will also contribute to hypokalemia. Hypokalemia may be avoided or treated by the use of potassium supplements or foods with a high potassium content.

Continued on next page

Lopressor HCT—Cont.

Any chloride deficit is generally mild and usually does not require specific treatment, except under extraordinary circumstances (as in liver disease or renal disease). Dilutional hyponatremia may occur in edematous patients in hot weather; appropriate therapy is water restriction, rather than administration of salt, except in rare instances when the hyponatremia is life-threatening. In cases of actual salt depletion, appropriate replacement is the therapy of choice. Hyperuricemia may occur or frank gout may be precipitated in certain patients receiving thiazide therapy.

Latent diabetes may become manifest during thiazide administration (see Drug/Drug Interactions).

The antihypertensive effects of the drug may be enhanced in the postsympathectomy patient.

If progressive renal impairment becomes evident, withholding or discontinuing diuretic therapy should be considered. Calcium excretion is decreased by thiazides. Pathological changes in the parathyroid gland with hypercalcemia and hypophosphatemia have been observed in a few patients on prolonged thiazide therapy. The common complications of hyperparathyroidism, such as renal lithiasis, bone resorption, and peptic ulceration, have not been seen.

Thiazide diuretics have been shown to increase the urinary excretion of magnesium; this may result in hypomagnesemia.

Information for Patients

Patients should be advised to take Lopressor HCT regularly and continuously, as directed, with or immediately following meals. If a dose should be missed, the patient should take only the next scheduled dose (without doubling it). Patients should not discontinue Lopressor HCT without consulting the physician.

Patients should be advised (1) to avoid operating automobiles and machinery or engaging in other tasks requiring alertness until the patient's response to therapy with Lopressor has been determined; (2) to contact the physician if any difficulty in breathing occurs; (3) to inform the physician or dentist before any type of surgery that he or she is taking Lopressor HCT.

Laboratory Tests

Lopressor. Clinical laboratory findings may include elevated levels of serum transaminase, alkaline phosphatase, and lactate dehydrogenase.

Hydrochlorothiazide. Initial and periodic determinations of serum electrolytes to detect possible electrolyte imbalance should be performed at appropriate intervals.

Serum and urine electrolyte determinations are particularly important when the patient is vomiting excessively or receiving parenteral fluids.

Drug/Drug Interactions

Lopressor. Catecholamine-depleting drugs (e.g., reserpine) may have an additive effect when given with beta-blocking agents. Patients treated with Lopressor plus a catecholamine depletor should therefore be closely observed for evidence of hypotension or marked bradycardia, which may produce vertigo, syncope, or postural hypotension.

Risk of Anaphylactic Reaction. While taking beta-blockers, patients with a history of severe anaphylactic reaction to a variety of allergens may be more reactive to repeated challenge, either accidental, diagnostic, or therapeutic. Such patients may be unresponsive to the usual doses of epinephrine used to treat allergic reaction.

Hydrochlorothiazide. Hypokalemia can sensitize or exaggerate the response of the heart to the toxic effects of digitalis (e.g., increased ventricular irritability).

Hypokalemia may develop during concomitant use of steroids or ACTH.

Insulin requirements in diabetic patients may be increased, decreased, or unchanged.

Thiazides may decrease arterial responsiveness to norepinephrine, but not enough to preclude effectiveness of the pressor agent for therapeutic use.

Thiazides may increase the responsiveness to tubocurarine.

Lithium renal clearance is reduced by thiazides, increasing the risk of lithium toxicity.

There have been rare reports in the literature of hemolytic anemia occurring with the concomitant use of hydrochlorothiazide and methyldopa.

Concurrent administration of some nonsteroidal antiinflammatory agents may reduce the diuretic, natriuretic and antihypertensive effects of thiazide diuretics.

Cholestyramine and colestipol resins: Absorption of hydrochlorothiazide is impaired in the presence of anionic exchange resins. Single doses of either cholestyramine or colestipol resins bind the hydrochlorothiazide and reduce its absorption from the gastrointestinal tract by up to 85% and 43%, respectively.

Drug/Laboratory Test Interactions

Hydrochlorothiazide. Thiazides may decrease serum levels of protein-bound iodine without signs of thyroid disturbance. Thiazides should be discontinued before tests for parathyroid function are made. (See PRECAUTIONS, General, *Hydrochlorothiazide*, Calcium excretion.)

Carcinogenesis, Mutagenesis, Impairment of Fertility

Lopressor HCT. Carcinogenicity and mutagenicity studies have not been conducted with Lopressor HCT. Lopressor HCT produced no evidence of impaired fertility in male or female rats administered gavaged doses up to 200/50 mg/kg (100/50 times the maximum recommended daily human dose) prior to mating and throughout gestation and rearing of young.

Lopressor. Long-term studies in animals have been conducted to evaluate carcinogenic potential. In a 2-year study in rats at three oral dosage levels of up to 800 mg/kg per day, there was no increase in the development of spontaneously occurring benign or malignant neoplasms of any type. The only histologic changes that appeared to be drug related were an increased incidence of generally mild focal accumulation of foamy macrophages in pulmonary alveoli and a slight increase in biliary hyperplasia. In a 21-month study in Swiss albino mice at three oral dosage levels of up to 750 mg/kg per day, benign lung tumors (small adenomas) occurred more frequently in female mice receiving the highest dose than in untreated control animals. There was no increase in malignant or total (benign plus malignant) lung tumors, nor in the overall incidence of tumors or malignant tumors. This 21-month study was repeated in CD-1 mice, and no statistically or biologically significant differences were observed between treated and control mice of either sex for any type of tumor.

All mutagenicity tests performed (a dominant lethal study in mice, chromosome studies in somatic cells, a *Salmonella*/mammalian-microsome mutagenicity test, and a nucleus anomaly test in somatic interphase nuclei) were negative.

No evidence of impaired fertility due to Lopressor was observed in a study performed in rats at doses up to 55.5 times the maximum daily human dose of 450 mg.

Hydrochlorothiazide. Two-year feeding studies in mice and rats conducted under the auspices of the National Toxicology Program (NTP) uncovered no evidence of a carcinogenic potential of hydrochlorothiazide in female mice (at doses up to approximately 600 mg/kg/day) or in male and female rats (at doses up to approximately 100 mg/kg/day). The NTP, however, found equivocal evidence for hepatocarcinogenicity in male mice.

Hydrochlorothiazide was not genotoxic in in vitro assays using strains TA 98, TA 100, TA 1535, TA 1537, and TA 1538 of *Salmonella typhimurium* (Ames assay) and in the Chinese Hamster Ovary (CHO) test for chromosomal aberrations, or in in vivo assays using mouse germinal cell chromosomes, Chinese hamster bone marrow chromosomes, and the *Drosophila* sex-linked recessive lethal trait gene. Positive test results were obtained only in the in vitro CHO Sister Chromatid Exchange (clastogenicity) and in the Mouse Lymphoma Cell (mutagenicity) assays, using concentrations of hydrochlorothiazide from 43 to 1300 µg/mL, and in the *Aspergillus nidulans* nondisjunction assay at an unspecified concentration.

Hydrochlorothiazide had no adverse effects on the fertility of mice and rats of either sex in studies wherein these species were exposed, via their diet, to doses of up to 100 and 4 mg/kg/day, respectively, prior to mating and throughout gestation.

Pregnancy: Teratogenic Effects. Pregnancy Category C

Lopressor HCT. No evidence of adverse effects on pregnancy or the fetus were observed in rats when dams were administered gavaged doses up to 200/50 mg/kg of Lopressor HCT (100/50 times the maximum recommended daily human dose) during the period of organogenesis. Increased postimplantation loss and decreased postnatal survival were observed with these doses when administered later in pregnancy (gestation days 15-21). In rabbits, increased fetal loss was observed with oral doses of 25/6.25 mg/kg of Lopressor HCT (12/6 times the maximum recommended daily human dose), but not with lower doses. There are no adequate and well-controlled studies of Lopressor HCT in pregnant women. Lopressor HCT should be used during pregnancy only if the potential benefit justifies the potential risk to the fetus.

Lopressor. Lopressor has been shown to increase postimplantation loss and decrease neonatal survival in rats at doses up to 55.5 times the maximum daily human dose of 450 mg. Distribution studies in mice confirm exposure of the fetus when Lopressor is administered to the pregnant animal. These studies have revealed no evidence of teratogenicity.

Hydrochlorothiazide. Studies in which hydrochlorothiazide was orally administered to pregnant mice and rats during their respective periods of major organogenesis at doses up to 3000 and 1000 mg/kg/day, respectively, provided no evidence of harm to the fetus.

Nonteratogenic Effects

Hydrochlorothiazide. Thiazides cross the placental barrier and appear in cord blood, and there is a risk of fetal or neonatal jaundice, thrombocytopenia, and possibly other adverse reactions that have occurred in adults.

Nursing Mothers

Lopressor is excreted in breast milk in very small quantity. An infant consuming 1 liter of breast milk daily would receive a dose of metoprolol of less than 1 mg. Thiazides are also excreted in breast milk. If the use of Lopressor HCT is deemed essential, the patient should stop nursing.

Pediatric Use

Safety and effectiveness in pediatric patients have not been established.

ADVERSE REACTIONS

Lopressor HCT

The following adverse reactions were reported in controlled clinical studies of the combination of Lopressor and hydrochlorothiazide.

Body as a Whole: Fatigue or lethargy and flu syndrome have each been reported in about 10 in 100 patients.

Nervous System: Dizziness or vertigo, drowsiness or somnolence, and headache have each occurred in about 10 in 100 patients. Nightmare has occurred in 1 in 100 patients.

Cardiovascular: Bradycardia has occurred in about 6 in 100 patients. Decreased exercise tolerance and dyspnea have each occurred in about 1 of 100 patients.

Digestive: Diarrhea, digestive disorder, dry mouth, nausea or vomiting, and constipation have each occurred in about 1 in 100 patients.

Metabolic and Nutritional: Hypokalemia has occurred in fewer than 10 in 100 patients. Edema, gout, and anorexia have each occurred in 1 in 100 patients.

Special Senses: Blurred vision, tinnitus, and earache have each been reported in 1 in 100 patients.

Skin: Sweating and purpura have each occurred in 1 in 100 patients.

Urogenital: Impotence has occurred in 1 in 100 patients.

Musculoskeletal: Muscle pain has occurred in 1 in 100 patients.

Lopressor

Most adverse effects have been mild and transient.

Central Nervous System: Tiredness and dizziness have occurred in about 10 of 100 patients. Depression has been reported in about 5 of 100 patients. Mental confusion and short-term memory loss have been reported. Headache, nightmares, and insomnia have also been reported, but a drug relationship is not clear.

Cardiovascular: Shortness of breath and bradycardia have occurred in approximately 3 of 100 patients. Cold extremities; arterial insufficiency, usually of the Raynaud type; palpitations; and congestive heart failure have been reported. (See CONTRAINDICATIONS, WARNINGS, and PRECAUTIONS).

Respiratory: Wheezing (bronchospasm) has been reported in fewer than 1 of 100 patients (see WARNINGS).

Gastrointestinal: Diarrhea has occurred in about 5 of 100 patients. Nausea, gastric pain, constipation, flatulence, and heartburn have been reported in 1 of 100, or fewer, patients.

Hypersensitive Reactions: Pruritus has occurred in fewer than 1 of 100 patients. Rash has been reported.

Miscellaneous: Peyronie's disease has been reported in fewer than 1 of 100,000 patients. Alopecia has been reported.

The oculomucocutaneous syndrome associated with the beta blocker practolol has not been reported with Lopressor.

Potential Adverse Reactions

A variety of adverse reactions not listed above have been reported with other beta-adrenergic blocking agents and should be considered potential adverse reactions to Lopressor.

Central Nervous System: Reversible mental depression progressing to catatonia; visual disturbances; hallucinations; an acute reversible syndrome characterized by disorientation for time and place, short-term memory loss, emotional lability, slightly clouded sensorium, and decreased performance on neuropsychometrics.

Cardiovascular: Intensification of AV block (see CONTRAINDICATIONS).

Hematologic: Agranulocytosis, nonthrombocytopenic purpura, thrombocytopenic purpura.

Hypersensitive Reactions: Fever combined with aching and sore throat, laryngospasm, and respiratory distress.

Hydrochlorothiazide

The following adverse reactions have been observed, but there has not been enough systematic collection of data to support an estimate of their frequency. Consequently the reactions are categorized by organ systems and are listed in decreasing order of severity and not frequency.

Digestive: Pancreatitis, jaundice (intrahepatic cholestatic), sialadenitis, vomiting, diarrhea, cramping, nausea, gastric irritation, constipation, anorexia.

Cardiovascular: Orthostatic hypotension (may be potentiated by alcohol, barbiturates, or narcotics).

Neurologic: Vertigo, dizziness, transient blurred vision, headache, paresthesia, xanthopsia, weakness, restlessness.

Musculoskeletal: Muscle spasm.

Hematologic: Aplastic anemia, agranulocytosis, leukopenia, thrombocytopenia.

Metabolic: Hyperglycemia, glycosuria, hyperuricemia.

Hypersensitive Reactions: Necrotizing angiitis, Stevens-Johnson syndrome, respiratory distress including pneumonitis and pulmonary edema, purpura, urticaria, rash, photosensitivity.

OVERDOSAGE

Acute Toxicity

Several cases of overdosage with Lopressor have been reported, some leading to death. No deaths have been reported with hydrochlorothiazide.

Oral LD_{50}'s (mg/kg): mice, 1158 (Lopressor); rats, 3090 (Lopressor), 2750 (hydrochlorothiazide).

Signs and Symptoms

Lopressor. Potential signs and symptoms associated with overdosage with Lopressor are bradycardia, hypotension, bronchospasm, and cardiac failure.

Hydrochlorothiazide. The most prominent feature of poisoning is acute loss of fluid and electrolytes.

Cardiovascular: Tachycardia, hypotension, shock.

Neuromuscular: Weakness, confusion, dizziness, cramps of the calf muscles, paresthesia, fatigue, impairment of consciousness.

Digestive: Nausea, vomiting, thirst.

Renal: Polyuria, oliguria, or anuria (due to hemoconcentration).

Laboratory Findings: Hypokalemia, hyponatremia, hypochloremia, alkalosis; increased BUN (especially in patients with renal insufficiency).

Combined Poisoning: Signs and symptoms may be aggravated or modified by concomitant intake of antihypertensive medication, barbiturates, curare, digitalis (hypokalemia), corticosteroids, narcotics, or alcohol.

Treatment

There is no specific antidote.

On the basis of the pharmacologic actions of Lopressor and hydrochlorothiazide, the following general measures should be employed:

Elimination of the Drug: Inducement of vomiting, gastric lavage, and activated charcoal.

Bradycardia: Atropine should be administered. If there is no response to vagal blockade, isoproterenol should be administered cautiously.

Hypotension: The patient's legs should be elevated, and lost fluid and electrolytes (potassium, sodium) should be replaced. A vasopressor should be administered, e.g., levarterenol or dopamine.

Bronchospasm: A $beta_2$-stimulating agent and/or a theophylline derivative should be administered.

Cardiac Failure: A digitalis glycoside and diuretic should be administered. In shock resulting from inadequate cardiac contractility, administration of dobutamine, isoproterenol, or glucagon may be considered.

Surveillance: Fluid and electrolyte balance (especially serum potassium) and renal function should be monitored until conditions become normal.

DOSAGE AND ADMINISTRATION

Dosage should be determined by individual titration (see INDICATIONS AND USAGE).

Hydrochlorothiazide is usually given at a dosage of 12.5 to 50 mg per day. The usual initial dosage of Lopressor is 100 mg daily in single or divided doses. Dosage may be increased gradually until optimum blood pressure control is achieved. The effective dosage range is 100 to 450 mg per day. While once-daily dosing is effective and can maintain a reduction in blood pressure throughout the day, lower doses (especially 100 mg) may not maintain a full effect at the end of the 24-hour period, and larger or more frequent daily doses may be required. This can be evaluated by measuring blood pressure near the end of the dosing interval to determine whether satisfactory control is being maintained throughout the day. $Beta_1$ selectivity diminishes as dosage of Lopressor is increased.

The following dosage schedule may be used to administer from 100 to 200 mg of Lopressor per day and from 25 to 50 mg of hydrochlorothiazide per day:

Lopressor HCT	***Dosage***
Tablets of 50/25	2 tablets per day in single or divided doses
Tablets of 100/25	1 to 2 tablets per day in single or divided doses
Tablets of 100/50	1 tablet per day in single or divided doses

Dosing regimens that exceed 50 mg of hydrochlorothiazide per day are not recommended. When necessary, another antihypertensive agent may be added gradually, beginning with 50% of the usual recommended starting dose to avoid an excessive fall in blood pressure.

HOW SUPPLIED

Tablets 50/25–capsule-shaped, white and blue, scored (imprinted Geigy on one side and 35 twice on the scored side), 50 mg of metoprolol tartrate and 25 mg of hydrochlorothiazide

Bottles of 100 .... NDC 0028-0035-01

Tablets 100/25–apsule-shaped, white and pink, scored (imprinted Geigy on one side and 53 twice on the scored side), 100 mg of metoprolol tartrate and 25 mg of hydrochlorothiazide

Bottles of 100 .... NDC 0028-0053-01

Tablets 100/50–capsule-shaped, white and yellow, scored (imprinted Geigy on one side and 73 twice on the scored side), 100 mg of metoprolol tartrate and 50 mg of hydrochlorothiazide

Bottles of 100 .... NDC 0028-0073-01

Store between 59°–86°F (15°–30°C). Protect from moisture.

Dispense in tight, light-resistant container (USP).

C98-4 (Rev. 1/98)

Shown in Product Identification Guide, page 325

LOTENSIN® ℞

[*lō tĕn sĭn*]

benazepril hydrochloride

Tablets

Rx only

The following prescribing information is based on official labeling in effect on October 1, 1998.

Prescribing Information

Use in Pregnancy

When used in pregnancy during the second and third trimesters, ACE inhibitors can cause injury and even death to the developing fetus. When pregnancy is detected, Lotensin should be discontinued as soon as possible. See **WARNINGS, Fetal/Neonatal Morbidity and Mortality.**

DESCRIPTION

Benazepril hydrochloride is a white to off-white crystalline powder, soluble (>100 mg/mL) in water, in ethanol, and in methanol. Benazepril's chemical name is 3-[[1-(ethoxycarbonyl)-3-phenyl-(1S)-propyl]amino]-2,3,4,5-tetrahydro-2-oxo-1*H*-1-(3S)-benzazepine-1-acetic acid monohydrochloride; its structural formula is

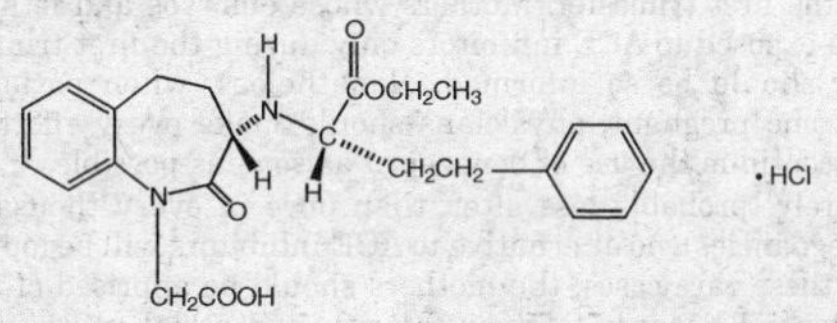

Its empirical formula is $C_{24}H_{28}N_2O_5 \bullet HCl$, and its molecular weight is 460.96.

Benazeprilat, the active metabolite of benazepril, is a non-sulfhydryl angiotensin-converting enzyme inhibitor. Benazepril is converted to benazeprilat by hepatic cleavage of the ester group.

Lotensin is supplied as tablets containing 5 mg, 10 mg, 20 mg, and 40 mg of benazepril for oral administration. The inactive ingredients are cellulose compounds, colloidal silicon dioxide, crospovidone, hydrogenated castor oil (5-mg, 10-mg, and 20-mg tablets), iron oxides, lactose, magnesium stearate (40-mg tablets), polysorbate 80, propylene glycol (5-mg and 40-mg tablets), starch, talc, and titanium dioxide.

CLINICAL PHARMACOLOGY

Mechanism of Action

Benazepril and benazeprilat inhibit angiotensin-converting enzyme (ACE) in human subjects and animals. ACE is a peptidyl dipeptidase that catalyzes the conversion of angiotensin I to the vasoconstrictor substance, angiotensin II. Angiotensin II also stimulates aldosterone secretion by the adrenal cortex.

Inhibition of ACE results in decreased plasma angiotensin II, which leads to decreased vasopressor activity and to decreased aldosterone secretion. The latter decrease may result in a small increase of serum potassium. Hypertensive patients treated with Lotensin alone for up to 52 weeks had elevations of serum potassium of up to 0.2 mEq/L. Similar patients treated with Lotensin and hydrochlorothiazide for up to 24 weeks had no consistent changes in their serum potassium (see PRECAUTIONS).

Removal of angiotensin II negative feedback on renin secretion leads to increased plasma renin activity. In animal studies, benazepril had no inhibitory effect on the vasopressor response to angiotensin II and did not interfere with the hemodynamic effects of the autonomic neurotransmitters acetylcholine, epinephrine, and norepinephrine.

ACE is identical to kininase, an enzyme that degrades bradykinin. Whether increased levels of bradykinin, a potent vasodepressor peptide, play a role in the therapeutic effects of Lotensin remains to be elucidated.

While the mechanism through which benazepril lowers blood pressure is believed to be primarily suppression of the renin-angiotensin-aldosterone system, benazepril has an antihypertensive effect even in patients with low-renin hypertension (see INDICATIONS AND USAGE).

Pharmacokinetics and Metabolism

Following oral administration of Lotensin, peak plasma concentrations of benazepril are reached within 0.5–1.0 hours. The extent of absorption is at least 37% as determined by urinary recovery and is not significantly influenced by the presence of food in the GI tract.

Cleavage of the ester group (primarily in the liver) converts benazepril to its active metabolite, benazeprilat. Peak plasma concentrations of benazeprilat are reached 1–2 hours after drug intake in the fasting state and 2–4 hours after drug intake in the nonfasting state. The serum protein binding of benazepril is about 96.7% and that of benazeprilat about 95.3%, as measured by equilibrium dialysis; on the basis of in vitro studies, the degree of protein binding should be unaffected by age, hepatic dysfunction, or concentration (over the concentration range of 0.24–23.6 μmol/L).

Benazepril is almost completely metabolized to benazeprilat, which has much greater ACE inhibitory activity than benazepril, and to the glucuronide conjugates of benazepril and benazeprilat. Only trace amounts of an administered dose of Lotensin can be recovered in the urine as unchanged benazepril, while about 20% of the dose is excreted as benazeprilat, 4% as benazepril glucuronide, and 8% as benazeprilat glucuronide.

The kinetics of benazepril are approximately dose-proportional within the dosage range of 10–80 mg.

The effective half-life of accumulation of benazeprilat following multiple dosing of benazepril hydrochloride is 10–11 hours. Thus, steady-state concentrations of benazeprilat should be reached after 2 or 3 doses of benazepril hydrochloride given once daily.

The kinetics did not change, and there was no significant accumulation during chronic administration (28 days) of once-daily doses between 5 mg and 20 mg. Accumulation ratios based on AUC and urinary recovery of benazeprilat were 1.19 and 1.27, respectively.

When dialysis was started two hours after ingestion of 10 mg of benazepril, approximately 6% of benazeprilat was removed in 4 hours of dialysis. The parent compound, benazepril, was not detected in the dialysate.

The disposition of benazepril and benazeprilat in patients with mild-to-moderate renal insufficiency (creatinine clearance >30 mL/min) is similar to that in patients with normal renal function. In patients with creatinine clearance ≤30 mL/min, peak benazeprilat levels and the initial (alpha phase) half-life increase, and time to steady state may be delayed (see DOSAGE AND ADMINISTRATION).

Benazepril and benazeprilat are cleared predominantly by renal excretion in healthy subjects with normal renal function. Nonrenal (i.e., biliary) excretion accounts for approximately 11%–12% of benazeprilat excretion in healthy subjects. In patients with renal failure, biliary clearance may compensate to an extent for deficient renal clearance.

In patients with hepatic dysfunction due to cirrhosis, levels of benazeprilat are essentially unaltered. The pharmacokinetics of benazepril and benazeprilat do not appear to be influenced by age.

In studies in rats given ^{14}C-benazepril, benazepril and its metabolites crossed the blood-brain barrier only to an extremely low extent. Multiple doses of benazepril did not result in accumulation in any tissue except the lung, where, as with other ACE inhibitors in similar studies, there was a slight increase in concentration due to slow elimination in that organ.

Some placental passage occurred when the drug was administered to pregnant rats.

Pharmacodynamics

Single and multiple doses of 10 mg or more of Lotensin cause inhibition of plasma ACE activity by at least 80%–90% for at least 24 hours after dosing. Pressor responses to exogenous angiotensin I were inhibited by 60%–90% (up to 4 hours post-dose) at the 10-mg dose.

Administration of Lotensin to patients with mild-to-moderate hypertension results in a reduction of both supine and standing blood pressure to about the same extent with no compensatory tachycardia. Symptomatic postural hypotension is infrequent, although it can occur in patients who are salt- and/or volume-depleted (see WARNINGS).

In single-dose studies, Lotensin lowered blood pressure within 1 hour, with peak reductions achieved 2–4 hours after dosing. The antihypertensive effect of a single dose persisted for 24 hours. In multiple-dose studies, once daily doses of 20–80 mg decreased seated pressure (systolic/diastolic) 24 hours after dosing by about 6–12/4–7 mmHg. The trough values represent reductions of about 50% of that seen at peak.

Four dose-response studies using once-daily dosing were conducted in 470 mild-to-moderate hypertensive patients not using diuretics. The minimal effective once-daily dose of Lotensin was 10 mg; but further falls in blood pressure, especially at morning trough, were seen with higher doses in the studied dosing range (10–80 mg). In studies compar-

Continued on next page

Lotensin—Cont.

ing the same daily dose of Lotensin given as a single morning dose or as a twice-daily dose, blood pressure reductions at the time of morning trough blood levels were greater with the divided regimen.

During chronic therapy, the maximum reduction in blood pressure with any dose is generally achieved after 1–2 weeks. The antihypertensive effects of Lotensin have continued during therapy for at least two years. Abrupt withdrawal of Lotensin has not been associated with a rapid increase in blood pressure.

In patients with mild-to-moderate hypertension, Lotensin 10–20 mg was similar in effectiveness to captopril, hydrochlorothiazide, nifedipine SR, and propranolol.

The antihypertensive effects of Lotensin were not appreciably different in patients receiving high- or low-sodium diets. In hemodynamic studies in dogs, blood pressure reduction was accompanied by a reduction in peripheral arterial resistance, with an increase in cardiac output and renal blood flow and little or no change in heart rate. In normal human volunteers, single doses of benazepril caused an increase in renal blood flow but had no effect on glomerular filtration rate.

Use of Lotensin in combination with thiazide diuretics gives a blood-pressure-lowering effect greater than that seen with either agent alone. By blocking the renin-angiotensin-aldosterone axis, administration of Lotensin tends to reduce the potassium loss associated with the diuretic.

INDICATIONS AND USAGE

Lotensin is indicated for the treatment of hypertension. It may be used alone or in combination with thiazide diuretics. In using Lotensin, consideration should be given to the fact that another angiotensin-converting enzyme inhibitor, captopril, has caused agranulocytosis, particularly in patients with renal impairment or collagen-vascular disease. Available data are insufficient to show that Lotensin does not have a similar risk (see WARNINGS).

Black patients receiving ACE-inhibitors have been reported to have a higher incidence of angioedema compared to nonblacks. It should also be noted that in controlled clinical trials ACE inhibitors have an effect on blood pressure that is less in black patients than in nonblacks.

CONTRAINDICATIONS

Lotensin is contraindicated in patients who are hypersensitive to this product or to any other ACE inhibitor.

WARNINGS

Anaphylactoid and Possibly Related Reactions

Presumably because angiotensin-converting enzyme inhibitors affect the metabolism of eicosanoids and polypeptides, including endogenous bradykinin, patients receiving ACE inhibitors (including Lotensin) may be subject to a variety of adverse reactions, some of them serious.

Angioedema: Angioedema of the face, extremities, lips, tongue, glottis, and larynx has been reported in patients treated with angiotensin-converting enzyme inhibitors. In U.S. clinical trials, symptoms consistent with angioedema were seen in none of the subjects who received placebo and in about 0.5% of the subjects who received Lotensin. Angioedema associated with laryngeal edema can be fatal. If laryngeal stridor or angioedema of the face, tongue, or glottis occurs, treatment with Lotensin should be discontinued and appropriate therapy instituted immediately. **Where there is involvement of the tongue, glottis, or larynx, likely to cause airway obstruction, appropriate therapy, e.g., subcutaneous epinephrine injection 1:1000 (0.3 mL to 0.5 mL) should be promptly administered (see ADVERSE REACTIONS).**

Anaphylactoid Reactions During Desensitization: Two patients undergoing desensitizing treatment with hymenoptera venom while receiving ACE inhibitors sustained life-threatening anaphylactoid reactions. In the same patients, these reactions were avoided when ACE inhibitors were temporarily withheld, but they reappeared upon inadvertent rechallenge.

Anaphylactoid Reactions During Membrane Exposure: Anaphylactoid reactions have been reported in patients dialyzed with high-flux membranes and treated concomitantly with an ACE inhibitor. Anaphylactoid reactions have also been reported in patients undergoing low-density lipoprotein apheresis with dextran sulfate absorption (a procedure dependent upon devices not approved in the United States).

Hypotension

Lotensin can cause symptomatic hypotension. Like other ACE inhibitors, benazepril has been only rarely associated with hypotension in uncomplicated hypertensive patients. Symptomatic hypotension is most likely to occur in patients who have been volume- and/or salt-depleted as a result of prolonged diuretic therapy, dietary salt restriction, dialysis, diarrhea, or vomiting. Volume- and/or salt-depletion should be corrected before initiating therapy with Lotensin.

In patients with congestive heart failure, with or without associated renal insufficiency, ACE inhibitor therapy may cause excessive hypotension, which may be associated with

oliguria or azotemia and, rarely, with acute renal failure and death. In such patients, Lotensin therapy should be started under close medical supervision; they should be followed closely for the first 2 weeks of treatment and whenever the dose of benazepril or diuretic is increased.

If hypotension occurs, the patient should be placed in a supine position, and, if necessary, treated with intravenous infusion of physiological saline. Lotensin treatment usually can be continued following restoration of blood pressure and volume.

Neutropenia/Agranulocytosis

Another angiotensin-converting enzyme inhibitor, captopril, has been shown to cause agranulocytosis and bone marrow depression, rarely in uncomplicated patients, but more frequently in patients with renal impairment, especially if they also have a collagen-vascular disease such as systemic lupus erythematosus or scleroderma. Available data from clinical trials of benazepril are insufficient to show that benazepril does not cause agranulocytosis at similar rates. Monitoring of white blood cell counts should be considered in patients with collagen-vascular disease, especially if the disease is associated with impaired renal function.

Fetal/Neonatal Morbidity and Mortality

ACE inhibitors can cause fetal and neonatal morbidity and death when administered to pregnant women. Several dozen cases have been reported in the world literature. When pregnancy is detected, ACE inhibitors should be discontinued as soon as possible.

The use of ACE inhibitors during the second and third trimesters of pregnancy has been associated with fetal and neonatal injury, including hypotension, neonatal skull hypoplasia, anuria, reversible or irreversible renal failure, and death. Oligohydramnios has also been reported, presumably resulting from decreased fetal renal function; oligohydramnios in this setting has been associated with fetal limb contractures, craniofacial deformation, and hypoplastic lung development. Prematurity, intrauterine growth retardation, and patent ductus arteriosus have also been reported, although it is not clear whether these occurrences were due to the ACE inhibitor exposure.

These adverse effects do not appear to have resulted from intrauterine ACE inhibitor exposure that has been limited to the first trimester. Mothers whose embryos and fetuses are exposed to ACE inhibitors only during the first trimester should be so informed. Nonetheless, when patients become pregnant, physicians should make every effort to discontinue the use of benazepril as soon as possible.

Rarely (probably less often than once in every thousand pregnancies), no alternative to ACE inhibitors will be found. In these rare cases, the mothers should be apprised of the potential hazards to their fetuses, and serial ultrasound examinations should be performed to assess the intraamniotic environment.

If oligohydramnios is observed, benazepril should be discontinued unless it is considered life-saving for the mother. Contraction stress testing (CST), a nonstress test (NST), or biophysical profiling (BPP) may be appropriate, depending upon the week of pregnancy. Patients and physicians should be aware, however, that oligohydramnios may not appear until after the fetus has sustained irreversible injury.

Infants with histories of in utero exposure to ACE inhibitors should be closely observed for hypotension, oliguria, and hyperkalemia. If oliguria occurs, attention should be directed toward support of blood pressure and renal perfusion. Exchange transfusion or dialysis may be required as means of reversing hypotension and/or substituting for disordered renal function. Benazepril, which crosses the placenta, can theoretically be removed from the neonatal circulation by these means; there are occasional reports of benefit from these maneuvers with another ACE inhibitor, but experience is limited.

No teratogenic effects of Lotensin were seen in studies of pregnant rats, mice, and rabbits. On a mg/m² basis, the doses used in these studies were 60 times (in rats), 9 times (in mice), and more than 0.8 times (in rabbits) the maximum recommended human dose (assuming a 50-kg woman). On a mg/kg basis these multiples are 300 times (in rats), 90 times (in mice) and more than 3 times (in rabbits) the maximum recommended human dose.

Hepatic Failure

Rarely, ACE inhibitors have been associated with a syndrome that starts with cholestatic jaundice and progresses to fulminant hepatic necrosis and (sometimes) death. The mechanism of this syndrome is not understood. Patients receiving ACE inhibitors who develop jaundice or marked elevations of hepatic enzymes should discontinue the ACE inhibitor and receive appropriate medical follow-up.

PRECAUTIONS

General

Impaired Renal Function: As a consequence of inhibiting the renin-angiotensin-aldosterone system, changes in renal function may be anticipated in susceptible individuals. In patients with severe congestive heart failure whose renal function may depend on the activity of the renin-angiotensin-aldosterone system, treatment with

angiotensin-converting enzyme inhibitors, including Lotensin, may be associated with oliguria and/or progressive azotemia and (rarely) with acute renal failure and/or death. In a small study of hypertensive patients with renal artery stenosis in a solitary kidney or bilateral renal artery stenosis, treatment with Lotensin was associated with increases in blood urea nitrogen and serum creatinine; these increases were reversible upon discontinuation of Lotensin or diuretic therapy, or both. When such patients are treated with ACE inhibitors, renal function should be monitored during the first few weeks of therapy. Some hypertensive patients with no apparent preexisting renal vascular disease have developed increases in blood urea nitrogen and serum creatinine, usually minor and transient, especially when Lotensin has been given concomitantly with a diuretic. This is more likely to occur in patients with preexisting renal impairment. Dosage reduction of Lotensin and/or discontinuation of the diuretic may be required. **Evaluation of the hypertensive patient should always include assessment of renal function (see DOSAGE AND ADMINISTRATION).**

Hyperkalemia: In clinical trials, hyperkalemia (serum potassium at least 0.5 mEq/L greater than the upper limit of normal) occurred in approximately 1% of hypertensive patients receiving Lotensin. In most cases, these were isolated values which resolved despite continued therapy. Risk factors for the development of hyperkalemia include renal insufficiency, diabetes mellitus, and the concomitant use of potassium-sparing diuretics, potassium supplements, and/or potassium-containing salt substitutes, which should be used cautiously, if at all, with Lotensin (see Drug Interactions).

Cough: Presumably due to the inhibition of the degradation of endogenous bradykinin, persistent nonproductive cough has been reported with all ACE inhibitors, always resolving after discontinuation of therapy. ACE inhibitor-induced cough should be considered in the differential diagnosis of cough.

Impaired Liver Function: In patients with hepatic dysfunction due to cirrhosis, levels of benazeprilat are essentially unaltered (see WARNINGS, Hepatic Failure).

Surgery/Anesthesia: In patients undergoing surgery or during anesthesia with agents that produce hypotension, benazepril will block the angiotensin II formation that could otherwise occur secondary to compensatory renin release. Hypotension that occurs as a result of this mechanism can be corrected by volume expansion.

Information for Patients

Pregnancy: Female patients of childbearing age should be told about the consequences of second- and third-trimester exposure to ACE inhibitors, and they should also be told that these consequences do not appear to have resulted from intrauterine ACE inhibitor exposure that has been limited to the first trimester. These patients should be asked to report pregnancies to their physicians as soon as possible.

Angioedema: Angioedema, including laryngeal edema, can occur at any time with treatment with ACE inhibitors. Patients should be so advised and told to report immediately any signs or symptoms suggesting angioedema (swelling of face, eyes, lips, or tongue, or difficulty in breathing) and to take no more drug until they have consulted with the prescribing physician.

Symptomatic Hypotension: Patients should be cautioned that lightheadedness can occur, especially during the first days of therapy, and it should be reported to the prescribing physician. Patients should be told that if syncope occurs, Lotensin should be discontinued until the prescribing physician has been consulted.

All patients should be cautioned that inadequate fluid intake or excessive perspiration, diarrhea, or vomiting can lead to an excessive fall in blood pressure, with the same consequences of lightheadedness and possible syncope.

Hyperkalemia: Patients should be told not to use potassium supplements or salt substitutes containing potassium without consulting the prescribing physician.

Neutropenia: Patients should be told to promptly report any indication of infection (e.g., sore throat, fever), which could be a sign of neutropenia.

Drug Interactions

Diuretics: Patients on diuretics, especially those in whom diuretic therapy was recently instituted, may occasionally experience an excessive reduction of blood pressure after initiation of therapy with Lotensin. The possibility of hypotensive effects with Lotensin can be minimized by either discontinuing the diuretic or increasing the salt intake prior to initiation of treatment with Lotensin. If this is not possible, the starting dose should be reduced (see DOSAGE AND ADMINISTRATION).

Potassium Supplements and Potassium-Sparing Diuretics: Lotensin can attenuate potassium loss caused by thiazide diuretics. Potassium-sparing diuretics (spironolactone, amiloride, triamterene, and others) or potassium supplements can increase the risk of hyperkalemia. Therefore, if concomitant use of such agents is indicated, they should be given with caution, and the patient's serum potassium should be monitored frequently.

Oral Anticoagulants: Interaction studies with warfarin and acenocoumarol failed to identify any clinically important effects on the serum concentrations or clinical effects of these anticoagulants.

Lithium: Increased serum lithium levels and symptoms of lithium toxicity have been reported in patients receiving ACE inhibitors during therapy with lithium. These drugs should be coadministered with caution, and frequent monitoring of serum lithium levels is recommended. If a diuretic is also used, the risk of lithium toxicity may be increased.

Other: No clinically important pharmacokinetic interactions occurred when Lotensin was administered concomitantly with hydrochlorothiazide, chlorthalidone, furosemide, digoxin, propranolol, atenolol, naproxen, or cimetidine.

Lotensin has been used concomitantly with beta-adrenergic-blocking agents, calcium-channel-blocking agents, diuretics, digoxin, and hydralazine, without evidence of clinically important adverse interactions. Benazepril, like other ACE inhibitors, has had less than additive effects with beta-adrenergic blockers, presumably because both drugs lower blood pressure by inhibiting parts of the renin-angiotensin system.

Carcinogenesis, Mutagenesis, Impairment of Fertility

No evidence of carcinogenicity was found when benazepril was administered to rats and mice for up to two years at doses of up to 150 mg/kg/day. When compared on the basis of body weights, this dose is 110 times the maximum recommended human dose. When compared on the basis of body surface areas, this dose is 18 and 9 times (rats and mice, respectively) the maximum recommended human dose (calculations assume a patient weight of 60 kg). No mutagenic activity was detected in the Ames test in bacteria (with or without metabolic activation), in an in vitro test for forward mutations in cultured mammalian cells, or in a nucleus anomaly test. In doses of 50–500 mg/kg/day (6–60 times the maximum recommended human dose based on mg/m^2 comparison and 37–375 times the maximum recommended human dose based on a mg/kg comparison), Lotensin had no adverse effect on the reproductive performance of male and female rats.

Pregnancy Categories C (first trimester) and D (second and third trimesters)

See WARNINGS, Fetal/Neonatal Morbidity and Mortality.

Nursing Mothers

Minimal amounts of unchanged benazepril and of benazeprilat are excreted into the breast milk of lactating women treated with benazepril. A newborn child ingesting entirely breast milk would receive less than 0.1% of the mg/kg maternal dose of benazepril and benazeprilat.

Geriatric Use

Of the total number of patients who received benazepril in U.S. clinical studies of Lotensin, 18% were 65 or older while 2% were 75 or older. No overall differences in effectiveness or safety were observed between these patients and younger patients, and other reported clinical experience has not identified differences in responses between the elderly and younger patients, but greater sensitivity of some older individuals cannot be ruled out.

Pediatric Use

Safety and effectiveness in pediatric patients have not been established.

ADVERSE REACTIONS

Lotensin has been evaluated for safety in over 6000 patients with hypertension; over 700 of these patients were treated for at least one year. The overall incidence of reported adverse events was comparable in Lotensin and placebo patients.

The reported side effects were generally mild and transient, and there was no relation between side effects and age, duration of therapy, or total dosage within the range of 2 to 80 mg. Discontinuation of therapy because of a side effect was required in approximately 5% of U.S. patients treated with Lotensin and in 3% of patients treated with placebo.

The most common reasons for discontinuation were headache (0.6%) and cough (0.5%) (see PRECAUTIONS, Cough).

The side effects considered possibly or probably related to study drug that occurred in U.S. placebo-controlled trials in more than 1% of patients treated with Lotensin are shown below.

PATIENTS IN U.S. PLACEBO-CONTROLLED STUDIES

	LOTENSIN (N=964)		PLACEBO (N=496)	
	N	%	N	%
Headache	60	6.2	21	4.2
Dizziness	35	3.6	12	2.4
Fatigue	23	2.4	11	2.2
Somnolence	15	1.6	2	0.4
Postural Dizziness	14	1.5	1	0.2
Nausea	13	1.3	5	1.0
Cough	12	1.2	5	1.0

Other adverse experiences reported in controlled clinical trials (in less than 1% of benazepril patients), and rarer events seen in postmarketing experience, include the following (in some, a causal relationship to drug use is uncertain):

Cardiovascular: Symptomatic hypotension was seen in 0.3% of patients, postural hypotension in 0.4%, and syncope in 0.1%; these reactions led to discontinuation of therapy in 4 patients who had received benazepril monotherapy and in 9 patients who had received benazepril with hydrochlorothiazide (see PRECAUTIONS and WARNINGS). Other reports included angina pectoris, palpitations, and peripheral edema.

Renal: Of hypertensive patients with no apparent preexisting renal disease, about 2% have sustained increases in serum creatinine to at least 150% of their baseline values while receiving Lotensin, but most of these increases have disappeared despite continuing treatment. A much smaller fraction of these patients (less than 0.1%) developed simultaneous (usually transient) increases in blood urea nitrogen and serum creatinine.

Fetal/Neonatal Morbidity and Mortality: See WARNINGS, Fetal/Neonatal Morbidity and Mortality.

Angioedema: Angioedema has been reported in patients receiving ACE inhibitors. During clinical trials in hypertensive patients with benazepril, 0.5% of patients experienced edema of the lips or face without other manifestations of angioedema. Angioedema associated with laryngeal edema and/or shock may be fatal. If angioedema of the face, extremities, lips, tongue, or glottis and/or larynx occurs, treatment with Lotensin should be discontinued and appropriate therapy instituted immediately (see WARNINGS).

Dermatologic: Stevens-Johnson syndrome, pemphigus, apparent hypersensitivity reactions (manifested by dermatitis, pruritus, or rash), photosensitivity, and flushing.

Gastrointestinal: Pancreatitis, constipation, gastritis, vomiting, and melena.

Hematologic: Thrombocytopenia and hemolytic anemia.

Neurologic and Psychiatric: Anxiety, decreased libido, hypertonia, insomnia, nervousness, and paresthesia.

Other: Asthma, bronchitis, dyspnea, sinusitus, urinary tract infection, infection, arthritis, impotence, alopecia, arthralgia, myalgia, asthenia, and sweating.

Another potentially important adverse experience, eosinophilic pneumonitis, has been attributed to other ACE inhibitors.

Clinical Laboratory Test Findings

Creatinine and Blood Urea Nitrogen: Of hypertensive patients with no apparent preexisting renal disease, about 2% have sustained increases in serum creatinine to at least 150% of their baseline values while receiving Lotensin, but most of these increases have disappeared despite continuing treatment. A much smaller fraction of these patients (less than 0.1%) developed simultaneous (usually transient) increases in blood urea nitrogen and serum creatinine. None of these increases required discontinuation of treatment. Increases in these laboratory values are more likely to occur in patients with renal insufficiency or those pretreated with a diuretic and, based on experience with other ACE inhibitors, would be expected to be especially likely in patients with renal artery stenosis (see PRECAUTIONS, General).

Potassium: Since benazepril decreases aldosterone secretion, elevation of serum potassium can occur. Potassium supplements and potassium-sparing diuretics should be given with caution, and the patient's serum potassium should be monitored frequently (see PRECAUTIONS).

Hemoglobin: Decreases in hemoglobin (a low value and a decrease of 5 g/dL) were rare, occurring in only 1 of 2014 patients receiving Lotensin alone and in 1 of 1357 patients receiving Lotensin plus a diuretic. No U.S. patients discontinued treatment because of decreases in hemoglobin.

Other (causal relationships unknown): Clinically important changes in standard laboratory tests were rarely associated with Lotensin administration. Elevations of uric acid, blood glucose, serum bilirubin, and liver enzymes (see WARNINGS) have been reported, as have scattered incidents of hyponatremia, electrocardiographic changes, leukopenia, eosinophilia, and proteinuria. In U.S. trials, less than 0.5% of patients discontinued treatment because of laboratory abnormalities.

OVERDOSAGE

Single oral doses of 3 g/kg benazepril were associated with significant lethality in mice. Rats, however, tolerated single oral doses of up to 6 g/kg. Reduced activity was seen at 1 g/kg in mice and at 5 g/kg in rats. Human overdoses of benazepril have not been reported, but the most common manifestation of human benazepril overdosage is likely to be hypotension.

Laboratory determinations of serum levels of benazepril and its metabolites are not widely available, and such determinations have, in any event, no established role in the management of benazepril overdose.

No data are available to suggest physiological maneuvers (e.g., maneuvers to change the pH of the urine) that might accelerate elimination of benazepril and its metabolites. Benazepril is only slightly dialyzable, but dialysis might be considered in overdosed patients with severely impaired renal function (see WARNINGS).

Angiotensin II could presumably serve as a specific antagonist-antidote in the setting of benazepril overdose, but angiotensin II is essentially unavailable outside of scattered research facilities. Because the hypotensive effect of benazepril is achieved through vasodilation and effective hypovolemia, it is reasonable to treat benazepril overdose by infusion of normal saline solution.

DOSAGE AND ADMINISTRATION

The recommended initial dose for patients not receiving a diuretic is 10 mg once-a-day. The usual maintenance dosage range is 20–40 mg per day administered as a single dose or in two equally divided doses. A dose of 80 mg gives an increased response, but experience with this dose is limited. The divided regimen was more effective in controlling trough (pre-dosing) blood pressure than the same dose given as a once-daily regimen. Dosage adjustment should be based on measurement of peak (2–6 hours after dosing) and trough responses. If a once-daily regimen does not give adequate trough response, an increase in dosage or divided administration should be considered. If blood pressure is not controlled with Lotensin alone, a diuretic can be added.

Total daily doses above 80 mg have not been evaluated.

Concomitant administration of Lotensin with potassium supplements, potassium salt substitutes, or potassium-sparing diuretics can lead to increases of serum potassium (see PRECAUTIONS).

In patients who are currently being treated with a diuretic, symptomatic hypotension occasionally can occur following the initial dose of Lotensin. To reduce the likelihood of hypotension, the diuretic should, if possible, be discontinued two to three days prior to beginning therapy with Lotensin (see WARNINGS). Then, if blood pressure is not controlled with Lotensin alone, diuretic therapy should be resumed.

If the diuretic cannot be discontinued, an initial dose of 5 mg Lotensin should be used to avoid excessive hypotension.

Dosage Adjustment in Renal Impairment

For patients with a creatinine clearance <30 mL/min/1.73 m^2 (serum creatinine >3 mg/dL), the recommended initial dose is 5 mg Lotensin once daily. Dosage may be titrated upward until blood pressure is controlled or to a maximum total daily dose of 40 mg (see WARNINGS).

HOW SUPPLIED

Lotensin is available in tablets of 5 mg, 10 mg, 20 mg, and 40 mg, packaged with a desiccant in bottles of 90 and 100 tablets. Lotensin is also supplied in blister packages (1 tablet/blister), in Accu-Pak® Unit Dose boxes containing 10 strips of 10 blisters each.

Each tablet is imprinted with LOTENSIN on one side and the tablet strength ("5", "10", "20", or "40") on the other.

The National Drug Codes for the various packages are:

[See table above]

Dose	Tablet Color	Bottle of 90	Bottle of 100	Accu-Pak® of 100
5 mg	light yellow	NDC 0083-0059-90	NDC 0083-0059-30	NDC 0083-0059-32
10 mg	dark yellow	NDC 0083-0063-90	NDC 0083-0063-30	NDC 0083-0063-32
20 mg	tan	NDC 0083-0079-90	NDC 0083-0079-30	NDC 0083-0079-32
40 mg	dark rose	NDC 0083-0094-90	NDC 0083-0094-30	NDC 0083-0094-32

Storage: Do not store above 30°C (86°F). Protect from moisture.

Dispense in tight container (USP).

Distributed by
Novartis Pharmaceuticals Corporation
East Hanover, New Jersey 07936

C98-30 (Rev. 8/98)

Shown in Product Identification Guide, page 325

LOTENSIN HCT® ℞

[*lō tĕn sĭn*]

benazepril hydrochloride and hydrochlorothiazide USP Combination Tablets

5 mg/6.25 mg
10 mg/12.5 mg
20 mg/12.5mg
20 mg/25 mg

The following prescribing information is based on official labeling in effect on August 1, 1998.

USE IN PREGNANCY

When used in pregnancy during the second and third trimesters, ACE inhibitors can cause injury and even death to the developing fetus. When pregnancy is

Continued on next page

Lotensin HCT—Cont.

detected, Lotensin HCT should be discontinued as soon as possible. See **WARNINGS, Fetal/Neonatal Morbidity and Mortality.**

DESCRIPTION

Benazepril hydrochloride is a white to off-white crystalline powder, soluble (>100 mg/mL) in water, in ethanol, and in methanol. Benazepril hydrochloride's chemical name is 3-[[1-(ethoxycarbonyl)-3-phenyl-(1S)-propyl]amino]-2,3,4,5-tetrahydro-2-oxo-1*H*-1-(3S)-benzazepine-1-acetic acid monohydrochloride; its structural formula is

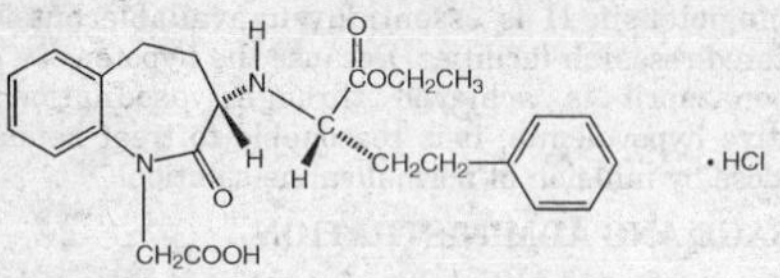

Its empirical formula is $C_{24}H_{28}N_2O_5 \cdot HCl$, and its molecular weight is 460.96.

Benazeprilat, the active metabolite of benazepril, is a non-sulfhydryl angiotensin-converting enzyme inhibitor. Benazepril is converted to benazeprilat by hepatic cleavage of the ester group.

Hydrochlorothiazide USP is a white, or practically white, practically odorless, crystalline powder. It is slightly soluble in water; freely soluble in sodium hydroxide solution, in *n*-butylamine, and in dimethylformamide; sparingly soluble in methanol; and insoluble in ether, in chloroform, and in dilute mineral acids. Hydrochlorothiazide's chemical name is 6-chloro-3,4-dihydro-2*H*-1,2,4-benzothiadiazine-7-sulfonamide 1,1-dioxide; its structural formula is

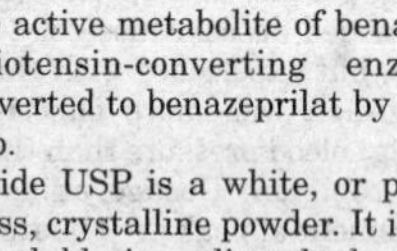

Its empirical formula is $C_7H_8ClN_3O_4S_2$, and its molecular weight is 297.73. Hydrochlorothiazide is a thiazide diuretic.

Lotensin HCT is a combination of benazepril hydrochloride and hydrochlorothiazide USP. The tablets are formulated for oral administration with a combination of 5, 10, or 20 mg of benazapril hydrochloride and 6.25, 12.5, or 25 mg of hydrochlorothiazide USP. The inactive ingredients of the tablets are cellulose compounds, crospovidone, hydrogenated castor oil, iron oxides (10/12.5-mg, 20/12.5-mg, and 20/25-mg tablets), lactose, polyethylene glycol, talc, and titanium dioxide.

CLINICAL PHARMACOLOGY

Mechanism of Action

Benazepril and benazeprilat inhibit angiotensin-converting enzyme (ACE) in human subjects and in animals. ACE is a peptidyl dipeptidase that catalyzes the conversion of angiotensin I to the vasoconstrictor substance, angiotensin II. Angiotensin II also stimulates aldosterone secretion by the adrenal cortex.

Inhibition of ACE results in decreased plasma angiotensin II, which leads to decreased vasopressor activity and to decreased aldosterone secretion. The latter decrease may result in a small increase of serum potassium. Hypertensive patients treated with benazepril alone for up to 52 weeks had elevations of serum potassium of up to 0.2 mEq/L. Similar patients treated with benazepril and hydrochlorothiazide for up to 24 weeks had no consistent changes in their serum potassium (see PRECAUTIONS).

Removal of angiotensin II negative feedback on renin secretion leads to increased plasma renin activity. In animal studies, benazepril had no inhibitory effect on the vasopressor response to angiotensin II and did not interfere with the hemodynamic effects of the autonomic neurotransmitters acetylcholine, epinephrine, and norepinephrine.

ACE is identical to kininase, an enzyme that degrades bradykinin. Whether increased levels of bradykinin, a potent vasodepressor peptide, play a role in the therapeutic effects of Lotensin HCT remains to be elucidated.

While the mechanism through which benazepril lowers blood pressure is believed to be primarily suppression of the renin-angiotensin-aldosterone system, benazepril has an antihypertensive effect even in patients with low-renin hypertension.

Hydrochlorothiazide is a thiazide diuretic. Thiazides affect the renal tubular mechanisms of electrolyte reabsorption, directly increasing excretion of sodium and chloride in approximately equivalent amounts. Indirectly, the diuretic action of hydrochlorothiazide reduces plasma volume, with consequent increases in plasma renin activity, increases in aldosterone secretion, increases in urinary potassium loss, and decreases in serum potassium. The renin-aldosterone link is mediated by angiotensin, so coadministration of an ACE inhibitor tends to reverse the potassium loss associated with these diuretics.

The mechanism of the antihypertensive effect of thiazides is unknown.

Pharmacokinetics and Metabolism

Following oral administration of Lotensin HCT, peak plasma concentrations of benazepril are reached within 0.5-1.0 hours. As determined by urinary recovery, the extent of absorption is at least 37%. The absorption of hydrochlorothiazide is somewhat slower (1-2.5 hours) and somewhat more complete (50%-80%). In fasting subjects, the rate and extent of absorption of benazepril and hydrochlorothiazide from Lotensin HCT are not different, respectively, from the rate and extent of absorption of benazepril and hydrochlorothiazide from immediate-release monotherapy formulations.

The absorption of benazepril from Lotensin® tablets is not influenced by the presence of food in the gastrointestinal tract, but possible effects of food upon absorption of either component from Lotensin HCT tablets have not been studied. The reported studies of food effects on hydrochlorothiazide absorption have been inconclusive. The absorption of hydrochlorothiazide is increased by agents that reduce gastrointestinal motility, but it is reported to be reduced by 50% in patients with congestive heart failure.

Cleavage of the ester group (primarily in the liver) converts benazepril to its active metabolite, benazeprilat. Peak plasma concentrations of benazeprilat are reached 1-2 hours after drug intake in the fasting state and 2-4 hours after drug intake in the nonfasting state. The serum protein binding of benazepril is about 96.7% and that of benazeprilat about 95.3%, as measured by equilibrium dialysis; on the basis of in vitro studies, the degree of protein binding should be unaffected by age, hepatic dysfunction, or-over the concentration range of 0.24-23.6 µmol/L-concentration.

Hydrochlorothiazide is not metabolized. Its apparent volume of distribution is 3.6-7.8 L/kg, and its measured plasma protein binding is 67.9%. The drug also accumulates in red blood cells, so that whole blood levels are 1.6-1.8 times those measured in plasma.

In studies of rats given ^{14}C-benazepril, benazepril and its metabolites crossed the blood-brain barrier only to an extremely low extent. Multiple doses of benazepril did not result in accumulation in any tissue except the lung, where, as with other ACE inhibitors in similar studies, there was a slight increase in concentration due to slow elimination in that organ.

Some placental passage occurred when benazepril was administered to pregnant rats. In humans, hydrochlorothiazide crosses the placenta freely, and levels in umbilical-cord blood are similar to those in the maternal circulation.

Benazepril is almost completely metabolized to benazeprilat, which has much greater ACE inhibitory activity than benazepril, and to the glucuronide conjugates of benazepril and benazeprilat. Only trace amounts of an administered dose of benazepril can be recovered unchanged in the urine; about 20% of the dose is excreted as benazeprilat, 4% as benazepril glucuronide, and 8% as benazeprilat glucuronide.

In patients with hepatic dysfunction due to cirrhosis, levels of benazeprilat are essentially unaltered. Similarly, the pharmacokinetics of benazepril and benazeprilat do not appear to be influenced by age.

The kinetics of benazepril are dose-proportional within the dosage range of 5-20 mg. Small deviations from dose proportionality were observed when the broader range of 2-80 mg was studied, possibly due to the saturable binding of the compound to ACE.

The effective half-life of accumulation of benazeprilat following multiple dosing of benazepril hydrochloride is 10-11 hours. Thus, steady-state concentrations of benazeprilat should be reached after 2 or 3 doses of benazepril hydrochloride given once daily.

During chronic administration (28 days) of once-daily doses of benazepril between 5 mg and 20 mg, the kinetics did not change, and there was no significant accumulation. Accumulation ratios based on AUC and urinary recovery of benazeprilat were 1.19 and 1.27, respectively.

When dialysis was started 2 hours after ingestion of 10 mg of benazepril, approximately 6% of benazeprilat was removed in 4 hours of dialysis. The parent compound, benazepril, was not detected in the dialysate.

Benazepril and benazeprilat are cleared predominantly by renal excretion in healthy subjects with normal renal function. Nonrenal (i.e., biliary) excretion accounts for approximately 11%-12% of benazeprilat excretion in healthy subjects. In patients with renal failure, biliary clearance may compensate to an extent for deficient renal clearance.

The disposition of benazepril and benazeprilat in patients with mild-to-moderate renal insufficiency (creatinine clearance >30 mL/min) is similar to that in patients with normal renal function. In patients with creatinine clearance ≤30 mL/min, peak benazeprilat levels and the initial (alpha phase) half-life increase, and time to steady state may be delayed (see DOSAGE AND ADMINISTRATION).

Thiazide diuretics are eliminated by the kidney, with a terminal half-life of 5-15 hours. In a study of patients with impaired renal function (mean creatinine clearance of 19 mL/min), the half-life of hydrochlorothiazide elimination was lengthened to 21 hours.

Pharmacodynamics

Single and multiple doses of 10 mg or more of **benazepril** cause inhibition of plasma ACE activity by at least 80%-90% for at least 24 hours after dosing. For up to 4 hours after a 10-mg dose, pressor responses to exogenous angiotensin I were inhibited by 60%-90%.

Administration of benazepril to patients with mild-to-moderate hypertension results in a reduction of both supine and standing blood pressure to about the same extent, with no compensatory tachycardia. Symptomatic postural hypotension is infrequent, although it can occur in patients who are salt and/or volume depleted (see WARNINGS, Hypotension).

In single-dose studies, benazepril lowered blood pressure within 1 hour, with peak reductions achieved 2-4 hours after dosing. The antihypertensive effect of a single dose persisted for 24 hours. In multiple-dose studies, once-daily doses of 20-80 mg decreased seated pressure (systolic/diastolic) 24 hours after dosing by about 6-12/4-7 mmHg. The reductions at trough are about 50% of those seen at peak.

Four dose-response studies of benazepril monotherapy using once-daily dosing were conducted in 470 mild-to-moderate hypertensive patients not using diuretics. The minimal effective once-daily dose of benazepril was 10 mg; further falls in blood pressure, especially at morning trough, were seen with higher doses in the studied dosing range (10-80 mg). In studies comparing the same daily dose of benazepril given as a single morning dose or as a twice-daily dose, blood pressure reductions at the time of morning trough blood levels were greater with the divided regimen.

During chronic therapy with benazepril, the maximum reduction in blood pressure with any given dose is generally achieved after 1-2 weeks. The antihypertensive effects of benazepril have continued during therapy for at least 2 years. Abrupt withdrawal of benazepril has not been associated with a rapid increase in blood pressure.

In patients with mild-to-moderate hypertension, total daily doses of Lotensin 20-40 mg were similar in effectiveness to total daily doses of captopril 50-100 mg, hydrochlorothiazide 25-50 mg, nifedipine SR 40-80 mg, and propranolol 80-160 mg.

The antihypertensive effects of benazepril were not appreciably different in patients receiving high- or low-sodium diets.

In hemodynamic studies in dogs, blood pressure reduction was accompanied by a reduction in peripheral arterial resistance, with an increase in cardiac output and renal blood flow and little or no change in heart rate. In normal human volunteers, single doses of benazepril caused an increase in renal blood flow but had no effect on glomerular filtration rate.

In clinical trials of **benazepril/hydrochlorothiazide** using benazepril doses of 5-20 mg and hydrochlorothiazide doses of 6.25-25 mg, the antihypertensive effects were sustained for at least 24 hours, and they increased with increasing dose of either component. Although benazepril monotherapy is somewhat less effective in blacks than in nonblacks, the efficacy of combination therapy appears to be independent of race.

By blocking the renin-angiotensin-aldosterone axis, administration of benazepril tends to reduce the potassium loss associated with the diuretic. In clinical trials of Lotensin HCT, the average change in serum potassium was near zero in subjects who received 5/6.25 mg or 20/12.5 mg, but the average subject who received 10/12.5 mg or 20/25 mg experienced a mild reduction in serum potassium, similar to that experienced by the average subject receiving the same dose of hydrochlorothiazide monotherapy.

INDICATIONS AND USAGE

Lotensin HCT is indicated for the treatment of hypertension.

This fixed combination drug is not indicated for the initial therapy of hypertension (see DOSAGE AND ADMINISTRATION).

In using Lotensin HCT, consideration should be given to the fact that another angiotensin-converting enzyme inhibitor, captopril, has caused agranulocytosis, particularly in patients with renal impairment or collagen-vascular disease. Available data are insufficient to show that benazepril does not have a similar risk (see WARNINGS, Neutropenia/Agranulocytosis).

Black patients receiving ACE inhibitors have been reported to have a higher incidence of angioedema compared to nonblacks.

CONTRAINDICATIONS

Lotensin HCT is contraindicated in patients who are anuric. Lotensin HCT is also contraindicated in patients who are hypersensitive to benazepril, to any other ACE inhibitor, to hydrochlorothiazide, or to other sulfonamide-derived drugs. Hypersensitivity reactions are more likely to occur in patients with a history of allergy or bronchial asthma.

WARNINGS

Anaphylactoid and Possibly Related Reactions

Presumably because angiotensin-converting enzyme inhibitors affect the metabolism of eicosanoids and polypeptides, including endogenous bradykinin, patients receiving ACE inhibitors (including Lotensin HCT) may be subject to a variety of adverse reactions, some of them serious.

Angioedema: Angioedema of the face, extremities, lips, tongue, glottis, and larynx has been reported in patients treated with angiotensin-converting enzyme inhibitors. In U.S. clinical trials, symptoms consistent with angioedema were seen in none of the subjects who received placebo and in about 0.5% of the subjects who received benazepril. Angioedema associated with laryngeal edema can be fatal. If laryngeal stridor or angioedema of the face, tongue, or glottis occurs, treatment with Lotensin HCT should be discontinued and appropriate therapy instituted immediately. *When involvement of the tongue, glottis, or larynx appears likely to cause airway obstruction, appropriate therapy, e.g., subcutaneous epinephrine injection 1:1000 (0.3-0.5 mL) should be promptly administered* (see PRECAUTIONS and ADVERSE REACTIONS).

Anaphylactoid Reactions During Desensitization: Two patients undergoing desensitizing treatment with hymenoptera venom while receiving ACE inhibitors sustained life-threatening anaphylactoid reactions. In the same patients, these reactions were avoided when ACE inhibitors were temporarily withheld, but they reappeared upon inadvertent rechallenge.

Anaphylactoid Reactions During Membrane Exposure: Anaphylactoid reactions have been reported in patients dialyzed with high-flux membranes and treated concomitantly with an ACE inhibitor. Anaphylactoid reactions have also been reported in patients undergoing low-density lipoprotein apheresis with dextran sulfate absorption.

Hypotension

Lotensin HCT can cause symptomatic hypotension. Like other ACE inhibitors, benazepril has been only rarely associated with hypotension in uncomplicated hypertensive patients. Symptomatic hypotension is most likely to occur in patients who have been volume and/or salt depleted as a result of prolonged diuretic therapy, dietary salt restriction, dialysis, diarrhea, or vomiting. Volume and/or salt depletion should be corrected before initiating therapy with Lotensin HCT.

Lotensin HCT should be used cautiously in patients receiving concomitant therapy with other antihypertensives. The thiazide component of Lotensin HCT may potentiate the action of other antihypertensive drugs, especially ganglionic or peripheral adrenergic-blocking drugs. The antihypertensive effects of the thiazide component may also be enhanced in the postsympathectomy patient.

In patients with congestive heart failure, with or without associated renal insufficiency, ACE inhibitor therapy may cause excessive hypotension, which may be associated with oliguria, azotemia, and (rarely) with acute renal failure and death. In such patients, Lotensin HCT therapy should be started under close medical supervision; they should be followed closely for the first 2 weeks of treatment and whenever the dose of benazepril or diuretic is increased.

If hypotension occurs, the patient should be placed in a supine position, and, if necessary, treated with intravenous infusion of physiological saline. Lotensin HCT treatment usually can be continued following restoration of blood pressure and volume.

Impaired Renal Function

Lotensin HCT should be used with caution in patients with severe renal disease. Thiazides may precipitate azotemia in such patients, and the effects of repeated dosing may be cumulative.

When the renin-angiotensin-aldosterone system is inhibited by benazepril, changes in renal function may be anticipated in susceptible individuals. In patients with **severe congestive heart failure**, whose renal function may depend on the activity of the renin-angiotensin-aldosterone system, treatment with angiotensin-converting enzyme inhibitors (including benazepril) may be associated with oliguria and/or progressive azotemia and (rarely) with acute renal failure and/or death.

In a small study of hypertensive patients with **unilateral or bilateral renal artery stenosis**, treatment with benazepril was associated with increases in blood urea nitrogen and serum creatinine; these increases were reversible upon discontinuation of benazepril therapy, concomitant diuretic therapy, or both. When such patients are treated with Lotensin HCT, renal function should be monitored during the first few weeks of therapy.

Some benazepril-treated hypertensive patients with **no apparent preexisting renal vascular disease** have developed increases in blood urea nitrogen and serum creatinine, usually minor and transient, especially when benazepril has been given concomitantly with a diuretic. Dosage reduction of Lotensin HCT may be required. **Evaluation of the hypertensive patient should always include assessment of renal function** (see DOSAGE AND ADMINISTRATION).

Neutropenia/Agranulocytosis

Another angiotensin-converting enzyme inhibitor, captopril, has been shown to cause agranulocytosis and bone marrow depression, rarely in uncomplicated patients (incidence probably less than once per 10,000 exposures) but more frequently (incidence possibly as great as once per 1000 exposures) in patients with renal impairment, especially those who also have collagen-vascular diseases such as systemic lupus erythematosus or scleroderma. Available data from clinical trials of benazepril are insufficent to show that benazepril does not cause agranulocytosis at similar rates. Monitoring of white blood cell counts should be considered in patients with collagen-vascular disease, especially if the disease is associated with impaired renal function.

Fetal/Neonatal Morbidity and Mortality

ACE inhibitors can cause fetal and neonatal morbidity and death when administered to pregnant women. Several dozen cases have been reported in the world literature. When pregnancy is detected, Lotensin HCT should be discontinued as soon as possible.

The use of ACE inhibitors during the second and third trimesters of pregnancy has been associated with fetal and neonatal injury, including hypotension, neonatal skull hypoplasia, anuria, reversible or irreversible renal failure, and death. Oligohydramnios has also been reported, presumably resulting from decreased fetal renal function; oligohydramnios in this setting has been associated with fetal limb contractures, craniofacial deformation, and hypoplastic lung development. Prematurity, intrauterine growth retardation, and patent ductus arteriosus have also been reported, although it is not clear whether these occurrences were due to the ACE-inhibitor exposure.

These adverse effects do not appear to have resulted from intrauterine ACE-inhibitor exposure that has been limited to the first trimester. Mothers whose embryos and fetuses are exposed to ACE inhibitors only during the first trimester should be so informed. Nonetheless, when patients become pregnant, physicians should make every effort to discontinue the use of benazepril as soon as possible.

Rarely (probably less often than once in every thousand pregnancies), no alternative to ACE inhibitors will be found. In these rare cases, the mothers should be apprised of the potential hazards to their fetuses, and serial ultrasound examinations should be performed to assess the intra-amniotic environment.

If oligohydramnios is observed, benazepril should be discontinued unless it is considered life-saving for the mother. Contraction stress testing (CST), a nonstress test (NST), or biophysical profiling (BPP) may be appropriate, depending upon the week of pregnancy. Patients and physicians should be aware, however, that oligohydramnios may not appear until after the fetus has sustained irreversible injury.

Infants with histories of in utero exposure to ACE inhibitors should be closely observed for hypotension, oliguria, and hyperkalemia. If oliguria occurs, attention should be directed toward support of blood pressure and renal perfusion. Exchange transfusion or peritoneal dialysis may be required as means of reversing hypotension and/or substituting for disordered renal function. Benazepril, which crosses the placenta, can theoretically be removed from the neonatal circulation by these means; there are occasional reports of benefit from these maneuvers, but experience is limited.

Intrauterine exposure to thiazide diuretics is associated with fetal or neonatal jaundice, thrombocytopenia, and possibly other adverse reactions that have occurred in adults. No teratogenic effects were seen when benazepril and hydrochlorothiazide were administered to pregnant rats at a dose ratio of 4:5. On a mg/kg basis, the doses used were up to 167 times the maximum recommended human dose. Similarly, no teratogenic effects were seen when benazepril and hydrochlorothiazide were administered to pregnant mice at total doses up to 160 mg/kg/day, with benazepril:hydrochlorothiazide ratios of 15:1. When hydrochlorothiazide was orally administered without benazepril to pregnant mice and rats during their respective periods of major organogenesis, at doses up to 3000 and 1000 mg/kg/day respectively, there was no evidence of harm to the fetus. Similarly, no teratogenic effects of benazepril were seen in studies of pregnant rats, mice, and rabbits; on a mg/kg basis, the doses used in these studies were 300 times (in rats), 90 times (in mice), and more than 3 times (in rabbits) the maximum recommended human dose.

Hepatic Failure

Rarely, ACE inhibitors have been associated with a syndrome that starts with cholestatic jaundice and progresses to fulminant hepatic necrosis and (sometimes) death. The mechanism of this syndrome is not understood. Patients receiving ACE inhibitors who develop jaundice or marked elevations of hepatic enzymes should discontinue the ACE inhibitor and receive appropriate medical follow-up.

Impaired Hepatic Function

Lotensin HCT should be used with caution in patients with impaired hepatic function or progressive liver disease, since minor alterations of fluid and electrolyte balance may precipitate hepatic coma (see Hepatic Failure, above). In patients with hepatic dysfunction due to cirrhosis, levels of benazeprilat are essentially unaltered. No formal pharmacokinetic studies have been carried out in hypertensive patients with impaired liver function.

Systemic Lupus Erythematosus

Thiazide diuretics have been reported to cause exacerbation or activation of systemic lupus erythematosus.

PRECAUTIONS

General

Derangements of Serum Electrolytes: In clinical trials of benazepril monotherapy, hyperkalemia (serum potassium at least 0.5 mEq/L greater than the upper limit of normal) occurred in approximately 1% of hypertensive patients receiving benazepril. In most cases, these were isolated values which resolved despite continued therapy. Risk factors for the development of hyperkalemia included renal insufficiency, diabetes mellitus, and the concomitant use of potassium-sparing diuretics, potassium supplements, and/or potassium-containing salt substitutes.

Conversely, treatment with thiazide diuretics has been associated with hypokalemia, hyponatremia, and hypochloremic alkalosis. These disturbances have sometimes been manifest as one or more of dryness of mouth, thirst, weakness, lethargy, drowsiness, restlessness, muscle pains or cramps, muscular fatigue, hypotension, oliguria, tachycardia, nausea, and vomiting. Hypokalemia can also sensitize or exaggerate the response of the heart to the toxic effects of digitalis. The risk of hypokalemia is greatest in patients with cirrhosis of the liver, in patients experiencing a brisk diuresis, in patients who are receiving inadequate oral intake of electrolytes, and in patients receiving concomitant therapy with corticosteroids or ACTH.

The opposite effects of benazepril and hydrochlorothiazide on serum potassium will approximately balance each other in many patients, so that no net effect upon serum potassium will be seen. In other patients, one or the other effect may be dominant. Initial and periodic determinations of serum electrolytes to detect possible electrolyte imbalance should be performed at appropriate intervals.

Chloride deficits are generally mild and require specific treatment only under extraordinary circumstances (e.g., in liver disease or renal disease). Dilutional hyponatremia may occur in edematous patients; appropriate therapy is water restriction rather than administration of salt, except in rare instances when the hyponatremia is life-threatening. In actual salt depletion, appropriate replacement is the therapy of choice.

Calcium excretion is decreased by thiazides. In a few patients on prolonged thiazide therapy, pathological changes in the parathyroid gland have been observed, with hypercalcemia and hypophosphatemia. More serious complications of hyperparathyroidism (renal lithiasis, bone resorption, and peptic ulceration) have not been seen.

Thiazides increase the urinary excretion of magnesium, and hypomagnesemia may result.

Other Metabolic Disturbances: Thiazide diuretics tend to reduce glucose tolerance and to raise serum levels of cholesterol, triglycerides, and uric acid. These effects are usually minor, but frank gout or overt diabetes may be precipitated in susceptible patients.

Cough: Presumably due to the inhibition of the degradation of endogenous bradykinin, persistent nonproductive cough has been reported with all ACE inhibitors, always resolving after discontinuation of therapy. ACE inhibitor-induced cough should be considered in the differential diagnosis of cough.

Surgery/Anesthesia: In patients undergoing surgery or during anesthesia with agents that produce hypotension, benazepril will block the angiotensin II formation that could otherwise occur secondary to compensatory renin release. Hypotension that occurs as a result of this mechanism can be corrected by volume expansion.

Information for Patients

Angioedema: Angioedema, including laryngeal edema, can occur at any time with treatment with ACE inhibitors. A patient receiving Lotensin HCT should be told to report immediately any signs or symptoms suggesting angioedema (swelling of face, eyes, lips, or tongue, or difficulty in breathing) and to take no more drug until after consulting with the prescribing physician.

Pregnancy: Female patients of childbearing age should be told about the consequences of second- and third-trimester exposure to ACE inhibitors, and they should also be told that these consequences do not appear to have resulted from intrauterine ACE-inhibitor exposure that has been limited to the first trimester. These patients should be asked to report pregnancies to their physicians as soon as possible.

Symptomatic Hypotension: A patient receiving Lotensin HCT should be cautioned that lightheadedness can occur, especially during the first days of therapy, and that it should be reported to the prescribing physician. The patient should be told that if syncope occurs, Lotensin HCT should be discontinued until the physician has been consulted.

Continued on next page

Lotensin HCT—Cont.

All patients should be cautioned that inadequate fluid intake, excessive perspiration, diarrhea, or vomiting can lead to an excessive fall in blood pressure, with the same consequences of lightheadedness and possible syncope.

Hyperkalemia: A patient receiving Lotensin HCT should be told not to use potassium supplements or salt substitutes containing potassium without consulting the prescribing physician.

Neutropenia: Patients should be told to promptly report any indication of infection (e.g., sore throat, fever), which could be a sign of neutropenia.

Laboratory Tests

The hydrochlorothiazide component of Lotensin HCT may decrease serum PBI levels without signs of thyroid disturbance.

Therapy with Lotensin HCT should be interrupted for a few days before carrying out tests of parathyroid function.

Drug Interactions

Potassium Supplements and Potassium-Sparing Diuretics: As noted above (Derangements of Serum Electrolytes), the net effect of Lotensin HCT may be to elevate a patient's serum potassium, to reduce it, or to leave it unchanged. Potassium-sparing diuretics (spironolactone, amiloride, triamterene, and others) or potassium supplements can increase the risk of hyperkalemia. If concomitant use of such agents is indicated, they should be given with caution, and the patient's serum potassium should be monitored frequently.

Lithium: Increased serum lithium levels and symptoms of lithium toxicity have been reported in patients receiving ACE inhibitors during therapy with lithium. Because renal clearance of lithium is reduced by thiazides, the risk of lithium toxicity is presumably raised further when, as in therapy with Lotensin HCT, a thiazide diuretic is coadministered with the ACE inhibitor. Lotensin HCT and lithium should be coadministered with caution, and frequent monitoring of serum lithium levels is recommended.

Other: Benazepril has been used concomitantly with beta-adrenergic-blocking agents, calcium-blocking agents, cimetidine, diuretics, digoxin, hydralazine, and naproxen without evidence of clinically important adverse interactions. Other ACE inhibitors have had less than additive effects with beta-adrenergic blockers, presumably because drugs of both classes lower blood pressure by inhibiting parts of the renin-angiotensin system.

Interaction studies with warfarin and acenocoumarol have failed to identify any clinically important effects of benazepril on the serum concentrations or clinical effects of these anticoagulants.

Insulin requirements in diabetic patients may be increased, decreased, or unchanged.

Thiazides may decrease arterial responsiveness to norepinephrine, but not enough to preclude effectiveness of the pressor agent for therapeutic use.

Thiazides may increase the responsiveness to tubocurarine.

The diuretic, natriuretic, and antihypertensive effects of thiazide diuretics may be reduced by concurrent administration of nonsteroidal anti-inflammatory agents.

Cholestyramine and colestipol resins: Absorption of hydrochlorothiazide is impaired in the presence of anionic exchange resins. Single doses of either cholestyramine or colestipol resins bind the hydrochlorothiazide and reduce its absorption from the gastrointestinal tract by up to 85% and 43%, respectively.

Carcinogenesis, Mutagenesis, Impairment of Fertility

No evidence of carcinogenicity was found when **benazepril** was given to rats and mice for 104 weeks at doses up to 150 mg/kg/day. On a body-weight basis, this dose is over 100 times the maximum recommended human dose; on a body-surface-area basis, this dose is 18 times (rats) and 9 times (mice) the maximum recommended human dose. No mutagenic activity was detected in the Ames test in bacteria (with or without metabolic activation), in an in vitro test for forward mutations in cultured mammalian cells, or in a nucleus anomaly test. At doses of 50-500 mg/kg/day (38-375 times the maximum recommended human dose on a body-weight basis; 6-61 times the maximum recommended dose on a body-surface-area basis), benazepril had no adverse effect on the reproductive performance of male and female rats.

Under the auspices of the National Toxicology Program, rats and mice received **hydrochlorothiazide** in their feed for two years, at doses up to 600 mg/kg/day in mice and up to 100 mg/kg/day in rats. These studies uncovered no evidence of a carcinogenic potential of hydrochlorothiazide in rats or female mice, but there was equivocal evidence of hepatocarcinogenicity in male mice. Hydrochlorothiazide was not genotoxic in in vitro assays using strains TA 98, TA 100, TA 1535, TA 1537, and TA 1538 of *Salmonella typhimurium* (the Ames test); in the Chinese Hamster Ovary (CHO) test for chromosomal aberrations; or in in vivo assays using mouse germinal cell chromosomes, Chinese hamster bone marrow chromosomes; and the *Drosophila* sex-linked reces-

sive lethal trait gene. Positive test results were obtained in the in vitro CHO Sister Chromatid Exchange (clastogenicity) test and in the Mouse Lymphoma Cell (mutagenicity) assays, using concentrations of hydrochlorothiazide of 43-1300 µg/mL. Positive test results were also obtained in the *Aspergillus nidulans* nondisjunction assay, using an unspecified concentration of hydrochlorothiazide.

Hydrochlorothiazide had no adverse effects on the fertility of mice and rats of either sex in studies wherein these species were exposed, via their diets, to doses up to 100 and 4 mg/kg/day, respectively, prior to mating and throughout gestation.

Pregnancy

Pregnancy Categories C (first trimester) and D (second and third trimesters): See WARNINGS, Fetal/Neonatal Morbidity and Mortality.

Nursing Mothers

Minimal amounts of unchanged benazepril and of benazeprilat are excreted into the breast milk of lactating women treated with benazepril, so that a newborn child ingesting nothing but breast milk would receive less than 0.1% of the maternal doses of benazepril and benazeprilat. Thiazides, on the other hand, are definitely excreted into breast milk. Because of the potential for serious adverse reactions in nursing infants from hydrochlorothiazide and the unknown effects of benazepril in infants, a decision should be made whether to discontinue nursing or to discontinue Lotensin HCT, taking into account the importance of the drug to the mother.

Geriatric Use

Of the total number of patients who received Lotensin HCT in U.S. clinical studies of Lotensin HCT, 19% were 65 or older while about 1.5% were 75 or older. Overall differences in effectiveness or safety were not observed between these patients and younger patients, and other reported clinical experience has not identified differences in responses between the elderly and younger patients, but greater sensitivity of some older individuals cannot be ruled out.

Pediatric Use

Safety and effectiveness in pediatric patients have not been established.

ADVERSE REACTIONS

Lotensin HCT has been evaluated for safety in over 2500 patients with hypertension; over 500 of these patients were treated for at least 6 months, and over 200 were treated for more than 1 year.

The reported side effects were generally mild and transient, and there was no relationship between side effects and age, sex, race, or duration of therapy. Discontinuation of therapy due to side effects was required in approximately 7% of U.S. patients treated with Lotensin HCT and in 4% of patients treated with placebo.

The most common reasons for discontinuation of therapy with Lotensin HCT in U.S. studies were cough (1.0%; see PRECAUTIONS), "dizziness" (1.0%), headache (0.6%), and fatigue (0.6%).

The side effects considered possibly or probably related to study drug that occurred in U.S. placebo-controlled trials in more than 1% of patients treated with Lotensin HCT are shown in the table below.

Reactions Possibly or Probably Drug Related Patients in U.S. Placebo-Controlled Studies				
	LOTENSIN HCT N=655		Placebo N=235	
	N	%	N	%
"Dizziness"	41	6.3	8	3.4
Fatigue	34	5.2	6	2.6
Postural Dizziness	23	3.5	1	0.4
Headache	20	3.1	10	4.3
Cough	14	2.1	3	1.3
Hypertonia	10	1.5	3	1.3
Vertigo	10	1.5	2	0.9
Nausea	9	1.4	2	0.9
Impotence	8	1.2	0	0.0
Somnolence	8	1.2	1	0.4

Other side effects considered possibly or probably related to study drug that occurred in U.S. placebo-controlled trials in 0.3% to 1.0% of patients treated with Lotensin HCT were the following:

Angioedema: Edema of the lips or face without other manifestations of angioedema (0.3%). See WARNINGS, Angioedema.

Cardiovascular: Hypotension (seen in 0.6% of patients), postural hypotension (0.3%), palpitations, and flushing.

Gastrointestinal: Vomiting, diarrhea, dyspepsia, anorexia, and constipation.

Neurologic and Psychiatric: Insomnia, nervousness, paresthesia, libido decrease, dry mouth, taste perversion, and tinnitus.

Dermatologic: Rash and sweating.

Other: Gout, urinary frequency, arthralgia, myalgia, asthenia, and pain (including chest pain and abdominal pain).

Other adverse experiences reported in 0.3% or more of Lotensin HCT patients in U.S. controlled clinical trials, and rarer events seen in postmarketing experience, were the following; asterisked entries occurred in more than 1% of patients (in some, a causal relationship to Lotensin HCT is uncertain).

Angioedema: Edema of the lips or face without other manifestations of angioedema. See WARNINGS, Angioedema.

Cardiovascular: Syncope, peripheral vascular disorder, and tachycardia.

Body as a Whole: Infection, back pain,* flu syndrome,* fever, chills, and neck pain.

Dermatologic: Photosensitivity and pruritus. There have been rare reports of pemphigus in patients receiving ACE inhibitors.

Gastrointestinal: Gastroenteritis, flatulence, and tooth disorder. There have been rare reports of pancreatitis in patients receiving ACE inhibitors.

Hematologic: There have been rare reports of hemolytic anemia in patients receiving ACE inhibitors.

Neurologic and Psychiatric: Hypesthesia, abnormal vision, abnormal dreams, and retinal disorder.

Respiratory: Upper respiratory infection,* epistaxis, bronchitis, rhinitis,* sinusitis,* and voice alteration.

Other: Conjunctivitis, arthritis, urinary tract infection, and urinary frequency.*

Fetal/Neonatal Morbidity and Mortality: See WARNINGS, Fetal/Neonatal Morbidity and Mortality.

Monotherapy with **benazepril** has been evaluated for safety in over 6000 patients. In clinical trials, the observed adverse reactions to benazepril were similar to those seen in trials of Lotensin HCT. In postmarketing experience with benazepril, there have been rare reports of Stevens-Johnson syndrome and thrombocytopenia.

Hydrochlorothiazide has been extensively prescribed for many years, but there has not been enough systematic collection of data to support an estimate of the frequency of the observed adverse reactions. Within organ-system groups, the reported reactions are listed here in decreasing order of severity, without regard to frequency.

Cardiovascular: Orthostatic hypotension (may be potentiated by alcohol, barbiturates, or narcotics).

Digestive: Pancreatitis, jaundice (intrahepatic cholestatic) (see WARNINGS), sialadenitis, vomiting, diarrhea, cramping, nausea, gastric irritation, constipation, and anorexia.

Neurologic: Vertigo, lightheadedness, transient blurred vision, headache, paresthesia, xanthopsia, weakness, and restlessness.

Musculoskeletal: Muscle spasm.

Hematologic: Aplastic anemia, agranulocytosis, leukopenia, and thrombocytopenia.

Metabolic: Hyperglycemia, glycosuria, and hyperuricemia.

Hypersensitivity: Necrotizing angiitis, Stevens-Johnson syndrome, respiratory distress (including pneumonitis and pulmonary edema), purpura, urticaria, rash, and photosensitivity.

Clinical Laboratory Test Findings

Serum Electrolytes: See PRECAUTIONS.

Creatinine: Minor reversible increases in serum creatinine were observed in patients with essential hypertension treated with Lotensin HCT. Such increases occurred most frequently in patients with renal artery stenosis (see PRECAUTIONS).

PBI and Tests of Parathyroid Function: See PRECAUTIONS.

Other (Causal Relationships Unknown): Other clinically important changes in standard laboratory tests were rarely associated with Lotensin HCT administration. Elevations in blood urea nitrogen, uric acid, glucose, SGOT, and SGPT (see WARNINGS) have been reported. In the somewhat larger patient population exposed to benazepril monotherapy in U.S. trials, the same abnormalities were reported, together with scattered accounts of hyponatremia, melena, electrocardiographic changes, leukopenia, eosinophilia, and proteinuria.

OVERDOSAGE

No specific information is available on the treatment of overdosage with Lotensin HCT; treatment should be symptomatic and supportive. Therapy with Lotensin HCT should be discontinued, and the patient should be observed. Dehydration electrolyte imbalance, and hypotension should be treated by established procedures.

Single oral doses of 1 g/kg of benazepril caused reduced activity in mice, and doses of 3 g/kg were associated with significant lethality. Reduction of activity in rats was not seen until they had received doses of 5 g/kg, and doses of 6 g/kg were not lethal. In single-dose studies of hydrochlorothiazide, most rats survived doses up to 2.75 g/kg.

Data from human overdoses of benazepril are scanty, but the most common manifestation of human benazepril over-

dosage is likely to be hypotension. In human hydrochlorothiazide overdose, the most common signs and symptoms observed have been those of dehydration and electrolyte depletion (hypokalemia, hypochloremia, hyponatremia). If digitalis has also been administered, hypokalemia may accentuate cardiac arrhythmias.

Laboratory determinations of serum levels of benazepril and its metabolites are not widely available, and such determinations have, in any event, no established role in the management of benazepril overdose.

No data are available to suggest physiological maneuvers (e.g., maneuvers to change the pH of the urine) that might accelerate elimination of benazepril and its metabolites. Benazeprilat is only slightly dialyzable, but dialysis might be considered in overdosed patients with severely impaired renal function (see WARNINGS).

Angiotensin II could presumably serve as a specific antagonist-antidote in the setting of benazepril overdose, but angiotensin II is essentially unavailable outside of scattered research facilities. Because the hypotensive effect of benazepril is achieved through vasodilation and effective hypovolemia, it is reasonable to treat benazepril overdose by infusion of normal saline solution.

DOSAGE AND ADMINISTRATION

Benazepril is an effective treatment of hypertension in once-daily doses of 10-80 mg, while hydrochlorothiazide is effective in doses of 12.5-50 mg per day. In clinical trials of benazepril/hydrochlorothiazide combination therapy using benazepril doses of 5-20 mg and hydrochlorothiazide doses of 6.25-25 mg, the antihypertensive effects increased with increasing dose of either component.

The side effects (see WARNINGS) of benazepril are generally rare and apparently independent of dose; those of hydrochlorothiazide are a mixture of dose-dependent phenomena (primarily hypokalemia) and dose-independent phenomena (e.g., pancreatitis), the former much more common than the latter. Therapy with any combination of benazepril and hydrochlorothiazide will be associated with both sets of dose-independent side effects, but regimens in which benazepril is combined with low doses of hydrochlorothiazide produce minimal effects on serum potassium. In clinical trials of Lotensin HCT, the average change in serum potassium was near zero in subjects who received 5/6.25 mg or 20/12.5 mg, but the average subject who received 10/12.5 mg or 20/25 mg experienced a mild reduction in serum potassium, similar to that experienced by the average subject receiving the same dose of hydrochlorothiazide monotherapy.

To minimize dose-independent side effects, it is usually appropriate to begin combination therapy only after a patient has failed to achieve the desired effect with monotherapy.

Dose Titration Guided by Clinical Effect: A patient whose blood pressure is not adequately controlled with benazepril monotherapy may be switched to Lotensin HCT 10/12.5 or Lotensin HCT 20/12.5. Further increases of either or both components could depend on clinical response. The hydrochlorothiazide dose should generally not be increased until 2-3 weeks have elapsed. Patients whose blood pressures are adequately controlled with 25 mg of daily hydrochlorothiazide, but who experience significant potassium loss with this regimen, may achieve similar blood-pressure control without electrolyte disturbance if they are switched to Lotensin HCT 5/6.25.

Replacement Therapy: The combination may be substituted for the titrated individual components.

Use in Renal Impairment: Regimens of therapy with Lotensin HCT need not take account of renal function as long as the patient's creatinine clearance is >30 mL/min/1.73m^2 (serum creatinine roughly ≤3 mg/dL or 265 µmol/L). In patients with more severe renal impairment, loop diuretics are preferred to thiazides, so Lotensin HCT is not recommended (see WARNINGS).

HOW SUPPLIED

Lotensin HCT is available in tablets of four different strengths:

Benazepril	Hydrochlorothiazide	Tablet Color
5 mg	6.25 mg	white
10 mg	12.50 mg	light pink
20 mg	12.50 mg	grayish-violet
20 mg	25.00 mg	red

Tablets of each strength are supplied in bottles that contain a desiccant and 100 tablets.

The National Drug Codes for the various packages are

Dose	Bottle of 100
5/6.25	NDC 0083-0057-30
10/12.5	NDC 0083-0072-30
20/12.5	NDC 0083-0074-30
20/25	NDC 0083-0075-30

Tablets are oblong and scored, with "Lotensin HCT" on one side and a portion of the NDC code ("57," "72," "74," or "75") on the other.

Storage: Do not store above 86°F (30°C). Protect from moisture and light. *Dispense in tight, light-resistant container (USP).*

C97-3 (Rev. 2/97)

Dist. by:
Ciba-Geigy Corporation
Pharmaceuticals Division
Summit, New Jersey 07901

Shown in Product Identification Guide, page 325

LOTREL® ℞

[lō-trĕl]

amlodipine and benazepril hydrochloride
Combination Capsules
2.5 mg/10 mg
5 mg/10 mg
5mg/20 mg

Rx only

The following prescribing information is based on official labeling in effect on October 1, 1998.

> **USE IN PREGNANCY**
> **When used in pregnancy during the second and third trimesters, ACE inhibitors can cause injury and even death to the developing fetus.** When pregnancy is detected, Lotrel should be discontinued as soon as possible. See **WARNINGS, Fetal/Neonatal Morbidity and Mortality.**

DESCRIPTION

Benazepril hydrochloride is a white to off-white crystalline powder, soluble (>100 mg/mL) in water, in ethanol, and in methanol. Benazepril hydrochloride's chemical name is 3-[[1-(ethoxycarbonyl)-3-phenyl-(1S)-propyl]amino]-2,3,4,5-tetrahydro-2-oxo-1*H*-1-(3S)-benzazepine-1-acetic acid monohydrochloride; its structural formula is

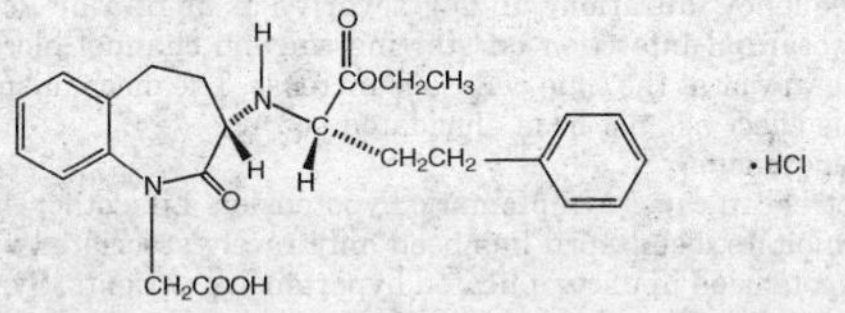

Its empirical formula is $C_{24}H_{28}N_2O_5$•HCl, and its molecular weight is 460.96.

Benazeprilat, the active metabolite of benazepril, is a non-sulfhydryl angiotensin-converting enzyme (ACE) inhibitor. Benazepril is converted to benazeprilat by hepatic cleavage of the ester group.

Amlodipine besylate is a white crystalline powder, slightly soluble in water and sparingly soluble in ethanol. Its chemical name is (R,S) 3-ethyl-5-methyl-2-(2-aminoethoxymethyl)-4-(2-chlorophenyl)-1,4-dihydro-6-methyl-3,5-pyridinedicarboxylate benzenesulfonate; its structural formula is

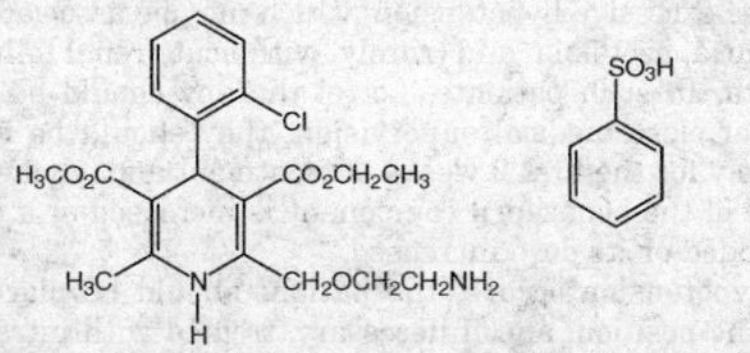

Its empirical formula is $C_{20}H_{25}ClN_2O_5$•$C_6H_6O_3S$, and its molecular weight is 567.1.

Amlodipine besylate is the besylate salt of amlodipine, a dihydropyridine calcium channel blocker.

Lotrel is a combination of amlodipine besylate and benazepril hydrochloride. The capsules are formulated for oral administration with a combination of amlodipine besylate equivalent to 2.5 mg or 5 mg of amlodipine and 10 mg or 20 mg of benazepril hydrochloride. The inactive ingredients of the capsules are calcium phosphate, cellulose compounds, colloidal silicon dioxide, crospovidone, gelatin, hydrogenated castor oil, iron oxides, lactose, magnesium stearate, polysorbate 80, silicon dioxide, sodium lauryl sulfate, sodium starch glycolate, starch, talc, and titanium dioxide.

CLINICAL PHARMACOLOGY

Mechanism of Action

Benazepril and benazeprilat inhibit angiotensin-converting enzyme (ACE) in human subjects and in animals. ACE is a peptidyl dipeptidase that catalyzes the conversion of angiotensin I to the vasoconstrictor substance angiotensin II. Angiotensin II also stimulates aldosterone secretion by the adrenal cortex.

Inhibition of ACE results in decreased plasma angiotensin II, which leads to decreased vasopressor activity and to decreased aldosterone secretion. The latter decrease may result in a small increase of serum potassium. Hypertensive patients treated with benazepril and amlodipine for up to 56 weeks had elevations of serum potassium up to 0.2 mEq/L (see PRECAUTIONS).

Removal of angiotensin II negative feedback on renin secretion leads to increased plasma renin activity. In animal studies, benazepril had no inhibitory effect on the vasopressor response to angiotensin II and did not interfere with the hemodynamic effects of the autonomic neurotransmitters acetylcholine, epinephrine, and norepinephrine.

ACE is identical to kininase, an enzyme that degrades bradykinin. Whether increased levels of bradykinin, a potent vasodepressor peptide, play a role in the therapeutic effects of Lotrel remains to be elucidated.

While the mechanism through which benazepril lowers blood pressure is believed to be primarily suppression of the renin-angiotensin-aldosterone system, benazepril has an antihypertensive effect even in patients with low-renin hypertension.

Amlodipine is a dihydropyridine calcium antagonist (calcium ion antagonist or slow channel blocker) that inhibits the transmembrane influx of calcium ions into vascular smooth muscle and cardiac muscle. Experimental data suggest that amlodipine binds to both dihydropyridine and non-dihydropyridine binding sites. The contractile processes of cardiac muscle and vascular smooth muscle are dependent upon the movement of extracellular calcium ions into these cells through specific ion channels. Amlodipine inhibits calcium ion influx across cell membranes selectively, with a greater effect on vascular smooth muscle cells than on cardiac muscle cells. Negative inotropic effects can be detected in vitro but such effects have not been seen in intact animals at therapeutic doses. Serum calcium concentration is not affected by amlodipine. Within the physiologic pH range, amlodipine is an ionized compound (pKa=8.6), and its kinetic interaction with the calcium channel receptor is characterized by a gradual rate of association and dissociation with the receptor binding site, resulting in a gradual onset of effect.

Amlodipine is a peripheral arterial vasodilator that acts directly on vascular smooth muscle to cause a reduction in peripheral vascular resistance and reduction in blood pressure.

Pharmacokinetics and Metabolism

The rate and extent of absorption of benazepril and amlodipine from Lotrel are not significantly different, respectively, from the rate and extent of absorption of benazepril and amlodipine from individual tablet formulations. Absorption from the individual tablets is not influenced by the presence of food in the gastrointestinal tract; food effects on absorption from Lotrel have not been studied. Following oral administration of Lotrel, peak plasma concentrations of benazepril are reached in 0.5-2 hours. Cleavage of the ester group (primarily in the liver) converts benazepril to its active metabolite, benazeprilat, which reaches peak plasma concentrations in 1.5-4 hours. The extent of absorption of benazepril is at least 37%.

Peak plasma concentrations of amlodipine are reached 6-12 hours after administration of Lotrel; the extent of absorption is 64%-90%.

The apparent volumes of **distribution** of amlodipine and benazeprilat are about 21 L/kg and 0.7 L/kg, respectively. Approximately 93% of circulating amlodipine is bound to plasma proteins, and the bound fraction of benazeprilat is slightly higher. On the basis of in vitro studies, benazeprilat's degree of protein binding should be unaffected by age, by hepatic dysfunction, or—over the therapeutic concentration range—by concentration.

Benazeprilat has much greater ACE-inhibitory activity than benazepril, and the **metabolism** of benazepril to benazeprilat is almost complete. Only trace amounts of an administered dose of benazepril can be recovered unchanged in the urine; about 20% of the dose is excreted as benazeprilat, 8% as benazeprilat glucuronide, and 4% as benazepril glucuronide.

Amlodipine is extensively metabolized in the liver, with 10% of the parent compound and 60% of the metabolites excreted in the urine. In patients with hepatic dysfunction, decreased clearance of amlodipine may increase the area-under-the-plasma-concentration curve by 40%-60%, and dosage reduction may be required (see DOSAGE AND ADMINISTRATION). In patients with renal impairment, the pharmacokinetics of amlodipine are essentially unaffected.

Benazeprilat's effective **elimination** half-life is 10-11 hours, while that of amlodipine is about 2 days, so steady-state levels of the two components are achieved after about a week of once-daily dosing. The clearance of benazeprilat from the plasma is primarily renal, but biliary excretion accounts for 11%-12% of benazepril elimination in normal subjects. In patients with severe renal insufficiency (creatinine clearance less than 30 mL/min), peak benazeprilat levels and the time to steady state may be increased (see DOSAGE AND

Continued on next page

Lotrel—Cont.

ADMINISTRATION). In patients with hepatic impairment, on the other hand, the pharmacokinetics of benazeprilat are essentially unaffected.

Although the pharmacokinetics of benazepril and benazeprilat are unaffected by **age**, clearance of amlodipine is decreased in the elderly, with resulting increases of 35%-70% in peak plasma levels, elimination half-life, and area-under-the-plasma-concentration curve. Dose adjustment may be required.

Pharmacodynamics

Single and multiple doses of 10 mg or more of **benazepril** cause inhibition of plasma ACE activity by at least 80%-90% for at least 24 hours after dosing. For up to 4 hours after a 10-mg dose, pressor responses to exogenous angiotensin I were inhibited by 60%-90%.

Administration of benazepril to patients with mild-to-moderate hypertension results in a reduction of both supine and standing blood pressure to about the same extent, with no compensatory tachycardia. Symptomatic postural hypotension is infrequent, although it can occur in patients who are salt and/or volume depleted (see WARNINGS, Hypotension).

The antihypertensive effects of benazepril were not appreciably different in patients receiving high- or low-sodium diets.

In normal human volunteers, single doses of benazepril caused an increase in renal blood flow but had no effect on glomerular filtration rate.

Following administration of therapeutic doses to patients with hypertension, **amlodipine** produces vasodilation resulting in a reduction of supine and standing blood pressures. These decreases in blood pressure are not accompanied by a significant change in heart rate or plasma catecholamine levels with chronic dosing. Plasma concentrations correlate with effect in both young and elderly patients.

As with other calcium channel blockers, hemodynamic measurements of cardiac function at rest and during exercise (or pacing) in patients with normal ventricular function treated with amlodipine have generally demonstrated a small increase in cardiac index without significant influence on dP/dt or on left ventricular end diastolic pressure or volume. In hemodynamic studies, amlodipine has not been associated with a negative inotropic effect when administered in the therapeutic dose range to intact animals and humans, even when coadministered with beta blockers to humans.

Amlodipine does not change sinoatrial (SA) nodal function or atrioventricular (AV) conduction in intact animals or humans. In clinical studies in which amlodipine was administered in combination with beta blockers to patients with either hypertension or angina, no adverse effects on electrocardiographic parameters were observed.

Over 700 patients received Lotrel once daily in five double-blind, placebo-controlled studies. Lotrel lowered blood pressure within 1 hour, with peak reductions achieved 2-8 hours after dosing. The antihypertensive effect of a single dose persisted for 24 hours.

Once-daily doses of benazepril/amlodipine using benazepril doses of 10-20 mg and amlodipine doses of 2.5-5 mg decreased seated pressure (systolic/diastolic) 24 hours after dosing by about 10-25/6-13 mmHg.

Combination therapy was effective in blacks and nonblacks. Both components contributed to the antihypertensive efficacy in nonblacks, but virtually all of the antihypertensive effect in blacks could be attributed to the amlodipine component. Among nonblack patients in placebo-controlled trials comparing Lotrel to the individual components, the blood pressure lowering effects of the combination were shown to be additive and in some cases synergistic.

During chronic therapy with Lotrel, the maximum reduction in blood pressure with any given dose is generally achieved after 1-2 weeks. The antihypertensive effects of Lotrel have continued during therapy for at least 1 year. Abrupt withdrawal of Lotrel has not been associated with a rapid increase in blood pressure.

INDICATIONS AND USAGE

Lotrel is indicated for the treatment of hypertension.

This fixed combination drug is not indicated for the initial therapy of hypertension (see DOSAGE AND ADMINISTRATION).

In using Lotrel, consideration should be given to the fact that an ACE inhibitor, captopril, has caused agranulocytosis, particularly in patients with renal impairment or collagen-vascular disease. Available data are insufficient to show that benazepril does not have a similar risk (see WARNINGS, Neutropenia/Agranulocytosis).

Black patients receiving ACE inhibitors have been reported to have a higher incidence of angioedema compared to nonblacks.

CONTRAINDICATIONS

Lotrel is contraindicated in patients who are hypersensitive to benazepril, to any other ACE inhibitor, or to amlodipine.

WARNINGS

Anaphylactoid and Possibly Related Reactions

Presumably because angiotensin-converting enzyme inhibitors affect the metabolism of eicosanoids and polypeptides, including endogenous bradykinin, patients receiving ACE inhibitors (including Lotrel) may be subject to a variety of adverse reactions, some of them serious. These reactions usually occur after one of the first few doses of the ACE inhibitor, but they sometimes do not appear until after months of therapy.

Angioedema: Angioedema of the face, extremities, lips, tongue, glottis, and larynx has been reported in patients treated with ACE inhibitors. In U.S. clinical trials, symptoms consistent with angioedema were seen in none of the subjects who received placebo and in about 0.5% of the subjects who received benazepril. Angioedema associated with laryngeal edema can be fatal. If laryngeal stridor or angioedema of the face, tongue, or glottis occurs, treatment with Lotrel should be discontinued and appropriate therapy instituted immediately. *When involvement of the tongue, glottis, or larynx appears likely to cause airway obstruction, appropriate therapy, e.g., subcutaneous epinephrine injection 1:1000 (0.3-0.5 mL), should be promptly administered (see ADVERSE REACTIONS).*

Anaphylactoid Reactions During Desensitization: Two patients undergoing desensitizing treatment with hymenoptera venom while receiving ACE inhibitors sustained life-threatening anaphylactoid reactions. In the same patients, these reactions were avoided when ACE inhibitors were temporarily withheld, but they reappeared upon inadvertent rechallenge.

Anaphylactoid Reactions During Membrane Exposure: Anaphylactoid reactions have been reported in patients dialyzed with high-flux membranes and treated concomitantly with an ACE inhibitor. Anaphylactoid reactions have also been reported in patients undergoing low-density lipoprotein apheresis with dextran sulfate absorption.

Increased Angina and/or Myocardial Infarction: Rarely, patients, particularly those with severe obstructive coronary artery disease, have developed documented increased frequency, duration, and/or severity of angina or acute myocardial infarction on starting calcium channel blocker therapy or at the time of dosage increase. The mechanism of this effect has not been elucidated.

Hypotension

Lotrel can cause symptomatic hypotension. Like other ACE inhibitors, benazepril has been only rarely associated with hypotension in uncomplicated hypertensive patients. Symptomatic hypotension is most likely to occur in patients who have been volume and/or salt depleted as a result of prolonged diuretic therapy, dietary salt restriction, dialysis, diarrhea, or vomiting. Volume and/or salt depletion should be corrected before initiating therapy with Lotrel.

Since the vasodilation induced by amlodipine is gradual in onset, acute hypotension has rarely been reported after oral administration of amlodipine. Nonetheless, caution should be exercised when administering Lotrel as with any other peripheral vasodilator, particularly in patients with severe aortic stenosis.

In patients with congestive heart failure, with or without associated renal insufficiency, ACE inhibitor therapy may cause excessive hypotension, which may be associated with oliguria, azotemia, and (rarely) with acute renal failure and death. In such patients, Lotrel therapy should be started under close medical supervision; they should be followed closely for the first 2 weeks of treatment and whenever the dose of the benazepril component is increased or a diuretic is added or its dose increased.

If hypotension occurs, the patient should be placed in a supine position, and if necessary, treated with intravenous infusion of physiologic saline. Lotrel treatment usually can be continued following restoration of blood pressure and volume.

Neutropenia/Agranulocytosis

Another ACE inhibitor, captopril, has been shown to cause agranulocytosis and bone marrow depression, rarely in uncomplicated patients (incidence probably less than once per 10,000 exposures) but more frequently (incidence possibly as great as once per 1000 exposures) in patients with renal impairment, especially those who also have collagen-vascular diseases such as systemic lupus erythematosis or scleroderma. Available data from clinical trials of benazepril are insufficient to show that benazepril does not cause agranulocytosis at similar rates. Monitoring of white blood cell counts should be considered in patients with collagen-vascular disease, especially if the disease is associated with impaired renal function.

Fetal/Neonatal Morbidity and Mortality

ACE inhibitors can cause fetal and neonatal morbidity and death when administered to pregnant women. Several dozen cases have been reported in the world literature. When pregnancy is detected, Lotrel should be discontinued as soon as possible.

The use of ACE inhibitors during the second and third trimesters of pregnancy has been associated with fetal and neonatal injury, including hypotension, neonatal skull hypo-

plasia, anuria, reversible or irreversible renal failure, and death. Oligohydramnios has also been reported, presumably resulting from decreased fetal renal function; oligohydramnios in this setting has been associated with fetal limb contractures, craniofacial deformation, and hypoplastic lung development. Prematurity, intrauterine growth retardation, and patent ductus arteriosus have also been reported, although it is not clear whether these occurrences were due to the ACE inhibitor exposure.

These adverse effects do not appear to have resulted from intrauterine ACE inhibitor exposure that has been limited to the first trimester. Mothers whose embryos and fetuses are exposed to ACE inhibitors only during the first trimester should be so informed. Nonetheless, when patients become pregnant, physicians should make every effort to discontinue the use of benazepril as soon as possible.

Rarely (probably less often than once in every thousand pregnancies), no alternative to ACE inhibitors will be found. In these rare cases, the mothers should be apprised of the potential hazards to their fetuses, and serial ultrasound examinations should be performed to assess the intraamniotic environment.

If oligohydramnios is observed, benazepril should be discontinued unless it is considered life-saving for the mother. Contraction stress testing (CST), a nonstress test (NST), or biophysical profiling (BPP) may be appropriate, depending upon the week of pregnancy. Patients and physicians should be aware, however, that oligohydramnios may not appear until after the fetus has sustained irreversible injury.

Infants with histories of in utero exposure to ACE inhibitors should be closely observed for hypotension, oliguria, and hyperkalemia. If oliguria occurs, attention should be directed toward support of blood pressure and renal perfusion. Exchange transfusion or peritoneal dialysis may be required as means of reversing hypotension and/or substituting for disordered renal function. Benazepril, which crosses the placenta, can theoretically be removed from the neonatal circulation by these means; there are occasional reports of benefit from these maneuvers, but experience is limited.

Lotrel has not been adequately studied in pregnant women. When rats received benazepril:amlodipine at doses ranging from 5:2.5 to 50:25 mg/kg/day, dystocia was observed with increasing dose-related incidence at all doses tested. On a mg/m^2 basis, the 2.5 mg/kg/day dose of amlodipine is 3.6 times the amlodipine dose delivered when the maximum recommended dose of Lotrel is given to a 50-kg woman. Similarly, the 5 mg/kg/day dose of benazepril is approximately 2 times the benazepril dose delivered when the maximum recommended dose of Lotrel is given to a 50-kg woman.

No teratogenic effects were seen when benazepril and amlodipine were administered in combination to pregnant rats or rabbits. Rats received dose ratios up to 50:25 mg/kg/day (benazepril:amlodipine) (24 times the maximum recommended human dose on a mg/m^2 basis, assuming a 50-kg woman). Rabbits received doses of up to 1.5:0.75 (benazepril:amlodipine) mg/kg/day; on a mg/m^2 basis, this is 0.97 times the size of a maximum recommended dose of Lotrel given to a 50-kg woman.

Similar results were seen in animal studies involving benazepril alone and amlodipine alone.

Hepatic Failure

Rarely, ACE inhibitors have been associated with a syndrome that starts with cholestatic jaundice and progresses to fulminant hepatic necrosis and (sometimes) death. The mechanism of this syndrome is not understood. Patients receiving ACE inhibitors who develop jaundice or marked elevations of hepatic enzymes should discontinue the ACE inhibitor and receive appropriate medical follow-up.

PRECAUTIONS

General

Impaired Renal Function: Lotrel should be used with caution in patients with severe renal disease.

When the renin-angiotensin-aldosterone system is inhibited by benazepril, changes in renal function may be anticipated in susceptible individuals. In patients with **severe congestive heart failure**, whose renal function may depend on the activity of the renin-angiotensin-aldosterone system, treatment with ACE inhibitors (including benazepril) may be associated with oliguria and/or progressive azotemia and (rarely) with acute renal failure and/or death.

In a small study of hypertensive patients with **unilateral or bilateral renal artery stenosis**, treatment with benazepril was associated with increases in blood urea nitrogen and serum creatinine; these increases were reversible upon discontinuation of benazepril therapy, concomitant diuretic therapy, or both. When such patients are treated with Lotrel, renal function should be monitored during the first few weeks of therapy.

Some benazepril-treated hypertensive patients with **no apparent preexisting renal vascular disease** have developed increases in blood urea nitrogen and serum creatinine, usually minor and transient, especially when benazepril has been given concomitantly with a diuretic. Dosage reduc-

tion of Lotrel may be required. **Evaluation of the hypertensive patient should always include assessment of renal function** (see DOSAGE AND ADMINISTRATION).

Hyperkalemia: In U.S. placebo-controlled trials of Lotrel, hyperkalemia (serum potassium at least 0.5 mEq/L greater than the upper limit of normal) not present at baseline occurred in approximately 1.5% of hypertensive patients receiving Lotrel. Increases in serum potassium were generally reversible. Risk factors for the development of hyperkalemia include renal insufficiency, diabetes mellitus, and the concomitant use of potassium-sparing diuretics, potassium supplements, and/or potassium-containing salt substitutes.

Patients With Congestive Heart Failure: Although hemodynamic studies and a controlled trial in patients with NYHA Class II-III heart failure have shown that amlodipine did not lead to clinical deterioration as measured by exercise tolerance, left ventricular ejection fraction, and clinical symptomatology, studies have not been performed in patients with NYHA Class IV heart failure. In general, all calcium channel blockers should be used with caution in patients with heart failure.

Patients With Hepatic Failure: In patients with hepatic dysfunction due to cirrhosis, levels of benazeprilat are essentially unaltered. However, since amlodipine is extensively metabolized by the liver and the plasma elimination half-life ($t_{1/2}$) is 56 hours in patients with impaired hepatic function, caution should be exercised when administering Lotrel to patients with severe hepatic impairment (see also WARNINGS).

Cough: Presumably due to the inhibition of the degradation of endogenous bradykinin, persistent nonproductive cough has been reported with all ACE inhibitors, always resolving after discontinuation of therapy. ACE inhibitor-induced cough should be considered in the differential diagnosis of cough.

Surgery/Anesthesia: In patients undergoing surgery or during anesthesia with agents that produce hypotension, benazepril will block the angiotensin II formation that could otherwise occur secondary to compensatory renin release. Hypotension that occurs as a result of this mechanism can be corrected by volume expansion.

Drug Interactions

Diuretics: Patients on diuretics, especially those in whom diuretic therapy was recently instituted, may occasionally experience an excessive reduction of blood pressure after initiation of therapy with Lotrel. The possibility of hypotensive effects with Lotrel can be minimized by either discontinuing the diuretic or increasing the salt intake prior to initiation of treatment with Lotrel.

Potassium Supplements and Potassium-Sparing Diuretics: Benazepril can attenuate potassium loss caused by thiazide diuretics. Potassium-sparing diuretics (spironolactone, amiloride, triamterene, and others) or potassium supplements can increase the risk of hyperkalemia. If concomitant use of such agents is indicated, they should be given with caution, and the patient's serum potassium should be monitored frequently.

Lithium: Increased serum lithium levels and symptoms of lithium toxicity have been reported in patients receiving ACE inhibitors during therapy with lithium. Lotrel and lithium should be coadministered with caution, and frequent monitoring of serum lithium levels is recommended.

Other: Benazepril has been used concomitantly with oral anticoagulants, beta-adrenergic-blocking agents, calcium-blocking agents, cimetidine, diuretics, digoxin, hydralazine, and naproxen without evidence of clinically important adverse interactions.

In clinical trials, amlodipine has been safely administered with thiazide diuretics, beta blockers, ACE inhibitors, long-acting nitrates, sublingual nitroglycerin, digoxin, warfarin, nonsteroidal anti-inflammatory drugs, antibiotics, and oral hypoglycemic drugs.

In vitro data in human plasma indicate that amlodipine has no effect on the protein binding of drugs tested (digoxin, phenytoin, warfarin, and indomethacin). Special studies have indicated that the coadministration of amlodipine with digoxin did not change serum digoxin levels or digoxin renal clearance in normal volunteers; that coadministration with cimetidine did not alter the pharmacokinetics of amlodipine; and that coadministration with warfarin did not change the warfarin-induced prothrombin response time.

Carcinogenesis, Mutagenesis, Impairment of Fertility

No evidence of carcinogenicity was found when **benazepril** was given, via dietary administration, to rats and mice for 104 weeks at doses up to 150 mg/kg/day. On a body-weight basis, this dose is over 100 times the maximum recommended human dose; on a body-surface-area basis, this dose is 18 times (rats) and 9 times (mice) the maximum recommended human dose. No mutagenic activity was detected in the Ames test in bacteria, in an in vitro test for forward mutations in cultured mammalian cells, or in a nucleus anomaly test. At doses of 50-500 mg/kg/day (38-375 times the maximum recommended human dose on a body-weight basis; 6-61 times the maximum recommended dose on a body-surface-area basis), benazepril had no adverse effect on the reproductive performance of male and female rats.

Rats and mice treated with amlodipine in the diet for 2 years, at concentrations calculated to provide daily dosage levels of 0.5, 1.25, and 2.5 mg/kg/day, showed no evidence of carcinogenicity. For mice, but not for rats, the highest dose was close to the maximum tolerated dose. On a mg/m^2 basis, this dose given to mice was approximately equal to the maximum recommended clinical dose. On the same basis, the same dose given to rats was approximately twice the maximum recommended clinical dose.

Mutagenicity studies with amlodipine revealed no drug-related effects at either the gene or chromosome levels.

There was no effect on the fertility of rats treated with amlodipine (males for 64 days and females for 14 days prior to mating) at doses up to 10 mg/kg/day (8 times the maximum recommended human dose of 10 mg on a mg/m^2 basis, assuming a 50-kg person).

No adverse effects on fertility occurred when the benazepril:amlodipine combination was given orally to rats of either sex at dose ratios up to 15:7.5 mg/kg/day (benazepril:amlodipine), prior to mating and throughout gestation.

Pregnancy

Pregnancy Categories C (first trimester) and D (second and third trimesters): See WARNINGS, Fetal/Neonatal Morbidity and Mortality.

Nursing Mothers

Minimal amounts of unchanged benazepril and of benazeprilat are excreted into the breast milk of lactating women treated with benazepril, so that a newborn child ingesting nothing but breast milk would receive less than 0.1% of the maternal doses of benazepril and benazeprilat. It is not known whether amlodipine is excreted in human milk. In the absence of this information, it is recommended that nursing be discontinued while Lotrel is administered.

Geriatric Use

Of the total number of patients who received Lotrel in U.S. clinical studies of Lotrel, 19% were 65 or older while about 2% were 75 or older. Overall differences in effectiveness or safety were not observed between these patients and younger patients. Clinical experience has not identified differences in responses between the elderly and younger patients, but greater sensitivity of some older individuals cannot be ruled out.

Pediatric Use

Safety and effectiveness in pediatric patients have not been established.

ADVERSE REACTIONS

Lotrel has been evaluated for safety in over 1600 patients with hypertension; over 500 of these patients were treated for at least 6 months, and over 400 were treated for more than 1 year.

The reported side effects were generally mild and transient, and there was no relationship between side effects and age, sex, race, or duration of therapy. Discontinuation of therapy due to side effects was required in approximately 4% of patients treated with Lotrel and in 3% of patients treated with placebo.

The most common reasons for discontinuation of therapy with Lotrel in U.S. studies were cough and edema.*

The side effects considered possibly or probably related to study drug that occurred in U.S. placebo-controlled trials in more than 1% of patients treated with Lotrel are shown in the table below.

PERCENT INCIDENCE IN U.S. PLACEBO-CONTROLLED TRIALS

	Benazepril/ Amlodipine N=760	Benazepril N=554	Amlodipine N=475	Placebo N=408
Cough	3.3	1.8	0.4	0.2
Headache	2.2	3.8	2.9	5.6
Dizziness	1.3	1.6	2.3	1.5
Edema*	2.1	0.9	5.1	2.2

*Edema refers to all edema, such as dependent edema, angioedema, facial edema.

The incidence of edema was statistically greater in patients treated with amlodipine monotherapy than in patients treated with the combination. Edema and certain other side effects are associated with amlodipine monotherapy in a dose-dependent manner, and appear to affect women more than men. The addition of benazepril resulted in lower incidences as shown in the following table; the protective effect of benazepril was independent of race and (within the range of doses tested) of dose.

[See table above]

PERCENT INCIDENCE BY SEX OF CERTAIN ADVERSE EVENTS

	Benazepril/ Amlodipine		Benazepril		Amlodipine		Placebo	
	Male N=329	Female N=431	Male N=269	Female N=285	Male N=277	Female N=198	Male N=217	Female N=191
Edema	0.6	3.2	0.0	1.8	2.2	9.1	1.4	3.1
Flushing	0.3	0.0	0.0	0.7	0.4	2.0	0.5	0.0
Palpitations	0.3	0.5	0.4	1.4	0.4	2.0	0.5	0.5
Somnolence	0.3	0.0	0.4	0.4	0.4	0.5	0.0	0.0

Other side effects considered possibly or probably related to study drug that occurred in U.S. placebo-controlled trials of patients treated with Lotrel were the following:

Angioedema: Includes edema of the lips or face without other manifestations of angioedema (see WARNINGS, Angioedema).

Body as a Whole: Asthenia and fatigue.

CNS: Insomnia, nervousness, anxiety, tremor, and decreased libido.

Dermatologic: Flushing, hot flashes, rash, skin nodule, and dermatitis.

Digestive: Dry mouth, nausea, abdominal pain, constipation, diarrhea, dyspepsia, and esophagitis.

Metabolic and Nutritional: Hypokalemia.

Musculoskeletal: Back pain, musculoskeletal pain, cramps, and muscle cramps.

Respiratory: Pharyngitis.

Urogenital: Sexual problems such as impotence, and polyuria.

Other infrequently reported events were seen in clinical trials (causal relationship unlikely) or in postmarketing experience. These included chest pain, ventricular extrasystole, gout, neuritis, tinnitus, and alopecia.

Fetal/Neonatal Morbidity and Mortality: See WARNINGS, Fetal/Neonatal Morbidity and Mortality.

Monotherapies of benazepril and amlodipine have been evaluated for safety in clinical trials in over 6000 and 11,000 patients, respectively. The observed adverse reactions to the monotherapies in these trials were similar to those seen in trials of Lotrel. In postmarketing experience with benazepril, there have been rare reports of Stevens-Johnson syndrome, pancreatitis, hemolytic anemia, pemphigus, and thrombocytopenia. Jaundice and hepatic enzyme elevations (mostly consistent with cholestasis) severe enough to require hospitalization have been reported in association with use of amlodipine. Other potentially important adverse experiences attributed to other ACE inhibitors and calcium channel blockers include: eosinophilic pneumonitis (ACE inhibitors) and gynecomastia (CCB's).

Clinical Laboratory Test Findings

Serum Electrolytes: See PRECAUTIONS.

Creatinine: Minor reversible increases in serum creatinine were observed in patients with essential hypertension treated with Lotrel. Increases in creatinine are more likely to occur in patients with renal insufficiency or those pretreated with a diuretic and, based on experience with other ACE inhibitors, would be expected to be especially likely in patients with renal artery stenosis (see PRECAUTIONS, General).

Other (causal relationships unknown): Clinically important changes in standard laboratory tests were rarely associated with Lotrel administration. Elevations of serum bilirubin and uric acid have been reported as have scattered incidents of elevations of liver enzymes.

OVERDOSAGE

Only a few cases of human overdose with amlodipine have been reported. One patient was asymptomatic after a 250-mg ingestion; another, who combined 70 mg of amlodipine with an unknown large quantity of a benzodiazepine, developed refractory shock and died.

Human overdoses with any combination of amlodipine and benazepril have not been reported. In scattered reports of human overdoses with benazepril and other ACE inhibitors, there are no reports of death.

When mice were given single oral doses of benazepril/amlodipine, mortality was 20% at 50:25 mg/kg, 10% at 100:50 mg/kg, and 100% at 500:250 mg/kg. In rats, mortality was 25% (pooling two studies) at 500:250 mg/kg and 100% at 900:450 mg/kg.

Treatment: To obtain up-to-date information about the treatment of overdose, a good resource is your certified Regional Poison-Control Center. Telephone numbers of certified poison-control centers are listed in the *Physicians'*

Continued on next page

Lotrel—Cont.

Desk Reference (PDR). In managing overdose, consider the possibilities of multiple-drug overdoses, drug-drug interactions, and unusual drug kinetics in your patient.
The most likely effect of overdose with Lotrel is vasodilation, with consequent hypotension and tachycardia. Simple repletion of central fluid volume (Trendelenburg positioning, infusion of crystalloids) may be sufficient therapy, but pressor agents (norepinephrine or high-dose dopamine) may be required. Overdoses of other dihydropyridine calcium channel blockers are reported to have been treated with calcium chloride and glucagon, but evidence of a dose-response relation has not been seen, and these interventions must be regarded as unproven. With abrupt return of peripheral vascular tone, overdoses of other dihydropyridine calcium channel blockers have sometimes progressed to pulmonary edema, and patients must be monitored for this complication.
Analyses of bodily fluids for concentrations of amlodipine, benazepril, or their metabolites are not widely available. Such analyses are, in any event, not known to be of value in therapy or prognosis.
No data are available to suggest physiologic maneuvers (e.g., maneuvers to change the pH of the urine) that might accelerate elimination of amlodipine, benazepril, or their metabolites. Benazeprilat is only slightly dialyzable; attempted clearance of amlodipine by hemodialysis or hemoperfusion has not been reported, but amlodipine's high protein binding makes it unlikely that these interventions will be of value.
Angiotensin II could presumably serve as a specific antagonist-antidote to benazepril, but angiotensin II is essentially unavailable outside of scattered research laboratories.

DOSAGE AND ADMINISTRATION

Amlodipine is an effective treatment of hypertension in once-daily doses of 2.5-10 mg while benazepril is effective in doses of 10-80 mg. In clinical trials of amlodipine/benazepril combination therapy using amlodipine doses of 2.5-5 mg and benazepril doses of 10-20 mg, the antihypertensive effects increased with increasing dose of amlodipine in all patient groups, and the effects increased with increasing dose of benazepril in nonblack groups. All patient groups benefited from the reduction in amlodipine-induced edema (see below).
The hazards (see WARNINGS) of benazepril are generally independent of dose; those of amlodipine are a mixture of dose-dependent phenomena (primarily peripheral edema) and dose-independent phenomena, the former much more common than the latter. When benazepril is added to a regimen of amlodipine, the incidence of edema is substantially reduced. Therapy with any combination of amlodipine and benazepril will thus be associated with both sets of dose-independent hazards, but the incidence of edema will generally be less than that seen with similar (or higher) doses of amlodipine monotherapy.
Rarely, the dose-independent hazards of benazepril are serious. To minimize dose-independent hazards, it is usually appropriate to begin therapy with Lotrel only after a patient has either (a) failed to achieve the desired antihypertensive effect with one or the other monotherapy, or (b) demonstrated inability to achieve adequate antihypertensive effect with amlodipine therapy without developing edema.

Dose Titration Guided by Clinical Effect: A patient whose blood pressure is not adequately controlled with amlodipine (or another dihydropyridine) alone or with benazepril (or another ACE inhibitor) alone may be switched to combination therapy with Lotrel. The addition of benazepril to a regimen of amlodipine should not be expected to provide additional antihypertensive effect in African-Americans. However, all patient groups benefit from the reduction in amlodipine-induced edema. Dosage must be guided by clinical response; steady-state levels of benazepril and amlodipine will be reached after approximately 2 and 7 days of dosing, respectively.
In patients whose blood pressures are adequately controlled with amlodipine but who experience unacceptable edema, combination therapy may achieve similar (or better) blood-pressure control without edema. Especially in nonblacks, it may be prudent to minimize the risk of excessive response by reducing the dose of amlodipine as benazepril is added to the regimen.

Replacement Therapy: For convenience, patients receiving amlodipine and benazepril from separate tablets may instead wish to receive capsules of Lotrel containing the same component doses.

Use in Patients With Metabolic Impairments: Regimens of therapy with Lotrel need not take account of renal function as long as the patient's creatinine clearance is >30 mL/min/1.73m^2 (serum creatinine roughly ≤3 mg/dL or 265 μmol/L). In patients with more severe renal impairment, the recommended initial dose of benazepril is 5 mg. Lotrel is not recommended in these patients.
In small, elderly, frail, or hepatically impaired patients, the recommended initial dose of amlodipine, as monotherapy or as a component of combination therapy, is 2.5 mg.

HOW SUPPLIED

Lotrel is available as capsules containing amlodipine/benazepril HCl 2.5/10 mg, 5/10 mg, and 5/20 mg. All three strengths are packaged with a desiccant in bottles of 100 capsules.
Capsules are imprinted with "Lotrel" and a portion of the NDC code.

Dose	Capsule Color	NDC Code Bottle of 100
2.5/10 mg	white capsule with 2 gold bands	NDC 0083-2255-30
5/10 mg	light brown capsule with 2 white bands	NDC 0083-2260-30
5/20 mg	pink capsule with 2 white bands	NDC 0083-2265-30

Storage: Do not store above 86°F (30°C). Protect from moisture and light.
Dispense in tight, light-resistant container (USP).
C98-26 (Rev. 6/98)

Distributed by
Novartis Pharmaceuticals Corporation
East Hanover, New Jersey 07936
Shown in Product Identification Guide, page 325

MIACALCIN® ℞
[*mī "ă-kal 'sin*]
***(calcitonin-salmon)* INJECTION, SYNTHETIC**

CAUTION: Federal law prohibits dispensing without prescription.
The following prescribing information is based on official labeling in effect on August 1, 1998.

DESCRIPTION

Calcitonin is a polypeptide hormone secreted by the parafollicular cells of the thyroid gland in mammals and by the ultimobranchial gland of birds and fish.
Miacalcin® (calcitonin-salmon) Injection, Synthetic is a synthetic polypeptide of 32 amino acids in the same linear sequence that is found in calcitonin of salmon origin. This is shown by the following graphic formula:

H-Cys-Ser-Asn-Leu-Ser-Thr-Cys-Val-Leu-
1 2 3 4 5 6 7 8 9

Gly-Lys-Leu-Ser-Gln-Glu-Leu-His-Lys-Leu-
10 11 12 13 14 15 16 17 18 19

Gln-Thr-Tyr-Pro-Arg-Thr-Asn-Thr-Gly-Ser-
20 21 22 23 24 25 26 27 28 29

Gly-Thr-Pro-NH_2
30 31 32

It is provided in sterile solution for subcutaneous or intramuscular injection. Each milliliter contains: calcitonin-salmon 200 I.U.; acetic acid, USP, 2.25 mg; phenol, USP, 5.0 mg; sodium acetate trihydrate, USP, 2.0 mg; sodium chloride, USP, 7.5 mg; water for injection, USP, qs to 1.0 mL.
The activity of Miacalcin® (calcitonin-salmon) is stated in International Units based on bioassay in comparison with the International Reference Preparation of calcitonin-salmon for Bioassay, distributed by the National Institute for Biological Standards and Control, Holly Hill, London.

CLINICAL PHARMACOLOGY

Calcitonin acts primarily on bone, but direct renal effects and actions on the gastrointestinal tract are also recognized. Calcitonin-salmon appears to have actions essentially identical to calcitonins of mammalian origin, but its potency per mg is greater and it has a longer duration of action. The actions of calcitonin on bone and its role in normal human bone physiology are still incompletely understood.
Bone—Single injections of calcitonin cause a marked transient inhibition of the ongoing bone resorptive process. With prolonged use, there is a persistent, smaller decrease in the rate of bone resorption. Histologically, this is associated with a decreased number of osteoclasts and an apparent decrease in their resorptive activity. Decreased osteocytic resorption may also be involved. There is some evidence that initially bone formation may be augmented by calcitonin through increased osteoblastic activity. However, calcitonin will probably not induce a long-term increase in bone formation.
Animal studies indicate that endogenous calcitonin, primarily through its action on bone, participates with parathyroid hormone in the homeostatic regulation of blood calcium. Thus, high blood calcium levels cause increased secretion of calcitonin which, in turn, inhibits bone resorption. This reduces the transfer of calcium from bone to blood and tends to return blood calcium to the normal level. The importance of this process in humans has not been determined. In normal adults, who have a relatively low rate of bone resorption, the administration of exogenous calcitonin results in only a slight decrease in serum calcium. In normal children and in patients with generalized Paget's disease, bone resorption is more rapid and decreases in serum calcium are more pronounced in response to calcitonin.
Paget's Disease of Bone (osteitis deformans)—Paget's disease is a disorder of uncertain etiology characterized by abnormal and accelerated bone formation and resorption in one or more bones. In most patients only small areas of bone are involved and the disease is not symptomatic. In a small fraction of patients, however, the abnormal bone may lead to bone pain and bone deformity, cranial and spinal nerve entrapment, or spinal cord compression. The increased vascularity of the abnormal bone may lead to high output congestive heart failure.
Active Paget's disease involving a large mass of bone may increase the urinary hydroxyproline excretion (reflecting breakdown of collagen-containing bone matrix) and serum alkaline phosphatase (reflecting increased bone formation).
Calcitonin-salmon, presumably by an initial blocking effect on bone resorption, causes a decreased rate of bone turnover with a resultant fall in the serum alkaline phosphatase and urinary hydroxyproline excretion in approximately 2/3 of patients treated. These biochemical changes appear to correspond to changes toward more normal bone, as evidenced by a small number of documented examples of: 1) radiologic regression of Pagetic lesions, 2) improvement of impaired auditory nerve and other neurologic function, 3) decreases (measured) in abnormally elevated cardiac output. These improvements occur extremely rarely, if ever, spontaneously (elevated cardiac output may disappear over a period of years when the disease slowly enters a sclerotic phase; in the cases treated with calcitonin, however, the decreases were seen in less than one year.)
Some patients with Paget's disease who have good biochemical and/or symptomatic responses initially, later relapse. Suggested explanations have included the formation of neutralizing antibodies and the development of secondary hyperparathyroidism, but neither suggestion appears to explain adequately the majority of relapses.
Although the parathyroid hormone levels do appear to rise transiently during each hypocalcemic response to calcitonin, most investigators have been unable to demonstrate persistent hypersecretion of parathyroid hormone in patients treated chronically with calcitonin-salmon.
Circulating antibodies to calcitonin after 2–18 months' treatment have been reported in about half of the patients with Paget's disease in whom antibody studies were done, but calcitonin treatment remained effective in many of these cases. Occasionally, patients with high antibody titers are found. These patients usually will have suffered a biochemical relapse of Paget's disease and are unresponsive to the acute hypocalcemic effects of calcitonin.
Hypercalcemia—In clinical trials, calcitonin-salmon has been shown to lower the elevated serum calcium of patients with carcinoma (with or without demonstrated metastases), multiple myeloma or primary hyperparathyroidism (lesser response). Patients with higher values for serum calcium tend to show greater reduction during calcitonin therapy. The decrease in calcium occurs about 2 hours after the first injection and lasts for about 6–8 hours. Calcitonin-salmon given every 12 hours maintained a calcium lowering effect for about 5–8 days, the time period evaluated for most patients during the clinical studies. The average reduction of 8-hour post-injection serum calcium during this period was about 9 percent.
Kidney—Calcitonin increases the excretion of filtered phosphate, calcium, and sodium by decreasing their tubular reabsorption. In some patients, the inhibition of bone resorption by calcitonin is of such magnitude that the consequent reduction of filtered calcium load more than compensates for the decrease in tubular reabsorption of calcium. The result in these patients is a decrease rather than an increase in urinary calcium.
Transient increases in sodium and water excretion may occur after the initial injection of calcitonin. In most patients, these changes return to pretreatment levels with continued therapy.
Gastrointestinal Tract—Increasing evidence indicates that calcitonin has significant actions on the gastrointestinal tract. Short-term administration results in marked transient decreases in the volume and acidity of gastric juice and in the volume and the trypsin and amylase content of pancreatic juice. Whether these effects continue to be elicited after each injection of calcitonin during chronic therapy has not been investigated.
Metabolism—The metabolism of calcitonin-salmon has not yet been studied clinically. Information from animal studies with calcitonin-salmon and from clinical studies with calcitonins of porcine and human origin suggest that calcitonin-salmon is rapidly metabolized by conversion to smaller inactive fragments, primarily in the kidneys, but

also in the blood and peripheral tissues. A small amount of unchanged hormone and its inactive metabolites are excreted in the urine.

It appears that calcitonin-salmon cannot cross the placental barrier and its passage to the cerebrospinal fluid or to breast milk has not been determined.

INDICATIONS AND USAGE

Miacalcin® (calcitonin-salmon) Injection, Synthetic is indicated for the treatment of symptomatic Paget's disease of bone, for the treatment of hypercalcemia, and for the treatment of postmenopausal osteoporosis.

Paget's Disease—At the present time, effectiveness has been demonstrated principally in patients with moderate to severe disease characterized by polyostotic involvement with elevated serum alkaline phosphatase and urinary hydroxyproline excretion.

In these patients, the biochemical abnormalities were substantially improved (more than 30% reduction) in about 2/3 of patients studied, and bone pain was improved in a similar fraction. A small number of documented instances of reversal of neurologic deficits has occurred, including improvement in the basilar compression syndrome, and improvement of spinal cord and spinal nerve lesions. At present, there is too little experience to predict the likelihood of improvement of any given neurologic lesion. Hearing loss, the most common neurologic lesion of Paget's disease, is improved infrequently (4 of 29 patients studied audiometrically).

Patients with increased cardiac output due to extensive Paget's disease have had measured decreases in cardiac output while receiving calcitonin. The number of treated patients in this category is still too small to predict how likely such a result will be.

The large majority of patients with localized, especially monostotic disease do not develop symptoms and most patients with mild symptoms can be managed with analgesics. There is no evidence that the prophylactic use of calcitonin is beneficial in asymptomatic patients, although treatment may be considered in exceptional circumstances in which there is extensive involvement of the skull or spinal cord with the possibility of irreversible neurologic damage. In these instances, treatment would be based on the demonstrated effect of calcitonin on Pagetic bone, rather than on clinical studies in the patient population in question.

Hypercalcemia—Miacalcin® (calcitonin-salmon) Injection, Synthetic is indicated for early treatment of hypercalcemic emergencies, along with other appropriate agents, when a rapid decrease in serum calcium is required, until more specific treatment of the underlying disease can be accomplished. It may also be added to existing therapeutic regimens for hypercalcemia such as intravenous fluids and furosemide, oral phosphate or corticosteroids, or other agents.

Postmenopausal Osteoporosis—Miacalcin® (calcitonin-salmon) Injection, Synthetic is indicated for the treatment of postmenopausal osteoporosis in conjunction with adequate calcium and vitamin D intake to prevent the progressive loss of bone mass. No evidence currently exists to indicate whether or not Miacalcin® (calcitonin-salmon) decreases the risk of vertebral crush fractures or spinal deformity. A recent controlled study, which was discontinued prior to completion because of questions regarding its design and implementation, failed to demonstrate any benefit of salmon calcitonin on fracture rate. No adequate controlled trials have examined the effect of salmon calcitonin injection on vertebral bone mineral density beyond 1 year of treatment. Two placebo-controlled studies with salmon calcitonin have shown an increase in total body calcium at 1 year, followed by a trend to decreasing total body calcium (still above baseline) at 2 years. The minimum effective dose of Miacalcin® (calcitonin-salmon) for prevention of vertebral bone mineral density loss has not been established. It has been suggested that those postmenopausal patients having increased rates of bone turnover may be more likely to respond to anti-resorptive agents such as Miacalcin® (calcitonin-salmon).

CONTRAINDICATIONS

Clinical allergy to synthetic calcitonin-salmon.

WARNINGS

Allergic Reactions

Because calcitonin is protein in nature, the possibility of a systemic allergic reaction exists. **Administration of calcitonin-salmon has been reported in a few cases to cause serious allergic-type reactions (e.g. bronchospasm, swelling of the tongue or throat, and anaphylactic shock), and in one case, death attributed to anaphylaxis.** The usual provisions should be made for the emergency treatment of such a reaction should it occur. Allergic reactions should be differentiated from generalized flushing and hypotension.

For patients with suspected sensitivity to calcitonin, skin testing should be considered prior to treatment utilizing a dilute, sterile solution of Miacalcin® (calcitonin-salmon) Injection, Synthetic. Physicians may wish to refer patients who require skin testing to an allergist. A detailed skin testing protocol is available from the Medical Services Department of Sandoz Pharmaceuticals Corporation.

The incidence of osteogenic sarcoma is known to be increased in Paget's disease. Pagetic lesions, with or without therapy, may appear by X-ray to progress markedly, possibly with some loss of definition of periosteal margins. Such lesions should be evaluated carefully to differentiate these from osteogenic sarcoma.

PRECAUTIONS

1. General

The administration of calcitonin possibly could lead to hypocalcemic tetany under special circumstances although no cases have yet been reported. Provisions for parenteral calcium administration should be available during the first several administrations of calcitonin.

2. Laboratory Tests

Periodic examinations of urine sediment of patients on chronic therapy are recommended.

Coarse granular casts and casts containing renal tubular epithelial cells were reported in young adult volunteers at bed rest who were given calcitonin-salmon to study the effect of immobilization on osteoporosis. There was no other evidence of renal abnormality and the urine sediment became normal after calcitonin was stopped. Urine sediment abnormalities have not been reported by other investigators.

3. Instructions for the Patient

Careful instruction in sterile injection technique should be given to the patient, and to other persons who may administer Miacalcin® (calcitonin-salmon) Injection, Synthetic.

4. Carcinogenesis, Mutagenesis, and Impairment of Fertility

An increased incidence of pituitary adenomas has been observed in one-year toxicity studies in Sprague-Dawley rats administered calcitonin-salmon at dosages of 20 and 80 I.U. kg/day and in Fisher 344 rats given 80 I.U./kg/day. The relevance of these findings to humans is unknown. Calcitonin-salmon was not mutagenic in tests using *Salmonella typhimurium, Escherichia coli,* and Chinese Hamster V79 cells.

5. Pregnancy: Teratogenic Effects

Category C

Calcitonin-salmon has been shown to cause a decrease in fetal birth weights in rabbits when given in doses 14–56 times the dose recommended for human use. Since calcitonin does not cross the placental barrier, this finding may be due to metabolic effects on the pregnant animal. There are no adequate and well-controlled studies in pregnant women. Miacalcin® (calcitonin-salmon) Injection, Synthetic should be used during pregnancy only if the potential benefit justifies the potential risk to the fetus.

6. Nursing Mothers

It is not known whether this drug is excreted in human milk. As a general rule, nursing should not be undertaken while a patient is on this drug since many drugs are excreted in human milk. Calcitonin has been shown to inhibit lactation in animals.

7. Pediatric Use

Disorders of bone in children referred to as juvenile Paget's disease have been reported rarely. The relationship of these disorders to adult Paget's disease has not been established and experience with the use of calcitonin in these disorders is very limited. There is no adequate data to support the use of Miacalcin® (calcitonin-salmon) Injection, Synthetic in children.

ADVERSE REACTIONS

Gastrointestinal System

Nausea with or without vomiting has been noted in about 10% of patients treated with calcitonin. It is most evident when treatment is first initiated and tends to decrease or disappear with continued administration.

Dermatologic/Hypersensitivity

Local inflammatory reactions at the site of subcutaneous or intramuscular injection have been reported in about 10% of patients. Flushing of face or hands occurred in about 2–5% of patients. Skin rashes, nocturia, pruritus of the ear lobes, feverish sensation, pain in the eyes, poor appetite, abdominal pain, edema of feet, and salty taste have been reported in patients treated with calcitonin-salmon. Administration of calcitonin-salmon has been reported in a few cases to cause serious allergic-type reactions (e.g. bronchospasm, swelling of the tongue or throat, and anaphylactic shock), and in one case, death attributed to anaphylaxis (*see WARNINGS*).

OVERDOSAGE

A dose of 1000 I.U. subcutaneously may produce nausea and vomiting as the only adverse effects. Doses of 32 units per kg per day for 1–2 days demonstrate no other adverse effects.

Data on chronic high dose administration are insufficient to judge toxicity.

DOSAGE AND ADMINISTRATION

Paget's Disease—The recommended starting dose of calcitonin-salmon in Paget's disease is 100 I.U. (0.5 mL) per day administered subcutaneously (preferred for outpatient self-administration) or intramuscularly. Drug effect should be monitored by periodic measurement of serum alkaline phosphatase and 24-hour urinary hydroxyproline (if available) and evaluations of symptoms. A decrease toward normal of the biochemical abnormalities is usually seen, if it is going to occur, within the first few months. Bone pain may also decrease during that time. Improvement of neurologic lesions, when it occurs, requires a longer period of treatment, often more than one year.

In many patients, doses of 50 I.U. (0.25 mL) per day or every other day are sufficient to maintain biochemical and clinical improvement. At the present time, however, there are insufficient data to determine whether this reduced dose will have the same effect as the higher dose on forming more normal bone structure. It appears preferable, therefore, to maintain the higher dose in any patient with serious deformity or neurological involvement.

In any patient with a good response initially who later relapses, either clinically or biochemically, the possibility of antibody formation should be explored. The patient may be tested for antibodies by an appropriate specialized test or evaluated for the possibility of antibody formation by critical clinical evaluation.

Patient compliance should also be assessed in the event of relapse.

In patients who relapse, whether because of antibodies or for unexplained reasons, a dosage increase beyond 100 I.U. per day does not usually appear to elicit an improved response.

Hypercalcemia—The recommended starting dose of Miacalcin® (calcitonin-salmon) Injection, Synthetic in hypercalcemia is 4 I.U./kg body weight every 12 hours by subcutaneous or intramuscular injection. If the response to this dose is not satisfactory after one or two days, the dose may be increased to 8 I.U./kg every 12 hours. If the response remains unsatisfactory after two more days, the dose may be further increased to a maximum of 8 I.U./kg every 6 hours.

Postmenopausal Osteoporosis—The minimum effective dose of salmon calcitonin for the prevention of vertebral bone mineral density loss has not been established. Data from a single one-year placebo-controlled study with salmon calcitonin injection suggested that 100 I.U. (subcutaneously or intramuscularly) every other day might be effective in preserving vertebral bone mineral density. Baseline and interval monitoring of biochemical markers of bone resorption/turnover (e.g., fasting AM, second-voided urine hydroxyproline to creatinine ratio) and of bone mineral density may be useful in achieving the minimum effective dose. Patients should also receive supplemental calcium such as calcium carbonate 1.5 g daily and an adequate vitamin D intake (400 units daily). An adequate diet is also essential.

If the volume of Miacalcin® (calcitonin-salmon) Injection, Synthetic to be injected exceeds 2 mL, intramuscular injection is preferable and multiple sites of injection should be used.

Parenteral drug products should be inspected visually for particulate matter and discoloration prior to administration whenever solution and container permit.

HOW SUPPLIED

Miacalcin® (calcitonin-salmon) Injection, Synthetic is available as a sterile solution in individual 2 mL vials containing 200 I.U. per mL (NDC 0078-0149-23).

Store in Refrigerator—Between 2°–8°C (36°–46°F).

Manufactured by
Sandoz Pharma Ltd.
Basle, Switzerland for
Sandoz Pharmaceuticals Corporation
East Hanover, NJ 07936

[REV: February 1997 30167403]

MIACALCIN® ℞

[*mī "ă-kal 'sin*]
(calcitonin-salmon)
Nasal Spray

Caution: Federal law prohibits dispensing without prescription.

The following prescribing information is based on official labeling in effect on August 1, 1998.

DESCRIPTION

Calcitonin is a polypeptide hormone secreted by the parafollicular cells of the thyroid gland in mammals and by the ultimobranchial gland of birds and fish.

Miacalcin® (calcitonin-salmon) Nasal Spray is a synthetic polypeptide of 32 amino acids in the same linear sequence

Continued on next page

Miacalcin Nasal Spray—Cont.

that is found in calcitonin of salmon origin. This is shown by the following graphic formula:

H-Cys-Ser-Asn-Leu-Ser-Thr-Cys-Val-Leu-
1 2 3 4 5 6 7 8 9

Gly-Lys-Leu-Ser-Gln-Glu-Leu-His-Lys-Leu-
10 11 12 13 14 15 16 17 18 19

Gln-Thr-Tyr-Pro-Arg-Thr-Asn-Thr-Gly-Ser-
20 21 22 23 24 25 26 27 28 29

Gly-Thr-Pro-NH_2
30 31 32

It is provided in 2 mL fill glass bottles as a solution for nasal administration. This is sufficient medication for at least 14 doses. Each milliliter contains calcitonin-salmon 2200 I.U. (corresponding to 200 I.U. per 0.09 mL actuation), sodium chloride 8.5 mg, benzalkonium chloride 0.10 mg, nitrogen, hydrochloric acid (added as necessary to adjust pH) and purified water.
The activity of Miacalcin® (calcitonin-salmon) Nasal Spray is stated in International Units based on bioassay in comparison with the International Reference Preparation of calcitonin-salmon for Bioassay, distributed by the National Institute of Biologic Standards and Control, Holly Hill, London.

CLINICAL PHARMACOLOGY

Calcitonin acts primarily on bone, but direct renal effects and actions on the gastrointestinal tract are also recognized. Calcitonin-salmon appears to have actions essentially identical to calcitonins of mammalian origin, but its potency per mg is greater and it has a longer duration of action.
The information below, describing the clinical pharmacology of calcitonin, has been derived from studies with *injectable* calcitonin. The mean bioavailability of Miacalcin® (calcitonin-salmon) Nasal Spray is approximately 3% of that of injectable calcitonin in normal subjects and, therefore, the conclusions concerning the *CLINICAL PHARMACOLOGY* of this preparation may be different.
The actions of calcitonin on bone and its role in normal human bone physiology are still not completely elucidated, although calcitonin receptors have been discovered in osteoclasts and osteoblasts.
Single injections of calcitonin cause a marked transient inhibition of the ongoing bone resorptive process. With prolonged use, there is a persistent, smaller decrease in the rate of bone resorption. Histologically, this is associated with a decreased number of osteoclasts and an apparent decrease in their resorptive activity. *In vitro* studies have shown that calcitonin-salmon causes inhibition of osteoclast function with loss of the ruffled osteoclast border responsible for resorption of bone. This activity resumes following removal of calcitonin-salmon from the test system. There is some evidence from the *in vitro* studies that bone formation may be augmented by calcitonin through increased osteoblastic activity.
Animal studies indicate that endogenous calcitonin, primarily through its action on bone, participates with parathyroid hormone in the homeostatic regulation of blood calcium. Thus, high blood calcium levels cause increased secretion of calcitonin which, in turn, inhibits bone resorption. This reduces the transfer of calcium from bone to blood and tends to return blood calcium towards the normal level. The importance of this process in humans has not been determined. In normal adults, who have a relatively low rate of bone resorption, the administration of exogenous calcitonin results in only a slight decrease in serum calcium in the limits of the normal range. In normal children and in patients with Paget's disease in whom bone resorption is more rapid, decreases in serum calcium are more pronounced in response to calcitonin.
Bone biopsy and radial bone mass studies at baseline and after 26 months of daily injectable calcitonin indicate that calcitonin therapy results in formation of normal bone.
Postmenopausal Osteoporosis – Osteoporosis is a disease characterized by low bone mass and architectural deterioration of bone tissue leading to enhanced bone fragility and a consequent increase in fracture risk as patients approach or fall below a bone mineral density associated with increased frequency of fracture. The most common type of osteoporosis occurs in postmenopausal females. Osteoporosis is a result of a disproportionate rate of bone resorption compared to bone formation which disrupts the structural integrity of bone, rendering it more susceptible to fracture. The most common sites of these fractures are the vertebrae, hip, and distal forearm (Colles' fractures). Vertebral fractures occur with the highest frequency and are associated with back pain, spinal deformity and a loss of height.
Calcitonin, given by the intranasal route, has been shown to increase spinal bone mass in postmenopausal women with established osteoporosis but not in early postmenopausal women.
Calcium Homeostasis – In two clinical studies designed to evaluate the pharmacodynamic response to Miacalcin® (calcitonin-salmon) Nasal Spray, administration of 100–1600 I.U. to healthy volunteers resulted in rapid and sustained small decreases (but still within the normal range) in both total serum calcium and serum ionized calcium. Single doses greater than 400 I.U. did not produce any further biological response to the drug. The development of hypocalcemia has not been reported in studies in healthy volunteers or postmenopausal females.
Kidney – Studies with injectable calcitonin show increases in the excretion of filtered phosphate, calcium, and sodium by decreasing their tubular reabsorption. Comparable studies have not been carried out with Miacalcin® (calcitonin-salmon) Nasal Spray.
Gastrointestinal Tract – Some evidence from studies with injectable preparations suggest that calcitonin may have significant actions on the gastrointestinal tract. Short-term administration of injectable calcitonin results in marked transient decreases in the volume and acidity of gastric juice and in the volume and the trypsin and amylase content of pancreatic juice. Whether these effects continue to be elicited after each injection of calcitonin during chronic therapy has not been investigated. These studies have not been conducted with Miacalcin® (calcitonin-salmon) Nasal Spray.

Pharmacokinetics and Metabolism
The data on bioavailability of Miacalcin® (calcitonin-salmon) Nasal Spray obtained by various investigators using different methods show great variability. Miacalcin® (calcitonin-salmon) Nasal Spray is absorbed rapidly by the nasal mucosa. Peak plasma concentrations of drug appear 31–39 minutes after nasal administration compared to 16–25 minutes following parenteral dosing. In normal volunteers approximately 3% (range 0.3%–30.6%) of a nasally administered dose is bioavailable compared to the same dose administered by intramuscular injection. The half-life of elimination of calcitonin-salmon is calculated to be 43 minutes. There is no accumulation of the drug on repeated nasal administration at 10 hour intervals for up to 15 days. Absorption of nasally administered calcitonin has not been studied in postmenopausal women.

INDICATION AND USAGE

Postmenopausal Osteoporosis – Miacalcin® (calcitonin-salmon) Nasal Spray is indicated for the treatment of postmenopausal osteoporosis in females greater than 5 years postmenopause with low bone mass relative to healthy premenopausal females. Miacalcin® (calcitonin-salmon) Nasal Spray should be reserved for patients who refuse or cannot tolerate estrogens or in whom estrogens are contraindicated. Use of Miacalcin® (calcitonin-salmon) Nasal Spray is recommended in conjunction with an adequate calcium (at least 1000 mg elemental calcium per day) and vitamin D (400 I.U. per day) intake to retard the progressive loss of bone mass. The evidence of efficacy is based on increases in spinal bone mineral density observed in clinical trials.
Two randomized, placebo controlled trials were conducted in 325 postmenopausal females [227 Miacalcin® (calcitonin-salmon) Nasal Spray treated and 98 placebo treated] with spinal, forearm or femoral bone mineral density (BMD) at least one standard deviation below normal for healthy premenopausal females. These studies conducted over two years demonstrated that 200 I.U. daily of Miacalcin® (calcitonin-salmon) Nasal Spray increases lumbar vertebral BMD relative to baseline and relative to placebo in osteoporotic females who were greater than 5 years postmenopause. Miacalcin® (calcitonin-salmon) Nasal Spray produced statistically significant increases in lumbar vertebral BMD compared to placebo as early as six months after initiation of therapy with persistence of this level for up to 2 years of observation.
No effects of Miacalcin® (calcitonin-salmon) Nasal Spray on cortical bone of the forearm or hip were demonstrated. However, in one study, BMD of the hip showed a statistically significant increase compared with placebo in a region composed of predominantly trabecular bone after one year of treatment changing to a trend at 2 years that was no longer statistically significant.

CONTRAINDICATIONS

Clinical allergy to calcitonin-salmon.

WARNINGS

Allergic Reactions
Because calcitonin is a polypeptide, the possibility of a systemic allergic reaction exists. A few cases of allergic-type reactions have been reported in patients receiving Miacalcin® (calcitonin-salmon) Nasal Spray, including one case of anaphylactic shock, which appears to have been due to the preservative because the patient could tolerate injectable calcitonin-salmon without incident. With injectable calcitonin-salmon there have been a few reports of serious allergic-type reactions (e.g., bronchospasm, swelling of the tongue or throat, anaphylactic shock, and in one case death attributed to anaphylaxis). The usual provisions should be made for the emergency treatment of such a reaction should it occur. Allergic reactions should be differentiated from generalized flushing and hypotension.
For patients with suspected sensitivity to calcitonin, skin testing should be considered prior to treatment utilizing a dilute, sterile solution of Miacalcin® (calcitonin-salmon) Injection, Synthetic. Physicians may wish to refer patients who require skin testing to an allergist. A detailed skin testing protocol is available from the Medical Services Department of Sandoz Pharmaceuticals Corporation.

PRECAUTIONS

1. Drug Interactions
Formal studies designed to evaluate drug interactions with calcitonin-salmon have not been done. No drug interaction studies have been performed with Miacalcin® (calcitonin-salmon) Nasal Spray ingredients.
Currently, no drug interactions with calcitonin-salmon have been observed. The effects of prior use of diphosphonates in postmenopausal osteoporosis patients have not been assessed; however, in patients with Paget's Disease prior diphosphonate use appears to reduce the anti-resorptive response to Miacalcin® (calcitonin-salmon) Nasal Spray.

2. Periodic Nasal Examinations
Periodic nasal examinations with visualization of the nasal mucosa, turbinates, septum and mucosal blood vessel status are recommended.
The development of mucosal alterations or transient nasal conditions occurred in up to 9% of patients who received Miacalcin® (calcitonin-salmon) Nasal Spray and in up to 12% of patients who received placebo nasal spray in studies in postmenopausal females. The majority of patients (approximately 90%) in whom nasal abnormalities were noted also reported nasally related complaints/symptoms as adverse events. Therefore, a nasal examination should be performed prior to start of treatment with nasal calcitonin and at any time nasal complaints occur.
In all postmenopausal patients treated with Miacalcin® (calcitonin-salmon) Nasal Spray, the most commonly reported nasal adverse events included rhinitis (12%), epistaxis (3.5%), and sinusitis (2.3%). Smoking was shown not to have any contributory effect on the occurrence of nasal adverse events. One patient (0.3%) treated with Miacalcin® (calcitonin-salmon) Nasal Spray who was receiving 400 I.U. daily developed a small nasal wound. In clinical trials in another disorder (Paget's Disease), 2.8% of patients developed nasal ulcerations.
If severe ulceration of the nasal mucosa occurs, as indicated by ulcers greater than 1.5 mm in diameter or penetrating below the mucosa, or those associated with heavy bleeding, Miacalcin® (calcitonin-salmon) Nasal Spray should be discontinued. Although smaller ulcers often heal without withdrawal of Miacalcin® (calcitonin-salmon) Nasal Spray, medication should be discontinued temporarily until healing occurs.

3. Information for Patients
Careful instructions on pump assembly, priming of the pump and nasal introduction of Miacalcin® (calcitonin-salmon) Nasal Spray should be given to the patient. Although instructions for patients are supplied with individual bottles, procedures for use should be demonstrated to each patient. Patients should notify their physician if they develop significant nasal irritation.
Patients should be advised of the following:

- Store new, unassembled bottles in the refrigerator between 36°–46°F (2°–8°C).
- Protect the product from freezing.
- Before priming the pump and using a new bottle, allow it to reach room temperature.
- Store bottle in use at room temperature in an upright position, for up to 30 days. Each bottle contains at least 14 doses.
- Store second bottle in refrigerator until ready to use. Protect from freezing.
- Discard all unrefrigerated bottles after 30 days.
- See *DOSAGE AND ADMINISTRATION, Priming (Activation) of Pump* for complete instructions on priming the pump and administering Miacalcin® (calcitonin-salmon) Nasal Spray.

4. Carcinogenicity, Mutagenicity, and Impairment of Fertility
An increased incidence of non-functioning pituitary adenomas has been observed in one-year toxicity studies in Sprague-Dawley and Fischer 344 Rats administered (subcutaneously) calcitonin-salmon at dosages of 80 I.U. per kilogram per day (16–19 times the recommended human parenteral dose and about 130–160 times the human intranasal dose based on body surface area). The findings suggest that calcitonin-salmon reduced the latency period for development of pituitary adenomas that do not produce hormones, probably through the perturbation of physiologic processes involved in the evolution of this commonly occurring endocrine lesion in the rat. Although administration of calcitonin-salmon reduces the

latency period of the development of nonfunctional proliferative lesions in rats, it did not induce the hyperplastic/neoplastic process.

Calcitonin-salmon was tested for mutagenicity using *Salmonella typhimurium* (5 strains) and *Escherichia coli* (2 strains), with and without rat liver metabolic activation, and found to be non-mutagenic. The drug was also not mutagenic in a chromosome aberration test in mammalian V79 cells of the Chinese Hamster *in vitro*.

5. Laboratory Tests

Urine sediment abnormalities have not been reported in ambulatory volunteers treated with Miacalcin® (calcitonin-salmon) Nasal Spray. Coarse granular casts containing renal tubular epithelial cells were reported in young adult volunteers at bed rest who were given injectable calcitonin-salmon to study the effect of immobilization on osteoporosis. There was no evidence of renal abnormality and the urine sediment became normal after calcitonin was stopped. Periodic examinations of urine sediment should be considered.

6. Pregnancy

Teratogenic Effects

Category C

Calcitonin-salmon has been shown to cause a decrease in fetal birth weights in rabbits when given by injection in doses 8–33 times the parenteral dose and 70–278 times the intranasal dose recommended for human use based on body surface area.

Since calcitonin does not cross the placental barrier, this finding may be due to metabolic effects on the pregnant animal. There are no adequate and well controlled studies in pregnant women with calcitonin-salmon. Miacalcin® (calcitonin-salmon) Nasal Spray is *not* indicated for use in pregnancy.

7. Nursing Mothers

It is not known whether this drug is excreted in human milk. As a general rule, nursing should not be undertaken while a patient is on this drug since many drugs are excreted in human milk. Calcitonin has been shown to inhibit lactation in animals.

8. Geriatric Use

Clinical trials using Miacalcin® (calcitonin-salmon) Nasal Spray have included postmenopausal patients up to 77 years of age. No unusual adverse events or increased incidence of common adverse events have been noted in patients over 65 years of age.

9. Pediatric Use

There are no data to support the use of Miacalcin® (calcitonin-salmon) Nasal Spray in children. Disorders of bone in children referred to as idiopathic juvenile osteoporosis have been reported rarely. The relationship of these disorders to postmenopausal osteoporosis has not been established and experience with the use of calcitonin in these disorders is very limited.

ADVERSE REACTIONS

The incidence of adverse reactions reported in studies involving postmenopausal osteoporotic patients chronically exposed to Miacalcin® (calcitonin-salmon) Nasal Spray (N=341) and to placebo nasal spray (N=131) and reported in greater than 3% of Miacalcin® (calcitonin-salmon) Nasal Spray treated patients are presented below in the following table. Most adverse reactions were mild to moderate in severity. Nasal adverse events were most common with 70% mild, 25% moderate, and 5% severe in nature (placebo rates were 71% mild, 27% moderate, and 2% severe).

Adverse Reactions Occurring in at Least 3% of Postmenopausal Patients Treated Chronically

Adverse Reaction	Miacalcin® (calcitonin-salmon) Nasal Spray N=341 % of Patients	Placebo N=131 % of Patients
Rhinitis	12.0	6.9
Symptom of Nose†	10.6	16.0
Back Pain	5.0	2.3
Arthralgia	3.8	5.3
Epistaxis	3.5	4.6
Headache	3.2	4.6

†Symptom of nose includes: nasal crusts, dryness, redness or erythema, nasal sores, irritation, itching, thick feeling, soreness, pallor, infection, stenosis, runny/blocked, small wound, bleeding wound, tenderness, uncomfortable feeling and sore across bridge of of nose.

In addition, the following adverse events were reported in fewer than 3% of patients during chronic therapy with Miacalcin® (calcitonin-salmon) Nasal Spray. Adverse events reported in 1%-3% of patients are identified with an asterisk(*). The remainder occurred in less than 1% of patients. Other than flushing, nausea, possible allergic reactions, and possible local irritative effects in the respiratory tract, a relationship to Miacalcin® (calcitonin-salmon) Nasal Spray has not been established.

Body as a whole – General Disorders: influenza-like symptoms*, fatigue*, periorbital edema, fever

Integumentary: erythematous rash*, skin ulceration, eczema, alopecia, pruritus, increased sweating

Musculoskeletal/Collagen: arthrosis*, myalgia*, arthritis, polymyalgia rheumatica, stiffness

Respiratory/Special Senses: sinusitis*, upper respiratory tract infection*, bronchospasm*, pharyngitis, bronchitis, pneumonia, coughing, dyspnea, taste perversion, parosmia

Cardiovascular: hypertension*, angina pectoris*, tachycardia, palpitation, bundle branch block, myocardial infarction

Gastrointestinal: dyspepsia*, constipation*, abdominal pain*, nausea*, diarrhea*, vomiting, flatulence, increased appetite, gastritis, dry mouth

Liver/Metabolic: cholelithiasis, hepatitis, thirst, weight increase

Endocrine: goiter, hyperthyroidism

Urinary System: cystitis*, pyelonephritis, hematuria, renal calculus

Central and Peripheral Nervous System: dizziness*, paresthesia*, vertigo, migraine, neuralgia, agitation

Hearing/Vestibular: tinnitus, hearing loss, earache

Vision: abnormal lacrimation*, conjunctivitis*, blurred vision, vitreous floater

Vascular: flushing, cerebrovascular accident, thrombophlebitis

Hematologic/Resistance Mechanisms: lymphadenopathy*, infection*, anemia

Psychiatric: depression*, insomnia, anxiety, anorexia

Common adverse reactions associated with the use of injectable calcitonin-salmon occurred less frequently in patients treated with Miacalcin® (calcitonin-salmon) Nasal Spray than in those patients treated with injectable calcitonin. Nausea, with or without vomiting, which occurred in 1.8% of patients treated with the nasal spray (and 1.5% of those receiving placebo nasal spray) occurs in about 10% of patients who take injectable calcitonin-salmon. Flushing, which occurred in less than 1% of patients treated with the Nasal Spray, occurs in 2%–5% of patients treated with injectable calcitonin-salmon. Although the administered dosages of injectable and nasal spray calcitonin-salmon are comparable (50–100 units daily of injectable versus 200 units daily of nasal spray), the nasal dosage form has a mean bioavailability of about 3% (range 0.3%–30.6%) and therefore provides less drug to the systemic circulation, possibly accounting for the decrease in frequency of adverse reactions.

The collective foreign marketing experience with Miacalcin® (calcitonin-salmon) Nasal Spray does not show evidence of any notable difference in the incidence profile of reported adverse reactions when compared with that seen in the clinical trials.

OVERDOSAGE

No instances of overdose with Miacalcin® (calcitonin-salmon) Nasal Spray have been reported and no serious adverse reactions have been associated with high doses. There is no known potential for drug abuse for calcitonin-salmon.

Single doses of Miacalcin® (calcitonin-salmon) Nasal Spray up to 1600 I.U., doses up to 800 I.U. per day for three days and chronic administration of doses up to 600 I.U. per day have been studied without serious adverse effects. A dose of 1000 I.U. of Miacalcin® (calcitonin-salmon) injectable solution given subcutaneously may produce nausea and vomiting. A dose of Miacalcin® (calcitonin-salmon) injectable solution of 32 I.U. per kg per day for one or two days demonstrated no additional adverse effects.

There have been no reports of hypocalcemic tetany. However, the pharmacologic actions of Miacalcin® (calcitonin-salmon) Nasal Spray suggest that this could occur in overdose. Therefore, provisions for parenteral administration of calcium should be available for the treatment of overdose.

DOSAGE AND ADMINISTRATION

The recommended dose of Miacalcin® (calcitonin-salmon) Nasal Spray in postmenopausal osteoporotic females is one spray (200 I.U.) per day administered intranasally, alternating nostrils daily.

Drug effect may be monitored by periodic measurements of lumbar vertebral bone mass to document stabilization of bone loss or increases in bone density. Effects of Miacalcin® (calcitonin-salmon) Nasal Spray on biochemical markers of bone turnover have not been consistently demonstrated in studies in postmenopausal osteoporosis. Therefore, these parameters should not be solely utilized to determine clinical response to Miacalcin® (calcitonin-salmon) Nasal Spray therapy in these patients.

Priming (Activation) of Pump

Before the first dose and administration, Miacalcin® (calcitonin-salmon) Nasal Spray should be at room temperature. To prime the pump, the bottle should be held upright and the two white side arms of the pump depressed toward the bottle until a full spray is produced. The pump is primed once the first full spray is emitted. To administer, the nozzle should be carefully placed into the nostril with the head in the upright position, and the pump firmly depressed toward the bottle. The pump should not be primed before each daily dose.

HOW SUPPLIED

Miacalcin® (calcitonin-salmon) Nasal Spray

Available as a metered dose solution in 2 mL fill glass bottles. It is available in a dosage strength of 200 I.U. per activation (0.09 mL/spray). Screw-on pumps are provided. The pumps, following priming, will deliver 0.09 mL of solution. Miacalcin® (calcitonin-salmon) Nasal Spray contains 2200 I.U./mL calcitonin-salmon and is provided in individual boxes containing two glass bottles and two screw-on pumps (NDC 0078-0311-90).

Store and Dispense

Store unopened bottle(s) in refrigerator between 36°–46°F (2°–8°C). Protect from freezing.

Store bottle in use at room temperature in an upright position, for up to 30 days. Each bottle contains at least 14 doses.

Store second bottle in refrigerator until ready to use. Protect from freezing.

Discard all unrefrigerated bottles after 30 days.

REV: JANUARY 1997 30367904

Shown in Product Identification Guide, page 325

MIGRANAL® ℞

[mī grā năl]

(dihydroergotamine mesylate, USP)

Nasal Spray

The solution used in Migranal® (dihydroergotamine mesylate, USP) Nasal Spray (4 mg/mL) is intended for intranasal use and must not be injected.

Caution: Federal law prohibits dispensing without prescription.

The following prescribing information is based on official labeling in effect on August 1, 1998.

DESCRIPTION

Migranal® is ergotamine hydrogenated in the 9,10 position as the mesylate salt. Migranal® is known chemically as ergotaman-3′,6′,18-trione,9,10-dihydro-12′-hydroxy-2′-methyl-5′-(phenylmethyl)-,(5′α)-,monomethanesulfonate. Its molecular weight is 679.80 and its empirical formula is $C_{33}H_{37}N_5O_5 \cdot CH_4O_3S$. The chemical structure is:

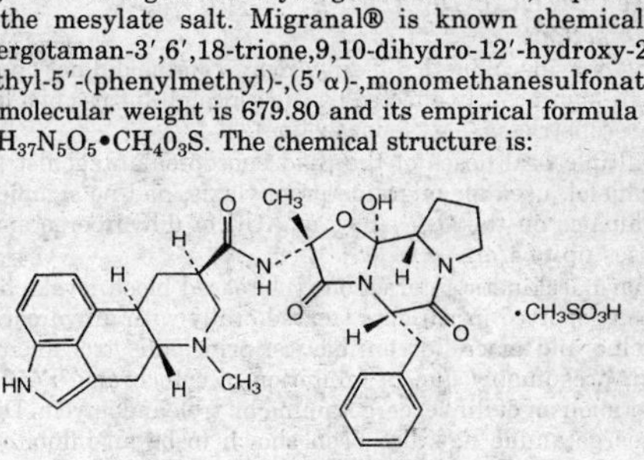

Dihydroergotamine mesylate

$C_{33}H_{37}N_5O_5 \cdot CH_4O_3S$ Mol. wt. 679.80

Migranal® (dihydroergotamine mesylate, USP) Nasal Spray is provided for intranasal administration as a clear, colorless to faintly yellow solution in an amber glass ampul containing:

dihydroergotamine mesylate, USP	4.0 mg
caffeine, anhydrous, USP	10.0 mg
dextrose, anhydrous, USP	50.0 mg
carbon dioxide	qs
water for injection, USP	qs 1.0 mL

CLINICAL PHARMACOLOGY

Mechanism of Action

Dihydroergotamine binds with high affinity to $5\text{-}HT_{1D\alpha}$ and $5\text{-}HT_{1D\beta}$ receptors. It also binds with high affinity to serotonin $5\text{-}HT_{1A}$, $5\text{-}HT_{2A}$, and $5\text{-}HT_{2C}$ receptors, noradrenaline α_{2A}, α_{2B} and α_1 receptors, and dopamine D_{2L} and D_3 receptors.

The therapeutic activity of dihydroergotamine in migraine is generally attributed to the agonist effect at $5\text{-}HT_{1D}$ receptors. Two current theories have been proposed to explain the efficacy of $5\text{-}HT_{1D}$ receptor agonists in migraine. One theory suggests that activation of $5\text{-}HT_{1D}$ receptors located on intracranial blood vessels, including those on arterio-venous anastomoses, leads to vasoconstriction, which correlates with the relief of migraine headache. The alternative hypothesis suggests that activation of $5\text{-}HT_{1D}$ receptors on sensory nerve endings of the trigeminal system results in the inhibition of pro-inflammatory neuropeptide release. In addition, dihydroergotamine possesses oxytocic properties. (See *CONTRAINDICATIONS*)

Continued on next page

Migranal—Cont.

Pharmacokinetics

Absorption

Dihydroergotamine mesylate is poorly bioavailable following oral administration. Following intranasal administration, however, the mean bioavailability of dihydroergotamine mesylate is 32% relative to the injectable administration. Absorption is variable, probably reflecting both intersubject differences of absorption and the technique used for self-administration.

Distribution

Dihydroergotamine mesylate is 93% plasma protein bound. The apparent steady-state volume of distribution is approximately 800 liters.

Metabolism

Four dihydroergotamine mesylate metabolites have been identified in human plasma following oral administration. The major metabolite, 8′-β-hydroxydihydroergotamine, exhibits affinity equivalent to its parent for adrenergic and 5-HT receptors and demonstrates equivalent potency in several venoconstrictor activity models, *in vivo* and *in vitro*. The other metabolites, i.e., dihydrolysergic acid, dihydrolysergic amide and a metabolite formed by oxidative opening of the proline ring are of minor importance. Following nasal administration, total metabolites represent only 20%-30% of plasma AUC. The systemic clearance of dihydroergotamine mesylate following I.V. and I.M. administration is 1.5 L/min. Quantitative pharmacokinetic characterization of the four metabolites has not been performed.

Excretion

The major excretory route of dihydroergotamine is via the bile in the feces. After intranasal administration the urinary recovery of parent drug amounts to about 2% of the administered dose compared to 6% after I.M. administration. The total body clearance is 1.5 L/min which reflects mainly hepatic clearance. The renal clearance (0.1 L/min) is unaffected by the route of dihydroergotamine administration. The decline of plasma dihydroergotamine is biphasic with a terminal half-life of about 10 hours.

Subpopulations

No studies have been conducted on the effect of renal or hepatic impairment, gender, race, or ethnicity on dihydroergotamine pharmacokinetics. Migranal® (dihydroergotamine mesylate, USP) Nasal Spray is contraindicated in patients with severely impaired hepatic or renal function. (See *CONTRAINDICATIONS*)

Interactions

The pharmacokinetics of dihydroergotamine did not appear to be significantly affected by the concomitant use of a local vasoconstrictor (e.g., fenoxazoline).

Multiple oral doses of the β-adrenoceptor antagonist propranolol, used for migraine prophylaxis, had no significant influence on the C_{max}, T_{max} or AUC of dihydroergotamine doses up to 4 mg.

Pharmacokinetic interactions (increased blood levels) have been reported in patients treated orally with dihydroergotamine and macrolide antibiotics, principally troleandomycin, presumably due to inhibition of cytochrome P450 3A metabolism of dihydroergotamine by troleandomycin. Dihydroergotamine has also been shown to be an inhibitor of cytochrome P450 3A catalyzed reactions. No pharmacokinetic interactions involving other cytochrome P450 isoenzymes are known.

Clinical Trials

The efficacy of Migranal® (dihydroergotamine mesylate, USP) Nasal Spray for the acute treatment of migraine headaches was evaluated in four randomized, double blind, placebo controlled studies in the U.S. The patient population for the trials was predominantly female (87%) and Caucasian (95%) with a mean age of 39 years (range 18 to 65 years). Patients treated a single moderate to severe migraine headache with a single dose of study medication and assessed pain severity over the 24 hours following treatment. Headache response was determined 0.5, 1, 2, 3 and 4 hours after dosing and was defined as a reduction in headache severity to mild or no pain. In studies 1 and 2, a four-point pain intensity scale was utilized; in studies 3 and 4, a five-point scale was used that included both pain response and restoration of function for "severe" or "incapacitating" pain, a less clear endpoint. Although rescue medication was allowed in all four studies, patients were instructed not to use them during the four hour observation period. In studies 3 and 4, a total dose of 2 mg was compared to placebo. In studies 1 and 2, doses of 2 and 3 mg were evaluated, and showed no advantage of the higher dose for a single treatment. In all studies, patients received a regimen consisting of 0.5 mg in each nostril, repeated in 15 minutes (and again in another 15 minutes for the 3 mg dose in studies 1 and 2).

The percentage of patients achieving headache response 4 hours after treatment was significantly greater in patients receiving 2 mg doses of Migranal® (dihydroergotamine mesylate, USP) Nasal Spray compared to those receiving placebo in 3 of the 4 studies (see Tables 1 & 2 and Figures 1 & 2).

Table 1: Studies 1 and 2: Percentage of patients with headache response[a] 2 and 4 hours following a single treatment of study medication [Migranal® (dihydroergotamine mesylate, USP) Nasal Spray or Placebo]

		N	2 hours	4 hours
Study 1	Migranal®	105	61%**	70%**
	Placebo	98	23%	28%
Study 2	Migranal®	103	47%	56%*
	Placebo	102	33%	35%

[a] Headache response was defined as a reduction in headache severity to mild or no pain. Headache response was based on pain intensity as interpreted by the patient using a four-point pain intensity scale.
*p value < 0.01
**p value < 0.001

Table 2: Studies 3 and 4: Percentage of patients with headache response[a] 2 and 4 hours following a single treatment of study medication [Migranal® (dihydroergotamine mesylate, USP) Nasal Spray or Placebo]

		N	2 hours	4 hours
Study 3	Migranal®	50	32%	48%
	Placebo	50	20%	22%
Study 4	Migranal®	47	30%	47%
	Placebo	50	20%	30%

[a] Headache response was defined as a reduction in headache severity to mild or no pain. Headache response was evaluated on a five-point scale that included both pain response and restoration of function for "severe" or "incapacitating" pain.
* p value < 0.01

Comparisons of drug performance based upon results obtained in different clinical trials are never reliable. Because studies are conducted at different times, with different samples of patients, by different investigators, employing different criteria and/or different interpretations of the same criteria, under different conditions (dose, dosing regimen, etc.), quantitative estimates of treatment response and the timing of response may be expected to vary considerably from study to study.

The Kaplan-Meier plots below (Figures 1 & 2) provides an estimate of the probability that a patient will have responded to a single 2 mg dose of Migranal® (dihydroergotamine mesylate, USP) Nasal Spray as a function of the time elapsed since initiation of treatment.

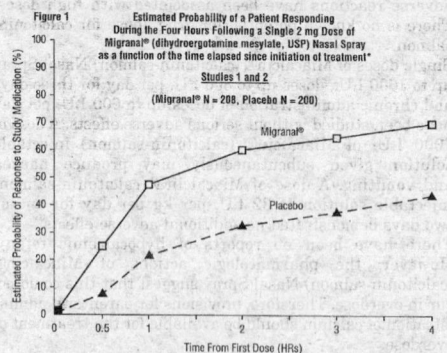

Figure 1
Estimated Probability of a Patient Responding During the Four Hours Following a Single 2 mg Dose of Migranal® (dihydroergotamine mesylate, USP) Nasal Spray as a function of the time elapsed since initiation of treatment*
Studies 1 and 2
(Migranal® N = 208, Placebo N = 200)

*The figure shows the probability over time of obtaining a response following treatment with Migranal® (dihydroergotamine mesylate, USP) Nasal Spray. Headache response was based on pain intensity as interpreted by the patient using a four-point pain intensity scale. Patients not achieving response within 4 hours were censored to 4 hours.

[See figure 2 at top of next column]

For patients with migraine-associated nausea, photophobia, and phonophobia at baseline, there was a lower incidence of these symptoms at 2 and 4 hours following administration of Migranal® (dihydroergotamine mesylate, USP) Nasal Spray compared to placebo.

Patients were not allowed to use additional treatments for eight hours prior to study medication dosing and during the four hour observation period following study treatment. Following the 4 hour observation period, patients were allowed to use additional treatments. For all studies, the estimated probability of patients using additional treatments for their

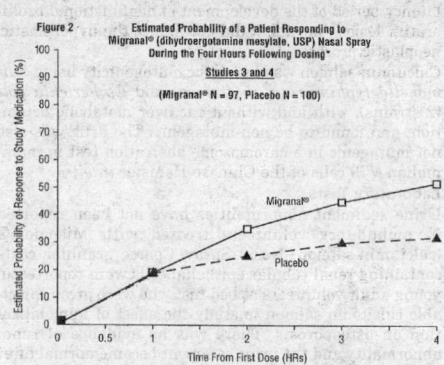

Figure 2
Estimated Probability of a Patient Responding to Migranal® (dihydroergotamine mesylate, USP) Nasal Spray During the Four Hours Following Dosing*
Studies 3 and 4
(Migranal® N = 97, Placebo N = 100)

*The figure shows the probability over time of obtaining a response following treatment with Migranal® (dihydroergotamine mesylate, USP) Nasal Spray. Headache response was evaluated on a five-point scale that confounded pain response and restoration of function for "severe" or "incapacitating" pain. Patients not achieving response within 4 hours were censored to 4 hours.

migraines over the 24 hours following the single 2 mg dose of study treatment is summarized in Figure 3 below.

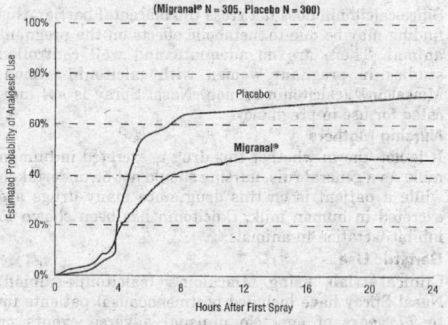

Figure 3
Estimated Probability of Patients Using Additional Treatments for Migraine Over the 24 Hours Following Either Migranal® (dihydroergotamine mesylate, USP) Nasal Spray 2 mg (or placebo)*
(Migranal® N = 305, Placebo N = 300)

*Kaplan-Meier plot based on data obtained from all studies with patients not using additional treatments censored to 24 hours. All patients received a single treatment of study medication for their migraine attack. The plot also includes patients who had no response to the initial dose.

Neither age nor sex appear to effect the patient's response to Migranal® (dihydroergotamine mesylate, USP) Nasal Spray. While patients with menstrual migraine, migraine with aura, and migraine without aura by medical history were included in the clinical evaluation of Migranal® (dihydroergotamine mesylate, USP) Nasal Spray, patients were not required to report the specific type of migraine treated with study medication. Thus, neither the effect of menses on migraine nor the presence or the absence of aura were assessed. The racial distribution of patients was insufficient to determine the effect of race on the efficacy of Migranal® (dihydroergotamine mesylate, USP) Nasal Spray.

INDICATIONS AND USAGE

Migranal® (dihydroergotamine mesylate, USP) Nasal Spray is indicated for the acute treatment of migraine headaches with or without aura.
Migranal® (dihydroergotamine mesylate, USP) Nasal Spray is not intended for the prophylactic therapy of migraine or for the management of hemiplegic or basilar migraine.

CONTRAINDICATIONS

Migranal® (dihydroergotamine mesylate, USP) Nasal Spray should not be given to patients with ischemic heart disease (angina pectoris, history of myocardial infarction, or documented silent ischemia) or to patients who have clinical symptoms or findings consistent with coronary artery vasospasm including Prinzmetal's variant angina. (See WARNINGS)
Because Migranal® (dihydroergotamine mesylate, USP) Nasal Spray may increase blood pressure, it should not be given to patients with uncontrolled hypertension.
Migranal® (dihydroergotamine mesylate, USP) Nasal Spray, 5-HT₁ agonists (e.g., sumatriptan), ergotamine-containing or ergot-type medications or methysergide should not be used within 24 hours of each other.
Migranal® (dihydroergotamine mesylate, USP) Nasal Spray should not be administered to patients with hemiplegic or basilar migraine.
In addition to those conditions mentioned above, Migranal® (dihydroergotamine mesylate, USP) Nasal Spray is also contraindicated in patients with known peripheral arterial disease, sepsis, following vascular surgery, and severely impaired hepatic or renal function.
Migranal® (dihydroergotamine mesylate, USP) Nasal Spray may cause fetal harm when administered to a pregnant woman. Dihydroergotamine possesses oxytocic

properties and, therefore, should not be administered during pregnancy. If this drug is used during pregnancy, or if the patient becomes pregnant while taking this drug, the patient should be apprised of the potential hazard to the fetus.

There are no adequate studies of dihydroergotamine in human pregnancy, but developmental toxicity has been demonstrated in experimental animals. In embryofetal development studies of dihydroergotamine mesylate nasal spray, intranasal administration to pregnant rats throughout the period of organogenesis resulted in decreased fetal body weights and/or skeletal ossification at doses of 0.16 mg/day (associated with maternal plasma dihydroergotamine exposures [AUC] approximately 0.4-1.2 times the exposures in humans receiving the MRDD of 4 mg) or greater. A no effect level for embryo-fetal toxicity was not established in rats. Delayed skeletal ossification was also noted in rabbit fetuses following intranasal administration of 3.6 mg/day (maternal exposures approximately 7 times human exposures at the MRDD) during organogenesis. A no effect level was seen at 1.2 mg/day (maternal exposures approximately 2.5 times human exposures at the MRDD). When dihydroergotamine mesylate nasal spray was administered intranasally to female rats during pregnancy and lactation, decreased body weights and impaired reproductive function (decreased mating indices) were observed in the offspring at doses of 0.16 mg/day or greater. A no effect level was not established. Effects on development occurred at doses below those that produced evidence of significant maternal toxicity in these studies. Dihydroergotamine-induced intrauterine growth retardation has been attributed to reduced uteroplacental blood flow resulting from prolonged vasoconstriction of the uterine vessels and/or increased myometrial tone.

Migranal® (dihydroergotamine mesylate, USP) Nasal Spray is contraindicated in patients who have previously shown hypersensitivity to ergot alkaloids.

Dihydroergotamine mesylate should not be used by nursing mothers. (See PRECAUTIONS)

Dihydroergotamine mesylate should not be used with peripheral and central vasoconstrictors because the combination may result in additive or synergistic elevation of blood pressure.

WARNINGS

Migranal® (dihydroergotamine mesylate, USP) Nasal Spray should only be used where a clear diagnosis of migraine headache has been established.

Risk of Myocardial Ischemia and/or Infarction and Other Adverse Cardiac Events:

Migranal® (dihydroergotamine mesylate, USP) Nasal Spray should not be used by patients with documented ischemic or vasospastic coronary artery disease. (See CONTRAINDICATIONS) It is strongly recommended that Migranal® (dihydroergotamine mesylate, USP) Nasal Spray not be given to patients in whom unrecognized coronary artery disease (CAD) is predicted by the presence of risk factors (e.g., hypertension, hypercholesterolemia, smoker, obesity, diabetes, strong family history of CAD, females who are surgically or physiologically postmenopausal, or males who are over 40 years of age) unless a cardiovascular evaluation provides satisfactory clinical evidence that the patient is reasonably free of coronary artery and ischemic myocardial disease or other significant underlying cardiovascular disease. The sensitivity of cardiac diagnostic procedures to detect cardiovascular disease or predisposition to coronary artery vasospasm is modest, at best. If, during the cardiovascular evaluation, the patient's medical history or electrocardiographic investigations reveal findings indicative of or consistent with coronary artery vasospasm or myocardial ischemia, Migranal® (dihydroergotamine mesylate, USP) Nasal Spray should not be administered. (See CONTRAINDICATIONS)

For patients with risk factors predictive of CAD who are determined to have a satisfactory cardiovascular evaluation, it is strongly recommended that administration of the first dose of Migranal® (dihydroergotamine mesylate, USP) Nasal Spray take place in the setting of a physician's office or similar medically staffed and equipped facility unless the patient has previously received dihydroergotamine mesylate. Because cardiac ischemia can occur in the absence of clinical symptoms, consideration should be given to obtaining on the first occasion of use an electrocardiogram (ECG) during the interval immediately following Migranal® (dihydroergotamine mesylate, USP) Nasal Spray, in these patients with risk factors.

It is recommended that patients who are intermittent long-term users of Migranal® (dihydroergotamine mesylate, USP) Nasal Spray and who have or acquire risk factors predictive of CAD, as described above, undergo periodic interval cardiovascular evaluation as they continue to use Migranal® (dihydroergotamine mesylate, USP) Nasal Spray.

The systematic approach described above is currently recommended as a method to identify patients in whom

Migranal® (dihydroergotamine mesylate, USP) Nasal Spray may be used to treat migraine headaches with an acceptable margin of cardiovascular safety.

Cardiac Events and Fatalities

No deaths have been reported in patients using Migranal® (dihydroergotamine mesylate, USP) Nasal Spray. However, the potential for adverse cardiac events exists. Serious adverse cardiac events, including acute myocardial infarction, life-threatening disturbances of cardiac rhythm, and death have been reported to have occurred following the administration of dihydroergotamine mesylate injection (e.g., D.H.E. 45® Injection). Considering the extent of use of dihydroergotamine mesylate in patients with migraine, the incidence of these events is extremely low.

Drug-Associated Cerebrovascular Events and Fatalities

Cerebral hemorrhage, subarachnoid hemorrhage, stroke, and other cerebrovascular events have been reported in patients treated with D.H.E. 45® Injection; and some have resulted in fatalities. In a number of cases, it appears possible that the cerebrovascular events were primary, the D.H.E. 45® Injection having been administered in the incorrect belief that the symptoms experienced were a consequence of migraine, when they were not. It should be noted that patients with migraine may be at increased risk of certain cerebrovascular events (e.g., stroke, hemorrhage, transient ischemic attack).

Other Vasospasm Related Events

Migranal® (dihydroergotamine mesylate, USP) Nasal Spray, like other ergot alkaloids, may cause vasospastic reactions other than coronary artery vasospasm. Myocardial and peripheral vascular ischemia have been reported with Migranal® (dihydroergotamine mesylate, USP) Nasal Spray.

Migranal® (dihydroergotamine mesylate, USP) Nasal Spray associated vasospastic phenomena may also cause muscle pains, numbness, coldness, pallor, and cyanosis of the digits. In patients with compromised circulation, persistent vasospasm may result in gangrene or death, Migranal® (dihydroergotamine mesylate, USP) Nasal Spray should be discontinued immediately if signs or symptoms of vasoconstriction develop.

Increase in Blood Pressure

Significant elevation in blood pressure has been reported on rare occasions in patients with and without a history of hypertension treated with Migranal® (dihydroergotamine mesylate, USP) Nasal Spray and dihydroergotamine mesylate injection. Migranal® (dihydroergotamine mesylate, USP) Nasal Spray is contraindicated in patients with uncontrolled hypertension. (See CONTRAINDICATIONS)

An 18% increase in mean pulmonary artery pressure was seen following dosing with another $5HT_1$ agonist in a study evaluating subjects undergoing cardiac catheterization.

Local Irritation

Approximately 30% of patients using Migranal® (dihydroergotamine mesylate, USP) Nasal Spray (compared to 9% of placebo patients) have reported irritation in the nose, throat, and/or disturbances in taste. Irritative symptoms include congestion, burning sensation, dryness, paraesthesia, discharge, epistaxis, pain, or soreness. The symptoms were predominantly mild to moderate in severity and transient. In approximately 70% of the above mentioned cases, the symptoms resolved within four hours after dosing with Migranal® (dihydroergotamine mesylate, USP) Nasal Spray. Examinations of the nose and throat in a small subset (N = 66) of study participants treated for up to 36 months (range 1-36 months) did not reveal any clinically noticeable injury. Other than this limited number of patients, the consequences of extended and repeated use of Migranal® (dihydroergotamine mesylate, USP) Nasal Spray on the nasal and/or respiratory mucosa have not been systematically evaluated in patients.

Nasal tissue in animals treated with dihydroergotamine mesylate daily at nasal cavity surface area exposures (in mg/mm²) that were equal to or less than those achieved in humans receiving the maximum recommended daily dose of 0.08 mg/kg/day showed mild mucosal irritation characterized by mucous cell and transitional cell hyperplasia and squamous cell metaplasia. Changes in rat nasal mucosa at 64 weeks were less severe than at 13 weeks. Local effects on respiratory tissue after chronic intranasal dosing in animals have not been evaluated.

PRECAUTIONS

General

Migranal® (dihydroergotamine mesylate, USP) Nasal Spray may cause coronary artery vasospasm; patients who experience signs or symptoms suggestive of angina following its administration should, therefore, be evaluated for the presence of CAD or a predisposition to variant angina before receiving additional doses. Similarly, patients who experience other symptoms or signs suggestive of decreased arterial flow, such as ischemic bowel syndrome or Raynaud's syndrome following the use of any 5-HT agonist are candidates for further evaluation. (See WARNINGS)

Information for Patients

The text of a patient information sheet is printed at the end of this insert. To assure safe and effective use of Migranal®

(dihydroergotamine mesylate, USP) Nasal Spray, the information and instructions provided in the patient information sheet should be discussed with patients.

Once the nasal spray applicator has been prepared, it should be discarded (with any remaining drug) after 8 hours.

Patients should be advised to report to the physician immediately any of the following: numbness or tingling in the fingers and toes, muscle pain in the arms and legs, weakness in the legs, pain in the chest, temporary speeding or slowing of the heart rate, swelling, or itching.

Prior to the initial use of the product by a patient, the prescriber should take steps to ensure that the patient understands how to use the product as provided. (See Patient Information Sheet and product packaging)

Drug Interactions

Vasoconstrictors

Migranal® (dihydroergotamine mesylate, USP) Nasal Spray should not be used with peripheral vasoconstrictors because the combination may cause synergistic elevation of blood pressure.

Sumatriptan

Sumatriptan has been reported to cause coronary artery vasospasm, and its effect could be additive with Migranal® (dihydroergotamine mesylate, USP) Nasal Spray. Sumatriptan and Migranal® (dihydroergotamine mesylate, USP) Nasal Spray should not be taken within 24 hours of each other. (See CONTRAINDICATIONS)

Beta Blockers

Although the results of a clinical study did not indicate a safety problem associated with the administration of Migranal® (dihydroergotamine mesylate, USP) Nasal Spray to subjects already receiving propranolol, there have been reports that propranolol may potentiate the vasoconstrictive action of ergotamine by blocking the vasodilating property of epinephrine.

Nicotine

Nicotine may provoke vasoconstriction in some patients, predisposing to a greater ischemic response to ergot therapy.

Macrolide Antibiotics (e.g., erythromycin and troleandomycin)

Agents of the ergot alkaloid class, of which Migranal® (dihydroergotamine mesylate, USP) Nasal Spray is a member, have been shown to interact with antibiotics of the macrolide class, resulting in increased plasma levels of unchanged alkaloids and peripheral vasoconstriction. Vasospastic reactions have been reported with therapeutic doses of ergotamine-containing drugs when co-administered with these antibiotics.

SSRI's

Weakness, hyperreflexia, and incoordination have been reported rarely when $5HT_1$ agonists have been co-administered with SSRI's (e.g., fluoxetine, fluvoxamine, paroxetine, sertraline). There have been no reported cases from spontaneous reports of drug interaction between SSRI's and Migranal® (dihydroergotamine mesylate, USP) Nasal Spray or D.H.E. 45®.

Oral Contraceptives

The effect of oral contraceptives on the pharmacokinetics of Migranal® (dihydroergotamine mesylate, USP) Nasal Spray has not been studied.

Carcinogenesis, Mutagenesis, Impairment of Fertility

Carcinogenesis

Assessment of the carcinogenic potential of dihydroergotamine mesylate in mice and rats is ongoing.

Mutagenesis

Dihydroergotamine mesylate was clastogenic in two in vitro chromosomal aberration assays, the V79 Chinese hamster cell assay with metabolic activation and the cultured human peripheral blood lymphocyte assay. There was no evidence of mutagenic potential when dihydroergotamine mesylate was tested in the presence or absence of metabolic activation in two gene mutation assays (the Ames test and the in vitro mammalian Chinese hamster V79/HGPRT assay) and in an assay for DNA damage (the rat hepatocyte unscheduled DNA synthesis test). Dihydroergotamine was not clastogenic in the in vivo mouse and hamster micronucleus tests.

Impairment of Fertility

There was no evidence of impairment of fertility in rats given intranasal doses of Migranal® (dihydroergotamine mesylate, USP) Nasal Spray up to 1.6 mg/day (associated with mean plasma dihydroergotamine mesylate exposures [AUC] approximately 9 to 11 times those in humans receiving the MRDD of 4 mg).

Pregnancy

Pregnancy Category X. See CONTRAINDICATIONS.

Nursing Mothers

Ergot drugs are known to inhibit prolactin. It is likely that Migranal® (dihydroergotamine mesylate, USP) Nasal Spray is excreted in human milk, but there are no data on the concentration of dihydroergotamine in human milk. It is known that ergotamine is excreted in breast milk and may

Continued on next page

Migranal—Cont.

cause vomiting, diarrhea, weak pulse, and unstable blood pressure in nursing infants. Because of the potential for these serious adverse events in nursing infants exposed to Migranal® (dihydroergotamine mesylate, USP) Nasal Spray, nursing should not be undertaken with the use of Migranal® (dihydroergotamine mesylate, USP) Nasal Spray. (See CONTRAINDICATIONS)

Pediatric Use

Safety and effectiveness in pediatric patients have not been established.

Use in the Elderly

There is no information about the safety and effectiveness of Migranal® (dihydroergotamine mesylate, USP) Nasal Spray in this population because patients over age 65 were excluded from the controlled clinical trials.

ADVERSE REACTIONS

During clinical studies and the foreign postmarketing experience with Migranal® (dihydroergotamine mesylate, USP) Nasal Spray there have been no fatalities due to cardiac events.

Serious cardiac events, including some that have been fatal, have occurred following use of the parenteral form of dihydroergotamine mesylate (D.H.E. 45® Injection), but are extremely rare. Events reported have included coronary artery vasospasm, transient myocardial ischemia, myocardial infarction, ventricular tachycardia, and ventricular fibrillation. (See CONTRAINDICATIONS, WARNINGS, and PRECAUTIONS)

Incidence in Controlled Clinical Trials

Of the 1,796 patients and subjects treated with Migranal® (dihydroergotamine mesylate, USP) Nasal Spray doses 2 mg or less in U.S. and foreign clinical studies, 26 (1.4%) discontinued because of adverse events.

The adverse events associated with discontinuation were, in decreasing order of frequency: rhinitis 13, dizziness 2, facial edema 2, and one each due to cold sweats, accidental trauma, depression, elective surgery, somnolence, allergy, vomiting, hypotension, and paraesthesia.

The most commonly reported adverse events associated with the use of Migranal® (dihydroergotamine mesylate, USP) Nasal Spray during placebo-controlled, double-blind studies for the treatment of migraine headache and not reported at an equal incidence by placebo-treated patients were rhinitis, altered sense of taste, application site reactions, dizziness, nausea, and vomiting. The events cited reflect experience gained under closely monitored conditions of clinical trials in a highly selected patient population. In actual clinical practice or in other clinical trials, these frequency estimates may not apply, as the conditions of use, reporting behavior, and the kinds of patients treated may differ.

Migranal® (dihydroergotamine mesylate, USP) Nasal Spray was generally well tolerated. In most instances these events were transient and self-limited and did not result in patient discontinuation from a study. The following table summarizes the incidence rates of adverse events reported by at least 1% of patients who received Migranal® (dihydroergotamine mesylate, USP) Nasal Spray for the treatment of migraine headaches during placebo-controlled, double-blind clinical studies and were more frequent than in those patients receiving placebo.

Table 3: Adverse events reported by at least 1% of the Migranal® (dihydroergotamine mesylate, USP) Nasal Spray treated patients and occurred more frequently than in the placebo-group in the migraine placebo-controlled trials

	Migranal® N=597	Placebo N=631
Respiratory System		
Rhinitis	26%	7%
Pharyngitis	3%	1%
Sinusitis	1%	1%
Gastrointestinal System		
Nausea	10%	4%
Vomiting	4%	1%
Diarrhea	2%	<1%
Special Senses, Other		
Altered Sense of Taste	8%	1%
Application Site		
Application Site Reaction	6%	2%
Central and Peripheral Nervous System		
Dizziness	4%	2%
Somnolence	3%	2%
Paraesthesia	2%	2%
Body as a Whole, General		
Hot Flushes	1%	<1%
Fatigue	1%	1%
Asthenia	1%	0%
Autonomic Nervous System		
Mouth Dry	1%	1%
Musculoskeletal System		
Stiffness	1%	<1%

Other Adverse Events During Clinical Trials

In the paragraphs that follow, the frequencies of less commonly reported adverse clinical events are presented. Because the reports include events observed in open and uncontrolled studies, the role of Migranal® (dihydroergotamine mesylate, USP) Nasal Spray in their causation cannot be reliably determined. Furthermore, variability associated with adverse event reporting, the terminology used to describe adverse events, etc., limit the value of the quantitative frequency estimates provided. Event frequencies are calculated as the number of patients who used Migranal® (dihydroergotamine mesylate, USP) Nasal Spray in placebo-controlled trials and reported an event divided by the total number of patients (n=1796) exposed to Migranal® (dihydroergotamine mesylate, USP) Nasal Spray. All reported events are included except those already listed in the previous table, those too general to be informative, and those not reasonably associated with the use of the drug. Events are further classified within body system categories and enumerated in order of decreasing frequency using the following definitions: frequent adverse events are defined as those occurring in at least 1/100 patients; infrequent adverse events are those occurring in 1/100 to 1/1,000 patients; and rare adverse events are those occurring in fewer than 1/1,000 patients.

Skin and Appendages: Infrequent: petechia, pruritus, rash, cold clammy skin; Rare: papular rash, urticaria, herpes simplex.

Musculoskeletal: Infrequent: cramps, myalgia, muscular weakness, dystonia; Rare: arthralgia, involuntary muscle contractions, rigidity.

Central and Peripheral Nervous System: Infrequent: confusion, tremor, hypoesthesia, vertigo; Rare: speech disorder, hyperkinesia, stupor, abnormal gait, aggravated migraine.

Autonomic Nervous System: Infrequent: increased sweating.

Special Senses: Infrequent: sense of smell altered, photophobia, conjunctivitis, abnormal lacrimation, abnormal vision, tinnitus, earache; Rare: eye pain.

Psychiatric: Infrequent: nervousness, euphoria, insomnia, concentration impaired; Rare: anxiety, anorexia, depression.

Gastrointestinal: Infrequent: abdominal pain, dyspepsia, dysphagia, hiccup; Rare: increased salivation, esophagospasm.

Cardiovascular: Infrequent: edema, palpitation, tachycardia; Rare: hypotension, peripheral ischemia, angina.

Respiratory System: Infrequent: dyspnea, upper respiratory tract infections; Rare: bronchospasm, bronchitis, pleural pain, epistaxis.

Urinary System: Infrequent: increased frequency of micturition, cystitis.

Reproductive, Female: Rare: pelvic inflammation, vaginitis.

Body as a Whole—General: Infrequent: feeling cold, malaise, rigors, fever, periorbital edema; Rare: flu-like symptoms, shock, loss of voice, yawning.

Application Site: Infrequent: local anesthesia.

Post-introduction Reports

Voluntary reports of adverse events temporally associated with dihydroergotamine products used in the management of migraine that have been received since the introduction of the injectable formulation are included in this section save for those already listed above. Because of their source (open and uncontrolled clinical use), whether or not events reported in association with the use of dihydroergotamine are causally related to it cannot be determined.

There have been reports of pleural and retroperitoneal fibrosis in patients following prolonged daily use of injectable dihydroergotamine mesylate. Migranal® (dihydroergotamine mesylate, USP) Nasal Spray is not recommended for prolonged daily use. (See DOSAGE AND ADMINISTRATION)

DRUG ABUSE AND DEPENDENCE

Currently available data have not demonstrated drug abuse or psychological dependence with dihydroergotamine. However, cases of drug abuse and psychological dependence in patients on other forms of ergot therapy have been reported. Thus, due to the chronicity of vascular headaches, it is imperative that patients be advised not to exceed recommended dosages.

OVERDOSAGE

To date, there have been no reports of acute overdosage with this drug. Due to the risk of vascular spasm, exceeding the recommended dosages of Migranal® (dihydroergotamine mesylate, USP) Nasal Spray is to be avoided. Excessive doses of dihydroergotamine may result in peripheral signs and symptoms of ergotism. Treatment includes discontinu-

ance of the drug, local application of warmth to the affected area, the administration of vasodilators, and nursing care to prevent tissue damage.

In general, the symptoms of an acute Migranal® (dihydroergotamine mesylate, USP) Nasal Spray overdose are similar to those of an ergotamine overdose, although there is less pronounced nausea and vomiting with Migranal® (dihydroergotamine mesylate, USP) Nasal Spray. The symptoms of an ergotamine overdose include the following: numbness, tingling, pain, and cyanosis of the extremities associated with diminished or absent peripheral pulses; respiratory depression; an increase and/or decrease in blood pressure, usually in that order; confusion, delirium, convulsions, and coma; and/or some degree of nausea, vomiting, and abdominal pain.

In laboratory animals, significant lethality occurs when dihydroergotamine is given at I.V. doses of 44 mg/kg in mice, 130 mg/kg in rats, and 37 mg/kg in rabbits.

Up-to-date information about the treatment of overdosage can often be obtained from a certified Regional Poison Control Center. Telephone numbers of certified Poison Control Centers are listed in the Physicians' Desk Reference® (PDR).*

DOSAGE AND ADMINISTRATION

The solution used in Migranal® (dihydroergotamine mesylate, USP) Nasal Spray (4 mg/mL) is intended for intranasal use and must not be injected.

In clinical trials, Migranal® (dihydroergotamine mesylate, USP) Nasal Spray has been effective for the acute treatment of migraine headaches with or without aura. One spray (0.5 mg) of Migranal® (dihydroergotamine mesylate, USP) Nasal Spray should be administered in each nostril. Fifteen minutes later, an additional one spray (0.5 mg) of Migranal® (dihydroergotamine mesylate, USP) Nasal Spray should be administered in each nostril, for a total dosage of four sprays (2.0 mg) of Migranal® (dihydroergotamine mesylate, USP) Nasal Spray. Studies have shown no additional benefit from acute doses greater than 2.0 mg for a single migraine administration. The safety of doses greater than 3.0 mg in a 24 hour period and 4.0 mg in a 7 day period has not been established.

Prior to administration, the pump must be primed (i.e., squeeze 4 times) before use. (See Patient Information Sheet or Patient Instruction Booklet)

Once the nasal spray applicator has been prepared, it should be discarded (with any remaining drug in opened ampul) after 8 hours.

HOW SUPPLIED

Migranal® (dihydroergotamine mesylate, USP) Nasal Spray is available (as a clear, colorless to faintly yellow solution) in 1 mL amber glass ampuls containing 4 mg of dihydroergotamine mesylate, USP (NDC 0078-0245-98).

Migranal® (dihydroergotamine mesylate, USP) Nasal Spray is provided in individual kits. The kits consist of four unit dose trays, a patient instruction booklet, one assembly case, and one patient information sheet packed in a carton. Each unit dose tray contains one ampul, a nasal spray applicator, and a breaker cap on the ampul.

Store below 77°F (25°C). Do not refrigerate or freeze.

Patient Information

Information for the Patient

Migranal® (dihydroergotamine mesylate, USP) Nasal Spray.

The solution used in Migranal® (dihydroergotamine mesylate, USP) Nasal Spray (4 mg/mL) is intended for intranasal use and must not be injected.

Please read this information carefully before using your Migranal® (dihydroergotamine mesylate, USP) Nasal Spray for the first time. Keep this information handy for future reference. This leaflet does not contain all of the information on Migranal® (dihydroergotamine mesylate, USP) Nasal Spray. Your pharmacist and/or health care provider can provide more detailed information.

Migranal® (dihydroergotamine mesylate, USP) Nasal Spray has been evaluated in a limited number of patients long term (e.g., 1 year or longer).

Purpose of your Medication

Migranal® (dihydroergotamine mesylate, USP) Nasal Spray is intended to treat an active migraine headache. Do not try to use it to prevent a headache if you have no symptoms. Do not use it to treat common tension headache or a headache that is not at all typical of your usual migraine headache.

Do not use Migranal® (dihydroergotamine mesylate, USP) Nasal Spray if you:
- are pregnant or nursing.
- have any disease affecting your heart, arteries, or circulation.

Important questions to consider before using Migranal® (dihydroergotamine mesylate, USP) Nasal Spray

Please answer the following questions before you use your Migranal® (dihydroergotamine mesylate, USP) Nasal Spray. If you answer YES to any of these questions or are

unsure of the answer, you should talk to your doctor before using Migranal® (dihydroergotamine mesylate, USP) Nasal Spray.

- Do you have high blood pressure?
- Do you have chest pain, shortness of breath, heart disease, or have you had any surgery on your heart arteries?
- Do you have risk factors for heart disease (such as high blood pressure, high cholesterol, obesity, diabetes, smoking, strong family history of heart disease, or you are postmenopausal or a male over 40)?
- Do you have any problems with blood circulation in your arms or legs, fingers, or toes?
- Are you pregnant? Do you think you might be pregnant? Are you trying to become pregnant? Are you sexually active and not using birth control? Are you breast feeding?
- Have you ever had to stop taking this or any other medication because of an allergy or bad reaction?
- Are you taking any other migraine medications, erythromycin or other antibiotics, or medications for blood pressure prescribed by your doctor, or other medicines obtained from your drugstore without a doctor's prescription?
- Do you smoke?
- Have you had, or do you have, any disease of the liver or kidney?
- Is this headache different from your usual migraine attacks?

REMEMBER TO TELL YOUR DOCTOR IF YOU HAVE ANSWERED YES TO ANY OF THESE QUESTIONS BEFORE YOU USE MIGRANAL® (dihydroergotamine mesylate, USP) NASAL SPRAY.

Side Effects To Watch Out For

In clinical trials, most migraine patients have used Migranal® (dihydroergotamine mesylate, USP) Nasal Spray without serious side effects. You may experience some nasal congestion or irritation, altered sense of taste, sore throat, nausea, vomiting, dizziness, and fatigue after using Migranal® (dihydroergotamine mesylate, USP) Nasal Spray. These side effects are temporary and usually do not require you to stop using Migranal® (dihydroergotamine mesylate, USP) Nasal Spray. Although the following reactions rarely occur, they can be serious and should be reported to your physician immediately:

- Numbness or tingling in your fingers and toes
- Pain, tightness, or discomfort in your chest
- Muscle pain or cramps in your arms and legs
- Weakness in your legs
- Temporary speeding or slowing of your heart rate
- Swelling or itching

Dosing Information

- Each ampul contains one complete dose of Migranal® (dihydroergotamine mesylate, USP) Nasal Spray, which is 1 spray in each nostril followed in 15 minutes by an additional spray in each nostril, for a total of 4 sprays.
- Studies have shown no benefit from acute doses greater than 2.0 mg (4 sprays) for a single administration. The safety of doses greater than 3.0 mg in a 24 hour period has not been established.
- The safety of doses greater than 4.0 mg in a 7-day period has not been established.

Learn what to do in case of an Overdose

If you have used more medication than you have been instructed, contact your doctor, hospital emergency department, or nearest poison control center immediately.

How to use the Migranal® (dihydroergotamine mesylate, USP) Nasal Spray

1. Use available training materials.
   - Read and follow the instructions in the patient instruction booklet which is provided with the Migranal® (dihydroergotamine mesylate, USP) Nasal Spray package before attempting to use the product.
   - If there are any questions concerning the use of your Migranal® (dihydroergotamine mesylate, USP) Nasal Spray, ask your doctor or pharmacist, or call the Migranal® (dihydroergotamine mesylate, USP) Nasal Spray Information Line at 1-888-MY-RELIEF (1-888-697-3543) for training in the use of the spray.
2. Check the contents of the package.
   - Assembly Case
   - Well (which is part of the Assembly Case)
   - Unit Dose Tray
   - Brown (amber) glass ampul with yellow breaker cap
   - Nasal Sprayer with cover
3. Assemble the sprayer.

   Assemble your Nasal Sprayer only when you are ready to use it.
   - Tap top of ampul until all medication is in the bottom.
   - Place ampul upright and straight in well of the Assembly Case with breaker cap pointing up.
   - Push down the Assembly Case lid slowly but firmly, until you hear ampul snap open.
   - Without removing ampul from well, push Nasal Sprayer onto ampul until it clicks. (To ensure that the ampul fits properly into the Nasal Sprayer, first look at the tube through the bottom of sprayer to make sure it is straight. If it is curved, straighten it with your finger.)
4. Using the sprayer:
   - Remove cover from the Nasal Sprayer.
   - Pump the Nasal Sprayer 4 times before using. (Point the Nasal Sprayer up and away from your face when pumping.) *Do not* prime the Nasal Sprayer more than 4 times. Although some medication will spray out, there is enough medication in each ampul to allow you to prepare your sprayer properly and still receive a full dose of Migranal® (dihydroergotamine mesylate, USP) Nasal Spray.
   - Spray once in each nostril. You should not tilt head back or inhale through your nose while spraying.
   - Wait 15 minutes, then spray once in each nostril again.
5. After completing these instructions:
   - Carefully dispose of the Nasal Sprayer containing the ampul and the breaker cap containing the top of the ampul.
   - Load a new Unit Dose Tray into your Assembly Case.
   - Keep the Assembly Case for a maximum of 4 treatments, then discard it along with the Unit Dose Tray.

Important Notes:

- Once a Migranal® (dihydroergotamine mesylate, USP) Nasal Spray ampul has been opened, it must be thrown away after 8 hours.
- You should not sniff or tilt your head back when using Migranal® (dihydroergotamine mesylate, USP) Nasal Spray.

Storing Migranal® (dihydroergotamine mesylate, USP) Nasal Spray

- Keep medication in a safe place away from children.
- Keep Migranal® (dihydroergotamine mesylate, USP) Nasal Spray away from heat and light.
  - — Do not expose Migranal® (dihydroergotamine mesylate, USP) Nasal Spray to temperatures over 77°F.
  - — Never refrigerate or freeze Migranal® (dihydroergotamine mesylate, USP) Nasal Spray.
- Keep Migranal® (dihydroergotamine mesylate, USP) Nasal Spray components in the Unit Dose Tray.
- Keep the Unit Dose Tray loaded in the Assembly Case.
- Do not keep an opened Migranal® (dihydroergotamine mesylate, USP) Nasal Spray ampul for more than 8 hours.

  Check the expiration date printed on the ampul containing medication. If the expiration date has passed, do not use it.

Answers to patients' questions about Migranal® (dihydroergotamine mesylate, USP) Nasal Spray

What if I need help in using my Migranal® (dihydroergotamine mesylate, USP) Nasal Spray?

If you have any questions or if you need help in opening, putting together, or using Migranal® (dihydroergotamine mesylate, USP) Nasal Spray, speak to your doctor or pharmacist, or call the Migranal® (dihydroergotamine mesylate, USP) Nasal Spray Information Line at 1-888-MY-RELIEF (1-888-697-3543).

How much medication should I use and how often?

Each ampul contains one complete dose of Migranal® (dihydroergotamine mesylate, USP) Nasal Spray, which is 1 spray in each nostril, followed by an additional spray in each nostril 15 minutes later for a total of 4 sprays. Do not use more than this amount unless instructed to do so by your doctor.

Why do I have to prime or pump the Nasal Sprayer 4 times before using? Am I wasting the medication?

You have to prime the Nasal Sprayer 4 times to make sure that you get the proper amount of medication when you use it. Although you will see some medication spray out, there is still enough medication in each ampul to allow you to prepare your sprayer properly and still receive a full dose of Migranal® (dihydroergotamine mesylate, USP) Nasal Spray.

Can I load the medication ampul into the Nasal Sprayer so it is ready before I need to use it?

No. The brown (amber) glass ampul containing your medication must remain unopened until you are ready to use it. It may not be fully effective if opened and not used within 8 hours. However, after each migraine attack, you should load a new plastic Unit Dose Tray containing an unopened Migranal® (dihydroergotamine mesylate, USP) Nasal Spray ampul and Nasal Sprayer into the Migranal® (dihydroergotamine mesylate, USP) Nasal Spray Assembly Case, so you will be prepared for your next migraine attack.

Can I reuse my Migranal® (dihydroergotamine mesylate, USP) Nasal Sprayer?

No. After completing the full dose, you must carefully dispose of your Migranal® (dihydroergotamine mesylate, USP) Nasal Sprayer containing the opened ampul. Each Unit Dose Tray contains a new Nasal Sprayer, an ampul of Migranal® (dihydroergotamine mesylate, USP) Nasal Spray medication, and a breaker cap on the ampul. But you should keep your Assembly Case and load it with a new Unit Dose Tray after each migraine so you are ready to treat your next migraine attack.

Can I use Migranal® (dihydroergotamine mesylate, USP) Nasal Spray if I have a stuffy nose, cold, or allergies?

Yes. Migranal® (dihydroergotamine mesylate, USP) Nasal Spray can be used if you have a stuffy nose, cold, or allergies. However, if you are taking any medications for your cold, or allergies, even those you can buy without a doctor's prescription, speak with your doctor before using Migranal® (dihydroergotamine mesylate, USP) Nasal Spray.

Do I need to sniff the medication when I spray it in my nostril?

No, you should not sniff because Migranal® (dihydroergotamine mesylate, USP) Nasal Spray should remain in the nose so that it can be absorbed into the bloodstream through the lining of the nose.

If you have any other unanswered question about Migranal® (dihydroergotamine mesylate, USP) Nasal Spray, consult your doctor or pharmacist.

*Trademark of Medical Economics Company, Inc.

DECEMBER 1997 30721901

NEORAL® Soft Gelatin Capsules ℞
(cyclosporine capsules for microemulsion)

NEORAL® Oral Solution
(cyclosporine oral solution for microemulsion)
[*nē ŏ 'răl*]

Caution: Federal law prohibits dispensing without prescription.

The following prescribing information is based on official labeling in effect on August 1, 1998.

WARNING

Only physicians experienced in management of systemic immunosuppressive therapy for the indicated disease should prescribe Neoral®. At doses used in solid organ transplantation, only physicians experienced in immunosuppressive therapy and management of organ transplant recipients should prescribe Neoral®. Patients receiving the drug should be managed in facilities equipped and staffed with adequate laboratory and supportive medical resources. The physician responsible for maintenance therapy should have complete information requisite for the follow-up of the patient.

Neoral®, a systemic immunosuppressant, may increase the susceptibility to infection and the development of neoplasia. In kidney, liver, and heart transplant patients Neoral® may be administered with other immunosuppressive agents. Increased susceptibility to infection and the possible development of lymphoma and other neoplasms may result from the increase in the degree of immunosuppression in transplant patients.

Neoral® Soft Gelatin Capsules (cyclosporine capsules for microemulsion) and Neoral® Oral Solution (cyclosporine oral solution for microemulsion) have increased bioavailability in comparison to Sandimmune® Soft Gelatin Capsules (cyclosporine capsules, USP) and Sandimmune® Oral Solution (cyclosporine oral solution, USP). Neoral® and Sandimmune® are not bioequivalent and cannot be used interchangeably without physician supervision. For a given trough concentration, cyclosporine exposure will be greater with Neoral® than with Sandimmune®. If a patient who is receiving exceptionally high doses of Sandimmune® is converted to Neoral®, particular caution should be exercised. Cyclosporine blood concentrations should be monitored in transplant and rheumatoid arthritis patients taking Neoral® to avoid toxicity due to high concentrations. Dose adjustments should be made in transplant patients to minimize possible organ rejection due to low concentrations. Comparison of blood concentrations in the published literature with blood concentrations obtained using current assays must be done with detailed knowledge of the assay methods employed.

For Psoriasis Patients *(See also Boxed WARNINGS above)*

Psoriasis patients previously treated with PUVA and to a lesser extent, methotrexate or other immunosuppressive agents, UVB, coal tar, or radiation therapy, are at an increased risk of developing skin malignancies when taking Neoral®.

Cyclosporine, the active ingredient in Neoral®, in recommended dosages, can cause systemic hypertension

Continued on next page

Neoral—Cont.

and nephrotoxicity. The risk increases with increasing dose and duration of cyclosporine therapy. Renal dysfunction, including structural kidney damage, is a potential consequence of cyclosporine, and therefore, renal function must be monitored during therapy.

DESCRIPTION

Neoral® is an oral formulation of cyclosporine that immediately forms a microemulsion in an aqueous environment.
Cyclosporine, the active principle in Neoral®, is a cyclic polypeptide immunosuppressant agent consisting of 11 amino acids. It is produced as a metabolite by the fungus species *Beauveria nivea*.
Chemically, cyclosporine is designated as [*R*-[*R**,*R**-(*E*)]]-cyclic-(L-alanyl-D-alanyl-*N*-methyl-L-leucyl-*N*-methyl-L-leucyl-*N*-methyl-L-valyl-3-hydroxy-*N*,4-dimethyl-L-2-amino-6-octenoyl-L-α-amino-butyryl-*N*-methylglycyl-*N*-methyl-L-leucyl-L-valyl-*N*-methyl-L-leucyl).
Neoral® Soft Gelatin Capsules (cyclosporine capsules for microemulsion) are available in 25 mg and 100 mg strengths.
Each 25 mg capsule contains:
cyclosporine .... 25 mg
alcohol, USP dehydrated .... 11.9% v/v (9.5% wt/vol.)
Each 100 mg capsule contains:
cyclosporine .... 100 mg
alcohol, USP dehydrated .... 11.9% v/v (9.5% wt/vol.)
Inactive Ingredients: Corn oil-mono-di-triglycerides, polyoxyl 40 hydrogenated castor oil NF, DL-α-tocopherol USP, gelatin NF, glycerol, iron oxide black, propylene glycol USP, titanium dioxide USP, carmine, and other ingredients.
Neoral® Oral Solution (cyclosporine oral solution for microemulsion) is available in 50 mL bottles.
Each mL contains:
cyclosporine .... 100 mg/mL
alcohol, USP dehydrated .... 11.9% v/v (9.5% wt/vol.)
Inactive Ingredients: Corn oil-mono-di-triglycerides, polyoxyl 40 hydrogenated castor oil NF, DL-α-tocopherol USP, propylene glycol USP.
The chemical structure of cyclosporine (also known as cyclosporin A) is:

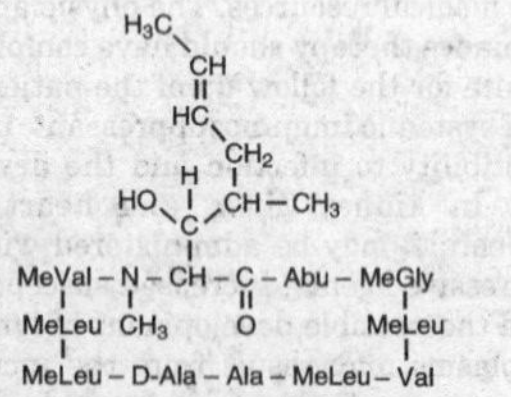
H3C
CH
HC
CH2
HO
CH—CH3
MeVal – N – CH – C – Abu – MeGly
MeLeu CH3 O MeLeu
MeLeu – D-Ala – Ala – MeLeu – Val

$C_{62}H_{111}N_{11}O_{12}$ Mol. Wt. 1202.63

CLINICAL PHARMACOLOGY

Cyclosporine is a potent immunosuppressive agent that in animals prolongs survival of allogeneic transplants involving skin, kidney, liver, heart, pancreas, bone marrow, small intestine, and lung. Cyclosporine has been demonstrated to suppress some humoral immunity and to a greater extent, cell-mediated immune reactions such as allograft rejection, delayed hypersensitivity, experimental allergic encephalomyelitis, Freund's adjuvant arthritis, and graft vs. host disease in many animal species for a variety of organs.
The effectiveness of cyclosporine results from specific and reversible inhibition of immunocompetent lymphocytes in the G_0- and G_1-phase of the cell cycle. T-lymphocytes are preferentially inhibited. The T-helper cell is the main target, although the T-suppressor cell may also be suppressed. Cyclosporine also inhibits lymphokine production and release including interleukin-2.
No effects on phagocytic function (changes in enzyme secretions, chemotactic migration of granulocytes, macrophage migration, carbon clearance *in vivo*) have been detected in animals. Cyclosporine does not cause bone marrow suppression in animal models or man.
Pharmacokinetics: The immunosuppressive activity of cyclosporine is primarily due to parent drug. Following oral administration, absorption of cyclosporine is incomplete. The extent of absorption of cyclosporine is dependent on the individual patient, the patient population, and the formulation. Elimination of cyclosporine is primarily biliary with only 6% of the dose (parent drug and metabolites) excreted in urine. The disposition of cyclosporine from blood is generally biphasic, with a terminal half-life of approximately 8.4 hours (range 5-18 hours). Following intravenous administration, the blood clearance of cyclosporine (assay: HPLC) is approximately 5-7 mL/min/kg in adult recipients of renal or liver allografts. Blood cyclosporine clearance appears to be slightly slower in cardiac transplant patients.

The Neoral® Soft Gelatin Capsules (cyclosporine capsules for microemulsion) and Neoral® Oral Solution (cyclosporine oral solution for microemulsion) are bioequivalent.
The relationship between administered dose and exposure (area under the concentration versus time curve, AUC) is linear within the therapeutic dose range. The intersubject variability (total, %CV) of cyclosporine exposure (AUC) when Neoral® or Sandimmune® is administered ranges from approximately 20% to 50% in renal transplant patients. This intersubject variability contributes to the need for individualization of the dosing regimen for optimal therapy *(see DOSAGE AND ADMINISTRATION)*. Intrasubject variability of AUC in renal transplant recipients (%CV) was 9%-21% for Neoral® and 19%-26% for Sandimmune®. In the same studies, intrasubject variability of trough concentrations (%CV) was 17%-30% for Neoral® and 16%-38% for Sandimmune®.
Absorption: Neoral® has increased bioavailability compared to Sandimmune®. The absolute bioavailability of cyclosporine administered as Sandimmune® is dependent on the patient population, estimated to be less than 10% in liver transplant patients and as great as 89% in some renal transplant patients. The absolute bioavailability of cyclosporine administered as Neoral® has not been determined in adults. In studies of renal transplant, rheumatoid arthritis and psoriasis patients, the mean cyclosporine AUC was approximately 20% to 50% greater and the peak blood cyclosporine concentration (C_{max}) was approximately 40% to 106% greater following administration of Neoral® compared to following administration of Sandimmune®. The dose normalized AUC in *de novo* liver transplant patients administered Neoral® 28 days after transplantation was 50% greater and C_{max} was 90% greater than in those patients administered Sandimmune®. AUC and C_{max} are also increased (Neoral® relative to Sandimmune®) in heart transplant patients, but data are very limited. Although the AUC and C_{max} values are higher on Neoral® relative to Sandimmune®, the pre-dose trough concentrations (dose-normalized) are similar for the two formulations.
Following oral administration of Neoral®, the time to peak blood cyclosporine concentrations (T_{max}) ranged from 1.5-2.0 hours. The administration of food with Neoral® decreases the cyclosporine AUC and C_{max}. A high fat meal (669 kcal, 45 grams fat) consumed within one-half hour before Neoral® administration decreased the AUC by 13% and C_{max} by 33%. The effects of a low fat meal (667 kcal, 15 grams fat) were similar.
The effect of T-tube diversion of bile on the absorption of cyclosporine from Neoral® was investigated in eleven *de novo* liver transplant patients. When the patients were administered Neoral® with and without T-tube diversion of bile, very little difference in absorption was observed, as measured by the change in maximal cyclosporine blood concentrations from pre-dose values with the T-tube closed relative to when it was open: 6.9±41% (range -55% to 68%).
[See table below]
Distribution: Cyclosporine is distributed largely outside the blood volume. The steady state volume of distribution during intravenous dosing has been reported as 3-5 L/kg in solid organ transplant recipients. In blood, the distribution is concentration dependent. Approximately 33%-47% is in plasma, 4%-9% in lymphocytes, 5%-12% in granulocytes, and 41%-58% in erythrocytes. At high concentrations, the binding capacity of leukocytes and erythrocytes becomes saturated. In plasma, approximately 90% is bound to proteins, primarily lipoproteins. Cyclosporine is excreted in human milk. *(See PRECAUTIONS, Nursing Mothers)*
Metabolism: Cyclosporine is extensively metabolized by the cytochrome P-450 III-A enzyme system in the liver, and to a lesser degree in the gastrointestinal tract, and the kidney. The metabolism of cyclosporine can be altered by the coadministration of a variety of agents. *(See PRECAUTIONS, Drug Interactions)*
At least 25 metabolites have been identified from human bile, feces, blood, and urine. The biological activity of the metabolites and their contributions to toxicity are considerably less than those of the parent compound. The major metabolites (M1, M9, and M4N) result from oxidation at the 1-beta, 9-gamma, and 4-N-demethylated positions, respectively. At steady state following the oral administration of Sandimmune®, the mean AUCs for blood concentrations of M1, M9, and M4N are about 70%, 21%, and 7.5% of the AUC for blood cyclosporine concentrations, respectively. Based on blood concentration data from stable renal transplant patients (13 patients administered Neoral® and Sandimmune® in a crossover study), and bile concentration data from *de novo* liver transplant patients (4 administered Neoral®, 3 administered Sandimmune®), the percentage of dose present as M1, M9, and M4N metabolites is similar when either Neoral® or Sandimmune® is administered.
Excretion: Only 0.1% of a cyclosporine dose is excreted unchanged in the urine. Elimination is primarily biliary with only 6% of the dose (parent drug and metabolites) excreted in the urine. Neither dialysis nor renal failure alter cyclosporine clearance significantly.
Drug Interactions: *(See PRECAUTIONS, Drug Interactions)* When diclofenac or methotrexate was co-administered with cyclosporine in rheumatoid arthritis patients, the AUC of diclofenac and methotrexate, each was significantly increased. *(See PRECAUTIONS, Drug Interactions)* No clinically significant pharmacokinetic interactions occurred between cyclosporine and aspirin, ketoprofen, piroxicam, or indomethacin.
Special Populations: ***Pediatric Population:*** Pharmacokinetic data from pediatric patients administered Neoral® or Sandimmune® are very limited. In 15 renal transplant patients aged 3-16 years, cyclosporine whole blood clearance after IV administration of Sandimmune® was 10.6±3.7 mL/min/kg (assay: Cyclo-trac specific RIA). In a study of 7 renal transplant patients aged 2-16, the cyclosporine clearance ranged from 9.8-15.5 mL/min/kg. In 9 liver transplant patients aged 0.6-5.6 years, clearance was 9.3±5.4 mL/min/kg (assay: HPLC).
In the pediatric population, Neoral® also demonstrates an increased bioavailability as compared to Sandimmune®. In 7 liver *de novo* transplant patients aged 1.4-10 years, the absolute bioavailability of Neoral® was 43% (range 30%-68%) and for Sandimmune® in the same individuals absolute bioavailability was 28% (range 17%-42%).
[See table at top of next page]
Geriatric Population: Comparison of single dose data from both normal elderly volunteers (N=18, mean age 69 years) and elderly rheumatoid arthritis patients (N=16, mean age 68 years) to single dose data in young adult volunteers (N=16, mean age 26 years) showed no significant difference in the pharmacokinetic parameters.

Pharmacokinetic Parameters (mean±SD)

Patient Population	Dose/day[1] (mg/d)	Dose/ weight (mg/kg/d)	AUC[2] (ng·hr/mL)	C_{max} (ng/mL	Trough[3] (ng/mL)	CL/F (mL/min)	CL/F (mL/min/kg)
De novo renal transplant[4] Week 4 (N=37)	597±174	7.95±2.81	8772±2089	1802±428	361±129	593±204	7.8±2.9
Stable renal transplant[4] (N=55)	344±122	4.10±1.58	6035±2194	1333±469	251±116	492±140	5.9±2.1
De novo liver transplant[5] Week 4 (N=18)	458±190	6.89±3.68	7187±2816	1555±740	268±101	577±309	8.6±5.7
De novo rheumatoid arthritis[6] (N=23)	182±55.6	2.37±0.36	2641±877	728±263	96.4±37.7	613±196	8.3±2.8
De novo psoriasis[6] Week 4 (N=18)	189±69.8	2.48±0.65	2324±1048	655±186	74.9±46.7	723±186	10.2±3.9

[1] Total daily dose was divided into two doses administered every 12 hours
[2] AUC was measured over one dosing interval
[3] Trough concentration was measured just prior to the morning Neoral® dose, approximately 12 hours after the previous dose
[4] Assay: TDx specific monoclonal fluorescence polarization immunoassay
[5] Assay: Cyclo-trac specific monoclonal radioimmunoassay
[6] Assay: INCSTAR specific monoclonal radioimmunoassay

Pediatric Parmacokinetic Parameters (mean±SD)

Patient Population	Dose/day (mg/d)	Dose/weight (mg/kg/d)	AUC[1] (ng·hr/mL)	C_max (ng/mL)	CL/F (mL/min)	CL/F (mL/min/kg)
Stable liver transplant[2]						
Age 2–8, Dosed TID (N=9)	101±25	5.95±1.32	2163±801	629±219	285±94	16.6±4.3
Age 8–15, Dosed BID (N=8)	188±55	4.96±2.09	4272±1462	975±281	378±80	10.2±4.0
Stable liver transplant[3]						
Age 3, Dosed BID (N=1)	120	8.33	5832	1050	171	11.9
Age 8–15, Dosed BID (N=5)	158±55	5.51±1.91	4452±2475	1013±635	328±121	11.0±1.9
Stable renal transplant[3]						
Age 7–15, Dosed BID (N=5)	328±83	7.37±4.11	6922±1988	1827±487	418±143	8.7±2.9

[1] AUC was measured over one dosing interval
[2] Assay: Cyclo-trac specific monoclonal radioimmunoassay
[3] Assay: TDx specific monoclonal fluorescence polarization immunoassay

CLINICAL TRIALS

Rheumatoid Arthritis: The effectiveness of Sandimmune® (cyclosporine) and Neoral® (cyclosporine for microemulsion) in the treatment of severe rheumatoid arthritis was evaluated in 5 clinical studies involving a total of 728 cyclosporine treated patients and 273 placebo treated patients. A summary of the results is presented for the "responder" rates per treatment group, with a responder being defined as a patient having *completed* the trial with a 20% improvement in the tender and the swollen joint count and a 20% improvement in 2 of 4 of investigator global, patient global, disability, and erythrocyte sedimentation rates (ESR) for the Studies 651 and 652 and 3 of 5 of investigator global, patient global, disability, visual analog pain, and ESR for Studies 2008, 654 and 302.

Study 651 enrolled 264 patients with active rheumatoid arthritis with at least 20 involved joints, who had failed at least one major RA drug, using a 3:3:2 randomization to one of the following three groups: (1) cyclosporine dosed at 2.5-5 mg/kg/day, (2) methotrexate at 7.5-15 mg/week, or (3) placebo. Treatment duration was 24 weeks. The mean cyclosporine dose at the last visit was 3.1 mg/kg/day. See Graph below.

Study 652 enrolled 250 patients with active RA with >6 active painful or tender joints who had failed at least one major RA drug. Patients were randomized using a 3:3:2 randomization to 1 of 3 treatment arms: (1) 1.5-5 mg/kg/day of cyclosporine, (2) 2.5-5 mg/kg/day of cyclosporine, and (3) placebo. Treatment duration was 16 weeks. The mean cyclosporine dose for group 2 at the last visit was 2.92 mg/kg/day. See Graph below.

Study 2008 enrolled 144 patients with active RA and >6 active joints who had unsuccessful treatment courses of aspirin and gold or Penicillamine. Patients were randomized to 1 of 2 treatment groups (1) cyclosporine 2.5-5 mg/kg/day with adjustments after the first month to achieve a target trough level and (2) placebo. Treatment duration was 24 weeks. The mean cyclosporine dose at the last visit was 3.63 mg/kg/day. See Graph below.

Study 654 enrolled 148 patients who remained with active joint counts of 6 or more despite treatment with maximally tolerated methotrexate doses for at least three months. Patients continued to take their current dose of methotrexate and were randomized to receive, in addition, one of the following medications: (1) cyclosporine 2.5 mg/kg/day with dose increases of 0.5 mg/kg/day at weeks 2 and 4 if there was no evidence of toxicity and further increases of 0.5 mg/kg/day at weeks 8 and 16 if a <30% decrease in active joint count occurred without any significant toxicity; dose

decreases could be made at any time for toxicity or (2) placebo. Treatment duration was 24 weeks. The mean cyclosporine dose at the last visit was 2.8 mg/kg/day (range: 1.3-4.1). See Graph below.

Study 302 enrolled 299 patients with severe active RA, 99% of whom were unresponsive or intolerant to at least one prior major RA drug. Patients were randomized to 2 treatment groups (1) Neoral® and (2) cyclosporine, both of which were started at 2.5 mg/kg/day and increased after 4 weeks for inefficacy in increments of 0.5 mg/kg/day to a maximum of 5 mg/kg/day and decreased at any time for toxicity. Treatment duration was 24 weeks. The mean cyclosporine dose at the last visit was 2.91 mg/kg/day (range: 0.72-5.17) for Neoral® and 3.27 mg/kg/day (range: 0.73-5.68) for cyclosporine. See Graph below.

[See graphic below]

INDICATIONS AND USAGE

Kidney, Liver, and Heart Transplantation: Neoral® is indicated for the prophylaxis of organ rejection in kidney, liver, and heart allogeneic transplants. Neoral® has been used in combination with azathioprine and corticosteroids.

Rheumatoid Arthritis: Neoral® is indicated for the treatment of patients with severe active, rheumatoid arthritis where the disease has not adequately responded to methotrexate. Neoral® can be used in combination with methotrexate in rheumatoid arthritis patients who do not respond adequately to methotrexate alone.

Psoriasis: Neoral® is indicated for the treatment of *adult, nonimmunocompromised* patients with severe (i.e., extensive and/or disabling), recalcitrant, plaque psoriasis who have failed to respond to at least one systemic therapy (eg., PUVA, retinoids, or methotrexate) or in patients for whom other systemic therapies are contraindicated, or cannot be tolerated.

While rebound rarely occurs, most patients will experience relapse with Neoral® as with other therapies upon cessation of treatment.

CONTRAINDICATIONS

General: Neoral® is contraindicated in patients with a hypersensitivity to cyclosporine or to any of the ingredients of the formulation.

Rheumatoid Arthritis: Rheumatoid arthritis patients with abnormal renal function, uncontrolled hypertension, or malignancies should not receive Neoral®.

Psoriasis: Psoriasis patients who are treated with Neoral® should not receive concomitant PUVA or UVB therapy, methotrexate or other immunosuppressive agents, coal tar

or radiation therapy. Psoriasis patients with abnormal renal function, uncontrolled hypertension, or malignancies should not receive Neoral®.

WARNINGS (See also Boxed WARNING)

All Patients: Cyclosporine, the active ingredient of Neoral®, can cause nephrotoxicity and hepatotoxicity. The risk increases with increasing doses of cyclosporine. Renal dysfunction including structural kidney damage is a potential consequence of Neoral® and therefore renal function must be monitored during therapy. **Care should be taken in using cyclosporine with nephrotoxic drugs. (See PRECAUTIONS)** Patients receiving Neoral® require frequent monitoring of serum creatinine. (See Special Monitoring under DOSAGE AND ADMINISTRATION) Elderly patients should be monitored with particular care, since decreases in renal function also occur with age. If patients are not properly monitored and doses are not properly adjusted, cyclosporine therapy can be associated with the occurrence of structural kidney damage and persistent renal dysfunction.

An increase in serum creatinine and BUN may occur during Neoral® therapy and reflect a reduction in the glomerular filtration rate. Impaired renal function at any time requires close monitoring, and frequent dosage adjustment may be indicated. The frequency and severity of serum creatinine elevations increase with dose and duration of cyclosporine therapy. These elevations are likely to become more pronounced without dose reduction or discontinuation.

Because Neoral® is not bioequivalent to Sandimmune®, conversion from Neoral® to Sandimmune® using a 1:1 ratio (mg/kg/day) may result in lower cyclosporine blood concentrations. Conversion from Neoral® to Sandimmune® should be made with increased monitoring to avoid the potential of underdosing.

Kidney, Liver, and Heart Transplant: Cyclosporine, the active ingredient of Neoral®, can cause nephrotoxicity and hepatotoxicity when used in high doses. It is not unusual for serum creatinine and BUN levels to be elevated during cyclosporine therapy. These elevations in renal transplant patients do not necessarily indicate rejection, and each patient must be fully evaluated before dosage adjustment is initiated.

Based on the historical Sandimmune® experience with oral solution, nephrotoxicity associated with cyclosporine had been noted in 25% of cases of renal transplantation, 38% of cases of cardiac transplantation, and 37% of cases of liver transplantation. Mild nephrotoxicity was generally noted 2-3 months after renal transplant and consisted of an arrest in the fall of the pre-operative elevations of BUN and creatinine at a range of 35-45 mg/dl and 2.0-2.5 mg/dl respectively. These elevations were often responsive to cyclosporine dosage reduction.

More overt nephrotoxicity was seen early after transplantation and was characterized by a rapidly rising BUN and creatinine. Since these events are similar to renal rejection episodes, care must be taken to differentiate between them. This form of nephrotoxicity is usually responsive to cyclosporine dosage reduction.

Although specific diagnostic criteria which reliably differentiate renal graft rejection from drug toxicity have not been found, a number of parameters have been significantly associated with one or the other. It should be noted however, that up to 20% of patients may have simultaneous nephrotoxicity and rejection.

[See table at top of next page]

A form of a cyclosporine-associated nephropathy is characterized by serial deterioration in renal function and morphologic changes in the kidneys. From 5%-15% of transplant recipients who have received cyclosporine will fail to show a reduction in rising serum creatinine despite a decrease or discontinuation of cyclosporine therapy. Renal biopsies from these patients will demonstrate one or several of the following alterations: tubular vacuolization, tubular microcalcifications, peritubular capillary congestion, arteriolopathy, and a striped form of interstitial fibrosis with tubular atrophy. Though none of these morphologic changes is entirely specific, a diagnosis of cyclosporine-associated structural nephrotoxicity requires evidence of these findings.

When considering the development of cyclosporine-associated nephropathy, it is noteworthy that several authors have reported an association between the appearance of interstitial fibrosis and higher cumulative doses or persistently high circulating trough levels of cyclosporine. This is particularly true during the first 6 post-transplant months when the dosage tends to be highest and when, in kidney recipients, the organ appears to be most vulnerable to the toxic effects of cyclosporine. Among other contributing factors to the development of interstitial fibrosis in these patients are prolonged perfusion time, warm ischemia time, as well as episodes of acute toxicity, and acute and chronic rejection. The reversibility of interstitial fibrosis and its correlation to renal function have not yet been determined. Reversibility of arteriolopathy has been reported after stopping cyclosporine or lowering the dosage.

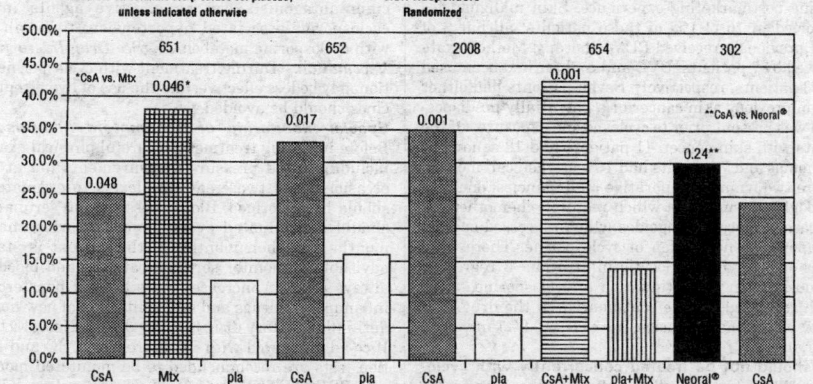

numbers on columns are p-values vs. placebo, unless indicated otherwise

ACR Responders Randomized

CsA vs. Mtx ; 651: 0.046; 0.048; 0.017; 652; 0.001; 2008; 0.001; 654; 0.24** ; **CsA vs. Neoral® ; 302

CsA | Mtx | pla | CsA | pla | CsA | pla | CsA+Mtx | pla+Mtx | Neoral® | CsA

Neoral—Cont.

Impaired renal function at any time requires close monitoring, and frequent dosage adjustment may be indicated.

In the event of severe and unremitting rejection, when rescue therapy with pulse steroids and monoclonal antibodies fail to reverse the rejection episode, it may be preferable to switch to alternative immunosuppressive therapy rather than increase the Neoral® dose to excessive levels.

Occasionally patients have developed a syndrome of thrombocytopenia and microangiopathic hemolytic anemia which may result in graft failure. The vasculopathy can occur in the absence of rejection and is accompanied by avid platelet consumption within the graft as demonstrated by Indium 111 labeled platelet studies. Neither the pathogenesis nor the management of this syndrome is clear. Though resolution has occurred after reduction or discontinuation of cyclosporine and 1) administration of streptokinase and heparin or 2) plasmapheresis, this appears to depend upon early detection with Indium 111 labeled platelet scans. *(See ADVERSE REACTIONS)*

Significant hyperkalemia (sometimes associated with hyperchloremic metabolic acidosis) and hyperuricemia have been seen occasionally in individual patients.

Hepatotoxicity associated with cyclosporine use had been noted in 4% of cases of renal transplantation, 7% of cases of cardiac transplantation, and 4% of cases of liver transplantation. This was usually noted during the first month of therapy when high doses of cyclosporine were used and consisted of elevations of hepatic enzymes and bilirubin. The chemistry elevations usually decreased with a reduction in dosage.

As in patients receiving other immunosuppressants, those patients receiving cyclosporine are at increased risk for development of lymphomas and other malignancies, particularly those of the skin. The increased risk appears related to the intensity and duration of immunosuppression rather than to the use of specific agents. Because of the danger of oversuppression of the immune system resulting in increased risk of infection or malignancy, a treatment regimen containing multiple immunosuppressants should be used with caution.

There have been reports of convulsions in adult and pediatric patients receiving cyclosporine, particularly in combination with high dose methylprednisolone.

Care should be taken in using cyclosporine with nephrotoxic drugs. *(See PRECAUTIONS)*

Rheumatoid Arthritis: Cyclosporine nephropathy was detected in renal biopsies of 6 out of 60 (10%) rheumatoid arthritis patients after the average treatment duration of 19 months. Only one patient, out of these 6 patients, was treated with a dose ≤4 mg/kg/day. Serum creatinine improved in all but one patient after discontinuation of cyclosporine. The "maximal creatinine increase" appears to be a factor in predicting cyclosporine nephropathy.

There is a potential, as with other immunosuppressive agents, for an increase in the occurrence of malignant lymphomas with cyclosporine. It is not clear whether the risk with cyclosporine is greater than that in Rheumatoid Arthritis patients or in Rheumatoid Arthritis patients on cytotoxic treatment for this indication. Five cases of lymphoma were detected: four in a survey of approximately 2,300 patients treated with cyclosporine for rheumatoid arthritis, and another case of lymphoma was reported in a clinical trial. Although other tumors (12 skin cancers, 24 solid tumors of diverse types, and 1 multiple myeloma) were also reported in this survey, epidemiologic analyses did not support a relationship to cyclosporine other than for malignant lymphomas.

Patients should be thoroughly evaluated before and during Neoral® treatment for the development of malignancies. Moreover, use of Neoral® therapy with other immunosuppressive agents may induce an excessive immunosuppression which is known to increase the risk of malignancy.

Psoriasis: *(See also Boxed WARNINGS for Psoriasis)* Since cyclosporine is a potent immunosuppressive agent with a number of potentially serious side effects, the risks and benefits of using Neoral® should be considered before treatment of patients with psoriasis. Cyclosporine, the active ingredient in Neoral®, can cause nephrotoxicity and hypertension *(see PRECAUTIONS)* and the risk increases with increasing dose and duration of therapy. Patients who may be at increased risk such as those with abnormal renal function, uncontrolled hypertension or malignancies, should not receive Neoral®.

Renal dysfunction is a potential consequence of Neoral® therefore renal function must be monitored during therapy. Patients receiving Neoral® require frequent monitoring of serum creatinine. *(See Special Monitoring under DOSAGE AND ADMINISTRATION)* Elderly patients should be monitored with particular care, since decreases in renal function also occur with age. If patients are not properly monitored and doses are not properly adjusted, cyclosporine therapy can cause structural kidney damage and persistent renal dysfunction.

Nephrotoxicity vs. Rejection

Parameter	Nephrotoxicity	Rejection
History	Donor >50 years old or hypotensive Prolonged kidney preservation Prolonged anastomosis time Concomitant nephrotoxic drugs	Anti-donor immune response Retransplant patient
Clinical	Often >6 weeks postop[b] Prolonged initial nonfunction (acute tubular necrosis)	Often < 4 weeks postop[b] Fever >37.5°C Weight gain >0.5 kg Graft swelling and tenderness Decrease in daily urine volume >500 mL (or 50%)
Laboratory	CyA serum trough level >200 ng/mL Gradual rise in Cr (< 0.15 mg/dl/day)[a] Cr plateau <25% above baseline BUN/Cr ≥ 20	CyA serum trough level < 150 ng/mL Rapid rise in Cr (>0.3 mg/dl/day)[a] Cr >25% above baseline BUN/Cr <20
Biopsy	Arteriolopathy (medial hypertrophy[a], hyalinosis, nodular deposits, intimal thickening, endothelial vacuolization, progressive scarring)	Endovasculitis[c] (proliferation[a], initmal arteritis[b], necrosis, sclerosis)
	Tubular atrophy, isometric vacuolization, isolated calcifications	Tubulitis with RBC[b] and WBC[b] casts, some irregular vacuolization
	Minimal edema	Interstitial edema[c] and hemorrhage[b]
	Mild focal infiltrates[c]	Diffuse moderate to severe mononuclear infiltrates[d]
	Diffuse interstitial fibrosis, often striped form	Glomerulitis (mononuclear cells)[c]
Aspiration Cytology	CyA deposits in tubular and endothelial cells Fine isometric vacuolization of tubular cells	Inflammatory infiltrate with mononuclear phagocytes, macrophages, lymphoblastoid cells, and activated T-cells These strongly express HLA-DR antigens
Urine Cytology	Tubular cells with vacuolization and granularization	Degenerative tubular cells, plasma cells, and lymphocyturia >20 % of sediment
Manometry	Intracapsular pressure < 40 mm Hg[b]	Intracapsular pressure >40 mm Hg[b]
Ultrasonography	Unchanged graft cross sectional area	Increase in graft cross sectional area AP diameter ≥ Transverse diameter
Magnetic Resonance Imagery	Normal appearance	Loss of distinct corticomedullary junction, swelling image intensity of parachyma approaching that of psoas, loss of hilar fat
Radionuclide Scan	Normal or generally decreased perfusion Decrease in tubular function (^{131} I-hippuran) >decrease in perfusion (^{99m} Tc DTPA)	Patchy arterial flow Decrease in perfusion >decrease in tubular function Increased uptake of Indium 111 labeled platelets or Tc-99m in colloid
Therapy	Responds to decreased cyclosporine	Responds to increased steroids or antilymphocyte globulin

$^a p < 0.05$, $^b p < 0.01$, $^c p < 0.001$, $^d p < 0.0001$

An increase in serum creatinine and BUN may occur during Neoral® therapy and reflects a reduction in the glomerular filtration rate.

Kidney biopsies from 86 psoriasis patients treated for a mean duration of 23 months with 1.2-7.6 mg/kg/day of cyclosporine showed evidence of cyclosporine nephropathy in 18/86 (21%) of the patients. The pathology consisted of renal tubular atrophy and interstitial fibrosis. On repeat biopsy of 13 of these patients maintained on various dosages of cyclosporine for a mean of 2 additional years, the number with cyclosporine induced nephropathy rose to 26/86 (30%). The majority of patients (19/26) were on a dose of ≥5.0 mg/kg/day (the highest recommended dose is 4 mg/kg/day). The patients were also on cyclosporine for greater than 15 months (18/26) and/or had a clinically significant increase in serum creatinine for greater than 1 month (21/26). Creatinine levels returned to normal range in 7 of 11 patients in whom cyclosporine therapy was discontinued.

There is an increased risk for the development of skin and lymphoproliferative malignancies in cyclosporine-treated psoriasis patients. The relative risk of malignancies is comparable to that observed in psoriasis patients treated with other immunosuppressive agents.

Tumors were reported in 32 (2.2%) of 1439 psoriasis patients treated with cyclosporine worldwide from clinical trials. Additional tumors have been reported in 7 patients in cyclosporine postmarketing experience. Skin malignancies were reported in 16 (1.1%) of these patients; all but 2 of them had previously received PUVA therapy. Methotrexate was received by 7 patients. UVB and coal tar had been used by 2 and 3 patients, respectively. Seven patients had either a history of previous skin cancer or a potentially predisposing lesion was present prior to cyclosporine exposure. Of the 16 patients with skin cancer, 11 patients had 18 squamous cell carcinomas and 7 patients had 10 basal cell carcinomas. There were two lymphoproliferative malignancies; one case of non-Hodgkin's lymphoma which required chemotherapy, and one case of mycosis fungoides which regressed spontaneously upon discontinuation of cyclosporine. There were four cases of benign lymphocytic infiltration: 3 regressed spontaneously upon discontinuation of cyclosporine, while the fourth regressed despite continuation of the drug. The remainder of the malignancies, 13 cases (0.9%), involved various organs.

Patients should not be treated concurrently with cyclosporine and PUVA or UVB, other radiation therapy, or other immunosuppressive agents, because of the possibility of excessive immunosuppression and the subsequent risk of malignancies. *(See CONTRAINDICATIONS)* Patients should also be warned to protect themselves appropriately when in the sun, and to avoid excessive sun exposure. Patients should be thoroughly evaluated before and during treatment for the presence of malignancies remembering that malignant lesions may be hidden by psoriatic plaques. Skin lesions not typical of psoriasis should be biopsied before starting treatment. Patients should be treated with Neoral® only after complete resolution of suspicious lesions, and only if there are no other treatment options. *(See Special Monitoring for Psoriasis Patients)*

PRECAUTIONS

General: *Hypertension:* Cyclosporine is the active ingredient of Neoral®. Hypertension is a common side effect of cyclosporine therapy which may persist. *(See ADVERSE REACTIONS and DOSAGE AND ADMINISTRATION for monitoring recommendations)* Mild or moderate hypertension is encountered more frequently than severe hypertension and the incidence decreases over time. In recipients of kidney, liver, and heart allografts treated with cyclosporine, antihypertensive therapy may be required. *(See Special Monitoring of Rheumatoid Arthritis and Psoriasis Patients)* However, since cyclosporine may cause hyperkalemia, potassium-sparing diuretics should not be used. While calcium antagonists can be effective agents in treating cyclosporine-associated hypertension, they can interfere with cyclosporine metabolism. *(See Drug Interactions)*

Vaccination: During treatment with cyclosporine, vaccination may be less effective; and the use of live attenuated vaccines should be avoided.

Special Monitoring of Rheumatoid Arthritis Patients: Before initiating treatment, a careful physical examination, including blood pressure measurements (on at least two occasions) and two creatinine levels to estimate baseline should be performed. Blood pressure and serum creatinine should be evaluated every 2 weeks during the initial 3 months and then monthly if the patient is stable. It is advisable to monitor serum creatinine and blood pressure always after an increase of the dose of nonsteroidal anti-inflammatory drugs and after initiation of new nonsteroidal anti-inflammatory drug therapy during Neoral® treatment. If co-administered with methotrexate, CBC and liver function tests are recommended to be monitored monthly. *(See also PRECAUTIONS, General, Hypertension)*

In patients who are receiving cyclosporine, the dose of Neoral® should be decreased by 25%-50% if hypertension occurs. If hypertension persists, the dose of Neoral® should be further reduced or blood pressure should be controlled with antihypertensive agents. In most cases, blood pressure has returned to baseline when cyclosporine was discontinued.

In placebo-controlled trials of rheumatoid arthritis patients, systolic hypertension (defined as an occurrence of two systolic blood pressure readings >140 mmHg) and diastolic hypertension (defined as two diastolic blood pressure readings >90 mmHg) occurred in 33% and 19% of patients treated with cyclosporine, respectively. The corresponding placebo rates were 22% and 8%.

Special Monitoring for Psoriasis Patients: Before initiating treatment, a careful dermatological and physical examination, including blood pressure measurements (on at least two occasions) should be performed. Since Neoral® is an immunosuppressive agent, patients should be evaluated for the presence of occult infection on their first physical examination and for the presence of tumors initially, and throughout treatment with Neoral®. Skin lesions not typical for psoriasis should be biopsied before starting Neoral®. Patients with malignant or premalignant changes of the skin should be treated with Neoral® only after appropriate treatment of such lesions and if no other treatment option exists.

Baseline laboratories should include serum creatinine (on two occasions), BUN, CBC, serum magnesium, potassium, uric acid, and lipids.

The risk of cyclosporine nephropathy is reduced when the starting dose is low (2.5 mg/kg/day), the maximum dose does not exceed 4.0 mg/kg/day, serum creatinine is monitored regularly while cyclosporine is administered, and the dose of Neoral® is decreased when the rise in creatinine is greater than or equal to 25% above the patients pretreatment level. The increase in creatinine is generally reversible upon timely decrease of the dose of Neoral® or its discontinuation.

Serum creatinine and BUN should be evaluated every 2 weeks during the initial 3 months of therapy and then monthly if the patient is stable. If the serum creatinine is greater than or equal to 25% above the patient's pretreatment level, serum creatinine should be repeated within two weeks. If the change in serum creatinine remains greater than or equal to 25% above baseline, Neoral® should be reduced by 25%-50%. If at **any time** the serum creatinine increases by greater than or equal to 50% above pretreatment level, Neoral® should be reduced by 25%-50%. Neoral® should be discontinued if reversibility (within 25% of baseline) of serum creatinine is not achievable after two dosage modifications. It is advisable to monitor serum creatinine after an increase of the dose of nonsteroidal anti-inflammatory drug and after initiation of new nonsteroidal anti-inflammatory therapy during Neoral® treatment.

Blood pressure should be evaluated every 2 weeks during the initial 3 months of therapy and then monthly if the patient is stable, or more frequently when dosage adjustments are made. Patients without a history of previous hypertension before initiation of treatment with Neoral®, should have the drug reduced by 25%-50% if found to have sustained hypertension. If the patient continues to be hypertensive despite multiple reductions of Neoral®, then Neoral® should be discontinued. For patients with treated hypertension, before the initiation of Neoral® therapy, their medication should be adjusted to control hypertension while on Neoral®. Neoral® should be discontinued if a change in hypertension management is not effective or tolerable.

CBC, uric acid, potassium, lipids, and magnesium should also be monitored every 2 weeks for the first 3 months of therapy, and then monthly if the patient is stable or more frequently when dosage adjustments are made. Neoral® dosage should be reduced by 25%-50% for any abnormality of clinical concern.

In controlled trials of cyclosporine in psoriasis patients, cyclosporine blood concentrations did not correlate well with either improvement or with side effects such as renal dysfunction.

Information for Patients: Patients should be advised that any change of cyclosporine formulation should be made cautiously and only under physician supervision because it may result in the need for a change in dosage.

Patients should be informed of the necessity of repeated laboratory tests while they are receiving cyclosporine. Patients should be advised of the potential risks during pregnancy and informed of the increased risk of neoplasia. Patients should also be informed of the risk of hypertension and renal dysfunction.

Patients should be advised that during treatment with cyclosporine, vaccination may be less effective and the use of live attenuated vaccines should be avoided.

Patients should be given careful dosage instructions. Neoral® Oral Solution (cyclosporine oral solution for microemulsion) should be diluted, preferably with orange or apple juice that is at room temperature. The combination of Neoral® Oral Solution (cyclosporine oral solution for microemulsion) with milk can be unpalatable.

Patients should be advised to take Neoral® on a consistent schedule with regard to time of day and relation to meals. Grapefruit and grapefruit juice affect metabolism, increasing blood concentration of cyclosporine, thus should be avoided.

Laboratory Tests: In all patients treated with cyclosporine, renal and liver functions should be assessed repeatedly by measurement of serum creatinine, BUN, serum bilirubin, and liver enzymes. Serum lipids, magnesium, and potassium should also be monitored. Cyclosporine blood concentrations should be routinely monitored in transplant patients *(see DOSAGE AND ADMINISTRATION, Blood Concentration Monitoring in Transplant Patients)*, and periodically monitored in rheumatoid arthritis patients.

Drug Interactions: All of the individual drugs cited below are well substantiated to interact with cyclosporine. In addition, concomitant non-steroidal anti-inflammatory drugs, particularly in the setting of dehydration, may potentiate renal dysfunction.

Drugs That May Potentiate Renal Dysfunction

Antibiotics	*Anti-inflammatory Drugs*
gentamicin	azapropazon
tobramycin	diclofenac
vancomycin	naproxen
trimethoprim with sulfamethoxazole	sulindac
	Gastrointestinal Agents
Antineoplastics	cimetidine
melphalan	ranitidine
Antifungals	*Immunosuppressives*
amphotericin B	tacrolimus
ketoconazole	

Drugs That Alter Cyclosporine Concentrations: Cyclosporine is extensively metabolized. Cyclosporine concentrations may be influenced by drugs that affect microsomal enzymes, particularly cytochrome P-450 III-A. Substances that inhibit this enzyme could decrease metabolism and increase cyclosporine concentrations. Substances that are inducers of cytochrome P-450 activity could increase metabolism and decrease cyclosporine concentrations. Monitoring of circulating cyclosporine concentrations and appropriate Neoral® dosage adjustment are essential when these drugs are used concomitantly. *(See Blood Concentration Monitoring)*

Drugs That Increase Cyclosporine Concentrations

Calcium Channel Blockers	*Antibiotics*
diltiazem	clarithromycin
nicardipine	erythromycin
varapamil	*Glucocorticoids*
Antifungals	methylprednisolone
fluconazole	*Other Drugs*
itraconazole	allopurinol
ketoconazole	bromocriptine
	danazol
	metoclopramide

The HIV protease inhibitors (e.g., indinavir, nelfinavir, ritonavir, and saquinavir) are known to inhibit cytochrome P-450 III-A and increase the concentrations of drugs metabolized by the cytochrome P-450 system. The interaction between HIV protease inhibitors and cyclosporine has not been studied. Care should be exercised when these drugs are administered concomitantly.

Grapefruit and grapefruit juice affect metabolism, increasing blood concentrations of cyclosporine, thus should be avoided.

Drugs That Decrease Cyclosporine Concentrations

Antibiotics	*Other Drugs*
nafcillin	octreotide
rifampin	ticlopidine
Anticonvulsants	
carbamazepine	
phenobarbital	
phenytoin	

Rifabutin is known to increase the metabolism of other drugs metabolized by the cytochrome P-450 system. The interaction between rifabutin and cyclosporine has not been studied. Care should be exercised when these two drugs are administered concomitantly.

Nonsteroidal Anti-inflammatory Drug (NSAID) Interactions: Clinical status and serum creatinine should be closely monitored when cyclosporine is used with nonsteroidal anti-inflammatory agents in rheumatoid arthritis patients. *(See WARNINGS)*

Pharmacodynamic interactions have been reported to occur between cyclosporine and both naproxen and sulindac, in that concomitant use is associated with additive decreases in renal function, as determined by ^{99m}Tc-diethylenetriaminepentaacetic acid (DTPA) and (*p*-aminohippuric acid) PAH clearances. Although concomitant administration of diclofenac does not affect blood levels of cyclosporine, it has been associated with approximate doubling of diclofenac blood levels and occasional reports of reversible decreases in renal function. Consequently, the dose of diclofenac should be in the lower end of the therapeutic range.

Methotrexate Interaction: Preliminary data indicate that when methotrexate and cyclosporine were co-administered to rheumatoid arthritis patients (N=20), methotrexate concentrations (AUCs) were increased approximately 30% and the concentrations (AUCs) of its metabolite, 7-hydroxy methotrexate, were decreased by approximately 80%. The clinical significance of this interaction is not known. Cyclosporine concentrations do not appear to have been altered (N=6).

Other Drug Interactions: Reduced clearance of prednisolone, digoxin, and lovastatin has been observed when these drugs are administered with cyclosporine. In addition, a decrease in the apparent volume of distribution of digoxin has been reported after cyclosporine administration. Severe digitalis toxicity has been seen within days of starting cyclosporine in several patients taking digoxin. Cyclosporine should not be used with potassium-sparing diuretics because hyperkalemia can occur.

During treatment with cyclosporine, vaccination may be less effective. The use of live vaccines should be avoided. Myositis has occurred with concomitant lovastatin, frequent gingival hyperplasia with nifedipine, and convulsions with high dose methylprednisolone.

Psoriasis patients receiving other immunosuppressive agents or radiation therapy (including PUVA and UVB) should not receive concurrent cyclosporine because of the possibility of excessive immunosuppression.

Carcinogenesis, Mutagenesis, and Impairment of Fertility: Carcinogenicity studies were carried out in male and female rats and mice. In the 78-week mouse study, evidence of a statistically significant trend was found for lymphocytic lymphomas in females, and the incidence of hepatocellular carcinomas in mid-dose males significantly exceeded the control value. In the 24-month rat study, pancreatic islet cell adenomas significantly exceeded the control rate in the low dose level. Doses used in the mouse and rat studies were 0.01 to 0.16 times the clinical maintenance dose (6 mg/kg). The hepatocellular carcinomas and pancreatic islet cell adenomas were not dose related. Published reports indicate that co-treatment of hairless mice with UV irradiation and cyclosporine or other immunosuppressive agents shorten the time to skin tumor formation compared to UV irradiation alone.

Cyclosporine was not mutagenic in appropriate test systems. Cyclosporine has not been found to be mutagenic/genotoxic in the Ames Test, the V79-HGPRT Test, the micronucleus test in mice and Chinese hamsters, the chromosome-aberration tests in Chinese hamster bone-marrow, the mouse dominant lethal assay, and the DNA-repair test in sperm from treated mice. A recent study analyzing sister chromatid exchange (SCE) induction by cyclosporine using human lymphocytes *in vitro* gave indication of a positive effect (i.e., induction of SCE), at high concentrations in this system.

No impairment in fertility was demonstrated in studies in male and female rats.

Widely distributed papillomatosis of the skin was observed after chronic treatment of dogs with cyclosporine at 9 times the human initial psoriasis treatment dose of 2.5 mg/kg, where doses are expressed on a body surface area basis. This papillomatosis showed a spontaneous regression upon discontinuation of cyclosporine.

An increased incidence of malignancy is a recognized complication of immunosuppression in recipients of organ transplants and patients with rheumatoid arthritis and psoriasis. The most common forms of neoplasms are non-Hodgkin's lymphoma and carcinomas of the skin. The risk of malignancies in cyclosporine recipients is higher than in the normal, healthy population but similar to that in patients receiving other immunosuppressive therapies. Reduction or discontinuance of immunosuppression may cause the lesions to regress.

In psoriasis patients on cyclosporine, development of malignancies, especially those of the skin has been reported. *(See WARNINGS)* Skin lesions not typical for psoriasis should be biopsied before starting cyclosporine treatment. Patients with malignant or premalignant changes of the skin should be treated with cyclosporine only after appropriate treatment of such lesions and if no other treatment option exists.

Pregnancy: *Pregnancy Category C.* Cyclosporine was not teratogenic in appropriate test systems. Only at dose levels toxic to dams, were adverse effects seen in reproduction studies in rats. Cyclosporine has been shown to be embryo- and fetotoxic in rats and rabbits following oral administration at maternally toxic doses. Fetal toxicity was noted in rats at 0.8 and rabbits at 5.4 times the transplant doses in humans of 6.0 mg/kg, where dose corrections are based on body surface area. Cyclosporine was embryo- and fetotoxic as indicated by increased pre- and postnatal mortality and reduced fetal weight together with related skeletal retardation.

There are no adequate and well-controlled studies in pregnant women. Neoral® should be used during pregnancy only if the potential benefit justifies the potential risk to the fetus.

Continued on next page

Neoral—Cont.

The following data represent the reported outcomes of 116 pregnancies in women receiving cyclosporine during pregnancy, 90% of whom were transplant patients, and most of whom received cyclosporine throughout the entire gestational period. The only consistent patterns of abnormality were premature birth (gestational period of 28 to 36 weeks) and low birth weight for gestational age. Sixteen fetal losses occurred. Most of the pregnancies (85 of 100) were complicated by disorders; including, pre-eclampsia, eclampsia, premature labor, abruptio placentae, oligohydramnios, Rh incompatibility, and fetoplacental dysfunction. Pre-term delivery occurred in 47%. Seven malformations were reported in 5 viable infants and in 2 cases of fetal loss. Twenty-eight percent of the infants were small for gestational age. Neonatal complications occurred in 27%. Therefore, the risks and benefits of using Neoral® during pregnancy should be carefully weighed.

Because of the possible disruption of maternal-fetal interaction, the risk/benefit ratio of using Neoral® in psoriasis patients during pregnancy should carefully be weighed with serious consideration for discontinuation of Neoral®.

Nursing Mothers: Since cyclosporine is excreted in human milk, breast-feeding should be avoided.

Pediatric Use: Although no adequate and well-controlled studies have been completed in children, transplant recipients as young as one year of age have received Neoral® with no unusual adverse effects. The safety and efficacy of Neoral® treatment in children with juvenile rheumatoid arthritis or psoriasis below the age of 18 have not been established.

Geriatric Use: In rheumatoid arthritis clinical trials with cyclosporine, 17.5% of patients were age 65 or older. These patients were more likely to develop systolic hypertension on therapy, and more likely to show serum creatinine rises ≥50% above the baseline after 3-4 months of therapy.

ADVERSE REACTIONS

Kidney, Liver, and Heart Transplantation: The principal adverse reactions of cyclosporine therapy are renal dysfunction, tremor, hirsutism, hypertension, and gum hyperplasia. Hypertension, which is usually mild to moderate, may occur in approximately 50% of patients following renal transplantation and in most cardiac transplant patients.

Glomerular capillary thrombosis has been found in patients treated with cyclosporine and may progress to graft failure. The pathologic changes resembled those seen in the hemolytic-uremic syndrome and included thrombosis of the renal microvasculature, with platelet-fibrin thrombi occluding glomerular capillaries and afferent arterioles, microan-giopathic hemolytic anemia, thrombocytopenia, and decreased renal function. Similar findings have been observed when other immunosuppressives have been employed post-transplantation.

Hypomagnesemia has been reported in some, but not all, patients exhibiting convulsions while on cyclosporine therapy. Although magnesium-depletion studies in normal subjects suggest that hypomagnesemia is associated with neurologic disorders, multiple factors, including hypertension, high dose methylprednisolone, hypocholesterolemia, and nephrotoxicity associated with high plasma concentrations of cyclosporine appear to be related to the neurological manifestations of cyclosporine toxicity.

In controlled studies, the nature, severity, and incidence of the adverse events that were observed in 493 transplanted patients treated with Neoral® were comparable with those observed in 208 transplanted patients who received Sandimmune® in these same studies when the dosage of the two drugs was adjusted to achieve the same cyclosporine blood trough concentrations.

Based on the historical experience with Sandimmune®, the following reactions occurred in 3% or greater of 892 patients involved in clinical trials of kidney, heart, and liver transplants.

[See first table below]

Among 705 kidney transplant patients treated with cyclosporine oral solution (Sandimmune®) in clinical trials, the reason for treatment discontinuation was renal toxicity in 5.4%, infection in 0.9%, lack of efficacy in 1.4%, acute tubular necrosis in 1.0%, lymphoproliferative disorders in 0.3%, hypertension in 0.3%, and other reasons in 0.7% of the patients.

The following reactions occurred in 2% or less of Sandimmune®-treated patients: allergic reactions, anemia, anorexia, confusion, conjunctivitis, edema, fever, brittle fingernails, gastritis, hearing loss, hiccups, hyperglycemia, muscle pain, peptic ulcer, thrombocytopenia, tinnitus.

The following reactions occurred rarely: anxiety, chest pain, constipation, depression, hair breaking, hematuria, joint pain, lethargy, mouth sores, myocardial infarction, night sweats, pancreatitis, pruritus, swallowing difficulty, tingling, upper GI bleeding, visual disturbance, weakness, weight loss.

[See second table below]

Rheumatoid Arthritis: The principal adverse reactions associated with the use of cyclosporine in rheumatoid arthritis are renal dysfunction (see WARNINGS), hypertension (see PRECAUTIONS), headache, gastrointestinal disturbances, and hirsutism/hypertrichosis.

In rheumatoid arthritis patients treated in clinical trials within the recommended dose range, cyclosporine therapy was discontinued in 5.3% of the patients because of hypertension and in 7% of the patients because of increased creatinine. These changes are usually reversible with timely dose decrease or drug discontinuation. The frequency and severity of serum creatinine elevations increase with dose and duration of cyclosporine therapy. These elevations are likely to become more pronounced without dose reduction or discontinuation.

The following adverse events occurred in controlled clinical trials:

[See table at top of next page]

In addition, the following adverse events have been reported in 1% to <3% of the rheumatoid arthritis patients in the cyclosporine treatment group in controlled clinical trials.

Autonomic Nervous System: dry mouth, increased sweating;

Body as a Whole: allergy, asthenia, hot flushes, malaise, overdose, procedure NOS*, tumor NOS*, weight decrease, weight increase;

Cardiovascular: abnormal heart sounds, cardiac failure, myocardial infarction, peripheral ischemia;

Central and Peripheral Nervous System: hypoesthesia, neuropathy, vertigo;

Endocrine: goiter;

Gastrointestinal: constipation, dysphagia, enanthema, eructation, esophagitis, gastric ulcer, gastroenteritis, gingival bleeding, glossitis, peptic ulcer, salivary gland enlargement, tongue disorder, tooth disorder;

Infection: abscess, bacterial infection, cellulitis, folliculitis, fungal infection, herpes simplex, herpes zoster, renal abscess, moniliasis, tonsillitis, viral infection;

Hematologic: anemia, epistaxis, leukopenia, lymphadenopathy;

Liver and Biliary System: bilirubinemia;

Metabolic and Nutritional: diabetes mellitus, hyperkalemia, hyperuricemia, hypoglycemia;

Musculoskeletal System: arthralgia, bone fracture, bursitis, joint dislocation, myalgia, stiffness, synovial cyst, tendon disorder;

Neoplasms: breast fibroadenosis, carcinoma;

Psychiatric: anxiety, confusion, decreased libido, emotional lability, impaired concentration, increased libido, nervousness, paroniria, somnolence;

Reproductive (Female): breast pain, uterine hemorrhage;

Respiratory System: abnormal chest sounds, bronchospasm;

Skin and Appendages: abnormal pigmentation, angioedema, dermatitis, dry skin, eczema, nail disorder, pruritus, skin disorder, urticaria;

Special Senses: abnormal vision, cataract, conjunctivitis, deafness, eye pain, taste perversion, tinnitus, vestibular disorder;

Urinary System: abnormal urine, hematuria, increased BUN, micturition urgency, nocturia, polyuria, pyelonephritis, urinary incontinence.

*NOS = Not Otherwise Specified.

Psoriasis: The principal adverse reactions associated with the use of cyclosporine in patients with psoriasis are renal dysfunction, headache, hypertension, hypertriglyceridemia, hirsutism/hypertrichosis, paresthesia or hyperesthesia, influenza-like symptoms, nausea/vomiting, diarrhea, abdominal discomfort, lethargy, and musculoskeletal or joint pain.

In psoriasis patients treated in US controlled clinical studies within the recommended dose range, cyclosporine therapy was discontinued in 1.0% of the patients because of hypertension and in 5.4% of the patients because of increased creatinine. In the majority of cases, these changes were reversible after dose reduction or discontinuation of cyclosporine.

There has been one reported death associated with the use of cyclosporine in psoriasis. A 27 year old male developed renal deterioration and was continued on cyclosporine. He had progressive renal failure leading to death.

Frequency and severity of serum creatinine increases with dose and duration of cyclosporine therapy. These elevations are likely to become more pronounced and may result in irreversible renal damage without dose reduction or discontinuation.

[See table at bottom of page 2070]

The following events occurred in 1% to less than 3% of psoriasis patients treated with cyclosporine:

Body as a Whole: fever, flushes, hot flushes; **Cardiovascular:** chest pain; **Central and Peripheral Nervous System:** appetite increased, insomnia, dizziness, nervousness, vertigo; **Gastrointestinal:** abdominal distention, constipation, gingival bleeding; **Liver and Biliary System:** hyperbilirubinemia; **Neoplasms:** skin malignancies [squamous cell (0.9%) and basal cell (0.4%) carcinomas]; **Reticuloendothelial:** platelet, bleeding, and clotting disorders, red blood cell disorder; **Respiratory:** infection, viral and other infection; **Skin and Appendages:** acne, folliculitis, keratosis, pruritus, rash, dry skin; **Urinary System:** micturition frequency; **Vision:** abnormal vision.

| Body System | Adverse Reactions | Randomized Kidney Patients | | Cyclosporine Patients (Sandimmune®) | | |
		Sandimmune® (N=227) %	Azathioprine (N=228) %	Kidney (N=705) %	Heart (N=112) %	Liver (N=75) %
Genitourinary	Renal Dysfunction	32	6	25	38	37
Cardiovascular	Hypertension	26	18	13	53	27
	Cramps	4	<1	2	<1	0
Skin	Hirsuitism	21	<1	21	28	45
	Acne	6	8	2	2	1
Central Nervous System	Tremor	12	0	21	31	55
	Convulsions	3	1	1	4	5
	Headache	2	<1	2	15	4
Gastrointestinal	Gum Hyperplasia	4	0	9	5	16
	Diarrhea	3	<1	3	4	8
	Nausea/Vomiting	2	<1	4	10	4
	Hepatotoxicity	<1	<1	4	7	4
	Abdominal Discomfort	<1	0	<1	7	0
Autonomic Nervous System	Paresthesia	3	0	1	2	1
	Flushing	<1	0	4	0	4
Hematopoietic	Leukopenia	2	19	1	6	0
	Lymphoma	<1	0	1	6	1
Respiratory	Sinusitis	<1	0	4	3	7
Miscellaneous	Gynecomastia	<1	0	<1	4	3

Infectious Complications in Historical Randomized Studies in Renal Transplant Patients Using Sandimmune®

Complication	Cyclosporine Treatment (N=227) % of Complications	Azathioprine with Steroids* (N=228) % of Complications
Septicemia	5.3	4.8
Abscesses	4.4	5.3
Systemic Fungal Infection	2.2	3.9
Local Fungal Infection	7.5	9.6
Cytomegalovirus	4.8	12.3
Other Viral Infections	15.9	18.4
Urinary Tract Infections	21.1	20.2
Wound and Skin Infections	7.0	10.1
Pneumonia	6.2	9.2

* Some patients also received ALG.

Neoral®/Sandimmune® Rheumatoid Arthritis
Percentage of Patients with Adverse Events ≥3% in any Cyclosporine Treated Group

Body System	Preferred term	Studies 651+652+2008 Sandimmune®† (N=269)	Study 302 Sandimmune® (N=155)	Study 654 Methotrexate & Sandimmune® (N=74)	Study 654 Methotrexate & Placebo (N=73)	Study 302 Neoral® (N=143)	Studies 651+652+2008 Placebo (N=201)
Autonomic Nervous System Disorders							
	Flushing	2%	2%	3%	0%	5%	2%
Body As a Whole–General Disorders							
	Accidental Trauma	0%	1%	10%	4%	4%	0%
	Edema NOS*	5%	14%	12%	4%	10%	<1%
	Fatigue	6%	3%	8%	12%	3%	7%
	Fever	2%	3%	0%	0%	2%	4%
	Influenza-like symptoms	<1%	6%	1%	0%	3%	2%
	Pain	6%	9%	10%	15%	13%	4%
	Rigors	1%	1%	4%	0%	3%	1%
Cardiovascular Disorders							
	Arrhythmia	2%	5%	5%	6%	2%	1%
	Chest Pain	4%	5%	1%	1%	6%	1%
	Hypertension	8%	26%	16%	12%	25%	2%
Central and Peripheral Nervous System Disorders							
	Dizziness	8%	6%	7%	3%	8%	3%
	Headache	17%	23%	22%	11%	25%	9%
	Migraine	2%	3%	0%	0%	3%	1%
	Paresthesia	8%	7%	8%	4%	11%	1%
	Tremor	8%	7%	7%	3%	13%	4%
Gastrointestinal System Disorders							
	Abdominal Pain	15%	15%	15%	7%	15%	10%
	Anorexia	3%	3%	1%	0%	3%	3%
	Diarrhea	12%	12%	18%	15%	13%	8%
	Dyspepsia	12%	12%	10%	8%	8%	4%
	Flatulence	5%	5%	5%	4%	4%	1%
	Gastrointestinal Disorder NOS*	0%	2%	1%	4%	4%	0%
	Gingivitis	4%	3%	0%	0%	3%	1%
	Gum Hyperplasia	2%	4%	1%	3%	4%	1%
	Nausea	23%	14%	24%	15%	18%	14%
	Rectal Hemorrhage	0%	3%	0%	0%	1%	1%
	Stomatitis	7%	5%	16%	12%	6%	8%
	Vomiting	9%	8%	14%	7%	6%	5%
Hearing and Vestibular Disorders							
	Ear Disorder NOS*	0%	5%	0%	0%	1%	0%
Metabolic and Nutritional Disorders							
	Hypomagnesemia	0%	4%	0%	0%	6%	0%
Musculoskeletal System Disorders							
	Arthropathy	0%	5%	0%	1%	4%	0%
	Leg Cramps/Involuntary Muscle Contractions	2%	11%	11%	3%	12%	1%
Psychiatric Disorders							
	Depression	3%	6%	1%	1%	1%	2%
	Insomnia	4%	1%	1%	0%	3%	2%
Renal							
	Creatinine elevations ≥30%	43%	39%	55%	19%	48%	13%
	Creatinine elevations ≥50%	24%	18%	26%	8%	18%	3%
Reproduction Disorders, Female							
	Leukorrhea	1%	0%	4%	0%	1%	0%
	Menstrual Disorder	3%	2%	1%	0%	1%	1%
Respiratory System Disorders							
	Bronchitis	1%	3%	1%	0%	1%	3%
	Coughing	5%	3%	5%	7%	4%	4%
	Dyspnea	5%	1%	3%	3%	1%	2%
	Infection NOS*	9%	5%	0%	7%	3%	10%
	Pharyngitis	3%	5%	5%	6%	4%	4%
	Pneumonia	1%	0%	4%	0%	0%	1%
	Rhinitis	0%	3%	11%	10%	1%	0%
	Sinusitis	4%	4%	8%	4%	3%	3%
	Upper Respiratory Tract	0%	14%	23%	15%	13%	0%
Skin and Appendages Disorders							
	Alopecia	3%	0%	1%	1%	4%	4%
	Bullous Eruption	1%	0%	4%	1%	1%	1%
	Hypertrichosis	19%	17%	12%	0%	15%	3%
	Rash	7%	12%	10%	7%	8%	10%
	Skin Ulceration	1%	1%	3%	4%	0%	2%
Urinary System Disorders							
	Dysuria	0%	0%	11%	3%	1%	2%
	Micturition Frequency	2%	4%	3%	1%	2%	2%
	NPN, Increased	0%	19%	12%	0%	18%	0%
	Urinary Tract Infection	0%	3%	5%	4%	3%	0%
Vascular (Extracardiac) Disorders							
	Purpura	3%	4%	1%	1%	2%	0%

†Includes patients in 2.5 mg/kg/day dose group only. *NOS = Not Otherwise Specified.

Mild hypomagnesemia and hyperkalemia may occur but are asymptomatic. Increases in uric acid may occur and attacks of gout have been rarely reported.

A minor and dose related hyperbilirubinemia has been observed in the absence of hepatocellular damage. Cyclosporine therapy may be associated with a modest increase of serum triglycerides or cholesterol. Elevations of triglycerides (>750 mg/dL) occur in about 15% of psoriasis patients; elevations of cholesterol (>300 mg/dL) are observed in less than 3% of psoriasis patients. Generally these laboratory abnormalities are reversible upon dose reduction or discontinuation of cyclosporine.

OVERDOSAGE

There is a minimal experience with cyclosporine overdosage. Forced emesis can be of value up to 2 hours after administration of Neoral®. Transient hepatotoxicity and nephrotoxicity may occur which should resolve following drug withdrawal. General supportive measures and symptomatic treatment should be followed in all cases of overdosage. Cyclosporine is not dialyzable to any great extent, nor is it cleared well by charcoal hemoperfusion. The oral dosage at which half of experimental animals are estimated to die is 31 times, 39 times, and >54 times the human maintenance dose for transplant patients (6mg/kg; corrections based on body surface area) in mice, rats, and rabbits.

DOSAGE AND ADMINISTRATION

Neoral® Soft Gelatin Capsules (cyclosporine capsules for microemulsion) and Neoral® Oral Solution (cyclosporine oral solution for microemulsion)
Neoral® has increased bioavailability in comparison to Sandimmune®. Neoral® and Sandimmune® are not bioequivalent and cannot be used interchangeably without physician supervision.
The daily dose of Neoral® should always be given in two divided doses (BID). It is recommended that Neoral® be administered on a consistent schedule with regard to time of day and relation to meals. Grapefruit and grapefruit juice affect metabolism, increasing blood concentration of cyclosporine, thus should be avoided.
Newly Transplanted Patients: The initial oral dose of Neoral® can be given 4–12 hours prior to transplantation or be given postoperatively. The initial dose of Neoral® varies depending on the transplanted organ and the other immunosuppressive agents included in the immunosuppressive protocol. In newly transplanted patients, the initial oral dose of Neoral® is the same as the initial oral dose of Sandimmune®. Suggested initial doses are available from the results of a 1994 survey of the use of Sandimmune® in US transplant centers. The mean ± SD initial doses were 9±3 mg/kg/day for renal transplant patients (75 centers), 8±4 mg/kg/day for liver transplant patients (30 centers), and 7±3 mg/kg/day for heart transplant patients (24 centers). Total daily doses were divided into two equal daily doses. The Neoral® dose is subsequently adjusted to achieve a pre-defined cyclosporine blood concentration. (*See Blood Concentration Monitoring in Transplant Patients, below*) If cyclosporine trough blood concentrations are used, the target range is the same for Neoral® as for Sandimmune®. Using the same trough concentration target range for Neoral® as for Sandimmune® results in greater cyclosporine exposure when Neoral® is administered. (*See Pharmacokinetics, Absorption*) Dosing should be titrated based on clinical assessments of rejection and tolerability. Lower Neoral® doses may be sufficient as maintenance therapy.
Adjunct therapy with adrenal corticosteroids is recommended initially. Different tapering dosage schedules of prednisone appear to achieve similar results. A representative dosage schedule based on the patient's weight started with 2.0 mg/kg/day for the first 4 days tapered to 1.0 mg/kg/day by 1 week, 0.6 mg/kg/day by 2 weeks, 0.3 mg/kg/day by 1 month, and 0.15 mg/kg/day by 2 months and thereafter as a maintenance dose. Steroid doses may be further tapered on an individualized basis depending on status of patient and function of graft. Adjustments in dosage of prednisone must be made according to the clinical situation.
Conversion from Sandimmune® to Neoral® in Transplant Patients: In transplanted patients who are considered for conversion to Neoral® from Sandimmune®, Neoral® should be started with the same daily dose as was previously used with Sandimmune® (1:1 dose conversion). The Neoral® dose should subsequently be adjusted to attain the pre-conversion cyclosporine blood trough concentration. Using the same trough concentration target range for Neoral® as for Sandimmune® results in greater cyclosporine exposure when Neoral® is administered. (*See Pharmacokinetics, Absorption*) Patients with suspected poor absorption of Sandimmune® require different dosing strategies. (*See Transplant Patients with Poor Absorption of Sandimmune®, below*) In some patients, the increase in blood trough concentration is more pronounced and may be of clinical significance.
Until the blood trough concentration attains the pre-conversion value, it is strongly recommended that the cyclosporine blood trough concentration be monitored every 4 to 7 days after conversion to Neoral®. In addition, clinical safety parameters such as serum creatinine and blood pressure should be monitored every two weeks during the first two months after conversion. If the blood trough concentrations are outside the desired range and/or if the clinical safety parameters worsen, the dosage of Neoral® must be adjusted accordingly.
Transplant Patients with Poor Absorption of Sandimmune®: Patients with lower than expected cyclosporine blood trough concentrations in relation to the oral dose of Sandimmune® may have poor or inconsistent absorption

Continued on next page

Neoral—Cont.

of cyclosporine from Sandimmune®. After conversion to Neoral®, patients tend to have higher cyclosporine concentrations. **Due to the increase in bioavailability of cyclosporine following conversion to Neoral®, the cyclosporine blood trough concentration may exceed the target range. Particular caution should be exercised when converting patients to Neoral® at doses greater than 10 mg/kg/day.** The dose of Neoral® should be titrated individually based on cyclosporine trough concentrations, tolerability, and clinical response. In this population the cyclosporine blood trough concentration should be measured more frequently, at least twice a week (daily, if initial dose exceeds 10 mg/kg/day) until the concentration stabilizes within the desired range.

Rheumatoid Arthritis: The initial dose of Neoral® is 2.5 mg/kg/day, taken twice daily as a divided (BID) oral dose. Salicylates, nonsteroidal anti-inflammatory agents, and oral corticosteroids may be continued. *(See WARNINGS and PRECAUTIONS: Drug Interactions)* Onset of action generally occurs between 4 and 8 weeks. If insufficient clinical benefit is seen and tolerability is good (including serum creatinine less than 30% above baseline), the dose may be increased by 0.5-0.75 mg/kg/day after 8 weeks and again after 12 weeks to a maximum of 4 mg/kg/day. If no benefit is seen by 16 weeks of therapy, Neoral® therapy should be discontinued.

Dose decreases by 25%-50% should be made at any time to control adverse events, e.g., hypertension elevations in serum creatinine (30% above patient's pretreatment level) or clinically significant laboratory abnormalities. *(See WARNINGS and PRECAUTIONS)*

If dose reduction is not effective in controlling abnormalities or if the adverse event or abnormality is severe, Neoral® should be discontinued. The same initial dose and dosage range should be used if Neoral® is combined with the recommended dose of methotrexate. Most patients can be treated with Neoral® doses of 3 mg/kg/day or below when combined with methotrexate doses of up to 15 mg/week. *(See CLINICAL PHARMACOLOGY, Clinical Trials)*

There is limited long-term treatment data. Recurrence of rheumatoid arthritis disease activity is generally apparent within 4 weeks after stopping cyclosporine.

Psoriasis: The initial dose of Neoral® should be 2.5 mg/kg/day. Neoral® should be taken twice daily, as a divided (1.25 mg/kg BID) oral dose. Patients should be kept at that dose for at least 4 weeks, barring adverse events. If significant clinical improvement has not occurred in patients by that time, the patient's dosage should be increased at 2 week intervals. Based on patient response, dose increases of approximately 0.5 mg/kg/day should be made to a maximum of 4.0 mg/kg/day.

Dose decreases by 25%-50% should be made at any time to control adverse events, e.g., hypertension, elevations in serum creatinine (≥25% above the patient's pretreatment level), or clinically significant laboratory abnormalities. If dose reduction is not effective in controlling abnormalities, or if the adverse event or abnormality is severe, Neoral® should be discontinued. *(See Special Monitoring of Psoriasis Patients)*

Patients generally show some improvement in the clinical manifestations of psoriasis in 2 weeks. Satisfactory control and stabilization of the disease may take 12-16 weeks to achieve. Results of a dose-titration clinical trial with Neoral® indicate that an improvement of psoriasis by 75% or more (based on PASI) was achieved in 51% of the patients after 8 weeks and in 79% of the patients after 12 weeks. Treatment should be discontinued if satisfactory response cannot be achieved after 6 weeks at 4 mg/kg/day or the patient's maximum tolerated dose. Once a patient is adequately controlled and appears stable the dose of Neoral® should be lowered, and the patient treated with the lowest dose that maintains an adequate response (this should not necessarily be total clearing of the patient). In clinical trials, cyclosporine doses at the lower end of the recommended dosage range were effective in maintaining a satisfactory response in 60% of the patients. Doses below 2.5 mg/kg/day may also be equally effective.

Upon stopping treatment with cyclosporine, relapse will occur in approximately 6 weeks (50% of the patients) to 16 weeks (75% of the patients). In the majority of patients rebound does not occur after cessation of treatment with cyclosporine. Thirteen cases of transformation of chronic plaque psoriasis to more severe forms of psoriasis have been reported. There were 9 cases of pustular and 4 cases of erythrodermic psoriasis. Long term experience with Neoral® in psoriasis patients is limited and continuous treatment for extended periods greater than one year is not recommended. Alternation with other forms of treatment should be considered in the long term management of patients with this life long disease.

Neoral® Oral Solution (cyclosporine oral solution for microemulsion)–Recommendations for Administration: To make Neoral® Oral Solution (cyclosporine oral solution for microemulsion) more palatable, it should be diluted preferably with orange or apple juice that is at room temperature. Grapefruit juice affects metabolism of cyclosporine and should be avoided. The combination of Neoral® solution with milk can be unpalatable.

Take the prescribed amount of Neoral® Oral Solution (cyclosporine oral solution for microemulsion) from the container using the dosing syringe supplied, after removal of the protective cover, and transfer the solution to a glass of orange or apple juice. Stir well and drink at once. Do not allow diluted oral solution to stand before drinking. Use a glass container (not plastic). Rinse the glass with more diluent to ensure that the total dose is consumed. After use, dry the outside of the dosing syringe with a clean towel and replace the protective cover. Do not rinse the dosing syringe with water or other cleaning agents. If the syringe requires cleaning, it must be completely dry before resuming use.

Blood Concentration Monitoring in Transplant Patients: Transplant centers have found blood concentration monitoring of cyclosporine to be an essential component of patient management. Of importance to blood concentration analysis are the type of assay used, the transplanted organ, and other immunosuppressant agents being administered. While no fixed relationship has been established, blood concentration monitoring may assist in the clinical evaluation of rejection and toxicity, dose adjustments, and the assessment of compliance.

Various assays have been used to measure blood concentrations of cyclosporine. Older studies using a nonspecific assay often cited concentrations that were roughly twice those of the specific assays. Therefore, comparison between concentrations in the published literature and an individual patient concentration using current assays must be made with detailed knowledge of the assay methods employed. Current assay results are also not interchangeable and their use should be guided by their approved labeling. A discussion of the different assay methods is contained in *Annals of Clinical Biochemistry* 1994;31:420-446. While several assays and assay matrices are available, there is a consensus that parent-compound-specific assays correlate best with clinical events. Of these, HPLC is the standard reference, but the monoclonal antibody RIAs and the monoclonal antibody FPIA offer sensitivity, reproducibility, and convenience. Most clinicians base their monitoring on trough cyclosporine concentrations. *Applied Pharmacokinetics, Principles of Therapeutic Drug Monitoring*(1992) contains a broad discussion of cyclosporine pharmacokinetics and drug monitoring techniques. Blood concentration monitoring is not a replacement for renal function monitoring or tissue biopsies.

HOW SUPPLIED

Neoral® Soft Gelatin Capsules (cyclosporine capsules for microemulsion)
25 mg
Oval, blue-gray imprinted in red, "NEORAL" over "25 mg."
Packages of 30 unit-dose blisters (NDC 0078-0246-15).
100 mg
Oblong, blue-gray imprinted in red, "NEORAL" over "100 mg."
Packages of 30 unit-dose blisters (NDC 0078-0248-15).
Store and Dispense: In the original unit-dose container at controlled room temperature 68°-77°F (20°-25°C).
Neoral® Oral Solution (cyclosporine oral solution for microemulsion): A clear, yellow liquid supplied in 50 mL bottles containing 100 mg/mL (NDC 0078-0274-22).
Store and Dispense: In the original container at controlled room temperature 68°-77°F (20°-25°C). Do not store in the refrigerator. Once opened, the contents must be used within two months. At temperatures below 68°F (20°C) the solution may gel; light flocculation or the formation of a light sediment may also occur. There is no impact on product performance or dosing using the syringe provided. Allow to warm to room temperature 77°F (25°C) to reverse these changes.
Neoral® Soft Gelatin Capsules (cyclosporine capsules for microemulsion)
Manufactured by R.P. Scherer GmbH, EBERBACH/BADEN, GERMANY
Manufactured for Novartis Pharmaceuticals Corporation, East Hanover, NJ 07936
Neoral® Oral Solution (cyclosporine oral solution for microemulsion)
Manufactured by Novartis Pharma AG, Basle, Switzerland
Manufactured for Novartis Pharmaceuticals Corporation, East Hanover, NJ 07936
REV: MARCH 1998   30771905
Shown in Product Identification Guide, page 325

PAMELOR®   ℞

[pam 'ah-lar"]
(nortriptyline HCl) capsules, USP
(nortriptyline HCl) oral solution, USP

CAUTION: Federal law prohibits dispensing without prescription.
The following prescribing information is based on official labeling in effect on August 1, 1998.

DESCRIPTION

Pamelor® (nortriptyline HCl) is 1-Propanamine, 3-(10,11-dihydro-5H-dibenzo[a,d]cyclohepten-5-ylidene)-N-methyl-, hydrochloride.
The structural formula is as follows:

$CH-CH_2-CH_2-NH-CH_3$ ·HCl

$C_{19}H_{21}N \cdot HCl$ Mol. wt. 299.8

Adverse Events Occurring in 3% or More of Psoriasis Patients in Controlled Clinical Trials

Body System* Preferred Term	Neoral® (N=182)	Sandimmune® (N=185)
Infection or Potential Infection	24.7%	24.3 %
Influenza-like Symptoms	9.9%	8.1%
Upper Respiratory Tract Infections	7.7%	11.3%
Cardiovascular System	28.0%	25.4%
Hypertension**	27.5%	25.4%
Urinary System	24.2%	16.2%
Increased Creatinine	19.8%	15.7%
Central and Peripheral Nervous System	26.4%	20.5%
Headache	15.9%	14.0%
Paresthesia	7.1%	4.8%
Musculoskeletal System	13.2%	8.7%
Arthralgia	6.0%	1.1%
Body As a Whole–General	29.1%	22.2%
Pain	4.4%	3.2%
Metabolic and Nutritional	9.3%	9.7%
Reproductive, female	8.5% (4 of 47 females)	11.5% (6 of 52 females)
Resistance Mechanism	18.7%	21.1%
Skin and Appendages	17.6%	15.1%
Hypertrichosis	6.6%	5.4%
Respiratory System	5.0%	6.5%
Bronchospasm, coughing, dyspnea, rhinitis	5.0%	4.9%
Psychiatric	5.0%	3.8%
Gastrointestinal System	19.8%	28.7%
Abdominal pain	2.7%	6.0%
Diarrhea	5.0%	5.9%
Dyspepsia	2.2%	3.2%
Gum hyperplasia	3.8%	6.0%
Nausea	5.5%	5.9%
White cell and RES	4.4%	2.7%

*Total percentage of events within the system
**Newly occurring hypertension = SBP≥160 mm Hg and/or DBP≥90 mm Hg

10 mg, 25 mg, 50 mg, and 75 mg Capsules
Active Ingredient: nortriptyline HCl, USP
10 mg, 25 mg, and 75 mg Capsules
Inactive Ingredients: D&C Yellow #10, FD&C Yellow #6, gelatin, silicone fluid, sodium lauryl sulfate, starch, and titanium dioxide.
May Also Include: benzyl alcohol, butylparaben, edetate calcium disodium, methylparaben, propylparaben, silicon dioxide, and sodium propionate.
50 mg Capsules
Inactive Ingredients: gelatin, silicone fluid, sodium lauryl sulfate, starch, and titanium dioxide.
May Also Include: benzyl alcohol, butylparaben, edetate calcium disodium, methylparaben, propylparaben, silicon dioxide, sodium bisulfite (capsule shell only), and sodium propionate.
Solution
Active Ingredient: nortriptyline HCl, USP
Inactive Ingredients: alcohol, benzoic acid, flavoring, purified water, and sorbitol.

ACTIONS

The mechanism of mood elevation by tricyclic antidepressants is at present unknown. Pamelor® (nortriptyline HCl) is not a monoamine oxidase inhibitor. It inhibits the activity of such diverse agents as histamine, 5-hydroxytryptamine, and acetylcholine. It increases the pressor effect of norepinephrine but blocks the pressor response of phenethylamine. Studies suggest that Pamelor® (nortriptyline HCl) interferes with the transport, release, and storage of catecholamines. Operant conditioning techniques in rats and pigeons suggest that Pamelor® (nortriptyline HCl) has a combination of stimulant and depressant properties.

INDICATIONS

Pamelor® (nortriptyline HCl) is indicated for the relief of symptoms of depression. Endogenous depressions are more likely to be alleviated than are other depressive states.

CONTRAINDICATIONS

The use of Pamelor® (nortriptyline HCl) or other tricyclic antidepressants concurrently with a monoamine oxidase (MAO) inhibitor is contraindicated. Hyperpyretic crises, severe convulsions, and fatalities have occurred when similar tricyclic antidepressants were used in such combinations. It is advisable to have discontinued the MAO inhibitor for at least two weeks before treatment with Pamelor® (nortriptyline HCl) is started. Patients hypersensitive to Pamelor® (nortriptyline HCl) should not be given the drug.
Cross-sensitivity between Pamelor® (nortriptyline HCl) and other dibenzazepines is a possibility.
Pamelor® (nortriptyline HCl) is contraindicated during the acute recovery period after myocardial infarction.

WARNINGS

Patients with cardiovascular disease should be given Pamelor® (nortriptyline HCl) only under close supervision because of the tendency of the drug to produce sinus tachycardia and to prolong the conduction time. Myocardial infarction, arrhythmia, and strokes have occurred. The antihypertensive action of guanethidine and similar agents may be blocked. Because of its anticholinergic activity, Pamelor® (nortriptyline HCl) should be used with great caution in patients who have glaucoma or a history of urinary retention. Patients with a history of seizures should be followed closely when Pamelor® (nortriptyline HCl) is administered, inasmuch as this drug is known to lower the convulsive threshold. Great care is required if Pamelor® (nortriptyline HCl) is given to hyperthyroid patients or to those receiving thyroid medication, since cardiac arrhythmias may develop.
Pamelor® (nortriptyline HCl) may impair the mental and/or physical abilities required for the performance of hazardous tasks, such as operating machinery or driving a car; therefore, the patient should be warned accordingly.
Excessive consumption of alcohol in combination with nortriptyline therapy may have a potentiating effect, which may lead to the danger of increased suicidal attempts or overdosage, especially in patients with histories of emotional disturbances or suicidal ideation.
The concomitant administration of quinidine and nortriptyline may result in a significantly longer plasma half-life, higher AUC, and lower clearance of nortriptyline.

Use in Pregnancy

Safe use of Pamelor® (nortriptyline HCl) during pregnancy and lactation has not been established; therefore, when the drug is administered to pregnant patients, nursing mothers, or women of childbearing potential, the potential benefits must be weighed against the possible hazards. Animal reproduction studies have yielded inconclusive results.

Pediatric Use

This drug is not recommended for use in children, since safety and effectiveness in the pediatric age group have not been established.

PRECAUTIONS

The use of Pamelor® (nortriptyline HCl) in schizophrenic patients may result in an exacerbation of the psychosis or

may activate latent schizophrenic symptoms. If the drug is given to overactive or agitated patients, increased anxiety and agitation may occur. In manic-depressive patients, Pamelor® (nortriptyline HCl) may cause symptoms of the manic phase to emerge.
Troublesome patient hostility may be aroused by the use of Pamelor® (nortriptyline HCl). Epileptiform seizures may accompany its administration, as is true of other drugs of its class.
When it is essential, the drug may be administered with electroconvulsive therapy, although the hazards may be increased. Discontinue the drug for several days, if possible, prior to elective surgery.
The possibility of a suicidal attempt by a depressed patient remains after the initiation of treatment; in this regard, it is important that the least possible quantity of drug be dispensed at any given time.
Both elevation and lowering of blood sugar levels have been reported.

Drug Interactions

Administration of reserpine during therapy with a tricyclic antidepressant has been shown to produce a "stimulating" effect in some depressed patients.
Close supervision and careful adjustment of the dosage are required when Pamelor® (nortriptyline HCl) is used with other anticholinergic drugs and sympathomimetic drugs.
Concurrent administration of cimetidine and tricyclic antidepressants can produce clinically significant increases in the plasma concentrations of the tricyclic antidepressant. The patient should be informed that the response to alcohol may be exaggerated.
A case of significant hypoglycemia has been reported in a type II diabetic patient maintained on chlorpropamide (250 mg/day), after the addition of nortriptyline (125 mg/day).
Drugs Metabolized by P450 2D6 – The biochemical activity of the drug metabolizing isozyme cytochrome P450 2D6 (debrisoquin hydroxylase) is reduced in a subset of the caucasian population (about 7%-10% of caucasians are so called "poor metabolizers"); reliable estimates of the prevalence of reduced P450 2D6 isozyme activity among Asian, African and other populations are not yet available. Poor metabolizers have higher than expected plasma concentrations of tricyclic antidepressants (TCAs) when given usual doses. Depending on the fraction of drug metabolized by P450 2D6, the increase in plasma concentration may be small, or quite large (8 fold increase in plasma AUC of the TCA).
In addition, certain drugs inhibit the activity of this isozyme and make normal metabolizers resemble poor metabolizers. An individual who is stable on a given dose of TCA may become abruptly toxic when given one of these inhibiting drugs as concomitant therapy. The drugs that inhibit cytochrome P450 2D6 include some that are not metabolized by the enzyme (quinidine; cimetidine) and many that are substrates for P450 2D6 (many other antidepressants, phenothiazines, and the Type 1C antiarrhythmics propafenone and flecainide). While all the selective serotonin reuptake inhibitors (SSRIs), e.g., fluoxetine, sertraline, and paroxetine, inhibit P450 2D6, they may vary in the extent of inhibition. The extent to which SSRI TCA interactions may pose clinical problems will depend on the degree of inhibition and the pharmacokinetics of the SSRI involved. Nevertheless, caution is indicated in the co-administration of TCAs with any of the SSRIs and also in switching from one class to the other. Of particular importance, sufficient time must elapse before initiating TCA treatment in a patient being withdrawn from fluoxetine, given the long half-life of the parent and active metabolite (at least 5 weeks may be necessary). Concomitant use of tricyclic antidepressants with drugs that can inhibit cytochrome P450 2D6 may require lower doses than usually prescribed for either the tricyclic antidepressant or the other drug. Furthermore, whenever one of these other drugs is withdrawn from co-therapy, an increased dose of tricyclic antidepressant may be required. It is desirable to monitor TCA plasma levels whenever a TCA is going to be co-administered with another drug known to be an inhibitor of P450 2D6.

ADVERSE REACTIONS

Note: Included in the following list are a few adverse reactions that have not been reported with this specific drug. However, the pharmacologic similarities among the tricyclic antidepressant drugs require that each of the reactions be considered when nortriptyline is administered.
Cardiovascular – Hypotension, hypertension, tachycardia, palpitation, myocardial infarction, arrhythmias, heart block, stroke.
Psychiatric – Confusional states (especially in the elderly) with hallucinations, disorientation, delusions; anxiety, restlessness, agitation; insomnia, panic, nightmares; hypomania; exacerbation of psychosis.
Neurologic – Numbness, tingling, paresthesias of extremities; incoordination, ataxia, tremors; peripheral neuropathy; extrapyramidal symptoms; seizures, alteration in EEG patterns; tinnitus.
Anticholinergic – Dry mouth and, rarely, associated sublingual adenitis; blurred vision, disturbance of accommodation, mydriasis; constipation, paralytic ileus; urinary retention, delayed micturition, dilation of the urinary tract.
Allergic – Skin rash, petechiae, urticaria, itching, photosensitization (avoid excessive exposure to sunlight); edema (general or of face and tongue), drug fever, cross-sensitivity with other tricyclic drugs.

Hematologic – Bone marrow depression, including agranulocytosis; eosinophilia; purpura; thrombocytopenia.
Gastrointestinal – Nausea and vomiting, anorexia, epigastric distress, diarrhea, peculiar taste, stomatitis, abdominal cramps, blacktongue.
Endocrine – Gynecomastia in the male; breast enlargement and galactorrhea in the female; increased or decreased libido, impotence; testicular swelling; elevation or depression of blood sugar levels; syndrome of inappropriate ADH (antidiuretic hormone) secretion.
Other – Jaundice (simulating obstructive), altered liver function; weight gain or loss; perspiration; flushing; urinary frequency, nocturia; drowsiness, dizziness, weakness, fatigue; headache; parotid swelling; alopecia.
Withdrawal Symptoms – Though these are not indicative of addiction, abrupt cessation of treatment after prolonged therapy may produce nausea, headache, and malaise.

DOSAGE AND ADMINISTRATION

Pamelor® (nortriptyline HCl) is not recommended for children.
Pamelor® (nortriptyline HCl) is administered orally in the form of capsules or liquid. Lower than usual dosages are recommended for elderly patients and adolescents. Lower dosages are also recommended for outpatients than for hospitalized patients who will be under close supervision. The physician should initiate dosage at a low level and increase it gradually, noting carefully the clinical response and any evidence of intolerance. Following remission, maintenance medication may be required for a longer period of time at the lowest dose that will maintain remission.
If a patient develops minor side effects, the dosage should be reduced. The drug should be discontinued promptly if adverse effects of a serious nature or allergic manifestations occur.
Usual Adult Dose — 25 mg three or four times daily; dosage should begin at a low level and be increased as required. As an alternate regimen, the total daily dosage may be given once a day. When doses above 100 mg daily are administered, plasma levels of nortriptyline should be monitored and maintained in the optimum range of 50-150 ng/mL. Doses above 150 mg/day are not recommended.
Elderly and Adolescent Patients — 30-50 mg/day, in divided doses, or the total daily dosage may be given once a day.

OVERDOSAGE

Deaths may occur from overdosage with this class of drugs. Multiple drug ingestion (including alcohol) is common in deliberate tricyclic antidepressant overdose. As the management is complex and changing, it is recommended that the physician contact a poison control center for current information on treatment. Signs and symptoms of toxicity develop rapidly after tricyclic antidepressant overdose, therefore, hospital monitoring is required as soon as possible.

Manifestations:

Critical manifestations of overdose include: cardiac dysrhythmias, severe hypotension, shock, congestive heart failure, pulmonary edema, convulsions, and CNS depression, including coma. Changes in the electrocardiogram, particularly in QRS axis or width, are clinically significant indicators of tricyclic antidepressant toxicity.
Other signs of overdose may include: confusion, restlessness, disturbed concentration, transient visual hallucinations, dilated pupils, agitation, hyperactive reflexes, stupor, drowsiness, muscle rigidity, vomiting, hypothermia, hyperpyrexia, or any of the acute symptoms listed under ADVERSE REACTIONS. There have been reports of patients recovering from nortriptyline overdoses of up to 525 mg.

Management:

General: Obtain an ECG and immediately initiate cardiac monitoring. Protect the patient's airway, establish an intravenous line and initiate gastric decontamination. A minimum of six hours of observation with cardiac monitoring and observation for signs of CNS or respiratory depression, hypotension, cardiac dysrhythmias and/or conduction blocks, and seizures is necessary. If signs of toxicity occur at any time during this period, extended monitoring is required. There are case reports of patients succumbing to fatal dysrhythmias late after overdose; these patients had clinical evidence of significant poisoning prior to death and most received inadequate gastrointestinal decontamination. Monitoring of plasma drug levels should not guide management of the patient.
Gastrointestinal Decontamination: All patients suspected of tricyclic antidepressant overdose should receive gastrointestinal decontamination. This should include large volume gastric lavage followed by activated charcoal. If consciousness is impaired, the airway should be secured prior to lavage. EMESIS IS CONTRAINDICATED.
Cardiovascular: A maximal limb-lead QRS duration of ≥0.10 seconds may be the best indication of the severity of the overdose. Intravenous sodium bicarbonate shoud be used to maintain the serum pH in the range of 7.45 to 7.55. If the pH response is inadequate, hyperventilation may also

Continued on next page

Pamelor—Cont.

be used. Concomitant use of hyperventilation and sodium bicarbonate should be done with extreme caution, with frequent pH monitoring. A pH >7.60 or a pCO_2 <20 mm Hg is undesirable. Dysrhythmias unresponsive to sodium bicarbonate therapy/hyperventilation may respond to lidocaine, bretylium or phenytoin. Type 1A and 1C antiarrhythmics are generally contraindicated (e.g., quinidine, disopyramide, and procainamide).
In rare instances, hemoperfusion may be beneficial in acute refractory cardiovascular instability in patients with acute toxicity. However, hemodialysis, peritoneal dialysis, exchange transfusions, and forced diuresis generally have been reported as ineffective in tricyclic antidepressant poisoning.
CNS: In patients with CNS depression, early intubation is advised because of the potential for abrupt deterioration. Seizures should be controlled with benzodiazepines, or if these are ineffective, other anticonvulsants (e.g., phenobarbital, phenytoin). Physostigmine is not recommended except to treat life-threatening symptoms that have been unresponsive to other therapies, and then only in consultation with a poison control center.
Psychiatric Follow-up: Since overdosage is often deliberate, patients may attempt suicide by other means during the recovery phase. Psychiatric referral may be appropriate.
Pediatric Management: The principles of management of child and adult overdosages are similar. It is strongly recommended that the physician contact the local poison control center for specific pediatric treatment.

HOW SUPPLIED

Pamelor® (nortriptyline HCl) Capsules, USP
Pamelor® (nortriptyline HCl) Capsules, USP, equivalent to 10 mg, 25 mg, 50 mg, and 75 mg base, are available in bottles of 100 (10 mg: NDC 0078-0086-05; 25 mg: NDC 0078-0087-05; 50 mg: NDC 0078-0078-05; 75 mg: NDC 0078-0079-05). 10 mg, 25 mg, and 50 mg are available in a unit dose package of 100 individually labeled blisters, each containing 1 capsule (10 mg: NDC 0078-0086-06; 25 mg: NDC 0078-0087-06; 50 mg: NDC 0078-0078-06). Pamelor® (nortriptyline HCl) Capsules, USP 25 mg is also available in bottles of 500 (NDC 0078-0087-08).
10 mg capsules branded "SANDOZ" on one half, "PAMELOR 10 mg" other half; 25 mg capsules branded "SANDOZ" on one half, "PAMELOR 25 mg" other half; 50 mg capsules branded "SANDOZ" on one half, "PAMELOR 50 mg" other half; and 75 mg capsules branded "SANDOZ" on one half, "PAMELOR 75 mg" other half.

Store and Dispense: Below 86°F (30°C); tight container.
Pamelor® (nortriptyline HCl) Solution, USP
Pamelor® (nortriptyline HCl) Solution, USP, equivalent to 10 mg base per 5 mL, is supplied in 16-fluid-ounce bottles (NDC 0078-0016-33). Alcohol content 4%.
Store and Dispense: Below 86°F (30°C); tight, light-resistant container.
[REV: AUGUST 1997 30275905]
Shown in Product Identification Guide, page 325

PARLODEL® ℞

[*par 'lō-del"*]
SnapTabs®
(*bromocriptine mesylate*) tablets, USP
(*bromocriptine mesylate*) capsules, USP

CAUTION: Federal law prohibits dispensing without prescription.
The following prescribing information is based on official labeling in effect on August 1, 1998.

DESCRIPTION

Parlodel® (bromocriptine mesylate) is an ergot derivative with potent dopamine receptor agonist activity. Each Parlodel® (bromocriptine mesylate) SnapTabs® tablet for oral administration contains 2½ mg and each capsule contains 5 mg bromocriptine (as the mesylate). Parlodel® (bromocriptine mesylate) is chemically designated as Ergotaman-3′,6′,18-trione,2-bromo-12′-hydroxy-2′-(1-methylethyl)-5′-(2-methylpropyl)-, (5′α)-monomethanesulfonate (salt).
The structural formula is:
[See chemical structure at top of next column]

2 ½ mg SnapTabs®
Active Ingredient: bromocriptine mesylate, USP
Inactive Ingredients: colloidal silicon dioxide, lactose, magnesium stearate, povidone, starch, and another ingredient
5 mg Capsules
Active Ingredient: bromocriptine mesylate, USP
Inactive Ingredients: colloidal silicon dioxide, gelatin, lactose, magnesium stearate, red iron oxide, silicon dioxide, sodium lauryl sulfate, starch, titanium dioxide, yellow iron oxide, and another ingredient

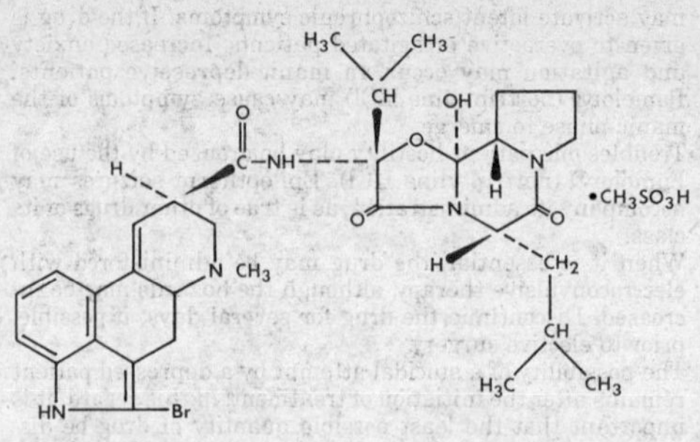

$C_{32}H_{40}BrN_5O_5 \bullet CH_4SO_3$ Mol. wt. 750.70

CLINICAL PHARMACOLOGY

Parlodel® (bromocriptine mesylate) is a dopamine receptor agonist, which activates post-synaptic dopamine receptors. The dopaminergic neurons in the tuberoinfundibular process modulate the secretion of prolactin from the anterior pituitary by secreting a prolactin inhibitory factor (thought to be dopamine); in the corpus striatum the dopaminergic neurons are involved in the control of motor function. Clinically, Parlodel® (bromocriptine mesylate) significantly reduces plasma levels of prolactin in patients with physiologically elevated prolactin as well as in patients with hyperprolactinemia. The inhibition of physiological lactation as well as galactorrhea in pathological hyperprolactinemic states is obtained at dose levels that do not affect secretion of other tropic hormones from the anterior pituitary. Experiments have demonstrated that bromocriptine induces long lasting stereotyped behavior in rodents and turning behavior in rats having unilateral lesions in the substantia nigra. These actions, characteristic of those produced by dopamine, are inhibited by dopamine antagonists and suggest a direct action of bromocriptine on striatal dopamine receptors.
Parlodel® (bromocriptine mesylate) is a nonhormonal, nonestrogenic agent that inhibits the secretion of prolactin in humans, with little or no effect on other pituitary hormones, except in patients with acromegaly, where it lowers elevated blood levels of growth hormone in the majority of patients.
In about 75% of cases of amenorrhea and galactorrhea, Parlodel® (bromocriptine mesylate) therapy suppresses the galactorrhea completely, or almost completely, and reinitiates normal ovulatory menstrual cycles.
Menses are usually reinitiated prior to complete suppression of galactorrhea; the time for this on average is 6-8 weeks. However, some patients respond within a few days, and others may take up to 8 months.
Galactorrhea may take longer to control depending on the degree of stimulation of the mammary tissue prior to therapy. At least a 75% reduction in secretion is usually observed after 8-12 weeks. Some patients may fail to respond even after 12 months of therapy.
In many acromegalic patients, Parlodel® (bromocriptine mesylate) produces a prompt and sustained reduction in circulating levels of serum growth hormone.
Parlodel® (bromocriptine mesylate) produces its therapeutic effect in the treatment of Parkinson's disease, a clinical condition characterized by a progressive deficiency in dopamine synthesis in the substantia nigra, by directly stimulating the dopamine receptors in the corpus striatum. In contrast, levodopa exerts its therapeutic effect only after conversion to dopamine by the neurons of the substantia nigra, which are known to be numerically diminished in this patient population.

Pharmacokinetics
The pharmacokinetics and metabolism of bromocriptine in human subjects were studied with the help of radioactively labeled drug. Twenty-eight percent of an oral dose was absorbed from the gastrointestinal tract. The blood levels following a 2½ mg dose were in the range of 2-3 ng equivalents/mL. Plasma levels were in the range of 4-6 ng equivalents/mL indicating that the red blood cells did not contain appreciable amounts of drug and/or metabolites. *In vitro* experiments showed that the drug was 90%-96% bound to serum albumin.
Bromocriptine was completely metabolized prior to excretion. The major route of excretion of absorbed drug was via the bile. Only 2.5%-5.5% of the dose was excreted in the urine. Almost all (84.6%) of the administered dose was excreted in the feces in 120 hours.

INDICATIONS AND USAGE

Hyperprolactinemia-Associated Dysfunctions
Parlodel® (bromocriptine mesylate) is indicated for the treatment of dysfunctions associated with **hyperprolactinemia** including **amenorrhea** with or without **galactorrhea, infertility or hypogonadism.** Parlodel® (bromocriptine mesylate) treatment is indicated in patients with **prolactin-secreting adenomas,** which may be the basic underlying endocrinopathy contributing to the above clinical presentations. **Reduction in tumor size** has been demonstrated in both male and female patients with macroadenomas. In cases where adenectomy is elected, a course of Parlodel® (bromocriptine mesylate) therapy may be used to reduce the tumor mass prior to surgery.

Acromegaly
Parlodel® (bromocriptine mesylate) therapy is indicated in the treatment of acromegaly. Parlodel® (bromocriptine mesylate) therapy, alone or as adjunctive therapy with pituitary irradiation or surgery, reduces serum growth hormone by 50% or more in approximately ½ of patients treated, although not usually to normal levels.
Since the effects of external pituitary radiation may not become maximal for several years, adjunctive therapy with Parlodel® (bromocriptine mesylate) offers potential benefit before the effects of irradiation are manifested.

Parkinson's Disease
Parlodel® (bromocriptine mesylate) SnapTabs® or capsules are indicated in the treatment of the signs and symptoms of idiopathic or postencephalitic Parkinson's disease. As adjunctive treatment to levodopa (alone or with a peripheral decarboxylase inhibitor), Parlodel® (bromocriptine mesylate) therapy may provide additional therapeutic benefits in those patients who are currently maintained on optimal dosages of levodopa, those who are beginning to deteriorate (develop tolerance) to levodopa therapy, and those who are experiencing "end of dose failure" on levodopa therapy. Parlodel® (bromocriptine mesylate) therapy may permit a reduction of the maintenance dose of levodopa and, thus may ameliorate the occurrence and/or severity of adverse reactions associated with long-term levodopa therapy such as abnormal involuntary movements (e.g., dyskinesias) and the marked swings in motor function ("on-off" phenomenon). Continued efficacy of Parlodel® (bromocriptine mesylate) therapy during treatment of more than 2 years has not been established.
Data are insufficient to evaluate potential benefit from treating newly diagnosed Parkinson's disease with Parlodel® (bromocriptine mesylate). Studies have shown, however, significantly more adverse reactions (notably nausea, hallucinations, confusion and hypotension) in Parlodel® (bromocriptine mesylate) treated patients than in levodopa/carbidopa treated patients. Patients unresponsive to levodopa are poor candidates for Parlodel® (bromocriptine mesylate) therapy.

CONTRAINDICATIONS

Uncontrolled hypertension and sensitivity to any ergot alkaloids. In patients being treated for hyperprolactinemia Parlodel® (bromocriptine mesylate) should be withdrawn when pregnancy is diagnosed *(see PRECAUTIONS, Hyperprolactinemic States).* In the event that Parlodel® (bromocriptine mesylate) is reinstituted to control a rapidly expanding macroadenoma *(see PRECAUTIONS, Hyperprolactinemic States)* and a patient experiences a hypertensive disorder of pregnancy, the benefit of continuing Parlodel® (bromocriptine mesylate) must be weighed against the possible risk of its use during a hypertensive disorder of pregnancy. When Parlodel® (bromocriptine mesylate) is being used to treat acromegaly, prolactinoma, or Parkinson's disease in patients who subsequently become pregnant, a decision should be made as to whether the therapy continues to be medically necessary or can be withdrawn. If it is continued, the drug should be withdrawn in those who may experience hypertensive disorders of pregnancy (including eclampsia, preeclampsia, or pregnancy-induced hypertension) unless withdrawal of Parlodel® (bromocriptine mesylate) is considered to be medically contraindicated.
The drug should not be used during the post-partum period in women with a history of coronary artery disease and other severe cardiovascular conditions unless withdrawal is considered medically contraindicated. If the drug is used in the post-partum period the patient should be observed with caution.

WARNINGS

Since hyperprolactinemia with amenorrhea/galactorrhea and infertility has been found in patients with pituitary tumors, a complete evaluation of the pituitary is indicated before treatment with Parlodel® (bromocriptine mesylate). If pregnancy occurs during Parlodel® (bromocriptine mesylate) administration, careful observation of these patients is mandatory. Prolactin-secreting adenomas may expand and compression of the optic or other cranial nerves may occur, emergency pituitary surgery becoming necessary. In most cases, the compression resolves following delivery. Reinitiation of Parlodel® (bromocriptine mesylate) treatment has been reported to produce improvement in the visual fields of patients in whom nerve compression has occurred during pregnancy. The safety of Parlodel® (bromocriptine mesylate) treatment during pregnancy to the mother and fetus has not been established.
Symptomatic hypotension can occur in patients treated with Parlodel® (bromocriptine mesylate) for any indication. In postpartum studies with Parlodel® (bromocriptine mesylate), decreases in supine systolic and diastolic pressures of greater than 20 mm and 10 mm Hg, respectively, have been observed in almost 30% of patients receiving

Parlodel® (bromocriptine mesylate). On occasion, the drop in supine systolic pressure was as much as 50-59 mm of Hg. **While hypotension during the start of therapy with Parlodel® (bromocriptine mesylate) occurs in some patients, in postmarketing experience in the U.S. in postpartum patients 89 cases of hypertension have been reported, sometimes at the initiation of therapy, but often developing in the second week of therapy; seizures have been reported in 72 cases (including 4 cases of status epilepticus), both with and without the prior development of hypertension; 30 cases of stroke have been reported mostly in postpartum patients whose prenatal and obstetric courses had been uncomplicated. Many of these patients experiencing seizures and/or strokes reported developing a constant and often progressively severe headache hours to days prior to the acute event. Some cases of strokes and seizures were also preceded by visual disturbances (blurred vision, and transient cortical blindness). Nine cases of acute myocardial infarction have been reported.**

Although a causal relationship between Parlodel® (bromocriptine mesylate) administration and hypertension, seizures, strokes, and myocardial infarction in postpartum women has not been established, use of the drug for prevention of physiological lactation, or in patients with uncontrolled hypertension is not recommended. In patients being treated for hyperprolactinemia Parlodel® (bromocriptine mesylate) should be withdrawn when pregnancy is diagnosed (see PRECAUTIONS, Hyperprolactinemic States). **In the event that Parlodel® (bromocriptine mesylate) is reinstituted to control a rapidly expanding macroadenoma** (see PRECAUTIONS, Hyperprolactinemia States) **and a patient experiences a hypertensive disorder of pregnancy, the benefit of continuing Parlodel® (bromocriptine mesylate) must be weighed against the possible risk of its use during a hypertensive disorder of pregnancy. When Parlodel® (bromocriptine mesylate) is being used to treat acromegaly or Parkinson's disease in patients who subsequently become pregnant, a decision should be made as to whether the therapy continues to be medically necessary or can be withdrawn. If it is continued, the drug should be withdrawn in those who may experience hypertensive disorders of pregnancy (including eclampsia, preeclampsia, or pregnancy-induced hypertension) unless withdrawal of Parlodel® (bromocriptine mesylate) is considered to be medically contraindicated. Because of the possibility of an interaction between Parlodel® (bromocriptine mesylate) and other ergot alkaloids, the concomitant use of these medications is not recommended. Particular attention should be paid to patients who have recently received other drugs that can alter the blood pressure.** Periodic monitoring of the blood pressure, particularly during the first weeks of therapy is prudent. If hypertension, severe, progressive, or unremitting headache (with or without visual disturbance), or evidence of CNS toxicity develops, drug therapy should be discontinued and the patient should be evaluated promptly.

Long-term treatment (6-36 months) with Parlodel® (bromocriptine mesylate) in doses ranging from 20-100 mg/day has been associated with pulmonary infiltrates, pleural effusion and thickening of the pleura in a few patients. In those instances in which Parlodel® (bromocriptine mesylate) treatment was terminated, the changes slowly reverted towards normal.

PRECAUTIONS
General
Safety and efficacy of Parlodel® (bromocriptine mesylate) have not been established in patients with renal or hepatic disease. Care should be exercised when administering Parlodel® (bromocriptine mesylate) therapy concomitantly with other medications known to lower blood pressure.

The drug should be used with caution in patients with a history of psychosis or cardiovascular disease. If acromegalic patients or patients with prolactinoma or Parkinson's disease are being treated with Parlodel® (bromocriptine mesylate) during pregnancy, they should be cautiously observed, particularly during the post-partum period if they have a history of cardiovascular disease.

Hyperprolactinemic States
The relative efficacy of Parlodel® (bromocriptine mesylate) versus surgery in preserving visual fields is not known. Patients with rapidly progressive visual field loss should be evaluated by a neurosurgeon to help decide on the most appropriate therapy. Since pregnancy is often the therapeutic objective in many hyperprolactinemic patients presenting with amenorrhea/galactorrhea and hypogonadism (infertility), a careful assessment of the pituitary is essential to detect the presence of a prolactin-secreting adenoma. Patients not seeking pregnancy, or those harboring large adenomas, should be advised to use contraceptive measures, other than oral contraceptives, during treatment with Parlodel® (bromocriptine mesylate). Since pregnancy may occur prior to reinitiation of menses, a pregnancy test is recommended at least every 4 weeks during the amenorrheic period, and, once menses are reinitiated, every time a patient misses a menstrual period. Treatment with Parlodel® (bromocriptine

mesylate) SnapTabs® or capsules should be discontinued as soon as pregnancy has been established. Patients must be monitored closely throughout pregnancy for signs and symptoms that may signal the enlargement of a previously undetected or existing prolactin-secreting tumor. Discontinuation of Parlodel® (bromocriptine mesylate) treatment in patients with known macroadenomas has been associated with rapid regrowth of tumor and increase in serum prolactin in most cases.

Acromegaly
Cold sensitive digital vasospasm has been observed in some acromegalic patients treated with Parlodel® (bromocriptine mesylate). The response, should it occur, can be reversed by reducing the dose of Parlodel® (bromocriptine mesylate) and may be prevented by keeping the fingers warm. Cases of severe gastrointestinal bleeding from peptic ulcers have been reported, some fatal. Although there is no evidence that Parlodel® (bromocriptine mesylate) increases the incidence of peptic ulcers in acromegalic patients, symptoms suggestive of peptic ulcer should be investigated thoroughly and treated appropriately. Patients with a history of peptic ulcer or gastrointestinal bleeding should be observed carefully during treatment with Parlodel® (bromocriptine mesylate).

Possible tumor expansion while receiving Parlodel® (bromocriptine mesylate) therapy has been reported in a few patients. Since the natural history of growth hormone secreting tumors is unknown, all patients should be carefully monitored and, if evidence of tumor expansion develops, discontinuation of treatment and alternative procedures considered.

Parkinson's Disease
Safety during long-term use for more than 2 years at the doses required for parkinsonism has not been established. As with any chronic therapy, periodic evaluation of hepatic, hematopoietic, cardiovascular, and renal function is recommended. Symptomatic hypotension can occur and, therefore, caution should be exercised when treating patients receiving antihypertensive drugs.

High doses of Parlodel® (bromocriptine mesylate) may be associated with confusion and mental disturbances. Since parkinsonian patients may manifest mild degrees of dementia, caution should be used when treating such patients.

Parlodel® (bromocriptine mesylate) administered alone or concomitantly with levodopa may cause hallucinations (visual or auditory). Hallucinations usually resolve with dosage reduction; occasionally, discontinuation of Parlodel® (bromocriptine mesylate) is required. Rarely, after high doses, hallucinations have persisted for several weeks following discontinuation of Parlodel® (bromocriptine mesylate).

As with levodopa, caution should be exercised when administering Parlodel® (bromocriptine mesylate) to patients with a history of myocardial infarction who have a residual atrial, nodal, or ventricular arrhythmia.

Retroperitoneal fibrosis has been reported in a few patients receiving long-term therapy (2-10 years) with Parlodel® (bromocriptine mesylate) in doses ranging from 30-140 mg daily.

Information for Patients
When initiating therapy, all patients receiving Parlodel® (bromocriptine mesylate) should be cautioned with regard to engaging in activities requiring rapid and precise responses, such as driving an automobile or operating machinery since dizziness (8%-16%), drowsiness (8%), faintness, fainting (8%), and syncope (less than 1%) have been reported early in the course of therapy. Patients receiving Parlodel® (bromocriptine mesylate) for hyperprolactinemic states associated with macroadenoma or those who have had previous transsphenoidal surgery, should be told to report any persistent watery nasal discharge to their physician. Patients receiving Parlodel® (bromocriptine mesylate) for treatment of a macroadenoma should be told that discontinuation of drug may be associated with rapid regrowth of the tumor and recurrence of their original symptoms.

Drug Interactions
The risk of using Parlodel® (bromocriptine mesylate) in combination with other drugs has not been systematically evaluated, but alcohol may potentiate the side effects of Parlodel® (bromocriptine mesylate). Parlodel® (bromocriptine mesylate) may interact with dopamine antagonists, butyrophenones, and certain other agents. Compounds in these categories result in a decreased efficacy of Parlodel® (bromocriptine mesylate): phenothiazines, haloperidol, metoclopramide, pimozide). Concomitant use of Parlodel® (bromocriptine mesylate) with other ergot alkaloids is not recommended.

Carcinogenesis, Mutagenesis, Impairment of Fertility
A 74-week study was conducted in mice using dietary levels of bromocriptine mesylate equivalent to oral doses of 10 and 50 mg/kg/day. A 100-week study in rats was conducted using dietary levels equivalent to oral doses of 1.7, 9.8, and 44 mg/kg/day. The highest doses tested in mice and rats were approximately 2.5 and 4.4 times, respectively, the maximum human dose administered in controlled clinical trials (100 mg/day) based on body surface area. Malignant

uterine tumors, endometrial and myometrial, were found in rats as follows: 0/50 control females, 2/50 females given 1.7 mg/kg daily, 7/49 females given 9.8 mg/kg daily, and 9/50 females given 44 mg/kg/daily. The occurrence of these neoplasms is probably attributable to the high estrogen/progesterone ratio which occurs in rats as a result of the prolactin-inhibiting action of bromocriptine mesylate. The endocrine mechanisms believed to be involved in the rats are not present in humans. There is no known correlation between uterine malignancies occurring in bromocriptine-treated rats and human risk. In contrast to the findings in rats, the uteri from mice killed after 74 weeks treatment did not exhibit evidence of drug-related changes.

Bromocriptine mesylate was evaluated for mutagenic potential in the battery of tests that included Ames bacterial mutation assay, mutagenic activity in vitro on V79 Chinese hamster fibroblasts, cytogenetic analysis of Chinese hamster bone marrow cells following in vivo treatment, and an in vivo micronucleus test for mutagenic potential in mice. No mutagenic effects were obtained in any of these tests.

Fertility and reproductive performance in female rats were not influenced adversely by treatment with bromocriptine beyond the predicted decrease in the weight of pups due to suppression of lactation. In males treated with 50 mg/kg of this drug, mating and fertility were within the normal range. Increased perinatal loss was produced in the subgroups of dams, sacrificed on day 21 postpartum (p.p.) after mating with males treated with the highest does (50 mg/kg).

Pregnancy
Category B: Administration of 10-30 mg/kg of bromocriptine to 2 strains of rats on days 6-15 post coitum (p.c.) as well as a single dose of 10 mg/kg on day 5 p.c., interfered with nidation. Three mg/kg given on days 6-15 were without effect on nidation, and did not produce any anomalies. In animals treated from day 8-15 p.c., i.e., after implantation, 30 mg/kg produced increased prenatal mortality in the form of increased incidence of embryonic resorption. One anomaly, aplasia of spinal vertebrae and ribs, was found in the group of 262 fetuses derived from the dams treated with 30 mg/kg bromocriptine. No fetotoxic effects were found in offspring of dams treated during the peri- or post-natal period.

Two studies were conducted in rabbits (2 strains) to determine the potential to interfere with nidation. Dose levels of 100 or 300 mg/kg/day from day 1 to day 6 p.c. did not adversely affect nidation. The high dose was approximately 63 times the maximum human dose administered in controlled clinical trials (100 mg/day), based on body surface area. In New Zealand white rabbits some embryo mortality occurred at 300 mg/kg which was a reflection of overt maternal toxicity. Three studies were conducted in 2 strains of rabbits to determine the teratological potential of bromocriptine at dose levels of 3, 10, 30, 100, and 300 mg/kg given from day 6 to day 18 p.c. In 2 studies with the Yellow-silver strain, cleft palate was found in 3 and 2 fetuses at maternally toxic doses of 100 and 300 mg/kg, respectively. One control fetus also exhibited this anomaly. In the third study conducted with New Zealand white rabbits using an identical protocol, no cleft palates were produced.

No teratological or embryo-toxic effects of bromocriptine were produced in any of 6 offspring from 6 monkeys at a dose level of 2 mg/kg.

Information concerning 1276 pregnancies in women taking bromocriptine has been collected. In the majority of cases, bromocriptine was discontinued within 8 weeks into pregnancy (mean 28.7 days), however, 8 patients received the drug continuously throughout pregnancy. The mean daily dose for all patients was 5.8 mg (range 1-40 mg).

Of these 1276 pregnancies, there were 1088 full term deliveries (4 stillborn), 145 spontaneous abortions (11.4%), and 28 induced abortions (2.2%). Moreover, 12 extrauterine gravidities and 3 hydatidiform moles (twice in the same patient) caused early termination of pregnancy. These data compare favorably with the abortion rate (11%-25%) cited for pregnancies induced by clomiphene citrate, menopausal gonadotropin, and chorionic gonadotropin.

Although spontaneous abortions often go unreported, especially prior to 20 weeks of gestation, their frequency has been estimated to be 15%.

The incidence of birth defects in the population at large ranges from 2%-4.5%. The incidence in 1109 live births from patients receiving bromocriptine is 3.3%.

There is no suggestion that bromocriptine contributed to the type or incidence of birth defects in this group of infants.

Nursing Mothers
Parlodel® (bromocriptine mesylate) should not be used during lactation in postpartum women.

Pediatric Use
Safety and effectiveness in pediatric patients under the age of 15 have not been established.

ADVERSE REACTIONS
Hyperprolactinemic Indications
The incidence of adverse effects is quite high (69%) but these are generally mild to moderate in degree. Therapy

Continued on next page

Parlodel—Cont.

was discontinued in approximately 5% of patients because of adverse effects. These in decreasing order of frequency are: nausea (49%), headache (19%), dizziness (17%), fatigue (7%), lightheadedness (5%), vomiting (5%), abdominal cramps (4%), nasal congestion (3%), constipation (3%), diarrhea (3%) and drowsiness (3%).

A slight hypotensive effect may accompany Parlodel® (bromocriptine mesylate) treatment. The occurrence of adverse reactions may be lessened by temporarily reducing dosage to ½ SnapTabs® tablet 2 or 3 times daily. A few cases of cerebrospinal fluid rhinorrhea have been reported in patients receiving Parlodel® (bromocriptine mesylate) for treatment of large prolactinomas. This has occurred rarely, usually only in patients who have received previous transsphenoidal surgery, pituitary radiation, or both, and who were receiving Parlodel® (bromocriptine mesylate) for tumor recurrence. It may also occur in previously untreated patients whose tumor extends into the sphenoid sinus.

Acromegaly

The most frequent adverse reactions encountered in acromegalic patients treated with Parlodel® (bromocriptine mesylate) were: nausea (18%), constipation (14%), postural/orthostatic hypotension (6%), anorexia (4%), dry mouth/nasal stuffiness (4%), indigestion/dyspepsia (4%), digital vasospasm (3%), drowsiness/tiredness (3%) and vomiting (2%).

Less frequent adverse reactions (less than 2%) were: gastrointestinal bleeding, dizziness, exacerbation of Raynaud's Syndrome, headache and syncope. Rarely (less than 1%) hair loss, alcohol potentiation, faintness, lightheadedness, arrhythmia, ventricular tachycardia, decreased sleep requirement, visual hallucinations, lassitude, shortness of breath, bradycardia, vertigo, paresthesia, sluggishness, vasovagal attack, delusional psychosis, paranoia, insomnia, heavy headedness, reduced tolerance to cold, tingling of ears, facial pallor and muscle cramps have been reported.

Parkinson's Disease

In clinical trials in which bromocriptine was administered with concomitant reduction in the dose of levodopa/carbidopa, the most common newly appearing adverse reactions were: nausea, abnormal involuntary movements, hallucinations, confusion, "on-off" phenomenon, dizziness, drowsiness, faintness/fainting, vomiting, asthenia, abdominal discomfort, visual disturbance, ataxia, insomnia, depression, hypotension, shortness of breath, constipation, and vertigo.

Less common adverse reactions which may be encountered include: anorexia, anxiety, blepharospasm, dry mouth, dysphagia, edema of the feet and ankles, erythromelalgia, epileptiform seizure, fatigue, headache, lethargy, mottling of skin, nasal stuffiness, nervousness, nightmares, paresthesia, skin rash, urinary frequency, urinary incontinence, urinary retention, and rarely, signs and symptoms of ergotism such as tingling of fingers, cold feet, numbness, muscle cramps of feet and legs or exacerbation of Raynaud's Syndrome.

Abnormalities in laboratory tests may include elevations in blood urea nitrogen, SGOT, SGPT, GGPT, CPK, alkaline phosphatase and uric acid, which are usually transient and not of clinical significance.

Adverse Events Observed in Other Conditions

Postpartum Patients

In postpartum studies with Parlodel® (bromocriptine mesylate) 23 percent of postpartum patients treated had at least 1 side effect, but they were generally mild to moderate in degree. Therapy was discontinued in approximately 3% of patients. The most frequently occurring adverse reactions were: headache (10%), dizziness (8%), nausea (7%), vomiting (3%), fatigue (1.0%), syncope (0.7%), diarrhea (0.4%), and cramps (0.4%). Decreases in blood pressure ($\geq$20 mm Hg systolic and $\geq$10 mm Hg diastolic) occurred in 28% of patients at least once during the first 3 postpartum days; these were usually of a transient nature. Reports of fainting in the puerperium may possibly be related to this effect. In postmarketing experience in the U.S. serious adverse reactions reported include 72 cases of seizures (including 4 cases of status epilepticus), 30 cases of stroke, and 9 cases of myocardial infarction among postpartum patients. Seizure cases were not necessarily accompanied by the development of hypertension. An unremitting and often progressively severe headache, sometimes accompanied by visual disturbance, often preceded by hours to days many cases of seizure and/or stroke. Most patients had shown no evidence of any of the hypertensive disorders of pregnancy including eclampsia, preeclampsia or pregnancy induced hypertension. One stroke case was associated with sagittal sinus thrombosis, and another was associated with cerebral and cerebellar vasculitis. One case of myocardial infarction was associated with unexplained disseminated intravascular coagulation and a second occurred in conjunction with use of another ergot alkaloid. The relationship of these adverse reactions to Parlodel® (bromocriptine mesylate) administration has not been established.

OVERDOSAGE

The most commonly reported signs and symptoms associated with acute Parlodel® (bromocriptine mesylate) overdose are: nausea, vomiting, constipation, diaphoresis, dizziness, pallor, severe hypotension, malaise, confusion, lethargy, drowsiness, delusions, hallucinations, and repetitive yawning. The lethal dose has not been established and the drug has a very wide margin of safety. However, one death occurred in a patient who committed suicide with an unknown quantity of Parlodel® (bromocriptine mesylate) and chloroquine.

Treatment of overdose consists of removal of the drug by emesis (if conscious), gastric lavage, activated charcoal, or saline catharsis. Careful supervision and recording of fluid intake and output is essential. Hypotension should be treated by placing the patient in the Trendelenburg position and administering I.V. fluids. If satisfactory relief of hypotension cannot be achieved by using the above measures to their fullest extent, vasopressors should be considered.

DOSAGE AND ADMINISTRATION

General

It is recommended that Parlodel® (bromocriptine mesylate) be taken with food. Patients should be evaluated frequently during dose escalation to determine the lowest dosage that produces a therapeutic response.

Hyperprolactinemic Indications

The initial dosage of Parlodel® (bromocriptine mesylate) is ½ to one 2½ mg SnapTabs® tablet daily. An additional 2½ mg SnapTabs® tablet may be added to the treatment regimen as tolerated every 3-7 days until an optimal therapeutic response is achieved. The therapeutic dosage usually is 5-7.5 mg and ranges from 2.5-15 mg/day.

In order to reduce the likelihood of prolonged exposure to Parlodel® (bromocriptine mesylate) should an unsuspected pregnancy occur, a mechanical contraceptive should be used in conjunction with Parlodel® (bromocriptine mesylate) therapy until normal ovulatory menstrual cycles have been restored. Contraception may then be discontinued in patients desiring pregnancy.

Thereafter, if menstruation does not occur within 3 days of the expected date, Parlodel® (bromocriptine mesylate) therapy should be discontinued and a pregnancy test performed.

Acromegaly

Virtually all acromegalic patients receiving therapeutic benefit from Parlodel® (bromocriptine mesylate) also have reductions in circulating levels of growth hormone. Therefore, periodic assessment of circulating levels of growth hormone will, in most cases, serve as a guide in determining the therapeutic potential of Parlodel® (bromocriptine mesylate). If, after a brief trial with Parlodel® (bromocriptine mesylate) therapy, no significant reduction in growth hormone levels has taken place, careful assessment of the clinical features of the disease should be made, and if no change has occurred, dosage adjustment or discontinuation of therapy should be considered.

The initial recommended dosage is ½ to one 2½ mg Parlodel® (bromocriptine mesylate) SnapTabs® tablet on retiring (with food) for 3 days. An additional ½ to 1 SnapTabs® tablet should be added to the treatment regimen as tolerated every 3-7 days until the patient obtains optimal therapeutic benefit. Patients should be reevaluated monthly and the dosage adjusted based on reductions of growth hormone or clinical response. The usual optimal therapeutic dosage range of Parlodel® (bromocriptine mesylate) varies from 20-30 mg/day in most patients. The maximal dosage should not exceed 100 mg/day.

Patients treated with pituitary irradiation should be withdrawn from Parlodel® (bromocriptine mesylate) therapy on a yearly basis to assess both the clinical effects of radiation on the disease process as well as the effects of Parlodel® (bromocriptine mesylate) therapy. Usually a 4-8 week withdrawal period is adequate for this purpose. Recurrence of the signs/symptoms or increases in growth hormone indicate the disease process is still active and further courses of Parlodel® (bromocriptine mesylate) should be considered.

Parkinson's Disease

The basic principle of Parlodel® (bromocriptine mesylate) therapy is to initiate treatment at a low dosage and, on an individual basis, increase the daily dosage slowly until a maximum therapeutic response is achieved. The dosage of levodopa during this introductory period should be maintained, if possible. The initial dose of Parlodel® (bromocriptine mesylate) is ½ of a 2½ mg SnapTabs® tablet twice daily with meals. Assessments are advised at 2-week intervals during dosage titration to ensure that the lowest dosage producing an optimal therapeutic response is not exceeded. If necessary, the dosage may be increased every 14-28 days by 2½ mg/day with meals. Should it be advisable to reduce the dosage of levodopa because of adverse reactions, the daily dosage of Parlodel® (bromocriptine mesylate), if increased, should be accomplished gradually in small (2½ mg) increments.

The safety of Parlodel® (bromocriptine mesylate) has not been demonstrated in dosages exceeding 100 mg/day.

HOW SUPPLIED

Parlodel® (bromocriptine mesylate) SnapTabs®

2½ mg

Round, white, scored SnapTabs®, each containing 2½ mg bromocriptine (as the mesylate). Engraved "PARLODEL 2½" on one side and scored on reverse side.

Packages of 30 (NDC 0078-0017-15)
Packages of 100 (NDC 0078-0017-05)

Parlodel® (bromocriptine mesylate) Capsules

5 mg

Caramel and white capsules, each containing 5 mg bromocriptine (as the mesylate). Imprinted "PARLODEL 5 mg" on one half and "S" on other half.

Packages of 30 (NDC 0078-0102-15)
Packages of 100 (NDC 0078-0102-05)

Store and Dispense

Below 77°F (25°C); tight, light-resistant container.

[REV: NOVEMBER 1996 30177907]

Shown in Product Identification Guide, page 325

REGITINE® ℞

[rej 'a-teen]

phentolamine mesylate for injection USP
Vials

Rx only

The following prescribing information is based on official labeling in effect on August 1, 1998.

DESCRIPTION

Regitine, phentolamine mesylate for injection, USP, is an antihypertensive, available in vials for intravenous and intramuscular administration. Each vial contains phentolamine mesylate USP, 5 mg, and mannitol USP, 25 mg, in sterile, lyophilized form.

Phentolamine mesylate is 4,5-dihydro-2-[N-(*m*-hydroxyphenyl)-N-(*p*-methylphenyl)aminomethyl]-1*H*-imidazole 1:1 methanesulfonate and its structural formula is:

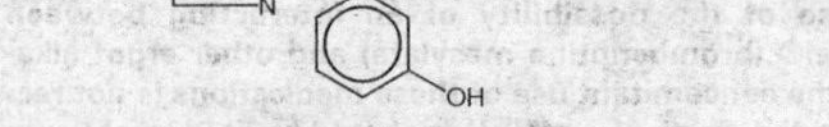

Phentolamine mesylate for injection, USP is a white or off-white, odorless crystalline powder with a molecular weight of 377.46. Its solutions are acid to litmus. It is freely soluble in water and in alcohol, and slightly soluble in chloroform. It melts at about 178°C.

CLINICAL PHARMACOLOGY

Regitine produces an alpha-adrenergic block of relatively short duration. It also has direct, but less marked, positive inotropic and chronotropic effects on cardiac muscle and vasodilator effects on vascular smooth muscle.

Regitine has a half-life in the blood of 19 minutes following intravenous administration. Approximately 13% of a single intravenous dose appears in the urine as unchanged drug.

INDICATIONS AND USAGE

Regitine is indicated for the prevention or control of hypertensive episodes that may occur in a patient with pheochromocytoma as a result of stress or manipulation during preoperative preparation and surgical excision.

Regitine is indicated for the prevention or treatment of dermal necrosis and sloughing following intravenous administration or extravasation of norepinephrine.

Regitine is also indicated for the diagnosis of pheochromocytoma by the Regitine blocking test.

CONTRAINDICATIONS

Myocardial infarction, history of myocardial infarction, coronary insufficiency, angina, or other evidence suggestive of coronary artery disease; hypersensitivity to phentolamine or related compounds.

WARNINGS

Myocardial infarction, cerebrovascular spasm, and cerebrovascular occlusion have been reported to occur following the administration of Regitine, usually in association with marked hypotensive episodes.

For screening tests in patients with hypertension, the generally available urinary assay of catecholamines or other biochemical assays have largely replaced the Regitine and other pharmacological tests for reasons of accuracy and safety. None of the chemical or pharmacological tests is infallible in the diagnosis of pheochromocytoma. The Regitine blocking test is not the procedure of choice and should be reserved for cases in which additional confirmatory evidence is necessary and the relative risks involved in conducting the test have been considered.

PRECAUTIONS

General

Tachycardia and cardiac arrhythmias may occur with the use of Regitine or other alpha-adrenergic blocking agents. When possible, administration of cardiac glycosides should be deferred until cardiac rhythm returns to normal.

Drug Interactions

See **DOSAGE AND ADMINISTRATION, Diagnosis of pheochromocytoma,** *Preparation.*

Carcinogenesis, Mutagenesis, Impairment of Fertility

Long-term carcinogenicity studies, mutagenicity studies, and fertility studies have not been conducted with Regitine.

Pregnancy Category C

Administration of Regitine to pregnant rats and mice at oral doses 24–30 times the usual daily human dose (based on a 60-kg human) resulted in slightly decreased growth and slight skeletal immaturity of the fetuses. Immaturity was manifested by increased incidence of incomplete or unossified calcanei and phalangeal nuclei of the hind limb and of incompletely ossified sternebrae. At oral doses 60 times the usual daily human dose (based on a 60-kg human), a slightly lower rate of implantation was found in the rat. Regitine did not affect embryonic or fetal development in the rabbit at oral doses 20 times the usual daily human dose (based on a 60-kg human). No teratogenic or embryotoxic effects were observed in the rat, mouse, or rabbit studies. There are no adequate and well-controlled studies in pregnant women. Regitine should be used during pregnancy only if the potential benefit justifies the potential risk to the fetus.

Nursing Mothers

It is not known whether this drug is excreted in human milk. Because many drugs are excreted in human milk and because of the potential for serious adverse reactions in nursing infants from Regitine, a decision should be made whether to discontinue nursing or to discontinue the drug, taking into account the importance of the drug to the mother.

Pediatric Use

See **DOSAGE AND ADMINISTRATION.**

ADVERSE REACTIONS

Acute and prolonged hypotensive episodes, tachycardia, and cardiac arrhythmias have been reported. In addition, weakness, dizziness, flushing, orthostatic hypotension, nasal stuffiness, nausea, vomiting, and diarrhea may occur.

OVERDOSAGE

Acute Toxicity

No deaths due to acute poisoning with Regitine have been reported.

Oral LD_{50}'s (mg/kg): mice, 1000; rats, 1250.

Signs and Symptoms

Overdosage with Regitine is characterized chiefly by cardiovascular disturbances, such as arrhythmias, tachycardia, hypotension, and possibly shock. In addition, the following might occur: excitation, headache, sweating, pupillary contraction, visual disturbances; nausea, vomiting, diarrhea; hypoglycemia.

Treatment

There is no specific antidote.

A decrease in blood pressure to dangerous levels or other evidence of shocklike conditions should be treated vigorously and promptly. The patient's legs should be kept raised and a plasma expander should be administered. If necessary, intravenous infusion of norepinephrine, titrated to maintain blood pressure at the normotensive level, and all available supportive measures should be included. Epinephrine should not be used, since it may cause a paradoxical reduction in blood pressure.

DOSAGE AND ADMINISTRATION

The reconstituted solution should be used upon preparation and should not be stored.

Note: Parenteral drug products should be inspected visually for particulate matter and discoloration prior to administration, whenever solution and container permit.

1. Prevention or control of hypertensive episodes in the patient with pheochromocytoma.

For preoperative reduction of elevated blood pressure, 5 mg of Regitine (1 mg for children) is injected intravenously or intramuscularly 1 or 2 hours before surgery, and repeated if necessary.

During surgery, Regitine (5 mg for adults, 1 mg for children) is administered intravenously as indicated, to help prevent or control paroxysms of hypertension, tachycardia, respiratory depression, convulsions, or other effects of epinephrine intoxication. (Postoperatively, norepinephrine may be given to control the hypotension that commonly follows complete removal of a pheochromocytoma.)

2. Prevention or treatment of dermal necrosis and sloughing following intravenous administration or extravasation of norepinephrine.

For Prevention: 10 mg of Regitine is added to each liter of solution containing norepinephrine. The pressor effect of norepinephrine is not affected.

For Treatment: 5–10 mg of Regitine in 10 ml of saline is injected into the area of extravasation within 12 hours.

3. Diagnosis of pheochromocytoma—Regitine blocking test.

The test is most reliable in detecting pheochromocytoma in patients with sustained hypertension and least reliable in those with paroxysmal hypertension. False-positive tests may occur in patients with hypertension without pheochromocytoma.

a. Intravenous

Preparation

The **CONTRAINDICATIONS**, **WARNINGS**, and **PRECAUTIONS** sections should be reviewed. Sedatives, analgesics, and all other medications except those that might be deemed essential (such as digitalis and insulin) are withheld for at least 24 hours, and preferably 48–72 hours, prior to the test. Antihypertensive drugs are withheld until blood pressure returns to the untreated, hypertensive level. This test is not performed on a patient who is normotensive.

Procedure

The patient is kept at rest in the supine position throughout the test, preferably in a quiet, darkened room. Injection of Regitine is delayed until blood pressure is stabilized, as evidenced by blood pressure readings taken every 10 minutes for at least 30 minutes.

Five milligrams of Regitine is dissolved in 1 ml of Sterile Water for Injection. The dose for adults is 5 mg; for children, 1 mg.

The syringe needle is inserted into the vein, and injection is delayed until pressor response to venipuncture has subsided.

Regitine is injected rapidly. Blood pressure is recorded immediately after injection, at 30-second intervals for the first 3 minutes, and at 60-second intervals for the next 7 minutes.

Interpretation

A positive response, suggestive of pheochromocytoma, is indicated when the blood pressure is reduced more than 35 mmHg systolic and 25 mmHg diastolic. A typical positive response is a reduction in pressure of 60 mmHg systolic and 25 mmHg diastolic. Usually, maximal effect is evident within 2 minutes after injection. A return to preinjection pressure commonly occurs within 15–30 minutes but may occur more rapidly.

If blood pressure decreases to a dangerous level, the patient should be treated as outlined under **OVERDOSAGE.**

A positive response should always be confirmed by other diagnostic procedures, preferably by measurement of urinary catecholamines or their metabolites.

A negative response is indicated when the blood pressure is elevated, unchanged, or reduced less than 35 mmHg systolic and 25 mmHg diastolic after injection of Regitine. A negative reponse to this test does not exclude the diagnosis of pheochromocytoma, especially in patients with paroxysmal hypertension in whom the incidence of false-negative responses is high.

b. Intramuscular

If the intramuscular test for pheochromocytoma is preferred, preparation is the same as for the intravenous test. Five milligrams of Regitine is then dissolved in 1 ml of Sterile Water for Injection. The dose for adults is 5 mg intramuscularly; for children, 3 mg. Blood pressure is recorded every 5 minutes for 30–45 minutes following injection. A positive response is indicated when the blood pressure is reduced 35 mmHg systolic and 25 mmHg diastolic, or more, within 20 minutes following injection.

HOW SUPPLIED

Vials—each containing 5 mg of phentolamine mesylate USP and 25 mg of mannitol USP, in lyophilized form

Cartons of 2 .... NDC 0083-6830-02

The reconstituted solution should be used upon preparation and should not be stored.

Store between 59° and 86°F.

Distributed by
Novartis Pharmaceuticals Corporation
East Hanover, New Jersey 07936

C98-25 (Rev. 6/98)

RESTORIL® CIV ℞

[res 'tah-ril "]

(temazepam) capsules, USP

CAUTION: Federal law prohibits dispensing without prescription.

The following prescribing information is based on official labeling in effect on August 1, 1998.

DESCRIPTION

Restoril® (temazepam) is a benzodiazepine hypnotic agent. The chemical name is 7-chloro-1,3-dihydro-3-hydroxy-1-methyl-5-phenyl-2*H*-1,4-benzodiazepin-2-one, and the structural formula is:

[See chemical structure at top of next column]

Temazepam is a white, crystalline substance, very slightly soluble in water and sparingly soluble in alcohol, USP.

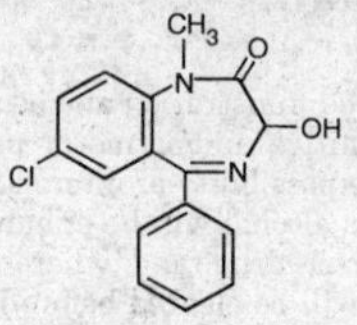

$C_{16}H_{13}ClN_2O_2$ Mol. wt. 300.74

Restoril® (temazepam) capsules, 7.5 mg, 15 mg, and 30 mg, are for oral administration.

7.5 mg, 15 mg, and 30 mg Capsules

Active Ingredient: temazepam, USP

7.5 mg Capsules

Inactive Ingredients: FD&C Blue #1, FD&C Red #3, gelatin, lactose, magnesium stearate, sodium lauryl sulfate, synthetic red ferric oxide, titanium dioxide, and other ingredients.

May also include: benzyl alcohol, butylparaben, carboxymethylcellulose sodium, edetate calcium disodium, methylparaben, propylparaben, silicon dioxide, and sodium propionate.

15 mg Capsules

Inactive Ingredients: FD&C Blue #1, FD&C Red #3, gelatin, lactose, magnesium stearate, sodium lauryl sulfate, synthetic red ferric oxide, titanium dioxide, and other ingredients.

May also include: benzyl alcohol, butylparaben, carboxymethylcellulose sodium, edetate calcium disodium, methylparaben, propylparaben, silicon dioxide, and sodium propionate.

30 mg Capsules

Inactive Ingredients: FD&C Blue #1, FD&C Red #3, gelatin, lactose, magnesium stearate, sodium lauryl sulfate, titanium dioxide, and other ingredients.

May also include: benzyl alcohol, butylparaben, carboxymethylcellulose sodium, edetate calcium disodium, methylparaben, propylparaben, silicon dioxide, and sodium propionate.

CLINICAL PHARMACOLOGY

Pharmacokinetics

In a single and multiple dose absorption, distribution, metabolism, and excretion (ADME) study, using ^3H labeled drug, Restoril® (temazepam) was well absorbed and found to have minimal (8%) first pass metabolism. There were no active metabolites formed and the only significant metabolite present in blood was the O-conjugate. The unchanged drug was 96% bound to plasma proteins. The blood level decline of the parent drug was biphasic with the short half-life ranging from 0.4-0.6 hours and the terminal half-life from 3.5-18.4 hours (mean 8.8 hours), depending on the study population and method of determination. Metabolites were formed with a half-life of 10 hours and excreted with a half-life of approximately 2 hours. Thus, formation of the major metabolite is the rate limiting step in the biodisposition of temazepam. There is no accumulation of metabolites. A dose-proportional relationship has been established for the area under the plasma concentration/time curve over the 15-30 mg dose range.

Temazepam was completely metabolized through conjugation prior to excretion; 80%-90% of the dose appeared in the urine. The major metabolite was the O-conjugate of temazepam (90%); the O-conjugate of N-desmethyl temazepam was a minor metabolite (7%).

Bioavailability, Induction, and Plasma Levels

Following ingestion of a 30 mg Restoril® (temazepam) capsule, measurable plasma concentrations were achieved 10-20 minutes after dosing with peak plasma levels ranging from 666-982 ng/mL (mean 865 ng/mL) occurring approximately 1.2-1.6 hours (mean 1.5 hours) after dosing.

In a 7 day study, in which subjects were given a 30 mg Restoril® (temazepam) capsule 1 hour before retiring, steady-state (as measured by the attainment of maximal trough concentrations) was achieved by the third dose. Mean plasma levels of temazepam (for days 2-7) were 260 ± 210 ng/mL at 9 hours and 75 ± 80 ng/mL at 24 hours after dosing. A slight trend toward declining 24 hour plasma levels was seen after day 4 in the study, however, the 24 hour plasma levels were quite variable.

At a dose of 30 mg once-a-day for 8 weeks, no evidence of enzyme induction was found in man.

Elimination Rate of Benzodiazepine Hypnotics and Profile of Common Untoward Effects

The type and duration of hypnotic effects and the profile of unwanted effects during administration of benzodiazepine hypnotics may be influenced by the biologic half-life of the administered drug and for some hypnotics, the half-life of any active metabolites formed. Benzodiazepine hypnotics have a spectrum of half-lives from short (<4 hours) to long (>20 hours). When half-lives are long, drug (and for some drugs their active metabolites) may accumulate during

Continued on next page

Restoril—Cont.

periods of nightly administration and be associated with impairments of cognitive and/or motor performance during waking hours; the possibility of interaction with other psychoactive drugs or alcohol will be enhanced. In contrast, if half-lives are shorter, drug (and, where appropriate, its active metabolites) will be cleared before the next dose is ingested, and carry-over effects related to excessive sedation or CNS depression should be minimal or absent. However, during nightly use for an extended period, pharmacodynamic tolerance or adaptation to some effects of benzodiazepine hypnotics may develop. If the drug has a short elimination half-life, it is possible that a relative deficiency of the drug, or, if appropriate, its active metabolites (i.e., in relationship to the receptor site) may occur at some point in the interval between each night's use. This sequence of events may account for 2 clinical findings reported to occur after several weeks of nightly use of rapidly eliminated benzodiazepine hypnotics, namely, increased wakefulness during the last third of the night, and the appearance of increased signs of daytime anxiety.

Controlled Trials Supporting Efficacy

Restoril® (temazepam) improved sleep parameters in clinical studies. Residual medication effects ("hangover") were essentially absent. Early morning awakening, a particular problem in the geriatric patient, was significantly reduced. Patients with chronic insomnia were evaluated in 2 week, placebo controlled sleep laboratory studies with Restoril® (temazepam) at doses of 7.5 mg, 15 mg, and 30 mg, given 30 minutes prior to bedtime. There was a linear dose-response improvement in total sleep time and sleep latency, with significant drug-placebo differences at 2 weeks occurring only for total sleep time at the 2 higher doses, and for sleep latency only at the highest dose.

In these sleep laboratory studies, REM sleep was essentially unchanged and slow wave sleep was decreased. No measurable effects on daytime alertness or performance occurred following Restoril® (temazepam) treatment or during the withdrawal period, even though a transient sleep disturbance in some sleep parameters was observed following withdrawal of the higher doses. There was no evidence of tolerance development in the sleep laboratory parameters when patients were given Restoril® (temazepam) nightly for at least 2 weeks.

In addition, normal subjects with transient insomnia associated with first night adaptation to the sleep laboratory were evaluated in 24 hour, placebo controlled sleep laboratory studies with Restoril® (temazepam) at doses of 7.5 mg, 15 mg, and 30 mg, given 30 minutes prior to bedtime. There was a linear dose-response improvement in total sleep time, sleep latency and number of awakenings, with significant drug-placebo differences occurring for sleep latency at all doses, for total sleep time at the 2 higher doses and for number of awakenings only at the 30 mg dose.

INDICATIONS AND USAGE

Restoril® (temazepam) is indicated for the short-term treatment of insomnia (generally 7-10 days). For patients in whom the drug is used for more than 2-3 weeks, periodic reevaluation is recommended to determine whether there is a continuing need. *(See WARNINGS)*

For patients with short-term insomnia, instructions in the prescription should indicate that Restoril® (temazepam) should be used for short periods of time (7-10 days).

Restoril® (temazepam) should not be prescribed in quantities exceeding a 1-month supply.

Insomnia is characterized by complaints of difficulty in falling asleep, frequent nocturnal awakenings, and/or early morning awakenings. Both sleep laboratory and outpatient studies provide support for the effectiveness of Restoril® (temazepam) administered 30 minutes before bedtime in decreasing sleep latency and improving sleep maintenance in patients with chronic insomnia. In addition, sleep laboratory studies have confirmed similar effects in normal subjects with transient insomnia *(see CLINICAL PHARMACOLOGY)*.

CONTRAINDICATIONS

Benzodiazepines may cause fetal damage when administered during pregnancy. An increased risk of congenital malformations associated with the use of diazepam and chlordiazepoxide during the first trimester of pregnancy has been suggested in several studies. Transplacental distribution has resulted in neonatal CNS depression following the ingestion of therapeutic doses of a benzodiazepine hypnotic during the last weeks of pregnancy.

Reproduction studies in animals with temazepam were performed in rats and rabbits. In a perinatal-postnatal study in rats, oral doses of 60 mg/kg/day resulted in increasing nursling mortality. Teratology studies in rats demonstrated increased fetal resorptions at doses of 30 and 120 mg/kg in one study and increased occurrence of rudimentary ribs, which are considered skeletal variants, in a second study at doses of 240 mg/kg or higher. In rabbits, occasional abnormalities such as exencephaly and fusion or asymmetry of ribs were

reported without dose relationship. Although these abnormalities were not found in the concurrent control group, they have been reported to occur randomly in historical controls. At doses of 40 mg/kg or higher, there was an increased incidence of the 13th rib variant when compared to the incidence in concurrent and historical controls.

Restoril® (temazepam) is contraindicated in pregnant women. If there is a likelihood of the patient becoming pregnant while receiving temazepam, she should be warned of the potential risk to the fetus. Patients should be instructed to discontinue the drug prior to becoming pregnant. The possibility that a woman of childbearing potential may be pregnant at the time of institution of therapy should be considered.

WARNINGS

Sleep disturbance may be the presenting manifestation of an underlying physical and/or psychiatric disorder. Consequently, a decision to initiate symptomatic treatment of insomnia should only be made after the patient has been carefully evaluated.

The failure of insomnia to remit after 7-10 days of treatment may indicate the presence of a primary psychiatric and/or medical illness.

Worsening of insomnia may be the consequence of an unrecognized psychiatric or physical disorder as may the emergence of new abnormalities of thinking or behavior. Such abnormalities have also been reported to occur in association with the use of drugs with central nervous system depressant activity, including those of the benzodiazepine class. Some of these changes may be characterized by decreased inhibition, e.g., aggressiveness and extroversion that seem out of character, similar to that seen with alcohol. Other kinds of behavioral changes can also occur, for example, bizarre behavior, agitation, hallucinations, depersonalization, and, in primarily depressed patients, the worsening of depression, including suicidal thinking. In controlled clinical trials involving 1076 patients on Restoril® (temazepam) and 783 patients on placebo, reports of hallucinations, agitation, and overstimulation occurred at rates less than 1 in 100 patients. Hallucinations were reported in 2 Restoril® (temazepam) patients and 1 placebo patient; agitation was reported in 1 Restoril® (temazepam) patient; 2 Restoril® (temazepam) patients reported overstimulation. There were no reports of worsening of depression or suicidal ideation, aggressiveness, extroversion, bizarre behavior or depersonalization in these controlled clinical trials.

It can rarely be determined with certainty whether a particular instance of the abnormal behaviors listed above is drug induced, spontaneous in origin, or a result of an underlying psychiatric or physical disorder. Nonetheless, the emergence of any new behavioral sign or symptom of concern requires careful and immediate evaluation.

Because some of the worrisome adverse effects of benzodiazepines, including Restoril® (temazepam), appear to be dose related *(see PRECAUTIONS and DOSAGE AND ADMINISTRATION)*, it is important to use the lowest possible effective dose. Elderly patients are especially at risk.

Patients receiving Restoril® (temazepam) should be cautioned about possible combined effects with alcohol and other CNS depressants.

Withdrawal symptoms (of the barbiturate type) have occurred after the abrupt discontinuation of benzodiazepines *(see DRUG ABUSE AND DEPENDENCE)*.

PRECAUTIONS

General

Since the risk of the development of oversedation, dizziness, confusion, and/or ataxia increases substantially with larger doses of benzodiazepines in elderly and debilitated patients, 7.5 mg of Restoril® (temazepam) is recommended as the initial dosage for such patients.

Restoril® (temazepam) should be administered with caution in severely depressed patients or those in whom there is any evidence of latent depression; it should be recognized that suicidal tendencies may be present and protective measures may be necessary.

The usual precautions should be observed in patients with impaired renal or hepatic function and in patients with chronic pulmonary insufficiency.

If Restoril® (temazepam) is to be combined with other drugs having known hypnotic properties or CNS-depressant effects, consideration should be given to potential additive effects.

The possibility of a synergistic effect exists with the co-administration of Restoril® (temazepam) and diphenhydramine. One case of stillbirth at term has been reported 8 hours after a pregnant patient received Restoril® (temazepam) and diphenhydramine. A cause and effect relationship has not yet been determined. *(See CONTRAINDICATIONS)*

Information for Patients

The text of a patient package insert is printed at the end of this insert. To assure safe and effective use of Restoril® (temazepam), the information and instructions provided in this patient package insert should be discussed with patients.

Laboratory Tests

The usual precautions should be observed in patients with impaired renal or hepatic function and in patients with chronic pulmonary insufficiency. Abnormal liver function tests as well as blood dyscrasias have been reported with benzodiazepines.

Drug Interactions

The pharmacokinetic profile of temazepam does not appear to be altered by orally administered cimetidine dosed according to labeling.

Carcinogenesis, Mutagenesis, Impairment of Fertility

Carcinogenicity studies were conducted in rats at dietary temazepam doses up to 160 mg/kg/day for 24 months and in mice at dietary dose of 160 mg/kg/day for 18 months. No evidence of carcinogenicity was observed although hyperplastic liver nodules were observed in female mice exposed to the highest dose. The clinical significance of this finding is not known.

Fertility in male and female rats was not adversely affected by Restoril® (temazepam).

No mutagenicity tests have been done with temazepam.

Pregnancy

Pregnancy Category X *(see CONTRAINDICATIONS)*.

Nursing Mothers

It is not known whether this drug is excreted in human milk. Because many drugs are excreted in human milk, caution should be exercised when Restoril® (temazepam) is administered to a nursing woman.

Pediatric Use

Safety and effectiveness in pediatric patients have not been established.

ADVERSE REACTIONS

During controlled clinical studies in which 1076 patients received Restoril® (temazepam) at bedtime, the drug was well tolerated. Side effects were usually mild and transient. Adverse reactions occurring in 1% or more of patients are presented in the following table:

	Restoril® (temazepam) % Incidence (n=1076)	Placebo % Incidence (n=783)
Drowsiness	9.1	5.6
Headache	8.5	9.1
Fatigue	4.8	4.7
Nervousness	4.6	8.2
Lethargy	4.5	3.4
Dizziness	4.5	3.3
Nausea	3.1	3.8
Hangover	2.5	1.1
Anxiety	2.0	1.5
Depression	1.7	1.8
Dry Mouth	1.7	2.2
Diarrhea	1.7	1.1
Abdominal Discomfort	1.5	1.9
Euphoria	1.5	0.4
Weakness	1.4	0.9
Confusion	1.3	0.5
Blurred Vision	1.3	1.3
Nightmares	1.2	1.7
Vertigo	1.2	0.8

The following adverse events have been reported less frequently (0.5-0.9%):

Central Nervous System – anorexia, ataxia, equilibrium loss, tremor, increased dreaming

Cardiovascular – dyspnea, palpitations

Gastrointestinal – vomiting

Musculoskeletal – backache

Special Senses – hyperhidrosis, burning eyes

Amnesia, hallucinations, horizontal nystagmus, and paradoxical reactions including restlessness, overstimulation and agitation were rare (less than 0.5%).

DRUG ABUSE AND DEPENDENCE

Controlled Substance

Restoril® (temazepam) is a controlled substance in Schedule IV.

Abuse and Dependence

Withdrawal symptoms, similar in character to those noted with barbiturates and alcohol (convulsions, tremor, abdominal, and muscle cramps, vomiting, and sweating), have occurred following abrupt discontinuance of benzodiazepines. The more severe withdrawal symptoms have usually been limited to those patients who received excessive doses over an extended period of time. Generally milder withdrawal symptoms (e.g., dysphoria and insomnia) have been reported following abrupt discontinuance of benzodiazepines taken continuously at therapeutic levels for several months. Consequently, after extended therapy at doses higher than 15 mg, abrupt discontinuation should generally be avoided and a gradual dosage tapering schedule followed. As with any hypnotic, caution must be exercised in administering Restoril® (temazepam) to individuals known to be

addiction-prone or to those whose history suggests they may increase the dosage on their own initiative. It is desirable to limit repeated prescriptions without adequate medical supervision.

OVERDOSAGE

Manifestations of acute overdosage of Restoril® (temazepam) can be expected to reflect the CNS effects of the drug and include somnolence, confusion, and coma, with reduced or absent reflexes, respiratory depression, and hypotension. The oral LD_{50} of Restoril® (temazepam) was 1963 mg/kg in mice, 1833 mg/kg in rats, and >2400 mg/kg in rabbits.

Treatment

If the patient is conscious, vomiting should be induced mechanically or with emetics. Gastric lavage should be employed utilizing concurrently a cuffed endotracheal tube if the patient is unconscious to prevent aspiration and pulmonary complications. Maintenance of adequate pulmonary ventilation is essential. The use of pressor agents intravenously may be necessary to combat hypotension. Fluids should be administered intravenously to encourage diuresis. The value of dialysis has not been determined. If excitation occurs, barbiturates should not be used. It should be borne in mind that multiple agents may have been ingested. Flumazenil (Romazicon®)*, a specific benzodiazepine receptor antagonist, is indicated for the complete or partial reversal of the sedative effects of benzodiazepines and may be used in situations when an overdose with a benzodiazepine is known or suspected. Prior to the administration of flumazenil, necessary measures should be instituted to secure airway, ventilation, and intravenous access. Flumazenil is intended as an adjunct to, not as a substitute for, proper management of benzodiazepine overdose. Patients treated with flumazenil should be monitored for re-sedation, respiratory depression, and other residual benzodiazepine effects for an appropriate period after treatment. **The prescriber should be aware of a risk of seizure in association with flumazenil treatment, particularly in long-term benzodiazepine users and in cyclic antidepressant overdose.** The complete flumazenil package insert including CONTRAINDICATIONS, WARNINGS, and PRECAUTIONS should be consulted prior to use.

Up-to-date information about the treatment of overdose can often be obtained from a certified Regional Poison Control Center. Telephone numbers of certified Regional Poison Control Centers are listed in the Physicians' Desk Reference®**.

DOSAGE AND ADMINISTRATION

While the recommended usual adult dose is 15 mg before retiring, 7.5 mg may be sufficient for some patients, and others may need 30 mg. In transient insomnia, a 7.5 mg dose may be sufficient to improve sleep latency. In elderly or debilitated patients, it is recommended that therapy be initiated with 7.5 mg until individual responses are determined.

HOW SUPPLIED

Restoril® (temazepam) Capsules, USP
7.5 mg
Blue and pink, imprinted "Restoril 7.5 mg" and "FOR SLEEP" twice on each capsule. Bottle of 100, NDC 0078-0140-05; and SandoPak® (unit-dose) package of 100 individually labeled blisters, each containing one capsule, NDC 0078-0140-06.
15 mg
Maroon and pink capsule imprinted "Restoril 15 mg" and "FOR SLEEP" twice on each capsule. Bottle of 100, NDC 0078-0098-05; bottle of 500, NDC 0078-0098-08; and SandoPak® (unit-dose) package of 100 individually labeled blisters, each containing one capsule, NDC 0078-0098-06.
30 mg
Maroon and blue capsule, imprinted "Restoril 30 mg" and "FOR SLEEP" twice on each capsule. Bottle of 100, NDC 0078-0099-05; bottle of 500, NDC 0078-0099-08; and SandoPak® (unit-dose) package of 100 individually labeled blisters, each containing one capsule, NDC 0078-0099-06.

Store and Dispense
Store in a tight, light-resistant container, below 86°F (30°C).

PATIENT INFORMATION

Introduction

Your doctor has prescribed Restoril® (temazepam) to help you sleep. The following information is intended to guide you in the safe use of this medicine. It is not meant to take the place of your doctor's instructions. If you have any questions about Restoril® (temazepam) capsules be sure to ask your doctor or pharmacist.

Restoril® (temazepam) is used to treat different types of sleep problems, such as:
• trouble falling asleep
• waking up too early in the morning
• waking up often during the night

Some people may have more than one of these problems. Restoril® (temazepam) belongs to a group of medicines known as the "benzodiazepines." There are many different benzodiazepine medicines used to help people sleep better. Sleep problems are usually temporary, requiring treatment

for only a short time, usually 7-10 days. However, if your sleep problems continue, consult your doctor. He/she will determine whether other measures are needed to overcome your sleep problems. Some people have chronic sleep problems that may require more prolonged use of sleep medicine. However, you should not use these medicines for long periods without talking with your doctor about the risks and benefits of prolonged use.

SIDE EFFECTS

Common Side Effects

All medicines have side effects. The most common side effects of benzodiazepine sleeping medicines include:
• drowsiness
• dizziness
• lightheadedness
• difficulty with coordination

You may find that these medicines make you sleepy during the day. How drowsy you feel depends upon how your body reacts to the medicine, which benzodiazepine sleeping medicine you are taking, and how large a dose your doctor has prescribed. Day-time drowsiness is best avoided by taking the lowest dose possible that will still help you to sleep at night. Your doctor will work with you to find the dose of Restoril® (temazepam) that is best for you.

To manage these side effects while you are taking this medicine:
• Use extreme care while doing anything that requires complete alertness, such as driving a car, operating machinery, or piloting an aircraft. As with any medicines used to help people sleep better, you should be very careful when you first start taking Restoril® (temazepam) until you know how the medicine will affect you.
• NEVER drink alcohol while you are being treated with Restoril® (temazepam) or any benzodiazepine medicine. Alcohol can increase the side effects of Restoril® (temazepam) or any other benzodiazepine medicine.
• Do not take any other medicines without asking your doctor first. This includes medicines you can buy without a prescription. Some medicines can cause drowsiness and are best avoided while taking Restoril® (temazepam).
• Always take the exact dose of Restoril® (temazepam) prescribed by your doctor. Never change your dose without talking to your doctor first.

SPECIAL CONCERNS

There are some special problems that may occur while taking benzodiazepine sleeping medicines.

Memory Problems

Benzodiazepine sleeping medicines may cause a special type of memory loss or "amnesia". When this occurs, a person may not remember what has happened for several hours after taking the medicine. This is usually not a problem since most people fall asleep after taking the medicine. Memory loss can be a problem, however, when sleeping medicines are taken while traveling, such as during an airplane flight and the person wakes up before the effect of the medicine is gone. This has been called "traveler's amnesia". Memory problems were noticed in fewer than 1 in 100 patients taking Restoril® (temazepam) in clinical trials. Memory problems can be avoided if you take Restoril® (temazepam) only when you are able to get a full night's sleep (7-8 hours) before you need to be active again. Be sure to talk to your doctor if you think you are having memory problems.

Tolerance

When benzodiazepine sleeping medicines are used every night for more than a few weeks, they may lose their effectiveness to help you sleep. This is known as "tolerance."
If tolerance to the medicine develops, other effects may occur depending upon which benzodiazepine sleeping medicine you are taking. Tolerance to benzodiazepine sleeping medicines that are shorter-acting may cause you to:
• wake up during the last third of the night
• become anxious or nervous while you are awake
These effects are less common with Restoril® (temazepam) because it is intermediate-acting.

Dependence

All the benzodiazepine sleeping medicines can cause dependence, especially when these medicines are used regularly for longer than a few weeks or at high doses. Some people develop a need to continue taking their medicines. This is known as dependence or "addiction."
When people develop dependence, they may have difficulty stopping the benzodiazepine sleeping medicine. If the medicine is suddenly stopped, the body is not able to function normally and unpleasant symptoms may occur (see Withdrawal). They may find they have to keep taking the medicine either at the prescribed dose or at increasing doses just to avoid withdrawal symptoms.
All people taking benzodiazepine sleeping medicines have some risk of becoming dependent on the medicine. However, people who have been dependent on alcohol or other drugs in the past may have a higher chance of becoming addicted to benzodiazepine medicines. This possibility must be considered before using these medicines for more than a few weeks.

If you have been addicted to alcohol or drugs in the past, it is important to tell your doctor before starting Restoril® (temazepam) or any benzodiazepine sleeping medicine.

Withdrawal

Withdrawal symptoms may occur when a benzodiazepine sleeping medicine is stopped suddenly after being used daily for a long time. But these symptoms can occur even if the medicine has been used for only a week or two.
In mild cases, withdrawal symptoms may include unpleasant feelings. In more severe cases, abdominal and muscle cramps, vomiting, sweating, shakiness, and rarely, seizures may occur. These more severe withdrawal symptoms are very uncommon.
Another problem that may occur when benzodiazepine sleeping medicines are stopped is known as "rebound insomnia". This means that a person may have more trouble sleeping the first few nights after the medicine is stopped than before starting the medicine. If you should experience rebound insomnia, do not get discouraged. This problem usually goes away on its own after 1 or 2 nights.
If you have been taking Restoril® (temazepam) or any other benzodiazepine sleeping medicine for more than 1 or 2 weeks, do not stop taking it on your own. Your doctor may give you special directions on how to gradually decrease your dose before stopping the medicine. Always follow your doctor's directions.

Changes in Behavior and Thinking

Some people using benzodiazepine sleeping medicines have experienced unusual changes in their thinking and/or behavior, including: more outgoing or aggressive behavior than normal; loss of personal identity; confusion; strange behavior; agitation; hallucinations; worsening of depression; and suicidal thoughts.
How often these effects occur depends on several factors, such as a person's general health or the use of other medicines. Clinical studies with Restoril® (temazepam) revealed that unusual behavior changes occurred in less than 1 in 100 patients.
It is also important to realize that it is rarely clear whether these behavior changes are caused by the medicine, an illness, or occur on their own. In fact, sleep problems that do not improve may be due to illnesses that were present before the medicine was used. If you or your family notice any changes in your behavior, or if you have any unusual or disturbing thoughts, call your doctor immediately.

Pregnancy

Certain benzodiazepines have been linked to birth defects when taken by a pregnant woman in the early months of pregnancy. These medicines can also cause sedation of the unborn baby when used during the last weeks of pregnancy. Restoril® (temazepam) should not be taken at any time during pregnancy. Be sure to tell your doctor if you are pregnant, if you are planning to become pregnant, or if you become pregnant while taking Restoril® (temazepam).

SAFE USE OF BENZODIAZEPINE SLEEPING MEDICINES

To ensure the safe and effective use of Restoril® (temazepam) or any other benzodiazepine sleeping medicine, you should observe the following cautions:
1. Restoril® (temazepam) is a prescription medicine and should be used ONLY as directed by your doctor. Follow your doctor's instructions about how to take, when to take, and how long to take Restoril® (temazepam).
2. Never use Restoril® (temazepam) or any other benzodiazepine sleeping medicine for longer than 1 or 2 weeks without first asking your doctor.
3. If you notice any unusual or disturbing thoughts or behavior during treatment with Restoril® (temazepam) or any other benzodiazepine sleeping medicine, contact your doctor.
4. Tell your doctor about any medicines you may be taking, including medicines you may buy without a prescription. You should also tell your doctor if you drink alcohol. DO NOT use alcohol while taking Restoril® (temazepam) or any other benzodiazepine sleeping medicine.
5. Do not take Restoril® (temazepam) or any other benzodiazepine sleeping medicine unless you are able to get a full night's sleep before you must be active again. For example, Restoril® (temazepam) or any other benzodiazepine sleeping medicine should not be taken on an overnight airplane flight of less than 7-8 hours since "traveler's amnesia" may occur.
6. Do not increase the prescribed dose of Restoril® (temazepam) or any other benzodiazepine sleeping medicine unless instructed by your doctor.
7. Use extreme care while doing anything that requires complete alertness, such as driving a car, operating machinery, or piloting an aircraft when you first start taking Restoril® (temazepam) or any other benzodi-

Continued on next page

Restoril—Cont.

azepine sleeping medicine until you know whether the medicine will still have some carryover effect in you the next day.

8. Be aware that you may have more sleeping problems (rebound insomnia) the first night or two after stopping Restoril® (temazepam) or any other benzodiazepine sleeping medicine.
9. Be sure to tell your doctor if you are pregnant, if you are planning to become pregnant, or if you become pregnant while taking Restoril® (temazepam). Restoril® (temazepam) or any other benzodiazepine sleeping medicine should not be taken at any time during pregnancy.
10. As with all prescription medicines, never share Restoril® (temazepam) or any other benzodiazepine sleeping medicine with anyone else. Always store Restoril® (temazepam) or any other benzodiazepine sleeping medicine in the original container out of reach of children.

[REV: OCTOBER 1996 30282902]

* Romazicon is the registered trademark of Roche Laboratories.

** Medical Economics Company, Inc.

Shown in Product Identification Guide, page 325

RITALIN® hydrochloride CII
[rit 'ah-lin]
methylphenidate hydrochloride
tablets USP
RITALIN-SR® CII
methylphenidate hydrochloride USP
sustained-release tablets

Caution: Federal law prohibits dispensing without prescription.

The following prescribing information is based on official labeling in effect August 1, 1998.

Prescribing Information

DESCRIPTION

Ritalin hydrochloride, methylphenidate hydrochloride USP, is a mild central nervous system (CNS) stimulant, available as tablets of 5, 10, and 20 mg for oral administration; Ritalin-SR is available as sustained-release tablets of 20 mg for oral administration. Methylphenidate hydrochloride is methyl α-phenyl-2-piperidineacetate hydrochloride, and its structural formula is

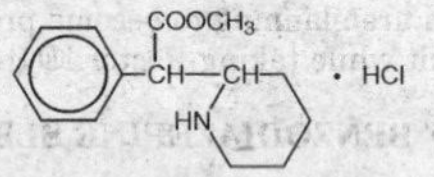
COOCH₃
CH—CH
· HCl
HN

Methylphenidate hydrochloride USP is a white, odorless, fine crystalline powder. Its solutions are acid to litmus. It is freely soluble in water and in methanol, soluble in alcohol, and slightly soluble in chloroform and in acetone. Its molecular weight is 269.77.

Inactive Ingredients. Ritalin tablets: D&C Yellow No. 10 (5-mg and 20-mg tablets), FD&C Green No. 3 (10-mg tablets), lactose, magnesium stearate, polyethylene glycol, starch (5-mg and 10-mg tablets), sucrose, talc, and tragacanth (20-mg tablets).

Ritalin-SR tablets: Cellulose compounds, cetostearyl alcohol, lactose, magnesium stearate, mineral oil, povidone, titanium dioxide, and zein.

CLINICAL PHARMACOLOGY

Ritalin is a mild central nervous system stimulant.

The mode of action in man is not completely understood, but Ritalin presumably activates the brain stem arousal system and cortex to produce its stimulant effect.

There is neither specific evidence which clearly establishes the mechanism whereby Ritalin produces its mental and behavioral effects in children, nor conclusive evidence regarding how these effects relate to the condition of the central nervous system.

Ritalin in the SR tablets is more slowly but as extensively absorbed as in the regular tablets. Relative bioavailability of the SR tablet compared to the Ritalin tablet, measured by the urinary excretion of Ritalin major metabolite (α-phenyl-2-piperidine acetic acid) was 105% (49%-168%) in children and 101% (85%-152%) in adults. The time to peak rate in children was 4.7 hours (1.3-8.2 hours) for the SR tablets and 1.9 hours (0.3-4.4 hours) for the tablets. An average of 67% of SR tablet dose was excreted in children as compared to 86% in adults.

In a clinical study involving adult subjects who received SR tablets, plasma concentrations of Ritalin's major metabolite appeared to be greater in females than in males. No gender differences were observed for Ritalin plasma concentration in the same subjects.

INDICATIONS

Attention Deficit Disorders, Narcolepsy

Attention Deficit Disorders (previously known as Minimal Brain Dysfunction in Children). Other terms being used to describe the behavioral syndrome below include: Hyperkinetic Child Syndrome, Minimal Brain Damage, Minimal Cerebral Dysfunction, Minor Cerebral Dysfunction.

Ritalin is indicated as an integral part of a total treatment program which typically includes other remedial measures (psychological, educational, social) for a stabilizing effect in children with a behavioral syndrome characterized by the following group of developmentally inappropriate symptoms: moderate-to-severe distractibility, short attention span, hyperactivity, emotional lability, and impulsivity. The diagnosis of this syndrome should not be made with finality when these symptoms are only of comparatively recent origin. Nonlocalizing (soft) neurological signs, learning disability, and abnormal EEG may or may not be present, and a diagnosis of central nervous system dysfunction may or may not be warranted.

Special Diagnostic Considerations

Specific etiology of this syndrome is unknown, and there is no single diagnostic test. Adequate diagnosis requires the use not only of medical but of special psychological, educational, and social resources.

Characteristics commonly reported include: chronic history of short attention span, distractibility, emotional lability, impulsivity, and moderate-to-severe hyperactivity; minor neurological signs and abnormal EEG. Learning may or may not be impaired. The diagnosis must be based upon a complete history and evaluation of the child and not solely on the presence of one or more of these characteristics.

Drug treatment is not indicated for all children with this syndrome. Stimulants are not intended for use in the child who exhibits symptoms secondary to environmental factors and/or primary psychiatric disorders, including psychosis. Appropriate educational placement is essential and psychosocial intervention is generally necessary. When remedial measures alone are insufficient, the decision to prescribe stimulant medication will depend upon the physician's assessment of the chronicity and severity of the child's symptoms.

CONTRAINDICATIONS

Marked anxiety, tension, and agitation are contraindications to Ritalin, since the drug may aggravate these symptoms. Ritalin is contraindicated also in patients known to be hypersensitive to the drug, in patients with glaucoma, and in patients with motor tics or with a family history or diagnosis of Tourette's syndrome.

WARNINGS

Ritalin should not be used in children under six years, since safety and efficacy in this age group have not been established.

Sufficient data on safety and efficacy of long-term use of Ritalin in children are not yet available. Although a causal relationship has not been established, suppression of growth (i.e., weight gain, and/or height) has been reported with the long-term use of stimulants in children. Therefore, patients requiring long-term therapy should be carefully monitored.

Ritalin should not be used for severe depression of either exogenous or endogenous origin. Clinical experience suggests that in psychotic children, administration of Ritalin may exacerbate symptoms of behavior disturbance and thought disorder.

Ritalin should not be used for the prevention or treatment of normal fatigue states.

There is some clinical evidence that Ritalin may lower the convulsive threshold in patients with prior history of seizures, with prior EEG abnormalities in absence of seizures, and, very rarely, in absence of history of seizures and no prior EEG evidence of seizures. Safe concomitant use of anticonvulsants and Ritalin has not been established. In the presence of seizures, the drug should be discontinued.

Use cautiously in patients with hypertension. Blood pressure should be monitored at appropriate intervals in all patients taking Ritalin, especially those with hypertension.

Symptoms of visual disturbances have been encountered in rare cases. Difficulties with accommodation and blurring of vision have been reported.

Drug Interactions

Ritalin may decrease the hypotensive effect of guanethidine. Use cautiously with pressor agents and MAO inhibitors.

Human pharmacologic studies have shown that Ritalin may inhibit the metabolism of coumarin anticoagulants, anticonvulsants (phenobarbital, diphenylhydantoin, primidone), phenylbutazone, and tricyclic drugs (imipramine, clomipramine, desipramine). Downward dosage adjustments of these drugs may be required when given concomitantly with Ritalin.

Usage in Pregnancy

Adequate animal reproduction studies to establish safe use of Ritalin during pregnancy have not been conducted. Therefore, until more information is available, Ritalin should not be prescribed for women of childbearing age unless, in the opinion of the physician, the potential benefits outweigh the possible risks.

Drug Dependence

Ritalin should be given cautiously to emotionally unstable patients, such as those with a history of drug dependence or alcoholism, because such patients may increase dosage on their own initiative.

Chronically abusive use can lead to marked tolerance and psychic dependence with varying degrees of abnormal behavior. Frank psychotic episodes can occur, especially with parenteral abuse. Careful supervision is required during drug withdrawal, since severe depression as well as the effects of chronic overactivity can be unmasked. Long-term follow-up may be required because of the patient's basic personality disturbances.

PRECAUTIONS

Patients with an element of agitation may react adversely; discontinue therapy if necessary.

Periodic CBC, differential, and platelet counts are advised during prolonged therapy.

Drug treatment is not indicated in all cases of this behavioral syndrome and should be considered only in light of the complete history and evaluation of the child. The decision to prescribe Ritalin should depend on the physician's assessment of the chronicity and severity of the child's symptoms and their appropriateness for his/her age. Prescription should not depend solely on the presence of one or more of the behavioral characteristics.

When these symptoms are associated with acute stress reactions, treatment with Ritalin is usually not indicated.

Long-term effects of Ritalin in children have not been well established.

Carcinogenesis/Mutagenesis

In a lifetime carcinogenicity study carried out in B6C3F1 mice, methylphenidate caused an increase in hepatocellular adenomas and, in males only, an increase in hepatoblastomas, at a daily dose of approximately 60 mg/kg/day. This dose is approximately 30 times and 2.5 times the maximum recommended human dose on a mg/kg and mg/m^2 basis, respectively. Hepatoblastoma is a relatively rare rodent malignant tumor type. There was no increase in total malignant hepatic tumors. The mouse strain used is sensitive to the development of hepatic tumors, and the significance of these results to humans is unknown.

Methylphenidate did not cause any increases in tumors in a lifetime carcinogenicity study carried out in F344 rats; the highest dose used was approximately 45 mg/kg/day, which is approximately 22 times and 4 times the maximum recommended human dose on a mg/kg and mg/m^2 basis, respectively.

Methylphenidate was not mutagenic in the in vitro Ames reverse mutation assay or in the in vitro mouse lymphoma cell forward mutation assay. Sister chromatid exchanges and chromosome aberrations were increased, indicative of a weak clastogenic response, in an in vitro assay in cultured Chinese Hamster Ovary (CHO) cells. The genotoxic potential of methylphenidate has not been evaluated in an in vivo assay.

ADVERSE REACTIONS

Nervousness and insomnia are the most common adverse reactions but are usually controlled by reducing dosage and omitting the drug in the afternoon or evening. Other reactions include hypersensitivity (including skin rash, urticaria, fever, arthralgia, exfoliative dermatitis, erythema multiforme with histopathological findings of necrotizing vasculitis, and thrombocytopenic purpura); anorexia; nausea; dizziness; palpitations; headache; dyskinesia; drowsiness; blood pressure and pulse changes, both up and down; tachycardia; angina; cardiac arrhythmia; abdominal pain; weight loss during prolonged therapy. There have been rare reports of Tourette's syndrome. Toxic psychosis has been reported. Although a definite causal relationship has not been established, the following have been reported in patients taking this drug: instances of abnormal liver function, ranging from transaminase elevation to hepatic coma; isolated cases of cerebral arteritis and/or occlusion; leukopenia and/or anemia; transient depressed mood; a few instances of scalp hair loss. Very rare reports of neuroleptic malignant syndrome (NMS) have been received, and, in most of these, patients were concurrently receiving therapies associated with NMS. In a single report, a ten year old boy who had been taking methylphenidate for approximately 18 months experienced an NMS-like event within 45 minutes of ingesting his first dose of venlafaxine. It is uncertain whether this case represented a drug-drug interaction, a response to either drug alone, or some other cause.

In children, loss of appetite, abdominal pain, weight loss during prolonged therapy, insomnia, and tachycardia may occur more frequently; however, any of the other adverse reactions listed above may also occur.

DOSAGE AND ADMINISTRATION

Dosage should be individualized according to the needs and responses of the patient.

Adults

Tablets: Administer in divided doses 2 or 3 times daily, preferably 30 to 45 minutes before meals. Average dosage is 20 to 30 mg daily. Some patients may require 40 to 60 mg daily. In others, 10 to 15 mg daily will be adequate. Patients who are unable to sleep if medication is taken late in the day should take the last dose before 6 p.m.

SR Tablets: Ritalin-SR tablets have a duration of action of approximately 8 hours. Therefore, Ritalin-SR tablets may be used in place of Ritalin tablets when the 8-hour dosage of Ritalin-SR corresponds to the titrated 8-hour dosage of Ritalin. Ritalin-SR tablets must be swallowed whole and never crushed or chewed.

Children (6 years and over)

Ritalin should be initiated in small doses, with gradual weekly increments. Daily dosage above 60 mg is not recommended.

If improvement is not observed after appropriate dosage adjustment over a one-month period, the drug should be discontinued.

Tablets: Start with 5 mg twice daily (before breakfast and lunch) with gradual increments of 5 to 10 mg weekly.

SR Tablets: Ritalin-SR tablets have a duration of action of approximately 8 hours. Therefore, Ritalin-SR tablets may be used in place of Ritalin tablets when the 8-hour dosage of Ritalin-SR corresponds to the titrated 8-hour dosage of Ritalin. Ritalin-SR tablets must be swallowed whole and never crushed or chewed.

If paradoxical aggravation of symptoms or other adverse effects occur, reduce dosage, or, if necessary, discontinue the drug.

Ritalin should be periodically discontinued to assess the child's condition. Improvement may be sustained when the drug is either temporarily or permanently discontinued.

Drug treatment should not and need not be indefinite and usually may be discontinued after puberty.

OVERDOSAGE

Signs and symptoms of acute overdosage, resulting principally from overstimulation of the central nervous system and from excessive sympathomimetic effects, may include the following: vomiting, agitation, tremors, hyperreflexia, muscle twitching, convulsions (may be followed by coma), euphoria, confusion, hallucinations, delirium, sweating, flushing, headache, hyperpyrexia, tachycardia, palpitations, cardiac arrhythmias, hypertension, mydriasis, and dryness of mucous membranes.

Consult with a Certified Poison Control Center regarding treatment for up-to-date guidance and advice.

Treatment consists of appropriate supportive measures. The patient must be protected against self-injury and against external stimuli that would aggravate overstimulation already present. Gastric contents may be evacuated by gastric lavage. In the presence of severe intoxication, use a carefully titrated dosage of a *short-acting* barbiturate before performing gastric lavage. Other measures to detoxify the gut include administration of activated charcoal and a cathartic.

Intensive care must be provided to maintain adequate circulation and respiratory exchange; external cooling procedures may be required for hyperpyrexia.

Efficacy of peritoneal dialysis or extracorporeal hemodialysis for Ritalin overdosage has not been established.

HOW SUPPLIED

Tablets 5 mg — round, yellow (imprinted CIBA 7)
Bottles of 100 .... NDC 0083-0007-30

Tablets 10 mg — round, pale green, scored (imprinted CIBA 3)
Bottles of 100 .... NDC 0083-0003-30

Tablets 20 mg — round, pale yellow, scored (imprinted CIBA 34)
Bottles of 100 .... NDC 0083-0034-30

Do not store above 30°C (86°F). Protect from light.
Dispense in tight, light-resistant container (USP).

SR Tablets 20 mg — round, white, coated (imprinted CIBA 16)
Bottles of 100 .... NDC 0083-0016-30

Note: SR Tablets are color-additive free.
Do not store above 30°C (86°F). Protect from moisture.
Dispense in tight, light-resistant container (USP).

C98-17 (Rev. 3/98)

Shown in Product Identification Guide, page 325

SANDIMMUNE® Soft Gelatin Capsules ℞
(cyclosporine capsules, USP)

SANDIMMUNE® Oral Solution ℞
(cyclosporine oral solution, USP)

SANDIMMUNE® Injection ℞
(cyclosporine concentrate for injection, USP)
FOR INFUSION ONLY

Caution: Federal law prohibits dispensing without prescription.

The following prescribing information is based on official labeling in effect on August 1, 1998.

WARNING

Only physicians experienced in immunosuppressive therapy and management of organ transplant patients should prescribe Sandimmune® (cyclosporine). Patients receiving the drug should be managed in facilities equipped and staffed with adequate laboratory and supportive medical resources. The physician responsible for maintenance therapy should have complete information requisite for the follow-up of the patient.

Sandimmune® (cyclosporine) should be administered with adrenal corticosteroids but not with other immunosuppressive agents. Increased susceptibility to infection and the possible development of lymphoma may result from immunosuppression.

Sandimmune® soft gelatin capsules (cyclosporine capsules, USP) and Sandimmune® oral solution (cyclosporine oral solution, USP) have decreased bioavailability in comparison to Neoral® soft gelatin capsules (cyclosporine capsules for microemulsion) and Neoral® oral solution (cyclosporine oral solution for microemulsion).

Sandimmune® and Neoral® are not bioequivalent and cannot be used interchangeably without physician supervision.

The absorption of cyclosporine during chronic administration of Sandimmune® soft gelatin capsules and oral solution was found to be erratic. It is recommended that patients taking the soft gelatin capsules or oral solution over a period of time be monitored at repeated intervals for cyclosporine blood levels and subsequent dose adjustments be made in order to avoid toxicity due to high levels and possible organ rejection due to low absorption of cyclosporine. This is of special importance in liver transplants. Numerous assays are being developed to measure blood levels of cyclosporine. Comparison of levels in published literature to patient levels using current assays must be done with detailed knowledge of the assay methods employed. *(See Blood Level Monitoring under DOSAGE AND ADMINISTRATION)*

DESCRIPTION

Cyclosporine, the active principle in Sandimmune® (cyclosporine) is a cyclic polypeptide immunosuppressant agent consisting of 11 amino acids. It is produced as a metabolite by the fungus species *Beauveria nivea*.

Chemically, cyclosporine is designated as [*R*-[*R**,*R**-(*E*)]]-cyclic(L-alanyl-D-alanyl-*N*-methyl-L-leucyl-*N*-methyl-L-leucyl-*N*-methyl-L-valyl-3-hydroxy-*N*,4-dimethyl-L-2-amino-6-octenoyl-L-α-amino-butyryl-*N*-methylglycyl-*N*-methyl-L-leucyl-L-valyl-*N*-methyl-L-leucyl).

Sandimmune® soft gelatin capsules (cyclosporine capsules, USP) are available in 25 mg, 50 mg, and 100 mg strengths.

Each 25 mg capsule contains:
cyclosporine, USP .... 25 mg
alcohol, USP dehydrated .... max 12.7% by volume

Each 50 mg capsule contains:
cyclosporine, USP .... 50 mg
alcohol, USP dehydrated .... max 12.7% by volume

Each 100 mg capsule contains:
cyclosporine, USP .... 100 mg
alcohol, USP dehydrated .... max 12.7% by volume

Inactive Ingredients: corn oil, gelatin, glycerol, Labrafil M 2125 CS (polyoxyethylated glycolysed glycerides), red iron oxide (25 mg and 100 mg capsules only), sorbitol, titanium dioxide, yellow iron oxide (50 mg capsule only), and other ingredients.

Sandimmune® oral solution (cyclosporine oral solution, USP) is available in 50 mL bottles.

Each mL contains:
cyclosporine, USP .... 100 mg
alcohol, Ph. Helv. .... 12.5% by volume

dissolved in an olive oil, Ph. Helv./Labrafil M 1944 CS (polyoxyethylated oleic glycerides) vehicle which must be further diluted with milk, chocolate milk, or orange juice before oral administration.

Sandimmune® injection (cyclosporine concentrate for injection, USP) is available in a 5 mL sterile ampul for I.V. administration.

Each mL contains:
cyclosporine, USP .... 50 mg
*Cremophor® EL
(polyoxyethylated castor oil) .... 650 mg
alcohol, Ph. Helv. .... 32.9% by volume
nitrogen .... qs

which must be diluted further with 0.9% Sodium Chloride Injection or 5% Dextrose Injection before use.

*Cremophor is the registered trademark of BASF Aktiengesellschaft.

The chemical structure of cyclosporine (also known as cyclosporin A) is:

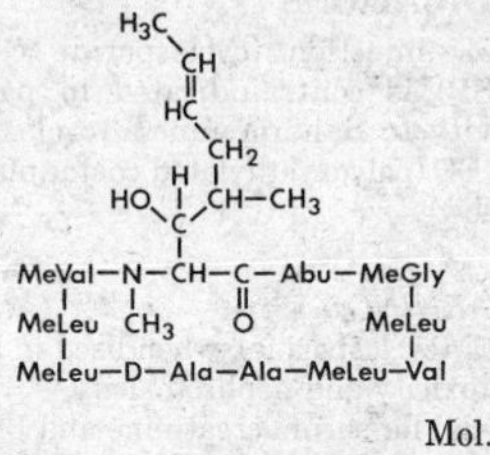

$C_{62}H_{111}N_{11}O_{12}$ Mol. Wt. 1202.63

CLINICAL PHARMACOLOGY

Sandimmune® (cyclosporine) is a potent immunosuppressive agent which in animals prolongs survival of allogeneic transplants involving skin, heart, kidney, pancreas, bone marrow, small intestine, and lung. Sandimmune® (cyclosporine) has been demonstrated to suppress some humoral immunity and to a greater extent, cell-mediated reactions such as allograft rejection, delayed hypersensitivity, experimental allergic encephalomyelitis, Freund's adjuvant arthritis, and graft vs. host disease in many animal species for a variety of organs.

Successful kidney, liver, and heart allogeneic transplants have been performed in man using Sandimmune® (cyclosporine).

The exact mechanism of action of Sandimmune® (cyclosporine) is not known. Experimental evidence suggests that the effectiveness of cyclosporine is due to specific and reversible inhibition of immunocompetent lymphocytes in the G_0- or G_1-phase of the cell cycle. T-lymphocytes are preferentially inhibited. The T-helper cell is the main target, although the T-suppressor cell may also be suppressed. Sandimmune® (cyclosporine) also inhibits lymphokine production and release including interleukin-2 or T-cell growth factor (TCGF).

No functional effects on phagocytic (changes in enzyme secretions not altered, chemotactic migration of granulocytes, macrophage migration, carbon clearance *in vivo*) or tumor cells (growth rate, metastasis) can be detected in animals. Sandimmune® (cyclosporine) does not cause bone marrow suppression in animal models or man.

The absorption of cyclosporine from the gastrointestinal tract is incomplete and variable. Peak concentrations (C_{max}) in blood and plasma are achieved at about 3.5 hours. C_{max} and area under the plasma or blood concentration/time curve (AUC) increase with the administered dose; for blood the relationship is curvilinear (parabolic) between 0 and 1400 mg. As determined by a specific assay, C_{max} is approximately 1.0 ng/mL/mg of dose for plasma and 2.7-1.4 ng/mL/mg of dose for blood (for low to high doses). Compared to an intravenous infusion, the absolute bioavailability of the oral solution is approximately 30% based upon the results in 2 patients. The bioavailability of Sandimmune® soft gelatin capsules (cyclosporine capsules, USP) is equivalent to Sandimmune® oral solution, (cyclosporine oral solution, USP).

Cyclosporine is distributed largely outside the blood volume. In blood the distribution is concentration dependent. Approximately 33%-47% is in plasma, 4%-9% in lymphocytes, 5%-12% in granulocytes, and 41%-58% in erythrocytes. At high concentrations, the uptake by leukocytes and erythrocytes becomes saturated. In plasma, approximately 90% is bound to proteins, primarily lipoproteins.

The disposition of cyclosporine from blood is biphasic with a terminal half-life of approximately 19 hours (range: 10-27 hours). Elimination is primarily biliary with only 6% of the dose excreted in the urine.

Cyclosporine is extensively metabolized but there is no major metabolic pathway. Only 0.1% of the dose is excreted in the urine as unchanged drug. Of 15 metabolites characterized in human urine, 9 have been assigned structures. The major pathways consist of hydroxylation of the Cγ-carbon of 2 of the leucine residues, Cη-carbon hydroxylation, and cyclic ether formation (with oxidation of the double bond) in the side chain of the amino acid 3-hydroxyl-*N*,4-dimethyl-L-2-amino-6-octenoic acid and *N*-demethylation of *N*-methyl leucine residues. Hydrolysis of the cyclic peptide chain or conjugation of the aforementioned metabolites do not appear to be important biotransformation pathways.

INDICATIONS AND USAGE

Sandimmune® (cyclosporine) is indicated for the prophylaxis of organ rejection in kidney, liver, and heart allogeneic transplants. It is always to be used with adrenal corticosteroids. The drug may also be used in the treatment of chronic rejection in patients previously treated with other immunosuppressive agents.

Because of the risk of anaphylaxis, Sandimmune® injection (cyclosporine concentrate for injection, USP) should be reserved for patients who are unable to take the soft gelatin capsules or oral solution.

Continued on next page

Sandimmune—Cont.

CONTRAINDICATIONS

Sandimmune® injection (cyclosporine concentrate for injection, USP) is contraindicated in patients with a hypersensitivity to Sandimmune® (cyclosporine) and/or Cremophor® EL (polyoxyethylated castor oil).

[See table below]

WARNINGS

(See boxed WARNINGs)

Sandimmune® (cyclosporine), when used in high doses, can cause hepatotoxicity and nephrotoxicity.

It is not unusual for serum creatinine and BUN levels to be elevated during Sandimmune® (cyclosporine) therapy. These elevations in renal transplant patients do not necessarily indicate rejection, and each patient must be fully evaluated before dosage adjustment is initiated.

Nephrotoxicity has been noted in 25% of cases of renal transplantation, 38% of cases of cardiac transplantation, and 37% of cases of liver transplantation. Mild nephrotoxicity was generally noted 2-3 months after transplant and consisted of an arrest in the fall of the preoperative elevations of BUN and creatinine at a range of 35-45 mg/dl and 2.0-2.5 mg/dl respectively. These elevations were often responsive to dosage reduction.

More overt nephrotoxicity was seen early after transplantation and was characterized by a rapidly rising BUN and creatinine. Since these events are similar to rejection episodes care must be taken to differentiate between them. This form of nephrotoxicity is usually responsive to Sandimmune® (cyclosporine) dosage reduction.

Although specific diagnostic criteria which reliably differentiate renal graft rejection from drug toxicity have not been found, a number of parameters have been significantly associated to one or the other. It should be noted however, that up to 20% of patients may have simultaneous nephrotoxicity and rejection.

A form of chronic progressive cyclosporine-associated nephrotoxicity is characterized by serial deterioration in renal function and morphologic changes in the kidneys. From 5%-15% of transplant recipients will fail to show a reduction in a rising serum creatinine despite a decrease or discontinuation of cyclosporine therapy. Renal biopsies from these patients will demonstrate an interstitial fibrosis with tubular atrophy. In addition, toxic tubulopathy, peritubular capillary congestion, arteriolopathy, and a striped form of interstitial fibrosis with tubular atrophy may be present. Though none of these morphologic changes is entirely specific, a histologic diagnosis of chronic progressive cyclosporine-associated nephrotoxicity requires evidence of these.

When considering the development of chronic nephrotoxicity it is noteworthy that several authors have reported an association between the appearance of interstitial fibrosis and higher cumulative doses or persistently high circulating trough levels of cyclosporine. This is particularly true during the first 6 post-transplant months when the dosage tends to be highest and when, in kidney recipients, the organ appears to be most vulnerable to the toxic effects of cyclosporine. Among other contributing factors to the development of interstitial fibrosis in these patients must be included, prolonged perfusion time, warm ischemia time, as well as episodes of acute toxicity, and acute and chronic rejection. The reversibility of interstitial fibrosis and its correlation to renal function have not yet been determined.

Impaired renal function at any time requires close monitoring, and frequent dosage adjustment may be indicated. In patients with persistent high elevations of BUN and creatinine who are unresponsive to dosage adjustments, consideration should be given to switching to other immunosuppressive therapy. In the event of severe and unremitting rejection, it is preferable to allow the kidney transplant to be rejected and removed rather than increase the Sandimmune® (cyclosporine) dosage to a very high level in an attempt to reverse the rejection.

Occasionally patients have developed a syndrome of thrombocytopenia and microangiopathic hemolytic anemia which may result in graft failure. The vasculopathy can occur in the absence of rejection and is accompanied by avid platelet consumption within the graft as demonstrated by Indium 111 labeled platelet studies. Neither the pathogenesis nor the management of this syndrome is clear. Though resolution has occurred after reduction or discontinuation of Sandimmune® (cyclosporine) and 1) administration of streptokinase and heparin or 2) plasmapheresis, this appears to depend upon early detection with Indium 111 labeled platelet scans. *(See ADVERSE REACTIONS)*

Significant hyperkalemia (sometimes associated with hyperchloremic metabolic acidosis) and hyperuricemia have been seen occasionally in individual patients.

Hepatotoxicity has been noted in 4% of cases of renal transplantation, 7% of cases of cardiac transplantation, and 4% of cases of liver transplantation. This was usually noted during the first month of therapy when high doses of Sandimmune® (cyclosporine) were used and consisted of elevations of hepatic enzymes and bilirubin. The chemistry elevations usually decreased with a reduction in dosage.

As in patients receiving other immunosuppressants, those patients receiving Sandimmune® (cyclosporine) are at increased risk for development of lymphomas and other malignancies, particularly those of the skin. The increased risk appears related to the intensity and duration of immunosuppression rather than to the use of specific agents. Because of the danger of oversuppression of the immune system, which can also increase susceptibility to infection, Sandimmune® (cyclosporine) should not be administered with other immunosuppressive agents except adrenal corticosteroids. The efficacy and safety of cyclosporine in combination with other immunosuppressive agents have not been determined.

There have been reports of convulsions in adult and pediatric patients receiving cyclosporine, particularly in combination with high dose methylprednisolone.

Rarely (approximately 1 in 1000), patients receiving Sandimmune® injection (cyclosporine concentrate for injection, USP) have experienced anaphylactic reactions. Although the exact cause of these reactions is unknown, it is believed to be due to the Cremophor® EL (polyoxyethylated castor oil) used as the vehicle for the I.V. formulation. These reactions have consisted of flushing of the face and upper thorax, acute respiratory distress with dyspnea and wheezing, blood pressure changes, and tachycardia. One patient died after respiratory arrest and aspiration pneumonia. In some cases, the reaction subsided after the infusion was stopped.

Patients receiving Sandimmune® injection (cyclosporine concentrate for injection, USP) should be under continuous observation for at least the first 30 minutes following the start of the infusion and at frequent intervals thereafter. If anaphylaxis occurs, the infusion should be stopped. An aqueous solution of epinephrine 1:1000 should be available at the bedside as well as a source of oxygen.

Anaphylactic reactions have not been reported with the soft gelatin capsules or oral solution which lack Cremophor® EL (polyoxyethylated castor oil). In fact, patients experiencing anaphylactic reactions have been treated subsequently with the soft gelatin capsules or oral solution without incident.

Care should be taken in using Sandimmune® (cyclosporine) with nephrotoxic drugs. *(See PRECAUTIONS)*

Because Sandimmune® is not bioequivalent to Neoral®, conversion from Neoral® to Sandimmune® using a 1:1 ratio (mg/kg/day) may result in a lower cyclosporine blood concentration. Conversion from Neoral® to Sandimmune® should be made with increased blood concentration monitoring to avoid the potential of underdosing.

PRECAUTIONS

General

Patients with malabsorption may have difficulty in achieving therapeutic levels with Sandimmune® soft gelatin capsules or oral solution.

Hypertension is a common side effect of Sandimmune® (cyclosporine) therapy. *(See ADVERSE REACTIONS)* Mild or moderate hypertension is more frequently encountered than severe hypertension and the incidence decreases over time. Antihypertensive therapy may be required. Control of blood pressure can be accomplished with any of the common antihypertensive agents. However, since cyclosporine may cause hyperkalemia, potassium-sparing diuretics should not be used. While calcium antagonists can be effective agents in treating cyclosporine-associated hypertension, care should be taken since interference with cyclosporine metabolism may require a dosage adjustment. *(See Drug Interactions)*

During treatment with Sandimmune® (cyclosporine), vaccination may be less effective; and the use of live attenuated vaccines should be avoided.

Information for Patients

Patients should be advised that any change of cyclosporine formulation should be made cautiously and only under physician supervision because it may result in the need for a change in dosage.

Patients should be informed of the necessity of repeated laboratory tests while they are receiving the drug. They should be given careful dosage instructions, advised of the potential risks during pregnancy, and informed of the increased risk of neoplasia.

Patients using cyclosporine oral solution with its accompanying syringe for dosage measurement should be cautioned not to rinse the syringe either before or after use. Introduction of water into the product by any means will cause variation in dose.

Nephrotoxicity vs Rejection

Parameter	Nephrotoxicity	Rejection
History	Donor >50 years old or hypotensive Prolonged kidney preservation Prolonged anastomosis time Concomitant nephrotoxic drugs	Antidonor immune response Retransplant patient
Clinical	Often >6 weeks postop[b] Prolonged initial nonfunction (acute tubular necrosis)	Often <4 weeks postop[b] Fever >37.5°C Weight gain >0.5 kg Graft swelling and tenderness Decrease in daily urine volume >500 mL (or 50%)
Laboratory	CyA serum trough level >200 ng/mL Gradual rise in Cr (<0.15 mg/dl/day[a] Cr plateau <25% above baseline BUN/Cr ≥20	CyA serum trough level <150 ng/mL Rapid rise in Cr (>0.3 mg/dl/day)[a] Cr >25% above baseline BUN/Cr<20
Biopsy	Arteriolopathy (medial hypertrophy[a], hyalinosis, nodular deposits, intimal thickening, endothelial vacuolization, progressive scarring)	Endovasculitis[c] (proliferation[a], intimal arteritis[b], necrosis, sclerosis)
	Tubular atrophy, isometric vacuolization, isolated calcifications	Tubulitis with RBC[b] and WBC[b] casts, some irregular vacuolization
	Minimal edema	Interstitial edema[c] and hemorrhage[b]
	Mild focal infiltrates[c]	Diffuse moderate to severe mononuclear infiltrates[d]
	Diffuse interstitial fibrosis, often striped form	Glomerulitis (mononuclear cells)[c]
Aspiration Cytology	CyA deposits in tubular and endothelial cells Fine isometric vacuolization of tubular cells	Inflammatory infiltrate with mononuclear phagocytes, macrophages, lymphoblastoid cells, and activated T-cells These strongly express HLA-DR antigens
Urine Cytology	Tubular cells with vacuolization and granularization	Degenerative tubular cells, plasma cells, and lymphocyturia >20% of sediment
Manometry	Intracapsular pressure <40 mm Hg[b]	Intracapsular pressure >40 mm Hg[b]
Ultrasonography	Unchanged graft cross sectional area	Increase in graft cross sectional area AP diameter ≥ Transverse diameter
Magnetic Resonance Imagery	Normal appearance	Loss of distinct corticomedullary junction, swelling image intensity of parachyma approaching that of psoas, loss of hilar fat
Radionuclide Scan	Normal or generally decreased perfusion Decrease in tubular function (^{131} I-hippuran) > decrease in perfusion (^{99m} Tc DTPA)	Patchy arterial flow Decrease in perfusion > decrease in tubular function Increased uptake of Indium 111 labeled platelets or Tc-99m in colloid
Therapy	Responds to decreased Sandimmune® (cyclosporine)	Responds to increased steroids or antilymphocyte globulin

[a]p <0.05, [b]p <0.01, [c]p <0.001, [d]p <0.0001

Laboratory Tests

Renal and liver functions should be assessed repeatedly by measurement of BUN, serum creatinine, serum bilirubin, and liver enzymes.

Drug Interactions

All of the individual drugs cited below are well substantiated to interact with Sandimmune® (cyclosporine).

Drugs That Exhibit Nephrotoxic Synergy

gentamicin	cimetidine
tobramycin	ranitidine
vancomycin	diclofenac
amphotericin B	trimethoprim
ketoconazole	with sulfamethoxazole
melphalan	azapropazon

Careful monitoring of renal function should be practiced when Sandimmune® (cyclosporine) is used with nephrotoxic drugs.

Drugs That Alter Cyclosporine Levels

Cyclosporine is extensively metabolized by the liver. Therefore, circulating cyclosporine levels may be influenced by drugs that affect hepatic microsomal enzymes, particularly the cytochrome P-450 system. Substances known to inhibit these enzymes will decrease hepatic metabolism and increase cyclosporine levels. Substances that are inducers of cytochrome P-450 activity will increase hepatic metabolism and decrease cyclosporine levels. Monitoring of circulating cyclosporine levels and appropriate Sandimmune® (cyclosporine) dosage adjustment are essential when these drugs are used concomitantly (*see Blood Level Monitoring*)

Drugs That Increase Cyclosporine Levels

diltiazem	danazol
nicardipine	bromocriptine
verapamil	metoclopramide
ketoconazole	erythromycin
fluconazole	methylprednisolone
itraconazole	

Drugs That Decrease Cyclosporine Levels

rifampin	phenobarbital
phenytoin	carbamazepine

Other Drug Interactions

Reduced clearance of prednisolone, digoxin, and lovastatin has been observed when these drugs are administered with Sandimmune® (cyclosporine). In addition, a decrease in the apparent volume of distribution of digoxin has been reported after Sandimmune® (cyclosporine) administration. Severe digitalis toxicity has been seen within days of starting cyclosporine in several patients taking digoxin. Sandimmune® (cyclosporine) should not be used with potassium-sparing diuretics because hyperkalemia can occur. During treatment with Sandimmune® (cyclosporine), vaccination may be less effective; and the use of live vaccines should be avoided. Myositis has occurred with concomitant lovastatin, frequent gingival hyperplasia with nifedipine, and convulsions with high dose methylprednisolone. Further information on drugs that have been reported to interact with Sandimmune® (cyclosporine) is available from Sandoz Pharmaceuticals Corporation.

Carcinogenesis, Mutagenesis, and Impairment of Fertility

Cyclosporine gave no evidence of mutagenic or teratogenic effects in appropriate test systems. Only at dose levels toxic to dams, were adverse effects seen in reproduction studies in rats. (See Pregnancy)

Carcinogenicity studies were carried out in male and female rats and mice. In the 78-week mouse study, at doses of 1, 4, and 16 mg/kg/day, evidence of a statistically significant trend was found for lymphocytic lymphomas in females, and the incidence of hepatocellular carcinomas in mid-dose males significantly exceeded the control value. In the 24-month rat study, conducted at 0.5, 2, and 8 mg/kg/day, pancreatic islet cell adenomas significantly exceeded the control rate in the low dose level. The hepatocellular carcinomas and pancreatic islet cell adenomas were not dose related.

No impairment in fertility was demonstrated in studies in male and female rats.

Cyclosporine has not been found mutagenic/genotoxic in the Ames Test, the V79-HGPRT Test, the micronucleus test in mice and Chinese hamsters, the chromosome-aberration tests in Chinese hamster bone-marrow, the mouse dominant lethal assay, and the DNA-repair test in sperm from treated mice. A recent study analyzing sister chromatid exchange (SCE) induction by cyclosporine using human lymphocytes *in vitro* gave indication of a positive effect (i.e., induction of SCE), at high concentrations in this system.

An increased incidence of malignancy is a recognized complication of immunosuppression in recipients of organ transplants. The most common forms of neoplasms are non-Hodgkin's lymphoma and carcinomas of the skin. The risk of malignancies in cyclosporine recipients is higher than in the normal, healthy population but similar to that in patients receiving other immunosuppressive therapies. It has been reported that reduction or discontinuance of immunosuppression may cause the lesions to regress.

Pregnancy

Pregnancy Category C. Sandimmune® oral solution (cyclosporine oral solution, USP) has been shown to be embryo- and fetotoxic in rats and rabbits when given in doses 2-5 times the human dose. At toxic doses (rats at 30 mg/kg/day and rabbits at 100 mg/kg/day), Sandimmune® (cyclosporine oral solution, USP) was embryo- and fetotoxic as indicated by increased pre- and postnatal mortality and reduced fetal weight together with related skeletal retardations. In the well-tolerated dose range (rats at up to 17 mg/kg/day and rabbits at up to 30 mg/kg/day), Sandimmune® oral solution (cyclosporine oral solution, USP) proved to be without any embryolethal or teratogenic effects.

There are no adequate and well-controlled studies in pregnant women. Sandimmune® (cyclosporine) should be used during pregnancy only if the potential benefit justifies the potential risk to the fetus.

The following data represent the reported outcomes of 116 pregnancies in women receiving Sandimmune® (cyclosporine) during pregnancy, 90% of whom were transplant patients, and most of whom received Sandimmune® (cyclosporine) throughout the entire gestational period. Since most of the patients were not prospectively identified, the results are likely to be biased toward negative outcomes. The only consistent patterns of abnormality were premature birth (gestational period of 28 to 36 weeks) and low birth weight for gestational age. It is not possible to separate the effects of Sandimmune® (cyclosporine) on these pregnancies from the effects of the other immunosuppressants, the underlying maternal disorders, or other aspects of the transplantation milieu. Sixteen fetal losses occurred. Most of the pregnancies (85 of 100) were complicated by disorders; including, pre-eclampsia, eclampsia, premature labor, abruptio placentae, oligohydramnios, Rh incompatibility and fetoplacental dysfunction. Preterm delivery occurred in 47%. Seven malformations were reported in 5 viable infants and in 2 cases of fetal loss. Twenty-eight percent of the infants were small for gestational age. Neonatal complications occurred in 27%. In a report of 23 children followed up to 4 years, postnatal development was said to be normal. More information on cyclosporine use in pregnancy is available from Sandoz Pharmaceuticals Corporation.

Nursing Mothers

Since Sandimmune® (cyclosporine) is excreted in human milk, nursing should be avoided.

Pediatric Use

Although no adequate and well controlled studies have been conducted in children, patients as young as 6 months of age have received the drug with no unusual adverse effects.

ADVERSE REACTIONS

The principal adverse reactions of Sandimmune® (cyclosporine) therapy are renal dysfunction, tremor, hirsutism, hypertension, and gum hyperplasia.

Hypertension, which is usually mild to moderate, may occur in approximately 50% of patients following renal transplantation and in most cardiac transplant patients.

Glomerular capillary thrombosis has been found in patients treated with cyclosporine and may progress to graft failure. The pathologic changes resemble those seen in the hemolytic-uremic syndrome and include thrombosis of the renal microvasculature, with platelet-fibrin thrombi occluding glomerular capillaries and afferent arterioles, microangiopathic hemolytic anemia, thrombocytopenia, and decreased renal function. Similar findings have been observed when other immunosuppressives have been employed post-transplantation.

Hypomagnesemia has been reported in some, but not all, patients exhibiting convulsions while on cyclosporine therapy. Although magnesium-depletion studies in normal subjects suggest that hypomagnesemia is associated with neurologic disorders, multiple factors, including hypertension, high dose methylprednisolone, hypocholesterolemia, and nephrotoxicity associated with high plasma concentrations of cyclosporine appear to be related to the neurological manifestations of cyclosporine toxicity.

The following reactions occurred in 3% or greater of 892 patients involved in clinical trials of kidney, heart, and liver transplants:

[See first table above]

The following reactions occurred in 2% or less of patients: allergic reactions, anemia, anorexia, confusion, conjunctivitis, edema, fever, brittle fingernails, gastritis, hearing loss, hiccups, hyperglycemia, muscle pain, peptic ulcer, thrombocytopenia, tinnitus.

Body System/ Adverse Reactions	Randomized Kidney Patients		All Sandimmune® (cyclosporine) Patients		
	Sandimmune® (N=227) %	Azathioprine (N=228) %	Kidney (N=705) %	Heart (N=112) %	Liver (N=75) %
Genitourinary					
Renal Dysfunction	32	6	25	38	37
Cardiovascular					
Hypertension	26	18	13	53	27
Cramps	4	<1	2	<1	0
Skin					
Hirsutism	21	<1	21	28	45
Acne	6	8	2	2	1
Central Nervous System					
Tremor	12	0	21	31	55
Convulsions	3	1	1	4	5
Headache	2	<1	2	15	4
Gastrointestinal					
Gum Hyperplasia	4	0	9	5	16
Diarrhea	3	<1	3	4	8
Nausea/Vomiting	2	<1	4	10	4
Hepatotoxicity	<1	<1	4	7	4
Abdominal Discomfort	<1	0	<1	7	0
Autonomic Nervous System					
Paresthesia	3	0	1	2	1
Flushing	<1	0	4	0	4
Hematopoietic					
Leukopenia	2	19	<1	6	0
Lymphoma	<1	0	1	6	1
Respiratory					
Sinusitis	<1	0	4	3	7
Miscellaneous					
Gynecomastia	<1	0	<1	4	3

Renal Transplant Patients in Whom Therapy Was Discontinued			
	Randomized Patients		All Sandimmune® Patients
Reason for Discontinuation	Sandimmune® (N=227) %	Azathioprine (N=228) %	(N=705) %
Renal Toxicity	5.7	0	5.4
Infection	0	0.4	0.9
Lack of Efficacy	2.6	0.9	1.4
Acute Tubular Necrosis	2.6	0	1.0
Lymphoma/Lymphoproliferative Disease	0.4	0	0.3
Hypertension	0	0	0.3
Hematological Abnormalities	0	0.4	0
Other	0	0	0.7

Sandimmune® (cyclosporine) was discontinued on a temporary basis and then restarted in 18 additional patients.

Continued on next page

Sandimmune—Cont.

The following reactions occurred rarely: anxiety, chest pain, constipation, depression, hair breaking, hematuria, joint pain, lethargy, mouth sores, myocardial infarction, night sweats, pancreatitis, pruritus, swallowing difficulty, tingling, upper GI bleeding, visual disturbance, weakness, weight loss.

[See second table at top of previous page]

[See table below]

Cremophor® EL (polyoxyethylated castor oil) is known to cause hyperlipemia and electrophoretic abnormalities of lipoproteins. These effects are reversible upon discontinuation of treatment but are usually not a reason to stop treatment.

OVERDOSAGE

There is a minimal experience with overdosage. Because of the slow absorption of Sandimmune® soft gelatin capsules or oral solution, forced emesis would be of value up to 2 hours after administration. Transient hepatotoxicity and nephrotoxicity may occur which should resolve following drug withdrawal. General supportive measures and symptomatic treatment should be followed in all cases of overdosage. Sandimmune® (cyclosporine) is not dialyzable to any great extent, nor is it cleared well by charcoal hemoperfusion. The oral LD_{50} is 2329 mg/kg in mice, 1480 mg/kg in rats, and >1000 mg/kg in rabbits. The I.V. LD_{50} is 148 mg/kg in mice, 104 mg/kg in rats, and 46 mg/kg in rabbits.

DOSAGE AND ADMINISTRATION

Sandimmune® Soft Gelatin Capsules (cyclosporine capsules, USP) and Sandimmune® Oral Solution (cyclosporine oral solution, USP)

Sandimmune® soft gelatin capsules (cyclosporine capsules, USP) and Sandimmune® oral solution (cyclosporine oral solution, USP) have decreased bioavailability in comparison to Neoral® soft gelatin capsules (cyclosporine capsules for microemulsion) and Neoral® oral solution (cyclosporine oral solution for microemulsion). Sandimmune® and Neoral® are not bioequivalent and cannot be used interchangeably without physician supervision.

The initial oral dose of Sandimmune® (cyclosporine) should be given 4-12 hours prior to transplantation as a single dose of 15 mg/kg. Although a daily single dose of 14-18 mg/kg was used in most clinical trials, few centers continue to use the highest dose, most favoring the lower end of the scale. There is a trend towards use of even lower initial doses for renal transplantation in the ranges of 10-14 mg/kg/day. The initial single daily dose is continued postoperatively for 1-2 weeks and then tapered by 5% per week to a maintenance dose of 5-10 mg/kg/day. Some centers have successfully tapered the maintenance dose to as low as 3 mg/kg/day in selected *renal* transplant patients without an apparent rise in rejection rate.

(See Blood Level Monitoring below)

In pediatric usage, the same dose and dosing regimen may be used as in adults although in several studies children have required and tolerated higher doses than those used in adults.

Adjunct therapy with adrenal corticosteroids is recommended. Different tapering dosage schedules of prednisone appear to achieve similar results. A dosage schedule based on the patient's weight started with 2.0 mg/kg/day for the first 4 days tapered to 1.0 mg/kg/day by 1 week, 0.6 mg/kg/day by 2 weeks, 0.3 mg/kg/day by 1 month, and 0.15 mg/kg/day by 2 months and thereafter as a maintenance dose. Another center started with an initial dose of 200 mg tapered by 40 mg/day until reaching 20 mg/day. After 2 months at this dose, a further reduction to 10 mg/day was made. Adjustments in dosage of prednisone must be made according to the clinical situation.

To make Sandimmune® oral solution (cyclosporine oral solution, USP) more palatable, the oral solution may be diluted with milk, chocolate milk, or orange juice preferably at room temperature. Patients should avoid switching diluents frequently. Sandimmune® soft gelatin capsules and oral solution should be administered on a consistent schedule with regard to time of day and relation to meals.

Take the prescribed amount of Sandimmune® (cyclosporine) from the container using the dosage syringe supplied after removal of the protective cover, and transfer the solution to a glass of milk, chocolate milk, or orange juice. Stir well and drink at once. Do not allow to stand before drinking. It is best to use a glass container and rinse it with more diluent to ensure that the total dose is taken. After use, replace the dosage syringe in the protective cover. Do not rinse the dosage syringe with water or other cleaning agents either before or after use. If the dosage syringe requires cleaning, it must be completely dry before resuming use. Introduction of water into the product by any means will cause variation in dose.

Sandimmune® Injection (cyclosporine concentrate for injection, USP)

FOR INFUSION ONLY

Note: Anaphylactic reactions have occurred with Sandimmune® injection (cyclosporine concentrate for injection, USP). *(See WARNINGS)*

Patients unable to take Sandimmune® soft gelatin capsules or oral solution pre- or postoperatively may be treated with the I.V. concentrate. **Sandimmune® injection (cyclosporine concentrate for injection, USP) is administered at 1/3 the oral dose.** The initial dose of Sandimmune® injection (cyclosporine concentrate for injection, USP) should be given 4-12 hours prior to transplantation as a single I.V. dose of 5-6 mg/kg/day. This daily single dose is continued postoperatively until the patient can tolerate the soft gelatin capsules or oral solution. Patients should be switched to Sandimmune® soft gelatin capsules or oral solution as soon as possible after surgery. In pediatric usage, the same dose and dosing regimen may be used, although higher doses may be required.

Adjunct steroid therapy is to be used. *(See aforementioned)*

Immediately before use, the I.V. concentrate should be diluted 1 mL Sandimmune® injection (cyclosporine concentrate for injection, USP) in 20 mL-100 mL 0.9% Sodium Chloride Injection or 5% Dextrose Injection and given in a slow intravenous infusion over approximately 2-6 hours.

Diluted infusion solutions should be discarded after 24 hours.

The Cremophor® EL (polyoxyethylated castor oil) contained in the concentrate for intravenous infusion can cause phthalate stripping from PVC.

Parenteral drug products should be inspected visually for particulate matter and discoloration prior to administration, whenever solution and container permit.

Blood Level Monitoring

Several study centers have found blood level monitoring of cyclosporine useful in patient management. While no fixed relationships have yet been established, in one series of 375 consecutive cadaveric renal transplant recipients, dosage was adjusted to achieve specific whole blood 24-hour trough levels of 100-200 ng/mL as determined by high-pressure liquid chromatography (HPLC).

Of major importance to blood level analysis is the type of assay used. The above levels are specific to the parent cyclosporine molecule and correlate directly to the new monoclonal specific radioimmunoassays (mRIA-sp). Nonspecific assays are also available which detect the parent compound molecule and various of its metabolites. Older studies often cited levels using a nonspecific assay which were roughly twice those of specific assays. Assay results are not interchangeable and their use should be guided by their approved labeling. If plasma specimens are employed, levels will vary with the temperature at the time of separation from whole blood. Plasma levels may range from 1/2-1/5 of whole blood levels. Refer to individual assay labeling for complete instructions. In addition, *Transplantation Proceedings* (June 1990) contains position papers and a broad consensus generated at the Cyclosporine-Therapeutic Drug Monitoring conference that year. Blood level monitoring is not a replacement for renal function monitoring or tissue biopsies.

Infectious Complications in the Randomized Renal Transplant Patients

Complication	Sandimmune® Treatment (N=227) % of Complications	Standard Treatment* (N=228) % of Complications
Septicemia	5.3	4.8
Abscesses	4.4	5.3
Systemic Fungal Infection	2.2	3.9
Local Fungal Infection	7.5	9.6
Cytomegalovirus	4.8	12.3
Other Viral Infections	15.9	18.4
Urinary Tract Infections	21.1	20.2
Wound and Skin Infections	7.0	10.1
Pneumonia	6.2	9.2

* Some patients also received ALG.

HOW SUPPLIED

Sandimmune® Soft Gelatin Capsules (cyclosporine capsules, USP)

25 mg

Oblong, pink, branded " 78/240". SandoPak® unit-dose packages of 30 capsules, 3 blister cards of 10 capsules (NDC 0078-0240-15).

50 mg

Oblong, corn-yellow, branded " 78/242". SandoPak® unit-dose packages of 30 capsules, 3 blister cards of 10 capsules (NDC 0078-0242-15).

100 mg

Oblong, dusty rose, branded " 78/241". SandoPak® unit-dose packages of 30 capsules, 3 blister cards of 10 capsules (NDC 0078-0241-15).

Store and Dispense

In the original unit-dose container at temperatures below 86°F (30°C). An odor may be detected upon opening the unit-dose container, which will dissipate shortly thereafter. This odor does not affect the quality of the product.

Sandimmune® Oral Solution (cyclosporine oral solution, USP)

Supplied in 50 mL bottles containing 100 mg of cyclosporine per mL (NDC 0078-0110-22). A dosage syringe is provided for dispensing.

Store and Dispense

In the original container at temperatures below 86°F (30°C). Do not store in the refrigerator. Protect from freezing. Once opened, the contents must be used within 2 months.

Sandimmune® Injection (cyclosporine concentrate for injection, USP)

FOR INTRAVENOUS INFUSION

Supplied as a 5 mL sterile ampul containing 50 mg of cyclosporine per mL, in boxes of 10 ampuls (NDC 0078-0109-01).

Store and Dispense

At temperatures below 86°F (30°C) and protected from light.

Sandimmune® Soft Gelatin Capsules (cyclosporine capsules, USP)

Manufactured by
R.P. Scherer GmbH, EBERBACH/BADEN, GERMANY
Manufactured for
Sandoz Pharmaceuticals Corporation,
East Hanover, NJ 07936

Sandimmune® Oral Solution (cyclosporine oral solution, USP) and Sandimmune® Injection (cyclosporine concentrate for injection, USP)

FOR INFUSION ONLY

Manufactured by
SANDOZ PHARMA LTD., Basle, Switzerland
Manufactured for
Sandoz Pharmaceuticals Corporation,
East Hanover, NJ 07936

[REV: NOVEMBER 1996 38425911]

Shown in Product Identification Guide, page 325

IMMUNE GLOBULIN INTRAVENOUS (HUMAN) SANDOGLOBULIN® ℞

Lyophilized Preparation

CAUTION: US Federal law prohibits dispensing without prescription.

The following prescribing information is based on official labeling in effect on August 1, 1998.

DESCRIPTION

Immune Globulin Intravenous (Human)*, Sandoglobulin®, is a sterile, highly purified polyvalent antibody product containing in concentrated form all the IgG antibodies which regularly occur in the donor population (1). This immunoglobulin preparation is produced by cold alcohol fractionation from the plasma of over 16,000 volunteer US donors. Part of the fractionation may be performed by another US-licensed manufacturer. The total viral reduction from plasma to the immune globulin fraction by the Kistler-Nitschmann cold ethanol fractionation procedure has been documented as greater than 10^8 for HIV, and greater than 10^5 for hepatitis B, vesicular stomatitis and sindbis virus (Hamamoto et al, 1987; Henin et al, 1988; Wells et al, 1986). Sandoglobulin® (IGIV) is made suitable for intravenous use by treatment at acid pH in the presence of trace amounts of pepsin (2,3). Moreover, viral reduction of 10^6 due to the effect of acid pH treatment has been demonstrated for HIV, herpes simplex virus type I, cytomegalovirus, Semliki Forest virus (a model for hepatitis C) and vesicular stomatitis virus (Kempf et al, 1991). The preparation contains at least 96% of IgG and after reconstitution with a neutral unbuffered diluent has a pH of 6.6 ± 0.2. Most of the immunoglobulins are monomeric (7 S) IgG; the remainder consists of dimeric IgG and a small amount of polymeric IgG, traces of IgA and IgM and immunoglobulin fragments (4). The distribution of the IgG subclasses corresponds to that of normal serum (5,6,7,8). Final container lyophilized

units are prepared so as to contain 1, 3, 6, or 12 g protein with 1.67 g sucrose and less than 20 mg NaCl per gram of protein. The lyophilized preparation is devoid of any preservatives and may be reconstituted with sterile water, 5% dextrose or 0.9% saline to a solution with protein concentrations ranging from 3%-12%. The patient's fluid, electrolyte and caloric requirements should be considered in selecting an appropriate diluent and concentration.
*Hereinafter referred to as IGIV.

Table 1
Calculated Sandoglobulin® (IGIV) Osmolality (mOsm/kg)

	Concentration			
Diluent	**3%**	**6%**	**9%**	**12%**
0.9% NaCl	498	690	882	1074
5% Dextrose	444	636	828	1020
Sterile Water	192	384	576	768

CLINICAL PHARMACOLOGY

This product contains a broad spectrum of antibody specificities against bacterial, viral, parasitic, and mycoplasma antigens, that are capable of both opsonization and neutralization of microbes and toxins. The 3 week half-life of Immune Globulin Intravenous (Human), Sandoglobulin®, corresponds to that of Immune Globulin (Human) for intramuscular use, although individual variations in half-life have been observed (9,10). Appropriate doses of Sandoglobulin® (IGIV) restore abnormally low immunoglobulin G levels to the normal range. One hundred percent of the infused dose is available in the recipient's circulation immediately after infusion. After approximately 6 days, an equilibrium is reached between the intra- and extravascular compartments, with immunoglobulin G being distributed approximately 50% intravascular and 50% extravascular. In comparison, after the intramuscular injection of immune globulin, the IgG requires 2-5 days to reach its maximum concentration in the intravascular compartment. This concentration corresponds to about 40% of the injected dose (10).

While Sandoglobulin® (IGIV) has been shown to be effective in some cases of Immune Thrombocytopenic Purpura (ITP) *(see INDICATIONS AND USAGE)*, the mechanism of action in ITP has not been fully elucidated.

Toxicity from overdose has not been observed on regimens of 0.4 g/kg body weight each day for 5 days (11,12,13). Sucrose is added to Sandoglobulin® (IGIV) for reasons of stability, solubility, and safety.

The intravenous administration of the sucrose used for stabilizing Immune Globulin Intravenous (Human), Sandoglobulin®, is considered to be innocuous (14). Because sucrose is excreted unchanged in the urine when given intravenously, Immune Globulin Intravenous (Human), Sandoglobulin®, may be given to diabetics without compensatory changes in insulin dosage regimen.

INDICATIONS AND USAGE

Immunodeficiency

Sandoglobulin® (IGIV) is indicated for the maintenance treatment of patients with primary immunodeficiencies, e.g., in common variable immunodeficiency, severe combined immunodeficiency, and primary immunoglobulin deficiency syndromes such as X-linked agammaglobulinemia (12,15,16,17). Sandoglobulin® (IGIV) is preferable to intramuscular Immune Globulin (Human) preparations in treating patients who require an immediate and large increase in the intravascular immunoglobulin level (10), in patients with limited muscle mass, and in patients with bleeding tendencies for whom intramuscular injections are contraindicated. The infusions must be repeated at regular intervals.

Immune Thrombocytopenic Purpura (ITP)

Acute

A controlled study was performed in children in which Sandoglobulin® (IGIV) was compared with steroids for the treatment of acute (defined as less than 6 months duration) ITP. In this study sequential platelet levels of 30,000, 100,000, and 150,000/µl were all achieved faster with Sandoglobulin® (IGIV) than with steroids and without any of the side effects associated with steroids (11,18). However, it should be noted that many cases of acute ITP in childhood resolve spontaneously within weeks to months. Immune Globulin Intravenous (Human), Sandoglobulin®, has been used with good results in the treatment of acute ITP in adult patients (19,20,21). In a study involving 10 adults with ITP of less than 16 weeks duration, Sandoglobulin® (IGIV) therapy raised the platelet count to the normal range after a 5 day course. This effect lasted a mean of over 173 days, ranging from 30-372 days (22).

Chronic

Children and adults with chronic (defined as greater than 6 months duration) ITP have also shown an increase (sometimes temporary) in platelet counts upon administration of Immune Globulin Intravenous (Human), Sandoglobulin® (18,22,23,24,25,26). Therefore, in situations that require a rapid rise in platelet count, for example prior to surgery or to control excessive bleeding, use of Sandoglobulin® (IGIV) should be considered. In children with chronic ITP, Sandoglobulin® (IGIV) therapy resulted in a mean rise in platelet count of 312,000/µl with a duration of increase ranging from 2-6 months (23,26). Sandoglobulin® (IGIV) therapy may be considered as a means to defer or avoid splenectomy (25,26,27). In adults, Sandoglobulin® (IGIV) therapy has been shown to be effective in maintaining the platelet count in an acceptable range with or without periodic booster therapy. The mean rise in platelet count was 93,000/µl and the average duration of the increase was 20-24 days (22,23). However, it should be noted that not all patients will respond. Even in those patients who do respond, this treatment should not be considered to be curative.

CONTRAINDICATIONS

As with all blood products containing IgA, Sandoglobulin® (IGIV) is contraindicated in patients with selective IgA deficiency, who possess antibody to IgA. It may also be contraindicated in patients who have had severe systemic reactions to the intravenous or intramuscular administration of human immune globulin.

WARNINGS

Patients with agamma- or extreme hypogammaglobulinemia who have never before received immunoglobulin substitution treatment or whose time from last treatment is greater than 8 weeks, may be at risk of developing inflammatory reactions on rapid infusion of Immune Globulin Intravenous (Human), Sandoglobulin®, (over 20 drops [1 mL] per minute). These reactions are manifested by a rise in temperature, chills, nausea, and vomiting. The patient's vital signs should be monitored continuously and he should be carefully observed throughout the infusion, since these reactions on rare occasions may lead to shock. Epinephrine should be available for treatment of an acute anaphylactic reaction. Particular care should be exercised when Immune Globulin Intravenous (Human), Sandoglobulin®, is administered to patients with paraproteins (17).

PRECAUTIONS

Please see *DOSAGE AND ADMINISTRATION* below, for important information on Sandoglobulin® (IGIV) compatibility with other medications or fluids.

Pregnancy

Pregnancy Category C: Animal reproduction studies have not been conducted with Sandoglobulin® (IGIV). It is also not known whether Sandoglobulin® (IGIV) can cause fetal harm when administered to a pregnant woman or can affect reproduction capacity. Sandoglobulin® (IGIV) should be given to a pregnant woman only if clearly needed (21).

Intact immune globulins such as those contained in Sandoglobulin® (IGIV) cross the placenta from maternal circulation increasingly after 30 weeks gestation (28,29). In cases of maternal ITP where Sandoglobulin® (IGIV) was administered to the mother prior to delivery, the platelet response and clinical effect were similar in the mother and neonate (21,29-38).

Pediatric Use

High dose administration of Immune Globulin Intravenous (Human), Sandoglobulin®, in children with acute or chronic Immune Thrombocytopenic Purpura did not reveal any pediatric-specific hazard (11).

Antibodies in Immune Globulin Intravenous (Human) may interfere with the response to live viral vaccines such as measles, mumps, and rubella. Immunizing physicians should be informed of recent therapy with Immune Globulin Intravenous (Human) so that appropriate precautions may be taken.

Aseptic Meningitis Syndrome

An aseptic meningitis syndrome (AMS) has been reported to occur infrequently in association with Immune Globulin Intravenous (Human) (IGIV) treatment. The syndrome usually begins within several hours to two days following IGIV treatment. It is characterized by symptoms and signs including severe headache, nuchal rigidity, drowsiness, fever, photophobia, painful eye movements, and nausea and vomiting. Cerebrospinal fluid studies are frequently positive with pleocytosis up to several thousand cells per cu.mm., predominantly from the granulocytic series, and elevated protein levels up to several hundred mg/dl. Patients exhibiting such symptoms and signs should receive a thorough neurological examination, including CSF studies, to rule out other causes of meningitis. AMS may occur more frequently in association with high dose (2 g/kg) IGIV treatment. Discontinuation of IGIV treatment has resulted in remission of AMS within several days without sequelae.

ADVERSE REACTIONS

Adverse reactions to Sandoglobulin® (IGIV) are rare and occur in less than 1% of patients who are not immunodeficient. Agammaglobulinemic and hypogammaglobulinemic patients who have never received immunoglobulin substitution therapy before or whose time from last treatment is greater than 8 weeks may show adverse reactions if the initial infusion rate exceeds 20 drops (1 mL) per minute. This occurs in approximately 10% of such cases.

These reactions, which generally become apparent only 30 minutes to 1 hour after the beginning of the infusion, are as follows: flushing of the face, feelings of tightness in the chest, chills, fever, dizziness, nausea, diaphoresis, and hypotension. In such cases the infusion should be temporarily stopped until the symptoms have subsided. Immediate anaphylactoid and hypersensitivity reactions due to previous sensitization of the recipient to certain antigens, most commonly IgA, may be observed in exceptional cases, described under *CONTRAINDICATIONS* (12,13,39).

In patients with ITP, who receive higher doses (0.4 g/kg/day or greater) 2.9% of infusions may result in adverse reactions (18). Headache, generally mild, is the most common symptom noted, occurring during or following 2% of infusions.

A few cases of usually mild hemolysis have been reported after infusion of intravenous immunoglobulin products (Brox et al, 1987, Kim et al, 1988). These were attributed to transferral of blood group (e.g., anti-D) antibodies (Copelan et al, 1986, Nicholls et al, 1989).

DOSAGE AND ADMINISTRATION

It is generally advisable not to dilute plasma derivatives with other infusable drugs. Immune Globulin Intravenous (Human), Sandoglobulin®, should be given by a separate infusion line. No other medications or fluids should be mixed with the Sandoglobulin® (IGIV) preparation.

Adult and Child Substitution Therapy

The usual dose of Sandoglobulin® (IGIV) in immunodeficiency syndromes is 0.2 g/kg of body weight administered once a month by intravenous infusion. If the clinical response is inadequate, the dose may be increased to 0.3 g/kg of body weight or the infusion may be repeated more frequently than once a month (12,15,16,17).

The first infusion of Immune Globulin Intravenous (Human), Sandoglobulin®, in previously untreated agammaglobulinemic or hypogammaglobulinemic patients must be given as a 3% immunoglobulin solution (use the total volume of fluid provided, or see *Table 2*, to reconstitute the lyophilized product). Start with a flow rate of 10-20 drops (0.5-1.0 mL) per minute. After 15-30 minutes the rate of infusion may be further increased to 30-50 drops (1.5-2.5 mL) per minute.

After the first bottle of 3% solution is infused and the patient shows good tolerance, subsequent infusions may be administered at a higher rate or concentration. Such increases should be made gradually allowing 15-30 minutes before each increment.

Infusion of Immune Globulin Intravenous (Human), Sandoglobulin®, at rates up to 30 mg/kg/min has been achieved without any increase in the number or degree of adverse reactions observed (13). The first infusion of Sandoglobulin® (IGIV) in previously untreated agammaglobulinemic and hypogammaglobulinemic patients may lead to systemic side effects. Some of the effects may occur as a result of the reaction between the antibodies administered and free antigens in the blood and tissues of the immunodeficient recipient (39,41). When free antigen is no longer present, further administration of Sandoglobulin® (IGIV) to immunodeficient patients as well as to normal individuals usually does not cause further untoward side effects.

Therapy of Idiopathic Thrombocytopenic Purpura (ITP)

Induction

0.4 g/kg of body weight on 2-5 consecutive days.

Acute ITP–Childhood

In acute ITP of childhood, if an initial platelet count response to the first two doses is adequate (30-50,000/µl), therapy may be discontinued after the second day of the 5 day course (18).

Maintenance–Chronic ITP

In adults and children, if after induction therapy the platelet count falls to less than 30,000/µl and/or the patient manifests clinically significant bleeding, 0.4 g/kg of body weight may be given as a single infusion. If an adequate response does not result, the dose can be increased to 0.8-1.0 g/kg of body weight given as a single infusion (19, 40).

Reconstitution

For a 3% solution using the transfer set

1. Tear off the protective caps from the bottle containing the solvent and the Immune Globulin Intravenous (Human), Sandoglobulin®. Disinfect both rubber stoppers with alcohol.
2. Remove the protective cover from one end of the transfer set and insert the needle through the rubber stopper into the bottle containing the solvent.
3. Remove the cover from the other needle and plunge the inverted Immune Globulin Intravenous (Human), Sandoglobulin®, bottle onto it, as shown in 3.

Continued on next page

Sandoglobulin—Cont.

4. Invert the two bottles so that the solvent flows into the Sandoglobulin® (IGIV) bottle until the required amount (see *Table 2*, below) has been transferred.
5. Discard any unused solvent and the transfer set.

For a 6% solution using the transfer set
1. Follow steps 1-3 aforementioned.
2. Invert the two bottles so that the solvent flows into the Immune Globulin Intravenous (Human), Sandoglobulin®, bottle. Use the appropriate amount (see *Table 2*, below) of solvent by removing the solvent bottle with transfer needle as soon as the fluid reaches the 6% mark printed on the Sandoglobulin® (IGIV) label.
3. Discard any unused solvent and the transfer set.

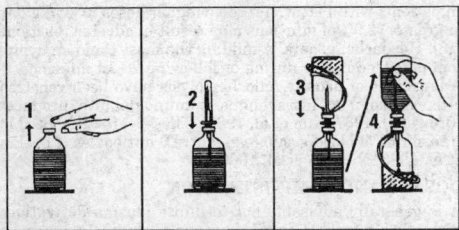

To reconstitute Sandoglobulin® (IGIV) from the multivial bulk pack, or when using other diluents or higher concentrations, *Table 2* indicates the volume of sterile diluent required. Observing aseptic technique, this volume should be drawn into a sterile hypodermic syringe and needle. The diluent is then injected into the corresponding Immune Globulin Intravenous (Human), Sandoglobulin®, vial size.

Table 2
Required Diluent Volume

Concentration	1 g Vial	3 g Vial	6 g Vial	12 g Vial
3%	33.0 cc	100 cc	200 cc	*
6%	16.5 cc	50 cc	100 cc	200 cc
9%	11.0 cc	33 cc	66 cc	132 cc
12%	8.3 cc	25 cc	50 cc	100 cc

*Container not large enough to permit this concentration

If large doses of Sandoglobulin® (IGIV) are to be administered, several reconstituted vials of identical concentration and diluent may be pooled in an empty sterile glass or plastic i.v. infusion container using aseptic technique.
Sandoglobulin® (IGIV) normally dissolves within a few minutes, though in exceptional cases it may take up to 20 minutes.
DO NOT SHAKE! Excessive shaking will cause foaming.
Any undissolved particles should respond to careful rotation of the bottle. Avoid foaming. Parenteral drug products should be inspected visually for particulate matter and discoloration prior to administration, whenever solution and container permit.
Filtering of Immune Globulin Intravenous (Human), Sandoglobulin®, is acceptable but not required. Pore sizes of 15 microns or larger will be less likely to slow infusion, especially with higher Sandoglobulin® (IGIV) concentrations. Antibacterial filters (0.2 microns) may be used.
When reconstitution of Sandoglobulin® (IGIV) occurs outside of sterile laminar air flow conditions, administration must begin promptly with partially used vials discarded. When reconstitution is carried out in a sterile laminar flow hood using aseptic technique, administration may begin within 24 hours provided the solution has been refrigerated during that time. Do not freeze Sandoglobulin® (IGIV) solution.
PROCEED WITH INFUSION ONLY IF SOLUTION IS CLEAR AND AT APPROXIMATELY ROOM TEMPERATURE!

HOW SUPPLIED

Immune Globulin Intravenous (Human), Sandoglobulin®, is available as a white lyophilized powder in 1, 3, 6, and 12 g size vials. The only diluents which may be used to reconstitute the product are sterile (0.9%) Sodium Chloride Injection USP, 5% Dextrose, or Sterile Water.
Sandoglobulin® (IGIV) is available in bulk packs of ten vials and individual vial packages.

1 g
Individual vial package (NDC 0078-0120-94)
3 g
Bulk pack (NDC 0078-0122-19)
Individual vial package (NDC 0078-0122-95)
6 g
Bulk pack (NDC 0078-0124-19)
Individual vial package (NDC 0078-0124-96)
12 g
Bulk pack (NDC 0078-0244-19)
Individual vial package (NDC 0078-0244-93)
Please see *Table 1* for Calculated Sandoglobulin® (IGIV) Osmolality (mOsm/kg).
Store and Dispense
Immune Globulin Intravenous (Human), Sandoglobulin®, should be stored at room temperature not exceeding 30°C (86°F). The preparation should not be used after the expiration date printed on the label.

References

1. Gardi A: Quality control in the production of an immunoglobulin for intravenous use. *Blut* **48**:337-344, 1984.
2. Römer J, Morgenthaler JJ, Scherz R, et al: Characterization of various immunoglobulin-preparations for intravenous application. I. Protein composition and antibody content. *Vox Sang* **42**:62-73, 1982.
3. Römer J, Späth PJ, Skvaril F, et al: Characterization of various immunoglobulin preparations for intravenous application. II. Complement activation and binding to Staphylococcus protein A. *Vox Sang* **42**:74-80, 1982.
4. Römer J, Späth PJ: Molecular composition of immunoglobulin preparations and its relation to complement activation, in Nydegger UE (ed): *Immunohemotherapy: A Guide to Immunoglobulin Prophylaxis and Therapy.* London, Academic Press, 1981, p 123.
5. Skvaril F, Roth-Wicky B, and Barandun S: IgG subclasses in human-γ-globulin preparations for intravenous use and their reactivity with Staphylococcus protein A. *Vox Sang* **38**:147, 1980.
6. Skvaril F: Qualitative and quantitative aspects of IgG subclasses in i.v. immunoglobulin preparations, in Nydegger UE (ed): *Immunohemotherapy: A Guide to Immunoglobulin Prophylaxis and Therapy.* London, Academic Press, 1981, p 113.
7. Skvaril F, and Barandun S: In vitro characterization of immunoglobulins for intravenous use, in Alving BM, Finlayson JS (eds): *Immunoglobulins: Characteristics and Uses of Intravenous Preparations*, DHHS Publication No. (FDA)-80-9005. US Government Printing Office, 1980, pp 201-206.
8. Burckhardt JJ, Gardi A, Oxelius V, et al: Immunoglobulin G subclass distribution in three human intravenous immunoglobulin preparations. *Vox Sang* **57**:10-14, 1989.
9. Morell A, and Skvaril F: Struktur und biologische Eigenschaften von Immunoglobulinen und γ-Globulin-Präparaten. II. Eigenschaften von γ-Globulin-Präparaten. *Schweiz Med Wochenschr* **110**:80, 1980.
10. Morell A, Schürch B, Ryser D, et al: In vivo behavior of gamma globulin preparations. *Vox Sang* **38**:272, 1980.
11. Imbach P, Barandun S, d'Apuzzo V, et al: High-dose intravenous gamma globulin for idiopathic thrombocytopenic purpura in childhood. *Lancet* **1**:1228, 1981.
12. Barandun S, Morell A, Skvaril F: Clinical experiences with immunoglobulin for intravenous use, in Alving BM, Finlayson JS (eds): *Immunoglobulins: Characteristics and Uses of Intravenous Preparations.* DHHS Publication No. (FDA)-80-9005. US Government Printing Office, 1980, pp 31-35.
13. Schiff R, Sedlak D, Buckley R: Rapid infusion of Sandoglobulin® in patients with primary humoral immunodeficiency. *J Allergy Clin Immunol* **88**:61, 1991.
14. Wade A (ed): *Martindale: The Extra Pharmacopoeia*, ed 27. London, The Pharmaceutical Press, 1979, p 65.
15. Joller PW, Barandun S, Hitzig WH: Neue Möglichkeiten der Immunoglobulin-Ersatztherapie bei Antikörpermangel. Syndrom. *Schweiz Med Wochenschr* **110**:1451, 1980.
16. Barandun S, Imbach P, Morell A, et al: Clinical indications for immunoglobulin infusion, in Nydegger UE (ed): *Immunohemotherapy: A Guide to Immunoglobulin Prophylaxis and Therapy.* London, Academic Press, 1981, p 275.
17. Cunningham-Rundles C, Smithwick EM, Siegal FP, et al: Treatment of primary humoral immunodeficiency disease with intravenous (pH 4.0 treated) gamma globulin, in Nydegger UE (ed): *Immunohemotherapy: A Guide to Immunoglobulin Prophylaxis and Therapy.* London, Academic Press, 1981, p 283.
18. Imbach P, Wagner HP, Berchtold W, et al: Intravenous immunoglobulin versus oral corticosteroids in acute immune thrombocytopenic purpura in childhood. *Lancet* **2**:464, 1985.
19. Fehr J, Hofmann V, Kappeler U: Transient reversal of thrombocytopenia in idiopathic thrombocytopenic purpura by high-dose intravenous gamma globulin. *N Engl J Med* **306**:1254, 1982.
20. Müeller-Eckhardt C, Küenzlen E, Thilo-Körner D, et al: High-dose intravenous immunoglobulin for posttransfusion purpura. *N Engl J Med* **308**:287, 1983.
21. Wenske G, Gaedicke G, Küenzlen E, et al: Treatment of idiopathic thrombocytopenic purpura in pregnancy by high-dose intravenous immunoglobulin. *Blut* **46**:347-353, 1983.
22. Newland AC, Treleaven JG, Minchinton B, et al: High-dose intravenous IgG in adults with autoimmune thrombocytopenia. *Lancet* **1**:84-87, 1983.
23. Bussel JB, Kimberly RP, Inman RD, et al: Intravenous gammaglobulin for chronic idiopathic thrombocytopenic purpura. *Blood* **62**:480-486, 1983.
24. Abe T, Matsuda J, Kawasugi K, et al: Clinical effect of intravenous immunoglobulin in chronic idiopathic thrombocytopenic purpura. *Blut* **47**:69-75, 1983.
25. Bussel JB, Schulman I, Hilgartner MW, et al: Intravenous use of gamma globulin in the treatment of chronic immune thrombocytopenic purpura as a means to defer splenectomy. *J Pediatr* **103**:651-654, 1983.
26. Imholz B, et al: Intravenous immunoglobulin (i.v. IgG) for previously treated acute or for chronic idiopathic thrombocytopenic purpura (ITP) in childhood: A prospective multicenter study. *Blut* **56**:63-68, 1988.
27. Lusher JM, and Warrier I: Use of intravenous gamma globulin in children with idiopathic thrombocytopenic purpura and other immune thrombocytopenias. *Am J Med* **83(suppl 4A)**:10-16, 1987.
28. Hammarstrom L, and Smith CI: Placental transfer of intravenous immunoglobulin. *Lancet* **1**:681, 1986.
29. Sidiropoulos D, et al: Transplacental passage of intravenous immunoglobulin in the last trimester of pregnancy. *J Pediatr* **109**:505-508, 1986.
30. Wenske G, et al: Idiopathic thrombocytopenic purpura in pregnancy and neonatal period. *Blut* **48**:377-382, 1984.
31. Fabris P, et al: Successful treatment of a steroid-resistant form of idiopathic thrombocytopenic purpura in pregnancy with high doses of intravenous immunoglobulins. *Acta Haemat* **77**:107-110, 1987.
32. Coller BS, et al: Management of severe ITP during pregnancy with intravenous immunoglobulin (IVIgG). *Clin Res* **33**:545A, 1985.
33. Tchernia G, et al: Management of immune thrombocytopenia in pregnancy: Response to infusions of immunoglobulins. *Am J Obstet Gynecol* **148**:225-226, 1984.
34. Newland AC, et al: Intravenous IgG for autoimmune thrombocytopenia in pregnancy. *N Engl J Med* **310**:261-262, 1984.
35. Morgenstern GR, et al: Autoimmune thrombocytopenia in pregnancy: New approach to management. *Br Med J* **287**:584, 1983.
36. Ciccimarra F, et al: Treatment of neonatal passive immune thrombocytopenia. *J Pediat* **105**:677-678, 1984.
37. Rose VL, and Gordon LI: Idiopathic thrombocytopenic purpura in pregnancy. Successful management with immunoglobulin infusion. *JAMA* **254**:2626-2628, 1985.
38. Gounder MP, et al: Intravenous gammaglobulin therapy in the management of a patient with idiopathic thrombocytopenic purpura and a warm autoimmune erythrocyte panagglutinin during pregnancy. *Obstet Gynecol* **67**:741-746, 1986.
39. Cunningham-Rundles C, Day NK, Wahn V, et al: Reactions to intravenous gamma globulin infusions and immune complex formation, in Nydegger UE (ed): *Immunohemotherapy: A Guide to Immunoglobulin Prophylaxis and Therapy.* London, Academic Press, 1981, p 447.
40. Bussel JB, Pham LC, Hilgartner MW, et al: Long-term maintenance of adults with ITP using intravenous gamma globulin. Abstract, *American Society of Hematology*. New Orleans, December, 1985.
41. Barandun S, Morell A: Adverse reactions to immunoglobulin preparations, in Nydegger UE (ed): *Immunohemotherapy: A Guide to Immunoglobulin Prophylaxis and Therapy.* London, Academic Press, 1981, p 223.
42. Hamamoto Y, Harada S, Yamamoto N, et al: Elimination of viruses (human immunodeficiency, hepatitis B, vesicular stomatitis and sindbis viruses) from an intravenous immunoglobulin preparation. *Vox Sang* **53**:65-69, 1987.
43. Henin Y, Marechal V, Barre-Sinoussi F, et al: Inactivation and partition of human immunodeficiency virus during Kistler and Nitschmann fractionation of human blood plasma. *Vox Sang* **54**:78-83, 1988.
44. Wells MA, Wittek AE, Epstein JS, et al: Inactivation and partition of human T-cell lymphotropic virus, type III, during ethanol fractionation of plasma. *Transfusion* **26**:394-397, 1986.
45. Kempf C, Jentsch P, Poirier B, et al: Virus inactivation during production of intravenous immunoglobulin. *Transfusion* **31**:423-427, 1991.
46. Brox AG, Cournoyer D, et al: Hemolytic anemia following intravenous gamma globulin administration. *Am J Med* **82**:633-635, 1987.
47. Kim HC, Park CL, Cowan JH, et al: Massive intravascular hemolysis associated with intravenous immunoglobulin in bone marrow transplant recipients. *Am J Ped Hematol/Oncol* **10**:67-74, 1988.

48. Nicholls MD, Cummins JC, et al: Hemolysis induced by intravenously-administered immunoglobulin. *Med J of Australia* **150**:404-406, 1989.
49. Copelan EA, et al: Hemolysis following intravenous immune globulin therapy. *Transfusion* **26**:410-412, 1986.

Manufactured by:
CENTRAL LABORATORY
BLOOD TRANSFUSION SERVICE
SWISS RED CROSS
Wankdorfstrasse 10, 3000 Berne 22, Switzerland
US License No. 647
Distributed by:
SANDOZ PHARMACEUTICALS CORPORATION
East Hanover, NJ 07936
REV. AUGUST 1996 30184903

Shown in Product Identification Guide, page 325

SANDOSTATIN® ℞

[*săn dō stăt ĭn*]
octreotide acetate/SANDOZ
INJECTION

CAUTION: Federal law prohibits dispensing without a prescription.

The following prescribing information is based on official labeling in effect on August 1, 1998.

DESCRIPTION

Sandostatin® (octreotide acetate) Injection, a cyclic octapeptide prepared as a clear sterile solution of octreotide, acetate salt, in a buffered lactic acid solution for administration by deep subcutaneous (intrafat) or intravenous injection. Octreotide acetate, known chemically as L-Cysteinamide, D-phenylalanyl -L- cysteinyl -L- phenylalanyl-D-tryptophyl-L -lysyl- L- threonyl - N - [2 - hydroxy - 1 - (hydroxymethyl) propyl] -, cyclic (2→7)-disulfide; [R-(R*, R*)] acetate salt, is a long-acting octapeptide with pharmacologic actions mimicking those of the natural hormone somatostatin.

Sandostatin® (octreotide acetate) Injection is available as: sterile 1 mL ampuls in 3 strengths, containing 50, 100, or 500 mcg octreotide (as acetate), and sterile 5 mL multi-dose vials in 2 strengths, containing 200 and 1000 mcg/mL of octreotide (as acetate).

Each ampul also contains:

lactic acid, USP	3.4 mg
mannitol, USP	45 mg
sodium bicarbonate, USP	qs to pH 4.2 ± 0.3
water for injection, USP	qs to 1 mL

Each mL of the multi-dose vials also contains:

lactic acid, USP	3.4 mg
mannitol, USP	45 mg
phenol, USP	5.0 mg
sodium bicarbonate, USP	qs to pH 4.2 ± 0.3
water for injection, USP	qs to 1 mL

Lactic acid and sodium bicarbonate are added to provide a buffered solution, pH to 4.2 ± 0.3.

The molecular weight of octreotide acetate is 1019.3 (free peptide, $C_{49}H_{66}N_{10}O_{10}S_2$) and its amino acid sequence is:

H-D-Phe-Cys-Phe-D-Trp-Lys-Thr-Cys-Thr-ol,
x CH_3COOH where x = 1.4 to 2.5

CLINICAL PHARMACOLOGY

Sandostatin® (octreotide acetate) exerts pharmacologic actions similar to the natural hormone, somatostatin. It is an even more potent inhibitor of growth hormone, glucagon, and insulin than somatostatin. Like somatostatin, it also suppresses LH response to GnRH, decreases splanchnic blood flow, and inhibits release of serotonin, gastrin, vasoactive intestinal peptide, secretin, motilin, and pancreatic polypeptide.

By virtue of these pharmacological actions, Sandostatin® (octreotide acetate) has been used to treat the symptoms associated with metastatic carcinoid tumors (flushing and diarrhea), and Vasoactive Intestinal Peptide (VIP) secreting adenomas (watery diarrhea).

Sandostatin® (octreotide acetate) substantially reduces growth hormone and/or IGF-I (somatomedin C) levels in patients with acromegaly.

Single doses of Sandostatin (octreotide acetate) have been shown to inhibit gallbladder contractility and to decrease bile secretion in normal volunteers. In controlled clinical trials the incidence of gallstone or biliary sludge formation was markedly increased *(See WARNINGS)*.

Sandostatin® (octreotide acetate) suppresses secretion of thyroid stimulating hormone (TSH).

Pharmacokinetics

After subcutaneous injection, octreotide is absorbed rapidly and completely from the injection site. Peak concentrations of 5.2 ng/mL (100 mcg dose) were reached 0.4 hours after dosing. Using a specific radioimmunoassay, intravenous and subcutaneous doses were found to be bioequivalent. Peak concentrations and area under the curve values were dose proportional both after subcutaneous or intravenous single doses up to 400 mcg and with multiple doses of 200 mcg t.i.d. (600 mcg/day). Clearance was reduced by about 66% suggesting non-linear kinetics of the drug at daily doses of 600 mcg/day as compared to 150 mcg/day. The relative decrease in clearance with doses above 600 mcg/day is not defined.

In healthy volunteers the distribution of octreotide from plasma was rapid ($t\alpha 1/2$ = 0.2 h), the volume of distribution (Vdss) was estimated to be 13.6 L, and the total body clearance was 10 L/hr.

In blood, the distribution into the erythrocytes was found to be negligible and about 65% was bound in the plasma in a concentration-independent manner. Binding was mainly to lipoprotein and, to a lesser extent, to albumin.

The elimination of octreotide from plasma had an apparent half-life of 1.7 hours compared with 1-3 minutes with the natural hormone. The duration of action of Sandostatin® (octreotide acetate) is variable but extends up to 12 hours depending upon the type of tumor. About 32% of the dose is excreted unchanged into the urine. In an elderly population, dose adjustments may be necessary due to a significant increase in the half-life (46%) and a significant decrease in the clearance (26%) of the drug.

In patients with acromegaly, the pharmacokinetics differ somewhat from those in healthy volunteers. A mean peak concentration of 2.8 ng/mL (100 mcg dose) was reached in 0.7 hours after subcutaneous dosing. The volume of distribution (Vdss) was estimated to be 21.6 ± 8.5 L and the total body clearance was increased to 18 L/h. The mean percent of the drug bound was 41.2%. The disposition and elimination half-lives were similar to normals.

In patients with severe renal failure requiring dialysis, clearance was reduced to about half that found in normal subjects (from approximately 10 L/h to 4.5 L/h). The effect of hepatic diseases on the disposition of octreotide is unknown.

INDICATIONS AND USAGE

Acromegaly

Sandostatin® (octreotide acetate) is indicated to reduce blood levels of growth hormone and IGF-I (somatomedin C) in acromegaly patients who have had inadequate response to or cannot be treated with surgical resection, pituitary irradiation, and bromocriptine mesylate at maximally tolerated doses. The goal is to achieve normalization of growth hormone and IGF-I (somatomedin C) levels *(See DOSAGE AND ADMINISTRATION)*. In patients with acromegaly, Sandostatin® (octreotide acetate) reduces growth hormone to within normal ranges in 50% of patients and reduces IGF-I (somatomedin C) to within normal ranges in 50%-60% of patients. Since the effects of pituitary irradiation may not become maximal for several years, adjunctive therapy with Sandostatin® (octreotide acetate) to reduce blood levels of growth hormone and IGF-I (somatomedin C) offers potential benefit before the effects of irradiation are manifested.

Improvement in clinical signs and symptoms or reduction in tumor size or rate of growth were not shown in clinical trials performed with Sandostatin® (octreotide acetate); these trials were not optimally designed to detect such effects.

Carcinoid Tumors

Sandostatin® (octreotide acetate) is indicated for the symptomatic treatment of patients with metastatic carcinoid tumors where it suppresses or inhibits the severe diarrhea and flushing episodes associated with the disease.

Sandostatin® (octreotide acetate) studies were not designed to show an effect on the size, rate of growth or development of metastases.

Vasoactive Intestinal Peptide Tumors (VIPomas)

Sandostatin® (octreotide acetate) is indicated for the treatment of the profuse watery diarrhea associated with VIP-secreting tumors. Sandostatin® (octreotide acetate) studies were not designed to show an effect on the size, rate of growth or development of metastases.

CONTRAINDICATIONS

Sensitivity to this drug or any of its components.

WARNINGS

Single doses of Sandostatin® (octreotide acetate) have been shown to inhibit gallbladder contractility and decrease bile secretion in normal volunteers. In clinical trials (primarily patients with acromegaly or psoriasis), the incidence of biliary tract abnormalities was 63% (27% gallstones, 24% sludge without stones, 12% biliary duct dilatation). The incidence of stones or sludge in patients who received Sandostatin® (octreotide acetate) for 12 months or longer was 52%. Less than 2% of patients treated with Sandostatin® (octreotide acetate) for 1 month or less developed gallstones. The incidence of gallstones did not appear related to age, sex or dose. Like patients without gallbladder abnormalities, the majority of patients developing gallbladder abnormalities on ultrasound had gastrointestinal symptoms. The symptoms were not specific for gallbladder disease. A few patients developed acute cholecystitis, ascending cholangitis, biliary obstruction, cholestatic hepatitis, or pancreatitis during Sandostatin® (octreotide acetate) therapy or following its withdrawal. One patient developed ascending cholangitis during Sandostatin® (octreotide acetate) therapy and died.

PRECAUTIONS

General

Sandostatin® (octreotide acetate) alters the balance between the counter-regulatory hormones, insulin, glucagon and growth hormone, which may result in hypoglycemia or hyperglycemia. Sandostatin® (octreotide acetate) also suppresses secretion of thyroid stimulating hormone, which may result in hypothyroidism. Cardiac conduction abnormalities have also occurred during treatment with Sandostatin® (octreotide acetate). However, the incidence of these adverse events during long-term therapy was determined vigorously only in acromegaly patients who, due to their underlying disease and/or the subsequent treatment they receive, are at an increased risk for the development of diabetes mellitus, hypothyroidism, and cardiovascular disease. Although the degree to which these abnormalities are related to Sandostatin® (octreotide acetate) therapy is not clear, new abnormalities of glycemic control, thyroid function and ECG developed during Sandostatin® (octreotide acetate) therapy as described below.

The hypoglycemia or hyperglycemia which occurs during Sandostatin® (octreotide acetate) therapy is usually mild, but may result in overt diabetes mellitus or necessitate dose changes in insulin or other hypoglycemic agents. Hypoglycemia and hyperglycemia occurred on Sandostatin® (octreotide acetate) in 3% and 16% of acromegalic patients, respectively. Severe hyperglycemia, subsequent pneumonia, and death following initiation of Sandostatin® (octreotide acetate) therapy was reported in one patient with no history of hyperglycemia.

In acromegalic patients, 12% developed biochemical hypothyroidism only, 8% developed goiter, and 4% required initiation of thyroid replacement therapy while receiving Sandostatin® (octreotide acetate). Baseline and periodic assessment of thyroid function (TSH, total and/or free T_4) is recommended during chronic therapy.

In acromegalics, bradycardia (<50 bpm) developed in 25%; conduction abnormalities occurred in 10% and arrhythmias occurred in 9% of patients during Sandostatin® (octreotide acetate) therapy. Other EKG changes observed included QT prolongation, axis shifts, early repolarization, low voltage, R/S transition, and early R wave progression. These ECG changes are not uncommon in acromegalic patients. Dose adjustments in drugs such as beta-blockers that have bradycardia effects may be necessary. In one acromegalic patient with severe congestive heart failure, initiation of Sandostatin® (octreotide acetate) therapy resulted in worsening of CHF with improvement when drug was discontinued. Confirmation of a drug effect was obtained with a positive rechallenge.

Several cases of pancreatitis have been reported in patients receiving Sandostatin® (octreotide acetate) therapy.

Sandostatin® (octreotide acetate) may alter absorption of dietary fats in some patients.

In patients with severe renal failure requiring dialysis, the half-life of Sandostatin® (octreotide acetate) may be increased, necessitating adjustment of the maintenance dosage.

Depressed vitamin B_{12} levels and abnormal Schilling's tests have been observed in some patients receiving Sandostatin® (octreotide acetate) therapy, and monitoring of vitamin B_{12} levels is recommended during chronic Sandostatin® (octreotide acetate) therapy.

Information for Patients

Careful instruction in sterile subcutaneous injection technique should be given to the patients and to other persons who may administer Sandostatin® (octreotide acetate) Injection.

Laboratory Tests

Laboratory tests that may be helpful as biochemical markers in determining and following patient response depend on the specific tumor. Based on diagnosis, measurement of the following substances may be useful in monitoring the progress of therapy:

Acromegaly:	Growth Hormone, IGF-I (somatomedin C)
	Responsiveness to Sandostatin® (octreotide acetate) may be evaluated by determining growth hormone levels at 1-4 hour intervals for 8-12 hours post dose. Alternatively, a single measurement of IGF-I (somatomedin C) level may be made two weeks after drug initiation or dosage change.
Carcinoid:	5-HIAA (urinary 5-hydroxyindole acetic acid), plasma serotonin, plasma Substance P
VIPoma:	VIP (plasma vasoactive intestinal peptide)

Continued on next page

Sandostatin—Cont.

Baseline and periodic total and/or free T_4 measurements should be performed during chronic therapy *(see PRECAUTIONS — General)*.

Drug Interactions

Sandostatin® (octreotide acetate) has been associated with alterations in nutrient absorption, so it may have an effect on absorption of orally administered drugs. Concomitant administration of Sandostatin® (octreotide acetate) with cyclosporine may decrease blood levels of cyclosporine and result in transplant rejection.

Patients receiving insulin, oral hypoglycemic agents, beta blockers, calcium channel blockers, or agents to control fluid and electrolyte balance, may require dose adjustments of these therapeutic agents.

Drug Laboratory Test Interactions

No known interference exists with clinical laboratory tests, including amine or peptide determinations.

Carcinogenesis/Mutagenesis/Impairment of Fertility

Studies in laboratory animals have demonstrated no mutagenic potential of Sandostatin® (octreotide acetate).

No carcinogenic potential was demonstrated in mice treated subcutaneously for 85-99 weeks at doses up to 2000 mcg/kg/day (8× the human exposure based on body surface area). In a 116-week subcutaneous study in rats, a 27% and 12% incidence of injection site sarcomas or squamous cell carcinomas was observed in males and females, respectively, at the highest dose level of 1250 mcg/kg/day (10× the human exposure based on body surface area) compared to an incidence of 8%-10% in the vehicle control groups. The increased incidence of injection site tumors was most probably caused by irritation and the high sensitivity of the rat to repeated subcutaneous injections at the same site. Rotating injection sites would prevent chronic irritation in humans. There have been no reports of injection site tumors in patients treated with Sandostatin® (octreotide acetate) for up to 5 years. There was also a 15% incidence of uterine adenocarcinomas in the 1250 mcg/kg/day females compared to 7% in the saline control females and 0% in the vehicle control females. The presence of endometritis coupled with the absence of corpora lutea, the reduction in mammary fibroadenomas, and the presence of uterine dilatation suggest that the uterine tumors were associated with estrogen dominance in the aged female rats which does not occur in humans.

Sandostatin® (octreotide acetate) did not impair fertility in rats at doses up to 1000 mcg/kg/day, which represents 7× the human exposure based on body surface area.

Pregnancy Category B

Reproduction studies have been performed in rats and rabbits at doses up to 16 times the highest human dose based on body surface area and have revealed no evidence of impaired fertility or harm to the fetus due to Sandostatin® (octreotide acetate). There are, however, no adequate and well-controlled studies in pregnant women. Because animal reproduction studies are not always predictive of human response, this drug should be used during pregnancy only if clearly needed.

Nursing Mothers

It is not known whether this drug is excreted in human milk. Because many drugs are excreted in milk, caution should be exercised when Sandostatin® (octreotide acetate) is administered to a nursing woman.

Pediatric Use

Experience with Sandostatin® (octreotide acetate) in the pediatric population is limited. The youngest patient to receive the drug was 1 month old. Doses of 1-10 mcg/kg body weight were well tolerated in the young patients. A single case of an infant (nesidioblastosis) was complicated by a seizure thought to be independent of Sandostatin® (octreotide acetate) therapy.

ADVERSE REACTIONS

Gallbladder Abnormalities

Gallbladder abnormalities, especially stones and/or biliary sludge, frequently develop in patients on chronic Sandostatin® (octreotide acetate) therapy *(See WARNINGS)*.

Cardiac

In acromegalics, sinus bradycardia (<50 bpm) developed in 25%; conduction abnormalities occurred in 10% and arrhythmias developed in 9% of patients during Sandostatin® (octreotide acetate) therapy *(see PRECAUTIONS — General)*.

Gastrointestinal

Diarrhea, loose stools, nausea and abdominal discomfort were each seen in 34%-61% of acromegalic patients in US studies although only 2.6% of the patients discontinued therapy due to these symptoms. These symptoms were seen in 5%-10% of patients with other disorders.

The frequency of these symptoms was not dose-related, but diarrhea and abdominal discomfort generally resolved more quickly in patients treated with 300 mcg/day than in those treated with 750 mcg/day. Vomiting, flatulence, abnormal stools, abdominal distention, and constipation were each seen in less than 10% of patients.

Hypo/Hyperglycemia

Hypoglycemia and hyperglycemia occurred in 3% and 16% of acromegalic patients, respectively, but only in about 1.5% of other patients. Symptoms of hypoglycemia were noted in approximately 2% of patients.

Hypothyroidism

In acromegalics, biochemical hypothyroidism alone occurred in 12% while goiter occurred in 6% during Sandostatin® (octreotide acetate) therapy *(see PRECAUTIONS — General)*. In patients without acromegaly, hypothyroidism has only been reported in several isolated patients and goiter has not been reported.

Other Adverse Events

Pain on injection was reported in 7.7%, headache in 6% and dizziness in 5%. Pancreatitis was also observed *(see WARNINGS and PRECAUTIONS)*.

Other Adverse Events 1%-4%

Other events (relationship to drug not established), each observed in 1%-4% of patients, included fatigue, weakness, pruritus, joint pain, backache, urinary tract infection, cold symptoms, flu symptoms, injection site hematoma, bruise, edema, flushing, blurred vision, pollakiuria, fat malabsorption, hair loss, visual disturbance and depression.

Other Adverse Events <1%

Events reported in less than 1% of patients and for which relationship to drug is not established are listed: *Gastrointestinal:* hepatitis, jaundice, increase in liver enzymes, GI bleeding, hemorrhoids, appendicitis, gastric/peptic ulcer, gallbladder polyp; *Integumentary:* rash, cellulitis, petechiae, urticaria, basal cell carcinoma; *Musculoskeletal:* arthritis, joint effusion, muscle pain, Raynaud's phenomenon; *Cardiovascular:* chest pain, shortness of breath, thrombophlebitis, ischemia, congestive heart failure, hypertension, hypertensive reaction, palpitations, orthostatic BP decrease, tachycardia; *CNS:* anxiety, libido decrease, syncope, tremor, seizure, vertigo, Bell's Palsy, paranoia, pituitary apoplexy, increased intraocular pressure, amnesia, hearing loss, neuritis; *Respiratory:* pneumonia, pulmonary nodule, status asthmaticus; *Endocrine:* galactorrhea, hypoadrenalism, diabetes insipidus, gynecomastia, amenorrhea, polymenorrhea, oligomenorrhea, vaginitis; *Urogenital:* nephrolithiasis, hematuria; *Hematologic:* anemia, iron deficiency, epistaxis; *Miscellaneous:* otitis, allergic reaction, increased CK, weight loss.

Evaluation of 20 patients treated for at least 6 months has failed to demonstrate titers of antibodies exceeding background levels. However, antibody titers to Sandostatin® (octreotide acetate) were subsequently reported in three patients and resulted in prolonged duration of drug action in two patients. Anaphylactoid reactions, including anaphylactic shock, have been reported in several patients receiving Sandostatin® (octreotide acetate).

OVERDOSAGE

No frank overdose has occurred in any patient to date. Intravenous bolus doses of 1 mg (1000 mcg) given to healthy volunteers and of 30 mg (30,000 mcg) IV over 20 minutes and of 120 mg (120,000 mcg) IV over 8 hours to research patients have not resulted in serious ill effects.

Up-to-date information about the treatment of overdose can often be obtained from a certified Regional Poison Control Center. Telephone numbers of certified Regional Poison Control Centers are listed in the Physicians' Desk Reference®.*

Mortality occurred in mice and rats given 72 mg/kg and 18 mg/kg IV, respectively.

*Medical Economics Company, Inc.

Drug Abuse and Dependence

There is no indication that Sandostatin® (octreotide acetate) has potential for drug abuse or dependence. Sandostatin® (octreotide acetate) levels in the central nervous system are negligible, even after doses up to 30,000 mcg.

DOSAGE AND ADMINISTRATION

Sandostatin® (octreotide acetate) may be administered subcutaneously or intravenously. Subcutaneous injection is the usual route of administration of Sandostatin® (octreotide acetate) for control of symptoms. Pain with subcutaneous administration may be reduced by using the smallest volume that will deliver the desired dose. Multiple subcutaneous injections at the same site within short periods of time should be avoided. Sites should be rotated in a systematic manner.

Parenteral drug products should be inspected visually for particulate matter and discoloration prior to administration. **Do not use if particulates and/or discoloration are observed.** Proper sterile technique should be used in the preparation of parenteral admixtures to minimize the possibility of microbial contamination. **Sandostatin® (octreotide acetate) is not compatible in Total Parenteral Nutrition (TPN) solutions because of the formation of a glycosyl octreotide conjugate which may decrease the efficacy of the product.**

Sandostatin® (octreotide acetate) is stable in sterile isotonic saline solutions or sterile solutions of dextrose 5% in water for 24 hours. It may be diluted in volumes of 50-200 mL and infused intravenously over 15-30 minutes or administered by IV push over 3 minutes. In emergency situations (e.g.: carcinoid crisis) it may be given by rapid bolus.

The initial dosage is usually 50 mcg administered twice or three times daily. Upward dose titration is frequently required. Dosage information for patients with specific tumors follows.

Acromegaly

Dosage may be initiated at 50 mcg t.i.d. Beginning with this low dose may permit adaptation to adverse gastrointestinal effects for patients who will require higher doses. IGF-I (somatomedin C) levels every 2 weeks can be used to guide titration. Alternatively, multiple growth hormone levels at 0-8 hours after Sandostatin® (octreotide acetate) administration permit more rapid titration of dose. The goal is to achieve growth hormone levels less than 5 ng/mL or IGF-I (somatomedin C) levels less than 1.9 U/mL in males and less than 2.2 U/mL in females. The dose most commonly found to be effective is 100 mcg t.i.d., but some patients require up to 500 mcg t.i.d. for maximum effectiveness. Doses greater than 300 mcg/day seldom result in additional biochemical benefit, and if an increase in dose fails to provide additional benefit, the dose should be reduced. IGF-I (somatomedin C) or growth hormone levels should be reevaluated at 6 month intervals.

Sandostatin® (octreotide acetate) should be withdrawn yearly for approximately 4 weeks from patients who have received irradiation to assess disease activity. If growth hormone or IGF-I (somatomedin C) levels increase and signs and symptoms recur, Sandostatin® (octreotide acetate) therapy may be resumed.

Carcinoid Tumors

The suggested daily dosage of Sandostatin® (octreotide acetate) during the first 2 weeks of therapy ranges from 100-600 mcg/day in 2-4 divided doses (mean daily dosage is 300 mcg). In the clinical studies, the **median** daily maintenance dosage was approximately 450 mcg, but clinical and biochemical benefits were obtained in some patients with as little as 50 mcg, while others required doses up to 1500 mcg/day. However, experience with doses above 750 mcg/day is limited.

VIPomas

Daily dosages of 200-300 mcg in 2-4 divided doses are recommended during the initial 2 weeks of therapy (range 150-750 mcg) to control symptoms of the disease. On an individual basis, dosage may be adjusted to achieve a therapeutic response, but usually doses above 450 mcg/day are not required.

HOW SUPPLIED

Sandostatin® (octreotide acetate) Injection is available in 1 mL ampuls and 5 mL multi-dose vials as follows:

Ampuls

50 mcg/mL octreotide (as acetate)
Package of 20 ampuls (NDC 0078-0180-03)
Package of 50 ampuls (NDC 0078-0180-04)

100 mcg/mL octreotide (as acetate)
Package of 20 ampuls (NDC 0078-0181-03)
Package of 50 ampuls (NDC 0078-0181-04)

500 mcg/mL octreotide (as acetate)
Package of 20 ampuls (NDC 0078-0182-03)
Package of 50 ampuls (NDC 0078-0182-04)

Multi-Dose Vials

200 mcg/mL octreotide (as acetate)
Box of one (NDC 0078-0183-25)

1000 mcg/mL octreotide (as acetate)
Box of one (NDC 0078-0184-25)

Storage

For prolonged storage, Sandostatin® (octreotide acetate) ampuls and multi-dose vials should be stored at refrigerated temperatures 2°-8°C (36°-46°F) and protected from light. At room temperature, (20°-30°C or 70°-86°F), Sandostatin® (octreotide acetate) is stable for 14 days if protected from light. The solution can be allowed to come to room temperature prior to administration. Do not warm artificially. After initial use, multiple dose vials should be discarded within 14 days. Ampuls should be opened just prior to administration and the unused portion discarded.

The ampuls and multi-dose are manufactured by
SANDOZ PHARMA LTD., Basle, Switzerland
for SANDOZ PHARMACEUTICALS CORPORATION,
East Hanover, New Jersey 07936

[REV: JANUARY 1997 30283903]

Shown in Product Identification Guide, page 325

SIMULECT® ℞

[*sĭ mu lɘct*]
(basiliximab)
For Injection
Rx only

The following prescribing information is based on official labeling in effect August 1, 1998.

WARNING

Only physicians experienced in immunosuppression therapy and management of organ transplantation patients should prescribe Simulect® (basiliximab). The physician responsible for Simulect® administration should have complete information requisite for the follow-up of the patient. Patients receiving the drug should be managed in facilities equipped and staffed with adequate laboratory and supportive medical resources.

DESCRIPTION

Simulect® (basiliximab) is a chimeric (murine/human) monoclonal antibody (IgG_{1k}), produced by recombinant DNA technology, that functions as an immunosuppressive agent, specifically binding to and blocking the interleukin-2 receptor α-chain (IL-2Rα, also known as CD25 antigen) on the surface of activated T-lymphocytes. Based on the amino acid sequence, the calculated molecular weight of the protein is 144 kilodaltons. It is a glycoprotein obtained from fermentation of an established mouse myeloma cell line genetically engineered to express plasmids containing the human heavy and light chain constant region genes and mouse heavy and light chain variable region genes encoding the RFT5 antibody that binds selectively to the IL-2Rα.

The active ingredient, basiliximab, is water soluble. The drug product, Simulect®, is a sterile lyophilisate which is available in 6 mL colorless glass vials. Each vial contains 20 mg basiliximab, 7.21 mg monobasic potassium phosphate, 0.99 mg disodium hydrogen phosphate (anhydrous), 1.61 mg sodium chloride, 20 mg sucrose, 80 mg mannitol and 40 mg glycine, to be reconstituted in 5 mL of Sterile Water for Injection, USP. No preservatives are added.

CLINICAL PHARMACOLOGY

General

Mechanism of action: Basiliximab functions as an IL-2 receptor antagonist by binding with high affinity ($K_a = 1 \times 10^{10}\ M^{-1}$) to the alpha chain of the high affinity IL-2 receptor complex and inhibiting IL-2 binding. Basiliximab is specifically targeted against IL-2Rα, which is selectively expressed on the surface of activated T-lymphocytes. This specific high affinity binding of Simulect® (basiliximab) to IL-2Rα competitively inhibits IL-2-mediated activation of lymphocytes, a critical pathway in the cellular immune response involved in allograft rejection.

While in the circulation, Simulect® impairs the response of the immune system to antigenic challenges. Whether the ability to respond to repeated or ongoing challenges with those antigens returns to normal after Simulect® is cleared is unknown. *(See PRECAUTIONS)*

Pharmacokinetics

Adults: Single-dose and multiple-dose pharmacokinetic studies have been conducted in patients undergoing first kidney transplantation. Cumulative doses ranged from 15 mg up to 150 mg. Peak mean ± SD serum concentration following intravenous infusion of 20 mg over 30 minutes is 7.1 ± 5.1 mg/L. There is a dose-proportional increase in C_{max} and AUC up to the highest tested single dose of 60 mg. The volume of distribution at steady state is 8.6 ± 4.1 L. The extent and degree of distribution to various body compartments have not been fully studied. The terminal half-life is 7.2 ± 3.2 days. Total body clearance is 41 ± 19 mL/h. No clinically relevant influence of body weight or gender on distribution volume or clearance has been observed in adult patients. Elimination half-life was not influenced by age (20-69 years), gender or race. *(See DOSAGE AND ADMINISTRATION)*

Pediatric: The pharmacokinetics of Simulect® were assessed in 12 pediatric renal transplantation patients, children (2-11 years of age, n=8) and adolescents (12-15 years of age, n=4). These data indicate that in children, the volume of distribution at steady state was 5.2 ± 2.8 L, half-life was 11.5 ± 6.3 days and clearance was 17 ± 6 mL/h. Distribution volume and clearance are reduced by about 50% compared to adult renal transplantation patients. Disposition parameters were not influenced to a clinically relevant extent by age, body weight (9-37 kg) or body surface area (0.44-1.20 m^2) in this age group. In adolescents, the volume of distribution at steady state was 10.1 ± 7.6 L, half-life was 7.2 ± 3.6 days and clearance was 45 ± 25 mL/h. Disposition in adolescents was similar to that in adult renal transplantation patients. *(See DOSAGE AND ADMINISTRATION)*

Pharmacodynamics

Complete and consistent binding to IL-2Rα in adults is maintained as long as serum Simulect® levels exceed 0.2 µg/mL. As concentrations fall below this threshold, the IL-2Rα sites are no longer fully bound and the number of T-cells expressing unbound IL-2Rα returns to pretherapy values within 1–2 weeks. The relationship between serum concentration and receptor saturation was assessed in two pediatric patients (2 and 12 years of age) and was similar to that characterized in adult renal transplantation patients. *In vitro* studies using human tissues indicate that Simulect® binds only to lymphocytes.

At the recommended dosing regimen, the mean ± SD duration of basiliximab saturation of IL-2Rα was 36 ± 14 days *(see DOSAGE AND ADMINISTRATION)*. The duration of clinically significant IL-2 receptor blockade after the recommended course of Simulect® is not known. No significant changes to circulating lymphocyte numbers or cell phenotypes were observed by flow cytometry. Cytokine release syndrome has not been reported after Simulect® administration.

Clinical Studies

The safety and efficacy of Simulect® for the prophylaxis of acute organ rejection in adults following first cadaveric- or living-donor renal transplantation were assessed in two randomized, double-blind, placebo-controlled, multicenter trials. These studies compared two 20 mg doses of Simulect® with placebo when each was administered intravenously as part of a standard immunosuppressive regimen comprised of cyclosporine for microemulsion and corticosteroids, administered starting on Day 0, to prevent acute renal allograft rejection. The first dose of Simulect® or placebo was administered within 2 hours prior to transplantation surgery (Day 0) and the second dose administered on Day 4 post-transplantation. The regimen of Simulect® was chosen to provide 30-45 days of IL-2Rα saturation. 729 patients were enrolled in the two studies, of which 363 Simulect®-treated patients and 358 placebo-treated patients underwent transplantation. One study was conducted at 21 sites in Europe and Canada (EU/CAN Study); the second was conducted at 21 sites in the USA (US Study). Patients 18-75 years of age undergoing first cadaveric (EU/CAN and US Studies) or living-donor (US only) renal transplantation, with ≥1 HLA mismatch, were enrolled.

The primary efficacy endpoint in both studies was the incidence of death, graft loss or an episode of acute rejection during the first 6 months post-transplantation. Secondary efficacy endpoints included the primary efficacy variable measured during the first 12 months post-transplantation, the incidence of biopsy-confirmed acute rejection during the first 6 and 12 months post-transplantation, and patient survival and graft survival, each measured at 12 months post-transplantation. Table 1 summarizes the results of these studies. Figure 1 displays the Kaplan-Meier estimates of the percentage of patients by treatment group experiencing the primary efficacy endpoint during the first 12 months post-transplantation for the US study. Patients in both studies receiving Simulect® experienced a significantly lower incidence of biopsy-confirmed rejection episodes at both 6 and 12 months post-transplantation. There was no difference in the rate of delayed graft function, patient survival, or graft survival between Simulect®-treated patients and placebo-treated patients in either study.

There was no evidence that the clinical benefit of Simulect® was limited to specific subpopulations based on age, gender, race, donor type (cadaveric or living-donor allograft) or history of diabetes mellitus.

Table 1
Efficacy Parameters (Percentage of Patients)

	EU/CAN Study			US Study		
	Placebo (N=185)	Simulect® (N=190)	p-value	Placebo (N=173)	Simulect® (N=173)	p-value
Primary endpoint						
Death, graft loss or acute rejection episode (0-6 months)	57%	42%	0.003	55%	38%	0.002
Secondary endpoints						
Death, graft loss or acute rejection episode (0-12 months)	60%	46%	0.007	58%	41%	0.001
Biopsy-confirmed rejection episode (0-6 months)	44%	30%	0.007	46%	33%	0.015
Biopsy-confirmed rejection episode (0-12 months)	46%	32%	0.005	49%	35%	0.009
Patient survival (12 months)	97%	95%	0.29	96%	97%	0.56
Patients with functioning graft (12 months)	87%	88%	0.70	93%	95%	0.50

[See figure at top of next column]

INDICATIONS AND USAGE

Simulect® (basiliximab) is indicated for the prophylaxis of acute organ rejection in patients receiving renal transplantation when used as part of an immunosuppressive regimen that includes cyclosporine and corticosteroids.

Figure 1
Kaplan-Meier Estimate of the Percentage of Subjects with Death, Graft Loss or First Rejection Episode
Month: 0 – 12

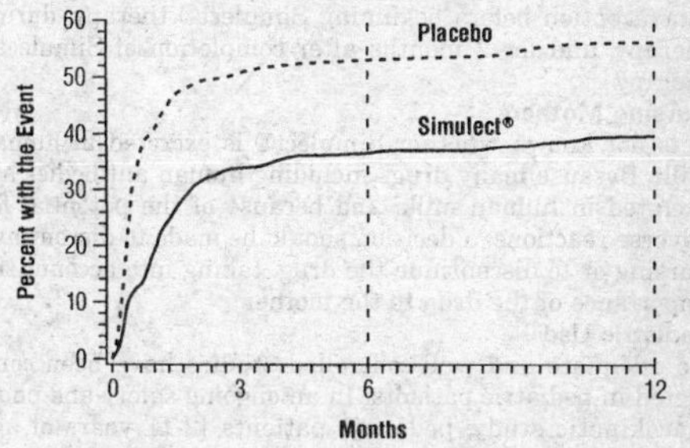

CONTRAINDICATIONS

Simulect® (basiliximab) is contraindicated in patients with known hypersensitivity to basiliximab or any other component of the formulation. See composition of Simulect® under *DESCRIPTION.*

WARNINGS: *See Boxed WARNING.*

General

Simulect® (basiliximab) should be administered under qualified medical supervision. Patients should be informed of the potential benefits of therapy and the risks associated with administration of immunosuppressive therapy. Anaphylactoid reactions following the administration of Simulect® have not been observed but can occur following the administration of proteins. Medications for the treatment of severe hypersensitivity reactions should be available for immediate use.

While neither the incidence of lymphoproliferative disorders nor opportunistic infections was higher in Simulect®-treated patients than in placebo-treated patients, patients on immunosuppressive therapy are at increased risk for developing these complications and should be monitored accordingly.

PRECAUTIONS

General

It is not known whether Simulect® (basiliximab) use will have a long-term effect on the ability of the immune system to respond to antigens first encountered during Simulect®-induced immunosuppression.

Re-administration of Simulect® after an initial course of therapy has not been studied in humans. The potential risks of such re-administration, specifically those associated with immunosuppression and/or the occurrence of anaphylaxis/anaphylactoid reactions, are not known.

Immunogenicity

Of renal transplantation patients treated with Simulect® (basiliximab) and tested for anti-idiotype antibodies, 1/246 developed an anti-idiotype antibody response, with no deleterious clinical effect upon the patient. In the US Study, the incidence of human anti-murine antibody (HAMA) in renal transplantation patients treated with Simulect® was 2/138 in patients not exposed to muromonab-CD3 and 4/34 in patients who subsequently received muromonab-CD3. The available clinical data on the use of muromonab-CD3 in patients previously treated with Simulect® suggest that subsequent use of muromonab-CD3 or other murine antilymphocytic antibody preparations is not precluded.

Drug Interactions

No formal drug-drug interaction studies have been conducted. The following medications have been administered in clinical trials with Simulect® (basiliximab) with no incremental increase in adverse reactions: ATG/ALG, azathioprine, corticosteroids, cyclosporine, mycophenolate mofetil, and muromonab-CD3.

Carcinogenesis, Mutagenesis and Impairment of Fertility

No mutagenic potential of Simulect® was observed in the *in vitro* assays with Salmonella (Ames) and V79 Chinese hamster cells. No long-term or fertility studies in laboratory animals have been performed to evaluate the potential of Simulect® to produce carcinogenicity or fertility impairment, respectively.

Pregnancy Category B

There are no adequate and well-controlled studies in pregnant women. No maternal toxicity, embryotoxicity, or teratogenicity was observed in cynomolgus monkeys 100 days post coitum following dosing with basiliximab during the organogenesis period; blood levels in pregnant monkeys were 13-fold higher than those seen in human patients. Immunotoxicology studies have not been performed in the offspring. Because IgG molecules are known to cross the placental barrier, because IL-2 receptor may play an important role in development of the immune system, and because animal reproduction studies are not always predictive of human response, Simulect® should only be used in pregnant women

Continued on next page

Simulect—Cont.

when the potential benefit justifies the potential risk to the fetus. Women of childbearing potential should use effective contraception before beginning Simulect® therapy, during therapy, and for 2 months after completion of Simulect® therapy.

Nursing Mothers

It is not known whether Simulect® is excreted in human milk. Because many drugs including human antibodies are excreted in human milk, and because of the potential for adverse reactions, a decision should be made to discontinue nursing or to discontinue the drug, taking into account the importance of the drug to the mother.

Pediatric Use

No adequate and well-controlled studies have been completed in pediatric patients. In an ongoing safety and pharmacokinetic study, pediatric patients [2-11 years of age (n=8), 12-15 years of age (n=4), median age 9.5 years] were treated with Simulect® via intravenous bolus injection in addition to standard immunosuppressive agents including cyclosporine, corticosteroids, azathioprine, and mycophenolate mofetil. Preliminary results indicate that 16.7% (2/12) of patients had experienced an acute rejection episode by 3 months post-transplantation. The most frequently reported adverse events were fever and urinary tract infections (41.7% each). Overall, the adverse event profile was consistent with general clinical experience in the pediatric renal transplantation population and with the profile in the controlled adult renal transplantation studies. The available pharmacokinetic data in children and adolescents are described in *CLINICAL PHARMACOLOGY* and *DOSAGE AND ADMINISTRATION*.

It is not known whether the immune response to vaccines, infection, and other antigenic stimuli administered or encountered during Simulect® therapy is impaired or whether such response will remain impaired after Simulect® therapy.

Geriatric Use

Controlled clinical studies of Simulect® have included a small number of patients 65 years and older (Simulect® 15; placebo 19). From the available data comparing Simulect®- and placebo-treated patients, the adverse event profile in patients ≥65 years of age is not different from patients <65 years of age and no age-related dosing adjustment is required. Caution must be used in giving immunosuppressive drugs to elderly patients.

ADVERSE REACTIONS

The incidence of adverse events for Simulect® (basiliximab) was determined in two randomized comparative double-blind trials for the prevention of renal allograft rejection. A total of 721 patients received renal allografts, of which 363 received Simulect® and 358 received placebo. All patients received concomitant cyclosporine for microemulsion and corticosteroids.

Simulect® did not appear to add to the background of adverse events seen in organ transplantation patients as a consequence of their underlying disease and the concurrent administration of immunosuppressants and other medications. Adverse events were reported by 99% of the patients in the placebo-treated group and 99% of the patients in the Simulect®-treated group. Simulect® did not increase the incidence of serious adverse events observed compared with placebo. The most frequently reported adverse events were gastrointestinal disorders, reported in 75% of Simulect®-treated patients and 73% of placebo-treated patients.

The incidence and types of adverse events were similar in Simulect®-treated and placebo-treated patients. The following adverse events occurred in ≥10% of Simulect®-treated patients: ***Gastrointestinal System:*** constipation, nausea, diarrhea, abdominal pain, vomiting, dyspepsia, moniliasis; ***Metabolic and Nutritional:*** hyperkalemia, hypokalemia, hyperglycemia, hyperuricemia, hypophosphatemia, hypocalcemia, weight increase, hypercholesterolemia, acidosis; ***Central and Peripheral Nervous System:*** headache, tremor, dizziness; ***Urinary System:*** dysuria, increased non-protein nitrogen, urinary tract infection; ***Body as a Whole–General:*** pain, peripheral edema, edema, fever, viral infection, leg edema, asthenia; ***Cardiovascular Disorders–General:*** hypertension; ***Respiratory System:*** dyspnea, upper respiratory tract infection, coughing, rhinitis, pharyngitis; ***Skin and Appendages:*** surgical wound complications, acne; ***Psychiatric:*** insomnia; ***Musculoskeletal System:*** leg pain, back pain; ***Red Blood Cell:*** anemia.

The following adverse events, not mentioned above, were reported with an incidence of ≥3% and <10% in patients treated with Simulect® in the two controlled clinical trials: ***Body as a Whole:*** accidental trauma, chest pain, increased drug level, face edema, fatigue, infection, malaise, generalized edema, rigors, sepsis; ***Cardiovascular:*** angina pectoris, cardiac failure, chest pain, abnormal heart sounds, aggravated hypertension, hypotension; ***Nervous System:*** hypoesthesia, neuropathy, paraesthesia; ***Endocrine:*** increased glucocorticoids; ***Gastrointestinal:*** enlarged abdomen, flatulence, gastrointestinal disorder, gastroenteritis, GI hemorrhage, gum hyperplasia, melena, esophagitis, ulcerative stomatitis; ***Heart Rate and Rhythm:*** arrhythmia, atrial fibrillation, tachycardia; ***Metabolic and Nutritional:*** dehydration, diabetes mellitus, fluid overload, hypercalcemia, hyperlipemia, hypoglycemia, hypoproteinemia, hypomagnesemia; ***Musculoskeletal:*** arthralgia, arthropathy, bone fracture, cramps, hernia, myalgia; ***Nervous System:*** paraesthesia, hypoesthesia; ***Platelet and Bleeding:*** hematoma, hemorrhage, purpura, thrombocytopenia, thrombosis; ***Psychiatric:*** agitation, anxiety, depression; ***Red Blood Cell:*** polycythemia; ***Reproductive Disorders, Male:*** impotence, genital edema; ***Respiratory:*** bronchitis, bronchospasm, abnormal chest sounds, pneumonia, pulmonary disorder, pulmonary edema, sinusitis; ***Skin and Appendages:*** cyst, herpes simplex, herpes zoster, hypertrichosis, pruritus, rash, skin disorder, skin ulceration; ***Urinary:*** albuminuria, bladder disorder, hematuria, frequent micturition, oliguria, abnormal renal function, renal tubular necrosis, surgery, ureteral disorder, urinary retention; ***Vascular Disorders:*** vascular disorder; ***Vision Disorders:*** cataract, conjunctivitis, abnormal vision.

Incidence of Malignancies: The overall incidence of malignancies among all patients in the two 12-month controlled trials was not significantly different between the Simulect® and placebo treatment groups. Overall, lymphoma/lymphoproliferative disease occurred in 1 patient (0.3%) in the Simulect® group compared with 2 patients (0.6%) in the placebo group. Other malignancies were reported among 5 patients (1.4%) in the Simulect® group compared with 7 patients (1.9%) in patients treated with placebo.

Incidence of Infectious Episodes: Cytomegalovirus infection was reported in 14% of Simulect®-treated patients and 18% of placebo-treated patients. The rates of infections, serious infections, and infectious organisms were similar in the Simulect® and placebo treatment groups.

OVERDOSAGE

There have not been any reports of overdoses with Simulect® (basiliximab). A maximum tolerated dose has not been determined in patients. In clinical studies, Simulect® has been administered to renal transplantation patients in single doses of up to 60 mg without any associated serious adverse events.

DOSAGE AND ADMINISTRATION

Simulect® (basiliximab) is used as part of an immunosuppressive regimen that includes cyclosporine and corticosteroids. Simulect® is for central or peripheral intravenous administration only. Reconstituted Simulect® (20 mg in 5 mL) should be diluted to a volume of 50 mL with normal saline or dextrose 5% and administered as an intravenous infusion over 20 to 30 minutes.

Adult: In adult patients, the recommended regimen is two doses of 20 mg each. The first 20 mg dose should be given within 2 hours prior to transplantation surgery. The second 20 mg dose should be given 4 days after transplantation.

Pediatric: For children and adolescents from 2 up to 15 years of age, the recommended regimen is two doses of 12 mg/m^2 each, up to a maximum of 20 mg/dose. The first dose should be given within 2 hours prior to transplantation surgery. The second dose should be given 4 days after transplantation.

RECONSTITUTION OF 20 mg Simulect® (basiliximab) VIAL

To prepare the infusion solution, add 5 mL of Sterile Water for Injection, USP, using aseptic technique, to the vial containing the Simulect® (basiliximab) powder. Shake the vial gently to dissolve the powder.

The reconstituted solution is isotonic and should be diluted to a volume of 50 mL with normal saline or dextrose 5% for infusion. When mixing the solution, gently invert the bag in order to avoid foaming; DO NOT SHAKE.

Parenteral drug products should be inspected visually for particulate matter and discoloration before administration. After reconstitution, Simulect® should be a clear to opalescent, colorless solution. If particulate matter is present or the solution is colored, do not use.

Care must be taken to assure sterility of the prepared solution because the drug product does not contain any antimicrobial preservatives or bacteriostatic agents.

It is recommended that after reconstitution the solution should be used immediately. If not used immediately, it can be stored at 2°C to 8°C for 24 hours or at room temperature for 4 hours. Discard the reconstituted solution if not used within 24 hours.

No incompatibility between Simulect® and polyvinyl chloride bags or infusion sets has been observed. No data are available on the compatibility of Simulect® with other intravenous substances. Other drug substances should not be added or infused simultaneously through the same intravenous line.

HOW SUPPLIED

Simulect® (basiliximab) is supplied in a single use glass vial containing 20 mg of basiliximab. Each box contains 1 Simulect® vial (NDC 0078-0331-84). Store lyophilized Simulect® under refrigerated conditions (2°C to 8°C; 36°F to 46°F). Do not use beyond the expiration date stamped on the vial.

Distributed by:
Novartis Pharmaceuticals Corporation
East Hanover, New Jersey 07936

US License No. 1244

REV: MAY 1998 30154901

Shown in Product Identification Guide, page 325

TEGRETOL® ℞

[*tĕ-grĕ-tōl*]

carbamazepine USP

Chewable Tablets of 100 mg – red-speckled, pink

Tablets of 200 mg – pink

Suspension of 100 mg/5 mL

TEGRETOL®-XR ℞

(carbamazepine extended-release tablets)

100 mg, 200 mg, 400 mg

Caution: Federal law prohibits dispensing without prescription.

The following prescribing information is based on official labeling in effect on August 1, 1998.

Prescribing Information

> **WARNING**
> APLASTIC ANEMIA AND AGRANULOCYTOSIS HAVE BEEN REPORTED IN ASSOCIATION WITH THE USE OF TEGRETOL. DATA FROM A POPULATION-BASED CASE CONTROL STUDY DEMONSTRATE THAT THE RISK OF DEVELOPING THESE REACTIONS IS 5-8 TIMES GREATER THAN IN THE GENERAL POPULATION. HOWEVER, THE OVERALL RISK OF THESE REACTIONS IN THE UNTREATED GENERAL POPULATION IS LOW, APPROXIMATELY SIX PATIENTS PER ONE MILLION POPULATION PER YEAR FOR AGRANULOCYTOSIS AND TWO PATIENTS PER ONE MILLION POPULATION PER YEAR FOR APLASTIC ANEMIA.
> ALTHOUGH REPORTS OF TRANSIENT OR PERSISTENT DECREASED PLATELET OR WHITE BLOOD CELL COUNTS ARE NOT UNCOMMON IN ASSOCIATION WITH THE USE OF TEGRETOL, DATA ARE NOT AVAILABLE TO ESTIMATE ACCURATELY THEIR INCIDENCE OR OUTCOME. HOWEVER, THE VAST MAJORITY OF THE CASES OF LEUKOPENIA HAVE NOT PROGRESSED TO THE MORE SERIOUS CONDITIONS OF APLASTIC ANEMIA OR AGRANULOCYTOSIS.
> BECAUSE OF THE VERY LOW INCIDENCE OF AGRANULOCYTOSIS AND APLASTIC ANEMIA, THE VAST MAJORITY OF MINOR HEMATOLOGIC CHANGES OBSERVED IN MONITORING OF PATIENTS ON TEGRETOL ARE UNLIKELY TO SIGNAL THE OCCURRENCE OF EITHER ABNORMALITY. NONETHELESS, COMPLETE PRETREATMENT HEMATOLOGICAL TESTING SHOULD BE OBTAINED AS A BASELINE. IF A PATIENT IN THE COURSE OF TREATMENT EXHIBITS LOW OR DECREASED WHITE BLOOD CELL OR PLATELET COUNTS, THE PATIENT SHOULD BE MONITORED CLOSELY. DISCONTINUATION OF THE DRUG SHOULD BE CONSIDERED IF ANY EVIDENCE OF SIGNIFICANT BONE MARROW DEPRESSION DEVELOPS.

Before prescribing Tegretol, the physician should be thoroughly familiar with the details of this prescribing information, particularly regarding use with other drugs, especially those which accentuate toxicity potential.

DESCRIPTION

Tegretol, carbamazepine USP, is an anticonvulsant and specific analgesic for trigeminal neuralgia, available for oral administration as chewable tablets of 100 mg, tablets of 200 mg, XR tablets of 100, 200, and 400 mg, and as a suspension of 100 mg/5 mL (teaspoon). Its chemical name is 5*H*-dibenz[*b,f*]azepine-5-carboxamide, and its structural formula is

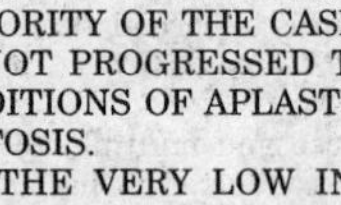

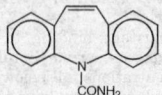

Carbamazepine USP is a white to off-white powder, practically insoluble in water and soluble in alcohol and in acetone. Its molecular weight is 236.27.

Inactive Ingredients. Tablets: Colloidal silicon dioxide, D&C Red No. 30 Aluminum Lake (chewable tablets only), FD&C Red No. 40 (200-mg tablets only), flavoring (chewable tablets only), gelatin, glycerin, magnesium stearate,

sodium starch glycolate (chewable tablets only), starch, stearic acid, and sucrose (chewable tablets only). Suspension: Citric acid, FD&C Yellow No. 6, flavoring, polymer, potassium sorbate, propylene glycol, purified water, sorbitol, sucrose, and xanthan gum. Tegretol-XR tablets: cellulose compounds, dextrates, iron oxides, magnesium stearate, mannitol, polyethylene glycol, sodium lauryl sulfate, titanium dioxide (200-mg tablets only).

CLINICAL PHARMACOLOGY

In controlled clinical trials, Tegretol has been shown to be effective in the treatment of psychomotor and grand mal seizures, as well as trigeminal neuralgia.

Mechanism of Action

Tegretol has demonstrated anticonvulsant properties in rats and mice with electrically and chemically induced seizures. It appears to act by reducing polysynaptic responses and blocking the post-tetanic potentiation. Tegretol greatly reduces or abolishes pain induced by stimulation of the infraorbital nerve in cats and rats. It depresses thalamic potential and bulbar and polysynaptic reflexes, including the linguomandibular reflex in cats. Tegretol is chemically unrelated to other anticonvulsants or other drugs used to control the pain of trigeminal neuralgia. The mechanism of action remains unknown.

The principal metabolite of Tegretol, carbamazepine-10, 11-epoxide, has anticonvulsant activity as demonstrated in several in vivo animal models of seizures. Though clinical activity for the epoxide has been postulated, the significance of its activity with respect to the safety and efficacy of Tegretol has not been established.

Pharmacokinetics

In clinical studies, Tegretol suspension, conventional tablets, and XR tablets delivered equivalent amounts of drug to the systemic circulation. However, the suspension was absorbed somewhat faster, and the XR tablet slightly slower, than the conventional tablet. The bioavailability of the XR tablet was 89% compared to suspension. Following a b.i.d. dosage regimen, the suspension provides higher peak levels and lower trough levels than those obtained from the conventional tablet for the same dosage regimen. On the other hand, following a t.i.d. dosage regimen, Tegretol suspension affords steady-state plasma levels comparable to Tegretol tablets given b.i.d. when administered at the same total mg daily dose. Following a b.i.d. dosage regimen, Tegretol-XR tablets afford steady-state plasma levels comparable to conventional Tegretol tablets given q.i.d., when administered at the same total mg daily dose. Tegretol in blood is 76% bound to plasma proteins. Plasma levels of Tegretol are variable and may range from 0.5-25 μg/mL, with no apparent relationship to the daily intake of the drug. Usual adult therapeutic levels are between 4 and 12 μg/mL. In polytherapy, the concentration of Tegretol and concomitant drugs may be increased or decreased during therapy, and drug effects may be altered (see PRECAUTIONS, Drug Interactions). Following chronic oral administration of suspension, plasma levels peak at approximately 1.5 hours compared to 4-5 hours after administration of conventional Tegretol tablets, and 3-12 hours after administration of Tegretol-XR tablets. The CSF/serum ratio is 0.22, similar to the 24% unbound Tegretol in serum. Because Tegretol induces its own metabolism, the half-life is also variable. Autoinduction is completed after 3-5 weeks of a fixed dosing regimen. Initial half-life values range from 25-65 hours, decreasing to 12-17 hours on repeated doses. Tegretol is metabolized in the liver. Cytochrome P450 3A4 was identified as the major isoform responsible for the formation of carbamazepine-10, 11-epoxide from Tegretol. After oral administration of ^{14}C-carbamazepine, 72% of the administered radioactivity was found in the urine and 28% in the feces. This urinary radioactivity was composed largely of hydroxylated and conjugated metabolites, with only 3% of unchanged Tegretol.

The pharmacokinetic parameters of Tegretol disposition are similar in children and in adults. However, there is a poor correlation between plasma concentrations of carbamazepine and Tegretol dose in children. Carbamazepine is more rapidly metabolized to carbamazepine-10, 11-epoxide (a metabolite shown to be equipotent to carbamazepine as an anticonvulsant in animal screens) in the younger age groups than in adults. In children below the age of 15, there is an inverse relationship between CBZ-E/CBZ ratio and increasing age (in one report from 0.44 in children below the age of 1 year to 0.18 in children between 10-15 years of age).

The effects of race and gender on carbamazepine pharmacokinetics have not been systematically evaluated.

INDICATIONS AND USAGE

Epilepsy

Tegretol is indicated for use as an anticonvulsant drug. Evidence supporting efficacy of Tegretol as an anticonvulsant was derived from active drug-controlled studies that enrolled patients with the following seizure types:

1. Partial seizures with complex symptomatology (psychomotor, temporal lobe). Patients with these seizures appear to show greater improvement than those with other types.
2. Generalized tonic-clonic seizures (grand mal).
3. Mixed seizure patterns which include the above, or other partial or generalized seizures. Absence seizures (petit mal) do not appear to be controlled by Tegretol (see PRECAUTIONS, General).

Trigeminal Neuralgia

Tegretol is indicated in the treatment of the pain associated with true trigeminal neuralgia.

Beneficial results have also been reported in glossopharyngeal neuralgia.

This drug is not a simple analgesic and should not be used for the relief of trivial aches or pains.

CONTRAINDICATIONS

Tegretol should not be used in patients with a history of previous bone marrow depression, hypersensitivity to the drug, or known sensitivity to any of the tricyclic compounds, such as amitriptyline, desipramine, imipramine, protriptyline, nortriptyline, etc. Likewise, on theoretical grounds its use with monoamine oxidase inhibitors is not recommended. Before administration of Tegretol, MAO inhibitors should be discontinued for a minimum of 14 days, or longer if the clinical situation permits.

WARNINGS

Patients with a history of adverse hematologic reaction to any drug may be particularly at risk.

Severe dermatologic reactions, including toxic epidermal necrolysis (Lyell's syndrome) and Stevens-Johnson syndrome, have been reported with Tegretol. These reactions have been extremely rare. However, a few fatalities have been reported.

Tegretol has shown mild anticholinergic activity; therefore, patients with increased intraocular pressure should be closely observed during therapy.

Because of the relationship of the drug to other tricyclic compounds, the possibility of activation of a latent psychosis and, in elderly patients, of confusion or agitation should be borne in mind.

Usage in Pregnancy

Carbamazepine can cause fetal harm when administered to a pregnant woman.

Epidemiological data suggest that there may be an association between the use of carbamazepine during pregnancy and congenital malformations, including spina bifida. In treating or counseling women of childbearing potential, the prescribing physician will wish to weigh the benefits of therapy against the risks. If this drug is used during pregnancy, or if the patient becomes pregnant while taking this drug, the patient should be apprised of the potential hazard to the fetus.

Retrospective case reviews suggest that, compared with monotherapy, there may be a higher prevalence of teratogenic effects associated with the use of anticonvulsants in combination therapy. Therefore, if therapy is to be continued, monotherapy may be preferable for pregnant women.

In humans, transplacental passage of carbamazepine is rapid (30-60 minutes), and the drug is accumulated in the fetal tissues, with higher levels found in liver and kidney than in brain and lung.

Carbamazepine has been shown to have adverse effects in reproduction studies in rats when given orally in dosages 10-25 times the maximum human daily dosage (MHDD) of 1200 mg on a mg/kg basis or 1.5-4 times the MHDD on a mg/m^2 basis. In rat teratology studies, 2 of 135 offspring showed kinked ribs at 250 mg/kg and 4 of 119 offspring at 650 mg/kg showed other anomalies (cleft palate, 1; talipes, 1; anophthalmos, 2). In reproduction studies in rats, nursing offspring demonstrated a lack of weight gain and an unkempt appearance at a maternal dosage level of 200 mg/kg.

Antiepileptic drugs should not be discontinued abruptly in patients in whom the drug is administered to prevent major seizures because of the strong possibility of precipitating status epilepticus with attendant hypoxia and threat to life. In individual cases where the severity and frequency of the seizure disorder are such that removal of medication does not pose a serious threat to the patient, discontinuation of the drug may be considered prior to and during pregnancy, although it cannot be said with any confidence that even minor seizures do not pose some hazard to the developing embryo or fetus.

Tests to detect defects using currently accepted procedures should be considered a part of routine prenatal care in childbearing women receiving carbamazepine.

There have been a few cases of neonatal seizures and/or respiratory depression associated with maternal Tegretol and other concomitant anticonvulsant drug use. A few cases of neonatal vomiting, diarrhea, and/or decreased feeding have also been reported in association with maternal Tegretol use. These symptoms may represent a neonatal withdrawal syndrome.

PRECAUTIONS

General

Before initiating therapy, a detailed history and physical examination should be made.

Tegretol should be used with caution in patients with a mixed seizure disorder that includes atypical absence seizures, since in these patients Tegretol has been associated with increased frequency of generalized convulsions (see INDICATIONS AND USAGE).

Therapy should be prescribed only after critical benefit-to-risk appraisal in patients with a history of cardiac, hepatic, or renal damage; adverse hematologic reaction to other drugs; or interrupted courses of therapy with Tegretol.

Since a given dose of Tegretol suspension will produce higher peak levels than the same dose given as the tablet, it is recommended that patients given the suspension be started on lower doses and increased slowly to avoid unwanted side effects (see DOSAGE AND ADMINISTRATION).

Information for Patients

Patients should be made aware of the early toxic signs and symptoms of a potential hematologic problem, such as fever, sore throat, rash, ulcers in the mouth, easy bruising, petechial or purpuric hemorrhage, and should be advised to report to the physician immediately if any such signs or symptoms appear.

Since dizziness and drowsiness may occur, patients should be cautioned about the hazards of operating machinery or automobiles or engaging in other potentially dangerous tasks.

Laboratory Tests

Complete pretreatment blood counts, including platelets and possibly reticulocytes and serum iron, should be obtained as a baseline. If a patient in the course of treatment exhibits low or decreased white blood cell or platelet counts, the patient should be monitored closely. Discontinuation of the drug should be considered if any evidence of significant bone marrow depression develops.

Baseline and periodic evaluations of liver function, particularly in patients with a history of liver disease, must be performed during treatment with this drug since liver damage may occur. The drug should be discontinued immediately in cases of aggravated liver dysfunction or active liver disease.

Baseline and periodic eye examinations, including slit-lamp, funduscopy, and tonometry, are recommended since many phenothiazines and related drugs have been shown to cause eye changes.

Baseline and periodic complete urinalysis and BUN determinations are recommended for patients treated with this agent because of observed renal dysfunction.

Monitoring of blood levels (see CLINICAL PHARMACOLOGY) has increased the efficacy and safety of anticonvulsants. This monitoring may be particularly useful in cases of dramatic increase in seizure frequency and for verification of compliance. In addition, measurement of drug serum levels may aid in determining the cause of toxicity when more than one medication is being used.

Thyroid function tests have been reported to show decreased values with Tegretol administered alone.

Hyponatremia has been reported in association with Tegretol use, either alone or in combination with other drugs.

Interference with some pregnancy tests has been reported.

Drug Interactions

There has been a report of a patient who passed an orange rubbery precipitate in his stool the day after ingesting Tegretol suspension immediately followed by Thorazine® solution. Subsequent testing has shown that mixing Tegretol suspension and chlorpromazine solution (both generic and brand name) as well as Tegretol suspension and liquid Mellaril® resulted in the occurrence of this precipitate. Because the extent to which this occurs with other liquid medications is not known. Tegretol suspension should not be administered simultaneously with other liquid medicinal agents or diluents (See Dosage and Administration).

Clinically meaningful drug interactions have occurred with concomitant medications and include, but are not limited to, the following:

Agents That May Affect Tegretol Plasma Levels

CYP 3A4 inhibitors inhibit Tegretol metabolism and can thus increase plasma carbamazepine levels. Drugs that have been shown, or would be expected, to increase plasma carbamazepine levels include

cimetidine, danazol, diltiazem, macrolides, erythromycin, troleandomycin, clarithromycin, fluoxetine, loratadine, terfenadine, isoniazid, niacinamide, nicotinamide, propoxyphene, ketaconazole, itraconazole, verapamil, valproate.*

CYP 3A4 inducers can increase the rate of Tegretol metabolism. Drugs that have been shown, or that would be expected, to decrease plasma carbamazepine levels include

cisplatin, doxorubicin HCl, felbamate,† rifampin, phenobarbital, phenytoin, primidone, theophylline.

*increased levels of the active 10, 11-epoxide

†decreased levels of carbamazepine and increased levels of the 10, 11-epoxide

Continued on next page

Tegretol—Cont.

Effect of Tegretol on Plasma Levels of Concomitant Agents

Increased levels: clomipramine HCl, phenytoin, primidone
Tegretol induces hepatic CYP activity. Tegretol causes, or would be expected to cause, decreased levels of the following:

acetaminophen, alprazolam, clonazepam, clozapine, dicumarol, doxycycline, ethosuximide, haloperidol, methsuximide, oral contraceptives, phensuximide, phenytoin, theophylline, valproate, warfarin.

Concomitant administration of carbamazepine and lithium may increase the risk of neurotoxic side effects.
Alterations of thyroid function have been reported in combination therapy with other anticonvulsant medications.
Breakthrough bleeding has been reported among patients receiving concomitant oral and subdermal implant contraceptives and their reliability may be adversely affected.

Carcinogenesis, Mutagenesis, Impairment of Fertility

Carbamazepine, when administered to Sprague-Dawley rats for two years in the diet at doses of 25, 75, and 250 mg/kg/day, resulted in a dose-related increase in the incidence of hepatocellular tumors in females and of benign interstitial cell adenomas in the testes of males. Carbamazepine must, therefore, be considered to be carcinogenic in Sprague-Dawley rats. Bacterial and mammalian mutagenicity studies using carbamazepine produced negative results. The significance of these findings relative to the use of carbamazepine in humans is, at present, unknown.

Usage in Pregnancy

Pregnancy Category D (See WARNINGS).

Labor and Delivery

The effect of Tegretol on human labor and delivery is unknown.

Nursing Mothers

Tegretol and its epoxide metabolite are transferred to breast milk. The ratio of the concentration in breast milk to that in maternal plasma is about 0.4 for Tegretol and about 0.5 for the epoxide. The estimated doses given to the newborn during breast feeding are in the range of 2-5 mg daily for Tegretol and 1-2 mg daily for the epoxide.
Because of the potential for serious adverse reactions in nursing infants from carbamazepine, a decision should be made whether to discontinue nursing or to discontinue the drug, taking into account the importance of the drug to the mother.

Pediatric Use

Substantial evidence of Tegretol's effectiveness for use in the management of children with epilepsy (see Indications for specific seizure types) is derived from clinical investigations performed in adults and from studies in several in vitro systems which support the conclusion that (1) the pathogenetic mechanisms underlying seizure propagation are essentially identical in adults and children, and (2) the mechanism of action of carbamazepine in treating seizures is essentially identical in adults and children.
Taken as a whole, this information supports a conclusion that the generally accepted therapeutic range of total carbamazepine in plasma (i.e., 4-12 mcg/mL) is the same in children and adults.

The evidence assembled was primarily obtained from short-term use of carbamazepine. The safety of carbamazepine in children has been systematically studied up to 6 months. No longer-term data from clinical trials is available.

Geriatric Use

No systematic studies in geriatric patients have been conducted.

ADVERSE REACTIONS

If adverse reactions are of such severity that the drug must be discontinued, the physician must be aware that abrupt discontinuation of any anticonvulsant drug in a responsive epileptic patient may lead to seizures or even status epilepticus with its life-threatening hazards.
The most severe adverse reactions have been observed in the hemopoietic system (see boxed WARNING), the skin, and the cardiovascular system.
The most frequently observed adverse reactions, particularly during the initial phases of therapy, are dizziness, drowsiness, unsteadiness, nausea, and vomiting. To minimize the possibility of such reactions, therapy should be initiated at the low dosage recommended.
The following additional adverse reactions have been reported:

Hemopoietic System: Aplastic anemia, agranulocytosis, pancytopenia, bone marrow depression, thrombocytopenia, leukopenia, leukocytosis, eosinophilia, acute intermittent porphyria.

Skin: Pruritic and erythematous rashes, urticaria, toxic epidermal necrolysis (Lyell's syndrome) (see WARNINGS), Stevens-Johnson syndrome (see WARNINGS), photosensitivity reactions, alterations in skin pigmentation, exfoliative dermatitis, erythema multiforme and nodosum, purpura, aggravation of disseminated lupus erythematosus, alopecia, and diaphoresis. In certain cases, discontinuation of therapy may be necessary. Isolated cases of hirsutism have been reported, but a causal relationship is not clear.

Cardiovascular System: Congestive heart failure, edema, aggravation of hypertension, hypotension, syncope and collapse, aggravation of coronary artery disease, arrhythmias and AV block, thrombophlebitis, thromboembolism, and adenopathy or lymphadenopathy.
Some of these cardiovascular complications have resulted in fatalities. Myocardial infarction has been associated with other tricyclic compounds.

Liver: Abnormalities in liver function tests, cholestatic and hepatocellular jaundice, hepatitis.

Pancreatic: Pancreatitis.

Respiratory System: Pulmonary hypersensitivity characterized by fever, dyspnea, pneumonitis, or pneumonia.

Genitourinary System: Urinary frequency, acute urinary retention, oliguria with elevated blood pressure, azotemia, renal failure, and impotence. Albuminuria, glycosuria, elevated BUN, and microscopic deposits in the urine have also been reported.
Testicular atrophy occurred in rats receiving Tegretol orally from 4-52 weeks at dosage levels of 50-400 mg/kg/day. Additionally, rats receiving Tegretol in the diet for 2 years at dosage levels of 25, 75, and 250 mg/kg/day had a dose-related incidence of testicular atrophy and aspermatogenesis. In dogs, it produced a brownish discoloration, pre-

sumably a metabolite, in the urinary bladder at dosage levels of 50 mg/kg and higher. Relevance of these findings to humans is unknown.

Nervous System: Dizziness, drowsiness, disturbances of coordination, confusion, headache, fatigue, blurred vision, visual hallucinations, transient diplopia, oculomotor disturbances, nystagmus, speech disturbances, abnormal involuntary movements, peripheral neuritis and paresthesias, depression with agitation, talkativeness, tinnitus, and hyperacusis.
There have been reports of associated paralysis and other symptoms of cerebral arterial insufficiency, but the exact relationship of these reactions to the drug has not been established.
Isolated cases of neuroleptic malignant syndrome have been reported with concomitant use of psychotropic drugs.

Digestive System: Nausea, vomiting, gastric distress and abdominal pain, diarrhea, constipation, anorexia, and dryness of the mouth and pharynx, including glossitis and stomatitis.

Eyes: Scattered punctate cortical lens opacities, as well as conjunctivitis, have been reported. Although a direct causal relationship has not been established, many phenothiazines and related drugs have been shown to cause eye changes.

Musculoskeletal System: Aching joints and muscles, and leg cramps.

Metabolism: Fever and chills. Inappropriate antidiuretic hormone (ADH) secretion syndrome has been reported. Cases of frank water intoxication, with decreased serum sodium (hyponatremia) and confusion, have been reported in association with Tegretol use (see PRECAUTIONS, Laboratory Tests). Decreased levels of plasma calcium have been reported.

Other: Isolated cases of a lupus erythematosus-like syndrome have been reported. There have been occasional reports of elevated levels of cholesterol, HDL cholesterol, and triglycerides in patients taking anticonvulsants.
A case of aseptic meningitis, accompanied by myoclonus and peripheral eosinophilia, has been reported in a patient taking carbamazepine in combination with other medications. The patient was successfully dechallenged, and the meningitis reappeared upon rechallenge with carbamazepine.

DRUG ABUSE AND DEPENDENCE

No evidence of abuse potential has been associated with Tegretol, nor is there evidence of psychological or physical dependence in humans.

OVERDOSAGE

Acute Toxicity

Lowest known lethal dose: adults, 3.2 g (a 24-year-old woman died of a cardiac arrest and a 24-year-old man died of pneumonia and hypoxic encephalopathy); children 4 g (a 14-year-old girl died of a cardiac arrest), 1.6 g (a 3-year-old girl died of aspiration pneumonia).
Oral LD_{50} in animals (mg/kg): mice, 1100-3750; rats, 3850-4025; rabbits, 1500-2680; guinea pigs, 920.

Signs and Symptoms

The first signs and symptoms appear after 1-3 hours. Neuromuscular disturbances are the most prominent. Cardio-

Dosage Information

Indication	Initial Dose Tablet*	Initial Dose XR†	Initial Dose Suspension	Subsequent Dose Tablet*	Subsequent Dose XR†	Subsequent Dose Suspension	Maximum Daily Dose Tablet*	Maximum Daily Dose XR†	Maximum Daily Dose Suspension
Epilepsy Under 6 yr	10-20 mg/kg/day b.i.d. or t.i.d.		10-20 mg/kg/day q.i.d.	Increase weekly to achieve optimal clinical response, t.i.d. or q.i.d.		Increase weekly to achieve optimal clinical response, t.i.d. or q.i.d.	35 mg/kg/24 hr (see Dosage and Administration section above)		35 mg/kg/24 hr (see Dosage and Administration section above)
6-12 yr	100 mg b.i.d. (200 mg/day)	100 mg b.i.d. (200 mg/day)	½ tsp q.i.d. (200 mg/day)	Add up to 100 mg/day at weekly intervals, t.i.d. or q.i.d.	Add 100 mg/day at weekly intervals b.i.d.	Add up to 1 tsp (100 mg)/day at weekly intervals, t.i.d. or q.i.d.		1000 mg/24 hr	
Over 12 yr	200 mg b.i.d. (400 mg/day)	200 mg b.i.d. (400 mg/day)	1 tsp q.i.d. (400 mg/day)	Add up to 200 mg/day at weekly intervals, t.i.d. or q.i.d.	Add up to 200 mg/day at weekly intervals, b.i.d.	Add up to 2 tsp (200 mg)/day at weekly intervals, t.i.d. or q.i.d.		1000 mg/24 hr (12–15 yr) 1200 mg/24 hr (>15 yr) 1600 mg/24 hr (adults, in rare instances)	
Trigeminal Neuralgia	100 mg b.i.d. (200 mg/day)	100 mg b.i.d. (200 mg/day)	½ tsp q.i.d. (200 mg/day)	Add up to 200 mg/day in increments of 100 mg every 12 hr	Add up to 200 mg/day in increments of 100 mg every 12 hr	Add up to 2 tsp (200 mg)/day in increments of 50 mg (½ tsp) q.i.d.		1200 mg/24 hr	

* Tablet = Chewable or conventional tablets
† XR = Tegretol®-XR extended-release tablets

Information will be superseded by supplements and subsequent editions

vascular disorders are generally milder, and severe cardiac complications occur only when very high doses (> 60 g) have been ingested.

Respiration: Irregular breathing, respiratory depression.

Cardiovascular System: Tachycardia, hypotension or hypertension, shock, conduction disorders.

Nervous System and Muscles: Impairment of consciousness ranging in severity to deep coma. Convulsions, especially in small children. Motor restlessness, muscular twitching, tremor, athetoid movements, opisthotonos, ataxia, drowsiness, dizziness, mydriasis, nystagmus, adiadochokinesia, ballism, psychomotor disturbances, dysmetria. Initial hyperreflexia, followed by hyporeflexia.

Gastrointestinal Tract: Nausea, vomiting.

Kidneys and Bladder: Anuria or oliguria, urinary retention.

Laboratory Findings: Isolated instances of overdosage have included leukocytosis, reduced leukocyte count, glycosuria, and acetonuria. EEG may show dysrhythmias.

Combined Poisoning: When alcohol, tricyclic antidepressants, barbiturates, or hydantoins are taken at the same time, the signs and symptoms of acute poisoning with Tegretol may be aggravated or modified.

Treatment

The prognosis in cases of severe poisoning is critically dependent upon prompt elimination of the drug, which may be achieved by inducing vomiting, irrigating the stomach, and by taking appropriate steps to diminish absorption. If these measures cannot be implemented without risk on the spot, the patient should be transferred at once to a hospital, while ensuring that vital functions are safeguarded. There is no specific antidote.

Elimination of the Drug: Induction of vomiting.

Gastric lavage. Even when more than 4 hours have elapsed following ingestion of the drug, the stomach should be repeatedly irrigated, especially if the patient has also consumed alcohol.

Measures to Reduce Absorption: Activated charcoal, laxatives.

Measures to Accelerate Elimination: Forced diuresis.

Dialysis is indicated only in severe poisoning associated with renal failure. Replacement transfusion is indicated in severe poisoning in small children.

Respiratory Depression: Keep the airways free; resort, if necessary, to endotracheal intubation, artificial respiration, and administration of oxygen.

Hypotension, Shock: Keep the patient's legs raised and administer a plasma expander. If blood pressure fails to rise despite measures taken to increase plasma volume, use of vasoactive substances should be considered.

Convulsions: Diazepam or barbiturates.

Warning: Diazepam or barbiturates may aggravate respiratory depression (especially in children), hypotension, and coma. However, barbiturates should not be used if drugs that inhibit monoamine oxidase have also been taken by the patient either in overdosage or in recent therapy (within 1 week).

Surveillance: Respiration, cardiac function (ECG monitoring), blood pressure, body temperature, pupillary reflexes, and kidney and bladder function should be monitored for several days.

Treatment of Blood Count Abnormalities: If evidence of significant bone marrow depression develops, the following recommendations are suggested: (1) stop the drug, (2) perform daily CBC, platelet, and reticulocyte counts, (3) do a bone marrow aspiration and trephine biopsy immediately and repeat with sufficient frequency to monitor recovery.

Special periodic studies might be helpful as follows: (1) white cell and platelet antibodies, (2) ^{59}Fe-ferrokinetic studies, (3) peripheral blood cell typing, (4) cytogenetic studies on marrow and peripheral blood, (5) bone marrow culture studies for colony-forming units, (6) hemoglobin electrophoresis for A_2 and F hemoglobin, and (7) serum folic acid and B_{12} levels.

A fully developed aplastic anemia will require appropriate, intensive monitoring and therapy, for which specialized consultation should be sought.

DOSAGE AND ADMINISTRATION

[See table at bottom of previous page]

Tegretol suspension in combination with liquid chlorpromazine or thioridazine results in precipitate formation, and, in the case of chlorpromazine, there has been a report of a patient passing an orange rubbery precipitate in the stool following coadministration of the two drugs. (See Drug Interactions). Because the extent to which this occurs with other liquid medications is not known, Tegretol suspension should not be administered simultaneously with other liquid medications or diluents.

Monitoring of blood levels has increased the efficacy and safety of anticonvulsants (see PRECAUTIONS, Laboratory Tests). Dosage should be adjusted to the needs of the individual patient. A low initial daily dosage with a gradual increase is advised. As soon as adequate control is achieved, the dosage may be reduced very gradually to the minimum effective level. Medication should be taken with meals.

Since a given dose of Tegretol suspension will produce higher peak levels than the same dose given as the tablet, it is recommended to start with low doses (children 6-12 years: $^1/_2$ teaspoon q.i.d.) and to increase slowly to avoid unwanted side effects.

Conversion of patients from oral Tegretol tablets to Tegretol suspension: Patients should be converted by administering the same number of mg per day in smaller, more frequent doses (i.e., b.i.d. tablets to t.i.d. suspension).

Tegretol-XR is an extended-release formulation for twice-a-day administration. When converting patients from Tegretol conventional tablets to Tegretol-XR, the same total daily mg dose of Tegretol-XR should be administered.

Tegretol-XR tablets must be swallowed whole and never crushed or chewed. Tegretol-XR tablets should be inspected for chips or cracks. Damaged tablets should not be consumed. Tegretol-XR tablet coating is not absorbed and is excreted in the feces; these coatings may be noticeable in the stool.

Epilepsy (see INDICATIONS AND USAGE)

Adults and children over 12 years of age—Initial: Either 200 mg b.i.d. for tablets and XR tablets, or 1 teaspoon q.i.d. for suspension (400 mg/day). Increase at weekly intervals by adding up to 200 mg/day using a b.i.d. regimen of Tegretol-XR or a t.i.d. or q.i.d. regimen of the other formulations until the optimal response is obtained. Dosage generally should not exceed 1000 mg daily in children 12-15 years of age, and 1200 mg daily in patients above 15 years of age. Doses up to 1600 mg daily have been used in adults in rare instances. ***Maintenance:*** Adjust dosage to the minimum effective level, usually 800-1200 mg daily.

Children 6-12 years of age - Initial: Either 100 mg b.i.d. for tablets or XR tablets, or $^1/_2$ teaspoon q.i.d. for suspension (200 mg/day). Increase at weekly intervals by adding up to 100 mg/day using a b.i.d. regimen of Tegretol-XR or a t.i.d. or q.i.d. regimen of the other formulations until the optimal response is obtained. Dosage generally should not exceed 1000 mg daily. ***Maintenance:*** Adjust dosage to the minimum effective level, usually 400-800 mg daily.

Children under 6 years of age-Initial: 10-20 mg/kg/day b.i.d. or t.i.d. as tablets, or q.i.d. as suspension. Increase weekly to achieve optimal clinical response administered t.i.d. or q.i.d. ***Maintenance:*** Ordinarily, optimal clinical response is achieved at daily doses below 35 mg/kg. If satisfactory clinical response has not been achieved, plasma levels should be measured to determine whether or not they are in the therapeutic range. No recommendation regarding the safety of carbamazepine for use at doses above 35 mg/kg/24 hours can be made.

Combination Therapy: Tegretol may be used alone or with other anticonvulsants. When added to existing anticonvulsant therapy, the drug should be added gradually while the other anticonvulsants are maintained or gradually decreased, except phenytoin, which may have to be increased (see PRECAUTIONS, Drug Interactions, and Pregnancy Category C).

Trigeminal Neuralgia (see INDICATIONS AND USAGE)

Initial: On the first day, either 100 mg b.i.d. for tablets or XR tablets, or $^1/_2$ teaspoon q.i.d. for suspension, for a total daily dose of 200 mg. This daily dose may be increased by up to 200 mg/day using increments of 100 mg every 12 hours for tablets or XR tablets, or 50 mg ($^1/_2$ teaspoon) q.i.d. for suspension, only as needed to achieve freedom from pain. Do not exceed 1200 mg daily. ***Maintenance:*** Control of pain can be maintained in most patients with 400-800 mg daily. However, some patients may be maintained on as little as 200 mg daily, while others may require as much as 1200 mg daily. At least once every 3 months throughout the treatment period, attempts should be made to reduce the dose to the minimum effective level or even to discontinue the drug.

HOW SUPPLIED

Chewable Tablets 100 mg-round, red-speckled, pink, single-scored (imprinted Tegretol on one side and 52 twice on the scored side)

Bottles of 100 .... NDC 0083-0052-30
Unit Dose (blister pack)
Box of 100 (strips of 10) .... NDC 0083-0052-32

Do not store above 30°C (86°F). *Protect from light and moisture. Dispense in tight, light-resistant container (USP).*

Tablets 200 mg-capsule-shaped, pink, single-scored (imprinted Tegretol on one side and 27 twice on the partially scored side)

Bottles of 100 .... NDC 0083-0027-30
Bottles of 1000 .... NDC 0083-0027-40
Unit Dose (blister pack)
Box of 100 (strips of 10) .... NDC 0083-0027-32

Do not store above 30°C (86°F). *Protect from moisture. Dispense in tight container (USP).*

XR Tablets 100 mg-round, yellow, coated (imprinted T on one side and 100 mg on the other), release portal on one side

Bottles of 100 .... NDC 0083-0061-30
Unit Dose (blister pack)
Box of 100 (strips of 10) .... NDC 0083-0061-32

XR Tablets 200 mg-round, pink, coated (imprinted T on one side and 200 mg on the other), release portal on one side

Bottles of 100 .... NDC 0083-0062-30
Unit Dose (blister pack)
Box of 100 (strips of 10) .... NDC 0083-0062-32

XR Tablets 400 mg-round, brown, coated (imprinted T on one side and 400 mg on the other), release portal on one side

Bottles of 100 .... NDC 0083-0060-30
Unit Dose (blister pack)
Box of 100 (strips of 10) .... NDC 0083-0060-32

Store at controlled room temperature 15°-30°C (59°F-86°F). *Protect from moisture. Dispense in tight container (USP).*

Samples, when available, are identified by the word *SAMPLE* appearing on each tablet.

Suspension 100 mg/5 mL (teaspoon)-yellow-orange, citrus-vanilla flavored

Bottles of 450 mL .... NDC 0083-0019-76

Shake well before using.

Because of the possibility of component interaction, Tegretol suspension should not be administered simultaneously with other liquid medicinal agents or diluents.

Do not store above 30°C (86°F). *Dispense in tight, light-resistant container (USP).*

C98-12 (Rev. 2/98)

Tegretol Suspension Manufactured by
Novartis Pharmaceuticals Canada Inc.
Dorval, (Quebec) H9R 4P5

Shown in Product Identification Guide, pages 325 and 326

TOFRANIL–PM® ℞

imipramine pamoate
Capsules of 75 mg
Capsules of 100 mg
Capsules of 125 mg
Capsules of 150 mg
For oral administration

Caution: Federal law prohibits dispensing without prescription.

The following prescribing information is based on official labeling in effect on October 1, 1998.

DESCRIPTION

Tofranil-PM, imipramine pamoate, is a tricyclic antidepressant, available as capsules for oral administration. The 75-, 100-, 125-, and 150-mg capsules contain imipramine pamoate equivalent to 75, 100, 125, and 150 mg of imipramine hydrochloride. Imipramine pamoate is 5-[3-(dimethylamino)propyl]-10,11-dihydro-5*H*-dibenz[b,f]azepine 4,4′-methylenebis-(3-hydroxy-2-naphthoate) (2:1), and its structural formula is

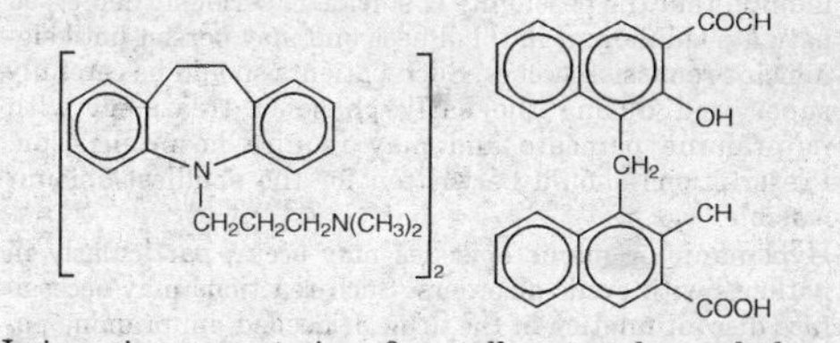

Imipramine pamoate is a fine, yellow, tasteless, odorless powder. It is soluble in ethanol, in acetone, in ether, in chloroform, and in carbon tetrachloride, and is insoluble in water. Its molecular weight is 949.21.

Inactive Ingredients. D&C Red No. 28, FD&C Blue No. 1, FD&C Yellow No. 6, D&C Yellow No. 10 (100 mg and 125 mg capsules only), gelatin, magnesium stearate, parabens, silicon dioxide, sodium lauryl sulfate, starch, talc, and titanium dioxide.

CLINICAL PHARMACOLOGY

The mechanism of action of imipramine is not definitely known. However, it does not act primarily by stimulation of the central nervous system. The clinical effect is hypothesized as being due to potentiation of adrenergic synapses by blocking uptake of norepinephrine at nerve endings.

INDICATIONS AND USAGE

For the relief of symptoms of depression. Endogenous depression is more likely to be alleviated than other depressive states. One to three weeks of treatment may be needed before optimal therapeutic effects are evident.

CONTRAINDICATIONS

The concomitant use of monoamine oxidase inhibiting compounds is contraindicated. Hyperpyretic crises or severe convulsive seizures may occur in patients receiving such combinations. The potentiation of adverse effects can be serious, or even fatal. When it is desired to substitute Tofranil-PM in patients receiving a monoamine oxidase inhibitor, as long an interval should elapse as the clinical situation will allow, with a minimum of 14 days. Initial dosage should be low and increases should be gradual and cautiously prescribed.

The drug is contraindicated during the acute recovery period after a myocardial infarction. Patients with a known hypersensitivity to this compound should not be given the drug. The possibility of cross-sensitivity to other dibenzazepine compounds should be kept in mind.

Continued on next page

Tofranil-PM—Cont.

WARNINGS

Extreme caution should be used when this drug is given to: patients with cardiovascular disease because of the possibility of conduction defects, arrhythmias, congestive heart failure, myocardial infarction, strokes and tachycardia. These patients require cardiac surveillance at all dosage levels of the drug; patients with increased intraocular pressure, history of urinary retention, or history of narrow-angle glaucoma because of the drug's anticholinergic properties; hyperthyroid patients or those on thyroid medication because of the possibility of cardiovascular toxicity; patients with a history of seizure disorder because this drug has been shown to lower the seizure threshold; patients receiving guanethidine, clonidine, or similar agents, since imipramine pamoate may block the pharmacologic effects of these drugs; patients receiving methylphenidate hydrochloride. Since methylphenidate hydrochloride may inhibit the metabolism of imipramine pamoate, downward dosage adjustment of imipramine pamoate may be required when given concomitantly with methylphenidate hydrochloride.

Since imipramine pamoate may impair the mental and/or physical abilities required for the performance of potentially hazardous tasks, such as operating an automobile or machinery, the patient should be cautioned accordingly.

Tofranil-PM may enhance the CNS depressant effects of alcohol. Therefore, it should be borne in mind that the dangers inherent in a suicide attempt or accidental overdosage with the drug may be increased for the patient who uses excessive amounts of alcohol. (See PRECAUTIONS.)

Usage in Children: Tofranil-PM should not be used in children of any age because of the increased potential for acute overdosage due to the high unit potency (75 mg, 100 mg, 125 mg, and 150 mg). Each capsule contains imipramine pamoate equivalent to 75 mg, 100 mg, 125 mg, or 150 mg imipramine hydrochloride.

PRECAUTIONS
General

An ECG recording should be taken prior to the initiation of larger-than-usual doses of imipramine pamoate and at appropriate intervals thereafter until steady state is achieved. (Patients with any evidence of cardiovascular disease require cardiac surveillance at all dosage levels of the drug. See WARNINGS.) Elderly patients and patients with cardiac disease or a prior history of cardiac disease are at special risk of developing the cardiac abnormalities associated with the use of imipramine pamoate. It should be kept in mind that the possibility of suicide in seriously depressed patients is inherent in the illness and may persist until significant remission occurs. Such patients should be carefully supervised during the early phase of treatment with imipramine pamoate and may require hospitalization. Prescriptions should be written for the smallest amount feasible.

Hypomanic or manic episodes may occur, particularly in patients with cyclic disorders. Such reactions may necessitate discontinuation of the drug. If needed, imipramine pamoate may be resumed in lower dosage when these episodes are relieved. Administration of a tranquilizer may be useful in controlling such episodes.

An activation of the psychosis may occasionally be observed in schizophrenic patients and may require reduction of dosage and the addition of a phenothiazine.

Concurrent administration of imipramine pamoate with electroshock therapy may increase the hazards: such treatment should be limited to those patients for whom it is essential, since there is limited clinical experience.

Patients taking imipramine pamoate should avoid excessive exposure to sunlight since there have been reports of photosensitization.

Both elevation and lowering of blood sugar levels have been reported with imipramine pamoate use.

Imipramine pamoate should be used with caution in patients with significantly impaired renal or hepatic function.

Patients who develop a fever and a sore throat during therapy with imipramine pamoate should have leukocyte and differential blood counts performed.

Imipramine pamoate should be discontinued if there is evidence of pathological neutrophil depression.

Prior to elective surgery, imipramine pamoate should be discontinued for as long as the clinical situation will allow.

Drug Interactions

Drugs Metabolized by P450 2D6: The biochemical activity of the drug metabolizing isozyme cytochrome P450 2D6 (debrisoquin hydroxylase) is reduced in a subset of the Caucasian population (about 7%-10% of Caucasians are so-called "poor metabolizers"); reliable estimates of the prevalence of reduced P450 2D6 isozyme activity among Asian, African, and other populations are not yet available. Poor metabolizers have higher than expected plasma concentrations of tricyclic antidepressants (TCAs) when given usual doses. Depending on the fraction of drug metabolized by

P450 2D6, the increase in plasma concentration may be small, or quite large (8-fold increase in plasma AUC of the TCA).

In addition, certain drugs inhibit the activity of this isozyme and make normal metabolizers resemble poor metabolizers. An individual who is stable on a given dose of TCA may become abruptly toxic when given one of these inhibiting drugs as concomitant therapy. The drugs that inhibit cytochrome P450 2D6 include some that are not metabolized by the enzyme (quinidine; cimetidine) and many that are substrates for P450 2D6 (many other antidepressants, phenothiazines, and the Type 1C antiarrhythmics propafenone and flecainide). While all the selective serotonin reuptake inhibitors (SSRIs), e.g., fluoxetine, sertraline, and paroxetine, inhibit P450 2D6, they may vary in the extent of inhibition. The extent to which SSRI-TCA interactions may pose clinical problems will depend on the degree of inhibition and the pharmacokinetics of the SSRI involved. Nevertheless, caution is indicated in the co-administration of TCAs with any of the SSRIs and also in switching from one class to the other. Of particular importance, sufficient time must elapse before initiating TCA treatment in a patient being withdrawn from fluoxetine, given the long half-life of the parent and active metabolite (at least 5 weeks may be necessary).

Concomitant use of tricyclic antidepressants with drugs that can inhibit cytochrome P450 2D6 may require lower doses than usually prescribed for either the tricyclic antidepressant or the other drug. Furthermore, whenever one of these other drugs is withdrawn from co-therapy, an increased dose of tricyclic antidepressant may be required. It is desirable to monitor TCA plasma levels whenever a TCA is going to be co-administered with another drug known to be an inhibitor of P450 2D6.

The plasma concentration of imipramine may increase when the drug is given concomitantly with hepatic enzyme inhibitors (e.g., cimetidine, fluoxetine) and decrease by concomitant administration with hepatic enzyme inducers (e.g., barbiturates, phenytoin), and adjustment of the dosage of imipramine may therefore be necessary.

In occasional susceptible patients or in those receiving anticholinergic drugs (including antiparkinsonism agents) in addition, the atropine-like effects may become more pronounced (e.g., paralytic ileus). Close supervision and careful adjustment of dosage is required when imipramine pamoate is administered concomitantly with anticholinergic drugs.

Avoid the use of preparations, such as decongestants and local anesthetics, that contain any sympathomimetic amine (e.g., epinephrine, norepinephrine), since it has been reported that tricyclic antidepressants can potentiate the effects of catecholamines.

Caution should be exercised when imipramine pamoate is used with agents that lower blood pressure. Imipramine pamoate may potentiate the effects of CNS depressant drugs.

Patients should be warned that imipramine pamoate may enhance the CNS depressant effects of alcohol. (See WARNINGS.)

Pregnancy

Animal reproduction studies have yielded inconclusive results. (See also ANIMAL PHARMACOLOGY & TOXICOLOGY.)

There have been no well-controlled studies conducted with pregnant women to determine the effect of imipramine on the fetus. However, there have been clinical reports of congenital malformations associated with the use of the drug. Although a causal relationship between these effects and the drug could not be established, the possibility of fetal risk from the maternal ingestion of imipramine cannot be excluded. Therefore, imipramine should be used in women who are or might become pregnant only if the clinical condition clearly justifies potential risk to the fetus.

Nursing Mothers

Limited data suggest that imipramine is likely to be excreted in human breast milk. As a general rule, a woman taking a drug should not nurse since the possibility exists that the drug may be excreted in breast milk and be harmful to the child.

Pediatric Use

See WARNINGS.

ADVERSE REACTIONS

Note: Although the listing which follows includes a few adverse reactions which have not been reported with this specific drug, the pharmacological similarities among the tricyclic antidepressant drugs require that each of the reactions be considered when imipramine is administered.

Cardiovascular: Orthostatic hypotension, hypertension, tachycardia, palpitation, myocardial infarction, arrhythmias, heart block, ECG changes, precipitation of congestive heart failure, stroke.

Psychiatric: Confusional states (especially in the elderly) with hallucinations, disorientation, delusions; anxiety, restlessness, agitation; insomnia and nightmares; hypomania; exacerbation of psychosis.

Neurological: Numbness, tingling, paresthesias of extremities; incoordination, ataxia, tremors; peripheral neuropathy; extrapyramidal symptoms; seizures, alterations in EEG patterns; tinnitus.

Anticholinergic: Dry mouth, and, rarely, associated sublingual adenitis; blurred vision, disturbances of accommodation, mydriasis; constipation, paralytic ileus; urinary retention, delayed micturition, dilation of the urinary tract.

Allergic: Skin rash, petechiae, urticaria, itching, photosensitization; edema (general or of face and tongue); drug fever; cross-sensitivity with desipramine.

Hematologic: Bone marrow depression including agranulocytosis; eosinophilia; purpura; thrombocytopenia.

Gastrointestinal: Nausea and vomiting, anorexia, epigastric distress, diarrhea; peculiar taste, stomatitis, abdominal cramps, black tongue.

Endocrine: Gynecomastia in the male; breast enlargement and galactorrhea in the female; increased or decreased libido, impotence; testicular swelling; elevation or depression of blood sugar levels; inappropriate antidiuretic hormone (ADH) secretion syndrome.

Other: Jaundice (simulating obstructive); altered liver function; weight gain or loss; perspiration; flushing; urinary frequency; drowsiness, dizziness, weakness and fatigue; headache; parotid swelling; alopecia; proneness to falling.

Withdrawal Symptoms: Though not indicative of addiction, abrupt cessation of treatment after prolonged therapy may produce nausea, headache and malaise.

DOSAGE AND ADMINISTRATION

The following recommended dosages for Tofranil-PM should be modified as necessary by the clinical response and any evidence of intolerance.

Initial Adult Dosage:

Outpatients — Therapy should be initiated at 75 mg/day. Dosage may be increased to 150 mg/day which is the dose level at which optimum response is usually obtained. If necessary, dosage may be increased to 200 mg/day.

Dosage higher than 75 mg/day may also be administered on a once-a-day basis after the optimum dosage and tolerance have been determined. The daily dosage may be given at bedtime. In some patients it may be necessary to employ a divided-dose schedule.

As with all tricyclics, the antidepressant effect of imipramine may not be evident for one to three weeks in some patients.

Hospitalized Patients — Therapy should be initiated at 100-150 mg/day and may be increased to 200 mg/day. If there is no response after two weeks, dosage should be increased to 250-300 mg/day.

Dosage higher than 150 mg/day may also be administered on a once-a-day basis after the optimum dosage and tolerance have been determined. The daily dosage may be given at bedtime. In some patients it may be necessary to employ a divided-dose schedule.

As with all tricyclics, the antidepressant effect of imipramine may not be evident for one to three weeks in some patients.

Adult Maintenance Dosage: Following remission, maintenance medication may be required for a longer period of time at the lowest dose that will maintain remission after which the dosage should gradually be decreased.

The usual maintenance dosage is 75-150 mg/day. The total daily dosage can be administered on a once-a-day basis, preferably at bedtime. In some patients it may be necessary to employ a divided-dose schedule.

In cases of relapse due to premature withdrawal of the drug, the effective dosage of imipramine should be reinstituted.

Adolescent and Geriatric Patients: Therapy in these age groups should be initiated with Tofranil®, brand of imipramine hydrochloride, tablets at a total daily dosage of 25-50 mg, since Tofranil-PM capsules are not available in these strengths. Dosage may be increased according to response and tolerance, but it is generally unnecessary to exceed 100 mg/day in these patients. Tofranil-PM capsules may be used when total daily dosage is established at 75 mg or higher.

The total daily dosage can be administered on a once-a-day basis, preferably at bedtime. In some patients it may be necessary to employ a divided-dose schedule.

As with all tricyclics, the antidepressant effect of imipramine may not be evident for one to three weeks in some patients.

Adolescent and geriatric patients can usually be maintained at lower dosage. Following remission, maintenance medication may be required for a longer period of time at the lowest dose that will maintain remission after which the dosage should gradually be decreased.

The total daily maintenance dosage can be administered on a once-a-day basis, preferably at bedtime.

In some patients it may be necessary to employ a divided-dose schedule.

In cases of relapse due to premature withdrawal of the drug, the effective dosage of imipramine should be reinstituted.

OVERDOSAGE

Deaths may occur from overdosage with this class of drugs. Multiple drug ingestion (including alcohol) is common in deliberate tricyclic overdose. As the management is complex and changing, it is recommended that the physician contact a poison control center for current information on treatment. Signs and symptoms of toxicity develop rapidly after tricyclic overdose. Therefore, hospital monitoring is required as soon as possible.

Children have been reported to be more sensitive than adults to an acute overdosage of imipramine pamoate. An acute overdose of any amount in infants or young children, especially, must be considered serious and potentially fatal.

Manifestations

These may vary in severity depending upon factors such as the amount of drug absorbed, the age of the patient, and the interval between drug ingestion and the start of treatment. Critical manifestations of overdose include cardiac dysrhythmias, severe hypotension, convulsions, and CNS depression including coma. Changes in the electrocardiogram, particularly in QRS axis or width, are clinically significant indicators of tricyclic toxicity.

Other CNS manifestations may include drowsiness, stupor, ataxia, restlessness, agitation, hyperactive reflexes, muscle rigidity, athetoid and choreiform movements.

Cardiac abnormalities may include tachycardia, and signs of congestive failure. Respiratory depression, cyanosis, shock, vomiting, hyperpyrexia, mydriasis, and diaphoresis may also be present.

Management

Obtain an ECG and immediately initiate cardiac monitoring. Protect the patient's airway, establish an intravenous line, and initiate gastric decontamination. A minimum of 6 hours of observation with cardiac monitoring and observation for signs of CNS or respiratory depression, hypotension, cardiac dysrhythmias and/or conduction blocks, and seizures is necessary. If signs of toxicity occur at any time during this period, extended monitoring is required. There are case reports of patients succumbing to fatal dysrhythmias late after overdose; these patients had clinical evidence of significant poisoning prior to death and most received inadequate gastrointestinal decontamination. Monitoring of plasma drug levels should not guide management of the patient.

Gastrointestinal Decontamination: All patients suspected of tricyclic overdose should receive gastrointestinal decontamination. This should include large volume gastric lavage followed by activated charcoal. If consciousness is impaired, the airway should be secured prior to lavage. Emesis is contraindicated.

Cardiovascular: A maximal limb-lead QRS duration of ≥0.10 seconds may be the best indication of the severity of the overdose. Intravenous sodium bicarbonate should be used to maintain the serum pH in the range of 7.45 to 7.55. If the pH response is inadequate, hyperventilation may also be used. Concomitant use of hyperventilation and sodium bicarbonate should be done with extreme caution, with frequent pH monitoring. A pH >7.60 or a P_{CO_2} <20 mmHg is undesirable. Dysrhythmias unresponsive to sodium bicarbonate therapy/hyperventilation may respond to lidocaine, bretylium, or phenytoin. Type 1A and 1C antiarrhythmics are generally contraindicated (e.g., quinidine, disopyramide, and procainamide).

In rare instances, hemoperfusion may be beneficial in acute refractory cardiovascular instability in patients with acute toxicity. However, hemodialysis, peritoneal dialysis, exchange transfusions, and forced diuresis generally have been reported as ineffective in tricyclic poisoning.

CNS: In patients with CNS depression, early intubation is advised because of the potential for abrupt deterioration. Seizures should be controlled with benzodiazepines, or if these are ineffective, other anticonvulsants (e.g., phenobarbital, phenytoin). Physostigmine is not recommended except to treat life-threatening symptoms that have been unresponsive to other therapies, and then only in consultation with a poison control center.

Psychiatric Follow-up: Since overdosage is often deliberate, patients may attempt suicide by other means during the recovery phase. Psychiatric referral may be appropriate.

Pediatric Management: The principles of management of child and adult overdosages are similar. It is strongly recommended that the physician contact the local poison control center for specific pediatric treatment.

HOW SUPPLIED

Capsules 75 mg — coral (imprinted black Geigy 20) equivalent to 75 mg imipramine hydrochloride

Bottles of 30 .... NDC 0028-0020-26
Bottles of 100 .... NDC 0028-0020-01

Capsules 100 mg — dark yellow/coral (imprinted black Geigy 40) equivalent to 100 mg imipramine hydrochloride

Bottles of 30 .... NDC 0028-0040-26
Bottles of 100 .... NDC 0028-0040-01

Capsules 125 mg — ivory/coral (imprinted black Geigy 45) equivalent to 125 mg imipramine hydrochloride

Bottles of 30 .... NDC 0028-0045-26
Bottles of 100 .... NDC 0028-0045-01

Capsules 150 mg — coral (imprinted black Geigy 22) equivalent to 150 mg imipramine hydrochloride

Bottles of 30 .... NDC 0028-0022-26
Bottles of 100 .... NDC 0028-0022-01

Do not store above 30°C (86°F).

Dispense in tight container (USP).

ANIMAL PHARMACOLOGY & TOXICOLOGY

A. *Acute:* Oral LD_{50}:

Mouse	2185 mg/kg
Rat (F)	1142 mg/kg
(M)	1807 mg/kg
Rabbit	1016 mg/kg
Dog	693 mg/kg (Emesis ED_{50})

B. *Subacute:*

Two three-month studies in dogs gave evidence of an adverse drug effect on the testes, but only at the highest dose level employed, i.e., 90 mg/kg (10 times the maximum human dose). Depending on the histological section of the testes examined, the findings consisted of a range of degenerative changes up to and including complete atrophy of the seminiferous tubules, with spermatogenesis usually arrested.

Human studies show no definitive effect on sperm count, sperm motility, sperm morphology or volume of ejaculate.

Rat

One three-month study was done in rats at dosage levels comparable to those of the dog studies. No adverse drug effect on the testes was noted in this study, as confirmed by histological examination.

C. *Reproduction/Teratogenic:*

Oral: Imipramine pamoate was fed to male and female albino rats for 28 weeks through two breeding cycles at dose levels of 15 mg/kg/day and 40 mg/kg/day (equivalent to $2^1/_2$ and 7 times the maximum human dose).

No abnormalities which could be related to drug administration were noted in gross inspection. Autopsies performed on pups from the second breeding likewise revealed no pathological changes in organs or tissues; however, a decrease in mean litter size from both matings was noted in the drug-treated groups and significant growth suppression occurred in the nursing pups of both sexes in the high group as well as in the females of the low-level group. Finally, the lactation index (pups weaned divided by number left to nurse) was significantly lower in the second litter of the high-level group.

C98-15 (Rev. 2/98)

Shown in Product Identification Guide, page 326

TRANSDERM-NITRO® ℞

[trans 'derm nye 'trow]

nitroglycerin

Transdermal Therapeutic System

Caution: Federal law prohibits dispensing without prescription.

The following prescribing information is based on official labeling in effect on October 1, 1998.

Prescribing Information

DESCRIPTION

Nitroglycerin is 1,2,3-propanetriol, trinitrate, an organic nitrate whose structural formula is

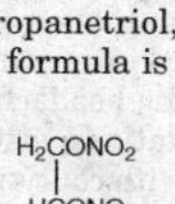
H2CONO2
HCONO2
H2CONO2

and whose molecular weight is 227.09. The organic nitrates are vasodilators, active on both arteries and veins.

The Transderm-Nitro (nitroglycerin) transdermal system is a flat unit designed to provide continuous controlled release of nitroglycerin through intact skin.

The rate of release of nitroglycerin is linearly dependent upon the area of the applied system; each cm^2 of applied system delivers approximately 0.02 mg of nitroglycerin per hour. Thus, the 5-, 10-, 20-, and 30-cm^2 systems deliver approximately 0.1, 0.2, 0.4, and 0.6 mg of nitroglycerin per hour, respectively.

The remainder of the nitroglycerin in each system serves as a reservoir and is not delivered in normal use. After 12 hours, for example, each system has delivered 10% of its original content of nitroglycerin.

The Transderm-Nitro system comprises four layers as shown below. Proceeding from the visible surface towards the surface attached to the skin, these layers are: 1) a tan-colored backing layer (aluminized plastic) that is impermeable to nitroglycerin; 2) a drug reservoir containing nitroglycerin adsorbed on lactose, colloidal silicon dioxide, and silicone medical fluid; 3) an ethylene-vinyl acetate copolymer membrane that is permeable to nitroglycerin; and 4) a layer of hypoallergenic silicone adhesive. Prior to use, a protective peel strip is removed from the adhesive surface. Cross section of the system:

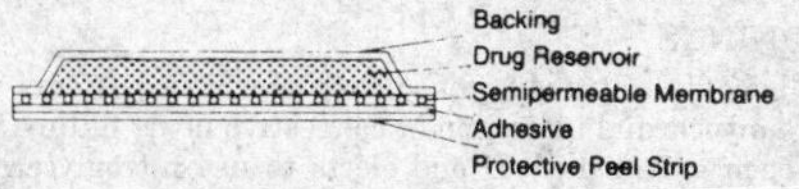
Backing
Drug Reservoir
Semipermeable Membrane
Adhesive
Protective Peel Strip

CLINICAL PHARMACOLOGY

The principal pharmacological action of nitroglycerin is relaxation of vascular smooth muscle, and consequent dilatation of peripheral arteries and veins, especially the latter. Dilatation of the veins promotes peripheral pooling of blood and decreases venous return to the heart, thereby reducing left ventricular end-diastolic pressure and pulmonary capillary wedge pressure (preload). Arteriolar relaxation reduces systemic vascular resistance, systolic arterial pressure, and mean arterial pressure (afterload). Dilatation of the coronary arteries also occurs. The relative importance of preload reduction, afterload reduction, and coronary dilatation remains undefined.

Dosing regimens for most chronically used drugs are designed to provide plasma concentrations that are continuously greater than a minimally effective concentration. This strategy is inappropriate for organic nitrates. Several well-controlled clinical trials have used exercise testing to assess the antianginal efficacy of continuously-delivered nitrates. In the large majority of these trials, active agents were indistinguishable from placebo after 24 hours (or less) of continuous therapy. Attempts to overcome nitrate tolerance by dose escalation, even to doses far in excess of those used acutely, have consistently failed. Only after nitrates had been absent from the body for several hours was their antianginal efficacy restored.

Pharmacokinetics

The volume of distribution of nitroglycerin is about 3 L/kg, and nitroglycerin is cleared from this volume at extremely rapid rates, with a resulting serum half-life of about 3 minutes. The observed clearance rates (close to 1 L/kg/min) greatly exceed hepatic blood flow. Known sites of extrahepatic metabolism include red blood cells and vascular walls. The first products in the metabolism of nitroglycerin are inorganic nitrate and the 1,2- and 1,3-dinitroglycerols. The dinitrates are less effective vasodilators than nitroglycerin, but they are longer-lived in the serum, and their net contribution to the overall effect of chronic nitroglycerin regimens is not known. The dinitrates are further metabolized to (nonvasoactive) mononitrates and, ultimately, to glycerol and carbon dioxide.

To avoid development of tolerance to nitroglycerin, drug-free intervals of 10-12 hours are known to be sufficient; shorter intervals have not been well studied. In one well-controlled clinical trial, subjects receiving nitroglycerin appeared to exhibit a rebound or withdrawal effect, so that their exercise tolerance at the end of the daily drug-free interval was *less* than that exhibited by the parallel group receiving placebo.

In healthy volunteers, steady-state plasma concentrations of nitroglycerin are reached by about two hours after application of a patch and are maintained for the duration of wearing the system (observations have been limited to 24 hours). Upon removal of the patch, the plasma concentration declines with a half-life of about an hour.

Clinical Trials

Regimens in which nitroglycerin patches were worn for 12 hours daily have been studied in well-controlled trials up to 4 weeks in duration. Starting about 2 hours after application and continuing until 10-12 hours after application, patches that deliver at least 0.4 mg of nitroglycerin per hour have consistently demonstrated greater antianginal activity than placebo. Lower-dose patches have not been as well studied, but in one large, well-controlled trial in which higher-dose patches were also studied, patches delivering 0.2 mg/hr had significantly less antianginal activity than placebo.

It is reasonable to believe that the rate of nitroglycerin absorption from patches may vary with the site of application, but this relationship has not been adequately studied.

The onset of action of transdermal nitroglycerin is not sufficiently rapid for this product to be useful in aborting an acute anginal episode.

INDICATIONS AND USAGE

Transdermal nitroglycerin is indicated for the prevention of angina pectoris due to coronary artery disease. The onset of action of transdermal nitroglycerin is not sufficiently rapid for this product to be useful in aborting an acute attack.

CONTRAINDICATIONS

Allergic reactions to organic nitrates are extremely rare, but they do occur. Nitroglycerin is contraindicated in patients who are allergic to it. Allergy to the adhesives used in nitro-

Continued on next page

Transderm-Nitro—Cont.

glycerin patches has also been reported, and it similarly constitutes a contraindication to the use of this product.

WARNINGS

The benefits of transdermal nitroglycerin in patients with acute myocardial infarction or congestive heart failure have not been established. If one elects to use nitroglycerin in these conditions, careful clinical or hemodynamic monitoring must be used to avoid the hazards of hypotension and tachycardia.

A cardioverter/defibrillator should not be discharged through a paddle electrode that overlies a Transderm-Nitro patch. The arcing that may be seen in this situation is harmless in itself, but it may be associated with local current concentration that can cause damage to the paddles and burns to the patient.

PRECAUTIONS

General

Severe hypotension, particularly with upright posture, may occur with even small doses of nitroglycerin. This drug should therefore be used with caution in patients who may be volume depleted or who, for whatever reason, are already hypotensive. Hypotension induced by nitroglycerin may be accompanied by paradoxical bradycardia and increased angina pectoris.

Nitrate therapy may aggravate the angina caused by hypertrophic cardiomyopathy.

As tolerance to other forms of nitroglycerin develops, the effect of sublingual nitroglycerin on exercise tolerance, although still observable, is somewhat blunted.

In industrial workers who have had long-term exposure to unknown (presumably high) doses of organic nitrates, tolerance clearly occurs. Chest pain, acute myocardial infarction, and even sudden death have occurred during temporary withdrawal of nitrates from these workers, demonstrating the existence of true physical dependence.

Several clinical trials in patients with angina pectoris have evaluated nitroglycerin regimens which incorporated a 10-12 hour nitrate-free interval. In some of these trials, an increase in the frequency of anginal attacks during the nitrate-free interval was observed in a small number of patients. In one trial, patients demonstrated decreased exercise tolerance at the end of the nitrate-free interval. Hemodynamic rebound has been observed only rarely; on the other hand, few studies were so designed that rebound, if it had occurred, would have been detected. The importance of these observations to the routine, clinical use of transdermal nitroglycerin is unknown.

Information for Patients

Daily headaches sometimes accompany treatment with nitroglycerin. In patients who get these headaches, the headaches may be a marker of the activity of the drug. Patients should resist the temptation to avoid headaches by altering the schedule of their treatment with nitroglycerin, since loss of headache may be associated with simultaneous loss of antianginal efficacy.

Treatment with nitroglycerin may be associated with lightheadedness on standing, especially just after rising from a recumbent or seated position. This effect may be more frequent in patients who have also consumed alcohol.

After normal use, there is enough residual nitroglycerin in discarded patches that they are a potential hazard to children and pets.

A patient leaflet is supplied with the systems.

Drug Interactions

The vasodilating effects of nitroglycerin may be additive with those of other vasodilators. Alcohol, in particular, has been found to exhibit additive effects of this variety.

Marked symptomatic orthostatic hypotension has been reported when calcium channel blockers and organic nitrates were used in combination. Dose adjustments of either class of agents may be necessary.

Carcinogenesis, Mutagenesis, Impairment of Fertility

Animal carcinogenesis studies with topically applied nitroglycerin have not been performed.

Rats receiving up to 434 mg/kg/day of dietary nitroglycerin for 2 years developed dose-related fibrotic and neoplastic changes in liver, including carcinomas, and interstitial cell tumors in testes. At high dose, the incidences of hepatocellular carcinomas in both sexes were 52% vs. 0% in controls, and incidences of testicular tumors were 52% vs. 8% in controls. Lifetime dietary administration of up to 1058 mg/kg/day of nitroglycerin was not tumorigenic in mice.

Nitroglycerin was weakly mutagenic in Ames tests performed in two different laboratories. Nevertheless, there was no evidence of mutagenicity in an in vivo dominant lethal assay with male rats treated with doses up to about 363 mg/kg/day, p.o., or in in vitro cytogenetic tests in rat and dog tissues.

In a three-generation reproduction study, rats received dietary nitroglycerin at doses up to about 434 mg/kg/day for six months prior to mating of the F_0 generation with treatment continuing through successive F_1 and F_2 generations. The high dose was associated with decreased feed intake and body weight gain in both sexes at all matings. No specific effect on the fertility of the F_0 generation was seen. Infertility noted in subsequent generations, however, was attributed to increased interstitial cell tissue and aspermatogenesis in the high-dose males. In this three-generation study there was no clear evidence of teratogenicity.

Pregnancy Category C

Animal teratology studies have not been conducted with nitroglycerin transdermal systems. Teratology studies in rats and rabbits, however, were conducted with topically applied nitroglycerin ointment at doses up to 80 mg/kg/day and 240 mg/kg/day, respectively. No toxic effects on dams or fetuses were seen at any dose tested. There are no adequate and well-controlled studies in pregnant women. Nitroglycerin should be given to a pregnant woman only if clearly needed.

Nursing Mothers

It is not known whether nitroglycerin is excreted in human milk. Because many drugs are excreted in human milk, caution should be exercised when nitroglycerin is administered to a nursing woman.

Pediatric Use

Safety and effectiveness in pediatric patients have not been established.

ADVERSE REACTIONS

Adverse reactions to nitroglycerin are generally dose-related, and almost all of these reactions are the result of nitroglycerin's activity as a vasodilator. Headache, which may be severe, is the most commonly reported side effect. Headache may be recurrent with each daily dose, especially at higher doses. Transient episodes of lightheadedness, occasionally related to blood pressure changes, may also occur. Hypotension occurs infrequently, but in some patients it may be severe enough to warrant discontinuation of therapy. Syncope, crescendo angina, and rebound hypertension have been reported but are uncommon.

Allergic reactions to nitroglycerin are also uncommon, and the great majority of those reported have been cases of contact dematitis or fixed drug eruptions in patients receiving nitroglycerin in ointments or patches. There have been a few reports of genuine anaphylactoid reactions, and these reactions can probably occur in patients receiving nitroglycerin by any route.

Extremely rarely, ordinary doses of organic nitrates have caused methemoglobinemia in normal-seeming patients. Methemoglobinemia is so infrequent at these doses that further discussion of its diagnosis and treatment is deferred (see OVERDOSAGE).

Application-site irritation may occur but is rarely severe.

In two placebo-controlled trials of intermittent therapy with nitroglycerin patches at 0.2 to 0.8 mg/hr, the most frequent adverse reactions among 307 subjects were as follows:

	Placebo	Patch
Headache	18%	63%
Lightheadedness	4%	6%
Hypotension, and/or syncope	0%	4%
Increased angina	2%	2%

OVERDOSAGE

Hemodynamic Effects

The ill effects of nitroglycerin overdose are generally the result of nitroglycerin's capacity to induce vasodilatation, venous pooling, reduced cardiac output, and hypotension. These hemodynamic changes may have protean manifestations, including increased intracranial pressure, with any or all of persistent throbbing headache, confusion, and moderate fever; vertigo; palpitations; visual disturbances; nausea and vomiting (possibly with colic and even bloody diarrhea); syncope (especially in the upright posture); air hunger and dyspnea, later followed by reduced ventilatory effort; diaphoresis, with the skin either flushed or cold and clammy; heart block and bradycardia; paralysis; coma; seizures; and death.

Laboratory determinations of serum levels of nitroglycerin and its metabolites are not widely available, and such determinations have, in any event, no established role in the management of nitroglycerin overdose.

No data are available to suggest physiological maneuvers (e.g., maneuvers to change the pH of the urine) that might accelerate elimination of nitroglycerin and its active metabolites. Similarly, it is not known which, if any, of these substances can usefully be removed from the body by hemodialysis.

No specific antagonist to the vasodilator effects of nitroglycerin is known, and no intervention has been subject to controlled study as a therapy of nitroglycerin overdose.

Because the hypotension associated with nitroglycerin overdose is the result of venodilatation and arterial hypovolemia, prudent therapy in this situation should be directed toward an increase in central fluid volume. Passive elevation of the patient's legs may be sufficient, but intravenous infusion of normal saline or similar fluid may also be necessary.

The use of epinephrine or other arterial vasoconstrictors in this setting is likely to do more harm than good.

In patients with renal disease or congestive heart failure, therapy resulting in central volume expansion is not without hazard. Treatment of nitroglycerin overdose in these patients may be subtle and difficult, and invasive monitoring may be required.

Methemoglobinemia

Nitrate ions liberated during metabolism of nitroglycerin can oxidize hemoglobin into methemoglobin. Even in patients totally without cytochrome b_5 reductase activity, however, and even assuming that the nitrate moieties of nitroglycerin are quantitatively applied to oxidation of hemoglobin, about 1 mg/kg of nitroglycerin should be required before any of these patients manifests clinically significant ($\geq$10%) methemoglobinemia. In patients with normal reductase function, significant production of methemoglobin should require even larger doses of nitroglycerin. In one study in which 36 patients received 2-4 weeks of continuous nitroglycerin therapy at 3.1 to 4.4 mg/hr, the average methemoglobin level measured was 0.2%; this was comparable to that observed in parallel patients who received placebo.

Notwithstanding these observations, there are case reports of significant methemoglobinemia in association with moderate overdoses of organic nitrates. None of the affected patients had been thought to be unusually susceptible.

Methemoglobin levels are available from most clinical laboratories. The diagnosis should be suspected in patients who exhibit signs of impaired oxygen delivery despite adequate cardiac output and adequate arterial pO_2. Classically, methemoglobinemic blood is described as chocolate brown, without color change on exposure to air.

When methemoglobinemia is diagnosed, the treatment of choice is methylene blue, 1-2 mg/kg intravenously.

DOSAGE AND ADMINISTRATION

The suggested starting dose is between 0.2 mg/hr*, and 0.4 mg/hr*. Doses between 0.4 mg/hr* and 0.8 mg/hr* have shown continued effectiveness for 10-12 hours daily for at least one month (the longest period studied) of intermittent administration. Although the minimum nitrate-free interval has not been defined, data show that a nitrate-free interval of 10-12 hours is sufficient (see CLINICAL PHARMACOLOGY). Thus, an appropriate dosing schedule for nitroglycerin patches would include a daily patch-on period of 12-14 hours and a daily patch-off period of 10-12 hours.

Although some well-controlled clinical trials using exercise tolerance testing have shown maintenance of effectiveness when patches are worn continuously, the large majority of such controlled trials have shown the development of tolerance (i.e., complete loss of effect) within the first 24 hours after therapy was initiated. Dose adjustment, even to levels much higher than generally used, did not restore efficacy.

PATIENT INSTRUCTIONS FOR APPLICATION OF SYSTEM

A patient leaflet is supplied with each carton.

HOW SUPPLIED

Nitroglycerin Transdermal System 0.1 mg/hr–tan, round (imprinted Transderm-Nitro 0.1 mg/hr), supplied in a foil-lined pouch

30 Systems .... NDC 0078-0332-85

Nitroglycerin Transdermal System 0.2 mg/hr–tan, oblong (imprinted Transderm-Nitro 0.2 mg/hr), supplied in a foil-lined pouch

30 Systems .... NDC 0078-0333-85

Nitroglycerin Transdermal System 0.4 mg/hr–tan, oblong (imprinted Transderm-Nitro 0.4 mg/hr), supplied in a foil-lined pouch

30 Systems .... NDC 0078-0334-85

Nitroglycerin Transdermal System 0.6 mg/hr–tan, oblong (imprinted Transderm-Nitro 0.6 mg/hr), supplied in a foil-lined pouch

30 Systems .... NDC 0078-0335-85

*Rated release in vivo. Release rates were formerly described in terms of drug delivered per 24 hours. In these terms, the supplied Transderm-Nitro systems would be rated at 2.5 mg/24 hr (0.1 mg/hr), 5 mg/24 hr (0.2 mg/hr), 10 mg/24 hr (0.4 mg/hr), 15 mg/24 hr (0.6 mg/hr), and 20 mg/24 hr (0.8 mg/hr).

Do not store above 30°C (86°F).

Do not store unpouched. Apply immediately upon removal from the pouch.

How to use
TRANSDERM-NITRO®
nitroglycerin
Transdermal Therapeutic System
for the prevention of angina

Transderm-Nitro is easy to use–it has a clear plastic backing, and a special adhesive that keeps the system firmly in place.

Where to place Transderm-Nitro

Select any area of skin on the body, EXCEPT the extremities below the knee or elbow. The chest is the preferred site. The area should be clean, dry, and hairless. If hair is likely to interfere with system adhesion or removal, it can be

clipped, but not shaved. Take care to avoid areas with cuts or irritations. Do NOT apply the system immediately after showering or bathing. It is best to wait until you are certain the skin is completely dry.

How to apply Transderm-Nitro® nitroglycerin

1. Each Transderm-Nitro system is individually sealed in a protective pouch. Tear open this pouch at the indicated indentations. Carefully pick up the system lengthwise with the tab up, and the clear plastic backing facing you. You should be able to see the white cream containing nitroglycerin. (On very rare occasions, you may find a system without any white medication in it. Do not use it. Simply apply another system.)

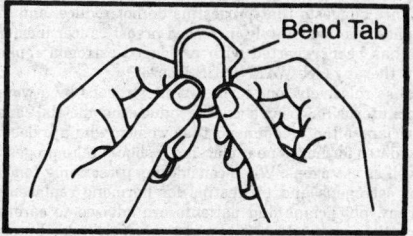

Figure A

2. Firmly bend the tab forward with the thumb (Figure A). With both thumbs, begin to remove the clear plastic backing from the system at the tab (Figure B). Do not touch the inside of the exposed system, because the adhesive covers the entire surface.

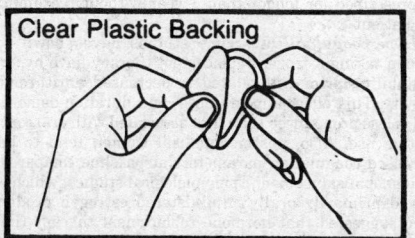

Figure B

3. Continue to remove the clear plastic backing slowly along the length of the system, allowing the system to rest on the outside of your fingers (Figure C).

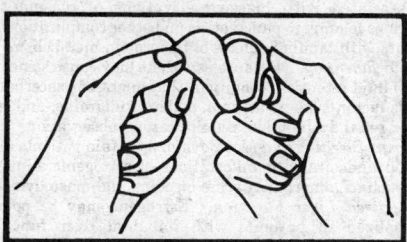

Figure C

4. Place the exposed, adhesive side of the system on the chosen skin site. Press firmly in place with the palm of your hand (Figure D). Once the system is in place, do not test the adhesion by pulling on it.

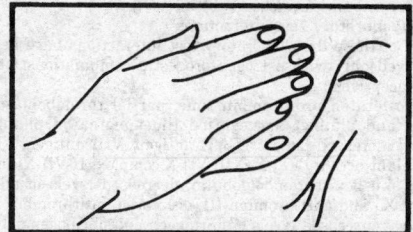

Figure D

When Transderm-Nitro is applied to your body, the nitroglycerin contained in the system begins to flow onto your skin through a unique rate-controlling membrane. This membrane allows the nitroglycerin to be released and available for absorption through your skin at a uniform rate.

5. At the time recommended by your doctor, remove and discard the system.

6. Place a new system on a different skin site, following Steps 1-4, according to your doctor's instructions.

Please note

Contact with water, as in bathing, swimming, or showering will not affect the system. In the unlikely event that a system falls off, discard it and put a new one on a different skin site.

PRECAUTIONS

The most common side effect is headache, which often decreases as therapy is continued, but may require treatment with a mild analgesic. Although uncommon, faintness, flushing, and dizziness may occur, especially when suddenly rising from the recumbent (lying horizontal) position. If these symptoms occur, remove the system and notify your physician.

Skin irritation may occur. If it persists, consult your physician.

Keep these systems and all drugs out of the reach of children.

Important

Your doctor may decide to increase or decrease the size of the system, or prescribe a combination of systems, to suit your particular needs. The dose may vary depending on your individual response to the system.

This system is to be used for preventing angina, not for treating an acute attack.

Do not store above 30°C (86°F) .

Do not store unpouched. Apply immediately upon removal from the protective pouch.

Distributed by
Novartis Pharmaceuticals Corporation
East Hanover, New Jersey 07936

C98-2 (Rev. 1/98)

Shown in Product Identification Guide, page 326

VIVELLE®   ℞
estradiol transdermal system
Continuous delivery for twice-weekly application

Rx only
The following prescribing information is based on official labeling in effect on August 1, 1998.
Prescribing Information

> **1. ESTROGENS HAVE BEEN REPORTED TO INCREASE THE RISK OF ENDOMETRIAL CARCINOMA IN POSTMENOPAUSAL WOMEN.**
> Close clinical surveillance of all women taking estrogens is important. Adequate diagnostic measures, including endometrial sampling when indicated, should be undertaken to rule out malignancy in all cases of undiagnosed persistent or recurring abnormal vaginal bleeding. There is no evidence that "natural" estrogens are more or less hazardous than "synthetic" estrogens at equiestrogenic doses.
> **2. ESTROGENS SHOULD NOT BE USED DURING PREGNANCY.**
> Estrogen therapy during pregnancy is associated with an increased risk of congenital defects in the reproductive organs of the fetus, and possibly other birth defects. Studies of women who received diethylstilbestrol (DES) during pregnancy have shown that female offspring have an increased risk of vaginal adenosis, squamous cell dysplasia of the uterine cervix, and clear cell vaginal cancer later in life; male offspring have an increased risk of urogenital abnormalities and possibly testicular cancer later in life. The 1985 DES Task Force concluded that use of DES during pregnancy is associated with a subsequent increased risk of breast cancer in the mothers, although a causal relationship remains unproven and the observed level of excess risk is similar to that for a number of other breast cancer risk factors.
> There is no indication for estrogen therapy during pregnancy or during the immediate postpartum period. Estrogens are ineffective for the prevention or treatment of threatened or habitual abortion. Estrogens are not indicated for the prevention of postpartum breast engorgement.

DESCRIPTION

The Vivelle estradiol transdermal system contains estradiol in a multipolymeric adhesive. The system is designed to release 17β-estradiol continuously upon application to intact skin.

Four systems are available to provide nominal in vivo delivery of 0.0375, 0.05, 0.075, or 0.1 mg of estradiol per day via skin of average permeability. Each corresponding system having an active surface area of 11.0, 14.5, 22.0, or 29.0 cm^2 contains 3.28, 4.33, 6.57, or 8.66 mg of estradiol USP, respectively. The composition of the systems per unit area is identical.

Estradiol USP (17β-estradiol) is a white, crystalline powder, chemically described as estra-1,3,5(10)-triene-3,17β-diol. The structural formula is

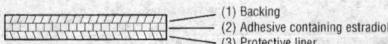

The molecular formula of estradiol is C$_{18}$H$_{24}$O$_2$. The molecular weight is 272.39.

The Vivelle system comprises three layers. Proceeding from the visible surface toward the surface attached to the skin, these layers are (1) a translucent flexible film consisting of an ethylene vinyl alcohol copolymer film, a polyurethane film, urethane polymer and epoxy resin, (2) an adhesive formulation containing estradiol, acrylic adhesive, polyisobutylene, ethylene vinyl acetate copolymer, 1,3 butylene glycol, styrene-butadiene rubber, oleic acid, lecithin, propylene glycol, bentonite, mineral oil, and dipropylene glycol, and (3) a polyester release liner that is attached to the adhesive surface and must be removed before the system can be used.

[See Figure below.]

(1) Backing
(2) Adhesive containing estradiol
(3) Protective liner

The active component of the system is estradiol. The remaining components of the system are pharmacologically inactive.

CLINICAL PHARMACOLOGY

The Vivelle system releases estradiol, the major estrogenic hormone secreted by the human ovary. Although circulating estrogens exist in a dynamic equilibrium of metabolic interconversions, estradiol is the principal intracellular human estrogen and is substantially more potent than estrone or estriol at the receptor level.

Vivelle provides systemic estrogen replacement therapy. Estrogen receptors have been identified in tissues of the reproductive tract, breast, pituitary, hypothalamus, liver, and bone of women. Among numerous effects, estradiol is largely responsible for the development and maintenance of the female reproductive system and secondary sex characteristics. By a direct action, it causes growth and development of the vagina, uterus, and fallopian tubes. With other hormones, such as pituitary hormones and progesterone, it causes enlargement of the breasts through promotion of ductal growth, stromal development, and the accretion of fat. Estrogens contribute to the shaping of the skeleton, to the maintenance of tone and elasticity of urogenital structures, to changes in the epiphyses of the long bones that allow for the pubertal growth spurt and its termination, to the growth of axillary and pubic hair, and pigmentation of the nipples and genitals.

Estrogens are intricately involved with other hormones, especially progesterone, in the processes of the ovulatory menstrual cycle and pregnancy, and affect the release of pituitary gonadotropins.

Loss of ovarian estradiol secretion after menopause can result in instability of thermoregulation, causing hot flushes associated with sleep disturbance and excessive sweating, and urogenital atrophy, causing dyspareunia and urinary incontinence. Estradiol replacement therapy alleviates many of these symptoms of estradiol deficiency in the menopausal woman.

Pharmacokinetics

Transdermal administration produces therapeutic plasma levels of estradiol with lower circulating levels of estrone and estrone conjugates and requires smaller total doses than does oral therapy. Studies conducted with the Vivelle system show the drug has an apparent mean half-life of 4.4±2.3 hours.

In a multiple-dose study consisting of three consecutive patch applications of the Vivelle system, which was conducted in 17 healthy, postmenopausal women, blood levels of estradiol and estrone were compared following application of these units to sites on the abdomen and buttocks in a crossover fashion. Patches that deliver nominal estradiol doses of approximately 0.0375 mg/day and 0.1 mg/day were applied to abdominal application sites while the 0.1 mg/day doses were also applied to sites on the buttocks. These systems increased estradiol levels above baseline within 4 hours and maintained mean respective levels of 25 and 79 pg/mL above baseline following application to the abdomen; slightly higher mean levels of 88 pg/mL above baseline were observed following application to the buttocks. At the same time, increases in estrone plasma concentrations averaged about 12 and 50 pg/mL, respectively, following application to the abdomen and 61 pg/mL for the buttocks.

Continued on next page

Vivelle—Cont.

While plasma concentrations of estradiol and estrone remained slightly above baseline at 12 hours following removal of the patches in this study, results from another study show these levels to return to baseline values within 24 hours following removal of the patches.

The graph illustrates the mean plasma concentrations of estradiol at steady-state during application of these patches at four different dosages.

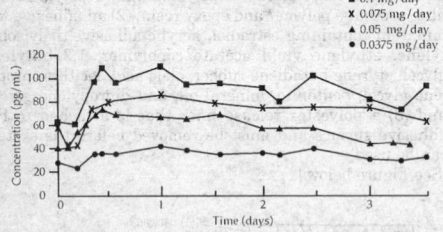

Steady-State Estradiol Plasma Concentrations for Systems Applied to the Abdomen
Nonbaseline-corrected levels

■ 0.1 mg/day
× 0.075 mg/day
▲ 0.05 mg/day
● 0.0375 mg/day

The corresponding pharmacokinetic parameters are summarized in the table below.

Steady-State Estradiol Pharmacokinetic Parameters for Systems Applied to the Abdomen (mean±standard deviation)
Nonbaseline-corrected data*

Dosage (mg/day)	C_{max}† (pg/mL)	C_{avg}‡ (pg/mL)	C_{min}(84 hr)§ (pg/mL)
0.0375	46±16	34±10	30±10
0.05	83±41	57± 23#	41± 11#
0.075	99±35	72±24	60±24
0.1	133±51	89±38	90±44
0.1¶	145±71	104±52	85±47

* Mean baseline estradiol concentration=11.7 pg/mL
† Peak plasma concentration
‡ Average plasma concentration
§ Minimum plasma concentration at 84 hr
# Measured over 80 hr
¶ Applied to the buttocks

INDICATIONS AND USAGE

Vivelle® (estradiol transdermal system) is indicated in the following:

1. Treatment of moderate-to-severe vasomotor symptoms associated with the menopause. There is no adequate evidence that estrogens are effective for nervous symptoms or depression that might occur during menopause and they should not be used to treat these conditions.
2. Treatment of vulval and vaginal atrophy.
3. Treatment of hypoestrogenism due to hypogonadism, castration, or primary ovarian failure.

CONTRAINDICATIONS

Patients with known hypersensitivity to any of the components of the therapeutic system should not use Vivelle. Estrogens should not be used in individuals with any of the following conditions:

1. Known or suspected pregnancy (see Boxed Warning). Estrogen may cause fetal harm when administered to a pregnant woman.
2. Undiagnosed abnormal genital bleeding.
3. Known or suspected cancer of the breast.
4. Known or suspected estrogen-dependent neoplasia.
5. Active thrombophlebitis or thromboembolic disorders, or a documented history of these conditions.

WARNINGS

1. Induction of Malignant Neoplasms. Some studies have suggested a possible increased incidence of breast cancer in those women taking estrogen therapy at higher doses or for prolonged periods of time. The majority of studies, however, have not shown an association with the usual doses used for estrogen replacement therapy. Women on this therapy should have regular breast examinations and should be instructed in breast self-examination. The reported endometrial cancer risk among unopposed estrogen users is about 2- to 12-fold greater than in nonusers and appears dependent on duration of treatment and on estrogen dose. Most studies show no significant increased risk associated with the use of estrogens for less than 1 year. The greatest risk appears associated with prolonged use with increased risks of 15- to 24-fold for 5 to 10 years or more. In three studies, persistence of risk was demonstrated for 8 to over 15 years after cessation of estrogen treatment. In one study, a significant decrease in the incidence of endometrial cancer occurred 6 months after estrogen withdrawal. Concurrent progestin therapy may offset this risk, but the overall health impact in postmenopausal women is not known (see PRECAUTIONS).

Estrogen therapy during pregnancy is associated with an increased risk of fetal congenital reproductive tract disorders. In female offspring, there is an increased risk of vaginal adenosis, squamous cell dysplasia of the cervix, and clear cell vaginal cancer later in life; in males, urogenital and possibly testicular abnormalities. Although some of these changes are benign, it is not known whether they are precursors of malignancy.

2. Gallbladder Disease. Two studies have reported a 2- to 4-fold increase in the risk of surgically confirmed gallbladder disease in postmenopausal women receiving oral estrogen replacement therapy, similar to the 2-fold increase previously noted in users of oral contraceptives.

3. Cardiovascular Disease. Large doses of estrogen (5 mg conjugated estrogens per day), comparable to those used to treat cancer of the prostate and breast, have been shown in a large prospective clinical trial in men to increase the risks of nonfatal myocardial infarction, pulmonary embolism, and thrombophlebitis. These risks cannot necessarily be extrapolated from men to women. However, to avoid the theoretical cardiovascular risk to women caused by high estrogen doses, the dose for estrogen replacement therapy should not exceed the lowest effective dose.

4. Elevated Blood Pressure. Occasional blood pressure increases during estrogen replacement therapy have been attributed to idiosyncratic reactions to estrogens. More often, blood pressure has remained the same or has dropped. Postmenopausal estrogen use does not increase the risk of stroke. Nonetheless, blood pressure should be monitored at regular intervals with estrogen use, especially if high doses are used. Ethinyl estradiol and conjugated estrogens have been shown to increase renin substrate. In contrast to these oral estrogens, transdermally administered estradiol does not affect renin substrate.

5. Hypercalcemia. Administration of estrogen may lead to severe hypercalcemia in patients with breast cancer and bone metastases. If this occurs, the drug should be stopped and appropriate measures taken to reduce the serum calcium level.

PRECAUTIONS

General

1. Addition of a Progestin. Studies of the addition of a progestin for 10 or more days of a cycle of estrogen administration have reported a lower incidence of endometrial hyperplasia than would be induced by estrogen treatment alone. Morphological and biochemical studies of endometria suggest that 10 to 14 days of progestin are needed to provide maximal maturation of the endometrium and to reduce the likelihood of hyperplastic changes.

There are, however, possible risks that may be associated with the use of progestins in estrogen replacement regimens. These include

(1) adverse effects on lipoprotein metabolism (lowering HDL and raising LDL), which could diminish the purported cardioprotective effect of estrogen therapy (see PRECAUTIONS, below);

(2) impairment of glucose tolerance; and

(3) possible enhancement of mitotic activity in breast epithelial tissue, although few epidemiologic data are available to address this point (see PRECAUTIONS, below).

The choice of progestin, its dose, and its regimen may be important in minimizing these adverse effects, but these issues will require further study before they are clarified.

2. Cardiovascular Risk. A causal relationship between estrogen replacement therapy and reduction of cardiovascular disease in postmenopausal women has not been proven. Furthermore, the effect of added progestins on this putative benefit is not yet known.

In recent years, many published studies have suggested that there may be a cause-effect relationship between postmenopausal oral estrogen replacement therapy *without added progestins* and a decrease in cardiovascular disease in women. Although most of the observational studies which assessed this statistical association have reported a 20% to 50% reduction in coronary heart disease risk and associated mortality in estrogen takers, the following should be considered when interpreting these reports:

(1) Because only one of these studies was randomized and it was too small to yield statistically significant results, all relevant studies were subject to selection bias. Thus, the apparently reduced risk of coronary artery disease cannot be attributed with certainty to estrogen replacement therapy. It may instead have been caused by life-style and medical characteristics of the women studied with the result that healthier women were selected for estrogen therapy. In general, treated women were of higher socioeconomic and educational status, more slender, more physically active, more likely to have undergone surgical menopause, and less likely to have diabetes than the untreated women. Although some studies attempted to control for these selection factors, it is common for properly designed randomized trials to fail to confirm benefits suggested by less rigorous study designs. Thus, ongoing and future large-scale randomized trials may fail to confirm this apparent benefit.

(2) Current medical practice often includes the use of concomitant progestin therapy in women with intact uteri (see PRECAUTIONS and WARNINGS). While the effects of added progestins on the risk of ischemic heart disease are not known, all available progestins reverse at least some of the favorable effects of estrogens on HDL and LDL levels.

(3) While the effects of added progestins on the risk of breast cancer are also unknown, available epidemiologic evidence suggests that progestins do not reduce, and may enhance, the moderately increased breast cancer incidence that has been reported with prolonged estrogen replacement therapy (see WARNINGS, above).

Because relatively long-term use of estrogens by a woman with a uterus has been shown to induce endometrial cancer, physicians often recommend that women who are deemed candidates for hormone replacement should take progestins as well as estrogens. When considering prescribing concomitant estrogens and progestins for hormone replacement therapy, physicians and patients are advised to carefully weigh the potential benefits and risks of the added progestin. Large-scale randomized, placebo-controlled, prospective clinical trials are required to clarify these issues.

3. Physical Examination. A complete medical and family history should be taken prior to the initiation of any estrogen therapy. The pretreatment and periodic physical examinations should include special reference to blood pressure, breasts, abdomen, and pelvic organs and should include a Papanicolaou smear. As a general rule, estrogen should not be prescribed for longer than 1 year without reexamining the patient.

4. Hypercoagulability. Some studies have shown that women taking estrogen replacement therapy have hypercoagulability, primarily related to decreased antithrombin activity. This effect appears dose- and duration-dependent and is less pronounced than that associated with oral contraceptive use. Also, postmenopausal women tend to have increased coagulation parameters at baseline compared to premenopausal women. Epidemiological studies, which employed primarily orally administered estrogen products, have suggested that hormone replacement therapy (HRT) may be associated with an increased relative risk of developing venous thromboembolism (VTE), i.e., deep venous thrombosis or pulmonary embolism. Risk/benefit should therefore be carefully weighed in consultation with the patient when prescribing either oral or transdermal HRT to women with a risk factor for VTE.

5. Familial Hyperlipoproteinemia. Estrogen therapy may be associated with massive elevations of plasma triglycerides leading to pancreatitis and other complications in patients with familial defects of lipoprotein metabolism.

6. Fluid Retention. Because estrogens may cause some degree of fluid retention, conditions that might be exacerbated by this factor, such as asthma, epilepsy, migraine, and cardiac or renal dysfunction, require careful observation.

7. Uterine Bleeding and Mastodynia. Certain patients may develop undesirable manifestations of estrogenic stimulation, such as abnormal uterine bleeding and mastodynia.

8. Impaired Liver Function. Estrogens may be poorly metabolized in patients with impaired liver function and should be administered with caution.

Information for the Patient

See text of Patient Package Insert, which appears after the HOW SUPPLIED section.

Laboratory Tests

Estrogen administration should generally be guided by clinical response at the smallest dose, rather than laboratory monitoring, for relief of symptoms for those indications in which symptoms are observable.

Drug/Laboratory Test Interactions

Some of these drug/laboratory test interactions have been observed only with estrogen-progestin combinations (oral contraceptives):

1. Accelerated prothrombin time, partial thromboplastin time, and platelet aggregation time; increased platelet count; increased factors II, VII antigen, VIII antigen, VIII coagulant activity, IX, X, XII, VII-X complex, II-VII-X complex; and beta-thromboglobulin; decreased levels of antifactor Xa and antithrombin III; decreased antithrombin III activity; increased levels of fibrinogen and fibrinogen activity; increased plasminogen antigen and activity.

2. Increased thyroid-binding globulin (TBG) leading to increased circulating total thyroid hormone, as measured by protein-bound iodine (PBI), T_4 levels (by column or by radioimmunoassay) or T_3 levels by radioimmunoassay. T_3 resin uptake is decreased, reflecting the elevated TBG. Free T_4 and free T_3 concentrations are unaltered.

3. Other binding proteins may be elevated in serum, i.e., corticosteroid binding globulin (CBG), sex hormone-binding globulin (SHBG), leading to increased circulating cortico-

steroids and sex steroids, respectively. Free or biologically active hormone concentrations are unchanged. Other plasma proteins may be increased (angiotensinogen/renin substrate, alpha-1-antitrypsin, ceruloplasmin).

4. Increased plasma HDL and HDL_2 subfraction concentrations, reduced LDL cholesterol concentration, increased triglyceride levels.

5. Impaired glucose tolerance.

6. Reduced response to metyrapone test.

7. Reduced serum folate concentration.

Carcinogenesis, Mutagenesis, Impairment of Fertility
Long-term, continuous administration of natural and synthetic estrogens in certain animal species increases the frequency of carcinomas of the breast, cervix, vagina, testis, and liver (see CONTRAINDICATIONS and WARNINGS).

Pregnancy Category X
Estrogens should not be used during pregnancy (see CONTRAINDICATIONS and Boxed Warning).

Nursing Mothers
As a general principle, the administration of any drug to nursing mothers should be done only when clearly necessary since many drugs are excreted in human milk. In addition, estrogen administration to nursing mothers has been shown to decrease the quantity and quality of the milk.

Pediatric Use
The safety and effectiveness in pediatric patients have not been established.

ADVERSE REACTIONS

See WARNINGS and Boxed Warning regarding the potential adverse effects on the fetus, the induction of malignant neoplasms, gallbladder disease, cardiovascular disease, elevated blood pressure, and hypercalcemia.

The most commonly reported systemic adverse event to the Vivelle system in controlled clinical trials was headache. This occurred in approximately 36% of patients treated with active systems and in 30% of patients treated with placebo. The most common topical adverse events in these trials were erythema and pruritus at the application site. Most cases were considered mild. Fewer than 5% of patients on active drug at the final visit of the study had reactions of greater than mild intensity. Rash was reported rarely in these trials. Two patients out of 356 were discontinued from the trials due to skin irritation/erythema.

The following additional adverse reactions have been reported with estrogen therapy:

1. Genitourinary System. Changes in vaginal bleeding pattern and abnormal withdrawal bleeding or flow; breakthrough bleeding, spotting; increase in size of uterine leiomyomata; vaginal candidiasis; change in amount of cervical secretion.

2. Breasts. Tenderness, enlargement.

3. Gastrointestinal. Nausea, vomiting; abdominal cramps, bloating; cholestatic jaundice; gallbladder disease.

4. Skin. Chloasma or melasma that may persist when drug is discontinued; erythema multiforme; erythema nodosum; hemorrhagic eruption; loss of scalp hair; hirsutism.

5. Eyes. Steepening of corneal curvature; intolerance to contact lenses.

6. Central Nervous System. Headache, migraine, dizziness; mental depression; chorea.

7. Miscellaneous. Increase or decrease in weight; reduced carbohydrate tolerance; aggravation of porphyria; edema; changes in libido.

OVERDOSAGE

Serious ill effects have not been reported following acute ingestion of large doses of estrogen-containing oral contraceptives by young children. Overdosage of estrogen may cause nausea and vomiting, and withdrawal bleeding may occur in females.

DOSAGE AND ADMINISTRATION

The adhesive side of the Vivelle system should be placed on a clean, dry area of the skin on the trunk of the body (including the abdomen or buttocks). *Vivelle should not be applied to the breasts.* The Vivelle system should be replaced twice weekly. The sites of application must be rotated, with an interval of at least 1 week allowed between applications to a particular site. The area selected should not be oily, damaged, or irritated. The waistline should be avoided, since tight clothing may rub the system off. The system should be applied immediately after opening the pouch and removing the protective liner. The system should be pressed firmly in place with the palm of the hand for about 10 seconds, making sure there is good contact, especially around the edges. In the unlikely event that a system should fall off, the same system may be reapplied. If necessary, a new system may be applied. In either case, the original treatment schedule should be continued.

Initiation of Therapy
For treatment of moderate-to-severe vasomotor symptoms and vulval and vaginal atrophy associated with the menopause, start therapy with the Vivelle estradiol transdermal system 0.05 mg/day applied to the skin twice weekly. In order to use the lowest dosage necessary for the control of symptoms, decisions to increase dosage should not be made until after the first month of therapy. Some women taking the 0.0375 mg/day dosage may experience a delayed onset of efficacy. Attempts to discontinue or taper medication should be made at 3-month to 6-month intervals.

In women not currently taking oral estrogens or in women switching from another estradiol transdermal therapy, treatment with the Vivelle estradiol transdermal system may be initiated at once. In women who are currently taking oral estrogens, treatment with the Vivelle estradiol transdermal system should be initiated 1 week after withdrawal of oral hormone replacement therapy, or sooner if menopausal symptoms reappear in less than 1 week.

Therapeutic Regimen
Vivelle may be given continuously in patients who do not have an intact uterus. In those patients with an intact uterus, Vivelle may be given on a cyclic schedule (e.g., 3 weeks on drug followed by 1 week off drug).

HOW SUPPLIED

Vivelle estradiol transdermal system 0.0375 mg/day - each 11.0 cm² system contains 3.28 mg of estradiol USP for nominal* delivery of 0.0375 mg of estradiol per day.
Patient Calendar Pack of
8 systems .... NDC 0083-2325-08
Carton of 6 Patient Calendar Packs
of 8 systems .... NDC 0083-2325-62
Carton of 24 systems .... NDC 0083-2325-25
Vivelle estradiol transdermal system 0.05 mg/day - each 14.5 cm² system contains 4.33 mg of estradiol USP for nominal* delivery of 0.05 mg of estradiol per day.
Patient Calendar Pack of
8 systems .... NDC 0083-2326-08
Carton of 6 Patient Calendar Packs
of 8 systems .... NDC 0083-2326-62
Carton of 24 systems .... NDC 0083-2326-25
Vivelle estradiol transdermal system 0.075 mg/day - each 22.0 cm² system contains 6.57 mg of estradiol USP for nominal* delivery of 0.075 mg of estradiol per day.
Patient Calendar Pack of
8 systems .... NDC 0083-2327-08
Carton of 6 Patient Calendar Packs
of 8 systems .... NDC 0083-2327-62
Carton of 24 systems .... NDC 0083-2327-25
Vivelle estradiol transdermal system 0.1 mg/day - each 29.0 cm² system contains 8.66 mg of estradiol USP for nominal* delivery of 0.1 mg of estradiol per day.
Patient Calendar Pack of
8 systems .... NDC 0083-2328-08
Carton of 6 Patient Calendar Packs
of 8 systems .... NDC 0083-2328-62
Carton of 24 systems .... NDC 0083-2328-25

*See DESCRIPTION.

Do not store above 86°F (30°C). Do not store unpouched. Apply immediately upon removal from the protective pouch.
C98-6 (Rev. 5/98)

Information for the Patient

VIVELLE®
estradiol transdermal system
Rx only

1. ESTROGENS INCREASE THE RISK OF CANCER OF THE UTERUS IN WOMEN WHO HAVE HAD THEIR MENOPAUSE ("CHANGE OF LIFE").
If you use any estrogen-containing drug, it is important to visit your doctor regularly and report any unusual vaginal bleeding right away. Vaginal bleeding after menopause may be a warning sign of uterine cancer. Your doctor should evaluate any unusual vaginal bleeding to find out the cause.
2. ESTROGENS SHOULD NOT BE USED DURING PREGNANCY.
Estrogens do not prevent miscarriage (spontaneous abortion) and are not needed in the days following childbirth. If you take estrogens during pregnancy, your unborn child has a greater than usual chance of having birth defects. The risk of developing these defects is small, but clearly larger than the risk in children whose mothers did not take estrogens during pregnancy. These birth defects may affect the baby's urinary system and sex organs. Daughters born to mothers who took DES (an estrogen drug) have a higher than usual chance of developing cancer of the vagina or cervix when they become teenagers or young adults. Sons may have a higher than usual chance of developing cancer of the testicles when they become teenagers or young adults.

INTRODUCTION

Your doctor has prescribed the Vivelle system for the treatment of your menopausal symptoms. During menopause, production of estrogen hormones by your body decreases well below the amounts normally produced during your fertile years. In many women, this decrease in estrogen production causes uncomfortable symptoms, most noticeably hot flushes and sleep disturbance. Estrogens can be given to reduce or eliminate these symptoms.

The Vivelle system that your doctor has prescribed for you releases small amounts of estradiol through the skin in a continuous way. Estradiol is the same hormone that your ovaries produce abundantly before menopause. The dose of estradiol you require will depend upon your individual response. The dose is adjusted by the size of the Vivelle system used; the systems are available in four sizes.

INFORMATION ABOUT VIVELLE

How Vivelle Works
Vivelle contains estradiol. When applied to the skin as directed below, the Vivelle system releases estradiol, which flows through the skin into the bloodstream.

How and Where to Apply Vivelle
Each system is individually sealed in a protective pouch. Tear open this pouch at the indentation (do not use scissors) and remove the system.

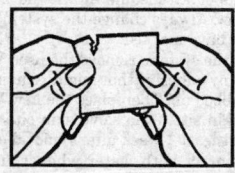

A stiff protective liner covers the adhesive side of the system—the side that will be placed against your skin. This liner must be removed before applying the system. Hold the unit with the protective liner facing you.

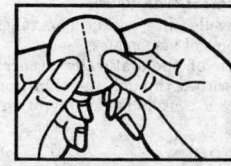

Peel off one side of the protective liner and discard it. Try to avoid touching the sticky side of the system with your fingers.

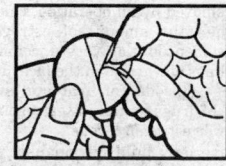

Using the other half of the liner as a handle, apply the sticky side of the system to a dry area of the skin on the trunk of the body (including the abdomen or buttocks). Press the sticky side on the skin and smooth down.

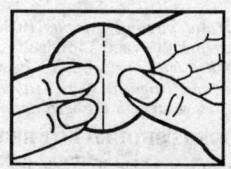

Fold back the remaining side of the system. Grasp the straight edge of the protective liner and pull it off the system.

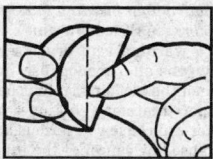

Press the system firmly in place.

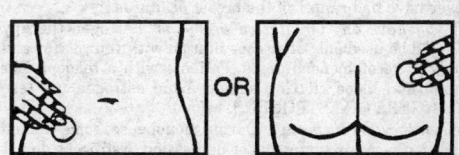

Some women may find that it is more comfortable to wear Vivelle on the buttocks. *Do not apply Vivelle to your breasts.*

Continued on next page

Vivelle—Cont.

The sites of application must be rotated, with an interval of at least 1 week allowed between applications to a particular site. The area selected should not be oily, damaged, or irritated. Avoid the waistline, since tight clothing may rub the system off. Apply the system immediately after opening the pouch and removing the protective liner. Press the system firmly in place with the palm of your hand for about 10 seconds, making sure there is good contact, especially around the edges.

The Vivelle system should be worn continuously until it is time to replace it with a new system. You may wish to experiment with different locations when applying a new system, to find ones that are most comfortable for you and where clothing will not rub on the system.

When to Apply Vivelle

The Vivelle system should be replaced twice weekly. Your Vivelle package contains a calendar checklist on the back to help you remember a schedule. Mark the 2-day schedule you plan to follow. Always change the system on the 2 days of the week you have marked.

When changing the system, remove the used Vivelle system and discard it. Any adhesive that might remain on your skin can be easily rubbed off. Then place the new Vivelle system on a different skin site. (The same skin site should not be used again for at least 1 week after removal of the system.) Please note: Contact with water when you are bathing, swimming, or showering will not affect the system. In the unlikely event that a system should fall off, put this same system back on and continue to follow your original treatment schedule. If necessary, you may apply a new system but continue to follow your original schedule.

Benefits of Treatment With Vivelle

Regular use of Vivelle twice weekly offers relief of moderate-to-severe symptoms of menopause.

Small quantities of the naturally occurring hormone estradiol are absorbed through the skin from the Vivelle system, ensuring a continuous supply of circulating hormone in the body.

USES OF ESTROGEN

To reduce moderate-to-severe menopausal symptoms. Estrogens are hormones produced by the ovaries. The decrease in the amount of estrogen that occurs in all women, usually between ages 45 and 55, causes the menopause. Sometimes the ovaries are removed by an operation, causing "surgical menopause." When the amount of estrogen begins to decrease, some women develop very uncomfortable symptoms, such as feelings of warmth in the face, neck, and chest or sudden intense episodes of heat and sweating ("hot flashes"). The use of drugs containing estrogens can help the body adjust to lower estrogen levels.

Some women have only mild menopausal symptoms, or none at all, and do not need estrogen therapy for these particular symptoms. Other women may need estrogens for a few months while their bodies adjust to lower estrogen levels. For the treatment of menopausal symptoms only, most women need estrogen replacement therapy for no longer than 6 months.

To treat vulval and vaginal atrophy (itching, burning, dryness in or around the vagina, difficulty or burning on urination) *associated with menopause.*

To treat certain conditions in which a young woman's ovaries do not produce enough estrogen naturally.

WHEN ESTROGENS SHOULD NOT BE USED

During pregnancy (see Boxed Warning). If you think you may be pregnant, do not use any form of estrogen-containing drug. Using estrogens while you are pregnant may cause your unborn child to have birth defects. Estrogens do not prevent miscarriage.

If you have unusual vaginal bleeding that has not been evaluated by your doctor (see Boxed Warning). Unusual vaginal bleeding can be a warning sign of cancer of the uterus, especially if it happens after menopause. Your doctor must find out the cause of the bleeding so that he or she can recommend the proper treatment. Taking estrogens without visiting your doctor can cause you serious harm if your vaginal bleeding is caused by cancer of the uterus.

If you have had cancer. Since estrogens increase the risk of certain types of cancer, you should not use estrogens if you ever have had cancer of the breast or uterus.

If you have any circulation problems. Estrogen therapy should be used only after consultation with your doctor and only in recommended doses. Patients with a tendency for abnormal blood clotting should avoid estrogen use (see DANGERS OF ESTROGENS, below).

When they are ineffective. During menopause, some women develop nervous symptoms or depression. Estrogens do not relieve these symptoms. You may have heard that taking estrogens for years after menopause will keep your skin soft and supple and keep you feeling young. There is no evidence for these claims and such long-term estrogen use may have serious risks.

After childbirth or when breastfeeding a baby. Estrogens should not be used to try to stop the breasts from filling with milk after a baby is born. Such treatment may increase the risk of developing blood clots (see DANGERS OF ESTROGENS, below).

If you are breastfeeding, you should avoid using any drugs because many drugs pass through to the baby in the milk. While nursing a baby, you should take drugs only on the advice of your healthcare provider.

DANGERS OF ESTROGENS

Cancer of the uterus. The risk of developing cancer of the uterus gets higher the longer estrogens are used and when larger doses are taken. One study showed that when estrogens are discontinued, this increased risk of cancer seems to fall off quickly. Three other studies showed that the risk for uterine cancer stayed high for 8 to more than 15 years after stopping estrogen treatment. Because of this risk, *it is important to take the lowest dose that works and to take it only as long as you need it.* Using progestin therapy together with estrogen therapy may reduce the higher risk of uterine cancer related to estrogen use (but see OTHER INFORMATION, below).

If you have had your uterus removed (total hysterectomy), there is no danger of developing cancer of the uterus.

Cancer of the breast. The majority of studies have shown no association between the usual doses used for estrogen replacement therapy and breast cancer. Some studies have suggested a possible increased incidence of breast cancer in those women taking estrogens for prolonged periods of time and especially if higher doses are used.

Regular breast examinations by a health professional and monthly self-examination are recommended for women receiving estrogen therapy, as they are for all women.

Gallbladder disease. Women who use estrogens after menopause are more likely to develop gallbladder disease needing surgery than women who do not use estrogens.

Abnormal blood clotting. Taking estrogens may increase the risk of blood clots. These clots can cause a stroke, heart attack, or pulmonary embolus, any of which may be fatal. However, most studies of low-dose estrogen usage by women do not show an increased risk of these complications.

SIDE EFFECTS

In addition to the risks listed above, the following side effects have been reported with estrogen use:

- Headache.
- Nausea and vomiting.
- Breast tenderness or enlargement.
- Enlargement of benign tumors ("fibroids") of the uterus.
- Retention of excess fluid. This may make some conditions worsen, such as asthma, epilepsy, migraine, heart disease, or kidney disease.
- A spotty darkening of the skin, particularly on the face. Skin irritation, redness, or rash may occur at the site of application.

REDUCING RISK OF ESTROGEN USE

If you use estrogens, you can reduce your risks by doing these things:

See your doctor regularly. While you are using estrogens, it is important to visit your doctor at least once a year for a check-up. If you develop vaginal bleeding while taking estrogens, you may need further evaluation. If members of your family have had breast cancer or if you have ever had breast lumps or an abnormal mammogram (breast x-ray), you may need to have more frequent breast examinations.

Reassess your need for estrogens. You and your doctor should reevaluate whether or not you still need estrogens at least every 6 months.

Be alert for signs of trouble. Report these or any other unusual side effects to your doctor immediately:

- Abnormal bleeding from the vagina.
- Pains in the calves or chest, sudden shortness of breath, or coughing blood (indicating possible clots in the legs, heart, or lungs).
- Severe headache, dizziness, faintness, or changes in vision (indicating possible clots in the brain or eye).
- Breast lumps.
- Yellowing of the skin or eyes.
- Pain, swelling, or tenderness in the abdomen.
- Skin irritation, redness, or rash.

OTHER INFORMATION

If your uterus has not been removed, your doctor may choose to prescribe a progestin, a different hormonal drug to be used in association with estrogen treatment. Progestins lower the risk of developing endometrial hyperplasia, a possible precancerous condition of the uterine lining, which may occur while using estrogen. There are possible additional risks that may be associated with the inclusion of a progestin in estrogen treatment. The possible risks include unfavorable effects on blood fats and sugars, as well as a possible further increase in breast cancer risk that may be associated with long-term estrogen use.

Some research has suggested that estrogen taken *without progestins* may protect women against developing heart disease. However, this effect of estrogen is not certain.

You are cautioned to discuss very carefully with your doctor or healthcare provider all the possible risks and benefits of long-term estrogen and progestin treatment, as they affect you personally.

Your doctor has prescribed this drug for you and you alone. Do not give the drug to anyone else.

Keep this and all drugs out of the reach of children. In case of overdose, remove the system and call your doctor, hospital, or poison control center immediately.

This leaflet provides a summary of the most important information about estrogens. If you want more information, ask your doctor or pharmacist to show you the professional labeling.

C98-7 (Rev. 5/98)
C98-6/C98-7 (Rev. 5/98)

Distributed by
Novartis Pharmaceuticals Corporation
East Hanover, New Jersey 07936
Shown in Product Identification Guide, page 326

Novo Nordisk Pharmaceuticals, Inc.

SUITE 200
100 OVERLOOK CENTER
PRINCETON, NJ 08540

Direct Inquiries to:
Novo Nordisk Pharmaceuticals, Inc.
(800) 727-6500
In Emergencies after hours and weekends:
609-987-5800

HUMAN INSULIN   OTC
NOVOLIN® 70/30
70% NPH, Human Insulin Isophane Suspension and
30% Regular, Human Insulin Injection
(recombinant DNA origin)
100 units/ml

WARNING

ANY CHANGE OF INSULIN SHOULD BE MADE CAUTIOUSLY AND ONLY UNDER MEDICAL SUPERVISION. CHANGES IN PURITY, STRENGTH, BRAND (MANUFACTURER), TYPE (REGULAR, NPH, LENTE®, ETC.), SPECIES (BEEF, PORK, BEEF-PORK, HUMAN) AND/OR METHOD OF MANUFACTURE (RECOMBINANT DNA VERSUS ANIMAL-SOURCE INSULIN) MAY RESULT IN THE NEED FOR A CHANGE IN DOSAGE.

SPECIAL CARE SHOULD BE TAKEN WHEN THE TRANSFER IS FROM A STANDARD BEEF OR MIXED SPECIES INSULIN TO A PURIFIED PORK OR HUMAN INSULIN. IF A DOSAGE ADJUSTMENT IS NEEDED, IT WILL USUALLY BECOME APPARENT EITHER IN THE FIRST FEW DAYS OR OVER A PERIOD OF SEVERAL WEEKS. ANY CHANGE IN TREATMENT SHOULD BE CAREFULLY MONITORED.

PLEASE READ THE SECTIONS "INSULIN REACTION AND SHOCK" AND "DIABETIC KETOACIDOSIS AND COMA" FOR SYMPTOMS OF HYPOGLYCEMIA (LOW BLOOD GLUCOSE) AND HYPERGLYCEMIA (HIGH BLOOD GLUCOSE).

INSULIN USE IN DIABETES

Your physician has explained that you have diabetes and that your treatment involves injections of insulin or insulin therapy combined with an oral antidiabetic medicine. Insulin is normally produced by the pancreas, a gland that lies behind the stomach. Without insulin, glucose (a simple sugar made from digested food) is trapped in the bloodstream and cannot enter the cells of the body. Some patients who don't make enough of their own insulin, or who cannot use the insulin they do make properly, must take insulin by injection in order to control their blood glucose levels.

Each case of diabetes is different and requires direct and continued medical supervision. Your physician has told you the type, strength and amount of insulin you should use and the time(s) at which you should inject it, and has also discussed with you a diet and exercise schedule. You should contact your physician if you experience any difficulties or if you have questions.

TYPES OF INSULINS

Standard and purified animal insulins as well as human insulins are available. Standard and purified insulins differ in their degree of purification and content of noninsulin material. Standard and purified insulins also vary in species source: they may be of beef, pork, or mixed beef and pork origin. Human insulin is identical in structure to the insulin produced by the human pancreas, and thus differs from an-

imal insulins. Insulins vary in time of action and in strength; see PRODUCT DESCRIPTION and SYRINGES for additional information.
Your physician has prescribed the insulin that is right for you; be sure you have purchased the correct insulin and check it carefully before you use it.

PRODUCT DESCRIPTION

This vial contains **Novolin® 70/30** which is a mixture of 70% NPH, Human Insulin Isophane Suspension (recombinant DNA origin) and 30% Regular, Human Insulin Injection (recombinant DNA origin). The concentration of this product is 100 units of insulin per milliliter. It is a cloudy or milky suspension of human insulin with protamine and zinc. The insulin substance (the cloudy material) settles at the bottom of the vial, therefore, the vial must be gently agitated or rotated so that the contents are uniformly mixed before a dose is withdrawn. **Novolin® 70/30** has an intermediate duration of action. The effect of **Novolin® 70/30** begins approximately $^1/_2$ hour after injection. The effect is maximal between 2 and approximately 12 hours. The full duration of action may last up to 24 hours after injection.
The time course of action of any insulin may vary considerably in different individuals, or at different times in the same individual. Because of this variation, the time periods listed here should be considered as general guidelines only.
This human insulin (recombinant DNA origin) is structurally identical to the insulin produced by the human pancreas. This human insulin is produced by recombinant DNA technology utilziing Saccharomyces cerevisiae (bakers' yeast) as the production organism.

STORAGE

Insulin should be stored in a cold place, preferably in a refrigerator, but not in the freezing compartment. **Do not let it freeze.** Keep the insulin vial in its carton so that it will stay clean and protected from light. If refrigeration is not possible, the bottle of insulin which you are currently using can be kept unrefrigerated as long as it is kept as cool as possible and away from heat and sunlight.
Never use **Novolin® 70/30** if the precipitate (the white deposit at the bottom of the vial) has become lumpy or granular in appearance or has formed a deposit of solid particles on the wall of the vial. This insulin should not be used if the liquid in the vial remains clear after the vial has been gently agitated.
Never use insulin after the expiration date which is printed on the vial label and carton.

SYRINGES

Use the Correct Syringe

Doses of insulin are measured in units. Some insulins are available in two strengths: U-100 and U-40. One milliliter (ml) of U-100 contains 100 units of insulin. One milliliter (ml) of U-40 contains 40 units of insulin. Be sure to use the proper syringe for the strength of the insulin prescribed for you. Syringes are clearly marked **"For use with U-100 insulin"** or **"For use with U-40 insulin"**. Low dose U-100 syringes are also available. Failure to use the proper syringe can lead to mistakes in dosage.

Disposable Syringes

Disposable syringes and needles require no sterilization provided the package is intact. They should be used only once and discarded.

Reusable Syringes

Reusable syringes and needles must be sterilized before each use.

1. Boil the syringe parts and needles in a pan of water for at least five minutes. Keep a special pan for this purpose. Heavily chlorinated water should not be used; distilled water is preferable.
   If boiling is not possible, the syringe parts and needles may be sterilized by immersion in 70% ethyl alcohol or 91% isopropyl alcohol for at least five minutes. **Do not use bathing, rubbing or medicated alcohol for sterilization.**
2. Assemble the syringe and fit the needle on the tip of the syringe being careful not to touch the surface of the plunger or needle.
3. Push the plunger in and out several times until the water (or alcohol) has been completely expelled. (The syringe should be thoroughly dried before its use.)

NEEDLE-FREE INJECTORS

This product may not be suitable for use with all needle-free injectors. You should consult the needle-free injector device manufacturer before using the device with this product.

IMPORTANT

Failure to comply with the above and the following antiseptic measures may lead to infections at the injection site.

PREPARING THE INJECTION

1. Clean your hands and the injection site with soap and water or with alcohol. Wipe the rubber stopper with an alcohol swab. (Note: remove the tamper-resistant cap at first use. If the cap has already been removed, do not use this product, return it to your pharmacy.)
2. For insulin suspensions, roll the vial of insulin gently in your hands to mix it. Vigorous shaking immediately before the dose is drawn into the syringe may result in the formation of bubbles or froth which could cause dosage errors.
3. Pull back the plunger until the black tip reaches the marking for the number of units you will inject.
4. Push the needle through the rubber stopper into the vial.
5. Push the plunger all the way in. This inserts air into the bottle.
6. Turn the vial and syringe upside down and slowly pull the plunger back to a few units beyond the correct dose.
7. If there are air bubbles, flick the syringe firmly with your finger to raise the air bubbles to the needle, then slowly push the plunger to the correct unit marking.
8. Lift the vial off the syringe.

GIVING THE INJECTION

1. The following areas are suitable for subcutaneous insulin injection: thighs, upper arms, buttocks, abdomen. Do not change areas without consulting your physician. The actual point of injection should be changed each time; injection sites should be about an inch apart.
2. The injection site should be clean and dry. Pinch up skin area to be injected and hold it firmly.
3. Hold the syringe like a pencil and push the needle quickly and firmly into the pinched-up area.
4. Release the skin and push the push-button all the way in to inject insulin beneath the skin. To ensure that all the insulin is injected keep the needle in the skin for several seconds after injection with your finger on the plunger. Do not inject into a muscle unless your physician has advised it. You should never inject insulin into a vein.
5. Remove needle. If slight bleeding occurs, press lightly with a dry cotton swab for a few seconds—**do not rub.**

Note:
The dose should be injected over 2–4 seconds. Preparations of insulin suspensions which are injected slowly may clog the tip of the needle, resulting in an inability to complete the injection. Syringe plugging does not occur when the drug is injected more rapidly. Use the injection technique recommended by your physician.

MIXING INSULIN

Novolin® 70/30 is a premixed insulin containing 70% NPH, Human Insulin Isophane Suspension, recombinant DNA origin (**Novolin® N**) and 30% Regular, Human Insulin Injection, recombinant DNA origin (**Novolin® R**). You should not attempt to change the ratio of this product by adding additional NPH or Regular insulin to this vial. If your physician has prescribed insulin mixed in a proportion other than 70% NPH and 30% Regular, you should use the separate insulin formulations (**Novolin® N** and **Novolin® R**) in the amounts recommended by your physician.

USAGE IN PREGNANCY

It is particularly important to maintain good control of your diabetes during pregnancy and special attention must be paid to your diet, exercise and insulin regimens. If you are pregnant or nursing a baby, consult your physician or nurse educator.

INSULIN REACTION AND SHOCK

Insulin reaction ("hypoglycemia") occurs when the blood glucose falls very low. This can happen if you take too much insulin, miss or delay a meal, exercise more than usual or work too hard without eating, or become ill (especially with vomiting or fever). Hypoglycemia can also happen if you combine insulin therapy and other medications that lower blood glucose, such as an oral antidiabetic agents or other prescription and over-the-counter drugs. The first symptoms of an insulin reaction usually come on suddenly. They may include a cold sweat, fatigue, nervousness or shakiness, rapid heartbeat, or nausea. Personality change or confusion may also occur. If you drink or eat something right away (a glass of milk or orange juice, or several sugar candies), you can often stop the progression of symptoms. If symptoms persist, call your physician — an insulin reaction can lead to unconsciousness. If a reaction results in loss of consciousness, emergency medical care should be obtained immediately. If you have had repeated reactions or if an insulin reaction has led to a loss of consciousness, contact your physician. Severe hypoglycemia can result in temporary or permanent impairment of brain function and death. **In certain cases, the nature and intensity of the warning symptoms of hypoglycemia may change. A few patients have reported that after being transferred to human insulin, the early warning symptoms of hypoglycemia were less pronounced than they had been with animal-source insulin.**

DIABETIC KETOACIDOSIS AND COMA

Diabetic ketoacidosis may develop if your body has too little insulin. The most common causes are acute illness or infection or failure to take enough insulin by injection. If you are ill you should check your urine for ketones. The symptoms of diabetic ketoacidosis usually come on gradually, over a period of hours or days, and include a drowsy feeling, flushed face, thirst and loss of appetite. Notify your physician right away if the urine test is positive for ketones (acetone) or if you have any of these symptoms. Fast, heavy breathing and rapid pulse are more severe symptoms and you should have medical attention right away. Severe, sustained hyperglycemia may result in diabetic coma and death.

ADVERSE REACTIONS

A few people with diabetes develop red, swollen and itchy skin where the insulin has been injected. This is called a "local reaction" and it may occur if the injection is not properly made, if the skin is sensitive to the cleansing solution, or if you are allergic to the insulin being used. If you have a local reaction, tell your physician.
Generalized insulin allergy occurs rarely, but when it does it may cause a serious reaction, including skin rash over the body, shortness of breath, fast pulse, sweating, and a drop in blood pressure. If any of these symptoms develop, you should seek emergency medical care.
If severe allergic reactions to insulin have occurred (i.e., generalized rash, swelling or breathing difficulties) you should be skin-tested with **each** new insulin preparation before it is used.

IMPORTANT NOTES

1. A change in the type, strength, species or purity of insulin could require a dosage adjustment. Any change in insulin should be made under medical supervision.
2. You may have learned how to test your urine or your blood for glucose. It is important to do these tests regularly and to record the results for review with your physician or nurse educator.
3. If you have an acute illness, especially with vomiting or fever, continue taking your insulin. If possible, stay on your regular diet. If you have trouble eating, drink fruit juices, regular soft drinks, or clear soups; if you can, eat small amounts of bland foods. Test your urine for glucose and ketones and, if possible, test your blood glucose. Note the results and contact your physician for possible insulin dose adjustment. If you have severe and prolonged vomiting, seek emergency medical care.
4. You should always carry identification which states that you have diabetes.
5. Always ask your physician or pharmacist before taking any drug.

Always consult your physician if you have any questions about your condition or the use of insulin.

Helpful information for people with diabetes is published by American Diabetes Association, 1660 Duke Street, Alexandria, VA 22314.

For information contact: Novo Nordisk Pharmaceuticals, Inc., Princeton, NJ 08540

Manufactured by Novo Nordisk A/S, DK-2880 Bagsvaerd, Denmark and by Novo Nordisk Pharmaceutical Industries, Inc., 3612 Powhatan Road, Clayton, NC. 27520
Date of issue: December 1995

HOW SUPPLIED

Vials, U-100, 100 units/mL, 10 mL, (List No. 183711) (1's)
Novolin 70/30 Prefilled® Syringe, U-100, 100 units/mL, 1.5 mL, (List No. 001771) (5's)
Novolin® 70/30 PenFill®, U-100, 100 units/mL, 1.5 mL, (List No. 183717) (5's)

NORDITROPIN® ℞

4 mg or 8 mg (approximately 12 or 24 IU) vials
Somatropin (rDNA origin) for injection
PRODUCT INFORMATION

DESCRIPTION

Norditropin® is the Novo Nordisk Pharmaceuticals, Inc. registered trademark for somatropin, a polypeptide hormone of recombinant DNA origin. The hormone is synthesized by a special strain of *E.coli* bacteria that has been modified by the addition of a plasmid which carries the gene for human growth hormone. Norditropin® contains the identical sequence of 191 amino acids constituting the naturally occurring pituitary human growth hormone with a molecular weight of about 22,000 Daltons.
Norditropin® is a sterile, almost white, lyophilized powder. It is a highly purified preparation intended for subcutaneous injection in the thighs after reconstitution with 2 mL diluent.
Each vial of lyophilized drug contains the following:

4 mg (approximately 12 IU) Vial

Somatropin	4 mg
Glycine	8.8 mg
Disodium Phosphate Dihydrate (Na_2HPO_4,$2H_2O$)	1.3 mg
Sodium Dihydrogen Phosphate Dihydrate (NaH_2PO_4,$2H_2O$)	1.1 mg
Mannitol	44 mg

Continued on next page

Norditropin—Cont.

8 mg (approximately 24 IU) Vial

Somatropin	8 mg
Glycine	8.8 mg
Disodium Phosphate Dihydrate ($Na_2HPO_4,2H_2O$)	1.3 mg
Sodium Dihydrogen Phosphate Dihydrate ($NaH_2PO_4,2H_2O$)	1.1 mg
Mannitol	44 mg

Each vial of lyophilized drug is supplied in a combination package which also contains a vial of diluent. Each mL contains 1.5% benzyl alcohol as preservative.
The pH of the reconstituted solution is about 7.3.

CLINICAL PHARMACOLOGY

a. Tissue Growth

The primary and most intensively studied action of somatropin is the stimulation of linear growth. This effect is demonstrated in patients with somatropin deficiency.

1. Skeletal growth – the measurable increase in bone length after administration of somatropin results from its effect on the cartilaginous growth areas of long bones. Studies *in vitro* have shown that the incorporation of sulfate into proteoglycans is not due to a direct effect of somatropin, but rather is mediated by the somatomedins or insulin-like growth factors (IGF). The somatomedins, among them somatomedin C, are polypeptide hormones which are synthesized in the liver, kidney, and various other tissue. Somatomedin C is low in the serum of hypopituitary dwarfs and hypophysectomized humans or animals, but its presence can be demonstrated after treatment with somatropin.

2. Cell growth – it has been shown that the total number of skeletal muscle cells is markedly decreased in short stature children lacking endogenous somatropin compared with normal children, and that treatment with somatropin results in an increase in both the number and size of muscle cells.

3. Organ growth – somatropin influences the size of internal organs, and it also increases red cell mass.

b. Protein Metabolism

Linear growth is facilitated in part by increased cellular protein synthesis. This synthesis and growth are reflected by nitrogen retention which can be quantitated by observing the decline in urinary nitrogen excretion and blood urea nitrogen following the initiation of somatropin therapy.

c. Carbohydrate Metabolism

Hypopituitary children sometimes experience fasting hypoglycemia that may be improved by treatment with somatropin. In healthy subjects, large doses of somatropin may impair glucose tolerance. Although the precise mechanism of the diabetogenic effect of somatropin is not known, it is attributed to blocking the action of insulin rather than blocking insulin secretion. Insulin levels in serum actually increase as somatropin levels increase.

d. Fat Metabolism

Somatropin stimulates intracellular lipolysis, and administration of somatropin leads to an increase in plasma free fatty acids, cholesterol, and triglycerides. Untreated growth hormone deficiency is associated with increased body fat stores including increased subcutaneous adipose tissue. On somatropin replacement a general reduction of fat stores and of subcutaneous tissue in particular takes place.

e. Mineral Metabolism

Administration of somatropin results in the retention of total body potassium and phosphorus and to a lesser extent sodium. This retention is thought to be the result of cell growth. Serum levels of phosphate increase in patients with growth hormone deficiency after somatropin therapy due to metabolic activity associated with bone growth. Serum calcium levels are not altered. Although calcium excretion in the urine is increased, there is a simultaneous increase in calcium absorption from the intestine. Negative calcium balance, however, may occasionally occur during somatropin treatment.

f. Connective Tissue Metabolism

Somatropin stimulates the synthesis of chondroitin sulfate and collagen as well as the urinary excretion of hydroxyproline.

g. Pharmacokinetics

A 180-min IV infusion of Norditropin® (33 ng/kg/min) was given to 9 GHD patients. A mean ($\pm$ SD) hGH steady-state serum level of approximately 23.1 ($\pm$ 15.0) ng/mL was reached at 150 min and a mean clearance rate of approximately 2.3 ($\pm$ 1.8) mL/min/kg or 139 ($\pm$ 105) mL/min for hGH was obtained. Following infusion, serum hGH levels had a biexponential decay with a terminal elimination half-life ($T_{1/2}$) of approximately 21.1 ($\pm$ 5.1) min.
In a study conducted in 18 GHD adult patients, where a SC dose of 0.024 mg/kg or 3 IU/m^2 was given in the thigh, the mean ($\pm$ SD) C_{max} values of 13.8 ($\pm$ 5.8) and 17.1 ($\pm$ 10.0) ng/mL were obtained for the 4 and 8 mg Norditropin® vials, respectively, at approximately 4 to 5 hr. post dose. The mean apparent terminal $T_{1/2}$ values were estimated to be approx-

imately 7 to 10 hr. However, the absolute bioavailability for Norditropin® after the SC route of administration is currently not known.

INDICATIONS AND USAGE

Norditropin® is indicated for the long-term treatment of children who have growth failure due to inadequate secretion of endogenous growth hormone.

CONTRAINDICATIONS

Norditropin® should not be used in subjects with closed epiphyses.
Norditropin® should not be used in hypopituitary children who have evidence of actively growing intracranial tumors. Therapy with somatropin should be discontinued if there is evidence of recurrent tumor growth.
Norditropin® should not be used in any subjects with known hypersensitivity to any of the constituents of the preparation.

WARNING

Benzyl alcohol as a preservative has been associated with toxicity in newborns. Norditropin® may be reconstituted in sterile water for injection. If Norditropin® is reconstituted in this manner, use only one dose per vial and discard the unused portion.

PRECAUTIONS

Norditropin® should be used only by physicians with experience in the diagnosis and management of patients with growth hormone deficiency.
Patients with growth hormone deficiency secondary to an intracranial lesion should be examined frequently for progression or recurrence of the underlying disease process.
Because growth hormone may induce a state of insulin resistance, patients should be observed for evidence of glucose intolerance.
Concomitant glucocorticoid therapy may inhibit the growth promoting effect of Norditropin®. Patients with coexisting ACTH deficiency should have their glucocorticoid replacement dose carefully adjusted to avoid an inhibitory effect on growth.
A state of hypothyroidism may develop during Norditropin® treatment. Since untreated hypothyroidism may interfere with the response to Norditropin®, patients should have a periodic thyroid function test and should be treated with thyroid hormone when indicated.
Patients with endocrine disorders, including growth hormone deficiency, may develop slipped capital epiphyses more frequently. Any child with the onset of a limp or complaints of hip or knee pain during growth hormone therapy should be evaluated.
Intracranial hypertension (IH) with papilledema, visual changes, headache, nausea and/or vomiting has been reported in a small number of patients treated with growth hormone products. Symptoms usually occurred within the first eight (8) weeks of the initiation of growth hormone therapy. In all reported cases, IH-associated signs and symptoms resolved after termination of therapy or a reduction of the growth hormone dose. Funduscopic examination of patients is recommended at the initiation and periodically during the course of growth hormone therapy.
Carcinogenesis, Mutagenesis, Impairment of Fertility: Long-term animal studies for carcinogenicity and impairment of fertility with Norditropin® have not been performed. There has been no evidence to date of Norditropin-induced mutagenicity.
Pregnancy: Pregnancy Category C. Reproduction studies have been performed in rats at doses up to 7 mg/m^2 or about 7 times the maximum recommended human dose on a body surface area basis (mg/m^2) and have revealed no evidence of impaired fertility or harm to the fetus due to Norditropin®. There are, however, no adequate and well-controlled studies in pregnant women. Because animal reproduction studies are not always predictive of human response, this drug should be used during pregnancy only if clearly needed.
Nursing Mothers: There have been no studies conducted with Norditropin® in nursing mothers. It is not known whether this drug is excreted in human milk. Because many drugs are excreted in human milk, caution should be exercised when Norditropin® is administered to a nursing woman.

ADVERSE REACTIONS

As with all protein drugs, a small percentage of patients may develop antibodies to the protein. Growth hormone antibody with binding capacity lower than 2 mg/L has not been associated with growth attenuation. In some cases, when binding capacity is greater than 2 mg/L, interference with growth response has been observed.
In clinical trials, patients receiving Norditropin® for up to 12 months have been tested for induction of antibodies and 0/358 patients developed antibodies with binding capacities above 2 mg/L. Among these patients, 165 had previously been treated with other preparations of growth hormone and 193 were previously untreated naive patients.

Since antibodies to somatropin have the potential to inhibit further linear growth, only patients failing to respond to treatment should be tested for antibodies.
The following adverse events have been reported from clinical studies: headache, localized muscle pain, weakness, mild hyperglycemia and glucosuria.
Leukemia has been reported in a small number of children who have been treated with growth hormone, including growth hormone of pituitary origin and recombinant somatrem and somatropin. On the basis of current evidence, experts cannot conclude that growth hormone therapy is responsible for these occurrences. If there is any risk to an individual patient, it is minimal.

OVERDOSAGE

The maximum dose generally recommended should not be exceeded due to the potential risk of side effects.

DOSAGE AND ADMINISTRATION

The Norditropin® dosage and schedule for administration must be individualized for each patient. Generally, subcutaneous administration in the evening, 6–7 times a week, is recommended. It is furthermore recommended to give the injections in the thighs and to vary the injection site on the thigh on a rotating basis. Dosage can be calculated according to body weight.

Generally recommended dosage:

Subcutaneous injection:
0.024–0.034 mg/kg body weight, 6–7 times a week.

Dissolution Procedure:

The Norditropin® solution for subcutaneous injection is prepared by adding the 2 mL diluent to the drug powder in the vial

1. Use a syringe and needle for injection. Before injection the rubber closures should be wiped with an antiseptic solution to prevent contamination of the contents after repeated needle insertions. Push the needle through the rubber closure on the top of the vial with the diluent. Draw up the diluent. It is easier to draw up the diluent if you have first injected air into the vial.

2. Pull out the needle. Take the vial with dry powder, push the needle through the rubber closure and inject the diluent into the vial aiming the stream of liquid against the glass wall.

3. Dissolve the dry powder completely by gently turning the vial upside down several times. DO NOT SHAKE the vial. The contents MUST NOT BE INJECTED if the solution is cloudy or contains particulate matter.

Measuring the Prescribed Dose:

4 mg (approximately 12 IU) Vial

After the dry powder has been dissolved, the solution contains 2 mg Norditropin® per mL. If the prescribed dose is e.g. 1 mg Norditropin®, draw up 0.5 mL of the solution into a syringe suitable for small volumes.

8 mg (approximately 24 IU) Vial

After the dry powder has been dissolved, the solution contains 4 mg Norditropin® per mL. If the prescribed dose is e.g. 1 mg Norditropin®, draw up 0.25 mL of the solution into a syringe suitable for small volumes.

Storage:

Before and after reconstitution with diluent Norditropin® must be stored at 2–8°C/36–46°F (refrigerator). Do not freeze. Avoid direct light.
Norditropin® retains its biological potency until the date of expiry indicated on the label. Reconstituted vials should be used within 14 days after dissolution.

HOW SUPPLIED

Norditropin® is supplied as 4 mg or 8 mg (approximately 12 or 24 IU) of lyophilized, sterile somatropin per vial.
Each 4 mg carton contains one vial of Norditropin® (4 mg per vial) and one vial of diluent (2 mL of Water for Injection USP with benzyl alcohol 1.5%).
NDC 0169-7774-11
Each 8 mg carton contains one vial of Norditropin® (8 mg per vial) and one vial of diluent (2 mL of Water for Injection USP with benzyl alcohol 1.5%).
NDC 0169-7778-12

© Novo Nordisk A/S, May 1995

For information contact:

Novo Nordisk
Pharmaceuticals, Inc.
100 Overlook Center, Suite 200
Princeton, New Jersey 08540
USA

Manufactured by:
Novo Nordisk A/S
2880 Bagsvaerd, Denmark

Shown in Product Identification Guide, page 326

NOVOLIN® N   **OTC**
NPH, Human Insulin Isophane Suspension
(recombinant DNA origin)
100 units/ml

PRODUCT DESCRIPTION

Novolin® N is commonly known as NPH, Human Insulin Isophane Suspension (recombinant DNA origin). The con-

centration of this product is 100 units of insulin per milliliter. It is a cloudy or milky suspension of human insulin with protamine and zinc. The insulin substance (the cloudy material) settles at the bottom of the vial, therefore, the vial must be gently agitated or rotated so that the contents are uniformly mixed before a dose is withdrawn. **Novolin® N** has an intermediate duration of action. The effect of **Novolin® N** begins approximately $1^1/_2$ hours after injection. The effect is maximal between 4 and 12 hours. The full duration of action may last up to 24 hours after injection. The time course of action of any insulin may vary considerably in different individuals, or at different times in the same individual. Because of this variation, the periods listed here should be considered as general guidelines only.

This human insulin (recombinant DNA origin) is structurally identical to the insulin produced by the human pancreas. This human insulin is produced by recombinant DNA technology utilizing *Saccharomyces cerevisiae* (bakers' yeast) as the production organism.

STORAGE

Insulin should be stored in a cold place, preferably in a refrigerator, but not in the freezing compartment. **Do not let it freeze.** Keep the insulin vial in its carton so that it will stay clean and protected from light. If refrigeration is not possible, the bottle of insulin which you are currently using can be kept unrefrigerated as long as it is kept as cool as possible and away from heat and sunlight.

Never use **Novolin® N** if the precipitate (the white deposit at the bottom of the vial) has become lumpy or granular in appearance or has formed a deposit of solid particles on the wall of the vial. This insulin should not be used if the liquid in the vial remains clear after the vial has been gently agitated.

Never use insulin after the expiration date which is printed on the vial label and carton.

MIXING TWO TYPES OF INSULIN

Different insulins should be mixed only under instruction from a physician. Hypodermic syringes may vary in the amount of space between the bottom line and the needle ("dead space"), so if you are mixing two types of insulin be sure to discuss any change in the model and brand of syringe you are using with your physician or pharmacist. When you are mixing two types of insulin, always draw the Regular (clear) insulin into the syringe first.

SEE NOVOLIN® 70/30 for complete package insert information on Warning: Insulin Use in Diabetes: Types of Insulin: Syringes: Needle-Free Injectors: Important Statement: Preparing the Injection: Giving the Injection: Usage in Pregnancy: Insulin Reaction and Shock; Diabetic Ketoacidosis and Coma: Adverse Reactions: Important Notes.

HOW SUPPLIED

Vials, U-100, 100 units/mL, 10 mL, (List No. 183411) (1's)
Novolin N Prefilled® Syringe, U-100, 100 units/mL, 1.5 mL, (List No. 004571) (5's)
Novolin® N PenFill®, U-100, 100 units/mL, 1.5 mL, (List No. 183417) (5's)
Manufactured by: Novo Nordisk A/S, DK-2880 Bagsvaerd, Denmark and by Novo Nordisk Pharmaceutical Industries, Inc., 3612 Powhatan Road, Clayton, NC. 27520
Date of Issue: December 1995

NOVOLIN® R OTC

Regular, Human Insulin Injection (recombinant DNA origin)
USP
100 units/ml

PRODUCT DESCRIPTION

Novolin® R is commonly known as Regular, Human Insulin Injection (recombinant DNA origin) USP. The concentration of this product is 100 units of insulin per milliliter. It is a clear, colorless solution which has a short duration of action. The effect of **Novolin® R** begins approximately $^1/_2$ hour after injection. The effect is maximal between $2^1/_2$ and 5 hours and ends approximately 8 hours after injection. The time course of action of any insulin may vary considerably in different individuals or at different times in the same individual. Because of this variation, the time periods listed here should be considered as general guidelines only.

This human insulin (recombinant DNA origin) is structurally identical to the insulin produced by the human pancreas. This human insulin is produced by recombinant DNA technology utilizing *Saccharomyces cerevisiae* (bakers' yeast) as the production organism.

STORAGE

Insulin should be stored in a cold place, preferably in a refrigerator, but not in the freezing compartment. **Do not let it freeze.** Keep the insulin vial in its carton so that it will stay clean and protected from light. If refrigeration is not possible, the bottle of insulin which you are currently using can be kept unrefrigerated as long as it is kept as cool as possible and away from heat and sunlight.

Never use **Novolin® R** if it becomes viscous (thickened) or cloudy; use it only if it is clear and colorless.

Never use insulin after the expiration date which is printed on the vial label and carton.

MIXING TWO TYPES OF INSULIN—SEE NOVOLIN® N.

IMPORTANT NOTES

1. Due to risk of precipitation in some pump catheters, Novolin® R is not recommended for use in insulin pumps.
2. A change in the type, strength, species or purity of insulin could require a dosage adjustment. Any change in insulin should be made under medical supervision.
3. You may have learned how to test your urine or your blood for glucose. It is important to do these tests regularly and to record the results for review with your physician or nurse educator.
4. If you have an acute illness, especially with vomiting or fever, continue taking your insulin. If possible, stay on your regular diet. If you have trouble eating, drink fruit juices, regular soft drinks, or clear soups; if you can, eat small amounts of bland foods. Test your urine for glucose and ketones and, if possible, test your blood glucose. Note the results and contact your physician for possible insulin dose adjustment. If you have severe and prolonged vomiting, seek emergency medical care.
5. You should always carry identification which states that you have diabetes.
6. Always ask your physician or pharmacist before taking any drug.

See Novolin® 70/30 for complete package insert information on Warning: Insulin use in Diabetes: Types of Insulin: Syringes: Needle-Free Injectors: Important Statement: Preparing the Injection: Giving the Injection: Usage in Pregnancy: Insulin Reaction and Shock: Diabetic Ketoacidosis and Coma: Adverse Reactions.

HOW SUPPLIED

Vials, U-100, 100 units/mL, 10 mL, (List No. 183311) (1's)
Novolin R Prefilled® Syringe, U-100, 100 units/mL, 1.5 mL, (List No. 004471) (5's)
Novolin® R PenFill®, U-100, 100 units/mL, 1.5 mL, (List No. 183317) (5's)
Manufactured by: Novo Nordisk A/S, DK 2880 Bagsvaerd, Denmark and by Novo Nordisk Pharmaceutical Industries, Inc., 3612 Powhatan Road, Clayton, NC. 27520
Date of Issue: October 1995

HUMAN INSULIN DELIVERY SYSTEMS

There are two types of Human Insulin Delivery Systems available from Novo Nordisk Pharmaceuticals, Inc.:

DURABLE INSULIN DELIVERY SYSTEM

For the durable insulin delivery system you will need the following items, which are sold separately:
1) **NovoPen® 3** Insulin Delivery Device
2) **NovoPen® 1.5** Insulin Delivery Device
3) **Novolin® PenFill®** Cartridges 1.5 mL and 3 mL
4) **NovoFine® 30** Disposable Needles

For information about obtaining NovoPen® Insulin Delivery Devices for patients, call 1-800-707-9856

DISPOSABLE INSULIN DELIVERY SYSTEM

For the disposable insulin delivery system you will need the following items, which are sold separately:
1) **Novolin Prefilled™ Syringes**
2) **NovoFine® 30** Disposable Needles

HUMAN INSULIN OTC
NOVOLIN® 70/30 PenFill®

70% NPH, Human Insulin Isophane Suspension and 30% Regular, Human Insulin Injection (recombinant DNA origin)
100 units/ml

NOVOLIN® N PenFill® OTC

NPH, Human Insulin Isophane Suspension
(recombinant DNA origin)
100 units/ml

NOVOLIN® R PenFill® OTC

Regular, Human Insulin Injection
(recombinant DNA origin)
100 units/ml

Insulin Information for the Patient

Please read this leaflet carefully before using this product. Please note the special directions under "PREPARING THE INJECTION".

Novolin® PenFill® cartridges are designed for use with **NovoPen®** and **NovolinPen® Insulin Delivery Devices** and **NovoFine®** disposable needles or other products specifically recommended by Novo Nordisk. PenFill® cartridge is for single person use only.

See Important Notes section.

WARNING

ANY CHANGE OF INSULIN SHOULD BE MADE CAUTIOUSLY AND ONLY UNDER MEDICAL SUPERVISION. CHANGES IN PURITY, STRENGTH, BRAND (MANUFACTURER), TYPE (REGULAR, NPH, LENTE®, ETC.), SPECIES (BEEF, PORK, BEEF-PORK, HUMAN), AND/OR METHOD OF MANUFACTURE (RECOMBINANT DNA VERSUS ANIMAL-SOURCE INSULIN) MAY RESULT IN THE NEED FOR A CHANGE IN DOSAGE.

SPECIAL CARE SHOULD BE TAKEN WHEN THE TRANSFER IS FROM A STANDARD BEEF OR MIXED SPECIES INSULIN TO A PURIFIED PORK OR HUMAN INSULIN. IF A DOSAGE ADJUSTMENT IS NEEDED, IT WILL USUALLY BECOME APPARENT EITHER IN THE FIRST FEW DAYS OR OVER A PERIOD OF SEVERAL WEEKS. ANY CHANGE IN TREATMENT SHOULD BE CAREFULLY MONITORED.

PLEASE READ THE SECTIONS "INSULIN REACTION AND SHOCK" AND "DIABETIC KETOACIDOSIS AND COMA" FOR SYMPTOMS OF HYPOGLYCEMIA (LOW BLOOD GLUCOSE) AND HYPERGLYCEMIA (HIGH BLOOD GLUCOSE).

INSULIN USE IN DIABETES

Your physician has explained that you have diabetes and that your treatment involves injections of insulin or insulin therapy combined with an oral antidiabetic medicine. Insulin is normally produced by the pancreas, a gland that lies behind the stomach. Without insulin, glucose (a simple sugar made from digested food) is trapped in the bloodstream and cannot enter the cells of the body. Some patients who don't make enough of their own insulin, or who cannot use properly the insulin they do make, must take insulin by injection in order to control their blood glucose levels. Each case of diabetes is different and requires direct and continued medical supervision. Your physician has told you the type, strength and amount of insulin you should use and the time(s) at which you should inject it, and has also discussed with you a diet and exercise schedule. You should contact your physician if you experience any difficulties or if you have questions.

TYPES OF INSULINS

Standard and purified animal insulins as well as human insulins are available. Standard and purified insulins differ in their degree of purification and content of noninsulin material. Standard and purified insulins also vary in species source: they may be of beef, pork, or mixed beef and pork origin. Human insulin is identical in structure to the insulin produced by the human pancreas, and thus differs from animal insulins. Insulins vary in time of action; see PRODUCT DESCRIPTION for additional information.

Your physician has prescribed the insulin that is right for you; be sure you have purchased the correct insulin and check it carefully before you use it.

PRODUCT DESCRIPTION

A package contains five (5) cartridges.

Novolin® 70/30 PenFill contain **Novolin® 70/30** which is a mixture of 70% NPH, Human Insulin Isophance Suspension (recombinant DNA origin) and 30% Regular, Human Insulin Injection (recombinant DNA origin) USP. The concentration of this product is 100 units of insulin per milliliter. It is a cloudy or milky suspension of human insulin with protamine and zinc. The insulin substance (the cloudy material) settles at the bottom of the cartridge, therefore, the cartridge must be rotated up and down as described under "PREPARING THE INJECTION" so that the contents are uniformly mixed before the dose is given.

Novolin® 70/30 has an intermediate duration of action. The effect of **Novolin® 70/30** begins approximately $^1/_2$ hour after injection. The effect is maximal between 2 and approximately 12 hours. The full duration of action may last up to 24 hours after injection.

The time course of action of any insulin may vary considerably in different individuals, or at different times in the same individual. Because of this variation, the time periods listed here should be considered as general guidelines only.

This human insulin (recombinant DNA origin) is structurally identical to the insulin produced by the human pancreas. This human insulin is produced by recombinant DNA technology utilizing Saccharomyces cerevisiae (bakers' yeast) as the production organism.

Novolin® N PenFill® cartridges contain **Novolin® N**, commonly known as NPH, Human Insulin Isophane Suspension (recombinant DNA origin). The concentration of this product is 100 units of insulin per milliliter. It is a cloudy or milky suspension of human insulin with protamine and zinc. The insulin substance (the cloudy material) settles at the bottom of the cartridge; therefore, the cartridge must be turned up and down at least 10 times or until the liquid appears uniformly white and cloudy (a glass ball inside the cartridge facilitates mixing).

Continued on next page

Novolin 70/30 Penfill—Cont.

Novolin® N has an intermediate duration of action. The effect of **Novolin® N** begins approximately 1½ hours after injection. The effect is maximal between 4 and 12 hours. The full duration of action may last up to 24 hours after injection. The time course of action of any insulin may vary considerably in different individuals, or at different times in the same individual. Because of this variation, the time periods listed here should be considered as general guidelines only. This human insulin (recombinant DNA origin) is structurally identical to the insulin produced by the human pancreas. This human insulin is produced by recombinant DNA technology utilizing *Saccharomyces cerevisiae* (bakers' yeast) as the production organism.
Novolin® R PenFill® cartridges contain **Novolin® R,** commonly known as Regular, Human Insulin (recombinant DNA origin). The concentration of this product is 100 units of insulin per milliliter. It is a clear, colorless solution which has a short duration of action. The effect of **Novolin® R** begins approximately ½ hour after injection. The effect is maximal between 2½ and 5 hours and ends approximately 8 hours after injection. The time course of action of any insulin may vary considerably in different individuals, or at different times in the same individual. Because of this variation, the time periods listed here should be considered as general guidelines only.
This human insulin (recombinant DNA origin) is structurally identical to the insulin produced by the human pancreas. This human insulin is produced by recombinant DNA technology utilizing *Saccharomyces cerevisiae* (bakers' yeast) as the production organism.

STORAGE

Insulin should be stored in a cold place, preferably in a refrigerator, but not in the freezing compartment. **Do not let it freeze.** Keep **Novolin® 70/30 PenFill®, Novolin® N PenFill®** and **Novolin® R PenFill®** cartridges in the carton so that they will stay clean and protected from light. **Novolin® 70/30 PenFill®,** and **Novolin® N PenFill®** cartridges can be kept unrefrigerated for one (1) week. **Novolin® R PenFill®** can be kept at unrefrigerated for one (1) month. Unrefrigerated cartridges must be used within this time period or discarded. Be sure to protect cartridges from sunlight and extreme heat or cold.
Never use any **Novolin® 70/30 PenFill®** or **Novolin® N PenFill®** cartridge if the precipitate (the white deposit), has become lumpy or granular in appearance or has formed a deposit of solid particles on the wall of the cartridge. This insulin should not be used if the liquid in the cartridge remains clear after it has been mixed.
Never use any **Novolin® R PenFill®** if it becomes viscous (thickened) or cloudy; use it only if it is clear and colorless.
Never use insulin after the expiration date which is printed on the label and carton.

IMPORTANT

Failure to comply with the following antiseptic measures may lead to infections at the injection site.
— **NovoFine® 30** disposable needles are for single use; they should be used only once and destroyed.
— Clean your hands and the injection site with soap and water or with alcohol.
— Wipe the rubber stopper on the insulin cartridge with an alcohol swab.

PREPARING THE INJECTION

Novolin® R PenFill®
Place a single-use on the device. Be sure there is sufficient insulin in the cartridge to complete the injection. Refer to the instruction manual for your insulin delivery device for assistance in estimating the amount of insulin remaining in the cartridge.
Novolin® 70/30 PenFill® and **Novolin® N PenFill®**
Never place a single-use needle on your insulin delivery device until you are ready to give an injection, and remove it immediately after each injection. If the needle is not removed, some liquid may be expelled from the cartridge causing a change in the insulin concentration (strength).
Place a single-use
The cloudy material in an insulin suspension will settle to the bottom of the cartridge, so the contents must be mixed before injection. These **Novolin® PenFill®** cartridges contain a glass ball to aid mixing.
When using a new cartridge, turn the cartridge up and down between positions A and B—See Figure 1. Do this at least 10 times until the liquid appears uniformly white and cloudy.
[See figure 1 at top of next column]
Assemble your insulin delivery device following the directions in your instruction manual.
For subsequent injections when a cartridge is already in the device, turn the device up and down between positions A and B—See Figure 2. Do this at least 10 times until the liquid appears uniformly white and cloudy. Follow the directions in your insulin delivery device instruction manual.

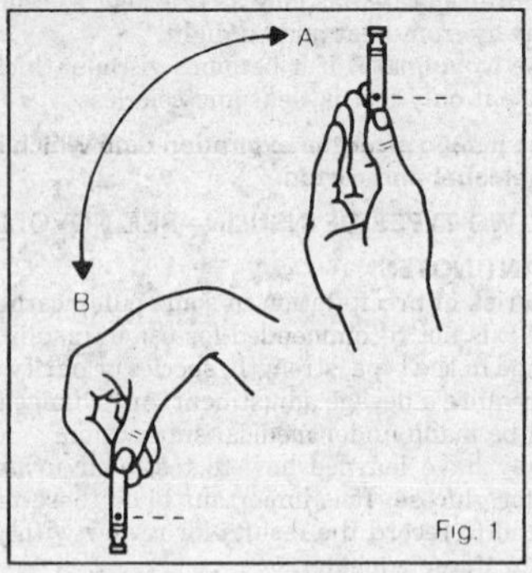

Fig. 1

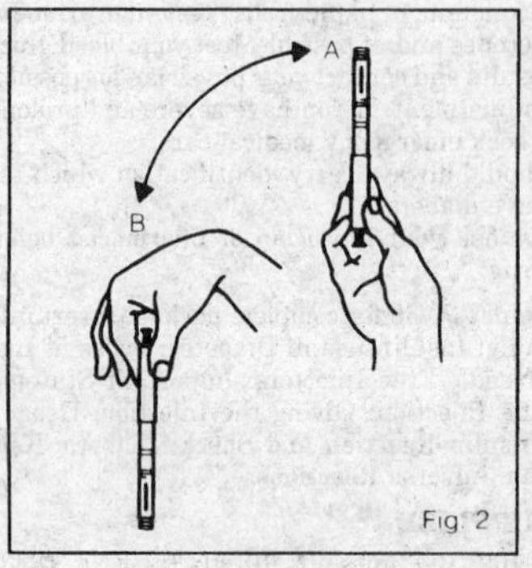

Fig. 2

Always be sure there is sufficient insulin in the cartridge to complete the injection. In order to help you estimate the amount of insulin in the cartridge, the width of the black band corresponds to 12 units of insulin.
Note: Never initiate a new injection unless there is sufficient insulin in the cartridge to ensure proper mixing (the glass ball needs adequate room for movement to mix the suspension). When using a **NovoPen®** device, never initiate a new injection once the leading edge of the plunger has passed the top edge of the black band.
Insulin Prefilled™ cartridges may contain a small amount of air. To prevent an injection of air and make certain insulin is delivered, an air shot must be done before each injection. Directions for performing an air shot are provided in your insulin delivery device instruction manual.

GIVING THE INJECTION

1. The following areas are suitable for subcutaneous insulin injection: thighs, upper arms, buttocks, abdomen. Do not change areas without consulting your physician. The actual point of injection should be changed each time; injection sites should be about an inch apart.
2. The injection site should be clean and dry. Pinch up skin area to be injected and hold it firmly.
3. Hold the device like a pencil and push the needle quickly and firmly into the pinched-up area.
4. Release the skin and push the push-button all the way in to inject insulin beneath the skin. To ensure that all the insulin is injected keep the needle in the skin for several seconds after injection with your thumb on the push-button. Do not inject into a muscle unless your physician has advised it. You should never inject insulin into a vein.
5. Do not inject into a muscle unless your physician has advised it. You should never inject insulin into a vein.
6. Remove needle. If slight bleeding occurs, press lightly with a dry cotton swab for a few seconds—**do not rub.**

For additional information see **GIVING THE INJECTION** on the reverse side of this insert.

USAGE IN PREGNANCY

It is particularly important to maintain good control of your diabetes during pregnancy and special attention must be paid to your diet, exercise and insulin regimens. If you are pregnant or nursing a baby, consult your physician or nurse educator.

INSULIN REACTION AND SHOCK

Insulin reaction (hypoglycemia) occurs when the blood glucose falls very low. This can happen if you take too much insulin, miss or delay a meal, exercise more than usual or work too hard without eating, or become ill (especially with vomiting or fever). Hypoglycemia can also happen if you combine insulin therapy and other medications that lower blood glucose, such as oral antidiabetic agents or other prescription and over-the-counter drugs. The first symptoms of an insulin reaction usually come on suddenly. They may include a cold sweat, fatigue, nervousness or shakiness, rapid heartbeat, or nausea. Personality change or confusion may also occur. If you drink or eat something right away (a glass of milk or orange juice, or several sugar candies), you can often stop the progression of symptoms. If symptoms persist, call your physician—an insulin reaction can lead to unconsciousness. If a reaction results in loss of consciousness, emergency medical care should be obtained immediately. If you have had repeated reactions or if an insulin reaction has led to a loss of consciousness, contact your physician. Severe hypoglycemia can result in temporary or permanent impairment of brain function and death.
In certain cases, the nature and intensity of the warning symptoms of hypoglycemia may change. A few patients have reported that after being transferred to human insulin, the early warning symptoms of hypoglycemia were less pronounced than they had been with animal-source insulin.

DIABETIC KETOACIDOSIS AND COMA

Diabetic ketoacidosis may develop if your body has too little insulin. The most common causes are acute illness or infection or failure to take enough insulin by injection. If you are ill you should check your urine for ketones. The symptoms of diabetic ketoacidosis usually come on gradually, over a period of hours or days, and include a drowsy feeling, flushed face, thirst and loss of appetite. Notify your physician right away if the urine test is positive for ketones (acetone) or if you have any of these symptoms. Fast, heavy breathing and rapid pulse are more severe symptoms and you should have medical attention right away. Severe, sustained hyperglycemia may result in diabetic coma and death.

ADVERSE REACTIONS

A few people with diabetes develop red, swollen and itchy skin where the insulin has been injected. This is called a "local reaction" and it may occur if the injection is not properly made, if the skin is sensitive to the cleansing solution, or if you are allergic to the insulin being used. If you have a local reaction, tell your physican.
Generalized insulin allergy occurs rarely, but when it does it may cause a serious reaction, including skin rash over the body, shortness of breath, fast pulse, sweating, and a drop in blood pressure. If any of these symptoms develop, you should seek emergency medical care.
If severe allergic reactions to insulin have occured (i.e., generalized rash, swelling or breathing difficulties) you should be skin-tested with **each** new insulin preparation before it is used.

IMPORTANT NOTES

1. A change in the type, strength, species or purity of insulin could require a dosage adjustment. Any change in insulin should be made under medical supervision.
2. To avoid possible transmission of disease, PenFill® cartridge is for single person use only.
3. You may have learned how to test your urine or your blood for glucose. It is important to do these tests regularly and to record the results for review with your physician or nurse educator.
4. If you have an acute illness, especially with vomiting or fever, continue taking your insulin. If possible, stay on your regular diet. If you have trouble eating, drink fruit juices, regular soft drinks, or clear soups; if you can, eat small amounts of bland foods. Test your urine for glucose and ketones and, if possible, test your blood glucose. Note the results and contact your physician for possible insulin dose adjustment. If you have severe and prolonged vomiting, seek emergency medical care.
5. You should always carry identification which states that you have diabetes.
6. Always ask your physician or pharmacist before taking any drug.

Always consult your physician if you have any questions about your conditon or the use of insulin.

Helpful information for people with diabetes is published by American Diabetes Association, 1660 Duke Street, Alexandria, VA 22314

For information contact:
Novo Nordisk Pharmaceuticals, Inc.,
Princeton, NJ 08540
Manufactured by
Novo Nordisk A/S
DK-2880 Bagsvaerd, Denmark
Novo Nordisk™, Novolin® PenFill®, NovoPen®, NovolinPen®, NovoFine® and Lente®
are trademarks owned by Novo Nordisk A/S
Date of issue: August 1994

HOW SUPPLIED

Novolin® 70/30 PenFill® cartridges, U-100, 100 units/mL, 1.5 mL, (List No. 183717) (5's)
Novolin® N PenFill® cartridges. U-100, 100 units/mL, 1.5 mL, (List No. 183417) (5's)

Novolin® R PenFill® cartridges, U-100, 100 units/mL, 1.5 mL, (List No. 183317) (5's)
Shown in Product Identification Guide, page 326

NovoFine® 30
Disposable Needle

℞

DESCRIPTION

The self contained disposable needle consists of a protective plastic outer cap, a smooth plastic needle cap and a protective tab. (The needle should not be used if the protective tab is missing or damaged.)
Each **NovoFine® 30** is 30 gauge, one-third ($^1/_3$) inch (8mm) in length and is intended for single use only. Each **NovoFine® 30** is cut to a sharp, low-angle point and coated with silicone for easier penetration.
NovoFine® 30 is for use with all Novo Nordisk™ Insulin Delivery Systems.
List# 185250
NovoFine® trademark owned by Novo Nordisk A/S.

HUMAN INSULIN
NOVOLIN 70/30 PREFILLED®
OTC
70% NPH, Human Insulin Isophane Suspension and
30% Regular,
Human Insulin Injection
(recombinant DNA origin)
in a 1.5 ml Prefilled Syringe
100 units/ml

NOVOLIN N PREFILLED®
NPH, Human Insulin Isophane
Suspension (recombinant DNA origin)
in a 1.5 ml Prefilled Syringe
100 units/ml

NOVOLIN R PREFILLED®
Regular, Human Insulin Injection
(recombinant DNA origin)
in a 1.5 ml Prefilled Syringe
100 units/ml

Insulin Information For The Patient
Please read both sides of this leaflet carefully before using this product.
Novolin Prefilled™ syringe is for single person use only. See Important Notes section.

WARNING
ANY CHANGE OF INSULIN SHOULD BE MADE CAUTIOUSLY AND ONLY UNDER MEDICAL SUPERVISION. CHANGES IN PURITY, STRENGTH, BRAND (MANUFACTURER), TYPE (REGULAR, NPH, LENTE® ETC.), SPECIES (BEEF, PORK, BEEF-PORK, HUMAN) AND/OR METHOD OF MANUFACTURE (RECOMBINANT DNA VERSUS ANIMAL-SOURCE INSULIN) MAY RESULT IN THE NEED FOR A CHANGE IN DOSAGE.
SPECIAL CARE SHOULD BE TAKEN WHEN THE TRANSFER IS FROM A STANDARD BEEF OR MIXED SPECIES INSULIN TO A PURIFIED PORK OR HUMAN INSULIN. IF A DOSAGE ADJUSTMENT IS NEEDED, IT WILL USUALLY BECOME APPARENT EITHER IN THE FIRST FEW DAYS OR OVER A PERIOD OF SEVERAL WEEKS, ANY CHANGE IN TREATMENT SHOULD BE CAREFULLY MONITORED.
PLEASE READ THE SECTIONS "INSULIN REACTION AND SHOCK" AND "DIABETIC KETOACIDOSIS AND COMA" FOR SYMPTOMS OF HYPOGLYCEMIA (LOW BLOOD GLUCOSE) AND HYPERGLYCEMIA (HIGH BLOOD GLUCOSE).

INSULIN USE IN DIABETES
Your physician has explained that you have diabetes and that your treatment involves injections of insulin or insulin therapy combined with an oral antidiabetic medicine. Insulin is normally produced by the pancreas, a gland that lies behind the stomach. Without insulin, glucose (a simple sugar made from digested food) is trapped in the bloodstream and cannot enter the cells of the body. Some patients who don't make enough of their own insulin, or who cannot properly use the insulin they do make, must take insulin by injection in order to control their blood glucose levels.
Each case of diabetes is different and requires direct and continued medical supervision. Your physician has told you the type, strength and amount of insulin you should use and the time(s) at which you should inject it, and has also discussed with you a diet and exercise schedule. You should contact your physician if you experience any difficulties or if you have questions.

TYPES OF INSULIN
Standard and purified animal insulin as well as human insulin are available. Standard and purified insulin differ in their degree of purification and content of noninsulin material. Standard and purified insulin also vary in species source: they may be of beef, pork, or mixed beef and pork origin. Human insulin is identical in structure to the insulin produced by the human pancreas, and thus differs from ani-

mals insulin. Insulin Products vary in time of action; see **PRODUCT DESCRIPTION** for additional information.
Your physician has prescribed the insulin that is right for you; be sure you have purchased the correct insulin and check it carefully before you use it.

PRODUCT DESCRIPTION
A package contains five (5) **Novolin Prefilled™** insulin syringes.
This human insulin (recombinant DNA origin) is structurally identical to the insulin produced by the human pancreas. This human insulin is produced by recombinant DNA technology utilizing *Saccharomyces cerevisiae* (bakers' yeast) as the production organism.
The time course of action of any insulin may vary considerably in different individuals, or at different times in the same individual. Because of the variation, the time periods listed here should be considered as general guidelines only.
Novolin 70/30 Prefilled® contains Novolin 70/30, a mixture of 70% NPH, Human Insulin Isophane Suspension (recombinant DNA origin) and 30% Regular, Human Insulin Injection (recombinant DNA origin) USP. The concentration of this product is 100 units of insulin per milliliter. It is a cloudy or milky suspension of human insulin with protamine and zinc. The insulin substance (the cloudy material) settles to the bottom of the insulin reservoir, therefore, the syringe must be rotated up and down so that the contents are uniformly mixed before a dose is given. Novolin® 70/30 has an intermediate duration of action. The effect of Novolin® 70/30 begins approximately $^1/_2$ hours after injection. The effect is maximal between 2 and approximately 12 hours. The full duration of action may last up to 24 hours after injection.
Novolin N Prefilled™ contains NPH, Human Insulin Isophane Suspension (recombinant DNA origin). The concentration of this product is 100 units of insulin per milliliter. It is a cloudy or milky suspension of human insulin with protamine and zinc. The insulin substance (the cloudy material) settles to the bottom of the insulin reservoir, therefore, the syringe must be rotated up and down so that the contents are uniformly mixed before a dose is given. Novolin® N has an intermediate duration of action. The effect of Novolin® N begins approximately $1^1/_2$ hours after injection. The effect is maximal between 4 and approximately 12 hours. The full duration of action may last up to 24 hours after injection.
Novolin R Prefilled® contains Regular, Human Insulin Injection (recombinant DNA origin) USP. The concentration of this product is 100 units of insulin per milliliter. It is a clear, colorless solution which has a short duration of action. The effect of Novolin® R begins approximately $^1/_2$ hour after injection. The effect is maximal between $2^1/_2$ and 5 hours and ends approximately 8 hours after injection.

STORAGE
Novolin Prefilled™ insulin syringes should be stored in a cold place, preferably in a refrigerator, but not in the freezing compartment. **Do not let it freeze.** Keep **Novolin Prefilled™** in the carton so that they will stay clean and protected from light. **Novolin 70/30 Prefilled®** and **Novolin N Prefilled®** can be kept unrefrigerated for one (1) week.
Novolin R Prefilled® can be kept unrefrigerated for (1) month. Unrefrigerated syringes must be used within this time period or discarded. Be sure to protect syringes from sunlight and extreme heat or cold.
Never use any **Novolin R Prefilled®** if the insulin becomes viscous (thickend or cloudy); use it only if it is clear and colorless. Never use any **Novolin 70/30 Prefilled®** or **Novolin N Prefilled®** if the precipitate (the white deposit) has become lumpy or granular in appearance or has formed a deposit of solid particles on the wall of the insulin reservoir. This insulin should not be used if the liquid in the insulin reservoir remains clear after it has been mixed.
Never use insulin after the expiration date which is printed on the label and carton.

IMPORTANT
Failure to comply with the following antiseptic measures may lead to infections at the injection site.
— Disposable needles are for single use; they should be used only once and discarded properly.
— Clean your hands and the injection site with soap and water or with alcohol.
— Wipe the rubber stopper with an alcohol swab.

PREPARING THE INJECTION
Never place a single-use needle on your insulin delivery device until you are ready to give an injection, and remove it immediately after each injection. If the needle is not removed, some liquid may be expelled from the syringe causing a change in the insulin concentration (strength).
For **Novolin N Prefilled®** & **Novolin 70/30 Prefilled®**, the cloudy material in an insulin suspension will settle to the bottom of the insulin reservoir, so the contents must be mixed before injection. These syringes contain a glass ball to aid mixing.

Rotate the syringe up and down so that the contents are uniformly mixed before the dose is given.
Follow the directions for use of this syringe on the reverse side of this insert.
Insulin Prefilled in cartridges may contain a small amount of air. To prevent an injection of air and make certain insulin is delivered an air shot must be done before each injection. Directions for performing an air shot are provided in your insulin delivery device instruction manual.

GIVING THE INJECTION
1. The following areas are suitable for subcutaneous insulin injection: thighs, upper arms, buttocks, abdomen. Do not change areas without consulting your physician. The actual point of injection should be changed each time; injection sites should be about an inch apart.
2. The injection site should be clean and dry. Pinch up skin area to be injected and hold it firmly.
3. Hold the device like a pencil and push the needle quickly and firmly into the pinched-up area.
4. Release the skin and push the push-button all the way in to inject insulin beneath the skin. To ensure that all the insulin is injected keep the needle in the skin for several seconds after injection with your thumb on the push-button. Do not inject into a muscle unless your physician has advised it. You should never inject insulin into a vein.
5. Remove needle. If slight bleeding occurs, press lightly with a dry cotton swab for a few seconds—**do not rub.**
For additional information see **GIVING THE INJECTION** on the reverse side of this insert.

USAGE IN PREGNANCY
It is particularly important to maintain good control of your diabetes during pregnancy and special attention must be paid to your diet, exercise and insulin regimens. If you are pregnant or nursing a baby, consult your physician or nurse educator.

INSULIN REACTION AND SHOCK
Insulin reaction (hypoglycemia) occurs when the blood glucose falls very low. This can happen if you take too much insulin, miss or delay a meal, exercise more than usual or work too hard without eating, or become ill (especially with vomiting or fever). Hypoglycemia can also happen if you combine insulin therapy and other medications that lower blood glucose, such as oral antidiabetic agents or other prescription and over-the-counter drugs. The first symptoms of an insulin reaction usually come on suddenly. They may include a cold sweat, fatigue, nervousness or shakiness, rapid heartbeat, or nausea. Personality change or confusion may also occur. If you drink or eat something right away (a glass of milk or orange juice, or several sugar candies), you can often stop the progression of symptoms. If symptoms persist, call your physician-an insulin reaction can lead to unconsciousness. If a reaction results in loss of consciousness, emergency medical care should be obtained immediately. If you have had repeated reactions or if an insulin reaction has led to a loss of consciousness, contact your physician. Severe hypoglycemia can result in temporary or permanent impairment of brain function and death.
In certain cases, the nature and intensity of the warning symptoms of hypoglycemia may change. A few patients have reported that after being transferred to human insulin, the early warning symptoms of hypoglycemia were less pronounced than they had been with animal-source insulin.

DIABETIC KETOACIDOSIS AND COMA
Diabetic ketoacidosis may develop if your body has too little insulin. The most common causes are acute illness or infection or failure to take enough insulin by injection. If you are ill you should check your urine for ketones. The symptoms of diabetic ketoacidosis usually come on gradually, over a period of hours or days, and include a drowsy feeling, flushed face, thirst and loss of appetite. Notify your physician right away if the urine test is positive for ketones (acetone) or if you have any of these symptoms. Fast, heavy breathing and rapid pulse are more severe symptoms and you should have medical attention right away. Severe sustained hyperglycemia may result in diabetic coma and death.

ADVERSE REACTIONS
A few people with diabetes develop red, swollen and itchy skin where the insulin has been injected. This is called a "local reaction" and it may occur if the injection is not properly made, if the skin is sensitive to the cleaning solution or if you are allergic to the insulin being used. If you have a local reaction, tell your physician.
Generalized insulin allergy occurs rarely, but when it does it may cause a serious reaction, including skin rash over the body, shortness of breath, fast pulse, sweating, and a drop in blood pressure. If any of these symptoms develop, you should seek emergency medical care.

Continued on next page

Novolin Prefilled—Cont.

If severe reactions to insulin have occurred (i.e. generalized rash, swelling or breathing difficulties) you should be skin-tested with each new insulin preparation before it is used.

IMPORTANT NOTES

1. A change in the type, strength, species or purity of insulin could require a dosage adjustment. Any change in insulin should be made under medical supervision.
2. To avoid possible transmission of disease, **Novolin Prefilled™** syringe is for single person use only.
3. You may have learned how to test your urine or your blood for glucose. It is important to do these tests regularly and to record the results for review with your physician or nurse educator.
4. If you have an acute illness, especially with vomiting or fever, continue taking your insulin. If possible, stay on your regular diet. If you have trouble eating, drink fruit juices, regular soft drinks, or clear soups; if you can, eat small amounts of bland foods. Test your urine for glucose and ketones and, if possible, test your blood glucose. Note the results and contact your physician for possible insulin dose adjustment. If you have severe and prolonged vomiting, seek emergency medical care.
5. You should always carry identification which states that you have diabetes.
6. Always ask your physician or pharmacist before taking any drug.

Always consult your physician if you have any questions about your condition or the use of insulin.

Helpful information for people with diabetes is published by American Diabetes Association, 1600 Duke Street, Alexandria, VA 22314.

Novolin Prefilled™, Novolin®, Novolin Prefilled®, Lente® and NovoFine® are trademarks of Novo Nordisk A/S
® 1998 Novo Nordisk Pharmaceuticals, Inc.
Date of Issue: May 1998

HOW SUPPLIED

Novolin 70/30 Prefilled® Syringe, U-100, 100 units/ml, 1.5 ml, (List No. 001771) (5's)

Novolin N Prefilled® Syringe, U-100, 100 units/ml, 1.5 ml, (List No. 004571) (5's)

Novolin R Prefilled® Syringe, U-100, 100 units/ml, 1.5 ml, (List No. 004471) (5's)

Prefilled syringe directions for use

This is a disposable dial-a-dose insulin delivery system able to deliver 2–58 units in increments of 2 units. **Novolin Prefilled™** syringe must only be used with **NovoFine®** single use needle or other products specifically recommended by Novo Nordisk. **Novolin Prefilled™** syringe is not recommended for the blind or visually impaired without the assistance of a sighted individual trained in the proper use of this product.

Please read these instructions completely before using this device.

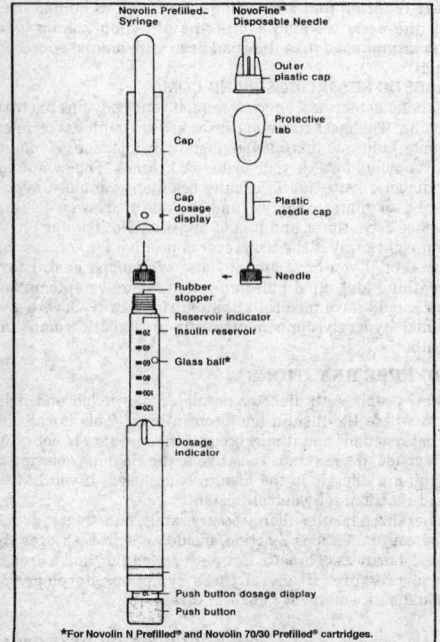

*For Novolin N Prefilled® and Novolin 70/30 Prefilled® cartridges.

1. Preparing the Syringe
Pull off the cap.

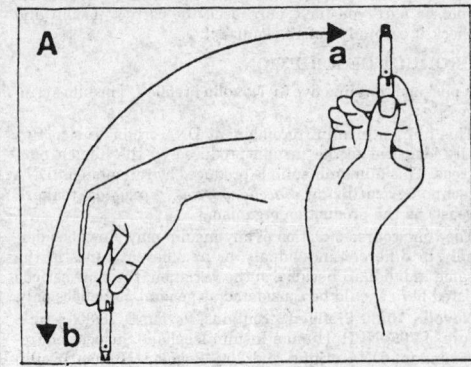

A. Turn the syringe up and down between **a** and **b** so the glass ball is moved from one end of the insulin reservoir to the other. Do this at least 10 times, until the liquid appears uniformly white and cloudy. Wipe rubber stopper with an alcohol swab. This step is not necessary with Novolin R Prefilled®.

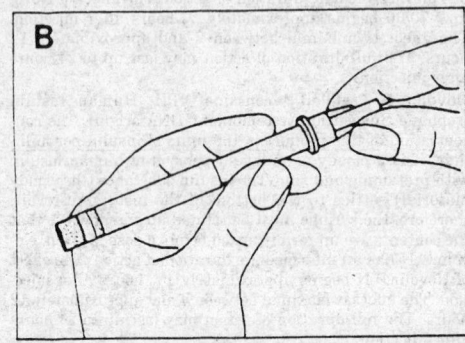

B. Remove the protective tab from disposable needle and screw the needle onto the syringe. Never place a disposable needle on your syringe until you are ready to give an injection. Remove the needle immediately after use. If the needle is not removed, some liquid may be expelled from the syringe causing a change in insulin concentration (strength).

Giving the air shot prior to each injection:
Small amounts of air may collect in the needle and insulin reservoir during normal use.

To avoid the injection of air and ensure proper dosing, hold the syringe with the needle upwards and tap the syringe gently with your finger so any air bubbles collect in the top of the reservoir. Remove both the plastic outer cap and the needle cap.

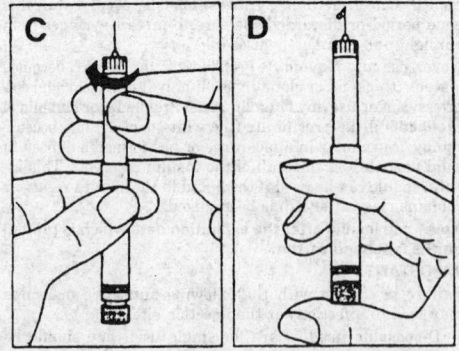

C. Holding the syringe with the needle pointing upwards, **slowly** turn the insulin reservoir clockwise (in the direction of the arrow, fig. C) to the first notch where resistance is felt ($^1/_5$ of a full rotation).

D. Still with the needle pointing upwards, press the push button as far as it will go and see if a drop of insulin appears at the needle tip (Fig. D).

Before the first use of Novolin Prefilled™ you may need to perform up to 6 air shots to get a droplet of insulin at the needle tip. If you need to make more than 6 air shots do not use and return the product to Novo Nordisk.

If not, repeat the procedure until insulin appears. A small air bubble may remain but it will not be injected because the operating mechanism prevents the reservoir from being completely emptied.

2. Setting the dose

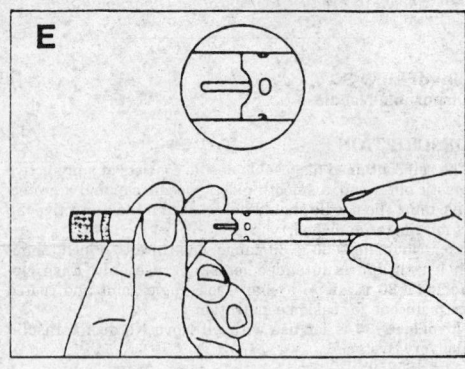

E. Replace the cap, so **0** is opposite the dosage indicator.

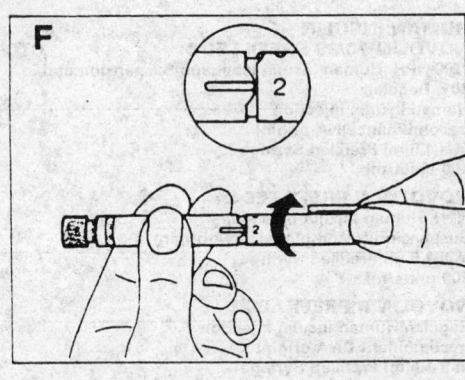

F. Hold the syringe horizontally and turn the cap in the direction of the arrow to set the required dose. Do not put your hand over the push button when dialing the dose. If the button is not allowed to rise freely, insulin will be pushed out of the needle. The dosage display on the cap shows **0, 2, 4, 6** and **8** units.

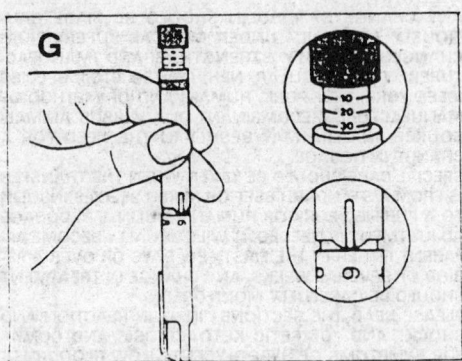

G. As the cap is turned, the push button rises. The dosage display below the push button shows **10, 20, 30, 40** and **50** units. Every time you fully turn the cap, 10 units will be set. To check the dose set, add the figure on the cap opposite the dosage indicator to the highest number showing on the push button display.

Dosage examples

- **8 units:**
  Turn the cap until **8** is opposite the dosage indicator.
- **36 units:**
  Turn the cap 3 full turns so **0** is opposite the dosage indicator. The 30-line will show on the push button display. Continue turning until **6** is opposite the dosage indicator (see **G**).

If you have set a wrong dose, simply turn the cap forwards or backwards until the right number of units has been set. **58 units is the maximum dose.** If you attempt to set a higher dose, insulin will be expelled from the needle and the dose will be wrong. If you set more than 58 units, turn the cap back as far as you can until resistance is felt and the push button is fully depressed. If the dosage indicator is not lined up with **0** when resistance is felt, remove the cap and replace it with **0** opposite the dosage indicator. Now start again, remembering that **58** units is the maximum dose. After the dose is set, remove the cap.

3. Giving the injection

Use the injection technique recommended by your doctor. Check that you have set the proper dose and depress the push button as far as it will go. When depressing the push button you may hear a clicking sound. Do not rely on this clicking sound as a means of determining or confirming your dose. After making the injection, replace the plastic outer cap. Unscrew the needle and discard appropriately. Replace the cap with 0 opposite the dosing indicator.

For additional information see **GIVING THE INJECTION** on the reverse side of this insert.

4. Subsequent Injections

Always check that the push button is fully depressed before using the syringe again. If not, turn the cap until the push button is completely down. Then proceed as stated under steps 1–3.

The numbers on the insulin reservoir can be used to estimate the amount of insulin left in the syringe. These numbers **are not** used for measuring the insulin dose.

You cannot set a dose greater then the number of units remaining in the reservoir.

If you are using Novolin N Prefilled® or Novolin 70/30 Prefilled® there must be at least 12 units left in the reservoir to give the glass ball space to move when mixing the insulin. If your dose is less than 12 units — and the reservoir is nearly empty — first dial up to 12 (to check that 12 units are left) and then set the desired dose. If 12 cannot be dialed, change to a new syringe. Discard the used syringe carefully, without the needle attached.

5. Important Notes

If you need to perform more than 6 air shots before the first use of Novolin Prefilled™ to get a droplet of insulin at the needle tip, do not use.

- Remember to perform an air shot before each injection. See Figures C and D.
- Care should be taken not to drop the syringe or subject it to impact.
- The compact size of this prefilled syringe makes it easy to use and convenient to carry. Remember to keep it with you; don't leave it in a car or other location where extremes of temperature can occur.
- Novolin Prefilled™ is for designed use with NovoFine® disposable needles or products specifically recommended by Novo Nordisk.
- Never place a disposable needle on this syringe until you are ready to use it. Remove the needle immediately after use. If the needle is not removed, some liquid may leak from the syringe causing a change in insulin concentration (strength).
- Always carry a spare Novolin Prefilled™ syringe with you in case your prefilled syringe is damaged or lost.
- Novo Nordisk cannot be held responsible for adverse reactions occurring as a consequence of using this insulin delivery system with products that are not recommended by Novo Nordisk.
- Keep this syringe out of the reach of children.

Call 800-727-6500 for additional information.

Novo Nordisk Pharmaceuticals, Inc.,
Princeton, NJ 08540

Manufactured by Novo Nordisk A/S,
DK-2880 Bagsvaerd, Denmark

Novo Nordisk™ Novolin®, Novolin Prefilled™, Lente® NovoFine® are trademarks of Novo Nordisk A/S.

Date of issue: May 1998

Shown in Product Identification Guide, page 326

VELOSULIN® BR   **OTC**
Buffered Regular
Human Insulin Injection
(semi-synthetic)
100 units/ml

FOR USE IN EXTERNAL INSULIN INFUSION PUMPS
OR WITH U-100 INSULIN SYRINGES
Please read this leaflet carefully.

WARNING

Any change of insulin should be made cautiously and only under medical supervision. Changes in purity, strength (U-40, U-100), brand (manufacturer), type (Lente®, NPH, regular etc.) and/or species source (beef, pork, beef/pork, human) may result in the need for a change in dosage. Adjustment may be needed with the first dose or over a period of several weeks. Be aware that symptoms of hypoglycemia (low blood glucose) or hyperglycemia (high blood glucose) may indicate the need for dosage adjustment. Please read sections entitled "Insulin Reaction" and "Diabetic Ketoacidosis and Coma".

Velosulin® BR should not be mixed with Lente®-type insulin products because the buffering agent in Velosulin® BR may interact with the other insulin and result in a change of activity. This change could lead to an unpredictable effect on blood glucose. When used with an external insulin infusion pump Velosulin® BR should not be mixed with any other insulin.

Velosulin® BR has been tested only in MiniMed® Model 504-S pumps, using the accompanying Model MMT-103 sy-

ringe as well as both MiniMed® Model MMT-106 Polyfin™ and MiniMed® Model 111 Sofset™ infusion sets. MiniMed® Model 504-S and Model 506 pumps are equivalent. Change the catheter tubing and the insulin in the reservoir every 48 hours.

INSULIN USE IN DIABETES

Your physician has explained that you have diabetes and that your treatment involves injections of insulin or insulin therapy combined with oral antidiabetic medicine. Insulin is normally produced by the pancreas, a gland that lies behind the stomach. Without insulin, glucose (a simple sugar made from digested food) is trapped in the bloodstream and cannot enter the cells of the body. Some patients who don't make enough of their own insulin, or who cannot use the insulin they do make properly, must take insulin by injection in order to control their blood glucose levels.

Each case of diabetes is different and requires direct and continued medical supervision. Your physician has told you the type, strength and amount of insulin you should use and the time(s) at which you should inject it, and has also discussed with you a diet and exercise schedule. You should contact your physician if you experience any difficulties or if you have questions.

TYPES OF INSULINS

Standard and purified animal insulins as well as human insulins are available. Standard and purified insulins differ in their degree of purification and content of noninsulin material.

Standard and purified insulins also vary in species source: they may be of beef, pork, or mixed beef and pork origin. Human insulin is identical in structure to the insulin produced by the human pancreas, and thus differs from animal insulins. Insulins vary in time of action and in strength; see PRODUCT DESCRIPTION and SYRINGES for additional information.

Your physician has prescribed the insulin that is right for you; be sure you have purchased the correct insulin and check it carefully before you use it.

PRODUCT DESCRIPTION

Velosulin® BR is a clear solution of insulin in a phosphate buffer. This human insulin is structurally identical to the insulin produced by the pancreas in the human body. This structural identity is obtained by enzymatic conversion of purified pork insulin. When a U-100 insulin syringe is used to deliver the insulin, Velosulin® BR has a rapid onset of action, approximately $1/2$ hour after the injection. The effect lasts up to approximately 8 hours with a maximal effect between the 1st and 3rd hour.

The time course of action of any insulin may vary considerably in different individuals, or at different times in the same individual, or if using an external insulin infusion pump to deliver the insulin.

Because of this variation, the time periods listed here should be considered as general guidelines only when using U-100 insulin syringes to deliver the insulin.

STORAGE

Insulin should be stored in a cold place, preferably in a refrigerator, but not in the freezing compartment. Do not let it freeze. Keep the insulin vial in its carton so that it will stay clean and protected from light. If refrigeration is not possible, the bottle of insulin which you are currently using can be kept unrefrigerated as long as it is kept as cool as possible and away from heat and sunlight.

Do not use the preparation if the color has become other than water clear or if the liquid has become viscous (thickened).

Never use insulin after expiration date which is printed on the vial label and carton.

EXTERNAL INSULIN INFUSION PUMPS

Read and follow the instructions that accompany your insulin infusion pump. It is important to follow the instructions from the manufacturer of the pump that you use.

Use the correct reservoir and catheter for the pump that you are using. Catheter clogging with insulin crystals has been known to occur.

You should change the catheter tubing and the insulin in the reservoir every 48 hours. Failure to do so may affect the amount of insulin you receive. This can cause serious problems for you, such as too little or too much glucose in the blood.

When used with an external insulin infusion pump, Velosulin® BR should not be mixed with any other insulin.

SYRINGES

Use the correct syringe

The volume of the dose depends on the number of units of insulin per ml. Velosulin® BR is only available in the U-100 strength (100 units per ml). Make sure that you understand the markings on your syringe and use only syringe marked for U-100.

Novo Nordisk insulin vials are intended for use with standard insulin syringes. Novo Nordisk has not evaluated the use of these vials with other devices for insulin delivery or with devices intended to aid in giving injections. Consult your doctor and the manufacturer of these devices before use with this product.

Disposable Syringes

Disposable syringes and needles require no sterilization provided the package is intact. They should be used only once and discarded.

Reusable Syringes

Reusable syringes and needles must be sterile when used. The best method of sterilization is to boil the syringe, plunger and needle in water for 5 minutes. If this is not possible, as when travelling, the parts may be sterilized by immersion for at least 5 minutes in a sterilizing liquid like ethyl alcohol, 70%. Do not use bathing, rubbing or medicated alcohol for sterilization.

Remove all liquid from the syringe by pushing the plunger in and out several times and leave it to dry if alcohol has been used for sterilization.

IMPORTANT

Failure to comply with the above and the following antiseptic measures may lead to infections at the injection site.

PREPARING THE INJECTION

1. Clean your hands and the injection site with soap and water or with alcohol.
   Wipe the rubber stopper with an alcohol swab. (Note: remove the tamper-resistant cap at first use. If the cap has already been removed, do not use this product, return it to your pharmacy.)
2. Pull back the plunger until the black tip reaches the marking for the number of units you will inject.
3. Push the needle through the rubber stopper into the vial.
4. Push the plunger all the way in. This inserts air into the bottle.
5. Turn the vial and syringe upside down and slowly pull the plunger back to a few units beyond the correct dose.
6. If there are air bubbles, flick the syringe firmly with your finger to raise the air bubbles to the needle, then slowly push the plunger to the correct unit marking.
7. Life the vial off the syringe.

GIVING THE INJECTION

1. The following areas are suitable for subcutaneous insulin injection: thighs, upper arms, buttocks, abdomen. Do not change areas without consulting your physician. The actual point of injection should be changed each time; injection sites should be about an inch apart.
2. The injection site should be clean and dry. Pinch up skin area to be injected and hold it firmly.
3. Hold the syringe like a pencil and push the needle quickly and firmly into the pinched-up area.
4. Release the skin and push plunger all the way in to inject insulin beneath the skin. To ensure that all the insulin is injected, keep the needle in the skin for several seconds after the injection with your finger on the plunger. Do not inject into a muscle unless your physician has advised it. You should never inject insulin into a vein.
5. Remove the needle. If slight bleeding occurs, press lightly with a dry cotton swab for a few seconds—do not rub.

Note: The dose should be injected over 2–4 seconds. Preparations of insulin suspensions which are injected slowly may clog the tip of the needle, resulting in an inability to complete the injection. Syringe plugging does not occur when the drug is injected more rapidly. Use the injection technique recommended by your physician.

**MIXING TWO TYPES OF INSULIN
(IN SYRINGES ONLY)**

When using U-100 Insulin Syringes, different insulins should be mixed only under instruction from a physician. Hypodermic syringes may vary in the amount of space between the bottom line and the needle ("dead space"), so if you are mixing two types of insulin be sure to discuss any change in the model and brand of syringe you are using with your physician or pharmacist. When you are mixing two types of insulin, always draw the Regular (clear) insulin into the syringe first.

Velosulin® BR should not be mixed with Lente®-type insulin products because the buffering agent in Velosulin® BR may interact with the other insulin and result in a change of activity. This change could lead to an unpredictable effect on blood glucose. When used with an external insulin infusion pump Velosulin® BR should not be mixed with any other insulin.

USAGE IN PREGNANCY

It is particularly important to maintain good control of your diabetes during pregnancy and special attention must be paid to your diet, exercise and insulin regimens. If you are pregnant or nursing a baby, consult your physician or nurse educator.

INSULIN REACTION

Insulin reaction (too little sugar in the blood, also called hypoglycemia) can occur if you take too much insulin, miss a meal or exercise or work harder than normal. Hypoglycemia can also happen if you combine insulin therapy and other medications that lower blood glucose, such as antidiabetic agents or other prescription and over-the-counter drugs. The symptoms, which usually come on suddenly, are hunger, dizziness, and sweating. Personality change or confusion may also occur. Eating sugar or a sugar-sweetened product will normally correct the condition.

If symptoms persist, call a physician; an insulin reaction can lead to unconsciousness. If a reaction results in loss of consciousness, emergency medical care should be obtained immediately. If you have had repeated reactions or if an insulin reaction had led to a loss of consciousness, contact

Continued on next page

Velosulin—Cont.

your physician. Severe hypoglycemia can result in temporary or permanent impairment of brain function and death. **In certain cases, the nature and intensity of the warning symptoms of hypoglycemia may change. A few patients have reported that after being transferred to human insulin, the early warning symptoms of hypoglycemia were less pronounced than they had been with animal-source insulin.**

DIABETIC KETOACIDOSIS AND COMA

Diabetic ketoacidosis may develop if your body has too little insulin. The most common causes are acute illness, infection or failure to take enough insulin by injection or catheter clogging when used with an external insulin infusion pump. If you are ill, you should check your urine for ketones. The symptoms of diabetic ketoacidosis usually come on gradually, over a period of hours or days, and include a drowsy feeling, fluschec face, thrist and loss of appetite. Notify a physician immediately if the urine test is positive for ketones (acetone) or if you have any of these symptoms. More severe symptoms are fast, heavy breathing and rapid pulse; if these symptoms occur, you should have medical attention right away. Severe, sustained hyperglycemia may result in diabetic coma and death.

ADVERSE REACTIONS

Insulin allergy occurs very rarely, but when it does, it may cause a serious reaction including a general skin rash over the body, shortness of breath, fast pulse, sweating and a drop in blood pressure. If any of these symptoms develop you should seek emergency medical care.

In a very few diabetics, the skin where insulin has been injected may become red, swollen and itchy. This is called a local reaction. It may occur if the injection is not properly made, if the skin is sentitive to the cleansing solution or if the patient is allergic to insulin. If you have a local reaction, notify your physician.

Patients with severe systemic allergic reactions to insulin (i.e. generalized urticaria, angioedema, anaphylaxis) should be skin tested with each new preparation to be used prior to initiation of therapy with that preparation.

IMPORTANT NOTES

1. A change in the type, strength, species or purity of insulin could require a dosage adjustment. Any change in insulin should be made under medical supervision.
2. You may have learned how to test your urine or your blood for glucose. It is important to do these tests regularly and to record the results for review with your physician or nurse educator.
3. If you have an illness, especially with vomiting or fever, continue taking your insulin. If possible, stay on your regular diet. If you have trouble eating, drink fruit juices, regular soft drinks, or clear soups; if you can, eat small amounts of bland foods. Test your urine for glucose and ketones and, if possible, test your blood glucose. Note the results and contact your physician for possible insulin dose adjustment. If you have severe and prolonged vomiting, seek emergency medical care.
4. You should always carry identification which states that you have diabetes.
5. Always ask your physician or pharmacist before taking any drug.

Always consult your physician if you have any questions about your condition or the use of insulin.

Helpful information for people with diabetes is published by American Diabetes Association, 1660 Duke St., Alexandria, VA 22314.

Novo Nordisk™, Velosulin® and Lente® are trademarks of Novo Nordisk A/S

MiniMed®, Polyfin™ and Sofset™ are trademarks of MiniMed Inc.

For information contact: Novo Nordisk Pharmaceuticals, Inc. Princeton, NJ 08540

Manufactured by: Novo Nordisk A/S, 2880 Bagsvaerd, Denmark

Date of issue: January 1995

HUMAN INSULIN OTC

NOVOLIN® L

Lente®, Human Insulin Zinc Suspension (recombinant DNA origin)
100 units/ml

PRODUCT DESCRIPTION

Novolin® L is commonly known as Lente® Human Insulin Zinc Suspension (recombinant DNA origin). The concentration of this product is 100 units of insulin per milliliter. It is a cloudy or milky suspension of 70% crystalline and 30% amorphous human insulin. The insulin substance (the cloudy material) settles at the bottom of the vial, therefore, the vial must be gently agitated or rotated so that the contents are uniformly mixed before a dose is withdrawn. **Novolin® L** has an intermediate duration of action. The effect of **Novolin® L** begins approximately $2^1/_2$ hours after injection. The effect is maximal between 7 and 15 hours and ends approximately 22 hours after injection. The time course of action of any insulin may vary considerably in different individuals or at different times in the same individual. Because of this variation, the periods listed here should be considered as general guidelines only.

This human insulin (recombinant DNA origin) is structurally identical to the insulin produced by the human pancreas. This human insulin is produced by recombinant DNA technology utilizing *Saccharomyces cerevisiae* (bakers' yeast) as the production organism.

STORAGE

Insulin should be stored in a cold place, preferably in a refrigerator, but not in the freezing compartment. **Do not let it freeze.** Keep the insulin vial in its carton so that it will stay clean and protected from light. If refrigeration is not possible, the bottle of insulin which you are currently using can be kept unrefrigerated as long as it is kept as cool as possible and away from heat and sunlight.

Never use **Novolin® L** if the precipitate (the white deposit at the bottom of the vial) has become lumpy or granular in appearance or has formed a deposit of solid particles on the wall of the vial. This insulin should not be used if the liquid in the vial remains clear after the vial has been gently agitated.

Never use insulin after the expiration date which is printed on the vial label and carton.

MIXING TWO TYPES OF INSULIN—SEE NOVOLIN® N

SEE NOVOLIN® 70/30 for complete package insert information on Warning: Insulin Use in Diabetes: Types of Insulins: Syringes: Needle-Free Injectors: Important Statement: Preparing the Injection: Giving the Injection: Usage in Pregnancy: Insulin Reaction and Shock: Diabetic Ketoacidosis and Coma: Adverse Reactions: Important Notes.

Date of Issue: December 1995

HOW SUPPLIED

Vials, U-100, 100 units/mL, 10 mL, (List No. 183511) (1's)

PURIFIED INSULIN OTC

LENTE® PURIFIED PORK INSULIN ZINC SUSPENSION USP 100 units/ml

PRODUCT DESCRIPTION

Lente® Purified Pork Insulin Zinc Suspension, USP, 100 units of insulin per milliliter, is a cloudy or milky suspension of 70% crystalline and 30% amorphous purified pork insulin. The insulin substance (the cloudy material) settles at the bottom of the vial, therefore, the vial must be gently agitated or rotated so that the contents are uniformly mixed before a dose is withdrawn. **Lente® Purified Insulin** has an intermediate duration of action. The effect of **Lente® Purified Insulin** begins approximately $2^1/_2$ hours after injection. The effect is maximal between 7 and 15 hours and ends approximately 22 hours after injection. The time course of action of any insulin may vary considerably in different individuals, or at different times in the same individual. Because of this variation, the time periods listed here should be considered as general guidelines only.

The word "purified" on the label indicates that this insulin differs from standard insulin in that it has undergone additional purification steps (i.e., molecular sieve and ion-exchange chromatography).

STORAGE

Insulin should be stored in a cold place, preferably in a refrigerator, but not in the freezing compartment. **Do not let it freeze.** Keep the insulin vial in its carton so that it will stay clean and protected from light. If refrigeration is not possible, the bottle of insulin which you are currently using can be kept unrefrigerated as long as it is kept as cool as possible and away from heat and sunlight.

Never use **Lente® Purified Insulin** if the precipitate (the white deposit at the bottom of the vial) has become lumpy or granular in appearance or has formed a deposit of solid particles on the wall of the vial. This insulin should not be used if the liquid in the vial remains clear after the vial has been gently agitated.

Never use insulin after the expiration date which is printed on the vial label and carton.

MIXING TWO TYPES OF INSULIN—See NOVOLIN® N

See NOVOLIN® 70/30 for package insert information on Warning: Insulin use in Diabetes: Types of Insulin: Syringes: Needle-Free Injectors: Important Statement: Preparing the Injection: Giving the Injection; Usage in Pregnancy: Insulin Reaction and Shock: Diabetic Ketoacidosis and Coma: Adverse Reactions: Important Notes.

Date of Issue: December 1995

HOW SUPPLIED

Vials, U-100, 100 units/mL, 10 mL, (List No. 244210) (1's)

NPH PURIFIED PORK ISOPHANE INSULIN SUSPENSION USP 100 units/ml OTC

PRODUCT DESCRIPTION

NPH Purified Pork Isophane Insulin Suspension, USP, 100 units of insulin per milliliter, is a cloudy or milky suspension of purified pork insulin with protamine and zinc. The insulin substance (the cloudy material) settles at the bottom of the vial, therefore, the vial must be gently agitated or rotated so that the contents are uniformly mixed before a dose is withdrawn. **NPH Purified Insulin** has an intermediate duration of action. The effect of **NPH Purified Insulin** begins approximately $1^1/_2$ hours after injection. The effect is maximal between 4 and 12 hours and ends approximately 24 hours after injection. The time course of action of any insulin may vary considerably in different individuals, or at different times in the same individual. Because of this variation, the time periods listed here should be considered as general guidelines only.

The word "purified" on the label indicates that this insulin differs from standard insulin in that it has undergone additional purification steps (i.e., molecular sieve and ion-exchange chromatography).

STORAGE

Insulin should be stored in a cold place, preferably in a refrigerator, but not in the freezing compartment. **Do not let it freeze.** Keep the insulin vial in its carton so that it will stay clean and protected from light. If refrigeration is not possible, the bottle of insulin which you are currently using can be kept unrefrigerated as long as it is kept as cool as possible and away from heat and sunlight.

Never use **NPH Purified Insulin** if the precipitate (the white deposit at the bottom of the vial) has become lumpy or granular in appearance or has formed a deposit of solid particles on the wall of the vial. This insulin should not be used if the liquid in the vial remains clear after the vial has been gently agitated.

Never use insulin after the expiration date which is printed on the vial label and carton.

MIXING TWO TYPES OF INSULIN—See NOVOLIN® N

See NOVOLIN® 70/30 for package insert information on Warning: Insulin use in Diabetes: Types of Insulin: Syringes: Needle-Free Injectors: Important Statement: Preparing the Injection: Giving the Injection: Usage in Pregnancy: Insulin Reaction and Shock: Diabetic Ketoacidosis and Coma: Adverse Reactions: Important Notes.

Date of Issue: December 1995

HOW SUPPLIED

Vials, U-100, 100 units/mL, 10 mL, (List No. 244710) (1's)

REGULAR PURIFIED PORK INSULIN INJECTION USP 100 units/ml OTC

PRODUCT DESCRIPTION

Regular Purified Pork Insulin Injection, USP, 100 units of insulin per milliliter, is a clear, colorless solution which has a short duration of action. The effect of **Regular Purified Insulin** begins approximately $^1/_2$ hour after injection. The effect is maximal between $2^1/_2$ and 5 hours and ends approximately 8 hours after injection. The time course of action of any insulin may vary considerably in different individuals, or at different times in the same individual. Because of this variation, the time periods listed here should be considered as general guidelines only.

The word "purified" on the label indicates that this insulin differs from standard insulin in that it has undergone additional purification steps (i.e., molecular sieve and ion-exchange chromatography).

STORAGE

Insulin should be stored in a cold place, preferably in a refrigerator, but not in the freezing compartment. **Do not let it freeze.** Keep the insulin vial in its carton so that it will stay clean and protected from light. If refrigeration is not possible, the bottle of insulin which you are currently using can be kept unrefrigerated as long as it is kept as cool as possible and away from heat and sunlight.

Never use Regular Purified Pork Insulin if it becomes viscous (thickened) or cloudy; use it only if it is clear and colorless.

Never use insulin after the expiration date which is printed on the vial label and carton.

IMPORTANT NOTES

1. Due to the risk of precipitation in some pump catheters, this regular purified pork insulin is not recommended for use in insulin pumps.

2. A change in the type, strength, species or purity of insulin could require a dosage adjustment. Any change in insulin should be made under medical supervision.

3. You may have learned how to test your urine or your blood for glucose. It is important to do these tests regularly and to record the results for review with your physician or nurse educator.

4. If you have an acute illness, especially with vomiting or fever, continue taking your insulin. If possible, stay on your regular diet. If you have trouble eating, drink fruit juices, regular soft drinks, or clear soups; if you can, eat small amounts of bland foods. Test your urine for glucose and ketones and, if possible, test your blood glucose. Note the results and contact your physician for possible insulin dose adjustment. If you have severe and prolonged vomiting, seek emergency medical care.

5. You should always carry identification which states that you have diabetes.

Always consult your physician if you have any questions about your condition or the use of insulin.

MIXING TWO TYPES OF INSULIN—See NOVOLIN® N

See NOVOLIN® 70/30 for package insert information on Warning: Insulin use in Diabetes: Types of Insulin: Syringes: Needle-Free Injectors: Important Statement: Preparing the Injection: Giving the Injection: Usage in Pregnancy: Insulin Reaction and Shock: Diabetic Ketoacidosis and Coma: Adverse Reactions.

Date of Issue: December 1995

HOW SUPPLIED

Vials, U-100, 100 units/mL, 10 mL, (List No. 244010) (1's)

PRANDIN™ ℞
(repaglinide) Tablets
(0.5, 1, and 2 mg)

DESCRIPTION

PRANDIN™ (repaglinide) is an oral blood glucose-lowering drug of the meglitinide class used in the management of type 2 diabetes mellitus (also known as non-insulin dependent diabetes mellitus or NIDDM). Repaglinide, S(+) 2-ethoxy-4(2((3-methyl-1-(2-(1-piperidinyl) phenyl)-butyl) amino)-2-oxoethyl) benzoic acid, is chemically unrelated to the oral sulfonylurea insulin secretagogues.

The structural formula is as shown below:

Repaglinide is a white to off-white powder with molecular formula $C_{27}H_{36}N_2O_4$ and a molecular weight of 452.6. PRANDIN™ tablets contain 0.5 mg, 1 mg, or 2 mg of repaglinide. In addition each tablet contains the following inactive ingredients: calcium hydrogen phosphate (anhydrous), microcrystalline cellulose, maize starch, polacrilin potassium, povidone, glycerol (85%), magnesium stearate, meglumine, and poloxamer. The 1 mg and 2 mg tablets contain iron oxides (yellow or red, respectively) as coloring agents.

CLINICAL PHARMACOLOGY
Mechanism of Action
Repaglinide lowers blood glucose levels by stimulating the release of insulin from the pancreas. This action is dependent upon functioning beta (β) cells in the pancreatic islets. Insulin release is glucose-dependent and diminishes at low glucose concentrations.

Repaglinide closes ATP-dependent potassium channels in the β-cell membrane by binding at characterizable sites. This potassium channel blockade depolarizes the β-cell, which leads to an opening of calcium channels. The resulting increased calcium influx induces insulin secretion. The ion channel mechanism is highly tissue selective with low affinity for heart and skeletal muscle.

Pharmacokinetics
Absorption: After oral administration, repaglinide is rapidly and completely absorbed from the gastrointestinal tract. After single and multiple oral doses in healthy subjects or in patients, peak plasma drug levels (C_{max}) occur within 1 hour (T_{max}). Repaglinide is rapidly eliminated from the blood stream with a half-life of approximately 1 hour. The mean absolute bioavailability is 56%. When repaglinide was given with food, the mean T_{MAX} was not changed, but the mean C_{MAX} and AUC (area under the time/plasma concentration curve) were decreased 20% and 12.4%, respectively.

Distribution: After intravenous (IV) dosing in healthy subjects, the volume of distribution at steady state (V_{ss}) was 31

L, and the total body clearance (CL) was 38 L/h. Protein binding and binding to human serum albumin was greater than 98%.

Metabolism: Repaglinide is completely metabolized by oxidative biotransformation and direct conjugation with glucuronic acid after either an IV or oral dose. The major metabolites are an oxidized dicarboxylic acid (M2), the aromatic amine (M1), and the acyl glucuronide (M7). The cytochrome P-450 enzyme system, specifically 3A4, has been shown to be involved in the N-dealkylation of repaglinide to M2 and the further oxidation to M1. Metabolites do not contribute to the glucose-lowering effect of repaglinide.

Excretion: Within 96 hours after dosing with ^{14}C-repaglinide as a single, oral dose, approximately 90% of the radiolabel was recovered in the feces and approximately 8% in the urine. Only 0.1% of the dose is cleared in the urine as parent compound. The major metabolite (M2) accounted for 60% of the administered dose. Less than 2% of parent drug was recovered in feces.

Pharmacokinetic parameters: The pharmacokinetic parameters of repaglinide obtained from a single-dose, crossover study in healthy subjects and from a multiple-dose, parallel, dose-proportionality (0.5, 1, 2 and 4 mg) study in patients with type 2 diabetes are summarized below:

Parameter	Patient with type 2 diabetes[a]
Dose	$AUC_{0-24 hr}$ Mean ±SD (ng/mL*hr):
0.5 mg	68.9 ± 154.4
1 mg	125.8 ± 129.8
2 mg	152.4 ± 89.6
4 mg	447.4 ± 211.3
Dose	$C_{max\ 0-5\ hr}$ Mean ±SD (ng/mL):
0.5 mg	9.8 ± 10.2
1 mg	18.3 ± 9.1
2 mg	26.0 ± 13.0
4 mg	65.8 ± 30.1
Dose	$T_{max\ 0-5\ hr}$ Means (SD)
0.5-4 mg	1.0-1.4 (0.3-0.5) hr
Dose	$T_{1/2}$ Means (Ind Range)
0.5-4 mg	1.0-1.4 (0.4-8.0) hr
Parameter	Healthy Subjects
CL based on i.v.	38± 16 L/hr
V_{ss} based on i.v.	31± 12 L
AbsBio	56± 9%

a: dosed preprandially with three meals
CL = Total body clearance
V_{ss} = Volume of distribution at steady state
AbsBio = Absolute bioavailability

These data indicate that repaglinide did not accumulate in serum. Clearance of oral repaglinide did not change over the 0.5-4 mg dose range, indicating a linear relationship between dose and plasma drug levels.

Variability of exposure: Repaglinide AUC after multiple doses of 0.25 to 4 mg with each meal varies over a wide range. The intra-individual and inter-individual coefficients of variation were 36% and 69%, respectively. AUC over the therapeutic dose range included 69 to 1005 ng/mL*hr, but AUC exposure up to 5417 ng/mL*hr was reached in dose escalation studies without apparent adverse consequences.

Special populations:
Geriatric. Healthy volunteers were treated with a regimen of 2 mg taken before each of 3 meals. There were no significant differences in repaglinide pharmacokinetics between the group of patients <65 years of age and a comparably

sized group of patients ≥65 years of age. (See **PRECAUTIONS, Geriatric Use**)

Pediatric. No studies have been performed in pediatric patients.

Gender. A comparison of pharmacokinetics in males and females showed the AUC over the 0.5 mg to 4 mg dose range to be 15% to 70% higher in females with type 2 diabetes. This difference was not reflected in the frequency of hypoglycemic episodes (male: 16%; female: 17%) or other adverse events. With respect to gender, no change in general dosage recommendation is indicated since dosage for each patient should be individualized to achieve optimal clinical response.

Race. No pharmacokinetic studies to assess the effects of race have been performed, but in a U.S. 1-year study in patients with type 2 diabetes, the blood glucose-lowering effect was comparable between Caucasians (n=297) and African-Americans (n=33). In a U.S. dose-response study, there was no apparent difference in exposure (AUC) between Caucasians (n=74) and Hispanics (n=33).

Renal insufficiency.
Single-dose and steady-state pharmacokinetics of repaglinide were evaluated in patients with various degrees of renal impairment. Measures of AUC and C_{max} after multiple dosing of 2 mg repaglinide were found to be higher in three groups of patients with reduced renal function ($AUC_{mild/moderate\ impairment}$: 90.8 ng/mL*hr to $AUC_{severe\ impairment}$: 137.7 ng/mL*hr versus $AUC_{healthy}$: 29.1 ng/mL*hr; $C_{max,\ mild/moderate\ impairment}$: 46.7 ng/mL to $C_{max,\ severe\ impairment}$: 44.0 ng/mL versus $C_{max,\ healthy}$: 20.6 ng/mL). Repaglinide AUC is only weakly correlated to creatinine clearance. Initial dosage adjustment does not appear to be necessary, but **subsequent increases in PRANDIN™ should be made carefully in patients with type 2 diabetes who have renal function impairment or renal failure requiring hemodialysis.**

Hepatic insufficiency.
A single-dose, open-label study was conducted in 12 healthy subjects and 12 patients with chronic liver disease (CLD) classified by caffeine clearance. Patients with moderate to severe impairment of liver function had higher and more prolonged serum concentrations of both total and unbound repaglinide than healthy subjects ($AUC_{healthy}$: 91.6 ng/mL*hr; $AUC_{CLD\ patients}$: 368.9 ng/mL*hr; $C_{max,\ healthy}$: 46.7 ng/mL; $C_{max,\ CLD\ patients}$: 105.4 ng/mL). AUC was statistically correlated with caffeine clearance. No difference in glucose profiles was observed across patient groups. Patients with impaired liver function may be exposed to higher concentrations of repaglinide and its associated metabolites than would patients with normal liver function receiving usual doses. Therefore, **PRANDIN™ should be used cautiously in patients with impaired liver function. Longer intervals between dose adjustments should be utilized to allow full assessment of response.**

Clinical Trials
A four-week, double-blind, placebo-controlled dose-response trial was conducted in 138 patients with type 2 diabetes using doses ranging from 0.25 to 4 mg taken with each of three meals. PRANDIN™ therapy resulted in dose-proportional glucose-lowering over the full dose range. Plasma insulin levels increased after meals and reverted toward baseline before the next meal. Most of the fasting blood glucose-lowering effect was demonstrated within 1–2 weeks.

In a double-blind, placebo-controlled, 3-month dose titration study, PRANDIN™ or placebo doses for each patient were increased weekly from 0.25 mg through 0.5, 1, and 2 mg, to a maximum of 4 mg, until a fasting plasma glucose (FPG) level <160 mg/dL was achieved or the maximum dose reached. The dose that achieved the targeted control or the maximum dose was continued to end of study. FPG and 2-hour post-prandial glucose (PPG) increased in patients receiving placebo and decreased in patients treated with repaglinide. Differences between the repaglinide- and placebo-treated groups were –61 mg/dL (FPG) and –104 mg/dL (PPG). The between-group change in HbA1c, which reflects long-term glycemic control, was 1.7% units.

[See table at top of page]

Prandin™ vs. Placebo Treatment: Mean FPG, PPG, and HbA1c Changes from baseline after 3 months of treatment:

	FPG	(mg/dL)	PPG	(mg/dL)	HbA1c	(%)
	PL	R	PL	R	PL	R
Baseline	215.3	220.2	245.2	261.7	8.1	8.5
Change from baseline (at last visit)	30.3	-31.0*	56.5	-47.6*	1.1	-0.6*

FPG = fasting plasma glucose
PPG = post-prandial glucose
PL = placebo (N=33)
R = repaglinide (N=66)
* p<0.05 for between group difference

Continued on next page

Prandin—Cont.

Another double-blind, placebo-controlled trial was carried out in 362 patients treated for 24 weeks. The efficacy of 1 and 4 mg preprandial doses was demonstrated by lowering of fasting blood glucose and by HbA$_{1C}$ at the end of the study. HbA$_{1C}$ for the PRANDIN™-treated groups (1 and 4 mg groups combined) at the end of the study was decreased compared to the placebo-treated group in previously naive patients and in patients previously treated with oral hypoglycemic agents by 2.1% units and 1.7% units, respectively. In this fixed-dose trial, patients who were naive to oral hypoglycemic agent therapy and patients in relatively good glycemic control at baseline (HbA$_{1c}$ below 8%) showed greater blood glucose-lowering including a higher frequency of hypoglycemia. Patients who were previously treated and who had baseline HbA$_{1c}$ ≥8% reported hypoglycemia at the same rate as patients randomized to placebo. There was no average gain in body weight when patients previously treated with oral hypoglycemic agents were switched to PRANDIN™. The average weight gain in patients treated with PRANDIN™ and not previously treated with sulfonylurea drugs was 3.3%.

The dosing of PRANDIN™ relative to meal-related insulin release was studied in three trials including 58 patients. Glycemic control was maintained during a period in which the meal and dosing pattern was varied (2, 3, or 4 meals per day; before meals × 2, 3 or 4) compared with a period of 3 regular meals and 3 doses per day (before meals × 3). It was also shown that PRANDIN™ can be administered at the start of a meal, 15 minutes before, or 30 minutes before the meal with the same blood glucose lowering effect.

PRANDIN™ was compared to other insulin secretagogues in 1-year controlled trials to demonstrate comparability of efficacy and safety. Hypoglycemia was reported in 16% of 1228 PRANDIN™ patients, 20% of 417 glyburide patients, and 19% of 81 glipizide patients. Of PRANDIN™ treated patients with symptomatic hypoglycemia, none developed coma or required hospitalization.

PRANDIN™ was studied in combination with metformin in 83 patients not satisfactorily controlled on exercise, diet, and metformin alone. Combination therapy with PRANDIN™ and metformin resulted in synergistic improvement in glycemic control compared to repaglinide or metformin monotherapy. HbA$_{1c}$ was improved by 1% unit and FPG decreased by an additional 35 mg/dL.

PRANDIN™ and Metformin Therapy:
Mean HbA$_{1C}$ and FPG
Changes from Baseline after 3 Months Treatment

	PRANDIN™	Combination	Metformin
N	28	27	27
HbA$_{1c}$ (% units)	-0.38	-1.41	-0.33
FPG (mg/dL)	8.8	-39.2	-4.5

INDICATIONS AND USAGE

PRANDIN™ is indicated as an adjunct to diet and exercise to lower the blood glucose in patients with type 2 diabetes mellitus (NIDDM) whose hyperglycemia cannot be controlled satisfactorily by diet and exercise alone.

PRANDIN™ is also indicated for use in combination with metformin to lower blood glucose in patients whose hyperglycemia cannot be controlled by exercise, diet, and either repaglinide or metformin alone. If glucose control has not been achieved after a suitable trial of combination therapy, consideration should be given to discontinuing these drugs and using insulin. Judgments should be based on regular clinical and laboratory evaluations.

In initiating treatment for patients with type 2 diabetes, diet and exercise should be emphasized as the primary form of treatment. Caloric restriction, weight loss, and exercise are essential in the obese diabetic patient. Proper dietary management and exercise alone may be effective in controlling the blood glucose and symptoms of hyperglycemia. In addition to regular physical activity, cardiovascular risk factors should be identified and corrective measures taken where possible.

If this treatment program fails to reduce symptoms and/or blood glucose, the use of an oral blood glucose-lowering agent or insulin should be considered. Use of PRANDIN™ must be viewed by both the physician and patient as a treatment in addition to diet, and not as a substitute for diet or as a convenient mechanism for avoiding dietary restraint. Furthermore, loss of blood glucose control on diet alone may be transient, thus requiring only short-term administration of PRANDIN™.

During maintenance programs, PRANDIN™ should be discontinued if satisfactory lowering of blood glucose is no longer achieved. Judgments should be based on regular clinical and laboratory evaluations.

The Diabetes Control and Complications Trial (DCCT) demonstrated, in patients with type 1 diabetes, that improved glycemic control, as reflected by HbA$_{1C}$ and fasting glucose levels, was associated with a reduction in the diabetic complications retinopathy, neuropathy, and nephropathy. In considering the use of PRANDIN™ or other antidiabetic therapies, it should be recognized that controlling the blood glucose in type 2 diabetes has not been established to be effective in preventing the long-term cardiovascular and neural complications of diabetes. It has not been shown that the implications of the DCCT results also apply to patients with type 2 diabetes. Nonetheless, improved glycemic control appears to be an important goal in many patients with non-insulin-dependent disease because it is presumed that the mechanisms by which glucose causes complications is the same in both forms of diabetes.

CONTRAINDICATIONS

PRANDIN™ is contraindicated in patients with:
1. Diabetic ketoacidosis, with or without coma. This condition should be treated with insulin.
2. Type 1 diabetes.
3. Known hypersensitivity to the drug or its inactive ingredients.

SPECIAL WARNING ON INCREASED RISK OF CARDIOVASCULAR MORTALITY

The administration of oral hypoglycemic drugs has been reported to be associated with increased cardiovascular mortality as compared to treatment with diet alone or diet plus insulin. This warning is based on the study conducted by the University Group Diabetes Program (UGDP), a long-term prospective clinical trial designed to evaluate the effectiveness of glucose-lowering drugs in preventing or delaying vascular complications in patients with type 2 diabetes (NIDDM). The study involved 823 patients who were randomly assigned to one of four treatment groups (Diabetes, 19 (Suppl. 2):747-830; 1970).

UGDP reported that patients treated for 5 to 8 years with diet plus a fixed dose of tolbutamide (1.5 grams per day) had a rate of cardiovascular mortality approximately 2$^{1}/_{2}$ times that of patients treated with diet alone. A significant increase in total mortality was not observed, but the use of tolbutamide was discontinued based on the increase in cardiovascular mortality. Despite controversy regarding the interpretation of these results, the findings of the UGDP study provide an adequate basis for this warning. The patient should be informed of the potential risks and advantages of repaglinide and of alternative modes of therapy. Although PRANDIN™ was not included in the UGDP study, it is prudent from a safety standpoint to consider that this warning may also apply to this oral hypoglycemic agent, in view of similarities in mode of action.

PRECAUTIONS

General: Hypoglycemia: All oral blood glucose-lowering drugs are capable of producing hypoglycemia. Proper patient selection, dosage, and instructions to the patients are important to avoid hypoglycemic episodes. Hepatic insufficiency may cause elevated repaglinide blood levels and may diminish gluconeogenic capacity, both of which increase the risk of serious hypoglycemia. Elderly, debilitated, or malnourished patients, and those with adrenal, pituitary, or hepatic insufficiency are particularly susceptible to the hypoglycemic action of glucose-lowering drugs.

Hypoglycemia may be difficult to recognize in the elderly and in people taking beta-adrenergic blocking drugs. Hypoglycemia is more likely to occur when caloric intake is deficient, after severe or prolonged exercise, when alcohol is ingested, or when more than one glucose-lowering drug is used.

The frequency of hypoglycemia is greater in patients with type 2 diabetes who have not been previously treated with oral blood glucose-lowering drugs (naive) or whose HbA$_{1C}$ is less than 8%. PRANDIN™ should be administered with meals to lessen the risk of hypoglycemia.

Loss of control of blood glucose: When a patient stabilized on any diabetic regimen is exposed to stress such as fever, trauma, infection, or surgery, a loss of glycemic control may occur. At such times, it may be necessary to discontinue PRANDIN™ and administer insulin. The effectiveness of any hypoglycemic drug in lowering blood glucose to a desired level decreases in many patients over a period of time, which may be due to progression of the severity of diabetes or to diminished responsiveness to the drug. This phenomenon is known as secondary failure, to distinguish it from primary failure in which the drug is ineffective in an individual patient when the drug is first given. Adequate adjustment of dose and adherence to diet should be assessed before classifying a patient as a secondary failure.

Information for Patients

Patients should be informed of the potential risks and advantages of PRANDIN™ and of alternative modes of therapy. They should also be informed about the importance of adherence to dietary instructions, of a regular exercise program, and of regular testing of blood glucose and HbA$_{1C}$. The risks of hypoglycemia, its symptoms and treatment, and conditions that predispose to its development and con-

comitant administration of other glucose-lowering drugs should be explained to patients and responsible family members. Primary and secondary failure should also be explained.

Patients should be instructed to take PRANDIN™ before meals (2, 3, or 4 times a day preprandially). Doses are usually taken within 15 minutes of the meal but time may vary from immediately preceding the meal to as long as 30 minutes before the meal. **Patients who skip a meal (or add an extra meal) should be instructed to skip (or add) a dose for that meal.**

Laboratory Tests

Response to all diabetic therapies should be monitored by periodic measurements of fasting blood glucose and glycosylated hemoglobin levels with a goal of decreasing these levels towards the normal range. During dose adjustment, fasting glucose can be used to determine the therapeutic response. Thereafter, both glucose and glycosylated hemoglobin should be monitored. Glycosylated hemoglobin may be especially useful for evaluating long-term glycemic control.

Drug Interactions

In vitro data indicate that repaglinide metabolism may be inhibited by antifungal agents like ketoconazole and miconazole, and antibacterial agents like erythromycin. Drugs that induce the cytochrome P-450 enzyme system 3A4 may increase repaglinide metabolism; such drugs include troglitazone, rifampicin, barbiturates, and carbamazepine. No systematically acquired data are available on increased or decreased plasma levels with 3A4 inhibitors or inducers.

Drug interaction studies performed in healthy volunteers show that PRANDIN™ had no clinically relevant effect on the pharmacokinetic properties of digoxin, theophylline, or warfarin. Thus, no dosage adjustment is required for digoxin, theophylline, or warfarin on coadministration of PRANDIN™. Co-administration of cimetidine with PRANDIN™ did not significantly alter the absorption and disposition of repaglinide.

The hypoglycemic action of oral blood glucose-lowering agents may be potentiated by certain drugs including nonsteroidal anti-inflammatory agents and other drugs that are highly protein bound, salicylates, sulfonamides, chloramphenicol, coumarins, probenecid, monoamine oxidase inhibitors, and beta adrenergic blocking agents. When such drugs are administered to a patient receiving oral blood glucose-lowering agents, the patient should be observed closely for hypoglycemia. When such drugs are withdrawn from a patient receiving oral blood glucose-lowering agents, the patient should be observed closely for loss of glycemic control. Certain drugs tend to produce hyperglycemia and may lead to loss of glycemic control. These drugs include the thiazides and other diuretics, corticosteroids, phenothiazines, thyroid products, estrogens, oral contraceptives, phenytoin, nicotinic acid, sympathomimetics, calcium channel blocking drugs, and isoniazid. When these drugs are administered to a patient receiving oral blood glucose-lowering agents, the patient should be observed for loss of glycemic control. When these drugs are withdrawn from a patient receiving oral blood glucose-lowering agents, the patient should be observed closely for hypoglycemia.

Carcinogenesis, Mutagenesis, and Impairment of Fertility

Long-term carcinogenicity studies were performed for 104 weeks at doses up to and including 120 mg/kg body weight/day (rats) and 500 mg/kg body weight/day (mice) or approximately 60 and 125 times clinical exposure, respectively, on a mg/m^2 basis. No evidence of carcinogenicity was found in mice or female rats. In male rats, there was an increased incidence of benign adenomas of the thyroid and liver. The relevance of these findings to humans is unclear. The no-effect doses for these observations in male rats were 30 mg/kg body weight/day for thyroid tumors and 60 mg/kg body weight/day for liver tumors, which are over 15 and 30 times, respectively, clinical exposure on a mg/m^2 basis.

Repaglinide was non-genotoxic in a battery of *in vivo* and *in vitro* studies: Bacterial mutagenesis (Ames test), *in vitro* forward cell mutation assay in V79 cells (HGPRT), *in vitro* chromosomal aberration assay in human lymphocytes, unscheduled and replicating DNA synthesis in rat liver, and *in vivo* mouse and rat micronucleus tests.

Fertility of male and female rats was unaffected by repaglinide administration at doses up to 80 mg/kg body weight/day (females) and 300 mg/kg body weight/day (males); over 40 times clinical exposure on a mg/m^2 basis.

Pregnancy

Pregnancy category C

Teratogenic Effects: Safety in pregnant women has not been established. Repaglinide was not teratogenic in rats or rabbits at doses 40 times (rats) and approximately 0.8 times (rabbit) clinical exposure (on a mg/m^2 basis) throughout pregnancy. Because animal reproduction studies are not always predictive of human response, PRANDIN™ should be used during pregnancy only if it is clearly needed.

Because recent information suggests that abnormal blood glucose levels during pregnancy are associated with a higher incidence of congenital abnormalities, many experts recommend that insulin be used during pregnancy to maintain blood glucose levels as close to normal as possible.

Nonteratogenic Effects: Offspring of rat dams exposed to repaglinide at 15 times clinical exposure on a mg/m^2 basis during days 17 to 22 of gestation and during lactation developed nonteratogenic skeletal deformities consisting of shortening, thickening, and bending of the humerus during the postnatal period. This effect was not seen at doses up to 2.5 times clinical exposure (on a mg/m^2 basis) on days 1 to 22 of pregnancy or at higher doses given during days 1 to 16 of pregnancy. Relevant human exposure has not occurred to date and therefore the safety of PRANDIN™ administration throughout pregnancy or lactation cannot be established.

Nursing Mothers

In rat reproduction studies, measurable levels of repaglinide were detected in the breast milk of the dams and lowered blood glucose levels were observed in the pups. Cross fostering studies indicated that skeletal changes (see **Nonteratogenic Effects**) could be induced in control pups nursed by treated dams, although this occurred to a lesser degree than those pups treated *in utero*. Although it is not known whether repaglinide is excreted in human milk some oral agents are known to be excreted by this route. Because the potential for hypoglycemia in nursing infants may exist, and because of the effects on nursing animals, a decision should be made as to whether PRANDIN™ should be discontinued in nursing mothers, or if mothers should discontinue nursing. If PRANDIN™ is discontinued and if diet alone is inadequate for controlling blood glucose, insulin therapy should be considered.

Pediatric Use

No studies have been performed in pediatric patients.

Geriatric Use

In repaglinide clinical studies of 24 weeks or greater duration, 415 patients were over 65 years of age. In one-year, active-controlled trials, no differences were seen in effectiveness or adverse events between these subjects and those less than 65 other than the expected age-related increase in cardiovascular events observed for PRANDIN™ and comparator drugs. There was no increase in frequency or severity of hypoglycemia in older subjects. Other reported clinical experience has not identified differences in responses between the elderly and younger patients, but greater sensitivity of some older individuals to PRANDIN™ therapy cannot be ruled out.

ADVERSE REACTIONS

Hypoglycemia: See **Precautions** and **Overdosage** Sections.

PRANDIN™ has been administered to 2931 individuals during clinical trials. Approximately 1500 of these individuals with type 2 diabetes have been treated for at least 3 months, 1000 for at least 6 months, and 800 for at least 1 year. The majority of these individuals (1228) received PRANDIN™ in one of five 1-year, active-controlled trials. The comparator drugs in these 1-year trials were oral sulfonylurea drugs (SU) including glyburide and glipizide. Over one year, 13% of PRANDIN™ patients were discontinued due to adverse events as were 14% of SU patients. The most common adverse events leading to withdrawal were hyperglycemia, hypoglycemia, and related symptoms (see **PRECAUTIONS**). Mild or moderate hypoglycemia occurred in 16% of PRANDIN™ patients, 20% glyburide patients, and 19% of glipizide patients.

The table below lists common adverse events for PRANDIN™ patients compared to both placebo (in trials less than 6 months duration) and to glyburide and glipizide in one year trials. The adverse event profile of PRANDIN™ was generally comparable to that for sulfonylurea drugs (SU).

[See table at top of page]

Cardiovascular events also occur commonly in patients with type 2 diabetes. In one-year comparator trials, the incidence of individual events was not greater than 1% except for chest pain (1.8%) and angina (1.8%). The overall incidence of other cardiovascular events (hypertension, abnormal EKG, myocardial infarction, arrhythmias, and palpitations) was ≤ 1% and not different for PRANDIN™ and the comparator drugs.

The incidence of serious cardiovascular adverse events added together, including ischemia, was slightly higher for repaglinide (4%) than for sulfonylurea drugs (3%) in controlled comparator clinical trials. In 1-year controlled trials, PRANDIN™ treatment was not associated with excess mortality rates compared to rates observed with other oral hypoglycemic agent therapies.

Commonly Reported Adverse Events (% of Patients)*

EVENT	PRANDIN N = 352	PLACEBO N = 108	PRANDIN N = 1228	SU N = 498
	Placebo controlled studies		Active controlled studies	
Metabolic				
Hypoglycemia	31**	7	16	20
Respiratory				
URI	16	8	10	10
Sinusitis	6	2	3	4
Rhinitis	3	3	7	8
Bronchitis	2	1	6	7
Gastrointestinal				
Nausea	5	5	3	2
Diarrhea	5	2	4	6
Constipation	3	2	2	3
Vomiting	3	3	2	1
Dyspepsia	2	2	4	2
Musculoskeletal				
Arthralgia	6	3	3	4
Back Pain	5	4	6	7
Other				
Headache	11	10	9	8
Paresthesia	3	3	2	1
Chest pain	3	1	2	1
Urinary tract infection	2	1	3	3
Tooth disorder	2	0	<1	<1
Allergy	2	0	1	<1

* Events ≥ 2% for the PRANDIN™ group in the placebo-controlled studies and ≥ events in the placebo group
** See trial description in **CLINICAL PHARMACOLOGY, Clinical Trials**

Summary of Serious Cardiovascular Events (% of total patients with events)

	PRANDIN™	SU*
Total Exposed	1228	498
Serious CV Events	4%	3%
Cardiac Ischemic Events	2%	2%
Deaths due to CV Events	0.1%	0.04%

* glyburide and glipizide

Infrequent adverse events (<1% of patients)

Less common adverse clinical or laboratory events observed in clinical trials included elevated liver enzymes, thrombocytopenia, leukopenia, and anaphylactoid reactions (one patient).

OVERDOSAGE

In a clinical trial, patients received increasing doses of PRANDIN™ up to 80 mg a day for 14 days. There were few adverse effects other than those associated with the intended effect of lowering blood glucose. Hypoglycemia did not occur when meals were given with these high doses. Hypoglycemic symptoms without loss of consciousness or neurologic findings should be treated aggressively with oral glucose and adjustments in drug dosage and/or meal patterns. Close monitoring may continue until the physician is assured that the patient is out of danger. Patients should be closely monitored for a minimum of 24 to 48 hours, since hypoglycemia may recur after apparent clinical recovery. There is no evidence that repaglinide is dialyzable using hemodialysis.

Severe hypoglycemic reactions with coma, seizure, or other neurological impairment occur infrequently, but constitute medical emergencies requiring immediate hospitalization. If hypoglycemic coma is diagnosed or suspected, the patient should be given a rapid intravenous injection of concentrated (50%) glucose solution. This should be followed by a continuous infusion of more dilute (10%) glucose solution at a rate that will maintain the blood glucose at a level above 100 mg/dL.

DOSAGE AND ADMINISTRATION

There is no fixed dosage regimen for the management of type 2 diabetes with PRANDIN™.

The patient's blood glucose should be monitored periodically to determine the minimum effective dose for the patient; to detect primary failure, i.e., inadequate lowering of blood glucose at the maximum recommended dose of medication; and to detect secondary failure, i.e., loss of an adequate blood glucose-lowering response after an initial period of effectiveness. Glycosylated hemoglobin levels are of value in monitoring the patient's longer term response to therapy.

Short-term administration of PRANDIN™ may be sufficient during periods of transient blood loss of control in patients usually well controlled on diet.

PRANDIN™ doses are usually taken within 15 minutes of the meal but time may vary from immediately preceding the meal to as long as 30 minutes before the meal.

Starting Dose

For patients not previously treated or whose HbA$_{1C}$ is <8%, the starting dose should be 0.5 mg. For patients previously treated with blood glucose-lowering drugs and whose HbA$_{1C}$ is ≥ 8%, the initial dose is 1 or 2 mg with each meal preprandially (see previous paragraph).

Dose Adjustment

Dosing adjustments should be determined by blood glucose response, usually fasting blood glucose. The preprandial dose should be doubled up to 4 mg until satisfactory blood glucose response is achieved. At least one week should elapse to assess response after each dose adjustment.

The recommended dose range is 0.5 mg to 4 mg taken with meals. PRANDIN™ may be dosed preprandially 2, 3, or 4 times a day in response to changes in the patient's meal pattern. The maximum recommended daily dose is 16 mg.

Patient Management

Long-term efficacy should be monitored by measurement of HbA$_{1c}$ levels approximately every 3 months. Failure to follow an appropriate dosage regimen may precipitate hypoglycemia or hyperglycemia. Patients who do not adhere to their prescribed dietary and drug regimen are more prone to exhibit unsatisfactory response to therapy including hypoglycemia.

Patients Receiving Other Oral Hypoglycemic Agents.

When PRANDIN™ is used to replace therapy with other oral hypoglycemic agents, PRANDIN™ may be started on the day after the final dose is given. Patients should then be observed carefully for hypoglycemia due to potential overlapping of drug effects. When transferred from longer half-life sulfonylurea agents (e.g., chloropropamide) to repaglinide, close monitoring may be indicated for up to one week or longer.

Combination Therapy

If PRANDIN™ monotherapy does not result in adequate glycemic control, metformin may be added. Or, if metformin therapy does not provide adequate control, PRANDIN™ may be added. The starting dose and dose adjustments for PRANDIN™ combination therapy is the same as for PRANDIN™ monotherapy. The dose of each drug should be carefully adjusted to determine the minimal dose required to achieve the desired pharmacologic effect. Failure to do so could result in an increase in the incidence of hypoglycemic episodes. Appropriate monitoring of FPG and HbA$_{1c}$ measurements should be used to ensure that the patient is not subjected to excessive drug exposure or increased probability of secondary drug failure.

Continued on next page

Prandin—Cont.

HOW SUPPLIED

PRANDIN™ (repaglinide) tablets are supplied as unscored, biconvex tablets available in 0.5 mg (white), 1 mg (yellow) and 2 mg (red) strengths. Tablets are embossed with the Novo Nordisk (Apis) bull symbol and colored to indicated strength.

0.5 mg tablets	Bottles of 100	NDC 00169-0081-81
(white)	Bottles of 500	NDC 00169-0081-82
	Bottles of 1000	NDC 00169-0081-83
1 mg tablets	Bottles of 100	NDC 00169-0082-81
(yellow)	Bottles of 500	NDC 00169-0082-82
	Bottles of 1000	NDC 00169-0082-83
2 mg tablets	Bottles of 100	NDC 00169-0084-81
(red)	Bottles of 500	NDC 00169-0084-82
	Bottles of 1000	NDC 00169-0084-83

Do not store above 25°C (77°F). Protect from moisture. Keep bottles tightly closed.
Dispense in tight containers with safety closures.
Caution
Federal law prohibits dispensing without a prescription.

PRANDIN™ is a trademark of Novo Nordisk A/S.

Manufactured in Germany for
Novo Nordisk
Pharmaceuticals, Inc.,
100 Overlook Center, Suite 200
Princeton, NJ 08540.
1-800-727-6500

Copyright © Novo Nordisk 1997
All rights reserved 12/28/97

EDUCATIONAL MATERIAL

PATIENT EDUCATION MATERIALS
NOVO NORDISK DIABETES CARE®
SERVICE PROGRAMS THAT
EDUCATE AND SUPPORT
Novo Nordisk Diabetes Care® is a comprehensive service program encompassing patient education materials, professional education programs and a wide variety of services to support health care professionals and their patients with diabetes.
Some of the items available from Novo Nordisk Diabetes Care® are:

Professional Education
• CME, CNE & CPE Programs
• Speakers Bureau

Patient Education
• Self-management materials
• Materials for individualized treatment
 — for children with diabetes and their parents
 — for patients with type 2 diabetes
 — for patients with complications
 — for patients who read Spanish
For additional information call 1-800-727-6500.

NOVOPHARM, USA INC.

165 EAST COMMERCE DRIVE
SCHAUMBURG, IL 60173-5326

Direct Inquiries to:
Robert J. Gunter, President & C.O.O.
(800) 635-5067
FAX: (847) 882-4232

The following list of Novopharm, Inc. products is provided to facilitate identification. It includes the color(s) and identification codes for all tablets and capsules. NDC Numbers are also provided for each product.

PRODUCT GENERIC NAME Description Color(s)	IDENTIFICATION CODE (Front/Back-Tablets) (Left/Right-Capsules) NDC NUMBER
ACYCLOVIR Capsules, 200mg Rx Blue Opaque	N 940/200 NDC: 55953-0940
ACYCLOVIR Tablets, 400mg Rx Deep Blue	N 943/400 NDC: 55953-0943
ACYCLOVIR Tablets, 800mg Rx White	N 947/800 NDC: 55953-0947
ALBUTEROL Tablets USP, 2MG Rx White	N 480/2 NDC: 55953-0480
ALBUTEROL Tablets USP, 2MG Rx White	N 480/2 NDC: 55953-0480
ALBUTEROL SULFATE Inhalation Aerosol 90 mcg	NDC: 55953-0051
AMANTADINE HCl Syrup, 50mg/5ml Rx Clear/Raspberry	NDC: 55953-0225
AMOXICILLIN Capsules USP, 250MG Rx Caramel/Buff	N 724/250 NDC: 55953-0724
AMOXICILLIN Capsules USP, 500mg Rx Buff/Buff	N 716/500 NDC: 55953-0716
AMOXICILLIN For Oral Suspension USP, 125MG/5ML, Rx	— NDC: 55953-0149
AMOXICILLIN For Oral Suspension USP, 250MG/5ML, Rx	— NDC: 55953-0130
AMOXICILLIN Tablets, 125mg, Chewable Rx Rose/Cherry	N 747/125 NDC: 55953-0747
AMOXICILLIN Rx Tablets, 250mg, Chewable Rose/Cherry	N 751/250 NDC: 55953-0751
ATENOLOL Tablets, 50mg Rx White	N 039/50 NDC: 55953-0039
ATENOLOL Tablets, 100mg Rx White	N 401/100 NDC: 55953-0401
CAPTOPRIL TABLETS White	
12.5 mg	N 132/12.5 55953-0132
25 mg	N 133/25 55953-0133
50 mg	N 134/50 55953-0134
100 mg	N 135/100 55953-0135
CEFACLOR Capsules, 250mg, Rx Lt Orange/White	N 253/250 NDC: 55953-0253
CEFACLOR Capsules, 500mg, Rx Lt Orange/Grey	N 251/500 NDC: 55953-0251
CEPHALEXIN Capsules USP, 250mg Rx Gray/Swedish Orange	N 084/250 NDC: 55953-0084
CEPHALEXIN Capsules USP, 500mg Rx Swedish Orange/Swedish Orange	N 114/500 NDC: 55953-0114
CEPHALEXIN For Oral Suspension USP 125MG/5ML Rx	— NDC: 55953-0106
CEPHALEXIN For Oral Suspension USP 250MG/5ML Rx	— NDC: 55953-0092
CIMETIDINE Tablets USP, 200mg Rx Green	N 181/200 NDC: 55953-0181
CIMETIDINE Tablets USP, 300mg Rx Green	N 192/300 NDC: 55953-0192
CIMETIDINE Tablets USP, 400mg Rx Green	N 204/400 NDC: 55953-0204
CIMETIDINE Tablets USP, 800mg Rx White	N 516/800 NDC: 55953-0516
CIMETIDINE Oral Sol. USP, 300mg/mL Rx Yellow Orange/Berry	NDC: 55953-0805
CLOFIBRATE Capsules, USP, 500MG Rx Yellow	N382 NDC: 55953-0382
DICLOFENAC SODIUM Tablets, 75mg Rx White	N 737/75 NDC: 55953-0737
FLURBIPROFEN Tablets, USP, 50mg Rx White	N 573/50 NDC: 55953-0573
FLURBIPROFEN Tablets, USP, 100mg Rx Deep Blue	N 577/100 NDC: 55953-0577
GLYBURIDE Tablets, USP, 1.25mg Rx White	N 342/1.25 NDC: 55953-0342
GLYBURIDE Tablets, USP, 2.5mg Rx Peach	N 343/2.5 NDC: 55953-0343
GLYBURIDE Tablets USP, 5mg Rx Lt. Green	N 344/5 NDC: 55953-0344
INDOMETHACIN Capsules USP, 25MG Rx Light Green/Light Green	N 420/25 NDC: 55953-0420
INDOMETHACIN Capsules USP, 50MG Rx Light Green/Light Green	N 439/50 NDC: 55953-0439
LOPERAMIDE HYDROCHLORIDE Capsules USP, 2MG Rx White Opaque/White Opaque	N 020/2 NDC: 55953-0020
METOPROLOL TARTRATE Tablets, USP 50mg, Rx White	N 727/50 NDC: 55953-0727
METOPROLOL TARTRATE Tablets, USP 100mg, Rx White	N 734/100 NDC: 55953-0734
MEXILETINE Capsules, USP 150mg Rx Lt. Orange/Tan	N 739/150 NDC: 55953-0739
MEXILETINE Capsules, USP 200mg Rx Lt. Orange/Lt. Orange	N 740/200 NDC: 55953-0740
MEXILETINE Capsules, USP 250mg Rx Lt. Orange/Dk. Green	N 741/250 NDC: 55953-0741
NAPROXEN Tablets USP, 250mg Rx Yellow/Peach	N 517/250 NDC: 55953-0517
NAPROXEN Tablets USP, 375mg Rx Pink	N 518/375 NDC: 55953-0518
NAPROXEN Tablets USP, 500mg Rx Yellow/Peach	N 520/500 NDC: 55953-0520
NAPROXEN SODIUM Tablets USP, 275mg Rx White	N 531/275 NDC: 55953-0531
NAPROXEN SODIUM Tablets USP, 550mg Rx White	N 533/550 NDC: 55953-0533
NIFEDIPINE Capsules USP, 10MG Rx Brown	N 171/10 NDC: 55953-0171
PINDOLOL Tablets USP, 5mg Rx White	N 088/5 NDC: 55953-0088
PINDOLOL Tablets USP, 10mg Rx White	N 093/10 NDC: 55953-0093
RANITIDINE HCl Tablets USP, 150mg Rx White	N 544/150 NDC: 55953-0544
RANITIDINE HCl Tablets USP, 300mg Rx White	N 547/300 NDC: 55953-0547
SELEGILINE HCl Tablets, 5mg, Rx White	N 179/5 NDC: 55953-0179
TIMOLOL MALEATE Tablets USP, 5MG Rx White	N 961/5 NDC: 55953-0961
TIMOLOL MALEATE Tablets USP, 10MG Rx White	N-972/10 NDC: 55953-0972
TIMOLOL MALEATE Tablets USP, 20MG Rx White	N 984/20 NDC: 55953-0984
TOLMETIN SODIUM Capsules USP, 400MG Rx Opaque Red/Opaque Red	N 815/400 NDC: 55953-0815

Nutramax Laboratories, Inc.
**5024 CAMPBELL BOULEVARD
BALTIMORE, MARYLAND 21236**

Direct Inquiries to:
Ph: 800-925-5187
Fax: (410) 931-4009

COSAMIN® DS   OTC

DESCRIPTION

Each Cosamin® DS Capsule Contains: **R.D.A.**

Glucosamine HCl 99+%	500mg	**
Sodium Chondroitin Sulfate 95+%	400mg	**
Ascorbate (Manganese Ascorbate)	66mg	110%
Manganese (Ascorbate)	10mg	**

R.D.A. - PERCENTAGE U.S. RECOMMENDED DAILY ALLOWANCE

**** NO R.D.A. ESTABLISHED**

Recommendation as a dietary supplement:

ACTIONS

Cosamin® is a patented combination of the following dietary ingredients of unparalleled purity. Each has its own primary function in connective tissue synthesis. Studies reported the following chondrometabolic effects*

- *Glucosamine HCl-In addition to being the main substrate for the biosynthesis of glycosaminoglycans and hyaluronic acid, the primary function of glucosamine is to stimulate the secretion of glycosaminoglycans in the articular cartilage. It was also found to provide natural protection against the cartilage-damaging effects of some NSAIDs*.*
- *Chondroitin sulfate-In addition to being the major glycosaminoglycans found in cartilage, its primary function is to inhibit degradative enzymes*. Degradative enzymes contribute to cartilage breakdown.*
- *Manganese-In addition to being a necessary cofactor in the body for the biosynthesis of glycosaminoglycans, it works as a cofactor for mitochondrial superoxide dismutase in the body.*
- *Ascorbate-It is necessary cofactor in the body for collagen biosynthesis. In case of its deficiency, collagen fibers cannot be cross-linked, greatly decreasing the tensile strength of the assembled fibers.*

[See figure above]

INDICATIONS

*The synergistic effect of glucosamine and chondroitin sulfate performing their primary functions **concurrently**, using manganese and ascorbate as cofactors, is what makes Cosamin® unique and the only true **broad-spectrum** cartilage matrix enhancer*. This overall matrix enhancement* will over time allow for lower maintenance dosing, thus making Cosamin® more economical to use the longer a person is on the product.*

> *These statements have not been evaluated by the Food and Drug Administration. This product is not intended to diagnose, treat, cure, or prevent any disease.*

DOSAGE

During the initial 60 day period: Adults weighing under 200 lbs. should take three (3) capsules daily (2 in the AM, 1 in the PM). Individuals weighing over 200 lbs. should take two (2) capsules twice a day. For children, consult your licensed health care professional. After 60 days, the number of capsules taken can be gradually decreased to a level that maintains the individual. The number of capsules may be increased at any time.
For individuals who have difficulty swallowing, capsules may be pulled apart and mixed with food or beverage. Regular Strength Cosamin® is also available in a smaller capsule size.

HOW SUPPLIED

Bottles of 90 & 180 capsules.
U.S. Patent Nos. 5,364,845 and 5,587,363.
NUTRAMAX LABORATORIES, INC.
5024 Campbell Boulevard • Baltimore, Maryland 21236
(410) 931 4000 • FAX (410) 931 4009
1-800-925-5187 U.S. & Canada
www.cosamin.com
Shown in Product Identification Guide, page 326

For your complimentary copies of Frequently Asked Questions booklets, please call 1-800-925-5187.

COSAMIN® DS   **MECHANISM OF ACTION**

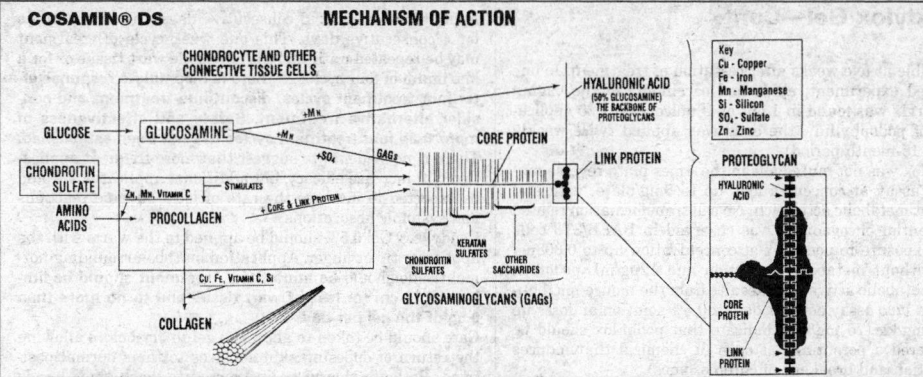

Oclassen Pharmaceuticals, Inc.
**A Division of
Watson Labs Inc.
CORONA, CA 91720**

Direct Inquiries to:
Customer Service Department
(800) 272-5525
Fax (909) 270-1096

For Medical Information Contact:
In Emergencies:
Customer Service Department
(800) 272-5525
Fax (909) 270-1096

CONDYLOX® Gel 0.5%   ℞
[cŏn 'dy-lox]
(podofilox gel)

DESCRIPTION

Podofilox is an antimitotic drug which can be chemically synthesized or purified from the plant families *Coniferae* and *Berberidaceae* (e.g. species of *Juniperus* and *Podophyllum*). Condylox® Gel 0.5% is formulated for topical administration. Each gram of gel contains 5mg of podofilox in a buffered alcoholic gel containing alcohol, glycerin, lactic acid, hydroxypropyl cellulose, sodium lactate, and butylated hydroxytoluene.
Podofilox has a molecular weight of 414.4 daltons, and is soluble in alcohol and sparingly soluble in water. Its chemical name is [5R-(5α,5aβ,8aα,9α)-5,8,8a,9-tetrahydro-9-hydroxy-5-(3,4,5-trimethoxyphenyl) furo[3',4':6,7]naphtho-[2,3,-d]-1,3-dioxol-6(5aH)-one.
Podofilox has the following structural formula:

CLINICAL PHARMACOLOGY

Mechanism of Action
Treatment of anogenital warts with podofilox results in necrosis of visible wart tissue. The exact mechanism of action is unknown.
Pharmacokinetics
In systemic absorption studies in 52 patients, topical application of 0.05mL of an ethanolic solution containing 0.5% podofilox to external genitalia did not result in detectable serum levels. Applications of 0.1 to 1.5mL resulted in peak serum levels of 1 to 17 ng/mL one to two hours after application. The elimination half-life ranged from 1.0 to 4.5 hours. The drug was not found to accumulate after multiple treatments.[1]

CLINICAL STUDIES

In the first multicenter clinical study in 326 patients with anogenital warts, Condylox® Gel 0.5% and its vehicle were applied in a double-blind fashion to comparable patient groups. Of the 260 patients with efficacy data, 176 were treated with Condylox® Gel 0.5%. Patients applied Condylox® Gel 0.5% twice daily for three consecutive days followed by a 4 day "rest" period.
At the end of 4 weeks, 38.4% of the patients had complete clearing of the wart tissue when treated with Condylox® Gel 0.5%.

In the second multicenter clinical trial in 108 evaluable patients with anogenital warts, Condylox® (podofilox) Topical Solution 0.5% was compared with Condylox® Gel 0.5% for efficacy. As in the first clinical trial, patients applied Condylox® Gel 0.5% twice daily for three consecutive days followed by a four day "rest" period.
Similar clearance rates were observed. At the end of 4 weeks, 25.6% of the patients had complete clearing of the wart tissue when treated with Condylox® Gel 0.5%.

INDICATIONS AND USAGE

Condylox® Gel 0.5% is indicated for the topical treatment of anogenital warts (external genital warts and perianal warts). This product is *not* indicated in the treatment of mucous membrane warts (see **PRECAUTIONS**).
Diagnosis
Although anogenital warts have a characteristic appearance, histopathologic confirmation should be obtained if there is any doubt of the diagnosis. Differentiating warts from squamous cell carcinoma and "Bowenoid papulosis" is of particular concern. Squamous cell carcinoma may also be associated with human papillomavirus which should not be treated with Condylox® Gel 0.5%.

CONTRAINDICATIONS

Condylox® Gel 0.5% is contraindicated for patients who develop hypersensitivity or intolerance to any components of the formulation.

WARNINGS

Correct diagnosis of the lesions to be treated is essential. See the **Diagnosis** subsection of the **INDICATIONS AND USAGE** section. Condylox® Gel 0.5% is intended for cutaneous use only. **Avoid contact with the eyes. If contact with the eyes occurs, patients should immediately flush the eyes with copious quantities of water and seek medical advice.**
Drug Product is Flammable. Keep Away From Open Flame.

PRECAUTIONS

General
Data are not available on the safe and effective use of this product for treatment of warts occurring on mucous membranes of the genital area (including the urethra, rectum and vagina). The recommended method of application, frequency of application, and duration of usage should not be exceeded (see **DOSAGE AND ADMINISTRATION**).
Information for Patients
Patients using Condylox® Gel 0.5% should receive the following information and instructions. This information is intended to aid in the safe and effective use of this medication. It is not intended to disclose all possible adverse or intended effects.
1) This medication should be used only as directed by the health care provider. Patients should be instructed to wash their hands thoroughly before and after each application. It is for external use only. Avoid contact with the eyes.
2) Patients should be advised not to use this medication for any disorder other than for which it was prescribed.
3) Patients should report any signs of adverse reactions to the health care provider.
4) If no improvement is observed after 4 weeks of treatment, discontinue the medication and consult the health care provider.
Carcinogenesis, Mutagenesis and Impairment of Fertility
An 80-week carcinogenicity study in the mouse was performed using a 0.5% podofilox solution applied dermally at 0.04, 0.2 and 1.0 mg/kg/day. There were no differences between the podofilox treated mice at any dose level and vehicle control in the incidence of neoplasia. Published animal studies, in general, have not shown the drug substance, podofilox, to be carcinogenic.[2,3,4,5,6] There are published reports that, in mouse studies, crude podophyllin resin (containing podofilox) applied topically to the cervix produced changes resembling carcinoma *in situ*.[7] These changes were

Continued on next page

Condylox Gel—Cont.

reversible at five weeks after cessation of treatment. In one reported experiment, epidermal carcinoma of the vagina and cervix was found in 1 out of 18 mice after 120 applications of podophyllin[8] (the drug was applied twice weekly over a 15-month period).

Podofilox was not mutagenic in the Ames plate reverse mutation assay at concentrations up to 5mg/plate, with and without metabolic activation. No cell transformation related to potential oncogenicity was observed in BALB/3T3 cells after exposure to podofilox at concentration up to 0.008µg/mL, without metabolic activation and 12µg/mL podofilox with metabolic activation. Results from the mouse micronucleus *in vivo* assay using podofilox 0.5% solution at doses up to 25 mg/kg (75 mg/m^2), indicate that podofilox should be considered a potential clastogen (a chemical that induces disruption and breakage of chromosomes).

Daily topical application of 0.5% podofilox solution at doses up to the equivalent of 0.2mg/kg (1.18 mg/m^2, approximately equivalent to the human daily dose) to rats throughout gametogenesis, mating, gestation, parturition and lactation for two generation demonstrated no impairment of fertility.

Pregnancy

Pregnancy Category C: 0.5% podofilox solution was not teratogenic in the rabbit following topical application of up to 0.21 mg/kg (2.85 mg/m^2, approximately 2 times the maximum human dose) once daily for 13 days. The scientific literature contains references that podofilox is embryotoxic in rats when administered intaperitoneally at a dose of 5 mg/kg (29.5 mg/m^2, approximately 19 times the recommended maximum human dose).[9] Teratogenicity and embryotoxicity have not been studies with intravaginal application. Many antimitotic drug products are known to be embryotoxic. There are no adequate and well-controlled studies in pregnant women. Condylox® Gel 0.5% should be used during pregnancy only if the potential benefit justifies the potential risk to the fetus.

Nursing Mothers

It is not known whether this drug is excreted in human milk. Because of the potential for serious adverse reactions in nursing infants from podofilox, a decision should be made whether to discontinue nursing or to discontinue the drug, taking into account the importance of the drug to the mother.

Pediatric Use

Safety and effectiveness in pediatric patients have not been established.

ADVERSE REACTIONS

In clinical trials with Condylox® Gel 0.5%, the following local adverse reactions were reported during the treatment of anogenital warts. The severity of local adverse reactions were predominantly mild or moderate and did not increase during the treatment period. Severe reactions were most frequent within the first 2 weeks of treatment.

Adverse Reaction	Mild	Moderate	Severe
Inflammation	32.2%	30.4%	9.3%
Burning	37.1%	25.9%	11.5%
Erosion	27.0%	20.8%	8.9%
Pain	23.7%	20.4%	11.5%
Itching	32.2%	16.0%	7.8%
Bleeding	19.2%	3.0%	0.7%

Other local adverse reactions reported included stinging (7%), and erythema (5%); less commonly reported local adverse events included desquamation, scabbing, discoloration, tenderness, dryness, crusting, fissures, soreness, ulceration, swelling/edema, tingling, rash, and blisters.

The most common systemic adverse event reported during the clinical studies was headache (7%).

OVERDOSAGE

Topically applied podofilox may be absorbed systemically (see **CLINICAL PHARMACOLOGY** section). Toxicity reported following systemic administration of podofilox in investigational use for cancer treatment included: nausea, vomiting, fever, diarrhea, bone marrow depression, and oral ulcers. Following 5 to 10 daily intravenous doses of 0.5 to 1 mg/kg/day, significant hematological toxicity occurred but was reversible.[10] Other toxicities occurred at lower doses. Toxicity reported following systemic administration of podophyllum resin included: nausea, vomiting, fever, diarrhea, peripheral neuropathy, altered mental status, lethargy, coma, tachypnea, respiratory failure, leukocytosis, pancytosis, hematuria, renal failure and seizures.[11] Treatment of topical overdosage should include washing the skin free of any remaining drug and symptomatic and supportive therapy.

DOSAGE AND ADMINISTRATION

The prescriber should ensure that the patients is fully aware of the correct method of therapy and identify which specific warts should be treated.

Apply twice daily for 3 consecutive days, then discontinue for 4 consecutive days. This one week cycle of treatment may be repeated until there is no visible wart tissue or for a maximum of four cycles. **If there is incomplete response after four treatment cycles, discontinue treatment and consider alternative treatment. Safety and effectiveness of more than four treatment cycles has not been established.** There is no evidence to suggest that more frequent application will increase efficacy, but additional applications would be expected to increase the rate of local adverse reactions and systemic absorptions.

Condylox® Gel 0.5% should be applied to the warts with the applicator tip or finger. Application on the surrounding normal tissue should be minimized. **Treatment should be limited to 10 cm^2 or less of wart tissue and to no more than 0.5g of the gel per day.**

Care should be taken to allow the gel to dry before allowing the return of opposing skin surfaces to their normal positions. Patients should be instructed to wash their hands thoroughly before and after each application.

HOW SUPPLIED

Condylox® Gel 0.5% is supplied as 3.5g of clear gel in aluminum tubes with an applicator tip. NDC 55515-102-01. Store at controlled room temperature between 15-30°C (59-86°F). **Avoid excessive heat. Do not freeze.**

Rx only

REFERENCES

1. von Krogh G. Podophyllotoxin in serum: Absorption subsequent to three day repeated applications of a 0.5% ethanolic preparation on condylomata acuminata. Sex Trans Disease 1982: 9: 26–33.
2. Berenblum I. The effect of podophyllotoxin on the skin of the mouse, with reference to carcinogenic, cocarcinogenic, and anticarcinogenic action. J Cancer Inst 11: 839–841, 1951.
3. Kaminetzky HA, Swerdlow M. Podophyllin and the mouse cervix: assessment of carcinogenic potential. Am J Obst Gyn 95:486–490, 1965.
4. McGrew EA, Kaminetzky HA. The genesis of experimental cervical epithelial dysplasia. Am J Clin Path 35: 538–545, 1961.
5. Roe FJC, Salaman MH. Further studies on incomplete carcinogenesis: triethylene melamine (T.E.M.) 1,2 benzanthracene and beta-propiolactone as initiators of skin tumor formation in the mouse. Brit J Cancer 9:177–203, 1955.
6. Taper HS. Induction of the deficient acid DNAase activity in mouse interfollicular epidermis by croton oil as a possible tumor promoting mechanism. Zeitschrift fur Krebsforschung and Klinisch Onkologie (Cancer Research and Clinical Oncology, Berlin) 90:197–210, 1977.
7. Kaminetzky HA, McGrew EA, Phillips RL. Experimental cervical epithelial dysplasia. J Obst Gyn 14:1–10, 1959.
8. Kaminetzky HA, McGrew EA: Podophyllin and mouse cervix: Effect of long term application. Arch Path 73: 481–485, 1962.
9. Thiersch JB. Effect of podophyllin (P) and podophylotoxine (PT.) on the rat litter in utero. Soc Exptl Biol Med Proc 113:124–27, 1963.
10. Savel H.: Clinical experience with intravenous podophyllotoxin. Proc Amer Assoc Cancer Res, 1964; 5: 56.
11. Cassidy DE, Dewry J and Fanning JP: Podophyllum toxicity: A report of a fatal case and a review of the literature. J Toxicol Clinic Toxicol 1982: 19:35–44.

Mfd. for
OCLASSEN PHARMACEUTICALS, INC.
a division of Watson Laboratories Inc.
Corona CA 91720
by DPT Laboratories, Inc.
San Antonio, TX 78215

Revised March 10, 1998
126963-0397

Shown in Product Identification Guide, page 326

CONDYLOX® ℞

[*con 'de-lox*]
(podofilox)
Topical Solution 0.5%

DESCRIPTION

Condylox® is the brand name of podofilox, an antimitotic drug which can be chemically synthesized or purified from the plant families *Coniferae* and *Berberidaceae* (e.g. species of *Juniperus* and *Podophyllum*). Condylox® 0.5% Solution is formulated for topical administration. Each milliliter of solution contains 5 mg of podofilox, in a vehicle containing lactic acid and sodium lactate in alcohol 95%, USP.

Podofilox has a molecular weight of 414.4 daltons, and is soluble in alcohol and sparingly soluble in water. Its chemical name is 5,8,8a,9-Tetrahydro-9-hydroxy-5- (3,4,5-trimethoxylphenyl)furo [3′,4′:6,7] naphtho [2,3,d] -1,3-dioxol-6(5aH)-one. Podofilox has the following structural formula:

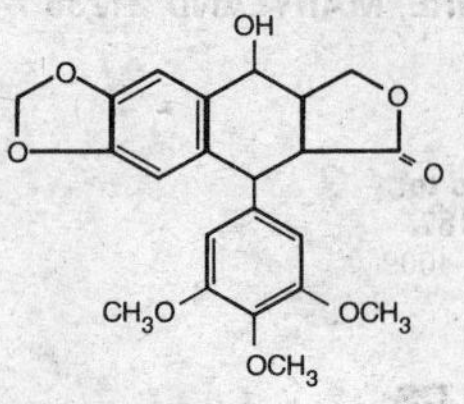

CLINICAL PHARMACOLOGY

Mechanism of Action

Treatment of genital warts with podofilox results in necrosis of visible wart tissue. The exact mechanism of action is unknown.

Pharmacokinetics

In systemic absorption studies in 52 patients, topical application of 0.05 mL of 0.5% podofilox solution to external genitalia did not result in detectable serum levels. Application of 0.1 to 1.5 mL resulted in peak serum levels of 1 to 17 ng/mL one to two hours after application. The elimination half-life ranged from 1.0 to 4.5 hours. The drug was not found to accumulate after multiple treatments.

CLINICAL STUDIES

In clinical studies with Condylox® Solution, the test product and its vehicle were applied in a double-blind fashion to comparable patient groups. Patients were treated for two to four weeks, and re-evaluated at a two-week follow-up examination. Although the number of patients and warts evaluated at each time period varied, the results among investigators were relatively consistent.

The following table represents the responses noted in terms of frequency of response by lesions treated and the overall response by patients. Data are presented for the 2-week follow-up only for those patients evaluated at that time point.

Responses in Treated Patients

	Initially Cleared*	Recurred after Clearing*	Cleared at 2-Week Follow-Up*
% Warts (n=524)	79% (412/524)	35% (146/412)	60% (269/449)
% Patients (n=70)	50% (35/70)	60% (21/35)	25% (14/57)

* Cleared and clearing mean no visible wart tissue remained at the treated sites

INDICATIONS AND USAGE

Condylox® 0.5% Solution is indicated for the topical treatment of external genital warts (Condyloma acuminatum). This product is *not* indicated in the treatment of perianal or mucous membrane warts (see **PRECAUTIONS**).

Diagnosis

Although genital warts have a characteristic appearance, histopathologic confirmation should be obtained if there is any doubt of the diagnosis. Differentiating warts from squamous cell carcinoma (so-called "Bowenoid papulosis") is of particular concern. Squamous cell carcinoma may also be associated with human papillomavirus but should not be treated with Condylox® 0.5% Solution.

CONTRAINDICATIONS

Condylox® 0.5% Solution is contraindicated for patients who develop hypersensitivity or intolerance to any component of the formulation.

WARNINGS

Correct diagnosis of the lesions to be treated is essential. See the "Diagnosis" subsection of the **INDICATIONS AND USAGE** statement.

Condylox® 0.5% Solution is intended for cutaneous use only. **Avoid contact with the eyes. If eye contact occurs, patients should immediately flush the eye with copious quantities of water and seek medical advice.**

PRECAUTIONS

General

Data are not available on the safe and effective use of this product for treatment of warts occurring in the perianal area or mucous membranes of the genital area (including the urethra, rectum and vagina). The recommended method of application, frequency of application, and duration of usage should not be exceeded (see **DOSAGE AND ADMINISTRATION**).

Information for Patients

The patient should be provided with a Patient Information leaflet when a Condylox® prescription is filled.

Carcinogenesis, Mutagenesis and Impairment of Fertility

Reports of lifetime carcinogenicity studies in mice are not available. Published animal studies, in general, have not

shown the drug substance, podofilox, to be carcinogenic.[1,2,3,4,5] There are published reports that, in mouse studies, crude podophyllin resin (containing podofilox) applied topically to the cervix produced changes resembling carcinoma *in situ*.[6] These changes were reversible at five weeks after cessation of treatment. In one reported experiment, epidermal carcinoma of the vagina and cervix was found in 1 out of 18 mice after 120 applications of podophyllin[7] (the drug was applied twice weekly over a 15-month period).

Podofilox was not mutagenic in the Ames plate reverse mutation assay at concentrations up to 5 mg/plate, with and without metabolic activation. No cell transformation related to potential oncogenicity was observed in BALB/3T3 cells after exposure to podofilox at concentrations up to 0.008 µg/mL without metabolic activation and 12 µg/mL podofilox with metabolic activation. Results from the mouse micronucleus in vivo assay using podofilox 0.5% solution in concentrations up to 25 mg/kg, indicate that podofilox should be considered a potential clastogen (a chemical that induces disruption and breakage of chromosomes).

Daily topical applications of Condylox® 0.5% Solution at doses up to the equivalent of 0.2 mg/kg (5 times the recommended maximum human dose) to rats throughout gametogenesis, mating, gestation, parturition and lactation for two generations demonstrated no impairment of fertility.

Pregnancy

Pregnancy Category C: Podofilox was not teratogenic in the rabbit following topical application of up to 0.21 mg/kg (5 times the maximum human dose) once daily for 13 days. The scientific literature contains references that podofilox is embryotoxic in rats when administered systemically in a dose approximately 250 times the recommended maximum human dose.[8,9] Teratogenicity and embryotoxicity have not been studied with intravaginal application. Many antimitotic drug products are known to be embryotoxic. There are no adequate and well-controlled studies in pregnant women. Podofilox should be used in pregnancy only if the potential benefit justifies the potential risk to the fetus.

Nursing Mothers

It is not known whether this drug is excreted in human milk. Because of the potential for serious adverse reactions in nursing infants from podofilox, a decision should be made whether to discontinue nursing or to discontinue the drug, taking into account the importance of the drug to the mother.

Pediatric Use

Safety and effectiveness in pediatric patients have not been established.

ADVERSE REACTIONS

In clinical trials, the following local adverse reactions were reported at some point during treatment.

Adverse Experience	Males	Females
Burning	64%	78%
Pain	50%	72%
Inflammation	71%	63%
Erosion	67%	67%
Itching	50%	65%

Reports of burning and pain were more frequent and of greater severity in women than in men.

Adverse effects reported in less than 5% of the patients included pain with intercourse, insomnia, tingling, bleeding, tenderness, chafing, malodor, dizziness, scarring, vesicle formation, crusting, edema, dryness/peeling, foreskin irretraction, hematuria, vomiting and ulceration.

OVERDOSAGE

Topically applied podofilox may be absorbed systemically (see **CLINICAL PHARMACOLOGY** section). Toxicity reported following systemic administration of podofilox in investigational use for cancer treatment included: nausea, vomiting, fever, diarrhea, bone marrow depression, and oral ulcers. Following 5 to 10 daily intravenous doses of 0.5 to 1 mg/kg/day, significant hematological toxicity occurred but was reversible. Other toxicities occurred at lower doses.

Toxicity reported following systemic administration of podophyllum resin included: nausea, vomiting, fever, diarrhea, peripheral neuropathy, altered mental status, lethargy, coma, tachypnea, respiratory failure, leukocytosis, pancytosis, hematuria, renal failure, and seizures. Treatment of topical overdosage should include washing the skin free of any remaining drug and symptomatic and supportive therapy.

DOSAGE AND ADMINISTRATION

In order to ensure that the patient is fully aware of the correct method of therapy and to identify which specific warts should be treated, the technique for initial application of the medication should be demonstrated by the prescriber.

Apply twice daily morning and evening (every 12 hours), for 3 consecutive days, then withhold use for 4 consecutive days. This one week cycle of treatment may be repeated up to four times until there is no visible wart tissue. **If there is incomplete response after four treatment weeks, alternative treatment should be considered. Safety and effectiveness of more than four treatment weeks have not been established.**

Condylox® 0.5% Solution is applied to the warts with a cotton-tipped applicator supplied with the drug. The drug-dampened applicator should be touched to the wart to be treated, applying the minimum amount of solution necessary to cover the lesion. **Treatment should be limited to less than 10 cm² of wart tissue and to no more than 0.5 mL of the solution per day.** There is no evidence to suggest that more frequent application will increase efficacy, but additional applications would be expected to increase the rate of local adverse reactions and systemic absorption.

Care should be taken to allow the solution to dry before allowing the return of opposing skin surfaces to their normal positions. After each treatment, the used applicator should be carefully disposed of and the patient should wash his or her hands.

HOW SUPPLIED

3.5 mL of Condylox® 0.5% Solution is supplied as a clear liquid in amber glass bottles with child-resistant screw caps. NDC #55515-101-01. Store at controlled room temperature between 15° and 30°C (59° and 86°F). **Avoid excessive heat. Do not freeze.**

Caution: Federal law prohibits dispensing without prescription.

REFERENCES

1. I. Berenblum, 1951. J. Natl. Cancer Inst. *11:* 839–841
2. H.A. Kaminetsky and M. Swerdlow, 1965. Am. J. Obst. Gyn. *95:* 486–490
3. E.A. McGrew and H.A. Kaminetsky. 1961. Am J. Clin. Pathol. *35:* 538–545
4. F.J.C. Roe and M.H. Salaman, 1955. Brit. J. Cancer. *9:* 177–203
5. H.S. Taper, 1977. Z. Kerbsforsch, *90:* 197–210
6. H.A. Kaminetsky and E.A. McGrew, and R.L. Phillips, 1959. Am. J. Obst. Gyn. *14:* 1–10
7. H.A. Kaminetsky and E.A. McGrew, 1962. Arch. Path. *73:* 481–485
8. K. Didcock, D. Jackson, and J.M. Robson, 1956. Brit. J. Pharmacol. *11:* 437–441
9. J. Thiersch, 1963. Soc. Exptl. Biol. Med. Proc. *113:* 124–127

Revised: March, 1998
127339-0398
Mfd. for
OCLASSEN PHARMACEUTICALS, INC.
A Division of Watson Labs., Inc., Carona, CA 91720
by DPT Labs, Ltd., San Antonio, TX 78215

03-4709-R4

Shown in Product Identification Guide, page 326

CORDRAN® Lotion, 0.05% Flurandrenolide Lotion, USP ℞

[*kōr 'drăn*]

DESCRIPTION

Cordran® (Flurandrenolide, USP) is a potent corticosteroid intended for topical use. Flurandrenolide occurs as white to off-white, fluffy, crystalline powder and is odorless. Flurandrenolide is practically insoluble in water and in ether. One g dissolves in 72 mL of alcohol and in 10 mL of chloroform. The molecular weight of flurandrenolide is 436.52.

The chemical name of flurandrenolide is Pregn-4-ene-3,20-dione, 6-fluoro-11,21-dihydroxy-16,17-[(1-methylethylidene)bis (oxy)]-, (6α, 11β, 16α)-; its empirical formula is $C_{24}H_{33}FO_6$. The structure is as follows:

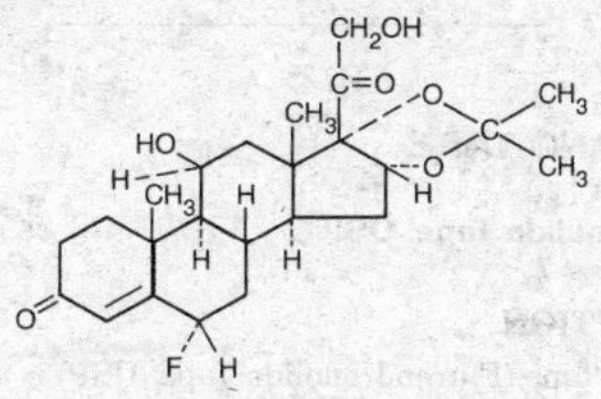

Each mL of Cordran Lotion contains 0.5 mg (1.145 µmol) (0.05%) flurandrenolide in an oil-in-water emulsion base composed of glycerin, cetyl alcohol, stearic acid, glyceryl monostearate, mineral oil, polyoxyl 40 stearate, menthol, benzyl alcohol, and purified water.

CLINICAL PHARMACOLOGY

Cordran is primarily effective because of its anti-inflammatory, antipruritic, and vasoconstrictive actions.

The mechanism of the anti-inflammatory effect of topical corticosteroids is not completely understood. Various laboratory methods, including vasoconstrictor assays, are used to compare and predict potencies and/or clinical efficacies of the topical corticosteroids. There is some evidence to suggest that a recognizable correlation exists between vasoconstrictor potency and therapeutic efficacy in man. Corticosteroids with anti-inflammatory activity may stabilize cellular and lysosomal membranes. There is also the suggestion that the effect on the membranes of lysosomes prevents the release of proteolytic enzymes and, thus, plays a part in reducing inflammation.

Evaporation of water from the lotion vehicle produces a cooling effect, which is often desirable in the treatment of acutely inflamed or weeping lesions.

Pharmacokinetics—The extent of percutaneous absorption of topical corticosteroids is determined by many factors, including the vehicle, the integrity of the epidermal barrier, and the use of occlusive dressings.

Topical corticosteroids can be absorbed from normal intact skin. Inflammation and/or other disease processes in the skin increase percutaneous absorption. Occlusive dressings substantially increase the percutaneous absorption of topical corticosteroids. Thus, occlusive dressings may be a valuable therapeutic adjunct for treatment of resistant dermatoses (*see* **DOSAGE AND ADMINISTRATION**).

Once absorbed through the skin, topical corticosteroids are handled through pharmacokinetic pathways similar to those of systematically administered corticosteroids. Corticosteroids are bound to plasma proteins in varying degrees. They are metabolized primarily in the liver and then excreted in the kidneys. Some of the topical corticosteroids and their metabolites are also excreted into the bile.

INDICATIONS AND USAGE

Cordran is indicated for the relief of the inflammatory and pruritic manifestations of corticosteroid-responsive dermatoses.

CONTRAINDICATIONS

Topical corticosteroids are contraindicated in patients with a history of hypersensitivity to any of the components of these preparations.

PRECAUTIONS

General—Systemic absorption of topical corticosteroids has produced reversible hypothalamic-pituitary-adrenal (HPA) axis suppression, manifestations of Cushing's syndrome, hyperglycemia, and glucosuria in some patients.

Conditions that augment systemic absorption include application of the more potent steroids, use over large surface areas, prolonged use, and the addition of occlusive dressings.

Therefore, patients receiving a large dose of a potent topical steroid applied to a large surface area or under an occlusive dressing should be evaluated periodically for evidence of HPA axis suppression using urinary-free cortisol and ACTH stimulation tests. If HPA axis suppression is noted, an attempt should be made to withdraw the drug, to reduce the frequency of application, or to substitute a less potent steroid.

Recovery of HPA axis function is generally prompt and complete on discontinuation of the drug. Infrequently, signs and symptoms of steroid withdrawal may occur, so that supplemental systemic corticosteroids are required.

Pediatric patients may absorb proportionately large amounts of topical corticosteroids and thus be more susceptible to systemic toxicity (*see Pediatric Use* under **PRECAUTIONS**).

If irritation develops, topical corticosteroids should be discontinued and appropriate therapy instituted.

In the presence of dermatologic infections, the use of an appropriate antifungal or antibacterial agent should be instituted. If a favorable response does not occur promptly, Cordran should be discontinued until the infection has been adequately controlled.

Information for the Patient—Patients using topical corticosteroids should receive the following information and instructions:

1. This medication is to be used as directed by the physician. It is for external use only. Avoid contact with the eyes.
2. Patients should be advised not to use this medication for any disorder other than that for which it was prescribed.
3. The treated skin area should not be bandaged or otherwise covered or wrapped in order to be occlusive unless the patient is directed to do so by the physician.
4. Patients should report any signs of local adverse reactions, especially under occlusive dressing.
5. Parents of pediatric patients should be advised not to use tight-fitting diapers or plastic pants on a patient being treated in the diaper area, because these garmets may constitute occlusive dressings.

Laboratory Tests—The following tests may be helpful in evaluating the HPA axis suppression:

Urinary-free cortisol test
ACTH stimulation test

Continued on next page

Cordran Lotion—Cont.

Carcinogenesis, Mutagenesis, and Impairment of Fertility—Long-term animal studies have not been performed to evaluate the carcinogenic potential or the effect on fertility of topical corticosteroids.
Studies to determine mutagenicity with prednisolone and hydrocortisone have revealed negative results.
Usage in Pregnancy—Pregnancy Category C—Corticosteroids are generally teratogenic in laboratory animals when administered systemically at relatively low dosage levels. The more potent corticosteroids have been shown to be teratogenic after dermal application in laboratory animals. There are no adequate and well-controlled studies in pregnant women on teratogenic effects from topically applied corticosteroids. Therefore, topical corticosteroids should be used during pregnancy only if the potential benefit justifies the potential risk to the fetus. Drugs of this class should not be used extensively for pregnant patients or in large amounts or for prolonged periods of time.
Nursing Mothers—It is not known whether topical administration of corticosteroids could result in sufficient systemic absorption to produce detectable quantities in breast milk. Systemically administered corticosteroids are secreted into breast milk in quantities *not* likely to have a deleterious effect on the infant. Nevertheless, caution should be exercised when topical corticosteroids are administered to a nursing woman.
Pediatric Use—Pediatric patients may demonstrate greater susceptibility to topical corticosteroid-induced HPA axis suppression and Cushing's syndrome than do mature patients because of a larger skin surface area to body weight ratio.
Hypothalamic-pituitary-adrenal (HPA) axis suppression, Cushing's syndrome, and intracranial hypertension have been reported in pediatric patients receiving topical corticosteroids. Manifestations of adrenal suppression in pediatric patients include linear growth retardation, delayed weight gain, low plasma cortisol levels, and absence of response to ACTH stimulation. Manifestations of intracranial hypertension include bulging fontanelles, headaches, and bilateral papilledema.
Administration of topical corticosteroids to pediatric patients should be limited to the least amount compatible with an effective therapeutic regimen. Chronic corticosteroid therapy may interfere with the growth and development of pediatric patients.

ADVERSE REACTIONS

The following local adverse reactions are reported infrequently with topical corticosteroids but may occur more frequently with the use of occlusive dressings. These reactions are listed in an approximate decreasing order of occurrence:

- Burning
- Itching
- Irritation
- Dryness
- Folliculitis
- Hypertrichosis
- Acneform eruptions
- Hypopigmentation
- Perioral dermatitis
- Allergic contact dermatitis

The following may occur more frequently with occlusive dressings:

- Maceration of the skin
- Secondary infection
- Skin atrophy
- Striae
- Miliaria

OVERDOSAGE

Topically applied corticosteroids can be absorbed in sufficient amounts to produce systemic effects (*see* **PRECAUTIONS**).

DOSAGE AND ADMINISTRATION

Topical corticosteroids are generally applied to the affected area as a thin film 1 to 4 times daily, depending on the severity of the condition.
A small quantity of Cordran Lotion should be rubbed gently into the affected area 2 or 3 times daily.
Occlusive dressings may be used for the management of psoriasis or recalcitrant conditions.
If an infection develops, the use of occlusive dressings should be discontinued and appropriate antimicrobial therapy instituted.

Use With Occlusive Dressings

The technique of occlusive dressings (for management of psoriasis and other persistant dermatoses) is as follows:

1. Remove as much as possible of the superficial scaling before applying Cordran Lotion. Soaking in a bath will help soften the scales and permit easier removal by brushing, picking, or rubbing.
2. Rub the lotion thoroughly into the affected areas.
3. Cover with an occlusive plastic film, such as polyethylene, Saran Wrap™, or Handi-Wrap®. (Added moisture may be provided by placing a slightly dampened cloth or gauze over the lesion before the plastic film is applied.)
4. Seal the edges to adjacent normal skin with tape or hold in place by a gauze wrapping.
5. For convenience, the patient may remove the dressing during the day. The dressing should then be reapplied each night.
6. For daytime therapy, the condition may be treated by rubbing Cordran Lotion sparingly into the affected areas.
7. In more resistant cases, leaving the dressing in place for 3 to 4 days at a time may result in a better response.
8. Thin polyethylene gloves are suitable for treatment of the hands and fingers; plastic garment bags may be utilized for treating lesions on the trunk or buttocks. A tight shower cap is useful in treating lesions on the scalp.

Occlusive Dressings Have the Following Advantages—

1. Percutaneous penetration of the corticosteroid is enhanced.
2. Medication is concentrated on the areas of skin where it is most needed.
3. This method of administration frequently is more effective in very resistant dermatoses than is the conventional application of Cordran.

Precautions to Be Observed in Therapy With Occlusive Dressings—Treatment should be continued for at least a few days after clearing of the lesions. If it is stopped too soon, a relapse may occur. Reinstitution of treatment frequently will cause remission.
Because of the increased hazard of secondary infection from resistant strains of staphylococci among hospitalized patients, it is suggested that the use of occlusive plastic films for corticosteroid therapy in such cases be restricted.
Generally, occlusive dressings should not be used on weeping, or exudative, lesions.
When large areas of the body are covered, thermal homeostasis may be impaired. If elevation of body temperature occurs, use of the occlusive dressing should be discontinued.
Rarely, a patient may develop miliaria, folliculitis, or a sensitivty to either the particular dressing material or a combination of Cordran and the occlusive dressing. If miliaria or folliculitis occurs, use of the occlusive dressing should be discontinued. Treatment by inunction with Cordran Lotion may be continued. If the sensitivity is caused by the particular material of the dressing, substitution of a different material may be tried.
Warnings—Some plastic films are readily flammable. Patients should be cautioned against the use of any such material.
When plastic films are used on pediatric patients, the persons caring for the patients must be reminded of the danger of suffocation if the plastic material accidentally covers the face.

HOW SUPPLIED

Lotion (Plastic squeeze bottles):
0.05% (UC 5352)—(15 mL) NDC 55515-052-15; (60 mL) NDC 55515-052-60
Store at controlled room temperature, 59° to 86°F (15° to 30°C).
Rx only
Literature revised June 12, 1998
PV 2681 UCP
Mfd. for
OCLASSEN PHARMACEUTICALS, INC.
a division of
Watson Laboratories Inc.
Corona CA 91720
by Eli Lily and Company
Indianapolis, IN 46285, U.S.A.
Shown in Product Identification Guide, page 326

CORDRAN® TAPE ℞

[*kōr 'drăn*]
Flurandrenolide Tape, USP

DESCRIPTION

Cordran® Tape (Flurandrenolide Tape, USP) is a transparent, inconspicuous, plastic surgical tape, impervious to moisture. It contains Cordran® (Flurandrenolide, USP), a potent corticosteroid for topical use. Flurandrenolide occurs as white to off-white, fluffy crystalline powder and is odorless. Flurandrenolide is practically insoluble in water and in ether. One g dissolves in 72 mL of alcohol and in 10 mL of chloroform. The molecular weight of flurandrenolide is 436.52.
The chemical name of flurandrenolide is Pregn-4-ene-3,20-dione, 6-fluoro-11,21-dihydroxy-16,17-[(1-methylethylidene)bis (oxy)]-, (6α, 11β, 16α)-; its empirical formula is $C_{24}H_{33}FO_6$. The structural formula is as follows:

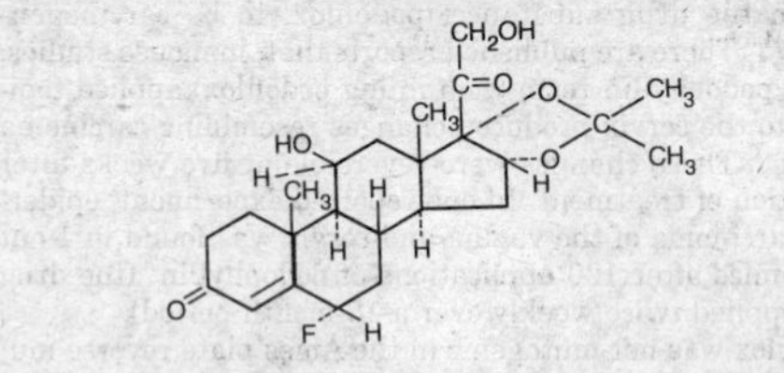

Each square centimeter contains 4 µg (0.00916 µmol) flurandrenolide uniformly distributed in the adhesive layer. The tape is made of a thin, matte-finish polyethylene film that is slightly elastic and highly flexible.
The adhesive is a synthetic copolymer of acrylate ester and acrylic acid that is free from substances of plant origin. The pressure-sensitive adhesive surface is covered with a protective paper liner to permit handling and trimming before application.

CLINICAL PHARMACOLOGY

Cordran is primarily effective because of its anti-inflammatory, antipruritic, and vasoconstrictive actions.
The mechanism of the anti-inflammatory effect of topical corticosteroids is not completely understood. Various laboratory methods, including vasoconstrictor assays, are used to compare and predict potencies and/or clinical efficacies of the topical corticosteroids. There is some evidence to suggest that a recognizable correlation exists between vasoconstrictor potency and therapeutic efficacy in man. Corticosteroids with anti-inflammatory activity may stabilize cellular and lysosomal membranes. There is also the suggestion that the effect on the membranes of lysosomes prevents the release of proteolytic enzymes and, thus, plays a part in reducing inflammation.
The tape serves as both a vehicle and an occlusive dressing. Retention of insensible perspiration by the tape results in hydration of the stratum corneum and improved diffusion of the medication. The skin is protected from scratching, rubbing, desiccation, and chemical irritation. The tape acts as a mechanical splint to fissured skin. Since it prevents removal of the medication by washing or the rubbing action of clothing, the tape formulation provides a sustained action.
Pharmacokinetics—The extent of percutaneous absorption of topical corticosteroids is determined by many factors, including the vehicle, the integrity of the epidermal barrier, and the use of occlusive dressings.
Topical corticosteroids can be absorbed from normal intact skin. Inflammation and/or other disease processes in the skin increase percutaneous absorption. Occlusive dressings substantially increase the percutaneous absorption of topical corticosteroids. Thus, occlusive dressings may be a valuable therapeutic adjunct for treatment of resistant dermatoses (*see* **DOSAGE AND ADMINISTRATION**).
Once absorbed through the skin, topical corticosteroids are handled through pharmacokinetic pathways similar to those of systematically administered corticosteroids. Corticosteroids are bound to plasma proteins in varying degrees. They are metabolized primarily in the liver and then excreted in the kidneys. Some of the topical corticosteroids and their metabolites are also excreted into the bile.

INDICATIONS AND USAGE

For relief of the inflammatory and pruritic manifestations of corticosteroid-responsive dermatoses, particularly dry, scaling localized lesions.

CONTRAINDICATIONS

Topical corticosteroids are contraindicated in patients with a history of hypersensitivity to any of the components of these preparations.
Use of Cordran Tape is not recommended for lesions exuding serum or in intertriginous areas.

PRECAUTIONS

General—Systemic absorption of topical corticosteroids has produced reversible hypothalamic-pituitary-adrenal (HPA) axis suppression, manifestations of Cushing's syndrome, hyperglycemia, and glucosuria in some patients.
Conditions that augment systemic absorption include application of the more potent steroids, use over large surface areas, prolonged use, and the addition of occlusive dressings.
Therefore, patients receiving a large dose of a potent topical steroid applied to a large surface area or under an occlusive dressing should be evaluated periodically for evidence of HPA axis suppression using urinary-free cortisol and ACTH stimulation tests. If HPA axis suppression is noted, an attempt should be made to withdraw the drug, to reduce the frequency of application, or to substitute a less potent steroid.
Recovery of HPA axis function is generally prompt and complete on discontinuation of the drug. Infrequently, signs and symptoms of steroid withdrawal may occur, so that supplemental systemic corticosteroids are required.

Pediatric patients may absorb proportionally large amounts of topical corticosteroids and thus be more susceptible to systemic toxicity (see Pediatric Use under **PRECAUTIONS**).

If irritation develops, topical corticosteroids should be discontinued and appropriate therapy instituted.

In the presence of dermatologic infections, the use of an appropriate antifungal or antibacterial agent should be instituted. If a favorable response does not occur promptly, Cordran should be discontinued until the infection has been adequately controlled.

Information for the Patient—Patients using topical corticosteroids should receive the following information and instructions:

1. This medication is to be used as directed by the physician. It is for external use only. Avoid contact with the eyes.
2. Patients should be advised not to use this medication for any disorder other than that for which it was prescribed.
3. The treated skin area should not be bandaged or otherwise covered or wrapped in order to be occlusive unless the patient is directed to do so by the physician.
4. Patients should report any signs of local adverse reactions, especially under occlusive dressing.
5. Parents of pediatric patients should be advised not to use tight-fitting diapers or plastic pants on a patient being treated in the diaper area, because these garments may constitute occlusive dressings.

Laboratory Tests—The following tests may be helpful in evaluating the HPA axis suppression:
  Urinary-free cortisol test
  ACTH stimulation test

Carcinogenesis, Mutagenesis, and Impairment of Fertility—Long-term animal studies have not been performed to evaluate the carcinogenic potential or the effect on fertility of topical corticosteroids.

Studies to determine mutagenicity with prednisolone and hydrocortisone have revealed negative results.

Usage in Pregnancy—Pregnancy Category C—Corticosteroids are generally teratogenic in laboratory animals when administered systemically at relatively low dosage levels. The more potent corticosteroids have been shown to be teratogenic after dermal application in laboratory animals. There are no adequate and well-controlled studies in pregnant women on teratogenic effects from topically applied corticosteroids. Therefore, topical corticosteroids should be used during pregnancy only if the potential benefit justifies the potential risk to the fetus. Drugs of this class should not be used extensively for pregnant patients or in large amounts or for prolonged periods of time.

Nursing Mothers—It is not known whether topical administration of corticosteroids could result in sufficient systemic absorption to produce detectable quantities in breast milk. Systemically administered corticosteroids are secreted into breast milk in quantities *not* likely to have a deleterious effect on the infant. Nevertheless, caution should be exercised when topical corticosteroids are administered to a nursing woman.

Pediatric Use—Pediatric patients may demonstrate greater susceptibility to topical corticosteroid-induced HPA axis suppression and Cushing's syndrome than do mature patients because of a larger skin surface area to body weight ratio.

Hypothalamic-pituitary-adrenal (HPA) axis suppression, Cushing's syndrome, and intracranial hypertension have been reported in pediatric patients receiving topical corticosteroids. Manifestations of adrenal suppression in pediatric patients include linear growth retardation, delayed weight gain, low plasma-cortisol levels, and absence of response to ACTH stimulation. Manifestations of intracranial hypertension include bulging fontanelles, headaches, and bilateral papilledema.

Administration of topical corticosteroids to pediatric patients should be limited to the least amount compatible with an effective therapeutic regimen. Chronic corticosteroid therapy may interfere with the growth and development of pediatric patients.

ADVERSE REACTIONS

The following local adverse reactions are reported infrequently with topical corticosteroids but may occur more frequently with the use of occlusive dressings. These reactions are listed in an approximate decreasing order of occurrence:
  Burning
  Itching
  Irritation
  Dryness
  Folliculitis
  Hypertrichosis
  Acneform eruptions
  Hypopigmentation
  Perioral dermatitis
  Allergic contact dermatitis
The following may occur more frequently with occlusive dressings:
  Maceration of the skin

  Secondary infection
  Skin atrophy
  Striae
  Miliaria

OVERDOSAGE

Topically applied corticosteroids can be absorbed in sufficient amounts to produce systemic effects (see **PRECAUTIONS**).

DOSAGE AND ADMINISTRATION

Occlusive dressings may be used for the management of psoriasis or recalcitrant conditions.

If an infection develops, the use of Cordran Tape and other occlusive dressings should be discontinued and appropriate antimicrobial therapy instituted.

Replacement of the tape every 12 hours produces the lowest incidence of adverse reactions, but it may be left in place for 24 hours if it is well tolerated and adheres satisfactorily. When necessary, the tape may be used at night only and removed during the day.

If ends of the tape loosen prematurely, they may be trimmed off and replaced with fresh tape.

The directions given below are included on a separate package insert for the patient to follow unless otherwise instructed by the physician.

APPLICATION OF
CORDRAN TAPE

> IMPORTANT: Skin should be clean and *dry* before tape is applied. Tape should always be cut, never torn.

DIRECTIONS FOR USE:
1. Prepare skin as directed by your physician or as follows: Gently clean the area to be covered to remove scales, crusts, dried exudates, and any previously used ointments or creams. A germicidal soap or cleanser should be used to prevent the development of odor under the tape. Shave or clip the hair in the treatment area to allow good contact with the skin and comfortable removal. If shower or tub bath is to be taken, it should be completed before the tape is applied. The skin should be dry before application of the tape.
2. Remove tape from package and cut a piece slightly larger than area to be covered. Round off corners.
3. Pull white paper from transparent tape. Be careful that tape does not stick to itself.
4. Apply tape, keeping skin smooth; press tape into place.
REPLACEMENT OF TAPE.
Unless instructed otherwise by your physician, replace tape after 12 hours. Cleanse skin and allow it to dry for 1 hour before applying new tape.
IF IRRITATION OR INFECTION DEVELOPS, REMOVE TAPE AND CONSULT PHYSICIAN.

HOW SUPPLIED
Tape:
4 mcg/sq cm (UC 5350)—small roll, 24 in × 3 in (60 cm × 7.5 cm) NDC 55515-014-24
4 mcg/sq cm (UC 5350)—large roll, 80 in × 3 in (200 cm × 7.5 cm) NDC 55515-014-80
4 mcg/sq cm (UC 5350)—12 patches, each 2 in × 3 in (5.1 cm × 7.5 cm) NDC 55515-014-12
Directions for the patient are included in each package.
Store at controlled room temperature, 59° to 86°F (15° to 30°C).
Rx only

REFERENCES
Bard JW: Flurandrenolide tape in the treatment of lichen simplex chronicus. *J Ky Med Assoc* 1969;67:668.
Baxter DL, Stoughton RB: Mitotic index of psoriatic lesions treated with anthralin, glucocorticosteroid and occlusion only. *J Invest Dermatol* 1970;54:410.
Compilation of clinical reports on Cordran Tape received by Eli Lilly and Company.
Halprin KM, Fukui K, Ohkawara A: Flurandrenolone (Cordran) tape and carbohydrate metabolizing enzymes. *Arch Dermatol* 1969;100:336.
Labow TA, Eisert J, Sanders SL: Flurandrenolide tape in treatment of psoriasis. *NY State J Med* 1969;69:3138.
Ronchese F: Flurandrenolone tape therapy. *RI Med J* 1969;52:389.
Sellers FM: Investigative study of flurandrenolone tape in a series of ambulatory outpatients. *J Indiana State Med Assoc* 1970;63:34.
Weiner MA: Flurandrenolone tape, a new preparation for occlusive therapy, *J Invest Dermatol* 1966;47:63.
Literature revised February 13, 1998   PV 3051 UCP
Mfd. for
**OCLASSEN
PHARMACEUTICALS INC.**
A Division of Watson Labs., Inc.
Corona, CA 91720

Mfg. by Minnesota Mining
and Manufacturing Company
St. Paul Minnesota 55101
Shown in Product Identification Guide, page 326

CORMAX™ OINTMENT 0.05%   ℞
[kor ´ măx]
**(Clobetasol Propionate Ointment, USP)
For Dermatologic Use Only—
Not For Ophthalmic Use.**

DESCRIPTION
Cormax™ Ointment (Clobetasol Propionate Ointment, USP) contains the active compound clobetasol propionate, a synthetic corticosteroid, for topical dermatologic use. Clobetasol, an analog of prednisolone, has a high degree of glucocorticoid activity and a slight degree of mineralocorticoid activity.
Chemically, clobetasol propionate is 21-chloro-9-fluoro-11β, 17-dihydroxy-16β-methylpregna-1, 4-diene-3,20-dione, 17-propionate, and it has the following structural formula:

Clobetasol propionate has the molecular formula $C_{25}H_{32}ClFO_5$ and a molecular weight of 467. It is a white to cream-colored crystalline powder insoluble in water.
Each gram of Cormax™ Ointment, contains 0.5 mg clobetasol propionate in a base composed of propylene glycol, sorbitan sesquioleate, and white petrolatum.

CLINICAL PHARMACOLOGY
The corticosteroids are a class of compounds comprising steroid hormones secreted by the adrenal cortex and their synthetic analogs. In pharmacologic doses, corticosteroids are used primarily for their anti-inflammatory and/or immunosuppressive effects. Topical corticosteroids such as clobetasol propionate are effective in the treatment of corticosteroid-responsive dermatoses primarily because of their anti-inflammatory, antipruritic, and vasoconstrictive actions. However, while the physiologic, pharmacologic, and clinical effects of the corticosteroids are well known, the exact mechanisms of their actions in each disease are uncertain. Clobetasol propionate, a corticosteroid, has been shown to have topical (dermatologic) and systemic pharmacologic and metabolic effects characteristic of this class of drugs.
Pharmacokinetics: The extent of percutaneous absorption of topical corticosteroids, including clobetasol propionate, is determined by many factors inclding the vehicle, the integrity of the epidermal barrier, and the use of occlusive dressings (see **DOSAGE AND ADMINISTRATION**).
As with all topical corticosteroids, clobetasol propionate can be absorbed from normal intact skin. Inflammation and/or other disease processes in the skin may increase percutaneous absorption. Occlusive dressings substantially increase the percutaneus absorption of topical corticosteroids (see **DOSAGE AND ADMINISTRATION**).
Once absorbed through the skin, topical corticosteroids enter pharmacokinetic pathways similarly to systemically administered corticosteroids.
Corticosteroids are bound to plasma proteins in varying degrees. Corticosteroids are metabolized primarily in the liver and are then excreted by the kidneys. Some of the topical corticosteroids, including clobetasol propionate and its metabolites, are also excreted into the bile.
Clobetasol propionate ointment has been shown to depress the plasma levels of adrenal cortical hormones following repeated nonocclusive application to diseased skin in patients with psoriasis and eczematous dermatitis. These effects have been shown to be transient and reversible upon completion of a two-week course of treatment.

INDICATIONS AND USAGE
Cormax™ Ointment (Clobetasol Propionate Ointment, USP) is indicated for short-term treatment of inflammatory and pruritic manifestations of moderate to severe corticosteroid-responsive dermatoses. Treatment beyond two consecutive weeks is not recommended, and the total dosage should not exceed 50 g per week because of the potential for the drug to suppress the hypothalamic-pituitary-adrenal (HPA) axis.
This product is not recommended for use in pediatric patients under 12 years of age.

Continued on next page

Cormax Ointment—Cont.

CONTRAINDICATIONS

Cormax™ Ointment (Clobetasol Propionate Ointment, USP) is contraindicated in patients who are hypersensitive to clobetasol propionate, to other corticosteroids, or to any ingredient in this preparation.

PRECAUTIONS

General: Clobetasol propionate is a highly potent topical corticosteroid that has been shown to suppress the HPA axis at doses as low as 2 g per day. Systemic absorption of topical corticosteroids has resulted in reversible HPA axis supression, manifestations of Cushing's syndrome, hyperglycemia, and glucosuria in some patients.

Conditions that augment systemic absorption include the application of more potent corticosteroids, use over large surface areas, prolonged use, and the addition of occlusive dressings. Therefore, patients receiving a large dose of a potent topical steroid applied to a large surface area should be evaluated periodically for evidence of HPA axis' suppression by using the urinary free cortisol and ACTH stimulation tests. If HPA axis suppression is noted, an attempt should be made to withdraw the drug, to reduce the frequency of application, or to substitute a less potent steroid.

Recovery of HPA axis function is generally prompt and complete upon discontinuation of the drug. Infrequently, signs and symptoms of steroid withdrawal may occur, requiring supplemental systemic corticosteroids.

Pediatric patients may absorb proportionally larger amounts of topical corticoteroids and thus be more susceptible to systemic toxicity (see **PRECAUTIONS: Pediatric Use**).

If irritation develops, topical corticosteroids should be discontinued and appropriate therapy instituted.

In the presence of dermatologic infections, the use of an appropriate antifungal or antibacterial agent should be instituted. If a favorable response does not occur promptly, the corticosteroid should be discontinued until the infection has been adequately controlled.

Certain areas of the body, such as the face, groin, and axillae, are more prone to atrophic changes than other areas of the body following treatment with corticosteroids. Frequent observations of the patient is important if these areas are to be treated.

As with other potent topical corticosteroids, Cormax™ Ointment (Clobetasol Propionate Ointment, USP) should not be used in the treatment of rosacea and perioral dermatitis. Topical corticosteroids in general should not be used in the treatment of acne or as a sole therapy in widespread plaque psoriasis.

Information for patients: Patients using Cormax™ Ointment (Clobetasol Propionate Ointment, USP) should receive the following information and instructions:

1. This medication is to be used as directed by the physician and should not be used longer than the prescribed time period. It is for external use only. Avoid contact with the eyes.
2. This medication should not be used for any disorder other than that for which it is prescribed.
3. The treated skin area should not be bandaged or otherwise covered or wrapped so as to be occlusive.
4. Patients should report any signs of local adverse reactions to the physician.

Laboratory Tests: The following tests may be helpful in evaluating HPA axis suppression:

Urinary free cortisol test
ACTH stimulation test

Carcinogenesis, Mutagenesis, Impairment of Fertility:

Long-term animal studies have not been performed to evaluate the carcinogenic potential or the effect on fertility of topical corticosteroids.

Studies to determine mutagenicity with prednisolone have revealed negative results.

Pregnancy: Teratogenic Effects: Pregnancy Category C: The more potent corticosteroids have been shown to be teratogenic in animals after dermal application. Clobetasol propionate has not been tested for teratogenicity by this route; however, it is absorbed percutaneously, and when administered subcutaneously it was a significant teratogen in both the rabbit and the mouse. Clobetasol propionate has greater teratogenic potential than steroids that are less potent.

There are no adequate and well-controlled studies of the teratogenic effects of topically applied corticosteroids, including clobetasol, in pregnant women. Therefore, clobetasol and other topical corticosteroids should be used during pregnancy only if the potential benefit justifies the potential risk to the fetus, and they should not be used extensively on pregnant patients, in large amounts, or for prolonged periods of time.

Nursing Mothers: It is not known whether topical administration of corticosteroids could result in sufficient systemic absorption to produce detectable quantities in breast milk. Systemically administered corticosteroids are secreted into breast milk in quantities **not** likely to have a deleterious effect on the infant. Nevertheless, caution should be exercised when topical corticosteroids are prescribed for a nursing woman.

Pediatric use: Use of Cormax™ Ointment, in pediatric patients is not recommended.

Pediatric patients may demonstrate greater susceptibility to topical corticosteroid-induced HPA axis suppression and Cushing's syndrome than mature patients because of a larger skin surface area to body weight ratio.

HPA axis suppression, Cushing's syndrome and intracranial hypertension have been reported in pediatric patients receiving topical corticosteroids. Manifestations of adrenal suppression in pediatric patients include linear growth retardation, delayed weight gain, low plasma cortisol levels, and absence of response to ACTH stimulation. Manifestations of intracranial hypertension include bulging fontanelles, headaches, and bilateral papilledema.

ADVERSE REACTIONS

Comax™ Ointment (Clobetasol Propionate Ointment, USP) is generally well tolerated when used for two-week treatment periods. The most frequent adverse reactions reported for clobetasol propionate ointment have been local and have included burning sensation, irritation, and itching. These occurred in approximately 0.5% of the patients. Less frequent adverse reactions wers stinging, cracking, erythema, folliculitis, numbness of fingers, skin atrophy, and telangiectasia, which occurred in approximately 0.3% of the patients.

The following local adverse reactions are reported infrequently when topical corticosteroids are used as recommended. These reactions are listed in an approximately decreasing order of occurrence: burning, itching, irritation, dryness, folliculitis, hypetrichosis, acneiform eruptions, hypopigmentation, perioral dermatitis, allergic contact dermatitis, maceration of the skin, secondary infection, skin atrophy, striae, miliaria. Systemic absorption of topical corticosteroids has produced reversible HPA axis suppression, manifestations of Cushing's syndrome, hyperglycemia, and glucosuria in some patients. In rare instances, treatment (or withdrawal of treatment) of psoriasis with corticosteroids is thought to have exacerbated the disease or provoked the pustular form of the disease, so careful patient supervision is recommended.

OVERDOSAGE

Topically applied Cormax™ Ointment (Clobetasol Propionate Ointment, USP) can be absorbed in sufficient amounts to produce systemic effects (see **PRECAUTIONS**).

DOSAGE AND ADMINISTRATION

A thin layer of Cormax™ Ointment (Clobetasol Propionate Ointment, USP) should be applied with gentle rubbing to the affected skin area twice daily, once in the morning and once at night.

Cormax™ Ointment is potent: therefore, **treatment must be limited to two consecutive weeks, and amounts greater than 50 g per week should not be used. Cormax™ Ointment is not to be used with occlusive dressings.**

HOW SUPPLIED

Cormax™ Ointment (Clobetasol Propionate Ointment, USP) 0.05% is supplied in 15 g (NDC 55515-410-15) and 45 g (NDC 55515-410-45) tubes.

Store at controlled room temperature 15°–30°C (59°–86°F). Do not refrigerate.

Rx only

Mfd. for
OCLASSEN PHARMACEUTICALS, INC.
a division of
Watson Laboratories Inc.
Corona CA 91720
by DPT Laboratories, Ltd.
San Antonio, TX 78215
Revised February 20, 1998.
127342-0298

Shown in Product Identification Guide, page 326

CORMAX™ ℞

[*kor ' māx*]

Scalp Application, 0.05% w/w
(Clobetasol Propionate Topical Solution, USP)
For Dermatologic Use Only
Not for Ophthalmic Use

DESCRIPTION

Cormax™ Scalp Application (Clobetasol Propionate Topical Solution, USP) contains the active compound clobetasol propionate, a synthetic corticosteroid, for topical dermatologic use. Clobetasol, an analog of prednisolone, has a high degree of glucocorticoid activity and a slight degree of mineralocorticoid activity.

Chemically, clobetasol propionate is 21-chloro-9-fluoro-11β, 17-dihydroxy-16β-methylpregna-1, 4-diene-3,20-dione 17-propionate, and it has the following structural formula:

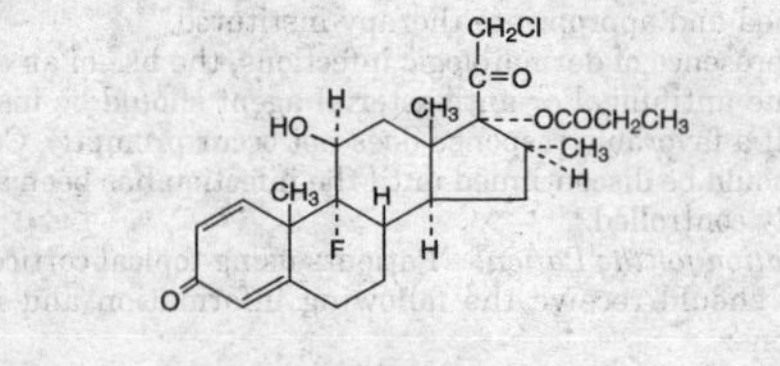

Clobetasol propionate has the molecular formula $C_{25}H_{32}ClFO_5$ and a molecular weight of 467. It is a white to cream-colored crystalline powder insoluble in water.

Each gram of Cormax™ Scalp Application contains 0.5 mg clobetasol propionate in a base composed of purified water, isopropyl alcohol (40% w/w), carbomer 934P, and sodium hydroxide.

CLINICAL PHARMACOLOGY

The corticosteroids are a class of compounds comprising steroid hormones secreted by the adrenal cortex and their synthetic analogs. In pharmacologic doses, corticosteroids are used primarily for their anti-inflammatory and/or immunosuppressive effects. Topical corticosteroids such as clobetasol propionate are effective in the treatment of corticosteroid-responsive dermatoses primarily because of their anti-inflammatory, antipruritic, and vasconstrictive actions. However, while the physiologic, pharmacologic, and clinical effects of the corticosteroids are well known, the exact mechanisms of their actions in each disease are uncertain. Clobetasol propionate, a corticosteroid, has been shown to have topical (dermatologic) and systemic pharmacologic and metabolic effects characteristic of this class of drugs.

Pharmacokinetics

The extent of percutaneous absorption of topical corticosteroids, including clobetasol propionate, is determined by many factors, including the vehicle, the integrity of the epidermal barrier, and the use of occlusive dressings (see **DOSAGE AND ADMINISTRATION**).

As with all topical corticosteroids, clobetasol propionate can be absorbed from normal intact skin. Inflammation and/or other disease processes in the skin may increase percutaneous absorption. Occlusive dressings substantially increase the percutaneous absorption of topical corticosteroids (see **DOSAGE AND ADMINISTRATION**).

As with all topical corticosteroids, clobetasol propionate can be absorbed from normal intact skin. Inflammation and/or other disease processes in the skin may increase percutaneous absorption. Occlusive dressings substantially increase the percutanous absorption of topical corticosteroids (see **DOSAGE AND ADMINISTRATION**).

Once absorbed through the skin, topical corticosteroids enter pharmacokinetic pathways similarly to systemically administered corticosteroids. Corticosteroids are bound to plasma proteins in varying degrees. Corticosteroids are metabolized primarily in the liver and are then excreted by the kidneys. Some of the topical corticosteroids, including clobetasol propionate and its metabolites, are also excreted in the bile.

Following repeated nonocclusive application in the treatment of scalp psoriasis, there is some evidence that Cormax™ Scalp Application (Clobetasol Propionate Topical Solution, USP) has the potential to depress plasma cortisol levels in some patients. However, hypothalamic-pituitary-adrenal (HPA) axis effects produced by systemically absorbed clobetasol propionate have been shown to be transient and reversible upon completion of a two-week course of treatment.

INDICATIONS AND USAGE

Cormax™ Scalp Application (Clobetasol Propionate Topical Solution, USP) is indicated for short-term topical treatment of inflammatory and pruritic manifestations of moderate to severe corticosteroid-responsive dermatoses of the scalp. Treatment beyond two consecutive weeks is not recommended, and the total dosage should not exceed 50 mL per week because of the potential for the drug to suppress the HPA axis.

This product is not recommended for use in pediatric patients under 12 years of age.

CONTRAINDICATIONS

Cormax™ Scalp Application (Clobetasol Propionate Topical Solution, USP) is contraindicated in patients with primary infections of the scalp, or in patients who are hypersensitive to clobetasol propionate, to other corticosteroids, or to any ingredient in this preparation.

PRECAUTIONS

General

Clobetasol propionate is a highly potent topical corticosteroid that has been shown to suppress the HPA axis at doses

as low as 2 g (of ointment) per day. Systemic absorption of topical corticosteroids has resulted in reversible HPA axis suppression, manifestations of Cushing's syndrome, hyperglycemia, and glucosuria in some patients.

Conditions that augment systemic absorption include the application of the more potent corticosteroids, use over large surface areas, prolonged use and the addition of occlusive dressings. Therefore, patients receiving a large dose of potent topical steroid applied to a large surface area should be evaluated periodically for evidence of HPA axis suppression by using the urinary free cortisol and ACTH stimulation tests. If HPA axis suppression is noted, an attempt should be made to withdraw the drug, to reduce the frequency of application, or to substitute a less potent steroid.

Recovery of HPA axis function is generally prompt and complete upon discontinuation of the drug. Infrequently, signs and symptoms of steroid withdrawal may occur, requiring supplemental systemic corticosteroids.

Pediatric patients may absorb proportionally larger amounts of topical corticosteroids and thus be more susceptible to systemic toxicity (see **PRECAUTIONS: Pediatric Use**).

If irritation develops, topical corticosteroids should be discontinued and appropriate therapy instituted. Irritation is possible if Cormax™ Scalp Application (Clobetasol Propionate Topical Solution, USP) contacts the eye. If that should occur, immediate flushing of the eye with a large volume of water is recommended.

In the presence of dermatologic infections, the use of an appropriate antifungal or antibacterial agent should be instituted. If a favorable response does not occur promptly, the corticosteroid should be discontinued until the infection has been adequately controlled.

Although Cormax™ Scalp Application (Clobetasol Propionate Topical Solution, USP) is intended for the treatment of inflammatory conditions of the scalp, it should be noted that certain areas of the body, such as the face, groin, and axillae, are more prone to atrophic changes than other areas of the body following treatment with corticosteroids. Frequent observation of the patient is important if these areas are to be treated.

As with other potent topical corticosteroids, Cormax™ Scalp Application should not be used in the treatment of rosacea and perioral dermatitits. Topical corticosteroids in general should not be used in the treatment of acne or as sole therapy in widespread plaque psoriasis.

Information for Patients

Patients using Cormax™ Scalp Application should receive the following information and instructions:

1. This medication is to be used as directed by the physician and should not be used longer than the prescribed time period. It is for external use only. Avoid contact with the eyes.
2. This medication should not be used for any disorder other than that for which it is prescribed.
3. The treated skin area should not be bandaged or otherwise covered or wrapped so as to be occlusive.
4. Patients should report any signs of local adverse reactions to the physician.

Laboratory Tests

The following tests may be helpful in evaluating HPA axis suppression:

Urinary free cortisol test
ACTH stimulation test

Carcinogenesis, Mutagenesis, Impairment of Fertility

Long-term animal studies have not been performed to evaluate the carcinogenic potential or the effect on fertility of topical corticosteroids.

Studies to determine mutagenicity with prednisolone have revealed negative results.

Pregnancy: Teratogenic Effects: Pregnancy Category C

The more potent corticosteroids have been shown to be teratogenic in animals after dermal application. Clobetasol propionate has not been tested for teratogenicity by this route; however, it is absorbed percutaneously, and when administered subcutaneously it was a significant teratogen in both the rabbit and the mouse. Clobetasol propionate has greater teratogenic potential than steroids that are less potent.

There are no adequate and well-controlled studies of the teratogenic effects of topically applied corticosteroids, including clobetasol, in pregnant women. Therefore, clobetasol and other topical corticosteroids should be used during pregnancy only if the potential benefit justifies the potential risk to the fetus, and they should not be used extensively on pregnant patients, in large amounts, or for prolonged periods of time.

Nursing Mothers

It is not known whether topical administration of corticosteroids could result in sufficient systemic absorption to produce detectable quantities in breast milk. Systemically administered corticosteroids are secreted into breast milk in quantities not likely to have a deleterious effect on the infant. Nevertheless, caution should be exercised when topical corticosteroids are prescribed for a nursing woman.

Pediatric Use

Use of Cormax™ Scalp Application in pediatric patients under 12 years of age is not recommended.

Pediatric patients may demonstrate greater susceptibility to topical corticosteroids-induced HPA axis suppression and Cushing's syndrome than mature patients because of a larger skin surface area to body weight ratio.

HPA axis suppression, Cushing's syndrome and intracranial hypertension have been reported in pediatric patients receiving topical corticosteroids. Manifestations of adrenal suppression in pediatric patients include linear growth retardation, delayed weight gain, low plasma cortisol levels, and absence of response to ACTH stimulation. Manifestations of intercranial hypertension include bulging fontanelles, headaches, and bilateral papilledema.

ADVERSE REACTIONS

Cormax™ Scalp Application (Clobetasol Propionate Topical Solution, USP) is generally well tolerated when used for two-week treatment periods.

The most frequent adverse events reported have been local and have included burning and/or stinging sensation, which occurred in approximately 10% of the patients; scalp pustules, which occurred in approximately 1% of the patients; and tingling, and folliculitis, each of which occurred in approximately 0.6% of the patients. Less frequent adverse events were itching and tightness of the scalp, dermatitis, tenderness, headache, hair loss, and eye irritation, each of which occurred in approximately 0.3% of the patients.

The following local adverse reactions are reported infrequently when topical corticosteroids are used as recommended. These reactions are listed in an approximately decreasing order of occurrence: burning, itching, irritation, dryness, folliculitis, hypertrichosis, acneiform eruptions, hypopigmentation, perioral dermatitis, allergic contact dermatitis, maceration of the skin, secondary infection, skin atrophy, striae and miliaria. Systemic absorption of topical corticosteroids has produced reversible HPA axis suppression, manifestations of Cushing's syndrome, hyperglycemia, and glucosuria in some patients. In rare instances, treatment (or withdrawal of treatment) of psoriasis with corticosteroids is thought to have exacerbated the disease or provoked the pustular form of the disease, so careful patient supervision is recommended.

OVERDOSAGE

Topically applied Cormax™ Scalp Application (Clobetasol Propionate Topical Solution, USP) can be absorbed in sufficient amounts to produce systemic effects (see **PRECAUTIONS**).

DOSAGE AND ADMINISTRATION

Cormax™ Scalp Application (Clobetasol Propionate Topical Solution, USP) should be applied to the affected scalp areas twice daily, once in the morning and once at night. Cormax™ Scalp Application is potent; therefore, **treatment must be limited to two consecutive weeks and amounts greater than 50mL per week should not be used. Cormax™ Scalp Application is not be used with occlusive dressings.**

HOW SUPPLIED

Cormax™ Scalp Application (Clobetasol Propionate Topical Solution, USP), 0.05% w/w is supplied in plastic squeeze bottles of 25 mL (NDC 55515-430-25), and 50 mL (NDC 55515-430-50). Store at controlled room temperature 15°–30° C (59°–86°F). Do not refrigerate. Do not use near an open flame.

Rx only

Mfd for
OCLASSEN PHARMACEUTICALS, INC.
a division of Watson Laboratories Inc.,
Corona CA 91720
by DPT Laboratories, Ltd.
San Antonio, TX 78215
Revised: February 21, 1998.
127138-0298

Shown in Product Identification Guide, page 326

MONODOX® ℞

DOXYCYCLINE MONOHYDRATE CAPSULES

[*mon 'o-dox*]

DESCRIPTION

Doxycycline is a broad-spectrum antibiotic synthetically derived from oxytetracycline. Monodox® 100 mg and 50 mg capsules contain doxycycline monohydrate equivalent to 100 mg or 50 mg of doxycycline for oral administration. The chemical designation of the light-yellow crystalline powder is alpha-6-deoxy-5-oxytetracycline.

Structural formula:

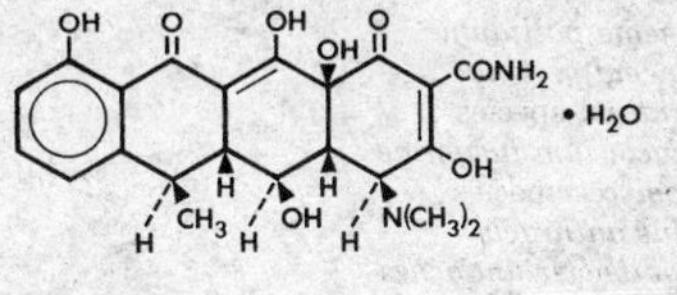

$C_{22}H_{24}N_2O_8 \cdot H_2O$ M.W.=462.46

Doxycycline has a high degree of lipid solubility and a low affinity for calcium binding. It is highly stable in normal human serum. Doxycycline will not degrade into an epianhydro form.

Inert Ingredients: colloidal silicon dioxide; hard gelatin capsule; magnesium stearate; microcrystalline cellulose; and sodium starch glycolate.

CLINICAL PHARMACOLOGY

Tetracyclines are readily absorbed and are bound to plasma proteins in varying degrees. They are concentrated by the liver in the bile and excreted in the urine and feces at high concentrations in a biologically active form. Doxycycline is virtually completely absorbed after oral administration.

Following a 200 mg dose of doxycycline monohydrate, 24 normal adult volunteers averaged the following serum concentration values:

[See table at bottom of next page]

	Average Observed Values
Maximum Concentration	3.61 mcg/mL (± 0.9 sd)
Time of Maximum Concentration	2.60 hr (± 1.10 sd)
Elimination Rate Constant	0.049 per hr (± 0.030 sd)
Half-Life	16.33 hr (± 4.53 sd)

Excretion of doxycycline by the kidney is about 40%/72 hours in individuals with normal function (creatinine clearance about 75 mL/min). This percentage excretion may fall as low as 1-5%/72 hours in individuals with severe renal insufficiency (creatinine clearance below 10 mL/min). Studies have shown no significant difference in serum half-life of doxycycline (range 18-22 hours) in individuals with normal and severely impaired renal function.

Hemodialysis does not alter serum half-life.

Microbiology: The tetracyclines are primarily bacteriostatic and are thought to exert their antimicrobial effect by the inhibition of protein synthesis. The tetracyclines, including doxycycline, have a similar antimicrobial spectrum of activity against a wide range of gram-positive and gram-negative organisms. Cross-resistance of these organisms to tetracyclines is common.

While *in vitro* studies have demonstrated the susceptibility of most strains of the following microorganisms, clinical efficacy for infections other than those included in the INDICATIONS AND USAGE section has not been documented.

GRAM-NEGATIVE BACTERIA:

- *Neisseria gonorrhoeae*
- *Haemophilus ducreyi*
- *Haemophilus influenzae*
- *Yersinia pestis* (formerly *Pasteurella pestis*)
- *Francisella tularensis* (formerly *Pasteurella tularensis*)
- *Vibrio cholerae* (formerly *Vibrio comma*)
- *Bartonella bacilliformis*
- *Brucella species*

Because many strains of the following groups of gram-negative microorganisms have been shown to be resistant to tetracyclines, culture and susceptibility testing are recommended:

- *Escherichia coli*
- *Klebsiella species*
- *Enterobacter aerogenes*
- *Shigella species*
- *Acinetobacter species* (formerly *Mima* species and *Herellea* species)
- *Bacteroides* species

GRAM-POSITIVE BACTERIA:

Because many strains of the following groups of gram-positive microorganisms have been shown to be resistant to tetracyclines, culture and susceptibility testing are recommended. Up to 44 percent of strains of *Streptococcus pyogenes* and 74 percent of *Streptococcus faecalis* have been found to be resistant to tetracycline drugs. Therefore, tetracyclines should not be used to treat streptococcal infections unless the organism has been demonstrated to be susceptible.

- *Streptococcus pyogenes*
- *Streptococcus pneumoniae*
- *Enterococcus* group (*Streptococcus faecalis* and *Streptococcus faecium*)
- *Alpha-hemolytic streptococci (viridans* group)

OTHER MICROORGANISMS:

- *Chlamydia psittaci*
- *Chlamydia trachomatis*
- *Ureaplasma urealyticum*
- *Borrelia recurrentis*

Continued on next page

Monodox—Cont.

- *Treponema pallidum*
- *Treponema pertenue*
- *Clostridium* species
- *Fusobacterium fusiforme*
- *Actinomyces* species
- *Bacillus anthracis*
- *Propionibacterium acnes*
- *Entamoeba* species
- *Balantidium coli*

Susceptibility tests: **Diffusion Techniques:** Quantitative methods that require measurement of zone diameters give the most precise estimate of the susceptibility of bacteria to antimicrobial agents.

One such standard procedure[1] which has been recommended for use with disks to test susceptibility of organisms to doxycycline uses the 30-mcg tetracycline-class disk or the 30-mcg doxycycline disk. Interpretation involves the correlation of the diameter obtained in the disk test with the minimum inhibitory concentration (MIC) for tetracycline or doxycycline, respectively.

Reports from the laboratory giving results of the standard single-disk susceptibility test with a 30-mcg tetracycline-class disk or the 30-mcg doxycycline disk should be interpreted according to the following criteria:

Zone Diameter (mm)		Interpretation
tetracycline	doxycycline	
≥19	≥16	Susceptible
15–18	13–15	Intermediate
≤14	≤12	Resistant

A report of "susceptible" indicates that the pathogen is likely to be inhibited by generally achievable blood levels. A report of "intermediate" suggests that the organism would be susceptible if a high dosage is used or if the infection is confined to tissues and fluids in which high antimicrobial levels are attained. A report of "resistant" indicates that achievable concentrations are unlikely to be inhibitory, and other therapy should be selected.

Standardized procedures require the use of laboratory control organisms. The 30-mcg tetracycline-class disk or the 30-mcg doxycycline disk should give the following zone diameters:

Organism	Zone Diameter	
	tetracycline	doxycycline
E. coli ATCC 25922	18–25	18–24
S. aureus ATCC 25923	19–28	23–29

Dilution Techniques:
Use a standardized dilution method[2] (broth, agar, microdilution) or equivalent with tetracycline powder. The MIC values obtained should be interpreted according to the following criteria:

MIC (mcg/mL)	Interpretation
≤4	Susceptible
8	Intermediate
≥16	Resistant

As with standard diffusion techniques, dilution methods require the use of laboratory control organisms. Standard tetracycline powder should provide the following MIC values:

Organism	MIC (mcg/mL)
S. aureus ATCC 29213	0.25–1
E. faecalis ATCC 29212	8–32
E. coli ATCC 25922	1–4
P. aeruginosa ATCC 27853	8–32

INDICATIONS AND USAGE
Doxycycline is indicated for the treatment of the following infections:

Rocky mountain spotted fever, typhus fever and the typhus group, Q fever, rickettsialpox, and tick fevers caused by Rickettsiae.

Respiratory tract infections caused by *Mycoplasma pneumoniae*.

Lymphogranuloma venereum caused by *Chlamydia trachomatis*.

Psittacosis (ornithosis) caused by *Chlamydia psittaci*.

Trachoma caused by *Chlamydia trachomatis*, although the infectious agent is not always eliminated as judged by immunofluorescence.

Inclusion conjunctivitis caused by *Chlamydia trachomatis*.

Uncomplicated urethral, endocervical or rectal infections in adults caused by *Chlamydia trachomatis*.

Nongonococcal urethritis caused by *Ureaplasma urealyticum*.

Relapsing fever due to *Borrelia recurrentis*.

Doxycycline is also indicated for the treatment of infections caused by the following gram-negative microorganisms:

Chancroid caused by *Haemophilus ducreyi*.

Plague due to *Yersinia pestis* (formerly *Pasteurella pestis*).

Tularemia due to *Francisella tularensis* (formerly *Pasteurella tularensis*).

Cholera caused by *Vibrio cholerae* (formerly *Vibrio comma*).

Campylobacter fetus infections caused by *Campylobacter fetus* (formerly *Vibrio fetus*).

Brucellosis due to *Brucella* species (in conjunction with streptomycin).

Bartonellosis due to *Bartonella bacilliformis*.

Granuloma inguinale caused by *Calymmatobacterium granulomatis*.

Because many strains of the following groups of microorganisms have been shown to be resistant to doxycycline, culture and susceptibility testing are recommended.

Doxycycline is indicated for treatment of infections caused by the following gram-negative microorganisms, when bacteriologic testing indicates appropriate susceptibility to the drug:

Escherichia coli

Enterobacter aerogenes (formerly *Aerobacter aerogenes*)

Shigella species

Acinetobacter species (formerly *Mima* species and *Herellea* species)

Respiratory tract infections caused by *Haemophilus influenzae*.

Respiratory tract and urinary tract infections caused by *Klebsiella* species.

Doxycycline is indicated for treatment of infections caused by the following gram-positive microorganisms when bacteriologic testing indicates appropriate susceptibility to the drug:

Upper respiratory infections caused by *Streptococcus pneumoniae* (formerly *Diplococcus pneumoniae*).

Skin and skin structure infections caused by *Staphylococcus aureus*. Doxycycline is not the drug of choice in the treatment of any type of staphylococcal infections.

When penicillin is contraindicated, doxycycline is an alternative drug in the treatment of the following infections:

Uncomplicated gonorrhea caused by *Neisseria gonorrhoeae*.

Syphilis caused by *Treponema pallidum*.

Yaws caused by *Treponema pertenue*.

Listeriosis due to Listeria monocytogenes.

Anthrax due to *Bacillus anthracis*.

Vincent's infection caused by *Fusobacterium fusiforme*.

Actinomycosis caused by *Actinomyces israelii*.

Infections caused by *Clostridium* species.

In acute intestinal amebiasis, doxycycline may be a useful adjunct to amebicides.

In severe acne, doxycycline may be useful adjunctive therapy.

CONTRAINDICATIONS
This drug is contraindicated in persons who have shown hypersensitivity to any of the tetracyclines.

WARNINGS
THE USE OF DRUGS OF THE TETRACYCLINE CLASS DURING TOOTH DEVELOPMENT (LAST HALF OF PREGNANCY, INFANCY, AND CHILDHOOD TO THE AGE OF 8 YEARS) MAY CAUSE PERMANENT DISCOLORATION OF THE TEETH (YELLOW-GRAY-BROWN). This adverse reaction is more common during long term use of the drugs but has been observed following repeated short-term courses. Enamel hypoplasia has also been reported. TETRACYCLINE DRUGS, THEREFORE, SHOULD NOT BE USED IN THIS AGE GROUP UNLESS OTHER DRUGS ARE NOT LIKELY TO BE EFFECTIVE OR ARE CONTRAINDICATED.

All tetracyclines form a stable calcium complex in any bone-forming tissue. A decrease in the fibula growth rate has been observed in prematures given oral tetracycline in doses of 25 mg/kg every six hours. This reaction was shown to be reversible when the drug was discontinued.

Results of animal studies indicate that tetracyclines cross the placenta, are found in fetal tissues, and can have toxic effects on the developing fetus (often related to retardation of skeletal development). Evidence of embryo toxicity has been noted in animals treated early in pregnancy. If any tetracycline is used during pregnancy or if the patient becomes pregnant while taking these drugs, the patient should be apprised of the potential hazard to the fetus.

The antianabolic action of the tetracyclines may cause an increase in BUN. Studies to date indicate that this does not occur with the use of doxycycline in patients with impaired renal function.

Photosensitivity manifested by an exaggerated sunburn reaction has been observed in some individuals taking tetracyclines. Patients apt to be exposed to direct sunlight or ultraviolet light should be advised that this reaction can occur with tetracycline drugs, and treatment should be discontinued at the first evidence of skin erythema.

PRECAUTIONS
General:
As with other antibiotic preparations, use of this drug may result in overgrowth of non-susceptible organisms, including fungi. If superinfection occurs, the antibiotic should be discontinued and appropriate therapy instituted.

Bulging fontanels in infants and benign intracranial hypertension in adults have been reported in individuals receiving tetracyclines. These conditions disappeared when the drug was discontinued.

Incision and drainage or other surgical procedures should be performed in conjunction with antibiotic therapy when indicated.

Laboratory tests: In venereal disease when coexistent syphilis is suspected, a dark-field examination should be done before treatment is started and the blood serology repeated monthly for at least four months.

In long-term therapy, periodic laboratory evaluations of organ systems, including hematopoietic, renal, and hepatic studies should be performed.

Drug interactions: Because tetracyclines have been shown to depress plasma prothrombin activity, patients who are on anticoagulant therapy may require downward adjustment of their anticoagulant dosage.

Since bacteriostatic drugs may interfere with the bactericidal action of penicillin, it is advisable to avoid giving tetracyclines in conjunction with penicillin.

Absorption of tetracyclines is impaired by antacids containing aluminum, calcium, or magnesium, and iron-containing preparations.

Barbiturates, carbamazepine, and phenytoin decrease the half-life of doxycycline.

The concurrent use of tetracycline and methoxyflurane has been reported to result in fatal renal toxicity.

Concurrent use of tetracycline may render oral contraceptives less effective.

Drug/laboratory test interactions: False elevations of urinary catecholamine levels may occur due to interference with the fluorescence test.

Carcinogenesis, mutagenesis, impairment of fertility: Long-term studies in animals to evaluate the carcinogenic potential of doxycycline have not been conducted. However, there has been evidence of oncogenic activity in rats in studies with related antibiotics, oxytetracycline (adrenal and pituitary tumors) and minocycline (thyroid tumors). Likewise, although mutagenicity studies of doxycycline have not been conducted, positive results in *in vitro* mammalian cell assays have been reported for related antibiotics (tetracycline, oxytetracycline). Doxycycline administered orally at dosage levels as high as 250 mg/kg/day had no apparent effect on the fertility of female rats. Effect on male fertility has not been studied.

Pregnancy: Pregnancy Category D. (See **WARNINGS**).
Labor and Delivery: The effect of tetracyclines on labor and delivery is unknown.
Nursing mothers: Tetracyclines are present in the milk of lactating women who are taking a drug in this class. Because of the potential for serious adverse reactions in nursing infants from the tetracyclines, a decision should be made whether to discontinue nursing or discontinue the drug, taking into account the importance of the drug to the mother. (See **WARNINGS**).
Pediatric Use: See **WARNINGS** and **DOSAGE AND ADMINISTRATION** sections.

ADVERSE REACTIONS
Due to oral doxycycline's virtually complete absorption, side effects to the lower bowel, particularly diarrhea, have been infrequent. The following adverse reactions have been observed in patients receiving tetracyclines.

Gastrointestinal: Anorexia, nausea, vomiting, diarrhea, glossitis, dysphagia, enterocolitis, and inflammatory lesions (with monilial overgrowth) in the anogenital region. These reactions have been caused by both the oral and parenteral administration of tetracyclines. Rare instances of esophagitis and esophageal ulcerations have been reported in patients receiving capsule and tablet forms of drugs in the tetracycline class. Most of these patients took medications immediately before going to bed. (See **DOSAGE AND ADMINISTRATION**).
Skin: Maculopapular and erythematous rashes. Exfoliative dermatitis has been reported but is uncommon. Photosensitivity is discussed above. (See **WARNINGS**.)
Renal toxicity: Rise in BUN has been reported and is apparently dose related. (See **WARNINGS**.)
Hypersensitivity reactions: Urticaria, angioneurotic edema, anaphylaxis, anaphylactoid purpura, pericarditis, and exacerbation of systemic lupus erythematosus.
Blood: Hemolytic anemia, thrombocytopenia, neutropenia, and eosinophilia have been reported with tetracyclines.
Other: Bulging fontanels in infants and intracranial hypertension in adults. (See **PRECAUTIONS—General**.)

Time (hr):	0.5	1.0	1.5	2.0	3.0	4.0	8.0	12.0	24.0	48.0	72.0
Conc. (mcg/mL)	1.02	2.26	2.67	3.01	3.16	3.03	2.03	1.62	0.95	0.37	0.15

When given over prolonged periods, tetracyclines have been reported to produce brown-black microscopic discoloration of the thyroid gland. No abnormalities of thyroid function are known to occur.

OVERDOSAGE

In case of overdosage, discontinue medication, treat symptomatically and institute supportive measures. Dialysis does not alter serum half-life, and it would not be of benefit in treating cases of overdosage.

DOSAGE AND ADMINISTRATION

THE USUAL DOSAGE AND FREQUENCY OF ADMINISTRATION OF DOXYCYCLINE DIFFERS FROM THAT OF THE OTHER TETRACYCLINES. EXCEEDING THE RECOMMENDED DOSAGE MAY RESULT IN AN INCREASED INCIDENCE OF SIDE EFFECTS.

Adults: The usual dose of oral doxycycline is 200 mg on the first day of treatment (administered 100 mg every 12 hours or 50 mg every 6 hours) followed by a maintenance dose of 100 mg/day. The maintenance dose may be administered as a single dose or as 50 mg every 12 hours. In the management of more severe infections (particularly chronic infections of the urinary tract), 100 mg every 12 hours is recommended.

For pediatric patients above eight years of age: The recommended dosage schedule for pediatric patients weighing 100 pounds or less is 2 mg/lb of body weight divided into two doses on the first day of treatment, followed by 1 mg/lb of body weight given as a single daily dose or divided into two doses, on subsequent days. For more severe infections, up to 2 mg/lb of body weight may be used. For pediatric patients over 100 lbs the usual adult dose should be used.

Uncomplicated gonococcal infections in adults (except anorectal infections in men): 100 mg by mouth, twice a day for 7 days. As an alternate single visit dose, administer 300 mg stat followed in one hour by a second 300 mg dose.

Acute epididymo-orchitis caused by *N. gonorrhoeae* : 100 mg, by mouth, twice a day for at least 10 days.

Primary and secondary syphilis: 300 mg a day in divided doses for at least 10 days.

Uncomplicated urethral, endocervical, or rectal infection in adults caused by *Chlamydia trachomatis*: 100 mg, by mouth, twice a day for at least 7 days.

Nongonococcal urethritis caused by *C. trachomatis* and *U. urealyticum*: 100 mg, by mouth, twice a day for at least 7 days.

Acute epididymo-orchitis caused by *C. trachomatis*: 100 mg, by mouth, twice a day for at least 10 days.

When used in streptococcal infections, therapy should be continued for 10 days.

Administration of adequate amounts of fluid along with capsule and tablet forms of drugs in the tetracycline class is recommended to wash down the drugs and reduce the risk of esophageal irritation and ulceration. (See **ADVERSE REACTIONS**). If gastric irritation occurs, doxycycline may be given with food. Ingestion of a high fat meal has been shown to delay the time to peak plasma concentrations by an average of one hour and 20 minutes. However, in the same study, food enhanced the average peak concentration by 7.5% and the area under the curve by 5.7%.

HOW SUPPLIED

MONODOX® 50 mg Capsules have a white opaque body with a yellow opaque cap. The capsule bears the inscription "MONODOX 50" in brown and "M 260" in brown. Each capsule contains doxycycline monohydrate equivalent to 50 mg doxycycline.

MONODOX® 50 mg is available in: Bottles of 100 capsules, NDC 55515-260-06. MONODOX® 100 mg Capsules have a yellow opaque body with a brown opaque cap. The capsule bears the inscription "MONODOX 100" in white and "M 259" in brown. Each capsule contains doxycycline monohydrate equivalent to 100 mg of doxycycline. MONODOX® 100 mg is available in: Bottles of 50 capsules, NDC 55515-259-04 and in bottles of 250 capsules, NDC 55515-259-07.

STORE AT CONTROLLED ROOM TEMPERATURE 15°–30°C (59°–86°F). PROTECT FROM LIGHT.

ANIMAL PHARMACOLOGY AND ANIMAL TOXICOLOGY

Hyperpigmentation of the thyroid has been produced by members of the tetracycline class in the following species: in rats by oxytetracycline, doxycycline, tetracycline PO_4, and methacycline; in minipigs by doxycycline, minocycline, tetracycline PO_4, and methacycline; in dogs by doxycycline and minocycline; in monkeys by minocycline.

Minocycline, tetracycline PO_4, methacycline, doxycycline, tetracycline base, oxytetracycline HCl and tetracycline HCl were goitrogenic in rats fed a low iodine diet. This goitrogenic effect was accompanied by high radioactive iodine uptake. Administration of minocycline also produced a large goiter with high radioiodine uptake in rats fed a relatively high iodine diet.

Treatment of various animal species with this class of drugs has also resulted in the induction of thyroid hyperplasia in the following: in rats and dogs (minocycline), in chickens (chlortetracycline) and in rats and mice (oxytetracycline). Adrenal gland hyperplasia has been observed in goats and rats treated with oxytetracycline.

REFERENCES:

1. National Committee for Clinical Laboratory Standards, *Performance Standards for Antimicrobial Disk Susceptibility Tests,* Fourth Edition. Approved Standard NCCLS Document M2-A4, Vol. 10, No. 7 NCCLS, Villanova, PA, April 1990.
2. National Committee for Clinical Laboratory Standards, *Methods for Dilution Antimicrobial Susceptibility Tests for Bacteria That Grow Aerobically,* Second Edition. Approved Standard NCCLS Document M7-A2, Vol. 10, No. 8 NCCLS, Villanova, PA, April 1990.

Rx Only

Manufactured for
OCLASSEN PHARMACEUTICALS, INC.
A Division of Watson Labs. Inc., Corona, CA 91720
by Vintage Pharmaceuticals, Inc., Charlotte, N.C.
Revised April 28, 1998 02-18391/R7

Shown in Product Identification Guide, page 326

OHMEDA

Pharmaceutical Products Division Inc.
(see BAXTER PHARMACEUTICAL PRODUCTS INC.)

Organon Inc.

375 MT. PLEASANT AVE.
WEST ORANGE, NJ 07052

Direct Inquiries to:
(973) 325-4500

Currently available products are listed below. For complete product line information and price lists, direct inquiries to Organon Inc. Customer Service. For specific product information, contact Organon Inc. Medical Services Department.

ARDUAN® ℞

(pipecuronium bromide) for injection

HOW SUPPLIED

10 mL vials/10 mg—boxes of 6 vials—NDC-0052-0446-36

TICE® BCG ℞

BCG VACCINE USP
(for Intravesical or Percutaneous use)

Distributed by Organon Inc.
(See page 2150 complete product information.)

CALDEROL® ℞

[*kal-dah 'rol*]
(calcifediol capsules, USP)

HOW SUPPLIED

20 µg (white, soft elastic capsules) bottle of 60
50 µg (orange, soft elastic capsules) bottle of 60

Shown in Product Identification Guide, page 326

CORTROSYN® ℞

[*cōr-trō-sin*]
(cosyntropin) for injection
FOR DIAGNOSTIC USE ONLY

DESCRIPTION

Cortrosyn® (cosyntropin) for injection is a sterile lyophilized powder in vials containing 0.25mg of Cortrosyn® and 10mg of mannitol to be reconstituted with 1mL sodium chloride for injection, USP as solvent. Administration is by intravenous or intramuscular injection. Cosyntropin is α 1–24 corticotropin, a synthetic subunit of ACTH. It is an open chain polypeptide containing, from the N terminus, the first 24 of the 39 amino acids of natural ACTH. The sequence of amino acids in the 1–24 compound is as follows:

Ser — Tyr — Ser — Met — Glu — His — Phe — Arg — Trp — Gly — Lys
1 2 3 4 5 6 7 8 9 10 11

Pro — Val — Gly — Lys — Lys — Arg — Arg — Pro — Val — Lys — Val
12 13 14 15 16 17 18 19 20 21 22

Tyr — Pro
23 24

CLINICAL PHARMACOLOGY

Cortrosyn® exhibits the full corticosteroidogenic activity of natural ACTH. Various studies have shown that the biologic activity of ACTH resides in the N-terminal portion of the molecule and that the 1–20 amino acid residue is the minimal sequence retaining full activity. Partial or complete loss of activity is noted with progressive shortening of the chain beyond 20 amino acid residue. For example, the decrement from 20 to 19 results in a 70% loss of potency.

The pharmacologic profile of Cortrosyn® is similar to that of purified natural ACTH. It has been established that 0.25 mg of Cortrosyn® will stimulate the adrenal cortex maximally and to the same extent as 25 units of natural ACTH. This dose of Cortrosyn® will produce maximal secretion of 17-OH corticosteroids, 17-ketosteroids and/or 17-ketogenic steroids.

The extra-adrenal effects which natural ACTH and Cortrosyn® have in common include increased melanotropic activity, increased growth hormone secretion and an adipokinetic effect. These are considered to be without physiological or clinical significance.

Animal, human and synthetic ACTH (1–39) which all contain 39 amino acids exhibit similar immunologic activity. This activity resides in the C-terminal portion of the molecule and the 22–39 amino acid residues exhibit the greatest degree of antigenicity. In contrast, synthetic polypeptides containing 1–19 or fewer amino acids have no detectable immunologic activity. Those containing 1–26, 1–24 or 1–23 amino acids have very little immunologic although full biologic activity. This property of Cortrosyn® assumes added importance in view of the known antigenicity of natural ACTH.

INDICATIONS AND USAGE

Cortrosyn® is intended for use as a diagnostic agent in the screening of patients presumed to have adrenocortical insufficiency. Because of its rapid effect on the adrenal cortex it may be utilized to perform a 30-minute test of adrenal function (plasma cortisol response) as an office or outpatient procedure, using only 2 venipunctures. (See DOSAGE AND ADMINISTRATION section for details.)

Severe hypofunction of the pituitary-adrenal axis is usually associated with subnormal plasma cortisol values but a low basal level is not per se evidence of adrenal insufficiency and does not suffice to make the diagnosis. Many patients with proven insufficiency will have normal basal levels and will develop signs of insufficiency only when stressed. For this reason the only criterion which should be used in establishing the diagnosis is the failure to respond to adequate corticotropin stimulation as provided by 0.25 mg of Cortrosyn® (cosyntropin) for injection. When presumptive adrenal insufficiency is diagnosed by a subnormal Cortrosyn® test, further studies are indicated to determine if it is primary or secondary.

Primary adrenal insufficiency (Addison's disease) is the result of an intrinsic disease process, such as tuberculosis within the gland. The production of adrenocortical hormones is deficient despite high ACTH levels (feedback mechanism). Secondary or relative insufficiency arises as the result of defective production of ACTH leading in turn to disuse atrophy of the adrenal cortex. It is commonly seen, for example, as a result of corticosteroid therapy, Sheehan's syndrome and pituitary tumors or ablation.

The differentiation of both types is based on the premise that a primarily defective gland cannot be stimulated by ACTH whereas a secondarily defective gland is potentially functional and will respond to adequate stimulation with ACTH. Patients selected for further study as the result of a subnormal Cortrosyn® test should be given a 3 or 4 day course of treatment with Repository Corticotropin Injection USP and then retested. Suggested doses are 40 USP units twice daily for 4 days or 60 USP units twice daily for 3 days. Under these conditions little or no increase in plasma cortisol levels will be seen in Addison's disease whereas higher or even normal levels will be seen in cases with secondary adrenal insufficiency.

CONTRAINDICATIONS

The only contraindication to Cortrosyn® is a history of a previous adverse reaction to it.

PRECAUTIONS

General: Cortrosyn® exhibits slight immunologic activity, does not contain foreign animal protein and is therefore less risky to use than natural ACTH. Patients known to be sensitized to natural ACTH with markedly positive skin tests will, with few exception, react negatively when tested intra-

Continued on next page

Cortrosyn—Cont.

dermally with Cortrosyn®. Further, most patients with a history of a previous hypersensitivity reaction to natural ACTH or a pre-existing allergic disease will tolerate Cortrosyn® without incident. Despite this however, Cortrosyn® is not completely devoid of immunologic activity and hypersensitivity reactions are possible, at least in susceptible patients. Therefore, the physician should be prepared, prior to injection, to treat any possible acute hypersensitivity reaction.

Drug Interactions: Corticotropin may accentuate the electrolyte loss associated with diuretic therapy.

Carcinogenesis, Mutagenesis, Impairment of Fertility: Long term studies in animals have not been performed to evaluate carcinogenic or mutagenic potential or impairment of fertility. A study in rats noted inhibition of reproductive function like natural ACTH.

Pregnancy: Pregnancy Category C. Animal reproduction studies have not been conducted with Cortrosyn®. It is also not known whether Cortrosyn® can cause fetal harm when administered to a pregnant woman or can affect reproduction capacity. Cortrosyn® should be given to a pregnant woman only if clearly needed.

Nursing Mothers: It is not known whether this drug is excreted in human milk. Because many drugs are excreted in human milk, caution should be exercised when Cortrosyn® is administered to a nursing woman.

Pediatric Usage: (See DOSAGE AND ADMINISTRATION section for details.)

ADVERSE REACTIONS

Since Cortrosyn® (cosyntropin) for injection is intended for diagnostic and not therapeutic use, adverse reactions other than a rare hypersensitivity reaction are not anticipated. To date only 3 such reactions have been reported in the literature and in each instance the patient had a pre-existing allergic disease and/or a previous reaction to natural ACTH. One investigator reported a single instance of slight whealing with splotchy erythema at the injection site. A similar but more marked reaction was also noted in the same patient following an injection of natural ACTH.

DOSAGE AND ADMINISTRATION

Cortrosyn® may be administered intramuscularly or as a direct intravenous injection when used as a rapid screening test of adrenal function. It may also be given as an intravenous infusion over a 4 to 8 hour period to provide a greater stimulus to the adrenal glands. Doses of Cortrosyn® 0.25 to 0.75 mg have been used in clinical studies and a maximal response noted with the smallest dose.

A suggested method for a rapid screening test of adrenal function has been described by Wood and associates(1). A control blood sample of 6 to 7 mL is collected in a heparinized tube. Reconstitute 0.25 mg of Cortrosyn® in solvent (ampul of 1 mL sodium chloride injection USP—0.9%) and inject intramuscularly. In children, aged 2 years or less, a dose of 0.125 mg will often suffice. A second blood sample is collected exactly 30 minutes later. Both blood samples should be refrigerated until sent to the laboratory for determination of the plasma cortisol response by some appropriate method. If it is not possible to send them to the laboratory or perform the fluorimetric procedure within 12 hours, then the plasma should be separated and refrigerated or frozen according to need.

The usual normal response in most cases is an approximate doubling of the basal level, provided that the basal level does not exceed the normal range. Patients taking inadvertent doses of cortisone or hydrocortisone on the test day and patients taking spironolactone or women taking drugs which contain estrogen may exhibit abnormally high basal plasma cortisol levels. A paradoxical response may be noted in the former group as seen in a decrease in plasma cortisol values following a stimulating dose of Cortrosyn®. In the latter group only a normal incremental response is to be expected. Many patients with normal adrenal function, however, do not respond to the expected degree so that the following criteria have been established to denote a normal response:

1. The control plasma cortisol level should exceed 5 micrograms/100 mL.
2. The 30-minute level should show an increment of at least 7 micrograms/100 mL above the basal level.
3. The 30-minute level should exceed 18 micrograms/100 mL. Comparable figures have been reported by Greig and co-workers (2). These criteria also apply when the drug is injected intravenously in 2 to 5 mL of saline over a 2-minute period.

Plasma cortisol levels usually peak about 45 to 60 minutes after an injection of Cortrosyn® (cosyntropin) for injection and some prefer the 60-minute interval for testing for this reason. While it is true that the 60-minute values are usually higher than the 30-minute values, the difference may not be significant enough in most cases to outweigh the disadvantage of a longer testing period. If the 60-minute test period is used, the criterion for a normal response is an approximate doubling of the basal plasma cortisol value.

When given as an intravenous infusion: Cortrosyn®, 0.25 mg may be added to glucose or saline solutions and given at the rate of approximately 40 micrograms per hour over a 6-hour period. It should not be added to blood or plasma as it is apt to be inactivated by enzymes. Adrenal response may be measured in the usual manner by determining urinary steroid excretion before and after treatment or by measuring plasma cortisol levels before and at the end of the infusion. The latter is preferable because the urinary steroid excretion does not always accurately reflect the adrenal or plasma control response to ACTH. Patients receiving cortisone, hydrocortisone or spironolactone should omit their pre-test doses on the day selected for testing. In patients with a raised plasma bilirubin or in patients where the plasma contains free hemoglobin, falsely high fluorescence measurements will result. The test may be performed at any time during the day but because of the physiological diurnal variation of plasma cortisol the criteria listed by Wood cannot apply. It has been shown that basal plasma cortisol levels and the post Cortrosyn® increment exhibit diurenal changes. However, the 30-minute plasma cortisol level remains unchanged throughout the day so that only this single criterion should be used (3).

Parenteral drug products should be inspected visually for particulate matter and discoloration whenever solution and container permit. Reconstituted Cortrosyn® should not be retained.

HOW SUPPLIED

Box containing: 10 vials of Cortrosyn® (cosyntropin) for injection 0.25mg
NDC # 0052-0731-10
10 ampuls of solvent (sodium chloride for injection, USP).
NDC # 0052-0318-01

CAUTION: Federal law prohibits dispensing without prescription.

References

1. Wood, J.B. et al. LANCET 1.243, 1965.
2. Greig, W.R. et al. J. ENDOCR 34.411, 1966.
3. McGill, P.E. et al. ANN RHEUM DIS 26.123, 1967.

Manufactured for ORGANON INC.
By BEN VENUE LABORATORIES, INC. • BEDFORD OHIO 44146
or by
ORGANON INC. • WEST ORANGE, NEW JERSEY 07052
731S 5310012 REVISED 6/89

COTAZYM® ℞

[*kōt 'a zīm*]
(pancrelipase capsules, USP)

DESCRIPTION

COTAZYM® (pancrelipase capsules, USP) contains pancrelipase obtained from the porcine pancreas. Pancrelipase is composed principally of lipase, amylase and protease and is used for oral digestive enzyme replacement. Each capsule contains not less than:

Lipase	8,000 USP Units
Protease	30,000 USP Units
Amylase	30,000 USP Units

At release, up to 25% more lipase may be present.

Each capsule also contains the inactive ingredients: cornstarch, precipitated calcium carbonate, gelatin, magnesium stearate, talc, titanium dioxide, FD&C Green #3 and D&C Yellow #10 as coloring.

CLINICAL PHARMACOLOGY

Pancrelipase, USP contains lipase, protease and amylase obtained from porcine pancreas. Normal pancreatic function includes secretion of proteolytic enzymes such as proteases (trypsin and chymotrypsin), nonproteolytic enzymes such as lipase and amylase, and electrolytes such as bicarbonate, chloride, sodium and potassium. Lipase, protease and amylase break down fat, protein, and starches, respectively, in the small intestine. Lipase hydrolyzes fats into glycerol and fatty acids. Protease converts proteins into proteoses and derived substances, while amylase converts starches into dextrins and sugars. Pancreatic enzymes are used to correct maldigestion, malabsorption and pain associated with pancreatic insufficiency. The major maldigestion/malabsorption problems arise from incomplete fat digestion. Exogenous pancrelipase reduces the amount of nitrogen and fat excreted in the stool. Activity of these products are dependent upon the amount of pancrelipase delivered to the small intestine. This delivery can be hampered by inactivation from low gastric pH, acidic precipitation of bile salts, and the proteolytic activity of the component protease. Pancreatic enzymes are more active at pH greater than 4, with lipase being the most sensitive of the pancreatic enzymes to inactivation by low pH. Malabsorption of fat is likely if an individual, ingesting 100 gm of fat per day, excretes more than 7 gm of fat (or 18 mmol) in a 24-hour period. Malabsorption of protein is likely if nitrogen excretion is greater than 2.5 gm per 24-hours (16% of protein by weight is nitrogen). In order for fat maldigestion to occur, a pancreas must secrete less than 10% of its normal output.

The enzymes contained in COTAZYM® (pancrelipase capsules, USP) are not absorbed systemically; therefore, pharmacokinetic studies of their absorption, distribution, metabolism, and excretion have not been conducted. The contents of COTAZYM® capsules are released in the stomach, whereupon some of the enzyme is inactivated by acid. The remaining enzymes traverse into the duodenum, where they facilitate digestion and subsequently are hydrolyzed to their constituent amino acids by proteases. Pancreatic extracts contain purines which are absorbed into the general circulation and are converted to uric acid. This uric acid could lead to hyperurticemia, hyperuticosuria, and possible kidney damage. Chymotrypsin activity in the stool is indicative of exocrine pancreatic function. Ingestion of pancrelipase enzymes result in an increase in chymotrypsin in the stool. Clinical bioactivity and bioavaliability studies in patients with exocrine pancreatic insufficiency from cystic fibrosis or chronic alcoholic pancreatitis have shown that the enzymes from COTAZYM® are released at the duodenojejunal junction.

A study was conducted in 6 patients (ages 43–58) with pancrelipase insufficiency secondary to chronic alcoholic pancreatitis. Four of the patients received 4 capsules of COTAZYM® with a standard test meal. The mean (±SEM) percent of ingested dose of lipase and trypsin delivered to the duodenum postprandially was 15.1% (±2.1) and 11.3% (±1.6), respectively. A randomized 3-way crossover study was also performed on this group of patients to further ascertain bioavaliability. Each patient received 10 PANCREATIN® tablets per meal, 4 COTAZYM® capsules per meal, and 4 or 8 PANCREASE® capsules per meal in a randomized order. In patients who received COTAZYM®, PANCREASE®, or PANCREATIN® while on a 100 gm fat/day diet, the fat excretions were 15.0 gm, 13.0 gm, and 19.0 gm per 24 hours, respectively, while fat excretion was 31.0 gm/24 hours in the no enzyme treatment group.[1] An investigation was also conducted in 8 cystic fibrosis patients (ages 18–29) with steatorrhea who were already on some type of enzyme replacement therapy. Two patients were given a test meal together with 4 capsules of COTAZYM®. The mean delivery of lipase and trypsin to the duodenum postprandially was 7.6% (3.5–11.7%) and 14.5% (12–17%) of intake, respectively. A randomized 2-way crossover study was performed on 7 of these 8 patients. Each patient received 4 COTAZYM® capsules per meal or 8 PANCREASE® capsules per meal, while on a 100 gm fat/day diet. Steatorrhea was controlled with 19.2% of fat excreted (as % of fat intake) for COTAZYM® and 5.9% of fat excreted for PANCREASE®, reduced from 28% fat excreted with previous treatments.[2]

SPECIAL POPULATIONS

Pediatric and Geriatric Patients

There is no evidence to suggest that the bioactivity or bioavailability of COTAZYM® would differ markedly in pediatric or geriatric patients from other patient populations.

CLINICAL STUDIES

Cystic Fibrosis

In a single center, unblinded, non-randomized, active-controlled, one sequence, 2-period (with no washout period) crossover Canadian study of 15 patients, under the age of 4 years, with exocrine pancreatic insufficiency secondary to cystic fibrosis, COTAZYM® (pancrelipase capsules, USP) was compared to another pancreatic enzyme preparation for the treatment of fat malabsorption.[3]

COTAZYM® significantly reduced fecal fat as a percentage of intake when compared to baseline as follows:

	Baseline Mean ± SEM	COTAZYM® Mean ± SEM
Fecal Fat (as % of intake)	29.5 ± 5.2	14.7 ± 1.8 P value = 0.088

In a single center, randomized, double-blind, placebo controlled, 2-period crossover, 5-day treatment U.S. study in 10 male patients, ages 10–16 years, with exocrine pancreatic insufficiency secondary to cystic fibrosis, COTAZYM® and other pancreatic enzyme preparation were compared to placebo for treatment of fat malabsorption.[4]

COTAZYM® significantly reduced fecal fat as compared to placebo as follows:

	Placebo Mean ± SEM	COTAZYM® Mean ± SEM
Fecal Fat Excretion (grams/day)	67.9± 13.1	29.9 ± 7.0 P value < 0.005

Chronic Pancreatitis

In a multicenter, randomized, unblinded, 3-period crossover, 6-day treatment U.S. study in 6 male patients, ages 43–58 years, with exocrine pancreatic insufficiency from chronic alcoholic pancreatitis, COTAZYM® (pancrelipase capsules, USP) and two other pancreatic enzyme preparations were compared to a no treatment control for the treatment of fat malabsorption.[1]

COTAZYM® significantly reduced fecal fat as compared to the no treatment control as follows:

	Control Mean ± SEM	COTAZYM® Mean ± SEM
Fecal Fat Excretion (grams/day)	3.10 ± 2.0	15.0 ± 2.0 P value < 0.005

INDICATIONS AND USAGE

COTAZYM® (pancrelipase capsules, USP) capsules are indicated for treatment of steatorrhea due to exocrine pancreatic enzyme deficiency in such conditions as cystic fibrosis and chronic pancreatitis.

CONTRAINDICATIONS

COTAZYM® (pancrelipase capsules, USP) is contraindicated in those individuals who are hypersensitive to antigens of porcine origin.

WARNINGS

(See PRECAUTIONS and DOSAGE AND ADMINISTRATION.)

PRECAUTIONS

General

Large doses of delayed release pancreatic enzyme preparations taken by patients with cystic fibrosis have been associated with fibrosing colonopathy (colonic stricture). While COTAZYM® (pancrelipase capsules, USP) is an immediate release product and such products have not generally been associated with the lesion, the dose recommended should not be exceeded unless justified by individual patient need and response (see DOSAGE AND ADMINISTRATION and ADVERSE REACTIONS). If capsules must be opened for any reason, care should be taken that the powder is not inhaled or spilled on hands; it may cause serious allergic reaction or be irritating to the skin or mucous membranes. A mask and gloves should be worn while handling opened capsules.

Folic acid supplementation during pregnancy is important. Daily oral supplementation with folic acid before conception and during pregnancy can substantially reduce the occurrence of neural tube defects (anencephaly and spina bifida). Women should take folic acid if they are pregnant, or are thinking of becoming pregnant during treatment with COTAZYM®.

Information for Patients

Physicians are advised to discuss the following issues with patients for whom they prescribe COTAZYM® (pancrelipase capsules, USP):

Taking the Capsules

Patients should be instructed not to increase their COTAZYM® (pancrelipase capsules, USP) dose without consulting their physician. If it becomes necessary to open the COTAZYM® capsules, inhalation of the powder or contact with the skin or mucous membranes should be avoided. It is suggested mask and gloves be worn when opening capsules. COTAZYM® should not be taken by patients with known hypersensitivity to antigens of porcine origin. Sensitive individuals may experience allergic reactions.

Folic acid supplementation during pregnancy is important. Daily oral supplementation with folic acid before conception and during pregnancy can substantially reduce the occurrence of neural tube defects (anencephaly and spina bifida). Women should take folic acid if they are pregnant, or are thinking of becoming pregnant during treatment with COTAZYM®.

Concomitant Medication

Patients should be advised not to take COTAZYM® (pancrelipase capsules, USP) together with a combination of calcium carbonate and magnesium hydroxide. Calcium carbonate and magnesium hydroxide may be found in certain antacids. Calcium carbonate can also be found in certain calcium or mineral supplements. COTAZYM® may interfere with the absorption of folic acid and iron. Patients should consult with their physician if taking folic acid or iron containing preparations.

Pregnancy

COTAZYM® (pancrelipase capsules, USP) may interfere with the absorption of folic acid. Folic acid supplementation during pregnancy is important. Daily oral supplementation with folic acid before conception and during pregnancy can substantially reduce the occurrence of neural tube defects (anencephaly and spina bifida). Patients should be advised to notify their physician if they are pregnant or are thinking of becoming pregnant during treatment with COTAZYM® (pancrelipase capsules, USP).

Nursing

Patients should be advised to notify their physician if they are breast-feeding an infant.

Drug Interactions

Antacids containing calcium carbonate and magnesium hydroxide should not be taken concurrently with pancrelipase. The combination of calcium carbonate and magnesium hydroxide with pancrelipase may precipitate glycine-conjugated bile acids and may form calcium and magnesium fatty acid soaps, causing a decrease in fat absorption and thus an increase in steatorrhea.

Carcinogenesis, Mutagenesis and Impairment of Fertility

Long-term animal studies for carcinogenesis and studies evaluating the potential for impairment of fertility of mutagenesis have not been performed with COTAZYM® (pancrelipase capsules, USP).

Pregnancy

Pregnancy Category C

Animal reproductive studies have not been conducted with COTAZYM® (pancrelipase capsules, USP). It is not known whether COTAZYM® can cause fetal harm when administered to a pregnant woman or can affect reproductive capacity. COTAZYM® should be given to a pregnant woman only if clearly needed.

Nursing Mothers

It is not known if COTAZYM® (pancrelipase capsules, USP) is excreted in human milk.

Because many products are excreted in human milk, caution should be exercised when COTAZYM® is administered to nursing mothers.

ADVERSE REACTIONS

Adverse reactions to COTAZYM® (pancrelipase capsules, USP) have been reported uncommonly. The most frequent adverse reactions reported during clinical use are diarrhea and stool abnormalities, such as green stools. Other reactions reported include pharyngitis, vomiting, abdominal pain, gastric burning, syncope, mouth irritation, mouth ulcers, mild anemia, abnormal smell and taste, stomach trouble and belching. Hyperuricosuria and/or hyperuricemia have been reported in patients taking high doses of COTAZYM®, pancreatic extracts have high purine content. Renal damage has not been reported. Hypersensitivity reactions, such as anaphylaxis, allergy, nasal irritation, coughing spells and episodes of bronchospasm, can occur in people exposed to the enzyme powder from opened capsules. High doses of the powder may cause mouth or perianal excoriation. In addition, pancreatic enzyme preparations may interfere with folic acid and iron absorption.

There is a report of a child with cystic fibrosis who developed fibrosing colonopathy, and who has been treated with delayed-release pancreatic enzyme preparations as well as COTAZYM® prior to detection of the lesion.

OVERDOSAGE

No cases of acute overdose have been reported with COTAZYM® (pancrelipase capsules, USP). Hyperuricemia and/or hyperuricosuria have been reported in patients chronically taking high doses of COTAZYM® (pancrelipase capsules, USP). The minimum effective dose of COTAZYM® should be determined and adhered to for each patient. Large doses of delayed-release pancreatic enzyme preparations taken by patients with cystic fibrosis have been associated with fibrosing colonopathy (see PRECAUTIONS).

DOSAGE AND ADMINISTRATION

Cystic Fibrosis

The dosage of COTAZYM® (pancrelipase capsules, USP) must be individualized according to the patient's remaining exocrine pancreatic function, pH of the gut lumen (if such measurements are routinely taken) and intake of fat and protein. Dosage should depend on nutritional intake as well as body weight, and varies with age. A high caloric diet with unrestricted fat appropriate to age and clinical status should be consumed. While the dose may need to be adjusted for control of steatorrhea, a total daily dose should not exceed 2500 lipase units/kg per meal without careful evaluation of the patient. A dose higher than 6000 lipase units/kg per meal should not be administered[5] (see PRECAUTIONS).

Prior to treatment, the patient's stool should be evaluated microscopically for the presence of fat droplets. If visible, a 72-hour fat balance study should be performed while monitoring nutrient intake, to determine the extent of malabsorption. In patients with meconium ileus, a fat balance study is not required prior to establishing a dosage and beginning treatment with COTAZYM®. Do not exceed recommended dosage. Based on 2500 lipase units/kg per meal, the maximum recommended dosage for a 70 kg patient would be 20 capsules per meal (60 capsules/day for 3 meals). Dosages greater than 2500 lipase units/kg per meal should only be used with caution and only if safely tolerated by the patient and documented to be effective by 3 day fecal fat measures that indicate a significantly improved coefficient of absorption.[5] Infants should be given a total of 2000 to 4000 lipase units for each 120 mL (4 oz.) of formula or each breast feeding. For other children less than 4 years of age, dosing should begin with 1000 lipase units/kg for each meal. For children 4 years of age or older, 500 lipase units/kg for each meal should be initiated. For a snack, half the dose for a meal should be given.

Chronic Pancreatitis

One or two capsules should be administered for control of symptoms and adjusted as needed.

HOW SUPPLIED

COTAZYM® (pancrelipase capsules, USP) are opaque green capsules imprinted with "Organon" and "381". COTAZYM® is supplied in bottles of 100, NDC# 0052-0381-91, and bottles of 500, NDC# 0052-0381-95.

Storage: Not to exceed 25°C (77°F). Store in dry place when opened.

Dispense: In tight container as defined in the USP.

REFERENCES

1. Dutta SK, Rubin J, Harvey J. Comparative Evaluation of the Therapeutic Efficacy of a pH-Sensitive Enteric Coated Pancreatic Enzyme Preparation with Conventional Pancreatic Enzyme Therapy in the Treatment of Exocrine Pancreatic Insufficiency. *Gastroenterology* 1983;84:476–482.
2. Dutta SK, Hubbard VS, Appler M. Critical examination of therapeutic efficacy of a pH-sensitive enteric-coated pancreatic enzyme preparation in treatment of exocrine pancreatic insufficiency secondary to cystic fibrosis. *Dig Dis and Sci* 1988;33:1237–1244.
3. Data on File at Organon Inc., W. Orange, NJ, USA
4. Mischler EH, Parrell S, Farrell PM, Odell GB. Comparison of effectiveness of pancreatic enzyme preparations in cystic fibrosis. *Am J Dis Child* 1982;136:1060–1063.
5. Borowitz DS, Grand RJ, Durie PR, and the Consensus Committee. Use of pancreatic enzyme supplements for patients with cystic fibrosis in the context of fibrosing colonopathy. *J Ped* 1995;127:681–684.

Caution: Federal law prohibits dispensing without a prescription.

Organon' Inc.
375 Mt. Pleasant Avenue
West Orange, NJ 07052

Shown in Product Identification Guide, page 326

COTAZYM®-S ℞

[kōt 'a zīm-s]

(pancrelipase, USP)

Enteric coated spheres

Each capsule contains not less than:

5,000	USP Units of Lipase
20,000	USP Units of Protease
20,000	USP Units of Amylase

HOW SUPPLIED

Bottles of 100 capsules

Bottles of 500 capsules

Shown in Product Identification Guide, page 326

DECA-DURABOLIN® Ⓒ ℞

(nandrolone decanoate injection, USP)

HOW SUPPLIED

100 mg/mL—2 mL vials—NDC-0052-0697-02

200 mg/mL—1 mL vials—NDC-0052-0698-01

DESOGEN® ℞

(desogestrel and ethinyl estradiol) Tablets

PATIENTS SHOULD BE COUNSELED THAT THIS PRODUCT DOES NOT PROTECT AGAINST HIV INFECTION (AIDS) AND OTHER SEXUALLY TRANSMITTED DISEASES.

Rx only

DESCRIPTION

Desogen® 28 Tablets provide an oral contraceptive regimen of 21 white round tablets each containing 0.15 mg desogestrel (13-ethyl-11- methylene-18,19-dinor-17 alpha-pregn- 4-en- 20-yn-17-ol) and 0.03 mg ethinyl estradiol (19-nor-17 alpha-pregna-1,3,5 (10)-trien-20-yne-3,17-diol). Inactive ingredients include vitamin E, corn starch, povidone, stearic acid, colloidal silicon dioxide, lactose, hydroxypropyl methylcellulose, polyethylene glycol, titanium dioxide and talc. Desogen® 28 also contains 7 green round tablets containing the following inactive ingredients: lactose, corn starch, magnesium stearate, FD&C Blue No. 2 aluminum lake, ferric oxide, hydroxypropyl methylcellulose, polyethylene glycol, titanium dioxide and talc.

Continued on next page

Desogen—Cont.

DESOGESTREL

DESOGESTREL

ETHINYL ESTRADIOL

CLINICAL PHARMACOLOGY

Pharmacodynamics

Combination oral contraceptives act by suppression of gonadotropins. Although the primary mechanism of this action is inhibition of ovulation, other alterations include changes in the cervical mucus, which increase the difficulty of sperm entry into the uterus, and changes in the endometrium which reduce the likelihood of implantation.

Receptor binding studies, as well as studies in animals and humans, have shown that 3-keto-desogestrel, the biologically active metabolite of desogestrel, combines high progestational activity with minimal intrinsic androgenicity (91,92). Desogestrel, in combination with ethinyl estradiol, does not counteract the estrogen-induced increase in SHBG, resulting in lower serum levels of free testosterone (96–99).

Pharmacokinetics

Desogestrel is rapidly and almost completely absorbed and converted into 3-keto-desogestrel, its biologically active metabolite. Following oral administration, the relative bioavailability of desogestrel, as measured by serum levels of 3-keto-desogestrel, is approximately 84%.

In the third cycle of use after a single dose of Desogen®, maximum concentrations of 3-keto-desogestrel of $2,805 \pm 1,203$ pg/mL (mean$\pm$SD) are reached at 1.4 ± 0.8 hours. The area under the curve (AUC$_{0-\infty}$) is $33,858 \pm 11,043$ pg/mL·hr after a single dose. At steady state, attained from at least day 19 onwards, maximum concentrations of $5,840 \pm 1,667$ pg/mL are reached at 1.4 ± 0.9 hours. The minimum plasma levels of 3-keto-desogestrel at steady state are $1,400 \pm 560$ pg/mL. The AUC$_{0-24}$ at steady state is $52,299 \pm 17,878$ pg/mL·hr. The mean AUC$_{0-\infty}$ for 3-keto-desogestrel at single dose is significantly lower than the mean AUC$_{0-24}$ at steady state. This indicates that the kinetics of 3-keto-desogestrel are non-linear due to an increase in binding of 3-keto-desogestrel to sex hormone-binding globulin in the cycle, attributed to increased sex hormone-binding globulin levels which are induced by the daily administration of ethinyl estradiol. Sex hormone-binding globulin levels increased significantly in the third treatment cycle from day 1 (150$\pm$64 nmol/L) to day 21 (230$\pm$59 nmol/L).

The elimination half-life for 3-keto-desogestrel is approximately 38 ± 20 hours at steady state. In addition to 3-keto-desogestrel, other phase I metabolites are 3α-OH-desogestrel, 3β-OH-desogestrel, and 3α-OH-5α-H-desogestrel. These other metabolites are not known to have any pharmacologic effects, and are further converted in part by conjugation (phase II metabolism) into polar metabolites, mainly sulfates and glucuronides.

Ethinyl estradiol is rapidly and almost completely absorbed. In the third cycle of use after a single dose of Desogen®, the relative bioavailability is approximately 83%.

In the third cycle of use after a single dose of Desogen®, maximum concentrations of ethinyl estradiol of 95 ± 34 pg/mL are reached at 1.5 ± 0.8 hours. The AUC$_{0-\infty}$ is $1,471 \pm 268$ pg/mL·hr after a single dose. At steady state, attained from at least day 19 onwards, maximum ethinyl estradiol concentrations of 141 ± 48 pg/mL are reached at about 1.4 ± 0.7 hours. The minimum serum levels of ethinyl estradiol at steady state are 24 ± 8.3 pg/mL. The AUC$_{0-24}$ at steady state is $1,117 \pm 302$ pg/mL·hr. The mean AUC$_{0-\infty}$ for ethinyl estradiol following a single dose during treatment cycle 3 does not significantly differ from the mean AUC$_{0-24}$ at steady state. This finding indicates linear kinetics for ethinyl estradiol.

The elimination half-life is 26 ± 6.8 hours at steady state. Ethinyl estradiol is subject to a significant degree of presystemic conjugation (phase II metabolism). Ethinyl estradiol escaping gut wall conjugation undergoes phase I metabolism and hepatic conjugation (phase II metabolism). Major phase I metabolites are 2-OH-ethinyl estradiol and 2-meth-

oxy-ethinyl estradiol. Sulfate and glucuronide conjugates of both ethinyl estradiol and phase I metabolites, which are excreted in bile, can undergo enterohepatic circulation.

INDICATIONS AND USAGE

Desogen® Tablets are indicated for the prevention of pregnancy in women who elect to use oral contraceptives as a method of contraception.

Oral contraceptives are highly effective. Table I lists the typical accidental pregnancy rates for users of combination oral contraceptives and other methods of contraception. The efficacy of these contraceptive methods, except sterilization, depends upon the reliability with which they are used. Correct and consistent use of these methods can result in lower failure rates.

TABLE I: LOWEST EXPECTED AND TYPICAL FAILURE RATES (%) DURING THE FIRST YEAR OF USE OF A CONTRACEPTIVE METHOD

Method	Lowest* Expected*	Typical**
Oral Contraceptives		3
combined	0.1	N/A
progestin only	0.5	N/A
Diaphragm with spermicidal cream or jelly	6	18
Spermicides alone (foam, creams, jellies and vaginal suppositories)	3	21
Vaginal Sponge		
nulliparous	6	18
parous	9	28
IUD (medicated)	2	3
Implant		
capsules	0.04	0.04
rods	0	0.03
Condom without spermicide	2.03	12
Cervical Cap	6	18
Periodic abstinence (all methods)	1–9	20
Female sterilization	0.2	0.4
Male sterilization	0.1	0.15
No contraception (planned pregnancy)	85	85

Adapted from J. Trussell, et al. Table 1, ref. #1.

N/A—Data not available.

* The author's best estimate of the percentage of women expected to experience an accidental pregnancy among couples who initiate a method (not necessarily for the first time) and who use it consistently and correctly during the first year, if they do not stop for any other reason.

** This term represents "typical" couples who initiate use of a method (not necessarily for the first time), who experience an accidental pregnancy during the first year, if they do not stop use for any other reason.

In clinical trials with Desogen®, 2,004 subjects completed 19,181 cycles and a total of 12 pregnancies were reported. This represents an overall user-efficacy pregnancy rate of 0.81 woman-years. This rate includes patients who did not take the drug correctly.

CONTRAINDICATIONS

Oral contraceptives should not be used in women who currently have the following conditions:

- Thrombophlebitis or thromboembolic disorders
- A past history of deep vein thrombophlebitis or thromboembolic disorders
- Cerebral vascular or coronary artery disease
- Known or suspected carcinoma of the breast
- Carcinoma of the endometrium or other known or suspected estrogen-dependent neoplasia
- Undiagnosed abnormal genital bleeding
- Cholestatic jaundice of pregnancy or jaundice with prior pill use
- Hepatic adenomas or carcinomas
- Known or suspected pregnancy

WARNINGS

Cigarette smoking increases the risk of serious cardiovascular side effects from oral contraceptive use. This risk increases with age and with heavy smoking (15 or more cigarettes per day) and is quite marked in women over 35 years of age. Women who use oral contraceptives should be strongly advised not to smoke.

The use of oral contraceptives is associated with increased risks of several serious conditions including myocardial infarction, thromboembolism, stroke, hepatic neoplasia, and gallbladder disease, although the risk of serious morbidity

or mortality is very small in healthy women without underlying risk factors. The risk of morbidity and mortality increases significantly in the presence of other underlying risk factors such as hypertension, hyperlipidemias, obesity and diabetes.

Practitioners prescribing oral contraceptives should be familiar with the following information relating to these risks. The information contained in this package insert is principally based on studies carried out in patients who used oral contraceptives with formulations of higher doses of estrogens and progestogens than those in common use today. The effect of long term use of the oral contraceptives with formulations of lower doses of both estrogens and progestogens remains to be determined.

Throughout this labeling, epidemiological studies reported are of two types: retrospective or case control studies and prospective or cohort studies. Case control studies provide a measure of the relative risk of a disease, namely, a ratio of the incidence of a disease among oral contraceptive users to that among nonusers. The relative risk does not provide information on the actual clinical occurrence of a disease. Cohort studies provide a measure of attributable risk, which is the *difference* in the incidence of disease between oral contraceptive users and nonusers. The attributable risk does provide information about the actual occurrence of a disease in the population (Adapted from refs. 2 and 3 with the author's permission). For further information, the reader is referred to a text on epidemiological methods.

1. THROMBOEMBOLIC DISORDERS AND OTHER VASCULAR PROBLEMS

a. Myocardial infarction

An increased risk of myocardial infarction has been attributed to oral contraceptive use. This risk is primarily in smokers or women with other underlying risk factors for coronary artery disease such as hypertension, hypercholesterolemia, morbid obesity, and diabetes. The relative risk of heart attack for current oral contraceptive users has been estimated to be two to six (4-10). The risk is very low in women under the age of 30.

Smoking in combination with oral contraceptive use has been shown to contribute substantially to the incidence of myocardial infarctions in women in their mid-thirties or older with smoking accounting for the majority of excess cases (11). Mortality rates associated with circulatory disease have been shown to increase substantially in smokers, especially in those 35 years of age and older among women who use oral contraceptives. (See Table II)

TABLE II: Circulatory disease mortality rates per 100,000 women-years by age, smoking status and oral contraceptive use

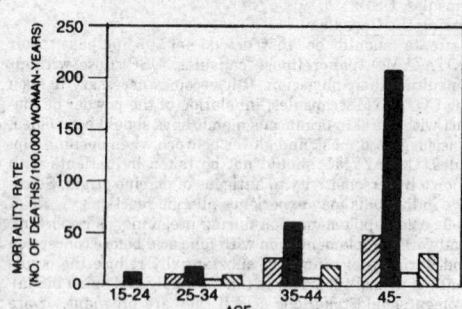

(Adapted from P.M. Layde and V. Beral, ref #12.)

Oral contraceptives may compound the effects of well-known risk factors, such as hypertension, diabetes, hyperlipidemias, age and obesity (13). In particular, some progestogens are known to decrease HDL cholesterol and cause glucose intolerance, while estrogens may create a state of hyperinsulinism (14–18). Oral contraceptives have been shown to increase blood pressure among users (see section 9 in WARNINGS). Similar effects on risk factors have been associated with an increased risk of heart disease. Oral contraceptives must be used with caution in women with cardiovascular disease risk factors. Desogestrel has minimal androgenic activity (see CLINICAL PHARMACOLOGY) and there is some evidence that the risk of myocardial infarction associated with oral contraceptives is lower when the progestogen has

minimal androgenic activity than when the activity is greater (100).

b. Thromboembolism

An increased risk of thromboembolic and thrombotic disease associated with the use of oral contraceptives is well established. Case control studies have found the relative risk of users compared to nonusers to be 3 for the first episode of superficial venous thrombosis, 4 to 11 for deep vein thrombosis or pulmonary embolism, and 1.5 to 6 for women with predisposing conditions for venous thromboembolic disease (2,3,19–24). Cohort studies have shown the relative risk to be somewhat lower, about 3 for new cases and about 4.5 for new cases requiring hospitalization (25). The risk of thromboembolic disease associated with oral contraceptives is not related to length of use and disappears after pill use is stopped (2).

In two case-control studies and one cohort study of venous thromboembolism, third generation oral contraceptives, including those containing desogestrel, were reported to have a relative risk between 1.5 and 2.4 when compared to certain second generation oral contraceptives (101–103). These risks are within the above-mentioned range for deep vein thrombosis and pulmonary embolism. A relative risk of 2 would translate into an additional 1–2 cases of non-fatal venous thromboembolism per 10,000 women-years of use. The risk of venous thromboembolic disease associated with oral contraceptives does not increase with length of use and disappears after pill use is stopped.

A two to four-fold increase in relative risk of postoperative thromboembolic complications has been reported with the use of oral contraceptives (9). The relative risk of venous thrombosis in women who have predisposing conditions is twice that of women without such medical conditions (26). If feasible, oral contraceptives should be discontinued at least four weeks prior to and for two weeks after elective surgery of a type associated with an increase in risk of thromboembolism and during and following prolonged immobilization. Since the immediate postpartum period is also associated with an increased risk of thromboembolism, oral contraceptives should be started no earlier than four weeks after delivery in women who elect not to breast feed.

c. Cerebrovascular diseases

Oral contraceptives have been shown to increase both the relative and attributable risks of cerebrovascular events (thrombotic and hemorrhagic strokes), although, in general, the risk is greatest among older (>35 years), hypertensive women who also smoke. Hypertension was found to be a risk factor for both users and nonusers, for both types of strokes, and smoking interacted to increase the risk of stroke (27–29).

In a large study, the relative risk of thrombotic strokes has been shown to range from 3 for normotensive users to 14 for users with severe hypertension (30). The relative risk of hemorrhagic stroke is reported to be 1.2 for non-smokers who used oral contraceptives, 2.6 for smokers who did not use oral contraceptives, 7.6 for smokers who used oral contraceptives, 1.8 for normotensive users and 25.7 for users with severe hypertension (30). The attributable risk is also greater in older women (3).

d. Dose-related risk of vascular disease from oral contraceptives

A positive association has been observed between the amount of estrogen and progestogen in oral contraceptives and the risk of vascular disease (31–33). A decline in serum high density lipoproteins (HDL) has been reported with many progestational agents (14–16). A decline in serum high density lipoproteins has been associated with an increased incidence of ischemic heart disease. Because estrogens increase HDL cholesterol, the net effect of an oral contraceptive depends on a balance achieved between doses of estrogen and progestogen and the nature and absolute amount of progestogens used in the contraceptives. The amount of both hormones should be considered in the choice of an oral contraceptive.

Minimizing exposure to estrogen and progestogen is in keeping with good principles of therapeutics. For any particular estrogen/progestogen combination, the dosage regimen prescribed should be one which contains the least amount of estrogen and progestogen that is compatible with a low failure rate and the needs of the individual patient. New acceptors of oral contraceptive agents should be started on preparations containing 0.035 mg or less of estrogen.

e. Persistence of risk of vascular disease

There are two studies which have shown persistence of risk of vascular disease for ever-users of oral contraceptives. In a study in the United States, the risk of developing myocardial infarction after discontinuing oral contraceptives persists for at least 9 years for women 40-49 years old who had used oral contraceptives for five or more years, but this increased risk was not demonstrated in other age groups (8). In another study in Great Britain, the risk of developing cerebrovascular disease persisted for at least 6 years after discontinuation of oral contraceptives, although excess risk was very small (34). However, both studies were performed with oral contraceptive formulations containing 0.050 mg or higher of estrogens.

TABLE III: ANNUAL NUMBER OF BIRTH-RELATED OR METHOD-RELATED DEATHS ASSOCIATED WITH CONTROL OF FERTILITY PER 100,000 NON-STERILE WOMEN, BY FERTILITY CONTROL METHOD ACCORDING TO AGE

Method of control and outcome	15–19	20–24	25–29	30–34	35–39	40–44
No fertility control methods*	7.0	7.4	9.1	14.8	25.7	28.2
Oral contraceptives non-smoker**	0.3	0.5	0.9	1.9	13.8	31.6
Oral contraceptives smoker**	2.2	3.4	6.6	13.5	51.1	117.2
IUD**	0.8	0.8	1.0	1.0	1.4	1.4
Condom*	1.1	1.6	0.7	0.2	0.3	0.4
Diaphragm/spermicide*	1.9	1.2	1.2	1.3	2.2	2.8
Periodic abstinence*	2.5	1.6	1.6	1.7	2.9	3.6

* Deaths are birth related
** Deaths are method related

(Adapted from H.W. Ory, ref. #35.)

2. ESTIMATES OF MORTALITY FROM CONTRACEPTIVE USE

One study gathered data from a variety of sources which have estimated the mortality rate associated with different methods of contraception at different ages (Table III). These estimates include the combined risk of death associated with contraceptive methods plus the risk attributable to pregnancy in the event of method failure. Each method of contraception has its specific benefits and risks. The study concluded that with the exception of oral contraceptive users 35 and older who smoke and 40 and older who do not smoke, mortality associated with all methods of birth control is low and below that associated with childbirth.

The observation of an increase in risk of mortality with age for oral contraceptive users is based on data gathered in the 1970's (35). Current clinical recommendation involves the use of lower estrogen dose formulations and a careful consideration of risk factors. In 1989, the Fertility and Maternal Health Drugs Advisory Committee was asked to review the use of oral contraceptives in women 40 years of age and over. The committee concluded that although cardiovascular disease risk may be increased with oral contraceptive use after age 40 in healthy non-smoking women (even with the newer low-dose formulations), there are also greater potential health risks associated with pregnancy in older women and with the alternative surgical and medical procedures which may be necessary if such women do not have access to effective and acceptable means of contraception. The Committee recommended that the benefits of low-dose oral contraceptive use by healthy non-smoking women over 40 may outweigh the possible risks.

Of course, older women, as all women who take oral contraceptives, should take an oral contraceptive which contains the least amount of estrogen and progestogen that is compatible with a low failure rate and individual patient needs.

[See table above]

3. CARCINOMA OF THE REPRODUCTIVE ORGANS AND BREASTS

Numerous epidemiological studies have been performed on the incidence of breast, endometrial, ovarian and cervical cancer in women using oral contraceptives. While there are conflicting reports most studies suggest that the use of oral contraceptives is not associated with an overall increase in the risk of developing breast cancer. Some studies have reported an increased relative risk of developing breast cancer, particularly at a younger age. This increased relative risk appears to be related to duration of use (36-43, 79-89).

Some studies suggest that oral contraceptive use has been associated with an increase in the risk of cervical intraepithelial neoplasia in some populations of women (45-48). However, there continues to be controversy about the extent to which such findings may be due to differences in sexual behavior and other factors.

4. HEPATIC NEOPLASIA

Benign hepatic adenomas are associated with oral contraceptive use, although the incidence of benign tumors is rare in the United States. Indirect calculations have estimated the attributable risk to be in the range of 3.3 cases/100,000 for users, a risk that increases after four or more years of use especially with oral contraceptives of higher dose (49). Rupture of rare, benign, hepatic adenomas may cause death through intra-abdominal hemorrhage (50,51).

Studies from Britain have shown an increased risk of developing hepatocellular carcinoma (52–54) in long-term (>8 years) oral contraceptive users. However, these cancers are rare in the U.S. and the attributable risk (the excess incidence) of liver cancers in oral contraceptive users approaches less than one per million users

5. OCULAR LESIONS

There have been clinical case reports of retinal thrombosis associated with the use of oral contraceptives. Oral contraceptives should be discontinued if there is unexplained partial or complete loss of vision; onset of proptosis or diplopia; papilledema; or retinal vascular lesions. Appropriate diagnostic and therapeutic measures should be undertaken immediately.

6. ORAL CONTRACEPTIVE USE BEFORE OR DURING EARLY PREGNANCY

Extensive epidemiological studies have revealed no increased risk of birth defects in women who have used oral contraceptives prior to pregnancy (56-57). The majority of recent studies also do not indicate a teratogenic effect, particularly in so far as cardiac anomalies and limb reduction defects are concerned (55, 56, 58, 59), when oral contraceptives are taken inadvertently during early pregnancy.

The administration of oral contraceptives to induce withdrawal bleeding should not be used as a test for pregnancy. Oral contraceptives should not be used during pregnancy to treat threatened or habitual abortion.

It is recommended that for any patient who has missed two consecutive periods, pregnancy should be ruled out before continuing oral contraceptive use. If the patient has not adhered to the prescribed schedule, the possibility of pregnancy should be considered at the time of the first missed period. Oral contraceptive use should be discontinued until pregnancy is ruled out.

7. GALLBLADDER DISEASE

Earlier studies have reported an increased lifetime relative risk of gallbladder surgery in users of oral contraceptives and estrogens (60,61). More recent studies, however, have shown that the relative risk of developing gallbladder disease among oral contraceptive users may be minimal (62-64). The recent findings of minimal risk may be related to the use of oral contraceptive formulations containing lower hormonal doses of estrogens and progestogens.

8. CARBOHYDRATE AND LIPID METABOLIC EFFECTS

Oral contraceptives have been shown to cause a decrease in glucose tolerance in a significant percentage of users (17). This effect has been shown to be directly related to estrogen dose (65). In general, progestogens increase insulin secretion and create insulin resistance, this effect varying with different progestational agents (17,66). In the nondiabetic woman, oral contraceptives appear to have no effect on fasting blood glucose (67). Because of these demonstrated effects, prediabetic and diabetic women should be carefully monitored while taking oral contraceptives.

A small proportion of women will have persistent hypertriglyceridemia while on the pill. As discussed earlier (see WARNINGS 1.a. and 1.d.), changes in serum triglycerides and lipoprotein levels have been reported in oral contraceptive users.

9. ELEVATED BLOOD PRESSURE

An increase in blood pressure has been reported in women taking oral contraceptives (68) and this increase is more likely in older oral contraceptive users (69) and with extended duration of use (61).

Data from the Royal College of General Practitioners (12) and subsequent randomized trials have shown that the incidence of hypertension increases with increasing progestational activity.

Women with a history of hypertension or hypertension-related diseases, or renal disease (70) should be encouraged to use another method of contraception. If women elect to use oral contraceptives, they should be monitored closely and if significant elevation of blood pressure occurs, oral contraceptive should be discontinued. For most women, elevated blood pressure will return to normal after stopping oral contraceptives (69), and there is no difference in the occurrence of hypertension among former and never users (68,70,71).

Continued on next page

Desogen—Cont.

10. HEADACHE

The onset or exacerbation of migraine or development of headache with a new pattern which is recurrent, persistent or severe requires discontinuation of oral contraceptives and evaluation of the cause.

11. BLEEDING IRREGULARITIES

Breakthrough bleeding and spotting are sometimes encountered in patients on oral contraceptives, especially during the first three months of use. Nonhormonal causes should be considered and adequate diagnostic measures taken to rule out malignancy or pregnancy in the event of breakthrough bleeding, as in the case of any abnormal vaginal bleeding. If pathology has been excluded, time or a change to another formulation may solve the problem. In the event of amenorrhea, pregnancy should be ruled out.

Some women may encounter post-pill amenorrhea or oligomenorrhea, especially when such a condition was pre-existent.

12. ECTOPIC PREGNANCY

Ectopic as well as intrauterine pregnancy may occur in contraceptive failures.

PRECAUTIONS

1. PHYSICAL EXAMINATION AND FOLLOW UP

It is good medical practice for all women to have annual history and physical examinations, including women using oral contraceptives. The physical examination, however, may be deferred until after initiation of oral contraceptives if requested by the woman and judged appropriate by the clinician. The physical examination should include special reference to blood pressure, breasts, abdomen and pelvic organs, including cervical cytology, and relevant laboratory tests. In case of undiagnosed, persistent or recurrent abnormal vaginal bleeding, appropriate measures should be conducted to rule out malignancy. Women with a strong family history of breast cancer or who have breast nodules should be monitored with particular care.

2. LIPID DISORDERS

Women who are being treated for hyperlipidemias should be followed closely if they elect to use oral contraceptives. Some progestogens may elevate LDL levels and may render the control of hyperlipidemias more difficult.

3. LIVER FUNCTION

If jaundice develops in any woman receiving such drugs, the medication should be discontinued. Steroid hormones may be poorly metabolized in patients with impaired liver function.

4. FLUID RETENTION

Oral contraceptives may cause some degree of fluid retention. They should be prescribed with caution, and only with careful monitoring, in patients with conditions which might be aggravated by fluid retention.

5. EMOTIONAL DISORDERS

Women with a history of depression should be carefully observed and the drug discontinued if depression recurs to a serious degree.

6. CONTACT LENSES

Contact lens wearers who develop visual changes or changes in lens tolerance should be assessed by an ophthalmologist.

7. DRUG INTERACTIONS

Reduced efficacy and increased incidence of breakthrough bleeding and menstrual irregularities have been associated with concomitant use of rifampin. A similar association, though less marked, has been suggested with barbiturates, phenylbutazone, phenytoin sodium, carbamazepine and possibly with griseofulvin, ampicillin and tetracyclines (72).

8. INTERACTIONS WITH LABORATORY TESTS

Certain endocrine and liver function tests and blood components may be affected by oral contraceptives:
a. Increased prothrombin and factors VII, VIII, IX and X; decreased antithrombin 3; increased norepinephrine-induced platelet aggregability.
b. Increased thyroid binding globulin (TBG) leading to increased circulating total thyroid hormone, as measured by protein-bound iodine (PBI), T4 by column or by radioimmunoassay. Free T3 resin uptake is decreased, reflecting the elevated TBG; free T4 concentration is unaltered.
c. Other binding proteins may be elevated in serum.
d. Sex-hormone binding globulins are increased and result in elevated levels of total circulating sex steroids; however, free or biologically active levels either decrease or remain unchanged.
e. High-density lipoprotein cholesterol (HDL-C) and triglycerides may be increased, while low-density lipoprotein cholesterol (LDL-C) and total cholesterol (Total-C) may be decreased or unchanged.
f. Glucose tolerance may be decreased.
g. Serum folate levels may be depressed by oral contraceptive therapy. This may be of clinical significance if a woman becomes pregnant

9. CARCINOGENESIS

See WARNINGS section.

10. PREGNANCY

Pregnancy Category X. See CONTRAINDICATIONS and WARNINGS sections.

11. NURSING MOTHERS

Small amounts of oral contraceptive steroids have been identified in the milk of nursing mothers and a few adverse effects on the child have been reported, including jaundice and breast enlargement. In addition, oral contraceptives given in the postpartum period may interfere with lactation by decreasing the quantity and quality of breast milk. If possible, the nursing mother should be advised not to use oral contraceptives but to use other forms of contraception until she has completely weaned her child.

12. GENERAL

PATIENTS SHOULD BE COUNSELED THAT THIS PRODUCT DOES NOT PROTECT AGAINST HIV INFECTION (AIDS) AND OTHER SEXUALLY TRANSMITTED DISEASES.

INFORMATION FOR THE PATIENT

See Patient Labeling Printed Below

ADVERSE REACTIONS

An increased risk of the following serious adverse reactions has been associated with the use of oral contraceptives (see WARNINGS section):
- Thrombophlebitis and venous thrombosis with or without embolism
- Arterial thromboembolism
- Pulmonary embolism
- Myocardial infarction
- Cerebral hemorrhage
- Cerebral thrombosis
- Hypertension
- Gallbladder disease
- Hepatic adenomas or benign liver tumors

The following adverse reactions have been reported in patients receiving oral contraceptives and are believed to be drug-related:
- Nausea
- Vomiting
- Gastrointestinal symptoms (such as abdominal cramps and bloating)
- Breakthrough bleeding
- Spotting
- Change in menstrual flow
- Amenorrhea
- Temporary infertility after discontinuation of treatment
- Edema
- Melasma which may persist
- Breast changes: tenderness, enlargement, secretion
- Change in weight (increase or decrease)
- Change in cervical erosion and secretion
- Diminution in lactation when given immediately postpartum
- Cholestatic jaundice
- Migraine
- Rash (allergic)
- Mental depression
- Reduced tolerance to carbohydrates
- Vaginal candidiasis
- Change in corneal curvature (steepening)
- Intolerance to contact lenses

The following adverse reactions have been reported in users of oral contraceptives and the association has been neither confirmed nor refuted:
- Pre-menstrual syndrome
- Cataracts
- Changes in appetite
- Cystitis-like syndrome
- Headache
- Nervousness
- Dizziness
- Hirsutism
- Loss of scalp hair
- Erythema multiforme
- Erythema nodosum
- Hemorrhagic eruption
- Vaginitis
- Porphyria
- Impaired renal function
- Hemolytic uremic syndrome
- Acne
- Changes in libido
- Colitis
- Budd-Chiari Syndrome

OVERDOSAGE

Serious ill effects have not been reported following acute ingestion of large doses of oral contraceptives by young children. Overdosage may cause nausea, and withdrawal bleeding may occur in females.

NON-CONTRACEPTIVE HEALTH BENEFITS

The following non-contraceptive health benefits related to the use of oral contraceptives are supported by epidemiological studies which largely utilized oral contraceptive formulations containing estrogen doses exceeding 0.035 mg of ethinyl estradiol or 0.05 mg of mestranol (73–78).
Effects on menses:
- increased menstrual cycle regularity
- decreased blood loss and decreased incidence of iron deficiency anemia
- decreased incidence of dysmenorrhea

Effects related to inhibition of ovulation:
- decreased incidence of functional ovarian cysts
- decreased incidence of ectopic pregnancies

Effects from long-term use:
- decreased incidence of fibroadenomas and fibrocystic disease of the breast
- decreased incidence of acute pelvic inflammatory disease
- decreased incidence of endometrial cancer
- decreased incidence of ovarian cancer

DESOGEN®

DOSAGE AND ADMINISTRATION

To achieve maximum contraceptive effectiveness, Desogen® must be taken exactly as directed and at intervals not exceeding 24 hours. Desogen® may be initiated using either a Sunday start or a Day 1 start.

NOTE: Each cycle pack dispenser is preprinted with the days of the week, starting with Sunday, to facilitate a Sunday start regimen. Six different "day label strips" are provided with each cycle pack dispenser in order to accommodate a Day 1 start regimen. In this case, the patient should place the self-adhesive "day label strip" that corresponds to her starting day over the preprinted days.

IMPORTANT: The possibility of ovulation and conception prior to initiation of use of Desogen® should be considered. The use of Desogen® for contraception may be initiated 4 weeks postpartum in women who elect not to breast feed. When the tablets are administered during the postpartum period, the increased risk of thromboembolic disease associated with the postpartum period must be considered. (See CONTRAINDICATIONS and WARNINGS concerning thromboembolic disease. See also PRECAUTIONS for "Nursing Mothers".)

If the patient starts on Desogen® postpartum, and has not yet had a period, she should be instructed to use another method of contraception until a white tablet has been taken daily for 7 days.

SUNDAY START

When initiating a Sunday start regimen, another method of contraception should be used until after the first 7 consecutive days of administration.

Using a Sunday start, tablets are taken without interruption as follows: The first white tablet should be taken on the first Sunday after menstruation begins (if menstruation begins on Sunday, the first white tablet is taken on that day). One white tablet is taken daily for 21 days, followed by 1 green (inert) tablet daily for 7 days. For all subsequent cycles, the patient then begins a new 28-tablet regimen on the next day (Sunday) after taking the last green tablet. [If switching from a Sunday start oral contraceptive, the first Desogen® tablet should be taken on the second Sunday after the last tablet of a 21 day regimen or should be taken on the first Sunday after the last inactive tablet of a 28 day regimen.]

If a patient misses 1 white tablet, she should take the missed tablet as soon as she remembers. If the patient misses 2 consecutive white tablets in Week 1 or Week 2, the patient should take 2 tablets the day she remembers and 2 tablets the next day; thereafter, the patient should keep taking 1 tablet daily until she finishes the cycle pack. The patient should be instructed to use a back-up method of birth control if she has intercourse in the 7 days after missing pills. If the patient misses 2 consecutive white tablets in the third week or misses 3 or more white tablets in a row at anytime during the cycle, the patient should keep taking 1 white tablet daily until the next Sunday. On Sunday the patient should throw out the rest of that cycle pack and start a new cycle pack that same day. The patient should be instructed to use a back-up method of birth control if she has intercourse in the 7 days after missing pills.

DAY 1 START

Counting the first day of menstruation as "Day 1 ", tablets are taken without interruption as follows: One white tablet daily for 21 days, then one green (inert) tablet daily for 7 days. For all subsequent cycles, the patient then begins a new 28-tablet regimen on the next day after taking the last green tablet. [If switching directly from another oral contra-

ceptive, the first white tablet should be taken on the first day of menstruation which begins after the last ACTIVE tablet of the previous product.]

If a patient misses 1 white tablet, she should take the missed tablet as soon as she remembers. If the patient misses 2 consecutive white tablets in Week 1 or Week 2, the patient should take 2 tablets the day she remembers and 2 tablets the next day; thereafter, the patient should resume taking 1 tablet daily until she finishes the cycle pack. The patient should be instructed to use a back-up method of birth control if she has intercourse in the 7 days after missing pills. If the patient misses 2 consecutive white tablets in the third week or misses 3 or more white tablets in a row at anytime during the cycle, the patient should throw out the rest of that cycle pack and start a new cycle pack that same day. The patient should be instructed to use a back-up method of birth control if she has intercourse in the 7 days after missing pills.

ALL ORAL CONTRACEPTIVES

Breakthrough bleeding, spotting, and amenorrhea are frequent reasons for patients discontinuing oral contraceptives. In breakthrough bleeding, as in all cases of irregular bleeding from the vagina, nonfunctional causes should be borne in mind. In undiagnosed persistent or recurrent abnormal bleeding from the vagina, adequate diagnostic measures are indicated to rule out pregnancy or malignancy. If both pregnancy and pathology have been excluded, time or a change to another preparation may solve the problem. Changing to an oral contraceptive with a higher estrogen content, while potentially useful in minimizing menstrual irregularity, should be done only if necessary since this may increase the risk of thromboembolic disease.

Use of oral contraceptives in the event of a missed menstrual period:

1. If the patient has not adhered to the prescribed schedule, the possibility of pregnancy should be considered at the time of the first missed period and oral contraceptive use should be discontinued until pregnancy is ruled out.

2. If the patient has adhered to the prescribed regimen and misses two consecutive periods, pregnancy should be ruled out before continuing oral contraceptive use.

HOW SUPPLIED

Desogen® 28 contains 21 round white tablets and 7 round green tablets in a blister card within a recyclable plastic dispenser. Each white tablet (debossed with "TR5" on one side and "Organon" on the other side) contains 0.15 mg desogestrel and 0.03 mg ethinyl estradiol. Each green tablet (debossed with "KH2" on one side and "Organon" on the other side) contains inert ingredients.

Boxes of 6 NDC#0052-0261-06.

STORAGE: Store below 86°F (30°C)

CAUTION: Federal law prohibits dispensing without a prescription.

REFERENCES

1. Reproduced with permission of the Population Council from J. Trussell and K. Kost: Contraceptive failure in the United States: A critical review of the literature. Studies in Family Planning, 18 (5), September–October 1987. 2. Stadel BV. Oral contraceptives and cardiovascular disease. (Pt.1). N Engl J Med 1981; 305: 612–618. 3. Stadel BV. Oral contraceptives and cardiovascular disease. (Pt. 2). N Engl J Med 1981; 305: 672–677. 4. Adam SA, Thorogood M. Oral contraception and myocardial infarction revisited: the effects of new preparations and prescribing patterns. Br J Obstet and Gynecol 1981; 88: 838–845. 5. Mann JI, Inman WH. Oral contraceptives and death from myocardial infarction. Br Med J 1975; 2(5965):245–248. 6. Mann JI, Vessey MP, Thorogood M, Doll R. Myocardial infarction in young women with special reference to oral contraceptive practice. Br Med J 1975 2(5956):241–245. 7. Royal College of General Practitioners' Oral Contraception Study: Further analyses of mortality in oral contraceptive users. Lancet 1981 1:541–546. 8. Sloan D, Shapiro S, Kaufman DW, Rosenberg L, Miettinen OS, Stolley PD. Risk of myocardial infarction in relation to current and discontinued use of oral contraceptives. N Engl J Med 1981; 305:420–424. 9. Vessey MP. Female hormones and vascular disease-an epidemiological overview. Br J Fam Plann 1980; 6:1–12. 10. Russell-Briefel RG, Ezzati TM, Fulwood R, Perlman JA, Murphy RS. Cardiovascular risk status and oral contraceptive use, United States, 1976-80. Prevent Med 1986; 15:352–362. 11. Goldbaum GM, Kendrick JS, Hogelin GC, Gentry EM. The relative impact of smoking and oral contraceptive use on women in the United States. JAMA 1987 258:1339–1342. 12. Layde PM, Beral V. Further analyses of mortality in oral contraceptive users: Royal College General Practitioners' Oral Contraception Study. (Table 5) Lancet 1981; 1:541–546. 13. Knopp RH. Arteriosclerosis risk: the roles of oral contraceptives and postmenopausal estrogens. J Reprod Med 1986; 31(9) (Supplement):913–921. 14. Krauss RM, Roy S, Mishell DR, Casagrande J, Pike MC. Effects of two low-dose oral contraceptives on serum lipids and lipoproteins: Differential changes in high-density lipoproteins subclasses. Am J Obstet 1983; 145:446–452. 15. Wahl P, Walden C, Knopp R, Hoover J, Wallace R, Heiss G, Rifkind B. Effect of estrogen/progestin potency on lipid/

lipoprotein cholesterol. N Engl J Med 1983; 308: 862–867. 16. Wynn V, Niththyananthan R. The effect of progestin in combined oral contraceptives on serum lipids with special reference to high-density lipoproteins. Am J Obstet Gynecol 1982; 142:766–771. 17. Wynn V, Godsland I. Effects of oral contraceptives and carbohydrate metabolism. J Reprod Med 1986; 31 (9) (Supplement):892–897. 18. LaRosa JC. Atherosclerotic risk factors in cardiovascular disease. J Reprod Med 1986; 31 (9) (Supplement):906–912. 19. Inman WH, Vessey MP. Investigation of death from pulmonary, coronary, and cerebral thrombosis and embolism in women of child-bearing age. Br Med J 1968; 2 (5599):193–199. 20. Maguire MG, Tonascia J, Sartwell PE, Stolley PD, Tockman MS. Increased risk of thrombosis due to oral contraceptives: a further report. Am J Epidemiol 1979; 110 (2):188–195. 21. Pettiti DB, Wingerd J, Pellegrin F, Ramacharan S. Risk of vascular disease in women: smoking, oral contraceptives, noncontraceptive estrogens, and other factors. JAMA 1979; 242:1150–1154. 22. Vessey MP, Doll R. Investigation of relation between use of oral contraceptives and thromboembolic disease. Br Med J 1968; 2 (5599):199–205. 23. Vessey MP, Doll R. Investigation of relation between use of oral contraceptives and thromboembolic disease. A further report. Br Med J 1969; 2 (5658):651–657. 24. Porter JB, Hunter JR, Danielson DA, Jick H, Stergachis A. Oral contraceptives and non-fatal vascular disease-recent experience. Obstet Gynecol 1982; 59 (3):299–302. 25. Vessey M, Doll R, Peto R, Johnson B, Wiggins P. A long-term follow-up study of women using different methods of contraception: an interim report. Biosocial Sci 1976; 8: 375–427. 26. Royal College of General Practitioners: Oral contraceptives, venous thrombosis, and varicose veins. J Royal Coll Gen Pract 1978; 28:393–399. 27. Collaborative Group for the Study of Stroke in Young Women: Oral contraception and increased risk of cerebral ischemia or thrombosis. N Engl J Med 1973; 288:871–878. 28. Petitti DB, Wingerd J. Use of oral contraceptives, cigarette smoking, and risk of subarachnoid hemorrhage. Lancet 1978; 2:234–236. 29. Inman WH. Oral contraceptives and fatal subarachnoid hemorrhage. Br Med J 1979; 2 (6203):1468–70. 30. Collaborative Group for the Study of Stroke in Young Women: Oral contraceptives and stroke in young women: associated risk factors. JAMA 1975; 231:718–722. 31. Inman WH, Vessey MP, Westerholm B, Engelund A. Thromboembolic disease and the steroidal content of oral contraceptives. A report to the Committee on Safety of Drugs. Br Med J 1970; 2:203–209. 32. Meade TW, Greenberg G, Thompson SG. Progestogens and cardiovascular reactions associated with oral contraceptives and a comparison of the safety of 50- and 35-mcg oestrogen preparations. Br Med J 1980; 280 (6224):1157–1161. 33. Kay CR. Progestogens and arterial disease-evidence from the Royal College of General Practitioners' Study. Am J Obstet Gynecol 1982; 142:762–765. 34. Royal College of General Practitioners: Incidence of arterial disease among oral contraceptive users. J Royal Coll Gen Pract 1983; 33:75–82. 35. Ory HW. Mortality associated with fertility and fertility control: 1983. Family Planning Perspectives 1983; 15: 50–56. 36. The Cancer and Steroid Hormone Study of the Centers for Disease Control and the National Institute of Child Health and Human Development: Oral-contraceptive use and the risk of breast cancer. N Engl J Med 1986; 315:405–411. 37. Pike MC, Henderson BE, Krailo MD, Duke A, Roy S. Breast cancer risk in young women and use of oral contraceptives: possible modifying effect of formulation and age at use. Lancet 1983; 2:926–929. 38. Paul C, Skegg DG, Spears GFS, Kaldor JM. Oral contraceptives and breast cancer: A national study. Br Med J 1986; 293: 723–725. 39. Miller DR, Rosenberg L, Kaufman DW, Schottenfeld D, Stolley PD, Shapiro S. Breast cancer risk in relation to early oral contraceptive use. Obstet Gynecol 1986; 68:863–868. 40. Olson H, Olson KL, Moller TR, Ranstam J, Holm P. Oral contraceptive use and breast cancer in young women in Sweden (letter). Lancet 1985; 2:748–749. 41. McPherson K, Vessey M, Neil A, Doll R, Jones L, Roberts M. Early contraceptive use and breast cancer: Results of another case-control study. Br J Cancer 1987; 56:653–660. 42. Huggins GR, Zucker PF. Oral contraceptives and neoplasia: 1987 update. Fertil Steril 1987; 47:733–761. 43. McPherson K, Drife JO. The pill and breast cancer: why the uncertainty? Br Med J 1986; 293:709–710. 44. Shapiro S. Oral contraceptives—time to take stock. N Engl J Med 1987; 315:450–451. 45. Ory H, Naib Z, Conger SB, Hatcher RA, Tyler CW. Contraceptive choice and prevalence of cervical dysplasia and carcinoma in situ. Am J Obstet Gynecol 1976; 124:573–577. 46. Vessey MP, Lawless M, McPherson K, Yeates D. Neoplasia of the cervix uteri and contraception: a possible adverse effect of the pill. Lancet 1983; 2:930. 47. Brinton LA, Huggins GR, Lehman HF, Malli K, Savitz DA, Trapido E, Rosenthal J, Hoover R. Long term use of oral contraceptives and risk of invasive cervical cancer. Int J Cancer 1986; 38: 339–344. 48. WHO Collaborative Study of Neoplasia and Steroid Contraceptives: Invasive cervical cancer and combined oral contraceptives. Br Med J 1985; 290:961–965. 49. Rooks JB, Ory HW, Ishak KG, Strauss LT, Greenspan JR, Hill AP, Tyler CW. Epidemiology of hepatocellular adenoma: the role of oral contraceptive use. JAMA 1979; 242:644–648.

50. Bein NN, Goldsmith HS. Recurrent massive hemorrhage from benign hepatic tumors secondary to oral contraceptives. Br J Surg 1977; 64:433–435. 51. Klatskin G. Hepatic tumors: possible relationship to use of oral contraceptives. Gastroenterology 1977; 73:386–394. 52. Henderson BE, Preston-Martin S, Edmondson HA, Peters RL, Pike MC. Hepatocellular carcinoma and oral contraceptives. Br J Cancer 1983; 48:437–440. 53. Neuberger J, Forman D, Doll R, Williams R. Oral contraceptives and hepatocellular carcinoma. Br Med J 1986; 292:1355–1357. 54. Forman D, Vincent TJ, Doll R. Cancer of the liver and oral contraceptives. Br Med J 1986; 292: 1357–1361. 55. Harlap S, Eldor J. Births following oral contraceptive failures. Obstet Gynecol 1980; 55:447–452. 56. Savolainen E, Saksela E, Saxen L. Teratogenic hazards of oral contraceptives analyzed in a national malformation register. Am J Obstet Gynecol 1981; 140:521–524. 57. Janerich DT, Piper JM, Glebatis DM. Oral contraceptives and birth defects. Am J Epidemiol 1980; 112:73–79. 58. Ferencz C, Matanoski GM, Wilson PD, Rubin JD, Neill CA, Gutberlet R. Maternal hormone therapy and congenital heart disease. Teratology 1980; 21:225–239. 59. Rothman KJ, Fyler DC, Goldbatt A, Kreidberg MB. Exogenous hormones and other drug exposures of children with congenital heart disease. Am J Epidemiol 1979; 109:433–439. 60. Boston Collaborative Drug Surveillance Program: Oral contraceptives and venous thromboembolic disease, surgically confirmed gallbladder disease, and breast tumors. Lancet 1973; 1:1399–1404. 61. Royal College of General Practitioners: Oral contraceptives and health. New York, Pittman, 1974. 62. Layde PM, Vessey MP, Yeates D. Risk of gallbladder disease: a cohort study of young women attending family planning clinics. J Epidemiol Community Health 1982; 36: 274–-278. 63. Rome Group for the Epidemiology and Prevention of Cholelithiasis (GREPCO): Prevalence of gallstone disease in an Italian adult female population. Am J Epidemiol 1984; 119:796–805. 64. Strom BL, Tamragouri RT, Morse ML, Lazar EL, West SL, Stolley PD, Jones JK. Oral contraceptives and other risk factors for gallbladder disease. Clin Pharmacol Ther 1986; 39:335–341. 65. Wynn V, Adams PW, Godsland IF, Melrose J, Niththyananthan R, Oakley NW, Seedj A. Comparison of effects of different combined oral-contraceptive formulations on carbohydrate and lipid metabolism. Lancet 1979; 1:1045–1049. 66. Wynn V. Effect of progesterone and progestins on carbohydrate metabolism. In Progesterone and Progestin. Edited by Bardin CW, Milgrom E,Mauvis-Jarvis P. New York, Raven Press, 1983 pp. 395–410. 67. Perlman JA, Roussell-Briefel RG, Ezzati TM, Lieberknecht G. Oral glucose tolerance and the potency of oral contraceptive progestogens. J Chronic Dis 1985; 38:857–864. 68. Royal College of General Practitioners' Oral Contraception Study: Effect on hypertension and benign breast disease of progestogen component incombined oral contraceptives. Lancet 1977; 1:624. 69. Fisch IR, Frank J. Oral contraceptives and blood pressure. JAMA 1977; 237:2499–2503. 70. Laragh AJ. Oral contraceptive induced hypertension-nine years later. Am J Obstet Gynecol 1976; 126:141–147. 71. Ramcharan S, Peritz E, Pellegrin FA, Williams WT. Incidence of hypertension in the Walnut Creek Contraceptive Drug Study cohort. In Pharmacology of Steroid Contraceptive Drugs. Garattini S, Berendes HW. Eds. New York, Raven Press, 1977 pp. 277–288. (Monographs of the Mario Negri Institute for Pharmacological Research, Milan). 72. Stockley I. Interactions with oral contraceptives. J Pharm 1976; 216:140–143. 73. The Cancer and Steroid Hormone Study of the Centers for Disease Control and the National Institute of Child Health and Human Development: Oral contraceptive use and the risk of ovarian cancer. JAMA 1983; 249:1596–1599. 74. The Cancer and Steroid Hormone Study of the Centers for Disease Control and the National Institute of Child Health and Human Development: Combination oral contraceptive use and the risk of endometrial cancer. JAMA 1987; 257: 796–800. 75. Ory HW. Functional ovarian cysts and oral contraceptives: negative association confirmed surgically. JAMA 1974; 228: 68–69. 76. Ory HW, Cole P, Macmahon B, Hoover R. Oral contraceptives and reduced risk of benign breast disease. N Engl J Med 1976; 294:419–422. 77. Ory HW. The noncontraceptive health benefits from oral contraceptive use. Fam Plann Perspect 1982;14:182–184. 78. Ory HW, Forrest JD, Lincoln R. Making Choices: Evaluating the health risks and benefits of birth control methods. New York, The Alan Guttmacher Institute, 1983; p. 1. 79. Schlesselman J, Stadel BV, Murray P, Lai S. Breast Cancer in relation to early use of oral contraceptives 1988; 259:1828–1833. 80. Hennekens CH, Speizer FE, Lipnick RJ, Rosner B, Bain C, Belanger C, Stampfer MJ, Willett W, Peto R. A case-controlled study of oral contraceptive use and breast cancer. JNCI 1984;72:39–42. 81. LaVecchia C, Decarli A, Fasoli M, Franceschi S, Gentile A, Negri E, Parazzini F, Tognoni G. Oral contraceptives and cancers of the breast and of the female genital tract. Interim results from a case-control study. Br. J. Cancer 1986; 54:311–317. 82. Meirik O, Lund E, Adami H, Bergstrom R, Christoffersen T, Bergsjo P. Oral contraceptive use in breast cancer in young women. A Joint National Case-

Continued on next page

Desogen—Cont.

control study in Sweden and Norway. Lancet 1986; 11:650–654. **83.** Kay CR, Hannaford PC. Breast cancer and the pill-A further report from the Royal College of General Practitioners' oral contraception study. Br. J. Cancer 1988; 58:675–680. **84.** Stadel BV, Lai S, Schlesselman JJ, Murray P. Oral contraceptives and premenopausal breast cancer in nulliparous women. Contraception 1988; 38:287–299. **85.** Miller DR, Rosenberg L, Kaufman DW, Stolley P, Warshauer ME, Shapiro S. Breast cancer before age 45 and oral contraceptive use: New Findings. Am. J. Epidemiol 1989; 129:269–280. **86.** The UK National Case-Control Study Group, Oral contraceptive use and breast cancer risk in young women. Lancet 1989; 1:973–982. **87.** Schlesselman JJ. Cancer of the breast and reproductive tract in relation to use of oral contraceptives. Contraception 1989; 40:1–38. **88.** Vessey MP, McPherson K, Villard-Mackintosh L, Yeates D. Oral contraceptives and breast cancer: latest findings in a large cohert study. Br. J. Cancer 1989; 59:613–617. **89.** Jick SS, Walker AM, Stergachis A, Jick H. Oral contraceptives and breast cancer. Br. J. Cancer 1989; 59:618–621. **90.** Godsland, I et al. The effects of different formulations of oral contraceptive agents on lipid and carbohydrate metabolism. N Engl J Med 1990;323:1375–81. **91.** Kloosterboer, HJ et al. Selectivity in progesterone and androgen receptor binding of progestogens used in oral contraception. Contraception, 1988;38:325–32. **92.** Van der Vies, J and de Visser, J. Endocrinological studies with desogestrel. Arzneim. Forsch./Drug Res., 1983;33(I),2:231–6. **93.** Data on file, Organon Inc.. **94.** Fotherby, K. Oral contraceptives, lipids and cardiovascular diseases. Contraception, 1985; Vol. 31; 4:367–94. **95.** Lawrence, DM et al. Reduced sex hormone binding globulin and derived free testosterone levels in women with severe acne. Clinical Endocrinology, 1981;15:87–91. **96.** Cullberg, G et al. Effects of a low-dose desogestrel-ethinyl estradiol combination on hirsutism, androgens and sex hormone binding globulin in women with a polycystic ovary syndrome. Acta Obstet Gynecol Scand, 1985;64:195–202. **97.** Jung-Hoffmann, C and Kuhl, H. Divergent effects of two low-dose oral contraceptives on sex hormone-binding globulin and free testosterone. AJOG, 1987;156:199–203. **98.** Hammond, G et al. Serum steroid binding protein concentrations, distribution of progestogens, and bioavailability of testosterone during treatment with contraceptives containing desogestrel or levonorgestrel. Fertil. Steril., 1984;42:44–51. **99.** Palatsi, R et al. Serum total and unbound testosterone and sex hormone binding globulin (SHBG) in female acne patients treated with two different oral contraceptives. Acta Derm Venereol, 1984; 64:517-23. **100.** Lewis M, Spitzer WO, Heinemann LAJ, MacRae KD, Bruppacher R, Thorogood M on behalf of Transnational Research Group on Oral Contraceptives and Health of Young Women. Third generation oral contraceptives and risk of myocardial infarction: an international case-control study. Br Med J, 1996: 312:88–90. **101.** Jick H, Jick SS, Gurewich V, Myers MW, Vasilakis C. Risk of idiopathic cardiovascular death and non-fatal venous thromboembolism in women using oral contraceptives with differing progestagen components. Lancet, 1995; 346:1589–93. **102.** World Health Organization Collaborative Study of Cardiovascular Disease and Steroid Hormone Contraception. Effect of different progestagens in low oestrogen oral contraceptives on venous thromboembolic disease. Lancet, 1995; 346:1582–88. **103.** Spitzer WO, Lewis MA, Heinemann LAJ, Thorogood M, MacRae KD on behalf of Transnational Research Group on Oral Contraceptives and Health of Young Women. Third generation oral contraceptives and risk of venous thromboembolic disorders: an international case-control study. Br Med J 1996; 312:83–88.

BRIEF SUMMARY
PATIENT PACKAGE INSERT

THIS PRODUCT (LIKE ALL ORAL CONTRACEPTIVES) IS INTENDED TO PREVENT PREGNANCY. IT DOES NOT PROTECT AGAINST HIV INFECTION (AIDS) AND OTHER SEXUALLY TRANSMITTED DISEASES.

Oral contraceptives, also known as "birth control pills" or "the pill", are taken to prevent pregnancy, and when taken correctly, have a failure rate of about 1% per year when used without missing any pills. The typical failure rate of large numbers of pill users is less than 3% per year when women who miss pills are included. For most women, oral contraceptives are also free of serious or unpleasant side effects. However, forgetting to take pills considerably increases the chances of pregnancy.

For the majority of women, oral contraceptives can be taken safely. But there are some women who are at high risk of developing certain serious diseases that can be life-threatening or may cause temporary or permanent disability. The risks associated with taking oral contraceptives increase significantly if you:

- smoke
- have high blood pressure, diabetes, high cholesterol
- have or have had clotting disorders, heart attack, stroke, angina pectoris, cancer of the breast or sex organs, jaundice or malignant or benign liver tumors

Although cardiovascular disease risks may be increased with oral contraceptive use after age 40 in healthy, nonsmoking women (even with the newer low-dose formulations), there are also greater potential health risks associated with pregnancy in older women.

You should not take the pill if you suspect you are pregnant or have unexplained vaginal bleeding.

Cigarette smoking increases the risk of serious cardiovascular side effects from oral contraceptive use. This risk increases with age and with heavy smoking (15 or more cigarettes per day) and is quite marked in women over 35 years of age. Women who use oral contraceptives are strongly advised not to smoke.

Most side effects of the pill are not serious. The most common such effects are nausea, vomiting, bleeding between menstrual periods, weight gain, breast tenderness, headache, and difficulty wearing contact lenses. These side effects, especially nausea and vomiting, may subside within the first three months of use.

The serious side effects of the pill occur very infrequently, especially if you are in good health and are young. However, you should know that the following medical conditions have been associated with or made worse by the pill:

1. Blood clots in the legs (thrombophlebitis) or lungs (pulmonary embolism), stoppage or rupture of a blood vessel in the brain (stroke), blockage of blood vessels in the heart (heart attack or angina pectoris) or other organs of the body. As mentioned above, smoking increases the risk of heart attacks and strokes, and subsequent serious medical consequences.
2. Liver tumors, which may rupture and cause severe bleeding. A possible but not definite association has been found with the pill and liver cancer. However, liver cancers are extremely rare. The chance of developing liver cancer from using the pill is thus even rarer.
3. High blood pressure, although blood pressure usually returns to normal when the pill is stopped.

The symptoms associated with these serious side effects are discussed in the detailed patient labeling given to you with your supply of pills. Notify your doctor or clinic if you notice any unusual physical disturbances while taking the pill. In addition, drugs such as rifampin, as well as some anticonvulsants and some antibiotics may decrease oral contraceptive effectiveness.

There is conflict among studies regarding breast cancer and oral contraceptive use. Some studies have reported an increase in the risk of developing breast cancer, particularly at a younger age. This increased risk appears to be related to duration of use. The majority of studies have found no overall increase in the risk of developing breast cancer. Some studies have found an increase in the incidence of cancer of the cervix in women who use oral contraceptives. However, this finding may be related to factors other than the use of oral contraceptives. There is insufficient evidence to rule out the possibility that pills may cause such cancers.

Taking the combination pill provides some important noncontraceptive benefits. These include less painful menstruation, less menstrual blood loss and anemia, fewer pelvic infections, and fewer cancers of the ovary and the lining of the uterus.

Be sure to discuss any medical condition you may have with your doctor or clinic. Your doctor or clinic will take a medical and family history before prescribing oral contraceptives and will examine you. The physical examination may be delayed to another time if you request it and your doctor or clinic believes that it is a good medical practice to postpone it. You should be reexamined at least once a year while taking oral contraceptives. The detailed patient information labeling gives you further information which you should read and discuss with your doctor or clinic.

DETAILED PATIENT LABELING

THIS PRODUCT (LIKE ALL ORAL CONTRACEPTIVES) IS INTENDED TO PREVENT PREGNANCY. IT DOES NOT PROTECT AGAINST HIV INFECTION (AIDS) AND OTHER SEXUALLY TRANSMITTED DISEASES.

PLEASE NOTE: This labeling is revised from time to time as important new medical information becomes available. Therefore, please review this labeling carefully.

The following oral contraceptive product contains a combination of progestogen and estrogen, the two kinds of female hormones:

Desogen® 28 Day Regimen

Each white tablet contains 0.15 mg desogestrel and 0.030 mg ethinyl estradiol. Each green tablet contains inert ingredients.

INTRODUCTION

Any woman who considers using oral contraceptives (the birth control pill or the pill) should understand the benefits and risks of using this form of birth control. This patient labeling will give you much of the information you will need to make this decision and will also help you determine if you are at risk of developing any of the serious side effects of the pill. It will tell you how to use the pill properly so that it will be as effective as possible. However, this labeling is not a replacement for a careful discussion between you and your doctor or clinic. You should discuss the information provided in this labeling with him or her, both when you first start taking the pill and during your revisits. You should also follow your doctor's or clinic's advice with regard to regular check-ups while you are on the pill.

EFFECTIVENESS OF ORAL CONTRACEPTIVES

Oral contraceptives or "birth control pills" or "the pill" are used to prevent pregnancy and are more effective than other non-surgical methods of birth control. When they are taken correctly, the chance of becoming pregnant is less than 1% (1 pregnancy per 100 women per year of use) when used perfectly, without missing any pills. Typical failure rates are actually 3% per year. The chance of becoming pregnant increases with each missed pill during a menstrual cycle.

In comparison, typical failure rates for other non-surgical methods of birth control during the first year of use are as follows:

IUD: 3%
Diaphragm with spermicides: 18%
Spermicides alone: 21%
Vaginal sponge: 18 to 28%
Implant: 0.03%
Condom alone: 12%
Periodic abstinence: 20%
No methods: 85%

WHO SHOULD NOT TAKE ORAL CONTRACEPTIVES

Cigarette smoking increases the risk of serious cardiovascular side effects from oral contraceptive use. This risk increases with age and with heavy smoking (15 or more cigarettesper day) and is quite marked in women over 35 years of age. Women who use oral contraceptives are strongly advised not to smoke.

Some women should not use the pill. For example, you should not take the pill if you are pregnant or think you may be pregnant. You should also not use the pill if you have any of the following conditions:

- A history of heart attack or stroke
- Blood clots in the legs (thrombophlebitis), lungs (pulmonary embolism), or eyes
- A history of blood clots in the deep veins of your legs
- Chest pain (angina pectoris)
- Known or suspected breast cancer or cancer of the lining of the uterus, cervix or vagina
- Unexplained vaginal bleeding (until a diagnosis is reached by your doctor)
- Yellowing of the whites of the eyes or of the skin (jaundice) during pregnancy or during previous use of the pill
- Liver tumor (benign or cancerous)
- Known or suspected pregnancy

Tell your doctor or clinic if you have ever had any of these conditions. Your doctor or clinic can recommend a safer method of birth control.

OTHER CONSIDERATIONS BEFORE TAKING ORAL CONTRACEPTIVES

Tell your doctor or clinic if you have or have had:

- Breast nodules, fibrocystic disease of the breast, an abnormal breast x-ray or mammogram
- Diabetes
- Elevated cholesterol or triglycerides
- High blood pressure
- Migraine or other headaches or epilepsy
- Mental depression
- Gallbladder, heart or kidney disease
- History of scanty or irregular menstrual periods

Women with any of these conditions should be checked often by their doctor or clinic if they choose to use oral contraceptives.

Also, be sure to inform your doctor or clinic if you smoke or are on any medications.

RISKS OF TAKING ORAL CONTRACEPTIVES

1. Risk of developing blood clots

Blood clots and blockage of blood vessels are one of the most serious side effects of taking oral contraceptives and can cause death or serious disability. In particular, a clot in one of the legs can cause thrombophlebitis and a clot that travels to the lungs can cause a sudden blocking of the vessel carrying blood to the lungs. These risks may be greater with desogestrel-containing oral contraceptives such as Desogen® than with certain other low-dose pills. Rarely, clots occur in the blood vessels of the eye and may cause blindness, double vision, or impaired vision.

If you take oral contraceptives and need elective surgery, need to stay in bed for a prolonged illness or have recently delivered a baby, you may be at risk of developing blood clots. You should consult your doctor or clinic about stopping oral contraceptives three to four weeks before surgery and

ANNUAL NUMBER OF BIRTH-RELATED OR METHOD-RELATED DEATHS ASSOCIATED WITH CONTROL OF FERTILITY PER 100,000 NON-STERILE WOMEN, BY FERTILITY CONTROL METHOD ACCORDING TO AGE

Method of control and outcome	15-19	20-24	25-29	30-34	35-39	40-44
No fertility control methods*	7.0	7.4	9.1	14.8	25.7	28.2
Oral contraceptives non-smoker**	0.3	0.5	0.9	1.9	13.8	31.6
Oral contraceptives smoker**	2.2	3.4	6.6	13.5	51.1	117.2
IUD**	0.8	0.8	1.0	1.0	1.4	1.4
Condom*	1.1	1.6	0.7	0.2	0.3	0.4
Diaphragm/spermicide*	1.9	1.2	1.2	1.3	2.2	2.8
Periodic abstinence*	2.5	1.6	1.6	1.7	2.9	3.6

* Deaths are birth related
** Deaths are method related

not taking oral contraceptives for two weeks after surgery or during bed rest. You should also not take oral contraceptives soon after delivery of a baby. It is advisable to wait for at least four weeks after delivery if you are not breast feeding or four weeks after a second trimester abortion. If you are breast feeding, you should wait until you have weaned your child before using the pill. (See also the section on Breast Feeding in General Precautions.)

The risk of circulatory disease in oral contraceptive users may be higher in users of high dose pills. The risk of venous thromboembolic disease associated with oral contraceptives does not increase with length of use and disappears after pill use is stopped. The risk of abnormal blood clotting increases with age in both users and nonusers of oral contraceptives, but the increased risk from the oral contraceptive appears to be present at all ages. For women aged 20 to 44 it is estimated that about 1 in 2,000 using oral contraceptives will be hospitalized each year because of abnormal clotting. Among nonusers in the same age group, about 1 in 20,000 would be hospitalized each year. For oral contraceptive users in general, it has been estimated that in women between the ages of 15 and 34 the risk of death due to a circulatory disorder is about 1 in 12,000 per year, whereas for nonusers the rate is about 1 in 50,000 per year. In the age group 35 to 44, the risk is estimated to be about 1 in 2,500 per year for oral contraceptive users and about 1 in 10,000 per year for non-users.

2. Heart attacks and strokes
Oral contraceptives may increase the tendency to develop strokes (stoppage or rupture of blood vessels in the brain) and angina pectoris and heart attacks (blockage of blood vessels in the heart). Any of these conditions can cause death or serious disability.
Smoking greatly increases the possibility of suffering heart attacks and strokes. Furthermore, smoking and the use of oral contraceptives greatly increase the chances of developing and dying of heart disease.

3. Gallbladder disease
Oral contraceptive users probably have a greater risk than nonusers of having gallbladder disease, although this risk may be related to pills containing high doses of estrogens.

4. Liver tumors
In rare cases, oral contraceptives can cause benign but dangerous liver tumors. These benign liver tumors can rupture and cause fatal internal bleeding. In addition, a possible but not definite association has been found with the pill and liver cancers in two studies, in which a few women who developed these very rare cancers were found to have used oral contraceptives for long periods. However, liver cancers are rare.

5. Cancer of the reproductive organs and breasts
There is conflict among studies regarding breast cancer and oral contraceptive use. Some studies have reported an increase in the risk of developing breast cancer, particularly at a younger age. This increased risk appears to be related to duration of use. The majority of studies have found no overall increase in the risk of developing breast cancer. Some studies have found an increase in the incidence of cancer of the cervix in women who use oral contraceptives. However, this finding may be related to factors other than the use of oral contraceptives. There is insufficient evidence to rule out the possibility that pills may cause such cancers.

ESTIMATED RISK OF DEATH FROM A BIRTH CONTROL METHOD OR PREGNANCY
All methods of birth control and pregnancy are associated with a risk of developing certain diseases which may lead to disability or death. An estimate of the number of deaths associated with different methods of birth control and pregnancy has been calculated and is shown in the following table.
[See table above]
In the above table, the risk of death from any birth control method is less than the risk of childbirth, except for oral contraceptive users over the age of 35 who smoke and pill users over the age of 40 even if they do not smoke. It can be seen in the table that for women aged 15 to 39, the risk of death was highest with pregnancy (7-26 deaths per 100,000 women, depending on age). Among pill users who do not smoke, the risk of death was always lower than that asso-

ciated with pregnancy for any age group, although over the age of 40, the risk increases to 32 deaths per 100,000 women, compared to 28 associated with pregnancy at that age. However, for pill users who smoke and are over the age of 35, the estimated number of deaths exceeds those for other methods of birth control. If a woman is over the age of 40 and smokes, her estimated risk of death is four times higher (117/100,000 women) than the estimated risk associated with pregnancy (28/100,000 women) in that age group. The suggestion that women over 40 who do not smoke should not take oral contraceptives is based on information from older, higher-dose pills. An Advisory Committee of the FDA discussed this issue in 1989 and recommended that the benefits of low-dose oral contraceptive use by healthy, nonsmoking women over 40 years of age may outweigh the possible risks.

WARNING SIGNALS
If any of these adverse effects occur while you are taking oral contraceptives, call your doctor or clinic immediately:
- Sharp chest pain, coughing of blood, or sudden shortness of breath (indicating a possible clot in the lung)
- Pain in the calf (indicating a possible clot in the leg)
- Crushing chest pain or heaviness in the chest (indicating a possible heart attack)
- Sudden severe headache or vomiting, dizziness or fainting, disturbances of vision or speech, weakness, or numbness in an arm or leg (indicating a possible stroke)
- Sudden partial or complete loss of vision (indicating a possible clot in the eye)
- Breast lumps (indicating possible breast cancer or fibrocystic disease of the breast; ask your doctor or clinic to show you how to examine your breasts)
- Severe pain or tenderness in the stomach area (indicating a possibly ruptured liver tumor)
- Difficulty in sleeping, weakness, lack of energy, fatigue, or change in mood (possibly indicating severe depression)
- Jaundice or a yellowing of the skin or eyeballs, accompanied frequently by fever, fatigue, loss of appetite, dark colored urine, or light colored bowel movements (indicating possible liver problems)

SIDE EFFECTS OF ORAL CONTRACEPTIVES
1. Vaginal bleeding
Irregular vaginal bleeding or spotting may occur while you are taking the pills. Irregular bleeding may vary from slight staining between menstrual periods to breakthrough bleeding which is a flow much like a regular period. Irregular bleeding occurs most often during the first few months of oral contraceptive use, but may also occur after you have been taking the pill for some time. Such bleeding may be temporary and usually does not indicate any serious problems. It is important to continue taking your pills on schedule. If the bleeding occurs in more than one cycle or lasts for more than a few days, talk to your doctor or clinic.

2. Contact lenses
If you wear contact lenses and notice a change in vision or an inability to wear your lenses, contact your doctor or clinic.

3. Fluid retention
Oral contraceptives may cause edema (fluid retention) with swelling of the fingers or ankles and may raise your blood pressure. If you experience fluid retention, contact your doctor or clinic.

4. Melasma
A spotty darkening of the skin is possible, particularly of the face, which may persist.

5. Other side effects
Other side effects may include nausea and vomiting, change in appetite, headache, nervousness, depression, dizziness, loss of scalp hair, rash, and vaginal infections.
If any of these side effects bother you, call your doctor or clinic.

GENERAL PRECAUTIONS
1. Missed periods and use of oral contraceptives before or during early pregnancy
There may be times when you may not menstruate regularly after you have completed taking a cycle of pills. If you

have taken your pills regularly and miss one menstrual period, continue taking your pills for the next cycle but be sure to inform your doctor or clinic before doing so. If you have not taken the pills daily as instructed and missed a menstrual period, you may be pregnant. If you missed two consecutive menstrual periods, you may be pregnant. Check with your doctor or clinic immediately to determine whether you are pregnant. Do not continue to take oral contraceptives until you are sure you are not pregnant, but continue to use another method of contraception.

There is no conclusive evidence that oral contraceptive use is associated with an increase in birth defects, when taken inadvertently during early pregnancy. Previously, a few studies had reported that oral contraceptives might be associated with birth defects, but these findings have not been seen in more recent studies. Nevertheless, oral contraceptives or any other drugs should not be used during pregnancy unless clearly necessary and prescribed by your doctor or clinic. You should check with your doctor or clinic about risks to your unborn child of any medication taken during pregnancy.

2. While breast feeding
If you are breast feeding, consult your doctor or clinic before starting oral contraceptives. Some of the drug will be passed on to the child in the milk. A few adverse effects on the child have been reported, including yellowing of the skin (jaundice) and breast enlargement. In addition, oral contraceptives may decrease the amount and quality of your milk. If possible, do not use oral contraceptives while breast feeding. You should use another method of contraception since breast feeding provides only partial protection from becoming pregnant and this partial protection decreases significantly as you breast feed for longer periods of time. You should consider starting oral contraceptives only after you have weaned your child completely.

3. Laboratory tests
If you are scheduled for any laboratory tests, tell your doctor or clinic you are taking birth control pills. Certain blood tests may be affected by birth control pills.

4. Drug interactions
Certain drugs may interact with birth control pills to make them less effective in preventing pregnancy or cause an increase in breakthrough bleeding. Such drugs include rifampin, drugs used for epilepsy such as barbiturates (for example, phenobarbital), anticonvulsants such as carbamazepine (Tegretol is one brand of this drug), phenytoin (Dilantin is one brand of this drug), phenylbutazone (Butazolidin is one brand), and possibly certain antibiotics. You may need to use additional contraception when you take drugs which can make oral contraceptives less effective.

THIS PRODUCT (LIKE ALL ORAL CONTRACEPTIVES) IS INTENDED TO PREVENT PREGNANCY. IT DOES NOT PROTECT AGAINST TRANSMISSION OF HIV (AIDS) AND OTHER SEXUALLY TRANSMITTED DISEASES SUCH AS CHLAMYDIA, GENITAL HERPES, GENITAL WARTS, GONORRHEA, HEPATITIS B, AND SYPHILIS.

HOW TO TAKE THE PILL

IMPORTANT POINTS TO REMEMBER
BEFORE YOU START TAKING YOUR PILLS:
1. BE SURE TO READ THESE DIRECTIONS:
   Before you start taking your pills.
   Anytime you are not sure what to do.
2. THE RIGHT WAY TO TAKE THE PILL IS TO TAKE ONE PILL EVERY DAY AT THE SAME TIME.
   If you miss pills you could get pregnant. This includes starting the pack late.
   The more pills you miss, the more likely you are to get pregnant.
3. MANY WOMEN HAVE SPOTTING OR LIGHT BLEEDING, OR MAY FEEL SICK TO THEIR STOMACH DURING THE FIRST 1–3 PACKS OF PILLS.
   If you feel sick to your stomach, do not stop taking the pill. The problem will usually go away. If it doesn't go away, check with your doctor or clinic.
4. MISSING PILLS CAN ALSO CAUSE SPOTTING OR LIGHT BLEEDING, even when you make up these missed pills. On the days you take 2 pills to make up for missed pills, you could also feel a little sick to your stomach.
5. IF YOU HAVE VOMITING OR DIARRHEA, for any reason, or IF YOU TAKE SOME MEDICINES, including some antibiotics, your pills may not work as well.
   Use a back-up method (such as condoms, foam, or sponge) until you check with your doctor or clinic.
6. IF YOU HAVE TROUBLE REMEMBERING TO TAKE THE PILL, talk to your doctor or clinic about how to make pill-taking easier or about using another method of birth control.
7. IF YOU HAVE ANY QUESTIONS OR ARE UNSURE ABOUT THE INFORMATION IN THIS LEAFLET, call your doctor or clinic.

Continued on next page

Desogen—Cont.

BEFORE YOU START TAKING YOUR PILLS:

1. DECIDE WHAT TIME OF DAY YOU WANT TO TAKE YOUR PILL. It is important to take it at about the same time every day.
2. LOOK AT YOUR PILL PACK TO SEE IF IT HAS 21 OR 28 PILLS:

   The **21-pill pack** has 21 "active" [white] pills (with hormones) to take for 3 weeks, followed by 1 week without pills.

   The **28-pill pack** has 21 "active" [white] pills (with hormones) to take for 3 weeks, followed by 1 week of reminder [green] pills (without hormones).
3. ALSO FIND:

   1) where on the pack to start taking the pills,
   2) in what order to take the pills (follow the arrows) and
   3) the week numbers printed on the pack.
4. BE SURE YOU HAVE READY AT ALL TIMES:

   ANOTHER KIND OF BIRTH CONTROL (such as condoms, foam or sponge) to use as a back-up in case you miss pills.

   AN EXTRA, FULL PILL PACK.

WHEN TO START THE FIRST PACK OF PILLS:

You have a choice of which day to start taking your first pack of pills. Decide with your doctor or clinic which is the best day for you. Pick a time of day which will be easy to remember.

DAY 1 START:

1. Pick the day label strip that starts with the first day of your period (this is the day you start bleeding or spotting, even if it is almost midnight when the bleeding begins.)
2. Place this day label strip in the cycle tablet dispenser over the area that has the days of the week (starting with Sunday) imprinted in the plastic.

   Note: If the first day of your period is a Sunday, you can skip steps #1 and #2.
3. Take the first "active" [white] pill of the first pack during the first 24 hours of your period.
4. You will not need to use a back-up method of birth control, since you are starting the pill at the beginning of your period.

SUNDAY START:

1. Take the first "active" [white] pill of the first pack on the Sunday after your period starts, even if you are still bleeding. If your period begins on Sunday, start the pack that same day.
2. Use another method of birth control as a back-up method if you have sex anytime from the Sunday you start your first pack until the next Sunday (7 days). Condoms, foam or the sponge are good back-up methods of birth control.

WHAT TO DO DURING THE MONTH:

1. **TAKE ONE PILL AT THE SAME TIME EVERY DAY UNTIL THE PACK IS EMPTY.**

   Do not skip pills even if you are spotting or bleeding between monthly periods or feel sick to your stomach (nausea).

   Do not skip pills even if you do not have sex very often.
2. **WHEN YOU FINISH A PACK OR SWITCH YOUR BRAND OF PILLS:**

   21 pills: Wait 7 days to start the next pack. You will probably have your period during that week. Be sure that no more than 7 days pass between 21-day packs.

   28 pills: Start the next pack on the day after your last "reminder" pill. Do not wait any days between packs.

WHAT TO DO IF YOU MISS PILLS:

If you **MISS 1** [white] "active" pill:

1. Take it as soon as you remember. Take the next pill at your regular time. This means you take 2 pills in 1 day.
2. You do not need to use a back-up birth control method if you have sex.

If you **MISS 2** [white] "active" pills in a row in **WEEK 1 OR WEEK 2** of your pack:

1. Take 2 pills on the day you remember and 2 pills the next day.
2. Then take 1 pill a day until you finish the pack.
3. You MAY BECOME PREGNANT if you have sex in the **7 days** after you miss pills. You MUST use another birth control method (such as condoms, foam, or sponge) as a back-up method for those 7 days.

If you **MISS 2** [white] "active" pills in a row in THE **3RD WEEK:**

1. *If you are a Day 1 Starter:*

   THROW OUT the rest of the pill pack and start a new pack that same day.

   If you are a Sunday Starter:

   Keep taking 1 pill every day until Sunday.

   On Sunday, THROW OUT the rest of the pack and start a new pack of pills that same day.
2. You may not have your period this month but this is expected. However, if you miss your period 2 months in a row, call your doctor or clinic because you might be pregnant.

3. You MAY BECOME PREGNANT if you have sex in the **7 days** after you miss pills.

   You MUST use another birth control method (such as condoms, foam, or sponge) as a back-up method for those 7 days.

If you **MISS 3** OR MORE [white] "active" pills in a row (during the first 3 weeks).

1. *If you are a Day 1 Starter:*

   THROW OUT the rest of the pill pack and start a new pack that same day.

   If you are a Sunday Starter:

   Keep taking 1 pill every day until Sunday.

   On Sunday, THROW OUT the rest of the pack and start a new pack of pills that same day.
2. You may not have your period this month but this is expected. However, if you miss your period 2 months in a row, call your doctor or clinic because you might be pregnant.
3. You MAY BECOME PREGNANT if you have sex in the **7 days** after you miss pills.

   You MUST use another birth control method (such as condoms, foam, or sponge) as a back-up method for those 7 days.

A REMINDER FOR THOSE ON 28-DAY PACKS:

If you forget any of the 7 [green] "reminder" pills in Week 4: THROW AWAY the pills you missed.

Keep taking 1 pill each day until the pack is empty.

You do not need a back-up method.

FINALLY, IF YOU ARE STILL NOT SURE WHAT TO DO ABOUT THE PILLS YOU HAVE MISSED:

Use a BACK-UP METHOD anytime you have sex.

KEEP TAKING ONE [WHITE] "ACTIVE" PILL EACH DAY until you can reach your doctor or clinic.

PREGNANCY DUE TO PILL FAILURE

The incidence of pill failure resulting in pregnancy is approximately one percent (i.e., one pregnancy per 100 women per year) if taken every day as directed, but more typical failure rates are about 3%. If failure does occur, the risk to the fetus is minimal.

PREGNANCY AFTER STOPPING THE PILL

There may be some delay in becoming pregnant after you stop using oral contraceptives, especially if you had irregular menstrual cycles before you used oral contraceptives. It may be advisable to postpone conception until you begin menstruating regularly once you have stopped taking the pill and desire pregnancy.

There does not appear to be any increase in birth defects in newborn babies when pregnancy occurs soon after stopping the pill.

OVERDOSAGE

Serious ill effects have not been reported following ingestion of large doses of oral contraceptives by young children. Overdosage may cause nausea and withdrawal bleeding in females. In case of overdosage, contact your doctor, clinic or pharmacist.

OTHER INFORMATION

Your doctor or clinic will take a medical and family history before prescribing oral contraceptives and will examine you. The physical examination may be delayed to another time if you request it and your doctor or clinic believes that it is a good medical practice to postpone it. You should be reexamined at least once a year. Be sure to inform your doctor or clinic if there is a family history of any of the conditions listed previously in this leaflet. Be sure to keep all appointments with your doctor or clinic because this is a time to determine if there are early signs of side effects of oral contraceptive use.

Do not use the drug for any condition other than the one for which it was prescribed. This drug has been prescribed specifically for you; do not give it to others who may want birth control pills.

HEALTH BENEFITS FROM ORAL CONTRACEPTIVES

In addition to preventing pregnancy, use of combination oral contraceptives may provide certain benefits. They are:

- menstrual cycles may become more regular
- blood flow during menstruation may be lighter and less iron may be lost. Therefore, anemia due to iron deficiency is less likely to occur.
- pain or other symptoms during menstruation may be encountered less frequently.
- ectopic (tubal) pregnancy may occur less frequently.
- noncancerous cysts or lumps in the breast may occur less frequently.
- acute pelvic inflammatory disease may occur less frequently.
- oral contraceptive use may provide some protection against developing two forms of cancer: cancer of the ovaries and cancer of the lining of the uterus.

If you want more information about birth control pills, ask your doctor, clinic or pharmacist. They have a more technical leaflet called the Professional Labeling, which you may

wish to read. The Professional Labeling is also published in a book entitled *Physicians' Desk Reference*, available in many book stores and public libraries.

©1996 Organon Inc.   5310130   Revised 4/98

Manufactured for Organon Inc.
West Orange, NJ 07052 USA
by N.V. Organon, Oss, Holland or
Organon (Ireland) Ltd, Swords, Co. Dublin, Ireland
Shown in Product Identification Guide, page 326

FOLLISTIM™   ℞
(follitropin beta for injection)

FOR SUBCUTANEOUS OR INTRAMUSCULAR USE ONLY

DESCRIPTION

Follistim™ (follitropin beta for injection) contains human follicle-stimulating hormone (hFSH), a glycoprotein hormone which is manufactured by recombinant DNA (rDNA) technology. Follitropin beta has a dimeric structure containing two glycoprotein subunits (alpha and beta). Both the 92 amino acid alpha-chain and the 111 amino acid beta-chain have complex heterogeneous structures arising from two N-linked oligosaccharide chains. Follitropin beta is synthesized in a Chinese hamster ovary (CHO) cell line that has been transfected with a plasmid containing the two subunit DNA sequences encoding for hFSH. The purification process results in a highly purified preparation with a consistent hFSH isoform profile and high specific activity[1]. The biological activity is determined by measuring the increase in ovary weight in female rats. The intrinsic luteinizing hormone (LH) activity in follitropin beta is less than 1 IU per 40,000 IU FSH. The compound is considered to contain no LH activity.

The amino acid sequence and tertiary structure of the product are indistinguishable from that of human follicle-stimulating hormone (hFSH) of urinary source. Also, based on available data derived from physio-chemical tests and bioassay, follitropin beta and follitropin alfa, another recombinant follicle-stimulating hormone product, are indistinguishable.

Follistim™ is presented as a sterile, freeze-dried cake, intended for SUBCUTANEOUS or INTRAMUSCULAR administration after reconstitution with 0.45% Sodium Chloride Injection, USP. Each vial of Follistim™ contains 75 IU of FSH activity plus 25.0 mg sucrose, NF; 7.35 mg sodium citrate dihydrate, USP; 0.10 mg polysorbate 20, NF, and hydrochloric acid, NF and/or sodium hydroxide, NF to adjust the pH in a sterile, lyophilized form. The pH of the reconstituted preparation is approximately 7.0. The recombinant protein in Follistim™ has been standardized for FSH *in vivo* bioactivity in terms of the First International Reference Preparation for human menopausal gonadotropins (code 70/45), issued by the World Health Organization Expert Committee on Biological Standardization (1982). Under current storage conditions, Follistim™ may contain up to 20% of oxidized follitropin beta.

In clinical trials with Follistim™, serum antibodies to FSH or anti-CHO cell derived proteins were not detected in any of the treated patients after exposure to Follistim™ for up to three cycles.

Therapeutic Class: Infertility.

[1]As determined by the Ph. Eur. Test for FSH *in vivo* bioactivity and on the basis of the molar extinction coefficient at 277 nm (ϵ_s:mg^{-1}cm^{-1}) = 1.066.

CLINICAL PHARMACOLOGY

Follistim™ (follitropin beta for injection) stimulates ovarian follicular growth in women who do not have primary ovarian failure. FSH, the active component of Follistim™, is required for normal follicular growth, maturation, and gonadal steroid production. In the female, the level of FSH is critical for the onset and duration of follicular development, and consequently for the timing and number of follicles reaching maturity. In order to effect the final phase of follicle maturation, resumption of meiosis and rupture of the follicle in the absence of an endogenous LH surge, human chorionic gonadotropin (hCG) must be given following the administration of Follistim™ when patient monitoring indicates that appropriate follicular development parameters have been reached.

Pharmacokinetics

Absorption: The bioavailablity of Follistim™ following subcutaneous and intramuscular administration was investigated in healthy, pituitary-suppressed, female subjects given a single 300 IU dose. After subcutaneous or intramuscular injection the apparent dose absorbed was 77.8% and 76.4%, respectively.

The subcutaneous (455.6 ± 141.4 IU*h/L) and intramuscular (445.7 ± 135.7 IU*h/L) routes of administration were equivalent with respect to area under the curve (AUC) in healthy, pituitary-suppressed, female subjects given a single 300 IU dose. However, equivalence could not be estab-

lished for C_{max} between the subcutaneous (5.41 ± 0.72 IU/L) and intramuscular (6.86 ± 2.90 IU/L) routes of administration.

The pharmacokinetics and pharmacodynamics of a single, intramuscular dose (300 IU) of Follistim™ were also investigated in a group of gonadotropin-deficient, but otherwise healthy women. Peak (C_{max}) serum FSH levels in these women were 4.3 ± 1.7 IU/L (mean ±SD) and it occurred approximately 27 hours after intramuscular administration.

A multiple, dose proportionality, pharmacokinetic study of Follistim™ was completed in healthy, pituitary-suppressed, female subjects given intramuscular doses of 75 IU, 150 IU or 225 IU for 7 days. Steady-state blood concentrations of FSH were reached with all doses after 4 days of treatment based on the minimum concentrations of FSH just prior to dosing (C_{min}). Peak blood concentrations with the 75 IU, 150 IU and 225 IU dose were 4.65 ± 1.49 IU/L, 9.46 ± 2.57 IU/L and 11.30 ± 1.77 IU/L, respectively.

A multiple, dose proportionality, pharmacokinetic study of Follistim™ was completed in healthy, pituitary-suppressed, female subjects given subcutaneous doses of 75 IU, 150 IU or 225 IU for 7 days. Steady-state blood concentrations of FSH were reached with all doses after 5 days of treatment based on the minimum concentrations of FSH just prior to dosing (C_{min}). Peak blood concentrations with the 75 IU, 150 IU and 225 IU dose were 4.30 ± 0.60 IU/L, 8.51 ± 1.16 IU/L and 13.92 ± 1.81 IU/L, respectively.

Distribution: The volume of distribution of Follistim™ in healthy, pituitary-suppressed, female subjects following intravenous administration of a 300 IU dose was approximately 8 L.

Metabolism: The recombinant FSH in Follistim™ is biochemically very similar to urinary FSH and it is therefore anticipated that it is metabolized in the same manner.

Elimination: The elimination half-life following a single intramuscular dose (300 IU) of Follistim™ in female subjects was 43.9 ± 14.1 hours (mean ± SD). The elimination half-life following a 7-day intramuscular treatment with 75 IU, 150 IU or 225 IU was 26.9 ± 7.8 hours (mean ± SD), 30.1 ± 6.2 and 28.9 ± 6.5, respectively.

Special Populations: The effect of body weight on the pharmacokinetics of Follistim™ was evaluated in a group of European and Japanese women who were significantly different in terms of body weight. The European subjects had a body weight of (mean ± SD) 67.4 ± 13.5 kg and the Japanese subjects were 46.8 ± 11.6 kg. Following a single intramuscular dose of 300 IU of Follistim™, the AUC (IU*h/L) was significantly smaller in European subjects (339 ± 105) than in Japanese subjects (544 ± 201). However, clearance per kg of body weight was essentially the same for the respective groups (0.014 and 0.13 $1*h^{-1}kg^{-1}$).

Clinical Studies

The efficacy of Follistim™ was established in four controlled, clinical studies [three studies for Assisted Reproductive Technologies (ART) and one study for Ovulation Induction], three of which are described below. In these comparative studies, there were no clinically significant differences between treatment groups in study outcomes.

Assisted Reproductive Technologies (ART): Results from a randomized, assessor-blind, group comparative, multicenter safety and efficacy study of Follistim™ (Protocol 37608) in 981 infertile women treated for one cycle with *in vitro* fertilization with Follistim™ or Metrodin® after pituitary suppression with a GnRH agonist are summarized in Table 1.
[See table 1 above]
[See table 2 above]
Results from a randomized, assessor-blind, group comparative, single center safety and efficacy study of Follistim™ (Protocol 37604) in 89 infertile women treated with *in vitro* fertilization with Follistim™ or Humegon™ without pituitary suppression with a GnRH agonist are summarized in Table 3.
[See table 3 above]
The outcomes of the 22 clinical pregnancies (14 in Follistim™ and 8 in Humegon™) are shown in Table 4:
[See table 4 at top of next page]
Ovulation Induction: Results from a randomized, assessor-blind, group comparative, multicenter safety and efficacy study of Follistim™ (Protocol 37609) in 172 chronic anovulatory women who failed to ovulate and/or conceive during clomiphene citrate treatment are summarized in Tables 5, 6, and 7.
[See table 5 on next page]
[See table 6 on next page]
The outcomes of the 56 clinical pregnancies (35 in Follistim™ and 21 in Metrodin®) are shown in Table 7:
[See table 7 on next page]

INDICATIONS AND USAGE

Follistim™ (follitropin beta for injection) is indicated for the development of multiple follicles in ovulatory patients participating in an Assisted Reproductive Technology (ART) program. Follistim™ is also indicated for the induction of ovulation and pregnancy in anovulatory infertile patients in whom the cause of infertility is functional and not due to primary ovarian failure.

Selection of Patients

Before treatment with Follistim™ is instituted:

Table 1. Results From a Randomized, Assessor-blind, Group Comparative, Multicenter Safety and Efficacy Study of Follistim™ (Protocol 37608) in Infertile Women Treated With *In Vitro* Fertilization With Follistim™ or Metrodin® After Pituitary Suppression With a GnRH Agonist[1]

Parameter	Follistim™ (n=585)	Metrodin® (n=396)
Total number of oocytes recovered	10.9	9.0
Number of mature oocytes recovered	9.1	7.3
Maximum serum estradiol before hCG (pmol/L)[2]	6637	5692
Treatment duration (days)	11.0 (range 1-29)	11.6 (range 1-21)
Ongoing[3] pregnancy rate/attempt	22.2%	18.2%
Ongoing[3] pregnancy rate/transfer[4]	26.0%	22.0%

[1] All values are means
[2] Conversion factor to pg/mL is 3.671
[3] A single vital or multiple vital pregnancy was termed ongoing when a pregnancy, at least 12 weeks after embryo transfer (ET), was confirmed by the investigator
[4] Transfers were limited to a maximum of three embryos
Metrodin® is a registered trademark of Serono Laboratories, Inc., Randolph, MA 02368.
The outcomes of the 286 clinical pregnancies (179 in Follistim™ and 107 in Metrodin®) are shown in Table 2:

Table 2. Outcome for All Clinical* Pregnancies

	Follistim™ (n=179)	Metrodin® (n=107)
Did not result in live birth	50 (28%)	35 (33%)
Single birth	87 (49%)	43 (40%)
Multiple birth	42 (23%)	29 (27%)

*Clinical pregnancies included ongoing pregnancies as well as miscarriages with or without proof of a vital fetus

Table 3. Results From a Randomized, Assessor-blind, Group Comparative, Single Center Safety and Efficacy Study of Follistim™ (Protocol 37604) in Infertile Women Treated With *In Vitro* Fertilization With Follistim™ or Humegon™ Without Pituitary Suppression With a GnRH Agonist[1]

Parameter	Follistim™ (n=54)	Humegon™ (n=35)
Total number of oocytes recovered	9.9	7.6
Number of mature oocytes recovered	9.4	6.9
Maximum serum estradiol before hCG (pmol/L)[2]	3791	3087
Treatment duration (days)	5.8 (range 1-9)	6.0 (range 2-10)
Ongoing[3] pregnancy rate/attempt	22.2%	17.1%
Ongoing[3] pregnancy rate/transfer[4]	30.8%	22.2%

[1] All values are means
[2] Conversion factor to pg/mL is 3.671
[3] A single vital or multiple vital pregnancy was termed ongoing when a pregnancy, at least 12 weeks after embryo transfer (ET), was confirmed by the investigator
[4] Transfers were limited to a maximum of three embryos

1. A thorough gynecologic and endocrinologic evaluation of the patient must be performed. The evaluation should include a hysterosalpingogram (to rule out uterine and tubal pathology) and documentation of anovulation by means of reviewing a patient's history, performing a physical examination, determining serum hormonal levels as indicated, and optionally performing an endometrial biopsy. Patients with tubal pathology should receive Follistim™ only if enrolled in an ART program.
2. Primary ovarian failure should be excluded by the determination of circulating gonadotropin levels.
3. Careful examination should be made to rule out early pregnancy.
4. Evaluation of the partner's fertility potential should be included in the workup procedure.

CONTRAINDICATIONS

Follistim™ (follitropin beta for injection) is contraindicated in women who exhibit:
1. Prior hypersensitivity to recombinant hFSH products.
2. A high circulating FSH level indicating primary ovarian failure.

3. Uncontrolled thyroid or adrenal dysfunction.
4. Tumor of the ovary, breast, uterus, hypothalamus or pituitary gland.
5. Pregnancy.
6. Heavy or irregular vaginal bleeding of undetermined origin.
7. Ovarian cysts or enlargement not due to polycystic ovary disease (PCOD).

WARNINGS

1. Follistim™ (follitropin beta for injection) should be used only by physicians who are experienced in infertility treatment. Follistim™ is a potent gonadotropic substance capable of causing Ovarian Hyperstimulation Syndrome (OHSS) (see **WARNINGS-Overstimulation of the Ovary During Follistim™ Therapy**) with or without pulmonary or vascular complications (see **WARNINGS-Pulmonary and Vascular Complications**) and multiple births (see **WARNINGS-Mul-**

Continued on next page

Follistim—Cont.

tiple Births). Gonadotropin therapy requires the availability of appropriate monitoring facilities (see **PRECAUTIONS-Laboratory Tests**).

2. Overstimulation of the Ovary During Follistim™ Therapy
In order to minimize the hazards associated with the occasional abnormal ovarian enlargement that may occur with Follistim™ therapy, the lowest effective dose should be used (see **DOSAGE AND ADMINISTRATION**). Use of ultrasound monitoring of ovarian response and/or measurement of serum estradiol levels can further minimize the risk of overstimulation.

If the ovaries are abnormally enlarged on the last day of Follistim™ therapy, hCG should not be administered in this course of treatment; this will reduce the chances of developing Ovarian Hyperstimulation Syndrome (OHSS).

The Ovarian Hyperstimulation Syndrome (OHSS): OHSS is a medical entity distinct from uncomplicated ovarian enlargement and may progress rapidly to become a serious medical event. OHSS is characterized by a dramatic increase in vascular permeability, which can result in a rapid accumulation of fluid in the peritoneal cavity, thorax, and potentially, the pericardium. The early warning signs of OHSS developing are severe pelvic pain, nausea, vomiting and weight gain. The following symptoms have been reported in cases of OHSS: abdominal pain, abdominal distension, gastrointestinal symptoms including nausea, vomiting and diarrhea, severe ovarian enlargement, weight gain, dyspnea, and oliguria. Clinical evaluation may reveal hypovolemia, hemoconcentration, electrolyte imbalances, ascites, hemoperitoneum, pleural effusions, hydrothorax, acute pulmonary distress, and thromboembolic events (see **WARNINGS-Pulmonary and Vascular Complications**).

During clinical trials with Follistim™ therapy, OHSS occurred in 53 (5.2%) of the 1,029 women treated and of these 29 (2.8%) were hospitalized. Cases of OHSS are more common, more severe, and more protracted if pregnancy occurs; therefore, patients should be followed for at least two weeks after hCG administration. Most often, OHSS occurs after treatment has been discontinued and it can develop rapidly, reaching its maximum about seven to ten days following treatment. Usually, OHSS resolves spontaneously with the onset of menses. If there is evidence that OHSS may be developing prior to hCG administration (see **PRECAUTIONS-Laboratory Tests**), the hCG must be withheld.

If serious OHSS occurs, treatment should be stopped and the patient should be hospitalized. Treatment is primarily symptomatic and should consist of bed rest, fluid and electrolyte management, and analgesics (if needed). Hemoconcentration associated with fluid loss into the peritoneal cavity, pleural cavity, and the pericardial cavity may occur and should be thoroughly assessed in the following manner: 1) fluid intake and output; 2) weight; 3) hematocrit; 4) serum and urinary electrolytes; 5) urine specific gravity; 6) BUN and creatinine; 7) total proteins with albumin: globulin ratio; 8) coagulation studies; 9) electrocardiogram to monitor for hyperkalemia and 10) abdominal girth. These determinations should be performed daily or more often based on clinical need.

OHSS increases the risk of injury to the ovary. The ascitic, pleural, and pericardial fluid should not be removed unless there is the necessity to relieve symptoms such as pulmonary or cardiac tamponade. Pelvic examination may cause rupture of an ovarian cyst, which may result in hemoperitoneum, and should therefore be avoided. If bleeding occurs and requires surgical intervention, the clinical objective should be to control the bleeding and retain as much ovarian tissue as possible. Intercourse should be prohibited in patients with significant ovarian enlargement after ovulation because of the danger of hemoperitoneum resulting from ruptured ovarian cysts.

The management of OHSS may be divided into three phases: an acute, a chronic, and a resolution phase. Because the use of diuretics can accentuate the diminished intravascular volume, diuretics should be avoided except in the late phase of resolution as described below.

Acute Phase: Management during the acute phase should be directed at preventing hemoconcentration due to loss of intravascular volume to the third space and minimizing the risk of thromboembolic phenomena and kidney damage. Treatment is intended to normalize electrolytes while maintaining an acceptable but somewhat reduced intravascular volume. Full correction of the intravascular volume deficit may lead to an unacceptable increase in the amount of third space fluid accumulation.

Management includes administration of limited intravenous fluids, electrolytes, human serum albumin and strict monitoring of fluid intake and output. Monitoring for the development of hyperkalemia is recommended.

Chronic Phase: After stabilizing the patient during the acute phase, excessive fluid accumulation in the third space should be limited by instituting severe potassium, sodium, and fluid restriction.

Resolution Phase: A fall in hematocrit and an increasing urinary output without an increased intake are observed due to the return of the third space fluid to the intravascular compartment. Peripheral and/or pulmonary edema may result if the kidneys are unable to excrete third space fluid as rapidly as it is mobilized. Diuretics may be indicated during the resolution phase, if necessary, to combat pulmonary edema.

Pulmonary and Vascular Complications
Serious pulmonary conditions (e.g., atelectasis, acute respiratory distress syndrome) have been reported in women treated with gonadotropins. In addition, thromboembolic events both in association with, and separate from, the Ovarian Hyperstimulation Syndrome have been reported following gonadotropin therapy. Intravascular thrombosis, which may originate in venous or arterial vessels, can result in reduced blood flow to vital organs or the extremities. Sequelae of such events have included venous thrombophlebitis, pulmonary embolism, pulmonary infarction, cerebral vascular occlusion (stroke), and arterial occlusion resulting in loss of limb. In rare cases, pulmonary complications and/or thromboembolic events have resulted in death.

Multiple Births
Reports of multiple births have been associated with Follistim™ treatment. The patient and her partner should be advised of the potential risk of multiple births before starting treatment. In clinical trials with Follistim™ and Metrodin®, multiple gestation rates in ART patients were 31% and 38%, respectively, and in ovulation induction patients, the rates were 8% in both groups.

PRECAUTIONS
General
Careful attention should be given to the diagnosis of infertility and in the selection of candidates for Follistim™ (follitropin beta for injection) therapy (see **INDICATIONS AND USAGE-Selection of Patients**).

Information for Patients
Prior to therapy with Follistim™, patients should be informed of the duration of treatment and monitoring procedures that will be required. The risks of Ovarian Hyperstimulation Syndrome and multiple births (see **WARNINGS**), and other possible adverse reactions (see **ADVERSE REACTIONS**) should be discussed.

Laboratory Tests
In most instances, treatment with Follistim™ will result only in follicular growth and maturation. In order to complete the final phase of follicular maturation and to induce ovulation, hCG must be given following the administration of Follistim™ or when clinical assessment of the patient indicates that sufficient follicular maturation has occurred. This may be directly estimated by sonographic visualization of the ovaries and endometrial lining and/or measuring serum estradiol levels. The combination of both ultrasonography and measurement of estradiol levels is useful for monitoring the growth and development of follicles, timing hCG administration, as well as minimizing the risk of OHSS and multiple gestations.

The clinical evaluation of estrogenic activity (changes in vaginal cytology, changes in appearance and volume of cervical mucus, spinnbarkeit, and ferning of the cervical mucus) provides an indirect estimate of the estrogenic effect upon the target organs, and therefore it should only be used adjunctively with more direct estimates of follicular development (e.g., ultrasonography and serum estradiol determinations).

The clinical confirmation of ovulation is obtained by direct and indirect indices of progesterone production. The indices most generally used are as follows:
a) A rise in basal body temperature,
b) Increase in serum progesterone, and
c) Menstruation following the shift in basal body temperature.

When used in conjunction with indices of progesterone production, sonographic visualization of the ovaries will assist in determining if ovulation has occurred. Sonographic evidence of ovulation may include the following:
a) Fluid in the cul-de-sac,
b) Follicle showing marked decrease in size, and
c) Collapsed follicle.

Drug Interactions
No drug/drug interaction studies have been performed.

Table 4. Outcome for All Clinical* Pregnancies

	Follistim™ (n=14)	Humegon™ (n=8)
Did not result in live birth	2 (14%)	2 (25%)
Single birth	7 (50%)	4 (50%)
Multiple birth	5 (36%)	2 (25%)

*Clinical pregnancies included ongoing pregnancies as well as miscarriages with or without proof of a vital fetus

Table 5. Cumulative Ovulation Rates From Protocol 37609

	Follistim™ (n=105)	Metrodin® (n=67)
First treatment cycle	72%	63%
Second treatment cycle	82%	79%
Third treatment cycle	85%	82%

Table 6. Cumulative Ongoing[1] Pregnancy Rates From Protocol 37609

	Follistim™ (n=105)	Metrodin® (n=67)
First treatment cycle	14%	10%
Second treatment cycle	19%	18%
Third treatment cycle	23%	19%

[1] All ongoing pregnancies were confirmed after at least 12 weeks after the hCG injection

Table 7. Outcome for All Clinical* Pregnancies

	Follistim™ (n=35)	Metrodin® (n=21)
Did not result in live birth	11 (31%)	8 (38%)
Single birth	22 (63%)	12 (57%)
Multiple birth	2 (6%)	1 (5%)

*Clinical pregnancies included ongoing pregnancies as well as miscarriages with or without proof of a vital fetus

Table 8. Incidence of Adverse Clinical Experiences (>1%) that Occurred in Protocol 37608

Adverse Event	Follistim™ (n=591)	Metrodin® (n=398)
Miscarriage	11.0%	11.3%
Ovarian Hyperstimulation Syndrome	5.2%	4.3%
Ectopic pregnancy	3.0%	3.8%
Abdominal pain	2.5%	2.3%
Injection site pain	1.7%	0.5%
Vaginal hemorrhage	1.5%	0.8%

Carcinogenesis and Mutagenesis, Impairment of Fertility
Long-term toxicity studies in animals have not been performed with Follistim™ to evaluate the carcinogenic potential of the drug. Follistim™ was not mutagenic in the Ames test using *S. typhimurium* and *E. coli* tester strains and did not produce chromosomal aberrations in an *in vitro* assay using human lymphocytes.

Pregnancy
Pregnancy Category X: See **CONTRAINDICATIONS**.

Nursing Mothers
It is not known whether this drug is excreted in human milk. Because many drugs are excreted in human milk and because of the potential for serious adverse reactions in the nursing infant from Follistim™, a decision should be made whether to discontinue nursing or to discontinue the drug, taking into account the importance of the drug to the mother.

Pediatric Use
Safety and effectiveness in pediatric patients have not been established.

ADVERSE REACTIONS

Assisted Reproductive Technologies (ART)
Rates of adverse events from a randomized, assessor-blind, group comparative, multicenter safety and efficacy study of Follistim™ (Protocol 37608) in 989 infertile women treated with *in vitro* fertilization with Follistim™ or Metrodin® after pituitary suppression with a GnRH agonist are summarized in Table 8.
[See table 8 above]

Ovulation Induction
Rates of adverse events from a randomized, assessor-blind, group comparative, multicenter safety and efficacy study of Follistim™ (Protocol 37609) in 172 chronic anovulatory women who failed to ovulate and/or conceive during clomiphene citrate treatment are summarized in Table 9.
[See table 9 below]
The following adverse events have been reported in women treated with gonadotropins: pulmonary and vascular complications (see **WARNINGS**), hemoperitoneum, adnexal torsion (as a complication of ovarian enlargement), dizziness, tachycardia, dyspnea, tachypnea, febrile reactions, flu-like symptoms including fever, chills, musculoskeletal aches, joint pains, nausea, headache and malaise, breast tenderness, and dermatological symptoms (dry skin, body rash, hair loss and hives).
There have been infrequent reports of ovarian neoplasms, both benign and malignant, in women who have undergone multiple drug regimens for ovulation induction; however, a causal relationship has not been established.

DRUG ABUSE AND DEPENDENCE
There have been no reports of abuse or dependence with Follistim™ (follitropin beta for injection).

OVERDOSAGE
Aside from the possibility of Ovarian Hyperstimulation Syndrome (see **WARNINGS-Overstimulation of the Ovary During Follistim™ Therapy**) and multiple gestations (see **WARNINGS-Multiple Births**), there is no additional information concerning the consequences of acute overdosage with Follistim™ (follitropin beta for injection).

DOSAGE AND ADMINISTRATION

Assisted Reproductive Technologies (ART)
Dosage: A starting dose of 150 to 225 IU of Follistim™ (follitropin beta for injection) is recommended for at least the first four days of treatment. After this, the dose may be adjusted for the individual patient based upon their ovarian response. In clinical studies with patients who are responding, it was shown that daily maintenance dosages ranging from 75 to 300 IU for six to twelve days are sufficient, although longer treatment may be necessary. However, in patients that were low or poor responders, maintenance doses of 375 to 600 IU were administered according to individual response. This later category comprised approximately 10% of the women evaluated during clinical studies. The maximum, individualized, daily dose of Follistim™ that has been used in clinical studies is 600 IU. When a sufficient number of follicles of adequate size are present, the final maturation of the follicles is induced by administering hCG at a dose of 5,000 IU to 10,000 IU. Oocyte (egg) retrieval is performed 34 to 36 hours later. The administration of hCG must be withheld in cases where the ovaries are abnormally enlarged on the last day of Follistim™ therapy; this will reduce the chance of developing OHSS.

Ovulation Induction
Dosage: There are a variety of treatment protocols available for ovulation induction. In studies using Follistim™, a stepwise gradually increasing dosing scheme was used. The starting dose was 75 IU of Follistim™ for up to 14 days. The dose was then increased by 37.5 IU of Follistim™ at weekly intervals until follicular growth and/or serum estradiol levels indicated an adequate response. The maximum, individualized, daily dose of Follistim™ that has been safely used for ovulation induction patients during clinical trials is 300 IU. The patient should be treated until ultrasonic visualizations and/or serum estradiol determinations indicate preovulatory conditions equivalent to or greater than those of the normal individual followed by hCG, 5,000 IU to 10,000 IU. If the ovaries are abnormally enlarged on the last day of Follistim™ therapy, hCG must be withheld during this course of treatment; this will reduce the chances of developing OHSS.
During treatment with Follistim™ and during a two week post-treatment period, patients should be examined at least every other day for signs of excessive ovarian stimulation. It is recommended that Follistim™ administration be stopped if the ovaries become abnormally enlarged or abdominal pain occurs. Most OHSS occurs after treatment has been discontinued and reaches its maximum at about seven to ten days post-ovulation.
For ovulation induction, the couple should be encouraged to have intercourse daily, beginning on the day prior to the administration of hCG and until ovulation becomes apparent from the indices employed for the determination of progestational activity (see **PRECAUTIONS-Laboratory Tests**).

Care should be taken to insure insemination. In the light of the foregoing indices and parameters mentioned, it should become obvious that, unless a physician is willing to devote considerable time to these patients and be familiar with and conduct these necessary laboratory studies, he/she should not use Follistim™.

Directions for using Follistim™
1. Wash hands thoroughly with soap and water.
2. Before injections, the septum tops of the vials should be wiped with an aseptic solution to prevent contamination of the contents.
3. To prepare the Follistim™ solution, inject 1 mL of 0.45% Sodium Chloride Injection, USP into the vial of Follistim™. **DO NOT SHAKE**, but gently swirl until the solution is clear. Generally, the Follistim™ dissolves immediately. Check the liquid in the container. If it is not clear or has particles in it, **DO NOT USE IT**.
4. For patients requiring a single injection from multiple vials of Follistim™, up to 4 vials can be reconstituted with 1 mL of 0.45% Sodium Chloride Injection, USP. This can be accomplished by reconstituting a single vial as described above (see step 3). Then draw the entire contents of the first vial into a syringe, and inject the contents into a second vial of lyophilized Follistim™. Gently swirl the second vial, as described above, once again checking to make sure the solution is clear and free of particles. This step can be repeated with 2 additional vials for a total of up to 4 vials of lyophilized Follistim™ into 1 mL of diluent.
5. Immediately **ADMINISTER** the reconstituted Follistim™ either **SUBCUTANEOUSLY** or **INTRAMUSCULARLY**. Any unused reconstituted material should be discarded.
6. Draw the reconstituted Follistim™ into an empty, sterile syringe.
7. Hold the syringe pointing upwards and gently tap the side to force any air bubbles to the top; then squeeze the plunger gently until all the air has been expelled and only Follistim™ solution is left in the syringe.
8. Follistim™ only works if it is injected **SUBCUTANEOUSLY** or **INTRAMUSCULARLY**. The most convenient sites for **SUBCUTANEOUS** injection are either in the abdomen around the navel where there is a lot of loose skin and layers of fatty tissue or in the upper thigh. Pinch up a large are of skin between the finger and thumb. You should vary the injection site a little with each injection.
The best site for **INTRAMUSCULAR** injection of Follistim™ is the upper outer quadrant of the buttock muscle. This area contains a large volume of muscle with few blood vessels and major nerves. Stretching the skin helps the needle to go in more easily and pushes the tissue beneath the skin out of the way. This helps the solution disperse correctly.
9. The injection site should be swabbed with a disinfectant to remove any surface bacteria. Clean about two inches around the point where the needle will go in and let the disinfectant dry for at least one minute before proceeding.
10. For **SUBCUTANEOUS** injection the needle should be inserted at the base of the pinched-up skin at an angle of 45° to the skin surface.
The needle for **INTRAMUSCULAR** injection should be inserted right up to the hilt at an angle of 90° to the skin surface. Pushing in with a quick thrust causes the least discomfort.
11. If the needle is correctly positioned it will be difficult to draw back on the plunger. Any blood drawn into the syringe means the needle tip has penetrated a vein or artery. If this happens, remove the syringe, cover the injection site with a swab containing disinfectant and apply pressure; the site should stop bleeding in a minute or two.
12. Once the needle is properly placed, depress the plunger **slowly** and steadily, so the solution is correctly injected and the skin or muscle tissue is not damaged.
13. Pull the syringe out quickly and apply pressure to the site with a swab containing disinfectant. A gentle massage of the site—while still maintaining pressure—helps disperse the Follistim™ solution and relieve any discomfort
14. Use the disposable syringe only once and dispose of it properly.

HOW SUPPLIED
Follistim™ (follitropin beta for injection) is supplied in a sterile, freeze-dried form, as a white to off-white cake or powder in vials containing 75 IU of FSH activity. The following package combinations are available:
—1 vial 75 IU Follistim™ and 1 vial 1 mL 0.45% Sodium Chloride Injection, USP.
NDC 0052-0306-17
—5 vials 75 IU Follistim™ and 5 vials 1 mL 0.45% Sodium Chloride Injection, USP.
NDC 0052-0306-21

Table 9. Incidence of Adverse Clinical Experiences (>1%) that Occurred in Protocol 37609

Adverse Event	Follistim™ (n=105)	Metrodin® (n=67)
Miscarriage	9.5%	9.0%
Ovarian Hyperstimulation Syndrome	7.6%	4.5%
Abdominal discomfort	2.9%	1.5%
Abdominal pain, lower	2.9%	1.5%
Abdominal pain	1.9%	3.0%
Ovarian cyst	2.9%	3.0%

Continued on next page

Follistim—Cont.

Lyophilized powder may be stored refrigerated or at room temperature (2°–25°C/36°–77°F). Protect from light. Use immediately after reconstitution. Discard unused material.
CAUTION: Federal law prohibits dispensing without prescription.

Manufactured by
ORGANON INC.
375 Mt. Pleasant Ave.
West Orange, NJ 07052

Printed in USA   5310164   Revised 9/97
Shown in Product Identification Guide, page 327

HUMEGON™   ℞
(menotropins for injection, USP)
FOR INTRAMUSCULAR INJECTION

DESCRIPTION

Humegon™ (menotropins for injection, USP) is a purified preparation of gonadotropins. Menotropins are extracted from the urine of postmenopausal females and possess follicle-stimulating hormone (FSH) and luteinizing hormone (LH) activity. The ratio of FSH bioactivity and LH bioactivity in menotropins is adjusted to approximate unity by the addition of human chorionic gonadotropin purified from the urine of pregnant women. Each vial of Humegon™ contains 75 IU or 150 IU of follicle-stimulating hormone activity and 75 IU or 150 IU of luteinizing hormone activity, respectively, plus 10.5 mg lactose, hydrous NF; 0.25 mg monosodium phosphate, monohydrate USP; 0.25 mg disodium phosphate, anhydrous USP; sodium hydroxide NF or phosphoric acid NF to adjust pH; in a sterile, lyophilized form. Humegon™ is administered by intramuscular injection.
Humegon™ is biologically standardized for FSH and LH gonadotropin activities and the potencies are based on the results of *in vivo* bioassays, which are in agreement with the recommendations of the World Health Organization Expert Committee on Biological Standardization (1982).
Both FSH and LH as well as hCG are glycoproteins that are acidic and water soluble.
Therapeutic class: Infertility.

CLINICAL PHARMACOLOGY

The geometric mean absolute bioavailability of FSH from the 150 IU intramuscular (IM) dose compared to the 150 IU intravenous (IV) dose was 76%. Following single dose IM injections of 75, 150, and 300 IU Humegon™ to healthy male volunteers, FSH dose response was less than proportional between the 75 and 150 IU doses and between the 150 and 300 IU doses. The mean FSH elimination half-lives of 75, 150, and 300 IU IM were 37 hrs, 30 hrs, and 36 hrs, respectively, and 31 hrs following 150 IU IV administration. Repeated daily IM administration of 150 IU Humegon™ to seven women on 8 consecutive days led to a gradual accumulation of FSH levels which plateaued in 3–4 days. It took 4–5 days for the elevated FSH levels to return to pretreatment levels. These findings underline the importance of very careful and frequent monitoring of the patient in order to reduce the danger of ovarian hyperstimulation.
Women:
Humegon™ administered for seven to twelve days produces ovarian follicular growth in women who do not have primary ovarian failure. Treatment with Humegon™ in most instances results only in follicular growth and maturation. In order to induce ovulation, human chorionic gonadotropin (hCG) must be given following the administration of Humegon™ when clinical assessment of the patient indicates that sufficient follicular maturation has occurred.
Men:
Humegon™ administered concomitantly with human chorionic gonadotropin (hCG) for at least three months induces spermatogenesis in men with primary or secondary pituitary hypofunction who have achieved adequate masculinization with prior hCG therapy.

INDICATIONS AND USAGE

Women:
Humegon™ and hCG given in a sequential manner are indicated for the induction of ovulation and pregnancy in the anovulatory infertile patient, in whom the cause of anovulation is functional and is not due to primary ovarian failure.
Humegon™ and hCG may also be used to stimulate the development of multiple follicles in ovulatory patients participating in an *in vitro* fertilization program.
Men:
Humegon™ with concomitant hCG is indicated for the stimulation of spermatogenesis in men who have primary or secondary hypogonadotropic hypogonadism, and idiopathic infertility.
Humegon™ with concomitant hCG has proven effective in inducing spermatogenesis in men with primary hypogonadotropic hypogonadism due to a congenital factor or prepu-

bertal hypophysectomy and in men with secondary hypogonadotropic hypogonadism due to hypophysectomy, craniopharyngioma, cerebral aneurysm, or chromophobe adenoma.

SELECTION OF PATIENTS

Women:
1. Before treatment with Humegon™ is instituted, a thorough gynecologic and endocrinologic evaluation must be performed. Except for those patients enrolled in an *in vitro* fertilization program, this should include a hysterosalpingogram (to rule out uterine and tubal pathology) and documentation of anovulation by means of basal body temperature, serial vaginal smears, examination of cervical mucus, determination of serum (or urinary) progesterone, urinary pregnanediol, and endometrial biopsy. Patients with tubal pathology should receive Humegon™ only if enrolled in an *in vitro* fertilization program.
2. Primary ovarian failure should be excluded by the determination of gonadotropin levels.
3. Careful examination should be made to rule out the presence of an early pregnancy.
4. Patients in late reproductive life have a greater predilection to endometrial carcinoma as well as a higher incidence of anovulatory disorders. Cervical dilation and curettage should always be done for diagnosis before starting Humegon™ therapy in such patients who demonstrate abnormal uterine bleeding or other signs of endometrial abnormalities.
5. Evaluation of the partner's fertility potential should be included in the workup.
Men:
Patient selection should be made based on a documented lack of pituitary function. Prior to hormonal therapy, these patients will have low testosterone levels and low or absent gonadotropin levels. Patients with primary hypogonadotropic hypogonadism will have a subnormal development of masculinization, and those with secondary hypogonadotropic hypogonadism will have decreased masculinization.

CONTRAINDICATIONS

Women:
Humegon™ is contraindicated in women who have:
1. A high FSH level indicating primary ovarian failure.
2. Uncontrolled thyroid and adrenal dysfunction.
3. An organic intracranial lesion such as a pituitary tumor.
4. The presence of any cause of infertility other than anovulation, unless they are candidates for *in vitro* fertilization.
5. Abnormal bleeding of undetermined origin.
6. Ovarian cysts or enlargement not due to polycystic ovary syndrome.
7. Prior hypersensitivity to menotropins.
8. Humegon™ is contraindicated in women who are pregnant and may cause fetal harm. There are limited human data on the effects of Humegon™ when administered during pregnancy.
Men:
Humegon™ is contraindicated in men who have:
1. Normal gonadotropin levels indicating normal pituitary function.
2. Elevated gonadotropin levels indicating primary testicular failure.
3. Infertility disorders other than hypogonadotropic hypogonadism.

WARNINGS

Humegon™ is a drug that should only be used by physicians who are thoroughly familiar with infertility problems. It is a potent gonadotropic substance capable of causing mild to severe adverse reactions in women. Gonadotropin therapy requires a certain time commitment by physicians and supportive health professionals, and its use requires the availability of appropriate monitoring facilities (see PRECAUTIONS/Laboratory Tests). In female patients it must be used with a great deal of care.

Overstimulation of the Ovary During Humegon™ Therapy:
Ovarian Enlargement: Mild to moderate uncomplicated ovarian enlargement which may be accompanied by abdominal distension and/or abdominal pain occurs in approximately 20% of those treated with Humegon™ and hCG, and generally regresses without treatment within two or three weeks.
In order to minimize the hazard associated with the occasional abnormal ovarian enlargement which may occur with Humegon™-hCG therapy, the lowest dose consistent with expectation of good results should be used. Careful monitoring of ovarian response can further minimize the risk of overstimulation.
If the ovaries are abnormally enlarged on the last day of Humegon™ therapy, hCG should not be administered in this course of therapy; this will reduce the chances of development of the Ovarian Hyperstimulation Syndrome.
The Ovarian Hyperstimulation Syndrome (OHSS): OHSS is a medical event distinct from uncomplicated ovarian enlargement. OHSS may progress rapidly to become a serious medical event. It is characterized by an apparent drama-

tic increase in vascular permeability which can result in a rapid accumulation of fluid in the peritoneal cavity, thorax, and potentially, the pericardium. The early warning signs of development of OHSS are severe pelvic pain, nausea, vomiting, and weight gain. The following symptomatology has been seen with cases of OHSS: abdominal pain, abdominal distension, gastrointestinal symptoms including nausea, vomiting and diarrhea, severe ovarian enlargement, weight gain, dyspnea, and oliguria. Clinical evaluation may reveal hypovolemia, hemoconcentration, electrolyte imbalances, ascites, hemoperitoneum, pleural effusions, hydrothorax, acute pulmonary distress, and thromboembolic events (see Pulmonary and Vascular Complications).
OHSS occurs in approximately 0.4% of patients when the recommended dose is administered and in 1.3% of patients when higher than recommended doses are administered. Cases of OHSS are more common, more severe and more protracted if pregnancy occurs. OHSS develops rapidly; therefore patients should be followed for at least two weeks after hCG administration. Most often, OHSS occurs after treatment has been discontinued and reaches its maximum at about seven to ten days following treatment. Usually, OHSS resolves spontaneously with the onset of menses. If there is evidence that OHSS may be developng prior to hCG administration (see PRECAUTIONS/Laboratory Tests), the hCG should be withheld.
If OHSS occurs, treatment should be stopped and the patient hospitalized. Treatment is primarily symptomatic, consisting of bed rest, fluid and electrolyte management, and analgesics if needed. The phenomenon of hemoconcentration associated with fluid loss into the peritoneal cavity, pleural cavity, and the pericardial cavity has been seen to occur and should be thoroughly assessed in the following manner: 1) fluid intake and output, 2) weight, 3) hematocrit, 4) serum and urinary electrolytes, 5) urine specific gravity, 6) BUN and creatinine, and 7) abdominal girth. These determinations are to be performed daily or more often if the need arises.
With OHSS there is an increased risk of injury to the ovary. The ascitic, pleural, and pericardial fluid should not be removed unless absolutely necessary to relieve symptoms such as pulmonary distress or cardiac tamponade. Pelvic examination may cause rupture of an ovarian cyst, which may result in hemoperitoneum, and should therefore be avoided. If this does occur, and if bleeding becomes such that surgery is required, the surgical treatment should be designed to control bleeding and to retain as much ovarian tissue as possible. Intercourse should be prohibited in those patients in whom significant ovarian enlargement occurs after ovulation because of the danger of hemoperitoneum resulting from ruptured ovarian cysts.
The management of OHSS may be divided into three phases; an acute, a chronic, and a resolution phase. Because the use of diuretics can accentuate the diminished intravascular volume, diuretics should be avoided except in the late phase of resolution as described below.
Acute Phase: Management during the acute phase should be designed to prevent hemoconcentration due to loss of intravascular volume to the third space and to minimize the risk of thromboembolic phenomena and kidney damage. Treatment is designed to normalize electrolytes while maintaining an acceptable but somewhat reduced intravascular volume. Full correction of the intravascular volume deficit may lead to an unacceptable increase in the amount of third space fluid accumulation. Management includes administration of limited intravenous fluids, electrolytes, and human serum albumin. Monitoring for the development of hyperkalemia is recommended.
Chronic Phase: After stabilizing the patient during the acute phase, excessive fluid accumulation in the third space should be limited by instituting severe potassium, sodium, and fluid restriction.
Resolution Phase: A fall in hematocrit and an increasing urinary output without an increased intake are observed due to the return of third space fluid to the intravascular compartment. Peripheral and/or pulmonary edema may result if the kidneys are unable to excrete third space fluid as rapidly as it is mobilized. Diuretics may be indicated during the resolution phase if necessary to combat pulmonary edema.

Pulmonary and Vascular Complications: Serious pulmonary conditions (e.g., atelectasis, acute respiratory distress syndrome) have been reported. In addition, thromboembolic events both in association with, and separate from, the Ovarian Hyperstimulation Syndrome have been reported following Humegon™ therapy. Intravascular thrombosis, which may originate in venous or arterial vessels, can result in reduced blood flow to vital organs or the extremities. Sequelae of such events have included venous thrombophlebitis, pulmonary embolism, pulmonary infarction, cerebral vascular occlusion (stroke), and arterial occlusion resulting in loss of limb. In rare cases, pulmonary complications and/or thromboembolic events have resulted in death.
Multiple Births: Data from a clinical trial revealed the following results regarding multiple births: Of the pregnancies following therapy with Humegon™ and hCG, 80% resulted

in single births. The patient and her partner should be advised of the frequency and potential hazards of multiple gestation before starting treatment.

PRECAUTIONS

General: Careful attention should be given to diagnosis in the selection of candidates for Humegon™ therapy (see INDICATIONS AND USAGE/SELECTION OF PATIENTS).

Information for Patients: Prior to therapy with Humegon™, patients should be informed of the duration of treatment and the monitoring of their condition that will be required. Possible adverse reactions (see ADVERSE REACTIONS) and the risk of multiple births should also be discussed.

Laboratory Tests:

Women:

Treatment for Induction of Ovulation

In most instances, treatment with Humegon™ results only in follicular growth and maturation. In order to induce ovulation, hCG must be given following the administration of Humegon™ when clinical assessment of the patient indicates that sufficient follicular maturation has occurred. This may be directly estimated by measuring serum (or urinary) estrogen levels and sonographic visualization of the ovaries. The combination of both estradiol levels and ultrasonography is useful for monitoring the growth and development of follicles, timing hCG administration, as well as minimizing the risk of the Ovarian Hyperstimulation Syndrome and multiple gestation.

Other clinical parameters which may have potential use for monitoring menotropins therapy include:

a) Changes in vaginal cytology;
b) Appearance and volume of cervical mucus;
c) Spinnbarkeit; and
d) Ferning of cervical mucus.

The above clinical indices provide an indirect estimate of the estrogenic effect upon the target organs, and therefore should only be used adjunctively with more direct estimates of follicular development, i.e., serum estradiol and ultrasonography.

The clinical confirmation of ovulation, with the exception of pregnancy, is obtained by direct and indirect indices of progesterone production. The indices most generally used are as follows:

a) A rise in basal body temperature;
b) Increase in serum progesterone; and
c) Menstruation following the shift in basal body temperature.

When used in conjunction with indices of progesterone production, sonographic visualization of the ovaries will assist in determining if ovulation has occurred. Sonographic evidence of ovulation may include the following:

a) Fluid in the cul-de-sac;
b) Ovarian stigmata; and
c) Collapsed follicle.

Because of the subjectivity of the various tests for the determination of follicular maturation and ovulation, it cannot be overemphasized that the physician should choose the test(s) with which he/she is thoroughly familiar.

Drug Interactions: No clinically significant drug/drug or drug/food adverse interactions have been reported during Humegon™ therapy.

Carcinogenesis, Mutagenesis, Impairment of Fertility: Long-term toxicity studies in animals have not been performed to evaluate the carcinogenic potential of Humegon™.

Pregnancy: Pregnancy Category X. See CONTRAINDICATIONS.

Males: No animal studies have been performed that examine the potential teratogenic effect associated with Humegon™ therapy when prescribed for male infertility.

Nursing Mothers: It is not known whether this drug is excreted in human milk. Because many drugs are excreted in human milk, caution should be exercised if Humegon™ is administered to a nursing woman.

ADVERSE REACTIONS

Women:

The following adverse reactions, reported during Humegon™ therapy, are listed in decreasing order of potential severity:

1. Pulmonary and vascular complications (see WARNINGS),
2. Ovarian Hyperstimulation Syndrome (see WARNINGS),
3. Hemoperitoneum,
4. Adnexal torsion (as a complication of ovarian enlargement),
5. Mild to moderate ovarian enlargement,
6. Ovarian cysts,
7. Abdominal pain,
8. Sensitivity to Humegon™,
   (Febrile reactions after the administration of Humegon™ have occurred. It is not clear whether or not these were pyrogenic responses or possible allergic reactions. In addition, reports of "flu-like symptoms" including fever, chills, musculoskeletal aches, joint pains, nausea, headache and malaise have been received.)
9. Gastrointestinal symptoms (nausea, vomiting, diarrhea, abdominal cramps, bloating),
10. Pain, rash, swelling and/or irritation at the site of injection,
11. Body rashes,
12. Dizziness, tachycardia, dyspnea, tachypnea.

The following medical events have been reported subsequent to pregnancies resulting from Humegon™ therapy:

1. Ectopic pregnancy
2. Congenital abnormalities
   From a large clinical trial comprising of 6,096 cycles (2,166 women) with 594 babies examined, the incidence of congenital malformation with Humegon™/hCG therapy was 1.7%. Of the major malformations (nine babies, 1.5%) there were two cases each of anencephaly and harelip, and one each of cleft palate, polydactyly, umbilical hernia, congenital dislocation of hip and equinovarus. There was one case (0.2%) of minor malformation (anomaly of auricle). The congenital anomaly rate after Humegon™ therapy is then no higher than that expected for the general population.

There have been infrequent reports of ovarian neoplasms, both benign and malignant, in women who have undergone multiple drug regimens for ovulation induction; however, a causal relationship has not been established.

Men:

Gynecomastia, breast pain, mastitis, nausea, abnormal lipoprotein fraction, abnormal SGOT and SGPT may occur occasionally during Humegon™- hCG therapy.

DRUG ABUSE AND DEPENDENCE

There have been no reports of abuse or dependence with Humegon™.

OVERDOSAGE

Aside from possible ovarian hyperstimulation (see WARNINGS), little is known concerning the consequences of acute overdosage with Humegon™.

DOSAGE AND ADMINISTRATION

Women:

1. Dosage:

The dose of Humegon™ to produce maturation of the follicle must be individualized for each patient. It is recommended that the initial dose to any patient should be 75 IU of FSH/LH per day, **ADMINISTERED INTRAMUSCULARLY,** for seven to twelve days followed by hCG, 5,000 U to 10,000 U, one day after the last dose of Humegon™. Administration of Humegon™ should not exceed 12 days in a single course of therapy. The patient should be treated until indices of estrogenic activity, as indicated under "Precautions" above, are equivalent to or greater than those of the normal individual. If serum or urinary estradiol determinations or ultrasonographic visualizations are available, they may be useful as a guide to therapy. If the ovaries are abnormally enlarged on the last day of Humegon™ therapy, hCG should not be administered in this course of therapy; this will reduce the chances of development of the Ovarian Hyperstimulation Syndrome. If there is evidence of ovulation but no pregnancy, repeat this dosage regime for at least two more courses before increasing the dose of Humegon™ to 150 IU of FSH/LH per day for seven to twelve days. As before, this dose should be followed by 5,000 U to 10,000 U of hCG one day after the last dose of Humegon™. A Humegon™ dose of 150 IU of FSH/LH per day has proven to be the most effective dose especially for *in vitro* fertilization. If evidence of ovulation is present, but pregnancy does not ensue, repeat the same dose for two more courses. Doses larger than this are not routinely recommended.

During treatment with both Humegon™ and hCG and during a two-week post-treatment period, patients should be examined at least every other day for signs of excessive ovarian stimulation. It is recommended that Humegon™ administration be stopped if the ovaries become abnormally enlarged or abdominal pain occurs. Most of the Ovarian Hyperstimulation Syndrome occurs after treatment has been discontinued and reaches its maximum at about seven to ten days post-ovulation. Patients should be followed for at least two weeks after hCG administration.

For ovulation induction, the couple should be encouraged to have intercourse daily, beginning on the day prior to the administration of hCG until ovulation becomes apparent from the indices employed for the determination of progestational activity. Care should be taken to insure insemination. In the light of the foregoing indices and parameters mentioned, it should become obvious that, unless a physician is willing to devote considerable time to these patients and be familiar with and conduct the necessary laboratory studies, he/she should not use Humegon™.

2. Administration:

Dissolve the contents of one vial of Humegon™ in one to two mL of sterile saline and **ADMINISTER INTRAMUSCULARLY** immediately. Any unused reconstituted material should be discarded. Parenteral drug products should be inspected visually for particulate matter and discoloration prior to administration, whenever solution and container permit.

Men:

1. Dosage:

Prior to concomitant therapy with Humegon™ and hCG, pretreatment with hCG alone (5,000 U three times a week) is required. Treatment should continue for a period sufficient to achieve serum testosterone levels within the normal range and masculinization as judged by the appearance of secondary sex characteristics. Such pretreatment may require four to six months, then the recommended dose of Humegon™ is 75 IU FSH/LH **ADMINISTERED INTRAMUSCULARLY, three times** a week and the recommended dose of hCG is 2,000 U **twice** a week. Therapy should be carried on for a minimum of four more months to insure detecting spermatozoa in the ejaculate, as it takes 74 ± 4 days in the human male for germ cells to reach the spermatozoa stage.

If the patient has not responded with evidence of increased spermatogenesis at the end of four months of therapy, treatment may continue with 75 IU FSH/LH **three times** a week, or the dose can be increased to 150 IU FSH/LH **three times** a week, with the hCG dose unchanged.

2. Administration:

Dissolve the contents of one vial of Humegon™ in one to two mL of sterile saline and **ADMINISTER INTRAMUSCULARLY** immediately. Any unused reconstituted material should be discarded. Parenteral drug products should be inspected visually for particulate matter and discoloration prior to administration, whenever solution and container permit.

HOW SUPPLIED

Humegon™ is supplied in sterile lyophilized form as a white to off-white powder in vials containing 75 IU or 150 IU FSH/LH activity. The following package combinations are available:

— 1 vial 75 IU Humegon™ and 1 vial 2 mL Sodium Chloride Injection, USP.
NDC 0052-0300-17
— 5 vials 75 IU Humegon™ and 5 vials 2 mL Sodium Chloride Injection, USP.
NDC 0052-0300-22
— 1 vial 150 IU Humegon™ and 1 vial 2 mL Sodium Chloride Injection, USP.
NDC 0052-0304-17

By biological assay, one IU of LH for the Second International Reference Preparation (2nd-IRP) for hMG is biologically equivalent to approximately 1/2 U of hCG.

Lyophilized powder may be stored refrigerated or at room temperature 2°–30°C (35°–86°F). Protect from light. Use immediately after reconstitution. Discard unused material.

CLINICAL STUDIES

Women:

The Induction of Ovulation

Results of clinical experience and effectiveness from the administration of Humegon™ to 2,682 patients in 7,204 courses of therapy are summarized below:

Patients Ovulating	73.2%†
Clinical Pregnancies	26.2%
Patients Aborting	22%*
Multiple Pregnancies	19.5%

† Data reported for 2,409 out of 2,682 patients
* Data reported for 678 out of 704 clinical pregnancies

IVF, GIFT, ZIFT

Results of clinical experience and effectiveness from the administration of Humegon™ in 1,081 cycles of therapy are summarized below:

% Cycles with Oocyte Retrieval	85†
% Cycles with Transfers	65.6*
# Clinical Pregnancies	182
% Clinical Pregnancy/Cycle	16.8
% Clincial Pregnancy/Retrieval	19.8
% Clinical Pregnancy/Transfer	25.6
% Abortion	32.7§

† Data reported for 773 cycles
* Data reported for 791 cycles
§ Data reported for 174 out of 182 clinical pregnancies

Men:

Clinical results of treatment of men with hypogonadotropic hypogonadism and idiopathic infertility were summarized from the medical literature. Efficacy was evaluated in 246 patients, 22 with hypogonadotropic hypogonadism and 224

Continued on next page

Humegon—Cont.

with idiopathic infertility. Treatment generally consisted of Humegon™, with or without concomitant administration of hCG 500–2,500 IU, two or three times per week for up to 48 months. Sperm count improved in 16 of 22 evaluable (73%) hypogonadotropic hypogonadism patients and in 86 of 224 evaluable (38%) idopathic infertility patients. Overall, seven of 14 (50%) evaluable hypogonadotropic hypogonadism patients and 26 of 224 (12%) idiopathic infertility patients impregnated their partners following Humegon™ treatment.

Caution: Federal law prohibits dispensing without prescription.

Organon Inc.
West Orange, New Jersey 07052
5310119   Iss. 8/95
Shown in Product Identification Guide, page 327

MIRCETTE™   Rx
(desogestrel/ethinyl estradiol and ethinyl estradiol) Tablets

Patients should be counseled that this product does not protect against HIV infection (AIDS) and other sexually transmitted diseases.

DESCRIPTION

Mircette™ (desogestrel/ethinyl estradiol and ethinyl estradiol) Tablets provide an oral contraceptive regimen of 21 white round tablets each containing 0.15 mg desogestrel (13-ethyl-11- methylene-18,19-dinor-17 alpha-pregn- 4-en-20-yn-17-ol), 0.02 mg ethinyl estradiol (19-nor-17 alpha-pregna-1,3,5 (10)-trien-20-yne-3,17-diol), and inactive ingredients which include vitamin E, corn starch, povidone, stearic acid, colloidal silicon dioxide, lactose, hydroxypropyl methylcellulose, polyethylene glycol, titanium dioxide and talc, followed by 2 green round tablets with the following inactive ingredients: lactose, corn starch, magnesium stearate, FD&C Blue No. 2 aluminum lake, yellow ferric oxide, hydroxypropyl methylcellulose, polyethylene glycol, titanium dioxide and talc. Mircette™ also contains 5 yellow round tablets containing 0.01 mg ethinyl estradiol (19-nor-17 alpha-pregna-1,3,5 (10)-trien-20-yne-3,17-diol) and inactive ingredients which include vitamin E, corn starch, povidone, stearic acid, colloidal silicon dioxide, lactose, hydroxypropyl methylcellulose, polyethylene glycol, titanium dioxide, talc, and yellow ferric oxide. The molecular weight for desogestrel and ethinyl estradiol are 310.48 and 296.41 respectively. The structural formulas are as follows:

DESOGESTREL

$C_{22}H_{30}O$

ETHINYL ESTRADIOL

$C_{20}H_{24}O_2$

CLINICAL PHARMACOLOGY

Combination oral contraceptives act by suppression of gonadotropins. Although the primary mechanism of this action is inhibition of ovulation, other alterations include changes in the cervical mucus (which increase the difficulty of sperm entry into the uterus) and the endometrium (which reduce the likelihood of implantation).
Receptor binding studies, as well as studies in animals, have shown that etonogestrel, the biologically active metabolite of desogestrel, combines high progestational activity with minimal intrinsic androgenicity (91,92).

Pharmacokinetics

Absorption
Desogestrel is rapidly and almost completely absorbed and converted into etonogestrel, its biologically active metabolite. Following oral administration, the relative bioavailability of desogestrel compared to a solution, as measured by serum levels of etonogestrel, is approximately 100%. Mircette™ (desogestrel/ethinyl estradiol and ethinyl estradiol) Tablets provide two different regimens of ethinyl estradiol;

TABLE I: MEAN (SD) PHARMACOKINETIC PARAMETERS OF Mircette™ OVER A 28-DAY DOSING PERIOD IN THE THIRD CYCLE (n=17).

Etonogestrel

Day	Dose mg	C_{max} pg/mL	T_{max} h	$t_{1/2}$ h	AUC_{0-24} pg/mL•hr	CL/F L/h
1	0.15	2503.6 (987.6)	2.4 (1.0)	29.8 (16.3)	17832 (5674)	5.4 (2.5)
21	0.15	4091.2 (1186.2)	1.6 (0.7)	27.8 (7.2)	39391 (12134)	4.4 (1.4)

Desogestrel

Ethinyl Estradiol

Day	Dose mg	C_{max} pg/mL	T_{max} h	$t_{1/2}$ h	AUC_{0-24} pg/mL•hr	CL/F L/h
1	0.02	51.9 (15.4)	2.9 (1.2)	16.5 (4.8)	566 (173)[a]	25.7 (9.1)
21	0.02	62.2 (25.9)	2.0 (0.8)	23.9 (25.5)	597 (127)[a]	35.1 (8.2)
24	0.01	24.6 (10.8)	2.4 (1.0)	18.8 (10.3)	246 (65)	43.6 (12.2)
28	0.01	35.3 (27.5)	2.1 (1.3)	18.9 (8.3)	312 (62)	33.2 (6.6)

[a]n=16
C_{max}—measured peak concentration
T_{max}—observed time of peak concentration
$t_{1/2}$—elimination half-life, calculated by $0.693/K_{elim}$
AUC_{0-24}—area under the concentration-time curve calculated by the linear trapezoidal rule (Time 0 to 24 hours)
CL/F—apparent clearance

0.02 mg in the combination tablet [white] as well as 0.01 mg in the yellow tablet. Ethinyl estradiol is rapidly and almost completely absorbed. After a single dose of Mircette™ combination tablet [white], the relative bioavailability of ethinyl estradiol is approximately 93% while the relative bioavailability of the 0.01 mg tablet [yellow] is 99%. The effect of food on the bioavailability of Mircette™ tablets following oral administration has not been evaluated.
The pharmacokinetics of etonogestrel and ethinyl estradiol following multiple dose administration of Mircette™ tablets was determined during the third cycle in 17 subjects. Plasma concentrations of etonogestrel and ethinyl estradiol reached steady-state by Day 21. The $AUC_{(0-24)}$ for etonogestrel at steady-state on Day 21 was approximately 2.2 times higher than $AUC_{(0-24)}$ on Day 1 of the third cycle. The pharmacokinetic parameters of etonogestrel and ethinyl estradiol during the third cycle following multiple dose administration of Mircette™ tablets are summarized in Table 1.
[See table above]

Distribution
Etonogestrel, the active metabolite of desogestrel was found to be 99% protein bound, primarily to sex hormone-binding globulin (SHBG). Ethinyl estradiol is approximately 98.3% bound, mainly to plasma albumin. Ethinyl estradiol does not bind to SHBG, but induces SHBG synthesis. Desogestrel, in combination with ethinyl estradiol, does not counteract the estrogen-induced increase in SHBG, resulting in lower serum levels of free testosterone (96–99).

Metabolism
Desogestrel: Desogestrel is rapidly and completely metabolized by hydroxylation in the intestinal mucosa and on first pass through the liver to etonogestrel. Other metabolites (i.e., 3α-OH-desogestrel, 3β-OH-desogestrel, and 3α-OH-5α-H-desogestrel) with no pharmacologic actions also have been identified and these metabolites may undergo glucuronide and sulfate conjugation.
Ethinyl estradiol: Ethinyl estradiol is subject to a significant degree of presystemic conjugation (phase II metabolism). Ethinyl estradiol escaping gut wall conjugation undergoes phase I metabolism and hepatic conjugation (phase II metabolism). Major phase I metabolites are 2-OH-ethinyl estradiol and 2-methoxy-ethinyl estradiol. Sulfate and glucuronide conjugates of both ethinyl estradiol and phase I metabolites, which are excreted in bile, can undergo enterohepatic circulation.

Excretion
Etonogestrel and ethinyl estradiol are excreted in urine, bile and feces. At steady state, on Day 21, the elimination half-life of etonogestrel is 27.8±7.2 hours and the elimination half-life of ethinyl estradiol for the combination tablet is 23.9±25.5 hours. For the 0.01 mg ethinyl estradiol tablet [yellow], the elimination half-life at steady state, Day 28, is 18.9±8.3 hours.

Special Populations
Race
There is no information to determine the effect of race on the pharmacokinetics of Mircette™ tablets.
Hepatic Insufficiency
No formal studies were conducted to evaluate the effect of hepatic disease on the disposition of Mircette™.
Renal Insufficiency
No formal studies were conducted to evaluate the effect of renal disease on the disposition of Mircette™.
Drug-Drug Interactions
Interactions between desogestrel/ethinyl estradiol and other drugs have been reported in the literature. No formal drug-drug interaction studies were conducted (see PRECAUTIONS section).

INDICATIONS AND USAGE

Mircette™ (desogestrel/ethinyl estradiol and ethinyl estradiol) Tablets are indicated for the prevention of pregnancy in women who elect to use this product as a method of contraception.
Oral contraceptives are highly effective. Table II lists the typical accidental pregnancy rates for users of combination oral contraceptives and other methods of contraception. The efficacy of these contraceptive methods, except sterilization, depends upon the reliability with which they are used. Correct and consistent use of these methods can result in lower failure rates.
[See table II at top of next page]

CONTRAINDICATIONS

Oral contraceptives should not be used in women who currently have the following conditions:
• Thrombophlebitis or thromboembolic disorders
• A past history of deep vein thrombophlebitis or thromboembolic disorders
• Cerebral vascular or coronary artery disease
• Known or suspected carcinoma of the breast
• Carcinoma of the endometrium or other known or suspected estrogen-dependent neoplasia
• Undiagnosed abnormal genital bleeding
• Cholestatic jaundice of pregnancy or jaundice with prior pill use
• Hepatic adenomas of carcinomas
• Known or suspected pregnancy

WARNINGS

> **Cigarette smoking increases the risk of serious cardiovascular side effects from oral contraceptive use. This risk increases with age and with heavy smoking (15 or more cigarettes per day) and is quite marked in women over 35 years of age. Women who use oral contraceptives should be strongly advised not to smoke.**

The use of oral contraceptives is associated with increased risks of several serious conditions including myocardial infarction, thromboembolism, stroke, hepatic neoplasia, and gallbladder disease, although the risk of serious morbidity or mortality is very small in healthy women without underlying risk factors. The risk of morbidity and mortality increases significantly in the presence of other underlying risk factors such as hypertension, hyperlipidemias, obesity and diabetes.
Practitioners prescribing oral contraceptives should be familiar with the following information relating to these risks. The information contained in this package insert is principally based on studies carried out in patients who used oral contraceptives with formulations of higher doses of estrogens and progestogens than those in common use today. The effect of long-term use of the oral contraceptives with formulations of lower doses of both estrogens and progestogens remains to be determined.
Throughout this labeling, epidemiological studies reported are of two types: retrospective or case control studies and prospective or cohort studies. Case control studies provide a measure of the relative risk of a disease, namely, a *ratio* of the incidence of a disease among oral contraceptive users to that among non-users. The relative risk does not provide information on the actual clinical occurrence of a disease. Cohort studies provide a measure of attributable risk, which is the *difference* in the incidence of disease between oral contraceptive users and non-users. The attributable risk does provide information about the actual occurrence of a disease

TABLE II: Percentage of women experiencing an unintended pregnancy during the first year of typical use and the first year of perfect use of contraception and the percentage continuing use at the end of the first year, United States

Method (1)	% of Women Experiencing an Unintended Pregnancy within the First Year of Use		% of Women Continuing Use at One Year[3] (4)
	Typical Use[1] (2)	Perfect Use[2] (3)	
Chance[4]	85	85	
Spermicides[5]	26	6	40
Periodic abstinence	25		63
Calendar		9	
Ovulation Method		3	
Sympto-Thermal[6]		2	
Post-Ovulation		1	
Withdrawal	19	4	
Cap[7]			
Parous Women	40	26	42
Nulliparous Women	20	9	56
Sponge			
Parous Women	40	20	42
Nulliparous Women	20	9	56
Diaphragm[7]	20	6	56
Condom[8]			
Female (Reality)	21	5	56
Male	14	3	61
Pill	5		71
Progestin Only		0.5	
Combined		0.1	
IUD			
Progesterone T	2.0	1.5	81
Copper T 380A	0.8	0.6	78
LNg 20	0.1	0.1	81
Depo-Provera	0.3	0.3	70
Norplant and Norplant-2	0.05	0.05	88
Female sterilization	0.5	0.5	100
Male sterilization	0.15	0.10	100

Adapted from Hatcher et al., 1998, Ref#1.

[1] Among *typical* couples who initiate use of a method (not necessarily for the first time), the percentage who experience an accidental pregnancy during the first year if they do not stop use for any other reason.

[2] Among couples who initiate use of a method (not necessarily for the first time) and who use it *perfectly* (both consistently and correctly), the percentage who experience an accidental pregnancy during the first year if they do not stop use for any other reason.

[3] Among couples attempting to avoid pregnancy, the percentage who continue to use a method for one year.

[4] The percents becoming pregnant in columns (2) and (3) are based on data from populations where contraception is not used and from women who cease using contraception in order to become pregnant. Among such populations, about 89% become pregnant within one year. This estimate was lowered slightly (to 85%) to represent the percent who would become pregnant within one year among women now relying on reversible methods of contraception if they abandoned contraception altogether.

[5] Foams, creams, gels, vaginal suppositories, and vaginal film.

[6] Cervical mucus (ovulation) method supplemented by calendar in the pre-ovulatory and basal body temperature in the post-ovulatory phases.

[7] With spermicidal cream or jelly.

[8] Without spermicides.

in the population (Adapted from refs. 2 and 3 with the author's permission). For further information, the reader is referred to a text on epidemiological methods.

1. THROMBOEMBOLIC DISORDERS AND OTHER VASCULAR PROBLEMS

a. Myocardial infarction

An increased risk of myocardial infarction has been attributed to oral contraceptive use. This risk is primarily in smokers or women with other underlying risk factors for coronary artery disease such as hypertension, hypercholesterolemia, morbid obesity, and diabetes. The relative risk of heart attack for current oral contraceptive users has been estimated to be two to six (4–10). The risk is very low in women under the age of 30.

Smoking in combination with oral contraceptive use has been shown to contribute substantially to the incidence of myocardial infarction in women in their mid-thirties or older with smoking accounting for the majority of excess cases (11). Mortality rates associated with circulatory disease have been shown to increase substantially in smokers, over the age of 35 and non-smokers over the age of 40 (Table III) among women who use oral contraceptives.

[See table III in next column]

Oral contraceptives may compound the effects of well-known risk factors, such as hypertension, diabetes, hyperlipidemias, age and obesity (13). In particular, some progestogens are known to decrease HDL cholesterol and cause glucose intolerance, while estrogens may create a state of hyperinsulinism (14–18). Oral contraceptives have been shown to increase blood pressure among users (see section 9 in WARNINGS). Similar effects on risk factors have been associated with an increased risk of heart disease. Oral contraceptives must be used with caution in women with cardiovascular disease risk factors.

b. Thromboembolism

An increased risk of thromboembolic and thrombotic disease associated with the use of oral contraceptives

TABLE III: CIRCULATORY DISEASE MORTALITY RATES PER 100,000 WOMAN-YEARS BY AGE, SMOKING STATUS AND ORAL CONTRACEPTIVE USE

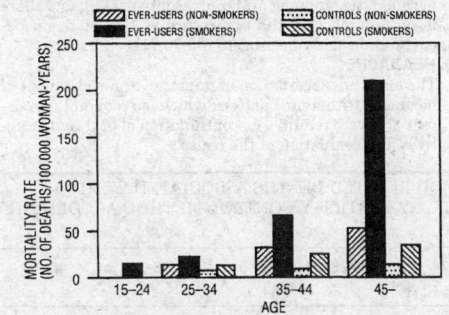

(Adapted from P.M. Layde and V. Beral, ref. #12.)

is well established. Case control studies have found the relative risk of users compared to non-users to be 3 for the first episode of superficial venous thrombosis, 4 to 11 for deep vein thrombosis or pulmonary embolism, and 1.5 to 6 for women with predisposing conditions for venous thromboembolic disease (2,3,19–24). Cohort studies have shown the relative risk to be somewhat lower, about 3 for new cases and about 4.5 for new cases requiring hospitalization (25). The risk of thromboembolic disease associated with oral contraceptives is not related to length of use and disappears after pill use is stopped (2).

A two- to four-fold increase in relative risk of postoperative thromboembolic complications has been reported with the use of oral contraceptives (9,26). The relative risk of venous thrombosis in women who have predisposing conditions is twice that of women without such medical conditions (9,26). If feasible, oral contra-

ceptives should be discontinued at least four weeks prior to and for two weeks after elective surgery of a type associated with an increase in risk of thromboembolism and during and following prolonged immobilization. Since the immediate postpartum period is also associated with an increased risk of thromboembolism, oral contraceptives should be started no earlier than four weeks after delivery in women who elect not to breast feed.

c. Cerebrovascular diseases

Oral contraceptives have been shown to increase both the relative and attributable risks of cerebrovascular events (thrombotic and hemorrhagic strokes), although, in general, the risk is greatest among older (>35 years), hypertensive women who also smoke. Hypertension was found to be a risk factor for both users and non-users, for both types of strokes, while smoking interacted to increase the risk for hemorrhagic strokes (27–29).

In a large study, the relative risk of thrombotic strokes has been shown to range from 3 for normotensive users to 14 for users with severe hypertension (30). The relative risk of hemorrhagic stroke is reported to be 1.2 for non-smokers who used oral contraceptives, 2.6 for smokers who did not use oral contraceptives, 7.6 for smokers who used oral contraceptives, 1.8 for normotensive users and 25.7 for users with severe hypertension (30). The attributable risk is also greater in older women (3).

d. Dose-related risk of vascular disease from oral contraceptives

A positive association has been observed between the amount of estrogen and progestogen in oral contraceptives and the risk of vascular disease (31–33). A decline in serum high-density lipoproteins (HDL) has been reported with many progestational agents (14–16). A decline in serum high-density lipoproteins has been associated with an increased incidence of ischemic heart disease. Because estrogens increase HDL cholesterol, the net effect of an oral contraceptive depends on a balance achieved between doses of estrogen and progestogen and the nature and absolute amount of progestogens used in the contraceptives. The amount of both hormones should be considered in the choice of an oral contraceptive.

Minimizing exposure to estrogen and progestogen is in keeping with good principles of therapeutics. For any particular estrogen/progestogen combination, the dosage regimen prescribed should be one which contains the least amount of estrogen and progestogen that is compatible with a low failure rate and the needs of the individual patient. New acceptors of oral contraceptive agents should be started on preparations containing the lowest estrogen content which produces satisfactory results in the individual.

e. Persistence of risk of vascular disease

There are two studies which have shown persistence of risk of vascular disease for ever-users of oral contraceptives. In a study in the United States, the risk for developing myocardial infarction after discontinuing oral contraceptives persists for at least 9 years for women 40–49 years old who had used oral contraceptives for five or more years, but this increased risk was not demonstrated in other age groups (8). In another study in Great Britain, the risk of developing cerebrovascular disease persisted for at least 6 years after discontinuation of oral contraceptives, although excess risk was very small (34). However, both studies were performed with oral contraceptive formulations containing 50 micrograms or more of estrogen.

2. ESTIMATES OF MORTALITY FROM CONTRACEPTIVE USE

One study gathered data from a variety of sources which have estimated the mortality rate associated with different methods of contraception at different ages (Table IV). These estimates include the combined risk of death associated with contraceptive methods plus the risk attributable to pregnancy in the event of method failure. Each method of contraception has its specific benefits and risks. The study concluded that with the exception of oral contraceptive users 35 and older who smoke and 40 and older who do not smoke, mortality associated with all methods of birth control is low and below that associated with childbirth.

The observation of a possible increase in risk of mortality with age for oral contraceptive users is based on data gathered in the 1970's—but not reported until 1983 (35). However, current clinical practice involves the use of lower estrogen formulations combined with careful consideration of risk factors.

Because of these changes in practice and, also, because of some limited new data which suggest that the risk of cardiovascular disease with the use of oral contraceptives may now be less than previously observed

Continued on next page

Mircette—Cont.

(100,101), the Fertility and Maternal Health Drugs Advisory Committee was asked to review the topic in 1989. The Committee concluded that although cardiovascular disease risks may be increased with oral contraceptive use after age 40 in healthy non-smoking women (even with the newer low-dose formulations), there are also greater potential health risks associated with pregnancy in older women and with the alternative surgical and medical procedures which may be necessary if such women do not have access to effective and acceptable means of contraception.

Therefore, the Committee recommended that the benefits of low-dose oral contraceptive use by healthy non-smoking women over 40 may outweigh the possible risks. Of course, older women, as all women who take oral contraceptives, should take the lowest possible dose formulation that is effective

[See table IV below]

3. CARCINOMA OF THE REPRODUCTIVE ORGANS AND BREASTS

Numerous epidemiological studies have been performed on the incidence of breast, endometrial, ovarian and cervical cancer in women using oral contraceptives. While there are conflicting reports, most studies suggest that the use of oral contraceptives is not associated with an overall increase in the risk of developing breast cancer. Some studies have reported an increased relative risk of developing breast cancer, particularly at a younger age. This increased relative risk appears to be related to duration of use (36–43, 79–89).

Some studies suggest that oral contraceptive use has been associated with an increase in the risk of cervical intra-epithelial neoplasia in some populations of women (45–48). However, there continues to be controversy about the extent to which such findings may be due to differences in sexual behavior and other factors.

4. HEPATIC NEOPLASIA

Benign hepatic adenomas are associated with oral contraceptive use, although the incidence of benign tumors is rare in the United States. Indirect calculations have estimated the attributable risk to be in the range of 3.3 cases/100,000 for users, a risk that increases after four or more years of use especially with oral contraceptives of higher dose (49). Rupture of rare, benign, hepatic adenomas may cause death through intra-abdominal hemorrhage (50,51).

Studies from Britain have shown an increased risk of developing hepatocellular carcinoma (52–54) in long-term (>8 years) oral contraceptive users. However, these cancers are extremely rare in the U.S. and the attributable risk (the excess incidence) of liver cancers in oral contraceptive users approaches less than one per million users.

5. OCULAR LESIONS

There have been clinical case reports of retinal thrombosis associated with the use of oral contraceptives. Oral contraceptives should be discontinued if there is unexplained partial or complete loss of vision; onset of proptosis or diplopia; papilledema; or retinal vascular lesions. Appropriate diagnostic and therapeutic measures should be undertaken immediately.

6. ORAL CONTRACEPTIVE USE BEFORE OR DURING EARLY PREGNANCY

Extensive epidemiological studies have revealed no increased risk of birth defects in women who have used oral contraceptives prior to pregnancy (55–57). Studies also do not suggest a teratogenic effect, particularly in so far as cardiac anomalies and limb reduction defects are concerned (55,56,58,59), when oral contraceptives are taken inadvertently during early pregnancy.

The administration of oral contraceptives to induce withdrawal bleeding should not be used as a test for pregnancy. Oral contraceptives should not be used during pregnancy to treat threatened or habitual abortion. It is recommended that for any patient who has missed two consecutive periods, pregnancy should be ruled out before continuing oral contraceptive use. If the patient has not adhered to the prescribed schedule, the possibility of pregnancy should be considered at the first missed period. Oral contraceptive use should be discontinued until pregnancy is ruled out.

7. GALLBLADDER DISEASE

Earlier studies have reported an increased lifetime relative risk of gallbladder surgery in users of oral contraceptives and estrogens (60,61). More recent studies, however, have shown that the relative risk of developing gallbladder disease among oral contraceptive users may be minimal (62–64). The recent findings of minimal risk may be related to the use of oral contraceptive formulations containing lower hormonal doses of estrogens and progestogens.

8. CARBOHYDRATE AND LIPID METABOLIC EFFECTS

Oral contraceptives have been shown to cause a decrease in glucose tolerance in a significant percentage of users (17). Oral contraceptives containing greater than 75 micrograms of estrogens cause hyperinsulinism, while lower doses of estrogen cause less glucose intolerance (65). Progestogens increase insulin secretion and create insulin resistance, this effect varying with different progestational agents (17,66). However, in the non-diabetic woman, oral contraceptives appear to have no effect on fasting blood glucose (67). Because of these demonstrated effects, prediabetic and diabetic women should be carefully monitored while taking oral contraceptives. A small proportion of women will have persistent hypertriglyceridemia while on the pill. As discussed earlier (see WARNINGS 1.a. and 1.d.), changes in serum triglycerides and lipoprotein levels have been reported in oral contraceptive users.

9. ELEVATED BLOOD PRESSURE

An increase in blood pressure has been reported in women taking oral contraceptives (68) and this increase is more likely in older oral contraceptive users (69) and with continued use (61). Data from the Royal College of General Practitioners (12) and subsequent randomized trials have shown that the incidence of hypertension increases with increasing quantities of progestogens. Women with a history of hypertension or hypertension-related diseases, or renal disease (70) should be encouraged to use another method of contraception. If women elect to use oral contraceptives, they should be monitored closely and if significant elevation of blood pressure occurs, oral contraceptives should be discontinued. For most women, elevated blood pressure will return to normal after stopping oral contraceptives (69), and there is no difference in the occurrence of hypertension between ever- and never-users (68,70,71).

10. HEADACHE

The onset or exacerbation of migraine or development of headache with a new pattern which is recurrent, persistent or severe requires discontinuation of oral contraceptives and evaluation of the cause.

11. BLEEDING IRREGULARITIES

Breakthrough bleeding and spotting are sometimes encountered in patients on oral contraceptives, especially during the first three months of use. Non-hormonal causes should be considered and adequate diagnostic measures taken to rule out malignancy or pregnancy in the event of breakthrough bleeding, as in the case of any abnormal vaginal bleeding. If pathology has been excluded, time or a change to another formulation may solve the problem. In the event of amenorrhea, pregnancy should be ruled out.

Some women may encounter post-pill amenorrhea or oligomenorrhea, especially when such a condition was pre-existent.

12. ECTOPIC PREGNANCY

Ectopic as well as intrauterine pregnancy may occur in contraceptive failures.

PRECAUTIONS

1. GENERAL

Patients should be counseled that this product does not protect against HIV infection (AIDS) and other sexually transmitted diseases.

2. PHYSICAL EXAMINATION AND FOLLOW UP

It is good medical practice for all women to have annual history and physical examinations, including women using oral contraceptives. The physical examination, however, may be deferred until after initiation of oral contraceptives if requested by the woman and judged appropriate by the clinician. The physical examination should include special reference to blood pressure, breasts, abdomen and pelvic organs, including cervical cytology, and relevant laboratory tests. In case of undiagnosed, persistent or recurrent abnormal vaginal bleeding, appropriate measures should be conducted to rule out malignancy. Women with a strong family history of breast cancer or who have breast nodules should be monitored with particular care.

3. LIPID DISORDERS

Women who are being treated for hyperlipidemias should be followed closely if they elect to use oral contraceptives. Some progestogens may elevate LDL levels and may render the control of hyperlipidemias more difficult.

4. LIVER FUNCTION

If jaundice develops in any woman receiving such drugs, the medication should be discontinued. Steroid hormones may be poorly metabolized in patients with impaired liver function.

5. FLUID RETENTION

Oral contraceptives may cause some degree of fluid retention. They should be prescribed with caution, and only with careful monitoring, in patients with conditions which might be aggravated by fluid retention.

6. EMOTIONAL DISORDERS

Women with a history of depression should be carefully observed and the drug discontinued if depression recurs to a serious degree.

7. CONTACT LENSES

Contact lens wearers who develop visual changes or changes in lens tolerance should be assessed by an ophthalmologist.

8. DRUG INTERACTIONS

Reduced efficacy and increased incidence of breakthrough bleeding and menstrual irregularities have been associated with concomitant use of rifampin. A similar association, though less marked, has been suggested with barbiturates, phenylbutazone, phenytoin sodium, carbamazepine and possibly with griseofulvin, ampicillin and tetracyclines (72).

9. INTERACTIONS WITH LABORATORY TESTS

Certain endocrine and liver function tests and blood components may be affected by oral contraceptives:

a. Increased prothrombin and factors VII, VIII, IX and X; decreased antithrombin 3; increased norepinephrine-induced platelet aggregability.

b. Increased thyroid binding globulin (TBG) lead to increased circulating total thyroid hormone, as measured by protein-bound iodine (PBI), T4 by column or by radioimmunoassay. Free T3 resin uptake is decreased, reflecting the elevated TBG; free T4 concentration is unaltered.

c. Other binding proteins may be elevated in serum.

d. Sex hormone-binding globulins are increased and result in elevated levels of total circulating sex steroids; however, free or biologically active levels either decrease or remain unchanged.

e. High-density lipoprotein cholesterol (HDL-C) and triglycerides may be increased, while low-density lipoprotein cholesterol (LDL-C) and total cholesterol (Total-C) may be decreased or unchanged.

f. Glucose tolerance may be decreased.

g. Serum folate levels may be depressed by oral contraceptive therapy. This may be of clinical significance if a woman becomes pregnant shortly after discontinuing oral contraceptives.

TABLE IV: ANNUAL NUMBER OF BIRTH-RELATED OR METHOD-RELATED DEATHS ASSOCIATED WITH CONTROL OF FERTILITY PER 100,000 NON-STERILE WOMEN, BY FERTILITY CONTROL METHOD ACCORDING TO AGE

Method of control and outcome	15–19	20–24	25–29	30–34	35–39	40–44
No fertility control methods*	7.0	7.4	9.1	14.8	25.7	28.2
Oral contraceptives non-smoker**	0.3	0.5	0.9	1.9	13.8	31.6
Oral contraceptives smoker**	2.2	3.4	6.6	13.5	51.1	117.2
IUD**	0.8	0.8	1.0	1.0	1.4	1.4
Condom*	1.1	1.6	0.7	0.2	0.3	0.4
Diaphragm/spermicide*	1.9	1.2	1.2	1.3	2.2	2.8
Periodic abstinence*	2.5	1.6	1.6	1.7	2.9	3.6

* Deaths are birth related
** Deaths are method related

Adapted from H.W. Ory, ref. #35.

10. CARCINOGENESIS
See WARNINGS section.

11. PREGNANCY
Pregnancy Category X. See CONTRAINDICATIONS and WARNINGS sections.

12. NURSING MOTHERS
Small amounts of oral contraceptive steroids have been identified in the milk of nursing mothers and few adverse effects on the child have been reported, including jaundice and breast enlargement. In addition, oral contraceptives given in the postpartum period may interfere with lactation by decreasing the quantity and quality of breast milk. If possible, the nursing mother should be advised not to use oral contraceptives but to use other forms of contraception until she has completely weaned her child.

13. PEDIATRIC USE
Safety and efficacy of Mircette™ (desogestrel/ethinyl estradiol and ethinyl estradiol) Tablets have been established in women of reproductive age. Safety and efficacy are expected to be the same for postpubertal adolescents under the age of 16 and for users 16 years and older. Use of this product before menarche is not indicated.

INFORMATION FOR THE PATIENT
See Patient Labeling Printed Below

ADVERSE REACTIONS

An increased risk of the following serious adverse reactions has been associated with the use of oral contraceptives (see WARNINGS section):

- Thrombophlebitis and venous thrombosis with or without embolism
- Arterial thromboembolism
- Pulmonary embolism
- Myocardial infarction
- Cerebral hemorrhage
- Cerebral thrombosis
- Hypertension
- Gallbladder disease
- Hepatic adenomas or benign liver tumors

There is evidence of an association between the following conditions and the use of oral contraceptives:

- Mesenteric thrombosis
- Retinal thrombosis

The following adverse reactions have been reported in patients receiving oral contraceptives and are believed to be drug-related:

- Nausea
- Vomiting
- Gastrointestinal symptoms (such as abdominal cramps and bloating)
- Breakthrough bleeding
- Spotting
- Change in menstrual flow
- Amenorrhea
- Temporary infertility after discontinuation of treatment
- Edema
- Melasma which may persist
- Breast changes: tenderness, enlargement, secretion
- Change in weight (increase or decrease)
- Change in cervical erosion and secretion
- Diminution in lactation when given immediately postpartum
- Cholestatic jaundice
- Migraine
- Rash (allergic)
- Mental depression
- Reduced tolerance to carbohydrates
- Vaginal candidiasis
- Change in corneal curvature (steepening)
- Intolerance to contact lenses

The following adverse reactions have been reported in users of oral contraceptives and the association has been neither confirmed nor refuted:

- Pre-menstrual syndrome
- Cataracts
- Changes in appetite
- Cystitis-like syndrome
- Headache
- Nervousness
- Dizziness
- Hirsutism
- Loss of scalp hair
- Erythema multiforme
- Erythema nodosum
- Hemorrhagic eruption
- Vaginitis
- Porphyria
- Impaired renal function
- Hemolytic uremic syndrome
- Acne
- Changes in libido
- Colitis
- Budd-Chiari Syndrome

OVERDOSAGE

Serious ill effects have not been reported following acute ingestion of large doses of oral contraceptives by young children. Overdosage may cause nausea, and withdrawal bleeding may occur in females.

NON-CONTRACEPTIVE HEALTH BENEFITS
The following non-contraceptive health benefits related to the use of oral contraceptives are supported by epidemiological studies which largely utilized oral contraceptive formulations containing estrogen doses exceeding 0.035 mg of ethinyl estradiol or 0.05 mg of mestranol (73–78).

Effects on menses:

- increased menstrual cycle regularity
- decreased blood loss and decreased incidence of iron deficiency anemia
- decreased incidence of dysmenorrhea

Effects related to inhibition of ovulation:

- decreased incidence of functional ovarian cysts
- decreased incidence of ectopic pregnancies

Effects from long-term use:

- decreased incidence of fibroadenomas and fibrocystic disease of the breast
- decreased incidence of acute pelvic inflammatory disease
- decreased incidence of endometrial cancer
- decreased incidence of ovarian cancer

DOSAGE AND ADMINISTRATION

To achieve maximum contraceptive effectiveness, Mircette™ (desogestrel/ethinyl estradiol and ethinyl estradiol) Tablets must be taken exactly as directed and at intervals not exceeding 24 hours. Mircette™ may be initiated using either a Sunday start or a Day 1 start.

NOTE: Each cycle pack dispenser is preprinted with the days of the week, starting with Sunday, to facilitate a Sunday start regimen. Six different "day label strips" are provided with each cycle pack dispenser in order to accommodate a Day 1 start regimen. In this case, the patient should place the self-adhesive "day label strip" that corresponds to her starting day over the preprinted days.

IMPORTANT: The possibility of ovulation and conception prior to initiation of use of Mircette™ should be considered. The use of Mircette™ for contraception may be initiated 4 weeks postpartum in women who elect not to breast feed. When the tablets are administered during the postpartum period, the increased risk of thromboembolic disease associated with the postpartum period, must be considered. (See CONTRAINDICATIONS and WARNINGS concerning thromboembolic disease. See also PRECAUTIONS for "Nursing Mothers".)

If the patient starts on Mircette™ postpartum, and has not yet had a period, she should be instructed to use another method of contraception until a white tablet has been taken daily for 7 days.

SUNDAY START
When initiating a Sunday start regimen, another method of contraception should be used until after the first 7 consecutive days of administration.

Using a Sunday start, tablets are taken daily without interruption as follows: The first white tablet should be taken on the first Sunday after menstruation begins (if menstruation begins on Sunday, the first white tablet is taken on that day). One white tablet is taken daily for 21 days, followed by 1 green (inert) tablet daily for 2 days and 1 yellow (active) tablet daily for 5 days. for all subsequent cycles, the patient then begins a new 28-tablet regimen on the next day (Sunday) after taking the last yellow tablet. [If switching from a Sunday Start oral contraceptive, the first Mircette™ (desogestrel/ethinyl estradiol and ethinyl estradiol) tablet should be taken on the second Sunday after the last tablet of a 21 day regimen or should be taken on the first Sunday after the last inactive tablet of a 28 day regimen.]

If a patient misses 1 white tablet, she should take the missed tablet as soon as she remembers. If the patient misses 2 consecutive white tablets in Week 1 or Week 2, the patient should take 2 tablets the day she remembers and 2 tablets the next day; thereafter, the patient should resume taking 1 tablet daily until she finishes the cycle pack. The patient should be instructed to use a back-up method of birth control if she has intercourse in the 7 days after missing pills. If the patient misses 2 consecutive white tablets in the third week or misses 3 or more white tablets in a row at any time during the cycle, the patient should keep taking 1 white tablet daily until the next Sunday. On Sunday the patient should throw out the rest of that cycle pack and start a new cycle pack that same day. The patient should be instructed to use a back-up method of birth control if she has intercourse in the 7 days after missing pills.

DAY 1 START
Counting the first day of menstruation as "Day 1", tablets are taken without interruption as follows: One white tablet daily for 21 fays, one green (inert) tablet daily for 2 days followed by 1 yellow (ethinyl estradiol) tablet daily for 5 days. For all subsequent cycles, the patient then begins a new 28-tablet regimen on the next day after taking the last yellow tablet. [If switching directly from another oral contraceptive, the first white tablet should be taken on the first day of menstruation which beings after the last ACTIVE tablet of the previous product.]

If a patient misses 1 white tablet, she should take the missed tablet as soon as she remembers. If the patient misses 2 consecutive white tablets in Week 1 or Week 2, the patient should take 2 tablets the day she remembers and 2 tablets the next day; thereafter, the patient should resume taking 1 tablet daily until she finishes the cycle pack. The patient should be instructed to use a back-up method of birth control if she has intercourse in the 7 days after missing pills. If the patient misses 2 consecutive white tablets in the third week or if the patient misses 3 or more white tablets in a row at any time during the cycle, the patient should throw out the rest of that cycle pack and start a new cycle pack that same day. The patient should be instructed to use a back-up method of birth control if she has intercourse in the 7 days after missing pills.

ALL ORAL CONTRACEPTIVES
Breakthrough bleeding, spotting, and amenorrhea are frequent reasons for patients discontinuing oral contraceptives. In breakthrough bleeding, as in all cases of irregular bleeding from the vagina, non-functional causes should be borne in mind. In undiagnosed persistent or recurrent abnormal bleeding from the vagina, adequate diagnostic measures are indicated to rule out pregnancy or malignancy. If both pregnancy and pathology have been excluded, time or a change to another preparation may solve the problem. Changing to an oral contraceptive with a higher estrogen content, while potentially useful in minimizing menstrual irregularity, should be done only if necessary since this may increase the risk of thromboembolic disease.

Use of oral contraceptives in the event of a missed menstrual period:

1. If the patient has not adhered to the prescribed schedule, the possibility of pregnancy should be considered at the time of the first missed period and oral contraceptive use should be discontinued until pregnancy is ruled out.
2. If the patient has adhered to the prescribed regimen and misses two consecutive periods, pregnancy should be ruled out before continuing oral contraceptive use.

HOW SUPPLIED

Mircette™ (desogestrel/ethinyl estradiol and ethinyl estradiol) Tablets contain 21 round white tablets, 2 round green tablets and 5 round yellow tablets in a blister card within a recyclable plastic dispenser. Each white tablet (debossed with "${}^{T}{}_{4}{}^{R}$" on one side and "Organon" on the other side) contains 0.15 mg desogestrel and 0.02 mg ethinyl estradiol. Each green tablet (debossed with "${}^{K}{}_{2}{}^{H}$" on one side and "Organon" on the other side) contains inert ingredients. Each yellow tablet (debossed with "${}^{K}{}_{2}{}^{S}$" on one side and "Organon" on the other side) contains 0.01 mg ethinyl estradiol.

Boxes of 6 NDC# 0052-0281-06

STORAGE: Store at controlled room temperature 20°–25°C (68°–77°F)

℞ **only**

REFERENCES

1. Hatcher RA, Trussell J, Stewart F et al. Contraceptive Technology: Seventeenth Revised Edition, New York: Irvington Publishers, 1998, in press. **2.** Stadel BV. Oral contraceptives and cardiovascular disease. (Pt. 1). N Engl J Med 1981; 305:612–618. **3.** Stadel BV. Oral contraceptives and cardiovascular disease. (Pt. 2). N Engl J Med 1981; 305: 672–677. **4.** Adam SA, Thorogood M. Oral contraception and myocardial infarction revisited: the effects of new preparations and prescribing patterns. Br J Obstet and Gynecol 1981; 88:838–845. **5.** Mann JI, Inman WH. Oral contraceptives and death from myocardial infarction. Br Med J 1975; 2(5965):245–248. **6.** Mann JI, Vessey MP, Thorogood M, Doll R. Myocardial infarction in young women with special reference to oral contraceptive practice. Br Med J 1975; 2(5956):241–245. **7.** Royal College of General Practitioners' Oral Contraception Study: Further analyses of mortality in oral contraceptive users. Lancet 1981; 1:541–546. **8.** Slone D, Shapiro S, Kaufman DW, Rosenberg L, Miettinen OS, Stolley PD. Risk of myocardial infarction in relation to current and discontinued use of oral contraceptives. N Engl J Med 1981; 305:420–424. **9.** Vessey MP. Female hormones and vascular disease—an epidemiological overview. Br J Fam Plann 1980; 6:1–12. **10.** Russell-Briefel RG, Ezzati TM, Fulwood R, Perlman JA, Murphy RS. Cardiovascular risk status and oral contraceptive use, United States, 1976–80. Prevent Med 1986; 15:352–362. **11.** Goldbaum GM, Kendrick JS, Hogelin GC, Gentry EM. The relative impact of smoking and oral contraceptive use on women in the United States. JAMA 1987; 258:1339–1342. **12.** Layde PM, Beral V. Further analyses of mortality in oral contraceptive users: Royal College General Practitioners' Oral Contraception Study. (Table 5) Lancet 1981; 1:541–546. **13.** Knopp RH. Arteriosclerosis risk: the roles of oral contraceptives and postmenopausal estrogens. J Reprod Med 1986; 31(9) (Supple-

Continued on next page

Mircette—Cont.

ment):913–921. **14.** Krauss RM, Roy S, Mishell DR, Casagrande J, Pike MC. Effects of two low-dose oral contraceptives on serum lipids and lipoproteins: Differential changes in high-density lipoproteins subclasses. Am J Obstet 1983; 145:446–452. **15.** Wahl P, Walden C, Knopp R, Hoover J, Wallace R, Heiss G, Rifkind B. Effect of estrogen/progestin potency on lipid/lipoprotein cholesterol. N Engl J Med 1983; 308:862–867. **16.** Wynn V, Niththyananthan R. The effect of progestin in combined oral contraceptives on serum lipids with special reference to high-density lipoproteins. Am J Obstet Gynecol 1982; 142:766–771. **17.** Wynn V, Godsland I. Effects of oral contraceptives and carbohydrate metabolism. J Reprod Med 1986; 31 (9) (Supplement):892–897. **18.** LaRosa JC. Atherosclerotic risk factors in cardiovascular disease. J Reprod Med 1986; 31 (9) (Supplement): 906–912. **19.** Inman WH, Vessey MP. Investigation of death from pulmonary, coronary, and cerebral thrombosis and embolism in women of child-bearing age. Br Med J 1968; 2 (5599):193–199. **20.** Maguire MG, Tonascia J, Sartwell PE, Stolley PD, Tockman MS. Increased risk of thrombosis due to oral contraceptives: a further report. Am J Epidemiol 1979; 110 (2):188–195. **21.** Pettiti DB, Wingerd J, Pellegrin F, Ramacharan S. Risk of vascular disease in women: smoking, oral contraceptives, noncontraceptive estrogens, and other factors. JAMA 1979; 242:1150–1154. **22.** Vessey MP, Doll R. Investigation of relation between use of oral contraceptives and thromboembolic disease. Br Med J 1968; 2 (5599):199–205. **23.** Vessey MP, Doll R. Investigation of relation between use of oral contraceptives and thromboembolic disease. A further report. Br Med J 1969; 2 (5658):651–657. **24.** Porter JB, Hunter JR, Danielson DA, Jick H, Stergachis A. Oral contraceptives and non-fatal vascular disease—recent experience. Obstet Gynecol 1982; 59 (3): 299–302. **25.** Vessey M, Doll R, Peto R, Johnson B, Wiggins P. A long-term follow-up study of women using different methods of contraception: an interim report. Biosocial Sci 1976; 8:375–427. **26.** Royal College of General Practitioners: Oral contraceptives, venous thrombosis, and varicose veins. J Royal Coll Gen Pract 1978; 28:393–399. **27.** Collaborative Group for the Study of Stroke in Young Women: Oral contraception and increased risk of cerebral ischemia or thrombosis. N Engl J Med 1973; 288:871–878. **28.** Pettiti DB, Wingerd J. Use of oral contraceptives, cigarette smoking, and risk of subarachnoid hemorrhage. Lancet 1978; 2:234–236. **29.** Inman WH. Oral contraceptives and fatal subarachnoid hemorrhage. Br Med J 1979; 2 (6203):1468–70. **30.** Collaborative Group for the Study of Stroke in Young Women: Oral contraceptives and stroke in young women: associated risk factors. JAMA 1975; 231:718–722. **31.** Inman WH, Vessey MP, Westerholm B, Engelund A. Thromboembolic disease and the steroidal content of oral contraceptives. A report to the Committee on Safety of Drugs. Br Med J 1970; 2:203–209. **32.** Meade TW, Greenberg G, Thompson SB. Progestogens and cardiovascular reactions associated with oral contraceptives and a comparison of the safety of 50- and 35-mcg oestrogen preparations. Br Med J 1980; 280 (6224):1157–1161. **33.** Kay CR. Progestogens and arterial disease—evidence from the Royal College of General Practitioners' Study. Am J Obstet Gynecol 1982; 142:762–765. **34.** Royal College of General Practitioners: Incidence of arterial disease among oral contraceptive users. J Royal Coll Gen Pract 1983; 33:75–82. **35.** Ory HW. Mortality associated with fertility and fertility control: 1983. Family Planning Perspectives 1983; 15:50–56. **36.** The Cancer and Steroid Hormone Study of the Centers for Disease Control and the National Institute of Child Health and Human Development: Oral-contraceptive use and the risk of breast cancer. N Engl J Med 1986; 315:405–411. **37.** Pike MC, Henderson BE, Krailo MD, Duke A, Roy S. Breast cancer risk in young women and use of oral contraceptives: possible modifying effect of formulation and age at use. Lancet 1983; 2:926–929. **38.** Paul C, Skegg DG, Spears GFS, Kaldor JM. Oral contraceptives and breast cancer: A national study. Br Med J 1986; 293:723–725. **39.** Miller DR, Rosenberg L, Kaufman DW, Schottenfeld D, Stolley PD, Shapiro S. Breast cancer risk in relation to early oral contraceptive use. Obstet Gynecol 1986; 68:863–868. **40.** Olson H, Olson KL, Moller TR, Ranstam J, Holm P. Oral contraceptive use and breast cancer in young women in Sweden (letter). Lancet 1985; 2:748–749. **41.** McPherson K, Vessey M, Neil A, Doll R, Jones L, Roberts M. Early contraceptive use and breast cancer: Results of another case-control study. Br J Cancer 1987; 56: 653–660. **42.** Huggins GR, Zucker PF. Oral contraceptives and neoplasia: 1987 update. Fertil Steril 1987; 47:733–761. **43.** McPherson K, Drife JO. The pill and breast cancer: why the uncertainty? Br Med J 1986; 293:709–710. **44.** Shapiro S. Oral contraceptives—time to take stock. N Engl J Med 1987; 315:450–451. **45.** Ory H, Naib Z, Conger SB, Hatcher RA, Tyler CW. Contraceptive choice and prevalence of cervical dysplasia and carcinoma in situ. Am J Obstet Gynecol 1976; 124:573–577. **46.** Vessey MP, Lawless M, McPherson K, Yeates D. Neoplasia of the cervix uteri and contraception: a possible adverse effect of the pill. Lancet 1983; 2:930. **47.** Brinton LA, Huggins GR, Lehman HF, Malli K, Savitz DA, Trapido E, Rosenthal J, Hoover R. Long-term use of oral contraceptives and risk of invasive cervical cancer. Int J Cancer 1986; 38:339–344. **48.** WHO Collaborative Study of Neoplasia and Steroid Contraceptives: Invasive cervical cancer and combined oral contraceptives. Br Med J 1985; 209:961–965. **49.** Rooks JB, Ory HW, Ishak KG, Strauss LT, Greenspan JR, Hill AP, Tyler CW. Epidemiology of hepatocellular adenoma: the role of oral contraceptive use. JAMA 1979; 242:644–648. **50.** Bein NN, Goldsmith HS. Recurrent massive hemorrhage from benign hepatic tumors secondary to oral contraceptives. Br J Surg 1977; 64:433–435. **51.** Klatskin G. Hepatic tumors: possible relationship to use of oral contraceptives. Gastroenterology 1977; 73:386–394. **52.** Henderson BE, Preston-Martin S, Edmondson HA, Peters RL, Pike MC. Hepatocellular carcinoma and oral contraceptives. Br J Cancer 1983; 48:437–440. **53.** Neuberger J, Forman D, Doll R, Williams R. Oral contraceptives and hepatocellular carcinoma. Br Med J 1986; 292:1355–1357. **54.** Forman D, Vincent TJ, Doll R. Cancer of the liver and oral contraceptives. Br Med J 1986; 292:1357–1361. **55.** Harlap S, Eldor J. Births following oral contraceptive failures. Obstet Gynecol 1980; 55:447–452. **56.** Savolainen E, Saksela E, Saxen L. Teratogenic hazards of oral contraceptives analyzed in a national malformation register. Am J Obstet Gynecol 1981; 140:521–524. **57.** Janerich DT, Piper JM, Glebatis DM. Oral contraceptives and birth defects. Am J Epidemiol 1980; 112:73–79. **58.** Ferencz C, Matanoski GM, Wilson PD, Rubin JD, Neill CA, Gutberlet R. Maternal hormone therapy and congenital heart disease. Teratology 1980; 21: 225–239. **59.** Rothman KJ, Fyler DC, Goldbatt A, Kreidberg MB. Exogenous hormones and other drug exposures of children with congenital heart disease. Am J Epidemiol 1979; 109:433–439. **60.** Boston Collaborative Drug Surveillance Program: Oral contraceptives and venous thromboembolic disease, surgically confirmed gallbladder disease, and breast tumors. Lancet 1973; 1:1399–1404. **61.** Royal College of General Practitioners: Oral contraceptives and health. New York, Pittman, 1974. **62.** Layde PM, Vessey MP, Yeates D. Risk of gallbladder disease: a cohort study of young women attending family planning clinics. J Epidemiol Community Health 1982; 36:274–278. **63.** Rome Group for the Epidemiology and Prevention of Cholelithiasis (GREPCO): Prevalence of gallstone disease in an Italian adult female population. Am J Epidemiol 1984; 119:796–805. **64.** Strom BL, Tamragouri RT, Morse ML, Lazar EL, West SL, Stolley PD, Jones JK. Oral contraceptives and other risk factors for gallbladder disease. Clin Pharmacol Ther 1986; 39:335–341. **65.** Wynn V, Adams PW, Godsland IF, Melrose J, Niththyananthan R, Oakley NW, Seedj A. Comparison of effects of different combined oral-contraceptive formulations on carbohydrate and lipid metabolism. Lancet 1979; 1:1045–1049. **66.** Wynn V. Effect of progesterone and progestins on carbohydrate metabolism. In Progesterone and Progestin. Edited by Bardin CW, Milgrom E, Mauvis-Jarvis P. New York, Raven Press, 1983 pp. 395–410. **67.** Perlman JA, Roussell-Briefel RG, Ezzati TM, Lieberknecht G. Oral glucose tolerance and the potency of oral contraceptive progestogens. J Chronic Dis 1985; 38:857–864. **68.** Royal College of General Practitioners' Oral Contraception Study: Effect on hypertension and benign breast disease of progestogen component in combined oral contraceptives. Lancet 1977; 1:624. **69.** Fisch IR, Frank J. Oral contraceptives and blood pressure. JAMA 1977; 237:2499–2503. **70.** Laragh AJ. Oral contraceptive induced hypertension—nine years later. Am J Obstet Gynecol 1976; 126:141–147. **71.** Ramcharan S, Peritz E, Pellegrin FA, Williams WT. Incidence of hypertension in the Walnut Creek Contraceptive Drug Study cohort. In Pharmacology of Steroid Contraceptive Drugs. Garattini S, Berendes HW. Eds. New York, Raven Press, 1977 pp. 277–288. (Monographs of the Mario Negri Institute for Pharmacological Research, Milan). **72.** Stockley I. Interactions with oral contraceptives. J Pharm 1976; 216:140–143. **73.** The Cancer and Steroid Hormone Study of the Centers for Disease Control and the National Institute of Child Health and Human Development: Oral contraceptive use and the risk of ovarian cancer. JAMA 1983; 249:1596–1599. **74.** The Cancer and Steroid Hormone Study of the Centers for Disease Control and the National Institute of Child Health and Human Development: Combination oral contraceptive use and the risk of endometrial cancer. JAMA 1987; 257:796–800. **75.** Ory HW. Functional ovarian cysts and oral contraceptives: negative association confirmed surgically. JAMA 1974; 228:68–69. **76.** Ory HW, Cole P, Macmahon B, Hoover R. Oral contraceptives and reduced risk of benign breast disease. N Engl J Med 1976; 294:419–422. **77.** Ory HW. The noncontraceptive health benefits from oral contraceptive use. Fam Plann Perspect 1982; 14:182–184. **78.** Ory HW, Forrest JD, Lincoln R. Making Choices: Evaluating the health risks and benefits of birth control methods. New York, The Alan Guttmacher Institute, 1983; p. 1. **79.** Schlesselman J, Stadel BV, Murray P, Lai S. Breast Cancer in relation to early use of oral contraceptives 1988; 259:1828–1833. **80.** Hennekens CH, Speizer FE, Lipnick RJ, Rosner B, Bain C, Belanger C, Stampfer MJ, Willett W, Peto R. A case-controlled study of oral contraceptive use and breast cancer. JNCI 1984; 72:39–42. **81.** LaVecchia C, Decarli A, Fasoli M, Franceschi S, Gentile A, Negri E, Parazzini F, Tognoni G. Oral contraceptives and cancers of the breast and of the female genital tract. Interim results from a case-control study. Br. J. Cancer 1986; 54:311–317. **82.** Meirik O, Lund E, Adami H, Bergstrom R, Christoffersen T, Bergsjo P. Oral contraceptive use in breast cancer in young women. A Joint National Case-control study in Sweden and Norway. Lancet 1986; 11:650–654. **83.** Kay CR, Hannaford PC. Breast cancer and the pill—A further report from the Royal College of General Practitioners' oral contraception study. Br. J. Cancer 1988; 58:675–680. **84.** Stadel BV, Lai S, Schlesselman JJ, Murray P. Oral contraceptives and premenopausal breast cancer in nulliparous women. Contraception 1988; 38:287–299. **85.** Miller DR, Rosenberg L, Kaufman DW, Stolley P, Warshauer ME, Shapiro S. Breast cancer before age 45 and oral contraceptive use: New Findings. Am. J. Epidemiol 1989; 129:269–280. **86.** The UK National Case-Control Study Group, Oral contraceptive use and breast cancer risk in young women. Lancet 1989; 1:973–982. **87.** Schlesselman JJ. Cancer of the breast and reproductive tract in relation to use of oral contraceptives. Contraception 1989; 40:1–38. **88.** Vessey MP, McPherson K, Villard-Mackintosh L, Yeates D. Oral contraceptives and breast cancer: latest findings in a large cohort study. Br. J. Cancer 1989; 59:613–617. **89.** Jick SS, Walker AM, Stergachis A, Jick H. Oral contraceptives and breast cancer. Br. J. Cancer 1989; 59:618–621. **90.** Godsland, I et al. The effects of different formulations of oral contraceptive agents on lipid and carbohydrate metabolism. N Engl J Med 1990; 323:1375–81. **91.** Kloosterboer, HJ et al. Selectivity in progesterone and androgen receptor binding of progestogens used in oral contraception. Contraception, 1988; 38:325–32. **92.** Van der Vies, J and de Visser, J. Endocrinological studies with desogestrel. Arzneim. Forsch./Drug Res., 1983; 33(l),2:231–6. **93.** Data on file, Organon Inc. **94.** Fotherby, K. oral contraceptives, lipids and cardiovascular diseases. Contraception, 1985; Vol. 31; 4:367–94. **95.** Lawrence, DM et al. Reduced sex hormone binding globulin and derived free testosterone levels in women with severe acne. Clinical Endocrinology, 1981; 15:87–91. **96.** Cullberg, G et al. Effects of a low-dose desogestrel-ethinyl estradiol combination on hirsutism, androgens and sex hormone binding globulin in women with a polycystic ovary syndrome. Acta Obstet Gynecol Scand, 1985; 64:195–202. **97.** Jung-Hoffmann, C and Kuhl, H. Divergent-effects of two low-dose oral contraceptives on sex hormone-binding globulin and free testosterone. AJOG, 1987; 156:199–203. **98.** Hammond, G et al. Serum steroid binding protein concentrations, distribution of progestogens, and bioavailability of testosterone during treatment with contraceptives containing desogestrel or levonorgestrel. Fertil. Steril., 1984; 42:44–51. **99.** Palatsi, R et al. Serum total and unbound testosterone and sex hormone binding globulin (SHBG) in female acne patients treated with two different oral contraceptives. Acta Derm Venereol, 1984; 64:517–23. **100.** Porter JB, Hunter J, Jick H et al. Oral contraceptives and nonfatal vascular disease. Obstet Gynecol 1985; 66:1–4. **101.** Porter JB, Jick H, Walker AM. Mortality among oral contraceptive users. Obstet Gynecol 1987; 7029–32.

PATIENT PACKAGE INSERT
BRIEF SUMMARY

Mircette™ (desogestrel/ethinyl estradiol and ethinyl estradiol) Tablets

This product (like all oral contraceptives) is intended to prevent pregnancy. It does not protect against HIV infection (AIDS) and other sexually transmitted diseases.

Oral contraceptives, also known as "birth control pills" or "the pill", are taken to prevent pregnancy, and when taken correctly, have a failure rate of about 1% per year when used without missing any pills. The typical failure rate of large numbers of pill users is less than 5% per year when women who miss pills are included. For most women, oral contraceptives are also free of serious or unpleasant side effects. However, forgetting to take pills considerably increases the chances of pregnancy.

For the majority of women, oral contraceptives can be taken safely. But there are some women who are at high risk of developing certain serious diseases that can be life-threatening or may cause temporary or permanent disability. The risks associated with taking oral contraceptives increase significantly if you:

- smoke
- have high blood pressure, diabetes, high cholesterol
- have or have had clotting disorders, heart attack, stroke, angina pectoris, cancer of the breast or sex organs, jaundice or malignant or benign liver tumors.

Although cardiovascular disease risks may be increased with oral contraceptive use after age 40 in healthy, nonsmoking women (even with the newer low-dose formulations), there are also greater potential health risks associated with pregnancy in older women.

Cigarette smoking increases the risk of serious cardiovascular side effects from oral contraceptive use.

This risk increases with age and with heavy smoking (15 or more cigarettes per day) and is quite marked in women over 35 years of age. Women who use oral contraceptives are strongly advised not to smoke.

You should not take the pill if you suspect you are pregnant or have unexplained vaginal bleeding. Most side effects of the pill are not serious. The most common such effects are nausea, vomiting, bleeding between menstrual periods, weight gain, breast tenderness, headache, and difficulty wearing contact lenses. These side effects, especially nausea and vomiting, may subside within the first three months of use:

The serious side effects of the pill occur very infrequently, especially if you are in good health and are young. However, you should know that the following medical conditions have been associated with or made worse by the pill:

1. Blood clots in the legs (thrombophlebitis) or lungs (pulmonary embolism), stoppage or rupture of a blood vessel in the brain (stroke), blockage of blood vessels in the heart (heart attack or angina pectoris) or other organs of the body. As mentioned above, smoking increases the risk of heart attacks and strokes, and subsequent serious medical consequences.
2. Liver tumors, which may rupture and cause severe bleeding. A possible but not definite association has been found with the pill and liver cancer. However, liver cancers are extremely rare. The chance of developing liver cancer from using the pill is thus even rarer.
3. High blood pressure, although blood pressure usually returns to normal when the pill is stopped.

The symptoms associated with these serious side effects are discussed in the detailed leaflet given to you with your supply of pills. Notify your doctor or health care provider if you notice any unusual physical disturbances while taking the pill. In addition, drugs such as rifampin, as well as some anticonvulsants and some antibiotics may decrease oral contraceptive effectiveness.

There is conflict among studies regarding breast cancer and oral contraceptive use. Some studies have reported an increase in the risk of developing breast cancer, particularly at a younger age.

This increased risk appears to be related to duration of use. The majority of studies have found no overall increase in the risk of developing breast cancer. Some studies have found an increase in the incidence of cancer of the cervix in women who use oral contraceptives. However, this finding may be related to factors other than the use of oral contraceptives. There is insufficient evidence to rule out the possibility that pills may cause such cancers.

Taking the pill provides some important non-contraceptive benefits. These include less painful menstruation, less menstrual blood loss and anemia, fewer pelvic infections, and fewer cancers of the ovary and the lining of the uterus.

Be sure to discuss any medical condition you may have with your doctor or health care provider. Your doctor or health care provider will take a medical and family history before prescribing oral contraceptives and will examine you. The physical examination may be delayed to another time if you request it and your doctor or health care provider believes that it is a good medical practice to postpone it. You should be reexamined at least once a year while taking oral contraceptives. The detailed patient information leaflet gives you further information which you should read and discuss with your doctor or health care provider.

This product (like all oral contraceptives) is intended to prevent pregnancy. It does not protect against transmission of HIV (AIDS) and other sexually transmitted diseases such as chlamydia, genital herpes, genital warts, gonorrhea, hepatitis B, and syphilis.

INSTRUCTIONS TO PATIENTS
HOW TO TAKE THE PILL

IMPORTANT POINTS TO REMEMBER

BEFORE YOU START TAKING YOUR PILLS:
1. BE SURE TO READ THESE DIRECTIONS:
   Before you start taking your pills.
   Anytime you are not sure what to do.
2. THE RIGHT WAY TO TAKE THE PILL IS TO TAKE ONE PILL EVERY DAY AT THE SAME TIME.
   If you miss pills you could get pregnant. This includes starting the pack late.
   The more pills you miss, the more likely you are to get pregnant.
3. MANY WOMEN HAVE SPOTTING OR LIGHT BLEEDING, OR MAY FEEL SICK TO THEIR STOMACH DURING THE FIRST 1–3 PACKS OF PILLS.
   If you feel sick to your stomach, do not stop taking the pill. The problem will usually go away. If it doesn't go away, check with your doctor or health care provider.
4. MISSING PILLS CAN ALSO CAUSE SPOTTING OR LIGHT BLEEDING, even when you make up these missed pills.

On the days you take 2 pills to make up for missed pills, you could also feel a little sick to your stomach.
5. IF YOU HAVE VOMITING OR DIARRHEA, for any reason, or IF YOU TAKE SOME MEDICINES, including some antibiotics, your pills may not work as well.
   Use a back-up method (such as condoms, foam, or sponge) until you check with your doctor or health care provider.
6. IF YOU HAVE TROUBLE REMEMBERING TO TAKE THE PILL, talk to your doctor or health care provider about how to make pill-taking easier or about using another method of birth control.
7. IF YOU HAVE ANY QUESTIONS OR ARE UNSURE ABOUT THE INFORMATION IN THIS LEAFLET, call your doctor or health care provider.

BEFORE YOU START TAKING YOUR PILLS

1. DECIDE WHAT TIME OF DAY YOU WANT TO TAKE YOUR PILL.
   It is important to take it at about the same time every day.
2. LOOK AT YOUR PILL PACK: IT WILL HAVE 28 PILLS:
   This 28-pill pack has 26 "active" [white and yellow] pills (with hormones) and 2 "inactive" [green] pills (without hormones).
3. ALSO FIND:
   1) where on the pack to start taking the pills,
   2) in what order to take the pills (follow the arrows) and
   3) the week numbers as shown in the picture below

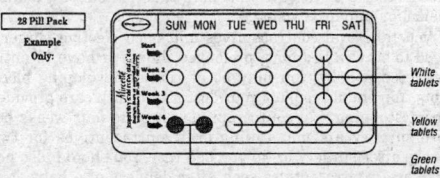

4. BE SURE YOU HAVE READY AT ALL TIMES:
   ANOTHER KIND OF BIRTH CONTROL (such as condoms, foam, or sponge) to use as a back-up in case you miss pills.
   AN EXTRA, FULL PILL PACK.

WHEN TO START THE FIRST PACK OF PILLS

You have a choice of which day to start taking your first pack of pills. Decide with your doctor or health care provider which is the best day for you. Pick a time of day which will be easy to remember.
DAY 1 START
1. Pick the day label strip that starts with the first day of your period (this is the day you start bleeding or spotting, even if it is almost midnight when the bleeding begins).
2. Place this day label strip in the cycle tablet dispenser over the area that has the days of the week (starting with Sunday) imprinted in the plastic.

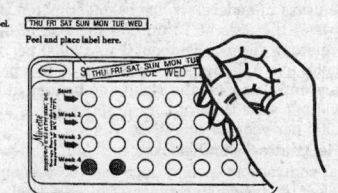

Note: If the first day of your period is a Sunday, you can skip steps #1 and #2.
3. Take the first "active" [white] pill of the first pack during the first 24 hours of your period.
4. You will not need to use a back-up method of birth control, since you are starting the pill at the beginning of your period.
SUNDAY START:
1. Take the first "active" [white] pill of the first pack on the Sunday after your period starts, even if you are still bleeding. If your period begins on Sunday, start the pack that same day.
2. Use another method of birth control as a back-up method if you have sex anytime from the Sunday you start your first pack until the next Sunday (7 days). Condoms, foam, or the sponge are good back-up methods of birth control.

WHAT TO DO DURING THE MONTH

1. TAKE ONE PILL AT THE SAME TIME EVERY DAY UNTIL THE PACK IS EMPTY.
   Do not skip pills even if you are spotting or bleeding between monthly periods or feel sick to your stomach (nausea).
   Do not skip pills even if you do not have sex very often.

2. WHEN YOU FINISH A PACK OR SWITCH YOUR BRAND OF PILLS:
   21 pills: Wait 7 days to start the next pack. You will probably have your period during that week. Be sure that no more than 7 days pass between 21-day packs.
   28 pills: Start the next pack on the day after your last pill. Do not wait any days between packs.

WHAT TO DO IF YOU MISS PILLS

If you MISS 1 [white] "active" pill:
1. Take it as soon as you remember. Take the next pill at your regular time. This means you take 2 pills in 1 day.
2. You do not need to use a back-up birth control method if you have sex.

If you MISS 2 [white] "active" pills in a row in WEEK 1 OR WEEK 2 of your pack:
1. Take 2 pills on the day you remember and 2 pills the next day.
2. Then take 1 pill a day until you finish the pack.
3. You MAY BECOME PREGNANT if you have sex in the 7 days after you miss pills.
   You MUST use another birth control method (such as condoms, foam, or sponge) as a back-up method for those 7 days.

If you MISS 2 [white] "active" pills in a row in THE 3RD WEEK:
1. If you are a Day 1 Starter:
   THROW OUT the rest of the pill pack and start a new pack that same day.
   If you are a Sunday Starter:
   Keep taking 1 pill every day until Sunday.
   On Sunday, THROW OUT the rest of the pack and start a new pack of pills that same day.
2. You may not have your period this month but this is expected. However, if you miss your period 2 months in a row, call your doctor or health care provider because you might be pregnant.
3. You MAY BECOME PREGNANT if you have sex in the 7 days after you miss pills. You MUST use another birth control method (such as condoms, foam, or sponge) as a back-up method for those 7 days.

If you MISS 3 OR MORE [white] "active" pills in a row (during the first 3 weeks):
1. If you are a Day 1 Starter:
   THROW OUT the rest of the pill pack and start a new pack that same day.
   If you are a Sunday Starter:
   Keep taking 1 pill every day until Sunday.
   On Sunday, THROW OUT the rest of the pack and start a new pack of pills that same day.
2. You may not have your period this month but this is expected. However, if you miss your period 2 months in a row, call your doctor or health care provider because you might be pregnant.
3. You MAY BECOME PREGNANT if you have sex in the 7 days after you miss pills. You MUST use another birth control method (such as condoms, foam, or sponge) as a back-up method for those 7 days.

A REMINDER FOR THOSE ON 28-DAY PACKS:

If you forget any of the 2 [green] or 5 [yellow] pills in Week 4:
THROW AWAY the pills you missed.
Keep taking 1 pill each day until the pack is empty.
You do not need a back-up method.

FINALLY, IF YOU ARE STILL NOT SURE WHAT TO DO ABOUT THE PILLS YOU HAVE MISSED:

Use a BACK-UP METHOD anytime you have sex.
KEEP TAKING ONE [WHITE] "ACTIVE" PILL EACH DAY until you can reach your doctor or health care provider.

DETAILED PATIENT PACKAGE INSERT

Mircette™ (desogestrel/ethinyl estradiol and ethinyl estradiol) Tablets

This product (like all oral contraceptives) is intended to prevent pregnancy. It does not protect against HIV infection (AIDS) and other sexually transmitted diseases.
R̸ only

PLEASE NOTE: This labeling is revised from time to time as important new medical information becomes available. Therefore, please review this labeling carefully.

DESCRIPTION

The following oral contraceptive product contains a combination of a progestin and estrogen, the two kinds of female hormones:

Each white tablet contains 0.15 mg desogestrel and 0.02 mg ethinyl estradiol. Each green tablet contains inert ingredients and each yellow tablet contains 0.01 mg ethinyl estradiol.

Continued on next page

Mircette—Cont.

INTRODUCTION

Any woman who considers using oral contraceptives (the birth control pill or the pill) should understand the benefits and risks of using this form of birth control. This leaflet will give you much of the information you will need to make this decision and will also help you determine if you are at risk of developing any of the serious side effects of the pill. It will tell you how to use the pill properly so that it will be as effective as possible. However, this leaflet is not a replacement for a careful discussion between you and your doctor or health care provider. You should discuss the information provided in this leaflet with him or her, both when you first start taking the pill and during your revisits. You should also follow your doctor's or health care provider's advice with regard to regular check-ups while you are on the pill.

EFFECTIVENESS OF ORAL CONTRACEPTIVES

Oral contraceptives or "birth control pills" or "the pill" are used to prevent pregnancy and are more effective than other non-surgical methods of birth control. When they are taken correctly, the chance of becoming pregnant is less than 1% (1 pregnancy per 100 women per year of use) when used perfectly, without missing any pills. Typical failure rates are actually 5% per year. The chance of becoming pregnant increases with each missed pill during a menstrual cycle.

In comparison, typical failure rates for other methods of birth control during the first year of use are as follows:

- Implants (2 or 6 capsules): <1%
- Injection: <1%
- IUD: <1 to 2%
- Diaphragm with spermicides: 20%
- Spermicides alone: 26%
- Vaginal sponge: 20 to 40%
- Female sterilization: <1%
- Male sterilization: <1%
- Cervical Cap with spermicides: 20 to 40%
- Condom alone (male): 14%
- Condom alone (female): 21%
- Periodic abstinence: 25%
- Withdrawal: 19%
- No methods: 85%

WHO SHOULD NOT TAKE ORAL CONTRACEPTIVES

> **Cigarette smoking increases the risk of serious cardiovascular side effects from oral contraceptive use. This risk increases with age and with heavy smoking (15 or more cigarettes per day) and is quite marked in women over 35 years of age. Women who use oral contraceptives are strongly advised not to smoke.**

Some women should not use the pill. For example, you should not take the pill if you are pregnant or think you may be pregnant. You should also not use the pill if you have any of the following conditions:

- A history of heart attack or stroke
- Blood clots in the legs (thrombophlebitis), lungs (pulmonary embolism), or eyes
- A history of blood clots in the deep veins of your legs
- Chest pain (angina pectoris)
- Known or suspected breast cancer or cancer of the lining of the uterus, cervix or vagina
- Unexplained vaginal bleeding (until a diagnosis is reached by your doctor)
- Yellowing of the whites of the eyes or of the skin (jaundice) during pregnancy or during previous use of the pill

- Liver tumor (benign or cancerous)
- Known or suspected pregnancy.

Tell your doctor or health care provider if you have ever had any of these conditions. Your doctor or health care provider can recommend another method of birth control.

OTHER CONSIDERATIONS BEFORE TAKING ORAL CONTRACEPTIVES

Tell your doctor or health care provider if you have:

- Breast nodules, fibrocystic disease of the breast, an abnormal breast x-ray or mammogram
- Diabetes
- Elevated cholesterol or triglycerides
- High blood pressure
- Migraine or other headaches or epilepsy
- Mental depression
- Gallbladder, heart or kidney disease
- History of scanty or irregular menstrual periods.

Women with any of these conditions should be checked often by their doctor or health care provider if they choose to use oral contraceptives.

Also, be sure to inform your doctor or health care provider if you smoke or are on any medications.

RISKS OF TAKING ORAL CONTRACEPTIVES

1. Risk of developing blood clots

Blood clots and blockage of blood vessels are one of the most serious side effects of taking oral contraceptives. In particular, a clot in the legs can cause thrombophlebitis and a clot that travels to the lungs can cause a sudden blocking of the vessel carrying blood to the lungs. Rarely, clots occur in the blood vessels of the eye and may cause blindness, double vision, or impaired vision.

If you take oral contraceptives and need elective surgery, need to stay in bed for a prolonged illness or have recently delivered a baby, you may be at risk of developing blood clots. You should consult your doctor or health care provider about stopping oral contraceptives three to four weeks before surgery and not taking oral contraceptives for two weeks after surgery or during bed rest. You should also not take oral contraceptives soon after delivery of a baby. it is advisable to wait for at least four weeks after delivery if you are not breast feeding or four weeks after a second trimester abortion. If you are breast feeding, you should wait until you have weaned your child before using the pill. (See also the section on Breast Feeding in General Precautions.)

The risk of circulatory disease in oral contraceptive users may be higher in users of high dose pills and may be greater with longer duration of oral contraceptive use. In addition, some of these increased risks may continue for a number of years after stopping oral contraceptives. The risk of venous thromboembolic disease associated with oral contraceptives does not increase with length of use and disappears after pill use is stopped. The risk of abnormal blood clotting increases with age in both users and non-users of oral contraceptives, but the increased risk from the oral contraceptive appears to be present at all ages. For women aged 20 to 44 it is estimated that about 1 in 2,000 using oral contraceptives will be hospitalized each year because of abnormal clotting. Among non-users in the same age group, about 1 in 20,000 would be hospitalized each year. For oral contraceptive users in general, it has been estimated that in women between the ages of 15 and 34 the risk of death due to a circulatory disorder is about 1 in 12,000 per year, whereas for non-users the rate is about 1 in 50,000 per year. In the age group 35 to 44, the risk is estimated to be about 1 in 2,500 per year for oral contraceptive users and about 1 in 10,000 per year for non-users.

2. Heart attacks and strokes

Oral contraceptives may increase the tendency to develop strokes (stoppage or rupture of blood vessels in the brain)

and angina pectoris and heart attacks (blockage of blood vessels in the heart). Any of these conditions can cause death or serious disability.

Smoking greatly increases the possibility of suffering heart attacks and strokes. Furthermore, smoking and the use of oral contraceptives greatly increase the chances of developing and dying of heart disease.

3. Gallbladder disease

Oral contraceptive users probably have a greater risk than non-users of having gallbladder disease, although this risk may be related to pills containing high doses of estrogens.

4. Liver tumors

In rare cases, oral contraceptives can cause benign but dangerous liver tumors. These benign liver tumors can rupture and cause fatal internal bleeding. In addition, a possible but not definite association has been found with the pill and liver cancers in two studies, in which a few women who developed these very rare cancers were found to have used oral contraceptives for long periods. However, liver cancers are extremely rare. The chance of developing liver cancer from using the pill is thus even rarer.

5. Cancer of the reproductive organs and breasts

There is conflict among studies regarding breast cancer and oral contraceptive use. Some studies have reported an increase in the risk of developing breast cancer, particularly at a younger age. This increased risk appears to be related to duration of use. The majority of studies have found no overall increase in the risk of developing breast cancer. Some studies have found an increase in the incidence of cancer of the cervix in women who use oral contraceptives. However, this finding may be related to factors other than the use of oral contraceptives. There is insufficient evidence to rule out the possibility that pills may cause such cancers.

ESTIMATED RISK OF DEATH FROM A BIRTH CONTROL METHOD OR PREGNANCY

All methods of birth control and pregnancy are associated with a risk of developing certain diseases which may lead to disability or death. An estimate of the number of deaths associated with different methods of birth control and pregnancy has been calculated and is shown in the following table.

[See table below]

In the above table, the risk of death from any birth control method is less than the risk of childbirth, except for oral contraceptive users over the age of 35 who smoke and pill users over the age of 40 even if they do not smoke. It can be seen in the table that for women aged 15 to 39, the risk of death was highest with pregnancy (7–26 deaths per 100,000 women, depending on age). Among pill users who do not smoke, the risk of death is always lower than that associated with pregnancy for any age group, although over the age of 40, the risk increases to 32 deaths per 100,000 women, compared to 28 associated with pregnancy at that age. However, for pill users who smoke and are over the age of 35, the estimated number of deaths exceeds those for other methods of birth control. If a woman is over the age of 40 and smokes, her estimated risk of death is four times higher (117/100,000 women) than the estimated risk associated with pregnancy (28/ 100,000 women) in that age group. The suggestion that women over 40 who do not smoke should not take oral contraceptives is based on information from older, high-dose pills and on less selective use of pills than is practiced today. An Advisory Committee of the FDA discussed this issue in 1989 and recommended that the benefits of oral contraceptive use by healthy, non-smoking women over 40 years of age may outweigh the possible risks. However, all women, especially older women, are cautioned to use the lowest dose pill that is effective.

WARNINGS SIGNALS

If any of these adverse effects occur while your are taking oral contraceptives, call your doctor or health care provider immediately:

- Sharp chest pain, coughing of blood, or sudden shortness of breath (indicating a possible clot in the lung)
- Pain in the calf (indicating a possible clot in the leg)
- Crushing chest pain or heaviness in the chest (indicating a possible heart attack)
- Sudden severe headache or vomiting, dizziness or fainting, disturbances of vision or speech, weakness, or numbness in an arm or leg (indicating a possible stroke)
- Sudden partial or complete loss of vision (indicating a possible clot in the eye)
- Breast lumps (indicating possible breast cancer or fibrocystic disease of the breast; ask your doctor or health care provider to show you how to examine your breasts)
- Severe pain or tenderness in the stomach area (indicating a possibly ruptured liver tumor)
- Difficulty in sleeping, weakness, lack of energy, fatigue, or change in mood (possibly indicating severe depression)
- Jaundice or a yellowing of the skin or eyeballs, accompanied frequently by fever, fatigue, loss of appetite, dark colored urine, or light colored bowel movements (indicating possible liver problems).

ANNUAL NUMBER OF BIRTH-RELATED OR METHOD-RELATED DEATHS ASSOCIATED WITH CONTROL OF FERTILITY PER 100,000 NONSTERILE WOMEN, BY FERTILITY CONTROL METHOD ACCORDING TO AGE

Method of control and outcome	15–19	20–24	25–29	30–34	35–39	40–44
No fertility control methods*	7.0	7.4	9.1	14.8	25.7	28.2
Oral contraceptives non-smoker**	0.3	0.5	0.9	1.9	13.8	31.6
Oral contraceptives smoker**	2.2	3.4	6.6	13.5	51.1	117.2
IUD**	0.8	0.8	1.0	1.0	1.4	1.4
Condom*	1.1	1.6	0.7	0.2	0.3	0.4
Diaphragm/spermicide*	1.9	1.2	1.2	1.3	2.2	2.8
Periodic abstinence*	2.5	1.6	1.6	1.7	2.9	3.6

* Deaths are birth related
** Deaths are method related

SIDE EFFECTS OF ORAL CONTRACEPTIVES

1. Vaginal bleeding

Irregular vaginal bleeding or spotting may occur while you are taking the pills. Irregular bleeding may vary from slight staining between menstrual periods to breakthrough bleeding which is a flow much like a regular period. Irregular bleeding occurs most often during the first few months of oral contraceptive use, but may also occur after you have been taking the pill for some time. Such bleeding may be temporary and usually does not indicated any serious problems. It is important to continue taking your pills on schedule. If the bleeding occurs in more than one cycle or lasts for more than a few days, talk to your doctor or health care provider.

2. Contact lenses

If you wear contact lenses and notice a change in vision or an inability to wear your lenses, contact your doctor or health care provider.

3. Fluid retention

Oral contraceptives may cause edema (fluid retention) with swelling of the fingers or ankles and may raise your blood pressure. If you experience fluid retention, contact your doctor or health care provider.

4. Melasma

A spotty darkening of the skin is possible, particularly of the face.

5. Other side effects

Other side effects may include nausea and vomiting, change in appetite, headache, nervousness, depression, dizziness, loss of scalp hair, rash, and vaginal infections.

If any of these side effects bother you, call your doctor or health care provider.

GENERAL PRECAUTIONS

1. Missed periods and use of oral contraceptives before or during early pregnancy

There may be times when you may not menstruate regularly after you have completed taking a cycle of pills. If you have taken your pills regularly and miss one menstrual period, continue taking your pills for the next cycle but be sure to inform your doctor or health care provider before doing so. If you have not taken the pills daily as instructed and missed an menstrual period, or if you missed two consecutive menstrual periods, you may be pregnant. Check with your doctor or health care provider immediately to determine whether you are pregnant. Do not continue to take oral contraceptives until you are sure you are not pregnant, but continue to use another method of contraception.

There is no conclusive evidence that oral contraceptive use is associated with an increase in birth defects, when taken inadvertently during early pregnancy. Previously, a few studies had reported that oral contraceptives might be associated with birth defects, but these studies have not been confirmed. Nevertheless, oral contraceptives or any other drugs should not be used during pregnancy unless clearly necessary and prescribed by your doctor or health care provider. You should check with your doctor or health care provider about risks to your unborn child of any medication taken during pregnancy.

2. While breast feeding

If you are breast feeding, consult your doctor or health care provider before starting oral contraceptives. Some of the drug will be passed on to the child in the milk. A few adverse effects on the child have been reported, including yellowing of the skin (jaundice) and breast enlargement. In addition, oral contraceptives may decrease the amount and quality of your milk. If possible, do not use oral contraceptives while breast feeding. You should use another method of contraception since breast feeding provides only partial protection from becoming pregnant and this partial protection decreases significantly as you breast feed for longer periods of time. You should consider starting oral contraceptives only after you have weaned your child completely.

3. Laboratory tests

If you are scheduled for any laboratory tests, tell your doctor or health care provider you are taking birth control pills. Certain blood tests may be affected by birth control pills.

4. Drug interactions

Certain drugs may interact with birth control pills to make them less effective in preventing pregnancy or cause an increase in breakthrough bleeding. Such drugs include rifampin, drugs used for epilepsy such as barbiturates (for example, phenobarbital), phenytoin (Dilantin is one brand of this drug), phenylbutazone (Butazolidin is one brand), and possibly certain antibiotics. You may need to use additional contraception when you take drugs which can make oral contraceptives less effective.

5. Sexually transmitted diseases

This product (like all oral contraceptives) is intended to prevent pregnancy. It does not protect against transmission of HIV (AIDS) and other sexually transmitted diseases such as chlamydia, genital herpes, genital warts, gonorrhea, hepatitis B, and syphilis.

HOW TO TAKE THE PILL

IMPORTANT POINTS TO REMEMBER

BEFORE YOU START TAKING YOUR PILLS:
1. BE SURE TO READ THESE DIRECTIONS:
   Before you start taking your pills.
   Anytime you are not sure what to do.
2. THE RIGHT WAY TO TAKE THE PILL IS TO TAKE ONE PILL EVERY DAY AT THE SAME TIME.
   If you miss pills you could get pregnant. This includes starting the pack late.
   The more pills you miss, the more likely you are to get pregnant.
3. MANY WOMEN HAVE SPOTTING OR LIGHT BLEEDING, OR MAY FEEL SICK TO THEIR STOMACH DURING THE FIRST 1–3 PACKS OF PILLS.
   If you feel sick to your stomach, do not stop taking the pill. The problem will usually go away. If it doesn't go away, check with your doctor or health care provider.
4. MISSING PILLS CAN ALSO CAUSE SPOTTING OR LIGHT BLEEDING, even when you make up these missed pills.
   On the days you take 2 pills to make up for missed pills, you could also feel a little sick to your stomach.
5. IF YOU HAVE VOMITING OR DIARRHEA, for any reason, or IF YOU TAKE SOME MEDICINES, including some antibiotics, your pills may not work as well.
   Use a back-up method (such as condoms, foam, or sponge) until you check with your doctor or health care provider.
6. IF YOU HAVE TROUBLE REMEMBERING TO TAKE THE PILL, talk to you doctor or health care provider about how to make pill-taking easier or about using another method of birth control.
7. IF YOU HAVE ANY QUESTIONS OR ARE UNSURE ABOUT THE INFORMATION IN THIS LEAFLET, call your doctor or health care provider.

BEFORE YOU START TAKING YOUR PILLS

1. DECIDE WHAT TIME OF DAY YOU WANT TO TAKE YOUR PILL.
   It is important to take it at about the same time every day.
2. LOOK AT YOUR PILL PACK: IT WILL HAVE 28 PILLS:
   This **28-pill pack** has 26 "active" [white and yellow] pills (with hormones) and 2 "inactive" [green] pills (without hormones).
3. ALSO FIND:
   1) where on the pack to start taking the pills,
   2) in what order to take the pills (follow the arrows) and
   3) the week numbers as shown in the picture below.

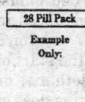 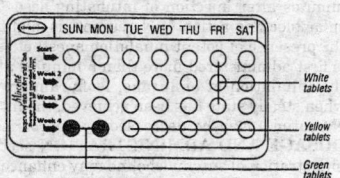

BE SURE YOU HAVE READY AT ALL TIMES ANOTHER KIND OF BIRTH CONTROL (such as condoms, foam or sponge) to use as a back-up in case you miss pills.
AN EXTRA FULL PILL PACK.

WHEN TO START THE FIRST PACK OF PILLS

You have a choice of which day to start taking your first pack of pills. Decide with your doctor or health care provider which is the best day for you. Pick a time of day which will be easy to remember.

DAY 1 START:
1. Pick the day label strip that starts with the first day of your period (this is the day you start bleeding or spotting, even if it is almost midnight when the bleeding begins).
2. Place this day label strip in the cycle tablet dispenser over the area that has the days of the week (starting with Sunday) imprinted in the plastic.

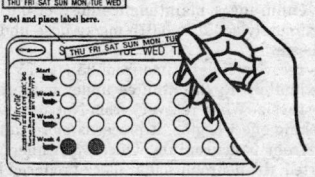

Note: If the first day of your period is a Sunday, you can skip steps #1 and #2.

3. Take the first "active" [white] pill of the first pack during the first 24 hours of your period.
4. You will not need to use a back-up method of birth control, since you are starting the pill at the beginning of your period.

SUNDAY START:
1. Take the first "active" [white] pill of the first pack on the Sunday after your period starts, even if you are still bleeding. If your period begins on Sunday, start the pack that same day.
2. Use another method of birth control as a back-up method if you have sex anytime from the Sunday you start your first pack until the next Sunday (7 days). Condoms, foam or the sponge are good back-up methods of birth control.

WHAT TO DO DURING THE MONTH

1. **TAKE ONE PILL AT THE SAME TIME EVERY DAY UNTIL THE PACK IS EMPTY.**
   Do not skip pills even if you are spotting or bleeding between monthly periods or feel sick to you stomach (nausea).
   Do not skip pills even if you do not have sex very often.
2. **WHEN YOU FINISH A PACK OR SWITCH YOUR BRAND OF PILLS:**
   21 pills: Wait 7 days to start the next pack. You will probably have your period during that week. Be sure that no more than 7 days pass between 21-day packs.
   28 pills: Start the next pack on the day after your last pill. Do not wait any days between packs.

WHAT TO DO IF YOU MISS PILLS

If you **MISS 1** [white] "active" pill:
1. Take it as soon as you remember. Take the next pill at your regular time. This means you take 2 pills in 1 day.
2. You do not need to use a back-up birth control method if you have sex.

If you **MISS 2** [white] "active" pills in a row in **WEEK 1 OR WEEK 2** of your pack:
1. Take 2 pills on the day you remember and 2 pills the next day.
2. Then take 1 pill a day until you finish the pack.
3. You MAY BECOME PREGNANT if you have sex in the **7 days** after you miss pills.
   You MUST use another birth control method (such as condoms, foam, or sponge) as a back-up method for those 7 days.

If you **MISS 2** [white] "active" pills in a row in **THE 3RD WEEK:**
1. *If you are a Day 1 Starter:*
   THROW OUT the rest of the pill pack and start a new pack that same day.
   If you are a Sunday Starter:
   Keep taking 1 pill every day until Sunday.
   On Sunday, THROW OUT the rest of the pack and start a new pack of pills that same day.
2. You may not have your period this month but this is expected. However, if you miss your period 2 months in a row, call your doctor or health care provider because you might be pregnant.
3. You MAY BECOME PREGNANT if you have sex in the **7 days** after you miss pills. You MUST use another birth control method (such as condoms, foam, or sponge) as a back-up method for those 7 days.

If you **MISS 3 OR MORE** [white] "active" pills in a row (during the first 3 weeks):
1. *If you are a Day 1 Starter:*
   THROW OUT the rest of the pill pack and start a new pack that same day.
   If you are a Sunday Starter:
   Keep taking 1 pill every day until Sunday.
   On Sunday, THROW OUT the rest of the pack and start a new pack of pills that same day.
2. You may not have your period this month but this is expected. However, if you miss your period 2 months in a row, call your doctor or health care provider because you might be pregnant.
3. You MAY BECOME PREGNANT if you have sex in the **7 days** after you miss pills. You MUST use another birth control method (such as condoms, foam, or sponge) as a back-up method for those 7 days.

A REMINDER FOR THOSE ON 28-DAY PACKS:

If you forget any of the 2 [green] or 5 [yellow] pills in Week 4:
THROW AWAY the pills you missed.
Keep taking 1 pill each day until the pack is empty.
You do not need a back-up method.

FINALLY, IF YOU ARE STILL NOT SURE WHAT TO DO ABOUT THE PILLS YOU HAVE MISSED:

Use a BACK-UP METHOD anytime you have sex.

Continued on next page

Mircette—Cont.

KEEP TAKING ONE [WHITE] "ACTIVE" PILL EACH DAY until you can reach your doctor or health care provider.

PREGNANCY DUE TO PILL FAILURE

The incidence of pill failure resulting in pregnancy is approximately one percent (i.e., one pregnancy per 100 women per year) if taken every day as directed, but more typical failure rates are about 5%. If failure does occur, the risk to the fetus is minimal.

PREGNANCY AFTER STOPPING THE PILL

There may be some delay in becoming pregnant after you stop using oral contraceptives, especially if you had irregular menstrual cycles before you used oral contraceptives. It may be advisable to postpone conception until you begin menstruating regularly once you have stopped taking the pill and desire pregnancy.

There does not appear to be any increase in birth defects in newborn babies when pregnancy occurs soon after stopping the pill.

OVERDOSAGE

Serious ill effects have not been reported following ingestion of large doses of oral contraceptives by young children. Overdosage may cause nausea and withdrawal bleeding in females. In case of overdosage, contact your doctor, health care provider or pharmacist.

OTHER INFORMATION

Your doctor or health care provider will take a medical and family history before prescribing oral contraceptives and will examine you. The physical examination may be delayed to another time if you request it and your doctor or the health care provider believes that it is a good medical practice to postpone it. You should be reexamined at least once a year. Be sure to inform your doctor or health care provider if there is a family history of any of the conditions listed previously in this leaflet. Be sure to keep all appointments with your doctor or health care provider, because this is a time to determine if there are early signs of side effects of oral contraceptive use.

Do not use the drug for any condition other than the one for which it was prescribed. This drug has been prescribed specifically for you; do not give it to others who may want birth control pills.

HEALTH BENEFITS FROM ORAL CONTRACEPTIVES

In addition to preventing pregnancy, use of combination oral contraceptives may provide certain benefits. They are:
- menstrual cycles may become more regular.
- blood flow during menstruation may be lighter and less iron may be lost. Therefore, anemia due to iron deficiency is less likely to occur.
- pain or other symptoms during menstruation may be encountered less frequently.
- ectopic (tubal) pregnancy may occur less frequently.
- non-cancerous cysts or lumps in the breast may occur less frequently.
- acute pelvic inflammatory disease may occur less frequently.
- oral contraceptive use may provide some protection against developing two forms of cancer; cancer of the ovaries and cancer of the lining of the uterus.

If you want more information about birth control pills, ask your doctor, health care provider, or pharmacist. They have a more technical leaflet called the Prescribing Information which you may wish to read.

Manufactured for Organon Inc.
West Orange, NJ 07052 USA
by N.V. Organon, Oss, The Netherlands
Ptd. in USA 281 ©1998 Organon Inc. 5310175 4/98
Shown in Product Identification Guide, page 327

NORCURON®
(vecuronium bromide) for injection

℞

> THIS DRUG SHOULD BE ADMINISTERED BY ADEQUATELY TRAINED INDIVIDUALS FAMILIAR WITH ITS ACTIONS, CHARACTERISTICS, AND HAZARDS.

DESCRIPTION

NORCURON® (vecuronium bromide) for injection is a nondepolarizing neuromuscular blocking agent of intermediate duration, chemically designated as piperidinium, 1-[(2β, 3α, 5α, 16β, 17β)-3, 17-bis(acetyloxy)-2-(1- piperidinyl) androstan-16-yl]-1-methyl-, bromide. The structural formula is:

[See chemical structure at top of next column]

Its chemical formula is $C_{34}H_{57}BrN_2O_4$ with molecular weight 637.74.

Norcuron® is supplied as a sterile nonpyrogenic freeze-dried buffered cake of very fine microscopic crystalline par-

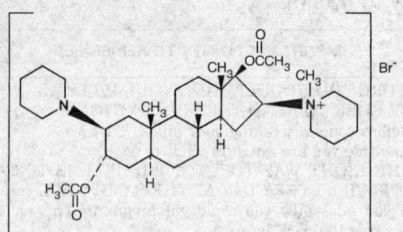

ticles for intravenous injection only. Each 10 mL vial contains 10 mg vecuronium bromide, 20.75 mg citric acid anhydrous, 16.25 mg sodium phosphate dibasic anhydrous, 97 mg mannitol (to adjust tonicity), sodium hydroxide and/or phosphoric acid to buffer and adjust to a pH of 4. Each 20 mL vial contains 20 mg of vecuronium bromide, 41.5 mg citric acid anhydrous, 32.5 mg sodium phosphate dibasic anhydrous, 194 mg mannitol (to adjust tonicity), sodium hydroxide and/or phosphoric acid to buffer and adjust to a pH of 4. Bacteriostatic water for injection, USP, when supplied, contains 0.9% w/v BENZYL ALCOHOL, WHICH IS NOT FOR USE IN NEWBORNS.

CLINICAL PHARMACOLOGY

Norcuron® (vecuronium bromide) for injection is a nondepolarizing neuromuscular blocking agent possessing all of the characteristic pharmacological actions of this class of drugs (curariform). It acts by competing for cholinergic receptors at the motor end-plate. The antagonism to acetylcholine is inhibited and neuromuscular block is reversed by acetylcholinesterase inhibitors such as neostigmine, edrophonium, and pyridostigmine. Norcuron® is about $^1/_3$ more potent than pancuronium; the duration of neuromuscular blockade produced by Norcuron® is shorter than that of pancuronium at initially equipotent doses. The time to onset of paralysis decreases and the duration of maximum effect increases with increasing Norcuron® doses. The use of a peripheral nerve stimulator is recommended in assessing the degree of muscular relaxation with all neuromuscular blocking drugs. The ED_{90} (dose required to produce 90% suppression of the muscle twitch response with balanced anesthesia) has averaged 0.057 mg/kg (0.049 to 0.062 mg/kg in various studies). An initial Norcuron® dose of 0.08 to 0.10 mg/kg generally produces first depression of twitch in approximately 1 minute, good or excellent intubation conditions within 2.5 to 3 minutes, and maximum neuromuscular blockade within 3 to 5 minutes of injection in most patients. Under balanced anesthesia, the time to recovery to 25% of control (clinical duration) is approximately 25 to 40 minutes after injection and recovery is usually 95% complete approximately 45–65 minutes after injection of intubating dose. The neuromuscular blocking action of Norcuron® is slightly enhanced in the presence of potent inhalation anesthetics. If Norcuron® is first administered more than 5 minutes after the start of the inhalation of enflurane, isoflurane, or halothane, or when steady state has been achieved, the intubating dose of Norcuron® may be decreased by approximately 15% (see **DOSAGE AND ADMINISTRATION** section). Prior administration of succinylcholine may enhance the neuromuscular blocking effect of Norcuron® and its duration of action. With succinylcholine as the intubating agent, initial doses of 0.04–0.06 mg/kg of Norcuron® will produce complete neuromuscular block with clinical duration of action of 25–30 minutes. If succinylcholine is used prior to Norcuron®, the administration of Norcuron® should be delayed until the patient starts recovering from succinylcholine-induced neuromuscular blockade. The effect of prior use of other nondepolarizing neuromuscular blocking agents on the activity of Norcuron® has not been studied (see **Drug Interactions**).

Repeated administration of maintenance doses of Norcuron® has little or no cumulative effect on the duration of neuromuscular blockade. Therefore, repeat doses can be administered at relatively regular intervals with predictable results. After an initial dose of 0.08 to 0.10 mg/kg under balanced anesthesia, the first maintenance dose (suggested maintenance dose is 0.010 to 0.015 mg/kg) is generally required within 25 to 40 minutes; subsequent maintenance doses, if required, may be administered at approximately 12 to 15 minute intervals. Halothane anesthesia increases the clinical duration of the maintenance dose only slightly. Under enflurane a maintenance dose of 0.010 mg/kg is approximately equal to 0.015 mg/kg dose under balanced anesthesia.

The recovery index (time from 25% to 75% recovery) is approximately 15–25 minutes under balanced or halothane anesthesia. When recovery from Norcuron® neuromuscular blocking effect begins, it proceeds more rapidly than recovery from pancuronium. Once spontaneous recovery has started, the neuromuscular block produced by Norcuron® is readily reversed with various anticholinesterase agents, e.g. pyridostigmine, neostigmine, or edrophonium in conjunction with an anticholinergic agent such as atropine or gly-

copyrrolate. Rapid recovery is a finding consistent with Norcuron® short elimination half-life, although there have been occasional reports of prolonged neuromuscular blockade in patients in the intensive care unit (See **PRECAUTIONS**). The administration of clinical doses of Norcuron® is not characterized by laboratory or clinical signs of chemically mediated histamine release. This does not preclude the possibility of rare hypersensitivity reactions (See ADVERSE REACTIONS).

Pharmacokinetics: At clinical doses of 0.04–0.10 mg/kg, 60–80% of Norcuron® is usually bound to plasma protein. The distribution half-life following a single intravenous dose (range 0.025–0.280 mg/kg) is approximately 4 minutes. Elimination half-life over this same dosage range is approximately 65–75 minutes in healthy surgical patients and in renal failure patients undergoing transplant surgery.

In late pregnancy, elimination half-life may be shortened to approximately 35–40 minutes. The volume of distribution at steady state is approximately 300–400 mL/kg; systemic rate of clearance is approximately 3–4.5 mL/minute/kg. In man, urine recovery of Norcuron® varies from 3–35% within 24 hours. Data derived from patients requiring insertion of a T-tube in the common bile duct suggests that 25–50% of a total intravenous dose of vecuronium may be excreted in bile within 42 hours. Only unchanged vecuronium has been detected in human plasma following use during surgery. In addition, one metabolite, 3-desacetyl vecuronium, has been rarely detected in human plasma following prolonged clinical use in the I.C.U. (See **PRECAUTIONS: Long Term Use in I.C.U.**). The 3-desacetyl vecuronium metabolite has been recovered in the urine of some patients in quantities that account for up to 10% of injected dose; 3-desacetyl vecuronium has also been recovered by T-tube in some patients accounting for up to 25% of the injected dose.

This metabolite has been judged by animal screening (dogs and cats) to have 50% or more of the potency of Norcuron®; equipotent doses are of approximately the same duration as Norcuron® in dogs and cats. Biliary excretion accounts for about half the dose of Norcuron® within 7 hours in the anesthetized rat. Circulatory bypass of the liver (cat preparation) prolongs recovery from Norcuron®. Limited data derived from patients with cirrhosis or cholestasis suggests that some measurements of recovery may be doubled in such patients. In patients with renal failure, measurements of recovery do not differ significantly from similar measurements in healthy patients.

Studies involving routine hemodynamic monitoring in good risk surgical patients reveal that the administration of Norcuron® in doses up to three times that needed to produce clinical relaxation (0.15 mg/kg) did not produce clinically significant changes in systolic, diastolic or mean arterial pressure. The heart rate, under similar monitoring, remained unchanged in some studies and was lowered by a mean of up to 8% in other studies. A large dose of 0.28 mg/kg administered during a period of no stimulation, while patients were being prepared for coronary artery bypass grafting, was not associated with alterations in rate-pressure-product or pulmonary capillary wedge pressure. Systemic vascular resistance was lowered slightly and cardiac output was increased insignificantly. (The drug has not been studied in patients with hemodynamic dysfunction secondary to cardiac valvular disease). Limited clinical experience with use of Norcuron® during surgery for pheochromocytoma has shown that administration of this drug is not associated with changes in blood pressure or heart rate.

Unlike other nondepolarizing skeletal muscle relaxants, Norcuron® has no clinically significant effects on hemodynamic parameters. Norcuron® will not counteract those hemodynamic changes or known side effects produced by or associated with anesthetic agents, other drugs or various other factors known to alter hemodynamics.

INDICATIONS AND USAGE

Norcuron® (vecuronium bromide) for Injection is indicated as an adjunct to general anesthesia, to facilitate endotracheal intubation and to provide skeletal muscle relaxation during surgery or mechanical ventilation.

CONTRAINDICATIONS

Norcuron® (vecuronium bromide) for Injection is contraindicated in patients known to have a hypersensitivity to it.

WARNINGS

NORCURON® (vecuronium bromide) for Injection SHOULD BE ADMINISTERED IN CAREFULLY ADJUSTED DOSAGE BY OR UNDER THE SUPERVISION OF EXPERIENCED CLINICIANS WHO ARE FAMILIAR WITH ITS ACTIONS AND THE POSSIBLE COMPLICATIONS THAT MIGHT OCCUR FOLLOWING ITS USE. THE DRUG SHOULD NOT BE ADMINISTERED UNLESS FACILITIES FOR INTUBATION, ARTIFICIAL RESPIRATION, OXYGEN THERAPY, AND REVERSAL AGENTS ARE IMMEDIATELY AVAILABLE. THE CLINICIAN MUST BE PREPARED TO ASSIST OR CONTROL RESPIRATION. TO REDUCE THE POSSIBILITY OF PROLONGED NEUROMUSCULAR BLOCKADE AND OTHER POSSIBLE COMPLICATIONS THAT MIGHT OCCUR

FOLLOWING LONG-TERM USE IN THE ICU, NORCURON® OR ANY OTHER NEUROMUSCULAR BLOCKING AGENT SHOULD BE ADMINISTERED IN CAREFULLY ADJUSTED DOSES BY OR UNDER THE SUPERVISION OF EXPERIENCED CLINICIANS WHO ARE FAMILIAR WITH ITS ACTIONS AND WHO ARE FAMILIAR WITH APPROPRIATE PERIPHERAL NERVE STIMULATOR MUSCLE MONITORING TECHNIQUES (see **PRECAUTIONS**). In patients who are known to have myasthenia gravis or the myasthenic (Eaton-Lambert) syndrome, small doses of Norcuron® may have profound effects. In such patients, a peripheral nerve stimulator and use of a small test dose may be of value in monitoring the response to administration of muscle relaxants.

PRECAUTIONS

Renal Failure: Norcuron® (vecuronium bromide) for Injection is well tolerated without clinically significant prolongation of neuromuscular blocking effect in patients with renal failure who have been optimally prepared for surgery by dialysis. Under emergency conditions in anephric patients some prolongation of neuromuscular blockade may occur; therefore, if anephric patients cannot be prepared for non-elective surgery, a lower initial dose of Norcuron® should be considered.

Altered Circulation Time: Conditions associated with slower circulation time in cardiovascular disease, old age, edematous states resulting in increased volume of distribution may contribute to a delay in onset time, therefore, dosage should not be increased.

Hepatic Disease: Experience in patients with cirrhosis or cholestasis has revealed prolonged recovery time in keeping with the role the liver plays in Norcuron® (vecuronium bromide) for Injection metabolism and excretion (**see Pharmacokinetics**). Data currently available do not permit dosage recommendations in patients with impaired liver function.

Long-term Use in I.C.U.: In the intensive care unit, long-term use of neuromuscular blocking drugs to facilitate mechanical ventilation may be associated with prolonged paralysis and/or skeletal muscle weakness, that may be first noted during attempts to wean such patients from the ventilator. Typically, such patients receive other drugs such as broad spectrum antibiotics, narcotics and/or steroids and may have electrolyte imbalance and diseases which lead to electrolyte imbalance, hypoxic episodes of varying duration, acid-base imbalance and extreme debilitation, any of which may enhance the actions of a neuromuscular blocking agent. Additionally, patients immobilized for extended periods frequently develop symptoms consistent with disuse muscle atrophy. The recovery picture may vary from regaining movement and strength in all muscles to initial recovery of movement of the facial and small muscles of the extremities then to the remaining muscles. In rare cases recovery may be over an extended period of time and may even, on occasion, involve rehabilitation. Therefore, when there is a need for long-term mechanical ventilation, the benefits-to-risk ratio of neuromuscular blockade must be considered.

Continuous infusion or intermittent bolus dosing to support mechanical ventilation, has not been studied sufficiently to support dosage recommendations. IN THE INTENSIVE CARE UNIT, APPROPRIATE MONITORING, WITH THE USE OF A PERIPHERAL NERVE STIMULATOR TO ASSESS THE DEGREE OF NEUROMUSCULAR BLOCKADE IS RECOMMENDED TO HELP PRECLUDE POSSIBLE PROLONGATION OF THE BLOCKADE. WHENEVER THE USE OF NORCURON® OR ANY NEUROMUSCULAR BLOCKING AGENT IS CONTEMPLATED IN THE ICU, IT IS RECOMMENDED THAT NEUROMUSCULAR TRANSMISSION BE MONITORED CONTINUOUSLY DURING ADMINISTRATION AND RECOVERY WITH THE HELP OF A NERVE STIMULATOR. ADDITIONAL DOSES OF NORCURON® OR ANY OTHER NEUROMUSCULAR BLOCKING AGENT SHOULD NOT BE GIVEN BEFORE THERE IS A DEFINITE RESPONSE TO T_1 OR TO THE FIRST TWITCH. IF NO RESPONSE IS ELICITED, INFUSION ADMINISTRATION SHOULD BE DISCONTINUED UNTIL A RESPONSE RETURNS.

Severe Obesity or Neuromuscular Disease: Patients with severe obesity or neuromuscular disease may pose airway and/or ventilatory problems requiring special care before, during and after the use of neuromuscular blocking agents such as Norcuron® (vecuronium bromide) for Injection.

Malignant Hyperthermia: Many drugs used in anesthetic practice are suspected of being capable of triggering a potentially fatal hypermetabolism of skeletal muscle known as malignant hyperthermia. There are insufficient data derived from screening in susceptible animals (swine) to establish whether or not Norcuron® (vecuronium bromide) for Injection is capable of triggering malignant hyperthermia.

C.N.S.: Norcuron® (vecuronium bromide) for Injection has no known effect on consciousness, the pain threshold or cerebration. Administration must be accompanied by adequate anesthesia or sedation.

Drug Interactions: Prior administration of succinylcholine may enhance the neuromuscular blocking effect of Norcuron® (vecuronium bromide) for injection and its duration of action. If succinycholine is used before Norcuron® the administration of Norcuron® should be delayed until the succinylcholine effect shows signs of wearing off. With succinylcholine as the intubating agent, initial doses of 0.04–0.06 mg/kg of Norcuron® may be administered to produce complete neuromuscular block with clinical duration of action of 25–30 minutes (see **CLINICAL PHARMACOLOGY**). The use of Norcuron® before succinylcholine, in order to attenuate some of the side effects of succinylcholine, has not been sufficiently studied.

Other nondepolarizing neuromuscular blocking agents (pancuronium, d-tubocurarine, metocurine, and gallamine) act in the same fashion as does Norcuron®, therefore, these drugs and Norcuron® may manifest an additive effect when used together. There are insufficient data to support concomitant use of Norcuron® and other competitive muscle relaxants in the same patient.

Inhalational Anesthetics: Use of volatile inhalational anesthetics such as enflurane, isoflurane, and halothane with Norcuron® (vecuronium bromide) for Injection will enhance neuromuscular blockade. Potentiation is most prominent with use of enflurane and isoflurane. With the above agents the initial dose of Norcuron® may be the same as with balanced anesthesia unless the inhalational anesthetic has been administered for a sufficient time at a sufficient dose to have reached clinical equilibrium (see **CLINICAL PHARMACOLOGY**).

Antibiotics: Parenteral/intraperitoneal administration of high doses of certain antibiotics may intensify or produce neuromuscular block on their own. The following antibiotics have been associated with various degrees of paralysis: aminoglycosides (such as neomycin, streptomycin, kanamycin, gentamicin, and dihydrostreptomycin); tetracyclines; bacitracin; polymyxin B; colistin; and sodium colistimethate. If these or other newly introduced antibiotics are used in conjunction with Norcuron®, unexpected prolongation of neuromuscular block should be considered a possibility.

Other: Experience concerning injection of quinidine during recovery from use of other muscle relaxants suggests that recurrent paralysis may occur. This possibility must also be considered for Norcuron® (vecuronium bromide) for Injection. Norcuron® induced neuromuscular blockade has been counteracted by alkalosis and enhanced by acidosis in experimental animals (cat). Electrolyte imbalance and diseases which lead to electrolyte imbalance, such as adrenal cortical insufficiency, have been shown to alter neuromuscular blockade. Depending on the nature of the imbalance, either enhancement or inhibition may be expected. Magnesium salts, administered for the management of toxemia of pregnancy may enhance the neuromuscular blockade.

Drug/laboratory test interactions: None known

Carcinogenesis, Mutagensis, Impairment of Fertility: Long-term studies in animals have not been performed to evaluate carcinogenic or mutagenic potential or impairment of fertility.

Pregnancy: Pregnancy Category C: Animal reproduction studies have not been conducted with Norcuron® (vecuronium bromide) for Injection. It is also not known whether Norcuron® can cause fetal harm when administered to a pregnant woman or can affect reproduction capacity. Norcuron® should be given to a pregnant woman only if clearly needed.

Pediatric Use: Infants under 1 year of age but older than 7 weeks also tested under halothane anesthesia, are moderately more sensitive to Norcuron® (vecuronium bromide) for Injection on a mg/kg basis than adults and take about $1^1/_2$ times as long to recover. See **Use in Pediatrics** subsection of **DOSAGE AND ADMINISTRATION** for recommendations for use in pediatric patients 7 weeks to 16 years of age. The safety and effectiveness of Norcuron® in pediatric patients less than 7 weeks of age have not been established.

ADVERSE REACTIONS

The most frequent adverse reaction to nondepolarizing blocking agents as a class consists of an extension of the drug's pharmacological action beyond the time period needed. This may vary from skeletal muscle weakness to profound and prolonged skeletal muscle paralysis resulting in respiration insufficiency or apnea.

Inadequate reversal of the neuromuscular blockade is possible with Norcuron® (vecuronium bromide) for Injection as with all curariform drugs. These adverse reactions are managed by manual or mechanical ventilation until recovery is judged adequate. Little or no increase in intensity of blockade or duration of action with Norcuron® is noted from the use of thiobarbiturates, narcotic analgesics, nitrous oxide, or droperidol. See **OVERDOSAGE** for discussion of other drugs used in anesthetic practice which also cause respiratory depression.

Prolonged to profound extensions of paralysis and/or muscle weakness as well as muscle atrophy have been reported after long-term use to support mechanical ventilation in the intensive care unit (see **PRECAUTIONS**). The administration of Norcuron® has been associated with rare instances of hypersensitivity reactions (bronchospasm, hypotension and/or tachycardia, sometimes associated with acute urticaria or erythema); (see also **CLINICAL PHARMACOLOGY**).

OVERDOSAGE

The possibility of iatrogenic overdosage can be minimized by carefully monitoring muscle twitch response to peripheral nerve stimulation.

Excessive doses of Norcuron® (vecuronium bromide) for Injection produced enhanced pharmacological effects. Residual neuromuscular blockade beyond the time period needed may occur with Norcuron® as with other neuromuscular blockers. This may be manifested by skeletal muscle weakness, decreased respiratory reserve, low tidal volume, or apnea. A peripheral nerve stimulator may be used to assess the degree of residual neuromuscular blockade from other causes of decreased respiratory reserve.

Respiratory depression may be due either wholly or in part to other drugs used during the conduct of general anesthesia such as narcotics, thiobarbiturates and other central nervous system depressants. Under such circumstances the primary treatment is maintenance of a patent airway and manual or mechanical ventilation until complete recovery of normal respiration is assured. Regonol® (pyridostigmine bromide) injection, neostigmine, or edrophonium, in conjunction with atropine or glycopyrrolate will usually antagonize the skeletal muscle relaxant action of Norcuron®. Satisfactory reversal can be judged by adequacy of skeletal muscle tone and by adequacy of respiration. A peripheral nerve stimulator may also be used to monitor restoration of twitch height. Failure of prompt reversal (within 30 minutes) may occur in the presence of extreme debilitation, carcinomatosis, and with concomitant use of certain broad spectrum antibiotics, or anesthetic agents and other drugs which enhance neuromuscular blockade or cause respiratory depression of their own. Under such circumstances the management is the same as that of prolonged neuromuscular blockade. Ventilation must be supported by artificial means until the patient has resumed control of his respiration. Prior to the use of reversal agents, reference should be made to the specific package insert of the reversal agent.

DOSAGE AND ADMINISTRATION

Norcuron® (vecuronium bromide) for injection is for intravenous use only.

This drug should be administered by or under the supervision of experienced clinicians familar with the use of neuromuscular blocking agents. Dosage must be individualized in each case. The dosage information which follows is derived from studies based upon units of drug per unit of body weight and is intended to serve as a guide only, especially regarding enhancement of neuromuscular blockade of Norcuron® by volatile anesthetics and by prior use of succinylcholine (see **PRECAUTIONS/Drug Interactions**). Parenteral drug products should be inspected visually for particulate matter and discoloration prior to administration whenever solution and container permit.

To obtain maximum clinical benefits of Norcuron® and to minimize the possibility of overdosage, the monitoring of muscle twitch response to peripheral nerve stimulation is advised.

The recommended initial dose of Norcuron® is 0.08 to 0.10 mg/kg (1.4 to 1.75 times the ED_{90}) given as an intravenous bolus injection. This dose can be expected to produce good or excellent non-emergency intubation conditions in 2.5 to 3 minutes after injection. Under balanced anesthesia, clinically required neuromuscular blockade lasts approximately 25–30 minutes, with recovery to 25% of control achieved approximately 25 to 40 minutes after injection and recovery to 95% of control achieved approximately 45–65 minutes after injection. In the presence of potent inhalation anesthetics, the neuromuscular blocking effect of Norcuron® is enhanced. If Norcuron® is first administered more than 5 minutes after the start of inhalation agent or when steady-state has been achieved, the initial Norcuron® dose may be reduced by approximately 15%, i.e., 0.060 to 0.085 mg/kg.

Prior administration of succinylcholine may enhance the neuromuscular blocking effect and duration of action of Norcuron®. If intubation is performed using succinylcholine, a reduction of initial dose of Norcuron® to 0.04–0.06 mg/kg with inhalation anesthesia and 0.05–0.06 mg/kg with balanced anesthesia may be required.

During prolonged surgical procedures, maintenance doses of 0.010 to 0.015 mg/kg of Norcuron® are recommended; after the initial Norcuron® injection, the first maintenance dose will generally be required within 25 to 40 minutes. However, clinical criteria should be used to determine the need for maintenance doses.

Since Norcuron® lacks clinically important cumulative effects, subsequent maintenance doses, if required, may be administered at relatively regular intervals for each patient, ranging approximately from 12 to 15 minutes under balanced anesthesia, slightly longer under inhalation agents. (If less frequent administration is desired, higher maintenance doses may be administered.)

Should there be reason for the selection of larger doses in individual patients, initial doses ranging from 0.15 mg/kg up to 0.28 mg/kg have been administered during surgery under halothane anesthesia without ill effects to the cardiovascular system being noted as long as ventilation is properly maintained (see **CLINICAL PHARMACOLOGY**).

Continued on next page

Norcuron—Cont.

Use by Continuous Infusion: After an intubating dose of 80–100 µg/kg, a continuous infusion of 1 µg/kg/min can be initiated approximately 20–40 min later. Infusion of Norcuron® should be initiated only after early evidence of spontaneous recovery from the bolus dose. Long-term intravenous infusion to support mechanical ventilation in the intensive care unit has not been studied sufficiently to support dosage recommendations. (see **PRECAUTIONS**).

The infusion of Norcuron® should be individualized for each patient. The rate of administration should be adjusted according to the patient's twitch response as determined by peripheral nerve stimulation. An initial rate of 1 µg/kg/min is recommended, with the rate of the infusion adjusted thereafter to maintain a 90% suppression of twitch response. Average infusion rates may range from 0.8 to 1.2 µg/kg/min.

Inhalation anesthetics, particularly enflurane and isoflurane may enhance the neuromuscular blocking action of nondepolarizing muscle relaxants. In the presence of steady-state concentrations of enflurane or isoflurane, it may be necessary to reduce the rate of infusion 25–60 percent, 45–60 min after the intubating dose. Under halothane anesthesia it may not be necessary to reduce the rate of infusion.

Spontaneous recovery and reversal of neuromuscular blockade following discontinuation of Norcuron® infusion may be expected to proceed at rates comparable to that following a single bolus dose (see **CLINICAL PHARMACOLOGY**).

Infusion solutions of Norcuron® can be prepared by mixing Norcuron® with an appropriate infusion solution such as 5% glucose in water, 0.9% NaCl, 5% glucose in saline, or Lactated Ringers. Unused portions of infusion solutions should be discarded.

Infusion rates of Norcuron® can be individualized for each patient using the following table:

Drug Delivery Rate	Infusion Delivery Rate	
(µg/kg/min)	(mL/kg/min)	
	0.1 mg/mL*	0.2 mg/mL†
0.7	0.007	0.0035
0.8	0.008	0.0040
0.9	0.009	0.0045
1.0	0.010	0.0050
1.1	0.011	0.0055
1.2	0.012	0.0060
1.3	0.013	0.0065

* 10 mg of Norcuron® in 100 mL solution
† 20 mg of Norcuron® in 100 mL solution

The following table is a guideline for mL/min delivery for a solution of 0.1 mg/mL (10 mg in 100 mL) with an infusion pump.

NORCURON® INFUSION RATE —mL/MIN

Amount of Drug µg/kg/min	Patient Weight—kg						
	40	50	60	70	80	90	100
0.7	0.28	0.35	0.42	0.49	0.56	0.63	0.70
0.8	0.32	0.40	0.48	0.56	0.64	0.72	0.80
0.9	0.36	0.45	0.54	0.63	0.72	0.81	0.90
1.0	0.40	0.50	0.60	0.70	0.80	0.90	1.00
1.1	0.44	0.55	0.66	0.77	0.88	0.99	1.10
1.2	0.48	0.60	0.72	0.84	0.96	1.08	1.20
1.3	0.52	0.65	0.78	0.91	1.04	1.17	1.30

NOTE: If a concentration of 0.2 mg/mL is used (20 mg in 100 mL), the rate should be decreased by one-half.

Use in Pediatrics: Older children (10 to 17 years of age) have approximately the same dosage requirements (mg/kg) as adults and may be managed the same way. Younger children (1 to 10 years of age) may require a slightly higher initial dose and may also require supplementation slightly more often than adults.

Infants under 1 year of age but older than 7 weeks are moderately more sensitive to Norcuron® (vecuronium bromide) for Injection on a mg/kg basis than adults and take about 1½ times as long to recover. See also subsection of **PRECAUTIONS** titled **Pediatric Use**. Information presently available does not permit recommendation on usage in pediatric patients less than 7 weeks of age (see **PRECAUTIONS**). There are insufficient data concerning continuous infusion of vecuronium in pediatric patients, therefore, no dosing recommendations can be made.

COMPATIBILITY

Norcuron® is compatible in solution with:
0.9% NaCl solution

5% glucose in water
Sterile water for injection
5% glucose in saline
Lactated Ringers
Use within 24 hours of mixing with the above solutions. Parenteral drug products should be inspected visually for particulate matter and discoloration prior to administration whenever solution and container permit.

HOW SUPPLIED

10 mL vials (10 mg of vecuronium bromide) and 10 mL pre-filled syringes of diluent (bacteriostatic water for injection, USP) 22g 1¼" needle.
Boxes of 10   NDC No. 0052-0441-60
10 mL vials (10 mg vecuronium bromide) and 10 mL vials of diluent (bacteriostatic water for injection, USP).
Boxes of 10   NDC No. 0052-0441-17
10 mL vials (10 mg vecuronium bromide) only; DILUENT NOT SUPPLIED.
Boxes of 10   NDC No. 0052-0441-15
20 mL vials (20 mg vecuronium bromide) only; DILUENT NOT SUPPLIED.
Boxes of 10   NDC No. 0052-0442-46

STORAGE

15–30°C (59–86°F). Protect from light.

AFTER RECONSTITUTION

- When reconstituted with supplied bacteriostatic water for injection: CONTAINS BENZYL ALCOHOL, WHICH IS NOT INTENDED FOR USE IN NEWBORNS. Use within 5 days. May be stored at room temperature or refrigerated.
- When reconstituted with sterile water for injection or other compatible I.V. solutions: Refrigerate vial. Use within 24 hours. Single use only. Discard unused portion.

Rx only

ORGANON INC.
WEST ORANGE, NEW JERSEY 07052
5310125 REVISED 2/98

ORGARAN®   ℞
(danaparoid sodium) Injection

SPINAL/EPIDURAL HEMATOMAS

When neuraxial anesthesia (epidural/spinal anesthesia) or spinal puncture is employed, patients anticoagulated or scheduled to be anticoagulated with low molecular weight heparins or heparinoids for prevention of thromboembolic complications are at risk of developing an epidural or spinal hematoma which can result in long-term or permanent paralysis.

The risk of these events is increased by the use of indwelling epidural catheters for administration of analgesia or by the concomitant use of drugs affecting hemostasis such as non steroidal anti-inflammatory drugs (NSAIDs), platelet inhibitors, or other anticoagulants. The risk also appears to be increased by traumatic or repeated epidural or spinal puncture.

Patient should be frequently monitored for signs and symptoms of neurological impairment. If neurologic compromise is noted, urgent treatment is necessary.

The physician should consider the potential benefit versus risk before intervention in patients anticoagulated or to be anticoagulated for thromboprophylaxis (see also WARNINGS, Hemorrhage and PRECAUTIONS, Drug Interactions).

DESCRIPTION

ORGARAN® (danaparoid sodium) Injection is a sterile, glycosaminoglycuronan antithrombotic agent. The active components of ORGARAN®, isolated from porcine intestinal mucosa, are heparan sulfate (84%), dermatan sulfate (12%) and a small amount of chondroitin sulfate (4%). The average molecular weight is approximately 5500 Daltons. ORGARAN® is intended for subcutaneous injection. Each prefilled syringe or ampule contains 750 anti-Xa units in 0.6 mL solution. ORGARAN® Injection is made isotonic with sodium chloride, adjusted to pH 7 with hydrochloric acid, or sodium hydroxide. ORGARAN® Injection contains 0.15% (w/v) sodium sulfite to prevent discoloration of the solution. The structural formula of the main repeating disaccharide units is as follows:
Structural Formula:
Main Repeating Disaccharide Units:

Heparan Sulfate: R_1 = H or SO_3^-

Heparan Sulfate: R_2 = $COCH_3$ or SO_3^-

Dermatan Sulfate
R = H or SO_3^-

Chondroitin Sulfate

CLINICAL PHARMACOLOGY

Pharmacodynamics: *Effect on Coagulation Factors:* ORGARAN® (danaparoid sodium) Injection is an antithrombotic agent. ORGARAN® prevents fibrin formation in the coagulation pathway via thrombin generation inhibition by anti-Xa and anti-IIa (thrombin) effects. The anti-Xa: anti-IIa activity ratio is greater than 22. Inactivation of factor Xa is mediated by antithrombin-III (AT-III) while factor IIa inactivation is mediated by both AT-III and heparin cofactor II (HC II). ORGARAN® has only minor effect on platelet function and platelet aggregability.

Measurements of Hemostasis: Because of its predominant anti-Xa activity, ORGARAN® (danaparoid sodium) has little effect on clotting assays (*e.g.*, prothrombin time [PT], partial thromboplastin time [PTT]). ORGARAN® has minimal effect on fibrinolytic activity and bleeding time.

Pharmacokinetics: The pharmacokinetics of ORGARAN® (danaparoid sodium) Injection have been described by monitoring its biological activity (plasma anti-Xa activity) since no specific chemical assay methods are currently available for the components of ORGARAN®.

By subcutaneous route of administration, ORGARAN® was approximately 100% bioavailable, compared with the same dose administered intravenously. The maximum anti-Xa activity (T_{max}) occurred at approximately two to five hours. For single subcutaneous doses of 750, 1500, 2250, and 3250 anti-Xa units of ORGARAN® the mean peak plasma anti-Xa activities were 102.4, 206.1, 283.9, and 403.4 mU/mL, respectively. The mean value for the terminal half-life ($T_{1/2}$) was about 24 hours and the clearance was 0.36 L/hour. Clearance was affected by body surface area in that the higher the body surface, the faster the clearance. ORGARAN® is mainly eliminated via the kidneys. In patients with severely impaired renal function, the half-life of elimination of plasma anti-Xa activity may be prolonged, therefore, monitoring such patients carefully is recommended.

Clinical Trials: In a European multicenter double-blind trial, ORGARAN® (danaparoid sodium) Injection was compared with placebo in 196 patients undergoing elective hip replacement surgery. The administration of ORGARAN® for 7 to 14 days post-operatively significantly reduced the overall incidence of DVT to 15% (15/98 patients) compared to the incidence of 57% (56/98 patients) observed with placebo.

Number (%) of Patients with DVT*
Intent-to-Treat

	ORGARAN® N=98	Placebo N=98	p-value[a]
Proximal; N (%)	8 (8)	26 (27)	0.001
Distal; N (%)	14 (14)	51 (52)	<0.001
Overall; N (%)	15 (15)	56 (57)	<0.001

* A patient may be counted more than once (proximal and/or distal)
[a] Using the Cochran Mantel-Haenszel test

In a United States multicenter trial, ORGARAN® was compared with warfarin in 396 patients undergoing elective hip replacement. A significant reduction in the overall incidence of DVT was observed with ORGARAN® (14.6%; 29/199 patients) compared with warfarin (26.9%; 53/197 patients), p=0.003.

Number (%) of Patients with DVT[a]
Intent-to-Treat

	ORGARAN® N=199	Warfarin N=197	p-value[b]
Proximal[c]; N (%)	3 (1.5)	8 (4.1)	0.13
Distal[d]; N (%)	28 (14.1)	49 (24.9)	0.007
Overall[e]; N (%)	29 (14.6)	53 (26.9)	0.003

[a] By positive venogram only
[b] Using the Cochran Mantel-Haenszel test
[c] Popliteal, iliac, and femoral
[d] Calf
[e] A patient may be counted more than once (proximal and distal)

INDICATIONS AND USAGE

ORGARAN® (danaparoid sodium) Injection is indicated for the prophylaxis of post-operative deep venous thrombosis (DVT), which may lead to pulmonary embolism (PE), in patients undergoing elective hip replacement surgery.

CONTRAINDICATIONS

ORGARAN® (danaparoid sodium) Injection is contraindicated in the following conditions: severe hemorrhagic diathesis, e.g., hemophilia and idiopathic thrombocytopenic purpura; active major bleeding state, including hemorrhagic stroke in the acute phase; hypersensitivity to ORGARAN®; Type II thrombocytopenia associated with a positive *in vitro* test for antiplatelet antibody in the presence of ORGARAN® Injection. ORGARAN® is contraindicated in patients with known hypersensitivity to pork products.

WARNINGS

General: ORGARAN® (danaparoid sodium) Injection is not intended for intramuscular administration. Since a specific standard for the anti-Xa activity of ORGARAN® is used, the anti-Xa unit activity of ORGARAN® is not equivalent to that described for heparin or low-molecular weight heparin. Therefore, ORGARAN® cannot be dosed interchangeably (unit for unit) with either heparin or any low molecular weight heparin.

Miscellaneous: ORGARAN® (danaparoid sodium) Injection contains sodium sulfite which may cause allergic-type reactions, including anaphylactic symptoms and life-threatening or less severe asthmatic episodes in certain susceptible people. The overall prevalence of sulfite sensitivity in the general population is unknown and probably low. Sulfite sensitivity is seen more frequently in asthmatic than in non-asthmatic patients.

Hemorrhage: Hemorrhage can occur at virtually any site in patients receiving ORGARAN® (danaparoid sodium) Injection. An unexplained fall in hematocrit and/or fall in blood pressure should lead to serious consideration of a hemorrhagic event. ORGARAN®, like anticoagulants, should be used with extreme caution in disease states in which there is increased risk of hemorrhage, such as severe uncontrolled hypertension, acute bacterial endocarditis, congenital or acquired bleeding disorders, active ulcerative and angiodysplastic gastrointestinal disease, non-hemorrhagic stroke, shortly after brain, spinal or ophthalmological surgery and post-operative indwelling epidural catheter use.

Spinal or epidural hematomas can occur with the associated use of low molecular weight heparins or heparinoids and neuraxial (spinal/epidural) anesthesia or spinal puncture which can result in long-term or permanent paralysis. The risk of these events is higher with the use of post-operative indwelling epidural catheters or concomitant use of additional drugs affecting hemostasis such as NSAIDs (see boxed WARNING).

PRECAUTIONS

General: The risks and benefits of ORGARAN® (danaparoid sodium) Injection should be carefully considered before use in patients with severely impaired renal function or hemorrhagic disorders (see **DOSAGE AND ADMINISTRATION**).

Laboratory Tests: ORGARAN® (danaparoid sodium) Injection has only a small effect on factor IIa (thrombin) activity, therefore, when administered at recommended prophylaxis doses routine coagulation tests (e.g., Prothrombin Time [PT], Activated Partial Thromboplastin Time [APTT], Kaolin Cephalin Clotting Time [KCCT], Whole Blood Clotting Time [WBCT], and Thrombin Time [TT]) are relatively insensitive measures of ORGARAN® activity and, therefore, unsuitable for monitoring.

Blood Loss and Transfusions
DVT and PE Prophylaxis for Orthopedic Hip Surgery
All Patients Treated

Blood Loss and Transfusions	Total N	ORGARAN®	Placebo	Warfarin	Other[2]
Total (728 Males: 1675 Females)		(N) Mean±SD	(N) Mean±SD	(N) Mean±SD	(N) Mean±SD
Intraoperative Blood Loss (mL)					
Males	596	(330) 694±555	(27) 586±737	(141) 689±499	(98) 754±661
Females	1259	(686) 486±430	(66) 416±252	(219) 471±306	(288) 530±456
Postoperative Blood Loss (mL)					
Males	580	(318) 954±879	(45) 908±812	(88) 817±585	(129) 1056±1055
Females	1256	(639) 700±778	(122) 715±520	(80) 619±352	(415) 798±779
Transfusions (units PRBCs)					
Males	462	(258) 2.6±1.8	(35) 2.7±1.4	(87) 2.5±1.4	(82) 2.9±2.1
Females	1152	(604) 2.6±1.7	(92) 2.8±1.4	(177) 2.1±1.1	(279) 2.8±2.0

[a] "Other" includes the following active reference agents: heparin, heparin/DHE, acetylsalicylic acid, dextran, and low-molecular weight heparins.
Total N = Total number of patients with available data across all treatment groups.
n = The number of patients with available data in each respective treatment group and by gender.

Incidence of Adverse Experiences (≥2%)
DVT and PE Prophylaxis for Elective Hip Surgery
All Patients Treated

Adverse Experience	ORGARAN® N=645 N(%)	Placebo N=135 N(%)	Warfarin N=243 N(%)	Other N=168 N(%)
Fever	143(22.2)	1(0.7)	138(56.8)	3(1.8)
Nausea	92(14.3)	3(2.2)	78(32.1)	8(4.8)
Constipation	73(11.3)	0(0.0)	70(28.8)	2(1.2)
Injection Site Pain	49(7.6)	4(3.0)	0(0.0)	34(20.2)
Rash	31(4.8)	0(0.0)	18(7.4)	2(1.2)
Pruritus	25(3.9)	1(0.7)	14(5.8)	0(0.0)
Peripheral Edema	21(3.3)	0(0.0)	19(7.8)	4(2.4)
Insomnia	20(3.1)	0(0.0)	32(13.2)	0(0.0)
Vomiting	19(2.9)	3(2.2)	20(8.2)	3(1.8)
Joint Disorder	17(2.6)	0(0.0)	15(6.2)	0(0.0)
Headache	17(2.6)	1(0.7)	13(5.3)	0(0.0)
Urinary Tract Infection	17(2.6)	1(0.7)	5(2.1)	5(3.0)
Edema	17(2.6)	0(0.0)	14(5.8)	2(1.2)
Asthenia	15(2.3)	0(0.0)	10(4.1)	1(0.6)
Dizziness	15(2.3)	0(0.0)	14(5.8)	0(0.0)
Anemia	14(2.2)	3(2.2)	5(2.1)	5(3.0)
Urinary Retention	13(2.0)	0(0.0)	14(5.8)	1(0.6)

Incidence of Adverse Experiences (≥2%)
DVT and PE Prophylaxis Indication
All Patients Treated

Adverse Experience	ORGARAN® N=2383 N(%)	Placebo N=276 N(%)	Warfarin N=421 N(%)	Other N=1163 N(%)
Injection Site Pain	327(13.7)	53(19.2)	0(0.0)	153(13.2)
Pain	207(8.7)	0(0.0)	202(48.0)	20(1.7)
Fever	173(7.3)	1(0.4)	150(35.6)	21(1.8)
Nausea	98(4.1)	3(1.1)	79(18.8)	13(1.1)
Urinary Tract Infection	96(4.0)	3(1.1)	27(6.4)	65(5.6)
Constipation	83(3.5)	0(0.0)	73(17.3)	3(0.3)
Rash	51(2.1)	0(0.0)	25(5.9)	5(0.4)
Infection	51(2.1)	3(1.1)	0(0.0)	47(4.0)

Periodic complete blood counts, including platelet count, and stool occult blood tests are recommended during the course of treatment with ORGARAN®.

Thrombocytopenia: ORGARAN® (danaparoid sodium) Injection shows a low cross-reactivity with antiplatelet antibodies in individuals with Type II heparin-induced thrombocytopenia. No cases of white clot syndrome or cases of Type II thrombocytopenia have been reported in clinical studies for the prophylaxis of DVT in patients receiving multiple doses of ORGARAN® up to 14 days.

Drug Interactions: In clinical studies for the prophylaxis of DVT, no clinically significant drug interactions have been noted in the following drugs: digoxin, cloxacillin, ticarcillin, chlorthalidone, and pentobarbital.

ORGARAN® (danaparoid sodium) Injection should be used with caution in patients receiving oral anticoagulants and/or platelet inhibitors. Monitoring of anticoagulant activity of oral anticoagulants by Prothrombin Time and Thrombotest is unreliable within 5 hours after ORGARAN® Injection administration.

Carcinogenesis, Mutagenesis, Impairment of Fertility: No long term studies in animals have been performed to eval-

Continued on next page

Orgaran—Cont.

uate the carcinogenic potential of ORGARAN® (danaparoid sodium) Injection. ORGARAN® was not genotoxic in the Ames test, the *in vitro* CHL/HGPRT forward gene mutation assay, the *in vitro* CHO cell chromosome aberration test, the *in vitro* HeLa cell unscheduled DNA synthesis (UDS) test or the *in vivo* mouse micronucleus test. ORGARAN® at intravenous doses of up to 1090 anti-Xa units/kg/day was found to have no effect on fertility or reproductive performance of male and female rats. This dose is 5.9 times the recommended human subcutaneous dose based on body surface area (50 kg body weight and 1.46 m^2 body surface area assumed).

Pregnancy: Teratogenic effects. Pregnancy Category B. Teratology studies have been performed in pregnant rats at intravenous doses up to 1600 anti-Xa units/kg/day (8.7 times the recommended human dose based on body surface area) and pregnant rabbits at intravenous doses up to 780 anti-Xa units/kg/day (6 times the recommended human dose based on body surface area) and have not revealed evidence of impaired fertility or harm to the fetus due to ORGARAN® (danaparoid sodium) Injection. There are, however, no adequate and well-controlled studies in pregnant women. Because animal reproduction studies are not always predictive of human response, this drug should be used during pregnancy only if clearly needed.

Nursing Mothers: It is not known whether ORGARAN® (danaparoid sodium) Injection is excreted in breast milk. Because many drugs are excreted in human milk, caution should be exercised when ORGARAN® is administered to a nursing woman.

Pediatric Use: Safety and effectiveness of ORGARAN® (danaparoid sodium) Injection in pediatric patients have not been established.

ADVERSE REACTIONS

The following table summarizes adverse bleeding events that occurred in clinical trials which studied ORGARAN® (danaparoid sodium) Injection compared to placebo, warfarin, and others (heparin, heparin/DHE, acetylsalicylic acid, dextran, and low-molecular weight heparins).

[See first table at top of previous page]

Other: The following table summarizes adverse events that occurred at a frequency greater than, or equal to, 2% of patients in clinical trials for the prophylaxis of DVT and PE following elective hip surgery which studied ORGARAN® (danaparoid sodium) Injection compared to placebo, warfarin, and others (dextran, heparin/DHE, aspirin).

[See second table at top of previous page]

In addition, the following table summarizes adverse events that occurred at a frequency greater than, or equal to, 2% of patients in clinical trials for the prophylaxis of DVT and PE which studied ORGARAN® (danaparoid sodium) Injection compared to placebo, warfarin, and others (heparin, heparin sodium, heparin calcium, enoxaparin, dalteparin, dextran, heparin/DHE, aspirin).

[See third table at top of previous page]

OVERDOSAGE

Symptoms/Treatment: Accidental overdosage following administration of ORGARAN® (danaparoid sodium) Injection may lead to bleeding complications. The effects of ORGARAN® on anti-Xa activity cannot be antagonized with any known agent at this time. Although protamine sulfate partially neutralizes the anti-Xa activity of ORGARAN® and can be safely co-administered, there is no evidence that protamine sulfate is capable of reducing severe non-surgical bleeding during treatment with ORGARAN®. In the event of serious bleeding, ORGARAN® should be stopped and blood or blood product transfusions should be administered as needed. Withdrawal of ORGARAN® may be expected to restore the coagulation balance without rebound phenomenon.

Single subcutaneous doses of ORGARAN® at 3800 anti-Xa units/kg (20.5 times the recommended human dose based on body surface area) and 15200 anti-Xa units/kg (82 times the recommended human dose based on body surface area) were lethal to female and male rats, respectively. Symptoms of acute toxicity after intravenous dosing were respiratory depression, prostration and twitching.

DOSAGE AND ADMINISTRATION

Usual Adult Dosage:

In patients undergoing hip replacement surgery, the recommended dose of ORGARAN® (danaparoid sodium) Injection is 750 anti-Xa units twice daily administered by subcutaneous injection beginning 1–4 hours pre-operatively, and then not sooner than two hours after surgery. Treatment should be continued throughout the period of post-operative care until the risk of deep vein thrombosis has diminished. The average duration of administration in clinical trials was 7 to 10 days, up to 14 days. Patients with serum creatinine ≥2.0 mg/dL should be carefully monitored.

Administration:

ORGARAN® (danaparoid sodium) Injection is intended for subcutaneous administration and should not be administered by intramuscular injection. Subcutaneous injection technique: Patients should be lying down and ORGARAN® Injection administered by deep subcutaneous injection using a fine needle (25 to 26 gauge) to minimize tissue trauma. Administration should be alternated between the left and right anterolateral and left and right posterolateral abdominal wall. The whole length of the needle should be introduced into a skin fold held gently between the thumb and forefinger; the skin fold should be held throughout the injection and should neither be pinched nor rubbed afterwards.

Parenteral drug products should be inspected visually for particulate matter and discoloration prior to administration whenever solution and container permit.

HOW SUPPLIED

ORGARAN® (danaparoid sodium) Injection is supplied in:

—Ampules containing 0.6 mL (750 anti-Xa units) of danaparoid sodium: boxes of 10, NDC 0052-0830-11.

—Disposable prefilled syringes containing 0.6 mL (750 anti-Xa) units of danaparoid sodium: boxes of 10, NDC 0052-0830-61. Each ORGARAN™ prefilled syringe is affixed with a 25 gauge ×5/8 inch needle.

Storage:

—Ampules should be stored at temperatures of 2°–30°C (36°–86°F).

—Syringes should be stored at a refrigerated temperature of 2°–8°C (36°–46°F).

—Protect from light.

Rx only

Organon Inc.
West Orange, N.J. 07052

5310150 1/98

Shown in Product Identification Guide, page 327

PAVULON® ℞

[pāv-u-lon]

(pancuronium bromide) injection

HOW SUPPLIED

2 mL ampuls—2 mg/mL—boxes of 25—NDC-0052-0444-26
5 mL ampuls—2 mg/mL—boxes of 25—NDC-0052-0444-25
10 mL vials—1 mg/mL—boxes of 25—NDC-0052-0443-25

PREGNYL® ℞

(chorionic gonadotropin for injection, U.S.P.)

DESCRIPTION

Human chorionic gonadotropin (HCG), a polypeptide hormone produced by the human placenta, is composed of an alpha and a beta sub-unit. The alpha sub-unit is essentially identical to the alpha sub-units of the human pituitary gonadotropins, luteinizing hormone (LH) and follicle-stimulating hormone (FSH), as well as to the alpha sub-unit of human thyroid-stimulating hormone (TSH). The beta sub-units of these hormones differ in amino acid sequence.

PREGNYL® (chorionic gonadotropin for injection, USP) is a highly purified pyrogen-free preparation obtained from the urine of pregnant females. It is standardized by a biological assay procedure. It is available for intramuscular injection in multiple dose vials containing 10,000 USP Units of sterile dried powder with 5 mg. monobasic sodium phosphate and 4.4 mg. dibasic sodium phosphate. If required, pH is adjusted with sodium hydroxide and/or phosphoric acid. Each package also contains a 10 mL vial of solvent (water for injection with 0.56% sodium chloride and 0.9% benzyl alcohol). If required, pH is adjusted with sodium hydroxide and/or hydrochloric acid.

CLINICAL PHARMACOLOGY

The action of HCG is virtually identical to that of pituitary LH although HCG appears to have a small degree of FSH activity as well. It stimulates production of gonadal steroid hormones by stimulating the interstitial cells, (Leydig cells) of the testis to produce androgens and the corpus luteum of the ovary to produce progesterone.

Androgen stimulation in the male leads to the development of secondary sex characteristics and may stimulate testicular descent when no anatomical impediment to descent is present. This descent is usually reversible when HCG is discontinued. During the normal menstrual cycle, LH participates with FSH in the development and maturation of the normal ovarian follicle and the mid-cycle LH surge triggers ovulation. HCG can substitute for LH in this function.

During a normal pregnancy, HCG secreted by the placenta maintains the corpus luteum after LH secretion decreases, supporting continued secretion of estrogen and progesterone and preventing menstruation. HCG HAS NO KNOWN EFFECT ON FAT MOBILIZATION, APPETITE OR SENSE OF HUNGER, OR BODY FAT DISTRIBUTION.

INDICATIONS

HCG HAS NOT BEEN DEMONSTRATED TO BE EFFECTIVE ADJUNCTIVE THERAPY IN THE TREATMENT OF OBESITY. THERE IS NO SUBSTANTIAL EVIDENCE THAT IT INCREASES WEIGHT LOSS BEYOND THAT RESULTING FROM CALORIC RESTRICTION, THAT IT CAUSES A MORE ATTRACTIVE OR "NORMAL" DISTRIBUTION OF FAT, OR THAT IT DECREASES THE HUNGER AND DISCOMFORT ASSOCIATED WITH CALORIE-RESTRICTED DIETS.

1. Prepubertal cryptorchidism not due to anatomical obstruction. In general, HCG is thought to induce testicular descent in situations when descent would have occurred at puberty. HCG thus may help predict whether or not orchioplexy will be needed in the future. Although, in some cases, descent following HCG administration is permanent, in most cases, the response is temporary. Therapy is usually instituted between the ages 4 and 9.
2. Selected cases of hypogonadotropic hypogonadism (hypogonadism secondary to a pituitary deficiency) in males.
3. Induction of ovulation and pregnancy in the anovulatory, infertile woman in whom the cause of anovulation is secondary and not due to primary ovarian failure and who has been appropriately pretreated with human menotropins.

CONTRAINDICATIONS

Precocious puberty, prostatic carcinoma or other androgen-dependent neoplasm, prior allergic reaction to HCG.

WARNINGS

HCG should be used in conjunction with human menopausal gonadotropins only by physicians experienced with infertility problems who are familiar with the criteria for patient selection, contraindications, warnings, precautions and adverse reactions described in the package insert for menotropins.

The principal serious adverse reactions during this use are: (1) Ovarian hyperstimulation, a syndrome of sudden ovarian enlargement, ascites with or without pain, and/or pleural effusion, (2) Rupture of ovarian cysts with resultant hemoperitoneum, (3) Multiple births, and (4) Arterial thromboembolism.

PRECAUTIONS

1. Induction of androgen secretion by HCG may induce precocious puberty in patients treated for cryptorchidism. Therapy should be discontinued if signs of precocious puberty occur.
2. Since androgens may cause fluid retention, HCG should be used with caution in patients with cardiac or renal disease, epilepsy, migraine, or asthma.

ADVERSE REACTIONS

Headache, irritability, restlessness, depression, fatigue, edema, precocious puberty, gynecomastia, pain at the site of injection.

DOSAGE AND ADMINISTRATION

For intramuscular use only. The dosage regimen employed in any particular case will depend upon the indication for use, the age and weight of the patient, and the physician's preference. The following regimens have been advocated by various authorities:

Prepubertal cryptorchidism not due to anatomical obstruction.

1. 4,000 U.S.P. Units three times weekly for three weeks.
2. 5,000 U.S.P. Units every second day for four injections.
3. 15 injections of 500 to 1,000 U.S.P. Units over a period of six weeks.
4. 500 U.S.P. Units three times weekly for four to six weeks. If this course of treatment is not successful, another series is begun one month later, giving 1,000 U.S.P. Units per injection.

Selected cases of hypogonadotropic hypogonadism in males.

1. 500 to 1,000 U.S.P. Units three times a week for three weeks, followed by the same dose twice a week for three weeks.
2. 4,000 U.S.P. Units three times weekly for six to nine months, following which the dosage may be reduced to 2,000 U.S.P. Units three times weekly for an additional three months.

Induction of ovulation and pregnancy in the anovulatory, infertile woman in whom the cause of anovulation is secondary and not due to primary ovarian failure and who has been appropriately pretreated with human menotropins. (See prescribing information for menotropins for dosage and administration for that drug product).

5,000 to 10,000 USP Units one day following the last dose of menotropins. (A dosage of 10,000 U.S.P. Units is recommended in the labeling for menotropins).

IMPORTANT: USE COMPLETELY AFTER RECONSTITUTION. RECONSTITUTED SOLUTION IS STABLE FOR 60 DAYS WHEN REFRIGERATED.

HOW SUPPLIED

Two-vial package containing:
1–10 mL lyophilized multiple dose vial containing:
10,000 USP Units chorionic gonadotropin per vial, NDC 0052-0315-10.
1–10 mL vial of solvent containing:
water for injection with sodium chloride 0.56% and benzyl alcohol 0.9%, NDC 0052-0325-10.
When reconstituted, each 10 mL vial contains:

Chorionic gonadotropin	10,000 USP Units
Monobasic sodium phosphate	5 mg.
Dibasic sodium phosphate	4.4 mg.
Sodium chloride	0.56%
Benzyl alcohol	0.9%

If required pH adjusted with sodium hydroxide and/or phosphoric acid.

STORAGE

Store at 15°–30°C (59°–86°F). Reconstituted material will remain stable for 60 days when refrigerated.

CAUTION

Federal law prohibits dispensing without prescription.

DIRECTIONS FOR RECONSTITUTION

Two vial package: Withdraw sterile air from lyophilized vial and inject into diluent vial. Remove 1–10 mL from diluent and add to lyophilized vial; agitate gently until powder is completely dissolved in solution.
Parenteral drug products should be inspected visually for particulate matter and discoloration prior to administration, whenever solution and container permit.
Organon Inc.
West Orange, NJ 07052
5310122 Revised 3/95

REGONOL® ℞

[*re-gō-nol*]
(pyridostigmine bromide) injection, USP

HOW SUPPLIED

5 mg/mL: 2 mL ampuls—boxes of 25—NDC-0052-0460-02
5 mg/mL: 5 mL vials— boxes of 25—NDC-0052-0460-05

REMERON® ℞

(mirtazapine) Tablets

5310179 7/97

DESCRIPTION

REMERON® (mirtazapine) is an antidepressant for oral administration. It has a tetracyclic chemical structure unrelated to selective serotonin reuptake inhibitors, tricyclics or monoamine oxidase inhibitors (MAOI). Mirtazapine belongs to the piperazino-azepine group of compounds. It is designated 1,2,3,4,10,14b-hexahydro-2-methylpyrazino [2,1-a]pyrido [2,3-c]benzazepine and has the empirical formula of $C_{17}H_{19}N_3$. Its molecular weight is 265.36. The structural formula is the following and it is the racemic mixture:

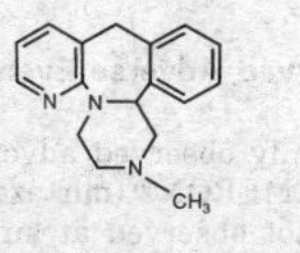

Mirtazapine is a white to creamy white crystalline powder which is slightly soluble in water.
REMERON® is supplied for oral administration as scored film-coated tablets containing 15 or 30 mg of mirtazapine. Each tablet also contains corn starch, hydroxypropyl cellulose, magnesium stearate, colloidal silicon dioxide, lactose and other inactive ingredients.

CLINICAL PHARMACOLOGY

Pharmacodynamics

The mechanism of action of REMERON® (mirtazapine), as with other antidepressants, is unknown.
Evidence gathered in preclinical studies suggests that mirtazapine enhances central noradrenergic and serotonergic activity. These studies have shown that mirtazapine acts as an antagonist at central presynaptic α_2 adrenergic inhibitory autoreceptors and heteroreceptors, an action that is postulated to result in an increase in central noradrenergic and serotonergic activity.
Mirtazapine is a potent antagonist of 5-HT_2 and 5-HT_3 receptors. Mirtazapine has no significant affinity for the 5-HT_{1A} and 5-HT_{1B} receptors.
Mirtazapine is a potent antagonist of histamine (H_1) receptors, a property that may explain its prominent sedative effects.
Mirtazapine is a moderate peripheral α_1 adrenergic antagonist, a property that may explain the occasional orthostatic hypotension reported in association with its use.
Mirtazapine is a moderate antagonist at muscarinic receptors, a property that may explain the relatively low incidence of anticholinergic side effects associated with its use.

Pharmacokinetics

REMERON® (mirtazapine) is rapidly and completely absorbed following oral administration and has a half-life of about 20–40 hours. Peak plasma concentrations are reached within about 2 hours following an oral dose. The presence of food in the stomach has a minimal effect on both the rate and extent of absorption and does not require a dosage adjustment.
Mirtazapine is extensively metabolized after oral administration. Major pathways of biotransformation are demethylation and hydroxylation followed by glucuronide conjugation. In vitro data from human liver microsomes indicate that cytochrome 2D6 and 1A2 are involved in the formation of the 8-hydroxy metabolite of mirtazapine, whereas cytochrome 3A is considered to be responsible for the formation of the N-desmethyl and N-oxide metabolite. Mirtazapine has an absolute bioavailability of about 50%. It is eliminated predominantly via urine (75%) with 15% in feces. Several unconjugated metabolites possess pharmacological activity but are present in the plasma at very low levels. The (−) enantiomer has an elimination half-life that is approximately twice as long as the (+) enantiomer and therefore achieves plasma levels that are about three times as high as that of the (+) enantiomer.
Plasma levels are linearly related to dose over a dose range of 15 to 80 mg. The mean elimination half-life of mirtazapine after oral administration ranges from approximately 20–40 hours across age and gender subgroups, with females of all ages exhibiting significantly longer elimination half-lives than males (mean half-life of 37 hours for females *vs.* 26 hours for males). Steady state plasma levels of mirtazapine are attained within 5 days, with about 50% accumulation (accumulation ratio = 1.5).
Mirtazapine is approximately 85% bound to plasma proteins over a concentration range of 0.01 to 10 μg/mL.

Population Subgroups

Liver Disease—Following a single 15 mg oral dose of mirtazapine, the oral clearance of mirtazapine was decreased by approximately 30% in hepatically impaired patients compared to subjects with normal hepatic function. Caution is indicated in administering REMERON® (mirtazapine) to patients with compromised hepatic function (see PRECAUTIONS and DOSAGE AND ADMINISTRATION).
Renal Disease—Following a single 15 mg oral dose of mirtazapine, patients with moderate [glomerular filtration rate (GFR) = 11–39 mL/min/1.73 m^2] and severe [GFR <10 mL/min/1.73 m^2] renal impairment had reductions in mean oral clearance of mirtazapine of about 30% and 50%, respectively, compared to normal subjects. Caution is indicated in administering REMERON® to patients with compromised renal function (see PRECAUTIONS and DOSAGE AND ADMINISTRATION).
Elderly Patients—Following oral administration of mirtazapine 20 mg/day for 7 days to subjects of varying ages (range, 25–74), oral clearance of mirtazapine was reduced in the elderly compared to the younger subjects. The differences were most striking in males, with a 40% lower clearance in elderly males compared to younger males, while the clearance in elderly females was only 10% lower compared to younger females. Caution is indicated in administering REMERON® to elderly patients (see PRECAUTIONS and DOSAGE AND ADMINISTRATION).

Clinical Trials Showing Effectiveness

The efficacy of REMERON® (mirtazapine) as a treatment for depression was established in four placebo-controlled, 6-week trials in adult outpatients meeting DSM-III criteria for major depression. Patients were titrated with mirtazapine from a dose range of 5 mg up to 35 mg/day. Overall, these studies demonstrated mirtazapine to be superior to placebo on at least three of the following four measures: 21-Item Hamilton Depression Rating Scale (HDRS) total score; HDRS Depressed Mood Item; CGI Severity score; and Montgomery and Asberg Depression Rating Scale (MADRS). Superiority of mirtazapine over placebo was also found for certain factors of the HDRS including anxiety/somatization factor and sleep disturbance factor. The mean mirtazapine dose for patients who completed these four studies ranged from 21 to 32 mg/day. A fifth study of similar design utilized a higher dose (up to 50 mg) per day and also showed effectiveness.
Examination of age and gender subsets of the population did not reveal any differential responsiveness on the basis of these subgroupings.

INDICATIONS AND USAGE

REMERON® (mirtazapine) Tablets are indicated for the treatment of depression.
The efficacy of REMERON® in the treatment of depression was established in six week controlled trials of outpatients whose diagnoses corresponded most closely to the Diagnostic and Statistical Manual of Mental Disorders–3rd edition (DSM-III) category of major depressive disorder (see CLINICAL PHARMACOLOGY).
A major depressive episode (DSM-IV) implies a prominent and relatively persistent (nearly every day for at least 2 weeks) depressed or dysphoric mood that usually interferes with daily functioning, and includes at least five of the following nine symptoms: depressed mood, loss of interest in usual activities, significant change in weight and/or appetite, insomnia or hypersomnia, psychomotor agitation or retardation, increased fatigue, feelings of guilt or worthlessness, slowed thinking or impaired concentration, a suicide attempt or suicidal ideation.
The antidepressant effectiveness of REMERON® (mirtazapine) in hospitalized depressed patients has not been adequately studied.
The effectiveness of REMERON® in long-term use, that is, for more than 6 weeks, has not been systematically evaluated in controlled trials. Therefore, the physician who elects to use REMERON® for extended periods should periodically evaluate the long-term usefulness of the drug for the individual patient.

CONTRAINDICATIONS

REMERON® (mirtazapine) Tablets are contraindicated in patients with a known hypersensitivity to mirtazapine.

WARNINGS

Agranulocytosis

In premarketing clinical trials, two (one with Sjögren's Syndrome) out of 2,796 patients treated with REMERON® (mirtazapine) Tablets developed agranulocytosis [absolute neutrophil count (ANC) <500/mm^3 with associated signs and symptoms, e.g., fever, infection, etc.] and a third patient developed severe neutropenia [ANC <500/mm^3 without any associated symptoms]. For these three patients, onset of severe neutropenia was detected on days 61, 9, and 14 of treatment, respectively. All three patients recovered after REMERON® was stopped. These three cases yield a crude incidence of severe neutropenia (with or without associated infection) of approximately 1.1 per thousand patients exposed, with a very wide 95% confidence interval, i.e., 2.2 cases per 10,000 to 3.1 cases per 1000. If a patient develops a sore throat, fever, stomatitis or other signs of infection, along with a low WBC count, treatment with REMERON® should be discontinued and the patient should be closely monitored.

MAO Inhibitors

In patients receiving other antidepressants in combination with a monoamine oxidase inhibitor (MAOI) and in patients who have recently discontinued an antidepressant drug and then are started on an MAOI, there have been reports of serious, and sometimes fatal, reactions, e.g., including nausea, vomiting, flushing, dizziness, tremor, myoclonus, rigidity, diaphoresis, hyperthermia, autonomic instability with rapid fluctuations of vital signs, seizures, and mental status changes ranging from agitation to coma. Although there are no human data pertinent to such an interaction with REMERON® (mirtazapine), it is recommended that REMERON® not be used in combination with an MAOI, or within 14 days of initiating or discontinuing therapy with an MAOI.

PRECAUTIONS

General

Somnolence

In U.S. controlled studies, somnolence was reported in 54% of patients treated with REMERON® (mirtazapine), compared to 18% for placebo and 60% for amitriptyline. In these studies, somnolence resulted in discontinuation for 10.4% of REMERON® treated patients, compared to 2.2% for placebo. It is unclear whether or not tolerance develops to the somnolent effects of REMERON®. Because of REMERON®'s potentially significant effects on impairment of performance, patients should be cautioned about engaging in activities requiring alertness until they have been able to assess the drug's effect on their own psychomotor performance (see Information for Patients).

Dizziness

In U.S. controlled studies, dizziness was reported in 7% of patients treated with REMERON® (mirtazapine), compared to 3% for placebo and 14% for amitriptyline. It is unclear whether or not tolerance develops to the dizziness observed in association with the use of REMERON®.

Increased Appetite/Weight Gain

In U.S. controlled studies, appetite increase was reported in 17% of patients treated with REMERON® (mirtazapine), compared to 2% for placebo and 6% for amitriptyline. In these same trials, weight gain of ≥7% of body weight was reported in 7.5% of patients treated with mirtazapine, compared to 0% for placebo and 5.9% for amitriptyline. In a pool of premarketing U.S. studies, including many patients in long-term, open label treatment, 8% of patients receiving REMERON® discontinued for weight gain.

Cholesterol/Triglycerides

In U.S. controlled studies, nonfasting cholesterol increases to ≥20% above the upper limits of normal were observed in 15% of patients treated with REMERON® (mirtazapine), compared to 7% for placebo and 8% for amitriptyline. In these same studies, nonfasting triglyceride increases to

Continued on next page

Remeron—Cont.

≥500 mg/dL were observed in 6% of patients treated with mirtazapine, compared to 3% for placebo and 3% for amitriptyline.

Transaminase Elevations

Clinically significant ALT (SGPT) elevations (≥3 times the upper limit of the normal range) were observed in 2.0% (8/424) of patients exposed to REMERON® (mirtazapine) in a pool of short-term U.S. controlled trials, compared to 0.3% (1/328) of placebo patients and 2.0% (3/181) of amitriptyline patients. Most of these patients with ALT increases did not develop signs or symptoms associated with compromised liver function. While some patients were discontinued for the ALT increases, in other cases, the enzyme levels returned to normal despite continued REMERON® treatment. Mirtazapine should be used with caution in patients with impaired hepatic function (see Pharmacokinetics section of CLINICAL PHARMACOLOGY, and DOSAGE AND ADMINISTRATION).

Activation of Mania/Hypomania

Mania/hypomania occurred in approximately 0.2% (3/1,299 patients) of REMERON® (mirtazapine) treated patients in U.S. studies. Although the incidence of mania/hypomania was very low during treatment with mirtazapine, it should be used carefully in patients with a history of mania/hypomania.

Seizure

In premarketing clinical trials only one seizure was reported among the 2,796 U.S. and non-U.S. patients treated with REMERON® (mirtazapine). However, no controlled studies have been carried out in patients with a history of seizures. Therefore, care should be exercised when mirtazapine is used in these patients.

Suicide

Suicidal ideation is inherent in depression and may persist until significant remission occurs. As with any patient receiving antidepressants, high-risk patients should be closely supervised during initial drug therapy. Prescriptions of REMERON® (mirtazapine) should be written for the smallest quantity consistent with good patient management, in order to reduce the risk of overdose.

Use in Patients with Concomitant Illness

Clinical experience with REMERON® (mirtazapine) in patients with concomitant systemic illness is limited. Accordingly, care is advisable in prescribing mirtazapine for patients with diseases or conditions that affect metabolism or hemodynamic responses.

Mirtazapine has not been systematically evaluated or used to any appreciable extent in patients with a recent history of myocardial infarction or other significant heart disease. Mirtazapine was not associated with clinically significant ECG abnormalities in U.S. and non-U.S. placebo controlled trials. Mirtazapine was associated with significant orthostatic hypotension in early clinical pharmacology trials with normal volunteers. Orthostatic hypotension was infrequently observed in clinical trials with depressed patients. REMERON® should be used with caution in patients with known cardiovascular or cerebrovascular disease that could be exacerbated by hypotension (history of myocardial infarction, angina, or ischemic stroke) and conditions that would predispose patients to hypotension (dehydration, hypovolemia, and treatment with antihypertensive medication).

Mirtazapine clearance is decreased in patients with moderate [glomerular filtration rate (GFR) = 11–39 mL/min/1.73 m²] and severe [GFR <10 mL/min/1.73 m²] renal impairment, and also in patients with hepatic impairment (see Pharmacokinetics subsection of CLINICAL PHARMACOLOGY). Caution is indicated in administering REMERON® to such patients (see DOSAGE AND ADMINISTRATION).

Information for Patients

Physicians are advised to discuss the following issues with patients for whom they prescribe REMERON® (mirtazapine):

Agranulocytosis

Patients who are to receive REMERON® (mirtazapine) should be warned about the risk of developing agranulocytosis. Patients should be advised to contact their physician if they experience any indication of infection such as fever, chills, sore throat, mucous membrane ulceration or other possible signs of infection. Particular attention should be paid to any flu-like complaints or other symptoms that might suggest infection.

Interference with Cognitive and Motor Performance

REMERON® (mirtazapine) may impair judgement, thinking, and, particularly, motor skills, because of its prominent sedative effect. The drowsiness associated with mirtazapine use may impair a patient's ability to drive, use machines or perform tasks that require alertness. Thus, patients should be cautioned about engaging in hazardous activities until they are reasonably certain that REMERON® therapy does not adversely affect their ability to engage in such activities.

Completing Course of Therapy

While patients may notice improvement with REMERON® (mirtazapine) therapy in 1 to 4 weeks, they should be advised to continue therapy as directed.

Concomitant Medication

Patients should be advised to inform their physician if they are taking, or intend to take, any prescription or over-the-counter drugs since there is a potential for REMERON® (mirtazapine) to interact with other drugs.

Alcohol

The impairment of cognitive and motor skills produced by REMERON® (mirtazapine) has been shown to be additive with those produced by alcohol. Accordingly, patients should be advised to avoid alcohol while taking mirtazapine.

Pregnancy

Patients should be advised to notify their physician if they become pregnant or intend to become pregnant during REMERON® (mirtazapine) therapy.

Nursing

Patients should be advised to notify their physician if they are breast-feeding an infant.

Laboratory Tests

There are no routine laboratory tests recommended.

Drug Interactions

As with other drugs, the potential for interaction by a variety of mechanisms (e.g., pharmacodynamic, pharmacokinetic inhibition or enhancement, etc.) is a possibility (see CLINICAL PHARMACOLOGY).

Drugs Affecting Hepatic Metabolism

The metabolism and pharmacokinetics of REMERON® (mirtazapine) may be affected by the induction or inhibition of drug-metabolizing enzymes.

Drugs that are Metabolized by and/or Inhibit Cytochrome P450 Enzymes

Many drugs are metabolized by and/or inhibit various cytochrome P450 enzymes, e.g., 2D6, 1A2, 3A4, etc. In vitro studies have shown that REMERON® (mirtazapine) is a substrate for several of these enzymes, including 2D6, 1A2, and 3A4. While in vitro studies have shown that mirtazapine is not a potent inhibitor of any of these enzymes, an indication that mirtazapine is not likely to have a clinically significant inhibitory effect on the metabolism of other drugs that are substrates for these cytochrome P450 enzymes, the concomitant use of mirtazapine with most other drugs metabolized by these enzymes has not been formally studied. Consequently, it is not possible to make any definitive statements about the risks of coadministration of mirtazapine with such drugs.

Alcohol

Concomitant administration of alcohol (equivalent to 60 g) had a minimal effect on plasma levels of REMERON® (mirtazapine) (15 mg) in 6 healthy male subjects. However, the impairment of cognitive and motor skills produced by REMERON® were shown to be additive with those produced by alcohol. Accordingly, patients should be advised to avoid alcohol while taking REMERON®.

Diazepam

Concomitant administration of diazepam (15 mg) had a minimal effect on plasma levels of mirtazapine (15 mg) in 12 healthy subjects. However, the impairment of motor skills produced by REMERON® (mirtazapine) has been shown to be additive with those caused by diazepam. Accordingly, patients should be advised to avoid diazepam and other similar drugs while taking REMERON®.

Carcinogenesis, Mutagenesis, Impairment of Fertility

Carcinogenesis

Carcinogenicity studies were conducted with REMERON® (mirtazapine) given in the diet at doses of 2, 20, and 200 mg/kg/day to mice and 2, 20, and 60 mg/kg/day to rats. The highest doses used are approximately 20 and 12 times the maximum recommended human dose (MRHD) of 45 mg/day on a mg/m² basis in mice and rats, respectively. There was an increased incidence of hepatocellular adenoma and carcinoma in male mice at the high dose. In rats, there was an increase in hepatocellular adenoma in females at the mid and high doses and in hepatocellular tumors and thyroid follicular adenoma/cystadenoma and carcinoma in males at the high dose. The data suggest that the above effects could possibly be mediated by non-genotoxic mechanisms, the relevance of which to humans is not known.

The doses used in the mouse study may not have been high enough to fully characterize the carcinogenic potential of REMERON®.

Mutagenesis

REMERON® (mirtazapine) was not mutagenic or clastogenic and did not induce general DNA damage as determined in several genotoxicity tests: Ames test, in vitro gene mutation assay in Chinese hamster V 79 cells, in vitro sister chromatid exchange assay in cultured rabbit lymphocytes, in vivo bone marrow micronucleus test in rats, and unscheduled DNA synthesis assay in HeLa cells.

Impairment of Fertility

In a fertility study in rats, REMERON® (mirtazapine) was given at doses up to 100 mg/kg (20 times the maximum recommended human dose (MRHD) on a mg/m² basis). Mating and conception were not affected by the drug, but estrous cycling was disrupted at doses that were 3 or more times the MRHD and pre-implantation losses occurred at 20 times the MRHD.

Pregnancy

Teratogenic Effects–Pregnancy Category C

Reproduction studies in pregnant rats and rabbits at doses up to 100 mg/kg and 40 mg/kg, respectively (20 and 17 times the maximum recommended human dose (MRHD) on a mg/m² basis, respectively), have revealed no evidence of teratogenic effects. However, in rats, there was an increase in post-implantation losses in dams treated with REMERON® (mirtazapine). There was an increase in pup deaths during the first 3 days of lactation and a decrease in pup birth weights. The cause of these deaths is not known. These effects occurred at doses that were 20 times the MRHD, but not at 3 times the MRHD, on a mg/m² basis. There are no adequate and well controlled studies in pregnant women. Because animal reproduction studies are not always predictive of human response, this drug should be used during pregnancy only if clearly needed.

Nursing Mothers

It is not known whether mirtazapine is excreted in human milk. Because many drugs are excreted in human milk, caution should be exercised when REMERON® (mirtazapine) Tablets are administered to nursing women.

Pediatric Use

Safety and effectiveness in pediatric patients have not been established.

Geriatric Use

Approximately 190 elderly individuals (≥65 years of age) participated in clinical studies with REMERON® (mirtazapine). No unusual adverse age-related phenomena were identified in this group. Pharmacokinetic studies revealed a decreased clearance in the elderly. Caution is indicated in administering REMERON® to elderly patients (see CLINICAL PHARMACOLOGY and DOSAGE AND ADMINISTRATION).

ADVERSE REACTIONS

Associated with Discontinuation of Treatment

Approximately 16 percent of the 453 patients who received REMERON® (mirtazapine) in U.S. 6-week controlled clinical trials discontinued treatment due to an adverse experience, compared to 7 percent of 361 placebo-treated patients in those studies. The most common events (≥1%) associated with discontinuation and considered to be drug related (i.e., those events associated with dropout at a rate at least twice that of placebo) included:

Common Adverse Events Associated with Discontinuation of Treatment in 6-Week U.S. REMERON® Trials

Adverse Event	Percentage of Patients Discontinuing with Adverse Event	
	REMERON® (n=453)	Placebo (n=361)
Somnolence	10.4%	2.2%
Nausea	1.5%	0%

Commonly Observed Adverse Events in U.S. Controlled Clinical Trials

The most commonly observed adverse events associated with the use of REMERON® (mirtazapine) (incidence of 5% or greater) and not observed at an equivalent incidence among placebo-treated patients (REMERON® incidence at least twice that for placebo) were:

Common Treatment-Emergent Adverse Events Associated with the Use of REMERON® in 6-Week U.S. Trials

Adverse Event	Percentage of Patients Reporting Adverse Event	
	REMERON® (n=453)	Placebo (n=361)
Somnolence	54%	18%
Increased Appetite	17%	2%
Weight Gain	12%	2%
Dizziness	7%	3%

Adverse Events Occurring at an Incidence of 1% or More Among REMERON® Treated Patients

The table that follows enumerates adverse events that occurred at an incidence of 1% or more, and were more frequent than in the placebo group, among REMERON® (mirtazapine)-treated patients who participated in short-term U.S. placebo-controlled trials in which patients were dosed in a range of 5 to 60 mg/day. This table shows the percentage of patients in each group who had at least one episode of

an event at some time during their treatment. Reported adverse events were classified using a standard COSTART-based dictionary terminology.

The prescriber should be aware that these figures cannot be used to predict the incidence of side effects in the course of usual medical practice where patient characteristics and other factors differ from those which prevailed in the clinical trials. Similarly, the cited frequencies cannot be compared with figures obtained from other investigations involving different treatments, uses and investigators. The cited figures, however, do provide the prescribing physician with some basis for estimating the relative contribution of drug and non-drug factors to the side effect incidence rate in the population studied.

INCIDENCE OF ADVERSE CLINICAL EXPERIENCES[1] (≥1%) IN SHORT-TERM U.S. CONTROLLED STUDIES

Body System / Adverse Clinical Experience	REMERON® (n=453)	Placebo (n=361)
Body as a Whole		
Asthenia	8%	5%
Flu Syndrome	5%	3%
Back Pain	2%	1%
Digestive System		
Dry Mouth	25%	15%
Increased Appetite	17%	2%
Constipation	13%	7%
Metabolic and Nutritional Disorders		
Weight Gain	12%	2%
Peripheral Edema	2%	1%
Edema	1%	0%
Musculoskeletal System		
Myalgia	2%	1%
Nervous System		
Somnolence	54%	18%
Dizziness	7%	3%
Abnormal Dreams	4%	1%
Thinking Abnormal	3%	1%
Tremor	2%	1%
Confusion	2%	0%
Respiratory System		
Dyspnea	1%	0%
Urogenital System		
Urinary Frequency	2%	1%

[1] Events reported by at least 1% of patients treated with REMERON® (mirtazapine) are included, except the following events which had an incidence on placebo ≥REMERON®: headache, infection, pain, chest pain, palpitation, tachycardia, postural hypotension, nausea, dyspepsia, diarrhea, flatulence, insomnia, nervousness, libido decreased, hypertonia, pharyngitis, rhinitis, sweating, amblyopia, tinnitus, taste perversion.

ECG Changes

In an analysis of ECGs obtained in U.S. placebo-controlled clinical trials, REMERON® (mirtazapine) and placebo-treated patients had a similar incidence of abnormal changes from baseline at 6–8 weeks of approximately 3%. The abnormalities were generally not considered clinically significant.

Other Adverse Events Observed During the Premarketing Evaluation of REMERON®

During its premarketing assessment, multiple doses of REMERON® (mirtazapine) were administered to 2,796 patients in clinical studies. The conditions and duration of exposure to mirtazapine varied greatly, and included (in overlapping categories) open and double-blind studies, uncontrolled and controlled studies, inpatient and outpatient studies, fixed dose and titration studies. Untoward events associated with this exposure were recorded by clinical investigators using terminology of their own choosing. Consequently, it is not possible to provide a meaningful estimate of the proportion of individuals experiencing adverse events without first grouping similar types of untoward events into a smaller number of standardized event categories.

In the tabulations that follow, reported adverse events were classified using a standard COSTART-based dictionary terminology. The frequencies presented, therefore, represent the proportion of the 2,796 patients exposed to multiple doses of REMERON® who experienced an event of the type cited on at least one occasion while receiving REMERON®. All reported events are included except those already listed in the previous table, those adverse experiences subsumed under COSTART terms that are either overly general or excessively specific so as to be uninformative, and those events for which a drug cause was very remote.

It is important to emphasize that, although the events reported occurred during treatment with REMERON®, they were not necessarily caused by it.

Events are further categorized by body system and listed in order of decreasing frequency according to the following definitions: frequent adverse events are those occurring on one or more occasions in at least 1/100 patients; infrequent adverse events are those occurring in 1/100 to 1/1000 patients; rare events are those occurring in fewer than 1/1000 patients. Only those events not already listed in the previous table appear in this listing. Events of major clinical importance are also described in the WARNINGS and PRECAUTIONS sections.

Body as a Whole: *frequent:* malaise, abdominal pain, abdominal syndrome acute; *infrequent:* chills, fever, face edema, ulcer, photosensitivity reaction, neck rigidity, neck pain, abdomen enlarged; *rare:* cellulitis, chest pain substernal.

Cardiovascular System: *frequent:* hypertension, vasodilatation; *infrequent:* angina pectoris, myocardial infarction, bradycardia, ventricular extrasystoles, syncope, migraine, hypotension; *rare:* atrial arrhythmia, bigeminy, vascular headache, pulmonary embolus, cerebral ischemia, cardiomegaly, phlebitis, left heart failure.

Digestive System: *frequent:* vomiting, anorexia; *infrequent:* eructation, glossitis, cholecystitis, nausea and vomiting, gum hemorrhage, stomatitis, colitis, liver function tests abnormal; *rare:* tongue discoloration, ulcerative stomatitis, salivary gland enlargement, increased salivation, intestinal obstruction, pancreatitis, aphthous stomatitis, cirrhosis of liver, gastritis, gastroenteritis, oral moniliasis, tongue edema.

Endocrine System: *rare:* goiter, hypothyroidism.

Hemic and Lymphatic System: *rare:* lymphadenopathy, leukopenia, petechia, anemia, thrombocytopenia, lymphocytosis, pancytopenia.

Metabolic and Nutritional Disorders: *frequent:* thirst; *infrequent:* dehydration, weight loss; *rare:* gout, SGOT increased, healing abnormal, acid phosphatase increased, SGPT increased, diabetes mellitus.

Musculoskeletal System: *frequent:* myasthenia, arthralgia; *infrequent:* arthritis, tenosynovitis; *rare:* pathological fracture, osteoporosis fracture, bone pain, myositis, tendon rupture, arthrosis, bursitis.

Nervous System: *frequent:* hypesthesia, apathy, depression, hypokinesia, vertigo, twitching, agitation, anxiety, amnesia, hyperkinesia, paresthesia; *infrequent:* ataxia, delirium, delusions, depersonalization, dyskinesia, extrapyramidal syndrome, libido increased, coordination abnormal, dysarthria, hallucinations, manic reaction, neurosis, dystonia, hostility, reflexes increased, emotional lability, euphoria, paranoid reaction; *rare:* aphasia, nystagmus, akathisia, stupor, dementia, diplopia, drug dependence, paralysis, grand mal convulsion, hypotonia, myoclonus, psychotic depression, withdrawal syndrome.

Respiratory System: *frequent:* cough increased, sinusitis; *infrequent:* epistaxis, bronchitis, asthma, pneumonia; *rare:* asphyxia, laryngitis, pneumothorax, hiccup.

Skin and Appendages: *frequent:* pruritus, rash; *infrequent:* acne exfoliative dermatitis, dry skin, herpes simplex, alopecia; *rare:* urticaria, herpes zoster, skin hypertrophy, seborrhea, skin ulcer.

Special Senses: *infrequent:* eye pain, abnormality of accommodation, conjunctivitis, deafness, keratoconjunctivitis, lacrimation disorder, glaucoma, hyperacusis, ear pain; *rare:* blepharitis, partial transitory deafness, otitis media, taste loss, parosmia.

Urogenital System: *frequent:* urinary tract infection; *infrequent:* kidney calculus, cystitis, dysuria, urinary incontinence, urinary retention, vaginitis, hematuria, breast pain, amenorrhea, dysmenorrhea, leukorrhea, impotence; *rare:* polyuria, urethritis, metrorrhagia, menorrhagia, abnormal ejaculation, breast engorgement, breast enlargement, urinary urgency.

DRUG ABUSE AND DEPENDENCE

Controlled Substance Class

REMERON® (mirtazapine) Tablets are not a controlled substance.

Physical and Psychological Dependence

REMERON® (mirtazapine) has not been systematically studied in animals or humans for its potential for abuse, tolerance or physical dependence. While clinical trials did not reveal any tendency for any drug-seeking behavior, these observations were not systematic and it is not possible to predict on the basis of this limited experience the extent to which a CNS-active drug will be misused, diverted and/or abused once marketed. Consequently, patients should be evaluated carefully for history of drug abuse, and such patients should be observed closely for signs of mirtazapine misuse or abuse (e.g., development of tolerance, incrementations of dose, drug-seeking behavior).

OVERDOSAGE

Human Experience

There is very limited experience with REMERON® (mirtazapine) overdose. In premarketing clinical studies, there were eight reports of mirtazapine overdose alone or in combination with other pharmacological agents. The only drug overdose death reported while taking REMERON® Tablets was in combination with amitriptyline and chlorprothixene in a non-U.S. clinical study. Based on plasma levels, the REMERON® dose taken was 30–45 mg, while plasma levels of amitriptyline and chlorprothixene were found to be at toxic levels. All other premarketing overdose cases resulted in full recovery. Signs and symptoms reported in association with overdose included disorientation, drowsiness, impaired memory, and tachycardia. There were no reports of ECG abnormalities, coma or convulsions following overdose with REMERON® alone.

Overdose Management

Treatment should consist of those general measures employed in the management of overdose with any antidepressant. There are no specific antidotes for REMERON® (mirtazapine). If the patient is unconscious, establish and maintain an airway to ensure adequate oxygenation and ventilation. Gastric evacuation either by the induction of emesis or lavage or both should be considered. Activated charcoal should also be considered in treatment of overdose. Cardiac and vital signs monitoring is recommended along with general symptomatic and supportive measures.

In managing overdosage, consider the possibility of multiple-drug involvement. The physician should consider contacting a poison control center for additional information on the treatment of any overdose.

DOSAGE AND ADMINISTRATION

Initial Treatment

The recommended starting dose for REMERON® (mirtazapine) is 15 mg/day, administered in a single dose, preferably in the evening prior to sleep. In the controlled clinical trials establishing the antidepressant efficacy of REMERON®, the effective dose range was generally 15–45 mg/day. While the relationship between dose and antidepressant response for REMERON® has not been adequately explored, patients not responding to the initial 15 mg dose may benefit from dose increases up to a maximum of 45 mg/day. REMERON® has an elimination half-life of approximately 20–40 hours; therefore, dose changes should not be made at intervals of less than one to two weeks in order to allow sufficient time for evaluation of the therapeutic response to a given dose.

Elderly and Patients with Renal or Hepatic Impairment

The clearance of mirtazapine is reduced in elderly patients and in patients with moderate to severe renal or hepatic impairment. Consequently, the prescriber should be aware that plasma mirtazapine levels may be increased in these patient groups, compared to levels observed in younger adults without renal or hepatic impairment (see Pharmacokinetics subsection of CLINICAL PHARMACOLOGY).

Maintenance/Extended Treatment

There is no body of evidence available from controlled trials to indicate how long the depressed patient should be treated with REMERON® (mirtazapine). It is generally agreed, however, that pharmacological treatment for acute episodes of depression should continue for up to six months or longer. Whether the dose of antidepressant needed to induce remission is identical to the dose needed to maintain euthymia is unknown.

Switching Patients To or From a Monoamine Oxidase Inhibitor

At least 14 days should elapse between discontinuation of an MAOI and initiation of therapy with REMERON® (mirtazapine). In addition, at least 14 days should be allowed after stopping REMERON® before starting an MAOI.

HOW SUPPLIED

REMERON® (mirtazapine) Tablets are supplied as:

15 mg Tablets—oval, scored, yellow, coated, with "Organon" embossed on one side and "TZ3" on the other side.

Bottles of 30	NDC# 0052-0105-30
Unit Dose, Box of 100	NDC# 0052-0105-90*

30 mg Tablets—oval, scored, red-brown, coated, with "Organon" embossed on one side and "TZ5" on the other side.

Bottles of 30	NDC# 0052-0107-30
Unit Dose, Box of 100	NDC# 0052-0107-90*

*Unit dose packs are provided as a blisterpack with 10 strips, each of which contains 10 tablets.

Store at controlled Room Temperature
20°–25°C (68°–77°F)

Dispense in a tight, light resistant container.

Caution: Federal law prohibits dispensing without prescription.

Manufactured for Organon Inc.
West Orange, NJ 07052
by N.V.Organon, OSS, Holland

Shown in Product Identification Guide, page 327

REVERSOL® ℞

(edrophonium chloride) injection, USP

HOW SUPPLIED

10 mg/mL: 10 mL Multiple Dose Vials-boxes of 25-NDC-0052-0466-34

Continued on next page

SUCCINYLCHOLINE CHLORIDE INJECTION, ℞
USP

HOW SUPPLIED

20 mg/mL: 10 mL vials-boxes of 25-NDC-0052-0445-10

TICE® BCG   ℞
BCG VACCINE USP
(for Intravesical or Percutaneous use)

DESCRIPTION

TICE® BCG, a BCG Vaccine for intravesical or percutaneous use, is an attenuated, live culture preparation of the Bacillus of Calmette and Guerin (BCG) strain *Mycobacterium bovis*.[1] The TICE strain was developed at the University of Illinois from a strain originated at the Pasteur Institute. The medium in which the BCG organism is grown for preparation of the freeze-dried cake is composed of the following ingredients: glycerin, asparagine, citric acid, potassium phosphate, magnesium sulfate, and iron ammonium citrate. The final preparation prior to freeze-drying also contains lactose. The freeze-dried BCG preparation is delivered in glass-sealed ampules, each containing 1 to 8×10^8 colony forming units (CFU) of TICE BCG which is equivalent to approximately 50 mg wet weight.
No preservatives have been added.

CLINICAL PHARMACOLOGY

Intravesical Use for Carcinoma In Situ of the Bladder. TICE BCG induces a granulomatous reaction at the local site of administration.[2] Intravesical TICE BCG has been used as a therapy for and prophylaxis against recurrent tumors in patients with carcinoma in situ (CIS) of the bladder. The precise mechanism of action is unknown. A variety of different treatment regimens have been used with the TICE[3-6] and other BCG substrains.[7-12]
An evaluation of intravesical administration of TICE BCG in patients with carcinoma in situ of the urinary bladder was recently completed. Bladder cancer patients were identified who had been treated with TICE BCG under six different Investigational New Drug (IND) applications in which the most important shared aspect was the use of an induction plus maintenance schedule. Comparison of demographic data between the six INDs revealed uniformity. Among these six studies were 119 evaluable patients who received intravesical treatment of CIS of the bladder. Patients with biopsy-proven CIS received TICE BCG (50 mg; $1–8 \times 10^8$ CFU) intravesically, once weekly for at least 6 weeks and once monthly thereafter for up to 12 months. A longer maintenance was given in some cases. Follow-up cystoscopies were performed at 3 month intervals, as were urine cytologies for most patients (71 of 119). Urine cytology was obtained at the time of the 1989 follow-up for all patients who responded to TICE BCG *treatment, (CR and CRNC, see below)*. The median time post treatment for these follow-up cytologies was 47 months.
The study population consisted of 153 patients; 132 males, 19 females and 2 unidentified as to gender. Thirty patients lacking baseline documentation of CIS and 4 patients lost to follow-up were not evaluable for treatment response. Therefore, 119 patients with biopsy or cystoscopy proven CIS prior to TICE BCG administration were available for efficacy evaluation. Some of these patients had undergone transurethral resection (TUR) one or more weeks prior to BCG, primarily for the treatment of papillomatous disease. The mean age for the CIS population was 68.8 ± 9.7 years s.d. (range: 38–97 years).
Sixty-three evaluable patients had received intravesical chemotherapy treatment for their bladder malignancy prior to TICE BCG treatment and had been diagnosed as treatment failures. The treatment had been as follows: thiotepa (30), mitomycin C (10), doxorubicin (1), mitomycin C and thiotepa (14), doxorubicin and thiotepa (1), doxorubicin and mitomycin C (1), thiotepa, mitomycin C and doxorubicin (2), interferon (1), interferon and thiotepa (1), cyclophosphamide IV (1), and cisplatin and thiotepa (1).
For the 119 patients with biopsy or cystoscopy proven CIS, the TICE BCG induction dosage consisted of a mean of 6.6 instillations (± 1.5 standard error of the mean). These patients also received a mean of 10.0 maintenance instillations after completing the induction phase. Twenty patients (16.8%) required TICE BCG reinduction at some point in the study. Nine patients in one of the six studies received a percutaneous dose along with intravesical instillation. Data from a recent study show that a percutaneous dose with CIS is unnecessary.[13]
Clinical response criteria were defined as follows:
Complete Histological Response (CR): Complete resolution of carcinoma in situ documented by biopsy or, if a biopsy was not obtained, then by negative cystoscopy. All patients in this category were required to have urine cytology tests that were negative upon examination.
Complete Clinical Response Without Cytology (CRNC): Patients in this category had an apparent complete disappear-

ance of tumor that was not confirmed by urine cytology tests. Complete resolution of carcinoma in situ documented by a biopsy or, if a biopsy was not obtained, then by negative cystoscopy.
Failure/Progression: Patients in this category had urine cytology tests that were found to be positive, although biopsy or cystoscopy was negative. This category also includes patients who continued to have evidence of malignant lesions, or a progression to a higher stage or grade; the appearance of new lesions; reappearance of old lesions.
A 75.6 percent response rate was reported for 119 evaluable patients (Table 1).

TABLE 1: RESPONSE OF PATIENTS TO TICE BCG IN CIS BLADDER CANCER

	Entered	Evaluable	CR	CRNC	Overall Response
No. of Patients	153	119	54	36	90
% Response	—		45.4%	30.2%	75.6%

The median duration of follow-up for the 1989 update, presented in Table 2, is 47 months. Of the 54 patients classified as CR in 1987, 30 remained without evidence of disease (CR) in 1989, whereas 6 patients died of unrelated disease and 18 relapsed. The 15 of 36 patients classified as CRNC in 1987 who remained without evidence of disease in 1989 were all found to meet the criteria of CR status on the basis of negative cytologies. In the interim, 4 CRNC patients died of unrelated diseases, 2 died of unknown causes, and 15 relapsed. Therefore, of the 90 overall responders (75.6%), 36.7 percent of patients relapsed, 13.3 percent died of other diseases, and 50 percent remained in CR. In addition, two patients who relapsed were reinduced in complete response by a second course of TICE BCG.

TABLE 2: THERAPEUTIC EFFICACY OF TICE BCG IN CIS BLADDER CANCER 1989 STATUS OF 90 RESPONDERS (CR OR CRNC)

Response	1987/CR n = 54	1987/CRNC n = 36	1987 Response n = 90	Percent
CR	30	15	45	50.0
CRNC	0	0	0	0.0
Unrelated Deaths	6	6	12	13.3
Failure	18	15	33	36.7

Among the 119 evaluable patients there was no significant difference in response rates between patients with or without prior intravesical chemotherapy: 45 of 63 (71%) versus 45 of 56 (80%), p >.05. Similarly, for the patients remaining in CR at the time of the 1989 evaluation, there was no significant difference between those with or without prior chemotherapy.
The median duration of response, calculated from the Kaplan-Meier curve as median time to recurrence, is estimated at 4 years or greater. The median duration of follow-up was 47 months. Of the total 90 responders, 45 patients (50%) remained without evidence of disease.
At a median follow-up of 47 months, 85 (71.4%) of the 119 evaluable patients remain alive. Thirteen patients (10.9%) died from causes unrelated to bladder cancer: cardiovascular disease (6 patients), second primary cancer (3 patients), and other (4 patients). Three patients died from unknown causes and bladder cancer cannot be ruled out. The bladder cancer related deaths were 18 (15%) of the 119. Historical data prior to the use of BCG, in a series of CIS patients treated usually with electrofulguration, indicate 82% of the patients recurred, 60% of the patients developed invasive cancer, and 34% of the patients died of their disease within 5 years.[14]
The incidence of cystectomy for 90 patients who achieved a complete response (CR or CRNC) with TICE BCG was 11%. For 29 patients who did not achieve CR or CRNC, the incidence of cystectomy was 55%, which is consistent with cystectomy rates reported in the literature for CIS patients who were not treated with intravesical therapies.[15]
The median time to cystectomy in patients who achieved a complete response (CR or CRNC) exceeded 74 months, whereas the median time to cystectomy for non-responders was 31 months.
Percutaneous Use for Immunization Against Tuberculosis. Immunization with BCG vaccine lowers the risk of serious complications of primary tuberculosis in children.[16-19] Estimates of efficacy from observational studies in areas where vaccination is performed at birth show that the incidence of tuberculous meningitis and miliary tuberculosis is 52%–100% lower and that the incidence of pulmonary tuberculosis is 2%–80% lower in vaccinated children less than 15 years of age than in unvaccinated controls.[16-21] However, estimates of vaccine efficacy may be distorted because of the

following: vaccination was not allocated randomly in observational studies; there were differences in BCG strains, methods, and routes of administration; and there were differences in the characteristics of the populations and environments in which the vaccines have been studied.[22]

INDICATIONS AND USAGE

Intravesical Use for Carcinoma In Situ of the Bladder. Intravesical instillation of TICE BCG is indicated for the treatment of carcinoma in situ of the bladder in the following situations: (1) primary treatment in the absence of an associated invasive cancer without papillary tumors or with papillary tumors after TUR, (2) secondary treatment in the absence of an associated invasive cancer, in patients failing to respond or relapsing after intravesical chemotherapy with other agents, (3) primary or secondary treatment in the absence of invasive cancer for patients with medical contraindications to radical surgery. TICE BCG is not indicated for the treatment of papillary tumors occurring alone.
Percutaneous Use for Immunization Against Tuberculosis. Exposed tuberculin skin test-negative infants and children: BCG vaccination is recommended for infants and children with negative tuberculin skin test who are (1) at high risk to intimate and prolonged exposure to persistently untreated or ineffectively treated patients with infectious pulmonary tuberculosis and who cannot be removed from the source of exposure and cannot be placed on long-term preventive therapy, or (2) continuously exposed to persons with tuberculosis who have bacilli resistant to isoniazid and rifampin.[22]
Groups with an excessive rate of new infections: BCG vaccination is also recommended for tuberculin-negative infants and children in groups in which the rate of new infections exceeds 1% per year and for whom the usual surveillance and treatment programs have been attempted but are not operationally feasible. These groups include persons without regular access to health care, those for whom usual health care is culturally or socially unacceptable, or groups who have demonstrated an inability to effectively use existing accessible care.
The US Immunization Practices Advisory Committee (ACIP) no longer recommends the use of BCG vaccination of health care workers at risk of repeated exposure to tuberculosis but recommends that these individuals be under tuberculin skin testing surveillance and receive isoniazid prophylaxis in case of tuberculin skin test conversion.[22]
For international travelers, the Centers for Disease Control (CDC) recommends that BCG vaccination be considered only for travelers with insignificant reaction to tuberculin skin test who will be in a high-risk environment for prolonged periods of time without access to tuberculin skin test surveillance.[22]

CONTRAINDICATIONS

Intravesical Use for Carcinoma In Situ of the Bladder. TICE BCG should not be used in immunosuppressed patients or persons with congenital or acquired immune deficiencies, whether due to concurrent disease (e.g., AIDS, leukemia, lymphoma) or cancer therapy (e.g., cytotoxic drugs, radiation). TICE BCG should be avoided in asymptomatic carriers with a positive HIV serology and in patients receiving steroids at immunosuppressive doses or other immunosuppressive therapies because of the possibility of the vaccine establishing a systemic infection.
Treatment should be postponed until resolution of a concurrent febrile illness, urinary tract infection, or gross hematuria. Seven to fourteen days should elapse before BCG is administered following biopsy, TUR, or traumatic catheterization.
A positive Mantoux test is a contraindication only if there is evidence of an active tuberculosis infection.
In the absence of safety data, intravesical TICE BCG should not be given to pregnant or lactating women.
Percutaneous Use for Immunization Against Tuberculosis. TICE BCG Vaccine for the prevention of tuberculosis should not be given to persons with impaired immune responses, whether they be congenital, disease produced, drug or therapy induced (i.e., cytotoxic drugs and radiation used in cancer therapy). The concurrent use of steroids requires caution because of the possibility of the vaccine establishing a systemic infection. If necessary, the infection can be treated with anti-tuberculous drugs.

WARNINGS

Intravesical Use for Carcinoma In Situ of the Bladder. TICE BCG is not a vaccine for the prevention of cancer.
There are currently no data on the effectiveness of intravesical installation of TICE BCG in the treatment of invasive bladder cancer.
The use of TICE BCG may cause tuberculin sensitivity. Since this is a valuable aid in the diagnosis of tuberculosis, it may therefore be useful to determine the tuberculin reactivity by PPD skin testing before treatment.
Intravesical instillations should be postponed in the presence of fever, suspected infection, or during treatment with antibiotics, since antimicrobial therapy may interfere with the effectiveness of TICE BCG.
Instillation of TICE BCG onto a bleeding mucosa may promote systemic BCG infection.[23] Death has been reported as a result of systemic BCG infection and sepsis. Patients should be monitored for the presence of symptoms and signs of toxicity after each intravesical treatment. Febrile epi-

sodes with flu-like symptoms lasting more than 48 hours, fever ≥103°F, systemic manifestations increasing in intensity with repeated instillations, or persistent abnormalities of liver function tests suggest systemic BCG infection and require anti-tuberculous therapy (see **ADVERSE REACTIONS** section).

Small bladder capacity has been associated with increased risk of severe local reactions and should be considered in deciding to use TICE BCG therapy.

Percutaneous Use for Immunization Against Tuberculosis. Administration should be percutaneous with the multiple puncture disc as described below. DO NOT INJECT INTRAVENOUSLY, SUBCUTANEOUSLY, OR INTRADERMALLY. TICE BCG Vaccine should not be used in infants, children, or adults with severe immune deficiency syndromes. Children with family history of immune deficiency disease should not be vaccinated. If they are, an infectious disease specialist should be consulted and anti-tuberculous therapy[24] administered if clinically indicated.

PRECAUTIONS

General: TICE BCG contains live bacteria and should be used with aseptic technique. All equipment, supplies, and receptacles in contact with TICE BCG should be handled and disposed of as biohazardous.

The possibility of allergic reactions should be assessed. TICE BCG administration should not be attempted in individuals with severe immune deficiency disease. TICE BCG Vaccine should be administered with caution to persons in groups at high risk for HIV infection.

Intravesical Use for Carcinoma In Situ of the Bladder.

General: Care should be taken not to traumatize the urinary tract or to introduce contaminants into the urinary system. Seven to fourteen days should elapse before BCG is administered following TUR, biopsy, or traumatic catheterization.

Information For Patients: TICE BCG is retained in the bladder 2 hours and then voided. Patients should void while seated for safety reasons following instillation of suspension. Within 6 hours after treatment, urine voided should be disinfected for 15 minutes with an equal volume of household bleach before flushing. Patients should be instructed to increase fluid intake to "flush" the bladder in the hours following BCG treatment. Patients may experience burning with the first void after treatment. Patients should be attentive to side effects, such as fever, chills, malaise, flu-like symptoms, or increased fatigue. If patient experiences severe urinary side effects, such as burning or pain on urination, urgency, frequency of urination, blood in urine, joint pain, cough, or skin rash, the physician should be notified.

Drug Interaction: Drug combinations containing immunosuppressants and/or bone marrow depressants and/or radiation interfere with the development of the immune response and should not be used in combination with TICE BCG. Antimicrobial therapy for other infections may interfere with the effectiveness of TICE BCG therapy.

Pregnancy Category C: Animal reproduction studies have not been conducted with TICE BCG. It is also not known whether TICE BCG can cause fetal harm when administered to a pregnant woman or can affect reproductive capacity. TICE BCG should be given to a pregnant woman only if clearly needed. Women should be advised not to become pregnant while on therapy.

Nursing Mothers: It is not known whether TICE BCG is excreted in human milk. Because many drugs are excreted in human milk and because of the potential for serious adverse reactions from TICE BCG in nursing infants, a decision should be made whether to discontinue nursing or to discontinue the drug, taking into account the importance of the drug to the mother.

Pediatric Use: Safety and effectiveness of carcinoma *in situ* of the urinary bladder in children have not been established.

Percutaneous Use for Immunization Against Tuberculosis.

Normal Reaction: The intensity and duration of the local reaction depends on the depth of penetration of the multiple-puncture disc and individual variations in patients' tissue reactions. The initial skin lesions usually appear within 10–14 days and consist of small red papules at the site. The papules reach maximum diameter (about 3 mm) after 4 to 6 weeks, after which they may scale and then slowly subside. Six months afterward there is usually no visible sign of the vaccination, but on occasion a faintly discernible pattern of the disc points may be visible. On people whose skin tends to keloid formation, there may be slightly more visible evidence of the vaccination.

Vaccination is recommended only for those who are tuberculin negative to a recent skin test with 5 tuberculin units (5TU). Otherwise, vaccination of persons highly sensitive to mycobacterial antigens can result in hypersensitivity reactions including fever, anorexia, myalgia, and neuralgia, which last a few days.

After TICE BCG vaccination, it is usually not possible to clearly distinguish between a tuberculin reaction caused by persistent postvaccination sensitivity and one caused by a virulent suprainfection. Caution is advised in attributing a positive skin test to TICE BCG vaccination. A sharp rise in the tuberculin reaction since the latest test should be further investigated (except in the immediate postvaccination period).

TABLE 3: SUMMARY OF ADVERSE EFFECTS SEEN IN 674 PATIENTS WITH SUPERFICIAL BLADDER CANCER, INCLUDING 153 WITH CARCINOMA IN SITU

Local Adverse Effects	Number of Patients	Percent (%)	Toxicity by Grade (%)* Mild	Moderate	Severe	Not Stated
Dysuria	401	59.5	28.2	18.1	10.7	2.5
Urinary Frequency	272	40.4	17.2	15.7	7.4	—
Hematuria	175	26.0	8.2	9.6	7.4	0.8
Cystitis	40	5.9	1.6	2.4	1.9	—
Urgency	39	5.8	1.2	1.8	1.3	1.5
Nocturia	30	4.5	1.3	1.8	0.6	0.7
Cramps/Pain	27	4.0	0.9	1.3	0.9	0.9
Urinary Incontinence	16	2.4	0.4	0.9	—	1.2
Urinary Debris	15	2.2	0.2	1.0	0.4	0.6
Genital Inflammation/ Abscess	12	1.8	0.3	0.4	0.4	0.6
Urinary Tract Infection	10	1.5	0.2	0.3	0.9	0.2
Urethritis	8	1.2	0.3	0.6	—	0.3
Pyuria	5	0.7	0.2	0.1	0.1	0.3
Epididymitis/Prostatitis	2	0.3	—	—	—	0.3
Urinary Obstruction	2	0.3	—	—	—	0.3
Contracted Bladder	1	0.2	—	—	—	0.2
Orchitis	1	0.2	—	—	—	0.2
Systemic Adverse Effects	**Number of Patients**	**Percent (%)**	**Toxicity by Grade (%)* Mild**	**Moderate**	**Severe**	**Not Stated**
Flu-like Syndrome**	224	33.2	9.3	10.9	9.0	4.0
Fever	134	19.9	6.1	5.3	7.6	0.9
Malaise/Fatigue	50	7.4	2.7	3.1	—	1.6
Shaking Chills	22	3.3	0.2	1.5	1.0	0.6
Nausea/Vomiting	20	3.0	1.0	1.6	0.3	—
Arthritis/Myalgia	18	2.7	0.3	1.0	0.4	0.9
Headache/Dizziness	16	2.4	0.3	0.9	—	1.2
Anorexia/Weight Loss	15	2.2	0.4	1.3	0.1	0.5
Allergic	14	2.1	0.6	0.7	0.4	0.3
Cardiac	13	1.9	—	0.3	1.3	0.3
Respiratory (Unclassified)	11	1.6	0.4	0.4	0.2	0.6
Abdominal Pain	10	1.5	—	0.6	0.6	0.3
Anemia	9	1.3	0.2	0.6	0.4	0.1
Diarrhea	8	1.2	0.2	0.6	0.1	0.3
Pneumonitis	8	1.2	0.2	—	0.6	0.4
Gastrointestinal (Unclassified)	7	1.0	0.2	0.1	—	0.7
Neurologic	6	0.9	0.1	—	0.3	0.4
Rash	4	0.6	—	0.4	0.2	—
BCG Sepsis	3	0.4	—	—	0.4	—
Coagulopathy	2	0.3	—	—	0.3	—
Leukopenia	2	0.3	0.2	0.1	—	—
Thrombocytopenia	2	0.3	0.2	0.1	—	—
Hepatic Granuloma	1	0.2	—	—	0.2	—
Hepatitis	1	0.2	—	—	0.2	—

* Grade was determined using ECOG scale of toxicity criteria, Mild = Grade 1, Moderate = Grade 2, Severe = Grade 3 or 4.

** Flu-like syndrome includes fever, shaking chills, malaise and myalgia.

Information For Patients: Keep the vaccination site clean until the local reaction has disappeared.

Drug Interaction: Antimicrobial or immunosuppressive agents may interfere with the development of the immune response and should be used only under medical supervision.

Pregnancy Category C: Animal reproduction studies have not been conducted with TICE BCG. It is also not known whether TICE BCG can cause fetal harm when administered to a pregnant woman or can affect reproduction capacity. TICE BCG should be given to a pregnant woman only if clearly needed.

Nursing Mothers: It is not known whether TICE BCG is excreted in human milk. Because many drugs are excreted in human milk and because of the potential for serious adverse reactions in nursing infants from TICE BCG, a decision should be made whether to discontinue nursing or not to vaccinate, taking into account the importance of tuberculosis vaccination to the mother.

Pediatric Use: See **Treatment and Schedule** under **DOSAGE AND ADMINISTRATION** section. Precautions should be taken with respect to infants vaccinated with BCG and exposed to persons with active tuberculosis.[25]

ADVERSE REACTIONS

Intravesical Use for Carcinoma In Situ of the Bladder. Adverse reactions are often localized to the bladder but may be accompanied by systemic manifestations. Symptoms of bladder irritability, related to the inflammatory response induced by intravesical TICE BCG, are reported in 60 percent of cases. They begin 3–4 hours after instillation and last 24–72 hours. The urinary side effects are usually seen after the third treatment and tend to increase in severity after each administration. There were, however, no long-term urinary complications in this group of patients.

A summary of adverse reactions seen with 674 patients with superficial bladder cancer, including 153 CIS patients treated intravesically with TICE BCG is shown in Table 3.[26] Irritative bladder adverse effects associated with BCG administration can be managed symptomatically with pyridium, propantheline bromide or oxybutynin chloride, and acetaminophen or ibuprofen.[27] Systemic adverse effects such as malaise, fever, and chills may reflect hypersensitivity reactions and can be treated with antihistamines.[27] The "flu-like" syndrome of 1–2 days' duration that frequently accompanies intravesical BCG administration should be managed by standard symptomatic treatment. Symptoms persisting longer than 2 days suggest continued infection, and consideration should be given to therapy with isoniazid. Localized (e.g., prostatitis, epididymitis) as well as systemic infection can occur with intravesical BCG administration. For systemic infection, an infectious diseases specialist should be consulted and the patient promptly treated with anti-tuberculous therapy as advised.[28] At least two deaths have been reported as a result of systemic BCG infection and sepsis.[27] There have been two cases of nephrogenic adenoma, a benign lesion of bladder epithelium, associated with intravesical BCG therapy.[29] In general, the adverse effects of BCG therapy in bladder carcinoma have been of short duration and moderate morbidity.

Percutaneous Use for Immunization Against Tuberculosis. Occasionally, lymphadenopathy of the regional lymph node, which spontaneously resolves itself, is seen in young children. Only rarely does the node create a fistula followed by a short period of drainage. The usual treatment is to maintain cleanliness of the site of drainage and allow the lesion to heal spontaneously without medical intervention.

Other rare events are osteomyelitis, lupoid reactions, disseminated BCG infection, and death. Osteomyelitis has been reported to occur at a rate of about 1 per 1,000,000 vaccinees.[22] Disseminated BCG infection and death are very rare (about 1 per 5,000,000 vaccinees)[30] and occur almost exclusively in children with impaired immune responses.

[See table above]

OVERDOSAGE

Intravesical Use for Carcinoma In Situ of the Bladder. Overdosage occurs if more than one vial of TICE BCG is administered per instillation. The patient should be closely monitored for signs of systemic BCG infection and treated with anti-tuberculous medication (see **ADVERSE REACTIONS** section).

Continued on next page

Tice BCG—Cont.

Percutaneous Use of Immunization Against Tuberculosis.
Accidental overdosages if treated immediately with anti-tuberculous drugs have not led to complications.[31] If the vaccination response is allowed to progress it can still be treated successfully with anti-tuberculous drugs but complications can include regional adenitis, lupus vulgaris, subcutaneous cold abscesses, ocular lesions, and others.[32]

DOSAGE AND ADMINISTRATION

Intravesical Use for Carcinoma In Situ of the Bladder. The intravesical dose consists of *one vial* of TICE BCG suspended in 50 mL preservative-free saline. **Preparation of Agent:** The preparation of the TICE BCG suspensions should be done using sterile technique. The pharmacist or individual responsible for mixing the agent should wear gloves, mask, and gown to avoid inadvertent exposure of open sores or inhalation of BCG organisms. Draw 1 mL of sterile, preservative-free saline (0.9% Sodium Chloride Injection USP) at 4°–25°C, into a small (e.g., 3 mL) syringe and add to one vial of TICE BCG to resuspend. Gently swirl the vial until a homogeneous suspension is obtained. Avoid forceful agitation which may cause clumping of mycobacteria. Dispense the cloudy BCG suspension into the top end of a catheter-tip syringe which contains 49 mL saline diluent bringing the total volume to 50 mL. Gently rotate the syringe. The suspended TICE BCG should be used immediately after preparation. Discard after 2 hours.
Note: DO NOT filter the contents of the TICE BCG vial. Precautions should be taken to avoid exposing the TICE BCG to sunlight. Bacteriostatic solutions must be avoided. In addition, use only sterile preservative-free saline, 0.9% Sodium Chloride Injection USP, as diluent and perform all mixing operations in sterile glass or thermosetting plastic containers and syringes.
Treatment and Schedule: Allow 7–14 days to elapse after bladder biopsy or TUR before TICE BCG is administered. Patients should not drink fluids for 4 hours before treatment and should empty their bladder prior to TICE BCG administration. The reconstituted TICE BCG is instilled into the bladder by gravity flow via the catheter. DO NOT depress plunger and force the flow of the TICE BCG. The TICE BCG is retained in the bladder 2 hours and then voided. Patients unable to retain the suspension for 2 hours should be allowed to void sooner, if necessary. While the TICE BCG is retained in the bladder, the patient may be repositioned from left side to right side and also may alternately lie upon the back and the abdomen, changing these positions every 15 minutes to maximize bladder surface exposure to the agent.
A standard treatment schedule consists of one intravesical instillation per week for 6 weeks. This schedule may be repeated once if tumor remission has not been achieved and if the clinical circumstances warrant. Thereafter, intravesical TICE BCG administration should continue at approximately monthly intervals for at least 6–12 months.
Percutaneous Use for Immunization Against Tuberculosis.
Preparation of Agent: Using sterile methods, 1 mL of sterile water for injection, USP at 4°–25°C, is added to one vial of vaccine (see **Pediatric Dose** below for pediatric use). Draw the mixture into a syringe and expel it back into the vial three times to ensure thorough mixing.
Parenteral drug products should be inspected visually for particulate matter and discoloration prior to administration, whenever solution and container permit. Reconstitution should result in a uniform suspension of the bacilli.
Treatment and Schedule: The vaccine is to be administered after fully explaining the risks and benefits to the vaccinee, parent, or guardian. Cleanse the skin area over the deltoid muscle and allow to dry completely. Position the subject's arm such that the deltoid area is parallel to the floor, presenting a flat, plane for vaccine application. After the vaccine is prepared, the immunizing dose of 0.2–0.3 mL is dropped-on the cleansed surface of the skin, and administered percutaneously utilizing a sterile multipuncture disc. The multipuncture disc is a thin wafer-like stainless steel plate from which 36 points protrude. The disc is attached to a plastic handle for use. Lower the disc to the skin surface. Using the edge of the disc, in a "hopping" motion, spread the vaccine evenly over the area to be punctured (avoid pushing the vaccine to the sides of the area). Coat the prongs of the disc by lightly dipping them into the spread vaccine. While continuing to hold the skin taut, press downward on the disc allowing the points of the disc to penetrate the skin. Apply firm pressure so that the points of the disc penetrate to their full depth of 2mm. Continue firm pressure for 5–10 seconds. Do not "rock" the disc. Remove the disc, and with the skin still taut use the long edge of the disc to re-spread the vaccine so that all puncture areas are filled. Additional vaccine may be dropped onto the site and re-spread if necessary to assure a "wet" vaccine site. Release the tension on the skin. With the arm held in the horizontal position, allow the vaccine to dry to the arm. A loose dressing may be applied for 24 hours. Multipuncture discs (part number 597279) may be acquired from Organon Teknika Corporation, 100 Akzo Avenue, Durham, NC 27712; telephone (800) 662-6842.

Pediatric Dose: In infants less than 1 month old the dosage of vaccine should be reduced by one half, by using 2 mL of sterile water when reconstituting. If a vaccinated infant remains tuberculin negative to 5TU on skin testing, and if indications for vaccination persist, the infant should receive a full dose after 1 year of age.

HOW SUPPLIED

TICE BCG vaccine is supplied in a box of one 2 mL vial of TICE BCG. Each vial contains 1 to 8×10^8 CFU, which is equivalent to approximately 50 mg (wet weight), as lyophilized (freeze-dried) powder, NDC 0052-0601-01.

STORAGE

Storage of the intact vials of TICE BCG should be at refrigerated temperatures of 2–8°C (36–46°F). This agent contains live bacteria and should be protected from light. The product should not be used after the expiration date printed on the label.

REFERENCES

1. Guerin C: The history of BCG. In: Rosenthal SR (ed); BCG Vaccine: Tuberculosis-Cancer. Littleton, MA, PSG Publishing Co., Inc. 1980, pp. 35–43.
2. Kelley DR, Haaff E, Becich M, et al.: Prognostic value of purified protein derivative skin test and granuloma formation in patients treated with intravesical bacillus Calmette-Guerin. J Urol 1986; 135:268–271.
3. Brosman SA: The use of bacillus Calmette-Guerin in the therapy of bladder carcinoma in situ. J Urol 1985; 134: 36–39.
4. DeKernion JB, Huang M, Linder A, et al.: The management of superficial bladder tumors and carcinoma in situ with intravesical bacillus Calmette-Guerin. J Urol 1985; 133:598–601.
5. Guinan P, Batenhorst R: BCG in the treatment of superficial bladder cancer (Abstract). J Urol 1987; 137:180A.
6. Soloway M, Perry A: Bacillus Calmette-Guerin for treatment of superficial transitional cell carcinoma of the bladder in patients who have failed thiotepa and/or mitomycin C. J Urol 1987; 137:871–873.
7. Morales A: Long-term results and complications of intracavitary bacillus Calmette-Guerin therapy for bladder cancer. J Urol 1984; 132:457–459.
8. Haaff E, Dresner SM, Ratliff TL, Catalona WJ: Two courses of intravesical bacillus Calmette-Guerin for transitional cell carcinoma of the bladder. J Urol 1986; 136:820–824.
9. Herr HW, Pinsky CM, Whitmore WF, et al.: Effect of intravesical bacillus Calmette-Guerin (BCG) on carcinoma in situ. Cancer 1983; 51:1323–1326.
10. Kelley DR, Ratliff T, Catalona WJ, et al.: Intravesical bacillus Calmette-Guerin therapy for superficial bladder cancer. Effect of bacillus Calmette-Guerin viability on treatment results. J Urol 1985; 134:48–53.
11. Schellhammer PF, Ladaga LE, Fillion MB: Bacillus Calmette-Guerin for therapy of superficial transitional cell carcinoma of the bladder. J Urol 1986; 135:261–264.
12. Lamm DL: BCG immunotherapy in bladder cancer. In: Urology Annual 1987. Vol. 1, Appleton & Lange, Norwalk, CT, 1987; pp. 67–86.
13. Lamm DL, Sarosdy MS, DeHaven JI: Percutaneous, oral, or intravesical BCG administration: What is the optimal route? EORTC Genitourinary Group Monograph 6: BCG in Superficial Bladder Cancer. Alan R. Liss, Inc., New York, NY, 1989; pp. 301–310.
14. Utz DC, Hanash KA, Farrow GM: The plight of the patient with carcinoma in situ of the bladder. J Urol 1970; 103: 160–164.
15. Herr HW, Pinsky CM, Whitmore WF Jr., et al.: Long-term effect of intravesical bacillus Calmette-Guerin on flat carcinoma in situ of the bladder. J Urol 1986; 135: 265–267.
16. Romanus V: Tuberculosis in bacillus Calmette-Guerin immunized and unimmunized children in Sweden: a ten-year evaluation following the cessation of general bacillus Calmette-Guerin immunization of the newborn in 1975. Pediatr Infect Dis 1987; 6:272–280.
17. Smith PG: Case-control studies of the efficacy of BCG against tuberculosis. In: International Union Against Tuberculosis, Proceedings of the XXXVIth IUAT World Conference on Tuberculosis and Respiratory Diseases, Singapore. Professional Postgraduate Services, International, Japan, 1987; 73–79.
18. Padungchan S, Konjanart S, Kasiratta S, et al.: The effectiveness of BCG vaccination of the newborn against childhood tuberculosis in Bangkok. Bull WHO 1986; 64: 247–258.
19. Tidjani O, Amedone A, ten Dam HG: The protective effect of BCG vaccination of the newborn against childhood tuberculosis in an African community. Tubercle 1986; 67:269–281.
20. Young TK, Hershfield ES: A case-control study to evaluate the effectiveness of mass neonatal BCG vaccination among Canadian Indians. Am J Public Health 1986; 76: 783–786.
21. Shapiro C, Cook N, Evans D, et al.: A case-control study of BCG and childhood tuberculosis in Cali, Columbia. Int H Epidemiol 1985; 14:441–446.
22. Morbidity and Mortality Weekly Report 37, No. 43 1988; pp. 663–675.
23. Rawls WH, Lamm DL, Eyolfson MF: Septic complications in the use of bacillus Calmette-Guerin (BCG) for noninvasive transitional cell carcinoma. Presented at: 1988 Annual Meeting, American Urological Association, Boston, MA.
24. Lorin MI, Hsu KHK, Jacob SC: Treatment of tuberculosis in children. In: Symposium on anti-infective therapy. Pediatric Clinics of North America, 1983; 30:333–348.
25. Report of the Committee on the Control of Infectious Diseases. American Academy of Pediatrics 1988; 21st Edition.
26. Data on file. Organon Teknika Corporation/Biotechnology Research Institute, Rockville, MD.
27. Lamm DL, Steg A, Boccon-Gibod L, et al.: Complications of bacillus Calmette-Guerin immunotherapy: Review of 2602 patients and comparison of chemotherapy complications. EORTC Genitourinary Group Monograph 6: BCG in Superficial Bladder Cancer. Alan R. Liss, Inc., New York, NY, 1989; pp. 335–355.
28. Standard Therapy for Tuberculosis, 1985. Presented at: National Consensus Conference on Tuberculosis. Chest, 1985; 87 (Suppl):117S–124S.
29. Oates R, Siroky M: Nephrogenic adenoma of urinary bladder due to intravesical BCG therapy. J Urol 1986; 135:186.
30. Mande R: BCG Vaccination. Dawsons, London, 1968.
31. Griffith AH: Ten cases of BCG overdose treated with isoniazid. Tubercle 1963; 44:247–250.
32. Watkins SM: Unusual complications of BCG vaccination. Brit Med J 1971; 1:442.

Manufactured by: Organon Teknika Corporation
100 Akzo Avenue
Durham, NC 27704
Distributed by: Organon Inc.
West Orange, NJ 07052
U.S. License
No. 956
TICE® is a trademark licensed from the University of Illinois.
RM 034.2   Issue Date: January 1998
Shown in Product Identification Guide, page 327

WIGRAINE®
(ergotamine tartrate and caffeine tablets, USP)

℞

DESCRIPTION

Wigraine® Tablets: Each tablet contains the following:
Ergotamine Tartrate, USP .... 1 mg
Caffeine, USP .... 100 mg
Each tablet also contains: Lactose, Magnesium Stearate, Microcrystalline Cellulose, Corn Starch, Glycerin, Acacia Powder, Colloidal Silicon Dioxide, and Purified Water as inactive ingredients.
Wigraine® tablets are uncoated and prepared to insure rapid disintegration (by an exclusive manufacturing process) and facilitate quick absorption. Rapid onset of effect is important for the satisfactory treatment of acute attacks of vascular headaches.

CLINICAL PHARMACOLOGY

Ergotamine is an alpha adrenergic blocking agent with a direct stimulating effect on the smooth muscle of peripheral and cranial blood vessels and produces depression of central vasomotor centers. The compound also has the properties of serotonin antagonism. In comparison to hydrogenated ergotamine, the adrenergic blocking actions are less pronounced and vasoconstrictive actions are greater. Caffeine, also a cranial vasoconstrictor, is added to further enhance the vasoconstrictive effect without the necessity of increasing ergotamine dosage.

INDICATIONS AND USAGE

Wigraine® (ergotamine tartrate and caffeine tablets, USP) is indicated as therapy to abort or prevent vascular headaches such as migraine, migraine variants, or so-called histamine cephalalgia.

CONTRAINDICATIONS

Wigraine® can cause fetal harm when administered to a pregnant women. It can produce prolonged uterine contractions which can result in abortion. Wigraine® is contraindicated in women who are or may become pregnant. If this is used during pregnancy, or if the patient becomes pregnant while taking this drug, the patient should be advised of the potential hazard to the fetus.
Peripheral vascular disease, coronary heart disease, hypertension, impaired hepatic or renal function, sepsis and hypersensitivity to any of the components.

PRECAUTIONS

Although signs and symptoms of ergotism rarely develop even after long term intermittent use of the orally administered drug, care should be exercised to remain within the limits of recommended dosage.

Pregnancy Category X. See Contraindications section.

Nursing Mothers. It is not known whether the ergotamine tartrate in Wigraine® is excreted in human milk. Because some ergot alkaloids have been found in the milk of nursing mothers resulting in symptoms of ergotism in their children, a decision should be made whether to discontinue nursing or to discontinue the drug, taking into account the importance of the drug to the mother.

Pediatric Usage. Safety and effectiveness in children have not been established.

ADVERSE REACTIONS

In order of decreasing severity; precordial distress and pain, muscle pains in the extremities, numbness and tingling in fingers and toes, transient tachycardia or bradycardia, vomiting, nausea, weakness in the legs, diarrhea, localized edema and itching.

DOSAGE AND ADMINISTRATION

Best results are obtained if the tablets are administered at the first sign of an attack.

The average adult dose is 2 tablets at the start of a vascular headache (migraine) attack; followed by 1 additional tablet every $1/2$ hour if needed, up to 6 tablets per attack. Total weekly dosage should not exceed 10 tablets.

OVERDOSAGE

The toxic effects of an acute overdosage of Wigraine® are due primarily to the ergotamine component. The amount of caffeine is such that its toxic effects will be overshadowed by those of ergotamine. Symptoms include vomiting, numbness, tingling, pain and cyanosis of the extremities associated with diminished or absent peripheral pulses, hypertension or hypotension, drowsiness, stupor, coma, convulsions and shock. Treatment consists of removal of the offending drug by induction of emesis, gastric lavage and catharsis. Maintenance of adequate pulmonary ventilation, correction of hypotension, and control of convulsions are important considerations. Treatment of peripheral vasospasm should consist of warmth, but not heat, and protection of the ischemic limbs. Vasodilators may be used with benefit but caution must be exercised to avoid aggravating an already existing hypotension. The LD50 limits of the various components as outlined in NIOSH 1978 Registry of Toxic Effects of Chemical Substances, published by U.S. Department of Health, Education and Welfare are as follows: Ergotamine Tartrate IV LD50 in rats = 80mg/Kg, Caffeine IV LD50 in rats = 105mg/Kg.

HOW SUPPLIED

Wigraine® tablets are white tablets embossed with "ORGANON 542" on one side. They are individually foil stripped and packaged in boxes of 20's NDC #0052-0542-20 and 100's NDC #0052-0542-91.

STORAGE

Wigraine® tablets should be stored at a maximum of 30°C (86°F).

CAUTION

R only

5310108   Revised 3/98

Organon Inc.

West Orange, NJ 07052

Shown in Product Identification Guide, page 327

ZEMURON™   R

(rocuronium bromide) injection

THIS DRUG SHOULD BE ADMINISTERED BY ADEQUATELY-TRAINED INDIVIDUALS FAMILIAR WITH ITS ACTIONS, CHARACTERISTICS, AND HAZARDS.

DESCRIPTION

ZEMURON™ (rocuronium bromide) Injection is a nondepolarizing neuromuscular blocking agent with a rapid to intermediate onset depending on dose and intermediate duration. Rocuronium bromide is chemically designated as 1-[17β-(acetyloxy)-3α-hydroxy-2β-(4-morpholinyl)-5α-androstan-16β-yl]-1-(2-propenyl)pyrrolidinium bromide.

The structural formula is:

[See chemical structure in next column]

The chemical formula is $C_{32}H_{53}BrN_2O_4$ with a molecular weight of 609.70. The partition coefficient of rocuronium bromide in n-octanol/water is 0.5 at 20°C.

ZEMURON™ (rocuronium bromide) Injection is supplied as a sterile, nonpyrogenic, isotonic solution for intravenous injection only. Each mL contains 10 mg rocuronium bromide and 2 mg sodium acetate. The aqueous solution is adjusted to isotonicity with sodium chloride and to a pH of 4 with acetic acid and/or sodium hydroxide.

Table 1. Intubating Conditions in Patients with Intubation Initiated at 60 to 70 seconds.
Percent, Median (Range)

ZEMURON™ Dose (mg/kg) Administered over 5 sec	Percent of patients with excellent or good intubating conditions	Time to completion of intubation (min)
Adults* 18–64 yr		
0.45 (n=43)	86%	1.6 (1.0–7.0)
0.6 (n=51)	96%	1.6 (1.0–3.2)
Infants 3 mo–1 yr		
0.6 (n=18)	100%	1.0 (1.0–1.5)
Pediatric 1–12 yr		
0.6 (n=12)	100%	1.0 (0.5–2.3)

* Excludes patients undergoing cesarean section

Excellent intubating conditions = jaw relaxed, vocal cords apart and immobile, no diaphragmatic movement.

Good intubating conditions = same as excellent but with some diaphragmatic movement.

Table 2. Time to Onset and Clinical Duration following Initial (intubating) Dose during Opioid/Nitrous Oxide/Oxygen Anesthesia (Adults) and Halothane Anesthesia (Children), Median (Range)

ZEMURON™ Dose (mg/kg) Administered over 5 sec	Time to ≥80% Block (min)	Time to Maximum Block (min)	Clinical Duration (min)
Adults 18–64 yr			
0.45 (n=50)	1.3 (0.8–6.2)	3.0 (1.3–8.2)	22 (12–31)
0.6 (n=142)	1.0 (0.4–6.0)	1.8 (0.6–13.0)	31 (15–85)
0.9 (n=20)	1.1 (0.3–3.8)	1.4 (0.8–6.2)	58 (27–111)
1.2 (n=18)	0.7 (0.4–1.9)	1.0 (0.6–4.7)	67 (38–160)
Geriatric ≥65 yr			
0.6 (n=31)	2.3 (1.0–8.3)	3.7 (1.3–11.3)	46 (22–73)
0.9 (n=5)	2.0 (1.0–3.0)	2.5 (1.2–5.0)	62 (49–75)
1.2 (n=7)	1.0 (0.8–3.5)	1.3 (1.2–4.7)	94 (64–138)
Infants 3 mo–1 yr			
0.6 (n=17)	—	0.8 (0.3–3.0)	41 (24–68)
0.8 (n=9)	—	0.7 (0.5–0.8)	40 (27–70)
Pediatric 1–12 yr			
0.6 (n=27)	0.8 (0.4–2.0)	1.0 (0.5–3.3)	26 (17–39)
0.8 (n=18)	—	0.5 (0.3–1.0)	30 (17–56)

n = the number of patients who had Time to Maximum Block recorded.

Clinical duration = time until return to 25% of control T_1. Patients receiving doses of 0.45 mg/kg who achieved less than 90% block (16% of these patients) had about 12 to 15 minutes to 25% recovery.

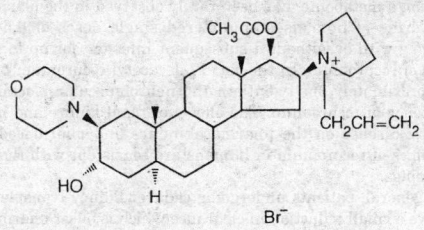

CLINICAL PHARMACOLOGY

ZEMURON™ (rocuronium bromide) Injection is a nondepolarizing neuromuscular blocking agent with a rapid to intermediate onset depending on dose and intermediate duration. It acts by competing for cholinergic receptors at the motor end-plate. This action is antagonized by acetylcholinesterase inhibitors, such as neostigmine and edrophonium.

Pharmacodynamics: The ED_{95} (dose required to produce 95% suppression of the first $[T_1]$ mechanomyographic [MMG] response of the adductor pollicis muscle [thumb] to indirect supramaximal train-of-four stimulation of the ulnar nerve) during opioid/nitrous oxide/oxygen anesthesia is approximately 0.3 mg/kg. Patient variability around the ED_{95} dose suggests that 50% of patients will exhibit T_1 depression of 91–97%.

Table 1 presents intubating conditions in patients with intubation initiated at 60 to 70 seconds.

[See table 1 above]

Table 2 presents the time to onset and clinical duration for the initial dose of ZEMURON™ (rocuronium bromide) under opioid/nitrous oxide/oxygen anesthesia in adults and geriatric patients, and under halothane anesthesia in children.

[See table 2 above]

The time to ≥80% block and clinical duration as a function of dose are presented in Figures 1 and 2.

[See figures 1 & 2 in next column]

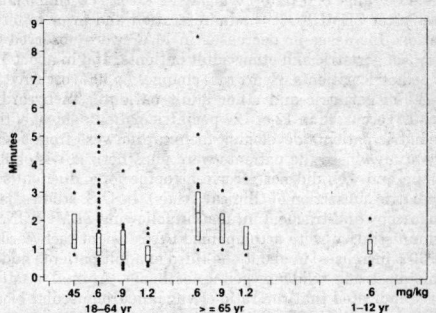

Figure 1. Time to ≥80% Block vs. Initial Dose of ZEMURON™ By Age Group (Median, 25th and 75th percentile, and individual values).

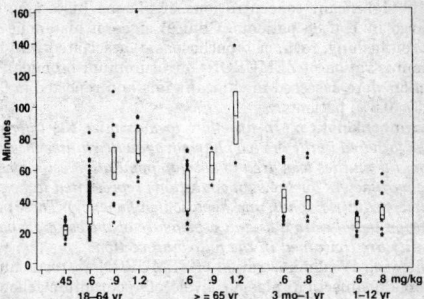

Figure 2. Duration of Clinical Effect vs. Initial Dose of ZEMURON™ By Age Group (Median, 25th and 75th percentile, and individual values).

The clinical durations for the first five maintenance doses, in patients receiving five or more maintenance doses are represented in Figure 3 (see also Maintenance Dosing subsection of DOSAGE AND ADMINISTRATION).

Continued on next page

Zemuron—Cont.

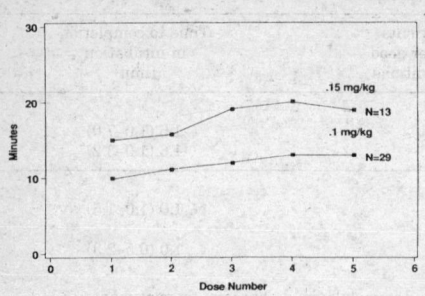

Figure 3. Duration of Clinical Effect *vs.* Number of ZEMU-RON™ Maintenance Doses, by Dose.

Once spontaneous recovery has reached 25% of control T_1, the neuromuscular block produced by ZEMURON™ is readily reversed with anticholinesterase agents, e.g., edrophonium or neostigmine.

The median spontaneous recovery from 25 to 75% T_1 was 13 minutes in adult patients. When neuromuscular block was reversed in 36 adults at a T_1 of 22–27%, recovery to a T_1 of 89 (50–132)% and T_4/T_1 of 69 (38–92)% was achieved within 5 minutes. Only five of 320 adults reversed received an additional dose of reversal agent. The median (range) dose of neostigmine was 0.04 (0.01 to 0.09) mg/kg and the median (range) dose of edrophonium was 0.5 (0.3 to 1.0) mg/kg. In geriatric patients (n=51) reversed with neostigmine, the median T_4/T_1 increased from 40 to 88% in 5 minutes. Pediatric patients (n=27) who received 0.5 mg/kg edrophonium had increases in the median T_4/T_1 from 37% at reversal to 93% after 2 minutes. Pediatric patients (n=58) who received 1 mg/kg edrophonium had increases in the median T_4/T_1 from 72% at reversal to 100% after 2 minutes. Infants (n=10) who were reversed with 0.03 mg/kg neostigmine recovered from 25 to 75% T_1 within 4 minutes.

There were no reports of less than satisfactory clinical recovery of neuromuscular function.

The neuromuscular blocking action of ZEMURON™ may be enhanced in the presence of potent inhalation anesthetics (see Inhalation Anesthetics subsection of PRECAUTIONS).

Hemodynamics: There were no dose-related effects on the incidence of changes from baseline ($\geq$30%) in mean arterial blood pressure (MAP) or heart rate associated with ZEMURON™ (rocuronium bromide) Injection administration over the dose range of 0.12 to 1.2 mg/kg ($4 \times ED_{95}$) within 5 minutes after ZEMURON™ administration and prior to intubation. Increases or decreases in MAP were observed in 2–5% of geriatric and other adult patients, and in about 1% of pediatric patients. Heart rate changes ($\geq$30%) occurred in 0–2% of geriatric and other adult patients. Tachycardia ($\geq$30%) occurred in 12 of 127 pediatric patients. Most of the pediatric patients developing tachycardia were from a single study where the patients were anesthetized with halothane and who did not receive atropine for induction (see Pediatric subsection of Clinical Trials). In U.S. studies, laryngoscopy and tracheal intubation following ZEMURON™ administration were accompanied by transient tachycardia ($\geq$30% increases) in about one-third of adult patients under opioid/nitrous oxide/oxygen anesthesia. Animal studies have indicated that the ratio of vagal:neuromuscular block following ZEMURON™ administration is less than vecuronium but greater than pancuronium. The tachycardia observed in some patients may result from this vagal blocking activity.

Histamine Release: In studies of histamine release, clinically significant concentrations of plasma histamine occurred in 1 of 88 patients. Clinical signs of histamine release (flushing, rash, or bronchospasm) associated with the administration of ZEMURON™ (rocuronium bromide) Injection were assessed in clinical trials and reported in 9 of 1137 (0.8%) patients.

Pharmacokinetics: *In an effort to maximize the information gathered in the in vivo pharmacokinetic studies the data from the studies was used to develop population estimates of the parameters for the subpopulations represented (e.g., geriatric, pediatric, renal, and hepatic insufficiency). These population based estimates and a measure of the estimate variability are contained in the following section.*

Following IV administration of ZEMURON™ (rocuronium bromide) Injection, plasma levels of rocuronium follow a three compartment open model. The rapid distribution half-life is 1–2 minutes and the slower distribution half-life is 14–18 minutes. Rocuronium is approximately 30% bound to human plasma proteins. In geriatric and other adult surgical patients undergoing either opioid/nitrous oxide/oxygen or inhalational anesthesia the observed pharmacokinetic profile was essentially unchanged.

[See table 3 above]

In general, studies with normal adult subjects did not reveal any differences in the pharmacokinetics of rocuronium due to gender.

Studies of distribution, metabolism, and excretion in cats and dogs indicate that rocuronium is eliminated primarily by the liver. The rocuronium analog 17-desacetyl-rocuronium, a metabolite, has been rarely observed in the plasma or urine of humans administered single doses of 0.5–1 mg/kg with or without a subsequent infusion (for up to 12 hr) of rocuronium. In the cat, 17-desacetyl-rocuronium has approximately one-twentieth the neuromuscular blocking potency of rocuronium. The effects of renal failure and hepatic disease on the pharmacokinetics and pharmacodynamics of rocuronium in humans are consistent with these findings.

In general, patients undergoing cadaver kidney transplant have a small reduction in clearance which is offset pharmacokinetically by a corresponding increase in volume, such that the net effect is an unchanged plasma half-life. Patients with demonstrated liver cirrhosis have a marked increase in their volume of distribution resulting in a plasma half-life approximately twice that of patients with normal hepatic function. Table 4 shows the pharmacokinetic parameters in subjects with either impaired renal or hepatic function.

[See table 4 above]

The net result of these findings is that subjects with renal failure have clinical durations that are similar to but somewhat more variable than the duration that one would expect in subjects with normal renal function. Hepatically impaired patients, due to the large increase in volume, may demonstrate clinical durations approaching 1.5 times that of subjects with normal hepatic function. In both populations the clinician should individualize the dose to the needs of the patient (see INDIVIDUALIZATION OF DOSAGE).

Tissue redistribution accounts for most (about 80%) of the initial amount of rocuronium administered. As tissue compartments fill with continued dosing (4–8 hours), less drug is redistributed away from the site of action and, for an infusion-only dose, the rate to maintain neuromuscular blockade falls to about 20% of the initial infusion rate. The use of a loading dose and a smaller infusion rate reduces the need for adjustment of dose.

Special Populations—Pediatrics: The clinical duration of effects of ZEMURON™ (rocuronium bromide) Injection did not vary with age in patients 4 months to 8 years of age. The terminal half-life and other pharmacokinetic parameters of rocuronium in these children are presented in Table 5.

[See table 5 above]

Clinical Trials

In U.S. clinical trials a total of 1,137 patients received ZEMURON™ (rocuronium bromide) Injection including 176 pediatric, 140 geriatric, 55 obstetric, and 766 other adults. Most patients (90%) were ASA physical status I or II, about 9% were ASA III, and 10 patients (undergoing coronary artery bypass grafting or valvular surgery) were ASA IV. In European clinical trials, a total of 1,394 patients received ZEMURON™ including 52 pediatric, 128 geriatric ($\geq$65 years) and 1,214 other adults.

Adult Patients: Intubation using doses of ZEMURON™ (rocuronium bromide) Injection 0.6 to 0.85 mg/kg was evaluated in 203 adults in 11 clinical trials. Excellent to good intubating conditions were generally achieved within 2 minutes and maximum block occurred within 3 minutes in most patients. Doses within this range provide clinical relaxation for a median (range) time of 33 (14–85) minutes under opioid/nitrous oxide/oxygen anesthesia. Larger doses (0.9 and 1.2 mg/kg) were evaluated in two trials with 19 and 16 patients under opioid/nitrous oxide/oxygen anesthesia and provided 58 (27–111) and 67 (38–160) minutes of clinical relaxation, respectively.

Cardiovascular Disease: In one clinical trial, 10 patients with clinically significant cardiovascular disease undergoing coronary artery bypass graft received an initial dose of 0.6 mg/kg ZEMURON™ (rocuronium bromide) Injection. Neuromuscular block was maintained during surgery with bolus maintenance doses of 0.3 mg/kg. Following induction, continuous 0.008 mg/kg/min infusion of ZEMURON™ produced relaxation sufficient to support mechanical ventilation for 6 to 12 hours in the surgical intensive care unit (SICU) while the patients were recovering from surgery. Hypertension and tachycardia were reported in some patients but these occurrences were less frequent in patients receiving beta or calcium channel blocking drugs. In 7 of these 10 patients ZEMURON™ was associated with transient increases ($\geq$30%) in pulmonary vascular resistance. In another clinical trial of 17 patients undergoing abdominal aortic surgery, transient increases ($\geq$30%) in pulmonary vascular resistance were observed in 4 of 17 patients receiving ZEMURON™ 0.6 or 0.9 mg/kg.

Rapid Sequence Intubation: Intubating conditions were assessed in 230 patients in six clinical trials where anesthesia was induced with either thiopental (3 to 6 mg/kg) or propofol (1.5 to 2.5 mg/kg) in combination with either fentanyl (2 to 5 mcg/kg) or alfentanil (1 mg). Most of the patients also received a premedication such as midazolam or temazepam. Most patients had intubation attempted within 60 to 90 seconds of administration of ZEMURON™ (rocuronium bro-

Table 3. Pharmacokinetic Parameters in Adults (n=22; ages 27–58 yr) and Geriatric (n=20; $\geq$65 yr) During Opioid/Nitrous Oxide/Oxygen Anesthesia (Mean $\pm$ SD)

PK Parameters	Adults (Ages 27–58 yr)	Geriatrics ($\geq$65 yr)
Clearance (L/kg/hr)	0.25 ± 0.08	0.21 ± 0.06
Volume of Distribution at Steady State (L/kg)	0.25 ± 0.04	0.22 ± 0.03
$T_{1/2}$ βElimination (hr)	1.4 ± 0.4	1.5 ± 0.4

Table 4. Pharmacokinetic Parameters in Adults with Normal Renal and Hepatic Function (n=10, ages 23–65), Renal Transplant Patients (n=10, ages 21–45) and Hepatic Dysfunction Patients (n=9, ages 31–67) During Isoflurane Anesthesia (Mean $\pm$ SD)

PK Parameters	Normal Renal and Hepatic Function	Renal Transplant Patients	Hepatic Dysfunction Patients
Clearance (L/kg/hr)	0.16 ± 0.05*	0.13 ± 0.04	0.13 ± 0.06
Volume of Distribution at Steady State (L/kg)	0.26 ± 0.03	0.34 ± 0.11	0.53 ± 0.14
$T_{1/2}$ β Elimination (hr)	2.4 ± 0.8*	2.4 ± 1.1	4.3 ± 2.6

* Differences in the calculated $T_{1/2}$ β and Cl between this study and the study in young adults vs. geriatrics ($\geq$65 years) is related to the different sample populations and anesthetic techniques.

Table 5. Pharmacokinetic Parameters of Rocuronium in Pediatric Patients (ages 3-<12 mo, n=6; 1-<3 yr, n=5; 3-<8 yr, n=7) During Halothane Anesthesia (Mean $\pm$SD)

PK Parameters	Patient Age Range		
	3-<12 mo	1-<3 yr	3-<8 yr
Clearance (L/kg/hr)	0.35 ± 0.08	0.32 ± 0.07	0.44 ± 0.16
Volume of Distribution at Steady State (L/kg)	0.30 ± 0.04	0.26 ± 0.06	0.21 ± 0.03
$T_{1/2}$ β Elimination (hr)	1.3 ± 0.5	1.1 ± 0.7	0.8 ± 0.3

mide) Injection 0.6 mg/kg or succinylcholine 1 to 1.5 mg/kg. Excellent or good intubating conditions were achieved in 119/120 (99% [95% confidence interval 95–99.9%]) patients receiving ZEMURON™ and in 108/110 (98% [94–99.8%]) patients receiving succinylcholine. The duration of action of ZEMURON™ 0.6 mg/kg is longer than succinylcholine and at this dose is approximately equivalent to the duration of other intermediate acting neuromuscular blocking drugs.

Geriatric Patients: ZEMURON™ (rocuronium bromide) Injection was evaluated in 55 geriatric patients (ages 65–80 years) in six clinical trials. Doses of 0.6 mg/kg provided excellent to good intubating conditions in a median (range) time of 2.3 (1–8) minutes. Recovery times from 25% to 75% after these doses were not prolonged in geriatric patients compared to other adult patients.

Pediatric Patients: ZEMURON™ (rocuronium bromide) Injection 0.6 or 0.8 mg/kg was evaluated for intubation in 75 pediatric patients (n=28; age 3–12 months, n=47; age 1–12 years) in three trials using halothane (1–5%) nitrous oxide (60–70%) in oxygen. Of the pediatric patients anesthetized with halothane who did not receive atropine for induction, about 80% experienced a transient increase (≥30%) in heart rate after intubation. One of the 19 infants anesthetized with halothane and fentanyl who received atropine for induction experienced this magnitude of change.

Obese Patients: ZEMURON™ (rocuronium bromide) Injection was dosed according to actual body weight (ABW) in most clinical trials. The administration of ZEMURON™ in the 47 of 330 (14%) patients who were at least 30% or more above their ideal body weight (IBW) was not associated with clinically significant differences in the onset, duration, recovery, or reversal of ZEMURON™-induced neuromuscular block.

In one clinical trial in obese patients, ZEMURON™ 0.6 mg/kg was dosed according to ABW (n=12) or IBW (n=11). Obese patients dosed according to IBW had a longer time to maximum block, a shorter clinical duration of 25 (14–29) minutes, and did not achieve intubating conditions comparable to those dosed based on ABW. These results support the recommendation that obese patients be dosed based on actual body weight.

Obstetric Patients: ZEMURON™ (rocuronium bromide) Injection 0.6 mg/kg was administered with thiopental, 3–4 mg/kg (n=13) or 4–6 mg/kg (n=42), for rapid sequence induction of anesthesia for cesarean section. No neonate had APGAR scores <7 at 5 minutes. The umbilical venous plasma concentrations were 18% of maternal concentrations at delivery. Intubating conditions were poor or inadequate in 5 of 13 women receiving 3–4 mg/kg thiopental when intubation was attempted 60 seconds after drug injection. Therefore, ZEMURON™ is not recommended for rapid sequence induction in cesarean section patients.

INDIVIDUALIZATION OF DOSAGE

DOSES OF ZEMURON™ (rocuronium bromide) INJECTION SHOULD BE INDIVIDUALIZED AND A PERIPHERAL NERVE STIMULATOR SHOULD BE USED TO MEASURE NEUROMUSCULAR FUNCTION DURING ZEMURON™ ADMINISTRATION IN ORDER TO MONITOR DRUG EFFECT, DETERMINE THE NEED FOR ADDITIONAL DOSES, AND CONFIRM RECOVERY FROM NEUROMUSCULAR BLOCK.

Based on the known actions of ZEMURON™, the following factors should be considered when administering ZEMURON™:

Renal or Hepatic Impairment: No differences from patients with normal hepatic and kidney function were observed for onset time at a dose of 0.6 mg/kg ZEMURON™ (rocuronium bromide) Injection. When compared to patients with normal renal and hepatic function, the mean clinical duration is similar in patients with end-stage renal disease undergoing renal transplant, and is about 1.5 times longer in patients with hepatic disease. Patients with renal failure may have a greater variation in duration of effect (see Pharmacokinetics subsection of CLINICAL PHARMACOLOGY and Renal Failure and Hepatic Disease subsections of PRECAUTIONS).

Reduced Plasma Cholinesterase Activity: No differences from patients with normal plasma cholinesterase activity is expected since rocuronium metabolism does not depend on plasma cholinesterase.

Drugs or Conditions Causing Potentiation of or Resistance to Neuromuscular Block: The neuromuscular blocking action of ZEMURON™ (rocuronium bromide) Injection is potentiated by isoflurane and enflurane anesthesia. Potentiation is minimal when administration of the recommended dose of ZEMURON™ occurs prior to the administration of these potent inhalation agents. The median clinical duration of a dose of 0.57–0.85 mg/kg was 34, 38, and 42 minutes under opioid/nitrous oxide/oxygen, enflurane and isoflurane maintenance anesthesia, respectively. During 1–2 hr of infusion, the infusion rate of ZEMURON™ required to maintain about 95% block was decreased by as much as 40% under enflurane and isoflurane anesthesia (see Inhalation Anesthetics subsection of PRECAUTIONS).

When ZEMURON™ is administered to patients chronically receiving anticonvulsant agents such as carbamazepine or phenytoin, shorter durations of neuromuscular block may occur and infusion rates may be higher due to the development of resistance to nondepolarizing muscle relaxants (see Anticonvulsants subsection of PRECAUTIONS).

Pulmonary Hypertension: ZEMURON™ (rocuronium bromide) Injection may be associated with increased pulmonary vascular resistance so caution is appropriate in patients with pulmonary hypertension or valvular heart disease (see Clinical Trials subsection of CLINICAL PHARMACOLOGY).

Obesity: In obese patients, the initial dose of ZEMURON™ (rocuronium bromide) Injection 0.6 mg/kg should be based upon the patient's actual body weight (see Obese Patients subsection of Clinical Trials).

Based on the known actions of other nondepolarizing neuromuscular blocking agents the following additional factors should be considered when administering ZEMURON™:

Drugs or Conditions Causing Potentiation of or Resistance to Neuromuscular Block: Resistance to nondepolarizing agents, consistent with up-regulation of skeletal muscle acetylcholine receptors, is associated with burns, disuse atrophy, denervation, and direct muscle trauma. Receptor up-regulation may also contribute to the resistance to nondepolarizing muscle relaxants which sometimes develops in patients with cerebral palsy, patients chronically receiving anticonvulsant agents such as carbamazepine or phenytoin or with chronic exposure to nondepolarizing agents (see PRECAUTIONS).

Other nondepolarizing neuromuscular blocking agents have been found to exhibit profound neuromuscular blocking effects in cachectic or debilitated patients, patients with neuromuscular diseases, and patients with carcinomatosis. In these or other patients in whom potentiation of neuromuscular block or difficulty with reversal may be anticipated, a decrease from the recommended initial dose should be considered.

Certain antibiotics, magnesium salts, lithium, local anesthetics, procainamide, and quinidine have been shown to increase the duration of neuromuscular block and decrease infusion requirements of other neuromuscular blocking agents. In patients in whom potentiation of neuromuscular block may be anticipated, a decrease from the recommended initial dose should be considered (see Antibiotics and Other subsections of PRECAUTIONS).

Severe acid-base and/or electrolyte abnormalities may potentiate or cause resistance to the neuromuscular blocking action of ZEMURON™ (rocuronium bromide) Injection (see Other subsection of PRECAUTIONS). No data are available in such patients and no dosing recommendations can be made.

Burns: Patients with burns are known to develop resistance to nondepolarizing neuromuscular blocking agents, probably due to up-regulation of post-synaptic skeletal muscle cholinergic receptors (see INDIVIDUALIZATION OF DOSAGE).

INDICATIONS AND USAGE

ZEMURON™ (rocuronium bromide) Injection is a nondepolarizing neuromuscular blocking agent with a rapid to intermediate onset depending on dose and intermediate duration and is indicated for inpatients and outpatients as an adjunct to general anesthesia to facilitate both rapid sequence and routine tracheal intubation, and to provide skeletal muscle relaxation during surgery or mechanical ventilation.

CONTRAINDICATIONS

ZEMURON™ (rocuronium bromide) Injection is contraindicated in patients known to have hypersensitivity to rocuronium bromide.

WARNINGS

ZEMURON™ (rocuronium bromide) INJECTION SHOULD BE ADMINISTERED IN CAREFULLY ADJUSTED DOSAGES BY OR UNDER THE SUPERVISION OF EXPERIENCED CLINICIANS WHO ARE FAMILIAR WITH THE DRUG'S ACTIONS AND THE POSSIBLE COMPLICATIONS OF ITS USE. THE DRUG SHOULD NOT BE ADMINISTERED UNLESS FACILITIES FOR INTUBATION, ARTIFICIAL RESPIRATION, OXYGEN THERAPY, AND AN ANTAGONIST ARE IMMEDIATELY AVAILABLE. IT IS RECOMMENDED THAT CLINICIANS ADMINISTERING NEUROMUSCULAR BLOCKING AGENTS SUCH AS ZEMURON™ EMPLOY A PERIPHERAL NERVE STIMULATOR TO MONITOR DRUG RESPONSE, NEED FOR ADDITIONAL RELAXANT, AND ADEQUACY OF SPONTANEOUS RECOVERY OR ANTAGONISM.

ZEMURON™ HAS NO KNOWN EFFECT ON CONSCIOUSNESS, PAIN THRESHOLD, OR CEREBRATION. THEREFORE, ITS ADMINISTRATION MUST BE ACCOMPANIED BY ADEQUATE ANESTHESIA OR SEDATION.

In patients with myasthenia gravis or myasthenic (Eaton-Lambert) syndrome, small doses of nondepolarizing neuromuscular blocking agents may have profound effects. In such patients, a peripheral nerve stimulator and use of a small test dose may be of value in monitoring the response to administration of muscle relaxants.

ZEMURON™, which has an acid pH, should not be mixed with alkaline solutions (e.g., barbiturate solutions) in the same syringe or administered simultaneously during intravenous infusion through the same needle.

PRECAUTIONS

Long-term Use in I.C.U.: ZEMURON™ (rocuronium bromide) Injection has not been studied for long-term use in the I.C.U. As with other nondepolarizing neuromuscular blocking drugs, apparent tolerance to ZEMURON™ may develop rarely during chronic administration in the I.C.U. While the mechanism for development of this resistance is not known, receptor up-regulation may be a contributing factor. It is STRONGLY RECOMMENDED THAT NEUROMUSCULAR TRANSMISSION BE MONITORED CONTINUOUSLY DURING ADMINISTRATION AND RECOVERY WITH THE HELP OF A NERVE STIMULATOR. ADDITIONAL DOSES OF ZEMURON™ OR ANY OTHER NEUROMUSCULAR BLOCKING AGENT SHOULD NOT BE GIVEN UNTIL THERE IS A DEFINITE RESPONSE (ONE TWITCH OF THE TRAIN-OF-FOUR) TO NERVE STIMULATION. Prolonged paralysis and/or skeletal muscle weakness may be noted during initial attempts to wean from the ventilator patients who have chronically received neuromuscular blocking drugs in the I.C.U. Therefore, ZEMURON™ should only be used in this setting if, in the opinion of the prescribing physician, the specific advantages of the drug outweigh the risk.

Labor and Delivery: The use of ZEMURON™ (rocuronium bromide) Injection in cesarean section has been studied in a limited number of patients. ZEMURON™ is not recommended for rapid sequence induction in cesarean section patients (see Clinical Trials subsection of CLINICAL PHARMACOLOGY).

Hepatic Disease: Since ZEMURON™ (rocuronium bromide) Injection is primarily excreted by the liver it should be used with caution in patients with clinically significant hepatic disease. ZEMURON™ 0.6 mg/kg has been studied in a limited number of patients (n=9) with clinically significant hepatic disease under steady-state isoflurane anesthesia. After ZEMURON™ 0.6 mg/kg, the median (range) clinical duration of 60 (35–166) minutes was moderately prolonged compared to 42 minutes in patients with normal hepatic function. The median recovery time of 53 minutes was also prolonged in patients with cirrhosis compared to 20 minutes in patients with normal hepatic function. Four of eight patients with cirrhosis, who received ZEMURON™ 0.6 mg/kg under opioid/nitrous oxide/oxygen anesthesia, did not achieve complete block. These findings are consistent with the increase in volume of distribution at steady state observed in patients with significant hepatic disease (see Pharmacokinetics subsection of CLINICAL PHARMACOLOGY). If used for rapid sequence induction in patients with ascites, an increased initial dosage may be necessary to assure complete block. Duration will be prolonged in these cases. The use of doses higher than 0.6 mg/kg has not been studied.

Renal Failure: Due to the limited role of the kidney in the excretion of ZEMURON™ (rocuronium bromide) Injection, usual dosing guidelines should be adequate. ZEMURON™ 0.6 mg/kg has been evaluated in three single center trials (n=30, ages 19–61 years) in patients undergoing renal transplant surgery, or shunt procedures in preparation for dialysis. After ZEMURON™ 0.6 mg/kg, the time to maximum block was about 1–2 minutes and was not different from patients without renal dysfunction. The mean ± SD clinical duration of 54 ± 22 minutes was not considered prolonged compared to 46 ± 12 minutes in normal patients; however, there was substantial variation (range, 22–90 minutes). The spontaneous recovery rate from 25 to 75% of control in renal dysfunction patients of 27 ± 11 minutes was similar to 28 ± 20 minutes in normal patients (see Pharmacokinetics subsection of CLINICAL PHARMACOLOGY).

Malignant Hyperthermia (MH): In an animal study in MH-susceptible swine, the administration of ZEMURON™ (rocuronium bromide) Injection did not appear to trigger malignant hyperthermia. ZEMURON™ has not been studied in MH-susceptible patients. Because ZEMURON™ is always used with other agents, and the occurrence of malignant hyperthermia during anesthesia is possible even in the absence of known triggering agents, clinicians should be familiar with early signs, confirmatory diagnosis and treatment of malignant hyperthermia prior to the start of any anesthetic.

Altered Circulation Time: Conditions associated with slower circulation time, e.g., cardiovascular disease or advanced age, may be associated with a delay in onset time. Because higher doses of ZEMURON™ (rocuronium bromide) Injection produce a longer duration of action, the initial dosage should usually not be increased in these patients to reduce onset time; instead, when feasible, more time should be allowed for the drug to achieve onset of effect.

Drug Interactions: The use of ZEMURON™ (rocuronium bromide) Injection before succinylcholine, for the purpose of attenuating some of the side effects of succinylcholine, has not been studied.

If ZEMURON™ is administered following administration of succinylcholine, it should not be given until recovery from succinylcholine has been observed. The median duration of action of ZEMURON™ 0.6 mg/kg administered after a 1 mg/kg dose of succinylcholine when T_1 returned to 75% of control was 36 minutes (range 14–57, n=12) *vs.* 28 minutes (17–51, n=12) without succinylcholine.

Continued on next page

Zemuron—Cont.

There are no controlled studies documenting the use of ZEMURON™ before or after other nondepolarizing muscle relaxants. Interactions have been observed when other nondepolarizing muscle relaxants have been administered in succession.

Inhalation Anesthetics: Use of inhalation anesthetics has been shown to enhance the activity of other neuromuscular blocking agents, enflurane > isoflurane > halothane.

Isoflurane and enflurane may also prolong the duration of action of initial and maintenance doses of ZEMURON™ (rocuronium bromide) Injection and decrease the average infusion requirement of ZEMURON™ by 40% compared to opioid/nitrous oxide/oxygen anesthesia. No definite interaction between ZEMURON™ and halothane has been demonstrated. In one study, use of enflurane in 10 patients resulted in a 20% increase in mean clinical duration of the initial intubating dose, and a 37% increase in the duration of subsequent maintenance doses, when compared in the same study to 10 patients under opioid/nitrous oxide/oxygen anesthesia. The clinical duration of initial doses of ZEMURON™ of 0.57–0.85 mg/kg under enflurane or isoflurane anesthesia, as used clinically, was increased by 11% and 23%, respectively. The duration of maintenance doses was affected to a greater extent, increasing by 30 to 50% under either enflurane or isoflurane anesthesia. Potentiation by these agents is also observed with respect to the infusion rates of ZEMURON™ required to maintain approximately 95% neuromuscular block. Under isoflurane and enflurane anesthesia, the infusion rates are decreased by approximately 40% compared to opioid/nitrous oxide/oxygen anesthesia. The median spontaneous recovery time (from 25 to 75% of control T_1) is not affected by halothane, but is prolonged by enflurane (15% longer) and isoflurane (62% longer). Reversal-induced recovery of ZEMURON™ neuromuscular block is minimally affected by anesthetic technique.

Intravenous Anesthetics: The use of propofol for induction and maintenance of anesthesia does not alter the clinical duration or recovery characteristics following recommended doses of ZEMURON™ (rocuronium bromide) Injection.

Anticonvulsants: In 2 of 4 patients receiving chronic anticonvulsant therapy apparent resistance to the effects of ZEMURON™ (rocuronium bromide) Injection was observed in the form of diminished magnitude of neuromuscular block, or shortened clinical duration. As with other nondepolarizing neuromuscular blocking drugs, if ZEMURON™ is administered to patients chronically receiving anticonvulsant agents such as carbamazepine or phenytoin, shorter durations of neuromuscular block may occur and infusion rates may be higher due to the development of resistance to non-depolarizing muscle relaxants. While the mechanism for development of this resistance is not known, receptor upregulation may be a contributing factor (see INDIVIDUALIZATION OF DOSAGE).

Antibiotics: Drugs which may enhance the neuromuscular blocking action of nondepolarizing agents such as ZEMURON™ (rocuronium bromide) Injection include certain antibiotics (e.g., aminoglycosides; vancomycin; tetracyclines; bacitracin; polymyxins; colistin; and sodium colistimethate). If these antibiotics are used in conjunction with ZEMURON™, prolongation of neuromuscular block should be considered a possibility.

Other: Experience concerning injection of quinidine during recovery from use of other muscle relaxants suggests that recurrent paralysis may occur. This possibility must also be considered for ZEMURON™ (rocuronium bromide) Injection.

ZEMURON™-induced neuromuscular blockade was modified by alkalosis and acidosis in experimental pigs. Both respiratory and metabolic acidosis prolonged the recovery time. The potency of ZEMURON™ was significantly enhanced in metabolic acidosis and alkalosis, but was reduced in respiratory alkalosis. In addition, experience with other drugs has suggested that acute (e.g., diarrhea) or chronic (e.g., adrenocortical insufficiency) electrolyte imbalance may alter neuromuscular blockade. Since electrolyte imbalance and acid-base imbalance are usually mixed, either enhancement or inhibition may occur. Magnesium salts, administered for the management of toxemia of pregnancy, may enhance neuromuscular blockade.

A local tolerance study in rabbits demonstrated that ZEMURON™ was well tolerated following intravenous, intra-arterial and perivenous administration with only a slight irritation of surrounding tissues observed after perivenous administration. In humans, if extravasation occurs it may be associated with signs or symptoms of local irritation; the injection or infusion should be terminated immediately and restarted in another vein (see DOSAGE AND ADMINISTRATION).

Drug/Laboratory Test Interactions: None known.

Carcinogenesis, Mutagenesis, Impairment of Fertility: Studies in animals have not been performed to evaluate carcinogenic potential or impairment of fertility. Mutagenicity studies (Ames test, analysis of chromosomal aberrations in mammalian cells, and micronucleus test) conducted with ZEMURON™ (rocuronium bromide) Injection did not suggest mutagenic potential.

Pregnancy Category B: A teratogenicity study has been conducted in rats using intravenously administered doses of ZEMURON™ (rocuronium bromide) Injection approximating the clinical dose in humans (0.3 mg/kg). No teratogenic effects were observed in this study. There are no adequate and well-controlled studies in pregnant women. ZEMURON™ should be used during pregnancy only if the potential benefit justifies the potential risk to the fetus.

Pediatric Use: The use of ZEMURON™ (rocuronium bromide) Injection in pediatric patients less than 3 months of age and greater than 14 years of age has not been studied. See Pharmacodynamics subsection of CLINICAL PHARMACOLOGY and Use in Pediatrics subsection of DOSAGE AND ADMINISTRATION for clinical experience and recommendations for use in pediatric patients and children 3 months to 14 years of age.

ADVERSE REACTIONS

Clinical studies in the U.S. (n=1,137) and Europe (n=1,394) totaled 2,531 patients. Prolonged neuromuscular block is associated with neuromuscular blockers as a class. Prolonged neuromuscular block (166 minutes) occurred after 0.6 mg/kg ZEMURON™ (rocuronium bromide) Injection in an obese 67 year-old female with hepatic dysfunction who had received gentamicin before surgery. The patients exposed in the U.S. clinical studies provide the basis for calculation of adverse reaction rates. The following adverse experiences were reported in patients administered ZEMURON™ (all events judged by investigators during the clinical trials to have a possible causal relationship):

Adverse experiences in greater than 1% patients:—NONE
Adverse experiences in less than 1% of patients Probably Related or Relationship Unknown:

Cardiovascular:	arrhythmia, abnormal electrocardiogram, tachycardia
Digestive:	nausea, vomiting
Respiratory:	asthma (bronchospasm, wheezing, or rhonchi), hiccup
Skin and Appendages:	rash, injection site edema, pruritus

In the European studies, the most commonly reported adverse experiences were transient hypotension (2%) and hypertension (2%); it is in greater frequency than the U.S. studies (0.1% and 0.1%). Changes in heart rate and blood pressure were defined differently from the U.S. studies in which changes in cardiovascular parameters were not considered as adverse events unless judged by the investigator as unexpected, clinically significant, or thought to be histamine related.

In clinical practice, there have been rare reports of allergic reactions (anaphylactic and anaphylactoid) with ZEMURON™ (rocuronium bromide) Injection.

OVERDOSAGE

No cases of significant accidental or intentional overdose with ZEMURON™ (rocuronium bromide) Injection have been reported. Overdosage with neuromuscular blocking agents may result in neuromuscular block beyond the time needed for surgery and anesthesia. The primary treatment is maintenance of a patent airway and controlled ventilation until recovery of normal neuromuscular function is assured. Once evidence of recovery from neuromuscular block is observed, further recovery may be facilitated by administration of an anticholinesterase agent (e.g., neostigmine, edrophonium) in conjunction with an appropriate anticholinergic agent (see Antagonism of Neuromuscular Blockade).

Antagonism of Neuromuscular Blockade
ANTAGONISTS (SUCH AS NEOSTIGMINE) SHOULD NOT BE ADMINISTERED PRIOR TO THE DEMONSTRATION OF SOME SPONTANEOUS RECOVERY FROM NEUROMUSCULAR BLOCKADE. THE USE OF A NERVE STIMULATOR TO DOCUMENT RECOVERY AND ANTAGONISM OF NEUROMUSCULAR BLOCKADE IS RECOMMENDED.

Patients should be evaluated for adequate clinical evidence of antagonism, e.g., 5 sec head lift, adequate phonation, ventilation, and upper airway maintenance. Ventilation must be supported until no longer required.

Antagonism may be delayed in the presence of debilitation, carcinomatosis, and concomitant use of certain broad spectrum antibiotics, or anesthetic agents and other drugs which enhance neuromuscular blockade or separately cause respiratory depression. Under such circumstances the management is the same as that of prolonged neuromuscular blockade.

DOSAGE AND ADMINISTRATION

ZEMURON™ (rocuronium bromide) INJECTION IS FOR INTRAVENOUS USE ONLY. THIS DRUG SHOULD BE ADMINISTERED BY OR UNDER THE SUPERVISION OF EXPERIENCED CLINICIANS FAMILIAR WITH THE USE OF NEUROMUSCULAR BLOCKING AGENTS. INDIVIDUALIZATION OF DOSAGE SHOULD BE CONSIDERED IN EACH CASE (see INDIVIDUALIZATION OF DOSAGE).

The dosage information which follows is derived from studies based upon units of drug per unit of body weight. It is expressed in this section in units of mg/kg to assist the clinician in calculating individual patient dosage requirements relative to the product as supplied for clinical use. It is intended to serve as an initial guide to clinicians familiar with other neuromuscular blocking agents to acquire experience with ZEMURON™. The monitoring of twitch response is recommended to evaluate recovery from ZEMURON™ and decrease the hazards of overdosage if additional doses are administered (see Pharmacodynamics subsection of CLINICAL PHARMACOLOGY and Maintenance Dosing subsection).

It is recommended that clinicians administering neuromuscular blocking agents such as ZEMURON™ employ a peripheral nerve stimulator to monitor drug response, determine the need for additional relaxant and adequacy of spontaneous recovery or antagonism.

Rapid Sequence Intubation: In appropriately premedicated and adequately anesthetized patients, ZEMURON™ (rocuronium bromide) Injection 0.6–1.2 mg/kg will provide excellent or good intubating conditions in most patients in less than 2 minutes (see Clinical Trials subsection of CLINICAL PHARMACOLOGY).

Dose for Tracheal Intubation: The recommended initial dose regardless of anesthetic technique is 0.6 mg/kg. Neuromuscular block sufficient for intubation (≥80% block) is attained in a median (range) time of 1 (0.4–6) minute(s) and most patients have intubation completed within 2 minutes. Maximum blockade is achieved in most patients in less than 3 minutes. This dose may be expected to provide 31 (15–85) minutes of clinical relaxation under opioid/nitrous oxide/oxygen anesthesia. Under halothane, isoflurane, and enflurane anesthesia, some extension of the period of clinical relaxation should be expected (see Inhalation Anesthetics subsection of PRECAUTIONS).

A lower dose of ZEMURON™ (rocuronium bromide) Injection (0.45 mg/kg) may be used. Neuromuscular block sufficient for intubation (≥80% block) is attained in a median (range) time of 1.3 (0.8–6.2) minute(s) and most patients have intubation completed within 2 minutes. Maximum blockade is achieved in most patients in less than 4 minutes. This dose may be expected to provide 22 (12–31) minutes of clinical relaxation under opioid/nitrous oxide/oxygen anesthesia. Patients receiving this low dose of 0.45 mg/kg who achieve less than 90% block (about 16% of these patients) may have a more rapid time to 25% recovery, 12–15 minutes.

Should there be reason for the selection of a larger bolus dose in individual patients, initial doses of 0.9 or 1.2 mg/kg can be administered during surgery under opioid/nitrous oxide/oxygen anesthesia without adverse effects to the cardiovascular system. These doses will provide ≥80% block in most patients in less than 2 minutes, with maximum blockade occurring in most patients in less than 3 minutes. Doses of 0.9 and 1.2 mg/kg may be expected to provide 58 (27–111) and 67 (38–160) minutes, respectively, of clinical relaxation under opioid/nitrous oxide/oxygen anesthesia.

Maintenance Dosing: Maintenance doses of 0.1, 0.15, and 0.2 mg/kg ZEMURON™ (rocuronium bromide) Injection, administered at 25% recovery of control T_1 (defined as 3 twiches of train-of-four), provide a median (range) of 12 (2–31), 17 (6–50) and 24 (7–69) minutes of clinical duration under opioid/nitrous oxide/oxygen anesthesia (see Pharmacodynamics subsection of CLINICAL PHARMACOLOGY). In all cases, dosing should be guided based on the clinical duration following initial dose or prior maintenance dose and not administered until recovery of neuromuscular function is evident. A clinically insignificant cumulation of effect with repetitive maintenance dosing has been observed (see Pharmacodynamics subsection of CLINICAL PHARMACOLOGY).

Use by Continuous Infusion: Infusion at an initial rate of 0.01 to 0.012 mg/kg/min of ZEMURON™ (rocuronium bromide) Injection should be initiated only after early evidence of spontaneous recovery from an intubating dose. Due to rapid redistribution (see Pharmacokinetics subsection of CLINICAL PHARMACOLOGY) and the associated rapid spontaneous recovery, initiation of the infusion after substantial return of neuromuscular function (more than 10% of control T_1), may necessitate additional bolus doses to maintain adequate block for surgery.

Upon reaching the desired level of neuromuscular block, the infusion of ZEMURON™ must be individualized for each patient. The rate of administration should be adjusted according to the patient's twitch response as monitored with the use of a peripheral nerve stimulator. In clinical trials, infusion rates have ranged from 0.004 to 0.016 mg/kg/min. Inhalation anesthetics, particularly enflurane and isoflurane may enhance the neuromuscular blocking action of nondepolarizing muscle relaxants. In the presence of

Table 6. Infusion Rates Using ZEMURON™ Injection (0.5 mg/mL)*

Patient Weight		Drug Delivery Rate (µg/kg/min)									
(kg)	(Lbs)	4	5	6	7	8	9	10	12	14	16
		Infusion Delivery Rate (mL/hr)									
10	22	4.8	6.0	7.2	8.4	9.6	10.8	12.0	14.4	16.8	19.2
15	33	7.2	9.0	10.8	12.6	14.4	16.2	18.0	21.6	25.2	28.8
20	44	9.6	12.0	14.4	16.8	19.2	21.6	24.0	28.8	33.6	38.4
25	55	12.0	15.0	18.0	21.0	24.0	27.0	30.0	36.0	42.0	48.0
35	77	16.8	21.0	25.2	29.4	33.6	37.8	42.0	50.4	58.8	67.2
50	110	24.0	30.0	36.0	42.0	48.0	54.0	60.0	72.0	84.0	96.0
60	132	28.8	36.0	43.2	50.4	57.6	64.8	72.0	86.4	100.8	115.2
70	154	33.6	42.0	50.4	58.8	67.2	75.6	84.0	100.8	117.6	134.4
80	176	38.4	48.0	57.6	67.2	76.8	86.4	96.0	115.2	134.4	153.6
90	198	43.2	54.0	64.8	75.6	86.4	97.2	108.0	129.6	151.2	172.8
100	220	48.0	60.0	72.0	84.0	96.0	108.0	120.0	144.0	168.0	192.0

steady-state concentrations of enflurane or isoflurane, it may be necessary to reduce the rate of infusion by 30 to 50%, at 45–60 minutes after the intubating dose.

Spontaneous recovery and reversal of neuromuscular blockade following discontinuation of ZEMURON™ infusion may be expected to proceed at rates comparable to that following comparable total doses administered by repetitive bolus injections (see Pharmacodynamics subsection of CLINICAL PHARMACOLOGY).

Infusion solutions of ZEMURON™ can be prepared by mixing ZEMURON™ with an appropriate infusion solution such as 5% glucose in water or Lactated Ringers (see Compatibility). Unused portions of infusion solutions should be discarded.

Infusion rates of ZEMURON™ can be individualized for each patient using the following tables as guidelines:
[See table 6 above]
[See table 7 below]

Use in Pediatrics: Initial doses of 0.6 mg/kg in pediatric patients under halothane anesthesia produce excellent to good intubating conditions within 1 minute. The median (range) time to maximum block was 1 (0.5–3.3) minute(s). This dose will provide a median (range) time of clinical relaxation of 41 (24–68) minutes in 3 months–1 year pediatric patients and 27 (17–41) minutes in 1–12 year-old pediatric patients. Maintenance doses of 0.075–0.125 mg/kg, administered upon return of T_1 to 25% of control, provide clinical relaxation for 7–10 minutes.

Spontaneous recovery proceeds at approximately the same rate in pediatric patients (3 months–1 year) as in adults, but is more rapid in pediatric patients (1–12 years) than adults (see Tables 2 and 4 in Pharmacodynamics subsection of CLINICAL PHARMACOLOGY). A continuous infusion of ZEMURON™ (rocuronium bromide) Injection initiated at a rate of 0.012 mg/kg/min upon return of T_1 to 10% of control (one twitch present in the train-of-four), may also be used to maintain neuromuscular blockade in children. The infusion of ZEMURON™ must be individualized for each patient. The rate of administration should be adjusted according to the patient's twitch response as monitored with the use of a peripheral nerve stimulator. Spontaneous recovery and reversal of neuromuscular blockade following discontinuation of ZEMURON™ infusion may be expected to proceed at rates comparable to that following similar total exposure to single bolus doses (see Pharmacodynamics subsection of CLINICAL PHARMACOLOGY).

Use in Obese Patients: An analysis across all U.S. controlled clinical studies indicates that the pharmacodynam-

ics of ZEMURON™ (rocuronium bromide) Injection are not different between obese and non-obese patients when dosed based upon their actual body weight.

Use in Geriatrics: Geriatric patients (≥65 year) exhibited a slightly prolonged median (range) clinical duration of 46 (22–73), 62 (49–75), and 94 (64–138) minutes under opioid/nitrous oxide/oxygen anesthesia following doses of 0.6, 0.9 and 1.2 mg/kg, respectively. Maintenance doses of 0.1 and 0.15 mg/kg ZEMURON™ (rocuronium bromide) Injection, administered at 25% recovery of T_1, provide approximately 13 and 33 minutes of clinical duration under opioid/nitrous oxide/oxygen anesthesia. The median (range) rate of spontaneous recovery of T_1 from 25 to 75% in geriatric patients is 17 (7–56) minutes which is not different from that in other adults (see Pharmacokinetics and Pharmacodynamics subsections of CLINICAL PHARMACOLOGY).

Compatibility: ZEMURON™ (rocuronium bromide) Injection is compatible in solution with:

0.9% NaCl solution	Sterile water for injection
5% glucose in water	Lactated Ringers
5% glucose in saline	

Use within 24 hours of mixing with the above solutions. Parenteral drug products should be inspected visually for particulate matter and clarity prior to administration whenever solution and container permit. Do not use solution if particulate matter is present.

Safety and Handling: There is no specific work exposure limit for ZEMURON™ (rocuronium bromide) Injection. In case of eye contact, flush with water for at least 10 minutes.

HOW SUPPLIED
ZEMURON™ (rocuronium bromide) Injection is available in the following forms:
ZEMURON™ 5 mL multiple dose vials containing 50 mg rocuronium bromide injection (10 mg/mL)
Boxes of 10   NDC No. 0052-0450-15
ZEMURON™ 10 mL multiple dose vials containing 100 mg rocuronium bromide injection (10 mg/mL)
Boxes of 10   NDC No. 0052-0450-16
Storage: ZEMURON™ (rocuronium bromide) Injection should be stored under refrigeration, 2 to 8°C (36 to 46°F). DO NOT FREEZE. Upon removal from refrigeration to room temperature storage conditions (25°C/77°F), use ZEMURON™ within 60 days. Use opened vials of ZEMURON™ within 30 days.

Caution: Federal law prohibits dispensing without prescription.
ORGANON INC. WEST ORANGE, NEW JERSEY 07052
5310153   7/97
Shown in Product Identification Guide, page 327

ZYMASE®
(pancrelipase, USP)
enteric coated spheres   ℞

DESCRIPTION
Zymase® capsules contain enteric coated spheres of pancrelipase, a substance containing enzymes, principally lipase, with amylase and protease obtained from the pancreas of the hog. Each capsule contains not less than:
Lipase—12,000 USP Units
Protease—24,000 USP Units
Amylase—24,000 USP Units
Each capsule also contains: Gelatin, purified water, starch, talc, titanium dioxide, FD&C Green #3, FD&C Yellow #10, and other inactive ingredients.

CLINICAL PHARMACOLOGY
Zymase® is protected against inactivation by gastric acidity, and active enzymes are released in the duodenum. The enzymes promote hydrolysis of fats into glycerol and fatty acids, protein into proteases and derived substances, and starch into dextrans and sugars.

INDICATIONS AND USAGE
Zymase® is indicated in conditions where pancreatic enzymes are either absent or deficient with resultant inadequate fat digestion. Such conditions include but are not limited to chronic pancreatitis, pancreatectomy, cystic fibrosis and steatorrhea of diverse etiologies.

CONTRAINDICATIONS
Known hypersensitivity to pork protein.

PRECAUTIONS
To maintain enteric coating integrity, do not chew or crush spheres.

ADVERSE REACTIONS
No adverse reactions have been reported. It should be noted, however, that extremely high doses of exogenous pancreatic enzymes have been associated with hyperuricosuria and hyperuricemia.

DOSAGE AND ADMINISTRATION
One to two capsules with each meal or snack. Individual cases may require higher dosage and dietary adjustment. Where swallowing of capsules is difficult, capsules may be opened and the spheres taken with liquids or soft foods which do not require chewing.

STORAGE
Not to exceed 25°C (77°F). Store in dry place when opened.

DISPENSE
In tight container as defined in the USP.
Revised 4/93
Shown in Product Identification Guide, page 327

Ortho Biotech Inc.
RARITAN, NJ 08869-0602

Direct Inquiries to:
(800) 325-7504
Prompt #1, Customer Service
Prompt #2, Medical Information
FAX: (908) 526-9230
(908) 526-6457

LEUSTATIN®
(cladribine) Injection
For Intravenous Infusion Only   ℞

WARNING
LEUSTATIN (cladribine) Injection should be administered under the supervision of a qualified physician experienced in the use of antineoplastic therapy. Suppression of bone marrow function should be anticipated. This is usually reversible and appears to be dose dependent. Serious neurological toxicity (including irreversible paraparesis and quadraparesis) has been reported in patients who received LEUSTATIN Injection by con-

Table 7. Infusion Rates Using ZEMURON™ Injection (1 mg/mL)**

Patient Weight		Drug Delivery Rate (µg/kg/min)									
(kg)	(Lbs)	4	5	6	7	8	9	10	12	14	16
		Infusion Delivery Rate (mL/hr)									
10	22	2.4	3.0	3.6	4.2	4.8	5.4	6.0	7.2	8.4	9.6
15	33	3.6	4.5	5.4	6.3	7.2	8.1	9.0	10.8	12.6	14.4
20	44	4.8	6.0	7.2	8.4	9.6	10.8	12.0	14.4	16.8	19.2
25	55	6.0	7.5	9.0	10.5	12.0	13.5	15.0	18.0	21.0	24.0
35	77	8.4	10.5	12.6	14.7	16.8	18.9	21.0	25.2	29.4	33.6
50	110	12.0	15.0	18.0	21.0	24.0	27.0	30.0	36.0	42.0	48.0
60	132	14.4	18.0	21.6	25.2	28.8	32.4	36.0	43.2	50.4	57.6
70	154	16.8	21.0	25.2	29.4	33.6	37.8	42.0	50.4	58.8	67.2
80	176	19.2	24.0	28.8	33.6	38.4	43.2	48.0	57.6	67.2	76.8
90	198	21.6	27.0	32.4	37.8	43.2	48.6	54.0	64.8	75.6	86.4
100	220	24.0	30.0	36.0	42.0	48.0	54.0	60.0	72.0	84.0	96.0

* 50 mg ZEMURON™ in 100 mL solution
** 100 mg ZEMURON™ in 100 mL solution

Continued on next page

Leustatin—Cont.

tinuous infusion at high doses (4 to 9 times the recommended dose for Hairy Cell Leukemia). Neurologic toxicity appears to demonstrate a dose relationship; however, severe neurological toxicity has been reported rarely following treatment with standard cladribine dosing regimens.

Acute nephrotoxicity has been observed with high doses of LEUSTATIN (4 to 9 times the recommended dose for Hairy Cell Leukemia), especially when given concomitantly with other nephrotoxic agents/therapies.

DESCRIPTION

LEUSTATIN (cladribine) Injection (also commonly known as 2-chloro-2'-deoxy-β-D-adenosine) is a synthetic antineoplastic agent for continuous intravenous infusion. It is a clear, colorless, sterile, preservative-free, isotonic solution. LEUSTATIN Injection is available in single-use vials containing 10 mg (1 mg/mL) of cladribine, a chlorinated purine nucleoside analog. Each milliliter of LEUSTATIN Injection contains 1 mg of the active ingredient and 9 mg (0.15 mEq) of sodium chloride as an inactive ingredient. The solution has a pH range of 5.5 to 8.0. Phosphoric acid and/or dibasic sodium phosphate may have been added to adjust the pH to 6.3±0.3.

The chemical name for cladribine is 2-chloro-6-amino-9-(2-deoxy-β-D-erythropento-furanosyl) purine and the structure is represented below:

cladribine

MW 285.7

CLINICAL PHARMACOLOGY

Cellular Resistance and Sensitivity:
The selective toxicity of 2-chloro-2'-deoxy-β-D-adenosine towards certain normal and malignant lymphocyte and monocyte populations is based on the relative activities of deoxycytidine kinase and deoxynucleotidase. Cladribine passively crosses the cell membrane. In cells with a high ratio of deoxycytidine kinase to deoxynucleotidase, it is phosphorylated by deoxycytidine kinase to 2-chloro-2'-deoxy-β-D-adenosine monophosphate (2-CdAMP). Since 2-chloro-2'-deoxy-β-D-adenosine is resistant to deamination by adenosine deaminase and there is little deoxynucleotide deaminase in lymphocytes and monocytes, 2-CdAMP accumulates intracellularly and is subsequently converted into the active triphosphate deoxynucleotide, 2-chloro-2'-deoxy-β-D-adenosine triphosphate (2-CdATP). It is postulated that cells with high deoxycytidine kinase and low deoxynucleotidase activities will be selectively killed by 2-chloro-2'-deoxy-β-D-adenosine as toxic deoxynucleotides accumulate intracellularly.

Cells containing high concentrations of deoxynucleotides are unable to properly repair single-strand DNA breaks. The broken ends of DNA activate the enzyme poly (ADP-ribose) polymerase resulting in NAD and ATP depletion and disruption of cellular metabolism. There is evidence, also, that 2-CdATP is incorporated into the DNA of dividing cells, resulting in impairment of DNA synthesis. Thus, 2-chloro-2'-deoxy-β-D-adenosine can be distinguished from other chemotherapeutic agents affecting purine metabolism in that it is cytotoxic to both actively dividing and quiescent lymphocytes and monocytes, inhibiting both DNA synthesis and repair.

HUMAN PHARMACOLOGY

In a clinical investigation, 17 patients with Hairy Cell Leukemia and normal renal function were treated for 7 days with the recommended treatment regimen of LEUSTATIN Injection (0.09 mg/kg/day) by continuous intravenous infusion. The mean steady-state serum concentration was estimated to be 5.7 ng/mL with an estimated systemic clearance of 663.5 mL/h/kg when LEUSTATIN was given by continuous infusion over 7 days. In Hairy Cell Leukemia patients, there does not appear to be a relationship between serum concentrations and ultimate clinical outcome.

In another study, 8 patients with hematologic malignancies received a two (2) hour infusion of LEUSTATIN Injection (0.12 mg/kg). The mean end-of-infusion plasma LEUSTATIN concentration was 48±19 ng/mL. For 5 of these patients, the disappearance of LEUSTATIN could be described by either a biphasic or triphasic decline. For these patients with normal renal function, the mean terminal half-life was

5.4 hours. Mean values for clearance and steady-state volume of distribution were 978±422 mL/h/kg and 4.5±2.8 L/kg, respectively.

Plasma concentrations are reported to decline multi-exponentially after intravenous infusions with terminal half-lives ranging from approximately 3-22 hours. In general, the apparent volume of distribution of cladribine is very large (mean approximately 9 L/kg), indicating an extensive distribution of cladribine in body tissues. The mean half-life of cladribine in leukemic cells has been reported to be 23 hours.

Cladribine penetrates into cerebrospinal fluid. One report indicates that concentrations are approximately 25% of those in plasma.

LEUSTATIN is bound approximately 20% to plasma proteins.

Except for some understanding of the mechanism of cellular toxicity, no other information is available on the metabolism of LEUSTATIN in humans. An average of 18% of the administered dose has been reported to be excreted in urine of patients with solid tumors during a 5-day continuous intravenous infusion of 3.5–8.1 mg/m²/day of LEUSTATIN. The effect of renal and hepatic impairment on the elimination of cladribine has not been investigated in humans.

Two single-center open label studies of LEUSTATIN (cladribine) have been conducted in patients with Hairy Cell Leukemia with evidence of active disease requiring therapy. In the study conducted at the Scripps Clinic and Research Foundation (Study A), 89 patients were treated with a single course of LEUSTATIN Injection given by continuous intravenous infusion for 7 days at a dose of 0.09 mg/kg/day. In the study conducted at the M.D. Anderson Cancer Center (Study B), 35 patients were treated with a 7-day continuous intravenous infusion of LEUSTATIN Injection at a comparable dose of 3.6 mg/m²/day. A complete response (CR) required clearing of the peripheral blood and bone marrow of hairy cells and recovery of the hemoglobin to 12 g/dL, platelet count to 100 × 10⁹/L, and absolute neutrophil count to 1500 × 10⁶/L. A good partial response (GPR) required the same hematologic parameters as a complete response, and that fewer than 5% hairy cells remain in the bone marrow. A partial response (PR) required that hairy cells in the bone marrow be decreased by at least 50% from baseline and the same response for hematologic parameters as for complete response. A pathologic relapse was defined as an increase in bone marrow hairy cells to 25% of pretreatment levels. A clinical relapse was defined as the recurrence of cytopenias, specifically, decreases in hemoglobin ≥2 g/dL, ANC ≥25% or platelet counts ≥50,000. Patients who met the criteria for a complete response but subsequently were found to have evidence of bone marrow hairy cells (<25% of pretreatment levels) were reclassified as partial responses and were not considered to be complete responses with relapse.

Among patients evaluable for efficacy (N=106), using the hematologic and bone marrow response criteria described above, the complete response rates in patients treated with LEUSTATIN Injection were 65% and 68% for Study A and Study B, respectively, yielding a combined complete response rate of 66%. Overall response rates (i.e., Complete plus Good Partial plus Partial Responses) were 89% and 86% in Study A and Study B, respectively, for a combined overall response rate of 88% in evaluable patients treated with LEUSTATIN Injection.

Using an intent-to-treat analysis (N=123) and further requiring no evidence of splenomegaly as a criterion for CR (i.e., no palpable spleen on physical examination and ≤13 cm on CT scan), the complete response rates for Study A and Study B were 54% and 53%, respectively, giving a combined CR rate of 54%. The overall response rates (CR + GPR + PR) were 90% and 85%, for Studies A and B, respectively, yielding a combined overall response rate of 89%.

RESPONSE RATES TO LEUSTATIN TREATMENT IN PATIENTS WITH HAIRY CELL LEUKEMIA

	CR	Overall
Evaluable Patients N=106	66%	88%
Intent-to-treat Population N=123	54%	89%

In these studies, 60% of the patients had not received prior chemotherapy for Hairy Cell Leukemia or had undergone splenectomy as the only prior treatment and were receiving LEUSTATIN as a first-line treatment. The remaining 40% of the patients received LEUSTATIN as a second-line treatment, having been treated previously with other agents, including α-interferon and/or deoxycoformycin. The overall response rate for patients without prior chemotherapy was 92%, compared with 84% for previously treated patients. LEUSTATIN is active in previously treated patients; however, retrospective analysis suggests that the overall re-

sponse rate is decreased in patients previously treated with splenectomy or deoxycoformycin and in patients refractory to α-interferon.

OVERALL RESPONSE RATES (CR + GPR + PR) TO LEUSTATIN TREATMENT IN PATIENTS WITH HAIRY CELL LEUKEMIA

	OVERALL RESPONSE (N=123)	NR + RELAPSE
No Prior Chemotherapy	68/74 92%	6 + 4 14%
Any Prior Chemotherapy	41/49 84%	8 + 3 22%
Previous Splenectomy	32/41* 78%	9 + 1 24%
Previous Interferon	40/48 83%	8 + 3 23%
Interferon Refractory	6/11* 55%	5 + 2 64%
Previous Deoxycoformycin	3/6* 50%	3 + 1 66%

NR = No Response
* P < 0.05

After a reversible decline, normalization of peripheral blood counts (Hemoglobin >12.0 g/dL, Platelets >100 × 10⁹/L, Absolute Neutrophil Count (ANC) >1500 × 10⁶/L) was achieved by 92% of evaluable patients. The median time to normalization of peripheral counts was 9 weeks from the start of treatment (Range: 2 to 72). The median time to normalization of Platelet Count was 2 weeks, the median time to normalization of ANC was 5 weeks and the median time to normalization of Hemoglobin was 8 weeks. With normalization of Platelet Count and Hemoglobin, requirements for platelet and RBC transfusions were abolished after Months 1 and 2, respectively, in those patients with complete response. Platelet recovery may be delayed in a minority of patients with severe baseline thrombocytopenia. Corresponding to normalization of ANC, a trend toward a reduced incidence of infection was seen after the third month, when compared to the months immediately preceding LEUSTATIN therapy. (see also WARNINGS, PRECAUTIONS, and ADVERSE REACTIONS)

LEUSTATIN TREATMENT IN PATIENTS WITH HAIRY CELL LEUKEMIA TIME TO NORMALIZATION OF PERIPHERAL BLOOD COUNTS

Parameter	Median Time to Normalization of Count*
Platelet Count	2 weeks
Absolute Neutrophil Count	5 weeks
Hemoglobin	8 weeks
ANC, Hemoglobin and Platelet Count	9 weeks

*Day 1 = First day of infusion

For patients achieving a complete response, the median time to response (i.e., absence of hairy cells in bone marrow and peripheral blood together with normalization of peripheral blood parameters), measured from treatment start, was approximately 4 months. Since bone marrow aspiration and biopsy were frequently not performed at the time of peripheral blood normalization, the median time to complete response may actually be shorter than that which was recorded. At the time of data cut-off, the median duration of complete response was greater than 8 months and ranged to 25+ months. Among 93 responding patients, seven had shown evidence of disease progression at the time of the data cut-off. In four of these patients, disease was limited to the bone marrow without peripheral blood abnormalities (pathologic progression), while in three patients there were also peripheral blood abnormalities (clinical progression). Seven patients who did not respond to a first course of LEUSTATIN received a second course of therapy. In the five patients who had adequate follow-up, additional courses did not appear to improve their overall response.

INDICATIONS FOR USE

LEUSTATIN Injection is indicated for the treatment of active Hairy Cell Leukemia as defined by clinically significant anemia, neutropenia, thrombocytopenia or disease-related symptoms.

CONTRAINDICATIONS

LEUSTATIN Injection is contraindicated in those patients who are hypersensitive to this drug or any of its components.

WARNINGS

Severe bone marrow suppression, including neutropenia, anemia and thrombocytopenia, has been commonly observed in patients treated with LEUSTATIN, especially at high doses. At initiation of treatment, most patients in the clinical studies had hematologic impairment as a manifestation of active Hairy Cell Leukemia. Following treatment with LEUSTATIN, further hematologic impairment occurred before recovery of peripheral blood counts began. During the first two weeks after treatment initiation, mean Platelet Count, ANC, and Hemoglobin concentration declined and subsequently increased with normalization of mean counts by Day 12, Week 5 and Week 8, respectively. The myelosuppressive effects of LEUSTATIN were most notable during the first month following treatment. Forty-four percent (44%) of patients received transfusions with RBCs and 14% received transfusions with platelets during Month 1. Careful hematologic monitoring, especially during the first 4 to 8 weeks after treatment with LEUSTATIN Injection, is recommended. (see PRECAUTIONS)

Fever (T≥100°F) was associated with the use of LEUSTATIN in approximately two-thirds of patients (131/196) in the first month of therapy. Virtually all of these patients were treated empirically with parenteral antibiotics. Overall, 47% (93/196) of all patients had fever in the setting of neutropenia (ANC ≤1000), including 62 patients (32%) with severe neutropenia (i.e., ANC ≤500).

In a Phase I investigational study using LEUSTATIN in high doses (4 to 9 times the recommended dose for Hairy Cell Leukemia) as part of a bone marrow transplant conditioning regimen, which also included high dose cyclophosphamide and total body irradiation, acute nephrotoxicity and delayed onset neurotoxicity were observed. Thirty-one (31) poor-risk patients with drug-resistant acute leukemia in relapse (29 cases) or non-Hodgkins Lymphoma (2 cases) received LEUSTATIN for 7 to 14 days prior to bone marrow transplantation. During infusion, 8 patients experienced gastrointestinal symptoms. While the bone marrow was initially cleared of all hematopoietic elements, including tumor cells, leukemia eventually recurred in all treated patients. Within 7 to 13 days after starting treatment with LEUSTATIN, 6 patients (19%) developed manifestations of renal dysfunction (e.g., acidosis, anuria, elevated serum creatinine, etc.) and 5 required dialysis. Several of these patients were also being treated with other medications having known nephrotoxic potential. Renal dysfunction was reversible in 2 of these patients. In the 4 patients whose renal function had not recovered at the time of death, autopsies were performed; in 2 of these, evidence of tubular damage was noted. Eleven (11) patients (35%) experienced delayed onset neurologic toxicity. In the majority, this was characterized by progressive irreversible motor weakness (paraparesis/quadriparesis), of the upper and/or lower extremities, first noted 35 to 84 days after starting high dose therapy with LEUSTATIN. Non-invasive testing (electromyography and nerve conduction studies) was consistent with demyelinating disease. Severe neurologic toxicity has also been noted with high doses of another drug in this class.

Axonal peripheral polyneuropathy was observed in a dose escalation study at the highest dose levels (approximately 4 times the recommended dose for Hairy Cell Leukemia) in patients not receiving cyclophosphamide or total body irradiation. Severe neurological toxicity has been reported rarely following treatment with standard cladribine dosing regimens.

In patients with Hairy Cell Leukemia treated with the recommended treatment regimen (0.09 mg/kg/day for 7 consecutive days), there have been no reports of nephrologic toxicities.

Of the 196 Hairy Cell Leukemia patients entered in the two trials, there were 8 deaths following treatment. Of these, 6 were of infectious etiology, including 3 pneumonias, and 2 occurred in the first month following LEUSTATIN therapy. Of the 8 deaths, 6 occurred in previously treated patients who were Refractory to α-interferon.

Benzyl alcohol is a constituent of the recommended diluent for the 7-day infusion solution. Benzyl alcohol has been reported to be associated with a fatal "Gasping Syndrome" in premature infants. (see DOSAGE AND ADMINISTRATION)

Pregnancy Category D: LEUSTATIN Injection should not be given during pregnancy.

Cladribine is teratogenic in mice and rabbits and consequently has the potential to cause fetal harm when administered to a pregnant woman. A significant increase in fetal variations was observed in mice receiving 1.5 mg/kg/day (4.5 mg/m²) and increased resorptions, reduced litter size and increased fetal malformations were observed when mice received 3.0 mg/kg/day (9 mg/m²). Fetal death and malformations were observed in rabbits that received 3.0 mg/kg/day (33.0 mg/m²). No fetal effects were seen in mice at 0.5 mg/kg/day (1.5 mg/m²) or in rabbits at 1.0 mg/kg/day (11.0 mg/m²).

Although there is no evidence of teratogenicity in humans due to LEUSTATIN, other drugs which inhibit DNA synthesis (e.g., methotrexate and aminopterin) have been reported to be teratogenic in humans. LEUSTATIN has been shown to be embryotoxic in mice when given at doses equivalent to the recommended dose.

There are no adequate and well controlled studies in pregnant women. If LEUSTATIN is used during pregnancy, or if the patient becomes pregnant while taking this drug, the patient should be apprised of the potential hazard to the fetus. Women of childbearing age should be advised to avoid becoming pregnant.

PRECAUTIONS

General: LEUSTATIN Injection is a potent antineoplastic agent with potentially significant toxic side effects. It should be administered only under the supervision of a physician experienced with the use of cancer chemotherapeutic agents. Patients undergoing therapy should be closely observed for signs of hematologic and non-hematologic toxicity. Periodic assessment of peripheral blood counts, particularly during the first 4 to 8 weeks post-treatment, is recommended to detect the development of anemia, neutropenia and thrombocytopenia and for early detection of any potential sequelae (e.g., infection or bleeding). As with other potent chemotherapeutic agents, monitoring of renal and hepatic function is also recommended, especially in patients with underlying kidney or liver dysfunction. (see WARNINGS and ADVERSE REACTIONS)

Fever was a frequently observed side effect during the first month on study. Since the majority of fevers occurred in neutropenic patients, patients should be closely monitored during the first month of treatment and empiric antibiotics should be initiated as clinically indicated. Although 69% of patients developed fevers, less than 1/3 of febrile events were associated with documented infection. Given the known myelosuppressive effects of LEUSTATIN, practitioners should carefully evaluate the risks and benefits of administering this drug to patients with active infections. (see WARNINGS and ADVERSE REACTIONS)

There are inadequate data on dosing of patients with renal or hepatic insufficiency. Development of acute renal insufficiency in some patients receiving high doses of LEUSTATIN has been described. Until more information is available, caution is advised when administering the drug to patients with known or suspected renal or hepatic insufficiency. (see WARNINGS)

Rare cases of tumor lysis syndrome have been reported in patients treated with cladribine with other hematologic malignancies having a high tumor burden.

LEUSTATIN Injection must be diluted in designated intravenous solutions prior to administration. (see DOSAGE AND ADMINISTRATION)

Laboratory Tests: During and following treatment, the patient's hematologic profile should be monitored regularly to determine the degree of hematopoietic suppression. In the clinical studies, following reversible declines in all cell counts, the mean Platelet Count reached 100×10^9/L by Day 12, the mean Absolute Neutrophil Count reached 1500×10^6/L by Week 5 and the mean Hemoglobin reached 12 g/dL by Week 8. After peripheral counts have normalized, bone marrow aspiration and biopsy should be performed to confirm response to treatment with LEUSTATIN. Febrile events should be investigated with appropriate laboratory and radiologic studies. Periodic assessment of renal function and hepatic function should be performed as clinically indicated.

Drug Interactions: There are no known drug interactions with LEUSTATIN Injection. Caution should be exercised if LEUSTATIN Injection is administered before, after, or in conjunction with other drugs known to cause immunosuppression or myelosuppression. (See WARNINGS)

Carcinogenesis: No animal carcinogenicity studies have been conducted with cladribine. However, its carcinogenic potential cannot be excluded based on demonstrated genotoxicity of cladribine.

Mutagenesis: As expected for compounds in this class, the actions of cladribine yield DNA damage. In mammalian cells in culture, cladribine caused the accumulation of DNA strand breaks. Cladribine was also incorporated into DNA of human lymphoblastic leukemia cells. Cladribine was not mutagenic *in vitro* (Ames and Chinese hamster ovary cell gene mutation tests) and did not induce unscheduled DNA synthesis in primary rat hepatocyte cultures. However, cladribine was clastogenic both *in vitro* (chromosome aberrations in Chinese hamster ovary cells) and *in vivo* (mouse bone marrow micronucleus test).

Impairment of Fertility: When administered intravenously to Cynomolgus monkeys, cladribine has been shown to cause suppression of rapidly generating cells, including testicular cells. The effect on human fertility is unknown.

Pregnancy: Pregnancy Category D: (see WARNINGS)

Nursing Mothers: It is not known whether this drug is excreted in human milk. Because many drugs are excreted in human milk and because of the potential for serious adverse reactions in nursing infants from cladribine, a decision should be made whether to discontinue nursing or discontinue the drug, taking into account the importance of the drug for the mother.

Pediatric Use: Safety and effectiveness in pediatric patients have not been established. In a Phase I study involving patients 1–21 years old with relapsed acute leukemia; LEUSTATIN was given by continuous intravenous infusion in doses ranging from 3 to 10.7 mg/m²/day for 5 days (one-half to twice the dose recommended in Hairy Cell Leukemia). In this study, the dose-limiting toxicity was severe myelosuppression with profound neutropenia and thrombocytopenia. At the highest dose (10.7 mg/m²/day), 3 of 7 patients developed irreversible myelosuppression and fatal systemic bacterial or fungal infections. No unique toxicities were noted in this study.[1] (see WARNINGS and ADVERSE REACTIONS)

ADVERSE REACTIONS

Safety data are based on 196 patients with Hairy Cell Leukemia: the original cohort of 124 patients plus an additional 72 patients enrolled at the same two centers after the original enrollment cutoff. In Month 1 of the Hairy Cell Leukemia clinical trials, severe neutropenia was noted in 70% of patients, fever in 69%, and infection was documented in 28%. Other adverse experiences reported frequently during the first 14 days after initiating treatment included: fatigue (45%), nausea (28%), rash (27%), headache (22%) and injection site reactions (19%). Most non-hematologic adverse experiences were mild to moderate in severity.

Myelosuppression was frequently observed during the first month after starting treatment. Neutropenia (ANC <500 × 10⁶/L) was noted in 70% of patients, compared with 26% in whom it was present initially. Severe anemia (Hemoglobin <8.5 g/dL) developed in 37% of patients, compared with 10% initially and thrombocytopenia (Platelets <20 × 10⁹/L) developed in 12% of patients, compared to 4% in whom it was noted initially.

During the first month, 54 of 196 patients (28%) exhibited documented evidence of infection. Serious infections (e.g., septicemia, pneumonia) were reported in 6% of all patients; the remainder were mild or moderate. Several deaths were attributable to infection and/or complications related to the underlying disease. During the second month, the overall rate of documented infection was 6%; these infections were mild to moderate and no severe systemic infections were seen. After the third month, the monthly incidence of infection was either less than or equal to that of the months immediately preceding LEUSTATIN therapy.

During the first month, 11% of patients experienced severe fever (i.e., ≥104°F). Documented infections were noted in fewer than one-third of febrile episodes. Of the 196 patients studied, 19 were noted to have a documented infection in the month prior to treatment. In the month following treatment, there were 54 episodes of documented infection: 23 (42%) were bacterial, 11 (20%) were viral and 11 (20%) were fungal. Seven (7) of 8 documented episodes of herpes zoster occurred during the month following treatment. Fourteen (14) of 16 episodes of documented fungal infections occurred in the first two months following treatment. Virtually all of these patients were treated empirically with antibiotics. (see WARNINGS and PRECAUTIONS)

Analysis of lymphocyte subsets indicates that treatment with cladribine is associated with prolonged depression of the CD4 counts. Prior to treatment, the mean CD4 count was 766/μL. The mean CD4 count nadir, which occurred 4 to 6 months following treatment, was 272/μL. Fifteen (15) months after treatment, mean CD4 counts remained below 500/μL. CD8 counts behaved similarly, though increasing counts were observed after 9 months. The clinical significance of the prolonged CD4 lymphopenia is unclear.

Another event of unknown clinical significance includes the observation of prolonged bone marrow hypocellularity. Bone marrow cellularity of <35% was noted after 4 months in 42 of 124 patients (34%) treated in the two pivotal trials. This hypocellularity was noted as late as day 1010. It is not known whether the hypocellularity is the result of disease related marrow fibrosis or if it is the result of cladribine toxicity. There was no apparent clinical effect on the peripheral blood counts.

The vast majority of rashes were mild and occurred in patients who were receiving or had recently been treated with other medications (e.g., allopurinol or antibiotics) known to cause rash.

Most episodes of nausea were mild, not accompanied by vomiting, and did not require treatment with antiemetics. In patients requiring antiemetics, nausea was easily controlled, most frequently with chlorpromazine.

Continued on next page

Leustatin—Cont.

Adverse reactions reported during the first 2 weeks following treatment initiation (regardless of relationship to drug) by >5% of patients included:

Body as a Whole: fever (69%), fatigue (45%), chills (9%), asthenia (9%), diaphoresis (9%), malaise (7%), trunk pain (6%)

Gastrointestinal: nausea (28%), decreased appetite (17%), vomiting (13%), diarrhea (10%), constipation (9%), abdominal pain (6%)

Hemic/Lymphatic: purpura (10%), petechiae (8%), epistaxis (5%)

Nervous System: headache (22%), dizziness (9%), insomnia (7%)

Cardiovascular System: edema (6%), tachycardia (6%)

Respiratory System: abnormal breath sounds (11%), cough (10%), abnormal chest sounds (9%), shortness of breath (7%)

Skin/Subcutaneous Tissue: rash (27%), injection site reactions (19%), pruritis (6%), erythema (6%)

Musculoskeletal System: myalgia (7%), arthralgia (5%)

Adverse experiences related to intravenous administration included: injection site reactions (9%) (i.e., redness, swelling, pain), thrombosis (2%), phlebitis (2%) and a broken catheter (1%). These appear to be related to the infusion procedure and/or indwelling catheter, rather than the medication or the vehicle.

From Day 15 to the last follow-up visit, the only events reported by >5% of patients were: fatigue (11%), rash (10%), headache (7%), cough (7%), and malaise (5%).

For a description of adverse reactions associated with use of high doses in non-Hairy Cell Leukemia patients, see WARNINGS.

The following additional adverse events have been reported since the drug became commercially available. These adverse events have been reported primarily in patients who received multiple courses of LEUSTATIN Injection:

Hematologic: bone marrow suppression with prolonged pancytopenia, including some reports of aplastic anemia; hemolytic anemia, which was reported in patients with lymphoid malignancies, occurring within the first few weeks following treatment.

Hepatic: reversible, generally mild increases in bilirubin and transaminases.

Nervous System: Neurological toxicity; however, severe neurotoxicity has been reported rarely following treatment with standard cladribine dosing regimens.

Respiratory System: pulmonary interstitial infiltrates; in most cases, an infectious etiology was identified.

Skin/Subcutaneous: urticaria, hypereosinophilia. In isolated cases Stevens-Johnson and toxic epidermal necrolysis have been reported in patients who were receiving or had recently been treated with other medications (e.g., allopurinol or antibiotics) known to cause these syndromes.

Opportunistic infections have occurred in the acute phase of treatment due to the immunosuppression mediated by LEUSTATIN Injection.

OVERDOSAGE

High doses of LEUSTATIN have been associated with: irreversible neurologic toxicity (paraparesis/quadriparesis), acute nephrotoxicity, and severe bone marrow suppression resulting in neutropenia, anemia and thrombocytopenia. (see WARNINGS) There is no known specific antidote to overdosage. Treatment of overdosage consists of discontinuation of LEUSTATIN, careful observation and appropriate supportive measures. It is not known whether the drug can be removed from the circulation by dialysis or hemofiltration.

DOSAGE AND ADMINISTRATION

Usual Dose:

The recommended dose and schedule of LEUSTATIN Injection for active Hairy Cell Leukemia is as a single course given by continuous infusion for 7 consecutive days at a dose of 0.09 mg/kg/day. Deviations from this dosage regimen are not advised. If the patient does not respond to the initial course of LEUSTATIN Injection for Hairy Cell Leukemia, it is unlikely that they will benefit from additional courses. Physicians should consider delaying or discontinuing the drug if neurotoxicity or renal toxicity occurs. (see WARNINGS)

Specific risk factors predisposing to increased toxicity from LEUSTATIN have not been defined. In view of the known toxicities of agents of this class, it would be prudent to proceed carefully in patients with known or suspected renal insufficiency or severe bone marrow impairment of any etiology. Patients should be monitored closely for hematologic and non-hematologic toxicity. (see WARNINGS and PRECAUTIONS).

Preparation and Administration of Intravenous Solutions:

LEUSTATIN Injection must be diluted with the designated diluent prior to administration. Since the drug product does not contain any anti-microbial preservative or bacteriostatic agent, **aseptic technique and proper environmental precautions must be observed in preparation of LEUSTATIN Injection solutions.**

To prepare a single daily dose: Add the calculated dose (0.09 mg/kg or 0.09 mL/kg) of LEUSTATIN Injection to an infusion bag containing 500 mL of 0.9% Sodium Chloride Injection, USP. Infuse continuously over 24 hours. Repeat daily for a total of 7 consecutive days. **The use of 5% dextrose as a diluent is not recommended because of increased degradation of cladribine.** Admixtures of LEUSTATIN Injection are chemically and physically stable for at least 24 hours at room temperature under normal room fluorescent light in Baxter Viaflex®† PVC infusion containers. **Since limited compatability data are available, adherence to the recommended diluents and infusion systems is advised.**

	Dose of LEUSTATIN Injection	Recommended Diluent	Quantity of Diluent
24-hour infusion method	1 (day) × 0.09 mg/kg	0.9% Sodium Chloride Injection, USP	500 mL

To prepare a 7-day infusion: The 7-day infusion solution should only be prepared with Bacteriostatic 0.9% Sodium Chloride Injection, USP (0.9% benzyl alcohol preserved). In order to minimize the risk of microbial contamination, both LEUSTATIN Injection and the diluent should be passed through a sterile 0.22µ disposable hydrophilic syringe filter as each solution is being introduced into the infusion reservoir. First add the calculated dose of LEUSTATIN Injection (7 days × 0.09 mg/kg or mL/kg) to the infusion reservoir through the sterile filter. Then add a calculated amount of Bacteriostatic 0.9% Sodium Chloride Injection, USP (0.9% benzyl alcohol preserved) also through the filter to bring the total volume of the solution to 100 mL. After completing solution preparation, clamp off the line, disconnect and discard the filter. Aseptically aspirate air bubbles from the reservoir as necessary using the syringe and a dry second sterile filter or a sterile vent filter assembly. Reclamp the line and discard the syringe and filter assembly. Infuse continuously over 7 days. Solutions prepared with Bacteriostatic Sodium Chloride Injection for individuals weighing more than 85 kg may have reduced preservative effectiveness due to greater dilution of the benzyl alcohol preservative. Admixtures for the 7-day infusion have demonstrated acceptable chemical and physical stability for at least 7 days in the SIMS Deltec MEDICATION CASSETTE™ Reservoir‡.

	Dose of LEUSTATIN Injection	Recommended Diluent	Quantity of Diluent
7-day infusion method (use sterile 0.22µ filter when preparing infusion solution)	7 (days) × 0.09 mg/kg	Bacteriostatic 0.9% Sodium Chloride Injection, USP (0.9% benzyl alcohol)	q.s. to 100 mL

Since limited compatibility data are available, adherence to the recommended diluents and infusion systems is advised. Solutions containing LEUSTATIN Injection should not be mixed with other intravenous drugs or additives or infused simultaneously via a common intravenous line, since compatibility testing has not been performed. Preparations containing benzyl alcohol should not be used in neonates. (see WARNINGS)

Care must be taken to assure the sterility of prepared solutions. Once diluted, solutions of LEUSTATIN Injection should be administered promptly or stored in the refrigerator (2° to 8°C) for no more than 8 hours prior to start of administration. Vials of LEUSTATIN Injection are for single-use only. Any unused portion should be discarded in an appropriate manner. (see Handling and Disposal)

Parenteral drug products should be inspected visually for particulate matter and discoloration prior to administration, whenever solution and container permit. A precipitate may occur during the exposure of LEUSTATIN Injection to low temperatures; it may be resolubilized by allowing the solution to warm naturally to room temperature and by shaking vigorously. **DO NOT HEAT OR MICROWAVE.**

Chemical Stability of Vials:

When stored in refrigerated conditions between 2° to 8°C (36° to 46°F) protected from light, unopened vials of LEUSTATIN Injection are stable until the expiration date indicated on the package. Freezing does not adversely affect the solution. If freezing occurs, thaw naturally to room temperature. DO NOT heat or microwave. Once thawed, the vial of LEUSTATIN Injection is stable until expiry if refrigerated. DO NOT refreeze. Once diluted, solutions containing LEUSTATIN Injection should be administered promptly or stored in the refrigerator (2° to 8°C) for no more than 8 hours prior to administration.

Handling and Disposal:

The potential hazards associated with cytotoxic agents are well established and proper precautions should be taken when handling, preparing, and administering LEUSTATIN Injection. The use of disposable gloves and protective garments is recommended. If LEUSTATIN Injection contacts the skin or mucous membranes, wash the involved surface immediately with copious amounts of water. Several guidelines on this subject have been published.[2–8] There is no general agreement that all of the procedures recommended in the guidelines are necessary or appropriate. Refer to your Institution's guidelines and all applicable state/local regulations for disposal of cytotoxic waste.

HOW SUPPLIED

LEUSTATIN Injection is supplied as a sterile, preservative-free, isotonic solution containing 10 mg (1 mg/mL) of cladribine as 10 mL filled into a single-use clear flint glass 20 mL vial. LEUSTATIN Injection is supplied in 10 mL (1 mg/mL) single-use vials (NDC 59676-201-01) available in a treatment set (case) of seven vials.

Store refrigerated 2° to 8°C (36° to 46°F). Protect from light during storage.

References:

1. Santana VM, Mirro J, Harwood FC, *et al:* A phase I clinical trial of 2-Chloro-deoxyadenosine in pediatric patients with acute leukemia. J. Clin. Onc., **9:** 416 (1991).
2. Recommendations for the Safe Handling of Parenteral Antineoplastic Drugs. NIH Publication No. 83–2621. For sale by the Superintendent of Documents, U. S. Government Printing Office, Washington, D.C. 20402.
3. AMA Council Report. Guidelines for Handling Parenteral Antineoplastics, JAMA, March 15 (1985).
4. National Study Commission on Cytotoxic Exposure—Recommendations for Handling Cytotoxic Agents. Available from Louis P. Jeffrey, Sc.D., Chairman, National Study Commission of Cytotoxic Exposure, Massachusetts College of Pharmacy and Allied Health Sciences, 179 Longwood Avenue, Boston, Massachusetts 02115.
5. Clinical Oncological Society of Australia: Guidelines and Recommendations for Safe Handling of Antineoplastic Agents, Med. J. Australia **1**:425 (1983).
6. Jones RB, *et al.* Safe Handling of Chemotherapeutic Agents: A Report from the Mount Sinai Medical Center. Ca—A Cancer Journal for Clinicians, Sept/Oct. 258–263 (1983).
7. American Society of Hospital Pharmacists Technical Assistance Bulletin on Handling Cytotoxic Drugs in Hospitals. Am. J. Hosp. Pharm., **42**:131 (1985).
8. OSHA Work-Practice Guidelines for Personnel Dealing with Cytotoxic (antineoplastic) Drugs. Am. J. Hosp. Pharm., **43**:1193 (1986).

CAUTION: Federal law prohibits dispensing without prescription.

† Viaflex® containers, manufactured by Baxter Healthcare Corporation - Code No. 2B8013 (testing in 1991)

‡ MEDICATION CASSETTE™ Reservoir, manufactured by SIMS Deltec, Inc. - Reorder No. 602100A (tested in 1991)

ORTHO BIOTECH INC.
Raritan, New Jersey 08869
©OBI 1996 638-10-940-5
Revised December 1996

Shown in Product Identification Guide, page 327

ORTHOCLONE OKT® 3 Sterile Solution ℞
(muromonab-CD3)
For Intravenous Use Only

WARNING

Only physicians experienced in immunosuppressive therapy and management of solid organ transplant patients should use ORTHOCLONE OKT3 (muromonab-CD3).

Anaphylactic or anaphylactoid reactions may occur following administration of any dose or course of ORTHOCLONE OKT3. Serious and occasionally life-threatening systemic, cardiovascular, and central nervous system reactions have been reported following administration of ORTHOCLONE OKT3. These have included: pulmonary edema, especially in patients with volume overload; shock; cardiovascular collapse; cardiac or respiratory arrest; seizures; and coma. Hence, a patient being treated with ORTHOCLONE OKT3 must be managed in a facility equipped and staffed for cardio-

pulmonary resuscitation. (see: WARNINGS: Cytokine Release Syndrome, Neuro-Psychiatric Events, Anaphylactic Reactions)

DESCRIPTION

ORTHOCLONE OKT3 (muromonab-CD3) Sterile Solution is a murine monoclonal antibody to the CD3 antigen of human T cells which functions as an immunosuppressant. It is for intravenous use only. The antibody is a biochemically purified IgG_{2a} immunoglobulin with a heavy chain of approximately 50,000 daltons and a light chain of approximately 25,000 daltons. It is directed to a glycoprotein with a molecular weight of 20,000 in the human T cell surface which is essential for T cell functions. Because it is a monoclonal antibody preparation, ORTHOCLONE OKT3 Sterile Solution is a homogeneous, reproducible antibody product with consistent, measurable reactivity to human T cells.

Each 5 mL ampule of ORTHOCLONE OKT3 Sterile Solution contains 5 mg (1 mg/mL) of muromonab-CD3 in a clear colorless solution which may contain a few fine translucent protein particles. Each ampule contains a buffered solution (pH 7.0 ±0.5) of monobasic sodium phosphate (2.25 mg), dibasic sodium phosphate (9.0 mg), sodium chloride (43 mg), and polysorbate 80 (1.0 mg) in water for injection.

The proper name, muromonab-CD3, is derived from the descriptive term murine monoclonal antibody. The CD3 designation identifies the specificity of the antibody as the Cell Differentiation (CD) cluster 3 defined by the First International Workshop on Human Leukocyte Differentiation Antigens.

CLINICAL PHARMACOLOGY

ORTHOCLONE OKT3 reverses graft rejection, most probably by blocking the function of all T cells which play a major role in acute allograft rejection. ORTHOCLONE OKT3 reacts with and blocks the function of a 20,000 dalton molecule (CD3) in the membrane of human T cells that has been associated *in vitro* with the antigen recognition structure of T cells and is essential for signal transduction. In *in vitro* cytolytic assays, ORTHOCLONE OKT3 blocks both the generation and function of effector cells. Binding of ORTHOCLONE OKT3 to T lymphocytes results in early activation of T cells, which leads to cytokine release, followed by blocking T cell functions. After termination of ORTHOCLONE OKT3 therapy, T cell function usually returns to normal within one week.

In vivo, ORTHOCLONE OKT3 reacts with most peripheral blood T cells and T cells in body tissues, but has not been found to react with other hematopoietic elements or other tissues of the body.

A rapid and concomitant decrease in the number of circulating CD2 positive, CD3 positive, CD4 positive, and CD8 positive T cells has been observed in patients studied within minutes after the administration of ORTHOCLONE OKT3. This decrease in the number of CD3 positive T cells results from the specific interaction between ORTHOCLONE OKT3 and the CD3 antigen on the surface of all T lymphocytes. T cell activation results in the release of numerous cytokines/lymphokines, which are felt to be responsible for many of the acute clinical manifestations seen following ORTHOCLONE OKT3 administration. (see: WARNINGS: Cytokine Release Syndrome, Neuro-Psychiatric Events)

While CD3 positive cells are not detectable between days two and seven, increasing numbers of circulating CD4 and CD8 positive cells have been observed. The presence of these CD4 and CD8 positive cells has not been shown to affect reversal of rejection. After termination of ORTHOCLONE OKT3 therapy, CD3 positive cells reappear rapidly and reach pre-treatment levels within a week. In some patients however, increasing numbers of CD3 positive cells have been observed prior to termination of ORTHOCLONE OKT3 therapy. This reappearance of CD3 positive cells has been attributed to the development of neutralizing antibodies to ORTHOCLONE OKT3, which in turn block its ability to bind to the CD3 antigen on T lypmphocytes. (see: PRECAUTIONS: Sensitization)

In the initial clinical trials using low doses of prednisone and azathioprine during ORTHOCLONE OKT3 therapy for renal allograft rejection, antibodies to ORTHOCLONE OKT3 were observed with an incidence of 21% (n=43) for IgM, 86% (n=43) for IgG and 29% (n=35) for IgE. The mean time of appearance of IgG antibodies was 20±2 (mean ±SD) days. Early IgG antibodies appeared towards the end of the second week of treatment in 3% (n=86) of the patients.

Subsequent clinical experience has shown that the dose, duration, and type of immunosuppressive medications used in combination with ORTHOCLONE OKT3 may affect both the incidence and magnitude of the host antibody response. Furthermore, immunosuppressive agents used concomitantly with ORTHOCLONE OKT3 (i.e., steroids, azathioprine, prednisone, or cyclosporine) have altered the time course of anti-mouse antibody development and the specificity of the antibodies formed (i.e., idiotypic, isotypic, allotypic).

Serum levels of ORTHOCLONE OKT3 are measurable using an enzyme-linked immunosorbent assay (ELISA). During the initial clinical trials in renal allograft rejection, in patients treated with 5 mg per day for 14 days, mean serum trough levels of the drug rose over the first three days and then averaged 900 ng/mL on days 3 to 14. Subsequent clinical experience has demonstrated that circulating serum levels greater than or equal to 800 ng/mL of ORTHOCLONE OKT3 blocks the function of cytotoxic T cells *in vitro* and *in vivo.* (see: PRECAUTIONS: Laboratory Tests)

Following administration of ORTHOCLONE OKT3 *in vivo,* leukocytes have been observed in cerebrospinal and peritoneal fluids. The mechanism for this effect is not completely understood, but probably is related to cytokines altering membrane permeability, rather than an active inflammatory process (see: WARNINGS: Cytokine Release Syndrome, Neuro-Psychiatric Events)

INDICATIONS AND USAGE

ORTHOCLONE OKT3 is indicated for the treatment of acute allograft rejection in renal transplant patients.

ORTHOCLONE OKT3 is also indicated for the treatment of steroid-resistant acute allograft rejection in cardiac and hepatic transplant patients.

Acute Renal Rejection:

In a controlled randomized clinical trial, ORTHOCLONE OKT3 was significantly more effective than conventional high-dose steroid therapy in reversing acute renal allograft rejection. In this trial, 122 evaluable patients undergoing acute rejection of cadaveric renal transplants were treated either with ORTHOCLONE OKT3 daily for a mean of 14 days, with concomitant lowering of the dosage of azathioprine and maintenance steroids (62 patients), or with conventional high-dose steroids (60 patients). ORTHOCLONE OKT3 reversed 94% of the rejections compared to a 75% reversal rate obtained with conventional high-dose steroid treatment (p=0.006). The one year Kaplan-Meier (actuarial) estimates of graft survival rates for these patients who had acute rejection were 62% and 45% for ORTHOCLONE OKT3 and steroid-treated patients, respectively (p=0.04). At two years the rates were 56% and 42%, respectively (p=0.06).

One- and two-year patient survivals were not significantly different between the two groups, being 85% and 75% for ORTHOCLONE OKT3 treated patients and 90% and 85% for steroid-treated patients.

In additional open clinical trials, the observed rate of reversal of acute renal allograft rejection was 92% (n=126) for ORTHOCLONE OKT3 therapy. ORTHOCLONE OKT3 was also effective in reversing acute renal allograft rejections in 65% (n=225) of cases where steroids and lymphocyte immune globulin preparations were contraindicated or were not successful (rescue).

Acute Cardiac or Hepatic Allograft Rejection:

ORTHOCLONE OKT3 has also been shown to be effective in reversing acute cardiac and hepatic allograft rejection in patients who are unresponsive to high-doses of steroids. Controlled randomized trials have not been conducted to evaluate the effectiveness of ORTHOCLONE OKT3 (muromonab-CD3) compared to conventional therapy as first line treatment for acute cardiac and hepatic allograft rejection.

The rate of reversal in acute cardiac allograft rejection was 90% (n=61) and was 83% for hepatic allograft rejection (n=124) in patients unresponsive to treatment with steroids.

The dosage of other immunosuppressive agents used in conjunction with ORTHOCLONE OKT3 should be reduced to the lowest level compatible with an effective therapeutic response. (see: WARNINGS and ADVERSE REACTIONS: Infections, Neoplasia; DOSAGE AND ADMINISTRATION)

CONTRAINDICATIONS

ORTHOCLONE OKT3 should not be given to patients who:

- are hypersensitive to this or any other product of murine origin;
- have anti-mouse antibody titers ≥1:1000;
- are in (uncompensated) heart failure or in fluid overload, as evidenced by chest X-ray or a greater than 3 percent weight gain within the week prior to planned ORTHOCLONE OKT3 administration;
- have a history of seizures, or are predisposed to seizures;
- are determined and/or suspected to be pregnant, or who are breast-feeding. (see: PRECAUTIONS: Pregnancy, Nursing Mothers)

WARNINGS

SEE BOXED WARNING

Cytokine Release Syndrome

Temporarily associated with the administration of the first few doses of ORTHOCLONE OKT3 (particularly, the first two to three doses), most patients have developed an acute clinical syndrome [i.e., Cytokine Release Syndrome (CRS)] that has been attributed to the release of cytokines by activated lymphocytes or monocytes. This clinical syndrome has ranged from a more frequently reported mild, self-limited, "flu-like" illness to a less frequently reported severe, life-threatening, shock-like reaction, which may include serious cardiovascular and central nervous system manifestations. The syndrome typically begins approximately 30 to 60 minutes after administration of a dose of ORTHOCLONE OKT3 (but may occur later) and may persist for several hours. The frequency and severity of this symptom complex is usually greatest with the first dose. With each successive dose of ORTHOCLONE OKT3, both the frequency and severity of the Cytokine Release Syndrome tends to diminish. Increasing the amount of a dose or resuming treatment after a hiatus may result in a reappearance of the CRS.

Common clinical manifestations of the Cytokine Release Syndrome may include: high (often spiking, up to 107°F) fever, chills/rigors, headache, tremor, nausea/vomiting, diarrhea, abdominal pain, malaise, muscle/joint aches and pains, and generalized weakness. Less frequently reported adverse experiences include: minor dermatologic reactions (e.g., rash, pruritus, etc.) and a spectrum of often serious, occasionally fatal, cardiorespiratory and neuro-psychiatric adverse experiences. (see: WARNINGS, PRECAUTIONS, and ADVERSE REACTIONS: Neuro-Psychiatric Events)

Cardiorespiratory findings may include: dyspnea, shortness of breath, bronchospasm/wheezing, tachypnea, respiratory arrest/failure/distress, cardiovascular collapse, cardiac arrest, angina/myocardial infarction, chest pain/tightness, tachycardia (including ventricular), hypertension, hemodynamic instability, hypotension including profound shock, heart failure, pulmonary edema (cardiogenic and non-cardiogenic), adult respiratory distress syndrome, hypoxemia, apnea, and arrhythmias. (see: BOXED WARNING; PRECAUTIONS; ADVERSE REACTIONS)

In the initial renal rejection studies, the most serious post-dose reaction-potentially fatal, severe *pulmonary edema*-occurred in 4.7% of the initial 107 patients. Fluid overload was present before treatment in all of these cases. However, it occurred in 0.0% of the subsequent 311 patients treated with first-dose volume/weight restrictions. In subsequent trials and in post-marketing experience, severe pulmonary edema has occurred in patients who appeared to be euvolemic. The pathogenesis of pulmonary edema may involve all or some of the following: volume overload; increased pulmonary vascular permeability; and/or reduced left ventricular compliance/contractility.

During the first 1 to 3 days of ORTHOCLONE OKT3 therapy, some patients have experienced an acute and transient decline in the glomerular filtration rate (GFR) and diminished urine output with a resulting *increase in the level of serum creatinine.* Massive release of cytokines appears to lead to reversible renal functional impairment and/or delayed renal allograft function.

Similarly, transient elevations in hepatic transaminases have been reported following administration of the first few doses of ORTHOCLONE OKT3 (muromonab-CD3).

Patients at risk for more serious complications of the Cytokine Release Syndrome may include those with the following conditions: unstable angina; recent myocardial infarction or symptomatic ischemic heart disease; heart failure of any etiology; pulmonary edema of any etiology; any form of chronic obstructive pulmonary disease; intravascular volume overload or depletion of any etiology (e.g., excessive dialysis, recent intensive diuresis, blood loss, etc.); cerebrovascular disease; patients with advanced symptomatic vascular disease or neuropathy; a history of seizures; and septic shock. Efforts should be made to correct or stabilize background conditions prior to the initiation of therapy.

Prior to administration of ORTHOCLONE OKT3, the patient's volume (fluid) status should be assessed carefully. It is imperative, especially prior to the first few doses, that there be no clinical evidence of volume overload or uncompensated heart failure, including a clear chest X-ray and weight restriction of ≤3% above the patient's minimum weight during the week prior to injection.

Manifestations of the Cytokine Release Syndrome may be prevented or minimized by pretreatment with 8 mg/kg of methylprednisolone (i.e., high-dose steroids), given 1 to 4 hours prior to administration of the first dose of ORTHOCLONE OKT3, and by closely following recommendations for dosage and treatment duration. (see: DOSAGE AND ADMINISTRATION)

The administration of ORTHOCLONE OKT3 should be performed in a facility that is equipped and staffed for cardiopulmonary resuscitation and where a patient can be closely monitored for an appropriate period based on the patient's status.

If any of the more serious presentations of the Cytokine Release Syndrome occur, intensive treatment including oxygen, intravenous fluids, corticosteroids, pressor amines, antihistamines, intubation, etc., may be required.

Anaphylactic Reactions

Serious and occasionally fatal, immediate (usually within 10 minutes) hypersensitivity (anaphylactic) reactions have been reported in patients treated with ORTHOCLONE OKT3. **Manifestations of anaphylaxis may appear similar to manifestations of the Cytokine Release Syndrome (described above). It may be impossible to determine the**

Continued on next page

Orthoclone—Cont.

mechanism responsible for any systemic reaction(s). Reactions attributed to hypersensitivity have been reported less frequently than those attributed to cytokine release. Acute hypersensitivity reactions may be characterized by: cardiovascular collapse, cardiorespiratory arrest, loss of consciousness, hypotension/shock, tachycardia, tingling, angioedema (including laryngeal, pharyngeal, or facial edema), airway obstruction, bronchospasm, dyspnea, urticaria, and pruritus.

Serious allergic events, including anaphylactic or anaphylactoid reactions, have been reported in patients re-exposed to ORTHOCLONE OKT3 subsequent to their initial course of therapy. Pretreatment with antihistamines and/or steroids may not reliably prevent anaphylaxis in this setting. Possible allergic hazards of retreatment should be weighed against expected therapeutic benefits and alternatives. If retreatment with ORTHOCLONE OKT3 is employed, epinephrine and other emergency life-support equipment should be available, and the patient should be monitored closely.

If hypersensitivity is suspected, discontinue the drug immediately, do not resume therapy or re-expose the patient to ORTHOCLONE OKT3. Serious acute hypersensitivity reactions may require emergency treatment with 0.3 mL to 0.5 mL aqueous epinephrine (1:1000 dilution) subcutaneously and other resuscitative measures including oxygen, intravenous fluids, antihistamines, corticosteroids, pressor amines, and airway management, as clinically indicated. (see: PRECAUTIONS: Cytokine Release Syndrome vs. Anaphylactic Reactions; ADVERSE REACTIONS: Hypersensitivity Reactions)

Neuro-Psychiatric Events

Seizures, encephalopathy, cerebral edema, aseptic meningitis, and headache have been reported, even following the first dose, during therapy with ORTHOCLONE OKT3, resulting in part from T cell activation and subsequent systemic release of cytokines.

Seizures, some accompanied by loss of consciousness or cardiorespiratory arrest, or death, have occurred independently or in conjunction with any of the neurologic syndromes described below. Patients predisposed to seizures may include those with the following conditions: acute tubular necrosis/uremia, fever, infection, a precipitous fall in serum calcium, fluid overload, hypertension, hypoglycemia, history of seizures, and electrolyte imbalances or those who are taking a medication concomitantly that may, by itself, cause seizures.

Between 1987 and 1992, 75 post-marketing reports described seizures, averaging about 12 per year, and including 23 fatalities. More than two-thirds of these reports (53) were of domestic spontaneous origin, and their age and sex distributions were broad. Post-licensure reports generally do not provide sufficient basis for estimation of actual risks (incidence rates for specific adverse events), due to the typically substantial but unknown extent of under-ascertainment of incident events. Nonetheless, the number and regularity of seizure reports with ORTHOCLONE OKT3 (muromonab-CD3) indicate that this hazard appears not to be rare. Convulsions should be anticipated clinically with appropriate patient monitoring.

Manifestations of encephalopathy may include: impaired cognition, confusion, obtundation, altered mental status, disorientation, auditory/visual hallucinations, psychosis (delirium, paranoia), mood changes (e.g., mania, agitation, combativeness, etc.), diffuse hypotonus, hyperreflexia, myoclonus, tremor, asterixis, involuntary movements, major motor seizures, lethargy/stupor/coma, and diffuse weakness. Approximately one-third of patients with a diagnosis of encephalopathy may have had coexisting aseptic meningitis syndrome.

Cerebral edema (and other signs of increased vascular permeability e.g., otitis media, nasal and ear stuffiness, etc.) has been seen in patients treated with ORTHOCLONE OKT3 and may accompany some of the other neurologic manifestations.

Signs and symptoms of the *aseptic meningitis syndrome* described in association with the use of ORTHOCLONE OKT3 have included: fever, headache, meningismus (stiff neck), and photophobia. In a post-marketing survey involving 214 renal transplant patients, the incidence of this syndrome was 6%. Fever (89%), headache (44%), neck stiffness (14%), and photophobia (10%) were the most commonly reported symptoms; a combination of these four symptoms occurred in 5% of patients. Diagnosis is confirmed by cerebrospinal fluid (CSF) analysis demonstrating leukocytosis with pleocytosis, elevated protein and normal or decreased glucose, with negative viral, bacterial, and fungal cultures. In any immunosuppressed transplant patient with clinical findings suggesting meningitis, the possibility of infection should be evaluated. Approximately one-third of the patients with a diagnosis of aseptic meningitis had coexisting signs and symptoms of encephalopathy. Most patients with the aseptic meningitis syndrome had a benign course and recovered without any permanent sequelae during therapy or subsequent to its completion or discontinuation.

Headache is frequently seen after any of the first few doses and may occur in any of the aforementioned neurologic syndromes or by itself.

The following additional neurologic events have each been reported occasionally in post-licensure reports: irreversible blindness, impaired vision, quadri- or paraparesis/plegia, cerebrovascular accident (hemiparesis/plegia), aphasia, transient ischemic attack, subarachnoid hemorrhage, palsy of the VI cranial nerve, and hearing loss.

Signs or symptoms of encephalopathy, meningitis, seizures, and cerebral edema, with or without headache, have typically been reversible. Headache, aseptic meningitis, seizures, and less severe forms of encephalopathy resolved in most patients despite continued treatment. However, some events have been irreversible.

Other neurologic events observed in patients treated with ORTHOCLONE OKT3 include: post-therapy encephalopathy with or without coexisting metabolic disturbances, post-therapy meningitis, CNS lymphoproliferative disorders and infections. Since these patients usually had both serious and multiple coexisting medical conditions and were also receiving multiple concomitant medications, the association of these events with ORTHOCLONE OKT3 treatment is unclear.

Patients who may be at greater risk for CNS adverse experiences include those: with known or suspected CNS disorders (e.g., history of seizure disorder, etc.); with cerebrovascular disease (small or large vessel); with conditions having associated neurologic problems (e.g., head trauma, uremia, etc.); with underlying vascular diseases; or who are receiving a medication concomitantly that may, by itself, affect the central nervous system. (see: WARNINGS, PRECAUTIONS and ADVERSE REACTIONS; Cytokine Release Syndrome; PRECAUTIONS: Drug Interactions)

Consequences of Immunosuppression

Serious and sometimes fatal infections and neoplasias have been reported in association with all immunosuppressive therapies, including those regimens containing ORTHOCLONE OKT3 (muromonab-CD-3).

Infections: ORTHOCLONE OKT3 is usually added to immunosuppressive therapeutic regimens, thereby augmenting the degree of immunosuppression. This increase in the total burden of immunosuppression may alter the spectrum of infections observed and increase the risk, the severity, and the potential gravity (morbidity) of infectious complications. During the first month post-transplant, patients are at greatest risk for the following infections: (1) those present prior to transplant, perhaps exacerbated by post-transplant immunosuppression; (2) infection conveyed by the donor organ; and (3) the usual post-operative urinary tract, intravenous line-related, wound, or pulmonary infections due to bacterial pathogens.

Approximately one to six months post-transplant, patients are at risk for viral infections [e.g., Cytomegalovirus (CMV), Epstein-Barr Virus (EBV), Herpes simplex virus (HSV), etc.] which produce serious systemic disease and which also increase the overall state of immunosuppression. Clinically significant infections (e.g., pneumonia, sepsis, etc.) may occur with any microorganisms including: *Pneumocystis carinii, Listeria monocytogenes, Aspergillus* species, *Candida* species, *Nocardia asteroides, Legionella,* mycobacteria, gram-negative rods, and gram-positive cocci (staphylococci and streptococci), etc. Opportunistic infections, related to decreased T cell function, are associated with all immunosuppressive modalities employed to treat transplant rejection. Multiple or intensive courses of any anti-T cell antibody preparation, including ORTHOCLONE OKT3, which produce profound impairment of cell-mediated immunity, further increase the risk of (opportunistic) infection, especially with the Herpes viruses (HSV, CMV, EBV) and fungi. Reactivation (1 to 4 months post-transplant) of EBV and CMV has been reported. Infectious syndromes due to CMV have included: fever of unknown origin, pneumonia, viremia, hepatitis, liver/renal dysfunction, gastritis or gastrointestinal ulcerations, pancreatitis, chorioretinitis, leukopenia, and thrombocytopenia. When administration of an antilymphocyte antibody, including ORTHOCLONE OKT3, is followed by an immunosuppressive regimen including cyclosporine, there is an increased risk of reactivating CMV and impaired ability to limit its proliferation, resulting in symptomatic and disseminated disease. EBV infection, either primary or reactivated, may play an important role in the development of post-transplant lymphoproliferative disorders. (see: WARNINGS and ADVERSE REACTIONS: Neoplasia)

Anti-infective prophylaxis may reduce the morbidity associated with certain potential pathogens and should be considered for high-risk patients. Judicious use of immunosuppressive drugs, including type, dosage, and duration, may limit the risk and seriousness of some opportunistic infections. It is also possible to reduce the risk of serious CMV or EBV infection by avoiding transplantation of a CMV-seropositive (donor) and/or EBV-seropositive (donor) organ into a seronegative patient.

Neoplasia: As a result of depressed cell-mediated immunity, organ transplant patients have an increased risk of developing malignancies. This risk is evidenced almost exclusively by the occurrence of lymphoproliferative disorders (LPD), lymphomas, and skin cancers. In immunosuppressed patients, T cell cytotoxicity is impaired allowing for transformation and proliferation of EBV-infected B lymphocytes. Transformed B lymphocytes are thought to initiate the oncogenic process that ultimately culminates in the development of most post-transplant lymphoproliferative disorders. (see: ADVERSE REACTIONS: Neoplasia)

Following the initiation of ORTHOCLONE OKT3 therapy, patients should be continuously monitored for evidence of LPD, through physical examination and histological evaluation of any suspect lymphoid tissue. Vigilant surveillance is advised, since early detection with subsequent reduction of total immunosuppression may result in regression of some of these lymphoproliferative disorders. Since the potential for the development of LPD is related to the duration and extent (intensity) of total immunosuppression, physicians are advised: to adhere to the recommended dosage and duration of ORTHOCLONE OKT3 therapy; to limit the number of courses of ORTHOCLONE OKT3 and other anti-T lymphocyte antibody preparations administered within a short period of time; and, if appropriate, to reduce the dosage(s) of immunosuppressive drugs used concomitantly to the lowest level compatible with an effective therapeutic response. (see: DOSAGE AND ADMINISTRATION) The long-term risk of neoplastic events in patients being treated with ORTHOCLONE OKT3 has not been determined.

PRECAUTIONS

General

Prior to Treatment with ORTHOCLONE OKT3 (muromonab-CD3)

Fluid Status: The patient's volume (fluid) status should be assessed carefully. It is imperative, especially prior to the first few doses, that there be no clinical evidence of volume overload, uncontrolled hypertension, or uncompensated heart failure, including a clear chest X-ray and weight restriction of ≤3% above the patient's minimum weight during the week prior to injection.

Fever: If the temperature of the patient exceeds 37.8°C (100°F), it should be lowered by antipyretics before administration of each dose of ORTHOCLONE OKT3. The possibility of infection should be evaluated.

Blood Tests: Periodic assessment of organ system functions (renal, hepatic, and hematopoietic) should be performed.

During therapy with ORTHOCLONE OKT3: Periodic monitoring to ensure plasma ORTHOCLONE OKT3 levels (≥800 ng/mL) or T cell clearance (CD3 positive T cells <25 cells/mm^3) is recommended.

Severe Cytokine Release Syndrome Versus Anaphylactic Reactions: **It may be very difficult, even impossible, to distinguish between an acute hypersensitivity reaction (e.g., anaphylaxis, angioedema, etc.) and the Cytokine Release Syndrome. Potentially serious signs and symptoms having an immediate onset (usually within 10 minutes) following administration of ORTHOCLONE OKT3 are more likely due to acute hypersensitivity; discontinue the drug immediately. If hypersensitivity is suspected, do not resume therapy or re-expose the patient** to ORTHOCLONE OKT3. Clinical manifestations beginning approximately 30 to 60 minutes (or later) following administration of ORTHOCLONE OKT3, are more likely cytokine-mediated. (see: WARNINGS: Cytokine Release Syndrome, Anaphylactic Reactions)

Neuro-Psychiatric Events: Since some seizures (and other serious central nervous system events) following ORTHOCLONE OKT3 administration have been life-threatening, anti-seizure precautions (e.g., an airway ready for use, if needed) should be taken. (see: WARNINGS and ADVERSE REACTIONS: Neuro-Psychiatric Events)

Infection/Viral-Induced Lymphoproliferative Disorders: Patients must be observed carefully for any signs and symptoms suggesting infection or viral-induced lymphoproliferative disorders (LPD). Anti-infective prophylaxis should be considered for patients at high risk. If infection or viral-induced LPD occur, culture or biopsy as soon as possible, institute promptly appropriate anti-infective therapy, and (if possible) reduce/discontinue immunosuppressive therapy.

When using combinations of immunosuppressive agents, the dose of each agent, including ORTHOCLONE OKT3, should be reduced to the lowest level compatible with an effective therapeutic response so as to reduce the potential for and severity of infections and malignant transformations (see: WARNINGS: Infections, Neoplasia)

Low Protein-Binding Filter: Use a low protein-binding 0.2 or 0.22 micrometer (μm) filter to prepare the injections. (see: ADMINISTRATION INSTRUCTIONS)

Sensitization: ORTHOCLONE OKT3 is a mouse (immunoglobulin) protein that can induce human anti-mouse antibody production (i.e., sensitization) in patients following exposure (See: CLINICAL PHARMACOLOGY). Monitoring for human antibody titers after ORTHOCLONE OKT3 therapy is strongly recommended. (see: CONTRAINDICATIONS)

Reduced T cell clearance or impaired ability to maintain adequate ORTHOCLONE OKT3 levels provides a basis for adjusting ORTHOCLONE OKT3 dosage or for discontinuing therapy. (see: WARNINGS: Anaphylactic Reactions; PRECAUTIONS: Laboratory Tests; ADVERSE REACTIONS: Hypersensitivity Reactions)

Intravascular Thrombosis: As with other immunosuppressive therapies, arterial or venous thromboses of allografts and other vascular beds (e.g., heart, lungs, brain, bowel, etc.) have been reported in patients treated with ORTHOCLONE OKT3. In addition, microangiopathic changes (e.g., platelet microthrombi) in the renal allograft associated in some patients with microangiopathic hemolytic anemia have been reported. This was observed in 5 of 93 (5%) patients receiving doses above the recommended dose (10 mg/day) Because a few cases have also been reported with the recommended dose, the relationship to dose remains uncertain. However, the relative risk appears to be greater with doses above the recommended dose. The decision to use ORTHOCLONE OKT3 in patients with a history of thrombotic events or underlying vascular disease should take these findings into consideration. Concomitant use of prophylactic anti-thrombotic interventions (e.g., mini-dose heparin, etc.) should be considered. (see: ADVERSE REACTIONS)

Information for Patients: Patients should be advised:

- of the signs and symptoms associated with the Cytokine Release Syndrome, including the potentially serious nature of this symptom complex (e.g., systemic, cardiovascular, neuro-psychiatric events).
- to seek medical attention at the first sign of skin rash, urticaria, rapid heartbeat, difficulty in swallowing and breathing, or any swelling that may suggest angioedema, or other allergic reaction.
- to know how they might react to ORTHOCLONE OKT3 (muromonab-CD-3) before operating an automobile or machinery, or engaging in activities requiring mental alertness and coordination.
- of the potential benefits and other risks attendant to the use of ORTHOCLONE OKT3. (see: BOXED WARNING; WARNINGS; PRECAUTIONS; ADVERSE REACTIONS)

Drug Interactions: The following medications are frequently used with ORTHOCLONE OKT3 and the information provided below may be helpful in evaluating any adverse events reported in ORTHOCLONE OKT3 treated patients.

With *indomethacin:* Encephalopathy and other CNS effects have been reported in patients treated with indomethacin alone and in conjunction with ORTHOCLONE OKT3. The mechanism of these effects is unknown.

With *corticosteroids:* Psychosis and infections have been seen in patients treated with corticosteroids alone and in conjunction with ORTHOCLONE OKT3.

With *azathioprine:* Infections or malignancies have been reported with azathioprine alone and in conjunction with ORTHOCLONE OKT3.

With *cyclosporine:* Seizures, encephalopathy, infections, malignancies, and thrombotic events have been reported in patients receiving cyclosporine alone and in conjunction with ORTHOCLONE OKT3.

Laboratory Tests: As with many potent drugs, periodic assessment of organ system functions should be performed during treatment with ORTHOCLONE OKT3.

The following tests should be monitored prior to and during ORTHOCLONE OKT3 therapy:

- Renal: BUN, serum creatinine, etc.:
- Hepatic: transaminases, alkaline phosphatase, bilirubin;
- Hematopoietic: WBCs and differential, platelet count, etc.;
- Chest X-ray within 24 hours before initiating ORTHOCLONE OKT3 treatment. *Recommendation: chest X-ray should be free of any evidence of heart failure or fluid overload.*

One of the following immunologic tests should be monitored **during** ORTHOCLONE OKT3 therapy:

- Plasma ORTHOCLONE OKT3 levels (as determined by an ELISA); *target ORTHOCLONE OKT3 levels should be ≥800 ng/mL;* or
- Quantitative T lymphocyte surface phenotyping (CD3, CD4, CD8); target CD3 positive T cells <25 cells/mm^3.

Testing for human-mouse antibody titers is strongly recommended; *a titer ≥1:1000 is a contraindication for use.* (see: CONTRAINDICATIONS; PRECAUTIONS: Sensitization)

Carcinogenesis: Long-term studies have not been performed in laboratory animals to evaluate the carcinogenic potential of ORTHOCLONE OKT3. (see: WARNINGS and ADVERSE REACTIONS: Neoplasia)

Pregnancy Category C: Animal reproductive studies have not been conducted with ORTHOCLONE OKT3. It is also not known whether ORTHOCLONE OKT3 can cause fetal harm when administered to a pregnant woman or can affect reproduction capacity. However, ORTHOCLONE OKT3 is an IgG antibody and may cross the human placenta. The effect on the fetus of the release of cytokines and/or immunosuppression after treatment with ORTHOCLONE OKT3 is not known. If this drug is used during pregnancy, or the patient becomes pregnant while taking this drug, the patient should be apprised of the potential hazard to the fetus. (see: CONTRAINDICATIONS, WARNINGS, and ADVERSE REACTIONS)

Nursing Mothers: It is not known whether ORTHOCLONE OKT3 is excreted in human milk. Because many drugs are excreted in human milk and because of the potential for serious adverse reactions/oncogenesis shown for ORTHOCLONE OKT3 in human studies, a decision should be made to discontinue nursing or to discontinue the drug, taking into account the importance of the drug to the mother. (see: CONTRAINDICATIONS)

Pediatric Use: Safety and effectiveness in children have not been established. No adequately controlled clinical studies have been conducted in children. Published literature[4,10] has reported the use of ORTHOCLONE OKT3 (muromonab-CD-3) infants/children, beginning with a dose of ≤5 mg. Based on immunologic monitoring, the dosage has been adjusted accordingly (See: PRECAUTIONS: Laboratory Tests). Pediatric recipients are reported to be significantly immunosuppressed for a prolonged period of time and therefore, require close monitoring post-therapy for opportunistic infections, particularly varicella (VZV), which poses an infectious complication unique to this population. Gastrointestinal fluid loss secondary to diarrhea and/or vomiting resulting from the Cytokine Release Syndrome may be significant when treating small children and may require parenteral hydration. It is unknown whether there may be significant long-term sequelae (e.g., neurodevelopmental language difficulties in infants under 1 year of age) related to the occurrence of seizures, high fever, CNS infections, aseptic meningitis, etc., following ORTHOCLONE OKT3 treatment. In cases where administration of ORTHOCLONE OKT3 would be deemed medically appropriate, more vigilant and frequent monitoring is required for children than in adults. (see: BOXED WARNING; WARNINGS; PRECAUTIONS; ADVERSE REACTIONS)

ADVERSE REACTIONS

Cytokine Release Syndrome

In controlled clinical trials for treatment of acute renal allograft rejection, patients treated with ORTHOCLONE OKT3 plus concomitant low-dose immunosuppressive therapy (primarily azathioprine and corticosteroids) were observed to have an increased incidence of adverse experiences during the first two days of treatment, as compared with the group of patients receiving azathioprine and high-dose steroid therapy. During this period the majority of patients experienced pyrexia (90%), of which 19% were 40.0°C (104°F) or above, and chills (59%). In addition, other adverse experiences occurring in 8% or more of the patients during the first two days of ORTHOCLONE OKT3 therapy included: dyspnea (21%), nausea (19%), vomiting (19%), chest pain (14%), diarrhea (14%), tremor (13%), wheezing (13%), headache (11%), tachycardia (10%), rigor (8%), and hypertension (8%). A similar spectrum of clinical manifestations has been observed in open clinical studies and in post-marketing experience involving patients treated with ORTHOCLONE OKT3 for rejection following renal, cardiac, and hepatic transplantation.

Additional serious and occasionally fatal cardiorespiratory manifestations have been reported following any of the first few doses. (see: WARNINGS: Cytokine Release Syndrome; ADVERSE REACTIONS: Cardiovascular, Respiratory)

In the acute renal allograft rejection trials, potentially fatal pulmonary edema had been reported following the first two doses in less than 2% of the patients treated with ORTHOCLONE OKT3. Pulmonary edema was usually associated with fluid overload. However, post-marketing experience revealed that pulmonary edema has occurred in patients who appeared to be euvolemic, presumably as a consequence of cytokine-mediated increased vascular permeability ("leaky capillaries") and/or reduced myocardial contractility/compliance (i.e., left ventricular dysfunction). (see: WARNINGS: Cytokine Release Syndrome; DOSAGE AND ADMINISTRATION)

Infections

In the controlled randomized renal rejection trial conducted during the pre-cyclosporine era, the most common infections during the first 45 days of ORTHOCLONE OKT3 therapy were due to Herpes simplex (27%) and cytomegalovirus (19%). Other severe and life-threatening infections were *Staphylococcus epidermidis* (4.8%), *Pneumocystis carinii* (3.1%), *Legionella* (1.6%), *Cryptococcus* (1.6%), *Serratia* (1.6%) and gram-negative bacteria (1.6%). The incidence of infections was similar in patients treated with ORTHOCLONE OKT3 and in patients treated with high-dose steroids.

In a clinical trial of acute hepatic rejection refractory to conventional treatment, the most common infections reported in patients treated with ORTHOCLONE OKT3 during the first 45 days of the study were cytomegalovirus (15.7% of patients, of which 43% of infections were severe), fungal infections (14.9% of patients, of which 30% were severe), and Herpes simplex (7.5% of patients, of which 10% were severe). Other severe and life-threatening infections were gram-positive infections (9.0% of patients), gram-negative infections (7.5% of patients), viral infections (1.5% of patients), and *Legionella* (0.7% of patients). In another hepatic rejection trial the incidence of fungal infections was 34% and infections with the Herpes simplex virus was 31%.

In a clinical trial of acute cardiac rejection refractory to conventional treatment, the most common infections reported in the ORTHOCLONE OKT3 (muromonab-CD3) group during the first 45 days of the study were Herpes simplex (5% of patients, of which 20% were severe), fungal infections (4% of patients, of which 75% were severe), and cytomegalovirus (3% of patients, of which 33% were severe). No other severe or life-threatening infections were reported during this period.

Clinically significant infections (e.g., pneumonia, sepsis, etc.) due to the following pathogens have been reported:

Bacterial: *Clostridium* species (including perfringens), *Corynebacterium,* Enterococcus, *Enterobacter aerogenes, Escherichia coli, Klebsiella* species, *Lactobacillus, Legionella, Listeria monocytogenes, Mycobacteria* species, *Nocardia asteroides, Proteus* species, *Providencia* species, *Pseudomonas aeruginosa, Serratia* species, *Staphylococcus* species, *Streptococcus* species, *Yersinia enterocolitica,* and other gram-negative bacteria.

Fungal: * *Aspergillus, Candida,* Cryptococcal, Dermatophytes.

Protozoa: *Pneumocystis carinii, Toxoplasma gondii.*

Viral: Cytomegalovirus* (CMV), Epstein-Barr virus* (EBV), Herpes simplex virus* (HSV), Hepatitis viruses, Varicella zoster virus (VZV).

As a consequence of being a potent immunosuppressive, the incidence and severity of infections with designated(*) pathogens, especially the Herpes family of viruses, may be increased. (see: WARNINGS: Infections)

Neoplasia

In patients treated with ORTHOCLONE OKT3 post-transplant lymphoproliferative disorders (LPD) reported have ranged from lymphadenopathy or benign polyclonal B cell hyperplasias to malignant and often fatal monoclonal B cell lymphomas. In post-marketing experience, approximately one-third of the lymphoproliferations reported were benign, and two-thirds were malignant. Classification of these lymphomas has included: B cell, large cell, polyclonal, non-Hodgkin's, lymphocytic, T cell, Burkitt's; the majority have not been classified histologically. When malignant lymphomas have been reported, they have appeared to develop early after transplantation, the majority within the first four months post-treatment. Many of these have been rapidly progressive, some fulminant involving the allografted organ, widely disseminated at time of diagnosis, and fatal. Carcinomas of the skin have included: basal cell, squamous cell, Kaposi's sarcoma, malanoma, and keratoacanthoma. Other neoplasms infrequently reported include: multiple myeloma, leukemia, carcinoma of the breast, adenocarcinoma, cholangiocarcinoma, and recurrences of pre-existing hepatoma and renal cell carcinoma. (see: WARNINGS: Neoplasia)

Hypersensitivity Reactions

Reported adverse reactions resulting from the formation of antibodies to ORTHOCLONE OKT3 have inlcuded antigen-antibody (immune complex) mediated syndromes and IgE-mediated reactions. Reported hypersensitivity reactions have ranged from a mild, self-limited rash or pruritus to severe, life-threatening anaphylactic reactions/shock or angioedema (including: swelling of lips, eyelids, laryngeal spasm and airway obstruction with hypoxia). (see: WARNINGS: Anaphylactic Reactions)

Other hypersensitivity reactions have included: ineffectiveness of treatment, serum sickness, arthritis, allergic interstitial nephritis, immune complex deposition resulting in glomerulonephritis, vasculitis, and temporal arteritis, and eosinophilia.

Clinical adverse events occurring in clinical trials and post-marketing experience are listed below by body system:

Body as a Whole: fever (including, spiking temperatures as high as 107°F), chills/rigors, flu-like syndrome, fatigue/malaise, generalized weakness, anorexia.

Cardiovascular: cardiac arrest, hypotension/shock, heart failure, cardiovascular collapse, angina/myocardial infarction, tachycardia, bradycardia, hemodynamic instability, hypertension, left ventricular dysfunction, arrhythmias, chest pain/tightness.

Respiratory: respiratory arrest, adult respiratory distress syndrome (ARDS), respiratory failure, pulmonary edema (cardiogenic or noncardiogenic), apnea, dyspnea, bronchospasm, wheezing, shortness of breath, hypoxemia, tachypnea/hyperventilation, abnormal chest sounds, and pneumonia/pneumonitis (bacterial, viral, *P. carinii,* etc.).

Dermatologic: rash, Stevens-Johnson syndrome, urticaria, pruritus, erythema, flushing, diaphoresis.

Gastrointestinal: diarrhea, nausea/vomiting, abdominal pain, bowel infarction, gastrointestinal hemorrhage.

Hematopoietic: pancytopenia, aplastic anemia, neutropenia, leukopenia, thrombocytopenia, lymphopenia, leukocy-

Continued on next page

Orthoclone—Cont.

tosis, lymphadenopathy; arterial and venous thrombosis of allografts and other vascular beds (e.g., heart, lung, brain, bowel, etc.); disturbances of coagulation, including disseminated intravascular coagulation; microangiopathic changes (e.g., platelet microthrombi); microangiopathic hemolytic anemia.

Hepatobiliary: increases in transaminases (SGOT, SGPT, etc.); hepato/splenomegaly or hepatitis, usually secondary to viral infection or lymphoma.

Neuro-Psychiatric: seizures, lethargy/stupor/coma, encephalopathy, psychotic reactions (delirium), encephalitis, meningitis, cerebral edema, headache, dizziness, tremor, aphasia, quadri- or paraparesis/plegia, obtundation, confusion, altered mental status (e.g., paranoia, etc.), impaired cognition, disorientation, auditory and visual hallucinations, agitation/combativeness, mood changes (e.g., mania, etc.), hypotonus, hyperreflexia, myoclonus, asterixis, involuntary movements, CNS infections, CNS malignancies, cerebrovascular accident/hemiparesis/plegia, transient ischemic attack, subarachnoid hemorrhage.

Musculoskeletal: arthralgia, arthritis, myalgia, stiffness/aches/pains.

Special Senses: blindness, blurred vision, diplopia, hearing loss, otitis media, tinnitus, vertigo, VI cranial nerve palsy, photophobia, conjunctivitis, nasal and ear stuffiness.

Renal: anuria/oliguria; delayed graft function; renal insufficiency/renal failure, usually transient and reversible, and occasionally in association with cytokine release syndrome; abnormal urinary cytology including exfoliation of damaged lymphocytes, collecting duct cells and cellular casts.

OVERDOSAGE

Symptoms of overdose with ORTHOCLONE OKT3 (muromonab-CD3) may include hyperthermia, severe chills, myalgia, vomiting, diarrhea, edema, oliguria, pulmonary edema and acute renal failure. A high incidence (5%) of microangiopathic hemolytic anemia/HUS syndrome in patients receiving 10 mg per day of ORTHOCLONE OKT3 was also reported. In the event of acute overdosage with ORTHOCLONE OKT3, the patient should be carefully observed and given symptomatic and supportive treatment.

DOSAGE AND ADMINISTRATION

The recommended dose of ORTHOCLONE OKT3 for the treatment of acute renal, steroid-resistant cardiac, or steroid-resistant hepatic allograft rejection is 5 mg per day in a single (**bolus**) intravenous injection for 10 to 14 days. For acute renal rejection, treatment should begin upon diagnosis. For steroid-resistant cardiac or hepatic allograft rejection, treatment should begin when the treating physician deems a rejection has not been reversed by an adequate course of corticosteroid therapy. (see: CLINICAL PHARMACOLOGY; PRECAUTIONS: Sensitization, Laboratory Tests)

For the first few doses, patients should be monitored in a facility equipped and staffed for cardiopulmonary resuscitation with frequent determinations of vital signs. With subsequent doses, the patient should be monitored following ORTHOCLONE OKT3 therapy in a facility equipped and staffed for CPR for an appropriate period of time based on the patient's clinical status. Since the Cytokine Release Syndrome may also occur following a treatment hiatus and resumption of therapy, as with the first few doses, exercise vigilant care.

Prior to the administration of any dose of ORTHOCLONE OKT3, the patient's temperature should be lowered to <37.8°C (100°F).

Prior to administration of ORTHOCLONE OKT3, the patient's volume status should be assessed carefully. It is imperative, especially prior to the first few doses, that there be no clinical evidence of volume overload or uncompensated heart failure, including a clear chest X-ray and weight restriction of ≤3% above the patient's minimum weight during the week prior to injection. (see: WARNINGS and ADVERSE REACTIONS: Cytokine Release Syndrome)

Intravenous methylprednisolone sodium succinate 8.0 mg/kg given 1 to 4 hours prior to administering the first dose of ORTHOCLONE OKT3 is strongly recommended to decrease the incidence and severity of reactions to the first dose, which have been attributed to the ORTHOCLONE OKT3 mediated Cytokine Release Syndrome.

Acetaminophen and antihistamines given concomitantly with ORTHOCLONE OKT3 (muromonab-CD-3) may also help to reduce some early reactions. (see: WARNINGS and ADVERSE REACTIONS: Cytokine Release Syndrome)

When using concomitant immunosuppressive drugs, the dose of each should be reduced to the lowest level compatible with an effective therapeutic response in order to reduce the potential for malignant transformations and the incidence and/or severity of infections. Maintenance immunosuppression should be resumed approximately three days prior to the cessation of ORTHOCLONE OKT3 therapy. (see: WARNINGS and ADVERSE REACTIONS: Infection, Neoplasia).

ADMINISTRATION INSTRUCTIONS

1. Prior to administration, parenteral drug products should be inspected visually for particulate matter and discoloration. Because ORTHOCLONE OKT3 is a protein solution, it may develop a few fine translucent particles which have been shown not to affect its potency.
2. No bacteriostatic agent is present in this product; adherence to aseptic technique is advised. Once the ampule is opened, use immediately and discard the unused portion.
3. Prepare ORTHOCLONE OKT3 for injection by drawing solution into a syringe through a low protein-binding 0.2 or 0.22 micrometer (μm) filter. Discard filter and attach a new needle for intravenous bolus injection.
4. Since no data is available on compatibility of ORTHOCLONE OKT3 with other intravenous substances or additives, other medications/substances should not be added or infused simultaneously through the same intravenous line. If the same intravenous line is used for sequential infusion of several different drugs, the line should be flushed with saline before and after infusion of ORTHOCLONE OKT3.
5. Administer ORTHOCLONE OKT3 as an intravenous bolus in less than one minute. Do **not** administer by intravenous infusion or in conjunction with other drug solutions.

HOW SUPPLIED

ORTHOCLONE OKT3 is supplied as a sterile solution in packages of 5 ampules (NDC 59676-101-01). Each 5 mL ampule contains 5 mg of muromonab-CD3.

Storage: Store in a refrigerator at 2° to 8°C (36° to 46°F). DO NOT FREEZE OR SHAKE.

REFERENCES

1. Adair JC, Woodley SL, O'Connell JB, *et al.* Aseptic Meningitis following Cardiac Transplantation: Clinical Characteristics and Relationship to Immunosuppressive Regimen. Neurology 41:249–252, 1991.
2. Chatenoud L, Legendre C, Ferran C, *et al.* Corticosteroid Inhibition of the OKT3–Induced Cytokine-Related Syndrome-Dosage and Kinetics Prerequisites. Transplantation 51:334–338, 1991.
3. Cockfield SM, Preiksaitis J, Harvey E, Jones C, Herbert D, Keown P, and Halloran PF. Is Sequential Use of ALG and OKT3 in Renal Transplants Associated With an Increased Incidence of Fulminant Post Transplant Lymphoproliferative Disorders? Transplant. Proc. 23: 1106–1107, 1991.
4. Ettenger RB, Marik J. Rosenthal JT, *et al.* OKT3 for Rejection Reversal in Pediatric Renal Transplantation. Clin. Transplantation 2:180–184, 1988.
5. Gaston RS, Deierhoi MH, Patterson T, *et al.* OKT3 First-Dose Reaction: Association with T Cell Subsets and Cytokine Release. Kid. International 39:141–148, 1991.
6. Goldman M, Abramowicz D, DePauw L, *et al.* OKT3-Induced Cytokine Released Attenuation by High-Dose Methylprednisolone. Lancet 2:802–803, 1989.
7. Ortho Multicenter Transplant Study Group. A Randomized Clinical Trial of OKT3 Monoclonal Antibody for Acute Rejection of Cadaveric Renal Transplants. N. Engl J. Med 313:337–342, 1985.
8. Penn I. The Changing Patterns of Posttransplant Malignancies. Transplant Proc. 23:1101–1103, 1991.
9. Rubin RH and Tolkoff-Rubin NE. The Impact of Infection on the Outcome of Transplantation. Transplant Proc. 23:2068–2074, 1991.
10. Schroeder TJ, Ryckman FC, Hurtubise PE, *et al.* Immunological Monitoring during and following OKT3 Therapy in Children. Clin. Transplantation 5:191–196, 1991.

ORTHO BIOTECH INC.
Raritan, New Jersey 08869
U.S.A.
©OBI 1986
631-10-191-9
Revised June 1995

PROCRIT® ℞
EPOETIN ALFA
PROCRIT registered trademark of distributor
FOR INJECTION

DESCRIPTION

Erythropoietin is a glycoprotein which stimulates red blood cell production. It is produced in the kidney and stimulates the division and differentiation of committed erythroid progenitors in the bone marrow. PROCRIT (Epoetin alfa), a 165 amino acid glycoprotein manufactured by recombinant DNA technology, has the same biological effects as endogenous erythropoietin.[1] It has a molecular weight of 30,400 daltons and is produced by mammalian cells into which the human erythropoietin gene has been introduced. The product contains the identical amino acid sequence of isolated natural erythropoietin.

PROCRIT is formulated as a sterile, colorless, liquid in an isotonic sodium chloride/sodium citrate buffered solution for intravenous (IV) or subcutaneous (SC) administration.

Single-Dose, Preservative-Free Vial: Each 1 mL of solution contains 2,000, 3,000, 4,000 or 10,000 Units of Epoetin alfa, 2.5 mg Albumin (Human), 5.8 mg sodium citrate, 5.8 mg sodium chloride, and 0.06 mg citric acid in Water for Injection, USP (pH 6.9±0.3). This formulation contains no preservative.

Multidose, Preserved Vial: 2 mL (20,000 Units, 10,000 Units/mL). Each 1 mL of solution contains 10,000 Units of Epoetin alfa, 2.5 mg Albumin (Human), 1.3 mg sodium citrate, 8.2 mg sodium chloride, 0.11 mg citric acid, and 1% benzyl alcohol as preservative in Water for Injection, USP (pH 6.1±0.3).

Multidose, Preserved Vial: 1 mL (20,000 Units/mL). Each 1 mL of solution contains 20,000 Units of Epoetin alfa, 2.5 mg Albumin (Human), 1.3 mg sodium citrate, 8.2 mg sodium chloride, 0.11 mg citric acid, and 1% benzyl alcohol as preservative in Water for Injection, USP (pH 6.1±0.3).

CLINICAL PHARMACOLOGY
Chronic Renal Failure Patients

Endogenous production of erythropoietin is normally regulated by the level of tissue oxygenation. Hypoxia and anemia generally increase the production of erythropoietin, which in turn stimulates erythropoiesis.[2] In normal subjects, plasma erythropoietin levels range from 0.01 to 0.03 Units/mL and increase up to 100- to 1000-fold during hypoxia or anemia.[2,3] In contrast, in patients with chronic renal failure (CRF), production of erythropoietin is impaired, and this erythropoietin deficiency is the primary cause of their anemia.[3,4]

Chronic renal failure is the clinical situation in which there is a progressive and usually irreversible decline in kidney function. Such patients may manifest the sequelae of renal dysfunction, including anemia, but do not necessarily require regular dialysis. Patients with end-stage renal disease (ESRD) are those patients with CRF who require regular dialysis or kidney transplantation for survival.

PROCRIT has been shown to stimulate erythropoiesis in anemic patients with CRF, including both patients on dialysis and those who do not require regular dialysis.[4-13] The first evidence of a response to the three times weekly (T.I.W.) administration of PROCRIT is an increase in the reticulocyte count within 10 days, followed by increases in the red cell count, hemoglobin, and hematocrit, usually within 2-6 weeks.[4,5] Because of the length of time required for erythropoiesis — several days for erythroid progenitors to mature and be released into the circulation — a clinically significant increase in hematocrit is usually not observed in less than 2 weeks and may require up to 6 weeks in some patients. Once the hematocrit reaches the suggested target range (30-36%), that level can be sustained by PROCRIT therapy in the absence of iron deficiency and concurrent illnesses.

The rate of hematocrit increase varies between patients and is dependent upon the dose of PROCRIT, within a therapeutic range of approximately 50-300 Units/kg (T.I.W.).[4] A greater biologic response is not observed at doses exceeding 300 Units/kg (T.I.W.).[6] Other factors affecting the rate and extent of response include availability of iron stores, the baseline hematocrit, and the presence of concurrent medical problems.

Zidovudine-treated HIV-infected Patients

Responsiveness to PROCRIT in HIV-infected patients is dependent upon the endogenous serum erythropoietin level prior to treatment. Patients with endogenous serum erythropoietin levels ≤ 500 mUnits/mL, and who are receiving a dose of zidovudine ≤ 4,200 mg/week, may respond to PROCRIT therapy. Patients with endogenous serum erythropoietin levels > 500 mUnits/mL do not appear to respond to PROCRIT therapy. In a series of four clinical trials involving 255 patients, 60% to 80% of HIV-infected patients treated with zidovudine had endogenous serum erythropoietin levels ≤ 500 mUnits/mL.

Response to PROCRIT in zidovudine-treated, HIV-infected patients is manifested by reduced transfusion requirements and increased hematocrit.

Cancer Patients on Chemotherapy

Anemia in cancer patients may be related to the disease itself or the effect of concomitantly administered chemotherapeutic agents. PROCRIT has been shown to increase hematocrit and decrease transfusion requirements after the first month of therapy (months 2 and 3), in anemic cancer patients undergoing chemotherapy.

A series of clinical trials enrolled 131 anemic cancer patients who were receiving cyclic cisplatin- or non cisplatin-containing chemotherapy. Endogenous baseline serum erythropoietin levels varied among patients in these trials with approximately 75% (N=83/110) having endogenous serum erythropoietin levels ≤ 132 mUnits/mL, and approximately 4% (N=4/110) of patients having endogenous serum erythropoietin levels > 500 mUnits/mL. In general, patients with lower baseline serum erythropoietin levels responded more vigorously to PROCRIT than patients with higher baseline erythropoietin levels. Although no specific serum erythropoietin level can be stipulated above which patients

would be unlikely to respond to PROCRIT therapy, treatment of patients with grossly elevated serum erythropoietin levels (e.g., > 200 mUnits/mL) is not recommended.

Pharmacokinetics

Intravenously administered PROCRIT is eliminated at a rate consistent with first order kinetics with a circulating half-life ranging from approximately 4 to 13 hours in patients with CRF. Within the therapeutic dose range, detectable levels of plasma erythropoietin are maintained for at least 24 hours.[7] After subcutaneous administration of PROCRIT to patients with CRF, peak serum levels are achieved within 5-24 hours after administration and decline slowly thereafter. There is no apparent difference in half-life between patients not on dialysis whose serum creatinine levels were greater than 3, and patients maintained on dialysis.

In normal volunteers, the half-life of intravenously administered PROCRIT is approximately 20% shorter than the half-life in CRF patients. The pharmacokinetics of PROCRIT have not been studied in HIV-infected patients.

INDICATIONS AND USAGE

Treatment of Anemia of Chronic Renal Failure Patients

PROCRIT is indicated in the treatment of anemia associated with chronic renal failure, including patients on dialysis (end-stage renal disease) and patients not on dialysis. PROCRIT is indicated to elevate or maintain the red blood cell level (as manifested by the hematocrit or hemoglobin determinations) and to decrease the need for transfusions in these patients.

Non-dialysis patients with symptomatic anemia considered for therapy should have a hematocrit less than 30%.

PROCRIT is not intended for patients who require immediate correction of severe anemia. PROCRIT may obviate the need for maintenance transfusions but is not a substitute for emergency transfusion.

Prior to initiation of therapy, the patient's iron stores should be evaluated. Transferrin saturation should be at least 20% and ferritin at least 100 ng/mL. Blood pressure should be adequately controlled prior to initiation of PROCRIT therapy, and must be closely monitored and controlled during therapy.

PROCRIT should be administered under the guidance of a qualified physician (see "DOSAGE and ADMINISTRATION").

Treatment of Anemia in Zidovudine-treated HIV-infected Patients

PROCRIT is indicated for the treatment of anemia related to therapy with zidovudine in HIV-infected patients. PROCRIT is indicated to elevate or maintain the red blood cell level (as manifested by the hematocrit or hemoglobin determinations) and to decrease the need for transfusions in these patients. PROCRIT is not indicated for the treatment of anemia in HIV-infected patients due to other factors such as iron or folate deficiencies, hemolysis or gastrointestinal bleeding, which should be managed appropriately.

PROCRIT, at a dose of 100 Units/kg three times per week, is effective in decreasing the transfusion requirement and increasing the red blood cell level of anemic, HIV-infected patients treated with zidovudine, when the endogenous serum erythropoietin level is ≤ 500 mUnits/mL and when patients are receiving a dose of zidovudine ≤ 4,200 mg/week.

Treatment of Anemia in Cancer Patients on Chemotherapy

PROCRIT is indicated for the treatment of anemia in patients with non-myeloid malignancies where anemia is due to the effect of concomitantly administered chemotherapy. PROCRIT is indicated to decrease the need for transfusions in patients who will be receiving concomitant chemotherapy for a minimum of 2 months. PROCRIT is not indicated for the treatment of anemia in cancer patients due to other factors such as iron or folate deficiencies, hemolysis or gastrointestinal bleeding which should be managed appropriately.

Reduction of Allogeneic Blood Transfusion in Surgery Patients

PROCRIT is indicated for the treatment of anemic patients (hemoglobin >10 to ≤13 g/dL) scheduled to undergo elective, noncardiac, nonvascular surgery to reduce the need for allogeneic blood transfusions.[14-15] PROCRIT is indicated for patients at high risk for perioperative transfusions with significant, anticipated blood loss. PROCRIT is not indicated for anemic patients who are willing to donate autologous blood. The safety of the perioperative use of PROCRIT has been studied only in patients who are receiving anticoagulant prophylaxis.

Clinical Experience: Response to PROCRIT

Chronic Renal Failure Patients

Response to PROCRIT was consistent across all studies. In the presence of adequate iron stores (see "Iron Evaluation"), the time to reach the target hematocrit is a function of the baseline hematocrit and the rate of hematocrit rise.

The rate of increase in hematocrit is dependent upon the dose of PROCRIT administered and individual patient variation. In clinical trials at starting doses of 50-150 Units/kg (T.I.W.), patients responded with an average rate of hematocrit rise of:

HEMATOCRIT INCREASE

STARTING DOSE (T.I.W. IV)	POINTS/DAY	POINTS/ 2 WEEKS
50 Units/kg	0.11	1.5
100 Units/kg	0.18	2.5
150 Units/kg	0.25	3.5

Over this dose range, approximately 95% of all patients responded with a clinically significant increase in hematocrit, and by the end of approximately 2 months of therapy virtually all patients were transfusion-independent. Changes in the quality of life of patients treated with PROCRIT were assessed as part of a Phase III clinical trial.[5,8] Once the target hematocrit (32-38%) was achieved, statistically significant improvements were demonstrated for most quality of life parameters measured, including energy and activity level, functional ability, sleep and eating behavior, health status, satisfaction with health, sex life, well-being, psychological effect, life satisfaction, and happiness. Patients also reported improvement in their disease symptoms. They showed a statistically significant increase in exercise capacity (VO_2 max), energy, and strength with a significant reduction in aching, dizziness, anxiety, shortness of breath, muscle weakness, and leg cramps.[8,17]

Patients On Dialysis: Thirteen clinical studies were conducted, involving intravenous administration to a total of 1,010 anemic patients on dialysis for 986 patient-years of PROCRIT therapy. In the three largest of these clinical trials, the median maintenance dose necessary to maintain the hematocrit between 30–36% was approximately 75 Units/kg (T.I.W.). In the U.S. multicenter Phase III study, approximately 65% of the patients required doses of 100 Units/kg (T.I.W.), or less, to maintain their hematocrit at approximately 35%. Almost 10% of patients required a dose of 25 Units/kg, or less, and approximately 10% required a dose of more than 200 Units/kg (T.I.W.) to maintain their hematocrit at this level.

A multicenter unit dose study was also conducted in 119 patients receiving peritoneal dialysis who self-administered PROCRIT subcutaneously for approximately 109 patient-years of experience. Patients responded to PROCRIT administered subcutaneously in a manner similar to patients receiving intravenous administration.[18]

Patients With CRF Not Requiring Dialysis: Four clinical trials were conducted in patients with CRF not on dialysis involving 181 patients treated with PROCRIT for approximately 67 patient-years of experience. These patients responded to PROCRIT therapy in a manner similar to that observed in patients on dialysis. Patients with CRF not on dialysis demonstrated a dose-dependent and sustained increase in hematocrit when PROCRIT was administered by either an intravenous (IV) or subcutaneous (SC) route, with similar rates of rise of hematocrit when PROCRIT was administered by either route. Moreover, PROCRIT doses of 75–150 Units/kg per week have been shown to maintain hematocrits of 36–38% for up to six months. Correcting the anemia of progressive renal failure will allow patients to remain active even though their renal function continues to decrease.[19–21]

Zidovudine-treated HIV-infected Patients

PROCRIT has been studied in four placebo-controlled trials enrolling 297 anemic (hematocrit < 30%) HIV-infected (AIDS) patients receiving concomitant therapy with zidovudine, (all patients were treated with Epoetin alfa manufactured by Amgen Inc.). In the subgroup of patients (89/125 PROCRIT, and 88/130 placebo) with prestudy endogenous serum erythropoietin levels ≤ 500 mUnits/mL PROCRIT reduced the mean cumulative number of units of blood transfused per patient by approximately 40%, as compared to the placebo group.[22] Among those patients who required transfusions at baseline, 43% of patients treated with PROCRIT versus 18% of placebo-treated patients were transfusion-independent during the second and third months of therapy. PROCRIT therapy also resulted in significant increases in hematocrit in comparison to placebo. When examining the results according to the weekly dose of zidovudine received during Month 3 of therapy, there was a statistically significant ($p < 0.003$) reduction in transfusion requirements in patients treated with PROCRIT (N=51) compared to placebo-treated patients (N=54) whose mean weekly zidovudine dose was ≤ 4,200 mg/week.[22]

Approximately 17% of the patients with endogenous serum erythropoietin levels ≤ 500 mUnits/mL receiving PROCRIT in doses from 100-200 Units/kg three times weekly (T.I.W.) achieved a hematocrit of 38% without administration of transfusions or a significant reduction in zidovudine dose. In the subgroup of patients whose prestudy endogenous serum erythropoietin levels were > 500 mUnits/mL, PROCRIT therapy did not reduce transfusion requirements or increase hematocrit, compared to the corresponding responses in placebo-treated patients.

In a six month open-label PROCRIT study, patients responded with decreased transfusion requirements and sustained increases in hematocrit and hemoglobin with doses of PROCRIT up to 300 Units/kg (T.I.W.).[21–23]

Responsiveness to PROCRIT therapy may be blunted by intercurrent infectious/inflammatory episodes and by an increase in zidovudine dosage. Consequently, the dose of PROCRIT must be titrated based on these factors to maintain the desired erythropoietic response.

Cancer Patients on Chemotherapy

PROCRIT has been studied in a series of placebo-controlled, double-blind trials in a total of 131 anemic cancer patients. Within this group, 72 patients were treated with concomitant noncisplatin-containing chemotherapy regimens and 59 patients were treated with concomitant cisplatin-containing chemotherapy regimens. Patients were randomized to PROCRIT 150 Units/kg or placebo subcutaneously (T.I.W.) for 12 weeks.

PROCRIT therapy was associated with a significantly ($p<0.008$) greater hematocrit response than in the corresponding placebo-treated patients (see TABLE).[22]

HEMATOCRIT (%): MEAN CHANGE FROM BASELINE TO FINAL VALUE[a]

STUDY	PROCRIT	PLACEBO
Chemotherapy	7.6	1.3
Cisplatin	6.9	0.6

[a] Significantly higher in PROCRIT patients than in placebo patients ($p < 0.008$)

In the two types of chemotherapy studies [utilizing a PROCRIT dose of 150 Units/kg (T.I.W.)] the mean number of units of blood transfused per patient after the first month of therapy was significantly ($p < 0.02$) lower in patients treated with PROCRIT (0.71 units in Months 2, 3) than in corresponding placebo-treated patients (1.84 units in Months 2, 3). Moreover, the proportion of patients transfused during Months 2 and 3 of therapy combined was significantly ($p < 0.03$) lower in the patients treated with PROCRIT than in the corresponding placebo-treated patients (22% versus 43%).[22]

Comparable intensity of chemotherapy in the PROCRIT and placebo groups in the chemotherapy trials was suggested by a similar area under the neutrophil time curve in patients treated with PROCRIT and placebo-treated patients as well as by a similar proportion of patients in groups treated with PROCRIT and placebo-treated groups whose absolute neutrophil counts fell below 1,000 cells/µL. Available evidence suggests that patients with lymphoid and solid cancers respond equivalently to PROCRIT therapy, and that patients with or without tumor infiltration of the bone marrow respond equivalently to PROCRIT therapy.

Surgery Patients

PROCRIT has been studied in a placebo-controlled, double-blind trial enrolling 316 patients scheduled for major, elective orthopedic hip or knee surgery who were expected to require ≥2 units of blood and who were not able or willing to participate in an autologous blood donation program. Based on previous studies which demonstrated that pretreatment hemoglobin is a predictor of risk of receiving transfusion[16,24], patients were stratified into one of three groups based on their pretreatment hemoglobin [≤10 (n=2), >10 to ≤13 (n=96), and >13 to ≤15 g/dL (n=218)] and then randomly assigned to receive 300 U/kg PROCRIT, 100 U/kg PROCRIT or placebo by subcutaneous injection for 10 days before surgery, on the day of surgery, and for four days after surgery[14]. All patients received oral iron and a low dose postoperative warfarin regimen.[14]

Treatment with PROCRIT 300 U/kg significantly (p=0.024) reduced the risk of allogeneic transfusion in patients with a pretreatment hemoglobin of >10 to ≤13 g/dL; 5/31 (16%) of PROCRIT 300 U/kg, 6/26 (23%) of PROCRIT 100 U/kg and 13/29 (45%) of placebo-treated patients were transfused.[14]

There was no significant difference in the number of patients transfused between PROCRIT (9% 300 U/kg, 6% 100 U/kg) and placebo (13%) in the >13 to ≤15 g/dL hemoglobin stratum. There were too few patients in the ≤10 g/dL group to determine if PROCRIT is useful in this hemoglobin strata.

In the >10 to ≤13 g/dL pretreatment stratum, the mean number of units transfused per PROCRIT-treated patient (0.45 units blood for 300 U/kg, 0.42 units blood for 100 U/kg) was less than the mean transfused per placebo-treated patient (1.14 units) (overall p=0.028). In addition, mean hemoglobin, hematocrit and reticulocyte counts increased significantly during the presurgery period in PROCRIT-treated patients.[25]

PROCRIT was also studied in an open-label, parallel-group trial enrolling 145 subjects with a pretreatment hemoglobin level of ≥10 to ≤13 g/dL who were scheduled for major orthopedic hip or knee surgery and who were not participating in an autologous program.[15] Subjects were randomly assigned to receive one of two subcutaneous dosing regimens of PROCRIT (600 U/kg once weekly for three weeks prior to

Continued on next page

Procrit—Cont.

surgery and on the day of surgery or 300 U/kg once daily for 10 days prior to surgery, on the day of surgery and for four days after surgery). All subjects received oral iron and appropriate pharmacologic anticoagulation therapy.

From pretreatment to presurgery, the mean increase in hemoglobin in 600 U/kg weekly group (1.44 g/dL) was greater than observed in the 300 U/kg daily group.[15] The mean increase in absolute reticulocyte count was smaller in the weekly group ($0.11 \times 10^6/mm^3$) compared to the daily group ($0.17 \times 10^6/mm^3$). Mean hemoglobin levels were similar for the two treatment groups throughout the postsurgical period.

The erythropoietic response observed in both treatment groups resulted in similar transfusion rates [11/69 (16%) in the 600 U/kg weekly group and 14/71 (20%) in the 300 U/kg daily group].[15] The mean number of units transfused per subject was approximately 0.3 units in both treatment groups.

CONTRAINDICATIONS

PROCRIT is contraindicated in patients with:

1) Uncontrolled hypertension.
2) Known hypersensitivity to mammalian cell-derived products.
3) Known hypersensitivity to Albumin (Human).

WARNINGS

Pediatric Use:

The multidose preserved formulation contains benzyl alcohol. Benzyl alcohol has been reported to be associated with an increased incidence of neurological and other complications in premature infants which are sometimes fatal. The safety and effectiveness of Epoetin alfa in children have not been established.

Thrombotic Events and Increased Mortality

A randomized, prospective trial of 1265 hemodialysis patients with clinically evident cardiac disease (ischemic heart disease or congestive heart failure) was conducted in which patients were assigned to PROCRIT treatment targeted to a maintenance hematocrit of either $42 \pm 3\%$ or $30 \pm 3\%$. Increased mortality was observed in 634 patients randomized to a target hematocrit of 42% [221 deaths (35% mortality)] compared to 631 patients targeted to remain at a hematocrit of 30% [185 deaths (29% mortality)]. The reason for increased mortality observed in these studies is unknown, however the incidence of non-fatal myocardial infarctions (3.1% vs. 2.3%), vascular access thrombosis (39% vs. 29%) and all other thrombotic events (22% vs. 18%) were also higher in the group randomized to achieve a hematocrit of 42%.

Increased mortality was observed in a randomized placebo-controlled study of PROCRIT in patients who did not have chronic renal failure who were undergoing coronary artery bypass surgery (7 deaths in 126 patients randomized to PROCRIT vs. no deaths among 56 patients receiving placebo). Four of these deaths occurred during the period of study drug administration and all 4 deaths were associated with thrombotic events. While the extent of the population affected is unknown, in patients at risk for thrombosis, the anticipated benefits of PROCRIT treatment should be weighed against the potential for increased risks associated with therapy.

Chronic Renal Failure Patients

Hypertension: Patients with uncontrolled hypertension should not be treated with PROCRIT; blood pressure should be controlled adequately before initiation of therapy. Up to 80% of patients with CRF have a history of hypertension.[25] Although there does not appear to be any direct pressor effects of PROCRIT, blood pressure may rise during PROCRIT therapy. During the early phase of treatment when the hematocrit is increasing, approximately 25% of patients on dialysis may require initiation of, or increases in, antihypertensive therapy. Hypertensive encephalopathy and seizures have been observed in patients with CRF treated with PROCRIT.

Special care should be taken to closely monitor and aggressively control blood pressure in patients treated with PROCRIT. Patients should be advised as to the importance of compliance with antihypertensive therapy and dietary restrictions. If blood pressure is difficult to control by initiation of appropriate measures, the hematocrit may be reduced by decreasing or withholding the dose of PROCRIT. A clinically significant decrease in hematocrit may not be observed for several weeks.

It is recommended that the dose of PROCRIT be decreased if the hematocrit increase exceeds 4 points in any two-week period, because of the possible association of excessive rate of rise of hematocrit with an exacerbation of hypertension. In chronic renal failure patients on hemodialysis with clinically evident ischemic heart disease or congestive heart failure, the hematocrit should be managed carefully, not to exceed 36%. (see "Thrombotic Events")

Seizures: Seizures have occurred in patients with CRF participating in PROCRIT clinical trials.

In patients on dialysis, there was a higher incidence of seizures during the first 90 days of therapy (occurring in approximately 2.5% of patients) as compared with later timepoints.

Given the potential for an increased risk of seizures during the first 90 days of therapy, blood pressure and the presence of premonitory neurologic symptoms should be monitored closely. Patients should be cautioned to avoid potentially hazardous activities such as driving or operating heavy machinery during this period.

While the relationship between seizures and the rate of rise of hematocrit is uncertain, it is recommended that the dose of PROCRIT be decreased if the hematocrit increase exceeds 4 points in any two-week period.

Thrombotic Events: During hemodialysis, patients treated with PROCRIT may require increased anticoagulation with heparin to prevent clotting of the artificial kidney. (See "ADVERSE REACTIONS" for more information about thrombotic events.)

Other thrombotic events (e.g., myocardial infarction, cerebrovascular accident, transient ischemic attack) have occurred in clinical trials at an annualized rate of less than 0.04 events per patient-year of PROCRIT therapy. These trials were conducted in patients with CRF (whether on dialysis or not) in whom the target hematocrit was 32-40%. However, the risk of thrombotic events, including vascular access thromboses, was significantly increased in patients with ischemic heart disease or congestive heart failure receiving PROCRIT therapy with the goal of reaching a normal hematocrit (42%) as compared to a target hematocrit of 30%. Patients with pre-existing cardiovascular disease should be monitored closely.

Zidovudine-treated HIV-infected Patients

In contrast to CRF patients, PROCRIT therapy has not been linked to exacerbation of hypertension, seizures, and thrombotic events in HIV-infected patients.

PRECAUTIONS

The parenteral administration of any biologic product should be attended by appropriate precautions in case allergic or other untoward reactions occur (see "CONTRAINDICATIONS"). In clinical trials, while transient rashes were occasionally observed concurrently with PROCRIT therapy, no serious allergic or anaphylactic reactions were reported. See "ADVERSE REACTIONS" for more information regarding allergic reactions.

The safety and efficacy of PROCRIT therapy have not been established in patients with a known history of a seizure disorder or underlying hematologic disease (e.g., sickle cell anemia, myelodysplastic syndromes, or hypercoagulable disorders).

In some female patients, menses have resumed following PROCRIT therapy; the possibility of pregnancy should be discussed and the need for contraception evaluated.

Hematology: Exacerbation of porphyria has been observed rarely in patients with CRF treated with PROCRIT. However, PROCRIT has not caused increased urinary excretion of porphyrin metabolites in normal volunteers, even in the presence of a rapid erythropoietic response. Nevertheless, PROCRIT should be used with caution in patients with known porphyria.

In preclinical studies in dogs and rats, but not in monkeys, PROCRIT therapy was associated with subclinical bone marrow fibrosis. Bone marrow fibrosis is a known complication of CRF in humans and may be related to secondary hyperparathyroidism or unknown factors. The incidence of bone marrow fibrosis was not increased in a study of patients on dialysis who were treated with PROCRIT for 12–19 months, compared to the incidence of bone marrow fibrosis in a matched group of patients who had not been treated with PROCRIT.

Hematocrit in CRF patients should be measured twice a week; zidovudine-treated HIV-infected and cancer patients should have hematocrit measured once a week until hematocrit has been stabilized, and measured periodically thereafter.

Delayed or Diminished Response: If the patient fails to respond or to maintain a response to doses within the recommended dosing range, the following etiologies should be considered and evaluated:

1) Iron deficiency: Virtually all patients will eventually require supplemental iron therapy. (See *"Iron Evaluation"*).
2) Underlying infectious, inflammatory, or malignant processes.
3) Occult blood loss.
4) Underlying hematologic diseases (i.e., thalassemia, refractory anemia, or other myelodysplastic disorders).
5) Vitamin deficiencies: folic acid or vitamin B12.
6) Hemolysis.
7) Aluminum intoxication.
8) Osteitis fibrosa cystica.

Iron Evaluation: During PROCRIT therapy, absolute or functional iron deficiency may develop. Functional iron deficiency, with normal ferritin levels but low transferrin saturation, is presumably due to the inability to mobilize iron stores rapidly enough to support increased erythropoiesis. Transferrin saturation should be at least 20% and ferritin should be at least 100 ng/mL.

Prior to and during PROCRIT therapy, the patient's iron status, including transferrin saturation (serum iron divided by iron binding capacity) and serum ferritin, should be evaluated. Virtually all patients will eventually require supplemental iron to increase or maintain transferrin saturation to levels which will adequately support erythropoiesis stimulated by PROCRIT. All surgery patients being treated with PROCRIT should receive adequate iron supplementation throughout the course of therapy in order to support erythropoiesis and avoid depletion of iron stores.

Drug Interactions: No evidence of interaction of PROCRIT with other drugs was observed in the course of clinical trials.

Carcinogenesis, Mutagenesis, and Impairment of Fertility: Carcinogenic potential of PROCRIT has not been evaluated. PROCRIT does not induce bacterial gene mutation (Ames Test), chromosomal aberrations in mammalian cells, micronuclei in mice, or gene mutation at the HGPRT locus. In female rats treated intravenously with PROCRIT, there was a trend for slightly increased fetal wastage at doses of 100 and 500 Units/kg.

Pregnancy Category C: PROCRIT has been shown to have adverse effects in rats when given in doses five times the human dose. There are no adequate and well-controlled studies in pregnant women. PROCRIT should be used during pregnancy only if potential benefit justifies the potential risk to the fetus.

In studies in female rats, there were decreases in body weight gain, delays in appearance of abdominal hair, delayed eyelid opening, delayed ossification, and decreases in the number of caudal vertebrae in the F1 fetuses of the 500 Units/kg group. In female rats treated intravenously, there was a trend for slightly increased fetal wastage at doses of 100 and 500 Units/kg. PROCRIT has not shown any adverse effect at doses as high as 500 Units/kg in pregnant rabbits (from day 6 to 18 of gestation).

Nursing Mothers: Postnatal observations of the live offspring (F1 generation) of female rats treated with PROCRIT during gestation and lactation revealed no effect of PROCRIT at doses of up to 500 Units/kg. There were, however, decreases in body weight gain, delays in appearance of abdominal hair, eyelid opening, and decreases in the number of caudal vertebrae in the F1 fetuses of the 500 Units/kg group. There were no effects related to PROCRIT on the F2 generation fetuses.

It is not known whether PROCRIT is excreted in human milk. Because many drugs are excreted in human milk, caution should be exercised when PROCRIT is administered to a nursing woman.

Pediatric Use: The safety and effectiveness of PROCRIT in children have not been established (See WARNINGS).

Chronic Renal Failure Patients

Patients with CRF Not Requiring Dialysis: Blood pressure and hematocrit should be monitored no less frequently than for patients maintained on dialysis. Renal function and fluid and electrolyte balance should be closely monitored, as an improved sense of well-being may obscure the need to initiate dialysis in some patients.

Hematology: Sufficient time should be allowed to determine a patient's responsiveness to a dosage of PROCRIT before adjusting the dose. Because of the time required for erythropoiesis and the red cell half-life, an interval of 2–6 weeks may occur between the time of a dose adjustment (initiation, increase, decrease, or discontinuation) and a significant change in hematocrit.

In order to avoid reaching the suggested target hematocrit too rapidly, or exceeding the suggested target range (hematocrit of 30–36%), the guidelines for dose and frequency of dose adjustments (see "DOSAGE AND ADMINISTRATION") should be followed.

For patients who respond to PROCRIT with a rapid increase in hematocrit (e.g., more than 4 points in any two-week period), the dose of PROCRIT should be reduced because of the possible association of excessive rate of rise of hematocrit with an exacerbation of hypertension.

The elevated bleeding time characteristic of CRF decreases toward normal after correction of anemia in patients treated with PROCRIT. Reduction of bleeding time also occurs after correction of anemia by transfusion.

Laboratory Monitoring: The hematocrit should be determined twice a week until it has stabilized in the suggested target range and the maintenance dose has been established. After any dose adjustment, the hematocrit should also be determined twice weekly for at least 2–6 weeks until it has been determined that the hematocrit has stabilized in response to the dose change. The hematocrit should then be monitored at regular intervals.

A complete blood count with differential and platelet count should be performed regularly. During clinical trials, mod-

est increases were seen in platelets and white blood cell counts. While these changes were statistically significant, they were not clinically significant and the values remained within normal ranges.

In patients with CRF, serum chemistry values [including blood urea nitrogen (BUN), uric acid, creatinine, phosphorus, and potassium] should be monitored regularly. During clinical trials in patients on dialysis, modest increases were seen in BUN, creatinine, phosphorus, and potassium. In some patients with CRF not on dialysis, treated with PROCRIT, modest increases in serum uric acid and phosphorus were observed. While changes were statistically significant, the values remained within the ranges normally seen in patients with CRF.

Diet: As the hematocrit increases and patients experience an improved sense of well-being and quality of life, the importance of compliance with dietary and dialysis prescriptions should be reinforced. In particular, hyperkalemia is not uncommon in patients with CRF. In U.S. studies in patients on dialysis, hyperkalemia has occurred at an annualized rate of approximately 0.11 episodes per patient-year of PROCRIT therapy, often in association with poor compliance to medication, diet and/or dialysis.

Dialysis Management: Therapy with PROCRIT results in an increase in hematocrit and a decrease in plasma volume which could affect dialysis efficiency. In studies to date, the resulting increase in hematocrit did not appear to adversely affect dialyzer function[9,10] or the efficiency of high flux hemodialysis.[11] During hemodialysis, patients treated with PROCRIT may require increased anticoagulation with heparin to prevent clotting of the artificial kidney.

Patients who are marginally dialyzed may require adjustments in their dialysis prescription. As with all patients on dialysis, the serum chemistry values (including BUN, creatinine, phosphorus, and potassium) in patients treated with PROCRIT should be monitored regularly to assure the adequacy of the dialysis prescription.

Information for Patients: In those situations in which the physician determines that a home dialysis patient can safely and effectively self-administer PROCRIT, the patient should be instructed as to the proper dosage and administration. Home dialysis patients should be referred to the full "INFORMATION FOR HOME DIALYSIS PATIENTS" section attached; it is not a disclosure of all possible effects. Patients should be informed of the signs and symptoms of allergic drug reaction and advised of appropriate actions. If home use is prescribed for a home dialysis patient, the patient should be thoroughly instructed in the importance of proper disposal and cautioned against the reuse of needles, syringes, or drug product. A puncture-resistant container for the disposal of used syringes and needles should be available to the patient. The full container should be disposed of according to the directions provided by the physician.

Renal Function: In patients with CRF not on dialysis, renal function and fluid and electrolyte balance should be closely monitored, as an improved sense of well-being may obscure the need to initiate dialysis in some patients. In patients with CRF not on dialysis, placebo-controlled studies of progression of renal dysfunction over periods of greater than one year have not been completed. In shorter-term trials in patients with CRF not on dialysis, changes in creatinine and creatinine clearance were not significantly different in patients treated with PROCRIT, compared with placebo-treated patients. Analysis of the slope of 1/serum creatinine vs. time plots in these patients indicates no significant change in the slope after the initiation of PROCRIT therapy.

Zidovudine-treated HIV-infected Patients
Hypertension: Exacerbation of hypertension has not been observed in zidovudine-treated HIV-infected patients treated with PROCRIT. However, PROCRIT should be withheld in these patients if pre-existing hypertension is uncontrolled, and should not be started until blood pressure is controlled. In double-blind studies, a single seizure has been experienced by a patient treated with PROCRIT.[22]

Cancer Patients on Chemotherapy
Hypertension: Hypertension, associated with a significant increase in hematocrit, has been noted rarely in cancer patients treated with PROCRIT. Nevertheless, blood pressure in patients treated with PROCRIT should be monitored carefully, particularly in patients with an underlying history of hypertension or cardiovascular disease.
Seizures: In double-blind, placebo-controlled trials, 3.2% (N=2/63) of patients treated with PROCRIT and 2.9% (N=2/68) of placebo-treated patients had seizures. Seizures in 1.6% (N=1/63) of patients treated with PROCRIT occurred in the context of a significant increase in blood pressure and hematocrit from baseline values. However, both patients treated with PROCRIT also had underlying CNS pathology which may have been related to seizure activity.
Thrombotic Events: In double-blind, placebo-controlled trials, 3.2% (N=2/63) of patients treated with PROCRIT and 11.8% (N=8/68) of placebo-treated patients had thrombotic events (e.g. pulmonary embolism, cerebrovascular accident).

Growth Factor Potential: PROCRIT is a growth factor that primarily stimulates red cell production. However, the possibility that PROCRIT can act as a growth factor for any tumor type, particularly myeloid malignancies, cannot be excluded.

Surgery Patients
Thrombotic/Vascular Events: In perioperative clinical trials with orthopedic patients, the overall incidence of thrombotic/vascular events was similar in Epoetin alfa and placebo-treated patients who had a pretreatment hemoglobin of >10 to ≤13 g/dL. In patients with a hemoglobin of >13 g/dL treated with 300 U/kg of Epoetin alfa, the possibility that PROCRIT treatment may be associated with an increased risk of postoperative thrombotic/vascular events cannot be excluded.[14–16,24]

In one study in which Epoetin alfa was administered in the perioperative period to patients undergoing coronary artery bypass graft surgery, there were seven deaths in the Epoetin alfa-treated groups (N=126) and no deaths in the placebo-treated group (N=56). Among the seven deaths in the Epoetin alfa-treated patients, four were at the time of therapy (between study day 2 and 8). The four deaths at the time of therapy (3%) were associated with thrombotic/vascular events. A causative role of Epoetin alfa cannot be excluded. (See "WARNINGS")

Hypertension: Blood pressure may rise in the perioperative period in patients being treated with PROCRIT. Therefore, blood pressure should be monitored carefully.

ADVERSE REACTIONS

Chronic Renal Failure Patients
Studies analyzed to date indicate that PROCRIT is generally well-tolerated. The adverse events reported are frequent sequelae of CRF and are not necessarily attributable to PROCRIT therapy. In double-blind, placebo-controlled studies involving over 300 patients with CRF, the events reported in greater than 5% of patients treated with PROCRIT during the blinded phase were:

PERCENT OF PATIENTS REPORTING EVENT

Event	Patients Treated with epoetin alfa (N=200)	PLACEBO-Treated Patients (N=135)
Hypertension	24%	19%
Headache	16%	12%
Arthralgias	11%	6%
Nausea	11%	9%
Edema	9%	10%
Fatigue	9%	14%
Diarrhea	9%	6%
Vomiting	8%	5%
Chest Pain	7%	9%
Skin Reaction (Administration Site)	7%	12%
Asthenia	7%	12%
Dizziness	7%	13%
Clotted Access	7%	2%

Significant adverse events of concern in patients with CRF treated in double-blinded, placebo-controlled trials occurred in the following percent of patients during the blinded phase of the studies:

Seizure	1.1%	1.1%
CVA / TIA	0.4%	0.6%
MI	0.4%	1.1%
Death	0	1.7%

In the U.S. PROCRIT studies in patients on dialysis (over 567 patients), the incidence (number of events per patient-year) of the most frequently reported adverse events were: hypertension (0.75), headache (0.40), tachycardia (0.31), nausea/vomiting (0.26), clotted vascular access (0.25), shortness of breath (0.14), hyperkalemia (0.11), and diarrhea (0.11). Other reported events occurred at a rate of less than 0.10 events per patient per year.

Events reported to have occurred within several hours of administration of PROCRIT were rare, mild, and transient, and included injection site stinging in dialysis patients and flu-like symptoms such as arthralgias and myalgias.

In all studies analyzed to date, PROCRIT administration was generally well-tolerated, irrespective of the route of administration.

Hypertension: Increases in blood pressure have been reported in clinical trials, often during the first 90 days of therapy. On occasion, hypertensive encephalopathy and seizures have been observed in patients with CRF treated with PROCRIT. When data from all patients in the U.S. Phase III multicenter trial were analyzed, there was an apparent trend of more reports of hypertensive adverse events in patients on dialysis with a faster rate of rise of hematocrit (greater than 4 hematocrit points in any two-week period). However, in a double-blind, placebo-controlled trial, hypertensive adverse events were not reported at an increased rate in the group treated with PROCRIT (150 Units/kg T.I.W.) relative to the placebo group.

Seizures: There have been 47 seizures in 1,010 patients on dialysis treated with PROCRIT in clinical trials, with an exposure of 986 patient-years for a rate of approximately 0.048 events per patient-year. However, there appeared to be a higher rate of seizures during the first 90 days of therapy (occurring in approximately 2.5% of patients) when compared to subsequent 90-day periods. The baseline incidence of seizures in the untreated dialysis population is difficult to determine; it appears to be in the range of 5–10% per patient-year.[26–28]

Thrombotic Events: In clinical trials where the maintenance hematocrit was 35 ± 3% on PROCRIT, clotting of the vascular access (A-V shunt) has occurred at an annualized rate of about 0.25 events per patient-year, and other thrombotic events (myocardial infarction, cerebrovascular accident, transient ischemic attack, and pulmonary embolism) occurred at a rate of 0.04 events per patient-year. In a separate study of 1,111 untreated dialysis patients, clotting of the vascular access occurred at a rate of 0.5 events per patient-year. However, in chronic renal failure patients on hemodialysis who also had clinically evident ischemic heart disease or congestive heart failure, the risk of A-V shunt thrombosis was higher (39% vs 29%, p<0.001), and myocardial infarction, vascular ischemic events, and venous thrombosis were increased in patients targeted to a hematocrit of 42 ± 3% compared to those maintained at 30 ± 3%. (see "WARNINGS")

In patients treated with commercial PROCRIT, there have been rare reports of serious or unusual thrombo-embolic events including migratory thrombophlebitis, microvascular thrombosis, pulmonary embolus, and thrombosis of the retinal artery, and temporal and renal veins. A causal relationship has not been established.

Allergic Reactions: There have been no reports of serious allergic reactions or anaphylaxis associated with PROCRIT administration during clinical trials. Skin rashes and urticaria have been observed rarely and when reported have generally been mild and transient in nature.

In over 125,000 patients treated with commercial PROCRIT, there have been rare reports of potentially serious allergic reactions including urticaria with associated respiratory symptoms or circumoral edema (<0.0001 events per patient-year), or urticaria alone (<0.0001 events per patient-year). Most reactions occurred in situations where a casual relationship could not be established. Many of these patients resumed PROCRIT therapy without recurrence of symptoms, some in conjunction with antihistamine pretreatment. However, symptoms recurred with rechallenge in a few instances, suggesting that allergic reactivity, although rare, may occasionally be associated with PROCRIT therapy.

There has been no evidence for development of antibodies to erythropoietin in patients tested to date, including those receiving PROCRIT for over 4 years. Nevertheless, if an anaphylactoid reaction occurs, PROCRIT should be immediately discontinued and appropriate therapy initiated.

Zidovudine-treated HIV-infected Patients
Adverse events reported in clinical trials with PROCRIT in zidovudine-treated HIV-infected patients were consistent with the progression of HIV infection. In double-blind, placebo-controlled studies of three-months duration involving approximately 300 zidovudine-treated HIV-infected patients, adverse events with an incidence of ≥10% in either patients treated with PROCRIT or placebo-treated patients were:

Percent of Patients Reporting Event

Event	Patients Treated with PROCRIT (N=144)	PLACEBO-Treated Patients (N=153)
Pyrexia	38%	29%
Fatigue	25%	31%
Headache	19%	14%
Cough	18%	14%
Diarrhea	16%	18%
Rash	16%	8%
Congestion, Respiratory	15%	10%

Continued on next page

Procrit—Cont.

Nausea	15%	12%
Shortness of Breath	14%	13%
Asthenia	11%	14%
Skin Reaction, (Administration Site)	10%	7%
Dizziness	9%	10%

There were no statistically significant differences between treatment groups in the incidence of the above events.

In the 297 patients studied, PROCRIT was not associated with significant increases in opportunistic infections or mortality.[22] In 71 patients from this group treated with PROCRIT at 150 Units/kg (T.I.W.), serum p24 antigen levels did not appear to increase.[23] Preliminary data showed no enhancement of HIV replication in infected cell lines in vitro.[22]

Peripheral white blood cell and platelet counts are unchanged following PROCRIT therapy.

Allergic Reactions: Two zidovudine-treated HIV-infected patients had urticarial reactions within 48 hours of their first exposure to study medication. One patient was treated with PROCRIT and one was treated with placebo (PROCRIT vehicle alone). Both patients had positive immediate skin tests against their study medication with a negative saline control. The basis for this apparent pre-existing hypersensitivity to components of the PROCRIT formulation is unknown, but may be related to HIV-induced immunosuppression or prior exposure to blood products.

Seizures: In double-blind and open-label trials of PROCRIT in zidovudine-treated HIV-infected patients, ten patients have experienced seizures.[22] In general, these seizures appear to be related to underlying pathology such as meningitis or cerebral neoplasms, not PROCRIT therapy.

Cancer Patients on Chemotherapy

Adverse experiences reported in clinical trials with PROCRIT in cancer patients were consistent with the underlying disease state. In double-blind, placebo-controlled studies of up to 3-months duration involving 131 cancer patients, adverse events with an incidence >10% in either patients treated with PROCRIT or placebo-treated patients were as indicated below.

Percent of Patients Reporting Event

Event	Patients Treated with PROCRIT (N=63)	PLACEBO-Treated Patients (N=68)
Pyrexia	29%	19%
Diarrhea	21%[a]	7%
Nausea	17%[b]	32%
Vomiting	17%	15%
Edema	17%[c]	1%
Asthenia	13%	16%
Fatigue	13%	15%
Shortness of Breath	13%	9%
Paresthesia	11%	6%
Upper Respiratory Infection	11%	4%
Dizziness	5%	12%
Trunk Pain	3%[d]	16%

[a] p = 0.041   [c] p = 0.0016
[b] p = 0.069   [d] p = 0.017

Although some statistically significant differences between patients treated with PROCRIT and placebo-treated patients were noted, the overall safety profile of PROCRIT appeared to be consistent with the disease process of advanced cancer. During double-blind and subsequent open-label therapy in which patients (N=72 for total exposure to PROCRIT) were treated for up to 32 weeks with doses as high as 927 Units/kg, the adverse experience profile of PROCRIT was consistent with the progression of advanced cancer.

Based on comparable survival data and on the percentage of patients treated with PROCRIT and placebo-treated patients who discontinued therapy due to death, disease progression or adverse experiences (22% and 13%, respectively; p = 0.25), the clinical outcome in patients treated with PROCRIT and placebo-treated patients appeared to be similar. Available data from animal tumor models and measurement of proliferation of solid tumor cells from clinical biopsy specimens in response to PROCRIT suggest that PROCRIT does not potentiate tumor growth. Nevertheless, as a growth factor, the possibility that PROCRIT may potentiate growth of some tumors, particularly myeloid tumors, cannot be excluded. A randomized controlled Phase IV study is currently ongoing to further evaluate this issue.

Percent of Patients Reporting Event

Event	Patients Treated with PROCRIT 300 U/kg (N=112)[a]	Patients Treated with PROCRIT 100 U/kg (N=101)[a]	PLACEBO-Treated Patients (N=103)[a]	PROCRIT 600 U/kg (N=73)[b]	PROCRIT 300 U/kg (N=72)[b]
Pyrexia	51%	50%	60%	47%	42%
Nausea	48%	43%	45%	45%	58%
Constipation	43%	42%	43%	51%	53%
Skin Reaction, (Administration Site)	25%	19%	22%	26%	29%
Vomiting	22%	12%	14%	21%	29%
Skin Pain	18%	18%	17%	5%	4%
Pruritus	16%	16%	14%	14%	22%
Insomnia	13%	16%	13%	21%	18%
Headache	13%	11%	9%	10%	19%
Dizziness	12%	9%	12%	14%	21%
Urinary Tract Infection	12%	3%	11%	11%	8%
Hypertension	10%	11%	10%	5%	10%
Diarrhea	10%	7%	12%	10%	6%
Deep Venous Thrombosis	10%	3%	5%	0%[c]	0%[c]
Dyspepsia	9%	11%	6%	7%	8%
Anxiety	7%	2%	11%	11%	4%
Edema	6%	11%	8%	11%	7%

[a] Study including patients undergoing orthopedic surgery treated with PROCRIT or placebo for 15 days
[b] Study including patients undergoing orthopedic surgery treated with PROCRIT 600 U/kg weekly × 4 or 300 U/kg daily × 15
[c] Determined by clinical symptoms

The mean peripheral white blood cell count was unchanged following PROCRIT therapy compared to the corresponding value in the placebo-treated group.

Surgery Patients
Adverse events with an incidence of ≥10% are shown in the following table:
[See table above]

Thrombotic/vascular events: In three double-blind, placebo-controlled orthopedic surgery studies, the rate of deep venous thrombosis (DVT) was similar among Epoetin alfa and placebo-treated patients in the recommended population of patients with a pretreatment hemoglobin of >10 to ≤13 g/dL.[14,16,24] However, in 2 of 3 orthopedic surgery studies the overall rate (all pretreatment hemoglobin groups combined) of DVTs detected by postoperative ultrasonography and/or surveillance venography was higher in the Epoetin alfa-treated group than in the placebo-treated group (11% vs. 6%). This finding was attributable to the difference in DVT rates observed in the subgroup of patients with pretreatment hemoglobin >13 g/dL. However, the incidence of DVTs was within the range of that reported in the literature for orthopedic surgery patients.

In the orthopedic surgery study of patients with pretreatment hemoglobin >10 to ≤13 g/dL which compared two dosing regimens (600 U/kg weekly × 4 and 300 U/kg daily × 15), four subjects in the 600 U/kg weekly PROCRIT group (5%) and no subjects in the 300 U/kg daily group had a thrombotic vascular event during the study period.[15]

In a study examining the use of Epoetin alfa in 182 patients scheduled for coronary artery bypass graft surgery, 23% of patients treated with Epoetin alfa and 29% treated with placebo experienced thrombotic/vascular events. There were 4 deaths among the Epoetin alfa-treated patients that were associated with a thrombotic/vascular event. A causative role of Epoetin alfa cannot be excluded. (See "WARNINGS")

OVERDOSAGE

The maximum amount of PROCRIT that can be safely administered in single or multiple doses has not been determined. Doses of up to 1,500 Units/kg (T.I.W.) for three to four weeks have been administered without any direct toxic effects of PROCRIT itself.[6] Therapy with PROCRIT can result in polycythemia if the hematocrit is not carefully monitored and the dose appropriately adjusted. If the suggested target range is exceeded, PROCRIT may be temporarily withheld until the hematocrit returns to the suggested target range; PROCRIT therapy may then be resumed using a lower dose (see "DOSAGE AND ADMINISTRATION"). If polycythemia is of concern, phlebotomy may be indicated to decrease the hematocrit.

DOSAGE AND ADMINISTRATION
Chronic Renal Failure Patients

Starting doses of PROCRIT over the range of 50–100 Units/kg three times weekly (T.I.W.) have been shown to be safe and effective in increasing hematocrit and eliminating transfusion dependency in patients with CRF (see "Clinical Experience"). The dose of PROCRIT should be reduced as the hematocrit approaches 36% or increases by more than 4 points in any 2-week period. The dosage of PROCRIT must be individualized to maintain the hematocrit within the suggested target range. At the physician's discretion, the suggested target hematocrit range may be expanded to achieve maximal patient benefit.

PROCRIT may be given either as an intravenous (IV) or subcutaneous (SC) injection. In patients on hemodialysis, PROCRIT usually has been administered as an IV bolus (T.I.W.). While the administration of PROCRIT is independent of the dialysis procedure, PROCRIT may be administered into the venous line at the end of the dialysis procedure to obviate the need for additional venous access. In patients with CRF not on dialysis, PROCRIT may be given either as an IV or SC injection.

Home hemodialysis patients who have been judged competent by their physicians to self-administer PROCRIT without medical or other supervision may give themselves either an IV or SC injection. The table below provides general therapeutic guidelines for patients with CRF:
[See table below]

During therapy, hematological parameters should be monitored regularly (see "Laboratory Monitoring").

Pre-Therapy Iron Evaluation: Prior to and during PROCRIT therapy, the patient's iron stores, including transferrin saturation (serum iron divided by iron binding capacity) and serum ferritin, should be evaluated. Transferrin saturation should be at least 20%, and ferritin should be at least 100 ng/mL. Virtually all patients will eventually require supplemental iron to increase or maintain transferrin saturation to levels that will adequately support erythropoiesis stimulated by PROCRIT.

Dose Adjustment: Following PROCRIT therapy, a period of time is required for erythroid progenitors to mature and be released into circulation resulting in an eventual increase in hematocrit. Additionally, red blood cell survival

Starting Dose	Reduce Dose If	Increase Dose When	Maintenance Dose	Suggested Hct. Range
50–100 Units/kg T.I.W.; IV or SC	1) Hct. approaches 36%, or 2) Hct. increases >4 points in any 2-week period	Hct. does not increase by 5–6 points after 8 weeks of therapy, and hct. is below suggested target range	Individually titrate	30–36%

time affects hematocrit and may vary due to uremia. As a result, the time required to elicit a clinically significant change in hematocrit (increase or decrease) following any dose adjustment may be 2–6 weeks.

Dose adjustment should not be made more frequently than once a month, unless clinically indicated. After any dose adjustment, the hematocrit should be determined twice weekly for at least 2–6 weeks (see "Laboratory Monitoring").

- If the hematocrit is increasing and approaching 36%, the dose should be reduced to maintain the suggested target hematocrit range. If the reduced dose does not stop the rise in hematocrit, and it exceeds 36%, doses should be temporarily withheld until the hematocrit begins to decrease, at which point therapy should be reinitiated at a lower dose.
- At any time, if the hematocrit increases by more than 4 points in a 2-week period, the dose should be immediately decreased. After the dose reduction, the hematocrit should be monitored twice weekly for 2–6 weeks, and further dose adjustments should be made as outlined in "Maintenance Dose".
- If a hematocrit increase of 5–6 points is not achieved after an 8-week period and iron stores are adequate (see "Delayed or Diminished Response"), the dose of PROCRIT may be incrementally increased. Further increases may be made at 4–6 week intervals until the desired response is attained.

Maintenance Dose: The maintenance dose must be individualized for each patient on dialysis. In the U.S. Phase III multicenter trial in patients on hemodialysis, the median maintenance dose was 75 Units/kg (T.I.W.), with a range from 12.5 to 525 Units/kg (T.I.W.). Almost 10% of the patients required a dose of 25 Units/kg, or less, and approximately 10% of the patients required more than 200 Units/kg (T.I.W.) to maintain their hematocrit in the suggested target range.

If the hematocrit remains below, or falls below, the suggested target range, iron stores should be re-evaluated. If the transferrin saturation is less than 20%, supplemental iron should be administered. If the transferrin saturation is greater than 20%, the dose of PROCRIT may be increased. Such dose increases should not be made more frequently than once a month, unless clinically indicated, as the response time of the hematocrit to a dose increase can be 2–6 weeks. Hematocrit should be measured twice weekly for 2–6 weeks following dose increases. In patients with CRF not on dialysis, the maintenance dose must also be individualized. PROCRIT doses of 75–150 Units/kg per week have been shown to maintain hematocrits of 36–38% for up to 6 months.

Delayed or Diminished Response: Over 95% of patients with CRF responded with clinically significant increases in hematocrit, and virtually all patients were transfusion-independent within approximately two months of initiation of PROCRIT therapy.

If a patient fails to respond or maintain a response, other etiologies should be considered and evaluated as clinically indicated. See "PRECAUTIONS" section for discussion of delayed or diminished response.

Zidovudine-treated HIV-infected Patients

Prior to beginning PROCRIT, it is recommended that the endogenous serum erythropoietin level be determined (prior to transfusion). Available evidence suggests that patients receiving zidovudine with endogenous serum erythropoietin levels > 500 mUnits/mL are unlikely to respond to therapy with PROCRIT.

Starting Dose: For patients with serum erythropoietin levels ≤ 500 mUnits/mL who are receiving a dose of zidovudine ≤ 4,200 mg/week, the recommended starting dose of PROCRIT is 100 Units/kg as an intravenous or subcutaneous injection three times weekly (T.I.W.) for 8 weeks.

Increase Dose: During the dose adjustment phase of therapy, the hematocrit should be monitored weekly. If the response is not satisfactory in terms of reducing transfusion requirements or increasing hematocrit after 8 weeks of therapy, the dose of PROCRIT can be increased by 50–100 Units/kg (T.I.W.). Response should be evaluated every 4–8 weeks thereafter and the dose adjusted accordingly by 50–100 Units/kg increments (T.I.W.). If patients have not responded satisfactorily to a PROCRIT dose of 300 Units/kg (T.I.W.), it is unlikely that they will respond to higher doses of PROCRIT.

Maintenance Dose: After attainment of the desired response (i.e., reduced transfusion requirements or increased hematocrit), the dose of PROCRIT should be titrated to maintain the response based on factors such as variations in zidovudine dose and the presence of intercurrent infectious or inflammatory episodes. If the hematocrit exceeds 40%, the dose should be discontinued until the hematocrit drops to 36%. The dose should be reduced by 25% when treatment is resumed and then titrated to maintain the desired hematocrit.

Cancer Patients on Chemotherapy

Baseline endogenous serum erythropoietin levels varied among patients in these trials with approximately 75% (N=83/110) having endogenous serum erythropoietin levels < 132 mUnits/mL, and approximately 4% (N=4/110) of patients having endogenous serum erythropoietin levels > 500 mUnits/mL. In general, patients with lower baseline serum erythropoietin levels responded more vigorously to PROCRIT than patients with higher erythropoietin levels. Although no specific serum erythropoietin level can be stipulated above which patients would be unlikely to respond to PROCRIT therapy, treatment of patients with grossly elevated serum erythropoietin levels (e.g., > 200 mUnits/mL) is not recommended. The hematocrit should be monitored on a weekly basis in patients receiving PROCRIT therapy until hematocrit becomes stable.

Starting Dose: The recommended starting dose of PROCRIT is 150 Units/kg subcutaneously (T.I.W.).

Dose Adjustment: If the response is not satisfactory in terms of reducing transfusion requirements or increasing hematocrit after 8 weeks of therapy, the dose of PROCRIT can be increased up to 300 Units/kg (T.I.W.). If patients have not responded satisfactorily to a PROCRIT dose of 300 Units/kg (T.I.W.), it is unlikely that they will respond to higher doses of PROCRIT. If the hematocrit exceeds 40%, the dose of PROCRIT should be withheld until the hematocrit falls to 36%. The dose of PROCRIT should be reduced by 25% when treatment is resumed and titrated to maintain the desired hematocrit. If the initial dose of PROCRIT includes a very rapid hematocrit response (e.g., an increase of more than 4 percentage points in any 2-week period), the dose of PROCRIT should be reduced.

Surgery Patients

Prior to initiating treatment with PROCRIT a hemoglobin should be obtained to establish that it is >10 to ≤13 g/dL.[14] The recommended dose of PROCRIT is 300 U/kg/day subcutaneously for 10 days before surgery, on the day of surgery, and for 4 days after surgery.[14]

An alternate dose schedule is 600 U/kg PROCRIT subcutaneously in once weekly doses (21, 14 and 7 days before surgery) plus a fourth dose on day of surgery.[15]

All patients should receive adequate iron supplementation. Iron supplementation should be initiated no later than the beginning of treatment with PROCRIT and should continue throughout the course of therapy.

PREPARATION AND ADMINISTRATION OF PROCRIT

1. DO NOT SHAKE. It is not necessary to shake PROCRIT. Prolonged vigorous shaking may denature any glycoprotein, rendering it biologically inactive.
2. Parenteral drug products should be inspected visually for particulate matter and discoloration prior to administration. Do not use any vials exhibiting particulate matter or discoloration.
3. Using aseptic techniques, attach a sterile needle to a sterile syringe. Remove the flip top from the vial containing PROCRIT, and wipe the septum with a disinfectant. Insert the needle into the vial, and withdraw into the syringe an appropriate volume of solution.
4. **Single-dose** 1 mL vial contains no preservative. Use one dose per vial; do not re-enter vial. Discard unused portions. **Multidose** 1 mL and 2 mL vials contain preservative. Store at 2 to 8°C after initial entry and between doses. Discard 21 days after initial entry.
5. Do not dilute or administer in conjunction with other drug solutions. However, at the time of subcutaneous administration, preservative-free PROCRIT from single-use vials may be admixed in a syringe with bacteriostatic 0.9% sodium chloride injection, USP, with benzyl alcohol 0.9% (bacteriostatic saline) at a 1:1 ratio using aseptic technique. The benzyl alcohol in the bacteriostatic saline acts as a local anesthetic which may ameliorate subcutaneous injection site discomfort. Admixing is not necessary when using the multidose vials of PROCRIT containing benzyl alcohol.

HOW SUPPLIED

PROCRIT, containing Epoetin alfa, is available in vials containing color coded labels.

1 mL **Single-Dose, Preservative-Free** Solution

Each dosage form is supplied in the following packages:

Cartons containing six (6) **single-dose** vials:

2,000 Units/mL (NDC 59676-302-01) (Purple)
3,000 Units/mL (NDC 59676-303-01) (Magenta)
4,000 Units/mL (NDC 59676-304-01) (Green)
10,000 Units/mL (NDC 59676-310-01) (Red)

Trays containing twenty-five (25) **single-dose** vials:

2,000 Units/mL (NDC 59676-302-02) (Purple)
3,000 Units/mL (NDC 59676-303-02) (Magenta)
4,000 Units/mL (NDC 59676-304-02) (Green)
10,000 Units/mL (NDC 59676-310-02) (Red)

2 mL **Multidose, Preserved** Solution

Cartons containing six (6) **multidose** vials:

10,000 Units/mL (NDC 59676-312-01) (Blue)

1 mL **Multidose, Preserved** Solution

Cartons containing six (6) **multidose** vials:

20,000 Units/mL (NDC 59676-320-01) (Lime)

STORAGE

Store at 2° to 8° C (36° to 46° F). Do not freeze or shake.

REFERENCES:

1. Egrie JC, Strickland TW, Lane J, *et al.*, (1986). "Characterization and Biological Effects of Recombinant Human Erythropoietin." *Immunobiol.* 72:213-224.
2. Graber SE and Krantz SB, (1978). "Erythropoietin and the Control of Red Cell Production." *Ann. Rev. Med.* 29:51-66.
3. Eschbach JW and Adamson JW, (1985). "Anemia of End-Stage Renal Disease (ESRD)." *Kidney Intl.* 28:1-5.
4. Eschbach JW, Egrie JC, Downing MR, Browne JK, and Adamson JW, (1987). "Correction of the Anemia of End-Stage Renal Disease with Recombinant Human Erythropoietin." *NEJM* 316:73-78.
5. Eschbach JW, Abdulhadi MH, Browne JK, *et al.*, (1989). "Recombinant Human Erythropoietin in Anemic Patients with End-Stage Renal Disease." *Ann. Intern. Med.* 111:12.
6. Eschbach JW, Egrie JC, Downing MR, Browne JK, Adamson JW, (1989). "The Use of Recombinant Human Erythropoietin (r-HuEPO): Effect in End-Stage Renal Disease (ESRD)," *Prevention Of Chronic Uremia*, (Friedman, Beyer, DeSanto, Giordano, eds.), Field and Wood Inc., Philadelphia, PA, pp 148-155.
7. Egrie JC, Eschbach JW, McGuire T, and Adamson JW, (1988). "Pharmacokinetics of Recombinant Human Erythropoietin (r-HuEPO) Administered to Hemodialysis (HD) Patients." *Kidney Intl.* 33:262.
8. Evans RW, Radar B, Manninen DL, *et al.*, (1990). "The Quality of Life of Hemodialysis Recipients Treated with Recombinant Human Erythropoietin." *JAMA* 263:6.
9. Paganini E, Garcia J, Ellis P, Bodnar D, and Magnussen M, (1988). "Clinical Sequelae of Correction of Anemia with Recombinant Human Erythropoietin (r-HuEPO); Urea Kinetics, Dialyzer Function and Reuse." *Am. J. Kid. Dis.* 11: 16.
10. Delano BG, Lundin AP, Golansky R, Quinn RM, Rao TKS, and Friedman EA, (1988). "Dialyzer Urea and Creatinine Clearances Not Significantly Changed in r-HuEPO Treated Maintenance Hemodialysis (MD) Patients." *Kidney Intl.* 33:219.
11. Stivelman J, Van Wyck D, and Ogden D, (1988). "Use of Recombinant Erythropoietin (r-HuEPO) with High Flux Dialysis (HFD) Does Not Worsen Azotemia or Shorten Access Survival." *Kidney Intl.* 33:239.
12. Lim VS, DeGowin RL, Zavala D, Kirchner PT, Abels R, Perry P, and Fangman J, (1989). "Recombinant Human Erythropoietin Treatment in Pre-Dialysis Patients: A Double-Blind Placebo-Controlled Trial." *Ann. Int. Med.* 110: 108-114.
13. Stone WJ, Graber SE, Krantz SB, et al., (1988). "Treatment of the Anemia of Pre-Dialysis Patients with Recombinant Human Erythropoietin: A Randomized, Placebo-Controlled Trial." *Am. J. Med. Sci.* 296:171-179.
14. de Andrade JR and Jove M, (1996). "Baseline Hemoglobin as a Predictor of Risk of Transfusion and Response to Epoetin alfa in Orthopedic Surgery Patients." Am. J. of Orthoped. 25(8): 533-542.
15. Goldberg MA and McCutchen JW, (1996). "A Safety and Efficacy Comparison Study of Two Dosing Regimens of Epoetin alfa in Patients Undergoing Major Orthopedic Surgery." *Am. J. of Orthoped.* 25 (8): 544-552.
16. Faris PM and Ritter MA, (1996). "The Effects of Recombinant Human Erythropoietin on Perioperative Transfusion Requirements in Patients Having a Major Orthopaedic Operation." *J. Bone and Joint Surg.* 78-A:62-72.
17. Lundin AP, Akerman MJH, Chesler RM, Delano BG, Goldberg N, Stein RA, and Friedman EA, (1991). "Exercise in Hemodialysis Patients after Treatment with Recombinant Human Erythropoietin" *Nephron.*, 58:315-319.
18. Data on file, Amgen Inc.
19. Eschbach JW, Kelly MR, Galey NR, Abels RI and Adamson JU (1989). "Treatment of the Anemia of Progressive Renal Failure with Recombinant Human Erythropoietin," *NEJM* 321:158-163.
20. The US Recombinant Human Erythropoietin Predialysis Study Group (1991). "Double-Blind, Placebo-Controlled Study of the Therapeutic Use of Recombinant Human Erythropoietin for Anemia Associated with Chronic Renal Failure in Predialysis Patients," *Am. J. Kid. Dis.* 18(1):50-59.
21. Danna RP, Rudnick SA, Abels RI, (1990). "Erythropoietin Therapy for the Anemia Associated with AIDS and AIDS Therapy and Cancer." *Erythropoietin in Clinical Applications—An International Perspective,* (MB Garnick, ed.), Marcel Dekker, New York, NY, pp. 301-324.
22. Data on file, Ortho Biologics, Inc.
23. Fischl M, Galpin JE, Levine JD, *et al.*, (1990). "Recombinant Human Erythropoietin for Patients with AIDS Treated with Zidovudine." *NEJM* 322:1488-1493.
24. Laupacis A, (1993). "Effectiveness of Perioperative Recombinant Human Erythropoietin in Elective Hip Replacement." *Lancet* 341:1228-1232.

Continued on next page

Procrit—Cont.

25. Kerr DN, (1979). "Chronic Renal Failure," *Cecil Textbook of Medicine*, (Beeson PB, McDermott W, Wyngaarden JB, eds.), W.B. Saunders, Philadelphia, PA, pp 1351-1367.

26. Raskin NH and Fishman RA, (1976). "Neurologic Disorders in Renal Failure (First of Two Parts)." *NEJM* 294:143-148.

27. Raskin NH and Fishman RA, (1976). "Neurologic Disorders in Renal Failure (Second of Two Parts)." *NEJM* 294: 204-210.

28. Messing RO and Simon RP,(1986). "Seizures as a Manifestation of Systemic Disease." *Neurologic Clinics 4:563-584.1.* Egrie JC, Strickland TW, Lane J, et al., (1986). "Characterization and Biological Effects of Recombinant Human Erythropoietin." *Immunobiol.* 72:213-224.

Manufactured by:
Amgen Inc.
U.S. Lic. # 1080
Thousand Oaks, California 91320-1789

Distributed by:
Ortho Biotech Inc.
Raritan, New Jersey 08869-0670   ORTHO BIOTECH
© OBI 1990   Revised February 1997   638-29-979-3
Printed in U.S.A.   6300G015

PROCRIT®
EPOETIN ALFA

INFORMATION FOR HOME DIALYSIS PATIENTS

What is PROCRIT and how does it work?

PROCRIT is a copy of human erythropoietin, a hormone produced primarily by healthy kidneys. PROCRIT replaces the erythropoietin that the failed kidneys can no longer produce, and signals the bone marrow to make the oxygen-carrying red blood cells once again. PROCRIT is produced in mammalian cells that have been genetically altered by the addition of a gene of the natural substance erythropoietin.

How should I take PROCRIT?

In those situations where your doctor has determined that you, as a home dialysis patient, can self-administer PROCRIT, you will receive instruction on how much PROCRIT to use, how to inject it, how often you should inject it, and how you should dispose of the unused portions of each vial.

You will be instructed to monitor your blood pressure carefully everyday and to report any changes outside of the guidelines that your doctor has given you. When the number of red blood cells increases, your blood pressure can also increase, so your doctor may prescribe some new or additional blood pressure medication. Be sure to follow your doctor's orders. You may also be instructed to have certain laboratory tests, such as additional hematocrit or iron level measurements, done more frequently. You may be asked to report these tests to your doctor or dialysis center. Also, your doctor may prescribe additional iron for you to take. Be sure to comply with your doctor's orders.

Continue to check your access, as your doctor or nurse has shown you, to make sure it is working. Be sure to let your health care professional know right away if there is a problem.

Allergy to PROCRIT

Patients occasionally experience redness, swelling, or itching at the site of injection of PROCRIT. This may indicate an allergy to the components of PROCRIT, or it may indicate a local reaction. If you have a local reaction, consult your doctor. A potentially more serious reaction would be a generalized allergy to PROCRIT, which could cause a rash over the whole body, shortness of breath, wheezing, reduction in blood pressure, fast pulse, or sweating. Severe cases of generalized allergy may be life-threatening. If you think you are having a generalized allergic reaction, stop taking PROCRIT and notify a doctor or emergency medical personnel immediately.

How will I know if PROCRIT is working?

The effectiveness of PROCRIT is measured by the increase in hematocrit (the amount of red blood cells in the blood) that results from PROCRIT therapy. The rise in hematocrit is not immediate. It usually takes about 2–6 weeks before the hematocrit starts to rise. The amount of time it takes, and the dose of PROCRIT that is needed to make the hematocrit increase, varies from patient to patient.

What is the most important information I should know about PROCRIT and CHRONIC RENAL FAILURE?

PROCRIT has been prescribed for you by your doctor because you:

1. Have anemia due to your kidney disease.
2. Are able to dialyze at home.
3. Have been determined to be able to administer PROCRIT without direct medical or other supervision.

A lack of energy or feeling of tiredness is the major symptom of anemia. Additional symptoms include shortness of breath, chest pain, and feeling cold all the time. The reason for these symptoms is that there is a lack of red blood cells.

Red blood cells carry oxygen, which is important for all of the body's functions. When there are fewer red blood cells, the body does not get all the oxygen it needs.

Kidneys remove toxins from the blood; they also measure the amount of oxygen in the blood. If there is not enough oxygen, the kidneys will produce a hormone called erythropoietin. Erythropoietin is released into the bloodstream and travels to the bone marrow where red blood cells are made. Erythropoietin signals the bone marrow to make more oxygen-carrying red blood cells.

As the kidneys fail, they stop cleansing toxins from your blood. They also make less erythropoietin than they should. Therefore, the bone marrow does not receive a strong-enough signal to make the oxygen-carrying red blood cells. Fewer red blood cells are produced so the muscles, brain, and other parts of the body do not get the oxygen they need to function properly.

Most patients treated with PROCRIT no longer need blood transfusions. However, certain medical conditions, or unexpected blood loss, may result in the need for a transfusion.

What do I need to know if I am giving myself PROCRIT injections?

When you receive your PROCRIT from the dialysis center, doctor's office or home dialysis supplier, always check to see that:

1. The name PROCRIT appears on the carton and vial label.
2. You will be able to use PROCRIT before the expiration date stamped on the package.

The PROCRIT solution in the vial should always be clear and colorless. Do not use PROCRIT if the contents of the vial appear discolored or cloudy, or if the vial appears to contain lumps, flakes, or particles. In addition, if the vial has been shaken vigorously, the solution may appear to be frothy and should not be used. Therefore, care should be taken not to shake the PROCRIT vial vigorously before use. Unless you have been prescribed Multidose PROCRIT (1 mL or 2 mL vials with a big "M" on the label, each containing a total of 20,000 Units of PROCRIT), vials of PROCRIT are for single use. Any unused portion of a vial should not be used. However, Multidose PROCRIT may be stored in the refrigerator between doses for up to 21 days, and can be used for multiple doses. Follow your dialysis center's instructions on what to do with the used vials.

How should I store PROCRIT?

PROCRIT should be stored in the refrigerator, but not in the freezing compartment. Do not let the vial freeze and do not leave it in direct sunlight. Do not use a vial of PROCRIT that has been frozen or after the expiration date that is stamped on the label. If you have any questions about the safety of a vial of PROCRIT that has been subjected to temperature extremes, be sure to check with your dialysis unit staff.

Always use the correct syringe.

Your doctor has instructed you on how to give yourself the correct dosage of PROCRIT. This dosage will usually be measured in Units per milliliter or cc's. It is important to use a syringe that is marked in tenths of milliliters (for example, 0.2 mL or cc). Failure to use the proper syringe can lead to a mistake in dosage, and you may receive too much or too little PROCRIT. Too little PROCRIT may not be effective in increasing your hematocrit, and too much PROCRIT may lead to a hematocrit that is too high. Only use disposable syringes and needles as they do not require sterilization; they should be used once and disposed of as instructed by your doctor.

IMPORTANT: TO HELP AVOID CONTAMINATION AND POSSIBLE INFECTION, FOLLOW THESE INSTRUCTIONS EXACTLY.

PREPARING THE DOSE

1. Wash your hands thoroughly with soap and water before preparing the medication.

2. Check the date on the PROCRIT vial to be sure that the drug has not expired.

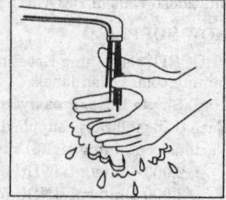

3. Remove the vial of PROCRIT from the refrigerator and allow it to reach room temperature. Each PROCRIT vial is designed to be used only once; do not reenter the vial. It is not necessary to shake PROCRIT. Prolonged vigorous shaking may damage the product. Assemble the other supplies you will need for your injection.

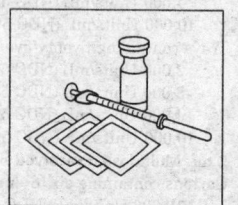

4. Hemodialysis patients should wipe off the venous port of the hemodialysis tubing with an antiseptic swab. Peritoneal dialysis patients should cleanse the skin with an antiseptic swab where the injection is to be made.

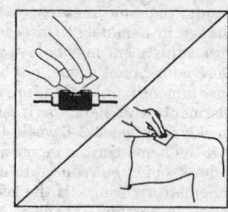

5. Flip off the red protective cap but do not remove the gray rubber stopper. Wipe the top of the gray rubber stopper with an antiseptic swab.

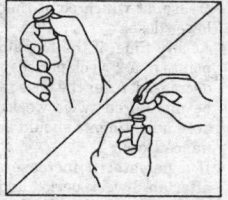

6. Using a syringe and needle designed for subcutaneous injection, draw air into the syringe by pulling back on the plunger. The amount of air should be equal to your PROCRIT dose.

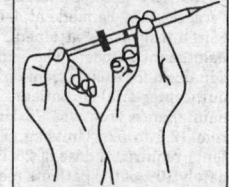

7. Carefully remove the needle cover. Put the needle through the gray rubber stopper of the PROCRIT vial.

8. Push the plunger in to discharge air into the vial. The air injected into the vial will allow PROCRIT to be easily withdrawn into the syringe.

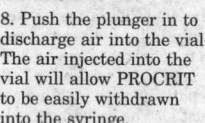

9. Turn the vial and syringe upside down in one hand. Be sure the tip of the needle is in the PROCRIT solution. Your other hand will be free to move the plunger. Draw back on the plunger slowly to draw the correct dose of PROCRIT into the syringe.

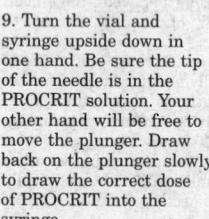
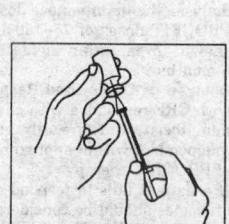

10. Check for air bubbles. The air is harmless, but too large an air bubble will reduce the PROCRIT dose. To remove air bubbles, gently tap the syringe to move the air bubbles to the top of the syringe, then use the plunger to push the solution and the air back into the vial. Then remeasure your correct dose of PROCRIT.

11. Double check your dose. Remove the needle from the vial. Do not lay the syringe down or allow the needle to touch anything.

INJECTING THE DOSE

Patients on home hemodialysis using the intravenous injection route:

1. Insert the needle of the syringe into the previously cleansed venous port and inject the PROCRIT.

2. Remove the syringe and dispose of the whole unit. Use the disposable syringe only once. Dispose of syringes and needles as directed by your doctor, by following these simple steps:

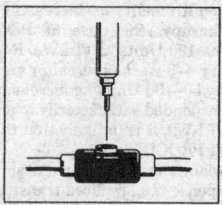

— Place all used needles and syringes in a hard plastic container with a screw-on-cap, or a metal container with a plastic lid, such as a coffee can properly labeled as to content. If a metal container is used, cut a small hole in the plastic lid and tape the lid to the metal container. If a hard-plastic container is used, always screw the cap on tightly after each use. When the container is full, tape around the cap or lid, and dispose of according to your doctor's instructions.

— Do not use glass or clear plastic containers, or any container that will be recycled or returned to a store.
— Always store the container out of the reach of children.
— Please check with your doctor, nurse, or pharmacist for other suggestions. There may be special state and local laws that they will discuss with you.

Patients on home peritoneal dialysis or home hemodialysis using the subcutaneous route:

1. With one hand, stabilize the previously cleansed skin by spreading it or by pinching up a large area with your free hand.

2. Hold the syringe with the other hand, as you would a pencil. Double check that the correct amount of PROCRIT is in the syringe. Insert the needle straight into the skin

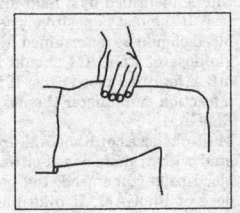

(90 degree angle). Pull the plunger back slightly. If blood comes into the syringe, do not inject PROCRIT, as the needle has entered a blood vessel; withdraw the syringe and inject at a different site. Inject the PROCRIT by pushing the plunger all the way down.

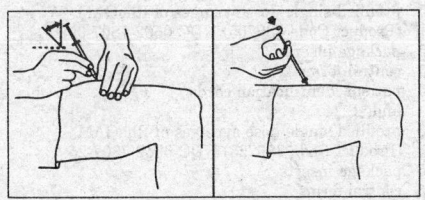

3. Hold an antiseptic swab near the needle and pull the needle straight out of the skin. Press the antiseptic swab over the injection site for several seconds.

4. **Use the disposable syringe only once.** Dispose of syringes and needles as directed by your doctor, by following these simple steps:

— Place all used needles and syringes in a hard plastic container with a screw-on-cap, or a metal container with a plastic lid, such as a coffee can properly labeled as to content. If a metal container is used, cut a small hole in the plastic lid and tape the lid to the metal container. If a hard-plastic container is used, always screw the cap on tightly after each use. When the container is full, tape around the cap or lid, and dispose of according to your doctor's instructions.
— Do not use glass or clear plastic containers, or any container that will be recycled or returned to a store.
— Always store the container out of the reach of children.
— Please check with your doctor, nurse, or pharmacist for other suggestions. There may be special state and local laws that they will discuss with you.

5. Always change the site for each injection as directed. Occasionally a problem may develop at the injection site. If you notice a lump, swelling, or bruising that doesn't go away, contact your doctor. You may wish to record the site just used so that you can keep track.

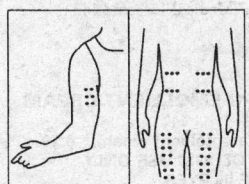

USAGE IN PREGNANCY
If you are pregnant or nursing a baby, consult your doctor before using PROCRIT.

IMPORTANT NOTES
Since you are a home dialysis patient and your doctor allows you to self-administer PROCRIT, please note the following:
1. Always follow the instructions of your doctor concerning the dosage and administration of PROCRIT. Do not change the dose or instructions for administration of PROCRIT without consulting your doctor.

2. Your doctor will tell you what to do if you miss a dose of PROCRIT. Always keep a spare syringe and needle on hand.
3. Always consult your doctor if you notice anything unusual about your condition or your use of PROCRIT.

Manufactured by:
Amgen Inc.
U.S. Lic. # 1080
Thousand Oaks, California 91320-1789

Distributed by:
Ortho Biotech Inc.
Raritan, New Jersey 08869-0670   ORTHO BIOTECH
© OBI 1994   Revised February 1997   638-29-979-3
Printed in U.S.A.   6300G015
Shown in Product Identification Guide, page 327

Ortho-Clinical Diagnostics, Inc.
A Johnson & Johnson Company
1001 U.S. HWY 202
RARITAN, NEW JERSEY 08869-0606

Direct Inquiries to:
Customer Service
(800) 322-6374

MICRhoGAM®   ℞
[mĭcrō gam]
Rh₀(D) Immune Globulin (Human)
Ultra-Filtered

Micro-dose for use *only* after spontaneous or induced abortion or termination of ectopic pregnancy up to and including 12 weeks' gestation.
Caution: Federal law prohibits dispensing without prescription.
For Intramuscular Injection Only

DESCRIPTION
MICRhoGAM $Rh_0(D)$ Immune Globulin (Human) is a sterile solution containing IgG anti-D(RH1) for use in preventing Rh immunization. A single dose of MICRhoGAM contains sufficient anti-D(RH1) (approximately 50 µg)† to suppress the immune response to 2.5 mL (or less) of Rh positive red blood cells.
All donors are carefully screened to reduce the risk of transmitting disease from individuals in high-risk groups. Fractionation of the plasma is performed by a modification of the cold alcohol procedure. Following fractionation, a viral-clearance filtration step is incorporated into the manufacturing process. This filtration step removes viruses via a size-exclusion mechanism utilizing a patented Viresolve* 180 ultrafiltration membrane with defined pore-size distribution. The filter is inert to the product. This virus removal process has been shown in laboratory spiking studies to reduce the levels of some viruses ranging from 18 to 200 nm in size, including enveloped viruses as well as non-enveloped viruses. Non-enveloped viruses are known to be resistant to chemical and physical inactivation.
The final product contains approximately $5\pm1\%$ gamma globulin, 2.9 mg/mL sodium chloride, 0.01% polysorbate 80 and 0.003% thimerosal (mercury derivative), with glycine (15 mg/mL) as a stabilizer.
This product is for intramuscular injection only.
† A full dose of $Rh_0(D)$ Immune Globulin (Human) has traditionally been referred to as a "300 µg" dose and this usage is employed here for convenience in terminology. *It should not be construed as the actual anti-D content.* Each full dose of $Rh_0(D)$ Immune Globulin (Human) must contain at least as much anti-D as 1 milliliter of the U.S. Reference $Rh_0(D)$ Immune Globulin (Human). Studies performed at the Food and Drug Administration have shown that the U.S. Reference contains 820 international units (IU) of anti-D per milliliter. When the conversion factor determined for the International (WHO) Reference Preparation is used, 820 IU per milliliter is equivalent to 164 µg per milliliter of anti-D. MICRhoGAM contains approximately one-sixth the amount of anti-D contained in the full dose.
*Viresolve is a trademark of Millipore Corporation.

CLINICAL PHARMACOLOGY
Intramuscular $Rh_0(D)$ human immune globulins prepared by cold alcohol fractionation have not been reported to transmit hepatitis or other infectious diseases.
MICRhoGAM acts by suppressing the immune response of Rh negative individuals to Rh positive red blood cells. The risk of immunization is related to the number of D positive red blood cells received. The risk was found to be 3% when 0.1 mL of fetal red blood cells is present in the mother and 65% when 5 mL is present. In the first 12 weeks of gestation, the total volume of red blood cells in the fetus is estimated at less than 2.5 mL.
Clinical studies demonstrated that administration of MICRhoGAM within three (3) hours following abortion was 100% effective in preventing Rh immunization. Studies showed MICRhoGAM to be effective when given as long as 72 hours after the infusion of Rh positive red cells. A lesser degree of protection is afforded if the antibody is administered beyond this time period.

INDICATIONS AND USAGE
MICRhoGAM is indicated for an Rh negative woman following spontaneous or induced abortion or termination of ectopic pregnancy up to and including 12 weeks' gestation, unless the father can be shown conclusively to be Rh negative.

CONTRAINDICATIONS
MICRhoGAM must not be used for any indication with continuation of pregnancy. RhoGAM® Rh₀(D) Immune Globulin (Human) is recommended for any indication beyond 12 weeks' gestation.
Individuals known to have had an anaphylactic or severe systemic reaction to human globulin should not receive MICRhoGAM or any other Rh₀(D) Immune Globulin (Human).

WARNINGS
Do not inject intravenously.
MICRhoGAM is made from human plasma. Products made from human plasma may contain infectious agents, such as viruses, that can cause disease. The risk that such products will transmit an infectious agent has been reduced by screening plasma donors for prior exposure to certain viruses, by testing for the presence of certain current viral infections and by removing certain viruses during the manufacturing process. Following fractionation, a viral-clearance filtration step is incorporated into the manufacturing process. This filtration step removes viruses via a size-exclusion mechanism utilizing a patented Viresolve 180 ultrafiltration membrane with defined pore-size distribution. The filter is inert to the product. This virus removal process has been shown in laboratory spiking studies to reduce the levels of some viruses ranging from 18 to 200 nm in size, including enveloped viruses as well as non-enveloped viruses. Despite these measures, such products can still potentially transmit disease. There is also the possibility that unknown infectious agents may be present in such products. ALL infections thought by a physician possibly to have been transmitted by this product should be reported by the physician or other healthcare provider in the U.S. to Ortho-Clinical Diagnostics, Inc. at 1-800-322-6374. Outside of the U.S., the company distributing this product should be contacted. The physician should discuss the risks and benefits of this product with the patient.

PRECAUTIONS
Pregnancy Category C
Animal reproduction studies have not been conducted with MICRhoGAM. It is also not known whether Rh₀(D) Immune Globulin (Human) can cause fetal harm when administered to a pregnant woman or can affect reproduction capacity. Rh₀(D) Immune Globulin (Human) should be given to a pregnant woman only if clearly needed.

ADVERSE REACTIONS
Systemic reactions associated with administration of MICRhoGAM are extremely rare. Discomfort at the site of injection has been reported and a small number of women have noted a slight elevation in temperature.

DOSAGE AND ADMINISTRATION
Parenteral drug products should be inspected visually for particulate matter and discoloration prior to administration, whenever solution and container permit.
A single dose (approximately 50 µg)† is contained in each prefilled syringe of MICRhoGAM. This will completely suppress the immune response to 2.5 mL of Rh positive red blood cells (packed cells, not whole blood).
Administer MICRhoGAM intramuscularly as soon as possible after termination of a pregnancy up to and including 12 weeks' gestation. At or beyond 13 weeks' gestation, it is recommended that a single dose of RhoGAM be given instead of MICRhoGAM. Do not inject intravenously.

†See footnote under Description

HOW SUPPLIED
MICRhoGAM is available in packages containing:
5	prefilled single-dose syringes of MICRhoGAM (Product Code 780805) NDC 0562-7808-05
5	package inserts
5	control forms
5	patient identification cards and
25	prefilled single-dose syringes of MICRhoGAM (Product Code 780825) NDC 0562-7808-25
25	package inserts
25	control forms
25	patient identification cards

STORAGE
Store at 2 to 8°C. Do not store frozen.

RhoGAM®   ℞
[rō gam]
Rh₀(D) Immune Globulin (Human)
Ultra-Filtered

Caution: Federal law prohibits dispensing without prescription.

Continued on next page

RhoGAM—Cont.

For Intramuscular Injection Only

DESCRIPTION

RhoGAM Rh$_o$(D) Immune Globulin (Human) is a sterile solution containing IgG anti-D(RH1) for use in preventing Rh immunization. A single dose of RhoGAM contains sufficient anti-D(RH1) (approximately 300 µg)† to suppress the immune response to 15 mL (or less) of Rh positive red blood cells.

All donors are carefully screened to reduce the risk of transmitting disease from individuals in high-risk groups. Fractionation of the plasma is performed by a modification of the cold alcohol procedure. Following fractionation, a viral-clearance filtration step is incorporated into the manufacturing process. This filtration step removes viruses via a size-exclusion mechanism utilizing a patented Viresolve* 180 ultrafiltration membrane with defined pore-size distribution. The filter is inert to the product. This virus removal process has been shown in laboratory spiking studies to reduce the levels of some viruses ranging from 18 to 200 nm in size, including enveloped viruses as well as non-enveloped viruses. Non-enveloped viruses are known to be resistant to chemical and physical inactivation.

The final product contains approximately 5±1% gamma globulin, 2.9 mg/mL sodium chloride, 0.01% polysorbate 80 and 0.003% thimerosal (mercury derivative), with glycine (15 mg/mL) as a stabilizer.

This product is for intramuscular injection only.

†A full dose of Rh$_o$(D) Immune Globulin (Human) has traditionally been referred to as a "300 µg" dose and this usage is employed here for convenience in terminology. *It should not be construed as the actual anti-D content.* Each full dose of Rh$_o$(D) Immune Globulin (Human) must contain at least as much anti-D as 1 milliliter of the U.S. Reference Rh$_o$(D) Immune Globulin (Human). Studies performed at the Food and Drug Administration have shown that the U.S. Reference contains 820 international units (IU) of anti-D per milliliter. When the conversion factor determined for the International (WHO) Reference Preparation is used, 820 IU per milliliter is equivalent to 164 µg per milliliter of anti-D.

*Viresolve is a trademark of Millipore Corporation.

CLINICAL PHARMACOLOGY

Intramuscular Rh$_o$(D) human immune globulins prepared by cold alcohol fractionation have not been reported to transmit hepatitis or other infectious diseases.

RhoGAM acts by suppressing the immune response of Rh negative individuals to Rh positive red blood cells.

The obstetrical patient may be exposed to red blood cells from her Rh positive fetus during the normal course of pregnancy. Clinical studies have proven that the incidence of Rh immunization as a result of pregnancy was reduced to 1–2% from 12–13% when RhoGAM was given within 72 hours following delivery. Further studies in which patients received Rh immune globulin, antepartum at 28 to 32 weeks and postpartum, reduced the risk of immunization to less than 0.1%.

An Rh negative individual transfused with one unit of Rh positive red blood cells has about an 80% likelihood of producing anti-D. Protection from Rh immunization is accomplished by administering the appropriate dose of RhoGAM.

INDICATIONS AND USAGE

Pregnancy and Other Obstetric Conditions

RhoGAM is indicated whenever it is known or suspected that fetal red blood cells have entered the circulation of an Rh negative mother unless the fetus or the father can be shown conclusively to be Rh negative.

Transfusion

RhoGAM is indicated for any Rh negative female of childbearing age who receives any Rh positive red blood cells or component such as platelets or granulocytes prepared from Rh positive blood.

CONTRAINDICATIONS

Individuals known to have had an anaphylactic or severe systemic reaction to human globulin should not receive RhoGAM or any other Rh$_o$(D) Immune Globulin (Human).

WARNINGS

Do not inject intravenously.

Do not inject infant.

RhoGAM is made from human plasma. Products made from human plasma may contain infectious agents, such as viruses, that can cause disease. The risk that such products will transmit an infectious agent has been reduced by screening plasma donors for prior exposure to certain viruses, by testing for the presence of certain current viral infections and by removing certain viruses during the manufacturing process. Following fractionation, a viral-clearance filtration step is incorporated into the manufacturing process. This filtration step removes viruses via a size-exclusion mechanism utilizing a patented Viresolve 180 ultrafiltration membrane with defined pore-size distribution. The filter is inert to the product. This virus removal process

has been shown in laboratory spiking studies to reduce the levels of some viruses ranging from 18 to 200 nm in size, including enveloped viruses as well as non-enveloped viruses. Despite these measures, such products can still potentially transmit disease. There is also the possibility that unknown infectious agents may be present in such products. ALL infections thought by a physician possibly to have been transmitted by this product should be reported by the physician or other healthcare provider in the U.S. to Ortho-Clinical Diagnostics, Inc. at 1-800-322-6374. Outside of the U.S., the company distributing this product should be contacted. The physician should discuss the risks and benefits of this product with the patient.

PRECAUTIONS

The presence of passively acquired anti-D in the maternal serum may cause a positive antibody screening test. This does not preclude further antepartum or postpartum prophylaxis.

Some babies born of women given Rh$_o$(D) Immune Globulin (Human) antepartum have weakly positive direct antiglobulin tests at birth.

Late in pregnancy or following delivery there may be sufficient fetal red blood cells in the maternal circulation to cause a positive antiglobulin test for weak D(D^u). When there is any doubt as to the patient's Rh type, RhoGAM should be administered.

Pregnancy Category C

Animal reproduction studies have not been conducted with RhoGAM. It is also not known whether Rh$_o$(D) Immune Globulin (Human) can cause fetal harm when administered to a pregnant woman or can affect reproduction capacity. Rh$_o$(D) Immune Globulin (Human) should be given to a pregnant woman only if clearly needed. However, use of Rh antibody during the third trimester in full doses of antibody has been reported to produce no evidence of hemolysis in the infant.

ADVERSE REACTIONS

Systemic reactions associated with administration of RhoGAM are extremely rare. Discomfort at the site of injection has been reported and a small number of women have noted a slight elevation in temperature. About one-quarter of a group of 22 individuals who were given multiple doses of RhoGAM to treat mismatched transfusions noted fever, myalgia and lethargy. Bilirubin levels of 0.4 to 6.8 mg/dL were observed in some of the treated individuals and one had splenomegaly.

DOSAGE AND ADMINISTRATION

Parenteral drug products should be inspected visually for particulate matter and discoloration prior to administration, whenever solution and container permit.

A single dose (approximately 300 µg)† is contained in each prefilled syringe of RhoGAM. This is the usual dose for the indications associated with pregnancy unless there is clinical or laboratory evidence of a fetal-maternal hemorrhage in excess of 15 mL of Rh positive red blood cells. The indications and recommended dosage for RhoGAM are summarized in the following table.

Indications and Recommended Dosage

Indication	Dose (approximately)
Threatened abortion at any stage of gestation with continuation of pregnancy	300 µg†
Abortion or termination of pregnancy at or beyond 13 weeks' gestation**	300 µg
Genetic amniocentesis, chorionic villus sampling (CVS) and percutaneous umbilical blood sampling (PUBS)	300 µg
Abdominal trauma	300 µg
Antepartum prophylaxis at 26 to 28 weeks' gestation††	300 µg
Postpartum (if newborn Rh positive)	300 µg

†See footnote under Description

**If abortion or termination of pregnancy occurs up to and including 12 weeks' gestation, a single dose of MICRhoGAM® Rh$_o$(D) Immune Globulin (Human) (approximately 50 µg)† may be used instead of RhoGAM.

††If antepartum prophylaxis is indicated, it is essential that the mother receive a postpartum dose if the infant is Rh positive.

If an adverse event requires the administration of RhoGAM early in the pregnancy, there is an obligation to maintain a level of passively acquired anti-D by administration of RhoGAM at 12-week intervals. RhoGAM should be given within 72 hours after delivery if the baby is Rh positive. If delivery occurs within three weeks after the last antepartum dose, the postpartum dose may be withheld, but a test

for fetal-maternal hemorrhage (FMH) should still be performed to determine a bleed greater than 15 mL of packed red blood cells.

Whenever there is a fetal-maternal hemorrhage in excess of 15 mL of Rh positive red blood cells, multiple doses of RhoGAM are required. A fetal-maternal hemorrhage of this magnitude is unlikely prior to the last trimester of pregnancy. Patients who may need multiple doses of RhoGAM can be identified by a fetal-maternal hemorrhage screening test. If the test is positive, the volume of the fetal-maternal bleed should be determined by a quantitative method. A single dose of RhoGAM should be administered for every 15 mL of fetal red blood cells. If the dose calculation results in a fraction, administer the next number of whole syringes of RhoGAM.

Multiple doses of RhoGAM are usual for indications associated with transfusion. For every 15 mL of Rh positive red blood cells transfused, the patient should receive a single dose of RhoGAM. If multiple doses are required, consult your pharmacy for pooling directions.

Administer RhoGAM intramuscularly. Do not inject intravenously. Multiple doses may be administered at the same time or at spaced intervals, as long as the total dose is administered within three days of exposure.

HOW SUPPLIED

RhoGAM is available in packages containing:

5	prefilled single-dose syringes of RhoGAM (Product Code 780705) NDC 0562-7807-05
5	package inserts
5	control forms
5	patient identification cards
	and
25	prefilled single-dose syringes of RhoGAM (Product Code 780725) NDC 0562-7807-25
25	package inserts
25	control forms
25	patient identification cards
	and
100	prefilled single-dose syringes of RhoGAM (Product Code 780795) NDC 0562-7807-10
100	package inserts
100	control forms
100	patient identification cards

STORAGE

Store at 2 to 8°C. Do not store frozen.

Ortho Pharmaceutical Corporation

See Ortho-McNeil Pharmaceutical

Ortho Dermatological

**199 GRANDVIEW ROAD
SKILLMAN, NJ 08558**

For Medical Information Contact:
Dermatological Medical Information
(800) 426-7762

DERMATOP® EMOLLIENT CREAM ℞
[dur' mə-täp]
**(prednicarbate emollient cream)* 0.1%
FOR DERMATOLOGIC USE ONLY.
NOT FOR USE IN EYES.**

Prescribing Information

DESCRIPTION

DERMATOP® Emollient Cream (prednicarbate emollient cream) 0.1% contains prednicarbate, a synthetic corticosteroid for topical dermatologic use. The chemical name of prednicarbate is 11β, 17, 21-trihydroxypregna-1,4-diene-3,20-dione 17-(ethyl carbonate) 21-propionate. Prednicarbate has the empirical formula $C_{27}H_{36}O_8$ and a molecular weight of 488.58. Topical corticosteroids constitute a class of primarily synthetic steroids used topically as anti-inflammatory and antipruritic agents.

The CAS Registry Number is 73771-04-7. The chemical structure is:

[See chemical structure at top of next column]

Prednicarbate is a practically odorless white to yellow-white powder insoluble to practically insoluble in water and freely soluble in ethanol.

Each gram of DERMATOP Emollient Cream 0.1% contains 1.0 mg of prednicarbate in a base consisting of white petro-

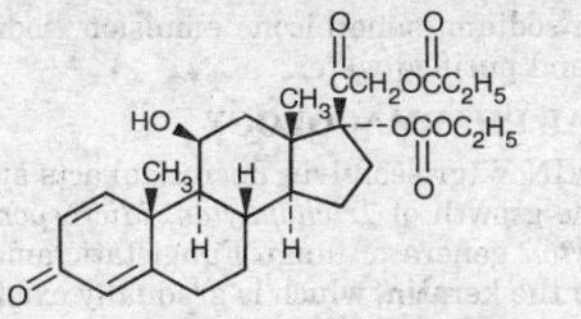

latum USP, purified water USP, isopropyl myristate NF, lanolin alcohols NF, mineral oil USP, cetostearyl alcohol NF, aluminum stearate, edetate disodium USP, lactic acid USP, and magnesium stearate DAB 9.

CLINICAL PHARMACOLOGY

In common with other topical corticosteroids, prednicarbate has anti-inflammatory, antipruritic, and vasoconstrictive properties. In general, the mechanism of the anti-inflammatory activity of topical steroids is unclear. However, corticosteroids are thought to act by the induction of phospholipase A_2 inhibitory proteins, collectively called lipocortins. It is postulated that these proteins control the biosynthesis of potent mediators of inflammation such as prostaglandins and leukotrienes by inhibiting the release of their common precursor arachidonic acid. Arachidonic acid is released from membrane phospholipids by phospholipase A_2.

Pharmacokinetics

The extent of percutaneous absorption of topical corticosteroids is determined by many factors, including the vehicle and the integrity of the epidermal barrier. Use of occlusive dressings with hydrocortisone for up to 24 hours have not been shown to increase penetration; however, occlusion of hydrocortisone for 96 hours does markedly enhance penetration. Topical corticosteroids can be absorbed from normal intact skin. Inflammation and/or other disease processes in the skin increase percutaneous absorption.

Studies performed with DERMATOP Emollient Cream (prednicarbate emollient cream) 0.1% indicate that the drug product is in the medium range of potency compared with other topical corticosteroids.

INDICATIONS AND USAGE

DERMATOP Emollient Cream 0.1% is a medium-potency corticosteroid indicated for the relief of the inflammatory and pruritic manifestations of corticosteroid-responsive dermatoses. DERMATOP Emollient Cream 0.1% may be used with caution in pediatric patients 1 year of age or older. The safety and efficacy of drug use for longer than 3 weeks in this population have not been established. Since safety and efficacy of DERMATOP Emollient Cream 0.1% have not been established in pediatric patients below 1 year of age, its use in this age group is not recommended.

CONTRAINDICATIONS

DERMATOP Emollient Cream 0.1% is contraindicated in those patients with a history of hypersensitivity to any of the components in the preparations.

PRECAUTIONS

General

Systemic absorption of topical corticosteroids can produce reversible hypothalamic-pituitary-adrenal (HPA) axis suppression with the potential for glucocorticosteroid insufficiency after withdrawal of treatment. Manifestations of Cushing's syndrome, hyperglycemia, and glucosuria can also be produced in some patients by systemic absorption of topical corticosteroids while on treatment.

Patients applying a topical steroid to a large surface area or under occlusion should be evaluated periodically for evidence of HPA-axis suppression. This may be done by using the ACTH stimulation, AM plasma cortisol, and urinary free cortisol tests.

DERMATOP Emollient Cream 0.1% did not produce significant HPA-axis suppression when used at a dose of 30 g/day for a week in 10 adult patients with extensive psoriasis or atopic dermatitis. DERMATOP Emollient Cream 0.1% did not produce HPA-axis suppression in any of 59 pediatric patients with extensive atopic dermatitis when applied BID for 3 weeks to >20% of the body surface (See PRECAUTIONS, Pediatric Use.)

If HPA-axis suppression is noted, an attempt should be made to withdraw the drug, to reduce the frequency of application, or to substitute a less potent corticosteroid. Recovery of HPA-axis function is generally prompt upon discontinuation of topical corticosteroids. Infrequently, signs and symptoms of glucocorticosteroid insufficiency may occur, requiring supplemental systemic corticosteroids. For information on systemic supplementation, see prescribing information for those products.

Pediatric patients may be more susceptible to systemic toxicity from equivalent doses due to their larger skin surface to body mass ratios. (See PRECAUTIONS, Pediatric Use.)

If irritation develops, DERMATOP Emollient Cream 0.1% should be discontinued and appropriate therapy instituted. Allergic contact dermatitis with corticosteroids is usually diagnosed by observing a *failure to heal* rather than noting a clinical exacerbation, as observed with most topical products not containing corticosteroids. Such an observation should be corroborated with appropriate diagnostic patch testing.

If concomitant skin infections are present or develop, an appropriate antifungal or antibacterial agent should be used. If a favorable response does not occur promptly, use of DERMATOP Emollient Cream 0.1% should be discontinued until the infection has been adequately controlled.

Information for Patients

Patients using topical corticosteroids should receive the following information and instructions:

1. This medication is to be used as directed by the physician. It is for external use only. Avoid contact with the eyes.
2. This medication should not be used for any disorder other than that for which it was prescribed.
3. The treated skin area should not be bandaged, otherwise covered or wrapped so as to be occlusive, unless directed by the physician.
4. Patients should report to their physician any signs of local adverse reactions.
5. Parents of pediatric patients should be advised not to use this medication in the treatment of diaper dermatitis. This medication should not be applied in the diaper area as diapers or plastic pants may constitute occlusive dressing. (See DOSAGE AND ADMINISTRATION.)
6. This medication should not be used on the face, underarms, or groin areas.
7. As with other corticosteroids, therapy should be discontinued when control is achieved. If no improvement is seen within two weeks, contact the physician.

Laboratory Tests

The following tests may be helpful in evaluating patients for HPA-axis suppression:

ACTH stimulation test
AM plasma cortisol test
Urinary free cortisol test

Carcinogenesis, Mutagenesis, and Impairment of Fertility

In a study of the effect of prednicarbate on fertility, pregnancy, and postnatal development in rats, no effect was noted on the fertility or pregnancy of the parent animals or postnatal development of the offspring after administration of up to 0.80 mg/kg of prednicarbate subcutaneously.

Prednicarbate has been evaluated in the Salmonella reversion test (Ames test) over a wide range of concentrations in the presence and absence of an S-9 liver microsomal fraction, and did not demonstrate mutagenic activity. Similarly, prednicarbate did not produce any significant changes in the numbers of micronuclei seen in erythrocytes when mice were given doses ranging from 1 to 160 mg/kg of the drug.

Pregnancy: Teratogenic Effects: Pregnancy Category C.

Corticosteroids have been shown to be teratogenic in laboratory animals when administered systemically at relatively low dosage levels. Some corticosteroids have been shown to be teratogenic after dermal application in laboratory animals.

Prednicarbate has been shown to be teratogenic and embryotoxic in Wistar rats and Himalayan rabbits when given subcutaneously during gestation at doses 1900 times and 45 times the recommended topical human dose, assuming a percutaneous absorption of approximately 3%.

In the rats, slightly retarded fetal development and an incidence of thickened and wavy ribs higher than the spontaneous rate were noted.

In rabbits, increased liver weights and slight increase in the fetal intrauterine death rate were observed. The fetuses that were delivered exhibited reduced placental weight, increased frequency of cleft palate, ossification disorders in the sternum, omphalocele, and anomalous posture of the forelimbs.

There are no adequate and well-controlled studies in pregnant women on teratogenic effects of prednicarbate. DERMATOP Emollient Cream (prednicarbate emollient cream) 0.1% should be used during pregnancy only if the potential benefit justifies the potential risk to the fetus.

Nursing Mothers

Systemically administered corticosteroids appear in human milk and could suppress growth, interfere with endogenous corticosteroid production, or cause other untoward effects. It is not known whether topical administration of corticosteroids could result in sufficient systemic absorption to produce detectable quantities in human milk. Because many drugs are excreted in human milk, caution should be exercised when DERMATOP Emollient Cream 0.1% is administered to a nursing woman.

Pediatric Use

DERMATOP Emollient Cream 0.1% may be used with caution in pediatric patients 1 year of age or older, although the safety and efficacy of drug use longer than 3 weeks have not been established. The use of DERMATOP Emollient Cream (prednicarbate emollient cream) 0.1% is supported by results of a three-week, uncontrolled study in 59 pediatric patients between the ages of 4 months and 12 years of age with atopic dermatitis. None of the 59 pediatric patients showed evidence of HPA-axis suppression. Safety and efficacy of DERMATOP Emollient Cream 0.1% in pediatric patients below 1 year of age have not been established, therefore use in this age group is not recommended. Because of a higher ratio of skin surface area to body mass, pediatric patients are at a greater risk than adults of HPA-axis suppression and Cushing's syndrome when they are treated with topical corticosteroids. They are therefore also at greater risk of adrenal insufficiency during and/or after withdrawal of treatment. In an uncontrolled study in pediatric patients with atopic dermatitis, the incidence of adverse reactions possibly or probably associated with the use of DERMATOP Emollient Cream 0.1% was limited. Mild signs of atrophy developed in 5 patients (5/59, 8%) during the clinical trial, with 2 patients exhibiting more than one sign. Two patients (2/59, 3%) developed shininess, and 2 patients (2/59, 3%) developed thinness. Three patients (3/59, 5%) were observed with mild telangectasia. It is unknown whether prior use of topical corticosteroids was a contributing factor in the development of telangectasia in 2 of the patients. Adverse effects including striae have also been reported with inappropriate use of topical corticosteroids in infants and children. Pediatric patients applying topical corticosteroids to greater than 20% of body surface are at higher risk for HPA-axis suppression.

HPA axis suppression, Cushing's syndrome, linear growth retardation, delayed weight gain and intracranial hypertension have been reported in children receiving topical corticosteroids. Manifestations of adrenal suppression in children include low plasma cortisol levels, and absence of response to ACTH stimulation. Manifestations of intracranial hypertension include bulging fontanelles, headaches, and bilateral papilledema.

DERMATOP Emollient Cream 0.1% should not be used in the treatment of diaper dermatitis.

ADVERSE REACTIONS

In controlled adult clinical studies, the incidence of adverse reactions probably or possibly associated with the use of DERMATOP Emollient Cream 0.1% was approximately 4%. Reported reactions included mild signs of skin atrophy in 1% of treated patients, as well as the following reactions which were reported in less than 1% of patients: pruritis, edema, paresthesia, urticaria, burning, allergic contact dermatitis and rash.

In an uncontrolled study in pediatric patients with atopic dermatitis, the incidence of adverse reactions possibly or probably associated with the use of DERMATOP Emollient Cream 0.1% was limited. Mild signs of atrophy developed in 5 patients (5/59, 8%) during the clinical trial, with 2 patients exhibiting more than one sign. Two patients (2/59, 3%) developed shininess, and 2 patients (2/59, 3%) developed thinness. Three patients (3/59, 5%) were observed with mild telangectasia. It is unknown whether prior use of topical corticosteroids was a contributing factor in the development of telangectasia in 2 of the patients (See PRECAUTIONS, Pediatric Use.)

The following additional local adverse reactions have been reported infrequently with topical corticosteroids, but may occur more frequently with the use of occlusive dressings. These reactions are listed in an approximate decreasing order of occurrence: folliculitis, acneiform eruptions, hypopigmentation, perioral dermatitis, secondary infection, striae and miliaria.

OVERDOSAGE

Topically applied corticosteroids can be absorbed in sufficient amounts to produce systemic effects. (See PRECAUTIONS.)

DOSAGE AND ADMINISTRATION

Apply a thin film of DERMATOP Emollient Cream (prednicarbate emollient cream) 0.1% to the affected skin areas twice daily. Rub in gently.

DERMATOP Emollient Cream (prednicarbate emollient cream) 0.1% may be used in pediatric patients 1 year of age or older. Safety and efficacy of DERMATOP Emollient cream 0.1% in pediatric patients for more than 3 weeks of use have not been established. Use in pediatric patients under 1 year of age is not recommended.

As with other corticosteroids, therapy should be discontinued when control is achieved. If no improvement is seen within 2 weeks, reassessment of the diagnosis may be necessary.

DERMATOP Emollient Cream 0.1% should not be used with occlusive dressings unless directed by the physician. DERMATOP Emollient Cream 0.1% should not be applied in the diaper area if the child still requires diapers or plastic pants as these garments may constitute occlusive dressing.

HOW SUPPLIED

DERMATOP Emollient Cream (prednicarbate emollient cream) 0.1% is supplied in 15 g (NDC 0062-0351-15) and 60 g (NDC 0062-0351-60) tubes.

Store between 41° and 77°F (5 and 25°C).

Prescribing Information as of February 1998

Dermatop REG TM HOECHST AG

Continued on next page

Dermatop—Cont.

U.S. Patent 4,242,334
Manufactured by:
Hoechst Marion Roussel
Deutschland GmbH
Distributed by:
Ortho Dermatological
Division of Ortho-McNeil Pharmaceutical, Inc.
Raritan, NJ
dercp0596p
Shown in Product Identification Guide, page 327

ERYCETTE® ℞
[ə 'ris-ət]
(erythromycin topical solution) 2%
For Dermatologic Use Only-
Not for Ophthalmic Use-

PRODUCT INFORMATION

DESCRIPTION

ERYCETTE® (erythromycin topical solution) 2% contains erythromycin ((3R*, 4S*,5S*,6R*,7R*,9R*,11R*,12R*, 13S*,14R*)-4-[(2,6-Dideoxy-3-C-methyl-3-O-methyl-α-L-*ribo*-hexopyranosyl)oxy]-14-ethyl-7,12,13-trihydroxy-3,5,7, 9,11,13-hexamethyl-6-[[3,4,6-trideoxy-3-(dimethylamino)-β-D-*xylo*-hexopyranosyl]-oxy]oxacyclotetradecane-2,10-dione), for topical dermatologic use. Erythromycin is a macrolide antibiotic produced from a strain of *Saccharopolyspora erythraea* (formerly *Streptomyces erythreus*). It is a base and readily forms salts with acids.
Chemically, erythromycin is $C_{37}H_{67}NO_{13}$.
It has the following structural formula:

Erythromycin has the molecular weight of 733.94. It is a white powder, is freely soluble in alcohols, acetone, chloroform, acetonitrile, ethyl acetate, and is moderately soluble in ether, ethylene dichloride, and amyl acetate.
Each milliliter of ERYCETTE contains 20 milligrams of erythromycin in a base of alcohol (66%) and propylene glycol, and may contain critic acid to adjust pH.

CLINICAL PHARMACOLOGY

The exact mechanism by which erythromycin reduces lesions of acne vulgaris is not fully known; however, the effect appears to be due in part to the antibacterial activity of the drug.

MICROBIOLOGY

Erythromycin acts by inhibition of protein synthesis in susceptible organisms by reversibly binding to 50 **S** ribosomal subunits, thereby inhibiting translocation of aminoacyl transfer-RNA and inhibiting polypeptide synthesis. Antagonism has been demonstrated *in vitro* between erythromycin, lincomycin, chloramphenicol, and clindamycin.

INDICATIONS AND USAGE

ERYCETTE is indicated for the topical treatment of acne vulgaris.

CONTRAINDICATIONS

ERYCETTE is contraindicated in those individuals who have shown hypersensitivity to any of its components.

WARNINGS

Pseudomembranous colitis has been reported with nearly all antibacterial agents, including erythromycin, and may range in severity from mild to life-threatening. Therefore, it is important to consider this diagnosis in patients who present with diarrhea subsequent to the administration of antibacterial agents.
Treatment with antibacterial agents alters the normal flora of the colon and may permit overgrowth of *clostridia*. Studies indicate that a toxin produced by *Clostridium difficile* is one primary cause of "antibiotic-associated colitis".
After the diagnosis of pseudomembranous colitis has been established, therapeutic measures should be initiated. Mild cases of pseudomembranous colitis usually respond to drug discontinuation alone. In moderate to severe cases, consideration should be given to management with fluids and electrolytes, protein supplementation and treatment with an antibacterial drug clinically effective against *C. difficile* colitis.

PRECAUTIONS

General: For topical use only; not for ophthalmic use. Concomitant topical acne therapy should be used with caution because a possible cumulative irritancy effect may occur, especially with the use of peeling, desquamating, or abrasive agents. The use of antibiotic agents may be associated with the overgrowth of antibiotic-resistant organisms. If this occurs, discontinue use and take appropriate measures. Avoid contact with eyes and all mucous membranes.
Information For Patients: Patients using ERYCETTE should receive the following information and instructions:
1. This medication is to be used as directed by the physician. It is for external use only. Avoid contact with the eyes, nose, mouth, and all mucous membranes.
2. This medication should not be used for any disorder other than that for which it was prescribed.
3. Patients should not use any other topical acne medication unless otherwise directed by their physician.
4. Patients should report to their physician any signs of local adverse reactions.
Carcinogenesis, mutagenesis, and impairment of fertility: No animal studies have been performed to evaluate the carcinogenic and mutagenic potential or effects on fertility of topical erythromycin. However, long-term (2-year) oral studies in rats with erythromycin ethylsuccinate and erythromycin base did not provide evidence of tumorigenicity. There was no apparent effect on male or female fertility in rats fed erythromycin (base) at levels up to 0.25% of diet.
Pregnancy: Teratogenic effects: Pregnancy Category B: There was no evidence of teratogenicity or any other adverse effect on reproduction in female rats fed erythromycin base (up to 0.25% diet) prior to and during mating, during gestation and through weaning of two successive litters.
There are, however, no adequate and well-controlled studies in pregnant women. Because animal reproduction studies are not always predictive of human response, this drug should be used in pregnancy only if clearly needed. Erythromycin has been reported to cross the placental barrier in humans, but fetal plasma levels are generally low.
Nursing Women: It is not known whether erythromycin is excreted in human milk after topical application. However, erythromycin is excreted in human milk following oral and parenteral erytromycin administration. Therefore, caution should be exercised when erythromycin is administered to a nursing woman.
Pediatric use: Safety and effectiveness of this product in pediatric patients have not been established.

ADVERSE REACTIONS

The following local adverse reactions have been reported occasionally: peeling, dryness, itching, erythema, and oiliness. Irritation of the eyes and tenderness of the skin have also been reported with topical use of erythromycin. Generalized urticarial reactions, possibly related to the use of erythromycin, which required systemic steroid therapy have been reported.

DOSAGE AND ADMINISTRATION

The ERYCETTE pledget should be rubbed over the affected area twice a day after the skin is thoroughly washed with warm water and soap and patted dry. Acne lesions on the face, neck, shoulder, chest, and back may be treated in this manner. Additional pledgets may be used, if needed. Each pledget should be used once and discarded.

HOW SUPPLIED

ERYCETTE (erythromycin topical solution) 2% is supplied as foil-covered saturated pledgets (swabs) in boxes of 60 (NDC 0062-1185-01). Each pledget is filled to contain 0.8 mL. ERYCETTE is not USP with regard to minimum volume.
Store below 25°C (77°F).
DERMATOLOGICAL DIVISION
ORTHO PHARMACEUTICAL
CORPORATION
Raritan, New Jersey 08869
© OPC 1984 PRINTED IN U.S.A.
REVISED AUGUST 1996
631-10-675-3
Shown in Product Identification Guide, page 327

GRIFULVIN V ® ℞
[gri 'fulvən]
(griseofulvin tablets) microsize
(griseofulvin oral suspension) microsize
Suspension and Tablets

DESCRIPTION

Griseofulvin is an antibiotic derived from a species of *Penicillium*. Each GRIFULVIN V Tablet contains either 250 mg or 500 mg of griseofulvin microsize, and also contains calcium stearate, colloidal silicon dioxide, starch, and wheat gluten. Additionally, the 250 mg tablet also contains dibasic calcium phosphate. Each 5 mL of GRIFULVIN V Suspension contains 125 mg of griseofulvin microsize and also contains alcohol 0.2%, docusate sodium, FD&C Red No. 40, FD&C Yellow No. 6, flavors, magnesium aluminium silicate, menthol, methylparaben, propylene glycol, propylparaben, saccharin sodium, simethicone emulsion, sodium alginate, sucrose, and purified water.

CLINICAL PHARMACOLOGY

GRIFULVIN V (griseofulvin microsize) acts systemically to inhibit the growth of *Trichophyton, Microsporum* and *Epidermophyton* genera of fungi. Fungistatic amounts are deposited in the keratin, which is gradually exfoliated and replaced by noninfected tissue.
Griseofulvin absorption from the gastrointestinal tract varies considerably among individuals, mainly because of insolubility of the drug in aqueous media of the upper G.I. tract. The peak serum level found in fasting adults given 0.5 g occurs at about four hours and ranges between 0.5 and 2.0 mcg/mL.
It should be noted that some individuals are consistently "poor absorbers" and tend to attain lower blood levels at all times. This may explain unsatisfactory therapeutic results in some patients. Better blood levels can probably be attained in most patients if the tablets are administered after a meal with a high fat content.

INDICATIONS AND USAGE

Major indications for GRIFULVIN V are:
Tinea capitis (ringworm of the scalp)
Tinea corporis (ringworm of the body)
Tinea pedis (athlete's foot)
Tinea unguium (onychomycosis; ringworm of the nails):
Tinea cruris (ringworm of the thigh)
Tinea barbae (barber's itch)
GRIFULVIN V inhibits the growth of those genera of fungi that commonly cause ringworm infections of the hair, skin, and nails, such as:
Trichophyton rubrum
Trichophyton tonsurans
Trichophyton mentagrophytes
Trichophyton interdigitalis
Trichophyton verrucosum
Trichophyton sulphureum
Trichophyton schoenleini
Microsporum audouini
Microsporum canis
Microsporum gypseum
Epidermophyton floccosum
Trichophyton megnini
Trichophyton gallinae
Trichophyton crateriform
Note: Prior to therapy, the type of fungi responsible for the infection should be identified. The use of the drug is not justified in minor or trivial infections which will respond to topical antifungal agents alone.
It is *not* effective in:
Bacterial infections
Candidiasis (Moniliasis)
Histoplasmosis
Actinomycosis
Sporotrichosis
Chromoblastomycosis
Coccidioidomycosis
North American Blastomycosis
Cryptococcosis (Torulosis)
Tinea versicolor
Nocardiosis

CONTRAINDICATIONS

This drug is contraindicated in patients with porphyria, hepatocellular failure, and in individuals with a history of hypersensitivity to griseofulvin.
Two cases of conjoined twins have been reported in patients taking griseofulvin during the first trimester of pregnancy. Griseofulvin should not be prescribed to pregnant patients.

WARNINGS

Prophylactic Usage: Safety and efficacy of prophylactic use of this drug have not been established.
Chronic feeding of griseofulvin, at levels ranging from 0.5-2.5% of the diet, resulted in the development of liver tumors in several strains of mice, particularly in males. Smaller particle sizes result in an enhanced effect. Lower oral dosage levels have not been tested. Subcutaneous administration of relatively small doses of griseofulvin once a week during the first three weeks of life has also been reported to induce hepatomata in mice. Although studies in other animal species have not yielded evidence of tumorigenicity, these studies were not of adequate design to form a basis for conclusions in this regard.
In subacute toxicity studies, orally administered griseofulvin produced hepatocellar necrosis in mice, but this has not been seen in other species. Disturbances in porphyrin metabolism have been reported in griseofulvin-treated laboratory animals. Griseofulvin has been reported to have a colchicine-like effect on mitosis and cocarcinogenicity with methyl cholanthrene in cutaneous tumor induction in laboratory animals.
Reports of animal studies in the Soviet literature state that a griseofulvin preparation was found to be embryotoxic and

teratogenic on oral administration to pregnant Wistar rats. Rat reproduction studies done in the United States and Great Britain were inconclusive in this regard. Pups with abnormalities have been reported in the litters of a few bitches treated with griseofulvin. Because the potential for adverse effects on the human fetus cannot be ruled out, additional contraceptive precautions should be taken during treatment with griseofulvin and for a month after termination of treatment. GRIFULVIN V should not be prescribed to women intending to become pregnant within one month following cessation of therapy.

Suppression of spermatogenesis has been reported to occur in rats but investigation in man failed to confirm this. Griseofulvin interferes with chromosomal distribution during cell division, causing aneuploidy in plant and mammalian cells. These effects have been demonstrated *in vitro* at concentrations that may be achieved in the serum with the recommended therapeutic dosage.

Since griseofulvin has demonstrated harmful effects *in vitro* on the genotype in bacteria, plants, and fungi, males should wait at least six months after completing griseofulvin therapy before fathering a child.

PRECAUTIONS

Patients on prolonged therapy with any potent medication should be under close observation. Periodic monitoring of organ system function, including renal, hepatic and hemopoietic, should be done.

Since griseofulvin is derived from species of penicillin, the possibility of cross sensitivity with penicillin exists; however, known penicillin-sensitive patients have been treated without difficulty.

Since a photosensitivity reaction is occasionally associated with griseofulvin therapy, patients should be warned to avoid exposure to intense natural or artificial sunlight. Should a photosensitivity reaction occur, lupus erythematosus may be aggravated.

Drug Interactions: Patients on warfarin-type anticoagulant therapy may require dosage adjustment of the anticoagulant during and after griseofulvin therapy. Concomitant use of barbiturates usually depresses griseofulvin activity and may necessitate raising the dosage.

The concomitant administration of griseofulvin has been reported to reduce the efficacy of oral contraceptives and to increase the incidence of breakthrough bleeding.

ADVERSE REACTIONS

When adverse reactions occur, they are most commonly of the hypersensitivity type such as skin rashes, urticaria and rarely, angioneurotic edema, or erythema multiforme-like drug reaction, and may necessitate withdrawal of therapy and appropriate countermeasures. Paresthesias of the hands and feet have been reported rarely after extended therapy. Other side effects reported occasionally are oral thrush, nausea, vomiting, epigastric distress, diarrhea, headache, fatigue, dizziness, insomnia, mental confusion and impairment of performance of routine activities.

Proteinuria and leukopenia have been reported rarely. Administration of the drug should be discontinued if granulocytopenia occurs.

When rare, serious reactions occur with griseofulvin, they are usually associated with high dosages, long periods of therapy, or both.

DOSAGE AND ADMINISTRATION

Accurate diagnosis of the infecting organism is essential. Identification should be made either by direct microscopic examination of a mounting of infected tissue in a solution of potassium hydroxide or by culture on an appropriate medium.

Medication must be continued until the infecting organism is completely eradicated as indicated by appropriate clinical or laboratory examination. Representative treatment periods are tinea capitis, 4 to 6 weeks; tinea corporis, 2 to 4 weeks; tinea pedis, 4 to 8 weeks; tinea unguium—depending on rate of growth—fingernails, at least 4 months; toenails, at least 6 months.

General measures in regard to hygiene should be observed to control sources of infection or reinfection. Concomitant use of appropriate topical agents is usually required, particularly in treatment of tinea pedis since in some forms of athlete's foot, yeasts and bacteria may be involved. Griseofulvin will not eradicate the bacterial or monilial infection.

Adults: A daily dose of 500 mg. will give a satisfactory response in most patients with tinea corporis, tinea cruris, and tinea capitis.

For those fungus infections more difficult to eradicate such as tinea pedis and tinea unguium, a daily dose of 1.0 g is recommended.

Children: Approximately 5 mg per pound of body weight per day is an effective dose for most children. On this basis the following dosage schedule for children is suggested:

Children weighing 30 to 50 pounds—125 mg to 250 mg daily.

Children weighing over 50 pounds—250 mg to 500 mg daily.

HOW SUPPLIED

GRIFULVIN V 250 mg Tablets in bottles of 100 (NDC 0062-0211-60) (white, scored, imprinted "ORTHO 211").

GRIFULVIN V 500 mg Tablets in bottles of 100 (NDC 0062-0214-60) and 500 (NDC 0062-0214-70) (white, scored, imprinted "ORTHO 214").

Dispense GRIFULVIN V Tablets in a tight container as defined in the USP.

GRIFULVIN V Suspension 125 mg per 5 mL in bottles of 4 fl oz (120mL) (NDC 0062-0206-04).

Dispense GRIFULVIN V Suspension in tight, light-resistant container as defined in the USP.

STORE AT ROOM TEMPERATURE

Revised January 1997

631-10-560-2

Shown in Product Identification Guide, page 327

MONISTAT-DERM® ℞

[*'män ə-stat-dərm*]

(miconazole nitrate 2%)
Cream
For Topical Use Only

DESCRIPTION

MONISTAT-DERM (miconazole nitrate 2%) Cream contains miconazole nitrate* 2%, formulated into a water-miscible base consisting of pegoxol 7 stearate, peglicol 5 oleate, mineral oil, benzoic acid, and butylated hydroxyanisole and purified water.

*Chemical name: 1-[2,4-dichloro-β-{(2,4-dichlorobenzyl)oxy} phenethyl] imidazole mononitrate.

ACTIONS

Miconazole nitrate is a synthetic antifungal agent which inhibits the growth of the common dermatophytes, *Trichophyton rubrum, Trichophyton mentagrophytes,* and *Epidermophyton floccosum,* the yeast-like fungus, *Candida albicans,* and the organism responsible for tinea versicolor *(Malassezia furfur).*

INDICATIONS

For topical application in the treatment of tinea pedis (athlete's foot), tinea cruris, and tinea corporis caused by *Trichophyton rubrum, Trichophyton mentagrophytes,* and *Epidermophyton floccosum,* in the treatment of cutaneous candidiasis (moniliasis), and in the treatment of tinea versicolor.

CONTRAINDICATIONS

MONISTAT-DERM (miconazole nitrate 2%) Cream has no known contraindications.

PRECAUTIONS

If a reaction suggesting sensitivity or chemical irritation should occur, use of the medication should be discontinued. For external use only. Avoid introduction of MONISTAT-DERM Cream into the eyes.

ADVERSE REACTIONS

There have been isolated reports of irritation, burning, maceration, and allergic contact dermatitis associated with application of MONISTAT-DERM.

DOSAGE AND ADMINISTRATION

Sufficient MONISTAT-DERM Cream should be applied to cover affected areas twice daily (morning and evening) in patients with tinea pedis, tinea cruris, tinea corporis, and cutaneous candidiasis, and once daily in patients with tinea versicolor. If MONISTAT-DERM Cream is used in intertriginous areas, it should be applied sparingly and smoothed in well to avoid maceration effects.

Early relief of symptoms (2 to 3 days) is experienced by the majority of patients and clinical improvement may be seen fairly soon after treatment is begun; however, *Candida* infections and tinea cruris and corporis should be treated for two weeks and tinea pedis for one month in order to reduce the possibility of recurrence. If a patient shows no clinical improvement after a month of treatment, the diagnosis should be redetermined. Patients with tinea versicolor usually exhibit clinical and mycological clearing after two weeks of treatment.

HOW SUPPLIED

MONISTAT-DERM (miconazole nitrate 2%) Cream containing miconazole nitrate at 2% strength is supplied in 15 g. (NDC 0062-5434-02), 1 oz. (NDC 0062-5434-01) and 3 oz. (NDC 0062-5434-03) tubes.

Shown in Product Identification Guide, page 327

RENOVA® ℞

[*rē' novă*]

(TRETINOIN EMOLLIENT CREAM) 0.05%
FOR TOPICAL USE ON THE FACE ONLY

Prescribing Information

DESCRIPTION

RENOVA (tretinoin emollient cream) 0.05% contains the active ingredient tretinoin (a retinoid) in an emollient cream base. Tretinoin is a yellow to light orange crystalline powder having a characteristic floral odor. Tretinoin is soluble in dimethylsulfoxide, slightly soluble in polyethylene glycol 400, octanol, and 100% ethanol. It is practically insoluble in water and mineral oil, and it is insoluble in glycerin. The chemical name for tretinoin is (all-E)-3,7-dimethyl-9-(2,6,6-trimethyl-1-cyclonexen-1-yl)-2,4,6,8-nonatetraenoic acid. Tretinoin is also referred to as all-*trans*-retinoic acid and has a molecular weight of 300.44. The structural formula is represented below.

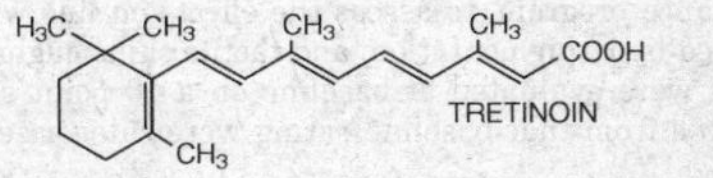

Tretinoin is available as RENOVA at a concentration of 0.05% w/w in a water in oil emulsion formulation consisting of light mineral oil, NF; sorbitol solution, USP; hydroxyoctacosanyl hydroxystearate; methoxy PEG-22/dodecyl glycol copolymer; PEG-45/dodecyl glycol copolymer; stearoxytrimethylsilane and stearyl alcohol; dimethicone 50 cs; methylparaben, NF; edetate disodium, USP; quaternium-15; butylated hydroxytoluene, NF; citric acid monohydrate, USP; fragrance; and purified water, USP.

CLINICAL PHARMACOLOGY

The exact mechanism of action of tretinoin is unknown although retinoids are believed to exert an effect on the growth and differentiation of various epithelial cells. When applied topically, however, there was no noted increase in desmosine, hydroxyproline, or elastin mRNA in human skin. In addition, the role of the irritative nature of this product in effecting the positive effects attributed to this product for its indication has not yet been fully determined. The transdermal absorption of tretinoin from various topical formulations ranged from 1% to 31% of applied dose, depending on whether it was applied to healthy skin or dermatitic skin. When percutaneous absorption of RENOVA was assessed in healthy male subjects (n=14) after a single application, as well as after repeated daily applications for 28 days, the absorption of tretinoin was less than 2% and endogenous concentrations of tretinoin and its major metabolites were unaltered.

INDICATIONS AND USAGE

(To understand fully the indication for this product, please read the entire INDICATIONS AND USAGE section of the labeling.)

RENOVA (tretinoin emollient cream) 0.05% is indicated as an adjunctive agent (see second bullet point below) for use in the mitigation (palliation) of fine wrinkles, mottled hyperpigmentation, and tactile roughness of facial skin in patients who do not achieve such palliation using comprehensive skin care and sun avoidance programs alone (see bullet point 3 for populations in which effectiveness has not been established). **RENOVA DOES NOT ELIMINATE WRINKLES, REPAIR SUN DAMAGED SKIN, REVERSE PHOTO-AGING, or RESTORE A MORE YOUTHFUL or YOUNGER DERMAL HISTOLOGIC PATTERN.** Many patients achieve desired palliative effects on fine wrinkling, mottled hyperpigmentation, and tactile roughness of facial skin with the use of comprehensive skin care and sun avoidance programs including sunscreens, protective clothing, and emollient creams NOT containing tretinoin.

- RENOVA has demonstrated NO MITIGATING EFFECT on significant signs of chronic sun exposure such as coarse or deep wrinkling, skin yellowing, lentigines, telangiectasia, skin laxity, keratinocytic atypia, melanocytic atypia, or dermal elastosis.
- RENOVA should only be used under medical supervision as an adjunct to a comprehensive skin care and sun avoidance program that includes the use of effective sunscreens (minimum SPF of 15) and protective clothing when desired results on fine wrinkles, mottled hyperpigmentation, and roughness of facial skin have not been achieved with a comprehensive skin care and sun avoidance program alone.
- The effectiveness of RENOVA in the mitigation of fine wrinkles, mottled hyperpigmentation, and tactile roughness of facial skin has not been established in people greater than 50 years of age OR in people with moderately to heavily pigmented skin. In addition, patients with visible actinic keratoses and patients with a history of skin cancer were excluded from clinical trials of RENOVA. Thus the effectiveness and safety of RENOVA in these populations are not known at this time.
- Neither the safety nor the effectiveness of RENOVA for the prevention or treatment of actinic keratoses or skin neoplasms has been established.
- Neither the safety nor the efficacy of using RENOVA daily for greater than 48 weeks has been established, and daily

Continued on next page

Renova—Cont.

use beyond 48 weeks has not been systematically and histologically investigated in adequate and well-controlled trials. (See **WARNINGS** section.)

CLINICAL TRIALS DATA:

Two adequate and well-controlled trials were conducted involving a total of 161 evaluable patients (under 50 years of age) treated with RENOVA and 154 evaluable patients treated with the vehicle emollient cream on the face for 24 weeks as an adjunct to a comprehensive skin care and sun avoidance program, to assess the effects on fine wrinkling, mottled hyperpigmentation, and tactile skin roughness. Patients were evaluated at baseline on a 10 point scale and changes from that baseline rating were categorized as follows:

No Improvement	No change or an increase of 1 unit or more.
Minimal Improvement	Reduction of 1 unit.
Moderate Improvement	Reduction of 2 units or more.

In these trials, the fine wrinkles, mottled hyperpigmentation, and tactile roughness of the facial skin were thought to be caused by multiple factors which included intrinsic aging or environmental factors, such as chronic sun exposure. The results of these assessments are as follows:
[See table below]

Most of the improvement in these signs was noted during the first 24 weeks of therapy. Thereafter, therapy primarily maintained the improvement realized during the first 24 weeks.

A majority of patients will lose most mitigating effects of RENOVA on fine wrinkles, mottled hyperpigmentation, and tactile roughness of facial skin with discontinuation of a comprehensive skin care and sun avoidance program including RENOVA; however, the safety and effectiveness of using RENOVA daily for greater than 48 weeks have not been established.

CONTRAINDICATIONS

This drug is contraindicated in individuals with a history of sensitivity reactions to any of its components. It should be discontinued if hypersensitivity to any of its ingredients is noted.

WARNINGS

* RENOVA is a dermal irritant, and the results of continued irritation of the skin for greater than 48 weeks in chronic, long term use are not known. There is evidence of atypical changes in melanocytes and keratinocytes, and of increased dermal elastosis in some patients treated with RENOVA for longer than 48 weeks. The significance of these findings is unknown.
* Safety and effectiveness of RENOVA in individuals with moderately or heavily pigmented skin have not been established.
* RENOVA should not be administered if the patient is also taking drugs known to be photosensitizers (e.g., thiazides, tetracyclines, fluoroquinolones, phenothiazines, sulfonamides) because of the possibility of augmented phototoxicity.

Because of heightened burning susceptibility, exposure to sunlight (including sunlamps) should be avoided or minimized during use of RENOVA. Patients must be warned to use sunscreens (minimum of SPF of 15) and protective clothing when using RENOVA. Patients with sunburn should be advised not to use RENOVA until fully recovered. Patients who may have considerable sun exposure due to their occupation and those patients with inherent sensitivity to sunlight should exercise particular caution when using RENOVA and assure that the precautions outlined in the Patient Package Insert are observed.

RENOVA should be kept out of the eyes, mouth, angles of the nose, and mucous membranes. Topical use may cause severe local erythema, pruritus, burning, stinging, and peeling at the site of application. If the degree of local irritation warrants, patients should be directed to use less medication, decrease the frequency of application, discontinue use temporarily or discontinue use altogether.

Tretinoin has been reported to cause severe irritation on eczematous skin and should be used only with utmost caution in patients with this condition.

Application of larger amounts of medication than recommended will not lead to more rapid or better results, and marked redness, peeling, or discomfort may occur.

PRECAUTIONS

General: RENOVA should only be used as an adjunct to a comprehensive skin care and sun avoidance program. (See **INDICATIONS AND USAGE** section.)

If a drug sensitivity, chemical irritation, or a systemic adverse reaction develops, use of RENOVA should be discontinued.

Weather extremes, such as wind or cold, may be more irritating to patients using RENOVA.

Information for Patients: See Patient Package Insert.

Drug Interactions: Concomitant topical medication, medicated or abrasive soaps, shampoos, cleansers, cosmetics with a strong drying effect, products with high concentration of alcohol, astringents, spices or lime, permanent wave solutions, electrolysis, hair depilatories or waxes, and products that may irritate the skin should be used with caution in patients being treated with RENOVA because they may increase irritation with RENOVA.

RENOVA should not be administered if the patient is also taking drugs known to be photosensitizers (e.g., thiazides, tetracyclines, fluoroquinolones, phenothiazines, sulfonamides) because of the possibility of augmented phototoxicity.

Carcinogenesis, Mutagenesis, Impairment of Fertility: In a life-time dermal study in CD-1 mice, at 100 and 200 times the average recommended human topical clinical dose, a few skin tumors in the female mice and liver tumors in male mice were observed. The biological significance of these findings is not clear because they occurred at doses that exceeded the dermal maximally tolerated dose (MTD) of tretinoin and because they were within the background natural occurrence rate for these tumors in this strain of mice. There was no evidence of carcinogenic potential when tretinoin was administered topically at a dose 5 times the average recommended human topical clinical dose. For purposes of comparisons of the animal exposure to human exposure, the "recommended human topical clinical dose" is defined as 500 mg of 0.05% RENOVA applied daily to a 50 kg person.

In a chronic, two-year bioassay of Vitamin A acid in mice performed by Tsubura and Yamamoto, generalized amyloid deposition was reported in all groups in the basal layer of the Vitamin A treated skin. In CD-1 mice, a similar study reported hyalinization at the treated skin sites and the incidence of this finding was 0/50, 3/50, 3/50, and 2/50 in male mice and 1/50, 0/50, 4/50, and 2/50 in female mice from the vehicle control, 0.25 mg/kg, 0.5 mg/kg, and 1 mg/kg groups, respectively.

Studies in hairless albino mice suggest that tretinoin may enhance the tumorigenic potential of carcinogenic doses of UVB and UVA light from a solar simulator. In other studies, when lightly pigmented hairless mice treated with tretinoin were exposed to carcinogenic doses of UVB light, the incidence and rate of development of skin tumors were either reduced or no effect was seen. Due to significantly different experimental conditions, no strict comparison of these disparate data is possible at this time. Although the significance of these studies to humans is not clear, patients should minimize exposure to sun.

The mutagenic potential of tretinoin was evaluated in the Ames assay and in the in vivo mouse micronucleus assay, both of which were negative.

Dermal Segment I and III studies with RENOVA have not been performed in any species. In oral Segment I and Segment III studies in rats with tretinoin, decreased survival of neonates and growth retardation were observed at doses in excess of 2 mg/kg/day (>400 times the average recommended human topical clinical dose).

Pregnancy:

Teratogenic effects: Pregnancy Category C.

ORAL tretinoin has been shown to be teratogenic in rats, mice, rabbits, hamsters, and subhuman primates. It was teratogenic and fetotoxic in rats when given orally in doses of 1000 times the average recommended human topical clinical dose. However, variations in teratogenic doses among various strains of rats have been reported. In the cynomolgus monkey, which, metabolically, is closer to humans for tretinoin than the other species examined, fetal malformations were reported at doses of 10 mg/kg/day or greater, but none were observed at 5 mg/kg/day (1000 times the average recommended human topical clinical dose), although increased skeletal variations were observed at all doses. A dose-related increased embryolethality and abortion was reported. Similar results have also been reported in pigtail macaques.

TOPICAL tretinoin in animal teratogenicity tests has generated equivocal results. There is evidence for teratogenicity (shortened or kinked tail) of topical tretinoin in Wistar rats at doses greater than 1 mg/kg/day (200 times the recommended human topical clinical dose). Anomalies (humerus: short 13%, bent 6%, os parietal incompletely ossified 14%) have also been reported when 10 mg/kg/day was dermally applied.

There are other reports in New Zealand White rabbits with doses of approximately 80 times the recommended human topical clinical dose of an increased incidence of domed head and hydrocephaly, typical of retinoid-induced fetal malformations in this species.

In contrast, several well-controlled animal studies have shown that dermally applied tretinoin was not teratogenic at doses of 100 and 200 times the recommended human topical clinical dose, in rats and rabbits, respectively.

With widespread use of any drug, a small number of birth defect reports associated temporally with the administration of the drug would be expected by chance alone. Thirty cases of temporally-associated congenital malformations have been reported during two decades of clinical use of another formulation of topical tretinoin (Retin-A). Although no definite pattern of teratogenicity and no causal association has been established from these cases, 5 of the reports describe the rare birth defect category holoprosencephaly (defects associated with incomplete midline development of the forebrain). The significance of these spontaneous reports in terms of risk to the fetus is not known.

Non-teratogenic effects:

Dermal tretinoin has been shown to be fetotoxic in rabbits when administered in doses 100 times the recommended topical human clinical dose. Oral tretinoin has been shown to be fetotoxic in rats when administered in doses 500 times the recommended topical human clinical dose.

There are, however, no adequate and well-controlled studies in pregnant women. RENOVA should not be used during pregnancy.

Nursing Mothers: It is not known whether this drug is excreted in human milk. Because many drugs are excreted in human milk, caution should be exercised when RENOVA is administered to a nursing women.

Pediatric Use: Safety and effectiveness in patients less than 18 years of age have not been established.

Geriatric Use: Safety and effectiveness in individuals older than 50 years of age have not been established.

ADVERSE REACTIONS

(See **WARNINGS** and **PRECAUTIONS** sections.)
In double-blind, vehicle-controlled studies involving 179 patients who applied RENOVA to their face, adverse reactions associated with the use of RENOVA were limited primarily

FINE WRINKLING

	NO IMPROVEMENT	MINIMAL IMPROVEMENT	MODERATE IMPROVEMENT
RENOVA +CSP*	36%	40%	24%
Vehicle + CSP	62%	30%	8%

MOTTLED HYPERPIGMENTATION

	NO IMPROVEMENT	MINIMAL IMPROVEMENT	MODERATE IMPROVEMENT
RENOVA +CSP	35%	27%	38%
Vehicle + CSP	53%	21%	27%

TACTILE SKIN ROUGHNESS

	NO IMPROVEMENT	MINIMAL IMPROVEMENT	MODERATE IMPROVEMENT
RENOVA +CSP	49%	35%	16%
Vehicle + CSP	67%	23%	10%

* CSP = Comprehensive skin protection and sun avoidance programs including use of sunscreens, protective clothing, and emollient cream.

to the skin. During these trials, 4% of patients had to discontinue use of RENOVA because of adverse reactions. These discontinuations were due to skin irritation or related cutaneous adverse reactions.

Local reactions such as peeling, dry skin, burning, stinging, erythema, and pruritus were reported by almost all subjects during therapy with RENOVA. These signs and symptoms were usually of mild to moderate severity and generally occurred early in therapy. In most patients the dryness, peeling, and redness recurred after an initial (24 week) decline.

OVERDOSAGE

Application of larger amounts of medication than recommended will not lead to more rapid or better results, and marked redness, peeling, or discomfort may occur. Oral ingestion of the drug may lead to the same side effects as those associated with excessive oral intake of Vitamin A.

DOSAGE AND ADMINISTRATION

- Do NOT use RENOVA if the patient is pregnant or is attempting to become pregnant or is at high risk of pregnancy,
- Do NOT use RENOVA if the patient is sunburned or if the patient has eczema or other chronic skin condition(s),
- Do NOT use RENOVA if the patient is inherently sensitive to sunlight,
- Do NOT use RENOVA if the patient is also taking drugs known to be photosensitizers (e.g., thiazides, tetracyclines, fluoroquinolones, phenothiazines, sulfonamides) because of the possibility of augmented phototoxicity.

Patients require detailed instruction to obtain maximal benefits and to understand all the precautions necessary to use this product with greatest safety. The physician should review the Patient Package Insert.

RENOVA should be applied to the face once a day before retiring using only enough to cover the entire affected area lightly. Patients should gently wash their face with a mild soap, pat the skin dry, and wait 20 to 30 minutes before applying RENOVA. The patient should apply a pea-sized amount of cream to cover the entire face lightly. Special caution should be taken when applying the cream to avoid the eyes, ears, nostrils, and mouth.

Application of RENOVA may cause a transitory feeling of warmth or slight stinging.

Mitigation (palliation) of facial fine wrinkling, mottled hyperpigmentation and tactile roughness may occur gradually over the course of therapy. Up to six months of therapy may be required before the effects are seen. Most of the improvement noted with RENOVA is seen during the first 24 weeks of therapy. Thereafter, therapy primarily maintains the improvement realized during the first 24 weeks.

With discontinuation of RENOVA therapy, a majority of patients will lose most mitigating effects of RENOVA on fine wrinkles, mottled hyperpigmentation, and tactile roughness of facial skin; **however, the safety and effectiveness of using RENOVA daily for greater than 48 weeks have not been established.**

Application of larger amounts of medication than recommended will not lead to more rapid or better results, and marked redness, peeling, or discomfort may occur.

Patients treated with RENOVA may use cosmetics but the areas to be treated should be cleansed thoroughly before the medication is applied. (See **PRECAUTIONS** section.)

HOW SUPPLIED

RENOVA is available in these sizes:

NDC 0062-0185-00	20 gram tube
NDC 0062-0185-05	40 gram tube
NDC 0062-0185-03	60 gram tube

Storage: Store between 15° and 25°C (59° and 77°F). DO NOT FREEZE.

QUESTIONS: Physicians and Pharmacists can call 1-800-426-7762, from 8:30 a.m. to 4:30 p.m. Eastern Time, Monday through Friday.

Rx only.

DERMATOLOGICAL DIVISION
ORTHO PHARMACEUTICAL CORPORATION
Raritan, New Jersey 08869

©OPC 1991 Revised February 1998

U.S. Patents 4,603,146, 4,423,041 and 4,877,805

653-10-870-5

Shown in Product Identification Guide, page 327

RETIN–A® ℞

[*'ret in-ā*]
(tretinoin)
Liquid • Cream • Gel
For Topical Use Only

DESCRIPTION

RETIN-A Gel, Cream and Liquid, containing tretinoin are used for the topical treatment of acne vulgaris. RETIN-A Gel contains tretinoin (retinoic acid, vitamin A acid) in either of two strengths. 0.025% or 0.01% by weight, in a gel vehicle of butylated hydroxytoluene, hydroxypropyl cellulose and alcohol (denatured with *tert*-butyl alcohol and brucine sulfate) 90% w/w. RETIN-A (tretinoin) Cream contains tretinoin in either of three strengths, 0.1%, 0.05%, or 0.025% by weight, in a hydrophilic cream vehicle of stearic acid, isopropyl myristate, polyoxyl 40 stearate, stearyl alcohol, xanthan gum, sorbic acid, butylated hydroxytoluene, and purified water. RETIN-A Liquid contains tretinoin 0.05% by weight, polyethylene glycol 400, butylated hydroxytoluene and alcohol (denatured with *tert*-butyl alcohol and brucine sulfate) 55%. Chemically, tretinoin is *all-trans*-retinoic acid and has the following structure:

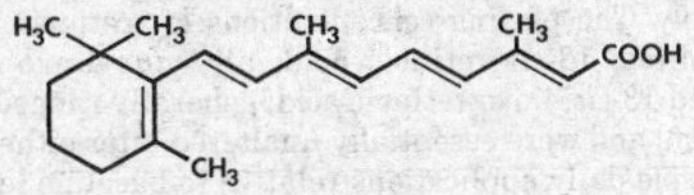

CLINICAL PHARMACOLOGY

Although the exact mode of action of tretinoin is unknown, current evidence suggests that topical tretinoin decreases cohesiveness of follicular epithelial cells with decreased microcomedo formation. Additionally, tretinoin stimulates mitotic activity and increased turnover of follicular epithelial cells causing extrusion of the comedones.

INDICATIONS AND USAGE

RETIN-A is indicated for topical application in the treatment of acne vulgaris. The safety and efficacy of the long-term use of this product in the treatment of other disorders have not been established.

CONTRAINDICATIONS

Use of the product should be discontinued if hypersensitivity to any of the ingredients is noted.

PRECAUTIONS

General: If a reaction suggesting sensitivity or chemical irritation occurs, use of the medication should be discontinued. Exposure to sunlight, including sunlamps, should be minimized during the use of RETIN-A, and patients with sunburn should be advised not to use the product until fully recovered because of heightened susceptibility to sunlight as a result of the use of tretinoin. Patients who may be required to have considerable sun exposure due to occupation and those with inherent sensitivity to the sun should exercise particular caution. Use of sunscreen products and protective clothing over treated areas is recommended when exposure cannot be avoided. Weather extremes, such as wind or cold, also may be irritating to patients under treatment with tretinoin.

RETIN-A (tretinoin) acne treatment should be kept away from the eyes, the mouth, angles of the nose, and mucous membranes. Topical use may induce severe local erythema and peeling at the site of application. If the degree of local irritation warrants, patients should be directed to use the medication less frequently, discontinue use temporarily, or discontinue use altogether. Tretinoin has been reported to cause severe irritation on eczematous skin and should be used with utmost caution in patients with this condition.

Drug Interactions: Concomitant topical medication, medicated or abrasive soaps and cleansers, soaps and cosmetics that have a strong drying effect, and products with high concentrations of alcohol, astringents, spices or lime should be used with caution because of possible interaction with tretinoin. Particular caution should be exercised in using preparations containing sulfur, resorcinol, or salicylic acid with RETIN-A. It also is advisable to "rest" a patient's skin until the effects of such preparations subside before use of RETIN-A is begun.

Carcinogenesis: Long-term animal studies to determine the carcinogenic potential of tretinoin have not been performed. Studies in hairless albino mice suggest that tretinoin may accelerate the tumorigenic potential of weakly carcinogenic light from a solar simulator. In other studies, when lightly pigmented hairless mice treated with tretinoin were exposed to carcinogenic doses of UVB light, the incidence and rate of development of skin tumors was reduced. Due to significantly different experimental conditions, no strict comparison of these disparate data is possible. Although the significance of these studies to man is not clear, patients should avoid or minimize exposure to sun.

Pregnancy: Teratogenic effects. Pregnancy Category C. *Oral* tretinoin has been shown to be teratogenic in rats when given in doses 1000 times the topical human dose. Oral tretinoin has been shown to be fetotoxic in rats when given in doses 500 times the topical human dose. *Topical* tretinoin has not been shown to be teratogenic in rats and rabbits when given in doses of 100 and 320 times the topical human dose, respectively (assuming a 50 kg adult applies 250 mg of 0.1% cream topically). However, at these topical doses, delayed ossification of a number of bones occurred in both species. These changes may be considered variants of normal development and are usually corrected after weaning. There are no adequate and well-controlled studies in pregnant women. Tretinoin should be used during pregnancy only if the potential benefit justifies the potential risk to the fetus.

Nursing mothers: It is not known whether this drug is excreted in human milk. Because many drugs are excreted in human milk, caution should be exercised when RETIN-A is administered to a nursing woman.

GELS ARE FLAMMABLE. Note: Keep away from heat and flame. Keep tube tightly closed.

ADVERSE REACTIONS

The skin of certain sensitive individuals may become excessively red, edematous, blistered, or crusted. If these effects occur, the medication should either be discontinued until the integrity of the skin is restored, or the medication should be adjusted to a level the patient can tolerate. True contact allergy to topical tretinoin is rarely encountered. Temporary hyper- or hypopigmentation has been reported with repeated application of RETIN-A. Some individuals have been reported to have heightened susceptibility to sunlight while under treatment with RETIN-A. To date, all adverse effects of RETIN-A have been reversible upon discontinuance of therapy (see Dosage and Administration Section).

OVERDOSAGE

If medication is applied excessively, no more rapid or better results will be obtained and marked redness, peeling, or discomfort may occur. Oral ingestion of the drug may lead to the same side effects as those associated with excessive oral intake of Vitamin A.

DOSAGE AND ADMINISTRATION

RETIN-A Gel, Cream or Liquid should be applied once a day, before retiring, to the skin where acne lesions appear, using enough to cover the entire affected area lightly. Liquid: The liquid may be applied using a fingertip, gauze pad or cotton swab. If gauze or cotton is employed, care should be taken not to oversaturate it to the extent that the liquid would run into areas where treatment is not intended. Gel: Excessive application results in "pilling" of the gel, which minimizes the likelihood of overapplication by the patient. Application may cause a transitory feeling of warmth or slight stinging. In cases where it has been necessary to temporarily discontinue therapy or to reduce the frequency of application, therapy may be resumed or frequency of application increased when the patients become able to tolerate the treatment.

Alterations of vehicle, drug concentration, or dose frequency should be closely monitored by careful observation of the clinical therapeutic response and skin tolerance.

During the early weeks of therapy, an *apparent* exacerbation of inflammatory lesions may occur. This is due to the action of the medication on deep, previously unseen lesions and should not be considered a reason to discontinue therapy.

Therapeutic results should be noticed after two to three weeks but more than six weeks of therapy may be required before definite beneficial effects are seen.

Once the acne lesions have responded satisfactorily, it may be possible to maintain the improvement with less frequent applications, or other dosage forms.

Patients treated with RETIN-A (tretinoin) acne treatment may use cosmetics, but the areas to be treated should be cleansed thoroughly before the medication is applied. **(See Precautions)**

HOW SUPPLIED

RETIN-A (tretinoin) is supplied as:

RETIN-A Cream

NDC Code	RETIN-A Strength/Form	RETIN-A Qty.
0062-0165-01	0.025% Cream	20g
0062-0165-02	0.025% Cream	45g
0062-0175-12	0.05% Cream	20g
0062-0175-13	0.05% Cream	45g
0062-0275-23	0.1% Cream	20g
0062-0275-01	0.1% Cream	45g

RETIN-A Gel

NDC Code	RETIN-A Strength/Form	RETIN-A Qty.
0062-0575-44	0.01% Gel	15g
0062-0575-46	0.01% Gel	45g
0062-0475-42	0.025% Gel	15g
0062-0475-45	0.025% Gel	45g

RETIN-A Liquid

NDC Code	RETIN-A Strength/Form	RETIN-A Qty.
0062-0075-07	0.05% Liquid	28 ml

Storage Conditions: RETIN-A Liquid, 0.05%, and RETIN-A Gel, 0.025% and 0.01%: store below 86°F. RETIN-A Cream, 0.1%, 0.05%, and 0.025%: store below 80°F.

Revised December 1996 643-11-339-2

Shown in Product Identification Guide, page 327

Continued on next page

RETIN-A® MICRO™ ℞
(tretinoin gel) microsphere, 0.1%

For Topical Use Only

DESCRIPTION
Retin-A Micro (tretinoin gel) microsphere, 0.1%, is a formulation containing 0.1% by weight tretinoin for the topical treatment of acne vulgaris. This formulation uses patented acrylates copolymer porous microspheres (MICROSPONGE® System) to enable inclusion of the active ingredient, tretinoin, in an aqueous gel. Other components of this formulation are purified water, carbomer 934P, glycerin, disodium EDTA, propylene glycol, sorbic acid, PPG-20 methyl glucose ether distearate, cyclomethicone and dimethicone copolyol, benzyl alcohol, trolamine, and butylated hydroxytoluene.
Chemically, tretinoin is all-*trans*-retinoic acid, also known as (all-E) 3,7-dimethyl-9-(2,6,6-trimethyl-1-cyclohexen-1-yl)-2,4,6,8-nonatetraenoic acid. It is a member of the retinoid family of compounds, and an endogenous metabolite of naturally occurring Vitamin A. Tretinoin has the following structure:

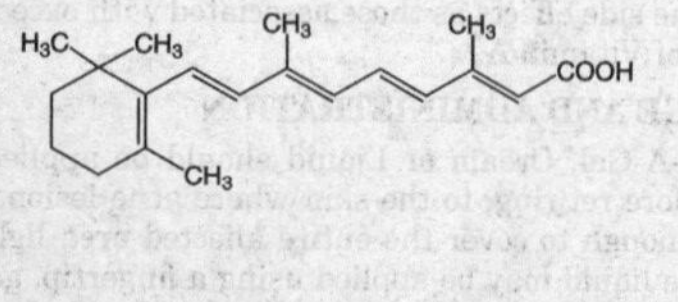

CLINICAL PHARMACOLOGY
Mode of Action: Although the exact mode of action of tretinoin is unknown, current evidence suggests that the effectiveness of tretinoin in acne is due primarily to its ability to modify abnormal follicular keratinization. Comedones form in follicles with an excess of keratinized epithelial cells. Tretinoin promotes detachment of cornified cells and the enhanced shedding of corneocytes from the follicle. By increasing the mitotic activity of follicular epithelia, tretinoin also increases the turnover rate of thin, loosely-adherent corneocytes. Through these actions, the comedo contents are extruded and the formation of the microcomedo, the precursor lesion of acne vulgaris, is reduced.
Additionally, tretinoin acts by modulating the proliferation and differentiation of epidermal cells. These effects are mediated by tretinoin's interaction with a family of nuclear retinoic acid receptors. Activation of these nuclear receptors causes changes in gene expression. The exact mechanisms whereby tretinoin-induced changes in gene expression regulate skin function are not understood.
Irritation Potential:
Acne clinical trial results
In clinical trials with acne patients treated with Retin-A Micro (tretinoin gel) microsphere, 0.1% analysis over the twelve week treatment period showed that cutaneous irritation scores for erythema, peeling, burning/stinging, or itching peaked during the initial 2 weeks of therapy, decreasing thereafter. Throughout, no more than 3% of patients had scores indicative of a severe irritation rating; although, 6% (14/224) of patients treated with Retin-A Micro (tretinoin gel) microsphere, 0.1%, discontinued treatment due to irritation. Of these 14 patients, four had severe irritation after 3 to 5 days of treatment, with blistering in one patient.
Results in studies of subjects without acne
In a half-face comparison trial conducted for up to 14 days in women with sensitive skin, but without acne, Retin-A Micro (tretinoin gel) microsphere, 0.1% was statistically less irritating than tretinoin cream, 0.1%. In addition, a cumulative 21 day irritation evaluation in subjects with normal skin showed that Retin-A Micro (tretinoin gel) microsphere, 0.1%, had a lower irritation profile than tretinoin cream, 0.1%. The clinical significance of these irritation studies for patients with acne is not established. Comparable effectiveness of Retin-A Micro (tretinoin gel) microsphere, 0.1%, and tretinoin cream, 0.1% has not been established. The lower irritancy of Retin-A Micro (tretinoin gel) microsphere, 0.1%, in subjects without acne may be attributable to the properties of its vehicle. The contribution to decreased irritancy by the MICROSPONGE® System has not been established.
Pharmacokinetics: Tretinoin is an endogenous metabolite of Vitamin A metabolism in man. Percutaneous absorption, as determined by the cumulative excretion of radiolabeled drug into urine and feces, was assessed in 44 healthy men and women. Estimates of in vivo bioavailability, mean (SD) %, following both single and multiple daily applications, for a period of 28 days, were 0.82 (0.11)% and 1.41 (0.54)%, respectively. The plasma concentrations of tretinoin and its metabolites, 13-*cis*-retinoic acid, all-*trans*-4-oxo-retinoic acid, and 13-*cis*-4-oxo-retinoic acid, generally ranged from 1 to 3 ng/ml and were essentially unaltered after either single or multiple daily applications relative to baseline levels.

INDICATIONS AND USAGE
Retin-A Micro (tretinoin gel) microsphere, 0.1%, is indicated for topical application in the treatment of acne vulgaris. The safety and efficacy of the use of this product in the treatment of other disorders have not been established.

CLINICAL STUDIES
In two vehicle-controlled clinical studies, Retin-A Micro (tretinoin gel) microsphere, 0.1%, applied once daily was significantly more effective than vehicle in reducing the severity of acne lesion counts. The mean reductions in lesion counts from baseline after treatment for 12 weeks are shown in the following table:
[See table below]
Retin-A Micro (tretinoin gel) microsphere, 0.1%, was also significantly superior to the vehicle in the investigator's global evaluation of the clinical response. In study #1, thirty-five percent (35%) of patients using Retin-A Micro (tretinoin gel) microsphere, 0.1%, achieved an excellent result compared to eleven percent (11%) of patients on vehicle control. In study #2, twenty-eight percent (28%) of patients using Retin-A Micro (tretinoin gel) microsphere, 0.1%, achieved an excellent result compared to nine percent (9%) of patients on vehicle control.

CONTRAINDICATIONS
This drug is contraindicated in individuals with a history of sensitivity reactions to any of its components. It should be discontinued if hypersensitivity to any of its ingredients is noted.

PRECAUTIONS
General: The skin of certain individuals may become excessively dry, red, swollen, or blistered. If the degree of irritation warrants, patients should be directed to temporarily reduce the amount or frequency of application of the medication, discontinue use temporarily, or discontinue use all together. Efficacy at reduced frequencies of application has not been established. If a reaction suggesting sensitivity occurs, use of the medication should be discontinued. Excessive skin dryness may also be experienced; if so, use of an appropriate emollient during the day may be helpful. Unprotected exposure to sunlight, including sunlamps, should be minimized during the use of Retin-A Micro (tretinoin gel) microsphere, 0.1%, and patients with sunburn should be advised not to use the product until fully recovered because of heightened susceptibility to sunlight as a result of the use of tretinoin. Patients who may be required to have considerable sun exposure due to their occupation and those with inherent sensitivity to the sun should exercise particular caution. Use of sunscreen products (SPF 15) and protective clothing over treated areas are recommended when exposure cannot be avoided. Weather extremes, such as wind or cold, also may be irritating to patients being treated with tretinoin. Retin-A Micro (tretinoin gel) microsphere, 0.1%, should be kept away from the eyes, the mouth, paranasal creases of the nose, and mucous membranes. Tretinoin has been reported to cause severe irritation on eczematous skin and should be used with utmost caution in patients with this condition.
Information for Patients: See Patient Information leaflet.
Drug Interactions: Concomitant topical medication, medicated or abrasive soaps and cleansers, products that have a strong drying effect, products with high concentrations of alcohol, astringents, or spices should be used with caution because of possible interaction with tretinoin. Avoid contact with the peel of limes. Particular caution should be exercised with the concomitant use of topical over-the-counter acne preparations containing benzoyl peroxide, sulfur, resorcinol, or salicylic acid with Retin-A Micro (tretinoin gel) microsphere, 0.1%. It also is advisable to allow the effects of such preparations to subside before use of Retin-A Micro (tretinoin gel) microsphere, 0.1%, is begun.
Carcinogenesis, Mutagenesis, Impairment of Fertility: In a life-time dermal study in CD-1 mice, there was no evidence of carcinogenic potential when tretinoin was administered topically at a dose of 1.25 times the recommended clinical dose. For purposes of comparisons of animal exposure to human exposure, the "recommended human clinical dose" is defined as 1.0 g of 0.1% Retin-A Micro (tretinoin gel) microsphere applied to a 50 kg person. In the same study, at 25 and 50 times the recommended human clinical dose, the dermal maximum tolerated dose (MTD) of tretinoin was exceeded, yet there were no biologically significant findings.
Dermal carcinogenicity testing has not been performed with the microspheres or Retin-A Micro (tretinoin gel) microsphere, 0.1%. The components of the microspheres have not demonstrated carcinogenic potential when evaluated individually. The components of the microspheres have shown mutagenic and teratogenic potential with chronic exposure at doses several orders of magnitude higher than the human clinical dose. The very low levels of these components in microsponge polymer (< 25 ppm), used in the drug formulation, indicate an insignificant human risk under usage conditions.
Studies in hairless albino mice suggest that tretinoin may enhance the tumorigenic potential of ultraviolet (UV) light from a solar simulator. In other studies, when lightly pigmented hairless mice treated with tretinoin were exposed to carcinogenic doses of UVA/UVB light, the incidence and rate of development of skin tumors were either reduced or no effect was seen. Due to significantly different experimental conditions, no strict comparison of these disparate data is possible. Although the significance of these studies to humans is not clear, patients should avoid or minimize exposure to sun.
Tretinoin had no mutagenic potential when evaluated in the Ames assay and the in vivo mouse micronucleus assay.
The microspheres had no mutagenic potential when evaluated in the Ames assay.
Dermal fertility and perinatal development studies with Retin-A Micro (tretinoin gel) microsphere, 0.1%, have not been performed in any species. In oral fertility and perinatal development studies in rats with tretinoin, decreased survival of neonates and growth retardation were observed at doses in excess of 2 mg/kg/day (> 100 times the recommended human clinical dose which is 1.0 g/50kg adult).
Pregnancy: Teratogenic effects. Pregnancy Category C. No teratogenic effects were seen in pregnant rats with topical application of Retin-A Micro (tretinoin gel) microsphere, 0.1%, at doses up to 50 times the recommended daily human topical dose. In one study in New Zealand white rabbits treated with Retin-A Micro (tretinoin gel) microsphere, 0.1%, where doses of 0.2, 0.5 and 1.0 mg/kg/day of tretinoin were administered topically for 24 hours a day to pregnant rabbits, there appeared to be an association of the dosages with increased incidences of domed head and hydrocephaly in some of the fetuses, typical of retinoid-induced fetal malformations in this species. No abnormalities were observed at 0.2 mg/kg/day, 10 times the normal human topical dose of tretinoin. In a repeat study of the highest topical dose (1.0 mg/kg/day) in pregnant rabbits, these effects were not seen. Other pregnant rabbits exposed to six hours of 0.5 or 1.0 mg/kg/day tretinoin with proper controls to prevent oral ingestion, did not show any teratogenic effects up to 50 times (1.0 mg/kg/day) the human topical dose. In addition, topical tretinoin in non Retin-A Micro (tretinoin gel) microsphere, 0.1%, formulations was not teratogenic in rats and rabbits when given in doses of 250 and 80 times the recommended human clinical topical dose, respectively, (assuming a 50 kg adult applied a daily dose of 1.0 g of 0.1% gel topically). At these topical doses, however, delayed ossification of several bones occurred in rabbits. In rats, a dose-dependent increase of supernumerary ribs was observed.
Oral tretinoin has been shown to be teratogenic in rats, mice, rabbits, hamsters, and subhuman primates. Tretinoin is teratogenic in rats when given orally in doses 500 times the human clinical topical dose. However, variations in teratogenic doses among various strains of rats have been reported. In the cynomolgus monkey, which metabolically is more similar to humans than other species in its handling of tretinoin, no malformations were reported at 5 mg/kg/day (250 times the recommended human clinical topical dose), although increased skeletal variations were observed. A dose-related increased embryolethality was also reported. Similar results have also been reported in pigtail macaques. There have been isolated reports of birth defects among babies born to women exposed to topical tretinoin during pregnancy. To date, there have been no adequate and well-controlled studies performed in pregnant women, and the ter-

Mean Percent Reduction In Lesion Counts

	Retin-A Micro (tretinoin gel) microsphere, 0.1%		Vehicle gel	
	Study #1 72 pts	Study #2 71 pts	Study #1 72 pts	Study #2 67 pts
Non-inflammatory lesion counts	49%	32%	22%	3%
Inflammatory lesion counts	37%	29%	18%	24%
Total lesion counts	45%	32%	23%	16%

atogenic blood level of tretinoin is not known. However, a well-conducted retrospective cohort study of babies born to women exposed to topical tretinoin during the first trimester of pregnancy found no excess birth defects among these babies when compared to babies born to women in the same cohort who were not similarly exposed. Nevertheless, topical tretinoin should be used during pregnancy only if the potential benefit justifies the potential risk to the fetus.

Pregnancy: Non-teratogenic Effects: Oral tretinoin has been shown to be fetotoxic in rats when administered in doses 125 times the recommended human clincal topical dose.

Preclinical toxicity studies: In male mice treated topically with Retin-A Micro (tretinoin gel) microsphere, 0.1%, at 0.5, 2.0 or 5.0 mg/kg/day tretinoin (25, 100 or 250 times the recommended human dose) for 90 days, a reduction in testicular weight, but with no pathological changes, was observed at 100 and 250 times the human topical dose. Similarly, in female mice, there was a reduction in ovarian weights, but without any underlying pathological changes, at 5.0 mg/kg/day (250 times the recommended human dose). In this study there was a dose-related increase in the plasma concentration of tretinoin 4 hours after the first dose. A separate toxicokinetic study in mice indicates that systemic exposure is greater after topical application to unrestrained animals than to restrained animals, suggesting that the systemic toxicity observed is probably related to oral ingestion. Male and female dogs treated with Retin-A Micro (tretinoin gel) microsphere, 0.1%, at 0.2, 0.5 or 1.0 mg/kg/day tretinoin (10, 25 or 50 times the human dose, respectively) for 90 days showed no evidence of reduced testicular or ovarian weights or pathological changes.

Nursing Mothers: It is not known whether this drug is excreted in human milk. Because many drugs are excreted in human milk, caution should be exercised when Retin-A Micro (tretinoin gel) microsphere, 0.1%, is administered to a nursing woman.

Pediatric Use: Safety and effectiveness in children below the age of 12 have not been established.

Geriatric Use: Safety and effectiveness in a geriatric population have not been established.

ADVERSE REACTIONS

The skin of certain sensitive individuals may become excessively red, edematous, blistered, or crusted. If these effects occur, the medication should be either discontinued until the integrity of the skin is restored, or the medication should be adjusted temporarily to a level the patient can tolerate. However, efficacy has not been established for lower dosing frequencies. True contact allergy to topical tretinoin is rarely encountered. Temporary hyper- or hypopigmentation has been reported with repeated application of tretinoin. Some individuals have been reported to have heightened susceptibility to sunlight while under treatment with tretinoin. To date, all adverse effects of tretinoin have been reversible upon discontinuance of therapy (see Dosage and Administration Section).

OVERDOSAGE

Retin-A Micro (tretinoin gel) microsphere, 0.1%, is intended for topical use only. If medication is applied excessively, no more rapid or better results will be obtained, and marked redness, peeling, or discomfort may occur. Oral ingestion of large amounts of the drug may lead to the same side effects as those associated with excessive oral intake of Vitamin A.

DOSAGE AND ADMINISTRATION

Retin-A Micro (tretinoin gel) microsphere, 0.1%, should be applied once a day, before retiring, to the skin areas where acne lesions appear, using enough to cover the entire affected area lightly. Application of excessive amounts of gel may result in "caking" of the gel, and will not provide incremental efficacy.

A transitory feeling of warmth or slight stinging may be noted on application. In cases where it has been necessary to temporarily discontinue therapy or to reduce the frequency of application, therapy may be resumed or the frequency of application increased as the patient becomes able to tolerate the treatment. Frequency of application should be closely monitored by careful observation of the clinical therapeutic response and skin tolerance. Efficacy has not been established for less than once daily dosing frequencies.

During the early weeks of therapy, an apparent exacerbation of inflammatory lesions may occur. If tolerated, this should not be considered a reason to discontinue therapy.

Therapeutic results may be noticed after two weeks, but more than seven weeks of therapy are required before consistent beneficial effects are observed.

Patients treated with Retin-A Micro (tretinoin gel) microsphere, 0.1%, may use cosmetics, but the areas to be treated should be cleansed thoroughly before the medication is applied.

HOW SUPPLIED

Retin-A Micro (tretinoin gel) microsphere, 0.1%, is supplied as:

20g (NDC 0062-0190-02) and 45g (NDC 0062-0190-03) tubes.

Storage Conditions: Store at 15°–25°C (59°–77°F).

Caution: Federal law prohibits dispensing without prescription.

DERMATOLOGICAL DIVISION
ORTHO PHARMACEUTICAL CORPORATION
Raritan, New Jersey 08869

 Issued February 1997 643-11-477-3

Retin-A® Micro™ is a trademark of Ortho Pharmaceutical Corporation.

MICROSPONGE® is a registered trademark of Advanced Polymer Systems, Inc., Redwood City, CA

Shown in Product Identification Guide, page 327

SPECTAZOLE® ℞

[*'spek-ti-zōl*]
(econazole nitrate 1%)
Cream
For Topical Use Only

DESCRIPTION

SPECTAZOLE Cream contains the antifungal agent, econazole nitrate 1%, in a water-miscible base consisting of pegoxol 7 stearate, peglicol 5 oleate, mineral oil, benzoic acid, butylated hydroxyanisole and purified water. The white to off-white soft cream is for topical use only.

Chemically, econazole nitrate is 1-[2-{(4-chlorophenyl) methoxy}-2-(2,4-dichlorophenyl)ethyl]-1H-imidazole mononitrate. Its structure is as follows:

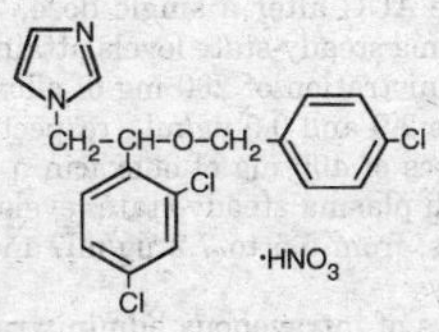

CLINICAL PHARMACOLOGY

After topical application to the skin of normal subjects, systemic absorption of econazole nitrate is extremely low. Although most of the applied drug remains on the skin surface, drug concentrations were found in the stratum corneum which, by far, exceeded the minimum inhibitory concentration for dermatophytes. Inhibitory concentrations were achieved in the epidermis and as deep as the middle region of the dermis. Less than 1% of the applied dose was recovered in the urine and feces.

Microbiology: Econazole nitrate has been shown to be active against most strains of the following microorganisms, both *in vitro* and in clinical infections as described in the INDICATIONS AND USAGE section.

Dermatophytes	**Yeasts**
Epidermophyton floccosum	*Candida albicans*
Microsporum audouini	*Malassezia furfur*
Microsporum canis	
Microsporum gypseum	
Trichophyton mentagrophytes	
Trichophyton rubrum	
Trichophyton tonsurans	

Econazole nitrate exhibits broad-spectrum antifungal activity against the following organisms *in vitro,* but the clinical significance of these data is unknown.

Dermatophytes	**Yeasts**
Trichophyton verrucosum	*Candida guillermondii*
	Candida parapsilosis
	Candida tropicalis

INDICATIONS AND USAGE

SPECTAZOLE Cream is indicated for topical application in the treatment of tinea pedis, tinea cruris, and tinea corporis caused by *Trichophyton rubrum, Trichophyton mentagrophytes, Trichophyton tonsurans, Microsporum canis, Microsporum audouini, Microsporum gypseum,* and *Epidermophyton floccosum,* in the treatment of cutaneous candidiasis, and in the treatment of tinea versicolor.

CONTRAINDICATIONS

SPECTAZOLE Cream is contraindicated in individuals who have shown hypersensitivity to any of its ingredients.

WARNINGS

SPECTAZOLE is not for ophthalmic use.

PRECAUTIONS

General: If a reaction suggesting sensitivity or chemical irritation should occur, use of the medication should be discontinued.

For external use only. Avoid introduction of SPECTAZOLE Cream into the eyes.

Carcinogenicity Studies: Long-term animal studies to determine carcinogenic potential have not been performed.

Fertility (Reproduction): Oral administration of econazole nitrate in rats has been reported to produce prolonged gestation. Intravaginal administration in humans has not shown prolonged gestation or other adverse reproductive effects attributable to econazole nitrate therapy.

Pregnancy: Pregnancy Category C. Econazole nitrate has not been shown to be teratogenic when administered orally to mice, rabbits or rats. Fetotoxic or embryotoxic effects were observed in Segment I oral studies with rats receiving 10 to 40 times the human dermal dose. Similar effects were observed in Segment II or Segment III studies with mice, rabbits and/or rats receiving oral doses 80 or 40 times the human dermal dose.

Econazole nitrate should be used in the first trimester of pregnancy only when the physician considers it essential to the welfare of the patient. The drug should be used during the second and third trimesters of pregnancy only if clearly needed.

Nursing Mothers: It is not known whether econazole nitrate is excreted in human milk. Following oral administration of econazole nitrate to lactating rats, econazole and/or metabolites were excreted in milk and were found in nursing pups. Also, in lactating rats receiving large oral doses (40 or 80 times the human dermal dose), there was a reduction in postpartum viability of pups and survival to weaning; however, at these high doses, maternal toxicity was present and may have been a contributing factor. Caution should be exercised when econazole nitrate is administered to a nursing woman.

ADVERSE REACTIONS

During clinical trials, approximately 3% of patients treated with econazole nitrate 1% cream reported side effects thought possibly to be due to the drug, consisting mainly of burning, itching, stinging and erythema. One case of pruritic rash has also been reported.

OVERDOSE

Overdosage of econazole nitrate in humans has not been reported to date. In mice, rats, guinea pigs and dogs, the oral LD 50 values were found to be 462, 668, 272, and > 160 mg/kg, respectively.

DOSAGE AND ADMINISTRATION

Sufficient SPECTAZOLE Cream should be applied to cover affected areas once daily in patients with tinea pedis, tinea cruris, tinea corporis, and tinea versicolor, and twice daily (morning and evening) in patients with cutaneous candidiasis.

Early relief of symptoms is experienced by the majority of patients and clinical improvement may be seen fairly soon after treatment is begun; however, candidal infections and tinea cruris and corporis should be treated for two weeks and tinea pedis for one month in order to reduce the possibility of recurrence. If a patient shows no clinical improvement after the treatment period, the diagnosis should be redetermined. Patients with tinea versicolor usually exhibit clinical and mycological clearing after two weeks of treatment.

HOW SUPPLIED

SPECTAZOLE (econazole nitrate 1%) Cream is supplied in tubes of 15 grams (NDC 0062-5460-02), 30 grams (NDC 0062-5460-01), and 85 grams (NDC 0062-5460-03).

Store SPECTAZOLE Cream below 86°F.

Revised June 1996 631-10-331-9

Shown in Product Identification Guide, page 327

Ortho-McNeil Pharmaceutical A Division of Ortho Pharmaceutical Corporation

RARITAN, NJ 08869-0602

For Medical Information Contact:
Generally:
(800) 682-6532
In Emergencies:
(908) 218-7325

ACI–JEL® Therapeutic Vaginal Jelly ℞

DESCRIPTION

ACI-JEL Vaginal Jelly is a bland, non-irritating, water-dispersible, buffered acid jelly for intravaginal use. ACI-JEL is classified as a Vaginal Therapeutic Jelly. ACI-JEL contains 0.921% glacial acetic acid ($C_2H_4O_2$), 0.025% oxyquinoline sulfate ($C_{18}H_{16}N_2O_6S$), 0.7% ricinoleic acid ($C_{18}H_{34}O_3$), and 5% glycerin ($C_3H_8O_3$) compounded with tragacanth,

Continued on next page

Aci-Jel—Cont.

acacia, propylparaben, potassium hydroxide, stannous chloride, egg albumen, potassium bitartrate, perfume and purified water. ACI-JEL is formulated to pH 3.9–4.1.

CLINICAL PHARMACOLOGY

ACI-JEL acts to restore and maintain normal vaginal acidity through its buffer action.

INDICATIONS AND USAGE

ACI-JEL is indicated as adjunctive therapy in those cases where restoration and maintenance of vaginal acidity are desirable.

CONTRAINDICATIONS

None known.

WARNINGS

No serious adverse reactions or potential safety hazards have been reported with the use of ACI-JEL.

PRECAUTIONS

General: No special care is required for the safe and effective use of ACI-JEL. *Drug Interactions:* No incidence of drug interactions have been reported with concomitant use of ACI-JEL and any other medications. *Laboratory Tests:* The monitoring of vaginal acidity (pH) may be helpful in following the patient's response. (The normal vaginal pH has been shown to be in the range of 4.0 to 5.0.) *Carcinogenesis:* No long-term studies in animals have been performed to evaluate carcinogenic potential. *Pregnancy:* Pregnancy Category C. Animal reproduction studies have not been conducted with ACI-JEL. It is also not known whether ACI-JEL can cause fetal harm when administered to a pregnant woman or can affect reproduction capacity. ACI-JEL should be given to a pregnant woman only if clearly needed. *Nursing Mothers:* It is not known whether this drug is excreted in human milk. Because many drugs are excreted in human milk, caution should be exercised when ACI-JEL is administered to a nursing woman.

ADVERSE REACTIONS

Occasional cases of local stinging and burning have been reported.

DOSAGE AND ADMINISTRATION

The usual dose is one applicatorful, administered intravaginally, morning and evening. Duration of treatment may be determined by the patient's response to therapy.

HOW SUPPLIED

85g Tube (NDC 0062-5421-01) with ORTHO® Measured-Dose Applicator.
Revised August 1996   643-10-310-2

DIENESTROL Cream   ℞

(See ORTHO® Dienestrol Cream.)

FLOXIN® I.V.   ℞
(ofloxacin injection)
FOR INTRAVENOUS INFUSION

Prescribing Information

DESCRIPTION

FLOXIN® (ofloxacin injection) I.V. is a synthetic, broad-spectrum antimicrobial agent for intravenous administration. Chemically, ofloxacin, a fluorinated carboxyquinolone, is the racemate, (±)-9-fluoro-2,3-dihydro-3-methyl-10-(4-methyl-1-piperazinyl)-7-oxo-7H-pyrido[1,2,3-de]-1,4-benzoxazine-6-carboxylic acid. The chemical structure is:

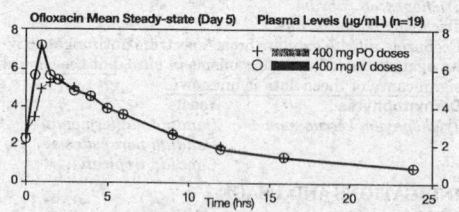

Its empirical formula is $C_{18}H_{20}FN_3O_4$, and its molecular weight is 361.4. Ofloxacin is an off-white to pale yellow crystalline powder. The relative solubility characteristics of ofloxacin at room temperature, as defined by USP nomenclature, indicate that ofloxacin is considered to be *soluble* in aqueous solutions with pH between 2 and 5. It is *sparingly* to *slightly soluble* in aqueous solutions with pH 7 (solubility falls to 4 mg/mL) and *freely soluble* in aqueous solutions with pH above 9. Ofloxacin has the potential to form stable coordination compounds with many metal ions. This *in vitro* chelation potential has the following formation order: Fe^{+3} > Al^{+3} > Cu^{+2} > Ni^{+2} > Pb^{+2} > Zn^{+2} > Mg^{+2} > Ca^{+2} > Ba^{+2}.

FLOXIN I.V. IN SINGLE-USE VIALS is a sterile, preservative-free aqueous solution of ofloxacin with pH ranging from 3.5 to 5.5. FLOXIN I.V. IN PRE-MIXED BOTTLES and IN PRE-MIXED FLEXIBLE CONTAINERS are sterile, preservative-free aqueous solutions of ofloxacin with pH ranging from 3.8 to 5.8. The color of FLOXIN I.V. may range from light yellow to amber. This does not adversely affect product potency. FLOXIN I.V. IN SINGLE-USE VIALS contains ofloxacin in Water for Injection. FLOXIN I.V. IN PRE-MIXED BOTTLES and IN PRE-MIXED FLEXIBLE CONTAINERS are dilute, non-pyrogenic, nearly isotonic pre-mixed solutions that contain ofloxacin in 5% Dextrose (D_5W). Hydrochloric acid and sodium hydroxide may have been added to adjust the pH.

The flexible container is fabricated from a specially formulated non-plasticized, thermoplastic copolyester (CR3). The amount of water that can permeate from the container into the overwrap is insufficient to affect the solution significantly. Solutions in contact with the flexible container can leach out certain of the container's chemical components in very small amounts within the expiration period. The suitability of the container material has been confirmed by tests in animals according to USP biological tests for plastic containers.

CLINICAL PHARMACOLOGY

Following a single 60-minute intravenous infusion of 200 mg or 400 mg of ofloxacin to normal volunteers, the mean maximum plasma concentrations attained were 2.7 and 4.0 μg/mL, respectively; the concentrations at 12 hours (h) after dosing were 0.3 and 0.7 μg/mL, respectively.

Steady-state concentrations were attained after four doses, and the area under the curve (AUC) was approximately 40% higher than the AUC after a single dose. The mean peak and trough plasma steady-state levels attained following intravenous administration of 200 mg of ofloxacin q 12 h for seven days were 2.9 and 0.5 μg/mL, respectively. Following intravenous doses of 400 mg of ofloxacin q 12 h, the mean peak and trough plasma steady-state levels ranged, in two different studies, from 5.5 to 7.2 μg/mL and 1.2 to 1.9 μg/mL, respectively.

Following 7 days of intravenous administration, the elimination half-life of ofloxacin was 6 h (range 5 to 10 h). The total clearance and the volume of distribution were approximately 15 L/h and 120 L, respectively.

Elimination of ofloxacin is primarily by renal excretion. Approximately 65% of a dose is excreted renally within 48 h. Studies indicate that <5% of an administered dose is recovered in the urine as the desmethyl or N-oxide metabolites. Four to eight percent of an ofloxacin dose is excreted in the feces. This indicates a small degree of biliary excretion of ofloxacin.

In vitro, approximately 32% of the drug in plasma is protein bound.

The single dose and steady-state plasma profiles of ofloxacin injection were comparable in extent of exposure (AUC) to those of ofloxacin tablets when the injectable and tablet formulations of ofloxacin were administered in equal doses (mg/mg). The mean $AUC_{(0-12)}$ attained after the intravenous administration of 400 mg over 60 min was 43.5 μg·h/mL; the mean $AUC_{(0-12)}$ attained after the oral administration of 400 mg was 41.2 μg•h/mL (two one-sided t-test, 90% confidence interval was 103–109). [See following chart.]

Ofloxacin Mean Steady-state (Day 5)   Plasma Levels (μg/mL) (n=19)
+ 400 mg PO doses
○ 400 mg IV doses
Time (hrs)

Between 0 and 6 h following the administration of a single 200 mg oral dose of ofloxacin to 12 healthy volunteers, the average urine ofloxacin concentration was approximately 220 μg/mL. Between 12 and 24 h after administration, the average urine ofloxacin level was approximately 34 μg/mL. Following oral administration of recommended therapeutic doses, ofloxacin has been detected in blister fluid, cervix, lung tissue, ovary, prostatic fluid, prostatic tissue, skin, and sputum. The mean concentration of ofloxacin in each of these various body fluids and tissues after one or more doses was 0.8 to 1.5 times the concurrent plasma level. Inadequate data are presently available on the distribution or levels of ofloxacin in the cerebrospinal fluid or brain tissue. Following the administration of oral doses of ofloxacin to healthy elderly volunteers (64–74 years of age) with normal renal function, the apparent half-life of ofloxacin was 7 to 8 h, as compared to approximately 6 h in younger adults. Clearance of ofloxacin is reduced in patients with impaired renal function (creatinine clearance ≤ 50 mL/min), and dosage adjustment is necessary. (See *PRECAUTIONS: General* and *DOSAGE AND ADMINISTRATION*.)

Microbiology

Ofloxacin has *in vitro* activity against a broad-spectrum of gram-positive and gram-negative aerobic and anaerobic bacteria. Ofloxacin is often bactericidal at concentrations equal to or slightly greater than inhibitory concentrations. Ofloxacin is thought to exert a bactericidal effect on susceptible microorganisms by inhibiting DNA gyrase, an essential enzyme that is a critical catalyst in the duplication, transcription, and repair of bacterial DNA.

Ofloxacin has been shown to be active against most strains of the following microorganisms, both in vitro and in clinical infections as described in the *INDICATIONS AND USAGE* section:

Gram-positive aerobes
Staphylococcus aureus   *Streptococcus pyogenes*
Streptococcus pneumoniae

Gram-negative aerobes
Citrobacter diversus	*Klebsiella pneumoniae*
Enterobacter aerogenes	*Neisseria gonorrhoeae*
Escherichia coli	*Proteus mirabilis*
Haemophilus influenzae	*Pseudomonas aeruginosa*

Other microorganisms
Chlamydia trachomatis

The following *in vitro* data are available, **but their clinical significance is unknown.**

Ofloxacin exhibits *in vitro* minimum inhibitory concentrations (MIC's) of 2 μg/mL or less against most (≥90%) strains of the following microorganisms; however, the safety and effectiveness of ofloxacin in treating clinical infections due to these microorganisms have not been established in adequate and well-controlled clinical trials:

[See table below]

Ofloxacin is not active against *Treponema pallidum*. (See *WARNINGS*.)

Many strains of other streptococcal species, *Enterococcus* species, and anaerobes are resistant to ofloxacin.

Resistance to ofloxacin due to spontaneous mutation *in vitro* is a rare occurrence (range: 10^{-9} to 10^{-11}). To date, emergence of resistance has been relatively uncommon in clinical practice. With the exception of *Pseudomonas aeruginosa* (10%), less than a 4% rate of resistance emergence has been reported for most other species. Although cross-resistance has been observed between ofloxacin and other fluoroquinolones, some organisms resistant to other quinolones may be susceptible to ofloxacin.

Susceptibility Tests
Dilution techniques:
Quantitative methods are used to determine antimicrobial minimal inhibitory concentrations (MIC's). These MIC's provide estimates of the susceptibility of bacteria to antimicrobial compounds. The MICs should be determined using a standardized procedure. Standardized procedures are based on a dilution method[1] (broth or agar) or equivalent with standardized inoculum concentrations and standardized

---

Gram-positive aerobes
Staphylococcus epidermidis (excluding methicillin-resistant strains)		*Staphylococcus haemolyticus*
		Staphylococcus saprophyticus

Gram-negative aerobes
Acinetobacter calcoaceticus	*Enterobacter cloacae*	*Proteus vulgaris*
Aeromonas caviae	*Haemophilus ducreyi*	*Providencia rettgeri*
Aeromonas hydrophila	*Klebsiella oxytoca*	*Providencia stuartii*
Bordetella parapertussis	*Moraxella catarrhalis*	*Serratia marcescens*
Bordetella pertussis	*Morganella morganii*	*Vibrio parahaemolyticus*
Citrobacter freundii		

Anaerobes
Clostridium perfringens	*Gardnerella vaginalis*	

Other organisms
Chlamydia pneumoniae	*Mycobacterium tuberculosis* (including multiple drug-resistant strains)	*Mycoplasma hominis*
Legionella pneumophila		*Mycoplasma pneumoniae*
		Ureaplasma urealyticum

concentrations of ofloxacin powder. The MIC values should be interpreted according to the following criteria:

MIC (µg/mL)	Interpretation
≤2	Susceptible (S)
4	Intermediate (I)
≥8	Resistant (R)

A report of "Susceptible" indicates that the pathogen is likely to be inhibited if the antimicrobial compound in the blood reaches the concentrations usually achievable. A report of "Intermediate" indicates that the result should be considered equivocal and, if the microorganism is not fully susceptible to alternative, clinically feasible drugs, the test should be repeated. This category implies possible clinical applicability in body sites where the drug is physiologically concentrated or in situations where high dosage of drug can be used. This category also provides a buffer zone which prevents small uncontrolled technical factors from causing major discrepancies in interpretation. A report of "Resistant" indicates that the pathogen is not likely to be inhibited if the antimicrobial compound in the blood reaches the concentrations usually achievable; other therapy should be selected.

Standardized susceptibility test procedures require the use of laboratory control microorganisms to control the technical aspects of the laboratory procedures. Standard ofloxacin powder should provide the following MIC values:

Microorganism		MIC (µg/mL)
Escherichia coli	ATCC 25922	0.015–0.12
Staphylococcus aureus	ATCC 29213	0.12–1.0
Pseudomonas aeruginosa	ATCC 27853	1.0–8.0
Haemophilus influenzae	ATCC 49247	0.016–0.06
Neisseria gonorrhoeae	ATCC 49226	0.004–0.016

Diffusion techniques:

Quantitative methods that require measurement of zone diameters also provide reproducible estimates of the susceptibility of bacteria to antimicrobial compounds. One such standardized procedure[2] requires the use of standardized inoculum concentrations. This procedure uses paper disks impregnated with 5-µg ofloxacin to test the susceptibility of microorganisms to ofloxacin.

Reports from the laboratory providing results of the standard single-disk susceptibility test with a 5-µg ofloxacin disk should be interpreted according to the following criteria:

Zone Diameter (mm)	Interpretation
≥16	Susceptible (S)
13–15	Intermediate (I)
≤12	Resistant (R)

Interpretation should be as stated above for results using dilution techniques. Interpretation involves correlation of the diameter obtained in the disk test with the MIC for ofloxacin.

As with standardized dilution techniques, diffusion methods require the use of laboratory control microorganisms that are used to control the technical aspects of the laboratory procedures. For the diffusion technique, the 5-µg ofloxacin disk should provide the following zone diameters in these laboratory test quality control strains:

Microorganism		Zone Diameter (mm)
Escherichia coli	ATCC 25922	29–33
Pseudomonas aeruginosa	ATCC 27853	17–21
Haemophilus influenzae	ATCC 49247	31–40
Neisseria gonorrhoeae	ATCC 49226	43–51
Staphylococcus aureus	ATCC 25923	24–28

INDICATIONS AND USAGE

FLOXIN (ofloxacin injection) I.V. is indicated for the treatment of adults with mild to moderate infections (unless otherwise indicated) caused by susceptible strains of the designated microorganisms in the infections listed below – when intravenous administration offers a route of administration advantageous to the patient, (e.g., patient cannot tolerate an oral dosage form). Please see *DOSAGE AND ADMINISTRATION* for specific recommendations.

The safety and effectiveness of the intravenous formulation in treating patients with severe infections have not been established.

NOTE: IN THE ABSENCE OF VOMITING OR OTHER FACTORS INTERFERING WITH THE ABSORPTION OF ORALLY ADMINISTERED DRUG, PATIENTS RECEIVE ESSENTIALLY THE SAME SYSTEMIC ANTIMICROBIAL THERAPY AFTER EQUIVALENT DOSES OF OFLOXACIN ADMINISTERED BY

EITHER THE ORAL OR THE INTRAVENOUS ROUTE. THEREFORE, THE INTRAVENOUS FORMULATION DOES NOT PROVIDE A HIGHER DEGREE OF EFFICACY OR MORE POTENT ANTIMICROBIAL ACTIVITY THAN AN EQUIVALENT DOSE OF THE ORAL FORMULATION OF OFLOXACIN.

Acute bacterial exacerbation of chronic bronchitis due to *Haemophilus influenzae* or *Streptococcus pneumoniae*.

Community-acquired Pneumonia due to *Haemophilus influenzae* or *Streptococcus pneumoniae*.

Uncomplicated skin and skin structure infections due to *Staphylococcus aureus, Streptococcus pyogenes*, or *Proteus mirabilis*.

Acute, uncomplicated urethral and cervical gonorrhea due to *Neisseria gonorrhoeae*. (See *WARNINGS*.)

Nongonococcal urethritis and cervicitis due to *Chlamydia trachomatis*. (See *WARNINGS*.)

Mixed infections of the urethra and cervix due to *Chlamydia trachomatis* and *Neisseria gonorrhoeae*. (See *WARNINGS*.)

Acute pelvic inflammatory disease (including severe infection) due to *Chlamydia trachomatis* and/or *Neisseria gonorrhoeae*. (See *WARNINGS*.)

NOTE: If anaerobic microorganisms are suspected of contributing to the infection, appropriate therapy for anaerobic pathogens should be administered.

Uncomplicated cystitis due to *Citrobacter diversus, Enterobacter aerogenes, Escherichia coli, Klebsiella pneumoniae, Proteus mirabilis*, or *Pseudomonas aeruginosa*.

Complicated urinary tract infections due to *Escherichia coli, Klebsiella pneumoniae, Proteus mirabilis, Citrobacter diversus**, or *Pseudomonas aeruginosa**.

Prostatitis due to *Escherichia coli*.

*= Although treatment of infections due to this organism in this organ system demonstrated a clinically significant outcome, efficacy was studied in fewer than 10 patients.

Appropriate culture and susceptibility tests should be performed before treatment in order to isolate and identify organisms causing the infection and to determine their susceptibility to ofloxacin. Therapy with ofloxacin may be initiated before results of these tests are known; once results become available, appropriate therapy should be continued. As with other drugs in this class, some strains of *Pseudomonas aeruginosa* may develop resistance fairly rapidly during treatment with ofloxacin. Culture and susceptibility testing performed periodically during therapy will provide information not only on the therapeutic effect of the antimicrobial agent but also on the possible emergence of bacterial resistance.

CONTRAINDICATIONS

FLOXIN (ofloxacin) is contraindicated in persons with a history of hypersensitivity associated with the use of ofloxacin or any member of the quinolone group of antimicrobial agents.

WARNINGS

THE SAFETY AND EFFICACY OF OFLOXACIN IN CHILDREN, ADOLESCENTS (UNDER THE AGE OF 18 YEARS), PREGNANT WOMEN, AND LACTATING WOMEN HAVE NOT BEEN ESTABLISHED. (SEE PEDIATRIC USE, USE IN PREGNANCY, AND NURSING MOTHERS SUBSECTIONS IN THE PRECAUTIONS SECTION.)

In the immature rat, the oral administration of ofloxacin at 5 to 16 times the recommended maximum human dose based on mg/kg or 1–3 times based on mg/m^2 increased the incidence and severity of osteochondrosis. The lesions did not regress after 13 weeks of drug withdrawal. Other quinolones also produce similar erosions in the weight-bearing joints and other signs of arthropathy in immature animals of various species. (See *ANIMAL PHARMACOLOGY*.)

Convulsions, increased intracranial pressure, and toxic psychosis have been reported in patients receiving quinolones, including ofloxacin. Quinolones, including ofloxacin, may also cause central nervous system stimulation which may lead to: tremors, restlessness/agitation, nervousness/anxiety, lightheadedness, confusion, hallucinations, paranoia and depression, nightmares, insomnia, and rarely suicidal thoughts or acts. These reactions may occur following the first dose. If these reactions occur in patients receiving ofloxacin, the drug should be discontinued and appropriate measures instituted. As with all quinolones, ofloxacin should be used with caution in patients with a known or suspected CNS disorder that may predispose to seizures or lower the seizure threshold (e.g., severe cerebral arteriosclerosis, epilepsy) or in the presence of other risk factors that may predispose to seizures or lower the seizure threshold (e.g., certain drug therapy, renal dysfunction). (See *PRECAUTIONS: General, Information for Patients, Drug Interactions* and *ADVERSE REACTIONS*.)

Serious and occasionally fatal hypersensitivity (anaphylactic/anaphylactoid) reactions have been reported in patients receiving therapy with quinolones, including ofloxacin. These reactions often occur following the first dose. Some reactions were accompanied by cardiovascular collapse, hypotension/shock, seizure, loss of consciousness, tingling, angioedema (including tongue, laryngeal, throat or facial edema/swelling), airway obstruction (including bronchospasm,

shortness of breath and acute respiratory distress), dyspnea, urticaria/hives, itching, and other serious skin reactions. A few patients had a history of hypersensitivity reactions. The drug should be discontinued immediately at the first appearance of a skin rash or any other sign of hypersensitivity. Serious acute hypersensitivity reactions may require treatment with epinephrine and other resuscitative measures, including oxygen, intravenous fluids, antihistamines, corticosteroids, pressor amines, and airway management, as clinically indicated. (See *PRECAUTIONS* and *ADVERSE REACTIONS*.)

Serious and sometimes fatal events, some due to hypersensitivity, and some due to uncertain etiology, have been reported in patients receiving therapy with quinolones, including ofloxacin. These events may be severe and generally occur following the administration of multiple doses. Clinical manifestations may include one or more of the following: fever, rash or severe dermatologic reactions (e.g., toxic epidermal necrolysis, Stevens-Johnson Syndrome); vasculitis; arthralgia; myalgia; serum sickness; allergic pneumonitis; interstitial nephritis; acute renal insufficiency/failure; hepatitis; jaundice; acute hepatic necrosis/failure; anemia, including hemolytic and aplastic; thrombocytopenia, including thrombotic thrombocytopenic purpura; leukopenia; agranulocytosis; pancytopenia; and/or other hematologic abnormalities. The drug should be discontinued immediately at the first appearance of a skin rash or any other sign of hypersensitivity and supportive measures instituted. (See *PRECAUTIONS: Information for Patients* and *ADVERSE REACTIONS*.)

Pseudomembranous colitis has been reported with nearly all antibacterial agents, including ofloxacin, and may range in severity from mild to life-threatening. Therefore, it is important to consider this diagnosis in patients who present with diarrhea subsequent to the administration of any antibacterial agent.

Treatment with antibacterial agents alters the normal flora of the colon and may permit overgrowth of clostridia. Studies indicate a toxin produced by *Clostridium difficile* is one primary cause of "antibiotic-associated colitis".

After the diagnosis of pseudomembranous colitis has been established, therapeutic measures should be initiated. Mild cases of pseudomembranous colitis usually respond to drug discontinuation alone. In moderate to severe cases, consideration should be given to management with fluids and electrolytes, protein supplementation, and treatment with an oral antibacterial drug clinically effective against *C. difficile* colitis. (See *ADVERSE REACTIONS*.)

Ruptures of the shoulder, hand, and Achilles tendons that required surgical repair or resulted in prolonged disability have been reported with ofloxacin and other quinolones. Ofloxacin should be discontinued if the patient experiences pain, inflammation, or rupture of a tendon. Patients should rest and refrain from exercise until the diagnosis of tendinitis or tendon rupture has been confidently excluded. Tendon rupture can occur at any time during or after therapy with ofloxacin.

Ofloxacin has not been shown to be effective in the treatment of syphilis. Antimicrobial agents used in high doses for short periods of time to treat gonorrhea may mask or delay the symptoms of incubating syphilis. All patients with gonorrhea should have a serologic test for syphilis at the time of diagnosis. Patients treated with ofloxacin for gonorrhea should have a follow-up serologic test for syphilis after three months and, if positive, treatment with an appropriate antimicrobial should be instituted.

PRECAUTIONS

General:

Because a rapid or bolus intravenous injection may result in hypotension, **OFLOXACIN INJECTION SHOULD ONLY BE ADMINISTERED BY SLOW INTRAVENOUS INFUSION OVER A PERIOD OF 60 MINUTES.** (See *DOSAGE AND ADMINISTRATION*.)

Adequate hydration of patients receiving ofloxacin should be maintained to prevent the formation of a highly concentrated urine.

Administer ofloxacin with caution in the presence of renal or hepatic insufficiency/impairment. In patients with known or suspected renal or hepatic insufficiency/impairment, careful clinical observation and appropriate laboratory studies should be performed prior to and during therapy since elimination of ofloxacin may be reduced. In patients with impaired renal function (creatinine clearance ≤ 50 mg/mL), alteration of the dosage regimen is necessary. (See *CLINICAL PHARMACOLOGY* and *DOSAGE AND ADMINISTRATION*.)

Moderate to severe phototoxicity reactions have been observed in patients exposed to direct sunlight while receiving some drugs in this class, including ofloxacin. Excessive sunlight should be avoided. Therapy should be discontinued if phototoxicity (e.g., a skin eruption) occurs.

As with other quinolones, ofloxacin should be used with caution in any patient with a known or suspected CNS disorder that may predispose to seizures or lower the seizure threshold (e.g., severe cerebral arteriosclerosis, epilepsy) or in the

Continued on next page

Floxin I.V.—Cont.

presence of other risk factors that may predispose to seizures or lower the seizure threshold (e.g., certain drug therapy, renal dysfunction). (See *WARNINGS* and *Drug Interactions*.)

A possible interaction between oral hypoglycemic drugs (e.g., glyburide/glibenclamide) or with insulin and fluoroquinolone antimicrobial agents have been reported resulting in a potentiation of the hypoglycemic action of these drugs. The mechanism for this interaction is not known. If a hypoglycemic reaction occurs in a patient being treated with ofloxacin, discontinue ofloxacin immediately and consult a physician. (See *Drug Interactions* and *ADVERSE REACTIONS*.)

As with any potent drug, periodic assessment of organ system functions, including renal, hepatic, and hematopoietic, is advisable during prolonged therapy. (See *WARNINGS* and *ADVERSE REACTIONS*.)

Information for Patients:
Patients should be advised:
— to drink fluids liberally if able to take fluids by the oral route;
— that ofloxacin may cause neurologic adverse effects (e.g., dizziness, lightheadedness) and that patients should know how they react to ofloxacin before they operate an automobile or machinery or engage in activities requiring mental alertness and coordination (See *WARNINGS* and *ADVERSE REACTIONS*);
— that ofloxacin may be associated with hypersensitivity reactions, even following the first dose, to discontinue the drug at the first sign of a skin rash, hives or other skin reactions, a rapid heartbeat, difficulty in swallowing or breathing, any swelling suggesting angioedema (e.g., swelling of the lips, tongue, face; tightness of the throat, hoarseness), or any other symptom of an allergic reaction (See *WARNINGS* and *ADVERSE REACTIONS*);
— to avoid excessive sunlight or artificial ultraviolet light while receiving ofloxacin and to discontinue therapy if phototoxicity (e.g., skin eruption) occurs;
— to discontinue treatment and inform their physician if they experience pain, inflammation, or rupture of a tendon, and to rest and refrain from exercise until the diagnosis of tendinitis or tendon rupture has been confidently excluded;
— that if they are diabetic and are being treated with insulin or an oral hypoglycemic agent, to discontinue ofloxacin immediately if a hypoglycemic reaction occurs and consult a physician (See *PRECAUTIONS: General* and *Drug Interactions*);
— that convulsions have been reported in patients taking quinolones, including ofloxacin, and to notify their physician before taking this drug if there is a history of this condition.

Drug Interactions:
Antacids, Sucralfate, Metal Cations, Multi-Vitamins: There are no data concerning an interaction of **intravenous** quinolones with **oral** antacids, sucralfate, multi-vitamins, or metal cations. However, no quinolone should be co-administered with any solution containing multivalent cations, e.g., magnesium, through the same intravenous line. (See *DOSAGE AND ADMINISTRATION*.)
Caffeine: Interactions between ofloxacin and caffeine have not been detected.
Cimetidine: Cimetidine has demonstrated interference with the elimination of some quinolones. This interference has resulted in significant increases in half-life and AUC of some quinolones. The potential for interaction between ofloxacin and cimetidine has not been studied.
Cyclosporine: Elevated serum levels of cyclosporine have been reported with concomitant use of cyclosporine with some other quinolones. The potential for interaction between ofloxacin and cyclosporine has not been studied.
Drugs metabolized by Cytochrome P450 enzymes: Most quinolone antimicrobial drugs inhibit cytochrome P450 enzyme activity. This may result in a prolonged half-life for some drugs that are also metabolized by this system (e.g., cyclosporine, theophylline/methylxanthines, warfarin) when co-administered with quinolones. The extent of this inhibition varies among different quinolones. (See other *Drug Interactions*.)
Non-steroidal anti-inflammatory drugs: The concomitant administration of a non-steroidal anti-inflammatory drug with a quinolone, including ofloxacin, may increase the risk of CNS stimulation and convulsive seizures. (See *WARNINGS* and *PRECAUTIONS: General*.)
Probenecid: The concomitant use of probenecid with certain other quinolones has been reported to affect renal tubular secretion. The effect of probenecid on the elimination of ofloxacin has not been studied.
Theophylline: Steady-state theophylline levels may increase when ofloxacin and theophylline are administered concurrently. As with other quinolones, concomitant administration of ofloxacin may prolong the half-life of theophylline, elevate serum theophylline levels, and increase the risk of theophylline-related adverse reactions. Theophylline

levels should be closely monitored and theophylline dosage adjustments made, if appropriate, when ofloxacin is co-administered. Adverse reactions (including seizures) may occur with or without an elevation in the serum theophylline level. (See *WARNINGS* and *PRECAUTIONS: General*.)
Warfarin: Some quinolones have been reported to enhance the effects of the oral anticoagulant warfarin or its derivatives. Therefore, if a quinolone antimicrobial is administered concomitantly with warfarin or its derivatives, the prothrombin time or other suitable coagulation test should be closely monitored.
Antidiabetic agents (e.g., insulin, glyburide/glibenclamide): Since disturbances of blood glucose, including hyperglycemia and hypoglycemia, have been reported in patients treated concurrently with quinolones and an antidiabetic agent, careful monitoring of blood glucose is recommended when these agents are used concomitantly (See *PRECAUTIONS: General* and *Information for Patients*.)
Carcinogenesis, Mutagenesis, Impairment of Fertility:
Long-term studies to determine the carcinogenic potential of ofloxacin have not been conducted.
Ofloxacin was not mutagenic in the Ames bacterial test, *in vitro* and *in vivo* cytogenetic assay, sister chromatid exchange (Chinese Hamster and Human Cell Lines), unscheduled DNA Repair (UDS) using human fibroblasts, dominant lethal assays, or mouse micronucleus assay. Ofloxacin was positive in the UDS test using rat hepatocytes and Mouse Lymphoma Assay.
Pregnancy: Teratogenic Effects. Pregnancy Category C.
Ofloxacin has not been shown to have any teratogenic effects at oral doses as high as 810 mg/kg/day (11 times the recommended maximum human dose based on mg/m^2 or 50 times based on mg/kg) and 160 mg/kg/day (4 times the recommended maximum human dose based on mg/m^2 or 10 times based on mg/kg) when administered to pregnant rats and rabbits, respectively. Additional studies in rats with oral doses up to 360 mg/kg/day (5 times the recommended maximum human dose based on mg/m^2 or 23 times based on mg/kg) demonstrated no adverse effect on late fetal development, labor, delivery, lactation, neonatal viability, or growth of the newborn. Doses equivalent to 50 and 10 times the recommended maximum human dose of ofloxacin (based on mg/kg) were fetotoxic (i.e., decreased fetal body weight and increased fetal mortality) in rats and rabbits, respectively. Minor skeletal variations were reported in rats receiving doses of 810 mg/kg/day, which is more than 10 times higher than the recommended maximum human dose based on mg/m^2.
There are, however, no adequate and well-controlled studies in pregnant women. Ofloxacin should be used during pregnancy only if the potential benefit justifies the potential risk to the fetus. (See *WARNINGS*.)
Nursing Mothers:
In lactating females, a single oral 200-mg dose of ofloxacin resulted in concentrations of ofloxacin in milk that were similar to those found in plasma. Because of the potential for serious adverse reactions from ofloxacin in nursing infants, a decision should be made whether to discontinue nursing or to discontinue the drug, taking into account the importance of the drug to the mother. (See *WARNINGS* and *ADVERSE REACTIONS*.)
Pediatric Use:
Safety and effectiveness in children and adolescents below the age of 18 years have not been established. Ofloxacin causes arthropathy (arthrosis) and osteochondrosis in juvenile animals of several species. (See *WARNINGS*.)

ADVERSE REACTIONS

The following is a compilation of the data for ofloxacin based on clinical experience with both the oral and intravenous formulations. The incidence of drug-related adverse reactions in patients during Phase 2 and 3 clinical trials was 11%. Among patients receiving multiple-dose therapy, 4% discontinued ofloxacin due to adverse experiences.
In clinical trials, the following events were considered likely to be drug-related in patients receiving multiple doses of ofloxacin:
nausea 3%, insomnia 3%, headache 1%, dizziness 1%, diarrhea 1%, vomiting 1%, rash 1%, pruritus 1%, external genital pruritus in women 1%, vaginitis 1%, dysgeusia 1%.
Local injection site reactions (phlebitis, swelling, erythema) were reported in approximately 2% of patients treated with the 3.63 mg/mL final infusion concentration of intravenous ofloxacin used in the clinical safety trials. The final infusion concentration of intravenous ofloxacin in the commercially available intravenous preparations is 4.0 mg/mL. To date, individuals administered the 4.0 mg/mL concentration of the intravenous ofloxacin have demonstrated clinically acceptable rates of local injection site reactions. Due to the small difference in concentration, significant differences in local site reactions are unexpected with the 4.0 mg/mL concentration.
In clinical trials, the most frequently reported adverse events, regardless of relationship to drug, were:

nausea 10%, headache 9%, insomnia 7%, external genital pruritus in women 6%, dizziness 5%, vaginitis 5%, diarrhea 4%, vomiting 4%.
In clinical trials, the following events, regardless of relationship to drug occurred in 1 to 3% of patients:
Abdominal pain and cramps, chest pain, decreased appetite, dry mouth, dysgeusia, fatigue, flatulence, gastrointestinal distress, nervousness, pharyngitis, pruritus, fever, rash, sleep disorders, somnolence, trunk pain, vaginal discharge, visual disturbances, and constipation.
Additional events, occurring in clinical trials at a rate of less than 1%, regardless of relationship to drug, were:

Body as a whole:	asthenia, chills, malaise, extremity pain, pain, epistaxis
Cardiovascular System:	cardiac arrest, edema, hypertension, hypotension, palpitations, vasodilation
Gastrointestinal System:	dyspepsia
Genital/Reproductive System:	burning, irritation, pain and rash of the female genitalia; dysmenorrhea; menorrhagia; metrorrhagia
Musculoskeletal System:	arthralgia, myalgia
Nervous System:	seizures, anxiety, cognitive change, depression, dream abnormality, euphoria, hallucinations, paresthesia, syncope, vertigo, tremor, confusion
Nutritional/Metabolic:	thirst, weight loss
Respiratory System:	respiratory arrest, cough, rhinorrhea
Skin/Hypersensitivity:	angioedema, diaphoresis, urticaria, vasculitis
Special Senses:	decreased hearing acuity, tinnitus, photophobia
Urinary System:	dysuria, urinary frequency, urinary retention

The following laboratory abnormalities appeared in ≥ 1.0% of patients receiving multiple doses of ofloxacin. It is not known whether these abnormalities were caused by the drug or the underlying conditions being treated.

Hematopoietic:	anemia, leukopenia, leukocytosis, neutropenia, neutrophilia, increased band forms, lymphocytopenia, eosinophilia, lymphocytosis, thrombocytopenia, thrombocytosis, elevated ESR
Hepatic:	elevated: alkaline phosphatase, AST (SGOT), ALT (SGPT)
Serum chemistry:	hyperglycemia, hypoglycemia, elevated creatinine, elevated BUN
Urinary:	glucosuria, proteinuria, alkalinuria, hyposthenuria, hematuria, pyuria

Post-Marketing Adverse Events:
Additional adverse events, regardless of relationship to drug, reported from worldwide marketing experience with quinolones, including ofloxacin:
Clinical:

Cardiovascular System:	cerebral thrombosis, pulmonary edema, tachycardia, hypotension/shock, syncope
Endocrine/Metabolic:	hyper- or hypoglycemia, especially in diabetic patients on insulin or oral hypoglycemic agents (See *PRECAUTIONS: General* and *Drug Interactions*.)
Gastrointestinal System:	hepatic dysfunction including: hepatic necrosis, jaundice (cholestatic or hepatocellular), hepatitis; intestinal perforation; pseudomembranous colitis (the onset of pseudomembranous colitis symptoms may occur during or after antimicrobial treatment), GI hemorrhage; hiccough, painful oral mucosa, pyrosis (See *WARNINGS*.)
Genitourinary System:	vaginal candidiasis
Hematopoietic:	anemia, including hemolytic and aplastic; hemorrhage, pancytopenia,

agranulocytosis, leukopenia, reversible bone marrow depression, thrombocytopenia, thrombotic thrombocytopenic purpura, petechiae, ecchymosis/bruising (See *WARNINGS*.)

Musculoskeletal:	tendinitis/rupture; weakness; rhabdomyolysis	
Nervous System:	nightmares; suicidal thoughts or acts, disorientation, psychotic reactions, paranoia; phobia, agitation, restlessness, aggressiveness/hostility, manic reaction, emotional lability; peripheral neuropathy, ataxia, incoordination; possible exacerbation of: myasthenia gravis and extrapyramidal disorders; dysphasia, lightheadedness (See *WARNINGS* and *PRECAUTIONS*.)	
Respiratory System:	dyspnea, bronchospasm, allergic pneumonitis, stridor (See *WARNINGS*.)	
Skin/Hypersensitivity:	anaphylactic (-toid) reactions/shock; purpura, serum sickness, erythema multiforme/Stevens-Johnson Syndrome, erythema nodosum, exfoliative dermatitis, hyperpigmentation, toxic epidermal necrolysis, conjunctivitis, photosensitivity, vesiculobullous eruption (See *WARNINGS* and *PRECAUTIONS*.)	
Special Senses:	diplopia, nystagmus, blurred vision, disturbances of: taste, smell, hearing and equilibrium, usually reversible following discontinuation	
Urinary System:	anuria, polyuria, renal calculi, renal failure, interstitial nephritis, hematuria (See *WARNINGS* and *PRECAUTIONS*.)	
Laboratory:		
Hematopoietic:	prolongation of prothrombin time	
Serum chemistry:	acidosis, elevation of: serum triglycerides, serum cholesterol, serum potassium, liver function tests including: GGTP, LDH, bilirubin	
Urinary:	albuminuria, candidiuria	

In clinical trials using multiple-dose therapy, ophthalmologic abnormalities, including cataracts and multiple punctate lenticular opacities, have been noted in patients undergoing treatment with other quinolones. The relationship of the drugs to these events is not presently established. CRYSTALLURIA and CYLINDRURIA HAVE BEEN REPORTED with other quinolones.

OVERDOSAGE

Information on overdosage with ofloxacin is limited. One incident of accidental overdosage has been reported. In this case, an adult female received 3 grams of ofloxacin intravenously over 45 minutes. A blood sample obtained 15 minutes after the completion of the infusion revealed an ofloxacin level of 39.3 µg/mL. In 7 h, the level had fallen to 16.2 µg/mL, and by 24 h to 2.7 µg/mL. During the infusion, the patient developed drowsiness, nausea, dizziness, hot and cold flushes, subjective facial swelling and numbness, slurring of speech, and mild to moderate disorientation. All complaints except the dizziness subsided within 1 h after discontinuation of the infusion. The dizziness, most bothersome while standing, resolved in approximately 9 h. Laboratory testing reportedly revealed no clinically significant changes in routine parameters in this patient.

In the event of acute overdose, the patient should be observed and appropriate hydration maintained. Ofloxacin is not efficiently removed by hemodialysis or peritoneal dialysis.

DOSAGE AND ADMINISTRATION

FLOXIN I.V. should only be administered by **intravenous** infusion. It is not for intramuscular, intrathecal, intraperitoneal, or subcutaneous administration.

Infection†	Unit Dose	Frequency	Duration	Daily Dose
Acute Bacterial Exacerbation of Chronic Bronchitis	400 mg	q12h	10 days	800 mg
Comm. Acquired Pneumonia	400 mg	q12h	10 days	800 mg
Uncomplicated Skin and Skin Structure Infections	400 mg	q12h	10 days	800 mg
Acute, Uncomplicated Urethral and Cervical Gonorrhea	400 mg	single dose	1 day	400 mg
Nongonococcal Cervicitis/Urethritis due to *C. trachomatis*	300 mg	q12h	7 days	600 mg
Mixed infection of the urethra and cervix due to *C. trachomatis* and *N. gonorrhoeae*	300 mg	q12h	7 days	600 mg
Acute Pelvic Inflammatory Disease	400 mg	q12h	10-14 days	800 mg
Uncomplicated Cystitis due to *E. coli* or *K. pneumoniae*	200 mg	q12h	3 days	400 mg
Uncomplicated Cystitis due to other approved pathogens	200 mg	q12h	7 days	400 mg
Complicated UTI's	200 mg	q12h	10 days	400 mg
Prostatitis due to *E. coli*	300 mg	q12h	6 wks‡	600 mg

†DUE TO THE DESIGNATED PATHOGENS (See *INDICATIONS AND USAGE*.)
‡BECAUSE THERE ARE NO SAFETY DATA PRESENTLY AVAILABLE TO SUPPORT THE USE OF THE INTRAVENOUS FORMULATION OF OFLOXACIN FOR MORE THAN 10 DAYS, THERAPY AFTER 10 DAYS SHOULD BE SWITCHED TO THE ORAL TABLET FORMULATION OR OTHER APPROPRIATE THERAPY.

Men: Creatinine clearance (mL/min) = $\dfrac{\text{Weight (kg)} \times (140\text{-age})}{72 \times \text{serum creatinine (mg/dL)}}$

Women: 0.85 × the value calculated for men.

CAUTION: RAPID OR BOLUS INTRAVENOUS INFUSION MUST BE AVOIDED. Ofloxacin injection should be infused intravenously slowly over a period of not less than 60 minutes. (See *PRECAUTIONS*.)

Single-use vials require dilution prior to administration. (See *PREPARATION FOR ADMINISTRATION*.)
The usual dose of FLOXIN (ofloxacin injection) I.V. is 200 mg to 400 mg administered by slow infusion over 60 minutes every 12 h as described in the following dosing chart. These recommendations apply to patients with mild to moderate infection and normal renal function (i.e., creatinine clearance >50 mL/min). For patients with altered renal function (i.e., creatinine clearance ≤50 mL/min), see the *Patients with Impaired Renal Function* subsection.
Patients with Normal Renal Function:
[See first table above]
Patients with Impaired Renal Function:
Dosage should be adjusted for patients with a creatinine clearance ≤ 50 mL/min. **After a normal initial dose,** dosage should be adjusted as follows:

Creatinine Clearance	Maintenance Dose	Frequency
20-50 mL/min	the usual recommended unit dose	q24h
<20 mL/min	1/2 the usual recommended unit dose	q24h

When only the serum creatinine is known, the following formula may be used to estimate creatinine clearance.
[See second table above]
The serum creatinine should represent a steady-state of renal function.
Patients with Cirrhosis:
The excretion of ofloxacin may be reduced in patients with severe liver function disorders (e.g., cirrhosis with or without ascites). A maximum dose of 400 mg of ofloxacin per day should therefore not be exceeded.
PREPARATION OF OFLOXACIN INJECTION FOR ADMINISTRATION
FLOXIN I.V. IN SINGLE-USE VIALS:
FLOXIN I.V. is supplied in single-use vials containing a concentrated ofloxacin solution with the equivalent of 400 mg of ofloxacin in Water for Injection. The 10 mL vials contain 40 mg of ofloxacin/mL. THESE FLOXIN I.V. SINGLE-USE VIALS MUST BE FURTHER DILUTED WITH AN APPROPRIATE SOLUTION PRIOR TO INTRAVENOUS ADMINISTRATION. (See COMPATIBLE INTRAVENOUS SOLUTIONS.) The concentration of the resulting diluted solution should be 4 mg/mL prior to administration.

This parenteral drug product should be inspected visually for discoloration and particulate matter prior to administration.
Since no preservative or bacteriostatic agent is present in this product, aseptic technique must be used in preparation of the final parenteral solution. **Since the vials are for single-use only, any unused portion should be discarded.**
Since only limited data are available on the compatibility of ofloxacin intravenous injection with other intravenous substances, **additives or other medications should not be added to FLOXIN I.V. in single-use vials or infused simultaneously through the same intravenous line.** If the same intravenous line is used for sequential infusion of several different drugs, the line should be flushed before and after infusion of FLOXIN I.V. with an infusion solution compatible with FLOXIN I.V. and with any other drug(s) administered via this common line.
Prepare the desired dosage of ofloxacin according to the following chart:

Desired Dosage Strength	From 10 mL Vial, Withdraw Volume	Volume of Diluent	Infusion Time
200 mg	5 mL	qs 50 mL	60 min
300 mg	7.5 mL	qs 75 mL	60 min
400 mg	10 mL	qs 100 mL	60 min

For example, to prepare a 200-mg dose using the 10 mL vial (40 mg/mL), withdraw 5 mL and dilute with a compatible intravenous solution to a total volume of 50 mL.
Compatible Intravenous Solutions:
Any of the following intravenous solutions may be used to prepare a 4 mg/mL ofloxacin solution with the approximate pH values:

Intravenous Fluids	pH of 4 mg/mL FLOXIN I.V. Solution
0.9% Sodium Chloride Injection, USP	4.69
5% Dextrose Injection, USP	4.57
5% Dextrose/0.9% NaCl Injection	4.56
5% Dextrose in Lactated Ringers	4.94
5% Sodium Bicarbonate Injection	7.95
Plasma-Lyte® 56/5% Dextrose Injection	5.02
5% Dextrose, 0.45% Sodium Chloride, and 0.15% Potassium Chloride Injection	4.64
Sodium Lactate Injection (M/6)	5.64
Water for Injection	4.66

Continued on next page

Floxin I.V.—Cont.

FLOXIN I.V. PRE-MIXED IN SINGLE-USE FLEXIBLE CONTAINERS:
FLOXIN I.V. is also supplied in 50 mL and 100 mL flexible containers containing a pre-mixed, ready-to-use ofloxacin solution in D_5W for single-use. **NO FURTHER DILUTION OF THIS PREPARATION IS NECESSARY. Each 50 mL pre-mixed flexible container already contains a dilute solution with the equivalent of 200 mg of ofloxacin (4 mg/mL) in 5% Dextrose (D_5W). Each 100 mL pre-mixed flexible container already contains a dilute solution with the equivalent of 400 mg of ofloxacin (4 mg/mL) in 5% Dextrose (D_5W).**
This parenteral drug product should be inspected visually for discoloration and particulate matter prior to administration.
Since no preservative or bacteriostatic agent is present in this product, aseptic technique must be used in preparation of the final parenteral solution. **Since the pre-mixed flexible containers are for single-use only, any unused portion should be discarded.**
Since only limited data are available on the compatibility of ofloxacin intravenous injection with other intravenous substances, **additives or other medications should not be added to FLOXIN I.V. in flexible containers or infused simultaneously through the same intravenous line.** If the same intravenous line is used for sequential infusion of several different drugs, the line should be flushed before and after infusion of FLOXIN I.V. with an infusion solution compatible with FLOXIN I.V. and with any other drug(s) administered via this common line.
Instructions for the Use of FLOXIN I.V. PRE-MIXED IN FLEXIBLE CONTAINERS:
To open:
1. Tear outer wrap at the notch and remove solution container.
2. Check the container for minute leaks by squeezing the inner bag firmly. If leaks are found, or if the seal is not intact, discard the solution, as the sterility may be compromised.
3. Do not use if the solution is cloudy or a precipitate is present.
4. Use sterile equipment.
5. **WARNING: Do not use flexible containers in series connections.** Such use could result in air embolism due to residual air being drawn from the primary container before administration of the fluid from the secondary container is complete.
Preparation for administration:
1. Close flow control clamp of administration set.
2. Remove cover from port at bottom of container.
3. Insert piercing pin of administration set into port with a twisting motion until the pin is firmly seated. **NOTE: See full directions on administration set carton.**
4. Suspend container from hanger.
5. Squeeze and release drip chamber to establish proper fluid level in chamber during infusion of FLOXIN I.V. IN PRE-MIXED FLEXIBLE CONTAINERS.
6. Open flow control clamp to expel air from set. Close clamp.
7. Regulate rate of administration with flow control clamp.
Stability of FLOXIN I.V. as Supplied:
When stored under recommended conditions, FLOXIN I.V., as supplied in 10 mL vials, and 50 mL and 100 mL flexible containers, is stable through the expiration date printed on the label.
Stability of FLOXIN I.V. Following Dilution:
FLOXIN I.V., when diluted in a compatible intravenous fluid to a concentration between 0.4 mg/mL and 4 mg/mL, is stable for 72 h when stored at or below 75°F or 24°C and for 14 days when stored under refrigeration at 41°F or 5°C in glass bottles or plastic intravenous containers. Solutions that are diluted in a compatible intravenous solution and frozen in glass bottles or plastic intravenous containers are stable for 6 months when stored at -4°F or -20°C. Once thawed, the solution is stable for up to 14 days, if refrigerated at 36°F to 46°F (2°C to 8°C). **THAW FROZEN SOLUTIONS AT ROOM TEMPERATURE (77°F OR 25°C) OR IN A REFRIGERATOR (46°F OR 8°C). DO NOT FORCE THAW BY MICROWAVE IRRADIATION OR WATER BATH IMMERSION. DO NOT REFREEZE AFTER INITIAL THAWING.**

HOW SUPPLIED

SINGLE-USE VIALS:
FLOXIN (ofloxacin injection) I.V. is supplied in single-use vials. Each vial contains a concentrated solution with the equivalent of 400 mg of ofloxacin.
40 mg/mL, 10 mL vials (NDC 0062-1550-01)
FLOXIN I.V. SINGLE-USE VIALS are manufactured for Ortho Pharmaceutical Corporation and McNeil Pharmaceutical by Schering-Plough Products, Inc., Manati, PR 00674.
PRE-MIXED IN FLEXIBLE CONTAINERS:
FLOXIN (ofloxacin injection) I.V. PRE-MIXED IN FLEXIBLE CONTAINERS is supplied as a single-use, pre-mixed solution in 50 mL and 100 mL flexible containers. Each contains a dilute solution with the equivalent of 200 mg or 400 mg of ofloxacin, respectively, in 5% Dextrose (D_5W).
4 mg/mL (200 mg), 50 mL flexible container (NDC 0062-1553-01)
4 mg/mL (400 mg), 100 mL flexible container (NDC 0062-1552-02)
FLOXIN I.V. PRE-MIXED IN FLEXIBLE CONTAINERS is manufactured for Ortho Pharmaceutical Corporation and McNeil Pharmaceutical by Abbott Laboratories, North Chicago, IL 60064.
FLOXIN (ofloxacin injection) I.V. in SINGLE-USE VIALS should be stored at controlled room temperature 59°F to 86°F (15°C to 30°C) and protected from light. FLOXIN I.V. PRE-MIXED IN FLEXIBLE CONTAINERS should be stored at or below 77°F or 25°C; however, brief exposure up to 104°F or 40°C does not adversely affect the product. Avoid excessive heat and protect from freezing and light.
Also Available:
TABLETS
Ofloxacin is also available as FLOXIN TABLETS (ofloxacin tablets) 200, 300 and 400 mg.

ANIMAL PHARMACOLOGY

Ofloxacin, as well as other drugs of the quinolone class, has been shown to cause arthropathies (arthrosis) in immature dogs and rats. In addition, these drugs are associated with an increased incidence of osteochondrosis in rats as compared to the incidence observed in vehicle-treated rats. (See ***WARNINGS***.) There is no evidence of arthropathies in fully mature dogs at intravenous doses up to 3 times the recommended maximum human dose (on a mg/m^2 basis or 5 times based on a mg/kg basis) for a one-week exposure period.
Long-term, high-dose systemic use of other quinolones in experimental animals has caused lenticular opacities; however, this finding was not observed in any animal studies with ofloxacin.
Reduced serum globulin and protein levels were observed in animals treated with other quinolones. In one ofloxacin study, minor decreases in serum globulin and protein levels were noted in female cynomolgus monkeys dosed orally with 40 mg/kg ofloxacin daily for one year. These changes, however, were considered to be within normal limits for monkeys.
Crystalluria and ocular toxicity were not observed in any animals treated with ofloxacin.
Caution: Federal (U.S.A.) law prohibits dispensing without prescription.
FLOXIN® is a trademark of Ortho Pharmaceutical Corporation. U.S. Patent No. 4,382,892

REFERENCES

1. National Committee for Clinical Laboratory Standards. Methods for Dilution Antimicrobial Susceptibility Tests for Bacteria That Grow Aerobically — Third Edition. Approved Standard NCCLS Document M7-A3, Vol. 13, No. 25, NCCLS, Villanova, PA, December, 1993.
2. National Committee for Clinical Laboratory Standards. Performance Standards for Antimicrobial Disk Susceptibility Tests — Fifth Edition. Approved Standard NCCLS Document M2-A5, Vol. 13, No. 24, NCCLS, Villanova, PA, December, 1993.

ORTHO PHARMACEUTICAL CORPORATION
Raritan, NJ USA 08869, and
McNEIL PHARMACEUTICAL
Spring House, PA USA 19477
© OPC 1991 Revised February 1997 635-10-291-3
17564129
Shown in Product Identification Guide, page 328

FLOXIN® TABLETS ℞
[ofloxacin tablets]

Prescribing Information

DESCRIPTION

FLOXIN® (ofloxacin tablets) Tablets is a synthetic broad-spectrum antimicrobial agent for oral administration. Chemically, ofloxacin, a fluorinated carboxyquinolone, is the racemate, (±)-9-fluoro-2,3-dihydro-3-methyl-10- (4-methyl-1-piperazinyl)-7-oxo-7H-pyrido[1,2,3-de]-1,4-benzoxazine-6-carboxylic acid. The chemical structure is:

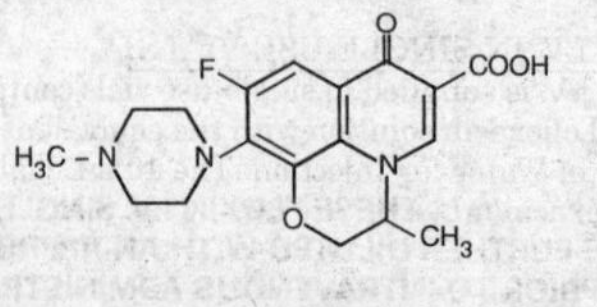

Its empirical formula is $C_{18}H_{20}FN_3O_4$, and its molecular weight is 361.4. Ofloxacin is an off-white to pale yellow crystalline powder. The molecule exists as a zwitterion at the pH conditions in the small intestine. The relative solubility characteristics of ofloxacin at room temperature, as defined by USP nomenclature, indicate that ofloxacin is considered to be *soluble* in aqueous solutions with pH between 2 and 5. It is *sparingly* to *slightly soluble* in aqueous solutions with pH 7 (solubility falls to 4 mg/mL) and *freely soluble* in aqueous solutions with pH above 9. Ofloxacin has the potential to form stable coordination compounds with many metal ions. This *in vitro* chelation potential has the following formation order: $Fe^{+3} > Al^{+3} > Cu^{+2} > Ni^{+2} > Pb^{+2} > Zn^{+2} > Mg^{+2} > Ca^{+2} > Ba^{+2}$.
FLOXIN Tablets contain the following inactive ingredients: anhydrous lactose, corn starch, hydroxypropyl cellulose, hydroxypropyl methylcellulose, magnesium stearate, polyethylene glycol, polysorbate 80, sodium starch glycolate, titanium dioxide and may also contain synthetic yellow iron oxide.

CLINICAL PHARMACOLOGY

Following oral administration, the bioavailability of ofloxacin in the tablet formulation is approximately 98%. Maximum serum concentrations are achieved one to two hours after an oral dose. Absorption of ofloxacin after single or multiple doses of 200 to 400 mg is predictable, and the amount of drug absorbed increases proportionately with the dose. Ofloxacin has biphasic elimination. Following multiple oral doses at steady-state administration, the half-lives are approximately 4–5 hours and 20–25 hours. However, the longer half-life represents less than 5% of the total AUC. Accumulation at steady-state can be estimated using a half-life of 9 hours. The total clearance and volume of distribution are approximately similar after single or multiple doses. Elimination is mainly by renal excretion. The following are mean peak serum concentrations in healthy 70–80 kg male volunteers after single oral doses of 200, 300, or 400 mg of ofloxacin or after multiple oral doses of 400 mg.

Oral Dose	Serum Concentration 2 hours after admin. (µg/mL)	Area Under the Curve ($AUC_{(0-\infty)}$) (µg•h/mL)
200 mg single dose	1.5	14.1
300 mg single dose	2.4	21.2
400 mg single dose	2.9	31.4
400 mg steady-state	4.6	61.0

Steady-state concentrations were attained after four oral doses, and the area under the curve (AUC) was approximately 40% higher than the AUC after single doses. Therefore, after multiple-dose administration of 200 mg and 300 mg doses, peak serum levels of 2.2 µg/mL and 3.6 µg/mL, respectively, are predicted at steady-state.
In vitro, approximately 32% of the drug in plasma is protein bound.
The single dose and steady-state plasma profiles of ofloxacin injection were comparable in extent of exposure (AUC) to those of ofloxacin tablets when the injectable and tablet formulations of ofloxacin were administered in equal doses (mg/mg) to the same group of subjects. The mean steady-state $AUC_{(0-12)}$ attained after the intravenous administration of 400 mg over 60 min was 43.5 µg•h/mL; the mean steady-state $AUC_{(0-12)}$ attained after the oral administration of 400 mg was 41.2 µg•h/mL (two one-sided t-test, 90% confidence interval was 103–109). (See following chart.)

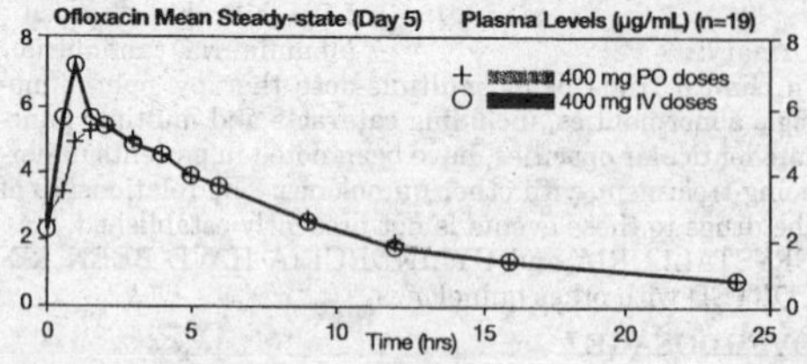

Between 0 and 6 h following the administration of a single 200 mg oral dose of ofloxacin to 12 healthy volunteers, the average urine ofloxacin concentration was approximately 220 µg/mL. Between 12 and 24 hours after administration, the average urine ofloxacin level was approximately 34 µg/mL.
Following oral administration of recommended therapeutic doses, ofloxacin has been detected in blister fluid, cervix, lung tissue, ovary, prostatic fluid, prostatic tissue, skin, and sputum. The mean concentration of ofloxacin in each of these various body fluids and tissues after one or more doses was 0.8 to 1.5 times the concurrent plasma level. Inadequate data are presently available on the distribution or levels of ofloxacin in the cerebrospinal fluid or brain tissue.
Ofloxacin has a pyridobenzoxazine ring that appears to decrease the extent of parent compound metabolism. Between 65% and 80% of an administered oral dose of ofloxacin is excreted unchanged via the kidneys within 48 hours of dosing. Studies indicate that less than 5% of an administered dose is recovered in the urine as the desmethyl or N-oxide metabolites. Four to eight percent of an ofloxacin dose is excreted in the feces. This indicates a small degree of biliary excretion of ofloxacin.

The administration of FLOXIN with food does not affect the C_{max} and AUC_{∞} of the drug, but T_{max} is prolonged.
Following the administration of oral doses of ofloxacin to healthy elderly volunteers (64–74 years of age) with normal renal function, the apparent half-life of ofloxacin was 7 to 8 hours, as compared to approximately 6 hours in younger adults. Drug absorption, however, appears to be unaffected by age.
Clearance of ofloxacin is reduced in patients with impaired renal function (creatinine clearance rate $\leq$ 50 mL/min), and dosage adjustment is necessary. (See ***PRECAUTIONS***: ***General*** and ***DOSAGE AND ADMINISTRATION***.)

Microbiology

Ofloxacin has *in vitro* activity against a broad-spectrum of gram-positive and gram-negative aerobic and anaerobic bacteria. Ofloxacin is often bactericidal at concentrations equal to or slightly greater than inhibitory concentrations. Ofloxacin is thought to exert a bactericidal effect on susceptible microorganisms by inhibiting DNA gyrase, an essential enzyme that is a critical catalyst in the duplication, transcription, and repair of bacterial DNA.
Ofloxacin has been shown to be active against most strains of the following microorganisms, both *in vitro* and in clinical infections as described in the ***INDICATIONS AND USAGE*** section:
[See first table above]
The following *in vitro* data are available, **but their clinical significance is unknown.**
Ofloxacin exhibits *in vitro* minimum inhibitory concentrations (MIC's) of 2 µg/mL or less against most ($\geq$ 90%) strains of the following microorganisms; however, the safety and effectiveness of ofloxacin in treating clinical infections due to these micro-organisms have not been established in adequate and well-controlled clinical trials:
[See second table above]
Ofloxacin is not active against *Treponema pallidum*. (See ***WARNINGS***.)
Many strains of other streptococcal species, *Enterococcus* species, and anaerobes are resistant to ofloxacin.
Resistance to ofloxacin due to spontaneous mutation *in vitro* is a rare occurrence (range: 10^{-9} to 10^{-11}). To date, emergence of resistance has been relatively uncommon in clinical practice. With the exception of *Pseudomonas aeruginosa* (10%), less than a 4% rate of resistance emergence has been reported for most other species. Although cross-resistance has been observed between ofloxacin and other fluoroquinolones, some organisms resistant to other quinolones may be susceptible to ofloxacin.

Susceptibility Tests

Dilution techniques:

Quantitative methods are used to determine antimicrobial minimal inhibitory concentrations (MIC's). These MIC's provide estimates of the susceptibility of bacteria to antimicrobial compounds. The MIC's should be determined using a standardized procedure. Standardized procedures are based on a dilution method[1] (broth or agar) or equivalent with standardized inoculum concentrations and standardized concentrations of ofloxacin powder. The MIC values should be interpreted according to the following criteria:

MIC (µg/mL)	Interpretation
$\leq$ 2	Susceptible (S)
4	Intermediate (I)
$\geq$ 8	Resistant (R)

A report of "Susceptible" indicates that the pathogen is likely to be inhibited if the antimicrobial compound in the blood reaches the concentrations usually achievable. A report of "Intermediate" indicates that the result should be considered equivocal, and, if the microorganism is not fully susceptible to alternative, clinically feasible drugs, the test should be repeated. This category implies possible clinical applicability in body sites where the drug is physiologically concentrated or in situations where high dosage of drug can be used. This category also provides a buffer zone which prevents small uncontrolled technical factors from causing major discrepancies in interpretation. A report of "Resistant" indicates that the pathogen is not likely to be inhibited if the antimicrobial compound in the blood reaches the concentrations usually achievable; other therapy should be selected.
Standardized susceptibility test procedures require the use of laboratory control microorganisms to control the technical aspects of the laboratory procedures. Standard ofloxacin powder should provide the following MIC values:

Microorganism		MIC (µg/mL)
Escherichia coli	ATCC 25922	0.015-0.12
Staphylococcus aureus	ATCC 29213	0.12-1.0
Pseudomonas aeruginosa	ATCC 27853	1.0-8.0
Haemophilus influenzae	ATCC 49247	0.016-0.06
Neisseria gonorrhoeae	ATCC 49226	0.004-0.016

Diffusion techniques:

Quantitative methods that require measurement of zone diameters also provide reproducible estimates of the susceptibility of bacteria to antimicrobial compounds. One such standardized procedure[2] requires the use of standard inoculum concentrations. This procedure uses paper disks impregnated with 5-µg ofloxacin to test the susceptibility of microorganisms to ofloxacin.

Gram-positive aerobes
Staphylococcus epidermidis
(excluding methicillin-resistant strains)
Staphylococcus haemolyticus
Staphylococcus saprophyticus
Gram-negative aerobes
Acinetobacter calcoaceticus
Aeromonas caviae
Aeromonas hydrophila
Bordetella parapertussis
Bordetella pertussis
Citrobacter freundii
Enterobacter cloacae
Haemophilus ducreyi
Klebsiella oxytoca
Moraxella catarrhalis
Morganella morganii
Gram-negative aerobes (continued)
Proteus vulgaris
Providencia rettgeri
Providencia stuartii
Serratia marcescens
Vibrio parahaemolyticus
Anaerobes
Clostridium perfringens
Gardnerella vaginalis
Other organisms
Chlamydia pneumoniae
Legionella pneumophila
Mycobacterium tuberculosis
(including multiple drug-resistant strains)
Mycoplasma hominis
Mycoplasma pneumoniae
Ureaplasma urealyticum

Gram-positive aerobes	Gram-negative aerobes	Other microorganisms
Staphylococcus aureus	*Citrobacter diversus*	*Chlamydia trachomatis*
Streptococcus pneumoniae	*Enterobacter aerogenes*	
Streptococcus pyogenes	*Escherichia coli*	
	Haemophilus influenzae	
	Klebsiella pneumoniae	
	Neisseria gonorrhoeae	
	Proteus mirabilis	
	Pseudomonas aeruginosa	

Reports from the laboratory providing results of the standard single-disk susceptibility test with a 5-µg ofloxacin disk should be interpreted according to the following criteria:

Zone Diameter (mm)	Interpretation
$\geq$ 16	Susceptible (S)
13-15	Intermediate (I)
$\leq$ 12	Resistant (R)

Interpretation should be as stated above for results using dilution techniques. Interpretation involves correlation of the diameter obtained in the disk test with the MIC for ofloxacin.
As with standardized dilution techniques, diffusion methods require the use of laboratory control microorganisms that are used to control the technical aspects of the laboratory procedures. For the diffusion technique, the 5-µg ofloxacin disk should provide the following zone diameters in these laboratory test quality control strains:

Microorganism		Zone Diameter (mm)
Escherichia coli	ATCC 25922	29-33
Pseudomonas aeruginosa	ATCC 27853	17-21
Haemophilus influenzae	ATCC 49247	31-40
Neisseria gonorrhoeae	ATCC 49226	43-51
Staphylococcus aureus	ATCC 25923	24-28

INDICATIONS AND USAGE

FLOXIN (ofloxacin tablets) Tablets are indicated for the treatment of adults with mild to moderate infections (unless otherwise indicated) caused by susceptible strains of the designated microorganisms in the infections listed below. Please see ***DOSAGE AND ADMINISTRATION*** for specific recommendations.

Acute bacterial exacerbations of chronic bronchitis due to *Haemophilus influenzae* or *Streptococcus pneumoniae*.
Community-acquired Pneumonia due to *Haemophilus influenzae* or *Streptococcus pneumoniae*.
Uncomplicated skin and skin structure infections due to *Staphylococcus aureus*, *Streptococcus pyogenes*, or *Proteus mirabilis*.
Acute, uncomplicated urethral and cervical gonorrhea due to *Neisseria gonorrhoeae*. (See ***WARNINGS***.)
Nongonococcal urethritis and cervicitis due to *Chlamydia trachomatis*. (See ***WARNINGS***.)
Mixed infections of the urethra and cervix due to *Chlamydia trachomatis* and *Neisseria gonorrhoeae*. (See ***WARNINGS***.)
Acute pelvic inflammatory disease (including severe infection) due to *Chlamydia trachomatis* and/or *Neisseria gonorrhoeae*. (See ***WARNINGS***.)
NOTE: If anaerobic microorganisms are suspected of contributing to the infection, appropriate therapy for anaerobic pathogens should be administered.
Uncomplicated cystitis due to *Citrobacter diversus, Enterobacter aerogenes, Escherichia coli, Klebsiella pneumoniae, Proteus mirabilis*, or *Pseudomonas aeruginosa*.
Complicated urinary tract infections due to *Escherichia coli, Klebsiella pneumoniae, Proteus mirabilis, Citrobacter diversus**, or *Pseudomonas aeruginosa**.
Prostatitis due to *Escherichia coli*.
* = Although treatment of infections due to this organism in this organ system demonstrated a clinically significant outcome, efficacy was studied in fewer than 10 patients.

Appropriate culture and susceptibility tests should be performed before treatment in order to isolate and identify organisms causing the infection and to determine their susceptibility to ofloxacin. Therapy with ofloxacin may be initiated before results of these tests are known; once results become available, appropriate therapy should be continued. As with other drugs in this class, some strains of *Pseudomonas aeruginosa* may develop resistance fairly rapidly during treatment with ofloxacin. Culture and susceptibility testing performed periodically during therapy will provide information not only on the therapeutic effect of the antimicrobial agent but also on the possible emergence of bacterial resistance.

CONTRAINDICATIONS

FLOXIN (ofloxacin tablets) Tablets is contraindicated in persons with a history of hypersensitivity associated with the use of ofloxacin or any member of the quinolone group of antimicrobial agents.

WARNINGS

THE SAFETY AND EFFICACY OF OFLOXACIN IN CHILDREN, ADOLESCENTS (UNDER THE AGE OF 18 YEARS), PREGNANT WOMEN, AND LACTATING WOMEN HAVE NOT BEEN ESTABLISHED. (SEE PEDIATRIC USE, USE IN PREGNANCY, AND NURSING MOTHERS SUBSECTIONS IN THE PRECAUTIONS SECTION.)
In the immature rat, the oral administration of ofloxacin at 5 to 16 times the recommended maximum human dose based on mg/kg or 1–3 times based on mg/m^2 increased the incidence and severity of osteochondrosis. The lesions did not regress after 13 weeks of drug withdrawal. Other quinolones also produce similar erosions in the weight-bearing joints and other signs of arthropathy in immature animals of various species. (See ***ANIMAL PHARMACOLOGY***.)
Convulsions, increased intracranial pressure, and toxic psychosis have been reported in patients receiving quinolones, including ofloxacin. Quinolones, including ofloxacin, may also cause central nervous system stimulation which may lead to: tremors, restlessness/agitation, nervousness/anxiety, lightheadedness, confusion, hallucinations, paranoia and depression, nightmares, insomnia, and rarely suicidal thoughts or acts. These reactions may occur following the first dose. If these reactions occur in patients receiving ofloxacin, the drug should be discontinued and appropriate measures instituted. As with all quinolones, ofloxacin should be used with caution in patients with a known or suspected CNS disorder that may predispose to seizures or lower the seizure threshold (e.g., severe cerebral arteriosclerosis, epilepsy) or in the presence of other risk factors that may predispose to seizures or lower the seizure threshold (e.g., certain drug therapy, renal dysfunction). (See ***PRECAUTIONS***: ***General, Information for Patients, Drug Interactions*** and ***ADVERSE REACTIONS***.)
Serious and occasionally fatal hypersensitivity (anaphylactic/anaphylactoid) reactions have been reported in patients receiving therapy with quinolones, including ofloxacin. These reactions often occur following the first dose. Some reactions were accompanied by cardiovascular collapse, hypotension/shock, seizure, loss of consciousness, tingling, an-

Continued on next page

Floxin Tablets—Cont.

gioedema (including tongue, laryngeal, throat or facial ede-ma/swelling), airway obstruction (including bronchospasm, shortness of breath and acute respiratory distress), dyspnea, urticaria/hives, itching, and other serious skin reactions. A few patients had a history of hypersensitivity reactions. The drug should be discontinued immediately at the first appearance of a skin rash or any other sign of hypersensitivity. Serious acute hypersensitivity reactions may require treatment with epinephrine and other resuscitative measures, including oxygen, intravenous fluids, antihistamines, corticosteroids, pressor amines, and airway management, as clinically indicated. (See *PRECAUTIONS* and *ADVERSE REACTIONS*.)

Serious and sometimes fatal events, some due to hypersensitivity, and some due to uncertain etiology, have been reported in patients receiving therapy with quinolones, including ofloxacin. These events may be severe and generally occur following the administration of multiple doses. Clinical manifestations may include one or more of the following: fever, rash or severe dermatologic reactions (e.g., toxic epidermal necrolysis, Stevens-Johnson Syndrome); vasculitis; arthralgia; myalgia; serum sickness; allergic pneumonitis; interstitial nephritis; acute renal insufficiency/failure; hepatitis; jaundice; acute hepatic necrosis/failure; anemia, including hemolytic and aplastic; thrombocytopenia, including thrombotic thrombocytopenic purpura; leukopenia; agranulocytosis; pancytopenia; and/or other hematologic abnormalities. The drug should be discontinued immediately at the first appearance of a skin rash or any other sign of hypersensitivity and supportive measures instituted. (See *PRECAUTIONS: Information for Patients* and *ADVERSE REACTIONS*.)

Pseudomembranous colitis has been reported with nearly all antibacterial agents, including ofloxacin, and may range in severity from mild to life-threatening. Therefore, it is important to consider this diagnosis in patients who present with diarrhea subsequent to the administration of any antibacterial agents.

Treatment with antibacterial agents alters the normal flora of the colon and may permit overgrowth of clostridia. Studies indicate a toxin produced by *Clostridium difficile* is one primary cause of "antibiotic-associated colitis".

After the diagnosis of pseudomembranous colitis has been established, therapeutic measures should be initiated. Mild cases of pseudomembranous colitis usually respond to drug discontinuation alone. In moderate to severe cases, consideration should be given to management with fluids and electrolytes, protein supplementation, and treatment with an antibacterial drug clinically effective against *C. difficile* colitis. (See *ADVERSE REACTIONS*.)

Ruptures of the shoulder, hand, and Achilles tendons that required surgical repair or resulted in prolonged disability have been reported with ofloxacin and other quinolones. Ofloxacin should be discontinued if the patient experiences pain, inflammation, or rupture of a tendon. Patients should rest and refrain from exercise until the diagnosis of tendinitis or tendon rupture has been confidently excluded. Tendon rupture can occur at any time during or after therapy with ofloxacin.

Ofloxacin has not been shown to be effective in the treatment of syphilis. Antimicrobial agents used in high doses for short periods of time to treat gonorrhea may mask or delay the symptoms of incubating syphilis. All patients with gonorrhea should have a serologic test for syphilis at the time of diagnosis. Patients treated with ofloxacin for gonorrhea should have a follow-up serologic test for syphilis after three months and, if positive, treatment with an appropriate antimicrobial should be instituted.

PRECAUTIONS
General:
Adequate hydration of patients receiving ofloxacin should be maintained to prevent the formation of a highly concentrated urine.

Administer ofloxacin with caution in the presence of renal or hepatic insufficiency/impairment. In patients with known or suspected renal or hepatic insufficiency/impairment, careful clinical observation and appropriate laboratory studies should be performed prior to and during therapy since elimination of ofloxacin may be reduced. In patients with impaired renal function (creatinine clearance ≤ 50 mg/mL), alteration of the dosage regimen is necessary. (See *CLINICAL PHARMACOLOGY* and *DOSAGE AND ADMINISTRATION*.)

Moderate to severe phototoxicity reactions have been observed in patients exposed to direct sunlight while receiving some drugs in this class, including ofloxacin. Excessive sunlight should be avoided. Therapy should be discontinued if phototoxicity (e.g., a skin eruption) occurs.

As with other quinolones, ofloxacin should be used with caution in any patient with a known or suspected CNS disorder that may predispose to seizures or lower the seizure threshold (e.g., severe cerebral arteriosclerosis, epilepsy) or in the presence of other risk factors that may predispose to sei-

zures or lower the seizure threshold (e.g., certain drug therapy, renal dysfunction). (See *WARNINGS* and *Drug Interactions*.)

A possible interaction between oral hypoglycemic drugs (e.g., glyburide/glibenclamide) or with insulin and fluoroquinolone antimicrobial agents have been reported resulting in a potentiation of the hypoglycemic action of these drugs. The mechanism for this interaction is not known. If a hypoglycemic reaction occurs in a patient being treated with ofloxacin, discontinue ofloxacin immediately and consult a physician. (See *Drug Interactions* and *ADVERSE REACTIONS*.)

As with any potent drug, periodic assessment of organ system functions, including renal, hepatic, and hematopoietic, is advisable during prolonged therapy. (See *WARNINGS* and *ADVERSE REACTIONS*.)

Information for Patients:
Patients should be advised:
— to drink fluids liberally;
— that mineral supplements, vitamins with iron or minerals, calcium-, aluminum- or magnesium-based antacids or sucralfate should not be taken within the two-hour period before or within the two-hour period after taking ofloxacin (See *Drug Interactions*);
— that ofloxacin can be taken without regard to meals;
— that ofloxacin may cause neurologic adverse effects (e.g., dizziness, lightheadedness) and that patients should know how they react to ofloxacin before they operate an automobile or machinery or engage in activities requiring mental alertness and coordination (See *WARNINGS* and *ADVERSE REACTIONS*);
— to discontinue treatment and inform their physician if they experience pain, inflammation, or rupture of a tendon, and to rest and refrain from exercise until the diagnosis of tendinitis or tendon rupture has been confidently excluded;
— that ofloxacin may be associated with hypersensitivity reactions, even following the first dose, to discontinue the drug at the first sign of a skin rash, hives or other skin reactions, a rapid heartbeat, difficulty in swallowing or breathing, any swelling suggesting angioedema (e.g., swelling of the lips, tongue, face; tightness of the throat, hoarseness), or any other symptom of an allergic reaction (See *WARNINGS* and *ADVERSE REACTIONS*);
— to avoid excessive sunlight or artificial ultraviolet light while receiving ofloxacin and to discontinue therapy if phototoxicity (e.g., skin eruption) occurs;
— that if they are diabetic and are being treated with insulin or an oral hypoglycemic drug, to discontinue ofloxacin immediately if a hypoglycemic reaction occurs and consult a physician (See *PRECAUTIONS: General* and *Drug Interactions*);
— that convulsions have been reported in patients taking quinolones, including ofloxacin, and to notify their physician before taking this drug if there is a history of this condition.

Drug Interactions:
Antacids, Sucralfate, Metal Cations, Multivitamins: Quinolones form chelates with alkaline earth and transition metal cations. Administration of quinolones with antacids containing calcium, magnesium, or aluminum, with sucralfate, with divalent or trivalent cations such as iron, or with multivitamins containing zinc may substantially interfere with the absorption of quinolones resulting in systemic levels considerably lower than desired. These agents should not be taken within the two-hour period before or within the two-hour period after ofloxacin administration. (See *DOSAGE AND ADMINISTRATION*.)

Caffeine: Interactions between ofloxacin and caffeine have not been detected.

Cimetidine: Cimetidine has demonstrated interference with the elimination of some quinolones. This interference has resulted in significant increases in half-life and AUC of some quinolones. The potential for interaction between ofloxacin and cimetidine has not been studied.

Cyclosporine: Elevated serum levels of cyclosporine have been reported with concomitant use of cyclosporine with some other quinolones. The potential for interaction between ofloxacin and cyclosporine has not been studied.

Drugs metabolized by Cytochrome P450 enzymes: Most quinolone antimicrobial drugs inhibit cytochrome P450 enzyme activity. This may result in a prolonged half-life for some drugs that are also metabolized by this system (e.g., cyclosporine, theophylline/methylxanthines, warfarin) when co-administered with quinolones. The extent of this inhibition varies among different quinolones. (See other **Drug Interactions**.)

Non-steroidal anti-inflammatory drugs: The concomitant administration of a non-steroidal anti-inflammatory drug with a quinolone, including ofloxacin, may increase the risk of CNS stimulation and convulsive seizures. (See *WARNINGS* and *PRECAUTIONS: General*.)

Probenecid: The concomitant use of probenecid with certain other quinolones has been reported to affect renal tubular secretion. The effect of probenecid on the elimination of ofloxacin has not been studied.

Theophylline: Steady-state theophylline levels may increase when ofloxacin and theophylline are administered concurrently. As with other quinolones, concomitant administration of ofloxacin may prolong the half-life of theophylline, elevate serum theophylline levels, and increase the risk of theophylline-related adverse reactions. Theophylline levels should be closely monitored and theophylline dosage adjustments made, if appropriate, when ofloxacin is co-administered. Adverse reactions (including seizures) may occur with or without an elevation in the serum theophylline level. (See *WARNINGS* and *PRECAUTIONS: General*.)

Warfarin: Some quinolones have been reported to enhance the effects of the oral anticoagulant warfarin or its derivatives. Therefore, if a quinolone antimicrobial is administered concomitantly with warfarin or its derivatives, the prothrombin time or other suitable coagulation test should be closely monitored.

Antidiabetic agents (e.g., insulin, glyburide/glibenclamide): Since disturbances of blood glucose, including hyperglycemia and hypoglycemia, have been reported in patients treated concurrently with quinolones and an antidiabetic agent, careful monitoring of blood glucose is recommended when these agents are used concomitantly. (See *PRECAUTIONS: General* and *Information for Patients*.)

Carcinogenesis, Mutagenesis, Impairment of Fertility:
Long-term studies to determine the carcinogenic potential of ofloxacin have not been conducted.

Ofloxacin was not mutagenic in the Ames bacterial test, *in vitro* and *in vivo* cytogenetic assay, sister chromatid exchange (Chinese Hamster and Human Cell Lines), unscheduled DNA Repair (UDS) using human fibroblasts, dominant lethal assays, or mouse micronucleus assay. Ofloxacin was positive in the UDS test using rat hepatocytes and Mouse Lymphoma Assay.

Pregnancy: Teratogenic Effects. Pregnancy Category C.
Ofloxacin has not been shown to have any teratogenic effects at oral doses as high as 810 mg/kg/day (11 times the recommended maximum human dose based on mg/m^2 or 50 times based on mg/kg) and 160 mg/kg/day (4 times the recommended maximum human dose based on mg/m^2 or 10 times based on mg/kg) when administered to pregnant rats and rabbits, respectively. Additional studies in rats with oral doses up to 360 mg/kg/day (5 times the recommended maximum human dose based on mg/m^2 or 23 times based on mg/kg) demonstrated no adverse effect on late fetal development, labor, delivery, lactation, neonatal viability, or growth of the newborn. Doses equivalent to 50 and 10 times the recommended maximum human dose of ofloxacin (based on mg/kg) were fetotoxic (i.e., decreased fetal body weight and increased fetal mortality) in rats and rabbits, respectively. Minor skeletal variations were reported in rats receiving doses of 810 mg/kg/day, which is more than 10 times higher than the recommended maximum human dose based on mg/m^2.

There are, however, no adequate and well-controlled studies in pregnant women. Ofloxacin should be used during pregnancy only if the potential benefit justifies the potential risk to the fetus. (See *WARNINGS*.)

Nursing Mothers:
In lactating females, a single oral 200-mg dose of ofloxacin resulted in concentrations of ofloxacin in milk that were similar to those found in plasma. Because of the potential for serious adverse reactions from ofloxacin in nursing infants, a decision should be made whether to discontinue nursing or to discontinue the drug, taking into account the importance of the drug to the mother. (See *WARNINGS* and *ADVERSE REACTIONS*.)

Pediatric Use:
Safety and effectiveness in children and adolescents below the age of 18 years have not been established. Ofloxacin causes arthropathy (arthrosis) and osteochondrosis in juvenile animals of several species. (See *WARNINGS*.)

ADVERSE REACTIONS
The following is a compilation of the data for ofloxacin based on clinical experience with both the oral and intravenous formulations. The incidence of drug-related adverse reactions in patients during Phase 2 and 3 clinical trials was 11%. Among patients receiving multiple-dose therapy, 4% discontinued ofloxacin due to adverse experiences.

In clinical trials, the following events were considered likely to be drug-related in patients receiving multiple doses of ofloxacin:

   nausea 3%, insomnia 3%, headache 1%, dizziness 1%, diarrhea 1%, vomiting 1%, rash 1%, pruritus 1%, external genital pruritus in women 1%, vaginitis 1%, dysgeusia 1%.

In clinical trials, the most frequently reported adverse events, regardless of relationship to drug, were:

   nausea 10%, headache 9%, insomnia 7%, external genital pruritus in women 6%, dizziness 5%, vaginitis 5%, diarrhea 4%, vomiting 4%.

In clinical trials, the following events, regardless of relationship to drug, occurred in 1 to 3% of patients:

Abdominal pain and cramps, chest pain, decreased appetite, dry mouth, dysgeusia, fatigue, flatulence, gastrointestinal distress, nervousness, pharyngitis, pruritus, fever, rash, sleep disorders, somnolence, trunk pain, vaginal discharge, visual disturbances, and constipation.

Additional events, occurring in clinical trials at a rate of less than 1%, regardless of relationship to drug, were:

Body as a whole:	asthenia, chills, malaise, extremity pain, pain, epistaxis
Cardiovascular System:	cardiac arrest, edema, hypertension, hypotension, palpitations, vasodilation
Gastrointestinal System:	dyspepsia
Genital/Reproductive System:	burning, irritation, pain and rash of the female genitalia; dysmenorrhea; menorrhagia; metrorrhagia
Musculoskeletal System:	arthralgia, myalgia
Nervous System:	seizures, anxiety, cognitive change, depression, dream abnormality, euphoria, hallucinations, paresthesia, syncope, vertigo, tremor, confusion
Nutritional/Metabolic:	thirst, weight loss
Respiratory System:	respiratory arrest, cough, rhinorrhea
Skin/Hypersensitivity:	angioedema, diaphoresis, urticaria, vasculitis
Special Senses:	decreased hearing acuity, tinnitus, photophobia
Urinary System:	dysuria, urinary frequency, urinary retention

The following laboratory abnormalities appeared in ≥ 1.0% of patients receiving multiple doses of ofloxacin. It is not known whether these abnormalities were caused by the drug or the underlying conditions being treated.

Hematopoietic:	anemia, leukopenia, leukocytosis, neutropenia, neutrophilia, increased band forms, lymphocytopenia, eosinophilia, lymphocytosis, thrombocytopenia, thrombocytosis, elevated ESR
Hepatic:	elevated: alkaline phosphatase, AST (SGOT), ALT (SGPT)
Serum chemistry:	hyperglycemia, hypoglycemia, elevated creatinine, elevated BUN
Urinary:	glucosuria, proteinuria, alkalinuria, hyposthenuria, hematuria, pyuria

Post-Marketing Adverse Events:

Additional adverse events, regardless of relationship to drug, reported from worldwide marketing experience with quinolones, including ofloxacin:

Clinical:

Cardiovascular System:	cerebral thrombosis, pulmonary edema, tachycardia, hypotension/shock, syncope
Endocrine/Metabolic:	hyper- or hypoglycemia, especially in diabetic patients on insulin or oral hypoglycemic agents (See **PRECAUTIONS: General** and **Drug Interactions.**)
Gastrointestinal System:	hepatic dysfunction including: hepatic necrosis, jaundice (cholestatic or hepatocellular), hepatitis; intestinal perforation; pseudomembranous colitis (the onset of pseudomembranous colitis symptoms may occur during or after antimicrobial treatment), GI hemorrhage; hiccough; painful oral mucosa, pyrosis (See **WARNINGS.**)
Genital/Reproductive System:	vaginal candidiasis
Hematopoietic:	anemia, including hemolytic and aplastic; hemorrhage, pancytopenia, agranulocytosis, leukopenia, reversible bone marrow depression, thrombocytopenia, thrombotic thrombocytopenic purpura, petechiae, ecchymosis/bruising (See **WARNINGS.**)

Infection†	Unit Dose	Frequency	Duration	Daily Dose
Acute Bacterial Exacerbation of Chronic Bronchitis	400 mg	q12h	10 days	800 mg
Comm. Acquired Pneumonia	400 mg	q12h	10 days	800 mg
Uncomplicated Skin and Skin Structure Infections	400 mg	q12h	10 days	800 mg
Acute, Uncomplicated Urethral and Cervical Gonorrhea	400 mg	single dose	1 day	400 mg
Nongonococcal Cervicitis/Urethritis due to C. trachomatis	300 mg	q12h	7 days	600 mg
Mixed Infection of the urethra and cervix due to C. trachomatis and N. gonorrhoeae	300 mg	q12h	7 days	600 mg
Acute Pelvic Inflammatory Disease	400 mg	q12h	10-14 days	800 mg
Uncomplicated Cystitis due to E. coli or K. pneumoniae	200 mg	q12h	3 days	400 mg
Uncomplicated Cystitis due to other approved pathogens	200 mg	q12h	7 days	400 mg
Complicated UTI's	200 mg	q12h	10 days	400 mg
Prostatitis due to E. coli	300 mg	q12h	6 weeks	600 mg

†DUE TO THE DESIGNATED PATHOGENS (See **INDICATIONS AND USAGE.**)

Creatinine Clearance	Maintenance Dose	Frequency
20-50 mL/min	the usual recommended unit dose	q24h
< 20 mL/min	1/2 the usual recommended unit dose	q24h

Musculoskeletal:	tendinitis/rupture: weakness; rhabdomyolysis
Nervous System:	nightmares; suicidal thoughts or acts, disorientation, psychotic reactions, paranoia; phobia, agitation, restlessness, aggressiveness/hostility, manic reaction, emotional lability; peripheral neuropathy, ataxia, incoordination; possible exacerbation of: myasthenia gravis and extrapyramidal disorders; dysphasia, lightheadedness (See **WARNINGS** and **PRECAUTIONS.**)
Respiratory System:	dyspnea, bronchospasm, allergic pneumonitis, stridor (See **WARNINGS.**)
Skin/Hypersensitivity:	anaphylactic (-toid) reactions/shock; purpura, serum sickness, erythema multiforme/Stevens-Johnson Syndrome, erythema nodosum, exfoliative dermatitis, hyperpigmentation, toxic epidermal necrolysis, conjunctivitis, photosensitivity, vesiculobullous eruption (See **WARNINGS** and **PRECAUTIONS.**)
Special Senses:	diplopia, nystagmus, blurred vision, disturbances of: taste, smell, hearing and equilibrium, usually reversible following discontinuation
Urinary System:	anuria, polyuria, renal calculi, renal failure, interstitial nephritis, hematuria (See **WARNINGS** and **PRECAUTIONS.**)
Laboratory:	
Hematopoietic:	prolongation of prothrombin time
Serum chemistry:	acidosis, elevation of: serum triglycerides, serum cholesterol, serum potassium, liver function tests including: GGTP, LDH, bilirubin
Urinary:	albuminuria, candiduria

In clinical trials using multiple-dose therapy, ophthalmologic abnormalities, including cataracts and multiple punctate lenticular opacities, have been noted in patients undergoing treatment with other quinolones. The relationship of the drugs to these events is not presently established.

CRYSTALLURIA and CYLINDRURIA HAVE BEEN REPORTED with other quinolones.

OVERDOSAGE

Information on overdosage with ofloxacin is limited. One incident of accidental overdosage has been reported. In this case, an adult female received 3 grams of ofloxacin intravenously over 45 minutes. A blood sample obtained 15 minutes after the completion of the infusion revealed an ofloxacin level of 39.3 μg/mL. In 7 h, the level had fallen to 16.2 μg/mL, and by 24 h to 2.7 μg/mL. During the infusion, the patient developed drowsiness, nausea, dizziness, hot and cold flushes, subjective facial swelling and numbness, slurring of speech, and mild to moderate disorientation. All complaints except the dizziness subsided within 1 h after discontinuation of the infusion. The dizziness, most bothersome while standing, resolved in approximately 9 h. Laboratory testing reportedly revealed no clinically significant changes in routine parameters in this patient.

In the event of an acute overdose, the stomach should be emptied. The patient should be observed and appropriate hydration maintained. Ofloxacin is not efficiently removed by hemodialysis or peritoneal dialysis.

DOSAGE AND ADMINISTRATION

The usual dose of FLOXIN (ofloxacin tablets) Tablets are 200 mg to 400 mg orally every 12 h as described in the following dosing chart. These recommendations apply to patients with normal renal function (i.e., creatinine clearance > 50 mL/min). For patients with altered renal function (i.e., creatinine clearance ≤ 50 mL/min), see the **Patients with Impaired Renal Function** subsection.

Patients with Normal Renal Function:

[See first table above]

Antacids containing calcium, magnesium, or aluminum; sucralfate; divalent or trivalent cations such as iron; or multivitamins containing zinc should not be taken within the two-hour period before, or within the two-hour period after ofloxacin administrations. (See **PRECAUTIONS.**)

Patients with Impaired Renal Function:

Dosage should be adjusted for patients with a creatinine clearance ≤ 50 mL/min.

After a normal initial dose, dosage should be adjusted as follows:

[See second table above]

When only the serum creatinine is known, the following formula may be used to estimate creatinine clearance.

Men: $\text{Creatinine clearance (mL/min)} = \dfrac{\text{Weight (kg)} \times (140 - \text{age})}{72 \times \text{serum creatinine (mg/dL)}}$

Women: 0.85 × the value calculated for men.

The serum creatinine should represent a steady-state of renal function.

Patients with Cirrhosis:

The excretion of ofloxacin may be reduced in patients with severe liver function disorders (e.g., cirrhosis with or without ascites). A maximum dose of 400 mg of ofloxacin per day should therefore not be exceeded.

HOW SUPPLIED

FLOXIN (ofloxacin tablets) Tablets are supplied as 200 mg light yellow, 300 mg white, and 400 mg pale gold film-coated tablets. Each tablet is distinguished by "FLOXIN" and the appropriate strength. FLOXIN Tablets are packaged in bottles and in unit-dose blister strips in the following configurations:

200 mg tablets — UROPAK unit-dose/6 tablets (NDC 0062-1540-09)

200 mg tablets — bottles of 50 (NDC 0062-1540-02)

200 mg tablets — unit-dose/100 tablets (NDC 0062-1540-05)

300 mg tablets — bottles of 50 (NDC 0062-1541-02)

300 mg tablets — unit-dose/100 tablets (NDC 0062-1541-05)

400 mg tablets — bottles of 100 (NDC 0062-1542-01)

400 mg tablets — unit-dose/100 tablets (NDC 0062-1542-05)

FLOXIN Tablets should be stored in well-closed containers. Store below 86°F (30°C).

Continued on next page

Floxin Tablets—Cont.

Also Available:
Ofloxacin is also available for intravenous administration in the following configurations:
FLOXIN (ofloxacin injection) I.V. IN SINGLE-USE VIALS (10 mL) containing a concentrated solution with the equivalent of 400 mg of ofloxacin.
FLOXIN (ofloxacin injection) I.V. PRE-MIXED IN FLEXIBLE CONTAINERS (50 mL and 100 mL) containing a dilute solution with the equivalent of 200 mg or 400 mg of ofloxacin, respectively, in 5% Dextrose (D_5W).

ANIMAL PHARMACOLOGY

Ofloxacin, as well as other drugs of the quinolone class, has been shown to cause arthropathies (arthrosis) in immature dogs and rats. In addition, these drugs are associated with an increased incidence of osteochondrosis in rats as compared to the incidence observed in vehicle-treated rats. (See ***WARNINGS***.) There is no evidence of arthropathies in fully mature dogs at intravenous doses up to 3 times the recommended maximum human dose (on a mg/m^2 basis or 5 times based on mg/kg basis), for a one-week exposure period.
Long-term, high-dose systemic use of other quinolones in experimental animals has caused lenticular opacities; however, this finding was not observed in any animal studies with ofloxacin.
Reduced serum globulin and protein levels were observed in animals treated with other quinolones. In one ofloxacin study, minor decreases in serum globulin and protein levels were noted in female cynomolgus monkeys dosed orally with 40 mg/kg ofloxacin for one year. These changes, however, were considered to be within normal limits for monkeys.
Crystalluria and ocular toxicity were not observed in any animals treated with ofloxacin.
Caution: Federal (U.S.A.) law prohibits dispensing without prescription.
FLOXIN® is a trademark of Ortho Pharmaceutical Corporation.
U.S. Patent No. 4,382,892

REFERENCES

1. National Committee for Clinical Laboratory Standards. Methods for Dilution Antimicrobial Susceptibility Tests for Bacteria That Grow Aerobically — Third Edition. Approved Standard NCCLS Document M7-A3, Vol. 13, No. 25, NCCLS, Villanova, PA, December, 1993.
2. National Committee for Clinical Laboratory Standards. Performance Standards for Antimicrobial Disk Susceptibility Tests — Fifth Edition. Approved Standard NCCLS Document M2-A5, Vol. 13, No. 24, NCCLS, Villanova, PA, December, 1993.

ORTHO PHARMACEUTICAL CORPORATION
Raritan, NJ USA 08869, and
McNEIL PHARMACEUTICAL
Spring House, PA USA 19477
 Revised April 1997 632-10-270-5
Shown in Product Identification Guide, pages 327 and 328

HALDOL® ℞
brand of
haloperidol
[hal 'dawl]
Tablets/Concentrate/Injection
(For Immediate Release)

DESCRIPTION

Haloperidol is the first of the butyrophenone series of major tranquilizers. The chemical designation is 4-[4-(p-chlorophenyl)-4-hydroxypiperidino]-4'-fluorobutyrophenone and it has the following structural formula:

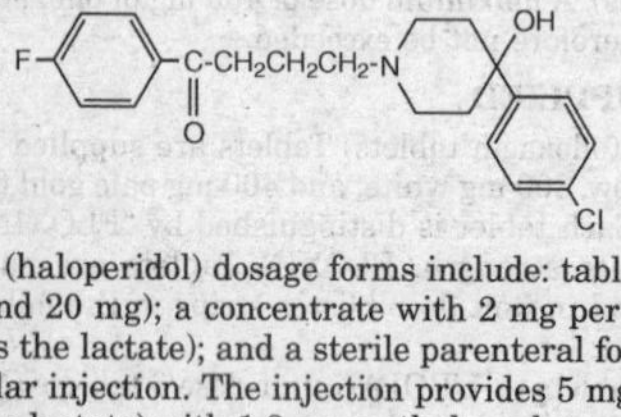

HALDOL (haloperidol) dosage forms include: tablets (½, 1, 2, 5, 10 and 20 mg); a concentrate with 2 mg per mL haloperidol (as the lactate); and a sterile parenteral form for intramuscular injection. The injection provides 5 mg haloperidol (as the lactate) with 1.8 mg methylparaben and 0.2 mg propylparaben per mL, and lactic acid for pH adjustment between 3.0–3.6.
Inactive ingredients: tablets—calcium phosphate, calcium stearate, corn starch and flavor—1mg contains D&C Yellow No. 10 and FD&C Red No. 40; 2mg contains D&C Red No. 33 and FD&C Blue No. 2; 5mg contains FD&C Blue No. 1, D&C Yellow No. 10 and D&C Red No. 30; 10 mg contains FD&C Blue No. 1, D&C Yellow No. 10 and D&C Red No. 30; and 20 mg contains FD&C Red No. 40; concentrate - lactic acid and methylparaben.

ACTIONS

The precise mechanism of action has not been clearly established.

INDICATIONS

HALDOL (haloperidol) is indicated for use in the management of manifestations of psychotic disorders.
HALDOL is indicated for the control of tics and vocal utterances of Tourette's Disorder in children and adults.
HALDOL is effective for the treatment of severe behavior problems in children of combative, explosive hyperexcitability (which cannot be accounted for by immediate provocation). HALDOL is also effective in the short-term treatment of hyperactive children who show excessive motor activity with accompanying conduct disorders consisting of some or all of the following symptoms: impulsivity, difficulty sustaining attention, aggressivity, mood lability and poor frustration tolerance. HALDOL should be reserved for these two groups of children only after failure to respond to psychotherapy or medications other than antipsychotics.

CONTRAINDICATIONS

HALDOL haloperidol is contraindicated in severe toxic central nervous system depression or comatose states from any cause and in individuals who are hypersensitive to this drug or have Parkinson's disease.

WARNINGS

Tardive Dyskinesia
A syndrome consisting of potentially irreversible, involuntary, dyskinetic movements may develop in patients treated with antipsychotic drugs. Although the prevalence of the syndrome appears to be highest among the elderly, especially elderly women, it is impossible to rely upon prevalence estimates to predict, at the inception of antipsychotic treatment, which patients are likely to develop the syndrome. Whether antipsychotic drug products differ in their potential to cause tardive dyskinesia is unknown.
Both the risk of developing tardive dyskinesia and the likelihood that it will become irreversible are believed to increase as the duration of treatment and the total cumulative dose of antipsychotic drugs administered to the patient increase. However, the syndrome can develop, although much less commonly, after relatively brief treatment periods at low doses.
There is no known treatment for established cases of tardive dyskinesia, although the syndrome may remit, partially or completely, if antipsychotic treatment is withdrawn. Antipsychotic treatment, itself, however, may suppress (or partially suppress) the signs and symptoms of the syndrome and thereby may possibly mask the underlying process. The effect that symptomatic suppression has upon the long-term course of the syndrome is unknown.
Given these considerations, antipsychotic drugs should be prescribed in a manner that is most likely to minimize the occurrence of tardive dyskinesia. Chronic antipsychotic treatment should generally be reserved for patients who suffer from a chronic illness that, 1) is known to respond to antipsychotic drugs, and 2) for whom alternative, equally effective, but potentially less harmful treatments are **not** available or appropriate. In patients who do require chronic treatment, the smallest dose and the shortest duration of treatment producing a satisfactory clinical response should be sought. The need for continued treatment should be reassessed periodically.
If signs and symptoms of tardive dyskinesia appear in a patient on antipsychotics, drug discontinuation should be considered. However, some patients may require treatment despite the presence of the syndrome.
(For further information about the description of tardive dyskinesia and its clinical detection, please refer to ADVERSE REACTIONS.)

Neuroleptic Malignant Syndrome (NMS)
A potentially fatal symptom complex sometimes referred to as Neuroleptic Malignant Syndrome (NMS) has been reported in association with antipsychotic drugs. Clinical manifestations of NMS are hyperpyrexia, muscle rigidity, altered mental status (including catatonic signs) and evidence of autonomic instability (irregular pulse or blood pressure, tachycardia, diaphoresis, and cardiac dysrhythmias). Additional signs may include elevated creatine phosphokinase, myoglobinuria (rhabdomyolysis) and acute renal failure.
The diagnostic evaluation of patients with this syndrome is complicated. In arriving at a diagnosis, it is important to identify cases where the clinical presentation includes both serious medical illness (e.g., pneumonia, systemic infection, etc.) and untreated or inadequately treated extrapyramidal signs and symptoms (EPS). Other important considerations in the differential diagnosis include central anticholinergic toxicity, heat stroke, drug fever and primary central nervous system (CNS) pathology.
The management of NMS should include 1) immediate discontinuation of antipsychotic drugs and other drugs not essential to concurrent therapy, 2) intensive symptomatic treatment and medical monitoring, and 3) treatment of any concomitant serious medical problems for which specific treatments are available. There is no general agreement about specific pharmacological treatment regimens for uncomplicated NMS.
If a patient requires antipsychotic drug treatment after recovery from NMS, the potential reintroduction of drug therapy should be carefully considered. The patient should be carefully monitored, since recurrences of NMS have been reported.
Hyperpyrexia and heat stroke, not associated with the above symptom complex, have also been reported with HALDOL.

Usage in Pregnancy
Rodents given 2 to 20 times the usual maximum human dose of haloperidol by oral or parenteral routes showed an increase in incidence of resorption, reduced fertility, delayed delivery and pup mortality. No teratogenic effect has been reported in rats, rabbits or dogs at dosages within this range, but cleft palate has been observed in mice given 15 times the usual maximum human dose. Cleft palate in mice appears to be a nonspecific response to stress or nutritional imbalance as well as to a variety of drugs, and there is no evidence to relate this phenomenon to predictable human risk for most of these agents.
There are no well controlled studies with HALDOL (haloperidol) in pregnant women. There are reports, however, of cases of limb malformations observed following maternal use of HALDOL along with other drugs which have suspected teratogenic potential during the first trimester of pregnancy. Causal relationships were not established in these cases. Since such experience does not exclude the possibility of fetal damage due to HALDOL, this drug should be used during pregnancy or in women likely to become pregnant only if the benefit clearly justifies a potential risk to the fetus. Infants should not be nursed during drug treatment.

Combined Use of HALDOL and Lithium
An encephalopathic syndrome (characterized by weakness, lethargy, fever, tremulousness and confusion, extrapyramidal symptoms, leukocytosis, elevated serum enzymes, BUN, and FBS) followed by irreversible brain damage has occurred in a few patients treated with lithium plus HALDOL. A causal relationship between these events and the concomitant administration of lithium and HALDOL has not been established; however, patients receiving such combined therapy should be monitored closely for early evidence of neurological toxicity and treatment discontinued promptly if such signs appear.

General
A number of cases of bronchopneumonia, some fatal, have followed the use of antipsychotic drugs, including HALDOL. It has been postulated that lethargy and decreased sensation of thirst due to central inhibition may lead to dehydration, hemoconcentration and reduced pulmonary ventilation. Therefore, if the above signs and symptoms appear, especially in the elderly, the physician should institute remedial therapy promptly.
Although not reported with HALDOL, decreased serum cholesterol and/or cutaneous and ocular changes have been reported in patients receiving chemically-related drugs.
HALDOL may impair the mental and/or physical abilities required for the performance of hazardous tasks such as operating machinery or driving a motor vehicle. The ambulatory patient should be warned accordingly.
The use of alcohol with this drug should be avoided due to possible additive effects and hypotension.

PRECAUTIONS

HALDOL (haloperidol) should be administered cautiously to patients:
— with severe cardiovascular disorders, because of the possibility of transient hypotension and/or precipitation of anginal pain. Should hypotension occur and a vasopressor be required, epinephrine should not be used since HALDOL may block its vasopressor activity and paradoxical further lowering of the blood pressure may occur. Instead, metaraminol, phenylephrine or norepinephrine should be used.
— receiving anticonvulsant medications, with a history of seizures, or with EEG abnormalities, because HALDOL may lower the convulsive threshold. If indicated, adequate anticonvulsant therapy should be concomitantly maintained.
— with known allergies, or with a history of allergic reactions to drugs.
— receiving anticoagulants, since an isolated instance of interference occurred with the effects of one anticoagulant (phenindione).

If concomitant antiparkinson medication is required, it may have to be continued after HALDOL is discontinued because of the difference in excretion rates. If both are discontinued simultaneously, extrapyramidal symptoms may occur. The physician should keep in mind the possible increase in intraocular pressure when anticholinergic drugs, including antiparkinson agents, are administered concomitantly with HALDOL.

As with other antipsychotic agents, it should be noted that HALDOL may be capable of potentiating CNS depressants such as anesthetics, opiates, and alcohol.

When HALDOL is used to control mania in cyclic disorders, there may be a rapid mood swing to depression.

Severe neurotoxicity (rigidity, inability to walk or talk) may occur in patients with thyrotoxicosis who are also receiving antipsychotic medication, including HALDOL.

No mutagenic potential of haloperidol was found in the Ames Salmonella microsomal activation assay. Negative or inconsistent positive findings have been obtained in *in vitro* and *in vivo* studies of effects of haloperidol on chromosome structure and number. The available cytogenetic evidence is considered too inconsistent to be conclusive at this time.

Carcinogenicity studies using oral haloperidol were conducted in Wistar rats (dosed at up to 5 mg/kg daily for 24 months) and in Albino Swiss mice (dosed at up to 5 mg/kg daily for 18 months). In the rat study survival was less than optimal in all dose groups, reducing the number of rats at risk for developing tumors. However, although a relatively greater number of rats survived to the end of the study in high dose male and female groups, these animals did not have a greater incidence of tumors than control animals. Therefore, although not optimal, this study does suggest the absence of a haloperidol related increase in the incidence of neoplasia in rats at doses up to 20 times the usual daily human dose for chronic or resistant patients.

In female mice at 5 and 20 times the highest initial daily dose for chronic or resistant patients, there was a statistically significant increase in mammary gland neoplasia and total tumor incidence; at 20 times the same daily dose there was a statistically significant increase in pituitary gland neoplasia. In male mice, no statistically significant differences in incidences of total tumors or specific tumor types were noted.

Antipsychotic drugs elevate prolactin levels; the elevation persists during chronic administration. Tissue culture experiments indicate that approximately one-third of human breast cancers are prolactin dependent *in vitro*, a factor of potential importance if the prescription of these drugs is contemplated in a patient with a previously detected breast cancer. Although disturbances such as galactorrhea, amenorrhea, gynecomastia, and impotence have been reported, the clinical significance of elevated serum prolactin levels is unknown for most patients. An increase in mammary neoplasms has been found in rodents after chronic administration of antipsychotic drugs. Neither clinical studies nor epidemiologic studies conducted to date, however, have shown an association between chronic administration of these drugs and mammary tumorigenesis; the available evidence is considered too limited to be conclusive at this time.

ADVERSE REACTIONS
CNS Effects:
Extrapyramidal Symptoms (EPS)—EPS during the administration of HALDOL (haloperidol) have been reported frequently, often during the first few days of treatment. EPS can be categorized generally as Parkinson-like symptoms, akathisia, or dystonia (including opisthotonos and oculogyric crisis). While all can occur at relatively low doses, they occur more frequently and with greater severity at higher doses. The symptoms may be controlled with dose reductions or administration of antiparkinson drugs such as benztropine mesylate USP or trihexyphenidyl hydrochloride USP. It should be noted that persistent EPS have been reported; the drug may have to be discontinued in such cases.
Withdrawal Emergent Neurological Signs—Generally, patients receiving short-term therapy experience no problems with abrupt discontinuation of antipsychotic drugs. However, some patients on maintenance treatment experience transient dyskinetic signs after abrupt withdrawal. In certain of these cases the dyskinetic movements are indistinguishable from the syndrome described below under "Tardive Dyskinesia" except for duration. It is not known whether gradual withdrawal of antipsychotic drugs will reduce the rate of occurrence of withdrawal emergent neurological signs but until further evidence becomes available, it seems reasonable to gradually withdraw use of HALDOL.
Tardive Dyskinesia—As with all antipsychotic agents HALDOL has been associated with persistent dyskinesias. Tardive dyskinesia, a syndrome consisting of potentially irreversible, involuntary, dyskinetic movements, may appear in some patients on long-term therapy or may occur after drug therapy has been discontinued. The risk appears to be greater in elderly patients on high-dose therapy, especially females. The symptoms are persistent and in some patients appear irreversible. The syndrome is characterized by rhythmical involuntary movements of tongue, face, mouth or jaw (e.g., protrusion of tongue, puffing of cheeks, puckering of mouth, chewing movements). Sometimes these may be accompanied by involuntary movements of extremities and the trunk.

There is no known effective treatment for tardive dyskinesia; antiparkinson agents usually do not alleviate the symptoms of this syndrome. It is suggested that all antipsychotic agents be discontinued if these symptoms appear. Should it

be necessary to reinstitute treatment, or increase the dosage of the agent, or switch to a different antipsychotic agent, this syndrome may be masked.

It has been reported that fine vermicular movement of the tongue may be an early sign of tardive dyskinesia and if the medication is stopped at that time the full syndrome may not develop.

Tardive Dystonia—Tardive dystonia, not associated with the above syndrome, has also been reported. Tardive dystonia is characterized by delayed onset of choreic or dystonic movements, is often persistent, and has the potential of becoming irreversible.

Other CNS Effects—Insomnia, restlessness, anxiety, euphoria, agitation, drowsiness, depression, lethargy, headache, confusion, vertigo, grand mal seizures, exacerbation of psychotic symptoms including hallucinations, and catatonic-like behavioral states which may be responsive to drug withdrawal and/or treatment with anticholinergic drugs.

Body as a Whole: Neuroleptic malignant syndrome (NMS), hyperpyrexia and heat stroke have been reported with HALDOL. (See WARNINGS for further information concerning NMS.)

Cardiovascular Effects: Tachycardia, hypotension, hypertension and ECG changes including prolongation of the Q-T interval and ECG pattern changes compatible with the polymorphous configuration of torsade de pointes.

Hematologic Effects: Reports have appeared citing the occurrence of mild and usually transient leukopenia and leukocytosis, minimal decreases in red blood cell counts, anemia, or a tendency toward lymphomonocytosis. Agranulocytosis has rarely been reported to have occurred with the use of HALDOL, and then only in association with other medication.

Liver Effects: Impaired liver function and/or jaundice have been reported.

Dermatologic Reactions: Maculopapular and acneiform skin reactions and isolated cases of photosensitivity and loss of hair.

Endocrine Disorders: Lactation, breast engorgement, mastalgia, menstrual irregularities, gynecomastia, impotence, increased libido, hyperglycemia, hypoglycemia and hyponatremia.

Gastrointestinal Effects: Anorexia, constipation, diarrhea, hypersalivation, dyspepsia, nausea and vomiting.

Autonomic Reactions: Dry mouth, blurred vision, urinary retention, diaphoresis and priapism.

Respiratory Effects: Laryngospasm, bronchospasm and increased depth of respiration.

Special Senses: Cataracts, retinopathy and visual disturbances.

Other: Cases of sudden and unexpected death have been reported in association with the administration of HALDOL. The nature of the evidence makes it impossible to determine definitively what role, if any, HALDOL played in the outcome of the reported cases. The possibility that HALDOL caused death cannot, of course, be excluded, but it is to be kept in mind that sudden and unexpected death may occur in psychotic patients when they go untreated or when they are treated with other antipsychotic drugs.

Postmarketing Events: Hyperammonemia has been reported in a 5$^{1}/_{2}$ year old child with citrullinemia, an inherited disorder of ammonia excretion, following treatment with HALDOL.

OVERDOSAGE
Manifestations
In general, the symptoms of overdosage would be an exaggeration of known pharmacologic effects and adverse reactions, the most prominent of which would be: 1) severe extrapyramidal reactions, 2) hypotension, or 3) sedation. The patient would appear comatose with respiratory depression and hypotension which could be severe enough to produce a shock-like state. The extrapyramidal reaction would be manifest by muscular weakness or rigidity and a generalized or localized tremor as demonstrated by the akinetic or agitans types respectively. With accidental overdosage, hypertension rather than hypotension occurred in a two-year old child. The risk of ECG changes associated with torsades de pointes should be considered. (For further information regarding torsades de pointes, please refer to ADVERSE REACTIONS.)

Treatment
Gastric lavage or induction of emesis should be carried out immediately followed by administration of activated charcoal. Since there is no specific antidote, treatment is primarily supportive. A patent airway must be established by use of an oropharyngeal airway or endotracheal tube or, in prolonged cases of coma, by tracheostomy. Respiratory depression may be counteracted by artificial respiration and mechanical respirators. Hypotension and circulatory collapse may be counteracted by use of intravenous fluids, plasma, or concentrated albumin, and vasopressor agents such as metaraminol, phenylephrine and norepinephrine. Epinephrine should not be used. In case of severe extrapyramidal reactions, antiparkinson medication should be administered. ECG and vital signs should be monitored especially

for signs of Q-T prolongation or dysrhythmias and monitoring should continue until the ECG is normal. Severe arrhythmias should be treated with appropriate anti-arrhythmic measures.

DOSAGE AND ADMINISTRATION
There is considerable variation from patient to patient in the amount of medication required for treatment. As with all antipsychotic drugs, dosage should be individualized according to the needs and response of each patient. Dosage adjustments, either upward or downward, should be carried out as rapidly as practicable to achieve optimum therapeutic control.

To determine the initial dosage, consideration should be given to the patient's age, severity of illness, previous response to other antipsychotic drugs, and any concomitant medication or disease state. Children, debilitated or geriatric patients, as well as those with a history of adverse reactions to antipsychotic drugs, may require less HALDOL haloperidol. The optimal response in such patients is usually obtained with more gradual dosage adjustments and at lower dosage levels, as recommended below.

Clinical experience suggests the following recommendations:

Oral Administration
Initial Dosage Range
Adults

Moderate Symptomatology	0.5 mg to 2.0 mg b.i.d. or t.i.d.
Severe Symptomatology	3.0 mg to 5.0 mg b.i.d. or t.i.d.

To achieve prompt control, higher doses may be required in some cases.

Geriatric or Debilitated Patients	0.5 mg to 2.0 mg b.i.d. or t.i.d.
Chronic or Resistant Patients	3.0 mg to 5.0 mg b.i.d. or t.i.d.

Patients who remain severely disturbed or inadequately controlled may require dosage adjustment. Daily dosages up to 100 mg may be necessary in some cases to achieve an optimal response. Infrequently, HALDOL has been used in doses above 100 mg for severely resistant patients; however, the limited clinical usage has not demonstrated the safety of prolonged administration of such doses.

Children
The following recommendations apply to children between the ages of 3 and 12 years (weight range 15 to 40 kg). HALDOL is not intended for children under 3 years old. Therapy should begin at the lowest dose possible (0.5 mg per day). If required, the dose should be increased by an increment of 0.5 mg at 5 to 7 day intervals until the desired therapeutic effect is obtained. (See chart below).
The total dose may be divided, to be given b.i.d. or t.i.d.

Psychotic Disorders	0.05 mg/kg/day to 0.15 mg/kg/day
Non-Psychotic Behavior Disorders and Tourette's Disorder	0.05 mg/kg/day to 0.075 mg/kg/day

Severely disturbed psychotic children may require higher doses. In severely disturbed, non-psychotic children or in hyperactive children with accompanying conduct disorders, who have failed to respond to psychotherapy or medications other than antipsychotics, it should be noted that since these behaviors may be short-lived, short-term administration of HALDOL may suffice. There is no evidence establishing a maximum effective dosage. There is little evidence that behavior improvement is further enhanced in dosages beyond 6 mg per day.

Maintenance Dosage
Upon achieving a satisfactory therapeutic response, dosage should then be gradually reduced to the lowest effective maintenance level.
Intramuscular Administration
Adults
Parenteral medication, administered intramuscularly in doses of 2 to 5 mg, is utilized for prompt control of the acutely agitated patient with moderately severe to very se-

Continued on next page

Haldol—Cont.

vere symptoms. Depending on the response of the patient, subsequent doses may be given, administered as often as every hour, although 4 to 8 hour intervals may be satisfactory.

Controlled trials to establish the safety and effectiveness of intramuscular administration in children have not been conducted.

Parenteral drug products should be inspected visually for particulate matter and discoloration prior to administration, whenever solution and container permit.

Switchover Procedure

The oral form should supplant the injectable as soon as practicable. In the absence of bioavailability studies establishing bioequivalence between these two dosage forms the following guidelines for dosage are suggested. For an initial approximation of the total daily dose required, the parenteral dose administered in the preceding 24 hours may be used. Since this dose is only an initial estimate, it is recommended that careful monitoring of clinical signs and symptoms, including clinical efficacy, sedation, and adverse effects, be carried out periodically for the first several days following the initiation of switchover. In this way, dosage adjustments, either upward or downward, can be quickly accomplished. Depending on the patient's clinical status, the first oral dose should be given within 12–24 hours following the last parenteral dose.

HOW SUPPLIED

HALDOL® brand of haloperidol Tablets with a cut-out "H" design, Scored, Imprinted "McNeil" and "HALDOL" with the mg strength of the tablet:

		Bottles Containing 100
1/2 mg, white	NDC 0045-0240-60	x
1 mg, yellow	NDC 0045-0241-60	x
2 mg, pink	NDC 0045-0242-60	x
5 mg, green	NDC 0045-0245-60	x
10 mg, aqua	NDC 0045-0246-60	x
20 mg, salmon	NDC 0045-0248-60	x

HALDOL® brand of haloperidol Concentrate 2 mg per mL (as the lactate) Colorless, Odorless, and Tasteless Solution—NDC 0045-0250-15, bottles of 15 mL and NDC 0045-0250-04, bottles of 120 mL.

HALDOL® brand of haloperidol Injection (For Immediate Release) 5 mg per mL (as the lactate)—NDC 0045-0255-01, units of 10 × 1 mL ampuls and NDC 0045-0255-49, 10 mL multiple-dose vial.

Store HALDOL® haloperidol Tablets at controlled room temperature (15°-30°C, 59°-86°F). Protect from light.

Store HALDOL® haloperidol Concentrate at controlled room temperature (15°-30°C, 59°-86°F). Protect from light. Do not freeze.

Store HALDOL® haloperidol Injection at controlled room temperature (15°-30°C, 59°-86°F). Protect from light. Do not freeze.

Dispense the HALDOL haloperidol tablets and concentrate in a tight, light-resistent container as defined in the official compendium.

McNEIL PHARMACEUTICAL
McNEILAB, INC.
SPRING HOUSE, PA 19477

643-94-066-3 Revised April 1997

Shown in Product Identification Guide, page 328

HALDOL® Decanoate 50 (haloperidol) ℞
HALDOL® Decanoate 100 (haloperidol) ℞

[hal 'dawl dek "ah-nō 'ōt]

For IM Injection Only

DESCRIPTION

Haloperidol decanoate is the decanoate ester of the butyrophenone, HALDOL haloperidol. It has a markedly extended duration of effect. It is available in sesame oil in sterile form for intramuscular (IM) injection. The structural formula of haloperidol decanoate, 4-(4-chlorophenyl)-1-[4-(4-fluorophenyl)-4-oxobutyl]-4 piperidinyl decanoate, is:

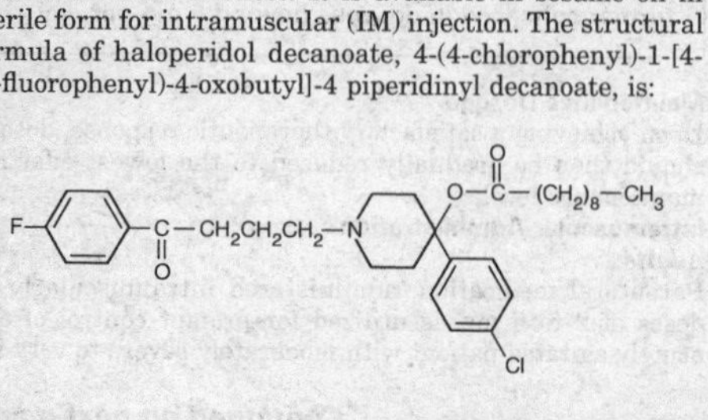

Haloperidol decanoate is almost insoluble in water (0.01 mg/mL), but is soluble in most organic solvents.

Each mL of HALDOL Decanoate 50 for IM injection contains 50 mg haloperidol (present as haloperidol decanoate 70.52 mg) in a sesame oil vehicle, with 1.2% (w/v) benzyl alcohol as a preservative.

Each mL of HALDOL Decanoate 100 for IM injection contains 100 mg haloperidol (present as haloperidol decanoate 141.04 mg) in a sesame oil vehicle, with 1.2% (w/v) benzyl alcohol as a preservative.

CLINICAL PHARMACOLOGY

HALDOL Decanoate 50 and HALDOL Decanoate 100 are the long-acting forms of HALDOL haloperidol. The basic effects of haloperidol decanoate are no different from those of HALDOL with the exception of duration of action. Haloperidol blocks the effects of dopamine and increases its turnover rate; however, the precise mechanism of action is unknown.

Administration of haloperidol decanoate in sesame oil results in slow and sustained release of haloperidol. The plasma concentrations of haloperidol gradually rise, reaching a peak at about 6 days after the injection, and falling thereafter, with an apparent half-life of about 3 weeks. Steady state plasma concentrations are achieved after the third or fourth dose. The relationship between dose of haloperidol decanoate and plasma haloperidol concentration is roughly linear for doses below 450 mg. It should be noted, however, that the pharmacokinetics of haloperidol decanoate following intramuscular injections can be quite variable between subjects.

INDICATIONS AND USAGE

HALDOL Decanoate 50 and HALDOL Decanoate 100 are long-acting parenteral antipsychotic drugs intended for use in the management of patients requiring prolonged parenteral antipsychotic therapy (e.g., patients with chronic schizophrenia).

CONTRAINDICATIONS

Since the pharmacologic and clinical actions of HALDOL Decanoate 50 and HALDOL Decanoate 100 are attributed to HALDOL haloperidol as the active medication, Contraindications, Warnings, and additional information are those of HALDOL, modified only to reflect the prolonged action.

HALDOL is contraindicated in severe toxic central nervous system depression or comatose states from any cause and in individuals who are hypersensitive to this drug or have Parkinson's disease.

WARNINGS

Tardive Dyskinesia

A syndrome consisting of potentially irreversible, involuntary, dyskinetic movements may develop in patients treated with antipsychotic drugs. Although the prevalence of the syndrome appears to be highest among the elderly, especially elderly women, it is impossible to rely upon prevalence estimates to predict, at the inception of antipsychotic treatment, which patients are likely to develop the syndrome. Whether antipsychotic drug products differ in their potential to cause tardive dyskinesia is unknown.

Both the risk of developing tardive dyskinesia and the likelihood that it will become irreversible are believed to increase as the duration of treatment and the total cumulative dose of antipsychotic drugs administered to the patient increase. However, the syndrome can develop, although much less commonly, after relatively brief treatment periods at low doses.

There is no known treatment for established cases of tardive dyskinesia, although the syndrome may remit, partially or completely, if antipsychotic treatment is withdrawn. Antipsychotic treatment, itself, however, may suppress (or partially suppress) the signs and symptoms of the syndrome and thereby may possibly mask the underlying process. The effect that symptomatic suppression has upon the long-term course of the syndrome is unknown.

Given these considerations, antipsychotic drugs should be prescribed in a manner that is most likely to minimize the occurrence of tardive dyskinesia. Chronic antipsychotic treatment should generally be reserved for patients who suffer from a chronic illness that 1) is known to respond to antipsychotic drugs, and 2) for whom alternative, equally effective, but potentially less harmful treatments are **not** available or appropriate. In patients who do require chronic treatment, the smallest dose and the shortest duration of treatment producing a satisfactory clinical response should be sought. The need for continued treatment should be reassessed periodically.

If signs and symptoms of tardive dyskinesia appear in a patient on antipsychotics, drug discontinuation should be considered. However, some patients may require treatment despite the presence of the syndrome. (For further information about the description of tardive dyskinesia and its clinical detection, please refer to ADVERSE REACTIONS.)

Neuroleptic Malignant Syndrome (NMS)

A potentially fatal symptom complex sometimes referred to as Neuroleptic Malignant Syndrome (NMS) has been reported in association with antipsychotic drugs. Clinical manifestations of NMS are hyperpyrexia, muscle rigidity, altered mental status (including catatonic signs) and evidence of autonomic instability (irregular pulse or blood pressure, tachycardia, diaphoresis, and cardiac dysrhythmias). Additional signs may include elevated creatine phosphokinase, myoglobinuria (rhabdomyolysis) and acute renal failure.

The diagnostic evaluation of patients with this syndrome is complicated. In arriving at a diagnosis, it is important to identify cases where the clinical presentation includes both serious medical illness (e.g., pneumonia, systemic infection, etc.) and untreated or inadequately treated extrapyramidal signs and symptoms (EPS). Other important considerations in the differential diagnosis include central anticholinergic toxicity, heat stroke, drug fever and primary central nervous system (CNS) pathology.

The management of NMS should include 1) immediate discontinuation of antipsychotic drugs and other drugs not essential to concurrent therapy, 2) intensive symptomatic treatment and medical monitoring, and 3) treatment of any concomitant serious medical problems for which specific treatments are available. There is no general agreement about specific pharmacological treatment regimens for uncomplicated NMS.

If a patient requires antipsychotic drug treatment after recovery from NMS, the potential reintroduction of drug therapy should be carefully considered. The patient should be carefully monitored, since recurrences of NMS have been reported.

Hyperpyrexia and heat stroke, not associated with the above symptom complex, have also been reported with HALDOL.

General

A number of cases of bronchopneumonia, some fatal, have followed the use of antipsychotic drugs, including HALDOL (haloperidol). It has been postulated that lethargy and decreased sensation of thirst due to central inhibition may lead to dehydration, hemoconcentration and reduced pulmonary ventilation. Therefore, if the above signs and symptoms appear, especially in the elderly, the physician should institute remedial therapy promptly.

Although not reported with HALDOL, decreased serum cholesterol and/or cutaneous and ocular changes have been reported in patients receiving chemically-related drugs.

PRECAUTIONS

HALDOL Decanoate 50 and HALDOL Decanoate 100 should be administered cautiously to patients:

— with severe cardiovascular disorders, because of the possibility of transient hypotension and/or precipitation of anginal pain. Should hypotension occur and a vasopressor be required, epinephrine should not be used since HALDOL (haloperidol) may block its vasopressor activity, and paradoxical further lowering of the blood pressure may occur. Instead, metaraminol, phenylephrine or norepinephrine should be used.

— receiving anticonvulsant medications, with a history of seizures, or with EEG abnormalities, because HALDOL may lower the convulsive threshold. If indicated, adequate anticonvulsant therapy should be concomitantly maintained.

— with known allergies, or with a history of allergic reactions to drugs.

— receiving anticoagulants, since an isolated instance of interference occurred with the effects of one anticoagulant (phenindione).

If concomitant antiparkinson medication is required, it may have to be continued after HALDOL Decanoate 50 or HALDOL Decanoate 100 is discontinued because of the prolonged action of haloperidol decanoate. If both drugs are discontinued simultaneously, extrapyramidal symptoms may occur. The physician should keep in mind the possible increase in intraocular pressure when anticholinergic drugs, including antiparkinson agents, are administered concomitantly with haloperidol decanoate.

In patients with thyrotoxicosis who are also receiving antipsychotic medication, including haloperidol decanoate, severe neurotoxicity (rigidity, inability to walk or talk) may occur.

When HALDOL is used to control mania in bipolar disorders, there may be a rapid mood swing to depression.

Information for Patients

Haloperidol decanoate may impair the mental and/or physical abilities required for the performance of hazardous tasks such as operating machinery or driving a motor vehicle. The ambulatory patient should be warned accordingly. The use of alcohol with this drug should be avoided due to possible additive effects and hypotension.

Drug Interactions

An encephalopathic syndrome (characterized by weakness, lethargy, fever, tremulousness and confusion, extrapyramidal symptoms, leukocytosis, elevated serum enzymes, BUN, and FBS) followed by irreversible brain damage has occurred in a few patients treated with lithium plus HALDOL. A causal relationship between these events and the concomitant administration of lithium and HALDOL

has not been established; however, patients receiving such combined therapy should be monitored closely for early evidence of neurological toxicity and treatment discontinued promptly if such signs appear.

As with other antipsychotic agents, it should be noted that HALDOL may be capable of potentiating CNS depressants such as anesthetics, opiates, and alcohol.

Carcinogenesis, Mutagenesis, and Impairment of Fertility
No mutagenic potential of haloperidol decanoate was found in the Ames Salmonella microsomal activation assay. Negative or inconsistent positive findings have been obtained in *in vitro* and *in vivo* studies of effects of short-acting haloperidol on chromosome structure and number. The available cytogenetic evidence is considered too inconsistent to be conclusive at this time.

Carcinogenicity studies using oral haloperidol were conducted in Wistar rats (dosed at up to 5 mg/kg daily for 24 months) and in Albino Swiss mice (dosed at up to 5 mg/kg daily for 18 months). In the rat study survival was less than optimal in all dose groups, reducing the number of rats at risk for developing tumors. However, although a relatively greater number of rats survived to the end of the study in high dose male and female groups, these animals did not have a greater incidence of tumors than control animals. Therefore, although not optimal, this study does suggest the absence of a haloperidol related increase in the incidence of neoplasia in rats at doses up to 20 times the usual daily human dose for chronic or resistant patients.

In female mice at 5 and 20 times the highest initial daily dose for chronic or resistant patients, there was a statistically significant increase in mammary gland neoplasia and total tumor incidence; at 20 times the same daily dose there was a statistically significant increase in pituitary gland neoplasia. In male mice, no statistically significant differences in incidences of total tumors or specific tumor types were noted.

Antipsychotic drugs elevate prolactin levels; the elevation persists during chronic administration. Tissue culture experiments indicate that approximately one-third of human breast cancers are prolactin dependent *in vitro*, a factor of potential importance if the prescription of these drugs is contemplated in a patient with a previously detected breast cancer. Although disturbances such as galactorrhea, amenorrhea, gynecomastia, and impotence have been reported, the clinical significance of elevated serum prolactin levels is unknown for most patients.

An increase in mammary neoplasms has been found in rodents after chronic administration of antipsychotic drugs. Neither clinical studies nor epidemiologic studies conducted to date, however, have shown an association between chronic administration of these drugs and mammary tumorigenesis; the available evidence is considered too limited to be conclusive at this time.

Usage in Pregnancy
Pregnancy Category C. Rodents given up to 3 times the usual maximum human dose of haloperidol decanoate showed an increase in incidence of resorption, fetal mortality, and pup mortality. No fetal abnormalities were observed.

Cleft palate has been observed in mice given oral haloperidol at 15 times the usual maximum human dose. Cleft palate in mice appears to be a non-specific response to stress or nutritional imbalance as well as to a variety of drugs, and there is no evidence to relate this phenomenon to predictable human risk for most of these agents.

There are no adequate and well-controlled studies in pregnant women. There are reports, however, of cases of limb malformations observed following maternal use of HALDOL along with other drugs which have suspected teratogenic potential during the first trimester of pregnancy. Causal relationships were not established with these cases. Since such experience does not exclude the possibility of fetal damage due to HALDOL, haloperidol decanoate should be used during pregnancy or in women likely to become pregnant only if the benefit clearly justifies a potential risk to the fetus.

Nursing Mothers
Since haloperidol is excreted in human breast milk, infants should not be nursed during drug treatment with haloperidol decanoate.

Pediatric Use
Safety and effectiveness of haloperidol decanoate in children have not been established.

ADVERSE REACTIONS

Adverse reactions following the administration of HALDOL Decanoate 50 or HALDOL Decanoate 100 are those of HALDOL (haloperidol). Since vast experience has accumulated with HALDOL, the adverse reactions are reported for that compound as well as for haloperidol decanoate. As with all injectable medications, local tissue reactions have been reported with haloperidol decanoate.

CNS Effects:
Extrapyramidal Symptoms (EPS) —EPS during the administration of HALDOL (haloperidol) have been reported frequently, often during the first few days of treatment. EPS

can be categorized generally as Parkinson-like symptoms, akathisia, or dystonia (including opisthotonos and oculogyric crisis). While all can occur at relatively low doses, they occur more frequently and with greater severity at higher doses. The symptoms may be controlled with dose reductions or administration of antiparkinson drugs such as benztropine mesylate USP or trihexyphenidyl hydrochloride USP. It should be noted that persistent EPS have been reported; the drug may have to be discontinued in such cases.

Withdrawal Emergent Neurological Signs —Generally, patients receiving short term therapy experience no problems with abrupt discontinuation of antipsychotic drugs. However, some patients on maintenance treatment experience transient dyskinetic signs after abrupt withdrawal. In certain of these cases the dyskinetic movements are indistinguishable from the syndrome described below under "Tardive Dyskinesia" except for duration. Although the long acting properties of haloperidol decanoate provide gradual withdrawal, it is not known whether gradual withdrawal of antipsychotic drugs will reduce the rate of occurrence of withdrawal emergent neurological signs.

Tardive Dyskinesia —As with all antipsychotic agents HALDOL has been associated with persistent dyskinesias. Tardive dyskinesia, a syndrome consisting of potentially irreversible, involuntary, dyskinetic movements, may appear in some patients on long-term therapy with haloperidol decanoate or may occur after drug therapy has been discontinued. The risk appears to be greater in elderly patients on high-dose therapy, especially females. The symptoms are persistent and in some patients appear irreversible. The syndrome is characterized by rhythmical involuntary movements of tongue, face, mouth, or jaw (e.g., protrusion of tongue, puffing of cheeks, puckering of mouth, chewing movements). Sometimes these may be accompanied by involuntary movements of extremities and the trunk.

There is no known effective treatment for tardive dyskinesia; antiparkinson agents usually do not alleviate the symptoms of this syndrome. It is suggested that all antipsychotic agents be discontinued if these symptoms appear. Should it be necessary to reinstitute treatment, or increase the dosage of the agent, or switch to a different antipsychotic agent, this syndrome may be masked.

It has been reported that fine vermicular movement of the tongue may be an early sign of tardive dyskinesia and if the medication is stopped at that time the full syndrome may not develop.

Tardive Dystonia —Tardive dystonia, not associated with the above syndrome, has also been reported. Tardive dystonia is characterized by delayed onset of choreic or dystonic movements, is often persistent, and has the potential of becoming irreversible.

Other CNS effects —Insomnia, restlessness, anxiety, euphoria, agitation, drowsiness, depression, lethargy, headache, confusion, vertigo, grand mal seizures, exacerbation of psychotic symptoms including hallucinations, and catatonic-like behavioral states which may be responsive to drug withdrawal and/or treatment with anticholinergic drugs.

Body as a Whole: Neuroleptic malignant syndrome (NMS), hyperpyrexia and heat stroke have been reported with HALDOL. (See WARNINGS for further information concerning NMS.)

Cardiovascular Effects: Tachycardia, hypotension, hypertension and ECG changes including prolongation of the Q-T interval and ECG pattern changes compatible with the polymorphous configuration of torsades de pointes.

Hematologic Effects: Reports have appeared citing the occurrence of mild and usually transient leukopenia and leukocytosis, minimal decreases in red blood cell counts, anemia, or a tendency toward lymphomonocytosis. Agranulocytosis has rarely been reported to have occurred with the use of HALDOL, and then only in association with other medication.

Liver Effects: Impaired liver function and/or jaundice have been reported.

Dermatologic Reactions: Maculopapular and acneiform skin reactions and isolated cases of photosensitivity and loss of hair.

Endocrine Disorders: Lactation, breast engorgement, mastalgia, menstrual irregularities, gynecomastia, impotence, increased libido, hyperglycemia, hypoglycemia and hyponatremia.

Gastrointestinal Effects: Anorexia, constipation, diarrhea, hypersalivation, dyspepsia, nausea and vomiting.

Autonomic Reactions: Dry mouth, blurred vision, urinary retention, diaphoresis and priapism.

Respiratory Effects: Laryngospasm, bronchospasm and increased depth of respiration.

Special Senses: Cataracts, retinopathy and visual disturbances.

Other: Cases of sudden and unexpected death have been reported in association with the administration of HALDOL. The nature of the evidence makes it impossible to determine definitively what role, if any, HALDOL played in the outcome of the reported cases. The possibility that HALDOL caused death cannot, of course, be excluded, but it

is to be kept in mind that sudden and unexpected death may occur in psychotic patients when they go untreated or when they are treated with other antipsychotic drugs.

Postmarketing Events: Hyperammonemia has been reported in a 5¹/₂ year old child with citrullinemia, an inherited disorder of ammonia excretion, following treatment with HALDOL.

OVERDOSAGE

While overdosage is less likely to occur with a parenteral than with an oral medication, information pertaining to HALDOL (haloperidol) is presented, modified only to reflect the extended duration of action of haloperidol decanoate.

Manifestations —In general, the symptoms of overdosage would be an exaggeration of known pharmacologic effects and adverse reactions, the most prominent of which would be: 1) severe extrapyramidal reactions, 2) hypotension, or 3) sedation. The patient would appear comatose with respiratory depression and hypotension which could be severe enough to produce a shock-like state. The extrapyramidal reactions would be manifested by muscular weakness or rigidity and a generalized or localized tremor, as demonstrated by the akinetic or agitans types, respectively. With accidental overdosage, hypertension rather than hypotension occurred in a two-year old child. The risk of ECG changes associated with torsades de pointes should be considered. (For further information regarding torsades de pointes, please refer to ADVERSE REACTIONS.)

Treatment —Since there is no specific antidote, treatment is primarily supportive. A patent airway must be established by use of an oropharyngeal airway or endotracheal tube or, in prolonged cases of coma, by tracheostomy. Respiratory depression may be counteracted by artificial respiration and mechanical respirators. Hypotension and circulatory collapse may be counteracted by use of intravenous fluids, plasma, or concentrated albumin, and vasopressor agents such as metaraminol, phenylephrine and norepinephrine. Epinephrine should not be used. In case of severe extrapyramidal reactions, antiparkinson medication should be administered, and should be continued for several weeks, and then withdrawn gradually as extrapyramidal symptoms may emerge. ECG and vital signs should be monitored especially for signs of Q-T prolongation or dysrhythmias and monitoring should continue until the ECG is normal. Severe arrhythmias should be treated with appropriate anti-arrhythmic measures.

DOSAGE AND ADMINISTRATION

HALDOL Decanoate 50 and HALDOL Decanoate 100 should be administered by deep intramuscular injection. A 21 gauge needle is recommended. The maximum volume per injection site should not exceed 3 mL. DO NOT ADMINISTER INTRAVENOUSLY.

Parenteral drug products should be inspected visually for particulate matter and discoloration prior to administration, whenever solution and container permit.

HALDOL Decanoate 50 and HALDOL Decanoate 100 are intended for use in chronic psychotic patients who require prolonged parenteral antipsychotic therapy. These patients should be previously stabilized on antipsychotic medication before considering a conversion to haloperidol decanoate. Furthermore, it is recommended that patients being considered for haloperidol decanoate therapy have been treated with, and tolerate well, short-acting HALDOL (haloperidol) in order to reduce the possibility of an unexpected adverse sensitivity to haloperidol. Close clinical supervision is required during the initial period of dose adjustment in order to minimize the risk of overdosage or reappearance of psychotic symptoms before the next injection. During dose adjustment or episodes of exacerbation of psychotic symptoms, haloperidol decanoate therapy can be supplemented with short-acting forms of haloperidol.

The dose of HALDOL Decanoate 50 or HALDOL Decanoate 100 should be expressed in terms of its haloperidol content. The starting dose of haloperidol decanoate should be based on the patient's age, clinical history, physical condition, and response to previous antipsychotic therapy. The preferred approach to determining the minimum effective dose is to begin with lower initial doses and to adjust the dose upward as needed. For patients previously maintained on low doses of antipsychotics (e.g. up to the equivalent of 10 mg/day oral haloperidol), it is recommended that the initial dose of haloperidol decanoate be 10–15 times the previous daily dose in oral haloperidol equivalents; limited clinical experience suggests that lower initial doses may be adequate.

Initial Therapy
Conversion from oral haloperidol to haloperidol decanoate can be achieved by using an initial dose of haloperidol decanoate that is 10 to 20 times the previous daily dose in oral haloperidol equivalents.

In patients who are elderly, debilitated, or stable on low doses of oral haloperidol (e.g. up to the equivalent of 10 mg/day oral haloperidol), a range of 10 to 15 times the previous daily dose in oral haloperidol equivalents is appropriate for initial conversion.

Continued on next page

Haldol Decanoate—Cont.

In patients previously maintained on higher doses of antipsychotics for whom a low dose approach risks recurrence of psychiatric decompensation and in patients whose long term use of haloperidol has resulted in a tolerance to the drug, 20 times the previous daily dose in oral haloperidol equivalents should be considered for initial conversion, with downward titration on succeeding injections.

The initial dose of haloperidol decanoate should not exceed 100 mg regardless of previous antipsychotic dose requirements. If, therefore, conversion requires more than 100 mg of haloperidol decanoate as an initial dose, that dose should be administered in two injections, i.e. a maximum of 100 mg initially followed by the balance in 3 to 7 days.

Maintenance Therapy

The maintenance dosage of haloperidol decanoate must be individualized with titration upward or downward based on therapeutic response. The usual maintenance range is 10 to 15 times the previous daily dose in oral haloperidol equivalents dependent on the clinical response of the patient.

HALDOL DECANOATE DOSING RECOMMENDATIONS MONTHLY

PATIENTS	1ST MONTH	MAINTENANCE
Stabilized on low daily oral doses (up to 10 mg/day)	10–15 x Daily Oral Dose	10–15 x Previous Daily Oral Dose
Elderly or Debilitated		
High dose	20 x Daily Oral Dose	10–15 x Previous Daily Oral Dose
Risk of relapse		
Tolerant to oral HALDOL®		

Close clinical supervision is required during initiation and stabilization of haloperidol decanoate therapy.

Haloperidol decanoate is usually administered monthly or every 4 weeks. However, variation in patient response may dictate a need for adjustment of the dosing interval as well as the dose (See CLINICAL PHARMACOLOGY).

Clinical experience with haloperidol decanoate at doses greater than 450 mg per month has been limited.

HOW SUPPLIED

HALDOL® (haloperidol) Decanoate 50 for IM injection, 50 mg haloperidol as 70.5 mg per mL haloperidol decanoate—NDC 0045-0253, 10 × 1 mL ampuls, 3 × 1 mL ampuls and 5 mL multiple dose vials.

HALDOL® (haloperidol) Decanoate 100 for IM injection, 100 mg haloperidol as 141.04 mg per mL haloperidol decanoate—NDC 0045-0254, 5 × 1 mL ampuls and 5 mL multiple dose vials.

Store at controlled room temperature (15°–30°C, 59°–86°F). Do not refrigerate or freeze.

Protect from light.

McNeil Pharmaceutical, McNEILAB, INC., Spring House, PA 19477

643-94-253-2   Revised April 1997

Shown in Product Identification Guide, page 328

LEVAQUIN® injection   ℞
(levofloxacin injection)

DESCRIPTION

LEVAQUIN® (levofloxacin injection) is a synthetic broad spectrum antibacterial agent for intravenous administration. Chemically, levofloxacin, a chiral fluorinated carboxyquinolone, is the pure (-)-(S)-enantiomer of the racemic drug substance ofloxacin. The chemical name is (-)-(S)-9-fluoro-2,3-dihydro-3-methyl-10-(4-methyl-1-piperazinyl)-7-oxo-7H-pyrido [1,2,3-de]-1,4-benzoxazine-6-carboxylic acid hemihydrate.

The chemical structure is:

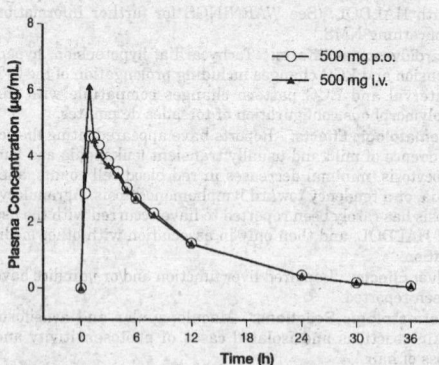

Its empirical formula is $C_{18}H_{20}FN_3O_4 \cdot \frac{1}{2}H_2O$ and its molecular weight is 370.38. Levofloxacin is a light yellowish-white to yellow-white crystal or crystalline powder. The molecule exists as a zwitterion at the pH conditions in the small intestine.

The data demonstrate that from pH 0.6 to 5.8, the solubility of levofloxacin is essentially constant (approximately 100 mg/mL). Levofloxacin is considered *soluble to freely soluble* in this pH range, as defined by USP nomenclature. Above pH 5.8, the solubility increases rapidly to its maximum at pH 6.7 (272 mg/mL) and is considered *freely soluble* in this range. Above pH 6.7, the solubility decreases and reaches a minimum value (about 50 mg/mL) at a pH of approximately 6.9.

Levofloxacin has the potential to form stable coordination compounds with many metal ions. This *in vitro* chelation potential has the following formation order: $Al^{+3} > Cu^{+2} > Zn^{+2} > Mg^{+2} > Ca^{+2}$.

LEVAQUIN INJECTION IN SINGLE-USE VIALS is a sterile, preservative-free aqueous solution of levofloxacin with pH ranging from 3.8 to 5.8. LEVAQUIN INJECTION IN PREMIX FLEXIBLE CONTAINERS is a sterile, preservative-free aqueous solution of levofloxacin with pH ranging from 3.8 to 5.8. The appearance of LEVAQUIN Injection may range from a clear yellow to a greenish-yellow solution. This does not adversely affect product potency.

LEVAQUIN INJECTION IN SINGLE-USE VIALS contains levofloxacin in Water for Injection. LEVAQUIN INJECTION IN PREMIX FLEXIBLE CONTAINERS is a dilute, non-pyrogenic, nearly isotonic premixed solution that contains levofloxacin in 5% Dextrose (D_5W). Solutions of hydrochloric acid and sodium hydroxide may have been added to adjust the pH.

The flexible container is fabricated from a specially formulated non-plasticized, thermoplastic copolyester (CR3). The amount of water that can permeate from the container into the overwrap is insufficient to affect the solution significantly. Solutions in contact with the flexible container can leach out certain of the container's chemical components in very small amounts within the expiration period. The suitability of the container material has been confirmed by tests in animals according to USP biological tests for plastic containers.

CLINICAL PHARMACOLOGY
Absorption

Following a single 60-minute intravenous infusion of 500-mg of levofloxacin to healthy volunteers, the mean peak plasma concentration attained was 6.2 µg/mL. Levofloxacin pharmacokinetics are linear and predictable after single and multiple i.v. dosing regimens. Steady-state is reached within 48 hours following a 500-mg once-daily regimen. The peak and trough plasma concentrations attained following multiple once-daily i.v. 500-mg regimens were approximately 6.4 and 0.6 µg/mL, respectively.

The plasma concentration profile of levofloxacin after i.v. administration is similar and comparable in extent of exposure (AUC) to that observed for levofloxacin tablets when equal doses (mg/mg) are administered. Therefore, the oral and i.v. routes of administration can be considered interchangeable. (See following chart.)

Mean Levofloxacin Plasma Concentration: Time Profiles

Distribution

The mean volume of distribution of levofloxacin generally ranges from 89 to 112 L after single and multiple 500-mg doses, indicating widespread distribution into body tissues. Penetration of levofloxacin into blister fluid is rapid and extensive. The blister fluid to plasma AUC ratio is approximately 1. Levofloxacin also penetrates well into lung tissues. Lung tissue concentrations were generally 2- to 5- fold higher than plasma concentrations and ranged from approximately 2.4 to 11.3 µg/g over a 24-hour period after a single 500-mg oral dose.

In vitro, over a clinically relevant range (1 to 10 µg/mL) of serum/plasma levofloxacin concentrations, levofloxacin is approximately 24 to 38% bound to serum proteins across all species studied, as determined by the equilibrium dialysis method. Levofloxacin is mainly bound to serum albumin in humans. Levofloxacin binding to serum proteins is independent of the drug concentration.

Metabolism

Levofloxacin is stereochemically stable in plasma and urine and does not invert metabolically to its enantiomer, D-flofloxacin. Levofloxacin undergoes limited metabolism in humans and is primarily excreted as unchanged drug in the urine. Following oral administration, approximately 87% of an administered dose was recovered as unchanged drug in urine within 48 hours, whereas less than 4% of the dose was recovered in feces in 72 hours. Less than 5% of an administered dose was recovered in the urine as the desmethyl and N-oxide metabolites, the only metabolites identified in humans. These metabolites have little relevant pharmacological activity.

Excretion

Levofloxacin is excreted largely as unchanged drug in the urine. The mean terminal plasma elimination half-life of levofloxacin ranges from approximately 6 to 8 hours following single or multiple doses of levofloxacin given orally or intravenously. The mean apparent total body clearance and renal clearance range from approximately 144 to 226 mL/min and 96 to 142 mL/min, respectively. Renal clearance in excess of the glomerular filtration rate suggests that tubular secretion of levofloxacin occurs in addition to its glomerular filtration. Concomitant administration of either cimetidine or probenecid results in approximately 24% and 35% reduction in the levofloxacin renal clearance, respectively, indicating that secretion of levofloxacin occurs in the renal proximal tubule. No levofloxacin crystals were found in any of the urine samples freshly collected from subjects receiving levofloxacin.

Special Populations
Geriatric

There are no significant differences in levofloxacin pharmacokinetics between young and elderly subjects when the subjects' differences in creatinine clearance are taken into consideration. Following a 500-mg oral dose of levofloxacin to healthy elderly subjects (66-80 years of age), the mean terminal plasma elimination half-life of levofloxacin was about 7.6 hours, as compared to approximately 6 hours in younger adults. The difference was attributable to the variation in renal function status of the subjects and was not believed to be clinically significant. Drug absorption appears to be unaffected by age. Levofloxacin dose adjustment based on age alone is not necessary.

Pediatric

The pharmacokinetics of levofloxacin in pediatric subjects have not been studied.

Gender

There are no significant differences in levofloxacin pharmacokinetics between male and female subjects when subjects' differences in creatinine clearance are taken into consideration. Following a 500-mg oral dose of levofloxacin to healthy male subjects, the mean terminal plasma elimination half-life of levofloxacin was about 7.5 hours, as compared to approximately 6.1 hours in female subjects. This difference was attributable to the variation in renal function status of the male and female subjects and was not believed to be clinically significant. Drug absorption appears to be unaffected by the gender of the subjects. Dose adjustment based on gender alone is not necessary.

Race

The effect of race on levofloxacin pharmacokinetics was examined through a covariate analysis performed on data from 72 subjects: 48 white and 24 nonwhite. The apparent total body clearance and apparent volume of distribution were not affected by the race of the subjects.

Renal insufficiency

Clearance of levofloxacin is reduced and plasma elimination half-life is prolonged in patients with impaired renal function (creatinine clearance ≤80 mL/min), requiring dosage adjustment in such patients to avoid accumulation. Neither hemodialysis nor continuous ambulatory peritoneal dialysis (CAPD) is effective in removal of levofloxacin from the body, indicating that supplemental doses of levofloxacin are not required following hemodialysis or CAPD. (See **PRECAUTIONS: General** and **DOSAGE AND ADMINISTRATION.**)

Hepatic insufficiency

Pharmacokinetic studies in hepatically impaired patients have not been conducted. Due to the limited extent of levofloxacin metabolism, the pharmacokinetics of levofloxacin are not expected to be affected by hepatic impairment.

Bacterial infection

The pharmacokinetics of levofloxacin in patients with serious community-acquired bacterial infections are comparable to those observed in healthy subjects.

Drug-drug interactions

The potential for pharmacokinetic drug interactions between levofloxacin and theophylline, warfarin, cyclosporine, digoxin, probenecid, cimetidine, sucralfate, and antacids has been evaluated. (See **PRECAUTIONS: Drug Interactions.**)

Regimen	C_{max} (μg/mL)	T_{max} (h)	AUC (μg·h/mL)	CL/F[1] (mL/min)	Vd/F[2] (L)	$t_{1/2}$ (h)	CL_R (mL/min)
Single dose							
250 mg p.o.[3]*	2.8 ± 0.4	1.6 ± 1.0	27.2 ± 3.9	156 ± 20	ND	7.3 ± 0.9	142 ± 21
500 mg p.o.[3]*	5.1 ± 0.8	1.3 ± 0.6	47.9 ± 6.8	178 ± 28	ND	6.3 ± 0.6	103 ± 30
500 mg i.v.[3]	6.2 ± 1.0	1.0 ± 0.1	48.3 ± 5.4	175 ± 20	90 ± 11	6.4 ± 0.7	112 ± 25
Multiple dose							
500 mg q24h p.o.[3]	5.7 ± 1.4	1.1 ± 0.4	47.5 ± 6.7	175 ± 25	102 ± 22	7.6 ± 1.6	116 ± 31
500 mg q24h i.v.[3]	6.4 ± 0.8	ND	54.6 ± 11.1	158 ± 29	91 ± 12	7.0 ± 0.8	99 ± 28
500 mg or 250 mg q24h i.v., patients with bacterial infection[4]	8.7 ± 4.0[5]	ND	72.5 ± 51.2[5]	154 ± 72	111 ± 58	ND	ND
500 mg p.o. single dose, effects of gender and age:							
male[6]	5.5 ± 1.1	1.2 ± 0.4	54.4 ± 18.9	166 ± 44	89 ± 13	7.5 ± 2.1	126 ± 38
female[7]	7.0 ± 1.6	1.7 ± 0.5	67.7 ± 24.2	136 ± 44	62 ± 16	6.1 ± 0.8	106 ± 40
young[8]	5.5 ± 1.0	1.5 ± 0.6	47.5 ± 9.8	182 ± 35	83 ± 18	6.0 ± 0.9	140 ± 33
elderly[9]	7.0 ± 1.6	1.4 ± 0.5	74.7 ± 23.3	121 ± 33	67 ± 19	7.6 ± 2.0	91 ± 29
500 mg p.o. single dose, patients with renal insufficiency:							
CL_{CR} 50–80 mL/min	7.5 ± 1.8	1.5 ± 0.5	95.6 ± 11.8	88 ± 10	ND	9.1 ± 0.9	57 ± 8
CL_{CR} 20–49 mL/min	7.1 ± 3.1	2.1 ± 1.3	182.1 ± 62.6	51 ± 19	ND	27 ± 10	26 ± 13
CL_{CR} <20 mL/min	8.2 ± 2.6	1.1 ± 1.0	263.5 ± 72.5	33 ± 8	ND	35 ± 5	13 ± 3
hemodialysis	5.7 ± 1.0	2.8 ± 2.2	ND	ND	ND	76 ± 42	ND
CAPD	6.9 ± 2.3	1.4 ± 1.1	ND	ND	ND	51 ± 24	ND

[1] clearance/bioavailability
[2] volume of distribution/bioavailability
[3] healthy males 18–53 years of age
[4] 500 mg q48h for patients with moderate renal impairment (CL_{CR} 20–50 mL/min) and infections of the respiratory tract or skin
[5] dose-normalized values (to 500 mg dose), estimated by population pharmacokinetic modeling
[6] healthy males 22–75 years of age
[7] healthy females 18–80 years of age
[8] young healthy male and female subjects 18–36 years of age
[9] healthy elderly male and female subjects 66–80 years of age
* Absolute bioavailability; F = 0.99 ± 0.08; ND = not determined.

The mean (± SD) pharmacokinetic parameters of levofloxacin determined under single and steady state conditions following oral (p.o.) or intravenous (i.v.) doses of levofloxacin are summarized as follows:
[See table above]

MICROBIOLOGY

Levofloxacin is the L-isomer of the racemate, ofloxacin, a quinolone antimicrobial agent. The antibacterial activity of ofloxacin resides primarily in the L-isomer. The mechanism of action of levofloxacin and other fluoroquinolone antimicrobials involves inhibition of DNA gyrase (bacterial topoisomerase II), an enzyme required for DNA replication, transcription, repair and recombination.

Levofloxacin has in vitro activity against a wide range of gram-negative and gram-positive microorganisms. Levofloxacin is often bactericidal at concentrations equal to or slightly greater than inhibitory concentrations.

Fluoroquinolones differ in chemical structure and mode of action from β-lactam antibiotics. Fluoroquinolones may, therefore, be active against bacteria resistant to β-lactam antibiotics.

Resistance to levofloxacin due to spontaneous mutation in vitro is a rare occurrence (range: 10^{-9} to 10^{-10}). Although cross-resistance has been observed between levofloxacin and some other fluoroquinolones, some microorgansims resistant to other fluoroquinolones may be susceptible to levofloxacin.

Levofloxacin has been shown to be active against most strains of the following microorganisms both in vitro and in clinical infections are described in the **INDICATIONS AND USAGE** section:

Aerobic gram-positive microorganisms
Enterococcus faecalis
Staphylococcus aureus
Streptococcus pneumoniae
Streptococcus pyogenes

Aerobic gram-negative microorganisms
Enterobacter cloacae
Escherichia coli
Haemophilus influenzae
Haemophilus parainfluenzae
Klebsiella pneumoniae
Legionella pneumophila
Moraxella catarrhalis
Proteus mirabilis
Pseudomonas aeruginosa

As with other drugs in this class, some strains of Pseudomonas aeruginosa may develop resistance fairly rapidly during treatment with levofloxacin.

Other microorganisms
Chlamydia pneumoniae
Mycoplasma pneumoniae

The following in vitro data are available, **but their clinical significance is unknown.**

Levofloxacin exhibits in vitro minimum inhibitory concentrations (MIC's) of 2μg/mL or less against most strains of the following microorganisms; however, the safety and effectiveness of levofloxacin in treating clinical infections due to these microorganisms have not been established in adequate and well-controlled trials.

Aerobic gram-positive microorganisms
Staphylococcus epidermidis
Streptococcus (Group C/F)
Streptococcus (Group G)
Staphylococcus saprophyticus
Streptococcus agalactiae
Viridans group streptococci

Aerobic gram-negative microorganisms
Acinetobacter anitratus
Acinetobacter baumannii
Acinetobacter calcoaceticus
Acinetobacter lwoffii
Bordetella pertussis
Citrobacter diversus
Citrobacter freundii
Enterobacter aerogenes
Enterobacter agglomerans
Enterobacter sakazakii
Klebsiella oxytoca
Morganella morganii
Proteus vulgaris
Providencia rettgeri
Providencia stuartii
Pseudomonas fluorescens
Serratia marcescens

Anaerobic gram-positive microorganisms
Clostridium perfringens

Susceptibility Tests
Susceptibility testing for levofloxacin should be performed, as it is the optimal predictor of activity. However, until levofloxacin susceptibility testing is available, the susceptibility of the organism to ofloxacin may be used to predict susceptibility to levofloxacin. While ofloxacin susceptible organisms will be susceptible to levofloxacin, ofloxacin intermediate or resistant organisms may be susceptible to levofloxacin.

Dilution techniques:
Quantitative methods are used to determine antimicrobial minimal inhibitory concentrations (MICs). These MICs provide estimates of the susceptibility of bacteria to antimicrobial compounds. The MICs should be determined using a standardized procedure. Standardized procedures are based on a dilution method[1] (broth or agar) or equivalent with standardized inoculum concentrations and standardized concentrations of levofloxacin powder. The MIC values should be interpreted according to the following criteria:
For testing aerobic microorgansims other than Haemophilus influenzae, Haemophilus parainfluenzae, and Streptococcus pneumoniae:

MIC (μg/mL)	Interpretation
≤2	Susceptible (S)
4	Intermediate (I)
≥8	Resistant (R)

For testing Haemophilus influenzae and Haemophilus parainfluenzae:[a]

MIC (μg/mL)	Interpretation
≤2	Susceptible (S)

[a] These interpretive standards are applicable only to broth microdilution susceptibility testing with Haemophilus influenza and Haemophilus parainfluenzae using Haemophilus Test Medium.[1]

The current absence of data on resistant strains precludes defining any categories other than "Susceptible". Strains yielding MIC results suggestive of a "nonsusceptible" category should be submitted to a reference laboratory for further testing.

For testing Streptococcus pneumoniae:[b]

MIC (μg/mL)	Interpretation
≤2	Susceptible (S)
4	Intermediate (I)
≥8	Resistant (R)

[b] These interpretive standards are applicable only to broth microdilution susceptibility tests using cation-adjusted Mueller-Hinton broth with 2–5% lysed horse blood.

A report of "Susceptible" indicates that the pathogen is likely to be inhibited if the antimicrobial compound in the blood reaches the concentrations usually achievable. A report of "Intermediate" indicates that the result should be considered equivocal, and, if the microorganism is not fully susceptible to alternative, clinically feasible drugs, the test should be repeated. This category implies possible clinical applicability in body sites where the drug is physiologically concentrated or in situations where a high dosage of drug can be used. This category also provides a buffer zone which prevents small uncontrolled technical factors from causing major discrepancies in interpretation. A report of "Resistant" indicates that the pathogen is not likely to be inhibited if the antimicrobial compound in the blood reaches the concentrations usually achievable; other therapy should be selected.

Standardized susceptibility test procedures require the use of laboratory control microorganisms to control the technical aspects of the laboratory procedures. Standard levofloxacin powder should give the following MIC values:

Microorganism		MI (μg/mL)
Enterococcus faecalis	ATCC 29212	0.25-2
Escherichia coli	ATCC 25922	0.008-0.06
Escherichia coli	ATCC 35218	0.015-0.06
Pseudomonas aeruginosa	ATCC 27853	0.5-4
Staphylococcus aureus	ATCC 29213	0.06-0.5
Haemophilus influenzae	ATCC 49247[c]	0.008-0.03
Streptococcus pneumoniae	ATCC 49619[d]	0.5-2

[c] This quality control range is applicable to only H. influenzae ATCC 49247 tested by a broth microdilution procedure using Haemophilus Test Medium (HTM).

[d] This quality control range is applicable to only S. pneumoniae ATCC 49619 tested by a broth microdilution procedure using cation-adjusted Mueller-Hinton broth with 2-5% lysed horse blood.

Diffusion techniques:
Quantitative methods that require measurement of zone diameters also provide reproducible estimates of the susceptibility of bacteria to antimicrobial compounds. One such standardized procedure[2] requires the use of standardized inoculum concentrations. This procedure uses paper disks impregnated with 5-μg levofloxacin to test the susceptibility of microorganisms to levofloxacin.

Reports from the laboratory providing results of the standard single-disk susceptibility test with a 5-μg levofloxacin disk should be interpreted according to the following criteria:
For aerobic microorganisms other than Haemophilus influenzae, Haemophilus parainfluenzae, and Streptococcus pneumoniae:

Zone diameter (mm)	Interpretation
≥17	Susceptible (S)
14–16	Intermediate (I)
≤13	Resistant (R)

For Haemophilus influenzae and Haemophilus parainfluenzae:[e]

Zone diameter (mm)	Interpretation
≥17	Susceptible (S)

[e] These interpretive standards are applicable only to disk diffusion susceptibility testing with Haemophilus influenza and Haemophilus parainfluenzae using Haemophilus Test Medium.[2]

Continued on next page

Levaquin Inj.—Cont.

The current absence of data on resistant strains precludes defining any categories other than "Susceptible". Strains yielding zone diameter results suggestive of a "nonsusceptible" category should be submitted to a reference laboratory for further testing.

For *Streptococcus pneumoniae:* [f]

Zone diameter (mm)	Interpretation
≥17	Susceptible (S)
14–16	Intermediate (I)
≤13	Resistant (R)

[f] These zone diameter standards for *Streptococcus pneumoniae* apply only to tests performed using Mueller-Hinton agar supplemented with 5% sheep blood and incubated in 5% CO_2.

Interpretation should be as stated above for results using dilution techniques. Interpretation involves correlation of the diameter obtained in the disk test with the MIC for levofloxacin.

As with standardized dilution techniques, diffusion methods require the use of laboratory control microorganisms to control the technical aspects of the laboratory procedures. For the diffusion technique, the 5-μg levofloxacin disk should provide the following zone diameters in these laboratory test quality control strains:

Microorganism		Zone Diameter (mm)
Escherichia coli	ATCC 25922	29–37
Pseudomonas aeruginosa	ATCC 27853	19–26
Staphylococcus aureus	ATCC 25923	25–30
Haemophilus influenzae	ATCC 49247[g]	32–40
Streptococcus pneumoniae	ATCC 49619[h]	20–25

[g] This quality control range is applicable to only *H. influenzae* ATCC 49247 tested by a disk diffusion procedure using Haemophilus Test Medium (HTM).[2]

[h] This quality control range is applicable to only *S. pneumoniae* ATCC 49619 tested by a disk diffusion procedure using Mueller-Hinton agar supplemented with 5% sheep blood and incubated in 5% CO_2.

INDICATIONS AND USAGE

LEVAQUIN Injection is indicated for the treatment of adults (≥18 years of age) with mild, moderate, and severe infections caused by susceptible strains of the designated microorganisms in the conditions listed below, when intravenous administration offers a route of administration advantageous to the patient (e.g., patient cannot tolerate an oral dosage form). Please see **DOSAGE AND ADMINISTRATION** for specific recommendations.

Acute maxillary sinusitis due to *Streptococcus pneumoniae, Haemophilus influenzae*, or *Moraxella catarrhalis*.

Acute bacterial exacerbation of chronic bronchitis due to *Staphylococcus aureus, Streptococcus pneumoniae, Haemophilus influenzae, Haemophilus parainfluenzae*, or *Moraxella catarrhalis*.

Community-acquired pneumonia due to *Staphylococcus aureus, Streptococcus pneumoniae, Haemophilus influenzae, Haemophilus parainfluenzae, Klebsiella pneumoniae, Moraxella catarrhalis, Chlamydia pneumoniae, Legionella pneumophila*, or *Mycoplasma pneumoniae*. (See **CLINICAL STUDIES.**)

Uncomplicated skin and skin structure infections (mild to moderate) including abscesses, cellulitis, furuncles, impetigo, pyoderma, wound infections, due to *Staphylococcus aureus*, or *Streptococcus pyogenes*.

Complicated urinary tract infections (mild to moderate) due to *Enterococcus faecalis, Enterobacter cloacae, Escherichia coli, Klebsiella pneumoniae, Proteus mirabilis*, or *Pseudomonas aeruginosa*.

Acute pyelonephritis (mild to moderate) caused by *Escherichia coli*.

Appropriate culture and susceptibility tests should be performed before treatment in order to isolate and identify organisms causing the infection and to determine their susceptibility to levofloxacin. Therapy with levofloxacin may be initiated before results of these tests are known; once results become available, appropriate therapy should be selected.

As with other drugs in this class, some strains of *Pseudomonas aeruginosa* may develop resistance fairly rapidly during treatment with levofloxacin. Culture and susceptibility testing performed periodically during therapy will provide information about the continued susceptibility of the pathogens to the antimicrobial agent and also the possible emergence of bacterial resistance.

CONTRAINDICATIONS

Levofloxacin is contraindicated in persons with a history of hypersensitivity to levofloxacin, quinolone antimicrobial agents, or any other components of this product.

WARNINGS

THE SAFETY AND EFFICACY OF LEVOFLOXACIN IN CHILDREN, ADOLESCENTS (UNDER THE AGE OF 18 YEARS), PREGNANT WOMEN, AND NURSING WOMEN HAVE NOT BEEN ESTABLISHED. (See **PRECAUTIONS: Pediatric Use, Pregnancy,** and **Nursing Mothers** subsections.)

In immature rats and dogs, the oral and intravenous administration of levofloxacin increased the incidence and severity of osteochondrosis. Other fluoroquinolones also produce similar erosions in the weight bearing joints and other signs of arthropathy in immature animals of various species. (See **ANIMAL PHARMACOLOGY.**)

Convulsions and toxic psychoses have been reported in patients receiving quinolones, including levofloxacin. Quinolones may also cause increased intracranial pressure and central nervous system stimulation which may lead to tremors, restlessness, anxiety, lightheadedness, confusion, hallucinations, paranoia, depression, nightmares, insomnia, and, rarely, suicidal thoughts or acts. These reactions may occur following the first dose. If these reactions occur in patients receiving levofloxacin, the drug should be discontinued and appropriate measures instituted. As with other quinolones, levofloxacin should be used with caution in patients with a known or suspected CNS disorder that may predispose to seizures or lower the seizure threshold (e.g., severe cerebral arteriosclerosis, epilepsy) or in the presence of other risk factors that may predispose to seizures or lower the seizure threshold (e.g., certain drug therapy, renal dysfunction.) (See **PRECAUTIONS: General, Information for Patients, Drug Interactions** and **ADVERSE REACTIONS.)**

Serious and occasionally fatal hypersensitivity and/or anaphylactic reactions have been reported in patients receiving therapy with quinolones. These reactions often occur following the first dose. Some reactions have been accompanied by cardiovascular collapse, hypotension/shock, seizure, loss of consciousness, tingling, angioedema (including tongue, laryngeal, throat, or facial edema/swelling), airway obstruction (including bronchospasm, shortness of breath, and acute respiratory distress), dyspnea, urticaria, itching, and other serious skin reactions. Levofloxacin should be discontinued immediately at the first appearance of a skin rash or any other sign of hypersensitivity. Serious acute hypersensitivity reactions may require treatment with epinephrine and other resuscitative measures, including oxygen, intravenous fluids, antihistamines, corticosteroids, pressor amines, and airway management, as clinically indicated. (See **PRECAUTIONS** and **ADVERSE REACTIONS.)**

Serious and sometimes fatal events, some due to hypersensitivity, and some due to uncertain etiology, have been reported rarely in patients receiving therapy with quinolones. These events may be severe and generally occur following the administration of multiple doses. Clinical manifestations may include one or more of the following: fever, rash or severe dermatologic reactions (e.g., toxic epidermal necrolysis, Stevens-Johnson Syndrome); vasculitis; arthralgia; myalgia; serum sickness; allergic pneumonitis; interstitial nephritis; acute renal insufficiency or failure; hepatitis; jaundice; acute hepatic necrosis or failure; anemia, including hemolytic and aplastic; thrombocytopenia, including thrombotic thrombocytopenic purpura; leukopenia; agranulocytosis; pancytopenia; and/or other hematologic abnormalities. The drug should be discontinued immediately at the first appearance of a skin rash or any other sign of hypersensitivity and supportive measures instituted. (See **PRECAUTIONS: Information for Patients** and **ADVERSE REACTIONS.)**

Pseudomembranous colitis has been reported with nearly all antibacterial agents, including levofloxacin, and may range in severity from mild to life-threatening. Therefore it is important to consider this diagnosis in patients who present with diarrhea subsequent to the administration of any antibacterial agent.

Treatment with antibacterial agents alters the normal flora of the colon and may permit overgrowth of clostridia. Studies indicate that a toxin produced by *Clostridium difficile* is one primary cause of "antibiotic-associated colitis".

After the diagnosis of pseudomembranous colitis has been established, therapeutic measures should be initiated. Mild cases of pseudomembranous colitis usually respond to drug discontinuation alone. In moderate to severe cases, consideration should be given to management with fluids and electrolytes, protein supplementation, and treatment with an antibacterial drug clinically effective against *C. difficile* colitis. (See **ADVERSE REACTIONS.)**

Ruptures of the shoulder, hand, and Achilles tendons that required surgical repair or resulted in prolonged disability have been reported in patients receiving quinolones. Levofloxacin should be discontinued if the patient experiences pain, inflammation, or rupture of a tendon. Patients should rest and refrain from exercise until the diagnosis of tendinitis or tendon rupture has been confidently excluded. Tendon rupture can occur during or after therapy with quinolones, including levofloxacin.

PRECAUTIONS

General

Because a rapid or bolus intravenous injection may result in hypotension, LEVOFLOXACIN INJECTION SHOULD ONLY BE ADMINISTERED BY SLOW INTRAVENOUS INFUSION OVER A PERIOD OF 60 MINUTES. (See **DOSAGE AND ADMINISTRATION.)**

Although levofloxacin is more soluble than other quinolones, adequate hydration of patients receiving levofloxacin should be maintained to prevent the formation of a highly concentrated urine.

Administer levofloxacin with caution in the presence of renal insufficiency. Careful clinical observation and appropriate laboratory studies should be performed prior to and during therapy since elimination of levofloxacin may be reduced. In patients with impaired renal function (creatinine clearance ≤ 80 mL/min), adjustment of the dosage regimen is necessary to avoid the accumulation of levofloxacin due to decreased clearance. (See **CLINICAL PHARMACOLOGY** and **DOSAGE AND ADMINISTRATION.)**

Moderate to severe phototoxicity reactions have been observed in patients exposed to direct sunlight while receiving drugs in this class. Excessive exposure to sunlight should be avoided. However, in clinical trials with levofloxacin, phototoxicity has been observed in less than 0.1% of patients. Therapy should be discontinued if phototoxicity (e.g., a skin eruption) occurs.

As with other quinolones, levofloxacin should be used with caution in any patient with a known or suspected CNS disorder that may predispose to seizures or lower the seizure threshold (e.g., severe cerebral arteriosclerosis, epilepsy) or in the presence of other risk factors that may predispose to seizures or lower the seizure threshold (e.g., certain drug therapy, renal dysfunction). (See **WARNINGS** and **Drug Interactions.)**

As with other quinolones, disturbances of blood glucose, including symptomatic hyper- and hypoglycemia, have been reported, usually in diabetic patients receiving concomitant treatment with an oral hypoglycemic agent (e.g., glyburide/glibenclamide) or with insulin. In these patients, careful monitoring of blood glucose is recommended. If a hypoglycemic reaction occurs in a patient being treated with levofloxacin, levofloxacin should be discontinued immediately and appropriate therapy should be initiated immediately. (See **Drug Interactions** and **ADVERSE REACTIONS.)**

As with any potent antimicrobial drug, periodic assessment of organ system functions, including renal, hepatic, and hematopoietic, is advisable during therapy. (See **WARNINGS** and **ADVERSE REACTIONS.)**

Information for Patients

Patients should be advised:

- to drink fluids liberally;
- that levofloxacin may cause neurologic adverse effects (e.g., dizziness, lightheadedness) and that patients should know how they react to levofloxacin before they operate an automobile or machinery or engage in other activities requiring mental alertness and coordination. (See **WARNINGS** and **ADVERSE REACTIONS**);
- to discontinue treatment and inform their physician if they experience pain, inflammation, or rupture of a tendon, and to rest and refrain from exercise until the diagnosis of tendinitis or tendon rupture has been confidently excluded;
- that levofloxacin may be associated with hypersensitivity reactions, even following the first dose, and to discontinue the drug at the first sign of a skin rash, hives or other skin reactions, a rapid heartbeat, difficulty in swallowing or breathing, any swelling suggesting angioedema (e.g., swelling of the lips, tongue, face, tightness of the throat, hoarseness), or other symptoms of an allergic reaction. (See **WARNINGS** and **ADVERSE REACTIONS**);
- to avoid excessive sunlight or artificial ultraviolet light while receiving levofloxacin and to discontinue therapy if phototoxicity (i.e., skin eruption) occurs;
- that if they are diabetic and are being treated with insulin or an oral hypoglycemic agent and a hypoglycemic reaction occurs, they should discontinue levofloxacin and consult a physician. (See **PRECAUTIONS: General** and **Drug Interactions.)**

Drug Interactions

Antacids, Sucralfate, Metal Cations, Multi-Vitamins: There are no data concerning an interaction of intravenous levofloxacin with oral antacids, sucralfate, multi-vitamins, or metal cations. However, levofloxacin should not be co-administered with any solution containing multivalent cations, e.g., magnesium, through the same intravenous line. (See **DOSAGE AND ADMINISTRATION.)**

Theophylline: No significant effect of levofloxacin on the plasma concentrations, AUC, and other disposition param-

eters for theophylline was detected in a clinical study involving 14 healthy volunteers. Similarly, no apparent effect of theophylline on levofloxacin absorption and disposition was observed. However, concomitant administration of other quinolones with theophylline has resulted in prolonged elimination half-life, elevated serum theophylline levels, and a subsequent increase in the risk of theophylline-related adverse reactions in the patient population. Therefore, theophylline levels should be closely monitored and appropriate dosage adjustments made when levofloxacin is co-administered. Adverse reactions, including seizures, may occur with or without an elevation in serum theophylline levels. (See **WARNINGS** and **PRECAUTIONS: General.**)

Warfarin: No significant effect of levofloxacin on the peak plasma concentrations, AUC, and other disposition parameters for R- and S- warfarin was detected in a clinical study involving healthy volunteers. No significant change in prothrombin time was noted in the presence of levofloxacin. Similarly, no apparent effect of warfarin on levofloxacin absorption and disposition was observed. However, since some quinolones have been reported to enhance the effects of oral anticoagulant warfarin or its derivatives in the patient population, the prothrombin time or other suitable coagulation test should be closely monitored if a quinolone antimicrobial is administered concomitantly with warfarin or its derivatives.

Cyclosporine: No significant effect of levofloxacin on the peak plasma concentrations, AUC, and other disposition parameters for cyclosporine was detected in a clinical study involving healthy volunteers. However, elevated serum levels of cyclosporine have been reported in the patient population when co-administered with some other quinolones. Levofloxacin C_{max} and k_e were slightly lower while T_{max} and $t_{1/2}$ were slightly longer in the presence of cyclosporine than those observed in other studies without concomitant medication. The differences, however, are not considered to be clinically significant. Therefore, no dosage adjustment is required for levofloxacin or cyclosporine when administered concomitantly.

Digoxin: No significant effect of levofloxacin on the peak plasma concentrations, AUC, and other disposition parameters for digoxin was detected in a clinical study involving healthy volunteers. Levofloxacin absorption and disposition kinetics were similar in the presence or absence of digoxin. Therefore, no dosage adjustment for levofloxacin or digoxin is required when administered concomitantly.

Probenecid and Cimetidine: No significant effect of probenecid or cimetidine on the rate and extent of levofloxacin absorption was observed in a clinical study involving healthy volunteers. The AUC and $t_{1/2}$ of levofloxacin were 27–38% and 30% higher, respectively, while CL/F and CL_R were 21–35% lower during concomitant treatment with probenecid or cimetidine compared to levofloxacin alone. Although these differences were statistically significant, the changes were not high enough to warrant dosage adjustment for levofloxacin when probenecid or cimetidine is co-administered.

Non-steroidal anti-inflammatory drugs: The concomitant administration of a non-steroidal anti-inflammatory drug with a quinolone, including levofloxacin, may increase the risk of CNS stimulation and convulsive seizures. (See **WARNINGS** and **PRECAUTIONS: General.**)

Antidiabetic agents: Disturbances of blood glucose, including hyperglycemia and hypoglycemia, have been reported in patients treated concomitantly with quinolones and an antidiabetic agent. Therefore, careful monitoring of blood glucose is recommended when these agents are co-administered.

Carcinogenesis, Mutagenesis, Impairment of Fertility: In a long term carcinogenicity study in rats, levofloxacin exhibited no carcinogenic or tumorigenic potential following daily dietary administration for 2 years; the highest dose was 2 or 10 times the recommended human dose based on surface area or body weight, respectively.

Levofloxacin was not mutagenic in the following assays; Ames bacterial mutation assay (*S. typhimurium* and *E. coli*), CHO/HGPRT forward mutation assay, mouse micronucleus test, mouse dominant lethal test, rat unscheduled DNA synthesis assay, and the mouse sister chromatid exchange assay. It was positive in the *in vitro* chromosomal aberration (CHL cell line) and sister chromatid exchange (CHL/IU cell line) assays.

Levofloxacin caused no impairment of fertility or reproductive performance in rats at oral doses as high as 360 mg/kg/day (2124 mg/m^2), corresponding to 3.0 or 18 times the recommended maximum human dose based on surface area or body weight, respectively, and intravenous doses as high as 100 mg/kg/day (590 mg/m^2), corresponding to 1.0 or 5 times the recommended maximum human dose based on surface area or body weight, respectively.

Pregnancy: Teratogenic Effects. Pregnancy Category C. Levofloxacin was not teratogenic in rats at oral doses as high as 810 mg/kg/day (4779 mg/m^2), which corresponds to 14 or 82 times the recommended maximum human dose based on surface area or body weight, respectively, or at intravenous doses as high as 160 mg/kg/day (944 mg/m^2) corresponding to 2.7 or 16 times the recommended maximum human dose based on surface area or body weight, respectively. Doses equivalent to 26 or 81 times the recommended maximum human dose of levofloxacin (based on surface area or body weight, respectively) caused decreased fetal body weight and increased fetal mortality in rats when administered orally at 810 mg/kg/day (8910 mg/m^2). No teratogenicity was observed when rabbits were dosed orally as high as 50 mg/kg/day (550 mg/m^2) which corresponds to 1.6 or 5.0 times the recommended maximum human dose based on surface area or body weight, respectively, or when dosed intravenously as high as 25 mg/kg/day (275 mg/m^2), corresponding to 0.8 or 2.5 times the maximum recommended human dose based on surface area or body weight, respectively.

There are, however, no adequate and well-controlled studies in pregnant women. Levofloxacin should be used during pregnancy only if the potential benefit justifies the potential risk to the fetus. (See **WARNINGS.**)

Nursing Mothers: Levofloxacin has not been measured in human milk. Based upon data from ofloxacin, it can be presumed that levofloxacin will be excreted in human milk. Because of the potential for serious adverse reactions from levofloxacin in nursing infants, a decision should be made whether to discontinue nursing or to discontinue the drug, taking into account the importance of the drug to the mother.

Pediatric Use: Safety and effectiveness in children and adolescents below the age of 18 years have not been established. Quinolones, including levofloxacin, cause arthropathy and osteochondrosis in juvenile animals of several species. (See **WARNINGS.**)

ADVERSE REACTIONS

The incidence of drug-related adverse reactions in patients during Phase 2 and 3 clinical trials conducted in North America was 6.2%. Among patients receiving multiple-dose therapy, 3.7% discontinued therapy with levofloxacin due to adverse experiences.

In clinical trials, the following events were considered likely to be drug-related in patients receiving multiple doses of levofloxacin: diarrhea 1.2%, nausea 1.2%, vaginitis 0.8%, flatulence 0.5%, pruritus 0.5%, rash 0.3%, abdominal pain 0.3%, genital moniliasis 0.3%, dizziness 0.3%, dyspepsia 0.3%, insomnia 0.3%, taste perversion 0.2%, vomiting 0.2%, anorexia 0.1%, anxiety 0.1%, constipation 0.1%, edema 0.1%, fatigue 0.1%, headache 0.1%, increased sweating 0.1%, leukorrhea 0.1%, malaise 0.1%, nervousness 0.1%, sleep disorders 0.1%, tremor 0.1%, urticaria 0.1%.

In clinical trials, the most frequently reported adverse events occurring in > 3% of the study population regardless of drug relationship, were:
nausea 6.6%, injection site reaction 5.6%, diarrhea 5.4%, headache 5.4%, constipation 3.1%.

In clinical trials, the following events occurred in 1 to 3% of patients, regardless of drug relationship:
insomnia 2.9%, injection site pain 2.7%, dizziness 2.5%, vomiting 2.1%, abdominal pain 2.0%, dyspepsia 2.0%, rash 1.7%, vaginitis 1.8%, flatulence 1.6%, pruritus 1.6%, injection site inflammation 1.5%, pain 1.4%, chest pain 1.1%, back pain 1.0%.

The following adverse events occurred in clinical trials at a rate of 0.5 to less than 1%, regardless of drug relationship:
agitation, anorexia, anxiety, arthralgia, dry mouth, edema, fatigue, fever, genital pruritus, increased sweating, nervousness, pharyngitis, rhinitis, skin disorder, somnolence, taste perversion.

Additional adverse events occurring in clinical trials at a rate of 0.3 to less than 0.5% regardless of drug relationship include:
cardiac failure, hypertension, leukorrhea, myocardial infarction, myalgia, purpura, tinnitus, tremor, urticaria.

Events occurring at a frequency lower than 0.3% regardless of drug relationship but considered medically important include: abnormal coordination, abnormal dreaming, abnormal hepatic function, abnormal platelets, abnormal renal function, abnormal vision, acute renal failure, aggravated diabetes mellitus, aggressive reaction, anemia, angina pectoris, ARDS, arrhythmia, arthritis, asthma, bradycardia, cardiac arrest, cerebrovascular disorder, circulatory failure, coma, confusion, convulsions (seizures), coronary thrombosis, delirium, depression, diplopia, embolism-blood clot, emotional lability, erythema nodosum, G.I. hemorrhage, granulocytopenia, hallucination, heart block, hepatic coma, hypoglycemia, hypotension, impaired concentration, increased LDH, jaundice, leukocytosis, leukopenia, lymphadenopathy, manic reaction, mental deficiency, muscle weakness, pancreatitis, paralysis, paranoia, postural hypotension, pseudomembranous colitis, rhabdomyolysis, sleep disorders, speech disorder, stupor, syncope, tachycardia, tendinitis, thrombocytopenia, vertigo, weight decrease, WBC abnormal not otherwise specified.

In clinical trials using multiple-dose therapy, ophthalmologic abnormalities, including cataracts and multiple punctate lenticular opacities, have been noted in patients undergoing treatment with other quinolones. The relationship of the drugs to these events is not presently established.

Crystalluria and cylindruria have been reported with other quinolones.

The following laboratory abnormalities appeared in 1.9% of patients receiving multiple doses of levofloxacin. It is not known whether these abnormalities were caused by the drug or the underlying condition being treated.

Blood Chemistry: decreased glucose, decreased lymphocytes

Post-Marketing Adverse Reactions:

Additional serious adverse events reported from the marketing experience with levofloxacin outside of the United States regardless of drug relationship include:
allergic pneumonitis, anaphylactic shock, anaphylactoid reaction, dysphonia, abnormal EEG, encephalopathy, eosinophilia, erythema multiforme, hemolytic anemia, multi-system organ failure, palpitation, paresthesia, Stevens-Johnson Syndrome, tendon rupture, vasodilation.

OVERDOSAGE

Levofloxacin exhibits a low potential for acute toxicity. Mice, rats, dogs and monkeys exhibited the following clinical signs after receiving a single high dose of levofloxacin: ataxia, ptosis, decreased locomotor activity, dyspnea, prostration, tremors, and convulsions. Doses in excess of 1500 mg/kg orally and 250 mg/kg i.v. produced significant mortality in rodents. In the event of an acute overdosage, the stomach should be emptied. The patient should be observed and appropriate hydration maintained. Levofloxacin is not efficiently removed by hemodialysis or peritoneal dialysis.

DOSAGE AND ADMINISTRATION

LEVAQUIN Injection should only be administered by intravenous infusion. It is not for intramuscular, intrathecal, intraperitoneal, or subcutaneous administration.

CAUTION: RAPID OR BOLUS INTRAVENOUS INFUSION MUST BE AVOIDED. Levofloxacin Injection should be infused intravenously slowly over a period of not less than 60 minutes. (See **PRECAUTIONS.**)

Single-use vials require dilution prior to administration. (See **PREPARATION FOR ADMINISTRATION.**)

The usual dose of LEVAQUIN Injection is 500 mg administered by slow infusion over 60 minutes every 24 h or as described in the following dosing chart. These recommendations apply to patients with normal renal function (i.e., creatinine clearance > 80 mL/min). For patients with altered renal function (i.e., creatinine clearance ≤ 80 mL/min), see the **Patients with Impaired Renal Function** subsection.

[See table above]

[See table at top of next page]

Patients with Normal Renal Function:

Infection*	Unit Dose	Freq.	Duration**	Daily Dose
Acute Bacterial Exacerbation of Chronic Bronchitis	500 mg	q24h	7 days	500 mg
Comm. Acquired Pneumonia	500 mg	q24h	7–14 days	500 mg
Acute Maxillary Sinusitis	500 mg	q24h	10–14 days	500 mg
Uncomplicated SSSI	500 mg	q24h	7–10 days	500 mg
Complicated UTI	250 mg	q24h	10 days	250 mg
Acute pyelonephritis	250 mg	q24h	10 days	250 mg

*DUE TO THE DESIGNATED PATHOGENS (See **INDICATIONS AND USAGE.**)
Sequential therapy (intravenous to oral) may be instituted at the discretion of the physician (See **DOSAGE AND ADMINISTRATION section of LEVAQUIN Tablets package insert.)

When only the serum creatinine is known, the following formula may be used to estimate creatinine clearance.

Men: Creatinine Clearance (mL/min) =
$$\frac{\text{Weight (kg)} \times (140\text{–age})}{72 \times \text{serum creatinine (mg/dL)}}$$
Women: 0.85 × the value calculated for men.

The serum creatinine should represent a steady state of renal function.

Continued on next page

Levaquin Inj.—Cont.

PREPARATION OF LEVOFLOXACIN INJECTION FOR ADMINISTRATION

LEVAQUIN INJECTION IN SINGLE-USE VIALS:
LEVAQUIN Injection is supplied in single-use vials containing a concentrated levofloxacin solution with the equivalent of 500 mg of levofloxacin in Water for Injection. The 20 mL vials contain 25 mg of levofloxacin/mL. **THESE LEVAQUIN INJECTION SINGLE-USE VIALS MUST BE FURTHER DILUTED WITH AN APPROPRIATE SOLUTION PRIOR TO INTRAVENOUS ADMINISTRATION.** (See **COMPATIBLE INTRAVENOUS SOLUTIONS.**) The concentration of the resulting diluted solution should be 5 mg/mL prior to administration. This intravenous drug product should be inspected visually for particulate matter prior to administration. Samples containing visible particles should be discarded.

Since no preservative or bacteriostatic agent is present in this product, aseptic technique must be used in preparation of the final intravenous solution. **Since the vials are for single-use only, any unused portion remaining in the vial should be discarded. When used to prepare two 250 mg doses, the full content of the vial should be withdrawn at once using a single-entry procedure, and a second dose should be prepared and stored for subsequent use.** (See **Stability of LEVAQUIN Injection Following Dilution.**)

Since only limited data are available on the compatibility of levofloxacin intravenous injection with other intravenous substances, **additives or other medications should not be added to LEVAQUIN Injection in single-use vials or infused simultaneously through the same intravenous line.** If the same intravenous line is used for sequential infusion of several different drugs, the line should be flushed before and after infusion of LEVAQUIN Injection with an infusion solution compatible with LEVAQUIN Injection and with any other drug(s) administered via this common line.

Prepare the desired dosage of levofloxacin according to the following chart:
[See second table above]

Compatible Intravenous Solutions: Any of the following intravenous solutions may be used to prepare a 5 mg/mL levofloxacin solution with the approximate pH values:

Intravenous Fluids	Final pH of LEVAQUIN Solution
0.9% Sodium Chloride Injection, USP	4.71
5% Dextrose Injection, USP	4.58
5% Dextrose/0.9% NaCl Injection	4.62
5% Dextrose in Lactated Ringers	4.92
Plasma-Lyte® 56/5% Dextrose Injection	5.03
5% Dextrose, 0.45% Sodium Chloride, and 0.15% Potassium Chloride Injection	4.61
Sodium Lactate Injection (M/6)	5.54

LEVAQUIN INJECTION PREMIX IN SINGLE-USE FLEXIBLE CONTAINERS:

LEVAQUIN Injection is also supplied in 100 mL flexible containers containing a premixed, ready-to-use levofloxacin solution in D₅W for single-use. The fill volume is either 50 or 100 mL. **NO FURTHER DILUTION OF THIS PREPARATION IS NECESSARY.** Consequently each 100 mL PREMIX flexible container already contains a dilute solution with the equivalent of either 250 mg or 500 mg of levofloxacin (5 mg/mL) in 5% Dextrose (D₅W).

This parenteral drug product should be inspected visually for particulate matter prior to administration. Samples containing visible particles should be discarded.

Since the PREMIX flexible containers are for single-use only, any unused portion should be discarded.

Since only limited data are available on the compatibility of levofloxacin intravenous injection with other intravenous substances, **additives or other medications should not be added to LEVAQUIN Injection in flexible containers or infused simultaneously through the same intravenous line.** If the same intravenous line is used for sequential infusion of several different drugs, the line should be flushed before and after infusion of LEVAQUIN Injection with an infusion solution compatible with LEVAQUIN Injection and with any other drug(s) administered via this common line.

Instructions for the Use of LEVAQUIN INJECTION PREMIX IN FLEXIBLE CONTAINERS:
To open:
1. Tear outer wrap at the notch and remove solution container.
2. Check the container for minute leaks by squeezing the inner bag firmly. If leaks are found, or if the seal is not intact, discard the solution, as the sterility may be compromised.
3. Do not use if the solution is cloudy or a precipitate is present.

4. Use sterile equipment.
5. **WARNING: Do not use flexible containers in series connections.** Such use could result in air embolism due to residual air being drawn from the primary container before administration of the fluid from the secondary container is complete.

Preparation for administration:
1. Close flow control clamp of administration set.
2. Remove cover from port at bottom of container.
3. Insert piercing pin of administration set into port with a twisting motion until the pin is firmly seated. **NOTE: See full directions on administration set carton.**
4. Suspend container from hanger.
5. Squeeze and release drip chamber to establish proper fluid level in chamber during infusion of LEVAQUIN INJECTION IN PREMIX FLEXIBLE CONTAINERS.
6. Open flow control clamp to expel air from set. Close clamp.
7. Regulate rate of administration with flow control clamp.

Stability of LEVAQUIN Injection as Supplied: When stored under recommended conditions, LEVAQUIN Injection, as supplied in 20 mL vials and 100 mL flexible containers, is stable through the expiration date printed on the label.

Stability of LEVAQUIN Injection Following Dilution: LEVAQUIN Injection, when diluted in a compatible intravenous fluid to a concentration of 5 mg/mL, is stable for 72 h when stored at or below 25°C (77°F) and for 14 days when stored under refrigeration at 5°C (41°F) in plastic intravenous containers. Solutions that are diluted in a compatible intravenous solution and frozen in glass bottles or plastic intravenous containers are stable for 6 months when stored at -20°C (-4°F). **THAW FROZEN SOLUTIONS AT ROOM TEMPERATURE 25°C (77°F) OR IN A REFRIGERATOR 8°C (46°F). DO NOT FORCE THAW BY MICROWAVE IRRADIATION OR WATER BATH IMMERSION. DO NOT REFREEZE AFTER INITIAL THAWING.**

HOW SUPPLIED

SINGLE-USE VIALS:
LEVAQUIN (levofloxacin injection) injection is supplied in single-use vials. Each vial contains a concentrated solution with the equivalent of 500 mg of levofloxacin.
25 mg/mL, 20 mL vials (NDC 0045-0069-51)
LEVAQUIN INJECTION IN SINGLE-USE VIALS should be stored at controlled room temperature and protected from light.
LEVAQUIN INJECTION IN SINGLE-USE VIALS is manufactured for Ortho-McNeil Pharmaceutical, Inc. OMJ Pharmaceuticals, Inc., San German, Puerto Rico, 00683.
PREMIX IN FLEXIBLE CONTAINERS:
LEVAQUIN INJECTION PREMIX IN FLEXIBLE CONTAINERS is supplied as a single-use, premixed solution in flexible containers. Each bag contains a dilute solution with the equivalent of 250 mg or 500 mg of levofloxacin, respectively, in 5% Dextrose (D₅W).
5 mg/mL (250 mg), 50 mL flexible container (NDC 0045-0067-01)
5 mg/mL (500 mg), 100 mL flexible container (NDC 0045-0068-01)
LEVAQUIN INJECTION PREMIX IN FLEXIBLE CONTAINERS should be stored at or below 25°C (77°F); however, brief exposure up to 40°C (104°F) does not adversely affect the product. Avoid excessive heat and protect from freezing and light.
LEVAQUIN INJECTION PREMIX IN FLEXIBLE CONTAINERS is manufactured for Ortho-McNeil Pharm by ABBOTT Laboratories, North Chicago, IL 60064.

Patients with Impaired Renal Function:

Renal Status	Initial Dose	Subsequent Dose
Acute Bacterial Exacerbation of Chronic Bronchitis/ Comm. Acquired Pneumonia/Acute Maxillary Sinusitis/Uncomplicated SSSI		
CL$_{CR}$ from 50 to 80 mL/min		No dosage adjustment required
CL$_{CR}$ from 20 to 49 mL/min	500 mg	250 mg q24h
CL$_{CR}$ from 10 to 19 mL/min	500 mg	250 mg q48h
Hemodialysis	500 mg	250 mg q48h
CAPD	500 mg	250 mg q48h
Complicated UTI/Acute Pyelonephritis		
CL$_{CR}$ ≥20 mL/min		No dosage adjustment required
CL$_{CR}$ from 10 to 19 mL/min	250 mg	250 mg q48h

CL$_{CR}$=creatinine clearances
CAPD=chronic ambulatory peritoneal dialysis

Desired Dosage Strength	From 20 mL Vial, Withdraw Volume	Volume of Diluent	Infusion Time
250 mg	10 mL	40 mL	60 min
500 mg	20 mL	80 mL	60 min

For example, to prepare a 500-mg dose using the 20 mL vial (25 mg/mL), withdraw 20 mL and dilute with a compatible intravenous solution to a total volume of 100 mL.

Also Available:
TABLETS
Levofloxacin is also available as 250-mg and 500-mg LEVAQUIN Tablets.

CLINICAL STUDIES
Community-Acquired Bacterial Pneumonia
Adult inpatients and outpatients with a diagnosis of community-acquired bacterial pneumonia were evaluated in two pivotal clinical studies. In the first study, 590 patients were enrolled in a prospective, multi-center, unblinded randomized trial comparing levofloxacin 500 mg once daily orally or intravenously for 7 to 14 days to ceftriaxone 1 to 2 grams intravenously once or in equally divided doses twice daily followed by cefuroxime axetil 500 mg orally twice daily for a total of 7 to 14 days. Patients assigned to treatment with the control regimen were allowed to receive erythromycin (or doxycycline if intolerant of erythromycin) if an infection due to atypical pathogens was suspected or proven. Clinical and microbiologic evaluations were performed during treatment, 5 to 7 days posttherapy, and 3 to 4 weeks posttherapy. Clinical success (cure plus improvement) with levofloxacin at 5 to 7 days posttherapy, the primary efficacy variable in this study, was superior (95%) to the control group (83%) [95% CI of -19,-6]. In the second study, 264 patients were enrolled in a prospective, multi-center, noncomparative trial of 500 mg levofloxacin administered orally or intravenously once daily for 7 to 14 days. Clinical success for clinically evaluable patients was 93%. For both studies, the clinical success rate in patients with atypical pneumonia due to *Chlamydia pneumoniae, Mycoplasma pneumoniae,* and *Legionella pneumophila* were 96%, 96%, and 70%, respectively. Microbiologic eradication rates across both studies were as follows:

Pathogen	No. Pathogens	Microbiologic Eradication Rate (%)
H. influenzae	55	98
S. pneumoniae	83	95
S. aureus	17	88
M. catarrhalis	18	94
H. parainfluenzae	19	95
K. pneumoniae	10	100.0

ANIMAL PHARMACOLOGY
Levofloxacin and other quinolones have been shown to cause arthropathy in immature animals of most species tested. (See **WARNINGS.**) In immature dogs (4–5 months old), oral doses of 10 mg/kg/day for 7 days and intravenous doses of 4 mg/kg/day for 14 days of levofloxacin resulted in arthropathic lesions. Administration at oral doses of 300 mg/kg/day for 7 days and intravenous doses of 60 mg/kg/day for 4 weeks produced arthropathy in juvenile rats.

When tested in a mouse ear swelling bioassay, levofloxacin exhibited phototoxicity similar in magnitude to ofloxacin, but less phototoxicity than other quinolones.

While crystalluria has been observed in some intravenous rat studies, urinary crystals are not formed in the bladder, being present only after micturition and are not associated with nephrotoxicity.

In mice, the CNS stimulatory effect of quinolones is enhanced by concomitant administration of non-steroidal anti-inflammatory drugs.

In dogs, levofloxacin administered at 6 mg/kg or higher by rapid intravenous injection produced hypotensive effects. These effects were considered to be related to histamine release.

In vitro and *in vivo* studies in animals indicate that levofloxacin is neither an enzyme inducer or inhibitor in the human therapeutic plasma concentration range; therefore, no drug metabolizing enzyme-related interactions with other drugs or agents are anticipated.
Rx Only

REFERENCES

1. National Committee for Clinical Laboratory Standards. Methods for Dilution Antimicrobial Susceptibility Tests for Bacteria That Grow Aerobically Third Edition. Approved Standard NCCLS Document M7-A3, Vol. 13, No. 25, NCCLS, Villanova, PA, December, 1993.
2. National Committee for Clinical Laboratory Standards. Performance Standards for Antimicrobial Disk Susceptibility Tests Fifth Edition. Approved Standard NCCLS Document M2-A5, Vol. 13, No. 24, NCCLS, Villanova, PA, December, 1993.

LEVAQUIN is manufactured and distributed by:
Ortho-McNeil Pharmaceutical Inc.
Raritan, New Jersey 08869
U.S. Patent No. 4,382,892 and U.S. Patent No. 5,053,407.
 Revised April 1998 635-10-287-2

Shown in Product Identification Guide, page 328

LEVAQUIN® tablets ℞
(levofloxacin tablets)

DESCRIPTION

LEVAQUIN® (levofloxacin tablets) Tablets contain levofloxacin, a synthetic broad spectrum antibacterial agent for oral administration. Chemically, levofloxacin, a chiral fluorinated carboxyquinolone, is the pure (-)-(S)-enantiomer of the racemic drug substance ofloxacin. The chemical name is (-)-(S)-9-fluoro-2,3-dihydro-3-methyl -10-(4-methyl-1-piperazinyl)-7-oxo-7H-pyrido [1,2,3-de]-1,4-benzoxazine-6-carboxylic acid hemihydrate.
The chemical structure is:

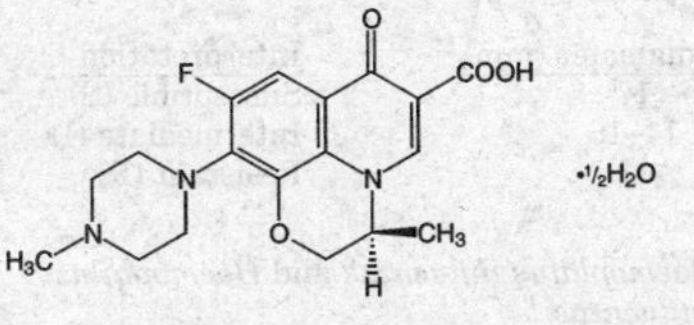

Its empirical formula is $C_{18}H_{20}FN_3O_4 \cdot {}^1/_2H_2O$ and its molecular weight is 370.38. Levofloxacin is a light yellowish-white to yellow-white crystal or crystalline powder. The molecule exists as a zwitterion at the pH conditions in the small intestine.
The data demonstrate that from pH 0.6 to 5.8, the solubility of levofloxacin is essentially constant (approximately 100 mg/mL). Levofloxacin is considered *soluble to freely soluble* in this pH range, as defined by USP nomenclature. Above pH 5.8, the solubility increases rapidly to its maximum at pH 6.7 (272 mg/mL) and is considered *freely soluble* in this range. Above pH 6.7, the solubility decreases and reaches a minimum value (about 50 mg/mL) at a pH of approximately 6.9.
Levofloxacin has the potential to form stable coordination compounds with many metal ions. This *in vitro* chelation potential has the following formation order: $Al^{+3} > Cu^{+2} > Zn^{+2} > Mg^{+2} > Ca^{+2}$.
LEVAQUIN Tablets are available as film-coated tablets and contain the following inactive ingredients:
250-mg (as expressed in the anhydrous form): hydroxypropyl methylcellulose, crospovidone, microcrystalline cellulose, magnesium stearate, polyethylene glycol, titanium dioxide, polysorbate 80 and synthetic red iron oxide.
500-mg (as expressed in the anhydrous form): hydroxypropyl methylcellulose, crospovidone, microcrystalline cellulose, magnesium stearate, polyethylene glycol, titanium dioxide, polysorbate 80 and synthetic red and yellow iron oxides.

CLINICAL PHARMACOLOGY

Absorption

Levofloxacin is rapidly and essentially completely absorbed after oral administration. Peak plasma concentrations are usually attained one to two hours after oral dosing. The absolute bioavailability of a 500-mg oral dose of levofloxacin is approximately 99%. Levofloxacin pharmacokinetics are linear and predictable after single and multiple oral dosing regimens. Steady-state is reached within 48 hours following a 500-mg once-daily regimen. The peak and trough plasma concentrations attained following multiple once-daily oral 500-mg regimens were approximately 5.7 and 0.5 μg/mL, respectively.
Oral administration with food slightly prolongs the time to peak concentration by approximately 1 hour and slightly decreases the peak concentration by approximately 14%. Therefore, levofloxacin can be administered without regard to food.
The plasma concentration profile of levofloxacin after i.v. administration is similar and comparable in extent of exposure (AUC) to that observed for levofloxacin tablets when equal doses (mg/mg) are administered. Therefore, the oral and i.v. routes of administration can be considered interchangeable. (See following chart.)

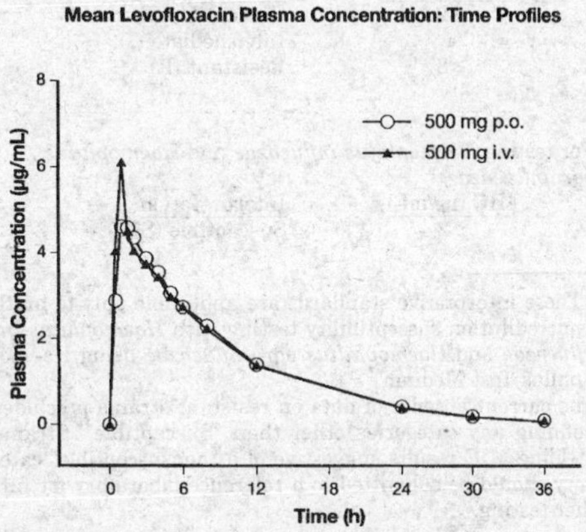

Mean Levofloxacin Plasma Concentration: Time Profiles
500 mg p.o.
500 mg i.v.
Plasma Concentration (μg/mL)
Time (h)
0
2
4
6
8
6
12
18
24
30
36

Distribution

The mean volume of distribution of levofloxacin generally ranges from 89 to 112 L after single and multiple 500-mg doses, indicating widespread distribution into body tissues. Penetration of levofloxacin into blister fluid is rapid and extensive. The blister fluid to plasma AUC ratio is approximately 1. Levofloxacin also penetrates well into lung tissues. Lung tissue concentrations were generally 2- to 5-fold higher than plasma concentrations and ranged from approximately 2.4 to 11.3 μg/g over a 24-hour period after a single 500-mg oral dose.
In vitro, over a clinically relevant range (1 to 10 μg/mL) of serum/plasma levofloxacin concentrations, levofloxacin is approximately 24 to 38% bound to serum proteins across all species studied, as determined by the equilibrium dialysis method. Levofloxacin is mainly bound to serum albumin in humans. Levofloxacin binding to serum proteins is independent of the drug concentration.

Metabolism

Levofloxacin is stereochemically stable in plasma and urine and does not invert metabolically to its enantiomer, D-ofloxacin. Levofloxacin undergoes limited metabolism in humans and is primarily excreted as unchanged drug in the urine. Following oral administration, approximately 87% of an administered dose was recovered as unchanged drug in urine within 48 hours, whereas less than 4% of the dose was recovered in feces in 72 hours. Less than 5% of an administered dose was recovered in the urine as the desmethyl and N-oxide metabolites, the only metabolites identified in humans. These metabolites have little relevant pharmacological activity.

Excretion

Levofloxacin is excreted largely as unchanged drug in the urine. The mean terminal plasma elimination half-life of levofloxacin ranges from approximately 6 to 8 hours following single or multiple doses of levofloxacin given orally or intravenously. The mean apparent total body clearance and renal clearance range from approximately 144 to 226 mL/min and 96 to 142 mL/min, respectively. Renal clearance in excess of the glomerular filtration rate suggests that tubular secretion of levofloxacin occurs in addition to its glomerular filtration. Concomitant administration of either cimetidine or probenecid results in approximately 24% and 35% reduction in the levofloxacin renal clearance, respectively, indicating that secretion of levofloxacin occurs in the renal proximal tubule. No levofloxacin crystals were found in any of the urine samples freshly collected from subjects receiving levofloxacin.

Special Populations

Geriatric

There are no significant differences in levofloxacin pharmacokinetics between young and elderly subjects when the subjects' differences in creatinine clearance are taken into consideration. Following a 500-mg oral dose of levofloxacin to healthy elderly subjects (66–80 years of age), the mean terminal plasma elimination half-life of levofloxacin was about 7.6 hours, as compared to approximately 6 hours in younger adults. The difference was attributable to the variation in renal function status of the subjects and was not believed to be clinically significant. Drug absorption appears to be unaffected by age. Levofloxacin dose adjustment based on age alone is not necessary.

Pediatric

The pharmacokinetics of levofloxacin in pediatric subjects have not been studied.

Gender

There are no significant differences in levofloxacin pharmacokinetics between male and female subjects when subjects' differences in creatinine clearance are taken into consideration. Following a 500-mg oral dose of levofloxacin to healthy male subjects, the mean terminal plasma elimination half-life of levofloxacin was about 7.5 hours, as compared to approximately 6.1 hours in female subjects. This difference was attributable to the variation in renal function status of the male and female subjects and was not believed to be clinically significant. Drug absorption appears to be unaffected by the gender of the subjects. Dose adjustment based on gender alone is not necessary.

Race

The effect of race on levofloxacin pharmacokinetics was examined through a covariate analysis performed on data from 72 subjects: 48 white and 24 nonwhite. The apparent total body clearance and apparent volume of distribution were not affected by the race of the subjects.

Renal Insufficiency

Clearance of levofloxacin is reduced and plasma elimination half-life is prolonged in patients with impaired renal function (creatinine clearance ≤80 mL/min), requiring dosage adjustment in such patients to avoid accumulation. Neither hemodialysis nor continuous ambulatory peritoneal dialysis (CAPD) is effective in removal of levofloxacin from the body, indicating that supplemental doses of levofloxacin are not required following hemodialysis or CAPD. (See **PRECAUTIONS: General** and **DOSAGE AND ADMINISTRATION.)**

Hepatic insufficiency

Pharmacokinetic studies in hepatically impaired patients have not been conducted. Due to the limited extent of levofloxacin metabolism, the pharmacokinetics of levofloxacin are not expected to be affected by hepatic impairment.

Bacterial infection

The pharmacokinetics of levofloxacin in patients with serious community-acquired bacterial infections are comparable to those observed in healthy subjects.

Drug-drug interactions

The potential for pharmacokinetic drug interactions between levofloxacin and theophylline, warfarin, cyclosporine, digoxin, probenecid, cimetidine, sucralfate, and antacids has been evaluated. (See **PRECAUTIONS: Drug Interactions.)**
The mean (±SD) pharmacokinetic parameters of levofloxacin determined under single and steady state conditions following oral (p.o.) or intravenous (i.v.) doses of levofloxacin are summarized as follows:
[See table at bottom of next page]

MICROBIOLOGY

Levofloxacin is the L-isomer of the racemate, ofloxacin, a quinolone antimicrobial agent. The antibacterial activity of ofloxacin resides primarily in the L-isomer. The mechanism of action of levofloxacin and other fluoroquinolone antimicrobials involves inhibition of DNA gyrase (bacterial topoisomerase II), an enzyme required for DNA replication, transcription, repair and recombination.
Levofloxacin has *in vitro* activity against a wide range of gram-negative and gram-positive microorganisms. Levofloxacin is often bactericidal at concentrations equal to or slightly greater than inhibitory concentrations.
Fluoroquinolones differ in chemical structure and mode of action from β-lactam antibiotics. Fluoroquinolones may, therefore, be active against bacteria resistant to β-lactam antibiotics.
Resistance to levofloxacin due to spontaneous mutation *in vitro* is a rare occurrence (range: 10^{-9} to 10^{-10}). Although cross-resistance has been observed between levofloxacin and some other fluoroquinolones, some microorganisms resistant to other fluoroquinolones may be susceptible to levofloxacin.
Levofloxacin has been shown to be active against most strains of the following microorganisms both *in vitro* and in clinical infections as described in the **INDICATIONS AND USAGE** section:

Aerobic gram-positive microorganisms
Enterococcus faecalis
Staphylococcus aureus
Streptococcus pneumoniae
Streptococcus pyogenes

Aerobic gram-negative microorganisms
Enterobacter cloacae
Escherichia coli
Haemophilus influenzae
Haemophilus parainfluenzae
Klebsiella pneumoniae
Legionella pneumophila
Moraxella catarrhalis
Proteus mirabilis
Pseudomonas aeruginosa

Continued on next page

Levaquin Tablets—Cont.

As with other drugs in this class, some strains of *Pseudomonas aeruginosa* may develop resistance fairly rapidly during treatment with levofloxacin.

Other microorganisms

Chlamydia pneumoniae
Mycoplasma pneumoniae
The following *in vitro* data are available, **but their clinical significance is unknown.**
Levofloxacin exhibits *in vitro* minimum inhibitory concentrations (MIC's) of 2 µg/mL or less against most strains of the following microorganisms; however, the safety and effectiveness of levofloxacin in treating clinical infections due to these microorganisms have not been established in adequate and well-controlled trials.

Aerobic gram-positive microorganisms

Staphylococcus epidermidis
Streptococcus (Group C/F)
Streptococcus (Group G)
Staphylococcus saprophyticus
Streptococcus agalactiae
Viridans group streptococci

Aerobic gram-negative microorganisms

Acinetobacter anitratus
Acinetobacter baumannii
Acinetobacter calcoaceticus
Acinetobacter lwoffii
Bordetella pertussis
Citrobacter diversus
Citrobacter freundii
Enterobacter aerogenes
Enterobacter agglomerans
Enterobacter sakazaki
Klebsiella oxytoca
Morganella morganii
Proteus vulgaris
Providencia rettgeri
Providencia stuartii
Pseudomonas fluorescens
Serratia marcescens

Anerobic gram-positive microorganisms

Clostridium perfringens

Susceptibility Tests

Susceptibility testing for levofloxacin should be performed, as it is the optimal predictor of activity. However, until levofloxacin susceptibility testing is available, the susceptibility of the organism to ofloxacin may be used to predict susceptibility to levofloxacin. While ofloxacin susceptible organisms will be susceptible to levofloxacin, ofloxacin intermediate or resistant organisms may be susceptible to levofloxacin.

Dilution techniques:

Quantitative methods are used to determine antimicrobial minimal inhibitory concentrations (MICs). These MICs provide estimates of the susceptibility of bacteria to antimicrobial compounds. The MICs should be determined using a standardized procedure. Standardized procedures are based on a dilution method[1] (broth or agar) or equivalent with standardized inoculum concentrations and standardized concentrations of levofloxacin powder. The MIC values should be interpreted according to the following criteria:
For testing aerobic microorganisms other than *Haemophilus influenzae*, *Haemophilus parainfluenzae*, and *Streptococcus pneumoniae*:

MIC (µg/mL)	Interpretation
≤2	Susceptible (S)
4	Intermediate (I)
≥8	Resistant (R)

For testing *Haemophilus influenzae* and *Haemophilus parainfluenzae*: [a]

MIC (µg/mL)	Interpretation
≤2	Susceptible (S)

[a] These interpretive standards are applicable only to broth microdilution susceptibility testing with *Haemophilus influenzae* and *Haemophilus parainfluenzae* using Haemophilus Test Medium.[1]
The current absence of data on resistant strains precludes defining any categories other than "Susceptible". Strains yielding MIC results suggestive of a "nonsusceptible" category should be submitted to a reference laboratory for further testing.

For testing *Streptococcus pneumoniae*: [b]

MIC (µg/mL)	Interpretation
≤2	Susceptible (S)
4	Intermediate (I)
≥8	Resistant (R)

[b] These interpretive standards are applicable only to broth microdilution susceptibility tests using cation-adjusted Mueller-Hinton broth with 2-5% lysed horse blood.
A report of "Susceptible" indicates that the pathogen is likely to be inhibited if the antimicrobial compound in the blood reaches the concentrations usually achievable. A report of "Intermediate" indicates that the result should be considered equivocal, and, if the microorganism is not fully susceptible to alternative, clinically feasible drugs, the test should be repeated. This category implies possible clinical applicability in body sites where the drug is physiologically concentrated or in situations where a high dosage of drug can be used. This category also provides a buffer zone which prevents small uncontrolled technical factors from causing major discrepancies in interpretation. A report of "Resistant" indicates that the pathogen is not likely to be inhibited if the antimicrobial compound in the blood reaches the concentrations usually achievable; other therapy should be selected.

Standardized susceptibility test procedures require the use of laboratory control microorganisms to control the technical aspects of the laboratory procedures. Standard levofloxacin powder should give the following MIC values:

Microorganism		MIC (µg/mL)
Enterococcus faecalis	ATCC 29212	0.25-2
Escherichia coli	ATCC 25922	0.008-0.06
Escherichia coli	ATCC 35218	0.015-0.06
Pseudomonas aeruginosa	ATCC 27853	0.5-4
Staphylococcus aureus	ATCC 29213	0.06-0.5
Haemophilus influenzae	ATCC 49247[c]	0.008-0.03
Streptococcus pneumoniae	ATCC 49619[d]	0.5-2

[c] This quality control range is applicable to only *H. influenzae* ATCC 49247 tested by a broth microdilution procedure using Haemophilus Test Medium (HTM).[1]
[d] This quality control range is applicable to only *S. pneumoniae* ATCC 49619 tested by a broth microdilution procedure using cation-adjusted Mueller-Hinton broth with 2-5% lysed horse blood.

Diffusion techniques:

Quantitative methods that require measurement of zone diameters also provide reproducible estimates of the susceptibility of bacteria to antimicrobial compounds. One such standardized procedure[2] requires the use of standardized inoculum concentrations. This procedure uses paper disks impregnated with 5-µg levofloxacin to test the susceptibility of microorganisms to levofloxacin.
Reports from the laboratory providing results of the standard single-disk susceptibility test with a 5-µg levofloxacin disk should be interpreted according to the following criteria:
For aerobic microorganisms other than *Haemophilus influenzae*, *Haemophilus parainfluenzae*, and *Streptococcus pneumoniae*:

Zone diameter (mm)	Interpretation
≥17	Susceptible (S)
14–16	Intermediate (I)
≤13	Resistant (R)

For *Haemophilus influenzae* and *Haemophilus parainfluenzae*: [e]

Zone diameter (mm)	Interpretation
≥17	Susceptible (S)

[e] These interpretive standards are applicable only to disk diffusion susceptibility testing with *Haemophilus influenzae* and *Haemophilus parainfluenzae* using Haemophilus Test Medium.[2]

The current absence of data on resistant strains precludes defining any categories other than "Susceptible". Strains yielding zone diameter results suggestive of a "nonsusceptible" category should be submitted to a reference laboratory for further testing.

For *Streptococcus pneumoniae*: [f]

Zone diameter (mm)	Interpretation
≥17	Susceptible (S)
14–16	Intermediate (I)
≤13	Resistant (R)

[f] These zone diameter standards for *Streptococcus pneumoniae* apply only to tests performed using Mueller-Hinton agar supplemented with 5% sheep blood and incubated in 5% CO_2.

Interpretation should be as stated above for results using dilution techniques. Interpretation involves correlation of the diameter obtained in the disk test with the MIC for levofloxacin.
As with standardized dilution techniques, diffusion methods require the use of laboratory control microorganisms to control the technical aspects of the laboratory procedures. For the diffusion technique, the 5-µg levofloxacin disk should provide the following zone diameters in these laboratory test quality control strains:

Microorganism		Zone Diameter (mm)
Escherichia coli	ATCC 25922	29–37
Pseudomonas aeruginosa	ATCC 27853	19–26
Staphylococcus aureus	ATCC 25923	25–30
Haemophilus influenzae	ATCC 49247[g]	32–40

Regimen	C_{max} (µg/mL)	T_{max} (h)	AUC (µg·h/mL)	CL/F[1] (mL/min)	Vd/F[2] (L)	$t_{1/2}$ (h)	CL_R (mL/min)
Single dose							
250 mg p.o.[3]	2.8 ± 0.4	1.6 ± 1.0	27.2 ± 3.9	156 ± 20	ND	7.3 ± 0.9	142 ± 21
500 mg p.o.[3]*	5.1 ± 0.8	1.3 ± 0.6	47.9 ± 6.8	178 ± 28	ND	6.3 ± 0.6	103 ± 30
500 mg i.v.[3]	6.2 ± 1.0	1.0 ± 0.1	48.3 ± 5.4	175 ± 20	90 ± 11	6.4 ± 0.7	112 ± 25
Multiple dose							
500 mg q24h p.o.[3]	5.7 ± 1.4	1.1 ± 0.4	47.5 ± 6.7	175 ± 25	102 ± 22	7.6 ± 1.6	116 ± 31
500 mg q24h i.v.[3]	6.4 ± 0.8	ND	54.6 ± 11.1	158 ± 29	91 ± 12	7.0 ± 0.8	99 ± 28
500 mg or 250 mg q24h i.v., patients with bacterial infection[4]	8.7 ± 4.0[5]	ND	72.5 ± 51.2[5]	154 ± 72	111 ± 58	ND	ND
500 mg p.o. single dose, effects of gender and age:							
male[6]	5.5 ± 1.1	1.2 ± 0.4	54.4 ± 18.9	166 ± 44	89 ± 13	7.5 ± 2.1	126 ± 38
female[7]	7.0 ± 1.6	1.7 ± 0.5	67.7 ± 24.2	136 ± 44	62 ± 16	6.1 ± 0.8	106 ± 40
young[8]	5.5 ± 1.0	1.5 ± 0.6	47.5 ± 9.8	182 ± 35	83 ± 18	6.0 ± 0.9	140 ± 33
elderly[9]	7.0 ± 1.6	1.4 ± 0.5	74.7 ± 23.3	121 ± 33	67 ± 19	7.6 ± 2.0	91 ± 29
500 mg p.o. single dose, patients with renal insufficiency:							
CL_{CR} 50–80 mL/min	7.5 ± 1.8	1.5 ± 0.5	95.6 ± 11.8	88 ± 10	ND	9.1 ± 0.9	57 ± 8
CL_{CR} 20–49 mL/min	7.1 ± 3.1	2.1 ± 1.3	182.1 ± 62.6	51 ± 19	ND	27 ± 0	26 ± 13
CL_{CR} <20 mL/min	8.2 ± 2.6	1.1 ± 1.0	263.5 ± 72.5	33 ± 8	ND	35 ± 5	13 ± 3
hemodialysis	5.7 ± 1.0	2.8 ± 2.2	ND	ND	ND	76.2 ± 42	ND
CAPD	6.9 ± 2.3	1.4 ± 1.1	ND	ND	ND	51 ± 24	ND

[1] clearance/bioavailability
[2] volume of distribution/bioavailability
[3] healthy males 18–53 years of age
[4] 500 mg q48h for patients with moderate renal impairment (CL_{CR} 20–50 mL/min) and infections of the respiratory tract or skin
[5] dose-normalized values (to 500 mg dose), estimated by population pharmacokinetic modeling
[6] healthy males 22–75 years of age
[7] healthy females 18–80 years of age
[8] young healthy male and female subjects 18–36 years of age
[9] healthy elderly male and female subjects 66–80 years of age
* Absolute bioavailability; F=0.99 ±0.08; ND=not determined.

Streptococcus pneumoniae	ATCC 49619[h]	20–25

[g] This quality control range is applicable to only *H. influenzae* ATCC 49247 tested by a disk diffusion procedure using Haemophilus Test Medium (HTM).[2]

[h] This quality control range is applicable to only *S. pneumoniae* ATCC 49619 tested by a disk diffusion procedure using Mueller-Hinton agar supplemented with 5% sheep blood and incubated in 5% CO_2.

INDICATIONS AND USAGE

LEVAQUIN Tablets are indicated for the treatment of adults (≥18 years of age) with mild, moderate, and severe infections caused by susceptible strains of the designated microorganisms in the conditions listed below:

Acute maxillary sinusitis due to *Streptococcus pneumoniae, Haemophilus influenzae,* or *Moraxella catarrhalis.*

Acute bacterial exacerbation of chronic bronchitis due to *Staphylococcus aureus, Streptococcus pneumoniae, Haemophilus influenzae, Haemophilus parainfluenzae,* or *Moraxella catarrhalis.*

Community-acquired pneumonia due to *Staphylococcus aureus, Streptococcus pneumoniae, Haemophilus influenzae, Haemophilus parainfluenzae, Klebsiella pneumoniae, Moraxella catarrhalis, Chlamydia pneumoniae, Legionella pneumophila,* or *Mycoplasma pneumoniae.* (See CLINICAL STUDIES.)

Uncomplicated skin and skin structure infections (mild to moderate) including abscesses, cellulitis, furuncles, impetigo, pyoderma, wound infections, due to *Staphylococcus aureus,* or *Streptococcus pyogenes.*

Complicated urinary tract infections (mild to moderate) due to *Enterococcus faecalis, Enterobacter cloacae, Echerichia coli, Klebsiella pneumoniae, Proteus mirabilis,* or *Pseudomonas aeruginosa.*

Acute pyelonephritis (mild to moderate) caused by *Escherichia coli.*

Appropriate culture and susceptibility tests should be performed before treatment in order to isolate and identify organisms causing the infection and to determine their susceptibility to levofloxacin. Therapy with levofloxacin may be initiated before results of these tests are known; once results become available, appropriate therapy should be selected.

As with other drugs in this class, some strains of *Pseudomonas aeruginosa* may develop resistance fairly rapidly during treatment with levofloxacin. Culture and susceptibility testing performed periodically during therapy will provide information about the continued susceptibility of the pathogens to the antimicrobial agent and also the possible emergence of bacterial resistance.

CONTRAINDICATIONS

Levofloxacin is contraindicated in persons with a history of hypersensitivity to levofloxacin, quinolone antimicrobial agents, or any other components of this product.

WARNINGS

THE SAFETY AND EFFICACY OF LEVOFLOXACIN IN CHILDREN, ADOLESCENTS (UNDER THE AGE OF 18 YEARS), PREGNANT WOMEN, AND NURSING WOMEN HAVE NOT BEEN ESTABLISHED. (See **PRECAUTIONS: Pediatric Use, Pregnancy,** and **Nursing Mothers** subsections.)

In immature rats and dogs, the oral and intravenous administration to levofloxacin increased the incidence and severity of osteochondrosis. Other fluoroquinolones also produce similar erosions in the weight bearing joints and other signs of arthropathy in immature animals of various species. (See **ANIMAL PHARMACOLOGY.**)

Convulsions and toxic psychoses have been reported in patients receiving quinolones, including levofloxacin. Quinolones may also cause increased intracranial pressure and central nervous system stimulation which may lead to tremors, restlessness, anxiety, lightheadedness, confusion, hallucinations, paranoia, depression, nightmares, insomnia, and, rarely, suicidal thoughts or acts. These reactions may occur following the first dose. If these reactions occur in patients receiving levofloxacin, the drug should be discontinued and appropriate measures instituted. As with other quinolones, levofloxacin should be used with caution in patients with a known or suspected CNS disorder that may predispose to seizures or lower the seizure threshold (e.g., severe cerebral arteriosclerosis, epilepsy) or in the presence of other risk factors that may predispose to seizures or lower the seizure threshold (e.g., certain drug therapy, renal dysfunction.) (See **PRECAUTIONS: General, Information for Patients, Drug Interactions** and **ADVERSE REACTIONS.**)

Serious and occasionally fatal hypersensitivity and/or anaphylactic reactions have been reported in patients receiving therapy with quinolones. These reactions often occur following the first dose. Some reactions have been accompanied by cardiovascular collapse, hypotension/shock, seizure, loss of consciousness, tingling, angioedema (including tongue, laryngeal, throat, or facial edema/swelling), airway obstruction (including bronchospasm, shortness of breath, and acute respiratory distress), dyspnea, urticaria, itching, and other serious skin reactions. Levofloxacin should be discontinued immediately at the first appearance of a skin rash or any other sign of hypersensitivity. Serious acute hypersensitivity reactions may require treatment with epinephrine and other resuscitative measures, including oxygen, intravenous fluids, antihistamines, corticosteroids, pressor amines, and airway management, as clinically indicated. (See **PRECAUTIONS** and **ADVERSE REACTIONS.**)

Serious and sometimes fatal events, some due to hypersensitivity, and some due to uncertain etiology, have been reported rarely in patients receiving therapy with quinolones. These events may be severe and generally occur following the administration of multiple doses. Clinical manifestations may include one or more of the following: fever, rash or severe dermatologic reactions (e.g., toxic epidermal necrolysis, Stevens-Johnson Syndrome); vasculitis; arthralgia; myalgia; serum sickness; allergic pneumonitis; interstitial nephritis; acute renal insufficiency or failure; hepatitis; jaundice; acute hepatic necrosis or failure; anemia, including hemolytic and aplastic; thrombocytopenia, including thrombotic thrombocytopenic purpura; leukopenia; agranulocytosis; pancytopenia; and/or other hematologic abnormalities. The drug should be discontinued immediately at the first appearance of a skin rash or any other sign of hypersensitivity and supportive measures instituted. (See **PRECAUTIONS: Information for Patients** and **ADVERSE REACTIONS.**)

Pseudomembranous colitis has been reported with nearly all antibacterial agents, including levofloxacin, and may range in severity from mild to life-threatening. Therefore, it is important to consider this diagnosis in patients who present with diarrhea subsequent to the administration of any antibacterial agent.

Treatment with antibacterial agents alters the normal flora of the colon and may permit overgrowth of clostridia. Studies indicate that a toxin produced by *Clostridium difficile* is one primary cause of "antibiotic-associated colitis".

After the diagnosis of pseudomembranous colitis has been established, therapeutic measures should be initiated. Mild cases of pseudomembranous colitis usually respond to drug discontinuation alone. In moderate to severe cases, consideration should be given to management with fluids and electrolytes, protein supplementation, and treatment with an antibacterial drug clinically effective against *C. difficile* colitis. (See **ADVERSE REACTIONS.**)

Ruptures of the shoulder, hand, and Achilles tendons that required surgical repair or resulted in prolonged disability have been reported in patients receiving quinolones. Levofloxacin should be discontinued if the patient experiences pain, inflammation, or rupture of a tendon. Patients should rest and refrain from exercise until the diagnosis of tendinitis or tendon rupture has been confidently excluded. Tendon rupture can occur during or after therapy with quinolones, including levofloxacin.

PRECAUTIONS

General: Although levofloxacin is more soluble than other quinolones, adequate hydration of patients receiving levofloxacin should be maintained to prevent the formation of a highly concentrated urine.

Administer levofloxacin with caution in the presence of renal insufficiency. Careful clinical observation and appropriate laboratory studies should be performed prior to and during therapy since elimination of levofloxacin may be reduced. In patients with impaired renal function (creatinine clearance ≤ 80 mL/min), adjustment of the dosage regimen is necessary to avoid the accumulation of levofloxacin due to decreased clearance. (See **CLINICAL PHARMACOLOGY** and **DOSAGE AND ADMINISTRATION.**)

Moderate to severe phototoxicity reactions have been observed in patients exposed to direct sunlight while receiving drugs in this class. Excessive exposure to sunlight should be avoided. However, in clinical trials with levofloxacin, phototoxicity has been observed in less than 0.1% of patients. Therapy should be discontinued if phototoxicity (e.g., a skin eruption) occurs.

As with other quinolones, levofloxacin should be used with caution in any patient with a known or suspected CNS disorder that may predispose to seizures or lower the seizure threshold (e.g., severe cerebral arteriosclerosis, epilepsy) or in the presence of other risk factors that may predispose to seizures or lower the seizure threshold (e.g., certain drug therapy, renal dysfunction). (See **WARNINGS** and **Drug Interactions.**)

As with other quinolones, disturbances of blood glucose, including symptomatic hyper- and hypoglycemia, have been reported, usually in diabetic patients receiving concomitant treatment with an oral hypoglycemic agent (e.g., glyburide/glibenclamide) or with insulin. In these patients, careful monitoring of blood glucose is recommended. If a hypoglycemic reaction occurs in a patient being treated with levofloxacin, levofloxacin should be discontinued immediately and appropriate therapy should be initiated immediately. (See **Drug Interactions** and **ADVERSE REACTIONS.**)

As with any potent antimicrobial drug, periodic assessment of organ system functions, including renal, hepatic, and hematopoietic, is advisable during therapy. (See **WARNINGS** and **ADVERSE REACTIONS.**)

Information for Patients:

Patients should be advised:

• to drink fluids liberally;

• that antacids containing magnesium, or aluminum, as well as sucralfate, metal cations such as iron, and multivitamin preparations with zinc should be taken at least two hours before or two hours after levofloxacin administration. (See **Drug Interactions**);

• that levofloxacin can be taken without regard to meals;

• that levofloxacin may cause neurologic adverse effects (e.g., dizziness, lightheadedness) and that patients should know how they react to levofloxacin before they operate an automobile or machinery or engage in other activities requiring mental alertness and coordination. (See **WARNINGS** and **ADVERSE REACTIONS**);

• to discontinue treatment and inform their physician if they experience pain, inflammation, or rupture of a tendon, and to rest and refrain from exercise until the diagnosis of tendinitis or tendon rupture has been confidently excluded;

• that levofloxacin may be associated with hypersensitivity reactions, even following the first dose, and to discontinue the drug at the first sign of a skin rash, hives or other skin reactions, a rapid heartbeat, difficulty in swallowing or breathing, any swelling suggesting angioedema (e.g., swelling of the lips, tongue, face, tightness of the throat, hoarseness), or other symptoms of an allergic reaction. (See **WARNINGS** and **ADVERSE REACTIONS**);

• to avoid excessive sunlight or artificial ultraviolet light while receiving levofloxacin and to discontinue therapy if phototoxicity (i.e., skin eruption) occurs;

• that if they are diabetic and are being treated with insulin or an oral hypoglycemic agent and a hypoglycemic reaction occurs, they should discontinue levofloxacin and consult a physician. (See **PRECAUTIONS: General** and **Drug Interactions.**)

Drug Interactions:

Antacids, Sucralfate, Metal Cations, Multi-Vitamins: While the chelation by divalent cations is less marked than with other quinolones, concurrent administration of LEVAQUIN Tablets with antacids containing magnesium, or aluminum, as well as sucralfate, metal cations such as iron, and multivitamin preparations with zinc may interfere with the gastrointestinal absorption of levofloxacin resulting in systemic levels considerably lower than desired. These agents should be taken at least two hours before or two hours after levofloxacin administration.

Theophylline: No significant effect of levofloxacin on the plasma concentrations, AUC, and other disposition parameters for theophylline was detected in a clinical study involving 14 healthy volunteers. Similarly, no apparent effect of theophylline on levofloxacin absorption and disposition was observed. However, concomitant administration of other quinolones with theophylline has resulted in prolonged elimination half-life, elevated serum theophylline levels, and a subsequent increase in the risk of theophylline-related adverse reactions in the patient population. Therefore, theophylline levels should be closely monitored and appropriate dosage adjustments made when levofloxacin is co-administered. Adverse reactions, including seizures, may occur with or without an elevation in serum theophylline levels. (See **WARNINGS** and **PRECAUTIONS: General.**)

Warfarin: No significant effect of levofloxacin on the peak plasma concentrations, AUC, and other disposition parameters for R- and S- warfarin was detected in a clinical study involving healthy volunteers. No significant change in prothrombin time was noted in the presence of levofloxacin. Similarly, no apparent effect of warfarin on levofloxacin absorption and disposition was observed. However, since some quinolones have been reported to enhance the effects of oral anticoagulant warfarin or its derivatives in the patient population, the prothrombin time or other suitable coagulation test should be closely monitored if a quinolone antimicrobial is administered concomitantly with warfarin or its derivatives.

Cyclosporine: No significant effect of levofloxacin on the peak plasma concentrations, AUC, and other disposition parameters for cyclosporine was detected in a clinical study involving healthy volunteers. However, elevated serum levels of cyclosporine have been reported in the patient population when co-administered with some other quinolones. Levofloxacin C_{max} and K_e were slightly lower while T_{max} and $t_{1/2}$ were slightly longer in the presence of cyclosporine than those observed in other studies without concomitant medication. The differences, however, are not considered to be clinically significant. Therefore, no dosage adjustment is required for levofloxacin or cyclosporine when administered concomitantly.

Continued on next page

Levaquin Tablets—Cont.

Digoxin: No significant effect of levofloxacin on the peak plasma concentrations, AUC, and other disposition parameters for digoxin was detected in a clinical study involving healthy volunteers. Levofloxacin absorption and disposition kinetics were similar in the presence or absence of digoxin. Therefore, no dosage adjustment for levofloxacin or digoxin is required when administered concomitantly.

Probenecid and Cimetidine: No significant effect of probenecid or cimetidine on the rate and extent of levofloxacin absorption was observed in a clinical study involving healthy volunteers. The AUC and $t_{1/2}$ of levofloxacin were 27–38% and 30% higher, respectively, while CL/F and CL_R were 21–35% lower during concomitant treatment with probenecid or cimetidine compared to levofloxacin alone. Although these differences were statistically significant, the changes were not high enough to warrant dosage adjustment for levofloxacin when probenecid or cimetidine is co-administered.

Non-steroidal anti-inflammatory drugs: The concomitant administration of a non-steroidal anti-inflammatory drug with a quinolone, including levofloxacin, may increase the risk of CNS stimulation and convulsive seizures. (See **WARNINGS** and **PRECAUTIONS: General.**)

Antidiabetic agents: Disturbances of blood glucose, including hyperglycemia and hypoglycemia, have been reported in patients treated concomitantly with quinolones and an antidiabetic agent. Therefore, careful monitoring of blood glucose is recommended when these agents are co-administered.

Carcinogenesis, Mutagenesis, Impairment of Fertility: In a long term carcinogenicity study in rats, levofloxacin exhibited no carcinogenic or tumorigenic potential following daily dietary administration for 2 years; the highest dose was 2 or 10 times the recommended human dose based on surface area or body weight, respectively.

Levofloxacin was not mutagenic in the following assays; Ames bacterial mutation assay (*S. typhimurium* and *E. coli*), CHO/HGPRT forward mutation assay, mouse micronucleus test, mouse dominant lethal test, rat unscheduled DNA synthesis assay, and the mouse sister chromatid exchange assay. It was positive in the *in vitro* chromosomal aberration (CHL cell line) and sister chromatid exchange (CHL/IU cell line) assays.

Levofloxacin caused no impairment of fertility or reproductive performance in rats at oral doses as high as 360 mg/kg/day (2124 mg/m^2), corresponding to 3.0 or 18 times the recommended maximum human dose based on surface area or body weight, respectively, and intravenous doses as high as 100 mg/kg/day (590 mg/m^2), corresponding to 1.0 or 5 times the recommended maximum human dose based on surface area or body weight, respectively.

Pregnancy: Teratogenic Effects. Pregnancy Category C. Levofloxacin was not teratogenic in rats at oral doses as high as 810 mg/kg/day (4779 mg/m^2), which corresponds to 14 or 82 times the recommended maximum human dose based on surface area or body weight, respectively, or at intravenous doses as high as 160 mg/kg/day (944 mg/m^2) corresponding to 2.7 or 16 times the recommended maximum human dose based on surface area or body weight, respectively. Doses equivalent to 26 or 81 times the recommended maximum human dose of levofloxacin (based on surface area or body weight, respectively) caused decreased fetal body weight and increased fetal mortality in rats when administered orally at 810 mg/kg/day (8910 mg/m^2). No teratogenicity was observed when rabbits were dosed orally as high as 50 mg/kg/day (550 mg/m^2) which corresponds to 1.6 or 5.0 times the recommended maximum human dose based on surface area or body weight, respectively, or when dosed intravenously as high as 25 mg/kg/day (275 mg/m^2), corresponding to 0.8 or 2.5 times the maximum recommended human dose based on surface area or body weight, respectively.

There are, however, no adequate and well-controlled studies in pregnant women. Levofloxacin should be used during pregnancy only if the potential benefit justifies the potential risk to the fetus. (See **WARNINGS.**)

Nursing Mothers: Levofloxacin has not been measured in human milk. Based upon data from ofloxacin, it can be presumed that levofloxacin will be excreted in human milk. Because of the potential for serious adverse reactions from levofloxacin in nursing infants, a decision should be made whether to discontinue nursing or to discontinue the drug, taking into account the importance of the drug to the mother.

Pediatric Use: Safety and effectiveness in children and adolescents below the age of 18 years have not been established. Quinolones, including levofloxacin, cause arthropathy and osteochondrosis in juvenile animals of several species. (See **WARNINGS.**)

ADVERSE REACTIONS

The incidence of drug-related adverse reactions in patients during Phase 2 and 3 clinical trials conducted in North America was 6.2%. Among patients receiving multiple-dose therapy, 3.7% discontinued therapy with levofloxacin due to adverse experiences.

Patients with Normal Renal Function:

Infection*	Unit Dose	Freq.	Duration	Daily Dose
Acute Bacterial Exacerbation of Chronic Bronchitis	500 mg	q24h	7 days	500 mg
Comm. Acquired Pneumonia	500 mg	q24h	7–14 days	500 mg
Acute Maxillary Sinusitis	500 mg	q24h	10–14 days	500 mg
Uncomplicated SSSI	500 mg	q24h	7–10 days	500 mg
Complicated UTI	250 mg	q24h	10 days	250 mg
Acute pyelonephritis	250 mg	q24h	10 days	250 mg

*** DUE TO THE DESIGNATED PATHOGENS** (See **INDICATIONS AND USAGE.**)

Patients with Impaired Renal Function:

Renal Status	Initial Dose	Subsequent Dose
Acute Bacterial Exacerbation of Chronic Bronchitis/ Comm. Acquired Pneumonia/ Acute Maxillary Sinusitus/Uncomplicated SSSI		
CL_{CR} from 50 to 80 mL/min		No dosage adjustment required
CL_{CR} from 20 to 49 mL/min	500 mg	250 mg q24h
CL_{CR} from 10 to 19 mL/min	500 mg	250 mg q48h
Hemodialysis	500 mg	250 mg q48h
CAPD	500 mg	250 mg q48h
Complicated UTI/Acute Pyelonephritis		
CL_{CR} ≥20 mL/min		No dosage adjustment required
CL_{CR} from 10 to 19 mL/min	250 mg	250 mg q48h

CL_{CR}=creatinine clearances
CAPD=chronic ambulatory peritoneal dialysis

In clinical trials, the following events were considered likely to be drug-related in patients receiving multiple doses of levofloxacin: diarrhea 1.2%, nausea 1.2%, vaginitis 0.8%, flatulence 0.5%, pruritus 0.5%, rash 0.3%, abdominal pain 0.3%, genital moniliasis 0.3%, dizziness 0.3%, dyspepsia 0.3%, insomnia 0.3%, taste perversion 0.2%, vomiting 0.2%, anorexia 0.1%, anxiety 0.1%, constipation 0.1%, edema 0.1%, fatigue 0.1%, headache 0.1%, increased sweating 0.1%, leukorrhea 0.1%, malaise 0.1%, nervousness 0.1%, sleep disorders 0.1%, tremor 0.1%, urticaria 0.1%.

In clinical trials, the most frequently reported adverse events occurring in > 3% of the study population regardless of drug relationship, were:
nausea 6.6%, diarrhea 5.4%, headache 5.4%, constipation 3.1%.

In clinical trials, the following events occurred in 1 to 3% of patients, regardless of drug relationship:
insomnia 2.9%, dizziness 2.5%, vomiting 2.1%, abdominal pain 2.0%, dyspepsia 2.0%, rash 1.7%, vaginitis 1.8%, flatulence 1.6%, pruritus 1.6%, pain 1.4%, chest pain 1.1%, back pain 1.0%.

The following adverse events occurred in clinical trials at a rate of 0.5 to less than 1%, regardless of drug relationship: agitation, anorexia, anxiety, arthralgia, dry mouth, dyspnea, edema, fatigue, fever, genital pruritus, increased sweating, nervousness, pharyngitis, rhinitis, skin disorder, somnolence, taste perversion.

Additional adverse events occurring in clinical trials at a rate of 0.3 to less than 0.5% regardless of drug relationship include:
cardiac failure, hypertension, leukorrhea, myocardial infarction, myalgia, purpura, tinnitus, tremor, urticaria.

Events occurring at a frequency lower than 0.3% regardless of drug relationship but considered medically important include: abnormal coordination, abnormal dreaming, abnormal hepatic function, abnormal platelets, abnormal renal function, abnormal vision, acute renal failure, aggravated diabetes mellitus, aggressive reaction, anemia, angina pectoris, ARDS, arrhythmia, arthritis, asthma, bradycardia, cardiac arrest, cerebrovascular disorder, circulatory failure, coma, confusion, convulsions (seizures), coronary thrombosis, delirium, depression, diplopia, embolism-blood clot, emotional lability, erythema nodosum, G.I. hemorrhage, granulocytopenia, hallucination, heart block, hepatic coma, hypoglycemia, hypotension, impaired concentration, increased LDH, jaundice, leukocytosis, leukopenia, lymphadenopathy, manic reaction, mental deficiency, muscle weakness, pancreatitis, paralysis, paranoia, postural hypotension, pseudomembranous colitis, rhabdomyolysis, sleep disorders, speech disorder, stupor, syncope, tachycardia, tendinitis, thrombocytopenia, vertigo, weight decrease, WBC abnormal not otherwise specified.

In clinical trials using multiple-dose therapy, ophthalmologic abnormalities, including cataracts and multiple punctate lenticular opacities, have been noted in patients undergoing treatment with other quinolones. The relationship of the drugs to these events is not presently established.

Crystalluria and cylindruria have been reported with other quinolones.

The following laboratory abnormalities appeared in 1.9% of patients receiving multiple doses of levofloxacin. It is not known whether these abnormalities were caused by the drug or the underlying condition being treated.

Blood Chemistry: decreased glucose, decreased lymphocytes

Post-Marketing Adverse Reactions: Additional serious adverse events reported from the marketing experience with levofloxacin outside of the United States regardless of drug relationship include:
allergic pneumonitis, anaphylactic shock, anaphylactoid reaction, dysphonia, abnormal EEG, encephalopathy, eosinophilia, erythema multiforme, hemolytic anemia, multi-system organ failure, palpitation, paresthesia, Stevens-Johnson Syndrome, tendon rupture, vasodilation.

OVERDOSAGE

Levofloxacin exhibits a low potential for acute toxicity. Mice, rats, dogs and monkeys exhibited the following clinical signs after receiving a single high dose of levofloxacin: ataxia, ptosis, decreased locomotor activity, dyspnea, prostration, tremors, and convulsions. Doses in excess of 1500 mg/kg orally and 250 mg/kg i.v. produced significant mortality in rodents. In the event of an acute overdosage, the stomach should be emptied. The patient should be observed and appropriate hydration maintained. Levofloxacin is not efficiently removed by hemodialysis or peritoneal dialysis.

DOSAGE AND ADMINISTRATION

The usual dose of LEVAQUIN Tablets is 500 mg orally every 24 hours as described in the following dosing chart. These recommendations apply to patients with normal renal function (i.e., CL_{CR} > 80 mL/min). For patients with altered renal function (i.e., $CL_{CR} \leq 80$ mL/min), see the **Patients with Impaired Renal Function** subsection. Oral doses should be administered at least two hours before or two hours after antacids containing magnesium, or aluminum, as well as sucralfate, metal cations such as iron, and multi-vitamin preparations with zinc.

[See first table above]
[See second table above]

When only the serum creatinine is known, the following formula may be used to estimate creatinine clearance.

Men: Creatinine Clearance (mL/min)=

$$\frac{\text{Weight (kg)} \times (140 - \text{age})}{72 \times \text{serum creatinine (mg/dL)}}$$

Women: 0.85 ×the value calculated for men.

The serum creatinine should represent a steady state of renal function.

HOW SUPPLIED

LEVAQUIN (levofloxacin tablets) Tablets are supplied as 250- and 500-mg modified rectangular, film-coated tablets. LEVAQUIN Tablets are packaged in bottles and in unit-dose blister strips in the following configurations:

250-mg tablets: color: terra cotta pink
 debossing: "LEVAQUIN" on side 1 and "250" on side 2
 bottles of 50 (NDC 0045-1520-50)
 unit-dose/100 tablets (NDC 0045-1520-10)

500-mg tablets: color: peach
 debossing: "LEVAQUIN" on side 1 and "500" on side 2
 bottles of 50 (NDC 0045-1525-50)
 unit-dose/100 tablets (NDC 0045-1525-10)

Storage
LEVAQUIN Tablets should be stored at 15° to 30°C (59° to 85°F) in well-closed containers.

Also available:
INJECTION
Levofloxacin is also available for intravenous administration in the following configurations:
LEVAQUIN INJECTION IN SINGLE-USE VIALS (20 mL) containing a concentrated solution with the equivalent of 500 mg of levofloxacin.
LEVAQUIN INJECTION PREMIX IN FLEXIBLE CONTAINERS containing a dilute solution with the equivalent of 250 or 500 mg of levofloxacin in 5% Dextrose (D_5W).

CLINICAL STUDIES

Community-Acquired Bacterial Pneumonia
Adult inpatients and outpatients with a diagnosis of community-acquired bacterial pneumonia were evaluated in two pivotal clinical studies. In the first study, 590 patients were enrolled in a prospective, multi-center, unblinded randomized trial comparing levofloxacin 500 mg once daily orally or intravenously for 7 to 14 days to ceftriaxone 1 to 2 grams intravenously once or in equally divided doses twice daily followed by cefuroxime axetil 500 mg orally twice daily for a total of 7 to 14 days. Patients assigned to treatment with the control regimen were allowed to receive erythromycin (or doxycycline if intolerant of erythromycin) if an infection due to atypical pathogens was suspected or proven. Clinical and microbiologic evaluations were performed during treatment, 5 to 7 days posttherapy, and 3 to 4 weeks posttherapy. Clinical success (cure plus improvement) with levofloxacin at 5 to 7 days posttherapy, the primary efficacy variable in this study, was superior (95%) to the control group (83%) [95% Cl of -19,-6]. In the second study, 264 patients were enrolled in a prospective, multi-center, noncomparative trial of 500 mg levofloxacin administered orally or intravenously once daily for 7 to 14 days. Clinical success for clinically evaluable patients was 93%. For both studies, the clinical success rate in patients with atypical pneumonia due to *Chlamydia pneumoniae*, *Mycoplasma pneumoniae*, and *Legionella pneumophila* were 96%, 96%, and 70%, respectively. Microbiologic eradication rates across both studies were as follows:

Pathogen	No. Pathogens	Microbiologic Eradication Rate (%)
H. influenzae	55	98
S. pneumoniae	83	95
S. aureus	17	88
M. catarrhalis	18	94
H. parainfluenzae	19	95
K. pneumoniae	10	100.0

ANIMAL PHARMACOLOGY

Levofloxacin and other quinolones have been shown to cause arthropathy in immature animals of most species tested. (See **WARNINGS.**) In immature dogs (4–5 months old), oral doses of 10 mg/kg/day for 7 days and intravenous doses of 4 mg/kg/day for 14 days of levofloxacin resulted in arthropathic lesions. Administration at oral doses of 300 mg/kg/day for 7 days and intravenous doses of 60 mg/kg/day for 4 weeks produced arthropathy in juvenile rats.
When tested in a mouse ear swelling bioassay, levofloxacin exhibited phototoxicity similar in magnitude to ofloxacin, but less phototoxicity than other quinolones.
While crystalluria has been observed in some intravenous rat studies, urinary crystals are not formed in the bladder, being present only after micturition and are not associated with nephrotoxicity.
In mice, the CNS stimulatory effect of quinolones is enhanced by concomitant administration of non-steroidal anti-inflammatory drugs.
In dogs, levofloxacin administered at 6 mg/kg or higher by rapid intravenous injection produced hypotensive effects. These effects were considered to be related to histamine release.
In vitro and *in vivo* studies in animals indicate that levofloxacin is neither an enzyme inducer or inhibitor in the human therapeutic plasma concentration range; therefore, no drug metabolizing enzyme-related interactions with other drugs or agents are anticipated.
℞ Only

REFERENCES

1. National Committee for Clinical Laboratory Standards. Methods for Dilution Antimicrobial Susceptibility Tests for Bacteria That Grow Aerobically Fourth Edition. Approved Standard NCCLS Document M7-A4, Vol. 17, No. 2, NCCLS, Wayne, PA, January 1997.
2. National Committee for Clinical Laboratory Standards. Performance Standards for Antimicrobial Disk Susceptibility Tests Sixth Edition. Approved Standard NCCLS Document M2-A6, Vol. 17, No. 1, NCCLS, Wayne, PA, January 1997.

LEVAQUIN is manufactured and distributed by:
Ortho-McNeil Pharmaceutical, Inc.
Raritan, NJ USA 08869

U.S. Patent No. 4,382,892 and U.S. Patent No. 5,053,407.
©OMP 1998 Revised March 1998 633-10-811-2
Shown in Product Identification Guide, page 328

MICRONOR® Tablets ℞
(norethindrone) 0.35 mg

Prescribing Information
Patients should be counseled that this product does not protect against HIV infection (AIDS) and other sexually transmitted diseases.

DESCRIPTION

MICRONOR® 28 Day Regimen
Each tablet contains 0.35 mg norethindrone. Inactive ingredients include D&C Green No. 5, D&C Yellow No. 10, lactose, magnesium stearate, povidone and starch.

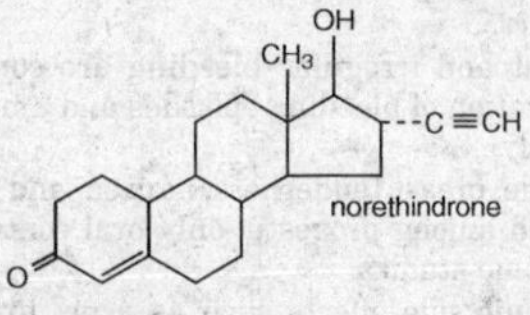

norethindrone

CLINICAL PHARMACOLOGY

1. MODE OF ACTION
MICRONOR progestin-only oral contraceptives prevent conception by suppressing ovulation in approximately half of users, thickening the cervical mucus to inhibit sperm penetration, lowering the midcycle LH and FSH peaks, slowing the movement of the ovum through the fallopian tubes, and altering the endometrium.
2. PHARMACOKINETICS
Serum progestin levels peak about two hours after oral administration, followed by rapid distribution and elimination. By 24 hours after drug ingestion, serum levels are near baseline, making efficacy dependent upon rigid adherence to the dosing schedule. There are large variations in serum levels among individual users. Progestin-only administration results in lower steady-state serum progestin levels and a shorter elimination half-life than concomitant administration with estrogens.

INDICATIONS AND USAGE

1. Indications
Progestin-only oral contraceptives are indicated for the prevention of pregnancy.
2. Efficacy
If used perfectly, the first-year failure rate for progestin-only oral contraceptives is 0.5%. However, the typical failure rate is estimated to be closer to 5%, due to late or omitted pills. Table 1 lists the pregnancy rates for users of all major methods of contraception
[See table I at bottom of next page]

CONTRAINDICATIONS

Progestin-only oral contraceptives (POPs) should not be used by women who currently have the following conditions:

- Known or suspected pregnancy
- Known or suspected carcinoma of the breast
- Undiagnosed abnormal genital bleeding
- Hypersensitivity to any component of this product
- Benign or malignant liver tumors
- Acute liver disease

WARNINGS

Cigarette smoking increases the risk of serious cardiovascular disease. Women who use oral contraceptives should be strongly advised not to smoke.
MICRONOR does not contain estrogen and, therefore, this insert does not discuss the serious health risks that have been associated with the estrogen component of combined oral contraceptives (COCs). The health care provider is referred to the prescribing information of combined oral contraceptives for a discussion of those risks. The relationship between progestin-only oral contraceptives and these risks is not fully defined. The physician should remain alert to the earliest manifestation of symptoms of any serious disease and discontinue oral contraceptive therapy when appropriate.
1. Ectopic Pregnancy
The incidence of ectopic pregnancies for progestin-only oral contraceptive users is 5 per 1000 woman-years. Up to 10% of pregnancies reported in clinical studies of progestin-only oral contraceptive users are extrauterine. Although symptoms of ectopic pregnancy should be watched for, a history of ectopic pregnancy need not be considered a contraindication to use of this contraceptive method. Health providers should be alert to the possibility of an ectopic pregnancy in women who become pregnant or complain of lower abdominal pain while on progestin-only oral contraceptives.
2. Delayed Follicular Atresia/Ovarian Cysts
If follicular development occurs, atresia of the follicle is sometimes delayed and the follicle may continue to grow beyond the size it would attain in a normal cycle. Generally these enlarged follicles disappear spontaneously. Often they are asymptomatic; in some cases they are associated with mild abdominal pain. Rarely they may twist or rupture, requiring surgical intervention.
3. Irregular Genital Bleeding
Irregular menstrual patterns are common among women using progestin-only oral contraceptives. If genital bleeding is suggestive of infection, malignancy or other abnormal conditions, such nonpharmacologic causes should be ruled out. If prolonged amenorrhea occurs, the possibility of pregnancy should be evaluated.
4. Carcinoma of the Breast and Reproductive Organs
Some epidemiological studies of oral contraceptive users have reported an increased relative risk of developing breast cancer, particularly at a younger age and apparently related to duration of use. These studies have predominantly involved combined oral contraceptives and there is insufficient data to determine whether the use of POPs similarly increases the risk.
A meta-analysis of 54 studies found a small increase in the frequency of having breast cancer diagnosed for women who were currently using combined oral contraceptives or had used them within the past ten years. This increase in the frequency of breast cancer diagnosis, within ten years of stopping use, was generally accounted for by cancers localized to the breast. There was no increase in the frequency of having breast cancer diagnosed ten or more years after cessation of use.
Women with breast cancer should not use oral contraceptives because the role of female hormones in breast cancer has not been fully determined.
Some studies suggest that oral contraceptive use has been associated with an increase in the risk of cervical intraepithealial neoplasia in some populations of women. However, there continues to be controversy about the extent to which such findings may be due to differences in sexual behavior and other factors. There is insufficient data to determine whether the use of POPs increases the risk of developing cervical intraepithelial neoplasia.
5. Hepatic Neoplasia
Benign hepatic adenomas are associated with combined oral contraceptive use, although the incidence of benign tumors is rare in the United States. Rupture of benign, hepatic adenomas may cause death through intraabdominal hemorrhage.
Studies have shown an increased risk of developing hepatocellular carcinoma in combined oral contraceptive users. However, these cancers are rare in the U.S. There is insufficient data to determine whether POPs increase the risk of developing hepatic neoplasia.

PRECAUTIONS

1. General
Patients should be counseled that this product does not protect against HIV infection (AIDS) and other sexually transmitted diseases.
2. Physical Examination and Follow up
It is considered good medical practice for sexually active women using oral contraceptives to have annual history and physical examinations. The physical examination may be deferred until after initiation of oral contraceptives if requested by the woman and judged appropriate by the clinician.
3. Carbohydrate and Lipid Metabolism
Some users may experience slight deterioration in glucose tolerance, with increases in plasma insulin but women with diabetes mellitus who use progestin-only oral contraceptives do not generally experience changes in their insulin requirements. Nonetheless, prediabetic and diabetic women in particular should be carefully monitored while taking POPs.
Lipid metabolism is occasionally affected in that HDL, HDL2, and apolipoprotein A-I and A-II may be decreased; hepatic lipase may be increased. There is usually no effect on total cholesterol, HDL_3, LDL, or VLDL.
4. Drug Interactions
The effectiveness of progestin-only pills is reduced by hepatic enzyme-inducing drugs such as the anticonvulsants phenytoin, carbamazepine, and barbiturates, and the antituberculosis drug rifampin. No significant interaction has been found with broad-spectrum antibiotics.
5. Interactions with Laboratory Tests
The following endocrine tests may be affected by progestin-only oral contraceptive use:

- Sex hormone-binding globulin (SHBG) concentrations may be decreased.
- Thyroxine concentrations may be decreased, due to a decrease in thyroid binding globulin (TBG).

6. Carcinogenesis
See WARNINGS section.

Continued on next page

Micronor—Cont.

7. Pregnancy

Many studies have found no effects on fetal development associated with long-term use of contraceptive doses of oral progestins. The few studies of infant growth and development that have been conducted have not demonstrated significant adverse effects. It is nonetheless prudent to rule out suspected pregnancy before initiating any hormonal contraceptive use.

8. Nursing Mothers

No adverse effects have been found on breastfeeding performance or on the health, growth or development of the infant. Small amounts of progestin pass into the breast milk, resulting in steroid levels in infant plasma of 1-6% of the levels of maternal plasma.

9. Pediatric Use

Safety and efficacy of MICRONOR Tablets have been established in women of reproductive age. Safety and efficacy are expected to be the same for postpubertal adolescents under the age of 16 and for users 16 years and older. Use of this product before menarche is not indicated.

10. Fertility Following Discontinuation

The limited available data indicate a rapid return of normal ovulation and fertility following discontinuation of progestin-only oral contraceptives.

11. Headache

The onset or exacerbation of migraine or development of severe headache with focal neurological symptoms which is recurrent or persistent requires discontinuation of progestin-only contraceptives and evaluation of the cause.

INFORMATION FOR THE PATIENT

1. See Detailed Patient Labeling for detailed information.
2. Counseling issues

The following points should be discussed with prospective users before prescribing progestin-only oral contraceptives:

- The necessity of taking pills at the same time every day, including throughout all bleeding episodes.
- The need to use a backup method such as condoms and spermicides for the next 48 hours whenever a progestin-only oral contraceptive is taken 3 or more hours late.
- The potential side effects of progestin-only oral contraceptives, particularly menstrual irregularities.
- The need to inform the clinician of prolonged episodes of bleeding, amenorrhea or severe abdominal pain.
- The importance of using a barrier method in addition to progestin-only oral contraceptives if a woman is at risk of contracting or transmitting STDs/HIV.

ADVERSE REACTIONS

Adverse reactions reported with the use of POPs include:

- Menstrual irregularity is the most frequently reported side effect.
- Frequent and irregular bleeding are common, while long duration of bleeding episodes and amenorrhea are less likely.
- Headache, breast tenderness, nausea, and dizziness are increased among progestin-only oral contraceptive users in some studies.
- Androgenic side effects such as acne, hirsutism, and weight gain occur rarely.

TABLE I: PERCENTAGE OF WOMEN EXPERIENCING AN UNINTENDED PREGNANCY DURING THE FIRST YEAR OF TYPICAL USE AND THE FIRST YEAR OF PERFECT USE OF CONTRACEPTION AND THE PERCENTAGE CONTINUING USE AT THE END OF THE FIRST YEAR. UNITED STATES.

Method (1)	% of Women Experiencing an Unintended Pregnancy within the First Year of Use		% of Women Continuing Use at One Year[3] (4)
	Typical Use[1] (2)	Perfect Use[2] (3)	
Chance[4]	85	85	
Spermicides[5]	26	6	40
Periodic abstinence	25		63
Calendar		9	
Ovulation method		3	
Sympto-Thermal[6]		2	
Post-Ovulation		1	
Withdrawal	19	4	
Cap[7]			
Parous Women	40	26	42
Nulliparous Women	20	9	56
Sponge			
Parous Women	40	20	42
Nulliparous Women	20	9	56
Diaphragm[7]	20	6	56
Condom[8]			
Female (Reality)	21	5	56
Male	14	3	61
Pill	5		71
Progestin Only		0.5	
Combined		0.1	
IUD			
Progesterone T	2.0	1.5	81
Copper T380A	0.8	0.6	78
LNg 20	0.1	0.1	81
Depo-Provera	0.3	0.3	70
Norplant and Norplant-2	0.05	0.05	88
Female Sterilization	0.5	0.5	100
Male Sterilization	0.15	0.10	100

Adapted from Trussel J. Contraceptive efficacy. In Hatcher RA, Trussel J, Stewart F, Cates W, Stewart GK, Kowal D, Guest F, Contraceptive Technology: Seventeenth Revised Edition. New York NY: Irvington Publishers, 1998, in press.

---

1. Among *typical* couples who initiate use of a method (not necessarily for the first time), the percentage who experience an accidental pregnancy during the first year if they do not stop use for any other reason.
2. Among couples who initiate use of a method (not necessarily for the first time) and who use it *perfectly* (both consistently and correctly), the percentage who experience an accidental pregnancy during the first year if they do not stop use for any other reason.
3. Among couples attempting to avoid pregnancy, the percentage who continue to use a method for one year.
4. The percents becoming pregnant in columns (2) and (3) are based on data from populations where contraception is not used and from women who cease using contraception in order to become pregnant. Among such populations, about 89% become pregnant within one year. This estimate was lowered slightly (to 85%) to represent the percent who would become pregnant within one year among women now relying on reversible methods of contraception if they abandoned contraception altogether.
5. Foams, creams, gels, vaginal suppositories, and vaginal film.
6. Cervical mucus (ovulation) method supplemented by calendar in the pre-ovulatory and basal body temperature in the post-ovulatory phases.
7. With spermicidal cream or jelly.
8. Without spermicides.

OVERDOSAGE

There have been no reports of serious ill effects from overdosage, including ingestion by children.

DOSAGE AND ADMINISTRATION

To achieve maximum contraceptive effectiveness, MICRONOR must be taken exactly as directed. One tablet is taken every day, at the same time. Administration is continuous, with no interruption between pill packs. See Detailed Patient Labeling for detailed instruction.

HOW SUPPLIED

MICRONOR Tablets are available in a DIALPAK® Tablet Dispenser
(NDC 0062-1411-01) containing 28 green tablets (0.35 mg norethindrone).
STORAGE: Store at controlled room temperature (15-30°C; 59-86°F).

REFERENCE

McCann M, and Potter L. Progestin-Only Oral Contraceptives: A Comprehensive Review. Contraception, 50:60 (Suppl. 1), December 1994.

MICRONOR® Tablets
(norethindrone) 0.35 mg
DETAILED PATIENT LABELING
MICRONOR® (norethindrone) Tablets
This product (like all oral contraceptives) is used to prevent pregnancy. It does not protect against HIV infection (AIDS) or other sexually transmitted diseases.

DESCRIPTION

MICRONOR® 28 Day Regimen
Each tablet contains 0.35 mg norethindrone. Inactive ingredients include D&C Green No. 5, D&C Yellow No. 10, lactose, magnesium stearate, povidone and starch.

INTRODUCTION

This leaflet is about birth control pills that contain one hormone, a progestin. Please read this leaflet before you begin to take your pills. It is meant to be used along with talking with your doctor or clinic.

Progestin-only pills are often called "POPs" or "the minipill". POPs have less progestin than the combined birth control pill (or "the pill") which contains both an estrogen and a progestin.

HOW EFFECTIVE ARE POPs?

About 1 in 200 POP users will get pregnant in the first year if they all take POPs perfectly (that is, on time, every day). About 1 in 20 "typical" POP users (including women who are late taking pills or miss pills) gets pregnant in the first year of use. Table 2 will help you compare the efficacy of different methods.

[See table II at top of next page]

HOW DO POPs WORK?

POPs can prevent pregnancy in different ways including:

- They make the cervical mucus at the entrance to the womb (the uterus) too thick for the sperm to get through to the egg.
- They prevent ovulation (release of the egg from the ovary) in about half of the cycles.
- They also affect other hormones, the fallopian tubes and the lining of the uterus.

YOU SHOULD NOT TAKE POPs

- If there is any chance you may be pregnant.
- If you have breast cancer.
- If you have bleeding between your periods that has not been diagnosed.
- If you are taking certain drugs for epilepsy (seizures) or for TB. (See "Using POPs with Other Medicines" below.)
- If you are hypersensitive, or allergic, to any component of this product.
- If you have liver tumors, either benign or cancerous.
- If you have acute liver disease.

RISKS OF TAKING POPs

Cigarette smoking greatly increases the possibility of suffering heart attacks and strokes. Women who use oral contraceptives are strongly advised not to smoke.

WARNING: If you have sudden or severe pain in your lower abdomen or stomach area, you may have an ectopic pregnancy or an ovarian cyst. If this happens, you should contact your doctor or clinic immediately.

Ectopic Pregnancy
An ectopic pregnancy is a pregnancy outside the womb. Because POPs protect against pregnancy, the chance of having a pregnancy outside the womb is very low. If you do get pregnant while taking POPs, you have a slightly higher chance that the pregnancy will be ectopic than do users of some other birth control methods.

Ovarian Cysts
These cysts are small sacs of fluid in the ovary. They are more common among POP users than among users of most other birth control methods. They usually disappear without treatment and rarely cause problems.

Cancer of the Reproductive Organs and Breasts
Some studies in women who use combined oral contraceptives that contain both estrogen and a progestin have re-

TABLE II: PERCENTAGE OF WOMEN EXPERIENCING AN UNINTENDED PREGNANCY DURING THE FIRST YEAR OF TYPICAL USE AND THE FIRST YEAR OF PERFECT USE OF CONTRACEPTION AND THE PERCENTAGE CONTINUING USE AT THE END OF THE FIRST YEAR. UNITED STATES.

Method (1)	% of Women Experiencing an Unintended Pregnancy within the First Year of Use		% of Women Continuing Use at One Year[3] (4)
	Typical Use[1] (2)	Perfect Use[2] (3)	
Chance[4]	85	85	
Spermicides[5]	26	6	40
Periodic abstinence	25		63
Calendar		9	
Ovulation method		3	
Sympto-Thermal[6]		2	
Post-Ovulation		1	
Withdrawal	19	4	
Cap[7]			
Parous Women	40	26	42
Nulliparous Women	20	9	56
Sponge			
Parous Women	40	20	42
Nulliparous Women	20	9	56
Diaphragm[7]	20	6	56
Condom[8]			
Female (Reality)	21	5	56
Male	14	3	61
Pill	5		71
Progestin Only		0.5	
Combined		0.1	
IUD			
Progesterone T	2.0	1.5	81
Copper T380A	0.8	0.6	78
LNg 20	0.1	0.1	81
Depo-Provera	0.3	0.3	70
Norplant and Norplant-2	0.05	0.05	88
Female Sterilization	0.5	0.5	100
Male Sterilization	0.15	0.10	100

Adapted from Trussel J. Contraceptive efficacy. In Hatcher RA, Trussel J, Stewart F, Cates W, Stewart GK, Kowal D, Guest F, Contraceptive Technology: Seventeenth Revised Edition. New York NY: Irvington Publishers, 1998, in press.

1. Among *typical* couples who initiate use of a method (not necessarily for the first time), the percentage who experience an accidental pregnancy during the first year if they do not stop use for any other reason.
2. Among couples who initiate use of a method (not necessarily for the first time) and who use it *perfectly* (both consistently and correctly), the percentage who experience an accidental pregnancy during the first year if they do not stop use for any other reason.
3. Among couples attempting to avoid pregnancy, the percentage who continue to use a method for one year.
4. The percents becoming pregnant in columns (2) and (3) are based on data from populations where contraception is not used and from women who cease using contraception in order to become pregnant. Among such populations, about 89% become pregnant within one year. This estimate is lowered slightly (to 85%) to represent the percent who would become pregnant within one year among women now relying on reversible methods of contraception if they abandoned contraception altogether.
5. Foams, creams, gels, vaginal suppositories, and vaginal film.
6. Cervical mucous (ovulation) method supplemented by calendar in the pre-ovulatory and basal body temperature in the post-ovulatory phases.
7. With spermicidal cream or jelly.
8. Without spermicides.

ported an increase in the risk of developing breast cancer, particularly at a younger age and apparently related to duration of use. There is insufficient data to determine whether the use of POPs similarly increases this risk.

A meta-analysis of 54 studies found a small increase in the frequency of having breast cancer diagnosed for women who were currently using combined oral contraceptives or had used them within the past ten years. This increase in the frequency of breast cancer diagnosis, within ten years of stopping use, was generally accounted for by cancers localized to the breast. There was no increase in the frequency of having breast cancer diagnosed ten or more years after cessation of use.

Some studies have found an increase in the incidence of cancer of the cervix in women who use oral contraceptives. However, this finding may be related to factors other than the use of oral contraceptives and there is insufficient data to determine whether the use of POPs increases the risk of developing cancer of the cervix.

Liver Tumors

In rare cases, combined oral contraceptives can cause benign but dangerous liver tumors. These benign liver tumors can rupture and cause fatal internal bleeding. In addition, some studies report an increased risk of developing liver cancer among women who use combined oral contraceptives. However, liver cancers are rare. There is insufficient data to determine whether POPs increase the risk of liver tumors.

Diabetic Women

Diabetic women taking POPs do not generally require changes in the amount of insulin they are taking. However, your physician may monitor you more closely under these conditions.

SEXUALLY TRANSMITTED DISEASES (STDs)

WARNING: POPs do not protect against getting or giving someone HIV (AIDS) or any other STD, such as chlamydia, gonorrhea, genital warts or herpes.

SIDE EFFECTS

Irregular Bleeding:

The most common side effect of POPs is a change in menstrual bleeding. Your periods may be either early or late, and you may have some spotting between periods. Taking pills late or missing pills can result in some spotting or bleeding.

Other Side Effects:

Less common side effects include headaches, tender breasts, nausea and dizziness. Weight gain, acne and extra hair on your face and body have been reported, but are rare.

If you are concerned about any of these side effects, check with your doctor or clinic.

USING POPs WITH OTHER MEDICINES

Before taking a POP, inform your health care provider of any other medication, including over-the-counter medicine, that you may be taking.

These medicines can make POPs less effective:

Medicines for seizures such as:
- Phenytoin (Dilantin)
- Carbamazepine (Tegretol)
- Phenobarbital

Medicine for TB:
- Rifampin (Rifampicin)

Before you begin taking any new medicines be sure your doctor or clinic knows you are taking a progestin-only birth control pill.

HOW TO TAKE POPs

IMPORTANT POINTS TO REMEMBER

- POPs must be taken at the same time every day, so choose a time and then take the pill at that same time every day. Every time you take a pill late, and especially if you miss a pill, you are more likely to get pregnant.
- Start the next pack the day after the last pack is finished. There is no break between packs. Always have your next pack of pills ready.
- You may have some menstrual spotting between periods. Do not stop taking your pills if this happens.
- If you vomit soon after taking a pill, use a backup method (such as a condom and/or a spermicide) for 48 hours.
- If you want to stop taking POPs, you can do so at any time, but, if you remain sexually active and don't wish to become pregnant, be certain to use another birth control method.
- If you are not sure about how to take POPs, ask your doctor or clinic.

STARTING POPs

- It's best to take your first POP on the first day of your menstrual period.
- If you decide to take your first POP on another day, use a backup method (such as a condom and/or a spermicide) every time you have sex during the next 48 hours.
- If you have had a miscarriage or an abortion, you can start POPs the next day.

IF YOU ARE LATE OR MISS TAKING YOUR POPs

- If you are more than 3 hours late or you miss one or more POPs:
  (1) **TAKE** a missed pill as soon as you remember that you missed it,
  (2) **THEN** go back to taking POPs at your regular time,
  (3) **BUT** be sure to use a backup method (such as a condom and/or a spermcide) every time you have sex for the next 48 hours.
- If you are not sure what to do about the pills you have missed, keep taking POPs and use a backup method until you can talk to your doctor or clinic.

IF YOU ARE BREASTFEEDING

- If you are fully breastfeeding (not giving your baby any food or formula), you may start your pills 6 weeks after delivery.
- If you are partially breastfeeding (giving your baby some food or formula), you should start taking pills by 3 weeks after delivery.

IF YOU ARE SWITCHING PILLS

- If you are switching from the combined pills to POPs, take the first POP the day after you finish the last active combined pill. Do not take any of the 7 inactive pills from the combined pill pack. You should know that many women have irregular periods after switching to POPs, but this is normal and to be expected.
- If you are switching from POPs to the combined pills, take the first active combined pill on the first day of your period, even if your POPs pack is not finished.
- If you switch to another brand of POPs, start the new brand anytime.
- If you are breastfeeding, you can switch to another method of birth control at any time, except do not switch to the combined pills until you stop breastfeeding or at least until 6 months after delivery.

PREGNANCY WHILE ON THE PILL

If you think you are pregnant, contact your physician. Even though research has shown that POPs do not cause harm to the unborn baby, it is always best not to take any drugs or medicines that you don't need when you are pregnant.

You should get a pregnancy test:
- If your period is late and you took one or more pills late or missed taking them and had sex without a backup method.
- Anytime it has been more than 45 days since the beginning of your last period.

WILL POPs AFFECT YOUR ABILITY TO GET PREGNANT LATER?

If you want to become pregnant, simply stop taking POPs. POPs will not delay your ability to get pregnant.

BREASTFEEDING

If you are breastfeeding, POPs will not affect the quality or amount of your breastmilk or the health of your nursing baby.

Continued on next page

Micronor—Cont.

OVERDOSE
No serious problems have been reported when many pills were taken by accident, even by a small child, so there is usually no reason to treat an overdose.

OTHER QUESTIONS OR CONCERNS
If you have any questions or concerns, check with your doctor or clinic. You can also ask for the more detailed "Professional Labeling" written for doctors and other health care providers.

HOW TO STORE YOUR POPs
Store your POPs at room temperature (between 59° and 86°F).
ORTHO-McNEIL
PHARMACEUTICAL, INC.
Raritan, New Jersey 08869
©OMP 1998
REVISED JUNE 1998   635-10-895-5
Shown in Product Identification Guide, page 328

ORTHO-CEPT®   ℞
(desogestrel and ethinyl estradiol) Tablets

Patients should be counseled that this product does not protect against HIV infection (AIDS) and other sexually transmitted diseases.

DESCRIPTION
ORTHO-CEPT 21 and ORTHO-CEPT 28 Tablets provide an oral contraceptive regimen of 21 orange round tablets each containing 0.15 mg desogestrel (13-ethyl-11-methylene-18,19-dinor-17 alpha-pregn-4-en-20-yn-17-ol) and 0.03 mg ethinyl estradiol (19-nor-17 alpha-pregna-1,3,5 (10)-trien-20-yne-3,17,diol). Inactive ingredients include vitamin E, pregelatinized starch, stearic acid, lactose, hydroxypropyl methylcellulose, polyethylene glycol, titanium dioxide, talc and ferric oxide. ORTHO-CEPT 28 also contains 7 green tablets containing the following inactive ingredients: lactose, pregelatinized starch, magnesium stearate, FD&C Blue No. 1 Aluminum Lake, ferric oxide, hydroxypropyl methylcellulose, polyethylene glycol, titanium dioxide and talc.

desogestrel

ethinyl estradiol

CLINICAL PHARMACOLOGY
Pharmacodynamics
Combination oral contraceptives act by suppression of gonadotropins. Although the primary mechanism of this action is inhibition of ovulation, other alterations include changes in the cervical mucus, which increase the difficulty of sperm entry into the uterus, and changes in the endometrium which reduce the likelihood of implantation.
Receptor binding studies, as well as studies in animals and humans, have shown that 3-keto-desogestrel, the biologically active metabolite of desogestrel, combines high progestational activity with minimal intrinsic androgenicity[91,92]. Desogestrel, in combination with ethinyl estradiol, does not counteract the estrogen-induced increases in SHBG, resulting in lower serum levels of free testosterone[96–99].
Pharmacokinetics
Desogestrel is rapidly and almost completely absorbed and converted into 3-keto-desogestrel, its biologically active metabolite. Following oral administration, the relative bioavailability of desogestrel, as measured by serum levels of 3-keto-desogestrel, is approximately 84%.
In the third cycle of use after a single dose of ORTHO-CEPT, maximum concentrations of 3-keto-desogestrel of $2,805\pm1,203$ pg/mL (mean$\pm$SD) are reached at 1.4 ± 0.8 hours. The area under the curve (AUC$_{0-\infty}$) is $33,858\pm11,043$ pg/mL·hr after a single dose. At steady state, attained from at least day 19 onwards, maximum concentrations of $5,840\pm1,667$ pg/mL are reached at 1.4 ± 0.9 hours. The minimum plasma levels of 3-keto-desogestrel at steady state are

$1,400\pm560$ pg/mL. The AUC$_{0-24}$ at steady state is $52,299\pm17,878$ pg/mL·hr. The mean AUC$_{0-\infty}$ for 3-keto-desogestrel at single dose is significantly lower than the mean AUC$_{0-24}$ at steady state. This indicates that the kinetics of 3-keto-desogestrel are non-linear due to an increase in binding of 3-keto-desogestrel to sex hormone-binding globulin in the cycle, attributed to increased sex hormone-binding globulin levels which are induced by the daily administration of ethinyl estradiol. Sex hormone-binding globulin levels increased significantly in the third treatment cycle from day 1 (150 ± 64 nmol/L) to day 21 (230 ± 59 nmol/L).
The elimination half-life for 3-keto-desogestrel is approximately 38 ± 20 hours at steady state. In addition to 3-keto-desogestrel, other phase I metabolites are 3α-OH-desogestrel, 3β-OH-desogestrel, and 3α-OH-5α-H-desogestrel. These other metabolites are not known to have any pharmacologic effects, and are further converted in part by conjugation (phase II metabolism) into polar metabolites, mainly sulfates and glucuronides.
Ethinyl estradiol is rapidly and almost completely absorbed. In the third cycle of use after a single dose of ORTHO-CEPT, the relative bioavailability is approximately 83%.
In the third cycle of use after a single dose of ORTHO-CEPT, maximum concentrations of ethinyl estradiol of 95 ± 34 pg/mL are reached at 1.5 ± 0.8 hours. The AUC$_{0-\infty}$ is $1,471\pm268$ pg/mL·hr after a single dose. At steady state, attained from at least day 19 onwards, maximum ethinyl estradiol concentrations of 141 ± 48 pg/mL are reached at about 1.4 ± 0.7 hours. The minimum serum levels of ethinyl estradiol at steady state are 24 ± 8.3 pg/mL. The AUC$_{0-24}$, at steady state is $1,117\pm302$ pg/mL·hr. The mean AUC$_{0-\infty}$ for ethinyl estradiol following a single dose during treatment cycle 3 does not significantly differ from the mean AUC$_{0-24}$ at steady state. This finding indicates linear kinetics for ethinyl estradiol.
The elimination half-life is 26 ± 6.8 hours at steady state. Ethinyl estradiol is subject to a significant degree of presystemic conjugation (phase II metabolism). Ethinyl estradiol escaping gut wall conjugation undergoes phase I metabolism and hepatic conjugation (phase II metabolism). Major phase I metabolites are 2-OH-ethinyl estradiol and 2-methoxy-ethinyl estradiol. Sulfate and glucuronide conjugates of both ethinyl estradiol and phase I metabolites, which are excreted in bile, can undergo enterohepatic circulation.

INDICATIONS AND USAGE
ORTHO-CEPT Tablets are indicated for the prevention of pregnancy in women who elect to use oral contraceptives as a method of contraception.
Oral contraceptives are highly effective. Table I lists the typical accidental pregnancy rates for users of combination oral contraceptives and other methods of contraception. The efficacy of these contraceptive methods, except sterilization, depends upon the reliability with which they are used. Correct and consistent use of these methods can result in lower failure rates.
[See table I below]
In a clinical trial with ORTHO-CEPT, 1,195 subjects completed 11,656 cycles and a total of 10 pregnancies were reported. This represents an overall user-efficacy (typical user-efficacy) pregnancy rate of 1.12 per 100 women-years. This rate includes patients who did not take the drug correctly.

CONTRAINDICATIONS
Oral contraceptives should not be used in women who currently have the following conditions:
- Thrombophlebitis or thromboembolic disorders
- A past history of deep vein thrombophlebitis or thromboembolic disorders
- Cerebral vascular or coronary artery disease
- Known or suspected carcinoma of the breast
- Carcinoma of the endometrium or other known or suspected estrogen-dependent neoplasia
- Undiagnosed abnormal genital bleeding
- Cholestatic jaundice of pregnancy or jaundice with prior pill use
- Hepatic adenomas or carcinomas
- Known or suspected pregnancy

WARNINGS

> **Cigarette smoking increases the risk of serious cardiovascular side effects from oral contraceptive use. This risk increases with age and with heavy smoking (15 or more cigarettes per day) and is quite marked in women over 35 years of age. Women who use oral contraceptives should be strongly advised not to smoke.**

TABLE I

LOWEST EXPECTED AND TYPICAL FAILURE RATES DURING THE FIRST YEAR OF CONTINUOUS USE OF A METHOD
% of Women Experiencing an Accidental Pregnancy in the First Year of Continuous Use

Method	Lowest Expected*	Typical**	
(No Contraceptive)	(85)	(85)	
Oral Contraceptives		3	
combined	0.1	N/A	***
progestin only	0.5	N/A	***
Diaphragm with spermicidal			
cream or jelly	6	18	
Spermicides alone (foams, creams, gels, jellies, vaginal suppositories, and vaginal film)	6	21	
Vaginal Sponge			
nulliparous	9	18	
parous	20	36	
Implant	0.09	0.09	
Injection: depot			
medroxyprogesterone acetate	0.3	0.3	
IUD			
progesterone	1.5	2.0	
copper T 380A	0.6	0.8	
Condom without spermicides			
female	5	21	
male	3	12	
Cervical Cap with spermicidal cream or jelly			
nulliparous	9	18	
parous	26	36	
Periodic abstinence			
(all methods)	1–9	20	
Female sterilization	0.4	0.4	
Male sterilization	0.10	0.15	

Adapted from RA Hatcher et al, Table 5–2, (1994) ref. #1.

---

* The authors' best guess of the percentage of women expected to experience an accidental pregnancy among couples who initiate a method (not necessarily for the first time) and who use it consistently and correctly during the first year if they do not stop for any other reason.

** This term represents "typical" couples who initiate use of a method (not necessarily for the first time), who experience an accidental pregnancy during the first year if they do not stop use for any other reason.

*** N/A—Data not available.

The use of oral contraceptives is associated with increased risks of several serious conditions including myocardial infarction, thromboembolism, stroke, hepatic neoplasia, and gallbladder disease, although the risk of serious morbidity or mortality is very small in healthy women without underlying risk factors. The risk of morbidity and mortality increases significantly in the presence of other underlying risk factors such as hypertension, hyperlipidemias, obesity and diabetes.

Practitioners prescribing oral contraceptives should be familiar with the following information relating to these risks. The information contained in this package insert is principally based on studies carried out in patients who used oral contraceptives with formulations of higher doses of estrogens and progestogens than those in common use today. The effect of long term use of the oral contraceptives with formulations of lower doses of both estrogens and progestogens remains to be determined.

Throughout this labeling, epidemiological studies reported are of two types: retrospective or case control studies and prospective or cohort studies. Case control studies provide a measure of the relative risk of a disease, namely, a *ratio* of the incidence of a disease among oral contraceptive users to that among nonusers. The relative risk does not provide information on the actual clinical occurrence of a disease. Cohort studies provide a measure of attributable risk, which is the *difference* in the incidence of disease between oral contraceptive users and nonusers. The attributable risk does provide information about the actual occurrence of a disease in the population (Adapted from refs. 2 and 3 with the author's permission). For further information, the reader is referred to a text on epidemiological methods.

1. THROMBOEMBOLIC DISORDERS AND OTHER VASCULAR PROBLEMS
a. Myocardial infarction
An increased risk of myocardial infarction has been attributed to oral contraceptive use. This risk is primarily in smokers or women with other underlying risk factors for coronary artery disease such as hypertension, hypercholesterolemia, morbid obesity, and diabetes. The relative risk of heart attack for current oral contraceptive users has been estimated to be two to six[4-10]. The risk is very low in women under the age of 30.

Smoking in combination with oral contraceptive use has been shown to contribute substantially to the incidence of myocardial infarctions in women in their mid-thirties or older with smoking accounting for the majority of excess cases[11]. Mortality rates associated with circulatory disease have been shown to increase substantially in smokers, especially in those 35 years of age and older among women who use oral contraceptives. (See Table II)

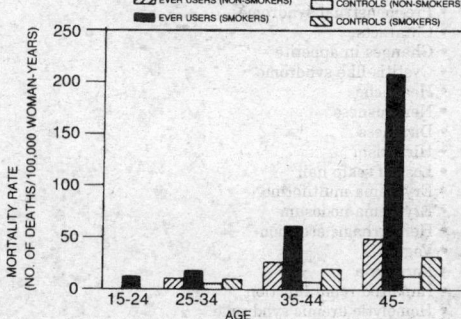

CIRCULATORY DISEASE MORTALITY RATES PER 100,000 WOMEN-YEARS BY AGE, SMOKING STATUS AND ORAL CONTRACEPTIVE USE

TABLE II. (Adapted from P.M. Layde and V. Beral, ref. #12.)

Oral contraceptives may compound the effects of well-known risk factors, such as hypertension, diabetes, hyperlipidemias, age and obesity.[13] In particular, some progestogens are known to decrease HDL cholesterol and cause glucose intolerance, while estrogens may create a state of hyperinsulinism[14-18]. Oral contraceptives have been shown to increase blood pressure among users (see section 9 in WARNINGS). Similar effects on risk factors have been associated with an increased risk of heart disease. Oral contraceptives must be used with caution in women with cardiovascular disease risk factors.

Desogestrel has minimum androgenic activity (See CLINICAL PHARMACOLOGY), and there is some evidence that the risk of myocardial infarction associated with oral contraceptives is lower when the progestogen has minimal androgenic activity than when the activity is greater.[100]
b. Thromboembolism
An increased risk of thromboembolic and thrombotic disease associated with the use of oral contraceptives is well established. Data from case-control and cohort studies report that oral contraceptives containing desogestrel (ORTHO-CEPT contains desogestrel) are associated with a two-fold increase in the risk of venous thromboembolic disease as compared to other low-dose (containing less than 50 mcg of estrogen) pills containing other progestins. According to these studies, this two-fold risk increases the yearly occurrence of venous thromboembolic disease by about 10-15 cases per 100,000 women.

Earlier case control studies on older formulations have found the relative risk of users compared to nonusers to be 3 for the first episode of superficial venous thrombosis, 4 to 11 for deep vein thrombosis or pulmonary embolism, and 1.5 to 6 for women with predisposing conditions for venous thromboembolic disease[2,3,19-24]. Cohort studies have shown the relative risk to be somewhat lower, about 3 for new cases and about 4.5 for new cases requiring hospitalization[25]. The risk of thromboembolic disease associated with oral contraceptives is not related to length of use and disappears after pill use is stopped[2].

A two- to four-fold increase in relative risk of post-operative thromboembolic complications has been reported with the use of oral contraceptives[9]. The relative risk of venous thrombosis in women who have predisposing conditions is twice that of women without such medical conditions[26]. If feasible, oral contraceptives should be discontinued at least four weeks prior to and for two weeks after elective surgery of a type associated with an increase in risk of thromboembolism and during and following prolonged immobilization. Since the immediate postpartum period is also associated with an increased risk of thromboembolism, oral contraceptives should be started no earlier than four weeks after delivery in women who elect not to breast feed.
c. Cerebrovascular diseases
Oral contraceptives have been shown to increase both the relative and attributable risks of cerebrovascular events (thrombotic and hemorrhagic strokes), although, in general, the risk is greatest among older (>35 years), hypertensive women who also smoke. Hypertension was found to be a risk factor for both users and nonusers, for both types of strokes, and smoking interacted to increase the risk of stroke[27-29].

In a large study, the relative risk of thrombotic strokes has been shown to range from 3 for normotensive users to 14 for users with severe hypertension[30]. The relative risk of hemorrhagic stroke is reported to be 1.2 for non-smokers who used oral contraceptives, 2.6 for smokers who did not use oral contraceptives, 7.6 for smokers who used oral contraceptives, 1.8 for normotensive users and 25.7 for users with severe hypertension[30]. The attributable risk is also greater in older women[3].
d. Dose-related risk of vascular disease from oral contraceptives
A positive association has been observed between the amount of estrogen and progestogen in oral contraceptives and the risk of vascular disease[31-33]. A decline in serum high density lipoproteins (HDL) has been reported with many progestational agents[14-16]. A decline in serum high density lipoproteins has been associated with an increased incidence of ischemic heart disease. Because estrogens increase HDL cholesterol, the net effect of an oral contraceptive depends on a balance achieved between doses of estrogen and progestogen and the nature and absolute amount of progestogens used in the contraceptives. The amount of both hormones should be considered in the choice of an oral contraceptive.

Minimizing exposure to estrogen and progestogen is in keeping with good principles of therapeutics. For any particular estrogen/progestogen combination, the dosage regimen prescribed should be one which contains the least amount of estrogen and progestogen that is compatible with a low failure rate and the needs of the individual patient. New acceptors of oral contraceptive agents should be started on preparations containing 0.035 mg or less of estrogen.

TABLE III—ANNUAL NUMBER OF BIRTH-RELATED OR METHOD-RELATED DEATHS ASSOCIATED WITH CONTROL OF FERTILITY PER 100,000 NON-STERILE WOMEN, BY FERTILITY CONTROL METHOD ACCORDING TO AGE

Method of control and outcome	15–19	20–24	25–29	30–34	35–39	40–44
No fertility control methods*	7.0	7.4	9.1	14.8	25.7	28.2
Oral contraceptives non-smoker**	0.3	0.5	0.9	1.9	13.8	31.6
Oral contraceptives smoker**	2.2	3.4	6.6	13.5	51.1	117.2
IUD**	0.8	0.8	1.0	1.0	1.4	1.4
Condom*	1.1	1.6	0.7	0.2	0.3	0.4
Diaphragm/spermicide*	1.9	1.2	1.2	1.3	2.2	2.8
Periodic abstinence*	2.5	1.6	1.6	1.7	2.9	3.6

* Deaths are birth-related
** Deaths are method-related

Adapted from H.W. Ory, ref. #35.

e. Persistence of risk of vascular disease
There are two studies which have shown persistence of risk of vascular disease for ever-users of oral contraceptives. In a study in the United States, the risk of developing myocardial infarction after discontinuing oral contraceptives persists for at least 9 years for women 40–49 years old who had used oral contraceptives for five or more years, but this increased risk was not demonstrated in other age groups[8]. In another study in Great Britain, the risk of developing cerebrovascular disease persisted for at least 6 years after discontinuation of oral contraceptives, although excess risk was very small[34]. However, both studies were performed with oral contraceptive formulations containing 0.050 mg or higher of estrogens.
2. ESTIMATES OF MORTALITY FROM CONTRACEPTIVE USE
One study gathered data from a variety of sources which have estimated the mortality rate associated with different methods of contraception at different ages (Table III). These estimates include the combined risk of death associated with contraceptive methods plus the risk attributable to pregnancy in the event of method failure. Each method of contraception has its specific benefits and risks. The study concluded that with the exception of oral contraceptive users 35 and older who smoke and 40 and older who do not smoke, mortality associated with all methods of birth control is low and below that associated with childbirth.

The observation of an increase in risk of mortality with age for oral contraceptive users is based on data gathered in the 1970's[35]. Current clinical recommendation involves the use of lower estrogen dose formulations and a careful consideration of risk factors. In 1989, the Fertility and Maternal Health Drugs Advisory Committee was asked to review the use of oral contraceptives in women 40 years of age and over. The Committee concluded that although cardiovascular disease risk may be increased with oral contraceptive use after age 40 in healthy non-smoking women (even with the newer low-dose formulations), there are also greater potential health risks associated with pregnancy in older women and with the alternative surgical and medical procedures which may be necessary if such women do not have access to effective and acceptable means of contraception. The Committee recommended that the benefits of low-dose oral contraceptive use by healthy non-smoking women over 40 may outweigh the possible risks.

Of course, older women, as all women who take oral contraceptives, should take an oral contraceptive which contains the least amount of estrogen and progestogen that is compatible with a low failure rate and individual patient needs. [See table III above]
3. CARCINOMA OF THE REPRODUCTIVE ORGANS AND BREASTS
Numerous epidemiological studies have been performed on the incidence of breast, endometrial, ovarian and cervical cancer in women using oral contraceptives. While there are conflicting reports most studies suggest that the use of oral contraceptives is not associated with an overall increase in the risk of developing breast cancer. Some studies have reported an increased relative risk of developing breast cancer, particularly at a younger age. This increased relative risk appears to be related to duration of use[36-44,79-89].

A meta-analysis of 54 studies reports that women who are currently using combined oral contraceptives or have used them in the past 10 years are at a slightly increased risk of having breast cancer diagnosed although the additional cancers tend to be localized to the breast. There is no evidence of an increased risk of having breast cancer diagnosed 10 or more years after cessation of use.[101]

Some studies suggest that oral contraceptive use has been associated with an increase in the risk of cervical intraepi-

Continued on next page

Ortho-Cept—Cont.

thelial neoplasia in some populations of women[45–48]. However, there continues to be controversy about the extent to which such findings may be due to differences in sexual behavior and other factors.

4. HEPATIC NEOPLASIA

Benign hepatic adenomas are associated with oral contraceptive use, although the incidence of benign tumors is rare in the United States. Indirect calculations have estimated the attributable risk to be in the range of 3.3 cases/100,000 for users, a risk that increases after four or more years of use especially with oral contraceptives of higher dose[49]. Rupture of benign, hepatic adenomas may cause death through intra-abdominal hemorrhage[50,51].

Studies have shown an increased risk of developing hepatocellular carcinoma[52–54,102] in oral contraceptive users. However, these cancers are rare in the U.S.

5. OCULAR LESIONS

There have been clinical case reports of retinal thrombosis associated with the use of oral contraceptives. Oral contraceptives should be discontinued if there is unexplained partial or complete loss of vision; onset of proptosis or diplopia; papilledema; or retinal vascular lesions. Appropriate diagnostic and therapeutic measures should be undertaken immediately.

6. ORAL CONTRACEPTIVE USE BEFORE OR DURING EARLY PREGNANCY

Extensive epidemiological studies have revealed no increased risk of birth defects in women who have used oral contraceptives prior to pregnancy[56–57]. The majority of recent studies also do not indicate a teratogenic effect, particularly in so far as cardiac anomalies and limb reduction defects are concerned[55,56,58,59], when oral contraceptives are taken inadvertently during early pregnancy.

The administration of oral contraceptives to induce withdrawal bleeding should not be used as a test for pregnancy. Oral contraceptives should not be used during pregnancy to treat threatened or habitual abortion.

It is recommended that for any patient who has missed two consecutive periods, pregnancy should be ruled out before continuing oral contraceptive use. If the patient has not adhered to the prescribed schedule, the possibility of pregnancy should be considered at the time of the first missed period. Oral contraceptive use should be discontinued until pregnancy is ruled out.

7. GALLBLADDER DISEASE

Earlier studies have reported an increased lifetime relative risk of gallbladder surgery in users of oral contraceptives and estrogens[60,61]. More recent studies, however, have shown that the relative risk of developing gallbladder disease among oral contraceptive users may be minimal[62–64]. The recent findings of minimal risk may be related to the use of oral contraceptive formulations containing lower hormonal doses of estrogens and progestogens.

8. CARBOHYDRATE AND LIPID METABOLIC EFFECTS

Oral contraceptives have been shown to cause a decrease in glucose tolerance in a significant percentage of users[17]. This effect has been shown to be directly related to estrogen dose[65]. In general, progestogens increase insulin secretion and create insulin resistance, this effect varying with different progestational agents[17,66]. In the nondiabetic woman, oral contraceptives appear to have no effect on fasting blood glucose[67]. Because of these demonstrated effects, prediabetic and diabetic women should be carefully monitored while taking oral contraceptives.

A small proportion of women will have persistent hypertriglyceridemia while on the pill. As discussed earlier (see WARNINGS 1.a. and 1.d.), changes in serum triglycerides and lipoprotein levels have been reported in oral contraceptive users.

9. ELEVATED BLOOD PRESSURE

An increase in blood pressure has been reported in women taking oral contraceptives[68] and this increase is more likely in older oral contraceptive users[69] and with extended duration of use[61]. Data from the Royal College of General Practitioners[12] and subsequent randomized trials have shown that the incidence of hypertension increases with increasing progestational activity.

Women with a history of hypertension or hypertension-related diseases, or renal disease[70] should be encouraged to use another method of contraception. If women elect to use oral contraceptives, they should be monitored closely and if significant elevation of blood pressure occurs, oral contraceptives should be discontinued. For most women, elevated blood pressure will return to normal after stopping oral contraceptives[69], and there is no difference in the occurrence of hypertension among former and never users[68,70,71].

10. HEADACHE

The onset or exacerbation of migraine or development of headache with a new pattern which is recurrent, persistent or severe requires discontinuation of oral contraceptives and evaluation of the cause.

11. BLEEDING IRREGULARITIES

Breakthrough bleeding and spotting are sometimes encountered in patients on oral contraceptives, especially during the first three months of use. Nonhormonal causes should be considered and adequate diagnostic measures taken to rule out malignancy or pregnancy in the event of breakthrough bleeding, as in the case of any abnormal vaginal bleeding. If pathology has been excluded, time or a change to another formulation may solve the problem. In the event of amenorrhea, pregnancy should be ruled out.

Some women may encounter post-pill amenorrhea or oligomenorrhea, especially when such a condition was pre-existent.

12. ECTOPIC PREGNANCY

Ectopic as well as intrauterine pregnancy may occur in contraceptive failures.

PRECAUTIONS

1. PHYSICAL EXAMINATION AND FOLLOW UP

It is good medical practice for all women to have annual history and physical examinations, including women using oral contraceptives. The physical examination, however, may be deferred until after initiation of oral contraceptives if requested by the woman and judged appropriate by the clinician. The physical examination should include special reference to blood pressure, breasts, abdomen and pelvic organs, including cervical cytology, and relevant laboratory tests. In case of undiagnosed, persistent or recurrent abnormal vaginal bleeding, appropriate measures should be conducted to rule out malignancy. Women with a strong family history of breast cancer or who have breast nodules should be monitored with particular care.

2. LIPID DISORDERS

Women who are being treated for hyperlipidemias should be followed closely if they elect to use oral contraceptives. Some progestogens may elevate LDL levels and may render the control of hyperlipidemias more difficult.

3. LIVER FUNCTION

If jaundice develops in any woman receiving such drugs, the medication should be discontinued. Steroid hormones may be poorly metabolized in patients with impaired liver function.

4. FLUID RETENTION

Oral contraceptives may cause some degree of fluid retention. They should be prescribed with caution, and only with careful monitoring, in patients with conditions which might be aggravated by fluid retention.

5. EMOTIONAL DISORDERS

Women with a history of depression should be carefully observed and the drug discontinued if depression recurs to a serious degree.

6. CONTACT LENSES

Contact lens wearers who develop visual changes or changes in lens tolerance should be assessed by an ophthalmologist.

7. DRUG INTERACTIONS

Reduced efficacy and increased incidence of breakthrough bleeding and menstrual irregularities have been associated with concomitant use of rifampin. A similar association, though less marked, has been suggested with barbiturates, phenylbutazone, phenytoin sodium, carbamazepine and possibly with griseofulvin, ampicillin and tetracyclines[72].

8. INTERACTIONS WITH LABORATORY TESTS

Certain endocrine and liver function tests and blood components may be affected by oral contraceptives:

a. Increased prothrombin and factors VII, VIII, IX and X; decreased antithrombin 3; increased norepinephrine-induced platelet aggregability.

b. Increased thyroid binding globulin (TBG) leading to increased circulating total thyroid hormone, as measured by protein-bound iodine (PBI), T4 by column or by radioimmunoassay. Free T3 resin uptake is decreased, reflecting the elevated TBG; free T4 concentration is unaltered.

c. Other binding proteins may be elevated in serum.

d. Sex hormone binding globulins are increased and result in elevated levels of total circulating sex steroids however, free or biologically active levels either decrease or remain unchanged.

e. High-density lipoprotein (HDL-C) and triglycerides may be increased, while low-density lipoprotein cholesterol (LDL-C) and total cholesterol (Total-C) may be decreased or unchanged.

f. Glucose tolerance may be decreased.

g. Serum folate levels may be depressed by oral contraceptive therapy. This may be of clinical significance if a woman becomes pregnant shortly after discontinuing oral contraceptives.

9. CARCINOGENESIS

See WARNINGS section.

10. PREGNANCY

Pregnancy Category X. See CONTRAINDICATIONS and WARNINGS sections.

11. NURSING MOTHERS

Small amounts of oral contraceptive steroids have been identified in the milk of nursing mothers and a few adverse effects on the child have been reported, including jaundice and breast enlargement. In addition, oral contraceptives given in the postpartum period may interfere with lactation by decreasing the quantity and quality of breast milk. If possible, the nursing mother should be advised not to use oral contraceptives but to use other forms of contraception until she has completely weaned her child.

12. SEXUALLY TRANSMITTED DISEASES

Patients should be counseled that this product does not provide against HIV infection (AIDS) and other sexually transmitted diseases.

INFORMATION FOR THE PATIENT

See Patient Labeling Printed Below

ADVERSE REACTIONS

An increased risk of the following serious adverse reactions has been associated with the use of oral contraceptives (see WARNINGS section).

- Thrombophlebitis and venous thrombosis with or without embolism
- Arterial thromboembolism
- Pulmonary embolism
- Myocardial infarction
- Cerebral hemorrhage
- Cerebral thrombosis
- Hypertension
- Gall bladder disease
- Hepatic adenomas or benign liver tumors

The following adverse reactions have been reported in patients receiving oral contraceptives and are believed to be drug-related:

- Nausea
- Vomiting
- Gastrointestinal symptoms (such as abdominal cramps and bloating)
- Breakthrough bleeding
- Spotting
- Change in menstrual flow
- Amenorrhea
- Temporary infertility after discontinuation of treatment
- Edema
- Melasma which may persist
- Breast changes: tenderness, enlargement, secretion
- Change in weight (increase or decrease)
- Change in cervical erosion and secretion
- Diminution in lactation when given immediately postpartum
- Cholestatic jaundice
- Migraine
- Rash (allergic)
- Mental depression
- Reduced tolerance to carbohydrates
- Vaginal candidiasis
- Change in corneal curvature (steepening)
- Intolerance to contact lenses

The following adverse reactions have been reported in users of oral contraceptives and the association has been neither confirmed nor refuted:

- Pre-menstrual syndrome
- Cataracts
- Changes in appetite
- Cystitis-like syndrome
- Headache
- Nervousness
- Dizziness
- Hirsutism
- Loss of scalp hair
- Erythema multiforme
- Erythema nodosum
- Hemorrhagic eruption
- Vaginitis
- Porphyria
- Impaired renal function
- Hemolytic uremic syndrome
- Acne
- Changes in libido
- Colitis
- Budd-Chiari Syndrome

OVERDOSAGE

Serious ill effects have not been reported following acute ingestion of large doses of oral contraceptives by young children. Overdosage may cause nausea, and withdrawal bleeding may occur in females.

NON-CONTRACEPTIVE HEALTH BENEFITS

The following non-contraceptive health benefits related to the use of oral contraceptives are supported by epidemiological studies which largely utilized oral contraceptive formulations containing estrogen doses exceeding 0.035 mg of ethinyl estradiol or 0.05 mg of mestranol[73–78].

Effects on menses:

- increased menstrual cycle regularity
- decreased blood loss and decreased incidence of iron deficiency anemia
- decreased incidence of dysmenorrhea

Effects related to inhibition of ovulation:

- decreased incidence of functional ovarian cysts

- decreased incidence of ectopic pregnancies

Effects from long-term use:

- decreased incidence of fibroadenomas and fibrocystic disease of the breast
- decreased incidence of acute pelvic inflammatory disease
- decreased incidence of endometrial cancer
- decreased incidence of ovarian cancer

DOSAGE AND ADMINISTRATION

To achieve maximum contraceptive effectiveness, ORTHO-CEPT must be taken exactly as directed and at intervals not exceeding 24 hours. ORTHO-CEPT is available in the DIALPAK® Tablet Dispenser which is preset for a Sunday Start. Day 1 start is also provided.

21-Day Regimen (Day 1 Start)

The dosage of ORTHO-CEPT 21 for the initial cycle of therapy is one tablet administered daily from the 1st day through the 21st day of the menstrual cycle, counting the first day of menstrual flow as "Day 1". For subsequent cycles, no tablets are taken for 7 days, then a new course is started of one tablet a day for 21 days. The dosage regimen then continues with 7 days of no medication, followed by 21 days of medication, instituting a three-weeks-on, one-week-off dosage regimen.

The use of ORTHO-CEPT 21 for contraception may be initiated 4 weeks postpartum in women who elect not to breast feed. When the tablets are administered during the postpartum period, the increased risk of thromboembolic disease associated with the postpartum period must be considered. (See CONTRAINDICATIONS and WARNINGS concerning thromboembolic disease. See also PRECAUTIONS for "Nursing Mothers".) If the patient starts on ORTHO-CEPT postpartum, and has not yet had a period, she should be instructed to use another method of contraception until an orange tablet has been taken daily for 7 days. The possibility of ovulation and conception prior to initiation of medication should be considered. If the patient misses one (1) active tablet in Weeks 1, 2, or 3, the tablet should be taken as soon as she remembers. If the patient misses two (2) active tablets in Week 1 or Week 2, the patient should take two (2) tablets the day she remembers and two (2) tablets the next day; and then continue taking one (1) tablet a day until she finishes the pack. The patient should be instructed to use a back-up method of birth control if she has sex in the seven (7) days after missing pills. If the patient misses two (2) active tablets in the third week or misses three (3) or more active tablets in a row, the patient should throw out the rest of the pack and start a new pack that same day. The patient should be instructed to use a back-up method of birth control if she has sex in the seven (7) days after missing pills.

21-Day Regimen (Sunday Start)

When taking ORTHO-CEPT 21, the first orange tablet should be taken on the first Sunday after menstruation begins. If period begins on Sunday, the first orange tablet is taken on that day. If switching directly from another oral contraceptive, the first orange tablet should be taken on the first Sunday after the last ACTIVE tablet of the previous product. One orange tablet is taken daily for 21 days. For subsequent cycles, no tablets are taken for seven days, then a new course is started of one tablet a day for 21 days instituting a 3-weeks-on, one-week-off dosage regimen. When initiating a Sunday start regimen, another method of contraception should be used until after the first 7 consecutive days of administration.

The use of ORTHO-CEPT 21 for contraception may be initiated 4 weeks postpartum in women who elect not to breast feed. When the tablets are administered during the postpartum period, the increased risk of thromboembolic disease associated with the postpartum period must be considered. (See CONTRAINDICATIONS and WARNINGS concerning thromboembolic disease. See also PRECAUTIONS for "Nursing Mothers".) If the patient starts on ORTHO-CEPT postpartum, and has not yet had a period, she should be instructed to use another method of contraception until an orange tablet has been taken daily for 7 days. The possibility of ovulation and conception prior to initiation of medication should be considered. If the patient misses one (1) active tablet in Weeks 1, 2, or 3, the tablet should be taken as soon as she remembers. If the patient misses two (2) active tablets in Week 1 or Week 2, the patient should take two (2) tablets the day she remembers and two (2) tablets the next day; and then continue taking one (1) tablet a day until she finishes the pack. The patient should be instructed to use a back-up method of birth control if she has sex in the seven (7) days after missing pills. If the patient misses two (2) active tablets in the third week or misses three (3) or more tablets in a row, the patient should continue taking one tablet every day until Sunday. On Sunday the patient should throw out the rest of the pack and start a new pack that same day. The patient should be instructed to use a back-up method of birth control if she has sex in the seven (7) days after missing pills.

28-Day Regimen (Day 1 Start)

The dosage of ORTHO-CEPT 28 for the initial cycle of therapy is one tablet administered daily from the 1st day through 21st day of the menstrual cycle, counting the first day of menstrual flow as "Day 1". Tablets are taken without interruption as follows: One orange tablet daily for 21 days, then one green tablet daily for 7 days. After 28 tablets have been taken, a new course is started and an orange tablet is taken the next day.

The use of ORTHO-CEPT 28 for contraception may be initiated 4 weeks postpartum in women who elect not to breast feed. When the tablets are administered during the postpartum period, the increased risk of thromboembolic disease associated with the postpartum period must be considered. (See CONTRAINDICATIONS and WARNINGS concerning thromboembolic disease. See also PRECAUTIONS for "Nursing Mothers".) If the patient starts on ORTHO-CEPT postpartum, and has not yet had a period, she should be instructed to use another method of contraception until an orange tablet has been taken daily for 7 days. The possibility of ovulation and conception prior to initiation of medication should be considered. If the patient misses one (1) active tablet in Weeks 1, 2, or 3, the tablet should be taken as soon as she remembers. If the patient misses two (2) active tablets in Week 1 or Week 2, the patient should take two (2) tablets the day she remembers and two (2) tablets the next day; and then continue taking one (1) tablet a day until she finishes the pack. The patient should be instructed to use a back-up method of birth control if she has sex in the seven (7) days after missing pills. If the patient misses two (2) active tablets in the third week or misses three (3) or more active tablets in a row, the patient should throw out the rest of the pack and start a new pack that same day. The patient should be instructed to use a back-up method of birth control if she has sex in the seven (7) days after missing pills.

28-Day Regimen (Sunday Start)

When taking ORTHO-CEPT 28, the first orange tablet should be taken on the first Sunday after menstruation begins. If period begins on Sunday, the first orange tablet is taken on that day. If switching directly from another oral contraceptive, the first orange tablet should be taken on the first Sunday after the last ACTIVE tablet of the previous product. Tablets are taken without interruption as follows: One orange tablet daily for 21 days, then one green tablet daily for 7 days. After 28 tablets have been taken, a new course is started and an orange tablet is taken the next day (Sunday). When initiating a Sunday start regimen, another method of contraception should be used until after the first 7 consecutive days of administration.

The use of ORTHO-CEPT 28 for contraception may be initiated 4 weeks postpartum. When the tablets are administered during the postpartum period, the increased risk of thromboembolic disease associated with the postpartum period must be considered. (See CONTRAINDICATIONS and WARNINGS concerning thromboembolic disease. See also PRECAUTIONS for "Nursing Mothers".) If the patient starts on ORTHO-CEPT postpartum, and has not yet had a period, she should be instructed to use another method of contraception until an orange tablet has been taken daily for 7 days. The possibility of ovulation and conception prior to initiation of medication should be considered. If the patient misses one (1) active tablet in Weeks 1, 2, or 3, the tablet should be taken as soon as she remembers. If the patient misses two (2) active tablets in Week 1 or Week 2, the patient should take two (2) tablets the day she remembers and two (2) tablets the next day; and then continue taking one (1) tablet a day until she finishes the pack. The patient should be instructed to use a back-up method of birth control if she has sex in the seven (7) days after missing pills. If the patient misses two (2) active tablets in the third week or misses three (3) or more tablets in a row, the patient should continue taking one tablet every day until Sunday. On Sunday the patient should throw out the rest of the pack and start a new pack that same day. The patient should be instructed to use a back-up method of birth control if she has sex in the seven (7) days after missing pills.

ALL ORAL CONTRACEPTIVES

Breakthrough bleeding, spotting, and amenorrhea are frequent reasons for patients discontinuing oral contraceptives. In breakthrough bleeding, as in all cases of irregular bleeding from the vagina, nonfunctional causes should be borne in mind. In undiagnosed persistent or recurrent abnormal bleeding from the vagina, adequate diagnostic measures are indicated to rule out pregnancy or malignancy. If pathology has been excluded, time or a change to another formulation may solve the problem. Changing to an oral contraceptive with a higher estrogen content, while potentially useful in minimizing menstrual irregularity, should be done only if necessary since this may increase the risk of thromboembolic disease.

Use of oral contraceptives in the event of a missed menstrual period:

1. If the patient has not adhered to the prescribed schedule, the possibility of pregnancy should be considered at the time of the first missed period and oral contraceptive use should be discontinued until pregnancy is ruled out.
2. If the patient has adhered to the prescribed regimen and misses two consecutive periods, pregnancy should be ruled out before continuing oral contraceptive use.

HOW SUPPLIED

ORTHO-CEPT® 21 Tablets are available in a DIALPAK® Tablet Dispenser (NDC 0062-1795-15) containing 21 orange tablets (0.15 mg desogestrel and 0.03 mg ethinyl estradiol) which are unscored with "ORTHO" on one side and "D 150" on the opposite side.

ORTHO-CEPT 21 is available for clinic usage in a VERIDATE® Tablet Dispenser (unfilled) and VERIDATE Refills (NDC 0062-1795-20).

ORTHO-CEPT 28 Tablets are available in a DIALPAK Tablet Dispenser (NDC 0062-1796-15) containing 28 tablets, as follows: 21 orange tablets as described under ORTHO-CEPT 21, and 7 green tablets containing inert ingredients.

ORTHO-CEPT 28 is available for clinic usage in a VERIDATE Tablet Dispenser (unfilled) and VERIDATE Refills (NDC 0062-1796-20).

STORAGE: Store before 86° F (30° C).

CAUTION

Federal law prohibits dispensing without prescription.

REFERENCES

1. Hatcher, RA, et al. 1994 Contraceptive Technology. Sixteenth Edition. New York; Irvington Publisher. **2.** Stadel BV. Oral contraceptives and cardiovascular disease. (Pt. 1). N Engl J Med 1981; 305:612–618. **3.** Stadel BV. Oral contraceptives and cardiovascular disease. (Pt. 2). N Engl J Med 1981; 305:672–677. **4.** Adam SA, Thorogood M. Oral contraception and myocardial infarction revisited: the effects of new preparations and prescribing patterns. Br J Obstet and Gynecol 1981; 88:838–845. **5.** Mann JI, Inman WH. Oral contraceptives and death from myocardial infarction. Br Med J 1975; 2(5965):245–248. **6.** Mann JI, Vessey MP, Thorogood M. Doll R. Myocardial infarction in young women with special reference to oral contraceptive practice. Br Med J 1975; 2(5956):241–245. **7.** Royal College of General Practitioners' Oral Contraception Study: Further analyses of mortality in oral contraceptive users. Lancet 1981;1:541–546. **8.** Slone D, Shapiro S, Kaufman DW, Rosenberg L, Miettinen OS, Stolley PD. Risk of myocardial infarction in relation to current and discontinued use of oral contraceptives. N Engl J Med 1981; 305:420–424. **9.** Vessey MP. Female hormones and vascular disease—an epidemiological overview. Br J Fam Plann 1980; 6:1–12. **10.** Russell-Briefel RG, Ezzati TM. Fulwood R, Perlman JA, Murphy RS. Cardiovascular risk status and oral contraceptive use, United States, 1976–80. Prevent Med 1986; 15:352–362. **11.** Goldbaum GM, Kendrick JS, Hogelin GC, Gentry EM. The relative impact of smoking and oral contraceptive use on women in the United States. JAMA 1987; 258:1339–1342. **12.** Layde PM, Beral V. Further analyses of mortality in oral contraceptive users: Royal College General Practitioners' Oral Contraception Study. (Table 5) Lancet 1981; 1:541–546. **13.** Knopp RH. Arteriosclerosis risk: the roles of oral contraceptives and postmenopausal estrogens. J Reprod Med 1986; 31(9) (Supplement):913–921. **14.** Krauss RM, Roy S, Mishell DR, Casagrande J, Pike MC. Effects of two low-dose oral contraceptives on serum lipids and lipoproteins: Differential changes in high-density lipoproteins subclasses. Am J Obstet 1983; 145:446–452. **15.** Wahl P, Walden C, Knopp R, Hoover J, Wallace R, Heiss G, Rifkind B. Effect of estrogen/progestin potency on lipid/lipoprotein cholesterol. N Engl J Med 1983; 308:862–867. **16.** Wynn V, Niththyananthan R. The effect of progestin in combined oral contraceptives on serum lipids with special reference to high-density lipoproteins. Am J Obstet Gynecol 1982; 142:766–771. **17.** Wynn V, Godsland I. Effects of oral contraceptives and carbohydrate metabolism. J Reprod Med 1986; 31 (9) (Supplement):892–897. **18.** LaRosa JC, Atherosclerotic risk factors in cardiovascular disease. J Reprod Med 1986;31 (9) (Supplement): 906–912. **19.** Inman WH, Vessey MP. Investigation of death from pulmonary, coronary, and cerebral thrombosis and embolism in women of childbearing age. Br Med J 1968; 2 (5599):193–199. **20.** Maguire MG, Tonascia J, Sartwell PE, Stolley PD, Tockman MS. Increased risk of thrombosis due to oral contraceptives: a further report. Am J Epidemiol 1979; 110(2):188–195. **21.** Pettiti DB, Wingerd J, Pellegrin F, Ramacharan S. Risk of vascular disease in women: smoking, oral contraceptives, noncontraceptive estrogens, and other factors. JAMA 1979; 242:1150–1154. **22.** Vessey MP, Doll R. Investigation of relation between use of oral contraceptives and thromboembolic disease. Br Med J 1968; 2(5599):199–205. **23.** Vessey MP, Doll R. Investigation of relation between use of oral contraceptives and thromboembolic disease. A further report. Br Med J 1969; 2 (5658):651–657. **24.** Porter JB, Hunter JR, Danielson DA, Jick H, Stergachis A. Oral contraceptives and non-fatal vascular disease—recent experience. Obstet Gynecol 1982; 59 (3): 299–302. **25.** Vessey M, Doll R, Peto R. Johnson B, Wiggins P. A long-term follow-up study of women using different methods of contraception: an interim report. J Biosocial Sci 1976; 8:375–427. **26.** Royal College of General Practitioners: Oral contraceptives, venous thrombosis, and varicose veins.

Continued on next page

Ortho-Cept—Cont.

J Royal Coll Gen Pract 1978; 28:393–399. **27.** Collaborative Group for the Study of Stroke in Young Women: Oral contraception and increased risk of cerebral ischemia or thrombosis. N Engl J Med 1973; 288:871–878. **28.** Petitti DB, Wingerd J. Use of oral contraceptives, cigarette smoking, and risk of subarachnoid hemorrhage. Lancet 1978; 2:234–236. **29.** Inman WH. Oral contraceptives and fatal subarachnoid hemorrhage. Br Med J 1979; 2 (6203):1468–70. **30.** Collaborative Group for the study of Stroke in Young Women: Oral contraceptives and stroke in young women: associated risk factors. JAMA 1975; 231:718–722. **31.** Inman WH, Vessey MP, Westerholm B, Engelund A. Thromboembolic disease and the steroidal content of oral contraceptives. A report to the Committee on Safety of Drugs. Br Med J 1970; 2:203–209. **32.** Meade TW, Greenberg G, Thompson SG. Progestogens and cardiovascular reactions associated with oral contraceptives and a comparison of the safety of 50- and 35-mcg oestrogen preparations. Br Med J 1980; 280 (6224):1157–1161. **33.** Kay, CR. Progestogens and arterial disease—evidence from the Royal College of General Practitioners' Study. Am J Obstet Gynecol 1982; 142:762–765. **34.** Royal College of General Practitioners: Incidence of arterial disease among oral contraceptive users. J Royal Coll Gen Pract 1983; 33:75–82. **35.** Ory HW. Mortality associated with fertility and fertility control: 1983. Family Planning Perspectives 1983; 15:50–56. **36.** The Cancer and Steroid Hormone Study of the Centers for Disease Control and the National Institute of Child Health and Human Development: Oral-contraceptive use and the risk of breast cancer. N Engl J Med 1986; 315:405–411. **37.** Pike MC, Henderson BE, Krailo MD, Duke A, Roy S. Breast cancer risk in young women and use of oral contraceptives: possible modifying effect of formulation and age at use. Lancet 1983; 2:926–929. **38.** Paul C, Skegg DG, Spears GFS, Kaldor JM. Oral contraceptives and breast cancer: A national study. Br Med J 1986; 293:723–725. **39.** Miller DR, Rosenberg L, Kaufman DW, Schottenfeld D, Stolley PD, Shapiro S. Breast cancer risk in relation to early oral contraceptive use. Obstet Gynecol 1986; 68:863–868. **40.** Olson H, Olson KL, Moller TR, Ranstam J, Holm P. Oral contraceptive use and breast cancer in young women in Sweden (letter). Lancet 1985; 2:748–749. **41.** McPherson K, Vessey M, Neil A, Doll R, Jones L, Roberts M. Early contraceptive use and breast cancer: Results of another case-control study. Br J Cancer 1987; 56: 653–660. **42.** Huggins GR, Zucker PF. Oral contraceptives and neoplasia: 1987 update. Fertil Steril 1987; 47:733–761. **43.** McPherson K, Drife JO. The pill and breast cancer: why the uncertainty? Br Med J 1986; 293:709–710. **44.** Shapiro S. Oral contraceptives—time to take stock. N Engl J Med 1987; 315:450–451. **45.** Ory H, Naib Z, Conger SB, Hatcher RA, Tyler CW. Contraceptive choice and prevalence of cervical dysplasia and carcinoma in situ. Am J Obstet Gynecol 1976;124:573–577. **46.** Vessey MP, Lawless M, McPherson K, Yeates D. Neoplasia of the cervix uteri and contraception: a possible adverse effect of the pill. Lancet 1983; 2:930. **47.** Brinton LA, Huggins GR, Lehman HF, Malli K, Savitz DA, Trapido E, Rosenthal J, Hoover R. Long term use of oral contraceptives and risk of invasive cervical cancer. Int J Cancer 1986; 38:339–344. **48.** WHO Collaborative Study of Neoplasia and Steroid Contraceptives: Invasive cervical cancer and combined oral contraceptives. Br Med J 1985; 290:961–965. **49.** Rooks JB, Ory HW, Ishak KG, Strauss LT, Greenspan JR, Hill AP, Tyler CW. Epidemiology of hepatocellular adenoma: the role of oral contraceptive use. JAMA 1979; 242:644–648. **50.** Bein NN, Goldsmith HS. Recurrent massive hemorrhage from benign hepatic tumors secondary to oral contraceptives. Br J Surg 1977; 64:433–435. **51.** Klatskin G. Hepatic tumors: possible relationship to use of oral contraceptives. Gastroenterology 1977; 73:386–394. **52.** Henderson BE, Preston-Martin S, Edmondson HA, Peters RL, Pike MC. Hepatocellular carcinoma and oral contraceptives. Br J Cancer 1983; 48:437–440. **53.** Neuberger J, Forman D, Doll R, Williams R. Oral contraceptives and hepatocellular carcinoma. Br Med J 1986; 292:1355–1357. **54.** Forman D, Vincent TJ, Doll R. Cancer of the liver and oral contraceptives. Br Med J 1986; 292:1357–1361. **55.** Harlap S, Eldor J. Births following oral contraceptive failures. Obstet Gynecol 1980; 55:447–452. **56.** Savolainen E, Saksela E, Saxen L. Teratogenic hazards of oral contraceptives analyzed in a national malformation register. Am J Obstet Gynecol 1981; 140:521–524. **57.** Janerich DT, Piper JM, Glebatis DM. Oral contraceptives and birth defects. Am J Epidemiol 1980; 112:73–79. **58.** Ferencz C, Matanoski GM, Wilson PD, Rubin JD, Neill CA, Gutberlet R. Maternal hormone therapy and congenital heart disease. Teratology 1980; 21: 225–239. **59.** Rothman KJ, Fyler DC, Goldbatt A, Kreidberg MB. Exogenous hormones and other drug exposures of children with congenital heart disease. Am J Epidemiol 1979; 109:433–439. **60.** Boston Collaborative Drug Surveillance Program: Oral contraceptives and venous thromboembolic disease, surgically confirmed gall-bladder disease, and breast tumors. Lancet 1973; 1:1399–1404. **61.** Royal College of General Practitioners: Oral contraceptives and health. New York, Pittman, 1974. **62.** Layde PM, Vessey MP, Yeates D. Risk of gall bladder disease: a cohort study of young women attending family planning clinics. J Epidemiol Community Health 1982; 36:274–278. **63.** Rome Group for the Epidemiology and Prevention of Cholelithiasis (GREPCO): Prevalence of gallstone disease in an Italian adult female population. Am J Epidemiol 1984; 119:796–805. **64.** Strom BL, Tamragouri RT, Morse ML, Lazar EL, West SL, Stolley PD, Jones JK. Oral contraceptives and other risk factors for gall bladder disease. Clin Pharmacol Ther 1986; 39:335–341. **65.** Wynn V, Adams PW, Godsland IF, Melrose J, Niththyananthan R, Oakley NW, Seedj A. Comparison of effects of different combined oral-contraceptive formulations on carbohydrate and lipid metabolism. Lancet 1979; 1:1045–1049. **66.** Wynn V. Effect of progesterone and progestins on carbohydrate metabolism. In Progesterone and Progestin. Edited by Bardin CW, Milgrom E, Mauvis-Jarvis P. New York, Raven Press, 1983 pp. 395–410. **67.** Perlman JA, Roussell-Briefel RG, Ezzati TM, Lieberknecht G. Oral glucose tolerance and the potency of oral contraceptive progestogens. J Chronic Dis 1985; 38:857–864. **68.** Royal College of General Practitioners' Oral Contraception Study: Effect on hypertension and benign breast disease of progestogen component in combined oral contraceptives. Lancet 1977; 1:624. **69.** Fisch IR, Frank J. Oral contraceptives and blood pressure. JAMA 1977; 237:2499–2503. **70.** Laragh AJ. Oral contraceptive induced hypertension—nine years later. Am J Obstet Gynecol 1976; 126:141–147. **71.** Ramcharan S, Peritz E, Pellegrin FA, Williams WT. Incidence of hypertension in the Walnut Creek Contraceptive Drug Study cohort. In Pharmacology of Steroid Contraceptive Drugs. Garattini S, Berendes HW. Eds. New York, Raven Press, 1977 pp. 277–278. (Monographs of the Mario Negri Institute for Pharmacological Research, Milan). **72.** Stockley I. Interactions with oral contraceptives. J Pharm 1976; 216:140–143. **73.** The Cancer and Steroid Hormone Study of the Centers for Disease Control and the National Institute of Child Health and Human Development: Oral contraceptive use and the risk of ovarian cancer. JAMA 1983; 249:1596–1599. **74.** The Cancer and Steroid Hormone Study of the Centers for Disease Control and the National Institute of Child Health and Human Development: Combination oral contraceptive use and the risk of endometrial cancer. JAMA 1987; 257:796–800. **75.** Ory HW. Functional ovarian cysts and oral contraceptives: negative association confirmed surgically. JAMA 1974; 228:68–69. **76.** Ory HW. Cole P. Macmahon B, Hoover R. Oral contraceptives and reduced risk of benign breast disease. N Engl J Med 1976; 294:419–422. **77.** Ory HW. The noncontraceptive health benefits from oral contraceptive use. Fam Plann Perspect 1982; 14:182–184. **78.** Ory HW, Forrest JD, Lincoln R. Making Choices: Evaluating the health risks and benefits of birth control methods. New York, The Alan Guttmacher Institute, 1983; p. 1. **79.** Schlesselman J, Stadel BV, Murray P, Lai S. Breast Cancer in relation to early use of oral contraceptives 1988; 259: 1828–1833. **80.** Hennekens CH, Speizer FE, Lipnick RJ, Rosner B, Bain C, Belanger C, Stampfer MJ, Willett W, Peto R. A case-controlled study of oral contraceptive use and breast cancer. JNCI 1984;72:39–42. **81.** LaVecchia C, Decarli A, Fasoli M, Franceschi S, Gentile A, Negri E, Parazzini F, Tognoni G. Oral contraceptives and cancers of the breast and of the female genital tract. Interim results from a case-control study. Br J Cancer 1986; 54:311–317. **82.** Meirik O, Lund E, Adami H, Bergstrom R, Christoffersen T, Bergsjo P. Oral contraceptive use in breast cancer in young women. A Joint National Case-control study in Sweden and Norway. Lancet 1986; 11:650–654. **83.** Kay CR, Hannaford PC. Breast cancer and the pill—A further report from the Royal College of General Practitioners' oral contraception study. Br J Cancer 1988; 58:675–680. **84.** Stadel BV, Lai S, Schlesselman JJ, Murray P. Oral contraceptives and premenopausal breast cancer in nulliparous women. Contraception 1988; 38:287–299. **85.** Miller DR, Rosenberg L, Kaufman DW, Stolley P, Warshauer ME, Shapiro S. Breast cancer before age 45 and oral contraceptive use: New Findings. Am J Epidemiol 1989; 129:269–280. **86.** The UK National Case-Control Study Group, Oral contraceptive use and breast cancer risk in young women. Lancet 1989; 1:973–982. **87.** Schlesselman JJ. Cancer of the breast and reproductive tract in relation to use of oral contraceptives. Contraception 1989; 40:1–38. **88.** Vessey MP, McPherson K, Villard-Mackintosh L, Yeates D. Oral contraceptives and breast cancer: latest findings in a large cohort study. Br J Cancer 1989; 59:613–617. **89.** Jick SS, Walker AM, Stergachis A, Jick H. Oral contraceptives and breast cancer. Br J Cancer 1989; 59:618–621. **90.** Godsland, I et al. The effects of different formulations of oral contraceptive agents on lipid and carbohydrate metabolism. N Engl J Med 1990;323: 1375–81. **91.** Kloosterboer, HJ et al. Selectivity in progesterone and androgen receptor binding of progestogens used in oral contraception. Contraception, 1988;38:325–32. **92.** Van der Vies, J and de Visser, J. Endocrinological studies with desogestrel. Arzneim. Forsch./Drug Res., 1983;33(l),2: 231–6. **93.** Data on file, Organon Inc. **94.** Fotherby, K. Oral contraceptives, lipids and cardiovascular diseases. Contraception, 1985; Vol. 31; 4:367–94. **95.** Lawrence, DM et al. Reduced sex hormone binding globulin and derived free testosterone levels in women with severe acne. Clinical Endocrinology, 1981; 15:87–91. **96.** Cullberg, G et al. Effects of a low-dose desogestrel-ethinyl estradiol combination on hirsutism, androgens and sex hormone binding globulin in women with a polycystic ovary syndrome. Acta Obstet Gynecol Scand, 1985;64:195–202. **97.** Jung-Hoffmann, C and Kuhl, H. Divergent effects of two low-dose oral contraceptives on sex hormone-binding globulin and free testosterone. AJOG, 1987; 156:199–203. **98.** Hammond, G et al. Serum steroid binding protein concentrations, distribution of progestogens, and bioavailability of testosterone during treatment with contraceptives containing desogestrel or levonorgestrel. Fertil Steril, 1984;42:44–51. **99.** Palatsi, R et al. Serum total and unbound testosterone and sex hormone binding globulin (SHBG) in female acne patients treated with two different oral contraceptives. Acta Derm Venereol, 1984; 64:517–23. **100.** Lewis M, Spitzer WO, Heinemann LAJ, MacRae KD, Bruppacher R, Thorogood M on behalf of Transnational Research Group on Oral Contraceptives and Health of Young Women. Third generation oral contraceptives and risk of myocardial infarction: an international case-control study. Br Med J 1996; 312:88–90. **101.** Collaborative Group on Hormonal Factors in Breast Cancer. Breast Cancer and hormonal contraceptives: collaborative reanalysis of individual data on 53 297 women with breast cancer and 100 239 women without breast cancer from 54 epidemiological studies. Lancet 1996; 347:1713–1727. **102.** Palmer JR, Rosenberg L, Kaufman DW, Warshauer ME, Stolley P, Shapiro S. Oral Contraceptive Use and Liver Cancer. Am J Epidemiol 1989; 130:878–882.

BRIEF SUMMARY PATIENT PACKAGE INSERT

Oral contraceptives, also known as "birth control pills" or "the pill", are taken to prevent pregnancy, and when taken correctly, have a failure rate of about 1% per year when used without missing any pills. The typical failure rate of large numbers of pill users is less than 3% per year when women who miss pills are included. For most women, oral contraceptives are also free of serious or unpleasant side effects. However, forgetting to take pills considerably increases the chances of pregnancy.

For the majority of women, oral contraceptives can be taken safely. But there are some women who are at high risk of developing certain serious diseases that can be life-threatening or may cause temporary or permanent disability. The risks associated with taking oral contraceptives increase significantly if you:

- smoke
- have high blood pressure, diabetes, high cholesterol
- have or have had clotting disorders, heart attack, stroke, angina pectoris, cancer of the breast or sex organs, jaundice or malignant or benign liver tumors

Although cardiovascular disease risks may be increased with oral contraceptive use after age 40 in healthy, non-smoking women (even with the newer low-dose formulations), there are also greater potential health risks associated with pregnancy in older women.

You should not take the pill if you suspect you are pregnant or have unexplained vaginal bleeding.

Cigarette smoking increases the risk of serious cardiovascular side effects from oral contraceptive use. This risk increases with age and with heavy smoking (15 or more cigarettes per day) and is quite marked in women over 35 years of age. Women who use oral contraceptives are strongly advised not to smoke.

Most side effects of the pill are not serious. The most common such effects are nausea, vomiting, bleeding between menstrual periods, weight gain, breast tenderness, headache, and difficulty wearing contact lenses. These side effects, especially nausea and vomiting, may subside within the first three months of use.

The serious side effects of the pill occur very infrequently, especially if you are in good health and are young. However, you should know that the following medical conditions have been associated with or made worse by the pill:

1. Blood clots in the legs (thrombophlebitis) or lungs (pulmonary embolism), stoppage or rupture of a blood vessel in the brain (stroke), blockage of blood vessels in the heart (heart attack or angina pectoris) or other organs of the body. As mentioned above, smoking increases the risk of heart attacks and strokes, and subsequent serious medical consequences.
2. In rare cases, oral contraceptives can cause benign but dangerous liver tumors. The benign liver tumors can rupture and cause fatal internal bleeding. In addition, some studies report an increased risk of developing liver cancer. However, liver cancers are rare.
3. High blood pressure, although blood pressure usually returns to normal when the pill is stopped.

The symptoms associated with these serious side effects are discussed in the detailed patient labeling given to you with

ANNUAL NUMBER OF BIRTH-RELATED OR METHOD-RELATED DEATHS ASSOCIATED WITH CONTROL OF FERTILITY PER 100,000 NONSTERILE WOMEN, BY FERTILITY CONTROL METHOD ACCORDING TO AGE

Method of control and outcome	15–19	20–24	25–29	30–34	35–39	40–44
No fertility control methods*	7.0	7.4	9.1	14.8	25.7	28.2
Oral contraceptives non-smoker**	0.3	0.5	0.9	1.9	13.8	31.6
Oral contraceptives smoker**	2.2	3.4	6.6	13.5	51.1	117.2
IUD**	0.8	0.8	1.0	1.0	1.4	1.4
Condom*	1.1	1.6	0.7	0.2	0.3	0.4
Diaphragm/spermicide*	1.9	1.2	1.2	1.3	2.2	2.8
Periodic abstinence*	2.5	1.6	1.6	1.7	2.9	3.6

* Deaths are birth-related
** Deaths are method-related

your supply of pills. Notify your doctor or clinic if you notice any unusual physical disturbances while taking the pill. In addition, drugs such as rifampin, as well as some anticonvulsants and some antibiotics may decrease oral contraceptive effectiveness.

There is conflict among studies regarding breast cancer and oral contraceptive use. Some studies have reported an increase in the risk of developing breast cancer, particularly at a younger age. This increased risk appears to be related to duration of use. The majority of studies have found no overall increase in the risk of developing breast cancer. Some studies have found an increase in the incidence of cancer of the cervix in women who use oral contraceptives. However, this finding may be related to factors other than the use of oral contraceptives. There is insufficient evidence to rule out the possibility that pills may cause such cancers. Taking the pill provides some important non-contraceptive benefits. These include less painful menstruation, less menstrual blood loss and anemia, few pelvic infections, and fewer cancers of the ovary and the lining of the uterus.

Be sure to discuss any medical condition you may have with your doctor or clinic. Your doctor or clinic will take a medical and family history before prescribing oral contraceptives and will examine you. The physical examination may be delayed to another time if you request it and the health care provider believes that it is good medical practice to postpone it. You should be reexamined at least once a year while taking oral contraceptives. The detailed patient information labeling gives you further information which you should read and discuss with your doctor or clinic.

This product (like all oral contraceptives) is intended to prevent pregnancy. It does not protect against transmission of HIV (AIDS) and other sexually transmitted diseases such as chlamydia, genital herpes, genital warts, gonorrhea, hepatitis B, and syphilis.

DETAILED PATIENT LABELING

PLEASE NOTE: This labeling is revised from time to time as important new medical information becomes available. Therefore, please review this labeling carefully.

The following oral contraceptive products contain a combination of a progestogen and estrogen, the two kinds of female hormones:

ORTHO-CEPT® □ 21 Day Regimen
ORTHO-CEPT® □ 28 Day Regimen

Each orange tablet contains 0.15 mg desogestrel and 0.03 mg ethinyl estradiol. Each green tablet in the ORTHO-CEPT 28 day regimen contains inert ingredients.

INTRODUCTION

Any woman who considers using oral contraceptives (the birth control pill or the pill) should understand the benefits and risks of using this form of birth control. This patient labeling will give you much of the information you will need to make this decision and will also help you determine if you are at risk of developing any of the serious side effects of the pill. It will tell you how to use the pill properly so that it will be as effective as possible. However, this labeling is not a replacement for a careful discussion between you and your doctor or clinic. You should discuss the information provided in this labeling with him or her, both when you first start taking the pill and during your revisits. You should also follow your doctor's or clinic's advice with regard to regular check-ups while you are on the pill.

EFFECTIVENESS OF ORAL CONTRACEPTIVES

Oral contraceptives or "birth control pills" or "the pill" are used to prevent pregnancy and are more effective than other non-surgical methods of birth control. When they are taken correctly, the chance of becoming pregnant is less than 1% (1 pregnancy per 100 women per year of use) when used perfectly, without missing any pills. Typical failure rates are actually 3% per year. The chance of becoming pregnant increases with each missed pill during a menstrual cycle.

In comparison, typical failure rates for other non-surgical methods of birth control during the first year of use are as follows:

Implant: <1%
Injection: <1%
IUD: 1 to 2%
Diaphragm with spermicides: 18%
Spermicides alone: 21%
Vaginal sponge: 18 to 36%
Cervical Cap: 18 to 36%
Condom alone (male): 12%
Condom alone (female): 21%
Periodic abstinence: 20%
No methods: 85%

WHO SHOULD NOT TAKE ORAL CONTRACEPTIVES

Cigarette smoking increases the risk of serious cardiovascular side effects from oral contraceptive use. This risk increases with age and with heavy smoking (15 or more cigarettes per day) and is quite marked in women over 35 years of age. Women who use oral contraceptives are strongly advised not to smoke.

Some women should not use the pill. For example, you should not take the pill if you are pregnant or think you may be pregnant. You should also not use the pill if you have any of the following conditions:
• A history of heart attack or stroke
• Blood clots in the legs (thrombophlebitis), lungs (pulmonary embolism), or eyes
• A history of blood clots in the deep veins of your legs
• Chest pain (angina pectoris)
• Known or suspected breast cancer or cancer of the lining of the uterus, cervix or vagina
• Unexplained vaginal bleeding (until a diagnosis is reached by your doctor)
• Yellowing of the whites of the eyes or of the skin (jaundice) during pregnancy or during previous use of the pill
• Liver tumor (benign or cancerous)
• Known or suspected pregnancy

Tell your doctor or clinic if you have ever had any of these conditions. Your doctor or clinic can recommend another method of birth control.

OTHER CONSIDERATIONS BEFORE TAKING ORAL CONTRACEPTIVES

Tell your doctor or clinic if you have or have had:
• Breast nodules, fibrocystic disease of the breast, an abnormal breast x-ray or mammogram
• Diabetes
• Elevated cholesterol or triglycerides
• High blood pressure
• Migraine or other headaches or epilepsy
• Mental depression
• Gallbladder, heart or kidney disease
• History of scanty or irregular menstrual periods

Women with any of these conditions should be checked often by their doctor or clinic if they choose to use oral contraceptives.

Also, be sure to inform your doctor or clinic if you smoke or are on any medications.

RISKS OF TAKING ORAL CONTRACEPTIVES

1. Risk of developing blood clots

Blood clots and blockage of blood vessels are one of the most serious side effects of taking oral contraceptives and can cause death or serious disability. In particular, a clot in the legs can cause thrombophlebitis and a clot that travels to the lungs can cause a sudden blocking of the vessel carrying blood to the lungs. These risks are greater with desogestrel–containing oral contraceptives, such as ORTHO-CEPT, than with other low-dose pills. Rarely, clots occur in the blood vessels of the eye and may cause blindness, double vision, or impaired vision.

If you take oral contraceptives and need elective surgery, need to stay in bed for a prolonged illness or have recently delivered a baby, you may be at risk of developing blood clots. You should consult your doctor or clinic about stopping oral contraceptives three to four weeks before surgery and

not taking oral contraceptives for two weeks after surgery or during bed rest. You should also not take oral contraceptives soon after delivery of a baby. It is advisable to wait for at least four weeks after delivery if you are not breast feeding or four weeks after a second trimester abortion. If you are breast feeding, you should wait until you have weaned your child before using the pill. (See also the section on Breast Feeding in General Precautions.)

The risk of circulatory disease in oral contraceptive users may be higher in users of high dose pills and may be greater with longer duration of oral contraceptive use. In addition, some of these increased risks may continue for a number of years after stopping oral contraceptives. The risk of abnormal blood clotting increases with age in both users and nonusers of oral contraceptives, but the increased risk from the oral contraceptive appears to be present at all ages. For women aged 20 to 44 it is estimated that about 1 in 2,000 using oral contraceptives will be hospitalized each year because of abnormal clotting. Among nonusers in the same age group, about 1 in 20,000 would be hospitalized each year. For oral contraceptive users in general, it has been estimated that in women between the ages of 15 and 34 the risk of death due to a circulatory disorder is about 1 in 12,000 per year, whereas for nonusers the rate is about 1 in 50,000 per year. In the age group 35 to 44, the risk is estimated to be about 1 in 2,500 per year for oral contraceptive users and about 1 in 10,000 per year for nonusers.

2. Heart attacks and strokes

Oral contraceptives may increase the tendency to develop strokes (stoppage or rupture of blood vessels in the brain) and angina pectoris and heart attacks (blockage of blood vessels in the heart). Any of these conditions can cause death or serious disability.

Smoking greatly increases the possibility of suffering heart attacks and strokes. Furthermore, smoking and the use of oral contraceptives greatly increase the chances of developing and dying of heart disease.

3. Gallbladder disease

Oral contraceptive users probably have a greater risk than nonusers of having gallbladder disease, although this risk may be related to pills containing high doses of estrogens.

4. Liver tumors

In rare cases, oral contraceptives can cause benign but dangerous liver tumors. These benign liver tumors can rupture and cause fatal internal bleeding. In addition, some studies report an increased risk of developing liver cancer. However, liver cancers are rare.

5. Cancer of the reproductive organs and breasts

There is conflict among studies regarding breast cancer and oral contraceptive use. Some studies have reported an increase in the risk of developing breast cancer, particularly at a younger age. This increased risk appears to be related to duration of use. The majority of studies have found no overall increase in the risk of developing breast cancer.

An analysis of 54 studies reports that women who are currently using combined oral contraceptives or have used them in the past 10 years are at a slightly increased risk of having breast cancer diagnosed although the additional cancers tend to be localized to the breast. There is no evidence of an increased risk of having breast cancer diagnosed 10 or more years after stopping use.

Some studies have found an increase in the incidence of cancer of the cervix in women who use oral contraceptives. However, this finding may be related to factors other than the use of oral contraceptives. There is insufficient evidence to rule out the possibility that pills may cause such cancers.

ESTIMATED RISK OF DEATH FROM A BIRTH CONTROL METHOD OR PREGNANCY

All methods of birth control and pregnancy are associated with a risk of developing certain diseases which may lead to disability or death. An estimate of the number of deaths associated with different methods of birth control and pregnancy has been calculated and is shown in the following table.

[See table above]

In the above table, the risk of death from any birth control method is less than the risk of childbirth, except for oral contraceptive users over the age of 35 who smoke and pill users over the age of 40 even if they do not smoke. It can be seen in the table that for women aged 15 to 39, the risk of death was highest with pregnancy (7–26 deaths per 100,000 women, depending on age). Among pill users who do not smoke, the risk of death is always lower than that associated with pregnancy for any age group, although over the age of 40, the risk increases to 32 deaths per 100,000 women, compared to 28 associated with pregnancy at that age. However, for pill users who smoke and are over the age of 35, the estimated number of deaths exceeds those for other methods of birth control. If a woman is over the age of 40 and smokes, her estimated risk of death is four times higher (117/100,000 women) than the estimated risk associated with pregnancy (28/100,000 women) in that age group.

Continued on next page

Ortho-Cept—Cont.

The suggestion that women over 40 who do not smoke should not take oral contraceptives is based on information from older, higher-dose pills. An Advisory Committee of the FDA discussed this issue in 1989 and recommended that the benefits of low-dose oral contraceptive use by healthy, non-smoking women over 40 years of age may outweigh the possible risks.

WARNING SIGNALS

If any of these adverse effects occur while you are taking oral contraceptives, call your doctor or clinic immediately:

- Sharp chest pain, coughing of blood, or sudden shortness of breath (indicating a possible clot in the lung)
- Pain in the calf (indicating a possible clot in the leg)
- Crushing chest pain or heaviness in the chest (indicating a possible heart attack)
- Sudden severe headache or vomiting, dizziness or fainting, disturbances of vision or speech, weakness, or numbness in an arm or leg (indicating a possible stroke)
- Sudden partial or complete loss of vision (indicating a possible clot in the eye)
- Breast lumps (indicating possible breast cancer or fibrocystic disease of the breast; ask your doctor or clinic to show you how to examine your breasts)
- Severe pain or tenderness in the stomach area (indicating a possibly ruptured liver tumor)
- Difficulty in sleeping, weakness, lack of energy, fatigue, or change in mood (possibly indicating severe depression)
- Jaundice or a yellowing of the skin or eyeballs, accompanied frequently by fever, fatigue, loss of appetite, dark colored urine, or light colored bowel movements (indicating possible liver problems)

SIDE EFFECTS OF ORAL CONTRACEPTIVES

1. Vaginal bleeding
Irregular vaginal bleeding or spotting may occur while you are taking the pills. Irregular bleeding may vary from slight staining between menstrual periods to breakthrough bleeding which is a flow much like a regular period. Irregular bleeding occurs most often during the first few months of oral contraceptive use, but may also occur after you have been taking the pill for some time. Such bleeding may be temporary and usually does not indicate any serious problems. It is important to continue taking your pills on schedule. If the bleeding occurs in more than one cycle or lasts for more than a few days, talk to your doctor or clinic.

2. Contact lenses
If you wear contact lenses and notice a change in vision or an inability to wear your lenses, contact your doctor or clinic.

3. Fluid retention
Oral contraceptives may cause edema (fluid retention) with swelling of the fingers or ankles and may raise your blood pressure. If you experience fluid retention, contact your doctor or clinic.

4. Melasma
A spotty darkening of the skin is possible, particularly of the face, which may persist.

5. Other side effects
Other side effects may include nausea and vomiting, change in appetite, headache, nervousness, depression, dizziness, loss of scalp hair, rash, and vaginal infections.
If any of these side effects bother you, call your doctor or clinic.

GENERAL PRECAUTIONS

1. Missed periods and use of oral contraceptives before or during early pregnancy
There may be times when you may not menstruate regularly after you have completed taking a cycle of pills. If you have taken your pills regularly and miss one menstrual period, continue taking your pills for the next cycle but be sure to inform your doctor or clinic before doing so. If you have not taken the pills daily as instructed and missed a menstrual period, you may be pregnant. If you missed two consecutive menstrual periods, you may be pregnant. Check with your doctor or clinic immediately to determine whether you are pregnant. Do not continue to take oral contraceptives until you are sure you are not pregnant, but continue to use another method of contraception.

There is no conclusive evidence that oral contraceptive use is associated with an increase in birth defects, when taken inadvertently during early pregnancy. Previously, a few studies had reported that oral contraceptives might be associated with birth defects, but these findings have not been seen in more recent studies. Nevertheless, oral contraceptives or any other drugs should not be used during pregnancy unless clearly necessary and prescribed by your doctor or clinic. You should check with your doctor or clinic about risks to your unborn child of any medication taken during pregnancy.

2. While breast feeding
If you are breast feeding, consult your doctor or clinic before starting oral contraceptives. Some of the drug will be passed on to the child in the milk. A few adverse effects on the child

have been reported, including yellowing of the skin (jaundice) and breast enlargement. In addition, oral contraceptives may decrease the amount and quality of your milk. If possible, do not use oral contraceptives while breast feeding. You should use another method of contraception since breast feeding provides only partial protection from becoming pregnant and this partial protection decreases significantly as you breast feed for longer periods of time. You should consider starting oral contraceptives only after you have weaned your child completely.

3. Laboratory tests
If you are scheduled for any laboratory tests, tell your doctor or clinic you are taking birth control pills. Certain blood tests may be affected by birth control pills.

4. Drug interactions
Certain drugs may interact with birth control pills to make them less effective in preventing pregnancy or cause an increase in breakthrough bleeding. Such drugs include rifampin, drugs used for epilepsy such as barbiturates (for example, phenobarbital), anticonvulsants such as carbamazepine (Tegretol is one brand of this drug), phenytoin (Dilantin is one brand of this drug), phenylbutazone (Butazolidin is one brand), and possibly certain antibiotics. You may need to use additional contraception when you take drugs which can make oral contraceptives less effective.

5. Sexually transmitted diseases
This product (like all oral contraceptives) is intended to prevent pregnancy. It does not protect against transmission of HIV (AIDS) and other sexually transmitted diseases such as chlamydia, genital herpes, genital warts, gonorrhea, hepatitis B, and syphilis.

HOW TO TAKE THE PILL

IMPORTANT POINTS TO REMEMBER

BEFORE YOU START TAKING YOUR PILLS:
1. BE SURE TO READ THESE DIRECTIONS:
Before you start taking your pills.
Anytime you are not sure what to do.
2. THE RIGHT WAY TO TAKE THE PILL IS TO TAKE ONE PILL EVERY DAY AT THE SAME TIME.
If you miss pills you could get pregnant. This includes starting the pack late. The more pills you miss, the more likely you are to get pregnant.
3. MANY WOMEN HAVE SPOTTING OR LIGHT BLEEDING, OR MAY FEEL SICK TO THEIR STOMACH DURING THE FIRST 1–3 PACKS OF PILLS. If you feel sick to your stomach, do not stop taking the pill. The problem will usually go away. If it doesn't go away, check with your doctor or clinic.
4. MISSING PILLS CAN ALSO CAUSE SPOTTING OR LIGHT BLEEDING, even when you make up these missed pills.
On the days you take 2 pills to make up for missed pills, you could also feel a little sick to your stomach.
5. IF YOU HAVE VOMITING OR DIARRHEA, for any reason, or IF YOU TAKE SOME MEDICINES, including some antibiotics, your pills may not work as well.
Use a back-up method (such as condoms, foam, or sponge) until you check with your doctor or clinic.
6. IF YOU HAVE TROUBLE REMEMBERING TO TAKE THE PILL, talk to your doctor or clinic about how to make pill-taking easier or about using another method of birth control.
7. IF YOU HAVE ANY QUESTIONS OR ARE UNSURE ABOUT THE INFORMATION IN THIS LEAFLET, call your doctor or clinic.

BEFORE YOU START TAKING YOUR PILLS

1. DECIDE WHAT TIME OF DAY YOU WANT TO TAKE YOUR PILL.
It is important to take it at about the same time every day.
2. LOOK AT YOUR PILL PACK TO SEE IF IT HAS 21 OR 28 PILLS:
The 21-pill pack has 21 "active" orange pills (with hormones) to take for 3 weeks, followed by 1 week without pills.
The 28-pill pack has 21 "active" orange pills (with hormones) to take for 3 weeks, followed by 1 week of "reminder" green pills (without hormones).
3. ALSO FIND:
    1) where on the pack to start taking pills,
    2) in what order to take the pills.
CHECK PICTURE OF PILL PACK AND ADDITIONAL INSTRUCTIONS FOR USING THIS PACKAGE IN THE BRIEF SUMMARY PATIENT PACKAGE INSERT.
4. BE SURE YOU HAVE READY AT ALL TIMES:
ANOTHER KIND OF BIRTH CONTROL (such as condoms, foam, or sponge) to use as a back-up method in case you miss pills.
AN EXTRA, FULL PILL PACK

WHEN TO START THE FIRST PACK OF PILLS

You have a choice of which day to start taking your first pack of pills. ORTHO-CEPT is available in the DIALPAK® Tablet Dispenser which is preset for a Sunday Start. Day 1 start is also provided. Decide with your doctor or clinic which is the best day for you. Pick a time of day which will be easy to remember.

DAY 1 START:
1. Take the first "active" orange pill of the first pack during the first 24 hours of your period.
2. You will not need to use a back-up method of birth control, since you are starting the pill at the beginning of your period.

SUNDAY START:
1. Take the first "active" orange pill of the first pack on the Sunday after your period starts, even if you are still bleeding. If your period begins on Sunday, start the pack that same day.
2. Use another method of birth control as a back-up method if you have sex anytime from the Sunday you start your first pack until the next Sunday (7 days). Condoms, foam, or the sponge are good back-up methods of birth control.

WHAT TO DO DURING THE MONTH

1. TAKE ONE PILL AT THE SAME TIME EVERY DAY UNTIL THE PACK IS EMPTY.
Do not skip pills even if you are spotting or bleeding between monthly periods or feel sick to your stomach (nausea).
Do not skip pills even if you do not have sex very often.
2. WHEN YOU FINISH A PACK OR SWITCH YOUR BRAND OF PILLS:
21 pills: Wait 7 days to start the next pack. You will probably have your period during that week. Be sure that no more than 7 days pass between 21-day packs.
28 pills: Start the next pack on the day after your last "reminder" pill. Do not wait any days between packs.

WHAT TO DO IF YOU MISS PILLS

If you MISS 1 orange "active" pill:
1. Take it as soon as you remember. Take the next pill at your regular time. This means you may take 2 pills in 1 day.
2. You do not need to use a back-up birth control method if you have sex.
If you MISS 2 orange "active" pills in a row in WEEK 1 OR WEEK 2 of your pack:
1. Take 2 pills on the day you remember and 2 pills the next day.
2. Then take 1 pill a day until you finish the pack.
3. You MAY BECOME PREGNANT if you have sex in the 7 days after you miss pills. You MUST use another birth control method (such as condoms, foam, or sponge) as a back-up method for those 7 days.
If you MISS 2 orange "active" pills in a row in THE 3RD WEEK:
1. If you are a Day 1 Starter:
THROW OUT the rest of the pill pack and start a new pack that same day.
If you are a Sunday Starter:
Keep taking 1 pill every day until Sunday. On Sunday, THROW OUT the rest of the pack and start a new pack of pills that same day.
2. You may not have your period this month but this is expected. However, if you miss your period 2 months in a row, call your doctor or clinic because you might be pregnant.
3. You MAY BECOME PREGNANT if you have sex in the 7 days after you miss pills. You MUST use another birth control method (such as condoms, foam, or sponge) as a back-up method for those 7 days.
If you MISS 3 OR MORE orange "active" pills in a row (during the first 3 weeks):
1. If you are a Day 1 Starter:
THROW OUT the rest of the pill pack and start a new pack that same day.
If you are a Sunday Starter:
Keep taking 1 pill every day until Sunday. On Sunday, THROW OUT the rest of the pack and start a new pack of pills that same day.
2. You may not have your period this month but this is expected. However, if you miss your period 2 months in a row, call your doctor or clinic because you might be pregnant.
3. You MAY BECOME PREGNANT if you have sex in the 7 days after you miss pills. You MUST use another birth control method (such as condoms, foam, or sponge) as a back-up method for those 7 days.

A REMINDER FOR THOSE ON 28-DAY PACKS:
If you forget any of the 7 green "reminder" pills in Week 4:
THROW AWAY the pills you missed.

Keep taking 1 pill each day until the pack is empty. You do not need a back-up method.

FINALLY, IF YOU ARE STILL NOT SURE WHAT TO DO ABOUT THE PILLS YOU HAVE MISSED:

Use a BACK-UP METHOD anytime you have sex. KEEP TAKING ONE "ACTIVE" PILL EACH DAY until you can reach your doctor or clinic.

PREGNANCY DUE TO PILL FAILURE

The incidence of pill failure resulting in pregnancy is approximately one percent (i.e., one pregnancy per 100 women per year) if taken every day as directed, but more typical failure rates are about 3%. If failure does occur, the risk to the fetus is minimal.

PREGNANCY AFTER STOPPING THE PILL

There may be some delay in becoming pregnant after you stop using oral contraceptives, especially if you had irregular menstrual cycles before you used oral contraceptives. It may be advisable to postpone conception until you begin menstruating regularly once you have stopped taking the pill and desire pregnancy.

There does not appear to be any increase in birth defects in newborn babies when pregnancy occurs soon after stopping the pill.

OVERDOSAGE

Serious ill effects have not been reported following ingestion of large doses of oral contraceptives by young children. Overdosage may cause nausea and withdrawal bleeding in females. In cases of overdosage, contact your doctor, clinic or pharmacist.

OTHER INFORMATION

Your doctor or clinic will take a medical and family history before prescribing oral contraceptives and will examine you. The physical examination may be delayed to another time if you request it and the health care provider believes that it is a good medical practice to postpone it. You should be re-examined at least once a year. Be sure to inform your doctor or clinic if there is a family history of any of the conditions listed previously in this leaflet. Be sure to keep all appointments with your doctor or clinic because this is a time to determine if there are early signs of side effects of oral contraceptive use.

Do not use the drug for any condition other than the one for which it was prescribed. This drug has been prescribed specifically for you; do not give it to others who may want birth control pills.

HEALTH BENEFITS FROM ORAL CONTRACEPTIVES

In addition to preventing pregnancy, use of combination oral contraceptives may provide certain benefits. They are:
- menstrual cycles may become more regular
- blood flow during menstruation may be lighter and less iron may be lost. Therefore, anemia due to iron deficiency is less likely to occur.
- pain or other symptoms during menstruation may be encountered less frequently
- ectopic (tubal) pregnancy may occur less frequently
- noncancerous cysts or lumps in the breast may occur less frequently
- acute pelvic inflammatory disease may occur less frequently
- oral contraceptive use may provide some protection against developing two forms of cancer: cancer of the ovaries and cancer of the lining of the uterus.

If you want more information about birth control pills, ask your doctor, clinic or pharmacist. They have a more technical leaflet called the Professional Labeling, which you may wish to read. The professional labeling is also published in a book entitled *Physicians' Desk Reference*, available in many book stores and public libraries.

ORTHO PHARMACEUTICAL CORPORATION
Raritan, New Jersey 08869

©OPC 1992   Issued April 1997   PO7-220
    631-70-840-1

Shown in Product Identification Guide, page 328

ORTHO® DIAPHRAGM KITS   ℞
This product contains dry natural rubber.

DESCRIPTION

ORTHO Diaphragm Kits include two different types in a variety of sizes.
1. The ALL-FLEX® Arcing Spring Diaphragm is a molded, buff-colored, natural rubber vaginal diaphragm containing a distortion-free, dual spring-within-a-spring which provides unique arcing action no matter where the rim is compressed. It is appropriate not only where ordinary diaphragms are indicated, but also in patients with mild cystocele, rectocele or retroversion.

2. The ORTHO® Coil Spring Diaphragm is a molded natural rubber vaginal diaphragm. The rim encases a tension-adjusted spring which allows for compressibility in one plane only, thus allowing insertion with the ORTHO UNIVERSAL INTRODUCER.

ORTHO Diaphragms should be used in conjunction with spermicides, e.g., ORTHO OPTIONS™ GYNOL II® Original Formula Contraceptive Jelly or ORTHO OPTIONS™ ORTHO-GYNOL Contraceptive Jelly, in preventing pregnancy.

ACTION

These Diaphragms when properly fitted serve two purposes:
a. To stop the sperm from entering the cervical canal;
b. To hold the spermicide.

INDICATIONS

ORTHO Diaphragms, in conjunction with an appropriate spermicide, are indicated for the prevention of pregnancy in women who elect to use diaphragms as a method of contraception.

CONTRAINDICATIONS

Known hypersensitivity to natural rubber products and prior history of Toxic Shock Syndrome (TSS).

WARNINGS

An association has been reported between diaphragm use and toxic shock syndrome (TSS), a serious condition which can be fatal.

For contraceptive effectiveness, the diaphragm should remain in place for six hours after intercourse and should be removed as soon as possible thereafter.

Continuous wearing of a contraceptive diaphragm for more than twenty-four hours is not recommended. Removal of the diaphragm before six hours may increase the risk of becoming pregnant. Retention of the diaphragm for any period of time may encourage the growth of certain bacteria in the vaginal tract. It has been suggested that under certain as yet unestablished conditions, overgrowth of these bacteria may lead to symptoms of toxic shock syndrome.

Primary symptoms of TSS are sudden high fever (usually 102° or more), and vomiting, diarrhea, fainting or near fainting when standing up, dizziness or a rash that looks like sunburn. There may also be other signs of TSS such as aching of muscles and joints, redness of the eyes, sore throat and weakness. Patients should be instructed that if they experience sudden high fever and one or more of the other symptoms, they should remove the diaphragm and consult their physician immediately.

PRECAUTIONS

Diaphragm users should be instructed to consult their physician or health care provider:
1. If they are not sure about the insertion and placement of the diaphragm.
2. If they or their partner feel or are made uncomfortable by the presence of the diaphragm.
3. If the diaphragm slips out of place when walking, coughing, or straining.
4. If the diaphragm no longer fits snugly above the pubic bone.
5. If at times other than menstruation there is blood on the diaphragm when it is removed.
6. If there are any holes, tears or other deterioration of the diaphragm.
7. If unable to remove the diaphragm.
8. IMPORTANT—For contraceptive effectiveness, the diaphragm should remain in place for six hours after intercourse and should be removed as soon as possible thereafter. Continuous wearing of a contraceptive diaphragm for more than twenty-four hours is not recommended. Removal of the diaphragm before six hours may increase the risk of becoming pregnant. Retention of the diaphragm for any period of time may encourage the growth of certain bacteria in the vaginal tract. It has been suggested that under certain as yet unestablished conditions, overgrowth of these bacteria may lead to symptoms of toxic shock syndrome. Primary symptoms of TSS are sudden high fever (usually 102° or more), and vomiting, diarrhea, fainting or near fainting when standing up, dizziness or a rash that looks like a sunburn. There may also be other signs of TSS such as aching of muscles and joints, redness of the eyes, sore throat and weakness. If the patient has a sudden high fever and one or more of the other symptoms, the diaphragm should be removed immediately and TSS should be considered.
9. Diaphragm users should have another diaphragm fitting if they have lost or gained more than ten pounds, have had the diaphragm for more than a year, or have had a baby or an abortion. As a matter of routine, each time a pelvic examination is performed, refitting should be done. The size and shape of the vagina changes and this may require a new size diaphragm. Even if the diaphragm size does not change, it is advisable to replace the diaphragm every two years or sooner.

10. Diaphragms may increase the risk of urinary tract infections especially if not properly fitted. Patients should be instructed to consult their physician if they experience any of the signs or symptoms of this type of infection which include pain on urination, blood in the urine, elevated temperature, frequent urination, or a sensation of obstruction while urinating.
11. Persons sensitive to dry natural rubber may have an allergic reaction to diaphragm use.
12. Persons sensitive to spermicides used with the diaphragm should discontinue use.
13. Petroleum jelly, mineral oil, vegetable oil and cold cream lubricants should not be used concurrently with the diaphragm.

INSTRUCTIONS

1. Proper placement of the diaphragm is vital for effectiveness.
2. To be fully effective the diaphragm should never be used without contraceptive cream or jelly. The contraceptive cream or jelly must be spread around the inner surface of the diaphragm as well as around the rim.
3. To avoid pregnancy the diaphragm must be used every time there is intercourse.
4. The diaphragm may be inserted up to six hours before intercourse. If more than six hours has elapsed between insertion of the diaphragm and intercourse, additional contraceptive jelly or cream must be inserted. The diaphragm should not be removed to insert this additional cream or jelly.

The following Patient Instructions for insertion and removal are contained in the booklet "After Your Doctor Prescribes your Ortho Diaphragm" which is included in each Ortho Diaphragm Kit.

Preparing for insertion

1. It is recommended that you urinate and wash your hands before inserting the diaphragm.
2. Prior to inserting your diaphragm, put an applicatorful (about a teaspoon) of contraceptive jelly into the cup of the dome of the diaphragm. You may elect to simply squeeze the tube or use the applicator provided with the starter kit of contraceptive cream or jelly.
3. Spread a small amount around the edge with your fingertip, (if the amount applied to the rim is excessive, it will be difficult to control the diaphragm during insertion) then insert.

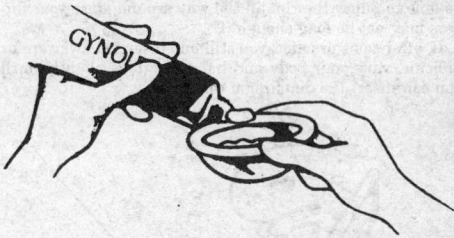

4. You can insert the diaphragm while you are standing with one leg up, squatting, or lying down. The position of the cervix and the walls of the vagina will be different depending on your position. If you are used to one position and then change to another, take extra care in positioning the diaphragm to be sure the cervix is covered.

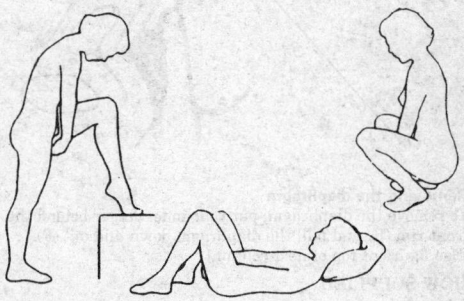

Inserting the diaphragm

1. Hold the diaphragm with the dome down (spermicide up) and press the opposite sides of the rim together between your thumb and third finger (A-1 and A-2). The diaphragm can be held from above or below.
2. Spread the lips of your vagina with your free hand. Hold the compressed diaphragm dome down (spermicide up) and push it gently inward along the rear wall of the vagina as far as it can go. Your index finger, kept on the outer rim of the diaphragm, helps you guide the diaphragm into place (B-1 and B-2).
[See figure at top of next column]

Continued on next page

Ortho Diaphragm—Cont.

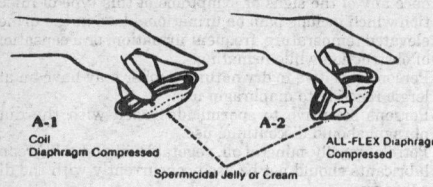

A-1 Coil Diaphragm Compressed

Spermicidal Jelly or Cream

A-2 ALL-FLEX Diaphragm Compressed

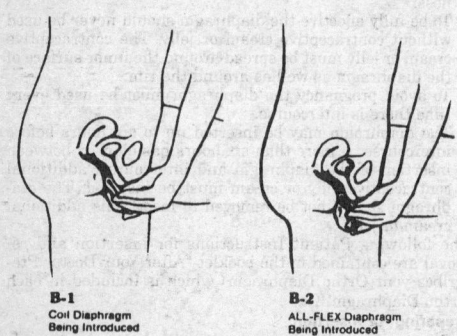

B-1 Coil Diaphragm Being Introduced

B-2 ALL-FLEX Diaphragm Being Introduced

3. With your index finger, push the front rim of the the diaphragm up until it is locked in place just above the pubic bone (C).

4. Check with your index finger to be sure the diaphragm is in place and is holding the contraceptive jelly or cream over the cervix. It is important that the cervix be covered by the diaphragm and spermicide and that the diaphragm be locked in place between the upper edge of the pubic bone and the rear wall of the vagina. You should be able to feel your cervix through the rubber shield. You can feel the front rim of the diaphragm above the pubic bone, but you may not be able to follow the rim all the way around since your fingers may not be long enough (D).

5. If, after some practice, you still find insertion awkward or difficult, vary your body and hand positions slightly until you can insert the diaphragm comfortably.

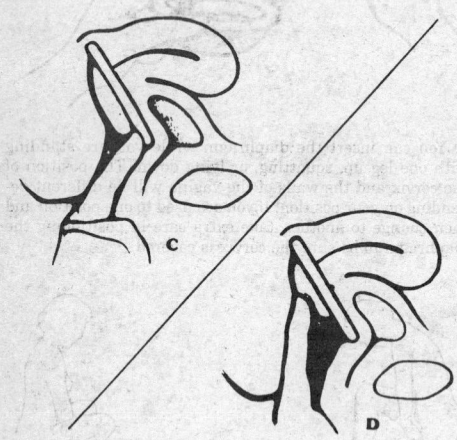

C

D

Removing the diaphragm

To remove the diaphragm, put your index finger behind the front rim (E) and pull the diaphragm down and out (F). [See figure at top of next column]

HOW SUPPLIED

All ORTHO Diaphragm Kits are available individually and contain a tube of ORTHO OPTIONS™ GYNOL II Original Formula Contraceptive Jelly.

1. The ALL-FLEX Arcing Spring Diaphragm is available in sizes 55mm through 95mm in 5mm increments.
2. The ORTHO Coil Spring Diaphragm is available in sizes 55mm through 100mm in 5mm increments.

HOW TO FIT ORTHO DIAPHRAGMS

1. To measure for diaphragm size:
Hold index and middle fingers together and insert into vagina up to the posterior fornix. Raise hand to bring surface of index finger to contact with pubic arch.
Use tip of thumb to mark the point directly beneath the inferior margin of the pubic bone and withdraw finger in this position.

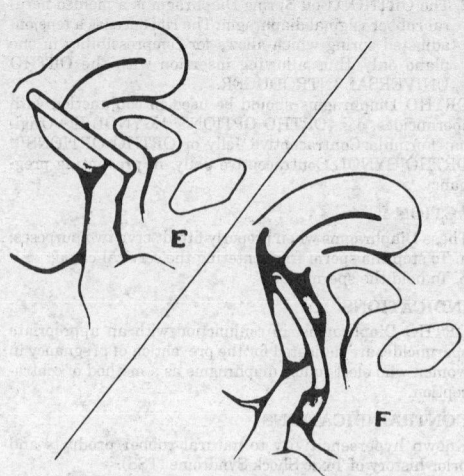

E

F

2. To determine diaphragm size:
Place one end of rim of fitting diaphragm or ring on tip of middle finger. The opposite end should lie just in front of the thumb tip. This is the approximate diameter of the diaphragm needed.
Insert a fitting diaphragm or ring of the appropriate size into the vagina.
Try both a larger and a smaller size before making a decision.
Revised May 1998
Shown in Product Identification Guide, page 327

ORTHO® Dienestrol Cream   Rx

1. ESTROGENS HAVE BEEN REPORTED TO INCREASE THE RISK OF ENDOMETRIAL CARCINOMA.

Three independent case control studies have shown an increased risk of endometrial cancer in postmenopausal women exposed to exogenous estrogens for prolonged periods.[1–3] This risk was independent of the other known risk factors for endometrial cancer. These studies are further supported by the finding that incidence rates of endometrial cancer have increased sharply since 1969 in eight different areas of the United States with population-based cancer reporting systems, an increase which may be related to the rapidly expanding use of estrogens during the last decade.[4]

The three case control studies reported that the risk of endometrial cancer in estrogen users was about 4.5 to 13.9 times greater than in nonusers. The risk appears to depend on both duration of treatment[1] and on estrogen dose.[3] In view of these findings, when estrogens are used for the treatment of menopausal symptoms, the lowest dose that will control symptoms should be utilized and medication should be discontinued as soon as possible. When prolonged treatment is medically indicated, the patient should be reassessed on at least a semiannual basis to determine the need for continued therapy. Although the evidence must be considered preliminary, one study suggests that cyclic administration of low doses of estrogen may carry less risk than continuous administration;[3] it therefore appears prudent to utilize such a regimen.

Close clinical surveillance of all women taking estrogens is important. In all cases of undiagnosed persistent or recurring abnormal vaginal bleeding, adequate diagnostic measures should be undertaken to rule out malignancy.

There is no evidence at present that "natural" estrogens are more or less hazardous than "synthetic" estrogens at equiestrogenic doses.

2. ESTROGENS SHOULD NOT BE USED DURING PREGNANCY

The use of female sex hormones, both estrogens and progestogens, during early pregnancy may seriously damage the offspring. It has been shown that females exposed *in utero* to diethylstilbestrol, a non-steroidal estrogen, have an increased risk of developing in later life a form of vaginal or cervical cancer that ordinarily is extremely rare.[5,6] This risk has been estimated as not greater than 4 per 1000 exposures.[7] Furthermore, a high percentage of such exposed women (from 30 to 90 percent) have been found to have vaginal adenosis,[8–12] epithelial changes of the vagina and cervix. Although these changes are histologically benign, it is not known whether they are precursors of malignancy. Although

similar data are not available with the use of other estrogens, it cannot be presumed they would not induce similar changes.

Several reports suggest an association between intrauterine exposure to female sex hormones and congenital anomalies, including congenital heart defects and limb reduction defects.[13–16] One case control study[16] estimated a 4.7 fold increased risk of limb reduction defects in infants exposed in utero to sex hormones (oral contraceptives, hormone withdrawal tests for pregnancy, or attempted treatment for threatened abortion). Some of these exposures were very short and involved only a few days of treatment. The data suggest that the risk of limb reduction defects in exposed fetuses is somewhat less than 1 per 1000.

In the past, female sex hormones have been used during pregnancy in an attempt to treat threatened or habitual abortion. There is considerable evidence that estrogens are ineffective for these indications, and there is no evidence from well controlled studies that progestogens are effective for these uses.

If ORTHO Dienestrol Cream is used during pregnancy, or if the patient becomes pregnant while using this drug, she should be apprised of the potential risks to the fetus, and the advisability of pregnancy continuation.

DESCRIPTION

ORTHO Dienestrol Cream
Cream for Intravaginal use only
Active ingredient: Dienestrol 0.01%.
Dienestrol is a synthetic, non-steroidal estrogen. It is compounded in a cream base suitable for intravaginal use only. The cream base is composed of glyceryl monostearate, peanut oil, glycerin, benzoic acid, glutamic acid, butylated hydroxyanisole, citric acid, sodium hydroxide and water. The pH is approximately 4.3.

4.4′-(Diethylideneethylene)diphenol

CLINICAL PHARMACOLOGY

Systemic absorption and mode of action of dienestrol are undetermined.

INDICATIONS AND USAGE

ORTHO Dienestrol Cream is indicated in the treatment of atrophic vaginitis and kraurosis vulvae.
ORTHO DIENESTROL CREAM HAS NOT BEEN SHOWN TO BE EFFECTIVE FOR ANY PURPOSE DURING PREGNANCY AND ITS USE MAY CAUSE SEVERE HARM TO THE FETUS (SEE BOXED WARNING).

CONTRAINDICATIONS

Estrogens may cause fetal harm when administered to a pregnant woman (see Boxed Warning). Estrogens are contraindicated in women who are or may become pregnant. If this drug is used during pregnancy, or if the patient becomes pregnant while using this drug, the patient should be apprised of the potential hazard to the fetus.
Estrogens should also not be used in women with any of the following conditions:
1. Known or suspected cancer of the breast.
2. Known or suspected estrogen-dependent neoplasia.
3. Undiagnosed abnormal genital bleeding.
4. Active thrombophlebitis or thromboembolic disorders.
5. A past history of thrombophlebitis, thrombosis, or thromboembolic disorders associated with previous estrogen use.

WARNINGS

1. *Induction of malignant neoplasms.* Long-term continuous administration of natural and synthetic estrogens in certain animal species increases the frequency of carcinomas of the breast, cervix, vagina, and liver. There is now evidence that estrogens increase the risk of carcinoma of the endometrium in humans. (*See* Boxed Warning.)
At the present time there is no satisfactory evidence that estrogens given to postmenopausal women increase the risk of cancer of the breast,[18] although a recent long-term followup of a single physician's practice has raised this possibility.[18a] Because of the animal data, there is a need for caution in prescribing estrogens for women with a strong family history of breast cancer or who have breast nodules, fibrocystic disease, or abnormal mammograms.
2. *Gallbladder disease.* A recent study has reported a 2- to 3-fold increase in the risk of surgically confirmed gall bladder disease in women receiving postmenopausal estrogens,[18] similar to the 2-fold increase previously noted in users of oral contraceptives.[19,24] In the case of oral contraceptives the increased risk appeared after two years of use.[24]
3. *Effects similar to those caused by estrogen-progestogen oral contraceptives.* There are several serious adverse effects of oral contraceptives, most of which have not, up to now, been documented as consequences of postmenopausal

estrogen therapy. This may reflect the comparatively low doses of estrogen used in postmenopausal women. It would be expected that the larger doses of estrogen used to treat prostatic or breast cancer or postpartum breast engorgement are more likely to result in these adverse effects, and, in fact, it has been shown that there is an increased risk of thrombosis in men receiving estrogens for prostatic cancer and women for postpartum breast engorgement.[20-23]

a. *Thromboembolic disease.* It is now well established that users of oral contraceptives have an increased risk of various thromboembolic and thrombotic vascular diseases, such as thrombophlebitis, pulmonary embolism, stroke, and myocardial infarction.[24-31] Cases of retinal thrombosis, mesenteric thrombosis, and optic neuritis have been reported in oral contraceptive users. There is evidence that the risk of several of these adverse reactions is related to the dose of the drug.[32,33] An increased risk of postsurgery thromboembolic complications has also been reported in users of oral contraceptives.[34,35] If feasible, estrogen should be discontinued at least 4 weeks before surgery of the type associated with an increased risk of thromboembolism, or during periods of prolonged immobilization.

While an increased rate of thromboembolic and thrombotic disease in postmenopausal users of estrogens has not been found,[18,36] this does not rule out the possibility that such an increase may be present or that subgroups of women who have underlying risk factors or who are receiving relatively large doses of estrogens may have increased risk. Therefore estrogens should not be used in persons with active thrombophlebitis or thromboembolic disorders, and they should not be used (except in treatment of malignancy) in persons with a history of such disorders in association with estrogen use. They should be used with caution in patients with cerebral vascular or coronary artery disease and only for those in whom estrogens are clearly needed.

Large doses of estrogen (5 mg conjugated estrogens per day), comparable to those used to treat cancer of the prostate and breast, have been shown in a large prospective clinical trial in men to increase the risk of nonfatal myocardial infarction, pulmonary embolism and thrombophlebitis. When estrogen doses of this size are used, any of the thromboembolic and thrombotic adverse effects associated with oral contraceptive use should be considered a clear risk.

b. *Hepatic adenoma.* Benign hepatic adenomas appear to be associated with the use of oral contraceptives.[38-40] Although benign, and rare, these may rupture and may cause death through intra-abdominal hemorrhage. Such lesions have not yet been reported in association with other estrogen or progestogen preparations but should be considered in estrogen users having abdominal pain and tenderness, abdominal mass, or hypovolemic shock. Hepatocellular carcinoma has also been reported in women taking estrogen-containing oral contraceptives.[39] The relationship of this malignancy to these drugs is not known at this time.

c. *Elevated blood pressure.* Increased blood pressure is not uncommon in women using oral contraceptives. There is now a report that this may occur with use of estrogens during menopause.[41] Blood pressure should be monitored with estrogen use, especially if high doses are used.

d. *Glucose tolerance.* A worsening of glucose tolerance has been observed in a significant percentage of patients on estrogen-containing oral contraceptives. For this reason, diabetic patients should be carefully observed while receiving estrogen.

4. *Hypercalcemia.* Administration of estrogens may lead to severe hypercalcemia in patients with breast cancer and bone metastases. If this occurs, the drug should be stopped and appropriate measures taken to reduce the serum calcium level.

PRECAUTIONS

A. General

1. A complete medical and family history should be taken prior to the initiation of any estrogen therapy. The pretreatment and periodic physical examinations should include special reference to blood pressure, breasts, abdomen, and pelvic organs, and should include a Papanicolaou smear. As a general rule, estrogen should not be prescribed for longer than one year without another physical examination being performed.

2. Fluid retention—Because estrogens may cause some degree of fluid retention, conditions which might be influenced by this factor such as epilepsy, migraine, and cardiac or renal dysfunction, require careful observation.

3. Certain patients may develop undesirable manifestations of excessive estrogenic stimulation, such as abnormal or excessive uterine bleeding, mastodynia, etc.

4. Oral contraceptives appear to be associated with an increased incidence of mental depression.[24] Although it is not clear whether this is due to the estrogenic or progestogenic component of the contraceptive, patients with a history of depression should be carefully observed.

5. Preexisting uterine leiomyomata may increase in size during estrogen use.

6. The pathologist should be advised of estrogen therapy when relevant specimens are submitted.

7. Patients with a past history of jaundice during pregnancy have an increased risk of recurrence of jaundice while receiving estrogen-containing oral contraceptive therapy. If jaundice develops in any patient receiving estrogen, the medication should be discontinued while the cause is investigated.

8. Estrogens may be poorly metabolized in patients with impaired liver function and they should be administered with caution in such patients.

9. Because estrogens influence the metabolism of calcium and phosphorus, they should be used with caution in patients with metabolic bone diseases that are associated with hypercalcemia or in patients with renal insufficiency.

10. Because of the effects of estrogens on epiphyseal closure, they should be used judiciously in young patients in whom bone growth is not complete.

11. The lowest effective dose appropriate for the specific indication should be utilized. Studies of the addition of a progestin for seven or more days of a cycle of estrogen administration have reported a lowered incidence of endometrial hyperplasia. Morphological and biochemical studies of endometrium suggest that 10 to 13 days of progestin are needed to provide maximal maturation of the endometrium and to eliminate any hyperplastic changes. Whether this will provide protection from endometrial carcinoma has not been clearly established. There are possible additional risks which may be associated with the inclusion of progestin in estrogen replacement regimens.The potential risks include adverse effects on carbohydrate and lipid metabolism. The choice of progestin and dosage may be important in minimizing these adverse effects.

B. Information for Patients: See text of Patient Package Information which is reproduced below.

C. Drug/Laboratory Test Interactions

Certain endocrine and liver function tests may be affected by estrogen-containing oral contraceptives. The following similar changes may be expected with larger doses of estrogen:

1. Increased sulfobromophthalein retention.

2. Increased prothrombin and factors VII, VIII, IX and X; decreased antithrombin 3; increased norepinephrine-induced platelet aggregability.

3. Increased thyroid-binding globulin (TBG) leading to increased circulating total thyroid hormone, as measured by PBI, T4 by column, or T4 by radioimmunoassay. Free T3 resin uptake is decreased, reflecting the elevated TBG; free T4 concentration is unaltered.

4. Impaired glucose tolerance.

5. Decreased pregnanediol excretion.

6. Reduced response to metyrapone test.

7. Reduced serum folate concentration.

8. Increased serum triglyceride and phospholipid concentration.

D. Carcinogenesis, Mutagenesis, Impairment of Fertility: See "Warnings" section for information on carcinogenesis, mutagenesis and impairment of fertility.

E. Pregnancy:

Teratogenic Effects.

Pregnancy Category X.

See "Contraindications" section.

F. Nursing Mothers: It is not known whether this drug is excreted in human milk. Because many drugs are excreted in human milk, caution should be exercised when estrogens are administered to a nursing woman.

ADVERSE REACTIONS

(See Warnings regarding induction of neoplasia, adverse effects on the fetus, increased incidence of gall bladder disease, and adverse effects similar to those of oral contraceptives, including thromboembolism.) The following additional adverse reactions have been reported with estrogenic therapy, including oral contraceptives:

1. *Genitourinary system.*

Increase in size of uterine fibromyomata.

Vaginal candidiasis.

Breakthrough bleeding, spotting, change in menstrual flow.

Dysmenorrhea.

Premenstrual-like syndrome.

Amenorrhea during and after treatment.

Change in cervical eversion and in degree of cervical secretion.

Cystitis-like syndrome.

2. *Breasts.*

Tenderness, enlargement, secretion.

3. *Gastrointestinal.*

Cholestatic jaundice.

Nausea, vomiting.

Abdominal cramps, bloating.

4. *Skin.*

Erythema multiforme.

Erythema nodosum.

Hemorrhagic eruption.

Loss of scalp hair.

Hirsutism.

Chloasma or melasma which may persist when drug is discontinued.

5. *Eyes.*

Steepening of corneal curvature.

Intolerance to contact lenses.

6. *CNS.*

Mental depression.

Headache, migraine, dizziness.

Chorea.

7. *Miscellaneous.*

Reduced carbohydrate tolerance.

Aggravation of porphyria.

Edema.

Changes in libido.

Increase or decrease in weight.

OVERDOSAGE

Numerous reports of ingestion of large doses of estrogen-containing oral contraceptives by young children indicate that serious ill effects do not occur. Overdosage of estrogen may cause nausea, and withdrawal bleeding may occur in females.

DOSAGE AND ADMINISTRATION

Given cyclically for short term use only:

For treatment of atrophic vaginitis, or kraurosis vulvae associated with the menopause.

The lowest dose that will control symptoms should be chosen and medication should be discontinued as promptly as possible.

Attempts to discontinue or taper medication should be made at 3 to 6 month intervals.

The usual dosage range is one or two applicatorsful per day for one or two weeks, then gradually reduced to one half initial dosage for a similar period. A maintenance dosage of one applicatorful, one to three times a week, may be used after restoration of the vaginal mucosa has been achieved. Treated patients with an intact uterus should be monitored closely for signs of endometrial cancer and appropriate diagnostic measures should be taken to rule out malignancy in the event of persistent or recurring abnormal vaginal bleeding.

HOW SUPPLIED

Available in 2.75 oz. (78g) tubes with or without ORTHO® Measured Dose Applicator.

With applicator: NDC 0062-5450-77

Without applicator: NDC 0062-5450-00

Store at controlled room temperature.

REFERENCES

1. Ziel, H.K. and W.D. Finkle, "Increased Risk of Endometrial Carcinoma Among Users of Conjugated Estrogens," *New England Journal of Medicine,* 293:1167–1170, 1975.

2. Smith, D.C., R. Prentice, D.J. Thompson, and W.L. Hermann, "Association of Exogenous Estrogen and Endometrial Carcinoma," *New England Journal of Medicine,* 293:1164–1167, 1975.

3. Mack, T.M., M.C. Pike, B.E. Henderson, R.I. Pfeffer, V.R. Gerkins, M. Arthur, and S.E. Brown, "Estrogens and Endometrial Cancer in a Retirement Community," *New England Journal of Medicine,* 294:1267–1287, 1976.

4. Weiss, N.S., D.R. Szekely and D.F. Austin, "Increasing Incidence of Endometrial Cancer in the United States," *New England Journal of Medicine,* 294:1259–1262, 1976.

5. Herbst, A.L., H. Ulfelder and D.C. Poskanzer, "Adenocarcinoma of Vagina," *New England Journal of Medicine,* 284:878–881, 1971.

6. Greenwald, P., J. Barlow, P. Nasca, and W. Burnett, "Vaginal Cancer after Maternal Treatment with Synthetic Estrogens," *New England Journal of Medicine,* 285:390–392, 1971.

7. Lanier, A., K. Noller, D. Decker, L. Elveback, and L. Kurland, "Cancer and Stilbestrol. A Follow-up of 1719 Persons Exposed to Estrogens in Utero and Born 1943–1959," *Mayo Clinic Proceedings,* 48:793–799, 1973.

8. Herbst, A., R. Kurman, and R. Scully, "Vaginal and Cervical Abnormalities After Exposure to Stilbestrol In Utero," *Obstetrics and Gynecology,* 40:287–298, 1972.

9. Herbst, A., S. Robboy, G. Macdonald, and R. Scully, "The Effects of Local Progesterone on Stilbestrol-Associated Vaginal Adenosis," *American Journal of Obstetrics and Gynecology* 118:607–615, 1974.

10. Herbst, A., D. Poskanzer, S. Robboy, L. Friedlander, and R. Scully, "Prenatal Exposure to Stilbestrol, A Prospective Comparison of Exposed Female Offspring with Unexposed Controls," *New England Journal of Medicine,* 292:334–339, 1975.

11. Staffi, A., R. Mattingly, D. Foley, and W. Fetherston, "Clinical Diagnosis of Vaginal Adenosis," *Obstetrics and Gynecology,* 43:118–128, 1974.

12. Sherman, A.I., M. Goldrath, A. Berlin, V. Vakhariya, F. Banooni, W. Michaels, P. Goodman, S. Brown, "Cervical-Vaginal Adenosis After In Utero Exposure to Synthetic Estrogens," *Obstetrics and Gynecology,* 44:531–545, 1974.

13. Gal, I., B. Kirman, and J. Stern, "Hormone Pregnancy Tests and Congenital Malformation," *Nature,* 216:83, 1967.

Continued on next page

Ortho Dienestrol—Cont.

14. Levy, E.P., A. Cohen, and F.C. Fraser, "Hormone Treatment During Pregnancy and Congenital Heart Defects," *Lancet,* 1:611, 1973.

15. Nora, J. and A. Nora, "Birth Defects and Oral Contraceptives," *Lancet,* 1:941–942, 1973.

16. Janerich, D.T., J.M. Piper, and D.M. Glebatis, "Oral Contraceptives and Congenital Limb-Reduction Defects," *New England Journal of Medicine,* 291:697–700, 1974.

17. "Estrogens for Oral or Parenteral Use," *Federal Register,* 40:8212, 1975.

18. Boston Collaborative Drug Surveillance Program, "Surgically Confirmed Gall Bladder Disease, Venous Thromboembolism and Breast Tumors in Relation to Post-Menopausal Estrogen Therapy," *New England Journal of Medicine,* 290:15–19, 1974.

18a. Hoover, R., L.A. Gray, Sr., P. Cole, and B. MacMahon, "Menopausal Estrogens and Breast Cancer," *New England Journal of Medicine,* 295:401–405, 1976.

19. Boston Collaborative Drug Surveillance Program, "Oral Contraceptives and Venous Thromboembolic Disease, Surgically Confirmed Gall Bladder Disease, and Breast Tumors," *Lancet* 1:1399–1404, 1973.

20. Daniel, D.G., H. Campbell, and A.C. Turnbull, "Puerperal Thromboembolism and Suppression of Lactation," *Lancet,* 2:287–289, 1967.

21. The Veterans Administration Cooperative Urological Research Group, "Carcinoma of the Prostate: Treatment Comparisons," *Journal of Urology,* 98:516–522, 1967.

22. Bailer, J.C., "Thromboembolism and Oestrogen Therapy," *Lancet,* 2:560, 1967.

23. Blackard, C., R. Doe, G. Mellinger, and D. Byar, "Incidence of Cardiovascular Disease and Death In Patients Receiving Diethylstilbestrol for Carcinoma of the Prostate," *Cancer,* 26:249–256, 1970.

24. Royal College of General Practitioners, "Oral Contraception and Thromboembolic Disease," *Journal of the Royal College of General Practitioners,* 13:267–279, 1967.

25. Inman, W.H.W. and M.P. Vessey, "Investigation of Deaths from Pulmonary, Coronary, and Cerebral Thrombosis and Embolism in Women of Child-Bearing Age," *British Medical Journal,* 2:193–199, 1968.

26. Vessey, M.P. and R. Doll, "Investigation of Relation Between Use of Oral Contraceptives and Thromboembolic Disease, A Further Report," *British Medical Journal,* 2:651–657, 1969.

27. Sartwell, P.E., A.T. Masi, F.G. Arthes, G.R. Greene, and H.E. Smith, "Thromboembolism and Oral Contraceptives: An Epidemiological Case Control Study," *American Journal of Epidemiology,* 90:365–380, 1969.

28. Collaborative Group for the Study of Stroke In Young Women, "Oral Contraception and Increased Risk of Cerebral Ischemia or Thrombosis," *New England Journal of Medicine,* 288:871–878, 1973.

29. Collaborative Group for the Study of Stroke in Young Women, "Oral Contraceptives and Stroke in Young Women: Associated Risk Factors," *Journal of the American Medical Association,* 231:718–722, 1975.

30. Mann, J.I. and W.H.W. Inman, "Oral Contraceptives and Death from Myocardial Infarction," *British Medical Journal,* 2:245–248, 1975.

31. Mann, J.I., M.P. Vessey, M. Thorogood, and R. Doll., "Myocardial Infarction in Young Women with Special Reference to Oral Contraceptive Practice," *British Medical Journal,* 2:241–245, 1975.

32. Inman, W.H.W., V.P. Vessey, B. Westerholm, and A. Engelund, "Thromboembolic Disease and the Steroidal Content of Oral Contraceptives," *British Medical Journal,* 2:203–209, 1970.

33. Stolley, P.D., J.A. Tonascia, M.S. Tockman, P.E. Sartwell, A.H. Rutledge, and M.P. Jacobs, "Thrombosis with Low-Estrogen Oral Contraceptives," *American Journal of Epidemiology,* 102:197–208, 1975.

34. Vessey, M.P., R. Doll, A.S. Fairbairn, and G. Glober, "Post-Operative Thromboembolism and the Use of the Oral Contraceptives," *British Medical Journal,* 3:123–126, 1970.

35. Greene, G.R. and P.E. Sartwell, "Oral Contraceptive Use in Patients with Thromboembolism Following Surgery, Trauma or Infection," *American Journal of Public Health,* 62:680–685, 1972.

36. Rosenberg, L., M.B. Armstrong and H. Jick, "Myocardial Infarction and Estrogen Therapy in Postmenopausal Women," *New England Journal of Medicine,* 294:1256–1259, 1976.

37. Coronary Drug Project Research Group, "The Coronary Drug Project: Initial Findings Leading to Modifications of Its Research Protocol," *Journal of the American Medical Association,* 214:1303–1313, 1970.

38. Baum, J., F. Holtz, J.J. Bookstein, and E.W. Klein, "Possible Association between Benign Hepatomas and Oral Contraceptives," *Lancet,* 2:926–928, 1973.

39. Mays, E.T., W.M. Christopherson, M.M. Mahr, and H.C. Williams, "Hepatic Changes in Young Women Ingesting Contraceptive Steroids, Hepatic Hemorrhage and Primary Hepatic Tumors." *Journal of the American Medical Association,* 235:730–782, 1976.

40. Edmondson, H.A., B. Henderson, and B. Benton, "Liver Cell Adenomas Associated with the Use of Oral Contraceptives," *New England Journal of Medicine,* 294:470–472, 1976.

41. Pfeffer, R.I. and S. Van Den Noore, "Estrogen Use and Stroke Risk in Postmenopausal Women," *American Journal of Epidemiology,* 103:445–456, 1976.

PATIENT INFORMATION ABOUT ESTROGENS

Estrogens are female hormones produced by the ovaries. The ovaries make several different kinds of estrogens. In addition, scientists have been able to make a variety of synthetic estrogens. As far as we know, all these synthetic estrogens have similar properties and therefore much the same usefulness, side effects, and risks. This leaflet is intended to help you understand what estrogens are used for, some of the risks involved in their use, and to help minimize these risks.

This leaflet includes important information about estrogens, but not all the information. If you want to know more, you can ask your doctor or pharmacist to let you read the package insert prepared for the doctor.

USES OF ESTROGEN

THERE IS NO PROPER USE OF ESTROGENS IN A PREGNANT WOMAN

Estrogens are prescribed by doctors for a number of purposes, including:

1. To provide estrogen during a period of adjustment when a woman's ovaries no longer produce it, in order to prevent certain uncomfortable symptoms of estrogen deficiency. (All women normally decrease the production of estrogens, generally between the ages of 45 and 55; this is called the menopause.)

2. To prevent symptoms of estrogen deficiency when a woman's ovaries have been removed surgically before the natural menopause.

3. To prevent pregnancy. (Estrogens are given along with a progestogen, another female hormone; these combinations are called oral contraceptives or birth control pills. Patient labeling is available to women taking oral contraceptives and they will not be discussed in this leaflet.)

4. To treat certain cancers in women and men.

5. To prevent painful swelling of the breasts after pregnancy in women who choose not to nurse their babies.

ESTROGENS IN THE MENOPAUSE

In the natural course of their lives, all women eventually experience a decrease in estrogen production. This usually occurs between ages 45 and 55 but may occur earlier or later. Sometimes the ovaries may need to be removed by an operation before natural menopause, producing a "surgical menopause."

When the amount of estrogen in the blood begins to decrease, many women may develop typical symptoms: Feelings of warmth in the face, neck, and chest or sudden intense episodes of heat and sweating throughout the body (called "hot flashes" or "hot flushes"). These symptoms are sometimes very uncomfortable. A few women eventually develop changes in the vagina (called "atrophic vaginitis") which cause discomfort, especially during and after intercourse.

Estrogens can be prescribed to treat these symptoms of the menopause. It is estimated that considerably more than half of all women undergoing the menopause have only mild symptoms or no symptoms at all and therefore do not need estrogens. Other women may need estrogens for a few months, while their bodies adjust to lower estrogen levels. Sometimes the need will be for periods longer than six months. In an attempt to avoid over-stimulation of the uterus (womb), estrogens are usually given cyclically during each month of use, that is three weeks of pills followed by one week without pills.

Sometimes women experience nervous symptoms or depression during menopause. There is no evidence that estrogens are effective for such symptoms and they should not be used to treat them, although other treatment may be needed.

You may have heard that taking estrogens for long periods (years) after the menopause will keep your skin soft and supple and keep you feeling young. There is no evidence that this is so, however, and such long-term treatment carries important risks.

ESTROGENS TO PREVENT SWELLING OF THE BREASTS AFTER PREGNANCY

If you do not breast-feed your baby after delivery, your breasts may fill up with milk and become painful and engorged. This usually begins about three to four days after delivery and may last for a few days to up to a week or more. Sometimes the discomfort is severe, but usually it is not and can be controlled by pain-relieving drugs such as aspirin and by binding the breasts up tightly. Estrogens can be used to try to prevent the breasts from filling up. While this treatment is sometimes successful, in many cases the breasts fill up to some degree in spite of treatment. The dose of estrogens needed to prevent pain and swelling of the breasts is much larger than the dose needed to treat symptoms of the menopause and this may increase your chances of developing blood clots in the legs or lungs (see below). Therefore, it is important that you discuss the benefits and the risks of estrogen use with your doctor if you have decided not to breast-feed your baby.

SOME OF THE DANGERS OF ESTROGEN

1. *Cancer of the uterus.* If estrogens are used in the postmenopausal period for more than a year, there is an increased risk of *endometrial cancer* (cancer of the uterus). Women taking estrogens have roughly five to ten times as great a chance of getting this cancer as women who take no estrogens. To put this another way, while a postmenopausal woman not taking estrogens has one chance in 1,000 each year of getting cancer of the uterus, a woman taking estrogens has five to ten chances in 1,000 each year. For this reason *it is important to take estrogens only when you really need them.*

The risk of this cancer is greater the longer estrogens are used and also seems to be greater when larger doses are taken. For this reason *it is important to take the lowest dose of estrogen that will control symptoms and to take it only as long as it is needed.* If estrogens are needed for longer periods of time, your doctor will want to reevaluate your need for estrogens at least every six months.

Women using estrogens should report any irregular vaginal bleeding to their doctors; such bleeding may be of no importance, but it can be an early warning of cancer of the uterus. If you have undiagnosed vaginal bleeding, you should not use estrogens until a diagnosis is made and you are certain there is no cancer of the uterus.

If you have had your uterus completely removed (total hysterectomy), there is no danger of developing cancer of the uterus.

2. *Other possible cancers.* Estrogens can cause development of other tumors in animals, such as tumors of the breast, cervix, vagina, or liver, when given for a long time. At present there is no good evidence that women using estrogen in the menopause have an increased risk of such tumors, but there is no way yet to be sure they do not; and one study raises the possibility that use of estrogens in the menopause may increase the risk of breast cancer many years later. This is a further reason to use estrogens only when clearly needed. While you are taking estrogens, it is important that you go to your doctor at least once a year for a physical examination. Also, if members of your family have had breast cancer or if you have breast nodules or abnormal mammograms (breast x-rays), your doctor may wish to carry out more frequent examinations of your breasts.

3. *Gall bladder disease.* Women who use estrogens after menopause are more likely to develop gall bladder disease needing surgery than women who do not use estrogens. Birth control pills have a similar effect.

4. *Abnormal blood clotting.* Oral contraceptives, some of which contain estrogens, increase the risk of blood clotting in various parts of the body. This can result in a stroke (if the clot is in the brain), a heart attack (clot in a blood vessel of the heart), or a pulmonary embolus (a clot which forms in the legs or pelvis, then breaks off and travels to the lungs). Any of these can be fatal. Blood clots may result in the loss of a limb, paralysis or loss of sight, depending on where the blood clot is formed or lodges if it breaks loose.

The larger doses of estrogen used to prevent swelling of the breasts after pregnancy have been reported to cause clotting in the legs and lungs.

It is recommended that if you have had any blood clotting disorders including clotting in the legs or lungs, or a heart attack or stroke, you should not use estrogens.

SPECIAL WARNING ABOUT PREGNANCY

You should not receive estrogen if you are pregnant. If this should occur, there is a greater than usual chance that the developing child will be born with a birth defect, although the possibility remains fairly small. A female child may have an increased risk of developing cancer of the vagina or cervix later in life (in the teens or twenties). Every possible effort should be made to avoid exposure to estrogens during pregnancy. If exposure occurs, see your doctor.

SOME OTHER EFFECTS OF ESTROGENS

In addition to the serious known risks of estrogens described above, estrogens have the following side effects and potential risks:

1. *Nausea and vomiting.* The most common side effect of estrogen therapy is nausea. Vomiting is less common.

2. *Effects on breasts.* Estrogens may cause breast tenderness or enlargement and may cause the breasts to secrete a liquid.

3. *Effects on the uterus.* Estrogens may cause benign fibroid tumors of the uterus to get larger.

Some women will have menstrual bleeding when estrogens are stopped. But if the bleeding occurs on days you are still taking estrogens you should report this to your doctor.

4. *Effects on liver.* Women taking estrogens develop on rare occasions a tumor of the liver which can rupture and bleed into the abdomen. You should report any swelling or unusual pain or tenderness in the abdomen to your doctor immediately.

Women with a past history of jaundice (yellowing of the skin and white parts of the eyes) may get jaundice again during estrogen use.

5. *Other effects.* Estrogens may cause excess fluid to be retained in the body. This may make some conditions worse, such as epilepsy, migraine, heart disease, or kidney disease. If any of the above occur, stop taking estrogens and call your doctor.

SUMMARY

Estrogens have important uses, but they have serious risks as well. You must decide, with your doctor, whether the risks are acceptable to you in view of the benefits of treatment. Except where your doctor has prescribed estrogens for use in special cases of cancer of the breast or prostate, you should not use estrogens if you have cancer of the breast or uterus, are pregnant, have undiagnosed abnormal vaginal bleeding, blood clotting disorders including clotting in the legs or lungs, or have had a stroke, heart attack or angina.

You must understand that your doctor will require regular physical examinations while you are taking them and will try to discontinue the drug as soon as possible and use the smallest dose possible. You can help minimize the risk by being alert for signs of trouble including:

1. Abnormal bleeding from the vagina.
2. Pains in the calves or chest or sudden shortness of breath, or coughing blood (indicating possible clots in the legs, heart or lungs).
3. Severe headache, dizziness, faintness, or changes in vision (indicating possible developing clots in the brain or eye).
4. Breast lumps (you should ask your doctor how to examine your own breasts).
5. Jaundice (yellowing of the skin).
6. Mental depression.
7. *Any* other unusual condition or problem.

Based on his or her assessment of your medical needs, your doctor has prescribed this drug for you. Do not give the drug to anyone else.

HOW SUPPLIED

Available in 2.75 oz. (78g) tubes with or without ORTHO® Measured-Dose Applicator.
With applicator: NDC 0062-5450-77
Without applicator: NDC 0062-5450-00
Store at controlled room temperature.

ORTHO-NOVUM® 1/50 tablets ℞
(norethindrone/mestranol)

Patients should be counseled that this product does not protect against HIV infection (AIDS) and other sexually transmitted diseases.

DESCRIPTION

Each of the following products is a combination oral contraceptive containing the progestational compound norethindrone and the estrogenic compound mestranol:
ORTHO-NOVUM 1/50 □ 21 Tablets and ORTHO-NOVUM 1/50 □ 28 Tablets: Each yellow tablet contains 1 mg norethindrone and 0.05 mg of mestranol. Inactive ingredients include D&C Yellow No. 10, lactose, magnesium stearate and pregelatinized starch. Each green tablet in the ORTHO-NOVUM 1/50 □ 28 package contains only inert ingredients, as follows: D&C Yellow No. 10 Aluminum Lake, FD&C Blue No. 2 Aluminum Lake, lactose, magnesium stearate, microcrystalline cellulose and pregelatinized starch.
The chemical name for norethindrone is 17-hydroxy-19-nor-17α-pregn-4-en-20-yn-3-one, and for mestranol is 3-methoxy-19-nor-17α-pregna-1,3,5(10)-trien-20-yn-17-ol. Their structural formulas are as follows:

norethindrone

mestranol

TABLE 1: LOWEST EXPECTED AND TYPICAL FAILURE RATES DURING THE FIRST YEAR OF CONTINUOUS USE OF A METHOD
% of Women Experiencing an Accidental Pregnancy in the First Year of Continuous Use

Method	Lowest Expected*	Typical**
(No Contraceptive)	(85)	(85)
Oral contraceptives		3
combined	0.1	N/A***
progestin only	0.5	N/A***
Diaphragm with spermicidal cream or jelly	6	18
Spermicides alone (foams, creams, gels, jellies, vaginal suppositories, and vaginal film)	6	21
Vaginal sponge		
nulliparous	9	18
parous	20	36
Implant	0.09	0.09
Injection: depot medroxyprogesterone acetate	0.3	0.3
IUD		
progesterone	1.5	2.0
copper T 380A	0.6	0.8
Condom without spermicides		
female	5	21
male	3	12
Cervial Cap with spermicidal cream or jelly		
nulliparous	9	18
parous	26	36
Periodic abstinence (all methods)	1-9	20
Female sterilization	0.4	0.4
Male sterilization	0.10	0.15

Adapted from RA Hatcher et al., Table 5-2, (1994) ref. #1.
*The authors' best guess of the percentage of women expected to experience an accidental pregnancy among couples who initiate a method (not necessarily for the first time) and who use it consistently and correctly during the first year if they do not stop for any other reason.
**This term represents "typical" couples who initiate use of a method (not necessarily for the first time), who experience an accidental pregnancy during the first year if they do not stop use for any other reason.
***N/A – Data not available.

CLINICAL PHARMACOLOGY
COMBINATION ORAL CONTRACEPTIVES

Combination oral contraceptives act by suppression of gonadotropins. Although the primary mechanism of this action is inhibition of ovulation, other alterations include changes in the cervical mucus (which increase the difficulty of sperm entry into the uterus) and the endometrium (which reduce the likelihood of implantation).

INDICATIONS AND USAGE

Oral contraceptives are indicated for the prevention of pregnancy in women who elect to use this product as a method of contraception. Oral contraceptive products such as ORTHO-NOVUM 1/50 □ 28-Day and ORTHO-NOVUM 1/50 □ 21-Day, which contain 50 mcg of estrogen, should not be used unless medically indicated.
Oral contraceptives are highly effective. Table I lists the typical accidental pregnancy rates for users of combination oral contraceptives and other methods of contraception. The efficacy of these contraceptive methods, except sterilization, depends upon the reliability with which they are used. Correct and consistent use of methods can result in lower failure rates.
[See table 1 above]

CONTRAINDICATIONS

Oral contraceptives should not be used in women who currently have the following conditions:
• Thrombophlebitis or thromboembolic disorders
• A past history of deep vein thrombophlebitis or thromboembolic disorders
• Cerebral vascular or coronary artery disease.
• Known or suspected carcinoma of the breast
• Carcinoma of the endometrium or other known or suspected estrogen-dependent neoplasia
• Undiagnosed abnormal genital bleeding
• Cholestatic jaundice of pregnancy or jaundice with prior pill use.
• Hepatic adenomas or carcinomas
• Known or suspected pregnancy

WARNINGS

Cigarette smoking increases the risk of serious cardiovascular side effects from oral contraceptive use. This risk increases with age and with heavy smoking (15 or more cigarettes per day) and is quite marked in women over 35 years of age. Women who use oral contraceptives should be strongly advised not to smoke.

The use of oral contraceptives is associated with increased risks of several serious conditions including myocardial infarction, thromboembolism, stroke, hepatic neoplasia, and gallbladder disease, although the risk of serious morbidity or mortality is very small in healthy women without underlying risk factors. The risk of morbidity and mortality increases significantly in the presence of other underlying risk factors such as hypertension, hyperlipidemias, obesity and diabetes.

Practitioners prescribing oral contraceptives should be familiar with the following information relating to these risks. The information contained in this package insert is principally based on studies carried out in patients who used oral contraceptives with higher formulations of estrogens and progestogens than those in common use today. The effect of long-term use of the oral contraceptives with lower formulations of both estrogens and progestogens remains to be determined.

Throughout this labeling, epidemiological studies reported are of two types: retrospective or case control studies and prospective or cohort studies. Case control studies provide a measure of the relative risk of a disease, namely, a *ratio* of the incidence of a disease among oral contraceptive users to that among nonusers. The relative risk does not provide information on the actual clinical occurrence of a disease. Cohort studies provide a measure of attributable risk, which is the *difference* in the incidence of disease between oral contraceptive users and nonusers. The attributable risk dose provide information about the actual occurrence of a disease in the population (adapted from refs. 2 and 3 with the author's permission). For further information, the reader is referred to a text on epidemiological methods.

1. THROMBOEMBOLIC DISORDERS AND OTHER VASCULAR PROBLEMS

a. Myocardial Infarction
An increased risk of myocardial infarction has been attributed to oral contraceptive use. This risk is primarily in smokers or women with other underlying risk factors for coronary artery disease such as hypertension, hypercholesterolemia, morbid obesity, and diabetes. The relative risk of heart attack for current oral contraceptive users has been estimated to be two to six.[4-10] The risk is very low under the age of 30.

Smoking in combination with other oral contraceptive use has been shown to contribute substantially to the incidence of myocardial infarctions in women in their mid-thirties or older with smoking accounting for the majority of excess cases.[11] Mortality rates associated with circulatory disease have been shown to increase substantially in smokers, especially in those 35 years of age and older among women who use oral contraceptives.
[See table II at top of next column]
Oral contraceptives may compound the effects of well-known risk factors, such as hypertension, diabetes, hyperlipidemias, age and obesity.[13] In particular, some progestogens are known to decrease HDL cholesterol and cause glu-

Continued on next page

Ortho-Novum 1/50—Cont.

TABLE II: CIRCULATORY DISEASE MORTALITY RATES PER 100,000 WOMAN-YEARS BY AGE, SMOKING STATUS AND ORAL CONTRACEPTIVE USE

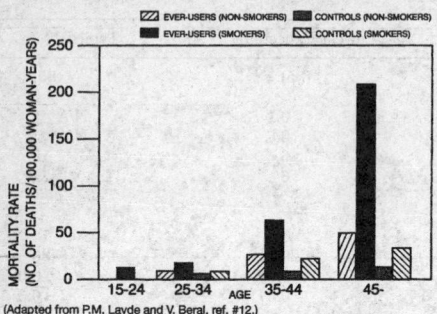

(Adapted from P.M. Layde and V. Beral, ref. #12.)

cose intolerance, while estrogens may create a state of hyperinsulinism.[14-18] Oral contraceptives have been shown to increase blood pressure among users (see Section 9 in WARNINGS). Similar effects on risk factors have been associated with an increased risk of heart disease. Oral contraceptives must be used with caution in women with cardiovascular disease risk factors.

b. Thromboembolism

An increased risk of thromboembolic and thrombotic disease associated with the use of oral contraceptives is well established. Case control studies have found the relative risk of users compared to nonusers to be 3 for the first episode of superficial venous thrombosis, 4 to 11 for deep vein thrombosis or pulmonary embolism, and 1.5 to 6 for women with predisposing conditions for venous thromboembolic disease.[2,3,19-24]

Cohort studies have shown the relative risk to be somewhat lower, about 3 for new cases and about 4.5 new cases requiring hospitalization.[25] The risk of thromboembolic disease associated with oral contraceptives is not related to length of use and disappears after pill use is stopped.[2]

A two- to four-fold increase in relative risk of post-operative thromboembolic complications has been reported with the use of oral contraceptives.[9] The relative risk of venous thrombosis in women who have predisposing conditions is twice that of women without such medical conditions.[26] If feasible, oral contraceptives should be discontinued at least four weeks prior to and for two weeks after elective surgery of a type associated with an increase in risk of thromboembolism and during and following prolonged immobilization. Since the immediate postpartum period is also associated with an increased risk of thromboembolism, oral contraceptives should be started no earlier than four weeks after delivery in women who elect not to breast feed or four weeks after a second trimester abortion.

c. Cerebrovascular diseases

Oral contraceptives have been shown to increase both the relative and attributable risks of cerebrovascular events (thrombotic and hemorrhagic strokes), although, in general, the risk is greatest among older (>35 years), hypertensive women who also smoke. Hypertension was found to be a risk factor for both users and nonusers, for both types of strokes, and smoking interacted to increase the risk of stroke.[27-29]

In a large study, the relative risk of thrombotic strokes has been shown to range from 3 for normotensive users to 14 for users with severe hypertension.[30] The relative risk of hemorrhagic stroke is reported to be 1.2 for non-smokers who used oral contraceptives, 2.6 for smokers who did not use oral contraceptives, 7.6 for smokers who used oral contraceptives, 1.8 for normotensive users and 25.7 for users with severe hypertension.[30] The attributable risk is also greater in older women.[3]

d. Dose-related risk of vascular disease from oral contraceptives

A positive association has been observed between the amount of estrogen and progestogen in oral contraceptives and the risk of vascular disease.[31-33] A decline in serum high density lipoproteins (HDL) has been reported with many progestational agents.[14-16] A decline in serum high density lipoproteins has been associated with an increased incidence of ischemic heart disease. Because estrogens increase HDL cholesterol, the net effect of an oral contraceptive depends on a balance achieved between doses of estrogen and progestogen and the activity of the progestogen used in the contraceptives. The activity and amount of both hormones should be considered in the choice of an oral contraceptive.

Minimizing exposure to estrogen and progestogen is in keeping with good principles of therapeutics. For any particular estrogen/progestogen combination, the dosage regimen prescribed should be one which contains the least amount of estrogen and progestogen that is compatible with

a low failure rate and the needs of the individual patient. New acceptors of oral contraceptive agents should be started on preparations containing 0.035 mg or less of estrogen. Products containing 50 mcg estrogen should be used only when medically indicated.

e. Persistence of risk of vascular disease

There are two studies which have shown persistence of risk of vascular disease for ever-users of oral contraceptives. In a study in the United States, the risk of developing myocardial infarction after discontinuing oral contraceptives persists for at least 9 years for women 40–49 years who had used oral contraceptives for five or more years, but this increased risk was not determined in other age groups.[8] In another study in Great Britain, the risk of developing cerebrovascular disease persisted for at least 6 years after discontinuation of oral contraceptives, although excess risk was very small.[34] However, both studies were performed with oral contraceptive formulations containing 50 micrograms or higher of estrogens.

2. ESTIMATES OF MORTALITY FROM CONTRACEPTIVE USE

One study gathered data from a variety of sources which have estimated the mortality rate associated with different methods of contraception at different ages (Table III). These estimates include the combined risk of death associated with contraceptive methods plus the risk attributable to pregnancy in the event of method failure. Each method of contraception has its specific benefits and risks. The study concluded that with the exception of oral contraceptive users 35 and older who smoke, and 40 and older who do not smoke, mortality associated with all methods of birth control is low and below that associated with childbirth. The observation of an increase in risk of morality with age for oral contraceptive users is based on data gathered in the 1970's.[35] Current clinical recommendation involves the use of lower estrogen dose formulations and a careful consideration of risk factors. In 1989, the Fertility and Maternal Health Drugs Advisory Committee was asked to review the use of oral contraceptives in women 40 years of age and over. The Committee concluded that although cardiovascular disease risks may be increased with oral contraceptive use after age 40 in healthy non-smoking women (even with the newer low-dose formulations), there are also greater potential health risks associated with pregnancy in older women and with the alternative surgical and medical procedures which may be necessary if such women do not have access to effective and acceptable means of contraception. The Committee recommended that the benefits of low-dose oral contraceptive use by healthy non-smoking women over 40 may outweigh the possible risks.

Of course, older women, as all women who take oral contraceptives, should take an oral contraceptive which contains the least amount of estrogen and progestogen that is compatible with a low failure rate and individual patient needs. [See table III below]

3. CARCINOMA OF THE REPRODUCTIVE ORGANS AND BREASTS

Numerous epidemiological studies have been performed on the incidence of breast, endometrial, ovarian and cervical cancer in women using oral contraceptives. While there are conflicting reports, most studies suggest that use of oral contraceptives is not associated with an overall increase in the risk of developing breast cancer. Some studies have reported an increased relative risk of developing breast cancer

particularly at a younger age. This increased relative risk has been reported to be related to duration of use.[36-44,79-89] A meta-analysis of 54 studies reports that women who are currently using combined oral contraceptives or have used them in the past 10 years are at a slightly increased risk of having breast cancer diagnosed although the additional cancers tend to be localized to the breast. There is no evidence of an increased risk of having breast cancer diagnosed 10 or more years after cessation of use.[90]

Some studies suggest that oral contraceptive use has been associated with an increase in the risk of cervical neoplasia in some populations of women.[45-48] However, there continues to be controversy about the extent to which such findings may be due to differences in sexual behavior and other factors.

4. HEPATIC NEOPLASIA

Benign hepatic adenomas are associated with oral contraceptive use, although the incidence of benign tumors is rare in the United States. Indirect calculations have estimated the attributable risk to be in the range of 3.3 cases/100,000 for users, a risk that increases after four or more years of use especially with oral contraceptives of higher dose.[49] Rupture of benign, hepatic adenomas may cause death through intra-abdominal hemorrhage.[50,51]

Studies have shown an increased risk of developing hepatocellular carcinoma[52-54,91] in oral contraceptive users. However, these cancers are rare in the U.S.

5. OCULAR LESIONS

There have been clinical case reports of retinal thrombosis associated with the use of oral contraceptives. Oral contraceptives should be discontinued if there is unexplained partial or complete loss of vision; onset of proptosis or diplopia; papilledema; or retinal vascular lesions. Appropriate diagnostic and therapeutic measures should be undertaken immediately.

6. ORAL CONTRACEPTIVE USE BEFORE OR DURING EARLY PREGNANCY

Extensive epidemiological studies have revealed no increased risk of birth defects in women who have used oral contraceptives prior to pregnancy.[56,57] The majority of recent studies also do not indicate a teratogenic effect, particularly in so far as cardiac anomalies and limb reduction defects are concerned,[55,56,58,59] when taken inadvertently during early pregnancy.

The administration of oral contraceptives to induce withdrawal bleeding should not be used as a test for pregnancy. Oral contraceptives should not be used during pregnancy to treat threatened or habitual abortion.

It is recommended that for any patient who has missed two consecutive periods, pregnancy should be ruled out before continuing oral contraceptive use. If the patient has not adhered to the prescribed schedule, the possibility of pregnancy should be considered at the time of the first missed period. Oral contraceptive use should be discontinued until pregnancy is ruled out.

7. GALLBLADDER DISEASE

Earlier studies have reported an increased lifetime relative risk of gallbladder surgery in users of oral contraceptives and estrogens.[60,61] More recent studies, however, have shown that the relative risk of developing gallbladder disease among oral contraceptive users may be minimal.[62-64]

TABLE III: ANNUAL NUMBER OF BIRTH-RELATED OR METHOD-RELATED DEATHS ASSOCIATED WITH CONTROL OF FERTILITY PER 100,000 NONSTERILE WOMEN, BY FERTILITY CONTROL METHOD ACCORDING TO AGE

Method of control and outcome	15–19	20–24	25–29	30–34	35–39	40–44
No fertility control methods*	7.0	7.4	9.1	14.8	25.7	28.2
Oral contraceptives non-smoker**	0.3	0.5	0.9	1.9	13.8	31.6
Oral contraceptives smoker**	2.2	3.4	6.6	13.5	51.1	117.2
IUD**	0.8	0.8	1.0	1.0	1.4	1.4
Condom	1.1	1.6	0.7	0.2	0.3	0.4
Diaphragm/ spermicide*	1.9	1.2	1.2	1.3	2.2	2.8
Periodic abstinence*	2.5	1.6	1.6	1.7	2.9	3.6

*Deaths are birth-related
** Deaths are method-related

Adapted from H.W. Ory, ref. #35.

The recent findings of minimal risk may be related to the use of oral contraceptive formulations containing lower hormonal doses of estrogens and progestogens.

8. CARBOHYDRATE AND LIPID METABOLIC EFFECTS

Oral contraceptives have been shown to cause a decrease in glucose tolerance in a significant percentage of users.[17] This effect has been shown to be directly related to estrogen dose.[65] Progestogens increase insulin secretion and create insulin resistance, this effect varying with different progestational agents.[17,66] However, in the non-diabetic woman, oral contraceptives appear to have no effect on fasting blood glucose.[67] Because of these demonstrated effects, prediabetic and diabetic women in particular should be carefully monitored while taking oral contraceptives.

A small proportion of women will have persistent hypertriglyceridemia while on the pill. As discussed earlier (see WARNINGS 1a and 1d), changes in serum triglycerides and lipoprotein levels have been reported in oral contraceptive users.

9. ELEVATED BLOOD PRESSURE

An increase in blood pressure has been reported in women taking oral contraceptives[68] and this increase is more likely in older oral contraceptive users[69] and with extended duration of use.[61] Data from the Royal College of General Practitioners[12] and subsequent randomized trials have shown that the incidence of hypertension increases with increasing progestational activity.

Women with a history of hypertension or hypertension-related diseases, or renal disease[70] should be encouraged to use another method of contraception. If women elect to use oral contraceptives, they should be monitored closely and if significant elevation of blood pressure occurs, oral contraceptives should be discontinued. For most women, elevated blood pressure will return to normal after stopping oral contraceptives, and there is no difference in the occurrence of hypertension between former and never users.[68–71]

10. HEADACHE

The onset or exacerbation of migraine or development of headache with a new pattern which is recurrent, persistent or severe requires discontinuation of oral contraceptives and evaluation of the cause.

11. BLEEDING IRREGULARITIES

Breakthrough bleeding and spotting are sometimes encountered in patients on oral contraceptives, especially during the first three months of use. Nonhormonal causes should be considered and adequate diagnostic measures taken to rule out malignancy or pregnancy in the event of breakthrough bleeding, as in the case of any abnormal vaginal bleeding. If pathology has been excluded, time or a change to another formulation may solve the problem. In the event of amenorrhea, pregnancy should be ruled out.

Some women may encounter post-pill amenorrhea or oligomennorrhea, especially when such a condition was preexistent.

12. ECTOPIC PREGNANCY

Ectopic as well as intrauterine pregnancy may occur in contraceptive failures.

PRECAUTIONS

1. PHYSICAL EXAMINATION AND FOLLOW UP

It is good medical practice for all women to have annual history and physical examinations, including women using oral contraceptives. The physical examination, however, may be deferred until after initiation of oral contraceptives if requested by the woman and judged appropriate by the clinician. The physical examination should include special reference to blood pressure, breasts, abdomen and pelvic organs, including cervical cytology, and relevant laboratory tests. In case of undiagnosed, persistent or recurrent abnormal vaginal bleeding, appropriate measures should be conducted to rule out malignancy. Women with a strong family history of breast cancer who have breast nodules should be monitored with particular care.

2. LIPID DISORDERS

Women who are being treated for hyperlipidemias should be followed closely if they elect to use oral contraceptives. Some progestogens may elevate LDL levels and may render the control of hyperlipidemias more difficult.

3. LIVER FUNCTION

If jaundice develops in any woman receiving such drugs, the medication should be discontinued. Steroid hormones may be poorly metabolized in patients with impaired liver function.

4. FLUID RETENTION

Oral contraceptives may cause some degree of fluid retention. They should be prescribed with caution, and only with careful monitoring, in patients with conditions which might be aggravated by fluid retention.

5. EMOTIONAL DISORDERS

Women with a history of depression should be carefully observed and the drug discontinued if depression recurs to a serious degree.

6. CONTACT LENSES

Contact lens wearers who develop visual changes or changes in lens tolerance should be assessed by an ophthalmologist.

7. DRUG INTERACTIONS

Reduced efficacy and increased incidence of breakthrough bleeding and menstrual irregularities have been associated with concomitant use of rifampin. A similar association, though less marked, has been suggested with barbiturates, phenylbutazone, phenytoin sodium, carbamazepine, and possibly with griseofulvin, ampicillin and tetracyclines.[72]

8. INTERACTIONS WITH LABORATORY TESTS

Certain endocrine and liver function tests and blood components may be affected by oral contraceptives:

a. Increased prothrombin and factors, VII, VIII, IX, and X; decreased antithrombin 3; increased norepinephrine-induced platelet aggregability.
b. Increased thyroid binding globulin (TBG) leading to increased circulating total thyroid hormone, as measured by protein-bound iodine (PBI), T4 by column or by radioimmunoassay. Free T3 resin uptake is decreased, reflecting the elevated TBG, free T4 concentration is unaltered.
c. Other binding proteins may be elevated in serum.
d. Sex-binding globulins are increased and result in elevated levels of total circulating sex steroids and corticoids; however, free or biologically active levels remain unchanged.
e. Triglycerides may be increased.
f. Glucose tolerance may be decreased.
g. Serum folate levels may be depressed by oral contraceptive therapy. This may be of clinical significance if a woman becomes pregnant shortly after discontinuing oral contraceptives.

9. CARCINOGENESIS

See WARNINGS Section.

10. PREGNANCY

Pregnancy Category X. See CONTRAINDICATIONS and WARNINGS Sections.

11. NURSING MOTHERS

Small amounts of oral contraceptive steroids have been identified in the milk of nursing mothers and a few adverse effects on the child have been reported, including jaundice and breast enlargement. In addition, oral contraceptives given in the post-partum period may interfere with lactation by decreasing the quantity and quality of breast milk. If possible, the nursing mother should be advised not to use oral contraceptives but to use other forms of contraception until she has completely weaned her child.

12. SEXUALLY TRANSMITTED DISEASES

Patients should be counseled that this product does not protect against HIV infection (AIDS) and other sexually transmitted diseases.

INFORMATION FOR THE PATIENT

See Patient Labeling printed below.

ADVERSE REACTIONS

An increased risk of the following serious adverse reactions has been associated with the use of oral contraceptives (See WARNINGS Section).

- Thrombophlebitis and venous thrombosis with or without embolism
- Arterial thromboembolism
- Pulmonary embolism
- Myocardial infarction
- Cerebral hemorrhage
- Cerebral thrombosis
- Hypertension
- Gallbladder disease
- Hepatic ademonas or benign liver tumors

The following adverse reactions have been reported in patients receiving oral contraceptives and are believed to be drug-related:

- Nausea
- Vomiting
- Gastrointestinal symptoms (such as abdominal cramps and bloating)
- Breakthrough bleeding
- Spotting
- Change in menstrual flow
- Amenorrhea
- Temporary infertility after discontinuation of treatment
- Edema
- Melasma which may persist
- Breast changes: tenderness, enlargement, secretion
- Change in weight (increase or decrease)
- Change in cervical erosion and secretion
- Diminution in lactation when given immediately postpartum
- Cholestatic jaundice
- Migraine
- Rash (allergic)
- Mental depression
- Reduced tolerance to carbohydrates
- Vaginal candidiasis
- Change in corneal curvature (steepening)
- Intolerance to contact lenses

The following adverse reactions have been reported in users of oral contraceptives and the association has been neither confirmed nor refuted:

- Pre-menstrual syndrome
- Cataracts
- Changes in appetite
- Cystitis-like syndrome
- Headache
- Nervousness
- Dizziness
- Hirsutism
- Loss of scalp hair
- Erythema multiforme
- Erythema nodosum
- Hemorrhagic eruption
- Vaginitis
- Porphyria
- Impaired renal function
- Hemolytic uremic syndrome
- Acne
- Changes in libido
- Colitis
- Budd-Chiari Syndrome

OVERDOSAGE

Serious ill effects have not been reported following acute ingestion of large doses of oral contraceptives by young children. Overdosage may cause nausea, and withdrawal bleeding may occur in females.

NON-CONTRACEPTIVE HEALTH BENEFITS

The following non-contraceptive health benefits related to the use of combination oral contraceptives are supported by epidemiological studies which largely utilized oral contraceptive formulations containing estrogen doses exceeding 0.035 mg of ethinyl estradiol or 0.05 mg mestranol.[73–76]

Effects on menses:
- increased menstrual cycle regularity
- decreased blood loss and decreased incidence of iron deficiency anemia
- decreased incidence of dysmenorrhea

Effects related to inhibition of ovulation:
- decreased incidence of functional ovarian cysts
- decreased incidence of ectopic pregnancies

Other effects:
- decreased incidence of fibroademonas and fibrocystic disease of the breast
- decreased incidence of acute pelvic inflammatory disease
- decreased incidence of endometrial cancer
- decreased incidence of ovarian cancer

DOSAGE AND ADMINISTRATION

To achieve maximum contraceptive effectiveness, ORTHO-NOVUM 1/50 Tablets must be taken exactly as directed and at intervals not exceeding 24 hours. ORTHO-NOVUM 1/50 Tablets are available in the DIALPAK® Tablet Dispenser which is preset for a Sunday Start. Day 1 Start is also available.

21-Day Regimen (Sunday Start)

When taking ORTHO-NOVUM 1/50 □ 21, the first tablet should be taken on the first Sunday after menstruation begins. If period begins on Sunday, the first tablet is taken on that day. One tablet is taken daily for 21 days. For subsequent cycles, no tablets are taken for 7 days, then a tablet is taken the next day (Sunday). For the first cycle of a Sunday Start regimen, another method of contraception should be used until after the first 7 consecutive days of administration.

If the patient misses one (1) active tablet in Weeks 1, 2, or 3, the tablet should be taken as soon as she remembers. If the patient misses two (2) active tablets in Week 1 or Week 2, the patient should take two (2) tablets the day she remembers and two (2) tablets the next day; and then continue taking one (1) tablet a day until she finishes the pack. The patient should be instructed to use a back-up method of birth control if she has sex in the seven (7) days after missing pills. If the patient misses (2) active tablets in the third week or misses three (3) or more active tablets in a row, the patient should continue taking one tablet every day until Sunday. On Sunday the patient should throw out the rest of the pack and start a new pack that same day. The patient should be instructed to use a back-up method of birth control if she has sex in the seven (7) days after missing pills. Complete instructions to facilitate patient counseling on proper pill usage may be found in the Detailed Patient Labeling ("How to Take the Pill" section).

21-Day Regimen (Day 1 Start)

The dosage of ORTHO-NOVUM 1/50 □ 21, for the initial cycle of therapy is one tablet administered daily from the 1st day through the 21st day of the menstrual cycle, counting the first day of menstrual flow as "Day 1." For subsequent cycles, no tablets are taken for 7 days, then a new course is started of one tablet a day for 21 days. The dosage regimen then continues with 7 days of no medication, followed by 21 days of medication, instituting a three-weeks-on, one-week-off dosage regimen.

If the patient misses one (1) active tablet in Weeks 1, 2, or 3, the tablet should be taken as soon as she remembers. If the patient misses two (2) active tablets in Week 1 or Week 2,

Continued on next page

Ortho-Novum 1/50—Cont.

the patient should take two (2) tablets the day she remembers and two (2) tablets the next day; and then continue taking one (1) tablet a day until she finishes the pack. The patient should be instructed to use a back-up method of birth control if she has sex in the seven (7) days after missing pills. If the patient misses two (2) active tablets in the third week or misses three (3) or more active tablets in a row, the patient should throw out the rest of the pack and start a new pack that same day. The patient should be instructed to use a back-up method of birth control if she has sex in the seven (7) days after missing pills.

Complete instructions to facilitate patient counseling on proper pill usage may be found in the Detailed Patient Labeling ("How to Take the Pill" section).

28-Day Regimen (Sunday Start)

When taking ORTHO-NOVUM 1/50 □ 28, the first tablet should be taken on the first Sunday after menstruation begins. If period begins on Sunday, the first tablet should be taken that day. Take one active tablet daily for 21 days followed by one green placebo tablet daily for 7 days. After 28 tablets have been taken, a new course is started the next day (Sunday). For the first cycle of a Sunday Start regimen, another method of contraception should be used until after the first 7 consecutive days of administration.

If the patient misses one (1) active tablet in Weeks 1, 2, or 3, the tablet should be taken as soon as she remembers. If the patient misses two (2) active tablets in Week 1 or Week 2, the patient should take two (2) tablets the day she remembers and two (2) tablets the next day; and then continue taking one (1) tablet a day until she finishes the pack. The patient should be instructed to use a back-up method of birth control if she has sex in the seven (7) days after missing pills. If the patient misses two (2) active tablets in the third week or misses three (3) or more active tablets in a row, the patient should continue taking one tablet every day until Sunday. On Sunday the patient should throw out the rest of the pack and start a new pack that same day. The patient should be instructed to use a back-up method of birth control if she has sex in the seven (7) days after missing pills.

Complete instructions to facilitate patient counseling on proper pill usage may be found in the Detailed Patient Labeling ("How to Take the Pill" section).

28-Day Regimen (Day 1 Start)

The dosage of ORTHO-NOVUM 1/50 □ 28, for the initial cycle of therapy is one active tablet administered daily from the 1st through the 21st day of the menstrual cycle, counting the first day of menstrual flow as "Day 1" followed by one green tablet daily for 7 days. Tablets are taken without interruption for 28 days. After 28 tablets have been taken, a new course is started the next day.

If the patient misses one (1) active tablet in Weeks 1, 2, or 3, the tablet should be taken as soon as she remembers. If the patient misses two (2) active tablets in Week 1 or Week 2, the patient should take two (2) tablets the day she remembers and two (2) tablets the next day; and then continue taking one (1) tablet a day until she finishes the pack. The patient should be instructed to use a back-up method of birth control if she has sex in the seven (7) days after missing pills. If the patient misses two (2) active tablets in the third week or misses three (3) or more active tablets in a row, the patient should throw out the rest of the pack and start a new pack that same day. The patient should be instructed to use a back-up method of birth control if she has sex in the seven (7) days after missing pills.

Complete instructions to facilitate patient counseling on proper pill usage may be found in the Detailed Patient Labeling ("How to Take the Pill" section).

The use of ORTHO-NOVUM 1/50 for contraception may be initiated 4 weeks postpartum in women who elect not to breast feed. When the tablets are administered during the postpartum period, the increased risk of thromboembolic disease associated with the postpartum period must be considered. (See CONTRAINDICATIONS and WARNINGS concerning thromboembolic disease. See also PRECAUTIONS for "Nursing Mothers.") The possibility of ovulation and conception prior to initiation of medication should be considered.

(See Discussion of Dose-Related Risk of Vascular Disease from Oral Contraceptives.

ADDITIONAL INSTRUCTIONS FOR ALL DOSING REGIMENS

Breakthrough bleeding, spotting, and amenorrhea are frequent reasons for patients discontinuing oral contraceptives. In breakthrough bleeding, as in all cases of irregular bleeding from the vagina, nonfunctional causes should be borne in mind. In undiagnosed persistent or recurrent abnormal bleeding from the vagina, adequate diagnostic measures are indicated to rule out pregnancy or malignancy. If pathology has been excluded, time or a change to another formulation may solve the problem. Changing to an oral contraceptive with a higher estrogen content, while potentially useful in minimizing menstrual irregularity, should be done only if necessary since this may increase the risk of thromboembolic disease.

Use of oral contraceptives in the event of a missed menstrual period:
1. If the patient has not adhered to the prescribed schedule, the possibility of pregnancy should be considered at the time of the first missed period and oral contraceptive use should be discontinued until pregnancy is ruled out.
2. If the patient has adhered to the prescribed regimen and misses two consecutive periods, pregnancy should be ruled out before continuing oral contraceptive use.

HOW SUPPLIED

ORTHO-NOVUM 1/50 □ 21 Tablets are available in a DIAL-PAK Tablet Dispenser (NDC 0062-1331-15) containing 21 yellow tablets (1 mg norethindrone and 0.05 mg mestranol) which are unscored with "Ortho" and "150" debossed on each side.

ORTHO-NOVUM 1/50 □ 21 is available for clinic usage in a VERIDATE Tablet Dispenser (unfilled) and VERIDATE Refills (NDC 0062-1331-20).

ORTHO-NOVUM 1/50 □ 28 Tablets are available in a DIAL-PAK Tablet Dispenser (NDC 0062-1332-15) containing 28 tablets, as follows: 21 yellow tablets as described under ORTHO-NOVUM 1/50 □ 21, and 7 green tablets containing inert ingredients.

ORTHO-NOVUM 1/50 □ 28 is available for clinic usage in a VERIDATE Tablet Dispenser (unfilled) and VERIDATE Refills (NDC 0062-1332-20).

Caution: Federal law prohibits dispensing without prescription.

REFERENCES

1. Hatcher RA, et al. 1994. Contraceptive Technology. Sixteenth Edition. New York: Irvington Publishers. **2.** Stadel BV, Oral contraceptives and cardiovascular disease. (Pt. 1). N Engl J Med 1981; 305:612-618. **3.** Stadel BV, Oral contraceptives and cardiovascular disease. (Pt. 2). N Engl J Med 1981; 305:672-677. **4.** Adam SA, Thorogood M. Oral contraception and myocardial infarction revisited: the effects of new preparations and prescribing patterns. Br J Obstet Gynaecol 1981; 88:838-845. **5.** Mann JI, Inman WH. Oral contraceptives and death from myocardial infarction. Br Med J 1975; 2(5965):245-248. **6.** Mann JI, Vessey MP, Thorogood M, Doll R. Myocardial infarction in young women with special reference to oral contraceptive practice. Br Med J 1975; 2(5956):241-245. **7.** Royal College of General Practitioners' Oral Contraception Study: further analyses of mortality in oral contraceptive users. Lancet 1981; 1:541-546. **8.** Slone D, Shapiro S, Kaufman DW, Rosenberg L, Miettinen OS, Stolley PD. Risk of myocardial infarction in relation to current and discounted use of oral contraceptives. N Engl J Med 1981; 305:420-424. **9.** Vessey MP. Female hormones and vascular disease – an epidemiological overview. Br J Fam Plann 1980; 6 (Supplement): 1-12. **10.** Russell-Briefel RG, Ezzati TM, Fulwood R, Perlman JA, Murphy RS. Cardiovascular risk status and oral contraceptive use, United States, 1976-80. Prevent Med 1986; 15:352-362. **11.** Goldbaum GM, Kendrick JS, Hogelin GC, Gentry EM. The relative impact of smoking and oral contraceptive use on women in the United States. JAMA 1987; 258:1339-1342. **12.** Layde PM, Beral V. Further analyses of mortality in oral contraceptive users; Royal College of General Practitioners' Oral Contraception Study. (Table 5) Lancet 1981; 1:541-546. **13.** Knopp RH. Arteriosclerosis risk: the roles of oral contraceptives and postmenopausal estrogens. J Reprod Med 1986; 31(9) (Supplement): 913-921. **14.** Krauss RM, Roy S, Mishell DR, Casagrande J, Pike MC. Effects of two low-dose oral contraceptives on serum lipids and lipoproteins: Differential changes in high-density lipoproteins subclasses. Am J Obstet 1983; 145:446-452. **15.** Wahl P, Walden C, Knopp R, Hoover J, Wallace R, Heiss G, Rifkind B. Effect of estrogen/progestin potency on lipid/lipoprotein cholesterol. N Engl J Med 1983; 308:862-867. **16.** Wynn V, Niththyananthan R. The effect of progestin in combined oral contraceptives on serum lipids with special reference to high density lipoproteins. Am J Obstet Gynecol 1982; 142:766-771. **17.** Wynn V, Godsland I. Effects of oral contraceptives on carbohydrate metabolism. J Reprod Med 1986; 31(9)(Supplement):892-897. **18.** LaRosa JC. Atherosclerotic risk factors in cardiovascular disease. J Reprod Med 1986; 31(9)(Supplement): 906-912. **19.** Inman WH, Vessey MP. Investigation of death from pulmonary, coronary, and cerebral thrombosis and embolism in women of child-bearing age. Br Med J 1968; 2(5599):193-199. **20.** Maguire MG, Tonascia J, Sartwell PE, Stolley PD, Tockman MS. Increased risk of thrombosis due to oral contraceptives: a further report. Am J Epidemiol 1979; 110(2):188-195. **21.** Petitti DB, Wingerd J, Pellegrin F, Ramacharan S. Risk of vascular disease in women: smoking, oral contraceptives, noncontraceptive estrogens, and other factors. JAMA 1979; 242:1150-1154. **22.** Vessey MP, Doll R. Investigation of relation between use of oral contraceptives and thromboembolic disease. Br Med J 1968; 2(5599):199-205. **23.** Vessey MP, Doll R. Investigation of relation between use of oral contraceptives and thromboembolic disease. A further report. Br Med J 1969; 2(5658):651-657. **24.** Porter JB, Hunter JR, Danielson DA, Jick H, Stergachis A. Oral contraceptives and non-fatal vascular disease

– recent experience. Obstet Gynecol 1982; 59(3):299-302. **25.** Vessey M, Doll R, Peto R, Johnson B, Wiggins P. A long-term follow-up study of women using different methods of contraception: an interim report. J Biosocial Sci 1976; 8:375-427. **26.** Royal College of General Practitioners: Oral Contraceptives, venous thrombosis, and varicose veins. J Royal Coll Gen Pract 1978; 28:393-399. **27.** Collaborative Group for the Study of Stroke in Young Women: Oral contraception and increased risk of cerebral ischemia or thrombosis. N Engl J Med 1973; 288:871-878. **28.** Petitti DB, Wingerd J. Use of oral contraceptives, cigarette smoking, and risk of subarachnoid hemorrhage. Lancet 1978; 2:234-236. **29.** Inman WH. Oral contraceptives and fatal subarachnoid hemorrhage. Br Med J 1979; 2(6203):1468-1470. **30.** Collaborative Group for the Study of Stroke in Young Women: Oral Contraceptives and stroke in young women: associated risk factors. JAMA 1975; 231:718-722. **31.** Inman WH, Vessey MP, Westerholm B, Engelund A. Thromboembolic disease and the steroidal content of oral contraceptives. A report to the Committee on Safety of Drugs. Br Med J 1970; 2:203-209. **32.** Meade TW, Greenberg G, Thompson SG. Progestogens and cardiovascular reactions associated with oral contraceptives and a comparison of the safety of 50- and 35-mcg oestrogen preparations. Br Med J 1980; 280(6224):1157-1161. **33.** Kay CR. Progestogens and arterial disease – evidence from the Royal College of General Practitioners' Study Am J Obstet Gynecol 1982; 142:762-765. **34.** Royal College of General Practitioners: incidence of arterial disease among oral contraceptive users. J Royal Coll Gen Pract 1983; 33:75-82. **35.** Ory HW. Mortality associated with fertility and fertility control: 1983. Family Planning Perspectives 1983; 15:50-56. **36.** The Cancer and Steroid Hormone Study of the Centers for Disease Control and the National Institute of Child Health and Human Development: Oral contraceptive use and the risk of breast cancer. N Engl J Med 1986; 315:405-411. **37.** Pike MC, Henderson BE, Krailo BE, Krailo MD, Duke A. Roy S. Breast cancer in young women and use of oral contraceptives: possible modifying effect of formulation and age at use. Lancet 1983; 2:926-929. **38.** Paul C, Skegg DG, Spears GFS, Kaldor JM. Oral contraceptives and breast cancer: A national study. Br Med J 1986; 293:723-725. **39.** Miller DR, Rosenberg L, Kaufman DW, Schottenfeld D, Stolley PD, Shapiro S. Breast cancer risk in relation to early oral contraceptive use. Obstet Gynecol 1986; 68:863-868. **40.** Olson H, Olson KL, Moller TR, Ranstam J, Holm P. Oral contraceptive use and breast cancer in young women in Sweden (letter). Lancet 1985; 2:748-749. **41.** McPherson K, Vessey M, Neil A, Doll R, Jones L, Roberts M. Early contraceptive use and breast cancer: Results of another case-control study. Br J Cancer 1987; 56:653-660. **42.** Huggins GR, Zucker PF. Oral contraceptives and neoplasia: 1987 update. Fertil Steril 1987; 47:733-761. **43.** McPherson K, Drife JO. The pill and breast cancer: why the uncertainty? Br Med J 1986; 293:709-710. **44.** Shapiro S. Oral contraceptives – time to take stock. N Engl J Med 1987; 315: 450-451. **45.** Ory H, Naib Z, Conger SB, Hatcher RA, Tyler CW. Contraceptive choice and prevalence of cervical dysplasia and carcinoma in situ. Am J Obstet Gynecol 1976; 124: 573-577. **46.** Vessey MP, Lawless M, McPherson K, Yeates D. Neoplasia of the cervix uteri and contraception: a possible adverse effect of the pill. Lancet 1983; 2:930. **47.** Brinton LA, Huggins GR, Lehman HF, Malli K, Savitz DA, Trapido E, Rosenthal J, Hoover R. Long term use of oral contraceptives and risk of invasive cervical cancer. Int J Cancer 1986; 38:339-344. **48.** WHO Collaborative Study of Neoplasia and Steroidal Contraceptives: Invasive cervical cancer and combined oral contraceptives. Br Med J 1985; 290:961-965. **49.** Rooks JB, Ory HW, Ishak KG, Strauss LT, Greenspan JR, Hill AP, Tyler CW. Epidemiology of hepatocellular adenoma: the role of oral contraceptive use. JAMA 1979; 242:644-648. **50.** Bein NN, Goldsmith HS. Recurrent massive hemorrhage from benign hepatic tumors secondary to oral contraceptives. Br J Surg 1977; 64:433-435. **51.** Klatskin G. Hepatic tumors: possible relationship to use of oral contraceptives. Gastroenterology 1977; 73:386-394. **52.** Henderson BE, Preston-Martin S, Edmondson HA, Peters RL, Pike MC. Hepatocellular carcinoma and oral contraceptives. Br J Cancer 1983; 48:437-440. **53.** Neuberger J, Forman D, Doll R, Williams R. Oral contraceptives and hepatocellular carcinoma. Br Med J 1986; 292:1355-1357. **54.** Forman D, Vincent TJ, Doll R. Cancer of the liver and oral contraceptives. Br Med J 1986; 292:1357-1361. **55.** Harlap S, Eldor J. Births following oral contraceptive failures. Obstet Gynecol 1980; 55:447-452. **56.** Savolainen E, Saksela L, Saxen, L. Teratogenic hazards of oral contraceptives analyzed in a national malformation register. Am J Obstet Gynecol 1981; 140:521-524. **57.** Janerich DT, Piper JM, Glebatis DM. Oral contraceptives and birth defects. Am J Epidemiol 1980; 112:73-79. **58.** Ferencz C, Matanoski GM, Wilson PD, Rubin JD, Neill CA, Gutberlet R. Maternal hormone therapy and congenital heart disease. Teratology 1980; 21:225-239. **59.** Rothman KJ, Fyler DC, Goldblatt A, Kreidberg MB. Exogenous hormones and other drug exposures of children with congenital heart disease. Am J Epidemiol 1979; 109:433-439. **60.** Boston Collaborative Drug Surveillance Program: Oral contraceptives and venous thromboembolic disease, surgically

comfirmed gallbladder disease, and breast tumors. Lancet 1973; 1:1399-1404. **61.** Royal College of General Practitioners: Oral contraceptives and health. New York, Pittman 1974. **62.** Layde PM, Vessey MP, Yeates D. Risk of gallbladder disease: a cohort study of young women attending family planning clinics. J Epidemiol Community Health 1982; 36:274-278. **63.** Rome Group for Epidemiology and Prevention of Cholelithiasis (GREPCO): Prevalence of gallstone disease in an Italian adult female population. Am J Epidemiol 1984; 119:796-805. **64.** Storm BL, Tamragouri RT, Morse ML, Lazar EL, West SL, Stolley PD, Jones JK. Oral contraceptives and other risk factors for gallbladder disease. Clin Pharmacol Ther 1986; 39:335-341. **65.** Wynn V, Adams PW, Godsland IF, Melrose J, Niththyananthan R, Oakley NW, Seedj A. Comparison of effects of different combined oral contraceptive formulations on carbohydrate and lipid metabolism. Lancet 1979; 1:1045-1049. **66.** Wynn V. Effect of progesterone and progestins on carbohydrate metabolism. In: Progesterone and Progestin. Bardin CW, Milgrom E, Mauvis-Jarvis P. eds. New York, Raven Press, 1983; pp. 395-410. **67.** Perlman JA, Roussell-Briefel RG, Ezzati TM, Lieberknecht G. Oral glucose tolerance and the potency of oral contraceptive progestogens. J Chronic Dis 1985; 38: 857-864. **68.** Royal College of General Practitioners' Oral Contraception Study: Effect on hypertension and benign breast disease of progestogen component in combined oral contraceptives. Lancet 1977; 1:624. **69.** Fisch IR, Frank J. Oral contraceptives and blood pressure. JAMA 1977; 237: 2499-2503. **70.** Laragh AJ. Oral contraceptive induced hypertension – nine years later. Am J Obstet Gynecol 1976; 126:141-147. **71.** Ramcharan S, Peritz E, Pellegrin FA, Williams WT. Incidence of hypertension in the Walnut Creek Contraceptive Drug Study cohort: In: Pharmacology of steroid contraceptive drugs. Garattini S, Berendes HW. Eds. New York, Raven Press, 1977; pp. 277-288, (Monographs of the Mario Negri Institute for Pharmacological Research Milan.) **72.** Stockley I. Interactions with oral contraceptives. J Pharm 1976; 216:140-143. **73.** The Cancer and Steroid Hormone Study of the Centers for Disease Control and the National Institute of Child Health and Human Development: Oral contraceptive use and the risk of ovarian cancer. JAMA 1983; 249:1596-1599. **74.** The Cancer and Steroid Hormone Study of the Centers for Disease Control and the National Institute of Child Health and Human Development: Combination oral contraceptive use and the risk of endometrial cancer. JAMA 1987; 257:796-800. **75.** Ory HW. Functional ovarian cysts and oral contraceptives: negative association confirmed surgically. JAMA 1974; 228:68-69. **76.** Ory HW, Cole P, MacMahon B, Hoover R. Oral contraceptives and reduced risk of benign breast disease. N Engl J Med 1976; 294:419-422. **77.** Ory HW. The noncontraceptive health benefits from oral contraceptive use. Fam Plann Perspect 1982; 14:182-184. **78.** Ory HW, Forrest JD, Lincoln R. Making choices: Evaluating the health risks and benefits of birth control methods. New York, The Alan Guttmacher Institute, 1983; p. 1. **79.** Schlesselman J, Stadel BV, Murray P, Lai S. Breast cancer in relation to early use of oral contraceptives. JAMA 1988; 259:1828-1833. **80.** Hennekens CH, Speizer FE, Lipnick RJ, Rosner B, Bain C, Belanger C, Stampfer MJ, Willett W, Peto R. A case-control study of oral contraceptive use and breast cancer. JNCI 1984; 72:39-42. **81.** LaVecchia C, Decarli A, Fasoli M, Franceschi S, Gentile A, Negri E, Parazzini R, Tognoni G. Oral contraceptives and cancers of the breast and of the female genital tract. Interim results from a case-control study. Br J Cancer 1986; 54:311-317. **82.** Meirik O, Lund E, Adami H, Bergstrom R, Christoffersen T, Bergsjo P. Oral contraceptive use and breast cancer in young women. A Joint National Case-control study in Sweden and Norway. Lancet 1986; 11:650-654. **83.** Kay CR, Hannaford PC. Breast cancer and the pill – A further report from the Royal College of General Practitioners' oral contraception study. Br J Cancer 1988; 58:675-680. **84.** Stadel BV, Lai S, Schlesselman JJ, Murray P. Oral contraceptives and premenopausal breast cancer in nulliparous women. Contraception 1988; 38:287-299. **85.** Miller DR, Rosenberg L, Kaufman DW, Stolley P. Warshauer ME, Shapiro S. Breast cancer before age 45 and oral contraceptive use: New Findings. Am J Epidemiol 1989; 129:269-280. **86.** The UK National Case-Control Study Group, Oral contraceptive use and breast cancer in young women. Lancet 1989; 1:973-982. **87.** Schlesselman JJ. Cancer of the breast and reproductive tract in relation to the use of oral contraceptives. Contraception 1989; 40:1-38. **88.** Vessey MP, McPherson K, Villard-Mackintosh L, Yeates D. Oral contraceptives and breast cancer: latest findings in a large cohort study. Br J Cancer 1989; 59:613-617. **89.** Jick SS, Walker AM, Stergachis A, Jick H. Oral contraceptives and breast cancer. Br J Cancer 1989; 59:618-621. **90.** Collaborative Group on Hormonal Factors in Breast Cancer. Breast cancer and hormonal contraceptives: collaborative reanalysis of individual data on 53 297 women with breast cancer and 100 239 women without breast cancer from 54 epidemiological studies. Lancet 1996; 347:1713-1727. **91.** Palmer JR, Rosenberg L, Kaufman DW, Warshauer ME, Stolley P, Shapiro S. Oral Contraceptive Use and Liver Cancer. Am J Epidemiol 1989; 130:878-882.

BRIEF SUMMARY PATIENT PACKAGE INSERT

Oral contraceptives, also known as "birth control pills" or "the pill," are taken to prevent pregnancy and when taken correctly, have a failure rate of less than 1% per year when used without missing any pills. The typical failure rate of large numbers of pill users is less than 3% per year when women who miss pills are included. For most women oral contraceptives are also free of serious or unpleasant side effects. However, forgetting to take pills considerably increases the chances of pregnancy.

For the majority of women, oral contraceptives can be taken safely. But there are some women who are at high risk of developing certain serious diseases that can be fatal or may cause temporary or permanent disability. The risks associated with taking oral contraceptives increases significantly if you:

- smoke
- have high blood pressure, diabetes, high cholesterol
- have or have had clotting disorders, heart attack, stroke, angina pectoris, cancer of the breast or sex organs, jaundice or malignant or benign liver tumors.

Although cardiovascular disease risks may be increased with oral contraceptive use after age 40 in healthy, nonsmoking women (even with the newer low-dose formulations), there are also greater potential health risks associated with pregnancy in older women.

You should not take the pill if you suspect you are pregnant or have unexplained vaginal bleeding.

Cigarette smoking increases the risk of serious cardiovascular side effects from oral contraceptive use. This risk increases with age and with heavy smoking (15 or more cigarettes per day) and is quite marked in women over 35 years of age. Women who use oral contraceptives are strongly advised not to smoke.

Most side effects of the pill are not serious. The most common side effects are nausea, vomiting, bleeding between menstrual periods, weight gain, breast tenderness, and difficulty wearing contact lenses. These side effects, especially nausea and vomiting, may subside within the first three months of use.

The serious side effects of the pill may occur very infrequently, especially if you are in good health and are young. However, you should know that the following medical conditions have been associated with or made worse by the pill:

1. Blood clots in the legs (thrombophlebitis), lungs (pulmonary embolism), stoppage or rupture of a blood vessel in the brain (stroke), blockage of blood vessels in the heart (heart attack or angina pectoris) or other organs of the body. As mentioned above, smoking increases the risk of heart attacks and strokes and subsequent serious medical consequences.
2. In rare cases, oral contraceptives can cause benign but dangerous liver tumors. These benign liver tumors can rupture and cause fatal internal bleeding. In addition, some studies report an increased risk of developing liver cancer. However, liver cancers are rare.
3. High blood pressure, although blood pressure usually returns to normal when the pill is stopped.

The symptoms associated with these serious side effects are discussed in the detailed leaflet given to you with your supply of pills. Notify your doctor or health care provider if you notice any unusual physical disturbances while taking the pill. In addition, drugs such as rifampin, as well as some anticonvulsants and some antibiotics may decrease oral contraceptive effectiveness.

There is conflict among studies regarding breast cancer and oral contraceptive use. Some studies have reported an increase in the risk of developing breast cancer, particularly at a younger age. This increased risk appears to be related to duration of use. The majority of studies have found no overall increase in the risk of developing breast cancer. Some studies have found an increase in the incidence of cancer of the cervix in women who use oral contraceptives. However, this finding may be related to factors other than the use of oral contraceptives. There is insufficient evidence to rule out the possibility that pills may cause such cancers.

Taking the combination pill provides some important noncontraceptive benefits. These include less painful menstruation, less menstrual blood loss and anemia, fewer pelvic infections, and fewer cancers of the ovary and the lining of the uterus.

Be sure to discuss any medical condition you may have with your health care provider. Your health care provider will take a medical and family history before prescribing oral contraceptives and will examine you. The physical examination may be delayed to another time if you request it and the health care provider believes that it is a good medical practice to postpone it. You should be reexamined at least once a year while taking oral contraceptives. Your pharmacist should have given you the detailed patient information labeling which gives you further information which you should read and discuss with your health care provider.

This product (like all oral contraceptives) is intended to prevent pregnancy. It does not protect against transmission of HIV (AIDS) and other sexually transmitted diseases such as chlamydia, genital herpes, genital warts, gonorrhea, hepatitis B, and syphilis.

DETAILED PATIENT LABELING

PLEASE NOTE: This labeling is revised from time to time as important new medical information becomes available. Therefore, please review this labeling carefully.

The following oral contraceptive product contains a combination of estrogen and progestogen, the two kinds of female hormones:

Each yellow tablet contains 1 mg norethindrone and 0.05 mg mestranol. Each green tablet in ORTHO-NOVUM 1/50 □ 28 Day Regimen contains inert ingredients.

INTRODUCTION

You should not use ORTHO-NOVUM 1/50 □ 28-Day and ORTHO-NOVUM 1/50 □ 21-Day, which contains higher doses of estrogen than other oral contraceptives, unless specifically recommended by your health care provider. Any woman who considers using oral contraceptives (the birth control pill or the pill) should understand the benefits and risks of using this form of birth control. This patient labeling will give you much of the information you will need to make this decision and will also help you determine if you are at risk of developing any of the serious side effects of the pill. It will tell you how to use the pill properly so that it will be as effective as possible. However, this labeling is not a replacement for a careful discussion between you and your health care provider. You should discuss the information provided in this labeling with him or her, both when you first start taking the pill and during your revisits. You should also follow your health care provider's advice with regard to regular check-ups while you are on the pill.

EFFECTIVENESS OF ORAL CONTRACEPTIVES

Oral contraceptives or "birth control pills" or "the pill" are used to prevent pregnancy and are more effective than other non-surgical methods of birth control. When they are taken correctly, the chance of becoming pregnant is less than 1% (1 pregnancy per 100 women per year of use) when used perfectly, without missing any pills. Typical failure rates are actually 3% per year. The chance of becoming pregnant increases with each missed pill during a menstrual cycle.

In comparison, typical failure rates for other non-surgical methods of birth control during the first year of use are as follows:

Implant: <1%	Cervical Cap 18 to 36%
Injection: <1%	Condom alone (male): 12%
IUD: 1 to 2%	Condom alone (female): 21%
Diaphragm with spermicides: 18%	Periodic abstinence: 20%
Spermicides alone: 21%	No methods: 85%
Vaginal sponge: 18 to 36%	

WHO SHOULD NOT TAKE ORAL CONTRACEPTIVES

Cigarette smoking increases the risk of serious cardiovascular side effects from oral contraceptive use. This risk increases with age and with heavy smoking (15 or more cigarettes per day) and is quite marked in women over 35 years of age. Women who use oral contraceptives are strongly advised not to smoke.

Some women should not use the pill. For example, you should not take the pill if you are pregnant or think you may be pregnant. You should also not use the pill if you have any of the following conditions:

- A history of heart attack or stroke
- Blood clots in the legs (thrombophlebitis), lungs (pulmonary embolism), or eyes
- A history of blood clots in the deep veins of your legs
- Chest pain (angina pectoris)
- Known or suspected breast cancer or cancer of the lining of the uterus, cervix or vagina
- Unexplained vaginal bleeding (until a diagnosis is reached by your doctor)
- Yellowing of the whites of the eyes or of the skin (jaundice) during pregnancy or during previous use of the pill
- Liver tumor (benign or cancerous)
- Known or suspected pregnancy

Tell your health care provider if you have ever had any of these conditions. Your health care provider can recommend a safer method of birth control.

OTHER CONSIDERATIONS BEFORE TAKING ORAL CONTRACEPTIVES

Tell your health care provider if you have or have had:

- Breast nodules, fibrocystic disease of the breast, an abnormal breast x-ray or mammogram
- Diabetes

Continued on next page

Ortho-Novum 1/50—Cont.

- Elevated cholesterol or triglycerides
- High blood pressure
- Migraine or other headaches or epilepsy
- Mental depression
- Gallbladder, heart or kidney disease
- History of scanty or irregular menstrual periods

Women with any of these conditions should be checked often by their health care provider if they choose to use oral contraceptives.

Also, be sure to inform your doctor or health care provider if you smoke or are on any medications.

RISKS OF TAKING ORAL CONTRACEPTIVES

1. Risk of developing blood clots

Blood clots and blockage of blood vessels are one of the most serious side effects of taking oral contraceptives and can cause death or serious disability. In particular, a clot in the legs can cause thrombophlebitis and a clot that travels to the lungs can cause a sudden blocking of the vessel carrying blood to the lungs. Rarely, clots occur in the blood vessels of the eye and may cause blindness, double vision, or impaired vision.

If you take oral contraceptives and need elective surgery, need to stay in bed for a prolonged illness or have recently delivered a baby, you may be at risk of developing blood clots. You should consult your doctor about stopping oral contraceptives three to four weeks before surgery and not taking oral contraceptives for two weeks after surgery or during bed rest. You should also not take oral contraceptives soon after delivery of a baby. It is advisable to wait for at least four weeks after delivery if you are not breast feeding or four weeks after a second trimester abortion. If you are breast feeding, you should wait until you have weaned your child before using the pill. (See also in the section on Breast Feeding in General Precautions.)

The risk of circulatory disease in oral contraceptive users may be higher in users of high dose pills and may be greater with longer duration of oral contraceptive use. In addition, some of these increased risks may continue for a number of years after stopping oral contraceptives. The risk of abnormal blood clotting increases with age in both users and nonusers of oral contraceptives, but the increased risk from the oral contraceptive appears to be present at all ages. For women aged 20 to 44, it is estimated that about 1 in 2,000 using oral contraceptives will be hospitalized each year because of abnormal clotting. Among nonusers in the same age group, about 1 in 20,000 would be hospitalized each year. For oral contraceptive users in general, it has been estimated that in women between the ages of 15 and 34 the risk of death due to a circulatory disorder is about 1 in 12,000 per year, whereas for nonusers the rate is about 1 in 50,000 per year. In the age group 35 to 44, the risk is estimated to be about 1 in 2,500 per year for oral contraceptive users and about 1 in 10,000 per year for nonusers.

2. Heart attacks and strokes

Oral contraceptives may increase the tendency to develop strokes (stoppage or rupture of blood vessels in the brain) and angina pectoris and heart attacks (blockage of blood vessels in the heart). Any of these conditions can cause death or serious disability.

Smoking greatly increases the possibility of suffering heart attacks and strokes. Furthermore, smoking and the use of oral contraceptives greatly increase the chances of developing and dying of heart disease

3. Gallbladder disease

Oral contraceptive users probably have a greater risk than nonusers of having gallbladder disease, although this risk may be related to pills containing high doses of estrogens.

4. Liver tumors

In rare cases, oral contraceptives can cause benign but dangerous liver tumors. These benign liver tumors can rupture and cause fatal internal bleeding. In addition, some studies report an increased risk of developing liver cancer. However, liver cancers are rare.

5. Cancer of the reproductive organs and breast

There is conflict among studies regarding breast cancer and oral contraceptive use. Some studies have reported an increase in the risk of developing breast cancer, particularly at a younger age. This increased risk appears to be related to duration of use. The majority of studies have found no overall increase in the risk of developing breast cancer.

An analysis of 54 studies reports that women who are currently using combined oral contraceptives or have used them in the past 10 years are at a slightly increased risk of having breast cancer diagnosed although the additional cancers tend to be localized to the breast. There is no evidence of an increased risk of having breast cancer diagnosed 10 or more years after stopping use.

Some studies have found an increase in the incidence of cancer of the cervix in women who use oral contraceptives. However, this finding may be related to factors other than the use of oral contraceptives. There is insufficient evidence to rule out the possibility that pills may cause such cancers.

ESTIMATED RISK OF DEATH FROM A BIRTH CONTROL METHOD OR PREGNANCY

All methods of birth control and pregnancy are associated with a risk of developing certain diseases which may lead to disability or death. An estimate of the number of deaths associated with different methods of birth control and pregnancy has been calculated and is shown in the following table.

[See table below]

In the above table, the risk of death from any birth control method is less than the risk of childbirth, except for oral contraceptive users over the age of 35 who smoke and pill users over the age of 40 even if they do not smoke. It can be seen in the table that for women aged 15 to 39, the risk of death was highest with pregnancy (7–26 deaths per 100,000 women, depending on age). Among pill users who do not smoke, the risk of death was always lower than that associated with pregnancy for any age group, although over the age of 40, the risk increases to 32 deaths per 100,000 women, compared to 28 associated with pregnancy at that age. However, for pill users who smoke and are over the age of 35, the estimated number of deaths exceed those for other methods of birth control. If a woman is over the age of 40 and smokes, her estimated risk of death is four times higher (117/100,000 women) than the estimated risk associated with pregnancy (28/100,000 women) in that age group.

The suggestion that women over 40 who do not smoke should not take oral contraceptives is based on information

from older, higher-dose pills. An Advisory Committee of the FDA discussed this issue in 1989 and recommended that the benefits of low-dose oral contraceptive use by healthy, nonsmoking women over 40 years of age may outweigh the possible risks.

WARNINGS SIGNALS

If any of these adverse effects occur while you are taking oral contraceptives, call your doctor immediately:

- Sharp chest pain, coughing of blood, or sudden shortness of breath (indicating a possible clot in the lung)
- Pain in the calf (indicating a possible clot in the leg)
- Crushing chest pain or heaviness in the chest (indicating a possible heart attack)
- Sudden severe headache or vomiting, dizziness, or fainting, disturbances of vision or speech, weakness, or numbness in an arm or leg (indicating a possible stroke)
- Sudden partial or complete loss of vision (indicating a possible clot in the eye)
- Breast lumps (indicating possible breast cancer or fibrocystic disease of the breast; ask your doctor or health care provider to show you how to examine your breasts)
- Severe pain or tenderness in the stomach area (indicating a possibly ruptured liver tumor)
- Difficulty in sleeping, weakness, lack of energy, fatigue, or change in mood (possibly indicating severe depression)
- Jaundice or yellowing of the skin or eyeballs, accompanied frequently by fever, fatigue, loss of appetite, dark colored urine, or light brown colored bowel movements (indicating possible liver problems)

SIDE EFFECTS OF ORAL CONTRACEPTIVES

1. Vaginal bleeding

Irregular vaginal bleeding or spotting may occur while you are taking the pills. Irregular bleeding may vary from slight staining between menstrual periods to breakthrough bleeding which is a flow much like a regular period. Irregular bleeding occurs most often during the first few months of oral contraceptive use, but may also occur after you have been taking the pill for some time. Such bleeding may be temporary and usually does not indicate any serious problems. It is important to continue taking your pills on schedule. If the bleeding occurs in more than one cycle or last for more than a few days, talk to your doctor or health care provider.

2. Contact lenses

If you wear contact lenses and notice a change in vision or an inability to wear your lenses, contact your doctor or health care provider.

3. Fluid retention

Oral contraceptives may cause edema (fluid retention) with swelling of the fingers or ankles and may raise your blood pressure. If you experience fluid retention, contact your doctor or health care provider.

4. Melasma

A spotty darkening of the skin is possible, particularly of the face, which may persist.

5. Other side effects

Other side effects may include nausea and vomiting, change in appetite, headache, nervousness, depression, dizziness, loss of scalp hair, rash, and vaginal infections.

If any of these side effects bother you, call your doctor or health care provider.

GENERAL PRECAUTIONS

1. Missed periods and use of oral contraceptives before or during early pregnancy

There may be times when you may not menstruate regularly after you have completed taking a cycle of pills. If you have taken your pills regularly and miss one menstrual period, continue taking your pills for the next cycle but be sure to inform your health care provider before doing so. If you have not taken the pills daily as instructed and missed a menstrual period, you may be pregnant. If you missed two consecutive menstrual periods, you may be pregnant. Check with your health care provider immediately to determine whether you are pregnant. Do not continue to take oral contraceptives until you are sure you are not pregnant, but continue to use another method of contraception.

There is no conclusive evidence that oral contraceptive use is associated with an increase in birth defects, when taken inadvertently during early pregnancy. Previously, a few studies had reported that oral contraceptives might be associated with birth defects, but these findings have not been seen in more recent studies. Nevertheless, oral contraceptives or any other drugs should not be used during pregnancy unless clearly necessary and prescribed by your doctor. You should check with your doctor about risks to your unborn child of any medication taken during pregnancy.

2. While breast feeding

If you are beast feeding, consult your doctor before starting oral contraceptives. Some of the drug will be passed on to the child in the milk. A few adverse effects on the child have been reported, including yellowing of the skin (jaundice) and breast enlargement. In addition, oral contraceptives may decrease the amount and quality of your milk. If possible, do not use oral contraceptives while breast feeding. You should use another method of contraception since

ANNUAL NUMBER OF BIRTH-RELATED OR METHOD-RELATED DEATHS ASSOCIATED WITH CONTROL OF FERTILITY PER 100,000 NONSTERILE WOMEN, BY FERTILITY CONTROL METHOD ACCORDING TO AGE

Method of control and outcome	15–19	20–24	25–29	30–34	35–39	40–44
No fertility control methods*	7.0	7.4	9.1	14.8	25.7	28.2
Oral contraceptives non-smoker**	0.3	0.5	0.9	1.9	13.8	31.6
Oral contraceptives smoker**	2.2	3.4	6.6	13.5	51.1	117.2
IUD**	0.8	0.8	1.0	1.0	1.4	1.4
Condom*	1.1	1.6	0.7	0.2	0.3	0.4
Diaphragm/ spermicide*	1.9	1.2	1.2	1.3	2.2	2.8
Periodic abstinence*	2.5	1.6	1.6	1.7	2.9	3.6

*Deaths are birth-related
**Deaths are method-related

breast feeding provides only partial protection from becoming pregnant and this partial protection decreases significantly as you breast feed for longer periods of time. You should consider starting oral contraceptives only after you have weaned your child completely.

3. Laboratory tests

If you are scheduled for any laboratory tests, tell your doctor you are taking birth control pills. Certain blood tests may be affected by birth control pills.

4. Drug interactions

Certain drugs may interact with birth control pills to make them less effective in preventing pregnancy or cause an increase in breakthrough bleeding. Such drugs include rifampin, drugs used for epilepsy such as barbiturates (for example, phenobarbital), anticonvulsants such as carbamazepine (Tegretol is one brand of this drug), phenytoin (Dilantin is one brand of this drug), phenylbutazone (Butazolidin is one brand), and possibly certain antibiotics. You may need to use additional contraception when you take drugs which can make oral contraceptives less effective.

5. Sexually transmitted diseases

This product (like all oral contraceptives) is intended to prevent pregnancy. It does not protect against transmission of HIV (AIDS) and other sexually transmitted diseases such as chlamydia, genital herpes, genital warts, gonorrhea, hepatitis B, and syphilis.

HOW TO TAKE THE PILL

IMPORTANT POINTS TO REMEMBER

BEFORE YOU START TAKING YOUR PILLS:

1. BE SURE TO READ THESE DIRECTIONS:

Before you start taking your pills.

Anytime you are not sure what to do.

2. THE RIGHT WAY TO TAKE THE PILL IS TO TAKE ONE PILL EVERY DAY AT THE SAME TIME.

If you miss pills you could get pregnant. This includes starting the pack late.

The more pills you miss, the more likely you are to get pregnant.

3. MANY WOMEN HAVE SPOTTING OR LIGHT BLEEDING, OR MAY FEEL SICK TO THEIR STOMACH DURING THE FIRST 1–3 PACKS OF PILLS. If you feel sick to your stomach, do not stop taking the pill. The problem will usually go away. If it doesn't go away, check with your doctor or clinic.

4. MISSING PILLS CAN ALSO CAUSE SPOTTING OR LIGHT BLEEDING, even when you make up these missed pills.

On the days you take 2 pill to make up for missed pills, you could also feel a little sick to your stomach.

5. IF YOU HAVE VOMITING OR DIARRHEA, for any reason, or IF YOU TAKE SOME MEDICINES, including some antibiotics, your pills may not work as well. Use a back-up method (such as condoms, foam, or sponge) until you check with your doctor or clinic.

6. IF YOU HAVE TROUBLE REMEMBERING TO TAKE THE PILL, talk to your doctor or clinic about how to make pill-taking easier or about using another method of birth control.

7. IF YOU HAVE ANY QUESTIONS OR ARE UNSURE ABOUT THE INFORMATION IN THIS LEAFLET, call your doctor or clinic.

BEFORE YOU START TAKING YOUR PILLS

1. DECIDE WHAT TIME OF DAY YOU WANT TO TAKE YOUR PILL.

It is important to take it at about the same time every day.

2. LOOK AT YOUR PILL PACK TO SEE IF IT HAS 21 OR 28 PILLS:

The 21-pill pack has 21 yellow "active" pills (with hormones) to take for 3 weeks. This is followed by 1 week without pills.

The 28-pill pack has 21 yellow "active" pills (with hormones) to take for 3 weeks. This is followed by 1 week of "reminder" green pills (without hormones).

3. ALSO FIND:

1) where on the pack to start taking the pills,

2) in what order to take the pills.

CHECK PICTURE OF PILL PACK AND ADDITIONAL INSTRUCTIONS FOR USING THIS PACKAGE IN THE BRIEF SUMMARY PATIENT PACKAGE INSERT.

4. BE SURE YOU HAVE READY AT ALL TIMES:

ANOTHER KIND OF BIRTH CONTROL (such as condoms, foam, or sponge) to use as a back-up method in case you miss pills.

AN EXTRA, FULL PILL PACK.

WHEN TO START THE FIRST PACK OF PILLS

You have a choice of which day to start taking your first pack of pills. ORTHO-NOVUM 1/50 is available in the DIALPAK® Tablet Dispenser which is preset for a Sunday

Start. Day 1 Start is also provided. Decide with your doctor or clinic which is the best day for you. Pick a time of day which will be easy to remember.

SUNDAY START:

Take the first "active" yellow pill of the first pack on the Sunday after your period starts, even if you are still bleeding If your period begins on Sunday, start the pack the same day.

Use another method of birth control as a back-up method if you have sex anytime from the Sunday you start your first pack of until the next Sunday (7 days). Condoms, foam, or the sponge are good back-up methods of birth control.

DAY 1 START:

Take the first "active" yellow pill of the first pack during the first 24 hours of your period.

You will not need to use a back-up method of birth control, since you are starting the pill at the beginning of your period.

WHAT TO DO DURING THE MONTH

1. TAKE ONE PILL AT THE SAME TIME EVERY DAY UNTIL THE PACK IS EMPTY.

Do not skip pills even if you are spotting or bleeding between monthly periods or feel sick to your stomach (nausea).

Do not skip pills even if you do not have sex very often.

2. WHEN YOU FINISH A PACK OR SWITCH YOUR BRAND OF PILLS:

21 pills: Wait 7 days to start the next pack. You will probably have your period during that week. Be sure that no more than 7 days pass between 21-day packs.

28 pills: Start the next pack on the day after your last "reminder" pill. Do not wait any days between packs.

WHAT TO DO IF YOU MISS PILLS

If you **MISS 1** yellow "active" pill.

1. Take it as soon as you remember. Take the next pill at your regular time. This means you may take 2 pills in 1 day.

2. You do not need to use a back-up birth control method if you have sex.

If you **MISS 2** yellow "active" pills in a row in **WEEK 1 OR WEEK 2** of your pack:

1. Take 2 pills on the day you remember and 2 pills the next day.

2. Then take 1 pill a day until you finish the pack.

3. You MAY BECOME PREGNANT if you have sex in the 7 days after you miss pills. You MUST use another birth control method (such as condoms, foam or sponge) as a back-up method for those 7 days.

If you **MISS 2** yellow "active" pills in a row in **THE 3RD WEEK:**

1. If you are a Sunday Starter:

Keep taking 1 pill every day until Sunday. On Sunday, THROW OUT the rest of the pack and start a new pack of pills that same day.

If you are a Day 1 Starter:

THROW OUT the rest of the pill pack and start a new pack that same day.

2. You may not have our period this month but this is expected. However, if you miss your period 2 months in a row, call your doctor or clinic because you might be pregnant.

3. You MAY BECOME PREGNANT if you have sex in the 7 days after you miss pills. You MUST use another birth control method (such as condoms, foam, or sponge) as a back-up method for those 7 days.

If you **MISS 3 OR MORE** yellow "active" pills in a row (during the first 3 weeks):

1. If you are a Sunday Starter:

Keep taking 1 pill every day until Sunday. On Sunday, THROW OUT the rest of the pack and start a new pack of pills that same day.

If you are a Day 1 Starter:

THROW OUT the rest of the pill pack and start a new pack that same day.

2. You may not have your period this month but this is expected. However, if you miss your period 2 months in a row, call your doctor or clinic because you might be pregnant.

3. You MAY BECOME PREGNANT if you have sex in the 7 days after you miss pills. You MUST use another birth control method (such as condoms, foam, or sponge) as a back-up method for those 7 days.

A REMINDER FOR ON 28-DAY PACKS:

If you forget any of the 7 green "reminder" pills in Week 4:

THROW AWAY the pills you missed.

Keep taking 1 pill each day until the pack is empty.

You do not need a back-up method.

FINALLY, IF YOU ARE STILL NOT SURE WHAT TO DO ABOUT THE PILLS YOU HAVE MISSED:

Use a BACK-UP METHOD anytime you have sex.

KEEP TAKING ONE "ACTIVE" PILL EACH DAY until you can reach your doctor or clinic.

PREGNANCY DUE TO PILL FAILURE

Combination Oral Contraceptives

The incidence of pill failure resulting in pregnancy is approximately one percent (i.e., one pregnancy per 100 women per year) if taken every day as directed, but more typical failure rates are about 3%. If failure does occur, the risk to the fetus is minimal.

PREGNANCY AFTER STOPPING THE PILL

There may be some delay in becoming pregnant after you stop using oral contraceptives, especially if you had irregular menstrual cycles before you used oral contraceptives. It may be advisable to postpone conception until you begin menstruating regularly once you have stopped taking the pill and desire pregnancy.

There does not appear to be any increase in birth defects in newborn babies when pregnancy occurs soon after stopping the pill.

OVERDOSAGE

Serious ill effects have not been reported following ingestion of large doses of oral contraceptives by young children. Overdosage may cause nausea and withdrawal bleeding in females. In case of overdosage, contact your health care provider or pharmacist.

OTHER INFORMATION

Your health care provider will take a medical and family history before prescribing oral contraceptives and will examine you. The physical examination may be delayed to another time if you request it and the health care provider believes that it is a good medical practice to postpone it. You should be reexamined at least once a year. Be sure to inform your health provider if there is a family history of any of the conditions listed previously in this leaflet. Be sure to keep all appointments with your health care provider, because this is a time to determine if there are early signs of side effects of oral contraceptive use.

Do not use the drug for any condition other than the one for which it was prescribed. This drug has been prescribed specifically for you; do not give it to others who may want birth control pills.

HEALTH BENEFITS FROM ORAL CONTRACEPTIVES

In addition to preventing pregnancy, use of combination oral contraceptives may provide certain benefits. They are:

• menstrual cycles may become more regular

• blood flow during menstruation may be lighter and less iron may be lost. Therefore, anemia due to iron deficiency is less likely to occur.

• pain or other symptoms during menstruation may be encountered less frequently

• ectopic (tubal) pregnancy may occur less frequently

• noncancerous cysts or lumps in the breast may occur less frequently

• acute pelvic inflammatory disease may occur less frequently

• oral contraceptive use may provide some protection against developing two forms of cancer: cancer of the ovaries and cancer of the lining of the uterus.

If you want more information about birth control pills, ask your doctor or pharmacist. They have a more technical leaflet called the Professional Labeling, which you may wish to read. The professional labeling is also published in a book called *Physicians' Desk Reference*, available in many book stores and public libraries.

ORTHO PHARMACEUTICAL CORPORATION

Raritan, NJ 08869

© OPC 1993   635-50-800-2

Shown in Product Identification Guide, page 328

ORTHO–NOVUM® Tablets   ℞
(norethindrone/ethinyl estradiol)

and MODICON® Tablets   ℞
(norethindrone/ethinyl estradiol)

Prescribing Information

Patients should be counseled that this product does not protect against HIV infection (AIDS) and other sexually transmitted diseases.

COMBINATION ORAL CONTRACEPTIVES

Each of the following products is a combination oral contraceptive containing the progestational compound norethindrone and the estrogenic compound ethinyl estradiol.

ORTHO-NOVUM 7/7/7 □ 21 Tablets and ORTHO-NOVUM 7/7/7 □ 28 Tablets: Each white tablet contains 0.5 mg of norethindrone and 0.035 mg of ethinyl estradiol. Inactive ingredients include lactose, magnesium stearate and pregelatinized starch. Each light peach tablet contains 0.75 mg of norethindrone and 0.035 mg of ethinyl estradiol. Inactive ingredients include FD&C Yellow No. 6, lactose, magnesium

Continued on next page

Ortho-Novum Tablets—Cont.

stearate and pregelatinized starch. Each peach tablet contains 1 mg of norethindrone and 0.035 mg of ethinyl estradiol. Inactive ingredients include FD&C Yellow No. 6, lactose, magnesium stearate and pregelatinized starch. Each green tablet in the ORTHO-NOVUM 7/7/7 □ 28 package contains only inert ingredients, as follows: D&C Yellow No. 10 Aluminum Lake, FD&C Blue No. 2 Aluminum Lake, lactose, magnesium stearate, microcrystalline cellulose and pregelatinized starch.

ORTHO-NOVUM 10/11 □ 21 Tablets and ORTHO-NOVUM 10/11 □ 28 Tablets: Each white tablet contains 0.5 mg of norethindrone and 0.035 mg of ethinyl estradiol. Inactive ingredients include lactose, magnesium stearate and pregelatinized starch. Each peach tablet contains 1 mg norethindrone and 0.035 mg ethinyl estradiol. Inactive ingredients include FD&C Yellow No. 6, lactose, magensium stearate and pregelatinized starch. Each green tablet in the ORTHO-NOVUM 10/11 □ 28 package contains only inert ingredients, as listed under green tablets in ORTHO-NOVUM 7/7/7 □ 28.

ORTHO-NOVUM 1/35 □ 21 Tablets and ORTHO-NOVUM 1/35 □ 28 Tablets: Each peach tablet contains 1 mg of norethindrone and 0.035 mg of ethinyl estradiol. Inactive ingredients include FD&C Yellow No. 6, lactose, magnesium stearate and pregelatinized starch. Each green tablet in the ORTHO-NOVUM 1/35 □ 28 package contains only inert ingredients, as listed under green tablets in ORTHO-NOVUM 7/7/7 □ 28.

MODICON 21 Tablets and MODICON 28 Tablets: Each white tablet contains 0.5 mg of norethindrone and 0.035 mg of ethinyl estradiol. Inactive ingredients include lactose, magnesium stearate and pregelatinized starch. Each green tablet in the MODICON 28 package contains only inert ingredients, as listed under green tablets in ORTHO-NOVUM 7/7/7 □ 28.

The chemical name for norethindrone is 17-hydroxy-19-nor-17α-pregn-4-en-20-yn-3-one, for ethinyl estradiol is 19-nor-17α-pregna-1,3,5(10)-trien-20-yne-3, 17-diol. Their structural formulas are as follows:

norethindrone

ethinyl estradiol

CLINICAL PHARMACOLOGY

COMBINATION ORAL CONTRACEPTIVES

Combination oral contraceptives act by suppression of gonadotropins. Although the primary mechanism of this action is inhibition of ovulation, other alterations include changes in the cervical mucus (which increase the difficulty of sperm entry into the uterus) and the endometrium (which reduce the likelihood of implantation).

INDICATIONS AND USAGE

ORTHO-NOVUM 7/7/7 □ 21, ORTHO-NOVUM 7/7/7 □ 28, ORTHO-NOVUM 10/11 □ 21, ORTHO-NOVUM 10/11 □ 28, ORTHO-NOVUM 1/35 □ 21, ORTHO-NOVUM 1/35 □ 28, MODICON 21, and **MODICON 28** are indicated for the prevention of pregnancy in women who elect to use this product as a method of contraception.

Oral contraceptives are highly effective. Table I lists the typical accidental pregnancy rates for users of combination oral contraceptives and other methods of contraception. The efficacy of these contraceptive methods, except sterilization, depends upon the reliability with which they are used. Correct and consistent use of methods can result in lower failure rates.

[See table I above]

CONTRAINDICATIONS

Oral contraceptives should not be used in women who currently have the following conditions:

- Thrombophlebitis or thromboembolic disorders
- A past history of deep vein thrombophlebitis or thromboembolic disorders
- Cerebral vascular or coronary artery disease
- Known or suspected carcinoma of the breast
- Carcinoma of the endometrium or other known or suspected estrogen-dependent neoplasia
- Undiagnosed abnormal genital bleeding

- Cholestatic jaundice of pregnancy or jaundice with prior pill use
- Hepatic adenomas or carcinomas
- Known or suspected pregnancy

WARNINGS

Cigarette smoking increase the risk of serious cardiovascular side effects from oral contraceptive use. This risk increases with age and with heavy smoking (15 or more cigarettes per day) and is quite marked in women over 35 years of age. Women who use oral contraceptives should be strongly advised not to smoke.

The use of oral contraceptives is associated with increased risks of several serious conditions including myocardial infarction, thromboembolism, stroke, hepatic neoplasia, and gallbladder disease, although the risk of serious morbidity or mortality is very small in healthy women without underlying risk factors. The risk of morbidity and mortality increases significantly in the presence of other underlying risk factors such as hypertension, hyperlipidemias, obesity and diabetes.

Practitioners prescribing oral contraceptives should be familiar with the following information relating to these risks. The information contained in this package insert is principally based on studies carried out in patients who used oral contraceptives with higher formulations of estrogens and progestogens than those in common use today. The effect of long-term use of the oral contraceptives with lower formulations of both estrogens and progestogens remains to be determined.

Throughout this labeling, epidemiological studies reported are of two types: retrospective or case control studies and prospective or cohort studies. Case control studies provide a measure of the relative risk of disease, namely, a *ratio* of the

TABLE I: PERCENTAGE OF WOMEN EXPERIENCING AN UNINTENDED PREGNANCY DURING THE FIRST YEAR OF TYPICAL USE AND THE FIRST YEAR OF PERFECT USE OF CONTRACEPTION AND THE PERCENTAGE CONTINUING USE AT THE END OF THE FIRST YEAR. UNITED STATES.

Method (1)	% of Women Experiencing an Unintended Pregnancy within the First Year of Use		% of Women Continuing Use at One Year[3] (4)
	Typical Use[1] (2)	Perfect Use[2] (3)	
Chance[4]	85	85	
Spermicides[5]	26	6	40
Periodic abstinence	25		63
Calender		9	
Ovulation Method		3	
Sympto-Thermal[6]		2	
Post-Ovulation		1	
Withdrawal	19	4	
Cap[7]			
Parous Women	40	26	42
Nulliparous Women	20	9	56
Sponge			
Parous Women	40	20	42
Nulliparous Women	20	9	56
Diaphragm[7]	20	6	56
Condom[8]			
Female (Reality)	21	5	56
Male	14	3	61
Pill	5		71
Progestin Only		0.5	
Combined		0.1	
IUD			
Progesterone T	2.0	1.5	81
Copper T380A	0.8	0.6	78
LNg 20	0.1	0.1	81
Depo-Provera	0.3	0.3	70
Norplant and Norplant-2	0.05	0.05	88
Female Sterilization	0.5	0.5	100
Male Sterilization	0.15	0.10	100

Adapted from Hatcher et al., 1998 Ref. #1.

[1]Among *typical* couples who initiate use of a method (not necessarily for the first time), the percentage who experience an accidental pregnancy during the first year if they do not stop use for any other reason.

[2]Among couples who initiate use of a method (not necessarily for the first time) and who use it *perfectly* (both consistently and correctly), the percentage who experience an accidental pregnancy during the first year if they do not stop use for any other reason.

[3]Among couples attempting to avoid pregnancy, the percentage who continue to use a method for one year.

[4]The percents becoming pregnant in columns (2) and (3) are based on data from populations where contraception is not used and from women who cease using contraception in order to become pregnant. Among such populations, about 89% become pregnant within one year. This estimate was lowered slightly (to 85%) to represent the percent who would become pregnant within one year among women now relying on reversible methods of contraception if they abandoned contraception altogether.

[5]Foams, creams gels, vaginal suppositories, and vaginal film.

[6]Cervical mucus (ovulation) method supplemented by calendar in the pre-ovulatory and basal body temperature in the post-ovulatory phases.

[7]With spermicidal cream or jelly.

[8]Without spermicides.

incidence of disease among oral contraceptive users to that among nonusers. The relative risk does not provide information on the actual clinical occurrence of a disease. Cohort studies provide a measure of attributable risk, which is the *difference* in the incidence of disease between oral contraceptive users and nonusers. The attributable risk does provide information about the actual occurrence of a disease in the population (adapted from refs. 2 and 3 with the author's permission). For further information, the reader is referred to a text on epidemiological methods.

1. THROMBOEMBOLIC DISORDERS AND OTHER VASCULAR PROBLEMS

a. Myocardial Infarction

An increased risk of myocardial infarction has been attributed to oral contraceptive use. This risk is primarily in smokers or women with other underlying risk factors for coronary artery disease such as hypertension, hypercholesterolemias, morbid obesity, and diabetes. The relative risk of heart attack for current oral contraceptive users has been estimated to be two to six.[4-10] The risk is very low under the age of 30.

Smoking in combination with oral contraceptive use has been shown to contribute substantially to the incidence of myocardial infarctions in women in their mid-thirties or older with smoking accounting for the majority of excess cases.[11] Mortality rates associated with circulatory disease have been shown to increase substantially in smokers, especially in those 35 years of age and older among women who use oral contraceptives.

[See table II at top of next column]

Oral contraceptives may compound the effects of well-known risk factors, such as hypertension, diabetes, hyperlipidemias, age and obesity.[13] In particular, some progestogens are known to decrease HDL cholesterol and cause glucose intolerance, while estrogens may create a state of hyperinsulinism.[14-18] Oral contraceptives have been shown to increase blood pressure among users (see Section 9 in

TABLE II: CIRCULATORY DISEASE MORTALITY RATES PER 100,000
WOMAN-YEARS BY AGE, SMOKING STATUS AND ORAL
CONTRACEPTIVE USE

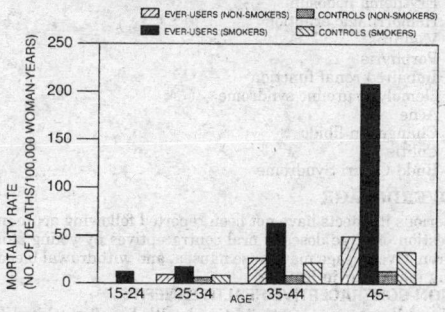

(Adapted from P.M. Layde and V. Beral, ref. #12.)

WARNINGS). Similar effects on risk factors have been associated with an increased risk of heart disease. Oral contraceptives must be used with caution in women with cardiovascular disease risk factors.

b. Thromboembolism

An increased risk of thromboembolic and thrombotic disease associated with the use of oral contraceptives is well established. Case control studies have found the relative risk of users compared to nonusers to be 3 for the first episode of superficial venous thrombosis, 4 to 11 for deep vein thrombosis or pulmonary embolism, and 1.5 to 6 for women with predisposing conditions for venous thromboembolic disease.[2,3,19-24] Cohort studies have shown the relative risk to be somewhat lower, about 3 for new cases and about 4.5 for new cases requiring hospitalization.[25] The risk of thromboembolic disease associated with oral contraceptives is not related to length of use and disappears after pill use is stopped.[2]

A two- to four-fold increase in relative risk of post-operative thromboembolic complications has been reported with the use of oral contraceptives.[9] The relative risk of venous thrombosis in women who have predisposing conditions is twice that of women without such medical conditions.[26] If feasible, oral contraceptives should be discontinued at least four weeks prior to and for two weeks after elective surgery of a type associated with an increase in risk of thromboembolism and during and following prolonged immobilization. Since the immediate postpartum period is also associated with an increased risk of thromboembolism, oral contraceptives should be started no earlier than four weeks after delivery in women who elect not to breast feed or four weeks after a second trimester abortion.

c. Cerebrovascular diseases

Oral contraceptives have been shown to increase both the relative and attributable risks of cerebrovascular events (thrombotic and hemorrhagic strokes), although, in general, the risk is greatest among older (>35 years), hypertensive women who also smoke. Hypertension was found to be a risk factor for both users and nonusers, for both types of strokes, and smoking interacted to increase the risk of stroke.[27-29]

In a large study, the relative risk of thrombotic strokes has been shown to range from 3 for normotensive users to 14 for users with severe hypertension.[30] The relative risk of hemorrhagic stroke is reported to be 1.2 for non-smokers who used oral contraceptives, 2.6 for smokers who did not use oral contraceptives, 7.6 for smokers who used oral contraceptives, 1.8 for normotensive users and 25.7 for users with severe hypertension.[30] The attributable risk is also greater in older women.[3]

d. Dose-related risk of vascular disease from oral contraceptives

A positive association has been observed between the amount of estrogen and progestogen in oral contraceptives and the risk of vascular disease.[31-33] A decline in serum high density lipoproteins (HDL) has been reported with many progestational agents.[14-16] A decline in serum high density lipoproteins has been associated with an increased incidence of ischemic heart disease. Because estrogens increase HDL cholesterol, the net effect of an oral contraceptive depends on a balance achieved between doses of estrogen and progestogen and the activity of the progestogen used in the contraceptives. The activity and amount of both hormones should be considered in the choice of an oral contraceptive.

Minimizing exposure to estrogen and progestogen is in keeping with good principles of therapeutics. For any particular estrogen/progestogen combination, the dosage regimen prescribed should be one which contains the least amount of estrogen and progestogen that is compatible with a low failure rate and the needs of the individual patient. New acceptors of oral contraceptive agents should be started on preparations containing 0.035 mg or less of estrogen.

e. Persistence of risk of vascular disease

There are two studies which have shown persistence of risk of vascular disease for ever-users of oral contraceptives. In a study in the United States, the risk of developing myocardial infarction after discontinuing oral contraceptives persists for at least 9 years for women 40-49 years who had used oral contraceptives for five or more years, but this increased risk was not demonstrated in other age groups.[8] In another study in Great Britain, the risk of developing cerebrovascular disease persisted for at least 6 years after discontinuation of oral contraceptives, although excess risk was very small.[34] However, both studies were performed with oral contraceptive formulations containing 50 micrograms or higher of estrogens.

2. ESTIMATES OF MORTALITY FROM CONTRACEPTIVE USE

One study gathered data from a variety of sources which have estimated the mortality rate associated with different methods of contraception at different ages (Table III). These estimates include the combined risk of death associated with contraceptive methods plus the risk attributable to pregnancy in the event of method failure. Each method of contraception has its specific benefits and risks. The study concluded that with the exception of oral contraceptive users 35 and older who smoke, and 40 and older who do not smoke, mortality associated with all methods of birth control is low and below that associated with childbirth. The observation of an increase in risk of mortality with age for oral contraceptive users is based on data gathered in the 1970's.[35] Current clinical recommendation involves the use of lower estrogen dose formulations and a careful consideration of risk factors. In 1989, the Fertility and Maternal Health Drugs Advisory Committee was asked to review the use of oral contraceptive in women 40 years of age and over. The committee concluded that although cardiovascular disease risks may be increased with oral contraceptive use after age 40 in healthy non-smoking women (even with the newer low-dose formulations), there are also greater potential health risks associated with pregnancy in older women and with the alternative surgical and medical procedures which may be necessary if such women do not have access to effective and acceptable means of contraception. The Committee recommended that the benefits of low-dose oral contraceptive use by healthy non-smoking women over 40 may outweigh the possible risks.

Of course, older women, as all women who take oral contraceptives, should take an oral contraceptive which contains the least amount of estrogen and progestogen that is compatible with a low failure rate and individual patient needs. [See table III below]

3. CARCINOMA OF THE REPRODUCTIVE ORGANS AND BREASTS

Numerous epidemiological studies have been performed on the incidence of breast, endometrial, ovarian and cervical cancer in women using oral contraceptives. While there are conflicting reports, most studies suggest that use of oral contraceptives is not associated with an overall increase in the risk of developing breast cancer. Some studies have reported an increased relative risk of developing breast cancer particularly at a younger age. This increased relative risk has been reported to be related to duration of use.[36-44,79-89]

A meta-analysis of 54 studies found a small increase in the frequency of having breast cancer diagnosed for women who were currently using combined oral contraceptives or had used them within the past ten years. This increase in the frequency of breast cancer diagnosis, within ten years of stopping use, was generally accounted for by cancers localized to the breast. There was no increase in the frequency of having breast cancer diagnosed ten or more years after cessation of use.[90]

Some studies suggest that oral contraceptive use has been associated with an increase in the risk of cervical intraepithelial neoplasia in some populations of women.[45-48] However, there continues to be controversy about the extent to which such findings may be due to differences in sexual behavior and other factors.

4. HEPATIC NEOPLASIA

Benign hepatic adenomas are associated with oral contraceptive use, although the incidence of benign tumors is rare in the United States. Indirect calculations have estimated the attributable risk to be in the range of 3.3 cases/100,000 for users, a risk that increases after four or more years of use especially with oral contraceptives of higher dose.[49] Rupture of benign, hepatic adenomas may cause death through intra-abdominal hemorrhage.[50,51] Studies have shown an increased risk of developing hepatocellular carcinoma[52-54,91] in oral contraceptive users. However, these cancers are rare in the U.S.

5. OCULAR LESIONS

There have been clinical case reports of retinal thrombosis associated with the use of oral contraceptives. Oral contraceptives should be discontinued if there is unexplained partial or complete loss of vision; onset of proptosis or diplopia; papilledema; or retinal vascular lesions. Appropriate diagnostic and therapeutic measures should be undertaken immediately.

6. ORAL CONTRACEPTIVE USE BEFORE OR DURING EARLY PREGNANCY

Extensive epidemiological studies have revealed no increased risk of birth defects in women who have used oral contraceptives prior to pregnancy.[56,57] The majority of recent studies also do not indicate a teratogenic effect, particularly in so far as cardiac anomalies and limb reduction defects are concerned,[55,56,58,59] when taken inadvertently during early pregnancy.

The administration of oral contraceptives to induce withdrawal bleeding should not be used as a test for pregnancy. Oral contraceptives should not be used during pregnancy to treat threatened or habitual abortion.

It is recommended that for any patient who has missed two consecutive periods, pregnancy should be ruled out before continuing oral contraceptive use. If the patient has not adhered to the prescribed schedule, the possibility of pregnancy should be considered at the time of the first missed period. Oral contraceptive use should be discontinued until pregnancy is ruled out.

7. GALLBLADDER DISEASE

Earlier studies have reported an increased lifetime relative risk of gallbladder surgery in users of oral contraceptives and estrogens.[60,61] More recent studies, however, have shown that the relative risk of developing gallbladder disease among oral contraceptive users may be minimal.[62-64] The recent findings of minimal risk may be related to the use of oral contraceptive formulations containing lower hormonal doses of estrogens and progestogens.

8. CARBOHYDRATE AND LIPID METABOLIC EFFECTS

Oral contraceptives have been shown to cause a decrease in glucose tolerance in a significant percentage of users.[17] This effect has been shown to be directly related to estrogen dose.[65] Progestogens increase insulin secretion and create insulin resistance, this effect varying with different progestational agents.[17,66] However, in the non-diabetic woman, oral contraceptives appear to have no effect on fasting blood glucose.[67] Because of these demonstrated effects, prediabetic and diabetic women in particular should be carefully monitored while taking oral contraceptives.

A small proportion of women will have persistent hypertriglyceridemia while on the pill. As discussed earlier (see

Continued on next page

TABLE III: ANNUAL NUMBER OF BIRTH-RELATED OR METHOD-RELATED DEATHS
ASSOCIATED WITH CONTROL OF FERTILITY PER 100,000 NONSTERILE WOMEN,
BY FERTILITY CONTROL METHOD ACCORDING TO AGE

Method of control and outcome	15-19	20-24	25-29	30-34	35-39	40-44
No fertility control methods*	7.0	7.4	9.1	14.8	25.7	28.2
Oral contraceptives non-smoker**	0.3	0.5	0.9	1.9	13.8	31.6
Oral contraceptives smoker**	2.2	3.4	6.6	13.5	51.1	117.2
IUD**	0.8	0.8	1.0	1.0	1.4	1.4
Condom*	1.1	1.6	0.7	0.2	0.3	0.4
Diaphragm/ spermicide*	1.9	1.2	1.2	1.3	2.2	2.8
Periodic abstinence*	2.5	1.6	1.6	1.7	2.9	3.6

*Deaths are birth-related
**Deaths are method-related

Adapted from H.W. Ory, ref. #35.

Ortho-Novum Tablets—Cont.

WARNINGS 1a and 1d), changes in serum triglycerides and lipoprotein levels have been reported in oral contraceptive users.

9. ELEVATED BLOOD PRESSURE

An increase in blood pressure has been reported in women taking oral contraceptives[68] and this increase is more likely in older oral contraceptive users[69] and with extended duration of use.[61] Data from the Royal College of General Practitioners[12] and subsequent randomized trials have shown that the incidence of hypertension increases with increasing progestational activity.

Women with a history of hypertension or hypertension-related diseases, or renal disease[70] should be encouraged to use another method of contraception. If women elect to use oral contraceptives, they should be monitored closely and if significant elevation of blood pressure occurs, oral contraceptives should be discontinued. For most women, elevated blood pressure will return to normal after stopping oral contraceptives, and there is no difference in the occurrence of hypertension between former and never users.[68–71]

10. HEADACHE

The onset or exacerbation of migraine or development of headache with a new pattern which is recurrent, persistent or severe requires discontinuation of oral contraceptives and evaluation of the cause.

11. BLEEDING IRREGULARITIES

Breakthrough bleeding and spotting are sometimes encountered in patients on oral contraceptives, especially during the first three months of use. Nonhormonal causes should be considered and adequate diagnostic measures taken to rule out malignancy or pregnancy in the event of breakthrough bleeding, as in the case of any abnormal vaginal bleeding. If pathology has been excluded, time or a change to another formulation may solve the problem. In the event of amenorrhea, pregnancy should be ruled out.

Some women may encounter post-pill amenorrhea or oligomenorrhea, especially when such a condition was preexistent.

12. ECTOPIC PREGNANCY

Ectopic as well as intrauterine pregnancy may occur in contraceptive failures.

PRECAUTIONS

1. PHYSICAL EXAMINATION AND FOLLOW UP

It is good medical practice for all women to have annual history and physical examinations, including women using oral contraceptives. The physical examination, however, may be deferred until after initiation of oral contraceptives if requested by the woman and judged appropriate by the clinician. The physical examination should include special reference to blood pressure, breasts, abdomen and pelvic organs, including cervical cytology, and relevant laboratory tests. In case of undiagnosed, persistent or recurrent abnormal vaginal bleeding, appropriate measures should be conducted to rule out malignancy. Women with a strong family history of breast cancer or who have breast nodules should be monitored with particular care.

2. LIPID DISORDERS

Women who are being treated for hyperlipidemias should be followed closely if they elect to use oral contraceptives. Some progestogens may elevate LDL levels and may render the control of hyperlipidemias more difficult.

3. LIVER FUNCTION

If jaundice develops in any woman receiving such drugs, the medication should be discontinued. Steroid hormones may be poorly metabolized in patients with impaired liver function.

4. FLUID RETENTION

Oral contraceptives may cause some degree of fluid retention. They should be prescribed with caution, and only with careful monitoring, in patients with conditions which might be aggravated by fluid retention.

5. EMOTIONAL DISORDERS

Women with a history of depression should be carefully observed and the drug discontinued if depression recurs to a serious degree.

6. CONTACT LENSES

Contact lens wearers who develop visual changes or changes in lens tolerance should be assessed by an ophthalmologist.

7. DRUG INTERACTIONS

Reduced efficacy and increased incidence of breakthrough bleeding and menstrual irregularities have been associated with concomitant use of rifampin. A similar association, though less marked, has been suggested with barbiturates, phenylbutazone, phenytoin sodium, carbamazepine, and possibly with griseofulvin, ampicillin and tetracyclines.[72]

8. INTERACTIONS WITH LABORATORY TESTS

Certain endocrine and liver function tests and blood components may be affected by oral contraceptives:

a. Increased prothrombin and factors VII, VIII, IX, and X; decreased antithrombin 3; increased norepinephrine-induced platelet aggregability.

b. Increased thyroid binding globulin (TBG) leading to increased circulating total thyroid hormone, as measured by protein-bound iodine (PBI), T4 by column or by radioimmunoassay. Free T3 resin uptake is decreased, reflecting the elevated TBG, free T4 concentration is unaltered.

c. Other binding proteins may be elevated in serum.

d. Sex-binding globulins are increased and result in elevated levels of total circulating sex steroids and corticoids; however, free or biologically active levels remain unchanged.

e. Triglycerides may be increased.

f. Glucose tolerance may be decreased.

g. Serum folate levels may be depressed by oral contraceptive therapy. This may be of clinical significance if a woman becomes pregnant shortly after discontinuing oral contraceptives.

9. CARCINOGENESIS

See WARNINGS Section.

10. PREGNANCY

Pregnancy Category X. See CONTRAINDICATIONS and WARNINGS Sections.

11. NURSING MOTHERS

Small amounts of oral contraceptive steroids have been identified in the milk of nursing mothers and a few adverse effects on the child have been reported, including jaundice and breast enlargement. In addition, combination oral contraceptives given in the postpartum period may interfere with lactation by decreasing the quantity of breast milk. If possible, the nursing mother should be advised not to use combination oral contraceptives but to use other forms of contraception until she has completely weaned her child.

12. PEDIATRIC USE

Safety and efficacy of ORTHO-NOVUM Tablets and MODICON Tablets has been established in women of reproductive age. Safety and efficacy are expected to be the same for postpubertal adolescents under the age of 16 and for users 16 years and older. Use of this product before menarche is not indicated.

13. SEXUALLY TRANSMITTED DISEASES

Patients should be counseled that this product does not protect against HIV infection (AIDS) and other sexually transmitted diseases.

INFORMATION FOR THE PATIENT

See Patient Labeling printed below.

ADVERSE REACTIONS

An increased risk of the following serious adverse reactions has been associated with the use of oral contraceptives (See WARNINGS Section).

- Thrombophlebitis and venous thrombosis with or without embolism.
- Arterial thromboembolism
- Pulmonary embolism
- Myocardial infarction
- Cerebral hemorrhage
- Cerebral thrombosis
- Hypertension
- Gallbladder disease
- Hepatic adenomas or benign liver tumors

The following adverse reactions have been reported in patients receiving oral contraceptives and are believed to be drug-related:

- Nausea
- Vomiting
- Gastrointestinal symptoms (such as abdominal cramps and bloating)
- Breakthrough bleeding
- Spotting
- Change in menstrual flow
- Amenorrhea
- Temporary infertility after discontinuation of treatment
- Edema
- Melasma which may persist
- Breast changes: tenderness, enlargement, secretion
- Change in weight (increase or decrease)
- Change in cervical erosion and secretion
- Diminution in lactation when given immediately postpartum
- Cholestatic jaundice
- Migraine
- Rash (allergic)
- Mental depression
- Reduced tolerance to carbohydrates
- Vaginal candidiasis
- Change in corneal curvature (steepening)
- Intolerance to contact lenses

The following adverse reactions have been reported in users of oral contraceptives and the association has been neither confirmed nor refuted:

- Pre-menstrual syndrome
- Cataracts
- Changes in appetite
- Cystitis-like syndrome
- Headache
- Nervousness
- Dizziness

- Hirsutism
- Loss of scalp hair
- Erythema multiforme
- Erythema nodosum
- Hemorrhagic eruption
- Vaginitis
- Porphyria
- Impaired renal function
- Hemolytic uremic syndrome
- Acne
- Changes in libido
- Colitis
- Budd-Chiari Syndrome

OVERDOSAGE

Serious ill effects have not been reported following acute ingestion of large doses of oral contraceptives by young children. Overdosage may cause nausea, and withdrawal bleeding may occur in females.

NON-CONTRACEPTIVE HEALTH BENEFITS

The following non-contraceptive health benefits related to the use of combination oral contraceptives are supported by epidemiological studies which largely utilized oral contraceptive formulations containing estrogen doses exceeding 0.035 mg of ethinyl estradiol or 0.05 mg mestranol.[73–78]

Effect on menses:
- increased menstrual cycle regularity
- decreased blood loss and decreased incidence of iron deficiency anemia
- decreased incidence of dysmenorrhea

Effects related to inhibition of ovulation:
- decreased incidence of functional ovulation cysts
- decreased incidence of ectopic pregnancies

Other effects:
- decreased incidence of fibroadenomas and fibrocystic disease of the breast
- decreased incidence of acute pelvic inflammatory disease
- decreased incidence of endometrial cancer
- decreased incidence of ovarian cancer

DOSAGE AND ADMINISTRATION

To achieve maximum contraceptive effectiveness, ORTHO-NOVUM Tablets and MODICON Tablets must be taken exactly as directed and in intervals not exceeding 24 hours. ORTHO-NOVUM Tablets and MODICON Tablets are available in the DIALPAK® Tablet Dispenser which is preset for a Sunday Start. Day 1 Start is also available.

21-Day Regimen (Sunday Start)

When taking ORTHO-NOVUM 7/7/7 □ 21, ORTHO-NOVUM 10/11 □ 21, ORTHO-NOVUM 1/35 □ 21, and MODICON 21, the first tablet should be taken on the first Sunday after menstruation begins. If period begins on Sunday, the first tablet is taken on that day. One tablet is taken daily for 21 days. For subsequent cycles, no tablets are taken for 7 days, then a tablet is taken the next day (Sunday). For the first cycle of a Sunday Start regimen, another method of contraception should be used until after the first 7 consecutive days of administration.

If the patient misses one (1) active tablet in Weeks 1, 2, or 3, the tablet should be taken as soon as she remembers. If the patient misses two (2) active tablets in Week 1 or Week 2, the patient should take two (2) tablets the day she remembers and two (2) tablets the next day; and then continue taking one (1) tablet a day until she finishes the pack. The patient should be instructed to use a back-up method of birth control if she has sex in the seven (7) days after missing pills. If the patient misses two (2) active tablets in the third week or misses three (3) or more active tablets in a row, the patient should continue taking one tablet every day until Sunday. On Sunday the patient should throw out the rest of the pack and start a new pack that same day. The patient should be instructed to use a back-up method of birth control if she has sex in the seven (7) days after missing pills. Complete instructions to facilitate patient counseling on proper pill usage may be found in the Detailed Patient Labeling ("How to Take the Pill" section).

21-Day Regimen (Day 1 Start)

The dosage of ORTHO-NOVUM 7/7/7 □ 21, ORTHO-NOVUM 10/11 □ 21, ORTHO-NOVUM 1/35 □ 21, and MODICON 21, for the initial cycle of therapy is one tablet administered daily from the 1st day through the 21st day of the menstrual cycle, counting the first day of menstrual flow as "Day 1." For subsequent cycles, no tablets are taken for 7 days, then a new course is started of one tablet a day for 21 days. The dosage regimen then continues with 7 days of no medication, followed by 21 days of medication, instituting a three-weeks-on, one-week-off dosage regimen.

If the patient misses one (1) active tablet in Weeks 1, 2, or 3, the tablet should be taken as soon as she remembers. If the patient misses two (2) active tablets in Week 1 or Week 2, the patient should take two (2) tablets the day she remembers and two (2) tablets the next day; and then continue taking one (1) tablet a day until she finishes the pack. The patient should be instructed to use a back-up method of birth control if she has sex in the seven (7) days after missing pills. If the patient misses two (2) active tablets in the third week or misses three (3) or more active tablets in a row, the patient should throw out the rest of the pack and start a

new pack that same day. The patient should be instructed to use a back-up method of birth control if she has sex in the seven (7) days after missing pills.

Complete instructions to facilitate patient counseling on proper pill usage may be found in the Detailed Patient Labeling ("How to Take the Pill" section).

28-Day Regimen (Sunday Start)

When taking ORTHO-NOVUM 7/7/7 □ 28, ORTHO-NOVUM 10/11 □ 28, ORTHO-NOVUM 1/35 □ 28, and MODICON 28, the first tablet should be taken on the first Sunday after menstruation begins. If period begins on Sunday, the first tablet should be taken that day. Take one active tablet daily for 21 days followed by one green placebo tablet daily for 7 days. After 28 tablets have been taken, a new course is started the next day (Sunday). For the first cycle of a Sunday Start regimen, another method of contraception should be used until after the first 7 consecutive days of administration.

If the patient misses one (1) active tablet in Weeks 1, 2, or 3, the tablet should be taken as soon as she remembers. If the patient misses two (2) active tablets in Week 1 or Week 2, the patient should take two (2) tablets the day she remembers and two (2) tablets the next day; and then continue taking one (1) tablet a day until she finishes the pack. The patient should be instructed to use a back-up method of birth control if she has sex in the seven (7) days after missing pills. If the patient misses two (2) active tablets in the third week or misses three (3) or more active tablets in a row, the patient should continue taking one tablet every day until Sunday. On Sunday the patient should throw out the rest of the pack and start a new pack that same day. The patient should be instructed to use a back-up method of birth control if she has sex in the seven (7) days after missing pills.

Complete instructions to facilitate patient counseling on proper pill usage may be found in the Detailed Patient Labeling ("How to Take the Pill" section).

28-Day Regimen (Day 1 Start)

The dosage of ORTHO-NOVUM 7/7/7 □ 28, ORTHO-NOVUM 10/11 □ 28, ORTHO-NOVUM 1/35 □ 28, and MODICON 28, for the first initial cycle of therapy is one active tablet administered daily from the 1st through the 21st day of the menstrual cycle, counting the first day of menstrual flow as "Day 1" followed by one green tablet daily for 7 days. Tablets are taken without interruption for 28 days. After 28 tablets have been taken, a new course is started the next day.

If the patient misses one (1) active tablet in Weeks 1, 2, or 3, the tablet should be taken as soon as she remembers. If the patient misses two (2) active tablets in Week 1 or Week 2, the patient should take two (2) tablets the day she remembers and two (2) tablets the next day; and then continue taking one (1) tablet a day until she finishes the pack. The patient should be instructed to use a back-up method of birth control if she has sex in the seven (7) days after missing pills. If the patient misses two (2) active tablets in the third week or misses three (3) or more active tablets in a row, the patient should throw out the rest of the pack and start a new pack that same day. The patient should be instructed to use a back-up method of birth control if she has sex in the seven (7) days after missing pills.

Complete instructions to facilitate patient counseling on proper pill usage may be found in the Detailed Patient Labeling ("How to Take the Pill" section).

The use of ORTHO-NOVUM 7/7/7, ORTHO-NOVUM 10/11, ORTHO-NOVUM 1/35, and MODICON for contraception may be initiated 4 weeks postpartum in women who elect not to breast feed. When the tablets are administered during the postpartum period, the increased risk of thromboembolic disease associated with the postpartum period must be considered. (See CONTRAINDICATIONS and WARNINGS concerning thromboembolic disease. See also PRECAUTIONS for "Nursing Mothers.") The possibility of ovulation and conception prior to initiation of medication should be considered.

(See Discussion of Dose-Related Risk of Vascular Disease from Oral Contraceptives.)

ADDITIONAL INSTRUCTIONS FOR ALL DOSING REGIMENS

Breakthrough bleeding, spotting, and amenorrhea are frequent reasons for patients discontinuing oral contraceptives. In breakthrough bleeding, as in all cases of irregular bleeding from the vagina, nonfunctional causes should be borne in mind. In undiagnosed persistent or recurrent abnormal bleeding from the vagina, adequate diagnostic measures are indicated to rule out pregnancy or malignancy. If pathology has been excluded, time or a change to another formulation may solve the problem. Changing to an oral contraceptive with a higher estrogen content, while potentially useful in minimizing menstrual irregularity, should be done only if necessary since this may increase the risk of thromboembolic disease.

Use of oral contraceptives in the event of a missed menstrual period:

1. If the patient has not adhered to the prescribed schedule, the possibility of pregnancy should be cosidered at the time of the first missed period and oral contraceptive use should be discontinued until pregnancy is ruled out.

2. If the patient has adhered to the prescribed regimen and misses two consecutive periods, pregnancy should be ruled out before continuing oral contraceptive use.

HOW SUPPLIED

ORTHO-NOVUM 7/7/7 □ 21 Tablets are available in a DIALPAK® Tablet Dispenser (NDC 0062-1780-15) containing 21 tablets, as follows: 7 white tablets (0.5 mg norethindrone and 0.035 mg ethinyl estradiol), 7 light peach tablets (0.75 mg norethindrone and 0.035 mg ethinyl estradiol) and 7 peach tablets (1 mg norethindrone and 0.035 mg ethinyl estradiol). The white tablets are unscored with "Ortho" and "535" debossed on each side; the light peach tablets are unscored with "Ortho" and "75" debossed on each side; the peach tablets are unscored with "Ortho" and "135" debossed on each side.

ORTHO-NOVUM 7/7/7 □ 21 is available for clinic usage in a VERIDATE® Tablet Dispenser (unfilled) and VERIDATE Refills (NDC 0062-1780-20).

ORTHO-NOVUM 7/7/7 □ 28 Tablets are available in a DIALPAK Tablet Dispenser (NDC 0062-1781-15) containing 28 tablets, as follows: 7 white, 7 light peach and 7 peach tablets as described under ORTHO-NOVUM 7/7/7 □ 21, and 7 green tablets containing inert ingredients.

ORTHO-NOVUM 7/7/7 □ 28 is available for clinic usage in a VERIDATE Tablet Dispenser (unfilled) and VERIDATE Refills (NDC 0062-1781-20).

ORTHO-NOVUM 10/11 □ 21 Tablets are available in a DIALPAK Tablet Dispenser (NDC 0062-1770-15) containing 21 tablets, as follows: 10 white tablets (0.5 mg norethindrone and 0.035 mg ethinyl estradiol) and 11 peach tablets (1 mg norethindrone and 0.035 mg ethinyl estradiol). The white tablets are unscored with "Ortho" and "535" debossed on each side; the peach tablets are unscored with "Ortho" and "135" debossed on each side.

ORTHO-NOVUM 10/11 □ 28 Tablets are available in a DIALPAK Tablet Dispenser (NDC 0062-1771-15) containing 28 tablets, as follows: 10 white and 11 peach tablets as described under ORTHO-NOVUM 10/11 □ 21, and 7 green tablets containing inert ingredients.

ORTHO-NOVUM 10/11 □ 28 is avalable for clinic usage in a VERIDATE Tablet Dispenser (unfilled) and VERIDATE Refills (NDC 0062-1771-20).

ORTHO-NOVUM 1/35 □ 21 Tablets are available in a DIALPAK Tablet Dispenser (NDC 0062-1760-15) containing 21 peach tablets (1 mg norethindrone and 0.035 mg ethinyl estradiol) which are unscored with "Ortho" and "135" debossed on each side.

ORTHO-NOVUM 1/35 □ 21 is available for clinic usage in a VERIDATE Tablet Dispenser (unfilled) and VERIDATE Refills (NDC 0062-1760-20).

ORTHO-NOVUM 1/35 □ 28 Tablets are available in a DIALPAK Tablet Dispenser (NDC 0062-1761-15) containing 28 tablets, as follows: 21 peach tablets as described under ORTHO-NOVUM 1/35 □ 21, and 7 green tablets containing inert ingredients.

ORTHO-NOVUM 1/35 □ 28 is available for clinic usage in a VERIDATE Tablet Dispenser (unfilled) and VERIDATE Refills (NDC 0062-1761-20).

MODICON 21 Tablets are available in a DIALPAK Tablet Dispenser (NDC 0062-1712-15) containing 21 white tablets (0.5 mg norethindrone and 0.035 mg ethinyl estradiol) which are unscored with "Ortho" and "535" debossed on each side.

MODICON 28 Tablets are available in a DIALPAK Tablet Dispenser (NDC 0062-1714-15) containing 28 tablets, as follows: 21 white tablets as described under MODICON 21, and 7 green tablets containing inert ingredients.

MODICON 28 is available for clinic usage in a VERIDATE Tablet Dispenser (unfilled) and VERIDATE Refills (NDC 0062-1714-20).

Rx only

REFERENCES

1. Trussel J. Contraceptive efficacy. In Hatcher RA, Trussel J, Stewart F, Cates W, Stewart GK, Kowal D, Guest F, Contraceptive Technology: Seventeenth Revised Edition. New York NY: Irvington Publishers, 1998, in press **2.** Stadel BV, Oral contraceptives and cardiovascular disease. (Pt. 1). N Engl J Med 1981; 305:612–618. **3.** Stadel BV, Oral contraceptives and cardiovascular disease. (Pt. 2). N Engl J Med 1981; 305:672–677. **4.** Adam SA, Thorogood M. Oral contraception and myocardial infarction revisited: the effects of new preparations and prescribing patterns. Br J Obstet Gynaecol 1981; 88:838–845. **5.** Mann JI, Inman WH. Oral contraceptives and death from myocardial infarction. Br Med J 1975; 2(5965):245–248. **6.** Mann JI, Vessey MP, Thorogood M, Doll R. Myocardial infarction in young women with special reference to oral contraceptive practice. Br Med J 1975; 2(5956):241–245. **7.** Royal College of General Practitioners' Oral Contraception Study: further analyses of mortality in oral contraceptive users. Lancet 1981; 1:541–546. **8.** Slone D, Shapiro S, Kaufman DW, Rosenberg L, Miettinen OS, Stolley PD. Risk of myocardial infarction in relation to current and discontinued use of oral contraceptives. N Engl J Med 1981; 305:420–424. **9.** Vessey MP. Female hormones and vascular disease—an epidemiological overview. Br J Fam Plann 1980; 6 (Supplement): 1–12. **10.** Russel-Briefel RG, Ezzati TM, Fulwood R, Perlman JA, Murphy RS. Cardiovascular risk satus and oral contraceptive use, United States, 1976–80. Prevent Med 1986; 15:352–362. **11.** Goldbaum GM, Kendrick JS, Hogelin GC, Gentry EM. The relative impact of smoking and oral contraceptive use on women in the United States. JAMA 1987; 258:1339–1342. **12.** Layde PM, Beral V. Further analyses of mortality in oral contraceptive users; Royal College of General Practitioners' Oral Contraception Study. (Table 5) Lancet 1981; 1:541–546. **13.** Knopp RH. Arteriosclerosis risk: the roles of oral contraceptives and postmenopausal estrogens. J Reprod Med 1986; 31(9) (Supplement): 913–921. **14.** Krauss RM, Roy S, Mishell DR, Casagrande J, Pike MC. Effects of two low-dose oral contraceptives on serum lipids and lipoproteins: Differential changes in high-density lipoproteins subclasses. Am J Obstet 1983; 145:446–452. **15.** Wahl P, Walden C, Knopp R, Hoover J, Wallace R, Heiss G, Rifkind B. Effect of estrogen/progestin potency on lipid/lipoprotein cholesterol. N Engl J Med 1983; 308:862–867. **16.** Wynn V. Niththyananthan R. The effect of progestin in combined oral contraceptives on serum lipids with special reference to high density lipoproteins. Am J Obstet Gynecol 1982; 142:766–771. **17.** Wynn V, Godsland I. Effects of oral contraceptives on carbohydrate metabolism. J Reprod Med 1986; 31(9)(Supplement):892–897. **18.** LaRosa JC. Atherosclerotic risk factors in cardiovascular disease. J Reprod Med 1986; 31(9)(Supplement): 906–912. **19.** Inman WH, Vessey MP. Investigation of death from pulmonary, coronary, and cerebral thrombosis and embolism in women of child-bearing age. Br Med J 1968; 2(5599):193–199. **20.** Maguire MG, Tonascia J, Sartwell PE, Stolley PD, Tockman MS. Increased risk of thrombosis due to oral contraceptives: a further report. Am J Epidemiol 1979; 110(2):188–195. **21.** Petitti DB, Wingerd J, Pellegrin F, Ramacharan S. Risk of vascular disease in women: smoking, oral contraceptives, noncontraceptive estrogens, and other factors, JAMA 1979; 242:1150–1154. **22.** Vessey MP, Doll R. Investigation of relation between use of oral contraceptives and thromboembolic disease. Br Med J 1968; 2(5599):199–205. **23.** Vessey MP, Doll R. Investigation of relation between use of oral contraceptives and thromboembolic disease. A further report. Br Med J 1969; 2(5658):651–657. **24.** Porter JB, Hunter JR, Danielson DA, Jick H, Stergachis A. Oral contraceptives and non-fatal vascular disease—recent experience. Obstet Gynecol 1982; 59(3): 299–302. **25.** Vessey M, Doll R, Peto R, Johnson B, Wiggins P. A long-term follow-up study of women using different methods of contraception: an interim report. J Biosocial Sci 1976; 8:375–427. **26.** Royal College of General Practitioners: Oral Contraceptives, venous thrombosis, and varicose veins. J Royal Coll Gen Pract 1978; 28:393–399. **27.** Collaborative Group for the Study of Stroke in Young Women: Oral contraception and increased risk of cerebral ischemia or thrombosis. N Engl J Med 1973; 288:871–878. **28.** Petitti DB, Wingerd J. Use of oral contraceptives, cigarette smoking, and risk of subarachnoid hemorrhage. Lancet 1978; 2:234–236. **29.** Inman WH. Oral contraceptives and fatal subarachnoid hemorrhage. Br Med J 1979; 2(6203):1468–1470. **30.** Collaborative Group for the Study of Stroke in Young Women: Oral Contraceptives and stroke in young women: associated risk factors. JAMA 1975; 231:718–722. **31.** Inman WH, Vessey MP, Westerholm B, Engelund A. Thromboembolic disease and the steroidal content of oral contraceptives. A report to the Committee on Safety of Drugs. Br Med J 1970; 2:203–209. **32.** Meade TW, Greenberg G, Thompson SG. Progestogens and cardiovascular reactions associated with oral contraceptives and a comparison of the safety of 50- and 35-mcg oestrogen preparations. Br Med J 1980; 280(6224):1157–1161. **33.** Kay CR. Progestogens and arterial disease—evidence from the Royal College of General Practitioners' Study. Am J Obstet Gynecol 1982; 142:762–765. **34.** Royal College of General Practitioners: Incidence of arterial disease among oral contraceptive users. J Royal Coll Gen Pract 1983; 33:75–82. **35.** Ory HW. Mortality associated with fertility and fertility control: 1983. Family Planning Perspectives 1983; 15:50–56. **36.** The Cancer and Steroid Hormone Study of the Centers for Disease Control and the National Institute of Child Health and Human Development: Oral contraceptive use and the risk of breast cancer. N Engl J Med 1986; 315:405–411. **37.** Pike MC, Henderson BE, Krailo MD, Duke A, Roy S. Breast cancer in young women and use of oral contraceptives: possible modifying effect of formulation and age at use. Lancet 1983; 2:926–929. **38.** Paul C, Skegg DG, Spears GFS, Kaldor JM. Oral contraceptives and breast cancer: A national study. Br Med J 1986; 293:723–725. **39.** Miller DR, Rosenberg L, Kaufman DW, Shottenfeld D, Stolley PD, Shapiro S. Breast cancer risk in relation to early oral contraceptive use. Obstet Gynecol 1986; 68:863–868. **40.** Olson H, Olson KL, Moller TR, Ranstam J, Holm P. Oral contraceptive use and breast cancer in young women in Sweden (letter). Lancet 1985; 2:748–749. **41.** McPherson K, Vessey M, Neil A, Doll R, Jones L, Roberts M. Early contraceptive use and breast cancer: Results of another case-control study. Br J Cancer 1987; 56:

Continued on next page

Ortho-Novum Tablets—Cont.

653–660. **42.** Huggins GR, Zucker PF. Oral contraceptives and neoplasia: 1987 update. Fertil Steril 1987; 47:733–761. **43.** McPherson K, Drife JO. The pill and breast cancer: why the uncertainty? Br J Med 1986; 293:709–710. **44.** Shapiro S. Oral contraceptives—time to take stock. N Engl J Med 1987; 315:450–451. **45.** Ory H, Naib Z, Conger SB, Hatcher RA, Tyler CW. Contraceptive choice and prevalence of cervical dysplasia and carcinoma in situ. Am J Obstet Gynecol 1976; 124:573–577. **46.** Vessey MP, Lawless M, McPherson K, Yeates D. Neoplasia of the cervix uteri and contraception: a possible adverse effect of the pill. Lancet 1983; 2:930. **47.** Brinton LA, Huggins GR, Lehman HF, Malli K, Savitz DA, Trapido E, Rosenthal J, Hoover R. Long term use of oral contraceptives and risk of invasive cervical cancer. Int J Cancer 1986; 38:339–344. **48.** WHO Collaborative Study of Neoplasia and Steroid Contraceptives: Invasive cervical cancer and combined oral contraceptives. Br Med J 1985; 290:961–965. **49.** Rooks JB, Ory HW, Ishak KG, Strauss LT, Greenspan JR, Hill AP, Tyler CW. Epidemiology of hepatocellular adenoma: the role of oral contraceptive use. JAMA 1979; 242:644–648. **50.** Bein NN, Goldsmith HS. Recurrent massive hemorrhage from benign hepatic tumors secondary to oral contraceptives. Br J Surg 1977; 64:433–435. **51.** Klatskin G. Hepatic tumors: possible relationship to use of oral contraceptives. Gastroenterology 1977; 73:386–394. **52.** Henderson BE, Preston-Martin S, Edmondson HA, Peters RL, Pike MC. Hepatocellular carcinoma and oral contraceptives. Br J Cancer 1983; 48:437–440. **53.** Neuberger J, Forman D, Doll R, Williams R. Oral contraceptives and hepatocellular carcinoma. Br Med J 1986; 292:1355–1357. **54.** Forman D, Vincent TJ, Doll R. Cancer of the liver and oral contraceptives. Br Med J 1986; 292:1357–1361. **55.** Harlap S, Eldor J. Births following oral contraceptive failures. Obstet Gynecol 1980; 55:447–452. **56.** Savolainen E, Saksela E, Saxen L. Teratogenic hazards of oral contraceptives analyzed in a national malformation register. Am J Obstet Gynecol 1981; 140:521–524. **57.** Janerick DT, Piper JM, Glebatis DM. Oral contraceptives and birth defects. Am J Epidemiol 1980; 112:73–79. **58.** Ferencz C, Matanoski GM, Wilson PD, Rubin JD, Neill CA, Gutberlet R. Maternal hormone therapy and congenital heart disease. Teratology 1980; 21: 225–239. **59.** Rothman KJ, Fyler DC, Goldblatt A, Kreidberg MB. Exogenous hormones and other drug exposures of children with congenital heart disease. Am J Epidemiol 1979; 109:433–439. **60.** Boston Collaborative Drug Surveillance Program: Oral contraceptives and venous thromboembolic disease, surgicaly confirmed gallbladder disease, and breast tumors. Lancet 1973; 1:1399–1404. **61.** Royal College of General Practitioners: Oral contraceptives and health. New York, Pittman 1974. **62.** Layde PM, Vessey MP, Yeates D. Risk of gallbladder disease: a cohort study of young women attending family planning clinics. J Epidemiol Community Health 1982; 36:274–278. **63.** Rome Group for Epidemiology and Prevention of Cholelithiasis (GREPCO): Prevalence of gallstone disease in an Italian adult female population. Am J Epidemiol 1984; 119:796–805. **64.** Storm BL, Tamragouri RT, Morse ML, Lazar El, West SL, Stolley PD, Jones JK. Oral contraceptives and other risk factors for gallbladder disease. Clin Pharmacol Ther 1986; 39:335–341. **65.** Wynn V, Adams PW, Godsland IF, Melrose J. Niththyananthan R, Oakley NW, Seedj A. Comparison of effects of different combined oral contraceptive formulations on carbohydrate and lipid metabolism. Lancet 1979; 1:1045–1049. **66.** Wynn V. Effect of progesterone and progestins on carbohydrate metabolism. In: Progesterone and Progestin. Bardin CW, Milgrom E, Mauvis-Jarvis P. eds. New York, Raven Press, 1983; pp. 395–410. **67.** Perlman JA, Roussell-Briefel RG, Ezzati TM, Lieberknecht G. Oral glucose tolerance and the potency of oral contraceptive progestogens. J Chronic Dis 1985; 38: 857–864. **68.** Royal College of General Practitioners' Oral Contraception Study: Effect on hypertension and benign breast disease of progestogen component in combined oral contraceptives. Lancet 1977; 1:624. **69.** Fisch IR, Frank J. Oral contraceptives and blood pressure. JAMA 1977; 237: 2499–2503. **70.** Laragh AJ. Oral contraceptive induced hypertension—nine years later. Am J Obstet Gynecol 1976; 126:141–147. **71.** Ramcharan S, Peritz E, Pellegrin FA, Williams WT. Incidence of hypertension in the Walnut Creek Contraceptive Drug Study cohort: In: Pharmacology of steroid contraceptive drugs. Garattini S, Berendes HW. Eds. New York, Raven Press, 1977; pp. 277–288, (Monographs of the Mario Negri Institute for Pharmacological Research Milan.) **72.** Stockley I. Interactions with oral contraceptives. J Pharm 1976; 216:140–143. **73.** The Cancer and Steroid Hormone Study of the Centers for Disease Control and the National Institute of Child Health and Human Development: Oral contraceptive use and the risk of ovarian cancer. JAMA 1983; 249:1596–1599. **74.** The Cancer and Steroid Hormone Study of the Centers for Disease Control and the National Institute of Child Health and Human Development: Combination oral contraceptive use and the risk of endometrial cancer. JAMA 1987; 257:796–800. **75.** Ory HW. Functional ovarian cysts and oral contraceptives: negative association confirmed surgically. JAMA 1974; 228:68–69. **76.** Ory HW, Cole P, MacMahon B, Hoover R. Oral contraceptives and reduced risk of benign breast disease. N Engl J Med 1976; 294:419–422. **77.** Ory HW. The noncontraceptive health benefits from oral contraceptive use. Fam Plann Perspect 1982; 14:182–184. **78.** Ory HW, Forrest JD, Lincoln R. Making choices: Evaluating the health risks and benefits of birth control methods. New York, The Alan Guttmacher Institute, 1983; p. 1. **79.** Schlesselman J, Stadel BV, Murray P, Lai S. Breast cancer in relation to early use of oral contraceptives. JAMA 1988; 259:1828–1833. **80.** Hennekens CH, Speizer FE, Lipnick RJ, Rosner B, Bain C, Belanger C, Stampfer MJ, Willett W, Peto R. A case-control study of oral contraceptive use and breast cancer. JNCI 1984; 72:39–42. **81.** LaVecchia C, Decarli A, Fasoli M, Franceschi S, Gentile A, Negri E, Parazzini F, Tognoni G. Oral contraceptives and cancers of the breast and of the female genital tract. Interim results from a case-control study. Br J Cancer 1986; 54:311–317. **82.** Meirik O, Lund E, Adami H, Bergstrom R, Christoffersen T, Bergsjo P. Oral contraceptive use and breast cancer in young women. A Joint National Case-control study in Sweden and Norway. Lancet 1986; 11:650–654. **83.** Kay CR, Hannaford PC. Breast cancer and the pill—A further report from the Royal College of General Practitioners' oral contraception study. Br J Cancer 1988; 58:675–680. **84.** Stadel BV, Lai S, Schlesselman JJ, Murray P. Oral contraceptives and premenopausal breast cancer in nulliparous women. Contraception 1988; 38:287–299. **85.** Miller DR, Rosenberg L, Kaufman DW, Stolley P, Warshauer ME, Shapiro S. Breast cancer before age 45 and oral contraceptive use: New Findings. Am J Epidemiol 1989; 129:269–280. **86.** The UK National Case-Control Study Group, Oral contraceptive use and breast cancer risk in young women. Lancet 1989; 1:973–982. **87.** Schlesselman JJ. Cancer of the breast and reproductive tract in relation to use of oral contraceptives. Contraception 1989; 40:1–38. **88.** Vessey MP, McPherson K, Villard-Mackintosh L, Yeates D. Oral contraceptives and breast cancer: latest findings in large cohort study. Br J Cancer 1989; 59:613–617. **89.** Jick SS, Walker AM, Stergachis A, Jick H. Oral contraceptives and breast cancer. Br J Cancer 1989; 59:618–621. **90.** Collaborative Group on Hormonal Factors in Breast Cancer. Breast cancer and hormonal contraceptives: collaborative reanalysis of individual data on 53 297 women with breast cancer and 100 239 women without breast cancer from 54 epidemiological studies. Lancet 1996; 347:1713–1727. **91.** Palmer JR, Rosenberg L, Kaufman DW, Warshauer ME, Stolley P, Shapiro S. Oral Contraceptive Use and Liver Cancer. Am J Epidemiol 1989; 130:878–882.

BRIEF SUMMARY PATIENT PACKAGE INSERT

Oral contraceptives, also known as "birth control pill" or "the pill," are taken to prevent pregnancy and when taken correctly, have a failure rate of less than 1% per year when used without missing any pills. The typical failure rate of large numbers of pill users is less than 3% per year when women who miss pills are included. For most women oral contraceptives are also free of serious or unpleasant side effects. However, forgetting to take pills considerably increases the chances of pregnancy.

For the majority of women, oral contraceptives can be taken safely. But there are some women who are at high risk of developing certain serious diseases that can be fatal or may cause temporary or permanent disability. The risks associated with taking oral contraceptives increase significantly if you:

- smoke
- have high blood pressure, diabetes, high cholesterol
- have or have had clotting disorders, heart attack, stroke, angina pectoris, cancer of the breast or sex organs, jaundice or malignant or benign liver tumors.

Although cardiovascular disease risks may be increased with oral contraceptive use after age 40 in healthy, nonsmoking women (even with the newer low-dose formulations), there are also greater potential health risks associated with pregnancy in older women.

You should not take the pill if you suspect you are pregnant or have unexplained vaginal bleeding.

Cigarette smoking increases the risk of serious cardiovascular side effects from oral contraceptive use. This risk increases with age and with heavy smoking (15 or more cigarettes per day) and is quite marked in women over 35 years of age. Women who use oral contraceptives are strongly advised not to smoke.

Most side effects of the pill are not serious. The most common such effects are nausea, vomiting, bleeding between menstrual periods, weight gain, breast tenderness, and difficulty wearing contact lenses. These side effects, especially nausea and vomiting, may subside within the first three months of use.

The serious side effects of the pill occur very infrequently, especially if you are in good health and are young. However, you should know that the follwing medical conditions have been associated with or made worse by the pill:

1. Blood clots in the legs (thrombophlebitis), lungs (pulmonary embolism), stoppage or rupture of a blood vessel in the brain (stroke), blockage of blood vessels in the heart (heart attack or angina pectoris) or other organs of the body. As mentioned above, smoking increases the risk of heart attacks and strokes and subsequent serious medical consequences.
2. In rare cases, oral contraceptives can cause benign but dangerous liver tumors. These benign liver tumors can rupture and cause fatal internal bleeding. In addition, some studies report an increased risk of developing liver cancer. However, liver cancers are rare.
3. High blood pressure, although blood pressure usually returns to normal when the pill is stopped.

The symptoms associated with these serious side effects are discussed in the detailed leaflet given to you with your supply of pills. Notify your doctor or health care provider if you notice any unusual physical disturbances while taking the pill. In addition, drugs such as rifampin, as well as some anticonvulsants and some antibiotics may decrease oral contraceptive effectiveness.

There is conflict among studies regarding breast cancer and oral contraceptive use. Some studies have reported an increase in the risk of developing breast cancer, particularly at a younger age. This increased risk appears to be related to duration of use. The majority of studies have found no overall increase in the risk of developing breast cancer. Some studies have found an increase in the incidence of cancer of the cervix in women who use oral contraceptives. However, this finding may be related to factors other than the use of oral contraceptives. There is insufficient evidence to rule out the possibility that pills may cause such cancers.

Taking the combination pill provides some important noncontraceptive benefits. These include less painful menstruation, less menstrual blood loss and anemia, fewer pelvic infections, and fewer cancers of the ovary and the lining of the uterus.

Be sure to discuss any medical condition you may have with your health care provider. Your health care provider will take a medical and family history before prescribing oral contraceptives and will examine you. The physical examination may be delayed to another time if you request it and the health care provider believes that it is a good medical practice to postpone it. You should be reexamined at least once a year while taking oral contraceptives. Your pharmacist should have given you the detailed patient information labeling which gives you further information which you should read and discuss with your health care provider.

This product (like all oral contraceptives) is intended to prevent pregnancy. It does not protect against transmission of HIV (AIDS) and other sexually transmitted diseases such as chlamydia, genital herpes, genital warts, gonorrhea, hepatitis B, and syphilis.

DETAILED PATIENT LABELING

PLEASE NOTE: This labeling is revised from time to time as important new medical information becomes available. Therefore, please review this labeling carefully.

The following oral contraceptive products contain a combination of an estrogen and progestogen, the two kinds of female hormones:

ORTHO-NOVUM 7/7/7 □ 21 Day Regimen and ORTHO-NOVUM 7/7/7 □ 28 Day Regimen

Each white tablet contains 0.5 mg norethindrone and 0.035 mg ethinyl estradiol. Each light peach tablet contains 0.75 mg norethindrone and 0.035 mg ethinyl estradiol. Each peach tablet contains 1 mg norethindrone and 0.035 mg ethinyl estradiol. Each green tablet in ORTHO-NOVUM 7/7/7 □ 28 Day Regimen contains inert ingredients.

ORTHO-NOVUM 10/11 □ 21 Day Regimen and ORTHO-NOVUM 10/11 □ 28 Day Regimen

Each white tablet contains 0.5 mg norethindrone and 0.035 mg ethinyl estradiol. Each peach tablet contains 1 mg norethindrone and 0.035 mg ethinyl estradiol. Each green tablet in ORTHO-NOVUM 10/11 □ 28 Day Regimen contains inert ingredients.

ORTHO-NOVUM 1/35 □ 21 Day Regimen and ORTHO-NOVUM 1/35 □ 28 Day Regimen

Each peach tablet contains 1 mg norethindrone and 0.035 mg ethinyl estradiol. Each green tablet in ORTHO-NOVUM 1/35 □ 28 Day Regimen contains inert ingredients.

MODICON 21 Day Regimen and MODICON 28 Day Regimen

Each white tablet contains 0.5 mg norethindrone and 0.035 mg ethinyl estradiol. Each green tablet in MODICON 28 Day Regimen contains inert ingredients.

INTRODUCTION

Any woman who considers using oral contraceptives (the birth control pill or the pill) should understand the benefits and the risks of using this form of birth control. This patient labeling will give you much of the information you will need to make this decision and will also help you determine if you are at risk of developing any of the serious side effects of the pill. It will tell you how to use the pill properly so that it will be as effective as possible. However, this labeling is not a replacement for a careful discussion between you and your health care provider. You should discuss the information

provided in this labeling with him or her, both when you first start taking the pill and during your revisits. You should also follow your health care provider's advice with regard to regular check-ups while you are on the pill.

EFFECTIVENESS OF ORAL CONTRACEPTIVES

Oral contraceptives or "birth control pills" or "the pill" are used to prevent pregnancy and are more effective than other non-surgical methods of birth control. When they are taken correctly, the chance of becoming pregnant is less than 1% (1 pregnancy per 100 women per year of use) when used perfectly, without missing any pills. Typical failure rates are actually 3% per year. The chance of becoming pregnant increases with each missed pill during a menstrual cycle.

In comparison, typical failure rates for other non-surgical methods of birth control during the first year of use are as follows:

Implant: <1%
Injection: <1%
IUD: 1 to 2%
Diaphragm with spermicides: 18%
Spermicides alone: 21%
Vaginal sponge: 18 to 36%
Cervical Cap: 18 to 36%
Condom alone (male): 12%
Condom alone (female): 21%
Periodic abstinence: 20%
No methods: 85%

WHO SHOULD NOT TAKE ORAL CONTRACEPTIVES

Cigarette smoking increases the risk of serious cardiovascular side effects from oral contraceptive use. This risk increases with age and with heavy smoking (15 or more cigarettes per day) and is quite marked in women over 35 years of age. Women who use oral contraceptives are strongly advised not to smoke.

Some women should not use the pill. For example, you should not take the pill if you are pregnant or think you may be pregnant. You should also not use the pill if you have any of the following conditions:

• A history of heart attack or stroke
• Blood clots in the legs (thrombophlebitis), lungs (pulmonary embolism), or eyes
• A history of blood clots in the deep veins of your legs
• Chest pain (angina pectoris)
• Known or suspected breast cancer or cancer of the lining of the uterus, cervix or vagina
• Unexplained vaginal bleeding (until a diagnosis is reached by your doctor)
• Yellowing of the whites of the eyes or of the skin (jaundice) during pregnancy or during previous use of the pill
• Liver tumor (benign or cancerous)
• Known or suspected pregnancy

Tell your health care provider if you have ever had any of these conditions. Your health care provider can recommend a safer method of brith control.

OTHER CONSIDERATIONS BEFORE TAKING ORAL CONTRACEPTIVES

Tell your health care provider if you have or have had:

• Breast nodules, fibrocystic disease of the breast, an abnormal breast x-ray or mammogram
• Diabetes
• Elevated cholesterol or triglycerides
• High blood pressure
• Migraine or other headaches or epilepsy
• Mental depression
• Gallbladder, heart or kidney disease
• History of scanty or irregular menstrual periods

Women with any of these conditions should be checked often by their health care provider if they choose to use oral contraceptives.

Also, be sure to inform your doctor or health care provider if you smoke or are on any medications.

RISKS OF TAKING ORAL CONTRACEPTIVES

1. Risk of developing blood clots

Blood clots and blockage of blood vessels are one of the most serious side effects of taking oral contraceptives and can cause death or serious disability. In particular, a clot in the legs can cause thrombophlebitis and a clot that travels to the lungs can cause a sudden blocking of the vessel carrying blood to the lungs. Rarely, clots occur in the blood vessels of the eye and may cause blindness, double vision, or impaired vision.

If you take oral contraceptives and need elective surgery, need to stay in bed for a prolonged illness or have recently delivered a baby, you may be at risk of develping blood clots. You should consult your doctor about stopping oral contraceptives three to four weeks before surgery and not taking oral contraceptives for two weeks after surgery or during bed rest. You should also not take oral contraceptives soon after delivery of a baby. It is advisable to wait for at least four weeks after delivery if you are not breast feeding or four weeks after a second trimester abortion. If you are breast feeding, you should wait until you have weaned your child before using the pill. (See also the section on Breast Feeding in General Precautions.)

The risk of circulatory disease in oral contraceptive users may be higher in users of high dose pills and may be greater with longer duration of oral contraceptive use. In addition, some of these increased risks may continue for a number of years after stopping oral contraceptives. The risk of abnormal blood clotting increases with age in both users and nonusers of oral contraceptives, but the increased risk from the oral contraceptive appears to be present at all ages. For women aged 20 to 44, it is estimated that about 1 in 2,000 using oral contraceptives will be hospitalized each year because of abnormal clotting. Among nonusers in the same age group, about 1 in 20,000 would be hospitalized each year. For oral contraceptive users in general, it has been estimated that in women between the ages of 15 and 34 the risk of death due to a circulatory disorder is about 1 in 12,000 per year, whereas for nonusers the rate is about 1 in 50,000 per year. In the age group 35 to 44, the risk is estimated to be about 1 in 2,500 per year for oral contraceptive users and about 1 in 10,000 per year for nonusers.

2. Heart attacks and strokes

Oral contraceptives may increase the tendency to develop strokes (stoppage or rupture of blood vessels in the brain) and angina pectoris and heart attacks (blockage of blood vessels in the heart). Any of these conditions can cause death or serious disability.

Smoking greatly increases the possibility of suffering heart attacks and strokes. Furthermore, smoking and the use of oral contraceptives greatly increase the chances of developing and dying of heart disease.

3. Gallbladder disease

Oral contraceptive users probably have a greater risk than nonusers of having gallbladder disease, although this risk may be related to pills containing high doses of estrogens.

4. Liver tumors

In rare cases, oral contraceptives can cause benign but dangerous liver tumors. These benign liver tumors can rupture and cause fatal internal bleeding. In addition, some studies report an increased risk of developing liver cancer. However, liver cancers are rare.

5. Cancer of the reproductive organs and breasts

There is conflict among studies regarding breast cancer and oral contraceptive use. Some studies have reported an increase in the risk of developing breast cancer, particularly at a younger age. This increased risk appears to be related to duration of use. The majority of studies have found no overall increase in the risk of developing breast cancer.

A meta-analysis of 54 studies found a small increase in the frequency of having breast cancer diagnosed for women who were currently using combined oral contraceptives or had used them within the past ten years. This increase in the frequency of breast cancer diagnosis, within ten years of stopping use, was generally accounted for by cancers localized to the breast. There was no increase in the frequency of having breast cancer diagnosed ten or more years after cessation of use.

Some studies have found an increase in the incidence of cancer of the cervix in women who use oral contraceptives. However, this finding may be related to factors other than the use of oral contraceptives. There is insufficient evidence to rule out the possibility that pills may cause such cancers.

ESTIMATED RISK OF DEATH FROM A BIRTH CONTROL METHOD OR PREGNANCY

All methods of birth control and pregnancy are associated with a risk of developing certain diseases which may lead to disability or death. An estimate of the number of deaths associated with different methods of birth control and pregnancy has been calculated and is shown in the following table.

ANNUAL NUMBER OF BIRTH-RELATED OR METHOD-RELATED DEATHS ASSOCIATED WITH CONTROL OF FERTILITY PER 100,000 NONSTERILE WOMEN, BY FERTILITY CONTROL METHOD ACCORDING TO AGE

Method of control and outcome	15-19	20-24	25-29	30-34	35-39	40-44
No fertility control methods*	7.0	7.4	9.1	14.8	25.7	28.2
Oral contraceptives non-smoker**	0.3	0.5	0.9	1.9	13.8	31.6
Oral contraceptives smoker**	2.2	3.4	6.6	13.5	51.1	117.2
IUD**	0.8	0.8	1.0	1.0	1.4	1.4
Condom*	1.1	1.6	0.7	0.2	0.3	0.4
Diaphragm/ spermicide*	1.9	1.2	1.2	1.3	2.2	2.8
Periodic abstinence*	2.5	1.6	1.6	1.7	2.9	3.6

*Deaths are birth-related
**Deaths are method-related

[See table above]

In the above table, the risk of death from any birth control method is less than the risk of childbirth, except for oral contraceptive users over the age of 35 who smoke and pill users over the age of 40 even if they do not smoke. It can be seen in the table that for women aged 15 to 39, the risk of death was highest with pregnancy (7–26 deaths per 100,000 women, depending on age). Among pill users who do not smoke, the risk of death was always lower than that associated with pregnancy for any age group, although over the age of 40, the risk increases to 32 deaths per 100,000 women, compared to 28 associated with pregnancy at that age. However, for pill users who smoke and are over the age of 35, the estimated number of deaths exceed those for other methods of birth control. If a woman is over the age of 40 and smokes, her estimated risk of death is four times higher (117/100,000 women) than the estimated risk associated with pregnancy (28/100,000 women) in that age group.

The suggestion that women over 40 who do not smoke should not take oral contraceptives is based on information from older, higher-dose pills. An Advisory Committee of the FDA discussed this issue in 1989 and recommended that the benefits of low-dose oral contraceptive use by healthy, non-smoking women over 40 years of age may outweigh the possible risks.

WARNING SIGNALS

If any of these adverse effects occur while you are taking oral contraceptives, call your doctor immediately:

• Sharp chest pain, coughing of blood, or sudden shortness of breath (indicating a possible clot in the lung)
• Pain in the calf (indicating a possible clot in the leg)
• Crushing chest pain or heaviness in the chest (indicating a possible heart attack)
• Sudden severe headache or vomiting, dizziness or fainting, disturbances of vision or speech, weakness, or numbness in an arm or leg (indicating a possible stroke)
• Sudden partial or complete loss of vision (indicating a possible clot in the eye)
• Breast lumps (indicating possible breast cancer or fibrocystic disease of the breast; ask your doctor or health care provider to show you how to examine your breasts)
• Severe pain or tenderness in the stomach area (indicating a possibly ruptured liver tumor)
• Difficulty in sleeping, weakness, lack of energy, fatigue, or change in mood (possibly indicating severe depression)
• Jaundice or a yellowing of the skin or eyeballs, accompanied frequently by fever, fatigue, loss of appetite, dark colored urine, or light colored bowel movements (indicating possible liver problems)

SIDE EFFECTS OF ORAL CONTRACEPTIVES

1. Vaginal bleeding

Irregular vaginal bleeding or spotting may occur while you are taking the pills. Irregular bleeding may vary from slight staining between menstrual periods to breakthrough bleeding which is a flow much like regular period. Irregular bleeding occurs most often during the first few months of oral contraceptive use, but may also occur after you have been taking the pill for some time. Such bleeding may be temporary and usually does not indicate any serious problems. It is important to continue taking your pills on schedule. If the bleeding occurs in more than one cycle or lasts for more than a few days, talk to your doctor or health care provider.

2. Contact lenses

If you wear contact lenses and notice a change in vision or an inability to wear your lenses, contact your doctor or health care provider.

Continued on next page

Ortho-Novum Tablets—Cont.

3. Fluid retention
Oral contraceptives may cause edema (fluid retention) with swelling of the fingers or ankles and may raise your blood pressure. If you experience fluid retention, contact your doctor or health care provider.

4. Melasma
A spotty darkening of the skin is possible, particularly of the face, which may persist.

5. Other side effects
Other side effects may include nausea and vomiting, change in appetite, headache, nervousness, depression, dizziness, loss of scalp hair, rash, and vaginal infections.
If any of these side effects bother you, call your doctor or health care provider.

GENERAL PRECAUTIONS

1. Missed periods and use of oral contraceptives before or during early pregnancy
There may be times when you may not menstruate regularly after you have completed taking a cycle of pills. If you have taken your pills regularly and miss one menstrual period, continue taking your pills for the next cycle but be sure to inform your health care provider before doing so. If you have not taken the pills daily as instructed and missed a menstrual period, you may be pregnant. If you missed two consecutive menstrual periods, you may be pregnant. Check with your health care provider immediately to determine whether you are pregnant. Do not continue to take oral contraceptives until you are sure you are not pregnant, but continue to use another method of contraception.
There is no conclusive evidence that oral contraceptive use is associated with an increase in birth defects, when taken inadvertently during early pregnancy. Previously, a few studies had reported that oral contraceptives might be associated with birth defects, but these findings have not been seen in more recent studies. Nevertheless, oral contraceptives or any other drugs should not be used during pregnancy unless clearly necessary and prescribed by your doctor. You should check with your doctor about risks to your unborn child of any medication taken during pregnancy.

2. While breast feeding
If you are breast feeding, consult your doctor before starting oral contraceptives. Some of the drug will be passed on to the child in the milk. A few adverse effects on the child have been reported, including yellowing of the skin (jaundice) and breast enlargement. In addition, combination oral contraceptives may decrease the amount and quality of your milk. If possible, do not use combination oral contraceptives while breast feeding. You should use another method of contraception since breast feeding provides only partial protection from becoming pregnant and this partial protection decreases significantly as you breast feed for longer periods of time. You should consider starting combination oral contraceptives only after you have weaned your child completely.

3. Laboratory tests
If you are scheduled for any laboratory tests, tell your doctor you are taking birth control pills. Certain blood tests may be affected by birth control pills.

4. Drug interactions
Certain drugs may interact with birth control pills to make them less effective in preventing pregnancy or cause an increase in breakthrough bleeding. Such drugs include rifampin, drugs used for epilepsy such as barbiturates (for example, phenobarbital), anticonvulsants such as carbamazepine (Tegretol is one brand of this drug), phenytoin (Dilantin is one brand of this drug), phenylbutazone (Butazolidin is one brand), and possibly certain antibiotics. You may need to use addtional contraception when you take drugs which can make oral contraceptives less effective.

5. Sexually transmitted diseases
This product (like all oral contraceptives) is intended to prevent pregnancy. It does not protect against transmission of HIV (AIDS) and other sexually transmitted diseases such as chlamydia, genital herpes, genital warts, gonorrhea, hepatitis B, and syphilis.

HOW TO TAKE THE PILL

IMPORTANT POINTS TO REMEMBER

BEFORE YOU START TAKING YOUR PILLS:
1. BE SURE TO READ THESE DIRECTIONS:
Before you start taking your pills.
Anytime you are not sure what to do.
2. THE RIGHT WAY TO TAKE THE PILL IS TO TAKE ONE PILL EVERY DAY AT THE SAME TIME.
If you miss pills you could get pregnant. This includes starting the pack late.
The more pills you miss, the more likely you are to get pregnant.
3. MANY WOMEN HAVE SPOTTING OR LIGHT BLEEDING, OR MAY FEEL SICK TO THEIR STOMACH DURING THE FIRST 1–3 PACKS OF PILLS: If you feel sick to

your stomach, do not stop taking the pill. The problem will usually go away. If it doesn't go away, check with your doctor or clinic.
4. MISSING PILLS CAN ALSO CAUSE SPOTTING OR LIGHT BLEEDING, even when you make up these missed pills.
On the days you take 2 pills to make up for missed pills, you could also feel a little sick to your stomach.
5. IF YOU HAVE VOMITING OR DIARRHEA, for any reason, or IF YOU TAKE SOME MEDICINES, including some antibiotics, your pills may not work as well. Use a back-up method (such as condoms, foam, or sponge) until you check with your doctor or clinic.
6. IF YOU HAVE TROUBLE REMEMBERING TO TAKE THE PILL, talk to your doctor or clinic about how to make pill-taking easier or about using another method of birth control.
7. IF YOU HAVE ANY QUESTIONS OR ARE UNSURE ABOUT THE INFORMATION IN THIS LEAFLET, call your doctor or clinic.

BEFORE YOU START TAKING YOUR PILLS

1. DECIDE WHAT TIME OF DAY YOU WANT TO TAKE YOUR PILL.
It is important to take it at about the same time every day.
2. LOOK AT YOUR PILL PACK TO SEE IF IT HAS 21 OR 28 PILLS:
The 21-pill pack has 21 "active" pills (with hormones) to take for 3 weeks. This is followed by 1 week without pills.
The 28-pill pack has 21 "active" pills (with hormones) to take for 3 weeks. This is followed by 1 week of "reminder" green pills (without hormones).
ORTHO-NOVUM 7/7/7: There are 7 white "active" pills, 7 light peach "active" pills, and 7 peach "active" pills.
ORTHO–NOVUM 10/11: There are 10 white "active" pills and 11 peach "active" pills.
ORTHO-NOVUM 1/35: There are 21 peach "active" pills.
MODICON: There are 21 white "active" pills.
3. ALSO FIND:
1) where on the pack to start taking pills,
2) in what order to take the pills.
CHECK PICTURE OF PILL PACK AND ADDITIONAL INSTRUCTIONS FOR USING THIS PACKAGE IN THE BRIEF SUMMARY PATIENT PACKAGE INSERT.
4. BE SURE YOU HAVE READY AT ALL TIMES.
ANOTHER KIND OF BIRTH CONTROL (such as condoms, foam, or sponge) to use as a back-up method in case you miss pills.
AN EXTRA, FULL PILL PACK.

WHEN TO START THE FIRST PACK OF PILLS

You have a choice of which day to start taking your first pack of pills. ORTHO-NOVUM 7/7/7, ORTHO-NOVUM 10/11, ORTHO-NOVUM 1/35, and MODICON are available in the DIALPAK® Tablet Dispenser which is preset for a Sunday Start. Day 1 Start is also provided. Decide with your doctor or clinic which is the best day for you. Pick a time of day which will be easy to remember.
SUNDAY START:
ORTHO-NOVUM 7/7/7: Take the first "active" white pill of the first pack on the Sunday after your period starts, even if you are still bleeding. If your period begins on Sunday, start the pack the same day.
ORTHO-NOVUM 10/11: Take the first "active" white pill of the first pack on the Sunday after your period starts, even if you are still bleeding. If your period begins on Sunday, start the pack the same day.
ORTHO-NOVUM 1/35: Take the first "active" peach pill of the first pack on the Sunday after your period starts, even if you are still bleeding. If your period begins on Sunday, start the pack the same day.
MODICON: Take the first "active" white pill of the first pack on the Sunday after your period starts, even if you are still bleeding. If your period begins on Sunday, start the pack the same day.
Use another method of birth control as a back-up method if you have sex anytime from the Sunday you start your first pack until the next Sunday (7 days). Condoms, foam, or the sponge are good back-up methods of birth control.
DAY 1 START:
ORTHO-NOVUM 7/7/7: Take the first "active" white pill of the first pack during the first 24 hours of your period.
ORTHO-NOVUM 10/11: Take the first "active" white pill of the first pack during the first 24 hours of your period.
ORTHO-NOVUM 1/35: Take the first "active" peach pill of the first pack during the first 24 hours of your period.
MODICON: Take the first "active" white pill of the first pack during the first 24 hours of your period.
You will not need to use a back-up method of birth control, since you are starting the pill at the beginning of your period.

WHAT TO DO DURING THE MONTH

1. TAKE ONE PILL AT THE SAME TIME EVERY DAY UNTIL THE PACK IS EMPTY.
Do not skip pills even if you are spotting or bleeding between monthly periods or feel sick to your stomach (nausea).
Do not skip pills even if you do not have sex very often.
2. WHEN YOU FINISH A PACK OR SWITCH YOUR BRAND OF PILLS:
21 pills: Wait 7 days to start the next pack. You will probably have your period during that week. Be sure that no more than 7 days pass between 21-day packs.
28 pills: Start the next pack on the day after your last "reminder" pill. Do not wait any days between packs.

WHAT TO DO IF YOU MISS PILLS

ORTHO-NOVUM 7/7/7:
If you **MISS 1** white, light peach, or peach "active" pill:
1. Take it as soon as you remember. Take the next pill at your regular time. This means you may take 2 pills in 1 day.
2. You do not need to use a back-up birth control method if you have sex.
If you **MISS 2** white or light peach "active" pills in a row in **WEEK 1 OR WEEK 2** of your pack:
1. Take 2 pills on the day you remember and 2 pills the next day.
2. Then take 1 pill a day until you finish the pack.
3. You MAY BECOME PREGNANT if you have sex in the 7 days after you miss pills. You MUST use another birth control method (such as condoms, foam, or sponge) as a back-up method for those 7 days.
If you **MISS 2** peach "active" pills in a row in **THE 3RD WEEK:**
1. If you are a Sunday Starter:
Keep taking 1 pill every day until Sunday. On Sunday, THROW OUT the rest of the pack and start a new pack of pills that same day.
If you are a Day 1 Starter:
THROW OUT the rest of the pill pack and start a new pack that same day.
2. You may not have your period this month but this is expected. However, if you miss your period 2 months in a row, call your doctor or clinic because you might be pregnant.
3. You MAY BECOME PREGNANT if you have sex in the 7 days after you miss pills. You MUST use another birth control method (such as condoms, foam, or sponge) as a back-up method for those 7 days.
If you **MISS 3 OR MORE** white, light peach, or peach "active" pills in a row (during the first 3 weeks):
1. If you are a Sunday Starter:
Keep taking 1 pill every day until Sunday. On Sunday, THROW OUT the rest of the pack and start a new pack of pills that same day.
If you are a Day 1 Starter:
THROW OUT the rest of the pill pack and start a new pack that same day.
2. You may not have your period this month but this is expected. However, if you miss your period 2 months in a row, call your doctor or clinic because you might be pregnant.
3. You MAY BECOME PREGNANT if you have sex in the 7 days after you miss pills. You MUST use another birth control method (such as condoms, foam, or sponge) as a back-up method for those 7 days.
ORTHO-NOVUM 10/11:
If you **MISS 1** white or peach "active" pill:
1. Take it as soon as you remember. Take the next pill at your regular time. This means you may take 2 pills in 1 day.
2. You do not need to use a back-up birth control method if you have sex.
If you **MISS 2** white or peach "active" pills in a row in **WEEK 1 OR WEEK 2** of your pack:
1. Take 2 pills on the day you remember and 2 pills the next day.
2. Then take 1 pill a day until you finish the pack.
3. You MAY BECOME PREGNANT if you have sex in the 7 days after you miss pills. You MUST use another birth control method (such as condoms, foam, or sponge) as a back-up method for those 7 days.
If you **MISS 2** peach "active" pills in a row in **THE 3RD WEEK:**
1. If you are a Sunday Starter:
Keep taking 1 pill every day until Sunday. On Sunday, THROW OUT the rest of the pack and start a new pack of pills that same day.
If you are a Day 1 Starter:
THROW OUT the rest of the pill pack and start a new pack that same day.
2. You may not have your period this month but this is expected. However, if you miss your period 2 months in a row, call your doctor or clinic because you might be pregnant.
3. You MAY BECOME PREGNANT if you have sex in the 7 days after you miss pills. You MUST use another birth control method (such as condoms, foam, or sponge) as a back-up method for those 7 days.

If you **MISS 3 OR MORE** white or peach "active" pills in a row (during the first 3 weeks):

1. **If you are a Sunday Starter:**
Keep taking 1 pill every day until Sunday. On Sunday, THROW OUT the rest of the pack and start a new pack of pills that same day.

If you are a Day 1 Starter:
THROW OUT the rest of the pill pack and start a new pack that same day.
2. You may not have your period this month but this is expected. However, if you miss your period 2 months in a row, call your doctor or clinic because you might be pregnant.
3. You MAY BECOME PREGNANT if you have sex in the 7 days after you miss pills. You MUST use another birth control method (such as condoms, foam, or sponge) as a back-up method for those 7 days.

ORTHO-NOVUM 1/35:
If you **MISS 1** peach "active" pill:
1. Take it as soon as you remember. Take the next pill at your regular time. This means you may take 2 pills in 1 day.
2. You do not need to use a back-up birth control method if you have sex.
If you **MISS 2** peach "active" pills in a row in **WEEK 1 OR WEEK 2** of your pack:
1. Take 2 pills on the day you remember and 2 pills the next day.
2. Then take 1 pill a day until you finish the pack.
3. You MAY BECOME PREGNANT if you have sex in the 7 days after you miss pills. You MUST use another birth control method (such as condoms, foam, or sponge) as a back-up method for those 7 days.
If you **MISS 2** peach "active" pills in a row in **THE 3RD WEEK:**

1. **If you are a Sunday Starter:**
Keep taking 1 pill every day until Sunday. On Sunday, THROW OUT the rest of the pack and start a new pack of pills that same day.

If you are a Day 1 Starter:
THROW OUT the rest of the pill pack and start a new pack that same day.
2. You may not have your period this month but this is expected. However, if you miss your period 2 months in a row, call your doctor or clinic because you might be pregnant.
3. You MAY BECOME PREGNANT if you have sex in the 7 days after you miss pills. You MUST use another birth control method (such as condoms, foam, or sponge) as a back-up method for those 7 days.
If you **MISS 3 OR MORE** peach "active" pills in a row (during the first 3 weeks):

1. **If you are a Sunday Starter:**
Keep taking 1 pill every day until Sunday. On Sunday, THROW OUT the rest of the pack and start a new pack of pills that same day.

If you are a Day 1 Starter:
THROW OUT the rest of the pill pack and start a new pack that same day.
2. You may not have your period this month but this is expected. However, if you miss your period 2 months in a row, call your doctor or clinic because you might be pregnant.
3. You MAY BECOME PREGNANT if you have sex in the 7 days after you miss pills. You MUST use another birth control method (such as condoms, foam, or sponge) as a back-up method for those 7 days.

MODICON:
If you **MISS 1** white "active" pill:
1. Take it as soon as you remember. Take the next pill at your regular time. This means you may take 2 pills in 1 day.
2. You do not need to use a back-up birth control method if you have sex.
If you **MISS 2** white "active" pills in a row in **WEEK 1 OR WEEK 2** of your pack:
1. Take 2 pills on the day you remember and 2 pills the next day.
2. Then take 1 pill a day until you finish the pack.
3. You MAY BECOME PREGNANT if you have sex in the 7 days after you miss pills. You MUST use another birth control method (such as condoms, foam, or sponge) as a back-up method for those 7 days.
If you **MISS 2** white "active" pills in a row in **THE 3RD WEEK:**

1. **If you are a Sunday Starter:**
Keep taking 1 pill every day until Sunday. On Sunday, THROW OUT the rest of the pack and start a new pack of pills that same day.

If you are a Day 1 Starter:
THROW OUT the rest of the pill pack and start a new pack that same day.
2. You may not have your period this month but this is expected. However, if you miss your period 2 months in a row, call your doctor or clinic because you might be pregnant.
3. You MAY BECOME PREGNANT if you have sex in the 7 days after you miss pills. You MUST use another birth control method (such as condoms, foam, or sponge) as a back-up method for those 7 days.
If you **MISS 3 OR MORE** white "active" pills in a row (during the first 3 weeks):

1. **If you are a Sunday Starter:**
Keep taking 1 pill every day until Sunday. On Sunday, THROW OUT the rest of the pack and start a new pack of pills that same day.

If you are a Day 1 Starter:
THROW OUT the rest of the pill pack and start a new pack that same day.
2. You may not have your period this month but this is expected. However, if you miss your period 2 months in a row, call your doctor or clinic because you might be pregnant.
3. You MAY BECOME PREGNANT if you have sex in the 7 days after you miss pills. You MUST use another birth control method (such as condoms, foam, or sponge) as a back-up method for those 7 days.

A REMINDER FOR THOSE ON 28-DAY PACKS:
If you forget any of the 7 green "reminder" pills in Week 4: THROW AWAY the pills you missed.
Keep taking 1 pill each day until the pack is empty.
You do not need a back-up method.

FINALLY, IF YOU ARE STILL NOT SURE WHAT TO DO ABOUT THE PILLS YOU HAVE MISSED:
Use a BACK-UP METHOD anytime you have sex.
KEEP TAKING ONE "ACTIVE" PILL EACH DAY until you can reach your doctor or clinic.

PREGNANCY DUE TO PILL FAILURE

Combination Oral Contraceptives
The incidence of pill failure resulting in pregnancy is approximately one percent (i.e., one pregnancy per 100 women per year) if taken every day as directed, but more typical failure rates are about 3%. If failure does occur, the risk to the fetus is minimal.

PREGNANCY AFTER STOPPING THE PILL

There may be some delay in becoming pregnant after you stop using oral contraceptives, especially if you had irregular menstrual cycles before you used oral contraceptives. It may be advisable to postpone conception until you begin menstruating regularly once you have stopped taking the pill and desire pregnancy.

There does not appear to be any increase in birth defects in newborn babies when pregnancy occurs soon after stopping the pill.

OVERDOSAGE

Serious ill effects have not been reported following ingestion of large doses of oral contraceptives by young children. Overdosage may cause nausea and withdrawal bleeding in females. In case of overdosage, contact your health care provider or pharmacist.

OTHER INFORMATION

Your health care provider will take a medical and family history before prescribing oral contraceptives and will examine you. The physical examination may be delayed to another time if you request it and the health care provider believes that it is a good medical practice to postpone it. You should be reexamined at least once a year. Be sure to inform your health care provider if there is a family history of any of the conditions listed previously in this leaflet. Be sure to keep all appointments with your health care provider, because this is a time to determine if there are early signs of side effects of oral contraceptive use.

Do not use the drug for any condition other than the one for which it was prescribed. This drug has been prescribed specifically for you; do not give it to others who may want birth control pills.

HEALTH BENEFITS FROM ORAL CONTRACEPTIVES

In addition to preventing pregnancy, use of combination oral contraceptives may provide certain benefits. They are:
• menstrual cycles may become more regular
• blood flow during menstruation may be lighter and less iron may be lost. Therefore, anemia due to iron deficiency is less likely to occur.
• pain or other symptoms during menstruation may be encountered less frequently
• ectopic (tubal) pregnancy may occur less frequently
• noncancerous cysts or lumps in the breast may occur less frequently
• acute pelvic inflammatory disease may occur less frequently
• oral contraceptive use may provide some protection against developing two forms of cancer: cancer of the ovaries and cancer of the lining of the uterus.

If you want more information about birth control pills, ask your doctor or pharmacist. They have a more technical leaflet called the Professional Labeling, which you may wish to read. The professional labeling is also published in a book entitled *Physicians' Desk Reference*, available in many book stores and public libraries.

ORTHO-McNEIL PHARMACEUTICAL, INC.
Raritan, New Jersey 08869

© OMP 1998   REVISED MAY 1998   635-50-700-3
Shown in Product Identification Guide, page 328

ORTHO TRI-CYCLEN® Tablets   ℞
ORTHO-CYCLEN® Tablets
(norgestimate/ethinyl estradiol)

Prescribing Information
Patients should be counseled that this product does not protect against HIV infection (AIDS) and other sexually transmitted diseases.

DESCRIPTION

Each of the following products is a combination oral contraceptive containing the progestational compound norgestimate and the estrogenic compound ethinyl estradiol.
ORTHO TRI-CYCLEN □ 21 Tablets and ORTHO TRI-CYCLEN □ 28 Tablets.
Each white tablet contains 0.180 mg of the progestational compound, norgestimate (18, 19-Dinor-17-pregn-4-en-20-yn-3-one, 17-(acetyloxy)-13-ethyl-,oxime,(17α)-(+)-) and 0.035 mg of the estrogenic compound, ethinyl estradiol (19-nor-17α-pregna, 1,3,5(10)-trien-20-yne-3, 17-diol). Inactive ingredients include lactose, magnesium stearate, and pregelatinized starch.
Each light blue tablet contains 0.215 mg of the progestational compound norgestimate (18, 19-Dinor-17-pregn-4-en-20-yn-3-one, 17-(acetyloxy)-13-ethyl-, oxime, (17α)-(+)-) and 0.035 mg of the estrogenic compound, ethinyl estradiol (19-nor-17α-pregna, 1,3,5(10)-trien-20-yne-3, 17-diol). Inactive ingredients include FD&C Blue No. 2 Aluminum Lake, lactose, magnesium stearate, and pregelatinized starch.
Each blue tablet contains 0.250 mg of the progestational compound norgestimate (18, 19-Dinor-17-pregn-4-en-20-yn-3-one, 17-(acetyloxy)-13-ethyl-, oxime, (17α)-(+)-) and 0.035 mg of the estrogenic compound, ethinyl estradiol (19-nor-17α-pregna, 1,3,5(10)-trien-20-yne-3, 17-diol). Inactive ingredients include FD&C Blue No. 2 Aluminum Lake, lactose, magnesium stearate, and pregelatinized starch.
Each green tablet in the ORTHO TRI-CYCLEN □ 28 package contains only inert ingredients, as follows: D&C Yellow No. 10 Aluminum Lake, FD&C Blue No. 2 Aluminum Lake, lactose, magnesium stearate, microcrystalline cellulose and pregelatinized starch.
ORTHO-CYCLEN □ 21 Tablets and ORTHO-CYCLEN □ 28 Tablets.
Each blue tablet contains 0.250 mg of the progestational compound norgestimate (18, 19-Dinor-17-pregn-4-en-20-yn-3-one, 17-(acetyloxy)-13-ethyl-, oxime, (17α)-(+)-) and 0.035 mg of the estrogenic compound, ethinyl estradiol (19-nor-17α-pregna, 1,3,5(10)-trien-20-yne-3, 17-diol). Inactive ingredients include FD&C Blue No. 2 Aluminum Lake, lactose, magnesium stearate, and pregelatinized starch.
Each green tablet in the ORTHO-CYCLEN □ 28 package contains only inert ingredients, as follows: D&C Yellow No. 10 Aluminum Lake, FD&C Blue No. 2 Aluminum Lake, lactose, magnesium stearate, microcrystalline cellulose and pregelatinized starch.

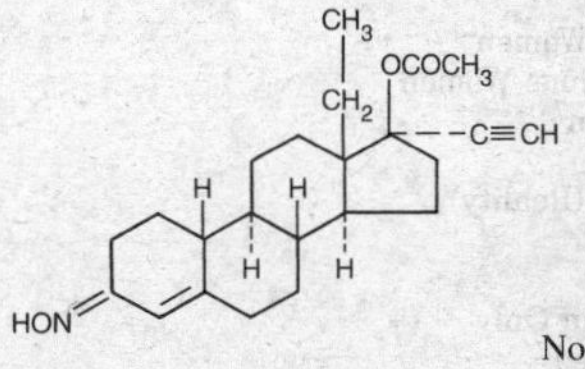

Norgestimate

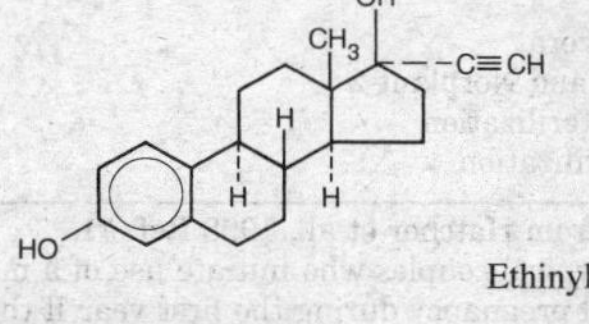

Ethinyl Estradiol

CLINICAL PHARMACOLOGY
ORAL CONTRACEPTION
Combination oral contraceptives act by suppression of gonadotropins. Although the primary mechanism of this action is inhibition of ovulation, other alterations include changes in the cervical mucus (which increase the difficulty of sperm entry into the uterus) and the endometrium (which reduce he likelihood of implantation).
Receptor binding studies, as well as studies in animals and humans, have shown that norgestimate and 17-deacetyl norgestimate, the major serum metabolite, combine high progestational activity with minimal intrinsic androgenici-

Continued on next page

Continued on next page

Left column middle

1. **If you are a Sunday Starter:**
Keep taking 1 pill every day until Sunday. On Sunday, THROW OUT the rest of the pack and start a new pack of pills that same day.
If you are a Day 1 Starter:
THROW OUT the rest of the pill pack and start a new pack that same day.
2. You may not have your period this month but this is expected. However, if you miss your period 2 months in a row, call your doctor or clinic because you might be pregnant.
3. You MAY BECOME PREGNANT if you have sex in the 7 days after you miss pills. You MUST use another birth control method (such as condoms, foam, or sponge) as a back-up method for those 7 days.

Ortho Tri-Cyclen—Cont.

ty.[90–93] Norgestimate, in combination with ethinyl estradiol, does not counteract the estrogen-induced increases in sex hormone binding globulin (SHBG), resulting in lower serum testosterone.[90,91,94]

ACNE

Acne is a skin condition with a multifactorial etiology. The combination of ethinyl estradiol and norgestimate may increase sex hormone binding globulin (SHBG) and decrease free testosterone resulting in a decrease in the severity of facial acne in otherwise healthy women with this skin condition.

Norgestimate and ethinyl estradiol are well absorbed following oral administration of ORTHO-CYCLEN and ORTHO TRI-CYCLEN. On the average, peak serum concentrations of norgestimate and ethinyl estradiol are observed within two hours (0.5–2.0 hr for norgestimate and 0.75–3.0 hr for ethinyl estradiol) after administration followed by a rapid decline due to distribution and elimination. Although norgestimate serum concentrations following single or multiple dosing were generally below assay detection within 5 hours, a major norgestimate serum metabolite, 17-deacetyl norgestimate, (which exhibits a serum half-life ranging from 12 to 30 hours) appears rapidly in serum with concentrations greatly exceeding that of norgestimate. The 17-deacetylated metabolite is pharmacologically active and the pharmacologic profile is similar to that of norgestimate. The elimination half-life of ethinyl estradiol ranged from approximately 6 to 14 hours.

Both norgestimate and ethinyl estradiol are extensively metabolized and eliminated by renal and fecal pathways. Following administration of ^{14}C-norgestimate, 47% (45–49%) and 37% (16–49%) of the administered radioactivity was eliminated in the urine and feces, respectively. Unchanged norgestimate was not detected in the urine. In addition to 17-deacetyl norgestimate, a number of metabolites of norgestimate have been identified in human urine following administration of radiolabeled norgestimate. These include 18, 19-Dinor-17-pregn-4-en-20-yn-3-one, 17-hydroxy-13-ethyl,(17α)-(-); 18, 19-Dinor-5β-17-pregnan-20-yn,3α,17β-dihydroxy-13-ethyl,(17α), various hydroxylated metabolites and conjugates of these metabolites. Ethinyl estradiol is metabolized to various hydroxylated products and their glucuronide and sulfate conjugates.

INDICATIONS AND USAGE

ORTHO-CYCLEN and ORTHO TRI-CYCLEN Tablets are indicated for the prevention of pregnancy in women who elect to use oral contraceptives as a method of contraception.

ORTHO TRI-CYCLEN is indicated for the treatment of moderate acne vulgaris in females, ≥ 15 years of age, who have no known contraindications to oral contraceptive therapy, desire contraception, have achieved menarche and are unresponsive to topical anti-acne medications.

Oral contraceptives are highly effective. Table I lists the typical accidental pregnancy rates for users of combination oral contraceptives and other methods of contraception. The efficacy of these contraceptive methods, except sterilization, depends up on the reliability with which they are used. Correct and consistent use of methods can result in lower failure rates.

[See table I below]

In clinical trials with ORTHO-CYCLEN, 1,651 subjects completed 24,272 cycles and a total of 18 pregnancies were reported. This represents an overal use-efficacy (typical user efficacy) pregnancy rate of 0.96 per 100 women-years. This rate includes patients who did not take the drug correctly. In four clinical trials with ORTHO TRI-CYCLEN, the use-efficacy pregnancy rate ranged from 0.68 to 1.47 per 100 women-years. In total, 4,756 subjects completed 45,244 cycles and a total of 42 pregnancies were reported. This rep-

resents an overall use-efficacy rate of 1.21 per 100 women-years. One of these 4 studies was a randomized comparative clinical trial in which 4,633 subjects completed 22,312 cycles. Of the 2,312 patients on ORTHO TRI-CYCLEN, 8 pregnancies were reported. This represents an overall use-efficacy pregnancy rate of 0.94 per 100 women-years.

In two double-blind, placebo-controlled, six month, multicenter clinical trials, ORTHO TRI-CYCLEN showed a statistically significant decrease in inflammatory lesion count and total lesion count (Table II). The adverse reaction profile of ORTHO TRI-CYCLEN from these two controlled clinical trials is consistent with what has been noted from previous studies involving ORTHO TRI-CYCLEN and are the known risks associated with oral contraceptives.

TABLE II: Acne Vulgaris Indication Combined Results: Two Multicenter, Placebo-Controlled Trials Primary Efficacy Variables: Evaluable-for-Efficacy Population

	ORTHO TRI-CYCLEN®	Placebo
	N = 163	N = 161
Mean Age at Enrollment	27.3 years	28.0
Inflammatory Lesions– Mean Percent Reduction	56.6	36.6
Total Lesions– Mean Percent Reduction	49.6	30.3

CONTRAINDICATIONS

Oral contraceptives should not be used in women who currently have the following conditions:
- Thrombophlebitis or thromboembolic disorders
- A past history of deep vein thrombophlebitis or thromboembolic disorders
- Cerebral vascular or coronary artery disease
- Known or suspected carcinoma of the breast
- Carcinoma of the endometrium or other known or suspected estrogen-dependent neoplasia
- Undiagnosed abnormal genital bleeding
- Cholestatic jaundice of pregnancy or jaundice with prior pill use
- Hepatic adenomas or carcinomas
- Known or suspected pregnancy

WARNINGS

> Cigarette smoking increases the risk of serious cardiovascular side effects from oral contraceptive use. This risk increases with age and with heavy smoking (15 or more cigarettes per day) and is quite marked in women over 35 years of age. Women who use oral contraceptives should be strongly advised not to smoke.

The use of oral contraceptives is associated with increased risks of several serious conditions including myocardial infarction, thromboembolism, stroke, hepatic neoplasia, and gallbladder disease, although the risk of serious morbidity or mortality is very small in healthy women without underlying risk factors. The risk of morbidity and mortality increases significantly in the presence of other underlying risk factors such as hypertension, hyperlipidemias, obesity and diabetes.

Practitioners prescribing oral contraceptives should be familiar with the following information relating to these risks. The information contained in this package insert is principally based on studies carried out in patients who used oral contraceptives with higher formulations of estrogens and progestogens than those in common use today. The effect of long-term use of the oral contraceptives with lower formulations of both estrogens and progestogens remains to be determined.

Throughout this labeling, epidemiological studies reported are of two types: retrospective or case control studies and prospective or cohort studies. Case control studies provide a measure of the relative risk of a disease, namely, a *ratio* of the incidence of a disease among oral contraceptive users to that among nonusers. The relative risk doe not provide information on the actual clinical occurrence of a disease. Cohort studies provide a measure of attributable risk, which is the *difference* in the incidence of disease between oral contraceptive users and nonusers. The attributable risk does provide information about the actual occurrence of a disease in the population (adapted from refs. 2 and 3 with the author's permission). For further information, the reader is referred to a text on epidemiological methods.

1. THROMBOEMBOLIC DISORDERS AND OTHER VASCULAR PROBLEMS
a. Myocardial Infarction
An increased risk of myocardial infarction has been attributed to oral contraceptive use. This risk is primarily in

TABLE I: PERCENTAGE OF WOMEN EXPERIENCING AN UNINTENDED PREGNANCY DURING THE FIRST YEAR OF TYPICAL USE AND THE FIRST YEAR OF PERFECT USE OF CONTRACEPTION AND THE PERCENTAGE CONTINUING USE AT THE END OF THE FIRST YEAR, UNITED STATES.

Method (1)	% of Women Experiencing an Unintended Pregnancy within the First Year of Use Typical Use[1] (2)	Perfect Use[2] (3)	% of Women Continuing Use at One Year[3] (4)
Chance [4]	85	85	
Spermicides[5]	26	6	40
Periodic abstinence	25		63
Calendar		9	
Ovulation Method		3	
Sympto-Thermal[6]		2	
Post-Ovulation		1	
Withdrawal	19	4	
Cap[7]			
Parous Women	40	26	42
Nulliparous Women	20	9	56
Sponge			
Parous Women	40	20	42
Nulliparous Women	20	9	56
Diaphragm[7]	20	6	56
Condom[8]			
Female (Reality)	21	5	56
Male	14	3	61
Pill	5		71
Progestin Only		0.5	
Combined		0.1	
IUD			
Progesterone T	2.0	1.5	81
Copper T380A	0.8	0.6	78
LNg 20	0.1	0.1	81
Depo-Provera	0.3	0.3	70
Norplant and Norplant-2	0.05	0.05	88
Female Sterilization	0.5	0.5	100
Male Sterilization	0.15	0.10	100

Adapted from Hatcher et al., 1998 Ref. #1.
[1]Among typical couples who initiate use of a method (not necessarily for the first time), the percentage who experience an accidental pregnancy during the first year if they do not stop use for any other reason.
[2]Among couples who initiate use of a method (not necessarily for the first time) and who use it perfectly (both consistently and correctly), the percentage who experience an accidental pregnancy during the first year if they do not stop use for any other reason.
[3]Among couples attempting to avoid pregnancy, the percentage who continue to use a method for one year.
[4]The percents becoming pregnant in columns (2) and (3) are based on data from populations where contraception is not used and from women who cease using contraception in order to become pregnant. Among such populations, about 89% become pregnant within one year. This estimate was lowered slightly (to 85%) to represent the percent who would become pregnant within one year among women now relying on reversible methods of contraception if they abandoned contraception altogether.
[5]Foams, creams, gels, vaginal suppositories, and vaginal film.
[6]Cervical mucus (ovulation) method supplemented by calendar in the pre-ovulatory and basal body temperature in the post-ovulatory phases.
[7]With spermicidal cream or jelly.
[8]Without spermicides.

smokers or women with other underlying risk factors for coronary artery disease such as hypertension, hypercholesterolemia, morbid obesity, and diabetes. The relative risk of heart attack for current oral contraceptive users has been estimated to be two to six.[4-10] The risk is very low under the age of 30.

Smoking in combination with oral contraceptive use has been shown to contribute substantially to the incidence of myocardial infarctions in women in their mid-thirties or older with smoking accounting for the majority of excess cases.[11] Mortality rates associated with circulatory disease have been shown to increase substantially in smokers, especially in those 35 years of age and older among women who use oral contraceptives.

CIRCULATORY DISEASE MORTALITY RATES PER 100,000 WOMAN-YEARS
BY AGE, SMOKING STATUS AND ORAL CONTRACEPTIVE USE

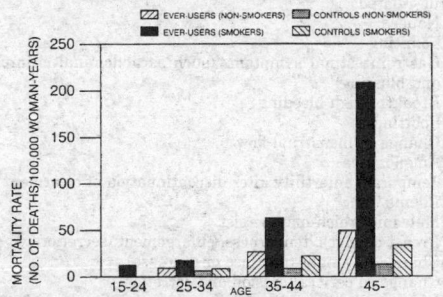

TABLE III. (Adapted from P.M. Layde and V. Beral, ref. #12.)

Oral contraceptives may compound the effects of well-known risk factors, such as hypertension, diabetes, hyperlipidemias, age and obesity.[13] In particular, some progestogens are known to decrease HDL cholesterol and cause glucose intolerance, while estrogens may create a state of hyperinsulinism.[14-18] Oral contraceptives have been shown to increase blood pressure among users (see Section 9 in WARNINGS). Similar effects on risk factors have been associated with an increased risk of heart disease. Oral contraceptives must be used with caution in women with cardiovascular disease risk factors.

Norgestimate has minimal androgenic activity (see CLINICAL PHARMACOLOGY), and there is some evidence that the risk of myocardial infarction associated with oral contraceptives is lower when the progestogen has minimal androgenic activity than when the activity is greater[97].

b. Thromboembolism

An increased risk of thromboembolic and thrombotic disease associated with the use of oral contraceptives is well established. Case control studies have found the relative risk of users compared to nonusers to be 3 for the first episode of superficial venous thrombosis, 4 to 11 for deep vein thrombosis or pulmonary embolism, and 1.5 to 6 for women with predisposing conditions for venous thromboembolic disease.[2,3,19-24] Cohort studies have shown the relative risk to be somewhat lower, about 3 for new cases and about 4.5 for new cases requiring hospitalization.[25] The risk of thromboembolic disease associated with oral contraceptives is not related to length of use and disapears after pill use is stopped.[2]

A two- to four-fold increase in relative risk of post-operative thromboembolic complications has been reported with the use of oral contraceptives.[9] The relative risk of venous thrombosis in women who have predisposing conditions is twice that of women without such medical conditions.[26] If feasible, oral contraceptives should be discontinued at least four weeks prior to and for two weeks after elective surgery of a type associated with an increase in risk of thromboembolism and during and following prolonged immobilization. Since the immediate postpartum period is also associated with an increased risk of thromboembolism, oral contraceptives should be started no earlier than four weeks after delivery in women who elect not to breast feed or four weeks after a second trimester abortion.

c. Cerebrovascular diseases

Oral contraceptives have been shown to increase both the relative and attributable risks of cerebrovascular events (thrombotic and hemorrhagic strokes), although, in general, the risk is greatest among older (>35 years), hypertensive women who also smoke. Hypertension was found to be a risk factor for both users and nonusers, for both types of strokes, and smoking interacted to increase the risk of stroke.[27-29]

In a large study, the relative risk of thrombotic strokes has been shown to range from 3 or normotensive users to 14 for users with severe hypertension.[30] The relative risk of hemorrhagic stroke is reported to be 1.2 for non-smokers who used oral contraceptives, 2.6 for smokers who did not use oral contraceptives, 7.6 for smokers who used oral contraceptives, 1.8 for normotensive users and 25.7 for users with severe hypertension.[30] The attributable risk is also greater in older women.[3]

TABLE IV: ANNUAL NUMBER OF BIRTH-RELATED OR METHOD-RELATED DEATHS ASSOCIATED WITH CONTROL OF FERTILITY PER 100,000 NON-STERILE WOMEN, BY FERTILITY CONTROL METHOD ACCORDING TO AGE

Method of control and outcome	15–19	20–24	25–29	30–34	35–39	40–44
No fertility control methods*	7.0	7.4	9.1	14.8	25.7	28.2
Oral contraceptives non-smoker**	0.3	0.5	0.9	1.9	13.8	31.6
Oral contraceptives smoker**	2.2	3.4	6.6	13.5	51.1	117.2
IUD**	0.8	0.8	1.0	1.0	1.4	1.4
Condom*	1.1	1.6	0.7	0.2	0.3	0.4
Diaphragm/ spermicide*	1.9	1.2	1.2	1.3	2.2	2.8
Periodic abstinence*	2.5	1.6	1.6	1.7	2.9	3.6

*Deaths are birth-related
**Deaths are method-related

Adapted from H.W. Ory, ref. #35.

d. Dose-related risk of vascular disease from oral contraceptives

A positive association has been observed between the amount of estrogen and progestogen in oral contraceptives and the risk of vascular disese.[31-33] A decline in serum high density lipoproteins (HDL) has been reported with many progestational agents.[14-16] A decline in serum high density lipoproteins has been associated with an increased incidence of ischemic heart disease. Because estrogens increase HDL cholesterol, the net efect or an oral contraceptive depends on a balance achieved between doses of estrogen and progestogen and the activity of the progestogen used in the contraceptives. The activity and amount of both hormones should be considered in the choice of an oral contraceptive. Minimizing exposure to estrogen and progestogen is in keeping with good principles of therapeutics. For any particular estrogen/progestogen combination, the dosage regimen prescribed should be one which contains the least amount of estrogen and progestogen that is compatible with a low failure rate and the needs of the individual patient. New acceptors of oral contraceptive agents should be started on preparations containing 0.035 mg or less of estrogen.

e. Persistence of risk of vascular disease

There are two studies which have shown persistence of risk of vascular disease for ever-users of oral contraceptives. In a study in the United States, the risk of developing myocardial infarction after discontinuing oral contraceptives persists for at least 9 years for women 40–49 years who had used oral contraceptives for five or more years, but this increased risk was not demonstrated in other age groups.[8] In another study in Great Britain, the risk of developing cerebrovascular disease persisted for at least 6 years after discontinuation of oral contraceptives, although excess risk was very small.[34] However, both studies were performed with oral contraceptive formulations containing 50 micrograms or higher of estrogens.

2. ESTIMATES OF MORTALITY FROM CONTRACEPTIVE USE

One study gathered data from a variety of sources which have estimated the mortality rate associated with different methods of contraception at different ages (Table IV). These estimates include the combined risk of death associated with contraceptive methods plus the risk attributable to pregnancy in the event of method failure. Each method of contraception has its specific benefits and risks. The study concluded that with the exception of oral contraceptive users 35 and older who smoke, and 40 and older who do not smoke, mortality associated with all methods of birth control is low and below that associated with childbirth. The observation of an increase in risk of mortality with age for oral contraceptive users is based on data gathered in the 1970's.[35] Current clinical recommendations involves the use of lower estrogen dose formulations and a careful consideration of risk factors. In 1989, the Fertility and Maternal Health Drugs Advisory Committee was asked to review the use of oral contraceptives in women 40 years of age and over. The Committee concluded that although cardiovascular disease risks may be increased with oral contraceptive use after age 40 in healthy non-smoking women (even with the newer low-dose formulations), there are also greater potential health risks associated with pregnancy in older women and with the alternative surgical and medical procedures which may be necessary if such women do not have access to effective and acceptable means of contraception. The Committee recommended that the benefits of low-dose oral contraceptive use by healthy non-smoking women over 40 may outweigh the possible risks.

Of course, older women, as all women, who take oral contraceptives, should take an oral contraceptive which contains the least amount of estrogen and progestogen that is compatible with a low failure rate and individual patient needs.

[See table IV above]

3. CARCINOMA OF THE REPRODUCTIVE ORGANS AND BREASTS

Numerous epidemiological studies have been performed on the incidence of breast, endometrial, ovarian, and cervical cancer in women using oral contraceptives. While there are conflicting reports, most studies suggest that use of oral contraceptives is not associated with an overall increase in the risk of developing breast cancer. Some studies have reported an increased relative risk of developing breast cancer, particularly at a younger age. This increased relative risk has been reported to be related to duration of use.[36-44,79-89]

A meta-analysis of 54 studies found a small increase in the frequency of having breast cancer diagnosed for women who were currently using combined oral contraceptives or had used them within the past ten years. This increase in the frequency of breast cancer diagnosis, within ten years of stopping use, was generally accounted for by cancers localized to the breast. There was no increase in the frequency of having breast cancer diagnosed ten or more years after cessation of use.[95]

Some studies suggest that oral contraceptive use has been associated with an increase in the risk of cervical intraepithelial neoplasia in some populations of women.[45-48] However, there continues to be controversy about the extent to which such findings may be due to differences in sexual behavior and other factors.

4. HEPATIC NEOPLASIA

Benign hepatic adenomas are associated with oral contraceptive use, although the incidence of benign tumors is rare in the United States. Indirect calculations have estimated the attributable risk to be in the range of 3.3 cases/100,000 for users, a risk that increases after four or more years of use especially with oral contraceptives of higher dose.[49] Rupture of benign, hepatic adenomas may cause death through intra-abdominal hemorrhage.[50,51] Studies have shown an increased risk of developing hepatocellular carcinoma[52-54, 96] in oral contraceptive users. However, these cancers are rare in the U.S.

5. OCULAR LESIONS

There have been clinical case reports of retinal thrombosis associated with the use of oral contraceptives. Oral contraceptives should be discontinued if there is unexplained partial or complete loss of vision; onset of proptosis or diplopia; papilledema; or retinal vascular lesions. Appropriate diagnostic and therapeutic measures should be undertaken immediately.

6. ORAL CONTRACEPTIVE USE BEFORE OR DURING EARLY PREGNANCY

Extensive epidemiological studies have revealed no increased risk of birth defects in women who have used oral contraceptives prior to pregnancy.[56,57] The majority of recent studies also do not indicate a teratogenic effect, particularly in so far as cardiac anomalies and limb reduction defects are concerned,[55,56,58,59] when taken inadvertently during early pregnancy.

The administration of oral contraceptives to induce withdrawal bleeding should not be used as a test for pregnancy. Oral contraceptives should not be used during pregnancy to treat threatened or habitual abortion.

Continued on next page

Ortho Tri-Cyclen—Cont.

It is recommended that for any patient who has missed two consecutive periods, pregnancy should be ruled out before continuing oral contraceptive use. If the patient has not adhered to the prescribed schedule, the possibility of pregnancy should be considered at the time of the first missed period. Oral contraceptive use should be discontinued until pregnancy is ruled out.

7. GALLBLADDER DISEASE
Earlier studies have reported an increased lifetime relative risk of gallbladder surgery in users of oral contraceptives and estrogens.[60,61] More recent studies, however, have shown that the relative risk of developing gallbladder disease among oral contraceptive users may be minimal.[62–64] The recent findings of minimal risk may be related to the use of oral contraceptive formulations containing lower hormonal doses of estrogens and progestogens.

8. CARBOHYDRATE AND LIPID METABOLIC EFFECTS
Oral contraceptives have been shown to cause a decrease in glucose tolerance in a significant percentage of users.[17] This effect has been shown to be directly related to estrogen dose.[65] Progestogens increase insulin secretion and create insulin resistance, this effect varying with different progestational agents.[17,66] However, in the non-diabetic woman, oral contraceptives appear to have no effect on fasting blood glucose.[67] Because of these demonstrated effects, prediabetic and diabetic women in particular should be carefully monitored while taking oral contraceptives.

A small proportion of women will have persistent hypertriglyceridemia while on the pill. As discussed earlier (see WARNINGS 1a and 1d), changes in serum triglycerides and lipoprotein levels have been reported in oral contraceptive users.

In clinical studies with ORTHO-CYCLEN there were no clinically significant changes in fasting blood glucose levels. No statistically significant changes in mean fasting blood glucose levels were observed over 24 cycles of use. Glucose tolerance tests showed minimal, clinically insignificant changes from baseline to cycles 3, 12, and 24.

In clinical studies with ORTHO TRI-CYCLEN there were no clinically significant changes in fasting blood glucose levels. Minimal statistically significant changes were noted in glucose levels over 24 cycles of use. Glucose tolerance tests showed no clinically significant changes from baseline to cycles 3, 12, and 24.

9. ELEVATED BLOOD PRESSURE
An increase in blood pressure has been reported in women taking oral contraceptives[68] and this increase is more likely in older oral contraceptive users[69] and with extended duration of use.[61] Data from the Royal College of General Practitioners[12] and subsequent randomized trials have shown that the incidence of hypertension increases with increasing progestational activity.

Women with a history of hypertension or hypertension-related diseases, or renal disease[70] should be encouraged to use another method of contraception. If women elect to use oral contraceptives, they should be monitored closely and if significant elevation of blood pressure occurs, oral contraceptives should be discontinued. For most women, elevated blood pressure will return to normal after stopping oral contraceptives, and there is no difference in the occurrence of hypertension between former and never users.[68–71] It should be noted that in two separate large clinical trials (N = 633 and N = 911), no statistically significant changes in mean blood pressure were observed with ORTHO-CYCLEN.

10. HEADACHE
The onset or exacerbation of migraine or development of headache with a new pattern which is recurrent, persistent or severe requires discontinuation of oral contraceptives and evaluation of the cause.

11. BLEEDING IRREGULARITIES
Breakthrough bleeding and spotting are sometimes encountered in patients on oral contraceptives, especially during the first three months of use. Non-hormonal causes should be considered and adequate diagnostic measures taken to rule out malignancy or pregnancy in the event of breakthrough bleeding, as in the case of any abnormal vaginal bleeding. If pathology has been excluded, time or a change to another formulation may solve the problem. In the event of amenorrhea, pregnancy should be ruled out.

Some women may encounter post-pill amenorrhea or oligomenorrhea, especially when such a condition was preexistent.

12. ECTOPIC PREGNANCY
Ectopic as well as intrauterine pregnancy may occur in contraceptive failures.

PRECAUTIONS
1. PHYSICAL EXAMINATION AND FOLLOW UP
It is good medical practice for all women to have annual history and physical examinations, including women using oral contraceptives. The physical examination, however, may be deferred until after initiation of oral contraceptives if requested by the woman and judged appropriate by the clinician. The physical examination should include special reference to blood pressure, breasts, abdomen and pelvic organs, including cervical cytology, and relevant laboratory tests. In case of undiagnosed, persistent or recurrent abnormal vaginal bleeding, appropriate measures should be conducted to rule out malignancy. Women with a strong family history of breast cancer or who have breast nodules should be monitored with particular care.

2. LIPID DISORDERS
Women who are being treated for hyperlipidemias should be followed closely if they elect to use oral contraceptives. Some progestogens may elevate LDL levels and may render the control of hyperlipidemias more difficult.

3. LIVER FUNCTION
If jaundice develops in any woman receiving such drugs, the medication should be discontinued. Steroid hormones may be poorly metabolized in patients with impaired liver function.

4. FLUID RETENTION
Oral contraceptives may cause some degree of fluid retention. They should be prescribed with caution, and only with careful monitoring, in patients with conditions which might be aggravated by fluid retention.

5. EMOTIONAL DISORDERS
Women with a history of depression should be carefully observed and the drug discontinued if depression recurs to a serious degree.

6. CONTACT LENSES
Contact lens wearers who develop visual changes or changes in lens tolerance should be assessed by an ophthalmologist.

7. DRUG INTERACTIONS
Reduced efficacy and increased incidence of breakthrough bleeding and menstrual irregularities have been associated with concomitant use of rifampin. A similar association, though less marked, has been suggested with barbiturates, phenylbutazone, phenytoin sodium, carbamazepine, and possibly with griseofulvin, ampicillin and tetracyclines.[72]

8. INTERACTIONS WITH LABORATORY TESTS
Certain endocrine and liver function tests and blood components may be affected by oral contraceptives:

a. Increased prothrombin and factors VII, VIII, IX, and X; decreased antithrombin 3; increased norepinephrine-induced platelet aggregability.

b. Increased thyroid binding globulin (TBG) leading to increased circulation total thyroid hormone, as measured by protein-bound iodine (PBI), T4 by column or by radioimmunoassay. Free T3 resin uptake is decreased, reflecting the elevated TBG, free T4 concentration is unaltered.

c. Other binding proteins may be elevated in serum.

d. Sex hormone binding globulins are increased and result in elevated levels of total circulating sex steroids; however, free or biologically active levels either decrease or remain unchanged.

e. High-density lipoprotein (HDL-C) and total cholesterol (Total-C) may be increased, low-density lipoprotein (LDL-C) may be increased or decreased, while LDL-C/HDL-C ratio may be decreased and triglycerides may be unchanged.

f. Glucose tolerance may be decreased.

g. Serum folate levels may be depressed by oral contraceptive therapy. This may be of clinical significance if a woman becomes pregnant shortly after discontinuing oral contraceptives.

9. CARCINOGENESIS
See WARNINGS Section.

10. PREGNANCY
Pregnancy Category X. See CONTRAINDICATIONS and WARNINGS Sections.

11. NURSING MOTHERS
Small amounts of oral contraceptive steroids have been identified in the milk of nursing mothers and a few adverse effects on the child have been reported, including jaundice and breast enlargement. In addition, combination oral contraceptives given in the postpartum period may interfere with lactation by decreasing the quantity and quality of breast milk. If possible, the nursing mother should be advised not to use combination oral contraceptives but to use other forms of contraception until she has completely weaned her child.

12. PEDIATRIC USE
Safety and efficacy of ORTHO-CYCLEN Tablets and ORTHO TRI-CYCLEN Tablets has been established in women of reproductive age. Safety and efficacy are expected to be the same for postpubertal adolescents under the age of 16 and for users 16 years and older. Use of this product before menarche is not indicated.

13. SEXUALLY TRANSMITTED DISEASES
Patients should be counseled that this product does not protect against HIV infection (AIDS) and other sexually transmitted diseases.

INFORMATION FOR THE PATIENT
See Patient Labeling printed below.

ADVERSE REACTIONS
An increased risk of the following serious adverse reactions has been associated with the use of oral contraceptives (See WARNINGS Section).

- Thrombophlebitis and venous thrombosis with or without embolism
- Arterial thromboembolism
- Pulmonary embolism
- Myocardial infarction
- Cerebral hemorrhage
- Cerebral thrombosis
- Hypertension
- Gallbladder disease
- Hepatic adenomas or benign liver tumors

The following adverse reactions have been reported in patients receiving oral contraceptives and are believed to be drug-related:

- Nausea
- Vomiting
- Gastrointestinal symptoms (such as abdominal cramps and bloating)
- Breakthrough bleeding
- Spotting
- Change in menstrual flow
- Amenorrhea
- Temporary infertility after discontinuation of treatment
- Edema
- Melasma which may persist
- Breast changes: tenderness, enlargement, secretion
- Change in weight (increase or decrease)
- Change in cervical erosion and secretion
- Diminution in lactation when given immediately postpartum
- Cholestatic jaundice
- Migraine
- Rash (allergic)
- Mental depression
- Reduced tolerance to carbohydrates
- Vaginal candidiasis
- Change in corneal curvature (steepening)
- Intolerance to contact lenses

The following adverse reactions have been reported in users of oral contraceptives and the association has been neither confirmed nor refuted:

- Pre-menstrual syndrome
- Cataracts
- Changes in appetite
- Cystitis-like syndrome
- Headache
- Nervousness
- Dizziness
- Hirsutism
- Loss of scalp hair
- Erythema multiforme
- Erythema nodosum
- Hemorrhagic eruption
- Vaginitis
- Porphyria
- Impaired renal function
- Hemolytic uremic syndrome
- Acne
- Changes in libido
- Colitis
- Budd-Chiari Syndrome

OVERDOSAGE
Serious ill effects have not been reported following acute ingestion of large doses of oral contraceptives by young children. Overdosage may cause nausea and withdrawal bleeding may occur in females.

NON-CONTRACEPTIVE HEALTH BENEFITS
The following non-contraceptive health benefits related to the use of combination oral contraceptives are supported by epidemiological studies which largely utilized oral contraceptive formulations containing estrogen doses exceeding 0.035 mg of ethinyl estradiol or 0.05 mg mestranol.[73–78]

Effects on menses:
- increased menstrual cycle regularity
- decreased blood loss and decreased incidence of iron deficiency anemia
- decreased incidence of dysmenorrhea

Effects related to inhibition of ovulation:
- decreased incidence of functional ovarian cysts
- decreased incidence of ectopic pregnancies

Other effects:
- decreased incidence of fibroadenomas and fibrocystic disease of the breast
- decreased incidence of acute pelvic inflammatory disease
- decreased incidence of endometrial cancer
- decreased incidence of ovarian cancer

DOSAGE AND ADMINISTRATION
ORAL CONTRACEPTION
To achieve maximum contraceptive effectiveness, ORTHO TRI-CYCLEN Tablets and ORTHO-CYCLEN Tablets must be taken exactly as directed and at intervals not exceeding

24 hours. ORTHO TRI-CYCLEN and ORTHO-CYCLEN are available in the DIALPAK® Tablet Dispenser which is preset for a Sunday Start. Day 1 Start is also provided.

21-Day Regimen (Sunday Start)

When taking ORTHO TRI-CYCLEN □ 21 and ORTHO-CYCLEN □ 21, the first tablet should be taken on the first Sunday after menstruation begins. If period begins on Sunday, the first tablet is taken on that day. One tablet is taken daily for 21 days. For subsequent cycles, no tablets are taken for 7 days, then a tablet is taken the next day (Sunday). For the first cycle of a Sunday Start regimen, another method of contraception should be used until after the first 7 consecutive days of administration.

If the patient misses one (1) active tablet in Weeks 1, 2, or 3, the tablet should be taken as soon as she remembers. If the patient misses two (2) active tablets in Week 1 or Week 2, the patient should take two (2) tablets the day she remembers and two (2) tablets the next day; and then continue taking one (1) tablet a day until she finishes the pack. The patient should be instructed to use a back-up method of birth control if she has sex in the seven (7) days after missing pills. If the patient misses two (2) active tablets in the third week or misses three (3) or more active tablets in a row, the patient should continue taking one tablet every day until Sunday. On Sunday the patient should throw out the rest of the pack and start a new pack that same day. The patient should be instructed to use a back-up method of birth control if she has sex in the seven (7) days after missing pills.

Complete instructions to facilitate patient counseling on proper pill usage may be found in the Detailed Patient Labeling ("How to Take the Pill" section).

21-Day Regimen (Day 1 Start)

The dosage of ORTHO TRI-CYCLEN □ 21 and ORTHO-CYCLEN □ 21, for the initial cycle of therapy is one tablet administered daily from the 1st day through the 21st day of the menstrual cycle, counting the first day of menstrual flow as "Day 1." For subsequent cycles, no tablets are taken for 7 days, then a new course is started of one tablet a day for 21 days. The dosage regimen then continues with 7 days of no medication, followed by 21 days of medication, instituting a three-weeks-on, one-week-off dosage regimen.

If the patient misses one (1) active tablet in Weeks 1, 2, or 3, the tablet should be taken as soon as she remembers. If the patient misses two (2) active tablets in Week 1 or Week 2, the patient should take two (2) tablets the day she remembers and two (2) tablets the next day; and then continue taking one (1) tablet a day until she finishes the pack. The patient should be instructed to use a back-up method of birth control if she has sex in the seven (7) days after missing pills. If the patient misses two (2) active tablets in the third week or misses three (3) or more active tablets in a row, the patient should throw out the rest of the pack and start a new pack that same day. The patient should be instructed to use a back-up method of birth control if she has sex in the seven (7) days after missing pills.

Complete instructions to facilitate patient counseling on proper pill usage may be found in the Detailed Patient Labeling ("How to Take the Pill" section).

28-Day Regimen (Sunday Start)

When taking ORTHO TRI-CYCLEN □ 28 and ORTHO-CYCLEN □ 28 the first tablet should be taken on the first Sunday after menstruation begins. If period begins on Sunday, the first tablet should be taken that day. Take one active tablet daily for 21 days followed by one green tablet daily for 7 days. After 28 tablets have been taken, a new course is started the next day (Sunday). For the first cycle of a Sunday Start regimen, another method of contraception should be used until after the first 7 consecutive days of administration.

If the patient misses one (1) active tablet in Weeks 1, 2, or 3, the tablet should be taken as soon as she remembers. If the patient misses two (2) active tablets in Week 1 or Week 2, the patient should take two (2) tablets the day she remembers and two (2) tablets the next day; and then continue taking one (1) tablet a day until she finishes the pack. The patient should be instructed to use a back-up method of birth control if she has sex in the seven (7) days after missing pills. If the patient misses two (2) active tablets in the third week or misses three (3) or more active tablets in a row, the patient should continue taking one tablet every day until Sunday. On Sunday the patient should throw out the rest of the pack and start a new pack that same day. The patient should be instructed to use a back-up method of birth control if she has sex in the seven (7) days after missing pills.

Complete instructions, to facilitate patient counseling on proper pill usage may be found in the Detailed Patient Labeling ("How to Take the Pill" section).

28-Day Regimen (Day 1 Start)

The dosage of ORTHO TRI-CYCLEN □ 28 and ORTHO-CYCLEN □ 28, for the initial cycle of therapy is one active tablet administered daily from the 1st day through the 21st day of the menstrual cycle, counting the first day of menstrual flow as "Day 1" followed by one green tablet daily for 7 days. Tablets are taken without interruption for 28 days. After 28 tablets have been taken, a new course is started the next day.

If the patient misses one (1) active tablet in Weeks 1, 2, or 3, the tablet should be taken as soon as she remembers. If the patient misses two (2) active tablets in Week 1 or Week 2, the patient should take two (2) tablets the day she remembers and two (2) tablets the next day; and then continue taking one (1) tablet a day until she finishes the pack. The patient should be instructed to use a back-up method of birth control if she has sex in the seven (7) days after missing pills. If the patient misses two (2) active tablets in the third week or misses three (3) or more active tablets in a row, the patient should throw out the rest of the pack and start a new pack that same day. The patient should be instructed to use a back-up method of birth control if she has sex in the seven (7) days after missing pills.

Complete instructions to facilitate patient counseling on proper pill usage may be found in the Detailed Patient Labeling ("How to Take the Pill" section).

The use of ORTHO TRI-CYCLEN and ORTHO-CYCLEN for contraception may be initiated 4 weeks postpartum in women who elect not to breast feed. When the tablets are administered during the postpartum period, the increased risk of thromboembolic disease associated with the postpartum period must be considered. (See CONTRAINDICATIONS and WARNINGS concerning thromboembolic disease. See also PRECAUTIONS for "Nursing Mothers.") The possibility of ovulation and conception prior to initiation of medication should be considered.

(See Discussion of Dose-Related Risk of Vascular Disease from Oral Contraceptives.)

ADDITIONAL INSTRUCTIONS FOR ALL DOSING REGIMENS

Breakthrough bleeding, spotting, and amenorrhea are frequent reasons for patients discontinuing oral contraceptives. In breakthrough bleeding, as in all cases of irregular bleeding from the vagina, nonfunctional causes should be borne in mind. In undiagnosed persistent or recurrent abnormal bleeding from the vagina, adequate diagnostic measures are indicated to rule out pregnancy or malignancy. If pathology has been excluded, time or a change to another formulation may solve the problem. Changing to an oral contraceptive with a higher estrogen content, while potentially useful in minimizing menstrual irregularity, should be done only if necessary since this may increase the risk of thromboembolic disease.

Use of oral contraceptives in the event of a missed menstrual period:

1. If the patient has not adhered to the prescribed schedule, the possibility of pregnancy should be considered at the time of the first missed period and oral contraceptive use should be discontinued until pregnancy is ruled out.
2. If the patient has adhered to the prescribed regimen and misses two consecutive periods, pregnancy should be ruled out before continuing oral contraceptive use.

ACNE

The timing of initiation of dosing with ORTHO TRI-CYCLEN for acne should follow the guidelines for use of ORTHO TRI-CYCLEN as an oral contraceptive. **Consult the DOSAGE AND ADMINISTRATION section for oral contraceptives.** The dosage regimen for ORTHO TRI-CYCLEN for treatment of facial acne, as available in a DIALPAK® Tablet Dispenser, utilizes a 21-day active and a 7-day placebo schedule. Take one active tablet daily for 21 days followed by one green tablet for 7 days. After 28 tablets have been taken, a new course is started the next day.

HOW SUPPLIED

ORTHO TRI-CYCLEN □ 21 Tablets are available in a DIALPAK® Tablet Dispenser (NDC 0062-1902-15) containing 21 tablets. Each white tablet contains 0.180 mg of the progestational compound, norgestimate, together with 0.035 mg of the estrogenic compound, ethinyl estradiol. Each light blue tablet contains 0.215 mg of the progestational compound, norgestimate, together with 0.035 mg of the estrogenic compound, ethinyl estradiol. Each blue tablet contains 0.250 mg of the progestational compound, norgestimate, together with 0.035 mg of the estrogenic compound, ethinyl estradiol.

The white tablets are unscored, with "Ortho" and "180" debossed on each side; the light blue tablets are unscored with "Ortho" and "215" debossed on each side; the blue tablets are unscored with "Ortho" and "250" debossed on each side.

ORTHO TRI-CYCLEN □ 21 Tablets are available for clinic usage in a VERIDATE® Tablet Dispenser (unfilled) and VERIDATE Refills (NDC 0062-1902-20).

ORTHO TRI-CYCLEN □ 28 Tablets are available in a DIALPAK® Tablet Dispenser (NDC 0062-1903-15) containing 28 tablets. Each white tablet contains 0.180 mg of the progestational compound, norgestimate, together with 0.035 mg of the estrogenic compound, ethinyl estradiol. Each light blue tablet contains 0.215 mg of the progestational compound, norgestimate, together with 0.035 mg of the estrogenic compound, ethinyl estradiol. Each blue tablet contains 0.250 mg of the progestational compound, norgestimate, together with 0.035 mg of the estrogenic compound, ethinyl estradiol. Each green tablet contains inert ingredients.

The white tablets are unscored, with "Ortho" and "180" debossed on each side; the light blue tablets are unscored with "Ortho" and "215" debossed on each side; the blue tablets are unscored with "Ortho" and "250" debossed on each side.

ORTHO TRI-CYCLEN □ 28 Tablets are available for clinic usage in a VERIDATE® Tablet Dispenser (unfilled) and VERIDATE Refills (NDC 0062-1903-20).

ORTHO CYCLEN □ 21 Tablets are available in a DIALPAK® Tablet Dispenser (NDC 0062-1900-15) containing 21 tablets. Each blue tablet contains 0.250 mg of the progestational compound, norgestimate, together with 0.035 mg of the estrogenic compound, ethinyl estradiol which are unscored with "Ortho" and "250" debossed on each side.

ORTHO CYCLEN □ 21 Tablets are available for clinic usage in a VERIDATE® Tablet Dispenser (unfilled) and VERIDATE Refills (NDC 0062-1900-20).

ORTHO CYCLEN □ 28 Tablets are available in a DIALPAK® Tablet Dispenser (NDC 0062-1901-15) containing 28 tablets as follows: 21 blue tablets as described under ORTHO CYCLEN □ 21 Tablets, and 7 green tablets containing inert ingredients.

ORTHO CYCLEN □ 28 Tablets are available for clinic usage in a VERIDATE® Tablet Dispenser (unfilled) and VERIDATE Refills (NDC 0062-1901-20).

Rx only.

REFERENCES

1. Trussel J. Contraceptive efficacy. In Hatcher RA, Trussel J, Stewart F, Cates W, Stewart GK, Kowal D, Guest F, Contraceptive Technology: Seventeenth Revised Edition. New York NY: Irvington Publishers, 1998, in press. **2.** Stadel BV, Oral contraceptives and cardiovascular disease. (Pt. 1). N Engl J Med 1981; 305:612-618. **3.** Stadel BV, Oral contraceptives and cardiovascular disease. (Pt. 2). N Engl J Med 1981; 305:672-677. **4.** Adam SA, Thorogood M. Oral contraception and myocardial infarction revisited: the effects of new preparations and prescribing patterns. Br J Obstet Gynaecol 1981; 88:838-845. **5.** Mann JI, Inman WH. Oral contraceptives and death from myocardial infarction. Br Med J 1975; 2(5965):245-248. **6.** Mann JI, Vessey MP, Thorogood M, Doll R. Myocardial infarction in young women with special reference to oral contraceptive practice. Br Med J 1975; 2(5956):241-245. **7.** Royal College of General Practitioners' Oral Contraception Study: further analyses of mortality in oral contraceptive users. Lancet 1981; 1:541-546. **8.** Slone D, Shapiro S, Kaufman DW, Rosenberg L, Miettinen OS, Stolley PD. Risk of myocardial infarction in relation to current and discontinued use of oral contraceptives. N Engl J Med 1981; 305:420-424. **9.** Vessey MP. Female hormones and vascular disease–an epidemiological overview. Br J Fam Plann 1980; 6 (Supplement): 1–12 **10.** Russell-Briefel RG, Ezzati TM, Fulwood R, Perlman JA, Murphy RS. Cardiovascular risk status and oral contraceptive use, United States, 1976–80. Prevent Med 1986; 15:352-362. **11.** Goldbaum GM, Kendrick JS, Hogelin GC, Gentry EM. The relative impact of smoking and oral contraceptive use on women in the United States. JAMA 1987; 258:1339-1342. **12.** Layde PM, Beral V. Further analyses of mortality in oral contraceptive users: Royal College of General Practitioners' Oral Contraception Study. (Table 5) Lancet 1981; 1:541-546. **13.** Knopp RH. Arteriosclerosis risk: the roles of oral contraceptives and postmenopausal estrogens. J Reprod Med 1986; 31(9)(Supplement): 913-921. **14.** Krauss RM, Roy S, Mishell DR, Casagrande J, Pike MC. Effects of two low-dose oral contraceptives on serum lipids and lipoproteins: Differential changes in high-density lipoproteins subclasses. Am J Obstet 1983; 145:446-452. **15.** Wahl P, Walden C, Knopp R, Hoover J, Wallace R, Heiss G, Rifkind B. Effect of estrogen-progestin potency on lipid/lipoprotein cholesterol. N Engl J Med 1983; 308:862-867. **16.** Wynn V, Niththyananthan R. The effect of progestin in combined oral contraceptives on serum lipids with special reference to high density lipoproteins. Am J Obstet Gynecol 1982; 142:766-771. **17.** Wynn V, Godsland I. Effects of oral contraceptives on carbohydrate metabolism. J Reprod Med 1986; 31(9)(Supplement):892-897. **18.** LaRosa JC. Atherosclerotic risk factors in cardiovascular disease. J Reprod Med 1986; 31(9)(Supplement): 906-912. **19.** Inman WH, Vessey MP. Investigation of death from pulmonary, coronary, and cerebral thrombosis and embolism in women of child-bearing age. Br Med J 1968; 2(5599):193-199. **20.** Maguire MG, Tonascia J, Startwell PE, Stolley PD, Tockman MS. Increased risk of thrombosis due to oral contraceptives: a further report. Am J Epidemiol 1979; 110(2):188-195. **21.** Petitti DB, Wingerd J, Pellegrin F, Ramacharan S. Risk of vascular disease in women: smoking, oral contraceptives, noncontraceptive estrogens, and other factors. JAMA 1979;242:1150-1154. **22.** Vessey MP, Doll R. Investigation of relation between use of oral contraceptives and thromboembolic disease. Br Med J 1968;2(5599):199-205. **23.** Vessey MP, Doll R. Investigation of relation between use of oral contraceptives and thromboembolic disease. A further report. Br Med J 1969; 2(5658): 651-657. **24.** Porter JB, Hunter JR, Danielson DA, Jick H. Stergachis A. Oral contraceptives and non-fatal vascular

Continued on next page

Ortho Tri-Cyclen—Cont.

disease–recent experience. Obstet Gynecol 1982; 59(3):299–302. **25.** Vessey M, Doll R, Peto R, Johnson B, Wiggins P. A long-term follow-up study of women using different methods of contraception: an interim report. J Biosocial Sci 1976; 8:375-427. **26.** Royal College of General Practitioners: Oral Contraceptives, venous thrombosis, and varicose veins. J Royal Coll Gen Pract 1978; 28:393-399. **27.** Collaborative Group for the Study of Stroke in Young Women: Oral contraception and increased risk of cerebral ischemia or thrombosis. N Engl J Med 1973; 288:871-878. **28.** Petitti DB, Wingerd J. Use of oral contraceptives, cigarette smoking, and risk of subarachnoid hemorrhage. Lancet 1978; 2:234-236. **29.** Inman WH. Oral contraceptives and fatal subarachnoid hemorrhage. Br Med J 1979; 2(6203):1468-1470. **30.** Collaborative Group for the Study of Stroke in Young Women: Oral Contraceptives and stroke in young women: associated risk factors. JAMA 1975; 231:718-722. **31.** Inman WH, Vessey MP, Westerholm B, Engelund A. Thromboembolic disease and the steroidal content of oral contraceptives. A report to the Committee on Safety of Drugs. Br Med J 1970;2:203-209. **32.** Meade TW, Greenberg G, Thompson SG. Progestogens and cardiovascular reactions associated with oral contraceptives and a comparison of the safety of 50- and 35-mcg oestrogen preparations. Br Med J 1980; 280(6224):1157-1161. **33.** Kay CR. Progestogens and arterial disease–evidence from the Royal College of General Practitioners' Study. Am J Obstet Gynecol 1982; 142:762-765. **34.** Royal College of General Practitioners: Incidence of arterial disease among oral contraceptive users. J Royal Coll Gen Pract 1983; 33:75-82. **35.** Ory HW. Mortality associated with fertility and fertility control: 1983. Family Planning Perspectives 1983; 15:50-56. **36.** The Cancer and Steroid Hormone Study of the Centers for Disease Control and the National Institute of Child Health and Human Development: Oral contraceptive use and the risk of breast cancer. N Engl J Med 1986; 315:405-411. **37.** Pike MC, Henderson BE, Krailo MD, Duke A, Roy S. Breast cancer in young women and use of oral contraceptives: possible modifying effect of formulation and age at use. Lancet 1983; 2:926-929. **38.** Paul C, Skegg DG, Spears GFS, Kaldor JM. Oral contraceptives and breast cancer: A national study. Br Med J 1986; 293:723-725. **39.** Miller DR, Rosenberg L, Kaufman DW, Schottenfeld D, Stolley PD, Shapiro S. Breast cancer risk in relation to early oral contraceptive use. Obstet Gynecol 1986; 68:863-868. **40.** Olson H, Olson KL, Moller TR, Ranstam J, Holm P. Oral contraceptive use and breast cancer in young women in Sweden (letter). Lancet 1985; 2:748-749. **41.** McPherson K, Vessey M, Neil A, Doll R, Jones L, Roberts M. Early contraceptive use and breast cancer: Results of another case-control study. Br J Cancer 1987; 56:653-660. **42.** Huggins GR, Zucker PF. Oral contraceptives and neoplasia: 1987 update. Fertil Steril 1987; 47:733-761. **43.** McPherson K, Drife JO. The pill and breast cancer: why the uncertainty? Br Med J 1986; 293:709-710. **44.** Shapiro S. Oral contraceptives–time to take stock. N Engl J Med 1987; 315: 450-451. **45.** Ory H, Naib Z, Conger SB, Hatcher RA, Tyler CW. Contraceptive choice and prevalence of cervical dysplasia and carcinoma in situ. Am J Obstet Gynecol 1976; 124: 573-577. **46.** Vessey MP, Lawless M, McPherson K, Yeates D. Neoplasia of the cervix uteri and contraception: a possible adverse effect of the pill. Lancet 1983; 2:930. **47.** Brinton LA, Huggins GR, Lehman HF, Malli K, Savitz DA, Trapido E, Rosenthal J, Hoover R. Long term use of oral contraceptives and risk of invasive cervical cancer. Int J Cancer 1986; 38:339-344. **48.** WHO Collaborative Study of Neoplasia and Steroid Contraceptives: Invasive cervical cancer and combined oral contraceptives. Br Med J 1985; 290:961-965. **49.** Rooks JB, Ory HW, Ishak KG, Strauss LT, Greenspan JR, Hill AP, Tyler CW. Epidemiology of hepatocellular adenoma: the role of oral contraceptive use. JAMA 1979; 242:644-648. **50.** Bein NN, Goldsmith HS. Recurrent massive hemorrhage from benign hepatic tumors secondary to oral contraceptives. Br J Surg 1977; 64:433-435. **51.** Klatskin G. Hepatic tumors: possible relationship to use of oral contraceptives. Gastroenterology 1977; 73:386-394. **52.** Henderson BE, Preston-Martin S, Edmondson HA, Peters RL, Pike MC. Hepatocellular carcinoma and oral contraceptives. Br J Cancer 1983; 48:437-440. **53.** Neuberger J, Forman D, Doll R, Williams R. Oral contraceptives and hepatocellular carcinoma. Br Med J 1986; 292:1355-1357. **54.** Forman D, Vincent TJ, Doll R. Cancer of the liver and oral contraceptives. Br Med J 1986; 292:1357-1361. **55.** Harlap S, Eldor J. Births following oral contraceptive failures. Obstet Gynecol 1980; 55:447-452. **56.** Savolainen E, Saksela E, Saxen L. Teratogenic hazards of oral contraceptives analyzed in a national malformation register. Am J Obstet Gynecol 1981; 140:521-524. **57.** Janerich DT, Piper JM, Glebatis DM. Oral contraceptives and birth defects. Am J Epidemiol 1980; 112:73-79. **58.** Ferencz C, Matanoski GM, Wilson PD, Rubin JD, Neill CA, Gutberlet R. Maternal hormone therapy and congenital heart disease. Teratology 1980; 21:225-239. **59.** Rothman KJ, Fyler DC, Goldblatt A, Kreidberg MB. Exogenous hormones and other drug exposures of children with congenital heart disease. Am J Epidemiol 1979; 109:433-439. **60.** Boston Collaborative Drug Surveillance Program: Oral contraceptives and venous thromboembolic disease, surgically confirmed gallbladder disease, and breast tumors. Lancet 1973; 1:1399-1404. **61.** Royal College of General Practitioners: Oral contraceptives and health. New York, Pittman 1974. **62.** Layde PM, Vessey MP, Yeates D. Risk of gallbladder disease: a cohort study of young women attending family planning clinics. J Epidemiol Community Health 1982; 36:274-278. **63.** Rome Group for Epidemiology and Prevention of Cholelithiasis (GREPCO): Prevalence of gallstone disease in an Italian adult female population. Am J Epidemiol 1984; 119:796-805. **64.** Storm BL, Tamragouri RT, Morse ML, Lazar EL, West SL, Stolley PD, Jones JK. Oral contraceptives and other risk factors for gallbladder disease. Clin Pharmacol Ther 1986; 39:335-341. **65.** Wynn V, Adams PW, Godsland IF, Melrose J, Niththyananthan R, Oakley NW, Seedj A. Comparison of effects of different combined oral contraceptive formulations on carbohydrate and lipid metabolism. Lancet 1979; 1:1045-1049. **66.** Wynn V. Effect of progesterone and progestins on carbohydrate metabolism. In: Progesterone and Progestin. Bardin CW, Milgrom E. Mauvis-Jarvis P. eds. New York, Raven Press 1983; pp. 395-410. **67.** Perlman JA, Roussell-Briefel RG, Ezzati TM, Lieberknecht G. Oral glucose tolerance and the potency of oral contraceptive progestogens. J Chronic Dis 1985; 38:857-864. **68.** Royal College of General Practitioners' Oral Contraception Study: Effect on hypertension and benign breast disease of progestogen component in combined oral contraceptives. Lancet 1977; 1:624. **69.** Fisch IR, Frank J. Oral contraceptives and blood pressure. JAMA 1977; 237:2499-2503. **70.** Laragh AJ. Oral contraceptive induced hypertension–nine years later. Am J Obstet Gynecol 1976; 126:141-147. **71.** Ramcharan S. Peritz E, Pellegrin FA, Williams WT. Incidence of hypertension in the Walnut Creek Contraceptive Drug Study cohort: In: Pharmacology of steroid contraceptive drugs. Garattini S, Berendes HW. eds. New York, Raven Press, 1977; pp. 277-288, (Monographs of the Mario Negri Institute for Pharmacological Research Milan.) **72.** Stockley I. Interactions with oral contraceptives. J Pharm 1976; 216: 140-143. **73.** The Cancer and Steroid Hormone Study of the Centers for Disease Control and the National Institute of Child Health and Human Development: Oral contraceptive use and the risk of ovarian cancer. JAMA 1983; 249:1596-1599. **74.** The Cancer and Steroid Hormone Study of the Centers for Disease Control and the National Institute of Child Health and Human Development: Combination oral contraceptive use and the risk of endometrial cancer. JAMA 1987; 257:796-800. **75.** Ory HW. Functional ovarian cysts and oral contraceptives: negative association confirmed surgically. JAMA 1974; 228:68-69. **76.** Ory HW, Cole P, MacMahon B, Hoover R. Oral contraceptives and reduced risk of benign breast disease. N Engl J Med 1976; 294:419-422. **77.** Ory HW. The noncontraceptive health benefits from oral contraceptive use. Fam Plann Perspect 1982; 14:182-184. **78.** Ory HW, Forrest JD, Lincoln R. Making choices: evaluating the health risks and benefits of birth control methods. New York, The Alan Guttmacher Institute, 1983; p. 1. **79.** Schlesselman J. Stadel BV, Murray P, Lai S. Breast cancer in relation to early use of oral contraceptives. JAMA 1988; 259:1828-1833. **80.** Hennekens CH, Speizer FE, Lipnick RJ, Rosner B, Bain C, Belanger C, Stampfer MJ, Willett W, Peto R. A case-control study of oral contraceptive use and breast cancer. JNCI 1984; 72:39-42. **81.** LaVecchia C, Decarli A, Fasoli M, Franceschi S, Gentile A, Negri E, Parazzini F, Tognoni G. Oral contraceptives and cancers of the breast and of the female genital tract. Interim results from a case-control study. Br J Cancer 1986; 54:311-317. **82.** Meirik O, Lund E, Adami H, Bergstrom R, Christoffersen T, Bergsjo P. Oral contraceptive use and breast cancer in young women. A Joint National Case-control study in Sweden and Norway. Lancet 1986; 11:650-654. **83.** Kay CR, Hannaford PC. Breast cancer and the pill–A further report from the Royal College of General Practitioners' oral contraception study. Br J Cancer 1988; 58:675-680. **84.** Stadel BV, Lai S, Schlesselman JJ, Murray P. Oral contraceptives and premenopausal breast cancer in nulliparous women. Contraception 1988; 38:287-299. **85.** Miller DR, Rosenberg L, Kaufman DW, Stolley P, Warshauer ME, Shapiro S. Breast cancer before age 45 and oral contraceptive use: New findings. Am J Epidemiol 1989; 129:269-280. **86.** The UK National Case-Control Study Group, Oral contraceptive use and breast cancer risk in young women. Lancet 1989; 1:973-982. **87.** Schlesselman JJ. Cancer of the breast and reproductive tract in relation to use of oral contraceptives. Contraception 1989; 40:1-38. **88.** Vessey MP, McPherson K, Villard-Mackintosh L, Yeates D. Oral contraceptives and breast cancer: latest findings in a large cohort study. Br J Cancer 1989; 59:613-617. **89.** Jick SS, Walker AM, Stergachis A, Jick H. Oral contraceptives and breast cancer. Br J Cancer 1989; 59:618-621. **90.** Anderson FD. Selectivity and minimal androgenicity of norgestimate in monophasic and triphasic oral contraceptives. Acta Obstet Gynecol Scand 1992; 156 (Supplement):15-21. **91.** Chapdelaine A, Desmaris J-L, Derman RJ. Clinical evidence of minimal androgenic activity of norgestimate. Int J Fertil 1989; 34(51):347-352. **92.** Phillips A, Demarest K, Hahn DW, Wong F, McGuire JL. Progestational and androgenic receptor binding affinities and in vivo activities of norgestimate and other progestins. Contraception 1989; 41(4):399-409. **93.** Phillips A, Hahn DW, Klimek S, McGuire JL. A comparison of the potencies and activities of progestogens used in contraceptives. Contraception 1987;36(2):181-192. **94.** Janaud A, Rouffy J, Upmalis D, Dain M-P. A comparison study of lipid and androgen metabolism with triphasic oral contraceptive formulations containing norgestimate or levonorgestrel. Acta Obstet Gynecol Scand 1992; 156 (Supplement):34-38. **95.** Collaborative Group on Hormonal Factors in Breast Cancer. Breast cancer and hormonal contraceptives: collaborative reanalysis of individual data on 53 297 women with breast cancer and 100 239 women without breast cancer from 54 epidemiological studies. Lancet 1996;347:1713-1727. **96.** Palmer JR, Rosenberg L, Kaufman DW, Warshauer ME, Stolley P, Shapiro S. Oral Contraceptive Use and Liver Cancer. Am J Epidemiol 1989; 130:878-882. **97.** Lewis M, Spitzer WO, Heinemann LAJ, MacRae KD, Bruppacher R, Thorogood M, on behalf of Transnational Research Group on Oral Contraceptives and Health of Young Women. Third generation oral contraceptives and risk of myocardial infarction: an international case-control study. Br Med J 1996; 312:88-90.

BRIEF SUMMARY PATIENT PACKAGE INSERT

Oral contraceptives, also known as "birth control pills" or "the pill," are taken to prevent pregnancy. ORTHO TRI-CYCLEN may also be taken to treat moderate acne in females who are able to use the pill. When taken correctly to prevent pregnancy, oral contraceptives have a failure rate of less than 1% per year when used without missing any pills. The typical failure rate of large numbers of pill users is less than 3% per year when women who miss pills are included. For most women oral contraceptives are also free of serious or unpleasant side effects. However, forgetting to take pills considerably increases the chances of pregnancy.

For the majority of women, oral contraceptives can be taken safely. But there are some women who are at high risk of developing certain serious diseases that can be fatal or may cause temporary or permanent disability. The risks associated with taking oral contraceptives increase significantly if you:

- smoke
- have high blood pressure, diabetes, high cholesterol
- have or have had clotting disorders, heart attack, stroke, angina pectoris, cancer of the breasts or sex organs, jaundice or malignant or benign liver tumors.

Although cardiovascular disease risks may be increased with oral contraceptive use after age 40 in healthy, non-smoking women (even with the newer low-dose formulations), there are also greater potential health risks associated with pregnancy in older women.

You should not take the pill if you suspect you are pregnant or have unexplained vaginal bleeding.

> **Cigarette smoking increases the risk of serious cardiovascular side effects from oral contraceptive use. This risk increases with age and with heavy smoking (15 or more cigarettes per day) and is quite marked in women over 35 years of age. Women who use oral contraceptives are strongly advised not to smoke.**

Most side effects of the pill are not serious. The most common such effects are nausea, vomiting, bleeding between menstrual periods, weight gain, breast tenderness, and difficulty wearing contact lenses. These side effects, especially nausea and vomiting, may subside within the first three months of use.

The serious side effects of the pill occur very infrequently, especially if you are in good health and are young. However, you should know that the following medical conditions have been associated with or made worse by the pill:

1. Blood clots in the legs (thrombophlebitis), lungs (pulmonary embolism), stoppage or rupture of a blood vessel in the brain (stroke), blockage of blood vessels in the heart (heart attack or angina pectoris) or other organs of the body. As mentioned above, smoking increases the risk of heart attacks and strokes and subsequent serious medical consequences.

2. In rare cases, oral contraceptives can cause benign but dangerous liver tumors. These benign liver tumors can rupture and cause fatal internal bleeding. In addition, some studies report an increased risk of developing liver cancer. However, live cancers are rare.

3. High blood pressure, although blood pressure usually returns to normal when the pill is stopped.

The symptoms associated with these serious side effects are discussed in the detailed leaflet given to you with your supply of pills. Notify your doctor or health care provider if you notice any unusual physical disturbances while taking the pill. In addition, drugs such as rifampin, as well as some anticonvulsants and some antibiotics may decrease oral contraceptive effectiveness.

ANNUAL NUMBER OF BIRTH-RELATED OR METHOD-RELATED DEATHS ASSOCIATED WITH CONTROL OF FERTILITY PER 100,000 NON-STERILE WOMEN, BY FERTILITY CONTROL METHOD ACCORDING TO AGE

Method of control and outcome	15–19	20–24	25–29	30–34	35–39	40–44
No fertility control methods*	7.0	7.4	9.1	14.8	25.7	28.2
Oral contraceptives non-smoker**	0.3	0.5	0.9	1.9	13.8	31.6
Oral contraceptives smoker**	2.2	3.4	6.6	13.5	51.1	117.2
IUD**	0.8	0.8	1.0	1.0	1.4	1.4
Condom*	1.1	1.6	0.7	0.2	0.3	0.4
Diaphragm/ spermicide*	1.9	1.2	1.2	1.3	2.2	2.8
Periodic abstinence*	2.5	1.6	1.6	1.7	2.9	3.6

*Deaths are birth-related
**Deaths are method-related

Adapted from H.W. Ory, ref. #35.

There is conflict among studies regarding breast cancer and oral contraceptive use. Some studies have reported an increase in the risk of developing breast cancer, particularly at a younger age. This increased risk appears to be related to duration of use. The majority of studies have found no overall increase in the risk of developing breast cancer. Some studies have found an increase in the incidence of cancer of the cervix in women who use oral contraceptives. However, this finding may be related to factors other than the use of oral contraceptives. There is insufficient evidence to rule out the possibility pills may cause such cancers.

Taking the combination pill provides some important non-contraceptive benefits. These include less painful menstruation, less menstrual blood loss and anemia, fewer pelvic infections, and fewer cancers of the ovary and the lining of the uterus.

Be sure to discuss any medical condition you may have with your health care provider. Your health care provider will take a medical and family history before prescribing oral contraceptives and will examine you. The physical examination may be delayed to another time if you request it and the health care provider believes that it is a good medical practice to postpone it. You should be reexamined at least once a year while taking oral contraceptives. Your pharmacist should have given you the detailed patient information labeling which gives you further information which you should read and discuss with your health care provider.

ORTHO-CYCLEN and ORTHO TRI-CYCLEN (like all oral contraceptives) are intended to prevent pregnancy. ORTHO TRI-CYCLEN is also used to treat moderate acne in females who are able to take oral contraceptives. Oral contraceptives do not protect against transmission of HIV (AIDS) and other sexually transmitted diseases such as chlamydia, genital herpes, genital warts, gonorrhea, hepatitis B, and syphilis.

DETAILED PATIENT LABELING

PLEASE NOTE: This labeling is revised from time to time as important new medical information becomes available. Therefore, please review this labeling carefully.

ORTHO TRI-CYCLEN □ 21 Day Regimen and
ORTHO TRI-CYCLEN □ 28 Day Regimen
Each white tablet contains 0.180 mg norgestimate and 0.035 mg ethinyl estradiol. Each light blue tablet contains 0.215 mg norgestimate and 0.035 mg ethinyl estradiol. Each blue tablet contains 0.250 mg norgestimate and 0.035 mg ethinyl estradiol. Each green tablet in ORTHO TRI-CYCLEN □ 28 Day Regimen contains inert ingredients.
ORTHO-CYCLEN □ 21 Day Regimen and
ORTHO-CYCLEN □ 28 Day Regimen
Each blue tablet contains 0.250 mg norgestimate and 0.035 mg ethinyl estradiol. Each green tablet in ORTHO-CYCLEN □ 28 Day Regimen contains inert ingredients.

INTRODUCTION

Any woman who considers using oral contraceptives (the birth control pill or the pill) should understand the benefits and risks of using this form of birth control. This patient labeling will give you much of the information you will need to make this decision and will also help you determine if you are at risk of developing any of the serious side effects of the pill. It will tell you how to use the pill properly so that it will be as effective as possible. However, this labeling is not a replacement for a careful discussion between you and your health care provider. You should discuss the information provided in this labeling with him or her, both when you first start taking the pill and during your revisits. You should also follow your health care provider's advice with regard to regular check-ups while you are on the pill.

EFFECTIVENESS OF ORAL CONTRACEPTIVES FOR CONTRACEPTION

Oral contraceptives or "birth control pills" or "the pill" are used to prevent pregnancy and are more effective than other non-surgical methods of birth control. When they are taken correctly, the chance of becoming pregnant is less than 1% (1 pregnancy per 100 women per year of use) when used perfectly, without missing any pills. Typical failure rates are actually 3% per year. The chance of becoming pregnant increases with each missed pill during a menstrual cycle.

In comparison, typical failure rates for other non-surgical methods of birth control during the first year of use are as follows:

Implant: <1%
Injection: <1%
IUD: 1 to 2%
Diaphragm with spermicides: 18%
Spermicides alone: 21%
Vaginal sponge: 18 to 36%
Cervical Cap: 18 to 36%
Condom alone (male): 12%
Condom alone (female): 21%
Periodic abstinence: 20%
No methods: 85%

WHO SHOULD NOT TAKE ORAL CONTRACEPTIVES

Cigarette smoking increases the risk of serious cardiovascular side effects from oral contraceptive use. This risk increases with age and with heavy smoking (15 or more cigarettes per day) and is quite marked in women over 35 years of age. Women who use oral contraceptives are strongly advised not to smoke.

Some women should not use the pill. For example, you should not take the pill if you are pregnant or think you may be pregnant. You should also not use the pill if you have any of the following conditions:

• A history of heart attack or stroke
• Blood clots in the legs (thrombophlebitis), lungs (pulmonary embolism), or eyes
• A history of blood clots in the deep veins of your legs
• Chest pain (angina pectoris)
• Known or suspected breast cancer or cancer of the lining of the uterus, cervix or vagina
• Unexplained vaginal bleeding (until a diagnosis is reached by your doctor)
• Yellowing of the whites of the eyes or of the skin (jaundice) during pregnancy or during previous use of the pill
• Liver tumor (benign or cancerous)
• Known or suspected pregnancy

Tell your health care provider if you have ever had any of these conditions. Your health care provider can recommend a safer method of birth control.

OTHER CONSIDERATIONS BEFORE TAKING ORAL CONTRACEPTIVES

Tell your health care provider if you have or have had:
• Breast nodules, fibrocystic disease of the breast, an abnormal breast x-ray or mammogram
• Diabetes
• Elevated cholesterol or triglycerides
• High blood pressure
• Migraine or other headaches or epilepsy
• Mental depression
• Gallbladder, heart or kidney disease
• History of scanty or irregular menstrual periods

Women with any of these conditions should be checked often by their health care provider if they choose to use oral contraceptives.

Also, be sure to inform your doctor or health care provider if you smoke or are on any medications.

RISKS OF TAKING ORAL CONTRACEPTIVES

1. Risk of developing blood clots
Blood clots and blockage of blood vessels are one of the most serious side effects of taking oral contraceptives and can cause death or serious disability. In particular, a clot in the legs can cause thrombophlebitis and a clot that travels to the lungs can cause a sudden blocking of the vessel carrying blood to the lungs. Rarely, clots occur in the blood vessels of the eye and may cause blindness, double vision, or impaired vision.

If you take oral contraceptives and need elective surgery, need to stay in bed for a prolonged illness or have recently delivered a baby, you may be at risk of developing blood clots. You should consult your doctor about stopping oral contraceptives four weeks before surgery and not taking oral contraceptives for two weeks after surgery or during bed rest. You should also not take oral contraceptives soon after delivery of a baby. It is advisable to wait for at least four weeks after delivery if you are not breast feeding or four weeks after a second trimester abortion. If you are breast feeding, you should wait until you have weaned your child before using the pill. (See also the section on Breast Feeding in General Precautions.)

The risk of circulatory disease in oral contraceptive users may be higher in users of high-dose pills and may be greater with longer duration of oral contraceptive use. In addition, some of these increased risks may continue for a number of years after stopping oral contraceptives. The risk of abnormal blood clotting increases with age in both users and nonusers of oral contraceptives, but the increased risk from the oral contraceptive appears to be present at all ages. For women aged 20 to 44 it is estimated that about 1 in 2,000 using oral contraceptives will be hospitalized each year because of abnormal clotting. Among nonusers in the same age group, about 1 in 20,000 would be hospitalized each year. For oral contraceptive users in general, it has been estimated that in women between the ages of 15 and 34 the risk of death due to a circulatory disorder is about 1 in 12,000 per year, whereas for nonusers the rate is about 1 in 50,000 per year. In the age group 35 to 44, the risk is estimated to be about 1 in 2,500 per year for oral contraceptive users and about 1 in 10,000 per year for nonusers.

2. Heart attacks and strokes
Oral contraceptives may increase the tendency to develop strokes (stoppage or rupture of blood vessels in the brain) and angina pectoris and heart attacks (blockage of blood vessels in the heart). Any of these conditions can cause death or serious disability.

Smoking greatly increases the possibility of suffering heart attacks and strokes. Furthermore, smoking and the use of oral contraceptives greatly increase the chances of developing and dying of heart disease.

3. Gallbladder disease
Oral contraceptive users probably have a greater risk than nonusers of having gallbladder disease, although the risk may be related to pills containing high doses of estrogens.

4. Liver tumors
In rare cases, oral contraceptives can cause benign but dangerous liver tumors. These benign liver tumors can rupture and cause fatal internal bleeding. In addition, some studies report an increased risk of developing liver cancer. However, liver cancers are rare.

5. Cancer of the reproductive organs and breasts
There is conflict among studies regarding breast cancer and oral contraceptive use. Some studies have reported an increase in the risk of developing breast cancer, particularly at a younger age. This increased risk appears to be related to duration of use. The majority of studies have found no overall increase in the risk of developing breast cancer.

A meta-analysis of 54 studies found a small increase in the frequency of having breast cancer diagnosed for women who were currently using combined oral contraceptives or had used them within the past ten years. This increase in the frequency of breast cancer diagnosis, within ten years of stopping use, was generally accounted for by cancers localized to the breast. There was no increase in the frequency of having breast cancer diagnosed ten or more years after cessation of use.

Some studies have found an increase in the incidence of cancer of the cervix in women who use oral contraceptives. However, this finding may be related to factors other than the use of oral contraceptives. There is insufficient evidence to rule out the possibility that pills may cause such cancers.

ESTIMATED RISK OF DEATH FROM A BIRTH CONTROL METHOD OR PREGNANCY

All methods of birth control and pregnancy are associated with a risk of developing certain diseases which may lead to disability or death. An estimate of the number of deaths associated with different methods of birth control and pregnancy has been calculated and is shown in the following table.
[See table above]

Continued on next page

Ortho Tri-Cyclen—Cont.

In the above table, the risk of death from any birth control method is less than the risk of childbirth, except for oral contraceptive users over the age of 35 who smoked and pill users over the age of 40 even if they do not smoke. It can be seen in the table that for women aged 15 to 39, the risk of death was highest with pregnancy (7–26 deaths per 100,000 women, depending on age). Among pill users who do not smoke, the risk of death was always lower than that associated with pregnancy for any age group, although over the age of 40, the risk increases to 32 deaths per 100,000 women, compared to 28 associated with pregnancy at that age. However, for pill users who smoke and are over the age of 35, the estimated number of deaths exceed those for other methods of birth control. If a woman is over the age of 40 and smokes, her estimated risk of death is four times higher (117/100,000 women) than the estimated risk associated with pregnancy (28/100,000 women) in that age group.

The suggestion that women over 40 who do not smoke should not take oral contraceptives is based on information from older, higher-dose pills. An Advisory Committee of the FDA discussed this in 1989 and recommended that the benefits of low-dose oral contraceptive use by healthy, non-smoking women over 40 years of age may outweigh the possible risks.

WARNING SIGNALS

If any of these adverse effects occur while you are taking oral contraceptives, call your doctor immediately:

- Sharp chest pain, coughing of blood, or sudden shortness of breath (indicating a possible clot in the lung)
- Pain in the calf (indicating a possible clot in the leg)
- Crushing chest pain or heaviness in the chest (indicating a possible heart attack)
- Sudden severe headache or vomiting, dizziness or fainting, disturbances of vision or speech, weakness, or numbness in an arm or leg (indicating a possible stroke)
- Sudden partial or complete loss of vision (indicating a possible clot in the eye)
- Breast lumps (indicating possible breast cancer or fibrocystic disease of the breast; ask your doctor or health care provider to show you how to examine your breasts)
- Severe pain or tenderness in the stomach area (indicating a possibly ruptured liver tumor)
- Difficulty in sleeping, weakness, lack of energy, fatigue, or change in mood (possibly indicating severe depression)
- Jaundice or a yellowing of the skin or eyeballs, accompanied frequently by fever, fatigue, loss of appetite, dark colored urine, or light colored bowel movements (indicating possible liver problems)

SIDE EFFECTS OF ORAL CONTRACEPTIVES

1. Vaginal bleeding

Irregular vaginal bleeding or spotting may occur while you are taking the pills. Irregular bleeding may vary from slight staining between menstrual periods to breakthrough bleeding which is a flow much like a regular period. Irregular bleeding occurs most often during the first few months of oral contraceptive use, but may also occur after you have been taking the pill for some time. Such bleeding may be temporary and usually does not indicate any serious problems. It is important to continue taking your pills on schedule. If the bleeding occurs in more than one cycle or lasts for more than a few days, talk to your doctor or health care provider.

2. Contact lenses

If you wear contact lenses and notice a change in vision or an inablity to wear your lenses, contact your doctor or health care provider.

3. Fluid retention

Oral contraceptives may cause edema (fluid retention) with swelling of the fingers or ankles and may raise your blood pressure. If you experience fluid retention, contact your doctor or health care provider.

4. Melasma

A spotty darkening of the skin is possible, particularly of the face, which may persist.

5. Other side effects

Other side effects may include nausea and vomiting, change in appetite, headache, nervousness, depression, dizziness, loss of scalp hair, rash, and vaginal infections.

If any of these side effects bother you, call your doctor or health care provider.

GENERAL PRECAUTIONS

1. Missed periods and use of oral contraceptives before or during early pregnancy

There may be times when you may not menstruate regularly after you have completed taking a cycle of pills. If you have taken your pills regularly and miss one menstrual period, continue taking your pills for the next cycle but be sure to inform your health care provider before doing so. If you have not taken the pills daily as instructed and missed a menstrual period, you may be pregnant. If you missed two consecutive menstrual periods, you may be pregnant. Check with your health care provider immediately to determine

whether you are pregnant. Do not continue to take oral contraceptives until you are sure you are not pregnant, but continue to use another method of contraception.

There is no conclusive evidence that oral contraceptive use is associated with an increase in birth defects, when taken inadvertently during early pregnancy. Previously, a few studies had reported that oral contraceptives might be associated with birth defects, but these findings have not been seen in more recent studies. Nevertheless, oral contraceptives or any other drugs should not be used during pregnancy unless clearly necessary and prescribed by your doctor. You should check with your doctor about risks to your unborn child of any medication taken during pregnancy.

2. While breast feeding

If you are breast feeding, consult your doctor before starting oral contraceptives. Some of the drug will be passed on to the child in the milk. A few adverse effects on the child have been reported, including yellowing of the skin (jaundice) and breast enlargement. In addition, combination oral contraceptives may decrease the amount and quality of your milk. If possible, do not use combination oral contraceptives while breast feeding. You should use another method of contraception since breast feeding provides only partial protection from becoming pregnant and this partial protection decreases significantly as you breast feed for longer periods of time. You should consider starting combination oral contraceptives only after you have weaned your child completely.

3. Laboratory tests

If you are scheduled for any laboratory tests, tell your doctor you are taking birth control pills. Certain blood tests may be affected by birth control pills.

4. Drug interactions

Certain drugs may interact with birth control pills to make them less effective in preventing pregnancy or cause an increase in breakthrough bleeding. Such drugs include rifampin, drugs used for epilepsy such as barbiturates (for example, phenobarbital), anticonvulsants such as carbamazepine (Tegretol is one brand of this drug), phenytoin (Dilantin is one brand of this drug), phenylbutazone (Butazolidin is one brand) and possibly certain antibiotics. You may need to use additional contraception when you take drugs which can make oral contraceptives less effective.

5. Sexually transmitted diseases

ORTHO-CYCLEN and ORTO TRI-CYCLEN (like all oral contraceptives) are intended to prevent pregnancy. ORTHO TRI-CYCLEN is also used to treat moderate acne in females who are able to take oral contraceptives. Oral contraceptives do not protect against transmission of HIV (AIDS) and other sexually transmitted diseases such as chlamydia, genital herpes, genital warts, gonorrhea, hepatitis B, and syphilis.

HOW TO TAKE THE PILL

IMPORTANT POINTS TO REMEMBER

BEFORE YOU START TAKING YOUR PILLS:
1. BE SURE TO READ THESE DIRECTIONS:
Before you start taking your pills.
Anytime you are not sure what to do.
2. THE RIGHT WAY TO TAKE THE PILL IS TO TAKE ONE PILL EVERY DAY AT THE SAME TIME.
If you miss pills you could get pregnant. This includes starting the pack late. The more pills you miss, the more likely you are to get pregnant.
3. MANY WOMEN HAVE SPOTTING OR LIGHT BLEEDING, OR MAY FEEL SICK TO THEIR STOMACH DURING THE FIRST 1–3 PACKS OF PILLS. If you feel sick to your stomach, do not stop taking the pill. The problem will usually go away. If it doesn't go away, check with your doctor or clinic.
4. MISSING PILLS CAN ALSO CAUSE SPOTTING OR LIGHT BLEEDING, even when you make up these missed pills.
On the days you take 2 pills to make up for missed pills, you could also fee a little sick to your stomach.
5. IF YOU HAVE VOMITING OR DIARRHEA, for any reason, or IF YOU TAKE SOME MEDICINES, including some antibiotics, your pills may not work as well. Use a back-up method (such as condoms, foam, or sponge) until you check with your doctor or clinic.
6. IF YOU HAVE TROUBLE REMEMBERING TO TAKE THE PILL, talk to your doctor or clinic about how to make pill-taking easier or about using another method of birth control.
7. IF YOU HAVE ANY QUESTIONS OR ARE UNSURE ABOUT THE INFORMATION IN THIS LEAFLET, call your doctor or clinic.

BEFORE YOUR START TAKING YOUR PILLS

1. DECIDE WHAT TIME OF DAY YOU WANT TO TAKE YOUR PILL.
It is important to take it at about the same time every day.
2. LOOK AT YOUR PILL PACK TO SEE IF IT HAS 21 OR 28 PILLS:

The 21-pill pack has 21 "active" pills (with hormones) to take for 3 weeks. This is followed by 1 week without pills.
The 28-pill pack has 21 "active" pills (with hormones) to take for 3 weeks. This is followed by 1 week of "reminder" green pills (without hormones).
ORTHO TRI-CYCLEN: There are 7 white "active" pills, 7 light blue "active" pills, and 7 blue "active" pills.
ORTHO CYCLEN: There are 21 blue "active" pills.
3. ALSO FIND:
1) where on the pack to start taking pills,
2) in what order to take the pills.
CHECK PICTURE OF PILL PACK AND ADDITIONAL INSTRUCTIONS FOR USING THIS PACKAGE IN THE BRIEF SUMMARY PATIENT PACKAGE INSERT.
4. BE SURE YOU HAVE READY AT ALL TIMES:
ANOTHER KIND OF BIRTH CONTROL (such as condoms, foam, or sponge) to use as a back-up method in case you miss pills.
AN EXTRA, FULL PILL PACK.

WHEN TO START THE FIRST PACK OF PILLS

You have a choice of which day to start taking your first pack of pills. ORTHO TRI-CYCLEN and ORTHO-CYCLEN are available in the DIALPAK® Tablet Dispenser which is preset for a Sunday Start. Day 1 Start is also provided. Decide with your doctor or clinic which is the best day for you. Pick a time of day which will be easy to remember.
SUNDAY START:
ORTHO TRI-CYCLEN: Take the first "active" white pill of the first pack on the Sunday after your period starts, even if you are still bleeding. If your period begins on Sunday, start the pack that same day.
ORTHO-CYCLEN: Take the first "active" blue pill of the first pack on the Sunday after your period starts, even if you are still bleeding. If your period begins on Sunday, start the pack that same day.
Use another method of birth control as a back-up if you have sex anytime from the Sunday you start your first pack until the next Sunday (7 days). Condoms, foam, or the sponge are good back-up methods of birth control.
DAY 1 START:
ORTHO TRI-CYCLEN: Take the first "active" white pill of the first pack during the first 24 hours of your period.
ORTHO-CYCLEN: Take the first "active" blue pill of the first pack during the first 24 hours of your period.
You will not need to use a back-up method of birth control, since you are starting the pill at the beginning of your period.

WHAT TO DO DURING THE MONTH

1. TAKE ONE PILL AT THE SAME TIME EVERY DAY UNTIL THE PACK IS EMPTY.
Do not skip pills even if you are spotting or bleeding between monthly periods or feel sick to your stomach (nausea).
Do not skip pills even if you do not have sex very often.
2. WHEN YOU FINISH A PACK OR SWITCH YOUR BRAND OF PILLS:
21 pills: Wait 7 days to start the next pack. You will probably have your period during that week. Be sure that no more than 7 days pass between 21-day packs.
28 pills: Start the next pack on the day after your last "reminder" pill. Do not wait any days between packs.

WHAT TO DO IF YOU MISS PILLS

ORTHO TRI-CYCLEN:
If you **MISS 1** white, light blue, or blue "active" pill:
1. Take it as soon as you remember. Take the next pill at your regular time. This means you may take 2 pills in 1 day.
2. You do not need to use a back-up birth control method if you have sex.
If you **MISS 2** white or light blue "active" pills in a row in **WEEK 1 OR WEEK 2** of your pack:
1. Take 2 pills on the day you remember and 2 pills the next day.
2. Then take 1 pill a day until you finish the pack.
3. You MAY BECOME PREGNANT if you have sex in the 7 days after you miss pills. You MUST use another birth control method (such as condoms, foam, or sponge) as a back-up method for those 7 days.
If you **MISS 2** blue "active" pills in a row in **THE 3RD WEEK:**
1. **If you are a Sunday Starter:**
Keep taking 1 pill every day until Sunday. On Sunday, THROW OUT the rest of the pack and start a new pack of pills that same day.
If you are a Day 1 Starter:
THROW OUT the rest of the pill pack and start a new pack that same day.
2. You may not have your period this month but this is expected. However, if you miss your period 2 months in a row, call your doctor or clinic because you might be pregnant.

3. You MAY BECOME PREGNANT if you have sex in the 7 days after you miss pills. You MUST use another birth control method (such as condoms, foam, or sponge) as a back-up method for those 7 days.
If you **MISS 3 OR MORE** white, light blue, or blue "active" pills in a row (during the first 3 weeks):
1. **If you are a Sunday Starter:**
Keep taking 1 pill every day until Sunday. On Sunday, THROW OUT the rest of the pack and start a new pack of pills that same day.
If you are a Day 1 Starter:
THROW OUT the rest of the pill pack and start a new pack that same day.
2. You may not have your period this month but this is expected. However, if you miss your period 2 months in a row, call your doctor or clinic because you might be pregnant.
3. You MAY BECOME PREGNANT if you have sex in the 7 days after you miss pills. You MUST use another birth control method (such as condoms, foam, or sponge) as a back-up method for those 7 days.

ORTHO-CYCLEN:
If you **MISS 1** blue "active" pill:
1. Take it as soon as you remember. Take the next pill at your regular time. This means you may take 2 pills in 1 day.
2. You do not need to use a back-up birth control method if you have sex.
If you **MISS 2** blue "active" pills in a row in **WEEK 1 OR WEEK 2** of your pack:
1. Take 2 pills on the day you remember and 2 pills the next day.
2. Then take 1 pill a day until you finish the pack.
3. You MAY BECOME PREGNANT if you have sex in the 7 days after you miss pills. You MUST use another birth control method (such as condoms, foam, or sponge) as a back-up method for those 7 days.
If you **MISS 2** blue "active" pills in a row in **THE 3RD WEEK:**
1. **If you are a Sunday Starter:**
Keep taking 1 pill every day until Sunday. On Sunday, THROW OUT the rest of the pack and start a new pack of pills that same day.
If you are a Day 1 Starter:
THROW OUT the rest of the pill pack and start a new pack that same day.
2. You may not have your period this month but this is expected. However, if you miss your period 2 months in a row, call your doctor or clinic because you might be pregnant.
3. You MAY BECOME PREGNANT if you have sex in the 7 days after you miss pills. You MUST use another birth control method (such as condoms, foam, or sponge) as a back-up method for those 7 days.
If you **MISS 3 OR MORE** blue "active" pills in a row (during the first 3 weeks):
1. **If you are a Sunday Starter:**
Keep taking 1 pill every day until Sunday. On Sunday, THROW OUT the rest of the pack and start a new pack of pills that same day.
If you are a Day 1 Starter:
THROW OUT the rest of the pill pack and start a new pack that same day.
2. You may not have your period this month but this is expected. However, if you miss your period 2 months in a row, call your doctor or clinic because you might be pregnant.
3. You MAY BECOME PREGNANT if you have sex in the 7 days after you miss pills. You MUST use another birth control method (such as condoms, foam, or sponge) as a back-up method for those 7 days.

A REMINDER FOR THOSE ON 28-DAY PACKS:
If you forget any of the 7 green "reminder" pills in Week 4:
THROW AWAY the pills you missed.
Keep taking 1 pill each day until the pack is empty.
You do not need a back-up method.

FINALLY, IF YOU ARE STILL NOT SURE WHAT TO DO ABOUT THE PILLS YOU HAVE MISSED:
Use a BACK-UP METHOD anytime you have sex.
KEEP TAKING ONE "ACTIVE" PILL EACH DAY until you can reach your doctor or clinic.

PREGNANCY DUE TO PILL FAILURE
The incidence of pill failure resulting in pregnancy is approximately one percent (i.e., one pregnancy per 100 women per year) if taken every day as directed, but more typical failure rates are about 3%. If failure does occur, the risk to the fetus is minimal.

PREGNANCY AFTER STOPPING THE PILL
There may be some delay in becoming pregnant after you stop using oral contraceptives, especially if you had irregular menstrual cycles before you used oral contraceptives. It may be advisable to postpone conception until you begin menstruating regularly once you have stopped taking the pill and desire pregnancy.
There does not appear to be any increase in birth defects in newborn babies when pregnancy occurs soon after stopping the pill.

OVERDOSAGE
Serious ill effects have not been reported following ingestion of large doses of oral contraceptives by young children. Overdosage may cause nausea and withdrawal bleeding in females. In case of overdosage, contact your health care provider or pharmacist.

OTHER INFORMATION
Your health care provider will take a medical and family history before prescribing oral contraceptives and will examine you. The physical examination may be delayed to another time if you request it and the health care provider believes that it is a good medical practice to postpone it. You should be reexamined at least once a year. Be sure to inform your health care provider if there is a family history of any of the conditions listed previously in this leaflet. Be sure to keep all appointments with your health care provider, because this is a time to determine if there are early signs of side effects of oral contraceptive use.
Do not use the drug for any condition other than the one for which it was prescribed. This drug has been prescribed specifically for you; do not give it to others who may want birth control pills.

HEALTH BENEFITS FROM ORAL CONTRACEPTIVES
In addition to preventing pregnancy, use of combination oral contraceptives may provide certain benefits. They are:
- menstrual cycles may become more regular
- blood flow during menstruation may be lighter and less iron may be lost. Therefore, anemia due to iron deficiency is less likely to occur.
- pain or other symptoms during menstruation may be encountered less frequently
- ectopic (tubal) pregnancy may occur less frequently
- noncancerous cysts or lumps in the breast may occur less frequently
- acute pelvic inflammatory disease may occur less frequently
- oral contraceptive use may provide some protection against developing two forms of cancer: cancer of the ovaries and cancer of the lining of the uterus.

If you want more information about birth control pills, ask your doctor/health care provider or pharmacist. They have a more technical leaflet called the Professional Labeling, which you may wish to read. The professional labeling is also published in a book entitled *Physicians' Desk Reference*, available in many book stores and public libraries.
ORTHO-McNEIL PHARMACEUTICAL, INC.
Raritan, New Jersey 08869
©OMP 1998
REVISED MAY 1998 **635-50-900-4**
Shown in Product Identification Guide, page 328

PANCREASE® ℞
[pan 'kre-āce]
brand of PANCRELIPASE
ENTERIC COATED MICROSPHERES
Capsules

DESCRIPTION
PANCREASE® (pancrelipase) Capsules are a pancreatic enzyme supplement for oral administration. Pancrelipase, the active ingredient in PANCREASE Capsules, is a natural product harvested by extraction from the pancreas of the hog. Pancrelipase powder is a slightly brown amorphous powder with a faint characteristic odor. It is partly soluble in water and practically insoluble in alcohol or ether.
PANCREASE Capsules contain enteric-coated microspheres of porcine pancreatic enzyme concentrate in the following theoretical quantities:

Lipase	4,500 U.S.P. Units
Amylase	20,000 U.S.P. Units
Protease	25,000 U.S.P. Units

Inactive ingredients are povidone, sodium starch glycolate, sugar (sucrose) spheres, cellulose acetate phthalate, diethyl phthalate, talc, corn starch, titanium dioxide, gelatin, and other trace ingredients.

PRECLINICAL
Studies in a small number of rats administered indomethacin or ibuprofen and pancrelipase enzymes concomitantly revealed intestinal and liver lesions. The clinical significance of these findings is not known.

CLINICAL PHARMACOLOGY
The enteric-coated microspheres contained PANCREASE Capsules resist gastric inactivation and deliver enzymes into the duodenum. The enzymes in PANCREASE act locally in the gastrointestinal tract. The enzymes are present in the form of pH-sensitive enteric-coated microspheres of less than 3 mm in diameter which are filled into gelatin capsules. The microspheres, which are released from the capsule into the stomach, are enteric coated to resist inactivation at low pH. Once released the microspheres are distributed into the stomach and pass into the duodenum where, when the pH reaches approximately 5.5, the enteric coating begins to dissolve and the release of the enzymes is initiated. The enzymes catalyze the hydrolysis of fats into glycerol and fatty acids, protein into proteoses and derived substances, and starch into dextrins and sugars. Duodenal availability studies in adults indicate that following oral administration of PANCREASE to adults, measurable levels of enzymes are present in the duodenum. Once thay have accomplished their digestive function the enzymes may be digested in the intestine. The constituents may be partially absorbed and subsequently excreted in the urine. Any undigested enzymes are excreted in the feces.

INDICATIONS AND USAGE
PANCREASE is indicated for the treatment of steatorrhea secondary to pancreatic insufficiency such as cystic fibrosis or chronic alcoholic pancreatitis.

CONTRAINDICATIONS
PANCREASE Capsules are contraindicated in patients known to be hypersensitive to pork protein or any other component of this product.

WARNINGS
Cases of fibrotic strictures in the colon have been reportedly primarily in cystic fibrosis patients with the use of enzyme supplements, generally at dosages above the recommended range. Some cases required surgery including resection of the bowel. If symptoms suggestive of gastrointestinal obstruction occur, the possibility of bowel strictures should be considered.
Any change in pancreatic enzyme replacement therapy (e.g., dose or brand of medication) should be made cautiously and only under medical supervision. It is recommended that therapy be initiated at a low dose, followed by titration to an effective dose. The titration schedule should be guided by measured changes in 3-day fecal fat excretion. (See **DOSAGE AND ADMINISTRATION.**)

PRECAUTIONS
General
TO PROTECT THE ENTERIC COATING, MICROSPHERES SHOULD NOT BE CRUSHED OR CHEWED. Intact capsules should be swallowed with liquids at mealtime. If an intact capsule can not be swallowed, it may be opened and the contents taken with small amounts of food that do not require chewing. (See **DOSAGE AND ADMINISTRATION.**)
Information for Patients
Patients should be advised that:
- PANCREASE Capsules must not be crushed or chewed;
- intact capsules should be swallowed with liquid at mealtimes;
- the microspheres from opened capsules should be swallowed immediately and not be retained in the mouth;
- doses should only be taken with meals or snacks;
- fluids should be consumed liberally while dosing with PANCREASE;
- any change in pancreatic enzyme replacement therapy (e.g., dose or brand of medication) should be made only under medical supervision.

Pregnancy: Teratogenic Effects
Pregnancy Category B
Reproduction studies have been conducted in rats and rabbits at doses 0.44 times and 0.35 times the maximum daily human dose, respectively, and have revealed no evidence of impaired fertility or harm to the fetus due to PANCREASE. No fertility or peri-/postnatal studies have been performed in animals. There are, however, no adequate and well-controlled studies in pregnant women. Because animal reproduction studies are not always predictive of human response, this drug should be used during pregnancy only if clearly needed.
Nursing Mothers
Pancreatic enzymes act locally in the gastrointestinal tract and are not likely to be systematically absorbed. Some of the constituent amino and nucleic acids are likely to be absorbed along with dietary proteins. The possibility of the protein constituents appearing in the breast milk can not be excluded.
Pediatric Use
Colonic strictures, particularly in children with cystic fibrosis, have been associated with doses generally above the recommended dosing range (See **WARNINGS.**) Patients currently receiving doses >2,500 lipase units/kg/meal or 4,000 lipase units/gm fat/day should be re-evaluated and the dosage either immediately decreased or titrated downward to the lowest effective clinical dose as assessed by 3-day fecal fat excretion.
Geriatric Use
Studies on the relationship or age to the effects of pancrelipase have not been conducted. However, geriatric-specific problems that would limit the usefulness of this medication in the elderly are not expected.

Continued on next page

Pancrease—Cont.

ADVERSE REACTIONS

Clinical evidence indicates that PANCREASE Capsules are well-tolerated.

The most frequently reported adverse events resulting from the post-marketing experience with PANCREASE were gastrointestinal and include diarrhea, abdominal pain, intestinal obstruction, vomiting, flatulence, nausea, constipation, melena, and perianal irritation. Frequently reported adverse events in other body systems included weight decrease and pain. Hyperuricemia and hyperuricosuria have been reported with the use of pancrelipase products, primarily with non-enteric coated formulations. Cases of fibrosing colonopathy have been reported primarily in cystic fibrosis. (See **WARNINGS**)

OVERDOSAGE

There have been no reports of acute overdosage.

DOSAGE AND ADMINISTRATION

General

Patients with pancreatic insufficiency should consume a high-calorie diet with unrestricted fat which is appropriate for age and clinical status. A nutritional assessment should be performed regularly as a component of routine care and additionally, when dosing of pancreatic enzyme replacement is altered.

Dosage should be individualized and determined by the degree of steatorrhea and the fat content of the diet. Therapy should be initiated at the lowest possible dose and gradually increased until the desired control of steatorrhea is obtained. Dosage should be adjusted based on 3-day fecal fat studies. PANCREASE Capsules should only be taken with meals or snacks.

It is important to ensure that patients ingest a liberal amount of liquids to maintain adequate hydration while dosing with PANCREASE.

Whenever possible, PANCREASE Capsules should be swallowed intact with generous amounts of liquid. However, if swallowing of capsules is difficult, they may be opened and the microspheres sprinkled onto a small quantity of soft food on a teaspoon or tablespoon and ingested immediately. Foods which do not require chewing and have a pH lower than 7.3 are recommended. Examples of such foods are apricot, banana and sweet potato baby foods, applesauce, instant pudding and gelatin snacks. Contact of the microspheres with foods having a pH greater than 7.3 (e.g., milk, custard, ice cream, and many other dairy products) can dissolve the protective enteric coating and destroy enzyme activity.

To avoid irritation of the mouth, lips, and tongue, opened PANCREASE Capsules should be swallowed immediately before regular feedings or meals to minimize the likelihood that the microspheres are retained in the mouth. Proteolytic enzymes present in pancrelipase, when retained in the mouth, may begin to digest the mucous membranes and cause ulcerations.

There is considerable variation among individuals in response to enzymes with respect to control of steatorrhea; therefore, a range of doses is suggested.

Infants: (up to 12 months)

Fat-consumption scheme

2,000–4000 U.S.P. lipase units per 120 mL of formula or per breast feeding. This provides approximately 450–900 lipase units per gram of fat ingested (based on 4.5 grams of fat per 120 mL standard cow's milk-based infant formula).

Higher doses are used in infants because on average, infants ingest 5 grams of fat per kilogram of body weight per day, whereas adults tend to ingest about 2 grams of fat per kilogram per day.

Children and Older

Weight-based scheme

< 4 yrs: Begin with 1,000 U.S.P. lipase units/kg/meal to a maximum of 2,500 lipase units/kg/meal.

> 4 yrs: Begin with 400 U.S.P. lipase units/kg/meal to a maximum of 2,500 units/kg/meal.

Enzyme doses, expressed as lipase units/kg/meal, should be decreased in older patients since they weigh more but tend to ingest less fat per kilogram. Usually, half the mealtime dose is given with a snack. The total daily dose reflects approximately three meals and two to three snacks per day. If doses greater than 2,500 lipase units/kg/meal (4,000 lipase units/gm fat/day) are required to control malabsorption, further investigation is warranted to rule out other causes of malabsorption. Doses greater than 2,500 lipase units/kg/meal should be used with caution and only if they are documented to be effective by 3-day fecal fat measures. It is unknown whether doses above 2,500 lipase units/kg/meal are safe.

Colonic strictures, particularly in children with cystic fibrosis, have been associated with doses generally above the recommended dosing range (See **WARNINGS**.) Patients currently receiving doses >2,500 lipase units/kg/meal or 4,000 lipase units/gm/fat/day should be re-evaluated and the dos-

age either immediately decreased or titrated downward to the lowest effective clinical dose as assessed by 3-day fecal fat excretion.

HOW SUPPLIED

PANCREASE (pancrelipase) Capsules are supplied as white body, clear cap, dye-free capsules. PANCREASE Capsules are imprinted with "McNEIL" and "Pancrease" and are packaged in bottles of:

    100–(NDC 0045-0095-60)
    250–(NDC 0045-0095-69)

Storage

PANCREASE Capsules should be stored in a dry place below 25° C (77° F) in well-closed containers. Do not refrigerate.

Rx only.

PANCREASE is manufactured and distributed by:

McNEIL PHARMACEUTICAL
McNEILAB, INC.
SPRING HOUSE, PA 19477
©McNEILAB, Inc. — 1992
Patent No. 4,079,125
Revised 6/98   643-10-106-4
Shown in Product Identification Guide, page 328

PANCREASE® MT   ℞

[pan 'kre-āce MT]
brand of PANCRELIPASE
ENTERIC COATED MICROTABLETS
Capsules

Prescribing Information

DESCRIPTION

PACREASE® MT (pancrelipase) Capsules are a pancreatic enzyme supplement for oral administration. Pancrelipase, the active ingredient in PANCREASE MT Capsules, is a natural product harvested by extraction from the pancreas of the hog. Pancrelipase powder is a slightly brown amorphous powder with a faint characteristic odor. It is partly soluble in water and practically insoluble in alcohol or ether. PANCREASE MT Capsules contain enteric-coated microtablets of porcine pancreatic enzyme concentrate in the following theoretical quantities:

PANCREASE MT 4 Capsules:	
Lipase	4,000 U.S.P. Units
Amylase	12,000 U.S.P. Units
Protease	12,000 U.S.P. Units
PANCREASE MT 10 Capsules:	
Lipase	10,000 U.S.P. Units
Amylase	30,000 U.S.P. Units
Protease	30,000 U.S.P. Units
PANCREASE MT 16 Capsules:	
Lipase	16,000 U.S.P. Units
Amylase	48,000 U.S.P. Units
Protease	48,000 U.S.P. Units
PANCREASE MT 20 Capsules:	
Lipase	20,000 U.S.P. Units
Amylase	56,000 U.S.P. Units
Protease	44,000 U.S.P. Units

Inactive ingredients are cellulose, crospovidone, magnesium stearate, colloidal silicon dioxide, methacrylic acid copolymer, triethyl citrate, talc, polydimethylsiloxane, wax, gelatin, iron oxide, polysorbate 80, sodium lauryl sulfate, titanium dioxide, and other trace ingredients.

PRECLINICAL

Studies in small number of rats administered indomethacin or ibuprofen and pancrelipase enzymes concomitantly revealed intestinal and liver lesions. The clinical significance of these findings is not known.

CLINICAL PHARMACOLOGY

The enteric-coated microtablets contained in PANCREASE MT Capsules resist gastric inactivation and deliver enzymes into the duodenum. The enzymes in PANCREASE MT act locally in the gastrointestinal tract. The enzymes are present in the form of pH-sensitive enteric-coated microtablets of less than 3 mm in diameter which are filled into gelatin capsules. The microtablets, which are released from the capsule into the stomach, are enteric coated to resist inactivation at low pH. Once released, the microtablets are distributed into the stomach and pass into the duodenum where, when the pH reaches approximately 5.5, the enteric coating begins to dissolve and release of the enzymes is initiated. The enzymes catalyze the hydrolysis of fats into glycerol and fatty acids, protein into proteoses and derived substances, and starch into dextrins and sugars. Duodenal availability studies in adults indicate that following oral administration of PANCREASE MT to adults, measurable levels of enzymes are present in the duodenum. Once they have accomplished their digestive function the enzymes

may be digested in the intestine. The constituents may be partially absorbed and subsequently excreted in the urine. Any undigested enzymes are excreted in the feces.

INDICATIONS AND USAGE

PANCREASE MT is indicated for the treatment of steatorrhea secondary to pancreatic insufficiency such as cystic fibrosis or chronic alcoholic pancreatitis.

CONTRAINDICATIONS

PANCREASE MT Capsules are contraindicated in patients known to be hypersensitive to pork protein or any other component of this product.

WARNINGS

Cases of fibrotic strictures in the colon have been reported primarily in cystic fibrosis patients with the use of enzyme supplements, generally at dosages above the recommended range. Some cases required surgery including resection of the bowel. If symptoms suggestive of gastrointestinal obstruction occur, the possibility of bowel strictures should be considered.

Any change in pancreatic enzyme replacement therapy (e.g., dose or brand of medication) should be made cautiously and only under medical supervision. It is recommended that therapy be initiated at a low dose, followed by titration to an effective dose. The titration schedule should be guided by measured changes in 3-day fecal fat excretion. (See **DOSAGE AND ADMINISTRATION**.)

PRECAUTIONS

General

TO PROTECT THE ENTERIC COATING, MICROTABLETS SHOULD NOT BE CRUSHED OR CHEWED. Intact capsules should be swallowed with liquids at mealtime. If an intact capsule can not be swallowed, it may be opened and the contents taken with small amounts of food that do not require chewing. (See **DOSAGE AND ADMINISTRATION**.)

Information for Patients

Patients should be advised that:

• PANCREASE MT Capsules must not be crushed or chewed;
• intact capsules should be swallowed with liquid at mealtimes;
• the microtablets from opened capsules should be swallowed immediately and not be retained in the mouth;
• doses should only be taken with meals or snacks;
• fluids should be consumed liberally while dosing with PANCREASE MT;
• any change in pancreatic enzyme replacement therapy (e.g., dose or brand of medication) should be made only under medical supervision.

Pregnancy: Teratogenic Effects

Pregnancy Category B

Reproduction studies have been conducted in rats and rabbits at doses 0.44 times and 0.35 times the maximum daily human dose, respectively, and have revealed no evidence of impaired fertility or harm to the fetus due to PANCREASE MT. No fertility or peri-/postnatal studies have been performed in animals. There are, however, no adequate and well-controlled studies in pregnant women. Because animal reproduction studies are not always predictive of human response, this drug should be used during pregnancy only if clearly needed.

Nursing Mothers

Pancreatic enzymes act locally in the gastrointestinal tract and are not likely to be systemically absorbed. Some of the constituent amino and nucleic acids are likely to be absorbed along with dietary proteins. The possibility of the protein constituents appearing in the breast milk can not be excluded.

Pediatric Use

Colonic strictures, particularly in children with cystic fibrosis, have been associated with doses generally above the recommended dosing range. (See **WARNINGS**.) Patients currently receiving doses >2,500 lipase units/kg/meal or 4,000 lipase units/gm fat/day should be re-evaluated and the dosage either immediately decreased or titrated downward to the lowest effective clinical dose as assessed by 3-day fecal fat excretion.

Geriatric Use

Studies on the relationship of age to the effects of pancrelipase have not been conducted. However, geriatric-specific problems that would limit the usefulness of this medication in the elderly are not expected.

ADVERSE REACTIONS

Clinical evidence indicates that PANCREASE MT Capsules are well-tolerated.

The most frequently reported adverse events resulting from the post-marketing experience with PANCREASE MT were gastrointestinal in nature and include diarrhea, abdominal pain, intestinal obstruction, vomiting, intestinal stenosis, and constipation. Frequently reported adverse events in other body systems include dermatitis. Hyperuricemia and hyperuricosuria have been reported with the use of pancre-

lipase products, primarily with non-enteric coated formulations. Cases of fibrosing colonopathy have been reported primarily in cystic fibrosis patients. (See **WARNINGS**.)

OVERDOSAGE

There have been no reports of acute overdosage.

DOSAGE AND ADMINISTRATION

General

Patients with pancreatic insufficiency should consume a high-calorie diet with unrestricted fat which is appropriate for age and clinical status. A nutritional assessment should be performed regularly as a component of routine care and additionally, when dosing of pancreatic enzyme replacement is altered.

Dosage should be individualized and determined by the degree of steatorrhea and the fat content of the diet. Therapy should be initiated at the lowest possible dose and gradually increased until the desired control of steatorrhea is obtained. Dosage should be adjusted based on 3-day fecal fat studies.

PANCREASE MT Capsules should only be taken with meals or snacks.

It is important to ensure that patients ingest a liberal amount of liquids to maintain adequate hydration while dosing with PANCREASE MT.

Whenever possible, PANCREASE MT Capsules should be swallowed intact with generous amounts of liquid. However, if swallowing of capsules is difficult, they may be opened and the microtablets sprinkled onto a small quantity of soft food on a teaspoon or tablespoon and ingested immediately. Foods which do not require chewing and have a pH lower than 7.3 are recommended. Examples of such foods are apricot, banana and sweet potato baby foods, applesauce, instant pudding and gelatin snacks. Contact of the microtablets with foods having a pH greater than 7.3 (e.g., milk, custard, ice cream, and many other dairy products) can dissolve the protective enteric coating and destroy the enzyme activity.

To avoid irritation of the mouth, lips, and tongue, opened PANCREASE MT Capsules should be swallowed immediately before regular feedings or meals to minimize the likelihood that the microtablets are retained in the mouth. Proteolytic enzymes present in pancrealipase, when retained in the mouth, may begin to digest the mucous membranes and cause ulcerations.

There is considerable variation among individuals in response to enzymes with respect to control of steatorrhea; therefore, a range of doses is suggested.

Infants: (up to 12 months)

Fat-consumption scheme

2,000–4,000 U.S.P. lipase units per 120 mL of formula or per breast feeding. This provides approximately 450–900 lipase units per gram of fat ingested (based on 4.5 grams of fat per 120 mL standard cow's milk-based infant formula).

Higher doses are used in infants because on average, infants ingest 5 grams of fat per kilogram of body weight per day, whereas adults tend to ingest about 2 grams of fat per kilogram per day.

Children and Older

Weight-based scheme

<4 yrs: Begin with 1,000 U.S.P. lipase units/kg/meal to a maximum of 2,500 lipase units/kg/meal. >4 yrs: Begin with 400 U.S.P. lipase units/kg/meal to a maximum of 2,500 lipase units/kg/meal.

Enzyme doses, expressed as lipase units/kg/meal, should be decreased in older patients since they weigh more but tend to ingest less fat per kilogram. Usually, half the mealtime dose is given with a snack. The total daily dose reflects approximately three meals and two to three snacks per day.

If doses greater than 2,500 lipase units/kg/meal (4,000 lipase units/gm fat/day) are required to control malabsorption, further investigation is warranted to rule out other causes of malabsorption. Doses greater than 2,500 lipase units/kg/meal should be used with caution and only if they are documented to be effective by 3-day fecal fat measures. It is unknown whether doses above 2,500 lipase units/kg/meal are safe.

Colonic strictures, particularly in children with cystic fibrosis, have been associated with doses generally above the recommended dosing range. (See **WARNINGS**.) Patients currently receiving doses >2,500 lipase units/kg/meal or 4,000 lipase units/gm fat/day should be re-evaluated and the dosage either immediately decreased or titrated downward to the lowest effective clinical dose as assessed by 3-day fecal fat excretion.

HOW SUPPLIED

PANCREASE MT 4 (pancrelipase) Capsules are supplied as yellow opaque body, clear cap capsules imprinted with "McNEIL" and "PANCREASE MT 4" and packaged in bottles of 100–(NDC 0045-0341-60).

PANCREASE MT 10 (pancrelipase) Capsules are supplied as pink opaque body, clear cap capsules imprinted with "McNEIL" and "PANCREASE MT 10" and packaged in bottles of 100–(NDC 0045-0342-60).

PANCREASE MT 16 (pancrelipase) Capsules are supplied as salmon opaque body, clear cap capsules imprinted with "McNEIL" and "PANCREASE MT 16" and packaged in bottles of 100–(NDC 0045-0343-60).

PANCREASE MT 20 (pancrelipase) Capsules are supplied as white opaque body, cap with yellow band capsules imprinted with "McNEIL" and "PANCREASE MT 20" and packaged in bottles of 100–(NDC 0045-0346-60).

Storage

PANCREASE MT Capsules should be stored in a dry place below 25° C (77° F) in well-closed containers. Do not refrigerate.

Rx only.

Microtablets manufactured by Knoll AG Uetersen, Germany.

McNEIL PHARMACEUTICAL
McNEILAB, INC.
SPRING HOUSE, PA 19477
©McNEILAB, Inc.—1994
Revised 6/98 643-10-104-4

Shown in Product Identification Guide, page 328

PARAFON FORTE® DSC ℞

[par 'a-fahn for 'ta]
(chlorzoxazone) Caplets 500 mg
NSN 6505-01-264-4453—100's
NSN 6505-01-288-0524—100's (10x10)

DESCRIPTION

Each caplet (capsule shaped tablet) contains:
Chlorzoxazone* .... 500 mg

Inactive ingredients: FD&C Blue No. 1, microcrystalline cellulose, docusate sodium, lactose (hydrous), magnesium stearate, sodium benzoate, sodium starch glycolate, pregelatinized corn starch, D&C Yellow No. 10.

*5-chlorobenzoxazolinone

ACTIONS

Chlorzoxazone is a centrally-acting agent for painful musculoskeletal conditions. Data available from animal experiments as well as human study indicate that chlorzoxazone acts primarily at the level of the spinal cord and subcortical areas of the brain where it inhibits multisynaptic reflex arcs involved in producing and maintaining skeletal muscle spasm of varied etiology. The clinical result is a reduction of the skeletal muscle spasm with relief of pain and increased mobility of the involved muscles. Blood levels of chlorzoxazone can be detected in people during the first 30 minutes and peak levels may be reached, in the majority of the subjects, in about 1 to 2 hours after oral administration of chlorzoxazone. Chlorzoxazone is rapidly metabolized and is excreted in the urine, primarily in a conjugated form as the glucuronide. Less than one percent of a dose of chlorzoxazone is excreted unchanged in the urine in 24 hours.

INDICATIONS

PARAFON FORTE DSC chlorzoxazone is indicated as an adjunct to rest, physical therapy, and other measures for the relief of discomfort associated with acute, painful musculoskeletal conditions. The mode of action of this drug has not been clearly identified, but may be related to its sedative properties. Chlorzoxazone does not directly relax tense skeletal muscles in man.

CONTRAINDICATIONS

PARAFON FORTE DSC chlorzoxazone is contraindicated in patients with known intolerance to the drug.

WARNINGS

Serious (including fatal) hepatocellular toxicity has been reported rarely in patients receiving chlorzoxazone. The mechanism is unknown but appears to be idiosyncratic and unpredictable. Factors predisposing patients to this rare event are not known. Patients should be instructed to report early signs and/or symptoms of hepatotoxicity such as fever, rash, anorexia, nausea, vomiting, fatigue, right upper quandrant pain, dark urine, or jaundice. Chlorzoxazone should be discontinued immediately and a physician consulted if any of these signs or symptoms develop. Chlorzoxazone use should also be discontinued if a patient develops abnormal liver enzymes (eg. AST, ALT, alkaline phosphatase and bilirubin).

The concomitant use of alcohol or other central nervous system depressants may have an additive effect.

Usage in Pregnancy: The safe use of PARAFON FORTE DSC chlorzoxazone has not been established with respect to the possible adverse effects upon fetal development. Therefore, it should be used in women of childbearing potential only when, in the judgment of the physician, the potential benefits outweigh the possible risks.

PRECAUTIONS

PARAFON FORTE DSC chlorzoxazone should be used with caution in patients with known allergies or with a history of allergic reactions to drugs. If a sensitivity reaction occurs such as urticaria, redness, or itching of the skin, the drug should be stopped.

If any signs or symptoms suggestive of liver dysfunction are observed, the drug should be discontinued.

ADVERSE REACTIONS

Chlorzoxazone containing products are usually well tolerated. It is possible in rare instances that chlorzoxazone may have been associated with gastrointestinal bleeding. Drowsiness, dizziness, light-headedness, malaise, or overstimulation may be noted by an occasional patient. Rarely, allergic-type skin rashes, petechiae, or ecchymoses may develop during treatment. Angioneurotic edema or anaphylactic reactions are extremely rare. There is no evidence that the drug will cause renal damage. Rarely, a patient may note discoloration of the urine resulting from a phenolic metabolite of chlorzoxazone. This finding is of no known clinical significance.

DOSAGE AND ADMINISTRATION

Usual Adult Dosage: One caplet three or four times daily. If adequate reponse is not obtained with this dose, it may be increased to $1^1/_2$ caplets (750 mg) three or four times daily. As improvement occurs dosage can usually be reduced.

OVERDOSAGE

Symptoms: Initially, gastrointestinal disturbances such as nausea, vomiting, or diarrhea together with drowsiness, dizziness, lightheadedness or headache may occur. Early in the course there may be malaise or sluggishness followed by marked loss of muscle tone, making voluntary movement impossible. The deep tendon reflexes may be decreased or absent. The sensorium remains intact, and there is no peripheral loss of sensation. Respiratory depression may occur with rapid, irregular respiration and intercostal and substernal retraction. The blood pressure is lowered, but shock has not been observed.

Treatment: Gastric lavage or induction of emesis should be carried out, followed by administration of activated charcoal. Thereafter, treatment is entirely supportive. If respirations are depressed, oxygen and artificial respiration should be employed and a patent airway assured by use of an oropharyngeal airway or endotracheal tube. Hypotension may be counteracted by use of dextran, plasma, concentrated albumin or a vasopressor agent such as norepinephrine. Cholinergic drugs or analeptic drugs are of no value and should not be used.

HOW SUPPLIED

PARAFON FORTE® DSC (chlorzoxazone) 500 mg caplets, (capsule shaped tablet, colored light green, imprinted "PARAFON FORTE DSC" and "McNEIL", scored).

NDC 0045-0325, bottles of 100, 500 and unit dose 100's.

Dispense in a tight container as defined in the official compendium.

Store at controlled room temperature (15°–30°C, 59°–86°F).

Revised 3/01/95 643-10-098-2

McNeil Pharmaceutical, McNEILAB, Inc.
Spring House, PA 19477

Shown in Product Identification Guide, page 328

PARAGARD® T 380A ℞

Intrauterine Copper Contraceptive

Patients should be counseled that this product does not protect against HIV Infection (AIDS) and other sexually transmitted diseases.

CAUTION: Federal law prohibits dispensing without prescription.

NOTICE

You have received a Patient Package Insert that Federal Regulations (21 CFR 310.502) require you to furnish to each patient who is considering the use of the ParaGard® T 380A.

The Patient Package Insert contains information on the safety and efficacy of the ParaGard® T 380A. Before inserting the ParaGard® T 380A:

- You should read the physician prescription labeling and be familiar with all the information it contains.
- You should counsel the patient and answer her questions about contraception, the ParaGard® T 380A, and the information in the Patient Package Insert.
- You and the patient should read each section of the Patient Package Insert, and if the patient agrees, she may sign a consent form provided for your convenience.

The Patient Package Insert is also available in Spanish and other foreign languages. Address requests to Ortho Pharmaceutical Corporation or telephone 1-800-322-4966.

[See figure at top of next column]

Continued on next page

Paragard T—Cont.

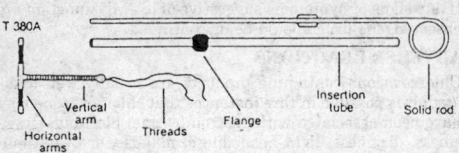

T 380A

Vertical arm / Threads / Flange / Insertion tube / Solid rod / Horizontal arms

DESCRIPTION

The polyethylene body of the ParaGard® T 380A is wound with approximately 176 mg of copper wire and carries a copper collar of approximately 68.7 mg of copper on each of its transverse arms. The exposed surface areas of copper are 380 ± 23 mm^2. The dimensions of the ParaGard® T 380A are 36 mm in the vertical direction and 32 mm in the horizontal direction. The tip of the vertical arm of the ParaGard® T 380A is enlarged to form a bulb having a diameter of 3 mm. The ParaGard® T 380A is equipped with a monofilament polyethylene thread which is tied through the bulb, resulting in two threads at the tip to aid in removal of the IUD. The ParaGard® T 380A contains barium sulfate to render it radiopaque.

The ParaGard® T 380A is packaged together with an insertion tube and solid rod in a Tyvek®-polyethylene pouch and then sterilized. The insertion tube is equipped with a movable flange to aid in gauging the depth to which the insertion tube is inserted through the cervical canal and into the uterine cavity.

CLINICAL PHARMACOLOGY

Available data indicate that the contraceptive effectiveness of the ParaGard® T 380A is enhanced by copper being released continuously from the copper coil and sleeves into the uterine cavity. The exact mechanism by which metallic copper enhances the contraceptive effect of an IUD has not been conclusively demonstrated. Various hypotheses have been advanced, including interference with sperm transport, fertilization, and implantation. Clinical studies with copper-bearing IUDs also suggest that fertilization is prevented either due to an altered number or lack of viability of spermatozoa.[1]

INDICATIONS AND USAGE

The ParaGard® T 380A is indicated for intrauterine contraception. ParaGard® T 380A is highly effective. Table II and Table III list an expected pregnancy rate for one year between 0.7 and 0.5, respectively. ParaGard® T 380A should not be kept in place longer than 10 years.

RECOMMENDED PATIENT PROFILE

The ParaGard® T 380A is recommended for women who have had at least one child, are in a stable, mutually monogamous relationship, and have no history of pelvic inflammatory disease.

CONTRAINDICATIONS

The ParaGard® T 380A should not be inserted when one or more of the following conditions exist:
1. Pregnancy or suspicion of pregnancy.
2. Abnormalities of the uterus resulting in distortion of the uterine cavity.
3. Acute pelvic inflammatory disease or a history of pelvic inflammatory disease.
4. Postpartum endometritis or infected abortion in the past 3 months.
5. Known or suspected uterine or cervical malignancy, including unresolved, abnormal "Pap" smear.
6. Genital bleeding of unknown etiology.
7. Untreated acute cervicitis or vaginitis, including bacterial vaginosis, until infection is controlled.
8. Copper-containing IUDs should not be inserted in the presence of diagnosed Wilson's disease.
9. Known allergy to copper.
10. Patient or her partner has multiple sexual partners.
11. Conditions associated with increased susceptibility to infections with micro-organisms. Such conditions include, but are not limited to, leukemia, acquired immune deficiency syndrome (AIDS), and I.V. drug abuse.
12. Genital actinomycosis.
13. A previously inserted IUD that has not been removed.

WARNINGS
1. PREGNANCY
Effects on the offspring when pregnancy occurs with the ParaGard® T 380A in place are unknown.

a. Septic Abortion
Reports indicate an increased incidence of septic abortion with septicemia, septic shock, and death in patients becoming pregnant with an IUD in place. Most of these reports have been associated with, but not limited to, the mid-trimester of pregnancy. In some cases, the initial symptoms have been insidious and not easily recognized. If pregnancy should occur with an IUD *in situ*, the IUD

should be removed if the string is visible and removal is easily accomplished. Of course, manipulation may result in spontaneous abortion. If removal proves to be difficult, or if threads are not visible, interruption of the pregnancy should be considered and offered as an option. Rates of mortality with and without contraception are shown in Table 1.

b. Continuation of Pregnancy
If the patient elects to maintain the pregnancy and the IUD remains *in situ,* she should be warned that there is an increased risk of spontaneous abortion and sepsis. In addition, she is at increased risk of premature labor and delivery. As a consequence of premature birth, the fetus is at increased risk of damage. She should be followed more closely than the usual obstetrical patient. The patient must be advised to report immediately all abnormal symptoms, such as flu-like syndrome, fever, abdominal cramping or pain, bleeding or vaginal discharge, because generalized symptoms of septicemia may be insidious.

2. ECTOPIC PREGNANCY
a. Patients with a history of ectopic pregnancy are at an increased risk of subsequent pregnancies being ectopic. Although current data indicate that there is no increased risk of ectopic pregnancy in patients using the ParaGard® T 380A and some data suggest there may be a lower risk than the general population using no method of contraception, a pregnancy which occurs with the ParaGard® T 380A in place is more likely to be ectopic than a pregnancy occurring without the ParaGard® T 380A[2–4]. Therefore, patients who become pregnant while using the ParaGard® T 380A should be carefully evaluated for the possibility of an ectopic pregnancy.

b. Special attention should be directed to patients with delayed menses, slight metrorrhagia and/or unilateral pelvic pain, and to those patients who wish to terminate a pregnancy because of IUD failure, to determine whether ectopic pregnancy has occurred.

3. PELVIC INFECTION (PELVIC INFLAMMATORY DISEASE, PID)
The ParaGard® T 380A is contraindicated in the presence of PID or in women with a history of PID. Use of all IUDs, including the ParaGard® T 380A, has been associated with an increased incidence of PID. Therefore, a decision to use the ParaGard® T 380A must include consideration of the risks of PID. The highest rate of PID has been reported to occur after insertion and up to four months thereafter. A study suggests that the highest incidence occurs within 20 days postinsertion, then falls, remaining constant thereafter.[5] Administration of prophylactic antibiotics has been reported, although studies do not confirm the utility of this prophylactic measure in reducing PID. PID can necessitate hysterectomy and can also lead to tubo-ovarian abscesses, tubal occlusion and infertility, and tubal damage that can predispose to ectopic pregnancy. PID can result in peritonitis and, infrequently, in death. The effect of PID on fertility is especially important for women who may wish to have children at a later date.

a. Women at special risk of PID
The risk of PID appears to be greater for women who have multiple sexual partners and also for those women whose sexual partners have multiple sexual partners, as PID is most frequently caused by sexually transmitted diseases.

b. PID warning to ParaGard® T 380A users
All women who choose the ParaGard® T 380A must be informed prior to insertion that IUD use has been associated with an increased incidence of PID and that PID can necessitate hysterectomy, can cause tubal damage leading to ectopic pregnancy or infertility or, in infrequent cases, can cause death. Patients must be taught to recognize and report to their physician promptly any symptoms of pelvic inflammatory disease. These symptoms include development of menstrual disorders (prolonged or heavy bleeding), unusual vaginal discharge, abdominal or pelvic pain or tenderness, dyspareunia, chills, and fever.

c. Asymptomatic PID
PID may be asymptomatic but still result in tubal damage and its sequelae.[6,7]

d. Treatment of PID
Following diagnosis of PID, or suspected PID, bacteriologic specimens should be obtained and antibiotic therapy should be initiated promptly. Removal of the ParaGard® T 380A after initiation of antibiotic therapy is usually appropriate. Time should be allowed for therapeutic blood levels to be reached prior to removal. Guidelines for PID treatment are available from the Center for Disease Control (CDC), Atlanta, Georgia. A copy of the printed guidelines has been provided to you by Ortho Pharmaceutical Corporation. The guidelines were established after deliberation by a group of experts and staff of the CDC, but they should not be construed as rules suitable for use in all patients. Adequate PID treatment requires the application of current standards of therapy prevailing at the time of occurrence of the infection with

reference to the prescription labeling of the antibiotic selected.

Genital actinomycosis has been associated primarily with long-term IUD use. If actinomycosis occurs, promptly institute appropriate antibiotic therapy and remove the ParaGard® T 380A.

4. EMBEDMENT
Partial penetration or embedment of the ParaGard® T 380A in the endometrium or myometrium can result in difficult removal. In some cases this can result in breakage of the IUD, necessitating surgical removal.

5. PERFORATION
Partial or total perforation of the uterine wall or cervix may occur with use of the ParaGard® T 380A. The rate of perforation in randomized trials of the ParaGard® T 380A has been 1 in 1,360. Insertions immediately after the expulsion of the placenta are not known to be associated with increased risks of perforation, but insertion later in the first postpartum month, particularly during lactation, has been associated with an increased risk of perforation.[8,9] Thus, unless performed immediately postpartum, insertion should be delayed to the second postpartum month. IUD insertion immediately postabortion in the first trimester is not known to be associated with increased risks of perforation, but insertion after second trimester abortion should be delayed until the second postabortion month.

The possibility of perforation must be kept in mind during insertion and at the time of any subsequent examination. If perforation occurs, the ParaGard® T 380A should be removed as soon as possible. A surgical procedure may be required. Abdominal adhesions, intestinal penetration, intestinal obstruction, and local inflammatory reaction with abscess formation and erosion of adjacent viscera may result if the ParaGard® T 380A is left in the peritoneal cavity. There are reports of migration after insertion.

6. MEDICAL DIATHERMY
The use of medical diathermy (short-wave and microwave) in a patient with a metal-containing IUD may cause heat injury to the surrounding tissue. Therefore, medical diathermy to the abdominal and sacral areas should not be used on patients with a ParaGard® T 380A in place.

7. EFFECTS OF COPPER
Additional amounts of copper available to the body from the ParaGard® T 380A may precipitate symptoms in women with Wilson's disease. The incidence of Wilson's disease is approximately 1 in 200,000. The long-term effects of intrauterine copper to a child conceived in the presence of an IUD are unknown.

8. RISKS OF MORTALITY
The available data from a variety of sources have been analyzed to estimate the risk of death associated with various methods of contraception. The estimates of risk of death include the combined risk of the contraceptive method plus the risk of pregnancy or abortion in the event of method failure. The findings of the analysis are shown in Table I.[10]
[See table I at top of next page]

PRECAUTIONS

Patients should be counseled that this product does not protect against HIV Infection (AIDS) and other sexually transmitted diseases.

1. Patient Counseling
Prior to insertion, the physician, nurse, or other trained health professional must provide the patient with the Patient Package Insert. The patient should be given the opportunity to read the information and discuss fully any questions she may have concerning the ParaGard® T 380A as well as other methods of contraception.

2. Patient Evaluation and Clinical Considerations
a. A complete medical and social history, including that of the partner, should be obtained to determine conditions that might influence the selection of an IUD. A physical examination should include a pelvic examination, a "Pap" smear, and appropriate tests for any other forms of genital disease, such as gonorrhea and chlamydia laboratory evaluations, if indicated. If actinomyces-like organisms are detected on the Pap smear, they should be cultured to determine whether genital actinomyces is present. The physician should determine that the patient is not pregnant.

b. The uterus should be carefully sounded prior to the insertion to determine the degree of patency of the endocervical canal and the internal os, and the direction and depth of the uterine cavity. In occasional cases, severe cervical stenosis may be encountered. Do not use excessive force to overcome this resistance.

c. The uterus should sound to a depth of 6 to 9 centimeters (cm). Insertion of an IUD into a uterine cavity measuring less than 6.0 cm by sounding may increase the incidence of expulsion, bleeding, pain, perforation, and possibly, pregnancy.

d. Clinicians are cautioned that it is imperative for them to become thoroughly familiar with the instructions for use before attempting placement of the ParaGard® T 380A. To reduce the possibility of insertion in the presence of

TABLE I—Annual Number of Birth-Related or Method-Related Deaths Associated with Control of Fertility per 100,000 Non-sterile Women by Fertility Control Method, by Age.

Methods	Age Group					
	15–19	20–24	25–29	30–34	35–39	40–44
No Birth Control Method/Term	4.7	5.4	4.8	6.3	11.7	20.6
No Birth Control Method/AB	2.1	2.0	1.6	1.9	2.8	5.3
IUD	0.2	0.3	0.2	0.1	0.3	0.6
Periodic Abstinence	1.4	1.3	0.7	1.0	1.0	1.9
Withdrawal	0.9	1.7	0.9	1.3	0.8	1.5
Condom	0.6	1.2	0.6	0.9	0.5	1.0
Diaphragm/Cap	0.6	1.1	0.6	0.9	1.6	3.1
Sponge	0.8	1.5	0.8	1.1	2.2	4.1
Spermicides	1.6	1.9	1.4	1.9	1.5	2.7
Oral Contraceptives	0.8	1.3	1.1	1.8	1.0	1.9
Implants/Injectables	0.2	0.6	0.5	0.8	0.5	0.6
Tubal Sterilization	1.3	1.2	1.1	1.1	1.2	1.3
Vasectomy	0.1	0.1	0.1	0.1	0.1	0.2

an existing undetermined pregnancy, the optimal time for insertion is the latter part of the menstrual period, or one or two days thereafter. The ParaGard® T 380A should not be inserted postpartum or postabortion until involution of the uterus is complete. The incidence of perforation and expulsion is greater if involution is not complete. Data also suggest that there may be an increased risk of perforation and expulsion if the woman is lactating.[8,9] Other recent studies report no increased incidence of perforation or expulsion in lactating women.[11,12]

The ParaGard® T 380A should be placed at the fundus of the uterine cavity. Proper placement enhances contraceptive effectiveness and helps avoid perforation and partial or complete expulsion that could result in pregnancy.

e. Patients experiencing menorrhagia and/or metrorrhagia following IUD insertion may be at risk for the development of hypochromic microcytic anemia. Careful consideration of this risk must be given before insertion in patients with anemia or a history of menorrhagia or hypermenorrhea. Patients receiving anticoagulants or having a coagulopathy may have a greater risk of menorrhagia or hypermenorrhea.

f. Syncope, bradycardia, or other neurovascular episodes may occur during insertion or removal of IUDs, especially in patients with a previous disposition to these conditions or cervical stenosis.

g. Use of an IUD in patients with cervicitis should be postponed until treatment has eradicated the infection.

h. Patients with valvular or congenital heart disease are more prone to develop subacute bacterial endocarditis than patients who do not have valvular or congenital heart disease. Use of an IUD in these patients may represent a potential source of septic emboli. Patients with known congenital heart disease who may be at increased risk should be treated with appropriate antibiotics at the time of insertion.

i. Patients requiring chronic corticosteroid therapy or insulin for diabetes should be monitored with special care for infection.

j. Since the ParaGard® T 380A may be partially or completely expelled, patients should be reexamined and evaluated shortly after the first postinsertion menses, but no later than 3 months afterwards. Thereafter, annual examination with appropriate evaluation, including a "Pap" smear, should be carried out. The ParaGard® T 380A should be kept in place no longer than 10 years.

k. The patient should be told that some bleeding or cramps may occur during the first few weeks after insertion. If these symptoms continue or are severe she should report them to her physician. She should be instructed on how to check to make certain that the threads still protrude from the cervix and cautioned that there is no contraceptive protection if the ParaGard® T 380A has been expelled. She should check frequently, at least after each menstrual period. She should be cautioned not to dislodge the ParaGard® T 380A by pulling on the thread. If a partial expulsion occurs, removal is indicated.

l. Rarely, a copper-induced urticarial allergic skin reaction may develop in women using a copper-containing IUD. If the symptoms of such an allergic response occur, the patient should be instructed to tell the consulting physician that a copper-containing device is being used.

m. The effect of magnetic resonance imaging of the pelvis was investigated in one study[13] in women with the CU-7® (Intrauterine Copper Contraceptive) and the LIPPES LOOP™ IUD. The CU-7® has a different configuration and contains less copper than the ParaGard® T 380A. The results of the study indicate that neither the CU-7® nor the LIPPES LOOP™ were moved under the influence of the magnetic field nor did they heat during the spin-echo sequences usually employed for pelvic imaging.

3. Insertion Prophylaxis

Observe strict asepsis at insertion; clean the endocervix with an antiseptic solution, because the presence of organisms capable of establishing PID cannot be determined by appearance, and because IUD insertion may be associated with introduction of vaginal bacteria into the uterus. Data do not confirm the utility of prophylactic administration of antibiotics in reducing the incidence of PID, and their use in nursing women is not recommended.

4. Requirements for Continuation and Removal

a. The ParaGard® T 380A must be replaced before the end of the tenth year of use. There is no evidence of decreasing contraceptive efficacy with time before ten years, but the contraceptive effectiveness at longer times has not been established; therefore, the patient should be informed of the known duration of contraceptive efficacy and be advised to return in 10 years for removal and possible insertion of a new ParaGard® T 380A.

b. The ParaGard® T 380A should be removed for the following medical reasons: menorrhagia- and/or metrorrhagia-producing anemia; pelvic infection; genital actinomycosis; intractable pelvic pain; dyspareunia; pregnancy; endometrial or cervical malignancy; uterine or cervical perforation; increase in length of the threads extending from the cervix, or any other indication of partial expulsion. Insertions immediately following placental delivery or first trimester abortion may result in threads becoming slightly longer as the uterus involutes and may not represent expulsion or partial expulsion.

c. If the retrieval threads cannot be visualized, they may have retracted into the uterus or have been broken, or the ParaGard® T 380A may have been broken, or the ParaGard® T 380A may have been expelled. Localization may be made by feeling with a probe, X-ray, or sonography. When the physician elects to recover a ParaGard® T 380A with the threads not visible, the removal instructions should be reviewed.

d. Should the patient's relationship cease to be mutually monogamous, or should her partner become HIV positive, or acquire a sexually transmitted disease, she should be instructed to report this change to her clinician immediately. It may be advisable to recommend the use of a barrier method as a partial protection against acquiring sexually transmitted diseases until the ParaGard® T 380A can be removed.

5. Continuing Care of Patients Using ParaGard® T 380A

a. Any inquiries regarding pain, odorous discharge, bleeding, fever, genital lesions or sores, or a missed period should be promptly responded to and prompt examination is recommended.

b. If examination during visits subsequent to insertion reveals that the length of the threads has visibly or palpably changed from their length at time of insertion, the ParaGard® T 380A should be considered displaced and should be removed. A new ParaGard® T 380A may be inserted at that time or during the next menses if it is certain that conception has not occurred. Under no circumstances should reinsertion with an expelled ParaGard® T 380A be attempted. A new ParaGard® T 380A should be inserted.

c. Since the ParaGard® T 380A may be partially or completely expelled, patients should be reexamined and evaluated shortly after the first postinsertion menses, but no later than 3 months afterwards. Thereafter, at least annual examination with appropriate evaluation, including a "Pap" smear, and if indicated, gonococcal and chlamydial laboratory evaluations, should be carried out. The ParaGard® T 380A should be kept in place no longer than 10 years.

d. In the event a pregnancy is confirmed during ParaGard® T 380A use, the following steps should be taken:
- Determine whether pregnancy is ectopic and take appropriate measures if it is.

- Inform patient of the risks of leaving an IUD *in situ* or removing it during pregnancy, and of the lack of data on the long term effects of the ParaGard® T 380A on the offspring of women who have had it *in utero* during conception or gestation (see WARNINGS). This information should include the risk of septic spontaneous abortion with the IUD *in situ*.
- If possible, the ParaGard® T 380A should be removed after the patient has been warned of the risks of removal. If removal is difficult, the patient should be counseled about and offered pregnancy termination.
- If the ParaGard® T 380A is left in place, the patient's course should be followed closely.

ADVERSE REACTIONS

These adverse reactions are not listed in any order of frequency or severity.

Reported adverse reactions with intrauterine contraceptives include: endometritis; spontaneous abortion; septic abortion; septicemia; perforation of the uterus and cervix; embedment; fragmentation of the IUD; pelvic infection; tubo-ovarian abscess; tubal damage; vaginitis; leukorrhea; cervical erosion; pregnancy; ectopic pregnancy; fetal damage; difficult removal; complete or partial expulsion of the IUD, particularly in those patients with uteri measuring less than 6.0 cm by sounding; menstrual spotting; prolongation of menstrual flow; anemia; amenorrhea or delayed menses; pain and cramping; dysmenorrhea; backaches; dyspareunia; neurovascular episodes, including bradycardia and syncope secondary to insertion. Uterine perforation and IUD displacement into the abdomen have been followed by peritonitis, abdominal adhesions, intestinal penetration, intestinal obstruction, and cystic masses in the pelvis. (Certain of these adverse reactions can lead to loss of fertility, partial or total removal of reproductive organs, hormonal imbalance, or death). Urticarial allergic skin reaction may occur.

CLINICAL STUDIES

Different event rates have been reported with the use of different intrauterine contraceptives. Inasmuch as these rates are usually derived from separate studies conducted by different investigators in several populations, they cannot be compared with precision. Considerably different rates are likely to be obtained because event rates per unit of time tend to decrease as studies are extended, since more susceptible subjects discontinue due to expulsions, adverse reactions, or pregnancy, leaving the study population richer in less susceptible subjects. In clinical trials conducted by The Population Council[14,15] and WHO, use-effectiveness of the ParaGard® T 380A as calculated by the life table method was determined through ten (10) years of use.

Data suggest a higher pregnancy rate in women under 20.[14,15,17]

[See table II at top of next page]

TABLE III

GROSS ANNUAL EVENT RATES PER 100 CONTINUING USERS BY YEAR AND PARITY

	1 Year Parous
Pregnancy	0.5
Expulsion	2.3
Bleeding/Pain	3.4
Infection	0.3
Other Medical	0.5
Planning Pregnancy	0.6
Other Personal	0.7
Continuation	92.1
No. Completed	1842.0

Rates were calculated by combining the experience on a weighted basis from both an international study by the World Health Organization (2110 women) and a U.S. study by GynoPharma Inc. (230 women).

The lowest expected and typical failure rates during the first year of continuous use of all contraceptive methods are listed in Table IV. (Adapted from Reference 16.)

[See table IV on next page]

HOW SUPPLIED

Available in cartons of one (NDC 54765-380-01) or five (NDC 54765-380-05) sterile units. Each ParaGard® T 380A is packaged in a Tyvek®-polyethylene pouch, together with an insertion tube and solid rod.

INSTRUCTIONS FOR USE
Paragard®T 380A
(Intrauterine Copper Contraceptive)
CLINICIANS SHOULD HAVE DEMONSTRATED CLINICAL COMPETENCE IN PARAGARD® T 380A INSERTIONS RE-

Continued on next page

Paragard T—Cont.

CEIVED UNDER SUPERVISION. PREVIOUS EDUCATION RE: SURGICAL PROCEDURES WILL REQUIRE VARYING LEVELS OF EXPERIENCE.

The ParaGard® T 380A (Intrauterine Copper Contraceptive) represents a different design in intrauterine contraceptives. Physicians are, therefore, cautioned that they should become thoroughly familiar with instructions for insertion before attempting placement of the ParaGard® T 380A. The insertion technique is different in several respects from that employed with other intrauterine contraceptives and the physician should pay particular attention to the drawings and commentary accompanying these instructions.

A single ParaGard® T 380A is placed at the fundus of the uterine cavity.

The ParaGard® T 380A may be inserted at any time during the cycle. However, it is essential that pregnancy be ruled out before insertion.

The ParaGard® T 380A is indicated for use up to 10 years. Therefore, the ParaGard® T 380A must be removed and a new one inserted on or before 10 years from the date of insertion.

PRELIMINARY PREPARATION AND INSERTION

1. Before insertion, you and the patient will want to review the Patient Package Insert. If the patient agrees, she may sign the Consent Form provided for your records.
2. Take a medical and social history.
3. Refer to CONTRAINDICATIONS, WARNINGS, and PRECAUTIONS.
4. Pelvic examination is to be performed prior to insertion of the ParaGard® T 380A, including a cervical "Pap" smear, and gonococcal and chlamydial evaluations, if indicated, and any other necessary specific tests.
5. If appropriate, commence antibiotic prophylaxis one hour before insertion.
6. Use of aseptic technique during insertion is essential.
7. The endocervix should be cleansed with an antiseptic solution and a tenaculum applied to the cervix with downward traction for correction of the angulation as well as stabilization of the cervix.
8. With a speculum in place, gently insert a sterile sound to determine the depth and direction of the uterine canal. Be sure to determine the position of the uterus before insertion.

CAUTION

Any intrauterine procedure can result in severe pain, bradycardia, and syncope.

It is generally believed that perforations, if they occur, are encountered at the time of insertion, although the perforation may not be detected until some time later. The position of the uterus should be determined during the preinsertion examination. Great care must be exercised during the pre-insertion sounding and subsequent insertion. No attempt should be made to force the insertion.

HOW TO LOAD AND INSERT ParaGard® T 380A
STEP 1

To minimize chance of introducing contamination, do not remove the ParaGard® T 380A from the inserter tube prior to placement in the uterus. Do not bend the arms of the ParaGard® T 380A earlier than 5 minutes before it is to be introduced into the uterus.

In the absence of sterile gloves, this can be accomplished without destroying sterility by folding the arms in the partially opened package. Place the partially opened package on a flat surface and pull the solid rod partially from the package so it will not interfere with assembly. Place thumb and index finger on top of package on ends of the horizontal arms. Push insertion tube against arms of ParaGard® T 380A as indicated by arrow in Fig. 1A to start arms folding.

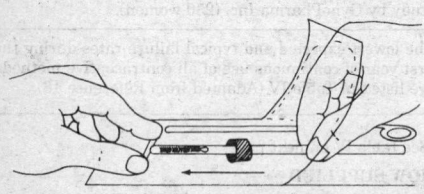

Fig. 1A

Complete the bending by bringing thumb and index finger together using the other hand to maneuver the insertion tube to pick up the arms of the ParaGard® T 380A (Fig. 1B). Insert no further than necessary to insure retention of the arms. Introduce the solid rod into the insertion tube from the bottom alongside the threads until it touches the bottom of the ParaGard® T 380A.

[See figure at top of next page]

TABLE II
ParaGard® T 380A
(Intrauterine Copper Contraceptive)
GROSS ANNUAL TERMINATION AND CONTINUATION RATES PER 100* USERS
All Copper T 380A IUD Acceptors
Combined Population Council and WHO Studies

RATE OF ITEM	YEAR									
	1	2	3	4	5	6	7	8	9	10
Pregnancy	0.7	0.3	0.6	0.2	0.3	0.2	0.0	0.4	0.0	0.0
Expulsion	5.7	2.5	1.6	1.2	0.3	0.0	0.6	1.7	0.2	0.4
Bleeding/Pain	11.9	9.8	7.0	3.5	3.7	2.7	3.0	2.5	2.2	3.7
Other Medical	2.5	2.1	1.6	1.7	0.1	0.3	1.0	0.4	0.7	0.3
Continuation	76.8	78.3	81.2	86.2	89.0	91.9	87.9	88.1	92.0	91.8
No. of Women:										
At Start of Year	4932	3149	2018	1121	872	621	563	483	423	325
At End of Year	3149	2018	1121	872	621	563	483	423	325	230

* Rates were calculated by weighing the annual rates by the number of subjects starting each year for each of the Population Council (3536 acceptors) and the World Health Organization (1396 acceptors) trials.

TABLE IV—Percentage of women experiencing a contraceptive failure during the first year of typical use and the first year of perfect use and the percentage continuing use at the end of the first year, United States.[16]

Method	% of Women Experiencing an Accidental Pregnancy Within the First Year of Use		% of Women Continuing Use at One Year[3]
	Typical Use[1]	Perfect Use[2]	
Chance[4]	85	85	
Spermicides[5]	21	6	43
Periodic Abstinence	20		67
Calendar		9	
Ovulation Method		3	
Sympto-Thermal[6]		2	
Post-Ovulation		1	
Withdrawal	19	4	
Cap[7]			
Parous Women	36	26	45
Nulliparous Women	18	9	58
Sponge			
Parous Women	36	20	45
Nulliparous Women	18	9	58
Diaphragm[7]	18	6	58
Condom[8]			
Female (Reality)	21	5	56
Male	12	3	63
Pill	3		72
Progestin Only		0.5	
Combined		0.1	
IUD			
Progesterone T	2.0	1.5	81
Copper T 380A (ParaGard® T 380A)	0.8	0.6	78
Depo-Provera®	0.3	0.3	70
Norplant® (6 Capsules)	0.09	0.09	85
Female Sterilization	0.4	0.4	100
Male Sterilization	0.15	0.10	100

Emergency Contraceptive Pills: Treatment initiated within 72 hours after unprotected intercourse reduces the risk of pregnancy by at least 75%[9].

Lactational Amenorrhea Method: LAM is a highly effective temporary method of contraception.[10]

Footnotes to Table IV

1. Among *typical* couples who initiate use of a method (not necessarily for the first time), the percentage who experience an accidental pregnancy during the first year if they do not stop use for any other reason.
2. Among couples who initiate use of a method (not necessarily for the first time) and who use it *perfectly* (both consistently and correctly), the percentage who experience an accidental pregnancy during the first year if they do not stop use for any other reason.
3. Among couples attempting to avoid pregnancy, the percentage who continue to use a method for one year.
4. The percentages failing in columns (2) and (3) are based on data from populations where contraception is not used and from women who cease using contraception in order to become pregnant. Among such populations, about 89% become pregnant within one year. This estimate was lowered slightly (to 85%) to represent the percentage who would become pregnant within 1 year among women now relying on reversible methods of contraception if they abandoned contraception altogether.
5. Foams, creams, gels, vaginal suppositories, and vaginal film.
6. Cervical mucus (ovulation) method supplemented by calendar in the pre-ovulatory and basal body temperature in the post-ovulatory phases.
7. With spermicidal cream or jelly.
8. Without spermicides.
9. The treatment schedule is one dose as soon as possible (but no more than 72 hours) after unprotected intercourse, and a second dose 12 hours after the first dose. The hormones that have been studied in the clinical trials of postcoital hormonal contraception are found in Nordette, Levlen, Lo/Orval (1 dose is 4 pills), Triphasil, Tri-Levlin (1 dose is 4 yellow pills), and Ovral (1 dose is 2 pills).
10. However, to maintain effective protection against pregnancy, another method of contraception must be used as soon as menstruation resumes, the frequency or duration of breastfeeds is reduced, bottle feeds are introduced, or the baby reaches 6 months of age.

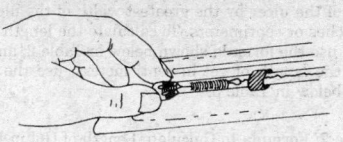

Fig. 1B

STEP 2
Adjust the movable flange so that it indicates the depth to which the ParaGard® T 380A should be inserted and the direction in which the arms of the ParaGard® T 380A will open. At this point, make certain that the horizontal arms of the ParaGard® T 380A and the long axis of the flange lie in the same horizontal plane. Introduce the loaded insertion tube through the cervical canal and upwards until the ParaGard® T 380A lies in contact with the fundus. The movable flange should be at the cervix (Fig. 2).
DO NOT FORCE THE INSERTION.

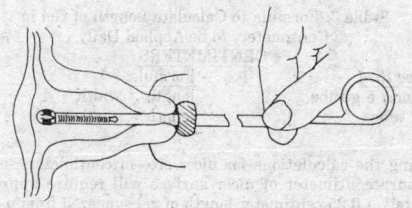

Fig. 2

STEP 3
To release the arms of the ParaGard® T 380A, withdraw the insertion tube not more than $1/2$ inch while the solid rod is not permitted to move. This releases the arms of the ParaGard® T 380A (Fig. 3).

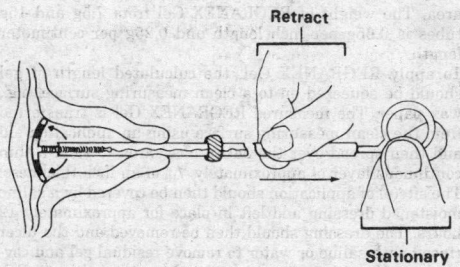

Retract

Stationary

Fig. 3

STEP 4
After the arms are released, the insertion tube should be moved upward gently until the resistance of the fundus is felt. This will assure placement of the T at the highest possible position within the endometrial cavity (Fig. 4).

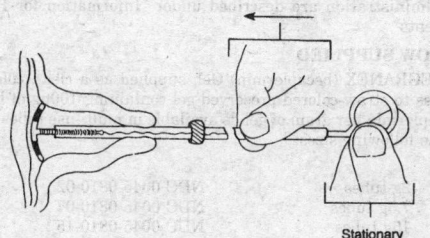

Stationary

Fig. 4

STEP 5
Withdraw the solid rod while holding the insertion tube stationary (Fig. 5).

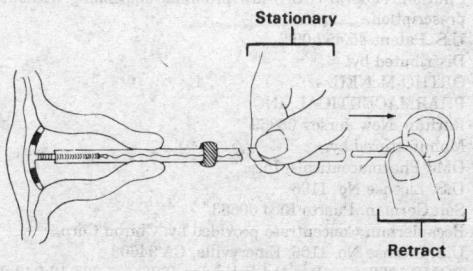

Stationary

Retract

Fig. 5

STEP 6
Withdraw the insertion tube from the cervix. Be sure sufficient length of the threads are visible (approximately 1 in. or 2.5 cm.) to facilitate checking for the presence of the ParaGard® T 380A (Fig. 6). Notation of length of the threads should be made in patient record.

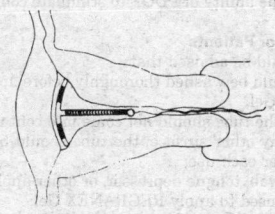

Fig. 6

HOW TO REMOVE ParaGard® T 380A
To remove the ParaGard® T 380A, pull gently on the exposed threads. The arms of the ParaGard® T 380A will fold upwards as it is withdrawn from the uterus. Even if removal proves difficult, the ParaGard® T 380A should not remain in the uterus after 10 years.

REFERENCES
1. Alvarez F et al: New insights on the mode of action on intrauterine contraceptives in women. *Fertil Steril* 1988; 49:768–773.
2. World Health Organization's Special Programme of Research, Development and Research Training in Human Reproduction: A multinational case-control study of ectopic pregnancy. *Clin Reprod Fertil* 1985; 3:131–143.
3. Ory HW, Women's Health Study: Ectopic pregnancy and intrauterine contraceptive devices: New perspectives. *Obstet Gynecol* 1981; 57:137–144.
4. Marchbanks PA et al: Risk factors for ectopic pregnancy: A population-based study. *JAMA* 1988; 259:1823–1827.
5. Farley TMM et al: Intrauterine devices and pelvic inflammatory disease: An international perspective. *Lancet* 1992; 339:785–788.
6. Cramer DW et al: Tubal infertility and the intrauterine device. *N Engl J Med* 1985; 312:941–947.
7. Daling JR et al: Primary tubal infertility in relation to the use of an intrauterine device. *N Engl J Med* 1985; 312:937–941.
8. Heartwell SF, Schlesselman S: Risk of uterine perforation among users of intrauterine devices. *Obstet Gynecol* 1983; 61:31–36.
9. Chi I-C, Kelly E: Is lactation a risk factor of IUD and sterilization-related uterine perforations? A hypothesis. *Int J Gynaecol Obstet* 1984; 22:315–317.
10. Harlap S, Kost K, Forrest JD: Preventing pregnancy, protecting health: a new look at birth control choices in the United States. The Alan Guttmacher Institute 1991; 1–129.
11. Chi I-C et al: Performance of the Copper T 380A Intrauterine device in breast feeding women. *Contraception* 1989; 39:603–618.
12. Farr G. Rivera R: Interactions between intrauterine contraceptive device use and breast-feeding status at time of intrauterine contraceptive device insertion. Analysis of TCu-380A acceptors in developing countries. *Am J Obstet Gynecol* 1992; 167:144–151.
13. Mark AS, Hricak H: Intrauterine contraceptive devices: MR imaging. *Radiology* 1987; 311–314.
14. Sivin, I, Stern J: Long-acting, more effective Copper T IUDs: A summary of US experience, 1970–1975, *Stud Fam Plann* 1979; 10:263–281.
15. Sivin I, Schmidt F: Effectiveness of IUDs: A review. *Contraception* 1987; 36:55–84.
16. Trussell J: The Essentials of Contraception, in R.A. Hatcher, et al: *Contraceptive Technology*, 16th Revised Ed., New York, Irvington, 1994, 113–114.
17. World Health Organization (WHO): Mechanism of action, safety, and efficacy of intrauterine devices. Report of a WHO Scientific Group. Technical Report Series 753. Geneva; World Health Organization, 1987, p. 22.

Manufactured for

Shown in Product Identification Guide, page 328

REGRANEX® GEL 0.01%   ℞
[rĕ gran 'x]
(becaplermin)

Prescribing Information

DESCRIPTION
REGRANEX® Gel contains becaplermin, a recombinant human platelet-derived growth factor (rhPDGF-BB) for topical administration. Becaplermin is produced by recombinant DNA technology by insertion of the gene for the B chain of platelet-derived growth factor (PDGF) into the yeast, *Saccharomyces cerevisiae*. Becaplermin has a molecular weight of approximately 25 KD and is a homodimer composed of two identical polypeptide chains that are bound together by disulfide bonds. Becaplermin Concentrate is produced by Chiron Corp. and supplied to OMJ Pharmaceuticals under a shared manufacturing arrangement. REGRANEX Gel is a non-sterile, low bioburden, preserved, sodium carboxymethylcellulose-based (CMC) topical gel, containing the active ingredient becaplermin and the following inactive ingredients: sodium chloride, sodium acetate trihydrate, glacial acetic acid, water for injection, and methylparaben, propylparaben, and m-cresol as preservatives and l-lysine hydrochloride as a stabilizer. Each gram of REGRANEX Gel contains 100 µg of becaplermin.

CLINICAL PHARMACOLOGY
REGRANEX has biological activity similar to that of endogenous platelet-derived growth factor, which includes promoting the chemotactic recruitment and proliferation of cells involved in wound repair and enhancing the formation of granulation tissue.

Pharmacokinetics
Ten patients with Stage III or IV (as defined in the International Association of Enterostomal Therapy (IAET) guide to chronic wound staging, *J. Enterostomal Ther* 15:4, 1988 and *Decubitis* 2:24, 1989) lower extremity diabetic ulcers received topical applications of becaplermin gel 0.01% at a dose range of 0.32–2.95 µg/kg (7µg/cm²) daily for 14 days. Six patients had non-quantifiable PDGF levels at baseline and throughout the study, two patients had PDGF levels at baseline which did not increase substantially, and two patients had PDGF levels that increased sporadically above their baseline values during the 14 day study period.
Systemic bioavailability of becaplermin was less than 3% in rats with full thickness wounds receiving single or multiple (5 days) topical applications of 127 µg/kg (20.1 µg/cm² of wound area) of becaplermin gel.

Clinical Studies
The effects of REGRANEX Gel on the incidence of and time to complete healing in lower extremity diabetic ulcers were assessed in four randomized controlled studies. Of 922 patients studied, 478 received either REGRANEX Gel 0.003% or 0.01%. All study participants had lower extremity diabetic neuropathic ulcers that extended into the subcutaneous tissue or beyond (Stages III and IV of the IAET guide to chronic wound staging). Ninety-three percent of the patients enrolled in these four trials had foot ulcers. The remaining 7% of the patients had ankle or leg ulcers. The diabetic ulcers were of at least 8 weeks duration and had an adequate blood supply (defined as $T_cpO_2 > 30$ mm Hg). In the four trials, ninety-five percent of the ulcers measured in area up to 10 cm², and the median ulcer size at baseline ranged from 1.4 cm² to 3.5 cm². All treatment groups received a program of good ulcer care consisting of initial complete sharp debridement, a non-weight-bearing regimen, systemic treatment for wound-related infection if present, moist saline dressings changed twice a day, and additional debridement as necessary. REGRANEX Gel 0.003% or 0.01% or placebo gel was applied once a day and covered with a saline moistened dressing. After approximately 12 hours, the gel was gently rinsed off and a saline moistened dressing was then applied for the remainder of the day. Patients were treated until complete healing, or for a period of up to 20 weeks. Patients were considered a treatment failure if their ulcer did not show an approximately 30% reduction in initial ulcer area after eight to ten weeks of REGRANEX Gel therapy.
The primary endpoint, incidence of complete ulcer closure within 20 weeks, for all treatment arms is shown in Figure 1. In each study, REGRANEX Gel in conjunction with good ulcer care was compared to placebo gel plus good ulcer care or good ulcer care alone.
In Study 1, a multicenter, double-blind, placebo controlled trial of 118 patients, the incidence of complete ulcer closure for REGRANEX Gel 0.003% (n=61) was 48% versus 25% for placebo gel (n=57; p=0.02, logistic regression analysis).
In Study 2, a multicenter, double-blind, placebo controlled trial of 382 patients, the incidence of complete ulcer closure for REGRANEX Gel 0.01% (n=123), was 50% versus 36% for REGRANEX Gel 0.003% (n=132), and 35% for placebo gel (n=127). Only REGRANEX Gel 0.01% was significantly different from placebo gel (p=0.01, logistic regression analysis).

Continued on next page

Regranex—Cont.

The primary goal of Study 3, a multicenter controlled trial of 172 patients, was to assess the safety of vehicle gel (placebo; n=70) compared to good ulcer care alone (n=68). The study included a small (n=34) REGRANEX Gel 0.01% arm. Incidences of complete ulcer closure were 44% for REGRANEX Gel, 36% for placebo gel and 22% for good ulcer care alone.

In Study 4, a multicenter, evaluator-blind, controlled trial of 250 patients, the incidences of complete ulcer closure in the REGRANEX Gel 0.01% arm (n=128) (36%) and good ulcer care alone (n=122) (32%) were not statistically different.

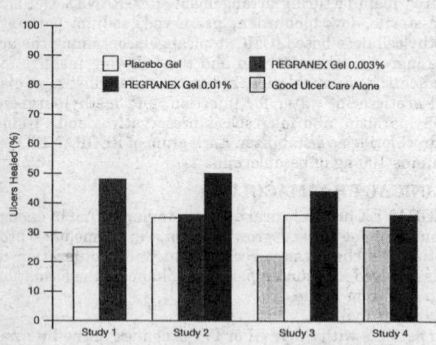

Figure 1: Incidence of Complete Healing

In general, where REGRANEX Gel was associated with higher incidences of complete ulcer closure, differences in the incidence first became apparent after approximately 10 weeks and increased with continued treatment (Table 1).

Table 1: Life Table Estimates of the Incidence (%) of Complete Healing Over Time for Study 2

	REGRANEX Gel 0.01% (%)	Placebo Gel (%)
Week 2	1	0
Week 4	6	2
Week 6	9	6
Week 8	16	14
Week 10	23	18
Week 12	34	25
Week 14	37	28
Week 16	43	33
Week 18	46	34
Week 20	50	37

In a 3-month follow-up period where no standardized regimen of preventative care was utilized, the incidence of ulcer recurrence was approximately 30% in all treatment groups, demonstrating that the durability of ulcer closure was comparable in all treatment groups.

The efficacy of REGRANEX Gel for the treatment of non-diabetic ulcers is under evaluation.

INDICATIONS AND USAGE

REGRANEX Gel is indicated for the treatment of lower extremity diabetic neuropathic ulcers that extend into the subcutaneous tissue or beyond and have an adequate blood supply. When used as an adjunct to, and not a substitute for, good ulcer care practices including initial sharp debridement, pressure relief and infection control, REGRANEX Gel increases the incidence of complete healing of diabetic ulcers.

The efficacy of REGRANEX Gel for the treatment of diabetic neuropathic ulcers that do not extend through the dermis into subcutaneous tissue (Stage I or II, IAET staging classification) or ischemic diabetic ulcers has not been evaluated.

CONTRAINDICATIONS

REGRANEX Gel is contraindicated in patients with:
— known hypersensitivity to any component of this product (e.g., parabens);
— known neoplasm(s) at the site(s) of application.

WARNINGS

REGRANEX (becaplermin) Gel is a non-sterile, low bioburden preserved product. Therefore, it should not be used in wounds that close by primary intention.

PRECAUTIONS

For external use only.
If application site reactions occur, the possibility of sensitization or irritation caused by parabens or m-cresol should be considered.

The effects of becaplermin on exposed joints, tendons, ligaments, and bone have not been established in humans. In pre-clinical studies, rats injected at the metatarsals with 3 or 10 µg/site (approximately 60 or 200 µg/kg) of becaplermin every other day for 13 days displayed histological changes indicative of accelerated bone remodeling consisting of periosteal hyperplasia and subperiosteal bone resorption and exostosis. The soft tissue adjacent to the injection site had fibroplasia with accompanying mononuclear cell infiltration reflective of the ability of PDGF to stimulate connective tissue growth.

Information for Patients

Patients should be advised that:
— hands should be washed thoroughly before applying REGRANEX Gel;
— the tip of the tube should not come into contact with the ulcer or any other surface; the tube should be recapped tightly after each use;
— a cotton swab, tongue depressor, or other application aid should be used to apply REGRANEX Gel;
— REGRANEX Gel should only be applied once a day in a carefully measured quantity (see Dosage and Administration section). The measured quantity of gel should be spread evenly over the ulcerated area to yield a thin continuous layer of approximately $^1/_{16}$ of an inch thickness. The measured length of the gel to be squeezed from the tube should be adjusted according to the size of the ulcer. The amount of REGRANEX Gel to be applied daily should be recalculated at weekly or biweekly intervals by the physician or wound care giver;

Step-by-step instructions for application of REGRANEX Gel are as follows:
• Squeeze the calculated length of gel on to a clean, firm, non-absorbable surface, e.g., wax paper.
• With a clean cotton swab, tongue depressor, or similar application aid, spread the measured REGRANEX Gel over the ulcer surface to obtain an even layer.
• Cover with a saline moistened gauze dressing.
— after approximately 12 hours, the ulcer should be gently rinsed with saline or water to remove residual gel and covered with a saline-moistened gauze dressing (without REGRANEX Gel);
— it is important to use REGRANEX Gel together with a good ulcer care program, including a strict non-weight-bearing program;
— excess application of REGRANEX Gel has not been shown to be beneficial;
— REGRANEX Gel should be stored in the refrigerator. Do not freeze REGRANEX Gel;
— REGRANEX Gel should not be used after the expiration date on the bottom, crimped end of the tube.

Drug Interactions

It is not known if REGRANEX Gel interacts with other topical medications applied to the ulcer site. The use of REGRANEX Gel with other topical drugs has not been studied.

Carcinogenesis, Mutagenesis, Impairment of Fertility

Becaplermin was not genotoxic in a battery of in vitro assays, (including those for bacterial and mammalian cell point mutation, chromosomal aberration, and DNA damage/repair). Becaplermin was also not mutagenic in an in vivo assay for the induction of micronuclei in mouse bone marrow cells.

Carcinogenesis and reproductive toxicity studies have not been conducted with REGRANEX Gel.

Pregnancy: Category C

Animal reproduction studies have not been conducted with REGRANEX Gel. It is also not known whether REGRANEX Gel can cause fetal harm when administered to a pregnant woman or can affect reproductive capacity. REGRANEX Gel should be given to pregnant women only if clearly needed.

Nursing Mothers

It is not known whether becaplermin is excreted in human milk. Because many drugs are secreted in human milk, caution should be exercised when REGRANEX Gel is administered to nursing women.

Pediatric Use

Safety and effectiveness of REGRANEX Gel in pediatric patients below the age of 16 years have not been established.

ADVERSE REACTIONS

Patients receiving REGRANEX Gel, placebo gel, and good ulcer care alone had a similar incidence of ulcer-related adverse events such as infection, cellulitis, or osteomyelitis. However, erythematous rashes occurred in 2% of patients treated with REGRANEX Gel and placebo, and none in patients receiving good ulcer care alone. The incidence of cardiovascular, respiratory, musculoskeletal and central and peripheral nervous system disorders was not different across all treatment groups. Mortality rates were also similar across all treatment groups. Patients treated with REGRANEX Gel did not develop neutralizing antibodies against becaplermin.

DOSAGE AND ADMINISTRATION

The amount of REGRANEX Gel to be applied will vary depending upon the size of the ulcer area. To calculate the length of gel to apply to the ulcer, measure the greatest length of the ulcer by the greatest width of the ulcer in either inches or centimeters. To calculate the length of gel in inches, use the formula shown below in Table 2, and to calculate the length of gel in centi meters, use the formula shown below in Table 3.

Table 2: Formula to Calculate Length of Gel in Inches to be Applied Daily
INCHES

Tube Size	Formula
15 or 7.5 g tube	length × width × 0.6
2 g tube	length × width × 1.3

Using the calculation, each square inch of ulcer surface will require approximately $^2/_3$ inch length of gel squeezed from a 15g or 7.5g tube, or approximately $1^1/_3$ inch length of the gel from a 2g tube. For example, if the ulcer measures 1 inch by 2 inches, then a 1¼ inch length of gel should be used for 15g or 7.5g tubes (1 × 2 × 0.6 = 1¼) and 2¾ inch gel length should be used for 2g tube (1 × 2 × 1.3 = 2¾).

Table 3: Formula to Calculate Length of Gel in Centimeters to be Applied Daily
CENTIMETERS

Tube Size	Formula
15 or 7.5 g tube	length × width ÷ 4
2 g tube	length × width ÷ 2

Using the calculations for ulcer size in centimeters, each square centimeter of ulcer surface will require approximately a 0.25 centimeter length of gel squeezed from 15g or 7.5g tube, or approximately a 0.5 centimeter length of gel from a 2g tube. For example, if the ulcer measures 4 cm by 2 cm, then a 2 centimeter length of gel should be used for 15g or 7.5g tube [(4 × 2) ÷ 4 = 2] and a 4 centimeter length of gel should be used for 2g tube [(4 × 2) ÷ 2 = 4].

The amount of REGRANEX Gel to be applied should be recalculated by the physician or wound care giver at weekly or biweekly intervals depending on the rate of change in ulcer area. The weight of REGRANEX Gel from 7.5g and 15g tubes is 0.65g per inch length and 0.25g per centimeter length.

To apply REGRANEX Gel, the calculated length of gel should be squeezed on to a clean measuring surface, e.g., wax paper. The measured REGRANEX Gel is transferred from the clean measuring surface using an application aid and then spread over the entire ulcer area to yield a thin continuous layer of approximately $^1/_{16}$ of an inch thickness. The site(s) of application should then be covered by a saline moistened dressing and left in place for approximately 12 hours. The dressing should then be removed and the ulcer rinsed with saline or water to remove residual gel and covered again with a second moist dressing (without REGRANEX Gel) for the remainder of the day. REGRANEX Gel should be applied once daily to the ulcer until complete healing has occurred. If the ulcer does not decrease in size by approximately 30% after 10 weeks of treatment or complete healing has not occurred in 20 weeks, continued treatment with REGRANEX Gel should be reassessed. The step-by-step instructions for applying REGRANEX Gel for home administration are described under "Information for Patients".

HOW SUPPLIED

REGRANEX (becaplermin) Gel, supplied as a clear, colorless to straw-colored preserved gel containing 100µg of becaplermin per gram of gel, is available in multi-use tubes in the following sizes:

2g tubes	NDC 0045-0810-02
7.5g tubes	NDC 0045-0810-07
15g tubes	NDC 0045-0810-15

REGRANEX Gel is for external use only.

Storage

Store refrigerated, 2–8° C (36–46° F). DO NOT FREEZE. DO NOT USE THE GEL AFTER THE EXPIRATION DATE AT THE BOTTOM OF THE TUBE.

Caution: Federal (USA) law prohibits dispensing without prescription.

U.S. Patent #5,457,093
Distributed by:
ORTHO-McNEIL
PHARMACEUTICAL, INC.
Raritan, New Jersey 08869
Manufactured by:
OMJ Pharmaceuticals, Inc.
U.S. License No. 1196
San German, Puerto Rico 00683
Becaplermin Concentrate provided by: Chiron Corp.,
U.S. License No. 1106, Emeryville, CA 94608
©OMP 1998   Revised February 1998   635-10-240-2
Shown in Product Identification Guide, page 328

SULTRIN® Triple Sulfa Cream ℞
(sulfathiazole/sulfacetamide/ sulfabenzamide)

DESCRIPTION

SULTRIN Cream contains sulfathiazole (Benzenesulfonamide,4-amino-N-2-thiazolyl-N[1]-2-thiazolylsulfanilamide) 3.42%, sulfacetamide (Acetamide,N-[(4-aminophenyl) sulfonyl]-N-Sulfanilylacetamide) 2.86%, and sulfabenzamide (Benzamide,N-[(4-aminophenyl) sulfonyl]-N-Sulfanilylbenzamide) 3.7%, compounded with cetyl alcohol 2%, cholesterol, diethylaminoethyl stearamide, glyceryl monostearate, lanolin, lecithin, methylparaben, peanut oil, phosphoric acid, propylene glycol, propylparaben, purified water, stearic acid and urea.
Each SULTRIN Tablet contains sulfathiazole (Benzenesulfonamide,4-amino-N -2- thiazolyl-N[1]-2-thiazolylsulfanilamide) 172.5 mg, sulfacetamide (Acetamide,N-[(4-aminophenyl)sulfonyl] -N- Sulfanilylacetamide) 143.75 mg and sulfabenzamide (Benzamide,N-[(4-aminophenyl)sulfonyl]-N-Sulfanilylbenzamide) 184.0 mg, compounded with guar gum, lactose, magnesium stearate, starch and urea.
SULTRIN Cream is a topical antibacterial preparation available for intravaginal administration.

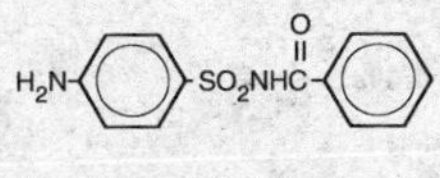

Sulfabenzamide

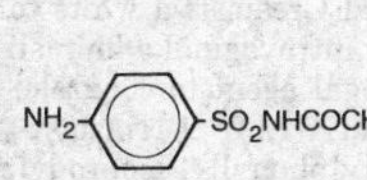

Sulfacetamide

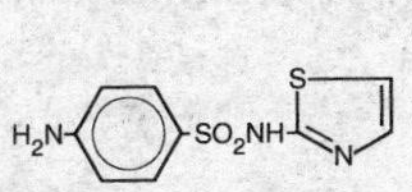

Sulfathiazole

CLINICAL PHARMACOLOGY

The mode of action of SULTRIN is not completely known. SULTRIN Cream is a topical antibacterial preparation used intravaginally against *Haemophilus (Gardnerella) vaginalis* bacteria. Indirect effects, such as lowering the vaginal pH, may be equally important mechanisms.

INDICATIONS AND USAGE

SULTRIN Cream is indicated for the treatment of vaginitis caused by *Haemophilus (Gardnerella) vaginalis* bacteria.
The diagnosis of a *Haemophilus (Gardnerella) vaginalis* vaginitis should be firmly established before initiation of treatment with SULTRIN.

CONTRAINDICATIONS

SULTRIN is contraindicated in the following circumstances: kidney disease; hypersensitivity to sulfonamides; in pregnancy at term and during the nursing period because sulfonamides cross the placenta, are excreted in breast milk and may cause Kernicterus.

WARNINGS

Deaths associated with the administration of sulfonamides have been reported from hypersensitivity reactions, agranulocytosis, aplastic anemia and other blood dyscrasias.
The presence of clinical signs such as sore throat, fever, pallor, purpura or jaundice may be early indications of serious blood disorders.

PRECAUTIONS

Because sulfonamides may be absorbed from the vaginal mucosa, the usual precautions for oral sulfonamides apply. Patients should be observed for skin rash or evidence of systemic toxicity, and if these develop, the medications should be discontinued.
Laboratory tests: Standard office diagnostic procedures for vaginitis are usually sufficient to establish the diagnosis of *Haemophilus (Gardnerella) vaginalis* and to rule out a trichomonal or monilial infection. These include noting a fish-like odor upon addition of 10% KOH to vaginal discharge and microscopic identification of "clue cells" in a wet mount preparation. If cultures are obtained, care must be taken to use appropriate media and methods for *Haemophilus (Gardnerella) vaginalis*.
Carcinogenesis, mutagenesis, impairment of fertility: The sulfonamides bear certain chemical similarities to some goitrogens. Rats appear to be especially susceptible to the goitrogenic effects of sulfonamides, and long-term administration has produced thyroid malignancies in this species.
Pregnancy:
Teratogenic Effects: Pregnancy Category C: The safe use of sulfonamides in pregnancy has not been established. The teratogenicity potential of most sulfonamides has not been thoroughly investigated in either animals or humans. However, a significant increase in the incidence of cleft palate and other bony abnormalities of offspring has been observed when certain sulfonamides of the short, intermediate and long-acting types were given to pregnant rats and mice at high oral doses (7 to 25 times the human therapeutic dose).
Nursing Mothers: Because of the potential for serious adverse reactions in nursing infants from SULTRIN, a decision should be made whether to discontinue nursing or to discontinue the drug, taking into account the importance of the drug to the mother. See CONTRAINDICATIONS.
Pediatric use: Safety and effectiveness in children have not been established.

ADVERSE REACTIONS

There has been one reported case of Agranulocytosis in a patient receiving SULTRIN Cream. The most frequent adverse reactions to SULTRIN are localized irritation and/or allergy including rare reports of Stevens Johnson syndrome which may be fatal.

DOSAGE AND ADMINISTRATION

SULTRIN Cream. One full applicator intravaginally twice daily for four to six days. This course of therapy may be repeated if necessary; the dosage may be reduced one-half to one-quarter.

HOW SUPPLIED

Cream—78 g tubes with the ORTHO* Measured-Dose Applicator.
NDC 0062-5440-77; SULTRIN Cream
REVISED November 1996 643-10-380-7

TERAZOL® 3 ℞
VAGINAL CREAM 0.8%
(terconazole)

DESCRIPTION

TERAZOL® 3 (terconazole) Vaginal Cream 0.8% is a white to off-white, water washable cream for intravaginal administration containing 0.8% of the antifungal agent terconazole, *cis* -1-[*p*-[[2-(2,4-Dichlorophenyl)-2-(1H-1,2,4-triazol-1-ylmethyl)-1,3-dioxolan-4-yl] methoxy] phenyl]-4-isopropylpiperazine, compounded in a cream base consisting of butylated hydroxyanisole, cetyl alcohol, isopropyl myristate, polysorbate 60, polysorbate 80, propylene glycol, stearyl alcohol, and purified water.
The structural formula of terconazole is as follows:

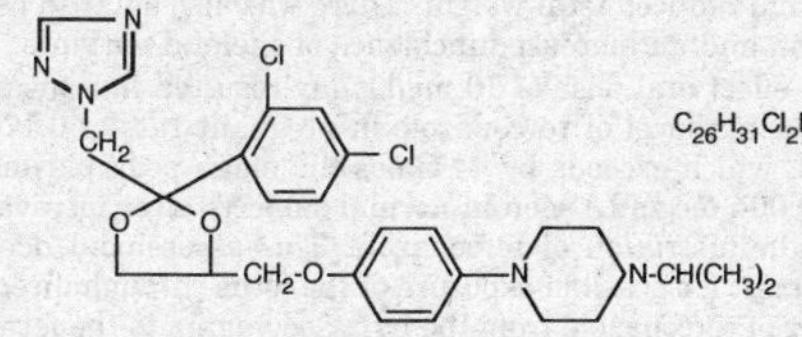

$C_{26}H_{31}Cl_2N_5O_3$

Terconazole, a triazole derivative, is a white to almost white powder with a molecular weight of 532.47. It is insoluble in water; sparingly soluble in ethanol; and soluble in butanol.

CLINICAL PHARMACOLOGY

Following daily intravaginal administration of 0.8% terconazole 40 mg (0.8% cream × 5 g) for seven days to normal humans, plasma concentrations were low and gradually rose to a daily peak (mean of 5.9 ng/mL or 0.006 mcg/mL) at 6.6 hours. Results from similar studies in patients with vulvovaginal candidiasis indicate that the slow rate of absorption, the lack of accumulation, and the mean peak plasma concentration of terconazole was not different from that observed in healthy women. The absorption characteristics of terconazole 0.8% in pregnant or non-pregnant patients with vulvovaginal candidiasis were also similar to those found in normal volunteers.
Following oral (30 mg) administration of ^{14}C-labelled terconazole, the harmonic half-life of elimination from the blood for the parent terconazole was 6.9 hours (range 4.0–11.3). Terconazole is extensively metabolized; the plasma AUC for terconazole compared to the AUC for total radioactivity was 0.6%. Total radioactivity was eliminated from the blood with a harmonic half-life of 52.2 hours (range 44–60). Excretion of radioactivity was both by renal (32–56%) and fecal (47–52%) routes.
In vitro, terconazole is highly protein bound (94.9%) and the degree of binding is independent of the drug concentration. Photosensitivity reactions were observed in some normal volunteers following repeated dermal application of terconazole 2.0% and 0.8% creams under conditions of filtered artificial ultraviolet light. Photosensitivity reactions have not been observed in U.S. and foreign clinical trials in patients who were treated with terconazole 0.8% vaginal cream.
Microbiology: Terconazole exhibits fungicidal activity *in vitro* against *Candida albicans.* Antifungal activity also has been demonstrated against other fungi. The MIC values for terconazole against most species of lactic acid bacteria typically found in the human vagina were ≥128 mcg/mL. The exact pharmacologic mode of action of terconazole is uncertain; however, it may exert its antifungal activity by the disruption of normal fungal cell membrane permeability. No resistance to terconazole has developed during successive passages of *C. albicans.*

INDICATIONS AND USAGE

TERAZOL 3 Vaginal Cream is indicated for the local treatment of vulvovaginal candidiasis (moniliasis). As TERAZOL 3 Vaginal Cream is effective only for vulvovaginitis caused by the genus *Candida,* the diagnosis should be confirmed by KOH smears and/or cultures.

CONTRAINDICATIONS

Patients known to be hypersensitive to terconazole or to any of the components of the cream.

WARNINGS

None.

PRECAUTIONS

General: Discontinue use and do not retreat with terconazole if sensitization, irritation, fever, chills or flu-like symptoms are reported during use.
Laboratory Tests: If there is lack of response to TERAZOL 3 Vaginal Cream, appropriate microbiologic studies (standard KOH smear and/or cultures) should be repeated to confirm the diagnosis and rule out other pathogens.
Drug Interactions: The levels of estradiol (E2) and progesterone did not differ significantly when 0.8% terconazole vaginal cream was administered to healthy female volunteers established on a low dose oral contraceptive.
Carcinogenesis, Mutagenesis, Impairment of Fertility:
Carcinogenesis: Studies to determine the carcinogenic potential of terconazole have not been performed.
Mutagenicity: Terconazole was not mutagenic when tested *in vitro* for induction of microbial point mutations (Ames test) or for inducing cellular transformation, or *in vivo* for chromosome breaks (micronucleus test) or dominant lethal mutations in mouse germ cells.
Impairment of Fertility: No impairment of fertility occurred when female rats were administered terconazole orally up to 40 mg/kg/day for a three month period.
PREGNANCY: Teratogenic Effects.
Pregnancy Category C.
There was no evidence of teratogenicity when terconazole was administered orally up to 40 mg/kg/day or subcutaneously up to 20 mg/kg/day in rats. Dosages at or below 10 mg/kg/day produced no embryotoxicity; however, there was a delay in fetal ossification at 10 mg/kg/day in rats. There was some evidence of embryotoxicity in rabbits and rats at 20–40 mg/kg. In rats, this was reflected as a decrease in litter size and number of viable young and reduced fetal weight. There was also delay in ossification and an increased incidence of skeletal variants. The no-effect oral dose of 10/mg/kg/day resulted in a mean peak plasma level of terconazole in pregnant rats of 0.176 mcg/mL which exceeds by 30 times the mean peak plasma level (0.006 mcg/mL) seen in normal subjects after intravaginal administration of terconazole 0.8% vaginal cream. This safety assessment does not account for possible exposure of the fetus through direct transfer of terconazole from the irritated vagina by diffusion across amniotic membranes. Since terconazole is absorbed from the human vagina, it should not be used in the first trimester of pregnancy unless the physician considers it essential to the welfare of the patient.
Nursing Mothers: It is not known whether this drug is excreted in human milk. Animal studies have shown that rat offspring exposed via the milk of treated (40 mg/kg/orally) dams showed decreased survival during the first few postpartum days, but overall pup weight and weight gain were comparable to or greater than controls throughout lactation. Because many drugs are excreted in human milk, and because of the potential for adverse reaction in nursing infants from terconazole, a decision should be made whether to discontinue nursing or to discontinue the drug, taking into account the importance of the drug to the mother.
Pediatric Use: Safety and efficacy in children have not been established.

ADVERSE REACTIONS

During controlled clinical studies conducted in the United States, patients with vulvovaginal candidiasis were treated with terconazole 0.8% vaginal cream for three days. Based on comparative analyses with placebo and a standard agent, the adverse experiences considered most likely related to terconazole 0.8% vaginal cream were headache (21% vs. 16% with placebo) and dysmenorrhea (6% vs. 2% with placebo). Genital complaints in general, and burning and itching in particular, occurred less frequently in the ter-

Continued on next page

Terazol 3 Cream—Cont.

conazole 0.8% vaginal cream 3 day regimen (5% vs. 6%–9% with placebo). Other adverse experiences reported with terconazole 0.8% vaginal cream were abdominal pain (3.4% vs. 1% with placebo) and fever (1% vs. 0.3% with placebo). The therapy related dropout rate was 2.0% for the terconazole 0.8% vaginal cream. The adverse drug experience most frequently causing discontinuation of therapy was vulvovaginal itching, 0.7% with the terconazole 0.8% vaginal cream group and 0.3% with the placebo group.

OVERDOSAGE

Overdose of terconazole in humans has not been reported to date. In the rat, the oral LD 50 values were found to be 1741 and 849 mg/kg for the male and female, respectively. The oral LD 50 values for the male and female dog were ≅1280 and ≥640 mg/kg, respectively.

DOSAGE AND ADMINISTRATION

One full applicator (5 g) of TERAZOL 3 Vaginal Cream (40 mg terconazole) should be administered intravaginally once daily at bedtime for three consecutive days. Before prescribing another course of therapy, the diagnosis should be reconfirmed by smears and/or cultures and other pathogens commonly associated with vulvovaginitis ruled out. The therapeutic effect of TERAZOL 3 Vaginal Cream is not affected by menstruation.

HOW SUPPLIED

TERAZOL 3 (terconazole) Vaginal Cream 0.8% is available in 20 g (NDC 0062-5356-01) tubes with an ORTHO® Measured-Dose Applicator. Store at controlled room temperature 15–30°C (59–86°F).
Caution: Federal (U.S.A.) law prohibits dispensing without prescription.
631-11-314-3 Revised March 1995
Shown in Product Identification Guide, page 328

TERAZOL® 3 ℞
Vaginal Suppositories 80 mg
(terconazole)

DESCRIPTION

TERAZOL 3 Vaginal Suppositories are white to offwhite suppositories for intravaginal administration containing 80 mg of the antifungal agent terconazole, *cis* -1-[*p*-[[2-(2,4-Dichlorophenyl)-2-(1H-1,2,4-triazol-1-ylmethyl)-1,3-dioxolan-4-yl]methoxy]phenyl]-4-isopropylpiperazine, in triglycerides derived from coconut and/or palm kernel oil (a base of hydrogenated vegetable oils) and butylated hydroxyanisole.
TERCONAZOLE

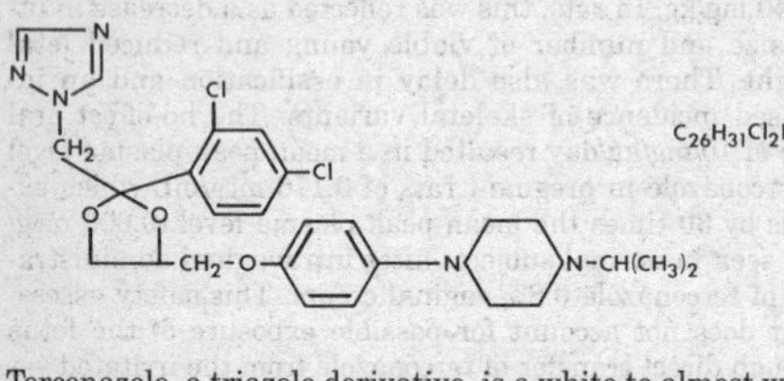

$C_{26}H_{31}Cl_2N_5O_3$

Terconazole, a triazole derivative, is a white to almost white powder with a molecular weight of 532.47. It is insoluble in water; sparingly soluble in ethanol; and soluble in butanol.

CLINICAL PHARMACOLOGY

Microbiology: Terconazole exhibits fungicidal activity *in vitro* against *Candida albicans.* The MIC values for terconazole against most species of lactic acid bacteria typically found in the human vagina were ≥128 mcg/mL, therefore, these beneficial bacteria are not affected by drug treatment.
The exact pharmacologic mode of action of terconazole is uncertain; however, it may exert its antifungal activity by the disruption of normal fungal cell membrane permeability. No resistance to terconazole has developed during successive passages of *C. albicans.*
Human Pharmacology: Following intravaginal administration of terconazole in humans, absorption ranged from 5–8% in three hysterectomized subjects and 12–16% in two non-hysterectomized subjects with tubal ligations. Following oral (30 mg) administration of ^{14}C-labelled terconazole, the half-life of elimination from the blood for the parent terconazole was 6.9 hours (range 4.0–11.3). Terconazole is extensively metabolized; the plasma AUC for terconazole compared to the AUC for total radioactivity was 0.6%. Total radioactivity was eliminated from the blood with a half-life of 52.2 hours (range 44–60). Excretion of radioactivity was both by renal (32–56%) and fecal (47–52%) routes.
Photosensitivity reactions were observed in some normal volunteers following repeated dermal application of terconazole 2.0% and 0.8% creams under conditions of filtered artificial ultraviolet light.
Photosensitivity reactions have not been observed in U.S. and foreign clinical trials in patients who were treated vaginally with terconazole suppositories or cream.

INDICATIONS AND USAGE

TERAZOL 3 Vaginal Suppositories are indicated for the local treatment of vulvovaginal candidiasis (moniliasis). As TERAZOL 3 Vaginal Suppositories are effective only for vulvovaginitis caused by the genus *Candida,* the diagnosis should be confirmed by KOH smears and/or cultures.

CONTRAINDICATIONS

Patients known to be hypersensitive to terconazole or to any components of the suppository.

WARNINGS

None.

PRECAUTIONS

General: Discontinue use and do not retreat with terconazole if sensitization, irritation, fever, chills or flu-like symptoms are reported during use. The base contained in the suppository formulation may interact with certain rubber or latex products, such as those used in vaginal contraceptive diaphragms, therefore concurrent use is not recommended.
If there is lack of response to TERAZOL 3 Vaginal Suppositories, appropriate microbiological studies (standard KOH smear and/or cultures) should be repeated to confirm the diagnosis and rule out other pathogens.
Drug Interactions: The therapeutic effect of TERAZOL 3 Vaginal Suppositories is not affected by oral contraceptive usage.
Carcinogenesis, Mutagenesis, Impairment of Fertility
Carcinogenesis: Studies to determine the carcinogenic potential of terconazole have not been performed.
Mutagenicity: Terconazole was not mutagenic when tested *in vitro* for induction of microbial point mutations (Ames test), or for inducing cellular transformation, or *in vivo* for chromosome breaks (micronucleus test) or dominant lethal mutations in mouse germ cells.
Impairment of Fertility: No impairment of fertility occurred when female rats were administered terconazole orally up to 40 mg/kg/day.
Pregnancy: Pregnancy Category C
There was no evidence of teratogenicity when terconazole was administered orally up to 40 mg/kg/day (25 × the recommended intravaginal human dose) in rats, or 20 mg/ kg/ day in rabbits, or subcutaneously in rats up to 20 mg/kg/ day. Dosages at or below 10 mg/kg/day produced no embryotoxicity; however, there was a delay in fetal ossification at 10 mg/kg/day in rats. There was some evidence of embryotoxicity in rabbits and rats at 20–40 mg/kg. In rats this was reflected as a decrease in litter size and number of viable young and reduced fetal weight. There was also delay in ossification and an increased incidence of skeletal variants.
The no-effect oral dose of 10 mg/kg/day resulted in a mean peak plasma level of terconazole in pregnant rats of 0.176 mcg/mL which exceeds by 44 times the mean peak plasma level (0.004 mcg/mL) seen in normal subjects after intravaginal administration of terconazole. This assessment does not account for possible exposure of the fetus through direct transfer of terconazole from the irritated vagina to the fetus by diffusion across amniotic membranes.
Since terconazole is absorbed from the human vagina, it should not be used in the first trimester of pregnancy unless the physician considers it essential to the welfare of the patient.
Nursing Mothers: It is not known whether terconazole is excreted in human milk. Animal studies have shown that rat off-spring exposed via the milk of treated (40 mg/kg/ orally) dams showed decreased survival during the first few post-partum days. Because many drugs are excreted in human milk, and because of the potential for adverse reaction in nursing infants from terconazole, a decision should be made whether to discontinue nursing or to discontinue the drug, taking into account the importance of the drug to the mother.
Pediatric Use: Safety and efficacy in children have not been established.

ADVERSE REACTIONS

During controlled clinical studies conducted in the United States, 284 patients with vulvovaginal candidiasis were treated with terconazole 80 mg vaginal suppositories. Based on comparative analyses with placebo (295 patients) the adverse experiences considered adverse reactions most likely related to terconazole 80 mg vaginal suppositories were headache (30.3% vs 20.7% with placebo) and pain of the female genitalia (4.2% vs 0.7% with placebo). Adverse reactions that were reported but were not statistically significantly different from placebo were burning (15.2% vs 11.2% with placebo) and body pain (3.9% vs 1.7% with placebo). Fever (2.8% vs 1.4% with placebo) and chills (1.8% vs 0.7% with placebo) have also been reported. The therapy-related dropout rate was 3.5% and the placebo therapy-related dropout rate was 2.7%. The adverse drug experience on terconazole most frequently causing discontinuation was burning (2.5% vs 1.4% with placebo) and pruritus (1.8% vs 1.4% with placebo).

DOSAGE AND ADMINISTRATION

One TERAZOL 3 Vaginal Suppository (80 mg terconazole) is administered intravaginally once daily at bedtime for three consecutive days. Before prescribing another course of therapy, the diagnosis should be reconfirmed by smears and/or cultures and other pathogens commonly associated with vulvovaginitis ruled out. The therapeutic effect of TERAZOL 3 Vaginal Suppositories is not affected by menstruation.

HOW SUPPLIED

TERAZOL 3 (terconazole) Vaginal Suppositories 80 mg are available as 2.5 g, elliptically shaped white to off-white suppositories in packages of three (NDC 0062-5351-01) with a vaginal applicator. Store at Controlled Room Temperature 15°–30°C (59°–86°F)
Caution: Federal (USA) law prohibits dispensing without a prescription.
631-11-303-7 REVISED March 1995
Shown in Product Identification Guide, page 328

TERAZOL® 7 ℞
Vaginal Cream 0.4%
(terconazole)

DESCRIPTION

TERAZOL 7 Vaginal Cream is a white to off-white, water washable cream for intravaginal administration containing 0.4% of the antifungal agent terconazole, *cis* -1-[*p*-[[2-(2,4-Dichlorophenyl)-2-(1H-1, 2, 4-triazol-1-ylmethyl)-1,3-dioxolan-4-yl]methoxy]phenyl]-4-isopropylpiperazine, compounded in a cream base consisting of butylated hydroxyanisole, cetyl alcohol, isopropyl myristate, polysorbate 60, polysorbate 80, propylene glycol, stearyl alcohol, and purified water.
TERCONAZOLE

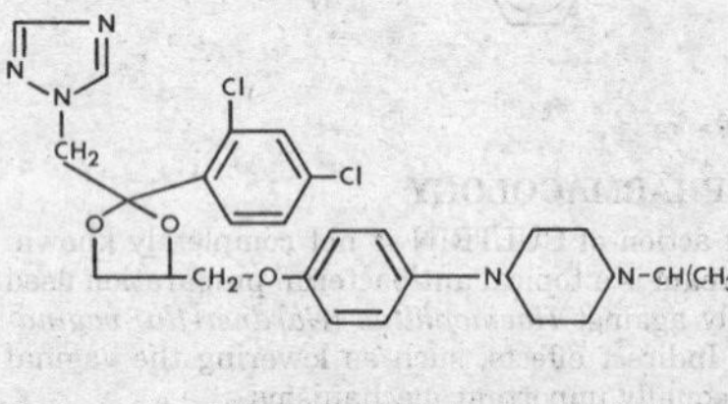

$C_{26}H_{31}Cl_2N_5O_3$

Terconazole, a triazole derivative, is a white to almost white powder with a molecular weight of 532.47. It is insoluble in water; sparingly soluble in ethanol; and soluble in butanol.

CLINICAL PHARMACOLOGY

Microbiology: Terconazole exhibits fungicidal activity *in vitro* against *Candida albicans.* Antifungal activity also has been demonstrated against other fungi. The MIC values for terconazole against most species of lactic acid bacteria typically found in the human vagina were ≥128 mcg/mL, therefore these beneficial bacteria are not affected by drug treatment.
The exact pharmacologic mode of action of terconazole is uncertain; however, it may exert its antifungal activity by the disruption of normal fungal cell membrane permeability. No resistance to terconazole has developed during successive passages of *C. albicans.*
Human Pharmacology: Following intravaginal administration of terconazole in humans, absorption ranged from 5–8% in three hysterectomized subjects and 12–16% in two non-hysterectomized subjects with tubal ligations.
Following oral (30 mg) administration of ^{14}C-labelled terconazole, the half-life of elimination from the blood for the parent terconazole was 6.9 hours (range 4.0–11.3). Terconazole is extensively metabolized; the plasma AUC for terconazole compared to the AUC for total radioactivity was 0.6%. Total radioactivity was eliminated from the blood with a half-life of 52.2 hours (range 44–60). Excretion of radioactivity was both by renal (32–56%) and fecal (47–52%) routes.
Photosensitivity reactions were observed in some normal volunteers following repeated dermal application of terconazole 2.0% and 0.8% creams under conditions of filtered artificial ultraviolet light. Photosensitivity reactions have not been observed in U.S. and foreign clinical trials in patients who were treated with terconazole 0.4% vaginal cream.

INDICATIONS AND USAGE

TERAZOL 7 Vaginal Cream is indicated for the local treatment of vulvovaginal candidiasis (moniliasis). As TERAZOL 7 Vaginal Cream is effective only for vulvovaginitis caused by the genus *Candida,* the diagnosis should be confirmed by KOH smears and/or cultures.

CONTRAINDICATIONS

Patients known to be hypersensitive to terconazole or to any of the components of the cream.

WARNINGS

None.

PRECAUTIONS

General: Discontinue use and do not retreat with terconazole if sensitization, irritation, fever, chills or flu-like symptoms are reported during use. If there is lack of response to TERAZOL 7 Vaginal Cream, appropriate microbiological studies (standard KOH smear and/or cultures) should be repeated to confirm the diagnosis and rule out other pathogens.

Drug Interactions: The therapeutic effect of TERAZOL 7 Vaginal Cream is not affected by oral contraceptive usage.

Carcinogenesis, Mutagenesis, Impairment of Fertility:

Carcinogenesis: Studies to determine the carcinogenic potential of terconazole have not been performed.

Mutagenicity: Terconazole was not mutagenic when tested *in vitro* for induction of microbial point mutations (Ames test) or for inducing cellular transformation, or *in vivo* for chromosome breaks (micronucleus test) or dominant lethal mutations in mouse germ cells.

Impairment of Fertility: No impairment of fertility occurred when female rats were administered terconazole orally up to 40 mg/kg/day.

Pregnancy: Pregnancy Category C.

There was no evidence of teratogenicity when terconazole was administered orally up to 40 mg/kg/day (100 × the recommended intravaginal human dose) in rats, or 20 mg/kg/day in rabbits, or subcutaneously in rats up to 20 mg/kg/day. Dosages at or below 10 mg/kg/day produced no embryotoxicity; however, there was a delay in fetal ossification at 10 mg/kg/day in rats. There was some evidence of embryotoxicity in rabbits and rats at 20–40 mg/kg. In rats this was reflected as a decrease in litter size and number of viable young and reduced fetal weight. There was also delay in ossification and an increased incidence of skeletal variants.

The no-effect oral dose of 10 mg/kg/day resulted in a mean peak plasma level of terconazole in pregnant rats of 0.176 mcg/mL which exceeds by 44 times the mean peak plasma levels (0.004 mcg/mL) seen in normal subjects after intravaginal administration of terconazole. This safety assessment does not account for possible exposure of the fetus through direct transfer of terconazole from the irritated vagina to the fetus by diffusion across amniotic membranes. Since terconazole is absorbed from the human vagina, it should not be used in the first trimester of pregnancy unless the physician considers it essential to the welfare of the patient.

Nursing Mothers: It is not known whether this drug is excreted in human milk. Animal studies have shown that rat off-spring exposed via the milk of treated (40 mg/kg/orally) dams showed decreased survival during the first few postpartum days, but overall pup weight and weight gain were comparable to or greater than controls throughout lactation. Because many drugs are excreted in human milk, and because of the potential for adverse reaction in nursing infants from terconazole, a decision should be made whether to discontinue nursing or to discontinue the drug, taking into account the importance of the drug to the mother.

Pediatric Use: Safety and efficacy in children have not been established.

ADVERSE REACTIONS

During controlled clinical studies conducted in the United States, 521 patients with vulvovaginal candidiasis were treated with terconazole 0.4% vaginal cream. Based on comparative analyses with placebo, the adverse experiences considered most likely related to terconazole 0.4% vaginal cream were headaches (26% *vs* 17% with placebo) and body pain (2.1% *vs* 0% with placebo). Vulvovaginal burning (5.2%), itching (2.3%) or irritation (3.1%) occurred less frequently with terconazole 0.4% vaginal cream than with the vehicle placebo. Fever (1.7% *vs* 0.5% with placebo) and chills (0.4% *vs* 0.0% with placebo) have also been reported. The therapy-related dropout rate was 1.9%. The adverse drug experience on terconazole most frequently causing discontinuation was vulvovaginal itching (0.6%), which was lower than the incidence for placebo (0.9%).

OVERDOSAGE

Overdose of terconazole in humans has not been reported to date. In the rat, the oral LD 50 values were found to be 1741 and 849 mg/kg for the male and female, respectively. The oral LD 50 values for the male and female dog were ≅1280 and ≥640 mg/kg, respectively.

DOSAGE AND ADMINISTRATION

One full applicator (5 g) of TERAZOL 7 Vaginal Cream (20 mg terconazole) is administered intravaginally once daily at bedtime for seven consecutive days. Before prescribing another course of therapy, the diagnosis should be reconfirmed by smears and/or cultures and other pathogens commonly associated with vulvovaginitis ruled out. The therapeutic effect of TERAZOL 7 Vaginal Cream is not affected by menstruation.

HOW SUPPLIED

TERAZOL® 7 (terconazole) Vaginal Cream 0.4% is available in 45 g (NDC 0062-5350-01) tubes with an ORTHO® Measured-Dose Applicator. Store at controlled room temperature 15°–30°C (59°–86°F).

Caution: Federal (USA) law prohibits dispensing without a prescription.

631-11-301-6 Revised September 1996

Shown in Product Identification Guide, page 328

TOLECTIN® 200 (tolmetin sodium) ℞

[*to-lek 'tin*]

200 mg Tablets

NSN 6505-01-038-7460—100's

TOLECTIN® DS (tolmetin sodium) ℞

400 mg Capsules

NSN 6505-01-091-9624—100's

NSN 6505-01-039-4469—U/D 100's

TOLECTIN® 600 (tolmetin sodium) ℞

600 mg Tablets

NSN 6505-01-322-8539—100's

For Oral Administration

DESCRIPTION

TOLECTIN 200 (tolmetin sodium) tablets for oral administration contain tolmetin sodium as the dihydrate in an amount equivalent to 200 mg of tolmetin (scored for 100 mg). Each tablet contains 18 mg (0.784 mEq) of sodium and the following inactive ingredients: cellulose, magnesium stearate, silicon dioxide, corn starch and talc.

TOLECTIN DS (tolmetin sodium) capsules for oral administration contain tolmetin sodium as the dihydrate in an amount equivalent to 400 mg of tolmetin. Each capsule contains 36 mg (1.568 mEq) of sodium and the following inactive ingredients: gelatin, magnesium stearate, corn starch, talc, FD&C Red No. 3, FD&C Yellow No. 6 and titanium dioxide.

TOLECTIN 600 (tolmetin sodium) tablets for oral administration contain tolmetin sodium as the dihydrate in an amount equivalent to 600 mg of tolmetin. Each tablet contains 54 mg (2.35 mEq) of sodium and the following inactive ingredients: cellulose, silicon dioxide, crospovidone, hydroxypropyl methyl cellulose, magnesium stearate, polyethylene glycol, corn starch, titanium dioxide, FD&C Yellow No. 6 and D&C Yellow No. 10.

The pKa of tolmetin is 3.5 and tolmetin sodium is freely soluble in water.

Tolmetin sodium is a nonsteroidal anti-inflammatory agent. The structural formula is:

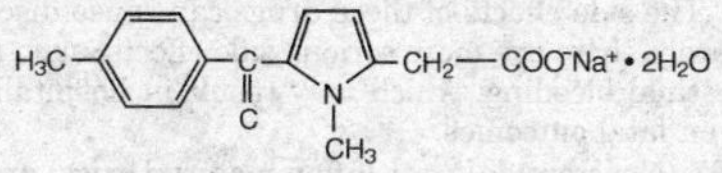

Sodium 1-methyl-5-(4-methylbenzoyl)-1*H* -pyrrole-2-acetate dihydrate.

CLINICAL PHARMACOLOGY

Studies in animals have shown TOLECTIN (tolmetin sodium) to possess anti-inflammatory, analgesic and antipyretic activity. In the rat, TOLECTIN prevents the development of experimentally induced polyarthritis and also decreases established inflammation.

The mode of action of TOLECTIN is not known. However, studies in laboratory animals and man have demonstrated that the anti-inflammatory action of TOLECTIN is *not* due to pituitary-adrenal stimulation. TOLECTIN inhibits prostaglandin synthetase *in vitro* and lowers the plasma level of prostaglandin E in man. This reduction in prostaglandin synthesis may be responsible for the anti-inflammatory action. TOLECTIN does not appear to alter the course of the underlying disease in man.

In patients with rheumatoid arthritis and in normal volunteers, tolmetin sodium is rapidly and almost completely absorbed with peak plasma levels being reached within 30–60 minutes after an oral therapeutic dose. In controlled studies, the time to reach peak tolmetin plasma concentration is approximately 20 minutes longer following administration of a 600 mg tablet, compared to an equivalent dose given as 200 mg tablets. The clinical meaningfulness of this finding, if any, is unknown. Tolmetin displays a biphasic elimination from the plasma consisting of a rapid phase with a half-life of one to 2 hours followed by a slower phase with a half-life of about 5 hours. Peak plasma levels of approximately 40 μg/mL are obtained with a 400 mg oral dose. Essentially all of the administered dose is recovered in the urine in 24 hours either as an inactive oxidative metabolite or as conjugates of tolmetin. An 18-day multiple dose study demonstrated no accumulation of tolmetin when compared with a single dose.

In two fecal blood loss studies of 4 to 6 days duration involving 15 subjects each, TOLECTIN did not induce an increase in blood loss over that observed during a 4-day drug-free control period. In the same studies, aspirin produced a greater blood loss than occurred during the drug-free control period, and a greater blood loss than occurred during the TOLECTIN treatment period. In one of the two studies, indomethacin produced a greater fecal blood loss than occurred during the drug-free control period; in the second study, indomethacin did not induce a significant increase in blood loss.

TOLECTIN is effectve in treating both the acute flares and in the long term management of the symptoms of rheumatoid arthritis, osteoarthritis and juvenile rheumatoid arthritis.

In patients with either rheumatoid arthritis or osteaoarthritis, TOLECTIN is as effective as aspirin and indomethacin in controlling disease activity, but the frequency of the milder gastrointestinal adverse effects and tinnitus was less than in aspirin-treated patients, and the incidence of central nervous system adverse effects was less than in indomethacin-treated patients.

In patients with juvenile rheumatoid arthritis, TOLECTIN is as effective as aspirin in controlling disease activity, with a similar incidence of adverse reactions. Mean SGOT values, initially elevated in patients on previous aspirin therapy, remained elevated in the aspirin group and decreased in the TOLECTIN group.

TOLECTIN has produced additional therapeutic benefit when added to a regimen of gold salts and, to a lesser extent, with corticosteroids. TOLECTIN should not be used in conjunction with salicylates since greater benefit from the combination is not likely, but the potential for adverse reactions is increased.

INDICATIONS AND USAGE

TOLECTIN (tolmetin sodium) is indicated for the relief of signs and symptoms of rheumatoid arthritis and osteoarthritis. TOLECTIN is indicated in the treatment of acute flares and the long-term management of the chronic disease.

TOLECTIN is also indicated for treatment of juvenile rheumatoid arthritis. The safety and effectiveness of TOLECTIN have not been established in children under 2 years of age (see PRECAUTIONS—Pediatric Use and DOSAGE AND ADMINISTRATION).

CONTRAINDICATIONS

Anaphylactoid reactions have been reported with TOLECTIN as with other nonsteroidal anti-inflammatory drugs. Because of the possibility of cross-sensitivity to other nonsteroidal anti-inflammatory drugs, particularly zomepirac sodium, anaphylactoid reactions may be more likely to occur in patients who have exhibited allergic reactions to these compounds. For this reason, TOLECTIN should not be given to patients in whom aspirin and other nonsteroidal anti-inflammatory drugs induce symptoms of asthma, rhinitis, urticaria and other symptoms of allergic or anaphylactoid reactions. Patients experiencing anaphylactoid reactions on TOLECTIN should be treated with conventional therapy, such as epinephrine, antihistamines and/or steroids.

WARNINGS

Risk of GI Ulceration, Bleeding and Perforation with NSAID Therapy:

Serious gastrointestinal toxicity such as bleeding, ulceration, and perforation, can occur at any time, with or without symptoms, in patients treated chronically with NSAID (Nonsteroidal Anti-Inflammatory Drug) therapy. Although minor upper gastrointestinal problems, such as dyspepsia, are common, usually developng early in therapy, physicians should remain alert for ulceration and bleeding in patients treated chronically with NSAID's even in the absence of previous GI tract symptoms. In patients observed in clinical trials of several months to two years duration, symptomatic upper GI ulcers, gross bleeding or perforation appear to occur in approximately 1% of patients treated for 3–6 months, and in about 2–4% of patients treated for one year. Physicians should inform patients about the signs and/or symptoms of serious GI toxicity and what steps to take if they occur.

Studies to date have not identified any subset of patients not at risk of developing peptic ulceration and bleeding. Except for a prior history of serious GI events and other risk factors known to be associated with peptic ulcer disease, such as alcoholism, smoking, etc., no risk factor (e.g., age, sex) have been associated with increased risk. Elderly or debilitated patients seem to tolerate ulceration or bleeding less well than other individuals and most spontaneous reports of fatal GI events are in this population. Studies to date are inconclusive concerning the relative risk of various NSAID's in causing such reactions. High doses of any NSAID probably carry a greater risk of these reactions, although controlled clinical trials showing this do not exist in

Continued on next page

Tolectin—Cont.

most cases. In considering the use of relatively large doses (within the recommended dosage range), sufficient benefit should be anticipated to offset the potential increased risk of GI toxicity.

PRECAUTIONS
General
Because of ocular changes observed in animals and reports of adverse eye findings with nonsteroidal anti-inflammatory agents, it is recommended that patients who develop visual disturbances during treatment with TOLECTIN have ophthalmologic evaluations.

As with other nonsteroidal anti-inflammatory drugs, long-term administration of tolmetin to animals has resulted in renal papillary necrosis and other abnormal renal pathology. In humans, there have been reports of acute interstitial nephritis with hematuria, proteinuria, and occasionally nephrotic syndrome.

A second form of renal toxicity has been seen in patients with prerenal conditions leading to a reduction in renal blood flow or blood volume, where the renal prostaglandins have a supportive role in the maintenance of renal perfusion. In these patients administration of an NSAID may cause a dose dependent reduction in prostaglandin formation and may precipitate overt renal decompensation. Patients at greatest risk of this reaction are those with heart failure, liver dysfunction, those taking diuretics, and the elderly. Discontinuation of NSAID therapy is typically followed by recovery to the pretreatment state.

Since TOLECTIN and its metabolites are eliminated primarily by the kidneys, patients with impaired renal function should be closely monitored, and it should be anticipated that they will require lower doses.

TOLECTIN prolongs bleeding time. Patients who may be adversely affected by prolongation of bleeding time should be carefully observed when TOLECTIN is administered.

In patients receiving concomitant TOLECTIN-steroid therapy, any reduction in steroid dosage should be gradual to avoid the possible complications of sudden steroid withdrawal.

Peripheral edema has been reported in some patients receiving TOLECTIN therapy. Therefore, as with other nonsteroidal anti-inflammatory drugs, TOLECTIN should be used with caution in patients with compromised cardiac function, hypertension, or other conditions predisposing to fluid retention.

The antipyretic and anti-inflammatory activities of the drug may reduce fever and inflammation, thus diminishing their utility as diagnostic signs in detecting complications of presumed non-infectious, non-inflammatory painful conditions.

As with other nonsteroidal anti-inflammatory drugs, borderline elevations of one or more liver tests may occur in up to 15% of patients. These abnormalities may progress, may remain essentially unchanged, or may be transient with continued therapy. The SGPT (ALT) test is probably the most sensitive indicator of liver dysfunction. Meaningful (3 times the upper limit of normal) elevations of SGPT or SGOT (AST) occurred in controlled clinical trials in less than 1% of patients. A patient with symptoms and/or signs suggesting liver dysfunction, or in whom an abnormal liver test has occurred, should be evaluated for evidence of the development of more severe hepatic reaction while on therapy with TOLECTIN. Severe hepatic reactions, including jaundice and fatal hepatitis, have been reported with TOLECTIN as with other nonsteroidal anti-inflammatory drugs. Although such reactions are rare, if abnormal liver tests persist or worsen, if clinical signs and symptoms consistent with liver disease develop, or if systemic manifestations occur (e.g. eosinophilia, rash, etc.), TOLECTIN should be discontinued.

Carcinogenesis, Mutagenesis, Impairment of Fertility
Tolmetin sodium did not possess any carcinogenic liability in the following long-term studies: a 24-month study in rats at doses as high as 75 mg/kg/day, and an 18-month study in mice at doses as high as 50 mg/kg/day.

No mutagenic potential of tolmetin sodium was found in the Ames Salmonella-Microsomal Activation Test.

Reproductive studies revealed no impairment of fertility in animals. Effects on parturition have been shown, however, as with other prostaglandin inhibitors. This information is detailed in the Pregnancy section below.

Pregnancy
Pregnancy Category C. Reproduction studies in rats and rabbits at doses up to 50 mg/kg (1.5 times the maximum clinical dose based on a body weight of 60 kg) revealed no evidence of teratogenesis or impaired fertility due to TOLECTIN. However, TOLECTIN is an inhibitor of prostaglandin synthetase. Drugs in this class have known effects on the fetal cardiovascular system which may cause constriction of the ductus arteriosus in utero during the third trimester of pregnancy, which may result in persistent pulmonary hypertension of the newborn.

There are no adequate and well-controlled studies in pregnant women. TOLECTIN should be used during pregnancy only if the potential benefit justifies the potential risk to the fetus.

Non-Teratogenic Effects
Prostaglandin inhibitors have also been shown to increase the incidence of dystocia and delayed parturition in animals.

Nursing Mothers
TOLECTIN has been shown to be secreted in human milk. Because of the possible adverse effects of prostaglandin inhibiting drugs on neonates, use in nursing mothers should be avoided.

Pediatric Use
The safety and effectiveness of TOLECTIN in children under 2 years of age have not been established.

Drug Interactions
The in vitro binding of warfarin to human plasma proteins is unaffected by tolmetin, and tolmetin does not alter the prothrombin time of normal volunteers. However, increased prothrombin time and bleeding have been reported in patients on concomitant TOLECTIN and warfarin therapy. Therefore, caution should be exercised when administering TOLECTIN to patients on anticoagulants.

In adult diabetic patients under treatment with either sulfonylureas or insulin there is no change in the clinical effects of either TOLECTIN or the hypoglycemic agents.

Caution should be used if TOLECTIN is administered concomitantly with methotrexate. TOLECTIN and other nonsteroidal anti-inflammatory drugs have been reported to reduce the tubular secretion of methotrexate in an animal model, possibly enhancing the toxicity of methotrexate.

Laboratory Tests
Because serious GI tract ulceration and bleeding can occur without warning symptoms, physicians should follow chronically treated patients for the signs and symptoms of ulceration and bleeding and should inform them of the importance of this follow-up (see WARNINGS—Risk of GI Ulceration, Bleeding and Perforation with NSAID Therapy).

Drug/Laboratory Test Interaction
The metabolites of tolmetin sodium in urine have been found to give positive tests for proteinuria using tests which rely on acid precipitation as their endpoint (e.g. sulfosalicylic acid). No interference is seen in the tests for proteinuria using dye-impregnated commercially available reagent strips (e.g., Albustix®, Uristix®, etc.).

Drug-Food Interaction
In a controlled single dose study, administration of TOLECTIN with milk had no effect on peak plasma tolmetin concentrations, but decreased total tolmetin bioavailability by 16%. When TOLECTIN was taken immediately after a meal, peak plasma tolmetin concentrations were reduced by 50% while total bioavailability was again decreased by 16%.

Information for Patients
TOLECTIN, like other drugs of its class, is not free of side effects. The side effects of these drugs can cause discomfort and, rarely, there are more serious side effects, such as gastrointestinal bleeding, which may result in hospitalization and even fatal outcomes.

NSAID's (Nonsteroidal Anti-Inflammatory Drugs) are often essential agents in the management of arthritis, but they also may be commonly employed for conditions which are less serious.

Physicians may wish to discuss with their patients the potential risks (see WARNINGS, PRECAUTIONS, and ADVERSE REACTIONS sections) and likely benefits of NSAID treatment, particularly when the drugs are used for less serious conditions where treatment without NSAID's may represent an acceptable alternative to both the patient and physician.

ADVERSE REACTIONS

The adverse reactions which have been observed in clinical trials encompass observations in about 4370 patients treated with TOLECTIN (tolmetin sodium), over 800 of whom have undergone at least one year of therapy. These adverse reactions, reported below by body system, are among those typical of nonsteroidal anti-inflammatory drugs and, as expected, gastrointestinal complaints were most frequent. In clinical trials with TOLECTIN, about 10% of patients dropped out because of adverse reactions, mostly gastrointestinal in nature.

Incidence Greater Than 1%
The following adverse reactions which occurred more frequently than 1 in 100 were reported in controlled clinical trials.

Gastrointestinal: Nausea (11%), dyspepsia,* gastrointestinal distress,* abdominal pain,* diarrhea,* flatulence,* vomiting,* constipation, gastritis, and peptic ulcer. Forty percent of the ulcer patients had a prior history of peptic ulcer disease and/or were receiving concomitant anti-inflammatory drugs including corticosteroids, which are known to produce peptic ulceration.

Body as a Whole: Headache,* asthenia,* chest pain

Cardiovascular: Elevated blood pressure,* edema*

Central Nervous System: Dizziness,* drowsiness, depression

Metabolic/Nutritional: Weight gain,* weight loss*

Dermatologic: Skin irritation

Special Senses: Tinnitus, visual disturbance

Hematologic: Small and transient decreases in hemoglobin and hematocrit not associated with gastrointestinal bleeding have occurred. These are similar to changes reported with other nonsteroidal anti-inflammatory drugs.

Urogenital: Elevated BUN, urinary tract infection

*Reactions occurring in 3% to 9% of patients treated with TOLECTIN. Reactions occurring in fewer than 3% of the patients are unmarked.

Incidence Less Than 1%
(Causal Relationship Probable)
The following adverse reactions were reported less frequently than 1 in 100 in controlled clinical trials or were reported since marketing. The probability exists that there is a causal relationship between TOLECTIN and these adverse reactions.

Gastrointestinal: Gastrointestinal bleeding with or without evidence of peptic ulcer, perforation, glossitis, stomatitis, hepatitis, liver function abnormalities

Body as a Whole: Anaphylactoid reactions, fever, lymphadenopathy, serum sickness

Hematologic: Hemolytic anemia, thrombocytopenia, granulocytopenia, agranulocytosis

Cardiovascular: Congestive heart failure in patients with marginal cardiac function

Dermatologic: Urticaria, purpura, erythema multiforme, toxic epidermal necrolysis

Urogenital: Hematuria, proteinuria, dysuria, renal failure

Incidence Less Than 1%
(Causal Relationship Unknown)
Other adverse reactions were reported less frequently than 1 in 100 in controlled clinical trials or were reported since marketing, but a causal relationship between TOLECTIN and the reaction could not be determined. These rarely reported reactions are being listed as alerting information for the physician since the possibility of a causal relationship cannot be excluded.

Body as Whole: Epistaxis

Special Senses: Optic neuropathy, retinal and macular changes

MANAGEMENT OF OVERDOSAGE

In the event of overdosage, the stomach should be emptied by inducing vomiting or by gastric lavage followed by the administration of activated charcoal.

DOSAGE AND ADMINISTRATION

In adults with rheumatoid arthritis or osteoarthritis, the recommended starting dose is 400 mg three times daily (1200 mg daily), preferably including a dose on arising and a dose at bedtime. To achieve optimal therapeutic effect the dose should be adjusted according to the patient's response after one to two weeks. Control is usually achieved at doses of 600–1800 mg daily in divided doses (generally t.i.d.). Doses larger than 1800 mg/kg have not been studied and are not recommended.

The recommended starting dose for children (2 years and older) is 20 mg/kg/day in divided doses (t.i.d. or q.i.d.). When control has been achieved, the usual dose ranges from 15 to 30 mg/kg/day. Doses higher than 30 mg/kg/day have not been studied and, therefore, are not recommended.

A therapeutic response to TOLECTIN (tolmetin sodium) can be expected in a few days to a week. Progressive improvement can be anticipated during succeeding weeks of therapy. If gastrointestinal symptoms occur, TOLECTIN can be administered with antacids other than sodium bicarbonate. TOLECTIN bioavailability and pharmacokinetics are not significantly affected by acute or chronic administration of magnesium and aluminum hydroxides; however, bioavailability is affected by food or milk (see PRECAUTIONS—Drug-Food Interaction).

HOW SUPPLIED

TOLECTIN® 200 (tolmetin sodium) tablets 200 mg (white, scored, imprinted "TOLECTIN," "200" and "McNEIL"), NDC 0045-0412, bottles of 100.

TOLECTIN® DS (tolmetin sodium) capsules 400 mg (colored orange opaque, with contrasting parallel bands, imprinted "TOLECTIN DS" and "McNEIL"), NDC 0045-0414, bottles of 100, 500.

TOLECTIN® 600 (tolmetin sodium) tablets 600 mg (colored orange, film coated, imprinted "TOLECTIN 600" and "McNEIL"), NDC 0045-0416, bottles of 100 and 500.

Dispense in tight, light-resistant container as defined in the official compendium.

Store at controlled room temperature (15°–30°C, 59°–86°F). Protect from light.

McNeil Pharmaceutical, McNEILAB, Inc.
Spring House, PA 19477
Revised June 1997   643-10-089-2
Shown in Product Identification Guide, pages 328 and 329

TOPAMAX® ℞

[tō'-pă-măx]
(topiramate) tablets

Prescribing Information

DESCRIPTION

TOPAMAX® (topiramate) is a sulfamate-substituted monosaccharide that is intended for use as an antiepileptic drug. It is available as 25 mg, 100 mg, and 200 mg round tablets for oral administration.

Topiramate is a white crystalline powder with a bitter taste. Topiramate is most soluble in alkaline solutions containing sodium hydroxide or sodium phosphate and having a pH of 9 to 10. It is freely soluble in acetone, chloroform, dimethylsulfoxide, and ethanol. The solubility in water is 9.8 mg/mL. Its saturated solution has a pH of 6.3. Topiramate has the molecular formula $C_{12}H_{21}NO_8S$ and a molecular weight of 339.36. Topiramate is designated chemically as 2,3:4,5-bis-*O*-(1-methylethylidene)-β-D-fructopyranose sulfamate and has the following structural formula:

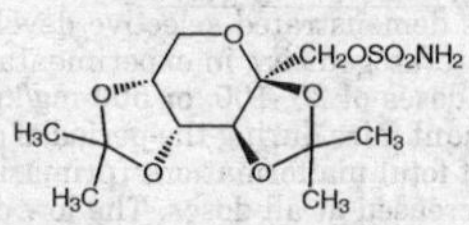

TOPAMAX® (topiramate) Tablets contain the following inactive ingredients: lactose monohydrate, pregelatinized starch, microcrystalline cellulose, sodium starch glycolate, magnesium stearate, purified water, carnauba wax, hydroxypropyl methylcellulose, titanium dioxide, polyethylene glycol, synthetic iron oxide (100 and 200 mg tablets) and polysorbate 80.

CLINICAL PHARMACOLOGY

Mechanism of Action:

The precise mechanism by which topiramate exerts its antiseizure effect is unknown; however, electrophysiological and biochemical studies of the effects of topiramate on cultured neurons have revealed three properties that may contribute to topiramate's antiepileptic efficacy. First, action potentials elicited repetitively by a sustained depolarization of the neurons are blocked by topiramate in a time-dependent manner, suggestive of a state-dependent sodium channel blocking action. Second, topiramate increases the frequency at which γ-aminobutyrate (GABA) activates $GABA_A$ receptors, and enhances the ability of GABA to induce a flux of chloride ions into neurons, suggesting that topiramate potentiates the activity of this inhibitory neurotransmitter. This effect was not blocked by flumazenil, a benzodiazepine antagonist, nor did topiramate increase the duration of the channel open time, differentiating topiramate from barbiturates that modulate $GABA_A$ receptors. Third, topiramate antagonizes the ability of kainate to activate the kainate/AMPA (α-amino-3-hydroxy-5- methylisoxazole-4-propionic acid, non-NMDA) subtype of excitatory amino acid (glutamate) receptor, but has no apparent effect on the activity of N-methyl-D-aspartate (NMDA) at the NMDA receptor subtype. These effects of topiramate are concentration-dependent within the range of 1 µM to 200 µM.

Topiramate also inhibits some isoenzymes of carbonic anhydrase (CA-II and CA-IV). This pharmacologic effect is generally weaker than that of acetazolamide, a known carbonic anhydrase inhibitor, and is not thought to be a major contributing factor to topiramate's antiepileptic activity.

Pharmacodynamics:

Topiramate has anticonvulsant activity in rat and mouse maximal electroshock seizure (MES) tests. Topiramate is only weakly effective in blocking clonic seizures induced by the $GABA_A$ receptor antagonist, pentylenetetrazole. Topiramate is also effective in rodent models of epilepsy, which include tonic and absence-like seizures in the spontaneous epileptic rat (SER) and tonic and clonic seizures induced in rats by kindling of the amygdala or by global ischemia.

Pharmacokinetics:

Absorption of topiramate is rapid, with peak plasma concentrations occurring at approximately 2 hours following a 400 mg oral dose. The relative bioavailability of topiramate from the tablet formulation is about 80% compared to a solution. The bioavailability of topiramate is not affected by food.

The pharmacokinetics of topiramate are linear with dose proportional increases in plasma concentration over the dose range studied (200 to 800 mg/day). The mean plasma elimination half-life is 21 hours after single or multiple doses. Steady state is thus reached in about 4 days in patients with normal renal function. Topiramate is 13–17% bound to human plasma proteins over the concentration range of 1–250 µg/mL.

Metabolism and Excretion:

Topiramate is not extensively metabolized and is primarily eliminated unchanged in the urine (approximately 70% of an administered dose). Six metabolites have been identified in humans, none of which constitutes more than 5% of an administered dose. The metabolites are formed via hydroxylation, hydrolysis, and glucuronidation. There is evidence

Table 1: Topiramate Dose Summary During the Stabilization Periods of Each of Five Double-Blind, Placebo-Controlled, Add-On Trials

Protocol	Stabilization Dose	Placebo[a]	Target Topiramate Dosage (mg/day) 200	400	600	800	1,000
YD	N	42	42	40	41	-	-
	Mean Dose	5.9	200	390	556	-	-
	Median Dose	6.0	200	400	600	-	-
YE	N	44	-	-	40	45	40
	Mean Dose	9.7	-	-	544	739	796
	Median Dose	10.0	-	-	600	800	1,000
Y1	N	23	-	19	-	-	-
	Mean Dose	3.8	-	395	-	-	-
	Median Dose	4.0	-	400	-	-	-
Y2	N	30	-	-	28	-	-
	Mean Dose	5.7	-	-	522	-	-
	Median Dose	6.0	-	-	600	-	-
Y3	N	28	-	-	-	25	-
	Mean Dose	7.9	-	-	-	568	-
	Median Dose	8.0	-	-	-	600	-

[a]Placebo dosages are given as the number of tablets. Placebo target dosages were as follows: Protocol Y1, 4 tablets/day; Protocols YD and Y2, 6 tablets/day; Protocol Y3, 8 tablets/day; Protocols YE, 10 tablets/day.

of renal tubular reabsorption of topiramate. In rats, given probenecid to inhibit tubular reabsorption, along with topiramate, a significant increase in renal clearance of topiramate was observed. This interaction has not been evaluated in humans. Overall, plasma clearance is approximately 20 to 30 mL/min in humans following oral administration.

Pharmacokinetic Interactions (see also Drug Interactions):
Antiepileptic Drugs

Potential interactions between topiramate and standard AEDs were assessed in controlled clincal pharmacokinetic studies in patients with epilepsy. The effect of these interactions on mean plasma AUCs are summarized under **PRECAUTIONS (Table 3).**

Special Populations:

Renal Impairment:

The clearance of topiramate was reduced by 42% in moderately renally impaired (creatinine clearance 30–69 mL/min/$1.73m^2$) and by 54% in severely renally impaired subjects (creatinine clearance <30 mL/min/$1.73m^2$) compared to normal renal function subjects (creatinine clearance >70 mL/min/$1.73m^2$). Since topiramate is presumed to undergo significant tubular reabsorption, it is uncertain whether this experience can be generalized to all situations of renal impairment. It is conceivable that some forms of renal disease could differentially affect glomerular filtration rate and tubular reabsorption resulting in a clearance of topiramate not predicted by creatinine clearance. In general, however, use of one-half the usual dose is recommended in patients with moderate or severe renal impairment.

Hemodialysis:

Topiramate is cleared by hemodialysis. Using a high efficiency, counterflow, single pass-dialysate hemodialysis procedure, topiramate dialysis clearance was 120 mL/min with blood flow through the dialyzer at 400 mL/min. This high clearance (compared to 20–30 mL/min total oral clearance in healthy adults) will remove a clinically significant amount of topiramate from the patient over the hemodialysis treatment period. Therefore, a dose adjustment may be required (see **DOSAGE AND ADMINISTRATION**).

Hepatic Impairment:

In hepatically impaired subjects, the clearance of topiramate may be decreased; the mechanism underlying the decrease is not well understood.

Age, Gender, and Race:

Clearance of topiramate was not affected by age (18–67 years), gender, or race.

Pediatric Pharmacokinetics:

Pharmacokinetics of topiramate were evaluated in patients ages 4 to 17 years receiving one or two other antiepileptic drugs. Pharmacokinetic profiles were obtained after one week at doses of 1, 3, and 9 mg/kg/day. Clearance was independent of dose. Although the relationship between age and clearance among patients of pediatric age has not been systematically evaluated, it appears that the weight adjusted clearance of topiramate is higher in pediatric patients than in adults.

CLINICAL STUDIES

The effectiveness of topiramate as an adjunctive treatment for partial onset seizures was established in five multicenter, randomized, double-blind, placebo-controlled trials, two comparing several dosages of topiramate and placebo and three comparing a single dosage with placebo, in patients with a history of partial onset seizures, with or without secondarily generalization.

Patients in these studies were permitted a maximum of two antiepileptic drugs (AEDs) in addition to TOPAMAX® or placebo. In each study, patients were stabilized on optimum dosages of their concomitant AEDs during an 8–12 week baseline phase. Patients who experienced at least 12 (or 8, for 8–week baseline studies) partial onset seizures, with or without secondarily generalization, during the baseline phase were randomly assigned to placebo or a specified dose of TOPAMAX® in addition to their other AEDs.

Following randomization, patients began the double-blind phase of treatment. Patients received active drug beginning at 100 mg per day; the dose was then increased by 100 mg or 200 mg/day increments weekly or every other week until the assigned dose was reached, unless intolerance prevented increases. After titration, patients entered an 8 or 12–week stabilization period. The numbers of patients randomized to each dose, and the actual mean, and median doses in the stabilization period are shown in Table 1.

[See table 1 above]

In all add-on trials, the reduction in seizure rate from baseline during the entire double-blind phase was measured. Responder rate (fraction of patients with at least a 50% reduction) was also measured. The median percent reductions in seizure rates and the responder rates by treatment group for each study are shown in Table 2.

[See table 2 at bottom of next page]

Subset analyses of the antiepileptic efficacy of TOPAMAX® in these studies showed no differences as a function of gender, race, age, baseline seizure rate, or concomitant AED.

INDICATIONS AND USAGE

TOPAMAX® (topiramate) is indicated as adjunctive therapy for the treatment of adults with partial onset seizures.

CONTRAINDICATIONS

TOPAMAX® (topiramate) is contraindicated in patients with a history of hypersensitivity to any component of this product.

WARNINGS

Withdrawal of AEDs

Antiepileptic drugs, including TOPAMAX® (topiramate), should be withdrawn gradually to minimize the potential of increased seizure frequency.

Cognitive/Neuropsychiatric Adverse Events

Adverse events most often associated with the use of TOPAMAX® were central nervous system-related. The most significant of these can be classified into two general categories: 1) psychomotor slowing, difficulty with concentration, and speech or language problems, in particular, word-finding difficulties and 2) somnolence or fatigue. Additional nonspecific CNS effects occasionally observed with topiramate as add-on therapy include dizziness or imbalance, confusion, memory problems, and exacerbation of mood disturbances (e.g., irritability and depression).

Reports of psychomotor slowing, speech and language problems, and difficulty with concentration and attention were common. Although in some cases these events were mild to moderate, they at times led to withdrawal from treatment. The incidence of psychomotor slowing is only marginally dose-related, but both language problems and difficulty with concentration or attention clearly increased in frequency with increasing dosage in the five double-blind trials [see **ADVERSE REACTIONS, Table 5**].

Somnolence and fatigue were the most frequently reported adverse events during clincal trials with TOPAMAX®. These events were generally mild to moderate and occurred early in therapy. While the incidence of somnolence does not appear to be dose-related, that of fatigue increases at dosages above 400 mg/day.

Continued on next page

Topamax—Cont.

Sudden Unexplained Death in Epilepsy (SUDEP)

During the course of premarketing development of TOPAMAX® (topiramate), 10 sudden and unexplained deaths were recorded among a cohort of treated patients (2,796 subject years of exposure).

This represents an incidence of 0.0035 deaths per patient year. Although this rate exceeds that expected in a healthy population matched for age and sex, it is within the range of estimates for the incidence of sudden unexplained deaths in patients with epilepsy not receiving TOPAMAX (ranging from 0.0005 for the general population of patients with epilepsy, to 0.003 for a clinical trial population similar to that in the TOPAMAX program, to 0.005 for patients with refractory epilepsy).

PRECAUTIONS

General:

Kidney Stones

A total of 32/2,086 (1.5%) of patients exposed to topiramate during its development reported the occurrence of kidney stones, an incidence about 2–4 times that expected in a similar, untreated population. As in the general population, the incidence of stone formation among topiramate treated patients was higher in men.

An explanation for the association of TOPAMAX® and kidney stones may lie in the fact that topiramate is a weak carbonic anhydrase inhibitor. Carbonic anhydrase inhibitors, e.g., acetazolamide or dichlorphenamide, promote stone formation by reducing urinary citrate excretion and by increasing urinary pH. The concomitant use of TOPAMAX® with other carbonic anhydrase inhibitors may create a physiological environment that increases the risk of kidney stone formation, and should therefore be avoided.

Increased fluid intake increases the urinary output, lowering the concentration of substances involved in stone formation. Hydration is recommended to reduce new stone formation.

Paresthesia

Paresthesia, an effect associated with the use of other carbonic anhydrase inhibitors, appears to be a common effect of TOPAMAX®.

Adjustment of Dose in Renal Failure

The major route of elimination of unchanged topiramate and its metabolites is via the kidney. Dosage adjustment may be required (see **DOSAGE AND ADMINISTRATION**).

Decreased Hepatic Function

In hepatically impaired patients, topiramate should be administered with caution as the clearance of topiramate may be decreased.

Information for Patients:

Patients, particularly those with predisposing factors, should be instructed to maintain an adequate fluid intake in order to minimize the risk of renal stone formation [see **PRECAUTIONS: General**, for support regarding hydration as a preventative measure].

Patients should be warned about the potential for somnolence, dizziness, confusion, and difficulty concentrating and advised not to drive or operate machinery until they have gained sufficient experience on topiramate to gauge whether it adversely affects their mental and/or motor performance.

Drug Interactions:

Antiepileptic Drugs

Potential interactions between topiramate and standard AEDs were assessed in controlled clinical pharmacokinetic studies in patients with epilepsy. The effect of these interactions on mean plasma AUCs are summarized in the following table:

In Table 3, the second column (AED concentration) describes what happens to the concentration of the AED listed in the first column when topiramate is added.

The third column (topiramate concentration) describes how the coadministration of a drug listed in the first column modifies the concentration of topiramate in experimental settings when TOPAMAX® was given alone.

Table 3: Summary of AED Interactions with TOPAMAX®

AED Co-administered	AED Concentration	Topiramate Concentration
Phenytoin	NC or 25% increase[a]	48% decrease
Carbamazepine (CBZ)	NC	40% decrease
CBZ epoxide[b]	NC	NE
Valproic acid	11% decrease	14% decrease
Phenobarbital	NC	NE
Primidone	NC	NE

a = Plasma concentration increased 25% in some patients, generally those on a b.i.d. dosing regimen of phenytoin.
b = is not administered but is an active metabolite of carbamazepine.
NC = Less than 10% change in plasma concentration.
AED = Antiepileptic drug.
NE = Not Evaluated.

Other Drug Interactions

Digoxin: In a single-dose study, serum digoxin AUC was decreased by 12% with concomitant TOPAMAX® administration. The clinical relevance of this observation has not been established.

CNS Depressants: Concomitant administration of TOPAMAX® and alcohol or other CNS depressant drugs has not been evaluated in clinical studies. Because of the potential of topiramate to cause CNS depression, as well as other cognitive and/or neuropsychiatric adverse events, topiramate should be used with extreme caution if used in combination with alcohol and other CNS depressants.

Oral Contraceptives: In an interaction study with oral contraceptives using a combination product containing norethindrone and ethinyl estradiol, TOPAMAX® did not significantly affect the clearance of norethindrone. The mean total exposure to the estrogenic component decreased by 18%, 21%, and 30% at daily doses of 200, 400, and 800 mg/day, respectively. Therefore, efficacy of oral contraceptives may be compromised by topiramate. Patients taking oral contraceptives should be asked to report any change in their bleeding patterns. The effect of oral contraceptives on the pharmacokinetics of topiramate is not known.

Others: Concomitant use of TOPAMAX®, a weak carbonic anhydrase inhibitor, with other carbonic anhydrase inhibitors, e.g., acetazolamide or dichlorphenamide, may create a physiological environment that increases the risk of renal stone formation, and should therefore be avoided.

Laboratory Tests: There are no known interactions of topiramate with commonly used laboratory tests.

Carcinogenesis, Mutagenesis, Impairment of Fertility:

An increase in urinary bladder tumors was observed in mice given topiramate (20, 75, and 300 mg/kg) in the diet for 21 months. The elevated bladder tumor incidence, which was statistically significant in males and females receiving 300 mg/kg, was primarily due to the increased occurrence of a smooth muscle tumor considered histomorphologically unique to mice. Plasma exposures in mice receiving 300 mg/kg were approximately 0.5 to 1 times steady state exposures measured in patients receiving topiramate monotherapy at the recommended human dose (RHD) of 400 mg, and 1.5 to 2 times steady state topiramate exposures in patients receiving 400 mg of topiramate plus phenytoin. The relevance of this finding to human carcinogenic risk is uncertain. No evidence of carcinogenicity was seen in rats following oral administration of topiramate for 2 years at doses up to 120 mg/kg (approximately 3 times the RHD on a mg/m² basis).

Topiramate did not demonstrate genotoxic potential when tested in a battery of *in vitro* and *in vivo* assays. Topiramate was not mutagenic in the Ames test or the *in vitro* mouse lymphoma assay; it did not increase unscheduled DNA synthesis in rat hepatocytes *in vitro*; and it did not increase chromosomal aberrations in human lymphocytes *in vitro* or in rat bone marrow *in vivo*.

No adverse effects on male or female fertility were observed in rats at doses up to 100 mg/kg (2.5 times the RHD on a mg/m² basis).

Pregnancy: Pregnancy Category C.

Topiramate has demonstrated selective developmental toxicity, including teratogenicity, in experimental animal studies. When oral doses of 20, 100, or 500 mg/kg were administered to pregnant mice during the period of organogenesis, the incidence of fetal malformations (primarily craniofacial defects) was increased at all doses. The low dose is approximately 0.2 times the recommended human dose (RHD=400 mg/day) on a mg/m² basis. Fetal body weights and skeletal ossification were reduced at 500 mg/kg in conjunction with decreased maternal body weight gain.

In rat studies (oral doses of 20, 100, and 500 mg/kg or 0.2, 2.5, 30 and 400 mg/kg), the frequency of limb malformations (ectrodactyly, micromelia, and amelia) was increased among the offspring of dams treated with 400 mg/kg (10 times the RHD on a mg/m² basis) or greater during the organogenesis period of pregnancy. Embryotoxicity (reduced fetal body weights, increased incidence of structural variations) was observed at doses as low as 20 mg/kg (0.5 times the RHD on a mg/m² basis). Clinical signs of maternal toxicity were seen at 400 mg/kg and above, and maternal body weight gain was reduced during treatment with 100 mg/kg or greater.

In rabbit studies (20, 60, and 180 mg/kg or 10, 35, and 120 mg/kg orally during organogenesis), embryo/fetal mortality was increased at 35 mg/kg (2 times the RHD on a mg/m² basis) or greater, and teratogenic effects (primarily rib and vertebral malformations) were observed at 120 mg/kg (6 times the RHD on a mg/m² basis). Evidence of maternal toxicity (decreased body weight gain, clinical signs, and/or mortality) was seen at 35 mg/kg and above.

When female rats were treated during the latter part of gestation and throughout lactation (0.2, 4, 20, and 100 mg/kg or 2, 20, and 200 mg/kg), offspring exhibited decreased viability and delayed physical development at 200 mg/kg (5 times the RHD on a mg/m² basis) and reductions in pre- and/or postweaning body weight gain at 2 mg/kg (0.05 times the RHD on a mg/m² basis) and above. Maternal toxicity (decreased body weight gain, clinical signs) was evident at 100 mg/kg or greater.

In a rat embryo/fetal development study with a postnatal component (0.2, 2.5, 30 or 400 mg/kg during organogenesis; noted above), pups exhibited delayed physical development at 400 mg/kg (10 times the RHD on a mg/m² basis) and persistent reductions in body weight gain at 30 mg/kg (1 times the RHD on a mg/m² basis) and higher.

There are no studies using TOPAMAX® (topiramate) in pregnant women. TOPAMAX® should be used during pregnancy only if the potential benefit outweighs the potential risk to the fetus.

Labor and Delivery:

In studies of rats where dams were allowed to deliver pups naturally, no drug-related effects on gestation length or parturition were observed at dosage levels up to 200 mg/kg/day. The effect of TOPAMAX® (topiramate) on labor and delivery in humans is unknown.

Nursing Mothers:

Topiramate is excreted in the milk of lactating rats. It is not known if topiramate is excreted in human milk. Since many drugs are excreted in human milk, and because the potential for serious adverse reactions in nursing infants to TOPAMAX® (topiramate) is unknown, the potential benefit to the mother should be weighed against the potential risk to the infant when considering recommendations regarding nursing.

Pediatric Use:

Safety and effectiveness in children have not been established. The pharmacokinetic profile of TOPAMAX® was studied in patients between the ages of 4 and 17 years [see **CLINICAL PHARMACOLOGY; Pediatric Pharmacokinetics**].

Geriatric Use:

In clinical trials, 2% of patients were over 60. No age related difference in effectiveness or adverse effects were seen. There were no pharmacokinetic differences related to age alone, although the possibility of age-associated renal functional abnormalities should be considered.

Table 2: Median Percent Seizure Rate Reduction and Percent Responders in Five Double-Blind, Placebo-Controlled, Add-On Trials

Protocol Efficacy Results		Placebo	Target Topiramate Dosage (mg/day) 200	400	600	800	1,000
YD	N	45	45	45	46	-	-
	Median % Reduction	11.6	27.2[a]	47.5[b]	44.7[c]	-	-
	% Responders	18	24	44[d]	46[d]	-	-
YE	N	47	-	-	48	48	47
	Median % Reduction	1.7	-	-	40.8[c]	41.0[c]	36.0[c]
	% Responders	9	-	-	40[c]	41[c]	36[d]
Y1	N	24	-	23	-	-	-
	Median % Reduction	1.1	-	40.7[e]	-	-	-
	% Responders	8	-	35[d]	-	-	-
Y2	N	30	-	-	30	-	-
	Median % Reduction	-12.2	-	-	46.4[f]	-	-
	% Responders	10	-	-	47[c]	-	-
Y3	N	28	-	-	-	28	-
	Median % Reduction	-20.6	-	-	-	24.3[c]	-
	% Responders	0	-	-	-	43[c]	-

Comparisons with placebo: [a] p = 0.080, [b] p≤0.010; [c] p≤0.001; [d] p≤0.050; [e] p=0.065; [f] p≤0.005

Table 4: Incidence (%) of Treatment-Emergent Adverse Events in Placebo-Controlled, Add-On Trials[a,b] (Events that occurred in at least 1% of topiramate-treated patients and occurred more frequently in topiramate-treated than placebo-treated patients)

Body System/ Adverse Event[c]	Placebo (N=174)	200-400 (N=113)	600-1,000 (N=247)
Body as a Whole - General Disorders			
Asthenia	1.1	8.0	4.5
Back Pain	4.0	6.2	2.0
Chest Pain	2.3	4.4	2.0
Influenza-Like Symptoms	2.9	3.5	3.2
Leg Pain	2.3	3.5	2.4
Hot Flushes	1.7	2.7	0.8
Body Odor	0.0	1.8	0.0
Edema	1.1	1.8	1.2
Rigors	0.0	1.8	0.4
Central & Peripheral Nervous System Disorders			
Dizziness	14.4	28.3	32.4
Ataxia	6.9	21.2	17.0
Speech Disorders/ Related Speech Problems	2.9	16.8	13.8
Nystagmus	11.5	15.0	15.0
Paresthesia	3.4	15.0	14.6
Tremor	6.3	10.6	13.8
Language Problems	0.6	6.2	11.7
Coordination Abnormal	1.7	5.3	3.6
Hypoaesthesia	1.1	2.7	0.8
Gastrointestinal System Disorders			
Nausea	6.3	11.5	13.8
Dyspepsia	5.2	8.0	5.7
Abdominal Pain	2.9	5.3	7.3
Constipation	0.6	5.3	3.2
Dry Mouth	1.1	2.7	3.2
Gingivitis	0.0	1.8	0.4
Hearing and Vestibular Disorders			
Hearing Decreased	1.1	1.8	1.6
Metabolic and Nutritional Disorders			
Weight Decrease	2.3	7.1	12.6
Musculoskeletal System Disorders			
Myalgia	1.1	1.8	1.2
Platelet, Bleeding and Clotting Disorders			
Epistaxis	1.1	1.8	0.8
Psychiatric Disorders			
Somnolence	10.3	30.1	25.9
Psychomotor Slowing	2.3	16.8	25.1
Nervousness	7.5	15.9	20.6
Difficulty with Memory	2.9	12.4	12.6
Confusion	5.2	9.7	15.0
Depression	6.3	8.0	13.4
Difficulty with Concentration/Attention	1.1	8.0	15.4
Anorexia	4.0	5.3	11.3
Agitation	1.7	4.4	4.0
Mood Problems	1.7	3.5	10.1
Aggressive Reaction	0.6	2.7	4.0
Apathy	0.0	1.8	4.5
Depersonalization	0.6	1.8	1.6
Emotional Lability	1.1	1.8	2.4
Reproduction Disorders, Female	(N=39)	(N=24)	(N=42)
Breast Pain, Female	0.0	8.3	0.0
Dysmenorrhea	2.6	8.3	0.0
Menstrual Disorder	0.0	4.2	0.0
Respiratory System Disorders			
Upper Respiratory Infection	11.5	12.4	12.1
Pharyngitis	2.9	7.1	2.8
Sinusitis	4.0	4.4	4.0
Dyspnea	1.1	1.8	3.2
Skin and Appendages Disorders			
Rash	4.0	4.4	3.2
Pruritus	1.1	1.8	3.2
Sweating Increased	0.0	1.8	0.4
Urinary System Disorders			
Hematuria	0.6	1.8	0.8
Vision Disorders			
Diplopia	6.3	14.2	14.6
Vision Abnormal	2.9	14.2	10.5
Eye Pain	1.1	1.8	2.0
White Cell and Res Disorders			
Leukopenia	0.6	2.7	1.6

[a] Patients in these add-on trials were receiving 1 to 2 concomitant antiepileptic drugs in addition to TOPAMAX or placebo.

[b] Values represent the percentage of patients reporting a given adverse event. Patients may have reported more than one adverse event during the study and can be included in more than one adverse event category.

[c] Adverse events reported by at least 1% of patients in the TOPAMAX 200-400 mg/day group and more common than in the placebo group are listed in this table.

Race and Gender Effects:

Evaluation of efficacy and safety in clinical trials has shown no race or gender related effects.

ADVERSE REACTIONS

The most commonly observed adverse events associated with the use of topiramate at dosages of 200 to 400 mg/day in controlled trials, that were seen at greater frequency in topiramate-treated patients and did not appear to be dose-related were: somnolence, dizziness, ataxia, speech disorders and related speech problems, psychomotor slowing, nystagmus, and paresthesia [see Table 4]. The most common dose-related adverse events at dosages of 200 to 1,000 mg/day were: fatigue, nervousness, difficulty with concentration or attention, confusion, depression, anorexia, language problems, anxiety, mood problems, cognitive problems not otherwise specified, weight decreased, and tremor [see Table 5].

In controlled clinical trials, 11% of patients receiving topiramate 200 to 400 mg/day as adjunctive therapy discontinued due to adverse events. This rate appeared to increase at dosages above 400 mg/day. Adverse events associated with discontinuing therapy included somnolence, dizziness, anxiety, difficulty with concentration or attention, fatigue, and paresthesia and increased at dosages above 400 mg/day.

Approximately 28% of the 1,715 individuals with epilepsy who received topiramate at dosages of 200 to 1,600 mg/day in clinical studies discontinued treatment because of adverse events; an individual patient could have reported more than one adverse event. These adverse events were: psychomotor slowing (4.1%), difficulty with memory (3.3%), fatigue (3.3%), confusion (3.2%), somnolence (3.2%), difficulty with concentration/attention (2.9%), anorexia (2.9%), depression (2.6%), dizziness (2.6%), weight decrease (2.5%), nervousness (2.2%), ataxia (2.2%), paresthesia (2.0%), and language problems (2.0%).

Incidence in Controlled Clinical Trials – Add-On Therapy

Table 4 lists treatment-emergent adverse events that occurred in at least 1% of patients treated with 200 to 400 mg/day topiramate in controlled trials that were numerically more common at this dose than in the patients treated with placebo. In general, most patients who experienced adverse events during the first eight weeks of these trials no longer experienced them by their last visit.

The prescriber should be aware that these data were obtained when TOPAMAX® was added to concurrent antiepileptic drug therapy and cannot be used to predict the frequency of adverse events in the course of usual medical practice where patient characteristics and other factors may differ from those prevailing during clinical studies. Similarly, the cited frequencies cannot be directly compared with data obtained from other clinical investigations involving different treatments, uses, or investigators. Inspection of these frequencies, however, does not provide the prescribing physician with a basis to estimate the relative contribution of drug and non-drug factors to the adverse event incidences in the population studied.

[See table 4 above]

[See table 5 at bottom of next page]

Other Adverse Events Observed

Other events that occurred in more than 1% of patients treated with 200 to 400 mg of topiramate in placebo-controlled trials but with equal or greater frequency in the placebo group were: fatigue, headache, injury, anxiety, rash, pain, convulsions aggravated, coughing, gastroenteritis, rhinitis, back pain, hot flushes, bronchitis, abnormal gait, involuntary muscle contractions, and epistaxis.

Other Adverse Events Observed During All Clinical Trials

Topiramate, initiated as adjunctive therapy, has been administered to 1,715 patients with epilepsy during all clinical studies. During these studies, all adverse events were recorded by the clinical investigators using terminology of their own choosing. To provide a meaningful estimate of the proportion of individuals having adverse events, similar types of events were grouped into a smaller number of standardized categories using modified WHOART dictionary terminology. The frequencies presented represent the proportion of 1,715 topiramate-treated patients who experienced an event of the type cited on at least one occasion while receiving topiramate. Reported events are included except those already listed in the previous table, those too general to be informative, and those not reasonably associated with the use of the drug.

Events are classified within body system categories and enumerated in order of decreasing frequency using the following definitions: *frequent* occurring in at least 1/100 patients; *infrequent* occurring in 1/100 to 1/1000 patients; *rare* occurring in fewer than 1/1000 patients.

Autonomic Nervous System Disorders: *Infrequent:* vasodilation.

Body as a Whole: *Frequent:* fatigue, fever, malaise. *Infrequent:* syncope, halitosis, abdomen enlarged. *Rare:* alcohol intolerance, substernal chest pain, sudden death.

Cardiovascular Disorders, General: *Infrequent:* hypertension, hypotension, postural hypotension.

Central & Peripheral Nervous System Disorders: *Frequent:* hypokinesia, vertigo, stupor, convulsions grand mal, hyper-

Continued on next page

Topamax—Cont.

kinesea, hypertonia. *Infrequent:* leg cramps, hyporeflexia, neuropathy, migraine, apraxia, hyperaesthesia, dyskinesia, hyperreflexia, dysphonia, scotoma, ptosis, dystonia, visual field defect, coma, encephalopathy, fecal incontinence, upper motor neuron lesion. *Rare:* cerebellar syndrome, EEG abnormal, tongue paralysis.

Endocrine Disorders: *Infrequent:* goiter. *Rare:* thyroid disorder.

Gastrointestinal System Disorders: *Frequent:* diarrhea, vomiting, flatulence, gastroenteritis. *Infrequent:* gum hyperplasia, hemorrhoids, tooth caries, stomatitis, dysphagia, melena, gastritis, saliva increased, hiccough, gastroesophageal reflux, tongue edema, esophagitis. *Rare:* eructation.

Hearing and Vestibular Disorders: *Frequent:* tinnitus. *Rare:* earache, hyperacusis.

Heart Rate and Rhythm Disorders: *Frequent:* palpitation. *Infrequent:* AV block bradycardia, bundle branch block. *Rare:* arrhythmia, arrhythmia atrial, fibrillation atrial.

Liver and Biliary System Disorders: *Infrequent:* SGPT increased, SGOT increased, gall bladder disorder. *Rare:* gamma-GT increased.

Metabolic and Nutritional Disorders: *Frequent:* weight increase. *Infrequent:* thirst, hypokalemia, alkaline phosphatase increased, dehydration, hypocalcemia, hyperlipemia, acidosis, hyperglycemia, creatinine increased, hyperchloremia, xerophthalmia. *Rare:* diabetes mellitus, hypernatremia, abnormal serum folate, hyponatremia, hypocholesterolemia, hypoglycemia, hypophosphatemia.

Musculoskeletal System Disorders: *Frequent:* arthralgia, muscle weakness. *Infrequent:* arthrosis, osteoporosis.

Myo-, Endo-, Pericardial & Valve Disorders: *Infrequent:* angina pectoris.

Neoplasms: *Infrequent:* basal cell carcinoma, thrombocythemia. *Rare:* polycythemia.

Platelet, Bleeding, and Clotting Disorders: *Infrequent:* gingival bleeding, purpura, thrombocytopenia, pulmonary embolism.

Psychiatric Disorders: *Frequent:* insomnia, personality disorder, impotence, hallucination, euphoria, psychosis, libido decreased, suicide attempt. *Infrequent:* paranoid reaction, appetite increased, delusion, paranoia, delirium, abnormal dreaming, neurosis. *Rare:* libido increased, manic reaction.

Red Blood Cell Disorders: *Frequent:* anemia. *Rare:* marrow depression, pancytopenia.

Reproductive Disorders, Female: *Frequent:* intermenstrual bleeding, leukorrhea, menorrhagia, vaginitis, amenorrhea.

Reproductive Disorders, Male: *Infrequent:* ejaculation disorder, breast discharge.

Respiratory System Disorders: *Frequent:* coughing, bronchitis. *Infrequent:* asthma, bronchospasm. *Rare:* laryngismus.

Skin and Appendages Disorders: *Frequent:* acne, alopecia. *Infrequent:* dermatitis, nail disorder, folliculitis, dry skin, urticaria, skin discoloration, eczema, photosensitivity reaction, erythematous rash, seborrhoea, sweating decreased, abnormal hair texture. *Rare:* chloasma.

Special Senses Other, Disorders: *Frequent:* taste perversion. *Infrequent:* taste loss, parosmia.

Urinary System Disorders: *Frequent:* urinary tract infection, micturition frequency, urinary incontinence, dysuria, renal calculus. *Infrequent:* urinary retention, face edema, renal pain, nocturia, albuminuria, polyuria, oliguria.

Vascular (Extracardiac) Disorders: *Infrequent:* flushing, deep vein thrombosis, phlebitis. *Rare:* vasospasm.

Vision Disorders: *Frequent:* conjunctivitis. *Infrequent:* abnormal accommodation, photophobia, abnormal lacrimation, strabismus, color blindness, myopia, mydriasis. *Rare:* cataract, corneal opacity, iritis.

White Cell and Reticuloendothelial System Disorders: *Infrequent:* lymphadenopathy, eosinophilia, lymphopenia, granulocytopenia, lymphocytosis.

DRUG ABUSE AND DEPENDENCE

The abuse and dependence potential of TOPAMAX® (topiramate) has not been evaluated in human studies.

OVERDOSAGE

In acute TOPAMAX® (topiramate) overdose, if the ingestion is recent, the stomach should be emptied immediately by lavage or by induction of emesis. Activated charcoal has not been shown to adsorb topiramate *in vitro*. Therefore, its use in overdosage is not recommended. Treatment should be appropriately supportive. Hemodialysis is an effective means of removing topiramate from the body. However, in the few cases of acute overdosage reported, hemodialysis has not been necessary.

DOSAGE AND ADMINISTRATION

In the controlled add-on trials, no correlation has been demonstrated between trough plasma concentrations of topiramate and clinical efficacy. No evidence of tolerance has been demonstrated in humans. Doses above 400 mg/day (600, 800, and 1000 mg/day) have not been shown to improve responses.

The recommended total daily dose of TOPAMAX® (topiramate) as adjunctive therapy is 400 mg/day in two divided doses. A daily dose of 200 mg/day has inconsistent effects and is less effective than 400 mg/day. It is recommended that therapy be initiated at 50 mg/day followed by titration to an effective dose. Daily doses above 1,600 mg have not been studied.

The recommended titration rate for topiramate is:

	AM DOSE	PM DOSE
Week 1	none	50 mg
Week 2	50 mg	50 mg
Week 3	50 mg	100 mg
Week 4	100 mg	100 mg
Week 5	100 mg	150 mg
Week 6	150 mg	150 mg
Week 7	150 mg	200 mg
Week 8	200 mg	200 mg

It is not necessary to monitor topiramate plasma concentrations to optimize TOPAMAX® therapy. On occasion, the addition of TOPAMAX® to phenytoin may require an adjustment of the dose of phenytoin to achieve optimal clinical outcome. Addition or withdrawal of phenytoin and/or carbamazepine during adjunctive therapy with TOPAMAX® may require adjustment of the dose of TOPAMAX®. Because of the bitter taste, tablets should not be broken. TOPAMAX® can be taken without regard to meals.

Patients with Renal Impairment:
In renally impaired subjects (creatinine clearance less than 70 mL/min/1.73m²), one half of the usual adult dose is recommended. Such patients will require a longer time to reach steady-state at each dose.

Patients Undergoing Hemodialysis:
Topiramate is cleared by hemodialysis at a rate that is 4 to 6 times greater than a normal individual. Accordingly, a prolonged period of dialysis may cause topiramate concentration to fall below that required to maintain an antiseizure effect. To avoid rapid drops in topiramate plasma concentration during hemodialysis a supplemental dose of topiramate may be required. The actual adjustment should take into account 1) the duration of dialysis period, 2) the clearance rate of the dialysis system being used, and 3) the effective renal clearance of topiramate in the patient being dialyzed.

Patients with Hepatic Disease:
In hepatically impaired patients topiramate plasma concentrations may be increased. The mechanism is not well understood.

HOW SUPPLIED

TOPAMAX® (topiramate) is available as debossed, coated, round tablets in the following strengths and colors:

25 mg white (coded "TOP" on one side; "25" on the other)
100 mg yellow (coded "TOPAMAX" on one side; "100" on the other)
200 mg salmon (coded "TOPAMAX" on one side; "200" on the other)
They are supplied as follows:
25 mg tablets – bottles of 60 count with desiccant (NDC 0045-0639-65)
100 mg tablets – bottles of 60 count with desiccant (NDC 0045-0641-65)
200 mg tablets – bottles of 60 count with desiccant (NDC 0045-0642-65)
TOPAMAX® (topiramate) Tablets should be stored in tightly-closed containers at controlled room temperature, (59 to 86°F, 15 to 30°C). Protect from moisture.
CAUTION: Federal law prohibits dispensing without a prescription.
TOPAMAX® (topiramate) is a trademark of ORTHO-MCNEIL PHARMACEUTICAL, INC.
ORTHO-McNEIL PHARMACEUTICAL, INC.
Raritan, NJ 08869
© OMP 1998   Revised March 1998   643-10-443-4
Shown in Product Identification Guide, page 329

TYLENOL® with Codeine   ℞
[*ti 'len-awl co 'dēn*]
(acetaminophen and codeine phosphate tablets and oral solution USP)
TabletsⅢ **and Elixir**Ⅴ
No. 3-NSN 6505-00-400-2054—100's
No. 3-NSN 6505-00-147-8347—500's
No. 3-NSN 6505-01-086-2993—U/D 500's
No. 3-NSN 6505-00-372-3032—1000's
Elixir-NSN 6505-01-035-1963—Pints

DESCRIPTION

Each tablet contains:
No. 2 Codeine Phosphate* .... 15 mg
　Acetaminophen .... 300 mg
No. 3 Codeine Phosphate* .... 30 mg
　Acetaminophen .... 300 mg
No. 4 Codeine Phosphate* .... 60 mg
　Acetaminophen .... 300 mg
Each 5 mL of elixir contains:
　Codeine Phosphate* .... 12 mg
　Acetaminophen .... 120 mg
　Alcohol 7%
*Warning—May be habit forming.
Inactive ingredients: tablets—powdered cellulose, magnesium stearate, sodium metabisulfite†, pregelatinized starch, starch (corn); elixir—alcohol, citric acid, propylene glycol, sodium benzoate, saccharin sodium, sucrose, natural and artificial flavors, FD&C Yellow No.6.
Acetaminophen, 4'-hydroxyacetanilide, is a non-opiate, non-salicylate analgesic and antipyretic which occurs as a white, odorless, crystalline powder, possessing a slightly bitter taste. Its structure is as follows:

C_8H_9NO M.W. 151.16

Codeine is an alkaloid, obtained from opium or prepared from morphine by methylation. Codeine phosphate occurs as fine, white, needle-shaped crystals, or white, crystalline powder. It is affected by light. Its chemical name is 7,8-didehydro- 4,5α-epoxy-3-methoxy-17- methylmorphinan-6α-ol phosphate (1:1) (salt) hemihydrate. Its structure is as follows:

$C_{18}H_{21}NO_3 \cdot H_3PO_4 \cdot \frac{1}{2}H_2O$ M.W. 406.37

†See WARNINGS

CLINICAL PHARMACOLOGY

TYLENOL with Codeine (acetaminophen and codeine phosphate tablets and oral solution USP) combine the analgesic effects of a centrally acting analgesic, codeine, with a peripherally acting analgesic, acetaminophen. Both ingredients are well absorbed orally. The plasma elimination half-life ranges from 1 to 4 hours for acetaminophen, and from 2.5 to 3 hours for codeine.
Codeine retains at least one-half of its analgesic activity when administered orally. A reduced first-pass metabolism

Table 5: Incidence (%) of Dose-Related Adverse Events From Five Placebo-Controlled, Add-On Trials

Adverse Event	TOPAMAX® Dosage (mg/day)			
	Placebo (N=174)	200 (N=45)	400 (N=68)	600-1,000 (N=247)
Fatigue	14.4	11.1	11.8	30.8
Nervousness	7.5	13.3	17.6	20.6
Difficulty with Concentration/Attention	1.1	6.7	8.8	15.4
Confusion	5.2	8.9	10.3	15.0
Depression	6.3	8.9	7.4	13.4
Anorexia	4.0	4.4	5.9	11.3
Language problems	0.6	2.2	8.8	11.7
Anxiety	5.2	2.2	2.9	9.3
Mood problems	1.7	0.0	5.9	10.1
Cognitive problems NOS	0.6	0.0	0.0	4.0
Weight decrease	2.3	4.4	8.8	12.6
Tremor	6.3	13.3	8.8	13.8

of codeine by the liver accounts for the greater oral efficacy of codeine when compared to most other morphine-like narcotics. Following absorption, codeine is metabolized by the liver and metabolic products are excreted in the urine. Approximately 10 percent of the administered codeine is demethylated to morphine, which may account for its analgesic activity.

Acetaminophen is distributed throughout most fluids of the body, and is metabolized primarily in the liver. Little unchanged drug is excreted in the urine, but most metabolic products appear in the urine within 24 hours.

INDICATIONS AND USAGE

TYLENOL with Codeine tablets (acetaminophen and codeine phosphate tablets) are indicated for the relief of mild to moderately severe pain.

TYLENOL with Codeine elixir (acetaminophen and codeine phosphate oral solution USP) is indicated for the relief of mild to moderate pain.

CONTRAINDICATIONS

TYLENOL with Codeine tablets or elixir (acetaminophen and codeine phosphate tablets and oral solution USP) should not be administered to patients who have previously exhibited hypersensitivity to any component.

WARNINGS

TYLENOL with Codeine tablets (acetaminophen and codeine phosphate tablets) contain sodium metabisulfite, a sulfite that may cause allergic-type reactions including anaphylactic symptoms and life-threatening or less severe asthmatic episodes in certain susceptible people. The overall prevalence of sulfite sensitivity in the general population is unknown and probably low. Sulfite sensitivity is seen more frequently in asthmatic than in nonasthmatic people.

PRECAUTIONS
General

Head Injury and Increased Intracranial Pressure: The respiratory depressant effects of narcotics and their capacity to elevate cerebrospinal fluid pressure may be markedly exaggerated in the presence of head injury, other intracranial lesions or a pre-existing increase in intracranial pressure. Furthermore, narcotics produce adverse reactions which may obscure the clinical course of patients with head injuries.

Acute Abdominal Conditions: The administration of this product or other narcotics may obscure the diagnosis or clinical course of patients with acute abdominal conditions.

Special Risk Patients: This drug should be given with caution to certain patients such as the elderly or debilitated, and those with severe impairment of hepatic or renal function, hypothyroidism, Addison's disease, and prostatic hypertrophy or urethral stricture.

Information for Patients

Codeine may impair the mental and/or physical abilities required for the performance of potentially hazardous tasks such as driving a car or operating machinery. The patient using this drug should be cautioned accordingly.

The patient should understand the single-dose and 24 hour dose limits, and the time interval between doses.

Drug Interactions

Patients receiving other narcotic analgesics, antipsychotics, antianxiety agents, or other CNS depressants (including alcohol) concomitantly with this drug may exhibit an additive CNS depression. When such combined therapy is contemplated, the dose of one or both agents should be reduced.

The concurrent use of anticholinergics with codeine may produce paralytic ileus.

Carcinogenesis, Mutagenesis, Impairment of Fertility

No long-term studies in animals have been performed with acetaminophen or codeine to determine carcinogenic potential or effects on fertility.

Acetaminophen and codeine have been found to have no mutagenic potential using the Ames Salmonella-Microsomal Activation test, the Basc test on Drosophila germ cells, and the Micronucleus test on mouse bone marrow.

Pregnancy

Teratogenic Effects: Pregnancy Category C.

Codeine: A study in rats and rabbits reported no teratogenic effect of codeine administered during the period of organogenesis in doses ranging from 5 to 120 mg/kg. In the rat, doses at the 120 mg/kg level, in the toxic range for the adult animal, were associated with an increase in embryo resorption at the time of implantation. In another study a single 100 mg/kg dose of codeine administered to pregnant mice reportedly resulted in delayed ossification in the offspring. There are no studies in humans, and the significance of these findings to humans, if any, is not known.

TYLENOL with Codeine (acetaminophen and codeine phosphate tablets and oral solution USP) should be used during pregnancy only if the potential benefit justifies the potential risk to the fetus.

Nonteratogenic Effects:

Dependence has been reported in newborns whose mothers took opiates regularly during pregnancy. Withdrawal signs include irritability, excessive crying, tremors, hyperreflexia, fever, vomiting, and diarrhea. These signs usually appear during the first few days of life.

Labor and Delivery

Narcotic analgesics cross the placental barrier. The closer to delivery and the larger the dose used, the greater the possibility of respiratory depression in the newborn. Narcotic analgesics should be avoided during labor if delivery of a premature infant is anticipated. If the mother has received narcotic analgesics during labor, newborn infants should be observed closely for signs of respiratory depression. Resuscitation may be required (see OVERDOSAGE). The effect of codeine, if any, on the later growth, development, and functional maturation of the child is unknown.

Nursing Mothers

Some studies, but not others, have reported detectable amounts of codeine in breast milk. The levels are probably not clinically significant after usual therapeutic dosage. The possibility of clinically important amounts being excreted in breast milk in individuals abusing codeine should be considered.

Pediatric Use

Safe dosage of TYLENOL with Codeine elixir (acetaminophen and codeine phosphate oral solution USP) has not been established in children below the age of three years.

ADVERSE REACTIONS

The most frequently observed adverse reactions include lightheadedness, dizziness, sedation, shortness of breath, nausea and vomiting. These effects seem to be more prominent in ambulatory than in non-ambulatory patients, and some of these adverse reactions may be alleviated if the patient lies down. Other adverse reactions include allergic reactions, euphoria, dysphoria, constipation, abdominal pain and pruritus.

At higher doses, codeine has most of the disadvantages of morphine including respiratory depression.

DRUG ABUSE AND DEPENDENCE

TYLENOL with Codeine tablets (acetaminophen and codeine phosphate tablets) are a Schedule III controlled substance.

TYLENOL with Codeine elixir (acetaminophen and codeine phosphate oral solution USP) is a Schedule V controlled substance.

Codeine can produce drug dependence of the morphine type and, therefore, has the potential for being abused. Psychic dependence, physical dependence and tolerance may develop upon repeated administration of this drug, and it should be prescribed and administered with the same degree of caution appropriate to the use of other oral narcotic-containing medications.

OVERDOSAGE
Acetaminophen

Signs and Symptoms: In acute acetaminophen overdosage, dose-dependent, potentially fatal hepatic necrosis is the most serious adverse effect. Renal tubular necrosis, hypoglycemic coma and thrombocytopenia may also occur.

In adults, hepatic toxicity has rarely been reported with acute overdoses of less than 10 grams and fatalities with less than 15 grams. Importantly, young children seem to be more resistant than adults to the hepatotoxic effect of an acetaminophen overdose. Despite this, the measures outlined below should be initiated in any adult or child suspected of having ingested an acetaminophen overdose.

Early symptoms following a potentially hepatotoxic overdose may include: nausea, vomiting, diaphoresis and general malaise. Clinical and laboratory evidence of hepatic toxicity may not be apparent until 48 to 72 hours postingestion.

Treatment: The stomach should be emptied promptly by lavage or by induction of emesis with syrup of ipecac. Patients' estimates of the quantity of a drug ingested are notoriously unreliable. Therefore, if an acetaminophen overdose is suspected, a serum acetaminophen assay should be obtained as early as possible, but no sooner than four hours following ingestion. Liver function studies should be obtained initially and repeated at 24-hour intervals.

The antidote, N-acetylcysteine, should be administered as early as possible, preferably within 16 hours of the overdose ingestion for optimal results, but in any case, within 24 hours. Following recovery, there are no residual, structural or functional hepatic abnormalities.

Codeine

Signs and Symptoms: Serious overdose with codeine is characterized by respiratory depression (a decrease in respiratory rate and/or tidal volume, Cheyne-Stokes respiration, cyanosis), extreme somnolence progressing to stupor or coma, skeletal muscle flaccidity, cold and clammy skin, and sometimes bradycardia and hypotension. In severe overdosage, apnea, circulatory collapse, cardiac arrest and death may occur.

Treatment: Primary attention should be given to the reestablishment of adequate respiratory exchange through provision of a patent airway and the institution of assisted or controlled ventilation. The narcotic antagonist naloxone is a specific antidote against respiratory depression which may result from overdosage or unusual sensitivity to narcotics, including codeine. Therefore, an appropriate dose of naloxone hydrochloride (see package insert) should be administered, preferably by the intravenous route, and simultaneously with efforts at respiratory resuscitation. Since the duration of action of codeine may exceed that of the antagonist, the patient should be kept under continued surveillance and repeated doses of the antagonist should be administered as needed to maintain adequate respiration.

An antagonist should not be administered in the absence of clinically significant respiratory or cardiovascular depression. Oxygen, intravenous fluids, vasopressors and other supportive measures should be employed as indicated. Gastric emptying may be useful in removing unabsorbed drug.

DOSAGE AND ADMINISTRATION

Dosage should be adjusted according to severity of pain and response of the patient.

It should be kept in mind, however, that tolerance to codeine can develop with continued use and that the incidence of untoward effects is dose related. Adult doses of codeine higher than 60 mg fail to give commensurate relief of pain but merely prolong analgesia and are associated with an appreciably increased incidence of undesirable side effects. Equivalently high doses in children would have similar effects.

The usual adult dosage for tablets is:

	Single Doses (Range)	Maximum 24 Hour Dose
Codeine Phosphate	15mg–60mg	360mg
Acetaminophen	300mg–1000mg	4000mg

Doses may be repeated up to every 4 hours.

The prescriber must determine the number of tablets per dose, and the maximum number of tablets per 24 hours, based upon the above dosage guidance. This information should be conveyed in the prescription.

For children, the dose of codeine phosphate is 0.5 mg/kg. TYLENOL with Codeine elixir (acetaminophen and codeine phosphate oral solution USP) contains 120 mg of acetaminophen and 12 mg of codeine phosphate/5 mL and is given orally.

The usual doses are:

Children: (7 to 12 years): 10 mL (2 teaspoonfuls)
　　　　 3 or 4 times daily.
　　　　 (3 to 6 years): 5 mL (1 teaspoonful)
　　　　 3 or 4 times daily.
　　　　 (under 3 years): safe dosage has not been established.

Adults: 15 mL (1 tablespoonful) every 4 hours as needed.

HOW SUPPLIED

TYLENOL with Codeine tablets (acetaminophen and codeine phosphate tablets): (round, white, imprinted "McNEIL," "TYLENOL CODEINE" and either "2," "3," "4"): No.2 – NDC 0045-0511–60 bottles of 100, NDC 0045-0511–72 unit dose (20 × 25); No. 3 – NDC 0045-0513–60 bottles of 100, NDC 0045-0513–70 bottles of 500, NDC 0045-0513–80 bottles of 1000, NDC 0045-0513–72 unit dose (20 × 25); No. 4 — NDC 0045-0515–60 bottles of 100, NDC 0045-0515–70 bottles of 500, NDC 0045-0515–72 unit dose (20 × 25).

TYLENOL with Codeine elixir (acetaminophen and codeine phosphate oral solution USP) contains 120 mg acetaminophen and 12 mg codeine phosphate/5 mL (colored amber, cherry flavored) — NDC 0045-0508-16, bottles of 1 pint.

Store TYLENOL with Codeine tablets at controlled room temperature (15–30°C, 59–86°F).

Store TYLENOL with Codeine elixir at controlled room temperature (15–30°C, 59–86°F). Protect from light. Do not refrigerate. Do not freeze.

Dispense in tight, light-resistant container as defined in the official compendium.

McNeil Pharmaceutical, McNEILAB, INC., Spring House, PA 19477

633–10–057–1　　　　　　　　　　 Revised 6/23/95

Shown in Product Identification Guide, page 329

TYLOX® Capsules　　　　　　　　　 ℂ ℞
[ti 'lox]
(oxycodone and acetaminophen capsules USP)
NSN 6505-01-210-4450-100's
NSN 6505-01-211-6803-Unit Dose (100's)

DESCRIPTION

Each capsule of TYLOX (oxycodone and acetaminophen capsules USP) contains:
　Oxycodone Hydrochloride USP　　　　　 5 mg*
　Warning—May be habit forming.
　Acetaminophen USP　　　　　　　　　 500 mg

Continued on next page

Tylox—Cont.

Inactive ingredients: docusate sodium, gelatin, magnesium stearate, sodium benzoate, sodium metabisulfite†, corn starch, FD&C Blue No. 1, FD&C Red No. 3, FD&C Red No. 40, and titanium dioxide.
Acetaminophen occurs as a white, odorless crystalline powder, possessing a slightly bitter taste.
The oxycodone component is 14-hydroxydihydrocodeinone, a white, odorless crystalline powder having a saline, bitter taste. It is derived from the opium alkaloid thebaine, and may be represented by the following structural formula:

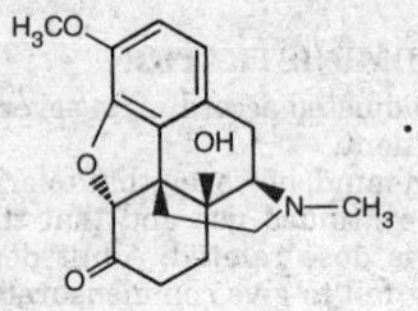

*5 mg oxycodone hydrochloride is equivalent to 4.4815 mg oxycodone
†See WARNINGS

CLINICAL PHARMACOLOGY

The principal ingredient, oxycodone, is a semisynthetic narcotic analgesic with multiple actions qualitatively similar to those of morphine; the most prominent of these involve the central nervous system and organs composed of smooth muscle. The principal actions of therapeutic value of the oxycodone in TYLOX (oxycodone and acetaminophen capsules) are analgesia and sedation.
Oxycodone is similar to codeine and methadone in that it retains at least one-half of its analgesic activity when administered orally.
Acetaminophen is a non-opiate, non-salicylate analgesic and antipyretic.

INDICATIONS AND USAGE

TYLOX (oxycodone and acetaminophen capsules) are indicated for the relief of moderate to moderately severe pain.

CONTRAINDICATIONS

TYLOX (oxycodone and acetaminophen capsules) should not be administered to patients who are hypersensitive to any component.

WARNINGS

Contains sodium metabisulfite, a sulfite that may cause allergic-type reactions including anaphylactic symptoms and life-threatening or less severe asthmatic episodes in certain susceptible people. The overall prevalence of sulfite sensitivity in the general population is unknown and probably low. Sulfite sensitivity is seen more frequently in asthmatic than in nonasthmatic people.

Drug Dependence

Oxycodone can produce drug dependence of the morphine type and, therefore, has the potential for being abused. Psychic dependence, physical dependence and tolerance may develop upon repeated administration of TYLOX (oxycodone and acetaminophen capsules), and it should be prescribed and administered with the same degree of caution appropriate to the use of other oral narcotic-containing medications. Like other narcotic-containing medications, TYLOX is subject to the Federal Control Substances Act (Schedule II).

PRECAUTIONS

General

Head Injury and Increased Intracranial Pressure: The respiratory depressant effects of narcotics and their capacity to elevate cerebrospinal fluid pressure may be markedly exaggerated in the presence of head injury, other intracranial lesions or a pre-existing increase in intracranial pressure. Furthermore, narcotics produce adverse reactions which may obscure the clinical course of patients with head injuries.
Acute Abdominal Conditions: The administration of TYLOX (oxycodone and acetaminophen capsules) or other narcotics may obscure the diagnosis or clinical course in patients with acute abdominal conditions.
Special Risk Patients: TYLOX should be given with caution to certain patients such as the elderly or debilitated, and those with severe impairment of hepatic or renal function, hypothyroidism, Addison's disease, and prostatic hypertrophy or urethral stricture.

Information for Patients

Oxycodone may impair the mental and/or physical abilities required for the performance of potentially hazardous tasks such as driving a car or operating machinery. The patient using TYLOX should be cautioned accordingly.

Drug Interactions

Patients receiving other narcotic analgesics, general anesthetics, phenothiazines, other tranquilizers, sedative-hypnotics or other CNS depressants (including alcohol) concomitantly with TYLOX may exhibit an additive CNS depression. When such combined therapy is contemplated, the dose of one or both agents should be reduced.
The concurrent use of anticholinergics with narcotics may produce paralytic ileus.

Usage in Pregnancy

Pregnancy Category C. Animal reproductive studies have not been conducted with TYLOX. It is also not known whether TYLOX can cause fetal harm when administered to a pregnant woman or can affect reproductive capacity. TYLOX should not be given to a pregnant woman unless in the judgment of the physician, the potential benefits outweigh the possible hazards.
Nonteratogenic Effects: Use of narcotics during pregnancy may produce physical dependence in the neonate.

Labor and Delivery

As with all narcotics, administration of TYLOX to the mother shortly before delivery may result in some degree of respiratory depression in the newborn and the mother, especially if higher doses are used.

Nursing Mothers

It is not known whether the components of TYLOX are excreted in human milk. Because many drugs are excreted in human milk, caution should be exercised when TYLOX is administered to a nursing woman.

Pediatric Use

Safety and effectiveness in children have not been established.

ADVERSE REACTIONS

The most frequently observed adverse reactions include lightheadedness, dizziness, sedation, nausea and vomiting. These effects seem to be more prominent in ambulatory than in non-ambulatory patients, and some of these adverse reactions may be alleviated if the patient lies down.
Other adverse reactions include allergic reactions, euphoria, dysphoria, constipation, skin rash and pruritus. At higher doses, oxycodone has most of the disadvantages of morphine including respiratory depression.

DRUG ABUSE AND DEPENDENCE

TYLOX capsules are a Schedule II controlled substance. Oxycodone can produce drug dependence and has the potential for being abused. (See WARNINGS)

OVERDOSAGE

Acetaminophen

Signs and Symptoms: In acute acetaminophen overdosage, dose-dependent potentially fatal hepatic necrosis is the most serious adverse effect. Renal tubular necrosis, hypoglycemic coma and thrombocytopenia may also occur.
In adults, hepatic toxicity has rarely been reported with acute overdoses of less than 10 grams and fatalities with less than 15 grams. Importantly, young children seem to be more resistant than adults to the hepatotoxic effect of an acetaminophen overdose. Despite this, the measures outlined below should be initiated in any adult or child suspected of having ingested an acetaminophen overdose.
Early symptoms following a potentially hepatotoxic overdose may include: nausea, vomiting, diaphoresis, and general malaise. Clinical and laboratory evidence of hepatic toxicity may not be apparent until 48 to 72 hours post-ingestion.
Treatment: The stomach should be emptied promptly by lavage or by induction of emesis with syrup of ipecac. Patients' estimates of the quantity of a drug ingested are notoriously unreliable. Therefore, if an acetaminophen overdose is suspected, a serum acetaminophen assay should be obtained as early as possible, but no sooner than four hours following ingestion. Liver function studies should be obtained initially and repeated at 24-hour intervals.
The antidote, N-acetylcysteine, should be administered as early as possible, and within 16 hours of the overdose ingestion for optimal results. Following recovery, there are no residual, structural, or functional hepatic abnormalities.

Oxycodone

Signs and symptoms: Serious overdosage with oxycodone is characterized by respiratory depression (a decrease in respiratory rate and/or tidal volume, Cheyne-Stokes respiration, cyanosis), extreme somnolence progressing to stupor or coma, skeletal muscle flaccidity, cold and clammy skin, and sometimes bradycardia and hypotension. In severe overdosage, apnea, circulatory collapse, cardiac arrest, and death may occur.
Treatment: Primary attention should be given to the reestablishment of adequate respiratory exchange through provision of a patent airway and the institution of assisted or controlled ventilation. The narcotic antagonist naloxone hydrochloride is a specific antidote against respiratory depression which may result from overdosage or unusual sensitivity to narcotics, including oxycodone. Therefore, an appropriate dose of naloxone hydrochloride (usual initial adult dose 0.4 mg to 2 mg) should be admininstered preferably by the intravenous route and simultaneously with efforts at respiratory resuscitation (see package insert). Since the duration of action of oxycodone may exceed that of the antagonist, the patient should be kept under continued surveillance and repeated doses of the antagonist should be administered as needed to maintain adequate respiration.
An antagonist should not be administered in the absence of clinically significant respiratory or cardiovascular depression. Oxygen, intravenous fluids, vasopressors and other supportive measures should be employed as indicated.
Gastric emptying may be useful in removing unabsorbed drug.

DOSAGE AND ADMINISTRATION

Dosage should be adjusted according to the severity of the pain and the response of the patient. However, it should be kept in mind that tolerance to oxycodone can develop with continued use and that the incidence of untoward effects is dose related. This product is inappropriate even in high doses for severe or intractable pain.
TYLOX (oxycodone and acetaminophen capsules) are given orally. The usual adult dosage is one TYLOX capsule every 6 hours as needed for pain.

HOW SUPPLIED

TYLOX (oxycodone and acetaminophen capsules USP): (colored red, imprinted "TYLOX" "McNEIL") NDC 0045-0526—bottles of 100 and unit dose 100's.
Dispense in tight, light-resistant container as defined in the official compendium.
Store at controlled room temperature (15°–30° C, 59°–86° F). Protect from moisture.
McNeil Pharmaceutical, McNEILAB, Inc.
Spring House, PA 19477
Revised June 1997 643-10-561-3
Shown in Product Identification Guide, page 329

ULTRAM® ℞
(tramadol hydrochloride tablets)

Prescribing Information

DESCRIPTION

ULTRAM® (tramadol hydrochloride tablets) is a centrally acting analgesic. The chemical name for tramadol hydrochloride is (±)*cis*-2-[(dimethylamino)methyl]-1-(3-methoxyphenyl) cyclohexanol hydrochloride. Its structural formula is:

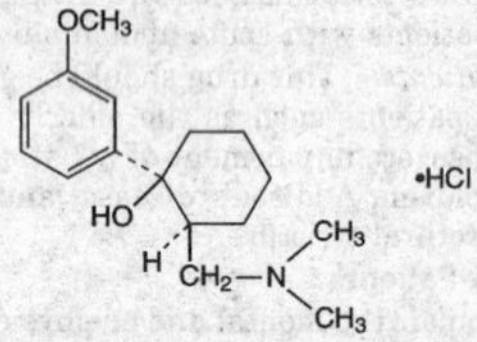

The molecular weight of tramadol hydrochloride is 299.8. Tramadol hydrochloride is a white, bitter, crystalline and odorless powder. It is readily soluble in water and ethanol and has a pKa of 9.41. The water/n-octanol partition coefficient is 1.35 at pH 7. ULTRAM tablets contain 50 mg of tramadol hydrochloride and are white in color. Inactive ingredients in the tablet are corn starch, hydroxypropyl methylcellulose, lactose, magnesium stearate, microcrystalline cellulose, polyethylene glycol, polysorbate 80, sodium starch glycolate, titanium dioxide and wax.

CLINICAL PHARMACOLOGY

Pharmacodynamics

ULTRAM is a centrally acting synthetic analgesic compound. Although its mode of action is not completely understood, from animal tests, at least two complementary mechanisms appear applicable: binding of parent and M1 metabolite to μ-opioid receptors and weak inhibition of reuptake of norepinephrine and serotonin. Opioid activity is due to both low affinity binding of the parent compound and higher affinity binding of the O-demethylated metabolite M1 to μ-opioid receptors. In animal models, M1 is up to 6 times more potent than tramadol in producing analgesia and 200 times more potent in μ-opioid binding. Tramadol-induced analgesia is only partially antagonized by the opiate antagonist naloxone in several animal tests. The relative contribution of both tramadol and M1 to human analgesia is dependent upon the plasma concentrations of each compound (see CLINICAL PHARMACOLOGY, Pharmacokinetics).
Tramadol has been shown to inhibit reuptake of norepinephrine and serotonin *in vitro*, as have some other opioid analgesics. These mechanisms may contribute independently to the overall analgesic profile of ULTRAM. Analgesia in humans begins approximately within one hour after administration and reaches a peak in approximately two to three hours.
Apart from analgesia, ULTRAM administration may produce a constellation of symptoms (including dizziness, somnolence, nausea, constipation, sweating and pruritus) simi-

lar to that of an opioid. However, tramadol causes less respiratory depression than morphine at recommended doses (see OVERDOSAGE). In contrast to morphine, tramadol has not been shown to cause histamine release. At therapeutic doses, ULTRAM has no effect on heart rate, left-ventricular function or cardiac index. Orthostatic hypotension has been observed.

Pharmacokinetics

The analgesic activity of ULTRAM is due to both parent drug and the M1 metabolite (see CLINICAL PHARMACOLOGY, Pharmacodynamics). Tramadol is administered as a racemate and both the [−] and [+] forms of both tramadol and M1 are detected in the circulation. Tramadol is well absorbed orally with an absolute bioavailability of 75%. Tramadol has a volume of distribution of approximately 2.7L/kg and is only 20% bound to plasma proteins. Tramadol is extensively metabolized by a number of pathways, including CYP2D6 and CYP3A4, as well as by conjugation of parent and metabolites. One metabolite, M1, is pharmacologically active in animal models. The formation of M1 is dependent upon Cytochrome P-450(2D6) and as such is subject to both metabolic induction and inhibition which may affect the therapeutic response (see PRECAUTIONS- Drug Interactions). Tramadol and its metabolites are excreted primarily in the urine with observed plasma half-lives of 6.3 and 7.4 hours for tramadol and M1, respectively. Linear pharmacokinetics have been observed following multiple doses of 50 and 100 mg to steady-state.

Absorption:

Racemic tramadol is rapidly and almost completely absorbed after oral administration. The mean absolute bioavailability of a 100 mg oral dose is approximately 75%. The mean peak plasma concentration of racemic tramadol and M1 occurs at two and three hours, respectively, after administration in healthy adults. In general, both enantiomers of tramadol and M1 follow a parallel time course in the body following single and multiple doses although small differences (~10%) exist in the absolute amount of each enantiomer present.

Steady-state plasma concentrations of both tramadol and M1 are achieved within two days with q.i.d. dosing. There is no evidence of self-induction (see Figure 1 and Table 1 below).

Figure 1: Mean Tramadol and M1 Plasma Concentration Profiles after a Single 100 mg Oral Dose and after Twenty-Nine 100 mg Oral Doses of Tramadol HCl given q.i.d.

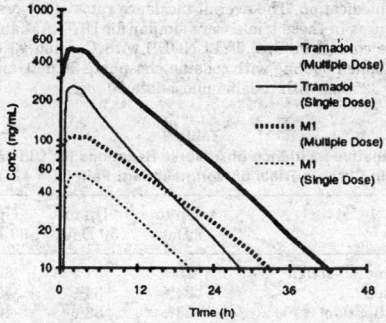

[See table 1 above]

Food Effects: Oral administration of ULTRAM with food does not significantly affect its rate or extent of absorption, therefore, ULTRAM can be administered without regard to food.

Distribution:

The volume of distribution of tramadol was 2.6 and 2.9 liters/kg in male and female subjects, respectively, following a 100 mg intravenous dose. The binding of tramadol to human plasma proteins is approximately 20% and binding also appears to be independent of concentration up to 10 µg/mL. Saturation of plasma protein binding occurs only at concentrations outside the clinically relevant range. Although not confirmed in humans, tramadol has been shown in rats to cross the blood-brain barrier.

Metabolism:

Tramadol is extensively metabolized after oral administration. Approximately 30% of the dose is excreted in the urine as unchanged drug, whereas 60% of the dose is excreted as metabolites. The remainder is excreted either as unidentified or as unextractable metabolites. The major metabolic pathways appear to be N- and O-demethylation and glucuronidation or sulfation in the liver. One metabolite (O-desmethyltramadol, denoted M1) is pharmacologically active in animal models. Production of M1 is dependent on the CYP2D6 isoenzyme of cytochrome P-450 and as such is subject to both metabolic induction and inhibition which may affect the therapeutic response (see PRECAUTIONS— Drug Interaction).

Table 1
Mean (%CV) Pharmacokinetic Parameters for Racemic Tramadol and M1 Metabolite

Population/ Dosage Regimen[a]	Parent Drug/ Metabolite	Peak Conc. (ng/mL)	Time to Peak (hrs)	Clearance/F[b] (mL/min/Kg)	$t_{1/2}$ (hrs)
Healthy Adults, 100 mg qid, MD p.o.	Tramadol	592 (30)	2.3 (61)	5.90 (25)	6.7 (15)
	M1	110 (29)	2.4 (46)	c	7.0 (14)
Healthy Adults, 100 mg SD p.o.	Tramadol	308 (25)	1.6 (63)	8.50 (31)	5.6 (20)
	M1	55.0 (36)	3.0 (51)	c	6.7 (16)
Geriatric, (>75 yrs) 50 mg SD p.o.	Tramadol	208 (31)	2.1 (19)	6.89 (25)	7.0 (23)
	M1	d	d	c	d
Hepatic Impaired, 50 mg SD p.o.	Tramadol	217 (11)	1.9 (16)	4.23 (56)	13.3 (11)
	M1	19.4 (12)	9.8 (20)	c	18.5 (15)
Renal Impaired, CL_{cr} 10-30 mL/min 100 mg SD i.v.	Tramadol	c	c	4.23 (54)	10.6 (31)
	M1	c	c	c	11.5 (40)
Renal Impaired, CL_{cr}<5 mL/min 100 mg SD i.v.	Tramadol	c	c	3.73 (17)	11.0 (29)
	M1	c	c	c	16.9 (18)

a SD = Single dose, MD = Multiple dose, p.o. = Oral administration, i.v. = Intravenous administration, qid = Four times daily
b F represents the oral bioavailability of tramadol
c Not applicable
d Not measured

Approximately 7% of the population has reduced activity of the CYP2D6 isoenzyme of cytochrome P-450. These individuals are "poor metabolizers" of debrisoquine, dextromethorphan, tricyclic antidepressants, among other drugs. After a single oral dose of tramadol, concentrations of tramadol were only slightly higher in "poor metabolizers" versus "extensive metabolizers", while M1 concentrations were lower. Concomitant therapy with inhibitors of CYP2D6 such as fluoxetine, paroxetine, and quinidine could result in significant drug interactions. In vitro drug interaction studies in human liver microsomes indicate that inhibitors of CYP2D6 such as fluoxetine and its metabolite norfluoxetine, amitriptyline and quinidine inhibit the metabolism of tramadol to various degrees, suggesting that concomitant administration of these compounds could result in increases in tramadol concentrations and decreased concentrations of M1. The pharmacological impact of these alterations in terms of either efficacy or safety is unknown.

Elimination:

The mean terminal plasma elimination half-lives of racemic tramadol and racemic M1 are 6.3 ± 1.4 and 7.4 ± 1.4 hours, respectively. The plasma elimination half-life of racemic tramadol increased from approximately six hours to seven hours upon multiple dosing.

Special Populations

Renal:

Impaired renal function results in a decreased rate and extent of excretion of tramadol and its active metabolite, M1. In patients with creatinine clearances of less than 30 mL/min, adjustment of the dosing regimen is recommended (see DOSAGE AND ADMINISTRATION). The total amount of tramadol and M1 removed during a 4-hour dialysis period is less than 7% of the administered dose.

Hepatic:

Metabolism of tramadol and M1 is reduced in patients with advanced cirrhosis of the liver, resulting in both a larger area under the concentration time curve for tramadol and longer tramadol and M1 elimination half-lives (13 hrs. for tramadol and 19 hrs. for M1). In cirrhotic patients, adjustment of the dosing regimen is recommended (see DOSAGE AND ADMINISTRATION).

Age:

Healthy elderly subjects aged 65 to 75 years have plasma tramadol concentrations and elimination half-lives comparable to those observed in healthy subjects less than 65 years of age. In subjects over 75 years, maximum serum concentrations are slightly elevated (208 vs. 162 ng/mL) and the elimination half-life is slightly prolonged (7 vs. 6 hours) compared to subjects 65 to 75 years of age. Adjustment of the daily dose is recommended for patients older than 75 years (see DOSAGE AND ADMINISTRATION).

Gender:

The absolute bioavailability of tramadol was 73% in males and 79% in females. The plasma clearance was 6.4 mL/min/kg in males and 5.7 mL/min/kg in females following a 100 mg IV dose of tramadol. Following a single oral dose, and after adjusting for body weight, females had a 12% higher peak tramadol concentration and a 35% higher area under the concentration-time curve compared to males. The clinical significance of this difference is unknown.

Clinical Studies

ULTRAM has been given in single oral doses of 50, 75, 100, 150 and 200 mg to patients with pain following surgical procedures and pain following oral surgery (extraction of impacted molars).

In single-dose models of pain following oral surgery, pain relief was demonstrated in some patients at doses of 50 mg and 75 mg. A dose of 100 mg ULTRAM tended to provide analgesia superior to codeine sulfate 60 mg, but it was not as effective as the combination of aspirin 650 mg with codeine phosphate 60 mg. In single-dose models of pain following surgical procedures, 150 mg provided analgesia generally comparable to the combination of acetaminophen 650 mg with propoxyphene napsylate 100 mg, with a tendency toward later peak effect.

ULTRAM has been studied in three long-term controlled trials involving a total of 820 patients, with 530 patients receiving ULTRAM. Patients with a variety of chronic painful conditions were studied in double-blind trials of one to three months duration. Average daily doses of approximately 250 mg of ULTRAM in divided doses were generally comparable to five doses of acetaminophen 300 mg with codeine phosphate 30 mg (TYLENOL® with Codeine #3) daily, five doses of aspirin 325 mg with codeine phosphate 30 mg daily, or two to three doses of acetaminophen 500 mg with oxycodone hydrochloride 5 mg (TYLOX®) daily.

INDICATIONS AND USAGE

ULTRAM is indicated for the management of moderate to moderately severe pain.

CONTRAINDICATIONS

ULTRAM should not be administered to patients who have previously demonstrated hypersensitivity to tramadol, any other component of this product or opioids. It is also contraindicated in cases of acute intoxication with alcohol, hypnotics, centrally acting analgesics, opioids or psychotropic drugs.

WARNINGS

Seizure Risk

Seizures have been reported in patients receiving ULTRAM within the recommended dosage range. Spontaneous post-marketing reports indicate that seizure risk is increased with doses of ULTRAM above the recommended range. Concomitant use of ULTRAM increases the seizure risk in patients taking:

- **Selective serotonin reuptake inhibitors (SSRI antidepressants or anoretics),**
- **Tricyclic antidepressants (TCAs), and other tricyclic compounds (e.g., cyclobenzaprine, promethazine, etc.), or**
- **Opioids.**

Administration of ULTRAM may enhance the seizure risk in patients taking:

- **MAO inhibitors (see also WARNINGS— Use with MAO Inhibitors),**
- **Neuroleptics, or**
- **Other drugs that reduce the seizure threshold.**

Continued on next page

Ultram—Cont.

Risk of convulsions may also increase in patients with epilepsy, those with a history of seizures, or in patients with a recognized risk for seizure (such as head trauma, metabolic disorders, alcohol and drug withdrawal, CNS infections). In ULTRAM overdose, naloxone administration may increase the risk of seizure.

Anaphylactoid Reactions

Serious and rarely fatal anaphylactoid reactions have been reported in patients receiving therapy with ULTRAM. These reactions often occur following the first dose. Other reported reactions include pruritus, hives, bronchospasm, and angioedema. Patients with a history of anaphylactoid reactions to codeine and other opioids may be at increased risk and therefore should not receive ULTRAM (see CONTRAINDICATIONS).

Use in Opioid-dependent Patients

ULTRAM should not be used in opioid-dependent patients. ULTRAM has been shown to reinitiate physical dependence in some patients that have been previously dependent on other opioids. Consequently, in patients with a tendency to opioid abuse or opioid dependence, treatment with ULTRAM is not recommended.

Use with CNS Depressants

ULTRAM should be used with caution and in reduced dosages when administered to patients receiving CNS depressants such as alcohol, opioids, anesthetic agents, phenothiazines, tranquilizers or sedative hypnotics.

Use with MAO Inhibitors

Use ULTRAM with great caution in patients taking monoamine oxidase inhibitors, because animal studies have shown increased deaths with combined administration.

PRECAUTIONS

Respiratory Depression

Administer ULTRAM cautiously in patients at risk for respiratory depression. When large doses of ULTRAM are administered with anesthetic medications or alcohol, respiratory depression may result. Treat such cases as an overdose. If naloxone is to be administered, use cautiously because it may precipitate seizures (see WARNINGS, Seizure Risk and OVERDOSAGE).

Increased Intracranial Pressure or Head Trauma

ULTRAM should be used with caution in patients with increased intracranial pressure or head injury. Pupillary changes (miosis) from tramadol may obscure the existence, extent, or course of intracranial pathology. Clinicians should also maintain a high index of suspicion for adverse drug reaction when evaluating altered mental status in these patients if they are receiving ULTRAM.

Acute Abdominal Conditions

The administration of ULTRAM may complicate the clinical assessment of patients with acute abdominal conditions.

Withdrawal

Withdrawal symptoms may occur if ULTRAM is discontinued abruptly. These symptoms may include: anxiety, sweating, insomnia, rigors, pain, nausea, tremors, diarrhoea, upper respiratory symptoms, piloerection, and rarely hallucinations. Clinical experience suggests that withdrawal symptoms may be relieved by tapering the medication.

Patients Physically Dependent on Opioids

ULTRAM is not recommended for patients who are dependent on opioids. Patients who have recently taken substantial amounts of opioids may experience withdrawal symptoms. Because of the difficulty in assessing dependence in patients who have previously received substantial amounts of opioid medication, administer ULTRAM cautiously to such patients.

Use in Renal and Hepatic Disease

Impaired renal function results in a decreased rate and extent of excretion of tramadol and its active metabolite, M1. In patients with creatinine clearances of less than 30 mL/min, dosing reduction is recommended (see DOSAGE AND ADMINISTRATION).

Metabolism of tramadol and M1 is reduced in patients with advanced cirrhosis of the liver. In cirrhotic patients, dosing reduction is recommended (see DOSAGE AND ADMINISTRATION).

With the prolonged half-life in these conditions, achievement of steady-state is delayed, so that it may take several days for elevated plasma concentrations to develop.

Information for Patients

- ULTRAM may impair mental or physical abilities required for the performance of potentially hazardous tasks such as driving a car or operating machinery.
- ULTRAM should not be taken with alcohol containing beverages.
- ULTRAM should be used with caution when taking medications such as tranquilizers, hypnotics or other opiate containing analgesics.
- The patient should be instructed to inform the physician if they are pregnant, think they might become pregnant, or are trying to become pregnant (see PRECAUTIONS: Labor and Delivery).
- The patient should understand the single-dose and 24-hour dose limit and the time interval between doses, since exceeding these recommendations can result in respiratory depression and seizures.

Drug Interactions

Tramadol does not appear to induce its own metabolism in humans, since observed maximal plasma concentrations after multiple oral doses are higher than expected based on single-dose data. Tramadol is a mild inducer of selected drug metabolism pathways measured in animals.

Use with Carbamazepine

Concomitant administration of ULTRAM with **carbamazepine** causes a significant increase in tramadol metabolism, presumably through metabolic induction by carbamazepine. Patients receiving chronic carbamazepine doses of up to 800 mg daily may require up to twice the recommended dose of ULTRAM.

Use with Quinidine

Tramadol is metabolized to M1 by the CYP2D6 P-450 isoenzyme. **Quinidine** is a selective inhibitor of that isoenzyme; so that concomitant administration of quinidine and ULTRAM results in increased concentrations of tramadol and reduced concentrations of M1. The clinical consequences of these findings are unknown. In vitro drug interaction studies in human liver microsomes indicate that tramadol has no effect on quinidine metabolism.

Use with Inhibitors of CYP2D6

In vitro drug interaction studies in human liver microsomes indicate that concomitant administration with inhibitors of CYP2D6 such as fluoxetine, paroxetine, and amitriptyline could result in some inhibition of the metabolism of tramadol.

Use with Cimetidine

Concomitant administration of ULTRAM with **cimetidine** does not result in clinically significant changes in tramadol pharmacokinetics. Therefore, no alteration of the ULTRAM dosage regimen is recommended.

Use with MAO Inhibitors

Interactions with **MAO Inhibitors**, due to interference with detoxification mechanisms, have been reported for some centrally acting drugs (see WARNINGS, Use with MAO Inhibitors).

Use with Digoxin and Warfarin

Post-marketing surveillance has revealed rare reports of digoxin toxicity and alteration of warfarin effect, including elevation of prothrombin times.

Carcinogenesis, Mutagenesis, Impairment of Fertility

Tramadol was not mutagenic in the following assays: Ames *Salmonella* microsomal activation test, CHO/HPRT mammalian cell assay, mouse lymphoma assay (in the absence of metabolic activation), dominant lethal mutation tests in mice, chromosome aberration test in Chinese hamsters, and bone marrow micronucleus tests in mice and Chinese hamsters. Weakly mutagenic results occurred in the presence of metabolic activation in the mouse lymphoma assay and micronucleus test in rats. Overall, the weight of evidence from these tests indicates that tramadol does not pose a genotoxic risk to humans.

A slight, but statistically significant, increase in two common murine tumors, pulmonary and hepatic, was observed in a mouse carcinogenicity study, particularly in aged mice (dosing orally up to 30 mg/kg for approximately two years, although the study was not done with the Maximum Tolerated Dose). This finding is not believed to suggest risk in humans. No such finding occurred in a rat carcinogenicity study.

No effects on fertility were observed for tramadol at oral dose levels up to 50 mg/kg in male rats and 75 mg/kg in female rats.

Pregnancy, Teratogenic Effects: *Pregnancy Category C*

There are no adequate and well-controlled studies in pregnant women. ULTRAM should be used during pregnancy only if the potential benefit justifies the potential risk to the fetus.

Tramadol has been shown to be embryotoxic and fetotoxic in mice, rats and rabbits at maternally toxic doses 3 to 15 times the maximum human dose or higher (120 mg/kg in mice, 25 mg/kg or higher in rats and 75 mg/kg or higher in rabbits), but was not teratogenic at these dose levels. No harm to the fetus due to tramadol was seen at doses that were not maternally toxic.

No drug-related teratogenic effects were observed in progeny of mice, rats or rabbits treated with tramadol by various routes (up to 140 mg/kg for mice, 80 mg/kg for rats or 300 mg/kg for rabbits). Embryo and fetal toxicity consisted primarily of decreased fetal weights, skeletal ossification and increased supernumerary ribs at maternally toxic dose levels. Transient delays in developmental or behavioral parameters were also seen in pups from rat dams allowed to deliver. Embryo and fetal lethality were reported only in one rabbit study at 300 mg/kg, a dose that would cause extreme maternal toxicity in the rabbit.

In peri- and post-natal studies in rats, progeny of dams receiving oral (gavage) dose levels of 50 mg/kg or greater had decreased weights, and pup survival was decreased early in lactation at 80 mg/kg (6 to 10 times the maximum human dose). No toxicity was observed for progeny of dams receiving 8, 10, 20, 25 or 40 mg/kg. Maternal toxicity was observed at all dose levels, but effects on progeny were evident only at higher dose levels where maternal toxicity was more severe.

Labor and Delivery

ULTRAM should not be used in pregnant women prior to or during labor unless the potential benefits outweigh the risks. Safe use in pregnancy has not been established. Chronic use during pregnancy may lead to physical dependence and post-partum withdrawal symptoms in the newborn. Tramadol has been shown to cross the placenta. The mean ratio of serum tramadol in the umbilical veins compared to maternal veins was 0.83 for 40 women given tramadol during labor.

The effect of ULTRAM, if any, on the later growth, development, and functional maturation of the child is unknown.

Nursing Mothers

ULTRAM is not recommended for obstetrical preoperative medication or for post-delivery analgesia in nursing mothers because its safety in infants and newborns has not been studied. Following a single IV 100 mg dose of tramadol, the cumulative excretion in breast milk within 16 hours postdose was 100 µg of tramadol (0.1% of the maternal dose) and 27 µg of M1.

Pediatric Use

The pediatric use of ULTRAM is not recommended because safety and efficacy in patients under 16 years of age have not been established.

Use in the Elderly

In subjects over the age of 75 years, serum concentrations are slightly elevated and the elimination half-life is slightly prolonged. The aged also can be expected to vary more widely in their ability to tolerate adverse drug effects. Daily doses in excess of 300 mg are not recommended in patients over 75 (see DOSAGE AND ADMINISTRATION).

ADVERSE REACTIONS

ULTRAM was administered to 550 patients during the double-blind or open-label extension periods in U.S. studies of chronic nonmalignant pain. Of these patients, 375 were 65 years old or older. Table 2 reports the cumulative incidence rate of adverse reactions by 7, 30 and 90 days for the most frequent reactions (5% or more by 7 days). The most frequently reported events were in the central nervous system and gastrointestinal system. Although the reactions listed in the table are felt to be probably related to ULTRAM administration, the reported rates also include some events that may have been due to underlying disease or concomitant medication. The overall incidence rates of adverse experiences in these trials were similar for ULTRAM and the active control groups, TYLENOL® with Codeine #3 (acetaminophen 300 mg with codeine phosphate 30 mg), and aspirin 325 mg with codeine phosphate 30 mg.

Table 2
Cumulative Incidence of Adverse Reactions for ULTRAM in Chronic Trials of Nonmalignant Pain (N = 427)

	Up to 7 Days	Up to 30 Days	Up to 90 Days
Dizziness/Vertigo	26%	31%	33%
Nausea	24%	34%	40%
Constipation	24%	38%	46%
Headache	18%	26%	32%
Somnolence	16%	23%	25%
Vomiting	9%	13%	17%
Pruritus	8%	10%	11%
"CNS Stimulation"[1]	7%	11%	14%
Asthenia	6%	11%	12%
Sweating	6%	7%	9%
Dyspepsia	5%	9%	13%
Dry Mouth	5%	9%	10%
Diarrhea	5%	6%	10%

[1] "CNS Stimulation" is a composite of nervousness, anxiety, agitation, tremor, spasticity, euphoria, emotional lability and hallucinations.

Incidence 1% to less than 5%, possibly causally related: the following lists adverse reactions that occurred with an incidence of 1% to less than 5% in clinical trials, and for which the possibility of a causal relationship with ULTRAM exists.

Body as a Whole: Malaise.

Cardiovascular: Vasodilation.

Central Nervous System: Anxiety, Confusion, Coordination disturbance, Euphoria, Nervousness, Sleep disorder.

Gastrointestinal: Abdominal pain, Anorexia, Flatulence.

Musculoskeletal: Hypertonia.

Skin: Rash.

Special Senses: Visual disturbance.

Urogenital: Menopausal symptoms, Urinary frequency, Urinary retention.

Incidence less than 1%, possibly causally related: the following lists adverse reactions that occurred with an incidence of less than 1% in clinical trials and/or reported in post-marketing experience.

Body as a Whole: Accidental injury, Allergic reaction, Anaphylaxis, Suicidal tendency, Weight loss.

Cardiovascular: Orthostatic hypotension, Syncope, Tachycardia.

Central Nervous System: Abnormal gait, Amnesia, Cognitive dysfunction, Depression, Difficulty in concentration, Hallucinations, Paresthesia, Seizure (See WARNINGS), Tremor.

Respiratory: Dyspnea.

Skin: Stevens-Johnson syndrome/Toxic epidermal necrolysis, Urticaria, Vesicles.

Special Senses: Dysgeusia.

Urogenital: Dysuria, Menstrual disorder.

Other adverse experiences, causal relationship unknown: A variety of other adverse events were reported infrequently in patients taking ULTRAM during clinical trials and/or reported in post-marketing experience. A causal relationship between ULTRAM and these events has not been determined. However, the most significant events are listed below as alerting information to the physician.

Cardiovascular: Abnormal ECG, Hypertension, Hypotension, Myocardial ischemia, Palpitations.

Central Nervous System: Migraine, Speech disorders.

Gastrointestinal: Gastrointestinal bleeding, Hepatitis, Stomatitis.

Laboratory Abnormalities: Creatinine increase, Elevated liver enzymes, Hemoglobin decrease, Proteinuria.

Sensory: Cataracts, Deafness, Tinnitus.

Skin: Pruritis.

DRUG ABUSE AND DEPENDENCE

ULTRAM has a potential to cause psychic and physical dependence of the morphine-type (μ-opioid). The drug has been associated with craving, drug-seeking behavior and tolerance development. Cases of abuse and dependence on ULTRAM have been reported. ULTRAM should not be used in opioid-dependent patients. ULTRAM can reinitiate physical dependence in patients that have been previously dependent or chronically using other opioids. In patients with a tendency to drug abuse, a history of drug dependence, or are chronically using opioids, treatment with ULTRAM is not recommended.

DOSAGE AND ADMINISTRATION

For the treatment of painful conditions, ULTRAM 50 mg to 100 mg can be administered as needed for relief every four to six hours, **not to exceed 400 mg per day.** For moderate pain, ULTRAM 50 mg may be adequate as the initial dose, and for more severe pain, ULTRAM 100 mg is usually more effective as the initial dose.

Individualization of Dose

Available data do not suggest that a dosage adjustment is necessary in elderly patients 65 to 75 years of age unless they also have renal or hepatic impairment. For elderly patients **over 75 years old,** not more than 300 mg/day in divided doses as above is recommended. In all patients with **creatinine clearance less than 30 mL/min,** it is recommended that the dosing interval of ULTRAM be increased to 12 hours, with a maximum daily dose of 200 mg. Since only 7% of an administered dose is removed by hemodialysis, **dialysis patients** can receive their regular dose on the day of dialysis. The recommended dose for patients with **cirrhosis** is 50 mg every 12 hours. Patients receiving chronic **carbamazepine** doses up to 800 mg daily may require up to twice the recommended dose of ULTRAM.

OVERDOSAGE

Cases of overdose with tramadol have been reported. Estimates of ingested dose in foreign fatalities have been in the range of 3 to 5 g. A 3 g intentional overdose by a patient in the clinical studies produced emesis and no sequelae. The lowest dose reported to be associated with fatality was possibly between 500 and 1000 mg in a 40 kg woman, but details of the case are not completely known.

Serious potential consequences of overdosage are respiratory depression and seizure. In treating an overdose, primary attention should be given to maintaining adequate ventilation along with general supportive treatment. While naloxone will reverse some, but not all, symptoms caused by overdosage with ULTRAM the risk of seizures is also increased with naloxone administration. In animals convulsions following the administration of toxic doses of tramadol could be suppressed with barbiturates or benzodiazepines but were increased with naloxone. Naloxone administration did not change the lethality of an overdose in mice. Hemodialysis is not expected to be helpful in an overdose because it removes less than 7% of the administered dose in a 4-hour dialysis period.

HOW SUPPLIED

ULTRAM (tramadol hydrochloride tablets) Tablets - 50 mg (white, film-coated capsule-shaped tablet) engraved "McNeil" on one side and "659" on the other side.

100's - NDC 0045-0659-60 bottles of 100 tablets
500's - NDC 0045-0659-70 bottles of 500 tablets
packages of 100 unit doses in blister packs - NDC 0045-0659-10 (10 cards of 10 tablets each).

Dispense in a tight container. Store at controlled room temperature (up to 25°C, 77°F).

Rx only

ORTHO-McNEIL PHARMACEUTICAL, INC.
Raritan, New Jersey 08869
U.S. Patents 3,652,589 and 3,830,934

 Revised April 1998 635-10-225-3

Shown in Product Identification Guide, page 329

VASCOR® ℞
(bepridil hydrochloride)
Tablets
For Oral Administration

DESCRIPTION

VASCOR (bepridil hydrochloride) is a calcium channel blocker that has well characterzied anti-anginal properties and known but poorly characterized type 1 anti-arrhythmic and anti-hypertensive properties. It has inhibitory effects on both the slow calcium and fast sodium inward currents in myocardial and vascular smooth muscle, interferes with calcium binding to calmodulin, and blocks both voltage and receptor operated calcium channels. It is not related chemically to other calcium channel blockers such as diltiazem hydrochloride, nifedipine and verapamil hydrochloride.

Bepridil hydrochloride monohydrate is a white to off-white, crystalline powder with a bitter taste. It is slightly soluble in water, very soluble in ethanol, methanol and chloroform, and freely soluble in acetone. The molecular weight of bepridil hydrochloride monohydrate is 421.02. Its molecular formula is $C_{24}H_{34}N_2O{\cdot}HCl{\cdot}H_2O$. The structural formula is:

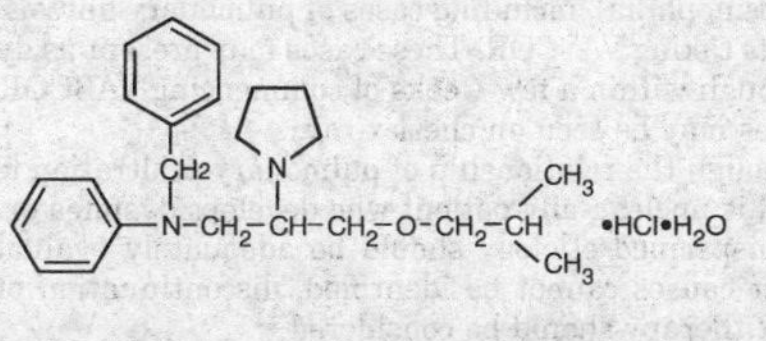

(±)-β-[(2-Methylpropoxy)methyl]-*N*-(phenylmethyl)-1-pyrrolidineethanamine monohydrochloride monohydrate

VASCOR is available as film-coated tablets for oral use containing 200, 300, or 400 mg of bepridil hydrochloride monohydrate. Inactive ingredients: hydroxypropyl methylcellulose, lactose, magnesium stearate, microcrystalline cellulose, polyethylene glycol, silicon dioxide, pregelatinized corn starch, corn starch, titanium dioxide, FD&C Blue #1.

CLINICAL PHARMACOLOGY

VASCOR (bepridil hydrochloride) inhibits the transmembrane influx of calcium ions into cardiac and vascular smooth muscle. This has been demonstrated in isolated myocardial and vascular smooth muscle preparations in which both the slope of the calcium dose response curve and the maximum calcium-induced inotropic response were significantly reduced by bepridil hydrochloride. In cardiac myocytes *in vitro,* bepridil hydrochloride was shown to be tightly bound to actin. A negative inotropic effect can be seen in the isolated guinea pig atria.

In *in vitro* studies, bepridil hydrochloride has also been demonstrated to inhibit the sodium inward current. Reductions in the maximal upstroke velocity and the amplitude of the action potential, as well as increases in the duration of the normal action potential, have been observed. Additionally, bepridil hydrochloride has been shown to possess local anesthetic activity in isolated myocardial preparations. It effects electrophysiological changes that are observed with several classes of anti-arrhythmic agents.

Clinical Studies

In controlled clinical studies with 200–400 mg of VASCOR, given as a once daily dose, exercise tolerance was improved and angina frequency and daily nitroglycerin use was reduced compared to placebo. Improvement in exercise performance was dose related. In one controlled clinical study, VASCOR was added to propranolol in daily doses of up to 240 mg. The 200–400 mg dose of VASCOR was well tolerated [patients entered were not allowed to be in NYHA Class III or IV heart failure] and there was an added effect of VASCOR on exercise tolerance.

In another controlled clinical study, VASCOR in doses of up to 400 mg/day, significantly improved exercise tolerance compared to diltiazem hydrochloride in patients refractory to diltiazem hydrochloride therapy.

Mechanism of Action: The precise mechanism of action for VASCOR as an anti-anginal agent remains to be fully determined, but is believed to include the following mechanisms: VASCOR regularly reduces heart rate and arterial pressure at rest and at a given level of exercise by dilating peripheral arterioles and reducing total peripheral resistance (afterload) against which the heart works. In exercise tolerance tests in patients with stable angina the heart rate/blood pressure product was reduced with VASCOR for a given work load.

Hemodynamic Effects: VASCOR produces dose dependent slowing of the heart, and reflex tachycardia is not seen. The mean decrease in heart rate in US clinical trials was 3 b.p.m. Orally administered VASCOR also produces modest decreases (less than 5 mm Hg) in systolic and diastolic blood pressure in normotensive patients and somewhat larger decreases in hypertensive patients.

Intravenous administration of VASCOR is associated with a modest reduction in left ventricular contractility (dP/dt), and increased filling pressure, but radionuclide cineangiography studies in angina patients demonstrated improvement in ejection fraction at rest and during exercise following oral VASCOR therapy. Patients with impaired cardiac function [overt heart failure] were not included in these studies.

Electrophysiological Effects: Intravenous administration of VASCOR in man prolongs the effective refractory periods of the atria and ventricles, and the functional refractory period of the AV node. There was a tendency for the AV node effective refractory period and A-H interval to be increased as well. Intravenous and oral administration of VASCOR slow heart rate, prolong the QT and QTc intervals, and alter the morphology of the T-wave (indentation). In clinical trials with angina patients, the mean percent prolongation of the QTc interval was approximately 8%, and of QT about 10%. The prolongation of QT is dose related, varying from about 0.030 sec at doses of 200 mg once a day to 0.055 sec at 400 mg once a day. Upon cessation of therapy, the ECG gradually normalizes. No instances of greater than first-degree heart block have been observed in US controlled or open clinical studies with VASCOR, and first-degree heart block occurred in 0.2% of patients in these studies.

Pulmonary Function: In healthy subjects and asthmatic patients, intravenous VASCOR did not cause bronchoconstriction. VASCOR has been safely used in asthmatic patients and in patients with chronic obstructive lung disease.

Pharmacokinetics and Metabolism: In studies with healthy volunteers, VASCOR is rapidly and completely absorbed after oral administration. The time to peak bepridil plasma concentration is about 2 to 3 hours. Over a ten day period, approximately 70% of a single dose of VASCOR is excreted in the urine and 22% in the feces, as metabolites of bepridil. Excretion of unmetabolized drug is negligible. In healthy male volunteers, the relationship between dose and steady-state blood levels of bepridil was linear over the range of 200 to 400 mg/day. Elimination of bepridil is biphasic, with a distribution half-life of about 2 hours. The terminal elimination half-life following the cessation of multiple dosing averaged 42 hours (range 26–64 hours). However, during a given dosing interval, decay from the peak concentration occurs relatively rapidly indicating a dosing interval half-life shorter than 24 hours. Following once-daily dosing with therapeutic doses, steady-state was reached in about 8 days in healthy volunteers. The clearance of bepridil decreases after multiple dosing.

Clearance of bepridil in angina patients was lower than that in healthy volunteers, resulting in higher average plasma bepridil concentrations. At steady state, maximum bepridil concentrations averaged 2332 ng/ml (range 1451 to 3609) and mean minimum concentrations were 1174 ng/ml (range 226 to 2639) in angina patients following 300 mg/day doses of VASCOR.

Bepridil is more than 99% bound to plasma proteins. Administration of VASCOR after a meal resulted in a clinically insignificant delay in time to peak concentration, but neither peak bepridil plasma levels nor the extent of absorption was changed.

Bepridil passes through the placental barrier. Bepridil may cause uterine hypotonia.

INDICATIONS AND USAGE

Chronic Stable Angina (Classic Effort-Associated Angina)

VASCOR (bepridil hydrochloride) is indicated for the treatment of chronic stable angina (classic effort-associated angina). Because VASCOR has caused serious ventricular arrhythmias, including torsades de pointes type ventricular tachycardia, and the occurrence of cases of agranulocytosis associated with its use (see **WARNINGS**), it should be reserved for patients who have failed to respond optimally to, or are intolerant of, other anti-anginal medication.

VASCOR may be used alone or in combination with beta blockers and/or nitrates. Controlled clinical studies have shown an added effect when VASCOR is administered to patients already receiving propranolol.

CONTRAINDICATIONS

VASCOR (bepridil hydrochloride) is contraindicated in patients with a known sensitivity to bepridil hydrochloride.

VASCOR is contraindicated in (1) patients with a history of serious ventricular arrhythmias (see **WARNINGS**—Induc-

Continued on next page

Vascor—Cont.

tion of New Serious Arrhythmias), (2) patients with sick sinus syndrome or patients with second- or third-degree AV block, except in the presence of a functioning ventricular pacemaker, (3) patients with hypotension (less than 90 mm Hg systolic), (4) patients with uncompensated cardiac insufficiency, (5) patients with congenital QT interval prolongation (see **WARNINGS**), and (6) patients taking other drugs that prolong QT interval (see **PRECAUTIONS**-Drug Interactions).

WARNINGS

Induction of New Serious Arrhythmias

VASCOR (bepridil hydrochloride) has Class 1 anti-arrhythmic properties and, like other such drugs, can induce new arrhythmias, including VT/VF. In addition, because of its ability to prolong the QT interval, VASCOR can cause torsades de pointes type ventricular tachycardia. Because of these properties VASCOR should be reserved for patients in whom other anti-anginal agents do not offer a satisfactory effect.

In US clinical trials, the QT and QTc intervals were commonly prolonged by VASCOR in a dose-related fashion. While the mean prolongation of QTc was 8% and of QT was 10%. Increases of 25% or more were not uncommon, occurring in 5% of the studied population for QTc and 8.7% of the studied population for QT. Increased QT and QTc may be associated with torsades de pointes type VT, which was seen at least briefly, in about 1.0% of patients in US trials; in many cases, however, patients with marked prolongation of QTc were taken off VASCOR therapy. All of the US patients with torsades de pointes had a prolonged QT interval and relatively low serum potassium. French marketing experience has reported over one hundred verified cases of torsades de pointes. While this number, based on total use, represents a rate of only 0.01%, the true rate is undoubtedly much higher, as spontaneous reporting systems all suffer from substantial under reporting.

Torsades de pointes is a polymorphic ventricular tachycardia often but not always associated with a prolonged QT interval, and often drug induced. The relation between the degree of QT prolongation and the development of torsades de pointes is not linear and the likelihood of torsades appears to be increased by hypokalemia, use of potassium wasting diuretics, and the presence of antecedent bradycardia. While the safe upper limit of QT is not defined, it is suggested that the interval not be permitted to exceed 0.52 seconds during treatment. If dose reduction does not eliminate the excessive prolongation, VASCOR should be stopped.

Because most domestic and foreign cases of torsades have developed in patients with hypokalemia, usually related to diuretic use or significant liver disease, if concomitant diuretics are needed, low doses and addition or primary use of a potassium sparing diuretic should be considered and serum potassium should be monitored.

VASCOR has been associated with the usual range of pro-arrhythmic effects characteristic of Class 1 anti-arrhythmics (increased premature ventricular contraction rates, new sustained VT, and VT/VF that is more resistant to sinus rhythm conversion). Use in patients with severe arrhythmias (who are most susceptible to certain pro-arrhythmic effects) has been limited, so that risk in these patients is not defined.

In the National Heart, Lung and Blood Institute's Cardiac Arrhythmia Suppression Trial (CAST), a long-term, multi-centered, randomized, double-blind study in patients with asymptomatic non-life-threatening ventricular arrhythmias who had myocardial infarctions more than six days but less than two years previously, an excess mortality/non-fatal cardiac arrest rate was seen in patients treated with encainide or flecainide (56/730) compared with that seen in patients assigned to matched placebo-treated groups (22/725). The applicability of these results to other populations (e.g., those without recent myocardial infarction) or to other anti-arrhythmic drugs is uncertain, but at present it is prudent to consider any drug documented to provoke new serious arrhythmias or worsening of pre-existing arrhythmias as having a similar risk and to avoid their use in the post-infarction period.

Agranulocytosis: In US clinical trials of over 800 patients treated with VASCOR for up to five years, two cases of marked leukopenia and neutropenia were reported. Both patients were diabetic and elderly. One died with overwhelming gram-negative sepsis, itself a possible cause of marked leukopenia. The other patient recovered rapidly when VASCOR was stopped.

Congestive Heart Failure: Congestive heart failure has been observed infrequently (about 1%) during US controlled clinical trials, but experience with the use of VASCOR in patients with significantly impaired ventricular function is limited. There is little information on the effect of concomitant administration of VASCOR and digoxin; therefore, caution should be exercised in treating patients with congestive heart failure.

Hepatic Enzyme Elevation: In US clinical studies with VASCOR in about 1000 patients and subjects, clinically significant (at least 2 times the upper limit of normal) transaminase elevations were observed in approximately 1% of the patients. None of these patients became clinically symptomatic or jaundiced and values returned to normal when the drug was stopped.

Hypokalemia: In clinical trials VASCOR has not been reported to reduce serum potassium levels. Because hypokalemia has been associated with ventricular arrhythmias, potassium insufficiency should be corrected before VASCOR therapy is initiated and normal potassium concentrations should be maintained during VASCOR therapy. Serum potassium should be monitored periodically.

PRECAUTIONS

General

Caution should be exercised when using VASCOR (bepridil hydrochloride) in patients with left bundle branch block or sinus bradycardia (less than 50 b.p.m.). Care should also be exercised in patients with serious hepatic or renal disorders because such patients have not been studied and bepridil is highly metabolized, with metabolites excreted primarily in the urine.

Recent Myocardial Infarction

In US clinical trials with VASCOR, patients with myocardial infarctions within three months prior to initiation of drug treatment were excluded. The initiation of VASCOR therapy in such patients, therefore, cannot be recommended.

Pulmonary Infiltration

There have been cases of noninfective, noncardiogenic pulmonary interstitial infiltrates (with or without the presence of eosinophilia), including cases of pulmonary fibrosis in patients taking VASCOR. These cases may present as dyspnea or cough within a few weeks of commencing VASCOR; infiltrates may be seen on chest x-ray.

Although the relationship of pulmonary infiltration to VASCOR is unclear, any patient who develops dyspnea or cough of unspecified etiology should be adequately evaluated. If other causes cannot be identified, discontinuation of VASCOR therapy should be considered.

Information for Patients

Since QT prolongation is not associated with defined symptomatology, patients should be instructed on the importance of maintaining any potassium supplementation or potassium sparing diuretic, and the need for routine electrocardiograms and periodic monitoring of serum potassium.

The following Patient Information is printed on the carton label of each unit of use bottle of 30 tablets:

> As with any medication that you take, you should notify your physician of any changes in your overall condition. Be sure to follow your physician's instructions regarding follow-up visits. Please notify any physician who treats you for a medical condition that you are taking VASCOR® (bepridil hydrochloride), as well as any other medications.

Drug Interactions

Nitrates: The concomitant use of VASCOR with long- and short-acting nitrates has been safely tolerated in patients with stable angina pectoris. Sublingual nitroglycerin may be taken if necessary for the control of acute angina attacks during VASCOR therapy.

Beta-blocking Agents: The concomitant use of VASCOR and beta-blocking agents has been well tolerated in patients with stable angina. Available data are not sufficient, however, to predict the effects of concomitant medication on patients with impaired ventricular function or cardiac conduction abnormalities (see **CLINICAL PHARMACOLOGY** and **DOSAGE AND ADMINISTRATION**).

Digoxin: In controlled studies in healthy volunteers, bepridil hydrochloride either had no effect (one study) or was associated with modest increases, about 30% (two studies) in steady-state serum digoxin concentrations. Limited clinical data in angina patients receiving concomitant bepridil hydrochloride and digoxin therapy indicate no discernible changes in serum digoxin levels. Available data are neither sufficient to rule out possible increases in serum digoxin with concomitant treatment in some patients, nor other possible interactions, particularly in patients with cardiac conduction abnormalities (Also see **WARNINGS**-Congestive Heart Failure).

Oral Hypoglycemics: VASCOR has been safely used in diabetic patients without significantly lowering their blood glucose levels or altering their need for insulin or oral hypoglycemic agents.

General Interactions: Certain drugs could increase the likelihood of potentially serious adverse effects with bepridil hydrochloride. In general, these are drugs that have one or more pharmacologic activities similar to bepridil hydrochloride, including anti-arrhythmic agents such as quinidine and procainamide, cardiac glycosides and tricyclic anti-depressants. Anti-arrhythmics and tricyclic anti-depressants could exaggerate the prolongation of the QT interval observed with bepridil hydrochloride. Cardiac glycosides could exaggerate the depression of AV nodal conduction observed with bepridil hydrochloride.

Carcinogenesis, Mutagenesis, Impairment of Fertility

No evidence of carcinogenicity was revealed in one lifetime study in mice at dosages up to 60 times (for a 60 kg subject) the maximum recommended dosage in man. Unilateral follicular adenomas of the thyroid were observed in a study in rats following lifetime administration of high doses of bepridil hydrochloride, i.e., ≥ 100 mg/kg/day (20 times the usual recommended dose in man). No mutagenic or other genotoxic potential of bepridil hydrochloride was found in the following standard laboratory tests: the Micronucleus Test for Chromosomal Effects, the Liver Microsome Activated Bacterial Assay for Mutagenicity, the Chinese Hamster Ovary Cell Assay for Mutagenicity, and the Sister Chromatid Exchange Assay. No intrinsic effect on fertility by bepridil hydrochloride was demonstrated in rats.

In monkeys, at 200 mg/kg/day, there was a decrease in testicular weight and spermatogenesis. There were no systematic studies in man related to this point. In rats, at doses up to 300 mg/kg/day, there was no observed alteration of mating behavior nor of reproductive performance.

Usage in Pregnancy

Pregnancy Category C. Reproductive studies (fertility and peri-postnatal) have been conducted in rats. Reduced litter

Adverse Experiences by Body System and Treatment in Greater Than 2% of Bepridil Patients in Controlled Trials

Adverse Reaction	Bepridil HCl (N = 529)	Nifedipine (N = 50)	Propranolol (N = 88)	Diltiazem (N = 41)	Placebo (N = 190)
Body as a Whole					
Asthenia	9.83	22.00	22.73	12.20	7.37
Headache	11.34	22.00	13.64	7.32	14.21
Flu Syndrome	2.08	8.00	2.27	—[α]	1.05
Cardiovascular/Respiratory					
Palpitations	2.27	6.00	2.27	0.00	1.58
Dyspnea	3.59	4.00	5.68	4.88	2.11
Respiratory Infection	2.84	4.00	3.41	4.88	3.68
Gastrointestinal					
Dyspepsia	6.81	4.00	5.68	4.88	1.58
G.I. Distress	4.35	10.00	6.82	—[α]	2.11
Nausea	12.29	14.00	11.36	2.44	3.68
Dry Mouth	3.40	0.00	0.00	2.44	2.63
Anorexia	3.02	0.00	2.27	0.00	1.58
Diarrhea	7.75	2.00	9.09	2.44	2.63
Abdominal Pain	3.02	4.00	1.14	—[α]	3.16
Constipation	2.84	6.00	1.14	4.88	2.11
Central Nervous System					
Drowsy	3.78	4.00	4.55	—[α]	3.68
Insomnia	2.65	6.00	3.41	—[α]	1.05
Dizziness	14.74	30.00	10.23	4.88	9.47
Tremor	4.91	4.00	0.00	—[α]	1.05
Tremor of Hand	3.02	4.00	0.00	—[α]	0.53
Paresthesia	2.46	2.00	1.14	4.88	3.16
Psychiatric					
Nervous	7.37	16.00	1.14	2.44	3.68

[α] No data available.

Adverse Experiences by Body System and Treatment In Greater Than 5% of Bepridil Patients in Controlled Trials

Adverse Reaction	Bepridil HCl 200 mg (N = 43)	Bepridil HCl 300 mg (N = 46)	Bepridil HCl 400 mg (N = 44)	Placebo (N = 44)
Body as a Whole				
Asthenia	13.95	6.52	11.36	2.27
Headache	6.98	8.70	13.64	15.91
Cardiovascular/ Respiratory				
Palpitations	0.00	6.52	4.55	0.00
Dyspnea	2.33	8.70	0.00	2.27
Gastrointestinal				
G.I. Distress	6.98	0.00	4.55	4.55
Nausea	6.98	26.09	18.18	2.27
Anorexia	0.00	2.17	6.82	2.27
Diarrhea	0.00	10.87	6.82	0.00
Central Nervous System				
Drowsy	6.98	6.52	0.00	4.55
Dizziness	11.63	15.22	27.27	6.82
Tremor	6.98	0.00	4.55	0.00
Tremor of Hand	9.30	0.00	4.55	0.00
Psychiatric				
Nervous	11.63	8.70	11.36	0.00
Special Senses				
Tinnitus	0.00	6.52	2.27	2.27

Most Common Events Resulting in Discontinuation

Adverse Reaction	Bepridil (N = 515) n (%)	Placebo (N = 288) n (%)	Positive Control (N = 119) n (%)
Dizziness	5 (0.97)	0 (0.0)	2 (1.68)
Gastrointestinal Symptoms	5 (0.97)	0 (0.0)	5 (4.20)
Ventricular Arrhythmia	5 (0.97)	0 (0.0)	0 (0.0)
Syncope	3 (0.58)	0 (0.0)	0 (0.0)

size at birth and decreased pup survival during lactation was observed at maternal dosages 37 times (on a mg/kg basis) the maximum daily recommended therapeutic dosage. In teratology studies, no effects were observed in rats or rabbits at these same dosages.

There are no well-controlled studies in pregnant women. Use VASCOR in pregnant or nursing women only if the potential benefit justifies the potential risk.

Nursing Mothers

Bepridil is excreted in human milk. Bepridil concentration in human milk is estimated to reach about one third the concentration in serum. Because of the potential for serious adverse reactions in nursing infants from VASCOR a decision should be made whether to discontinue nursing or to discontinue the drug, taking into account the importance of the drug to the mother.

Pediatric Use

The safety and effectiveness of VASCOR in children have not been established.

ADVERSE REACTIONS

Adverse reactions were assessed in placebo and active-drug controlled trials of 4–12 weeks duration and longer-term uncontrolled studies. The most common side effects occurring more frequently than in control groups were upper gastrointestinal complaints (nausea, dyspepsia or GI distress) in about 22%, diarrhea in about 8%, dizziness in about 15%, asthenia in about 10% and nervousness in about 7%. The adverse reactions seen in at least 2% of bepridil patients in controlled trials are shown in the following table.

[See table at bottom of previous page]

In one twelve week controlled study, daily doses of 200, 300, and 400 mg were compared to placebo. The following table shows the rates of more common reactions (at least 5% in at least one bepridil group).

[See first table above]

Adverse experiences in long-term open studies were generally similar to those seen in controlled trials.

Although adverse experiences were frequent (at least one being reported in 71% of patients participating in controlled clinical trials), most were well-tolerated. About 15% of patients however, discontinued bepridil treatment because of adverse experiences. In controlled clinical trials, these were principally gastrointestinal (1.0%), dizziness (1.0%) ventricular arrhythmias (1.0%) and syncope (0.6%). The major reasons for discontinuation, with comparison to control agents, are shown below.

[See second table above]

Across all controlled and uncontrolled trials, VASCOR was evaluated in over 800 patients with chronic angina. In addition to the adverse reactions noted above, the following were observed in 0.5 to 2.0% of the VASCOR patients or are rarer, but potentially important events seen in clinical stud-

ies or reported in post marketing experience. In most cases it is not possible to determine whether there is a causal relationship to bepridil treatment.

Body as a Whole: Fever, pain, myalgic asthenia, superinfection, flu syndrome.

Cardiovascular/Respiratory: Sinus tachycardia, sinus bradycardia, hypertension, vasodilation, edema, ventricular premature contractions, ventricular tachycardia, prolonged QT interval, rhinitis, cough, pharyngitis.

Gastrointestinal: Flatulence, gastritis, appetite increase, dry mouth, constipation.

Musculoskeletal: Arthritis.

Central Nervous System: Fainting, vertigo, akathisia, drowsiness, insomnia, tremor.

Psychiatric: Depression, anxiousness, adverse behavior effect.

Skin: Rash, sweating, skin irritation.

Special Senses: Blurred vision, tinnitus, taste change.

Urogenital: Loss of libido, impotence.

Abnormal Lab Values: Abnormal liver function test, SGPT increase.

In postmarketing experience with other calcium blockers, gynecomastia has been rarely observed.

Certain cardiovascular events, such as acute myocardial infarction (about 3% of patients) worsened heart failure (1.9%), worsened angina (4.5%), severe arrhythmia (about 2.4% VT/VF) and sudden death (1.6%) have occurred in patients receiving bepridil, but have not been included as adverse events because they appear to be, and cannot be distinguished from, manifestations of the patient's underlying cardiac disease. Such events as torsades de pointes arrhythmias, prolonged QT/QTc, bradycardia, first degree heart block, which are probably related to bepridil, are included in the tables.

OVERDOSAGE

In the event of overdosage, we recommend close observation in a cardiac care facility for a minimum of 48 hours and use of appropriate supportive measures in addition to gastric lavage. Beta-adrenergic stimulation or parenteral administration of calcium solutions may increase transmembrane calcium ion influx. Clinically significant hypotensive reactions or high-degree AV block should be treated with vasopressor agents or cardiac pacing. Ventricular tachycardia should be handled by cardioversion and, if persistent, by overdrive pacing.

In a few reported cases, overdose with calcium channel blockers has been associated with hypotension and bradycardia, initially refractory to atropin but becoming more responsive to this treatment when the patients received large doses (close to 1 gram/hour for more than 24 hours) of calcium chloride.

There has been one experience with overdosage in which a patient inadvertently took a single dose of 1600 mg of VAS-

COR (bepridil hydrochloride). The patient was observed for 72 hours in intensive care, but no significant adverse experiences were noted.

DOSAGE AND ADMINISTRATION

Therapy with VASCOR (bepridil hydrochloride) should be individualized according to each patient's response and the physician's clinical judgement. The usual starting dose of VASCOR is 200 mg once daily. After 10 days, dosage may be adjusted upward depending upon the patient's response (e.g., ability to perform activities of daily living, QT interval, heart rate, and frequency and severity of angina). This long interval for dosage adjustment is needed because steady-state blood levels are not achieved until 8 days of therapy. In clinical trials, most patients were maintained at a dose of VASCOR of 300 mg once daily. The maximum daily dose of VASCOR is 400 mg and the established minimum effective dose is 200 mg daily.

The starting dose for elderly patients does not differ from that for young patients. After therapeutic response is demonstrated, however, elderly patients may require more frequent monitoring.

Food does not interfere with the absorption of VASCOR. (see **CLINICAL PHARMACOLOGY**—Pharmacokinetics and Metabolism). If nausea is experienced with VASCOR, the drug may be given at meals or at bedtime.

VASCOR has not been studied adequately in patients with impaired hepatic or renal function. It is therefore possible that dosage adjustments may be necessary in these patients.

Concomitant Use with Other Agents

The concomitant use of VASCOR and beta-blocking agents in patients without heart failure is safely tolerated. Physicians wishing to switch patients from beta-blocker therapy to VASCOR therapy may initiate VASCOR before terminating the beta blocker in the usual gradual fashion (see **CLINICAL PHARMACOLOGY** and **PRECAUTIONS**).

HOW SUPPLIED

VASCOR® (bepridil hydrochloride) tablets 200 mg (film coated light blue, scored, printed VASCOR and 200), 90 tablets (3 bottles of 30) (NDC 0045-0682-33) and unit dose of 100s (NDC 0045-0682-10) for hospital use.

VASCOR® (bepridil hydrochloride) tablets 300 mg (film coated blue, printed VASCOR and 300), 90 tablets (3 bottles of 30) (NDC 0045-0683-33).

Store at 15°–25° C (59°–77° F). Protect from light.

633–10–692–3

McNEIL PHARMACEUTICAL
MCNEILAB, INC.
SPRING HOUSE, PA 19477-0776

Shown in Product Identification Guide, page 329

EDUCATIONAL MATERIAL

FLOXIN® (ofloxacin tablets/injection)
"AUA Video Library"
"Simple Answers About UTI's" (English and Spanish)
Both are available free to physicians and pharmacists through representatives or directly from Ortho-McNeil Pharmaceutical (908) 218–6000.

PANCREASE® (pancrelipase) and **PANCREASE® MT**
"Tree of Life" film and brochure—film available in $1/2$" videotape.
"The Adventures of Mr. Enzyme" Nutritional Video
Target 100%—Growth and Nutrition brochure—for CF patients and families.
Guide to CF for Patients and Families video and workbook. (English and Spanish)
"Living with CF-Family Guide to Nutrition"
"This is Paul"-book for children with CF
Available free to physicians and pharmacists through representatives or directly from Ortho-McNeil Pharmaceutical (908) 218-6000.

PARAFON FORTE® DSC (chlorzoxazone)
"Exercises for Low Back Pain" (English and Spanish)
"Exercises for Cervical Sprain" (English and Spanish)
Both are available free to physicians and pharmacists through McNeil representatives or directly from Ortho-McNeil Pharmaceutical (908) 218-6000.

ULTRAM® (tramadol hydrochloride tablets)
"Exercises for Low Back Pain" (English and Spanish)
"Exercises for the Painful Neck and Shoulder (English and Spanish)
Both are available free to physicians and pharmacists through representatives or directly from Ortho-McNeil Pharmaceutical (908) 218–6000.

VASCOR® (bepridil hydrochloride) "Patients' Guide" brochure

Continued on next page

Educational Info.—Cont.

Available free to physicians and pharmacists through representatives or directly from Ortho-McNeil Pharmaceutical (908) 218-6000.

Paddock Laboratories, Inc.

3940 QUEBEC AVENUE NORTH
MINNEAPOLIS, MN 55427

Direct Inquiries to:
(800) 328-5113

For Medical Information Contact:
Medical Department
(800) 328-5113

ACTIDOSE with SORBITOL™ OTC

[act 'ĭ –dose]
(Activated Charcoal with Sorbitol Suspension)

DESCRIPTION

Actidose with Sorbitol is supplied in bottles and tubes. Each 120 mL package contains 25 grams of activated charcoal in suspension and 48 grams of sorbitol. Each 240 mL package contains 50 grams of activated charcoal in suspension and 96 grams of sorbitol. Each milliliter contains 208 mg (0.208 gram) activated in charcoal and 400 mg (0.4 gram) sorbitol.

HOW SUPPLIED

25 g unit-of-use bottle NDC 0574-0120-04
50 g unit-of-use bottle NDC 0574-0120-08
25 g unit-of-use tube NDC 0574-0120-74
50 g unit-of-use tube NDC 0574-0120-76

ACTIDOSE–AQUA™ OTC

[act 'ĭ 'dose a–qua]
(Activated Charcoal Suspension)

DESCRIPTION

Actidose-Aqua is supplied in bottles and tubes. Each 72 mL package contains 15 grams of activated charcoal in suspension, each 120 mL package contains 25 grams of activated charcoal in suspension and each 240 mL package contains 50 grams of activated charcoal in suspension. Each milliliter contains 208 mg (0.208 gram) activated charcoal.

HOW SUPPLIED

25 g unit-of-use bottle NDC 0574-0121-04
50 g unit-of-use bottle NDC 0574-0121-08
15 g unit-of-use tube NDC 0574-0121-25
25 g unit-of-use tube NDC 0574-0121-74
50 g unit-of-use tube NDC 0574-0121-76

DIABE-TUSS DM™ Syrup OTC

(Dextromethorphan Hydrobromide USP)

DESCRIPTION

Cherry flavored cough suppressant in an alcohol-free, sugar-free, dye-free base. Each teaspoonful (5 mL) contains Dextromethorphan Hydrobromide USP 15 mg.

INDICATIONS

Temporarily relieves cough due to minor throat and bronchial irritation associated with the common cold.

DOSAGE AND ADMINISTRATION

Do not exceed four doses in a 24-hour period.
Adults and children over 12 years: 2 teaspoonfuls every 6 hours.
Children 6 to 12 years: 1 teaspoonful every 6 hours.
Children 2 to 6 years: $^1/_2$ teaspoonful every 6 hours.
Children under 2: Consult a doctor.

HOW SUPPLIED

DIABE-TUSS DM is available in 118 mL (4 Fl Oz) bottles. NDC: 0574-0022-04

GLUTOSE 15™ GLUTOSE 45™ OTC

(Oral Glucose Gel)

DESCRIPTION

Glutose gel is a lemon-flavored, dye-free oral glucose gel for treatment of insulin reaction or hypoglycemia. Glutose gel contains Dextrose (d-glucose) USP 40%.

HOW SUPPLIED

Glutose 15: 3 x 15g unit-of-use tubes per package NDC 0574-0069-30
Glutose 45: 1 x 45g multi-use tube per package NDC 0574-0069-45

KIONEX™ ℞

[ky-onĕx]
Sodium Polystyrene Sulfonate, USP

Cation-Exchange Resin

DESCRIPTION

Kionex™ brand of sodium polystyrene sulfonate is a benzene, diethenyl-, polymer with ethenylbenzene, sulfonated, sodium salt.
The drug is a light brown to brown finely ground, powdered form of sodium polystyrene sulfonate, a cation-exchange resin prepared in the sodium phase with an *in vitro* exchange capacity of approximately 3.1 mEq (*in vivo* approximately 1 mEq) of potassium per gram. The sodium content is approximately 100 mg (4.1 mEq) per gram of the drug. It can be administered orally or in an enema.

CLINICAL PHARMACOLOGY

As the resin passes along the intestine or is retained in the colon after administration by enema, the sodium ions from the resin are partially released and are replaced by potassium ions. For the most part, this action occurs in the large intestine, which excretes potassium ions to a greater degree than does the small intestine. The efficiency of this process is limited and unpredictably variable. It commonly approximates the order of 33 percent but the range is so large that definitive indices of electrolyte balance must be clearly monitored. Metabolic data are unavailable.

INDICATIONS AND USAGE

Kionex is indicated for the treatment of hyperkalemia.

CONTRAINDICATIONS

Kionex is contraindicated in patients with hypokalemia or those patients who are hypersensitive to it.

WARNINGS

Alternative Therapy in Severe Hyperkalemia: Since effective lowering of serum potassium with this product may take hours to days, treatment with this drug alone may be insufficient to rapidly correct severe hyperkalemia associated with states of rapid tissue breakdown (e.g., burns and renal failure) or hyperkalemia so marked as to constitute a medical emergency. Therefore, other definitive measures, including dialysis, should always be considered and may be imperative.
Hypokalemia: Serious potassium deficiency can occur from therapy with Kionex. The effect must be carefully controlled by frequent serum potassium determinations within each 24 hour period. Since intracellular potassium deficiency is not always reflected by serum potassium levels, the level at which treatment with Kionex should be discontinued must be determined individually for each patient. Important aids in making this determination are the patient's clinical condition and electrocardiogram. Early clinical signs of severe hypokalemia include a pattern of irritable confusion and delayed thought processes. Electrocardiographically, severe hypokalemia is often associated with a lengthened Q-T interval, widening, flattening, or inversion of the T wave, and prominent U waves. Also, cardiac arrhythmias may occur, such as premature atrial, nodal, and ventricular contractions, and supraventricular and ventricular tachycardias. The toxic effects of digitalis are likely to be exaggerated. Marked hypokalemia can also be manifested by severe muscle weakness, at times extending into frank paralysis.
Electrolyte Disturbances: Like all cation-exchange resins, Kionex is not totally selective (for potassium) in its actions, and small amounts of other cations such as calcium and magnesium can also be lost during treatment. Accordingly patients receiving Kionex should be monitored for all applicable electrolyte disturbances.
Systemic Alkalosis: Systemic alkalosis has been reported after cation-exchange resins were administered orally in combination with nonabsorbable cation-donating antacids and laxatives such as magnesium hydroxide and aluminum carbonate. Magnesium hydroxide should not be administered with Kionex. One case of grand mal seizure has been reported in a patient with chronic hypocalcemia of renal failure who was given sodium polystyrene sulfonate with magnesium hydroxide as a laxative. (See PRECAUTIONS, Drug Interactions.)

PRECAUTIONS

Caution is advised when Kionex is administered to patients who cannot tolerate even a small increase in sodium loads (i.e., severe congestive heart failure, severe hypertension, or marked edema). In such instances, compensatory restriction of sodium intake from other sources may be indicated. If constipation occurs, patients should be treated with sorbitol (from 10 to 20 mL of 70 percent syrup every two hours or as needed to produce 1 or 2 watery stools daily), a measure which also reduces any tendency to fecal impaction.
Drug Interactions
Antacids: The simultaneous oral administration of Kionex with nonabsorbable cation-donating antacids and laxatives may reduce the resin's potassium exchange capability.
Systemic alkalosis has been reported after cation-exchange resins were administered orally in combination with nonabsorbable cation-donating antacids and laxatives such as magnesium hydroxide and aluminum carbonate. Magnesium hydroxide should not be administered with Kionex. One case of grand mal seizure has been reported in a patient with chronic hypocalcemia of renal failure who was given sodium polystyrene sulfonate with magnesium hydroxide as a laxative.
Intestinal obstruction due to concretions of aluminum hydroxide when used in combination with sodium polystyrene sulfonate has been reported.
Digitalis: The toxic effects of digitalis on the heart, especially various ventricular arrhythmias and A-V nodal dissociation, are likely to be exaggerated by hypokalemia, even in the face of serum digoxin concentrations in the "normal range". (See WARNINGS.)
Carcinogenesis, Mutagenesis, Impairment of Fertility
Studies have not been performed.
Pregnancy Category C
Animal reproduction studies have not been conducted with Kionex. It is also not known whether Kionex can cause fetal harm when administered to a pregnant woman or can affect reproduction capacity. Kionex should be given to a pregnant woman only if clearly needed.
Nursing Mothers
It is not known whether this drug is excreted in human milk. Because many drugs are excreted in human milk, caution should be exercised when Kionex is administered to a nursing woman.

ADVERSE REACTIONS

Kionex may cause some degree of gastric irritation. Anorexia, nausea, vomiting, and constipation may occur especially if high doses are given. Also, hypokalemia, hypocalcemia, and significant sodium retention may occur. Occasionally diarrhea develops. Large doses in elderly individuals may cause fecal impaction (see PRECAUTIONS). This effect may be obviated through usage of the resin in enemas as described under DOSAGE AND ADMINISTRATION. Rare instances of colonic necrosis have been reported. Intestinal obstruction due to concretions of aluminum hydroxide, when used in combination with sodium polystyrene sulfonate, has been reported.

DOSAGE AND ADMINISTRATION

Suspension of this drug should be freshly prepared and not stored beyond 24 hours.
The average daily adult dose of the resin is 15 g to 60 g. This is best provided by administering 15 grams (approximately 4 *level teaspoons*) of Kionex one to four times daily. One gram of Kionex contains 4.1 mEq of sodium; one level teaspoon contains approximately 3.5 grams of Kionex and 15 mEq of sodium. (A heaping teaspoon may contain as much as 10 to 12 grams of Kionex.) Since the *in vivo* efficiency of sodium-potassium exchange resins is approximately 33 percent, about one third of the resin's actual sodium content is being delivered to the body.
In smaller children and infants, lower doses should be employed by using as a guide a rate of 1 mEq of potassium per gram of resin as the basis for calculation.
Each dose should be given as a suspension in a small quantity of water or, for greater palatability, in syrup. The amount of fluid usually ranges from 20 to 100 mL, depending on the dose, or may be simply determined by allowing 3 to 4 mL per gram resin. Sorbitol may be administered in order to combat constipation.
The resin may be introduced into the stomach through a plastic tube and, if desired, mixed with a diet appropriate for a patient in renal failure.
The resin may also be given, although with less effective results, in an enema consisting (for adults) of 30 g to 50 g every six hours. Each dose is administered as a warm emulsion (at body temperature) in 100 mL of aqueous vehicle, such as sorbitol. The emulsion should be agitated gently during administration. The enema should be retained as long as possible and followed by a cleansing enema.
After an initial cleansing enema, a soft, large size (French 28) rubber tube is inserted into the rectum for a distance of about 20 cm, with the tip well into the sigmoid colon, and taped in place. The resin is then suspended in the appropriate amount of aqueous vehicle at body temperature and introduced by gravity, while the particles are kept in suspension by stirring. The suspension is flushed with 50 mL or 100 mL of fluid, following which the tube is clamped and left in place. If back leakage occurs, the hips are elevated on pillows or a knee-chest position is taken temporarily. A

somewhat thicker suspension may be used, but care should be taken that no paste is formed, because the latter has a greatly reduced exchange surface and will be particularly ineffective if deposited in the rectal ampulla. The suspension is kept in the sigmoid colon for several hours, if possible. Then the colon is irrigated with nonsodium containing solution at body temperature in order to remove the resin. Two quarts of flushing solution may be necessary. The returns are drained constantly through a Y tube connection. Particular attention should be paid to this cleansing enema when sorbitol has been used.

The intensity and duration of therapy depend upon the severity and resistance of hyperkalemia.

HOW SUPPLIED

Store at controlled room temperature 15–30°C (59–86°F). Kionex should not be heated for to do so may alter the exchange properties of the resin.

Dispense in a tight, light-resistant container as defined in the USP.

Rx only

Kionex™ (Sodium Polystyrene Sulfonate, USP) is available as a powder in containers of:

1 Pound (454 grams)   NDC 0574-2004-16

Packaged by:
**PADDOCK
LABORATORIES, INC.**
Minneapolis, Minnesota 55427
Revised April 1993   124142 (04.93)

NYSTATIN PADDOCK™

NYSTATIN, USP   ℞
**For Extemporaneous Preparation
of Oral Suspension**

DESCRIPTION

Nystatin USP is an antifungal antibiotic obtained from *Streptomyces noursei*. It is known to be a mixture, but the composition has not been completely elucidated. Nystatin A is closely related to amphotericin B. Each is a macrocyclic lactone containing a ketal ring, an all-*trans* polyene system, and a mycosamine (3-amino-3-deoxy-rhamnose) moiety. Nystatin A has a molecular formula of $C_{47}H_{75}NO_{17}$ and a molecular weight of 926.11.

Nystatin USP is a ready-to-use, non-sterile powder for oral administration which contains no excipients or preservatives. It is available in containers of 50 million, 150 million, 500 million, 2 billion, and 5 billion units. Each mg contains a minimum of 5,000 units.

HOW SUPPLIED

Product Code (NDC)	Size (units)	Approx. Weight (grams)
0574-0404-05	50 million	8.3 – 10
0574-0404-15	150 million	25 – 30
0574-0404-50	500 million	83 – 100
0574-0404-02	2 billion	333 – 400
0574-0404-00	5 billion	833 – 1,000

Storage: Store in a refrigerator. 2°–8°C (36°–46°F). Protect from light.

NYSTOP™   ℞
Nystatin Topical Powder USP
For topical use only.
Not for ophthalmic use.

DESCRIPTION

Nystatin Topical Powder USP is for dermatologic use. Nystatin Topical Powder USP provides, in each gram, 100,000 USP nystatin units dispersed in talc.

CLINICAL PHARMACOLOGY

Nystatin is an antifungal antibiotic which is both fungistatic and fungicidal *in vitro* against a wide variety of yeasts and yeast-like fungi. It probably acts by binding to sterols in the cell membrane of the fungus with a resultant change in membrane permeability allowing leakage of intracellular components. Nystatin is a polyene antibiotic of undetermined structural formula that is obtained from *Streptomyces noursei*, and is the first well tolerated antifungal antibiotic of dependable efficacy for the treatment of cutaneous, oral and intestinal infections caused by *Candida* (Monilia) *albicans* and other Candida species. It exhibits no appreciable activity against bacteria.

Nystatin provides specific therapy for all localized forms of candidiasis. Symptomatic relief is rapid, often occurring within 24 to 72 hours after the initiation of treatment. Cure is effected both clinically and mycologically in most cases of localized candidiasis.

INDICATIONS AND USAGE

Nystatin Topical Powder is indicated in the treatment of cutaneous or mucocutaneous mycotic infections caused by *Candida* (Monilia) *albicans* and other Candida species.

CONTRAINDICATIONS

Nystatin Topical Powder is contraindicated in patients with a history of hypersensitivity to any of its components.

PRECAUTIONS

Should a reaction of hypersensitivity occur the drug should be immediately withdrawn and appropriate measures taken.

This preparation is not for ophthalmic use.

ADVERSE REACTIONS

Nystatin is virtually nontoxic and nonsensitizing and is well tolerated by all age groups including debilitated infants, even on prolonged administration. If irritation on topical application should occur, discontinue medication.

DOSAGE AND ADMINISTRATION

The powder should be applied to candidal lesions two or three times daily until lesions have healed. For fungal infection of the feet caused by Candida species, the powder should be dusted freely on the feet as well as in shoes and socks.

Nystatin Topical Powder does not stain skin or mucous membranes and provides a simple, convenient means of treatment. The cream is usually preferred to the ointment in candidiasis involving intertriginous areas; very moist lesions, however, are best treated with topical dusting powder.

HOW SUPPLIED

Nystatin Topical Powder USP is supplied in 15 gram plastic squeeze bottles providing, in each gram, 100,000 USP nystatin units.

Nystatin Topical Powder USP 15 grams NDC 0574–2008–15
Keep tightly closed. Store at controlled room temperature 15°-30° C (59°-86° F); avoid excessive heat (40° C; 104° F).
Rx only

PODOCON-25™   ℞
(25% podophyllin in benzoin tincture)

DESCRIPTION

Podocon-25™ is composed of Podophyllin (Podophyllum Resin, American) 25% in Benzoin Tincture. Podophyllum Resin is the powdered mixture of resins removed from the May apple or Mandrake (*Podophyllum peltatum Linne'*), a perennial plant of northern and middle United States[1]. The podophyllum resin used in this product is exclusively the American podophyllin (rather than the Indian resin). American podophyllin typically has a reduced level of podophyllotoxin (see below).

CLINICAL PHARMACOLOGY

Podophyllin is a cytotoxic agent that has been used topically in the treatment of genital warts. It arrests mitosis in metaphase, an effect it shares with other cytotoxic agents such as the vinca alkaloids[2]. The active agent is podophyllotoxin, whose concentration varies with the type of podophyllin used; the American source normally containing one-fourth the amount of podophyllotoxin as the Indian source[3].

NOTE: PODOCON-25 IS TO BE APPLIED ONLY BY A PHYSICIAN. IT IS NOT TO BE DISPENSED TO THE PATIENT.

INDICATIONS

Podocon-25 (25% podophyllin in benzoin tincture) is indicated for the removal of soft genital (venereal) warts (condylomata acuminata)[4].

CONTRAINDICATIONS

Podocon-25 is contraindicated in diabetics, patients using steroids or with poor blood circulation. **Podocon-25** should not be used on bleeding warts, moles, birthmarks or unusual warts with hair growing from them. It is recommended that **Podocon-25** not be used during pregnancy (see Pregnancy warning below).

WARNINGS

Podophyllin is a powerful caustic and severe irritant. Keep away from the eyes; if eye contact occurs, flush with copious amounts of warm water and consult physician or poison control center immediately for advice.

PRECAUTIONS

Do not use **Podocon-25** if wart or surrounding tissue is inflamed or irritated. Do not use on bleeding warts, moles, birthmarks or unusual warts with hair growing from them.

ADVERSE REACTIONS

The use of topical podophyllin has been known to result in paresthesia, polyneuritis, paralytic ileus, pyrexia, leukopenia, thrombocytopenia, coma and death[5].

Pregnancy: There have been reports of complications associated with the topical use of podophyllin on condylomata of pregnant patients including birth defects, fetal death and stillbirth[6]. In the absence of controlled safety studies, podophyllin remains® contraindicated for use on pregnant patients.

Nursing Mothers: It is not known whether podophyllin is excreted in human milk following topical application. In the absence of controlled safety studies, podophyllin remains contraindicated for use on nursing patients.

DOSAGE AND ADMINISTRATION

PODOCON-25 IS TO BE APPLIED ONLY BY A PHYSICIAN. IT IS NOT TO BE DISPENSED TO THE PATIENT. Thoroughly cleanse affected area. Use supplied applicator to apply **Podocon-25** sparingly to lesion. Avoid contact with healthy tissue. Allow to dry thoroughly. Only intact (no bleeding) lesions should be treated. As podophyllin is a powerful caustic and severe irritant, it is recommended the first application of **Podocon-25** be left in contact for only a short time (30 to 40 minutes) to determine patient's sensitivity. To avoid systemic absorption, time of contact should be minimum time necessary to produce the desired result (1 to 4 hours, depending on conditition of lesion and of patient), the physician developing his/her own experience and technique. Large areas or numerous warts should not be treated at once.

After treatment time has elapsed, remove dried **Podocon-25** thoroughly with alcohol or soap and water.

HOW SUPPLIED

Podocon-25 is available in 15-mL bottles with tapered tip applicator attached inside cap. **NDC 0574-0601-15**
Store at room temperature 15°–30° C (59°–86° F) in tight, light-resistant containers.
Rx only

1) Blumgarten, A.F.: Text Book of Materia Medica, Pharmacology and Therapeutics; Ed. 7, New York, The Macmillan Company, 1937, pp. 220 and 223.
2) Green, L.K., Klima, M., Burns, T.; Arch Dermatol. Vol 124, Nov 1988, p. 1718.
3) Martindale, 28th Ed. London, 1982, pp. 1366, 1367.
4) Medical Letter; Vol 26, New Rochelle, N.Y., 1984, p10.
5) Fisher: Severe Systemic and Local Reactions to Topical Podophyllum Resins; Cutis, Volume 28, 1981.
6) Zackheim: Hazards of Topical Mitotic-Blocking Agents; Arch. Dermat. Volume 113, 1977.

VIOKASE   ℞
Pancrealipase, USP
Tablets, Powder

For full prescribing information, see listing under Axcan Pharma.

Par Pharmaceutical, Inc.
ONE RAM RIDGE ROAD
SPRING VALLEY, NY 10977

Direct Inquiries to:
Customer Service
(800) 828-9393
(914) 425-7100

The following is a listing of products currently available from Par Pharmaceutical, Inc.

NDC # 49884-	Product
602	Allopurinol Tablets 100 mg
603	Allopurinol Tablets 300 mg
448	Alprazolam Tablets 0.25 mg
449	Alprazolam Tablets 0.5 mg
450	Alprazolam Tablets 1 mg
117	Amiloride HCl Tablets 5 mg
568	Amoxicillin Capsules 250 mg
569	Amoxicillin Capsules 500 mg
570	Amoxicillin Oral Suspension 125 mg
571	Amoxicillin Oral Suspension 250 mg
574	Ampicillin Capsules 250 mg
575	Ampicillin Capsules 500 mg
576	Ampicillin Oral Suspension 125 mg
577	Ampicillin Oral Suspension 250 mg
456	Atenolol Tablets 50 mg
457	Atenolol Tablets 100 mg
164	Benztropine Mesylate Tablets 0.5 mg
165	Benztropine Mesylate Tablets 1 mg
166	Benztropine Mesylate Tablets 2 mg

Continued on next page

Product Listing—Cont.

246	Carisoprodol and Aspirin Tablets 200 mg/325 mg
495	Clonazepam Tablets 0.5 mg
496	Clonazepam Tablets 1 mg
497	Clonazepam Tablets 2 mg
083	Dexamethasone Tablets 0.25 mg
084	Dexamethasone Tablets 0.5 mg
085	Dexamethasone Tablets 0.75 mg
086	Dexamethasone Tablets 1.5 mg
087	Dexamethasone Tablets 4 mg
129	Dexamethasone Tablets 6 mg
217	Doxepin HCl Capsules 10 mg
218	Doxepin HCl Capsules 25 mg
219	Doxepin HCl Capsules 50 mg
220	Doxepin HCl Capsules 75 mg
221	Doxepin HCl Capsules 100 mg
222	Doxepin HCl Capsules 150 mg
061	Fluphenazine HCl Tablets 1 mg
062	Fluphenazine HCl Tablets 2.5 mg
076	Fluphenazine HCl Tablets 5 mg
064	Fluphenazine HCl Tablets 10 mg
193	Flurazepam HCl Capsules 15 mg
194	Flurazepam HCl Capsules 30 mg
223	Haloperidol Tablets 0.5 mg
224	Haloperidol Tablets 1 mg
225	Haloperidol Tablets 2 mg
226	Haloperidol Tablets 5 mg
227	Haloperidol Tablets 10 mg
029	Hydralazine HCl Tablets 10 mg
027	Hydralazine HCl Tablets 25 mg
028	Hydralazine HCl Tablets 50 mg
121	Hydralazine HCl Tablets 100 mg
143	Hydra-Zide (Hydralazine HCl and Hydrochlorothiazide) Capsules 25 mg/25 mg
144	Hydra-Zide (Hydralazine HCl and Hydrochlorothiazide) Capsules 50 mg/50 mg
145	Hydra-Zide (Hydralazine HCl and Hydrochlorothiazide) Capsules 100 mg/50 mg
200	Ibuprofen Tablets 200 mg
162	Ibuprofen Tablets 400 mg
467	IBU (Ibuprofen Tablets) 400 mg
163	Ibuprofen Tablets 600 mg
468	IBU (Ibuprofen Tablets) 600 mg
216	Ibuprofen Tablets 800 mg
469	IBU (Ibuprofen Tablets) 800 mg
494	Ibuprofen Suspension 100 mg/5 ml
054	Imipramine HCl Tablets 10 mg
055	Imipramine HCl Tablets 25 mg
056	Imipramine HCl Tablets 50 mg
020	Isosorbide Dinitrate Tablets 5 mg
021	Isosorbide Dinitrate Tablets 10 mg
022	Isosorbide Dinitrate Tablets 20 mg
009	Isosorbide Dinitrate Tablets 30 mg
034	Meclizine HCl Tablets 12.5 mg
035	Meclizine HCl Tablets 25 mg
289	Megestrol Acetate Tablets 20 mg
290	Megestrol Acetate Tablets 40 mg
478	Melatonin Caplets 1.5 mg
479	Melatonin Tablets 500 mcg
480	Melatonin CR Capsules 3 mg
249	Methocarbamol and Aspirin Tablets 400 mg/325 mg
490	Methylprednisolone Tablets 4 mg
256	Minoxidil Tablets 2.5 mg
257	Minoxidil Tablets 10 mg
498	Nicardipine Capsules 20 mg
499	Nicardipine Capsules 30 mg
058	Nicotine Patch 7 mg
059	Nicotine Patch 14 mg
063	Nicotine Patch 21 mg
119	Nystatin Tablets 500,000 Units
578	Penicillin V Potassium Tablets 250 mg
579	Penicillin V Potassium Tablets 500 mg
580	Penicillin V Potassium Susp 125 mg
581	Penicillin V Potassium Susp 250 mg
442	Pindolol Tablets 5 mg
443	Pindolol Tablets 10 mg
440	Piroxicam Capsules 10 mg
441	Piroxicam Capsules 20 mg
549	Prochlorperazine Tablets 5 mg
550	Prochlorperazine Tablets 10 mg
600	SSD (1% Silver Sulfadiazine) Cream
601	SSD AF (1% Silver Sulfadiazine) Cream
240	Temazepam Capsules 15 mg
241	Temazepam Capsules 30 mg
486	TransZone Controlled Release Melatonin Capsules 3 mg
453	Triazolam Tablets 0.125 mg
454	Triazolam Tablets 0.25 mg
057	Zorprin Tablets 800 mg

Parkedale Pharmaceuticals

**870 PARKDALE ROAD
ROCHESTER, MI 48307**

Direct Inquiries to:
888-401-2879
FAX: 423-989-6279
Medical Emergency Contact:
Henry Richards, M.D.
800-546-4906
FAX: 423-989-6137

APLISOL® ℞
[ăp' lĭsŏl]
**(Tuberculin Purified Protein Derivative, Diluted [Stabilized Solution])
Diagnostic Antigen
For Intradermal Injection Only**

DESCRIPTION

Aplisol (tuberculin PPD, diluted) is a sterile aqueous solution of purified protein fraction for intradermal administration as an aid in the diagnosis of tuberculosis. The solution is stabilized with polysorbate (Tween)80, buffered with potassium and sodium phosphates and contains approximately 0.35% phenol as a preservative. This product is ready for immediate use without further dilution.

The purified protein fraction is isolated from culture media filtrates of a human strain of *Mycobacterium tuberculosis* by the method of F.B. Seibert.[1,2] Tuberculin PPD, diluted, is prepared from Tuberculin PPD Powder Master Lot 154616 which is clinically bioequivalent in potency to the standard PPD-S* (5 TU** per 0.1mL) of the U.S. Public Health Service, National Centers for Disease Control. This product is made from a single master lot (No. 154616) to eliminate lot to lot variation inherent in manufacturing.

The potency of each lot of tuberculin PPD, diluted is determined in sensitized guinea pigs.

CLINICAL PHARMACOLOGY

In the United States, the prevalence of *Mycobacterium tuberculosis* infection and active disease varies for different segments of the population; however, the risk for *M. tuberculosis* infection in the overall population is low. Tuberculosis (TB) case rates declined steadily for decades in the United States. However, in 1985 the TB case rate stabilized and subsequently increased through 1992, accompanied by a 14% increase in the TB mortality rate in 1988. This has been attributed to several complex social and medical factors, including the human immunodeficiency virus (HIV) epidemic, the occurrence of TB in foreign-born persons from countries that have a high prevalence of TB, the emergence of drug-resistant strains of TB, and the transmission of *M. tuberculosis* in congregate settings. (e.g., health-care facilities, correctional facilities, drug-treatment centers, and homeless shelters). Because the overall risk of acquiring M. tuberculosis is low for the total U.S. population, the primary strategy for preventing and controlling TB in the United States is to minimize the risk transmission by the early identification and treatment of patients who have active infectious TB, finding screening persons who have been in contact with active infectious TB patients and screening high-risk populations.

Tuberculin PPD is recommended by the American Lung Association as an aid in the detection of infection with *Mycobacterium tuberculosis*.[3,4] After a person becomes infected with mycobacteria, T lymphocytes proliferate and become sensitized. These sensitized T cells enter the bloodstream and circulate for months or years. This sensitization process occurs principally in the regional lymph nodes and may take 2–10 weeks to develop following infection. Once acquired, tuberculin sensitivity tends to persist, although it often wanes with time and advancing age. The injection of tuberculin into the skin stimulates the lymphocytes and activates a series of events leading to a delayed-type hypersensitivity (DTH) response. This response is called "delayed" because the reaction becomes evident hours after injection. Dermal reactivity involves vasodilation, edema, and the infiltration of lymphocytes, basophils, monocytes, and neutrophils into the site of antigen injection. Antigen-specific T lymphocytes proliferate and release lymphokines, which mediate the accumulation of other cells at the site. The area of induration reflects DTH activity.[5] In most tuberculin-sensitive individuals, the delayed hypersensitivity reaction is evident 5–6 hours after administration of a tuberculin skin test and is maximal 48–72 hours. In geriatric patients or in patients receiving a tuberculin skin test for the first time, the reaction may develop more slowly and may not be maximal until after 72 hours.[6] Because their immune systems are immature, many neonates and infants < 6 weeks of age, who are infected with *M. tuberculosis*, do not react at all to tuberculin tests.[5]

Immediate erythematous or other hypersensitivity reactions to tuberculin or the constituents of the diluent may occur at the injection site. A possible decrease in responsiveness to skin testing may occur in the presence of tuberculous infections including viral infections, live virus vaccination, overwhelming tuberculosis, other bacterial infections, drugs and malignancy.

Tuberculin skin-test results are also less reliable as CD4 counts decline in HIV infected individuals.[3]

The 5TU dose of Tuberculin PPD intradermally (Mantoux) is recommended as the standard tuberculin test, and Tuberculin PPD is recommended by the American Lung Association as an aid in the detection of infection with *Mycobacterium tuberculosis*. Reactions to the Mantoux test are interpreted on the basis of a quantitative measurement of the response to a specific dose (5 TU PPD-S or equivalent) of Tuberculin PPD[7].

To determine that Tuberculin PPD Master Lot 154616 is clinically bioequivalent in potency to standard 5TU PPD-S*, 3 dose-response studies were conducted in the following populations (1) persons with a history of bacteriologically confirmed TB; (2) healthy volunteers in a geographical region of low endemicity of atypical mycobacterial infection; and (3) healthy volunteers in a geographical location of high endemicity of atypical mycobacterial infection.

---

*PPD-S (No. 49608) World Health Organization International PPD-Tuberculin Standard (PPD-S is a dried powder from which WHO and U.S. Standard tuberculin solutions are made.)

**U.S. Tuberculin Unit

INDICATIONS AND USAGE

Tuberculin PPD is recommended by the American Lung Association as an aid in the detection of infection with *Mycobacterium tuberculosis*. The standard tuberculin test recommended employs the intradermal (Mantoux) test using a 5TU dose of tuberculin PPD.[7] The 0.1-mL test dose of Aplisol (tuberculin PPD, diluted) is equivalent to the 5 TU dose recommended as clinically established and standardized with PPD-S. Tuberculin skin testing is not contraindicated for persons who have been vaccinated with BCG and the skin-test results of such persons are used to support or exclude the diagnosis of *M. tuberculosis* infections.[4]

HIV infection is a strong risk factor for the development of TB disease in persons having TB infection. All HIV-infected persons should receive a PPD-tuberculin skin test.[3]

CONTRAINDICATIONS

Aplisol is contraindicated in patients with known hypersensitivity or allergy to Aplisol or any of its components. Aplisol should not be administered to persons who have previously experienced a severe reaction (e.g., vesiculation, ulceration, or necrosis) because of the severity of reactions that may occur at the test site.

WARNINGS

Tuberculin should be administered with caution to known tuberculin-positive reactors because of the severity of reactions (e.g., vesiculation, ulceration, or necrosis) that may occur at the test site in very sensitive individuals.

Not all infected persons will have a delayed hypersensitivity reaction to a tuberculin test. A number of factors have been reported to cause a decreased ability to respond to the tuberculin test, such as the presence of tuberculous infection or viral infections (measles, mumps chickenpox, and HIV), live virus vaccination (measles, mumps, rubella, oral polio and yellow fever), overwhelming tuberculosis, other bacterial infections, drugs (corticosteroids and other immunosuppressive agents) and malignancy.[8,9]

Any condition that impairs or attenuates cell mediated immunity potentially can cause a false negative reaction.

Tuberculin skin test results are less reliable in HIV-infected individuals as CD4 counts decline (see CLINICAL PHARMACOLOGY).[3]

Aplisol should not be administered to persons who previously experienced a severe reaction (e.g., vesiculation, ulceration, or necrosis) because of the severity of reactions that may occur at the test site (see CONTRAINDICATIONS).

Avoid injecting tuberculin subcutaneously. If this occurs, no local reaction develops, but a general febrile reaction and/or acute inflammation around old tuberculous lesions may occur in highly sensitive individuals.

PRECAUTIONS
General

The predictive value of the tuberculin skin test depends on the prevalence of infection with *M. tuberculosis* and the relative prevalence of cross-reactions with nontuberculous mycobacteria.[9,10]

A separate, sterile, single-use disposable syringes and needles should be used for each individual patient to prevent possible transmission of serum hepatitis virus and other infectious agents from one person to another.

Special care should be taken to ensure that the product is injected intradermally and not into a blood vessel.

Before administration of Aplisol, a review of the patient's history with respect to possible immediate-type hypersensitivity to the product, determination of previous use of Aplisol and the presence of any contraindication to the test should be made (see CONTRAINDICATIONS). As with any biological product, epinephrine should be immediately available in case an anaphylactoid or acute hypersensitivity reaction occurs.

Failure to store and handle Aplisol as recommended may result in a loss of potency and inaccurate test results.[11,8]

Reactivity to the test may be depressed or suppressed for as long as 5–6 weeks in individuals following immunization with certain live viral vaccines, viral infections or discontinuation of corticosteroids or immunosuppressive agents.[8,9]

Information to Patients

Patients should be instructed to report adverse events such as vesiculation, ulceration or necrosis which may occur at the test site in highly sensitive individuals. Patients should be informed that pain, pruritus and discomfort may occur at injection site.

Patient should be informed of the need to return to their physician or health care provider for the reading of the test and of the need to keep and maintain a personal immunization record.

Drug Interactions

In patients who are receiving corticosteroids or immunosuppressive agents, reactivity to the test may be depressed or suppressed. This reduced reactivity may present for as long as 5–6 weeks after discontinuation of therapy (see PRECAUTIONS-General).[9]

The reactivity to PPD may be temporarily depressed by certain live virus vaccines. Therefore, if a tuberculin test is to be performed, it should be administered either before or simultaneously with the use of oral polio and/or injection of measles, mumps and rubella vaccines in combined form or as separate antigens, or testing should be postponed for 4–6 weeks.[10]

Carcinogenesis, Mutagenesis, Impairment of Fertility

No long term studies have been conducted in animals or in humans to evaluate carcinogenic or mutagenic potential or effects on fertility with Aplisol.

Pregnancy

Teratogenic effects: Pregnancy Category C. Animal reproduction studies have not been conducted with Aplisol. It is also not known whether Aplisol can cause fetal harm when administered to a pregnant woman or can affect the reproduction capacity. Aplisol should be given to a pregnant woman only if clearly needed.

However, the risk of unrecognized tuberculosis and the postpartum contact between a mother with active disease and an infant leaves the infant in grave danger of tuberculosis and complications such as tuberculous meningitis. Although there have not been any reported adverse effects upon the fetus recognized as being due to tuberculosis skin testing, the prescribing physician will want to consider if the potential benefits outweigh the possible risks for performing the tuberculin test on a pregnant woman or a woman of childbearing age, particularly in certain high risk populations.

ADVERSE REACTIONS

In highly sensitive individuals, strongly positive reactions including vesiculation, ulceration or necrosis may occur at the test site. Cold packs or topical steroid preparations may be employed for symptomatic relief of the associated pain, pruritus and discomfort.

Strongly positive test reactions may result in scarring at the test site. Immediate erythematous or other reactions may occur at the injection site.

DOSAGE AND ADMINISTRATION

Aplisol vials should be inspected visually for both particulate matter and discoloration prior to administration and discarded of either is seen. Vials in use for more than 30 days should be discarded.

Standard Method (Mantoux Test)

The Mantoux test is performed by **intradermally** injecting with a syringe and needle exactly 0.1mL of Aplisol. The result is read 48 to 72 hours later and **induration only is considered in interpreting the test.**

Induration is a hard, raised area with clearly defined margins at and around the injection site. Erythema may develop at the injection site but has no diagnostic value. The standard test is performed as follows:

1. The site of the test is usually the flexor or dorsal surface of the forearm about 4″ below the elbow. Other skin sites may be used, but the flexor surface of the forearm is preferred. The use of a skin area free of lesions and away from any veins is recommended.[7]
2. The skin at the injection site is cleansed with 70% alcohol and allowed to dry.
3. The test material is administered with a tuberculin syringe (0.5 or 1.0mL) fitted with a short (1/2″) 26 or 27 gauge needle.
4. A separate, sterile, single-use disposable syringe and needles should be used for each individual patient.
5. The diaphragm of the vial-stopper should be wiped with 70% alcohol.
6. The needle is inserted through the stopper diaphragm of the inverted vial. Exactly 0.1 mL is filled into the syringe with care being taken to exclude air bubbles and to maintain the lumen of the needle filled.
7. The point of the needle is inserted into the most superficial layers of the skin with the needle bevel pointed upward. **As the tuberculin solution is injection, a pale bleb 6 to 10mm in size (1/3) will rise over the point of the needle.** This is quickly absorbed and no dressing is required.

In the event the injection is delivered subcutaneously (i.e., no bleb will form), or if a significant part of the dose leaks from the injection site, the test should be repeated immediately at another site at least 5cm (2") removed.

The Mantoux test is the standard of comparison for all other tuberculin tests.

Interpretation of tuberculin Reaction

Readings of Mantoux reactions should be made during the period from 48 to 72 hours after the injection. **Induration only should be considered in interpreting the test.** The diameter of induration should be measured transversely to the long axis of the forearm and recorded in millimeters. Erythema has no diagnostic value and should be disregarded. The presence and size of necrosis and edema if present should be recorded although not used in the interpretation of the test. In the absence of induration, an area of erythema greater than 10 mm is diameter may indicate the injection was made too deeply and retesting is indicated.

Reactions should be interpreted as follows:

Positive—A positive reaction to the tuberculin skin test may not be seen until 2–10 weeks after the infection.[7] Based in current guidelines,[3,12] interpretation of positive reactions (depending on the age, immune status or risk factors of the persons tested) is:

1. An induration of ≥5mm is classified as positive in the following:
   - Person who have had recent close contact with persons who have active TB;
   - Persons who have human immunodeficiency virus (HIV) infection or risk factors for HIV infection but unknown HIV status;
   - Persons who have fibrotic chest radiographs consistent with healed TB.
2. An induration of ≥10mm is classified as positive in all persons who do not meet any of the above criteria, but who belong to one or more of the following groups at high risk for TB:
   - Injecting-drug users known to be HIV seronegative;
   - Persons who have other medical conditions that have been reported to increase the risk for progressing from latent TB infection to active TB infection. These medical conditions include diabetes mellitus, conditions requiring prolonged high-dose corticosteroid therapy and other immunosuppressive therapy (including bone marrow and organ transplantation), chronic renal failure, some hematologic disorders (e.g., leukemias and lymphomas), other specific malignancies (e.g., carcinoma of the head or neck), weight loss of ≥10% below ideal body weight, silicosis, gastrectomy, jejunileal bypass;
   - Residents and employees of high-risk congregate settings; prisons and jails, nursing homes and other long-term facilities for the elderly, health-care facilities (including some residential mental health facilities), and homeless shelters;
   - Foreign-born persons recently arrived (i.e., within the last 5 years) from countries having a high prevalence or incidence of TB;
   - Some medically underserved, low-income populations, including migrant farm workers and homeless persons;
   - High-risk racial or ethnic minority populations, as defined locally;
   - Children <4 years of age or infants, children and adolescents exposed to adults in high-risk categories.
3. An induration of ≥ 15mm is classified as positive in persons who do not meet any of the above criteria.

Negative—Induration of less than 5 mm. This indicates a lack of hypersensitivity to tuberculoprotein and tuberculous infection is highly unlikely.

Booster Effect—Infection of an individual with tubercle bacilli or other mycobacteria or BCG vaccination results in a delayed hypersensitivity response to tuberculin which is demonstrated by the skin test. The delayed hypersensitivity response may gradually wane over a period of years. If a person receives a tuberculin test at this time, a significant reaction may not be detected. However, the stimulus of the test may boost or increase the size of the reaction to a second test, sometimes causing an apparent conversion or development of sensitivity. This booster effect can be seen on a second test done one week after the initial stimulating test and can persist for a year, and perhaps longer. When routine periodic tuberculin testing of adults is done, initially two-stage testing should be considered to minimize the likelihood of interpreting a boosted reaction as a conversion.[13,14]

It should be noted that reactivity to tuberculin may be depressed or suppressed for as long as 5–6 weeks by viral infections, live virus vaccines (i.e., measles, smallpox, polio, rubella and mumps), or after discontinuation of therapy with corticosteroids or immunosuppressive agents.

Malnutrition may also have a similar effect. When of diagnostic importance, a negative test should be accepted as proof that hypersensitivity is absent only after normal reactivity to non-specific irritants has been demonstrated. A primary injection of tuberculin may possibly have a boosting effect on subsequent tuberculin reactions.

A pediatric patient who is known to have been exposed to a person with tuberculosis must not be adjudged free of infection until that patient has a negative tuberculin reaction at least ten weeks after contact with tuberculous person has ceased.[15] Annual testing is generally recommended for pediatric patients in high risk populations, such as persons from countries with a high prevalence of tuberculosis and low-income groups.[16]

A positive tuberculin reaction does not necessarily signify the presence of active disease. Further diagnostic procedures (e.g., chest radiograph, sputum smear and/or culture examination) should be carried out before a diagnosis of tuberculosis is made. A small percentage of responders may not have been infected with *M. tuberculosis* but by some other mycobacterium. The negative tuberculin skin test should never be used to exclude the possibility of active tuberculosis among persons for whom the diagnosis is being considered (symptoms compatible with tuberculosis).

HOW SUPPLIED

Tuberculin PPD-Aplisol bioequivalent to 5US units (TU) PPD-S per test dose (0.1mL) is available in the following presentations:

NDC 64029-4525-3 (Bio. 1525)

1 mL (10 tests) - rubber-diaphragm-capped vial

NDC 64029-4525-4 (Bio. 1607)

5 mL (50 tests) - rubber-diaphragm-capped vial

This product is ready for use without further dilution.

Storage

DO NOT FREEZE

This product should be stored at 2°–8°C (36°–46°F) and protected from light.

Vials in use more than 30 days should be discarded due to possible oxidation and degradation which may affect potency.

REFERENCES

1 Seibert, F.B.: Am Rev Tuberc, 30:713, 1934
2 Seibert, F.B., and Glenn, J.T.: Am Rev Tuberc, 44:9, 1941
3 MMWR, 1995:44 RR-11
4 MMWR, 1996:45 RR-4
5 Huebner RE, Shein MF, Bass JB, The Tuberculin Skin Test, *Clin Infect Dis*, 1993;17:968-75
6 AHFS Drug Information, 1997, 36:84 pp 1962-1968
7 American Thoracic Society: Diagnostic Standards and classification of tuberculosis, 1990 Am Rev Respir Dis, 142:725-735
8 Am Rev Respir Dis, 1985;886
9 Brickman HF et.Al., The Timing of Tuberculin Tests in Relation to Immunization with Live Viral Vaccines, *Pediatrics*; 1975;55:392
10 Red Book Report of the Committee on Infectious Disease, (1994)
11 Landi S, Held HR, Stability of a dilute solution of tuberculin purified derivative at extreme temperatures, *J Biol Stand*, 1981; 9:195
12 Diagnosis of TB Infection and TB Disease, Centers For Disease Control and Prevention(CDC), March 21, 1996, Doc#2250102
13 Sewell, E.M., O'Hare, D., and Kendig, E.L., Jr.: The Tuberculin Test, Pediatrics, Vol.54, No. 5, Nov.1974.
14 Advisory Committee of Elimination of Tuberculosis (ACET/CDC: Prevention and control of tuberculosis in facilities providing long-term care to the elderly, 1990. MMWR 39(10): 7–13,15.
15 ACET(CDC): The use of preventative therapy therapy for tuberculosis infection in the United States, 1990. MMWR 39(8):9–12.
16 ACET(CDC): Screening for tuberculosis and tuberculosis infection in high risk populations. Recommendations of the ACET, 1990. MMWR 39(8):1–7.

Rx only.

Rev. 7/98

0932906

Manufactured by: Parkedale Pharmaceuticals, Inc.

Rochester, MI 48307

Shown in Product Identification Guide, page 329

INFLUENZA VIRUS VACCINE, TRIVALENT, TYPES A AND B

FLUOGEN® ℞

Subvirion Vaccine/Immunizing Antigen, Ether Extracted

DESCRIPTION

Fluogen (Influenza Virus Vaccine, Trivalent, Types A and B) is a sterile product for intramuscular injection composed of

Continued on next page

Fluogen—Cont.

the antigens of the strains of influenza virus recommended for vaccine use during the 1998–1999 season by the US Public Health Service. It is formulated to contain no less than 45 micrograms of hemagglutinin antigen (HA) content per 0.5 mL dose in the recommended ratio of 15μg of HA of the A influenza virus component representative of A/Beijing/262/95 (H1N1), 15 μg of HA of the A influenza virus component representative of A/Sydney/5/97 (H3N2), and 15 μg of HA of the B influenza virus component representative of B/Harbin/07/94 (B/Beijing/184/93-like).

Influenza virus is propagated in embryonated chicken eggs using an inoculum containing approximately 1 mg/mL streptomycin sulfate. The allantoic fluids containing the virus are harvested, clarified by filtration, and concentrated and refined by ultracentrifugation and zonal centrifugation. Polysorbate 80, USP, is added to the refined concentrate, which is subsequently extracted with ethyl ether to disrupt the virus and allow removal of a high proportion of pyrogenic substances. The extracted concentrate is inactivated with formaldehyde. The vaccine is diluted to its final volume with phosphate-buffered-saline solution. Thimerosal (mercury derivative) 0.01% is added as a preservative. Streptomycin sulfate is undetectable (less than the limit of detection of the assay) in the final product.

Treatment of the influenza virus with ethyl ether results in disruption or "splitting" of the virus. The active immunizing antigens, hemagglutinin and neuraminidase, are retained while a high proportion of egg protein and pyrogenic substances are removed. The resultant split-virus vaccine has been shown to be less reactogenic than whole-virus vaccines in younger age groups.

CLINICAL PHARMACOLOGY

The inoculation of antigen prepared from inactivated influenza virus stimulates the production of specific antibodies. Protection is afforded only against those strains of virus from which the vaccine is prepared or closely related strains.

The effectiveness of influenza vaccine in preventing or attenuating illness varies, depending primarily on the age and immunocompetence of the vaccine recipient and the degree of similarity between the virus strains included in the vaccine and those that circulate during the influenza season. When a good match exists between vaccine and circulating viruses, influenza vaccine has been shown to prevent illness in approximately 70%–90% of healthy persons aged less than 65 years. Under these circumstances, studies also have indicated that the effectiveness of influenza vaccine in preventing hospitalization for pneumonia and influenza among elderly persons living in settings other than nursing homes or similar chronic-care facilities ranges from 30%–70%.

Among elderly persons residing in nursing homes, influenza vaccine is most effective in preventing severe illness, secondary complications, and death. Studies in this population have indicated that the vaccine can be 50%–60% effective in preventing hospitalization and pneumonia and 80% effective in preventing death, even though efficacy in preventing influenza illness may often be in the range of 30%–40% among the frail elderly. Achieving a high rate of vaccination among nursing home residents can reduce the spread of infection in a facility, thus preventing disease through herd immunity. Vaccination of health care workers in nursing homes has also been demonstrated to reduce the impact of influenza among residents.

Based on the most recent epidemiological and laboratory data, the US Public Health Service anticipates that the strains prevalent in 1998–1999 will be closely related to A/Beijing/262/95 (H1N1), A/Sydney/5/97 (H3N2), and B/Harbin/07/94 (B/Beijing/184/93-like). Therefore, these strains will be included in the influenza virus vaccine for use during the 1998–1999 season.

INDICATIONS AND USAGE

Fluogen is indicated for the production of immunity to influenza virus containing antigens related to those in the vaccine.

Influenza vaccine is strongly recommended for any person 6 months of age or older who, because of age or underlying medical condition, is at increased risk for complications of influenza. Health-care workers and others (including household members) in close contact with persons in high-risk groups should also be vaccinated. In addition, influenza vaccine may be administered to any person who wishes to reduce the chance of becoming infected with influenza. Guidelines for the use of vaccine among certain patient populations follow.[1]

TARGET GROUPS FOR SPECIAL VACCINATION PROGRAMS

To maximize protection of high-risk persons, they and their close contacts should be targeted for organized vaccination programs.

Groups at increased risk for influenza-related complications:

1. Persons 65 years of age or older.

2. Residents of nursing homes and other chronic-care facilities that house persons of any age with chronic medical conditions.
3. Adults and pediatric patients with chronic disorders of the pulmonary or cardiovascular systems, including pediatric patients with asthma.
4. Adults and pediatric patients who have required regular medical follow-up or hospitalization during the preceding year because of chronic metabolic diseases (including diabetes mellitus), renal dysfunction, hemoglobinopathies, or immunosuppression (including immunosuppression caused by medications).
5. Pediatric patients and young adults (6 months to 18 years of age) who are receiving long-term aspirin therapy and, therefore, may be at risk for developing Reye syndrome after influenza.

Groups that can transmit influenza to persons at high risk: Persons who are clinically or subclinically infected and who care for or live with members of high-risk groups can transmit influenza virus to them. Some persons at high risk (eg, the elderly, transplant recipients, and persons with acquired immunodeficiency syndrome [AIDS]) can have a low antibody response to influenza vaccine. Efforts to protect these members of high-risk groups against influenza might be improved by reducing the likelihood of influenza exposure from their caregivers.

Therefore, the following groups should be vaccinated:

1. Physicians, nurses, and other personnel in both hospital and outpatient-care settings.
2. Employees of nursing homes and chronic-care facilities who have contact with patients or residents.
3. Providers of home care to persons at high risk (eg, visiting nurses, volunteer workers).
4. Household-members (including the pediatric population 6 months of age or older) of persons in high-risk groups.

VACCINATION OF OTHER GROUPS

General population: Physicians should administer influenza vaccine to any person greater than or equal to age 6 months who wishes to reduce the likelihood of becoming ill with influenza. Persons who provide essential community services should be considered for vaccination to minimize disruption of essential activities during influenza outbreaks. Students or other persons in institutional settings, such as those who reside in dormitories, should be encouraged to receive vaccine to minimize the disruption of routine activities during epidemics.

Pregnant women: Influenza-associated excess mortality among pregnant women has not been documented except during the pandemics of 1918–19 and 1957–58. However, because death-certificate data often do not indicate whether a woman was pregnant at the time of death, studies conducted during interpandemic periods may underestimate the impact of influenza in this population. Case reports and limited studies suggest that pregnancy may increase the risk for serious medical complications of influenza as a result of increases in heart rate, stroke volume and oxygen consumption, decreases in lung capacity, and changes in immunologic function. A recent study of the impact of influenza during 17 interpandemic influenza seasons documented that the relative risk of hospitalization for selected cardiorespiratory conditions among pregnant women increased from 1.4 during weeks 14–20 of gestation to 4.7 during weeks 37–42 compared with rates among women who were 1–6 months postpartum. Women in their third trimester of pregnancy were hospitalized at a rate comparable to that of nonpregnant women who have high-risk medical conditions for whom influenza vaccine was traditionally recommended. Physicians generally avoid prescribing unnecessary drugs and biologics for pregnant women especially in the first trimester; however, there are no data specifically to contraindicate vaccination with the available killed virus vaccine in pregnant women who have underlying high-risk conditions. (See also PRECAUTIONS.)

Persons infected with human immunodeficiency virus (HIV): Limited information exists regarding the frequency and severity of influenza illness among human immunodeficiency virus (HIV)-infected persons, but reports suggest that symptoms might be prolonged and the risk for complications increased for some HIV-infected persons. Because influenza can result in serious illness and complications, vaccination is a prudent precaution and may result in protective antibody levels in many HIV-infected persons. However, the antibody response to vaccine can be low in persons with advanced HIV-disease and low CD4+ T-lymphocyte cell counts; a booster dose of vaccine does not improve the immune response for these persons.

Foreign travelers: The risk for exposure to influenza during foreign travel varies, depending on season and destination. In the tropics, influenza can occur throughout the year; in the Southern Hemisphere, most activity occurs from April through September. Because of the short incubation period for influenza, exposure to the virus during travel can result in clinical illness that begins while travelling, an inconvenience or potential danger, especially for persons at increased risk for complications. Persons preparing to travel to the tropics at any time of year or to the Southern Hemi-

sphere from April through September should review their influenza vaccination histories. If they were not vaccinated the previous fall/winter, they should consider influenza vaccination before travel. Persons in the high-risk categories should be especially encouraged to receive the most current vaccine. Persons at high risk who received the previous season's vaccine before travel should be revaccinated in the fall/winter with the current vaccine.

TIMING OF INFLUENZA VACCINATION ACTIVITIES

Beginning each September, when vaccine for the upcoming influenza season becomes available, persons at high risk who are seen by health-care providers for routine care or as a result of hospitalization should be offered influenza vaccine. Opportunities to vaccinate persons at high risk for complications of influenza should not be missed.

The optimal time for organized vaccination campaigns for persons in high-risk groups is usually the period from the beginning of October through mid-November. In the United States, influenza activity generally peaks between late December and early March. High levels of influenza activity infrequently occur in the contiguous 48 states before December. Administering vaccine too far in advance of the influenza season should be avoided in facilities such as nursing homes because antibody levels might begin to decline within a few months of vaccination. Vaccination programs can be undertaken as soon as current vaccine is available if regional influenza activity is expected to begin earlier than December.

Pediatric patients under 9 years of age who have not been vaccinated previously should receive two doses of vaccine at least one month apart to maximize the likelihood of a satisfactory antibody response to all three vaccine antigens. The second dose should be administered before December, if possible. Vaccine should be offered to both the pediatric and adult populations up to and even after influenza virus activity is documented in a community.

The degree of protection afforded by immunization with any vaccine may not be sufficient to prevent the disease if the exposure to the influenza virus strains is overwhelming or if the virus strains are not closely related antigenically to those used in the production of vaccine.

CONTRAINDICATIONS

Influenza virus vaccine should not be administered to individuals with a history of hypersensitivity (allergy) to chicken eggs or to other components of influenza virus vaccine, including thimerosal (see Adverse reactions).

In persons suspected of having an allergic condition, immunization procedures should be preceded by a scratch test or an intradermal injection (0.05 to 0.1 mL) of vaccine diluted 1:100 in sterile saline to determine possible sensitivity to the minute residual egg protein that may be present in the vaccine. A positive skin reaction contraindicates immunization with the vaccine. See PRECAUTIONS.

Immunization should be deferred in the presence of any acute respiratory disease or other active infection.

WARNING

Persons being given immunosuppressive therapy or other immunosuppressed individuals may experience a lower than expected antigenic response.

The packaging of this product contains natural rubber latex which may cause allergic reactions. Proper precautions should be taken for persons with known sensitivity to latex.

PRECAUTIONS

General

A separate sterile syringe and needle should be used for each patient to prevent transmission of hepatitis B virus or other infectious agents from one person to another.

Although current influenza vaccines contain only a minute quantity of egg protein, they do, on rare occasions, provoke anaphylactic hypersensitivity reactions. Epinephrine 1 mg/mL (1:1000) should be available and ready for immediate use should such reactions occur.

Because of the possibility of a febrile reaction following immunization with influenza virus vaccine, the wisdom of attempting to immunize patients with a history of febrile convulsion should be given careful consideration. Persons with acute febrile illnesses usually should not be vaccinated until their temporary symptoms have abated.

Drug Interactions

Although influenza vaccination can inhibit the clearance of warfarin and theophylline, studies have failed to show any adverse clinical effects attributable to these drugs in patients receiving influenza vaccine.

Concomitant influenza vaccination and immunosuppressive therapy (eg, corticosteroids, chemotherapy) may be associated with impaired immune response to the vaccine.

Pregnancy

Pregnancy Category C:

Animal reproduction studies have not been conducted with influenza vaccine. It is also not known whether influenza vaccine can cause fetal harm when administered to a preg-

nant woman or can affect reproduction capacity. Influenza vaccine should be given to a pregnant woman only if clearly needed. (See also INDICATIONS AND USAGE.)

Nursing Mothers

Influenza vaccine does not affect the safety of breastfeeding for mothers or infants. Breastfeeding does not adversely affect immune response and is not a contraindication for vaccination.

Pediatric Use

The safety and effectiveness of Fluogen in infants below the age of 6 months have not been established.

ADVERSE REACTIONS

Side effects of influenza vaccine are generally inconsequential in adults and occur at low frequency. The most frequent side effect of vaccination is soreness at the vaccination site that lasts for up to two days. Severe reactions are uncommon in adults, and truly disabling effects appear to be exceedingly rare.

The following types of systemic reactions to influenza vaccine have occurred:

Fever, malaise, myalgia, and other systemic symptoms of toxicity occurring 6 to 12 hours after vaccination and persisting one or two days. These responses to influenza vaccine are usually attributed to characteristics of the influenza virus antigens (even though the virus is inactivated) and represent the bulk of the side effects of influenza vaccination. Such effects occur most frequently in persons who have had no exposure to the influenza virus antigen in the vaccine (eg, young children).

Immediate, presumably allergic, responses, such as hives, angioedema, allergic asthma, and systemic anaphylaxis, are expressions of hypersensitivity. These reactions occur rarely after influenza vaccination. They probably derive from exquisite sensitivity to some vaccine component, most likely to residual egg protein.

Neurologic disorders, including such central nervous system conditions as encephalopathy, have a temporal association with influenza vaccination.

Although the 1976 swine influenza vaccine was associated with an increased frequency of Guillain-Barre syndrome (GBS), evidence for a casual relationship of GBS with subsequent vaccines prepared from other virus strains is less clear. However, it is difficult to obtain strong evidence for a possible small increase in risk for a rare condition such as GBS, which has an annual background incidence of only 10 to 20 cases per million adult population. During three of four seasons studied between 1977 through 1991, the point estimates of the overall relative risks of GBS after influenza vaccination were slightly elevated, but were not statistically significant in any of these studies. However, a recent study of the 1992–93 and 1993–94 seasons found an elevation in the overall relative risk of 1.83 (95% confidence Interval 1.12–3.00) during the 6 weeks following vaccination, representing an excess of an estimated 1–2 cases per million persons vaccinated; the combined number of GBS cases peaked 2 weeks after vaccination. The increase in the relative risk and the increased number of cases in the second week after vaccination may be the result of vaccination but also could be due to other factors (e.g., confounding or diagnostic bias) rather than a true vaccine-related risk.

Among persons who received the swine influenza vaccine in 1976, the rate of GBS that exceeded the background rate was slightly less than 10 cases per million vaccinations. Even if GBS were a true side effect in subsequent years, the estimated risk for GBS of 1–2 cases per million vaccinations is substantially less than the risk for severe influenza, which could be prevented by vaccination among, especially for persons aged ≥65 years and those who have medical indications for influenza vaccination. During different epidemics occurring from 1972–1981, estimated rates of influenza-associated hospitalization have ranged from approximately 200–300 hospitalizations per million in previously healthy persons age 5–44 years to 2000≥10,000 hospitalizations per million in persons aged 65 and older. During epidemics from 1972–73 through 1994–95, estimates of influenza-associated death rates have ranged from approximately 300–1500 per million in persons aged 65 and older, who account for more than 90% of all influenza-associated deaths. The potential benefits of influenza vaccination clearly outweigh the possible risks for vaccine-associated GBS.

The average case-fatality ratio for GBS is approximately 6% and increases with age. However, no evidence indicates that the case-fatality ratio for GBS differs among vaccinated persons and those not vaccinated.

Whereas the incidence of GBS in the general population is very low, persons with a history of GBS have a substantially greater likelihood of subsequently developing GBS than persons without such a history. Thus, the likelihood of coincidentally developing GBS after influenza vaccination is expected to be greater among persons with a history of GBS than among persons with no history of this syndrome. Whether influenza vaccination might be causally associated with this risk for recurrence is not known. Avoiding subse-

quent influenza vaccination in persons known to have developed GBS within 6 weeks of a previous influenza vaccination seems prudent. However, for most persons with a history of GBS who are at high risk for severe complication from influenza, many experts believe the established benefits of influenza vaccination justify yearly vaccination.

DOSAGE AND ADMINISTRATION

Although the current influenza vaccine can contain one or more of the antigens administered in previous years, annual vaccination with the current vaccine is necessary because immunity declines in the year following vaccination. **Because the 1998–1999 vaccine differs from the 1997–1998 vaccine, supplies of 1997–1998 vaccine should not be administered to provide protection for the 1998–1999 influenza season.**[1]

Two doses administered at least one month apart may be required for satisfactory antibody responses among pediatric patients under 9 years of age who are receiving influenza vaccine for the first time. (See timing for vaccination under INDICATIONS AND USAGE.) To minimize febrile reactions, only subvirion or purified-surface-antigen preparations should be used for pediatric patients 6 months to 12 years of age.[1] Studies of vaccines similar to those being used currently have indicated little or no improvement in antibody response when a second dose is administered to adults during the same season.[1]

Data on inactivated influenza vaccine immunogenicity and reactogenicity have been obtained when vaccine is administered by the intramuscular (deltoid) route. Because of lack of adequate evaluation of other routes, the preferred route of vaccination for adults and older pediatric patients is the deltoid muscle whenever possible. The preferred site for infants and young pediatric patients is the anterolateral aspect of the thigh musculature.[1] *Do Not Inject Intravenously.*

Parenteral drug products should be inspected visually for particulate matter and discoloration prior to administration whenever solution and containers permit.

The dosage may be administered by the intramuscular route as follows:

1. Persons 9 years and older, a single injection of 0.5 mL.
2. Persons 3 years through 8 years, one or two injections of 0.5 mL*.
3. Persons 6 months through 35 months, one or two injections of 0.25 mL.*†

---

*Two doses administered at least one month apart are recommended for children under 9 years of age who are receiving influenza virus vaccine for the first time.

†Note: based on limited data. Because the likelihood of febrile convulsions is greater in this age group, special care should be taken in weighing risks and benefits.

HOW SUPPLIED

NDC 64029-4098-2—5 mL multiple-dose vials (Steri-Vial®)*.

NDC 64029-4098-1—0.5 mL disposable syringes (Steri-Dose®)*. Supplied in packages of 10.

Storage—Store at temperature between 2 and 8°C (36 and 46°F).

Freezing destroys potency.

Shake before use.

REFERENCES

1. Centers for Disease Control and Prevention. Recommendations of the Public Health Service Advisory Committee on Immunization Practices—Prevention and Control of Influenza. *MMWR*, Vol. 47, No. RR-6 (May 1, 1998).
2. Centers for Disease Control. Recommendation of the Public Health Service Immunization Practices Advisory Committee—Influenza Vaccines, 1983–1984. *MMWR*, Vol. 32, No. 26 (July 8, 1983).

IMPORTANT INFORMATION for Group Immunization Programs

If any portion of this product is to be used in an immunization program sponsored by any organization WHERE A TRADITIONAL PHYSICIAN/PATIENT RELATIONSHIP DOES NOT EXIST, each recipient (or legal guardian) should be made aware of the benefits and risks, including a possible risk of a form of paralysis sometimes known as Guillain-Barré syndrome. These are summarized in the current labeling, and informed consent should be obtained from the recipient (or legal guardian) before immunization.

PLEASE CONTACT YOUR LOCAL MONARCH REPRESENTATIVE for copies of the following group immunization forms:

1. Group immunization acknowledgment form
2. Group immunization patient informed consent form (sample)
3. Posters announcing the group immunization program

Rx only.

---

* Registered trademark of Warner-Lambert Co.
Manufactured by: Parkedale Pharmaceuticals, Inc.
Rochester, MI 48307

Shown in Product Identification Guide, page 329

Parke-Davis
Division of Warner-Lambert Company
201 TABOR ROAD
MORRIS PLAINS, NEW JERSEY 07950

For Medical Information Contact:
Generally:
Customer Service
Product/Medical Information
(800) 223-0432
FAX: (973) 540-2248
After Hours and Weekend Emergencies:
(973) 540-6089

PARCODE®
(Parke-Davis Accurate Recognition Code)

Code Number	Product Name
001-006	*Unassigned*
007	**Dilantin® Infatabs®** Each tablet contains 50 mg phenytoin, USP.
008-154	*Unassigned*
155	**Lipitor® Tablets** Each tablet contains atorvastatin calcium equivalent to 10 mg atorvastatin.
156	**Lipitor® Tablets** Each tablet contains atorvastatin calcium equivalent to 20 mg atorvastatin.
157	**Lipitor® Tablets** Each tablet contains atorvastatin calcium equivalent to 40 mg atorvastatin.
158-236	*Unassigned*
237	**Zarontin® Capsules** Each capsule contains 250 mg ethosuximide, USP.
238-269	*Unassigned*
270	**Nardil® Tablets** Each tablet contains 15 mg phenelzine sulfate, USP.
271-351	*Unassigned*
352	**Rezulin® Tablets** Each tablet contains 200 mg troglitazone.
353	**Rezulin® Tablets** Each tablet contains 400 mg troglitazone.
354-356	*Unassigned*
357	**Rezulin® Tablets** Each tablet contains 300 mg troglitazone.
358-361	*Unassigned*
362	**Dilantin® Kapseals®** Each Kapseal contains 100 mg extended phenytoin sodium, USP. The Kapseal is a No. 3 capsule with Orange band. (The Orange band on White capsule is a trademark registered in the US Patent Office.)
363-364	*Unassigned*
365	**Dilantin® Kapseals®** Each Kapseal contains 30 mg extended phenytoin sodium, USP. The Kapseal is a No. 4 capsule with Pink opaque band.
366-424	Unassigned
425	**Estrostep® Tablets** Each tablet contains 1 mg norethindrone acetate and 30 mcg ethinyl estradiol.
426	*Unassigned*
427	**Estrostep® Tablets** Each tablet contains 1 mg norethindrone acetate and 20 mcg ethinyl estradiol.
428-524	*Unassigned*
525	**Celontin® Kapseals®** Each Kapseal contains 300 mg methsuximide, USP. The Kapseal is a Yellow Tint No. 2 capsule with Orange band.

Continued on next page

This product information was prepared in June 1998. On these and other Parke-Davis Products, information may be obtained by addressing PARKE-DAVIS, Division of Warner-Lambert Company, Morris Plains, New Jersey 07950.

Product Listing—Cont.

526	*Unassigned*
527	**Accupril® Tablets**
	Each tablet contains quinapril hydrochloride equivalent to 5 mg quinapril.
528-	
529	*Unassigned*
530	**Accupril® Tablets**
	Each tablet contains quinapril hydrochloride equivalent to 10 mg quinapril.
531	*Unassigned*
532	**Accupril® Tablets**
	Each tablet contains quinapril hydrochloride equivalent to 20 mg quinapril.
533-	
534	*Unassigned*
535	**Accupril® Tablets**
	Each tablet contains quinapril hydrochloride equivalent to 40 mg quinapril.
536	*Unassigned*
537	**Celontin® Kapseals®**
	Each Kapseal contains 150 mg methsuximide, USP.
538-	
539	*Unassigned*
540	**Ponstel® Kapseals®**
	Each Kapseal contains 250 mg mefenamic acid. The Kapseal is an Ivory opaque No. 1 capsule with Light Blue opaque band. The blue band on ivory capsule combination is a Parke-Davis trademark.
541-	
554	*Unassigned*
555	**Estrostep® Tablets**
	Each tablet contains 1 mg norethindrone acetate and 35 mcg ethinyl estradiol.
556-	
621	*Unassigned*
622	**Ferrous Fumarate Tablets**
	Each tablet contains 75 mg ferrous fumarate.
623-	
736	*Unassigned*
737	**Lopid® Tablets**
	Each tablet contains 600 mg gemfibrozil.
738-	
914	*Unassigned*
915	**Loestrin® 1/20 Tablets**
	Each tablet contains norethindrone acetate, 1 mg; ethinyl estradiol, 20 mcg.
916	**Loestrin® 1.5/30 Tablets**
	Each tablet contains norethindrone acetate, 1.5 mg; ethinyl estradiol, 30 mcg.
917-	
999	*Unassigned*

ACCUPRIL®
(Quinapril Hydrochloride Tablets) ℞

USE IN PREGNANCY
When used in pregnancy during the second and third trimesters, ACE inhibitors can cause injury and even death to the developing fetus. When pregnancy is detected, ACCUPRIL should be discontinued as soon as possible. See WARNINGS, Fetal/Neonatal Morbidity and Mortality.

DESCRIPTION
ACCUPRIL® (quinapril hydrochloride) is the hydrochloride salt of quinapril, the ethyl ester of a nonsulfhydryl, angiotensin-converting enzyme (ACE) inhibitor, quinaprilat. Quinapril hydrochloride is chemically described as [3S-[2[R*(R*)], 3R*]]-2-[2-[[1-(ethoxycarbonyl)-3-phenylpropyl]amino] -1- oxopropyl]-1,2,3,4- tetrahydro -3- isoquinolinecarboxylic acid, monohydrochloride. Its empirical formula is $C_{25}H_{30}N_2O_5 \cdot HCl$.
Quinapril hydrochloride is a white to off-white amorphous powder that is freely soluble in aqueous solvents.
ACCUPRIL tablets contain 5 mg, 10 mg, 20 mg, or 40 mg of quinapril for oral administration. Each tablet also contains candelilla wax, crospovidone, gelatin, lactose, magnesium carbonate, magnesium stearate, synthetic red iron oxide, and titanium dioxide.

CLINICAL PHARMACOLOGY
Mechanism of Action: Quinapril is deesterified to the principal metabolite, quinaprilat, which is an inhibitor of ACE activity in human subjects and animals. ACE is a peptidyl dipeptidase that catalyzes the conversion of angiotensin I to the vasoconstrictor, angiotensin II. The effect of quinapril in hypertension and in congestive heart failure (CHF) appears to result primarily from the inhibition of circulating and tissue ACE activity, thereby reducing angiotensin II formation. Quinapril inhibits the elevation in blood pressure caused by intravenously administered angiotensin I, but has no effect on the pressor response to angiotensin II, norepinephrine or epinephrine. Angiotensin II also stimulates the secretion of aldosterone from the adrenal cortex, thereby facilitating renal sodium and fluid reabsorption. Reduced aldosterone secretion by quinapril may result in a small increase in serum potassium. In controlled hypertension trials, treatment with ACCUPRIL alone resulted in mean increases in potassium of 0.07 mmol/L (see PRECAUTIONS). Removal of angiotensin II negative feedback on renin secretion leads to increased plasma renin activity (PRA).
While the principal mechanism of antihypertensive effect is thought to be through the renin-angiotensin-aldosterone system, quinapril exerts antihypertensive actions even in patients with low renin hypertension. ACCUPRIL was an effective antihypertensive in all races studied, although it was somewhat less effective in blacks (usually a predominantly low renin group) than in nonblacks. ACE is identical to kininase II, an enzyme that degrades bradykinin, a potent peptide vasodilator; whether increased levels of bradykinin play a role in the therapeutic effect of quinapril remains to be elucidated.
Pharmacokinetics and Metabolism: Following oral administration, peak plasma quinapril concentrations are observed within one hour. Based on recovery of quinapril and its metabolites in urine, the extent of absorption is at least 60%. The rate and extent of quinapril absorption are diminished moderately (approximately 25–30%) when ACCUPRIL tablets are administered during a high-fat meal. Following absorption, quinapril is deesterified to its major active metabolite, quinaprilat (about 38% of oral dose), and to other minor inactive metabolites. Following multiple oral dosing of ACCUPRIL, there is an effective accumulation half-life of quinaprilat of approximately 3 hours, and peak plasma quinaprilat concentrations are observed approximately 2 hours post-dose. Quinaprilat is eliminated primarily by renal excretion, up to 96% of an IV dose, and has an elimination half-life in plasma of approximately 2 hours and a prolonged terminal phase with a half-life of 25 hours. The pharmacokinetics of quinapril and quinaprilat are linear over a single-dose range of 5–80 mg doses and 40–160 mg in multiple daily doses. Approximately 97% of either quinapril or quinaprilat circulating in plasma is bound to proteins.
In patients with renal insufficiency, the elimination half-life of quinaprilat increases as creatinine clearance decreases. There is a linear correlation between plasma quinaprilat clearance and creatinine clearance. In patients with end-stage renal disease, chronic hemodialysis or continuous ambulatory peritoneal dialysis has little effect on the elimination of quinapril and quinaprilat. Elimination of quinaprilat may be reduced in elderly patients (≥65 years) and in those with heart failure; this reduction is attributable to decrease in renal function (see DOSAGE AND ADMINISTRATION). Quinaprilat concentrations are reduced in patients with alcoholic cirrhosis due to impaired deesterification of quinapril. Studies in rats indicate that quinapril and its metabolites do not cross the blood-brain barrier.
Pharmacodynamics and Clinical Effects
Hypertension: Single doses of 20 mg of ACCUPRIL provide over 80% inhibition of plasma ACE for 24 hours. Inhibition of the pressor response to angiotensin I is shorter-lived, with a 20 mg dose giving 75% inhibition for about 4 hours, 50% inhibition for about 8 hours, and 20% inhibition at 24 hours. With chronic dosing, however, there is substantial inhibition of angiotensin II levels at 24 hours by doses of 20–80 mg.
Administration of 10 to 80 mg of ACCUPRIL to patients with mild to severe hypertension results in a reduction of sitting and standing blood pressure to about the same extent with minimal effect on heart rate. Symptomatic postural hypotension is infrequent although it can occur in patients who are salt- and/or volume-depleted (see WARNINGS). Antihypertensive activity commences within 1 hour with peak effects usually achieved by 2 to 4 hours after dosing. During chronic therapy, most of the blood pressure lowering effect of a given dose is obtained in 1–2 weeks. In multiple-dose studies, 10–80 mg per day in single or divided doses lowered systolic and diastolic blood pressure throughout the dosing interval, with a trough effect of about 5–11/3–7 mm Hg. The trough effect represents about 50% of the peak effect. While the dose-response relationship is relatively flat, doses of 40–80 mg were somewhat more effective at trough than 10–20 mg, and twice daily dosing tended to give a somewhat lower trough blood pressure than once daily dosing with the same total dose. The antihypertensive effect of ACCUPRIL continues during long-term therapy, with no evidence of loss of effectiveness.
Hemodynamic assessments in patients with hypertension indicate that blood pressure reduction produced by quinapril is accompanied by a reduction in total peripheral resistance and renal vascular resistance with little or no change in heart rate, cardiac index, renal blood flow, glomerular filtration rate, or filtration fraction.
Use of ACCUPRIL with a thiazide diuretic gives a blood-pressure lowering effect greater than that seen with either agent alone.
In patients with hypertension, ACCUPRIL 10–40 mg was similar in effectiveness to captopril, enalapril, propranolol, and thiazide diuretics.
Therapeutic effects appear to be the same for elderly (≥65 years of age) and younger adult patients given the same daily dosages, with no increase in adverse events in elderly patients.
Heart Failure: In a placebo-controlled trial involving patients with congestive heart failure treated with digitalis and diuretics, parenteral quinaprilat, the active metabolite of quinapril, reduced pulmonary capillary wedge pressure and systemic vascular resistance and increased cardiac output/index. Similar favorable hemodynamic effects were seen with oral quinapril in baseline-controlled trials, and such effects appeared to be maintained during chronic oral quinapril therapy. Quinapril reduced renal hepatic vascular resistance and increased renal and hepatic blood flow with glomerular filtration rate remaining unchanged.
A significant dose response relationship for improvement in maximal exercise tolerance has been observed with ACCUPRIL therapy. Beneficial effects on the severity of heart failure as measured by New York Heart Association (NYHA) classification and Quality of Life and on symptoms of dyspnea, fatigue, and edema were evident after 6 months in a double blind, placebo controlled study. Favorable effects were maintained for up to two years of open label therapy. The effects of quinapril on long-term mortality in heart failure have not been evaluated.

INDICATIONS AND USAGE
Hypertension
ACCUPRIL is indicated for the treatment of hypertension. It may be used alone or in combination with thiazide diuretics.
Heart Failure
ACCUPRIL is indicated in the management of heart failure as adjunctive therapy when added to conventional therapy including diuretics and/or digitalis.
In using ACCUPRIL, consideration should be given to the fact that another angiotensin converting enzyme inhibitor, captopril, has caused agranulocytosis, particularly in patients with renal impairment or collagen vascular disease. Available data are insufficient to show that ACCUPRIL does not have a similar risk (see WARNINGS).
Angioedema in black patients:
Black patients receiving ACE inhibitor monotherapy have been reported to have a higher incidence of angioedema compared to non-blacks. It should also be noted that in controlled clinical trials ACE inhibitors have an effect on blood pressure that is less in black patients than in non-blacks.

CONTRAINDICATIONS
ACCUPRIL is contraindicated in patients who are hypersensitive to this product and in patients with a history of angioedema related to previous treatment with an ACE inhibitor.

WARNINGS
Anaphylactoid and Possibly Related Reactions
Presumably because angiotensin-converting inhibitors affect the metabolism of eicosanoids and polypeptides, including endogenous bradykinin, patients receiving ACE inhibitors (including Accupril) may be subject to a variety of adverse reactions, some of them serious.
Angioedema: Angioedema of the face, extremities, lips, tongue, glottis, and larynx has been reported in patients treated with ACE inhibitors and has been seen in 0.1% of patients receiving ACCUPRIL.
In two similarly sized U.S. postmarketing trials that, combined, enrolled over 3,000 black patients and over 19,000 non-blacks, angioedema was reported in 0.30% and 0.55% of blacks (in study 1 and 2 respectively) and 0.39% and 0.17% of non-blacks.
Angioedema associated with laryngeal edema can be fatal. If laryngeal stridor or angioedema of the face, tongue, or glottis occurs, treatment with ACCUPRIL should be discontinued immediately, the patient treated in accordance with accepted medical care, and carefully observed until the swelling disappears. In instances where swelling is confined to the face and lips, the condition generally resolves without treatment; antihistamines may be useful in relieving symptoms. **Where there is involvement of the tongue, glottis, or larynx likely to cause airway obstruction, emergency therapy including, but not limited to, subcutaneous epinephrine solution 1:1000 (0.3 to 0.5 mL) should be promptly administered** (see ADVERSE REACTIONS).
Patients with a history of angioedema: Patients with a history of angioedema unrelated to ACE inhibitor therapy may be at increased risk of angioedema while receiving an ACE inhibitor (see also CONTRAINDICATIONS).
Anaphylactoid reactions during desensitization: Two patients undergoing desensitizing treatment with hymenoptera venom while receiving ACE inhibitors sustained life-threatening anaphylactoid reactions. In the same patients,

these reactions were avoided when ACE inhibitors were temporarily withheld, but they reappeared upon inadvertent rechallenge.

Anaphylactoid reactions during membrane exposure: Anaphylactoid reactions have been reported in patients dialyzed with high-flux membranes and treated concomitantly with an ACE inhibitor. Anaphylactoid reactions have also been reported in patients undergoing low-density lipoprotein apheresis with dextran sulfate absorption.

Hepatic Failure: Rarely, ACE inhibitors have been associated with a syndrome that starts with cholestatic jaundice and progresses to fulminant hepatic necrosis and (sometimes) death. The mechanism of this syndrome is not understood. Patients receiving ACE inhibitors who develop jaundice or marked elevations of hepatic enzymes should discontinue the ACE inhibitor and receive appropriate medical follow-up.

Hypotension: Excessive hypotension is rare in patients with uncomplicated hypertension treated with ACCUPRIL alone. Patients with heart failure given ACCUPRIL commonly have some reduction in blood pressure, but discontinuation of therapy because of continuing symptomatic hypotension usually is not necessary when dosing instructions are followed. Caution should be observed when initiating therapy in patients with heart failure (see DOSAGE AND ADMINISTRATION). In controlled studies, syncope was observed in 0.4% of patients (N=3203); this incidence was similar to that observed for captopril (1%) and enalapril (0.8%). Patients at risk of excessive hypotension, sometimes associated with oliguria and/or progressive azotemia, and rarely with acute renal failure and/or death, include patients with the following conditions or characteristics: heart failure, hyponatremia, high dose diuretic therapy, recent intensive diuresis or increase in diuretic dose, renal dialysis, or severe volume and/or salt depletion of any etiology. It may be advisable to eliminate the diuretic (except in patients with heart failure), reduce the diuretic dose or cautiously increase salt intake (except in patients with heart failure) before initiating therapy with ACCUPRIL in patients at risk for excessive hypotension who are able to tolerate such adjustments.

In patients at risk of excessive hypotension, therapy with ACCUPRIL should be started under close medical supervision. Such patients should be followed closely for the first two weeks of treatment and whenever the dose of ACCUPRIL and/or diuretic is increased. Similar considerations may apply to patients with ischemic heart or cerebrovascular disease in whom an excessive fall in blood pressure could result in a myocardial infarction or a cerebrovascular accident.

If excessive hypotension occurs, the patient should be placed in the supine position and, if necessary, receive an intravenous infusion of normal saline. A transient hypotensive response is not a contraindication to further doses of ACCUPRIL, which usually can be given without difficulty once the blood pressure has stabilized. If symptomatic hypotension develops, a dose reduction or discontinuation of ACCUPRIL or concomitant diuretic may be necessary.

Neutropenia/Agranulocytosis: Another ACE inhibitor, captopril, has been shown to cause agranulocytosis and bone marrow depression rarely in patients with uncomplicated hypertension, but more frequently in patients with renal impairment, especially if they also have a collagen vascular disease, such as systemic lupus erythematosus or scleroderma. Agranulocytosis did occur during ACCUPRIL treatment in one patient with a history of neutropenia during previous captopril therapy. Available data from clinical trials of ACCUPRIL are insufficient to show that, in patients without prior reactions to other ACE inhibitors, ACCUPRIL does not cause agranulocytosis at similar rates. As with other ACE inhibitors, periodic monitoring of white blood cell counts in patients with collagen vascular disease and/or renal disease should be considered.

Fetal/Neonatal Morbidity and Mortality: ACE inhibitors can cause fetal and neonatal morbidity and death when administered to pregnant women. Several dozen cases have been reported in the world literature. When pregnancy is detected, ACE inhibitors should be discontinued as soon as possible.

The use of ACE inhibitors during the second and third trimesters of pregnancy has been associated with fetal and neonatal injury, including hypotension, neonatal skull hypoplasia, anuria, reversible or irreversible renal failure, and death. Oligohydramnios has also been reported, presumably resulting from decreased fetal renal function; oligohydramnios in this setting has been associated with fetal limb contractures, craniofacial deformation, and hypoplastic lung development. Prematurity, intrauterine growth retardation, and patent ductus arteriosus have also been reported, although it is not clear whether these occurrences were due to the ACE inhibitor exposure.

These adverse effects do not appear to have resulted from intrauterine ACE inhibitor exposure that has been limited to the first trimester. Mothers whose embryos and fetuses are exposed to ACE inhibitors only during the first trimes-

ter should be so informed. Nonetheless, when patients become pregnant, physicians should make every effort to discontinue the use of ACCUPRIL as soon as possible.

Rarely (probably less often than once in every thousand pregnancies), no alternative to ACE inhibitors will be found. In these rare cases, the mothers should be apprised of the potential hazards to their fetuses, and serial ultrasound examinations should be performed to assess the intraamniotic environment.

If oligohydramnios is observed, ACCUPRIL should be discontinued unless it is considered life-saving for the mother. Contraction stress testing (CST), a non-stress test (NST), or biophysical profiling (BPP) may be appropriate, depending upon the week of pregnancy. Patients and physicians should be aware, however, that oligohydramnios may not appear until after the fetus has sustained irreversible injury.

Infants with histories of *in utero* exposure to ACE inhibitors should be closely observed for hypotension, oliguria, and hyperkalemia. If oliguria occurs, attention should be directed toward support of blood pressure and renal perfusion. Exchange transfusion or dialysis may be required as a means of reversing hypotension and/or substituting for disordered renal function. Removal of ACCUPRIL, which crosses the placenta, from the neonatal circulation is not significantly accelerated by these means.

No teratogenic effects of ACCUPRIL were seen in studies of pregnant rats and rabbits. On a mg/kg basis, the doses used were up to 180 times (in rats) and one time (in rabbits) the maximum recommended human dose.

PRECAUTIONS

General

Impaired renal function: As a consequence of inhibiting the renin-angiotensin-aldosterone system, changes in renal function may be anticipated in susceptible individuals. In patients with severe heart failure whose renal function may depend on the activity of the renin-angiotensin-aldosterone system, treatment with ACE inhibitors, including ACCUPRIL, may be associated with oliguria and/or progressive azotemia and rarely acute renal failure and/or death.

In clinical studies in hypertensive patients with unilateral or bilateral renal artery stenosis, increases in blood urea nitrogen and serum creatinine have been observed in some patients following ACE inhibitor therapy. These increases were almost always reversible upon discontinuation of the ACE inhibitor and/or diuretic therapy. In such patients, renal function should be monitored during the first few weeks of therapy.

Some patients with hypertension or heart failure with no apparent preexisting renal vascular disease have developed increases in blood urea and serum creatinine, usually minor and transient, especially when ACCUPRIL has been given concomitantly with a diuretic. This is more likely to occur in patients with preexisting renal impairment. Dosage reduction and/or discontinuation of any diuretic and/or ACCUPRIL may be required.

Evaluation of patients with hypertension or heart failure should always include assessment of renal function (see DOSAGE AND ADMINISTRATION).

Hyperkalemia and potassium-sparing diuretics: In clinical trials, hyperkalemia (serum potassium ≥5.8 mmol/L) occurred in approximately 2% of patients receiving ACCUPRIL. In most cases, elevated serum potassium levels were isolated values which resolved despite continued therapy. Less than 0.1% of patients discontinued therapy due to hyperkalemia. Risk factors for the development of hyperkalemia include renal insufficiency, diabetes mellitus, and the concomitant use of potassium-sparing diuretics, potassium supplements, and/or potassium-containing salt substitutes, which should be used cautiously, if at all, with ACCUPRIL (see PRECAUTIONS, Drug Interactions).

Cough: Presumably due to the inhibition of the degradation of endogenous bradykinin, persistent nonproductive cough has been reported with all ACE inhibitors, always resolving after discontinuation of therapy. ACE inhibitor-induced cough should be considered in the differential diagnosis of cough.

Surgery/anesthesia: In patients undergoing major surgery or during anesthesia with agents that produce hypotension, ACCUPRIL will block angiotensin II formation secondary to compensatory renin release. If hypotension occurs and is considered to be due to this mechanism, it can be corrected by volume expansion.

Information for Patients

Pregnancy: Female patients of childbearing age should be told about the consequences of second- and third-trimester exposure to ACE inhibitors, and they should also be told that these consequences do not appear to have resulted from intrauterine ACE-inhibitor exposure that has been limited to the first trimester. These patients should be asked to report pregnancies to their physicians as soon as possible.

Angioedema: Angioedema, including laryngeal edema, can occur with treatment with ACE inhibitors, especially following the first dose. Patients should be so advised and told to report immediately any signs or symptoms suggesting angioedema (swelling of face, extremities, eyes, lips,

tongue, difficulty in swallowing or breathing) and to stop taking the drug until they have consulted with their physician (see WARNINGS).

Symptomatic hypotension: Patients should be cautioned that lightheadedness can occur, especially during the first few days of ACCUPRIL therapy, and that it should be reported to a physician. If actual syncope occurs, patients should be told to not take the drug until they have consulted with their physician (see WARNINGS).

All patients should be cautioned that inadequate fluid intake or excessive perspiration, diarrhea, or vomiting can lead to an excessive fall in blood pressure because of reduction in fluid volume, with the same consequences of lightheadedness and possible syncope.

Patients planning to undergo any surgery and/or anesthesia should be told to inform their physician that they are taking an ACE inhibitor.

Hyperkalemia: Patients should be told not to use potassium supplements or salt substitutes containing potassium without consulting their physician (see PRECAUTIONS).

Neutropenia: Patients should be told to report promptly any indication of infection (eg, sore throat, fever) which could be a sign of neutropenia.

NOTE: As with many other drugs, certain advice to patients being treated with ACCUPRIL is warranted. This information is intended to aid in the safe and effective use of this medication. It is not a disclosure of all possible adverse or intended effects.

Drug Interactions

Concomitant diuretic therapy: As with other ACE inhibitors, patients on diuretics, especially those on recently instituted diuretic therapy, may occasionally experience an excessive reduction of blood pressure after initiation of therapy with ACCUPRIL. The possibility of hypotensive effects with ACCUPRIL may be minimized by either discontinuing the diuretic or cautiously increasing salt intake prior to initiation of treatment with ACCUPRIL. If it is not possible to discontinue the diuretic, the starting dose of quinapril should be reduced (see DOSAGE AND ADMINISTRATION).

Agents increasing serum potassium: Quinapril can attenuate potassium loss caused by thiazide diuretics and increase serum potassium when used alone. If concomitant therapy of ACCUPRIL with potassium-sparing diuretics (eg, spironolactone, triamterene, or amiloride), potassium supplements, or potassium-containing salt substitutes is indicated, they should be used with caution along with appropriate monitoring of serum potassium (see PRECAUTIONS).

Tetracycline and other drugs that interact with magnesium: Simultaneous administration of tetracycline with ACCUPRIL reduced the absorption of tetracycline by approximately 28% to 37%, possibly due to the high magnesium content in ACCUPRIL tablets. This interaction should be considered if coprescribing ACCUPRIL and tetracycline or other drugs that interact with magnesium.

Lithium: Increased serum lithium levels and symptoms of lithium toxicity have been reported in patients receiving concomitant lithium and ACE inhibitor therapy. These drugs should be coadministered with caution and frequent monitoring of serum lithium levels is recommended. If a diuretic is also used, it may increase the risk of lithium toxicity.

Other agents: Drug interaction studies of ACCUPRIL with other agents showed:

- Multiple dose therapy with propranolol or cimetidine has no effect on the pharmacokinetics of single doses of ACCUPRIL.
- The anticoagulant effect of a single dose of warfarin (measured by prothrombin time) was not significantly changed by quinapril coadministration twice-daily.
- ACCUPRIL treatment did not affect the pharmacokinetics of digoxin.
- No pharmacokinetic interaction was observed when single doses of ACCUPRIL and hydrochlorothiazide were administered concomitantly.

Carcinogenesis, Mutagenesis, Impairment of Fertility

Quinapril hydrochloride was not carcinogenic in mice or rats when given in doses up to 75 or 100 mg/kg/day (50 to 60 times the maximum human daily dose, respectively, on an mg/kg basis and 3.8 to 10 times the maximum human daily dose when based on an mg/m² basis) for 104 weeks. Female rats given the highest dose level had an increased incidence of mesenteric lymph node hemangiomas and skin/subcutaneous lipomas. Neither quinapril nor quinaprilat were mutagenic in the Ames bacterial assay with or without metabolic activation. Quinapril was also negative in the follow-

Continued on next page

This product information was prepared in June 1998. On these and other Parke-Davis Products, information may be obtained by addressing PARKE-DAVIS, Division of Warner-Lambert Company, Morris Plains, New Jersey 07950.

Accupril—Cont.

ing genetic toxicology studies: *in vitro* mammalian cell point mutation, sister chromatid exchange in cultured mammalian cells, micronucleus test with mice, *in vitro* chromosome aberration with V79 cultured lung cells, and in an *in vivo* cytogenetic study with rat bone marrow. There were no adverse effects on fertility or reproduction in rats at doses up to 100 mg/kg/day (60 and 10 times the maximum daily human dose when based on mg/kg and mg/m², respectively).

Pregnancy

Pregnancy Categories C (first trimester) and D (second and third trimesters): See WARNINGS, Fetal/Neonatal Morbidity and Mortality.

Nursing Mothers

Because ACCUPRIL is secreted in human milk, caution should be exercised when this drug is administered to a nursing woman.

Geriatric Use

Elderly patients exhibited increased area under the plasma concentration time curve (AUC) and peak levels for quinaprilat compared to values observed in younger patients; this appeared to relate to decreased renal function rather than to age itself. In controlled and uncontrolled studies of ACCUPRIL where 918 (21%) patients were 65 years and older, no overall differences in effectiveness or safety were observed between older and younger patients. However, greater sensitivity of some older individual patients cannot be ruled out.

Pediatric Use

The safety and effectiveness of ACCUPRIL in pediatric patients have not been established.

ADVERSE REACTIONS

Hypertension

ACCUPRIL has been evaluated for safety in 4960 subjects and patients. Of these, 3203 patients, including 655 elderly patients, participated in controlled clinical trials. ACCUPRIL has been evaluated for long-term safety in over 1400 patients treated for 1 year or more.

Adverse experiences were usually mild and transient.

In placebo-controlled trials, discontinuation of therapy because of adverse events was required in 4.7% of patients with hypertension.

Adverse experiences probably or possibly related to therapy or of unknown relationship to therapy occurring in 1% or more of the 1563 patients in placebo-controlled hypertension trials who were treated with ACCUPRIL are shown below.

Adverse Events in Placebo-Controlled Trials

	Accupril (N=1563) Incidence (Discontinuance)	Placebo (N=579) Incidence (Discontinuance)
Headache	5.6 (0.7)	10.9 (0.7)
Dizziness	3.9 (0.8)	2.6 (0.2)
Fatigue	2.6 (0.3)	1.0
Coughing	2.0 (0.5)	0.0
Nausea and/or Vomiting	1.4 (0.3)	1.9 (0.2)
Abdominal Pain	1.0 (0.2)	0.7

Heart Failure

Accupril has been evaluated for safety in 1222 ACCUPRIL treated patients. Of these, 632 patients participated in controlled clinical trials. In placebo-controlled trials, discontinuation of therapy because of adverse events was required in 6.8% of patients with congestive heart failure.

Adverse experiences probably or possibly related or of unknown relationship to therapy occurring in 1% or more of the 585 patients in placebo-controlled congestive heart failure trials who were treated with ACCUPRIL are shown below.

	Accupril (N=585) Incidence (Discontinuance)	Placebo (N=295) Incidence (Discontinuance)
Dizziness	7.7 (0.7)	5.1 (1.0)
Coughing	4.3 (0.3)	1.4
Fatigue	2.6 (0.2)	1.4
Nausea and/or Vomiting	2.4 (0.2)	0.7
Chest Pain	2.4	1.0
Hypotension	2.9 (0.5)	1.0
Dyspnea	1.9 (0.2)	2.0
Diarrhea	1.7	1.0
Headache	1.7	1.0 (0.3)
Myalgia	1.5	2.0
Rash	1.4 (0.2)	1.0
Back Pain	1.2	0.3

See PRECAUTIONS. Cough.

Hypertension and/or Heart Failure

Clinical adverse experiences probably, possibly, or definitely related, or of uncertain relationship to therapy occurring in 0.5% to 1.0% (except as noted) of the patients with CHF or hypertension treated with ACCUPRIL (with or without concomitant diuretic) in controlled or uncontrolled trials (N=4847) and less frequent, clinically significant events seen in clinical trials or post-marketing experience (the rarer events are in italics) include (listed by body system):

General: back pain, malaise, viral infections

Cardiovascular: palpitation, vasodilation, tachycardia, *heart failure, hyperkalemia, myocardial infarction, cerebrovascular accident, hypertensive crisis, angina pectoris, orthostatic hypotension, cardiac rhythm disturbances, cardiogenic shock*

Hematology: *hemolytic anemia*

Gastrointestinal: dry mouth or throat, constipation, *gastrointestinal hemorrhage, pancreatitis, abnormal liver function tests*

Nervous/Psychiatric: somnolence, vertigo, syncope, nervousness, depression, insomnia, paresthesia

Integumentary: alopecia, increased sweating, pemphigus, pruritus, *exfoliative dermatitis, photosensitivity reaction, dermatopolymyositis*

Urogenital: impotence, *acute renal failure, worsening renal failure*

Respiratory: *eosinophilic pneumonitis*

Other: amblyopia, pharyngitis, *agranulocytosis, hepatitis, thrombocytopenia*

Fetal/Neonatal Morbidity and Mortality

See WARNINGS, Fetal/Neonatal Morbidity and Mortality.

Angioedema

Angioedema has been reported in patients receiving ACCUPRIL (0.1%). Angioedema associated with laryngeal edema may be fatal. If angioedema of the face, extremities, lips, tongue, glottis, and/or larynx occurs, treatment with ACCUPRIL should be discontinued and appropriate therapy instituted immediately. (See WARNINGS.)

Clinical Laboratory Test Findings

Hematology: (See WARNINGS)

Hyperkalemia: (See PRECAUTIONS)

Creatinine and Blood Urea Nitrogen: Increases (>1.25 times the upper limit of normal) in serum creatinine and blood urea nitrogen were observed in 2% and 2%, respectively, of all patients treated with ACCUPRIL alone. Increases are more likely to occur in patients receiving concomitant diuretic therapy than in those on ACCUPRIL alone. These increases often remit on continued therapy. In controlled studies of heart failure, increases in blood urea nitrogen and serum creatinine were observed in 11% and 8%, respectively, of patients treated with ACCUPRIL; most often these patients were receiving diuretics with or without digitalis.

OVERDOSAGE

No data are available with respect to overdosage in humans. Doses of 1440 to 4280 mg/kg of quinapril cause significant lethality in mice and rats.

The most likely clinical manifestation would be symptoms attributable to severe hypotension.

Laboratory determinations of serum levels of quinapril and its metabolites are not widely available, and such determinations have, in any event, no established role in the management of quinapril overdose.

No data are available to suggest physiological maneuvers (eg, maneuvers to change pH of the urine) that might accelerate elimination of quinapril and its metabolites.

Hemodialysis and peritoneal dialysis have little effect on the elimination of quinapril and quinaprilat. Angiotensin II could presumably serve as a specific antagonist-antidote in the setting of quinapril overdose, but angiotensin II is essentially unavailable outside of scattered research facilities. Because the hypotensive effect of quinapril is achieved through vasodilation and effective hypovolemia, it is reasonable to treat quinapril overdose by infusion of normal saline solution.

DOSAGE AND ADMINISTRATION

Hypertension

Monotherapy: The recommended initial dose of ACCUPRIL in patients not on diuretics is 10 or 20 mg once daily. Dosage should be adjusted according to blood pressure response measured at peak (2–6 hours after dosing) and trough (predosing). Generally, dosage adjustments should be made at intervals of at least 2 weeks. Most patients have required dosages of 20, 40, or 80 mg/day, given as a single dose or in two equally divided doses. In some patients treated once daily, the antihypertensive effect may diminish toward the end of the dosing interval. In such patients an increase in dosage or twice daily administration may be warranted. In general, doses of 40–80 mg and divided doses give a somewhat greater effect at the end of the dosing interval.

Concomitant Diuretics: If blood pressure is not adequately controlled with ACCUPRIL monotherapy, a diuretic may be added. In patients who are currently being treated with a diuretic, symptomatic hypotension occasionally can occur following the initial dose of ACCUPRIL. To reduce the likelihood of hypotension, the diuretic should, if possible, be discontinued 2 to 3 days prior to beginning therapy with ACCUPRIL (see WARNINGS). Then, if blood pressure is not controlled with ACCUPRIL alone, diuretic therapy should be resumed.

If the diuretic cannot be discontinued, an initial dose of 5 mg ACCUPRIL should be used with careful medical supervision for several hours and until blood pressure has stabilized.

The dosage should subsequently be titrated (as described above) to the optimal response (see WARNINGS, PRECAUTIONS, and Drug Interactions).

Renal Impairment: Kinetic data indicate that the apparent elimination half-life of quinaprilat increases as creatinine clearance decreases. Recommended starting doses, based on clinical and pharmacokinetic data from patients with renal impairment, are as follows:

Creatinine Clearance	Maximum Recommend Initial Dose
>60 mL/min	10 mg
30–60 mL/min	5 mg
10–30 mL/min	2.5 mg
<10 mL/min	Insufficient data for dosage recommendation

Patients should subsequently have their dosage titrated (as described above) to the optimal response.

Elderly (≥65 years): The recommended initial dosage of ACCUPRIL in elderly patients is 10 mg given once daily followed by titration (as described above) to the optimal response.

Heart Failure

ACCUPRIL is indicated as adjunctive therapy when added to conventional therapy including diuretics and/or digitalis. The recommended starting dose is 5 mg twice daily. This dose may improve symptoms of heart failure, but increases in exercise duration have generally required higher doses. Therefore, if the initial dosage of ACCUPRIL is well tolerated, patients should then be titrated at weekly intervals until an effective dose, usually 20 to 40 mg daily given in two equally divided doses, is reached or undesirable hypotension, orthostasis, or azotemia (see WARNINGS) prohibit reaching this dose.

Following the initial dose of ACCUPRIL, the patient should be observed under medical supervision for at least two hours for the presence of hypotension or orthostasis and, if present, until blood pressure stabilizes. The appearance of hypotension, orthostasis, or azotemia early in dose titration should not preclude further careful dose titration. Consideration should be given to reducing the dose of concomitant diuretics.

DOSE ADJUSTMENTS IN PATIENTS WITH HEART FAILURE AND RENAL IMPAIRMENT OR HYPONATREMIA

Pharmacokinetic data indicate that quinapril elimination is dependent on level of renal function. In patients with heart failure and renal impairment, the recommended initial dose of ACCUPRIL is 5 mg in patients with a creatinine clearance above 30 mL/min and 2.5 mg in patients with a creatinine clearance of 10 to 30 mL/min. There is insufficient data for dosage recommendation in patients with a creatinine clearance less than 10 mL/min. (See DOSAGE AND ADMINISTRATION, Heart Failure, WARNINGS, and PRECAUTIONS, Drug Interactions.)

If the initial dose is well tolerated, ACCUPRIL may be administered the following day as a twice daily regimen. In the absence of excessive hypotension or significant deterioration of renal function, the dose may be increased at weekly intervals based on clinical and hemodynamic response.

HOW SUPPLIED

ACCUPRIL tablets are supplied as follows:

5-mg tablets: brown, film-coated, elliptical, scored tablets, coded "PD 527" on one side and "5" on the other.

N0071-0527-23 bottles of 90 tablets

N0071-0527-40 10 × 10 unit dose blisters

10-mg tablets: brown, film-coated, triangular tablets, coded "PD 530" on one side and "10" on the other.

N0071-0530-23 bottles of 90 tablets

N0071-0530-40 10 × 10 unit dose blisters

20-mg tablets: brown, film-coated, round tablets, coded "PD 532" on one side and "20" on the other.

N0071-0532-23 bottles of 90 tablets

N0071-0532-40 10 × 10 unit dose blisters

40-mg tablets: brown, film-coated, elliptical tablets, coded "PD 535" on one side and "40" on the other.

N0071-0535-23 bottles of 90 tablets

Dispense in well-closed containers as defined in the USP.

Storage: Store at controlled room temperature 15°–30°C (59°–86°F). Protect from light.

PARKE-DAVIS
Div. of Warner-Lambert Co.
Morris Plains, NJ 07950 USA
Shown in Product Identification Guide, page 329

0527G075

BENADRYL® ℞
[bĕ 'nă-dril]
(Diphenhydramine Hydrochloride Injection, USP)

DESCRIPTION

Benadryl (diphenhydramine hydrochloride) is an antihistamine drug having the chemical name 2-(Diphenylmethoxy)-N, N-dimethylethylamine hydrochloride. It occurs as a white, crystalline powder, is freely soluble in water and alcohol and has a molecular weight of 291.82. The molecular formula is $C_{17}H_{21}NO·HCl$.
Benadryl in the parenteral form is a sterile, pyrogen-free solution available in a concentration of 50 mg of diphenhydramine hydrochloride per mL. The solutions for parenteral use have been adjusted to a pH between 5.0 and 6.0 with either sodium hydroxide or hydrochloric acid. The multidose Steri-Vials® contain 0.1 mg/mL benzethonium chloride as a germicidal agent.

CLINICAL PHARMACOLOGY

Diphenhydramine hydrochloride is an antihistamine with anticholinergic (drying) and sedative side effects. Antihistamines appear to compete with histamine for cell receptor sites on effector cells.
Benadryl in the injectable form has a rapid onset of action. Diphenhydramine hydrochloride is widely distributed throughout the body, including the CNS. A portion of the drug is excreted unchanged in the urine, while the rest is metabolized via the liver. Detailed information on the pharmacokinetics of Diphenhydramine Hydrochloride Injection is not available.

INDICATIONS AND USAGE

Benadryl in the injectable form is effective in adults and pediatric patients, other than premature infants and neonates, for the following conditions when Benadryl in the oral form is impractical.
Antihistaminic: For amelioration of allergic reactions to blood or plasma, in anaphylaxis as an adjunct to epinephrine and other standard measures after the acute symptoms have been controlled, and for other uncomplicated allergic conditions of the immediate type when oral therapy is impossible or contraindicated.
Motion Sickness: For active treatment of motion sickness.
Antiparkinsonism: For use in parkinsonism, when oral therapy is impossible or contraindicated, as follows: parkinsonism in the elderly who are unable to tolerate more potent agents, mild cases of parkinsonism in other age groups, and in other cases of parkinsonism in combination with centrally acting anticholinergic agents.

CONTRAINDICATIONS

Use in Neonates or Premature Infants
This drug should *not* be used in neonates or premature infants.
Use in Nursing Mothers
Because of the higher risk of antihistamines for infants generally, and for neonates and prematures in particular, antihistamine therapy is contraindicated in nursing mothers.
Use as a Local Anesthetic
Because of the risk of local necrosis, this drug should not be used as a local anesthetic.
Antihistamines are also contraindicated in the following conditions:
Hypersensitivity to diphenhydramine hydrochloride and other antihistamines of similar chemical structure.

WARNINGS

Antihistamines should be used with considerable caution in patients with narrow-angle glaucoma, stenosing peptic ulcer, pyloroduodenal obstruction, symptomatic prostatic hypertrophy, or bladder-neck obstruction.
Local necrosis has been associated with the use of subcutaneous or intradermal use of intravenous Benadryl.
Use in Pediatric Patients
In pediatric patients, especially, antihistamines in *overdosage* may cause hallucinations, convulsions, or death.
As in adults, antihistamines may diminish mental alertness in pediatric patients. In the young pediatric patient, particularly, they may produce excitation.
Use in the Elderly (approximately 60 years or older)
Antihistamines are more likely to cause dizziness, sedation, and hypotension in elderly patients.

PRECAUTIONS

General
Diphenhydramine hydrochloride has an atropine-like action and, therefore, should be used with caution in patients with a history of bronchial asthma, increased intraocular pressure, hyperthyroidism, cardiovascular disease or hypertension. Use with caution in patients with lower respiratory disease including asthma.
Information for Patients
Patients taking diphenhydramine hydrochloride should be advised that this drug may cause drowsiness and has an additive effect with alcohol.
Patients should be warned about engaging in activities requiring mental alertness such as driving a car or operating appliances, machinery, etc.
Drug Interactions
Diphenhydramine hydrochloride has additive effects with alcohol and other CNS depressants (hypnotics, sedatives, tranquilizers, etc.).
MAO inhibitors prolong and intensify the anticholinergic (drying) effects of antihistamines.
Carcinogenesis, Mutagenesis, Impairment of Fertility
Long-term studies in animals to determine mutagenic and carcinogenic potential have not been performed.
Pregnancy
Pregnancy Category B. Reproduction studies have been performed in rats and rabbits at doses up to 5 times the human dose and have revealed no evidence of impaired fertility or harm to the fetus due to diphenhydramine hydrochloride. There are, however, no adequate and well-controlled studies in pregnant women. Because animal reproduction studies are not always predictive of human response, this drug should be used during pregnancy only if clearly needed.
Pediatric Use
Benadryl should not be used in neonates and premature infants (see CONTRAINDICATIONS).
Benadryl may diminish mental alertness, or, in the young pediatric patient, cause excitation. Overdosage may cause hallucinations, convulsions, or death (see WARNINGS, and OVERDOSAGE).
See also DOSAGE AND ADMINISTRATION Section.

ADVERSE REACTIONS
The most frequent adverse reactions are underscored.
1. *General:* Urticaria, drug rash, anaphylactic shock, photosensitivity, excessive perspiration, chills, dryness of mouth, nose, and throat
2. *Cardiovascular System:* Hypotension, headache, palpitations, ta chycardia, extrasystoles
3. *Hematologic System:* Hemolytic anemia, thrombocytopenia, agranulocytosis
4. *Nervous System:* Sedation, sleepiness, dizziness, disturbed coordination, fatigue, confusion, restlessness, excitation, nervousness, tremor, irritability, insomnia, euphoria, paresthesia, blurred vision, diplopia, vertigo, tinnitus, acute labyrinthitis, neuritis, convulsions
5. *GI System:* Epigastric distress, anorexia, nausea, vomiting, diarrhea, constipation
6. *GU System:* Urinary frequency, difficult urination, urinary retention, early menses
7. *Respiratory System:* Thickening of bronchial secretions, tightness of chest or throat and wheezing, nasal stuffiness

OVERDOSAGE

Antihistamine overdosage reactions may vary from central nervous system depression to stimulation. Stimulation is particularly likely in pediatric patients. Atropine-like signs and symptoms, dry mouth; fixed, dilated pupils; flushing, and gastrointestinal symptoms may also occur.
Stimulants should not be used.
Vasopressors may be used to treat hypotension.

DOSAGE AND ADMINISTRATION

THIS PRODUCT IS FOR INTRAVENOUS OR INTRAMUSCULAR ADMINISTRATION ONLY.
Benadryl in the injectable form is indicated when the oral form is impractical.
Parenteral drug products should be inspected visually for particulate matter and discoloration prior to administration, whenever solution and container permit.
DOSAGE SHOULD BE INDIVIDUALIZED ACCORDING TO THE NEEDS AND THE RESPONSE OF THE PATIENT.
Pediatric Patients, other than premature infants and neonates: 5 mg/kg/24 hr or 150 mg/m²/24 hr. Maximum daily dosage is 300 mg. Divide into four doses, administered intravenously at a rate generally not exceeding 25 mg/min, or deep intramuscularly.
Adults: 10 to 50 mg intravenously at a rate generally not exceeding 25 mg/min, or deep intramuscularly, 100 mg if required; maximum daily dosage is 400 mg.

HOW SUPPLIED

Benadryl in parenteral form is supplied as:
Benadryl Steri-Vials®—Sterile, pyrogen-free solution containing 50 mg diphenhydramine hydrochloride in each milliliter of solution with 0.1 mg/mL benzethonium chloride as a germicidal agent. Available in 10-mL (N-0071-4402-10) Steri-Vials.
—sterile, pyrogen-free solution containing 50 mg diphenhydramine hydrochloride in each milliliter of solution. Available in packages of twenty-five 1-mL (N 0071-4259-13) Steri-Vials.
Benadryl Steri-Dose®—sterile, pyrogen-free solution containing 50 mg diphenhydramine hydrochloride in a 1-mL disposable syringe (Steri-Dose). Available in packages of ten syringes (N 0071-4259-45).
Benadryl Ampoule—sterile, pyrogen-free solution containing 50 mg diphenhydramine hydrochloride in a 1-mL ampoule. Available in packages of ten (N 0071-4259-03).

STORAGE CONDITIONS

Store at controlled room temperature 15°–30°C (59°–86°F). Protect from freezing and light.
Rx only
©1997–'98, Warner-Lambert Co.
Manufactured by:
Parkedale Pharmaceuticals, Inc.
Rochester, MI 48307
For:
PARKE-DAVIS
Div of Warner-Lambert Co.
Morris Plains, NJ 07950 USA
Revised April 1998   4259G444

CELONTIN® KAPSEALS® ℞
[cĕ "lŏn 'tĭn]
(methsuximide capsules, USP)

DESCRIPTION

Celontin (methsuximide) is an anticonvulsant succinimide, chemically designated as N,2-Dimethyl-2-phenylsuccinimide.
Each Celontin capsule contains 150 mg or 300 mg methsuximide, USP. Also contains starch, NF. The capsule and band contain citric acid, USP; colloidal silicon dioxide, NF; D&C yellow No. 10; FD&C red No. 3; FD&C yellow No. 6 (Sunset Yellow); gelatin, NF; glyceryl monooleate; sodium benzoate, NF; sodium lauryl sulfate NF. The 150-mg capsule and band also contain FD&C blue No. 1; titanium dioxide, USP. The 300-mg capsule and band also contain polyethylene glycol 200.

ACTION

Methsuximide suppresses the paroxysmal three cycle per second spike and wave activity associated with lapses of consciousness which is common in absence (petit mal) seizures. The frequency of epileptiform attacks is reduced, apparently by depression of the motor cortex and elevation of the threshold of the central nervous system to convulsive stimuli.

INDICATION

Celontin is indicated for the control of absence (petit mal) seizures that are refractory to other drugs.

CONTRAINDICATION

Methsuximide should not be used in patients with a history of hypersensitivity to succinimides.

WARNINGS

Blood dyscrasias, including some with fatal outcome, have been reported to be associated with the use of succinimides; therefore, periodic blood counts should be performed. Should signs and/or symptoms of infection (eg sore throat, fever) develop, blood counts should be considered at that point.
It has been reported that succinimides have produced morphological and functional changes in animal liver. For this reason, methsuximide should be administered with extreme caution to patients with known liver or renal disease. Periodic urinalysis and liver function studies are advised for all patients receiving the drug.
Cases of systemic lupus erythematosus have been reported with the use of succinimides. The physician should be alert to this possibility.

Continued on next page

This product information was prepared in June 1998. On these and other Parke-Davis Products, information may be obtained by addressing PARKE-DAVIS, Division of Warner-Lambert Company, Morris Plains, New Jersey 07950.

Celontin—Cont.

USAGE IN PREGNANCY

Reports suggest an association between the use of anticonvulsant drugs by women with epilepsy and an elevated incidence of birth defects in children born to these women. Data are more extensive with respect to phenytoin and phenobarbital, but these are also the most commonly prescribed anticonvulsants; less systematic or anecdotal reports suggest a possible similar association with the use of all known anticonvulsant drugs.

The reports suggesting an elevated incidence of birth defects in children of drug-treated epileptic women cannot be regarded as adequate to prove a definite cause and effect relationship. There are intrinsic methodologic problems in obtaining adequate data on drug teratogenicity in humans; the possibility also exists that other factors, eg, genetic factors or the epileptic condition itself, may be more important than drug therapy in leading to birth defects. The great majority of mothers on anticonvulsant medication deliver normal infants. It is important to note that anticonvulsant drugs should not be discontinued in patients in whom the drug is administered to prevent major seizures because of the strong possibility of precipitating status epilepticus with attendant hypoxia and threat to life. In individual cases where the severity and frequency of the seizure disorder are such that the removal of medication does not pose a serious threat to the patient, discontinuation of the drug may be considered prior to and during pregnancy, although it cannot be said with any confidence that even minor seizures do not pose some hazard to the developing embryo or fetus.

The prescribing physician will wish to weigh these considerations in treating or counseling epileptic women of childbearing potential.

PRECAUTIONS

General:

It is recommended that the physician withdraw the drug slowly on the appearance of unusual depression, aggressiveness, or other behavioral alterations.

As with other anticonvulsants, it is important to proceed slowly when increasing or decreasing dosage, as well as when adding or eliminating other medication. Abrupt withdrawal of anticonvulsant medication may precipitate absence (petit mal) status.

Methsuximide, when used alone in mixed types of epilepsy, may increase the frequency of grand mal seizures in some patients.

Information for Patients:

Methsuximide may impair the mental and/or physical abilities required for the performance of potentially hazardous tasks, such as driving a motor vehicle or other such activity requiring alertness, therefore, the patient should be cautioned accordingly.

Patients taking methsuximide should be advised of the importance of adhering strictly to the prescribed dosage regimen.

Patients should be instructed to promptly contact their physician if they develop signs and/or symptoms suggesting an infection (eg sore throat, fever).

ADVICE TO THE PHARMACIST AND PATIENT: Since methsuximide has a relatively low melting temperature (124°F), storage conditions which may promote high temperatures (closed cars, delivery vans, or storage near steam pipes) should be avoided. Do not dispense or use capsules that are not full or in which contents have melted. Effectiveness may be reduced. Protect from excessive heat (104°F).

Drug Interactions:

Since Celontin (methsuximide) may interact with concurrently administered antiepileptic drugs, periodic serum level determinations of these drugs may be necessary (eg methsuximide may increase the plasma concentrations of phenytoin and phenobarbital).

Pregnancy:

See WARNINGS.

Pediatric Use:

See DOSAGE AND ADMINISTRATION.

ADVERSE REACTIONS

Gastrointestinal System: Gastrointestinal symptoms occur frequently and have included nausea or vomiting, anorexia, diarrhea, weight loss, epigastric and abdominal pain, and constipation.

Hemopoietic System: Hemopoietic complications associated with the administration of methsuximide have included eosinophilia, leukopenia, monocytosis, and pancytopenia with or without bone marrow suppression.

Nervous System: Neurologic and sensory reactions reported during therapy with methsuximide have included drowsiness, ataxia or dizziness, irritability and nervousness, headache, blurred vision, photophobia, hiccups, and insomnia. Drowsiness, ataxia, and dizziness have been the most frequent side effects noted. Psychologic abnormalities have included confusion, instability, mental slowness, depression, hypochondriacal behavior, and aggressiveness. There have been rare reports of psychosis, suicidal behavior, and auditory hallucinations.

Integumentary System: Dermatologic manifestations which have occurred with the administration of methsuximide have included urticaria, Stevens-Johnson syndrome, and pruritic erythematous rashes.

Cardiovascular: Hyperemia.

Genitourinary system: Proteinuria, microscopic hematuria

Body as a Whole: Periorbital edema.

OVERDOSAGE

Acute overdoses may produce nausea, vomiting, and CNS depression including coma with respiratory depression. Methsuximide poisoning may follow a biphasic course. Following an initial comatose state, patients have awakened and then relapsed into a coma within 24 hours. It is believed that an active metabolite of methsuximide, N-desmethylmethsuximide, is responsible for this biphasic profile. It is important to follow plasma levels of N-desmethylmethsuximide in methsuximide poisonings. Levels greater than 40 µg/mL have caused toxicity and coma has been seen at levels of 150 µg/mL.

Treatment:

Treatment should include emesis (unless the patient is or could rapidly become obtunded, comatose, or convulsing) or gastric lavage, activated charcoal, cathartics, and general supportive measures. Charcoal hemoperfusion may be useful in removing the N-desmethyl metabolite of methsuximide. Forced diuresis and exchange transfusions are ineffective.

DOSAGE AND ADMINISTRATION

Optimum dosage of Celontin must be determined by trial. A suggested dosage schedule is 300 mg per day for the first week. If required, dosage may be increased thereafter at weekly intervals by 300 mg per day for the three weeks following to a daily dosage of 1.2 g. Because therapeutic effect and tolerance vary among patients, therapy with Celontin must be individualized according to the response of each patient. Optimal dosage is that amount of Celontin which is barely sufficient to control seizures so that side effects may be kept to a minimum. The smaller capsule (150 mg) facilitates administration to small children.

Celontin may be administered in combination with other anticonvulsants when other forms of epilepsy coexist with absence (petit mal).

HOW SUPPLIED

N 0071-0525-24 (P-D 525)—Celontin Kapseals, #1 capsule each containing 300 mg methsuximide; bottles of 100.

N 0071-0537-24 (P-D 537)—Celontin Kapseals, Half Strength, #3 capsule each containing 150 mg methsuximide, bottles of 100.

Store at controlled room temperature 15°–30°C (59°–86°F). Protect from light and moisture.

Protect from excessive heat (104°F).

Rx only

©1997–'98, Warner-Lambert Co.

Revised March 1998 0537G095

Shown in Product Identification Guide, page 329

CEREBYX® ℞

(Fosphenytoin Sodium Injection)

DESCRIPTION

Cerebyx® (fosphenytoin sodium injection) is a prodrug intended for parenteral administration; its active metabolite is phenytoin. Each Cerebyx vial contains 75 mg/mL fosphenytoin sodium (hereafter referred to as fosphenytoin) **equivalent to 50 mg/mL phenytoin sodium** after administration. Cerebyx is supplied in vials as a ready-mixed solution in Water for Injection, USP, and Tromethamine, USP (TRIS), buffer adjusted to pH 8.6 to 9.0 with either Hydrochloric Acid, NF, or Sodium Hydroxide, NF. Cerebyx is a clear, colorless to pale yellow, sterile solution.

The chemical name of fosphenytoin is 5,5-diphenyl-3-[(phosphonooxy)methyl]-2,4-imidazolidinedione disodium salt. The molecular structure of fosphenytoin is:

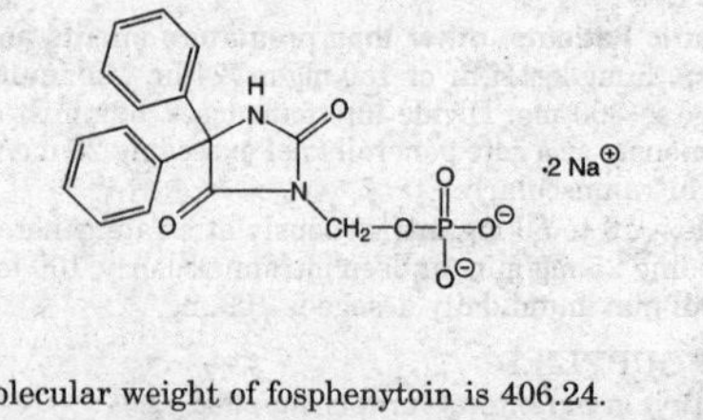

The molecular weight of fosphenytoin is 406.24.

IMPORTANT NOTE: Throughout all Cerebyx® product labeling, the amount and concentration of fosphenytoin is expressed in terms of phenytoin sodium equivalents (PE). Fosphenytoin's weight is expressed as phenytoin sodium equivalents to avoid the need to perform molecular weight-based adjustments when converting between fosphenytoin and phenytoin sodium doses. Cerebyx should always be prescribed and dispensed in phenytoin sodium equivalent units (PE) (see DOSAGE AND ADMINISTRATION**).**

CLINICAL PHARMACOLOGY

Introduction

Following parenteral administration of Cerebyx, fosphenytoin is converted to the anticonvulsant phenytoin. For every mmol of fosphenytoin administered, one mmol of phenytoin is produced. The pharmacological and toxicological effects of fosphenytoin include those of phenytoin. However, the hydrolysis of fosphenytoin to phenytoin yields two metabolites, phosphate and formaldehyde. Formaldehyde is subsequently converted to formate, which is in turn metabolized via a folate dependent mechanism. Although phosphate and formaldehyde (formate) have potentially important biological effects, these effects typically occur at concentrations considerably in excess of those obtained when Cerebyx is administered under conditions of use recommended in this labeling.

Mechanism of Action

Fosphenytoin is a prodrug of phenytoin and accordingly, its anticonvulsant effects are attributable to phenytoin.

After IV administration to mice, fosphenytoin blocked the tonic phase of maximal electroshock seizures at doses equivalent to those effective for phenytoin. In addition to its ability to suppress maximal electroshock seizures in mice and rats, phenytoin exhibits anticonvulsant activity against kindled seizures in rats, audiogenic seizures in mice, and seizures produced by electrical stimulation of the brainstem in rats. The cellular mechanisms of phenytoin thought to be responsible for its anticonvulsant actions include modulation of voltage-dependent sodium channels of neurons, inhibition of calcium flux across neuronal membranes, modulation of voltage-dependent calcium channels of neurons, and enhancement of the sodium-potassium ATPase activity of neurons and glial cells. The modulation of sodium channels may be a primary anticonvulsant mechanism because this property is shared with several other anticonvulsants in addition to phenytoin.

Pharmacokinetics and Drug Metabolism

Fosphenytoin

Absorption/Bioavailability: *Intravenous:* When Cerebyx is administered by IV infusion, maximum plasma fosphenytoin concentrations are achieved at the end of the infusion. Fosphenytoin has a half-life of approximately 15 minutes.

Intramuscular: Fosphenytoin is completely bioavailable following IM administration of Cerebyx. Peak concentrations occur at approximately 30 minutes postdose. Plasma fosphenytoin concentrations following IM administration are lower but more sustained than those following IV administration due to the time required for absorption of fosphenytoin from the injection site.

Distribution: Fosphenytoin is extensively bound (95% to 99%) to human plasma proteins, primarily albumin. Binding to plasma proteins is saturable with the result that the percent bound decreases as total fosphenytoin concentrations increase. Fosphenytoin displaces phenytoin from protein binding sites. The volume of distribution of fosphenytoin increases with Cerebyx dose and rate. and ranges from 4.3 to 10.8 liters.

Metabolism and Elimination: The conversion half-life of fosphenytoin to phenytoin is approximately 15 minutes. The mechanism of fosphenytoin conversion has not been determined, but phosphatases probably play a major role. Fosphenytoin is not excreted in urine. Each mmol of fosphenytoin is metabolized to 1 mmol of phenytoin, phosphate, and formate (see CLINICAL PHARMACOLOGY, Introduction and PRECAUTIONS, Phosphate Load for Renally Impaired Patients).

Phenytoin (after Cerebyx administration)

In general, IM administration of Cerebyx generates systemic phenytoin concentrations that are similar enough to oral phenytoin sodium to allow essentially interchangeable use.

The pharmacokinetics of fosphenytoin following IV administration of Cerebyx, however, are complex, and when used in an emergency setting (eg, status epilepticus), differences in rate of availability of phenytoin could be critical. Studies have therefore empirically determined an infusion rate for Cerebyx that gives a rate and extent of phenytoin systemic availability similar to that of a 50 mg/min phenytoin sodium infusion.

A dose of 15 to 20 mg PE/kg of Cerebyx infused at 100 to 150 mg PE/min yields plasma free phenytoin concentrations over time that approximate those achieved when an equivalent dose of phenytoin sodium (eg, parenteral Dilantin®) is administered at 50 mg/min (see DOSAGE AND ADMINISTRATION, WARNINGS).

[See figure at top of next column]

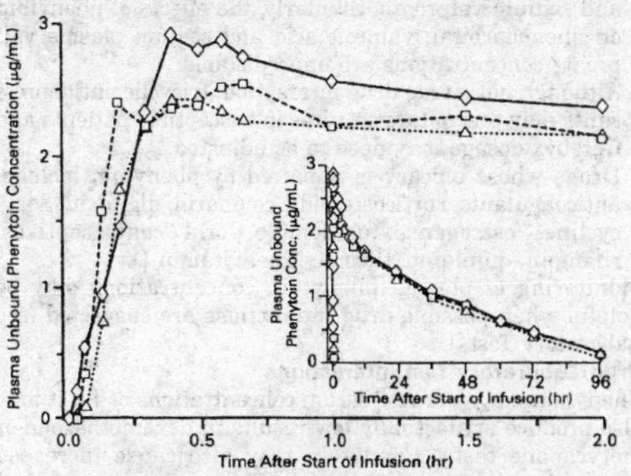

FIGURE 1. Mean plasma unbound phenytoin concentrations following IV administration of 1200 mg PE Cerebyx infused at 100 mg PE/min (triangles) or 150 mg PE/min (squares) and 1200 mg Dilantin infused at 50 mg/min (diamonds) to healthy subjects (N = 12). Inset shows time course for the entire 96-hour sampling period.

Following administration of single IV Cerebyx doses of 400 to 1200 mg PE, mean maximum total phenytoin concentrations increase in proportion to dose, but do not change appreciably with changes in infusion rate. In contrast, mean maximum unbound phenytoin concentrations increase with both dose and rate.

Absorption/Bioavailability: Fosphenytoin is completely converted to phenytoin following IV administration, with a half-life of approximately 15 minutes. Fosphenytoin is also completely converted to phenytoin following IM administration and plasma total phenytoin concentrations peak in approximately 3 hours.

Distribution: Phenytoin is highly bound to plasma proteins, primarily albumin, although to a lesser extent than fosphenytoin. In the absence of fosphenytoin, approximately 12% of total plasma phenytoin is unbound over the clinically relevant concentration range. However, fosphenytoin displaces phenytoin from plasma protein binding sites. This increases the fraction of phenytoin unbound (up to 30% unbound) during the period required for conversion of fosphenytoin to phenytoin (approximately 0.5 to 1 hour postinfusion).

Metabolism and Elimination: Phenytoin derived from administration of Cerebyx is extensively metabolized in the liver and excreted in urine primarily as 5-(p-hydroxyphenyl)-5-phenythydantoin and its glucuronide; little unchanged phenytoin (1%-5% of the Cerebyx dose) is recovered in urine. Phenytoin hepatic metabolism is saturable, and following administration of single IV Cerebyx doses of 400 to 1200 mg PE, total and unbound phenytoin AUC values increase disproportionately with dose. Mean total phenytoin half-life values (12.0 to 28.9 hr) following Cerebyx administration at these doses are similar to those after equal doses of parenteral Dilantin and tend to be greater at higher plasma phenytoin concentrations.

Special Populations

Patients with Renal or Hepatic Disease: Due to an increased fraction of unbound phenytoin in patients with renal or hepatic disease, or in those with hypoalbuminemia, the interpretation of total phenytoin plasma concentrations should be made with caution (see DOSAGE AND ADMINISTRATION). Unbound phenytoin concentrations may be more useful in these patient populations. After IV administration of Cerebyx to patients with renal and/or hepatic disease, or in those with hypoalbuminemia, fosphenytoin clearance to phenytoin may be increased without similar increase in phenytoin clearance. This has the potential to increase the frequency and severity of adverse events (see PRECAUTIONS).

Age: The effect of age was evaluated in patients 5 to 98 years of age. Patient age had no significant impact on fosphenytoin pharmacokinetics. Phenytoin clearance tends to decrease with increasing age (20% less in patients over 70 years of age relative to that in patients 20–30 years of age). Phenytoin dosing requirements are highly variable and must be individualized (see DOSAGE AND ADMINISTRATION).

Gender and Race: Gender and race have no significant impact on fosphenytoin or phenytoin pharmacokinetics.

Pediatrics: Only limited pharmacokinetic data are available in children (N=8; age 5 to 10 years). In these patients with status epilepticus who received loading doses of Cerebyx, the plasma fosphenytoin, total phenytoin, and unbound phenytoin concentration-time profiles did not signal any major differences from those in adult patients with status epilepticus receiving comparable doses.

Clinical Studies

Infusion tolerance was evaluated in clinical studies. One double-blind study assessed infusion-site tolerance of equivalent loading doses (15–20 mg PE/kg) of Cerebyx infused at 150 mg PE/min or phenytoin infused at 50 mg/min. The study demonstrated better local tolerance (pain and burning at the infusion site), fewer disruptions of the infusion, and a shorter infusion period for Cerebyx-treated patients (Table 1).

TABLE 1. Infusion Tolerance of Equivalent Loading Doses of IV Cerebyx and IV Phenytoin

	IV Cerebyx N=90	IV Phenytoin N=22
Local Intolerance	9%[a]	90%
Infusion Disrupted	21%	67%
Average Infusion Time	13 min	44 min

[a] Percent of patients.

Cerebyx-treated patients, however, experienced more systemic sensory disturbances (see PRECAUTIONS, Sensory Disturbances).

Infusion disruptions in Cerebyx-treated patients were primarily due to systemic burning, pruritus, and/or paresthesia while those in phenytoin-treated patients were primarily due to pain and burning at the infusion site (see Table 1).

In a double-blind study investigating temporary substitution of Cerebyx for oral phenytoin, IM Cerebyx was as well-tolerated as IM placebo. IM Cerebyx resulted in a slight increase in transient, mild to moderate local itching (23% of patients vs 11% of IM placebo-treated patients at any time during the study). This study also demonstrated that equimolar doses of IM Cerebyx may be substituted for oral phenytoin sodium with no dosage adjustments needed when initiating IM or returning to oral therapy. In contrast, switching between IM and oral phenytoin requires dosage adjustments because of slow and erratic phenytoin absorption from muscle.

INDICATIONS AND USAGE

Cerebyx is indicated for short-term parenteral administration when other means of phenytoin administration are unavailable, inappropriate, or deemed less advantageous. The safety and effectiveness of Cerebyx in this use has not been systematically evaluated for more than 5 days.

Cerebyx can be used for the control of generalized convulsive status epilepticus and prevention and treatment of seizures occurring during neurosurgery. It can also be substituted, short-term, for oral phenytoin.

CONTRAINDICATIONS

Cerebyx is contraindicated in patients who have demonstrated hypersensitivity to Cerebyx or its ingredients, or to phenytoin or other hydantoins.

Because of the effect of parenteral phenytoin on ventricular automaticity, Cerebyx is contraindicated in patients with sinus bradycardia, sino-atrial block, second and third degree A-V block, and Adams-Strokes syndrome.

WARNINGS

DOSES OF CEREBYX ARE EXPRESSED AS THEIR PHENYTOIN SODIUM EQUIVALENTS IN THIS LABELING (PE=phenytoin sodium equivalent).

DO NOT, THEREFORE, MAKE ANY ADJUSTMENT IN THE RECOMMENDED DOSES WHEN SUBSTITUTING CEREBYX FOR PHENYTOIN SODIUM OR VICE VERSA.

The following warnings are based on experience with Cerebyx or phenytoin.

Status Epilepticus Dosing Regimen

- **Do not administer Cerebyx at a rate greater than 150 mg PE/min.**

The dose of IV Cerebyx (15 to 20 mg PE/kg) that is used to treat status epilepticus is administered at a maximum rate of 150 mg PE/min. The typical Cerebyx infusion administered to a 50 kg patient would take between 5 and 7 minutes. Note that the delivery of an identical molar dose of phenytoin using parenteral Dilantin or generic phenytoin sodium injection cannot be accomplished in less than 15 to 20 minutes because of the untoward cardiovascular effects that accompany the direct intravenous administration of phenytoin at rates greater than 50 mg/min.

If rapid phenytoin loading is a primary goal, IV administration of Cerebyx is preferred because the time to achieve therapeutic plasma phenytoin concentrations is greater following IM than that following IV administration (see DOSAGE AND ADMINISTRATION).

Withdrawal Precipitated Seizure, Status Epilepticus

Antiepileptic drugs should not be abruptly discontinued because of the possibility of increased seizure frequency, including status epilepticus. When, in the judgement of the clinician, the need for dosage reduction, discontinuation, or substitution of alternative medication arises, this should be done gradually. However, in the event of an allergic or hypersensitivity reaction, rapid substitution of alternative therapy may be necessary. In this case, alternative therapy should be an antiepileptic drug not belonging to the hydantoin chemical class.

Cardiovascular Depression

Hypotension may occur, especially after IV administration at high doses and high rates of administration. Following administration of phenytoin, severe cardiovascular reactions and fatalities have been reported with atrial and ventricular conduction depression and ventricular fibrillation. Severe complications are most commonly encountered in elderly or gravely ill patients. Therefore, careful cardiac monitoring is needed when administering IV loading doses of Cerebyx. Reduction in rate of administration or discontinuation of dosing may be needed.

Cerebyx should be used with caution in patients with hypotension and severe myocardial insufficiency.

Rash

Cerebyx should be discontinued if a skin rash appears. If the rash is exfoliative, purpuric, or bullous, or if lupus erythematosus, Stevens-Johnson syndrome, or toxic epidermal necrolysis is suspected, use of this drug should not be resumed and alternative therapy should be considered. If the rash is of a milder type (measles-like scarlatiniform), therapy may be resumed after the rash has completely disappeared. If the rash recurs upon reinstitution, further Cerebyx or phenytoin administration is contraindicated.

Hepatic Injury

Cases of acute hepatotoxicity, including infrequent cases of acute hepatic failure, have been reported with phenytoin. These incidents have been associated with a hypersensitivity syndrome characterized by fever, skin eruptions, and lymphadenopathy, and usually occur within the first 2 months of treatment. Other common manifestations include jaundice, hepatomegaly, elevated serum transaminase levels, leukocytosis, and eosinophilia. The clinical course of acute phenytoin hepatotoxicity ranges from prompt recovery to fatal outcomes. In these patients with acute hepatotoxicity, Cerebyx should be immediately discontinued and not readministered.

Hemopoietic System

Hemopoietic complications, some fatal, have occasionally been reported in association with administration of phenytoin. These have included thrombocytopenia, leukopenia, granulocytopenia, agranulocytosis, and pancytopenia with or without bone marrow suppression.

There have been a number of reports that have suggested a relationship between phenytoin and the development of lymphadenopathy (local or generalized), including benign lymph node hyperplasia, pseudolymphoma, lymphoma, and Hodgkin's disease. Although a cause and effect relationship has not been established, the occurrence of lymphadenopathy indicates the need to differentiate such a condition from other types of lymph node pathology. Lymph node involvement may occur with or without symptoms and signs resembling serum sickness, eg, fever, rash, and liver involvement. In all cases of lymphadenopathy, follow-up observation for an extended period is indicated and every effort should be made to achieve seizure control using alternative antiepileptic drugs.

Alcohol Use

Acute alcohol intake may increase plasma phenytoin concentrations while chronic alcohol use may decrease plasma concentrations.

Usage in Pregnancy

Clinical:

A. *Risks to Mother.* An increase in seizure frequency may occur during pregnancy because of altered phenytoin pharmacokinetics. Periodic measurements of plasma phenytoin concentrations may be valuable in the management of pregnant women as a guide to appropriate adjustment of dosage (see PRECAUTIONS, Laboratory Tests). However, postpartum restoration of the original dosage will probably be indicated.

B. *Risks to the Fetus.* If this drug is used during pregnancy, or if the patient becomes pregnant while taking the drug, the patient should be apprised of the potential harm to the fetus.

Prenatal exposure to phenytoin may increase the risks for congenital malformations and other adverse developmental outcomes. Increased frequencies of major malformations (such as orofacial clefts and cardiac defects), minor anomalies (dysmorphic facial features, nail and digit hypoplasia), growth abnormalities (including microcephaly), and mental deficiency have been reported among children born to epileptic women who took phenytoin alone or in combination with other antiepileptic drugs during pregnancy. There have also been several reported cases of malignancies, including neuroblastoma, in children whose mothers received phenytoin during pregnancy. The overall incidence of malformations for children of epileptic women treated with antiepileptic drugs (phenytoin and/or others) during pregnancy is about 10%, or two-to three-fold that in the general population. However, the relative contributions of antiepi-

Continued on next page

This product information was prepared in June 1998. On these and other Parke-Davis Products, information may be obtained by addressing PARKE-DAVIS, Division of Warner-Lambert Company, Morris Plains, New Jersey 07950.

Cerebyx—Cont.

leptic drugs and other factors associated with epilepsy to this increased risk are uncertain and in most cases it has not been possible to attribute specific developmental abnormalities to particular antiepileptic drugs.

Patients should consult with their physicians to weigh the risks and benefits of phenytoin during pregnancy.

C. Postpartum Period. A potentially life-threatening bleeding disorder related to decreased levels of vitamin K-dependent clotting factors may occur in newborns exposed to phenytoin *in utero* . This drug-induced condition can be prevented with vitamin K administration to the mother before delivery and to the neonate after birth.

Preclinical: Increased frequencies of malformations (brain, cardiovascular, digit, and skeletal anomalies), death, growth retardation, and functional impairment (chromodacryorrhea, hyperactivity, circling) were observed among the offspring of rats receiving fosphenytoin during pregnancy. Most of the adverse effects of embryo-fetal development occurred at doses of 33 mg PE/kg or higher (approximately 30% of the maximum human loading dose or higher on a mg/m^2 basis), which produced peak maternal plasma phenytoin concentrations of approximately 20 µg/mL or greater. Maternal toxicity was often associated with these doses and plasma concentrations, however, there is no evidence to suggest that the developmental effects were secondary to the maternal effects. The single occurrence of a rare brain malformation at a non-maternotoxic dose of 17 mg PE/kg (approximately 10% of the maximum human loading dose on a mg/m^2 basis) was also considered drug-induced. The developmental effects of fosphenytoin in rats were similar to those which have been reported following administration of phenytoin to pregnant rats.

No effects on embryo-fetal development were observed when rabbits were given up to 33 mg PE/kg of fosphenytoin (approximately 50% of the maximum human loading dose on a mg/m^2 basis) during pregnancy. Increased resorption and malformation rates have been reported following administration of phenytoin doses of 75 mg/kg or higher (approximately 120% of the maximum human loading dose or higher on a mg/m^2 basis) to pregnant rabbits.

PRECAUTIONS

General: (Cerebyx specific)

Sensory Disturbances

Severe burning, itching, and/or paresthesia were reported by 7 of 16 normal volunteers administered IV Cerebyx at a dose of 1200 mg PE at the maximum rate of administration (150 mg PE/min). The severe sensory disturbance lasted from 3 to 50 minutes in 6 of these subjects and for 14 hours in the seventh subject. In some cases, milder sensory disturbances persisted for as long as 24 hours. The location of the discomfort varied among subjects with the groin mentioned most frequently as an area of discomfort. In a separate cohort of 16 normal volunteers (taken from 2 other studies) who were administered IV Cerebyx at a dose of 1200 mg PE at the maximum rate of administration (150 mg PE/min), none experienced severe disturbances, but most experienced mild to moderate itching or tingling.

Patients administered Cerebyx at doses of 20 mg PE/kg at 150 mg PE/min are expected to experience discomfort of some degree. The occurrence and intensity of the discomfort can be lessened by slowing or temporarily stopping the infusion.

The effect of continuing infusion unaltered in the presence of these sensations is unknown. No permanent sequelae have been reported thus far. The pharmacologic basis for these positive sensory phenomena is unknown, but other phosphate ester drugs, which deliver smaller phosphate loads, have been associated with burning, itching, and/or tingling predominantly in the groin area.

Phosphate Load

The phosphate load provided by Cerebyx (0.0037 mmol phosphate/mg PE Cerebyx) should be considered when treating patients who require phosphate restriction, such as those with severe renal impairment.

IV Loading in Renal and/or Hepatic Disease or in Those With Hypoalbuminemia

After IV administration to patients with renal and/or hepatic disease, or in those with hypoalbuminemia, fosphenytoin clearance to phenytoin may be increased without a similar increase in phenytoin clearance. This has the potential to increase the frequency and severity of adverse events (see CLINICAL PHARMACOLOGY: Special Populations, and DOSAGE AND ADMINISTRATION: Dosing in Special Populations).

General: (phenytoin associated)

Cerebyx is *not* indicated for the treatment of *absence seizures*.

A small percentage of individuals who have been treated with phenytoin have been shown to metabolize the drug slowly. *Slow metabolism* may be due to limited enzyme availability and lack of induction; it appears to be genetically determined.

Phenytoin and other hydantoins are contraindicated in patients who have experienced phenytoin hypersensitivity. Additionally, caution should be exercised if using structurally similar (eg, barbiturates, succinimides, oxazolidinediones, and other related compounds) in these same patients.

Phenytoin has been infrequently associated with the exacerbation of *porphyria.* Caution should be exercised when Cerebyx is used in patients with this disease.

Hyperglycemia, resulting from phenytoin's inhibitory effect on insulin release, has been reported. Phenytoin may also raise the serum glucose concentrations in diabetic patients. Plasma concentrations of phenytoin sustained above the optimal range may produce confusional states referred to as "delirium," "psychosis," or "encephalopathy," or rarely, irreversible cerebellar dysfunction. Accordingly, at the first sign of *acute toxicity,* determination of plasma phenytoin concentrations is recommended (see PRECAUTIONS: Laboratory Tests). Cerebyx dose reduction is indicated if phenytoin concentrations are excessive, if symptoms persist, administration of Cerebyx should be discontinued.

The liver is the primary site of biotransformation of phenytoin; patients with impaired liver function, elderly patients, or those who are gravely ill may show early signs of toxicity. Phenytoin and other hydantoins are not indicated for seizures due to hypoglycemic or other metabolic causes. Appropriate diagnostic procedures should be performed as indicated.

Phenytoin has the potential to lower serum folate levels.

Laboratory Tests

Phenytoin doses are usually selected to attain therapeutic plasma total phenytoin concentrations of 10 to 20 µg/mL, (unbound phenytoin concentrations of 1 to 2 µg/mL). Following Cerebyx administration, it is recommended that phenytoin concentrations not be monitored until conversion to phenytoin is essentially complete. This occurs within approximately 2 hours after the end of IV infusion and 4 hours after IM injection.

Prior to complete conversion, commonly used immunoanalytical techniques, such as TDx®/TDxFLx™ (fluorescence polarization) and Emit® 2000 (enzyme multiplied), may significantly overestimate plasma phenytoin concentrations because of cross-reactivity with fosphenytoin. The error is dependent on plasma phenytoin and fosphenytoin concentration (influenced by Cerebyx dose, route and rate of administration, and time of sampling relative to dosing), and analytical method. Chromatographic assay methods accurately quantitate phenytoin concentrations in biological fluids in the presence of fosphenytoin. Prior to complete conversion, blood samples for phenytoin monitoring should be collected in tubes containing EDTA as an anticoagulant to minimize *ex vivo* conversion of fosphenytoin to phenytoin. However, even with specific assay methods, phenytoin concentrations measured before conversion of fosphenytoin is complete will not reflect phenytoin concentrations ultimately achieved.

Drug Interactions

No drugs are known to interfere with the conversion of fosphenytoin to phenytoin. Conversion could be affected by alterations in the level of phosphatase activity, but given the abundance and wide distribution of phosphatases in the body it is unlikely that drugs would affect this activity enough to affect conversion of fosphenytoin to phenytoin. Drugs highly bound to albumin could increase the unbound fraction of fosphenytoin. Although, it is unknown whether this could result in clinically significant effects, caution is advised when administering Cerebyx with other drugs that significantly bind to serum albumin.

The pharmacokinetics and protein binding of fosphenytoin, phenytoin, and diazepam were not altered when diazepam and Cerebyx were concurrently administered in single submaximal doses.

The most significant drug interactions following administration of Cerebyx are expected to occur with drugs that interact with phenytoin. Phenytoin is extensively bound to serum plasma proteins and is prone to competitive displacement. Phenytoin is metabolized by hepatic cytochrome P450 enzymes and is particularly susceptible to inhibitory drug interactions because it is subject to saturable metabolism. Inhibition of metabolism may produce significant increases in circulating phenytoin concentrations and enhance the risk of drug toxicity. Phenytoin is a potent inducer of hepatic drug-metabolizing enzymes.

The most commonly occurring drug interactions are listed below:

- Drugs that may increase plasma phenytoin concentrations include: acute alcohol intake, amiodarone, chloramphenicol, chlordiazepoxide, cimetidine, diazepam, dicumarol, disulfiram, estrogens, ethosuximide, fluoxetine, H$_2$-antagonists, halothane, isoniazid, methylphenidate, phenothiazines, phenylbutazone, salicylates, succinimides, sulfonamides, tolbutamide, trazodone.
- Drugs that may decrease plasma phenytoin concentrations include: carbamazepine, chronic alcohol abuse, reserpine.
- Drugs that may either increase or decrease plasma phenytoin concentrations include: phenobarbital, valproic acid,

and sodium valproate. Similarly, the effects of phenytoin on phenobarbital, valproic acid and sodium plasma valproate concentrations are unpredictable.

- Although not a true drug interaction, tricyclic antidepressants may precipitate seizures in susceptible patients and Cerebyx dosage may need to be adjusted.
- Drugs whose efficacy is impaired by phenytoin include: anticoagulants, corticosteroids, coumarin, digitoxin, doxycycline, estrogens, furosemide, oral contraceptives, rifampin, quinidine, theophylline, vitamin D.

Monitoring of plasma phenytoin concentrations may be helpful when possible drug interactions are suspected (see Laboratory Tests).

Drug/Laboratory Test Interactions

Phenytoin may decrease serum concentrations of T$_4$. It may also produce artifactually low results in dexamethasone or metyrapone tests. Phenytoin may also cause increased serum concentrations of glucose, alkaline phosphatase, and gamma glutamyl transpeptidase (GGT).

Care should be taken when using immunoanalytical methods to measure plasma phenytoin concentrations following Cerebyx administration (see Laboratory Tests).

Carcinogenesis, Mutagenesis, Impairment of Fertility

The carcinogenic potential of fosphenytoin has not been studied. Assessment of the carcinogenic potential of phenytoin in mice and rats is ongoing.

Structural chromosome aberration frequency in cultured V79 Chinese hamster lung cells was increased by exposure to fosphenytoin in the presence of metabolic activation. No evidence of mutagenicity was observed in bacteria (Ames test) or Chinese hamster lung cells *in vitro,* and no evidence for clastogenic activity was observed in an *in vivo* mouse bone marrow micronucleus test.

No effects on fertility were noted in rats of either sex given fosphenytoin. Maternal toxicity and altered estrous cycles, delayed mating, prolonged gestation length, and developmental toxicity were observed following administration of fosphenytoin during mating, gestation, and lactation at doses of 50 mg PE/kg or higher (approximately 40% of the maximum human loading dose or higher on a mg/m^2 basis).

Pregnancy-Category D: (see WARNINGS)

Use in Nursing Mothers

It is not known whether fosphenytoin is excreted in human milk.

Following administration of Dilantin, phenytoin appears to be excreted in low concentrations in human milk. Therefore, breast-feeding is not recommended for women receiving Cerebyx.

Pediatric Use

The safety of Cerebyx in pediatric patients has not been established.

Geriatric Use

No systematic studies in geriatric patients have been conducted. Phenytoin clearance tends to decrease with increasing age (see CLINICAL PHARMACOLOGY: Special Populations).

ADVERSE REACTIONS

The more important adverse clinical events caused by the IV use of Cerebyx or phenytoin are cardiovascular collapse and/or central nervous system depression. Hypotension can occur when either drug is administered rapidly by the IV route. The rate of administration is very important; for Cerebyx, it should not exceed 150 mg PE/min.

The adverse clinical events most commonly observed with the use of Cerebyx in clinical trials were nystagmus, dizziness, pruritus, paresthesia, headache, somnolence, and ataxia. With two exceptions, these events are commonly associated with the administration of IV phenytoin. Paresthesia and pruritus, however, were seen much more often following Cerebyx administration and occurred more often with IV Cerebyx administration than with IM Cerebyx administration. These events were dose and rate related; most alert patients (41 of 64; 64%) administered doses of ≥15 mg PE/kg at 150 mg PE/min experienced discomfort of some degree. These sensations, generally described as itching, burning, or tingling, were usually not at the infusion site. The location of the discomfort varied with the groin mentioned most frequently as a site of involvement. The paresthesia and pruritus were transient events that occurred within several minutes of the start of infusion and generally resolved within 10 minutes after completion of Cerebyx infusion. Some patients experienced symptoms for hours. These events did not increase in severity with repeated administration.

Concurrent adverse events or clinical laboratory change suggesting an allergic process were not seen (see PRECAUTIONS, Sensory Disturbances).

Approximately 2% of the 859 individuals who received Cerebyx in premarketing clinical trials discontinued treatment because of an adverse event. The adverse events most commonly associated with withdrawal were pruritus (0.5%), hypotension (0.3%), and bradycardia (0.2%).

Dose and Rate Dependency of Adverse Events Following IV Cerebyx: The incidence of adverse events tended to increase as both dose and infusion rate increased. In particular, at

doses of ≥15 mg PE/kg and rates ≥150 mg PE/min, transient pruritus, tinnitus, nystagmus, somnolence, and ataxia occurred 2 to 3 times more often than at lower doses or rates.

Incidence in Controlled Clinical Trials

All adverse events were recorded during the trials by the clinical investigators using terminology of their own choosing. Similar types of events were grouped into standardized categories using modfied COSTART dictionary terminology. These categories are used in the tables and listings below with the frequencies representing the proportion of individuals exposed to Cerebyx or comparative therapy.

The prescriber should be aware that these figures cannot be used to predict the frequency of adverse events in the course of usual medical practice where patient characteristics and other factors may differ from those prevailing during clinical studies. Similarly, the cited frequencies cannot be directly compared with figures obtained from other clinical investigations involving different treatments, uses or investigators. An inspection of these frequencies, however, does provide the prescribing physician with one basis to estimate the relative contribution of drug and nondrug factors to the adverse event incidences in the population studied.

Incidence in Controlled Clinical Trials-IV Administration To Patients With Epilepsy or Neurosurgical Patients: Table 2 lists treatment-emergent adverse events that occurred in at least 2% of patients treated with IV Cerebyx at the maximum dose and rate in a randomized, double-blind, controlled clinical trial where the rates for phenytoin and Cerebyx administration would have resulted in equivalent systemic exposure to phenytoin.

TABLE 2. Treatment-Emergent Adverse Event Incidence Following IV Administration at the Maximum Dose and Rate to Patients With Epilepsy or Neurosurgical Patients

(Events in at Least 2% of Cerebyx-Treated Patients)

BODY SYSTEM Adverse Event	IV Cerebyx N=90	IV Phenytoin N=22
BODY AS A WHOLE		
Pelvic Pain	4.4	0.0
Asthenia	2.2	0.0
Back Pain	2.2	0.0
Headache	2.2	4.5
CARDIOVASCULAR		
Hypotension	7.7	9.1
Vasodilatation	5.6	4.5
Tachycardia	2.2	0.0
DIGESTIVE		
Nausea	8.9	13.6
Tongue Disorder	4.4	0.0
Dry Mouth	4.4	4.5
Vomiting	2.2	9.1
NERVOUS		
Nystagmus	44.4	59.1
Dizziness	31.1	27.3
Somnolence	20.0	27.3
Ataxia	11.1	18.2
Stupor	7.7	4.5
Incoordination	4.4	4.5
Paresthesia	4.4	0.0
Extrapyramidal Syndrome	4.4	0.0
Tremor	3.3	9.1
Agitation	3.3	0.0
Hypesthesia	2.2	9.1
Dysarthria	2.2	0.0
Vertigo	2.2	0.0
Brain Edema	2.2	4.5
SKIN AND APPENDAGES		
Pruritus	48.9	4.5
SPECIAL SENSES		
Tinnitus	8.9	9.1
Diplopia	3.3	0.0
Taste Perversion	3.3	0.0
Amblyopia	2.2	9.1
Deafness	2.2	0.0

Incidence in Controlled Trials-IM Administration to Patients With Epilepsy. Table 3 lists treatment-emergent adverse events that occurred in at least 2% of Cerebyx-treated patients in a double-bind, randomized controlled clinical trial of adult epilepsy patients receiving either IM Cerebyx substituted for oral Dilantin or continuing oral Dilantin. Both treatments were administered for 5 days.

TABLE 3. Treatment-Emergent Adverse Event Incidence Following Substitution of IM Cerebyx for Oral Dilantin in Patients With Epilepsy

(Events in at Least 2% of Cerebyx-Treated Patients)

BODY SYSTEM Adverse Event	IM Cerebyx N=179	Oral Dilantin N=61
BODY AS A WHOLE		
Headache	8.9	4.9
Asthenia	3.9	3.3
Accidental Injury	3.4	6.6
DIGESTIVE		
Nausea	4.5	0.0
Vomiting	2.8	0.0
HEMATOLOGIC AND LYMPHATIC		
Ecchymosis	7.3	4.9
NERVOUS		
Nystagmus	15.1	8.2
Tremor	9.5	13.1
Ataxia	8.4	8.2
Incoordination	7.8	4.9
Somnolence	6.7	9.8
Dizziness	5.0	3.3
Paresthesia	3.9	3.3
Reflexes Decreased	2.8	4.9
SKIN AND APPENDAGES		
Pruritus	2.8	0.0

Adverse Events During All Clinical Trials

Cerebyx has been administered to 859 individuals during all clinical trials. All adverse events seen at least twice are listed in the following, except those already included in previous tables and listings. Events are further classified within body system categories and enumerated in order of decreasing frequency using the following definitions: frequent adverse events are defined as those occurring in greater than 1/100 individuals; infrequent adverse events are those occurring in 1/100 to 1/1000 individuals.

Body As a Whole: *Frequent:* fever, injection-site reaction, infection, chills, face edema, injection-site pain; *Infrequent:* sepsis, injection-site inflammation, injection-site edema, injection-site hemorrhage, flu syndrome, malaise, generalized edema, shock, photosensitivity reaction, cachexia, cryptococcosis.

Cardiovascular: *Frequent:* hypertension; *Infrequent:* cardiac arrest, migraine, syncope, cerebral hemorrhage, palpitation, sinus bradycardia, atrial flutter, bundle branch block, cardiomegaly, cerebral infarct, postural hypotension, pulmonary embolus, QT interval prolongation, thrombophlebitis, ventricular extrasystoles, congestive heart failure.

Digestive: *Frequent:* constipation; *Infrequent:* dyspepsia, diarrhea, anorexia, gastrointestinal hemorrhage, increased salivation, liver function tests abnormal, tenesmus, tongue edema, dysphagia, flatulence, gastritis, ileus.

Endocrine: *Infrequent:* diabetes insipidus.

Hematologic and Lymphatic: *Infrequent:* thrombocytopenia, anemia, leukocytosis, cyanosis, hypochromic anemia, leukopenia, lymphadenopathy, petachia.

Metabolic and Nutritional: *Frequent:* hypokalemia; *Infrequent:* hyperglycemia, hypophosphatemia, alkalosis, acidosis, dehydration, hyperkalemia, ketosis.

Musculoskeletal: *Frequent:* myasthenia; *Infrequent:* myopathy, leg cramps, arthralgia, myalgia.

Nervous: *Frequent:* reflexes increased, speech disorder, dysarthria, intracranial hypertension, thinking abnormal, nervousness, hypesthesia; *Infrequent:* confusion, twitching, Babinski sign positive, circumoral paresthesia, hemiplegia, hypotonia, convulsion, extrapyramidal syndrome, insomnia, meningitis, depersonalization, CNS depression, depression, hypokinesia, hyperkinesia, brain edema, paralysis, psychosis, aphasia, emotional lability, coma, hyperesthesia, myoclonus, personality disorder, acute brain syndrome, encephalitis, subdural hematoma, encephalopathy, hostility, akathisia, amnesia, neurosis.

Respiratory: *Frequent:* pneumonia; *Infrequent:* pharyngitis, sinusitis, hyperventilation, rhinitis, apnea, aspiration pneumonia, asthma, dyspnea, atelectasis, cough increased, sputum increased, epistaxis, hypoxia, pneumothorax, hemoptysis, bronchitis.

Skin and Appendages: *Frequent:* rash; *Infrequent:* maculopapular rash, urticaria, sweating, skin discoloration, contact dermatitis, pustular rash, skin nodule.

Special Senses: *Frequent:* taste perversion; *Infrequent:* deafness, visual field defect, eye pain, conjunctivitis, photophobia, hyperacusis, mydriasis, parosmia, ear pain, taste loss.

Urogenital: *Infrequent:* urinary retention, oliguria, dysuria, vaginitis, albuminuria, genital edema, kidney failure, polyuria, urethral pain, urinary incontinence, vaginal moniliasis.

OVERDOSAGE

There is no experience with Cerebyx overdosage in humans. The median lethal dose of fosphenytoin given intravenously in mice and rats was 156 mg PE/kg and approximately 250 mg PE/kg, or about 0.6 and 2 times, respectively, the maximum human loading dose on a mg/m^2 basis. Signs of acute toxicity in animals included ataxia, labored breathing, ptosis, and hypoactivity.

Because Cerebyx is a prodrug of phenytoin, the following information may be helpful. Initial symptoms of acute phenytoin toxicity are nystagmus, ataxia, and dysarthria. Other signs include tremor, hyperreflexia, lethargy, slurred speech, nausea, vomiting, coma, and hypotension. Depression of respiratory and circulatory systems leads to death. There are marked variations among individuals with respect to plasma phenytoin concentrations where toxicity occurs. Lateral gaze nystagmus usually appears at 20 µg/mL, ataxia at 30 µg/mL, and dysarthria and lethargy appear when the plasma concentration is over 40 µg/mL. However, phenytoin concentrations as high as 50 µg/mL have been reported without evidence of toxicity. As much as 25 times the therapeutic phenytoin dose has been taken, resulting in plasma phenytoin concentrations over 100 µg/mL, with complete recovery.

Treatment is nonspecific since there is no known antidote to Cerebyx or phenytoin overdosage. The adequacy of the respiratory and circulatory systems should be carefully observed, and appropriate supportive measures employed. Hemodialysis can be considered since phenytoin is not completely bound to plasma proteins. Total exchange transfusion has been used in the treatment of severe intoxication in children. In acute overdosage the possibility of other CNS depressants, including alcohol, should be borne in mind.

Formate and phosphate are metabolites of fosphenytoin and therefore may contribute to signs of toxicity following overdosage. Signs of formate toxicity are similar to those of methanol toxicity and are associated with severe anion-gap metabolic acidosis. Large amounts of phosphate, delivered rapidly, could potentially cause hypocalcemia with paresthesia, muscle spasms, and seizures. Ionized free calcium levels can be measured and, if low, used to guide treatment.

DOSAGE AND ADMINISTRATION

The dose, concentration in dosing solutions, and infusion rate of IV Cerebyx is expressed as phenytoin sodium equivalents (PE) to avoid the need to perform molecular weight-based adjustments when converting between fosphenytoin and phenytoin sodium doses. Cerebyx should always be prescribed and dispensed in phenytoin sodium equivalent units (PE). Cerebyx has important differences in administration from those for parenteral phenytoin sodium (see below).

Products with particulate matter or discoloration should not be used. Prior to IV infusion, dilute Cerebyx in 5% dextrose or 0.9% saline solution for injection to a concentration ranging from 1.5 to 25 mg PE/mL.

Status Epilepticus

- The loading dose of Cerebyx is 15 to 20 mg PE/kg administered at 100 to 150 mg PE/min.
- Because of the risk of hypotension, fosphenytoin should be administered no faster than 150 mg PE/min. Continuous monitoring of the electrocardiogram, blood pressure, and respiratory function is essential and the patient should be observed throughout the period where maximal serum phenytoin concentrations occur, approximately 10 to 20 minutes after the end of Cerebyx infusions.
- Because the full antiepileptic effect of phenytoin, whether given as Cerebyx or parenteral phenytoin is not immediate, other measures, including concomitant administration of an IV benzodiazepine, will usually be necessary for the control of status epilepticus.
- The loading dose should be followed by maintenance doses of Cerebyx, or phenytoin either orally or parenterally.

If administration of Cerebyx does not terminate seizures, the use of other anticonvulsants and other appropriate measures should be considered.

IM Cerebyx should not be used in the treatment of status epilepticus because therapeutic phenytoin concentrations may not be reached as quickly as with IV administration. If IV access is impossible, loading doses of Cerebyx have been given by the IM route for other indications.

Nonemergent Loading and Maintenance Dosing

The loading dose of Cerebyx is 10-20 mg PE/kg given IV or IM. The rate of administration for IV Cerebyx should be no greater than 150 mg PE/min. Continuous monitoring of the

Continued on next page

This product information was prepared in June 1998. On these and other Parke-Davis Products, information may be obtained by addressing PARKE-DAVIS, Division of Warner-Lambert Company, Morris Plains, New Jersey 07950.

Cerebyx—Cont.

electrocardiogram, blood pressure, and respiratory function is essential and the patient should be observed throughout the period where maximal serum phenytoin concentrations occur, approximately 10 to 20 minutes after the end of Cerebyx infusions.

The initial daily maintenance dose of Cerebyx is 4-6 mg PE/kg/day.

IM or IV Substitution For Oral Phenytoin Therapy

Cerebyx can be substituted for oral phenytoin sodium therapy at the same total daily dose.

Dilantin capsules are approximately 90% bioavailable by the oral route. Phenytoin, supplied as Cerebyx, is 100% bioavailable by both the IM and IV routes. For this reason, plasma phenytoin concentrations may increase modestly when IM or IV Cerebyx is substituted for oral phenytoin sodium therapy.

The rate of administration for IV Cerebyx should be no greater than 150 mg PE/min.

In controlled trials, IM Cerebyx was administered as a single daily dose utilizing either 1 or 2 injection sites. Some patients may require more frequent dosing.

Dosing in Special Populations

Patients with Renal or Hepatic Disease: Due to an increased fraction of unbound phenytoin in patients with renal or hepatic disease, or in those with hypoalbuminemia, the interpretation of total phenytoin plasma concentrations should be made with caution (see CLINICAL PHARMACOLOGY: Special Populations). Unbound phenytoin concentrations may be more useful in these patient populations. After IV Cerebyx administration to patients with renal and/or hepatic disease, or in those with hypoalbuminemia, fosphenytoin clearance to phenytoin may be increased without a similar increase in phenytoin clearance. This has the potential to increase the frequency and severity of adverse events (see PRECAUTIONS).

Elderly Patients: Age does not have a significant impact on the pharmacokinetics of fosphenytoin following Cerebyx administration. Phenytoin clearance is decreased slightly in elderly patients and lower or less frequent dosing may be required.

Pediatric: The safety of Cerebyx in pediatric patients has not been established.

HOW SUPPLIED

Cerebyx Injection is supplied as follows:

10 mL per vial—Each vial contains fosphenytoin sodium 750 mg equivalent to 500 mg of phenytoin sodium:

N 0071-4008-10 Packages of 10.

2 mL per vial—Each vial contains fosphenytoin sodium 150 mg equivalent to 100 mg of phenytoin sodium:

N 0071-4007-05. Packages of 25.

Both sizes of vials contain Tromethamine, USP (TRIS), Hydrochloric Acid, NF, or Sodium Hydroxide, NF, and Water for Injection, USP.

Cerebyx should always be prescribed in phenytoin sodium equivalent units (PE) (see DOSAGE AND ADMINISTRATION).

Storage

Store under refrigeration at 2°C to 8°C (36°F to 46°F). The product should not be stored at room temperature for more than 48 hours. Vials that develop particulate matter should not be used.

Rx only

© 1996–'98, Warner-Lambert Co.

Revised April 1998

Manufactured by:

Parkedale Pharmaceuticals, Inc.

Rochester, MI 48307

For:

PARKE-DAVIS

Div of Warner-Lambert Co.

Morris Plains, NJ 07950 USA   4007G031

COGNEX®
(Tacrine Hydrochloride Capsules)   ℞

DESCRIPTION

Cognex® (tacrine hydrochloride) is a reversible cholinesterase inhibitor, known chemically as 1,2,3,4-tetrahydro-9-acridinamine monohydrochloride monohydrate. Tacrine hydrochloride is commonly referred to in the clinical and pharmacological literature as THA. It has an empirical formula of $C_{13}H_{14}N_2 \cdot HCl \cdot H_2O$ and a molecular weight of 252.74. Tacrine hydrochloride is a white solid and is freely soluble in distilled water, 0.1N hydrochloric acid, acetate buffer (pH 4.0), phosphate buffer (pH 7.0 to 7.4), methanol, dimethylsulfoxide (DMSO), ethanol, and propylene glycol. The compound is sparingly soluble in linoleic acid and PEG 400.

Each capsule of Cognex® contains tacrine as the hydrochloride. Inactive ingredients are hydrous lactose, magnesium stearate, and microcrystalline cellulose. The hard gelatin capsules contain gelatin, NF; silicon dioxide, NF; sodium

lauryl sulfate, NF; and the following dyes: 10 mg: D&C Yellow #10, FD&C Green #3, titanium dioxide; 20 mg: D&C Yellow #10, FD&C Blue #1, titanium dioxide; 30 mg: D&C Yellow #10, FD&C Blue #1, FD&C Red #40, titanium dioxide; 40 mg: D&C Yellow #10, FD&C Blue #1, FD&C Red #40, D&C Red #28, titanium dioxide.

Each 10-, 20-, 30-, and 40-mg Cognex® capsule for oral administration contains 12.75, 25.50, 38.25, and 51.00 mg of tacrine HCl, respectively.

CLINICAL PHARMACOLOGY

Although widespread degeneration of multiple CNS neuronal systems eventually occurs, early pathological changes in Alzheimer's Disease involve, in a relatively selective manner, cholinergic neuronal pathways that project from the basal forebrain to the cerebral cortex and hippocampus. The resulting deficiency of cortical acetylcholine is believed to account for some of the clinical manifestations of mild to moderate dementia. Tacrine, an orally bioavailable, centrally active, reversible cholinesterase inhibitor, presumably acts by elevating acetylcholine concentrations in the cerebral cortex by slowing the degradation of acetylcholine released by still intact cholinergic neurons. If this theoretical mechanism of action is correct, tacrine's effects may lessen as the disease process advances and fewer cholinergic neurons remain functionally intact. There is no evidence that tacrine alters the course of the underlying dementing process.

Clinical Trial Data

The conclusion that Cognex® is an effective treatment for Alzheimer's Disease derives from two adequate and well controlled clinical investigations that evaluated tacrine's effects in patients with probable Alzheimer's disease of mild to moderate severity (NINCDS criteria, Mini-Mental State Examination (MMSE) of Folstein, Folstein and McHugh scores of 10 to 26).

In each study, outcomes during treatment with tacrine and placebo were assessed on two primary measures: (1) the cognitive subscale of the Alzheimer's Disease Assessment Scale (ADAS cog) of Rosen, Mohs, and Davis and (2) a clinician's rated clinical global impression of change.

Study Endpoints

The ADAS cog is a multi-item test battery administered by a psychometrician that examines aspects of memory, attention, praxis, reason, and language. The worst possible score is 70. Elderly, normal adults may score as low as 0 or 1 unit, but individuals judged not to be demented can score higher. The mean score of patients entering each study was approximately 28 units (range 7 to 62). The ADAS cog score is reported to deteriorate at a rate of about 6 to 10 units per year for untreated patients at this stage of dementia.

The clinician's global assessments used in the two studies relied on a clinician's judgment about the overall clinical change observed in patients over the course of the study. Although the conditions for obtaining the clinical assessment differed in each study, the global assessment was rated on a 7-point scale in both studies. A rating of four (4) represents no change; lower ratings indicate improvement from baseline and higher ratings deterioration.

Twelve-Week Study

In one study of 12 weeks duration, patients were randomized to sequences that provided a comparison between placebo, 20, 40, and 80 mg/day by study's end. Statistically significant drug-placebo differences were detected on both primary outcome measures for the group titrated to 80 mg/day. Estimates of the size of the treatment effect varied between 2 and 4 ADAS cog units. The imprecision in these estimates reflects the fact that different analyses, conducted in attempts to account for the effects of the failure of a substantial fraction of the patients randomized to complete the full 12 weeks of the study, yielded different results.

The placebo-80 mg/day comparison also achieved statistical significance on the clinician's global impression of change (CGIC) with a 0.3 to 0.4 unit mean difference. The following diagram illustrates the percentages of patients falling into each global category at trial's end for the patients given placebo or 80 mg/day.

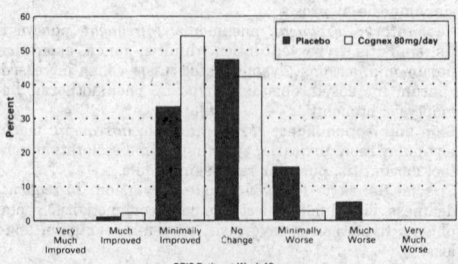

FIGURE 1: Percent of Patients in Each of the Seven Outcome Categories on the Clinician-Rated CGIC for Patients Completing 12 Weeks of Treatment (83% of patients randomized to placebo completed 12 weeks of treatment and are represented above; 56% of those randomized to the 80 mg/day Cognex® sequence completed 12 weeks)

Thirty-Week Study

The second study was 30 weeks long. Six hundred sixty-three patients were randomized to 4 treatment sequences (placebo and 3 drug groups) that called for the daily dose of tacrine to be increased at 6-week intervals, starting with a 40-mg/day dose. By study's end, a comparison between placebo, 80, 120, and 160 mg/day was possible. Patients in the 160 mg group received this dose for the final 12 weeks; the 120 mg group received that dose for 18 weeks.

The study showed statistically significant drug-placebo differences for the 80 and 120 mg/day groups at 18 weeks and for the 120 and 160 mg/day groups at 30 weeks on both a performance-based test of cognitive function (the ADAS cog) and a clinician's assessment of global change (Clinician Interview Based Impression: CIBI). Because many patients failed to complete 30 weeks on treatment, analyses that used each patient's last on-study value or retrieved patients' (see below) 30-week value, even if they were no longer in the study ("intent-to-treat" analysis) were also carried out. All analyses confirmed the effectiveness of tacrine, although the estimated mean treatment effect was different in each analysis.

Effects on ADAS Cog: The results for the ADAS cog are shown in Figure 2 for the subset of patients actually completing the full 30 weeks of the study. They show that individual patients, whether assigned to tacrine or to placebo, had a wide range of responses. This variability in response is illustrated in the display that follows (Figure 2).

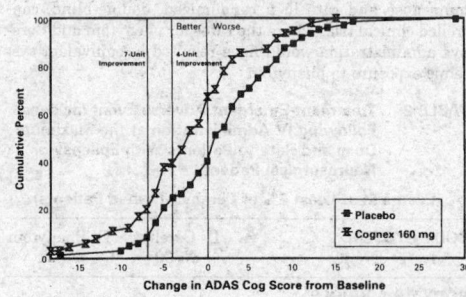

FIGURE 2. Cumulative Percent of Patients Completing 30 Weeks of Treatment Who Attained a Change in ADAS Cog Score From Baseline at Least as Large as the Value on the X Axis. The display is based on scores obtained from a subset of patients (ie, 64% of the 184 randomized to placebo and 27% of the 239 randomized to the 160 mg/day treatment group).

Figure 2 presents the cumulative percentage (Y axis) of patients assigned to placebo or 160 mg/day who actually completed 30 weeks on treatment and who attained a change in ADAS cog score from baseline at least as large as the ADAS cog change score value given on the X axis. A negative change from baseline represents improvement; a positive change deterioration. Thus, in a display of this type, the curve for an effective treatment is shifted to the left of the curve for placebo. The frequency in each group of any response, e.g., an improvement of 7 ADAS cog units, can be found by plotting the change on the X axis, then reading upward along the Y axis. The variability of response is apparent from the fact that the distribution of responses under both treatment conditions range from large negative to large positive values. Nonetheless, the mean drug-placebo ADAS cog difference for the 30-week 160 mg/day completer patients is 4.8 units, a statistically significant difference.

Effects on CIBI: The results on the CIBI are shown in Figure 3.

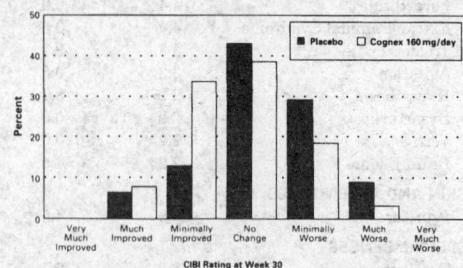

FIGURE 3. Percent of Patients in Each of the Seven Outcome Categories of the CIBI Among Those Completing 30 Weeks. The display is based on scores obtained from the same subset of patients as Figure 2.

Figure 3 is a histogram of the frequency distribution of CIBI scores attained by patients assigned to placebo or to the 160 mg/day tacrine dose group who actually completed the full 30 weeks of the study. The mean tacrine-placebo difference for this group of patients on the CIBI was 0.5 units and was statistically significant.

Expected Responses in Newly Treated Patients: Although the results described clearly document tacrine's effectiveness, they are based on only a fraction of the patients initially randomized to tacrine, those who could tolerate tacrine and remain on treatment uninterrupted for the full

Table 1. Proportion of Patients Attaining ≥7 Unit Improvement on the ADAS Cog at the Week 30 Assessment

Treatment Group N Randomized	I N (%) of Those Randomized	II N (%) of Those Completing Week 30	III N (%) of Those With Week 30 Assessments
Placebo (N = 184)	10/184(5.4)	10/117(8.5)	11/143[1](7.7)
160 mg/day (N = 239)	13/239(5.4)	13/64 (20.3)	25/172[2](14.5)

[1]: 13 of the 143 were receiving tacrine when evaluated.
[2]: 41 of the 172 were not receiving tacrine when evaluated.

30 weeks. In considering the expected outcome in a group of patients newly started on tacrine, account must be taken both of the likelihood of staying on therapy and the responses in patients who do so.

Table 1 provides 3 different estimates of the proportion of patients assigned to treatment with tacrine at 160 mg a day or with placebo who attained a particular measure of improvement (i.e., a 7 point improvement from baseline in ADAS cog score). The criterion has been chosen entirely for illustrative purposes.

[See table 1 above]

The first column of the table is based on all patients participating in the study. The proportion provides an estimate of the likelihood that a patient entering the study will (1) still be on his or her assigned treatment at week 30 **and** (2) will improve 7 or more ADAS cognitive points over his or her baseline score. The estimate of response derived in this manner is conservative because the rules under which the 30-week study was conducted required the withdrawal of patients with relatively low (>3 × ULN), asymptomatic, transaminase elevations. In actual clinical practice under the conditions of treatment recommended in the Dosage and Administration Section, a larger fraction of these patients would be able to remain on tacrine and the proportion of those improving 7 or more points on tacrine would be expected, therefore, to be increased (the third column illustrates this).

The second column of the table presents the proportion of 7 unit responders based on the number of patients who (1) were able to complete the full 30 weeks of the study and (2) attained an ADAS cognitive score at week 30 that was 7 or more points better than their baseline score. This analysis provides an optimistic estimate of tacrine's effects because it reflects experience gained only with the minority of patients who were able to remain on treatment to the study's end. The comparison between the proportions of placebo and 160 mg patients attaining a 7 or more point improvement is complicated further by the fact that a larger proportion of tacrine assigned patients withdrew prematurely.

The third column of the table presents the proportion of patients who had evaluations made at 30 weeks and had a 7-point or greater response. The analysis includes data from patients still on their assigned treatment at week 30 as well as patients who withdrew from the study prior to that time, but were retrieved for a week 30 evaluation. Because patients who withdrew prior to week 30 were permitted to receive tacrine under "open label" conditions, retrieved patients included in this analysis could be receiving either no treatment or treatment with tacrine. In this analysis, patients are considered under the treatment to which they were randomized, regardless of the treatment they were actually receiving at week 30. Thus, some placebo patients could have received tacrine and some tacrine patients could have been receiving no tacrine. Like the analysis based on percent randomized (column I), this analysis, therefore, tends to provide a conservative view of the expected effects of tacrine treatment.

Effects of Cognex® Over Time: Figure 4 shows for each dose group the time course of change from baseline in ADAS cog scores for patients completing 30 weeks of treatment. There appears to be a persistent difference between groups, but all groups, after initial improvement, deteriorate with time.

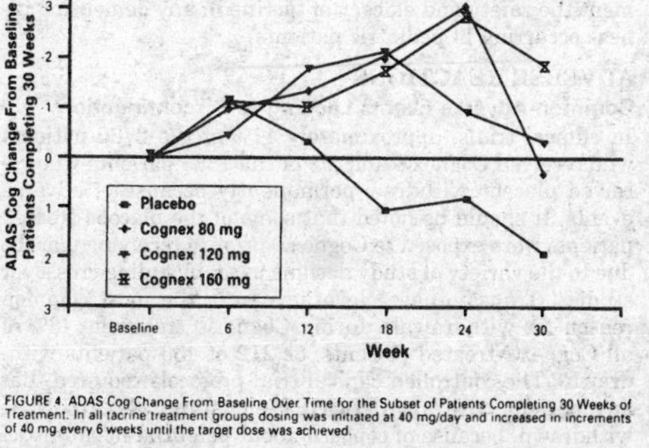

FIGURE 4. ADAS Cog Change From Baseline Over Time for the Subset of Patients Completing 30 Weeks of Treatment. In all tacrine treatment groups dosing was initiated at 40 mg/day and increased in increments of 40 mg every 6 weeks until the target dose was achieved.

Patient age, gender, and other baseline patient characteristics were not found to predict clinical outcome.

Clinical Pharmacokinetics (Absorption, Distribution, Metabolism, and Elimination)

Absorption: Cognex® is rapidly absorbed after oral administration; maximal plasma concentrations occur within 1 to 2 hours. The rate and extent of tacrine absorption following administration of tacrine capsules and solution are virtually indistinguishable. Absolute bioavailability of tacrine is approximately 17 (SD ± 13) %. Food reduces tacrine bioavailability by approximately 30–40%; however, there is no food effect if tacrine is administered at least an hour before meals. The effect of achlorhydria on the absorption of tacrine is unknown.

Distribution: Mean volume of distribution of tacrine is approximately 349 (SD ± 193) L. Tacrine is about 55% bound to plasma proteins. The extent and degree of tacrine's distribution within various body compartments has not been systematically studied. However, 336 hours after the administration of a single radiolabeled dose, approximately 25% of the radiolabel was not recovered in a mass balance study, suggesting the possibility that tacrine and/or one or more of its metabolites may be retained.

Metabolism: Tacrine is extensively metabolized by the cytochrome P450 system to multiple metabolites, not all of which have been identified. The vast majority of radiolabeled species present in the plasma following a single dose of ^{14}C radiolabeled tacrine are unidentified (ie, only 5% of radioactivity in plasma has been identified [tacrine and 3-hydroxylated metabolites; 1-, 2-, and 4-hydroxytacrine]). Studies utilizing human liver preparations demonstrated that cytochrome P450 IA2 is the principal isozyme involved in tacrine metabolism. These findings are consistent with the observation that tacrine and/or one of its metabolites inhibits the metabolism of theophylline in humans (see PRECAUTIONS: Drug-Drug Interactions: theophylline). Results from a study utilizing quinidine to inhibit cytochrome P450 IID6 indicate that tacrine is not metabolized extensively by this enzyme system.

Following aromatic ring hydroxylation, tacrine's metabolites undergo glucuronidation. Whether tacrine and/or its metabolites undergo biliary excretion or entero-hepatic circulation is unknown.

Special Populations: *Age:* Based on pooled pharmacokinetic studies (n = 192), there is no clinically relevant influence of age (50 to 84 years) on tacrine clearance. *Gender:* Average tacrine plasma concentrations are approximately 50% higher in females than in males. This is not explained by differences in body surface area or elimination half-life. The difference is probably due to higher systemic availability after oral dosing and may reflect the known lower activity of cytochrome P450 IA2 in women. *Race:* The effect of race on tacrine clearance has not been studied. *Smoking:* Mean plasma tacrine concentrations in current smokers are approximately one third the concentrations in nonsmokers. Cigarette smoking is known to induce cytochrome P450 IA2. *Renal disease:* Renal disease does not appear to affect the clearance of tacrine. *Liver disease:* Although studies in patients with liver disease have not been done, it is likely that functional hepatic impairment will reduce the clearance of tacrine and its metabolites.

Presystemic Clearance/Elimination/Excretion: Tacrine undergoes presystemic clearance (ie, first pass metabolism). The extent of this first pass metabolism depends upon the dose of tacrine administered. Because the enzyme system involved can be saturated at relatively low doses, a larger fraction of a high dose of tacrine will escape first pass elimination than of a smaller dose. Thus, when a 40 mg daily dose is increased by 40 mg, the average plasma concentration will be increased by approximately 6 ng/mL. However, when a daily dose of 80 or 120 mg is increased by 40 mg, the increment in average plasma concentration is approximately 10 ng/mL.

Elimination of tacrine from the plasma, however, is not dose dependent (ie, the half-life is independent of dose or plasma concentration). The elimination half-life is approximately 2 to 4 hours. Following initiation of therapy or a change in daily dose, steady state tacrine plasma concentration should be attained within 24 to 36 hours.

Drug Interactions (See PRECAUTIONS)

INDICATIONS AND USAGE

Cognex® (tacrine hydrochloride capsules) is indicated for the treatment of mild to moderate dementia of the Alzheimer's type.

Evidence of Cognex®'s effectiveness in the treatment of dementia of the Alzheimer's type derives from results of two adequate and well-controlled clinical investigations that compared tacrine and placebo on both a performance based measure of cognition and a clinician's global assessment of change. (See CLINICAL PHARMACOLOGY Section: Clinical Trial Data.)

CONTRAINDICATIONS

Cognex® is contraindicated in patients with known hypersensitivity to tacrine or acridine derivatives.

Cognex® is contraindicated in patients previously treated with Cognex® who developed treatment-associated jaundice: a serum bilirubin >3 mg/dL; and/or those exhibiting clinical signs or symptoms of hypersensitivity (eg, rash or fever) in association with ALT/SGPT elevations.

WARNINGS

Anesthesia

Cognex®, as a cholinesterase inhibitor, is likely to exaggerate succinylcholine-type muscle relaxation during anesthesia.

Cardiovascular Conditions

Because of its cholinomimetic action, Cognex® may have vagotonic effects on the heart rate (eg, bradycardia). This action may be particularly important to patients with conduction abnormalities, bradyarrhythmia, or a sick sinus syndrome.

Gastrointestinal Disease and Dysfunction

Cognex® is an inhibitor of cholinesterase and may be expected to increase gastric acid secretion due to increased cholinergic activity. Therefore, patients are at increased risk for developing ulcers. Those with a history of ulcer disease or those receiving concurrent nonsteroidal antiinflammatory drugs (NSAIDS) should be monitored closely for symptoms of active or occult gastrointestinal disease.

Cognex®, also as a predictable consequence of its pharmacological properties, can cause nausea, vomiting, and loose stools at recommended doses.

Liver Injury

Cognex® should be prescribed with care in patients with current evidence or history of abnormal liver function indicated by significant abnormalities in serum transaminase (ALT/SGPT; AST/SGOT), bilirubin, and gamma-glutamyl transpeptidase (GGT) levels (see PRECAUTIONS and DOSAGE AND ADMINISTRATION sections).

The use of tacrine in patients without a prior history of liver disease is commonly associated with serum aminotransferase elevations, some to levels ordinarily considered to indicate clinically important hepatic injury (see Table 2).

Experience gained in more than 12,000 patients who received tacrine in clinical studies and the treatment IND program indicates that if tacrine is promptly withdrawn following detection of these elevations, clinically evident signs and symptoms of liver injury are rare.

Long-term follow up of patients who experience transaminase elevations, however, is limited and it is impossible, therefore, to exclude, with certainty, the possibility of chronic sequelae.

Controlled Clinical Trials, Treatment IND and Post Marketing Experience:

Experience with tacrine in controlled trials and in a large, less closely monitored experience (a treatment IND) is summarized below:

Clinically evident liver toxicity: One of more than 12,000 patients exposed to tacrine in clinical studies and the treatment IND program had documented elevated bilirubin (5.3 × Upper Limit of Normal, ULN) and jaundice with transaminase levels (AST/SGOT) nearly 20 × ULN.

Rare cases of liver toxicity associated with jaundice, raised serum bilirubin, pyrexia, hepatitis and liver failure have been reported in post-marketing experience. Most of these cases have been reversible but some deaths have occurred. Since there was multiple pathology including infection, gallstones and carcinoma it was not possible to clearly establish the relationship to Cognex® treatment.

Blood chemistry signs of liver injury: Experience from the 30-week clinical study (described earlier) provides a representative estimate of the frequency of ALT/SGPT elevations expected for patients whose transaminase levels are moni-

Continued on next page

This product information was prepared in June 1998. On these and other Parke-Davis Products, information may be obtained by addressing PARKE-DAVIS, Division of Warner-Lambert Company, Morris Plains, New Jersey 07950.

Cognex—Cont.

tored weekly and who receive Cognex® according to the recommended regimen for dose introduction and titration (Table 2). A dosing regimen employing a more rapid escalation of the daily dose of tacrine may be associated with more serious clinical events (see *Monitoring of Liver function and the Management of the patient who develops transaminase elevations*).

Table 2. Cumulative Incidence of ALT/SGPT Elevations Based on Maximum Values with Weekly Monitoring During the 30-Week Study
[Number and (%) of Patients]

Maximum ALT	Males N=229	Females N=250	Total N=479
Within Normal Limits	121(53)	100(40)	221(46)
>ULN	108(47)	150(60)	258(54)
>2 times ULN	77(34)	104(42)	181(38)
>3 times ULN	58(25)	81(32)	139(29)
>10 times ULN	12 (5)	19 (8)	31 (6)
>20 times ULN	3 (1)	6 (2)	9 (2)

Experience in 2446 patients who participated in all clinical trials, including the 30-week study, indicates approximately 50% of patients treated with Cognex® can be expected to have at least 1 ALT/SGPT level above ULN; approximately 25% of patients are likely to develop elevations >3 × ULN, and about 7% of patients may develop elevations >10 × ULN. Data collected from the treatment IND program were consistent with those obtained during clinical studies, and showed 3% of 5665 patients experiencing an ALT/SGPT elevation >10 × ULN.

In clinical trials where transaminases were monitored weekly, the median time to onset of the first ALT/SGPT elevation above ULN was approximately 6 weeks, with maximum ALT/SGPT occurring 1 week later, even in instances when Cognex® treatment was stopped. Under the conditions of forced slow upwards dose titration (increases of 40 mg a day every 6 weeks) employed in clinical studies, 95% of transaminase elevations >3 × ULN occurred within the first 18 weeks of Cognex® therapy, and 99% of the 10-fold elevations occurred by the 12th week and on not more than 80 mg; note, however, that for most patients ALT was monitored weekly and Cognex® was stopped when liver enzymes exceeded 3 × ULN. A total of 276 patients were monitored for ALT/SGPT levels every other week in two double-blind clinical studies, an open-label study, and amended treatment IND. The incidence, severity, time to onset, peak and recovery of ALT/SGPT levels were similar to weekly monitoring. With less frequent monitoring than every other week or the less stringent discontinuation criteria recommended below (see DOSAGE AND ADMINISTRATION), it is possible that marked elevations might be more common. It must also be appreciated that experience with prolonged exposure to the high dose (160 mg/day) is limited. In all cases, transaminase levels returned to within normal limits upon discontinuation of Cognex® treatment or following dosage reduction, usually within 4 to 6 weeks.

This relatively benign experience may be the consequence of careful laboratory monitoring that facilitated the discontinuation of patients early on after the onset of their transaminase elevations. Consequently, frequent monitoring of serum transaminase levels is recommended (see DOSAGE AND ADMINISTRATION, WARNINGS: Liver Injury: Monitoring of Liver Function and the Management of the Patient Who Develops Transaminase Elevations, and PRECAUTIONS: Laboratory Tests).

Liver biopsy experience: Liver biopsy results in 7 patients who received tacrine (1 in a Parke-Davis sponsored study and 6 in studies reported in the literature) revealed hepatocellular necrosis in 6 patients, and granulomatous changes in the seventh. In all cases, liver function tests returned to normal with no evidence of persisting hepatic dysfunction.

Experience with the Rechallenge of Patients with Transaminase Elevations following recovery: Two hundred and twelve patients among the 866 patients assigned to tacrine in the 12 and 30 week studies were withdrawn because they developed transaminase elevations >3 × ULN. One hundred and forty-five of these patients were subsequently rechallenged with weekly monitoring of ALT/SGPT. During their initial exposure to tacrine, 20 of these 145 had experienced initial elevations >10 times ULN, while the remainder had experienced elevations between 3 and 10 × ULN. Upon rechallenge with an initial dose of 40 mg/day, only 48 (33%) of the 145 patients developed transaminase elevations greater than 3 × ULN. Of these patients, 44 had elevations that were between 3 and 10 × ULN and 4 had elevations that were >10 × ULN.

The mean time to onset of elevations occurred earlier on rechallenge than on initial exposure (22 versus 48 days). Of

the 145 patients rechallenged, 127 (88%) were able to continue Cognex® treatment, and 91 of these 127 patients titrated to doses higher than those associated with the initial transaminase elevation.

Predictors of the risk of transaminase elevations: The incidence of transaminase elevations is higher among females. There are no other known predictors of the risk of hepatocellular injury.

Monitoring of Liver function and the Management of the patient who develops transaminase elevations. (See also DOSAGE AND ADMINISTRATION and PRECAUTIONS: Laboratory Tests.)

Blood chemistries: Serum transaminase levels (specifically ALT/SGPT) should be monitored every other week from at least week 4 to week 16 following initiation of treatment, after which monitoring may be decreased to every 3 months. For patients who develop ALT/SGPT elevations greater than two times the upper limit of normal, the dose and monitoring regimen should be modified as described in Table 4 (see DOSAGE AND ADMINISTRATION).

A full monitoring sequence should be repeated in the event that a patient suspends treatment with tacrine for more than 4 weeks.

If ALT/SGPT elevations occur, the frequency of monitoring and the dose of Cognex® should be modified according to the table shown below in DOSAGE AND ADMINISTRATION.

Rechallenge: **Patients with clinical jaundice confirmed by a significant elevation in total bilirubin (>3 mg/dL) and/or those exhibiting clinical signs and/or symptoms of hypersensitivity (e.g. rash or fever) in association with ALT/SGPT elevations should immediately and permanently discontinue Cognex® and not be rechallenged.** Other patients who are required to discontinue Cognex® treatment because of ALT/SGPT elevations may be rechallenged once ALT/SGPT levels return to within normal limits. (See DOSAGE AND ADMINISTRATION.)

Rechallenge of patients with ALT/SGPT elevations less than 10 × ULN has not resulted in serious liver injury. However, because experience in the rechallenge of patients who had elevations greater than 10 × ULN is limited, the risks associated with the rechallenge of these patients are not well characterized. Careful, frequent (weekly) monitoring of serum ALT/SGPT should be undertaken when rechallenging such patients.

If rechallenged, patients should be given an initial dose of 40 mg/day (10 mg QID) and ALT/SGPT levels monitored weekly. If, after 6 weeks on 40 mg/day, the patient is tolerating the dosage with no unacceptable elevations in ALT/SGPT, recommended dose-titration may be resumed. Weekly monitoring of the ALT/SGPT levels should continue for a total of 16 weeks after which monitoring may be decreased to monthly for 2 months and every 3 months thereafter.

Liver biopsy: Liver biopsy is not indicated in cases of uncomplicated transaminase elevation.

Genitourinary
Cholinomimetics may cause bladder outflow obstruction.

Neurological Conditions
Seizures: Cholinomimetics are believed to have some potential to cause generalized convulsions; seizure activity may, however, also be a manifestation of Alzheimer's disease.

Sudden worsening of the degree of cognitive impairment: Worsening of cognitive function has been reported following abrupt discontinuation of Cognex® or after a large reduction in total daily dose (80 mg/day or more).

Pulmonary Conditions
Because of its cholinomimetic action, Cognex® should be prescribed with care to patients with a history of asthma.

PRECAUTIONS
General
Liver Injury: see WARNINGS
Hematology
An absolute neutrophil count (ANC) less than 500/µL occurred in 4 patients who received Cognex® during the course of clinical trials. Three of the 4 patients had concurrent medical conditions commonly associated with a low ANC; 2 of these patients remained on Cognex®. The fourth patient, who had a history of hypersensitivity (penicillin allergy), withdrew from the study as a result of a rash and also developed an ANC <500/µL, which returned to normal; this patient was not rechallenged and, therefore, the role played by Cognex® in this reaction is unknown.

Six patients had an absolute neutrophil count ≤1500/µL, associated with an elevation of ALT/SGPT.

The total clinical experience in more than 12,000 patients does not indicate a clear association between Cognex® treatment and serious white blood cell abnormalities.

Information for Patients and Caregivers
Patients and caregivers should be advised that the effect of Cognex® (brand of tacrine hydrochloride) therapy is thought to depend upon its administration at regular intervals, as directed.

The caregiver should be advised about the possibility of adverse effects. Two types should be distinguished: (1) those

occurring in close temporal association with the initiation of treatment or an increase in dose (eg, nausea, vomiting, loose stools, diarrhea, etc) and (2) those with a delayed onset (eg, rash, jaundice, changes in the color of stool—black, very dark or light [ie, acholic]).

Patients and caregivers should be encouraged to inform the physician about the emergence of new events or any increase in the severity of existing adverse clinical events.

Caregivers should be advised that abrupt discontinuation of Cognex® or a large reduction in total daily dose (80 mg/day or more) may cause a decline in cognitive function and behavioral disturbances. Unsupervised increases in the dose of tacrine may also have serious consequences. Consequently, changes in dose should not be undertaken in the absence of direct instruction of a physician.

Laboratory Tests (see WARNINGS: Liver Injury and DOSAGE AND ADMINISTRATION)
Serum transaminase levels (specifically ALT/SGPT) should be monitored in patients given Cognex® (see WARNINGS: Liver Injury).

Drug-Drug Interactions
Possible metabolic basis for interactions: Tacrine is primarily eliminated by hepatic metabolism via cytochrome P450 drug metabolizing enzymes. Drug-drug interactions may occur when Cognex® is given concurrently with agents such as theophylline that undergo extensive metabolism via cytochrome P450 IA2.

Theophylline. **Coadministration of tacrine with theophylline increased theophylline elimination half-life and average plasma theophylline concentrations by approximately 2-fold. Therefore, monitoring of plasma theophylline concentrations and appropriate reduction of theophylline dose are recommended in patients receiving tacrine and theophylline concurrently. The effect of theophylline on tacrine pharmacokinetics has not been assessed.**

Cimetidine. Cimetidine increased the Cmax and AUC of tacrine by approximately 54% and 64%, respectively.

Anticholinergics. Because of its mechanism of action, Cognex® has the potential to interfere with the activity of anticholinergic medications.

Cholinomimetics and Cholinesterase Inhibitors. A synergistic effect is expected when Cognex® is given concurrently with succinylcholine (see WARNINGS), cholinesterase inhibitors, or cholinergic agonists such as bethanechol.

Fluvoxamine. In a study of 13 healthy, male volunteers, a single 40 mg dose of tacrine added to fluvoxamine 100 mg/day administered at steady-state was associated with five- and eight-fold increases in tacrine Cmax and AUC, respectively, compared to the administration of tacrine alone. Five subjects experienced nausea, vomiting, sweating, and diarrhea following coadministration, consistent with the cholinergic effects of tacrine.

Other Interactions. Rate and extent of tacrine absorption were not influenced by the coadministration of an antacid containing magnesium and aluminum. Tacrine had no major effect on digoxin or diazepam pharmacokinetics or the anticoagulant activity of warfarin.

Carcinogenesis, Mutagenesis, Impairment of Fertility
Tacrine was mutagenic to bacteria in the Ames test. Unscheduled DNA synthesis was induced in rat and mouse hepatocytes *in vitro*. Results of cytogenetic (chromosomal aberration) studies were equivocal. Tacrine was not mutagenic in an *in vitro* mammalian mutation test. Overall, the results of these tests, along with the fact that tacrine belongs to a chemical class (acridines) containing some members which are animal carcinogens, suggest that tacrine may be carcinogenic.

Studies of the effects of tacrine on fertility have not been performed.

Pregnancy
Category C: Animal reproduction studies have not been conducted with tacrine. It is also not known whether Cognex® can cause fetal harm when administered to a pregnant woman or can affect reproductive capacity.

Nursing Mothers
It is not known whether this drug is excreted in human milk.

Pediatric Use
There are no adequate and well-controlled trials to document the safety and efficacy of tacrine in any dementing illness occurring in pediatric patients.

ADVERSE REACTIONS
Common Adverse Events Leading to Discontinuation
In clinical trials, approximately 17% of the 2706 patients who received Cognex® and 5% of the 1886 patients who received placebo withdrew permanently because of adverse events. It should be noted that some of the placebo-treated patients were exposed to Cognex® prior to receiving placebo due to the variety of study designs used, including crossover studies. Transaminase elevations were the most common reason for withdrawals during Cognex® treatment (8% of all Cognex®-treated patients, or 212 of 456 patients withdrawn). The controlled clinical trial protocols required that any patient with an ALT/SGPT elevation >3 × ULN be withdrawn, because of concern about potential hepatotoxic-

ity. Apart from withdrawals due to transaminase elevations, 244 patients (9%) withdrew for adverse events while receiving Cognex®.

Other adverse events that most frequently led to the withdrawal of tacrine-treated patients in clinical trials were nausea and/or vomiting (1.5%), agitation (0.9%), rash (0.7%), anorexia (0.7%), and confusion (0.5%). These adverse events also most frequently led to the withdrawal of placebo-treated patients, although at lower frequencies (0.1% to 0.2%).

Most Frequent Adverse Clinical Events Seen in Association With the Use of Tacrine

The events identified here are those that occurred at an absolute incidence of at least 5% of patients treated with Cognex®, and at a rate at least 2-fold higher in patients treated with Cognex® than placebo.

The most common adverse events associated with the use of Cognex® were elevated transaminases, nausea and/or vomiting, diarrhea, dyspepsia, myalgia, anorexia, and ataxia. Of these events, nausea and/or vomiting, diarrhea, dyspepsia, and anorexia appeared to be dose-dependent.

Adverse Events Reported in Controlled Trials

The events cited in the tables below reflect experience gained under closely monitored conditions of clinical trials with a highly selective patient population. In actual clinical practice or in other clinical trials, these frequency estimates may not apply, as the conditions of use, reporting behavior, and the kinds of patients treated may differ.

Table 3 lists treatment-emergent signs and symptoms that occurred in at least 2% of patients with Alzheimer's disease in placebo-controlled trials and who received the recommended regimen for dose introduction and titration of Cognex® (see DOSAGE AND ADMINISTRATION).

Table 3. Adverse Events Occurring in at Least 2% of Patients Receiving Cognex® at a Starting Dose of 40 mg/day with Titration in 40 mg/day Increments Every 6 Weeks

BODY SYSTEM/ Adverse Events	Cognex® N = 634		Placebo N = 342	
LABORATORY DEVIATIONS				
Elevated Transaminase[a]	184	(29)	5	(2)
BODY AS A WHOLE				
Headache	67	(11)	52	(15)
Fatigue	26	(4)	9	(3)
Chest Pain	24	(4)	18	(5)
Weight Decrease	21	(3)	4	(1)
Back Pain	15	(2)	14	(4)
Asthenia	15	(2)	7	(2)
DIGESTIVE SYSTEM				
Nausea and/or Vomiting	178	(28)	29	(9)
Diarrhea	99	(16)	18	(5)
Dyspepsia	57	(9)	22	(6)
Anorexia	54	(9)	11	(3)
Abdominal Pain	48	(8)	24	(7)
Flatulence	22	(4)	5	(2)
Constipation	24	(4)	8	(2)
HEMIC AND LYMPHATIC SYSTEM				
Purpura	15	(2)	8	(2)
MUSCULOSKELETAL SYSTEM				
Myalgia	54	(9)	18	(5)
NERVOUS SYSTEM				
Dizziness	73	(12)	39	(11)
Confusion	42	(7)	24	(7)
Ataxia	36	(6)	12	(4)
Insomnia	37	(6)	18	(5)
Somnolence	22	(4)	11	(3)
Tremor	14	(2)	2	(<1)
PSYCHOBIOLOGIC FUNCTION				
Agitation	43	(7)	30	(9)
Depression	22	(4)	14	(4)
Thinking Abnormal	17	(3)	14	(4)
Anxiety	16	(3)	7	(2)
Hallucination	15	(2)	12	(4)
Hostility	15	(2)	5	(2)
RESPIRATORY SYSTEM				
Rhinitis	51	(8)	22	(6)
Upper Respiratory Infection	18	(3)	11	(3)
Coughing	17	(3)	18	(5)
SKIN AND APPENDAGES				
Rash[b]	46	(7)	18	(5)
Facial Flushing, Skin Flushing	16	(3)	3	(<1)
UROGENITAL SYSTEM				
Urination Frequency	21	(3)	12	(4)
Urinary Tract Infection	21	(3)	20	(6)
Urinary Incontinence	16	(3)	9	(3)

[a] ALT or AST value of approximately 3 × ULN or greater or that resulted in a change in patient management. Patients were monitored weekly.
[b] Includes COSTART terms: rash, rash-erythematous, rash-maculopapular, urticaria, petechial rash, rash-vesiculobullous, and pruritus.

Other Adverse Events Observed During All Clinical Trials

Cognex® has been administered to 2706 individuals during clinical trials. A total of 1471 patients were treated for at least 3 months, 1137 for at least 6 months, and 773 for at least 1 year. Any untoward reactions that occurred during these trials were recorded as adverse events by the clinical investigators using terminology of their own choosing. To provide a meaningful estimate of the proportion of individuals having similar types of events, the events were grouped into a smaller number of standardized categories using a modified COSTART dictionary. These categories are used in the listing below. The frequencies represent the proportion of the 2706 individuals exposed to Cognex® who experienced that event while receiving Cognex®. All adverse events are included except those already listed on the previous table and those COSTART terms too general to be informative. Events are further classified by body system categories and listed using the following definitions: frequent adverse events are defined as those occurring in at least 1/100 patients; infrequent adverse events are those occurring in 1/100 to 1/1000 patients; and rare adverse events are those occurring in less than 1/1000 patients. These adverse events are not necessarily related to Cognex® treatment. Only rare adverse events deemed to be potentially important are included.

Body As a Whole: *Frequent:* Chill, fever, malaise, peripheral edema. *Infrequent:* Face edema, dehydration, weight increase, cachexia, edema (generalized), lipoma. *Rare:* Heat exhaustion, sepsis, cholingeric crisis, death.

Cardiovascular System: *Frequent:* Hypotension, hypertension. *Infrequent:* Heart failure, myocardial infarction, angina pectoris, cerebrovascular accident, transient ischemic attack, phlebitis, venous insufficiency, abdominal aortic aneurysm, atrial fibrillation or flutter, palpitation, tachycardia, bradycardia, pulmonary embolus, migraine, hypercholesterolemia. *Rare:* Heart arrest, premature atrial contractions, A-V block, bundle branch block.

Digestive System: *Infrequent:* Glossitis, gingivitis, mouth or throat dry, stomatitis, increased salivation, dysphagia, esophagitis, gastritis, gastroenteritis, GI hemorrhage, stomach ulcer, hiatal hernia, hemorrhoids, stools bloody, diverticulitis, fecal impaction, fecal incontinence, hemorrhage (rectum), cholelithiasis, cholecystitis, increased appetite. *Rare:* Duodenal ulcer, bowel obstruction.

Endocrine System: *Infrequent:* Diabetes. *Rare:* Hyperthyroid, hypothyroid.

Hemic and Lymphatic: *Infrequent:* Anemia, lymphadenopathy. *Rare:* Leukopenia, thrombocytopenia, hemolysis, pancytopenia.

Musculoskeletal: *Frequent:* Fracture, arthralgia, arthritis, hypertonia. *Infrequent:* Osteoporosis, tendinitis, bursitis, gout. *Rare:* Myopathy.

Nervous System: *Frequent:* Convulsions, vertigo, syncope, hyperkinesia, paresthesia. *Infrequent:* Dreaming abnormal, dysarthria, aphasia, amnesia, wandering, twitching, hypesthesia, delirium, paralysis, bradykinesia, movement disorder, cogwheel rigidity, paresis, neuritis, hemiplegia, Parkinson's disease, neuropathy, extrapyramidal syndrome, reflexes decreased/absent. *Rare:* Tardive dyskinesia, dysesthesia, dystonia, encephalitis, coma, apraxia, oculogyric crisis, akathisia, oral facial dyskinesia, Bell's palsy, exacerbation of Parkinson's disease.

Psychobiologic Function: *Frequent:* Nervousness. *Infrequent:* Apathy, increased libido, paranoia, neurosis. *Rare:* Suicidal, psychosis, hysteria.

Respiratory System: *Frequent:* Pharyngitis, sinusitis, bronchitis, pneumonia, dyspnea. *Infrequent:* Epistaxis, chest congestion, asthma, hyperventilation, lower respiratory infection. *Rare:* Hemoptysis, lung edema, lung cancer, acute epiglottitis.

Skin and Appendages: *Frequent:* Sweating increased. *Infrequent:* Acne, alopecia, dermatitis, eczema, skin dry, herpes zoster, psoriasis, cellulitis, cyst, furunculosis, herplex simplex, hyperkeratosis, basal cell carcinoma, skin cancer. *Rare:* Desquamation, seborrhea, squamous cell carcinoma, ulcer (skin), skin necrosis, melanoma.

Urogenital System: *Infrequent:* Hematuria, renal stone, kidney infection, glycosuria, dysuria, polyuria, nocturia, pyuria, cystitis, urinary retention, urination urgency, vaginal hemorrhage, pruritus (genital), breast pain, impotence, prostate cancer. *Rare:* Bladder tumor, renal tumor, renal failure, urinary obstruction, breast cancer, epididymitis, carcinoma (ovary).

Special Senses: *Frequent:* Conjunctivitis. *Infrequent:* Cataract, eyes dry, eye pain, visual field defect, diplopia, amblyopia, glaucoma, hordeolum, deafness, earache, tinnitus, inner ear infection, otitis media, unusual taste. *Rare:* Vision loss, ptosis, blepharitis, labyrinthitis, inner ear disturbance.

Postintroduction Reports

Voluntary reports of adverse events temporarily associated with Cognex® that have been received since market introduction, that are not listed above, and that may have no causal relationship with the drug include the following: pancreatitis, perforated peptic ulcer, and falling.

OVERDOSAGE

As in any case of overdose, general supportive measures should be utilized. Overdosage with cholinesterase inhibitors can cause a cholinergic crisis characterized by severe nausea/vomiting, salivation, sweating, bradycardia, hypotension, collapse, and convulsions. Increasing muscle weakness is a possibility and may result in death if respiratory muscles are involved.

Tertiary anticholinergics such as atropine may be used as an antidote for Cognex® overdosage. Intravenous atropine sulfate titrated to effect is recommended: in adults, initial dose of 1.0 to 2.0 mg IV with subsequent doses based on clinical response. In children, the usual IM or IV dose is 0.05 mg/kg, repeated every 10–30 minutes until muscarinic signs and symptoms subside and repeated if they reappear. Atypical increases in blood pressure and heart rate have been reported with other cholinomimetics when coadministered with quaternary anticholinergics such as glycopyrrolate.

It is not known whether Cognex® or its metabolites can be eliminated by dialysis (hemodialysis, peritoneal dialysis, or hemofiltration).

The estimated median lethal dose of tacrine following a single oral dose in rats is 40 mg/kg, or approximately 12 times the maximum recommended human dose of 160 mg/day. Dose-related signs of cholinergic stimulation were observed in animals and included vomiting, diarrhea, salivation, lacrimation, ataxia, convulsions, tremor, and stereotypic head and body movements.

DOSAGE AND ADMINISTRATION

The recommendations for dose titration are based on experience from clinical trials. The rate of dose escalation may be slowed if a patient is intolerant to the titration schedule recommended below. It is not advisable, however, to accelerate the dose incrementation plan.

Following initiation of therapy, or any dosage increase, patients should be observed carefully for adverse effects. Cognex® should be taken between meals whenever possible; however, if minor GI upset occurs, Cognex® may be taken with meals to improve tolerability. Taking Cognex® with meals can be expected to reduce plasma levels approximately 30% to 40%.

The initial dose of Cognex® brand of tacrine hydrochloride is 40 mg/day (10 mg Q.I.D.). This dose should be maintained for a minimum of 4 weeks with every other week monitoring of transaminase levels beginning 4 weeks after initiation of treatment. It is important that the dose not be increased during this period because of the potential for delayed onset of transaminase elevations.

Dose Titration

Following 4 weeks of treatment at 40 mg/day (10 mg Q.I.D.), the dose of Cognex® should then be increased to 80 mg/day (20 mg Q.I.D.), providing there are no significant transaminase elevations and the patient is tolerating treatment. Patients should be titrated to higher doses (120 and 160 mg/day, in divided doses on a Q.I.D. schedule) at 4-week intervals on the basis of tolerance.

Dose Adjustment

Serum ALT/SGPT should be monitored every other week from at least week 4 to week 16 following initiation of treatment, after which monitoring may be decreased to every 3 months. For patients who develop ALT/SGPT elevations greater than two times the upper limit of normal, the dose and monitoring regimen should be modified as described in Table 4.

A full monitoring and dose titration sequence must be repeated in the event that a patient suspends treatment with tacrine for more than 4 weeks.

Table 4. Recommended Dose amd Monitoring Regimen Modification in Response to ALT/SGPT Elevations

ALT/SGPT Level	Treatment and Monitoring Regimen
≤2 × ULN	Continue treatment according to recommended titration and monitoring schedule.
>2 to ≤3 × ULN	Continue treatment according to recommended titration. Monitor ALT/SGPT levels weekly until levels return to normal limits.
>3 to ≤5 × ULN	Reduce the daily dose of Cognex® by 40 mg/day. Monitor ALT/SGPT levels weekly. Resume dose titration and every other week monitoring when the levels of the ALT/SGPT return to normal limits.

Continued on next page

This product information was prepared in June 1998. On these and other Parke-Davis Products, information may be obtained by addressing PARKE-DAVIS, Division of Warner-Lambert Company, Morris Plains, New Jersey 07950.

Cognex—Cont.

| >5 × ULN | Stop Cognex® treatment. Monitor the patient closely for signs and symptoms associated with hepatitis and follow ALT/SGPT levels until within normal limits. See Rechallenge section below. Experience is limited in patients with ALT/SGPT >10 × ULN. The risk of rechallenge must be considered against demonstrated clinical benefit. **Patients with clinical jaundice confirmed by a significant elevation in total bilirubin (>3 mg/dL) and/or those exhibiting clinical signs and/or symptoms of hypersensitivity (e.g. rash or fever) in association with ALT/SGPT elevations should immediately and permanently discontinue Cognex® and not be rechallenged.** |

Rechallenge

Patients who are required to discontinue Cognex® treatment because of ALT/SGPT elevations may be rechallenged once ALT/SGPT levels return to normal limits.

Rechallenge of patients exposed to ALT/SGPT elevations less than 10 × ULN has not resulted in serious liver injury. However, because experience in the rechallenge of patients who had elevations greater than 10 × ULN is limited, the risks associated with the rechallenge of these patients are not well characterized. Careful, frequent (weekly) monitoring of serum ALT/SGPT should be undertaken when rechallenging such patients.

If rechallenged, patients should be given an initial dose of 40 mg/day (10 mg QID) and ALT/SGPT levels monitored weekly. If, after 6 weeks on 40 mg/day, the patient is tolerating the dosage with no unacceptable elevations in ALT/SGPT, the recommended dose-titration may be resumed. Weekly monitoring of the ALT/SGPT levels should continue for a total of 16 weeks after which monitoring may be decreased to monthly for 2 months and every 3 months thereafter.

HOW SUPPLIED

Cognex® is supplied as capsules of tacrine hydrochloride containing 10, 20, 30, and 40 mg of tacrine. The capsule logo is Cognex®, with the strength (eg, 10, 20, 30, or 40) printed underneath.

10 mg (yellow/dark green)	Bottles of 120 (N 0071-0096-25) Unit-dose package of 100 (10 × 10) (N 0071-0096-40)
20 mg (yellow/light blue)	Bottles of 120 (N 0071-0097-25) Unit-dose package of 100 (10 × 10) (N 0071-0097-40)
30 mg (yellow/swedish orange)	Bottles of 120 (N 0071-0095-25) Unit-dose package of 100 (10 × 10) (N 0071-0095-40)
40 mg (yellow/lavender)	Bottles of 120 (N 0071-0098-25) Unit-dose package of 100 (10 × 10) (N 0071-0098-40)

Storage

Store at controlled room temperature 15°C to 30°C (59°F to 86°F) away from moisture.

Rx only

Manufactured by:
Parke Davis Pharmaceuticals, Ltd.
Vega Baja, PR 00694
Distributed by:
PARKE-DAVIS
Div of Warner-Lambert Co.
Morris Plains, NJ 07950 USA
©1997-'98, PDPL
Revised May 1998   0096G025
Shown in Product Identification Guide, page 329

KAPSEALS®
DILANTIN®   ℞
[dĭ-lăn 'tĭn ']
(Extended Phenytoin Sodium Capsules, USP)

DESCRIPTION

Phenytoin Sodium is an antiepileptic drug. Phenytoin sodium is related to the barbiturates in chemical structure, but has a five-membered ring. The chemical name is sodium 5,5-diphenyl-2,4-imidazolidinedione.

Each Dilantin—*Extended Phenytoin Sodium Capsule* USP contains 30 mg or 100 mg phenytoin sodium USP. Also contains lactose, NF; confectioner's sugar, NF; talc, USP; and magnesium stearate, NF. The capsule shell and band contain colloidal silicon dioxide, NF; FD&C red No. 3; gelatin, NF; glyceryl monooleate; sodium lauryl sulfate, NF. The Dilantin 30-mg capsule shell and band also contain citric acid, USP; FD&C blue No. 1; sodium benzoate, NF; titanium dioxide, USP. The Dilantin 100-mg capsule shell and band also contain FD&C yellow no. 6; purified water, USP; polyethylene glycol 200. Product *in vivo* performance is characterized by a slow and extended rate of absorption with peak blood concentrations expected in 4 to 12 hours as contrasted to *Prompt Phenytoin Sodium Capsules* USP with a rapid rate of absorption with peak blood concentration expected in $1^1/_2$ to 3 hours.

CLINICAL PHARMACOLOGY

Phenytoin is an antiepileptic drug which can be useful in the treatment of epilepsy. The primary site of action appears to be *the motor cortex* where spread of seizure activity is inhibited. Possibly by promoting sodium efflux from neurons, phenytoin tends to *stabilize* the threshold against hyperexcitability caused by excessive stimulation or environmental changes capable of reducing membrane sodium gradient. This includes the reduction of posttetanic potentiation at synapses. Loss of posttetanic potentiation prevents cortical seizure foci from detonating adjacent cortical areas. Phenytoin reduces the maximal activity of brain stem centers responsible for the tonic phase of tonic-clonic (grand mal) seizures.

The plasma half-life in man after oral administration of phenytoin averages 22 hours, with a range of 7 to 42 hours. Steady-state therapeutic levels are achieved 7 to 10 days after initiation of therapy with recommended doses of 300 mg/day.

When serum level determinations are necessary, they should be obtained at least 5-7 half-lives after treatment initiation, dosage change, or addition or subtraction of another drug to the regimen so that equilibrium or steady-state will have been achieved. Trough levels provide information about clinically effective serum level range and confirm patient compliance and are obtained just prior to the patient's next scheduled dose. Peak levels indicate an individual's threshold for emergence of dose-related side effects and are obtained at the time of expected peak concentration. For Dilantin Kapseals peak serum levels occur 4-12 hours after administration.

Optimum control without clinical signs of toxicity occurs more often with serum levels between 10 and 20 mcg/ml, although some mild cases of tonic-clonic (grand mal) epilepsy may be controlled with lower serum levels of phenytoin.

In most patients maintained at a steady dosage, stable phenytoin serum levels are achieved. There may be wide interpatient variability in phenytoin serum levels with equivalent dosages. Patients with unusually low levels may be noncompliant or hypermetabolizers of phenytoin. Unusually high levels result from liver disease, congenital enzyme deficiency or drug interactions which result in metabolic interference. The patient with large variations in phenytoin plasma levels, despite standard doses, presents a difficult clinical problem. Serum level determinations in such patients may be particularly helpful. As phenytoin is highly protein bound, free phenytoin levels may be altered in patients whose protein binding characteristics differ from normal.

Most of the drug is excreted in the bile as inactive metabolites which are then reabsorbed from the intestinal tract and excreted in the urine. Urinary excretion of phenytoin and its metabolites occurs partly with glomerular filtration but more importantly, by tubular secretion. Because phenytoin is hydroxylated in the liver by an enzyme system which is saturable at high plasma levels, small incremental doses may increase the half-life and produce very substantial increases in serum levels, when these are in the upper range. The steady-state level may be disproportionately increased, with resultant intoxication, from an increase in dosage of 10% or more.

INDICATIONS AND USAGE

Dilantin is indicated for the control of generalized tonic-clonic (grand mal) and complex partial (psychomotor, temporal lobe) seizures and prevention and treatment of seizures occurring during or following neurosurgery.

Phenytoin serum level determinations may be necessary for optimal dosage adjustments (see Dosage and Administration and Clinical Pharmacology sections).

CONTRAINDICATIONS

Phenytoin is contraindicated in those patients who are hypersensitive to phenytoin or other hydantoins.

WARNINGS

Abrupt withdrawal of phenytoin in epileptic patients may precipitate status epilepticus. When, in the judgment of the clinician, the need for dosage reduction, discontinuation, or substitution of alternative antiepileptic medication arises, this should be done gradually. However, in the event of an allergic or hypersensitivity reaction, rapid substitution of alternative therapy may be necessary. In this case, alternative therapy should be an antiepileptic drug not belonging to the hydantoin chemical class.

There have been a number of reports suggesting a relationship between phenytoin and the development of lymphadenopathy (local or generalized) including benign lymph node hyperplasia, pseudolymphoma, lymphoma, and Hodgkin's Disease. Although a cause and effect relationship has not been established, the occurrence of lymphadenopathy indicates the need to differentiate such a condition from other types of lymph node pathology. Lymph node involvement may occur with or without symptoms and signs resembling serum sickness, eg, fever, rash and liver involvement.

In all cases of lymphadenopathy, follow-up observation for an extended period is indicated and every effort should be made to achieve seizure control using alternative antiepileptic drugs.

Acute alcoholic intake may increase phenytoin serum levels while chronic alcoholic use may decrease serum levels.

In view of isolated reports associating phenytoin with exacerbation of porphyria, caution should be exercised in using this medication in patients suffering from this disease.

Usage in Pregnancy:

A number of reports suggests an association between the use of antiepileptic drugs by women with epilepsy and a higher incidence of birth defects in children born to these women. Data are more extensive with respect to phenytoin and phenobarbital, but these are also the most commonly prescribed antiepileptic drugs; less systematic or anecdotal reports suggest a possible similar association with the use of all known antiepileptic drugs.

The reports suggesting a higher incidence of birth defects in children of drug-treated epileptic women cannot be regarded as adequate to prove a definite cause and effect relationship. There are intrinsic methodologic problems in obtaining adequate data on drug teratogenicity in humans; genetic factors or the epileptic condition itself may be more important than drug therapy in leading to birth defects. The great majority of mothers on antiepileptic medication deliver normal infants. It is important to note that antiepileptic drugs should not be discontinued in patients in whom the drug is administered to prevent major seizures, because of the strong possibility of precipitating status epilepticus with attendant hypoxia and threat to life. In individual cases where the severity and frequency of the seizure disorder are such that the removal of medication does not pose a serious threat to the patient, discontinuation of the drug may be considered prior to and during pregnancy, although it cannot be said with any confidence that even minor seizures do not pose some hazard to the developing embryo or fetus. The prescribing physician will wish to weigh these considerations in treating or counseling epileptic women of childbearing potential.

In addition to the reports of increased incidence of congenital malformation, such as cleft lip/palate and heart malformations in children of women receiving phenytoin and other antiepileptic drugs, there have more recently been reports of a fetal hydantoin syndrome. This consists of prenatal growth deficiency, microcephaly and mental deficiency in children born to mothers who have received phenytoin, barbiturates, alcohol, or trimethadione. However, these features are all interrelated and are frequently associated with intrauterine growth retardation from other causes.

There have been isolated reports of malignancies, including neuroblastoma, in children whose mothers received phenytoin during pregnancy.

An increase in seizure frequency during pregnancy occurs in a high proportion of patients, because of altered phenytoin absorption or metabolism. Periodic measurement of serum phenytoin levels is particularly valuable in the management of a pregnant epileptic patient as a guide to an appropriate adjustment of dosage. However, postpartum restoration of the original dosage will probably be indicated.

Neonatal coagulation defects have been reported within the first 24 hours in babies born to epileptic mothers receiving phenobarbital and/or phenytoin. Vitamin K has been shown to prevent or correct this defect and has been recommended to be given to the mother before delivery and to the neonate after birth.

PRECAUTIONS
General:

The liver is the chief site of biotransformation of phenytoin; patients with impaired liver function, elderly patients, or those who are gravely ill may show early signs of toxicity.

A small percentage of individuals who have been treated with phenytoin have been shown to metabolize the drug slowly. Slow metabolism may be due to limited enzyme availability and lack of induction; it appears to be genetically determined.

Phenytoin should be discontinued if a skin rash appears (see "Warnings" section regarding drug discontinuation). If the rash is exfoliative, purpuric, or bullous or if lupus erythematosus, Stevens-Johnson syndrome, or toxic epidermal necrolysis is suspected, use of the drug should not be resumed and alternative therapy should be considered. (See

ADVERSE REACTIONS section.) If the rash is of a milder type (measles-like or scarlatiniform), therapy may be resumed after the rash has completely disappeared. If the rash recurs upon reinstitution of therapy, further phenytoin medication is contraindicated.

Phenytoin and other hydantoins are contraindicated in patients who have experienced phenytoin hypersensitivity. Additionally, caution should be exercised if using structurally similar compounds (eg, barbiturates, succinimides, oxazolidinediones and other related compounds) in these same patients.

Hyperglycemia, resulting from the drug's inhibitory effects on insulin release, has been reported. Phenytoin may also raise the serum glucose level in diabetic patients.

Osteomalacia has been associated with phenytoin therapy and is considered to be due to phenytoin's interference with Vitamin D metabolism.

Phenytoin is not indicated for seizures due to hypoglycemic or other causes. Appropriate diagnostic procedures should be performed as indicated.

Phenytoin is not effective for absence (petit mal) seizures. If tonic-clonic (grand-mal) and absence (petit mal) seizures are present, combined drug therapy is needed.

Serum levels of phenytoin sustained above the optimal range may produce confusional states referred to as "delirium," "psychosis," or "encephalopathy," or rarely irreversible cerebellar dysfunction. Accordingly, at the first sign of acute toxicity, plasma levels are recommended. Dose reduction of phenytoin therapy is indicated if plasma levels are excessive; if symptoms persist, termination is recommended. (See Warnings section.)

Information for Patients:
Patients taking phenytoin should be advised of the importance of adhering strictly to the prescribed dosage regimen, and of informing the physician of any clinical condition in which it is not possible to take the drug orally as prescribed, eg, surgery, etc.

Patients should also be cautioned on the use of other drugs or alcoholic beverages without first seeking the physician's advice.

Patients should be instructed to call their physician if skin rash develops.

The importance of good dental hygiene should be stressed in order to minimize the development of gingival hyperplasia and its complications.

Laboratory Tests:
Phenytoin serum level determinations may be necessary to achieve optimal dosage adjustments.

Drug Interactions:
There are many drugs which may increase or decrease phenytoin levels or which phenytoin may affect. Serum level determinations for phenytoin are especially helpful when possible drug interactions are suspected. The most commonly occurring drug interactions are listed below.

1. Drugs which may increase phenytoin serum levels include: acute alcohol intake, amiodarone, chloramphenicol, chlordiazepoxide, diazepam, dicumarol, disulfiram, estrogens, H$_2$-antagonists, halothane, isoniazid, methylphenidate, phenothiazines, phenylbutazone, salicylates, succinimides, sulfonamides, tolbutamide, trazodone.
2. Drugs which may decrease phenytoin levels include: carbamazepine, chronic alcohol abuse, reserpine, and sucralfate. Moban® brand of molindone hydrochloride contains calcium ions which interfere with the absorption of phenytoin. Ingestion times of phenytoin and antacid preparations containing calcium should be staggered in patients with low serum phenytoin levels to prevent absorption problems.
3. Drugs which may either increase or decrease phenytoin serum levels include: phenobarbital, sodium valproate, and valproic acid. Similarly, the effect of phenytoin on phenobarbital, valproic acid and sodium valproate serum levels is unpredictable.
4. Although not a true drug interaction, tricyclic antidepressants may precipitate seizures in susceptible patients and phenytoin dosage may need to be adjusted.
5. Drugs whose efficacy is impaired by phenytoin include: corticosteroids, coumarin anticoagulants, digitoxin, doxycycline, estrogens, furosemide, oral contraceptives, quinidine, rifampin, theophylline, vitamin D.

Drug/Laboratory Test Interactions:
Phenytoin may cause decreased serum levels of protein-bound iodine (PBI). It may also produce lower than normal values for dexamethasone or metyrapone tests. Phenytoin may cause increased serum levels of glucose, alkaline phosphatase, and gamma glutamyl transpeptidase (GGT).

Carcinogenesis:
See 'Warnings' section for information on carcinogenesis.

Pregnancy:
See WARNINGS section.

Nursing Mothers:
Infant breast feeding is not recommended for women taking this drug because phenytoin appears to be secreted in low concentrations in human milk.

ADVERSE REACTIONS
Central Nervous System: The most common manifestations encountered with phenytoin therapy are referable to this system and are usually dose-related. These include nystagmus, ataxia, slurred speech, decreased coordination, and mental confusion. Dizziness, insomnia, transient nervousness, motor twitchings, and headaches have also been observed. There have also been rare reports of phenytoin induced dyskinesias, including chorea, dystonia, tremor and asterixis, similar to those induced by phenothiazine and other neuroleptic drugs.

A predominantly sensory peripheral polyneuropathy has been observed in patients receiving long-term phenytoin therapy.

Gastrointestinal System: Nausea, vomiting, constipation, toxic hepatitis and liver damage.

Integumentary System: Dermatological manifestations sometimes accompanied by fever have included scarlatiniform or morbilliform rashes. A morbilliform rash (measleslike) is the most common; other types of dermatitis are seen more rarely. Other more serious forms which may be fatal have included bullous, exfoliative or purpuric dermatitis, lupus erythematosus, Stevens-Johnson syndrome, and toxic epidermal necrolysis (see Precautions section).

Hemopoietic System: Hemopoietic complications, some fatal, have occasionally been reported in association with administration of phenytoin. These have included thrombocytopenia, leukopenia, granulocytopenia, agranulocytosis, and pancytopenia with or without bone marrow suppression. While macrocytosis and megaloblastic anemia have occurred, these conditions usually respond to folic acid therapy. Lymphadenopathy including benign lymph node hyperplasia, pseudolymphoma, lymphoma, and Hodgkin's Disease have been reported (see WARNINGS section).

Connective Tissue System: Coarsening of the facial features, enlargement of the lips, gingival hyperplasia, hypertrichosis, and Peyronie's Disease.

Cardiovascular: Periarteritis nodosa.

Immunologic: Hypersensitivity syndrome (which may include, but is not limited to, symptoms such as arthralgias, eosinophilia, fever, liver dysfunction, lymphadenopathy or rash), systemic lupus erythematosus, immunoglobulin abnormalities.

OVERDOSAGE
The lethal dose in pediatric patients is not known. The lethal dose in adults is estimated to be 2 to 5 grams. The initial symptoms are nystagmus, ataxia, and dysarthria. Other signs are tremor, hyperflexia, lethargy, slurred speech, nausea, vomiting. The patient may become comatose and hypotensive. Death is due to respiratory and circulatory depression.

There are marked variations among individuals with respect to phenytoin plasma levels where toxicity may occur. Nystagmus, on lateral gaze, usually appears at 20 mcg/ml, ataxia at 30 mcg/ml, dysarthria and lethargy appear when the plasma concentration is over 40 mcg/ml, but as high a concentration as 50 mcg/ml has been reported without evidence of toxicity. As much as 25 times the therapeutic dose has been taken to result in a serum concentration over 100 mcg/ml with complete recovery.

Treatment:
Treatment is nonspecific since there is no known antidote. The adequacy of the respiratory and circulatory systems should be carefully observed and appropriate supportive measures employed. Hemodialysis can be considered since phenytoin is not completely bound to plasma proteins. Total exchange transfusion has been used in the treatment of severe intoxication in pediatric patients.

In acute overdosage, the possibility of other CNS depressants, including alcohol, should be borne in mind.

DOSAGE AND ADMINISTRATION
Serum concentrations should be monitored in changing from extended Phenytoin Sodium Capsules USP (Dilantin) to Prompt Phenytoin Sodium Capsules USP, and from the sodium salt to the free acid form.

Dilantin® Kapseals® and Dilantin Parenteral are formulated with the sodium salt of phenytoin. The free acid form of phenytoin is used in Dilantin-125 Suspension and Dilantin Infatabs. Because there is approximately an 8% increase in drug content with the free acid form over that of the sodium salt, dosage adjustments and serum level monitoring may be necessary when switching from a product formulated with the free acid to a product formulated with the sodium salt and vice versa.

General:
Dosage should be individualized to provide maximum benefit. In some cases, serum blood level determinations may be necessary for optimal dosage adjustments—the clinically effective serum level is usually 10-20 mcg/ml. With recommended dosage, a period of seven to ten days may be required to achieve steady-state blood levels with phenytoin and changes in dosage (increase or decrease) should not be carried out at intervals shorter than seven to ten days.

Adult Dosage:
Divided Daily Dosage
Patients who have received no previous treatment may be started on one 100-mg Dilantin (Extended Phenytoin Sodium Capsule) three times daily and the dosage then adjusted to suit individual requirements. For most adults, the satisfactory maintenance dosage will be one capsule three to four times a day. An increase up to two capsules three times a day may be made, if necessary.

Once-a-Day Dosage:
In adults, if seizure control is established with divided doses of three 100 mg Dilantin capsules daily, once-a-day dosage with 300 mg of extended phenytoin sodium capsules may be considered. Studies comparing divided doses of 300 mg with a single daily dose of this quantity indicated absorption, peak plasma levels, biologic half-life, difference between peak and minimum values, and urinary recovery were equivalent. Once-a-day dosage offers a convenience to the individual patient or to nursing personnel for institutionalized patients and is intended to be used only for patients requiring this amount of drug daily. A major problem in motivating noncompliant patients may also be lessened when the patient can take this drug once a day. However, patients should be cautioned not to miss a dose, inadvertently.

Only extended phenytoin sodium capsules are recommended for once-a-day dosing. Inherent differences in dissolution characteristics and resultant absorption rates of phenytoin due to different manufacturing procedures and/or dosage forms preclude such recommendation for other phenytoin products. When a change in the dosage form or brand is prescribed, careful monitoring of phenytoin serum levels should be carried out.

Loading Dose:
Some authorities have advocated use of an oral loading dose of phenytoin in adults who require rapid steady-state serum levels and where intravenous administration is not desirable. This dosing regimen should be reserved for patients in a clinic or hospital setting where phenytoin serum levels can be closely monitored. Patients with a history of renal or liver disease should not receive the oral loading regimen. Initially, one gram of phenytoin capsules is divided into 3 doses (400 mg, 300 mg, 300 mg) and administered at two-hourly intervals. Normal maintenance dosage is then instituted 24 hours after the loading dose, with frequent serum level determinations.

Pediatric Dosage:
Initially, 5 mg/kg/day in two or three equally divided doses, with subsequent dosage individualized to a maximum of 300 mg daily. A recommended daily maintenance dosage is usually 4 to 8 mg/kg. Children over 6 years old and adolescents may require the minimum adult dose (300 mg/day).

HOW SUPPLIED
N 0071-0362 (Kapseal 362, transparent #3 capsule with an orange band)—Dilantin 100 mg; in 100's, 1,000's, and unit dose 100's.

N 0071-0365 (Kapseal 365, transparent #4 capsule with a pink band)—Dilantin 30 mg; in 100's.

Store below 30°C (86°F). Protect from light and moisture.
Also available as:
N 0071-2214—Dilantin-125® Suspension 125 mg phenytoin/5 ml with a maximum alcohol content not greater than 0.6 percent, available in 8-oz bottles. The minimum sales unit is 100 pouches.

N 0071-0007 (Tablet 7)—Dilantin Infatabs® each contain 50 mg phenytoin, 100's and unit dose 100's.

For Parenteral Use:
N 0071-4488-47 (Steri-Dose® 4488)-Dilantin ready-mixed solution containing 50 mg phenytoin sodium per milliliter is supplied in a 2-mL sterile disposable syringe (22 gauge × 1¼ inch needle). Packages of ten syringes.

N 0071-4488-45 Dilantin ready-mixed solution containing 50 mg phenytoin sodium per milliliter is supplied in 2-mL Steri-Vials.® Packages of twenty-five.

N 0071-4475-45 Dilantin ready-mixed solution containing 50 mg phenytoin sodium per milliliter is supplied in 5-mL Steri-Vials.® Packages of twenty-five.

Store below 30°C (86°F). Protect from light and moisture.
Revised September 1997
© 1997, Warner-Lambert Co. 0362G288
Shown in Product Identification Guide, page 329

Continued on next page

This product information was prepared in June 1998. On these and other Parke-Davis Products, information may be obtained by addressing PARKE-DAVIS, Division of Warner-Lambert Company, Morris Plains, New Jersey 07950.

INFATABS®
DILANTIN®
[dī-lăn'tĭn" ĭn'fă-tăbs"]
(Phenytoin Tablets, USP)

℞

NOT FOR ONCE A DAY DOSING

DESCRIPTION

Dilantin is an antiepileptic drug.

Dilantin (phenytoin) is related to the barbiturates in chemical structure, but has a five-membered ring. The chemical name is 5,5-diphenyl-2,4-imidazolidinedione.

Each Dilantin Infatab, for oral administration, contains 50 mg phenytoin, USP. Also contains: D&C yellow No. 10, Al lake; FD&C yellow No. 6, Al lake flavor; saccharin sodium, USP; sucrose, NF; talc, USP; and other ingredients.

CLINICAL PHARMACOLOGY

Phenytoin is an antiepileptic drug which can be useful in the treatment of epilepsy. The primary site of action appears to be the motor cortex where spread of seizure activity is inhibited. Possibly by promoting sodium efflux from neurons, phenytoin tends to stabilize the threshold against hyperexcitability caused by excessive stimulation or environmental changes capable of reducing membrane sodium gradient. This includes the reduction of posttetanic potentiation at synapses. Loss of posttetanic potentiation prevents cortical seizure foci from detonating adjacent cortical areas. Phenytoin reduces the maximal activity of brain stem centers responsible for the tonic phase of tonic-clonic (grand mal) seizures.

Clinical studies using Dilantin Infatabs have shown an average plasma half-life of 14 hours with a range of 7 to 29 hours. Steady-state therapeutic levels are achieved at least 7 to 10 days (5-7 half-lives) after initiation of therapy with recommended doses of 300 mg/day.

When serum level determinations are necessary, they should be obtained at least 5-7 half-lives after treatment initiation, dosage change, or addition or subtraction of another drug to the regimen so that equilibrium or steady-state will have been achieved. Trough levels provide information about clinically effective serum level range and confirm patient compliance and are obtained just prior to the patient's next scheduled dose. Peak levels indicate an individual's threshold for emergence of dose-related side effects and are obtained at the time of expected peak concentration. For Dilantin Infatabs peak levels occur 1$\frac{1}{2}$-3 hours after administration.

Optimum control without clinical signs of toxicity occurs more often with serum levels between 10 and 20 mcg/ml, although some mild cases of tonic-clonic (grand mal) epilepsy may be controlled with lower serum levels of phenytoin.

In most patients maintained at a steady dosage, stable phenytoin serum levels are achieved. There may be wide interpatient variability in phenytoin serum levels with equivalent dosages. Patients with unusually low levels may be noncompliant or hypermetabolizers of phenytoin. Unusually high levels result from liver disease, congenital enzyme deficiency or drug interactions which result in metabolic interference. The patient with large variations in phenytoin plasma levels, despite standard doses, presents a difficult clinical problem. Serum level determinations in such patients may be particularly helpful. As phenytoin is highly protein bound, free phenytoin levels may be altered in patients whose protein binding characteristics differ from normal.

Most of the drug is excreted in the bile as inactive metabolites which are then reabsorbed from the intestinal tract and excreted in the urine. Urinary excretion of phenytoin and its metabolites occurs partly with glomerular filtration but more importantly, by tubular secretion. Because phenytoin is hydroxylated in the liver by an enzyme system which is saturable at high plasma levels small incremental doses may increase the half-life and produce very substantial increases in serum levels, when these are in the upper range. The steady-state level may be disproportionately increased, with resultant intoxication, from an increase in dosage of 10% or more.

Clinical studies show that chewed and unchewed Dilantin Infatabs are bioequivalent, yield approximately equivalent plasma levels, and are more rapidly absorbed than 100-mg Dilantin Kapseals.®

INDICATIONS AND USAGE

Dilantin Infatabs (Phenytoin Tablets, USP) are indicated for the control of generalized tonic-clonic (grand mal) and complex partial (psychomotor, temporal lobe) seizures and prevention and treatment of seizures occurring during or following neurosurgery. Phenytoin serum level determinations may be necessary for optimal dosage adjustments (see Dosage and Administration and Clinical Pharmacology sections).

CONTRAINDICATIONS

Phenytoin is contraindicated in those patients who are hypersensitive to phenytoin or other hydantoins.

WARNINGS

Abrupt withdrawal of phenytoin in epileptic patients may precipitate status epilepticus. When, in the judgment of the clinician, the need for dosage reduction, discontinuation, or substitution of alternative antiepileptic medication arises, this should be done gradually. However, in the event of an allergic or hypersensitivity reaction, rapid substitution of alternative therapy may be necessary. In this case, alternative therapy should be an antiepileptic drug not belonging to the hydantoin chemical class.

There have been a number of reports suggesting a relationship between phenytoin and the development of lymphadenopathy (local or generalized) including benign lymph node hyperplasia, pseudolymphoma, lymphoma, and Hodgkin's Disease. Although a cause and effect relationship has not been established, the occurrence of lymphadenopathy indicates the need to differentiate such a condition from other types of lymph node pathology. Lymph node involvement may occur with or without symptoms and signs resembling serum sickness eg, fever, rash and liver involvement. In all cases of lymphadenopathy, follow-up observation for an extended period is indicated and every effort should be made to achieve seizure control using alternative antiepileptic drugs.

Acute alcoholic intake may increase phenytoin serum levels while chronic alcoholic use may decrease serum levels.

In view of isolated reports associating phenytoin with exacerbation of porphyria, caution should be exercised in using this medication in patients suffering from this disease.

Usage in Pregnancy

A number of reports suggest an association between the use of antiepileptic drugs by women with epilepsy and a higher incidence of birth defects in children born to these women. Data are more extensive with respect to phenytoin and phenobarbital, but these are also the most commonly prescribed antiepileptic drugs; less systematic or anecdotal reports suggest a possible similar association with the use of all known antiepileptic drugs.

The reports suggesting a higher incidence of birth defects in children of drug-treated epileptic women cannot be regarded as adequate to prove a definite cause and effect relationship. There are intrinsic methodologic problems in obtaining adequate data on drug teratogenicity in humans: genetic factors or the epileptic condition itself, may be more important than drug therapy in leading to birth defects. The great majority of mothers on antiepileptic medication deliver normal infants. It is important to note that antiepileptic drugs should not be discontinued in patients in whom the drug is administered to prevent major seizures, because of the strong possibility of precipitating status epilepticus with attendant hypoxia and threat to life. In individual cases where the severity and frequency of the seizure disorder are such that the removal of medication does not pose a serious threat to the patient, discontinuation of the drug may be considered prior to and during pregnancy, although it cannot be said with any confidence that even minor seizures do not pose some hazard to the developing embryo or fetus. The prescribing physician will wish to weigh these considerations in treating or counseling epileptic women of childbearing potential.

In addition to the reports of increased incidence of congenital malformations, such as cleft lip/palate and heart malformations in children of women receiving phenytoin and other antiepileptic drugs, there have more recently been reports of a fetal hydantoin syndrome. This consists of prenatal growth deficiency, microcephaly and mental deficiency in children born to mothers who have received phenytoin, barbiturates, alcohol, or trimethadione. However, these features are all interrelated and are frequently associated with intrauterine growth retardation from other causes.

There have been isolated reports of malignancies, including neuroblastoma, in children whose mothers received phenytoin during pregnancy.

An increase in seizure frequency during pregnancy occurs in a high proportion of patients, because of altered phenytoin absorption or metabolism. Periodic measurement of serum phenytoin levels is particularly valuable in the management of a pregnant epileptic patient as a guide to an appropriate adjustment of dosage. However, postpartum restoration of the original dosage will probably be indicated.

Neonatal coagulation defects have been reported within the first 24 hours in babies born to epileptic mothers receiving phenobarbital and/or phenytoin. Vitamin K has been shown to prevent or correct this defect and has been recommended to be given to the mother before delivery and to the neonate after birth.

PRECAUTIONS
General

The liver is the chief site of biotransformation of phenytoin; patients with impaired liver function, elderly patients, or those who are gravely ill may show early signs of toxicity.

A small percentage of individuals who have been treated with phenytoin have been shown to metabolize the drug slowly. Slow metabolism may be due to limited enzyme availability and lack of induction; it appears to be genetically determined.

Phenytoin should be discontinued if a skin rash appears (see "Warnings" section regarding drug discontinuation). If the rash is exfoliative, purpuric, or bullous or if lupus erythematosus, Stevens-Johnson syndrome, or toxic epidermal necrolysis is suspected, use of this drug should not be resumed, and alternative therapy should be considered (see Adverse Reactions). If the rash is of a milder type (measles-like or scarlatiniform), therapy may be resumed after the rash has completely disappeared. If the rash recurs upon reinstitution of therapy, further phenytoin medication is contraindicated.

Phenytoin and other hydantoins are contraindicated in patients who have experienced phenytoin hypersensitivity. Additionally, caution should be exercised if using structurally similar (eg barbiturates, succinimides, oxazolidinediones and other related compounds) in these same patients.

Hyperglycemia, resulting from the drug's inhibitory effects on insulin release, has been reported. Phenytoin may also raise the serum glucose level in diabetic patients.

Osteomalacia has been associated with phenytoin therapy and is considered to be due to phenytoin's interference with Vitamin D metabolism.

Phenytoin is not indicated for seizures due to hypoglycemic or other metabolic causes. Appropriate diagnostic procedures should be performed as indicated.

Phenytoin is not effective for absence (petit mal) seizures. If tonic-clonic (grand-mal) and absence (petit mal) seizures are present, combined drug therapy is needed.

Serum levels of phenytoin sustained above the optimal range may produce confusional states referred to as "delirium," "psychosis," or "encephalopathy," or rarely irreversible cerebellar dysfunction. Accordingly, at the first sign of acute toxicity, plasma levels are recommended. Dose reduction of phenytoin therapy is indicated if plasma levels are excessive; if symptoms persist, termination is recommended. (See Warnings).

Information for Patients

Patients taking phenytoin should be advised of the importance of adhering strictly to the prescribed dosage regimen, and of informing the physician of any clinical condition in which it is not possible to take the drug orally as prescribed, eg, surgery, etc.

Patients should also be cautioned on the use of other drugs or alcoholic beverages without first seeking the physician's advice.

Patients should be instructed to call their physician if skin rash develops.

The importance of good dental hygiene should be stressed in order to minimize the development of gingival hyperplasia and its complications.

Laboratory Tests

Phenytoin serum level determinations may be necessary to achieve optimal dosage adjustments.

Drug Interactions

There are many drugs which may increase or decrease phenytoin levels or which phenytoin may affect. Serum level determinations for phenytoin are especially helpful when possible drug interactions are suspected. The most commonly occurring drug interactions are listed below:

1. Drugs which may increase phenytoin serum levels include: acute alcohol intake, amiodarone, chloramphenicol, chlordiazepoxide, diazepam, dicumarol, disulfiram, estrogens, H$_2$-antagonists, halothane, isoniazid, methylphenidate, phenothiazines, phenylbutazone, salicylates, succinimides, sulfonamides, tolbutamide, trazodone.

2. Drugs which may decrease phenytoin serum levels include: carbamazepine, chronic alcohol abuse, reserpine, and sucralfate. Moban® brand of Molindone Hydrochloride contains calcium ions which interfere with the absorption of phenytoin. Ingestion times of phenytoin and antacid preparations containing calcium should be staggered in patients with low serum phenytoin levels to prevent absorption problems.

3. Drugs which may either increase or decrease phenytoin serum levels include: phenobarbital, sodium valproate, and valproic acid. Similarly, the effect of phenytoin on phenobarbital, valproic acid and sodium valproate serum levels is unpredictable.

4. Although not a true drug interaction, tricyclic antidepressants may precipitate seizures in susceptible patients and phenytoin dosage may need to be adjusted.

5. Drugs whose efficacy is impaired by phenytoin include: corticosteroids, coumarin anticoagulants, digitoxin, doxycycline, estrogens, furosemide, oral contraceptives, quinidine, rifampin, theophylline, vitamin D.

Drug/Laboratory Test Interactions

Phenytoin may cause decreased serum levels of protein-bound iodine (PBI). It may also produce lower than normal values for dexamethasone or metyrapone tests. Phenytoin may cause increased serum levels of glucose, alkaline phosphatase, and gamma glutamyl transpeptidase (GGT).

Carcinogenesis

See 'Warnings' section for information on carcinogenesis.

Pregnancy

See Warnings Section.

Nursing Mothers

Infant breast-feeding is not recommended for women taking this drug because phenytoin appears to be secreted in low concentrations in human milk.

ADVERSE REACTIONS

Central Nervous System: The most common manifestations encountered with phenytoin therapy are referable to this system and are usually dose-related. These include nystagmus, ataxia, slurred speech, decreased coordination and mental confusion. Dizziness, insomnia, transient nervousness, motor twitchings, and headache have also been observed.

There have also been rare reports of phenytoin induced dyskinesias, including chorea, dystonia, tremor and asterixis, similar to those induced by phenothiazine and other neuroleptic drugs.

A predominantly sensory peripheral polyneuropathy has been observed in patients receiving long-term phenytoin therapy.

Gastrointestinal System: Nausea, vomiting, constipation, toxic hepatitis and liver damage.

Integumentary System: Dermatological manifestations sometimes accompanied by fever have included scarlatiniform or morbilliform rashes. A morbilliform rash (measleslike) is the most common; other types of dermatitis are seen more rarely. Other more serious forms which may be fatal have included bullous, exfoliative or purpuric dermatitis, lupus erythematosus, Stevens-Johnson syndrome, and toxic epidermal necrolysis (see Precautions section).

Hemopoietic System: Hemopoietic complications, some fatal, have occasionally been reported in association with administration of phenytoin. These have included thrombocytopenia, leukopenia, granulocytopenia, agranulocytosis, and pancytopenia with or without bone marrow suppression. While macrocytosis and megaloblastic anemia have occurred, these conditions usually respond to folic acid therapy. Lymphadenopathy including benign lymph node hyperplasia, pseudolymphoma, lymphoma, and Hodgkin's Disease have been reported (see Warnings section).

Connective Tissue System: Coarsening of the facial features, enlargement of the lips, gingival hyperplasia, hypertrichosis, and Peyronie's Disease.

Cardiovascular: Periarteritis nodosa.

Immunologic: Hypersensitivity syndrome (which may include, but is not limited to, symptoms such as arthralgias, eosinophilia, fever, liver dysfunction, lymphadenopathy or rash), systemic lupus erythematosus, and immunoglobulin abnormalities.

OVERDOSAGE

The lethal dose in pediatric patients is not known. The lethal dose in adults is estimated to be 2 to 5 grams. The initial symptoms are nystagmus, ataxia, and dysarthria. Other signs are tremor, hyperflexia, lethargy, slurred speech, nausea, vomiting. The patient may become comatose and hypotensive. Death is due to respiratory and circulatory depression.

There are marked variations among individuals with respect to phenytoin plasma levels where toxicity may occur. Nystagmus on lateral gaze usually appears at 20 mcg/ml, ataxia at 30 mcg/ml; dysarthria and lethargy appear when the plasma concentration is over 40 mcg/ml, but as high a concentration as 50 mcg/ml has been reported without evidence of toxicity. As much as 25 times the therapeutic dose has been taken to result in a serum concentration over 100 mcg/ml with complete recovery.

Treatment

Treatment is nonspecific since there is no known antidote. The adequacy of the respiratory and circulatory systems should be carefully observed and appropriate supportive measures employed. Hemodialysis can be considered since phenytoin is not completely bound to plasma proteins. Total exchange transfusion has been used in the treatment of severe intoxication in pediatric patients.

In acute overdosage the possibility of other CNS depressants, including alcohol, should be borne in mind.

DOSAGE AND ADMINISTRATION

When given in equal doses, Dilantin Infatabs yield higher plasma levels than Dilantin Kapseals.® For this reason serum concentrations should be monitored and care should be taken when switching a patient from the sodium salt to the free acid form.

Dilantin® Kapseals,® Dilantin Parenteral, and Dilantin with Phenobarbital are formulated with the sodium salt of phenytoin. The free acid form of phenytoin is used in Dilantin-30 Pediatric and Dilantin-125 Suspensions and Dilantin Infatabs. Because there is approximately an 8% increase in drug content with the free acid form over that of the sodium salt, dosage adjustments and serum level monitoring may be necessary when switching from a product formulated with the free acid to a product formulated with the sodium salt and vice versa.

General

Not for once a day dosing.

Dosage should be individualized to provide maximum benefit. In some cases, serum blood level determinations may be necessary for optimal dosage adjustments—the clinically effective serum level is usually 10–20 mcg/ml. With recommended dosage, a period of seven to ten days may be required to achieve steady-state blood levels with phenytoin and changes in dosage (increase or decrease) should not be carried out at intervals shorter than seven to ten days.

Dilantin Infatabs can be either chewed thoroughly before being swallowed or swallowed whole.

Adult Dosage

Patients who have received no previous treatment may be started on two Infatabs three times daily, and the dose is then adjusted to suit individual requirements. For most adults, the satisfactory maintenance dosage will be six to eight Infatabs daily; an increase to twelve Infatabs daily may be made, if necessary.

Pediatric Dosage

Initially, 5 mg/kg/day in two or three equally divided doses, with subsequent dosage individualized to a maximum of 300 mg daily. A recommended daily maintenance dosage is usually 4 to 8 mg/kg. Children over 6 years old and adolescents may require the minimum adult dose (300 mg/day). If the daily dosage cannot be divided equally, the larger dose should be given before retiring.

HOW SUPPLIED

Dilantin Infatabs are supplied as:

N 0071-0007-24—Bottle of 100.

Store at a room temperature below 30°C (86°F).

N 0071-0007-40—Unit dose (10/10's).

Store at controlled room temperature 15°–30°C (59°–86°F). Protect from moisture.

Each tablet contains 50 mg phenytoin in a yellow triangular scored chewable tablet.

Dilantin is also supplied in the following forms:

N 0071-0362-24—Bottle of 100.

N 0071-0362-32—Bottle of 1000.

N 0071-0362-40—Unit dose (10/10's).

Each Kapseal® contains 100 mg phenytoin sodium.

N 0071-0365-24—Bottle of 100.

Each Kapseal® contains 30 mg phenytoin sodium.

N 0071-2214-20—8 oz bottle.

Each 5 ml of suspension contains 125 mg phenytoin with a maximum alcohol content not greater than 0.6 percent.

N 0071-4488-47—2-ml prefilled Steri-Dose® syringes.

A sterile solution for parenteral use containing 50 mg phenytoin sodium per mL in a disposable syringe (22 gauge × 1¼ inch needle). Supplied in packages of ten.

N 0071-4488-45 Dilantin ready-mixed solution containing 50 mg phenytoin sodium per milliliter is supplied in 2-mL Steri-Vials.® Packages of twenty-five.

N 0071-4475-45 Dilantin ready-mixed solution containing 50 mg phenytoin sodium per milliliter is supplied in 5 mL Steri-Vials.® Packages of twenty-five.

Caution—Federal law prohibits dispensing without prescription.

© 1996, Warner-Lambert Co.

Revised July 1996   0007G165

Shown in Product Identification Guide, page 329

DILANTIN-125®   ℞

[dī-lăn'tĭn]
**(Phenytoin Oral
Suspension, USP)**

DESCRIPTION

Dilantin (phenytoin) is related to the barbiturates in chemical structure, but has a five-membered ring. The chemical name is 5,5-diphenyl-2,4 imidazolidinedione.

Each teaspoonful of suspension contains 125 mg of phenytoin, USP with a maximum alcohol content not greater than 0.6 percent. Also contains carboxymethylcellulose sodium, USP; citric acid, anhydrous, USP; flavors; glycerin, USP; magnesium aluminum silicate, NF; polysorbate 40, NF; purified water, USP; sodium benzoate, NF; sucrose, NF; vanillin, NF; and FD&C yellow No. 6.

CLINICAL PHARMACOLOGY

Phenytoin is an antiepileptic drug which can be useful in the treatment of epilepsy. The primary site of action appears to be *the motor cortex* where spread of seizure activity is inhibited. Possibly by promoting sodium efflux from neurons, phenytoin tends to *stabilize* the threshold against hyperexcitability caused by excessive stimulation or environmental changes capable of reducing membrane sodium gradient. This includes the reduction of posttetanic potentiation at synapses. Loss of posttetanic potentiation prevents cortical seizure foci from detonating adjacent cortical areas. Phenytoin reduces the maximal activity of brain stem centers responsible for the tonic phase of tonic-clonic (grand mal) seizures.

The plasma half-life in man after oral administration of phenytoin averages 22 hours, with a range of 7 to 42 hours.

Steady-state therapeutic levels are achieved at least 7 to 10 days (5–7 half-lives) after initiation of therapy with recommended doses of 300 mg/day.

When serum level determinations are necessary, they should be obtained at least 5–7 half-lives after treatment initiation, dosage change, or addition or subtraction of another drug to the regimen so that equilibrium or steady-state will have been achieved. Trough levels provide information about clinically effective serum level range and confirm patient compliance and are obtained just prior to the patient's next scheduled dose. Peak levels indicate an individual's threshold for emergence of dose-related side effects and are obtained at the time of expected peak concentration. For Dilantin-125 Suspension peak levels occur 1½–3 hours after administration.

Optimum control without clinical signs of toxicity occurs more often with serum levels between 10 and 20 mcg/mL, although some mild cases of tonic-clonic (grand mal) epilepsy may be controlled with lower serum levels of phenytoin.

In most patients maintained at a steady dosage, stable phenytoin serum levels are achieved. There may be wide interpatient variability in phenytoin serum levels with equivalent dosages. Patients with unusually low levels may be noncompliant or hypermetabolizers of phenytoin. Unusually high levels result from liver disease, congenital enzyme deficiency or drug interactions which result in metabolic interference. The patient with large variations in phenytoin plasma levels, despite standard doses, presents a difficult clinical problem. Serum level determinations in such patients may be particularly helpful. As phenytoin is highly protein bound, free phenytoin levels may be altered in patients whose protein binding characteristics differ from normal.

Most of the drug is excreted in the bile as inactive metabolites which are then reabsorbed from the intestinal tract and excreted in the urine. Urinary excretion of phenytoin and its metabolites occurs partly with glomerular filtration but more importantly, by tubular secretion. Because phenytoin is hydroxylated in the liver by an enzyme system which is saturable at high plasma levels small incremental doses may increase the half-life and produce very substantial increases in serum levels, when these are in the upper range. The steady-state level may be disproportionately increased, with resultant intoxication, from an increase in dosage of 10% or more.

INDICATIONS AND USAGE

Dilantin (phenytoin) is indicated for the control of tonic-clonic (grand mal) and psychomotor (temporal lobe) seizures.

Phenytoin serum level determinations may be necessary for optimal dosage adjustments (see Dosage and Administration and Clinical Pharmacology sections).

CONTRAINDICATIONS

Dilantin is contraindicated in those patients with a history of hypersensitivity to phenytoin or other hydantoins.

WARNINGS

Abrupt withdrawal of phenytoin in epileptic patients may precipitate status epilepticus. When in the judgment of the clinician the need for dosage reduction, discontinuation, or substitution of alternative anticonvulsant medication arises, this should be done gradually. In the event of an allergic or hypersensitivity reaction, more rapid substitution of alternative therapy may be necessary. In this case, alternative therapy should be an anticonvulsant not belonging to the hydantion chemical class.

There have been a number of reports suggesting a relationship between phenytoin and the development of lymphadenopathy (local or generalized) including benign lymph node hyperplasia, pseudolymphoma, lymphoma, and Hodgkin's Disease. Although a cause and effect relationship has not been established, the occurrence of lymphadenopathy indicates the need to differentiate such a condition from other types of lymph node pathology. Lymph node involvement may occur with or without symptoms and signs resembling serum sickness eg, fever, rash and liver involvement.

In all cases of lymphadenopathy, follow-up observation for an extended period is indicated and every effort should be made to achieve seizure control using alternative antiepileptic drugs.

Acute alcoholic intake may increase phenytoin serum levels while chronic alcoholic use may decrease serum levels.

In view of isolated reports associating phenytoin with exacerbation of porphyria, caution should be exercised in using this medication in patients suffering from this disease.

Continued on next page

This product information was prepared in June 1998. On these and other Parke-Davis Products, information may be obtained by addressing PARKE-DAVIS, Division of Warner-Lambert Company, Morris Plains, New Jersey 07950.

Dilantin-125—Cont.

Usage in Pregnancy: A number of reports suggests an association between the use of antiepileptic drugs by women with epilepsy and a higher incidence of birth defects in children born to these women. Data are more extensive with respect to phenytoin and phenobarbital, but these are also the most commonly prescribed antiepileptic drugs; less systematic or anecdotal reports suggest a possible similar association with the use of all known antiepileptic drugs.

The reports suggesting a higher incidence of birth defects in children of drug-treated epileptic women cannot be regarded as adequate to prove a definite cause and effect relationship. There are intrinsic methodologic problems in obtaining adequate data on drug teratogenicity in humans; genetic factors or the epileptic condition itself may be more important than drug therapy in leading to birth defects. The great majority of mothers on antiepileptic medication deliver normal infants. It is important to note that antiepileptic drugs should not be discontinued in patients in whom the drug is administered to prevent major seizures, because of the strong possibility of precipitating status epilepticus with attendant hypoxia and threat to life. In individual cases where the severity and frequency of the seizure disorder are such that the removal of medication does not pose a serious threat to the patient, discontinuation of the drug may be considered prior to and during pregnancy, although it cannot be said with any confidence that even minor seizures do not pose some hazards to the developing embryo or fetus. The prescribing physician will wish to weigh these considerations in treating and counseling epileptic women of childbearing potential.

In addition to the reports of increased incidence of congenital malformation, such as cleft lip/palate and heart malformations in children of women receiving phenytoin and other antiepileptic drugs, there have more recently been reports of a fetal hydantoin syndrome. This consists of prenatal growth deficiency, microcephaly and mental deficiency in children born to mothers who have received phenytoin, barbiturates, alcohol, or trimethadione. However, these features are all interrelated and are frequently associated with intrauterine growth retardation from other causes.

There have been isolated reports of malignancies, including neuroblastoma, in children whose mothers received phenytoin during pregnancy.

An increase in seizure frequency during pregnancy occurs in a high proportion of patients, because of altered phenytoin absorption or metabolism. Periodic measurement of serum phenytoin levels is particularly valuable in the management of a pregnant epileptic patient as a guide to an appropriate adjustment of dosage. However, postpartum restoration of the original dosage will probably be indicated.

Neonatal coagulation defects have been reported within the first 24 hours in babies born to epileptic mothers receiving phenobarbital and/or phenytoin. Vitamin K has been shown to prevent or correct this defect and has been recommended to be given to the mother before delivery and the neonate after birth.

PRECAUTIONS

General: The liver is the chief site of biotransformation of phenytoin; patients with impaired liver function, elderly patients, or those who are gravely ill may show early signs of toxicity.

A small percentage of individuals who have been treated with phenytoin have been shown to metabolize the drug slowly. Slow metabolism may be due to limited enzyme availability and lack of induction; it appears to be genetically determined.

Phenytoin should be discontinued if a skin rash appears (see "Warnings" section regarding drug discontinuation). If the rash is exfoliative, purpuric, or bullous or if lupus erythematosus, Stevens-Johnson syndrome, or toxic epidermal necrolysis is suspected, use of this drug should not be resumed and alternative therapy should be considered. (See Adverse Reactions section). If the rash is of a milder type (measles-like or scarlatiniform), therapy may be resumed after the rash has completely disappeared. If the rash recurs upon reinstitution of therapy, further phenytoin medication is contraindicated. Phenytoin and other hydantoins are contraindicated in patients who have experienced phenytoin hypersensitivity. Additionally, caution should be exercised if using structurally similar (eg, barbiturates, succinamides, oxazolidinediones and other related compounds) in these same patients. Hyperglycemia, resulting from the drug's inhibitory effects on insulin release, has been reported. Phenytoin may also raise the serum glucose level in diabetic patients.

Osteomalacia has been associated with phenytoin therapy and is considered to be due to phenytoin's interference with Vitamin D metabolism.

Phenytoin is not indicated for seizures due to hypoglycemic or other metabolic causes. Appropriate diagnostic procedures should be performed as indicated.

Phenytoin is not effective for absence (petit mal) seizures. If tonic-clonic (grand mal) and absence (petit mal) seizures are present, combined drug therapy is needed.

Serum levels of phenytoin sustained above the optimal range may produce confusional states referred to as "delirium," "psychosis" or "encephalopathy," or rarely irreversible cerebellar dysfunction. Accordingly, at the first sign of acute toxicity, plasma levels are recommended. Dose reduction of phenytoin therapy is indicated if plasma levels are excessive; if symptoms persist, termination is recommended. (See Warnings section).

Information for Patients: Patients taking phenytoin should be advised of the importance of adhering strictly to the prescribed dosage regimen, and of informing the physician of any clinical condition in which it is not possible to take the drug orally as prescribed, eg, surgery, etc. Patients should be instructed to use an accurately calibrated measuring device when using this medication to ensure accurate dosing.

Patients should also be cautioned on the use of other drugs or alcoholic beverages without first seeking the physician's advice.

Patients should be instructed to call their physician if skin rash develops.

The importance of good dental hygiene should be stressed in order to minimize the development of gingival hyperplasia and its complications.

Laboratory Tests: Phenytoin serum level determinations may be necessary to achieve optimal dosage adjustments.

Drug Interactions: There are many drugs which may increase or decrease phenytoin levels or which phenytoin may affect. Serum level determinations for phenytoin are especially helpful when possible drug interactions are suspected. The most commonly occurring drug interactions are:

1. Drugs which may increase phenytoin serum levels include: acute alcohol intake, amiodarone, chloramphenicol, chlordiazepoxide, diazepam, dicumarol, disulfiram, estrogens, ethosuximide, fluoxetine, H$_2$-antagonists, halothane, isoniazid, methylphenidate, phenothiazines, phenylbutazone, salicylates, succinimides, sulfonamides, tolbutamide, trazodone.

2. Drugs which may decrease phenytoin levels include: carbamazepine, chronic alcohol abuse, reserpine and sucralfate. Moban® brand of molindone hydrochloride contains calcium ions which interfere with the absorption of phenytoin. Ingestion times of phenytoin and antacid preparations containing calcium should be staggered in patients with low serum phenytoin levels to prevent absorption problems.

3. Drugs which may either increase or decrease phenytoin serum levels include: phenobarbital, sodium valproate, and valproic acid. Similarly, the effect of phenytoin on phenobarbital, valproic acid and sodium valproate serum levels is unpredictable.

4. Although not a true drug interaction, tricyclic antidepressants may precipitate seizures in susceptible patients and phenytoin dosage may need to be adjusted.

5. Drugs whose efficacy is impaired by phenytoin include: corticosteroids, coumarin anticoagulants, digitoxin, doxycycline, estrogens, furosemide, oral contraceptives, quinidine, rifampin, theophylline, vitamin D.

Drug/Laboratory Test Interactions: Phenytoin may cause decreased serum levels of protein-bound iodine (PBI). It may also produce lower than normal values for dexamethasone or metyrapone tests. Phenytoin may cause increased serum levels of glucose, alkaline phosphatase, and gamma glutamyl transpeptidase (GGT).

Carcinogenesis: See 'Warnings' section for information on carcinogenesis.

Pregnancy: See Warnings section.

Nursing Mothers: Infant breast feeding is not recommended for women taking this drug because phenytoin appears to be secreted in low concentrations in human milk.

Pediatric Use: See DOSAGE AND ADMINISTRATION section.

ADVERSE REACTIONS

Central Nervous System: The most common manifestations encountered with phenytoin therapy are referable to this system and are usually dose-related. These include nystagmus, ataxia, slurred speech, decreased coordination, and mental confusion. Dizziness, insomnia, transient nervousness, motor twitchings, and headaches have also been observed. There have also been rare reports of phenytoin induced dyskinesias, including chorea, dystonia, tremor and asterixis, similar to those induced by phenothiazine and other neuroleptic drugs.

A predominantly sensory peripheral polyneuropathy has been observed in patients receiving long-term phenytoin therapy.

Gastrointestinal System: Nausea, vomiting, constipation, toxic hepatitis and liver damage.

Integumentary System: Dermatological manifestations sometimes accompanied by fever have included scarlatiniform or morbilliform rashes. A morbilliform rash (measles-like) is the most common; other types of dermatitis are seen more rarely. Other more serious forms which may be fatal

have included bullous, exfoliative or purpuric dermatitis, lupus erythematosus, Stevens-Johnson syndrome, and toxic epidermal necrolysis (see Precautions section).

Hemopoietic System: Hemopoietic complications, some fatal, have occasionally been reported in association with administration of phenytoin. These have included thrombocytopenia, leukopenia, granulocytopenia, agranulocytosis, and pancytopenia with or without bone marrow suppression. While macrocytosis and megaloblastic anemia have occurred, these conditions usually respond to folic acid therapy. Lymphadenopathy including benign lymph node hyperplasia, pseudolymphoma, lymphoma, and Hodgkin's Disease have been reported (see Warnings section).

Connective Tissue System: Coarsening of the facial features, enlargement of the lips, gingival hyperplasia, hypertrichosis, and Peyronie's Disease.

Cardiovascular: Periarteritis nodosa.

Immunologic: Hypersensitivity syndrome (which may include, but is not limited to, symptoms such as arthralgias, eosinophilia, fever, liver dysfunction, lymphadenopathy or rash), systemic lupus erythematosus, and immunoglobulin abnormalities.

OVERDOSAGE

The lethal dose in pediatric patients is not known. The lethal dose in adults is estimated to be 2 to 5 grams. The initial symptoms are nystagmus, ataxia, and dysarthria. Other signs are tremor, hyperflexia, lethargy, slurred speech, nausea, vomiting. The patient may become comatose and hypotensive. Death is due to respiratory and circulatory depression.

There are marked variations among individuals with respect to phenytoin plasma levels where toxicity may occur. Nystagmus, on lateral gaze, usually appears at 20 mcg/mL, ataxia at 30 mcg/mL, dysarthria and lethargy appear when the plasma concentration is over 40 mcg/mL, but as high a concentration as 50 mcg/mL has been reported without evidence of toxicity. As much as 25 times the therapeutic dose has been taken to result in a serum concentration over 100 mcg/mL with complete recovery.

Treatment: Treatment is nonspecific since there is no known antidote.

The adequacy of the respiratory and circulatory systems should be carefully observed and appropriate supportive measures employed. Hemodialysis can be considered since phenytoin is not completely bound to plasma proteins. Total exchange transfusion has been used in the treatment of severe intoxication in pediatric patients.

In acute overdosage the possibility of other CNS depressants, including alcohol, should be borne in mind.

DOSAGE AND ADMINISTRATION

Serum concentrations should be monitored and care should be taken when switching a patient from the sodium salt to the free acid form.

Dilantin® Kapseals®, Dilantin Parenteral, and Dilantin with Phenobarbital are formulated with the sodium salt of phenytoin. The free acid form of phenytoin is used in Dilantin-125 Suspension and Dilantin Infatabs. Because there is approximately an 8% increase in drug content with the free acid form over that of the sodium salt, dosage adjustments and serum level monitoring may be necessary when switching from a product formulated with the free acid to a product formulated with the sodium salt and vice versa.

General: Dosage should be individualized to provide maximum benefit. In some cases serum blood level determinations may be necessary for optimal dosage adjustments—the clinically effective serum level is usually 10–20 mcg/mL. With recommended dosage, a period of seven to ten days may be required to achieve steady-state blood levels with phenytoin and changes in dosage (increase or decrease) should not be carried out at intervals shorter than seven to ten days.

Adult Dose: Patients who have received no previous treatment may be started on one teaspoonful (5 mL) of Dilantin-125 Suspension three times daily, and the dose is then adjusted to suit individual requirements. An increase to five teaspoonfuls daily may be made, if necessary.

Pediatric Dose: Initially, 5 mg/kg/day in two or three equally divided doses, with subsequent dosage individualized to a maximum of 300 mg daily. A recommended daily maintenance dosage is usually 4 to 8 mg/kg. Children over 6 years and adolescents may require the minimum adult dose (300 mg/day).

HOW SUPPLIED

N 0071-2214—Dilantin-125® Suspension (phenytoin oral suspension, USP), 125 mg phenytoin/5 mL with a maximum alcohol content not greater than 0.6 percent, an orange suspension with an orange-vanilla flavor; available in 8-oz bottles.

Store below 30°C (86°F). Protect from freezing and light.

Also available as:

N 0071-0362 (Kapseal® 362)—Dilantin (extended phenytoin sodium capsules, USP) 100 mg; in 100's, 1000's, unit dose 100's.

N 0071-0365 (Kapseal 365)—Dilantin (extended phenytoin sodium capsules, USP) 30 mg, in 100's.
N 0071-0007 (Tablet 7)—Dilantin Infatabs® (phenytoin tablets, USP) each contain 50 mg phenytoin; 100's and unit dose 100's.

For Parenteral Use:
N 0071-4488-47 (Steri-Dose® 4488)-Dilantin ready-mixed solution containing 50 mg phenytoin sodium per milliliter is supplied in a 2-mL sterile disposable syringe (22 gauge × 1¹/₄ inch needle). Packages of ten syringes.
N 0071-4488-45 Dilantin ready-mixed solution containing 50 mg phenytoin sodium per milliliter is supplied in 2 mL Steri-Vials.® Packages of twenty-five.
N 0071-4475-45 Dilantin ready-mixed solution containing 50 mg phenytoin sodium per milliliter is supplied in 5 mL Steri-Vials.® Packages of twenty-five.
Storage: Store below 30° C (86° F). Protect from freezing and light.
Caution—Federal law prohibits dispensing without prescription.
© 1997, Warner-Lambert Co.
Revised January 1997   2214G129

ESTROSTEP®   ℞
[ĕs ′trō stĕp]
(Norethindrone Acetate and Ethinyl Estradiol Tablets, USP)
ESTROSTEP® 21
(Each white triangular tablet contains 1 mg norethindrone acetate and 20 mcg ethinyl estradiol; each white square tablet contains 1 mg norethindrone acetate and 30 mcg ethinyl estradiol; each white round tablet contains 1 mg norethindrone acetate and 35 mcg ethinyl estradiol.)

ESTROSTEP® Fe
(Each white triangular tablet contains 1 mg norethindrone acetate and 20 mcg ethinyl estradiol; each white square tablet contains 1 mg norethindrone acetate and 30 mcg ethinyl estradiol; each white round tablet contains 1 mg norethindrone acetate and 35 mcg ethinyl estradiol; each brown tablet contains 75 mg ferrous fumarate.)

Patients should be counseled that this product does not protect against HIV infection (AIDS) and other sexually transmitted diseases.

DESCRIPTION
Estrostep is a graduated estrophasic providing estrogen in a graduated sequence over a 21-day period with a constant dose of progestogen.
Estrostep **21** provides for a 21-day dosage regimen of oral contraceptive tablets.
Estrostep **Fe** provides for a continuous dosage regimen consisting of 21 oral contraceptive tablets and seven ferrous fumarate tablets. The ferrous fumarate tablets are present to facilitate ease of drug administration via a 28-day regimen, are non-hormonal, and do not serve any therapeutic purpose.
Each white triangle-shaped tablet contains 1 mg norethindrone acetate [(17 alpha)-17 (acetyloxy)-19-norpregna-4-en-20-yn-3-one] and 20 mcg ethinyl estradiol [(17 alpha)-19-norpregna-1,3,5(10)-trien-20-yne-3,17-diol]; each white square-shaped tablet contains 1 mg norethindrone acetate and 30 mcg ethinyl estradiol; and each white round tablet contains 1 mg norethindrone acetate, 35 mcg ethinyl estradiol. Each tablet also contains calcium stearate; lactose; microcrystalline cellulose; and starch.
The structural formulas are as follows:

Ethinyl Estradiol

Norethindrone Acetate

Each brown tablet contains microcrystalline cellulose; ferrous fumarate; magnesium stearate; povidone; sodium starch glycolate; sucrose with modified dextrins.
Each Estrostep **21** tablet dispenser contains five white triangular tablets, seven white square tablets, and nine white round tablets. These tablets are to be taken in the following

---

order: one triangular tablet each day for five days, followed by one square tablet each day for seven days, and then one round tablet each day for nine days.
Each Estrostep **Fe** tablet dispenser contains five white triangular tablets, seven white square tablets, nine white round tablets, and seven brown tablets. These tablets are to be taken in the following order: one triangular tablet each day for five days, then one square tablet each day for seven days, followed by one round tablet each day for nine days, and then one brown tablet each day for seven days.

CLINICAL PHARMACOLOGY
Combination oral contraceptives act by suppression of gonadotropins. Although the primary mechanism of this action is inhibition of ovulation, other alterations include changes in the cervical mucus (which increase the difficulty of sperm entry into the uterus) and the endometrium (which reduce the likelihood of implantation).
Pharmacokinetics
Norethindrone acetate and ethinyl estradiol are well absorbed and are subject to first-pass metabolism after oral dosing (1–3). Norethindrone acetate is completely and rapidly deacetylated to norethindrone after oral administration and thus the disposition of norethindrone acetate is indistinguishable from that of orally administered norethindrone (1). Plasma protein binding of both steroids is extensive (>95%); norethindrone binds to both albumin and sex hormone binding globulin, and ethinyl estradiol binds only to albumin (4). Volume of distribution for both compounds ranges from 2 to 4 L/kg (1–3). Plasma clearance values for norethindrone and ethinyl estradiol are also similar (approximately 0.4 L/hr/kg) (1–3). Norethindrone and ethinyl estradiol undergo extensive biotransformation via reduction, oxidation, and conjugation pathways, and are excreted in both urine and feces, primarily as metabolites (5,6). The effects of food and morning versus evening administration of Estrostep on the pharmacokinetics of norethindrone and ethinyl estradiol are unknown.

INDICATIONS AND USAGE
Estrostep is indicated for the prevention of pregnancy in women who elect to use oral contraceptives as a method of contraception.
Oral contraceptives are highly effective. Table I lists the typical accidental pregnancy rates for users of combination oral contraceptives and other methods of contraception. The efficacy of these contraceptive methods, except sterilization, depends upon the reliability with which they are used. Correct and consistent use of methods can result in lower failure rates.
[See table 1 above]

TABLE 1
LOWEST EXPECTED AND TYPICAL FAILURE RATES DURING THE FIRST YEAR
OF CONTINUOUS USE OF A METHOD
% of Women Experiencing an Accidental Pregnancy in the First Year of Continuous Use

Method	Lowest Expected*	Typical**
(No contraception)	(85)	(85)
Oral contraceptives		3
combined	0.1	N/A***
progestin only	0.5	N/A***
Diaphragm with spermicidal cream or jelly	6	18
Spermicides alone (foam, creams, gels, jellies, vaginal suppositories, and vaginal film)	6	21
Vaginal Sponge		
nulliparous	9	18
parous	20	36
Implant (6 capsules)	0.09	0.09
Injection: depot medroxyprogesterone acetate	0.3	0.3
IUD		
progesterone T	1.5	2.0
copper T 380A	0.6	0.8
LNg 20	0.1	0.1
Condom without spermicides		
female	5	21
male	3	12
Cervical Cap with spermicidal cream or jelly		
nulliparous	9	18
parous	26	36
Periodic abstinence (all methods)	1–9	20
Withdrawal	4	19
Female sterilization	0.4	0.4
Male sterilization	0.10	0.15

Adapted from RA Hatcher et al, Reference 7.

---

*The authors' best guess of the percentage of women expected to experience an accidental pregnancy among couples who initiate a method (not necessarily for the first time) and who use it consistently and correctly during the first year if they do not stop for any other reason.
**This term represents "typical" couples who initiate use of a method (not necessarily for the first time), who experience an accidental pregnancy during the first year if they do not stop use for any other reason.
***N/A—Data not available.

CONTRAINDICATIONS
Oral contraceptives should not be used in women who currently have the following conditions:
• Thrombophlebitis or thromboembolic disorders
• A past history of deep vein thrombophlebitis or thromboembolic disorders
• Cerebral vascular or coronary artery disease
• Known or suspected carcinoma of the breast
• Carcinoma of the endometrium or other known or suspected estrogen-dependent neoplasia
• Undiagnosed abnormal genital bleeding
• Cholestatic jaundice of pregnancy or jaundice with prior pill use
• Hepatic adenomas or carcinomas
• Known or suspected pregnancy

WARNINGS

> **Cigarette smoking increases the risk of serious cardiovascular side effects from oral contraceptive use. This risk increases with age and with heavy smoking (15 or more cigarettes per day) and is quite marked in women over 35 years of age. Women who use oral contraceptives should be strongly advised not to smoke.**

The use of oral contraceptives is associated with increased risks of several serious conditions including myocardial infarction, thromboembolism, stroke, hepatic neoplasia, and gallbladder disease, although the risk of serious morbidity or mortality is very small in healthy women without underlying risk factors. The risk of morbidity and mortality increases significantly in the presence of other underlying risk factors such as hypertension, hyperlipidemias, obesity, and diabetes.
Practitioners prescribing oral contraceptives should be familiar with the following information relating to these risks. The information contained in this package insert is principally based on studies carried out in patients who used oral contraceptives with higher formulations of estrogens and progestogens than those in common use today. The effect of

Continued on next page

This product information was prepared in June 1998. On these and other Parke-Davis Products, information may be obtained by addressing PARKE-DAVIS, Division of Warner-Lambert Company, Morris Plains, New Jersey 07950.

Estrostep—Cont.

long-term use of the oral contraceptives with lower formulations of both estrogens and progestogens remains to be determined.

Throughout this labeling, epidemiological studies reported are of two types: retrospective or case control studies and prospective or cohort studies. Case control studies provide a measure of the relative risk of a disease, namely, a *ratio* of the incidence of a disease among oral contraceptive users to that among nonusers. The relative risk does not provide information on the actual clinical occurrence of a disease. Cohort studies provide a measure of attributable risk, which is the *difference* in the incidence of disease between oral contraceptive users and nonusers. The attributable risk does provide information about the actual occurrence of a disease in the population (adapted from References 8 and 9 with the authors' permission). For further information, the reader is referred to a text on epidemiological methods.

1. Thromboembolic Disorders and Other Vascular Problems
a. Myocardial infarction

An increased risk of myocardial infarction has been attributed to oral contraceptive use. This risk is primarily in smokers or women with other underlying risk factors for coronary artery disease such as hypertension, hypercholesterolemia, morbid obesity, and diabetes. The relative risk of heart attack for current oral contraceptive users has been estimated to be two to six (10–16). The risk is very low under the age of 30.

Smoking in combination with oral contraceptive use has been shown to contribute substantially to the incidence of myocardial infarctions in women in their mid-thirties or older with smoking accounting for the majority of excess cases (17). Mortality rates associated with circulatory disease have been shown to increase substantially in smokers over the age of 35 and non-smokers over the age of 40 (Table II) among women who use oral contraceptives.

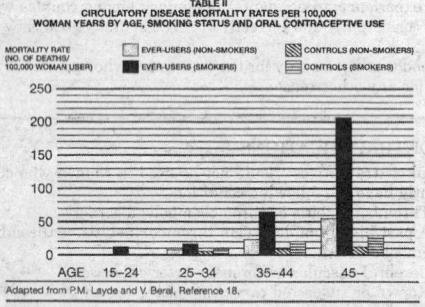

TABLE II
CIRCULATORY DISEASE MORTALITY RATES PER 100,000
WOMAN YEARS BY AGE, SMOKING STATUS AND ORAL CONTRACEPTIVE USE

Adapted from P.M. Layde and V. Beral, Reference 18.

Oral contraceptives may compound the effects of well-known risk factors, such as hypertension, diabetes, hyperlipidemias, age and obesity (19). In particular, some progestogens are known to decrease HDL cholesterol, and cause glucose intolerance, while estrogens may create a state of hyperinsulinism (20–24). Oral contraceptives have been shown to increase blood pressure among users (See Section 9 in WARNINGS). Similar effects on risk factors have been associated with an increased risk of heart disease. Oral contraceptives must be used with caution in women with cardiovascular disease risk factors.

b. Thromboembolism

An increased risk of thromboembolic and thrombotic disease associated with the use of oral contraceptives is well established. Case control studies have found the relative risk of users compared to nonusers to be 3 for the first episode of superficial venous thrombosis, 4 to 11 for deep vein thrombosis or pulmonary embolism, and 1.5 to 6 for women with predisposing conditions for venous thromboembolic disease (9, 10, 25–30). Cohort studies have shown the relative risk to be somewhat lower, about 3 for new cases and about 4.5 for new cases requiring hospitalization (31). The risk of thromboembolic disease due to oral contraceptives is not related to length of use and disappears after pill use is stopped (8).

A two- to four-fold increase in relative risk of postoperative thromboembolic complications has been reported with the use of oral contraceptives (15, 32). The relative risk of venous thrombosis in women who have predisposing conditions is twice that of women without such medical conditions (15, 32). If feasible, oral contraceptives should be discontinued at least 4 weeks prior to and for 2 weeks after elective surgery of a type associated with an increase in risk of thromboembolism and during and following prolonged immobilization. Since the immediate postpartum period is also associated with an increased risk of thromboembolism, oral contraceptives should be started no earlier than 4 to 6 weeks after delivery in women who elect not to breast feed.

c. Cerebrovascular disease

Oral contraceptives have been shown to increase both the relative and attributable risks of cerebrovascular events

(thrombotic and hemorrhagic strokes), although, in general, the risk is greatest among older (>35 years) hypertensive women who also smoke. Hypertension was found to be a risk factor for both users and nonusers, for both types of strokes, while smoking interacted to increase the risk for hemorrhagic strokes (33–35).

In a large study, the relative risk of thrombotic strokes has been shown to range from 3 for normotensive users to 14 for users with severe hypertension (36). The relative risk of hemorrhagic stroke is reported to be 1.2 for non-smokers who used oral contraceptives, 2.6 for smokers who did not use oral contraceptives, 7.6 for smokers who used oral contraceptives, 1.8 for normotensive users, and 25.7 for users with severe hypertension (36). The attributable risk is also greater in older women (9).

d. Dose-related risk of vascular disease from oral contraceptives

A positive association has been observed between the amount of estrogen and progestogen in oral contraceptives and the risk of vascular disease (37–39). A decline in serum high-density lipoproteins (HDL) has been reported with many progestational agents (20–22). A decline in serum high-density lipoproteins has been associated with an increased incidence of ischemic heart disease. Because estrogens increase HDL cholesterol, the net effect of an oral contraceptive depends on a balance achieved between doses of estrogen and progestin and the nature of the progestin used in the contraceptives. The amount and activity of both hormones should be considered in the choice of an oral contraceptive.

Minimizing exposure to estrogen and progestogen is in keeping with good principles of therapeutics. For any particular oral contraceptive, the dosage regimen prescribed should be one which contains the least amount of estrogen and progestogen that is compatible with the needs of the individual patient. New acceptors of oral contraceptive agents should be started on preparations containing the lowest dose of estrogen which produces satisfactory results for the patient.

e. Persistence of risk of vascular disease

There are two studies which have shown persistence of risk of vascular disease for ever-users of oral contraceptives. In a study in the United States, the risk of developing myocardial infarction after discontinuing oral contraceptives persists for at least 9 years for women 40–49 years who had used oral contraceptives for 5 or more years, but this increased risk was not demonstrated in other age groups (14). In another study in Great Britain, the risk of developing cerebrovascular disease persisted for at least 6 years after discontinuation of oral contraceptives, although excess risk was very small (40). However, both studies were performed with oral contraceptive formulations containing 50 mcg or higher of estrogens.

2. Estimates of Mortality from Contraceptive Use

One study gathered data from a variety of sources which have estimated the mortality rate associated with different methods of contraception at different ages (Table III). These estimates include the combined risk of death associated with contraceptive methods plus the risk attributable to pregnancy in the event of method failure. Each method of contraception has its specific benefits and risks. The study concluded that with the exception of oral contraceptive users 35 and older who smoke and 40 and older who do not smoke, mortality associated with all methods of birth control is low and below that associated with childbirth. The observation of a possible increase in risk of mortality with age for oral contraceptive users is based on data gathered in the 1970's but not reported until 1983 (41). However, current clinical practive involves the use of lower estrogen dose formulations combined with careful restriction of oral contraceptive use to women who do not have the various risk factors listed in this labeling.

Because of these changes in practice and, also, because of some limited new data which suggest that the risk of cardiovascular disease with the use of oral contraceptives may now be less than previously observed (Porter JB, Hunter J, Jick H, et al. Oral contraceptives and nonfatal vascular disease. Obstet Gynecol 1985;66:1–4; and Porter JB, Hershel J,

Walker AM, Mortality among oral contraceptive users. Obstet Gynecol 1987;70:29–32), the Fertility and Maternal Health Drugs Advisory Committee was asked to review the topic in 1989. The Committee concluded that although cardiovascular disease risks may be increased with oral contraceptive use after age 40 in healthy non-smoking women (even with the newer low-dose formulations), there are greater potential health risks associated with pregnancy in older women and with the alternative surgical and medical procedures which may be necessary if such women do not have access to effective and acceptable means of contraception.

Therefore, the Committee recommended that the benefits of oral contraceptive use by healthy non-smoking women over 40 may outweigh the possible risks. Of course, older women, as all women who take oral contraceptives, should take the lowest possible dose formulation that is effective.

[See table III below]

3. Carcinoma of the Reproductive Organs

Numerous epidemiological studies have been performed on the incidence of breast, endometrial, ovarian, and cervical cancer in women using oral contraceptives. Most of the studies on breast cancer and oral contraceptive use report that the use of oral contraceptives is not associated with an increase in the risk of developing breast cancer (42, 44, 89). Some studies have reported an increased risk of developing breast cancer in certain subgroups of oral contraceptive users, but the findings reported in these studies are not consistent (43, 45–49, 85–88).

Some studies suggest that oral contraceptive use has been associated with an increase in the risk of cervical intraepithelial neoplasia in some populations of women (51–54). However, there continues to be controversy about the extent to which such findings may be due to differences in sexual behavior and other factors.

In spite of many studies of the relationship between oral contraceptive use and breast and cervical cancers, a cause and effect relationship has not been established.

4. Hepatic Neoplasia

Benign hepatic adenomas are associated with oral contraceptive use, although the incidence of benign tumors is rare in the United States. Indirect calculations have estimated the attributable risk to be in the range of 3.3 cases/100,000 for users, a risk that increases after 4 or more years of use (55). Rupture of rare, benign, hepatic adenomas may cause death through intraabdominal hemorrhage (56,57).

Studies from Britain have shown an increased risk of developing hepatocellular carcinoma (58–60) in long-term (>8 years) oral contraceptive users. However, these cancers are extremely rare in the U.S., and the attributable risk (the excess incidence) of liver cancers in oral contraceptive users approaches less than one per million users.

5. Ocular Lesions

There have been clinical case reports of retinal thrombosis associated with the use of oral contraceptives. Oral contraceptives should be discontinued if there is unexplained partial or complete loss of vision; onset of proptosis or diplopia; papilledema; or retinal vascular lesions. Appropriate diagnostic and therapeutic measures should be undertaken immediately.

6. Oral Contraceptive Use Before and During Early Pregnancy

External epidemiological studies have revealed no increased risk of birth defects in women who have used oral contraceptives prior to pregnancy (61–63). Studies also do not suggest a teratogenic effect, particularly insofar as cardiac anomalies and limb reduction defects are concerned (61,62,64,65), when taken inadvertently during early pregnancy.

The administration of oral contraceptives to induce withdrawal bleeding should not be used as a test for pregnancy. Oral contraceptives should not be used during pregnancy to treat threatened or habitual abortion.

It is recommended that for any patient who has missed two consecutive periods, pregnancy should be ruled out before continuing oral contraceptive use. If the patient has not ad-

TABLE III
ANNUAL NUMBER OF BIRTH-RELATED OR METHOD-RELATED DEATHS ASSOCIATED WITH CONTROL OF FERTILITY PER 100,000 NONSTERILE WOMEN, BY FERTILITY CONTROL METHOD ACCORDING TO AGE

Method of control and outcome	15–19	20–24	25–29	30–34	35–39	40–44
No fertility control methods*	7.0	7.4	9.1	14.8	25.7	28.2
Oral contraceptives non-smoker**	0.3	0.5	0.9	1.9	13.8	31.6
Oral contraceptives smoker**	2.2	3.4	6.6	13.5	51.1	117.2
IUD**	0.8	0.8	1.0	1.0	1.4	1.4
Condom*	1.1	1.6	0.7	0.2	0.3	0.4
Diaphragm/spermicide*	1.9	1.2	1.2	1.3	2.2	2.8
Periodic abstinence*	2.5	1.6	1.6	1.7	2.9	3.6

*Deaths are birth related.
**Deaths are method related.

Adapted from H.W. Ory, Reference 41.

hered to the prescribed schedule, the possibility of pregnancy should be considered at the time of the first missed period. Oral contraceptive use should be discontinued if pregnancy is confirmed.

7. Gallbladder Disease

Earlier studies have reported an increased lifetime relative risk of gallbladder surgery in users of oral contraceptives and estrogens (66,67). More recent studies, however, have shown that the relative risk of developing gallbladder disease among oral contraceptive users may be minimal (68–70). The recent findings of minimal risk may be related to the use of oral contraceptive formulations containing lower hormonal doses of estrogens and progestogens.

8. Carbohydrate and Lipid Metabolic Effects

Oral contraceptives have been shown to cause glucose intolerance in a significant percentage of users (23). Oral contraceptives containing greater than 75 mcg of estrogens cause hyperinsulinism, while lower doses of estrogen cause less glucose intolerance (71). Progestogens increase insulin secretion and create insulin resistance, this effect varying with different progestational agents (23,72). However, in the non-diabetic woman, oral contraceptives appear to have no effect on fasting blood glucose (73). Because of these demonstrated effects, pre-diabetic and diabetic women should be carefully observed while taking oral contraceptives.

A small proportion of women will have persistent hypertriglyceridemia while on the pill. As discussed earlier (see WARNINGS 1a. and 1d.), changes in serum triglycerides and lipoprotein levels have been reported in oral contraceptive users.

9. Elevated Blood Pressure

An increase in blood pressure has been reported in women taking oral contraceptives (74) and this increase is more likely in older oral contraceptive users (75) and with continued use (74). Data from the Royal College of General Practitioners (18) and subsequent randomized trials have shown that the incidence of hypertension increases with increasing concentrations of progestogens.

Women with a history of hypertension or hypertension-related diseases or renal disease (76) should be encouraged to use another method of contraception. If women elect to use oral contraceptives, they should be monitored closely, and if significant elevation of blood pressure occurs, oral contraceptives should be discontinued. For most women, elevated blood pressure will return to normal after stopping oral contraceptives (75), and there is no difference in the occurrence of hypertension among ever and never users (74, 76, 77).

10. Headache

The onset or exacerbation of migraine or development of headache with a new pattern which is recurrent, persistent, or severe requires discontinuation of oral contraceptives and evaluation of the cause.

11. Bleeding Irregularities

Breakthrough bleeding and spotting are sometimes encountered in patients on oral contraceptives, especially during the first three months of use. Non-hormonal causes should be considered, and adequate diagnostic measures taken to rule out malignancy or pregnancy in the event of prolonged breakthrough bleeding, as in the case of any abnormal vaginal bleeding. If pathology has been excluded, time or a change to another formulation may solve the problem. In the event of amenorrhea, pregnancy should be ruled out.

Some women may encounter post-pill amenorrhea or oligomenorrhea, especially when such a condition was preexistent.

PRECAUTIONS

1. Patients should be counseled that this product does not protect against HIV infection (AIDS) and other sexually transmitted diseases.

2. Physical Examination and Follow-Up

It is good medical practice for all women to have annual history and physical examinations, including women using oral contraceptives. The physical examination, however, may be deferred until after initiation of oral contraceptives if requested by the woman and judged appropriate by the clinician. The physical examination should include special reference to blood pressure, breasts, abdomen and pelvic organs, including cervical cytology, and relevant laboratory tests. In case of undiagnosed, persistent or recurrent abnormal vaginal bleeding, appropriate measures should be conducted to rule out malignancy. Women with a strong family history of breast cancer or who have breast nodules should be monitored with particular care.

3. Lipid Disorders

Women who are being treated for hyperlipidemia should be followed closely if they elect to use oral contraceptives. Some progestogens may elevate LDL levels and may render the control of hyperlipidemias more difficult.

4. Liver Function

If jaundice develops in any woman receiving such drugs, the medication should be discontinued. Steroid hormones may be poorly metabolized in patients with impaired liver function.

5. Fluid Retention

Oral contraceptives may cause some degree of fluid retention. They should be prescribed with caution, and only with careful monitoring, in patients with conditions which might be aggravated by fluid retention.

6. Emotional Disorders

Women with a history of depression should be carefully observed, and the drug discontinued if depression recurs to a serious degree.

7. Contact Lenses

Contact lens wearers who develop visual changes or changes in lens tolerance should be assessed by an ophthalmologist.

8. Drug Interactions

Reduced efficacy and increased incidence of breakthrough bleeding and menstrual irregularities have been associated with concomitant use of rifampin. A similar association, though less marked, has been suggested with barbiturates, phenylbutazone, phenytoin sodium, and possibly with griseofulvin, ampicillin, and tetracyclines (78).

9. Interactions with Laboratory Tests

Certain endocrine and liver function tests and blood components may be affected by oral contraceptives:

a. Increased prothrombin and factors VII, VIII, IX, and X; decreased antithrombin 3; increased norepinephrine-induced platelet aggregability.

b. Increased thyroid binding globulin (TBG) leading to increased circulating total thyroid hormone, as measured by protein-bound iodine (PBI), T_4 by column or by radioimmunoassay. Free T_3 resin uptake is decreased, reflecting the elevated TBG; free T_4 concentration is unaltered.

c. Other binding proteins may be elevated in serum.

d. Sex-binding globulins are increased and result in elevated levels of total circulating sex steroids and corticoids; however, free or biologically active levels remain unchanged.

e. Triglycerides may be increased.

f. Glucose tolerance may be decreased.

g. Serum folate levels may be depressed by oral contraceptive therapy. This may be of clinical significance if a woman becomes pregnant shortly after discontinuing oral contraceptives.

10. Carcinogenesis

See **WARNINGS** section.

11. Pregnancy

Pregnancy Category X. See **CONTRAINDICATIONS** and **WARNINGS** sections.

12. Nursing Mothers

Small amounts of oral contraceptive steroids have been identified in the milk of nursing mothers, and a few adverse effects on the child have been reported, including jaundice and breast enlargement. In addition, oral contraceptives given in the postpartum period may interfere with lactation by decreasing the quantity and quality of breast milk. If possible, the nursing mother should be advised not to use oral contraceptives but to use other forms of contraception until she has completely weaned her child.

INFORMATION FOR THE PATIENT

See patient labeling printed below.

ADVERSE REACTIONS

An increased risk of the following serious adverse reactions has been associated with the use of oral contraceptives (see WARNINGS section):

- Thrombophlebitis
- Arterial thromboembolism
- Pulmonary embolism
- Myocardial infarction
- Cerebral hemorrhage
- Cerebral thrombosis
- Hypertension
- Gallbladder disease
- Hepatic adenomas or benign liver tumors

There is evidence of an association between the following conditions and the use of oral contraceptives, although additional confirmatory studies are needed:

- Mesenteric thrombosis
- Retinal thrombosis

The following adverse reactions have been reported in patients receiving oral contraceptives and are believed to be drug-related:

- Nausea
- Vomiting
- Gastrointestinal symptoms (such as abdominal cramps and bloating)
- Breakthrough bleeding
- Spotting
- Change in menstrual flow
- Amenorrhea
- Temporary infertility after discontinuation of treatment
- Edema
- Melasma which may persist
- Breast changes: tenderness, enlargement, secretion
- Change in weight (increase or decrease)
- Change in cervical erosion and secretion
- Diminution in lactation when given immediately postpartum
- Cholestatic jaundice
- Migraine
- Rash (allergic)
- Mental depression
- Reduced tolerance to carbohydrates
- Vaginal candidiasis
- Change in corneal curvature (steepening)
- Intolerance to contact lenses

The following adverse reactions have been reported in users of oral contraceptives and the association has been neither confirmed no refuted:

- Pre-menstrual syndrome
- Cataracts
- Changes in appetite
- Cystitis-like syndrome
- Headache
- Nervousness
- Dizziness
- Hirsutism
- Loss of scalp hair
- Erythema multiforme
- Erythema nodosum
- Hemorrhagic eruption
- Vaginitis
- Porphyria
- Impaired renal function
- Hemolytic uremic syndrome
- Budd-Chiari syndrome
- Acne
- Changes in libido
- Colitis

OVERDOSAGE

Serious ill effects have not been reported following acute ingestion of large doses of oral contraceptives by young children. Overdosage may cause nausea, and withdrawal bleeding may occur in females.

NON-CONTRACEPTIVE HEALTH BENEFITS

The following non-contraceptive health benefits related to the use of oral contraceptives are supported by epidemiological studies which largely utilized oral contraceptive formulations containing estrogen doses exceeding 0.035 mg of ethinyl estradiol or 0.05 mg of mestranol (79–84).

Effects on menses:

- Increase menstrual cycle regularity
- Decreased blood loss and decreased incidence of iron deficiency anemia
- Decreased incidence of dysmenorrhea

Effects related to inhibition of ovulation:

- Decreased incidence of functional ovarian cysts
- Decreased incidence of ectopic pregnancies

Effects from long-term use:

- Decreased incidence of fibroadenomas and fibrocystic disease of the breast
- Decreased incidence of acute pelvic inflammatory disease
- Decreased incidence of endometrial cancer
- Decreased incidence of ovarian cancer

DOSAGE AND ADMINISTRATION

The tablet dispenser has been designed to make oral contraceptive dosing as easy and as convenient as possible. The tablets are arranged in either three or four rows of seven tablets each, with the days of the week appearing on the tablet dispenser above the first row of tablets.

Important Notes: The patient should be instructed to use an additional method of protection until after the first week of administration in the initial cycle when utilizing the Sunday-Start Regimen.

The possibility of ovulation and conception prior to initiation of use should be considered.

Dosage and Administration for 21–Day Dosage Regimen

To achieve maximum contraceptive effectiveness, Estrostep **21** must be taken exactly as directed and at intervals not exceeding 24 hours. Estrostep **21** provides the patient with a convenient tablet schedule of "3 weeks on—1 week off." For the initial cycle of therapy, the patient begins her tablets according to a Sunday-Start Regimen. With this regimen, the patient takes one tablet daily for 21 consecutive days followed by 1 week of no tablets.

The patient begins taking tablets from the top row on the first Sunday after menstrual flow begins. When menstrual flow begins on Sunday, the first tablet is taken on the same day. The last tablet in the dispenser will then be taken on a Saturday, followed by no tablets for a week (7 days). For all subsequent cycles, the patient then begins a new 21–tablet

Continued on next page

This product information was prepared in June 1998. On these and other Parke-Davis Products, information may be obtained by addressing PARKE-DAVIS, Division of Warner-Lambert Company, Morris Plains, New Jersey 07950.

Consult 1999 PDR® supplements and future editions for revisions

Estrostep—Cont.

regimen on the eighth day, Sunday, after taking her last tablet. Following this regimen, of 21 days on—7 days off, the patient will start all subsequent cycles on a Sunday.

All tablets should be taken regularly with a meal or at bedtime. It should be stressed that efficacy of medication depends on strict adherence to the dosage schedule.

Special Notes on Administration

Menstruation usually begins two or three days, but may begin as late as the fourth or fifth day, after discontinuing medication. If spotting occurs while on the usual regimen of one tablet daily, the patient should continue medication without interruption.

If a patient forgets to take one or more *white* tablets, the following is suggested:

One tablet is missed
* take tablet as soon as remembered
* take next tablet at the regular time

Two consecutive tablets are missed (week 1 or week 2)
* take *two* tablets as soon as remembered
* take *two* tablets the next day
* use another birth control method for seven days following the missed tablets

Two consecutive tablets are missed (week 3)
* take *one* tablet daily until Sunday
* discard remaining tablets
* start new pack of tablets immediately (Sunday)
* use another birth control method for seven days following the missed tablets

Three (or more) consecutive tablets are missed
* take *one* tablet daily until Sunday
* discard remaining tablets
* start a new pack of tablets immediately (Sunday)
* use another birth control method for seven days following the missed tablets

The possibility of ovulation increases with each successive day that scheduled tablets are missed. While there is little likelihood of ovulation occurring if only one tablet is missed, the possibility of spotting or bleeding is increased. This is particularly likely to occur if two or more consecutive tablets are missed.

In the rare case of bleeding which resembles menstruation, the patient should be advised to discontinue medication and then begin taking tablets from a new tablet dispenser on the next Sunday. Persistent bleeding which is not controlled by this method indicates the need for reexamination of the patient, at which time nonfunctional causes should be considered.

Dosage and Administration for 28–Day Dosage Regimen

To achieve maximum contraceptive effectiveness, Estrostep **Fe** should be taken exactly as directed and at intervals not exceeding 24 hours.

Estrostep Fe provides a continuous administration regimen consisting of 21 white tablets of Estrostep and seven brown non-hormone containing tablets of ferrous fumarate. The ferrous fumarate tablets are present to facilitate ease of drug administration via a 28–day regimen and do not serve any therapeutic purpose. There is no need for the patient to count days between cycles because there are no "off-tablet days."

The patient begins taking the first white tablet in the top row of the dispenser (labeled Sunday) on the first Sunday after menstrual flow begins. When the menstrual flow begins on Sunday, the first white tablet is taken on the same day. The patient takes one tablet daily for 21 days. The last white tablet in the dispenser will be taken on a Saturday. Upon completion of all 21 white tablets, and without interruption, the patient takes one brown tablet daily for 7 days. Upon completion of this first course of tablets, the patient begins a second course of 28–day tablets without interruption the next day, Sunday, starting with the Sunday white tablet in the top row. Adhering to this regimen of one white tablet daily for 21 days, followed without interruption by one brown tablet daily for 7 days, the patient will start all subsequent cycles on a Sunday.

Tablets should be taken regularly with a meal or at bedtime. It should be stressed that efficacy of medication depends on strict adherence to the dosage schedule.

Special Notes on Administration

Menstruation usually begins two or three days, but may begin as late as the fourth or fifth day, after the brown tablets have been started. In any event, the next course of tablets should be started without interruption. If spotting occurs while the patient is taking white tablets, continue medication without interruption.

If a patient forgets to take one or more *white* tablets, the following is suggested:

One tablet is missed
* take tablet as soon as remembered
* take next tablet at the regular time

Two consecutive tablets are missed (week 1 or week 2)
* take *two* tablets as soon as remembered
* take *two* tablets the next day

* use another birth control method for seven days following the missed tablets

Two consecutive tablets are missed (week 3)
* take *one* tablet daily until Sunday
* discard remaining tablets
* start new pack of tablets immediately (Sunday)
* use another birth control method for seven days following the missed tablets

Three (or more) consecutive tablets are missed
* take *one* tablet daily until Sunday
* discard remaining tablets
* start a new pack of tablets immediately (Sunday)
* use another birth control method for seven days following the missed tablets

The possibility of ovulation occurring increases with each successive day that white tablets are missed. While there is little likelihood of ovulation occurring if only one white tablet is missed, the possibility of spotting or bleeding is increased. This is particularly likely to occur if two or more consecutive tablets are missed.

If the patient forgets to take any of the seven brown tablets in week four, those brown tablets that were missed are discarded and one brown tablet is taken each day until the pack is empty. A back up birth control method is not required during this time. A new pack of tablets should be started no later than the eighth day after the last white colored tablet was taken.

In the rare case of bleeding which resembles menstruation, the patient should be advised to discontinue medication and then begin taking tablets from a new tablet dispenser on the next Sunday. Persistent bleeding which is not controlled by this method indicates the need for reexamination of the patient, at which time nonfunctional causes should be considered.

Use of Oral Contraceptives in the Event of a Missed Menstrual Period

1. If the patient has not adhered to the prescribed dosage regimen, the possibility of pregnancy should be considered after the first missed period and oral contraceptives should be withheld until pregnancy has been ruled out.

2. If the patient has adhered to the prescribed regimen and misses two consecutive periods, pregnancy should be ruled out before continuing the contraceptive regimen.

After several months on treatment, bleeding may be reduced to a point of virtual absence. This reduced flow may occur as a result of medication, in which event it is not indicative of pregnancy.

HOW SUPPLIED

Estrostep **21** is available in dispensers each containing 21 white tablets. The first five triangle tablets each contain 1 mg of norethindrone acetate and 20 mcg of ethinyl estradiol; the next seven square tablets each contain 1 mg of norethindrone acetate and 30 mcg of ethinyl estradiol; the last nine round tablets each contain 1 mg of norethindrone acetate and 35 mcg of ethinyl estradiol. Available in boxes of five dispensers.

Estrostep **Fe** is available in dispensers each containing 21 white tablets. The first five triangle tablets each contain 1 mg of norethindrone acetate and 20 mcg of ethinyl estradiol; the next seven square tablets each contain 1 mg of norethindrone acetate and 30 mcg of ethinyl estradiol; the next nine round tablets each contain 1 mg of norethindrone acetate and 35 mcg of ethinyl estradiol; and the last seven (brown) tablets each contain 75 mg ferrous fumarate. Available in boxes of five dispensers.

Storage-Do not store above 25° C (77° F). Protect from light.

Store tablets inside pouch when not in use.

REFERENCES

1. Back DJ, Breckenridge AM, Crawford FE, McIver M, Orme ML'E, Rowe PH and Smith E: Kinetics of norethindrone in women II. Single-dose kinetics. Clin Pharmacol Ther 1978;24:448-453.

2. Hümpel M, Nieuweboer B, Wendt H and Speck U: Investigations of pharmacokinetics of ethinyloestradiol to specific consideration of a possible first-pass effect in women. Contraception 1979;19:421-432.

3. Back DJ, Breckenridge AM, Crawford FE, MacIver M, Orme ML'E, Rowe PH and Watts MJ. An investigation of the pharmacokinetics of ethynylestradiol in women using radioimmunoassay. Contraception 1979;20:263-273.

4. Hammond GL, Lähteenmäki PLA, Lähteenmäki P and Luukkainen T. Distribution and percentages of non-protein bound contraceptive steroids in human serum. J Steroid Biochem 1982;17:375-380.

5. Fotherby K. Pharmacokinetics and metabolism of progestins in humans, in Pharmacology of the contraceptive steroids, Goldzieher JW, Fotherby K (eds), Raven Press Ltd., New York, 1994, 99-126.

6. Goldzieher JW. Pharmacokinetics and metabolism of ethynyl estrogens, in Pharmacology of the contraceptive steroids, Goldzieher JW, Fotherby K (eds), Raven Press Ltd., New York, 1994, 127-151.

7. Hatcher, RA, et al. 1994. Contraceptive Technology, Sixteenth Edition. New York: Irvington Publishers.

8. Stadel, B.V.: Oral contraceptives and cardiovascular disease. (Pt. 1). *New England Journal of Medicine,*305:612-618, 1981.

9. Stadel, B.V.: Oral contraceptives and cardiovascular disease. (Pt. 2). *New England Journal of Medicine,*305:672-677, 1981.

10. Adam, S.A., and M. Thorogood: Oral contraception and myocardial infarction revisited: The effects of new preparations and prescribing patterns. *Brit. J. Obstet. and Gynec.,* 88:838-845, 1981.

11. Mann, J.I., and W.H. Inman: Oral contraceptives and death from myocardial infarction. *Brit. Med. J.,* 2(5965): 245-248, 1975.

12. Mann, J.I., M.P. Vessey, M. Thorogood, and R. Doll: Myocardial infarction in young women with special reference to oral contraceptive practice. *Brit. Med. J.,* 2(5965):241-245, 1975.

13. Royal College of General Practitioners' Oral Contraception Study: Further analyses of mortality in oral contraceptive users. *Lancet,* 1:541-546, 1981.

14. Slone, D., S. Shapiro, D.W. Kaufman, L. Rosenberg, O.S. Miettinen, and P.D. Stolley: Risk of myocardial infarction in relation to current and discontinued use of oral contraceptives. *N.E.J.M.,*305:420-424, 1981.

15. Vessey, M.P.: Female hormones and vascular disease: An epidemiological overview. *Brit. J. Fam. Plann.,* 6:1-12, 1980.

16. Russell-Briefel, R.G., T.M. Ezzati, R. Fulwood, J.A. Perlman, and R.S. Murphy: Cardiovascular risk status and oral contraceptive use, United States, 1976-80. *Preventive Medicine,* 15:352-362, 1986.

17. Goldbaum, G.M., J.S. Kendrick, G.C. Hogelin, and E.M. Gentry: The relative impact of smoking and oral contraceptive use on women in the United States. *J.A.M.A.,* 258:1339-1342, 1987.

18. Layde, P.M., and V. Beral: Further analyses of mortality in oral contraceptive users: Royal College General Practitioners' Oral Contraception Study. (Table 5) *Lancet,* 1:541-546, 1981.

19. Knopp, R.H.: Arteriosclerosis risk: The roles of oral contraceptives and postmenopausal estrogens; *J. of Reprod. Med.,* 31(9)(Supplement): 913-921, 1986.

20. Krauss, R.M., S. Roy, D.R. Mishell, J. Casagrande, and M.C. Pike: Effects of two low-dose oral contraceptives on serum lipids and lipoproteins: Differential changes in high-density lipoproteins subclasses. *Am. J. Obstet. Gyn.,* 145: 446-452, 1983.

21. Wahl, P., C. Walden, R. Knopp, J. Hoover, R. Wallace, G. Heiss, and B. Rifkind: Effect of estrogen/progestin potency on lipid/lipoprotein cholesterol. *N.E.J.M.,* 308:862-867, 1983.

22. Wynn, V., and R. Niththyananthan: The effect of progestin in combined oral contraceptives on serum lipids with special reference to high-density lipoproteins. *Am. J. Obstet. and Gyn.,* 142:766-771, 1982.

23. Wynn, V., and I. Godsland: Effects of oral contraceptives on carbohydrate metabolism. *J. Reprod. Medicine,* 31 (9)(Supplement): 892-897, 1986.

24. LaRosa, J.C.: Atherosclerotic risk factors in cardiovascular disease. *J. Reprod. Med.,* 31(9)(Supplement): 906-912, 1986.

25. Inman, W.H., and M.P. Vessey: Investigations of death from pulmonary, coronary, and cerebral thrombosis and embolism in women of child-bearing age. *Brit. Med. J.,* 2(5599): 193-199, 1968.

26. Maguire, M.G., J. Tonascia, P.E. Sartwell, P.D. Stolley, and M.S. Tockman: Increased risk of thrombosis due to oral contraceptives: A further report. *Am. J. Epidemiology,* 110(2): 188-195, 1979.

27. Pettiti, D.B., J. Wingerd, F. Pellegrin, and S. Ramacharan: Risk of vascular disease in women: Smoking, oral contraceptives, noncontraceptive estrogens, and other factors. *J.A.M.A.,* 242:1150-1154, 1979.

28. Vessey, M.P., and R. Doll: Investigation of relation between use of oral contraceptives and thromboembolic disease. *Brit. Med. J.,* 2(5599): 199-205, 1968.

29. Vessey, M.P., and R. Doll: Investigation of relation between use of oral contraceptives and thromboembolic disease. A further report. *Brit. Med. J.,* 2 (5658): 651-657, 1969.

30. Porter, J.B., J.R. Hunter, D.A. Danielson, H. Jick, and A. Stergachis: Oral contraceptives and non-fatal vascular disease: Recent experience. *Obstet. and Gyn.,* 59(3):299-302, 1982.

31. Vessey, M.P., and R. Doll, R. Peto, B. Johnson, and P. Wiggins: A long-term follow-up study of women using different methods of contraception: An interim report. *J Biosocial. Sci.,* 8:375-427, 1976.

32. Royal College of General Practitioners: Oral contraceptives, venous thrombosis, and varicose veins. *J. of Royal College of General Practitioners,* 28:393-399, 1978.

33. Collaborative Group for the study of stroke in young women: Oral contraception and increased risk of cerebral ischemia or thrombosis. *N.E.J.M.,* 288:871-878, 1973.

34. Petitti, D.B., and J. Wingerd: Use of oral contraceptives, cigarette smoking, and risk of subarachnoid hemorrhage. *Lancet,* 2:234-236, 1978.

35. Inman, W.H.: Oral contraceptives and fatal subarachnoid hemorrhage, *Brit. Med. J.*, 2(6203): 1468-70, 1979.
36. Collaborative Group for the study of stroke in young women: Oral contraceptives and stroke in young women: Associated risk factors. *J.A.M.A.*, 231:718-722, 1975.
37. Inman, W.H., M.P. Vessey, B. Westerholm, and A. Engelund: Thromboembolic disease and the steroidal content of oral contraceptives. A report to the Committee on Safety of Drugs. *Brit. Med. J.*, 2:203-209, 1970.
38. Meade, T.W., G. Greenberg, and S.G. Thompson: Progestogens and cardiovascular reactions associated with oral contraceptives and a comparison of the safety of 50- and 35-mcg oestrogen preparations. *Brit. Med. J.*, 280(6224): 1157-1161, 1980.
39. Kay, C.R.: Progestogens and arterial disease: Evidence from the Royal College of General Practitioners' study. *Amer. J. Obstet. Gyn.*, 142:762–765, 1982.
40. Royal College of General Practitioners: Incidence of arterial disease among oral contraceptive users. *J. Coll. Gen. Pract.*, 33:75–82, 1983.
41. Ory, H.W: Mortality associated with fertility and fertility control: 1983. *Family Planning Perspectives*, 15:50–56, 1983.
42. The Cancer and Steroid Hormone Study of the Centers for Disease Control and the National Institute of Child Health and Human Development: Oral-contraceptive use and the risk of breast cancer. *N.E.J.M.*, 315:405–411, 1986.
43. Pike, M.C., B.E. Henderson, M.D. Krailo, A. Duke, and S. Roy: Breast cancer in young women and use of oral contraceptives: Possible modifying effect of formulation and age at use. *Lancet*, 2:926–929, 1983.
44. Paul, C., D.G. Skegg, G.F.S. Spears, and J.M. Kaldor: Oral contraceptives and breast cancer: A national study. *Brit. Med. J.*,293:723–725, 1986.
45. Miller, D.R., L. Rosenberg, D.W. Kaufman, D. Schottenfeld, P.D. Stolley, and S. Shapiro: Breast cancer risk in relation to early oral contraceptive use. *Obstet. Gynec.*, 68: 863–868, 1986.
46. Olson, H. K.L. Olson, T.R. Moller, J. Ranstam, P. Holm: Oral contraceptive use and breast cancer in young women in Sweden (letter). *Lancet*, 2:748–749, 1985.
47. McPherson, K., M. Vessey, A. Neil, R. Doll, L. Jones, and M. Roberts: Early contraceptive use and breast cancer: Results of another case-control study. *Brit. J. Cancer*, 56:653–660, 1987.
48. Huggins, G.R., and P.F. Zucker: Oral contraceptives and neoplasia: 1987 update. *Fertil. Steril.*, 47:733–761, 1987.
49. McPherson, K., and J.O. Drife: The pill and breast cancer: Why the uncertainty? *Brit. Med. J.*, 293:709–710, 1986.
50. Shapiro, S.: Oral contraceptives: Time to take stock. *N.E.J.M.*, 315:450–451, 1987.
51. Ory, H., Z. Naib, S.B. Conger, R.A. Hatcher, and C.W. Tyler: Contraceptive choice and prevalence of cervical dysplasia and carcinoma in situ. *Am. J. Obstet. Gynec.*, 124: 573–577, 1976.
52. Vessey, M.P., M. Lawless, K. McPherson, D. Yeates: Neoplasia of the cervix uteri and contraception: A possible adverse effect of the pill. *Lancet*, 2:930, 1983.
53. Brinton, L.A., G.R. Huggins, H.F. Lehman, K. Malli, D.A. Savitz, E. Trapido, J. Rosenthal, and R. Hoover: Long-term use of oral contraceptives and risk of invasive cervical cancer. *Int. J. Cancer*, 38:339–344, 1986.
54. WHO Collaborative Study of Neoplasia and Steroid Contraceptives: Invasive cervical cancer and combined oral contraceptives. *Brit. Med. J.*, 290:961–965, 1985.
55. Rooks, J.B., H.W. Ory, K.G. Ishak, L.T. Strauss, J.R. Greenspan, A.P. Hill, and C.W. Tyler: Epidemiology of hepatocellular adenoma: The role of oral contraceptive use. *J.A.M.A.*,242:644–648, 1979.
56. Bein, N.N., and H.S. Goldsmith: Recurrent massive hemorrhage from benign hepatic tumors secondary to oral contraceptives. *Brit. J. Surg.*, 64:433–435, 1977.
57. Klatskin, G.: Hepatic tumors: Possible relationship to use of oral contraceptives. *Gastroenterology*, 73:386–394, 1977.
58. Henderson, B.E., S. Preston-Martin, H.A. Edmondson, R.L. Peters, and M.C. Pike: Hepatocellular carcinoma and oral contraceptives. *Brit. J. Cancer*, 48:437–440, 1983.
59. Neuberger, J., D. Forman, R. Doll, and R. Williams: Oral contraceptives and hepatocellular carcinoma. *Brit. Med. J.*, 292:1355–1357, 1986.
60. Forman, D., T.J. Vincent, and R. Doll: Cancer of the liver and oral contraceptives. *Brit. Med. J.*,292: 1357–1361, 1986.
61. Harlap, S., and J. Eldor: Births following oral contraceptive failures. *Obstet. Gynec.*, 55:447–452, 1980.
62. Savolainen, E., E. Saksela, and L. Saxen: Teratogenic hazards of oral contraceptives analyzed in a national malformation register. *Amer. J. Obstet. Gynec.*, 140:521–524, 1981.
63. Janerich, D.T., J.M. Piper, and D.M. Glebatis: Oral contraceptives and birth defects. *Am. J. Epidemiology*, 112:73–79, 1980.
64. Ferencz, C., G.M. Matanoski, P.D. Wilson, J.D. Rubin, C.A. Neill, and R. Gutberlet: Maternal hormone therapy and congenital heart disease. *Teratology*, 21:225–239, 1980.
65. Rothman, K.J., D.C. Fyler, A. Goldbatt, and M.B. Kreidberg: Exogenous hormones and other drug exposures of children with congenital heart disease. *Am. J. Epidemiology*, 109:433–439, 1979.
66. Boston Collaborative Drug Surveillance Program: Oral contraceptives and venous thromboembolic disease, surgically confirmed gallbladder disease, and breast tumors. *Lancet*, 1:1399–1404, 1973.
67. Royal College of General Practitioners: *Oral Contraceptives and Health.* New York, Pittman, 1974. 100p.
68. Layde, P.M., M.P. Vessey, and D. Yeates: Risk of gallbladder disease: A cohort study of young women attending family planning clinics. *J. Epidemiol. and Comm. Health*, 36: 274–278, 1982.
69. Rome Group for the Epidemiology and Prevention of Cholelithiasis (GREPCO): Prevalence of gallstone disease in an Italian adult female population. *Am. J. Epidemiol.*, 119: 796–805, 1984.
70. Strom, B.L., R.T. Tamragouri, M.L. Morse, E.L. Lazar, S.L. West, P.D. Stolley, and J.K. Jones: Oral contraceptives and other risk factors for gallbladder disease. *Clin. Pharmacol. Ther.*, 39:335–341, 1986.
71. Wynn, V., P.W. Adams, I.F. Godsland, J. Melrose, R. Niththyananthan, N.W. Oakley, and A. Seedj: Comparison of effects of different combined oral-contraceptive formulations on carbohydrate and lipid metabolism. *Lancet*,1:1045–1049, 1979.
72. Wynn, V.: Effect of progesterone and progestins on carbohydrate metabolism. In *Progesterone and Progestin.* Edited by C.W. Bardin, E. Milgrom, P. Mauvis-Jarvis. New York, Raven Press, 395–410, 1983.
73. Perlman, J.A., R.G. Roussell-Briefel, T.M. Ezzati, and G. Lieberknecht: Oral glucose tolerance and the potency of oral contraceptive progestogens. *J. Chronic Dis.*, 38:857–864, 1985.
74. Royal College of General Practitioners' Oral Contraception Study: Effect on hypertension and benign breast disease of progestogen component in combined oral contraceptives. *Lancet*, 1:624, 1977.
75. Fisch, I.R., and J. Frank: Oral contraceptives and blood pressure. *J.A.M.A.*, 237:2499–2503, 1977.
76. Laragh, A.J.: Oral contraceptive induced hypertension: Nine years later. *Amer. J. Obstet. Gynecol.*, 126:141–147, 1976.
77. Ramcharan, S., E. Peritz, F.A. Pellegrin, and W.T. Williams: Incidence of hypertension in the Walnut Creek Contraceptive Drug Study cohort. In *Pharmacology of Steroid Contraceptive Drugs.* Edited by S. Garattini and H.W. Berendes. New York, Raven Press, 277–288, 1977. (Monographs of the Mario Negri Institute for Pharmacological Research, Milan.)
78. Stockley, I.: Interactions with oral contraceptives. *Pharm. J.*, 216:140–143, 1976.
79. The Cancer and Steroid Hormone Study of the Centers for Disease Control and the National Institute of Child Health and Human Development: Oral contraceptive use and the risk of ovarian cancer. *J.A.M.A.*, 249:1596–1599, 1983.
80. The Cancer and Steroid Hormone Study of the Centers for Disease Control and the National Institute of Child Health and Human Development: Combination oral contraceptive use and the risk of endometrial cancer. *J.A.M.A.*, 257:796–800, 1987.
81. Ory, H.W.: Functional ovarian cysts and oral contraceptives: Negative association confirmed surgically. *J.A.M.A.*, 228:68–69, 1974.
82. Ory, H.W., P. Cole, B. Macmahon, and R. Hoover: Oral contraceptives and reduced risk of benign breast disease. *N.E.J.M.*, 294:41–422, 1976.
83. Ory, H.W.: The noncontraceptive health benefits from oral contraceptive use. *Fam. Plann. Perspectives*, 14:182–184, 1982.
84. Ory, H.W., J.D. Forrest, and R. Lincoln: Making Choices: Evaluating the health risks and benefits of birth control methods. New York, The Alan Guttmacher Institute, 1, 1983.
85. Miller, D.R., L. Rosenberg, D.W. Kaufman, P. Stolley, M.E. Warshauer, and S. Shapiro: Breast cancer before age 45 and oral contraceptive use: new findings. *Am. J. Epidemiol.*, 129:269–280, 1989.
86. Kay, C.R., and P.C. Hannaford: Breast cancer and the pill: a further report from the Royal College of General Practitioners Oral Contraception Study: *Br. J. Cancer*, 58: 675–680, 1988.
87. Stadel, B.V., S. Lai, J.J. Schlesselman, and P. Murray: Oral contraceptives and premenopausal breast cancer in nulliparous women. *Contraception*, 38:287–299, 1988.
88. UK National Case-Control Study Group: Oral contraceptive use and breast cancer risk in young women. *Lancet*, 973–982, 1989.
89. Romieu, I., W.C. Willett, G.A. Colditz, M.J. Stampfer, B. Rosner, C.H. Hennekens, and F.E. Speizer: Prospective study of oral contraceptive use and risk of breast cancer in women. *J. Natl. Cancer Inst.*, 81:1313–1321, 1989.

The patient labeling for oral contraceptive drug products is set forth below:

This product (like all oral contraceptives) is intended to prevent pregnancy. It does not protect against HIV infection (AIDS) and other sexually transmitted diseases.

BRIEF SUMMARY PATIENT PACKAGE INSERT

Oral contraceptives, also known as "birth control pills" or "the pill," are taken to prevent pregnancy and, when taken correctly, have a failure rate of about 1% per year when used without missing any pills. The typical failure rate of large numbers of pill users is less than 3% per year when women who miss pills are included. For most women oral contraceptives are also free of serious or unpleasant side effects. However, forgetting to take pills considerably increases the chances of pregnancy.

For the majority of women, oral contraceptives can be taken safely. But there are some women who are at high risk of developing certain serious diseases that can be life-threatening or may cause temporary or permanent disability. The risks associated with taking oral contraceptives increase significantly if you:

- Smoke
- Have high blood pressure, diabetes, high cholesterol
- Have or have had clotting disorders, heart attack, stroke, angina pectoris, cancer of the breast or sex organs, jaundice, or malignant or benign liver tumors.

You should not take the pill if you suspect you are pregnant or have unexplained vaginal bleeding.

Cigarette smoking increases the risk of serious cardiovascular side effects from oral contraceptive use. This risk increases with age and with heavy smoking (15 or more cigarettes per day) and is quite marked in women over 35 years of age. Women who use oral contraceptives are strongly advised not to smoke.

Most side effects of the pill are not serious. The most common side effects are nausea, vomiting, bleeding between menstrual periods, weight gain, breast tenderness, and difficulty wearing contact lenses. These side effects, especially nausea, vomiting, and breakthrough bleeding, may subside within the first three months of use.

The serious side effects of the pill occur very infrequently, especially if you are in good health and are young. However, you should know that the following medical conditions have been associated with or made worse by the pill:

1. Blood clots in the legs (thrombophlebitis), lungs (pulmonary embolism), stoppage or rupture of a blood vessel in the brain (stroke), blockage of blood vessels in the heart (heart attack or angina pectoris), or other organs of the body. As mentioned above, smoking increases the risk of heart attacks and strokes and subsequent serious medical consequences.
2. Liver tumors, which may rupture and cause severe bleeding. A possible but not definite association has been found with the pill and liver cancer. However, liver cancers are extremely rare. The chance of developing liver cancer from using the pill is thus even rarer.
3. High blood pressure, although blood pressure usually returns to normal when the pill is stopped.

The symptoms associated with these serious side effects are discussed in the detailed leaflet given to you with your supply of pills. Notify your doctor or health care provider if you notice any unusual physical disturbances while taking the pill. In addition, drugs such as rifampin, as well as some anticonvulsants and some antibiotics, may decrease oral contraceptive effectiveness.

Most of the studies to date on breast cancer and pill use have found no increase in the risk of developing breast cancer although some studies have reported an increased risk of developing breast cancer in certain groups of women. However, some studies have found an increase in the risk of developing cancer of the cervix in women taking the pill, but this finding may be related to differences in sexual behavior or other factors not related to use of the pill. Therefore, there is insufficient evidence to rule out the possibility that the pill may cause cancer of the breast or cervix.

Taking the pill provides some important non-contraceptive benefits. These include less painful menstruation, less menstrual blood loss and anemia, fewer pelvic infections, and fewer cancers of the ovary and the lining of the uterus.

Be sure to discuss any medical condition you may have with your health care provider. Your health care provider will take a medical and family history and examine you before prescribing oral contraceptives. The physical examination

Continued on next page

This product information was prepared in June 1998. On these and other Parke-Davis Products, information may be obtained by addressing PARKE-DAVIS, Division of Warner-Lambert Company, Morris Plains, New Jersey 07950.

Estrostep—Cont.

may be delayed to another time if you request it and your health care provider believes that it is a good medical practice to postpone it. You should be reexamined at least once a year while taking oral contraceptives. The detailed patient information leaflet gives you further information which you should read and discuss with your health care provider. **This product (like all oral contraceptives) is intended to prevent pregnancy. It does not protect against transmission of HIV (AIDS) and other sexually transmitted diseases such as chlamydia, genital herpes, genital warts, gonorrhea, hepatitis B and syphilis.**

INSTRUCTIONS TO PATIENT
TABLET DISPENSER

The ESTROSTEP® tablet dispenser has been designed to make oral contraceptive dosing as easy and as convenient as possible. The tablets are arranged in either three or four rows of seven tablets each with the days of the week appearing above the first row of tablets.

If your TABLET DISPENSER contains:	You are taking:
21 white tablets	ESTROSTEP 21
21 white tablets and 7 brown tablets	ESTROSTEP Fe

Each triangle *tablet* contains 1 mg norethindrone acetate and 20 mcg ethinyl estradiol.
Each *square* tablet contains 1 mg norethindrone acetate and 30 mcg ethinyl estradiol.
Each *round* tablet contains 1 mg norethindrone acetate and 35 mcg ethinyl estradiol.
Each *brown* tablet contains 75 mg ferrous fumarate and is intended to help you remember to take the tablets correctly. These brown tablets are not intended to have any health benefit.

DIRECTIONS

To remove a tablet, press down on it with your thumb or finger. The tablet will drop through the back of the tablet dispenser. Do not press with your thumbnail, fingernail, or any other sharp object.

HOW TO TAKE THE PILL

IMPORTANT POINTS TO REMEMBER

BEFORE YOU START TAKING YOUR PILLS:
1. BE SURE TO READ THESE DIRECTIONS:
Before you start taking your pills.
Anytime you are not sure what to do.
2. THE RIGHT WAY TO TAKE THE PILL IS TO TAKE ONE PILL EVERY DAY AT THE SAME TIME. If you miss pills you could get pregnant. This includes starting the pack late. The more pills you miss, the more likely you are to get pregnant.
3. MANY WOMEN HAVE SPOTTING OR LIGHT BLEEDING OR MAY FEEL SICK TO THEIR STOMACH DURING THE FIRST 1–3 PACKS OF PILLS. If you do have spotting or light bleeding or feel sick to your stomach, do not stop taking the pill. The problem will usually go away. If it doesn't go away, check with your doctor or clinic.
4. MISSING PILLS CAN ALSO CAUSE SPOTTING OR LIGHT BLEEDING, even when you make up these missed pills. On the days you take 2 pills to make up for missed pills, you could also feel a little sick to your stomach.
5. IF YOU HAVE VOMITING OR DIARRHEA, for any reason, or IF YOU TAKE SOME MEDICINES, including some antibiotics, your birth control pills may not work as well. Use a backup birth control method (such as condoms or foam) until you check with your doctor or clinic.
6. IF YOU HAVE TROUBLE REMEMBERING TO TAKE THE PILL, talk to your doctor or clinic about how to make pill-taking easier or about using another method of birth control.
7. IF YOU HAVE ANY QUESTIONS OR ARE UNSURE ABOUT THE INFORMATION IN THIS LEAFLET, call your doctor or clinic.

BEFORE YOU START TAKING YOUR PILLS

1. DECIDE WHAT TIME OF DAY YOU WANT TO TAKE YOUR PILL. It is important to take it at about the same time every day.
2. LOOK AT YOUR PILL PACK TO SEE IF IT HAS 21 OR 28 PILLS:
The 21-pill pack has 21 "active" white pills (with hormones) to take for 3 weeks, followed by 1 week without pills.
The 28-pill pack has 21 "active" white pills (with hormones) to take for 3 weeks, followed by 1 week of reminder brown pills (without hormones).

3. ALSO FIND:
1) where on the pack to start taking pills.
2) in what order to take the pills (follow the arrows), and
3) the week numbers as shown in the pictures below.

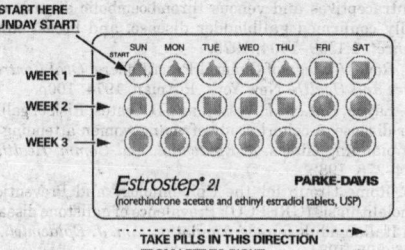

Each Estrostep 21 tablet dispenser contains five white triangular tablets, seven white square tablets, and nine white round tablets. These tablets are to be taken in the following order: one triangular tablet each day for five days, followed by one square tablet each day for seven days, and then one round tablet each day for nine days.
Estrostep 21 will contain : **ALL WHITE PILLS**

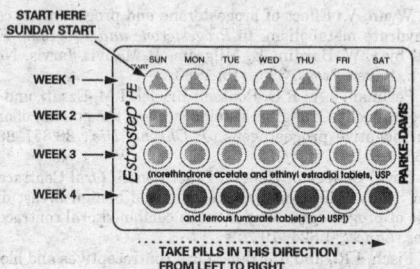

Each Estrostep Fe tablet dispenser contains five white triangular tablets, seven white square tablets, nine white round tablets, and seven brown tablets. These tablets are to be taken in the following order: one triangular tablet each day for five days, then one square tablet each day for seven days, followed by one round tablet each day for nine days, and then one brown tablet each day for seven days.
Estrostep Fe will contain: **21 WHITE PILLS** for **WEEKS 1, 2, and 3. WEEK 4** will contain **BROWN PILLS ONLY.**
4. BE SURE YOU HAVE READY AT ALL TIMES:
ANOTHER KIND OF BIRTH CONTROL (such as condoms or foam) to use as a back-up in case you miss pills.
An EXTRA, FULL PILL PACK.

WHEN TO START THE FIRST PACK OF PILLS

SUNDAY START:
1. Take the first "active" white pill of the first pack on the Sunday after your period starts, even if you are still bleeding. If your period begins on Sunday, start the pack that same day.
2. Use another method of birth control as a back-up method if you have sex anytime from the Sunday you start your first pack until the next Sunday (7 days). Condoms or foam are good back-up methods of birth control.

WHAT TO DO DURING THE MONTH

1. TAKE ONE PILL AT THE SAME TIME EVERY DAY UNTIL THE PACK IS EMPTY.
Do not skip pills even if you are spotting or bleeding between monthly periods or feel sick to your stomach (nausea).
Do not skip pills even if you do not have sex very often.
2. WHEN YOU FINISH A PACK OR SWITCH YOUR BRAND OF PILLS:
21 PILLS: Wait 7 days to start the next pack. You will probably have your period during that week. Be sure that no more than 7 days pass between 21-day packs.
28 PILLS: Start the next pack on the day after your last "reminder" pill. Do not wait any days between packs.

WHAT TO DO IF YOU MISS PILLS

If you **MISS 1** white "active" pill:
1. Take it as soon as you remember. Take the next pill at your regular time. This means you may take 2 pills in 1 day.
2. You do not need to use a back-up birth control method if you have sex.
If you **MISS 2** white "active" pills in a row in **WEEK 1 OR WEEK 2** of your pack:
1. Take 2 pills on the day you remember and 2 pills the next day.
2. Then take 1 pill a day until you finish the pack.

3. You COULD GET PREGNANT if you have sex in the 7 days after you miss pills. You MUST use another birth control method (such as condoms or foam) as a back-up method of birth control until you have taken a white "active" pill every day for 7 days.
If you **MISS 2** white "active" pills in a row in **THE 3rd WEEK:**
1. Keep taking 1 pill every day until Sunday. On Sunday, THROW OUT the rest of the pack and start a new pack of pills that same day.
2. You may not have your period this month, but this is expected. However, if you miss your period 2 months in a row, call your doctor or clinic because you might be pregnant.
3. You COULD GET PREGNANT if you have sex in the 7 days after you miss pills. You MUST use another birth control method (such as condoms or foam) as a back-up method of birth control until you have taken a white "active" pill every day for 7 days.
If you **MISS 3 OR MORE** white "active" pills in a row (during the first 3 weeks):
1. Keep taking 1 pill every day until Sunday. On Sunday, THROW OUT the rest of the pack and start a new pack of pills that same day.
2. You may not have your period this month, but this is expected. However, if you miss your period 2 months in a row, call your doctor or clinic because you might be pregnant.
3. You COULD GET PREGNANT if you have sex in the 7 days after you miss pills. You MUST use another birth control method (such as condoms or foam) as a back-up method of birth control until you have taken a white "active" pill every day for 7 days.

A REMINDER FOR THOSE ON 28-DAY PACKS:
IF YOU FORGET ANY OF THE 7 BROWN "REMINDER" PILLS IN WEEK 4:
THROW AWAY THE PILLS YOU MISSED.
KEEP TAKING 1 PILL EACH DAY UNTIL THE PACK IS EMPTY.
YOU DO NOT NEED A BACK-UP METHOD.

FINALLY, IF YOU ARE STILL NOT SURE WHAT TO DO ABOUT THE PILLS YOU HAVE MISSED:
Use a BACK-UP METHOD anytime you have sex.
KEEP TAKING ONE WHITE "ACTIVE" PILL EACH DAY until you can reach your doctor or clinic.

Based on his or her assessment of your medical needs, your doctor or health care provider has prescribed this drug for you. Do not give this drug to anyone else.
Keep this and all drugs out of the reach of children.
Caution—Federal law prohibits dispensing without prescription.
Storage—Do not store above 25° C (77° F).
Protect from light.
Store tablets inside pouch when not in use.
This product (like all oral contraceptives) is intended to prevent pregnancy. It does not protect against HIV infection (AIDS) and other sexually transmitted diseases.

DETAILED PATIENT PACKAGE INSERT
What You Should Know About Oral Contraceptives
Any woman who considers using oral contraceptives (the "birth control pill" or "the pill") should understand the benefits and risks of using this form of birth control. This leaflet will give you much of the information you will need to make this decision and will also help you determine if you are at risk of developing any of the serious side effects of the pill. It will tell you how to use the pill properly so that it will be as effective as possible. However, this leaflet is not a replacement for a careful discussion between you and your health care provider. You should discuss the information provided in this leaflet with him or her, both when you first start taking the pill and during your revisits. You should also follow your health care provider's advice with regard to regular check-ups while you are on the pill.

EFFECTIVENESS OF ORAL CONTRACEPTIVES

Oral contraceptives or "birth control pills" or "the pill" are used to prevent pregnancy and are more effective than other nonsurgical methods of birth control. When they are taken correctly, the chance of becoming pregnant is less than 1% (1 pregnancy per 100 women per year of use) when used perfectly, without missing any pills. Typical failure rates are actually 3% per year. The chance of becoming pregnant increases with each missed pill during a menstrual cycle.
In comparison, typical failure rates for other methods of birth control during the first year of use are as follows:
Implant (6 capsules): <1%
Injection: <1%
IUD: <1 to 2%
Diaphragm with spermicides: 18%
Spermicides alone: 21%
Vaginal Sponge: 18 to 36%
Female sterilization: <1%
Male sterilization: <1%
Cervical Cap: 18 to 36%
Condom alone (male): 12%
Condom alone (female): 21%

Periodic abstinence: 20%
Withdrawal: 19%
No method: 85%

WHO SHOULD NOT TAKE ORAL CONTRACEPTIVES

Cigarette smoking increases the risk of serious cardiovascular side effects from oral contraceptive use. This risk increases with age and with heavy smoking (15 or more cigarettes per day) and is quite marked in women over 35 years of age. Women who use oral contraceptives are strongly advised not to smoke.

Some women should not use the pill. For example, you should not take the pill if you are pregnant or think you may be pregnant. You should also not use the pill if you have any of the following conditions:
• A history of heart attack or stroke
• Blood clots in the legs (thrombophlebitis), lungs (pulmonary embolism), or eyes
• A history of blood clots in the deep veins of your legs
• Chest pain (angina pectoris)
• Known or suspected breast cancer or cancer of the lining of the uterus, cervix, or vagina
• Unexplained vaginal bleeding (until a diagnosis is reached by your doctor)
• Yellowing of the whites of the eyes or of the skin (jaundice) during pregnancy or during previous use of the pill
• Liver tumor (benign or cancerous)
• Known or suspected pregnancy
Tell your health care provider if you have ever had any of these conditions. Your health care provider can recommend a safer method of birth control.

OTHER CONSIDERATIONS BEFORE TAKING ORAL CONTRACEPTIVES
Tell your health care provider if you have:
• Breast nodules, fibrocystic disease of the breast, an abnormal breast x-ray or mammogram
• Diabetes
• Elevated cholesterol or triglycerides
• High blood pressure
• Migraine or other headaches or epilepsy
• Mental depression
• Gallbladder, heart, or kidney disease
• History of scanty or irregular menstrual periods
Women with any of these conditions should be checked often by their health care provider if they choose to use oral contraceptives.
Also, be sure to inform your doctor or health care provider if you smoke or are on any medications.

RISKS OF TAKING ORAL CONTRACEPTIVES
1. Risk of Developing Blood Clots
Blood clots and blockage of blood vessels are the most serious side effects of taking oral contraceptives; in particular, a clot in the leg can cause thrombophlebitis, and a clot that travels to the lungs can cause a sudden blocking of the vessel carrying blood to the lungs. Rarely, clots occur in the blood vessels of the eye and may cause blindness, double vision, or impaired vision.
If you take oral contraceptives and need elective surgery, need to stay in bed for a prolonged illness, or have recently delivered a baby, you may be at risk of developing blood clots. You should consult your doctor about stopping oral contraceptives three to four weeks before surgery and not taking oral contraceptives for two weeks after surgery or during bed rest. You should also not take oral contraceptives soon after delivery of a baby. It is advisable to wait for at least four weeks after delivery if you are not breast feeding. If you are breast feeding, you should wait until you have weaned your child before using the pill. (See also the section on Breast Feeding in GENERAL PRECAUTIONS.)
2. Heart Attacks and Strokes
Oral contraceptives may increase the tendency to develop strokes (stoppage or rupture of blood vessels in the brain) and angina pectoris and heart attacks (blockage of blood vessels in the heart). Any of these conditions can cause death or disability.
Smoking greatly increases the possibility of suffering heart attacks and strokes. Furthermore, smoking and the use of oral contraceptives greatly increase the chances of developing and dying of heart disease.
3. Gallbladder Disease
Oral contraceptive users probably have a greater risk than nonusers of having gallbladder disease, although this risk may be related to pills containing high doses of estrogens.
4. Liver Tumors
In rare cases, oral contraceptives can cause benign but dangerous liver tumors. These benign liver tumors can rupture and cause fatal internal bleeding. In addition, a possible but not definite association has been found with the pill and liver cancers in two studies, in which a few women who developed these very rare cancers were found to have used oral contraceptives for long periods. However, liver cancers are extremely rare. The chance of developing liver cancer from using the pill is thus even rarer.

ANNUAL NUMBER OF BIRTH-RELATED OR METHOD-RELATED DEATHS ASSOCIATED WITH CONTROL OF FERTILITY PER 100,000 NONSTERILE WOMEN, BY FERTILITY CONTROL METHOD ACCORDING TO AGE

Method of control and outcome	15–19	20–24	25–29	30–34	35–39	40–44
No fertility control methods*	7.0	7.4	9.1	14.8	25.7	28.2
Oral contraceptives non-smoker**	0.3	0.5	0.9	1.9	13.8	31.6
Oral contraceptives smoker**	2.2	3.4	6.6	13.5	51.1	117.2
IUD**	0.8	0.8	1.0	1.0	1.4	1.4
Condom*	1.1	1.6	0.7	0.2	0.3	0.4
Diaphragm/spermicide*	1.9	1.2	1.2	1.3	2.2	2.8
Periodic abstinence*	2.5	1.6	1.6	1.7	2.9	3.6

*Deaths are birth related.
**Deaths are method related.

5. Cancer of the Reproductive Organs and Breasts
There is, at present, no confirmed evidence that oral contraceptive use increases the risk of developing cancer of the reproductive organs. Studies to date of women taking the pill have reported conflicting findings on whether pill use increases the risk of developing cancer of the breast or cervix. Most of the studies on breast cancer and pill use have found no overall increase in the risk of developing breast cancer, although some studies have reported an increased risk of developing breast cancer in certain groups of women. Women who use oral contraceptives and have a strong family history of breast cancer or who have breast nodules or abnormal mammograms should be closely followed by their doctors.
Some studies have found an increase in the incidence of cancer of the cervix in women who use oral contraceptives. However, this finding may be related to factors other than the use of oral contraceptives.

ESTIMATED RISK OF DEATH FROM A BIRTH CONTROL METHOD OR PREGNANCY
All methods of birth control and pregnancy are associated with a risk of developing certain diseases which may lead to disability or death. An estimate of the number of deaths associated with different methods of birth control and pregnancy has been calculated and is shown in the following table.
[See table above]
In the table, the risk of death from any birth control method is less than the risk of childbirth, except for oral contraceptive users over the age of 35 who smoke and pill users over the age of 40 even if they do not smoke. It can be seen in the table that for women aged 15 to 39, the risk of death was highest with pregnancy (7 to 26 deaths per 100,000 women, depending on age). Among pill users who do not smoke, the risk of death was always lower than that associated with pregnancy for any age group, although over the age of 40, the risk increases to 32 deaths per 100,000 women, compared to 28 associated with pregnancy at that age. However, for pill users who smoke and are over the age of 35, the estimated number of deaths exceeds those for other methods of birth control. If a woman is over the age of 40 and smokers, her estimated risk of death is four times higher (117/100,000 women) than the estimated risk associated with pregnancy (28/100,000 women) in that age group.
The suggestion that women over 40 who don't smoke should not take oral contraceptives is based on information from older higher dose pills and on less selective use of pills than is practiced today. An Advisory Committee of the FDA discussed this issue in 1989 and recommended that the benefits of oral contraceptive use by healthy, non-smoking women over 40 years of age may outweigh the possible risks. However, all women, especially older women, are cautioned to use the lowest dose pill that is effective.

WARNING SIGNALS
If any of these adverse effects occur while you are taking oral contraceptives, call your doctor immediately:
• Sharp chest pain, coughing of blood, or sudden shortness of breath (indicating a possible clot in the lung)
• Pain in the calf (indicating a possible clot in the leg)
• Crushing chest pain or heaviness in the chest (indicating a possible heart attack)
• Sudden severe headache or vomiting, dizziness or fainting, disturbances or vision or speech, weakness, or numbness in an arm or leg (indicating a possible stroke)
• Sudden partial or complete loss of vision (indicating a possible clot in the eye)
• Breast lumps (indicating possible breast cancer or fibrocystic disease of the breast; ask you doctor or health care provider to show you how to examine your breasts)
• Severe pain or tenderness in the stomach area (indicating a possible ruptured liver tumor)
• Difficulty in sleeping, weakness, lack of energy, fatigue, or change in mood (possibly indicating severe depression)
• Jaundice or a yellowing of the skin or eyeballs, accompanied frequently by fever, fatigue, loss of appetite, dark colored urine, or light colored bowel movements (indicating possible liver problems)

SIDE EFFECTS OF ORAL CONTRACEPTIVES
1. Vaginal Bleeding
Irregular vaginal bleeding or spotting may occur while you are taking the pills. Irregular bleeding may vary from slight staining between menstrual periods to breakthrough bleeding which is a flow much like a regular period. Irregular bleeding occurs most often during the first few months of oral contraceptive use, but may also occur after you have been taking the pill for some time. Such bleeding may be temporary and usually does not indicate serious problems. It is important to continue taking your pills on schedule. If the bleeding occurs in more than one cycle or lasts for more than a few days, talk to your doctor or health care provider.
2. Contact Lenses
If you wear contact lenses and notice a change in vision or an inability to wear your lenses, contact your doctor or health care provider.
3. Fluid Retention
Oral contraceptives may cause edema (fluid retention) with swelling of the finger or ankles and may raise your blood pressure. If you experience fluid retention, contact you doctor or health care provider.
4. Melasma
A spotty darkening of the skin is possible, particularly of the face.
5. Other Side Effects
Other side effects may include change in appetite, headache, nervousness, depression, dizziness, loss of scalp hair, rash, and vaginal infections.
If any of these side effects bother you, call your doctor or health care provider.
GENERAL PRECAUTIONS
1. Missed Periods and Use of Oral Contraceptives Before or During Early Pregnancy
There may be times when you may not menstruate regularly after you have completed taking a cycle of pills. If you have taken your pills regularly and miss one menstrual period, continue taking your pills for the next cycle but be sure to inform your health care provider before doing so. If you have not taken the pills daily as instructed and missed a menstrual period, or if you missed two consecutive menstrual periods, you may be pregnant. Check with your health care provider immediately to determine whether you are pregnant. Do not continue to take oral contraceptives until you are sure you are not pregnant, but continue to use another method of contraception.
There is no conclusive evidence that oral contraceptive use is associated with an increase in birth defects, when taken inadvertently during early pregnancy. Previously, a few studies had reported that oral contraceptives might be associated with birth defects, but these studies have not been confirmed. Nevertheless, oral contraceptives or any other drugs should not be used during pregnancy unless clearly necessary and prescribed by your doctor. You should check with your doctor about risks to your unborn child of any medication taken during pregnancy.
2. While Breast Feeding
If you are breast feeding, consult your doctor before starting oral contraceptives. Some of the drug will be passed on to the child in the milk. A few adverse effects on the child have been reported, including yellowing of the skin (jaundice) and breast enlargement. In addition, oral contraceptives may decrease the amount and quality of your milk. If possible, do not use oral contraceptives while breast feeding. You should use another method of contraception since breast feeding provides only partial protection from becoming pregnant, and this partial protection decreases significantly as you breast feed for longer periods of time. You should consider starting oral contraceptives only after you have weaned your child completely.
3. Laboratory Tests
If you are scheduled for any laboratory tests, tell your doctor you are taking birth control pills. Certain blood tests may be affected by birth control pills.

Continued on next page

This product information was prepared in June 1998. On these and other Parke-Davis Products, information may be obtained by addressing PARKE-DAVIS, Division of Warner-Lambert Company, Morris Plains, New Jersey 07950.

Estrostep—Cont.

4. Drug Interactions

Certain drugs may interact with birth control pills to make them less effective in preventing pregnancy or cause an increase in breakthrough bleeding. Such drugs include rifampin, drugs used for epilepsy such as barbiturates (for example, phenobarbital) and phenytoin (Dilantin® is one brand of this drug), phenylbutazone (Butazolidin® is one brand), and possibly certain antibiotics. You may need to use additional contraception when you take drugs which can make oral contraceptives less effective.

5. This product (like all contraceptives) is intended to prevent pregnancy. It does not protect against transmission of HIV (AIDS) and other sexually transmitted diseases such as chlamydia, genital herpes, genital warts, gonorrhea, hepatitis B, and syphilis.

INSTRUCTIONS TO PATIENT

TABLET DISPENSER

The ESTROSTEP® tablet dispenser has been designed to make oral contraceptive dosing as easy and as convenient as possible. The tablets are arranged in either three or four rows of seven tablets each, with the days of the week appearing above the first row of tablets.

If your TABLET DISPENSER contains:	You are taking:
21 white tablets	ESTROSTEP 21
21 white tablets and 7 brown tablets	ESTROSTEP Fe

Each *triangle* tablet contains 1 mg norethindrone acetate and 20 mcg ethinyl estradiol.

Each *square* tablet contains 1 mg norethindrone acetate and 30 mcg ethinyl estradiol.

Each *round tablet* contains 1 mg norethindrone acetate and 35 mcg ethinyl estradiol.

Each *brown* tablet contains 75 mg ferrous fumarate and is intended to help you remember to take the tablets correctly. These brown tablets are not intended to have any health benefit.

DIRECTIONS

To remove a tablet, press down on it with your thumb or finger. The tablet will drop through the back of the tablet dispenser. Do not press with your thumbnail, fingernail, or any other sharp object.

HOW TO TAKE THE PILL

IMPORTANT POINTS TO REMEMBER

BEFORE YOU START TAKING YOUR PILLS:

1. BE SURE TO READ THESE DIRECTIONS:
Before you start taking your pills.
Anytime you are not sure what to do.

2. THE RIGHT WAY TO TAKE THE PILL IS TO TAKE ONE PILL EVERY DAY AT THE SAME TIME. If you miss pills you could get pregnant. This includes starting the pack late. The more pills you miss, the more likely you are to get pregnant.

3. MANY WOMEN HAVE SPOTTING OR LIGHT BLEEDING OR MAY FEEL SICK TO THEIR STOMACH DURING THE FIRST 1–3 PACKS OF PILLS. If you do have spotting or light bleeding or feel sick to your stomach, do not stop taking the pill. The problem will usually go away. If it doesn't go away, check with your doctor or clinic.

4. MISSING PILLS CAN ALSO CAUSE SPOTTING OR LIGHT BLEEDING, even when you make up these missed pills. On the days you take 2 pills to make up for missed pills, you could also feel a little sick to your stomach.

5. IF YOU HAVE VOMITING OR DIARRHEA, for any reason, or IF YOU TAKE SOME MEDICINES, including some antibiotics, your birth control pills may not work as well. Use a back-up birth control method (such as condoms or foam) until you check with your doctor or clinic.

6. IF YOU HAVE TROUBLE REMEMBERING TO TAKE THE PILL, talk to your doctor or clinic about how to make pill-taking easier or about using another method of birth control.

7. IF YOU HAVE ANY QUESTIONS OR ARE UNSURE ABOUT THE INFORMATION IN THIS LEAFLET, call your doctor or clinic.

BEFORE YOU START TAKING YOUR PILLS

1. DECIDE WHAT TIME OF DAY YOU WANT TO TAKE YOUR PILL. It is important to take it at about the same time every day.

2. LOOK AT YOUR PILL PACK TO SEE IF IT HAS 21 OR 28 PILLS:

The 21-pill pack has 21 "active" white pills (with hormones) to take for 3 weeks, followed by 1 week without pills.

The 28-pill pack has 21 "active" white pills (with hormones) to take for 3 weeks, followed by 1 week of reminder brown pills (without hormones).

3. ALSO FIND:

1) where on the pack to start taking pills,

2) in what order to take the pills (follow the arrows), and

3) the week numbers as shown in the pictures below.

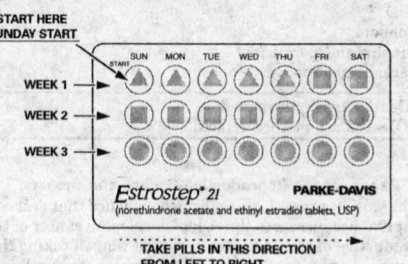

START HERE SUNDAY START

WEEK 1 / WEEK 2 / WEEK 3

Estrostep® 21   **PARKE-DAVIS**
(norethindrone acetate and ethinyl estradiol tablets, USP)

TAKE PILLS IN THIS DIRECTION FROM LEFT TO RIGHT

Each Estrostep® 21 tablet dispenser, contains five white triangular tablets, seven white square tablets, and nine white round tablets. These tablets are to be taken in the following order: one triangular tablet each day for five days, followed by one square tablet each day for seven days, and then one round tablet each day for nine days.

Estrostep 21 will contain: **ALL WHITE PILLS**

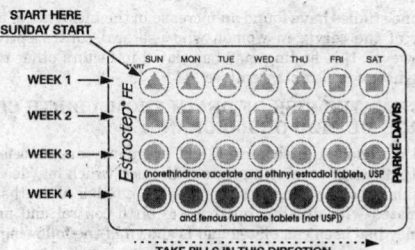

START HERE SUNDAY START

WEEK 1 / WEEK 2 / WEEK 3 / WEEK 4

Estrostep FE
(norethindrone acetate and ethinyl estradiol tablets, USP)
and ferrous fumarate tablets (not USP)
PARKE-DAVIS

TAKE PILLS IN THIS DIRECTION FROM LEFT TO RIGHT

Each Estrostep Fe tablet dispenser contains five white triangular tablets, seven white square tablets, nine white round tablets, and seven brown tablets. These tablets are to be taken in the following order: one triangular tablet each day for five days, then one square tablet each day for seven days, followed by one round tablet each day for nine days, and then one brown tablet each day for seven days.

Estrostep Fe will contain: **21 WHITE PILLS** for **WEEKS 1, 2, and 3. WEEK 4** will contain **BROWN PILLS ONLY.**

4. BE SURE YOU HAVE READY AT ALL TIMES:

ANOTHER KIND OF BIRTH CONTROL (such as condoms or foam) to use as a back-up in case you miss pills.

An EXTRA, FULL PILL PACK.

WHEN TO START THE FIRST PACK OF PILLS

SUNDAY START:

1. Take the first "active" white pill of the first pack on the Sunday after your period starts, even if you are still bleeding. If your period begins on Sunday, start the pack that same day.

2. Use another method of birth control as a back-up method if you have sex anytime from the Sunday you start your first pack until the next Sunday (7 days). Condoms or foam are good back-up methods of birth control.

WHAT TO DO DURING THE MONTH

1. TAKE ONE PILL AT THE SAME TIME EVERY DAY UNTIL THE PACK IS EMPTY.

Do not skip pills even if you are spotting or bleeding between monthly periods or feel sick to your stomach (nausea).

Do not skip pills even if you do not have sex very often.

2. WHEN YOU FINISH A PACK OR SWITCH YOUR BRAND OF PILLS:

21 PILLS: Wait 7 days to start the next pack. You will probably have your period during that week. Be sure that no more than 7 days pass between 21-day packs.

28 pills: Start the next pack on the day after your last "reminder" pill. Do not wait any days between packs.

WHAT TO DO IF YOU MISS PILLS

If you **MISS 1** white "active" pill:

1. Take it as soon as you remember. Take the next pill at your regular time. This means you may take 2 pills in 1 day.

2. You do not need to use a back-up birth control method if you have sex.

If you **MISS 2** white "active" pills in a row in **WEEK 1 OR WEEK 2** of your pack:

1. Take 2 pills on the day you remember and 2 pills the next day.

2. Then take 1 pill a day until you finish the pack.

3. You COULD GET PREGNANT if you have sex in the 7 days after you miss pills. You MUST use another birth control method (such as condoms or foam) as a back-up method of birth control until you have taken a white "active" pill every day for 7 days.

If you **MISS 2** white "active" pills in a row in **THE 3rd WEEK:**

1. Keep taking one pill every day until Sunday. On Sunday, THROW OUT the rest of the pack and start a new pack of pills that same day.

2. You may not have your period this month, but this is expected. However, if you miss your period 2 months in a row, call your doctor or clinic because you might be pregnant.

3. You COULD GET PREGNANT if you have sex in the 7 days after you miss pills You MUST use another birth control method (such as condoms or foam) as a back-up method of birth control until you have taken a white "active" pill every day for 7 days.

If you **MISS 3 OR MORE** white "active" pills in a row (during the first 3 weeks).

1. Keep taking 1 pill every day until Sunday. On Sunday, THROW OUT the rest of the pack and start a new pack of pills that same day.

2. You may not have your period this month, but this is expected. However, if you miss your period 2 months in a row, call your doctor or clinic because you might be pregnant.

3. You COULD GET PREGNANT if you have sex in the 7 days after you miss pills. You MUST use another birth control method (such as condoms or foam) as a back-up method of birth control until you have taken a white "active" pill every day for 7 days.

A REMINDER FOR THOSE ON 28-DAY PACKS:

IF YOU FORGET ANY OF THE 7 BROWN "REMINDER" PILLS IN WEEK 4:

THROW AWAY THE PILLS YOU MISSED.

KEEP TAKING 1 PILL EACH DAY UNTIL THE PACK IS EMPTY.

YOU DO NOT NEED A BACK-UP METHOD.

FINALLY, IF YOU ARE STILL NOT SURE WHAT TO DO ABOUT THE PILLS YOU HAVE MISSED:

Use a BACK-UP METHOD anytime you have sex.

KEEP TAKING ONE WHITE "ACTIVE" PILL EACH DAY until you can reach your doctor or clinic.

PREGNANCY DUE TO PILL FAILURE

The incidence of pill failure resulting in pregnancy is approximately 1% (i.e., one pregnancy per 100 women per year) if taken every day as directed, but more typical failure rates are about 3%. If failure does occur, the risk to the fetus is minimal.

PREGNANCY AFTER STOPPING THE PILL

There may be some delay in becoming pregnant after you stop using oral contraceptives, especially if you had irregular menstrual cycles before you used oral contraceptives. It may be advisable to postpone conception until you begin menstruating regularly once you have stopped taking the pill and desire pregnancy.

There does not appear to be any increase in birth defects in newborn babies when pregnancy occurs soon after stopping the pill.

OVERDOSAGE

Serious ill effects have not been reported following ingestion of large doses of oral contraceptives by young children. Overdosage may cause nausea and withdrawal bleeding in females. In case of overdosage, contact your health care provider or pharmacist.

OTHER INFORMATION

Your health care provider will take a medical and family history and examine you before prescribing oral contraceptives. The physical examination may be delayed to another time if you request it and your health care provider believes that it is a good medical practice to postpone it. You should be reexamined at least once a year. Be sure to inform your health care provider if there is a family history of any of the conditions listed previously in this leaflet. Be sure to keep all appointments with your health care provider, because this is a time to determine if there are early signs of side effects of oral contraceptive use.

Do not use the drug for any condition other than the one for which it was prescribed. This drug has been prescribed specifically for you; do not give it to others who may want birth control pills.

HEALTH BENEFITS FROM ORAL CONTRACEPTIVES

In addition to preventing pregnancy, use of oral contraceptives may provide certain benefits. They are:

• Menstrual cycles may become more regular.

• Blood flow during menstruation may be lighter and less iron may be lost. Therefore, anemia due to iron deficiency is less likely to occur.

• Pain or other symptoms during menstruation may be encountered less frequently.

• Ectopic (tubal) pregnancy may occur less frequently.

- Noncancerous cysts or lumps in the breast may occur less frequently.
- Acute pelvic inflammatory disease may occur less frequently.
- Oral contraceptive use may provide some protection against developing two forms of cancer; cancer of the ovaries and cancer of the lining of the uterus.

If you want more information about birth control pills, ask your doctor or pharmacist. They have a more technical leaflet called the "Physician Insert," which you may wish to read.

Remembering to take tablets according to schedule is stressed because of its importance in providing you the greatest degree of protection.

MISSED MENSTRUAL PERIODS FOR BOTH DOSAGE REGIMENS

At times there may be no menstrual period after a cycle of pills. Therefore, if you miss one menstrual period but have taken the pills *exactly as you were supposed to*, continue as usual into the next cycle. If you have not taken the pills correctly and miss a menstrual period, *you may be pregnant* and should stop taking oral contraceptives until your doctor or health care provider determines whether or not you are pregnant. Until you can get to your doctor, use another form of contraception. If two consecutive menstrual periods are missed, you should stop taking pills until it is determined whether or not you are pregnant. Although there does not appear to be any increase in birth defects in newborn babies, if you become pregnant while using oral contraceptives, you should discuss the situation with your doctor or health care provider.

Periodic Examination

Your doctor or health care provider will take a complete medical and family history before prescribing oral contraceptives. At that time and about once a year thereafter, he or she will generally examine your blood pressure, breasts, abdomen, and pelvic organs generally (including a Papanicolaou smear, i.e., test for cancer).

Keep this and all drugs out of the reach of children.

Caution—Federal law prohibits dispensing without prescription.

Storage: Do not store above 25°C (77°F).

Protect from light.

Store tablets inside pouch when not in use.

Revised June 1997

PARKE-DAVIS

Div of Warner-Lambert Co ©1996

Morris Plains, NJ 07950 USA

Direct Medical Inquiries to:

Parke-Davis

Warner-Lambert Company

201 Tabor Road, Morris Plains, NJ 07950

Attn: Medical Affairs Department   0928G251

Shown in Product Identification Guide, page 329

FEMPATCH®   ℞

[fěm 'păch]

(Estradiol Transdermal System)

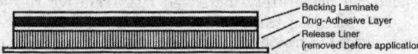

1. ESTROGENS HAVE BEEN REPORTED TO INCREASE THE RISK OF ENDOMETRIAL CARCINOMA IN POST-MENOPAUSAL WOMEN

Close clinical surveillance of all women taking estrogens is important. Adequate diagnostic measures, including endometrial sampling when indicated, should be undertaken to rule out malignancy in all cases of undiagnosed persistent or recurring abnormal vaginal bleeding. There is currently no evidence that "natural" estrogens are more or less hazardous than "synthetic" estrogens at equiestrogenic doses.

2. ESTROGENS SHOULD NOT BE USED DURING PREGNANCY

There is no indication for estrogen therapy during pregnancy or during the immediate postpartum period. Estrogens are ineffective for the prevention or treatment of threatened or habitual abortion. Estrogens are not indicated for the prevention of postpartum breast engorgement.

Estrogen therapy during pregnancy is associated with an increased risk of congenital defects in the reproductive organs of the fetus, and possibly other birth defects. Studies of women who received diethylstilbestrol (DES) during pregnancy have shown that female offspring have an increased risk of vaginal adenosis, squamous cell dysplasia of the uterine cervix, and clear cell vaginal cancer later in life; male offspring have an increased risk of urogenital abnormalities and possibly testicular cancer later in life. The 1985 DES Task Force concluded that use of DES during pregnancy is associated with a subsequent increased risk of breast cancer in the mothers, although a causal relationship remains unproven, and the ob-

served level of excess risk is similar to that for a number of other breast cancer risk factors.

DESCRIPTION

FemPatch® (estradiol transdermal system) is designed to release 17β-estradiol continuously during application to skin. The system delivers a nominal dose of 0.025 mg estradiol per day when applied to intact skin for a 7-day period. FemPatch is a translucent, thin, film laminate system comprising 2 layers (see below) and a release liner attached to the adhesive surface. The release liner must be removed before the system can be used.

[diagram: FemPatch cross-section]
Backing Laminate
Drug-Adhesive Layer
Release Liner
(removed before application)

The backing laminate is an elastic film with an adhesive formulation of polybutene, polyisobutylenes, and propylene glycol monolaurate between 2 layers of polyurethane film. The drug-adhesive layer consists of estradiol, USP and propylene glycol monolaurate in silicone adhesive. The release liner is a fluorocoated polyester. Estradiol is the active component of the system. All other components are pharmacologically inactive. The system contains 10.3 mg of estradiol, USP (17β-estradiol), a white, crystalline powder, chemically described as estra-1,3,5 (10)-triene-3, 17β-diol, and has a contact surface area of 30 cm^2.

Estradiol has an empirical formula of $C_{18}H_{24}O_2$ and molecular weight of 272.4.

The structural formula is:

[chemical structure of estradiol]

CLINICAL PHARMACOLOGY

Estrogen drug products act by regulating the transcription of a limited number of genes. Estrogens diffuse through cell membranes, distribute themselves throughout the cell, and bind to and activate the nuclear estrogen receptor, a DNA-binding protein which is found in estrogen-responsive tissues. The activated estrogen receptor binds to specific DNA sequences, or hormone-response elements, which enhance the transcription of adjacent genes and in turn lead to the observed effects. Estrogen receptors have been identified in tissues of the reproductive tract, breast, pituitary, hypothalamus, liver, and bone of women.

Estrogens are important in the development and maintenance of the female reproductive system and secondary sex characteristics. By a direct action, they cause growth and development of the uterus, fallopian tubes, and vagina. With other hormones, such as pituitary hormones and progesterone, they cause enlargement of the breasts through promotion of ductal growth, stromal development, and the accretion of fat. Estrogens are intricately involved with other hormones, especially progesterone, in the processes of the ovulatory menstrual cycle and pregnancy, and affect the release of pituitary gonadotropins. They also contribute to the shaping of the skeleton, maintenance of tone and elasticity of urogenital structures, changes in the epiphyses of the long bones that allow for the pubertal growth spurt and its termination, and pigmentation of the nipples and genitals.

Estrogens occur naturally in several forms. The primary source of estrogen in normally cycling adult women is the ovarian follicle, which secretes 70 to 500 μg of estradiol daily, depending on the phase of the menstrual cycle. This is converted primarily to estrone, which circulates in roughly equal proportion to estradiol, and to small amounts of estriol. After menopause, most endogenous estrogen is produced by conversion of androstenedione, secreted by the adrenal cortex, to estrone by peripheral tissues. Thus, estrone—especially in its sulfate ester form—is the most abundant circulating estrogen in postmenopausal women. Although circulating estrogens exist in a dynamic equilibrium of metabolic interconversions, estradiol is the principal intracellular human estrogen and is substantially more potent than estrone or estriol at the receptor.

Estrogens used in therapy are well absorbed through the skin, mucous membranes, and gastrointestinal tract. When applied for a local action, absorption is usually sufficient to cause systemic effects. When conjugated with aryl and alkyl groups for parenteral administration, the rate of absorption of oily preparations is slowed with a prolonged duration of action, such that a single intramuscular injection of estradiol valerate or estradiol cypionate is absorbed over several weeks.

Administered estrogens and their esters are handled within the body essentially the same as the endogenous hormones. Metabolic conversion of estrogens occurs primarily in the liver (first-pass effect), but also at local target tissue sites. Complex metabolic processes result in a dynamic equilib-

rium of circulating conjugated and unconjugated estrogenic forms which are continually interconverted, especially between estrone and estradiol and between esterified and nonesterified forms. Although naturally occurring estrogens circulate in the blood largely bound to sex hormone-binding globulin and albumin, only unbound estrogens enter target tissue cells. A significant proportion of the circulating estrogen exists as sulfate conjugates, especially estrone sulfate, which serves as a circulating reservoir for the formation of more active estrogenic species. A certain proportion of the estrogen is excreted into the bile and then reabsorbed from the intestine. During this enterohepatic recirculation, estrogens are desulfated and resulfated and undergo degradation through conversion to less active estrogens (estriol and other estrogens), oxidation to nonestrogenic substances (catecholestrogens, which interact with catecholamine metabolism, especially in the central nervous system), and conjugation with glucuronic acids (which are then rapidly excreted in the urine).

When given orally, naturally occurring estrogens and their esters are extensively metabolized (first-pass effect) and circulate primarily as estrone sulfate, with smaller amounts of other conjugated and unconjugated estrogenic species. This results in limited oral potency. By contrast, synthetic estrogens, such as ethinyl estradiol and the nonsteroidal estrogens, are degraded very slowly in the liver and other tissues, which results in their high intrinsic potency. Estrogen drug products administered by nonoral routes are not subject to first-pass metabolism, but also undergo significant hepatic uptake, metabolism, and enterohepatic recycling.

PHARMACOKINETICS

When FemPatch (estradiol transdermal system) was applied to the buttocks of 79 healthy postmenopausal women, serum estradiol concentrations increased steadily over the first 24 hours and then remained relatively constant for the remainder of the 7-day application period (Figure 1). Serum concentrations of approximately 22 pg/mL above baseline were achieved with a nominal estradiol delivery rate of 0.025 mg per day. When FemPatch was removed, serum estradiol concentrations declined to baseline within 24 hours (Figure 2).

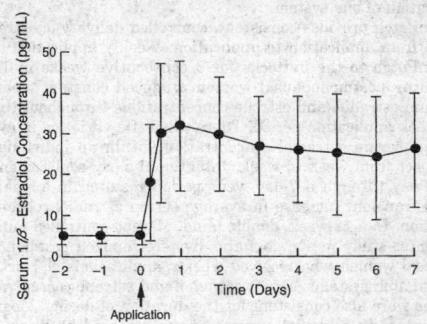

FIGURE 1. Serum Estradiol Concentrations Following Application of FemPatch to 79 Postmenopausal Healthy Volunteers in Three Pharmacokinetic Studies (average ± standard deviation)

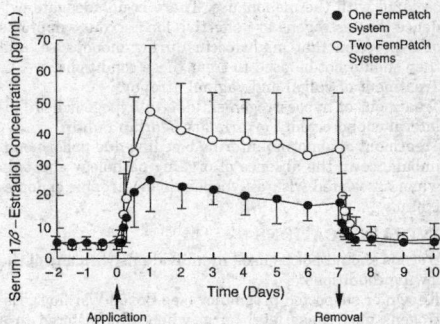

FIGURE 2. Serum Estradiol Concentrations Following Application of One and Two FemPatch Systems to 23 Postmenopausal Healthy Volunteers in a Single Pharmacokinetic Study (average ± standard deviation)

Continued on next page

This product information was prepared in June 1998. On these and other Parke-Davis Products, information may be obtained by addressing PARKE-DAVIS, Division of Warner-Lambert Company, Morris Plains, New Jersey 07950.

Fempatch—Cont.

The estradiol/estrone concentration ratio increased from an average baseline value of 0.3 to a value of 1.0 during application of FemPatch. This value is comparable to the ratio observed during the early follicular phase of the menstrual cycle in premenopausal women. A summary of estradiol pharmacokinetic parameters is presented in Table 1.

TABLE 1. Mean (SD) Estradiol and Estrone Pharmacokinetic Parameters for FemPatch Applied to the Buttocks

Estradiol Dose (mg/day)	Number of Women	Cmax (pg/mL)	Cmin (pg/mL)	Cavg (pg/mL)
ESTRADIOL				
Healthy Postmenopausal Women[a]				
0.025 (1 System)	79	39 (19)	20 (9)	27 (13)
Symptomatic, Hysterectomized Postmenopausal Women				
0.025 (1 System)	50	—	—	27 (13)
0.050 (2 Systems)	52	—	—	46 (21)
ESTRONE				
Healthy Postmenopausal Women[a]				
0.025 (1 System)	79	39 (12)	27 (7)	32 (9)
Symptomatic, Hysterectomized Postmenopausal Women				
0.025 (1 System)	50	—	—	39 (12)
0.050 (2 Systems)	52	—	—	48 (13)

Cmax = Maximum serum concentration.
Cavg = Average serum concentration.
Cmin = Minimum serum concentration.
[a] Week 1 of application

Dose proportionality was demonstrated for FemPatch in a study in 23 healthy postmenopausal women who received a 1-week application of 1 or 2 systems (Figure 2). The mean increase in serum estradiol concentrations over baseline during application of 2 systems was twice that during application of one system.

FemPatch provides consistent, controlled delivery of estradiol from application to application. Weekly application of FemPatch to the buttocks for 3 consecutive weeks in 18 healthy postmenopausal women produced constant mean serum estradiol and estrone concentrations throughout the 3-week application period. There was little variation in average serum estradiol concentration within an individual subject from week to week. Intentional early replacement midway through a 7-day wear period resulted in a small and transient increase in average serum estradiol concentration. In a 12-week, double-blind, placebo-controlled multicenter study in symptomatic, hysterectomized postmenopausal women who received weekly applications of 1 or 2 FemPatch systems, serum estradiol and estrone concentrations were also consistent for the duration of dosing. Mean increases in estradiol concentrations achieved by Week 1 were maintained over the remainder of the 12-week application period.

INDICATIONS AND USAGE

Estrogen drug products are indicated in the:
1. Treatment of moderate to severe vasomotor symptoms associated with the menopause. There is no adequate evidence that estrogens are effective for nervous symptoms or depression that might occur during menopause, and they should not be used to treat these conditions.
2. Treatment of vulval and vaginal atrophy.
3. Treatment of hypoestrogenism due to hypogonadism, bilateral oophorectomy, or primary ovarian failure.
4. Treatment of abnormal uterine bleeding due to hormonal imbalance in the absence of organic pathology and only when associated with a hypoplastic or atrophic endometrium.

CONTRAINDICATIONS

Estrogens should not be used in individuals with any of the following conditions:
1. Known or suspected pregnancy (see Boxed Warning). Estrogens may cause fetal harm when administered to a pregnant woman.
2. Undiagnosed abnormal genital bleeding.
3. Known or suspected cancer of the breast except in appropriately selected patients being treated for metastatic disease.
4. Known or suspected estrogen-dependent neoplasia.
5. Active thrombophlebitis or thromboembolic disorders.

WARNINGS

1. Induction of malignant neoplasms
Endometrial cancer: The reported endometrial cancer risk among unopposed estrogen users is about 2- to 12-fold greater than in nonusers, and appears dependent on duration of treatment and on estrogen dose. Most studies show no significant increased risk associated with use of

estrogens for less than 1 year. The greatest risk appears associated with prolonged use—with increased risks of 15- to 24-fold for 5 to 10 years or more. In 3 studies, persistence of risk was demonstrated for 8 to over 15 years after cessation of estrogen treatment. In 1 study, a significant decrease in the incidence of endometrial cancer occurred 6 months after estrogen withdrawal. Concurrent progestin therapy may offset this risk, but the overall health impact in postmenopausal women is not known (see PRECAUTIONS).

Breast cancer: While the majority of studies have not shown an increased risk of breast cancer in women who have ever used estrogen replacement therapy, some have reported a moderately increased risk (relative risks of 1.3–2.0) in those taking higher doses or those taking lower doses for prolonged periods of time, especially in excess of 10 years. Other studies have not shown this relationship.

Congenital lesions with malignant potential: Estrogen therapy during pregnancy is associated with an increased risk of fetal congenital reproductive tract disorders, and possibly other birth defects. Studies of women who received DES during pregnancy have shown that female offspring have an increased risk of vaginal adenosis, squamous cell dysplasia of the uterine cervix, and clear cell vaginal cancer later in life; male offspring have an increased risk of urogenital abnormalities and possibly testicular cancer later in life. Although some of these changes are benign, others are precursors of malignancy.

2. Gallbladder disease. Two studies have reported a 2- to 4-fold increase in the risk of gallbladder disease requiring surgery in women receiving postmenopausal estrogens.

3. Cardiovascular disease. Large doses of estrogen (5 mg conjugated estrogens per day), comparable to those used to treat cancer of the prostate and breast, have been shown in a large prospective clinical trial in men to increase the risks of nonfatal myocardial infarction, pulmonary embolism, and thrombophlebitis. These risks cannot necessarily be extrapolated from men to women. However, to avoid the theoretical cadiovascular risk to men or women caused by high estrogen doses, the dose for estrogen replacement therapy should not exceed the lowest effective dose.

4. Elevated blood pressure. Occasional blood pressure increases during estrogen replacement therapy have been attributed to idiosyncratic reactions to estrogens. More often, blood pressure has remained the same or has dropped. One study showed that postmenopausal estrogen users have higher blood pressure than nonusers. Two other studies showed slightly lower blood pressure among estrogen users compared to nonusers. Postmenopausal estrogen use does not increase the risk of stroke. Nonetheless, blood pressure should be monitored at regular intervals with estrogen use. Oral estrogens have been shown to increase renin substrate while transdermally administered estradiol has not been shown to affect renin substrate.

5. Hypercalcemia. Administration of estrogens may lead to severe hypercalcemia in patients with breast cancer and bone metastases. If this occurs, the drug should be stopped and appropriate measures taken to reduce the serum calcium level.

PRECAUTIONS
A. General
1. Addition of a progestin. Studies of the addition of a progestin for 10 or more days of a cycle of estrogen administration have reported a lowered incidence of endometrial hyperplasia than would be induced by estrogen treatment alone. Morphological and biochemical studies of endometria suggest that 10 to 14 days of progestin are needed to provide maximal maturation of the endometrium and to reduce the likelihood of hyperplastic changes. There are, however, possible risks which may be associated with the use of progestins in estrogen replacement regimens. These include:
a. Adverse effects on lipoprotein metabolism (lowering HDL and raising LDL) which could diminish the purported cardioprotective effect of estrogen therapy (see PRECAUTIONS below).
b. Impairment of glucose tolerance
c. Possible enhancement of mitotic activity in breast epithelial tissue, although few epidemiological data are available to address this point (see PRECAUTIONS below).
The choice of progestin, its dose, and its regimen may be important in minimizing these adverse effects, but these issues will require further study before they are clarified.

2. Cardiovascular risk. A causal relationship between estrogen replacement therapy and reduction of cardiovascular disease in postmenopausal women has not been proven. Furthermore, the effect of added progestins on this putative benefit is not yet known. In recent years, many published studies have suggested that there may be a cause-effect relationship

between postmenopausal oral estrogen replacement therapy **without added progestins** and a decrease in cardiovascular disease in women. Although most of the observational studies which assessed this statistical association have reported a 20% to 50% reduction in coronary heart disease risk and associated mortality in estrogen takers, the following should be considered when interpreting these reports:
a. Because only one of these studies was randomized and it was too small to yield statistically significant results, all relevant studies were subject to selection bias. Thus, the apparently reduced risk of coronary artery disease cannot be attributed with certainty to estrogen replacement therapy. It may instead have been caused by lifestyle and medical characteristics of the women studied with the result that healthier women were selected for estrogen therapy. In general, treated women were of higher socioeconomic and educational status, more slender, more physically active, more likely to have undergone surgical menopause, and less likely to have diabetes than the untreated women. Although some studies attempted to control for these selection factors, it is common for properly designed randomized trials to fail to confirm benefits suggested by less rigorous study designs. Thus, ongoing and future large-scale randomized trials may fail to confirm this apparent benefit.
b. Current medical practice often includes the use of concomitant progestin therapy in women with intact uteri (see PRECAUTIONS and WARNINGS). While the effects of added progestins on the risk of ischemic heart disease are not known, all available progestins reverse at least some of the favorable effects of estrogens on HDL and LDL levels.
c. While the effects of added progestins on the risk of breast cancer are also unknown, available epidemiological evidence suggests that progestins do not reduce, and may enhance, the moderately increased breast cancer incidence that has been reported with prolonged estrogen replacement therapy (see WARNINGS above).
Because relatively long-term use of estrogens by a woman with a uterus has been shown to induce endometrial cancer, physicians often recommend that women who are deemed candidates for hormone replacement should take progestins as well as estrogens. When considering prescribing concomitant estrogens and progestins for hormone replacement therapy, physicians and patients are advised to carefully weigh the potential benefits and risks of the added progestin. Large-scale randomized, placebo-controlled, prospective clinical trials are required to clarify these issues.

3. Physical examination. A complete medical and family history should be taken prior to the initiation of any estrogen therapy. Pretreatment and periodic physical examinations should include special reference to blood pressure, breasts, abdomen, and pelvic organs, and should include a Papanicolaou smear. As a general rule, estrogen should not be prescribed for longer than 1 year without reexamining the patient.

4. Hypercoagulability. Some studies have shown that women taking estrogen replacement therapy have hypercoagulability, primarily related to decreased antithrombin activity. This effect appears dose- and duration-dependent and is less pronounced than that associated with oral contraceptive use. Also, postmenopausal women tend to have increased coagulation parameters at baseline compared to premenopausal women. There is some suggestion that low-dose postmenopausal mestranol may increase the risk of thromboembolism, although the majority of studies (of primarily conjugated estrogen users) report no such increase. There is insufficient information on hypercoagulability in women who have had previous thromboembolic disease.

5. Familial hyperlipoproteinemia. Estrogen therapy may be associated with massive elevations of plasma triglycerides leading to pancreatitis and other complications in patients with familial defects of lipoprotein metabolism.

6. Fluid retention. Because estrogens may cause some degree of fluid retention, conditions which might be exacerbated by this factor, such as asthma, epilepsy, migraine, and cardiac or renal dysfunction, require careful observation.

7. Uterine bleeding and mastodynia. Certain patients may develop undesirable manifestations of estrogenic stimulation, such as abnormal uterine bleeding and mastodynia.

8. Impaired liver function. Estrogens may be poorly metabolized in patients with impaired liver function and should be administered with caution.

B. Information for Patients
See text of Patient Package insert after the HOW SUPPLIED section.

C. Laboratory Tests
Estrogen administration should generally be guided by clinical response at the smallest dose, rather than laboratory monitoring, for relief of symptoms for those indications in which symptoms are observable.

D. Drug/Laboratory Tests Interactions

1. Accelerated prothrombin time, partial thromboplastin time, and platelet aggregation time; increased platelet count; increased factors II, VII antigen, VIII antigen, VIII coagulant activity, IX, X, XII, VII-X complex, II-VII-X complex, and β-thromboglobulin; decreased levels of antifactor Xa and antithrombin III, decreased antithrombin III activity; increased levels of fibrinogen and fibrinogen activity; increased plasminogen antigen and activity.
2. Increased thyroid-binding globulin (TBG) leading to increased circulating total thyroid hormone, as measured by protein-bound iodine (PBI), T4 levels (by column or by radioimmunoassay), or T3 levels by radioimmunoassay. T3 resin uptake is decreased, reflecting the elevated TBG. Free T4 and free T3 concentrations are unaltered.
3. Other binding proteins may be elevated in serum, ie, corticosteroid binding globulin (CBG), sex-hormone binding globulin (SHBG), leading to increased circulating corticosteroids and sex steroids, respectively. Free or biologically active hormone concentrations are unchanged. Other plasma proteins may be increased (angiotensinogen/renin substrate, α-1-antitrypsin, ceruloplasmin).
4. Increased plasma HDL and HDL-2 subfraction concentrations, reduced LDL cholesterol concentration levels, increased triglyceride levels.
5. Impaired glucose tolerance.
6. Reduced response to metyrapone test.
7. Reduced serum folate concentration.

E. Carcinogenesis, Mutagenesis, Impairment of Fertility
Long-term continuous administration of natural and synthetic estrogens in certain animal species increases the frequency of carcinomas of the breast, uterus, cervix, vagina, testis, and liver. See CONTRAINDICATIONS and WARNINGS.

F. Pregnancy—Category X
Estrogens should not be used during pregnancy. See CONTRAINDICATIONS and Boxed Warnings.

G. Nursing Mothers
As a general principle, the administration of any drug to nursing mothers should be done only when clearly necessary since many drugs are excreted in human milk. In addition, estrogen administration to nursing mothers has been shown to decrease the quantity and quality of the milk.

H. Pediatric Use
Safety and effectiveness in pediatric patients have not been established.

ADVERSE REACTIONS

Incidence in Controlled Studies. Studies of the safety of FemPatch (estradiol transdermal system) have been conducted in 324 postmenopausal women. Nine (2.8%) patients discontinued treatment because of a skin effect, 7 (2.2%) were patients treated with placebo systems, and 2 (0.6%) were treated with FemPatch. A total of 5 (2.8%) patients treated with FemPatch withdrew from the controlled studies due to an adverse event (bloating, swelling, dizziness, depression, breast pain). An additional 4 (2.8%) patients treated with placebo systems withdrew from the studies because of an adverse event (vaginal bleeding, headache, arthralgia, and encephalitis).

The following additional adverse reactions have been reported with estrogen therapy (see WARNINGS regarding induction of neoplasia, adverse effects on the fetus, increased incidence of gallbladder disease, cardiovascular disease, elevated blood pressure, and hypercalcemia).

Genitourinary System. Changes in vaginal bleeding pattern and abnormal withdrawal bleeding or flow; breakthrough bleeding, spotting; increase in size of uterine leiomyomata; vaginal candidiasis; change in amount of cervical secretion.

Breasts. Tenderness, enlargement.

Gastrointestinal. Nausea, vomiting; abdominal cramps, bloating; cholestatic jaundice; increased incidence of gallbladder disease.

Skin. Chloasma or melasma that may persist when drug is discontinued; erythema multiforme; erythema nodosum; hemorrhagic eruption; loss of scalp hair; hirsutism.

Eyes. Steepening of corneal curvature; intolerance to contact lenses.

Central Nervous System. Headache, migraine, dizziness; mental depression; chorea.

Miscellaneous. Increase or decrease in weight; reduced carbohydrate tolerance; aggravation of porphyria; edema; changes in libido.

OVERDOSAGE

Serious ill effects have not been reported following acute ingestion of large doses of estrogen-containing oral contraceptives by young children. Overdosage of estrogen may cause nausea and vomiting, and withdrawal bleeding may occur in females.

DOSAGE AND ADMINISTRATION

For treatment of moderate to severe vasomotor symptoms, vulval and vaginal atrophy associated with the menopause, the lowest dose that will control symptoms should be chosen, and medication should be discontinued as promptly as possible. Attempts to discontinue or taper medication should be made at 3- to 6-month intervals.

Treatment should be initiated with 1 FemPatch (estradiol transdermal system) system applied to the skin on the buttocks once weekly. If symptoms are not relieved after 4 to 6 weeks, 2 FemPatch systems may be applied weekly. **FemPatch was not studied in women with a uterus.** It is recommended that FemPatch therapy be given continuously to patients who do not have a uterus. FemPatch may be given on a continuous or cyclic schedule (eg, 21 days on drug followed by 7 days off) to patients who have a uterus.

Each FemPatch has 2 protective plastic liners: One side has a wavy perforation in the middle and 1 side does not. The protective liner without the wavy perforation should be peeled from the patch and discarded. The other protective plastic liner (with the wavy perforation) must be removed, one-half at a time, exposing the adhesive surface, before the system can be used. The adhesive side of the FemPatch system should be placed on a clean, dry area horizontally on the upper outer quadrant of the buttocks above the gluteal cleft and below the sacroiliac crest in order to expose the system to the least amount of stretching. The area should not be oily, damaged, or irritated, and the waistline should be avoided, because friction from clothing may cause detachment. FemPatch should not be applied to the breasts. The sites of application must be rotated (eg, from left to right buttock), with an interval of at least 1 week allowed between applications to a recently used site. The system should be pressed firmly in place, making sure there is good contact with the skin, especially around the edges. At the end of a 7-day period, the system should be removed, folded in half with the adhesive sides touching, and disposed of in a trash receptacle.

Should wrinkling or minor detachment of FemPatch occur, the patient should attempt to smooth or reattach the system using minor pressure. In the event that FemPatch becomes more than 50% detached, it should be removed and a new system should be applied to a different skin site on the buttocks.

- If a patient is following a cyclic treatment regimen, it is recommended that the replacement system be removed when the system it replaced was scheduled for removal.
- If the patient is following a continuous treatment regimen, the replacement system should be removed when the system it replaced was scheduled for removal or the replacement system may be left in place for the full 7 days.

HOW SUPPLIED

Each FemPatch, estradiol transdermal system, contains 10.3 mg of estradiol USP for delivery of 0.025 mg per day for a 7-day period.

Carton of 4 systems .... N 0071-3006-03.

Store at 15°C to 30°C (59°F to 86°F). Extremes of temperature and/or humidity should be avoided. Do not store unpouched.

Caution: Federal law prohibits dispensing without prescription.

WARNING: CFC-113 is used in the manufacturing process. It is a substance which harms public health and environment by destroying ozone in the upper atmosphere. The final product does not contain CFC-113.

U.S. Pat. Nos. 4,906,463; 5,006,342

Issued January 1997

Distributed by:
PARKE-DAVIS
Div of Warner-Lambert Co ©1997
Morris Plains, NJ 07950 USA 3006G013

LIPITOR® ℞
(Atorvastatin Calcium) Tablets

DESCRIPTION

Lipitor® (atorvastatin calcium) is a synthetic lipid-lowering agent. Atorvastatin is an inhibitor of 3-hydroxy-3-methylglutaryl-coenzyme A (HMG-CoA) reductase. This enzyme catalyzes the conversion of HMG-CoA to mevalonate, an early and rate-limiting step in cholesterol biosynthesis.

Atorvastatin calcium is [R-(R*,R*)]-2-(4-fluorophenyl)-β, δ-dihydroxy-5-(1-methylethyl)-3-phenyl-4-[(phenylamino)carbonyl]-1H-pyrrole-1-heptanoic acid, calcium salt (2:1) trihydrate. The empirical formula of atorvastatin calcium is $(C_{33}H_{34}FN_2O_5)_2Ca \bullet 3H_2O$ and its molecular weight is 1209.42. Its structural formula is:

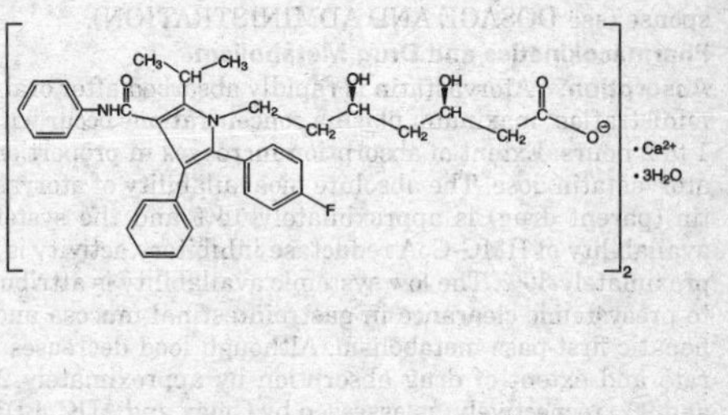

Atorvastatin calcium is a white to off-white crystalline powder that is insoluble in aqueous solution of pH 4 and below. Atorvastatin calcium is very slightly soluble in distilled water, pH 7.4 phosphate buffer, and acetonitrile, slightly soluble in ethanol, and freely soluble in methanol.

Lipitor tablets for oral administration contain 10, 20, or 40 mg atorvastatin and the following inactive ingredients: calcium carbonate, USP; candelilla wax, FCC; croscarmellose sodium, NF; hydroxypropyl cellulose, NF; lactose monohydrate, NF; magnesium stearate, NF; microcrystalline cellulose, NF; Opadry White YS-1-7040 (hydroxypropylmethylcellulose, polyethylene glycol, talc, titanium dioxide); polysorbate 80, NF; simethicone emulsion.

CLINICAL PHARMACOLOGY

Mechanism of Action

Atorvastatin is a selective, competitive inhibitor of HMG-CoA reductase, the rate-limiting enzyme that converts 3-hydroxy-3-methyl-glutaryl-coenzyme A to mevalonate, a precursor of sterols, including cholesterol. Cholesterol and triglycerides circulate in the bloodstream as part of lipoprotein complexes. With ultracentrifugation, these complexes separate into HDL (high-density lipoprotein), IDL (intermediate-density lipoprotein), LDL (low-density lipoprotein), and VLDL (very-low-density lipoprotein) fractions. Triglycerides (TG) and cholesterol in the liver are incorporated into VLDL and released into the plasma for delivery to peripheral tissues. LDL is formed from VLDL and is catabolized primarily through the high-affinity LDL receptor. Clinical and pathologic studies show that elevated plasma levels of total cholesterol (total-C), LDL-cholesterol (LDL-C), and apolipoprotein B (apo B) promote human atherosclerosis and are risk factors for developing cardiovascular disease, while increased levels of HDL-C are associated with a decreased cardiovascular risk.

In animal models, Lipitor lowers plasma cholesterol and lipoprotein levels by inhibiting HMG-CoA reductase and cholesterol synthesis in the liver and by increasing the number of hepatic LDL receptors on the cell-surface to enhance uptake and catabolism of LDL; Lipitor also reduces LDL production and the number of LDL particles. Lipitor reduces LDL-C in some patients with homozygous familial hypercholesterolemia (FH), a population that rarely responds to other lipid-lowering medication(s).

A variety of clinical studies have demonstrated that elevated levels of total-C, LDL-C, and apo B (a membrane complex for LDL-C) promote human atherosclerosis. Similarly, decreased levels of HDL-C (and its transport complex, apo A) are associated with the development of atherosclerosis. Epidemiologic investigations have established that cardiovascular morbidity and mortality vary directly with the level of total-C and LDL-C, and inversely with the level of HDL-C. Although frequently found in association with low HDL-C, elevated plasma TG has not been established as an independent risk factor for coronary heart disease. The independent effect of raising HDL-C or lowering TG on the risk for coronary and cardiovascular morbidity and mortality has not been established.

Lipitor reduces total-C, LDL-C, and apo B in patients with homozygous and heterozygous FH, nonfamilial forms of hypercholesterolemia, and mixed dyslipidemia. Lipitor also reduces VLDL-C and TG and produces variable increases in HDL-C and apolipoprotein A-1. The effect of Lipitor on cardiovascular morbidity and mortality has not been determined.

Pharmacodynamics

Atorvastatin as well as some of its metabolites are pharmacologically active in humans. The liver is the primary site of action and the principal site of cholesterol synthesis and

Continued on next page

This product information was prepared in June 1998. On these and other Parke-Davis Products, information may be obtained by addressing PARKE-DAVIS, Division of Warner-Lambert Company, Morris Plains, New Jersey 07950.

Lipitor—Cont.

LDL clearance. Drug dosage rather than systemic drug concentration correlates better with LDL-C reduction. Individualization of drug dosage should be based on therapeutic response (see DOSAGE AND ADMINISTRATION).

Pharmacokinetics and Drug Metabolism

Absorption: Atorvastatin is rapidly absorbed after oral administration; maximum plasma concentrations occur within 1 to 2 hours. Extent of absorption increases in proportion to atorvastatin dose. The absolute bioavailability of atorvastatin (parent drug) is approximately 14% and the systemic availability of HMG-CoA reductase inhibitory activity is approximately 30%. The low systemic availability is attributed to presystemic clearance in gastrointestinal mucosa and/or hepatic first-pass metabolism. Although food decreases the rate and extent of drug absorption by approximately 25% and 9%, respectively, as assessed by Cmax and AUC, LDL-C reduction is similar whether atorvastatin is given with or without food. Plasma atorvastatin concentrations are lower (approximately 30% for Cmax and AUC) following evening drug administration compared with morning. However, LDL-C reduction is the same regardless of the time of day of drug administration (see DOSAGE AND ADMINISTRATION).

Distribution: Mean volume of distribution of atorvastatin is approximately 381 liters. Atorvastatin is ≥98% bound to plasma proteins. A blood/plasma ratio of approximately 0.25 indicates poor drug penetration into red blood cells. Based on observation in rats, atorvastatin is likely to be secreted in human milk (see CONTRAINDICATIONS, Pregnancy and Lactation, and PRECAUTIONS, Nursing Mothers).

Metabolism: Atorvastatin is extensively metabolized to ortho- and parahydroxylated derivatives and various beta-oxidation products. *In vitro* inhibition of HMG-CoA reductase by ortho- and parahydroxylated metabolites is equivalent to that of atorvastatin. Approximately 70% of circulating inhibitory activity for HMG-CoA reductase is attributed to active metabolites. *In vitro* studies suggest the importance of atorvastatin metabolism by cytochrome P450 3A4, consistent with increased plasma concentrations of atorvastatin in humans following coadministration with erythromycin, a known inhibitor of this isozyme (see PRECAUTIONS, Drug Interactions). In animals, the ortho-hydroxy metabolite undergoes further glucuronidation.

Excretion: Atorvastatin and its metabolites are eliminated primarily in bile following hepatic and/or extrahepatic metabolism; however, the drug does not appear to undergo enterohepatic recirculation. Mean plasma elimination half-life of atorvastatin in humans is approximately 14 hours, but the half-life of inhibitory activity for HMG-CoA reductase is 20 to 30 hours due to the contribution of active metabolites. Less than 2% of a dose of atorvastatin is recovered in urine following oral administration.

Special Populations

Geriatric: Plasma concentrations of atorvastatin are higher (approximately 40% for Cmax and 30% for AUC) in healthy elderly subjects (age ≥65 years) than in young adults. LDL-C reduction is comparable to that seen in younger patient populations given equal doses of Lipitor.

Pediatric: Pharmacokinetic data in the pediatric population are not available.

Gender: Plasma concentrations of atorvastatin in women differ from those in men (approximately 20% higher for Cmax and 10% lower for AUC); however, there is no clinically significant difference in LDL-C reduction with Lipitor between men and women.

Renal Insufficiency: Renal disease has no influence on the plasma concentrations or LDL-C reduction of atorvastatin; thus, dose adjustment in patients with renal dysfunction is not necessary (see DOSAGE AND ADMINISTRATION).

Hemodialysis: While studies have not been conducted in patients with end-stage renal disease, hemodialysis is not expected to significantly enhance clearance of atorvastatin since the drug is extensively bound to plasma proteins.

Hepatic Insufficiency: In patients with chronic alcoholic liver disease, plasma concentrations of atorvastatin are markedly increased Cmax and AUC are each 4-fold greater in patients with Childs-Pugh A disease. Cmax and AUC are approximately 16-fold and 11-fold increased, respectively, in patients with Childs-Pugh B disease (see CONTRAINDICATIONS).

Clinical Studies

Hypercholesterolemia (Heterozygous Familial and Nonfamilial and Mixed Dyslipidemia (Fredrickson Types IIa and IIb)

Lipitor reduces total-C, LDL-C, VLDL-C, apo B, and TG, and increases HDL-C in patients with hypercholesterolemia and mixed dyslipidemia. Therapeutic response is seen within 2 weeks, and maximum response is usually achieved within 4 weeks and maintained during chronic therapy.

Lipitor is effective in a wide variety of patient populations with hypercholesterolemia, with and without hypertriglyc-

TABLE 1. Dose-Response in Patients With Primary Hypercholesterolemia (Adjusted Mean % Change From Baseline)[a]

Dose	N	TC	LDL-C	Apo B	TG	HDL-C	Non-HDL-C/ HDL-C
Placebo	21	4	4	3	10	−3	7
10	22	−29	−39	−32	−19	6	−34
20	20	−33	−43	−35	−26	9	−41
40	21	−37	−50	−42	−29	6	−45
80	23	−45	−60	−50	−37	5	−53

[a] Results are pooled from 2 dose-response studies

TABLE 2. Mean Percent Change From Baseline at End Point (Double-Blind, Randomized, Active-Controlled Trials)

Treatment (Daily Dose)	N	Total-C	LDL-C	Apo B	TG	HDL-C	Non-HDL-C/ HDL-C
Study 1							
Atorvastatin 10 mg	707	−27[a]	−36[a]	−28[a]	−17[a]	+7	−37[a]
Lovastatin 20 mg	191	−19	−27	−20	−6	+7	−28
95% CI for Diff[1]		−9.2, −6.5	−10.7, −7.1	−10.0, −6.5	−15.2, −7.1	−1.7, −2.0	−11.1, −7.1
Study 2							
Atorvastatin 10 mg	222	−25[b]	−35[b]	−27[b]	−17[b]	+6	−36[b]
Pravastatin 20 mg	77	−17	−23	−17	−9	+8	−28
95% CI for Diff[1]		−10.8, −6.1	−14.5, −8.2	−13.4, −7.4	−14.1, −0.7	−4.9, −1.6	−11.5, −4.1
Study 3							
Atorvastatin 10 mg	132	−29[c]	−37[c]	−34[c]	−23[c]	+7	−39[c]
Simvastatin 10 mg	45	−24	−30	−30	−15	+7	−33
95% CI for Diff[1]		−8.7, −2.7	−10.1, −2.6	−8.0, −1.1	−15.1, −0.7	−4.3, −3.9	−9.6, −1.9

[1] A negative value for the 95% CI for the difference between treatment favors atorvastatin for all except HDL-C, for which a positive value favors atorvastatin. If the range does not include 0, this indicates a statistically significant difference.
[a] Significantly different from lovastatin, ANCOVA, p ≤0.05
[b] Significantly different from pravastatin, ANCOVA, p ≤0.05
[c] Significantly different from simvastatin, ANCOVA, p ≤0.05

eridemia, in men and women, and in the elderly. Experience in pediatric patients has been limited to patients with homozygous FH.

In two multicenter, placebo-controlled, dose-response studies in patients with hypercholesterolemia, Lipitor given as a single dose over 6 weeks significantly reduced total-C, LDL-C, apo B, and TG (Pooled results are provided in Table 1).

[See table 1 above]

In three multicenter, double-blind studies in patients with hypercholesterolemia, Lipitor was compared to other HMG-CoA reductase inhibitors. After randomization, patients were treated for 16 weeks with either Lipitor 10 mg per day or a fixed dose of the comparative agent (Table 2).

[See table 2 above]

The impact on clinical outcomes of the differences in lipid-altering effects between treatments shown in Table 2 is not known. Table 2 does not contain data comparing the effects of atorvastatin 10 mg and higher doses of lovastatin, pravastatin, and simvastatin. The drugs compared in the studies summarized in the table are not necessarily interchangeable.

In a large clinical study, the number of patients meeting their National Cholesterol Education Program-Adult Treatment Panel (NCEP-ATP) II target LDL-C levels on 10 mg of Lipitor daily was assessed. After 16 weeks, 156/167 (93%) of patients with less than 2 risk factors for CHD and baseline LDL-C ≥ 190 mg/dL reached a target of ≤ 160 mg/dL; 141/218 (65%) of patients with 2 or more risk factors for CHD and LDL-C ≥ 160 mg/dL achieved a level of ≤130 mg/dL LDL-C, and 21/113 (19%) of patients with CHD and LDL-C ≥130 mg/dL reached a target level of ≤100 mg/dL LDL-C.

Homozygous Familial Hypercholesterolemia

In a study without a concurrent control group, 29 patients ages 6 to 37 years with homozygous FH received maximum daily doses of 20 to 80 mg of Lipitor. The mean LDL-C reduction in this study was 18%. Twenty-five patients with a reduction in LDL-C had a mean response of 20% (range of 7% to 53%, median of 24%); the remaining 4 patients had 7% to 24% increases in LDL-C. Five of the 29 patients had absent LDL-receptor function. Of these, 2 patients also had a portacaval shunt and had no significant reduction in LDL-C. The remaining 3 receptor-negative patients had a mean LDL-C reduction of 22%.

INDICATIONS AND USAGE

Lipitor is indicated as an adjunct to diet to reduce elevated total-C, LDL-C, apo B, and TG levels in patients with primary hypercholesterolemia (heterozygous familial and nonfamilial) and mixed dyslipidemia (*Fredrickson* Types IIa and IIb).

Lipitor is also indicated to reduce total-C and LDL-C in patients with homozygous familial hypercholesterolemia as an adjunct to other lipid-lowering treatments (eg, LDL apheresis) or if such treatments are unavailable.

Therapy with lipid-altering agents should be a component of multiple-risk-factor intervention in individuals at increased risk for atherosclerotic vascular disease due to hypercholesterolemia. Lipid-altering agents should be used in addition to a diet restricted in saturated fat and cholesterol only when the response to diet and other nonpharmacological measures has been inadequate (see *National Cholesterol Education Program (NCEP) Guidelines*, summarized in Table 3).

[See table 3 below]

TABLE 3. NCEP Guidelines for Lipid Management

Definite Atherosclerotic Disease[a]	Two or More Other Risk Factors[b]	LDL-Cholesterol mg/dL (mmol/L)	
		Initiation Level	Minimum Goal
No	No	≥190 (≥4.9)	<160 (<4.1)
No	Yes	≥160 (≥4.1)	<130 (<3.4)
Yes	Yes or No	≥130[c] (≥3.4)	≤100 (≤2.6)

[a] Coronary heart disease or peripheral vascular disease (including symptomatic carotid artery disease).
[b] Other risk factors for coronary heart disease (CHD) include: age (males: ≥45 years; females: ≥55 years or premature menopause without estrogen replacement therapy); family history of premature CHD; current cigarette smoking; hypertension; confirmed HDL-C <35 mg/dL (<0.91 mmol/L); and diabetes mellitus. Subtract 1 risk factor if HDL-C is ≥60 mg/dL (≥1.6 mmol/L).
[c] In CHD patients with LDL-C levels 100 to 129 mg/dL, the physician should exercise clinical judgment in deciding whether to initiate drug treatment.

At the time of hospitalization for an acute coronary event, consideration can be given to initiating drug therapy at discharge if the LDL-C level is ≥130 mg/dL (NCEP-ATP II). Prior to initiating therapy with Lipitor, secondary causes for hypercholesterolemia (eg, poorly controlled diabetes mellitus, hypothyroidism, nephrotic syndrome, dysproteinemias, obstructive liver disease, other drug therapy, and alcoholism) should be excluded, and a lipid profile performed to measure total-C, LDL-C, HDL-C, and TG. For patients with TG <400 mg/dL (<4.5 mmol/L), LDL-C can be estimated using the following equation: LDL-C = total-C − (0.20 × [TG] + HDL-C). For TG levels >400 mg/dL (>4.5 mmol/L), this equation is less accurate and LDL-C concentrations should be determined by ultracentrifugation.

CONTRAINDICATIONS

Active liver disease or unexplained persistent elevations of serum transaminases.
Hypersensitivity to any component of this medication.

Pregnancy and Lactation
Atherosclerosis is a chronic process and discontinuation of lipid-lowering drugs during pregnancy should have little impact on the outcome of long-term therapy of primary hypercholesterolemia. Cholesterol and other products of cholesterol biosynthesis are essential components for fetal development (including synthesis of steroids and cell membranes). Since HMG-CoA reductase inhibitors decrease cholesterol synthesis and possibly the synthesis of other biologically active substances derived from cholesterol, they may cause fetal harm when administered to pregnant women. Therefore, HMG-CoA reductase inhibitors are contraindicated during pregnancy and in nursing mothers. ATORVASTATIN SHOULD BE ADMINISTERED TO WOMEN OF CHILDBEARING AGE ONLY WHEN SUCH PATIENTS ARE HIGHLY UNLIKELY TO CONCEIVE AND HAVE BEEN INFORMED OF THE POTENTIAL HAZARDS. If the patient becomes pregnant while taking this drug, therapy should be discontinued and the patient apprised of the potential hazard to the fetus.

WARNINGS
Liver Dysfunction
HMG-CoA reductase inhibitors, like some other lipid-lowering therapies, have been associated with biochemical abnormalities of liver function. **Persistent elevations (>3 times the upper limit of normal [ULN] occurring on 2 or more occasions) in serum transaminases occurred in 0.7% of patients who received atorvastatin in clinical trials. The incidence of these abnormalities was 0.2%, 0.2%, 0.6%, and 2.3% for 10, 20, 40, and 80 mg, respectively.**
One patient in clinical trials developed jaundice. Increases in liver function tests (LFT) in other patients were not associated with jaundice or other clinical signs or symptoms. Upon dose reduction, drug interruption, or discontinuation, transaminase levels returned to or near pretreatment levels without sequelae. Eighteen of 30 patients with persistent LFT elevations continued treatment with a reduced dose of atorvastatin.
It is recommended that liver function tests be performed prior to and at 12 weeks following both the initiation of therapy and any elevation of dose, and periodically (e.g., semiannually) thereafter. Liver enzyme changes generally occur in the first 3 months of treatment with atorvastatin. Patients who develop increased transaminase levels should be monitored until the abnormalities resolve. Should an increase in ALT or AST of >3 times ULN persist, reduction of dose or withdrawal of atorvastatin is recommended.
Atorvastatin should be used with caution in patients who consume substantial quantities of alcohol and/or have a history of liver disease. Active liver disease or unexplained persistent transaminase elevations are contraindications to the use of atorvastatin (see CONTRAINDICATIONS).

Skeletal Muscle
Rhabdomyolysis with acute renal failure secondary to myoglobinuria has been reported with other drugs in this class.
Uncomplicated myalgia has been reported in atorvastatin-treated patients (see ADVERSE REACTIONS). Myopathy, defined as muscle aches or muscle weakness in conjunction with increases in creatine phosphokinase (CPK) values >10 times ULN, should be considered in any patient with diffuse myalgias, muscle tenderness or weakness, and/or marked elevation of CPK. Patients should be advised to report promptly unexplained muscle pain, tenderness or weakness, particularly if accompanied by malaise or fever. Atorvastatin therapy should be discontinued if markedly elevated CPK levels occur or myopathy is diagnosed or suspected.
The risk of myopathy during treatment with other drugs in this class is increased with concurrent administration of cyclosporine, fibric acid derivatives, erythromycin, niacin, or azole antifungals. Physicians considering combined therapy with atorvastatin and fibric acid derivatives, erythromycin, immunosuppressive drugs, azole antifungals, or lipid-lowering doses of niacin should carefully weigh the potential benefits and risks and should carefully monitor patients for any signs or symptoms of muscle pain, tenderness, or weakness,

particularly during the initial months of therapy and during any periods of upward dosage titration of either drug. Periodic creatine phosphokinase (CPK) determinations may be considered in such situations, but there is no assurance that such monitoring will prevent the occurrence of severe myopathy.
Atorvastatin therapy should be temporarily withheld or discontinued in any patient with an acute, serious condition suggestive of a myopathy or having a risk factor predisposing to the development of renal failure secondary to rhabdomyolysis (eg, severe acute infection, hypotension, major surgery, trauma, severe metabolic, endocrine and electrolyte disorders, and uncontrolled seizures).

PRECAUTIONS
General
Before instituting therapy with atorvastatin, an attempt should be made to control hypercholesterolemia with appropriate diet, exercise, and weight reduction in obese patients, and to treat other underlying medical problems (see INDICATIONS AND USAGE).

Information for Patients
Patients should be advised to report promptly unexplained muscle pain, tenderness, or weakness, particularly if accompanied by malaise or fever.

Drug Interactions
The risk of myopathy during treatment with other drugs of this class is increased with concurrent administration of cyclosporine, fibric acid derivatives, niacin (nicotinic acid), erythromycin, azole antifungals (see WARNINGS, Skeletal Muscle).
Antacid: When atorvastatin and Maalox® TC suspension were coadministered, plasma concentrations of atorvastatin decreased approximately 35%. However, LDL-C reduction was not altered.
Antipyrine: Because atorvastatin does not affect the pharmacokinetics of antipyrine, interactions with other drugs metabolized via the same cytochrome isozymes are not expected.
Colestipol: Plasma concentrations of atorvastatin decreased approximately 25% when colestipol and atorvastatin were coadministered. However, LDL-C reduction was greater when atorvastatin and colestipol were coadministered than when either drug was given alone.
Cimetidine: Atorvastatin plasma concentrations and LDL-C reduction were not altered by coadministration of cimetidine.
Digoxin: When multiple doses of atorvastatin and digoxin were coadministered, steady-state plasma digoxin concentrations increased by approximately 20%. Patients taking digoxin should be monitored appropriately.
Erythromycin: In healthy individuals, plasma concentrations of atorvastatin increased approximately 40% with coadministration of atorvastatin and erythromycin, a known inhibitor of cytochrome P450 3A4 (see WARNINGS, Skeletal Muscle).
Oral Contraceptives: Coadministration of atorvastatin and an oral contraceptive increased AUC values for norethindrone and ethinyl estradiol by approximately 30% and 20%. These increases should be considered when selecting an oral contraceptive for a woman taking atorvastatin.
Warfarin: Atorvastatin had no clinically significant effect on prothrombin time when administered to patients receiving chronic warfarin treatment.

Endocrine Function
HMG-CoA reductase inhibitors interfere with cholesterol synthesis and theoretically might blunt adrenal and/or gonadal steroid production. Clinical studies have shown that atorvastatin does not reduce basal plasma cortisol concentration or impair adrenal reserve. The effects of HMG-CoA reductase inhibitors on male fertility have not been studied in adequate numbers of patients. The effects, if any, on the pituitary-gonadal axis in premenopausal women are unknown. Caution should be exercised if an HMG-CoA reductase inhibitor is administered concomitantly with drugs that may decrease the levels or activity of endogenous steroid hormones, such as ketoconazole, spironolactone, and cimetidine.

CNS Toxicity
Brain hemorrhage was seen in a female dog treated for 3 months at 120 mg/kg/day. Brain hemorrhage and optic nerve vacuolation were seen in another female dog that was sacrificed in moribund condition after 11 weeks of escalating doses up to 280 mg/kg/day. The 120 mg/kg dose resulted in a systemic exposure approximately 16 times the human plasma area-under-the curve (AUC, 0–24 hours) based on the maximum human dose of 80 mg/day. A single tonic convulsion was seen in each of 2 male dogs (one treated at 10 mg/kg/day and one at 120 mg/kg/day) in a 2-year study. No CNS lesions have been observed in mice after chronic treatment for up to 2 years at doses up to 400 mg/kg/day or in rats at doses up to 100 mg/kg/day. These doses were 6 to 11 times (mouse) and 8 to 16 times (rat) the human AUC (0–24) based on the maximum recommended human dose of 80 mg/day.

CNS vascular lesions, characterized by perivascular hemorrhages, edema, and mononuclear cell infiltration of perivascular spaces, have been observed in dogs treated with other members of this class. A chemically similar drug in this class produced optic nerve degeneration (Wallerian degeneration of retinogeniculate fibers) in clinically normal dogs in a dose-dependent fashion at a dose that produced plasma drug levels about 30 times higher than the mean drug level in humans taking the highest recommended dose.
Carcinogenesis, Mutagenesis, Impairment of Fertility
In a 2-year carcinogenicity study in rats at dose levels of 10, 30, and 100 mg/kg/day, 2 rare tumors were found in muscle in high-dose females: in one, there was a rhabdomyosarcoma and, in another, there was a fibrosarcoma. This dose represents a plasma AUC (0–24) value of approximately 16 times the mean human plasma drug exposure after an 80 mg oral dose.
A 2-year carcinogenicity study in mice given 100, 200, or 400 mg/kg/day resulted in a significant increase in liver adenomas in high-dose males and liver carcinomas in high-dose females. These findings occurred at plasma AUC (0–24) values of approximately 6 times the mean human plasma drug exposure after an 80 mg oral dose.
In vitro, atorvastatin was not mutagenic or clastogenic in the following tests with and without metabolic activation: the Ames test with *Salmonella-typhimurium* and *Escherichia coli,* the HGPRT forward mutation assay in Chinese hamster lung cells, and the chromosomal aberration assay in Chinese hamster lung cells. Atorvastatin was negative in the *in vivo* mouse micronucleus test.
Studies in rats performed at doses up to 175 mg/kg (15 times the human exposure) produced no changes in fertility. There was aplasia and aspermia in the epididymis of 2 of 10 rats treated with 100 mg/kg/day of atorvastatin for 3 months (16 times the human AUC at the 80 mg dose); testis weights were significantly lower at 30 and 100 mg/kg and epididymal weight was lower at 100 mg/kg. Male rats given 100 mg/kg/day for 11 weeks prior to mating had decreased sperm motility, spermatid head concentration, and increased abnormal sperm. Atorvastatin caused no adverse effects on semen parameters, or reproductive organ histopathology in dogs given doses of 10, 40, or 120 mg/kg for two years.
Pregnancy
Pregnancy Category X
See CONTRAINDICATIONS
Safety in pregnant women has not been established. Atorvastatin crosses the rat placenta and reaches a level in fetal liver equivalent to that of maternal plasma. Atorvastatin was not teratogenic in rats at doses up to 300 mg/kg/day or in rabbits at doses up to 100 mg/kg/day. These doses resulted in multiples of about 30 times (rat) or 20 times (rabbit) the human exposure based on surface area (mg/m²).
In a study in rats given 20, 100, or 225 mg/kg/day, from gestation day 7 through to lactation day 21 (weaning), there was decreased pup survival at birth, neonate, weaning, and maturity in pups of mothers dosed with 225 mg/kg/day. Body weight was decreased on days 4 and 21 in pups of mothers dosed at 100 mg/kg/day; pup body weight was decreased at birth and at days 4, 21, and 91 at 225 mg/kg/day. Pup development was delayed (rotorod performance at 100 mg/kg/day and acoustic startle at 225 mg/kg/day; pinnae detachment and eye opening at 225 mg/kg/day). These doses correspond to 6 times (100 mg/kg) and 22 times (225 mg/kg) the human AUC at 80 mg/day.
Rare reports of congenital anomalies have been received following intrauterine exposure to HMG-CoA reductase inhibitors. There has been one report of severe congenital bony deformity, tracheo-esophageal fistula, and anal atresia (VATER association) in a baby born to a woman who took lovastatin with dextroamphetamine sulfate during the first trimester of pregnancy. Lipitor should be administered to women of child-bearing potential only when such patients are highly unlikely to conceive and have been informed of the potential hazards. If the woman becomes pregnant while taking Lipitor, it should be discontinued and the patient advised again as to the potential hazards to the fetus.
Nursing Mothers
Nursing rat pups had plasma and liver drug levels of 50% and 40%, respectively, of that in their mother's milk. Because of the potential for adverse reactions in nursing infants, women taking Lipitor should not breast-feed (see CONTRAINDICATIONS).
Pediatric Use
Treatment experience in a pediatric population is limited to doses of Lipitor up to 80 mg/day for 1 year in 8 patients with homozygous FH. No clinical or biochemical abnormalities were reported in these patients. None of these patients was below 9 years of age.

Continued on next page

This product information was prepared in June 1998. On these and other Parke-Davis Products, information may be obtained by addressing PARKE-DAVIS, Division of Warner-Lambert Company, Morris Plains, New Jersey 07950.

Consult 1999 PDR® supplements and future editions for revisions

Lipitor—Cont.

Geriatric Use

Treatment experience in adults age ≥70 years with doses of Lipitor up to 80 mg/day has been evaluated in 221 patients. The safety and efficacy of Lipitor in this population were similar to those of patients <70 years of age.

ADVERSE REACTIONS

Lipitor is generally well-tolerated. Adverse reactions have usually been mild and transient. In controlled clinical studies of 2502 patients, <2% of patients were discontinued due to adverse experiences attributable to atorvastatin. The most frequent adverse events thought to be related to atorvastatin were constipation, flatulence, dyspepsia, and abdominal pain.

Clinical Adverse Experiences

Adverse experiences reported in ≥2% of patients in placebo-controlled clinical studies of atorvastatin, regardless of causality assessment, are shown in Table 4.

[See table 4 below]

The following adverse events were reported, regardless of causality assessment in patients treated with atorvastatin in clinical trials. The events in italics occurred in ≥2% of patients and the events in plain type occurred in <2% of patients.

Body as a Whole: *Chest pain,* face edema, fever, neck rigidity, malaise, photosensitivity reaction, generalized edema.

Digestive System: *Nausea,* gastroenteritis, liver function tests abnormal, colitis, vomiting, gastritis, dry mouth, rectal hemorrhage, esophagitis, eructation, glossitis, mouth ulceration, anorexia, increased appetite, stomatitis, biliary pain, cheilitis, duodenal ulcer, dysphagia, enteritis, melena, gum hemorrhage, stomach ulcer, tenesmus, ulcerative stomatitis, hepatitis, pancreatitis, cholestatic jaundice.

Respiratory System: *Bronchitis, rhinitis,* pneumonia, dyspnea, asthma, epistaxis.

Nervous System: *Insomnia, dizziness,* paresthesia, somnolence, amnesia, abnormal dreams, libido decreased, emotional lability, incoordination, peripheral neuropathy, torticollis, facial paralysis, hyperkinesia, depression, hypesthesia, hypertonia.

Musculoskeletal System: *Arthritis,* leg cramps, bursitis, tenosynovitis, myasthenia, tendinous contracture, myositis.

Skin and Appendages: Pruritus, contact dermatitis, alopecia, dry skin, sweating, acne, urticaria, eczema, seborrhea, skin ulcer.

Urogenital System: *Urinary tract infection,* urinary frequency, cystitis, hematuria, impotence, dysuria, kidney calculus, nocturia, epididymitis, fibrocystic breast, vaginal hemorrhage, albuminuria, breast enlargement, metrorrhagia, nephritis, urinary incontinence, urinary retention, urinary urgency, abnormal ejaculation, uterine hemorrhage.

Special Senses: Amblyopia, tinnitus, dry eyes, refraction disorder, eye hemorrhage, deafness, glaucoma, parosmia, taste loss, taste perversion.

Cardiovascular System: Palpitation, vasodilatation, syncope, migraine, postural hypotension, phlebitis, arrhythmia, angina pectoris, hypertension.

Metabolic and Nutritional Disorders: *Peripheral edema,* hyperglycemia, creatine phosphokinase increased, gout, weight gain, hypoglycemia.

Hemic and Lymphatic System: Ecchymosis, anemia, lymphadenopathy, thrombocytopenia, petechia.

Postintroduction Reports

Adverse events associated with Lipitor that have been received since market introduction, that are not listed above, and that may have no causal relationship to drug include the following: anaphylaxis, angioneurotic edema and rhabdomyolysis.

OVERDOSAGE

There is no specific treatment for atorvastatin overdosage. In the event of an overdose, the patient should be treated symptomatically, and supportive measures as required. Due to extensive drug binding to plasma proteins, hemodialysis is not expected to significantly enhance atorvastatin clearance.

DOSAGE AND ADMINISTRATION

The patient should be placed on a standard cholesterol-lowering diet before receiving Lipitor and should continue on this diet during treatment with Lipitor.

Hypercholesterolemia (Heterozygous Familial and Nonfamilial) and Mixed Dyslipidemia (*Frederickson* Types IIa and IIb)

The recommended starting dose of Lipitor is 10 mg once daily. The dosage range is 10 to 80 mg once daily. Lipitor can be administered as a single dose at any time of the day, with or without food. Therapy should be individualized according to goal of therapy and response (see *NCEP Guidelines,* summarized in Table 3). After initiation and/or upon titration of Lipitor, lipid levels should be analyzed within 2 to 4 weeks and dosage adjusted accordingly.

Since the goal of treatment is to lower LDL-C, the NCEP recommends that LDL-C levels be used to initiate and assess treatment response. Only if LDL-C levels are not available, should total-C be used to monitor therapy.

Homozygous Familial Hypercholesterolemia

The dosage of Lipitor in patients with homozygous FH is 10 to 80 mg daily. Lipitor should be used as an adjunct to other lipid-lowering treatments (eg, LDL apheresis) in these patients or if such treatments are unavailable.

Concomitant Therapy

Atorvastatin may be used in combination with a bile acid binding resin for additive effect. The combination of HMG-CoA reductase inhibitors and fibrates should generally be avoided (see WARNINGS, Skeletal Muscle, and PRECAUTIONS, Drug Interactions for other drug-drug interactions).

Dosage in Patients With Renal Insufficiency

Renal disease does not affect the plasma concentrations nor LDL-C reduction of atorvastatin; thus, dosage adjustment in patients with renal dysfunction is not necessary (see CLINICAL PHARMACOLOGY, Pharmacokinetics).

HOW SUPPLIED

Lipitor is supplied as white, elliptical, film-coated tablets of atorvastatin calcium containing 10, 20, and 40 mg atorvastatin.

10 mg tablets: coded "PD 155" on one side and "10" on the other.

N0071-0155-23 bottles of 90
N0071-0155-34 bottles of 5000
N0071-0155-40 10 × 10 unit dose blisters

20 mg tablets: coded "PD 156" on one side and "20" on the other.

N0071-0156-23 bottles of 90
N0071-0156-40 10 × 10 unit dose blisters

40 mg tablets: coded "PD 157" on one side and "40" on the other.

N0071-0157-23 bottles of 90

Storage

Store at controlled room temperature 20°C to 25°C (68°F to 77°F) [see USP].

Rx only

Revised April 1998

Manufactured by:
Warner-Lambert Export, Ltd. © 1998
Dublin, Ireland

Distributed by:
PARKE-DAVIS
Div of Warner-Lambert Co
Morris Plains, NJ 07950 USA
MADE IN GERMANY

Marketed by:
PARKE-DAVIS
Div of Warner-Lambert Co and
PFIZER Inc.
New York, NY 10017

0155G026

Shown in Product Identification Guide, page 329

LOPID® ℞
[lō 'pĭd]
(Gemfibrozil Tablets, USP)

DESCRIPTION

Lopid® (gemfibrozil tablets, USP) is a lipid regulating agent. It is available as tablets for oral administration. Each tablet contains 600 mg gemfibrozil. Each also contains calcium stearate, NF; candelilla wax FCC; microcrystalline cellulose, NF; hydroxypropyl cellulose, NF: hydroxypropyl methylcellulose, USP; methylparaben, NF; Opaspray white; polyethylene glycol, NF; polysorbate 80, NF; propylparaben, NF; colloidal silicon dioxide, NF; pregelatinized starch, NF. The chemical name is 5-(2,5-dimethylphenoxy)-2,2-dimethylpentanoic acid.

The empirical formula is $C_{15}H_{22}O_3$ and the molecular weight is 250.35; the solubility in water and acid is 0.0019% and in dilute base it is greater than 1%. The melting point is 58°–61°C. Gemfibrozil is a white solid which is stable under ordinary conditions.

CLINICAL PHARMACOLOGY

Lopid (gemfibrozil tablets, USP) is a lipid regulating agent which decreases serum triglycerides and very low density lipoprotein (VLDL) cholesterol, and increases high density lipoprotein (HDL) cholesterol. While modest decreases in total and low density lipoprotein (LDL) cholesterol may be observed with Lopid therapy, treatment of patients with elevated triglycerides due to Type IV hyperlipoproteinemia often results in a rise in LDL-cholesterol. LDL-cholesterol levels in Type IIb patients with elevations of both serum LDL-cholesterol and triglycerides are, in general, minimally affected by Lopid treatment; however, Lopid usually raises HDL-cholesterol significantly in this group. Lopid increases levels of high density lipoprotein (HDL) subfractions HDL_2 and HDL_3, as well as apolipoproteins AI and AII. Epidemiological studies have shown that both low HDL-cholesterol and high LDL-cholesterol are independent risk factors for coronary heart disease.

In the primary prevention component of the Helsinki Heart Study (refs. 1,2), in which 4081 male patients between the ages of 40 and 55 were studied in a randomized, double-blind, placebo-controlled fashion, Lopid therapy was associated with significant reductions in total plasma triglycerides and a significant increase in high density lipoprotein cholesterol. Moderate reductions in total plasma cholesterol and low density lipoprotein cholesterol were observed for the Lopid treatment group as a whole, but the lipid response was heterogeneous, especially among different Frederickson types. The study involved subjects with serum non-HDL-cholesterol of over 200 mg/dL and no previous history of coronary heart disease. Over the 5-year study period, the Lopid group experienced a 1.4% absolute (34% relative) reduction in the rate of serious coronary events (sudden cardiac deaths plus fatal and nonfatal myocardial infarctions) compared to placebo, p = 0.04 (see Table I). There was a 37% relative reduction in the rate of nonfatal myocardial infarction compared to placebo, equivalent to a treatment-related difference of 13.1 events per thousand persons. Deaths from

---

TABLE 4. Adverse Events in Placebo-Controlled Studies (% of Patients)

BODY SYSTEM/ Adverse Event	Placebo N = 270	Atorvastatin 10 mg N = 863	Atorvastatin 20 mg N = 36	Atorvastatin 40 mg N = 79	Atorvastatin 80 mg N = 94
BODY AS A WHOLE					
Infection	10.0	10.3	2.8	10.1	7.4
Headache	7.0	5.4	16.7	2.5	6.4
Accidental Injury	3.7	4.2	0.0	1.3	3.2
Flu Syndrome	1.9	2.2	0.0	2.5	3.2
Abdominal Pain	0.7	2.8	0.0	3.8	2.1
Back Pain	3.0	2.8	0.0	3.8	1.1
Allergic Reaction	2.6	0.9	2.8	1.3	0.0
Asthenia	1.9	2.2	0.0	3.8	0.0
DIGESTIVE SYSTEM					
Constipation	1.8	2.1	0.0	2.5	1.1
Diarrhea	1.5	2.7	0.0	3.8	5.3
Dyspepsia	4.1	2.3	2.8	1.3	2.1
Flatulence	3.3	2.1	2.8	1.3	1.1
RESPIRATORY SYSTEM					
Sinusitis	2.6	2.8	0.0	2.5	6.4
Pharyngitis	1.5	2.5	0.0	1.3	2.1
SKIN AND APPENDAGES					
Rash	0.7	3.9	2.8	3.8	1.1
MUSCULOSKELETAL SYSTEM					
Arthralgia	1.5	2.0	0.0	5.1	0.0
Myalgia	1.1	3.2	5.6	1.3	0.0

Table I
Reduction in CHD Rates (events per 1000 patients) by Baseline Lipids[1] in the Helsinki Heart Study, Years 0–5[2]

	All Patients			LDL-C > 175; HDL-C > 46.4			LDL-C > 175; TG > 177			LDL-C > 175; TG > 200; HDL-C < 35		
	P	L	Dif[3]	P	L	Dif	P	L	Dif	P	L	Dif
Incidence of Evidents[4]	41	27	14	32	29	3	71	44	27	149	64	85

[1] lipid values in mg/dL at baseline
[2] P=placebo group; L=Lopid group
[3] difference in rates between placebo and Lopid groups
[4] fatal and nonfatal myocardial infarctions plus sudden cardiac deaths (events per 1000 patients over 5 years)

any cause during the double-blind portion of the study totaled 44 (2.2%) in the Lopid randomization group and 43 (2.1%) in the placebo group.
[See table I above]

Among Fredrickson types, during the 5-year double-blind portion of the primary prevention component of the Helsinki Heart Study, the greatest reduction in the incidence of serious coronary events occurred in Type IIb patients who had elevations of both LDL-cholesterol and total plasma triglycerides. This subgroup of Type IIb gemfibrozil group patients had a lower mean HDL-cholesterol level at baseline than the Type IIa subgroup that had elevations of LDL-cholesterol and normal plasma triglycerides. The mean increase in HDL-cholesterol among the Type IIb patients in this study was 12.6% compared to placebo. The mean change in LDL-cholesterol among Type IIb patients was −4.1% with Lopid compared to a rise of 3.9% in the placebo subgroup. The Type IIb subjects in the Helsinki Heart Study had 26 fewer coronary events per thousand persons over 5 years in the gemfibrozil group compared to placebo. The difference in coronary events was substantially greater between Lopid and placebo for that subgroup of patients with the triad of LDL-cholesterol >175 mg/dL (>4.5 mmol), triglycerides >200 mg/dL (>2.2 mmol), and HDL-cholesterol <35 mg/dL (<0.90 mmol) (see Table I).

Further information is available from a 3.5 year (8.5 year cumulative) follow-up of all subjects who had participated in the Helsinki Heart Study. At the completion of the Helsinki Heart study, subjects could choose to start, stop, or continue to receive Lopid; without knowledge of their own lipid values or double-blind treatment, 60% of patients originally randomized to placebo began therapy with Lopid and 60% of patients originally randomized to Lopid continued medication. After approximately 6.5 years following randomization, all patients were informed of their original treatment group and lipid values during the 5 years of the double-blind treatment. After further elective changes in Lopid treatment status, 61% of patients in the group originally randomized to Lopid were taking drug; in the group originally randomized to placebo, 65% were taking Lopid. The event rate per 1000 occurring during the open-label follow-up period is detailed in Table II.

Table II
Cardiac Events and All-Cause Mortality (events per 1000 patients) Occurring During the 3.5 Year Open-Label Follow-up to the Helsinki Heart Study[1]

Group:	PDrop N=215	PN N=494	PL N=1283	LDrop N=221	LN N=574	LL N=1207
Cardiac Events	38.8	22.9	22.5	37.2	28.3	25.4
All-Cause Mortality	41.9	22.3	15.6	72.3	19.2	24.9

[1] The six open-label groups are designated first by the original randomization (P = placebo, L = Lopid) and then by the drug taken in the follow-up period (N = Attend clinic but took no drug, L = Lopid, Drop = No attendance at clinic during open-label).

Cumulative mortality through 8.5 years showed a 20% relative excess of deaths in the group originally randomized to Lopid versus the originally randomized placebo group and a 20% relative decrease in cardiac events in the group originally randomized to Lopid versus the originally randomized placebo group (see Table III). This analysis of the originally randomized "intent-to-treat" population neglects the possible complicating effects of treatment switching during the open-label phase. Adjustment of hazard ratios taking into account open-label treatment status from years 6.5 to 8.5 could change the reported hazard ratios for mortality toward unity.

Table III
Cardiac Events, Cardiac Deaths, Non-Cardiac Deaths and All-Cause Mortality in the Helsinki Heart Study, Year 0–8.5.[1]

Event	Lopid at Study Start	Placebo at Study Start	Lopid: Placebo Hazard Ratio[2]	Cl Hazard[3] Ratio
Cardiac Events[4]	110	131	0.80	0.62–1.03
Cardiac Deaths	36	38	0.98	0.63–1.54
Non-Cardiac Deaths	65	45	1.40	0.95–2.05
All-Cause Mortality	101	83	1.20	0.90–1.61

[1] Intention-to-Treat Analysis of originally randomized patients neglecting the open-label treatment switches and exposure to study conditions.
[2] Hazard ratio for risk of event in the group originally randomized to Lopid compared to the group originally randomized to placebo neglecting open-label treatment switch and exposure to study condition.
[3] 95% confidence intervals of Lopid:placebo group hazard ratio.
[4] Fatal and non-fatal myocardial infarctions plus sudden cardiac deaths over the 8.5 year period.

It is not clear to what extent the findings of the primary prevention component of the Helsinki Heart Study can be extrapolated to other segments of the dyslipidemic population not studied (such as women, younger or older males, or those with lipid abnormalities limited solely to HDL-cholesterol) or to other lipid-altering drugs.

The secondary prevention component of the Helsinki Heart Study was conducted over 5 years in parallel and at the same centers in Finland in 628 middle-aged males excluded from the primary prevention component of the Helsinki Heart Study because of a history of angina, myocardial infarction or unexplained ECG changes (ref. 3). The primary efficacy endpoint of the study was cardiac events (the sum of fatal and non-fatal myocardial infarctions and sudden cardiac deaths). The hazard ratio (Lopid:placebo) for cardiac events was 1.47 (95% confidence limits 0.88–2.48, p = 0.14). Of the 35 patients in the Lopid group who experienced cardiac events, 12 patients suffered events after discontinuation from the study. Of the 24 patients in the placebo group with cardiac events, 4 patients suffered events after discontinuation from the study. There were 17 cardiac deaths in the Lopid group and 8 in the placebo group (hazard ratio 2.18; 95% confidence limits 0.94–5.05, p = 0.06). Ten of these deaths in the Lopid group and 3 in the placebo group occurred after discontinuation from therapy. In this study of patients with known or suspected coronary heart disease, no benefit from Lopid treatment was observed in reducing cardiac events or cardiac deaths. Thus, Lopid has shown benefit only in selected dyslipidemic patients *without* suspected or established coronary heart disease. Even in patients with coronary heart disease and the triad of elevated LDL-cholesterol, elevated triglycerides, plus low HDL-cholesterol, the possible effect of Lopid on coronary events has not been adequately studied.

No efficacy in the patients with established coronary heart disease was observed during the Coronary Drug Project with the chemically and pharmacologically related drug, clofibrate. The Coronary Drug Project was a 6-year randomized, double-blind study involving 1000 clofibrate, 1000 nicotinic acid, and 3000 placebo patients with known coronary heart disease. A clinically and statistically significant reduction in myocardial infarctions was seen in the concurrent nicotinic acid group compared to placebo; no reduction was seen with clofibrate.

The mechanism of action of gemfibrozil has not been definitely established. In man, Lopid has been shown to inhibit peripheral lipolysis and to decrease the hepatic extraction of free fatty acids, thus reducing hepatic triglyceride production. Lopid inhibits synthesis and increases clearance of VLDL carrier apolipoprotein B, leading to a decrease in VLDL production.

Animal studies suggest that gemfibrozil may, in addition to elevating HDL-cholesterol, reduce incorporation of long-chain fatty acids into newly formed triglycerides, accelerate turnover and removal of cholesterol from the liver, and increase excretion of cholesterol in the feces. Lopid is well absorbed from the gastrointestinal tract after oral administration. Peak plasma levels occur in 1 to 2 hours with a plasma half-life of 1.5 hours following multiple doses. Plasma levels appear proportional to dose and do not demonstrate accumulation across time following multiple doses.

Lopid mainly undergoes oxidation of a ring methyl group to successively form a hydroxymethyl and a carboxyl metabolite. Approximately seventy percent of the administered human dose is excreted in the urine, mostly as the glucuronide conjugate, with less than 2% excreted as unchanged gemfibrozil. Six percent of the dose is accounted for in the feces.

INDICATIONS AND USAGE

Lopid (gemfibrozil tablets, USP) is indicated as adjunctive therapy to diet for:

1. Treatment of adult patients with very high elevations of serum triglyceride levels (Types IV and V hyperlipidemia) who present a risk of pancreatitis and who do not respond adequately to a determined dietary effort to control them. Patients who present such risk typically have serum triglycerides over 2000 mg/dL and have elevations of VLDL-cholesterol as well as fasting chylomicrons (Type V hyperlipidemia). Subjects who consistently have total serum or plasma triglycerides below 1000 mg/dL are unlikely to present a risk of pancreatitis. Lopid therapy may be considered for those subjects with triglyceride elevations between 1000 and 2000 mg/dL who have a history of pancreatitis or of recurrent abdominal pain typical of pancreatitis. It is recognized that some Type IV patients with triglycerides under 1000 mg/dL may, through dietary or alcoholic indiscretion, convert to a Type V pattern with massive triglyceride elevations accompanying fasting chylomicronemia, but the influence of Lopid therapy on the risk of pancreatitis in such situations has not been adequately studied. Drug therapy is not indicated for patients with Type I hyperlipoproteinemia, who have elevations of chylomicrons and plasma triglycerides, but who have normal levels of very low density lipoprotein (VLDL). Inspection of plasma refrigerated for 14 hours is helpful in distinguishing Types I, IV, and V hyperlipoproteinemia (ref. 4).
2. Reducing the risk of developing coronary heart disease **only** in Type IIb patients without history of or symptoms of existing coronary heart disease who have had an inadequate response to weight loss, dietary therapy, exercise, and other pharmacologic agents (such as bile acid sequestrants and nicotinic acid, known to reduce LDL- and raise HDL-cholesterol **and** who have the following triad of lipid abnormalities: low HDL-cholesterol levels in addition to elevated LDL-cholesterol and elevated triglycerides (see WARNINGS, PRECAUTIONS, and CLINICAL PHARMACOLOGY). The National Cholesterol Education Program has defined a serum HDL-cholesterol value that is consistently below 35 mg/dL as constituting an independent risk factor for coronary heart disease (ref. 5). Patients with significantly elevated triglycerides should be closely observed when treated with gemfibrozil. In some patients with high triglyceride levels, treatment with gemfibrozil is associated with a significant increase in LDL-cholesterol. BECAUSE OF POTENTIAL TOXICITY SUCH AS MALIGNANCY, GALLBLADDER DISEASE, ABDOMINAL PAIN LEADING TO APPENDECTOMY AND OTHER ABDOMINAL SURGERIES, AN INCREASED INCIDENCE IN NONCORONARY MORTALITY, AND THE 44% RELATIVE INCREASE DURING THE TRIAL PERIOD IN AGE-ADJUSTED ALL-CAUSE MORTALITY SEEN WITH THE CHEMICALLY AND PHARMACOLOGICALLY RELATED DRUG, CLOFIBRATE, THE POTENTIAL BENEFIT OF GEMFIBROZIL IN TREATING TYPE IIA PATIENTS WITH ELEVATIONS OF LDL-CHOLESTEROL ONLY IS NOT LIKELY TO OUTWEIGH THE RISKS. LOPID IS ALSO NOT INDICATED FOR THE TREATMENT OF PATIENTS WITH LOW HDL-CHOLESTEROL AS THEIR ONLY LIPID ABNORMALITY.

In a subgroup analysis of patients in the Helsinki Heart Study with above-median HDL-cholesterol values at baseline (greater than 46.4 mg/dL), the incidence of serious coronary events was similar for gemfibrozil and placebo subgroups (see Table I).

Continued on next page

This product information was prepared in June 1998. On these and other Parke-Davis Products, information may be obtained by addressing PARKE-DAVIS, Division of Warner-Lambert Company, Morris Plains, New Jersey 07950.

Consult 1999 PDR® supplements and future editions for revisions

Lopid—Cont.

The initial treatment for dyslipidemia is dietary therapy specific for the type of lipoprotein abnormality. Excess body weight and excess alcohol intake may be important factors in hypertriglyceridemia and should be managed prior to any drug therapy. Physical exercise can be an important ancillary measure, and has been associated with rises in HDL-cholesterol. Diseases contributory to hyperlipidemia such as hypothyroidism or diabetes mellitus should be looked for and adequately treated. Estrogen therapy is sometimes associated with massive rises in plasma triglycerides, especially in subjects with familial hypertriglyceridemia. In such cases, discontinuation of estrogen therapy may obviate the need for specific drug therapy of hypertriglyceridemia. The use of drugs should be considered only when reasonable attempts have been made to obtain satisfactory results with nondrug methods. If the decision is made to use drugs, the patient should be instructed that this does not reduce the importance of adhering to diet.

CONTRAINDICATIONS

1. Hepatic or severe renal dysfunction, including primary biliary cirrhosis.
2. Preexisting gallbladder disease (see WARNINGS).
3. Hypersensitivity to gemfibrozil.

WARNINGS

1. Because of chemical, pharmacological, and clinical similarities between gemfibrozil and clofibrate, the adverse findings with clofibrate in two large clinical studies may also apply to gemfibrozil. In the first of those studies, the Coronary Drug Project, 1000 subjects with previous myocardial infarction were treated for 5 years with clofibrate. There was no difference in mortality between the clofibrate-treated subjects and 3000 placebo-treated subjects, but twice as many clofibrate-treated subjects developed cholelithiasis and cholecystitis requiring surgery. In the other study, conducted by the World Health Organization (WHO), 5000 subjects without known coronary heart disease were treated with clofibrate for 5 years and followed one year beyond. There was a statistically significant, 44%, higher age-adjusted total mortality in the clofibrate-treated than in a comparable placebo-treated control group during the trial period. The excess mortality was due to a 33% increase in noncardiovascular causes, including malignancy, post-cholecystectomy complications, and pancreatitis. The higher risk of clofibrate-treated subjects for gallbladder disease was confirmed.
   Because of the more limited size of the Helsinki Heart Study, the observed difference in mortality from any cause between the Lopid and placebo group is not statistically significantly different from the 29% excess mortality reported in the clofibrate group in the separate WHO study at the 9 year follow-up (see CLINICAL PHARMACOLOGY). Noncoronary heart disease related mortality showed an excess in the group originally randomized to Lopid primarily due to cancer deaths observed during the open-label extension.
   During the 5 year primary prevention component of the Helsinki Heart Study mortality from any cause was 44 (2.2%) in the Lopid group and 43 (2.1%) in the placebo group; including the 3.5 year follow-up period since the trial was completed, cumulative mortality from any cause was 101 (4.9%) in the Lopid group and 83 (4.1%) in the group originally randomized to placebo (hazard ratio 1.20 in favor of placebo). Because of the more limited size of the Helsinki Heart Study, the observed difference in mortality from any cause between the Lopid and placebo groups at year-5 or at year-8.5 is not statistically significantly different from the 29% excess mortality reported in the clofibrate group in the separate WHO study at the 9 year follow-up. Noncoronary heart disease related mortality showed an excess in the group originally randomized to Lopid at the 8.5 year follow-up (65 Lopid versus 45 placebo noncoronary deaths).
   The incidence of cancer (excluding basal cell carcinoma) discovered during the trial and in the 3.5 years after the trial was completed was 51 (2.5%) in both originally randomized groups. In addition, there were 16 basal cell carcinomas in the group originally randomized to Lopid and 9 in the group randomized to placebo (p = 0.22). There were 30 (1.5%) deaths attributed to cancer in the group originally randomized to Lopid and 18 (0.9%) in the group originally randomized to placebo (p = 0.11). Adverse outcomes, including coronary events, were higher in gemfibrozil patients in a corresponding study in men with a history of known or suspected coronary heart disease in the secondary prevention component of the Helsinki Heart Study. (See CLINICAL PHARMACOLOGY.)
2. A gallstone prevalence substudy of 450 Helsinki Heart Study participants showed a trend toward a greater prevalence of gallstones during the study within the Lopid treatment group (7.5% vs 4.9% for the placebo group, a 55% excess for the gemfibrozil group). A trend toward a greater incidence of gallbladder surgery was observed for the Lopid group (17 vs 11 subjects, a 54% excess). This result did not differ statistically from the increased incidence of cholecystectomy observed in the WHO study in the group treated with clofibrate. Both clofibrate and gemfibrozil may increase cholesterol excretion into the bile leading to cholelithiasis. If cholelithiasis is suspected, gallbladder studies are indicated. Lopid therapy should be discontinued if gallstones are found.
3. Since a reduction of mortality from coronary heart disease has not been demonstrated and because liver and interstitial cell testicular tumors were increased in rats, Lopid should be administered only to those patients described in the INDICATIONS AND USAGE section. If a significant serum lipid response is not obtained, Lopid should be discontinued.
4. Concomitant Anticoagulants—Caution should be exercised when anticoagulants are given in conjunction with Lopid. The dosage of the anticoagulant should be reduced to maintain the prothrombin time at the desired level to prevent bleeding complications. Frequent prothrombin determinations are advisable until it has been definitely determined that the prothrombin level has stabilized.
5. Concomitant therapy with Lopid and Mevacor® (lovastatin) has been associated with rhabdomyolysis, markedly elevated creatine kinase (CK) levels and myoglobinuria, leading in a high proportion of cases to acute renal failure. IN VIRTUALLY ALL PATIENTS WHO HAVE HAD AN UNSATISFACTORY LIPID RESPONSE TO EITHER DRUG ALONE, ANY POTENTIAL LIPID BENEFIT OF COMBINED THERAPY WITH LOVASTATIN AND GEMFIBROZIL DOES NOT OUTWEIGH THE RISKS OF SEVERE MYOPATHY, RHABDOMYOLYSIS, AND ACUTE RENAL FAILURE (see Drug Interactions). The use of fibrates alone, including Lopid, may occasionally be associated with myositis. Patients receiving Lopid and complaining of muscle pain, tenderness, or weakness should have prompt medical evaluation for myositis, including serum creatine kinase level determination. If myositis is suspected or diagnosed, Lopid therapy should be withdrawn.
6. Cataracts—Subcapsular bilateral cataracts occurred in 10% and unilateral in 6.3% of male rats treated with gemfibrozil at 10 times the human dose.

PRECAUTIONS

1. **Initial Therapy**—Laboratory studies should be done to ascertain that the lipid levels are consistently abnormal. Before instituting Lopid therapy, every attempt should be made to control serum lipids with appropriate diet, exercise, weight loss in obese patients, and control of any medical problems such as diabetes mellitus and hypothyroidism that are contributing to the lipid abnormalities.
2. **Continued Therapy**—Periodic determination of serum lipids should be obtained, and the drug withdrawn if lipid response is inadequate after 3 months of therapy.
3. **Drug Interactions—(A) HMG-CoA reductase inhibitors:** Rhabdomyolysis has occurred with combined gemfibrozil and lovastatin therapy. It may be seen as early as 3 weeks after initiation of combined therapy or after several months. In most subjects who have had an unsatisfactory lipid response to either drug alone, the possible benefit of combined therapy with lovastatin (or other HMG-CoA reductase inhibitors) and gemfibrozil does not outweigh the risks of severe myopathy, rhabdomyolysis, and acute renal failure. There is no assurance that periodic monitoring of creatine kinase will prevent the occurrence of severe myopathy and kidney damage.
   (B) **Anticoagulants:** CAUTION SHOULD BE EXERCISED WHEN ANTICOAGULANTS ARE GIVEN IN CONJUNCTION WITH LOPID. THE DOSAGE OF THE ANTICOAGULANT SHOULD BE REDUCED TO MAINTAIN THE PROTHROMBIN TIME AT THE DESIRED LEVEL TO PREVENT BLEEDING COMPLICATIONS. FREQUENT PROTHROMBIN DETERMINATIONS ARE ADVISABLE UNTIL IT HAS BEEN DEFINITELY DETERMINED THAT THE PROTHROMBIN LEVEL HAS STABILIZED.
4. **Carcinogenesis, Mutagenesis, Impairment of Fertility—Long-term studies have been conducted in rats at 0.2 and 2 times** the human dose (based on surface area, mg/meter^2). Based on two-week toxicokinetic studies, exposure (AUC) of the dose groups was estimated to be 0.2 and 1.3 times the human exposure. The incidence of benign liver nodules and liver carcinomas was significantly increased in high dose male rats. The incidence of liver carcinomas increased also in low dose males, but this increase was not statistically significant (p=0.1). Male rats had a dose-related and statistically significant increase of benign Leydig cell tumors. The higher dose female rats had a significant increase in the combined incidence of benign and malignant liver neoplasms.
   Long-term studies have been conducted in mice at 0.1 and 1 times the human dose (based on surface area). Based on two-week toxicokinetic studies, exposure (AUC) of the two dose groups was estimated to be 0.1 and 0.7 times the human exposure. There were no statistically significant differences from controls in the incidence of liver tumors, but the doses tested were lower than those shown to be carcinogenic with other fibrates.
   Electron microscopy studies have demonstrated a florid hepatic peroxisome proliferation following Lopid administration to the male rat. An adequate study to test for peroxisome proliferation has not been done in humans, but changes in peroxisome morphology have been observed. Peroxisome proliferation has been shown to occur in humans with either of two other drugs of the fibrate class when liver biopsies were compared before and after treatment in the same individual.
   Administration of approximately 0.6 and 2 times the human dose (based on surface area) to male rats for 10 weeks resulted in a dose-related decrease of fertility. Subsequent studies demonstrated that this effect was reversed after a drug-free period of about eight weeks, and it was not transmitted to the offspring.
5. **Pregnancy Category C**—Lopid has been shown to produce adverse effects in rats and rabbits at doses between 0.5 and 3 times the human dose (based on surface area) but no developmental toxicity or teratogenicity among offspring of either species. There are no adequate and well-controlled studies in pregnant women. Lopid should be used during pregnancy only if the potential benefit justifies the potential risk to the fetus.
   Administration of Lopid to female rats at 0.6 and 2 times the human dose (based on surface area) before and throughout gestation caused a dose-related decrease in conception rate and, at the high dose, an increase in stillborns and a slight reduction in pup weight during lactation. There were also dose-related increased skeletal variations. Anophthalmia occurred, but rarely.
   Administration of 0.6 and 2 times the human dose (based on surface area) of Lopid to female rats from gestation day 15 through weaning caused dose-related decreases in birth weight and suppressions of pup growth during lactation.
   Administration of 1 and 3 times the human dose (based on surface area) of Lopid to female rabbits during organogenesis caused a dose-related decrease in litter size and, at the high dose, an increased incidence of parietal bone variations.
6. **Nursing Mothers**—It is not known whether this drug is excreted in human milk. Because many drugs are excreted in human milk and because of the potential for tumorigenicity shown for Lopid in animal studies, a decision should be made whether to discontinue nursing or to discontinue the drug, taking into account the importance of the drug to the mother.
7. **Hematologic Changes**—Mild hemoglobin, hematocrit and white blood cell decreases have been observed in occasional patients following initiation of Lopid therapy. However, these levels stabilize during long-term administration. Rarely, severe anemia, leukopenia, thrombocytopenia, and bone marrow hypoplasia have been reported. Therefore, periodic blood counts are recommended during the first 12 months of Lopid administration.
8. **Liver Function**—Abnormal liver function tests have been observed occasionally during Lopid administration, including elevations of AST (SGOT), ALT (SGPT), LDH, bilirubin, and alkaline phosphatase. These are usually reversible when Lopid is discontinued. Therefore periodic liver function studies are recommended and Lopid therapy should be terminated if abnormalities persist.
9. **Kidney Function**—There have been reports of worsening renal insufficiency upon the addition of Lopid therapy in individuals with baseline plasma creatinine >2.0 mg/dL. In such patients, the use of alternative therapy should be considered against the risks and benefits of a lower dose of Lopid.
10. **Use in Pediatric Patients**—Safety and efficacy in pediatric patients have not been established.

ADVERSE REACTIONS

In the double-blind controlled phase of the primary prevention component of the Helsinki Heart Study, 2046 patients received Lopid for up to 5 years. In that study, the following adverse reactions were statistically more frequent in subjects in the Lopid group:

	LOPID (N=2046)	PLACEBO (N=2035)
	Frequency in percent of subjects	
Gastrointestinal reactions	34.2	23.8
Dyspepsia	19.6	11.9
Abdominal pain	9.8	5.6
Acute appendicitis (histologically confirmed in most cases where data were available)	1.2	0.6
Atrial fibrillation	0.7	0.1

	CAUSAL RELATIONSHIP PROBABLE	CAUSAL RELATIONSHIP NOT ESTABLISHED
General:		weight loss
Cardiac:		extrasystoles
Gastrointestinal:	cholestatic jaundice	pancreatitis
		hepatoma
		colitis
Central Nervous System:	dizziness	confusion
	somnolence	convulsions
	paresthesia	convulsions
	peripheral neuritis	syncope
	decreased libido	
	depression	
	headache	
Eye:	blurred vision	retinal edema
Genitourinary:	impotence	decreased male fertility
		renal dysfunction
Musculoskeletal:	myopathy	
	myasthenia	
	myalgia	
	painful extremities	
	arthralgia	
	synovitis	
	rhabdomyolysis (see WARNINGS and Drug Interactions under PRECAUTIONS)	
Clinical Laboratory:	increased creatine phosphokinase	positive antinuclear antibody
	increased bilirubin	
	increased liver transaminases (AST [SGOT], ALT [SGPT])	
	increased alkaline phosphatase	
Hematopoietic:	anemia	thrombocytopenia
	leukopenia	
	bone marrow hypoplasia	
	eosinophilia	
Immunologic:	angioedema	anaphylaxis
	aryngeal edema	Lupus-like syndrome
	urticaria	vasculitis
Integumentary:	exfoliative dermatitis	alopecia
	rash	
	dermatitis	
	pruritus	

Adverse events reported by more than 1% of subjects, but without a significant difference between groups:

Diarrhea	7.2	6.5
Fatigue	3.8	3.5
Nausea/Vomiting	2.5	2.1
Eczema	1.9	1.2
Rash	1.7	1.3
Vertigo	1.5	1.3
Constipation	1.4	1.3
Headache	1.2	1.1

Gallbladder surgery was performed in 0.9% of Lopid and 0.5% of placebo subjects in the primary prevention component, a 64% excess, which is not statistically different from the excess of gallbladder surgery observed in the clofibrate compared to the placebo group of the WHO study. Gallbladder surgery was also performed more frequently in the Lopid group compared to placebo (1.9% vs 0.3%, p = 0.07) in the secondary prevention component. A statistically significant increase in appendectomy in the gemfibrozil group was seen also in the secondary prevention component (6 on gemfibrozil vs 0 on placebo, p = 0.014).

Nervous system and special senses adverse reactions were more common in the Lopid group. These included hypesthesia, paresthesias, and taste perversion. Other adverse reactions that were more common among Lopid treatment group subjects but where a causal relationship were not established include cataracts, peripheral vascular disease, and intracerebral hemorrhage.

From other studies it seems probable that Lopid is causally related to the occurrence of MUSCULOSKELETAL SYMPTOMS (see WARNINGS), and to ABNORMAL LIVER FUNCTION TESTS and HEMATOLOGIC CHANGES (see PRECAUTIONS).

Reports of viral and bacterial infections (common cold, cough, urinary tract infections) were more common in gemfibrozil treated patients in other controlled clinical trials of 805 patients. Additional adverse reactions that have been reported for gemfibrozil are listed below by system. These are categorized according to whether a causal relationship to treatment with Lopid is probable or not established: [See table at top of page]

DOSAGE AND ADMINISTRATION

The recommended dose for adults is 1200 mg administered in two divided doses 30 minutes before the morning and evening meal.

OVERDOSAGE

There have been reported cases of overdosage with Lopid. In one case a 7 year old child recovered after ingesting up to 9 grams of Lopid. Symptomatic supportive measures should be taken should an overdose occur.

HOW SUPPLIED

Lopid (Tablet 737), white, elliptical, film-coated, scored tablets, each containing 600 mg gemfibrozil, are available as follows:
N 0071-0737-20: Bottles of 60
N 0071-0737-30: Bottles of 500
N 0071-0737-40: Unit dose packages of 100 (10 strips of 10 tablets each)
Parcode No. 737
Storage: Store below 30°C (86°F).

REFERENCES

1. Frick MH, Elo O, Haapa K, et al: Helsinki Heart Study: Primary prevention trial with gemfibrozil in middle-aged men with dyslipidemia. *N Engl J Med* 1987; 317:1237-1245.
2. Manninen V, Elo O, Frick MH, et al: Lipid alterations and decline in the incidence of coronary heart disease in the Helsinki Heart Study. *JAMA* 1988; 260:641-651.
3. Frick MH, Heinonen OP, et al: Efficacy of Gemfibrozil in Dyslipidemic Subjects with Suspected Heart Disease. An Ancillary Study in the Helsinki Heart Study Frame Population. *Annals of Medicine* 1993; 25:41-45.
4. Nikkila EA: Familial lipoprotein lipase deficiency and related disorders of chylomicron metabolism. In Stanbury J.B. et al. (eds.): *The Metabolic Basis of Inherited Disease,* 5th ed., McGraw-Hill, 1983, Chap. 30, pp. 622-642.
5. Report of the National Cholesterol Education Program Expert Panel on Detection, Evaluation, and Treatment of High Blood Cholesterol. *Arch Int Med* 1988;148:36-69.
Caution—Federal law prohibits dispensing without prescription.
Revised August 1996
© 1996, Warner-Lambert Co.   0737G300
Shown in Product Identification Guide, page 329

NARDIL®
(Phenelzine Sulfate Tablets, USP)   ℞

DESCRIPTION

Nardil® (phenelzine sulfate) is a potent inhibitor of monoamine oxidase (MAO). Phenelzine sulfate is a hydrazine derivative. It is a molecular weight of 234.27 and is chemically described as $C_8H_{12}N_2\cdot N_2SO_4$. Its chemical structure is shown below:

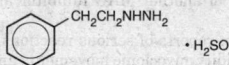

$\cdot H_2SO_4$

Molecular weight: 234.27

Each Nardil tablet for oral administration contains phenelzine sulfate equivalent to 15 mg of phenelzine base. Inactive ingredients include: acacia NF; calcium carbonate; carnauba wax, NF; corn-starch, NF; FD and C yellow No. 6; gelatin, NF; kaolin, USP; magnesium stearate, NF; mannitol, USP; pharmaceutical glaze, NF; povidone, USP; sucrose, NF; talc, USP; white wax, NF; white wheat flour.

CLINICAL PHARMACOLOGY

Monoamine oxidase is a complex enzyme system, widely distributed throughout the body. Drugs that inhibit monoamine oxidase in the laboratory are associated with a number of clinical effects. Thus, it is unknown whether MAO inhibition per se, other pharmacologic actions, or an interaction of both is responsible for the clinical effects observed. Therefore, the physician should become familiar with all the effects produced by drugs of this class.

INDICATIONS AND USAGE

Nardil has been found to be effective in depressed patients clinically characterized as "atypical," "nonendogenous," or "neurotic." These patients often have mixed anxiety and depression and phobic or hypochondriacal features. There is less conclusive evidence of its usefulness with severely depressed patients with endogenous features.

Nardil should rarely be the first antidepressant drug used. Rather, it is more suitable for use with patients who have failed to respond to the drugs more commonly used for these conditions.

CONTRAINDICATIONS

Nardil should not be used in patients who are hypersensitive to the drug or its ingredients, with pheochromocytoma, congestive heart failure, a history of liver disease, or abnormal liver function tests.

The potentiation of sympathomimetic substances and related compounds by MAO inhibitors may result in hypertensive crises (see WARNINGS). Therefore, patients being treated with Nardil should not take sympathomimetic drugs (including amphetamines, cocaine, methylphenidate, dopamine, epinephrine and norepinephrine) or related compounds (including methyldopa, L-dopa, L-tryptophan, L-tyrosine, and phenylalanine). Hypertensive crises during Nardil therapy may also be caused by the ingestion of foods with a high concentration of tyramine or dopamine. Therefore, patients being treated with Nardil should avoid high protein food that has undergone protein breakdown by aging, fermentation, pickling, smoking, or bacterial contamination. Patients should also avoid cheeses (especially aged varieties), pickled herring, beer, wine, liver, yeast extract (including brewer's yeast in large quantities), dry sausage (including Genoa salami, hard salami, pepperoni, and Lebanon bologna), pods of broad beans (fava beans), and yogurt. Excessive amounts of caffeine and chocolate may also cause hypertensive reactions.

Nardil should not be used in combination with dextromethorphan or with CNS depressants such as alcohol and certain narcotics. Excitation, seizures, delirium, hyperpyrexia, circulatory collapse, coma, and death have been reported in patients receiving MAOI therapy who have been given a single dose of meperidine. Nardil should not be administered together with or in rapid succession to other MAO inhibitors because HYPERTENSIVE CRISES and convulsive seizures, fever, marked sweating, excitation, delirium, tremor, coma, and circulatory collapse may occur.

A List of MAO Inhibitors by generic name follows:
pargyline hydrochloride
pargyline hydrochloride and methylclothiazide
furazolidone
isocarboxazid
procarbazine
tranylcypromine

Nardil should also not be used in combination with buspirone HCl, since several cases of elevated blood pressure have been reported in patients taking MAO inhibitors who were then given buspirone HCl. At least 10 days should elapse between the discontinuation of Nardil and the insti-

Continued on next page

This product information was prepared in June 1998. On these and other Parke-Davis Products, information may be obtained by addressing PARKE-DAVIS, Division of Warner-Lambert Company, Morris Plains, New Jersey 07950.

Nardil—Cont.

tution of another antidepressant or buspirone HCl, or the discontinuation of another MAO inhibitor and the institution of Nardil.

There have been reports of serious reactions (including hyperthermia, rigidity, myoclonic movements and death) when serotoninergic drugs (e.g., dexfenfluramine, fluoxetine, fluvoxamine, paroxetine, sertraline, venlafaxine) have been combined with an MAO inhibitor. Therefore the concomitant use of Nardil with serotoninergic agents is contraindicated (see PRECAUTIONS—*Drug Interactions*). Allow at least five weeks between discontinuation of fluoxetine and initiation of Nardil and at least 10 days between discontinuation of Nardil and initiation of fluoxetine, or other serotoninergic agents. Before initiating Nardil after using other serotoninergic agents, a sufficient amount of time must be allowed for clearance of the serotoninergic agent and its active metabolites.

The combination of MAO inhibitors and tryptophan has been reported to cause behavioral and neurologic syndromes including disorientation, confusion, amnesia, delirium, agitation, hypomanic signs, ataxia, myoclonus, hyperreflexia, shivering, ocular oscillations, and Babinski signs.

The concurrent administration of an MAO inhibitor and bupropion hydrochloride (Wellbutrin®) is contraindicated. At least 14 days should elapse between discontinuation of an MAO inhibitor and initiation of treatment with bupropion hydrochloride.

Patients taking Nardil should not undergo elective surgery requiring general anesthesia. Also, they should not be given cocaine or local anesthesia containing sympathomimetic vasoconstrictors. The possible combined hypotensive effects of Nardil and spinal anesthesia should be kept in mind. Nardil should be discontinued at least 10 days prior to elective surgery.

MAO inhibitors, including Nardil, are contraindicated in patients receiving guanethidine.

WARNINGS

The most serious reactions to Nardil involve changes in blood pressure.

Hypertensive Crises: The most important reaction associated with Nardil administration is the occurrence of hypertensive crises, which have sometimes been fatal.

These crises are characterized by some or all of the following symptoms: occipital headache which may radiate frontally, palpitation, neck stiffness or soreness, nausea, vomiting, sweating (sometimes with fever and sometimes with cold, clammy skin), dilated pupils, and photophobia. Either tachycardia or bradycardia may be present and can be associated with constricting chest pain.

NOTE: Intracranial bleeding has been reported in association with the increase in blood pressure.

Blood pressure should be observed frequently to detect evidence of any pressor response in all patients receiving Nardil. Therapy should be discontinued immediately upon the occurrence of palpitation or frequent headaches during therapy.

Recommended treatment in hypertensive crisis: If a hypertensive crisis occurs, Nardil should be discontinued immediately and therapy to lower blood pressure should be instituted immediately. On the basis of present evidence, phentolamine is recommended. (The dosage reported for phentolamine is 5 mg intravenously.) Care should be taken to administer this drug slowly in order to avoid producing an excessive hypotensive effect. Fever should be managed by means of external cooling.

Warning to the Patient: All patients should be warned that the following foods, beverages, and medications must be avoided while taking Nardil, and for two weeks after discontinuing use.

Foods and Beverages To Avoid

Meat and Fish

Pickled herring
Liver
Dry sausage (including Genoa salami, hard salami, pepperoni, and Lebanon bologna)

Vegetables

Broad bean pods (fava bean pods)
Sauerkraut

Dairy Products

Cheese (cottage cheese and cream cheese are allowed)
Yogurt

Beverages

Beer and wine
Alcohol-free and reduced-alcohol beer and wine products

Miscellaneous

Yeast extract (including brewer's yeast in large quantities)
Meat extract
Excessive amounts of chocolate and caffeine

Also, any spoiled or improperly refrigerated, handled, or stored protein-rich foods such as meats, fish, and dairy products, including foods that may have undergone protein changes by aging, pickling, fermentation, or smoking to improve flavor should be avoided.

OTC Medications To Avoid

Cold and cough preparations (including those containing dextromethorphan)
Nasal decongestants (tablets, drops, or spray)
Hay-fever medications
Sinus medications
Asthma inhalant medications
Antiappetite medicines
Weight-reducing preparations
"Pep" pills
L-tryptophan containing preparations

Also, certain prescription drugs should be avoided. Therefore, patients under the care of another physician or dentist should inform him/her they are taking Nardil.

Patients should be warned that the use of the above foods, beverages, or medications may cause a reaction characterized by headache and other serious symptoms due to a rise in blood pressure, with the exception of dextromethorphan which may cause reactions similar to those seen with meperidine. Also, there has been a report of an interaction between Nardil and dextromethorphan (ingested as a lozenge) causing drowsiness and bizarre behavior.

Patients should be instructed to report promptly the occurrence of headache or other unusual symptoms.

Concomitant Use with Dibenzazepine Derivative Drugs

If the decision is made to administer Nardil concurrently with other antidepressant drugs, or within less than 10 days after discontinuation of antidepressant therapy, the patient should be cautioned by the physician regarding the possibility of adverse drug interaction.

A List of Dibenzazepine Derivative Drugs by generic name follows:

nortriptyline hydrochloride
amitriptyline hydrochloride
amitriptyline hydrochloride
perphenazine and amitriptyline hydrochloride
perphenazine and amitriptyline hydrochloride
clomipramine hydrochloride
desipramine hydrochloride
desipramine hydrochloride
imipramine hydrochloride
doxepin
doxepin
carbamazepine
cyclobenzaprine HCl
amoxapine
maprotiline HCl
trimipremine maleate
protriptyline HCl
mirtazapine

Nardil should be used with caution in combination with antihypertensive drugs, including thiazide diuretics and β-blockers, since exaggerated hypotensive effects may result.

Use in Pregnancy: The safe use of Nardil during pregnancy or lactation has not been established. The potential benefit of this drug, if used during pregnancy, lactation, or in women of childbearing age, should be weighed against the possible hazard to the mother or fetus.

Doses of Nardil in pregnant mice well exceeding the maximum recommended human dose have caused a significant decrease in the number of viable offspring per mouse. In addition, the growth of young dogs and rats has been retarded by doses exceeding the maximum human dose.

Use in Pediatric Patients: Nardil is not recommended for pediatric patients under 16 years of age, since there are no controlled studies of safety in this age group. Nardil, as with other hydrazine derivatives, has been reported to induce pulmonary and vascular tumors in an uncontrolled lifetime study in mice.

PRECAUTIONS

In depressed patients, the possibility of suicide should always be considered and adequate precautions taken. It is recommended that careful observations of patients undergoing Nardil treatment be maintained until control of depression is achieved. If necessary, additional measures (ECT, hospitalization, etc) should be instituted.

All patients undergoing treatment with Nardil should be closely followed for symptoms of postural hypotension. Hypotensive side effects have occurred in hypertensive as well as normotensive and hypotensive patients. Blood pressure usually returns to pretreatment levels rapidly when the drug is discontinued or the dosage is reduced.

Because the effect of Nardil on the convulsive threshold may be variable, adequate precautions should be taken when treating epileptic patients.

Of the more severe side effects that have been reported with any consistency, hypomania has been the most common. This reaction has been largely limited to patients in whom disorders characterized by hyperkinetic symptoms coexist with, but are obscured by, depressive affect; hypomania usually appeared as depression improved. If agitation is present, it may be increased with Nardil. Hypomania and agitation have also been reported at higher than recommended doses or following long-term therapy.

Nardil may cause excessive stimulation in schizophrenic patients; in manic-depressive states it may result in a swing from a depressive to a manic phase.

MAO inhibitors, including Nardil, potentiate hexobarbital hypnosis in animals. Therefore, barbiturates should be given at a reduced dose with Nardil.

MAO inhibitors inhibit the destruction of serotonin and norepinephrine, which are believed to be released from tissue stores by rauwolfia alkaloids. Accordingly, caution should be exercised when rauwolfia is used concomitantly with an MAO inhibitor, including Nardil.

There is conflicting evidence as to whether or not MAO inhibitors affect glucose metabolism or potentiate hypoglycemic agents. This should be kept in mind if Nardil is administered to diabetics.

Drug Interactions

In patients receiving nonselective monoamine oxidase (MOA) inhibitors in combination with serotoninergic agents (e.g., dexfenfluramine, fluoxetine, fluvoxamine, paroxetine, sertraline, venlafexine) there have been reports of serious, sometimes fatal, reactions. Because Nardil is a monoamine oxidase (MAO) inhibitor, Nardil should not be used concomitantly with a serotoninergic agent (See CONTRAINDICATIONS).

ADVERSE REACTIONS

Nardil is a potent inhibitor of monoamine oxidase. Because this enzyme is widely distributed throughout the body, diverse pharmacologic effects can be expected to occur. When they occur, such effects tend to be mild or moderate in severity (see below), often subside as treatment continues, and can be minimized by adjusting dosage; rarely is it necessary to institute counteracting measures or to discontinue Nardil.

Common side effects include:

Nervous System —Dizziness, headache, drowsiness, sleep disturbances (including insomnia and hypersomnia), fatigue, weakness, tremors, twitching, myoclonic movements, hyperreflexia.

Gastrointestinal —Constipation, dry mouth, gastrointestinal disturbances, elevated serum transaminases (without accompanying signs and symptoms).

Metabolic —Weight gain.

Cardiovascular —Postural hypotension, edema.

Genitourinary —Sexual disturbances, eg, anorgasmia and ejaculatory disturbances and impotence.

Less common mild to moderate side effects (some of which have been reported in a single patient or by a single physician) include:

Nervous System —Jitteriness, palilalia, euphoria, nystagmus, paresthesias.

Genitourinary —Urinary retention.

Metabolic—Hypernatremia.

Dermatologic —Pruritus, Skin rash, sweating.

Special Senses —Blurred vision, glaucoma.

Although reported less frequently, and sometimes only once, additional severe side effects include:

Nervous System —Ataxia, shock-like coma, toxic delirium, manic reaction, convulsions, acute anxiety reaction, precipitation of schizophrenia, transient respiratory and cardiovascular depression following ECT.

Gastrointestinal —To date, fatal progressive necrotizing hepatocellular damage has been reported in a very few patients. Reversible jaundice.

Hematologic —Leukopenia.

Immunologic —Lupus-like syndrome.

Metabolic —Hypermetabolic syndrome (which may include, but is not limited to, hyperpyrexia, tachycardia, tachypnea, muscular rigidity, elevated CK levels, metabolic acidosis, hypoxia, coma and may resemble an overdose).

Respiratory —Edema of the glottis.

General —Fever associated with increased muscle tone.

Withdrawal may be associated with nausea, vomiting, and malaise.

An uncommon withdrawal syndrome following abrupt withdrawal of Nardil has been infrequently reported. Signs and symptoms of this syndrome generally commence 24 to 72 hours after drug discontinuation and may range from vivid nightmares with agitation to frank psychosis and convulsions. This syndrome generally responds to reinstitution of low-dose Nardil therapy followed by cautious downward titration and discontinuation.

DOSAGE AND ADMINISTRATION

Initial dose: The usual starting dose of Nardil is one tablet (15 mg) three times a day.

Early phase treatment: Dosage should be increased to at least 60 mg per day at a fairly rapid pace consistent with patient tolerance. It may be necessary to increase dosage up to 90 mg per day to obtain sufficient MAO inhibition. Many patients do not show a clinical response until treatment at 60 mg has been continued for at least 4 weeks.

Maintenance dose: After maximum benefit from Nardil is achieved, dosage should be reduced slowly over several weeks. Maintenance dose may be as low as one tablet, 15 mg, a day or every other day, and should be continued for as long as is required.

OVERDOSAGE

Note—For management of *hypertensive crises* see WARNINGS section.

Accidental or intentional overdosage may be more common in patients who are depressed. It should be remembered that multiple drugs and/or alcohol may have been ingested. Depending on the amount of overdosage with Nardil, a varying and mixed clinical picture may develop, including signs and symptoms of central nervous system and cardiovascular stimulation and/or depression. Signs and symptoms may be absent or minimal during the initial 12-hour period following ingestion and may develop slowly thereafter, reaching a maximum in 24–48 hours. Death has been reported following overdosage. Therefore, immediate hospitalization, with continuous patient observation and monitoring throughout this period, is essential.

Signs and symptoms of overdosage may include, alone or in combination, any of the following: drowsiness, dizziness, faintness, irritability, hyperactivity, agitation, severe headache, hallucinations, trismus, opisthotonus, rigidity, convulsions, and coma; rapid and irregular pulse, hypertension, hypotension, and vascular collapse; precordial pain, respiratory depression and failure, hyperpyrexia, diaphoresis, and cool, clammy skin.

Treatment: Intensive symptomatic and supportive treatment may be required. Induction of emesis or gastric lavage with instillation of charcoal slurry may be helpful in early poisoning, provided the airway has been protected against aspiration. Signs and symptoms of central nervous system stimulation, including convulsions, should be treated with diazepam, given slowly intravenously. Phenothiazine derivatives and central nervous system stimulants should be avoided. Hypotension and vascular collapse should be treated with intravenous fluids and, if necessary, blood pressure titration with an intravenous infusion of dilute pressor agent. It should be noted that adrenergic agents may produce a markedly increased pressor response.

Respiration should be supported by appropriate measures, including management of the airway, use of supplemental oxygen, and mechanical ventilatory assistance, as required. Body temperature should be monitored closely. Intensive management of hyperpyrexia may be required. Maintenance of fluid and electrolyte balance is essential.

There are no data on the lethal dose in man. The pathophysiologic effects of massive overdosage may persist for several days, since the drug acts by inhibiting physiologic enzyme systems. With symptomatic and supportive measures, recovery from *mild* overdosage may be expected within 3 to 4 days.

Hemodialysis, peritoneal dialysis, and charcoal hemoperfusion may be of value in massive overdosage, but sufficient data are not available to recommend their routine use in these cases.

Toxic blood levels of phenelzine have not been established, and assay methods are not practical for clinical or toxicological use.

HOW SUPPLIED

Each Nardil tablet is orange, biconvex, glossy sugar-coated, and imprinted with "P-D 270" in brown ink and contains phenelzine sulfate equivalent to 15 mg of phenelzine base. N 0071-0270-24 Bottles of 100

Storage: Store between 15°–30° C (59°–86°F).

Rx only

US Patent 3,314,855

Revised February 1998   0270G080

Shown in Product Identification Guide, page 329

NEURONTIN®   ℞
(Gabapentin Capsules)

DESCRIPTION

Neurontin® (gabapentin capsules) is supplied as imprinted hard shell capsules containing 100 mg, 300 mg, and 400 mg of gabapentin. The inactive ingredients are lactose, corn starch, and talc. The 100-mg capsule shell contains gelatin and titanium dioxide. The 300-mg capsule shell contains gelatin, titanium dioxide, and yellow iron oxide. The 400-mg capsule shell contains gelatin, red iron oxide, titanium dioxide, and yellow iron oxide. The imprinting ink contains FD&C Blue No. 2 and titanium dioxide.

Gabapentin is described as 1-(aminomethyl)cyclohexaneacetic acid with an empirical formula of $C_9H_{17}NO_2$ and a molecular weight of 171.24. The molecular structure of gabapentin is:

[See chemical structure at top of next column]

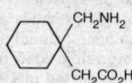

Gabapentin is a white to off-white crystalline solid. It is freely soluble in water and both basic and acidic aqueous solutions.

CLINICAL PHARMACOLOGY
Mechanism of Action

The mechanism by which gabapentin exerts its anticonvulsant action is unknown, but in animal test systems designed to detect anticonvulsant activity, gabapentin prevents seizures as do other marketed anticonvulsants. Gabapentin exhibits antiseizure activity in mice and rats in both the maximal electroshock and pentylenetetrazole seizure models and other preclinical models (e.g., strains with genetic epilepsy, etc.). The relevance of these models to human epilepsy is not known.

Gabapentin is structurally related to the neurotransmitter GABA (gamma-aminobutyric acid) but it does not interact with GABA receptors, it is not converted metabolically into GABA or a GABA agonist, and it is not an inhibitor of GABA uptake or degradation. Gabapentin was tested in radioligand binding assays at concentrations up to 100 μM and did not exhibit affinity for a number of other common receptor sites, including benzodiazepine, glutamate, N-methyl-D-aspartate (NMDA), quisqualate, kainate, strychnine-insensitive or strychnine-sensitive glycine, alpha 1, alpha 2, or beta adrenergic, adenosine A1 or A2, cholinergic, muscarinic or nicotinic, dopamine D1 or D2, histamine H1, serotonin S1 or S2, opiate mu, delta or kappa, voltage-sensitive calcium channel sites labeled with nitrendipine or diltiazem, or at voltage-sensitive sodium channel sites with batrachotoxinin A 20-alpha-benzoate.

Several test systems ordinarily used to assess activity at the NMDA receptor have been examined. Results are contradictory. Accordingly, no general statement about the effects, if any, of gabapentin at the NMDA receptor can be made.

In vitro studies with radiolabeled gabapentin have revealed a gabapentin binding site in areas of rat brain including neocortex and hippocampus. The identity and function of this binding site remain to be elucidated.

Pharmacokinetics and Drug Metabolism

All pharmacological actions following gabapentin administration are due to the activity of the parent compound; gabapentin is not appreciably metabolized in humans.

Oral Bioavailability: Gabapentin bioavailability is not dose proportional; i.e., as dose is increased, bioavailability decreases. A 400-mg dose, for example, is about 25% less bioavailable than a 100-mg dose. Over the recommended dose range of 300 to 600 mg T.I.D., however, the differences in bioavailability are not large, and bioavailability is about 60 percent. Food has no effect on the rate and extent of absorption of gabapentin.

Distribution: Gabapentin circulates largely unbound (<3%) to plasma protein. The apparent volume of distribution of gabapentin after 150 mg intravenous administration is 58±6 L (Mean ±SD). In patients with epilepsy, steady-state predose (Cmin) concentrations of gabapentin in cerebrospinal fluid were approximately 20% of the corresponding plasma concentrations.

Elimination: Gabapentin is eliminated from the systemic circulation by renal excretion as unchanged drug. Gabapentin is not appreciably metabolized in humans.

Gabapentin elimination half-life is 5 to 7 hours and is unaltered by dose or following multiple dosing. Gabapentin elimination rate constant, plasma clearance, and renal clearance are directly proportional to creatinine clearance (see Special Populations: Patients With Renal Insufficiency, below). In elderly patients, and in patients with impaired renal function, gabapentin plasma clearance is reduced. Gabapentin can be removed from plasma by hemodialysis. Dosage adjustment in patients with compromised renal function or undergoing hemodialysis is recommended (see DOSAGE AND ADMINISTRATION, Table 2).

Special Populations: *Patients With Renal Insufficiency:* Subjects (N=60) with renal insufficiency (mean creatinine clearance ranging from 13–114 mL/min) were administered single 400-mg oral doses of gabapentin. The mean gabapentin half-life ranged from about 6.5 hours (patients with creatinine clearance >60 mL/min) to 52 hours (creatinine clearance <30 mL/min) and gabapentin renal clearance from about 90 mL/min (>60 mL/min group) to about 10 mL/min (<30 mL/min). Mean plasma clearance (CL/F) decreased from approximately 190 mL/min to 20 mL/min.

Dosage adjustment in patients with compromised renal function is necessary (see DOSAGE AND ADMINISTRATION).

Hemodialysis: In a study in anuric subjects (N=11), the apparent elimination half-life of gabapentin on nondialysis days was about 132 hours; dialysis three times a week (4 hours duration) lowered the apparent half-life of gabapen-

tin by about 60%, from 132 hours to 51 hours. Hemodialysis thus has a significant effect on gabapentin elimination in anuric subjects.

Dosage adjustment in patients undergoing hemodialysis is necessary (see DOSAGE AND ADMINISTRATION).

Hepatic Disease: Because gabapentin is not metabolized, no study was performed in patients with hepatic impairment.

Age: The effect of age was studied in subjects 20–80 years of age. Apparent oral clearance (CL/F) of gabapentin decreased as age increased, from about 225 mL/min in those under 30 years of age to about 125 mL/min in those over 70 years of age. Renal clearance (CLr) and CLr adjusted for body surface area also declined with age; however, the decline in the renal clearance of gabapentin with age can largely be explained by the decline in renal function. Reduction of gabapentin dose may be required in patients who have age related compromised renal function. (See PRECAUTIONS, Geriatric Use, and DOSAGE AND ADMINISTRATION.)

Pediatric: No pharmacokinetic data are available in pediatric patients below the age of 18 years.

Gender: Although no formal study has been conducted to compare the pharmacokinetics of gabapentin in men and women, it appears that the pharmacokinetic parameters for males and females are similar and there are no significant gender differences.

Race: Pharmacokinetic differences due to race have not been studied. Because gabapentin is primarily renally excreted and there are no important racial differences in creatinine clearance, pharmacokinetic differences due to race are not expected.

Clinical Studies

The effectiveness of Neurontin® as adjunctive therapy (added to other antiepileptic drugs) was established in three multicenter placebo-controlled, double-blind, parallel-group clinical trials in 705 adults with refractory partial seizures. The patients enrolled had a history of at least 4 partial seizures per month in spite of receiving one or more antiepileptic drugs at therapeutic levels and were observed on their established antiepileptic drug regimen during a 12-week baseline period. In patients continuing to have at least 2 (or 4 in some studies) seizures per month, Neurontin® or placebo was then added on to the existing therapy during a 12-week treatment period. Effectiveness was assessed primarily on the basis of the percent of patients with a 50% or greater reduction in seizure frequency from baseline to treatment (the "responder rate") and a derived measure called response ratio, a measure of change defined as (T − B)/(T + B), where B is the patient's baseline seizure frequency and T is the patient's seizure frequency during treatment. Response ratio is distributed within the range −1 to +1. A zero value indicates no change while complete elimination of seizures would give a value of −1; increased seizure rates would give positive values. A response ratio of −0.33 corresponds to a 50% reduction in seizure frequency. The results given below are for all partial seizures in the intent-to-treat (all patients who received any doses of treatment) population in each study, unless otherwise indicated.

One study compared Neurontin® 1200 mg/day T.I.D. with placebo. Responder rate was 23% (14/61) in the Neurontin® group and 9% (6/66) in the placebo group; the difference between groups was statistically significant. Response ratio was also better in the Neurontin® group (−0.199) than in the placebo group (−0.044), a difference that also achieved statistical significance.

A second study compared primarily 1200 mg/day T.I.D. Neurontin® (N=101) with placebo (N=98). Additional smaller Neurontin® dosage groups (600 mg/day, N=53; 1800 mg/day, N=54) were also studied for information regarding dose response. Responder rate was higher in the Neurontin® 1200 mg/day group (16%) than in the placebo group (8%), but the difference was not statistically significant. The responder rate at 600 mg (17%) was also not significantly higher than in the placebo, but the responder rate in the 1800 mg group (26%) was statistically significantly superior to the placebo rate. Response ratio was better in the Neurontin® 1200 mg/day group (−0.103) than in the placebo group (−0.022); but this difference was also not statistically significant (p = 0.224). A better response was seen in the Neurontin® 600 mg/day group (−0.105) and 1800 mg/day group (−0.222) than in the 1200 mg/day group, with the 1800 mg/day group achieving statistical significance compared to the placebo group.

A third study compared Neurontin® 900 mg/day T.I.D. (N = 111) and placebo (N = 109). An additional Neurontin® 1200

Continued on next page

This product information was prepared in June 1998. On these and other Parke-Davis Products, information may be obtained by addressing PARKE-DAVIS, Division of Warner-Lambert Company, Morris Plains, New Jersey 07950.

Neurontin—Cont.

mg/day dosage group (N = 52) provided dose-response data. A statistically significant difference in responder rate was seen in the Neurontin® 900 mg/day group (22%) compared to that in the placebo group (10%). Response ratio was also statistically significantly superior in the Neurontin® 900 mg/day group (− 0.119) compared to that in the placebo group (= 0.027), as was response ratio in 1200 mg/day Neurontin® (−0.184) compared to placebo.

Analyses were also performed in each study to examine the effect of Neurontin® on preventing secondarily generalized tonic-clonic seizures. Patients who experienced a secondarily generalized tonic-clonic seizure in either the baseline or in the treatment period in all three placebo-controlled studies were included in these analyses. There were several response ratio comparisons that showed a statistically significant advantage for Neurontin® compared to placebo and favorable trends for almost all comparisons.

Analysis of responder rate using combined data from all three studies and all doses (N=162, Neurontin® ; N=89, placebo) also showed a significant advantage for Neurontin® over placebo in reducing the frequency of secondarily generalized tonic-clonic seizures.

In two of the three controlled studies, more than one dose of Neurontin® was used. Within each study the results did not show a consistently increased response to dose. However, looking across studies, a trend toward increasing efficacy with increasing dose is evident (see Figure 1).

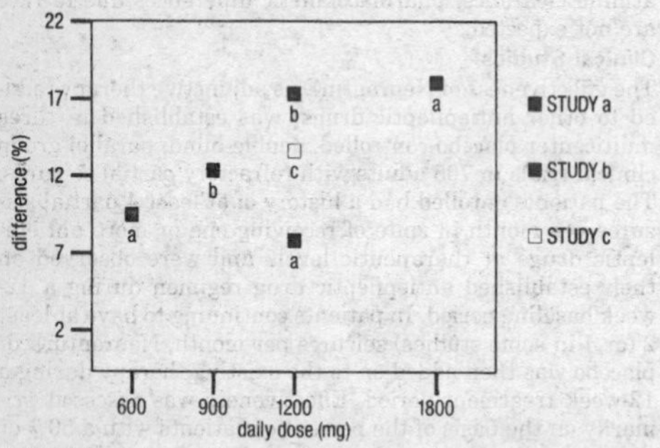

FIGURE 1. Responder Rate in Patients Receiving Neurontin® Expressed as a Difference from Placebo by Dose and Study

In the figure, treatment effect magnitude, measured on the Y axis in terms of the difference in the proportion of gabapentin and placebo assigned patients attaining a 50% or greater reduction in seizure frequency from baseline, is plotted against the daily dose of gabapentin administered (X axis).

Although no formal analysis by gender has been performed, estimates of response (Response Ratio) derived from clinical trials (398 men, 307 women) indicate no important gender differences exist. There was no consistent pattern indicating that age had any effect on the response to Neurontin® . There were insufficient numbers of patients of races other than Caucasian of permit a comparison of efficacy among racial groups.

INDICATIONS AND USAGE

Neurontin® (gabapentin) is indicated as adjunctive therapy in the treatment of partial seizures with and without secondary generalization in adults with epilepsy.

CONTRAINDICATIONS

Neurontin® is contraindicated in patients who have demonstrated hypersensitivity to the drug or its ingredients.

WARNINGS

Withdrawal Precipitated Seizure, Status Epilepticus

In the placebo-controlled studies, the incidence of status epilepticus in patients receiving Neurontin® was 0.6% (3 of 543) versus 0.5% in patients receiving placebo (2 of 378).

In the placebo-controlled studies, the incidence of status epilepticus in patients receiving Neurontin® was 0.6% (5 of 543) versus 0.5% in patients receiving placebo (2 of 378). Among the 2074 patients treated with Neurontin® across all studies (controlled and uncontrolled) 31 (1.5%) had status epilepticus. Of these, 14 patients had no prior history of status epilepticus either before treatment or while on other medications. Because adequate historical data are not available, it is impossible to say whether or not treatment with Neurontin® is associated with a higher or lower rate of status epilepticus than would be expected to occur in a similar population not treated with Neurontin®.

Tumorigenic Potential

In standard preclinical *in vivo* lifetime carcinogenicity studies, an unexpectedly high incidence of pancreatic acinar adenocarcinomas was indentified in male, but not female, rats. (See PRECAUTIONS: Carcinogenesis, Mutagenesis, Impairment of Fertility.) The clinical significance of this finding is unknown. Clinical experience during gabapentin's premarketing development provides no direct means to assess its potential for inducing tumors in humans.

In clinical studies comprising 2085 patient-years of exposure, new tumors were reported in 10 patients (2 breast, 3 brain, 2 lung, 1 adrenal, 1 non-Hodgkin's lymphoma, 1 endometrial carcinoma *in situ*), and preexisting tumors worsened in 11 patients (9 brain, 1 breast, 1 prostate) during or up to 2 years following discontinuation of Neurontin®. Without knowledge of the background incidence and recurrence in a similar population not treated with Neurontin®, it is impossible to know whether the incidence seen in this cohort is or is not affected by treatment.

Sudden and Unexplained Deaths

During the course of premarketing development of Neurontin®, 8 sudden and unexplained deaths were recorded among a cohort of 2203 patients treated (2103 patient-years of exposure).

Some of these could represent seizure-related deaths in which the seizure was not observed, e.g., at night. This represents an incidence of 0.0038 deaths per patient-year. Although this rate exceeds that expected in a healthy population matched for age and sex, it is within the range of estimates for the incidence of sudden unexplained deaths in patients with epilepsy not receiving Neurontin® (ranging from 0.0005 for the general population of epileptics, to 0.003 for a clinical trial population similar to that in the Neurontin® program, to 0.005 for patients with refractory epilepsy). Consequently, whether these figures are reassuring or raise further concern depends on comparability of the populations reported upon to the Neurontin® cohort and the accuracy of the estimates provided.

PRECAUTIONS

Information for Patients

Patients should be instructed to take Neurontin® only as prescribed.

Patients should be advised that Neurontin® may cause dizziness, somnolence and other symptoms and signs of CNS depression. Accordingly, they should be advised neither to drive a car nor to operate other complex machinery until they have gained sufficient experience on Neurontin® to gauge whether or not it affects their mental and/or motor performance adversely.

Laboratory Tests

Clinical trials data do not indicate that routine monitoring of clinical laboratory parameters is necessary for the safe use of Neurontin®. The value of monitoring Neurontin® blood concentrations has not been established. Neurontin® may be used in combination with other antiepileptic drugs without concern for alteration of the blood concentrations of gabapentin or of other antiepileptic drugs.

Drug Interactions

Gabapentin is not appreciably metabolized nor does it interfere with the metabolism of commonly coadministered antiepileptic drugs.

The drug interaction data described in this section were obtained from studies involving healthy adults and patients with epilepsy.

Phenytoin: In a single and multiple dose study of Neurontin® (400 mg T.I.D.) in epileptic patients (N=8) maintained on phenytoin monotherapy for at least 2 months, gabapentin had no effect on the steady-state trough plasma concentrations of phenytoin and phenytoin had no effect on gabapentin pharmacokinetics.

Carbamazepine: Steady-state trough plasma carbamazepine and carbamazepine 10, 11 epoxide concentrations were not affected by concomitant gabapentin (400 mg T.I.D.; N=12) administration. Likewise, gabapentin pharmacokinetics were unaltered by carbamazepine administration.

Valproic Acid: The mean steady-state trough serum valproic acid concentrations prior to and during concomitant gabapentin administration (400 mg T.I.D.; N=17) were not different and neither were gabapentin pharmacokinetics parameters affected by valproic acid.

Phenobarbital: Estimates of steady-state pharmacokinetic parameters for phenobarbital or gabapentin (300 mg T.I.D.; N=12) are identical whether the drugs are administered alone or together.

Cimetidine: In the presence of cimetidine at 300 mg Q.I.D. (N=12) the mean apparent oral clearance of gabapentin fell by 14% and creatinine clearance fell by 10%. Thus cimetidine appeared to alter the renal excretion of both gabapentin and creatinine, an endogenous marker of renal function. This small decrease in excretion of gabapentin by cimetidine is not expected to be of clinical importance. The effect of gabapentin on cimetidine was not evaluated.

Oral Contraceptive: Based on AUC and half-life, multiple-dose pharmacokinetic profiles of norethindrone and ethinyl estradiol following administration of tablets containing 2.5 mg of norethindrone acetate and 50 mcg of ethinyl estradiol were similar with and without coadministration of gabapentin (400 mg T.I.D.; N=13). The Cmax of norethindrone was 13% higher when it was coadministered with gabapentin; this interaction is not expected to be of clinical importance.

Antacid (Maalox®): Maalox reduced the bioavailability of gabapentin (N=16) by about 20%. This decrease in bioavailability was about 5% when gabapentin was administered 2 hours after Maalox. It is recommended that gabapentin be taken at least 2 hours following Maalox administration.

Effect of Probenecid: Probenecid is a blocker of renal tubular secretion. Gabapentin pharmacokinetic parameters without and with probenecid were comparable. This indicates that gabapentin does not undergo renal tubular secretion by the pathway that is blocked by probenecid.

Drug/Laboratory Tests Interactions

Because false positive readings were reported with the Ames N-Multistix SG® dipstick test for urinary protein when gabapentin was added to the other antiepileptic drugs, the more specific sulfosalicylic acid precipitation procedure is recommended to determine the presence of urine protein.

Carcinogenesis, Mutagenesis, Impairment of Fertility

Gabapentin was given in the diet to mice at 200, 600, and 2000 mg/kg/day and to rats at 250, 1000, and 2000 mg/kg/day for 2 years. A statistically significant increase in the incidence of pancreatic acinar cell adenomas and carcinomas was found in male rats receiving the high dose; the no-effect dose for the occurrence of carcinomas was 1000 mg/kg/day. Peak plasma concentrations of gabapentin in rats receiving the high dose of 2000 mg/kg were 10 times higher than plasma concentrations in humans receiving 3600 mg per day, and in rats receiving 1000 mg/kg/day peak plasma concentrations were 6.5 times higher than in humans receiving 3600 mg/day. The pancreatic acinar cell carcinomas did not affect survival, did not metastasize and were not locally invasive. Studies to attempt to define a mechanism by which this relatively rare tumor type is occurring are in progress. The relevance of this finding to carcinogenic risk in humans is unclear.

Gabapentin did not demonstrate mutagenic or genotoxic potential in three *in vitro* and two *in vivo* assays. It was negative in the Ames test and the *in vitro* HGPRT forward mutation assay in Chinese hamster lung cells; it did not produce significant increases in chromosomal aberrations in the *in vitro* Chinese hamster lung cell assay; it was negative in the *in vivo* chromosomal aberration assay and in the *in vivo* micronucleus test in Chinese hamster bone marrow.

No adverse effects on fertility or reproduction were observed in rats at doses up to 2000 mg/kg (approximately 5 times the maximum recommended human dose on an mg/m^2 basis).

Pregnancy

Pregnancy Category C: Gabapentin has beeen shown to be fetotoxic in rodents, causing delayed ossification of several bones in the skull, vertebrae, forelimbs, and hindlimbs. These effects occurred when pregnant mice received oral doses of 1000 or 3000 mg/kg/day during the period of organogeneis, or approximately 1 to 4 times the maximum dose of 3600 mg/day given to epileptic patients on a mg/m^2 basis. The no-effect level was 500 mg/kg/day or approximately $^1/_2$ of the human dose on a mg/m^2 basis.

When rats were dosed prior to and during mating, and throughout gestation, pups from all dose groups (500, 1000 and 2000 mg/kg/day) were affected. These doses are equivalent to less than approximately 1 to 5 times the maximum human dose on a mg/m^2 basis. There was an increased incidence of hydroureter and/or hydronephrosis in rats in a study of fertility and general reproductive performance at 2000 mg/kg/day with no effect at 1000 mg/kg/day, in a teratology study at 1500 mg/kg/day with no effect at 300 mg/kg/day, and in a perinatal and postnatal study at all doses studied (500, 1000 and 2000 mg/kg/day). The doses at which the effects occurred are approximately 1 to 5 times the maximum human dose of 3600 mg/day on a mg/m^2 basis; the no-effect doses were approximately 3 times (Fertility and General Reproductive Performance study) and approximately equal to (Teratogenicity study) the maximum human dose on a mg/m^2 basis. Other than hydroureter and hydronephrosis, the etiologies of which are unclear, the incidence of malformations was not increased compared to controls in offspring of mice, rats, or rabbits given doses up to 50 times (mice), 30 times (rats), and 25 times (rabbits) the human daily dose on a mg/kg basis, or 4 times (mice), 5 times (rats), or 8 times (rabbits) the human daily dose on a mg/m^2 basis.

In a teratology study in rabbits, an increased incidence of postimplantation fetal loss occurred in dams exposed to 60, 300 and 1500 mg/kg/day, or less than approximately $^1/_4$ to 8 times the maximum human dose on a mg/m^2 basis. There are no adequate and well-controlled studies in pregnant women. Because animal reproduction studies are not always predictive of human response, this drug should be used during pregnancy only if the potential benefit justifies the potential risk to the fetus.

Use in Nursing Mothers

It is not known if gabapentin is excreted in human milk and the effect on the nursing infant is unknown. However, because many drugs are excreted in human milk, Neurontin® should be used in women who are nursing only if the benefits clearly outweigh the risks.

Pediatric Use
Safety and effectiveness in pediatric patients below the age of 12 years have not been established.

Geriatric Use
No systematic studies in geriatric patients have been conducted. Adverse clinical events reported among 59 Neurontin® exposed patients over age 65 did not differ in kind from those reported for younger individuals. The small number of older individuals evaluated, however, limits the strength of any conclusions reached about the influence, if any, of age on the kind and incidence of adverse events or laboratory abnormality associated with the use of Neurontin®.

Because Neurontin® is eliminated primarily by renal excretion, the dose of Neurontin® should be adjusted as noted in DOSAGE AND ADMINISTRATION (Table 2) for elderly patients with compromised renal function. Creatinine clearance is difficult to measure in outpatients and serum creatinine may be reduced in the elderly because of decreased muscle mass. Creatinine clearance (C_{Cr}) can be reasonably well estimated using the equation of Cockcroft and Gault:

for females $C_{Cr} = (0.85)(140-\text{age})(\text{wt})/[(72)(S_{Cr})]$

for males $C_{Cr} = (140-\text{age})(\text{wt})/[(72)(S_{Cr})]$

where age is in years, wt is in kilograms and S_{Cr} is serum creatinine in mg/dL.

ADVERSE REACTIONS

The most commonly observed adverse events associated with the use of Neurontin® in combination with other antiepileptic drugs, not seen at an equivalent frequency among placebo-treated patients, were somnolence, dizziness, ataxia, fatique, and nystagmus.

Approximately 7% of the 2074 individuals who received Neurontin® in premarketing clinical trials discontinued treatment because of an adverse event. The adverse events most commonly associated with withdrawal were somnolence (1.2%), ataxia (0.8%), fatique (0.6%), nausea and/or vomiting (0.6%), and dizziness (0.6%).

Incidence in Controlled Clinical Trials
Table 1 lists treatment-emergent signs and symptoms that occurred in at least 1% of Neurontin®-treated patients with epilepsy participating in placebo-controlled trials and were numerically more common in the Neurontin® group. In these studies, either Neurontin® or placebo was added to the patient's current antiepileptic drug therapy. Adverse events were usually mild to moderate in intensity.

The prescriber should be aware that these figures, obtained when Neurontin® was added to concurrent antiepileptic drug therapy, cannot be used to predict the frequency of adverse events in the course of usual medical practice where patient characteristics and other factors may differ from those prevailing during clinical studies. Similarly, the cited frequences cannot be directly compared with figures obtained from other clinical investigations involving different treatments, uses, or investigators. An inspection of these frequencies, however, does provide the prescribing physician with one basis to estimate the relative contribution of drug and nondrug factors to the adverse event incidences in the population studied.

TABLE 1. Treatment-Emergent Adverse Event Incidence in Controlled Add-On Trials (Events in at least 1% of Neurontin patients and numerically more frequent than in the placebo group)

Body System/ Adverse Event	Neurontin®[a] N=543 %	Placebo[a] N=378 %
Body As A Whole		
Fatique	11.0	5.0
Weight Increase	2.9	1.6
Back Pain	1.8	0.5
Peripheral Edema	1.7	0.5
Cardiovascular		
Vasodilatation	1.1	0.3
Digestive System		
Dyspepsia	2.2	0.5
Mouth or Throat Dry	1.7	0.5
Constipation	1.5	0.8
Dental Abnormalities	1.5	0.3
Increased Appetite	1.1	0.8
Hematologic and Lymphatic Systems		
Leukopenia	1.1	0.5
Musculoskeletal System		
Myalgia	2.0	1.9
Fracture	1.1	0.8
Nervous System		
Somnolence	19.3	8.7
Dizziness	17.1	6.9
Ataxia	12.5	5.6
Nystagmus	8.3	4.0
Tremor	6.8	3.2
Nervousness	2.4	1.9
Dysarthria	2.4	0.5
Amnesia	2.2	0.0
Depression	1.8	1.1
Thinking Abnormal	1.7	1.3
Twitching	1.3	0.5
Coordination Abnormal	1.1	0.3
Respiratory System		
Rhinitis	4.1	3.7
Pharyngitis	2.8	1.6
Coughing	1.8	1.3
Skin and Appendages		
Abrasion	1.3	0.0
Pruritus	1.3	0.5
Urogenital System		
Impotence	1.5	1.1
Special Senses		
Diplopia	5.9	1.9
Amblyopia[b]	4.2	1.1
Laboratory Deviations		
WBC Decreased	1.1	0.5

[a] Plus background antiepileptic drug therapy
[b] Amblyopia was often described as blurred vision.

Other events in more than 1% of patients but equally or more frequent in the placebo group included: headache, viral infection, fever, nausea and/or vomiting, abdominal pain, diarrhea, convulsions, confusion, insomnia, emotional lability, rash, acne.

Among the treatment-emergent adverse events occurring at an incidence of at least 10% of Neurontin-treated patients, somnolence and ataxia appeared to exhibit a positive dose-response relationship.

The overall incidence of adverse events and the types of adverse events seen were similar among men and women treated with Neurontin®. The incidence of adverse events increased slightly with increasing age in patients treated with either Neurontin® or placebo. Because only 3% of patients (28/921) in placebo-controlled studies were identified as nonwhite (black or other), there are insufficient data to support a statement regarding the distribution of adverse events by race.

Other Adverse Events Observed During All Clinical Trials
Neurontin® has been administered to 2074 individuals during all clinical trials, only some of which were placebo-controlled. During these trials, all adverse events were recorded by the clinical investigators using terminology of their own choosing. To provide a meaningful estimate of the proportion of individuals having adverse events, similar types of events were grouped into a smaller number of standardized categories using modified COSTART dictionary terminology. These categories are used in the listing below. The frequencies presented represent the proportion of the 2074 individuals exposed to Neurontin® who experienced an event of the type cited on at least one occasion while receiving Neurontin®. All reported events are included except those already listed in the previous table, those too general to be informative, and those not reasonably associated with the use of the drug.

Events are further classified within body system categories and enumerated in order of decreasing frequency using the following definitions: frequent adverse events are defined as those occurring in at least 1/100 patients; infrequent adverse events are those occurring in 1/100 to 1/1000 patients; rare events are those occurring in fewer than 1/1000 patients.

Body As A Whole: *Frequent:* asthenia, malaise, face edema; *Infrequent:* allergy, generalized edema, weight decrease, chill; *Rare:* strange feelings, lassitude, alcohol intolerance, hangover effect.

Cardiovascular System: *Frequent:* hypertension; *Infrequent:* hypotension, angina pectoris, peripheral vascular disorder, palpitation, tachycardia, migraine, murmur; *Rare:* atrial fibrillation, heart failure, thrombophlebitis, deep thrombophlebitis, myocardial infarction, cerebrovascular accident, pulmonary thrombosis, ventricular extrasystoles, bradycardia, premature atrial contraction, pericardial rub, heart block, pulmonary embolus, hyperlipidemia, hypercholesterolemia, pericardial effusion, pericarditis.

Digestive System: *Frequent:* anorexia, flatulence, gingivitis; *Infrequent:* glossitis, gum hemorrhage, thirst, stomatitis, increased salivation, gastroenteritis, hemorrhoids, bloody stools, fecal incontinence, hepatomegaly; *Rare:* dysphagia, eructation, pancreatitis, peptic ulcer, colitis, blisters in mouth, tooth discolor, perleche, salivary gland enlarged, lip hemorrhage, esophagitis, hiatal hernia, hematemesis, proctitis, irritable bowel syndrome, rectal hemorrhage, esophageal spasm.

Endocrine System: ***Rate:*** hyperthyroid, hypothyroid, goiter, hypoestrogen, ovarian failure, epididymitis, swollen testicle, cushingoid appearance.

Hematologic and Lymphatic System: *Frequent:* purpura most often described as bruises resulting from physical trauma; *Infrequent:* anemia, thrombocytopenia, lymphadenopathy; *Rare:* WBC count increased, lymphocytosis, non-Hodgkin's lymphoma, bleeding time increased.

Musculoskeletal System: *Frequent:* arthralgia: *Infrequent:* tendinitis, arthritis, joint stiffness, joint swelling, positive Romberg test; *Rare:* costochondritis, osteoporosis, bursitis, contracture.

Nervous System: *Frequent:* vertigo, hyperkinesia, paresthesia, decreased or absent reflexes, increased reflexes, anxiety, hostility; *Infrequent:* CNS tumors, syncope, dreaming abnormal, aphasia, hypesthesia, intracranial hemorrhage, hypotonia, dysesthesia, paresis, dystonia, hemiplegia, facial paralysis, stupor, cerebellar dysfunction, positive Babinski sign, decreased position sense, subdural hematoma, apathy, hallucination, decrease or loss of libido, agitation, paranoia, depersonalization, euphoria, feeling high, doped-up sensation, suicidal, psychosis; *Rare:* choreoathetosis, orofacial dyskinesia, encephalopathy, nerve palsy, personality disorder, increased libido, subdued temperament, apraxia, fine motor control disorder, meningismus, local myoclonus, hyperesthesia, hypokinesia, mania, neurosis, hysteria, antisocial reaction, suicide gesture.

Respiratory System: *Frequent:* pneumonia; *Infrequent:* epistaxis, dyspnea, apnea; *Rare:* mucositis, aspiration pneumonia, hyperventilation, hiccup, laryngitis, nasal obstruction, snoring, bronchospasm, hypoventilation, lung edema.

Dermatological: *Infrequent:* alopecia, eczema, dry skin, increased sweating, urticaria, hirsutism, seborrhea, cyst, herpes simplex; *Rare:* herpes zoster, skin discolor skin papules photosensitive reaction, leg ulcer, scalp seborrhea, psoriasis, desquamation, maceration, skin nodules, subcutaneous nodule, melanosis, skin necrosis, local swelling.

Urogenital System: *Infrequent:* hematuria, dysuria, urination frequency, cystitis urinary retention, urinary incontinence, vaginal hemorrhage, amenorrhea, dysmenorrhea, menorrhagia, breast cancer, unable to climax, ejaculation abnormal; *Rare:* kidney pain, leukorrhea, pruritus genital, renal stone, acute renal failure, anuria, glycosuria, nephrosis, nocturia, pyuria, urination urgency, vaginal pain, breast pain, testicle pain.

Special Senses: *Frequent:* abnormal vision; *Infrequent:* cataract, conjunctivitis, eyes dry, eye pain, visual field defect, photophobia, bilateral or unilateral ptosis, eye hemorrhage, hordeolum, hearing loss, earache, tinnitus, inner ear infection, otitis, taste loss, unusual taste, eye twitching, ear fullness; *Rare:* eye itching, abnormal accommodation, perforated ear drum, sensitivity to noise, eye focusing problem, watery eyes, retinopathy, glaucoma, iritis, corneal disorders, lacrimal dysfunction, degenerative eye changes, blindness, retinal degeneration, miosis, chorioetinitis, strabismus, eustachian tube dysfunction, labyrinthitis, otitis externa, odd smell.

Postmarketing and Other Experience
In addition to the adverse experiences reported during clinical testing of Neurontin, the following adverse experiences have been reported in patients receiving marketed Neurontin. These adverse experiences have not been listed above and data are insufficient to support an estimate of their incidence or to establish causation. The listing is alphabetized: angioedema, blood glucose fluctuation, erythema multiforme, elevated liver function tests, fever, jaundice, Stevens-Johnson syndrome.

DRUG ABUSE AND DEPENDENCE

The abuse and dependence potential of Neurontin® has not been evaluated in human studies.

OVERDOSAGE

A lethal dose of gabapentin was not identified in mice and rats receiving single oral doses as high as 8000 mg/kg. Signs of acute toxicity in animals included ataxia, labored breathing, ptosis, sedation, hypoactivity, or excitation.

Acute oral overdoses of Neurontin® up to 49 grams have been reported. In these cases, double vision, slurred speech, drowsiness, lethargy and diarrhea were observed. All patients recovered with supportive care.

Gabapentin can be removed by hemodialysis. Although hemodialysis has not been performed in the few overdose cases reported, it may be indicated by the patient's clinical state or in patients with significant renal impairment.

DOSAGE AND ADMINISTRATION

Neurontin® is recommended for add-on therapy in patients over 12 years of age. Evidence bearing on its safety and effectiveness in pediatric patients below the age of 12 is not available.

Neurontin® is given orally with or without food.

The effective dose of Neurontin® is 900 to 1800 mg/day and given in divided doses (three times a day) using 300– or 400–mg capsules. Titration to an effective dose can take place rapidly, over a few days, giving 300 mg on Day 1, 300

Continued on next page

This product information was prepared in June 1998. On these and other Parke-Davis Products, information may be obtained by addressing PARKE-DAVIS, Division of Warner-Lambert Company, Morris Plains, New Jersey 07950.

Neurontin—Cont.

mg twice a day on Day 2, and 300 mg three times a day on Day 3. To minimize potential side effects, especially somnolence, dizziness, fatigue, and ataxia, the first dose on Day 1 may be administered at bedtime. If necessary, the dose may be increased using 300- or 400-mg capsules three times a day up to 1800 mg/day. Dosages up to 2400 mg/day have been well tolerated in long-term clinical studies. Doses of 3600 mg/day have also been administered to a small number of patients for a relatively short duration, and have been well tolerated. The maximum time between doses in the T.I.D. schedule should not exceed 12 hours.

It is not necessary to monitor gabapentin plasma concentrations to optimize Neurontin® therapy. Further, because there are no significant pharmacokinetic interactions among Neurontin® and other commonly used antiepileptic drugs, the addition of Neurontin® does not alter the plasma levels of these drugs appreciably.

If Neurontin® is discontinued and/or alternate anticonvulsant medication is added to the therapy, this should be done gradually over a minimum of 1 week.

Dosage adjustment in patients with compromised renal function or undergoing hemodialysis is recommended as follows:

TABLE 2. Neurontin® Dosage Based on Renal Function

Renal Function Creatinine Clearance (mL/min)	Total Daily Dose (mg/day)	Dose Regimen (mg)
<60	1200	400 T.I.D
30—60	600	300 B.I.D
15—30	300	300 Q.D
<15	150	300 Q.O.D.[a]
Hemodialysis	—	200–300[b]

[a] Every other day
[b] Loading dose of 300 to 400 mg in patients who have never received Neurontin®, then 200 to 300 mg Neurontin® following each 4 hours of hemodialysis.

HOW SUPPLIED

Neurontin® (gabapentin capsules) are supplied as follows:
100-mg capsules;
White hard gelatin capsules printed with "PD" on one side and "Neurontin®/100 mg" on the other; available in:
Bottles of 100: N 0071-0803-24
Unit dose 50's: N 0071-0803-40
300-mg capsules;
Yellow hard gelatin capsules printed with "PD" on one side and "Neurontin®/300 mg" on the other; available in:
Bottles of 100: N 0071-0805-24
Unit dose 50's: N 0071-0805-40
400-mg capsules;
Orange hard gelatin capsules printed with "PD" on one side and "Neurontin®/400 mg" on the other; available in:
Bottles of 100: N 0071-0806-24
Unit dose 50's: N 0071-0806-40
Storage
Store at controlled room temperature 15°–30°C (59°–86°F).
Rx only
Revised February 1998   0803G024
©1998
Shown in Product Identification Guide, page 329

NITROSTAT®
(Nitroglycerin Tablets, USP)   ℞

DESCRIPTION

Nitrostat is a stabilized sublingual nitroglycerin tablet manufactured by a process which prevents the migration of nitroglycerin by adding the nonvolatile fixing agent polyethylene glycol 3350. This stabilized formulation has been shown to be more stable and more uniform than conventional molded tablets. Nitrostat tablets contain 0.3 mg (1/200 grain), 0.4 mg (1/150 grain) and 0.6 mg (1/100 grain) nitroglycerin. Also contains lactose, NF; polyethylene glycol 3350, NF; sucrose, NF.
Nitroglycerin, an organic nitrate, is a vasodilating agent.

CLINICAL PHARMACOLOGY

Relaxation of vascular smooth muscle is the principal pharmacologic action of nitroglycerin. The mechanism by which nitroglycerin produces relaxation of smooth muscle is unknown. Although venous effects predominate, nitroglycerin produces, in a dose-related manner, dilation of both arterial and venous beds. Dilation of the postcapillary vessels, including large veins, promotes peripheral pooling of blood and decreases venous return to the heart, reducing left ventricular end-diastolic pressure (preload). Arteriolar relaxation reduces systemic vascular resistance and arterial pressure (afterload). Myocardial oxygen consumption or demand (as measured by the pressure-rate product, tension-time index and stroke-work index) is decreased by both the arterial and venous effects of nitroglycerin, and a more favorable supply-demand ratio can be achieved.

Nitroglycerin also dilates large epicardial coronary arteries; however, the extent to which this effect contributes to the relief of exertional angina is unclear.

Therapeutic doses of nitroglycerin may reduce systolic, diastolic and mean arterial blood pressure. Effective coronary perfusion pressure is usually maintained, but can be compromised if blood pressure falls excessively or increased heart rate decreases diastolic filling time.

Elevated central venous and pulmonary capillary wedge pressures, pulmonary vascular resistance and systemic vascular resistance are also reduced by nitroglycerin therapy. Heart rate is usually slightly increased, presumably a reflex response to the fall in blood pressure. Cardiac index may be increased, decreased, or unchanged. Patients with elevated left ventricular filling pressure and systemic vascular resistance values in conjunction with a depressed cardiac index are likely to experience an improvement in cardiac index. On the other hand, when filling pressures and cardiac index are normal, cardiac index may be slightly reduced by intravenous nitroglycerin.

Mechanism of Action
Nitroglycerin forms free radical nitric oxide (NO) which activates guanylate cyclase, resulting in an increase of guanosine 3'5' monophosphate (cyclic GMP) in smooth muscle and other tissues. This eventually leads to dephosphorylation of the light chain of myosin, which regulates the contractile state in smooth muscle, resulting in vasodilation.

Pharmacokinetics and Metabolism
Nitroglycerin is rapidly absorbed following sublingual administration. Its onset of action is approximately one to three minutes. Significant pharmacologic effects are present for 30 to 60 minutes following administration by the above route.

Nitroglycerin is rapidly metabolized to dinitrates and mononitrates, with a short half-life, estimated at 1 to 4 minutes. A liver reductase enzyme is of primary importance in the metabolism of nitroglycerin to glycerol nitrate metabolites and organic nitrate. Two active major metabolites 1,2- and 1,3-dinitroglycerols are less potent vasodilators and have longer half-lives than the parent compound. Dinitrates are metabolized to mononitrates and ultimately glycerol. The monohydrate is not considered biologically active with respect to cardiovascular effects.

At plasma concentrations of between 50 and 500 ng/mL, the binding of nitroglycerin to plasma proteins is approximately 60%, while that of 1,2 dinitroglycerin and 1,3 dinitroglycerin is 60% and 30%, respectively. The activity and half-life of 1,2 dinitroglycerin and 1,3 dinitroglycerin are not well characterized. The mononitrate is not active.

INDICATIONS AND USAGE

Nitroglycerin is indicated for the acute relief of an attack or prophylaxis of angina pectoris due to coronary artery disease.

CONTRAINDICATIONS

Sublingual nitroglycerin therapy is contraindicated in patients with early myocardial infarction, severe anemia, increased intracranial pressure and those with a known hypersensitivity to nitroglycerin.

WARNINGS

The use of nitroglycerin during the early course of acute myocardial infarction requires particular attention to hemodynamic monitoring and clinical status.

PRECAUTIONS

General: Only the smallest dose required for effective relief of the acute anginal attack should be used. Excessive use may lead to the development of tolerance. Nitrostat tablets are intended for sublingual or buccal administration and should not be swallowed.

Severe hypotension, particularly with upright posture, may occur even with small doses of nitroglycerin. The drug should be used cautiously in patients with volume depletion or low systolic blood pressure.

Paradoxical bradycardia and increased angina pectoris may accompany nitroglycerin-induced hypotension.

Nitrate therapy may aggravate angina caused by hypertrophic cardiomyopathy.

Tolerance to the vascular and antianginal effects of nitroglycerin and cross-tolerance to other nitrates and nitrites may occur.

The drug should be discontinued if blurring of vision or drying of the mouth occurs. Excessive dosage of nitroglycerin may produce severe headaches.

Information for Patients: If possible, patients should sit down when taking Nitrostat tablets. This eliminates the possibility of falling due to lightheadedness or dizziness.

Nitroglycerin may produce a burning or tingling sensation when administered sublingually; however, the ability to produce a burning or tingling sensation should not be considered a reliable method for determining the potency of the tablets.

Nitroglycerin should be kept in the original glass container, tightly capped. The cotton should be discarded once the bottle is opened.

Drug Interactions: Concomitant use of nitrates and alcohol may cause hypotension. Patients receiving antihypertensive drugs, beta-adrenergic blockers or phenothiazines and nitrates should be observed for possible additive hypotensive effects. Marked orthostatic hypotension has been reported when calcium channel blockers and organic nitrates were used concomitantly. Dose adjustment of either class of agent may be necessary.

Aspirin may decrease the clearance and enhance the hemodynamic effects of sublingual nitroglycerin.

A decrease in the therapeutic effect of sublingual nitroglycerin may result from use of long-acting nitrates.

Drug/Laboratory Test Interactions: Nitrates may interfere with the Zlatkis-Zak color reaction causing a false report of decreased serum cholesterol.

Carcinogenesis, Mutagenesis, Impairment of Fertility: No long-term studies in animals were performed to evaluate the carcinogenic potential of nitroglycerin.

Pregnancy Category C: Animal reproduction studies have not been conducted with nitroglycerin. It is also not known whether nitroglycerin can cause fetal harm when administered to a pregnant woman or can affect reproduction capacity. Nitroglycerin should be given to a pregnant woman only if clearly needed.

Nursing Mother: It is not known whether nitroglycerin is excreted in human milk. Because many drugs are excreted in human milk, caution should be exercised when intravenous nitroglycerin is administered to a nursing woman.

Pediatric Use: The safety and effectiveness of nitroglycerin in pediatric patients have not been established.

ADVERSE REACTIONS

Headache which may be severe and persistent may occur immediately after use. Vertigo, weakness, palpitation and other manifestations of postural hypotension may develop occasionally, particularly in erect, immobile patients. Marked sensitivity to the hypotensive effects of nitrates (manifested by nausea, vomiting, weakness, diaphoresis, pallor and collapse) may occur at therapeutic doses. Syncope due to nitrate vasodilation has been reported. Flushing, drug rash, and exfoliative dermatitis have been reported in patients receiving nitrate therapy.

OVERDOSAGE

Nitrate overdose may result in: severe hypotension, tachycardia, bradycardia, heart block, palpitation, death due to circulatory collapse, syncope, persistent throbbing headache, vertigo, visual disturbance, increased intracranial pressure, paralysis and coma followed by convulsions, flushing and diaphoresis, nausea and vomiting, colic and diarrhea, dyspnea and methemoglobinemia.

Since hypotension from nitroglycerin overdosage results from venodilation and arterial hypovolemia, therapy should be directed toward central volume expansion. Elevation of extremities may be sufficient, but intravenous infusion may also be necessary. Use of arterial vasoconstrictors may do more harm than good. Management of nitroglycerin overdose in patients with renal disease or congestive heart failure may require invasive monitoring.

If methemoglobinemia is present, intravenous administration of methylene blue 1–2 mg/kg of body weight may be required.

DOSAGE AND ADMINISTRATION

One tablet should be dissolved under the tongue or in the buccal pouch at the first sign of an acute anginal attack. The dose may be repeated approximately every five minutes, until relief is obtained. If the pain persists after a total of 3 tablets in a 15-minute period, prompt medical attention is recommended. Nitrostat may be used prophylactically 5 to 10 minutes prior to engaging in activities which might precipitate an acute attack.

During administration the patient should rest, preferably in the sitting position.

No dosage adjustment is required in patients with renal failure.

HOW SUPPLIED

Nitrostat is supplied in three strengths in bottles containing 100 tablets each, with color-coded labels, and in color-coded Patient Convenience Packages of four bottles of 25 tablets each.

0.3 mg (1/200 grain):	N 0071-0569-24—Bottle of 100 tablets
0.4 mg (1/150 grain):	N 0071-0570-13—Convenience Package
	N 0071-0570-24—Bottle of 100 tablets
0.6 mg (1/100 grain):	N 0071-0571-24—Bottle of 100 tablets

OMNICEF®   ℞
(Cefdinir) Capsules
[omnē-sĕf]

OMNICEF®
(Cefdinir) for Oral Suspension

DESCRIPTION

OMNICEF® (cefdinir) Capsules and OMNICEF® (cefdinir) for Oral Suspension contain the active ingredient cefdinir, an extended-spectrum, semisynthetic cephalosporin, for oral administration. Chemically, cefdinir is [6R-[6α,7β (Z)]]-7-[[(2-amino-4-thiazolyl)-(hydroxyimino)acetyl]amino]-3-ethenyl-8-oxo-5-thia-1-azabicyclo[4.2.0]oct-2-ene-2-carboxylic acid. Cefdinir is a white to slightly brownish-yellow solid. It is slightly soluble in dilute hydrochloric acid and sparingly soluble in 0.1 M pH 7.0 phosphate buffer. The empirical formula is $C_{14}H_{13}N_5O_5S_2$ and the molecular weight is 395.42. Cefdinir has the structural formula shown below:

OMNICEF Capsules contain 300 mg cefdinir and the following inactive ingredients: carboxymethylcellulose calcium, NF; polyoxyl 40 stearate, NF; magnesium stearate, NF; and silicon dioxide, NF. The capsule shells contain FD&C Blue #1; FD&C Red #40; D&C Red #28; titanium dioxide, NF; gelatin, NF; and sodium lauryl sulfate, NF.
OMNICEF for Oral Suspension, after reconstitution, contains 125 mg cefdinir per 5 mL and the following inactive ingredients: sucrose, NF; citric acid, USP; sodium citrate, USP; sodium benzoate, NF; xanthan gum, NF; guar gum, NF; artificial strawberry and cream flavors; silicon dioxide, NF; and magnesium stearate, NF.

CLINICAL PHARMACOLOGY
Pharmacokinetics and Drug Metabolism
Absorption:
Oral Bioavailability: Maximal plasma cefdinir concentrations occur 2 to 4 hours postdose following capsule or suspension administration. Plasma cefdinir concentrations increase with dose, but the increases are less than dose-proportional from 300 mg (7 mg/kg) to 600 mg (14 mg/kg). Following administration of suspension to healthy adults, cefdinir bioavailability is 120% relative to capsules. Estimated bioavailability of cefdinir capsules is 21% following administration of a 300 mg capsule dose, and 16% following administration of a 600 mg capsule dose. Estimated absolute bioavailability of cefdinir suspension is 25%.
Effect of Food: Although the rate (C_{max}) and extent (AUC) of cefdinir absorption from the capsules are reduced by 16% and 10%, respectively, when given with a high-fat meal, the magnitude of these reductions is not likely to be clinically significant. Therefore, cefdinir may be taken without regard to food.
Cefdinir Capsules: Cefdinir plasma concentrations and pharmacokinetic parameter values following administration of single 300- and 600-mg oral doses of cefdinir to adult subjects are presented in the following table:
[See first table above]
Cefdinir Suspension: Cefdinir plasma concentrations and pharmacokinetic parameter values following administration of single 7- and 14-mg/kg oral doses of cefdinir to pediatric subjects (age 6 months–12 years) are presented in the following table:
[See second table above]
Multiple Dosing: Cefdinir does not accumulate in plasma following once- or twice-daily administration to subjects with normal renal function.
Distribution: The mean volume of distribution (Vd_{area}) of cefdinir in adult subjects is 0.35 L/kg (±0.29); in pediatric subjects (age 6 months–12 years), cefdinir Vd_{area} is 0.67 L/kg (±0.38) Cefdinir is 60% to 70% bound to plasma proteins in both adult and pediatric subjects; binding is independent of concentration.
Skin Blister: In adult subjects, median (range) maximal blister fluid cefdinir concentrations of 0.65 (0.33–1.1) and 1.1 (0.49–1.9) μg/mL were observed 4 to 5 hours following administration of 300- and 600-mg doses, respectively.

Mean (±SD) Plasma Cedfinir Pharmacokinetic Parameter Values Following Administration of Capsules to Adult Subjects			
Dose	C_{max} (μg/mL)	t_{max} (hr)	AUC (μg•hr/mL)
300 mg	1.60 (0.55)	2.9 (0.89)	7.05 (2.17)
600 mg	2.87 (1.01)	3.0 (0.66)	11.1 (3.87)

Mean (±SD) Plasma Cedfinir Pharmacokinetic Parameter Values Following Administration of Suspension to Pediatric Subjects			
Dose	C_{max} (μg/mL)	t_{max} (hr)	AUC (μg•hr/mL)
7 mg/kg	2.30 (0.65)	2.2 (0.6)	8.31 (2.50)
14 mg/kg	3.86 (0.62)	1.8 (0.4)	13.4 (2.64)

Mean (±SD) blister C_{max} and AUC (0–∞) values were 48% (±13) and 91% (±18) of corresponding plasma values.
Tonsil Tissue: In adult patients undergoing elective tonsillectomy, respective median tonsil tissue cefdinir concentrations 4 hours after administration of single 300- and 600-mg doses were 0.25 (0.22–0.46) and 0.36 (0.22–0.80) μg/g. Mean tonsil tissue concentrations were 24% (±8) of corresponding plasma concentrations.
Sinus Tissue: In adult patients undergoing elective maxillary and ethmoid sinus surgery, respective median sinus tissue cefdinir concentrations 4 hours after administration of single 300- and 600-mg doses were <0.12 (<0.12–0.46) and 0.21 (<0.12–2.0) μg/g. Mean sinus tissue concentrations were 16% (±20) of corresponding plasma concentrations.
Lung Tissue: In adult patients undergoing diagnostic bronchoscopy, respective median bronchial mucosa cefdinir concentrations 4 hours after administration of single 300- and 600-mg doses were 0.78 (<0.06-1.33) and 1.14 (<0.06-1.92) μg/mL, and were 31% (±18) of corresponding plasma concentrations. Respective median epithelial lining fluid concentrations were 0.29 (<0.3-4.73) and 0.49 (<0.3-0.59) μg/mL, and were 35% (±83) of corresponding plasma concentrations.
Middle Ear Fluid: In 14 pediatric patients with acute bacterial otitis media, respective median middle ear fluid cefdinir concentrations 3 hours after administration of single 7- and 14-mg/kg doses were 0.21 (<0.09-0.94) and 0.72 (0.14-1.42) μg/mL. Mean middle ear fluid concentrations were 15% (±15) of corresponding plasma concentrations.
CSF: Data on cefdinir penetration into human cerebrospinal fluid are not available.
Metabolism and Excretion: Cefdinir is not appreciably metabolized. Activity is primarily due to parent drug. Cefdinir is eliminated principally via renal excretion with a mean plasma elimination half-life ($t_{1/2}$) of 1.7 (±0.6) hours. In healthy subjects with normal renal function, renal clearance is 2.0 (±1.0) mL/min/kg, and apparent oral clearance is 11.6 (±6.0) and 15.5 (±5.4) mL/min/kg following doses of 300- and 600-mg, respectively.
Mean percent of dose recovered unchanged in the urine following 300- and 600-mg doses is 18.4% (±6.4) and 11.6% (±4.6), respectively. Cefdinir clearance is reduced in patients with renal dysfunction (see **Special Populations:** *Patients with Renal Insufficiency*).
Because renal excretion is the predominant pathway of elimination, dosage should be adjusted in patients with markedly compromised renal function or who are undergoing hemodialysis (see **DOSAGE AND ADMINISTRATION**).
Special Populations:
Patients with Renal Insufficiency: Cefdinir pharmacokinetics were investigated in 21 adult subjects with varying degrees of renal function. Decreases in cefdinir elimination rate, apparent oral clearance (CL/F), and renal clearance were approximately proportional to the reduction in creatinine clearance (CL_{cr}). As a result, plasma cefdinir concentrations were higher and persisted longer in subjects with renal impairment than in those without renal impairment. In subjects with CL_{cr} between 30 and 60 mL/min, C_{max} and $t_{1/2}$ increased by approximately 2-fold and AUC by approximately 3-fold. In subjects with CL_{cr} <30 mL/min, C_{max} increased by approximately 2-fold, $t_{1/2}$ by approximately 5-fold, and AUC by approximately 6-fold. Dosage adjustment is recommended in patients with markedly compromised renal function (creatinine clearance <30 mL/min; see **DOSAGE AND ADMINISTRATION**).
Hemodialysis: Cefdinir pharmacokinetics were studied in 8 adult subjects undergoing hemodialysis. Dialysis (4 hours duration) removed 63% of cefdinir from the body and reduced apparent elimination $t_{1/2}$ from 16 (±3.5) to 3.2 (±1.2) hours. Dosage adjustment is recommended in this patient population (see **DOSAGE AND ADMINISTRATION**).

Hepatic Disease: Because cefdinir is predominantly renally eliminated and not appreciably metabolized, studies in patients with hepatic impairment were not conducted. It is not expected that dosage adjustment will be required in this population.
Geriatric Patients: The effect of age on cefdinir pharmacokinetics after a single 300-mg dose was evaluated in 32 subjects 19 to 91 years of age. Systemic exposure to cefdinir was substantially increased in older subjects (N=16), C_{max} by 44% and AUC by 86%. This increase was due to a reduction in cefdinir clearance. The apparent volume of distribution was also reduced, thus no appreciable alterations in apparent elimination $t_{1/2}$ were observed (elderly: 2.2 ± 0.6 hours vs young: 1.8 ± 0.4 hours). Since cefdinir clearance has been shown to be primarily related to changes in renal function rather than age, elderly patients do not require dosage adjustment unless they have markedly compromised renal function (creatinine clearance <30 mL/min, see *Patients with Renal Insufficiency*, above).
Gender and Race: The results of a meta-analysis of clinical pharmacokinetics (N=217) indicated no significant impact of either gender or race on cefdinir pharmacokinetics
Microbiology
As with other cephalosporins, bactericidal activity of cefdinir results from inhibition of cell wall synthesis. Cefdinir is stable in the presence of some, but not all, β-lactamase enzymes. As a result, many organisms resistant to penicillins and some cephalosporins are susceptible to cefdinir.
Cefdinir has been shown to be active against most strains of the following microorganisms, both *in vitro* and in clinical infections as described in the **INDICATIONS AND USAGE**.
Aerobic Gram-Positive Microorganisms:
Staphylococcus aureus (including β-lactamase producing strains)
NOTE: Cefdinir is inactive against methicillin-resistant staphylococci.
Streptococcus pneumoniae (penicillin-susceptible strains only)
Streptococcus pyogenes
Aerobic Gram-Negative Microorganisms:
Haemophilus influenzae (including β-lactamase producing strains)
Haemophilus parainfluenzae (including β-lactamase producing strains)
Moraxella catarrhalis (including β-lactamase producing strains)
The following *in vitro* data are available, **but their clinical significance is unknown.**
Cefdinir exhibits *in vitro* minimum inhibitory concentrations (MICs) of 1 μg/mL or less against (≥90%) strains of the following microorganisms; however, the safety and effectiveness of cefdinir in treating clinical infections due to these microorganisms have not been established in adequate and well-controlled clinical trials.
Aerobic Gram-Positive Microorganisms:
Staphylococcus epidermidis (methicillin-susceptible strains only)
Streptococcus agalactiae
Viridans group streptococci

NOTE: Cefdinir is inactive against *Enterococcus* and methicillin-resistant *Staphylococcus* species.

Continued on next page

This product information was prepared in June 1998. On these and other Parke-Davis Products, information may be obtained by addressing PARKE-DAVIS, Division of Warner-Lambert Company, Morris Plains, New Jersey 07950.

Omnicef—Cont.

Aerobic Gram-Negative Microorganisms:
Citrobacter diversus
Escherichia coli
Klebsiella pneumoniae
Proteus mirabilis
NOTE: Cefdinir is inactive against *Pseudomonas* and *Enterobacter* species.
Susceptibility Tests:

Dilution Techniques: Quantitative methods are used to determine antimicrobial minimum inhibitory concentrations (MICs). These MICs provide estimates of the susceptibility of bacteria to antimicrobial compounds. The MICs should be determined using a standardized procedure. Standardized procedures are based on a dilution method[1] (broth or agar) or equivalent with standardized inoculum concentrations and standardized concentrations of cefdinir powder. The MIC values should be interpreted according to the following criteria:

For organisms other than *Haemophilus* spp. and *Streptococcus* spp:

MIC (µg/mL)	Interpretation
≤1	Susceptible (S)
2	Intermediate (I)
≥4	Resistant (R)

For *Haemophilus* spp:[a]

MIC (µg/mL)	Interpretation[b]
≤1	Susceptible (S)

[a] These interpretive standards are applicable only to broth microdilution susceptibility tests with *Haemophilus* spp. using Haemophilus Test Medium (HTM).[1]
[b] The current absence of data on resistant strains precludes defining any results other than "Susceptible." Strains yielding MIC results suggestive of a "nonsusceptible" category should be submitted to a reference laboratory for further testing.

For *Streptococcus* spp:
Streptococcus pneumoniae that are susceptible to penicillin (MIC ≤0.06 µg/mL), or streptococci other than *S. pneumoniae* that are susceptible to penicillin (MIC ≤0.12 µg/mL), can be considered susceptible to cefdinir. Testing of cefdinir against penicillin-intermediate or penicillin-resistant isolates is not recommended. Reliable interpretive criteria for cefdinir are not available.
A report of "Susceptible" indicates that the pathogen is likely to be inhibited if the antimicrobial compound in the blood reaches the concentration usually achievable. A report of "Intermediate" indicates that the result should be considered equivocal, and, if the microorganism is not fully susceptible to alternative, clinically feasible drugs, the test should be repeated. This category implies possible clinical applicability in body sites where the drug is physiologically concentrated or in situations where high dosage of drug can be used. This category also provides a buffer zone which prevents small uncontrolled technical factors from causing major discrepancies in interpretation. A report of "Resistant" indicates that the pathogen is not likely to be inhibited if the antimicrobial compound in the blood reaches the concentrations usually achievable; other therapy should be selected.

Standardized susceptibility test procedures require the use of laboratory control microorganisms to control the technical aspects of laboratory procedures. Standard cefdinir powder should provide the following MIC values:

Microorganism	MIC Range (µg/mL)
Escherichia coli ATCC 25922	0.12–0.5
Haemophilus influenzae ATCC 49766[c]	0.12–0.5
Staphylococcus aureus ATCC 29213	0.12–0.5

[c] This quality control range is applicable only to *H. influenza* ATCC 49766 tested by a broth microdilution procedure using HTM.

Diffusion Techniques: Quantitative methods that require measurement of zone diameters also provide reproducible estimates of the susceptibility of bacteria to antimicrobial compounds. One such standardized procedure[2] requires the use of standardized inoculum concentrations. This procedure uses paper disks impregnated with 5-µg cefdinir to test the susceptibility of microorganisms to cefdinir.
Reports from the laboratory providing results of the standard single-disk susceptibility test with a 5-µg cefdinir disk should be interpreted according to the following criteria:

For organisms other than *Haemophilus* spp: and *Streptococcus* spp:[d]

Zone Diameter (mm)	Interpretation
≥20	Susceptible (S)
17–19	Intermediate (I)
≤16	Resistant (R)

[d] Because certain strains of *Citrobacter, Providencia,* and *Enterobacter* spp. have been reported to give false susceptible results with the cefdinir disk, strains of these genera should not be tested and reported with this disk.

For *Haemophilus* spp:[e]

Zone Diameter (mm)	Interpretation[f]
≥20	Susceptible

[e] These zone diameter standards are applicable only to tests with *Haemophilus* spp. using HTM.[2]
[f] The current absence of data on resistant strains precludes defining any results other than "Susceptible." Strains yielding MIC results suggestive of a "nonsusceptible" category should be submitted to a reference laboratory for further testing.

For *Streptococcus* spp:
Isolates of *Streptococcus pneumoniae* should be tested against a 1-µg oxacillin disk. Isolates with oxacillin zone sizes ≥20 mm are susceptible to penicillin and can be considered susceptible to cefdinir. Streptococci other than *S. pneumoniae* should be tested with a 10-unit penicillin disk. Isolates with penicillin zone sizes ≥28 mm are susceptible to penicillin and can be considered susceptible to cefdinir. Interpretation should be as stated above for results using dilution techniques. Interpretation involves correlation of the diameter obtained in the disk test with the MIC for cefdinir.
As with standardized dilution techniques, diffusion methods require the use of laboratory control microorganisms to control the technical aspects of laboratory procedures. For the diffusion technique, the 5-µg cefdinir disk should provide the following zone diameters in these laboratory quality control strains:

Organism	Zone Diameter (mm)
Escherichia coli ATCC 25922	24–28
Haemophilus influenzae ATCC 49766[g]	24–31
Staphylococcus aureus ATCC 25923	25–32

[g] This quality control range is applicable only to *H. influenza* ATCC 49766 using HTM.

INDICATIONS AND USAGE

OMNICEF (cefdinir) Capsules and OMNICEF (cefdinir) for Oral Suspension are indicated for the treatment of patients with mild to moderate infections caused by susceptible strains of the designated microorganisms in the conditions listed below.

Adults and Adolescents
Community-Acquired Pneumonia caused by *Haemophilus influenzae* (including β-lactamase producing strains), *Haemophilus parainfluenzae* (including β-lactamase producing strains), *Streptococcus pneumoniae* (penicillin-susceptible strains only), and *Moraxella catarrhalis* (including β-lactamase producing strains) (see **CLINICAL STUDIES**).
Acute Exacerbations of Chronic Bronchitis caused by *Haemophilus influenzae* (including β-lactamase producing strains), *Haemophilus parainfluenzae* (including β-lactamase producing strains), *Streptococcus pneumoniae* (penicillin-susceptible strains only), and *Moraxella catarrhalis* (including β-lactamase producing strains).
Acute Maxillary Sinusitis caused by *Haemophilus influenzae* (including β-lactamase producing strains), *Streptococcus pneumoniae* (penicillin-susceptible strains only), and *Moraxella catarrhalis* (including β-lactamase producing strains).
NOTE: For information on use in pediatric patients, See **Pediatric Use** and **DOSAGE AND ADMINISTRATION**.
Pharyngitis/Tonsillitis caused by *Streptococcus pyogenes* (see **CLINICAL STUDIES**).
NOTE: Cefdinir is effective in the eradication of *S. pyogenes* from the oropharynx. Cefdinir has not, however, been studied for the prevention of rheumatic fever following *S. pyogenes* pharyngitis/tonsillitis. Only intramuscular penicillin has been demonstrated to be effective for the prevention of rheumatic fever.
Uncomplicated Skin and Skin Structure Infections caused by *Staphylococcus aureus* (including β-lactamase producing strains) and *Streptococcus pyogenes*.

Pediatric Patients
Acute Bacterial Otitis Media caused by *Haemophilus influenzae* (including β-lactamase producing strains), *Streptococcus pneumoniae* (penicillin-susceptible strains only), and *Moraxella catarrhalis* (including β-lactamase producing strains).
Pharyngitis/Tonsillitis caused by *Streptococcus pyogenes* (see **CLINICAL STUDIES**).
NOTE: Cefdinir is effective in the eradication of *S. pyogenes* from the oropharynx. Cefdinir has not, however, been studied for the prevention of rheumatic fever following *S. pyogenes* pharyngitis/tonsillitis. Only intramuscular penicillin has been demonstrated to be effective for the prevention of rheumatic fever.
Uncomplicated Skin and Skin Structure Infections caused by *Staphylococcus aureus* (including β-lactamase producing strains) and *Streptococcus pyogenes*.

CONTRAINDICATIONS

OMNICEF (cefdinir) is contraindicated in patients with known allergy to the cephalosporin class of antibiotics.

WARNINGS

BEFORE THERAPY WITH OMNICEF (CEFDINIR) IS INSTITUTED, CAREFUL INQUIRY SHOULD BE MADE TO DETERMINE WHETHER THE PATIENT HAS HAD PREVIOUS HYPERSENSITIVITY REACTIONS TO CEFDINIR, OTHER CEPHALOSPORINS, PENICILLINS, OR OTHER DRUGS. IF CEFDINIR IS TO BE GIVEN TO PENICILLIN-SENSITIVE PATIENTS, CAUTION SHOULD BE EXERCISED BECAUSE CROSS-HYPERSENSITIVITY AMONG β-LACTAM ANTIBIOTICS HAS BEEN CLEARLY DOCUMENTED AND MAY OCCUR IN UP TO 10% OF PATIENTS WITH A HISTORY OF PENICILLIN ALLERGY. IF AN ALLERGIC REACTION TO CEFDINIR OCCURS, THE DRUG SHOULD BE DISCONTINUED. SERIOUS ACUTE HYPERSENSITIVITY REACTIONS MAY REQUIRE TREATMENT WITH EPINEPHRINE AND OTHER EMERGENCY MEASURES, INCLUDING OXYGEN, INTRAVENOUS FLUIDS, INTRAVENOUS ANTIHISTAMINES, CORTICOSTEROIDS, PRESSOR AMINES, AND AIRWAY MANAGEMENT, AS CLINICALLY INDICATED.
Pseudomembranous colitis has been reported with nearly all antibacterial agents, including cefdinir, and may range in severity from mild-to life-threatening. Therefore, it is important to consider this diagnosis in patients who present with diarrhea subsequent to the administration of antibacterial agents.
Treatment with antibacterial agents alters the normal flora of the colon and may permit overgrowth of clostridia. Studies indicate that a toxin produced by *Clostridium difficile* is a primary cause of "antibiotic-associated colitis."
After the diagnosis of pseudomembranous colitis has been established, appropriate therapeutic measures should be initiated. Mild cases of pseudomembranous colitis usually respond to drug discontinuation alone. In moderate to severe cases, consideration should be given to management with fluids and electrolytes, protein supplementation, and treatment with an antibacterial drug clinically effective against *Clostridium difficile*.

PRECAUTIONS
General
As with other broad-spectrum antibiotics, prolonged treatment may result in the possible emergence and overgrowth of resistant organisms. Careful observation of the patient is essential. If superinfection occurs during therapy, appropriate alternative therapy should be administered.
Cefdinir, as with other broad-spectrum antimicrobials (antibiotics), should be prescribed with caution in individuals with a history of colitis.
In patients with transient or persistent renal insufficiency (creatinine clearance <30 mL/min), the total daily dose of OMNICEF should be reduced because high and prolonged plasma concentrations of cefdinir can result following recommended doses (see **DOSAGE AND ADMINISTRATION**).

Information for Patients
Antacids containing magnesium or aluminum interfere with the absorption of cefdinir. If this type of antacid is required during OMNICEF therapy, OMNICEF should be taken at least 2 hours before or after the antacid.
Iron supplements, including multivitamins that contain iron, interfere with the absorption of cefdinir. If iron supplements are required during OMNICEF therapy, OMNICEF should be taken at least 2 hours before or after the supplement.
Iron-fortified infant formula does not significantly interfere with the absorption of cefdinir. Therefore, OMNICEF for Oral Suspension can be administered with iron-fortified infant formula.
If the patient is diabetic, he/she/the guardian should be aware that the oral suspension contains 2.86 g of sucrose per teaspoon.

Drug Interactions
Antacids: (aluminum- or magnesium-containing): Concomitant administration of 300-mg cefdinir capsules with 30 mL Maalox® TC suspension reduces rate (C_{max}) and extent (AUC) of absorption by approximately 40%. Time to reach C_{max} is also prolonged by 1 hour. There are no significant effects on cefdinir pharmacokinetics if the antacid is administered 2 hours before or 2 hours after cefdinir. If antacids are required during OMNICEF therapy, OMNICEF should be taken at least 2 hours before or after the antacid.

Probenecid: As with other β-lactam antibiotics, probenecid inhibits the renal excretion of cefdinir, resulting in an approximate doubling in AUC, a 54% increase in peak cefdinir plasma levels, and a 50% prolongation in the apparent elimination t½.

Iron Supplements and Foods Fortified With Iron: Concomitant administration of cefdinir with a therapeutic iron supplement containing 60 mg of elemental iron (as FeSO₄) or vitamins supplemented with 10 mg of elemental iron reduced extent of absorption by 80% and 31%, respectively. If iron supplements are required during OMNICEF therapy, OMNICEF should be taken at least 2 hours before or after the supplement.

The effect of foods highly fortified with elemental iron (primarily iron-fortified breakfast cereals) on cefdinir absorption has not been studied.

Concomitantly administered iron-fortified infant formula (2.2 mg elemental iron/6 oz) has no significant effect on cefdinir pharmacokinetics. Therefore, OMNICEF for Oral Suspension can be administered with iron-fortified infant formula.

There have been rare reports of reddish stools in patients who have received cefdinir in Japan. The reddish color is due to the formation of a nonabsorbable complex between cefdinir or its breakdown products and iron in the gastrointestinal tract.

Drug/Laboratory Test Interactions

A false-positive reaction for ketones in the urine may occur with tests using nitroprusside, but not with those using nitroferricyanide. The administration of cefdinir may result in a false-positive reaction for glucose in urine using Clinitest®, Benedict's solution, or Fehling's solution. It is recommended that glucose tests based on enzymatic glucose oxidase reactions (such as Clinistix® or Tes-Tape®) be used. Cephalosporins are known to occasionally induce a positive direct Coombs' test.

Carcinogenesis, Mutagenesis, Impairment of Fertility

The carcinogenic potential of cefdinir has not been evaluated. No mutagenic effects were seen in the bacterial reverse mutation assay (Ames) or point mutation assay at the hypoxanthine-guanine phosphoribosyltransferase locus (HGPRT) in V79 Chinese hamster lung cells No clastogenic effects were observed *in vitro* in the structural chromosome aberration assay in V79 Chinese hamster lung cells or *in vivo* in the micronucleus assay in mouse bone marrow. In rats, fertility and reproductive performance were not affected by cefdinir at oral doses up to 1000 mg/kg/day (70 times the human dose based on mg/kg/day, 11 times based on mg/m²/day).

Pregnancy—Teratogenic Effects

Pregnancy Category B: Cefdinir was not teratogenic in rats at oral doses up to 1000 mg/kg/day (70 times the human dose based on mg/kg/day, 11 times based on mg/m²/day) or in rabbits at oral doses up to 10 mg/kg/day (0.7 times the human dose based on mg/kg/day, 0.23 times based on mg/m²/day). Maternal toxicity (decreased body weight gain) was observed in rabbits at the maximum tolerated dose of 10 mg/kg/day without adverse effects on offspring. Decreased body weight occurred in rat fetuses at ≥100 mg/kg/day, and in rat offspring at ≥32 mg/kg/day. No effects were observed on maternal reproductive parameters or offspring survival, development, behavior, or reproductive function.

There are, however, no adequate and well-controlled studies in pregnant women. Because animal reproduction studies are not always predictive of human response, this drug should be used during pregnancy only if clearly needed.

Labor and Delivery

Cefdinir has not been studied for use during labor and delivery.

Nursing Mothers

Following administration of single 600-mg doses, cefdinir was not detected in human breast milk.

Pediatric Use

Safety and efficacy in neonates and infants less than 6 months of age have not been established. Use of cefdinir for the treatment of acute maxillary sinusitis in pediatric patients (age 6 months through 12 years) is supported by evidence from adequate and well-controlled studies in adults and adolescents, the similar pathophysiology of acute sinusitis in adult and pediatric patients, and comparative pharmacokinetic data in the pediatric population.

Geriatric Use

Efficacy is comparable in geriatric patients and younger adults. While cefdinir has been well-tolerated in all age groups, in clinical trials geriatric patients experienced a lower rate of adverse events, including diarrhea, than younger adults. Dose adjustment in elderly patients is not necessary unless renal function is markedly compromised (see **DOSAGE AND ADMINISTRATION**).

ADVERSE EVENTS

Clinical Trials—OMNICEF Capsules (Adult and Adolescent Patients):

In clinical trials, 4527 adult and adolescent patients (3275 US and 1252 non-US) were treated with the recommended dose of cefdinir capsules (600 mg/day). Most adverse events were mild and self-limiting in nature. No deaths or permanent disabilities were attributed to cefdinir. One hundred twenty-five of 4527 (3%) patients discontinued medication due to adverse events thought by the investigators to be possibly, probably, or definitely associated with cefdinir therapy. The discontinuations were primarily for gastrointestinal disturbances, usually diarrhea or nausea. Seventeen of 4527 (0.4%) patients were discontinued due to rash thought related to cefdinir administration.

In the US, the following adverse events were thought by the investigators to be possibly, probably, or definitely related to cefdinir capsules in multiple-dose clinical trials (N=3275 cefdinir-treated patients):

LABORATORY VALUE CHANGES OBSERVED WITH CEFDINIR CAPSULES US TRIALS IN ADULT AND ADOLESCENT PATIENTS (N=3275)

Incidence ≥ 1%	↑ Gamma-glutamyltransferase	1%
	↑ Urine protein	1%
	↑ Urine red blood cells	1%
Incidence <1% but >0.1%	↑ Glucose, ↓ Glucose	0.9, 0.2
	↑ Alanine aminotransferase (ALT)	0.9
	↑ Urine glucose	0.9
	↑ White blood cells, ↓ White blood cells	0.8, 0.7
	↓ Lymphocytes, ↑ Lymphocytes	0.8, 0.2
	↑ Urine specify gravity	0.8
	↓ Bicarbonate	0.6
	↑ Eosinophils	0.6
	↑ Phosphorus, ↓ Phosphorus	0.6, 0.3
	↑ Aspartate aminotransferase (AST)	0.4
	↑ Urine white blood cells	0.4
	↓ Hemoglobin	0.3
	↑ Alkaline phosphatase	0.2
	↑ Blood urea nitrogen (BUN)	0.2
	↑ Bilirubin	0.2
	↑ Lactate dehydrogenase	0.2
	↑ Platelets	0.2
	↓ Polymorphonuclear neutrophils (PMNs)	0.2
	↓ Potassium	0.2
	↑ Urine pH	0.2

ADVERSE EVENTS ASSOCIATED WITH CEFDINIR CAPSULES US TRIALS IN ADULT AND ADOLESCENT PATIENTS (N=3275)[a]

Incidence ≥1%	Diarrhea	16%
	Vaginal moniliasis	5% of women
	Nausea	3%
	Headache	2%
	Abdominal pain	1%
	Vaginitis	1% of women
Incidence <1% but >0.1%	Rash	0.9%
	Dyspepsia	0.8%
	Flatulence	0.6%
	Vomiting	0.6%
	Anorexia	0.3%
	Constipation	0.3%
	Abnormal stools	0.2%
	Asthenia	0.2%
	Dizziness	0.2%
	Insomnia	0.2%
	Leukorrhea	0.2% of women
	Pruritus	0.2%
	Somnolence	0.2%

[a] 1469 males, 1806 females

The following laboratory value changes of possible clinical significance, irrespective of relationship to therapy with cefdinir, were seen during clinical trials conducted in the US: [See table at top of page]

Clinical Trials—OMNICEF for Oral Suspension (Pediatric Patients):

In clinical trials, 1893 pediatric patients (1387 US and 506 non-US) were treated with the recommended dose of cefdinir suspension (14 mg/kg/day). Most adverse events were mild and self-limiting. No deaths or permanent disabilities were attributed to cefdinir. Thirty-nine of 1893 (2%) patients discontinued medication due to adverse events considered by the investigators to be possibly, probably, or definitely associated with cefdinir therapy. Discontinuations were primarily for gastrointestinal disturbances, usually diarrhea. Five of 1893 (0.3%) patients were discontinued due to rash thought related to cefdinir administration.

In the US, the following adverse events were thought by investigators to be possibly, probably, or definitely related to cefdinir suspension in multiple-dose clinical trials (N=1387 cefdinir-treated patients):

ADVERSE EVENTS ASSOCIATED WITH CEFDINIR SUSPENSION US TRIALS IN PEDIATRIC PATIENTS (N = 1387)[a]

Incidence ≥ 1%	Diarrhea	8%
	Rash	3%
	Cutaneous moniliasis	1%
	Vomiting	1%
Incidence <1% but > 0.1%	Abdominal pain	0.9%
	Leukopenia[b]	0.4%
	Nausea	0.3%
	Vaginal moniliasis	0.3% of girls
	Vaginitis	0.3% of girls
	Dyspepsia	0.2%
	Maculopapular rash	0.2%
	Increased AST[b]	0.2%

[a] 743 males, 644 females
[b] Laboratory changes were occasionally reported as adverse events.

The following laboratory value changes of possible clinical significance, irrespective of relationship to therapy with cefdinir, were seen during clinical trials conducted in the US: [See first table at top of next page]

Postmarketing Experience

The following adverse experiences and altered laboratory tests, regardless of their relationship to cefdinir, have been reported during extensive postmarketing experience, beginning with approval in Japan in 1991: Stevens-Johnson syndrome, toxic epidermal necrolysis, exfoliative dermatitis, erythema multiforme, erythema nodosum, conjunctivitis, stomatitis, acute hepatitis, cholestasis, fulminant hepatitis, hepatic failure, jaundice, increased amylase, shock, anaphylaxis, facial and laryngeal edema, feeling of suffocation, acute enterocolitis, bloody diarrhea, hemorrhagic colitis, melena, pseudomembranous colitis, pancytopenia, granulocytopenia, leukopenia, thrombocytopenia, idiopathic thrombocytopenic purpura, hemolytic anemia, acute respiratory failure, asthmatic attack, drug-induced pneumonia, eosinophilic pneumonia, idiopathic interstitial pneumonia, fever, acute renal failure, nephropathy, bleeding tendency, coagulation disorder, disseminated intravascular coagulation, upper GI bleed, peptic ulcer, ileus, loss of consciousness, allergic vasculitis, possible cefdinir-diclofenac interaction, cardiac failure, chest pain, myocardial infarction, hypertension, involuntary movements, and rhabdomyolysis.

Cephalosporin Class Adverse Events

The following adverse events and altered laboratory tests have been reported for cephalosporin-class antibiotics in general:

Allergic reactions, anaphylaxis, Stevens-Johnson syndrome, erythema multiforme, toxic epidermal necrolysis, renal dysfunction, toxic nephropathy, hepatic dysfunction

Continued on next page

This product information was prepared in June 1998. On these and other Parke-Davis Products, information may be obtained by addressing PARKE-DAVIS, Division of Warner-Lambert Company, Morris Plains, New Jersey 07950.

Omnicef—Cont.

including cholestasis, aplastic anemia, hemolytic anemia, hemorrhage, false-positive test for urinary glucose, neutropenia, pancytopenia, and agranulocytosis. Pseudomembranous colitis symptoms may begin during or after antibiotic treatment (see **WARNINGS**).

Several cephalosporins have been implicated in triggering seizures, particularly in patients with renal impairment when the dosage was not reduced (see **DOSAGE AND ADMINISTRATION** and **OVERDOSAGE**). If seizures associated with drug therapy occur, the drug should be discontinued. Anticonvulsant therapy can be given if clinically indicated.

OVERDOSAGE

Information on cefdinir overdosage in humans is not available. In acute rodent toxicity studies, a single oral 5600-mg/kg dose produced no adverse effects. Toxic signs and symptoms following overdosage with other β-lactam antibiotics have included nausea, vomiting, epigastric distress, diarrhea, and convulsions. Hemodialysis removes cefdinir from the body. This may be useful in the event of a serious toxic reaction from overdosage, particularly if renal function is compromised.

DOSAGE AND ADMINISTRATION

(see **INDICATIONS AND USAGE** for Indicated Pathogens)

Capsules

The recommended dosage and duration of treatment for infections in adults and adolescents are described in the following chart; the total daily dose for all infections is 600 mg. Once-daily dosing for 10 days is as effective as BID dosing. Once-daily dosing has not been studied in pneumonia or skin infections; therefore, OMNICEF Capsules should be administered twice daily in these infections. OMNICEF Capsules may be taken without regard to meals.
[See second table from top of page]

Powder for Oral Suspension

The recommended dosage and duration of treatment for infections in pediatric patients are described in the following chart; the total daily dose for all infections is 14 mg/kg, up to a maximum dose of 600 mg per day. Once-daily dosing for 10 days is as effective as BID dosing. Once-daily dosing has not been studied in skin infections; therefore, OMNICEF for Oral Suspension should be administered twice daily in this infection. OMNICEF for Oral Suspension may be administered without regard to meals.
[See third table from top of page]

OMNICEF FOR ORAL SUSPENSION PEDIATRIC DOSAGE CHART

Weight	125 mg/5 mL
9 kg/20 lbs	2.5 mL (½ tsp) q12h or 5 mL (1 tsp) q24h
18 kg/40 lbs	5 mL (1 tsp) q12h or 10 mL (2 tsp) q24h
27 kg/60 lbs	7.5 mL (1½ tsp) q12h or 15 mL (3 tsp) q24h
36 kg/80 lbs	10 mL (2 tsp) q12h or 20 mL (4 tsp) q24h
≥ 43 kg[a]/95 lbs	12 mL (2½ tsp) q12h or 24 mL (5 tsp) q24h

[a] Pediatric patients who weigh ≥43 kg should receive the maximum daily dose of 600 mg.

Patients With Renal Insufficiency

For adult patients with creatinine clearance <30 mL/min, the dose of cefdinir should be 300 mg given once daily. Creatinine clearance is difficult to measure in outpatients. However, the following formula may be used to estimate creatinine clearance (CL_{cr}) in adult patients. For estimates to be valid, serum creatinine levels should reflect steady-state levels of renal function.

$$\text{Males:} \quad CL_{cr} = \frac{(\text{weight})(140 - \text{age})}{(72)(\text{serum creatinine})}$$

$$\text{Females:} \quad CL_{cr} = 0.85 \times \text{above value}$$

where creatinine clearance is in mL/min, age is in years, weight is in kilograms, and serum creatinine is in mg/dL.[3] The following formula may be used to estimate creatinine clearance in pediatric patients:

$$CL_{cr} = K \times \frac{\text{body length or height}}{\text{serum creatinine}}$$

where K=0.55 for pediatric patients older than 1 year[4] and 0.45 for infants (up to 1 year)[5].

In the above equation, creatinine clearance is in mL/min/1.73 m², body length or height is in centimeters, and serum creatinine is in mg/dL.

For pediatric patients with a creatinine clearance of <30 mL/min/1.73 m², the dose of cefdinir should be 7 mg/kg (up to 300 mg) given once daily.

LABORATORY VALUE CHANGES OBSERVED WITH CEFDINIR SUSPENSION US TRIALS IN PEDIATRIC PATIENTS (N = 1387)

Incidence ≥1%	↑ Lactate dehydrogenase	2%
	↑ Alkaline phosphatase	1%
	↓ Bicarbonate	1%
	↑ Eosinophils	1%
	↑ Urine pH	1%
Incidence <1% but >0.1%	↑ Lymphocytes, ↓ Lymphocytes	0.9, 0.7
	↑ Phosphorus, ↓ Phosphorus	0.9, 0.4
	↓ White blood cells, ↑ White blood cells	0.9, 0.4
	↑ Urine protein	0.9
	↑ PMNs	0.8
	↓ Platelets	0.7
	↓ Calcium	0.5
	↑ AST	0.2
	↓ Hemoglobin	0.4
	↑ Potassium	0.3
	↑ ALT	0.2
	↓ Hematocrit	0.2
	↑ Urine specific gravity	0.2
	↑ Urine white blood cells	0.2

Adults and Adolescents (Age 13 Years and Older)

Type of Infection	Dosage	Duration
Community-Acquired Pneumonia	300 mg q12h	10 days
Acute Exacerbations of Chronic Bronchitis	300 mg q12h or 600 mg q24h	10 days 10 days
Acute Maxillary Sinusitis	300 mg q12h or 600 mg q24h	10 days 10 days
Pharyngitis/Tonsillitis	300 mg q12h or 600 mg q24h	5 to 10 days 10 days
Uncomplicated Skin and Skin Structure Infections	300 mg q12h	10 days

Pediatric Patients (Age 6 Months Through 12 Years)

Type of Infection	Dosage	Duration
Acute Bacterial Otitis Media	7 mg/kg q12h or 14 mg/kg q24h	10 days 10 days
Acute Maxillary Sinusitis	7 mg/kg q12h or 14 mg/kg q24h	10 days 10 days
Pharyngitis/Tonsillitis	7 mg/kg q12h or 14 mg/kg q24h	5 to 10 days 10 days
Uncomplicated Skin and Skin Structure Infections	7 mg/kg q12h	10 days

Patients on Hemodialysis

Hemodialysis removes cefdinir from the body. In patients maintained on chronic hemodialysis, the recommended initial dosage regimen is a 300-mg or 7-mg/kg dose every other day. At the conclusion of each hemodialysis session, 300 mg (or 7 mg/kg) should be given. Subsequent doses (300 mg or 7 mg/kg) are then administered every other day.

Directions for Mixing OMNICEF for Oral Suspension

[See first table top of next page]
After mixing, the suspension can be stored at room temperature (25°C/77°F). The container should be kept tightly closed, and the suspension should be shaken well before each administration. The suspension may be used for 10 days, after which any unused portion must be discarded.

HOW SUPPLIED

OMNICEF Capsules, containing 300 mg cefdinir, as lavender and turquoise capsules imprinted with the product name, are available as follows:

60 Capsules/Bottle   N 0071-0067-20

OMNICEF for Oral Suspension is a cream-colored powder formulation that, when reconstituted as directed, contains 125 mg cefdinir/5 mL. The reconstituted suspension has a cream color and strawberry flavor. The powder is available as follows:

60-mL bottles   N 0071-2006-16
100-mL bottles   N 0071-2006-18

Store the capsules and unsuspended powder at 25°C (77°F); excursions permitted to 15°-30°C (59°-86°F) [see

USP Controlled Room Temperature]. **Once reconstituted, the oral suspension can be stored at controlled room temperature for 10 days.**

CLINICAL STUDIES

Community-Acquired Bacterial Pneumonia

In a controlled, double-blind study in adults and adolescents conducted in the US, cefdinir BID was compared with cefaclor 500 mg TID. Using strict evaluability and microbiologic/clinical response criteria 6 to 14 days posttherapy, the following clinical cure rates, presumptive microbiologic eradication rates, and statistical outcomes were obtained:
[See second table from top of next page]

In a second controlled, investigator-blind study in adults and adolescents conducted primarily in Europe, cefdinir BID was compared with amoxicillin/clavulanate 500/125 mg TID. Using strict evaluability and clinical response criteria 6 to 14 days posttherapy, the following clinical cure rates, presumptive microbiologic eradication rates, and statistical outcomes were obtained:
[See third table from top of next page]

Streptococcal Pharyngitis/Tonsillitis

In four controlled studies conducted in the US, cefdinir was compared with 10 days of penicillin in adult, adolescent, and pediatric patients. Two studies (one in adults and adolescents, the other in pediatric patients) compared 10 days of cefdinir QD or BID to penicillin 250 mg or 10 mg/kg QID. Using strict evaluability and microbiologic/clinical response criteria 5 to 10 days posttherapy, the following clinical cure rates, microbiologic eradication rates, and statistical outcomes were obtained:

Final Concentration	Final Volume (mL)	Amount of Water	Directions
125 mg/5 mL	60	38 mL	Tap bottle to loosen powder, then add water in 2 portions. Shake well after each aliquot.
	100	63 mL	

Us Community-Acquired Pneumonia Study
Cefdinir vs Cefaclor

	Cefdinir BID	Cefaclor TID	Outcome
Clinical Cure Rates	150/187 (80%)	147/186 (79%)	Cefdinir equivalent to control
Eradication Rates			
Overall	177/195 (91%)	184/200 (92%)	Cefdinir equivalent to control
S. pneumoniae	31/31 (100%)	35/35 (100%)	
H. influenzae	55/65 (85%)	60/72 (83%)	
M. catarrhalis	10/10 (100%)	11/11 (100%)	
H. parainfluenzae	81/89 (91%)	78/82 (95%)	

European Community-Acquired Pneumonia Study
Cefdinir vs Amoxicillin/Clavulanate

	Cefdinir BID	Amoxicillin/ Clavulanate TID	Outcome
Clinical Cure Rates	83/104 (80%)	86/97 (89%)	Cefdinir not equivalent to control
Eradication Rates			
Overall	85/96 (89%)	84/90 (93%)	Cefdinir equivalent to control
S. pneumoniae	42/44 (95%)	43/44 (98%)	
H. influenzae	26/35 (74%)	21/26 (81%)	
M. catarrhalis	6/6 (100%)	8/8 (100%)	
H. parainfluenzae	11/11 (100%)	12/12 (100%)	

Pharyngitis/Tonsillitis Studies
Cefdinir (10 days) vs Penicillin (10 days)

Study	Efficacy Parameter	Cefdinir QD	Cefdinir BID	Penicillin QID	Outcome
Adults/ Adolescents	Eradication of S. pyogenes	192/210 (91%)	199/217 (92%)	181/217 (83%)	Cefdinir superior to control
	Clinical Cure Rates	199/210 (95%)	209/217 (96%)	193/217 (89%)	Cefdinir superior to control
Pediatric Patients	Eradication of S. pyogenes	215/228 (94%)	214/227 (94%)	159/227 (70%)	Cefdinir superior to control
	Clinical Cure Rates	222/228 (97%)	218/227 (96%)	196/227 (86%)	Cefdinir superior to control

Pharyngitis/Tonsillitis Studies
Cefdinir (5 days) vs Penicillin (10 days)

Study	Efficacy Parameter	Cefdinir BID	Penicillin QID	Outcome
Adults/ Adolescents	Eradication of S. pyogenes	193/218 (89%)	176/214 (82%)	Cefdinir equivalent to control
	Clinical Cure Rates	194/218 (89%)	181/214 (85%)	Cefdinir equivalent to control
Pediatric Patients	Eradication of S. pyogenes	176/196 (90%)	135/193 (70%)	Cefdinir superior to control
	Clinical Cure Rates	179/196 (91%)	173/193 (90%)	Cefdinir equivalent to control

[See fourth table above]
Two studies (one in adults and adolescents, the other in pediatric patients) compared 5 days of cefdinir BID to 10 days of penicillin 250 mg or 10 mg/kg QID. Using strict evaluability and microbiologic/clinical response criteria 4 to 10 days posttherapy, the following clinical cure rates, microbiologic eradication rates, and statistical outcomes were obtained:
[See fifth table above]

REFERENCES

1. National Committee for Clinical Laboratory Standards. Methods for Dilution Antimicrobial Susceptibility Tests for Bacteria That Grow Aerobically, 4th ed. Approved Standard, NCCLS Document M7-A4, vol 17(2). NCCLS, Villanova, PA, Jan 1997.
2. National Committee for Clinical Laboratory Standards Performance Standards for Antimicrobial Disk Susceptibility Tests, 6th ed. Approved Standard, NCCLS Document M2-A6, Vol 17(1). NCCLS, Villanova, PA, Jan 1997.
3. Cockcroft DW, Gault MH. Prediction of creatinine clearance from serum creatinine. Nephron, 1976;16:31-41.
4. Schwartz GJ, Haycock GB, Edelmann CM, Spitzer A. A simple estimate of glomerular filtration rate in children derived from body length and plasma creatinine. Pediatrics 1976;58:259-63.
5. Schwartz GJ, Feld LG, Langford DJ. A simple estimate of glomerular filtration rate in full-term infants during the first year of life. J Pediatrics 1984; 104:849-54.

Rx only
©1998, Warner-Lambert Co.
March 1998
Manufactured by:

Lilly del Caribe, Inc.
Carolina, Puerto Rico 00986
For:
PARKE-DAVIS
Div of Warner-Lambert Co
Morris Plains, NJ 07950 USA
Under License of
Fujisawa Pharmaceutical Co., Ltd.
Osaka, Japan
0067G050
Shown in Product Identification Guide, page 329

PONSTEL®
[pŏn 'stĕl]
(mefenamic acid)

℞

DESCRIPTION

Ponstel (mefenamic acid) is N-(2,3-xylyl)-anthranilic acid. It is an analgesic agent for oral administration. Ponstel is available in capsules containing 250 mg of mefenamic acid. Each capsule also contains lactose, NF. The capsule shell and/or band contains citric acid, USP; D&C yellow No. 10; FD&C blue No. 1; FD&C red No. 3; FD&C yellow No. 6; gelatin, NF; glycerol monooleate; silicon dioxide, NF; sodium benzoate, NF; sodium lauryl sulfate, NF; titanium dioxide, USP.
It is a white powder with a melting point of 230–231° C, molecular weight 241.28, and water solubility of 0.004% at pH 7.1.

CLINICAL PHARMACOLOGY

Ponstel is a nonsteroidal agent with demonstrated antiinflammatory, analgesic, and antipyretic activity in laboratory animals.[1,2] The mode of action is not known. In animal studies, Ponstel was found to inhibit prostaglandin synthesis and to compete for binding at the prostaglandin receptor site.[3]
Pharmacologic studies show Ponstel did not relieve morphine abstinence signs in abstinent, morphine-habituated monkeys.[1]
Following a single 1-gram oral dose, peak plasma levels of 10 µg/ml occurred in 2 to 4 hours with a half-life of 2 hours. Following multiple doses, plasma levels are proportional to dose with no evidence of drug accumulation. One gram of Ponstel given four times daily produces peak blood levels of 20 µg/ml by the second day of administration.[4]
Following a single dose, sixty-seven percent of the total dose is excreted in the urine as unchanged drug or as one of two metabolites. Twenty to twenty-five percent of the dose is excreted in the feces during the first three days.[4]
In controlled, double-blind, clinical trials, Ponstel was evaluated for the treatment of primary spasmodic dysmenorrhea. The parameters used in determining efficacy included pain assessment by both patient and investigator; the need for concurrent analgesic medication; and evaluation of change in frequency and severity of symptoms characteristic of spasmodic dysmenorrhea. Patients received either Ponstel, 500 mg (2 capsules) as an initial dose and 250 mg every 6 hours, or placebo at onset of bleeding or of pain, whichever began first. After three menstrual cycles, patients were crossed over to the alternate treatment for an additional three cycles. Ponstel was significantly superior to placebo in all parameters, and both treatments (drug and placebo) were equally tolerated.

INDICATIONS AND USAGE

Ponstel is indicated for the relief of moderate pain[5] when therapy will not exceed one week. Ponstel is also indicated for the treatment of primary dysmenorrhea.[5,6]
Studies in pediatric patients under 14 years of age have been inadequate to evaluate the safety and effectiveness of Ponstel.

CONTRAINDICATIONS

Ponstel should not be used in patients who have previously exhibited hypersensitivity to it.
Because the potential exists for cross-sensitivity to aspirin or other nonsteroidal antiinflammatory drugs, Ponstel should not be given to patients in whom these drugs induce symptoms of bronchospasm, allergic rhinitis, or urticaria. Ponstel is contraindicated in patients with active ulceration or chronic inflammation of either the upper or lower gastrointestinal tract.
Ponstel should be avoided in patients with preexisting renal disease.

WARNINGS

If diarrhea occurs, the dosage should be reduced or temporarily suspended (see Adverse Reactions and Dosage and Administration). Certain patients who develop diarrhea may be unable to tolerate the drug because of recurrence of the symptoms on subsequent exposure.

Continued on next page

This product information was prepared in June 1998. On these and other Parke-Davis Products, information may be obtained by addressing PARKE-DAVIS, Division of Warner-Lambert Company, Morris Plains, New Jersey 07950.

Ponstel—Cont.

Risk of GI Ulceration, Bleeding and Perforation with NSAID Therapy: Serious gastrointestinal toxicity such as bleeding, ulceration, and perforation, can occur at any time, with or without warning symptoms, in patients treated chronically with NSAID therapy. Although minor upper gastrointestinal problems, such as dyspepsia, are common, usually developing early in therapy, physicians should remain alert for ulceration and bleeding in patients treated chronically with NSAIDs even in the absence of previous GI tract symptoms. In patients observed in clinical trials of several months to two years duration, symptomatic upper GI ulcers, gross bleeding or perforation appear to occur in approximately 1% of patients treated for 3–6 months, and in about 2–4% of patients treated for one year. Physicians should inform patients about the signs and/or symptoms of serious GI toxicity and what steps to take if they occur.

Studies to date have not identified any subset of patients not at risk of developing peptic ulceration and bleeding. Except for a prior history of serious GI events and other risk factors known to be associated with peptic ulcer disease, such as alcoholism, smoking, etc., no risk factors (eg, age, sex) have been associated with increased risk. Elderly or debilitated patients seem to tolerate ulceration or bleeding less well than other individuals and most spontaneous reports of fatal GI events are in this population. Studies to date are inconclusive concerning the relative risk of various NSAIDs in causing such reactions. High doses of any NSAID probably carry a greater risk of these reactions, although controlled clinical trials showing this do not exist in most cases. In considering the use of relatively large doses (within the recommended dosage range), sufficient benefit should be anticipated to offset the potential increased risk of GI toxicity.

PRECAUTIONS

If rash occurs, administration of the drug should be stopped. A false-positive reaction for urinary bile, using the diazo tablet test, may result after mefenamic acid administration. If biliuria is suspected, other diagnostic procedures, such as the Harrison spot test, should be performed.

Renal Effects: As with other nonsteroidal antiinflammatory drugs, long-term administration of mefenamic acid to animals has resulted in renal papillary necrosis and other abnormal renal pathology. In humans, there have been reports of acute interstitial nephritis with hematuria, proteinuria and occasionally nephrotic syndrome.

A second form of renal toxicity has been seen in patients with prerenal conditions leading to a reduction in renal blood flow or blood volume, where the renal prostaglandins have a supportive role in the maintenance of renal perfusion. In these patients administration of an NSAID may cause a dose-dependent reduction in prostaglandin formation and may precipitate overt renal decompensation. Patients at greatest risk of this reaction are those with impaired renal function, heart failure, liver dysfunction, those taking diuretics, and the elderly Discontinuation of NSAID therapy is typically followed by recovery to the pretreatment state.

Since Ponstel is eliminated primarily by the kidneys, the drug should not be administered to patients with significantly impaired renal functions.

As with other nonsteroidal antiinflammatory drugs, borderline elevations of one or more liver tests may occur in some patients. These abnormalities may progress, may remain essentially unchanged, or may be transient with continued therapy. The SGPT (ALT) test is probably the most sensitive indicator of liver dysfunction. Meaningful (3 times the upper limit of normal) elevations of SGPT or SGOT (AST) occurred in controlled clinical trials in less than 1% of patients. A patient with symptoms and/or signs suggesting liver dysfunction, or in whom an abnormal liver test has occurred, should be evaluated for evidence of the development of more severe hepatic reaction while on therapy with Ponstel. Severe hepatic reactions, including jaundice and cases of fatal hepatitis, have been reported with other nonsteroidal antiinflammatory drugs. Although such reactions are rare, if abnormal liver tests persist or worsen, if clinical signs and symptoms consistent with liver disease develop, or if systemic manifestations occur (eg eosinophilia, rash, etc), Ponstel should be discontinued.

Information for Patients: Patients should be advised that if rash, diarrhea or other digestive problems arise, they should stop the drug and consult their physician.

Patients in whom aspirin or other nonsteroidal antiinflammatory drugs induce symptoms of bronchospasm, allergic rhinitis, or urticaria should be made aware that the potential exists for cross-sensitivity to Ponstel.

The long-term effects, if any, of intermittent Ponstel therapy for dysmenorrhea are not known. Women on such therapy should consult their physician if they should decide to become pregnant.

Ponstel, like other drugs of its class, is not free of side effects. The side effects of these drugs can cause discomfort and, rarely, there are more serious side effects, such as gastrointestinal bleeding, which may result in hospitalization and even fatal outcomes.

NSAIDs (nonsteroidal antiinflammatory drugs) are often essential agents in the management of arthritis and have a major role in the treatment of pain, but they also may be commonly employed for conditions which are less serious. Physicians may wish to discuss with their patients the potential risks (see WARNINGS, PRECAUTIONS, and ADVERSE REACTIONS sections) and likely benefits of NSAID treatment, particularly when the drugs are used for less serious conditions where treatment without NSAIDs may represent an acceptable alternative to both the patient and physician.

Laboratory Tests: Because serious GI tract ulceration and bleeding can occur without warning symptoms, physicians should follow chronically treated patients for the signs and symptoms of ulceration and bleeding and should inform them of the importance of this follow-up (see Risk of GI Ulcerations, Bleeding and Perforation with NSAID Therapy).

Drug Interactions: Ponstel may prolong prothrombin time.[5] Therefore, when the drug is administered to patients receiving oral anticoagulant drugs, frequent monitoring of prothrombin time is necessary.

Use in Pregnancy: Pregnancy Category C. Reproduction studies have been performed in rats, rabbits and dogs. Rats given up to 10 times the human dose showed decreased fertility, delay in parturition, and a decreased rate of survival to weaning. Rabbits at 2.5 times the human dose showed an increase in the number of resorptions. There were no fetal anomalies observed in these studies nor in dogs at up to 10 times the human dose.[5]

There are no adequate and well-controlled studies in pregnant women. Because animal reproduction studies are not always predictive of human response, this drug should be used only if clearly needed.

The use of Ponstel in late pregnancy is not recommended because of the effects on the fetal cardiovascular system of drugs of this class.

Nursing Mothers: Trace amounts of Ponstel may be present in breast milk and transmitted to the nursing infant[7]; thus Ponstel should not be taken by the nursing mother because of the effects on the infant cardiovascular system of drugs of this class.

Pediatric Use: Safety and effectiveness in pediatric patients below the age of 14 have not been established.

ADVERSE REACTIONS

Gastrointestinal: The most frequently reported adverse reactions associated with the use of Ponstel involve the gastrointestinal tract. In controlled studies for up to eight months, the following disturbances were reported in decreasing order of frequency: diarrhea (approximately 5% of patients), nausea with or without vomiting, other gastrointestinal symptoms, and abdominal pain.

In certain patients, the diarrhea was of sufficient severity to require discontinuation of medication. The occurrence of the diarrhea is usually dose related, generally subsides on reduction of dosage, and rapidly disappears on termination of therapy.

Other gastrointestinal reactions less frequently reported were anorexia, pyrosis, flatulence, and constipation.

Gastrointestinal ulceration with and without hemorrhage has been reported.

Hematopoietic: Cases of autoimmune hemolytic anemia have been associated with the continuous administration of Ponstel for 12 months or longer. In such cases the Coombs test results are positive with evidence of both accelerated RBC production and RBC destruction. The process is reversible upon termination of Ponstel administration.

Decreases in hematocrit have been noted in 2–5% of patients and primarily in those who have received prolonged therapy. Leukopenia, eosinophilia, thrombocytopenic purpura, agranulocytosis, pancytopenia, and bone marrow hypoplasia have also been reported on occasion.

Nervous System: Drowsiness, dizziness, nervousness, headache, blurred vision, and insomnia have occurred.

Integumentary: Urticaria, rash, and facial edema have been reported.

Renal: As with other nonsteroidal antiinflammatory agents, renal failure, including papillary necrosis, has been reported. In elderly patients renal failure has occurred after taking Ponstel for 2–6 weeks. The renal damage may not be completely reversible. Hematuria and dysuria have also been reported with Ponstel.

Other: Eye irritation, ear pain, perspiration, mild hepatic toxicity, and increased need for insulin in a diabetic have been reported. There have been rare reports of palpitation, dyspnea, and reversible loss of color vision.

OVERDOSAGE

Although doses up to 6000 mg/day have been given, no specific information is available on the management of acute massive overdosage.

Should accidental overdosage occur, the stomach should be emptied by inducing emesis or by careful gastric lavage followed by the administration of activated charcoal.[8] Laboratory studies indicate that Ponstel should be absorbed from the gastrointestinal tract by activated charcoal.[4] Vital functions should be monitored and supported. Because mefenamic acid and its metabolites are firmly bound to plasma proteins, hemodialysis and peritoneal dialysis may be of little value.[4]

DOSAGE AND ADMINISTRATION

Administration is by the oral route, preferably with food.

The recommended regimen in acute pain for adults and adolescents over 14 years of age is 500 mg as an initial dose followed by 250 mg every six hours as needed, usually not to exceed one week.[5]

For the treatment of primary dysmenorrhea, the recommended dosage is 500 mg as an initial dose followed by 250 mg every 6 hours, starting with the onset of bleeding and associated symptoms. Clinical studies indicate that effective treatment can be initiated with the start of menses and should not be necessary for more than 2 to 3 days.[6]

HOW SUPPLIED

N 0071-0540-24 (P-D 540) Ponstel (mefenamic acid) is available as 250 mg capsules in bottles of 100.

REFERENCES

1. Winder CV, et al: Antiinflammatory, antipyretic and antinociceptive properties of N-(2,3-xylyl) anthranilic acid (mefenamic acid). *J Pharmacol Exp Ther* 138: 405–413, 1962.
2. Wax J, et al: Comparative activities, tolerances and safety of nonsteroidal antiinflammatory agents in rats. *J Pharmacol Exp Ther* 192: 172–178, 1975.
3. Ferreira SH, Vane JR: Aspirin and prostaglandins, in *The Prostaglandins,* Ramwell PW Ed, Plenum Press, NY, vol. 2, 1974, pp 1–47.
4. Glazko AJ: Experimental observations of flufenamic, mefenamic, and meclofenamic acids. Part III. Metabolic disposition, in *Fenamates in Medicine.* A Symposium, London 1966; *Annals of Physical Medicine,* supplement, pp 23–36, 1967.
5. Data on file, Medical Affairs Dept, Parke-Davis.
6. Budoff PW: Use of mefenamic acid in the treatment of primary dysmenorrhea. *JAMA* 241: 2713–2716, 1979.
7. Buchanan RA, et al: The breast milk excretion of mefenamic acid. *Curr Ther Res* 10:592, 1968.
8. Corby DG, Decker WJ: Management of acute poisoning with activated charcoal. *Pediatrics* 54:324, 1974.

0540G154

Caution—Federal law prohibits dispensing without prescription.

Revised May 1997

© 1996, Warner-Lambert Co.

Shown in Product Identification Guide, page 329

REZULIN® ℞
(Troglitazone) Tablets

WARNINGS

Hepatic

Rare cases of severe idiosyncratic hepatocellular injury have been reported during marketed use (see ADVERSE REACTIONS). The hepatic injury is usually reversible, but very rare cases of hepatic failure, leading to death or liver transplant, have been reported. Injury has occurred after both short- and long-term troglitazone treatment.

During all clinical studies in North America, a total of 48 of 2510 (1.9%) Rezulin-treated patients and 3 of 475 (0.6%) placebo-treated patients had ALT levels greater than 3 times the upper limit of normal. Twenty of the Rezulin-treated and one of the placebo-treated patients were withdrawn from treatment. Two of the 20 Rezulin-treated patients developed reversible jaundice; one of these patients had a liver biopsy which was consistent with an idiosyncratic drug reaction. An additional Rezulin-treated patient had a liver biopsy which was also consistent with an idiosyncratic drug reaction. (See ADVERSE REACTIONS, Laboratory Abnormalities).

It is recommended that serum transaminase levels be checked at the start of therapy, monthly for the first six months of therapy, every two months for the remainder of the first year of troglitazone therapy, and periodically thereafter. Liver function tests also should be obtained for patients at the first symptoms suggestive of hepatic dysfunction, eg, nausea, vomiting, abdominal pain, fatigue, anorexia, dark urine. Rezulin therapy should not be initiated if the patient exhibits clinical or laboratory evidence of active liver disease (eg, ALT>3 times the upper limit of normal) and should be discontinued if the patient has jaundice or laboratory measurements suggest liver injury (eg, ALT>3 times the upper limit of normal).

DESCRIPTION

Rezulin® (troglitazone) is an oral antihyperglycemic agent which acts primarily by decreasing insulin resistance. Rezulin is used in the management of type II diabetes (noninsulin-dependent diabetes mellitis (NIDDM) also known as adult-onset diabetes). It improves sensitivity to insulin in muscle and adipose tissue and inhibits hepatic gluconeogenesis. Troglitazone (±-5-[[4-[(3,4-dihydro-6-hydroxy-2,5,7,8-tetramethyl-2H-1-benzopyran-2-yl)methoxy]phenyl]methyl]-2,4-thiazolidinedione) is not chemically or functionally related to either the sulfonylureas, the biguanides, or the α-glucosidase inhibitors. The molecule contains 2 chiral centers, with each of the 4 stereoisomers having similar pharmacologic effects. The structural formula is as shown:

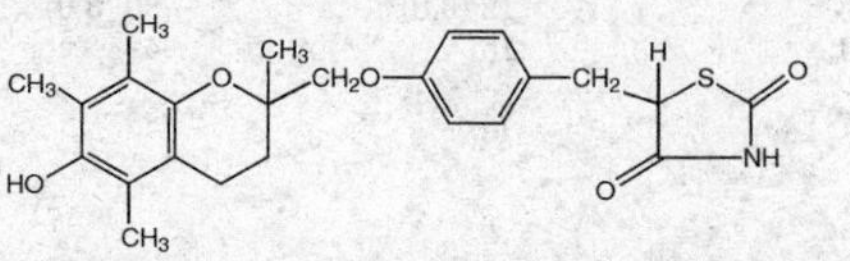

Troglitazone is a white to yellowish crystalline compound; it may have a faint, characteristic odor. Troglitazone has a molecular formula of $C_{24}H_{27}NO_5S$ and a molecular weight of 441.55 daltons. It is soluble in N,N-dimethylformamide or acetone; sparingly soluble in ethyl acetate; slightly soluble in acetonitrite, anhydrous ethanol, or ether; and practically insoluble in water.

Rezulin is available as 200, 300 and 400 mg tablets for oral administration formulated with the following excipients: croscarmellose sodium, hydroxypropyl methylcellulose, magnesium stearate, microcrystalline cellulose, polyethylene glycol 400, polysorbate 80, povidone, purified water, silicon dioxide, titanium dioxide, and synthetic iron oxides.

CLINICAL PHARMACOLOGY

Mechanism of Action

Troglitazone is a thiazolidinedione antidiabetic agent that lowers blood glucose by improving target cell response to insulin. It has a unique mechanism of action that is dependent on the presence of insulin for activity. Troglitazone decreases hepatic glucose output and increases insulin-dependent glucose disposal in skeletal muscle. Its mechanism of action is thought to involve binding to nuclear receptors (PPAR) that regulate the transcription of a number of insulin responsive genes critical for the control of glucose and lipid metabolism. Unlike sulfonylureas, troglitazone is not an insulin secretagogue.

In animal models of diabetes, troglitazone reduces the hyperglycemia, hyperinsulinemia, and hypertriglyceridemia characteristic of insulin-resistant states such as type II diabetes. Plasma lactate and ketone body formation are also decreased. The metabolic changes produced by troglitazone result from the increased responsiveness of insulin-dependent tissues and are observed in numerous animal models of insulin resistance. Treatment with troglitazone did not affect pancreatic weight, islet number or glucagon content, but did increase regranulation of the pancreatic beta cells in rodent models of insulin resistance.

Since troglitazone enhances the effects of circulating insulin (by decreasing insulin resistance), it does not lower blood glucose in animal models that lack endogenous insulin.

Pharmacokinetics and Drug Metabolism

Maximum plasma concentration (Cmax) and the area under plasma concentration-time curve (AUC) of troglitazone increase proportionally with increasing doses over the dose range of 200 to 600 mg/day (Table 1). Following daily drug administration, steady-state plasma concentrations of troglitazone are reached within 3 to 5 days.

TABLE 1. Mean (±1 SD) Steady-State Pharmacokinetics of Troglitazone in 21 Normal Volunteers

Dose (mg/day)	Cmax (µg/mL)	AUC (0-24) (µg-hr/mL)	CL/F* (mL/min)
200	0.90 (0.36)	7.4 (2.4)	500 (187)
400	1.61 (0.69)	13.4 (5.5)	601 (324)
600	2.82 (1.03)	22.1 (6.8)	496 (166)

*CL/F = Apparent oral clearance.

Absorption: Troglitazone is absorbed rapidly following oral administration; the time for maximum plasma concentration (tmax) occurs within 2 to 3 hours. Food increases the extent of absorption by 30% to 85%; thus Rezulin should be taken with a meal to enhance systemic drug availability.

Distribution: Mean apparent volume of distribution (V/F) of troglitazone following multiple-dose administration ranges from 10.5 to 26.5 L/kg of body weight. Troglitazone is extensively bound (>99%) to serum albumin. [^{14}C]troglitazone partitions into red blood cells (~5% of whole blood radioactivity).

Metabolism: In 6 healthy male volunteers given a single 400 mg dose of [^{14}C]troglitazone after 14 days of treatment with 400 mg troglitazone tablets, the major metabolites found in the plasma were the sulfate conjugate (Metabolite 1), followed by the quinone metabolite (Metabolite 3). Only 3.1% of the dose was detected in the urine; this was primarily in the form of glucuronide conjugate (Metabolite 2), which is present in negligible amounts in the plasma. In both normal volunteers and patients with type II diabetes, steady-state levels of Metabolite 1 are 6 to 7 times that of troglitazone and Metabolite 3.

Troglitazone incubated with expressed human P450 1A1, 1A2, 2A6, 2B6, 2D6, 2E1, and 3A4 in the presence and absence of known inhibitors of these enzymes showed no Metabolite 3 formation above levels in control samples. Studies in human microsomes suggest that Metabolite 3 is not subject to further metabolism by the major P450 isozymes. Troglitazone did not inhibit any of the major P450 enzymes at clinically relevent concentrations. The inhibitory characteristics of Metabolite 3 have not been investigated directly.

The results of human *in vivo* drug interaction trials suggest that troglitazone induces cytochrome P450 3A4 at clinically relevent doses (see Drug Interactions).

Excretion: Following oral administration of [^{14}C]troglitazone, approximately 88% of the radioactivity is recovered in feces (85%) and urine (3%). Unchanged troglitazone is not recovered in urine following oral administration. Mean plasma elimination half-life of troglitazone ranges from 16 to 34 hours.

Special Populations

Renal Insufficiency: In patients with various degrees of renal function, the apparent clearance of total and unbound troglitazone and the plasma elimination half-life of troglitazone, Metabolite 1, and Metabolite 3 do not correlate with creatinine clearance. Thus, dose adjustment in patients with renal dysfunction is not necessary (see DOSAGE AND ADMINISTRATION).

Hepatic Insufficiency: Troglitazone, Metabolite 1, and Metabolite 3 plasma concentrations in patients with chronic liver disease (Childs-Pugh Grade B or C) were increased by approximately 30%, 400% and 100%, respectively, compared to those in healthy subjects without hepatic dysfunction. There was no change in plasma protein binding. No adverse events were noted in any group that were attributed to drug. However, Rezulin therapy should not be initiated if the patient exhibits clinical or laboratory evidence of active liver disease (eg, ALT>3 times the upper limit of normal); see WARNINGS).

Geriatrics: Steady-state pharmacokinetics of troglitazone, Metabolite 1, and Metabolite 3 in healthy elderly subjects are comparable to those seen in young adults.

Pediatrics: Pharmacokinetic data in the pediatric population are not available.

Gender: Plasma concentrations of troglitazone and its metabolites are similar in men and women.

Ethnicity: Pharmacokinetics of troglitazone and its metabolites are similar among various ethnic groups.

Pharmacodynamics and Clinical Effects

Clinical studies demonstrate that Rezulin improves insulin sensitivity in insulin-resistant patients. Rezulin increases insulin-dependent glucose disposal, reduces hepatic gluconeogenesis, and enhances cellular responsiveness to insulin and thus, improves dysfunctional glucose homeostasis. In patients with type II diabetes, the decreased insulin resistance produced by Rezulin causes decreases in serum glucose, plasma insulin, and hemoglobin A_{1C}. Unlike sulfonylureas, Rezulin does not stimulate insulin secretion. Addition of Rezulin to a sulfonylurea has a synergistic effect since both agents act to improve glucose tolerance by different but complementary mechanisms. These effects occur without weight loss and persist for 52 weeks of Rezulin treatment.

In clinical trials of Rezulin as monotherapy or in combination, an increase in LDL (up to 13%), HDL (up to 16%), and total cholesterol (total-C) (up to 5%) occurred while total-C/HDL and LDL/HDL ratios did not change. The increase in total cholesterol is due to the increase in HDL and LDL cholesterol. Despite the observed increase in total and LDL cholesterol, ApoB fraction levels are not increased. Patients treated with Rezulin as monotherapy or in combination with other agents exhibited a reduction in fasting (-13% to -26%) and postprandial triglyceride levels. For patients on Rezulin and insulin, reduction in insulin doses may occur following Rezulin therapy and some attenuation of the triglyceride reduction may occur.

Pharmacokinetic estimators of systemic troglitazone exposure do not improve the prediction of pharmacodynamic response beyond that obtained based upon knowledge of the administered dose.

Rezulin has only been shown to exert its antihyperglycemic effect in the presence of insulin. Because Rezulin does not stimulate insulin secretion, hypoglycemia in patients treated with Rezulin alone is not to be expected. Because of this insulin-dependent mechanism of action, Rezulin should not be used in patients with type I diabetes.

Clinical Studies

Combination With Sulfonylureas

A 52-week, double-blind, placebo-controlled study of Rezulin and 12 mg micronized glyburide, alone and in combination, was conducted in patients with type II diabetes (N=552), who had failed to achieve adequate glycemic control (FSG of 224 mg/dL and HbA_{1C} of 9.6%) while on maximal doses of a sulfonylurea. Patients randomized to receive micronized glyburide showed mean increases in FSG and HbA_{1C}. [See table 2 above]

TABLE 2. Combination Therapy With Glyburide: Mean Difference From 12 mg Micronized Glyburide Monotherapy (1 yr)

	200 mg Rezulin + Glyburide	400 mg Rezulin + Glyburide	600 mg Rezulin + Glyburide
FSG (mg/dL)			
Mean Baseline	226	231	220
Adjusted Mean Change From Baseline	−31	−38	−56
Adjusted Mean Difference From Glyburide	−54**	−61**	−79**
HbA_{1C}(%)			
Mean Baseline	9.5	9.7	9.5
Adjusted Mean Change From Baseline	−0.7	−0.9	−1.8
Adjusted Mean Difference From Glyburide	−1.6**	−1.8**	−2.7**
Insulin (µU/mL)			
Mean Baseline	28.2	24.9	26.4
Adjusted Mean Change From Baseline	−3.8	−5.9	−6.1
Adjusted Mean Difference From Glyburide	−2.4	−4.4*	−4.6*

* p <0.05 compared to continuation of glyburide monotherapy.
** p <0.0001 compared to continuation of glyburide monotherapy.

TABLE 3. Combination Therapy With Glyburide: Percent of Patients Achieving Glycemic Control At End of Study (1 yr)

Rezulin (mg)	0	200	400	600
Glyburide (mg)	12	12	12	12
HbA_{1C} (%)				
≤7%	1	22	21	41
≤8%	10	33	33	60

A combination of 200, 400, or 600 mg of Rezulin with micronized glyburide achieved lower levels of fasting plasma glucose and HbA_{1C} levels than either agent achieved alone (see Tables 2 and 3). These improvements in glycemic control were associated with mean weight gains of 5.8 to 13.1 pounds. To eliminate weight as a confounding factor in this study, patients had been instructed to follow a diet to maintain current weight.

Combination With Insulin

Two clinical studies were conducted to evaluate the effects of Rezulin on glycemic control and insulin dose in patients with type II diabetes who were being treated with insulin. In one 6-month, double-blind, placebo-controlled study in insulin-treated type II diabetic patients receiving a mean of 73 (range 27–143) units/day of insulin with a mean baseline HbA_{1C} of 9.42 (range 7.04–12.48), Rezulin (200 or 600

Continued on next page

This product information was prepared in June 1998. On these and other Parke-Davis Products, information may be obtained by addressing PARKE-DAVIS, Division of Warner-Lambert Company, Morris Plains, New Jersey 07950.

Rezulin—Cont.

mg/day) or placebo was added to the insulin therapy. Investigators were instructed to reduce the insulin doses only if two consecutive FSGs were ≤100 mg/dL. Rezulin-treated patients showed a significant (p<0.0001) reduction in HbA_{1C} compared with patients who received placebo (see Table 4).

Thirty percent of patients treated with 200 mg Rezulin and 57% of patients treated with 600 mg Rezulin had an HbA_{1C} value below 8% at the end of the study compared with 11% of placebo-treated patients. Accompanying this improvement in glycemic control was a significant (p<0.0001) decrease in exogenous insulin dosage of 15% in the 200 mg Rezulin treatment group and 42% in the 600 mg Rezulin treatment group compared with 1% in the placebo group. HbA_{1C} values and insulin dose as a function of duration of Rezulin treatment are presented in Figures 1 and 2.

[See table 4 above]

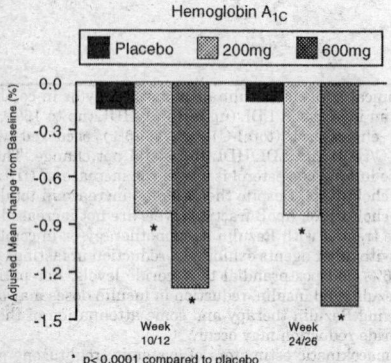

FIGURE 1: Combination Therapy With Insulin, Mean Change From Baseline for HbA_{1C}

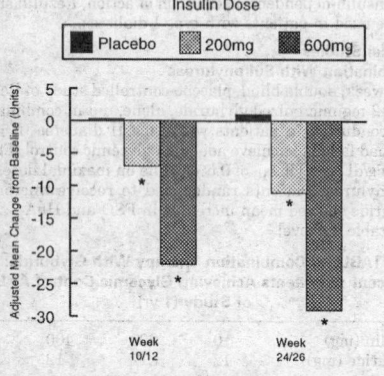

FIGURE 2: Combination Therapy With Insulin, Mean Change From Baseline for Insulin Dose

A second 6-month, double-blind, placebo-controlled study in insulin-treated type II diabetics who previously were poorly controlled on oral agents receiving 30 to 150 units insulin/day assessed the use of Rezulin in reducing exogenous insulin dosage while improving glycemic control as measured by capillary blood glucose.

Patients treated with 200 mg (N=75) and 400 mg (N=76) Rezulin had their insulin doses decreased by 41% and 58%, respectively, compared to a reduction of insulin dose in the placebo group (N=71) of 14% while maintaining or improving glycemic control. Forty-one percent of the patients in the 400 mg group decreased their insulin injection frequency an average from 3 to 1 injections per day; 19% of patients receiving placebo decreased their injection frequency an average from 3 to 2 injections per day. Insulin therapy was discontinued in 15% of patients in the 400 mg Rezulin group compared to 7% in the 200 mg group and 1.5% in the placebo group.

A greater than 50% reduction in insulin was achieved by 51% of patients on 200 mg and 70% on 400 mg once daily as compared to 17% on placebo.

Monotherapy

Three clinical trials, including 2 placebo-controlled studies with durations from 12 to 26 weeks have been conducted to study the use of Rezulin as monotherapy. These studies

TABLE 4. Combination Therapy with Insulin: Mean Change From Baseline at 6 Months

Parameter	Placebo	Troglitazone 200 mg	Troglitazone 600 mg
N	118	116	116
HbA_{1c}(%)			
Mean Baseline (SE)	9.43 (0.10)	9.51 (0.10)	9.32 (0.11)
Mean Change From Baseline (SE)[1]	−0.12 (0.10)	−0.84 (0.10)	−1.41 (0.10)
Adjusted Mean Difference From Placebo (SE)	--	−0.72 (0.14)*	−1.29 (0.14)*
Percent Mean Change From Baseline	−1.3	−8.8	−15.1
Insulin daily dosage (units)			
Mean Baseline (SE)	75 (3.3)	73 (3.4)	71 (2.9)
Mean Change From Baseline (SE)	1 (2.1)	−11 (2.1)	−29 (2.2)
Adjusted Mean Differene From Placebo (SE)	--	−12 (3.0)*	−30 (3.0)*
Percent Mean Change From Baseline	1	−15	−42

* p ≤0.0001
[1]Least squares mean adjusted for investigator center and baseline

have examined Rezulin doses from 100 to 600 mg/day in approximately 1500 patients. The patients studied have included patients previously treated with a sulfonylurea who were studied following prior therapy wash out (N=1265) and patients previously treated with diet only (N=230). In patients previously treated with a sulfonylurea, Rezulin treatment did not result in an improvement in glycemic control beyond that seen with the patients' prior therapy, although glucose lowering was significantly better than that seen with placebo treatment. For patients previously treated with diet, Rezulin doses of 200 mg, 400 mg and 600 mg/day were associated with improved FSG compared to placebo. However, only the 600 mg/day dose resulted in a difference compared with placebo that was statistically significant in both studies (see Table 5). At 600 mg per day, 58% of patients previously treated with diet in the 12-week study and 47% of patients previously treated with diet in the 26-week study (versus placebo values of 28% and 21%, respectively) had a response to Rezulin of ≥ 30 mg/dL reduction from baseline in fasting serum glucose.

TABLE 5. Glycemic Parameters in Diet-Failure Patients

	12 Week Study Placebo	200	400	600
N	19	23	20	33
FSG (mg/dL)				
Mean Baseline	168	169	181	196
Adjusted Mean Change From Baseline	14	−14	−20	−38
Adjusted Mean Difference From Placebo		−31*	−37*	−55*
HbA_{1c}(%)				
Mean Baseline	8	8.2	8.6	8.6
Adjusted Mean Change From Baseline	−0.1	−0.6	−0.6	−0.8
Adjusted Mean Difference From Placebo		−0.5	−0.6	−0.7*

	26 Week Study Placebo	200	400	600
N	18	18	19	15
FSG (mg/dL)				
Mean Baseline	202	191	201	201
Adjusted Mean Change From Baseline	−6	−24	−17	−48
Adjusted Mean Difference From Placebo		−18	−10	−42*
HbA_{1c}(%)				
Mean Baseline	8.7	8.3	8.5	8.6
Adjusted Mean Change From Baseline	0.4	−0.2	0.3	−1
Adjusted Mean Difference From Placebo		−0.6	−0.1	−1.4*

*p<0.05

INDICATIONS AND USAGE

Rezulin may be used concomitantly with a sulfonylurea or insulin to improve glycemic control. Rezulin, as monotherapy, is indicated as an adjunct to diet and exercise to lower blood glucose in patients with type II diabetes (see DOSAGE AND ADMINISTRATION). Rezulin should not be used as monotherapy in patients previously well-controlled on sulfonylurea therapy. For patients inadequately controlled with a sulfonylurea alone, Rezulin should be added to, not substituted for, the sulfonylurea.

Management of type II diabetes should include diet control. Caloric restriction, weight loss, and exercise are essential for the proper treatment of the diabetic patient. This is important not only in the primary treatment of type II diabetes, but in maintaining the efficacy of drug therapy. Prior to initiation of Rezulin therapy, secondary causes of poor glycemic control, eg, infection of poor injection technique, should be investigated and treated.

CONTRAINDICATIONS

Rezulin is contraindicated in patients with known hypersensitivity or allergy to Rezulin or any of its components.

WARNINGS

SEE BOXED WARNING.

PRECAUTIONS

General

Because of its mechanism of action, Rezulin is active only in the presence of insulin. Therefore, Rezulin should not be used in type I diabetes or for the treatment of diabetic keto-acidosis.

Hypoglycemia: Patients receiving Rezulin in combination with insulin or oral hypoglycemic agents may be at risk for hypoglycemia and a reduction in the dose of concomitant agent may be necesary. Hypoglycemia has not been observed during the administration of Rezulin as monotherapy and would not be expected based on the mechanism of action.

Ovulation: In premenopausal anovulatory patients with insulin resistance, Rezulin treatment may result in resumption of ovulation. **These patients may be at risk for pregnancy.**

Hematologic: Across all clinical studies, hemoglobin declined by 3 to 4% in troglitazone-treated patients compared with 1 to 2% in those treated with placebo. White blood cell counts also declined slightly in troglitazone-treated patients compared to those treated with placebo. These changes occurred within the first four to eight weeks of therapy. Levels stabilized and remained unchanged for up to two years of continuing therapy. These changes may be due to the dilutional effects of increased plasma volume and have not been associated with any significant hematologic clinical effects (see ADVERSE REACTIONS, Laboratory Abnormalities).

Use in Patients With Heart Failure

Heart enlargement without microscopic changes has been observed in rodents at exposures of parent compound and active metabolite exceeding 7 times the AUC of the 400 mg human dose (see PRECAUTIONS, Carcinogenesis, Mutagenesis, Impairment of Fertility, and Animal Toxicology). Serial echocardiographic evaluations in monkeys treated chronically at exposures at 4–9 times the human exposure to parent compound and active metabolite at the 400 mg dose did not reveal changes in heart size or function. In a 2-year echocardiographic clinical study using 600 to 800 mg/day of Rezulin in patients with type II diabetes, no increase in left ventricular mass or decrease in cardiac output was observed. The methodology employed was able to detect a change of about 10% or more in left ventricular mass.

In animal studies, troglitazone treatment was associated with increases of 6% to 15% in plasma volume. In a study of 24 normal volunteers, an increase in plasma volume of 6% to 8% compared to placebo was observed following 6 weeks of troglitazone treatment.

No increased incidence of adverse events potentially related to volume expansion (eg, congestive heart failure) have been observed during controlled clinical trials. However, patients with New York Heart Association (NYHA) Class III and IV

cardiac status were not studied during clinical trials. Therefore, Rezulin is not indicated unless the expected benefit is believed to outweigh the potential risk to patients with NYHA Class III or IV cardiac status.

Information for Patients

Rezulin should be taken with meals. If the dose is missed at the usual meal, it may be taken at the next meal. If the dose is missed on one day, the dose should not be doubled the following day.

It is important to adhere to dietary instructions and to regularly have blood glucose and glycosylated hemoglobin tested. During periods of stress such as fever, trauma, infection, or surgery, insulin requirements may change and patients should seek the advice of their physician.

Patients who develop nausea, vomiting, abdominal pain, fatigue, anorexia, dark urine or other symptoms suggestive of hepatic dysfunction or jaundice should immediately report these signs or symptoms to their physician.

When using combination therapy with insulin or oral hypoglycemic agents, the risks of hypoglycemia, its symptoms and treatment, and conditions that predispose to its development should be explained to patients and their family members.

Use of Rezulin can cause resumption of ovulation in women taking oral contraceptives and in patients with polycystic ovary disease. Therefore, a higher dose of an oral contraceptive or an alternative method of contraception should be considered.

Rezulin may affect other medications used in diabetic patients. Patients started on Rezulin should ask their physician to review their other medications to make sure that they are not affected by Rezulin.

Drug Interactions

Oral Contraceptives: Administration of Rezulin with an oral contraceptive containing ethinyl estradiol and norethindrone reduced the plasma concentrations of both by approximately 30%, which could result in loss of contraception. Therefore, a higher dose of oral contraceptive or an alternative method of contraception should be considered.

Terfenadine: Coadministration of Rezulin with terfenadine decreases the plasma concentration of both terfenadine and its active metabolite by 50–70% and may result in decreased efficacy of terfenadine.

Cholestyramine: Concomitant administration of cholestyramine with Rezulin reduces the absorption of troglitazone by 70%; thus, coadministration of cholestyramine and Rezulin is not recommended.

Glyburide: Coadministration of Rezulin and glyburide does not appear to alter troglitazone or glyburide pharmacokinetics.

Digoxin: Coadministration of Rezulin with digoxin does not alter the steady-state pharmacokinetics of digoxin.

Warfarin: Rezulin has no clinically significant effect on prothrombin time when administered to patients receiving chronic warfarin therapy.

Acetaminophen: Coadministration of acetaminophen and Rezulin does not alter the pharmacokinetics of either drug.

Metformin: No information is available on the use of Rezulin with metformin.

Ethanol: A single administration of a moderate amount of alcohol did not increase the risk of acute hypoglycemia in Rezulin-treated patients with type II diabetes mellitus.

The above interactions with terfenadine and oral contraceptives suggest that troglitazone may induce drug metabolism by CYP3A4. Studies have not been performed with other drugs metabolized by this enzyme such as: astemizole, calcium channel blockers, cisapride, corticosteroids, cyclosporine, HMG-CoA reductase inhibitors, tacrolimus, triazolam, and trimetrexate. The possibility of altered safety and efficacy should be considered when Rezulin is used concomitantly with these drugs.

Patients stable on one or more of these agents when Rezulin is started should be closely monitored and their therapy adjusted as necessary.

Carcinogenesis, Mutagenesis, Impairment of Fertility

Troglitazone was administered daily for 104 weeks to male rats at 100, 400, or 800 mg/kg and to female rats at 25, 50, or 200 mg/kg. No tumors of any type were increased at the low and mid doses. Plasma drug exposure based on AUC of parent compound and total metabolites at the low and mid doses was up to 24-fold higher than human exposure at 400 mg daily. The highest dose in each sex exceeded the maximum tolerated dose. In a 104-week study in mice given 50, 400, or 800 mg/kg, incidence of hemangiosarcoma was increased in females at 400 mg/kg and in both sexes at 800 mg/kg; incidence of hepatocellular carcinoma was increased in females at 800 mg/kg. The lowest dose associated with increased tumor incidence (400 mg/kg) was associated with AUC values of parent compound and total metabolites that were at least 2-fold higher than the human exposures at 400 mg daily. No tumors of any type were increased in mice at 50 mg/kg at exposures up to 40% of that in humans at 400 mg daily, based on AUC of parent compound and total metabolites.

Troglitazone was neither mutagenic in bacteria nor clastogenic in bone marrow of mice. Equivocal increases in chromosome aberrations were observed in an *in vitro* Chinese hamster lung cell assay. In mouse lymphoma cell gene mutations assays, results were equivocal when conducted with a microtiter technique and negative was an agar plate technique. A liver unscheduled DNA synthesis assay in rats was negative.

No adverse effects on fertility or reproduction were observed in male or female rats given 40, 200, or 1000 mg/kg daily prior to and throughout mating and gestation. AUC of parent compound at these doses was estimated to be 3- to 9-fold higher than the human exposure.

Animal Toxicology

Increased heart weights without microscopic changes were observed in mice and rats treated for up to 1 year at exposure (AUC) of parent and active metabolite exceeding 7 times the human AUC at 400 mg/day. These heart weight increases were reversible in 2- and 13-week studies, were prevented by coadministration of an ACE inhibitor, and 14 days of troglitazone administration to rats did not affect left ventricular performance. In the lifetime carcinogenicity studies, microscopic changes were noted in the hearts of rats but not mice. In control and treated rats, microscopic changes included myocardial inflammation and fibrosis and karyomegaly of atrial myocytes. The incidence of these changes in drug-treated rats was increased compared to controls at twice the AUC of the 400 mg human dose.

Pregnancy

Pregnancy Category B. Troglitazone was not teratogenic in rats given up to 2000 mg/kg or rabbits given up to 1000 mg/kg during organogenesis. Compared to human exposure of 400 mg daily, estimated exposures in rats (parent compound) and rabbits (parent compound and active metabolite) based on AUC at these doses were up to 9-fold and 3-fold higher, respectively. Body weights of fetuses and offspring of rats given 2000 mg/kg during gestation were decreased. Delayed postnatal development, attributed to decreased body weight, was observed in offspring of rats given 40, 200, or 1000 mg/kg during late gestation and lactation periods; no effects were observed in offspring of rats given 10 or 20 mg/kg.

There are no adequate and well-controlled studies in pregnant women. Rezulin should not be used during pregnancy unless the potential benefit justifies the potential risk to the fetus.

Because current information strongly suggests that abnormal blood glucose levels during pregnancy are associated with a higher incidence of congenital anomalies as well as increased neonatal morbidity and mortality, most experts recommend that insulin be used during pregnancy to maintain blood glucose levels as close to normal as possible.

Nursing Mothers

It is not known whether troglitazone is secreted in human milk. Troglitazone is secreted in the milk of lactating rats. Because many drugs are excreted in human milk, Rezulin should not be administered to a breast-feeding woman.

Pediatric Use

Safety and effectiveness in pediatric patients have not been established.

Geriatric Use

Twenty-two percent of patients in clinical trials of Rezulin were 65 and over. No differences in effectiveness and safety were observed between these patients and younger patients.

ADVERSE REACTIONS

Two patients in the clinical studies developed reversible jaundice; one of these patients had a liver biopsy which was consistent with an idiosyncratic drug reaction. An additional patient had a liver biopsy which was also consistent with an idiosyncratic drug reaction. Symptoms that are associated with hepatic dysfunction or hepatitis have been reported, including: nausea, vomiting, abdominal pain, fatigue, anorexia, dark urine, abnormal liver function tests (including increased ALT, AST, LDH, alkaline phosphatase, bilirubin). Also see WARNINGS.

The overall incidence and types of adverse reactions reported in placebo-controlled clinical trials for Rezulin-treated patients and placebo-treated patients are shown in Table 6. In patients treated with Rezulin in glyburide-controlled studies (N=550) or uncontrolled studies (N=510), the safety profile of Rezulin appeared similar to that displayed in Table 6. The incidence of withdrawals during clinical trials was similar for patients treated with placebo or Rezulin (4%).

TABLE 6. North American Placebo-Controlled Clinical Studies: Adverse Events Reported at a Frequency ≥ 5% of Rezulin-Treated Patients % of Patients

	Placebo N = 492	Rezulin N = 1450		Placebo N = 492	Rezulin N = 1450
Infection	22	18	Nausea	4	6
Headache	11	11	Rhinitis	7	5
Pain	14	10	Diarrhea	6	5
Accidental Injury	6	8	Urinary Tract Infection	6	5
Asthenia	5	6	Peripheral Edema	5	5
Dizziness	5	6	Pharyngitis	4	5
Back Pain	4	6			

[See table 6 above]

Types of adverse events seen when Rezulin was used concomitantly with insulin (N=543) were similar to those during Rezulin monotherapy (N=1731), although hypoglycemia occurred on insulin combination therapy (see PRECAUTIONS).

Laboratory Abnormalities

Hematologic: Small decreases in hemoglobin, hematocrit, and neutrophil counts (within the normal range) were more common in Rezulin-treated than placebo-treated patients and may be related to increased plasma volume observed with Rezulin treatment. Hemoglobin decreases to below the normal raange occurred in 5% of Rezulin-treated and 4% of placebo-treated patients.

Lipids: Small changes in serum lipids have been observed (see CLINICAL PHARMACOLOGY, Pharmacodynamics and Clinical Effects).

Serum Transaminase Levels: During all clinical studies in North America, a total of 48 of 2510 (1.9%) Rezulin-treated patients and 3 of 475 (0.6%) placebo-treated patients had ALT levels greater than 3 times the upper limit of normal. During controlled clinical trials, 2.2% of Rezulin-treated patients had reversible elevations in AST or ALT greater than 3 times the upper limit of normal, compared with 0.6% of patients receiving placebo. Hyperbilirubinemia (>1.25 upper limit of normal) was found in 0.7% of Rezulin-treated patients compared with 1.7% of patients receiving placebo. In the population of patients treated with Rezulin, mean and median values for bilirubin, AST, ALT, alkaline phosphatase, and GGT were decreased at the final visit compared with baseline, while values for LDH were increased slightly (see WARNINGS).

Postintroduction Reports

Adverse events associated with Rezulin that have been reported since market introduction, that are not listed above, and for which causal relationship to drug has not been established include the following: congestive heart failure, weight gain, edema, fever, abnormal lab tests including increased CPK and creatinine, hyperglycemia, syncope, anemia, malaise.

DOSAGE AND ADMINISTRATION

Rezulin should be taken with a meal.

Combination Therapy

Sulfonylureas: Rezulin in combination with a sulfonylurea should be initiated at 200 mg once daily. The current sulfonylurea dose should be continued upon initiation of Rezulin therapy. For patients not responding adequately, the Rezulin dose should be increased at 2 to 4 weeks. The maximum recommended dose is 600 mg once daily. The dose of sulfonylurea may require lowering to optimize therapy.

Insulin: The current insulin dose should be continued upon initiation of Rezulin therapy. Rezulin therapy should be initiated at 200 mg once daily in patients on insulin therapy. For patients not responding adequately, the dose of Rezulin should be increased after approximately 2 to 4 weeks. The usual dose of Rezulin is 400 mg once daily. The maximum recommended daily dose is 600 mg. It is recommended that the insulin dose be decreased by 10% to 25% when fasting plasma glucose concentrations decrease to less than 120 mg/dL in patients receiving concomitant insulin and Rezulin. Further adjustments should be individualized based on glucose-lowering response.

Monotherapy

Rezulin monotherapy in patients not adequately controlled with diet alone should be initiated at 400 or 600 mg once daily. For patients not responding to 400 mg once daily, the Rezulin dose should be increased to 600 mg after 6–8 weeks. For patients not responding adequately to 600 mg after 6–8

Continued on next page

This product information was prepared in June 1998. On these and other Parke-Davis Products, information may be obtained by addressing PARKE-DAVIS, Division of Warner-Lambert Company, Morris Plains, New Jersey 07950.

Rezulin—Cont.

weeks, Rezulin should be discontinued and alternative therapeutic options should be pursued. See CLINICAL PHARMACOLOGY, Clinical Studies, Monotherapy.

Patients With Renal Insufficiency
Dose adjustment in patients with renal insufficiency is not required (see CLINICAL PHARMACOLOGY, Pharmacokinetics and Drug Metabolism). Out of 2938 patients, 148 (5%) had a serum creatinine ≥ 1.5 at baseline. Of these 148 patients, 145 had creatinine levels between 1.5 and 2.0, inclusive; only 3 patients had levels >2.0. No consistent trend was seen in any of these adverse events, and no worsening of renal insufficiency was observed.

Patients With Hepatic Impairment
Rezulin therapy should not be initiated if the patient exhibits clinical or laboratory evidence of active liver disease (eg, ALT>3 times the upper limit of normal). See CLINICAL PHARMACOLOGY, Special Populations, Hepatic Insufficiency, and WARNINGS.

HOW SUPPLIED

Rezulin is available in 200, 300 and 400 mg tablets as follows:
200 mg Tablets: Yellow, oval, non-scored, film-coated tablet with "PD 352" debossed on one side, and "200" on the other, available in:
N 0071-0352-15 Bottles of 30
N 0071-0352-23 Bottles of 90
N 0071-0352-40 (10 × 10 unit-dose blisters)
300 mg Tablets: White, oval, non-scored, film-coated tablet with "PD 357" debossed on one side and "300" on the other, available in:
N 0071-0357-20 Bottles of 60
N 0071-0357-25 Bottles of 120
400 mg Tablets: Tan, oval, non-scored, film-coated tablet with "PD 353" debossed on one side, and "400" on the other, available in:
N 0071-0353-15 Bottles of 30
N 0071-0353-23 Bottles of 90
N 0071-0353-40 (10 × 10 unit-dose blisters)
Storage
Store at controlled room temperature 20°C–25°C (68°–77°F). Protect from moisture and humidity.
Rx only
©1997, PDPL
February 1998
Manufactured by:
Parke Davis Pharmaceuticals, Ltd.
Vega Baja, PR 00694
Distributed by
PARKE-DAVIS
Div of Warner-Lambert Co
Morris Plains, NJ 07950 USA
Marketed by:
PARKE-DAVIS
Div of Warner-Lambert Co and
SANKYO PARKE DAVIS
Parsippany, NJ 07054 USA

0352G203
Shown in Product Identification Guide, page 329

ZARONTIN® ℞
[ză "rŏn 'tĭn]
(ethosuximide, USP)
Capsules

DESCRIPTION

Zarontin (ethosuximide) is an anticonvulsant succinimide, chemically designated as alpha-ethyl-alpha-methyl-succinimide, with the following structural formula:

Each Zarontin capsule contains 250 mg ethosuximide, USP. Also contains: polyethylene glycol 400, NF. The capsule contains D&C yellow No. 10; FD&C red No. 3; gelatin, NF; glycerin, USP; and sorbitol.

CLINICAL PHARMACOLOGY

Ethosuximide suppresses the paroxysmal three cycle per second spike and wave activity associated with lapses of consciousness which is common in absence (petit mal) seizures. The frequency of epileptiform attacks is reduced, apparently by depression of the motor cortex and elevation of the threshold of the central nervous system to convulsive stimuli.

INDICATIONS AND USAGE

Zarontin is indicated for the control of absence (petit mal) epilepsy.

CONTRAINDICATION

Ethosuximide should not be used in patients with a history of hypersensitivity to succinimides.

WARNINGS

Blood dyscrasias, including some with fatal outcome, have been reported to be associated with the use of ethosuximide; therefore, periodic blood counts should be performed. Should signs and/or symptoms of infection (eg, sore throat, fever) develop, blood counts should be considered at that point.
Ethosuximide is capable of producing morphological and functional changes in the animal liver. In humans, abnormal liver and renal function studies have been reported. Ethosuximide should be administered with extreme caution to patients with known liver or renal diseases. Periodic urinalysis and liver function studies are advised for all patients receiving the drug.
Cases of systemic lupus erythematosus have been reported with the use of ethosuximide. The physician should be alert to this possibility.
Usage in Pregnancy: Reports suggest an association between the use of anticonvulsant drugs by women with epilepsy and an elevated incidence of birth defects in children born to these women. Data are more extensive with respect to phenytoin and phenobarbital, but these are also the most commonly prescribed anticonvulsants; less systematic or anecdotal reports suggest a possible similar association with the use of all known anticonvulsant drugs.
The reports suggesting an elevated incidence of birth defects in children of drug-treated epileptic women cannot be regarded as adequate to prove a definite cause and effect relationship. There are intrinsic methodological problems in obtaining adequate data on drug teratogenicity in humans; the possibility also exists that other factors, eg, genetic factors or the epileptic condition itself, may be more important than drug therapy in leading to birth defects. The great majority of mothers on anticonvulsant medication deliver normal infants. It is important to note that anticonvulsant drugs should not be discontinued in patients in whom the drug is administered to prevent major seizures because of the strong possibility of precipitating status epilepticus with attendant hypoxia and threat to life. In individual cases where the severity and frequency of the seizure disorder are such that the removal of medication does not pose a serious threat to the patient, discontinuation of the drug may be considered prior to and during pregnancy, although it cannot be said with any confidence that even minor seizures do not pose some hazard to the developing embryo or fetus.
The prescribing physician will wish to weigh these considerations in treating or counseling epileptic women of childbearing potential.

PRECAUTIONS
General
Ethosuximide, when used alone in mixed types of epilepsy, may increase the frequency of grand mal seizures in some patients.
As with other anticonvulsants, it is important to proceed slowly when increasing or decreasing dosage, as well as when adding or eliminating other medication. Abrupt withdrawal of anticonvulsant medication may precipitate absence (petit mal) status.
Information for Patients
Ethosuximide may impair the mental and/or physical abilities required for the performance of potentially hazardous tasks, such as driving a motor vehicle or other such activity requiring alertness; therefore, the patient should be cautioned accordingly.
Patients taking ethosuximide should be advised of the importance of adhering strictly to the prescribed dosage regimen.
Patients should be instructed to promptly contact their physician if they develop signs and/or symptoms (eg, sore throat, fever) suggesting an infection.
Drug Interactions
Since Zarontin (ethosuximide) may interact with concurrently administered antiepileptic drugs, periodic serum level determinations of these drugs may be necessary (eg, ethosuximide may elevate phenytoin serum levels and valproic acid has been reported to both increase and decrease ethosuximide levels).
Pregnancy
See WARNINGS.
Pediatric Use
Safety and effectiveness in pediatric patients below the age of 3 years have not been established. (See DOSAGE AND ADMINISTRATION section)

ADVERSE REACTIONS
Gastrointestinal System: Gastrointestinal symptoms occur frequently and include anorexia, vague gastric upset, nausea and vomiting, cramps, epigastric and abdominal pain, weight loss, and diarrhea. There have been reports of gum hypertrophy and swelling of the tongue.

Hemopoietic System: Hemopoietic complications associated with the administration of ethosuximide have included leukopenia, agranulocytosis, pancytopenia, with or without bone marrow suppression, and eosinophilia.
Nervous System: Neurologic and sensory reactions reported during therapy with ethosuximide have included drowsiness, headache, dizziness, euphoria, hiccups, irritability, hyperactivity, lethargy, fatigue, and ataxia. Psychiatric or psychological aberrations associated with ethosuximide administration have included disturbances of sleep, night terrors, inability to concentrate, and aggressiveness. These effects may be noted particularly in patients who have previously exhibited psychological abnormalities. There have been rare reports of paranoid psychosis, increased libido, and increased state of depression with overt suicidal intentions.
Integumentary System: Dermatologic manifestations which have occurred with the administration of ethosuximide have included urticaria, Stevens-Johnson syndrome, systemic lupus erythematosus, pruritic erythematous rashes, and hirsutism.
Special Senses: Myopia.
Genitourinary System: Vaginal bleeding, microscopic hematuria.

OVERDOSAGE

Acute overdoses may produce nausea, vomiting, and CNS depression including coma with respiratory depression. A relationship between ethosuximide toxicity and its plasma levels has not been established. The therapeutic range of serum levels is 40 mcg/mL to 100 mcg/mL, although levels as high as 150 mcg/mL have been reported without signs of toxicity.
Treatment:
Treatment should include emesis (unless the patient is or could rapidly become obtunded, comatose, or convulsing) or gastric lavage, activated charcoal, cathartics and general supportive measures. Hemodialysis may be useful to treat ethosuximide overdose. Forced diuresis and exchange transfusions are ineffective.

DOSAGE AND ADMINISTRATION

Zarontin is administered by the oral route. The *initial* dose for patients 3 to 6 years of age is one capsule (250 mg) per day; for patients 6 years of age and older, 2 capsules (500 mg) per day. The dose thereafter must be individualized according to the patient's response. Dosage should be increased by small increments. One useful method is to increase the daily dose by 250 mg every four to seven days until control is achieved with minimal side effects. Dosages exceeding 1.5 g daily, in divided doses, should be administered only under the strictest supervision of the physician. The *optimal* dose for most pediatric patients is 20 mg/kg/day. This dose has given average plasma levels within the accepted therapeutic range of 40 to 100 mcg/mL. Subsequent dose schedules can be based on effectiveness and plasma level determinations.
Zarontin may be administered in combination with other anticonvulsants when other forms of epilepsy coexist with absence (petit mal). The *optimal* dose for most pediatric patients is 20 mg/kg/day.

HOW SUPPLIED
Zarontin is supplied as:
N 0071-0237-24 Bottles of 100. Each capsule contains 250 mg ethosuximide.
Store at controlled room temperature 15°–30°C (59°–86°F).
Zarontin is also supplied as:
N 0071-2418-23—1 pint bottles. Each 5 mL of syrup contains 250 mg ethosuximide in a raspberry flavored base.
Caution—Federal law prohibits dispensing without prescription.
Revised May 1997   0237G200
©1997, Warner-Lambert Co.
Shown in Product Identification Guide, page 329

ZARONTIN® ℞
[ză "rŏn 'tĭn]
(ethosuximide)
Syrup

DESCRIPTION

Zarontin (ethosuximide) is an anticonvulsant succinimide, chemically designated as alpha-ethyl-alpha-methyl-succinimide, with the following structural formula:

Each teaspoonful (5 mL), for oral administration, contains 250 mg ethosuximide, USP. Also contains citric acid; anhydrous, USP; FD&C red No. 40; FD&C yellow No. 6; flavor; glycerin, USP; purified water, USP; saccharin sodium, USP; sodium benzoate, NF; sodium citrate, USP; sucrose, NF.

CLINICAL PHARMACOLOGY

Ethosuximide suppresses the paroxysmal three cycle per second spike and wave activity associated with lapses of consciousness which is common in absence (petit mal) seizures. The frequency of epileptiform attacks is reduced, apparently by depression of the motor cortex and elevation of the threshold of the central nervous system to convulsive stimuli.

INDICATION AND USAGE

Zarontin is indicated for the control of absence (petit mal) epilepsy.

CONTRAINDICATIONS

Ethosuximide should not be used in patients with a history of hypersensitivity to succinimides.

WARNINGS

Blood dyscrasias, including some with fatal outcome, have been reported to be associated with the use of ethosuximide; therefore, periodic blood counts should be performed. Should signs and/or symptoms of infection (eg, sore throat, fever) develop, blood counts should be considered at that point. Ethosuximide is capable of producing morphological and functional change in the animal liver. In humans, abnormal liver and renal function studies have been reported. Ethosuximide should be administered with extreme caution to patients with known liver or renal disease. Periodic urinalysis and liver function studies are advised for all patients receiving the drug.

Cases of systemic lupus erythematosus have been reported with the use of ethosuximide. The physician should be alert to this possibility.

Usage in Pregnancy: Reports suggest an association between the use of anticonvulsant drugs by women with epilepsy and an elevated incidence of birth defects in children born to these women. Data are more extensive with respect to phenytoin and phenobarbital, but these are also the most commonly prescribed anticonvulsants; less systematic or anecdotal reports suggest a possible similar association with the use of all known anticonvulsant drugs.

The reports suggesting an elevated incidence of birth defects in children of drug-treated epileptic women cannot be regarded as adequate to prove a definite cause and effect relationship. There are intrinsic methodologic problems in obtaining adequate data on drug teratogenicity in humans; the possibility also exists that other factors, eg. genetic factors or the epileptic condition itself, may be more important than drug therapy in leading to birth defects. The great majority of mothers on anticonvulsant medication deliver normal infants. It is important to note that anticonvulsant drugs should not be discontinued in patients in whom the drug is administered to prevent major seizures because of the strong possibility of precipitating status epilepticus with attendant hypoxia and threat to life. In individual cases where the severity and frequency of the seizure disorder are such that the removal of medication does not pose a serious threat to the patient, discontinuation of the drug may be considered prior to and during pregnancy, although it cannot be said with any confidence that even minor seizures do not pose some hazard to the developing embryo or fetus.

The prescribing physician will wish to weigh these considerations in treating or counseling epileptic women of childbearing potential.

PRECAUTIONS

General: Ethosuximide, when used alone in mixed types of epilepsy, may increase the frequency of grand mal seizures in some patients.

As with other anticonvulsants, it is important to proceed slowly when increasing or decreasing dosage, as well as when adding or eliminating other medication. Abrupt withdrawal of anticonvulsant medication may precipitate absence (petit mal) status.

Information for Patients: Ethosuximide may impair the mental and/or physical abilities required for the performance of potentially hazardous tasks such as driving a motor vehicle or other such activity requiring alertness; therefore, the patient should be cautioned accordingly.

Patients taking ethosuximide should be advised of the importance of adhering strictly to the prescribed dosage regimen. Patients should be instructed to promptly contact their physician when they develop signs and/or symptoms suggesting an infection (eg, sore throat, fever).

Drug Interactions: Since Zarontin (ethosuximide) may interact with concurrently administered antiepileptic drugs, periodic serum level determinations of both drugs are recommended (ethosuximide may elevate phenytoin serum levels and valproic acid has been reported to both increase and decrease ethosuximide levels).

Pregnancy: See WARNINGS

ADVERSE REACTIONS

Gastrointestinal System: Gastrointestinal symptoms occur frequently and include anorexia, vague gastric upset, nausea and vomiting, cramps, epigastric and abdominal pain, weight loss, and diarrhea. There have been reports of gum hypertrophy and swelling of the tongue.

Hemopoietic System: Hemopoietic complications associated with the administration of ethosuximide have included leukopenia, agranulocytosis, pancytopenia with or without bone marrow suppression, and eosinophilia.

Nervous System: Neurologic and sensory reactions reported during therapy with ethosuximide have included drowsiness, headache, dizziness, euphoria, hiccups, irritability, hyperactivity, lethargy, fatigue, and ataxia.

Psychiatric or psychological aberrations associated with ethosuximide administration have included disturbances of sleep, night terrors, inability to concentrate, and aggressiveness. These effects may be noted particularly in patients who have previously exhibited psychological abnormalities. There have been rare reports of paranoid psychosis, increased libido, and increased state of depression with overt suicidal intentions.

Integumentary System: Dermatologic manifestations which have occurred with the administration of ethosuximide have included urticaria, Stevens-Johnson syndrome, systemic lupus erythematosus, pruritic erythematous rashes, and hirsutism.

Special Senses: Myopia.

Genitourinary System: Vaginal bleeding, microscopic hematuria.

DOSAGE AND ADMINISTRATION

Zarontin is administered by the oral route. The *initial* dose for patients 3 to 6 years of age is one teaspoonful (250 mg) per day; for patients 6 years of age and older, 2 teaspoonfuls (500 mg) per day. The dose thereafter must be individualized according to the patient's response. Dosage should be increased by small increments. One useful method is to increase the daily dose by 250 mg every four to seven days until control is achieved with minimal side effects. Dosages exceeding 1.5 g daily, in divided doses, should be administered only under the strictest supervision of the physician. The *optimal* dose for most pediatric patients is 20 mg/kg/day. This dose has given average plasma levels within the accepted therapeutic range of 40 to 100 mcg/mL. Subsequent dose schedules can be based on effectiveness and plasma level determinations.

Zarontin may be administered in combination with other anticonvulsants when other forms of epilepsy coexist with absence (petit mal). The optimal dose for most pediatric patients is 20 mg/kg/day.

OVERDOSAGE

Acute overdoses produce CNS depression including coma with respiratory depression. A relationship between ethosuximide toxicity and its plasma levels has not been established. The therapeutic range of serum levels is 40 mcg/mL to 100 mcg/mL, although levels as high as 150 mcg/mL have been reported without signs of toxicity.

Treatment: Treatment should include emesis (unless the patient is, or could rapidly become, obtunded, comatose, or convulsing) or gastric lavage, activated charcoal, cathartics, and general supportive measures. Hemodialysis may be useful to treat ethosuximide overdose. Forced diuresis and exchange transfusions are ineffective.

HOW SUPPLIED

Zarontin is supplied as:
N0071-2418-23—1 pint bottles. Each 5 ml of syrup contains 250 mg ethosuximide in a raspberry flavored base.
Store below 30°C (86°F). Protect from freezing and light.
Zarontin is also supplied in the following form:
N0071-0237-24—Bottles of 100. Each capsule contains 250 mg ethosuximide.
Store at controlled room temperature 15°–30°C (59°–86°F).
Caution—Federal law prohibits dispensing without prescription.
Revised October 1996   2418G027
©1996, Warner-Lambert Co.

IDENTIFICATION PROBLEM?
Turn to the **Product Identification Guide**,
where you'll find more than
1600 products pictured in actual
size and full color.

Parnell Pharmaceuticals, Inc.
P.O. BOX 5130
LARKSPUR, CA 94977

Direct Inquiries to:
Customer Services
(800) 45-PHARM
(415) 256-1800
FAX: (415) 256-8099

Medical Emergency Contact:
Francis W. Parnell, M.D.
(415) 256-1800
FAX: (415) 256-8099

ADDITIONAL PRODUCTS

NDC 50930-	PRODUCT NAME	DESCRIPTION	SIZE
272-03 OTC	EarSol-HC™	anti-itch otic solution 1.0% hydrocortisone, alcohol, propylene glycol with Yerba Santa	30 ml (1 oz)
060-02 OTC	Feminease®	vaginal moisturizing and lubricating cream with Yerba Santa	60 ml (2 oz)
098-02 OTC	MouthKote®	oral moisturizer for dry mouth with Yerba Santa	60 ml (2 oz)
098-08 OTC	MouthKote®	oral moisturizer for dry mouth with Yerba Santa	237 ml (8 oz)
099-08 OTC	Oragesic®	oral analgesic/ anesthetic saline irrigating solution with Yerba Santa	237 ml (8 oz)
280-08 OTC	Pretz® Irrigation	moisturizing nasal irrigating solution glycerin in normal saline with Yerba Santa	237 ml (8 oz)
280-32 OTC	Pretz® Refill	moisturizing nasal solution glycerin in normal saline with Yerba Santa	1 quart (32 oz)
280-50 OTC	Pretz® Spray	moisturizing nasal spray glycerin in normal saline with Yerba Santa	50 ml (1.7 oz)
281-50 OTC	Pretz-D®	moisturizing decongestant nose spray with low-dose ephedrine sulfate (0.25%), glycerin, saline with Yerba Santa	50 ml (1.7 oz)

TAC®-3   ℞
(sterile triamcinolone acetonide suspension) 3mg/mL

NOT FOR INTRAVENOUS USE
FOR INTRALESIONAL AND INTRADERMAL USE

Each mL of aqueous suspension contains: **Active Ingredient:** triamcinolone acetonide 3 mg. **Inactive Ingredients:** benzyl alcohol 0.9% as preservative; carboxymethylcellulose sodium 7.5 mg; polysorbate 80 0.4 mg; sodium chloride 2 mg; in water for injection q.s. Sodium hydroxide and/or hydrochloric acid may have been used to adjust pH.

HOW SUPPLIED

Multiple dose vials of 5 mL containing triamcinolone acetonide 3 mg/mL.

NDC 50930-218-05.

Continued on next page

Tac-3—Cont.

Manufactured for Parnell Pharmaceuticals, Inc.
Larkspur, CA 94977, U.S.A.

by

Steris Laboratories, Inc.
Phoenix, AZ 85043

Pasteur Mérieux Connaught
SWIFTWATER, PA 18370

For Medical Information Contact:
Generally:
Medical Affairs
(800) VACCINE

(800) 822-2463
Adverse Drug Experiences:
Medical Director
(717) 839-7187

(800) 835-3592

Sales and Ordering:
Pasteur Mérieux Connaught
Customer Service
(800) VACCINE
(800) 822-2463
(717) 839-7187

HAEMOPHILUS b CONJUGATE VACCINE ℞
(Tetanus Toxoid Conjugate)
ActHIB®

Caution: Federal (USA) law prohibits dispensing without prescription.

NOTE: Haemophilus b Conjugate Vaccine (Tetanus Toxoid Conjugate) - ActHIB® is identical to Haemophilus b Conjugate Vaccine (Tetanus Toxoid Conjugate)-OmniHIB® (distributed by SmithKline Beecham Pharmaceuticals); and is manufactured by Pasteur Mérieux Sérums & Vaccins S.A.

DESCRIPTION

ActHIB®, Haemophilus b Conjugate Vaccine (Tetanus Toxoid Conjugate), produced by Pasteur Mérieux Sérums & Vaccins S.A., is a sterile, lyophilized powder which is reconstituted at the time of use with either saline diluent (0.4% Sodium Chloride) or Connaught Laboratories, Inc. (CLI) Diphtheria and Tetanus Toxoids and Pertussis Vaccine Adsorbed (whole-cell pertussis vaccine DTP) or Tripedia®, CLI Diphtheria and Tetanus Toxoids and Acellular Pertussis Vaccine Adsorbed (DTaP) (when reconstituted known as TriHIBit™) for intramuscular use only. The vaccine consists of the Haemophilus b capsular polysaccharide (polyribosyl-ribitol-phosphate, PRP), a high molecular weight polymer prepared from the *Haemophilus influenzae* type b strain 1482 grown in a semi-synthetic medium, covalently bound to tetanus toxoid.[1] The lyophilized ActHIB® powder and saline diluent contain no preservative. The tetanus toxoid is prepared by extraction, ammonium sulfate purification, and formalin inactivation of the toxin from cultures of *Clostridium tetani* (Harvard strain) grown in a modified Mueller and Miller medium.[2] The toxoid is filter sterilized prior to the conjugation process. Potency of ActHIB® is specified on each lot by limits on the content of PRP polysaccharide and protein in each dose and the proportion of polysaccharide and protein in the vaccine which is characterized as high molecular weight conjugate.

When ActHIB® is reconstituted with saline diluent, each single dose of 0.5 mL is formulated to contain 10 μg of purified capsular polysaccharide conjugated to 24 μg of inactivated tetanus toxoid, and 8.5% of sucrose.

When ActHIB® is combined with CLI DTP vaccine by reconstitution, each single dose (0.5 mL) is formulated to contain 10 μg of purified capsular polysaccharide conjugated to 24 μg of inactivated tetanus toxoid, 8.5% of sucrose, 6.7 Lf of diphtheria toxoid, 5 Lf of tetanus toxoid and an estimate of 4 protective units of pertussis vaccine. Thimerosal (mercury derivative) 1:10,000 is added as a preservative to CLI DTP vaccine. *(Refer to product insert for CLI whole-cell DTP.)*
When ActHIB® is combined with Tripedia® (TriHIBit™) by reconstitution **for booster dose**, each single dose (0.5 mL) is

formulated to contain 10 μg of purified capsular polysaccharide conjugated to 24 μg of inactivated tetanus toxoid, 8.5% of sucrose, 6.7 Lf of diphtheria toxoid, 5 Lf of tetanus toxoid and 46.8 μg of pertussis antigens. Thimerosal (mercury derivative) 1:10,000 is added as a preservative to Tripedia®.*(Refer to product insert for Tripedia®.)*
The reconstituted vaccine, using saline diluent, appears clear and colorless. The reconstituted vaccine, using CLI DTP vaccine, appears whitish in color. TriHIBit™, the reconstituted vaccine, using Tripedia®, is a homogenous white suspension.

CLINICAL PHARMACOLOGY

NOTE: Haemophilus b Conjugate Vaccine (Tetanus Toxoid Conjugate) - ActHIB® is identical to Haemophilus b Conjugate Vaccine (Tetanus Toxoid Conjugate) - OmniHIB® (distributed by SmithKline Beecham Pharmaceuticals); and is manufactured by Pasteur Mérieux Sérums & Vaccins S.A.

H influenzae type b was the leading cause of invasive bacterial disease among children in the United States prior to licensing of Haemophilus b conjugate vaccines. Based on its active surveillance areas, the Centers for Disease Control and Prevention (CDC) now estimate that *H influenzae* type b disease in children under the age of 5 years has been reduced by 95%.[3] Before effective vaccines were introduced, it was estimated that one in 200 children developed invasive *H influenzae* type b disease by the age of 5 years. In children less than 5 years of age, the mortality rate for invasive *H influenzae* type b disease ranged between 3% and 6%.[3] In more than 60% of these children, meningitis was the clinical syndrome and permanent sequelae ranging from mild hearing loss to mental retardation affecting 20% to 30% of all survivors.[3] Ninety-five percent of the cases of invasive *H influenzae* disease among children < 5 years of age were caused by organisms with the type b polysaccharide capsule. Approximately two-thirds of all cases of invasive *H influenzae* type b disease affected infants and children < 15 months of age, a group for which a vaccine was not available until late 1990.[4,5]
Incidence rates of invasive *H influenzae* type b disease have been shown to be increased in certain high-risk groups, such as native Americans (both American Indians and Eskimos), blacks, individuals of lower socioeconomic status, and patients with asplenia, sickle cell disease, Hodgkin's disease, and antibody deficiency syndromes.[5,6] Studies also have suggested that the risk of acquiring primary invasive *H influenzae* type b disease for children under 5 years of age appears to be greater for those who attend day-care facilities.[7,8,9,10]
The potential for person to person transmission of the organism among susceptible individuals has been recognized. Studies of secondary spread of disease in household contacts of index patients have shown a substantially increased risk among exposed household contacts under 4 years of age.[11] Adults can be colonized with *H influenzae* type b from children infected with the organism.[12]
The response to ActHIB® is typical of a T-dependent immune response to antigen. The prominent isotype of anti-capsular PRP antibody induced by ActHIB® is IgG.[13] A substantial booster response has been demonstrated in children 12 months of age or older who previously received two or three doses. Bactericidal activity against *H influenzae* type b is demonstrated in serum after immunization and statistically correlates with the anti-PRP antibody response induced by ActHIB®.[14]
Antibody to *H influenzae* capsular polysaccharide (anti-PRP) titers of > 1.0 μg/mL following vaccination with unconjugated PRP vaccine correlated with long-term protection against invasive *H influenzae* type b disease in children older than 24 months of age.[15] Although the relevance of this threshold to clinical protection after immunization with conjugate vaccines is not known, particularly in light of the induced, immunologic memory, this level continues to be considered as indicative of long-term protection.[4] The immunogenicity and safety of ActHIB® has been demonstrated in the United States and worldwide. ActHIB® induced, on average anti-PRP levels ≥ 1.0 μg/mL in 90% of infants after the primary series and in more than 98% of infants after a booster dose.[14]
Two clinical trials supported by the National Institutes of Health (NIH) have compared the anti-PRP antibody responses to three Haemophilus b conjugate vaccines in racially mixed populations of children. These studies were done in Tennessee[16] (Table 1) and in Minnesota, Missouri and Texas[17] (Table 2) in infants immunized with ActHIB® and other Haemophilus b conjugate vaccines at 2, 4 and 6 months of age. All Haemophilus b conjugate vaccines were administered concomitantly with Poliovirus Vaccine Live Oral and DTP vaccines at separate sites.

TABLE 1[16]
ANTI-PRP ANTIBODY RESPONSES IN 2-MONTH-OLD INFANTS NIH TRIAL IN TENNESSEE

VACCINE	N*	GEOMETRIC MEAN TITER (GMT) (μg/mL)			
		Pre-Immuni-zation	Post Second Immuni-zation	Post Third Immuni-zation	Post Third Immuni-zation % ≥1.0 μg/mL
PRP-T† (ActHIB®)	65	0.10	0.30	3.64	83%
PRP-OMP¶ (PedvaxHIB®)	64	0.11	0.84	N/A	50%**
HbOC‡ (HibTITER®)	61	0.07	0.13	3.08	75%

TABLE 2[17]
ANTI-PRP ANTIBODY RESPONSES IN 2-MONTH-OLD INFANTS NIH TRIAL IN MINNESOTA, MISSOURI AND TEXAS

VACCINE	N*	GEOMETRIC MEAN TITER (GMT) (μg/mL)			
		Pre-Immuni-zation	Post Second Immuni-zation	Post Third§ Immuni-zation	Post Third§ Immuni-zation % ≥1.0 μg/mL
PRP-T† (ActHIB®)	142	0.25	1.25	6.37	97%
PRP-OMP¶ (PedvaxHIB®)	149	0.18	4.00	N/A	85%**
HbOC‡ (HibTITER®)	167	0.17	0.45	6.31	90%

* N = Number of Children
§ Sera were obtained after the third dose from 86 and 110 infants, in PRP-T and HbOC vaccine groups, respectively.
† Haemophilus b Conjugate Vaccine (Tetanus Toxoid Conjugate)
¶ Haemophilus b Conjugate Vaccine (Meningococcal Protein Conjugate)
** Seroconversion after the recommended 2-dose primary immunization series is shown.
‡ Haemophilus b Conjugate Vaccine (Diphtheria CRM$_{197}$ Protein Conjugate)
N/A Not applicable in this comparison trial although third dose data have been published.[16,17]

Native American populations have had high rates of *H influenzae* type b disease and have been observed to have low immune responses to Haemophilus b conjugate vaccines. Following three doses of ActHIB® at six weeks, four and six months of age, 75% of Native Americans in Alaska showed an anti-PRP antibody titer of ≥ 1.0 μg/mL.[18]
Children 12 to 24 months of age who had not previously received Haemophilus b conjugate vaccination were immunized with a single dose of ActHIB®. GMT anti-PRP antibody responses were 5.12 μg/mL (90% responding with ≥ 1.0 μg/mL) for children 12 to 15 months of age and 4.4 μg/mL (82% responding with ≥ 1.0 μg/mL) for children 17 to 24 months of age.[18]
These trials demonstrated that ActHIB® consistently conferred an anti-PRP antibody response previously shown to correlate with protection, when administered either as a regimen of three doses at least four to eight weeks apart in infants 2 to 6 months of age or as a single dose in children 12 months of age and older.[18]
ActHIB® has been found to be immunogenic in children with sickle cell anemia, a condition which may cause increased susceptibility to Haemophilus b disease. Two doses of ActHIB® given at two-month intervals induced anti-PRP antibody titers of ≥ 1.0 μg/mL in 89% of these children with a mean age of 11 months. This is comparable to anti-PRP antibody levels demonstrated in normal children of similar age following two doses of ActHIB®.[19]

ActHIB® COMBINED WITH WHOLE-CELL PERTUSSIS VACCINE (DTP) BY RECONSTITUTION FOR PRIMARY IMMUNIZATION

Comparative clinical trials demonstrated that a similar anti-PRP response was achieved in infants as young as 2 months old when one dose of CLI whole-cell DTP vaccine was used to reconstitute lyophilized ActHIB® (Table 3).[14,18]

TABLE 3[18]

ANTI-PRP RESPONSES IN 2-MONTH-OLD INFANTS FOLLOWING IMMUNIZATION WITH ActHIB® COMBINED WITH CONNAUGHT LABORATORIES, INC. DTP BY RECONSTITUTION

		GEOMETRIC MEAN TITER (GMT) (µg/mL)			
STUDY SITE	N*	Pre-Immunization	Post Second Immunization	Post Third Immunization	Post Third Immunization % ≥1.0 µg/mL
US	45	0.13	0.55	4.49	91
US	135	0.12	0.43	4.46	85
Chile	94	0.09	4.31	6.94	96

* N = Number of Children

Antibody responses to diphtheria, tetanus and pertussis antigens were also measured in this trial. Post dose three antibody responses to all measured vaccine antigens were similar, within each study, when infants who received the combined vaccine were compared to infants who received whole-cell DTP and ActHIB® separately. Interference with the antibody response to the pertussis component has been suggested with a DTP vaccine unlicensed in the US.[20] Percentages of subjects achieving antibody titers over 1 µg/mL and GMT to PRP in 2-month-old infants following immunization with ActHIB® combined with CLI DTP by reconstitution was similar when compared to infants who received DTP and ActHIB® separately (84% versus 85% and 4.3 µg/mL versus 4.8 µg/mL).[14,18]

TriHIBit™, ActHIB® COMBINED WITH TRIPEDIA® VACCINE BY RECONSTITUTION FOR BOOSTER DOSE

Randomized comparative clinical trials demonstrated that the anti-PRP response achieved in 15 to 20-month-old children after one dose of TriHIBit™, Tripedia® and ActHIB® combination vaccine, was similar to that achieved when the two vaccines were given concomitantly at different sites with separate needles and syringes (Table 4).[18] All children had received three doses of a Haemophilus b conjugate vaccine (HibTITER® or ActHIB®) and three doses of a whole-cell DTP vaccine prior to entry into this clinical trial.

TABLE 4[18]

ANTI-PRP RESPONSES IN 15 TO 20-MONTH-OLD CHILDREN FOLLOWING IMMUNIZATION WITH TriHIBit™ COMPARED TO ActHIB® AND TRIPEDIA® GIVEN CONCOMITANTLY AT SEPARATE SITES

	IMMUNOGENICITY			
	Pre-Dose		Post-Dose	
	TriHIBit™	Separate Injections	TriHIBit™	Separate Injections
N*	88	94	93	98
Anti-PRP (µg/mL)	0.89	1.15	90.30	80.90
% >1 µg/mL	45.50	53.20	100.00	100.00

* N = Number of Children

Geometric mean titers in response to diphtheria, tetanus and pertussis (PT and FHA) were also similar between groups. ***(Refer to product insert for Tripedia®.)*** A difference in four-fold antibody response to FHA was noted in this trial. However, the clinical significance of this difference is not known at present.

INDICATIONS AND USAGE

NOTE: Haemophilus b Conjugate Vaccine (Tetanus Toxoid Conjugate)—ActHIB® is identical to Haemophilus b Conjugate Vaccine (Tetanus Toxoid Conjugate)—OmniHIB® (distributed by SmithKline Beecham Pharmaceuticals); and is manufactured by Pasteur Mérieux Sérums & Vaccins S.A.

ActHIB® or ActHIB® combined with CLI DTP vaccine by reconstitution is indicated for the active immunization of infants and children 2 through 18 months of age for the prevention of invasive disease caused by *H influenzae* type b and/or diphtheria, tetanus and pertussis.

TriHIBit™, ActHIB® combined with Tripedia® by reconstitution, is indicated for the active immunization of children 15 to 18 months of age for prevention of invasive disease caused by *H influenzae* type b and diphtheria, tetanus and pertussis.

Antibody levels associated with protection may not be achieved earlier than two weeks following the last recommended dose.

Only CLI whole-cell DTP, Tripedia® or 0.4% Sodium Chloride diluent may be used for reconstitution of lyophilized ActHIB®. TriHIBit™, ActHIB® combined with Tripedia® by reconstitution, should not be administered to infants younger than 15 months of age.

As with any vaccine, vaccination with ActHIB® reconstituted with CLI DTP or ActHIB® reconstituted with Tripedia® (TriHIBit™) or 0.4% Sodium Chloride diluent may not protect 100% of susceptible individuals.

A single injection containing diphtheria, tetanus, pertussis and Haemophilus b conjugate antigens may be more acceptable to parents and may increase compliance with vaccination programs. Therefore, in these situations it may be the judgment of the physician that it is of benefit to administer a single injection of whole-cell DTP or DTaP and Haemophilus b conjugate vaccines.

CONTRAINDICATIONS

ActHIB® IS CONTRAINDICATED IN CHILDREN WITH A HISTORY OF HYPERSENSITIVITY TO ANY COMPONENT OF THE VACCINE AND TO ANY COMPONENT OF DTP OR Tripedia® WHEN COMBINED BY RECONSTITUTION WITH THESE VACCINES. ANY CONTRAINDICATION FOR DTP IS A CONTRAINDICATION FOR ActHIB® RECONSTITUTED WITH DTP. ANY CONTRAINDICATION FOR Tripedia® IS A CONTRAINDICATION FOR TriHIBit™, ActHIB® RECONSTITUTED WITH Tripedia®. ***(Refer to product inserts for CLI whole-cell DTP and Tripedia®.)***

WARNINGS

If ActHIB® or ActHIB® reconstituted with CLI DTP or ActHIB® reconstituted with Tripedia® (TriHIBit™) is administered to immunosuppressed persons or persons receiving immunosuppressive therapy, the expected antibody responses may not be obtained. This includes patients with asymptomatic or symptomatic HIV-infection,[21] severe combined immunodeficiency, hypogammaglobulinemia, or agammaglobulinemia; altered immune states due to diseases such as leukemia, lymphoma, or generalized malignancy; or an immune system compromised by treatment with corticosteroids, alkylating drugs, antimetabolites or radiation.[22] ***(Refer to product inserts for CLI whole-cell DTP and Tripedia®.)***

TriHIBit™, ActHIB® combined with Tripedia® by reconstitution, should not be administered to infants younger than 15 months of age.

PRECAUTIONS

GENERAL

Care is to be taken by the health-care provider for the safe and effective use of this vaccine.

EPINEPHRINE INJECTION (1:1000) MUST BE IMMEDIATELY AVAILABLE SHOULD AN ANAPHYLACTIC OR OTHER ALLERGIC REACTIONS OCCUR DUE TO ANY COMPONENT OF THE VACCINE.

Prior to an injection of any vaccine, all known precautions should be taken to prevent adverse reactions. This includes a review of the patient's history with respect to possible sensitivity and any previous adverse reactions to the vaccine or similar vaccines, previous immunization history, current health status (see **CONTRAINDICATIONS; WARNINGS** sections), and a current knowledge of the literature concerning the use of the vaccine under consideration. ***(Refer to product inserts for CLI whole-cell DTP and Tripedia®.)***

The health-care provider should ask the parent or guardian about the recent health status of the infant or child to be immunized including the infant's or child's previous immunization history prior to administration of ActHIB®, CLI DTP and Tripedia®.

Minor illnesses such as upper respiratory infection with or without low-grade fever are not contraindications for use of ActHIB®.[23]

As reported with Haemophilus b polysaccharide vaccines,[24] cases of *H influenzae* type b disease may occur subsequent to vaccination and prior to the onset of protective effects of the vaccine.[18] (See **INDICATIONS AND USAGE** section.)

The evidence favors rejection of a causal relation between immunization with Hib conjugate vaccines and early-onset Hib disease.[25]

Antigenuria has been detected in some instances following receipt of ActHIB®; therefore, urine antigen detection may not have definitive diagnostic value in suspected *H influenzae* type b disease within one week of immunization.[26]

Special care should be taken to ensure that ActHIB® reconstituted with CLI DTP or Tripedia® or saline diluent (0.4% Sodium Chloride) is not injected into a blood vessel.

Administration of ActHIB® reconstituted with CLI DTP or ActHIB® reconstituted with Tripedia® (TriHIBit™) or saline diluent (0.4% Sodium Chloride) is not contraindicated in individuals with HIV infection.[22]

A separate, sterile syringe and needle or a sterile disposable unit should be used for each patient to prevent transmission of hepatitis or other infectious agents from person to person. Needles should not be recapped and should be properly disposed.

INFORMATION FOR PATIENT

The health-care provider should inform the parent or guardian of the benefits and risks of the vaccine.

Prior to administration of ActHIB® reconstituted with CLI DTP or ActHIB® reconstituted with Tripedia® (TriHIBit™) or saline diluent (0.4% Sodium Chloride), the parent or guardian should be asked about the recent health status of the infant or child to be immunized.

The physician should inform the parent or guardian about the significant adverse reactions that have been temporally associated with the administration of ActHIB® reconstituted with saline or DTP, or ActHIB® reconstituted with Tripedia® (TriHIBit™). The parent or guardian should be instructed to report any serious adverse reactions to their health-care provider.

As part of the child's immunization record, the date, lot number and manufacturer of the vaccine administered should be recorded.[27,28,29]

The US Department of Health and Human Services has established a new Vaccine Adverse Event Reporting System (VAERS) to accept all reports of suspected adverse events after the administration of any vaccine, including but not limited to the reporting of events required by the National Childhood Vaccine Injury Act of 1986.[27] The toll-free number for VAERS forms and information is 1-800-822-7967.

The National Vaccine Injury Compensation Program, established by the National Childhood Vaccine Injury Act of 1986, requires physicians and other health-care providers who administer vaccines to maintain permanent vaccination records and to report occurrences of certain adverse events to the US Department of Health and Human Services. Reportable events include those listed in the Act for each vaccine and events specified in the package insert as contraindications to further doses of the vaccine.[28,29]

The health-care provider should inform the parent or guardian of the importance of completing the immunization series.

The health-care provider should provide the Vaccine Information Materials (VIMs) which are required to be given with each immunization.

DRUG INTERACTIONS

When CLI DTP is used to reconstitute ActHIB® or Tripedia® is used to reconstitute ActHIB® (TriHIBit™) and administered to immunosuppressed persons or persons receiving immunosuppressive therapy, the expected antibody response may not be obtained.

Immunosuppressive therapies, including irradiation, antimetabolites, alkylating agents, cytotoxic drugs, and corticosteroids (used in greater than physiologic doses), may reduce the immune response to vaccines. Short-term (<2 weeks) corticosteroid therapy or intra-articular, bursal, or tendon injections with corticosteroids should not be immunosuppressive. Although no specific studies with pertussis vaccine are available, if immunosuppressive therapy will be discontinued shortly, it is reasonable to defer vaccination until the patient has been off therapy for one month; otherwise, the patient should be vaccinated while still on therapy.[23]

If ActHIB® reconstituted with CLI DTP or ActHIB® reconstituted with Tripedia® (TriHIBit™) has been administered to persons receiving immunosuppressive therapy, a recent injection of immunoglobulin or having an immunodeficiency disorder, an adequate immunologic response may not be obtained.

In clinical trials, ActHIB® was administered, at separate sites, concomitantly with one or more of the following vaccines: DTP, DTaP, Poliovirus Vaccine Live Oral (OPV), Measles, Mumps and Rubella vaccine (MMR), Hepatitis B vaccine and occasionally Inactivated Poliovirus Vaccine (IPV). No impairment of the antibody response to the individual antigens, diphtheria, tetanus and pertussis, was demonstrated when ActHIB® was given at the same time, at separate sites, with IPV or MMR.[18] In addition, more than 47,000 infants in Finland have received a third dose of ActHIB® concomitantly with MMR vaccine with no increase in serious or unexpected adverse events.[18]

No significant impairment of antibody response to Measles, Mumps and Rubella was noted in 15- 20-month-old children who received TriHIBit™, ActHIB® reconstituted with Tripedia®, concomitantly with MMR. No data are available to the manufacturer concerning the effects on immune response of OPV, IPV or Hepatitis B vaccine when given concurrently with ActHIB® reconstituted with 0.4% Sodium Chloride or CLI DTP or ActHIB® reconstituted with Tripedia® (TriHIBit™).[18]

As with other intramuscular injections, use with caution in patients on anticoagulant therapy.

Continued on next page

ActHIB—Cont.

CARCINOGENESIS, MUTAGENESIS, IMPAIRMENT OF FERTILITY

ActHIB® reconstituted with CLI DTP or ActHIB® reconstituted with Tripedia® (TriHIBit™) has not been evaluated for its carcinogenic, mutagenic potential or impairment of fertility.

PREGNANCY

REPRODUCTIVE STUDIES - PREGNANCY CATEGORY C

Animal reproduction studies have not been conducted with ActHIB® reconstituted with CLI DTP or ActHIB® reconstituted with Tripedia® (TriHIBit™) or saline diluent (0.4% Sodium Chloride). It is also not known whether ActHIB® reconstituted with CLI DTP or ActHIB® reconstituted with Tripedia® (TriHIBit™) or saline diluent (0.4% Sodium Chloride) can cause fetal harm when administered to a pregnant woman or can affect reproduction capacity. ActHIB® reconstituted with CLI DTP or ActHIB® reconstituted with Tripedia® (TriHIBit™) or saline diluent (0.4% Sodium Chloride) is NOT recommended for use in a pregnant woman and is not approved for use in children 5 years of age or older.

PEDIATRIC USE

SAFETY AND EFFECTIVENESS OF TriHIBit™, ActHIB® RECONSTITUTED WITH Tripedia®, IN INFANTS BELOW THE AGE OF 15 MONTHS HAVE NOT BEEN ESTABLISHED. (See DOSAGE AND ADMINISTRATION section.)

SAFETY AND EFFECTIVENESS OF ActHIB® RECONSTITUTED WITH CLI DTP OR SALINE DILUENT (0.4% SODIUM CHLORIDE) IN INFANTS BELOW THE AGE OF SIX WEEKS HAVE NOT BEEN ESTABLISHED. (See DOSAGE AND ADMINISTRATION section.)

ADVERSE REACTIONS

NOTE: Haemophilus b Conjugate Vaccine (Tetanus Toxoid Conjugate) - ActHIB® is identical to Haemophilus b Conjugate Vaccine (Tetanus Toxoid Conjugate) - OmniHIB® (distributed by SmithKline Beecham Pharmaceuticals); and is manufactured by Pasteur Mérieux Sérums & Vaccins S.A.

More than 7,000 infants and young children (≤ 2 years of age) have received at least one dose of ActHIB® during US clinical trials. Of these, 1,064 subjects 12 to 24 months of age who received ActHIB® alone reported no serious or life threatening adverse reactions.

Adverse reactions commonly associated with a first ActHIB® immunization of children 12 to 15 months of age who were previously unimmunized with any Haemophilus b conjugate vaccine, include local pain, redness and swelling at the injection site. Systemic reactions include fever, irritability and lethargy.[14,18]

In a multicenter trial, ActHIB® was administered to US infants at 2, 4, and 6 months of age concomitantly, at separate sites, with CLI DTP. The adverse events observed are summarized in Table 5.

[See table 5 above]

In general, the rates of minor systemic reactions after ActHIB® and DTP immunization were comparable to those usually reported after DTP vaccine alone.[30,31,32,33]

When ActHIB® reconstituted with CLI whole-cell DTP was administered in infants at 2, 4, and 6 months of age, the systemic adverse experience profile (Table 6) was comparable to that observed when the two vaccines were given separately (Table 5). An increase in the rates of local reactions was observed within the 24-hour period after immunization.[18]

[See table 6 above]

In a third US trial when ActHIB® was combined with DTP by reconstitution, approximately 1,450 doses were administered to infants starting at 2 months of age. Adverse reactions observed at 6 and 24 hours respectively after the first immunization (n = 498) were tenderness 66.9% and 30.7%; erythema (>1″) 8.6% and 2.2%; induration 38.2% and 21.7%; irritability 77.9% and 35.7%; drowsiness 63.7% and 34.1%; anorexia 26.1% and 12.9%; diarrhea 6.8% and 9.0%; and vomiting 3.4% and 3.8%.[18] One hypotonic/hyporesponsive episode (HHE) was seen in an infant following the second dose in this trial. This is consistent with the HHE incidence rate observed with DTP vaccination alone.[4]

Adverse reactions associated with ActHIB® generally subsided after 24 hours and usually do not persist beyond 48 hours after immunization.

No data are available on the safety of a booster dose of ActHIB® combined with CLI DTP vaccine by reconstitution given in 15 to 20-month-old children.

In a US trial, safety of TriHIBit™, ActHIB® combined with Tripedia® by reconstitution, in 110 children aged 15 to 20 months was compared to ActHIB® given with Tripedia® at separate sites to 110 children. All children received three doses of Haemophilus b conjugate vaccine (ActHIB® or Hib-TITER®) and three doses of whole-cell DTP at approximately 2, 4 and 6 months of age.

[See table 7 above]

TABLE 5[14]
PERCENTAGE OF INFANTS PRESENTING WITH LOCAL OR SYSTEMIC REACTIONS AT 6, 24, AND 48 HOURS OF IMMUNIZATION WITH ActHIB® ADMINISTERED SIMULTANEOUSLY, AT SEPARATE SITES, WITH CLI DTP VACCINE

REACTION	AGE AT IMMUNIZATION								
	2 Months (n=365)			4 Months (n=364)			6 Months (n=365)		
	6 Hrs.	24 Hrs.	48 Hrs.	6 Hrs.	24 Hrs.	48 Hrs.	6 Hrs.	24 Hrs.	48 Hrs.
Local§									
Tenderness	46.3%	11.5%	2.2%	23.4%	7.4%	1.1%	19.2%	6.0%	1.1%
Erythema	14.3%	4.1%	0.3%	8.8%	5.8%	0.6%	11.5%	6.9%	1.6%
Induration	22.5%	6.3%	1.9%	12.4%	4.7%	0.8%	9.6%	3.8%	1.1%
Systemic*									
Fever >100.8°F†	20.1%	1.3%	0.6%	14.6%	6.6%	1.4%	15.7%	8.8%	0.8%
Irritability	72.6%	21.9%	12.6%	48.4%	25.0%	13.2%	44.1%	25.2%	10.1%
Drowsiness	57.5%	29.9%	10.4%	44.2%	18.1%	7.4%	32.6%	13.4%	2.5%
Anorexia	15.3%	5.8%	4.9%	8.0%	5.0%	3.0%	5.5%	4.9%	2.2%
Diarrhea	4.4%	6.6%	5.2%	5.0%	4.7%	4.7%	4.7%	6.3%	3.6%
Vomiting	2.7%	4.1%	2.7%	2.5%	3.3%	2.8%	2.2%	2.7%	1.9%

Persistent Crying — Percentage of infants within 72 hours after immunization was 1.6% after dose one, 0.6% after dose two, and 0.3% after dose three.

§ Local reactions were evaluated at the ActHIB® injection site.
* The adverse reaction profile is defined by the concomitant use of CLI DTP vaccine.
† The number of individuals observed at each time point for fever varied from 357 to 363.

TABLE 6[18]
PERCENTAGE OF INFANTS PRESENTING WITH LOCAL OR SYSTEMIC REACTIONS AT 6, 24, AND 48 HOURS OF IMMUNIZATION WITH ActHIB® COMBINED WITH CLI DTP VACCINE BY RECONSTITUTION

REACTION	AGE AT IMMUNIZATION								
	2 Months (n=204)			4 Months (n=199)			6 Months (n=200)		
	6 Hrs.	24 Hrs.	48 Hrs.	6 Hrs.	24 Hrs.	48 Hrs.	6 Hrs.	24 Hrs.	48 Hrs.
Local									
Tenderness	47.1%	18.6%	3.4%	33.2%	17.6%	4.0%	25.0%	17.0%	3.5%
Erythema >1″	11.8%	2.5%	0.0%	11.6%	9.1%	2.5%	10.5%	13.5%	3.5%
Induration	31.4%	17.2%	3.9%	26.1%	20.1%	7.5%	28.5%	22.5%	10.0%
Systemic									
Fever >100.4°F	24.6%	2.0%	0.5%	15.8%	6.1%	3.6%	13.0%	10.3%	3.1%
Irritability	70.6%	22.1%	12.8%	56.8%	31.2%	19.1%	40.5%	28.2%	15.9%
Drowsiness	60.3%	23.5%	11.3%	42.2%	20.6%	9.6%	30.3%	12.3%	5.6%
Anorexia	17.7%	6.4%	2.9%	10.1%	7.5%	5.5%	5.1%	4.6%	4.1%
Diarrhea	2.5%	5.4%	1.5%	3.5%	3.5%	2.5%	2.6%	4.1%	5.6%
Vomiting	2.9%	5.4%	2.9%	3.0%	5.0%	3.0%	3.6%	3.6%	1.5%

Persistent Crying — Percentage of infants within 72 hours after immunization was 0.0% after dose one, 0.0% after dose two, and 0.005% after dose three.

TABLE 7[18]
PERCENTAGE OF 15 TO 20-MONTH-OLD CHILDREN PRESENTING WITH LOCAL OR SYSTEMIC REACTIONS AT 6, 24 AND 48 HOURS OF IMMUNIZATION WITH TriHIBit™ COMPARED TO ActHIB® AND TRIPEDIA® GIVEN CONCOMITANTLY AT SEPARATE SITES

REACTION	6 Hrs. Post-dose		24 Hrs. Post-dose		48 Hrs. Post-dose	
	Separate Injections*	TriHIBit™	Separate Injections*	TriHIBit™	Separate Injections*	TriHIBit™
Local	n=110	n=110	n=110	n=110	n=110	n=110
Tenderness	17.3/20.0	19.1	8.2/8.2	10.0	1.8/0.9	1.8
Erythema >1″	0.9/0.0	3.6	2.7/0.9	3.6	0.9/0.0	1.8
Induration**	3.6/5.5	2.7	2.7/3.6	8.2	4.5/0.9	3.6
Swelling	3.6/3.6	3.6	2.7/1.8	5.5	0.9/0.0	4.5
Systemic	n=103–110	n=102–109	n=105–110	n=103–108	n=104–110	n=103–109
Fever >102.2°F	0	2.0	1.0	1.9	1.9	0
Irritability	27.3	22.9	20.9	17.6	12.7	10.1
Drowsiness	36.4	30.3	17.3	13.9	12.7	11.0
Anorexia	12.7	9.2	10.0	6.5	6.4	2.8
Vomiting	0.9	1.8	0.9	1.9	0.9	2.8
Persistent Cry	0	0	0	0	0	0
Unusual Cry	0	0	0	0	0	0.9

*Tripedia® injection site/ActHIB® injection site.
**Induration is defined as hardness with or without swelling.

TriHIBit™, ActHIB® combined with Tripedia® by reconstitution, was administered to approximately 850 children, aged 15 to 20 months. All children received three doses of a Haemophilus b conjugate vaccine (ActHIB® or HibTITER®) and three doses of whole-cell DTP at approximately 2, 4, and 6 months of age. Local reactions were typically mild and usually resolved within the 24 to 48 hour period after immunization. The most common local reactions were pain and tenderness at the injection site. Systemic reactions occurring were usually mild and resolved within 72 hours of immunization. The reaction rates were similar to those observed in Table 7 when TriHIBit™, ActHIB® reconstituted with Tripedia® was administered and when Tripedia® was administered alone as a booster.[18]

In a randomized, double-blind US clinical trial, ActHIB® was given concomitantly with DTP to more than 5,000 infants and hepatitis B vaccine was given with DTP to a similar number. In this large study, deaths due to sudden infant death syndrome (SIDS) and other causes were observed but were not different in the two groups. In the first 48 hours following immunization, two definite and three possible seizures were observed after ActHIB® and DTP in comparison

with none after hepatitis B vaccine and DTP.[18] This rate of seizures following ActHIB® and DTP was not greater than previously reported in infants receiving DTP alone. ***(Refer to product insert for CLI DTP.)*** Other adverse reactions reported with administration of other Haemophilus b conjugate vaccines include urticaria, seizures, hives, renal failure and Guillain-Barré syndrome (GBS).[18,34] A cause and effect relationship among any of these events and the vaccination has not been established.

When ActHIB® was given with DTP and inactivated poliovirus vaccine to more than 100,000 Finnish infants, the rate and extent of serious adverse reactions were not different from those seen when other Haemophilus b conjugate vaccines were evaluated in Finland (i.e. HibTITER®, ProHIBiT®).[18]

However, the number of subjects studied with TriHIBit™, ActHIB® combined with Tripedia® by reconstitution, was inadequate to detect rare serious adverse events.

Reporting of Adverse Events

Reporting by the parent or guardian of all adverse events occurring after vaccine administration should be encouraged. Adverse events following immunization with vaccine should be reported by the health-care provider to the US Department of Health and Human Services (DHHS) Vaccine Adverse Event Reporting System (VAERS). Reporting forms and information about reporting requirements or completion of the form can be obtained from VAERS through a toll-free number 1-800-822-7967.[26,27,28]

Health-care providers also should report these events to the Director of Medical Affairs, Connaught Laboratories, Inc., Route 611, PO Box 187, Swiftwater, PA 18370 or call 1-800-822-2463.

DOSAGE AND ADMINISTRATION

NOTE: Haemophilus b Conjugate Vaccine (Tetanus Toxoid Conjugate) - ActHIB® is identical to Haemophilus b Conjugate Vaccine (Tetanus Toxoid Conjugate) - OmniHIB® (distributed by SmithKline Beecham Pharmaceuticals); and is manufactured by Pasteur Mérieux Sérums & Vaccins S.A.

Parenteral drug products should be inspected visually for particulate matter and/or discoloration prior to administration, whenever solution and container permit. If these conditions exist, the vaccine should not be administered.

RECONSTITUTION:

Using Connaught Laboratories, Inc. DTP, cleanse both the DTP and ActHIB® vial rubber stoppers with a suitable germicide prior to reconstitution. Thoroughly agitate the vial of CLI DTP then withdraw a 0.6 mL dose and inject into the vial of lyophilized ActHIB®. After reconstitution and thorough agitation, the combined vaccines will appear whitish in color. Withdraw and administer 0.5 mL dose of the combined vaccines intramuscularly. Vaccine should be used within 24 hours after reconstitution. Refer to Figures 1, 2, 3, 4, and 5.

To prepare TriHIBit™, cleanse both the Tripedia® and ActHIB® vial rubber stoppers with a suitable germicide prior to reconstitution. Thoroughly agitate the vial of CLI Tripedia® then withdraw a 0.6 mL dose and inject into the vial of lyophilized ActHIB®. After reconstitution and thorough agitation, the combined vaccines will appear whitish in color. Withdraw and administer 0.5 mL dose of the combined vaccines intramuscularly. Vaccine should be used immediately **(within 30 minutes)** after reconstitution. Refer to Figures 1, 2, 3, 4, and 5.

Using saline diluent (0.4% Sodium Chloride) cleanse the vaccine vial rubber stopper with a suitable germicide and inject the entire volume of diluent contained in the vial or syringe into the vial of lyophilized vaccine. Thorough agitation is advised to ensure complete reconstitution. The entire volume of reconstituted vaccine is then drawn back into the syringe before injecting one 0.5 mL dose intramuscularly. The vaccine will appear clear and colorless. Vaccine should be used within 24 hours after reconstitution. Refer to Figures 1, 2, 3, 4, and 5.

INSTRUCTIONS FOR RECONSTITUTION OF ActHIB® WITH CLI DTP OR RECONSTITUTION OF ActHIB® WITH TRIPEDIA® (TriHIBit™) OR SALINE DILUENT (0.4% SODIUM CHLORIDE):

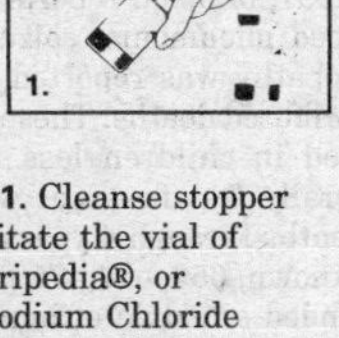

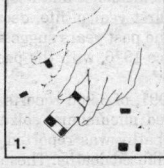

Figure 1. Cleanse stopper and agitate the vial of DTP, Tripedia®, or 0.4% Sodium Chloride used to reconstitute ActHIB®.

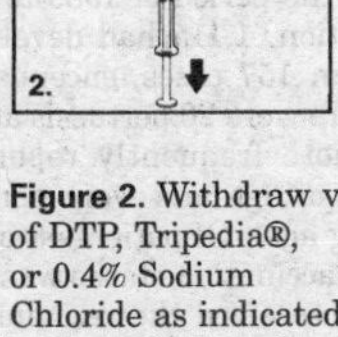

Figure 2. Withdraw volume of DTP, Tripedia®, or 0.4% Sodium Chloride as indicated.

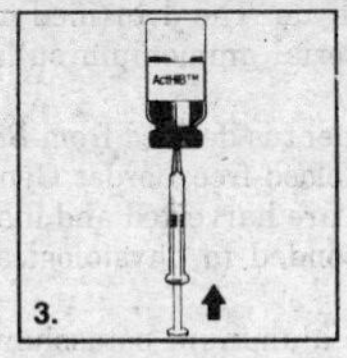

Figure 3. Cleanse the ActHIB® stopper, insert syringe needle through the rubber stopper and inject volume as directed.

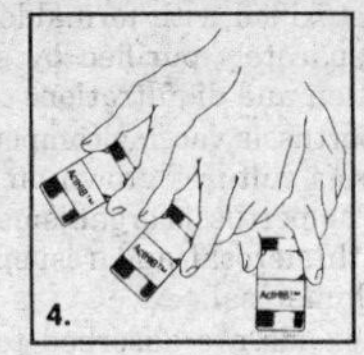

Figure 4. Agitate vial thoroughly.

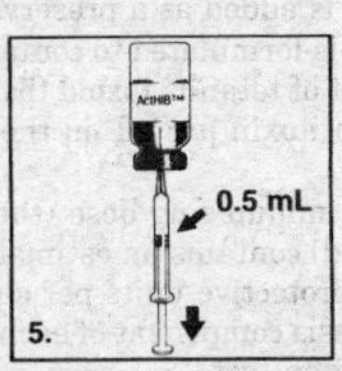

Figure 5. After reconstitution with either DTP, or reconstitution with Tripedia® (TriHIBit™) or with 0.4% Sodium Chloride withdraw 0.5 mL of reconstituted vaccine and administer **intramuscularly.**

Before injection, the skin over the site to be injected should be cleansed with a suitable germicide. After insertion of the needle, aspirate to ensure that the needle has not entered a blood vessel.

DO NOT INJECT INTRAVENOUSLY.

Each dose of ActHIB® reconstituted with CLI DTP or ActHIB® reconstituted with Tripedia® (TriHIBit™) or saline diluent (0.4% Sodium Chloride) is administered intramuscularly in the outer aspect of the vastus lateralis (midthigh) or deltoid. The vaccine should not be injected into the gluteal area or areas where there may be a nerve trunk. During the course of primary immunizations, injections should not be made more than once at the same site.

When ActHIB® is reconstituted with CLI DTP, the combined vaccines are indicated for infants and children 2 through 18 months of age for intramuscular administration in accordance with the schedule indicated in Table 8.[14]

When ActHIB® is reconstituted with Tripedia® (TriHIBit™), the combined vaccines are indicated for children 15 to 18 months of age for intramuscular administration in accordance with the schedule in Table 8.[14]

TABLE 8[14]

RECOMMENDED IMMUNIZATION SCHEDULE FOR ActHIB® AND DTP OR TRIPEDIA®

For Previously Unvaccinated Children

DOSE	AGE	IMMUNIZATION
First, Second and Third	At 2, 4 and 6 months	ActHIB® reconstituted with DTP or with saline diluent (0.4% Sodium Chloride)
Fourth	At 15 to 18 months	ActHIB® reconstituted with DTP or with Tripedia® (TriHIBit™) or with saline diluent (0.4% Sodium Chloride)
Fifth	At 4 to 6 years	DTP or Tripedia®

For Previously Unvaccinated Children

The number of doses of Haemophilus b Conjugate Vaccine indicated depends on the age at which immunization is begun. A child 7 to 11 months of age should receive 2 doses of Haemophilus b Conjugate Vaccine at 8-week intervals and a booster dose at 15 to 18 months of age. A child 12 to 14 months of age should receive 1 dose of Haemophilus b Conjugate Vaccine followed by a booster 2 months later.

Preterm infants should be vaccinated according to their chronological age from birth.[35]

Interruption of the recommended schedule with a delay between doses should not interfere with the final immunity achieved with ActHIB® reconstituted with CLI DTP or ActHIB® reconstituted with Tripedia® (TriHIBit™) or saline diluent (0.4% Sodium Chloride). There is no need to start the series over again, regardless of the time elapsed between doses.

It is acceptable to administer a booster dose of TriHIBit™, ActHIB® reconstituted with Tripedia®, following a primary series of Haemophilus b conjugate and whole-cell DTP vaccines, or a primary series of a combination vaccine containing whole-cell DTP.

HOW SUPPLIED

ActHIB® RECONSTITUTED WITH WHOLE-CELL DTP

Vial, 1 Dose, lyophilized vaccine (10 x 1 Dose vials per package), packaged with one 7.5 mL vial of Connaught Laboratories, Inc. Diphtheria and Tetanus Toxoids and Pertussis Vaccine as Diluent—Product No. 49281-549-10

ActHIB® RECONSTITUTED WITH 0.4% SODIUM CHLORIDE DILUENT

Vial, 1 Dose, lyophilized vaccine (5 x 1 Dose vials per package), packaged with 0.6 mL vial containing diluent (5 x 0.6 mL vials per package)—Product No. 49281-545-05

Administer vaccine within 24 hours after reconstitution.

TriHIBit™, ActHIB® RECONSTITUTED WITH TRIPEDIA®

Vial, 1 Dose, lyophilized vaccine (10 x 1 Dose vials per package), packaged with one 7.5 mL vial of Tripedia® as Diluent—Product No. 49281-557-10

Vial, 1 Dose, lyophilized vaccine (5 x 1 Dose vials per package), packaged with five 1 Dose vials of Tripedia® as Diluent—Product No. 49281-557-05

Administer vaccine immediately (within 30 minutes) after reconstitution.

STORAGE

Store lyophilized vaccine packaged with saline diluent, Diphtheria and Tetanus Toxoids and Pertussis or Tripedia® between 2°–8°C (35°–46°F). DO NOT FREEZE.

REFERENCES

1. Chu CY, et al. Further studies on the immunogenicity of *Haemophilus influenzae* type b and pneumococcal type 6A polysaccharide-protein conjugate. Infect Immun 40: 245-246, 1983
2. Mueller JH, et al. Production of diphtheria toxin of high potency (100 Lf) on a reproducible medium. J Immunol 40: 21-32, 1941
3. Adams WG, et al. Decline of Childhood *Haemophilus influenzae* Type b (Hib) Disease in the Hib Vaccine Era. JAMA 269: 221-226, 1993
4. Recommendations of the Immunization Practices Advisory Committee (ACIP). Haemophilus b conjugate vaccines for prevention of *Haemophilus influenzae* type b disease among infants and children two months of age and older. MMWR 40: No. RR-1, 1991
5. Broome CV. Epidemiology of *Haemophilus influenzae* type b infections in the United States. Pediatr Infect Dis J 6: 779-782, 1987
6. ACIP. Polysaccharide vaccine for prevention of *Haemophilus influenzae* type b disease. MMWR 34: 201-205, 1985
7. Istre GR, et al. Risk factors for primary invasive *Haemophilus influenzae* disease: Increased risk from day care attendance and school-aged household members. J Pediatr 106: 190-195, 1985
8. Redmond SR, et al. *Haemophilus influenzae* type b disease. An epidemiologic study with special reference to day-care centers. JAMA 252: 2581-2584, 1984
9. Murphy TV, et al. County-wide surveillance of invasive Haemophilus infections: Risk of associated cases in Child Care Programs (CCPs). Twenty-third Interscience Conference on Antimicrobial Agents and Chemotherapy (Abstract #788) 229, 1983
10. Fleming D, et al. *Haemophilus influenzae* b (Hib) disease - secondary spread in day care. Twenty-fourth Interscience Conference on Antimicrobial Agents and Chemotherapy (Abstract #967) 261, 1984
11. CDC. Prevention of secondary cases of *Haemophilus influenzae* type b disease. MMWR 31: 672-680, 1982
12. Michaels RH, et al. Pharyngeal colonization with *Haemophilus influenzae* type b: A longitudinal study of families with a child with meningitis or epiglottitis due to *H. influenzae* type b. J Infec Dis 136: 222-227, 1977
13. Holmes SJ, et al. Immunogenicity of four *Haemophilus influenzae* type b conjugate vaccines in 17- to 19-month-old children. J Pediatr 118: 364-371, 1991
14. Data on file, Pasteur Mérieux Sérums & Vaccins S.A.
15. Peltola H, et al. Prevention of *Haemophilus influenzae* type b bacteremic infections with the capsular polysaccharide vaccine. N Engl J Med 310: 1561-1566, 1984
16. Decker MD, et al. Comparative trial in infants of four conjugate *Haemophilus influenzae* type b vaccines. J Pediatr 120: 184-189, 1992
17. Granoff DM, et al. Differences in the immunogenicity of three *Haemophilus influenzae* type b conjugate vaccines in infants. J Pediatr 121: 187-194, 1992
18. Data on file, Connaught Laboratories, Inc.
19. Kaplan SL, et al. Immunogenicity of *Haemophilus influenzae* type b polysaccharide-tetanus protein conjugate vaccine in children with sickle hemoglobinopathy or malignancies, and after systemic *Haemophilus influenzae* type b infection. J Pediatr 120: 367-370, 1992
20. Clemens JD, et al. Impact of *Haemophilus influenzae* Type b Polysaccharide-Tetanus Protein Conjugate Vac-

Continued on next page

ActHIB—Cont.

cine on responses to concurrently administered Diphtheria-Tetanus-Pertussis Vaccine. JAMA 267: 673-678, 1992

21. Steinhoff MC, et al. Antibody responses to *Haemophilus influenzae* type b vaccines in men with human immunodeficiency virus infection. N Engl J Med 325 (26): 1837-1842, 1991

22. ACIP. General recommendations on immunization. MMWR 38: 205-227, 1989

23. ACIP. Diphtheria, Tetanus, and Pertussis: Recommendations for Vaccine Use and Other Preventive Measures. MMWR 40: No. RR-10, 1991

24. FDA Workshop on Haemophilus b Polysaccharide Vaccine - A Preliminary Report. MMWR 36: 529-531, 1987

25. IOM. Adverse Events Associated with Childhood Vaccines: Evidence Bearing on Causality. *Haemophilus influenzae* Type b Vaccines. In: Stratton KR, Howe CJ, Johnston Jr. RB, eds. 1993. National Academy Press. Washington DC, pp. 236-273, 1993

26. Rothstein EP, et al. Comparison of antigenuria after immunization with three *Haemophilus influenzae* type b conjugate vaccines. Pediatr Infect Dis J 10: 311-314, 1991

27. Vaccine Adverse Event Reporting System - United States. MMWR 39: 730-733, 1990

28. CDC. National Childhood Vaccine Injury Act: Requirements for permanent vaccination records and for reporting of selected events after vaccination. MMWR 37: 197-200, 1988

29. National Childhood Vaccine Injury Act of 1986 (Amended 1987)

30. Cody CL, et al. Nature and rates of adverse reactions associated with DTP and DT immunizations in infants and children. Pediatr 68: 650-660, 1981

31. Barkin RM, et al. Diphtheria-tetanus-pertussis vaccine: reactogenicity of commercial products. Pediatr 63: 256-260, 1979

32. Baraff LJ, et al. DTP-associated reactions: an analysis by injection site, manufacturer, prior reactions and dose. Pediatr 73: 31-39, 1984

33. Long SS, et al. Longitudinal study of adverse reactions following diphtheria-tetanus-pertussis vaccine in infancy. Pediatr 85: 294-302, 1990

34. D'Cruz OF, et al. Acute inflammatory demyelinating polyradiculoneuropathy (Guillain-Barré Syndrome) after immunization with *Haemophilus influenzae* type b conjugate vaccine. J Pediatr 115: 743-746, 1989

35. American Academy of Pediatrics. Immunization in Special Clinical Circumstances. In: Peter G, ed. 1994 Red Book: Report of the Committee on Infectious Diseases. 23rd ed. Elk Grove Village, IL 51-52, 1994

Product information
as of September 1996

Manufactured by:
PASTEUR MÉRIEUX Sérums & Vaccins S.A.
Lyon, France US License No. 384
Distributed by:
CONNAUGHT LABORATORIES, INC.
Swiftwater, Pennsylvania 18370, USA
1-800-VACCINE (1-800-822-2463)   3441
PASTEUR MÉRIEUX CONNAUGHT
RHÔNE-POULENC GROUP
Shown in Product Identification Guide, pages 329 and 330

ActHIB for reconstitution with Connaught DTP vaccine Haemophilus b Conjugate Vaccine (Tetanus Toxoid Conjugate) packaged with Diphtheria and Tetanus Toxoids and Pertussis Vaccine Adsorbed USP (For Pediatric Use) See package inserts for each component product.

DIPHTHERIA AND TETANUS TOXOIDS   ℞
and Pertussis Vaccine Adsorbed USP
(For Pediatric Use)

Caution: Federal (USA) law prohibits dispensing without prescription.

DESCRIPTION

Diphtheria and Tetanus Toxoids and Pertussis Vaccine Adsorbed USP (For Pediatric Use) combines diphtheria and tetanus toxoids adsorbed with pertussis vaccine, for intramuscular use, in a sterile isotonic sodium chloride solution containing sodium phosphate buffer to control pH. The vaccine, after shaking, is a turbid liquid, whitish-gray in color. When used to reconstitute Haemophilus b Conjugate Vaccine (Tetanus Toxoid Conjugate), ActHIB® or OmniHIB™, the combined vaccines appear whitish in color.
Corynebacterium diphtheriae cultures are grown in a modified Mueller and Miller medium.[1] *Clostridium tetani* cultures are grown in a peptone-based medium. Both toxins

are detoxified with formaldehyde. The detoxified materials are separately purified by serial ammonium sulfate fractionation and diafiltration.
The pertussis vaccine component is derived from *Bordetella pertussis* cultures grown on blood-free Bordet Gengou media. The pertussis organisms are harvested and inactivated with thimerosal and resuspended in physiological saline and thimerosal.
The toxoids are adsorbed to aluminum potassium sulfate (alum). The adsorbed diphtheria and tetanus toxoids are combined with pertussis vaccine concentrate, and diluted to a final volume using sterile phosphate-buffered physiological saline. Each 0.5 mL dose contains, by assay, not more than 0.17 mg of aluminum and not more than 100 µg (0.02%) of residual formaldehyde. Thimerosal (mercury derivative) 1:10,000 is added as a preservative.
Each 0.5 mL dose is formulated to contain 6.7 Lf of diphtheria toxoid and 5 Lf of tetanus toxoid (both toxoids induce at least 2 units of antitoxin per mL in the guinea pig potency test).
The total human immunizing dose (the first three 0.5 mL doses administered) contains an estimate of 12 units of pertussis vaccine (4 protective units per single dose).[2] The potency of the pertussis component of each lot of DTP is tested in a mouse protection test.
At the time when Connaught Laboratories, Inc. (CLI) DTP vaccine is used to reconstitute ActHIB® and OmniHIB™, each single dose of the 0.5 mL mixture is formulated to contain 6.7 Lf of diphtheria toxoid, 5 Lf of tetanus toxoid, an estimate of 4 protective units of pertussis vaccine, 10 µg of purified capsular polysaccharide conjugated to 24 µg of inactivated tetanus toxoid, and 8.5% of sucrose.
NOTE: Haemophilus b Conjugate Vaccine (Tetanus Toxoid Conjugate)—ActHIB® is identical to Haemophilus b Conjugate Vaccine (Tetanus Toxoid Conjugate)—OmniHIB™ (distributed by SmithKline Beecham Pharmaceuticals); both products are manufactured by Pasteur Mérieux Sérums & Vaccins S.A.

CLINICAL PHARMACOLOGY

DIPHTHERIA

Corynebacterium diphtheria may cause both localized and generalized disease. Systemic intoxication is caused by diphtheria exotoxin, an extracellular protein metabolite of toxigenic strains of *C. diphtheria*. Protection against disease is due to the development of neutralizing antibodies to diphtheria toxin.
At one time, diphtheria was common in the United States. More than 200,000 cases, primarily among young children, were reported in 1921. Approximately 5% to 10% of cases were fatal; the highest case-fatality ratios were recorded for the very young and the elderly. Reported cases of diphtheria of all types declined from 306 in 1975 to 59 in 1979; most were cutaneous diphtheria reported from a single state. After 1979, cutaneous diphtheria was no longer a notifiable disease. From 1980 to 1989, only 24 cases of respiratory diphtheria were reported; two cases were fatal, and 18 (75%) occurred among persons 20 years of age or older.[2]
Diphtheria is currently a rare disease in the United States primarily because of the high level of appropriate vaccination among children (97% of children entering school have received ≥ three doses of diphtheria and tetanus toxoids and pertussis vaccine adsorbed [DTP]) and because of an apparent reduction in the prevalence of toxigenic strains of *C. diphtheria*. Most cases occur among unvaccinated or inadequately immunized persons.[2]
Both toxigenic and nontoxigenic strains of *C. diphtheria* can cause disease, but only strains that produce toxin cause myocarditis and neuritis. Toxigenic strains are more often associated with severe or fatal illness in noncutaneous (respiratory or other mucosal surface) infections and are more commonly recovered in association with respiratory than from cutaneous infections.[2]
A complete vaccination series substantially reduces the risk of developing diphtheria, and vaccinated persons who develop disease have milder illness. Protection lasts at least 10 years. Vaccination does not, however, eliminate carriage of *C. diphtheriae* in the pharynx or nose or on the skin.[2]

TETANUS

Tetanus is an intoxication manifested primarily by neuromuscular dysfunction caused by a potent exotoxin elaborated by *Clostridium tetani*.
The occurrence of tetanus in the United States has decreased dramatically from 560 reported cases in 1947 to a record low of 48 reported cases in 1987. Tetanus in the United States is primarily a disease of older adults. Of 99 tetanus patients with complete information reported to the Centers for Disease Control and Prevention (CDC) during 1987 and 1988, 68% were ≥ 50 years of age, while only six were < 20 years of age. Overall, the case-fatality rate was 21%. In 1992, 45 cases were reported of which 82% were ≥ 50 years of age.[3] The disease continues to occur almost exclusively among persons who are unvaccinated or inadequately vaccinated or whose vaccination histories are unknown or uncertain.[2]

In 4% of tetanus cases reported during 1987 and 1988, no wound or other condition could be implicated. Non-acute skin lesions, such as ulcers, or medical conditions such as abscesses were reported in 14% of cases.[2]
Spores of *C. tetani* are ubiquitous. Serologic tests indicate that naturally acquired immunity to tetanus toxin does not occur in the United States.[2] Thus, universal primary vaccination, with subsequent maintenance of adequate antitoxin levels by means of appropriately timed boosters, is necessary to protect persons among all age-groups. Tetanus toxoid is a highly effective antigen, and a completed primary series generally induces protective levels of neutralizing antibodies to tetanus toxin that persist for ≥ 10 years.[2]
The potency of diphtheria and tetanus toxoids was determined on the basis of immunogenicity studies with a comparison to a serological correlate of protection (0.01 I.U./mL) established by the Panel on Review of Bacterial Vaccines & Toxoids.[4]

EFFICACY OF DIPHTHERIA AND TETANUS TOXOID VACCINES

Circulating protective levels of neutralizing antibodies to diphtheria and tetanus toxins can be induced by the administration of Diphtheria and Tetanus Toxoids Adsorbed USP (For Pediatric Use) (DT) or DTP.
A clinical study was performed in 20 children under one year of age to determine the serological responses and the adverse reactions when Connaught Laboratories, Inc. (CLI) DT was administered as a primary series of three doses. Protective levels of diphtheria and tetanus antitoxins that were equal to or greater than 0.01 I.U./mL were detected in 100% of the children following two doses of the vaccine. However, maternal antibody have contributed to the total neutralizing antibody in some of these infants. Protective levels of antitoxin were observed in 100% of these infants following three doses of DT. No local or systemic reactions were observed in approximately half of the infants and only mild or moderate reactions were observed in the remainder of the DT study group.[5]
Another clinical study to evaluate serological responses and adverse reactions of CLI DT was performed in 40 children under one year of age. One group of 20 children received 0.5 mL doses of DTP, DT, DTP at two, four and six months of age, respectively. The second group of 20 children received 0.5 mL doses of DTP, DTP, and DT, respectively, at the same ages. The immunologic protection against diphtheria and tetanus as measured by toxin neutralizing antibodies induced by DT was comparable when administered as either a second or third dose.[6] The reaction rates following CLI whole-cell DTP vaccination closely correlated with the rates observed with other commercially available whole-cell DTP vaccines.[7] The incidence of adverse reactions was significantly lower following DT administration (p < 0.05). Although the number of vaccinees was small, no persistent screaming episodes or severe neurological reactions such as seizures or encephalopathy were observed with either vaccine in this study.[6]

PERTUSSIS

Disease caused by *Bordetella pertussis* was once a major cause of infant and childhood morbidity and mortality in the United States. Pertussis (whooping cough) became a nationally notifiable disease in 1922, and reports reached a peak of 265,269 cases and 7,518 deaths in 1934. The highest number of reported pertussis deaths (9,269) occurred in 1923. The introduction and widespread use of standardized whole-cell pertussis vaccines combined with diphtheria and tetanus toxoids (DTP) in the late 1940s resulted in a substantial decline in pertussis disease, a decline which continued without interruption for nearly 30 years.[2]
By 1970, the annual reported incidence of pertussis had been reduced by 99%. During the 1970s the annual numbers of reported cases stabilized at an average of approximately 2,300 cases each year. During the 1980s, however, the annual numbers of reported cases gradually increased from 1,730 cases in 1980 to 4,517 cases in 1989. An average of eight pertussis-associated fatalities was reported each year throughout the 1980s.[2]
From 1989 to 1991, 11,446 cases of pertussis were reported for an unadjusted incidence per 100,000 population of 1.7 in 1989, 1.8 in 1990 and 1.1 in 1991. The incidence for 1992 was 1.6 per 100,000. Age specific incidence and hospitalization rates were highest in the first year of life, decreasing with increasing age. Trends of the past years suggest an increase in reported pertussis since 1976, with the peak year being 1990.[8]
During the period of 1989 to 1991, of 3,900 reports of hospitalization, 1,115 had developed pneumonia, seizures occurred in 157 cases, encephalopathy was reported for 12, and there were 20 pertussis attributed deaths. These events were more frequently reported in children less than 6 months of age and were generally less frequent with increasing age.[7] Of patients 3 months through 4 years of age, where vaccination status was known, 65% of 4,471 patients had not received the recommended schedule of immunization and 39% had not received any pertussis containing vaccine.[3]

Among older children and adults, including those previously vaccinated, *B. pertussis* infection may result in symptoms of bronchitis or upper-respiratory-tract infection. Pertussis may not be associated with classic signs, especially the inspiratory whoop. Older preschool children and school-age siblings who are not fully vaccinated and who develop pertussis can be important sources of infection for infants < 1 year of age. Adults also play an important role in the transmission of pertussis to unvaccinated or incompletely vaccinated infants and young children.[2]

EFFICACY OF PERTUSSIS VACCINE

Although DTP has been evaluated as a control vaccine in a number of clinical trials of "Acellular pertussis vaccines," no formal efficacy trial was performed prior to approval. Approval was based on historical and continuing evidence of protection (surveillance) in the population at risk. It was also shown that vaccines with acceptable mouse protection potencies induced protective serum agglutinin antibody titers.[4] The pertussis component of each lot of DTP is tested for potency by a mouse protection test.

In clinical trials, one dose of CLI whole-cell DTP vaccine was used to reconstitute one lyophilized single dose vial of ActHIB® or OmniHIB™ with no diminution of anti-PRP response or diphtheria, tetanus and pertussis responses.

INDICATIONS AND USAGE

Diphtheria and Tetanus Toxoids and Pertussis Vaccine Adsorbed USP (For Pediatric Use) is recommended for active immunization of children up to 7 years against diphtheria, tetanus, and pertussis (whooping cough) simultaneously. However, in instances where the pertussis vaccine component is contraindicated, or where the physician decides that pertussis vaccine is not to be administered, DT should be used. Immunization should be started at 6 weeks to 2 months of age and be completed before the seventh birthday.[2,9]

Persons recovering from confirmed pertussis do not need additional doses of DTP but should receive additional doses of DT to complete the series.[2]

Available data indicate that the appropriate age for institution of immunizations in prematurely born infants is the usual chronological age of 2 months. Vaccine doses should not be reduced for preterm infants.[2,9]

If passive immunization is required, Tetanus Immune Globulin (Human) (TIG) and/or equine Diphtheria Antitoxin are the products of choice for tetanus and diphtheria, respectively (see **DOSAGE AND ADMINISTRATION** section).

When CLI DTP vaccine is used to reconstitute ActHIB® or OmniHIB™, the combined vaccines are indicated for the active immunization of infants and children 2 months through 5 years of age for the prevention of invasive diseases caused by diphtheria, tetanus, pertussis and *H influenzae* type b.[10,11] ***(Refer to ActHIB® package insert.)***

A single injection containing diphtheria, tetanus, pertussis and Haemophilus b conjugate antigens may be more acceptable to parents and may increase compliance with vaccination programs. Therefore, in those situations where, in the judgment of the physician, it is of benefit to administer a single injection of whole-cell DTP vaccine and Haemophilus b conjugate vaccine concomitantly, ***only CLI whole-cell DTP vaccine may be used for reconstitution of lyophilized ActHIB® or OmniHIB™.*** Antibody levels associated with protection may not be achieved earlier than two weeks following the last recommended dose. (See **DOSAGE AND ADMINISTRATION** section.)

As with any vaccine, vaccination with DTP or combined vaccines CLI DTP and ActHIB® or OmniHIB™ may not protect 100% of susceptible individuals.

NOTE: Haemophilus b Conjugate Vaccine (Tetanus Toxoid Conjugate)—ActHIB® is identical to Haemophilus b Conjugate Vaccine (Tetanus Toxoid Conjugate)—OmniHIB™ (distributed by SmithKline Beecham Pharmaceuticals); both products are manufactured by Pasteur Mérieux Sérums & Vaccins S.A.

This vaccine is NOT to be used for the treatment of diphtheria, tetanus, pertussis or H influenzae type b infection.

This vaccine should NOT be used for immunizing persons 7 years of age and older.

CONTRAINDICATIONS

Hypersensitivity to any component of the vaccine, including thimerosal, a mercury derivative, is a contraindication for further use of this vaccine.

It is a contraindication to use this or any other related vaccine after an immediate anaphylactic reaction associated with a previous dose.

It is a contraindication to administer this vaccine in the presence of any evolving neurological condition.

Encephalopathy after a previous dose is a contraindication to further use.

Immunization should be deferred during the course of an acute illness. Vaccination of infants and children with severe, febrile illness should generally be deferred until these persons have recovered. However, the presence of minor illnesses such as mild upper respiratory infections with or without low-grade fever are not contraindications to further use.[2]

Elective immunization procedures should be deferred during an outbreak of poliomyelitis.[12]

WARNINGS

If any of the following events occur in temporal relation to receipt of DTP, the decision to give subsequent doses of vaccine containing the pertussis component should be carefully considered. There may be circumstances, such as a high incidence of pertussis, when the potential benefits outweigh possible risks, particularly since these events are not associated with permanent sequelae.[2]

THE FOLLOWING EVENTS WERE PREVIOUSLY CONSIDERED CONTRAINDICATIONS AND ARE NOW CONSIDERED WARNINGS:[2]

1. **Temperature of ≥40.5°C (105°F) within 48 hours not due to another identifiable cause:** Such a temperature is considered a warning because of the likelihood that fever following a subsequent dose of DTP vaccine also will be high. Because such febrile reactions are usually attributed to the pertussis component, vaccination with DT should not be discontinued.[2]
2. **Collapse or shock-like state (hypotonic-hyporesponsive episode) within 48 hours:** Although these uncommon events have not been recognized to cause death nor to induce permanent neurological sequelae, it is prudent to continue vaccination with DT, omitting the pertussis component.[2]
3. **Persistent, inconsolable crying lasting ≥3 hours, occurring within 48 hours:** Follow-up of infants who have cried inconsolably following DTP vaccination has indicated that this reaction, though unpleasant, is without long-term sequelae and not associated with other reactions of greater significance.[2] Evidence is insufficient to indicate whether pertussis vaccine-associated protracted, inconsolable, or high-pitched crying or screaming does, or does not, lead to chronic neurological damage.[13] Inconsolable crying occurs most frequently following the first dose and is less frequently reported following subsequent doses of DTP vaccine. However, crying for >30 minutes following DTP vaccination can be a predictor of increased likelihood of recurrence of persistent crying following subsequent doses. Children with persistent crying have had a higher rate of local reactions than children who had other DTP-associated reactions (including high fever, seizures, and hypotonic-hyporesponsive episodes), suggesting that prolonged crying was really a pain reaction.[2]
4. **Convulsions with or without fever occurring within three days:** Short-lived convulsions, with or without fever, have not been shown to cause permanent sequelae. Furthermore, the occurrence of prolonged febrile seizures (i.e., status epilepticus—any seizure lasting > 30 minutes or recurrent seizures lasting a total of 30 minutes without the child fully regaining consciousness), irrespective of their cause, involving an otherwise normal child does not substantially increase the risk for subsequent febrile (brief or prolonged) or afebrile seizures. The risk is significantly increased (p = 0.018) only among children who are neurologically abnormal before their episode of status epilepticus.[2] Accordingly, although a convulsion following DTP vaccination has previously been considered a contraindication to further doses, under certain circumstances subsequent doses may be indicated, particularly if the risk of pertussis in the community is high. If a child has a seizure following the first or second dose of DTP, it is desirable to delay subsequent doses until the child's neurological status is better defined. By the end of the first year of life, the presence of an underlying neurologic disorder has usually been determined, and appropriate treatment instituted. DT vaccine should not be administered before a decision has been made about whether to continue the DTP series. Regardless of which vaccine is given, it is prudent also to administer acetaminophen,[2] 15 mg/kg of body weight, at the time of vaccination and every 4 hours subsequently for 24 hours.

Persons who experience Arthus-type hypersensitivity reactions or a temperature of > 103°F (39.4°C) following a prior dose of tetanus toxoid usually have high serum tetanus antitoxin levels and should not be given even emergency doses of Td more frequently than every 10 years, even if they have a wound that is neither clean nor minor.[2]

DTP should not be given to children with any coagulation disorder, including thrombocytopenia, that would contraindicate intramuscular injection unless the potential benefit clearly outweighs the risk of administration.

Recent studies suggest that infants and children with a history of convulsions in first-degree family members (i.e., siblings and parents) have a 3.2-fold increased risk for neurologic events compared with those without such histories.[14] *However, the ACIP has concluded that a family history of convulsions in parents and siblings is not a contraindication to pertussis vaccination and that children with such family histories should receive pertussis vaccine according to the recommended schedule.*[2]

A recent review of all available data by the IOM found evidence is consistent with a causal relationship between DTP vaccination and acute encephalopathy, but that there is insufficient evidence to indicate a causal relation between DTP vaccine and permanent neurologic damage.[13]

Infants and children with recognized possible or potential underlying neurologic conditions seem to be at enhanced risk for the appearance of manifestations of the underlying neurologic disorder within two or three days following vaccination.[2] Whether to administer DTP to children with proven or suspected underlying neurologic disorders must be decided on an individual basis. Important considerations include the current local incidence of pertussis, the near absence of diphtheria in the United States and the low risk of infection with *C. tetani.*[2]

Although these events were considered absolute contraindications in previous ACIP recommendations, there may be circumstances, such as a high incidence of pertussis, in which the potential benefits outweigh possible risks, particularly because these events are not associated with permanent sequelae.[2]

The administration of DTP to children with proven or suspected underlying neurologic disorders that are not actively evolving must be decided on an individual basis.

Only full doses (0.5 mL) of DTP vaccine should be given; if a specific contraindication to DTP exists, the vaccine should not be given.[2] Controversy regarding the safety of pertussis vaccine during the 1970s led to several studies of the benefits and risks of this vaccination during the 1980s. These epidemiologic analyses clearly indicate that the benefits of pertussis vaccination outweigh any risks and have not shown a cause and effect with neurologic illness.[2,9]

Deaths have been reported in temporal association with the administration of DTP vaccine (see **ADVERSE REACTIONS** section). When CLI DTP vaccine is used alone or to reconstitute ActHIB® or OmniHIB™ and administered to immunosuppressed persons or persons receiving immunosuppressive therapy, the expected antibody responses may not be obtained. This includes patients with severe combined immunodeficiency, hypogammaglobulinemia, or agammaglobulinemia; altered immune states due to diseases such as leukemia, lymphoma, or generalized malignancy; or an immune system compromised by treatment with corticosteroids, alkylating drugs, antimetabolites or radiation.[15]

Administration of DTP and/or Haemophilus b Conjugate Vaccine (Tetanus Toxoid Conjugate) is not contraindicated in individuals with HIV infection.[11]

NOTE: Haemophilus b Conjugate Vaccine (Tetanus Toxoid Conjugate)—ActHIB® is identical to Haemophilus b Conjugate Vaccine (Tetanus Toxoid Conjugate)—OmniHIB™ (distributed by SmithKline Beecham Pharmaceuticals); both products are manufactured by Pasteur Mérieux Sérums & Vaccins S.A.

PRECAUTIONS

GENERAL

Care is to be taken by the health-care provider for the safe and effective use of DTP.

Epinephrine Injection (1:1000) must be immediately available should an acute anaphylactic reaction occur due to any component of the vaccine.

Prior to an injection of any vaccine, all known precautions should be taken to prevent adverse reactions. This includes a review of the patient's history with respect to possible sensitivity and any previous adverse reactions to the vaccine or similar vaccines, previous immunization history, current health status (see **CONTRAINDICATIONS**; **WARNINGS** sections), and a current knowledge of the literature concerning the use of the vaccine under consideration. Immunosuppressed patients may not respond.

Prior to administration of DTP, health-care personnel should inform the patient or guardian of the patient the benefits and risks of immunization, and also inquire about the recent health status of the patient to be injected.

Special care should be taken to ensure that the injection does not enter a blood vessel.

A separate, sterile syringe and needle or a sterile disposable unit should be used for each patient to prevent transmission of hepatitis or other infectious agents from person to person. Needles should not be recapped and should be properly disposed.

INFORMATION FOR PATIENTS

As part of the child's immunization record, the date, lot number and manufacturer of the vaccine administered MUST be recorded.[16,17,18]

The health-care provider should inform the parent or guardian of the patient about the potential for adverse reactions that have been temporally associated with DTP administration. Parents or guardians should be instructed to report any serious adverse reactions to their health-care provider.

IT IS EXTREMELY IMPORTANT WHEN THE CHILD RETURNS FOR THE NEXT DOSE IN THE SERIES, THAT THE PARENT OR GUARDIAN OF THE PATIENT SHOULD BE QUESTIONED CONCERNING OCCURRENCE OF ANY SYMPTOMS AND/OR SIGNS OF AN AD-

Continued on next page

Diphtheria/Tetanus Toxoids—Cont.

VERSE REACTION AFTER THE PREVIOUS DOSE (SEE **CONTRAINDICATIONS; ADVERSE REACTIONS** SECTIONS).

The health-care provider should inform the parent or guardian of the patient the importance of completing the immunization series.

The health-care provider should provide the Vaccine Information Materials (VIMs) which are required to be given with each immunization.

The US Department of Health and Human Services has established a Vaccine Adverse Event Reporting System (VAERS) to accept all reports of suspected adverse events after the administration of any vaccine, including but not limited to the reporting of events required by the National Childhood Vaccine Injury Act of 1986.[16] The toll-free number of VAERS forms and information is 1-800-822-7967.

The National Vaccine Injury Compensation Program, established by the National Childhood Vaccine Injury Act of 1986, requires physicians and other health-care providers who administer vaccines to maintain permanent records and to report occurrences of certain adverse events to the US Department of Health and Human Services. Reportable events include those listed in the Act for each vaccine and events specified in the package insert as contraindications to further doses of the vaccine.[17,18]

DRUG INTERACTIONS

If DTP and TIG or Diphtheria Antitoxin are administered concurrently, separate syringes and separate sites should be used.

As with other intramuscular injections, use with caution in patients on anticoagulant therapy.

Immunosuppressive therapies, including irradiation, antimetabolites, alkylating agents, cytotoxic drugs, and corticosteroids (used in greater than physiologic doses), may reduce the immune response to vaccines. Short-term (<2 weeks) corticosteroid therapy or intra-articular, bursal, or tendon injections with corticosteroids should not be immunosuppressive. Although no specific studies with pertussis vaccine are available, if immunosuppressive therapy will be discontinued shortly, it is reasonable to defer vaccination until the patient has been off therapy for one month; otherwise, the patient should be vaccinated while still on therapy.[2]

If DTP has been administered to persons receiving immunosuppressive therapy, a recent injection of immunoglobulin or having an immunodeficiency disorder, an adequate immunologic response may not be obtained.

CARCINOGENESIS, MUTAGENESIS, IMPAIRMENT OF FERTILITY

No studies have been performed to evaluate carcinogenicity, mutagenic potential, or impact on fertility.

PREGNANCY

THIS VACCINE IS NOT RECOMMENDED FOR PERSONS 7 YEARS OF AGE AND OLDER.

PEDIATRIC USE

SAFETY AND EFFECTIVENESS OF DTP VACCINE OR AT THE TIME WHEN DTP VACCINE IS USED TO RECONSTITUTE ActHIB® OR OmniHIB™ IN INFANTS BELOW THE AGE OF SIX WEEKS HAVE NOT BEEN ESTABLISHED. (See **DOSAGE AND ADMINISTRATION** section.)

This vaccine is recommended for immunizing children 6 weeks of age through 6 years of age (up to the seventh birthday). DTP is the preferred vaccine in this age group, but in those situations where an *absolute contraindication* to pertussis vaccination exists, or where in the opinion of the physician the pertussis vaccine should not be administered, DT is the appropriate alternative.

Full protection is achieved upon completion of primary immunization with either four doses of DTP, or three doses of DTP followed by a dose of an approved acellular DTP. A fifth dose of DTP or an approved acellular DTP is required.

THIS VACCINE IS NOT RECOMMENDED FOR PERSONS 7 YEARS OF AGE AND OLDER. For persons 7 years of age and older, the recommended vaccine is Tetanus and Diphtheria Toxoids Adsorbed for Adult Use (Td).

ADVERSE REACTIONS

Adverse reactions associated with the use of DTP include local redness, warmth, edema, induration with or without tenderness, as well as urticaria and rash. Some data suggest that febrile reactions are more likely to occur in those who have experienced such responses after prior doses.[6]

The frequency of local reactions and fever following DTP vaccination is significantly higher with increasing numbers of doses of DTP, while other mild to moderate systemic reactions (e.g., fretfulness, vomiting) are significantly less frequent.[19] If local redness 2.5 cm occurs, the likelihood of recurrence after another DTP dose increases significantly.[6]

Evidence does not indicate a causal relation between DTP vaccine and SIDS. Studies showing a temporal relation

between these events are consistent with the expected occurrence of SIDS over the age range in which DTP immunization typically occurs.[13]

Deaths due to causes other than SIDS, including deaths due to serious infections, have occurred in infants following the administration of DTP. No association has been shown for hospitalizations due to infectious disease and receipt of DTP.[20]

Approximate rates for adverse events following receipt of DTP vaccine (regardless of dose number in the series) are indicated in TABLE 1.[2]

[See table 1 below]

BODY SYSTEM AS A WHOLE

Mild systemic reactions such as fever, drowsiness, fretfulness, and anorexia, occur quite frequently. These reactions are significantly more common following administration of DTP than following DT, are usually self-limited, and need no therapy other than symptomatic treatment such as acetaminophen.[2]

Rarely, an anaphylactic reaction (i.e., hives, swelling of the mouth, difficulty breathing, hypotension, or shock) and death have been reported after receiving preparations containing diphtheria, tetanus, and/or pertussis antigens.[2]

Arthus-type hypersensitivity reactions, characterized by severe local reactions (generally starting 2 to 8 hours after an injection), may follow receipt of tetanus toxoid.[2]

Moderate to severe systemic events, include high fever (i.e., temperature of ≥40.5°C [≥ 105°F]) and persistent, inconsolable crying lasting ≥3 hours. These events occur infrequently and appear to be without sequelae.[2]

Occasionally, a nodule may be palpable at the injection site of adsorbed products for several weeks. Sterile abscesses at the site of injection have been reported (6 to 10 per million doses).[2]

NERVOUS SYSTEM

The following neurologic illnesses have been reported as temporally associated with vaccine containing tetanus toxoid; neurological complications[21,22] including cochlear lesion,[23] brachial plexus neuropathies,[23,24] paralysis of the radial nerve,[25] paralysis of the recurrent nerve,[23] accommodation paresis, and EEG disturbances with encephalopathy.[19] The report from the IOM suggests that there is a causal relation between Guillain-Barré syndrome (GBS) and vaccines containing tetanus toxoid.[26] In the differential diagnosis of polyradiculoneuropathies following administration of a vaccine containing tetanus toxoid should be considered as a possible etiology.[19,27]

Short-lived convulsions (usually febrile), or collapse (hypotonic-hyporesponsive episode) occur infrequently and appear to be without sequelae.[2]

More severe neurologic events, such as a prolonged convulsion, or encephalopathy, although rare, have been reported in temporal association with DTP administration. An analysis of these data failed to show any cause and effect association.[2]

In the National Childhood Encephalopathy Study (NCES), a large, case-control study in England, children 2 to 35 months of age with serious, acute neurologic disorders such as encephalopathy or complicated convulsion(s), were more likely to have received DTP in the 7 days preceding onset than their age-, sex-, and neighborhood-matched controls. Among children known to be neurologically normal before entering the study, the relative risk (estimated by odds ratio) of a neurologic illness occurring within the 7-day period following receipt of DTP dose, compared to children not receiving DTP in the 7-day period before onset of their illness, was 3.3 (p < 0.001).[2]

Within this 7-day period, the risk was significantly increased for immunized children only within 3 days of vaccination (relative risk 4.2, p < 0.001). The relative risk for illnesses occurring 4 to 7 days after vaccination was 2.1 (p < 0.1). Serious neurologic illnesses requiring hospitalization attributable to pertussis vaccine are rare. Final analysis of

a comprehensive case-control study has estimated that the attributable risk of such illnesses is 1 in 140,000 doses administered. An earlier analysis had estimated this risk at 1/110,000 doses. In contrast, final analysis of the case-control study found that the risk of serious neurologic illness following pertussis disease was 1/11,000 pertussis cases. Repeated evaluations have shown that benefits of vaccine outweigh the risks.[2,9]

The methods and results of the NCES have been thoroughly scrutinized since publication of the study. This reassessment by multiple groups has determined that the number of patients was too small and their classification subject to enough uncertainty to preclude drawing valid conclusions about whether a causal relation exists between pertussis vaccine and permanent neurologic damage. Preliminary data from a 10-year follow-up study of some of the children studied in the original NCES study also suggested a relation between symptoms following DTP vaccination and permanent neurologic disability. However, details are not available to evaluate this study adequately, and the same concerns remain about DTP vaccine precipitating initial manifestations of pre-existing neurologic disorders.[2]

An IOM report by the Committee to review the adverse consequences of pertussis and rubella vaccines concluded that evidence is consistent with a causal relation between DTP vaccine and acute encephalopathy, defined in the controlled studies reviewed as encephalopathy, encephalitis, or encephalomyelitis. On the basis of a review of the evidence bearing on this relation, the Committee concludes that the range of excess risk of acute encephalopathy following DTP immunization is consistent with that estimated for the NCES: 0.0 to 10.5 per million immunizations. The report also states that there is insufficient evidence to indicate a causal relation between DTP vaccine and permanent neurologic damage.[13]

Onset of infantile spasms has occurred in infants who have recently received DTP or DT. Analysis of data from the NCES on children with infantile spasms showed that receipt of DT or DTP was not causally related to infantile spasms.[28] The incidence of onset of infantile spasms increases at 3 to 9 months of age, the time period in which the second and third doses of DTP are generally given. Therefore, some cases of infantile spasms can be expected to be related by chance alone to recent receipt of DTP.[2]

A bulging fontanelle associated with increased intracranial pressure which occurred within 24 hours following DTP immunization has been reported. A causal relationship has not been established.[29,30,31]

CARDIOVASCULAR SYSTEM

An infant who developed myocarditis several hours after immunization has been reported.[32]

RESPIRATORY SYSTEM

Respiratory difficulties, including apnea, have been observed.

LOCAL

Rash and allergic reactions have been observed.

Sudden Infant Death Syndrome (SIDS) has temporally occurred in infants following administration of DTP. A large case-control study of SIDS in the United States showed that receipt of DTP was not causally related to SIDS.[33,34,35] It should be recognized that the first three primary immunizing doses of DTP are usually administered to infants 2 to 6 months of age and that approximately 85% of SIDS cases occur at ages 1 to 6 months, with the peak incidence occurring at 6 weeks to 4 months of age. By chance alone, some SIDS victims can be expected to have recently received DTP.[33,34,35]

When CLI whole-cell DTP was administered concomitantly (at separate sites with separate syringes) with ActHIB® or OmniHIB™, the systemic adverse experience profile was not different from that seen when CLI whole-cell DTP vaccine was administered alone.[10,11] *(Refer to ActHIB® package insert.)*

TABLE 1[2]   **ADVERSE EVENTS OCCURRING WITHIN 48 HOURS OF DTP VACCINATIONS**

Event	Frequency*
Local	
Redness	1/3 doses
Swelling	2/5 doses
Pain	1/2 doses
Systemic	
Fever ≥ 38°C (≥ 100.4°F)	1/2 doses
Drowsiness	1/3 doses
Fretfulness	1/2 doses
Vomiting	1/15 doses
Anorexia	1/5 doses
Persistent, inconsolable crying (duration ≥ 3 hours)	1/100 doses
Fever ≥ 40.5°C (≥ 105°F)	1/330 doses
Nervous System	
Collapse (hypotonic-hyporesponsive episode)	1/1,750 doses
Convulsions (with or without fever)	1/1,750 doses

* Rate per total number of doses regardless of dose number in DTP series.

TABLE 2[2] ROUTINE DIPHTHERIA, TETANUS, AND PERTUSSIS VACCINATION SCHEDULE
Summary For Children <7 Years Old — United States, 1991

Dose	Customary Age	Age/Interval†	Product
Primary 1	2 Months	6 weeks old or older	DTP†
Primary 2	4 Months	4–8 weeks after first dose*	DTP†
Primary 3	6 Months	4–8 weeks after second dose*	DTP†
Primary 4	15 Months	6–12 months after third dose*	DTP†
Booster	4–6 years old, before entering kindergarten or elementary school (not necessary if fourth primary vaccination dose administered after fourth birthday)		DTP†
Additional Boosters		Every 10 years after last dose	Td

* Use DT if pertussis vaccine is contraindicated. If the child is ≥1 year of age at the time that primary dose three is due, a third dose 6 to 12 months after the second dose completes primary vaccination with DT.
† Prolonging the interval does not require restarting series.

TABLE 3[10] RECOMMENDED IMMUNIZATION SCHEDULE
For Previously Unvaccinated Children

DOSE	AGE	IMMUNIZATION
First, Second and Third	At 2, 4 and 6 months	DTP or DTP/ActHIB® or DTP/OmniHIB™
Fourth	At 15 to 18 months	DTP or DTP ActHIB® or DTP/OmniHIB™ or Acellular Pertussis (DTaP)*
Fifth	At 4 to 6 years	DTP or Acellular Pertussis (DTaP)*

* Acellular Pertussis (DTaP) should NOT be used to reconstitute ActHIB®/OmniHIB™. When administering DTaP for the fourth dose, *Haemophilus influenzae* type b vaccine also should be administered at this time in a separate syringe at a different site.

In general, the rates of minor systemic reactions after DTP was used to reconstitute ActHIB® or OmniHIB™ were comparable to those usually reported after DTP vaccine alone.[6,19,36]

When CLI whole-cell DTP was used to reconstitute ActHIB® or OmniHIB™ and administered to infants at 2, 4, and 6 months of age, the systemic adverse experience profile was comparable to that observed when the two vaccines were given separately. An increase in the rate of local reactions was observed in some instances within the 24-hour period after immunization.[10,11] ***(Refer to ActHIB® package insert.)***

Reporting of Adverse Events

Reporting by parents or guardians of all adverse events occurring after vaccine administration should be encouraged. Adverse events following immunization with vaccine should be reported by health-care providers to the US Department of Health and Human Services (DHHS) Vaccine Adverse Event Reporting System (VAERS). Reporting forms and information about reporting requirements or completion of the form can be obtained from VAERS through a toll-free number 1-800-822-7967.[16,17,18]

Health-care providers also should report these events to the Director of Medical Affairs, Connaught Laboratories, Inc., a Pasteur Mérieux Connaught Company, Route 611, PO Box 187, Swiftwater, PA 18370 or cal 1-800-822-2463.

DOSAGE AND ADMINISTRATION

Parenteral drug products should be inspected visually for extraneous particulate matter and/or discoloration prior to administration whenever solution and container permit. If these conditions exist, the vaccine should not be administered.

SHAKE VIAL WELL *before withdrawing each dose. Vaccine contains a bacterial suspension. Vigorous agitation is required to resuspend the contents of the vial.* Discard if vaccine cannot be resuspended.

For Administration of DTP Vaccine Only:

The primary series for children less than 7 years of age is four doses of 0.5 mL each given intramuscularly. The customary age for the first dose is 2 months of age but may be given as young as 6 weeks of age and up to the seventh birthday.

Inject 0.5 mL intramuscularly only. The preferred injection sites are the anterolateral aspect of the thigh and the deltoid muscle of the upper arm. The vaccine should not be injected into the gluteal area or areas where there may be a major nerve trunk. During the course of primary immunizations, injections should not be made more than once at the same site.

The use of reduced volume (fractional doses) is not recommended. The effect of such practices on the frequency of serious adverse events and on protection against disease has not been determined.

Do NOT administer this product subcutaneously.

Special care should be taken to ensure that the injection does not enter a blood vessel.

PRIMARY IMMUNIZATION

This vaccine is recommended for children 6 weeks through 6 years (up to the seventh birthday) ideally beginning when the infant is 6 weeks to 2 months of age.

The primary series consists of four doses. For infants 6 weeks through 12 months of age, administer three 0.5 mL doses intramuscularly at least 4 to 8 weeks apart. The fourth dose is administered 6 to 12 months after the third injection.

BOOSTER IMMUNIZATION

For children between 4 and 6 years of age (preferably at time of kindergarten or elementary school entrance), a booster of 0.5 mL should be administered intramuscularly. Those who receive all four primary immunizing doses before their fourth birthday should receive a single dose of DTP just before entering kindergarten or elementary school. This booster dose is not necessary if the fourth dose in the primary series was administered after the fourth birthday. Thereafter, routine booster immunizations should be with Td, at intervals of 10 years. PERSONS 7 YEARS OF AGE AND OLDER SHOULD NOT BE IMMUNIZED WITH DIPHTHERIA AND TETANUS TOXOIDS AND PERTUSSIS VACCINE ADSORBED USP (FOR PEDIATRIC USE) (DTP).

[See table 2 above]

Preterm infants should be vaccinated according to their chronological age from birth.[2,9]

Interruption of the recommended schedule with a delay between doses does not interfere with the final immunity achieved with DTP. There is no need to start the series over again, regardless of the time elapsed between doses.

Diphtheria and Tetanus Toxoids and Acellular Pertussis Vaccine Adsorbed (DTaP) can be interchangeably used with DTP for the fourth and fifth doses. However, ActHIB® cannot be reconstituted with DTaP.

The simultaneous administration of DTP, oral polivirus vaccine (OPV), and measles-mumps-rubella vaccine (MMR) has resulted in seroconversion rates and rates of side effects similar to those observed when the vaccines are administered separately. Simultaneous vaccination (at separate sites with separate syringes) with DTP, MMR, OPV, or inactivated poliovirus vaccine (IPV), and Haemophilus b conjugate vaccine (HbCV) is also acceptable.[2] The ACIP recommends the simultaneous administration, at separate sites with separate syringes, of all vaccines appropriate to the age and previous vaccination status of the recipients including the special circumstances of simultaneous administration of DTP, OPV, HbCV, and MMR at ≥ 15 months of age.[2]

If passive immunization is needed for tetanus, TIG is the product of choice. It provides longer protection than antitoxin of animal origin and causes few adverse reactions. The currently recommended prophylactic dose of TIG for wounds of average severity is 250 units intramuscularly. When tetanus toxoid and TIG are administered concurrently, separate syringes and separate sites should be used. The ACIP recommends the use of only adsorbed toxoid in this situation.[2]

WHEN RECONSTITUTING HAEMOPHILUS b CONJUGATE VACCINE (TETANUS TOXOID CONJUGATE), ActHIB® or OmniHIB™

NOTE: Haemophilus b Conjugate Vaccine (Tetanus Toxoid Conjugate)—ActHIB® is identical to Haemophilus b Conjugate Vaccine (Tetanus Toxoid Conjugate)—OmniHIB™ (distributed by SmithKline Beecham Pharmaceuticals); both products are manufactured by Pasteur Mérieux Sérums & Vaccins S.A.

CLI whole-cell DTP vaccine also can be used for reconstitution of ActHIB® or OmniHIB™. Cleanse both the DTP and ActHIB® or OmniHIB™ vaccine vial rubber barriers with a suitable germicide prior to reconstitution. Thoroughly agitate the vial of CLI whole-cell DTP vaccine, then withdraw a 0.6 mL dose and inject into the vial of lyophilized ActHIB® or OmniHIB™. After reconstitution and thorough agitation, ActHIB® or OmniHIB™ will appear whitish in color. Withdraw and administer 0.5 mL dose of DTP/ActHIB® or OmniHIB™ vaccines.

When CLI whole-cell DTP vaccine is used to reconstitute ActHIB® or OmniHIB™, administer **intramuscularly only. Vaccine should be used within 24 hours after reconstitution.**

After reconstitution, each 0.5 mL dose is formulated to contain 6.7 Lf of diphtheria toxoid, 5 Lf of tetanus toxoid, an estimate of 4 protective units of pertussis vaccine, 10 µg of purified capsular polysaccharide conjugated to 24 µg of inactivated tetanus toxoid, and 8.5% of sucrose. ***(Refer to ActHIB® package insert.)***

Before injection, the skin over the site to be injected should be cleansed with a suitable germicide. After insertion of the needle, aspirate to ensure that the needle has not entered a blood vessel.

Each dose of DTP/ActHIB® or OmniHIB™ vaccines is administered intramuscularly in the outer aspect of the vastus lateralis (mid-thigh) or deltoid. The vaccine should not be injected into the gluteal area or areas where there may be a nerve trunk. During the course of primary immunizations, injections should not be made more than once at the same site.

When CLI DTP vaccine is used to reconstitute ActHIB® or OmniHIB™, the combined vaccines are indicated for infants and children 2 months through 5 years of age for intramuscular administration in accordance with the schedule indicated in Table 3.[10]

[See table 3 above]

For Previously Unvaccinated Children

Immunization schedules should be considered on an individual basis for children not vaccinated according to the recommended schedule. Three doses of a product containing DTP, given at approximately 2-month intervals, are required followed by a fourth dose of a product containing DTP or DTaP approximately 12 months later and a fifth dose of a product containing DTP or DTaP at 4 to 6 years of age. If the fourth dose of a pertussis-containing vaccine is not given until after the fourth birthday, no further doses of a pertussis-containing vaccine are necessary.

The number of doses of a product containing *H influenzae* type b conjugate vaccine indicated depends on the age that immunization is begun. A child 7 to 11 months of age should receive 3 doses of a product containing *H influenzae* type b conjugate vaccine. A child 12 to 14 months of age should receive 2 doses of a product containing *H influenzae* type b conjugate vaccine. A child 15 to 59 months of age should receive 1 dose of a product containing *H influenzae* type b conjugate vaccine.

Preterm infants should be vaccinated according to their chronological age from birth.[9]

Interruption of the recommended schedule with a delay between doses should not interfere with the final immunity achieved when CLI DTP vaccine is used to reconstitute ActHIB® or OmniHIB™. There is no need to start the series over again, regardless of the time elapsed between doses.

It is recommended that the same conjugate vaccine be used throughout each immunization schedule, consistent with the data supporting approval and licensure of the vaccine. Since ActHIB® and OmniHIB™ are the same vaccine, these may be used interchangeably.

DO NOT INJECT INTRAVENOUSLY.

HOW SUPPLIED

DTP Vial, 7.5 mL—Product No. 49281-280-84

One 7.5 mL vial of Connaught Laboratories, Inc. Diphtheria and Tetanus Toxoids and Pertussis Vaccine as Diluent packaged with Vial, 1 Dose lyophilized Haemophilus b Conjugate Vaccine (Tetanus Toxoid Conjugate) (10 × 1 Dose vials per package)—Product No. 49281-549-10

Administer vaccine within 24 hours after reconstitution.

STORAGE

Store between 2°–8°C (35°–46°F). DO NOT FREEZE. Temperature extremes may adversely affect resuspendability of this vaccine.

Store lyophilized vaccine packaged with vial containing Diphtheria and Tetanus Toxoids and Pertussis vaccine and reconstituted vaccine, when not in use, between 2°–8°C (35°–46°F). DO NOT FREEZE. Discard vaccine within 24 hours after reconstitution.

Continued on next page

Diphtheria/Tetanus Toxoids—Cont.

REFERENCES

1. Mueller JH, et al. Production of diphtheria toxin of high potency (100 Lf) on a reproducible medium. J Immunol 40: 21-32, 1941
2. Recommendations of the Immunization Practices Advisory Committee (ACIP). Diphtheria, Tetanus, and Pertussis: Recommendations for vaccine use and other preventive measures. MMWR 40: No. RR-10, 1991 (NOTE: Articles relevant to reference cited are listed in the MMWR publication.)
3. CDC. Summary of Notifiable Diseases, United States 1992. No. 55, 1993
4. Department of Health and Human Services, Food and Drug Administration. Biological Products; Bacterial Vaccines and Toxoids; Implementation of Efficacy Review; Proposed Rule. Federal Register Vol 50 No. 240, pp 51002-51117, 1985
5. Pichichero ME, et al. Pediatric diphtheria and tetanus toxoids-adsorbed vaccine: Immune response to the first booster following the diphtheria and tetanus toxoids vaccine primary series. Pediatr Infec Dis 5: 428-430, 1986
6. Barkin RM, et al. Pediatric diphtheria and tetanus toxoids (DT) vaccine: Clinical and immunologic response when administered as the primary series. J Pediatr 106: 779-781, 1985
7. Baraff L, et al. DTP—associated reactions: An analysis by injection site, manufacturer, prior reactions and dose. Pediatr 73: 31-36, 1984
8. Centers for Disease Control and Prevention (CDC). Tetanus Surveillance—United States, 1989-1990. Pertussis Surveillance—United States, 1989-1991. MMWR 41: No. SS-8, 1992
9. American Academy of Pediatrics. In: Peter G, ed. 1994 Red Book: Report of the Committee on Infectious Diseases. 23rd ed. Elk Grove Village, IL 1994
10. Data on file, Pasteur Mérieux Sérums & Vaccins S.A.
11. Data on file, Connaught Laboratories, Inc.
12. Wilson GS. The Hazards of Immunization. Provocation poliomyelitis. 270-274, 1967
13. Howson CP, et al. *Adverse Effects of Pertussis and Rubella Vaccines.* National Academy Press, Washington, DC, 1991
14. ACIP. Pertussis immunization: Family history of convulsions and use of antipyretics—supplementary ACIP statement. MMWR 36: 281–282, 1987
15. ACIP. General recommendations on immunization. MMWR 38: 205-227, 1989
16. CDC. Vaccine Adverse Event Reporting System—United States. MMWR 39: 730-733, 1990
17. CDC. National Childhood Vaccine Injury Act: requirements for permanent vaccination records and for reporting of selected events after vaccination. MMWR 37: 197-200, 1988
18. Food and Drug Administration. New reporting requirements for vaccine adverse events. FDA Drug Bull 18 (2), 16-18, 1988
19. Cody CL, et al. Nature and rates of adverse reactions associated with DTP and DT immunizations in infants and children. Pediatr 68: 650-660, 1981
20. Joffe LS, et al. Diphtheria-tetanus toxoids-pertussis vaccination does not increase the risk of hospitalization with an infectious illness. Pediatr Infect Dis J 11: 730-735, 1992
21. Rutledge SL, et al. Neurological complications of immunization. J Pediatr 109: 917-924, 1986
22. Walker AM, et al. Neurologic events following Diphtheria-Tetanus-Pertussis immunization. Pediatr 81: 345-349, 1988
23. Wilson GS. The Hazards of Immunization. Allergic manifestations: Post-Vaccinal neuritis. pp 153-156, 1967
24. Tsairis P, et al. Natural history of brachial plexus neuropathy. Arch Neurol 27: 109-117, 1972
25. Blumstein GI, et al. Peripheral neuropathy following tetanus toxoid administration. JAMA 198: 1030-1031, 1966
26. Stratton KR, et al. *Adverse Events Associated with Childhood Vaccines: Evidence Bearing on Causality.* National Academy Press, Washington, DC, 1993
27. Schlenska GK. Unusual neurological complications following tetanus toxoid administration. J Neurol 215: 299-302, 1977
28. Bellman MH, et al. Infantile spasms and pertussis immunization. Lancet, i: 1031-1034, 1983
29. Jacob J, et al. Increased intracranial pressure after diphtheria, tetanus and pertussis immunization. Am J Dis Child Vol 133: 217-218, 1979
30. Mathur R, et al. Bulging fontanel following triple vaccine. Indian Pediatr 19 (6): 417-418, 1981
31. Shendurnikar N, et al. Bulging fontanel following DTP vaccine. Indian Pediatr 23 (11): 960, 1986
32. CDC. *Adverse events following immunization.* Surveillance Report No. 3, 1985-1986, Issued February 1989
33. Griffin MR, et al. Risk of sudden infant death sydrome after immunization with the Diphtheria-Tetanus-Pertussis Vaccine. N Engl J Med 618-623, 1988
34. Hoffman HJ, et al. Diphtheria-Tetanus-Pertussis immunization and sudden infant death: Results of the National Institute of Child Health and Human Development Cooperative Epidemiological Study of Sudden Infant Death Syndrome Risk Factors. Pediatr 79: 598-611, 1987
35. Walker AM, et al. Diphtheria-Tetanus-Pertussis immunization and sudden infant death syndrome. Am J Public Health 77: 945-951, 1987
36. Long SS, et al. Longitudinal study of adverse reactions following diphtheria-tetanus-pertussis vaccine in infancy. Pediatr 85: 294-302, 1990

Product Information as of November 1994

Manufactured by:
CONNAUGHT LABORATORIES, INC.
Swiftwater, Pennsylvania 18370, USA 3261

INFLUENZA VIRUS VACCINE USP ℞
Trivalent Types A and B
(Zonal Purified, Subvirion)
1998–99 Formula—For 6 Months and Older
Rx only
FLUZONE®

SPECIAL NOTICE: *FOR USE IN IMMUNIZATION BY OR UNDER THE DIRECTION OF A PHYSICIAN.*
Caution: Federal (USA) law prohibits dispensing without a prescription.

DESCRIPTION

Fluzone®, Influenza Virus Vaccine USP, (Zonal Purified, Subviron) for intramuscular use, is a sterile suspension prepared from influenza viruses propagated in chicken embryos. The virus-containing fluids are harvested and inactivated with formaldehyde. Influenza virus is concentrated and purified in a linear sucrose density gradient solution using a continuous flow centrifuge. The virus is then chemically disrupted using Polyethelene Glycol p-Isooctylphenyl Ether (Triton® X-100—A registered trademark of Rohm and Haas, Co.) producing a "split-antigen." The split-antigen is then further purified by chemical means and suspended in sodium phosphate-buffered isotonic sodium chloride solution. Fluzone has been standardized according the USPHS requirements for the 1998–99 influenza season and is formulated to contain 45 micrograms (µg) hemagglutinin (HA) per 0.5 mL dose, in the recommended ratio of 15 µg HA each, representative of the following three prototype strains: A/Beijing/262/95 (H1N1), A/Sydney/05/97 (h3N2) and B/Harbin/07/94 (a B/Beijing/184/93-like strain).[1] Gelatin 0.05% is added as a stabilizer and thimerosal (mercury derivative) 1:10,000 is added as a preservative. Fluzone, after shaking syringe/vial well, is essentially clear and slightly opalescent in color.

ANTIBIOTICS ARE NOT USED IN THE MANUFACTURE OF FLUZONE.

CLINICAL PHARMACOLOGY

Influenza A viruses are classified into subtypes on the basis of two surface antigens: hemagglutinin (H) and neuraminidase (N). Three subtypes of hemagglutinin (H1, H2, H3) and two subtypes of neuraminidase (N1, N2) are recognized among influenza A viruses that have caused widespread human disease. Immunity to these antigens—especially to the hemagglutinin—reduces the likelihood of infection and lessens the severity of disease if infection occurs. Infection with a virus of one subtype confers little or no protection against viruses of other subtypes. Furthermore, over time, antigenic variation (antigenic drift) within a subtype may be so marked that infection or vaccination with one strain may not induce immunity to distantly related strains of the same subtype. Although influenza B viruses have shown more antigenic stability than influenza A viruses, antigenic variation does occur. For these reasons, major epidemics of respiratory disease caused by new variants of influenza continue to occur. The antigenic characteristics of circulating strains provide the basis for selecting the virus strains included in each year's vaccine.[1]

Formal subclassification utilizing neuraminidase antigens has not been done for influenza B viruses.

Influenza illness is characterized by abrupt onset of fever, myalgia, sore throat, and nonproductive cough. Unlike other common respiratory illnesses, influenza can cause severe malaise lasting several days. More severe illness can result if either primary influenza pneumonia or secondary bacterial pneumonia occurs. During influenza epidemics, high attack rates of acute illness result in both increased numbers of visits to physicians' offices, walk-in clinics, and emergency rooms and increased hospitalizations for management of lower-respiratory-tract complications.[1,2]

Elderly persons and persons with underlying health problems are at increased risk for complications of influenza infection. If they become ill with influenza, such members of high-risk groups (see Groups at Increased Risk for Influenza-Related Complications under Target Groups for Special Vaccination Programs) are more likely than the general population to require hospitalization. During major epidemics, hospitalization rates for persons at high-risk may increase substantially, depending on the age group. Previously healthy children and younger adults also may require hospitalization for influenza-related complications, but the relative increase in their hospitalization rates during epidemics is less than for persons who belong to high-risk groups. Estimated rates of influenza-associated hospitalization have varied substantially in studies of different influenza epidemics occurring from 1972 through 1981:

- Rates for persons greater than or equal to 65 years of age (all of whom are considered to be in a high-risk group) have ranged from approximately 200 to greater than 1,000 per 100,000 population.[1]
- Rates for persons 45 to 65 years of age have ranged from approximately 80 to 400 per 100,000 population for those with high-risk medical conditions from approximately 20 to 40 per 100,000 for those without high-risk conditions.[1]
- Rates for persons 15 to 44 years of age have ranged from approximately 40 to more than 60 per 100,000 population for those with high-risk conditions and from approximately 20 to 30 per 100,000 population for those without high-risk conditions.[1]
- Rates for children 5 to 14 years of age have ranged from approximately 200 per 100,000 population for those with high-risk conditions to 20 per 100,000 population for those without high-risk conditions.[1]
- Rates for children 0 to 4 years of age have ranged from approximately 500 per 100,000 population for those with high-risk conditions to 100 per 100,000 population for those without high-risk conditions.[1]

During influenza epidemics from 1969–70 through 1993–94, the estimated number of influenza-associated hospitalizations has ranged from approximately 20,000 to more than 300,000 per epidemic, with an average of approximately 130,000 to 170,000 per epidemic. The greatest numbers of influenza-associated hospitalizations have occurred during epidemics caused by type A(H3N2) viruses, with an estimated average of 160,000 to 200,000 excess hospitalizations per epidemic.[1]

Increased mortality results not only from influenza and pneumonia but also from cardiopulmonary and other chronic diseases that can be exacerbated by influenza. In studies of influenza epidemics occurring from 1972–73 through 1994–95, excess deaths associated with influenza occurred during 19 of 23 influenza epidemics. During those 19 influenza seasons, estimated rates of influenza-associated deaths ranged from approximately 25 to greater than 150 per 100,000 persons greater than 65 years of age, who account for more than 90% of the deaths attributed to pneumonia and influenza. An estimate of greater than 20,000 influenza-associated deaths occurring during each of 11 different US epidemics from 1972–73 through 1994–95, and greater than 40,000 influenza-associated deaths occurred during each of six of these 11 epidemics.[1]

Pneumonia and influenza deaths may be increasing because the number of elderly persons in the US population is increasing, as well as the number of persons less than 65 years of age at increased risk for influenza-related complications (e.g., organ-transplant recipients, neonates in intensive-care units, and persons who have cystic fibrosis and acquired immunodeficiency syndrome [AIDS], all of whom have longer life expectancies than in previous years).[1]

Vaccinating persons at high-risk each year before the influenza season is currently the most effective measure for reducing the impact of influenza. Vaccination can be highly effective when it is a) directed at persons who are most likely to experience complications or who are at increased risk for exposure and b) administered to persons at high-risk during hospitalizations or routine health-care visits before the influenza season, thus making special visits to physicians' offices or clinics unnecessary. When vaccine and epidemic strains of virus are well matched, achieving high vaccination rates amoung persons living in closed settings (e.g., nursing homes and other chronic-care facilities) can reduce the risk for outbreaks of influenza by inducing herd immunity.[1]

Other indications for vaccination include the desire to avoid becoming ill with influenza, reduce the severity of disease, or reduce the chance of transmitting influenza to close contacts who are members of high-risk groups.[1]

Each year's influenza vaccine contains three virus strains (usually two type A and one type B) representing the influenza viruses that are likely to circulate in the United States in the upcoming winter. The vaccine is made from highly purified, egg-grown viruses that have been made noninfectious (inactivated). Influenza vaccine rarely causes systemic or febrile reactions. Whole-virus and subvirion preparations are available.[1]

Most vaccinated children and young adults develop high post-vaccination hemagglutination-inhibition antibody titers. These antibody titers are protective against illness caused by strains similar to those in the vaccine or the re-

lated variants that may emerge during outbreak periods. Elderly persons and persons with certain chronic diseases may develop lower post-vaccination antibody titers than healthy young adults and may remain susceptible to influenza-related upper-respiratory-tract infection. However, even if such persons develop influenza illness despite vaccination, the vaccine can be effective in preventing lower-respiratory-tract involvement or other secondary complications, thereby reducing the risk for hospitalization and death.[1]

The effectiveness of influenza vaccine in preventing or attenuating illness varies, depending primarily on the age and immunocompetence of the vaccine recipient and the degree of similarity between the virus strains included in the vaccine and those that circulate during the influenza season. When a good match exists between vaccine and circulating viruses, influenza vaccine has been shown to prevent illness in approximately 70% to 90% of healthy persons less than 65 years of age. In these circumstances, studies also have indicated that the effectiveness of influenza vaccine in preventing hospitalization for pneumonia and influenza among elderly persons living in settings other than nursing homes or similar chronic-care facilities ranges from 30% to 70%.[1]

Among elderly persons residing in nursing homes, influenza vaccine is most effective in preventing severe illness, secondary complications, and death. Studies of this population have indicated that the vaccine can be 50% to 60% effective in preventing hospitalization and pneumonia and 80% effective in preventing death, even though efficacy in preventing influenza illness may often be in the range of 30% to 40% among the frail elderly. Achieving a high rate of vaccination among nursing home residents and staff can reduce the spread of infection in a facility, thus preventing disease through herd immunity. Vaccination of health care workers in nursing homes also has been demonstrated to reduce the impact of influenza among residents.[1]

INDICATIONS AND USAGE

Fluzone is indicated only for immunization against the selected virus strains contained in the vaccine (see **PRECAUTIONS** section).

Influenza vaccine (subvirion) is strongly recommended for any person greater than or equal to 6 months of age who—because of age or underlying medical conditions—is at increased risk for influenza complications. Health-care workers and others (including household members) in close contact with persons in high-risk groups also should be vaccinated. In addition, influenza vaccine may be administered to any person who wishes to reduce the chance of becoming infected with influenza.[1]

Dosage recommendations for the 1998–99 season are given in Table 1. Guidelines for the use of vaccine among certain patient populations are given below.[1]

Although the current influenza vaccine can contain one or more of the antigens administered in previous years, annual vaccination using the current vaccine is necessary because immunity declines in the year following vaccination.[1]

REMAINING 1997–98 VACCINE SHOULD NOT BE USED TO PROVIDE PROTECTION FOR THE 1998–99 INFLUENZA SEASON.[1]

Persons at high-risk who are seen by health-care providers for routine care or as a result of hospitalization should be offered influenza vaccine as early as September. (See Foreign Travelers section for foreign travel exceptions.) The optimal time for organized vaccination campaigns for persons in high-risk groups is usually the period from October through mid-November. In the United States, influenza activity generally peaks between late December and early March. High levels of influenza activity infrequently occur before December. Administering vaccine too far in advance of the influenza season should be avoided in facilities such as nursing homes, because antibody levels might begin to decline within a few months of vaccination. Vaccination programs can be undertaken as soon as current vaccine is available if regional influenza activity is expected to begin earlier than December.[1]

Vaccine should be offered to both children and adults up to and even after influenza virus activity is documented in a community.[1]

Two doses administered at least one month apart may be required for satisfactory antibody responses among previously unvaccinated children less than 9 years of age; however, studies of vaccines similar to those being used currently have indicated little or no improvement in antibody response when a second dose is administered to adults during the same season.[1]

During recent decades, data on influenza vaccine immunogenicity and side effects have been obtained for intramuscularly administered vaccine. Because recent influenza vaccines have not been adequately evaluated when administered by other routes, the intramuscular route is recommended. Adults and older children should be vaccinated in the deltoid muscle and infants and young children in the anterolateral aspect of the thigh.[1]

TARGET GROUPS FOR SPECIAL VACCINATION PROGRAMS

To maximize protection of high-risk persons, they and their close contacts should be selected for organized vaccination programs.[1]

Groups at Increased Risk for Influenza-Related Complications:[1]
- Persons greater than or equal 65 years of age
- Residents of nursing homes and other chronic-care facilities that house persons of any age with chronic medical conditions
- Adults and children with chronic disorders of the pulmonary or cardiovascular systems, including children with asthma
- Adults and children who have required regular medical follow-up or hospitalization during the preceding year because of chronic metabolic diseases (including diabetes mellitus), renal dysfunction, hemoglobinopathies, or immunosuppression (including immunosuppression caused by medications)
- Infants, children and teenagers (6 months to 18 years of age) who are receiving long-term aspirin therapy and therefore might be at risk for developing Reye syndrome after influenza[1,3,4]
- Women who will be in the second or third trimester of pregnancy during the influenza season

Also, persons who smoke tobacco products are at increased risk for influenza-related complications and therefore should receive influenza vaccine.[5,6,7]

Groups That Can Transmit Influenza to Persons at High-Risk:[1]

Persons who are clinically or subclinically infected can transmit influenza virus to persons at high risk that they care for or with whom they live. Some persons at high-risk (e.g., the elderly, transplant recipients, and persons with AIDS) can have a low antibody response to influenza vaccine. Efforts to protect these members of high-risk groups against influenza might be improved by reducing the likelihood of influenza exposure from their care givers. Therefore, the following groups should be vaccinated:
- physician, nurses, and other personnel in both hospital and outpatient-care settings;
- employees of nursing homes and chronic-care facilities who have contact with patients or residents;
- providers of home care to persons at high-risk (e.g., visiting nurses and volunteer workers); and
- household members (including children) of persons in high-risk groups.

General Population

Physicians should administer influenza vaccine to any person who wishes to reduce the likelihood of becoming ill with influenza (the vaccine can be administered to children as young as 6 months of age). Persons who provide essential community services should be considered for vaccination to minimize disruption of essential activities during influenza outbreaks. Students or other persons in institutional settings (e.g., those who reside in dormitories) should be encouraged to receive vaccine to minimize the disruption of routine activities during epidemics.[1]

Pregnant Women

Influenza-associated excess mortality among pregnant women has not been determined except during the pandemics of 1918–1919 and 1957–1958. However, because death-certificate data often do not indicate whether a woman was pregnant at the time of death, similar studies conducted during interpandemic periods may underestimate the impact of influenza in this population. Case reports and limited studies suggest that pregnancy may indeed increase the risk for serious medical complications as a result of increases in heart rate, stroke volume and oxygen consumption, decreases in lung capacity and changes in immunologic function. A recent study of the impact of influenza during 17 interpandemic influenza seasons found that the relative risk of hospitalization for selected cardiorespiratory conditions among pregnant women increased from 1.4 during weeks 14 to 20 of gestation to 4.7 during weeks 37 to 42 when their hospitalization rates were compared with rates among women who were 1 to 6 months post-partum. The risk during the third trimester was comparable to the risk for non-pregnant women with high-risk medical conditions for whom influenza vaccine has traditionally been recommended. It was estimated that immunizing 1,000 women who would be in their third trimester during influenza season would prevent one hospitalization.[1]

In view of these and other data which suggest that influenza infection may cause increased morbidity in women during the second and third trimesters of pregnancy, the ACIP recommends that health-care workers who provide care for pregnant women should consider administering influenza vaccine.[1] **(Refer to Pregnancy Category C statement.)**

Breastfeeding Mothers

Influenza vaccine does not affect the safety of breastfeeding for mothers or infants. Breastfeeding does not adversely affect immune response and is not a contraindication for vaccination.[1]

Persons Infected with Human Immunodeficiency Virus (HIV)

Limited information exists regarding the frequency and severity of influenza illness among HIV-infected persons, but reports suggest that symptoms might be prolonged and the risk for complications increased for some HIV-infected persons. Influenza vaccine has produced protective antibody titers against influenza in vaccinated HIV-infected persons who have minimal AIDS-related symptoms and high CD4+ T-lymphocyte cell counts. In patients who have advanced HIV disease and low CD4+ T-lymphocyte cell counts, however, influenza vaccine may not induce protective antibody titers; a second dose of vaccine does not improve the immune response for these persons.[1]

Recent studies have examined the effect of influenza vaccination on replication of HIV type I (HIV-1). Although some studies have demonstrated a transient (i.e., 2- to 4-week) increase in replication of HIV-1 in the plasma or peripheral blood mononuclear cells of HIV-infected persons after vaccine administration, other studies using similar laboratory techniques have not indicated any substantial increase in replication. Deterioration of CD4+ T-lymphocyte cell counts and progression of clinical HIV disease have not been demonstrated among HIV-infected persons who receive vaccine. Because influenza can result in serious illness and complications and because influenza and vaccination may result in protective antibody titers, vaccination will benefit many HIV-infected patients.[1]

Foreign Travelers

The risk for exposure to influenza during foreign travel varies, depending on season and destination. Because of the short incubation period for influenza, exposure to the virus during travel can result in clinical illness that begins while traveling, which is an inconvenience or potential danger, especially for persons at increased risk for complications. Persons preparing to travel to the tropics at any time of year or to the southern hemisphere from April through September should review their influenza vaccination histories. If they were not vaccinated the previous fall or winter, they should consider influenza vaccination before travel. Persons in the high-risk categories should be especially encouraged to receive the current vaccine. Persons at high-risk who received the previous seasons's vaccine before travel should be revaccinated in the fall or winter with the current vaccine.[1]

SIMULTANEOUS ADMINISTRATION OF OTHER VACCINES, INCLUDING CHILDHOOD VACCINES

CONCURRENT USE WITH PNEUMOCOCCAL VACCINE. Fluzone has been shown in clinical studies to be acceptable for concurrent use with pneumococcal vaccine using separate syringes at different sites. Although Influenza Virus Vaccine is recommended in certain patients for annual use, the pneumococcal vaccine should only be given once.[1,8,9]

Children at high-risk for influenza-related complications can receive influenza vaccine at the same time they receive other routine vaccinations, including pertussis vaccine (DTaP or DTP) using separate syringes at different sites. Because influenza vaccine can cause fever when administered to young children, DTaP (which is less frequently associated with fever and other adverse events) is preferable.[1]

CONTRAINDICATIONS

INFLUENZA VIRUS IS PROPAGATED IN EGGS FOR THE PREPARATION OF INFLUENZA VIRUS VACCINE. THEREFORE, FLUZONE SHOULD NOT BE ADMINISTERED TO ANYONE WITH A HISTORY OF HYPERSENSITIVITY (ALLERGY), ESPECIALLY ANAPHYLACTIC REACTIONS, TO EGGS OR EGG PRODUCTS. IT IS ALSO A CONTRAINDICATION TO ADMINISTER FLUZONE TO INDIVIDUALS KNOWN TO BE SENSITIVE TO THIMEROSAL. EPINEPHRINE INJECTION (1:1000) MUST BE IMMEDIATELY AVAILABLE SHOULD AN ACUTE ANAPHYLACTIC REACTION OCCUR DUE TO ANY COMPONENT OF FLUZONE.

Fluzone should not be administered to patients with acute respiratory or other active infections or illnesses.

Immunization should be delayed in a patient with an active neurologic disorder, but should be considered when the disease process has been stabilized.

WARNINGS

This product contains dry natural latex rubber as follows: The stopper to the vial contains dry natural latex rubber. In case of the syringe, the needle cover contains dry natural latex rubber, but the plunger for the syringe contains no rubber of any kind.

Fluzone should not be administered to individuals who have a prior history of Guillain-Barré syndrome (GBS).

If Fluzone is administered to immunosuppressed persons, the expected antibody response may not be obtained.

As with any vaccine, vaccination with Fluzone may not protect 100% of susceptible individuals.

PRECAUTIONS
GENERAL

Care is to be taken by the health-care provider for the safe and effective use of this vaccine.

Continued on next page

Fluzone—Cont.

EPINEPHRINE INJECTION (1:1000) MUST BE IMMEDIATELY AVAILABLE SHOULD AN ACUTE ANAPHYLACTIC REACTION OCCUR DUE TO ANY COMPONENT OF THIS VACCINE.

Influenza virus is remarkably capricious in that significant antigenic changes may occur from time-to-time. *It is known definitely that Influenza Virus Vaccine, as now constituted, is not effective against all possible strains of influenza virus. Protection is afforded most people only against those strains of virus from which the vaccine is prepared or against closely related strains.*

During the course of any febrile respiratory illness or other active infection, use of Influenza Virus Vaccine should be delayed.

Since the likelihood of febrile convulsions is greater in children 6 months through 35 months of age, special care should be taken in weighing relative risks and benefits of vaccination.

Prior to an injection of any vaccine, all known precautions should be taken to prevent side reactions. This includes a review of the patient's history with respect to possible sensitivity to the vaccine or similar vaccine, to possible sensitivity to dry natural latex rubber, previous immunization history, current health status (see **CONTRAINDICATIONS** and **WARNINGS** sections) and a knowledge of the current literature concerning the use of the vaccine under consideration.

Special care should be taken to prevent injection into a blood vessel.

A separate, sterile syringe and needle or a sterile disposable unit should be used for each patient to prevent transmission of hepatitis or other infectious agents from person to person. Needles should not be recapped and should be disposed of according to biohazard waste guidelines.

INFORMATION FOR PATIENT

Patients, parents or guardians should be fully informed by their health-care provider of the benefits and risks of immunization with Influenza Virus Vaccine.

Patients, parents or guardians should be instructed to report any serious adverse reaction to their health-care provider.

Drug Interaction:

Although influenza vaccination can inhibit the clearance of warfarin, theophylline, phenytoin, and aminopyrine therapy, studies have failed to show any adverse clinical effects attributable to these drugs in patients receiving influenza vaccine.[10,11,12,13,14,15,16]

If Fluzone is administered to immunosuppressed persons or persons receiving immunosuppressive therapy, the expected antibody response may not be obtained. This includes patients with asymptomatic HIV infection, AIDS or AIDS-Related Complex, severe combined immunodeficiency, hypogammaglobulinemia, or aggammaglobulinemia; altered immune states due to diseases such as leukemia, lymphoma, or generalized malignancy; or an immune system compromised by treatment with corticosteroids, alkylating drugs, antimetabolites or radiation.[17]

PREGNANCY

REPRODUCTIVE STUDIES—PREGNANCY CATEGORY C

Animal reproductive studies have not been conducted with Influenza Virus Vaccine USP Trivalent, Types A and B. It is not known whether Influenza Virus Vaccine can cause fetal harm when administered to a pregnant woman or can affect reproduction capacity. Influenza Virus Vaccine should be give to a pregnant women only if clearly needed (see **INDICATIONS AND USAGE**

PEDIATRIC USE

SAFETY AND EFFECTIVENESS OF FLUZONE (SUBVIRION) IN INFANTS BELOW THE AGE OF 6 MONTHS HAVE NOT BEEN ESTABLISHED.

ADVERSE REACTIONS

Because influenza vaccine contains only noninfectious viruses, it cannot cause influenza Respiratory disease after vaccination represents coincidental illness unrelated to influenza vaccination. The most frequent side effect of vaccination is soreness at the vaccination site that lasts up to 2 days. These local reactions generally are mild and rarely interfere with the ability to conduct daily activities.[1]

Two types of systemic reactions have occurred:

- Fever, malaise, myalgia, and other systemic symptoms can occur following vaccination and most often affect persons who have had no exposure to the influenza virus antigens in the vaccine (e.g., young children). These reactions begin 6 to 12 hours after vaccination and can persist for 1 or 2 days. Recent placebo-controlled trials suggest that in elderly persons and healthy young adults, split-virus influenza vaccine is not associated with higher rates of systemic symptoms (e.g., fever, malaise, myalgia, and headache) when compared with placebo injections.[1]
- Immediate—presumably allergic—reactions (e.g., hives, angioedema, allergic asthma, and systemic anaphylaxis) occur rarely after influenza vaccination. These reactions probably result from hypersensitivity to some vaccine component; the majority of reactions are most likely related to residual egg protein. Although current influenza vaccines contain only a small quantity of egg protein, this protein can induce immediate hypersensitivity reactions among persons who have severe egg allergy. Persons who have developed hives, have had swelling of the lips or tongue, or have experience acute respiratory distress or collapse after eating eggs should consult a physician for appropriate evaluation to help determine if vaccine should be administered. Persons who have documented immunoglobulin E(IgE)-mediated hypersensitivity to eggs—including those who have had occupational asthma or other allergic responses due to exposure to egg protein—also might be at increased risk for reactions from influenza vaccine, and similar consultation should be considered.[1,10,11,12,13,14,15,16]

The protocol for influenza vaccination developed by Murphy and Strunk may be considered for patients who have egg allergies and medical conditions that place them at increased risk for influenza-associated complications.[1,18]

Although the 1976 swine influenza vaccine was associated with an increased frequency of Guillain-Barré syndrome (GBS), evidence for a causal relationship of GBS with subsequent vaccines prepared from other virus strains is less clear.[1,19,20,21] However, obtaining strong evidence for a possible small increase in risk is difficult for a rare condition such as GBS, which has an annual background incidence of only 10 to 20 cases per million adults. During three of four influenza seasons studied from 1977 through 1991, the point estimates of the overall relative risks of GBS after influenza vaccination were slightly elevated; but were not statistically significant in any of these studies. However, a recent study in the 1992–93 and 1993–94 seasons, investigators found an elevation in the overall relative risk for GBS of 1.83 (95% Confidence Interval =1.12 to 3.00) during the 6 weeks following vaccination, representing an excess of an estimated 1 to 2 cases of GBS per million persons vaccinated; the combined number of GBS cases peaked 2 weeks after vaccination. The increase in relative risks and the increased number of cases in the second week after vaccination may be the result of vaccination but also could be the result of other factors (e.g., confounding or diagnostic bias) rather than a true vaccine-related risk.[1]

Among persons who received the swine influenza vaccine in 1976, the rate of GBS that exceeded the background rate was slightly less than 10 cases per million persons vaccinated. Even if GBS were a true side effect in subsequent years, the estimated risk for GBS of 1 to 2 cases per million persons vaccinated is substantially less than that for severe influenza, which could be prevented by vaccination in all age groups, especially persons greater than or equal to 65 years of age and those who have medical indications for influenza vaccination. During different epidemics occurring from 1972 through 1981, estimated rates of influenza-associated hospitalization have ranged from approximately 200 to 300 hospitalizations per million population for previously healthy persons 5 to 44 years of age and from 2,000 to greater than 10,000 hospitalizations per million population for persons greater than or equal to 65 years of age. During epidemics from 1972–73 through 1994–95, estimated rates of influenza-associated deaths have ranged from approximately 300 to greater than 1,500 per million persons greater than or equal to 65 years of age, who account for more than 90% of all influenza-associated deaths. The potential benefits of influenza vaccination clearly outweigh the possible risks for vaccine-associated GBS.[1]

The average case-fatality ratio for GBS is 6% and increases with age. However, no evidence indicates that the case-fatality ratio for GBS differs among vaccinated persons and those not vaccinated.[1]

Whereas the incidence of GBS in the general population is very low, persons, with a history of GBS have a substantially greater likelihood of subsequently developing GBS than persons without such a history. Thus, the likelihood of coincidently developing GBS after influenze vaccination is expected to be greater among persons with a history of GBS than among persons with no history of this syndrome. Whether influenza vaccination might be causally associated with this risk for recurrence is not known.[1]

Neurological disorders temporally associated with influenza vaccination such as encephalopathy, optic neuritis, partial facial paralysis, and brachial plexus neuropathy have been reported. However, no cause and effect has been established.[22,23] Almost all persons affected were adults, and the described clinical reactions began as soon as a few hours and as late as 2 weeks after vaccination. Full recovery was almost always reported.[24,25,26]

Reporting of Adverse Events

Reporting by patients, parents or guardians of all adverse events occurring after vaccine administration should be encouraged. Adverse events following immunization with vaccine should be reported by the health-care provider to the US Department of Health and Human Services (DHHS) Vaccine Adverse Event Reporting Systems (VAERS). Reporting forms and information about reporting requirements or completion of the form can be obtained from VAERS through a toll-free number 1-800-822-7967.[27]

The health-care provider also should report these events to the Director of Medical Affairs, Connaught Laboratories, Inc., a Pasteur Mérieux Connaught Company, Route 611, PO Box 187, Swiftwater, PA 18370 or call 1-800-822-2463.

DOSAGE AND ADMINISTRATION

Parenteral drug products should be inspected visually for particulate matter and/or discoloration prior to administration whenever solution and container permit. If either of these conditions exist, the vaccine should not be administered.

The syringe/vial should be well shaken before withdrawing each 0.5 mL dose.

Do NOT inject intravenously.

Injections of Influenza Virus Vaccine should be administered intramuscularly, preferable in the region of the deltoid muscle, in adults and older children. The preferred site for infants and young children is the anterolateral aspect of the thigh. Before injection, the skin over the site to be injected should be cleansed with a suitable germicide. After insertion of the needle, aspirate to assure that the needle has not entered a blood vessel.

Influenza vaccine should be offered beginning in September (see **INDICATIONS AND USAGE** section).

Children less than 9 years of age who have not previously been vaccinated should receive two doses of vaccine at least one month apart to maximize the likelihood of a satisfactory antibody response to all three vaccine antigens. The second dose should be administered before December, if possible.[1]

Fluzone (Subvirion) is to be used for persons 6 months of age and older. Fluzone (Subvirion) is NOT approved for infants under 6 months of age. The dosage is as follows:

Table 1[1] – Influenza Vaccine Dosage by Age Group 1998-1999 Season

Age Group	Vaccine†	Dosage	No. of Doses
6 – 35 months	Split virus only	0.25 mL	1 or 2*
3 – 8 years	Split virus only	0.50 mL	1 or 2*
9 – 12 years	Split virus only	0.50 mL	1
> 12 years	Whole or split virus	0.50 mL	1

† Because of the lower potential for causing febrile reactions, only split-virus (subvirion) vaccines should be used for children. Immunogenicity and side effects of split- and whole-virus vaccines are similar among adults when vaccines are administered at the recommended dosage.

* Two doses administered at least one month apart are recommended for children less than 9 years of age who are receiving influenza vaccine for the first time.

HOW SUPPLIED

Syringe, 0.5 mL. (Shake syringe well before administering.) **(Do not use for administering 0.25 mL.)** – Product No. 49281-362-11

Vial 5 mL, for administration with needle and syringe (NOT to be used with jet injector). (Shake vial well before withdrawing each dose.) – Product No. 49281-362-15

STORAGE

Store between 2° – 8°C (35° – 46°F). Potency is destroyed by freezing. **DO NOT USE FLUZONE IF IT HAS BEEN FROZEN.**

REFERENCES

1. Recommendations of the Advisory Committee on Immunization Practices (ACIP). Prevention and control of influenza. MMWR 47: No. RR-6, 1998.
2. Feigin RD, et al. Textbook of Pediatric Infectious Diseases. (Second Edition) Saunders: 1709–1729, 1987
3. CDC. Update: Influenza Activity-Micronesia, United States. MMWR 35: 685–687, 1986
4. CDC. Reye Syndrome-United States, 1985. MMWR 35: 66–74, 1986
5. Mulloy E. Management of Chronic Obstructive Pulmonary Disease. Ir Med J Vol 89 (6):202, 204, 1996
6. Zimmerman RK, et al. Adult immunizations – a practical approach for clinicians: Part II. Am Fam Physician 51 (4): 859–867, 1995
7. Rothbarth PH, et al. Sense and nonsense of influenza vaccination in asthma and chronic obstructive pulmonary disease. Am J Respir Crit Care Med 151: 1682–1686, 1995.
8. ACIP. Pneumococcal polysaccharide vaccine. MMWR 38: 64–76, 1989
9. DeStefano F, et al. Simultaneous administration of influenza and pneumococcal vaccines. JAMA 247: 2551–2554, 1982
10. Renton KW, et al. Decreased elimination of theophylline after influenza vaccination. Can Med Assoc J 123: 288–290, 1980

11. Fischer RG, et al. Influence of the trivalent influenza vaccine on serum theophylline levels. Can Med Assoc J 126: 1312–1313, 1982
12. Lipsky BA, et al. Influenza vaccination and warfarin anticoagulation. Ann Intern Med 100: 6: 835–837, 1984
13. Kramer P, et al. Effect of influenza vaccine on warfarin anticoagulation. Clin Pharmacol Ther Vol 35, #3: 416–418, 1984
14. Patriarca PA, et al. Influenza vaccination and warfarin or theophylline toxicity in nursing-home residents. New Engl J Med 308: 1601–1602, 1983
15. Levine M, et al. Increased serum phenytoin concentration following influenza vaccination. Clin Pharm 3: 505–509, 1984
16. Kilbourne ED. Inactivated Influenza Vaccines. Effects of influenza vaccination on drug metabolism. Vaccines (Plotkin and Mortimer eds.) Saunders Company: 429, 1988
17. ACIP. Immunization of children infected with human T-lymphotropic virus type III/lymphadenopathy-associated virus. MMWR 35: 595–606, 1986
18. Murphy KR, et al. Safe administration of influenza vaccine in asthmatic children hypersensitive to egg proteins. J Pediatr 106: 931–933, 1985
19. Schonberger LB, et al. Guillain-Barré syndrome following vaccination in the National Influenza Immunization Program, United States, 1976–1977. Am J Epid 110: 105–123, 1979
20. Schonberger LG, et al. Guillain-Barré Syndrome: Its epidemiology and associations with influenza vaccination. Ann Neurol 9 (Suppl.): 31–38, 1981
21. Kurland LT, et al. Swine influenza vaccine and Guillain-Barré syndrome. Epidemic or artifact? Arch Neurol, Vol 42, 1089–1090, 1985
22. CDC. Adverse Events Following Immunization. Surveillance Report No. 3, 1985–1986, Issued February 1989
23. Data on file, Connaught Laboratories, Inc.
24. Barry DW, et al. Comparative trial of influenza vaccines. II. Adverse reactions in children and adults. Am J Epid 104: 47–59, 1976
25. Retaillaiu HF, et al. Illness after influenza vaccination reported through a nationwide surveillance system, 1976–1977. Am J Epid III (3): 270–278, 1980
26. Guerrero IC, et al. No increased meningoencephalitis after influenza vaccine. N Engl J Med 300 (10): 565, 1979
27. CDC Vaccine Adverse Event Reporting System – United States. MMWR 39: 730–733, 1990

Product information
as of May 1998

Manufactured by:
CONNAUGHT LABORATORIES, INC.
Swiftwater, Pennsylvania 18370, USA
PASTEUR MÉRIEUX CONNAUGHT
RHÔNE-POULENC GROUP
3755/3756

Shown in Product Identification Guide, page 330

RABIES IMMUNE GLOBULIN (HUMAN) USP IMOGAM® RABIES – HT ℞

[*Im 'o-gam*]

Caution: Federal (USA) law prohibits dispensing without prescription.

DESCRIPTION

Rabies Immune Globulin (Human) USP, IMOGAM® RABIES – HT, is a sterile solution of antirabies immunoglobulin (10–18% protein) for intramuscular administration. It is prepared by cold alcohol fractionation from pooled venous plasma of individuals immunized with Rabies Vaccine prepared from human diploid cells (HDCV). The product is stabilized with 0.3 M glycine. The globulin solution has a pH of 6.8 ± 0.4 adjusted with sodium hydroxide or hydrochloric acid. No preservatives are added. IMOGAM® RABIES – HT is a colorless to light opalescent liquid.

A heat-treatment process step (58° to 60°C, 10 hours) to inactivate viruses has been added to further reduce any risk of blood-borne viral transmission. The inactivation and removal of model and laboratory strains of enveloped and nonenveloped viruses during the manufacture and heat treatment processes for IMOGAM® RABIES – HT has been validated by spiking experiments. Human immunodeficiency virus, type I (HIV-1) and type 2 (HIV-2) were selected as relevant viruses for plasma derived products. Bovine viral diarrhea virus and Sindbis virus were chosen to model hepatitis C virus. Porcine pseudorabies virus was selected to model hepatitis B virus and herpes virus. Avian reovirus was used to model non-enveloped RNA viruses and for its relative resistance to inactivation by chemical and physical methods. Finally, porcine parvovirus was selected to model human parvovirus B19 and its notable resistance to inactivation by heat treatment.

Removal and/or inactivation of the studied enveloped and non-enveloped model viruses was demonstrated at the precipitation III stage of manufacturing. In addition, inactivation was demonstrated to occur during the 10-hour (58° to 60°C) heat treatment process for the studied enveloped and non-enveloped viruses.

The product is standardized against the United States (US) Standard Rabies Immune Globulin. The US unit of potency is equivalent to the International Unit (IU) for rabies antibody. The average potency is 150 IU/mL.

CLINICAL PHARMACOLOGY

Following the marked decrease of rabies cases among domestic animals in the US in the 1940s and 1950s, indigenously acquired rabies among humans decreased to fewer than two cases per year in the 1960s and 1970s and fewer than one case per year during the 1980s.[1,2] In 1950, for example, 4,979 cases of rabies were reported among dogs and 18 were reported among human populations; in 1989, 160 cases were reported among dogs and one was reported among humans. Thus, the likelihood of human exposure to a rabid domestic animal has decreased greatly; however, the many possible exposures that result from frequent contact between domestic dogs and humans continue to be the basis of most antirabies treatments.[1,3]

Rabies among wild animals – especially skunks, raccoons, and bats – has become more prevalent since the 1950s accounting for > 85% of all reported cases of animal rabies every year since 1976.[1,2] Rabies among animals occurs throughout the continental US; only Hawaii remains consistently rabies-free. Wild animals now constitute the most important potential source of infection for both humans and domestic animals in the US. In much of the rest of the world, including most of Asia, Africa, and Latin America, the dog remains the major species with rabies and the major source of rabies among humans. Nine of the 13 human rabies deaths reported to CDC from 1980 through 1990 appear to have been related to exposure to rabid animals outside of the US.[1,4–10]

Although rabies among humans is rare in the US, every year approximately 18,000 persons receive rabies pre-exposure prophylaxis and an additional 10,000 receive postexposure prophylaxis. Appropriate management of persons possibly exposed to rabies depends on the interpretation of the risk of infection. Decisions about management must be made immediately. All available methods of systemic prophylactic treatment are complicated by occasional adverse reactions, but these are rarely severe.[1,11–15]

Data on the efficacy of active and passive rabies immunization have come from both human and animal studies. Evidence from laboratory and field experience in many areas of the world indicates that postexposure prophylaxis combining local wound treatment, passive immunization, and vaccination is uniformly effective when appropriately applied.[1,16–21]

Although no postexposure vaccine failures have occurred in the US during the 10 years that HDCV has been licensed, seven persons have contracted rabies after receiving postexposure treatment with both HRIG and HDCV outside the US. An additional six persons have contracted the disease after receiving postexposure prophylaxis with other cell culture-derived vaccines and HRIG or ARS (equine antirabies serum). However, in each of these cases, there was some deviation from the recommended postexposure treatment protocol.[1,22–24] Specifically, patients who contracted rabies after postexposure prophylaxis did not have their wounds cleansed with soap and water or other antiviral agents, did not receive their rabies vaccine injections in the deltoid area (i.e., vaccine was administered in the gluteal area), or did not receive passive vaccination around the wound site.[1]

Rabies antibody provides passive protection when given immediately to individuals exposed to rabies virus.[25,26] Rabies Immune Globulin (Human) [RIG(H)] of adequate potency[27] was used in conjunction with Rabies Vaccine of duck embryo origin.[27,28] When a globulin dose of 20 IU/kg of rabies antibody was given simultaneously with the first dose of vaccine, levels of passive rabies antibody were detected 24 hours after injection in all individuals. There was minimal or no interference with the immune response to the initial and subsequent doses of vaccine, including booster doses.

Studies of Rabies Immune Globulin (Human)[29] IMOGAM® RABIES given with the first of five doses of Pasteur Mérieux Sérums et Vaccins S.A. HDCV[1] confirmed that passive immunization with 20 IU/kg of Rabies Immune Globulin (Human) provides maximum circulating antibody with minimum interference of active immunization by HDCV.

A double-blind randomized trial[30] was conducted to compare the safety and antibody levels achieved following intramuscular injection of IMOGAM® RABIES – HT (heat treated) and Rabies Immune Globulin (Human), IMOGAM® RABIES (non-heat treated). Each globulin was administered on day 0, either alone or in combination with the human diploid cell Rabies Vaccine (IMOVAX® RABIES) using the standard post-exposure prophylactic schedule of day 0, 3, 7, 14, and 28.

Sixty-four healthy veterinary student volunteers were randomized into four parallel groups of 16 each to receive the following immune globulin and vaccine regimens.

IMOGAM® RABIES – HT	+	IMOVAX®
IMOGAM® RABIES	+	IMOVAX®
IMOGAM® RABIES – HT	+	placebo
IMOGAM® RABIES	+	placebo

The dosage corresponded to the post-exposure recommended dose of 20 IU/kg of rabies immune globulin and was administered in three, equally divided IM injections of under 5 mL in either gluteus. Serum rabies antibody levels were assessed before treatment and on days 3, 7, 14, 28, 35, and 42 by the Rabies Fluorescent Focus Inhibition Test (RFFIT).

Serum antibody levels were similar in the IMOGAM® RABIES – HT and IMOGAM® RABIES groups. By day three, 60% of each group had detectable antibody titers of ≥ 0.05 IU/mL. By day 14, the geometric mean titers (with 95% confidence interval) were 19 IU/mL (11–38) in the IMOGAM® RABIES – HT + vaccine group and 31 IU/mL (20–48) in the IMOGAM® RABIES + vaccine group. These differences were not statistically different.

Two subjects reported severe headaches, one in the IMOGAM® RABIES – HT + placebo group and one in the IMOGAM® Rabies + IMOVAX® Rabies group. One third of the volunteers had moderate systemic (headache and malaise) reactions. These were equally distributed among the 4 treatment groups with no significant differences between the groups.

Both IMOGAM® RABIES – HT + IMOGAM® RABIES were safe and without serious adverse events or allergic reactions. The safety profile did not differ between groups, although IMOGAM® RABIES – HT produced fewer and milder local reactions such as pain or tenderness at the injection site.

INDICATIONS AND USAGE

Rabies Immune Globulin (Human) IMOGAM® RABIES – HT is indicated for individuals suspected of exposure to rabies, particularly severe exposure, with one exception: persons who have been previously immunized with HDCV Rabies Vaccine in a pre or postexposure treatment series should receive only vaccine. Persons who have received Rabies Vaccines other than HDCV or RVA vaccines should have confirmed adequate rabies antibody titers if they are to receive only vaccine.[1]

IMOGAM® RABIES – HT should be injected as promptly as possible after exposure along with the first dose of vaccine. If initiation of treatment is delayed for any reason, IMOGAM® RABIES – HT and the first dose of vaccine should still be given, regardless of the interval between exposure and treatment IMOGAM® RABIES – HT may be given up to eight days after the first dose of vaccine was given.

Rabies virus is usually transmitted by the bit of a rabid animal but can occasionally penetrate abraded skin contaminated with the saliva of infected animals. Progress of the virus after exposure is believed to follow a neural pathway and the time between exposure and clinical rabies is a function of the proximity of the bite (or abrasion) to the central nervous system and the dose of virus injected. The incubation is usually 2 to 6 weeks but can be longer. After severe bites about the face and neck and arms, it may be as short as 10 days. After initiation of the vaccine series (human diploid cell origin), it takes approximately one week for development of immunity of rabies; therefore, the value of immediate passive immunization with rabies antibodies in the form of Rabies Immune Globulin (Human) cannot be overemphasized.

Recommendations for passive and/or active immunization after exposure to an animal suspected of having rabies have been outlined by the WHO[31] and by the United States Public Health Service Advisory Committee on Immunization Practices (ACIP).[1]

I. Rationale of Treatment

In the United States and Canada the following factors should be considered before specific antirabies treatment is indicated:

1. Species of Biting Animal

Carnivorous animals (especially skunks, foxes, coyotes, racccoons, dogs, bobcats, and cats) and bats are more likely to be infected with rabies than other animals. Rats, mice, squirrels, hamsters, guinea pigs, gerbils, chipmunks and other rodents or rabbits and hares are rarely infected with rabies and have not been known to cause human rabies in the United States. Their bites almost never call for antirabies prophylaxis; therefore, before initiating antirabies prophylaxis, the local state health department should be consulted.

Because some bat bites may be less severe, and therefore more difficult to recognize, than bites inflicted by larger mammalian carnivores, rabies postexposure treatment

Continued on next page

Imogam Rabies—Cont.

should be considered for any physical contact with bats when bite or mucous membrane contact cannot be excluded.[32,33]

2. Circumstances of Biting Incident
An UNPROVOKED attack is more likely than a provoked attack to indicate that the animal is rabid. Bites inflicted on a person attempting to feed or handle an apparently healthy animal should generally be regarded as PROVOKED.

3. Type of Exposure
Rabies is commonly transmitted by inoculation with infectious saliva. The likelihood that rabies infection will result from exposure to a rabid animal varies with the nature and extent of the exposure. Two categories of exposure should be considered:

Bite: Any penetration of the skin by teeth.

Nonbite: Scratches, abrasions, open wounds or mucous membranes contaminated with saliva or other potentially infectious material such as brain tissue from a rabid animal.

In addition, two cases of rabies have been attributed to airborne exposures in laboratories and two cases of rabies have been attributed to probable exposures to a bat-infested cave (Frio Cave, Texas).[1,34–36] Casual contact with a rabid animal, such as petting the animal (without a bite or nonbite exposure as described above) does not constitute an exposure and is not an indication for prophylaxis.

The only documented cases of rabies due to human-to-human transmission occurred in patients who received corneas transplanted from persons who died of rabies undiagnosed at the time of death.[1,37]

Each exposure to possible rabies infection must be individually evaluated. Local or state public health officials should be consulted if questions arise about the need for rabies prophylaxis.

4. Vaccination Status of Biting Animal
A properly immunized animal has only a minimal chance of developing rabies and transmitting the virus.

II. Postexposure Treatment of Rabies

1. Local Treatment of Wounds
Immediate and thorough local treatment of all bite wounds and scratches is perhaps the most effective preventive measure. The would should be thoroughly cleansed immediately with soap and water. Tetanus prophylaxis and measures to control bacterial infection should be given as indicated.

2. Specific Treatment
Postexposure antirabies treatment should always include both passive (preferably Rabies Immune Globulin—Human) and active (preferably Rabies Vaccine prepared from human diploid cells) immunization with one exception: persons who have been previously immunized with HDCV Rabies Vaccine in a pre or postexposure treatment series should receive only vaccine. Persons who have received Rabies Vaccines other than HDCV or RVA vaccines should have confirmed adequate rabies antibody titers if they are to receive only vaccine.[1] The combination of globulin and vaccine is recommended for both bite exposures and nonbite exposures (as described under "Rationale of Treatment") and regardless of the interval between exposure and treatment. The sooner treatment is begun after exposure, the better.

3. Postexposure Treatment Guide
The following recommendations are only a guide. They should be applied in conjunction with knowledge of the animal species involved, circumstances of the bite or other exposure, vaccination status of the animal, and presence of rabies in the region. Local and state public health officials should be consulted if questions arise about the need for rabies prophylaxis.
[See table 1 below]

CONTRAINDICATIONS

IMOGAM® RABIES – HT should NOT be administered in repeated doses once vaccine treatment has been initiated. Repeating the dose may interfere with maximum active immunity expected from the vaccine.

WARNINGS

Rabies Immune Globulin (Human) USP, IMOGAM® – HT, is made from human plasma. Products made from human plasma may contain infectious agents, such as viruses, that can cause disease. The risk that such products will transmit an infectious agent has been reduced by screening plasma donors for prior exposure to certain viruses, by testing for the presence of certain current virus infections, and by inactivating and/or removing certain viruses. An alcohol fractionation procedure used to purify the immunoglobulin component removes and/or inactivates both enveloped and non-enveloped viruses. An added heat treatment process (60°C, 10 hours) further inactivates both enveloped and non-enveloped viruses. Despite these measures, it is still theoretically possible that known or unknown infectious agents may be present. All infections thought by a physician possibly to have been transmitted by this product should be reported by the physician or other health-care provider to the Director of Medical Affairs, Connaught Laboratories, Inc., Telephone 1-800-822-2463. The physician should discuss the risks and benefits of this product with the patient.

IMOGAM® RABIES – HT should be given with caution to patients with a history of prior systemic allergic reactions following the administration of human immune globulin.

Persons with specific IgA deficiency have increased potential for developing antibodies to IgA and could have anaphylactic reactions to subsequent administration of blood products containing IgA.[38,39]

PRECAUTIONS

GENERAL

Care is to be taken by the health-care provider for the safe and effective use of this product.

EPINEPHRINE INJECTION (1:1000) MUST BE IMMEDIATELY AVAILABLE SHOULD AN ACUTE ANAPHYLACTIC REACTION OCCUR DUE TO ANY COMPONENT OF THIS PRODUCT.

IMOGAM® RABIES – HT should not be administered intravenously because of the potential for serious reactions. Injection should be made intramuscularly and care should be taken to draw back on the plunger of the syringe before injection in order to be certain that the needle is not in a blood vessel. Although systemic reactions to immunoglobulin preparations are rare, epinephrine should be available for treatment of acute anaphylactoid reactions. As with all preparations given intramuscularly, bleeding complications may be encouraged in patients with bleeding disorders.

HRIG should never be administered in the same syringe or into the same anatomical site as vaccine. Because HRIG may partially suppress active production of antibody, no more than the recommended dose should be given.[1]

A separate, sterile syringe and needle or a sterile disposable unit should be used for each patient to prevent transmission of hepatitis or other infectious agents from person to person. Needles should not be recapped and should be disposed of according to biohazard waste guidelines.

INFORMATION FOR PATIENT

Patients, parents or guardians should be fully informed by their health-care provider of the benefits and risks of administration of IMOGAM® RABIES – HT.

Patients, parents or guardians should be instructed to report any serious adverse reactions to their health-care provider.

DRUG INTERACTIONS
Live virus vaccine such as measles vaccines should not be given close to the time of IMOGAM® RABIES – HT administration because antibodies in the globulin preparation may interfere with the immune response to the vaccination. Immunization with live vaccines should not be given within three months after IMOGAM® RABIES – HT administration.

PREGNANCY
REPRODUCTIVE STUDIES—PREGNANCY CATEGORY C

Animal reproduction studies have not been conducted with IMOGAM® RABIES – HT. It is also not known whether IMOGAM® RABIES – HT can cause fetal harm when administered to a pregnant woman or can affect reproductive capacity. IMOGAM® RABIES – HT should be given to a pregnant woman only if clearly needed.

ADVERSE REACTIONS

In a recent clinical trial involving 16 volunteers in 4 treatment groups, two subjects reported severe headaches, one in the IMOGAM® RABIES – HT + placebo group and one in the IMOGAM® Rabies + IMOVAX® Rabies group, and one third of the volunteers reported moderate systemic (headache and malaise) reactions. These were equally distributed among the 4 treatment groups with no significant differences between the groups.[30]

Local adverse reactions such as tenderness, pain, soreness or stiffness of the muscles may occur at the injection site and may persist for several hours after injection. These may be treated symptomatically. Mild systemic adverse reactions to the globulin after intramuscular injection are uncommon.[30,40,41]

Although not reported specifically for HRIG, angioneurotic edema, nephrotic syndrome, and anaphylaxis have been reported after injection of immune globulin (IG). These reactions occur so rarely that a causal relationship between IG and these reactions is not clear.[1]

Reporting of Adverse Events
The National Vaccine Injury Compensation Program, established by the National Childhood Vaccine Injury Act of 1986, requires physicians and other health-care providers who administer vaccines to maintain permanent vaccination records and to report occurrences of certain adverse events to the US Department of Health and Human Services. Reportable events include those listed in the Act for each vaccine and events specified in the package insert as contraindications to further doses of that vaccine.[42,43,44]

Reporting by patients, parents or guardians of all adverse events occurring after HRIG administration should be encouraged. Adverse events following treatment with HRIG should be reported by the health-care provider to the US Department of Health and Human Services (DHHS) Vaccine Adverse Event Reporting Systems (VAERS). Reporting forms and information about reporting requirements or completion of the form can be obtained from VAERS through a toll-free number 1-800-822-7967.[42,43,44]

The health-care provider also should report these events to the Director of Medical Affairs, Connaught Laboratories, Inc., Route 611, PO Box 187, Swiftwater, PA 18370 or call 1-800-822-2463.

DOSAGE AND ADMINISTRATION

Parenteral drug products should be inspected visually for particulate matter and/or discoloration prior to administration, whenever solution and container permit. If either of these conditions exist, the vaccine should not be administered.

IMOGAM® RABIES – HT should be used in conjunction with Rabies Vaccine such as RABIES VACCINE IMOVAX® RABIES, for intramuscular immunization, vaccine prepared from human diploid cell cultures. The recommended dose of IMOGAM® RABIES – HT is 20 IU/kg (0.133 mL/kg) or 9 IU/lb (0.06 mL/lb) of body weight administered at time of the first vaccine dose.[27,28] As much as possible of the recommended dose should be infiltrated around the wound if anatomically feasible and the remaining HRIG should be administered intramuscularly in the gluteal region.[45] Two injections would be given in the gluteal region if the volume is greater than 5 mL.

HRIG should never be administered in the same syringe or into the same anatomical site as vaccine. Because HRIG may partially suppress active production of antibody, no more than the recommended dose should be given.[1]

HOW SUPPLIED

IMOGAM® RABIES – HT is supplied in 2 mL and 10 mL vials with average potency of 150 International Units per milliliter (IU/mL). The 2 mL vial contains 300 IU which is sufficient for a child weighing 15 kg (33 lb). Product No. 49281-190-20. The 10 mL vial contains a total of 1,500 IU which is sufficient for an adult weighing 75 kg (165 lb). Product No. 49281-190-10

STORAGE

IMOGAM® RABIES – HT should be stored in the refrigerator between 2° and 8°C (35° and 46°F). Do not freeze.

IMOGAM® RABIES – HT CONTAINS NO PRESERVATIVE AND UNUSED PORTION MUST BE DISCARDED IMMEDIATELY.

TABLE 1 RABIES POSTEXPOSURE PROPHYLAXIS GUIDE, UNITED STATES, 1991[1]

Animal Type	Evaluation and disposition of animal	Postexposure Prophylaxis Recommendations
Dogs and cats	Healthy and available for 10 days observation	Should not begin prophylaxis unless animal develops symptoms of rabies*
	Rabid or suspected rabid	Immediate vaccination
	Unknown (escaped)	Consult public health officials
Skunks, raccoons, bats, foxes, and most other carnivores; woodchucks	Regarded as rabid unless geographic area is known to be free of rabies or until animal proven negative by laboratory tests†	Immediate vaccination
Livestock, rodents, and lagomorphs (rabbits and hares)	Consider individually	Consult public health officials. Bites of squirrels, hamsters, guinea pigs gerbils, chipmunks, rats, mice, other rodents, rabbits, and hares almost never require antirabies treatment

* During the 10-day holding period, begin treatment with HRIG and HDCV or RVA at first sign of rabies in a dog or cat that has bitten someone. The symptomatic animal should be killed immediately and tested.

† The animal should be killed and tested as soon as possible. Holding for observation is not recommended. Discontinue vaccine if immunofluorescence test results of the animal are negative.

REFERENCES
1. Recommendation of the Advisory Committee on Immunization Practices (ACIP). Rabies prevention – United States, 1991. MMWR 40: No. RR-3, 1991
2. Reid-Sanden FL, et al. Rabies surveillance, United States during 1989. J Am Vet Med Assoc 197: 1571–1583, 1990
3. Helmick CG. The epidemiology of human rabies postexposure prophylaxis, 1980–1981. JAMA 250: 1990–1996, 1983
4. CDC. Human rabies diagnosed 2 months postmortem – Texas. MMWR 34: 700, 705–707, 1985
5. CDC. Human rabies acquired outside the United States. MMWR 34: 235–236, 1985
6. CDC. Human rabies – California, 1987. MMWR 37: 305–308, 1988
7. CDC. Human rabies – Oregon, 1989. MMWR 38: 335–337, 1989
8. CDC. Human rabies – Texas. MMWR 33: 469–470, 1984
9. CDC. Imported human rabies. MMWR 32: 78–80, 85–86, 1983
10. CDC. Human rabies acquired outside the United States from a dog bite. MMWR 30: 537–540, 1981
11. Bernard, KW, et al. Neuroparalytic illness and human diploid cell rabies vaccine. JAMA 248: 3136–3138, 1982
12. CDC. Systemic allergic reactions following immunization with human diploid cell rabies vaccine. MMWR 33: 185–187, 1984
13. Dreesen EW, et al. Immune complex-like disease in 23 persons following a booster dose of rabies human diploid cell vaccine. Vaccine 4: 45–49, 1986
14. Aoki FY, et al. Immunogenicity and acceptability of a human diploid-cell culture rabies vaccine in volunteers. Lancet 1: 660–662, 1975
15. Cox JH, et al. Prophylactic immunization of humans against rabies by intradermal inoculation of human diploid cell culture vaccine. J Clin Microbiol 3: 96–101, 1976
16. Anderson LJ, et al. Postexposure trial of a human diploid cell strain rabies vaccine. J Infect Dis 142: 133–138, 1980
17. Bahmanyar M, et al. Successful protection of humans exposed to rabies infection. Postexposure treatment with the new human diploid cell rabies vaccine and antirabies serum. JAMA 236: 2751–2754, 1976
18. Hattwick MAW. Human rabies. Public Health Rev 3: 229–274, 1974
19. Wiktor TJ, et al. Development and clinical trials of the new human rabies vaccine of tissue culture (human diploid cell) origin. Dev. Biol Stand 40: 3–9, 1978
20. World Health Organization. WHO expert committee on rabies. WHO Tech Rep Ser 709: 1–104, 1984
21. Kuwert EK, et al. Immunization against rabies with rabies immune globulin, human (RIGH) and a human diploid cell strain (HDCS) rabies vaccine. J Biol Stand 6: 211–219, 1978
22. CDC. Human rabies despite treatment with rabies immune globulin and human diploid cell rabies vaccine – Thailand. MMWR 36: 759–760, 765, 1987
23. Shill M, et al. Fatal rabies encephalitis despite appropriate post-exposure prophylaxis. A case report. N Engl J Med 316: 1257–1258, 1987
24. Wilde H, et al. Failure of rabies postexposure treatment in Thailand. Vaccine 7: 49–52, 1989
25. Baltazard M, et al. Essai pratique du serum antirabique chez les mordus par loups enrages. Bull WHO 13: 757–772, 1955
26. Habel K, et al. Laboratory data supporting clinical trial of antirabies serum in persons bitten by rabid wolf. Bull WHO 13: 773–779, 1955
27. Cabasso VJ, et al. Rabies immune globulin of human origin: preparation and dosage determination in non-exposed volunteer subjects. Bull WHO 45: 303–315, 1971
28. Loofbourow JC, et al. Rabies immune globulin (human). Clinical trials and dose determination. JAMA 217:1825–1831, 1971
29. Helmick CG, et al. A clinical study of Mérieux human rabies immune globulin. J Biol Stand 10:357–367 1982
30. Lang J, et al. A clinical evaluation of a new heat treated Rabies Immune Globulin (Human). VII Annual International Meeting on Research Advances & Rabies Control in the Americas. Centers for Disease Control & Prevention, Atlanta, Georgia, December 9–13, 1996
31. WHO Expert Committee on Rabies. WHO Tech Rep Ser 523: 50–51, 1973
32. ACIP. Human Rabies – California, 1994. MMWR 43: 455–457, 1994
33. Wilde H, et al. Failure of Postexposure Treatment of Rabies in Children. Clin Infect Dis 22: 228–232, 1996
34. Afshar A. A review of non-bite transmission of rabies virus infection. Br Vet J 135: 142–148, 1979
35. Winkler WG, et al. Airborne rabies transmission in a laboratory worker. JAMA 226: 1219–1221, 1973
36. CDC. Rabies in a laboratory worker – New York. MMWR 26: 183–184, 1977
37. Gode GR, et al. Two rabies deaths after corneal grafts from one donor {letter}. Lancet 2: 791, 1988
38. Fudenberg HH. Sensitization to immunoglobulins and hazards of gamma globulin therapy, pp 211–220 in Merler E, Editor Immunoglobulins: biologic aspects and clinical uses. National Academy of Sciences, Wash., DC. 1970
39. Pineda AA, et al. Transfusion reactions associated with anti-IgA antibodies: report of four cases and review of the literature. Transfusion 15:10–15, 1975
40. Janeway CA, et al. The gamma globulins. IV. Therapeutic uses of gamma globulins. N Engl J Med 275: 826–831, 1966
41. Kjellman H. Adverse reactions to human immune serum globulin in Sweden (1969–1978). pp 143–150. Immunoglobulins: characteristics and uses of intravenous preparations. Alving BM and Finlayson JS, Editors. US Dept. Health & Human Services, DHHS Publ. No. (FDA) 80–9005, Wash., DC. 1980
42. CDC. Vaccine Adverse Event Reporting System – United States. MMWR 39: 730–733, 1990
43. CDC. National Childhood Vaccine Injury Act. Requirements for permanent vaccination records and for reporting of selected events after vaccination. MMWR 37: 197–200, 1988
44. Food and Drug Administration. New Reporting Requirements for Vaccine Adverse Events. FDA Drug Bull 18(2), 16–18, 1988
45. World Health Organization. WHO expert committee on rabies. WHO Tech Rep Ser 824: 1992

Product Information
as of April 1997

Manufactured by:
PASTEUR MÉRIEUX Sérums & Vaccins S.A.
Lyon, France
US License No. 384
Distributed by:
CONNAUGHT LABORATORIES, INC.
Swiftwater, Pennsylvania 18370, USA
800-VACCINE (800-822-2463)

3439

Shown in Product Identification Guide, page 330

RABIES VACCINE ℞
IMOVAX® RABIES
[Im 'o-vaks]
WISTAR RABIES VIRUS STRAIN PM-1503-3M
GROWN IN HUMAN DIPLOID CELL STRUCTURES

DESCRIPTION
The Imovax® Rabies Vaccine produced by Pasteur Mérieux Sérums et Vaccins is a sterile, stable, freeze-dried suspension of rabies virus prepared from strain PM-1503-3M obtained from the Wistar Institute, Philadelphia, PA.
The virus is harvested from infected human diploid cells, MRC-5 strain, concentrated by ultrafiltration and is inactivated by beta propiolactone. One dose of reconstituted vaccine contains less than 100 mg albumin, less than 150 µg neomycin sulfate and 20 µg of phenol red indicator. This vaccine must only be used intramuscularly and as a single dose vial.
The vaccine contains no preservative or stabilizer. It should be used immediately after reconstitution, and if not administered promptly, discard contents.
The potency of one dose (1.0 ml) Merieux Imovax Rabies Vaccine is equal to or greater than 2.5 international units of rabies antigen.

CLINICAL PHARMACOLOGY
Pre-exposure immunization
High titer antibody responses of the Merieux Imovax Rabies Vaccine made in human diploid cells have been demonstrated in trials conducted in England (1), Germany (2, 3), France (4) and Belgium (5), Seroconversion was often obtained with only one dose. With two doses one month apart, 100% of the recipients developed specific antibody and the geometric mean titer of the group was approximately 10 international units. In the U.S., Merieux Imovax Rabies Vaccine resulted in geometric mean titers (GMT) of 12.9 I.U./ml at Day 49 and 5.1 I.U./ml at Day 90 when three doses were given intramuscularly during the course of one month. The range of antibody responses was 2.8 to 55.0 I.U./ml at Day 49 and 1.8 to 12.4 I.U. at Day 90. (6) The definition of a minimally accepted antibody titer varies among laboratories and is influenced by the type of test conducted. CDC currently specifies a 1:5 titer (complete inhibition) by the rapid fluorescent focus inhibition test (RFFIT) as acceptable. The World Health Organization (WHO) specifies a titer of 0.5 I.U.

Post-exposure immunization
Post-exposure efficacy of Merieux Imovax Rabies Vaccine was successfully proven during clinical experience in Iran (7) in conjunction with antirabies serum. Forty-five persons severely bitten by rabid dogs and wolves received Merieux vaccine within hours of and up to 14 days after the bites. All individuals were fully protected against rabies.
There have been reports of possible vaccine failure when the vaccine has been administered in the gluteal area. Presumably subcutaneous fat in the gluteal area may interfere with the immunogenicity of human diploid cell rabies vaccine (HDCV) (26, 29). For adults and children, Rabies Vaccine should be administered in the deltoid muscle. (See Dosage and Administration).

INDICATIONS AND USAGE
1. Rationale of treatment
Physicians must evaluate each possible rabies exposure. Local or state public health officials should be consulted if questions arise about the need for prophylaxis. (8)
In the United States and Canada, the following factors should be considered before antirabies treatment is initiated.

Species of biting animal
Carnivorous wild animals (especially skunks, raccoons, foxes, coyotes, and bobcats) and bats are the animals most commonly infected with rabies and have caused most of the indigenous cases of human rabies in the United States since 1960. Unless an animal is tested and shown not to be rabid, post-exposure prophylaxis should be initiated upon bite or nonbite exposure to the animals. (See definition in "Type of Exposure" below.) If treatment has been initiated and subsequent testing in a competent laboratory shows the exposing animal is not rabid, treatment can be discontinued. (8)
The likelihood that a domestic dog or cat is infected with rabies varies from region to region; hence the need for post-exposure prophylaxis also varies. (8)
Rodents (such as squirrels, hamsters, guinea pigs, gerbils, chipmunks, rats and mice) and lagomorphs (including rabbits and hares) are rarely found to be infected with rabies and have not been known to cause human rabies in the United States. In these cases, the state or local health department should be consulted before a decision is made to initiate post-exposure antirabies prophylaxis. (8)

Circumstances of biting incident
An UNPROVOKED attack is more likely than a provoked attack to indicate the animal is rabid. Bites inflicted on a person attempting to feed or handle an apparently healthy animal should generally be regarded as PROVOKED.

Type of exposure
Rabies is transmitted by introducing the virus into open cuts or wounds in skin or via mucous membranes. The likelihood of rabies infection varies with the nature and extent of exposure. Two categories of exposure should be considered.
Bite: Any penetration of the skin by teeth.
Nonbite: Scratches, abrasions, open wounds, or mucous membranes contaminated with saliva or other potentially infectious material, such as brain tissue, from a rabid animal. Casual contact, such as petting a rabid animal (without a bite or nonbite exposure as described above), does not constitute an exposure and is not an indication for prophylaxis. There have been two instances of airborne rabies acquired in laboratories and two probable airborne rabies cases acquired in a bat-infested cave in Texas. (8, 9)
The only documented cases for rabies from human-to-human transmission occured in four patients in the United States and overseas who received corneas transplanted from persons who died of rabies, undiagnosed at the time of death. (9,10) Stringent guidelines for acceptance of donor corneas should reduce this risk. Bite and nonbite exposure from humans with rabies theoretically could transmit rabies, although no cases of rabies acquired this way have been documented. Each potential exposure to human rabies should be carefully evaluated to minimize unnecessary rabies prophylaxis. (8, 11).

II. Pre- and post-exposure treatment of rabies
A. Pre-exposure—See Table 1
Pre-exposure immunization may be offered to persons in high risk groups, such as veterinarians, animal handlers, certain laboratory workers, and persons spending time (e.g. 1 month or more) in foreign countries where rabies is a constant threat. Persons whose vocational or avocational pursuits bring them into contact with potentially rabid dogs, cats, foxes, skunks, bats, or other species at risk of having rabies should also be considered for pre-exposure prophylaxis. (8)
Vaccination is recommended for children living in or visiting countries where exposure to rabid animals is a constant threat. Worldwide statistics indicate children are more at risk than adults.
Pre-exposure prophylaxis is given for several reasons. First, it may provide protection to persons with inapparent exposure to rabies. Secondly, it may protect persons whose post-exposure therapy might be expected to be delayed. Finally, although it does not eliminate the need for additional therapy after a rabies exposure, it simplifies therapy by eliminating the need for globulin and decreasing the number of

Continued on next page

Imovax Rabies—Cont.

doses of vaccine needed. This is of particular importance for persons at high risk of being exposed in countries where the available rabies immunizing products may carry a higher risk of adverse reactions.

Pre-exposure immunization does not eliminate the need for prompt prophylaxis following an exposure. It only reduces the post-exposure treatment regimen. (8)

PRE-EXPOSURE RABIES TREATMENT GUIDE

1. Pre-exposure immunization: Consists of the three doses of HDCV, 1.0 ml, intramuscularly (deltoid area), one each on Days 0,7 and 21 or 28. Administration of routine booster doses of vaccine depends on exposure risk category as noted in Table 1. Pre-exposure immunization of immunosuppressed persons is not recommended. (8)
[See table 1 below]

B. Post-exposure—See Table 2
The essential components of rabies post-exposure prophylaxis are local treatment of wounds and immunization, including administration, in most instances, of both globulin and vaccine (Table 2). (8, 13)

1. Local treatment of wounds: Immediate and thorough washing of all bite wounds and scratches with soap and water is perhaps the most effective measure for preventing rabies. In experimental animals, simple local wound cleansing has been shown to reduce markedly the likelihood of rabies. (8, 11)

Tetanus prophylaxis and measures to control bacterial infection should be given as indicated.

2. Specific treatment: Post-exposure antirabies immunization should always include administration of both antibody (preferably RIG) and vaccine, with one exception: persons who have been previously immunized with the recommended pre-exposure or post-exposure regimens with HDCV or who have been immunized with other types of vaccines and have a history of documented adequate rabies antibody titer should receive only vaccine. The combination of globulin and vaccine is recommended for both bite exposures and nonbite exposures regardless of the interval between exposure and treatment. (14,15) The sooner treatment is begun after exposure, the better. However, there have been instances in which the decision to begin treatment was made as late as 6 months or longer after the exposure due to delay in recognition that an exposure had occurred. (8, 13)

3. Treatment outside the United States: If post-exposure is begun outside the United States with locally produced biologics, it may be desirable to provide additional treatment when the patient reaches the U.S. State health departments should be contacted for specific advice in such cases. (8)

POST-EXPOSURE TREATMENT GUIDE

The following recommendations are only a guide. In applying them, take into account the animal species involved, the circumstances of the bite or other exposure, the vaccination status of the animal, and presence of rabies in the region.

Local or state public health officials should be consulted if questions arise about the need for rabies prophylaxis. (8)
[See table 2 below]

CONTRAINDICATIONS

For post-exposure treatment, there are no known specific contraindications to the use of Merieux Imovax Rabies Vaccine. In cases of pre-exposure immunization, there are no known specific contraindications other than situations such as developing febrile illness, etc.

WARNINGS

Rabies Vaccine in this package is a unit dose to be delivered intramuscularly in the deltoid area. (8)

This vaccine must not be used intradermally or as a multiple dose dispensing unit. In both pre-exposure and post exposure immunization, the full 1.0 ml dose should be given intramuscularly.

In the case of pre-exposure immunization, recently a significant increase has been noted in "immune complex-like" reactions in persons receiving booster doses of HDCV. (16) The illness characterized by onset 2–21 days post-booster, presents with a generalized urticaria and may also include arthralgia, arthritis, angioedema, nausea, vomiting, fever, and malaise. In no cases were the illnesses life-threatening. Preliminary data suggest this "immune complex-like" illness may occur in up to 6% of persons receiving booster vaccines and much less frequently in persons receiving primary immunization. Additional experience with this vaccine is needed to define more clearly the risk of these adverse reactions. (8, 17)

Two cases of neurologic illness resembling Guillain-Barre syndrome (18, 19), a transient neuroparalytic illness, that resolved without sequelae in 12 weeks and a focal subacute central nervous system disorder temporally associated with HDCV, have been reported. (20)

All serious systemic neuroparalytic or anaphylactic reactions to a rabies vaccine should be immediately reported to the state health department or Connaught Laboratories, Inc., 800-VACCINE/800-822-2463. (8)

PRECAUTIONS

IN ADULTS AND CHILDREN THE VACCINE SHOULD BE INJECTED INTO THE DELTOID MUSCLE. IN INFANTS AND SMALL CHILDREN THE MID-LATERAL ASPECT OF THE THIGH MAY BE PREFERABLE.

General
When a person with a history of hypersensitivity must be given rabies vaccine, antihistamines may be given; epinephrine (1:1000) should be readily available to counteract anaphylactic reactions, and the person should be carefully observed after immunization.

While the concentration of antibiotics in each dose of vaccine is extremely small, persons with known hypersensitivity to any of these agents could manifest an allergic reaction. While the risk is small, it should be weighed in light of the potential risk of contracting rabies.

Drug interactions
Corticosteroids, other immunosuppressive agents, and immunosuppressive illnesses can interfere with the development of active immunity and predispose the patient to developing rabies. Immunosuppressive agents should not be administered during post-exposure therapy, unless essential for the treatment of other conditions. When rabies post-exposure prophylaxis is administered to persons receiving steroids or other immunosuppressive therapy, it is especially important that serum be tested for rabies antibody to ensure than an adequate response has developed. (8)

Usage in pregnancy
Pregnancy Category C. Animal reproduction studies have not been conducted with Imovax Rabies Vaccine. It is also not known whether the product can cause fetal harm when administered to a pregnant woman or can affect reproductive capacity. Rabies vaccine should be given to a pregnant woman only if clearly needed.

Because of the potential consequences of inadequately treated rabies exposure and limited data that indicate that fetal abnormalities have not been associated with rabies vaccination, pregnancy is not considered a contraindication to post-exposure prophylaxis. (8, 21) If there is substantial risk of exposure to rabies, pre-exposure prophylaxis may also be indicated during pregnancy. (8)

Pediatric use
Both safety and efficacy in children have been established.

ADVERSE REACTIONS

ALSO SEE WARNINGS AND CONTRAINDICATIONS SECTIONS FOR ADDITIONAL STATEMENTS

Once initiated, rabies prophylaxis should not be interrupted or discontinued because of local or mild systemic adverse reactions to rabies vaccine. Usually such reactions can be successfully managed with anti-inflammatory and antipyretic agents (e.g. aspirin).

Reactions after vaccination with HDCV are less common than with previously available vaccines. (12,16,17) In a study using five doses of HDCV, local reactions, such as pain, erythema, and swelling or itching at the injection site were reported in about 25% of recipients of HDCV, and mild

---

TABLE 1 (8)

CRITERIA FOR PRE-EXPOSURE IMMUNIZATION

Risk category	Nature of risk	Typical populations	Pre-exposure regimen
Continuous	Virus present continuously often in high concentrations. Aerosol, mucus membrane, bite or nonbite exposure possible. Specific exposures may go unrecognized.	Rabies research lab workers* Rabies biologics production workers..	Primary pre-exposure immunization course. Serology every 6 months. Booster immunization when antibody titer falls below acceptable level*
Frequent	Exposure usually episodic, with source recognized, but exposure may also be unrecognized. Aerosol, mucous membrane, bite or nonbite exposure.	Rabies diagnostic lab workers*, spelunkers, veterinarians, and animal control and wildlife workers in rabies epizootic areas.	Primary pre-exposure immunization course. Booster immunization or serology every 2 years†
Infrequent (greater than population-at-large)	Exposure nearly always episodic with source recognized. Mucous membrane, bite or nonbite exposure.	Veterinarians and animal control and wildlife workers in areas of low rabies endemicity. Certain travelers to foreign rabies epizootic areas. Veterinary students.	Primary pre-exposure immunization course. No routine booster immunization or serology.
Rare (population-at-large)	Exposure always episodic, mucous membrane, or bite with source recognized.	U.S. population-at-large, including individuals in rabies epizootic areas.	No pre-exposure immunization.

* Judgement of relative risk and extra monitoring of immunization status of laboratory workers is the responsibility of the laboratory supervisor (see U.S. Department of Health and Human Service's Biosafety in Microbiological and Biomedical Laboratories, 1984).

† Pre-exposure booster immunization consists of one dose of HDCV, 1.0 ml/dose, IM (deltoid area). Acceptable antibody level is 1:5 titer (complete inhibition in RFFIT at 1:5 dilution). See Clinical Pharmacology. Boost if titer falls below 1:5.

TABLE 2 (8)

Animal species	Condition of animal at time of attack	Treatment of exposed person*
DOMESTIC: Dog and cat	Healthy and available for 10 days of observation Rabid or suspected rabid Unknown (escaped)	None unless animal develops rabies† RIG§ and HDCV Consult public health officials If treatment is indicated, give RIG§ and HDCV
WILD: Skunk, bat, fox, coyote, raccoon, bobcat and other carnivores	Regard as rabid unless proven negative by laboratory tests £	RIG§ and HDCV
OTHER: Livestock, rodents and lagomorphs (rabbits and hares)	Consider individually. Local and state public health officials should be consulted on questions about the need for rabies prophylaxis. Bites of squirrels, hamsters, guinea pigs, gerbils, chipmunks, rats, mice, other rodents, rabbits and hares, almost never call for antirabies prophylaxis.	

* All bites and wounds should immediately be thoroughly cleansed with soap and water. If antirabies treatment is indicated, both rabies immune globulin (RIG) and human diploid cell rabies vaccine (HDCV) should be given as soon as possible regardless of the interval from exposure. Local reactions to vaccines are common and do not contraindicate continuing treatment. Discontinue vaccine if fluorescent antibody tests of the animal are negative.

† During the usual holding period of 10 days, begin treatment with RIG and HDCV at first sign of rabies in a dog or cat that has bitten someone. The symptomatic animal should be killed immediately and tested.

§ If RIG is not available, use antirabies serum, equine (ARS). Do not use more than the recommended dosage.

£ The animal should be killed and tested as soon as possible. Holding for observation is not recommended.

systemic reactions such as headache, nausea, abdominal pain, muscle aches and dizziness were reported in about 20% of recipients. (8)

Serious systemic anaphylactic or neuroparalytic reactions occurring during the administration of rabies vaccines pose a dilemma for the attending physician. A patient's risk of developing rabies must be carefully considered before deciding to discontinue vaccination. Moreover, the use of corticosteroids to treat life-threatening neuroparalytic reactions carries the risk of inhibiting the development of active immunity to rabies. It is especially important in these cases that the serum of the patient be tested for rabies antibodies. Advice and assistance on the management of serious adverse reactions in persons receiving rabies vaccines may be sought from the state health department or Merieux Institute, Inc. (8)

DOSAGE AND ADMINISTRATION

Parenteral drug products should be inspected visually for particulate matter and discoloration prior to administration, whenever solution and container permit. Reconstitute the freeze-dried vaccine in its vial with the 1.0 ml of diluent supplied in the disposable syringe using the longer of the two needles. Gently swirl the contents until completely dissolved and withdraw the total amount of dissolved vaccine into the syringe by setting the vial in an upright position on the table. Remove the reconstitution needle and replace it with the smaller needle.

The reconstituted vaccine should be used immediately.

After preparation of the injection site, immediately inject the vaccine intramuscularly. For adults and children, the vaccine should be injected into the deltoid muscle (22 to 27, 29). In infants and small children, the mid lateral aspect of the thigh may be preferable. Care should be taken to avoid injection into or near blood vessels and nerves. After aspiration, if blood or any suspicious discoloration appears in the syringe, do not inject but discard contents and repeat procedure using a new dose of vaccine, at a different site.

NOTE: The freeze-dried vaccine is creamy white to orange. After reconstitution it is pink to red.

A. Pre-exposure dosage

1. Primary vaccination: In the United States, the Immunization Practices Avisory Committee (ACIP) recommends three injections of 1.0 ml each, one injection on Day 0 and one on Day 7 and one either on Day 21 or 28. (8)

2. Booster dose: Persons working with live rabies virus in research laboratories and in vaccine production facilities should have rabies antibody titers checked every six months and boosters given as needed to maintain an adequate titer. (For definition of adequate titer, see Clinical Pharmacology.) Only laboratory workers, such as those doing rabies diagnostic tests, spelunkers and veterinarians, animal control and wildlife officers in areas where rabies is epizootic should have boosters every 2 years or have their serum tested for rabies antibody every 2 years and, if the titer is inadequate, have a booster dose. Veterinarians and animal control and wildlife officers, if working in areas of low rabies endemicity, do not require routine booster doses of HDCV after completion of primary pre-exposure immunization (Table 1). (8)

Persons who have experienced "immune complex-like" hypersensitivity reactions should receive no further doses of HDCV unless they are exposed to rabies or they are truly likely to be inapparently and/or unavoidably exposed to rabies virus and have unsatisfactory antibody titers.

B. Post-exposure dosage

The World Health Organization established a recommendation for six intramuscular doses of human diploid cell vaccine (HDCV) based on studies in Germany and Iran. (3,7) Used in this way, a total of 6 injections of a 1.0 ml dose of vaccine are given according to the following schedule. On Day 0, 3, 7, 14, 30 and 90. The first dose should be accompanied by Rabies Immune Globulin (RIG) or Antirabies Serum (ARS). If possible, up to half the dose of RIG or ARS should be used to infiltrate the wound, and the rest administered intramuscularly, in a different site from the rabies vaccine, preferably in the gluteal region.

Studies conducted at the CDC in the United States have shown that a regimen of 1 dose of Rabies Immune Globulin (RIG) and 5 doses of HDCV induced an excellent antibody response in all recipients. Of 511 persons bitten by proven rabid animals and so treated, none developed rabies. (8)

Based on these data, the ACIP recommends a 5-dose regimen for post-exposure situations. Five 1.0 ml doses are given intramuscularly on Day 0, 3, 7, 14 and 28 in conjunction with RIG on Day 0. (8)

Because the antibody response following the recommended vaccination regimen with HDCV has been so satisfactory, routine post-vaccination serologic testing is not recommended. Serologic testing is indicated in unusual circumstances, as when the patient is known to be immunosuppressed. Contact state health department or CDC for recommendations. (8, 28)

C. Post-exposure therapy of previously immunized persons

When an immunized person who was vaccinated by the recommended regimen with HDCV or who had previously demonstrated rabies antibody is exposed to rabies, that person should receive two I.M. doses (1.0 ml each) of HDCV, one immediately and one 3 days later. RIG should not be given in these cases. If the immune status of a previously vaccinated person who did not receive the recommended HDCV regimen is not known, full primary post-exposure antirabies treatment (RIG plus 5 doses of HDCV) may be necessary. In such cases, if antibody can be demonstrated in a serum sample collected before vaccine is given, treatment can be discontinued after at least two doses of HDCV.-(8)

HOW SUPPLIED

IMOVAX RABIES VACCINE is supplied in a tamperproof unit dose plastic box with:

—One vial of freeze-dried vaccine containing a single dose.

—One disposable needle and syringe containing diluent for reconstitution.

—One smaller disposable needle for administration.

STORAGE

The freeze-dried vaccine is stable if stored in the refrigerator between 2°C and 8°C (36°F to 46°F). Do not freeze.

REFERENCES

1. Aoki FY, Tyrell DAJ, Hill LE. Immunogenicity and acceptability of a human diploid cell culture rabies vaccine in volunteers. The Lancet, March 22, pp. 660–2 (1975).
2. Cox JH, Schneider LG. Prophylactic immunization of humans against rabies by intradermal inoculation of human diploid cell culture vaccine. J Clin Microbiol 3:96–101 (1976).
3. Kuwert EK, Marcus 1, Werner J, Iwand A, Thraenhart O. Some experiences with human diploid cell strain—(HDCS) rabies vaccine in pre- and post-exposure vaccinated humans. Develop Biol Standard 40:79–88 (1978).
4. Ajjan N, Soulebot J-P, Stellmann C, Biron G, Charbonnier C, Triau R, Merieux C. Resultats de la vaccination antirabique preventive par le vaccin inactivé concentré souche rabies PM/W138-1503-3M cultivés sur cellules diploïdes humaines. Develop Biol Standard 40:89–199 (1978).
5. Coty-Berger F. Vaccination antirabique préventive par du vaccin préparé sur cellules diploïdes humaines. Develop Biol Standard 40:101–4 (1978).
6. Bernard KW, Roberts MA, Sumner J, Winkler WG, Mallonee J, Baer GM, Chaney R. Human diploid cell rabies vaccine JAMA 247:1138–42 (1982).
7. Bahmanyar M, Fayaz A, Nour-Salehi S, Mohammadi M, Koprowski H. Successful protection of humans exposed to rabies infection. JAMA 236: 2751–4 (1976).
8. CDC. Recommendations of the Immunization Practices Advisory Committee (ACIP). Rabies Prevention—United States, 1984, MMWR 33: 393–402, 407–8 (1984).
9. Anderson U.,Nicholson KG, Tauxe RV, Winkler WG. Human rabies in the United States, 1960 to 1979, epidemiology, diagnosis and prevention. Ann Intern Med 100: 728–35 (1984).
10. WHO. Sixth report of the Expert Committee on Rabies. Geneva Switzerland: World Health Organization. (WHO technical report No. 523) (1973).
11. Baer GM, ed. The natural history of rabies. New York: Academic Press. (1975).
12. Greenberg M, Childress J. Vaccination against rabies with duck-embryo and Semple vaccines. JAMA 173:333–7 (1960).
13. Helmick CG. The epidemiology of human rabies post-exposure prophylaxis. JAMA 250: 1990–6 (1983).
14. Devriendt J, Staroukine M, Costy F, Vanderhaegen, J-J Fatal encephalitis apparently due to rabies. JAMA 248: 2304–6 (1982).
15. DC. Human Rabies—Rwanda. MMWR 31: 135 (1982).C
16. CDC. Systemic allergic reactions following immunization with human diploid cell rabies vaccine. MMWR 33: 185–7 (1984).
17. Rubin RH, Hattwick MAW, Jones S, Gregg MB, Schwartz VD. Adverse reactions to duck embryo rabies vaccine. Ann Intern Med 78: 643–9 (1973).
18. Boe E, Nyland H. Guillain-Barre syndrome after vaccination with human diploid cell rabies vaccine. Scand J Infect Dis 12:231–2 (1980).
19. CDC. Adverse reactions to human diploid cell rabies vaccine. MMWR 29: 609–10 (1980).
20. Bernard KW, Smith PW, Kader FJ, Moran MJ. Neuroparalytic illness and human diploid cell rabies vaccine. JAMA 248: 3136–8 (1982).
21. Varner MW, McGuinness GA, Galask RP. Rabies vaccination in pregnancy. Am J of Obst and Gyn 143:717–18 (1982).
22. Cockshott WP, Thompson GT, Howlett U, Seely ET. Intramuscular or intralipomatous injections? N Eng J Med 307: 356–58 (1982).
23. CDC. General Recommendations on Immunization, ACIP. MMWR 32: 1–8, 13–17 (1983).
24. Committee on Immunization Council of Medical Societies, American College of Physicians. Guide for Adult Immunizations. (1985).
25. CDC. Rabies post-exposure prophylaxis with HDCV: Lower neutralizing antibody titers with Wyeth vaccine. MMWR 34: 90–92 (1985).
26. Shill M, Baynes RD, Miller SD. Fatal rabies encephalitis despite appropriate post-exposure prophylaxis. N Engl J Med 316:1257–58 (1987).
27. Baer GM, Fishbein DB. Rabies post-exposure prophylaxis. N Engl J Med 316: 1270–72 (1987).
28. CDC. Recommendations of the Immunization Practices Advisory Committee (ACIP). Supplementary statement on rabies vaccine and serologic testing. MMWR 30: 535–6 (1981).
29. CDC. Human rabies despite treatment with Rabies Immune Globulin and Human Diploid Cell Rabies Vaccine—Thailand. MMWR 36: 759–765 (1987).

Manufactured by:
PASTEUR MERIEUX Sérums & Vaccins S.A.
Lyon, France U.S. License No. 384
Distributed by:
CONNAUGHT LABORATORIES, INC.
Swiftwater, Pennsylvania 18370, U.S.A.
800-VACCINE (800-822-2463)
Revised: July 1991

Shown in Product Identification Guide, page 330

RABIES VACCINE ℞

IMOVAX® RABIES I.D.
Wistar Rabies Virus Strain PM–1503–3M
Grown in Human Diploid Cell Cultures

FOR PRE-EXPOSURE USE ONLY BY THE INTRADERMAL ROUTE (I.D.)

DESCRIPTION

The Imovax Rabies I.D., Rabies Vaccine, produced by Pasteur Mérieux Sérums et Vaccins is a sterile, stable, freeze-dried suspension of rabies virus prepared from strain PM-1503-3M obtained from the Wistar Institute, Philadelphia, PA.

The virus is harvested from infected human diploid cells, MRC-5 strain, concentrated by ultrafiltration and is inactivated by beta propiolactone. One dose of reconstituted vaccine contains less than 15 mg human albumin, less than 22 µg neomycin sulfate and 3 µg of phenol red indicator. *This vaccine dose is for intradermal use only.*

The vaccine contains no preservative or stabilizer. It should be used immediately after reconstitution.

The potency of Merieux Imovax Rabies I.D., Rabies Vaccine, is equal to or greater than 2.5 International Units/ml of rabies antigen. An intradermal dose contains at least 0.25 International Units (I.U.).

CLINICAL PHARMACOLOGY

Studies in Europe (1–6) and in the United States (7,8) to investigate the efficacy and safety of low dose intradermal vaccination schedules have shown that satisfactory levels of antibody were produced in all subjects with two or more inoculations.

Studies in the United States (7,8,9) using three doses of Merieux's Rabies Vaccine demonstrated adequate rabies antibody titers in 100% persons receiving intradermal injections. The geometric mean titer in these subjects 49 days after immunization was approximately 7.5 to 8.9 I.U. compared with 12.9 to 13.8 I.U. in controls receiving 1.0 ml of vaccine intramuscularly (7).

The definition of a minimally acceptable antibody titer varies both among laboratories and according to the purposes for which immunization is given. The Centers for Disease Control (CDC) currently specifies, complete virus neutralization at a 1:5 serum dilution in the rapid fluorescent focus inhibition test (RFFIT) as an acceptable response to pre-exposure immunization. After studies of post-exposure immunization, the World Health Organization (WHO) specifies a titer of 0.5 I.U. as an acceptable response.

INDICATIONS AND USAGE

For Pre-Exposure Use Only

Pre-exposure immunization should be considered for persons in high risk groups, such as veterinarians, animal handlers, certain laboratory workers, and those whose vocational or avocational pursuits bring them into contact with potentially rabid dogs, cats, foxes, skunks, bats, or other species at risk of having rabies. (See Table I).

For persons traveling abroad into endemic areas, Human Diploid Cell Vaccine (HDCV) may be administered by the I.D. dose and route if the 3 dose series is completed 30 days or more before departure. If pre-exposure vaccination is performed for travelers at other times, a vaccine intended for intramuscular use should be used.

Vaccination is recommended for children living in or visiting countries where exposure to rabid animals is a constant threat. Worldwide statistics indicate children are more at risk than adults.

Pre-exposure prophylaxis is given for several reasons. First, it may provide protection to persons with inapparent exposure to rabies. Secondly, it may protect persons, whose post-exposure therapy might be expected to be delayed. Finally, although it does not eliminate the need for additional therapy after a rabies exposure, it simplifies therapy by elimi-

Continued on next page

Imovax Rabies I.D.—Cont.

nating the need for globulin and decreasing the number of doses of vaccine needed. This is of particular importance for persons at high risk of being exposed in countries where the available rabies immunizating products may carry a higher risk of adverse reactions.

Pre-exposure immunization does not eliminate the need for prompt prophylaxis following an exposure. It only reduces the post-exposure treatment regimen.

Pre-Exposure Rabies Treatment Guide

Pre-exposure immunization consists of a total of three doses of HDCV given on Days 0, 7 and 21 or 28. Each dose is 0.1 given intradermally in the deltoid area of either arm. Administration of booster doses of vaccine following primary 3-dose immunization depends on exposure risk category as noted in Table I. Pre-exposure immunization of immunosuppressed persons is not recommended. (9)

[See table 1 at right]

CONTRAINDICATIONS

There are no known specific contraindications other than situations such as developing febrile illness, etc.

WARNINGS

SYRINGES IN THIS PACKAGE TO DELIVER INTRADERMALLY ONE DOSE (0.1 ML) OF IMOVAX RABIES I.D., RABIES VACCINE MUST NOT BE USED FOR POST-EXPOSURE IMMUNIZATION

The full 0.1 ml dose should be given intradermally.

Recently a significant increase has been noted of "immune complex-like" reactions in persons receiving booster doses of HDCV by the intradermal (0.1 ml) or intramuscular (1.0 ml) route. (10.11). The illness characterized by onset 2-21 days post-booster, presents with a generalized urticaria and may also include arthralgia, arthritis, angioedema, nausea, vomiting, fever and malaise. In no cases were the illnesses life-threatening. Preliminary data suggest this "immune complex-like" illness may occur in up to 6% of persons receiving booster doses of Rabies Vaccines and much less frequently in persons receiving primary immunization. There is preliminary evidence that beta propiolactone altered human albumin induces most of the allergic reactions. (9, 12)

Persons who travel from the U.S. to developing countries and receive their pre-exposure vaccination abroad or within 30 days before leaving should be immunized by the intramuscular (IM) route (3 × 1.0 ml).

Two cases of neurologic illness resembling Guillain-Barré syndrome (13, 14), a transient neuroparalytic illness, that resolved without sequelae in 12 weeks, and a focal subacute nervous system disorder temporarily associated with HDCV, have been reported. (15)

All serious systemic neuroparalytic or anaphylactic reactions to a Rabies Vaccine should be immediately reported to the state health department or the Division of Viral Diseases, Center for Infectious Diseases, CDC, 404-329-3095 during working hours, or 404-329-2888 at other times. (9)

Persons previously vaccinated successfully against rabies and who come in contact with a rabid or potentially rabid animal, should have the wounds cleansed and receive a post-exposure dose of 1.0 ml of Rabies Vaccine intramuscularly, followed by a second 1.0 ml dose on Day 3. Intradermal immunization must not be used. Rabies Immune Globulin should NOT be given.

PRECAUTIONS

General—When a person with a history of hypersensitivity must be given Rabies Vaccine, antihistamines may be given; epinephrine (1:1000) should be readily available to counteract anaphylactic reactions, and the person should be carefully observed after immunization.

While the concentration of antibiotics in each dose of vaccine is extremely small, persons with known hypersensitivity to any of these agents could manifest an allergic reaction. While the risk is small, it should be weighed in light of potential risk of contracting rabies.

Drug Interactions—Antimalarial drugs such as chloroquine have been associated with a reduction in the antibody response to Rabies Vaccine administered by the intradermal route. Although it is apparent that antimalarial agents are not the sole factor responsible for the reduced antibody response, it is recommended that persons on corticosteroids and other immunosuppressive drugs receive Rabies Vaccine (3 doses/1.0 ml each) by the intramuscular route until more definitive data is available. (16, 17, 18)

Pregnancy Category C—Animal reproduction studies have not been conducted with Imovax Rabies I.D., Rabies Vaccine. It is also not known whether the product can cause fetal harm when administered to a pregnant woman or can affect reproductive capacity. Rabies Vaccine should be given to a pregnant woman only if clearly needed. Pre-exposure immunization should be carefully considered and may be indicated if there is substantial risk of rabies exposure.

Pediatric Use—Although specific intradermal studies in children have not been conducted, vaccine given to children intramuscularly (1.0 ml) has been shown to be safe. There are no known specific hazards expected from intradermal use of the vaccine in children. (19)

Table I (9)

Criteria for Pre-exposure Immunization

Risk category	Nature at risk	Typical populations	Pre-esposure regimen
Continuous	Virus present continuously, often in high concentrations. Aerosol, mucous membrane, bite, or nonbite exposure possible. Specific exposures may go unrecognized.	Rabies research lab worker.* Rabies biologics production workers.	Primary pre-exposure immunization course. Serology every 6 months. Booster immunization when antibody titer alls below acceptable level.†
Frequent	Exposure usually episodic. with source recognized, but exposure may also be unrecognized. Aerosol, mucous, membrane, bite, or nonbite exposure.	Rabies diagnostic lab workers, * spelunkers, veterinarians, and animal control and wildlife workers in rabies epizootic areas.	Primary pre-exposure immunization course. Booster immunization or serology every 2 years.†
Infrequent (greater than population-at-large)	Exposure nearly always episodic with source recognized Mucous membrane, bite, or nonbite exposure.	Veterinarians and animal control and wildlife workers in areas of low rabies endemicity. Certain travelers to foreign rabies epizootic areas. Veterinary students.	Primary pre-exposure immunization course. No routine booster immunization or serology.
Rare (population-at-large).	Exposure always episodic, mucous membrane, or bite with source recognized.	U.S. population-at-large, including individuals in rabies epizootic areas.	No pre-exposure immunization.

* Judgment of relative risk and extra monitoring of immunization status of laboratory workers is the responsibility of the laboratory supervisor (see U.S. Department of Health and Human Service's Biosafety in Microbiological and Biomedical Laboratories, 1984).

† Pre-exposure booster immunization consists of one dose of HDCV, 0.1 ml I.D. or 1.0 ml I.M. (deltoid area). Acceptable antibody level is a titer of 1:5 (complete inhibition of infectious foci in RFFIT at 1:5 serum dilution). See Clinical Pharmacology. Boost if titer falls below 1:5.

ADVERSE REACTIONS

Also See Warnings and Contraindications Sections for Additional Statements

Reactions after vaccination with HDVC are less common than with previously available vaccines. (10, 12, 20). In a study using five doses of HDVC administered intramuscularly, local reactions such as pain, erythema and swelling or itching at the injection site were reported in about 25% of recipients; mild systemic reactions such as headache, nausea, abdominal pain, muscle aches and dizziness were reported in about 20% of recipients. (9)

Clinical experience with Merieux Imovax Rabies I.D., Rabies Vaccine, has resulted in a low incidence of adverse reactions comparable to those following intramuscular vaccination when administered by the intradermal route except that a slight increase in transient local reactions has been observed following intradermal vaccination, especially when the vaccine is given in the forearm rather than in the lateral aspect of the upper arm. Local reactions consist of redness, itching, mild pain and minimal swelling at the site of injection. Generalized reactions are uncommon.(7) Mild local or systemic reactions can be treated with anti-inflammatory, antipyretic agents, e.g., aspirin and antihistamines. Systemic allergic or anaphylactic reactions following primary immunization have been reported to be less than 1%.(14) If an anaphylactic reaction should occur, epinephrine is indicated.

For "immune complex-like" reactions in persons receiving booster doses of HDCV see WARNINGS.

Advice and assistance on the management of serious adverse reactions in persons receiving primary or booster rabies immunization may be sought from the state health department or CDC.(9)

DOSAGE AND ADMINISTRATION

PARENTERAL DRUG PRODUCTS SHOULD BE INSPECTED VISUALLY FOR PARTICULATE MATTER AND DISCOLORATION PRIOR TO ADMINISTRATION, WHENEVER SOLUTION AND CONTAINER PERMIT. THE FREEZE-DRIED VACCINE IS CREAMY WHITE TO ORANGE. AFTER RECONSTITUTION IT IS PINK TO RED.

Primary Vaccination—Based upon studies in Europe (3,4) and the United States (8,9) the Immunization Practices Advisory Committee (ACIP) recommends three injections of 0.1 ml each; one injection on Day 0, one on Day 7, and one either on Day 21 or 28. (9,21) The ACIP, in making this recommendation, cites studies conducted in the United States and Europe in which more than 1500 persons received 0.1 ml of vaccine intradermally as the 2 or 3-dose pre-exposure vaccination. All subjects developed antibody as shown by the rapid fluorescent focus inhibition test (RFFIT). The ACIP suggests that routine serologic testing to confirm a satisfactory antibody response is not necessary. (22)

Booster Dose—Persons working with live rabies virus in research laboratories and in vaccine production facilities should have rabies antibody titers checked every six months and boosters given as needed to maintain an adequate titer. (For definition of adequate titer, see Clinical Pharmacology.) Laboratory workers, such as those doing rabies diagnostic tests, spelunkers and veterinarians, animal control and wildlife officers in areas where rabies is epizootic should have boosters every 2 years or have their serum tested for rabies antibody every 2 years and, if the titer is inadequate, have a booster dose. Veterinarians and animal control and wildlife officers working in areas of low rabies endemicity do not require routine doses of HDCV after completion of primary pre-exposure immunization (Table 1).

Persons who have experienced "immune complex-like" hypersensitivity reactions should receive no further doses of HDCV unless they are exposed to rabies or they are truly likely to be inapparently and/or unavoidably exposed to rabies virus and have unsatisfactory antibody titers.

INSTRUCTIONS FOR USE—Please Read Carefully and Completely

This package contains:

A single dose syringe of freeze dried Imovax Rabies I.D., Rabies Vaccine, which after reconstitution must be completely given by the intradermal route.

If the intradermal inoculation was not performed satisfactorily (vaccine injected subcutaneously) another dose should be given intradermally at a different site.

One vial of diluent (Sterile Water for Injection USP). The quantity of diluent contained in the vial is in excess of the volume needed. The purpose of this excess is to permit withdrawal of diluent without introduction of air.

To Open Vial

1. Pull green metal flip top in direction of arrow. This will loosen outer seal enough to be removed. (Figure 1)
2. Remove gray stopper. (Figure 2)
3. Carefully slide syringe out of glass vial.

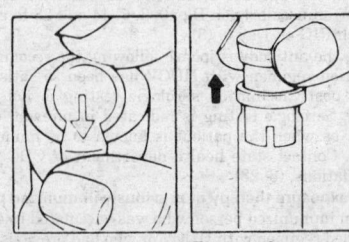

Figure 1   **Figure 2**

To Prepare Diluent
1. Remove center of green protective cover at perforation on diluent vial. (Figure 3)

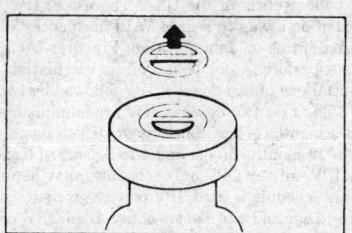

Figure 3

2. Disinfect pink stopper seal surface.
Reconstituting Vaccine
1. Remove protective rubber cap from needle. (Figure 4)

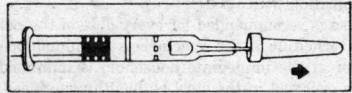

Figure 4

2. Push plunger so that the leading edge of the black stopper is even with the broken blue line (Figure 5).

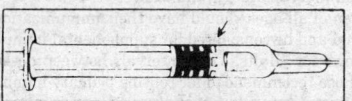

Figure 5

3. Insert needle into diluent bottle, keeping it upright. The needle must be in the liquid during withdrawal of the diluent to prevent air bubbles. (Fig. 6)
4. Withdraw diluent so that end of black stopper is at solid blue line. (Figure 7)

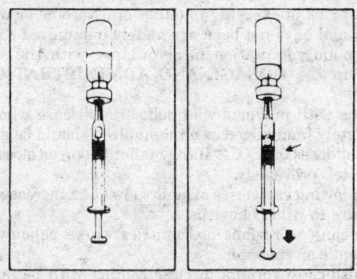

Figure 6   **Figure 7**

5. Replace protective rubber cap on needle and wait for freeze-dried vaccine to dissolve. Make sure that the freeze dried vaccine is completely dissolved. Shake if necessary. (Figure 8)

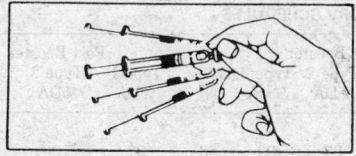

Figure 8

6. Remove protective cap and vaccine is ready to use.
After reconstitution, eliminate the air bubbles and bring together the droplets of vaccine either by flicking the syringe or, if necessary, grasp the covered needle end of the syringe and use a strong downward motion as indicated in Fig. 8 (as with a thermometer).
THE RECONSTITUTED VACCINE SHOULD BE USED IMMEDIATELY.
Remove the needle cover.
Push in the plunger to eliminate the air.
Disinfect the injection site.
Inject intradermally.
Destroy needle by clipping it off at the base of syringe.

HOW SUPPLIED

Imovax Rabies I.D., Rabies Vaccine—for pre-exposure use only by the intradermal route is supplied in a tamperproof unit with:
- One disposable syringe with integral needle containing a single dose of freeze-dried vaccine.

- One vial of Sterile Water for Injection USP for reconstitution.

STORAGE

The freeze-dried vaccine should be stored in the refrigerator between 2°C and 8°C (35°F to 47°F). Do not freeze.

REFERENCES

1. Aoki FY, Tyrell DA, Hill LE: Immunogenicity and acceptability of a human diploid cell rabies vaccine in volunteers. Lancet 1: 660-62(1975).
2. Turner GS, Aoki FY, Nicholson KG, Tyrrell DA, Hill LE: Human diploid cell strain rabies vaccine: Rapid prophylactic immunization of volunteers with small doses. Lancet 1: 1379-81 (1976).
3. Cox JH, Schneider LG: Prophylactic immunization of humans against rabies by intradermal inoculation of human diploid cell culture vaccine. J. Clin. Microbiol. 3: 96-101 (1976).
4. Nicholson KG, Turner GS, Aoki FY: Immunization with a human diploid cell strain of rabies virus vaccine: Two-year results, J. Infect. Dis. 137: 783-88 (1978).
5. Nicholson KG, Turner GS: Studies with human diploid cell strain rabies vaccine and human antirabies globulin in man. Dev. Biol. Stand. 40:115-20 (1978).
6. Ajjan N, Soulebot JP, Triau R, Biron G: Intradermal Immunization with rabies vaccine: Inactivated Wistar strain cultivated in human diploid cells. JAMA 244: 2528-31 (1980).
7. Bernard KW, Roberts MA, Sumner J, Winkler WG, Mallonee J, Baer GM, Chaney R: Human diploid cell rabies vaccine: Effectiveness of immunization with small intradermal or subcutaneous doses. JAMA 247: 1138-42 (1982).
8. Dreesen DW, Brown WJ, Kemp DT, Brown J, Reid FL, Baer GM: Pre-exposure rabies prophylaxis: efficacy of a new packaging and delivery system for intradermal administration of human diploid cell vaccine. Vaccine 2: 185-88 (1984).
9. CDC. Recommendations of the Immunization Practices Advisory Committee (ACIP). Rabies Prevention—United States, 1984. MMWR 33: 393-402, 407-8 (1984).
10. CDC. Systemic allergic reactions following immunization with human diploid cell rabies vaccine. MMWR 33: 185-87 (1984).
11. Dreesen DW, Bernard KW, Parker RA, Deutsch AJ, Brown J: Immune complex-like disease in 23 persons following a booster dose of rabies human diploid cell vaccine. Vaccine 4: 45-49 (1986).
12. Baer H, Anderson HC, Bernard K, Quinnan G: Beta propiolactone treated human serum albumin (BPL-HSA) an allergen for humans receiving rabies vaccine. (Abstract). J. Allergy and Clin. Immunol.75: (No. 1 Part 2 suppl) (1985).
13. Boe E, Nyland H: Guillain-Barré syndrome after vaccination with human diploid cell rabies vaccine. Scand. J. Infect. Dis. 12: 231-32 (1980).
14. CDC. Adverse reactions to human diploid cells rabies vaccine MMWR 29: 609-10 (1980).
15. Bernard KW, Smith PW, Kader FJ, Moran MJ: Neuroparalytic illness and human diploid cell rabies vaccine. JAMA 248: 3136-38 (1982).
16. Taylor DN, Wasi C, Bernard K: Chloroquine prophylaxis associated with a poor antibody reponse to human diploid cell rabies vaccine. Lancet 1: 1408 (1984).
17. Pappaioanou M, Fishbein DB, Dreesen DW, Schwartz IK, Campbell GH, Sumner JW, Patchen LC, Brown WJ: Antibody response to pre-exposure human diploid cell rabies vaccine given concurrently with chloroquine. N. Engl. J. Med. 314: 280-84 (1986).
18. Bernard KW, Fishbein DB, Miller KD, Parker RA, Waterman S, Sumner JW, Reid FL, Johnson BK, Rollins AJ, Oster CN, Schonberger LB, Baer GM, Winkler WG: Pre-exposure rabies immunization with human diploid cell vaccine. Decreased antibody reponses in persons immunized in developing countries. Am. J. Trop. Med. Hyg. 34: 633-47 (1985).
19. Fridell E, Grandien M, Johansson R: Pre-exposure prophylaxis against rabies in children by human diploid cell vaccine. Lancet 1: 623 (1984).
20. Greenberg M, Childress J: Vaccination against rabies with duck embryo and Semple vaccines. JAMA 173: 333-37 (1960).
21. CDC. ACIP Recommendations: Supplementary statement on pre-exposure rabies prophylaxis by the intradermal route. MMWR: 31: 279-85 (1982).
22. CDC. ACIP Recommendation: Supplementary statement on rabies vaccine and serologic testing. MMWR 30: 535-36 (1981).
A.H.F.S Category 80:12

Manufactured by:
PASTEUR MÉRIEUX Sérums & Vaccins S.A.
Lyon, France   U.S. License No. 384
Distributed by:
CONNAUGHT LABORATORIES, INC.
Swiftwater, Pennsylvania 18370, U.S.A.
800-VACCINE (800-822-2463)

CONNAUGHT
A PASTEUR MÉRIEUX COMPANY
Issued July 1991
Shown in Product Identification Guide, page 330

IPOL®   ℞
POLIOVIRUS VACCINE INACTIVATED

DESCRIPTION

IPOL®, Poliovirus Vaccine Inactivated, produced by Pasteur Mérieux Sérums & Vaccins S.A., is a sterile suspension of three types of poliovirus: Type 1 (Mahoney), Type 2 (MEF-1), and Type 3 (Saukett). IPOL® is a highly purified, inactivated poliovirus vaccine produced by microcarrier culture.[1,2] This culture technique and improvements in purification, concentration and standardization of poliovirus antigen produce a more potent and consistent immunogenic vaccine than the IPV available in the US prior to 1988. The viruses are grown in cultures of VERO cells, a continuous line of monkey kidney cells, by the microcarrier technique. The cells are grown in Eagle MEM modified medium, supplemented with newborn calf serum tested for adventitious agents prior to use, originated from countries free of bovine spongiform encephalopathy. For viral growth the culture medium is replaced by M-199, without calf serum.
After clarification and filtration, viral suspensions are concentrated by ultrafiltration, and purified by three liquid chromatography steps; one column of anion exchanger, one column of gel filtration and again one column of anion exchanger. After re-equilibration of the purified viral suspension, with Medium M-199 and adjustment of the antigen titer, the monovalent viral suspensions are inactivated at + 37°C for at least 12 days with 1:4000 formalin.
Each sterile immunizing dose (0.5 mL) of trivalent vaccine is formulated to contain 40 D antigen units of Type 1, 8 D antigen units of Type 2, and 32 D antigen units of Type 3 poliovirus. For each lot of IPOL®, D-antigen content is determined *in vitro* using the D-antigen ELISA assay and immunogenicity is determined by *in vivo* testing in animals. IPOL® is produced from vaccine concentrates diluted with M-199 medium. Also present are 0.5% of 2-phenoxyethanol and a maximum of 0.02% of formaldehyde per dose as preservatives. Neomycin, streptomycin and polymyxin B are used in vaccine production, and although purification procedures eliminate measurable amounts, less than 5 ng neomycin, 200 ng streptomycin and 25 ng polymyxin B per dose may still be present. The residual calf serum protein is less than 1 ppm in the final vaccine.
The vaccine is clear and colorless and should be administered intramuscularly or subcutaneously.

CLINICAL PHARMACOLOGY

Poliomyelitis is caused by poliovirus types 1, 2, or 3. It is primarily spread by the fecal-oral route of transmission but may also be spread by the pharyngeal route.
Approximately 90% to 95% of poliovirus infections are asymptomatic. Nonspecific illness with low-grade fever and sore throat (minor illness) occurs in 4% to 8% of infections. Aseptic meningitis occurs in 1% to 5% of patients a few days after the minor illness has resolved. Rapid onset of asymmetric acute flaccid paralysis occurs in 0.1% to 2% of infections, and residual paralytic disease involving motor neurons (paralytic poliomyelitis) occurs in approximately 1 per 1,000 infections.[3]
Prior to the introduction of conventional (non-enhanced) inactivated poliovirus vaccines in 1955, large outbreaks of poliomyelitis occurred each year in the United States (US). The annual incidence of paralytic disease of 11.4 cases/100,000 population declined to 0.5 cases by the time oral poliovirus vaccine (OPV) was introduced in 1961. Incidence continued to decline thereafter to its present rate of 0.002 to 0.005 cases per 100,000 population. Of the 127 cases of paralytic poliomyelitis reported in the US between 1980 and 1994, six were imported cases (caused by wild polioviruses), two were "indeterminant" cases, and 119 were vaccine associated paralytic poliomyelitis (VAPP) cases associated with the use of live, attenuated oral poliovirus vaccine (OPV).[4]
Poliovirus Vaccine Inactivated induces the production of neutralizing antibodies against each type of virus which are related to protective efficacy and induces antibody responses in most children after administering fewer doses[5] than the vaccine available in the United States prior to 1988.
Studies in developed[5] and developing[6,7] countries with a similar enhanced inactivated poliovirus vaccine produced by the same technology with the use of different cell substrate (primary kidney cells) have shown that a direct relationship exists between the antigenic content of the vaccine, the frequency of seroconversion, and resulting antibody titer. Approval in the US was based upon demonstration of immunogenicity and safety in US children.[8]

Continued on next page

Ipol—Cont.

In the US, 219 infants received three doses of IPV at two, four and eighteen months of age manufactured by the same process as IPOL® except the cell substrate for IPV was primary monkey kidney cells. Seroconversion to all three types of poliovirus was demonstrated in 99% of these infants after two doses of vaccine given at 2 and 4 months of age. Following the third dose of vaccine at 18 months of age, neutralizing antibodies were present at a level of ≥ 1:10 in 99.1% of children to Type 1 and 100% of children to Types 2 and 3 polioviruses.[9]

IPOL® was administered to more than 700 infants between 2 to 18 months of age during three clinical studies conducted in the US using IPV only schedules and sequential IPV-OPV schedules.[10,11] Seroprevalence rates for detectable serum neutralizing antibody (DA) at a ≥ 1:4 dilution were 95% to 100% (Type 1); 97% to 100% (Type 2) and 96% to 100% (Type 3) after two doses of IPOL® depending on studies.

[See table 1 below]

In one study,[11] the persistence of DA in infants receiving two doses of IPOL® at 2 and 4 months of age was 91% to 100% (Type 1), 97% to 100% (Type 2), and 93% to 94% (Type 3) at twelve months of age. In another study,[10] 86% to 100% (Type 1), 95% to 100% (Type 2), and 82% to 94% (Type 3) of infants still had DA at 18 months of age.

IPV ONLY SCHEDULES

Poliomyelitis vaccination based on IPV only schedules using IPOL® or other IPV vaccines implemented in numerous countries.[14,15] None of these countries use the schedule proposed for the US.

In trials and field studies conducted outside the US, IPOL®, or a combination vaccine containing IPOL® and DTP, was administered to more than 3,000 infants between 2 to 18 months of age using IPV only schedules and immunogenicity data are available from 1,485 infants. After two doses of vaccine given during the first year of life, seroprevalence rates for detectable serum neutralizing antibody (neutralizing titer ≥ 1:4) were 88% to 100% (Type 1); 84% to 100% (Type 2) and 94% to 100% (Type 3) of infants, depending on studies. When three doses were given during the first year of life, post-dose 3 DA ranged between 93% to 100% (Type 1); 89% to 100% (Type 2) and 97% to 100% (Type 3) and reached 100% for Types 1, 2, and 3 after the fourth dose given during the second year of life (12 to 18 months of age).[12]

In infants immunized with three doses of an unlicensed combination vaccine containing IPOL® and DTP given during the first year of life, and a fourth dose given during the second year of life, the persistence of detectable neutralizing antibodies was 96%, 96% and 97% against poliovirus types 1, 2, and 3, respectively, at six years of age. DA reached 100% for all types after a booster dose of IPOL® combined with DTP vaccine.[8] A survey of Swedish children and young adults given a Swedish IPV only schedule demonstrated persistence of detectable serum neutralizing antibody for at least 10 years to all three types of poliovirus.[13]

IPV is able to induce secretory antibody (IgA) produced in the pharynx and gut and reduces pharyngeal excretion of poliovirus type 1 from 75% in children with neutralizing antibodies at levels less than 1:8 to 25% in children with neutralizing antibodies at levels more than 1:64.[12,14-21] There is also evidence of induction of herd immunity with IPV,[13,22-25] and that this herd immunity is sufficiently maintained in a population vaccinated only with IPV.[25]

Paralytic polio and VAPP have not been reported in association with administration of IPOL®.

SEQUENTIAL IPV-OPV SCHEDULES

In an effort to obtain the benefits of both of the available poliomyelitis vaccines, several countries, including Denmark and Israel, have implemented schedules using IPV and OPV. Although none of these countries uses the sequential IPV-OPV schedule recommended for the US, certain general conclusions can be drawn from this experience, along with other, more limited studies of IPV-OPV schedules.

Induction of serum neutralizing antibody: It is expected, based on the overall experience with various schedules of IPV and OPV, that administration of two doses of IPV followed by two doses of OPV will induce detectable levels of serum neutralizing antibody against all three poliovirus types in at least 90% of recipients.

Induction of secretory antibody: It is expected, based on the overall experience with various schedules of IPV and OPV, that administration of two doses of IPV followed by two doses of OPV will induce higher levels of secretory antibody in the gut—and therefore potentially reduce virus excretion—when compared with schedules using IPV alone. One study comparing OPV alone with a sequential schedule of MRC-5 cell-derived IPV at 2 months and 4 months, followed by OPV at 6 and 15 months, found similar levels of virus excretion when subjects were challenged with OPV at 28 months of age.[26]

Potential reduction in recipient cases of VAPP: It is expected, based on high percentage levels of seroconversion following two doses of IPOL®, that the risk of recipient VAPP will be lower with the sequential schedule shown in Table 3 when compared to schedules using OPV alone. No recipient cases were reported in children who previously received two or more doses of "conventional" or non-enhanced IPV, and only one case was reported (in 1969) in a child who had previously received one dose of "conventional" IPV.[27] VAPP has also been reported prior to 1969 in a few OPV recipients who had previously received conventional IPV.[28] Effect on contact cases of VAPP: It is unknown whether the sequential IPV-OPV schedule will reduce the risk of contact VAPP. However, three studies conducted to date indicate that prior vaccination with IPV will not significantly increase the number of children excreting revertant poliovirus (as determined by genomic sequencing studies) after subsequent vaccination with OPV.[15,29,30]

Persistence of serum neutralizing antibody: It is expected, but not yet known, that sequential IPV-OPV schedules will provide a similar degree of long-term protection when compared with schedules using IPV or OPV alone.

INDICATIONS AND USAGE

IPOL® is indicated for active immunization of infants (as young as 6 weeks of age), children and adults for the prevention of poliomyelitis caused by poliovirus Types 1, 2, and 3.[31]

INFANTS, CHILDREN AND ADOLESCENTS

General Recommendations

It is recommended that all infants (as young as 6 weeks of age), unimmunized children and adolescents not previously immunized be vaccinated routinely against paralytic poliomyelitis.[32] Following the eradication of poliomyelitis caused by wild poliovirus from the Western Hemisphere (including North and South America)[33] VAPP is the only cause of paralytic poliomyelitis in the US.[34] The use of IPV has been suggested as a way to reduce VAPP incidence.[34] The Advisory Committee on Immunization Practices (ACIP) recommends a preference for poliomyelitis vaccination based on sequential use of two doses of IPV followed by two doses of OPV.[31] The first two doses of IPV are administered at two and four months of age. Subsequent OPV doses can be given at 12 to 18 months of age and 4 to 6 years of age. Alternatively, IPV only or OPV only schedules may be used. If an IPV only schedule is used, IPV may be given at 2, 4, 6 to 18 months of age and 4 to 6 years of age. If an OPV- only schedule is used, refer to the manufacturer's latest package insert for the appropriate administration schedule and all other issues related to the use of OPV.

Previous clinical poliomyelitis (usually due to only a single poliovirus type) or incomplete immunization with OPV are not contraindications to completing the primary series of immunization with IPOL®.

IPV also is recommended for every dose of the polio vaccination schedule if the vaccinee is immunodeficient or a member of the immediate household is immunodeficient. OPV is excreted in the stool by healthy vaccinees and can infect an immunocompromised household member, which may result in paralytic disease. In a household with an immunocompromised member, only IPV should be used for all those requiring poliovirus immunization.[31]

Children Incompletely Immunized

Children of all ages should have their immunization status reviewed and be considered for supplemental immunization as follows for adults. Time intervals between doses longer than those recommended for routine primary immunization do not necessitate additional doses as long as a final total of four doses is reached (see DOSAGE AND ADMINISTRATION section).

ADULTS

General Recommendations

Routine primary poliovirus vaccination of adults (generally those 18 years of age or older) residing in the US is not recommended. Unimmunized adults residing in a household when a child is receiving OPV and/or adults who have increased risk of exposure to either oral vaccine or wild poliovirus and have not been adequately immunized should receive polio vaccination in accordance with the schedule given in the DOSAGE AND ADMINISTRATION section.[31]

Persons with previous wild poliovirus disease who are incompletely immunized or unimmunized should be given additional doses of IPOL® if they fall into one or more categories listed previously.

The following categories of adults are at an increased risk of exposure to wild polioviruses:[31,35]

• Travelers to regions or countries where poliomyelitis is endemic or epidemic.
• Health-care workers in close contact with patients who may be excreting polioviruses.
• Laboratory workers handling specimens that may contain polioviruses.
• Members of communities or specific population groups with disease caused by wild polioviruses.

TABLE 1 U.S. STUDIES WITH IPOL® ADMINISTERED USING IPV ONLY OR SEQUENTIAL IPV-OPV SCHEDULES

Dose 1 (2)	Age (months) for Dose 2 (4)	Dose 3 (6)	12 to 18 Booster	N*	Post Dose 2 Type 1 %DA**	Type 2 %DA	Type 3 %DA	N*	Post Dose 3 Type 1 %DA	Type 2 %DA	Type 3 % DA	N*	Pre Booster Type 1 %DA	Type 2 %DA	Type 3 %DA	N*	Post Booster Type 1 %DA	Type 2 %DA	Type 3 %DA
STUDY 1[11¶]																			
I(s)	I(s)	NA†	I(s)	56	97	100	97	—	—	—		53	91	97	93	53	97	100	100
O	O	NA	O	22	100	100	100	—	—	—		22	78	91	78	20	100	100	100
I(s)	O	NA	O	17	95	100	95	—	—	—		17	95	100	95	17	100	100	100
I(s)	I(s)	NA	O	17	100	100	100	—	—	—		16	100	100	94	16	100	100	100
STUDY 2[10§]																			
I(c)	I(c)	NA	I(s)	94	98	97	96	—	—	—		100	92	95	88	97	100	100	100
I(s)	I(s)	NA	I(s)	68	99	100	99	—	—	—		72	100	100	94	75	100	100	100
I(c)	I(c)	NA	O	75	95	99	96	—	—	—		77	86	97	82	78	100	100	97
I(s)	I(s)	NA	O	101	99	99	95	—	—	—		103	99	97	89	107	100	100	100
STUDY 3[10§]																			
I(c)	I(c)	I(c)	O	91	98	99	100	91	100	100	100	41	100	100	100	40	100	100	100
I(c)	I(c)	O	O	96	100	98	99	94	100	100	99	47	100	100	100	45	100	100	100
I(c)	I(c)	I(c) + O	O	91	96	97	100	85	100	100	100	47	100	100	100	46	100	100	100

*N = Number of children from whom serum was available
**Detectable antibody (neutralizing titer ≥1:4)
† NA—No poliovirus vaccine administered
¶ IPOL® given subcutaneously
§ IPOL® given intramuscularly
I POL® given either separately in association with DTP in two sites (s) or combined (c) with DTP in a dual chambered syringeI
O OPV

- Incompletely vaccinated or unvaccinated adults in a household (or other close contacts) with children given OPV. The adult should be informed of the risk of VAPP associated with contact of those receiving OPV.

IMMUNODEFICIENCY AND ALTERED IMMUNE STATUS

Patients with recognized immunodeficiency are at greater risk of developing paralysis when exposed to live poliovirus than persons with a normal immune system. Under no circumstances should oral poliovirus vaccine be used in such patients or introduced into a household where such a patient resides.[31]

IPOL® should be used in all patients with immunodeficiency diseases and members of such patients' households when vaccination of such persons is indicated. This includes patients with asymptomatic HIV infection, AIDS or AIDS-Related Complex, severe combined immunodeficiency, hypogammaglobulinemia, or aggammaglobulinemia; altered immune states due to diseases such as leukemia, lymphoma, or generalized malignancy; or an immune system compromised by treatment with corticosteroids, alkylating drugs, antimetabolites or radiation. Immunogenicity of IPOL® in individuals receiving immunoglobulin could be impaired and patients with an altered immune state may or may not develop a protective response against paralytic poliomyelitis after administration of IPV.[36]

As with any vaccine, vaccination with IPOL® may not protect 100% of susceptible individuals.

Use with other vaccines: refer to **DOSAGE AND ADMINISTRATION** section for this information.

CONTRAINDICATIONS

IPOL® is contraindicated in persons with a history of hypersensitivity to any component of the vaccine, including neomycin, streptomycin and polymyxin B.

No further doses should be given if anaphylaxis or anaphylactic shock occurs within 24 hours of administration of one dose of vaccine.

Vaccination of persons with an acute, febrile illness should be deferred until after recovery; however, minor illness, such as mild upper respiratory infection, with or without low grade fever, are not reasons for postponing vaccine administration.

WARNINGS

Neomycin, streptomycin, and polymyxin B are used in the production of this vaccine. Although purification procedures eliminate measurable amounts of these substances, traces may be present (see **DESCRIPTION** section) and allergic reactions may occur in persons sensitive to these substances (see **CONTRAINDICATIONS** section).

Systemic adverse reactions reported in infants receiving IPV concomitantly at separate sites or combined with DTP have been similar to those associated with administration of DTP alone.[8] Local reactions are usually mild and transient in nature.

Although no causal relationship between IPOL® and Guillain-Barré Syndrome (GBS) has been established,[31] GBS has been temporally related to administration of another inactivated poliovirus vaccine. Deaths have been reported in temporal association with the administration of IPV (see **ADVERSE REACTIONS** section).

PRECAUTIONS

GENERAL

Before injection of the vaccine, the physician should carefully review the recommendations for vaccine use and the patient's medical history including possible hypersensitivities and side effects that may have occurred following previous doses of the vaccine.

Health-care providers should question the patient, parent or guardian about reactions to a previous dose of this product, or similar product.

Epinephrine Injection (1:1000) and other appropriate agents should be available to control immediate allergic reactions.

Health-care providers should obtain the previous immunization history of the vaccinee, and inquire about the current health status of the vaccinee.

Immunodeficient patients or patients under immunosuppressive therapy may not develop a protective immune response against paralytic poliomyelitis after administration of IPV.

Administration of IPOL® is not contraindicated in individuals infected with HIV.[37,38,39]

Special care should be taken to ensure that the injection does not enter a blood vessel.

A separate, sterile syringe and needle or a sterile disposable unit must be used for each patient to prevent transmission of hepatitis or other infectious agents from person to person. Needles should not be recapped and should be disposed of according to biohazard waste guidelines.

INFORMATION FOR PATIENTS

Patients, parents, or guardians should be instructed to report any serious adverse reactions to their health-care provider.

TABLE 2[10] PERCENTAGE OF INFANTS PRESENTING WITH LOCAL OR SYSTEMIC REACTIONS AT 6, 24, AND 48 HOURS OF IMMUNIZATION WITH IPOL® ADMINISTERED INTRAMUSCULARLY CONCOMITANTLY AT SEPARATE SITES WITH CLI WHOLE-CELL DTP VACCINE AT 2 AND 4 MONTHS OF AGE AND WITH CLI ACELLULAR PERTUSSIS VACCINE (TRIPEDIA®) AT 18 MONTHS OF AGE

	AGE AT IMMUNIZATION								
REACTION	2 Months (n=211)			4 Months (n=206)			18 Months† (n=74)		
	6 Hrs.	24 Hrs.	48 Hrs.	6 Hrs.	24 Hrs.	48 Hrs.	6 Hrs.	24 Hrs.	48 Hrs.
Local, IPOL® alone§									
Erythema >1″	0.5%	0.5%	0.5%	1.0%	0.0%	0.0%	1.4%	0.0%	0.0%
Swelling	11.4%	5.7%	0.9%	11.2%	4.9%	1.9%	2.7%	0.0%	0.0%
Tenderness	29.4%	8.5%	2.8%	22.8%	4.4%	1.0%	13.5%	4.1%	0.0%
Systemic*									
Fever >102.2°F	1.0%	0.5%	0.5%	2.0%	0.5%	0.0%	0.0%	0.0%	4.2%
Irritability	64.5%	24.6%	17.5%	49.5%	25.7%	11.7%	14.7%	6.7%	8.0%
Tiredness	60.7%	31.8%	7.1%	38.8%	18.4%	6.3%	9.3%	5.3%	4.0%
Anorexia	16.6%	8.1%	4.3%	6.3%	4.4%	2.4%	2.7%	1.3%	2.7%
Vomiting	1.9%	2.8%	2.8%	1.9%	1.5%	1.0%	1.3%	1.3%	0.0%
Persistent Crying	Percentage of infants within 72 hours after immunization was 0.0% after dose one, 1.4% after dose two, and 0.0% after dose three.								

§ Data are from the IPOL® administration site, given intramuscularly.

* The adverse reaction profile includes the concomitant use of CLI whole-cell DTP vaccine or Tripedia® with IPOL®. Rates are comparable in frequency and severity to that reported for whole-cell DTP given alone.

† Children vaccinated with Tripedia® vaccine.

The health-care provider should inform the patient, parent, or guardian of the benefits and risks of the vaccine.

If a sequential IPV-OPV schedule is used, before giving OPV, the health-care provider should question the patient, parent or guardian if the vaccinee is immunodeficient or a member of the immediate household is immunodeficient.

The health-care provider should inform the patient, parent, or guardian of the importance of completing the immunization series.

The health-care provider should provide the Vaccine Information Materials (VIMs) which are required to be given with each immunization.

DRUG INTERACTIONS

There are no known interactions of IPOL® with drugs or foods. Simultaneous administration, with separate syringes at separate sites, of other parenteral vaccines is not contraindicated. The first two doses of IPOL® may be administered at separate sites using separate syringes concomitantly with DTP, acellular pertussis, *Haemophilus influenzae* type b (Hib), and hepatitis B vaccines. From historical data on the antibody responses to diphtheria, tetanus, whole-cell or acellular pertussis, Hib, or hepatitis B vaccines used concomitantly or in combination with IPOL®, no interferences have been observed on the immunological end points accepted for clinical protection.[8,12,40] (See **DOSAGE AND ADMINISTRATION** section.)

If IPOL® has been administered to persons receiving immunosuppressive therapy, an adequate immunologic response may not be obtained. (See **PRECAUTIONS**—GENERAL section)

CARCINOGENESIS, MUTAGENESIS, IMPAIRMENT OF FERTILITY

Long-term studies in animals to evaluate carcinogenic potential or impairment of fertility have not been conducted.

PREGNANCY

REPRODUCTIVE STUDIES—PREGNANCY CATEGORY C

Animal reproduction studies have not been conducted with IPOL®. It is also not known whether IPOL® can cause fetal harm when administered to a pregnant woman or can affect reproduction capacity. IPOL® should be given to a pregnant woman only if clearly needed.

NURSING MOTHERS

It is not known whether IPOL® is excreted in human milk. Because many drugs are excreted in human milk, caution should be exercised when IPOL® is administered to a nursing woman.

PEDIATRIC USE

SAFETY AND EFFECTIVENESS OF IPOL® IN INFANTS BELOW SIX WEEKS OF AGE HAVE NOT BEEN ESTABLISHED.[10,19] (See **DOSAGE AND ADMINISTRATION** section.)

In the US, infants receiving two doses of IPV at 2 and 4 months of age, the seroconversion to all three types of poliovirus was demonstrated in 95% to 100% of these infants after two doses of vaccine.[10,11]

ADVERSE REACTIONS

BODY SYSTEM AS A WHOLE

In earlier studies with the vaccine grown in primary monkey kidney cells, transient local reactions at the site of injection were observed.[9] Erythema, induration and pain occurred in 3.2%, 1% and 13%, respectively, of vaccinees within 48 hours post-vaccination. Temperatures of ≥ 39°C (≥ 102°F) were reported in 38% of vaccinees. Other symptoms included irritability, sleepiness, fussiness, and crying. Because IPV was given in a different site but concurrently with Diphtheria and Tetanus Toxoids and Pertussis Vaccine Adsorbed (DTP), these systemic reactions could not be attributed to a specific vaccine. However, these systemic reactions were comparable in frequency and severity to that reported for DTP given alone without IPV.[10] Although no causal relationship has been established, deaths have occurred in temporal association after vaccination of infants with IPV.

Four additional US studies using IPOL® in more than 1,300 infants,[10] between two to eighteen months of age administered with DTP at the same time at separate sites or combined have demonstrated that local and systemic reactions were similar when DTP was given alone.

[See table 2 above]

DIGESTIVE SYSTEM

Anorexia and vomiting occurred with frequencies not significantly different as reported when DTP was given alone without IPV or OPV.[10]

NERVOUS SYSTEM

Although no causal relationship between IPOL® and GBS has been established,[32] GBS has been temporally related to administration of another inactivated poliovirus vaccine.

Reporting of Adverse Events

The National Vaccine Injury Compensation Program, established by the National Childhood Vaccine Injury Act of 1986, requires physicians and other health-care providers who administer vaccines to maintain permanent vaccination records and to report occurrences of certain adverse events to the US Department of Health and Human Services. Reportable events include those listed in the Act for each vaccine and events specified in the package insert as contraindications to further doses of that vaccine.[41,42,43]

Reporting by parents or guardians of all adverse events after vaccine administration should be encouraged. Adverse events following immunization with vaccine should be reported by health-care providers to the US Department of Health and Human Services (DHHS) Vaccine Adverse Event Reporting System (VAERS). Reporting forms and information about reporting requirements or completion of the form can be obtained from VAERS through a toll-free number 1-800-822-7967.[41,42,43]

Health-care providers also should report these events to the Director of Medical Affairs, Connaught Laboratories, Inc., Route 611, PO Box 187, Swiftwater, PA 18370 or call 1-800-822-2463.

DOSAGE AND ADMINISTRATION

Parenteral drug products should be inspected visually for particulate matter and/or discoloration prior to administration whenever solution and container permit. If these conditions exist, the vaccine should not be administered.

After preparation of the injection site, immediately administer IPOL® intramuscularly or subcutaneously. In infants and small children, the mid-lateral aspect of the thigh is the preferred site. In adults IPOL® should be administered intramuscularly or subcutaneously in the deltoid area.

Care should be taken to avoid administering the injection into or near blood vessels and nerves. After aspiration, if blood or any suspicious discoloration appears in the syringe, do not inject but discard contents and repeat procedures using a new dose of vaccine administered at a different site.

DO NOT ADMINISTER VACCINE INTRAVENOUSLY.

Continued on next page

Ipol—Cont.

Children

Primary Immunization

A primary series of IPOL® consists of two 0.5 mL doses administered intramuscularly or subcutaneously in accordance with the schedules indicated in Table 3.[31] The interval between the first two doses should be at least four weeks, but preferably eight weeks. The first two doses of IPOL® are usually administered at two and four months of age. The first immunization may be administered as early as six weeks of age.

If a sequential IPV-OPV schedule is used, OPV has been recommended by the ACIP to be given at 12 to 18 months of age and 4 to 6 years of age. The third dose of oral poliovirus vaccine, (OPV), should follow at least six months but not more than twelve months after the second IPOL® dose.

Patients with recognized immunodeficiency are at greater risk of developing paralysis when exposed to OPV than persons with a normal immune system. Under no circumstances should OPV be used in such patients or introduced in a household where such a patient resides.[31]

If a full (IPV only) IPOL® schedule is used, the third dose of IPOL® should be given at 6 to 18 months of age and 4 to 6 years of age. The third dose of IPOL® should follow at least two months but not more than 12 months after the second IPOL® dose. If this third dose is given at 6 months of age, it would be preferable to administer this dose two months after the second IPOL® dose simultaneously with DTP or acellular pertussis and Hib or hepatitis B vaccines using separate syringes at separate sites. From historical data on the antibody responses to diphtheria, tetanus, whole-cell or acellular pertussis, Hib, or hepatitis B vaccines used concomitantly or in combination with IPOL®, no interferences have been observed on the immunological end points accepted for clinical protection.[8,12,40] (See DRUG INTERACTIONS section.) If the third dose is given between 12 to 18 months of age, it may be desirable to administer this dose with Measles, Mumps, and Rubella (MMR) and other vaccines using separate syringes at separate sites,[31] but no data on the immunological interference between IPOL® and these vaccines exist. The fourth dose of IPOL® should be given before entering school at 4 to 6 years of age.

[See table 3 below]

The need to routinely administer additional doses is unknown at this time.[31]

Two doses of IPOL® followed by two doses of OPV (or alternatively four doses of IPV or four doses of OPV) are necessary to complete the ACIP recommended series of primary and booster doses. Children and adolescents with a previously incomplete series of IPOL®/OPV or IPOL® alone should receive sufficient additional doses of IPOL® or OPV to complete the series.

The preferred site of injection in infants and children is the mid lateral aspect of the thigh.

Interruption of the recommended schedule with a delay between doses does not interfere with the final immunity. There is no need to start the series over again, regardless of the time elapsed between doses.

Adults

Unvaccinated Adults

A primary series of IPOL® is recommended for unvaccinated adults at increased risk of exposure to poliovirus. While the responses of adults to primary series have not been studied, the recommended schedule for adults is two doses given at a 1 to 2 month interval and a third dose given 6 to 12 months later. If less than 3 months but more than 2 months are available before protection is needed, three doses of IPOL® should be given at least 1 month apart. Likewise, if only 1 or 2 months are available, two doses of IPOL® should be given at least 1 month apart. If less than 1 month is available, a single dose of IPOL® is recommended.[31]

Incompletely Vaccinated Adults

Adults who are at an increased risk of exposure to poliovirus and who have had at least one dose of OPV, fewer than three doses of conventional IPV or a combination of conventional IPV or OPV totaling fewer than three doses should receive at least one dose of IPOL®. Additional doses needed to complete a primary series should be given if time permits.[31]

Completely Vaccinated Adults

Adults who are at an increased risk of exposure to poliovirus and who have previously completed a primary series with one or a combination of polio vaccines can be given a dose of either OPV or IPOL®.[31]

The preferred injection site of IPOL® for adults is in the tissue of the deltoid area.

HOW SUPPLIED

Syringe, 0.5 mL with integrated needle (1 × 1 Dose package - Product No. 49281-860-51) (10 × 1 Dose package Product No. 49281-860-52)

Vial, 10 Dose - Product No. 49281-860-10

STORAGE

The vaccine is stable if stored in the refrigerator between 2°C and 8°C (35°F and 46°F). The vaccine must not be frozen.

REFERENCES

1. van Wezel AL, et al. Inactivated poliovirus vaccine: Current production methods and new developments. Rev Infect Dis 6 (Suppl 2): S335-S340, 1984
2. Montagnon BJ, et al. Industrial scale production of inactivated poliovirus vaccine prepared by culture of Vero cells on microcarrier. Rev Infect Dis 6 (Suppl 2): S341-S344, 1984
3. Sabin AB. Poliomyelitis. In Brande AI, Davis CE, Fierer J (eds) International Textbook of Medicine, Vol II. Infectious Diseases and Medical Microbiology. 2nd ed. Philadelphia, WBSaunders, 1986
4. Prevots DR, et al. Vaccine-associated paralytic poliomyelitis in the United States, l980-1994: current risk and potential impact of a proposed sequential schedule of IPV followed by OPV (Abstract #H90). In: Abstracts of the 36th Interscience Conference on Antimicrobial Agents and Chemotherapy. Washington, DC. American Society for Microbiology, 179, 1996
5. Salk J, et al. Antigen content of inactivated poliovirus vaccine for use in a one- or two-dose regimen. Ann Clin Res 14: 204-212, 1982
6. Salk J, et al. Killed poliovirus antigen titration in humans. Develop Biol Standard 41: 110-132, 1978
7. Salk J, et al. Theoretical and practical considerations in the application of killed poliovirus vaccine for the control of paralytic poliomyelitis. Develop Biol Standard 47: 181-198, 1981
8. Unpublished data available from Pasteur Mérieux Sérums & Vaccins S.A.
9. McBean AM, et al. Serologic response to oral polio vaccine and enhanced-potency inactivated polio vaccines. Am J Epidemiol 128: 615-628, 1988
10. Unpublished data available from Connaught Laboratories, Inc.
11. Faden H, et al. Comparative evaluation of immunization with live attenuated and enhanced potency inactivated trivalent poliovirus vaccines in childhood: Systemic and local immune responses. J Infect Dis 162: 1291-1297, 1990
12. Vidor E, et al. The place of DTP/eIPV vaccine in routine paediatric vaccination. Rev Med Virol 4: 261-277, 1994
13. Bottiger M. Long-term immunity following vaccination with killed poliovirus vaccine in Sweden, a country with no circulating poliovirus. Rev Infect Dis 6 (Suppl 2): S545-S551, 1984
14. Plotkin SA, et al. Inactivated polio vaccine for the United States: a missed vaccination opportunity. Pediatr Infect Dis J 14: 835-839, 1995
15. Murdin AD, et al. Inactivated poliovirus vaccine: past and present experience. Vaccine 8: 735-746, 1996
16. Marine WM, et al. Limitation of fecal and pharyngeal poliovirus excretion in Salk-vaccinated children. A family study during a Type 1 poliomyelitis epidemic. Amer J Hyg 76: 173-175, 1962
17. Bottiger M, et al. Vaccination with attenuated Type 1 poliovirus, the Chat strain. II. Transmission of virus in relation to age. Acta Paed Scand 55: 416-421, 1966
18. Dick GWA, et al. Vaccination against poliomyelitis with live virus vaccines. Effect of previous Salk vaccination on virus excretion. Brit Med J 2: 266-269, 1961
19. Wehrle PF, et al. Transmission of poliovirus; III. Prevalence of polioviruses in pharyngeal secretions of infected household contacts of patients with clinical disease. Pediatrics 27: 762-764, 1961
20. Adenyi-Jones SC, et al. Systemic and local immune responses to enhanced-potency inactivated poliovirus vaccine in premature and term infants. J Pediatr 120: No 5, 686-689, 1992
21. Chin TDY. Immunity induced by inactivated poliovirus vaccine and excretion of virus. Rev Infect Dis 6 (Suppl 2): S369-S370, 1984
22. Salk D. Herd effect and virus eradication with use of killed poliovirus vaccine. Develop Biol Standard 47: 247-255, 1981
23. Bijerk H. Surveillance and control of poliomyelitis in the Netherlands. Rev Infect Dis 6 (Suppl 2): S451-S456, 1984
24. Lapinleimu K. Elimination of poliomyelitis in Finland. Rev Infect Dis 6 (Suppl 2): S457-S460, 1984
25. Conyn van Spaendonck M, et al. Circulation of Poliovirus during the poliomyelitis outbreak in the Netherlands in 1992-1993—Amer J Epidemiology 143: 929-935, 1996
26. Modlin JF, et al. Serum neutralizing antibody response to three experimental sequential IPV-OPV immunization schedules. J Infec Dis (in press)
27. von Magnus H, et al. Vaccination with inactivated poliovirus vaccine and oral poliovirus vaccine in Denmark. Rev Infect Dis 6 (suppl): S471-S474, 1984
28. Henderson DA, et al. Paralytic disease associated with oral polio vaccines. JAMA 190:41-48, 1964
29. Ogra PL, et al. Effect of prior immunity on the shedding of virulent revertant virus in feces after oral immunization with live attenuated poliovirus vaccines. J Infect Dis 164: 191-194, 1991
30. Abraham R, et al. Shedding of virulent poliovirus revertants during immunization with oral poliovirus vaccine after immunization with inactivated polio vaccine. J Infect Dis 168: 1105-1109, 1993
31. Recommendations of the Advisory Committee on Immunization Practices (ACIP). Poliomyelitis Prevention in the United States: Introduction of a Sequential Vaccination Schedule of Inactivated Poliovirus Vaccine Followed by Oral Poliovirus Vaccine. MMWR 46: No. RR-3, 1997
32. WHO. Weekly Epidemiology Record 54: 82-83, 1979
33. Certification of poliomyelitis eradication—the Americas, 1994. MMWR 43: 720-722, 1994
34. Strebel PM, et al. Epidemiology of poliomyelitis in the United States one decade after the last reported case of indegenous wild virus associated disease. Clin Infect Dis 14: 568-579, 1992
35. Institute of Medicine. An evaluation of poliomyelitis vaccine policy options. Washington, DC. National Academy of Sciences, 1988
36. ACIP. Immunization of children infected with human T-lymphotropic virus type III/lymphadenopathy-associated virus. MMWR 35: 595-606, 1986
37. ACIP. General recommendations on immunization. MMWR 43: No. RR-1, 1994
38. Barbi M, et al. Antibody response to inactivated polio vaccine (eIPV) in children born to HIV positive mothers. Eur J Epidemiol 8: 211-216, 1992
39. Varon D, et al. Response to hemophilic patients to poliovirus vaccination: Correlation with HIV serology and with immunological parameters. J Med Virol 40: 91-95, 1993
40. Vidor E, et al. Fifteen-years experience with vero-produced enhanced potency inactivated poliovirus vaccine (eIPV). Ped Infect Dis J, 1997 (In Press)
41. CDC. Vaccine Adverse Event Reporting System—United States. MMWR 39: 730-733, 1990
42. CDC. National Childhood Vaccine Injury Act. Requirements for permanent vaccination records and for reporting of selected events after vaccination. MMWR 37: 197-200, 1988
43. Food & Drug Administration. New Reporting Requirements for Vaccine Adverse Events. FDA Drug Bull 18 (2), 16-18, 1988

A.H.F.S. Category 80:12

Product information
as of February 1997

Manufactured by:
PASTEUR MÉRIEUX Sérums & Vaccins S.A.
Lyon, France
U.S. License No. 384

Distributed by:
CONNAUGHT LABORATORIES, INC.
Swiftwater, Pennsylvania 18370, USA
1-800-VACCINE (1-800-822-2463) 2316

PASTEUR MÉRIEUX CONNAUGHT

Shown in Product Identification Guide, page 330

TABLE 3

PRIMARY IMMUNIZATION SCHEDULES

OPTION	2 MONTHS OF AGE	4 MONTHS OF AGE	6 to 12 MONTHS OF AGE	12 to 18 MONTHS OF AGE	4 to 6 YEARS OF AGE
Sequential IPOL®/OPV	IPOL®	IPOL®		OPV	OPV
IPOL® alone*	IPOL®	IPOL®	IPOL®		IPOL®

*This schedule should be used for individuals and household contacts who are immunocompromised (See **General Recommendations** section.)

JAPANESE ENCEPHALITIS VIRUS VACCINE INACTIVATED JE-VAX®

℞

CAUTION: Federal (USA) law prohibits dispensing without prescription.

DESCRIPTION

JE-VAX®, Japanese Encephalitis Virus Vaccine Inactivated, is a sterile, lyophilized vaccine for subcutaneous use, pre-

pared by inoculating mice intracerebrally with Japanese encephalitis (JE) virus, "Nakayama-NIH" strain, manufactured by The Research Foundation for Microbial Diseases of Osaka University ("BIKEN®"). Infected brains are harvested and homogenized in phosphate buffered saline, pH 8.0. The homogenate is centrifuged and the supernatant inactivated with formaldehyde, then processed to yield a partially purified, inactivated virus suspension. This is further purified by ultra-centrifugation through 40% w/v sucrose. The suspension is then lyophilized in final containers and sealed under dry nitrogen atmosphere. Thimerosal (mercury derivative) is added as a preservative to a final concentration of 0.007%. The diluent, Sterile Water for Injection, contains no preservative. Each 1.0 mL dose contains approximately 500 μg of gelatin, less than 100 μg of formaldehyde, and less than 0.0007% v/v Polysorbate 80, and less than 50 ng of mouse serum protein. No myelin basic protein can be detected at the detection threshold of the assay (< 2 ng/mL). Prior to reconstitution, the vaccine is a white caked powder, and after reconstitution the vaccine is a colorless transparent liquid. The potency of JE vaccine is determined by immunizing mice with either the test vaccine or the JE reference vaccine. Neutralizing antibodies are measured in a plaque neutralization assay performed on sera from the immunized mice. The potency of the test vaccine must be no less than that of the reference vaccine.

CLINICAL PHARMACOLOGY

Japanese encephalitis (JE), a mosquito-borne arboviral Flavivirus infection, is the leading cause of viral encephalitis in Asia.

Infection leads to overt encephalitis in 1 of 20 to 1000 cases. Encephalitis, usually is severe, resulting in a fatal outcome in 25% of cases and residual neuropsychiatric sequelae in 50% of cases. JE acquired during the first or second trimesters of pregnancy may cause intrauterine infection and miscarriage. Infections that occur during the third trimester of pregnancy have not been associated with adverse outcomes in newborns.[1]

The virus is transmitted in an enzootic cycle among mosquitoes and vertebrate amplifying hosts, chiefly domestic pigs and, in some areas, wild Ardeid (wading) birds. Viral infection rates in mosquitoes range from < 1% to 3%. These species are prolific in rural areas where their larvae breed in ground pools and flooded rice fields. Thus all elements of the transmission cycle are prevalent in rural areas of Asia and human infections occur principally in this setting. Because vertebrate amplifying hosts and agricultural activities may be situated within and at the periphery of cities, human cases occasionally are reported from urban locations.[1]

JE virus is transmitted seasonally in most areas of Asia. The seasonal patterns of viral transmission are correlated with the abundance of vector mosquitoes and of vertebrate amplifying hosts. Although the abundance of vector mosquitoes fluctuates with the amount of rainfall, and with the impact of the rainy season, in some tropical locations, irrigation associated with agricultural practices is a more important factor affecting vector abundance, and transmission may occur year-round. Thus the periods of greatest risk for JE viral transmission vary regionally and within countries, and from year to year.[1]

In areas where JE is endemic, annual incidence ranges from 1 to 10 per 10,000 people. Cases occur primarily in children under 10 years of age. Seroprevalence studies in these endemic areas indicate nearly universal exposure by adulthood (calculating from a ratio of asymptomatic to symptomatic infections of 200 to 1, approximately 10% of the susceptible population is infected per year). In addition to children < 10 years, an increase in JE incidence has been observed in the elderly.[1]

Challenge experiments in passively protected mice have defined the levels of neutralizing antibody that may be protective for humans.[2] Mice passively immunized to achieve a neutralizing antibody titer of ≥1:10 were protected from a JE virus challenge of $10^5 LD_{50}$, a viral dose thought to be transmitted by an infected mosquito.[2]

The efficacy of the BIKEN Nakayama-NIH strain Japanese Encephalitis Virus Vaccine Inactivated was demonstrated in a placebo-controlled, randomized clinical trial in Thai children, sponsored by the US Army.[3] In this trial, children between 1 and 14 years of age received BIKEN monovalent Nakayama-NIH strain (n = 21,628) or a bivalent vaccine containing the Nakayama-NIH and Beijing JE virus strains (n = 22,080) or tetanus toxoid as a placebo (n = 21,516). Immunization consisted of two (2) subcutaneous 1.0 mL doses of vaccine, *except in children under 3 years of age who received two 0.5 mL doses.* One case (5 cases/100,000) of JE occurred in the monovalent vaccine group, one case (5 cases/100,000) in the bivalent vaccine group, and 11 cases (51 cases/100,000) in the placebo group. The observed efficacy of both monovalent and bivalent vaccines was 91% (95% confidence interval, 54% to 98%). Side effects of vaccination, including headache, sore arm, rash, and swelling were reported at rates similar to those in the placebo group, usually less than 1%. Symptoms did not increase after the second dose. It should be noted that a schedule of two doses, separated by seven days, as employed in this trial, may be appropriate for use in residents of endemic or epidemic areas, where pre-existing exposure to Flaviviruses may contribute to the immune response.[3]

A three-dose vaccination schedule is recommended for U.S. travelers and military personnel, based on the Centers for Disease Control and Prevention (CDC) experience and on a controlled immunogenicity trial performed in US military personnel.[4,5] The CDC experience demonstrated that neutralizing antibody was produced in fewer than 80% of vaccinees following two doses of vaccine in US travelers and antibody levels declined substantially in most vaccinees within six months. The US Army studied the immunogenicity of JE-VAX in 538 volunteers. Two three-dose regimens were evaluated (Day 0, 7, and 14 or Day 0, 7, and 30). All vaccine recipients demonstrated neutralizing antibodies at 2 months and 6 months after initiation of vaccination. The schedule of Day 0, 7, and 30 produced higher antibody responses than the Day 0, 7, and 14 schedule. Two hundred and seventy-three of the original study participants were tested at 12 months post-vaccination and there was no longer a statistical difference in antibody titers between the two vaccination regimens.[5]

The full duration of protection is unknown. Of US Army volunteers completing a three-dose regimen, 252 agreed to receive a booster dose of vaccine one year after the primary series. All boosted participants still had antibody 12 months after the booster. Protective levels of neutralizing antibody persisted for 24 months (2 years) in all 21 persons who had not received a booster.[5] Definitive recommendations cannot be given on the timing of booster doses at this time.

INDICATIONS AND USAGE

JE-VAX is indicated for active immunization against JE for persons one year of age and older. For recommended primary immunization series see **DOSAGE AND ADMINISTRATION** section.

JE-VAX should be considered for use in persons who plan to reside in or travel to areas where JE is endemic or epidemic during a transmission season. ***JE-VAX is NOT recommended for all persons traveling to or residing in Asia.*** The incidence of JE in the location of intended stay, the conditions of housing, nature of activities, duration of stay, and the possibility of unexpected travel to high-risk areas are factors that should be considered in the decision to administer vaccine. In general, vaccine should be considered for use in persons spending a month or longer in epidemic or endemic areas during the transmission season, especially if travel will include rural areas. Depending on the epidemic circumstances, vaccine should be considered for persons spending less than 30 days whose activities, such as extensive outdoor activities in rural areas, place them at particularly high risk for exposure.[1]

In all instances, travelers are advised to take personal precautions to reduce exposure to mosquito bites. (See INFORMATION FOR PATIENTS section)

Current CDC advisories should be consulted with regard to JE epidemicity in specific locales.[1]

The decision to use JE-VAX should balance the risks for exposure to the virus and for developing illness, the availability and acceptability of repellents and other alternative measures, and the side effects of vaccination. Assessments should be interpreted cautiously because risk can vary within areas and from year to year and available data are incomplete. Estimates suggest that risk of JE in highly endemic areas during the transmission season can reach 1 per 5000 per month of exposure; risk for most short-term travelers may be 1 per million or less. Although JE vaccine is reactogenic, rates of serious allergic reactions (generalized urticaria and/or angioedema) are low (approximately 1–104 per 10,000).[1]

Advanced age may be a risk factor for developing symptomatic illness after infection. JE acquired during pregnancy carries the potential for intrauterine infection and fetal death. These factors should be considered when advising elderly persons and pregnant women who plan visits to JE endemic areas.

There are no data on the safety and efficacy of JE vaccine in infants under one year of age. Whenever possible, immunization of infants should be deferred until they are one year of age or older.[1]

Research laboratory workers:

Laboratory acquired JE has been reported in 22 cases. JE virus may be transmitted in a laboratory setting through needle sticks and other accidental exposures. Vaccine-derived immunity presumably protects against exposure through these percutaneous routes. Exposure to aerosolized JE virus, and particularly to high concentrations of virus, such as may occur during viral purification, potentially could lead to infection through mucous membranes and possibly directly into the central nervous system through the olfactory mucosa. It is unknown whether vaccine-derived immunity protects against such exposures, but immunization is recommended for all laboratory workers with a potential for exposure to infectious JE virus.[1]

As with any vaccine, vaccination with JE-VAX may not result in protection in all individuals. Long-term protection, as demonstrated by persistence of neutralizing antibody for more than two years, has not yet been shown.

CONTRAINDICATIONS

Adverse reactions to a prior dose of JE vaccine manifesting as generalized urticaria and angioedema are considered to be contraindications to further vaccination.

Patients who develop allergic or unusual adverse events after vaccination should be reported through the Vaccine Adverse Event Reporting System (VAERS) 1-800-822-7967.[1]

JE vaccine is produced in mouse brains and should not be administered to persons with a proven or suspected hypersensitivity to proteins of rodent or neural origin. ***HYPERSENSITIVITY TO THIMEROSAL IS A CONTRAINDICATION TO VACCINATION.***[1]

WARNINGS

Adverse reactions to JE vaccine manifesting as generalized urticaria or angioedema may occur within minutes following vaccination. A possibly related reaction has occurred as late as 17 days after vaccination. Most reactions occur within 10 days with the majority occurring within 48 hours.[1] (See ADVERSE REACTIONS section)

Vaccinees should be observed for 30 minutes after vaccination and warned about the possibility of delayed generalized urticaria, often in a generalized distribution or angioedema of the extremities, face and oropharynx, especially of the lips.[1]

Vaccinees should be advised to remain in areas where they have ready access to medical care for 10 days after receiving a dose of JE vaccine. *Vaccinees should be instructed to seek medical attention immediately upon onset of any reaction.*[1]

Persons should not embark on international travel within 10 days of JE-VAX immunization because of the possibility of delayed allergic reactions.[1]

Persons with a past history of urticaria after hymenoptera envenomation, drugs, physical or other provocations, or of idiopathic cause appear to have a greater risk of developing reactions to JE vaccine (relative risk 9.1, 95% confidence interval 1.8 to 50.9).[6] This history should be considered when weighing risks and benefits of the vaccine for an individual patient. When patients with such a history are offered JE vaccine, they should be alerted to their increased risk for reaction and monitored appropriately. There are no data supporting the efficacy of prophylactic antihistamines or steroids in preventing JE vaccine-ralated allergic reactions.[1]

Another case control study consisting of 5 cases and 15 controls identified an increased risk of hypersensitivity reactions to JE vaccine in individuals who had unusual alcohol consumption during the two days following vaccination (p=0.005)[7]. **Recipients should be advised to avoid more than the usual alcohol intake during the 48 hours following JE vaccination.**

In the same study an increased risk for hypersensitivity reactions was seen in individuals who received other vaccines within the 7-day period prior to receipt of JE vaccine. **Where possible JE vaccine should be administered concurrently with other vaccines.[7]**

Epinephrine and other medications and equipment to treat anaphylaxis should be available at vaccine administration centers.

PRECAUTIONS

GENERAL

Epinephrine Injection (1:1000) must be immediately available should an acute anaphylactic reaction occur due to any component of the vaccine.

Prior to injection of any vaccine, all known precautions should be taken to prevent adverse reactions. This includes a review of the patient's history with respect to possible sensitivity to this vaccine, a similar vaccine or allergic disorders in general (see **CONTRAINDICATIONS** section).

A separate, sterile syringe and needle or a disposable unit should be used for each patient to prevent transmission of infectious agents from person to person. Needles should not be recapped and should be disposed of according to biohazard waste guidelines.

Although substantial neutralizing antibody titers are elicited by JE-VAX in more than 90% of U.S. travelers without history of prior JE immunization or of prior exposure to JE, the precise relationship between antibody level and efficacy has not been established even though these titers persisted for at least two years after immunization.[8]

The decision to administer JE vaccine should balance the risks for exposure to the virus and for developing illness, the availability and acceptability of repellents and other alternative protective measures, and the side effects of vaccination.

INFORMATION FOR PATIENTS

Patients should be advised of the following:

- JE-VAX is given to provide immunization against Japanese encephalitis virus.

Continued on next page

Je-Vax—Cont.

- A three-dose immunizing series should be completed, except in unusual circumstances. (See **CONTRAINDICATIONS** and **DOSAGE AND ADMINISTRATION** sections)
- JE-VAX should be given to a pregnant women only if, in the opinion of a physician, withholding the vaccine entails even greater risk.
- Any adverse events following JE-VAX should be reported through the Vaccine Adverse Event Reporting System (VAERS) 1-800-822-7967 after contacting the physician immediately.
- If the patient has a past history of urticaria (hives) (following hymenoptera envenomation, drugs, physical or other provocation or of idiopathic origin), adverse effects are more likely.
- Adverse events consisting of arm soreness and local redness can occur shortly after vaccination.
- Adverse events consisting of headache, rash, edema and generalized urticaria or angioedema may occur shortly after vaccination or up to 17 days (usually within 10 days) following vaccination.
- International travel should not be initiated within 10 days of JE-VAX vaccination because of the possibility of delayed adverse reactions. Patients should be instructed to seek medical attention immediately upon onset of any adverse reaction.
- Personal precautions should be taken to avoid exposure to mosquito bites by the use of insect repellents, and protective clothing. Avoiding outdoor activity, especially during twilight periods and in the evening, will reduce risk even further.

DRUG INTERACTIONS

There are no data on the effect of concurrent administration of other vaccines, drugs (e.g. chloroquine, mefloquine) or biologicals on the safety and immunogenicity of JE vaccine.

CARCINOGENESIS, MUTAGENESIS, IMPAIRMENT OF FERTILITY

No studies have been performed to evaluate carcinogenicity, mutagenic potential, or impact on fertility.

PREGNANCY

REPRODUCTIVE STUDIES - PREGNANCY CATEGORY C

Animal reproduction studies have not been conducted with Japanese Encephalitis Virus Vaccine. It is not known whether Japanese Encephalitis Virus Vaccine can cause fetal harm when administered to a pregnant woman or can affect reproductive capacity. Pregnant women who must travel to an area where risk of JE is high should be immunized when the theoretical risks of immunization are outweighed by the risk of infection to the mother and developing fetus. Japanese Encephalitis Virus Vaccine should be given to a pregnant woman only if clearly needed.

NURSING MOTHERS

It is not known whether JE-VAX is excreted in human milk. Because many drugs are excreted in human milk, caution should be exercised when JE-VAX is administered to a nursing woman.

PEDIATRIC USE

SAFETY AND EFFECTIVENESS OF JE-VAX IN INFANTS UNDER ONE YEAR OF AGE HAVE NOT BEEN ESTABLISHED. (See **DOSAGE AND ADMINISTRATION** section.)

ADVERSE REACTIONS

JE vaccine is associated with a moderate frequency of local and mild systemic adverse effects.[3,4,5,9,10,11,12] Tenderness, redness, swelling and other local effects have been reported in about 20% of vaccinees (<1% to 31%). Systemic side effects, principally fever, headache, malaise, rash, and other reactions, such as chills, dizziness, myalgia, nausea, vomiting and abdominal pain have been reported in approximately 10% of vaccinees.

In a study conducted by the CDC less than 5% of the 1,756 US travelers immunized with a three-dose regimen of the vaccine reported headache, flu-like symptoms, fever, and other systemic complaints. Hives and facial swelling were reported in 0.2% and 0.1% of vaccinees, respectively. Local soreness occurred in 5.9% and local redness in 2.9%. There was no increase in the number or severity of reactions with increasing numbers of doses.[8]

The US Army studied 4,034 personnel from 1987 to 1989.[11] Using a two- or three-dose regimen of JE vaccine, arm soreness was described in 22.7%, local redness in 4.8%, headache in 15.2%, and a febrile episode in 5.5%. In another trial evaluating the safety and immunogenicity of a three-dose immunizing series (Day 0, 7, and 30 or Day 0, 7, and 14), performed in 538 adult volunteers in 1990, the Army determined that local soreness and redness occurred in 21% of vaccinees after the first dose, then decreased with subsequent injections (p <0.0001, Chi-square for downward trend). Systemic symptoms including feverishness, headache and rash occurred in 5% of vaccinees after the first dose, then decreased with subsequent injections (p <0.001, Chi-square for downward trend).[5] Participants who received the third dose on Day 14 reported more side effects than

those who received the injection on Day 30. Among these volunteers, 252 received a booster injection of vaccine one year after receiving the first dose of the primary series. Side effects reported after the booster injection included local symptoms of soreness (24.5%) and redness (6.1%) at the injection site and systemic complaints of headache (4.9%), fever (1.6%), and rash (0.8%). Less than 1% of all reported symptoms was graded as severe. No generalized urticaria or anaphylaxis was reported.

Since 1989, an apparently new pattern of adverse reactions has been reported among vaccinees in Europe, North America, and Australia.[12,13,14] The reactions have been characterized by urticaria, often in a generalized distribution, or angioedema of the extremities, face, especially of the lips and oropharynx. Three vaccine recipients developed respiratory distress. Distress or collapse due to hypotension or other causes led to hospitalization in several cases. Most reactions were treated successfully with antihistamines or oral steroids; however some patients were hospitalized for parenteral steroid therapy. Three patients developed an erythema multiforme or erythema nodosum and some patients have had joint swelling. Some vaccinees complained of generalized itching without objective evidence of a rash.

An important feature of the reactions has been the interval between vaccination and onset of symptoms. Reactions after a first vaccine dose occurred after a median of 12 hours after immunization (88% of reactions occurred within 3 days). The interval between administration of a second dose and onset of symptoms generally was longer, (median 3 days and possibly as long as 2 weeks). Reactions have occurred after a second or third dose, when preceding doses were received uneventfully.

Between November 1991 and May 1992, the US Navy immunized 35,253 US personnel (marines, other military and dependents) with JE-VAX on Okinawa. The overall reaction rate, 62.4 per 10,000 vaccinees (95% confidence interval 54.2 to 70.6) includes persons reporting urticaria, angioedema, generalized itching and wheezing. The reaction rate per 10,000 vaccinees was 26.7 (95% confidence interval 21.3 to 32.1), 30.8 (95% confidence interval 24.6 to 37.0) or 12.2 (95% confidence interval 7.9 to 16.5) after the first, second or third dose, respectively.[6] These reactions were generally mild to moderate in severity. Nine out of 35,253 persons immunized were hospitalized (2.6 per 10,000 vaccinees) primarily to allow administration of intravenous steroids for refractory urticaria. None of these reactions were considered life-threatening.

A case-control study conducted as part of the JE immunization campaign in Okinawa found that persons developing these reactions after JE vaccination were more likely to have had a past history of urticaria after hymenoptera envenomation, drugs, physical or other provocations or of idiopathic origins (relative risk 9.1, 95% confidence interval 1.8 to 50.9).[6] The vaccine constituents responsible for these adverse reactions have not been identified.

Other serious adverse events reported following vaccination include (1) one case of Guillain-Barré syndrome after JE vaccination has been reported in the United States since 1984 (this patient was diagnosed as having mononucleosis three weeks before the onset of weakness); (2) one case of urticaria, hepatitis and respiratory failure one week after dose 2 (this person showed effusion and infiltrate on chest x-ray and eosinophilia); (3) one case of respiratory and renal failure one week after a dose (this 26-month-old male had infiltrate on chest x-ray and acid fast bacilli in sputum); and (4) one case of newly diagnosed hypertension in a young adult male presenting with a headache several hours after receiving dose one. The relationship of JE-VAX to the etiology of these adverse events is unknown.

Optic neuritis has been reported for one patient. In addition to JE-VAX, this patient concurrently received a number of other vaccines.[15]

Fatal myocarditis has been reported in a patient who had recently been given meningococcal vaccine and at least one dose of JE vaccine. Any causal role for the vaccines is unclear.[15]

Sudden death occurred approximately 60 hours after receiving the first dose of JE vaccine in a 21-year-old US military person with a history of recurrent hypersensitivity and an episode of possible anaphylaxis. This person also received the third dose of plague vaccine approximately 12 to 15 hours prior to the death. There was no evidence of urticaria or angioedema. Cause of death was not established at autopsy.

Surveillance of JE vaccine related complications in Japan from 1965 to 1973 disclosed neurologic events (primarily encephalitis, encephalopathy, seizures, and peripheral neuropathy) in 1 to 2.3 per million vaccinees.[16,17] Very rarely, deaths occurred with vaccine-associated encephalitis. Between 1987 and 1989, two cases of neurologic dysfunction were reported from Japan; one of these was a transverse myelitis, while the second included seizures, cranial nerve paresis, cerebellar ataxia, and behavior disorder.[17] In 1992, two cases of acute disseminated encephalomyelitis were reported from Japan; one occurred 14 days after the second

dose and the second occurred 17 days after a booster dose of JE vaccine. Both cases recovered.[18] One case of Bell's Palsy was reported from Thailand.

Reporting of Adverse Events

The National Vaccine Injury Compensation Program, established by the National Childhood Vaccine Injury Act of 1986, requires physicians and other health-care providers who administer vaccines to maintain permanent vaccination records and to report occurrences of certain adverse events to the US Department of Health and Human Services. Reportable events include those listed in the Act for each vaccine and events specified in the package insert as contraindications to further doses of that vaccine.[19,20,21]

Reporting by parents and patients of all adverse events occurring after antigen administration should be encouraged. Adverse events following immunization with vaccine should be reported by the health-care provider to the US Department of Health and Human Services (DHHS) Vaccine Adverse Event Reporting System (VAERS). Reporting forms and information about reporting requirements or completion of the form can be obtained from VAERS through a toll-free number 1-800-822-7967.[19,20,21]

Health-care providers also should report these events to Director of Medical Affairs, Connaught Laboratories, Inc., Route 611, P.O. Box 187, Swiftwater, PA 18370 or call 1-800-822-2463.

DOSAGE AND ADMINISTRATION

Parenteral drug products should be inspected visually for extraneous particulate matter and/or discoloration prior to administration whenever solution and container permit. If either of these conditions exist, the vaccine should not be administered.

For persons 3 years of age and older, a single dose is 1.0 mL of vaccine. *For children 1 year to 3 years of age, a single dose is 0.5 mL of vaccine.* (See PRIMARY IMMUNIZATION SCHEDULE below.)

Single-Dose vial of lyophilized vaccine: Remove plastic tab of flip-off cap. DO NOT REMOVE RUBBER STOPPER. Cleanse stopper with a suitable disinfectant. Reconstitute only with the supplied 1.3 mL of diluent (Sterile Water for Injection). Shake vial thoroughly. After reconstitution the vaccine should be stored between 2°–8°C (35°–46°F) and used within 8 hours. DO NOT FREEZE RECONSTITUTED VACCINE.

10-Dose vial of lyophilized vaccine: Remove plastic tab of flip-off cap. DO NOT REMOVE RUBBER STOPPER. Cleanse stopper with a suitable disinfectant. Reconstitute only with the supplied 11 mL of diluent (Sterile Water for Injection). Shake vial thoroughly. After reconstitution the vaccine should be stored between 2°–8°C (35°–46°F) and used within 8 hours. DO NOT FREEZE RECONSTITUTED VACCINE.

The vaccine is to be given by subcutaneous administration only.

A separate, sterile syringe and needle or a sterile disposable unit should be used for each patient to prevent transmission of infectious agents from person to person. Needles should not be recapped and should be disposed of according to biohazard waste guidelines.

SHAKE VIAL WELL

PRIMARY IMMUNIZATION SCHEDULE[1]

The recommended primary immunization series is three doses of 1.0 mL each for individuals > 3 years of age given subcutaneously on days 0, 7, and 30. *For children 1 to 3 years of age a series of three doses of 0.5 mL each should be given subcutaneously on days 0, 7, and 30.* An abbreviated schedule of days 0, 7, and 14 can be used when the longer schedule is impractical because of time constraints. (When it is impossible to follow one of the above recommended schedules, two doses given a week apart will induce antibodies in approximately 80% of vaccinees; however, this two-dose regimen should not be used except under unusual circumstances.) The last dose should be given at least 10 days before the commencement of international travel to ensure an adequate immune response and access to medical care in the event of delayed adverse reactions.

A booster dose of 1.0 mL (*0.5 mL for children from 1 to 3 years of age*) may be given after two years. In the absence of firm data on the persistence of antibody after primary immunization, a definite recommendation cannot be made on the spacing of boosters beyond two years.

There are no data on the safety and efficacy of JE vaccine in infants under one year of age. Whenever possible, immunization of infants should be deferred until they are one year of age or older.[1]

The skin at the site of injection first should be cleansed and disinfected. Shake vial thoroughly before each use. Cleanse top of rubber stopper of the vial with a suitable antiseptic and wipe away all excess before withdrawing vaccine.

When JE-VAX and any other vaccines are given concurrently, separate syringes and separate sites should be used.

HOW SUPPLIED

Vial, Single Dose (3 per package) with vial of Diluent (3 per package) – Product No. 49281-680-30

Vial, 10 Dose with vial Diluent – Product No. 49281-680-20

For persons 3 years of age and older, a single dose is 1.0 mL of vaccine. *For children 1 year to 3 years of age, a single dose is 0.5 mL of vaccine.* (See PRIMARY IMMUNIZATION SCHEDULE above.)

STORAGE

The vaccine should be stored between 2°–8°C (35°–46°F). DO NOT FREEZE. After reconstitution the vaccine should be stored between 2°–8°C (35°–46°F) and used within 8 hours. DO NOT FREEZE RECONSTITUTED VACCINE.

REFERENCES

1. Recommendations of the Advisory Committee on Immunization Practices (ACIP). Inactivated Japanese Encephalitis Virus Vaccine. MMWR 42: 1–15, 1993
2. Oya A. Japanese Encephalitis Vaccine. Acta Paediatr Jpn 30: 175–184, 1988
3. Hoke CH, et al. Protection Against Japanese Encephalitis by Inactivated Vaccines. N Eng J Med 319: 608–614, 1988
4. Poland JD, et al. Evaluation of the Potency and Safety of Inactivated Japanese Encephalitis Vaccine in US Inhabitants. J Infect Dis 161: 878–882, 1990
5. DeFraites RF. Immunogenicity and Safety of Japanese Encephalitis Vaccine (Inactivated: Nakayama/BIKEN) in U.S. Army Soldiers: Evaluation of Three Consecutively Manufactured Lots of Vaccine Administered in Two Dosing Regimens. April 30, 1991, and November 12, 1992. Unpublished Data, on file with BIKEN and with Walter Reed Army Institute of Research, Washington, DC
6. Berg WS. Systemic Reactions in U.S. Marine Corps Personnel Who Received Japanese Encephalitis Vaccine. Clin Infect Dis 24:001–064, 1997
7. Robinson, P, et al. Australian Case-Control Study of Adverse Reactions to Japanese Encephalitis Vaccine, J Travel Med 2: 159–164, 1995
8. Unpublished data on file with "BIKEN" and CDC
9. Rojanasuphot S. et al. A field trial of Japanese encephalitis vaccine produced in Thailand. Southeast Asian J Trop Med Publ Health 20: 653–654, 1989
10. Rao Bhau LN, et al. Safety and efficacy of Japanese encephalitis vaccine produced in India. Indian J Med Res 88: 301–307, 1988
11. Sanchez JL, et al. Further Experience with Japanese Encephalitis Vaccine. Lancet 335: 972–973, 1990
12. Japanese Encephalitis Vaccine and Adverse Effects among Travelers. Canada Diseases Weekly Report. Vol. 17–32: 173–177, 1991
13. Anderson MM, et al. Side-Effects with Japanese Encephalitis Vaccine. Lancet 337: 1044, 1991
14. Ruff TA, et al. Adverse Reactions to Japanese Encephalitis Vaccine. Lancet 338: 881–882, 1991
15. Unpublished data on file with Connaught Laboratories, Inc.
16. Kitaoka M. Follow-up on use of vaccine in children in Japan, in McDHammon W, Kitaoka M, Downs WG eds. Immunization for Japanese encephalitis, Excerpta Medica, Amsterdam 275–277, 1972
17. Unpublished data on file with "BIKEN"
18. Ohtaki E, et al. Acute disseminated encephalomyelitis after Japanese B Encephalitis Vaccination. Pediatric Neurology Vol. 8 No. 2: 137–139, 1992
19. CDC. Vaccine Adverse Event Reporting System – United States. MMWR 39: 730–733, 1990
20. CDC. National Childhood Vaccine Injury Act. Requirements for permanent vaccination records and for reporting of selected events after vaccination. MMWR 37: 197–200, 1988
21. Food and Drug Administration. New Reporting Requirements for Vaccine Adverse Events, FDA Drug Bull 18(2), 16–18, 1988

Manufactured by:

The Research Foundation for Microbial Diseases of Osaka University

Suita, Osaka, Japan

"BIKEN ®"

Distributed by:

CONNAUGHT LABORATORIES, INC.

Swiftwater, PA 18370, USA

1-800-VACCINE (1-800-822-2463)

Product Information as of February 1997
3294

Shown in Product Identification Guide, page 330

MENOMUNE®—A/C/Y/W-135

[mĕn-ō-mūne]

MENINGOCOCCAL POLYSACCHARIDE VACCINE, GROUPS A, C, Y AND W-135 COMBINED

℞

Caution: Federal (U.S.A.) law prohibits dispensing without prescription.

For special instructions on use of Meningococcal Polysaccharide Vaccine Groups A, C, Y and W-135 Combined, for Jet Injector Use—see end of insert.

DESCRIPTION

Menomune®, Meningococcal Polysaccharide Vaccine, Groups A, C, Y and W-135 Combined, is a freeze-dried preparation of the group-specific polysaccharide antigens from *Neisseria meningitidis,* Group A, Group C, Group Y and Group W-135 for subcutaneous use. The diluent is sterile pyrogen-free distilled water to which thimerosal (mercury derivative) 1:10,000 is added as a preservative. After reconstitution with diluent as indicated on the label, each 0.5 ml dose contains 50 mcg of "isolated product" from each of Groups A, C, Y and W-135 in isotonic sodium chloride solution preserved with thimerosal (mercury derivative). Each dose of vaccine also contains 2.5 mg to 5 mg of lactose added as a stabilizer.[1] The vaccine when reconstituted is a clear colorless liquid.

THIS VACCINE CONFORMS TO WHO REQUIREMENTS.

CLINICAL PHARMACOLOGY

N. meningitidis causes both endemic and epidemic disease, principally meningitis and meningococcemia. It is the second most common cause of bacterial meningitis in the United States (approximately 20% of all cases), affecting an estimated 3,000–4,000 people each year. The case-fatality rate is approximately 10% for meningococcal meningitis and 20% for meningococcemia, despite therapy with antimicrobial agents, such as penicillin, to which all strains remain highly sensitive.[2]

Within the United States, serogroup B, for which a vaccine is not yet available, accounts for 50%–55% of all cases; serogroup C, for 20%–25%; and serogroup W-135, for 15%. Serogroups Y (10%) and A (1%–2%) account for nearly all remaining cases. Serogroup W-135 has emerged as a major cause of disease only since 1975. While serogroup A causes only a small proportion of endemic disease in the United States, it is the most common cause of epidemics elsewhere.[2]

A study performed using 4 lots of Meningococcal Polysaccharide Vaccine, Groups A, C, Y and W-135 Combined in 150 adults showed at least a 4-fold increase in bactericidal antibodies to all groups in greater than 90 percent of the subjects.[3,4]

A study was conducted in 73 children 2 to 12 years of age. Post-immunization sera were not obtained on four children. Therefore, the seroconversion rates were based on 69 paired samples. Seroconversion rates as measured by bactericidal antibody were: Group A—72 percent, Group C—58 percent, Group Y—90 percent and Group W-135—82 percent. Seroconversion rates as measured by a 2-fold rise in antibody titers based on Solid Phase Radioimmunoassay were: Group A—99 percent, Group C—99 percent, Group Y—97 percent and Group W-135—89 percent.[5]

As with any vaccine, vaccination with Meningococcal Polysaccharide Vaccine, Groups A, C, Y and W-135 Combined may not protect 100% of susceptible individuals.

Vaccine efficacy. Numerous studies have demonstrated the immunogenicity and clinical efficacy of the A and C vaccines. The serogroup A polysaccharide induces antibody in some children as young as 3 months of age, although a response comparable to that seen in adults is not achieved until 4 or 5 years of age; the serogroup C component does not induce a good antibody response before age 18–24 months. The serogroup A vaccine has been shown to have a clinical efficacy of 85%–95% and to be of use in controlling epidemics.[6] A similar level of clinical efficacy has been demonstrated for the serogroup C vaccine, both in American military recruits and in an epidemic. The group Y and W-135 polysaccharides have been shown to be safe and immunogenic in adults and in children over 2 years of age; clinical protection has not been demonstrated directly, but is assumed, based on the production of bactericidal antibody, which for group C has been correlated with clinical protection. The antibody responses to each of the four polysaccharides in the quadrivalent vaccine are serogroup-specific and independent.[2]

Duration of efficacy. Antibodies against the group A and C polysaccharides decline markedly over the first 3 years following a single dose of vaccine. This antibody decline is more rapid in infants and young children than in adults. Similarly, while vaccine-induced clinical protection probably persists in schoolchildren and adults for at least 3 years, a recent study in Africa has demonstrated a marked decline in the efficacy of the group A vaccine in young children over time. In this study, efficacy declined from greater than 90% to less than 10% over 3 years in those under 4 years of age at the time of vaccination; in older children, efficacy was still 67%, 3 years after vaccination.[2,7]

INDICATIONS AND USAGE

Meningococcal Polysaccharide Vaccine, Groups A, C, Y and W-135 Combined, is indicated for the following individuals:

1. Persons 2 years of age and above in epidemic or endemic areas as might be determined in a population delineated by neighborhood, school, dormitory, or other reasonable boundary. The prevalent serogroup in such a situation should match a serogroup in the vaccine.

2. Individuals at particular high-risk to include persons with terminal component complement deficiencies and those with anatomic or functional asplenia.

3. Travelers to countries recognized as having hyperendemic or epidemic disease such as the part of Sub-Saharan Africa known as the "meningitis belt", which extends from Mauritania in the west to Ethiopia in the east.

Vaccinations also should be considered for household or institutional contacts of persons with meningococcal disease as an adjunct to appropriate antibiotic chemoprophylaxis as well as medical and laboratory personnel at risk of exposure to meningococcal disease.

This vaccine will not stimulate protection against infections caused by organisms other than Groups A, C, Y and W-135 meningococci.

CONTRAINDICATIONS

Immunization should be deferred during the course of any acute illness. Pregnant women should not be immunized since effects of vaccine on the fetus are unknown.

IT IS A CONTRAINDICATION TO ADMINISTER MENOMUNE A/C/Y/W-135 TO INDIVIDUALS KNOWN TO BE SENSITIVE TO THIMEROSAL OR AN OTHER COMPONENT OF THE VACCINE.

WARNING

If the vaccine is used in persons receiving immunosuppressive therapy, the expected immune response may not be obtained.

PRECAUTIONS

GENERAL

Epinephrine Injection (1:1000) must be immediately available to combat unexpected anaphylactic or other allergic reactions.

Prior to an injection of any vaccine, all known precautions should be taken to prevent side reactions. This includes a review of the patient's history with respect to possible sensitivity to the vaccine or similar vaccines.

As with any vaccine, vaccination with Meningococcal Polysaccharide Vaccine, Groups A, C, Y and W-135 Combined may not protect 100% of susceptible individuals. Protective antibody levels may be achieved within 10–14 days after vaccination.[2]

Special care should be taken to avoid injecting the vaccine intradermally, intramuscularly, or intravenously since clinical studies have not been done to establish safety and efficacy of the vaccine using these routes of administration.

A separate, sterile syringe and needle or a sterile disposable unit should be used for each individual patient to prevent transmission of hepatitis and other infectious agents from one person to another.

During use it is possible that the nozzle of the Jet Injector Apparatus may become contaminated with blood or serum. In one instance, such contamination has been reported to be associated with transmission of hepatitis b disease. Therefore, if blood or serum contamination occurs, the nozzle should be disassembled, cleansed and sterilized before continued use to prevent the possibility of transmission of hepatitis or other infectious agents from one person to another.[8]

PREGNANCY[9]

REPRODUCTIVE STUDIES—PREGNANCY CATEGORY C

Animal reproduction studies have not been conducted with Meningococcal Polysaccharide Vaccine, Groups A, C, Y and W-135. It is also not known whether Meningococcal Polysaccharide Vaccine, Groups A, C, Y and W-135 can cause fetal harm when administered to a pregnant woman or can affect reproduction capacity.

EXPERIENCE IN HUMANS

There is no data on the safety of Menomune when administered to a pregnant woman. Therefore, Menomune should not be administered to a pregnant woman, particularly in the first trimester.

PEDIATRIC USE

THERE ARE NO DATA ON SAFETY AND EFFICACY OF MENOMUNE WHEN ADMINISTERED TO CHILDREN UNDER 2 YEARS OF AGE.

ADVERSE REACTIONS

Adverse reactions to meningococcal vaccine are mild and infrequent, consisting of localized erythema lasting 1–2 days. Up to 2% of young children develop fever transiently after vaccination.[2]

As with the administration of any vaccine, one should expect possible hypersensitivity reactions.

DOSAGE AND ADMINISTRATION

Parenteral drug products should be inspected visually for extraneous particulate matter and/or discoloration prior to administration whenever solution and container permit. If these conditions exist, vaccine should not be administered. Reconstitute the vaccine using only the diluent supplied for this purpose. Draw the volume of diluent shown on the dil-

Continued on next page

Menomune-A/C/Y/W-135—Cont.

uent label into a suitable size syringe and inject into the vial containing the vaccine. Shake vial until the vaccine is dissolved. Administer the vaccine subcutaneously.
The immunizing dose is a single injection of 0.5 ml given subcutaneously.

Primary Immunization

For both adults and children, vaccine is administered subcutaneously as a single 0.5 ml dose. The vaccine can be given at the same time as other immunizations, if needed. Protective antibody levels may be achieved within 10–14 days after vaccination.[2]

REVACCINATION

Revaccination may be indicated for individuals at high risk of infection, particularly children who were first immunized under 4 years of age; such children should be considered for revaccination after 2 or 3 years if they remain at high risk. The need for revaccination in older children and adults remains unknown.[2]

HOW SUPPLIED

Vial, 1 Dose, with 0.78 ml vial of diluent—Product No. 49281-489-01
Vial, 10 Dose, with 6 ml vial of diluent, for administration with needle and syringe (may be used with jet injector although the desired number of doses may not be obtained). Product No. 49281-489-91
Vial, 50 Dose, with 27.5 ml of diluent, for JET INJECTOR USE ONLY. Product No. 49281-489-95
Additional package sizes available on special order.

STORAGE

Store freeze-dried vaccine and reconstituted vaccine, when not in use, between 2°–8°C (35°–46°F). Discard remainder of multidose vials of vaccine within 5 days after reconstitution. The single dose vial should be used within 24 hours of reconstitution.

Special instructions for 50 Dose Vial of Meningococcal Polysaccharide Vaccine, A, C, Y and W-135 Combined, for Jet Injector Use.

DOSAGE AND ADMINISTRATION

Parenteral drug products should be inspected visually for extraneous particular matter and/or discoloration prior to administration whenever solution and container permit. If these conditions exist, vaccine should not be administered.
Using a suitable size syringe and needle and aseptic precautions, transfer the volume of diluent shown on the diluent label into the vial containing the vaccine. Shake vial until the vaccine is dissolved.
Administer ONLY with automatic hypodermic jet apparatus. 50 DOSE VIAL NOT TO BE UTILIZED IN NEEDLE AND SYRINGE METHOD OF IMMUNIZATION. If absolutely necessary, syringes and needles may be used with such containers with caution. However, due to coring of the stopper do NOT insert needle into vial more than 20 times. Discard partially used vial of vaccine. Immunization consists of a single injection of 0.5 ml given subcutaneously. Special care should be taken to avoid injecting the vaccine intradermally, intramuscularly, or intravenously by using the deltoid area, since clinical studies have not been done to establish the safety and efficacy of the vaccine using these routes of administration.
Any partially used reconstituted vaccine which has been administered with a Jet Injector Apparatus should NOT be reused and should be discarded.

CAUTION

During use it is possible that the nozzle of Jet Injector Apparatus may become contaminated with blood or serum. In one instance, such contamination has been reported to be associated with transmission of hepatitis b disease. Therefore, if blood or serum contamination occurs, the nozzle should be disassembled, cleansed and sterilized before continued use to prevent the possibility of transmission of hepatitis or other infectious agents from one person to another.[8]

REFERENCES

1. Tiesjema, R. H., et al: Enhanced stability of meningococcal polysaccharide vaccines by using lactose as a menstruum for lyophilization. Bull WHO 55: 43–48, 1977
2. Recommendation of the Immunization Practices Advisory Committee (ACIP). Meningococcal Vaccines. MMWR 34: 255–259, 1985
3. Hankins, W.A., et al: Clinical and serological evaluation of a meningococcal polysaccharide vaccine groups A, C, Y and W-135. Proc Soc Exper Biol Med 169: 54–57, 1982
4. Lepow, M. L., et al: Reactogenicity and immunogenicity of a quadrivalent combined meningococcal polysaccharide vaccine in children. J Infect Dis 154: 1033–1036, 1986
5. Unpublished data available from Connaught Laboratories, Inc., compiled 1982
6. Peltola, H., et al: Clinical efficacy of meningococcus Group A capsular polysaccharide vaccine in children three months to five years of age. N Engl J Med 297: 686–691, 1977
7. Reingold, A. L., et al: Age-specific differences in duration of clinical protection after vaccination with meningococcal polysaccharide A vaccine. Lancet. No. 8447: 114–118, 1985
8. CDC. Hepatitis B associated with jet gun injection—California. MMWR 35: 373–376, 1986
9. Code of Federal Regulations. 21CFR201.57 (f) (6) (c), 1989

CONNAUGHT© is a trademark owned by Connaught Laboratories Limited.
Manufactured by:
CONNAUGHT LABORATORIES, INC.
Swiftwater, Pennsylvania 18370, U.S.A.
Product Information as of July, 1990

1895

Shown in Product Identification Guide, page 330

TETANUS AND DIPHTHERIA TOXOIDS ADSORBED FOR ADULT USE ℞

Caution: Federal (USA) law prohibits dispensing without prescription.

For special instructions on use of Tetanus and Diphtheria Toxoids Adsorbed for Adult Use for JET INJECTOR USE—see other side of insert.

DESCRIPTION

Tetanus and Diphtheria Toxoids Adsorbed for Adult Use, for intramuscular use, is a sterile suspension of alum-precipitated (aluminum potassium sulfate) toxoid in an isotonic sodium chloride solution containing sodium phosphate buffer to control pH. The vaccine, after shaking, is a turbid liquid, whitish-gray in color.
Clostridium tetani culture is grown in a peptone-based medium. *Corynebacterium diphtheriae* culture is grown in a modified Mueller and Miller medium.[1] Both toxins are detoxified with formaldehyde. The detoxified materials are then separately purified by serial ammonium sulfate fractionation and diafiltration. Thimerosal (a mercury derivative) 1:10,000 is added as a preservative.
Each 0.5 mL dose is formulated to contain 5 Lf of tetanus toxoid, 2 Lf of diphtheria toxoid, and not more than 0.28 mg of aluminum by assay. The tetanus and diphtheria toxoids induce at least 2 units and 0.5 units of antitoxin per mL, respectively, in the guinea pig potency test.

HOW SUPPLIED

Syringe, 0.5 mL (10 × 0.5 mL syringes per package)—Product No. 49281-271-10
Vial, 5 mL—Product No. 49281-271-83
Vial, 30 mL for JET INJECTOR USE ONLY—Product No. 49281-271-92

TRIHIBIT® ℞

ActHIB® Haemophilus b Conjugate Vaccine (Tetanus Toxoid Conjugate) reconstituted with Tripedia® Diphtheria and Tetanus Toxoids and Acellular Pertussis Vaccine Adsorbed.
See package inserts for Acthib® and Tripedia®

Shown in Product Identification Guide, page 330

DIPHTHERIA AND TETANUS TOXOIDS AND ACELLULAR PERTUSSIS VACCINE ADSORBED TRIPEDIA® ℞

DESCRIPTION

Tripedia®, Diphtheria and Tetanus Toxoids and Acellular Pertussis Vaccine Adsorbed (DTaP), for intramuscular use, is a sterile preparation of diphtheria and tetanus toxoids adsorbed, with acellular pertussis vaccine in an isotonic sodium chloride solution containing thimerosal as a preservative and sodium phosphate to control pH. After shaking, the vaccine is a homogeneous white suspension. Tripedia® vaccine is distributed by Connaught Laboratories, Inc. (CLI).
The acellular pertussis vaccine components are isolated from culture fluids of Phase 1 *Bordetella pertussis* grown in a modified Stainer-Scholte medium.[1] After purification by salt precipitation, ultracentrifugation, and ultrafiltration, preparations containing varying amounts of both pertussis toxin (PT) and filamentous hemagglutinin (FHA) are combined to obtain a 1:1 ratio and treated with formaldehyde to inactivate PT. Thimerosal (mercury derivative) 1:10,000 is added as a preservative.
Corynebacterium diphtheriae cultures are grown in a modified Mueller and Miller medium.[2] *Clostridium tetani* cultures are grown in a peptone-based medium. Both toxins are detoxified with formaldehyde. The detoxified materials are then separately purified by serial ammonium sulfate fractionation and diafiltration.
The toxoids are adsorbed using aluminum potassium sulfate (alum). The adsorbed diphtheria and tetanus toxoids are combined with acellular pertussis concentrate, and diluted to a final volume using sterile phosphate-buffered physiological saline. Thimerosal (mercury derivative) 1:10,000 is added as a preservative. Each 0.5 mL dose contains, by assay, not more than 0.170 mg of aluminum and not more than 100 µg (0.02%) of residual formaldehyde. The vaccine contains gelatin and polysorbate 80 (Tween-80) which are used in the production of the pertussis concentrate.
Each 0.5 mL dose is formulated to contain 6.7 Lf of diphtheria toxoid and 5 Lf of tetanus toxoid (both toxoids induce at least 2 units of antitoxin per mL in the guinea pig potency test), and 46.8 µg of pertussis antigens. This is represented in the final vaccine as approximately 23.4 µg of inactivated PT (also referred to as lymphocytosis promoting factor or LPF) and 23.4 µg of FHA. The inactivated acellular pertussis component contributes not more than 50 endotoxin units (EU) to the endotoxin content of 1 mL of DTaP. The potency of the pertussis components is evaluated by measuring the antibody response to PT and FHA in immunized mice using an ELISA system.
Acellular Pertussis Vaccine Concentrates (For Further Manufacturing Use) are produced by The Research Foundation for Microbial Diseases of Osaka University (BIKEN), Osaka, Japan under United States (US) license, and are combined with diphtheria and tetanus toxoids manufactured by CLI. The Tripedia® vaccine is filled, labeled, packaged, and released by CLI.
TriHIBit™, when Tripedia® vaccine is used to reconstitute ActHIB® **for the fourth dose only**, each single dose of combined vaccine (0.5 mL) is formulated to contain 6.7 Lf of diphtheria toxoid, 5 Lf of tetanus toxoid (both toxoids induce at least 2 units of antitoxin per mL in the guinea pig potency test), 46.8 µg of pertussis antigens (approximately 23.4 µg of inactivated PT and 23.4 µg of FHA), 10 µg of purified *Haemophilus influenzae* type b capsular polysaccharide conjugated to 24 µg of inactivated tetanus toxoid, and 8.5% sucrose.

CLINICAL PHARMACOLOGY

Simultaneous immunization against diphtheria, tetanus, and pertussis, using a conventional "whole-cell" pertussis DTP vaccine (Diphtheria and Tetanus Toxoids and Pertussis Vaccine Adsorbed—For Pediatric Use), has been a routine practice during infancy and childhood in the US since the late 1940s. This practice has played a major role in markedly reducing the incidence rates of cases and deaths from each of these diseases.[3]
Tripedia® vaccine combines CLI's diphtheria and tetanus toxoids with purified pertussis antigens (inactivated PT and FHA). These pertussis antigens have been used routinely for childhood vaccination in Japan since 1981[4,5,6,7] and have been used for investigational purposes in Sweden,[1,8,9,10,11] as well as in the US and Germany.[1,12,13,14,15] In the US, since 1992, Tripedia® vaccine has been indicated for immunization of children 15 months to 7 years of age (prior to the seventh birthday) who have previously been immunized with three or four doses of whole-cell pertussis DTP.

DIPHTHERIA

Corynebacterium diphtheriae may cause both localized and generalized disease. The systemic intoxication is caused by diphtheria exotoxin, an extracellular protein metabolite of toxigenic strains of *C. diphtheriae*. Protection against disease is due to the development of neutralizing antibody to diphtheria toxin.
Both toxigenic and nontoxigenic strains of *C. diphtheriae* can cause disease, but only strains that produce diphtheria toxin cause severe manifestations, such as myocarditis and neuritis. Diphtheria remains a serious disease, with the highest case-fatality rates among infants and the elderly.[3]
At one time, diphtheria was common in the US. More than 200,000 cases, primarily among children, were reported in 1921. Approximately 5% to 10% of cases were fatal; the highest case-fatality rates were in the very young and the elderly. Reported cases of diphtheria of all types declined from 306 in 1975 to 59 in 1979; most were cutaneous diphtheria reported from a single state. After 1979, cutaneous diphtheria was no longer reportable.[3] From 1980 to 1989, only 24 cases of respiratory diphtheria were reported in the US; 2 cases were fatal and 18 (75%) occurred among persons ≥ 20 years of age.[3] From 1990 through 1994, 15 cases were reported.[16]
Diphtheria is currently a rare disease in the US primarily because of the high level of appropriate vaccination among children (97% of children entering school have received ≥

three doses of diphtheria and tetanus toxoids and pertussis vaccine adsorbed [DTP]) and because of an apparent reduction in the circulation of toxigenic strains of *C. diphtheriae*.[3] Most cases occur among unvaccinated or inadequately vaccinated persons.[3] Diphtheria remains a serious disease in some areas of the world as evidenced by the recent outbreak in the former Soviet Union.[17]

Complete immunization significantly reduces the risk of developing diphtheria, and immunized persons who develop disease have milder illness. Protection is thought to last at least 10 years. Immunization does not, however, eliminate carriage of *C. diphtheriae* in the pharynx, nose or on the skin.[3]

Efficacy of CLI's diphtheria toxoid used in Tripedia® vaccine was determined on the basis of immunogenicity studies, with a comparison to a serological correlate of protection (0.01 antitoxin units/mL) established by the Panel on Review of Bacterial Vaccines & Toxoids.[18]

TETANUS

Tetanus is an intoxication manifested primarily by neuromuscular dysfunction caused by a potent exotoxin elaborated by *Clostridium tetani*.

The occurrence of tetanus in the US has decreased dramatically from 560 reported cases in 1947 to an average of 57 cases reported annually from 1985-1994.[16] Tetanus in the US is primarily a disease of older adults. Of 99 tetanus patients with complete information reported to the Centers for Disease Control and Prevention (CDC) during 1987 and 1988, 68% were ≥ 50 years of age, while only six were < 20 years of age. Overall, the case-fatality rate was 21%. The disease continues to occur almost exclusively among persons who are unvaccinated or inadequately vaccinated or whose vaccination histories are unknown or uncertain.[3]

In 4% of tetanus cases reported during 1987 and 1988, no wound or other condition was implicated. Non-acute skin lesions, such as ulcers, or medical conditions, such as abscesses, were reported in 14% of cases.[3]

Spores of *C. tetani* are ubiquitous. Serological tests indicate that naturally acquired immunity to tetanus toxin does not occur in the US. Thus, universal primary immunization, with subsequent maintenance of adequate antitoxin levels by means of appropriately timed boosters, is necessary to protect all age groups. Tetanus toxoid is a highly effective antigen, and a completed primary series generally induces protective levels of serum antitoxin that persist for 10 or more years.[3]

Efficacy of CLI's tetanus toxoid used in Tripedia® vaccine was determined on the basis of immunogenicity studies, with a comparison to a serological correlate of protection (0.01 antitoxin units/mL) established by the Panel on Review of Bacterial Vaccines & Toxoids.[18]

PERTUSSIS

Since pertussis became a nationally reportable disease in 1922, the highest number of pertussis cases (approximately 266,000) was reported in 1934. Following the licensure of whole-cell pertussis DTP vaccine in 1949 and the widespread use of DTP among infants and children, the incidence of reported pertussis declined to a historical low of 1,010 cases in 1976. However, since the early 1980s, reported pertussis incidence has increased with cyclical peaks occurring in 1983, 1986, 1990, and 1993. Following the peak in reported cases in 1993, the number declined during 1994 and the first 2 quarters of 1995, a pattern consistent with the previously observed 3-4 year periodicity in pertussis incidence. National pertussis surveillance data for January 1992-December 1994 during which an average of 5,095 cases were reported annually, demonstrate the continued effectiveness of the current pertussis vaccination program.[19]

Pertussis (whooping cough) is a disease of the respiratory tract caused by *Bordetella pertussis*. This gram-negative coccobacillus produces a variety of biologically active components. The role of the different components produced by *B pertussis* in either the pathogenesis of, or the immunity to, pertussis is not well understood. However, efficacy has been demonstrated for this vaccine that contained both inactivated PT and FHA.

Pertussis is highly communicable (attack rates of >90% have been reported among unvaccinated household contacts[20]) and can cause severe disease, particularly among very young children. Of 10,749 patients < 1 year of age reported nationally as having pertussis during the period 1980 to 1989, 69% were hospitalized, 22% had pneumonia, 3.0% had one or more seizures, 0.9% had encephalopathy, and 0.6% died.[21]

In older children and adults, including some who were previously immunized, infection may result in nonspecific symptoms of bronchitis or an upper respiratory tract infection, and pertussis may not be diagnosed because classic signs, especially the inspiratory whoop, may be absent. Older preschool-aged children and school-aged siblings who are not fully immunized and develop pertussis may be important sources of infection for young infants, the group at highest risk of clinical disease and severe pertussis.[3] The infected adult may play a role in the transmission of pertussis.[22,23]

General use of whole-cell pertussis DTP vaccines has resulted in a substantial reduction in cases and deaths from pertussis disease.[20,24] The use of Tripedia® vaccine as a primary series evokes an antibody response with respect to PT and FHA and has been shown to be effective in clinical studies.[1]

Acellular pertussis vaccines have been used in Japan since 1981, mostly in 2-year-old children. Evidence for the efficacy of these vaccines, as a group, is demonstrated by the decline in pertussis disease with their routine use in that country.[4,20] In addition, a review of epidemiological studies of the Japanese acellular pertussis vaccines estimated that these vaccines, as a group, were 88% efficacious in protecting against clinical pertussis on household exposure, with a 95% confidence interval (CI) of 79% to 93%.[25]

Two clinical studies were conducted to assess the protective efficacy of these acellular pertussis components of Tripedia® vaccine. A randomized, controlled clinical trial in Sweden assessed efficacy after only two doses of the pertussis component in children 5 to 11 months of age.[10] A second study was conducted in Germany using a three-dose schedule to evaluate the protective efficacy of the Tripedia® vaccine in younger infants.

In 1986-1987, a double-blind, randomized, placebo-controlled efficacy trial of two BIKEN acellular pertussis vaccines was conducted in Sweden. One of the vaccines was a two-component vaccine comparable to the acellular pertussis components contained in Tripedia® vaccine. This prospective trial used a standardized case definition and active case ascertainment. In this trial, 1,389 children, 5 to 11 months of age (median 8.5 months), received two doses of the acellular pertussis vaccine 7 to 13 weeks apart and 954 received a placebo control. During the 15 months of follow-up from 30 days after the second dose, culture-confirmed whooping cough (cough of any duration and a positive culture of *B pertussis*) occurred in 40 placebo and 18 acellular pertussis vaccine recipients. The point estimate of protective efficacy for two doses of vaccine was 69% (95% CI; 47% to 82%) for all cases of culture-confirmed pertussis with any cough 1 day or longer and 79% (95% CI; 57% to 90%) using a secondary case definition of culture-confirmed cases with cough of over 30 days duration.[10] In a reanalysis of the Swedish data efficacy estimates increased with duration of coughing spasms and when the case definition included whoops and whoops plus at least nine coughing spasms a day.[26] Using a case definition of cough of 21 days or more of coughing spasms, confirmed by positive culture resulted in an efficacy estimate of 81% (95% CI; 61% to 90%).[26]

Using a passive reporting system, three-year unblinded follow-up of vaccine and placebo recipients from the above Swedish study has shown a post-trial efficacy of 77% (95% CI; 65% to 85%) for all culture-proven cases of pertussis, and an efficacy of 92% (95% CI; 84% to 96%) for culture-proven cases with a cough of over 30 days duration.[27]

A case-control study to evaluate the efficacy of Tripedia® vaccine was conducted in Germany. The study population consisted of patients in 63 pediatric practices who had no contraindications to pertussis immunization and were enrolled in the study between the ages of 6 and 17 weeks (actual range of age at first visit was up to 20 weeks for the DT group). By parental choice, infants received Tripedia® vaccine or whole-cell pertussis DTP (Behringwerke, Germany) at approximately 3, 5, and 7 months of age, or DT, or no vaccine. Cases of pertussis were identified by obtaining cultures for *B pertussis* from all patients between the ages of 2 and 24 months who presented to the physician's office with 7 or more days of cough. Identification of presumptive cases of pertussis was made by primary care physicians who were not blinded to the vaccine status of subjects. Cases were confirmed by positive culture in the subject or positive culture in a subject's household contact. Duration of cough in study subjects was determined at an office visit, by telephone, or by home visit 21-24 days after the onset of cough. Four age-matched controls were selected for each case from the same pediatric practice. Selection of controls was done without knowledge of vaccination status. The vaccine (or no vaccine) and number of doses which each case and control subject received subsequently was determined from medical records.

In order to adjust for potentially confounding variables, information on sex, race, day-care attendance, well-baby visits, sick-child visits, pertussis vaccination status of siblings, age of siblings, number of siblings, day-care attendance of siblings, and parental employment status was obtained through interview of parents. Information on erythromycin use was not obtained for the study population.

A total of 16,780 infants were enrolled in the study, of whom 74.6% received Tripedia® vaccine and 10.9%, 12.5%, and 2.1% received DTP, DT, or no vaccine, respectively, by nonrandom parental choice. A total of 11,017 cultures for *B pertussis* was obtained and 140 cases were identified using a primary case definition of cough ≥ 21 days, plus positive culture for *B pertussis* or household contact with a person with culture-positive pertussis. Of the 140 cases, 130 cases were diagnosed on the basis of a positive culture and 10 on the basis of household contact with a culture-positive case.

For the 140 cases, 543 controls were selected. Of the 140 cases, 29 (20.7%) received three doses of DTaP, 5 (3.6%) received two doses of DTaP, 44 (31.4%) received two or three doses of DT vaccine, 44 (31.4%) received one dose of either DTaP, whole-cell pertussis DTP or DT, and 18 (13%) received no vaccine. Of the 543 controls, 175 (32.2%) received three doses of DTaP, 67 (12.3%) received two doses of DTaP, 45 (8.3%) received two or three doses of whole-cell pertussis DTP, 73 (13.4%) received DT vaccine, 153 (28.2%) received one dose of either DT, DTP, or DTaP, and 30 (5.5%) received no vaccine. Adjusting for sibling age, sibling pertussis immunization by age group, siblings in day care, number of siblings in day care, and father's employment status, the vaccine efficacy of three doses of Tripedia® vaccine compared to two or three doses of DT was 80% (95% CI; 59% to 90%).[1]

In a clinical study conducted in 65 US and 89 German infants, a single lot of Tripedia® vaccine was administered at 2, 4 and 6 months of age for the purpose of comparing immune responses to PT and FHA. This study showed that US and German infants, who received three doses of Tripedia® vaccine, expressed similar antibody responses to these antigens. The percentage of infants demonstrating a four-fold or greater antibody response, was also similar for PT and FHA in both groups.[1]

In a clinical study, US infants received Tripedia®, ActHIB®, OPV, and hepatitis B vaccines simultaneously. In one of the study groups, Tripedia®, ActHIB® and OPV were administered at 2, 4, and 6 months of age and hepatitis B was given at 2 and 4 months of age. One hundred percent of the 69 children who received ActHIB® simultaneously with Tripedia® vaccine demonstrated anti-PRP antibodies ≥ 1 µg/mL. Sera from a subset of 12 infants who received hepatitis B simultaneously at 2 and 4 months of age showed that 93% had anti-HBs titers of > 10 mIU/mL. Sera from a subset of 20 infants who received OPV simultaneously at 2, 4, and 6 months of age showed that 100% had protective neutralizing antibody responses to all three polio virus types.

TRIPEDIA® COMBINED WITH ActHIB®, TriHIBit™, BY RECONSTITUTION

Clinical studies examined the immune response in 15- to 20-month-old children when Tripedia® vaccine was used to reconstitute one lyophilized single dose vial of ActHIB® (TriHIBit™). All children received three doses of Haemophilus b Conjugate Vaccine (ActHIB® or HibTITER®) and three doses of whole-cell DTP at approximately 2, 4, and 6 months of age. Table 1 shows the diphtheria, tetanus and pertussis responses when Tripedia® vaccine was used to reconstitute ActHIB® (TriHIBit™) compared to the two vaccines given concomitantly but at different sites. In children who received the vaccines separately or combined, 100% had an antibody response to the PRP component ≥ 1.0 µg/mL.[1]

[See table 1 at bottom of next page]

In clinical studies evaluating simultaneous administration of Tripedia® and ActHIB® with MMR vaccine to 15- to 20-month-old children, the data suggest that the combination vaccine does not interfere with the immunogenicity of the MMR vaccine. Overall seroconversion rates in children who received ActHIB® reconstituted with Tripedia® (TriHIBit™) vaccine were 98% (46/47), 98% (42/43) and 96% (43/45) for measles, mumps and rubella, respectively.

INDICATIONS AND USAGE

Tripedia® vaccine is indicated for active immunization against diphtheria, tetanus and pertussis (whooping cough) simultaneously in infants and children 6 weeks to 7 years of age (prior to seventh birthday). Because of the substantial risks of complications of the disease, completion of a primary series of pertussis vaccine early in life is strongly recommended.[3] However, in instances where the pertussis vaccine component is contraindicated, Diphtheria and Tetanus Toxoids Adsorbed (For Pediatric Use) (DT) should be used for each of the remaining doses. (See **CONTRAINDICATIONS** section.)

When Tripedia® vaccine is used to reconstitute ActHIB® (TriHIBit™), the combined vaccines are indicated for the active immunization of children 15 to 18 months of age who have previously been immunized against diphtheria, tetanus and pertussis with three doses consisting of either whole-cell pertussis DTP or acellular pertussis vaccine and three or fewer doses of ActHIB® (OmniHIB®) within the first year of life for the prevention of invasive diseases caused by *H influenzae* type b and caused by diphtheria, tetanus, and pertussis.[1] ***(Refer to ActHIB® package insert.)***

If passive immunization is required, Tetanus Immune Globulin (Human) (TIG) and/or equine Diphtheria Antitoxin should be used.

Persons who have recovered from culture-confirmed pertussis do not need additional doses of Tripedia® vaccine but should receive additional doses of DT to complete the series.

Tripedia® vaccine is not to be used for treatment of *B. pertussis, C. diphtheriae, or C. tetani* infections.

Continued on next page

Tripedia—Cont.

As with any vaccine, vaccination with Tripedia® vaccine may not protect 100% of susceptible individuals.

CONTRAINDICATIONS

Hypersensitivity to any component of the vaccine, including thimerosal and gelatin, is a contraindication.

It is a contraindication to use this vaccine after an immediate anaphylactic reaction temporally associated with a previous dose. Because of uncertainty as to which component of the vaccine might be responsible, no further vaccination with diphtheria, tetanus, or pertussis components should be carried out. Alternatively, because of the importance of tetanus vaccination, such individuals may be referred for evaluation by an allergist.[3]

Immunization should be deferred during the course of an acute febrile illness. The decision to administer or delay vaccination because of a current or recent febrile illness depends on the severity of symptoms and on the etiology of the disease. All vaccines can be administered to persons with mild illness such as diarrhea, mild upper-respiratory infection with or without low-grade fever, or other low grade febrile illness.[28]

Elective immunization procedures should be deferred during an outbreak of poliomyelitis.[29]

Encephalopathy not due to an identifiable cause, occurring within 7 days of a prior whole-cell pertussis DTP or DTaP immunization and consisting of major alterations of consciousness, unresponsiveness, generalized or focal seizures that persist for more than a few hours and failure to recover within 24 hours should be considered a contraindication to further use; this includes severe alterations in consciousness with generalized or focal neurologic signs. Even though causation cannot be established, no subsequent doses of pertussis vaccine should be given.[3]

WARNINGS

If any of the following events occurs in temporal relation with the receipt of either whole-cell pertussis DTP or DTaP, the decision to administer subsequent doses of vaccine containing the pertussis component should be carefully considered. Although these events were once considered contraindications to whole-cell pertussis DTP, there may be circumstances, such as high incidence of pertussis, in which the potential benefits outweigh the possible risks, particularly since the following events have not been proven to cause permanent sequelae:[3,30]

1. Temperature of ≥ 40.5°C (105°F) within 48 hours, not due to another identifiable cause.
2. Collapse or shock-like state (hypotonic-hyporesponsive episode) within 48 hours.
3. Persistent, inconsolable crying lasting ≥ 3 hours, occurring within 48 hours.
4. Convulsions with or without fever, occurring within 3 days.

A recent clinical study suggests that persistent, inconsolable crying lasting at least 3 hours following vaccination with Tripedia® vaccine may occur less frequently than has been observed historically for DTP vaccine.[1,31]

When a decision is made to withhold the pertussis component, immunization with DT should be continued.

Tripedia® vaccine should not be given to children with any coagulation disorder, including thrombocytopenia, that would contraindicate intramuscular injection unless the potential benefit clearly outweighs the risk of administration.

In the opinion of the manufacturer, seizure disorder in children before or after any immunization with Tripedia® is considered a warning against further immunization with this vaccine. Recent studies suggest that infants and children with a history of convulsions in first-degree family members (i.e., siblings and parents) have a 3.2-fold increased risk for neurologic events compared with those without such histories when given DTP.[25,32] However, the ACIP has concluded that a family history of convulsions in parents and siblings is not a contraindication to pertussis vaccination and that children with such family histories should receive pertussis vaccine according to the recommended schedule.[3,20,28]

In children with a history of febrile or non-febrile convulsions, acetaminophen should be given at the time of Tripedia® vaccination according to acetaminophen package insert recommended dosage to reduce the possibility of post-vaccination fever.[3,20,28]

A committee of the Institute of Medicine (IOM) has concluded that evidence is consistent with a causal relationship between DTP and acute neurologic illness, and under special circumstances, between DTP and chronic neurologic disease in the context of the NCES report.[33,34] However, the IOM committee concluded that the evidence was insufficient to indicate whether or not DTP increased the overall risk of chronic neurologic disease.[34] Acute encephalopathy or permanent neurological injury, have not been reported in temporal association after administration of Tripedia® vaccine but the experience with this vaccine is insufficient to rule this out. (See **ADVERSE REACTIONS** section).

Infants and children with recognized possible or potential underlying neurologic conditions seem to be at enhanced risk for the appearance of manifestations of the underlying neurologic disorder within two or three days following whole-cell pertussis vaccination.[3] Whether to administer Tripedia® vaccine to children with proven or suspected underlying neurologic disorders must be decided on an individual basis. Important considerations include the current local incidence of pertussis.[3]

Tripedia® vaccine should not be combined through reconstitution with any vaccine for administration to infants younger than 15 months of age. Tripedia® vaccine should not be reconstituted with any vaccine other than ActHIB® (OmniHIB®) for children 15 months of age or older.

PRECAUTIONS

GENERAL

Care is to be taken by the health-care provider for the safe and effective use of this vaccine.

EPINEPHRINE INJECTION (1:1000) MUST BE IMMEDIATELY AVAILABLE SHOULD AN ACUTE ANAPHYLACTIC REACTION OCCUR DUE TO ANY COMPONENT OF THE VACCINE.

Prior to an injection of any vaccine, all known precautions should be taken to prevent adverse reactions. This includes a review of the patient's history with respect to possible sensitivity and any previous adverse reactions to the vaccine or similar vaccines, previous immunization history, current health status (see **CONTRAINDICATIONS** section), and a current knowledge of the literature concerning the use of the vaccine under consideration. Immunosuppressed patients may not respond. Tripedia® vaccine is not contraindicated in patients with HIV infection.[3]

Special care should be taken to ensure that the injection does not enter a blood vessel.

A separate, sterile syringe and needle or a sterile disposable unit should be used for each patient to prevent transmission of hepatitis or other infectious agents from person to person. Needles should not be recapped but should be disposed of properly.

INFORMATION FOR PATIENT

Parents should be fully informed of the benefits and risks of immunization with Tripedia® vaccine.

The physician should inform the parents or guardians about the potential for adverse reactions that have been temporally associated with Tripedia® and other pertussis vaccine administration. The health-care provider should provide the Vaccine Information Materials (VIMs) which are required by the National Childhood Vaccine Injury Act of 1986 to be given with each immunization. Parents or guardians should be instructed to report any serious adverse reactions to their health-care provider.

IT IS EXTREMELY IMPORTANT WHEN A CHILD IS RETURNED FOR THE NEXT DOSE IN THE SERIES THAT THE PARENT SHOULD BE QUESTIONED CONCERNING OCCURRENCE OF ANY SYMPTOMS AND/OR SIGNS OF AN ADVERSE REACTION AFTER THE PREVIOUS DOSE OF THE SAME VACCINE (SEE **CONTRAINDICATIONS** AND **ADVERSE REACTIONS** SECTIONS).

The health-care provider should inform the parent or guardian of the importance of completing the pertussis immunization series, unless a contraindication to further immunization exists.

The US Department of Health and Human Services has established a Vaccine Adverse Event Reporting System (VAERS) to accept all reports of suspected adverse events after the administration of any vaccine, including but not limited to the reporting of events required by the National Childhood Vaccine Injury Act of 1986.[35] The toll-free number for VAERS forms and information is 1-800-822-7967.

The National Vaccine Injury Compensation Program, established by the National Childhood Vaccine Injury Act of 1986, requires physicians and other health-care providers who administer vaccines to maintain permanent vaccination records and to report occurrences of certain adverse events to the US Department of Health and Human Services. Reportable events include those listed in the Act (i.e. those listed in the vaccine injury table) for each vaccine and events specified in the package insert as contraindications to further doses of the vaccine.[36,37]

DRUG INTERACTIONS

As with other IM injections use with caution in patients on anticoagulant therapy.

Immunosuppressive therapies, including irradiation, antimetabolites, alkylating agents, cytotoxic drugs, and corticosteroids (used in greater than physiologic doses), may reduce the immune response to vaccines. Although no specific studies with pertussis vaccine are available, if immunosuppressive therapy will be discontinued shortly, it would be reasonable to defer immunization until the patient has been off therapy for one month; otherwise, the patient should be vaccinated while still on therapy.[3]

For information regarding simultaneous administration with other vaccines refer to **DOSAGE AND ADMINISTRATION** section.

If Tripedia® vaccine has been administered to persons receiving immunosuppressive therapy, a recent injection of immune globulin or having an immunodeficiency disorder, an adequate immunologic response may not be obtained.

Tetanus Immune Globulin, or Diphtheria Antitoxin, if used, should be given in a separate site, with a separate needle and syringe.

The combination of Tripedia® vaccine with other vaccines has not been evaluated for safety and immunogenicity in infants younger than 15 months of age. The combination of Tripedia® vaccine with any vaccine other than ActHIB® (OmniHIB®) has not been evaluated for safety and immunogenicity in infants 15 months of age or older.

CARCINOGENESIS, MUTAGENESIS, IMPAIRMENT OF FERTILITY

Tripedia® vaccine has not been evaluated for its carcinogenic or mutagenic potentials or impairment of fertility.

PREGNANCY

REPRODUCTIVE STUDIES—PREGNANCY CATEGORY C

Animal reproduction studies have not been conducted with Tripedia® vaccine. It is not known whether Tripedia® vaccine can cause fetal harm when administered to a pregnant woman or can affect reproductive capacity. Tripedia® vaccine is NOT recommended for use in a pregnant woman.

PEDIATRIC USE

SAFETY AND EFFECTIVENESS OF TRIPEDIA® VACCINE IN INFANTS BELOW SIX WEEKS OF AGE HAVE NOT BEEN ESTABLISHED. (SEE **DOSAGE AND ADMINISTRATION SECTION.**) *THIS VACCINE IS NOT RECOMMENDED FOR PERSONS 7 YEARS OF AGE AND OLDER.* Tetanus and Diphtheria Toxoids Adsorbed For Adult Use (Td) is to be used in individuals 7 years of age or older.

Tripedia® vaccine should **not** be combined through reconstitution with any vaccine for administration to infants younger than 15 months of age. Tripedia® vaccine can only be combined with ActHIB® (OmniHIB®) by reconstitution for children 15 months of age or older.

TABLE 1[1]

IMMUNE RESPONSES IN 15- TO 20-MONTH-OLD CHILDREN WHEN TRIPEDIA® VACCINE IS COMBINED WITH ActHIB® BY RECONSTITUTION (TriHIBit™) COMPARED TO THE VACCINES ADMINISTERED SEPARATELY

VACCINE GROUP	PRE-DOSE		POST-DOSE	
	TriHIBit™	Separate	TriHIBit™	Separate
N*	92–93	102–103	93	98
Anti-LPF				
GMT (ELISA units/mL)	26. 30	24. 56	471. 00	363. 90
% 4-Fold Rise	— —	87. 0	85. 7	
Anti-LPF				
GMT (CHO CELL)	33. 48	31. 78	806. 70	701. 60
% 4-Fold Rise	— —	92. 3	90. 6	
Anti-FHA				
GMT (ELISA units/mL)	3. 83	3. 61	44. 68	38. 81
% 4-Fold Rise	— —	68. 5**	80. 6	
Diphtheria Antitoxin				
GMT (units/mL)	0. 15	0. 16	6. 31	6. 65
>0.01 u/mL	— —	100. 00	100. 00	
Tetanus Antitoxin				
GMT (equivalents/mL)	0. 05	0. 06	1. 10	1. 15
>0.01 u/mL	— —	100. 00	100. 00	

*N = number of children

**The clinical significance of the difference in 4-fold rise of anti-FHA is unknown at present.

TABLE 2[1]

ADVERSE EVENTS OCCURRING WITHIN 72 HOURS FOLLOWING DIPHTHERIA AND TETANUS TOXOIDS AND ACELLULAR PERTUSSIS VACCINE ADSORBED (TRIPEDIA®) IMMUNIZATIONS GIVEN TO INFANTS 2 TO 6 MONTHS OF AGE

EVENT	FREQUENCY					
	TRIPEDIA® REACTION %			WHOLE-CELL PERTUSSIS DTP REACTION %		
	Dose 1	Dose 2	Dose 3	Dose 1	Dose 2	Dose 3
No. of Infants†	505	499	490	167	159	152
Local						
Erythema*	9.0	9.8	16.9	28.3	32.9	32.9
Erythema >1[11]*	1.2	1.8	2.2	7.8	8.4	7.4
Swelling*	6.4	4.5	6.5	28.3	23.9	27.5
Swelling >1[11]*	1.4	0.6	1.0	12.7	11.0	11.4
Tenderness*	11.8	6.7	7.1	50.6	44.2	42.6
Systemic						
Fever >101°F (rectal)*	0.4	1.6	3.5	3.6	7.5	11.2
Irritability*	35.3	30.1	27.1	72.9	71.8	57.7
Drowsiness*	39.4	17.6	15.9	59.6	45.2	25.5
Anorexia*	6.0	5.3	5.7	26.5	20.0	18.8
Vomiting	6.0**	5.5	3.7	10.8	7.1	2.7
High-pitched cry	2.4	1.0	1.4	10.8	5.8	3.4
Persistent cry	0.2	0.2	0.8	3.0	1.3	2.0

*p <0.01 when compared to whole-cell pertussis DTP for all doses.
**p <0.05 when compared to whole-cell pertussis DTP.
†For certain adverse events information was not available for a small number of infants.

TABLE 3[38]

PERCENT OF INFANTS WHO WERE REPORTED TO HAVE HAD THE INDICATED REACTION BY THE THIRD EVENING AFTER ANY OF THE FIRST THREE DOSES OF WHOLE-CELL PERTUSSIS DTP OR DTaP

	N¶	ERYTHEMA	SWELLING	PAIN†	FEVER* >101°F	ANOREXIA	VOMITING	DROWSINESS	FUSSINESS‡
Tripedia®	135	32.6**	20.0**	9.6**	5.2**	22.2**	7.4	41.5**	19.3**
Whole-Cell Pertussis DTP	371	72.7	60.9	40.2	15.9	35.0	13.7	62.0	41.5

*Rectal Temperatures
**p <0.01 when compared to whole-cell pertussis DTP.
† Moderate or severe = cried or protested to touch or when leg moved.
‡ Moderate or severe = prolonged or persistent crying that could not be comforted and refusal to play.
¶ N = Number of infants

TABLE 4[1,38]

ADVERSE EVENTS (%) OCCURRING WITHIN 72 HOURS FOLLOWING EACH DOSE OF DIPHTHERIA AND TETANUS TOXOID AND ACELLULAR PERTUSSIS VACCINE (TRIPEDIA®) VACCINATION IN CHILDREN IN WHICH ALL DOSES WERE TRIPEDIA® VACCINE

EVENT	PRIMARY (N =135 INFANTS)			BOOSTER	
				(N = 82 CHILDREN)	(N = 18 CHILDREN)
	DOSE 1 2 Months	DOSE 2 4 Months	DOSE 3 6 Months	DOSE 4 15 to 20 Months	DOSE 5 4 to 6 Years
Local					
Erythema	12.6	12.7	19.1	17.1	33.3
Swelling	8.8	8.2	10.7	15.9	27.8
Pain*	8.1	3.7	2.3	7.3	11.1
Systemic					
Fever >101°F†	0.7	1.4	3.1	2.4	0
Anorexia	8.1	9.7	9.9	8.5	0
Vomiting	5.2	1.5	2.3	2.4	0
Drowsiness	28.9	17.9	4.6	6.1	5.6
Fussiness**	8.1	7.4	7.6	3.7	0

*Moderate or severe = cried or protested to touch or when leg moved.
**Moderate or severe = prolonged or persistent crying that could not be comforted and refusal to play.
†Rectal temperatures for primary series, oral temperatures for Dose 4 and Dose 5.

ADVERSE REACTIONS

A total of 11,400 doses of Tripedia® vaccine has been administered in US clinical trials in children 2 to 6 months, 15 to 20 months of age or 4 to 6 years of age. When compared to CLI's whole-cell pertussis DTP vaccine, Tripedia® vaccine produced fewer local reactions such as erythema, swelling, and tenderness at the injection site and fewer systemic reactions such as fever, irritability, drowsiness, vomiting, anorexia and high-pitched unusual cry.[1] In a double-blind, comparative US trial, 673 infants were randomized to receive either 3 doses of Tripedia® vaccine or CLI's DTP vaccine (Table 2).[1] Safety data are available for 672 infants. Rates for all reported local reactions and other reactions such as fever >101°F, irritability, drowsiness, and anorexia were significantly less in Tripedia® vaccine recipients. In contrast to whole-cell pertussis DTP, no hypotonic-hyporesponsive episodes occurred in Tripedia® vaccine recipients. Reaction rates generally peaked within the first 24 hours, and decreased substantially over the next two days.[1,14,15]
[See table 2 above]

Adverse event data for Tables 2-6 were actively collected using patient diaries, phone call follow-up and/or by questioning the parent(s) at clinic visits. All data were recorded on standardized case report forms.
A similar reduction in adverse events was seen in a randomized, double-blind, comparative trial conducted in the US by the National Institutes of Health (NIH) when Tripedia® vaccine was compared to Lederle Laboratories whole-cell pertussis DTP vaccine (Table 3).[38] Each data point presented in Table 3 is a summary of the frequency of reactions following any of the three primary immunizing doses. Local adverse reactions which include pain, erythema, swelling, and systemic reactions such as fever, anorexia, vomiting, drowsiness and fussiness may occur following any of the three primary vaccinations.
[See table 3 above]
The frequency of adverse reactions following each dose in children who received only Tripedia® vaccine is shown in Table 4.[1,38] Of the 135 infants who received Tripedia® vac-

cine at 2, 4, and 6 months of age, a subset of 82 received a fourth dose of Tripedia® vaccine and a subset of 18 received a fifth dose of Tripedia® vaccine.
[See table 4 below]
In an open label US study additional safety data are available in 15- to 20-month-old children who had previously received three doses of either Tripedia® vaccine (n=109) or whole-cell pertussis DTP (n=30).[39] Reaction rates are presented in Table 5. Data on 738 children (a subset of the German case control study) receiving a fourth dose of Tripedia® vaccine in an open label study showed local and systemic reaction rates in the day following vaccination as follows: erythema (36.7%), erythema >1 inch (12.5%), swelling (20.2%), pain (14%), temperature ≥100.4°F (10.6%), irritability (14.6%), anorexia (8.4%), and persistent crying >3 hours (0.4%).[1]

TABLE 5

COMPARISON OF ADVERSE EVENTS (%) OCCURRING WITHIN 72 HOURS FOLLOWING VACCINATION WITH TRIPEDIA® VACCINE IN CHILDREN WHO HAD RECEIVED THREE PREVIOUS DOSES OF TRIPEDIA® VACCINE OR THREE DOSES OF WHOLE-CELL PERTUSSIS DTP

	N	ERYTHEMA ≥1 INCH	SWELLING ≥1 INCH	PAIN	TEMPERATURE ≥ 101°F	IRRITABILITY
Tripedia® Primed	109	30.3	29.4	19.3	5.5	19.3
Whole-Cell pertussis DTP Primed	30	23.3	20.0	10.3	3.3	13.3

Table 6 lists the frequency of adverse reactions in 372 US children who received Tripedia® vaccine at 15 to 20 months of age and 240 US children who received Tripedia® vaccine at 4 to 6 years of age in a study conducted from 1989-1990. These children had previously received three or four doses of whole-cell pertussis DTP vaccine at approximately 2, 4, 6, and 18 months of age.[1]

TABLE 6[1]

ADVERSE EVENTS (%) OCCURRING WITHIN 72 HOURS FOLLOWING DIPHTHERIA AND TETANUS TOXOIDS AND ACELLULAR PERTUSSIS VACCINE ADSORBED (TRIPEDIA®) IMMUNIZATIONS GIVEN AT 15 TO 20 MONTHS AND 4 TO 6 YEARS OF AGE IN CHILDREN WHO HAD RECEIVED THREE OR FOUR DOSES OF DTP

EVENT	15 to 20 MONTHS THREE PREVIOUS DTP DOSES REACTION % (N = 372 CHILDREN)	4 TO 6 YEARS FOUR PREVIOUS DTP DOSES REACTION % (N = 240 CHILDREN)
Local		
Erythema*	18.3	31.3
Swelling**	10.8	27.9
Tenderness	14.2	46.2
Systemic		
Fever >101°F	4.7	4.8
Diarrhea	6.3	0.8
Vomiting	2.2	1.7
Anorexia	7.8	5.4
Drowsiness	12.4	15.0
Irritability	21.2	15.8
High-pitched unusual cry	1.1	NA

* Includes all occurrences of erythema.
** Includes all occurrences of swelling.
NAData not collected in this age group.

The results of an open label, non-controlled clinical study, of 2,457 US children and targeted to evaluate less common and more severe adverse events following three doses of Tripedia® vaccine in the primary series are shown in Table 7.[1] Data were collected by parental interview at subsequent immunizations, chart review and telephone calls to the parents 60 days after the third dose.

TABLE 7[1]

MODERATELY SEVERE ADVERSE EVENTS OCCURRING WITHIN 48 HOURS FOLLOWING VACCINATION WITH TRIPEDIA® AT 2, 4, OR 6 MONTHS OF AGE (N = 7,102 DOSES)

EVENT	NUMBER	RATE/ 1,000 DOSES
Fever ≥105°F	2	0.28
Hypotonic/Hyporesponsive Episode	1	0.14

Continued on next page

Tripedia—Cont.

Persistent cry		
≥3 hours	4	0.56
Convulsions*	0	0

*One seizure episode was noted between 48 and 72 hours.

Adverse experiences that are more serious and less common than those reported in Table 7 are not known at this time. In the large German efficacy study that enrolled 16,780 infants, 12,514 of whom received 41,615 doses of Tripedia® vaccine, hospitalization rates and death rates were similar between Tripedia® vaccine and DT recipients.[1] Adverse events were monitored by spontaneous reporting by parents and a medical history obtained at each subsequent vaccination. Adverse events (rates per 1,000 doses) occurring within 7 days including those events interpreted by the investigator as related as well as those interpreted as unrelated to vaccination included; unusual cry (0.96), persistent cry >3 hours (0.12), febrile seizure (0.05), afebrile seizure (0.02) and hypotonic/hyporesponsive episodes (0.05). In contrast to the first Swedish pertussis efficacy trial conducted in 1986-87,[10] no deaths due to invasive bacterial infections were reported.

Rarely, an anaphylactic reaction (i.e., hives, swelling of the mouth, difficulty breathing, hypotension, or shock) has been reported after receiving preparations containing diphtheria, tetanus, and/or pertussis antigens.[3]

Arthus-type hypersensitivity reactions, characterized by severe local reactions (generally starting 2 to 8 hours after an injection), may follow receipt of tetanus toxoid. A few cases of peripheral neuropathy have been reported following tetanus toxoid administration, although the evidence is inadequate to accept or reject a causal relation.[40]

Whole-cell pertussis DTP has been associated with acute encephalopathy.[33] A 10-year follow-up to the National Childhood Encephalopathy Study (NCES) of children who experienced acute neurologic disorders in infancy concluded that serious acute neurologic illness increased the risk of chronic neurologic disease or death.[41] A committee of the Institute of Medicine (IOM) has concluded that, because DTP may cause acute neurologic illness, DTP may also cause chronic neurologic disease in the context of the NCES report.[34] However the IOM committee concluded that the evidence was insufficient to indicate whether or not DTP increased the overall risk of chronic neurologic disease.[34]

Sudden Infant Death Syndrome (SIDS) has occurred in infants following administration of whole-cell pertussis DTP and DTaP. Large case-control studies of SIDS in the US have shown that receipt of whole-cell pertussis DTP was not causally related to SIDS.[42,43,44] It should be recognized that the first three primary immunizing doses of whole-cell pertussis DTP and DTaP are usually administered to infants 2 to 6 months old and that approximately 85% of SIDS cases occur at ages 1 to 6 months, with the peak incidence occurring at 6 weeks to 4 months of age. By chance alone, some cases of SIDS can be expected to follow receipt of whole-cell pertussis DTP[44] and DTaP. A review by a committee of the IOM concluded that available evidence did not indicate a causal relation between DTP vaccine and SIDS.[33]

Onset of infantile spasms has occurred in infants who have recently received DTP or DT. Analysis of data from the NCES on children with infantile spasms showed that receipt of DT or DTP was not causally related to infantile spasms.[45] The incidence of onset of infantile spasms increases at 3 to 9 months of age, the time period in which the second and third doses of DTP are generally given. Therefore, some cases of infantile spasms can be expected to be related by chance alone to recent receipt of DTP.[3]

A bulging fontanelle associated with increased intracranial pressure which occurred within 24 hours following DTP immunization has been reported, although a causal relationship has not been established.[33,46,47,48]

The above findings regarding possible association of unusual neurologic events and SIDS relate only to DTP vaccine containing whole-cell pertussis. At this time there are insufficient data to determine their relevance to Tripedia® vaccine.

A review by the IOM found a causal relation between tetanus toxoid and brachial neuritis and Guillian-Barré syndrome.[40] The following illnesses have been reported as temporally associated with vaccine containing tetanus toxoid: neurological complications[49,50] including cochlear lesion,[51] brachial plexus neuropathies,[51,52] paralysis of the radial nerve,[53] paralysis of the recurrent nerve,[51] accommodation paresis, and EEG disturbances with encephalopathy.[17] In the differential diagnosis of polyradiculoneuropathies following administration of a vaccine containing tetanus toxoid, tetanus toxoid should be considered as a possible etiology.[54,55]

In the German case-control study and US open-label safety study in which 14,971 infants received Tripedia® vaccine, 13 deaths in Tripedia® vaccine recipients were reported to study investigators. Causes of deaths included; seven SIDS,

and one of each of the following; enteritis, Leigh Syndrome, adrenogenital syndrome, cardiac arrest, motor vehicle accident and accidental drowning. None of these events were determined to be vaccine-related and all occurred more than two weeks past immunization.[1] The rate of SIDS observed in the German case-control study was 0.4/1,000 vaccinated infants. The rate of SIDS observed in the US open-label safety study was 0.8/1,000 vaccinated infants and the reported rate of SIDS in the US from 1985-1991 was 1.5/1,000 live births.[56] By chance alone, some cases of SIDS can be expected to follow receipt of whole-cell pertussis DTP[44] and DTaP.

In the Swedish efficacy trial where 1,419 recipients received the pertussis components in Tripedia® vaccine, three deaths due to invasive bacterial infections occurred. Further investigation revealed no evidence for a causal relation between vaccination and altered resistance to invasive disease caused by encapsulated bacteria.[11] While the hypothesis that the two variables are related cannot be ruled out in the Swedish trial, deaths due to invasive bacterial infections have been monitored in other trials. In contrast to the Swedish trial, in the German case-control study and US open-label safety study, 14,971 infants received Tripedia® vaccine and no deaths due to invasive bacterial infections were reported.

When Tripedia® vaccine was used to reconstitute ActHIB® (TriHIBit™) and administered to children 15 to 20 months of age, the systemic adverse experience profile was comparable to that observed when the two vaccines were given separately. An increase in rates of minor local reactions was observed within the 24-hour period after immunization when compared to the Tripedia® and ActHIB® (OmniHIB®) vaccines administered separately. However, local adverse event rates of the combined vaccines were comparable when taking into consideration reactions observed at the ActHIB® site.[1] *(Refer to ActHIB® package insert; Table 7.)*

Reporting of Adverse Events

Reporting by parents and patients of all adverse events occurring after vaccine administration should be encouraged. Adverse events following immunization with vaccine should be reported by the health-care provider to the US Department of Health and Human Services (DHHS) Vaccine Adverse Event Reporting System (VAERS). Reporting forms and information about reporting requirements or completion of the form can be obtained from VAERS through a toll-free number 1-800-822-7967.[35,36,37]

The health-care provider also should report these events to the Director of Medical Affairs, Connaught Laboratories, Inc., Route 611, PO Box 187, Swiftwater, PA 18370 or call 1-800-822-2463.

DOSAGE AND ADMINISTRATION

Parenteral drug products should be inspected visually for extraneous particulate matter and/or discoloration prior to administration whenever solution and container permit. If these conditions exist, the vaccine should not be administered.

SHAKE VIAL WELL *before withdrawing each dose.* Inject 0.5 mL of Tripedia® vaccine intramuscularly only. The preferred injection sites are the anterolateral aspect of the thigh and the deltoid muscle of the upper arm. The vaccine should not be injected into the gluteal area or areas where there may be a major nerve trunk.

The primary series for children less than 7 years of age is three intramuscular doses of 0.5 mL. The customary age for the first dose is 2 months of age but may be given as early as 6 weeks of age and up to the seventh birthday.

Before injection, the skin over the site to be injected should be cleansed with a suitable germicide. After insertion of the needle, aspirate to ensure that the needle has not entered a blood vessel.

Fractional doses (doses < 0.5 mL) should not be given. The effect of fractional doses on the frequency of serious adverse events and on efficacy has not been determined.

Do NOT administer this product subcutaneously.

PRIMARY IMMUNIZATION

The primary series consists of three doses administered at intervals of 4 to 8 weeks. It is recommended that Tripedia® vaccine be given for all three doses since no interchangeability data on DTaP vaccines exist for the primary series.

Tripedia® vaccine may be used to complete the primary series in infants who have received one or two doses of whole-cell pertussis DTP. However, the safety and efficacy of Tripedia® vaccine in such infants has not been evaluated.

Tripedia® vaccine should not be combined through reconstitution with any other vaccine for administration to infants younger than 15 months of age. There are insufficient data at this time to support the use of Tripedia® vaccine to reconstitute ActHIB® (TriHIBit™) for primary immunization.

BOOSTER IMMUNIZATION

When Tripedia® vaccine is given for the primary series, a fourth dose is recommended at 15 to 20 months of age. The interval between the third and fourth dose should be at least 6 months. At this time, data are insufficient to establish frequencies of adverse events following a fifth dose of

Tripedia® vaccine in children who have previously received 4 doses of Tripedia® vaccine. (See **ADVERSE REACTIONS** section.)

If a child receives whole-cell pertussis DTP for one or more doses, Tripedia® vaccine may be given to complete the five-dose series. A fourth dose is recommended at 15 to 20 months of age. The interval between the third and fourth dose should be at least 6 months. Children four to six years of age (up to the seventh birthday) who received all four doses by the fourth birthday, including one or more doses of whole-cell pertussis DTP, should receive a single dose of Tripedia® vaccine before entering kindergarten or elementary school. This dose is not needed if the fourth dose was given on or after the fourth birthday.

Tripedia® vaccine combined with ActHIB® (TriHIBit™) by reconstitution, may be administered at 15 to 18 months of age for the fourth dose. *(Refer to ActHIB® package insert.)*

Tripedia® vaccine may be administered according to any of the following schedules for infants and children 6 weeks through 6 years of age (up to the 7th birthday).

Primary series
- Three doses administered at intervals of 4 to 8 weeks, beginning at 6 weeks of age
- To complete the primary series for infants who have received one or two doses of DTP

Booster doses
- As a 4th and/or 5th dose following a primary series of three doses of DTP
- As a 4th dose following a primary series of Tripedia® vaccine*
- As a 4th dose when used to reconstitute ActHIB® (TriHIBit™)**

---

* Data are insufficient to establish frequencies of adverse events following a fifth dose of Tripedia® vaccine in children who have previously received four doses of Tripedia® vaccine.

** Tripedia® vaccine should not be combined through reconstitution with any other vaccine.

If any recommended dose of pertussis vaccine cannot be given, DT (For Pediatric Use) should be given as needed to complete the series.

PERSONS 7 YEARS OF AGE AND OLDER SHOULD NOT BE IMMUNIZED WITH TRIPEDIA® VACCINE.[28]

Preterm infants should be vaccinated according to their chronological age from birth.[20]

Interruption of the recommended schedule with a delay between doses should not interfere with the final immunity achieved with Tripedia® vaccine. There is no need to start the series over again, regardless of the time between doses. Routine simultaneous administration of DTaP, OPV (or IPV), Haemophilus b conjugate vaccine, MMR, and hepatitis B vaccine is encouraged for children who are the recommended age to receive these vaccines and for whom no specific contraindications exist at the time of the visit, unless, in the judgment of the provider, complete vaccination of the child will not be compromised by administering different vaccines at different visits. Simultaneous administration is particularly important if the child might not return for subsequent vaccinations (see **CLINICAL PHARMACOLOGY** section).[28]

Data are unavailable to the manufacturer concerning the effects on immune response of IPV when given concurrently with ActHIB® reconstituted with Tripedia® (TriHIBit™).

If passive immunization is needed for tetanus prophylaxis, Tetanus Immune Globulin (Human) (TIG) is the product of choice. It provides longer protection than antitoxin of animal origin and causes few adverse reactions. The currently recommended prophylactic dose of TIG for wounds of average severity is 250 units intramuscularly. When tetanus toxoid and TIG are administered concurrently, separate syringes and separate sites should be used. The ACIP recommends the use of only adsorbed toxoid in this situation.

HOW SUPPLIED

Vial, 1 Dose (5 per package) - Product No. 49281-288-05
Vial, 15 Dose (7.5 mL) - Product No. 49281-288-15
TriHIBit™, One 7.5 mL vial of Tripedia® vaccine as Diluent packaged with Ten 1 Dose vials of lyophilized ActHIB® - Product No. 49281-557-10
TriHIBit™, Five 0.6 mL vials of Tripedia® vaccine as Diluent packaged with Five 1 Dose vials of lyophilized ActHIB® - Product No. 49281-557-05

STORAGE

Store between 2°–8°C (35°–46°F). DO NOT FREEZE. Temperature extremes may adversely affect resuspendability of this vaccine.

REFERENCES

1. Unpublished data available from Connaught Laboratories, Inc.
2. Mueller JH, et al. Production of diphtheria toxin of high potency (100 Lf) on a reproducible medium. J Immunol 40: 21-32, 1941

3. Recommendations of the Advisory Committee of Immunization Practices (ACIP). Diphtheria, Tetanus, and Pertussis: Recommendations for vaccine use and other preventive measures. MMWR 40: No RR-10, 1991

4. Kimura M, et al. Developments in pertussis immunization in Japan. The Lancet: 30-32, 1990

5. Kimura M, et al. Current epidemiology of pertussis in Japan. Pediatr Infect Dis J 9: 705-709, 1990

6. Aoyama T, et al. Efficacy and immunogenicity of acellular pertussis vaccine by manufacturer and patient age. Amer J Dis Child 143: 655-659, 1989

7. Aoyama T, et al. Efficacy of an acellular pertussis vaccine in Japan. J Pediatr 107: 180-183, 1985

8. Blennow M, et al. Preliminary data from a clinical trial (phase 2) of an Acellular Pertussis Vaccine, J NIH-6. Develop Biol Standard 65: 185-190, 1986

9. Blennow M, et al. Primary immunization of infants with an Acellular Pertussis Vaccine in a double-blind randomized clinical trial. Pediatr 82: 293-299, 1988

10. Kallings LO, et al. Placebo-controlled trial of two Acellular Pertussis Vaccines in Sweden - protective efficacy and adverse events. Lancet: 955-960, 1988

11. Storsaeter J, et al. Mortality and morbidity from invasive bacterial infections during a clinical trial of acellular pertussis vaccines in Sweden. Pediatr Infect Dis J 7: 637-645, 1988

12. Bernstein H, et al. Clinical reactions and immunogenicity of the BIKEN Acellular Diphtheria and Tetanus Toxoids and Pertussis Vaccine in 4- through 6-year-old US children. Amer J Dis Child 146: 556-559, 1992

13. Feldman S, et al. Comparison of acellular (B-Type) and whole-cell pertussis-component diphtheria-tetanus-pertussis vaccines as the first booster immunization in 15- to 24-month old children. J Pediatr 121: 857-861, 1992

14. Feldman S, et al. Comparison of two-component acellular and standard whole-cell pertussis vaccines, combined with diphtheria-tetanus toxoids, as the primary immunization series in infants. South Med J 86: 269-275, 284, 1993

15. Pichichero ME, et al. Acellular pertussis vaccination of 2-month-old infants in the United States. J Pediatr 89: 882-887, 1992

16. CDC. Summary of Notifiable Disease, United States, 1994. MMWR 43: No. 53, 1995

17. CDC. Diphtheria Epidemic - New Independent States of the Former Soviet Union, 1990-1994. MMWR 44: 177-181, 1995

18. Department of Health and Human Services, Food and Drug Administration. Biological Products; Bacterial Vaccines and Toxoids; Implementation of Efficacy Review; Proposed Rule. Federal Register Vol 50 No 240, pp 51002-51117, 1985

19. CDC - Pertussis - United States, January 1992-June 1995. MMWR 44: 525-529, 1995

20. Report of the Committee on Infectious Diseases. American Academy of Pediatrics, Evanston, Illinois. Twenty-third Edition, 1994

21. Farizo KM, et al. Epidemiologic features of pertussis in the United States, 1980-1989. Clin Infect Dis 14: 708-719, 1992

22. Nennig ME, et al. Prevalence and Incidence of Adult Pertussis in an Urban Population. JAMA (21) 275: 1672-1674, 1996

23. Linnemann CC, et al. Pertussis in the adult. Ann Rev Med 28: 179-185, 1977

24. CDC. Pertussis Surveillance - United States, 1986 and 1988. MMWR 39: 57-66, 1990

25. Noble GR, et al. Acellular and whole-cell pertussis vaccines in Japan. JAMA 257: 1351-1356, 1987

26. Blackwelder WC, et al., Acellular Pertussis Vaccines. Efficacy and evaluation of clinical case definitions. Am J Dis Child: 145 (11): 1285-1289, 1991

27. Olin P, et al. Relative efficacy of two acellular pertussis vaccines during three years of passive surveillance. Vaccine 10: pp 142-144, 1992

28. ACIP. General recommendations on immunization. MMWR 43: No. RR-1, 1994

29. Wilson GS. The Hazards of Immunization. Provocation poliomyelitis. pp 270-274, 1967

30. ACIP. Pertussis Vaccination: Acellular Pertussis Vaccine for Reinforcing and Booster Use - Supplementary ACIP Statement. MMWR 41: No. RR-1, 1992

31. Cody CL, et al. Nature and rates of adverse reactions associated with DTP and DT immunizations in infants and children. Pediatr 68: 650-660, 1981

32. ACIP. Pertussis immunization: Family history of convulsions and use of antipyretics - Supplementary ACIP statement. MMWR 36: 281-282, 1987

33. Howson CP, et al. Adverse Effects of Pertussis and Rubella Vaccines, Pertussis Vaccines and CNS Disorders. Institute of Medicine (IOM). National Academy Press, Washington, DC, 1991

34. IOM. DTP vaccine and chronic nervous system dysfunction: a new analysis. National Academy Press, Washington, DC, 1994 (Supplement)

35. CDC. Vaccine Adverse Event Reporting System - United States. MMWR 39: 730-733, 1990

36. CDC. National Childhood Vaccine Injury Act: requirements for permanent vaccination records and for reporting of selected events after vaccination. MMWR 37: 197-200, 1988

37. Food and Drug Administration. New reporting requirements for vaccine adverse events. FDA Drug Bull 18 (2), 16-18, 1988

38. Decker MD, et al. Comparison of 13 Acellular Pertussis Vaccines: Adverse Reactions. Pediatr 96: 557-566, 1995

39. Pichichero ME, et al. Safety and immunogenicity of an acellular pertussis vaccine booster in 15- to 20-month-old children previously immunized with acellular or whole-cell pertussis vaccine as infants. Pediatr 91: 756-760, 1993

40. Stratton KR, et al. Adverse Events Associated with Childhood Vaccines. Evidence Bearing on Causality. IOM. National Academy Press. Washington, DC, 1994

41. Miller D, et al. Pertussis immunisation and serious acute neurological illnesses in children. Academic Department of Public Health, St Mary's Hospital Medical School, University of London, 1993

42. Griffin MR, et al. Risk of sudden infant death syndrome after immunization with the Diphtheria-Tetanus-Pertussis vaccine. N Engl J Med 618-623, 1988

43. Hoffman HJ, et al. Diphtheria-tetanus-pertussis immunization and sudden infant death: Results of the National Institute of Child Health and Human Development Cooperative Epidemiological Study of Sudden Infant Death Syndrome Risk Factors. Pediatr 79: 598-611, 1987

44. Walker AM, et al. Diphtheria-tetanus-pertussis immunization and sudden infant death syndrome. Am J Public Health 77: 945-951, 1987

45. Bellman MH, et al. Infantile spasms and pertussis immunization. Lancet, i: 1031-1034, 1983

46. Jacob J, et al. Increased intracranial pressure after diphtheria, tetanus and pertussis immunization. Am J Dis Child Vol 133: 217-218, 1979

47. Mathur R, et al. Bulging fontanel following triple vaccine. Indian Pediatr 18 (6): 417-418, 1981

48. Shendurnikar N, et al. Bulging fontanel following DTP vaccine. Indian Pediatr 23 (11): 960, 1986

49. Rutledge SL, et al. Neurological complications of immunizations. J Pediatr 109: 917-924, 1986

50. Walker AM, et al. Neurologic events following diphtheria-tetanus-pertussis immunization. Pediatr 81: 345-349, 1988

51. Wilson GS. The Hazards of Immunization. Allergic manifestations: Post-vaccinal neuritis. pp 153-156, 1967

52. Tsairis P, et al. Natural history of brachial plexus neuropathy. Arch Neurol 27: 109-117, 1972

53. Blumstein GI, et al. Peripheral neuropathy following tetanus toxoid administration. JAMA 198: 1030-1031, 1966

54. CDC. Adverse events following immunization. Surveillance Report No. 3, 1985-1986, Issued February 1989

55. Schlenska GK. Unusual neurological complications following tetanus toxoid administration. J Neurol 215: 299-302, 1977

56. Willinger M, et al. Infant Sleep Position and Risk for Sudden Infant Death Syndrome: Report of Meeting Held January 13 and 14, 1994, National Institutes of Health, Bethesda, MD. Pediatr 93: 814-819, 1994

Product information
as of September 1996

Manufactured by:
CONNAUGHT LABORATORIES, INC
Swiftwater, Pennsylvania 18370, USA
and
The Research Foundation for Microbial
Diseases of Osaka University ("BIKEN®")
Suita, Osaka, Japan   3442
PASTEUR MÉRIEUX CONNAUGHT
RHÔNE-POULENC GROUP

Shown in Product Identification Guide, page 330

ProHIBiT®   ℞
HAEMOPHILUS b CONJUGATE VACCINE
(Diphtheria Toxoid-Conjugate)

Caution: Federal (U.S.A.) law prohibits dispensing without prescription.

DESCRIPTION

ProHIBiT®, Haemophilus b Conjugate Vaccine (Diphtheria Toxoid-Conjugate), for intramuscular use, is a sterile solution, prepared from the purified capsular polysaccharide, a polymer of ribose, ribitol and phosphate (PRP) of the Eagen *Haemophilus influenzae* type b strain covalently bound to diphtheria toxoid (D) and dissolved in sodium phosphate buffered isotonic sodium chloride solution. The polysaccharide-protein conjugate molecule is referred to as PRP-D. Thimerosal (mercury derivative) 1:10,000 is added as a preservative. The vaccine is a clear, colorless solution. Each single dose of 0.5 mL is formulated to contain 25 µg of purified capsular polysaccharide and 18 µg of diphtheria toxoid protein.

HOW SUPPLIED

Vial, 1 Dose (5 per package)—Product No. 49281-541-01
Vial, 5 Dose—Product No. 49281-541-05
Vial, 10 Dose—Product No. 49281-541-10

THERACYS®   ℞
BCG LIVE (INTRAVESICAL)
For Treatment of Carcinoma In-situ of the Urinary Bladder

DESCRIPTION

BCG Live (Intravesical), TheraCys®, as prepared by Connaught Laboratories Limited, is a freeze-dried suspension of an attenuated strain of *Mycobacterium bovis* (Bacillus Calmette and Guérin), which has been grown on Sauton medium (potato and glycerin based medium), used in the nonspecific active therapy of carcinoma in-situ of the urinary bladder. CAUTION: TheraCys® is NOT intended to be used as an immunizing agent for the prevention of tuberculosis. TheraCys® is NOT a vaccine for the prevention of cancer. TheraCys® is formulated to contain 81 mg (dry weight)/vial Bacillus of Calmette and Guérin (BCG) and 5% w/v monosodium glutamate. This product contains no preservative. A vial of TheraCys® is ready for use following reconstitution with the accompanying diluent (3.0 ml), which consists of approximately 0.85% sodium chloride, 0.025% Tween 80, 0.06% w/v sodium dihydrogen phosphate and 0.25% disodium hydrogen phosphate. The diluent contains no preservative. One dose consists of one vial of reconstituted material further diluted in sterile, preservative-free saline. The reconstituted product contains $10.5 \pm 8.7 \times 10^8$ colony-forming units (CFU) per vial when resuspended in the diluent provided.

To ensure viability of the product through to its labeled expiration date, it is very important that TheraCys® and diluent be stored continuously between 2° and 8°C (35° and 46°F) until use (see STORAGE). It should be used immediately after reconstitution.

CLINICAL PHARMACOLOGY

TheraCys® promotes a local inflammatory reaction with histiocytic and leukocytic infiltration in the urinary bladder.[1,2,3] The local inflammatory effects are associated with an apparent elimination or reduction of superficial cancerous lesions of the urinary bladder. The exact mechanism by which this is accomplished is unknown.

In a randomized, actively controlled multicenter study TheraCys® was compared to doxorubicin hydrochloride (Adriamycin®) in the treatment of carcinoma in-situ of the urinary bladder. The response of 114 eligible patients for evaluation is given in Table 1 below. Among the 54 patients receiving TheraCys®, 74% had a complete response (negative by cystoscopic examination and by urine cytology). The estimated median time to treatment failure (recurrence, progression or death) was 48.2 months (Table 2).[4]

TABLE 1: Response of Patients with Carcinoma In-Situ to Treatment with TheraCys® or Adriamycin®

	TheraCys® (n = 54)	Adriamycin® (n = 60)
Complete Response†	74%*	42%*
No Response††	11%	10%
Progressive Disease§	13%	42%
No Evaluation	2%	7%
Total	100%	100%

* Difference is statistically significant ($P < 0.01$).
† Confirmed by cytology and cystoscopic examination.
†† Less than a CR or stable disease.
§ Increase of stage or grade.

Continued on next page

Theracys BCG Live—Cont.

TABLE 2: Time to Recurrence, Progression or Death: Time to Treatment Failure (TTF)

Treatment	Number Studied	Number Failures	Median TTF
TheraCys®	54	27	48.2 months*
Adriamycin®	60	46	5.9 months*

* Difference is statistically significant (P<0.01 by stratified logrank test).

TABLE 3: Prior Versus No Prior Treatment

Prior Treatment*	Study Arm	Response Rate	Median TTF (# Events/N)
Yes	TheraCys®	81%	Not reached (11/26)
Yes	Adriamycin®	53%	7.0 months (22/30)
No	TheraCys®	68%	32.8 months (16/28)
No	Adriamycin®	30%	3.7 months (24/30)

* Other than TheraCys® and Adriamycin®.

The effect of chemotherapy (other than TheraCys® or Adriamycin®) prior to entry into the controlled study was analysed. Patients in the TheraCys® treated arm who had received prior chemotherapy had a complete response rate of 81% (11/26) as compared to 68% (16/28) in the group who had not received prior chemotherapy (Table 3). This difference was not statistically significant.

No survival advantage for TheraCys® therapy[4] over that for Adriamycin®[4,5,6] was demonstrated after a 40–72 month follow-up. The median time to death for each group was 23 months and 21 months for TheraCys® and Adriamycin® respectively.

The clinical trials carried out with TheraCys® included percutaneous administration of 0.5 ml of BCG Live (Intravesical) solution, which was reconstituted in the diluent provided and further diluted in 50 ml sterile preservative-free saline, with each intravesical dose.[4] Some studies have suggested that this may not be necessary[15] and if severe reactions, such as ulceration, occurred the percutaneous treatment was discontinued.

INDICATIONS AND USAGE

TheraCys® is indicated for intravesical use in the treatment of primary and relapsed carcinoma in-situ of the urinary bladder to eliminate residual tumor cells and to reduce the frequency of tumor recurrence. It is indicated for the treatment of carcinoma in-situ with or without associated papillary tumors. TheraCys® is not indicated for the treatment of papillary tumors occurring alone. TheraCys® is also indicated as a therapy for patients with carcinoma in-situ of the bladder following failure to respond to other treatment regimens. CAUTION: TheraCys® is NOT indicated as an immunizing agent for the prevention of tuberculosis. TheraCys® is NOT a vaccine for the prevention of cancer.

CONTRAINDICATIONS

Patients on immunosuppressive therapy or with compromised immune systems should not receive TheraCys® due to the risk of overwhelming systemic mycobacterial sepsis. TheraCys® should not be administered to patients with fever unless the cause of the fever is determined and evaluated. If the fever is due to an infection, TheraCys® should be withheld until the patient is afebrile and off all therapy. Patients with urinary tract infection should not receive TheraCys® treatment because administration may result in the risk of disseminated BCG infection or in an increased severity of bladder irritation.

TheraCys® should NOT be administered as an immunizing agent for the prevention of tuberculosis. TheraCys® is NOT a vaccine for the prevention of cancer.

WARNINGS

TheraCys® should NOT be administered as an immunizing agent for the prevention of tuberculosis. TheraCys® is NOT a vaccine for the prevention of cancer.

Since administration of intravesical TheraCys® causes an inflammatory response in the bladder and has been associated with hematuria, urinary frequency, dysuria and bacterial urinary tract infection, careful monitoring of urinary status is required. If there is an increase in the patient's existing symptoms, or if their symptoms persist or if any of these symptoms develop, the patient should be evaluated and managed for urinary tract infection or BCG toxicity.

Since death has occurred due to systemic BCG infection, patients should be closely monitored for symptoms of such an infection (see PRECAUTIONS). BCG therapy should be withheld upon any suspicion of systemic infection, e.g. granulomatous hepatitis.

Drug combinations containing bone marrow depressants and/or immunosuppressants and/or radiation may either impair the response to TheraCys® or increase the risk of osteomyelitis or disseminated BCG infection (see DRUG INTERACTIONS).

Patients undergoing antimicrobial therapy for other infections should be evaluated to assess whether the therapy will obviate the effects of TheraCys® actions.

For patients with small bladder capacity, increased risk of severity of local irritation should be considered in decisions to treat with TheraCys®.

Intravesical treatment with TheraCys® may induce a sensitivity to tuberculin which could complicate future interpretations of skin test reactions to tuberculin in the diagnosis of suspected mycobacterial infections. Determination of a patient's reactivity to tuberculin prior to administration of TheraCys® may be desirable in this regard.

PRECAUTIONS

General

Contains viable attenuated mycobacteria. Handle as infectious. Use aseptic technique.

The possibility of allergic reactions in individuals sensitive to the components of the product should be borne in mind. After usage all equipment and materials (e.g. syringes, catheters and containers that may have come into contact with TheraCys®) used for instillation of the product into the bladder, should be placed immediately into plastic bags which are labelled "Infectious Waste" and disposed of accordingly as biohazardous waste.

Aseptic technique must be used during administration of intravesical TheraCys® so as not to introduce contaminants into the urinary tract or to traumatize unduly the urinary mucosa.

Urine voided for 6 hours after instillation should be disinfected with an equal volume of 5% hypochlorite solution (undiluted household bleach) and allowed to stand for 15 minutes before flushing.

It is recommended that intravesical TheraCys® not be administered any sooner than one week following transurethral resection because fatalities due to disseminated BCG infection have been reported with use of TheraCys® after traumatic catheterization.

If the physician believes that the bladder catheterization has been traumatic (e.g., associated with bleeding or possible false passage), then TheraCys® should not be administered and there must be a treatment delay of at least one week. Subsequent treatment should be resumed as if no interruption in the schedule had occurred. That is, all doses of TheraCys® should be administered even after a temporary halt in administration.

If systemic BCG infection is suspected (i.e., if patients have fever over 39°C (103°F) or persistent fever above 38°C (101°F) over two days or severe malaise), an infectious disease specialist should be consulted and fast acting antituberculosis therapy should be initiated. It should be noted that BCG systemic infections are rarely evidenced by positive cultures.

INFORMATION FOR PATIENTS

Patients should be advised to check with their doctor as soon as possible if there is an increase in their existing symptoms, or if their symptoms persist even after receiving a number of treatments, or if any of the following symptoms develop:

More Common	Rare
Blood in Urine	Cough
Fever and Chills	Skin Rash
Frequent Urge to Urinate	
Increased Frequency of Urination	
Joint Pain	
Nausea and Vomiting	
Painful Urination	

A cough that develops after administration of TheraCys® could indicate a BCG systemic infection which is life-threatening. If systemic infection occurs it should be treated immediately with antituberculous antibiotics.

All patients should sit while voiding following instillation of solution.

Urine voided for 6 hours after instillation should be disinfected with an equal volume of 5% hypochlorite solution (undiluted household bleach) and allowed to stand for 15 minutes before flushing.

DRUG INTERACTIONS

Patients must also be advised that drug combinations containing bone marrow depressants and/or immunosuppressants and/or radiation may impair the response to TheraCys® or increase the risk of osteomyelitis or disseminated BCG infection.

TABLE 4: Local Reactions (1% OF 112 Patients)

Reaction	Total	Severe*
Dysuria	51.8	3.6
Frequency	40.2	1.8
Hematuria	39.3	17.0
Cystitis	29.5	0.0
Urgency	17.9	0.0
Urinary Tract Infection	17.9	1.0
Urinary Incontinence	6.3	0.0
Cramps/Pain	6.3	0.0
Decreased Bladder Capacity	5.4	0.0
Tissue in Urine	0.9	0.0
Local Infection	0.9	0.0

*Severe is defined as grade 3 (severe) or grade 4 (life threatening).

PREGNANCY

Pregnancy Category C. TheraCys®. Animal reproduction studies have not been conducted with TheraCys®. It is also not known whether TheraCys® can cause fetal harm when administered to a pregnant woman or can affect reproduction capacity. TheraCys® should be given to a pregnant woman only if clearly needed. Women should be advised not be become pregnant while on therapy.

NURSING MOTHERS

It is not known whether TheraCys® is excreted in human milk. Because many drugs are excreted in human milk, caution should be exercised when TheraCys® is administered to a nursing mother.

TABLE 5: Systemic Reactions (% of 112 Patients)

Reaction	Total	Severe*
Malaise	40.2	2.0
Fever (> 38°C)	38.4	2.6
Chills	33.9	2.6
Anemia	20.5	0.0
Nausea/Vomiting	16.1	0.0
Anorexia	10.7	0.0
Myalgia/Arthralgia/Arthritis	7.1	1.0
Diarrhea	6.3	0.0
Mild Liver Involvement	2.7	0.0
Mild Abdominal Pain	2.7	0.0
Systemic Infection**	2.7	2.0
Pulmonary Infection**	2.7	0.0
Cardiac	2.7	0.0
Headache	1.8	0.0
Hypersensitivity Skin Rash	1.8	0.0
Constipation	0.9	0.0
Dizziness	0.9	0.0
Fatigue	0.9	0.0
Leukopenia	5.4	0.0
Disseminated Intravascular Coagulation	2.7	0.0
Thrombocytopenia	0.9	0.0
Renal Toxicity	9.8	2.0
Genital Pain	9.8	0.0
Flank Pain	0.9	0.0

*Severe is defined as grade 3 (severe) or grade 4 (life threatening).
*Includes both BCG and other infections.

PEDIATRIC USE

Safety and effectiveness for carcinoma in-situ of the urinary bladder in children have not been established.

ADVERSE REACTIONS

TheraCys® therapy can affect several organs (or parts) of the body in addition to the cancer cells.

In a controlled multi-center clinical trial comparing BCG therapy and doxorubicin hydrochloride (Adriamycin®) for the intravesical treatment of superficial transitional cell carcinoma with and without carcinoma in-situ of the bladder, 112 patients received BCG.[4]

In another controlled study using TheraCys® for the treatment of superficial transitional cell carcinoma, with or without carcinoma in-situ, of the bladder, similar adverse reactions were observed.[13] However, two deaths were noted in this study which may have been associated with traumatic catheterization.

The incidence of adverse reactions associated with intravesical TheraCys® therapy is given below. Most local adverse

reactions occur following the third intravesical instillation. Symptoms usually begin two to four hours after instillation and persist for 24 to 72 hours. Systemic reactions usually last for 1–3 days after each intravesical instillation.[4,13,14]

No fatalities associated with the use of TheraCys® were reported in this study. Two fatalities have been reported with the use of TheraCys® in another study after traumatic catheterization or in the presence of urinary infection.[13]

An increased risk of additional primary malignancies has been reported following radiotherapy and chemotherapy for many types of malignancies. No increase in second primary malignancies after treatment with TheraCys® was reported in these studies.[4]

Irritative bladder symptoms associated with TheraCys® administration can be managed symptomatically with phenazopyridine hydrochloride (Pyridium), propantheline bromide (Pro-Banthine), and acetaminophen.[4]

Systemic side effects (such as malaise, fever and chills) may represent hypersensitivity reactions and can be treated with diphenhydramine hydrochloride.[4] Systemic infection as a result of the spread of BCG organisms has occasionally occurred with intravesical TheraCys® administration. The management of this condition is provided under PRECAUTIONS.

DOSAGE AND ADMINISTRATION

Intravesical treatment and prophylaxis for carcinoma in-situ of the urinary bladder should begin between 7 to 14 days after biopsy or transurethral resection if this procedure is done. A dose of TheraCys® is given intravesically under aseptic conditions once weekly for 6 weeks (induction therapy). Each dose (1 reconstituted vial) is further diluted in an additional 50 ml sterile, preservative-free saline for a total of 53 ml (see below). A urethral catheter is inserted into the bladder under aseptic conditions, the bladder drained and then 53 ml suspension of TheraCys® is instilled slowly by gravity following which the catheter is withdrawn. During the first hour following instillation, the patient should lie for 15 minutes each in the prone and supine positions and also on each side. The patient is then allowed to be up but retains the suspension for another 60 minutes for a total of 2 hours. All patients may not be able to retain the suspension for the 2 hours and should be instructed to void in less time if necessary. At the end of 2 hours all patients should void in a seated position for safety reasons. Patients should be instructed to maintain adequate hydration.

If the physician believes that the bladder catheterization has been traumatic (e.g., associated with bleeding or possible false passage), then TheraCys® should not be administered and there must be a treatment delay of at least one week. Subsequent treatment should be resumed as if no interruption in the schedule had occurred. That is, all doses of TheraCys® should be administered even after a temporary halt in administration.

The induction therapy should be followed by one treatment given 3, 6, 12, 18 and 24 months following the initial treatment.

After use, all equipment, materials and containers that may have come in contact with TheraCys® should be sterilized or disposed of properly as with any other biohazardous waste (see PRECAUTIONS).

Reconstitution of Freeze-Dried Product and Withdrawal from Rubber-Stoppered Vial.

TheraCys® SHOULD BE USED IMMEDIATELY AFTER RECONSTITUTION. KEEP REFRIGERATED UNTIL USE. DISCARD AFTER 2 HOURS.
DO NOT REMOVE THE RUBBER STOPPER FROM THE VIAL.
Reconstitute and dilute immediately prior to use.
Persons handling product should be masked and gloved.
TheraCys® should not be handled by persons with a known immunologic deficiency.
TheraCys® should be handled as infectious material.
Reconstitute and dilute using aseptic technique.
TheraCys® should be reconstituted only with the diluent provided to ensure proper dispersion of the organisms.

IMPORTANT RECONSTITUTION INSTRUCTIONS

Fig. (1) Apply a **sterile** pledget of cotton moistened with a suitable antiseptic to the surface of the rubber stoppers of vials of diluent and TheraCys®.

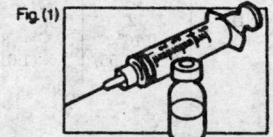

Fig. (2) Using a 5 ml **sterile** syringe and needle, draw into the syringe 3.0 ml of air. Pierce the center of the rubber stopper in the vial containing dilutent with the **sterile** needle of the syringe, invert the vial and slowly inject some of

the air in the syringe into the vial. Without removing the needle, alternately withdraw diluent and inject air into the vial until 3 ml of diluent has been withdrawn into the syringe. Then holding the syringe-plunger steady, withdraw the needle from the vial.

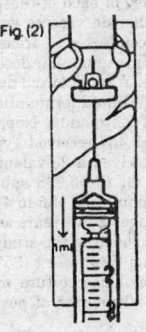

Fig. (3) Using the same syringe and needle, pierce the stopper in one vial of freeze-dried material with the needle.

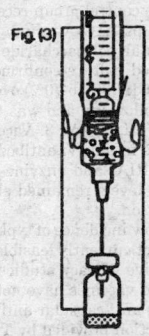

Fig. (4) Hold the vial of freeze-dried material upright and pull the plunger of the syringe back to the 5 ml marking on the barrel. This will create a mild vacuum in the vial.
Release the plunger and allow the vacuum to pull the diluent from the syringe into the vial of freeze-dried material. After all the diluent has passed into the vial of freeze-dried material, remove the needle and syringe.
Shake the vial gently until a fine, even suspension results.

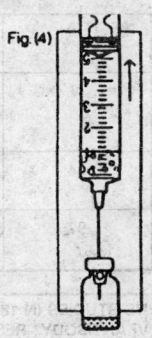

Fig. (5) Withdraw the entire contents of the reconstituted material from the vial again using the same 5 ml syringe. [See figure at top of next column]

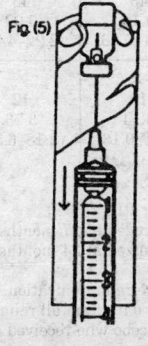

Fig. (6) Return the vial to an upright position before removing the syringe from the vial.
The reconstituted material from the vial (1 dose) is further diluted in an additional 50 ml **sterile**, preservative-free saline to a final volume of 53 ml for intravesical instillation (and percutaneous injection if it is given, see CLINICAL PHARMACOLOGY).

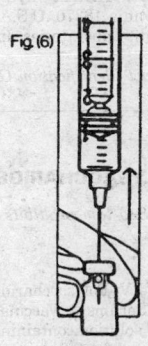

HOW SUPPLIED

TheraCys® is supplied in packages containing one vial of the freeze-dried product, containing 81 mg (dry weight) $(10.5 \pm 8.7 \times 10^8$ CFU), and one vial of diluent containing 3 ml. A 50 ml vial of Phosphate Buffered Saline is available for use as the final diluent.

STORAGE

TheraCys® and the accompanying diluent should be kept in a refrigerator at a temperature between 2°C and 8°C (35° and 46°F). It should not be used after the expiration date marked on the vial, otherwise it may be inactive. The product should be used **immediately** after reconstitution; however, it must not be used after 2 hours. Any reconstituted product which exhibits flocculation or clumping that cannot be dispersed with gentle shaking should not be used.
At no time should the freeze-dried or reconstituted TheraCys® be exposed to sunlight, direct or indirect. Exposure to artificial light should be kept to a minimum.[9]

REFERENCES

1. Old LJ, Clarke DA, Benacerraf B. Effect of bacillus Calmette-Guérin infection on transplanted tumors in the mouse. Nature 1959; 184: 291.
2. Lamm DL, Harris SC, Gittes RF. Bacillus Calmette-Guérin and dinitrochlorobenzene immunotherapy of chemically induced bladder tumors. Investigative Urology 1977; 14: 369.
3. Morales A. Ottenhof P, Emerson L. Treatment of residual non-infiltrating bladder cancer with bacillus Calmette-Guérin. J Urol 1979; 125: 649.
4. Unpublished clinical data available from Connaught Laboratories Limited.
5. Horn Y, Eidelman A, Walach N, Ilian M. Intravesical chemotherapy in controlled trial with thiotepa versus doxorubicin hydrochloride. J Urol 1981; 125: 652–654.
6. Zincke H, Utz DC, Taylor WF, Myers RP, Leary FJ. Influence of thiotepa and doxorubicin instillation at time of transurethral surgical treatment of bladder cancer on tumor recurrence: a prospective, randomized, double-blind, controlled trial. J Urol 1983; 129: 505–509.
7. Unpublished clinical data available from Connaught Laboratories Limited.
8. Lamm DL, et al. Complications of Bacillus Calmette-Guérin immunotherapy: review of 2602 patients and comparison of chemotherapy complications. EORTC GU Group Monograph 1989; 6: 335–355.
9. Landi S, Barbara C, Przykuta K, Held RH. Effect of light on freeze dried BCG Vaccines. J Biol Stand 1977; 5: 321–6.
10. Lamm DL, Blumenstein BA, Crawford ED, et al. South-West Oncology Group comparison of bacillus Calmette-Guérin and doxorubicin in the treatment and prophylaxis of superficial bladder cancer. J Urol 1987; 178A.
11. Mori K, Lamm DL, Crawford ED. A trial of Bacillus Calmette-Guérin versus Adriamycin in superficial bladder cancer: a South-West Oncology Group study. Urol Int 1986; 41: 254–259.
12. Soloway M. Evaluation and management of patients with superficial bladder cancer. Urol Clin North Am 1987; 14: 771.
13. Lamm DL, BCG in carcinoma in-situ and superficial bladder tumors. EORTC GU Group Monograph 1988; 5: 497.
14. Lamm DL. Complications of Bacillus Calmette-Guérin immunotherapy in 1,278 patients with bladder cancer. J Urol 1986; 135: 272.
15. Lamm DL, Sarodosy MS, DeHaven JI. Percutaneous, oral, or intravesical BCG administration: what is the optimal route? EORTC Genitourinary Group Monograph 6: BCG in Superficial Bladder Cancer. 1989; 301–310.

Continued on next page

Theracys BCG Live—Cont.

Manufactured by
CONNAUGHT LABORATORIES LIMITED
Willowdale, Ontario, Canada
Distributed by:
CONNAUGHT LABORATORIES, INC.
Swiftwater, Pennsylvania 18370, U.S.A.
©July 1993 Connaught Laboratories, Inc.
MKT 1916
Shown in Product Identification Guide, page 330

TYPHIM Vi™ ℞
TYPHOID Vi POLYSACCHARIDE VACCINE

Caution: Federal (USA) law prohibits dispensing without prescription.

DESCRIPTION

Typhim Vi™, Typhoid Vi Polysaccharide Vaccine, produced by Pasteur Mérieux Sérums & Vaccins S.A., for intramuscular use, is a sterile solution containing the cell surface Vi polysaccharide extracted from *Salmonella typhi* Ty2 strain. The organism is grown in a semi-synthetic medium without animal proteins. The capsular polysaccharide is precipitated from the concentrated culture supernatant by the addition of hexadecyltrimethylammonium bromide and the product is purified by differential centrifugation and precipitation. The potency of the purified polysaccharide is assessed by molecular size and O-acetyl content. Phenol, 0.25%, is added as a preservative. The vaccine contains residual polydimethylsiloxane or fatty-acid ester-based antifoam. The vaccine is a clear, colorless solution. Each single-dose of 0.5 mL is formulated to contain 25 µg of purified Vi polysaccharide in a colorless isotonic phosphate buffered saline (pH 7 ± 0.3), 4.150 mg of sodium chloride, 0.065 mg of disodium Phosphate ($2H_2O$), 0.023 mg of Monosodium Phosphate and 0.5 mL of Sterile Water for Injection.

CLINICAL PHARMACOLOGY

Typhoid fever is an infectious disease caused by *S. typhi*. Humans are the only natural host and reservoir for *S. typhi*; infections result from the consumption of food or water that has been contaminated by the excretions of an acute case or a carrier. *S.typhi* organisms efficiently invade the human intestinal mucosae ultimately leading to bacteremia following a typical 10- to 14-day incubation period, a systemic illness occurs. The clinical presentation of typhoid fever exhibits a broad range of severity and can be debilitating. Classical cases have fever, myalgia, anorexia, abdominal discomfort and headaches; the fever increases step-wise over a period of days and then may remain at 102°F to 106°F over 10 to 14 days before decreasing in a step-wise manner. Skin lesions known as rose spots may be present. Constipation is common in older children and adults, while diarrhea may occur in younger children. Among the less common but most severe complications are intestinal perforation and hemorrhage, and death. The course is typically more severe without appropriate antimicrobial therapy. The case fatality rate was reported to be approximately 10% to 20% in the pre-antibiotic era.[1,2,3] During the period of 1983 to 1991 in the US, the case fatality rate reported to the Centers for Disease Control and Prevention (CDC) was 0.2% (9/4010).[4]
Infection of the gallbladder can lead to the chronic carrier state.
Typhoid fever is still endemic in many countries of the world where it is predominantly a disease of school-age children and may be a major public health problem. Most cases of typhoid fever in the US are thought to be acquired during foreign travel. During the period of 1975 to 1984 and 1983 to 1984, respectively, 62% and 70% of the cases of typhoid fever reported to the CDC were acquired during foreign travel; this compares to 33% of cases during 1967-1972.[5]
In 1992, 414 cases of typhoid fever were reported to the CDC. Of these 414 cases, 1 (0.2%) case occurred in an infant under one year of age; 77 (18.6%) cases occurred in persons one to nine years of age; 81 (19.6%) cases occurred in persons 10 to 19 years of age; 251 (60.6%) cases occurred in individuals ≥20 years of age; the age was not available for 4 (1%) cases. One death was reported in 1991.[4] Domestic surveillance could underestimate the risk of typhoid fever in travelers since the disease is unlikely to be reported for persons who received diagnosis and treatment overseas.[6]
Approximately 2% to 4% of acute typhoid fever cases develop into a chronic carrier state. The chronic carrier state occurs more frequently with advanced age, and among females than males.[2,7] These non-symptomatic carriers are the natural reservoir for *S. typhi* and can serve to maintain the disease in its endemic state or to directly infect new individuals. Outbreaks of typhoid fever are often traced to food handlers who are asymptomatic carriers.[8]
Other vaccines used for the prevention of typhoid fever in selected populations include a parenteral vaccine containing killed *S. typhi* bacteria and an oral vaccine with live, attenuated *S. typhi*. Typhim Vi, consisting of purified *S. typhi* Vi capsular polysaccharide, is a different type of vaccine. Two formulations were utilized in studies of the typhoid Vi polysaccharide vaccine. These included the liquid formulation which is identical to Typhim Vi and lyophilized formulation.
The protective efficacy of each of these formulations of the typhoid Vi polysaccharide vaccine was assessed independently in two trials conducted in areas where typhoid fever is endemic. A single intramuscular dose of 25 µg was used in these efficacy studies. A randomized double-blind controlled trial with Typhim Vi (liquid formulation) was conducted in five villages west of Katmandu, Nepal. There were 6,908 vaccinated subjects: 3,454 received Typhim Vi and 3,454 in the control group received a 23-valent pneumococcal polysaccharide vaccine. Of the 6,908 subjects, 6,439 subjects were in the target population of 5 to 44 years of age. In addition, 165 children ages 2 to 4 years and 304 adults over 44 years of age were included in the study. The overall protective efficacy of Typhim Vi was 74% (95% confidence interval (CI): 49% to 87%) for blood culture confirmed cases of typhoid fever during 20 months of post-vaccination follow-up.[9,10,11]
The protective efficacy of the typhoid Vi polysaccharide vaccine, lyophilized formulation, was evaluated in a randomized double-blind controlled trial conducted in South Africa. There were 11,384 vaccinated children 5 to 15 years of age; 5,692 children received the Vi capsular polysaccharide vaccine and 5,692 in the control group received meningococcal polysaccharide (Groups A+C) vaccine. The protective efficacy for the Vi capsular polysaccharide (lyophilized formulation) group for blood culture confirmed cases of typhoid fever was 55% (95% CI: 30% to 70%) overall during 3 years of post-vaccination follow-up, and was 61%, 52% and 50%, respectively, for years 1, 2, and 3. Vaccination was associated with an increase in anti-Vi antibodies as measured by radioimmunoassay (RIA) and enzyme-linked immunosorbent assay. Antibody levels remained elevated at 6 and 12 months post-vaccination.[11,12]
Because of the very low incidence of typhoid fever in the US, efficacy studies are not currently feasible in this population. Controlled comparative efficacy studies of Typhim Vi and other types of typhoid vaccines have not been performed.
An increase in serum anti-capsular antibodies is thought to be the basis of protection provided by Typhim Vi. However, a specific correlation of post-vaccination antibody levels with subsequent protection is not available and the level of Vi antibody that will provide protection has not been determined. Also, limitations exist for comparing immunogenicity results from subjects in endemic areas, where some subjects have baseline serological evidence of prior *S. typhi* exposure, to naive populations such as most American travelers.
In endemic regions (Nepal, South Africa, Indonesia) where trials were conducted, pre-vaccination geometric mean antibody levels suggest that infection with *S. typhi* has previously occurred in a large percentage of the vaccinees. In these populations, specific antibody levels increased four-fold or greater in 68% to 87.5% of older children and adult subjects following vaccination. For 43 persons 15 to 44 years of age in the Nepal pilot study, geometric mean specific antibody levels pre- and 3 weeks post-vaccination were, respectively, 0.38 and 3..68 µg antibody/mL by RIA; 79% had a four-fold or greater rise in Vi antibody levels.[9,12]
Immunogenicity and safety trials were conducted in a racially mixed US population. A single dose of Typhim Vi vaccine induced a four-fold or greater increase in antibody levels in 88% and 96% of this adult population for 2 studies, respectively, following vaccination (see TABLE 1).[10,13]
[See table 1 below]
No studies of safety and immunogenicity have been conducted in US children. A double-blind randomized controlled trial testing the safety and immunogenicity of Typhim Vi was performed in 175 Indonesian children. The percentage of 2- to 5-year-old children achieving a four-fold or greater increase in antibody levels at 4 weeks post-vaccination was 96.3% (52/54) (95% CI: 87.3% to 99.6%), and in the study subset of 2-year-old children was 94.4% (17/18) (95% CI: 72.7% to 99.9%). The geometric mean levels (µg antibody/mL by RIA) for the 2-to 5-year-old children and the subset of 2-year-olds were, respectively, 5.81 (4.36 to 7.77) and 5.76 (3.48 to 9.53).[10,11]
In the US Reimmunization Study, adults previously immunized with Typhim Vi in other studies were reimmunized with a 25 µg dose at 27 or 34 months after the primary dose. Data on antibody response to primary immunization, decline following primary immunization, and response to reimmunization are presented in TABLE 2. Antibody levels attained following reimmunization at 27 or 34 months after the primary dose were similar to levels attained following the primary immunization.[10,13] This response is typical for a T-cell independent polysaccharide vaccine in that reimmunization does not elicit higher antibody levels than primary immunization. The safety of reimmunization was also evaluated in this study (see **ADVERSE REACTIONS** section).
[See table 2 below]

INDICATIONS AND USAGE

Typhim Vi vaccine is indicated for active immunization against typhoid fever for persons two years of age or older. Immunization with Typhim Vi should occur at least two weeks prior to expected exposure to *S. typhi*.
Routine immunization against typhoid fever is not recommended in the United States.[14]
Selective immunization against typhoid fever is recommended under the following circumstances: 1) travelers to

TABLE 1.[10,13] **Vi ANTIBODY LEVELS IN US ADULTS 18 TO 40 YEARS OF AGE GIVEN TYPHIM Vi**

	N	GEOMETRIC MEAN ANTIBODY LEVELS (µg antibody/mL by RIA) Pre (95% CI)	Post (4 weeks)	% ≥4 FOLD INCREASE (95% CI)
Trial 1 (1 lot)	54	0.16 (0.13 to 0.21)	3.23 (2.59 to 4.03)	96% (52/54) (87% to 100%)
Trial 2 (2 lots combined)	97	0.17 (0.14 to 0.21)	2.86 (2.26 to 3.62)	88% (85/97) (81% to 94%)

TABLE 2.[10,13] **US STUDIES IN 18- TO 40-YEAR-OLD ADULTS: KINETICS AND PERSISTENCE OF Vi ANTIBODY* RESPONSE TO PRIMARY IMMUNIZATION WITH TYPHIM Vi, AND RESPONSE TO REIMMUNIZATION AT 27 OR 34 MONTHS**

	PRE-DOSE 1	1 MONTH	11 MONTHS	18 MONTHS	27 MONTHS	34 MONTHS	1 MONTH POST-REIMMUNIZATION[e]
GROUP 1[a]							
N	43	43	39	ND[c]	43	ND	43
Level*	0.19	3.02	1.97		1.07[d]		3.04
95% CI	(0.14–0.26)	(2.22–4.06)	(1.31–3.00)		(0.71–1.62)		(2.17–4.26)
GROUP 2[b]							
N	12	12	ND	10	ND	12	12
Level	0.14	3.78		1.21		0.76[d]	3.31
95% CI	(0.11–0.18)	(2.18–6.56)		(0.63–2.35)		(0.37–1.55)	(1.61–6.77)

* µg antibody/mL by RIA
[a] Group 1: Reimmunized at 27 months following primary immunization.
[b] Group 2: Reimmunized at 34 months following primary immunization.
[c] Not Done
[d] Antibody levels pre-reimmunization.
[e] Includes available data from all reimmunized subjects (subjects initially randomized to Typhim Vi, and subjects initially randomized to placebo who received open label Typhim Vi two weeks later).

areas where a recognized risk of exposure to typhoid exists, particularly ones who will have prolonged exposure to potentially contaminated food and water, 2) persons with intimate exposure (i.e., continued household contact) to a documented typhoid carrier, and 3) workers in microbiology laboratories who frequently work with *S. typhi*.[14]

Typhoid vaccination is not required for international travel, but is recommended for travelers to areas where there is a recognized risk of exposure to *S. typhi*. *S. typhi* is prevalent in many countries of Africa, Asia, and Central and South America. Current CDC advisories should be consulted with regard to specific locales. Vaccination is particularly recommended for travelers who will have prolonged exposure to potentially contaminated food and water. However, even travelers who have been vaccinated should use caution in selecting food and water.[15]

Based on the available efficacy data, vaccination of Typhim Vi may not be expected to protect 100% of susceptible individuals.

There is no evidence to support the use of typhoid vaccine to control common source outbreaks, disease following natural disaster or in persons attending rural summer camps.[16]

An optimal reimmunization schedule has not been established. Reimmunization every two years under conditions of repeated or continued exposure to the *S. typhi* organism is recommended at this time.

Typhim Vi has efficacy against typhoid fever caused by *S. typhi* infection but will not afford protection against species of *Salmonella* and other than *S. typhi* or other bacteria that cause enteric disease.

For recommended primary immunization and reimmunization see **DOSAGE AND ADMINISTRATION** section.

Typhim Vi should not be used to treat a patient with typhoid fever or a chronic typhoid carrier.

CONTRAINDICATIONS

TYPHIM Vi IS CONTRAINDICATED IN PATIENTS WITH A HISTORY OF HYPERSENSITIVITY TO ANY COMPONENT OF THIS VACCINE

WARNINGS

Allergic reactions have been reported rarely in the French post-marketing experience (see **ADVERSE REACTIONS** section).

If Typhim Vi is administered to immunosuppressed persons or persons receiving immunosuppressive therapy, the expected immune response may not be obtained. This includes patients with asymptomatic or symptomatic HIV-infection, severe combined immunodeficiency, hypogammaglobulinemia, or agammaglobulinemia; altered immune states due to diseases such as leukemia, lymphoma, or generalized malignancy; or an immune system compromised by treatment with corticosteroids, alkylating drugs, antimetabolites or radiation.[17]

As with any intramuscular injection, Typhim Vi should be given with caution to individuals with thrombocytopenia or any coagulation disorder that would contraindicate intramuscular injection (see **DRUG INTERACTIONS** section).

PRECAUTIONS

GENERAL

Care is to be taken by the health-care provider for the safe and effective use of Typhim Vi.

EPINEPHRINE INJECTION (1:1000) MUST BE IMMEDIATELY AVAILABLE FOLLOWING IMMUNIZATION SHOULD AN ANAPHYLACTIC OR OTHER ALLERGIC REACTIONS OCCUR DUE TO ANY COMPONENT OF THE VACCINE.

Prior to an injection of any vaccine, all known precautions should be taken to prevent adverse reactions. This includes a review of the patient's history with respect to possible hypersensitivity to the vaccine or similar vaccines.

Acute infection or febrile illness may be reason for delaying use of Typhim Vi except when in the opinion of the physician, withholding the vaccine entails a greater risk.

A separate, sterile syringe and needle or a sterile disposable unit must be used for each patient to prevent the transmission of infectious agents from person to person. Needles should not be recapped and should be properly disposed.

Special care should be taken to ensure that Typhim Vi is not injected into a blood vessel.

Safety and immunogenicity data from controlled trials are not available for Typhim Vi following previous immunization with whole-cell typhoid or live, oral typhoid vaccine (see **ADVERSE REACTIONS** section).

INFORMATION FOR PATIENTS

Patients, parents or guardians should be fully informed of the benefits and risks of immunization with Typhim Vi.

Prior to administration of Typhim Vi, patients, parents and guardians should be asked about the recent health status of the patient to be immunized.

Typhim Vi is indicated in persons traveling to endemic or epidemic areas. Current CDC advisories should be consulted with regard to specific locales.

Travelers should take all necessary precautions to avoid contact with or ingestion of contaminated food and water.

TABLE 3.[10,11] **PERCENTAGE OF 18- TO 40-YEAR-OLD US ADULTS PRESENTING WITH LOCAL OR SYSTEMIC REACTIONS WITHIN 48 HOURS AFTER THE FIRST IMMUNIZATION WITH TYPHIM Vi**

REACTION	Trial 1 Placebo N = 54	Trial 1 Typhim Vi N = 54 (1 Lot)	Trial 2 Typhim Vi N = 98 (2 Lots combined)
Local			
Tenderness	7 (13.0%)	53 (98.0%)	95 (96.9%)
Pain	4 (7.4%)	22 (40.7%)	26 (26.5%)
Induration	0	8 (14.8%)	5 (5.1%)
Erythema	0	2 (3.7%)	5 (5.1%)
Systemic			
Malaise	8 (14.8%)	12 (24.0%)	4 (4.1%)
Headache	7 (13.0%)	11 (20.4%)	16 (16.3%)
Myalgia	0	4 (7.4%)	3 (3.1%)
Nausea	2 (3.7%)	1 (1.9%)	8 (8.2%)
Diarrhea	2 (3.7%)	0	3 (3.1%)
Feverish (subjective)	0	6 (11.1%)	3 (3.1%)
Fever ≥100°F	0	1 (1.9%)	0
Vomiting	0	1 (1.9%)	0

One dose of vaccine should be given at least 2 weeks prior to expected exposure.

An optimal reimmunization schedule has not been established. Reimmunization consisting of a single dose for US travelers every two years under conditions of repeated or continued exposure to the *S. typhi* organism is recommended at this time.

As part of the child's or adult's immunization record, the date, lot number and manufacturer of the vaccine administered should be recorded.[18]

The US Department of Health and Human Services has established a new Vaccine Adverse Event Reporting System (VAERS) to accept reports of suspected adverse events after the administration of any vaccine, including but not limited to the reporting of events required by the National Childhood Vaccine Injury Act of 1986.[19,20] The toll-free number for VAERS forms and information is 1-800-822-7967.[18]

DRUG INTERACTIONS

There are no known interactions with Typhim Vi with drugs or foods.

No studies have been conducted in the US to evaluate interactions or immunological interference between the concurrent use of Typhim Vi and drugs (including antibiotics and antimalarial drugs), immune globulins or common traveler's vaccines (e.g., vaccines for tetanus, poliomyelitis, yellow fever and meningococcus). (See **ADVERSE REACTIONS** section.)

As with other intramuscular injections, Typhim Vi should be given with caution to individuals on anticoagulant therapy.

CARCINOGENESIS, MUTAGENESIS, IMPAIRMENT OF FERTILITY

Typhim Vi has not been evaluated for its carcinogenic potential, mutagenic potential or impairment of fertility.

PREGNANCY

REPRODUCTIVE STUDIES—PREGNANCY CATEGORY C

Animal reproduction studies have not been conducted with Typhim Vi. It is not known whether Typhim Vi can cause fetal harm when administered to a pregnant woman or can affect reproduction capacity. Typhim Vi should be given to a pregnant woman only if clearly needed.[21]

When possible, delaying vaccination until the second or third trimester to minimize the possibility of teratogenicity is a reasonable precaution.[14]

NURSING MOTHERS

It is not known if Typhim Vi is excreted in human milk.

There is no data to warrant the use of this product in nursing mothers for passive antibody transfer to an infant.

PEDIATRIC USE

Safety and effectiveness of Typhim Vi have been established in children 2 years of age and older.[10,11] (See **DOSAGE AND ADMINISTRATION** section.) FOR CHILDREN BELOW THE AGE OF 2 YEARS, SAFETY AND EFFECTIVENESS HAVE NOT BEEN ESTABLISHED.

ADVERSE REACTIONS

Safety of Typhim Vi, the US licensed liquid formulation, has been assessed in clinical trials in more than 4,000 subjects both in countries of high and low endemicity. In addition, the safety of the lyophilized formulation has been assessed in more than 6,000 individuals. The adverse reactions were predominately minor and transient local reactions. Local reactions such as injection site pain, erythema and induration almost always resolved within 48 hours of vaccination. Elevated oral temperature, above 38°C (100.4°F), was observed in approximately 1% of vaccinees in all studies. No serious or life-threatening systemic events were reported in these clinical trials.[10,11]

Adverse reactions from two trials evaluating Typhim Vi lots in the US (18- to 40-year-old adults) are summarized in TABLE 3. No severe or unusual side effects were observed. Most subjects reported pain and/or tenderness (pain upon direct pressure). Local adverse experiences were generally limited to the first 48 hours.[10,11]

[See table 3 above]

No studies were conducted in US children. Adverse reactions from a trial in Indonesia in children one to twelve years of age are summarized in TABLE 4.[10,11] No severe or unusual side effects were observed.

TABLE 4.[10,11] PERCENTAGE OF INDONESIAN CHILDREN ONE TO TWELVE YEARS OF AGE PRESENTING WITH LOCAL OR SYSTEMIC REACTIONS WITHIN 48 HOURS AFTER THE FIRST IMMUNIZATION WITH TYPHIM Vi

REACTIONS	N=175
Local	
Soreness	23 (13.0%)
Pain	25 (14.3%)
Erythema	12 (6.9%)
Induration	5 (2.9%)
Impaired Limb Use	0
Systemic	
Feverishness*	5 (2.9%)
Headache	0
Decreased Activity	3 (1.7%)

*Subjective feeling of fever.

In the US Reimmunization Study, subjects who had received Typhim Vi 27 or 34 months earlier, and subjects who had never previously received a typhoid vaccination, were randomized to placebo or Typhim Vi, in a double-blind study. Safety data from the US Reimmunization Study are presented in TABLE 5.[10,11,13] In this study 5/30 (17%) primary immunization subjects and 10/45 (22%) reimmunization subjects had an objective local reaction. No severe or unusual side effects were observed. Most subjects reported pain and/or tenderness (pain upon direct pressure). Local adverse experiences were generally limited to the first 48 hours.[10,11,13]

[See table 5 at bottom of next page]

Post-marketing data from foreign countries are available. During the first 5.5 years following approval of Typhim Vi in France, approximately 3.89 million doses were distributed in France. An additional 10.8 million doses have been distributed to other countries worldwide. Reports of adverse events were received either by the French post-marketing surveillance system, which utilizes spontaneous reporting of adverse events, or directly by Pasteur Mérieux; 56 and 16 reports were received, respectively, from French and other foreign distribution. Local events reported included erythema, induration and/or pain at the injection site and lymphadenopathy. Systemic events reported included fever, flu-like episode, headache, cervical pain, vomiting, diarrhea, abdominal pain, tremor, hypotension, loss of consciousness, allergic type reactions including urticaria, and other events described below.[10,11]

In the French post-marketing experience, there was one report of diffuse arthralgias and fever two weeks post-vaccination in a 44-year-old female who had also received hepatitis B vaccine simultaneously; one report of glomerulonephritis seven days post-vaccination in a 23-year-old male who had also received BCG vaccine; one report of neutropenia in a 29-year-old female two days post-vaccination who had also received yellow fever vaccine; one report of bilateral retinitis three weeks post-vaccination in a 26-year-old male who had also received hepatitis B vaccine; and one report of polyarthritis four days post-vaccination in an 18-year-old male who had also received Meningococcal Groups

Continued on next page

Typhim VI—Cont.

A + C vaccine and DT Polio (Diphtheria Tetanus Poliomyelitis) vaccine combination manufactured by Pasteur Mérieux Sérums & Vaccins.[10,11]

In the French post-marketing experience, the most severe allergic-type reaction occurred in a 24-year-old female with known multiple allergies who had previously received two complete series with whole-cell typhoid vaccine; she experienced sweats, myalgia and difficulty breathing starting two hours after an IM injection (deltoid) of Typhim Vi. She received 10 mg hydrocortisone and did not require hospitalization.[10,11]

Reporting of Adverse Events

Reporting by parents and patients of all adverse events occurring after vaccine administration should be encouraged. Adverse events following immunization with vaccine should be reported by the health-care provider to the US Department of Health and Human Services (DHHS) Vaccine Adverse Event Reporting System (VAERS). Reporting forms and information about reporting requirements or completion of the form can be obtained from VAERS through a toll-free number 1-800-822-7967.[18]

Health-care providers also should report these events to the Director of Medical Affairs, Connaught Laboratories, Inc., Route 611, P.O. Box 187, Swiftwater, PA 18370, the US distributor, or call 1-800-822-2463.

DOSAGE AND ADMINISTRATION

Parenteral drug products should be inspected visually for particulate matter and/or discoloration prior to administration. If either of these conditions exist, the vaccine should not be administered.

For intramuscular use only. Do NOT inject intravenously. Typhim Vi vaccine is indicated for persons two years of age and older.

The immunizing dose for adults and children is a single injection of 0.5 mL. The dose for adults is given intramuscularly in the deltoid, and the dose for children is given IM either in the deltoid or the vastus lateralis. The vaccine should not be injected into the gluteal area or areas where there may be a nerve trunk.

A reimmunizing dose is 0.5 mL. An optimal reimmunization schedule has not been established. Reimmunization consisting of a single dose for US travelers every two years under conditions of repeated or continued exposure to the *S. typhi* organism is recommended at this time.

The skin at the site of injection first should be cleansed and disinfected. Tear off upper aluminum seal of cap. Cleanse top of rubber stopper of the vial with a suitable antiseptic and wipe away all excess antiseptic before withdrawing vaccine.

For single dose syringes, thread the plunger rod into stopper until the plunger rod bottoms out against the stopper and resistance is felt. Do not over tighten the plunger rod. A separate, sterile syringe and needle or a sterile disposable unit should be used for each patient to prevent transmission of infectious agents from person to person. Needles should not be recapped and should be properly disposed.

There are no data on the safety and efficacy of Typhim Vi administered with any jet injector apparatus and this method of delivery is not recommended.

HOW SUPPLIED

Syringe, 0.5 mL—Product No. 49281-790-01
Vial, 20 Dose (Available on special contract basis only.)—Product No. 49281-790-20
Vial, 50 Dose (Available on special contract basis only.)—Product No. 49281-790-20

STORAGE

Store between 2°–8°C (35°–46°F). DO NOT FREEZE.

REFERENCES

1. Levine MM, et al. New knowledge on pathogenesis of bacterial enteric infections as applied to vaccine development. Microbiol. Rev. 47:510–550, 1983.
2. Levine MM. Typhoid Fever Vaccines. p 333–361. In Vaccines, Plotkin SA, Mortimer EA, eds. W.B. Saunders, 1988
3. Levine MM, et al. Typhoid Fever Chapter 5, In: *Vaccines and Immunotherapy.* Stanley J. Cryz, Jr., Editor. pp 59–72, 1991
4. CDC. Summary of Notifiable Diseases, United States 1992. MMWR 41: No. 55, 1993
5. Ryan CA, et al. *Salmonella typhi* infections in the United States, 1975–1984: Increasing Role of Foreign Travel. Rev Infect Dis 11:1–8, 1989
6. Woodruff BA, et al. A new look at typhoid vaccination. Information for the practicing physician. JAMA 265: 756–759, 1991
7. Ames WR, et al. Age and sex as factors in the development of the typhoid carrier state, and a method for estimating carrier prevalence. Am J Public Health 33: 221–230, 1943
8. CDC. Typhoid fever—Skagit County, Washington. MMWR 39: 749–751, 1990
9. Acharya IL, et al. Prevention of typhoid fever in Nepal with the Vi capsular polysaccharide of *Salmonella typhi.* N Engl J Med 317: 1101–1104, 1987
10. Unpublished data available from Connaught Laboratories, Inc., compiled 1991
11. Unpublished data available from Pasteur Mérieux Sérums & Vaccins S.A.
12. Klugman KP, et al. Protective activity of Vi capsular polysaccharide vaccine against typhoid fever. The Lancet, 1165–1169, 1987
13. Keitel WA, et al. Clinical and serological responses following primary and booster immunization with *Salmonella typhi* Vi capsular polysaccharide vaccines. Vaccine 12: 195–199, 1994
14. Recommendations of the Advisor Committee on Immunization Practices (ACIP): Update on Adult Immunization. MMWR 40: No. RR-12, 1991
15. CDC. Health Information for International Travel 1992. U.S. Department of Health and Human Services, Public Health Service
16. Recommendations of the Immunization Practices Advisory Committee (ACIP). Typhoid Immunization. MMWR 39: No. RR-10, 1990
17. ACIP: Use of vaccines and immune globulins in persons with altered immunocompetence. MMWR 42: No. RR-4, 1993
18. CDC. Vaccine Adverse Event Reporting System—United States. MMWR 39:730–733, 1990
19. National Childhood Vaccine Injury Act: Requirements for permanent vaccination records and for reporting of selected events after vaccination. MMWR 37: 197–200, 1988
20. National Childhood Vaccine Injury Act of 1986 (Amended 1987)
21. Recommendations of the ACIP. General recommendations on immunization. MMWR 43: No. RR-14, 1994

Product Information as of June 1995

Manufactured by:
PASTEUR MÉRIEUX Sérums & Vaccins S.A.
Lyon, France   US License No. 384

Distributed by:
CONNAUGHT   LABORATORIES,   INC.
Swiftwater, Pennsylvania 18370, USA.
1-800-VACCINE (1-800-822-2463)

3029

Shown in Product Identification Guide, page 330

YF-VAX®
YELLOW FEVER VACCINE   ℞

Caution: Federal (U.S.A.) law prohibits dispensing without prescription.

> For special instructions on use of Yellow Fever for JET INJECTOR USE—see other side of insert.

DESCRIPTION

YF-VAX®, Yellow Fever Vaccine (for subcutaneous use), is prepared by culturing the 17D strain of yellow fever virus in living avian leukosis virus-free (ALV-free) chicken embryos. The vaccine, containing sorbitol and gelatin as a stabilizer, is lyophilized, and hermetically sealed under nitrogen. No preservative is added. The vaccine must be reconstituted immediately before use with the sterile diluent provided (Sodium Chloride Injection USP—contains no preservative). YF-VAX is formulated to contain not less than 5.04 Log_{10} Plaque Forming Units (PFU) per 0.5 mL dose. The vaccine appears slightly opalescent and light orange in color after reconstitution.

YF-VAX complies with official potency tests and other requirements of the U.S. Food and Drug Administration (FDA), and the World Health Organization (WHO).

HOW SUPPLIED

Vial, 1 Dose (5 per package) with vial of diluent (5 per package) for administration with needle and syringe. Product No. 49281-915-01
Vial, 5 Dose, with vial of diluent, for administration with needle and syringe. Product No. 49281-915-05
Vial, 20 Dose, with vial of diluent, for administration with needle and syringe or jet injector use. Product No. 49281-915-20
Vial, 100 Dose, with vial of diluent, for JET INJECTOR USE ONLY; *this package size and others available on special contract basis only.*

> YF-VAX® (Yellow Fever Vaccine) in the United States is supplied only to designated Yellow Fever Vaccination Centers authorized to issue valid certificates of Yellow Fever Vaccination. Location of the nearest Yellow Fever Vaccination Centers may be obtained from the Centers for Disease Control and Prevention Atlanta, GA 30333, state or local health departments, or the USPHS booklet "Immunization Information for International Travel" (obtainable from the Superintendent of Documents, U.S. Government Printing Office, Washington, D.C. 20402).

Shown in Product Identification Guide, page 330

PathoGenesis Corporation
**201 ELLIOTT AVENUE WEST
SEATTLE, WA 98119**

Direct Inquiries to:
Ph. 1-888-508-TOBI (8624)

TOBI   ℞
**Tobramycin Solution for Inhalation
Nebulizer Solution—For Inhalation Use Only**

PRESCRIBING INFORMATION

DESCRIPTION

TOBI® is a tobramycin solution for inhalation. It is a sterile, clear, slightly yellow, non-pyrogenic, aqueous solution with the pH and salinity adjusted specifically for administration by a compressed air driven reusable nebulizer. The chemical formula for tobramycin is $C_{18}H_{37}N_5O_9$ and the molecular weight is 467.52. Tobramycin is O-3-amino-3-deoxy-α-D-glucopyranosyl-(1→4)-O-[2,6-diamino-2,3,6-trideoxy-α-D-*ribo*-hexopyranosyl-(1→6)]-2-deoxy-L-streptamine. The structural formula for tobramycin is:
[See chemical structure at top of next column]
Each single-use 5 mL ampule contains 300 mg tobramycin and 11.25 mg sodium chloride in sterile water for injection. Sulfuric acid and sodium hydroxide are added to adjust the pH to 6.0. Nitrogen is used for sparging. All ingredients meet USP requirements. The formulation contains no preservatives.

TABLE 5.[10,11,13]   U. S. REIMMUNIZATION STUDY, SUBJECTS PRESENTING WITH LOCAL AND SYSTEMIC REACTIONS WITHIN 48 HOURS AFTER IMMUNIZATION WITH TYPHIM Vi

REACTIONS	PLACEBO (N=32)	FIRST IMMUNIZATION (N=30)	REIMMUNIZATION (N=45*)
Local			
Tenderness	2 (6%)	28 (93%)	44 (98%)
Pain	1 (3%)	13 (43%)	25 (56%)
Induration	0	5 (17%)	8 (18%)
Erythema	0	1 (3%)	5 (11%)
Systemic			
Malaise	1 (3%)	11 (37%)	11 (24%)
Headache	5 (16%)	8 (27%)	5 (11%)
Myalgia	0	2 (7%)	1 (2%)
Nausea	0	1 (3%)	1 (2%)
Diarrhea	0	0	1 (2%)
Feverish (subjective)	0	3 (10%)	2 (4%)
Fever ≥100°F	1 (3%)	0	1 (2%)
Vomiting	0	0	0

*At 27 or 34 months following a previous dose given in different studies.

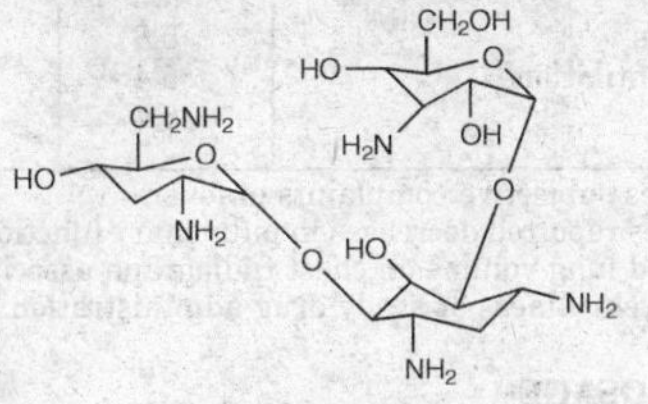

CLINICAL PHARMACOLOGY

TOBI is specifically formulated for administration by inhalation. When inhaled, tobramycin is concentrated in the airways.

Pharmacokinetics

TOBI contains tobramycin, a cationic polar molecule that does not readily cross epithelial membranes.[1] The bioavailability of TOBI may vary because of individual differences in nebulizer performance and airway pathology.[2] Following administration of TOBI, tobramycin remains concentrated primarily in the airways.

Sputum Concentrations: Ten minutes after inhalation of the first 300 mg dose of TOBI, the average concentration of tobramycin was 1237 µg/g (ranging from 35 to 7414 µg/g) in sputum. Tobramycin does not accumulate in sputum; after 20 weeks of therapy with the TOBI regimen, the average concentration of tobramycin at ten minutes after inhalation was 1154 µg/g (ranging from 39 to 8085 µg/g) in sputum. High variability of tobramycin concentration in sputum was observed. Two hours after inhalation, sputum concentrations declined to approximately 14% of tobramycin levels at ten minutes after inhalation.

Serum Concentrations: The average serum concentration of tobramycin one hour after inhalation of a single 300 mg dose of TOBI by cystic fibrosis patients was 0.95 µg/mL. After 20 weeks of therapy on the TOBI regimen, the average serum tobramycin concentration one hour after dosing was 1.05 µg/mL.

Elimination: The elimination half-life of tobramycin from serum is approximately 2 hours after intravenous (IV) administration. Assuming tobramycin absorbed following inhalation behaves similarly to tobramycin following IV administration, systemically absorbed tobramycin is eliminated principally by glomerular filtration. Unabsorbed tobramycin, following TOBI administration, is probably eliminated primarily in expectorated sputum.

Microbiology

Tobramycin is an aminoglycoside antibiotic produced by *Streptomyces tenebrarius*.[1] It acts primarily by disrupting protein synthesis, leading to altered cell membrane permeability, progressive disruption of the cell envelope, and eventual cell death.[3]

Tobramycin has *in vitro* activity against a wide range of gram-negative organisms including *Pseudomonas aeruginosa*. It is bactericidal at concentrations equal to or slightly greater than inhibitory concentrations.

Susceptibility Testing

A single sputum sample from a cystic fibrosis patient may contain multiple morphotypes of *Pseudomonas aeruginosa* and each morphotype may have a different level of *in vitro* susceptibility to tobramycin. Treatment for 6 months with TOBI in two clinical studies did not affect the susceptibility of the majority of *P. aeruginosa* isolates tested; however, increased minimum inhibitory concentrations (MICs) were noted in some patients. The clinical significance of this information has not been clearly established in the treatment of *P. aeruginosa* in cystic fibrosis patients. For additional information regarding the effects of TOBI on *P. aeruginosa* MIC values and bacterial sputum density, please refer to the **CLINICAL STUDIES** section.

The *in vitro* antimicrobial susceptibility test methods used for parenteral tobramycin therapy can be used to monitor the susceptibility of *P. aeruginosa* isolated from cystic fibrosis patients. If decreased susceptibility is noted, the results should be reported to the clinician.

Susceptibility breakpoints established for parenteral administration of tobramycin do not apply to aerosolized administration of TOBI. The relationship between *in vitro* susceptibility test results and clinical outcome with TOBI therapy is not clear.

INDICATIONS AND USAGE

TOBI is indicated for the management of cystic fibrosis patients with *P. aeruginosa*.

Safety and efficacy have not been demonstrated in patients under the age of 6 years, patients with FEV_1 <25% or >75% predicted, or patients colonized with *Burkholderia cepacia* (see **CLINICAL STUDIES**).

CONTRAINDICATIONS

TOBI is contraindicated in patients with a known hypersensitivity to any aminoglycoside.

WARNINGS

Caution should be exercised when prescribing TOBI to patients with known or suspected renal, auditory, vestibular, or neuromuscular dysfunction. Patients receiving concomitant parenteral aminoglycoside therapy should be monitored as clinically appropriate.

Aminoglycosides can cause fetal harm when administered to a pregnant woman. Aminoglycosides cross the placenta, and streptomycin has been associated with several reports of total, irreversible, bilateral congenital deafness in pediatric patients exposed *in utero*. Patients who use TOBI during pregnancy, or become pregnant while taking TOBI should be apprised of the potential hazard to the fetus.

Ototoxicity

Ototoxicity, as measured by complaints of hearing loss or by audiometric evaluations, did not occur with TOBI therapy during clinical studies. However, transient tinnitus occurred in eight TOBI-treated patients versus no placebo patients in the clinical studies. Tinnitus is a sentinel symptom of ototoxicity, and therefore the onset of this symptom warrants caution (see **ADVERSE REACTIONS**). Ototoxicity, manifested as both auditory and vestibular toxicity, has been reported with parenteral aminoglycosides. Vestibular toxicity may be manifested by vertigo, ataxia or dizziness.

Nephrotoxicity

Nephrotoxicity was not seen during TOBI clinical studies but has been associated with aminoglycosides as a class. If nephrotoxicity occurs in a patient receiving TOBI, tobramycin therapy should be discontinued until serum concentrations fall below 2 µg/mL.

Muscular Disorders

TOBI should be used cautiously in patients with muscular disorders, such as myasthenia gravis or Parkinson's disease, since aminoglycosides may aggravate muscle weakness because of a potential curare-like effect on neuromuscular function.

Bronchospasm

Bronchospasm can occur with inhalation of TOBI. In clinical studies of TOBI, changes in FEV_1 measured after the inhaled dose were similar in the TOBI and placebo groups. Bronchospasm should be treated as medically appropriate.

PRECAUTIONS

Information for Patients

NOTE: In addition to information provided below, a Patient Medication Guide providing instructions for proper use of TOBI is contained inside the package.

Safety Information

TOBI is in a class of antibiotics that, when given by injection, have caused hearing loss, dizziness, kidney damage, and harm to a fetus. Ringing in the ears and hoarseness were two symptoms that were seen in more patients taking TOBI than placebo in research studies. Patients with cystic fibrosis can have many symptoms. Some of these symptoms may be related to your medications. If you have new or worsening symptoms, you should tell your doctor.

Hearing: You should tell your doctor if you have ringing in the ears, dizziness, or any changes in hearing.

Kidney Damage: Inform your doctor if you have any history of kidney problems.

Pregnancy: If you want to become pregnant or are pregnant while on TOBI, you should talk with your doctor about the possibility of TOBI causing any harm.

Nursing Mothers: If you are nursing a baby, you should talk with your doctor before using TOBI.

TOBI Packaging

TOBI comes in a single dose, ready-to-use ampule containing 300 mg tobramycin. Each box of TOBI contains a 28-day supply - 56 ampules packaged in 14 foil pouches. Each foil pouch contains four ampules, for two days of TOBI therapy.

Dosage

The 300 mg dose of TOBI is the same for patients regardless of age or weight. TOBI has not been studied in patients less than six years old. Doses should be inhaled as close to 12 hours apart as possible and not less than six hours apart.

You should not mix TOBI with dornase alfa (PULMOZYME®, Genentech) in the nebulizer.

If you are taking several medications the recommended order is as follows: bronchodilator first, followed by chest physiotherapy, then other inhaled medications and, finally, TOBI.

Treatment Schedule

You should take TOBI in repeated cycles of 28 days on drug followed by 28 days off drug. You should take TOBI twice a day during the 28 day period on drug.

How to Administer TOBI

THIS INFORMATION IS NOT INTENDED TO REPLACE CONSULTATION WITH YOUR PHYSICIAN AND CF CARE TEAM ABOUT PROPERLY TAKING MEDICATION OR USING INHALATION EQUIPMENT.

TOBI is specially formulated for inhalation using a PARI LC PLUS™ reusable nebulizer and a DeVilbiss Pulmo-Aide® air compressor. TOBI can be taken at home, school, or at work. The following are instructions on how to use the DeVilbiss Pulmo-Aide Compressor and PARI LC PLUS reusable nebulizer to administer TOBI.

You will need the following supplies:

- TOBI plastic ampule (vial)
- DeVilbiss Pulmo-Aide Compressor
- PARI LC PLUS reusable nebulizer
- Tubing to connect the nebulizer and compressor
- Clean paper or cloth towels
- Nose clips (optional)

It is important that your nebulizer and compressor function properly before starting your TOBI therapy.

Note: Please refer to the manufacturers' care and use instructions for important information.

Preparing Your TOBI For Inhalation

1. Wash your hands thoroughly with soap and water.
2. TOBI is packaged with four ampules per foil pouch. Remove one ampule of TOBI from the foil pouch. Store all remaining ampules in the refrigerator as directed.
3. Lay out the contents of a PARI LC PLUS reusable nebulizer package on a clean, dry paper or cloth towel. You should have the following parts:
   - Nebulizer Top and Bottom (Nebulizer Cup) Assembly
   - Inspiratory Valve Cap
   - Mouthpiece with Valve
   - Tubing
4. Remove the Nebulizer Top from the Nebulizer Cup by twisting the Nebulizer Top counter-clock-wise, and then lifting. Place the Nebulizer Top on the clean paper towel or cloth towel. Stand the Nebulizer Cup upright on the towel.
5. Connect one end of the tubing to the compressor air outlet. The tubing should fit snugly. Plug in your compressor to an electrical outlet.
6. Open the TOBI ampule by holding the bottom tab with one hand and twisting off the top of the ampule with the other. Be careful not to squeeze the ampule until you are ready to empty its contents into the Nebulizer Cup.
7. Squeeze all the contents of the ampule into the Nebulizer Cup.
8. Replace the Nebulizer Top. Note: the Semi-Circle halfway down the stem of the Nebulizer Top should face the Nebulizer Outlet to reinsert into the Nebulizer Cup. Turn the Nebulizer Top clockwise until securely fastened to the Nebulizer Cup.
9. Attach the Mouthpiece to the Nebulizer Outlet. Then firmly push the Inspiratory Valve Cap in place on the Nebulizer Top. Note: the Inspiratory Valve Cap will fit snugly.
10. Connect the free end of the tubing to the Air Intake on the bottom of the nebulizer, making sure to keep the nebulizer upright. Press the tubing on the Air Intake firmly.

TOBI Treatment

1. Turn on the compressor.
2. Check for a steady mist from the Mouthpiece. If there is no mist, check all tubing connections and confirm that the compressor is working properly.
3. Sit or stand in an upright position that will allow you to breathe normally.
4. Place Mouthpiece between your teeth and on top of your tongue and breathe normally only through your mouth. Nose clips may help you breathe through your mouth and not through your nose. Do not block airflow with your tongue.
5. Continue treatment until all your TOBI is gone, and there is no longer any mist being produced. You may hear a sputtering sound when the Nebulizer Cup is empty. The entire TOBI treatment should take approximately 15 minutes to complete. Note: if you are interrupted, need to cough or rest during your TOBI treatment, turn off the compressor to save your medication. Turn the compressor back on when you are ready to resume your therapy.
6. Follow the nebulizer cleaning and disinfecting instructions after completing therapy.

Cleaning Your Nebulizer

To reduce the risk of infection, illness or injury from contamination, you must thoroughly clean all parts of the nebulizer as instructed after each treatment. Never use a nebulizer with a clogged nozzle. If the nozzle is clogged, no aerosol mist is produced, which will alter the effectiveness of the treatment. Replace the nebulizer if clogging occurs.

1. Remove tubing from nebulizer and disassemble nebulizer parts.
2. Wash all parts (except tubing) with warm water and liquid dish soap.
3. Rinse thoroughly with warm water and shake out water.
4. Air dry or hand dry nebulizer parts on a clean, lint-free cloth. Reassemble nebulizer when dry, and store.
5. You can also wash all parts of the nebulizer in a dishwasher (except tubing). Place the nebulizer parts in a dishwasher basket, then place on the top rack of the dishwasher. Remove and dry the parts when the cycle is complete.

Disinfecting Your Nebulizer

Your nebulizer is for your use only—Do not share your nebulizer with other people. You must regularly disinfect the nebulizer. Failure to do so could lead to serious or fatal illness.

1. Clean the nebulizer as described above. Every other treatment day, soak all parts of the nebulizer (except tubing) in a solution of 1 part distilled white vinegar and 3 parts hot tap water for 1 hour. You can substitute respi-

Continued on next page

TOBI—Cont.

ratory equipment disinfectants (such as Control III®) for distilled white vinegar (follow manufacturer's instructions for mixing). Rinse all parts of the nebulizer thoroughly with warm tap water and dry with a clean, lint-free cloth. Discard the vinegar solution when disinfection is complete.

2. The nebulizer parts (except tubing) may also be disinfected by boiling them in water for a full 10 minutes. Dry parts on a clean, lint-free cloth.

Care and Use of Your Pulmo-Aide Compressor

Follow the manufacturer's instructions for care and use of your compressor.

Filter Change:

1. DeVilbiss Compressor filters should be changed every six months or sooner if filter turns completely gray in color.

Compressor Cleaning:

1. With power switch in the "Off" position, unplug power cord from wall outlet.
2. Wipe outside of the compressor cabinet with a clean, damp cloth every few days to keep dust free.

Caution: Do not submerge in water: doing so will result in compressor damage.

Storage Instructions

You should store TOBI ampules in a refrigerator (2–8°C or 36–46°F). However, when you don't have a refrigerator available (e.g., transporting your TOBI), you may store the foil pouches (opened or unopened) at room temperature (up to 25°C/77°F) for up to 28 days.

Avoid exposing TOBI ampules to intense light.

Unrefrigerated TOBI, which is normally slightly yellow, may darken with age; however, the color change does not indicate any change in the quality of the product.

You should not use TOBI if it is cloudy, if there are particles in the solution, or if it has been stored at room temperature for more than 28 days. You should not use TOBI beyond the expiration date stamped on the ampule.

Additional Information

Nebulizer: 1-800-327-8632
Compressor: 1-800-338-1988
TOBI: 1-888-508-TOBI (8624)

Laboratory Tests

Audiograms

Clinical studies of TOBI did not identify hearing loss using audiometric tests which evaluated hearing up to 8000 Hz. Tinnitus may be a sentinel symptom of ototoxicity, and therefore the onset of this symptom warrants caution. Physicians should consider an audiogram for patients who show any evidence of auditory dysfunction, or who are at increased risk for auditory dysfunction.

Serum Concentrations

In patients with normal renal function treated with TOBI, serum tobramycin concentrations are approximately 1 μg/mL one hour after dose administration and do not require routine monitoring. Serum concentrations of tobramycin in patients with renal dysfunction or patients treated with concomitant parenteral tobramycin should be monitored at the discretion of the treating physician.

Renal Function

The clinical studies of TOBI did not reveal any imbalance in the percentage of patients in the TOBI and placebo groups who experienced at least a 50% rise in serum creatinine from baseline (see **ADVERSE REACTIONS**). Laboratory tests of urine and renal function should be conducted at the discretion of the treating physician.

Drug Interactions

In clinical studies of TOBI, patients taking TOBI concomitantly with dornase alfa (PULMOZYME®, Genentech), β-agonists, inhaled corticosteroids, other anti-pseudomonal antibiotics, or parenteral aminoglycosides demonstrated adverse experience profiles similar to the study population as a whole.

Concurrent and/or sequential use of TOBI with other drugs with neurotoxic or ototoxic potential should be avoided. Some diuretics can enhance aminoglycoside toxicity by altering antibiotic concentrations in serum and tissue. TOBI should not be administered concomitantly with ethacrynic acid, furosemide, urea, or mannitol.

Carcinogenesis, Mutagenesis, Impairment of Fertility

A two-year rat inhalation toxicology study to assess carcinogenic potential of TOBI is in progress.

TOBI has been evaluated for genotoxicity in a battery of *in vitro* and *in vivo* tests. The Ames bacterial reversion test, conducted with five tester strains, failed to show a significant increase in revertants with or without metabolic activation in all strains. Tobramycin was negative in the mouse lymphoma forward mutation assay, did not induce chromosomal aberrations in Chinese hamster ovary cells, and was negative in the mouse micronucleus test.

Subcutaneous administration of up to 100 mg/kg of tobramycin did not affect mating behavior or cause impairment of fertility in male or female rats.

Pregnancy

Teratogenic Effects—Pregnancy Category D

(See **WARNINGS**).

No reproduction toxicology studies have been conducted with TOBI. However, subcutaneous administration of tobramycin at doses of 100 or 20 mg/kg/day during organogenesis was not teratogenic in rats or rabbits, respectively. Doses of tobramycin ≥40 mg/kg/day were severely maternally toxic to rabbits and precluded the evaluation of teratogenicity. Aminoglycosides can cause fetal harm (e.g., congenital deafness) when administered to a pregnant woman. Ototoxicity was not evaluated in offspring during nonclinical reproduction toxicity studies with tobramycin. If TOBI is used during pregnancy, or if the patient becomes pregnant while taking TOBI, the patient should be apprised of the potential hazard to the fetus.

Nursing Mothers

It is not known if TOBI will reach sufficient concentrations after administration by inhalation to be excreted in human breast milk. Because of the potential for ototoxicity and nephrotoxicity in infants, a decision should be made whether to terminate nursing or discontinue TOBI.

Pediatric Use

The safety and efficacy of TOBI have not been studied in pediatric patients under 6 years of age.

ADVERSE REACTIONS

TOBI was generally well tolerated during two clinical studies in 258 cystic fibrosis patients ranging in age from 6 to 48 years. Patients received TOBI in alternating periods of 28 days on and 28 days off drug in addition to their standard cystic fibrosis therapy for a total of 24 weeks.

Voice alteration and tinnitus were the only adverse experiences reported by significantly more TOBI-treated patients. Thirty-three patients (13%) treated with TOBI complained of voice alteration compared to 17 (7%) placebo patients. Voice alteration was more common in the on-drug periods. Eight patients from the TOBI group (3%) reported tinnitus compared to no placebo patients. All episodes were transient, resolved without discontinuation of the TOBI treatment regimen, and were not associated with loss of hearing in audiograms. Tinnitus is one of the sentinel symptoms of cochlear toxicity, and patients with this symptom should be carefully monitored for high frequency hearing loss. The numbers of patients reporting vestibular adverse experiences such as dizziness were similar in the TOBI and placebo groups.

Nine (3%) patients in the TOBI group and nine (3%) patients in the placebo group had increases in serum creatinine of at least 50% over baseline. In all nine patients in the TOBI group, creatinine decreased at the next visit.

Table 1 lists the percent of patients with treatment-emergent adverse experiences (spontaneously reported and solicited) that occurred in >5% of TOBI patients during the two Phase III studies.

Table 1: Percent of Patients With Treatment Emergent Adverse Experiences Occurring in >5% of TOBI Patients

Adverse Event	TOBI (n=258) %	Placebo (n=262) %
Cough increased	46.1	47.3
Pharyngitis	38.0	39.3
Sputum increased	37.6	39.7
Asthenia	35.7	39.3
Rhinitis	34.5	33.6
Dyspnea	33.7	38.5
Fever[1]	32.9	43.5
Lung Disorder	31.4	31.3
Headache	26.7	32.1
Chest pain	26.0	29.8
Sputum discoloration	21.3	19.8
Hemoptysis	19.4	23.7
Anorexia	18.6	27.9
Lung Function decreased[2]	16.3	15.3
Asthma	15.9	20.2
Vomiting	14.0	22.1
Abdominal pain	12.8	23.7
Voice alteration	12.8	6.5
Nausea	11.2	16.0
Weight loss	10.1	15.3
Pain	8.1	12.6
Sinusitis	8.1	9.2
Ear pain	7.4	8.8
Back pain	7.0	8.0
Epistaxis	7.0	6.5
Taste perversion	6.6	6.9
Diarrhea	6.2	10.3
Malaise	6.2	5.3
Lower Resp. Tract Infection	5.8	8.0
Dizziness	5.8	7.6
Hyperventilation	5.4	9.9
Rash	5.4	6.1

[1] Includes subjective complaints of fever.
[2] Includes reported decreases in pulmonary function tests or decreased lung volume on chest radiograph associated with intercurrent illness or study drug administration.

OVERDOSAGE

Signs and symptoms of acute toxicity from overdosage of IV tobramycin might include dizziness, tinnitus, vertigo, loss of high-tone hearing acuity, respiratory failure, and neuromuscular blockade. Administration by inhalation results in low systemic bioavailability of tobramycin. Tobramycin is not significantly absorbed following oral administration. Tobramycin serum concentrations may be helpful in monitoring overdosage.

In all cases of suspected overdosage, physicians should contact the Regional Poison Control Center for information about effective treatment. In the case of any overdosage, the possibility of drug interactions with alterations in drug disposition should be considered.

DOSAGE AND ADMINISTRATION

The recommended dosage for both adults and pediatric patients 6 years of age and older is one single-use ampule (300 mg) administered BID for 28 days. Dosage is not adjusted by weight. All patients should be administered 300 mg BID. The doses should be taken as close to 12 hours apart as possible; they should not be taken less than six hours apart.

TOBI is inhaled while the patient is sitting or standing upright and breathing normally through the mouthpiece of the nebulizer. Nose clips may help the patient breathe through the mouth.

TOBI is administered BID in alternating periods of 28 days. After 28 days of therapy, patients should stop TOBI therapy for the next 28 days, and then resume therapy for the next 28 day on/28 day off cycle.

TOBI is supplied as a single-use ampule and is administered by inhalation, using a hand-held PARI LC PLUS reusable nebulizer with a DeVilbiss Pulmo-Aide compressor. TOBI is not for subcutaneous, intravenous or intrathecal administration.

Usage

TOBI is administered by inhalation over an approximate 15 minute period, using a hand-held PARI LC PLUS reusable nebulizer with a DeVilbiss Pulmo-Aide compressor. TOBI should not be diluted or mixed with dornase alfa (PULMOZYME®, Genentech) in the nebulizer.

During clinical studies, patients on multiple therapies were instructed to take them first, followed by TOBI.

HOW SUPPLIED

TOBI is supplied in single-use, low-density polyethylene plastic 5 mL ampules. TOBI is packaged in boxes of 56 ampules (14 flexible, laminated foil over-pouches, each containing 4 ampules).

Storage

TOBI should be stored under refrigeration at 2–8°C/36–46°F. Upon removal from the refrigerator, or if refrigeration is unavailable, TOBI pouches (opened or unopened) may be stored at room temperature (up to 25°C/77°F) for up to 28 days. TOBI should not be used beyond the expiration date stamped on the ampule when stored under refrigeration (2–8°C/36–46°F) or beyond 28 days when stored at room temperature (25°C/77°F).

TOBI ampules should not be exposed to intense light. The solution in the ampule is slightly yellow, but may darken with age if not stored in the refrigerator; however, the color change does not indicate any change in the quality of the product as long as it is stored within the recommended storage conditions.

NDC 63430-065-01

CLINICAL STUDIES

Two identically designed, double-blind, randomized, placebo-controlled, parallel group, 24-week clinical studies (Study 1 and Study 2) at a total of 69 cystic fibrosis centers in the United States were conducted in cystic fibrosis patients with *P. aeruginosa*. Subjects who were less than six years of age, had a baseline creatinine of > 2 mg/dL, or had *Burkholderia cepacia* isolated from sputum were excluded. All subjects had baseline FEV_1 % predicted between 25% and 75%. In these clinical studies, 258 patients received TOBI therapy on an outpatient basis (see Table 2) using a hand-held PARI LC PLUS reusable nebulizer with a DeVilbiss Pulmo-Aide compressor.

[See table 2 top of next page]

All patients received either TOBI or placebo (saline with 1.25 mg quinine for flavoring) in addition to standard treatment recommended for cystic fibrosis patients, which included oral and parenteral anti-pseudomonal therapy, β_2-agonists, cromolyn, inhaled steroids, and airway clearance techniques. In addition, approximately 77% of patients were concurrently treated with dornase alfa (PULMOZYME®, Genentech).

Table 2: Dosing Regimens in Clinical Studies

	Cycle 1		Cycle 2		Cycle 3	
	28 days	28 days	28 days	28 days	28 days	28 days
TOBI regimen n=258	TOBI 300 mg BID	no drug	TOBI 300 mg BID	no drug	TOBI 300 mg BID	no drug
Placebo regimen n=262	placebo BID	no drug	placebo BID	no drug	placebo BID	no drug

In each study, TOBI-treated patients experienced significant improvement in pulmonary function. Improvement was demonstrated in the TOBI group in Study 1 by an average increase in FEV_1% predicted of about 11% relative to baseline (Week 0) during 24 weeks compared to no average change in placebo patients. In Study 2, TOBI treated patients had an average increase of about 7% compared to an average decrease of about 1% in placebo patients. Figure 1 shows the average relative change in FEV_1% predicted over 24 weeks for both studies.

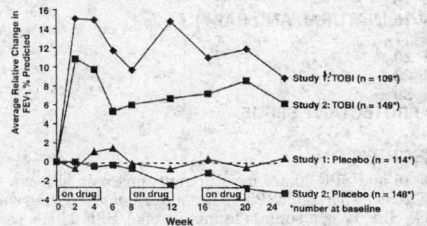

Figure 1: Relative Change From Baseline in FEV_1% Predicted

In each study, TOBI therapy resulted in a significant reduction in the number of *P. aeruginosa* colony forming units (CFUs) in sputum during the on-drug periods. Sputum bacterial density returned to baseline during the off-drug periods. Reductions in sputum bacterial density were smaller in each successive cycle (see Figure 2).

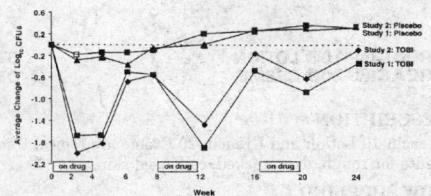

Figure 2: Absolute Change From Baseline in Log_{10} CFUs

Patients treated with TOBI were hospitalized for an average of 5.1 days compared to 8.1 days for placebo patients. Patients treated with TOBI required an average of 9.7 days of parenteral anti-pseudomonal antibiotic treatment compared to 14.1 days for placebo patients. During the six months of treatment, 40% of TOBI patients and 53% of placebo patients were treated with parenteral anti-pseudomonal antibiotics.

The relationship between *in vitro* susceptibility test results and clinical outcome with TOBI therapy is not clear. However, four TOBI patients who began the clinical trial with *P. aeruginosa* isolates having MIC values ≥128 µg/mL did not experience an improvement in FEV_1 or a decrease in sputum bacterial density.

Treatment with TOBI did not affect the susceptibility of the majority of *P. aeruginosa* isolates during the six month studies. However, some *P. aeruginosa* isolates did exhibit increased tobramycin MICs. The percentage of patients with *P. aeruginosa* isolates with tobramycin MICs ≥ 16 µg/mL was 13% at the beginning, and 23% at the end of six months of the TOBI regimen.

REFERENCES

1. Neu HC. Tobramycin: an overview. [Review]. J Infect Dis 1976; Suppl 134:S3-19.
2. Weber A, Smith A, Williams-Warren J et al. Nebulizer delivery of tobramycin to the lower respiratory tract. Pediatr Pulmonol 1994; 17 (5):331-9.
3. Bryan LE. Aminoglycoside resistance. Bryan LE, Ed. Antimicrobial drug resistance. Orlando, FL: Academic Press, 1984: 241-77.

Manufactured for
PathoGenesis Corporation
201 Elliott Avenue West, Seattle, WA 98119

by Automatic Liquid Packaging, Inc., Woodstock, IL 60098
Packaged by Packaging Coordinators Inc., Philadelphia, PA 19114-1123

DATE OF ISSUANCE 1/98
©PathoGenesis Corporation, 1998
Shown in Product Identification Guide, page 330

Pedinol Pharmacal Inc.
**30 BANFI PLAZA NORTH
FARMINGDALE, N.Y. 11735**

Direct Inquiries to:
Director of Professional Services
(516) 293-9500

BREEZEE MIST® FOOT POWDER   OTC

DESCRIPTION
Cooling formula soothes and helps keep feet dry and odor free.

HOW SUPPLIED
4 oz. (113g) aerosol can. 0884 0659-04
Store at controlled room temperature 15°–30°C (59°–86°F)

CASTELLANI PAINT Modified   OTC
CASTELLANI PAINT Modified–Colorless   OTC

DESCRIPTION
Castellani Paint Modified is a first aid antiseptic and drying agent. Care should be taken to avoid spilling. Guard against staining as Castellani Paint Modified will stain skin and clothing.

HOW SUPPLIED

Bottle Size	1 oz. (29.57 mL)	1 pt. (453.6 mL)
Color	NDC 0884-2893-01	NDC 0884-2893-16
Colorless	NDC 0884-2993-01	NDC 0884-2993-16

Store at controlled room temperature 15°–30°C (59°–86°F)

CITRADERM™   OTC
[*sitra-durm*]
L-Ascorbic Acid USP 10%

DESCRIPTION
FACIAL COMPLEX—The highest level of stable Vitamin C (L-Ascorbic Acid) available in a super emollient, quick absorbing, non-greasy formula.

DIRECTIONS
Apply sparingly and feather into skin as directed by your Dermatologist. Apply moisturizer or TI-SCREEN Sunscreen SPF 15 as usual.
Cap tightly after use.
CAUTION: FOR EXTERNAL USE ONLY. KEEP OUT OF THE REACH OF CHILDREN.
Keep away from open flame. Store in a cool, dry place, away from sunlight.

HOW SUPPLIED
FACIAL COMPLEX CREAM 0.5 oz   0884-5996-15

FORMALYDE-10® SPRAY   ℞

DESCRIPTION
Formalyde-10 Spray is a topical solution containing Formaldehyde 10% to safeguard against offensive odor and dry excessive moisture of the feet. Drying agent for pre & post-surgical removal of warts where dryness is required.

HOW SUPPLIED
Available in 2 oz. (59.14 mL) plastic spray bottle.
NDC 0884-4789-02
Store at controlled room temperature 15°–30°C (59°–86°F)

FUNGOID® CREME   ℞

DESCRIPTION
Fungoid Creme (Clotrimazole Cream USP, 1%) is indicated for the topical treatment of candidiasis due to Candida albicans and tinea versicolor due to Malassezia furfur.

HOW SUPPLIED
NDC 0884-2495-45
Fungoid® Creme is available in a 45 gram tube.
Store between 2°-30°C (36°-86°F).

FUNGOID® SOLUTION   ℞
Antifungal Solution

DESCRIPTION
Fungoid Solution (Clotrimazole Topical Solution USP, 1%) contains 10 mg Clotrimazole USP, a synthetic antifungal agent having the chemical name 1-(o-Chloro-a, α-diphenybenzyl) imidazole.
Clotrimazole is an odorless, white crystalline substance. It is practically insoluble in water, sparingly soluble in ether and very soluble in polyethylene glycol 400, ethanol and chloroform. Each mL of Fungoid Solution (Clotrimazole Topical Solution USP, 1%) contains 10 mg Clotrimazole USP in a nonaqueous vehicle of Polyethylene Glycol 400.
Prescription Fungoid Solution (Clotrimazole Topical Solution USP, 1%) product is indicated for the topical treatment of candidiasis due to *Candida albicans* and tinea versicolor due to *Malassezia furfur*.

HOW SUPPLIED
NDC 0884-3197-01
Available in a 1 oz (29.57 mL) plastic bottle with controlled dropper.
Store at controlled room temperature 15°–30°C (59°–86°F).

FUNGOID® TINCTURE   OTC

DESCRIPTION
A topical antifungal which is applied as a thin application twice a day (morning and night), to the affected area using the attached brush, **or as recommended by your physician.** Remove Fungoid Tincture from any untreated areas.

HOW SUPPLIED
1 oz. (29.57 mL) bottle with brush applicator NDC 0884-0293-01, 1 pt. (473.12 mL) bottle NDC 0884-0293-16.
FUNGOID TINCTURE TOPICAL ANTIFUNGAL TREATMENT KIT includes: 1 oz. (29.57 mL) FUNGOID TINCTURE, 2 oz. (56.7g) NAIL SCRUB, nail brush. NDC 0884-5493-01.
Store at controlled room temperature 15°–30°C (59°–86°F).
Protect from freezing.

HYDRISALIC® GEL   OTC

DESCRIPTION
HYDRISALIC GEL aids in the exfoliation of dry, scaly, calloused skin. Contains salicylic acid USP 5%.

HOW SUPPLIED
1 oz. (28.35 g) plastic tube. 0884-2296-01
Store at controlled room temperature 15°–30°C (59°–86°F)

HYDRISINOL® CREME and LOTION   OTC

DESCRIPTION
Both Hydrisinol Creme and Lotion contain Sulfonated Castor Oil in a Hydrogenated Vegetable Oil Base for application on dry, cracked, calloused skin and are particularly useful after a bath, shower, exposure to the sun or wind to help soften the skin by containing the moisture in the skin.

HOW SUPPLIED
Hydrisinol Cream is available in a 4 oz. (113.4g), 0884-0142-04 and 1 lb. (453.6g) jars, 0884-0142-16.
Hydrisinol Lotion is available in an 8 oz. (226.8g) plastic bottle w/pump, 0884-3042-08.

Continued on next page

LACTINOL-E® CREME ℞
LACTINOL® LOTION ℞

DESCRIPTION

Lactic acid has been reported as an effective naturally occurring humectant in the skin. It has beneficial effects on dry skin and on severe hyperkeratotic conditions. Vitamin E has been used as an aid to control dry or chapped skin. Vitamin E has also found application as an aid in the relief of minor skin disorders such as burns, sunburn, and irritated skin. It has antioxidant properties thus protecting the skin. Lactinol-E Creme and Lactinol Lotion which contain Lactic Acid 10%, is indicated for moisturizing and softening dry, scaly skin (xerosis), ichthyosis vulgaris and itching associated with these conditions.

HOW SUPPLIED

Lactinol-E Creme is available in a 4 oz. (113.4g) plastic jar. NDC 0884-4990-04
Lactinol Lotion is available in a 12 oz. (354.84 mL) bottle w/pump.
NDC 0884-5292-12
Store at controlled room temperature 15°–30°C (59°–86°F).

LAZERCREME® OTC

DESCRIPTION

The moisturizing ingredients Vitamin A and Vitamin E aid in the natural healing process of fissures, keratosis and dryness of the skin, post surgical regeneration of the skin and to revitalize lasered tissue.

HOW SUPPLIED

Available in 2 oz. (56.7g) plastic jar. 0884-3886-02

LAZERFORMALYDE® SOLUTION ℞

DESCRIPTION

Lazerformalyde Solution is a topical solution containing Formaldehyde 10% as a drying agent for pre and post surgical removal of warts or for non-surgical laser treatment of warts where dryness is required. Safeguards against offensive odor and dries excessive moisture of feet.

HOW SUPPLIED

Available in 3 oz. (88.71 mL) plastic bottle with roll-on applicator. NDC 0884-3986-03
Store at controlled room temperature 15°–30°C (59°–86°F).

LAZERSPORIN-C® SOLUTION ℞

DESCRIPTION

Lazersporin-C Solution is a combination of Neomycin Sulfate USP, Polymixin B Sulfate USP, and Hydrocortisone 1% USP for the treatment of superficial bacterial infections of the external auditory canal caused by organisms susceptible to the action of the antibiotics. **For otic use. Not for ophthalmic use.**

HOW SUPPLIED

10cc bottle with sterile dropper. NDC 0884-4086-10
Store at controlled room temperature 15°–30°C (59°–86°F).

NAIL SCRUB™ WITH BRUSH OTC

DESCRIPTION

Nail Scrub is a nail rejuvenator, cleanser and bleaching agent which is applied to the nail surface and scrubbed briskly with a nail brush. The nail scrub is then washed off and the nail dried. Nail scrub is useful for smoothing out rough, thickened nails and reduction of discoloration from fungus infections.

HOW SUPPLIED

Available in 2 oz. (56.7g) plastic bottle with applicator tip. 0884-4891-02

ONY-CLEAR® SOLUTION OTC

DESCRIPTION

Solution of Benzalkonium Chloride. Helps guard against bacterial contamination that potentially can cause skin infections and to help revitalize feet and nails when applied twice a day.

HOW SUPPLIED

Available in a 1 oz. (29.57 mL) bottle with brush cap. NDC 0884-4897-01
Store at controlled room temperature 15°–30°C (59°–86°F).

OSTIDERM®
OSTIDERM® ROLL-ON OTC

DESCRIPTION

Safeguards against offensive odor and dries excessive moisture of the feet. Provides comfort while absorbing moisture.
NOTE: For OSTIDERM (not OSTIDERM Roll-on): **If contents harden, add hot water and stir.**

HOW SUPPLIED

Ostiderm is available in a 1.5 oz. (42.5g) jar. 0884-2051-45.
Ostiderm Roll-On is available in a 3 oz. (88.71 mL) plastic bottle with roll-on applicator. 0884-2052-03
Store at Controlled Room Temperature 15°–30°C (59°–86°F).

PEDI-BORO® SOAK PAKS OTC

DESCRIPTION

Pedi-Boro makes a soothing wet dressing of a modified Burow's Solution, Buffered. A mild astringent solution to aid in the relief of minor skin irritations due to allergies, poison ivy, insect bites, or athlete's foot, and as an aid in the relief of swelling associated with minor bruises. Dissolve one or two paks in a pint of water and prepare fresh daily.

HOW SUPPLIED

Box of 12 NDC 0884-1773-27
Box of 100 NDC 0884-1773-10

PEDI-DRI® TOPICAL POWDER ℞

DESCRIPTION

Pedi-Dri Topical Powder provides in each gram 100,000 USP nystatin units dispersed in talc.
Nystatin is an antifungal antibiotic which is both fungistatic and fungicidal in vitro against a wide variety of yeasts and yeast-like fungus. It probably acts by binding to sterols in the cell membrane of the fungus with a resultant change in membrance permeability allowing leakage of intracellular compounds. Nystatin is a polyene antibiotic of undetermined structural formula that is obtained from Streptomyces noursei, and is the first well tolerated antifungal antibiotic of dependable efficacy for the treatment of cutaneous, oral and intestinal infections caused by Candida (Monilia) albicans and other candida species. It exhibits no appreciable activity against bacteria. Nystatin provides specific therapy for all localized forms of candidiasis. Symptomatic relief is rapid, often occurring within 24 to 48 hours after the initiation of treatment.
Pedi-Dri Topical Powder (Nystatin) is a topical preparation indicated in the treatment of cutaneous or mucocutaneous mycotic infections caused by Candida albicans and other Candida species.

HOW SUPPLIED

Available in a 2 oz. plastic bottle (56.7g) with shaker cap. NDC 0884-0396-02
Store at controlled room temperature 15°–30°C (59°–86°F).

PEDI-PRO® TOPICAL POWDER OTC

DESCRIPTION

PEDI-PRO is an antimicrobial topical powder for drying, absorbing and deodorizing.

HOW SUPPLIED

2 oz. (56.7g) plastic bottle with shaker cap. NDC 0884-3597-02.

SAL-ACID® PLASTERS OTC

DESCRIPTION

Medicated plaster of Salicylic Acid 40%, for the removal of common and plantar warts. The common wart can be easily recognized by the rough, cauliflower-like appearance of the surface. The plantar wart is recognized by its location only on the bottom of the foot, its tenderness and the interruption of the footprint pattern. The specialized gauze pad helps relieve painful pressure, while the SAL-ACID PLASTER medication remedies the wart. To be applied over the wart daily or as directed by your physician.

HOW SUPPLIED

SAL-ACID® PLASTERS are available 14 plasters per package, NDC 0884-4393-14.

SALACTIC® FILM OTC
SAL-PLANT® GEL

DESCRIPTION

Salactic Film and Sal-Plant Gel both contain Salicylic Acid 17% USP in a collodion-like vehicle, for the removal of common warts. The common wart is easily recognized by the rough cauliflower-like appearance of the surface.
For the removal of plantar warts on the bottom of the foot. The plantar wart is recognized by its location only on the bottom of the foot, its tenderness and the interruption of the footprint pattern.

HOW SUPPLIED

Salactic Film available in 0.5 oz (15 mL) bottle with brush applicator. NDC 0884-2592-15
Sal-Plant Gel available in a 0.5 oz (14g) tube with tip applicator. NDC 0884-5192-15

TI-SCREEN® OTC
SPF 15
SPF 16 (NATURAL AND BABY)
SPF 17
SPF 20
SPF 23
SPF 30
LIP PROTECTANT SPF 15

DESCRIPTION

SPF 15 and SPF 30 are moisturizing sunscreen lotions. SPF 20 is a sportsgel. SPF 16 is a natural moisturizing sunblock. SPF 17 is a sunless tanning creme. SPF 23 is a cooling sunscreen spray.
SPF 15 lip protectant sunscreen.

HOW SUPPLIED

TI-SCREEN SPF 15 Lotion 4 oz. bottle NDC 0884-1596-04
SPF 16 Lotion, 4 oz. bottle NDC 0884-1696-04
SPF 16 Baby 4 oz. bottle NDC 0884-6196-04
SPF 17 Creme, 4 oz. tube NDC 0884-6097-04
SPF 20 Gel 4 oz. bottle NDC 0884-2096-04
SPF 23 Spray, 4 oz. pump bottle, NDC 0884-2397-04
SPF 30 Lotion 4 oz. bottle NDC 0884-3096-04
SPF 15 Lip Prot. 0.15 oz. stick NDC 0884-1096-01

UREACIN-10® LOTION OTC
UREACIN-20® CREME OTC

DESCRIPTION

Ureacin-10 Lotion and Ureacin-20 Creme are topical treatments for rough, dry, cracked, calloused skin.

HOW SUPPLIED

Ureacin-10®, 8 oz. (226.8g) plastic bottle w/pump. 0884-3249-08.
Ureacin-20®, 4 oz. (113.4g) plastic jar 0884-0449-04.
Store at controlled room temperature 15°–30°C (59°–86°F)

Penederm Incorporated
320 LAKESIDE DRIVE, SUITE A
FOSTER CITY, CA 94404-1146

Direct Inquiries to:
800-395-DERM
650-358-0100
email: productinfo@penederm.com

ACTICIN™ ℞
[act' ĭ cĭn]
(permethrin) Cream 5%

DESCRIPTION

Acticin™ (permethrin) Cream 5% is a topical scabicidal agent for the treatment of infestation with Sarcoptes scabiei (scabies). It is available in an off-white, vanishing cream base. Acticin™ Cream is for topical use only.
Chemical Name: The permethrin used is an approximate 1:3 mixture of the cis and trans isomers of the pyrethroid (±)-3-phenoxybenzyl 3-(2,2-dichlorovinyl)-2,2-dimethylcyclopropanecarboxylate. Permethrin has a molecular formula of $C_{21}H_{20}Cl_2O_3$ and a molecular weight of 391.29. It is a yellow to light orange-brown, low melting solid or viscous liquid.
[See chemical structure at top of next column]

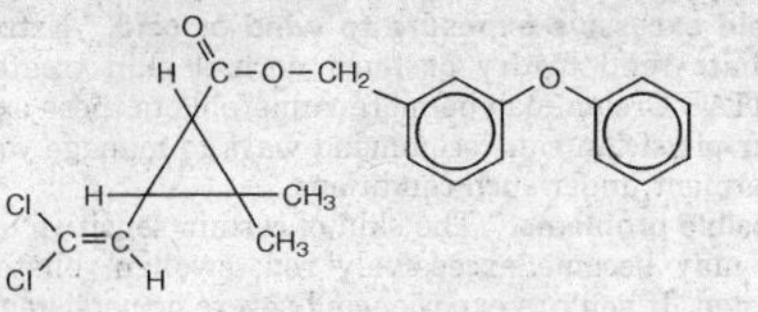

Each gram of Acticin™ Cream 5% contains permethrin 50 mg (5%) and the inactive ingredients butylated hydroxytoluene, carbomer 934P, coconut oil, glycerin, glyceryl stearate, isopropyl myristate, lanolin alcohols, light mineral oil, polyoxyethylene cetyl ethers, purified water, and sodium hydroxide. Formaldehyde 1 mg (0.1%) is added as a preservative.

CLINICAL PHARMACOLOGY

Permethrin, a pyrethroid, is active against a broad range of pests including lice, ticks, fleas, mites, and other arthropods. It acts on the nerve cell membrane to disrupt the sodium channel current by which the polarization of the membrane is regulated. Delayed repolarization and paralysis of the pests are the consequences of this disturbance.

Permethrin is rapidly metabolized by ester hydrolysis to inactive metabolites which are excreted primarily in the urine. Although the amount of permethrin absorbed after a single application of the 5% cream has not been determined precisely, data from studies with ^{14}C-labeled permethrin and absorption studies of the cream applied to patients with moderate to severe scabies indicate it is 2% or less of the amount applied.

INDICATIONS AND USAGE

Acticin™ Cream 5% is indicated for the treatment of infestation with *Sarcoptes scabiei* (scabies).

CONTRAINDICATIONS

Permethrin cream is contraindicated in patients with known hypersensitivity to any of its components, to any synthetic pyrethroid or pyrethrin.

WARNINGS

If hypersensitivity to permethrin cream occurs, discontinue use.

PRECAUTIONS

General: Scabies infestation is often accompanied by pruritis, edema and erythema. Treatment with permethrin cream may temporarily exacerbate these conditions.

Information for Patients: Patients with scabies should be advised that itching, mild burning and/or stinging may occur after application of permethrin cream. In clinical trials, approximately 75% of patients treated with permethrin cream who continued to manifest pruritis at 2 weeks had cessation by 4 weeks. If irritation persists, they should consult their physician. Permethrin cream may be very mildly irritating to the eyes. Patients should be advised to avoid contact with eyes during application and to flush with water immediately if permethrin cream gets in the eyes.

Carcinogenesis, Mutagenesis, Impairment of Fertility: Six carcinogenicity bioassays were evaluated with permethrin, three each in rats and mice. No tumorigenicity was seen in the rat studies. However, species-specific increases in pulmonary adenomas, a common benign tumor of mice of high spontaneous background incidence, were seen in the three mouse studies. In one of these studies there was an increased incidence of pulmonary alveolar-cell carcinomas and benign liver adenomas only in female mice when permethrin was given in their food at a concentration of 5000 ppm. Mutagenicity assays, which give useful correlative data for interpreting results from carcinogenicity bioassays in rodents, were negative. Permethrin showed no evidence of mutagenic potential in a battery of *in vitro* and *in vivo* genetic toxicity studies.

Permethrin did not have any adverse effect on reproductive function at a dose of 180 mg/kg/day orally in a three-generation rat study.

Pregnancy: *Teratogenic Effects:* Pregnancy Category B: Reproduction studies have been performed in mice, rats, and rabbits (200 to 400 mg/kg/day orally) and have revealed no evidence of impaired fertility or harm to the fetus due to permethrin. There are, however, no adequate and well-controlled studies in pregnant women. Because animal reproduction studies are not always predictive of human response, this drug should be used during pregnancy only if clearly needed.

Nursing Mothers: It is not known whether this drug is excreted in human milk. Because many drugs are excreted in human milk and because of the evidence for tumorigenic potential of permethrin in animal studies, consideration should be given to discontinuing nursing temporarily or withholding the drug while the mother is nursing.

Pediatric Use: Permethrin cream is safe and effective in pediatric patients two months of age and older. Safety and effectiveness in pediatric patients less than two months of age have not been established.

ADVERSE REACTIONS

In clinical trials, generally mild and transient burning and stinging followed application with permethrin cream in 10% of patients and was associated with the severity of infestation. Pruritis was reported in 7% of patients at various times post-application. Erythema, numbness, tingling, and rash were reported in 1 to 2% or less of patients (see PRECAUTIONS: General).

OVERDOSAGE

No instance of accidental ingestion of permethrin cream has been reported. If ingested, gastric lavage and general supportive measures should be employed.

DOSAGE AND ADMINISTRATION

Adults and children: Thoroughly massage Acticin™ (permethrin) Cream into the skin from the head to the soles of the feet. Scabies rarely infests the scalp of adults, although the hairline, neck, temple, and forehead may be infested in infants and geriatric patients. Usually 30 grams is sufficient for an average adult. The cream should be removed by washing (shower or bath) after 8 to 14 hours. Infants should be treated on the scalp, temple and forehead. ONE APPLICATION IS GENERALLY CURATIVE.

Patients may experience persistent pruritus after treatment. This is rarely a sign of treatment failure and is not an indication for retreatment. Demonstrable living mites after 14 days indicate that retreatment is necessary.

HOW SUPPLIED

Acticin™ (permethrin) Cream 5% (wt./wt.) is supplied in 60g tubes.

NDC Code	Strength	Quantity
25074-131-06	5%	60 g

Store at room temperature 15°–25°C (59°–77°F).

CAUTION: Federal (USA) law prohibits dispensing without prescription.

Distributed by: Penederm Incorporated
Foster City, CA 94404

Manufactured by: Alpharma USPD Inc.
Baltimore, MD 21244

PN402.01A
Rev.9/97 VC1350

AVITA® ℞

[ă vēt' ă]
(tretinoin cream)
CREAM, 0.025%
For Topical Use Only

DESCRIPTION

AVITA® Cream, a topical retinoid, contains tretinoin 0.025% by weight in a hydrophilic cream vehicle of stearic acid, polyolprepolymer-2, isopropyl myristate, polyoxyl 40 stearate, propylene glycol, stearyl alcohol, xanthan gum, sorbic acid, butylated hydroxytoluene, and purified water. Chemically, tretinoin is all-trans-retinoic acid (C20H2802; molecular weight 300.44 vitamin A acid) and has the following structural formula:

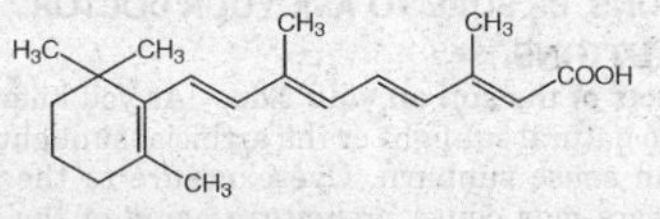

CLINICAL PHARMACOLOGY

Although the exact mode of action of tretinoin is unknown, current evidence suggests that topical tretinoin decreases cohesiveness of follicular epithelial cells with decreased microcomedo formation. Additionally, tretinoin stimulates mitotic activity and increased turnover of follicular epithelial cells causing extrusion of the comedones.

Pharmacokinetics:

In vitro and in vivo pharmacokinetic studies with AVITA® Cream indicate that less than 0.3% of the topically applied dose is bioavailable. Circulating plasma levels of both tretinoin and isotretinoin are only slightly elevated above those found in healthy normal controls.

CLINICAL STUDIES

In one vehicle-controlled clinical trial, AVITA® (tretinoin cream) Cream 0.025%, applied once daily was more effective than vehicle in the treatment of facial acne vulgaris of mild to moderate severity. Percent reductions in lesion count after treatment for 12 weeks in this study are shown in the following table:

	AVITA® Cream, 0.025%	Vehicle Cream
	N=75	N=58
Noninflammatory Lesions	45%	27%
Inflammatory Lesions	46%	32%
Total Lesions	46%	28%

N=Number of Subjects

INDICATIONS AND USAGE

AVITA® Cream is indicated for topical application in the treatment of acne vulgaris. The safety and efficacy of this product in the treatment of other disorders have not been established.

CONTRAINDICATIONS

The product should not be used if there is hypersensitivity to any of the ingredients.

PRECAUTIONS

General: If a reaction suggesting sensitivity or chemical irritation occurs, use of the medication should be discontinued. Exposure to sunlight, including sunlamps, should be minimized during the use of AVITA® Cream, and patients with sunburn should be advised not to use the product until fully recovered because of heightened susceptibility to sunlight as a result of the use of tretinoin. Patients who may be required to have considerable sun exposure due to occupation and those with inherent sensitivity to the sun should exercise particular caution. Use of sunscreen products and protective clothing over treated areas is recommended when exposure cannot be avoided. Whether extremes, such as wind or cold, also may be irritating to patients under treatment with tretinoin.

AVITA® Cream should be kept away from the eyes, the mouth, the paranasal creases, and mucous membranes. Topical use may induce severe local erythema and peeling at the site of application. If the degree of local irritation warrants, patients should be directed to temporarily use the medication less frequently, discontinue use temporarily, or discontinue use altogether. Efficacy at reduced frequencies of application has not been established. Tretinoin has been reported to cause severe irritation on eczematous skin and should be used with utmost caution in patients with this condition.

Information for Patients: See attached Patient Package Insert.

Drug Interactions: Concomitant topical medication, medicated or abrasive soaps and cleansers, soaps and cosmetics that have a strong drying effect, and products with high concentrations of alcohol, astringents, spices or lime should be used with caution because of possible interaction with tretinoin. Particular caution should be exercised in using preparations containing sulfur, resorcinol, or salicylic acid with AVITA® Cream. It also is advisable to "rest" a patient's skin until the effects of such preparations subside before use of AVITA® Cream is begun.

Carinogenesis Mutagenesis and Impairment of Fertility: In a life-time dermal study in CD-1 mice with another tretinoin cream, at 100 and 200 times the average recommended human topical clinical dose, and few skin tumors in the female mice and liver tumors in male mice were observed. The biological significance of these findings is not clear because they occurred at doses that exceeded the dermal maximally tolerated dose (MTD) of tretinoin and because they were within the background natural occurrence rate for these tumors in this strain of mice. There was no evidence of carcinogenic potential when tretinoin was administered topically at a dose five times the average recommended human topical clinical dose. For purposes of comparisons of the animal exposure to human exposure, the "recommended human topical clinical dose" is defined as 1.0 g of 0.025% AVITA® Cream applied daily to a 50 kg person. In a chronic, two-year bioassay of vitamin A acid in mice performed by Tsubura and Yamamoto, generalized amyloid deposition was reported in all vitamin A treated groups in the basal layer of the skin. In CD-1 mice, a similar study reported hyalinization at the treated skin sites and the incidence of this finding was 0/50, 3/50, 3/50, and 2/50 in male mice and 1/50, 0/50, 4/50, and 2/50 in female mice from the vehicle control, 0.25 mg/kg, 0.5 mg/kg, and 1 mg/kg groups, respectively.

Studies in hairless albino mice suggest that tretinoin may enhance the tumorigenic potential of carcinogenic doses of UVB and UVA light from a solar simulator. In other studies, when lightly pigmented hairless mice treated with tretinoin were exposed to carcinogenic doses of UVA/UVB light, the incidence and rate of development of skin tumors were either reduced or no effect was seen. Due to significantly different experimental conditions, no strict comparison of these disparate data is possible at this time. Although the significance of these studies to humans is not clear, patients should minimize exposure to sun.

The mutagenic potential of tretinoin was evaluated in the Ames assay and in the *in vivo* mouse micronucleus assay, both of which were negative.

Continued on next page

Avita Cream—Cont.

Dermal Segment I and III studies with AVITA® Cream have not been performed in any species. In oral Segment I and Segment III studies in rats with tretinoin, decreased survival of neonates and growth retardation were observed at doses in excess of 2 mg/kg/day (> 400 times the average recommended human topical clinical dose).

Pregnancy: Pregnancy Category C.

Teratogenic Effects: Oral tretinoin has been shown to be teratogenic in rats, mice, rabbits, hamsters, and subhuman primates. It was teratogenic and fetotoxic in rats when given orally in doses 1000 times the average recommended human topical clinical dose. However, variations in teratogenic doses among various strains of rats have been reported. In the cynomolgus monkey, which metabolically is closer to humans for tretinoin than other species examined, fetal malformations were reported at oral doses of 10 mg/kg/day or greater, but none were observed at 5 mg/kg/day (1000 times the average recommended human topical clinical dose), although increased skeletal variations were observed at all doses. Dose-related increased embryolethality and abortion were reported. Similar results have also been reported in pigtail macaques.

Topical tretinoin in animal teratogenicity tests has generated equivocal results. There is evidence for teratogenicity (shortened or kinked tail) of topical tretinoin in Wistar rats at doses greater than 1 mg/kg/day (200 times the recommended human topical clinical dose) Anomalies (humerus: short 13%, bent 6%; os parietal incompletely ossified 14%) have also been reported in rats when 10 mg/kg/day was dermally applied.

Topical tretinoin (AVITA® Cream, 0.1%) has been shown to be teratogenic in rabbits when given in doses 91 times the topical human dose for cream (assuming a 50 mg adult applied 1.0 g of 0.1% cream topically). In this study, increased incidence of cleft palate and hydrocephaly was reported in the tretinoin-treated animals.

There are other reports, in New Zealand White rabbits with doses of approximately 80 times the recommended human topical clinical dose, of an increased incidence of domed head and hydrocephaly, typical of retinoid induced fetal malformations in this species.

When given subcutaneously to rabbits, tretinoin was teratogenic at 2 mg/kg/day but not at 1 mg/kg/day. These doses are approximately 400 and 200 times, respectively, the human topical dose of tretinoin cream, 0.025% (assuming a 50 kg adult applies 1.0 g of 0.025% cream topically).

In contrast, several well-controlled animal studies have shown that dermally applied tretinoin was not teratogenic at doses of 100 and 200 times the recommended human topical clinical dose, in rats and rabbits, respectively.

With widespread use of any drug, a small number of birth defect reports associated temporally with the administration of the drug would be expected by chance alone. Thirty cases of temporally associated congenital malformations have been reported during two decades of clinical use of another formulation of topical tretinoin (Retin-A). Although no definite pattern of teratogenicity and no causal association have been established from these cases, five of the reports describe the rare birth defect category, holoprosencephaly (defects associated with incomplete midline development of the forebrain). The significance of these spontaneous reports in terms of risk to the fetus is not known.

Nonteratogenic Effects: Dermal tretinoin has been shown to be fetotoxic in rabbits when administered in doses 100 times the recommended topical human clinical dose. Oral tretinoin has been shown to be fetotoxic in rats when administered in doses 500 times the recommended topical human clinical dose. There are, however, no adequate and well-controlled studies in pregnant women. AVITA® Cream should not be used during pregnancy.

Nursing Mothers: It is not known whether this drug is excreted in human milk. Because many drugs are excreted in human milk, caution should be exercised when AVITA® Cream is administered to a nursing woman.

ADVERSE REACTIONS

The skin of certain sensitive individuals may become excessively red, edematous, blistered, or crusted. If these effects occur, the medication should either be discontinued until the integrity of the skin is restored, or the medication dosing frequency should be adjusted temporarily to a level the patient can tolerate. However, efficacy has not been established for lower dosing frequencies. True contact allergy to topical tretinoin is rarely encountered. Temporary hyper- or hypopigmentation has been reported with repeated application of AVITA® Cream. Some individuals have been reported to have heightened susceptiblity to sunlight while under treatment with AVITA® Cream. Adverse effects of AVITA® Cream have been reversible upon discontinuation of therapy (see Dosage and Administration Section).

OVERDOSAGE

If medication is applied excessively, no more rapid or better results will be obtained and marked redness, peeling, or discomfort may occur. Oral ingestion of the drug may lead to the same side effects as those associated with excessive oral intake of vitamin A.

DOSAGE AND ADMINISTRATION

AVITA® Cream should be applied once a day, in the evening, to the skin where acne lesions appear, using enough to cover the entire affected area lightly. Application may cause a transient feeling of warmth or slight stinging. In cases where it has been necessary to temporarily discontinue therapy or reduce the frequency of applications, therapy may be resumed or frequency of application increased when the patients become able to tolerate the treatment. Alterations of dose frequency should be closely monitored by careful observation of the clinical therapeutic response and skin tolerance. Efficacy has not been established for less than once-daily dosing frequencies.

During the early weeks of therapy, an apparent increase in number and exacerbation of inflammatory acne lesions may occur. This is due, in part, to the action of the medication on deep, previously unseen lesions and should not be considered a reason to discontinue therapy. Therapeutic results should be noticed after two to three weeks but more than six weeks of therapy may be required before definite beneficial effects are seen. Patients treated with AVITA® Cream may use cosmetics, but the areas to be treated should be cleansed thoroughly before the medication is applied (see Precautions Section).

HOW SUPPLIED

AVITA® (tretinoin cream) Cream, 0.025% is supplied as:

NDC Code	Strength	Quantity
25074-141-02	0.025%	20 g
25074-141-03	0.025%	45 g

Storage Conditions: Store below 30°C (86°F); avoid freezing.

CAUTION: Rx only

Manufactured By:
DPT Laboratories, Inc.
San Antonio, Texas 78215

Distributed By:
PENEDERM INCORPORATED
Foster City, California 94404
Revised February 1997

PN310.01B

Remove this portion before dispensing
AVITA®
(tretinoin cream)
CREAM, 0.025%

PATIENT INSTRUCTIONS
Acne Treatment
IMPORTANT
Read Directions Carefully Before Using

THIS LEAFLET TELLS YOU ABOUT AVITA® (TRETINOIN) CREAM ACNE TREATMENT AS PRESCRIBED BY YOUR PHYSICIAN. THIS PRODUCT IS TO BE USED ONLY ACCORDING TO YOUR DOCTOR'S INSTRUCTIONS, AND IT SHOULD NOT BE APPLIED TO OTHER AREAS OF THE BODY OR TO OTHER GROWTHS OR LESIONS. THE SAFETY AND EFFECTIVENESS OF THIS PRODUCT IN OTHER DISORDERS HAVE NOT BEEN EVALUATED. IF YOU HAVE ANY QUESTIONS, BE SURE TO ASK YOUR DOCTOR.

PRECAUTIONS

The effects of the sun on your skin. As you know, overexposure to natural sunlight or the artificial sunlight of a sunlamp can cause sunburn. Overexposure to the sun over many years may cause premature aging of the skin and even skin cancer. The chances of these effects occurring will vary depending on skin type, the climate and the care taken to avoid overexposure to the sun. Therapy with AVITA® Cream may make your skin more susceptible to sunburn and other adverse effects of the sun, so unprotected exposure to natural or artificial sunlight should be minimized.

Laboratory findings. *When laboratory mice are exposed to artificial sunlight, they often develop skin tumors. These sunlight-induced tumors may appear more quickly and in greater number if the mouse is also topically treated with the active ingredient in AVITA® Cream, tretinoin. In some studies, under different conditions, however, when mice treated with tretinoin were exposed to artificial sunlight, the incidence and rate of development of skin tumors was reduced. There is no evidence to date that tretinoin alone will cause the development of skin tumors in either laboratory animals or humans. However, investigations in this area are continuing.*

Use caution in the sun. When outside, even on hazy days, areas treated with AVITA® Cream should be protected. An effective sunscreen should be used any time you are outside (consult your physician for a recommendation of an SPF level which will provide you with the necessary high level of protection). For extended sun exposure, protective clothing, like a hat, should be worn. Do not use artificial sunlamps while you are using AVITA® Cream. If you do become sunburned, stop your therapy with AVITA® Cream until your skin has recovered.

Avoid excessive exposure to wind or cold. Extremes of climate tend to dry or burn normal skin treated with AVITA® Cream may be more vulnerable to these extremes. Your physician can recommend ways to manage your acne treatment under such conditions.

Possible problems. The skin of certain sensitive individuals may become excessively red, swollen, blistered, or crusted. If you are experiencing severe or persistent irritation, discontinue the use of AVITA® Cream and consult your physician.

There have been reports that, in some patients, areas treated with AVITA® Cream developed a temporary increase or decrease in the amount of skin pigment (color) present.

Use other medication only on your physician's advice. Only your physician knows which other medications may be helpful during treatment and will recommended them to you if necessary. Follow the physician's instructions carefully. In addition, you should avoid preparations that may dry or irritate your skin. These preparations may include certain astringents, toiletries containing alcohol, spices or lime, or certain medicated soaps, shampoos, and hair permanent solutions. Do not allow anyone else to use this medication.

Do not use other medications with AVITA® Cream which are not recommended by your doctor. The medications you have used in the past might cause unnecessary redness or peeling.

If you are pregnant, think you are pregnant, or are nursing an infant: No studies have been conducted in humans to establish the safety of AVITA® Cream in pregnant women. If you are pregnant, think you are pregnant, or are nursing a baby, consult your physician before using this medication.

AND WHILE YOU'RE ON AVITA® THERAPY

Use a mild non-medicated soap. avoid frequent washings and harsh scrubbing. Acne isn't caused by dirt, so no matter how hard you scrub, you can't wash it away. Washing too frequently or scrubbing too roughly may at times actually make your acne worse. Wash your skin gently with a mild, bland soap. Two or three times a day should be sufficient. Pat skin dry with a towel. Let the face dry 20 to 30 minutes before applying AVITA® Cream. Remember, excessive irritation such as rubbing, too much washing, use of other medications not suggested by your physician, etc., may worsen your acne.

HOW TO USE AVITA® (TRETINOIN) CREAM

To get the best results with AVITA® Cream therapy, it is necessary to use it properly. Forget about the instructions given for other products and the advice of friends. Just stick to the special plan your doctor has laid out for you and be patient. Remember, when AVITA® Cream is used properly, many users see improvement by 12 weeks. AGAIN FOLLOW INSTRUCTIONS – BE PATIENT – DON'T START AND STOP THERAPY ON YOUR OWN – IF YOU HAVE QUESTIONS, ASK YOUR DOCTOR.

To help you use the medication correctly, keep these simple instructions in mind.

- AVITA® Cream should be applied once a day, in the evening, or as directed by our physician, to the skin where acne lesions appear, using enough to cover the entire affected area lightly. First, wash with a mild soap and dry your skin gently. WAIT 20 to 30 MINUTES BEFORE APPLYING MEDICATION; it is important for skin to be completely dry in order to minimize possible irritation.
- It is better not to use more than the amount suggested by your physician or to apply more frequently than instructed. To much may irritate the skin, waste medication, and won't give faster or better results.
- Keep the medication away from the corners of the nose, mouth, eyes, and open wounds. *Spread away from these areas when applying.*
- *Cream:* Squeeze about a half inch or less of medications onto the fingertip. While that should be enough for your whole face, after you have had some experience with the medication you may find you need slightly more or less to do the job. The medications should become invisible almost immediately. If it is still visible, you are using too much. Cover the affected area lightly with AVITA® Cream by first dabbing it on your forehead, chin, and both cheeks, then spreading it over the entire affected area. Smooth gently into the skin.
- If needed, you may apply a moisturizer or a moisturizer with sunscreen that will not aggravate your acne (noncomedogenic) in the morning after you wash.

WHAT TO EXPECT WITH YOUR NEW TREATMENT

AVITA® Cream works deep inside your skin and this takes time. You cannot make AVITA® Cream work any faster by applying more than one dose each day, but an excess amount of AVITA® Cream may irritate your skin. Be patient.

There may be some discomfort or peeling during the early days of treatment. Some patients also notice that their skin begins to take on a blush.

These reactions do not happen to everyone. If they do, it is just skin adjusting to AVITA® Cream and this usually subsides within two to four weeks. These reactions can usually

be minimized by following instructions carefully. Should the effects become excessively troublesome, consult your doctor.

BY THREE TO SIX WEEKS, some patients notice an appearance of new blemishes (papules and pustules). At this stage it is important to continue using AVITA® Cream.

If AVITA® Cream is going to have a beneficial effect for you, you should notice an improvement in your appearance by 6 to 12 weeks of therapy. Don't be discouraged if you see no immediate improvement. Don't stop treatment at the first signs of improvement.

Once your acne is under control you should continue regular application of AVITA® Cream until your physician instructs otherwise.

Manufactured By:
DPT Laboratories, Inc.
San Antonio, Texas 78215

Distributed By:
PENEDERM INCORPORATED
Foster City, California 94404
Revised February 1997

AVITA® ℞
[ă vēt' ă]
(tretinoin gel)
GEL, 0.025%
For Topical Use Only

DESCRIPTION

AVITA® Gel, a topical retinoid, contains tretinoin 0.025% by weight in a gel vehicle of butylated hydroxytoluene, hydroxypropyl cellulose, polyolprepolymer-2, and ethanol (denatured with *tert*-butyl alcohol and brucine sulfate) 83% w/w. Chemically, tretinoin is all-*trans*-retinoic acid ($C_{20}H_{28}O_2$; molecular weight 300.44 vitamin A acid) and has the following structural formula:

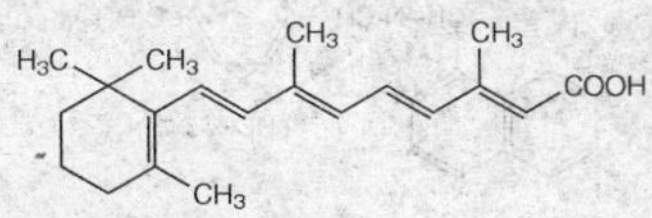

CLINICAL PHARMACOLOGY

Although the exact mode of action of tretinoin is unknown, current evidence suggests that topical tretinoin decreases cohesiveness of follicular epithelial cells with decreased microcomedo formation. Additionally, tretinoin stimulates mitotic activity and increased turnover of follicular epithelial cells causing extrusion of the comedones.

Pharmacokinetics:

In vitro and in vivo pharmacokinetic studies with AVITA® Gel indicate that less than 0.3% of the topically applied dose is bioavailable. Circulating plasma levels of both tretinoin and isotretinoin are only slightly elevated above those found in healthy normal controls.

CLINICAL STUDIES

In two large vehicle-controlled clinical trials, AVITA® (tretinoin gel) Gel 0.025%, applied once daily was more effective than vehicle in the treatment of facial acne vulgaris of mild to moderate severity. Percent reductions in lesion counts after treatment for 12 weeks in these studies are shown in the following Tables:

Study 1	AVITA® Gel, 0.025%	Vehicle Gel
	N = 198	N= 204
Noninflammatory Lesions	-36%	-27%
Inflammatory Lesions	-35%	-25%
Total Lesions	-36%	-27%

Study 2	AVITA® Gel, 0.025%	Vehicle Gel
	N = 58	N= 58
Noninflammatory Lesions	-42%	-26%
Inflammatory Lesions	-38%	-23%
Total Lesions	-41%	-26%

N = Number of Subjects

INDICATIONS AND USAGE

AVITA® Gel is indicated for topical application in the treatment of acne vulgaris. The safety and efficacy of this product in the treatment of other disorders have not been established.

CONTRAINDICATIONS

The product should not be used if there is hypersensitivity to any of the ingredients.

WARNINGS

GELS ARE FLAMMABLE. Note: Keep away from heat and flame. Keep tube tightly closed.

PRECAUTIONS

General: If a reaction suggesting sensitivity or chemical irritation occurs, use of the medication should be discontinued. Exposure to sunlight, including sunlamps, should be minimized during the use of AVITA® Gel, and patients with sunburn should be advised not to use the product until fully recovered because of heightened susceptibility to sunlight as a result of the use of tretinoin. Patients who may be required to have considerable sun exposure due to occupation and those with inherent sensitivity to the sun should exercise particular caution. Use of sunscreen products and protective clothing over treated areas is recommended when exposure cannot be avoided. Weather extremes, such as wind or cold, also may be irritating to patients under treatment with tretinoin.

AVITA® Gel should be kept away from the eyes, the mouth, the paranasal creases, and mucous membranes. Topical use may induce severe local erythema and peeling at the site of application. If the degree of local irritation warrants, patients should be directed to temporarily use the medication less frequently, discontinue use temporarily, or discontinue use altogether. Efficacy at reduced frequencies of application has not been established. Tretinoin has been reported to cause severe irritation on eczematous skin and should be used with utmost caution in patients with this condition.

Information for Patients: See attached Patient Package Insert.

Drug Interactions: Concomitant topical medication, medicated or abrasive soaps and cleansers, soaps and cosmetics that have a strong drying effect, and products with high concentrations of alcohol, astringents, spices or lime should be used with caution because of possible interaction with tretinoin. Particular caution should be exercised in using preparations containing sulfur, resorcinol, or salicylic acid with AVITA® Gel. It also is advisable to "rest" a patient's skin until the effects of such preparations subside before use of AVITA® Gel is begun.

Carcinogenesis Mutagenesis and Impairment of Fertility: In a life-time dermal study in CD-1 mice with another tretinoin gel, at 100 and 200 times the average recommended human topical clinical dose, a few skin tumors in the female mice and liver tumors in male mice were observed. The biological significance of these findings is not clear because they occurred at doses that exceeded the dermal maximally tolerated dose (MTD) of tretinoin and because they were within the background natural occurrence rate for these tumors in this strain of mice. There was no evidence of carcinogenic potential when tretinoin was administered topically at a dose 5 times the average recommended human topical clinical dose. For purposes of comparisons of the animal exposure to human exposure, the "recommended human topical clinical dose" is defined as 1.0 g of 0.025% AVITA® Gel applied daily to a 50 kg person. In a chronic, two-year bioassay of Vitamin A acid in mice performed by Tsubura and Yamamoto, generalized amyloid deposition was reported in all Vitamin A treated groups in the basal layer of the skin. In CD-1 mice, a similar study reported hyalinization at the treated skin sites and the incidence of this finding was 0/50, 3/50, 3/50, and 2/50 in male mice and 1/50, 0/50, 4/50, and 2/50 in female mice from the vehicle control, 0.25 mg/kg, 0.5 mg/kg, and 1 mg/kg groups, respectively.

Studies in hairless albino mice suggest that tretinoin may enhance the tumorigenic potential of carcinogenic doses of UVB and UVA light from a solar simulator. In other studies, when lightly pigmented hairless mice treated with tretinoin were exposed to carcinogenic doses of UVA/UVB light, the incidence and rate of development of skin tumors were either reduced or no effect was seen. Due to significantly different experimental conditions, no strict comparison of these disparate data is possible at this time. Although the significance of these studies to humans is not clear, patients should minimize exposure to sun.

The mutagenic potential of tretinoin was evaluated in the Ames assay and in the *in vivo* mouse micronucleus assay, both of which were negative.

Dermal Segment I and III studies with AVITA® Gel have not been performed in any species. In oral Segment I and Segment III studies in rats with tretinoin, decreased survival of neonates and growth retardation were observed at doses in excess of 2 mg/kg/day (> 400 times the average recommended human topical clinical dose).

Pregnancy: Pregnancy Category C.

Teratogenic Effects: Oral tretinoin has been shown to be teratogenic in rats, mice, rabbits, hamsters, and subhuman primates. It was teratogenic and fetotoxic in rats when given orally in doses 1000 times the average recommended human topical clinical dose. However, variations in teratogenic doses among various strains of rats have been reported. In the cynomolgus monkey, which metabolically is closer to humans for tretinoin than other species examined, fetal malformations were reported at oral doses of 10 mg/kg/day or greater, but none were observed at 5 mg/kg/day (1000 times the average recommended human topical clinical dose), although increased skeletal variations were observed at all doses. Dose-related increased embryolethality and abortion were reported. Similar results have also been reported in pigtail macaques.

Topical tretinoin in animal teratogenicity tests has generated equivocal results. There is evidence for teratogenicity (shortened or kinked tail) of topical tretinoin in Wistar rats at doses greater than 1 mg/kg/day (200 times the recommended human topical clinical dose). Anomalies (humerus: short 13%, bent 6%; os parietal incompletely ossified 14%) have also been reported in rats when 10 mg/kg/day was dermally applied.

Topical tretinoin (AVITA® Gel, 0.025%) has been shown to be teratogenic in rabbits when given in doses 364 times the topical human dose for gel (assuming a 50 kg adult applies 1.0 g of 0.025% gel topically). In this study, increased incidence of cleft palate and hydrocephaly was reported in the tretinoin-treated animals.

There are other reports, in New Zealand White rabbits with doses of approximately 80 times the recommended human topical clinical dose, of an increased incidence of domed head and hydrocephaly, typical of retinoid-induced fetal malformations in this species.

When given subcutaneously to rabbits, tretinoin was teratogenic at 2 mg/kg/day but not at 1 mg/kg/day. These doses are approximately 400 and 200 times, respectively, the human topical dose of tretinoin gel, 0.025% (assuming a 50 kg adult applies 1.0 g of 0.025% gel topically).

In contrast, several well-controlled animal studies have shown that dermally applied tretinoin was not teratogenic at doses of 100 and 200 times the recommended human topical clinical dose, in rats and rabbits, respectively.

With widespread use of any drug, a small number of birth defect reports associated temporally with the administration of the drug would be expected by chance alone. Thirty cases of temporally associated congenital malformations have been reported during two decades of clinical use of another formulation of topical tretinoin (Retin A). Although no definite pattern of teratogenicity and no causal association have been established from these cases, 5 of the reports describe the rare birth defect category, holoprosencephaly (defects associated with incomplete midline development of the forebrain). The significance of these spontaneous reports in terms of risk to the fetus is not known.

Nonteratogenic Effects: Dermal tretinoin has been shown to be fetotoxic in rabbits when administered in doses 100 times the recommended topical human clinical dose. Oral tretinoin has been shown to be fetotoxic in rats when administered in doses 500 times the recommended topical human clinical dose. There are, however, no adequate and well-controlled studies in pregnant women. AVITA® Gel should not be used during pregnancy.

Nursing Mothers: It is not known whether this drug is excreted in human milk, caution should be exercised when AVITA® Gel is administered to a nursing woman.

ADVERSE REACTIONS

The skin of certain sensitive individuals may become excessively red, edematous, blistered, or crusted. If these effects occur, the medication should either be discontinued until the integrity of the skin is restored, or the medication dosing frequency should be adjusted temporarily to a level the patient can tolerate. However, efficacy has not been established for lower dosing frequencies. True contact allergy to topical tretinoin is rarely encountered. Temporary hyper- or hypopigmentation has been reported with repeated application of AVITA® Gel. Some individuals have been reported to have heightened susceptibility to sunlight while under treatment with AVITA® Gel. Adverse effects of AVITA® Gel have been reversible upon discontinuation of therapy (see Dosage and Administration Section).

OVERDOSAGE

If medication is applied excessively, no more rapid or better results will be obtained and marked redness, peeling, or discomfort may occur. Oral ingestion of the drug may lead to the same side effects as those associated with excessive oral intake of Vitamin A.

DOSAGE AND ADMINISTRATION

AVITA® Gel should be applied once a day, in the evening, to the skin where acne lesions appear, using enough to cover the entire affected area lightly. Application may cause a transient feeling of warmth or slight stinging. In cases where it has been necessary to temporarily discontinue therapy or reduce the frequency of application, therapy may be resumed or frequency of application increased when the patients become able to tolerate the treatment. Alterations of dose frequency should be closely monitored by careful ob-

Continued on next page

Avita Gel—Cont.

servation of the clinical therapeutic response and skin tolerance. Efficacy has not been established for less than once-daily dosing frequencies.

During the early weeks of therapy, an *apparent* increase in number and exacerbation of inflammatory acne lesions may occur. This is due, in part, to the action of the medication on deep, previously unseen lesions and should not be considered a reason to discontinue therapy. Therapeutic results should be noticed after two to three weeks, but more than six weeks of therapy may be required before definite beneficial effects are seen. Patients treated with AVITA® Gel may use cosmetics, but the areas to be treated should be cleansed thoroughly before the medication is applied (see Precautions Section).

HOW SUPPLIED

AVITA® (tretinoin gel) Gel, 0.025% is supplied as:

NDC Code	Strength	Quantity
25074-140-02	0.025%	20 g
25074-140-03	0.025%	45 g

Storage Conditions: Store below 30°C (86°F); avoid freezing.

CAUTION: Federal (U.S.A.) law prohibits dispensing without prescription.

Manufactured By:
DPT LABORATORIES, INC.
San Antonio, Texas 78215

Distributed by:
Penederm Incorporated
Foster City, California 94404

December 1997 PN308.01A

Remove this portion before dispensing

AVITA®
(tretinoin gel)
GEL, 0.025%

PATIENT INSTRUCTIONS
Acne Treatment
IMPORTANT
Read Directions Carefully
Before Using

THIS LEAFLET TELLS YOU ABOUT AVITA® (TRETINOIN) ACNE TREATMENT AS PRESCRIBED BY YOUR PHYSICIAN. THIS PRODUCT IS TO BE USED ONLY ACCORDING TO YOUR DOCTOR'S INSTRUCTIONS, AND IT SHOULD NOT BE APPLIED TO OTHER AREAS OF THE BODY OR TO OTHER GROWTHS OR LESIONS. THE SAFETY AND EFFECTIVENESS OF THIS PRODUCT IN OTHER DISORDERS HAVE NOT BEEN EVALUATED. IF YOU HAVE ANY QUESTIONS, BE SURE TO ASK YOUR DOCTOR.

WARNINGS

GELS ARE FLAMMABLE. Note: Keep away from heat and flame. Keep tube tightly closed.

PRECAUTIONS

The effects of the sun on your skin. As you know, overexposure to natural sunlight or the artificial sunlight of a sunlamp can cause sunburn. Overexposure to the sun over many years may cause premature aging of the skin and even skin cancer. The chances of the these effects occurring will vary depending on skin type, the climate and the care taken to avoid overexposure to the sun. Therapy with AVITA® Gel may make your skin more susceptible to sunburn and other adverse effects of the sun, so unprotected exposure to natural or artificial sunlight should be minimized.

Laboratory findings. *When laboratory mice are exposed to artificial sunlight, they often develop skin tumors. These sunlight-induced tumors may appear more quickly and in greater number if the mouse is also topically treated with the active ingredient in AVITA® Gel, tretinoin. In some studies, under different conditions, however, when mice treated with tretinoin were exposed to artificial sunlight, the incidence and rate of development of skin tumors were reduced. There is no evidence to date that tretinoin alone will cause the development of skin tumors in either laboratory animals or humans. However, investigations in this area are continuing.*

Use caution in the sun. When outside, even on hazy days, areas treated with AVITA® Gel should be protected. An effective sunscreen should be used any time you are outside (consult your physician for a recommendation of an SPF level which will provide you with the necessary high level of protection). For extended sun exposure, protective clothing, like a hat, should be worn. Do not use artificial sunlamps while you are using AVITA® Gel. If you do become sunburned, stop your therapy with AVITA® Gel until your skin has recovered.

Avoid excessive exposure to wind or cold. Extremes of climate tend to dry or burn normal skin. Skin treated with AVITA® Gel may be more vulnerable to these extremes. Your physician can recommend ways to manage your acne treatment under such conditions.

Possible problems. The skin of certain sensitive individuals may become excessively red, swollen, blistered, or crusted. If you are experiencing severe or persistent irritation, discontinue the use of AVITA® Gel and consult your physician.

There have been reports that, in some patients, areas treated with AVITA® Gel developed a temporary increase or decrease in the amount of skin pigment (color) present.

Use other medication only on your physician's advice. Only your physician knows which other medications may be helpful during treatment and will recommend them to you if necessary. Follow the physician's instructions carefully. In addition, you should avoid preparations that may dry or irritate your skin. These preparations may include certain astringents, toiletries containing alcohol, spices or lime, or certain medicated soaps, shampoos, and hair permanent solutions. Do not allow anyone else to use this medication.

Do no use other medications with AVITA® Gel which are not recommended by your doctor. The medications you have used in the past might cause unnecessary redness or peeling.

If you are pregnant, think you are pregnant, or are nursing an infant: No studies have been conducted in humans to establish the safety of AVITA® Gel in pregnant women. If you are pregnant, think you are pregnant, or are nursing a baby, consult your physician before using this medication.

AND WHILE YOU'RE ON AVITA® THERAPY

Use a mild non-mediated soap. Avoid frequent washings and harsh scrubbing. Acne isn't caused by dirt, so no matter how hard you scrub, you can't wash it away. Washing too frequently or scrubbing too roughly may at times actually make your acne worse. Wash your skin gently with a mild, bland soap. Two or three times a day should be sufficient. Pat skin dry with a towel. Let the face dry 20 to 30 minutes before applying AVITA® Gel. Remember, excessive irritation such as rubbing, too much washing, use of other medications not suggested by your physician, etc., may worsen your acne.

HOW TO USE AVITA® (TRETINOIN) GEL

To get the best results with AVITA® Gel therapy, it is necessary to use it properly. Forget about the instructions given for other products and the advice of friends. Just stick to the special plan your doctor has laid out of you and be patient. Remember, when AVITA® Gel is *used properly*, many users see improvement by 12 weeks. AGAIN, FOLLOW INSTRUCTIONS – BE PATIENT – DON'T START AND STOP THERAPY ON YOUR OWN – IF YOU HAVE QUESTIONS, ASK YOUR DOCTOR.

To help you use the medication correctly, keep these simple instructions in mind.

- AVITA® Gel should be applied once a day, in the evening, or as directed by your physician, to the skin where acne lesions appear, using enough to cover the entire affected area lightly. First, wash with a mild soap and dry your skin gently. WAIT 20 to 30 MINUTES BEFORE APPLYING MEDICATION; it is important for skin to be completely dry in order to minimize possible irritation.
- It is better not to use more than the amount suggested by your physician or to apply more frequently than instructed. Too much may irritate the skin, waste medication, and won't give faster or better results.
- Keep the medication away from the corners of the nose, mouth, eyes, and open wounds. *Spread away from these areas when applying.*
- *Gel:* Squeeze about a half inch or less of medication onto the fingertip. While that should be enough for your whole face, after you have had some experience with the medication you may find you need slightly more or less to do the job. The medication should become invisible almost immediately. If it is still visible, or if dry flaking occurs from the gel *within a minute or so* you are using too much. Cover the affected area lightly with AVITA® Gel by first dabbing it on your forehead, chin, and both cheeks, then spreading it over the entire affected area. Smooth gently into the skin.
- If needed, you may apply a moisturizer or a moisturizer with sunscreen that will not aggravate your acne (noncomedogenic) in the morning after you wash.

WHAT TO EXPECT WITH YOUR NEW TREATMENT

AVITA® Gel works deep inside your skin and this takes time. You cannot make AVITA® Gel work any faster by applying more than one dose each day, but an excess amount of AVITA® Gel may irritate your skin. Be patient.

There may be some discomfort or peeling during the early days of treatment. Some patients also notice that their skin begins to take on a blush.

These reactions do not happen to everyone. If they do, it is just your skin adjusting to AVITA® Gel and this usually subsides within two to four weeks. These reactions can usually be minimized by following instructions carefully. Should the effects become excessively troublesome, consult your doctor.

BY THREE TO SIX WEEKS, some patients notice an appearance of new blemishes (papules and pustules). At this stage it is important to continue using AVITA® Gel.

If AVITA® Gel is going to have a beneficial effect for you, you should notice an improvement in your appearance by 6 to 12 weeks of therapy. Don't be discouraged if you see no immediate improvement. Don't stop treatment at the first signs of improvement.

Once your acne is under control you should continue regular application of AVITA® Gel until your physician instructs otherwise.

Manufactured By:
DPT LABORATORIES, INC.
San Antonio, Texas 78215

Distributed By:
Penederm Incorporated
Foster City, California 94404.

December 1997

MENTAX® ℞

[*měn-tax*]
(butenafine HCl cream)
Cream, 1%

CAUTION: Federal (USA) law prohibits dispensing without a prescription.

DESCRIPTION

Mentax® Cream, 1%, contains the synthetic antifungal agent, butenafine hydrochloride. Butenafine is a member of the class of antifungal compounds known as benzylamines which are structurally related to the allylamines.

Butenafine HCl is designated chemically as *N*-4-*tert*-butylbenzyl-*N*-methyl-1-naphthalenemethylamine hydrochloride. The compound has the empirical formula $C_{23}H_{27}N \cdot HCl$, a molecular weight of 353.93, and the following structural formula:

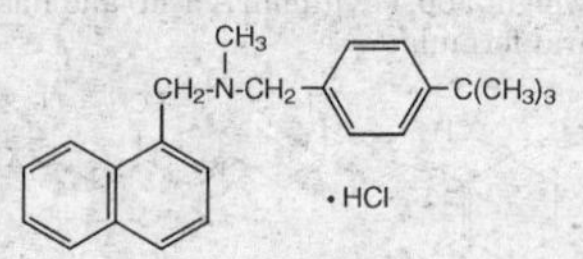

Butenafine HCl is a white, odorless, crystalline powder. It is freely soluble in methanol, ethanol, and chloroform, and slightly soluble in water. Each gram of Mentax® Cream, 1%, contains 10 mg of butenafine HCl in a white cream base of purified water USP, propylene glycol dicaprylate, glycerin USP, cetyl alcohol NF, glyceryl monostearate SE, white petrolatum USP, stearic acid NF, polyoxyethylene (23) cetyl ether, benzyl alcohol NF, diethanolamine NF, and sodium benzoate NF.

CLINICAL PHARMACOLOGY

Mechanism of Action

Butenafine HCl is a benzylamine derivative with a mode of action similar to that of the allylamine class of antifungal drugs. Butenafine HCl is hypothesized to act by inhibiting the epoxidation of squalene, thus blocking the biosynthesis of ergosterol, an essential component of fungal cell membranes. The benzylamine derivatives, like the allylamines, act at an earlier step in the ergosterol biosynthesis pathway than the azole class of antifungal drugs. Depending on the concentration of the drug and the fungal species tested, butenafine HCl may be fungicidal *in vitro*. However, the clinical significance of these *in vitro* data is unknown.

Pharmacokinetics

In one study conducted in healthy subjects for 14 days, 6 grams of Mentax® Cream, 1%, was applied once daily to the dorsal skin (3,000 cm^2) of 7 subjects, and 20 grams of the cream was applied once daily to the arms, trunk and groin areas (10,000 cm^2) of another 12 subjects. After 14 days of topical applications, the 6-gram dose group yielded a mean peak plasma butenafine HCl concentration, Cmax, of 1.4 ± 0.8 ng/mL, occurring at a mean time to the peak plasma concentration, Tmax, of 15 ± 8 hours, and a mean area under the plasma concentration-time curve, $AUC_{0-24\ hrs}$ of 23.9 ± 11.3 ng-hr/mL. For the 20-gram dose group, the mean Cmax was 5.0 ± 2.0 ng/mL, occurring at a mean Tmax of 6 ± 6 hours, and the mean $AUC_{0-24\ hrs}$ was 87.8 ± 45.3 ng-hr/mL. A biphasic decline of plasma butenafine HCl concentrations was observed with the half-lives estimated to be 35 hours and > 150 hours, respectively. At 72 hours after the last dose application, the mean plasma concentrations decreased to 0.3 ± 0.2 ng/mL for the 6-gram dose group and 1.1 ± 0.9 ng/mL for the 20-gram dose group. Low levels of butenafine HCl remained in the plasma 7 days after the last dose application (mean: 0.1 ± 0.2 ng/mL for the 6-gram dose group, and 0.7 ± 0.5 ng/mL for the 20-gram dose group). The total amount (or % dose) of butenafine HCl absorbed through the skin into the systemic circulation has not been quantitated. It was determined that the primary metabolite in urine was formed through hydroxylation at the terminal *t*-butyl side-chain.

In 11 patients with tinea pedis, Mentax® Cream, 1%, was applied by the patients to cover the affected and immedi-

Interdigital Tinea Pedis: 4 Week Dosing Regimen

Patient Outcome Category	WEEK 4 (End of Treatment)		WEEK 8 (4 Weeks Post-Treatment)	
	Butenafine	Vehicle	Butenafine	Vehicle
Mycological Cure	89% (83/93)	57% (51/90)	90% (66/73)	38% (25/66)
Effective Treatment	57% (53/93)	28% (25/90)	74% (54/73)	26% (17/66)
Overall Cure	15% (14/93)	8% (7/90)	25% (18/73)	9% (6/66)

Interdigital Tinea Pedis: 1 Week Dosing Regimen

Patient Outcome Category	WEEK 1 (End of Treatment)		WEEK 6 (5 Weeks Post-Treatment)	
	Butenafine	Vehicle	Butenafine	Vehicle
Mycological Cure	44% (111/253)	28% (75/265)	79% (200/253)	20% (54/265)
Effective Treatment	5% (12/253)	3% (7/265)	38% (95/253)	7% (18/265)
Overall Cure	0.4% (1/253)	0.4% (1/265)	*15% (37/253)	0.7% (2/265)

*The Overall Cure rate of 15% is calculated from a 9% rate in one trial and a 20% rate in the second trial.

Tinea Corporis

Patient Outcome Category	WEEK 2 (End of Treatment)		WEEK 6 (4 Weeks Post-Treatment)	
	Butenafine	Vehicle	Butenafine	Vehicle
Mycological Cure	88% (37/42)	28% (10/36)	88% (37/42)	17% (6/36)
Effective Treatment	60% (25/42)	17% (6/36)	81% (34/42)	14% (5/36)
Overall Cure	31% (13/42)	3% (1/36)	67% (28/42)	14% (5/36)

Tinea Cruris

Patient Outcome Category	WEEK 2 (End of Treatment)		WEEK 6 (4 Weeks Post-Treatment)	
	Butenafine	Vehicle	Butenafine	Vehicle
Mycological Cure	78% (29/37)	11% (4/38)	81% (30/37)	13% (5/39)
Effective Treatment	57% (21/37)	8% (3/39)	73% (27/37)	5% (2/39)
Overall cure	32% (12/37)	8% (3/39)	62% (23/37)	3% (1/39)

ately surrounding skin area once daily for 4 weeks, and a single blood sample was collected between 10 and 20 hours following dosing at 1, 2 and 4 weeks after treatment. The plasma butenafine HCl concentration ranged from undetectable to 0.3 ng/mL.

In 24 patients with tinea cruris, Mentax® Cream, 1 %, was applied by the patients to cover the affected and immediately surrounding skin area once daily for 2 weeks (mean average daily dose: 1.3 ± 0.2 g). A single blood sample was collected between 0.5 and 65 hours after the last dose, and the plasma butenafine HCl concentration ranged from undetectable to 2.52 ng/mL (mean $\pm$ SD: 0.91 ± 0.15 ng/mL). Four weeks after cessation of treatment, the plasma butenafine HCl concentration ranged from undetectable to 0.28 ng/mL.

Microbiology
Butenafine HCl has been shown to be active against most strains of the following microorganisms, both *in vitro* and in clinical infections as described in the INDICATIONS AND USAGE section:

Epidermophyton floccosum
Trichophyton mentagrophytes
Trichophyton rubrum
Trichophyton tonsurans

CLINICAL STUDIES
Interdigital Tinea Pedis
Once Daily Four Week Dosing
In the following data presentations, patients with interdigital tinea pedis in the absence of moccasin-type tinea pedis and onychomycosis were studied. The term **"Mycological Cure"** is defined as both negative KOH and culture. The term **"Effective Treatment"** refers to patients who had a "Mycological Cure" and an Investigator's Global of either "Excellent" (80% to 99% improvement) or "Cleared" (100% improvement). The term **"Overall Cure"** refers to patients who had both a "Mycological Cure" and an Investigator's Global Assessment of "Cleared" (100% improvement).
Data from the two controlled studies in which Mentax® Cream, 1%, was used once daily for 4 weeks have been combined in the table below. Patients were treated for 4 weeks

and evaluated 4 weeks post-treatment. In the "per protocol" analysis shown in the table below, statistical significance (Mentax® vs. vehicle) was assessed 4 weeks post-treatment.
[See first table above]

Twice Daily One Week Dosing
In the following data presentations, patients with interdigital tinea pedis in the absence of moccasin-type tinea pedis were studied. Patients with concurrent onychomycosis were not excluded. The term **"Mycological Cure"** is defined as both negative KOH and culture. The term **"Effective Treatment"** refers to patients who had a "Mycological Cure" and an Investigator's Global of either "Excellent" (90% to 99% improvement) or "Cleared" (100% improvement). The term **"Overall Cure"** refers to patients who had both a "Mycological Cure" and an Investigator's Global Assessment of "Cleared" (100% improvement).
Data from the two controlled studies in which Mentax® Cream, 1%, was used twice daily for 1 week have been combined in the table below. Patients were treated for 1 week and evaluated 5 weeks post-treatment. In the "modified-intent-to-treat" analysis shown in the table below, statistical significance (Mentax® vs. vehicle) was assessed 5 weeks post-treatment.
[See second table above]

Tinea Corporis and Tinea Cruris
In the following data presentations, patients with tinea corporis or tinea cruris were studied. The term **"Mycological Cure"** is defined as both negative KOH and culture. The term **"Effective Treatment"** refers to patients who had a "Mycological Cure" and an Investigator's Global of either "Excellent" (90% to 99% improvement) or "Cleared" (100% improvement). The term **"Overall Cure"** refers to patients who had both a "Mycological Cure" and an Investigator's Global Assessment of "Cleared" (100% improvement).
Separate studies compared Mentax® Cream to vehicle applied once daily for 2 weeks in the treatment of tinea corporis and tinea cruris. Patients were treated for 2 weeks and evaluated 4 weeks post-treatment. All subjects with a positive baseline exam (including positive culture and KOH) and who were dispensed medication were included in the

"modified intent-to-treat" analysis shown in the table below. Statistical significance (Mentax® vs. vehicle) was achieved for all patient outcome categories at Week 2 (end of treatment) and Week 6 (4 weeks post-treatment).
[See third & fourth tables below]

INDICATIONS AND USAGE
Mentax® (butenafine HCl cream) Cream, 1%, is indicated for the topical treatment of the following superficial dermatophytoses: interdigital tinea pedis (athlete's foot), tinea corporis (ringworm) and tinea cruris (jock itch) due to *E. floccosum, T. mentagrophytes, T. rubrum,* and *T. tonsurans.* Butenafine HCl cream was not studied in immunocompromised patients. (See DOSAGE AND ADMINISTRATION).

CONTRAINDICATIONS
Mentax® (butenafine HCl cream) Cream, 1%, is contraindicated in individuals who have known or suspected sensitivity to Mentax® Cream, 1%, or any of its components.

WARNINGS
Mentax® (butenafine HCl cream) Cream, 1%, is not for ophthalmic, oral, or intravaginal use.

PRECAUTIONS
General
Mentax® Cream, 1%, is for external use only. If irritation or sensitivity develops with the use of Mentax® Cream, 1%, treatment should be discontinued and appropriate therapy instituted. Diagnosis of the disease should be confirmed either by direct microscopic examination of infected superficial epidermal tissue in a solution of potassium hydroxide or by culture on an appropriate medium.
Patients who are known to be sensitive to allylamine antifungals should use Mentax® (butenafine HCl cream) Cream, 1%, with caution, since cross-reactivity may occur. Use Mentax® Cream, 1%, as directed by the physician, and avoid contact with the eyes, nose, and mouth, and other mucous membranes.
Information for Patients
The patient should be instructed to:
1. Use Mentax® Cream, 1%, as directed by the physician. The hands should be washed after applying the medication to the affected area(s). Avoid contact with the eyes, nose, mouth, and other mucous membranes. Mentax® Cream, 1%, is for external use only.
2. Dry the affected area(s) thoroughly before application, if you wish to apply Mentax® Cream, 1%, after bathing.
3. Use the medication for the full treatment time recommended by the physician, even though symptoms may have improved. Notify the physician if there is no improvement after the end of the prescribed treatment period, or sooner, if the condition worsens (see below).
4. Inform the physician if the area of application shows signs of increased irritation, redness, itching, burning, blistering, swelling, or oozing.
5. Avoid the use of occlusive dressings unless otherwise directed by the physician.
6. Do not use this medication for any disorder other than that for which it was prescribed.
Drug Interactions
Potential drug interactions between Mentax® (butenafine HCl cream) Cream, 1%, and other drugs have not been systematically evaluated.
Carcinogenesis, Mutagenesis, Impairment of Fertility
Long-term studies to evaluate the carcinogenic potential of Mentax® Cream, 1%, have not been conducted. Two *in vitro* assays (bacterial reverse mutation test and chromosome aberration test in Chinese hamster lymphocytes) and one *in vivo* study (rat micronucleus bioassay) revealed no mutagenic or clastogenic potential for butenafine. Reproductive studies were conducted in which approximately 150 mg/m²/day (25 mg/kg/day) of butenafine was administered subcutaneously, which is 5 times higher than the maximum recommended human topical dose (30 mg/m²/day) for the treatment of tinea pedis, and six times higher than the anticipated maximum human topical dose (24 mg/m²/day) for the treatment of tinea corporis or tinea cruris. At this dose in animals no adverse effects on male or female fertility were demonstrated.
Pregnancy
Teratogenic Effects: Pregnancy Category B
Subcutaneous or topical doses of butenafine at 150 to 300 mg/m²/day (25 to 50 mg/kg/day) (equivalent to 5 to 10 times the maximum potential exposure at the recommended human topical dose for the treatment of tinea pedis, or 6 to 12 times the anticipated maximum exposure at the human topical dose for the treatment of tinea corporis or tinea cruris) during organogenesis in rats and rabbits were not teratogenic. There are, however, no adequate and well-controlled studies that have been conducted of topically-applied butenafine in pregnant women. Because animal reproduction studies are not always predictive of human response, this drug should be used during pregnancy only if clearly needed.

Continued on next page

Mentax—Cont.

Nursing Mothers

It is not known if butenafine HCl is excreted in human milk. Because many drugs are excreted in human milk, caution should be exercised in prescribing Mentax® Cream, 1%, to a nursing women.

Pediatric Use

Safety and efficacy in pediatric patients below the age of 12 years have not been studied. Use of Mentax® Cream, 1%, in pediatric patients 12 to 16 years of age is supported by evidence from adequate and well-controlled studies of Mentax® Cream, 1%, in adults.

ADVERSE REACTIONS

In controlled clinical trials, 8 (approximately 1%) of 644 patients treated with Mentax® Cream, 1%, reported adverse events related to the skin. These included burning/stinging and worsening of the condition. No patient treated with Mentax® Cream, 1%, discontinued treatment due to an adverse event. In the vehicle-treated patients, two of 624 patients discontinued because of treatment site adverse events, one of which was severe burning/stinging and itching at the site of application.

In uncontrolled clinical trials, the most frequently reported adverse events in patients treated with Mentax® Cream, 1%, were: contact dermatitis, erythema, irritation, and itching, each occurring in less than 2% of patients.

OVERDOSAGE

Overdosage of butenafine HCl in humans has not been reported to date.

DOSAGE AND ADMINISTRATION

In the treatment of interdigital tinea pedis, Mentax® should be applied twice daily for 7 days OR once daily for 4 weeks (NOTE: in separate clinical trials, the 7 day dosing regimen was less efficacious than the 4 week regimen; see CLINICAL STUDIES. While the clinical significance of this difference is unknown, these data should be carefully considered before selecting the dosage regimen for patients at risk for the development of bacterial cellulitis of the lower extremity associated with interdigital cracking/fissuring).
Patients with tinea corporis or tinea cruris should apply Mentax® once daily for two weeks.
Sufficient Mentax® Cream should be applied to cover affected areas and immediately surrounding skin of patients with interdigital tinea pedis, tinea corporis, and tinea cruris. If a patient shows no clinical improvement after the treatment period, the diagnosis should be reviewed.

HOW SUPPLIED

Mentax® (butenafine HCl cream) Cream, 1%, is supplied in tubes in the following sizes:
15-gram tube (NDC 25074-151-02) 30-gram tube (NDC 25074-151-03)
STORE BETWEEN 5°C and 30°C (41° and 86°F).
Manufactured By: DPT LABORATORIES, INC.
San Antonio, Texas 78215
Distributed By: Penederm Incorporated
Foster City, California 94404
November 1997
PN341.02E

Persōn & Covey, Inc.
P.O. Box 25018
GLENDALE, CA 91221-5018

For Additional Information:
(818) 240-1030
(800) 423-2341

AQUANIL HC™ LOTION   OTC
Lipid-free with 1.0% Hydrocortisone
Non-comedogenic

INDICATIONS

AQUANIL HC Lotion contains 1.0% Hydrocortisone an effective anti-itch ingredient, in a gentle, free flowing, lipid-free (oil free), lotion, formulated for sensitive skin. It is indicated for the temporary relief of minor skin irritations, inflammations, itches and rashes due to seborrheic dermatitis, insect bites, eczema, psoriasis, soaps, detergents, cosmetics, jewelry, poison oak, poison ivy and poison sumac. Other uses of this product should be only under the advice and supervision of a physician.

DIRECTIONS

For adults and children 2 years of age and older: Apply to affected area not more than 3 to 4 times daily. For children under 2 years of age there is no recommended dosage except under the advice and supervision of a physician.

WARNINGS

For external use only. Avoid contact with eyes. If condition worsens, or if symptoms persist for more than 7 days or clear up and occur again within a few days, discontinue use of this product and do not begin use of any other hydrocortisone product unless you have consulted a physician. Do not use for diaper rash, consult a physician. Keep this and all drugs out of reach of children. In case of accidental ingestion, seek professional assistance or contact a Poison Control Center immediately.

Store at room temperature.
Shake well before using.

Active Ingredient: Hydrocortisone U.S.P. 1.0% (Micronized). Inactive Ingredients: Purified Water, Glycerin, Cetyl Alcohol, Stearyl Alcohol, Benzyl Alcohol. Sodium Laureth Sulfate, Simethicone, Xanthan Gum.

HOW SUPPLIED

Plastic bottle, 118.3 ml (4 fluid oz.) (NDC 0096-0732-04)

DHS™ Tar Shampoo and   OTC
DHS Tar Gel Shampoo (Scented)
Aids in the control of the scaling of seborrhea (dandruff) and psoriasis of the scalp.

DIRECTIONS

Wet hair thoroughly apply a liberal quantity of DHS Tar Shampoo and massage into a lather. Rinse thoroughly and repeat application. Allow lather to remain on scalp for about 5 minutes. Use DHS Tar Shampoo once or twice weekly, or as directed by your physician.

ACTIVE INGREDIENT

Tar, equivalent to 0.5% Coal Tar, inactive ingredients: TEA-Lauryl Sulfate, Purified Water, U.S.P., Sodium Chloride, PEG-8 Distearate, Cocamide DEA, Cocamide MEA, Citric Acid. DHS Tar Gel Shampoo also contains: Hydroxypropyl Methylcellulose and fragrance.

WARNINGS

For external use only. Avoid contact with eyes. If contact occurs, rinse eyes thoroughly with water. If condition worsens or does not improve after regular use of the product as directed consult a physician. Use caution in exposing skin to sunlight after applying this product. It may increase your tendency to sunburn for up to 24 hours after application. Do not use for prolonged periods without consulting a physician. Do not use this product with other forms of psoriasis therapy such as ultraviolet radiation or prescription drugs, unless directed to do so by a physician. If condition covers a large portion of the body, consult your physician before using this product. In rare instances, discoloration of gray, blond, bleach or tinted hair may occur. Store away from direct sunlight. Keep this and all drugs out of the reach of children. In case of accidental ingestion, seek professional assistance or contact a Poison Control Center immediately.

HOW SUPPLIED

DHS Tar Shampoo 4 oz Plastic bottle (NDC 0096-0728-04)
DHS Tar Shampoo 8 oz Plastic bottle (NDC 0096-0728-08)
DHS Tar Shampoo 16 oz Plastic bottle (NDC 0096-0728-16)
DHS Tar Gel Shampoo Plastic bottle (NDC 0096-0730-08)

DHS Zinc Shampoo
Aids in the control of dandruff/seborrheic dermatitis of the scalp.

DIRECTIONS

Shake well before using. Wet hair thoroughly; apply a liberal quantity of DHS Zinc Shampoo and massage into a lather. Rinse thoroughly and repeat application. Allow lather to remain on scalp for about 5 minutes. Use DHS Zinc Shampoo at least twice weekly for the first two weeks, then regularly thereafter, or as directed by your physician.

ACTIVE INGREDIENT

2% Zinc Pyrithione, inactive ingredients: Purified Water, U.S.P., TEA-Lauryl Sulfate, PEG-8 Distearate, Sodium Chloride, Cocamide DEA, Cocamide MEA, Magnesium Aluminum Silicate, Hydroxypropyl Methylcellulose, fragrance and FD&C yellow #6.

WARNINGS

For external use only. Avoid contact with eyes. If contact occurs, rinse eyes thoroughly with water. If condition worsens or does not improve after regular use of this product as directed, consult a physician. If condition covers a large portion of the body, consult your physician before using this product. **Keep this and all drugs out of the reach of children.** In case of accidental ingestion, seek professional assistance or contact a Poison Control Center immediately.

HOW SUPPLIED

8 oz Plastic bottle (NDC 0096-0729-08)
12 oz Plastic bottle (NDC 0096-0729-12)

DML™ FACIAL MOISTURIZER   OTC
Moisturizer with Sunscreen (SPF 15)
Hyaluronic Acid
Non-comedogenic
Fragrance Free

INDICATION

Contains special ingredients that help soothe dry, sensitive skin. Contains sunscreen agents with an SPF of 15 to protect from damaging effects of sunlight (UVA & UVB).

DIRECTIONS

Apply to face as needed or as directed by your dermatologist.

CAUTION

For external use only. Avoid contact with eyes. Keep out of reach of children.

ACTIVE INGREDIENT

Octyl Methoxycinnamate 7.5%, Oxybenzone USP 4%, Inactive ingredients: Purified Water, Propylene Glycol Dioctanoate, Petrolatum USP, Glycerin, Cetyl Phosphate (and) DEA-Cetyl Phosphate, Glyceryl Stearate (and) PEG-100 Stearate, Stearic Acid, Hyaluronic Acid, Benzyl Alcohol, Dimethicone, PVP/Eicosene Copolymer, Sodium Carbomer 941, Disodium EDTA, Magnesium Aluminum Silicate.

HOW SUPPLIED

Plastic tube, 1.5 oz.   (NDC 0096-0721-45)

DML-FORTE   OTC

DESCRIPTION

Moisturizing cream for severe dry skin.

HOW SUPPLIED

Plastic Tube 4 oz NDC 0096-0720-04

DML-LOTION   OTC

DESCRIPTION

Moisturizing lotion for dry skin.

HOW SUPPLIED

Plastic bottle 8 oz NDC 0096-0722-08
Plastic bottle 16 oz NDC 0096-0722-16

DRYSOL™   R

DESCRIPTION

A Solution of Aluminum Chloride (Hexahydrate) 20% w/v in Anhydrous Ethyl Alcohol (S.D. Alcohol 40) 93% v/v.

INDICATION

An aid in the management of hyperhidrosis.

DIRECTIONS

Apply Drysol to the affected area once a day, **only at bedtime**. To help prevent irritation, the area should be completely dry prior to application. Do not apply Drysol to broken, irritated or recently shaved skin.

FOR MAXIMUM EFFECT

Your doctor may instruct you to cover the treated area with saran wrap held in place by a snug fitting "T" or body shirt, mitten or sock. (Never hold saran in place with tape.) Wash the treated area the following morning. Excessive sweating may be stopped after two or more treatments. Thereafter, apply Drysol once or twice weekly or as needed.

NOTICE

Drysol may produce a burning or prickling sensation. Keep cap tightly closed when not in use to prevent evaporation.

WARNING

For external use only. Keep out of the reach of children. Avoid contact with the eyes. If irritation or sensitization occurs, discontinue use or consult with a physician. Drysol may be harmful to certain metals and fabrics. Keep away from open flame.

HOW SUPPLIED

37.5cc Plastic bottle (NDC 0096-0707-37)
35cc Plastic dab-O-Matic (NDC 0096-0707-35)
60cc Plastic dab-O-Matic (NDC 0096-0707-60)

SOLBAR® PF CREAM SPF 50†*+   OTC
Ultra protection sunscreen
Broad Spectrum UVA and UVB protection

CONTAINS
Oxybenzone Octyl Methoxycinnamate, Octocrylene

INDICATIONS
SOLBAR PF 50 Cream is specially formulated for ultra protection from the sun's burning and tanning rays.

HOW SUPPLIED
Plastic bottle, 4oz. (NDC 0096-0686-04).

SOLBAR® PF LIQUID SPF 30†*+   OTC
Ultra protection sunscreen
Broad Spectrum UVA and UVB protection

CONTAINS
Octocrylene, Octyl Methoxycinnamate, Oxybenzone and SD Alcohol 40.

INDICATIONS
SOLBAR PF 30 LIQUID is specially formulated for oily, acne prone skin ultra protection from the sun's burning and tanning rays.
WARNING: Keep away from open flame.

HOW SUPPLIED
Plastic bottle, 3.8 oz. (NDC 0096-0685-04)

* Caution: If irritation or sensitization occurs, discontinue use and consult a physician. Avoid contact with the eyes.
+ Warning: For external use only. Keep out of the reach of children.

XERAC™ AC   ℞
Aluminum Chloride Hexahydrate in
Anhydrous Ethyl Alcohol

DESCRIPTION
A solution of Aluminum Chloride (Hexahydrate) 6.25% (w/v) in Anhydrous Ethyl Alcohol (S.D. Alcohol 40) 96% (v/v).

INDICATION
For topical application as an antiperspirant (anhidrotic).

DIRECTIONS
Apply Xerac AC to the axillae at bedtime or as directed by physician. To help prevent irritation, the area should be completely dry prior to application. Do not apply Xerac AC to broken or irritated skin. Keep container tightly closed.

ADVERSE REACTIONS
Transient stinging or itching may occur. It is not evidence of contact sensitivity and may be prevented or reduced by applying Xerac AC only to skin which is completely dry or by removing the solution with soap and water.

WARNING
For external use only. Some users of this product will experience skin irritation. If this occurs, discontinue use. Avoid contact with the eyes. This product may be harmful to certain metals and fabrics. Keep the container tightly closed when not in use to prevent evaporation. Keep this and all medication out of the reach of children. Do not use near open flame.

HOW SUPPLIED
35cc bottle/Dab-O-Matic head (NDC 0096-0709-35)
60cc bottle/Dab-O-Matic head (NDC 0096-0709-60)

NOTICE
Before prescribing or administering
any product described in
PHYSICIANS' DESK REFERENCE
check the **PDR Supplements**
for revised information.

Pfizer Inc
Consumer Health Care
Group
235 E. 42nd STREET
NY, NY 10017-5755

DIRECT MEDICAL EMERGENCIES AND INQUIRIES TO:
Consumer Relations Group
(212) 573-5656
FAX: (212) 973-7437

BONINE®   OTC
(Meclizine hydrochloride)
Chewable Tablets

ACTION
BONINE (meclizine) is an H_1 histamine receptor blocker of the piperazine side chain group. It exhibits its action by an effect on the Central Nervous System (CNS), possibly by its ability to block muscarinic receptors in the brain.

INDICATIONS
BONINE is effective in the management of nausea, vomiting and dizziness associated with motion sickness.

CONTRAINDICATIONS
Do not take this product, unless directed by a doctor, if you have a breathing problem such as emphysema or chronic bronchitis, or if you have glaucoma or difficulty in urination due to enlargement of the prostate gland.

WARNINGS
May cause drowsiness; alcohol, sedatives and tranquilizers may increase the drowsiness effect. Avoid alcoholic beverages while taking this product. Do not take this product if you are taking sedatives or tranquilizers without first consulting your doctor. Do not drive or operate dangerous machinery while taking this medication.
Usage in Children:
Clinical studies establishing safety and effectiveness in children have not been done; therefore, usage is not recommended in children under 12 years of age.
Usage in Pregnancy:
As with any drug, if you are pregnant or nursing a baby, seek advice of a health care professional before taking this product.

ADVERSE REACTIONS
Drowsiness, dry mouth, and on rare occasions, blurred vision have been reported.

DOSAGE AND ADMINISTRATION
For motion sickness, take one or two tablets of Bonine once daily, one hour before travel starts, for up to 24 hours of protection against motion sickness. The tablet can be chewed with or without water or swallowed whole with water. Thereafter, the dose may be repeated every 24 hours for the duration of the travel.

HOW SUPPLIED
BONINE (meclizine HCl) is available in convenient packets of 8 chewable tablets of 25 mg. meclizine HCl.

INACTIVE INGREDIENTS
FD&C Red #40, Lactose, Magnesium Stearate, Purified Siliceous Earth, Raspberry Flavor, Saccharin Sodium, Starch, Talc.

UNISOM® SleepTabs™   OTC
[yu 'na-som]
Nighttime Sleep Aid
(doxylamine succinate)

PRODUCT OVERVIEW
KEY FACTS
Unisom is an ethanolamine antihistamine (doxylamine) which characteristically shows a high incidence of sedation. It produces a reduced latency to end of wakefulness and early onset of sleep.

MAJOR USES
Unisom has been shown to be clinically effective as a sleep aid when 1 tablet is given 30 minutes before retiring.

SAFETY INFORMATION
Unisom is contraindicated in pregnancy and nursing mothers. It is also contraindicated in patients with asthma, glaucoma, and enlargement of the prostate. Caution should be used if taken when alcohol is being consumed. Caution is

---

also indicated when taken concurrently with other medications due to the anticholinergic properties of antihistamines.

PROFESSIONAL INFORMATION

UNISOM®   OTC
[yu 'na-som]
Nighttime Sleep Aid
(doxylamine succinate)

DESCRIPTION
Pale blue oval scored tablets containing 25 mg. of doxylamine succinate, 2-[α-(2-dimethylaminoethoxy)α-methylbenzyl]pyridine succinate.

ACTIVE INGREDIENT
Doxylamine Succinate 25 mg.

ACTION AND USES
Doxylamine succinate is an antihistamine of the ethanolamine class, which characteristically shows a high incidence of sedation. In a comparative clinical study of over 20 antihistamines on more than 3000 subjects, doxylamine succinate 25 mg. was one of the three most sedating antihistamines, producing a significantly reduced latency to end of wakefulness and comparing favorably with established hypnotic drugs such as secobarbital and pentobarbital in sedation activity. It was chosen as the antihistamine, based on dosage, causing the earliest onset of sleep. In another clinical study, doxylamine succinate 25 mg. scored better than secobarbital 100 mg. as a nighttime hypnotic. Two additional, identical clinical studies, involving a total of 121 subjects demonstrated that doxylamine succinate 25 mg. reduced the sleep latency period by a third, compared to placebo. Duration of sleep was 26.6% longer with doxylamine succinate, and the quality of sleep was rated higher with the drug than with placebo. An EEG study on 6 subjects confirmed the results of these studies. In yet another study, no statistically significant difference was found between doxylamine succinate and flurazepam in the average time required for 200 patients with mild to moderate insomnia to fall asleep over 5 nights following a nightly dose of doxylamine succinate 25 mg. or flurazepam 30 mg., nor was any statistically significant difference found in the total time the 200 patients slept. Patients on doxylamine succinate awoke an average of 1.2 times per night while those on flurazepam awoke an average of 0.9 times per night. In either case the patients awoke rested the following morning. On a rating scale of 1 to 5, doxylamine succinate was given a 3.0, flurazepam a 3.4 by patients rating the degree of restfulness provided by their medication (5 represents "very well rested"). Although statistically significant, the difference between doxylamine succinate 25 mg. and flurazepam 30 mg. in the number of awakenings and degree of restfulness is clinically insignificant.

ADMINISTRATION AND DOSAGE
One tablet 30 minutes before retiring. Not for children under 12 years of age.

WARNINGS
Do not take this product, unless directed by a doctor, if you have a breathing problem such as emphysema or chronic bronchitis, or if you have glaucoma or difficulty in urination due to enlargement of the prostate gland.
Do not take this product if pregnant or nursing a baby.
- If sleeplessness persists continuously for more than two weeks, consult your doctor. Insomnia may be a symptom of serious underlying medical illness.
- Do not take this product if presently taking any other drug, without consulting you doctor or pharmacist.
- Take this product with caution if alcohol is being consumed.
- For adults only. Do not give to children under 12 years of age.
- Keep this and all medications out of the reach of children. This product contains an antihistamine and will cause drowsiness. It should be used only at bedtime.

HOW SUPPLIED
Boxes of 8, 16, 32 or 48 tablets.

INACTIVE INGREDIENTS
Dibasic Calcium Phosphate, FD&C Blue #1 Aluminum Lake, Magnesium Stearate, Microcrystalline Cellulose, Sodium Starch Glycolate.

MAXIMUM STRENGTH   OTC
UNISOM SleepGels®
Nighttime Sleep Aid

DESCRIPTION
Maximum Strength Unisom SleepGels are liquid-filled, blue soft gelatin capsules.

Continued on next page

Unisom Maximum Strength—Cont.

ACTIVE INGREDIENT

Diphenhydramine Hydrochloride 50 mg.

INACTIVE INGREDIENTS

FD&C Blue No. 1, Gelatin, Glycerin, Pharmaceutical Glaze, Polyethylene Glycol, Propylene Glycol, Purified Water, Sorbitol, Titanium Dioxide.

INDICATIONS

Helps to reduce difficulty falling asleep.

ACTION

Diphenhydramine Hydrochloride is an ethanolamine antihistamine with anticholinergic and sedative effects.

ADMINISTRATION AND DOSAGE

Adults and children 12 years of age and over: Oral dosage is one softgel (50 mg) at bedtime if needed, or as directed by a doctor.

WARNINGS

Do not take this product, unless directed by a doctor, if you have a breathing problem such as emphysema or chronic bronchitis, or if you have glaucoma or difficulty in urination due to enlargement of the prostate gland. Do not take this product if pregnant or nursing a baby.
• Do not give to children under 12 years of age.
• If sleeplessness persists continuously for more than two weeks, consult your doctor. Insomnia may be a symptom of serious underlying medical illness.
• Avoid alcoholic beverages while taking this product. Do not take this product if you are taking sedatives or tranquilizers, without first consulting your doctor.
• **Do Not Use:** with any other product containing diphenhydramine, including one applied topically.
• Keep this and all drugs out of the reach of children.
• In case of accidental overdose, seek professional assistance or contact a Poison Control Center immediately.

ATTENTION

Use only if softgel blister seals are unbroken.

HOW SUPPLIED

Boxes of 16 liquid filled softgels in child resistant blisters and boxes of 8 with non-child resistant packaging. Also in a 32 count easy to open child resistant bottle.
Store between 15° and 30°C (59° and 86°F)

UNISOM® WITH PAIN RELIEF®   OTC
[yu 'na-som]
Nighttime Sleep Aid and Pain Reliever

PRODUCT OVERVIEW

KEY FACTS

Unisom With Pain Relief (diphenhydramine sleep aid/acetaminophen pain relief formula) is a product with a dual antihistamine sleep aid/analgesic action to utilize the sedative effects of an antihistamine and relieve mild to moderate pain that may disturb normal sleep patterns. If patients have difficulty in falling asleep but are not experiencing pain at the same time, regular Unisom Sleep Aid which contains doxylamine succinate or Maximum Strength Unisom SleepGels which contains diphenhydramine is indicated.

MAJOR USES

One Unisom With Pain Relief is indicated 30 minutes before retiring to help reduce difficulty in falling asleep while relieving accompanying minor aches and pains, such as headache, muscle aches or menstrual discomfort.

SAFETY INFORMATION

Do not take this product, unless directed by a doctor, if you have a breathing problem such as emphysema or chronic bronchitis, or if you have glaucoma or difficulty in urination due to enlargement of the prostate gland. Unisom With Pain Relief is contraindicated in pregnancy or in nursing mothers. Excessive dosing may lead to liver damage. Product is intended for patients 12 years and older. Alcoholic beverages should be avoided while taking this product. This product should not be taken without first consulting a physician if sedatives or tranquilizers are being taken.

PRESCRIBING INFORMATION

UNISOM WITH PAIN RELIEF®
[yu 'na-som]
Nighttime Sleep Aid and Pain Reliever >

DESCRIPTION

Unisom With Pain Relief® is a pale blue, capsule-shaped, coated tablet.

ACTIVE INGREDIENTS

650 mg acetaminophen and 50 mg diphenhydramine HCl per tablet.

INDICATIONS

Unisom With Pain Relief is a special formula that helps reduce difficulty in falling asleep while relieving accompanying minor aches and pains such as headache, muscle ache or menstrual discomfort. If you have difficulty in falling asleep but are not experiencing pain at the same time, use regular Unisom sleep aid, which contains doxylamine succinate.

ADMINISTRATION AND DOSAGE

Take ONLY ONE TABLET 30 minutes before going to bed to aid sleep and relieve pain. Take once daily or as directed by physician.

WARNINGS

Do not take this product, unless directed by a doctor, if you have a breathing problem such as emphysema or chronic bronchitis, or if you have glaucoma or difficulty in urination due to enlargement of the prostate gland.
Do not take this product for treatment of arthritis except under the advice and supervision of a physican.
• Do not exceed recommended dosage because severe liver damage may occur.
• If symptoms persist continuously for more than ten days, consult your physician. Insomnia may be a symptom of serious underlying medical illness.
• Take this product with caution if alcohol is being consumed.
• Do not take this product if pregnant or nursing a baby.
• For adults only. Do not give to children under 12 years of age.
• Keep this and all medications out of reach of children. In case of accidental overdose seek professional advice or contact a poison control center immediately.

CAUTION

This product contains an antihistamine and will cause drowsiness. It should be used only at bedtime.

ATTENTION

Use only if tablet blister seals are unbroken. Child resistant packaging.

HOW SUPPLIED

Boxes of 8 and 16 tablets in child resistant blisters.

INACTIVE INGREDIENTS

Corn starch, FD&C Blue #1 Aluminum Lake, FD&C Blue #2 Aluminum Lake, Hydroxypropyl Methylcellulose, Magnesium Stearate, Polyethylene Glycol, Polysorbate 80, Povidone, Stearic Acid, Titanium Dioxide.

Pfizer Inc

235 EAST 42nd STREET
NEW YORK, NY 10017–5755

For Medical Information Contact:
(800) 438-1985
24 hours a day, seven days a week.

Product Identification Codes

To provide quick and positive identification of Pfizer Inc products, we have either a unique identifying number of the National Drug Code or the product name on all tablets or capsules.

In order that you may quickly identify a product by its code number, we have compiled below a numerical list of code numbers with their corresponding product names. We are also listing the code numbers by alphabetical order of products.

Numerical Listing

Product Ident. Number	Product
035	Spectrobid® (bacampicillin HCl) Tablets, 400 mg, equivalent to 280 mg ampicillin
092	Urobiotic®-250 (oxytetracycline HCl 250 mg with sulfamethizole 250 mg and phenazopyridine 50 mg) Capsules
094	Vibramycin® Hyclate (doxycycline hyclate) Capsules 50 mg
095	Vibramycin® Hyclate (doxycycline hyclate) Capsules 100 mg
099	Vibra-Tabs® (doxycycline hyclate) Film Coated Tablets 100 mg
143	Geocillin® (carbenicillin indanyl sodium) Tablets, equivalent to 382 mg carbenicillin
152	Norvasc® (amlodipine besylate) Tablets 2.5 mg
153	Norvasc® (amlodipine besylate) Tablets 5 mg
154	Norvasc® (amlodipine besylate) Tablets 10 mg
155	Glucotrol XL® (glipizide) Extended Release Tablets, 5 mg GITS
156	Glucotrol XL® (glipizide) Extended Release Tablets, 10 mg GITS
PD155	Lipitor® (atorvastatin calcium) Tablets, 10 mg
PD156	Lipitor® (atorvastatin calcium) Tablets, 20 mg
PD157	Lipitor® (atorvastatin calcium) Tablets, 40 mg
159	TAO® (troleandomycin) Capsules, 250 mg
210	Antivert® (meclizine HCl) Tablets, 12.5 mg
211	Antivert® /25 (meclizine HCl) Tablets, 25 mg
214	Antivert® /50 (meclizine HCl) Tablets, 50 mg
E245	Aricept® (donepezil HCl) Tablets, 5 mg
E246	Aricept® (donepezil HCl) Tablets, 10 mg
260	Procardia® (nifedipine) Capsules, 10 mg
261	Procardia® (nifedipine) Capsules, 20 mg
265	Procardia XL® (nifedipine) Extended Release Tablets, 30 mg GITS
266	Procardia XL® (nifedipine) Extended Release Tablets, 60 mg GITS
267	Procardia XL® (nifedipine) Extended Release Tablets, 90 mg GITS
275	Cardura® (doxazosin mesylate) Tablets, 1 mg
276	Cardura® (doxazosin mesylate) Tablets, 2 mg
277	Cardura® (doxazosin mesylate) Tablets, 4 mg
278	Cardura® (doxazosin mesylate) Tablets, 8 mg
305	Zithromax® (azithromycin) Capsules 250 mg
306	Zithromax® (azithromycin) Z-Pak™(6 × 250-mg Tablets)
306	Zithromax® (azithromycin) Tablets, 250 mg
308	Zithromax® (azithromycin) Tablets 600 mg
311	Zithromax® (azithromycin for oral suspension) 300 mg (100 mg/5 mL)
312	Zithromax® (azithromycin for oral suspension) 600 mg (200 mg/5 mL)
313	Zithromax® (azithromycin for oral suspension) 900 mg (200 mg/5 mL)
314	Zithromax® (azithromycin for oral suspension) 1200 mg (200 mg/5 mL)
315	Zithromax® (azithromycin) for injection, 500 mg vial
322	Feldene® (piroxicam) Capsules 10 mg
323	Feldene® (piroxicam) Capsules 20 mg
341	Diflucan® (fluconazole) Tablets, 50 mg
342	Diflucan® (fluconazole) Tablets, 100 mg
343	Diflucan® (fluconazole) Tablets, 200 mg
350	Diflucan® (fluconazole) Tablets, 150 mg
375	Rensese® (polythiazide) Tablets, 1 mg
376	Rensese® (polythiazide) Tablets, 2 mg
377	Rensese® (polythiazide) Tablets, 4 mg
378	Trovan™ (trovafloxacin mesylate) Tablets, 100 mg
379	Trovan™ (trovafloxacin mesylate) Tablets 200 mg
389	Trovan™ I.V. (alatrofloxacin mesylate injection) 200 mg for intravenous infusion
390	Trovan™ I.V. (alatrofloxacin mesylate injection) 300 mg for intravenous infusion
393	Diabinese® (chlorpropamide) Tablets 100 mg
394	Diabinese® (chlorpropamide) Tablets 250 mg
411	Glucotrol® (glipizide) Tablets, 5 mg
412	Glucotrol® (glipizide) Tablets, 10 mg
420	Viagra® (sildenafil citrate) Tablets, 25 mg
421	Viagra® (sildenafil citrate) Tablets, 50 mg
422	Viagra® (sildenafil citrate) Tablets, 100 mg
430	Minizide® 1 Capsules (1 mg prazosin HCl and 0.5 mg polythiazide)
431	Minipress® (prazosin HCl) Capsules 1 mg
432	Minizide® 2 Capsules (2 mg prazosin HCl and 0.5 mg polythiazide)

436 Minizide® 5 Capsules (5 mg prazosin HCl and 0.5 mg polythiazide)
437 Minipress® (prazosin HCl) Capsules 2 mg
438 Minipress® (prazosin HCl) Capsules 5 mg
490 Zoloft® (sertraline HCl) Tablets, 50 mg
491 Zoloft® (sertraline HCl) Tablets, 100 mg
496 Zoloft® (sertraline HCl) Tablets, 25 mg
534 Sinequan® (doxepin HCl) Capsules 10 mg
535 Sinequan® (doxepin HCl) Capsules 25 mg
536 Sinequan® (doxepin HCl) Capsules 50 mg
537 Sinequan® (doxepin HCl) Capsules 150 mg
538 Sinequan® (doxepin HCl) Capsules 100 mg
539 Sinequan® (doxepin HCl) Capsules 75 mg
541 Vistaril® (hydroxyzine pamoate) Capsules 25 mg
542 Vistaril® (hydroxyzine pamoate) Capsules 50 mg
543 Vistaril® (hydroxyzine pamoate) Capsules 100 mg
550 Zyrtec® (cetirizine hydrochloride) Tablets 5 mg
551 Zyrtec® (cetirizine hydrochloride) Tablets 10 mg
553 Zyrtec® (cetirizine hydrochloride) Syrup, 5 mg/5 mL
560 Atarax® (hydroxyzine HCl) Tablets, 10 mg
561 Atarax® (hydroxyzine HCl) Tablets, 25 mg
562 Atarax® (hydroxyzine HCl) Tablets, 50 mg
563 Atarax® (hydroxyzine HCl) Tablets, 100 mg
571 Navane® (thiothixene) Capsules, 1 mg
572 Navane® (thiothixene) Capsules, 2 mg
573 Navane® (thiothixene) Capsules, 5 mg
574 Navane® (thiothixene) Capsules, 10 mg
577 Navane® (thiothixene) Capsules, 20 mg

Alphabetical Listing

Prod. Ident.

Number	Product
210	Antivert® (meclizine HCl) Tablets, 12.5 mg
211	Antivert® /25 (meclizine HCl) Tablets, 25 mg
214	Antivert® /50 (meclizine HCl) Tablets, 50 mg
E245	Aricept® (donepezil HCl) Tablets, 5 mg
E246	Aricept® (donepezil HCl) Tablets, 10 mg
560	Atarax® (hydroxyzine HCl) Tablets, 10 mg
561	Atarax® (hydroxyzine HCl) Tablets, 25 mg
562	Atarax® (hydroxyzine HCl) Tablets, 50 mg
563	Atarax® (hydroxyzine HCl) Tablets, 100 mg
275	Cardura® (doxazosin mesylate) Tablets, 1 mg
276	Cardura® (doxazosin mesylate) Tablets, 2 mg
277	Cardura® (doxazosin mesylate) Tablets, 4 mg
278	Cardura® (doxazosin mesylate) Tablets, 8 mg
393	Diabinese® (chlorpropamide) Tablets 100 mg
394	Diabinese® (chlorpropamide) Tablets 250 mg
341	Diflucan® (fluconazole) Tablets 50 mg
342	Diflucan® (fluconazole) Tablets 100 mg
350	Diflucan® (fluconazole) Tablets 150 mg
343	Diflucan® (fluconazole) Tablets 200 mg

344 Diflucan® (fluconazole for oral suspension) 10 mg/mL
345 Diflucan® (fluconazole for oral suspension) 40 mg/mL
322 Feldene® (piroxicam) Capsules 10 mg
323 Feldene® (piroxicam) Capsules 20 mg
143 Geocillin® (carbenicillin indanyl sodium) Tablets equivalent to 382 mg carbenicillin
411 Glucotrol® (glipizide) Tablets 5 mg
412 Glucotrol® (glipizide) Tablets 10 mg
155 Glucotrol XL® (glipizide) Extended Release Tablets 5 mg GITS
156 Glucotrol XL® (glipizide) Extended Release Tablets 10 mg GITS
PD155 Lipitor® (atorvastatin calcium) Tablets, 10 mg
PD156 Lipitor® (atorvastatin calcium) Tablets, 20 mg
PD157 Lipitor® (atorvastatin calcium) Tablets, 40 mg
431 Minipress® (prazosin HCl) Capsules 1 mg
437 Minipress® (prazosin HCl) Capsules 2 mg
438 Minipress® (prazosin HCl) Capsules 5 mg
430 Minizide® 1 Capsules (1 mg prazosin HCl and 0.5 mg polythiazide)
432 Minizide® 2 Capsules (2 mg prazosin HCl and 0.5 mg polythiazide)
436 Minizide® 5 Capsules (5 mg prazosin HCl and 0.5 mg polythiazide)
571 Navane® (thiothixene) Capsules, 1 mg
572 Navane® (thiothixene) Capsules, 2 mg
573 Navane® (thiothixene) Capsules, 5 mg
574 Navane® (thiothixene) Capsules, 10 mg
577 Navane® (thiothixene) Capsules, 20 mg
152 Norvasc® (amlodipine besylate) Tablets 2.5 mg
153 Norvasc® (amlodipine besylate) Tablets 5 mg
154 Norvasc® (amlodipine besylate) Tablets 10 mg
260 Procardia® (nifedipine) Capsules, 10 mg
261 Procardia® (nifedipine) Capsules, 20 mg
265 Procardia XL® (nifedipine) Extended Release Tablets, 30 mg GITS
266 Procardia XL® (nifedipine) Extended Release Tablets, 60 mg GITS
267 Procardia XL® (nifedipine) Extended Release Tablets, 90 mg GITS
375 Rensese® (polythiazide) Tablets, 1 mg
376 Rensese® (polythiazide) Tablets, 2 mg
377 Rensese® (polythiazide) Tablets, 4 mg
378 Trovan™ (trovafloxacin mesylate) Tablets, 100 mg
379 Trovan™ (trovafloxacin mesylate) Tablets, 200 mg
389 Trovan™ I.V. (alatrofloxacin mesylate injection) 200 mg for intravenous infusion
390 Trovan™ I.V. (alatrofloxacin mesylate injection) 300 mg for intravenous infusion
420 Viagra® (sildenafil citrate) Tablets, 25 mg
421 Viagra® (sildenafil citrate) Tablets, 50 mg
422 Viagra® (sildenafil citrate) Tablets, 100 mg
534 Sinequan® (doxepin HCl) Capsules 10 mg
535 Sinequan® (doxepin HCl) Capsules 25 mg
536 Sinequan® (doxepin HCl) Capsules 50 mg
539 Sinequan® (doxepin HCl) Capsules 75 mg
538 Sinequan® (doxepin HCl) Capsules 100 mg
537 Sinequan® (doxepin HCl) Capsules 150 mg
035 Spectrobid® (bacampicillin HCl) Tablets, 400 mg, equivalent to 280 mg ampicillin

159 TAO® (troleandomycin) Capsules, 250 mg
092 Urobiotic®-250 (oxytetracycline HCl 250 mg with sulfamethizole 250 mg and phenazopyridine 50 mg) Capsules
094 Vibramycin® Hyclate (doxycycline hyclate) Capsules 50 mg
095 Vibramycin® Hyclate (doxycycline hyclate) Capsules 100 mg
099 Vibra-Tabs® (doxycycline hyclate) Film Coated Tablets 100 mg
541 Vistaril® (hydroxyzine pamoate) Capsules 25 mg
542 Vistaril® (hydroxyzine pamoate) Capsules 50 mg
543 Vistaril® (hydroxyzine pamoate) Capsules 100 mg
305 Zithromax® (azithromycin) Capsules 250 mg
306 Zithromax® (azithromycin) Z-PAK™ (6 × 250-mg Tablets)
306 Zithromax® (azithromycin) Tablets, 250-mg
308 Zithromax® (azithromycin) 600 mg Tablets
311 Zithromax® (azithromycin for oral suspension) 300 mg (100 mg/5 mL)
312 Zithromax® (azithromycin for oral suspension) 600 mg (200 mg/5 mL)
313 Zithromax® (azithromycin for oral suspension) 900 mg (200 mg/5 mL)
314 Zithromax® (azithromycin for oral suspension) 1200 mg (200 mg/5 mL)
315 Zithromax® Injection (azithromycin) 500 mg Vial
496 Zoloft® (sertraline HCl) Tablets, 25 mg
490 Zoloft® (sertraline HCl) Tablets, 50 mg
491 Zoloft® (sertraline HCl) Tablets, 100 mg
550 Zyrtec® (cetirizine hydrochloride) Tablets 5 mg
551 Zyrtec® (cetirizine hydrochloride) Tablets 10 mg
553 Zyrtec® (cetirizine hydrochloride) Syrup, 5 mg/5 mL

ANTIVERT® TABLETS ℞
[ăn 'tǐ-vert "]
(12.5 mg meclizine HCl)
ANTIVERT®/25 TABLETS ℞
(25 mg meclizine HCl)
ANTIVERT®/50 TABLETS ℞
(50 mg meclizine HCl)

DESCRIPTION

Chemically, Antivert® (meclizine HCl) is 1-(p-chloro-α-phenylbenzyl) -4- (m -methylbenzyl) piperazine dihydrochloride monohydrate.

Inert ingredients for the tablets are: dibasic calcium phosphate; magnesium stearate; polyethylene glycol; starch; sucrose. The 12.5 mg tablets also contain: Blue 1. The 25 mg tablets also contain: Yellow 6 Lake; Yellow 10 Lake. The 50 mg tablets also contain: Blue 1 Lake; Yellow 10 Lake.

ACTIONS

Antivert is an antihistamine which shows marked protective activity against nebulized histamine and lethal doses of intravenously injected histamine in guinea pigs. It has a marked effect in blocking the vasodepressor response to histamine, but only a slight blocking action against acetylcholine. Its activity is relatively weak in inhibiting the spasmogenic action of histamine on isolated guinea pig ileum.

INDICATIONS

Based on a review of this drug by the National Academy of Sciences-National Research Council and/or other information, FDA has classified the indications as follows:
Effective: Management of nausea and vomiting, and dizziness associated with motion sickness.

Continued on next page

Antivert—Cont.

Possibly Effective: Management of vertigo associated with diseases affecting the vestibular system.
Final classification of the less than effective indications requires further investigation.

CONTRAINDICATIONS

Meclizine HCl is contraindicated in individuals who have shown a previous hypersensitivity to it.

WARNINGS

Since drowsiness may, on occasion, occur with use of this drug, patients should be warned of this possibility and cautioned against driving a car or operating dangerous machinery.
Patients should avoid alcoholic beverages while taking this drug. Due to its potential anticholinergic action, this drug should be used with caution in patients with asthma, glaucoma, or enlargement of the prostate gland.

USAGE IN CHILDREN
Clinical studies establishing safety and effectiveness in children have not been done; therefore, usage is not recommended in children under 12 years of age.

USAGE IN PREGNANCY
Pregnancy Category B. Reproduction studies in rats have shown cleft palates at 25–50 times the human dose. Epidemiological studies in pregnant women, however, do not indicate that meclizine increases the risk of abnormalities when administered during pregnancy. Despite the animal findings, it would appear that the possibility of fetal harm is remote. Nevertheless, meclizine, or any other medication, should be used during pregnancy only if clearly necessary.

ADVERSE REACTIONS

Drowsiness, dry mouth and, on rare occasions, blurred vision have been reported.

DOSAGE AND ADMINISTRATION

Vertigo:
For the control of vertigo associated with diseases affecting the vestibular system, the recommended dose is 25 to 100 mg daily, in divided dosage, depending upon clinical response.

Motion Sickness:
The initial dose of 25 to 50 mg of Antivert should be taken one hour prior to embarkation for protection against motion sickness. Thereafter, the dose may be repeated every 24 hours for the duration of the journey.

HOW SUPPLIED

Antivert®—12.5 mg tablets:
Bottles of 100 (NDC 0662-2100-66), (NDC 0049-2100-66)
Bottles of 1000 (NDC 0662-2100-82), (NDC 0049-2100-82)
Antivert®/25—25 mg tablets:
Bottles of 100 (NDC 0662-2110-66), (NDC 0049-2110-66)
Bottles of 1000 (NDC 0662-2110-82), (NDC 0049-2110-82)
Antivert®/50—50 mg tablets:
Bottles of 100 (NDC 0662-2140-66), (NDC 0049-2140-66)
Revised June 1996 69-2148-00-8

ARICEPT® ℞
(Donepezil Hydrochloride Tablets)

DESCRIPTION

ARICEPT® (donepezil hydrochloride) is a reversible inhibitor of the enzyme acetylcholinesterase, known chemically as (±)-2,3-dihydro-5,6-dimethoxy-2-[[1- (phenylmethyl)-4-piperidinyl]methyl]-1*H*-inden-1-one hydrochloride. Donepezil hydrochloride is commonly referred to in the pharmacological literature as E2020. It has an empirical formula of $C_{24}H_{29}NO_3HCl$ and a molecular weight of 415.96. Donepezil hydrochloride is a white crystalline powder and is freely soluble in chloroform, soluble in water and in glacial acetic acid, slightly soluble in ethanol and in acetonitrile and practically insoluble in ethyl acetate and in n-hexane.

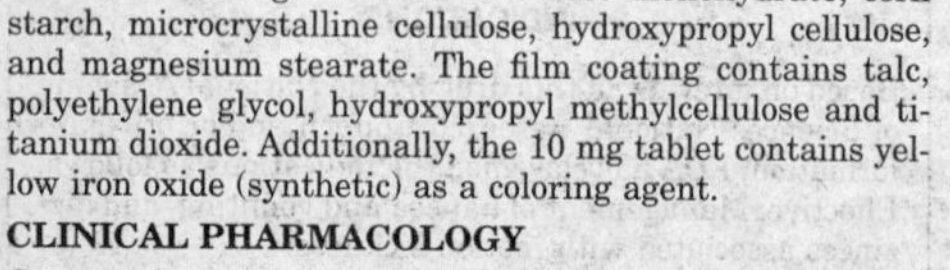

ARICEPT® is available for oral administration in film-coated tablets containing 5 or 10 mg donepezil hydrochloride. Inactive ingredients are lactose monohydrate, corn starch, microcrystalline cellulose, hydroxypropyl cellulose, and magnesium stearate. The film coating contains talc, polyethylene glycol, hydroxypropyl methylcellulose and titanium dioxide. Additionally, the 10 mg tablet contains yellow iron oxide (synthetic) as a coloring agent.

CLINICAL PHARMACOLOGY

Current theories on the pathogenesis of the cognitive signs and symptoms of Alzheimer's Disease attribute some of them to a deficiency of cholinergic neurotransmission. Donepezil hydrochloride is postulated to exert its therapeutic effect by enhancing cholinergic function. This is accomplished by increasing the concentration of acetylcholine through reversible inhibition of its hydrolysis by acetylcholinesterase. If this proposed mechanism of action is correct, donepezil's effect may lessen as the disease process advances and fewer cholinergic neurons remain functionally intact. There is no evidence that donepezil alters the course of the underlying dementing process.

Clinical Trial Data
The effectiveness of ARICEPT® as a treatment for Alzheimer's Disease is demonstrated by the results of two randomized, double-blind, placebo-controlled clinical investigations in patients with Alzheimer's Disease (diagnosed by NINCDS and DSM III-R criteria, Mini-Mental State Examination ≥ 10 and ≤ 26 and Clinical Dementia Rating of 1 or 2). The mean age of patients participating in ARICEPT® trials was 73 years with a range of 50 to 94. Approximately 62% of patients were women and 38% were men. The racial distribution was white 95%, black 3% and other races 2%.

Study Outcome Measures: In each study, the effectiveness of treatment with ARICEPT® was evaluated using a dual outcome assessment strategy.
The ability of ARICEPT® to improve cognitive performance was assessed with the cognitive subscale of the Alzheimer's Disease Assessment Scale (ADAS-cog), a multi-item instrument that has been extensively validated in longitudinal cohorts of Alzheimer's Disease patients. The ADAS-cog examines selected aspects of cognitive performance including elements of memory, orientation, attention, reasoning, language and praxis. The ADAS-cog scoring range is from 0 to 70, with higher scores indicating greater cognitive impairment. Elderly normal adults may score as low as 0 or 1, but it is not unusual for non-demented adults to score slightly higher.
The patients recruited as participants in each study had mean scores on the Alzheimer's Disease Assessment Scale (ADAS-cog) of approximately 26 units, with a range from 4 to 61. Experience gained in longitudinal studies of ambulatory patients with a mild to moderate Alzheimer's Disease suggest that they gain 6 to 12 units a year on the ADAS-cog. However, lesser degrees of change are seen in patients with very mild or very advanced disease because the ADAS-cog is not uniformly sensitive to change over the course of the disease. The annualized rate of decline in the placebo patients participating in ARICEPT® trials was approximately 2 to 4 units per year.
The ability of ARICEPT® to produce an overall clinical effect was assessed using a Clinician's Interview Based Impression of Change that required the use of caregiver information, the CIBIC plus. The CIBIC plus is not a single instrument and is not a standardized instrument like the ADAS-cog. Clinical trials for investigational drugs have used a variety of CIBIC formats, each different in terms of depth and structure. As such, results from a CIBIC plus reflect clinical experience from the trial or trials in which it was used and can not be compared directly with the results of CIBIC plus evaluations from other clinical trials. The CIBIC plus used in ARICEPT® trials was a semi-structured instrument that was intended to examine four major areas of patient function: General, Cognitive, Behavioral and Activities of Daily Living. It represents the assessment of a skilled clinician based upon his/her observations at an interview with the patient, in combination with information supplied by a caregiver familiar with the behavior of the patient and over the interval rated. The CIBIC plus is scored as a seven point categorical rating, ranging from a score of 1, indicating "markedly improved," to a score of 4, indicating "no change" to a score of 7, indicating "markedly worse." The CIBIC plus has not been systematically compared directly to assessments not using information from caregivers (CIBIC) or other global methods.

Thirty-Week Study
In a study of 30 weeks duration, 473 patients were randomized to receive single daily doses of placebo, 5 mg/day or 10 mg/day of ARICEPT®. The 30-week study was divided into a 24-week double-blind active treatment phase followed by a 6-week single-blind placebo washout period. The study was designed to compare 5 mg/day or 10 mg/day fixed doses of ARICEPT® to placebo. However, to reduce the likelihood of cholinergic effects, the 10 mg/day treatment was started following an initial 7-day treatment with 5 mg/day doses.

Effects on the ADAS-cog: Figure 1 illustrates the time course for the change from baseline in ADAS-cog scores for all three dose groups over the 30 weeks of the study. After 24 weeks of treatment, the mean differences in the ADAS-cog change scores for ARICEPT® treated patients compared to the patients on placebo were 2.8 and 3.1 units for the 5 mg/day and 10 mg/day treatments, respectively. These differences were statistically significant. While the treatment effect size may appear to be slightly greater for the 10 mg/day treatment, there was no statistically significant difference between the two active treatments.
Following 6 weeks of placebo washout, scores on the ADAS-cog for both ARICEPT® treatment groups were indistinguishable from those patients who had received only placebo for 30 weeks. This suggests that the beneficial effects of ARICEPT® abate over 6 weeks following discontinuation of treatment and do not represent a change in the underlying disease. There is no evidence of a rebound effect 6 weeks after abrupt discontinuation of therapy.

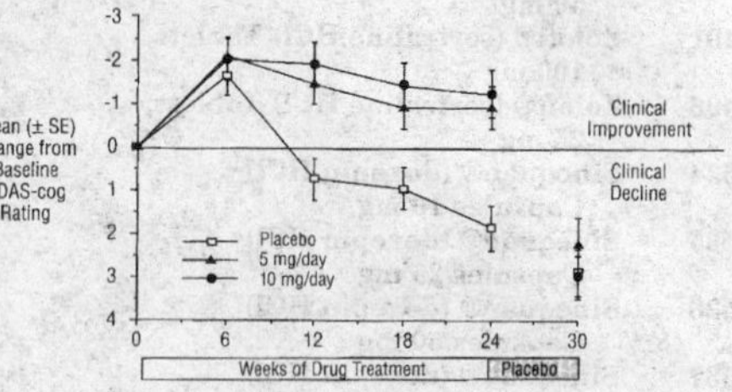

Figure 1. Time-course of the Change from Baseline in ADAS-cog Score for Patients Completing 24 Weeks of Treatment.

Figure 2 illustrates the cumulative percentages of patients from each of the three treatment groups who had attained the measure of improvement in ADAS-cog score shown on the X axis. Three change scores, (7-point and 4-point reductions from baseline or no change in score) have been identified for illustrative purposes and the percent of patients in each group achieving that result is shown in the inset table.
The curves demonstrate that both patients assigned to placebo and ARICEPT® have a wide range of responses, but that the active treatment groups are more likely to show the greater improvements. A curve for an effective treatment would be shifted to the left of the curve for placebo, while an ineffective or deleterious treatment would be superimposed upon or shifted to the right of the curve for placebo, respectively.

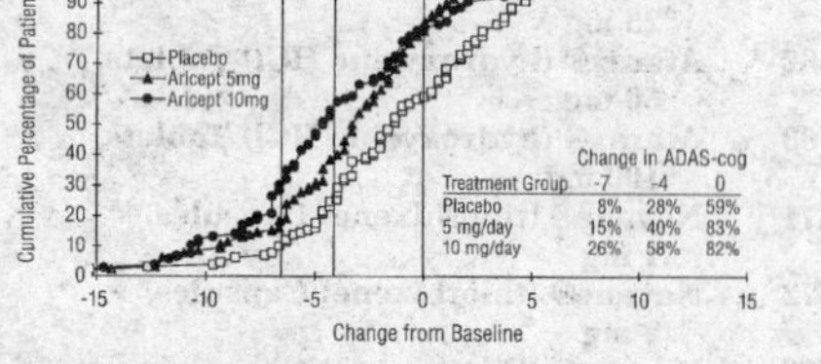

Figure 2. Cumulative Percentage of Patients Completing 24 Weeks of Double-blind Treatment with Specified Changes from Baseline ADAS-cog Scores. The Percentages of Randomized Patients who Completed the Study were: Placebo 80%, 5 mg/day 85% and 10 mg/day 68%.

Effects on the CIBIC plus: Figure 3 is a histogram of the frequency distribution of CIBIC plus scores attained by patients assigned to each of the three treatment groups who completed 24 weeks of treatment. The mean drug-placebo differences for these groups of patients were 0.35 units and 0.39 units for 5 mg/day and 10 mg/day of ARICEPT®, respectively. These differences were statistically significant. There was no statistically significant difference between the two active treatments.

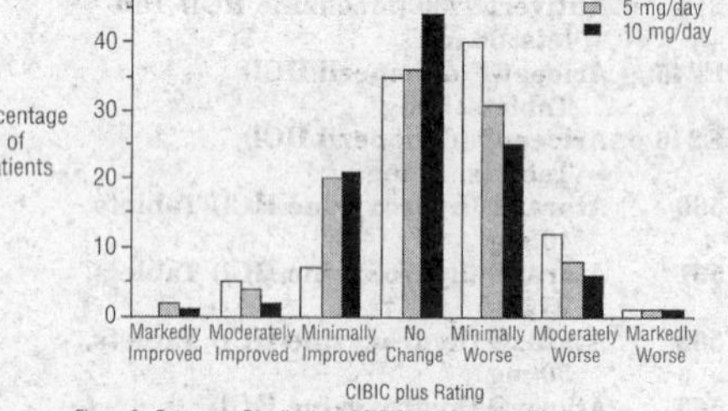

Figure 3. Frequency Distribution of CIBIC plus Scores at Week 24

Fifteen-Week Study
In a study of 15 weeks duration, patients were randomized to receive single daily doses of placebo or either 5 mg/day or 10 mg/day of ARICEPT® for 12 weeks, followed by a 3-week placebo washout period. As in the 30-week study, to avoid acute cholinergic effects, the 10 mg/day treatment followed an initial 7-day treatment with 5 mg/day doses.

Effects of the ADAS-Cog: Figure 4 illustrates the time course of the change from baseline in ADAS-cog scores for all three dose groups over the 15 weeks of the study. After 12 weeks of treatment, the differences in mean ADAS-cog change scores for the ARICEPT® treated patients compared to the patients on placebo were 2.7 and 3.0 units each, for the 5 and 10 mg/day ARICEPT® treatment groups respectively. These differences were statistically significant. The effect sized for the 10 mg/day group may appear to be slightly larger than that for 5 mg/day. However, the differences between active treatments were not statistically significant.

[See figure 4 at top of next coloumn]

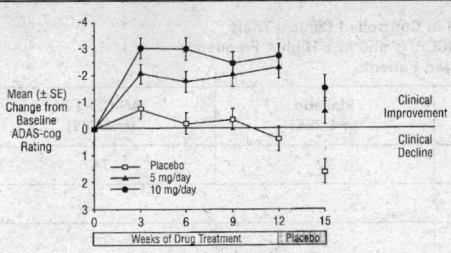

Figure 4. Time-course of the Change from Baseline in ADAS-cog Score for Patients Completing the 15-week Study.

Table 1. Most Frequent Adverse Events Leading to Withdrawal from Controlled Clinical Trials by Dose Group			
Dose Group	Placebo	5 mg/day ARICEPT®	10 mg/day ARICEPT®
Patients Randomized	355	350	315
Event/% Discontinuing			
Nausea	1%	1%	3%
Diarrhea	0%	<1%	3%
Vomiting	<1%	<1%	2%

Following 3 weeks of placebo washout, scores on the ADAS-cog for both the ARICEPT® treatment groups increased, indicating that discontinuation of ARICEPT® resulted in a loss of its treatment effect. The duration of this placebo washout period was not sufficient to characterize the rate of loss of the treatment effect, but, the 30-week study (see above) demonstrated that treatment effects associated with the use of ARICEPT® abate within 6 weeks of treatment discontinuation.

Figure 5 illustrates the cumulative percentages of patients from each of the three treatment groups who attained the measure of improvement in ADAS-cog score shown on the X axis. The same three change scores, (7-point and 4-point reductions from baseline or no change in score) as selected for the 30-week study have been used for this illustration. The percentages of patients achieving those results are shown in the inset table.

As observed in the 30-week study, the curves demonstrate that patients assigned to either placebo or to ARICEPT® have a wide range of responses, but that the ARICEPT® treated patients are more likely to show the greater improvements in cognitive performance.

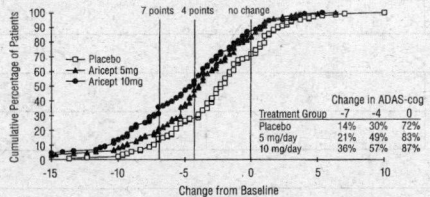

Figure 5. Cumulative Percentage of Patients with Specified Changes from Baseline ADAS-cog Scores. The Percentages of Randomized Patients Within Each Treatment Group Who Completed the Study Were: Placebo 93%, 5 mg/day 90% and 10 mg/day 82%.

Effects on the CIBIC plus: Figure 6 is a histogram of the frequency distribution of CIBIC plus scores attained by patients assigned to each of the three treatment groups who completed 12 weeks of treatment. The differences in mean scores for ARICEPT® treated patients compared to the patients on placebo at Week 12 were 0.36 and 0.38 units for the 5 mg/day and 10 mg/day treatment groups, respectively. These differences were statistically significant.

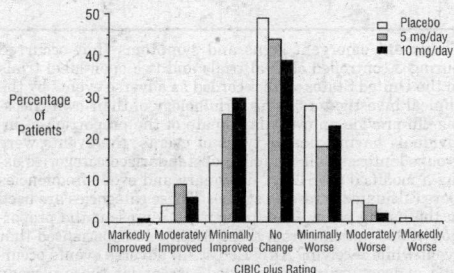

Figure 6. Frequency Distribution of CIBIC plus Scores at Week 12

In both studies, patient age, sex and race were not found to predict the clinical outcome of ARICEPT® treatment.

Clinical Pharmacokinetics
Donepezil is well absorbed with a relative oral bioavailability of 100% and reaches peak plasma concentrations in 3 to 4 hours. Pharmacokinetics are linear over a dose range of 1–10 mg given once daily. Neither food nor time of administration (morning vs. evening dose) influences the rate or extent of absorption. The elimination half-life of donepezil is about 70 hours and the mean apparent plasma clearance (Cl/F) is 0.13 L/hr/kg. Following multiple dose administration, donepezil accumulates in plasma by 4–7 fold and steady state is reached within 15 days. The steady state volume of distribution is 12 L/kg. Donepezil is approximately 96% bound to human plasma proteins, mainly to albumins (about 75%) and alpha₁-acid glycoprotein (about 21%) over the concentration range of 2–1000 ng/mL.
Donepezil is both excreted in the urine intact and extensively metabolized to four major metabolites, two of which are known to be active, and a number of minor metabolites, not all of which have been identified. Donepezil is metabo-

lized by CYP 450 isoenzymes 2D6 and 3A4 and undergoes glucuronidation. Following administration of ^{14}C-labeled donepezil, plasma radioactivity, expressed as a percent of the administered dose, was present primarily as intact donepezil (53%) and as 6-O-desmethyl donepezil (11%), which has been reported to inhibit AChE to the same extent as donepezil in vitro and was found in plasma concentrations equal to about 20% of donepezil. Approximately 57% and 15% of the total radioactivity was recovered in urine and feces, respectively, over a period of 10 days, while 28% remained unrecovered, with about 17% of the donepezil dose recovered in the urine as unchanged drug.

Special Populations:
Hepatic Disease: In a study of 10 patients with stable alcoholic cirrhosis, the clearance of ARICEPT® was decreased by 20% relative to 10 healthy age and sex matched subjects.
Renal Disease: In a study of 4 patients with moderate to severe renal impairment ($Cl_{Cr} < 22$ mL/min/1.73 m²) the clearance of ARICEPT® did not differ from 4 age and sex matched healthy subjects.
Age: No formal pharmacokinetic study was conducted to examine age related differences in the pharmacokinetics of ARICEPT®. However, mean plasma ARICEPT® concentrations measured during therapeutic drug monitoring of elderly patients with Alzheimer's Disease are comparable to those observed in young healthy volunteers.
Gender and Race: No specific pharmacokinetic study was conducted to investigate the effects of gender and race on the disposition of ARICEPT®. However, retrospective pharmacokinetic analysis indicates that gender and race (Japanese and Caucasians) did not affect the clearance of ARICEPT®.

Drug-Drug Interactions
Drugs Highly Bound to Plasma Proteins: Drug displacement studies have been performed in vitro between this highly bound drug (96%) and other drugs such as furosemide, digoxin, and warfarin. ARICEPT® at concentrations of 0.3–10 µg/mL did not affect the binding of furosemide (5 µg/mL), digoxin (2 ng/mL), and warfarin (3 µg/mL) to human albumin. Similarly, the binding of ARICEPT® to human binding was not affected by furosemide, digoxin and warfarin.
Effect of ARICEPT® on the Metabolism of Other Drugs: No in vivo clinical trials have investigated the effect of ARICEPT® on the clearance of drugs metabolized by CYP 3A4 (e.g. cisapride, terfenadine) or by CYP 2D6 (e.g. imipramine). However, in vitro studies show a low rate of binding to these enzymes (mean K_i about 50–130 µM), that, given the therapeutic plasma concentrations of donepezil (164 nM), indicates little likelihood of interference.
Whether ARICEPT® has any potential for enzyme induction is not known.
Formal pharmacokinetic studies evaluated the potential of ARICEPT® for interaction with theophylline, cimetidine, warfarin and digoxin. No significant effects on the pharmacokinetics of these drugs were observed.
Effects of Other Drugs on the Metabolism of ARICEPT®: Ketoconazole and quinidine, inhibitors of CYP450, 3A4 and 2D6, respectively, inhibit donepezil metabolism in vitro. Whether there is clinical effect of these inhibitors is not known. Inducers of CYP 2D6 and CYP 3A4 (e.g., phenytoin, carbamazepine, dexamethasone, rifampin, and phenobarbital) could increase the rate of elimination of ARICEPT®.
Formal pharmacokinetic studies demonstrated that the metabolism of ARICEPT® is not significantly affected by concurrent administration of digoxin or cimetidine.

INDICATIONS AND USAGE
ARICEPT® is indicated for the treatment of mild to moderate dementia of the Alzheimer's type.

CONTRAINDICATIONS
ARICEPT® is contraindicated in patients with known hypersensitivity to donepezil hydrochloride or to piperidine derivatives.

WARNINGS
Anesthesia: ARICEPT®, as a cholinesterase inhibitor, is likely to exaggerate succinylcholine-type muscle relaxation during anesthesia.
Cardiovascular Conditions: Because of their pharmacological action, cholinesterase inhibitors may have vagotonic effects on heart rate (e.g., bradycardia). The potential for this

action may be particularly important to patients with "sick sinus syndrome" or other supraventricular cardiac conduction conditions. Syncopal episodes have been reported in association with the use of ARICEPT®.
Gastrointestinal Conditions: Through their primary action, cholinesterase inhibitors would be expected to increase gastric acid secretion due to increased cholinergic activity. Therefore, patients should be monitored closely for symptoms of active or occult gastrointestinal bleeding, especially those at increased risk for developing ulcers, e.g., those with a history of ulcer disease or those receiving concurrent nonsteroidal anti-inflammatory drugs (NSAIDS). Clinical studies of ARICEPT® have shown no increase, relative to placebo, in the incidence of either peptic ulcer disease or gastrointestinal bleeding.
ARICEPT®, as a predictable consequence of its pharmacological properties, has been shown to produce diarrhea, nausea and vomiting. These effects, when they occur, appear more frequently with the 10 mg/day dose than with the 5 mg/day dose. In most case, these effects have been mild and transient, sometimes lasting one to three weeks, and have resolved during continued use of ARICEPT®.
Genitourinary: Although not observed in clinical trials of ARICEPT®, cholinomimetics may cause bladder outflow obstruction.
Neurological Conditions: Seizures: Cholinomimetics are believed to have some potential to cause generalized convulsions. However, seizure activity also may be a manifestation of Alzheimer's Disease.
Pulmonary Conditions: Because of their cholinomimetic actions, cholinesterase inhibitors should be prescribed with care to patients with a history of asthma or obstructive pulmonary disease.

PRECAUTIONS
Drug-Drug Interactions (see Clinical Pharmacology: Clinical Pharmacokinetics: Drug-drug Interactions)
Effect of ARICEPT® on the Metabolism of Other Drugs: No in vivo clinical trials have investigated the effect of ARICEPT® on the clearance of drugs metabolized by CYP 3A4 (e.g. cisapride, terfenadine) or by CYP 2D6 (e.g. imipramine). However, in vitro studies show a low rate of binding to these enzymes (mean K_i about 50-130 µM), that, given the therapeutic plasma concentrations of donepezil (164 nM), indicates little likelihood of interference.
Whether ARICEPT® has any potential for enzyme induction is not known.
Effect of Other Drugs on the Metabolism of ARICEPT®: Ketoconazole and quinidine, inhibitors of CYP450, 3A4 and 2D6, respectively, inhibit donepezil metabolism in vitro. Whether there is a clinical effect of these inhibitors is not known. Inducers of CYP 2D6 and CYP 3A4 (e.g., phenytoin, carbamazepine, dexamethasone, rifampin, and phenobarbital) could increase the rate of elimination of ARICEPT®.
Use with Anticholinergics: Because of their mechanism of action, cholinesterase inhibitors have the potential to interfere with the activity of anticholinergic medications.
Use with Cholinomimetics and Other Cholinesterase Inhibitors: A synergistic effect may be expected when cholinesterase inhibitors are given concurrently with succinylcholine, similar neuromuscular blocking agents or cholinergic agonists such as bethanechol.
Carcinogenesis, Mutagenesis, Impairment of Fertility
Carcinogenicity studies of donepezil have not been completed.
Donepezil was not mutagenic in the Ames reverse mutation assay in bacteria. In the chromosome aberration test in cultures of Chinese hamster lung (CHL) cells, some clastogenic effects were observed. Donepezil was not clastogenic in the in vivo mouse micronucleus test.
Donepezil had no effect on fertility in rats at doses up to 10 mg/kg/day (approximately 8 times the maximum recommended human dose on a mg/m² basis).
Pregnancy
Pregnancy Category C: Teratology studies conducted in pregnant rats at doses up to 16 mg/kg/day (approximately 13 times the maximum recommended human dose on a mg/m² basis) and in pregnant rabbits at doses up to 10 mg/kg/day (approximately 16 times the maximum recommended human dose on a mg/m² basis) did not disclose any

Continued on next page

Aricept—Cont.

evidence for a teratogenic potential of donepezil. However, in a study in which pregnant rats were given up to 10 mg/kg/day (approximately 8 times the maximum recommended human dose on a mg/m² basis) from day 17 of gestation through day 20 postpartum, there was a slight increase in still births and a slight decrease in pup survival through day 4 postpartum at this dose; the next lower dose tested was 3 mg/kg/day. There are no adequate or well-controlled studies in pregnant women. ARICEPT® should be used during pregnancy only if the potential benefit justifies the potential risk to the fetus.

Nursing Mothers
It is not known whether donepezil is excreted in human breast milk. ARICEPT® has no indication for use in nursing mothers.

Pediatric Use
There are no adequate and well-controlled trials to document the safety and efficacy of ARICEPT® in any illness occurring in children.

ADVERSE REACTIONS

Adverse Events Leading to Discontinuation
The rates of discontinuation from controlled clinical trials of ARICEPT® due to adverse events for the ARICEPT® 5 mg/day treatment groups were comparable to those of placebo-treatment groups at approximately 5%. The rate of discontinuation of patients who received 7-day escalations from 5 mg/day to 10 mg/day, was higher at 13%.

The most common adverse events leading to discontinuation, defined as those occurring in at least 2% of patients and at twice the incidence seen in placebo patients, are shown in Table 1.

[See table 1 at top of previous page]

Most Frequent Adverse Clinical Events Seen in Association with the Use of ARICEPT®
The most common adverse events, defined as those occurring at a frequency of at least 5% in patients receiving 10 mg/day and twice the placebo rate, are largely predicted by ARICEPT®'s cholinomimetic effects. These include nausea, diarrhea, insomnia, vomiting, muscle cramp, fatigue and anorexia. These adverse events were often of mild intensity and transient, resolving during continued ARICEPT® treatment without the need for dose modification.

There is evidence to suggest that the frequency of these common adverse events may be affected by the rate of titration. An open-label study was conducted with 269 patients who received placebo in the 15 and 30-week studies. These patients were titrated to a dose of 10 mg/day over a 6-week period. The rates of common adverse events were lower than those seen in patients titrated to 10 mg/day over one week in the controlled clinical trials and were comparable to those seen in patients on 5 mg/day.

See Table 2 for a comparison of the most common adverse events following one and six week titration regimens.

[See table 2 below]

Adverse Events Reported in Controlled Trials
The events cited reflect experience gained under closely monitored conditions of clinical trials in a highly selected patient population. In actual clinical practice or in other clinical trials, these frequency estimates may not apply, as the conditions of use, reporting behavior, and the kinds of patients treated may differ. Table 3 lists treatment emergent signs and symptoms that were reported in at least 2% of patients in placebo-controlled trials who received ARICEPT® and for which the rate of occurrence was greater for ARICEPT® assigned than placebo assigned patients. In general, adverse events occurred more frequently in female patients and with advancing age.

[See table 3 above]

Other Adverse Events Observed During Clinical Trials
ARICEPT® has been administered to over 1700 individuals during clinical trials worldwide. Approximately 1200 of these patients have been treated for at least 3 months and more than 1000 patients have been treated for at least 6 months. Controlled and uncontrolled trials in the United States included approximately 900 patients. In regards to the highest dose of 10 mg/day, this population includes 650 patients treated for 3 months, 475 patients treated for 6 months and 116 patients treated for over 1 year. The range of patient exposure is from 1 to 1214 days.

Treatment emergent signs and symptoms that occurred during 3 controlled clinical trials and two open-label trials in the United States were recorded as adverse events by the clinical investigators using terminology of their own choosing. To provide an overall estimate of the proportion of individuals having similar types of events, the events were grouped into a smaller number of standarized categories using a modified COSTART dictionary and event frequencies were calculated across all studies. These categories are used in the listing below. The frequencies represent the proportion of 900 patients from these trials who experienced that event while receiving ARICEPT®. All adverse events occurring at least twice are included, except for those already listed in Tables 2 or 3, COSTART terms too general to be informative, or events less likely to be drug caused. Events are classified by body system and listed using the following definitions: *frequent adverse events* - those occurring in at least 1/100 patients; *infrequent adverse events* - those occurring in 1/100 to 1,000 patients. These adverse events are not necessarily related to ARICEPT® treatment and in most cases were observed at a similar frequency in placebo-treated patients in the controlled studies. No important additional adverse events were seen in studies conducted outside the United States.

Body as a Whole: *Frequent:* influenza, chest pain, toothache; *Infrequent:* fever, edema face, periorbital edema, hernia hiatal, abscess, cellulitis, chills, generalized coldness, head fullness, listlessness.

Cardiovascular System: *Frequent:* hypertension, vasodilation, atrial fibrillation, hot flashes, hypotension; *Infrequent:* angina pectoris, postural hypotension, myocardial infarction, AV block (first degree), congestive heart failure, arteritis, bradycardia, peripheral vascular disease, supraventricular tachycardia, deep vein thrombosis.

Disgestive System: *Frequent:* fecal incontinence, gastrointestinal bleeding, bloating, epigastric pain; *Infrequent:*

Table 3. Adverse Events Reported in Controlled Clinical Trials in at Least 2% of Patients Receiving ARICEPT® and at a Higher Frequency than Placebo-treated Patients

Body System/Adverse Event	Placebo (n = 355)	ARICEPT® (n = 747)
Percent of Patients with any Adverse Event	72	74
Body as a Whole		
Headache	9	10
Pain, various locations	8	9
Accident	6	7
Fatigue	3	5
Cardiovascular System		
Syncope	1	2
Digestive System		
Nausea	6	11
Diarrhea	5	10
Vomiting	3	5
Anorexia	2	4
Hemic and Lymphatic System		
Ecchymosis	3	4
Metabolic and Nutritional Systems		
Weight Decrease	1	3
Musculoskeletal System		
Muscle Cramps	2	6
Arthritis	1	2
Nervous System		
Insomnia	6	9
Dizziness	6	8
Depression	<1	3
Abnormal Dreams	0	3
Somnolence	<1	2
Urogenital System		
Frequent Urination	1	2

Table 2. Comparison of rates of adverse events in patients titrated to 10 mg/day over 1 and 6 weeks

Adverse Event	No titration		One week titration	Six week titration
	Placebo (n = 315)	5 mg/day (n = 311)	10 mg/day (n = 315)	10 mg/day (n = 269)
Nausea	6%	5%	19%	6%
Diarrhea	5%	8%	15%	9%
Insomnia	6%	6%	14%	6%
Fatigue	3%	4%	8%	3%
Vomiting	3%	3%	8%	5%
Muscle cramps	2%	6%	8%	3%
Anorexia	2%	3%	7%	3%

eructation, gingivitis, increased appetite, flatulence, periodontal abscess, cholelithiasis, diverticulitis, drooling, dry mouth, fever sore, gastritis, irritable colon, tongue edema, epigastric distress, gastroenteritis, increased transaminases, hemorrhoids, ileus, increased thirst, jaundice, melena, polydypsia, duodenal ulcer, stomach ulcer.

Endocrine System: *Infrequent:* diabetes mellitus, goiter.

Hemic and Lymphatic System: *Infrequent:* anemia, thrombocythemia, thrombocytopenia, eosinophilia, erythrocytopenia.

Metabolic and Nutritional Disorders: *Frequent:* dehydration; *Infrequent:* gout, hypokalemia, increased creatine kinase, hyperglycemia, weight increase, increased lactate dehydrogenase.

Musculoskeletal System: *Frequent:* bone fracture; *Infrequent:* muscle weakness, muscle fasciculation.

Nervous System: *Frequent:* delusions, tremor, irritability, paresthesia, aggression, vertigo, ataxia, increased libido, restlessness, abnormal crying, nervousness, aphasia; *Infrequent:* cerebrovascular accident, intracranial hemorrhage, transient ischemic attack, emotional lability, neuralgia, coldness (localized), muscle spasm, dysphoria, gait abnormality, hypertonia, hypokinesia, neurodermatitis, numbness (localized), paranoia, dysarthria, dysphasia, hostility, decreased libido, melancholia, emotional withdrawal, nystagmus, pacing.

Respiratory System: *Frequent:* dyspnea, sore throat, bronchitis; *Infrequent:* epistaxis, post nasal drip, pneumonia, hyperventilation, pulmonary congestion, wheezing, hypoxia, pharyngitis, pleurisy, pulmonary collapse, sleep apnea, snoring.

Skin and Appendages: *Frequent:* pruritus, diaphoresis, urticaria; *Infrequent:* dermatitis, erythema, skin discoloration, hyperkeratosis, alopecia, fungal dermatitis, herpes zoster, hirsutism, skin striae, night sweats, skin ulcer.

Special Senses: *Frequent:* cataract, eye irritation, vision blurred; *Infrequent:* dry eyes, glaucoma, earache, tinnitus, blepharitis, decreased hearing, retinal hemorrhage, otitis externa, otitis media, bad taste, conjunctival hemorrhage, ear buzzing, motion sickness, spots before eyes.

Urogenital System: *Frequent:* urinary incontinence, nocturia; *Infrequent:* dysuria, hematuria, urinary urgency, metrorrhagia, cystitis, enuresis, prostate hypertrophy, pyelonephritis, inability to empty bladder, breast fibroadenosis, fibrocystic breast, mastitis, pyuria, renal failure, vaginitis.

Postintroduction Reports

Voluntary reports of adverse events temporally associated with ARICEPT® that have been received since market introduction that are not listed above, and that there is inadequate data to determine the causal relationship with the drug include the following: abdominal pain, agitation, cholecystitis, confusion, convulsions, hallucinations, hemolytic anemia, pancreatitis, and rash.

OVERDOSAGE

Because strategies for the management of overdose are continually evolving, it is advisable to contact a Poison Control Center to determine the latest recommendations for the management of an overdose of any drug.

As in any case of overdose, general supportive measures should be utilized. Overdosage with cholinesterase inhibitors can result in cholinergic crisis characterized by severe nausea, vomiting, salivation, sweating, bradycardia, hypotension, respiratory depression, collapse and convulsions. Increasing muscle weakness is a possibility and may result in death if respiratory muscles are involved. Tertiary anticholinergics such as atropine may be used as an antidote for ARICEPT® overdosage. Intravenous atropine sulfate titrated to effect is recommended: an initial dose of 1.0 to 2.0 mg IV with subsequent doses based upon clinical response. Atypical responses in blood pressure and heart rate have been reported with other cholinomimetics when co-administered with quaternary anticholinergics such as glycopyrrolate. It is not known whether ARICEPT® and/or its metabolites can be removed by dialysis (hemodialysis, peritoneal dialysis, or hemofiltration).

Dose-related signs of toxicity in animals included reduced spontaneous movement, prone position, staggering gait, lacrimation, clonic convulsions, depressed respiration, salivation, miosis, tremors, fasciculation and lower body surface temperature.

DOSAGE AND ADMINISTRATION

The dosages of ARICEPT® shown to be effective in controlled clinical trials are 5 mg and 10 mg administered once per day.

The higher dose of 10 mg did not provide a statistically significantly greater clinical benefit than 5 mg. There is a suggestion, however, based upon order of group mean scores and dose trend analyses of data from these clinical trials, that a daily dose of 10 mg of ARICEPT® might provide additional benefit for some patients. Accordingly, whether or not to employ a dose of 10 mg is a matter of prescriber and patient preference.

Evidence from the controlled trials indicates that the 10 mg dose, with a one week titration, is likely to be associated with a higher incidence of cholinergic adverse events than

the 5 mg dose. In open label trials using a 6 week titration, the frequency of these same adverse events was similar between the 5 mg and 10 mg dose groups. Therefore, because steady state is not achieved for 15 days and because the incidence of untoward effects may be influenced by the rate of dose escalation, treatment with a dose of 10 mg should not be contemplated until patients have been on a daily dose of 5 mg for 4 to 6 weeks.

ARICEPT® should be taken in the evening, just prior to retiring. ARICEPT® can be taken with or without food.

HOW SUPPLIED

ARICEPT® is supplied as film-coated, round tablets containing either 5 mg or 10 mg of donepezil hydrochloride. The 5 mg tablets are white. The strength, in mg (5), is debossed on one side and the medication code number (E 245) is debossed on the other side.

The 10 mg tablets are yellow and have the strength debossed on one side (10) and the medication code (E 246) on the other side.

5 mg (White)   Bottles of 30 (NDC# 62856-245-30)
              Unit Dose Blister Package 100 (10×10)
              (NDC # 62856-245-41)

10 mg (Yellow)   Bottles of 30 (NDC# 62856-246-30)
              Unit Dose Blister Package 100 (10×10)
              (NDC # 62856-246-41)

Storage: Store at controlled room temperature, 15°C to 30°C (59°F to 86°F).

Rx only

ARICEPT® is a registered trademark of Eisai Co., Ltd., Tokyo, Japan

Marketed by Eisai Inc., Teaneck, NJ 07666

Manufactured and Distributed/Marketed by

Roerig Division of Pfizer Inc, New York, NY 10017

©1998 Eisai Inc.

70-5210-00-3   Revised April, 1998

Shown in Product Identification Guide, page 330

ATARAX®   ℞
[ăt 'ā-raks"]
(hydroxyzine hydrochloride)
TABLETS AND SYRUP

DESCRIPTION

Hydroxyzine hydrochloride is designated chemically as 1-(p-chlorobenzhydryl) 4-[2-(2-hydroxyethoxy)-ethyl] piperazine dihydrochloride.

Inert ingredients for the tablets are: acacia; carnauba wax; dibasic calcium phosphate; gelatin; lactose; magnesium stearate; precipitated calcium carbonate; shellac; sucrose; talc; white wax. The 10 mg tablets also contain: sodium hydroxide; starch; titanium dioxide; Yellow 6 Lake. The 25 mg tablets also contain: starch, velo dark green. The 50 mg tablets also contain: starch; velo yellow. The 100 mg tablets also contain: alginic acid; Blue 1; polyethylene glycol; Red 3. The inert ingredients for the syrup are: alcohol; menthol; peppermint oil; sodium benzoate; spearmint oil; sucrose; water.

CLINICAL PHARMACOLOGY

Atarax is unrelated chemically to the phenothiazines, reserpine, meprobamate, or the benzodiazepines.

Atarax is not a cortical depressant, but its action may be due to a suppression of activity in certain key regions of the subcortical area of the central nervous system. Primary skeletal muscle relaxation has been demonstrated experimentally. Bronchodilator activity, and antihistaminic and analgesic effects have been demonstrated experimentally and confirmed clinically. An antiemetic effect, both by the apomorphine test and the veriloid test, has been demonstrated. Pharmacological and clinical studies indicate that hydroxyzine in therapeutic dosage does not increase gastric secretion or acidity and in most cases has mild antisecretory activity. Hydroxyzine is rapidly absorbed from the gastrointestinal tract and Atarax's clinical effects are usually noted within 15 to 30 minutes after oral administration.

INDICATIONS

For symptomatic relief of anxiety and tension associated with psychoneurosis and as an adjunct in organic disease states in which anxiety is manifested.

Useful in the management of pruritus due to allergic conditions such as chronic urticaria and atopic and contact dermatoses, and in histamine-mediated pruritus.

As a sedative when used as premedication and following general anesthesia, **Hydroxyzine may potentiate meperidine (Demerol®) and barbiturates,** so their use in pre-anesthetic adjunctive therapy should be modified on an individual basis. Atropine and other belladonna alkaloids are not affected by the drug. Hydroxyzine is not known to interfere with the action of digitalis in any way and it may be used concurrently with this agent.

The effectiveness of hydroxyzine as an antianxiety agent for long term use, that is more than 4 months, has not been

assessed by systematic clinical studies. The physician should reassess periodically the usefulness of the drug for the individual patient.

CONTRAINDICATIONS

Hydroxyzine, when administered to the pregnant mouse, rat, and rabbit, induced fetal abnormalities in the rat and mouse at doses substantially above the human therapeutic range. Clinical data in human beings are inadequate to establish safety in early pregnancy. Until such data are available, hydroxyzine is contraindicated in early pregnancy. Hydroxyzine is contraindicated for patients who have shown a previous hypersensitivity to it.

WARNINGS

Nursing Mothers: It is not known whether this drug is excreted in human milk. Since many drugs are so excreted, hydroxyzine should not be given to nursing mothers.

For Tablets Only: This product is manufactured with 1,1,1-trichloroethane, a substance which harms public health and the environment by destroying ozone in the upper atmosphere.

PRECAUTIONS

THE POTENTIATING ACTION OF HYDROXYZINE MUST BE CONSIDERED WHEN THE DRUG IS USED IN CONJUNCTION WITH CENTRAL NERVOUS SYSTEM DEPRESSANTS SUCH AS NARCOTICS, NON-NARCOTIC ANALGESICS AND BARBITURATES. Therefore when central nervous system depressants are administered concomitantly with hydroxyzine their dosage should be reduced.

Since drowsiness may occur with use of this drug, patients should be warned of this possibility and cautioned against driving a car or operating dangerous machinery while taking Atarax. Patients should be advised against the simultaneous use of other CNS depressant drugs, and cautioned that the effect of alcohol may be increased.

ADVERSE REACTIONS

Side effects reported with the administration of Atarax (hydroxyzine hydrochloride) are usually mild and transitory in nature.

Anticholinergic: Dry mouth.

Central Nervous System: Drowsiness is usually transitory and may disappear in a few days of continued therapy or upon reduction of the dose. Involuntary motor activity including rare instances of tremor and convulsions have been reported, usually with doses considerably higher than those recommended. Clinically significant respiratory depression has not been reported at recommended doses.

OVERDOSAGE

The most common manifestation of Atarax overdosage is hypersedation. As in the management of overdosage with any drug, it should be borne in mind that multiple agents may have been taken.

If vomiting has not occurred spontaneously, it should be induced. Immediate gastric lavage is also recommended. General supportive care, including frequent monitoring of the vital signs and close observation of the patient, is indicated. Hypotension, though unlikely, may be controlled with intravenous fluids and Levophed® (levarterenol), or Aramine® (metaraminol). Do not use epinephrine as Atarax counteracts its pressor action.

There is no specific antidote. It is doubtful that hemodialysis would be of any value in the treatment of overdosage with hydroxyzine. However, if other agents such as barbiturates have been ingested concomitantly, hemodialysis may be indicated. There is no practical method to quantitate hydroxyzine in body fluids or tissue after its ingestion or administration.

DOSAGE

For symptomatic relief of anxiety and tension associated with psychoneurosis and as an adjunct in organic disease states in which anxiety is manifested: in adults, 50–100 mg q.i.d.; children under 6 years, 50 mg daily in divided doses and over 6 years, 50–100 mg daily in divided doses.

For use in the management of pruritus due to allergic conditions such as chronic urticaria and atopic and contact dermatoses, and in histamine-mediated pruritus: in adults, 25 mg t.i.d. or q.i.d.; children under 6 years, 50 mg daily in divided doses and over 6 years, 50–100 mg daily in divided doses.

As a sedative when used as a premedication and following general anesthesia: 50–100 mg in adults, and 0.6 mg/kg in children.

When treatment is initiated by the intramuscular route of administration, subsequent doses may be administered orally.

As with all medications, the dosage should be adjusted according to the patient's response to therapy.

SUPPLY

Atarax Tablets

10 mg—orange tablets: 100's (NDC 0049-5600-66), 500's (NDC 0049-5600-73) Unit Dose 10 × 10's (NDC 0049-5600-41), and Unit of Use 40's (NDC 0049-5600-43)

Continued on next page

Atarax—Cont.

25 mg—green tablets: 100's (NDC 0049-5610-66), 500's (NDC 0049-5610-73) Unit Dose 10 × 10's (NDC 0049-5610-41), and Unit of Use 40's (NDC 0049-5610-43)
50 mg—yellow tablets: 100's (NDC 0049-5620-66), 500's (NDC 0049-5620-73) and Unit Dose 10 × 10's (NDC 0049-5620-41)
100 mg—red tablets: 100's (NDC 0049-5630-66) and Unit Dose 10 × 10's (NDC 0049-5630-41)
Atarax Syrup
10 mg per teaspoon (5 ml): 1 pint bottles (NDC 0049-5590-93)
Alcohol Content—Ethyl Alcohol—0.5% v/v

BIBLIOGRAPHY

Available on request.
69-0618-00-5   Revised Dec. 1993

CARDURA®   ℞
(doxazosin mesylate)
Tablets

DESCRIPTION

CARDURA® (doxazosin mesylate) is a quinazoline compound that is a selective inhibitor of the alpha$_1$ subtype of alpha adrenergic receptors. The chemical name of doxazosin mesylate is 1-(4-amino-6,7-dimethoxy-2-quinazolinyl)-4-(1,4-benzodioxan-2-ylcarbonyl) piperazine methanesulfonate. The empirical formula for doxazosin mesylate is $C_{23}H_{25}N_5O_5 \cdot CH_4O_3S$ and the molecular weight is 547.6. It has the following structure:

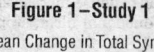

CARDURA® (doxazosin mesylate) is freely soluble in dimethylsulfoxide, soluble in dimethylformamide, slightly soluble in methanol, ethanol, and water (0.8% at 25°C), and very slightly soluble in acetone and methylene chloride. CARDURA® is available as colored tablets for oral use and contains 1 mg (white), 2 mg (yellow), 4 mg (orange) and 8 mg (green) of doxazosin as the free base.
The inactive ingredients for all tablets are: microcrystalline cellulose, lactose, sodium starch glycolate, magnesium stearate and sodium lauryl sulfate. The 2 mg tablet contains D & C yellow 10 and FD & C yellow 6; the 4 mg tablet contains FD & C yellow 6; the 8 mg tablet contains FD & C blue 10 and D & C yellow 10.

CLINICAL PHARMACOLOGY
Pharmacodynamics
A. Benign Prostatic Hyperplasia (BPH)

Benign prostatic hyperplasia (BPH) is a common cause of urinary outflow obstruction in aging males. Severe BPH may lead to urinary retention and renal damage. A static and a dynamic component contribute to the symptoms and reduced urinary flow rate associated with BPH. The static

component is related to an increase in prostate size caused, in part, by a proliferation of smooth muscle cells in the prostatic stroma. However, the severity of BPH symptoms and the degree of urethral obstruction do not correlate well with the size of the prostate. The dynamic component of BPH is associated with an increase in smooth muscle tone in the prostate and bladder neck. The degree of tone in this area is mediated by the alpha$_1$ adrenoceptor, which is present in high density in the prostatic stroma, prostatic capsule and bladder neck. Blockade of the alpha$_1$ receptor decreases urethral resistance and may relieve the obstruction and BPH symptoms. In the human prostate, CARDURA® antagonizes phenylephrine (alpha$_1$ agonist)-induced contractions, in vitro, and binds with high affinity to the alpha$_{1c}$ adrenoceptor. The receptor subtype is thought to be the predominant functional type in the prostate. CARDURA® acts within 1-2 weeks to decrease the severity of BPH symptoms and improve urinary flow rate. Since alpha$_1$ adrenoceptors are of low density in the urinary bladder (apart from the bladder neck), CARDURA® should maintain bladder contractility.
The efficacy of CARDURA® was evaluated extensively in over 900 patients with BPH in double-blind, placebo-controlled trials. CARDURA® treatment was superior to placebo in improving patient symptoms and urinary flow rate. Significant relief with CARDURA® was seen as early as one week into the treatment regimen, with CARDURA® treated patients (N=173) showing a significant (p<0.01) increase in maximum flow rate of 0.8 mL/sec compared to a decrease of 0.5 mL/sec in the placebo group (N=41). In long-term studies improvement was maintained for up to 2 years of treatment. In 66-71% of patients, improvements above baseline were seen in both symptoms and maximum urinary flow rate.
In three placebo-controlled studies of 14-16 weeks duration obstructive symptoms (hesitation, intermittency, dribbling, weak urinary stream, incomplete emptying of the bladder) and irritative symptoms (nocturia, daytime frequency, urgency, burning) of BPH were evaluated at each visit by patient-assessed symptom questionnaires. The bothersomeness of symptoms was measured with a modified Boyarsky questionnaire. Symptom severity/frequency was assessed using a modified Boyarsky questionnaire or an AUA-based questionnaire. Uroflowmetric evaluations were performed at times of peak (2-6 hours post-dose) and/or trough (24 hours post-dose) plasma concentrations of CARDURA®.
The results from the three placebo-controlled studies (N=609) showing significant efficacy with 4 mg and 8 mg doxazosin are summarized in Table 1. In all three studies, CARDURA® resulted in statistically significant relief of obstructive and irritative symptoms compared to placebo. Statistically significant improvements of 2.3-3.3 mL/sec in maximum flow rate were seen with CARDURA® in Studies 1 and 2, compared to 0.1-0.7 mL/sec with placebo.
[See table 1 below]
In one fixed dose study (study 2) CARDURA® (doxazosin mesylate) therapy (4-8 mg, once daily) resulted in a significant and sustained improvement in maximum urinary flow rate of 2.3-3.3 mL/sec (Table 1) compared to placebo (0.1 mL/sec). In this study, the only study in which weekly evaluations were made, significant improvement with CARDURA® vs. placebo was seen after one week. The proportion of patients who responded with a maximum flow rate improvement of ≥ 3 mL/sec was significantly larger with CARDURA® (34-42%) than placebo (13-17%). A significantly greater improvement was also seen in average flow rate with CARDURA® (1.6 mL/sec) than with placebo

(0.2 mL/sec). The onset and time course of symptom relief and increased urinary flow from study 1 are illustrated in Figure 1.

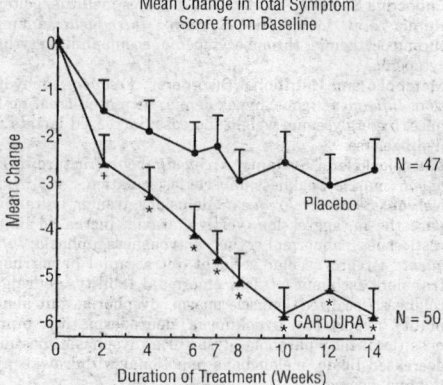

Figure 1–Study 1
Mean Change in Total Symptom Score from Baseline

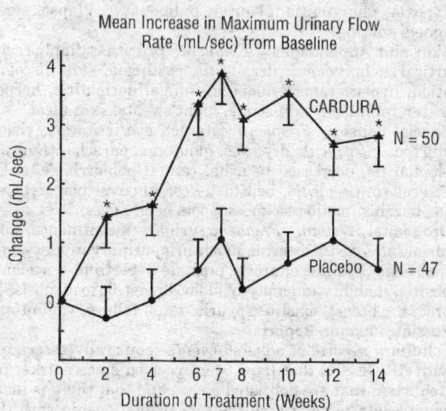

Mean Increase in Maximum Urinary Flow Rate (mL/sec) from Baseline

* p < 0.05 Compared to Placebo;   + p < 0.05 Compared to Baseline;   Doxazosin Titration to Maximum of 8 mg.

In BPH patients (N=450) treated for up to 2 years in open-label studies, CARDURA® therapy resulted in significant improvement above baseline in urinary flow rates and BPH symptoms. The significant effects of CARDURA® were maintained over the entire treatment period.
Although blockade of alpha$_1$ adrenoceptors also lowers blood pressure in hypertensive patients with increased peripheral vascular resistance, CARDURA® treatment of normotensive men with BPH did not result in a clinically significant blood pressure lowering effect (Table 2). The proportion of normotensive patients with a sitting systolic blood pressure less than 90 mmHg and/or diastolic blood pressure less than 60 mmHg at any time during treatment with CARDURA® 1-8 mg once daily was 6.7% with doxazosin and not significantly different (statistically) from that with placebo (5%).
[See table 2 at top of next page]

B. Hypertension

The mechanism of action of CARDURA® (doxazosin mesylate) is selective blockade of the alpha$_1$ (postjunctional) subtype of adrenergic receptors. Studies in normal human subjects have shown that doxazosin competitively antagonized the pressor effects of phenylephrine (an alpha$_1$ agonist) and the systolic pressor effect of norepinephrine. Doxazosin and prazosin have similar abilities to antagonize phenylephrine. The antihypertensive effect of CARDURA® results from a decrease in systemic vascular resistance. The parent compound doxazosin is primarily responsible for the antihypertensive activity. The low plasma concentrations of known active and inactive metabolites of doxazosin (2-piperazinyl, 6'- and 7'-hydroxy and 6- and 7-O-desmethyl compounds) compared to parent drug indicate that the contribution of even the most potent compound (6'-hydroxy) to the antihypertensive effect of doxazosin in man is probably small. The 6'- and 7'-hydroxy metabolites have demonstrated antioxidant properties at concentrations of 5 μM, in vitro.
Administration of CARDURA® results in a reduction in systemic vascular resistance. In patients with hypertension there is little change in cardiac output. Maximum reductions in blood pressure usually occur 2-6 hours after dosing and are associated with a small increase in standing heart rate. Like other alpha$_1$-adrenergic blocking agents, doxazosin has a greater effect on blood pressure and heart rate in the standing position.

TABLE 1
SUMMARY OF EFFECTIVENESS DATA IN PLACEBO-CONTROLLED TRIALS

		SYMPTOM SCORE[a]			MAXIMUM FLOW RATE (mL/sec)	
	N	MEAN BASELINE	MEAN[b] CHANGE	N	MEAN BASELINE	MEAN[c] CHANGE
STUDY 1 (Titration to maximum dose of 8 mg)[e]						
Placebo	47	15.6	-2.3	41	9.7	+0.7
CARDURA	49	14.5	-4.9**	41	9.8	+2.9**
STUDY 2 (Titration to fixed dose–14 weeks)[d]						
Placebo	37	20.7	-2.5	30	10.6	+0.1
CARDURA 4 mg	38	21.2	-5.0**	32	9.8	+2.3*
CARDURA 8 mg	42	19.9	-4.2*	36	10.5	+3.3**
STUDY 3 (Titration to fixed dose–12 weeks)						
Placebo	47	14.4	-4.7	44	9.9	+2.1
CARDURA 4 mg	46	16.6	-6.1*	46	9.6	+2.6

[a] AUA questionnaire (range 0-30) in studies 1 and 3. Modified Boyarsky Questionnaire (range 7-39) in study 2.
[b] Change is to endpoint.
[c] Change is to fixed-dose efficacy phase, 22-26 hours post-dose for studies 1 and 3 and 2-6 hours post-dose for study 2.
[d] Study in hypertensives with BPH
[e] 36 patients received a dose of 8 mg CARDURA®
*(**) p < 0.05 (0.01) compared to placebo mean change.

STUDY 2
Maximum Flow Rate
Maximum Flow Rate values: Placebo 0.1; 4 mg 2.3*; 8 mg 3.3**
Symptom Score values: Placebo -2.5; 4 mg -5.0**; 8 mg -4.2*

TABLE 2
Mean Changes in Blood Pressure from Baseline to the Mean of the Final Efficacy Phase in Normotensives (Diastolic BP <90 mmHg) in Two Double-blind, Placebo-controlled U.S. Studies with CARDURA® 1-8 mg once daily.

	PLACEBO (N=85)		CARDURA® (N=183)	
Sitting BP (mmHg)	**Baseline**	**Change**	**Baseline**	**Change**
Systolic	128.4	−1.4	128.8	−4.9*
Diastolic	79.2	−1.2	79.6	−2.4*
Standing BP (mmHg)	**Baseline**	**Change**	**Baseline**	**Change**
Systolic	128.5	−0.6	128.5	−5.3*
Diastolic	80.5	−0.7	80.4	−2.6*

*p ≤0.05 compared to placebo

In a pooled analysis of placebo-controlled hypertension studies with about 300 hypertensive patients per treatment group, doxazosin, at doses of 1–16 mg given once daily, lowered blood pressure at 24 hours by about 10/8 mmHg compared to placebo in the standing position and about 9/5 mmHg in the supine position. Peak blood pressure effects (1–6 hours) were larger by about 50–75% (i.e., trough values were about 55–70% of peak effect), with the larger peak-trough differences seen in systolic pressures. There was no apparent difference in the blood pressure response of Caucasians and blacks or of patients above and below age 65. In these predominantly normocholesterolemic patients doxazosin produced small reductions in total serum cholesterol (2–3%), LDL cholesterol (4%), and a similarly small increase in HDL/total cholesterol ratio (4%). The clinical significance of these findings is uncertain. In the same patient population, patients receiving CARDURA® gained a mean of 0.6 kg compared to a mean loss of 0.1 kg for placebo patients.

Pharmacokinetics

After oral administration of therapeutic doses, peak plasma levels of CARDURA® (doxazosin mesylate) occur at about 2–3 hours. Bioavailability is approximately 65%, reflecting first pass metabolism of doxazosin by the liver. The effect of food on the pharmacokinetics of CARDURA® was examined in a crossover study with twelve hypertensive subjects. Reductions of 18% in mean maximum plasma concentration and 12% in the area under the concentration-time curve occurred when CARDURA® was administered with food. Neither of these differences was statistically or clinically significant.

CARDURA® is extensively metabolized in the liver, mainly by O-demethylation of the quinazoline nucleus or hydroxylation of the benzodioxan moiety. Although several active metabolites of doxazosin have been identified, the pharmacokinetics of these metabolites have not been characterized. In a study of two subjects administered radiolabelled doxazosin 2 mg orally and 1 mg intravenously on two separate occasions, approximately 63% of the dose was eliminated in the feces and 9% of the dose was found in the urine. On average only 4.8% of the dose was excreted as unchanged drug in the feces and only a trace of the total radioactivity in the urine was attributed to unchanged drug. At the plasma concentrations achieved by therapeutic doses approximately 98% of the circulating drug is bound to plasma proteins.

Plasma elimination of doxazosin is biphasic, with a terminal elimination half-life of about 22 hours. Steady-state studies in hypertensive patients given doxazosin doses of 2–16 mg once daily showed linear kinetics and dose proportionality. In two studies, following the administration of 2 mg orally once daily, the mean accumulation ratios (steady-state AUC vs. first dose AUC) were 1.2 and 1.7. Enterohepatic recycling is suggested by secondary peaking of plasma doxazosin concentrations.

In a crossover study in 24 normotensive subjects, the pharmacokinetics and safety of doxazosin were shown to be similar with morning and evening dosing regimens. The area under the curve after morning dosing was, however, 11% less than that after evening dosing and the time to peak concentration after evening dosing occurred significantly later than that after morning dosing (5.6 hr vs. 3.5 hr).

The pharmacokinetics of CARDURA® (doxazosin mesylate) in young (<65 years) and elderly (≥65 years) subjects were similar for plasma half-life values and oral clearance. Pharmacokinetic studies in elderly patients and patients with renal impairment have shown no significant alterations compared to younger patients with normal renal function. Administration of a single 2 mg dose to patients with cirrhosis (Child-Pugh Class A) showed a 40% increase in exposure to doxazosin. There are only limited data on the effects of drugs known to influence the hepatic metabolism of doxazosin [e.g., cimetidine (see PRECAUTIONS)]. As with any drug wholly metabolized by the liver, use of CARDURA® in patients with altered liver function should be undertaken with caution.

In two placebo-controlled studies, of normotensive and hypertensive BPH patients, in which doxazosin was administered in the morning and the titration interval was two weeks and one week, respectively, trough plasma concentrations of CARDURA® were similar in the two populations. Linear kinetics and dose proportionality were observed.

INDICATIONS AND USAGE

A. ***Benign Prostatic Hyperplasia (BPH).*** CARDURA® is indicated for the treatment of both the urinary outflow obstruction and obstructive and irritative symptoms associated with BPH: obstructive symptoms (hesitation, intermittency, dribbling, weak urinary stream, incomplete emptying of the bladder) and irritative symptoms (nocturia, daytime frequency, urgency, burning). CARDURA® may be used in all BPH patients whether hypertensive or normotensive. In patients with hypertension and BPH, both conditions were effectively treated with CARDURA® monotherapy. CARDURA® provides rapid improvement in symptoms and urinary flow rate in 66–71% of patients. Sustained improvements with CARDURA® were seen in patients treated for up to 14 weeks in double-blind studies and up to 2 years in open-label studies.

B. ***Hypertension.*** CARDURA® (doxazosin mesylate) is also indicated for the treatment of hypertension. CARDURA® may be used alone or in combination with diuretics, beta-adrenergic blocking agents, calcium channel blockers or angiotensin-converting enzyme inhibitors.

CONTRAINDICATIONS

CARDURA® is contraindicated in patients with a known sensitivity to quinazolines (e.g., prazosin, terazosin).

WARNINGS

Syncope and "First-dose" Effect: Doxazosin, like other alpha-adrenergic blocking agents, can cause marked hypotension, especially in the upright position, with syncope and other postural symptoms such as dizziness. Marked orthostatic effects are most common with the first dose but can also occur when there is a dosage increase, or if therapy is interrupted for more than a few days. To decrease the likelihood of excessive hypotension and syncope, it is essential that treatment be initiated with the 1 mg dose. The 2, 4, and 8 mg tablets are not for initial therapy. Dosage should then be adjusted slowly (see DOSAGE AND ADMINISTRATION section) with evaluations and increases in dose every two weeks to the recommended dose. Additional antihypertensive agents should be added with caution.

Patients being titrated with doxazosin should be cautioned to avoid situations where injury could result should syncope occur, during both the day and night.

In an early investigational study of the safety and tolerance of increasing daily doses of doxazosin in normotensives beginning at 1 mg/day, only 2 of 6 subjects could tolerate more than 2 mg/day without experiencing symptomatic postural hypotension. In another study of 24 healthy normotensive male subjects receiving initial doses of 2 mg/day of doxazosin, seven (29%) of the subjects experienced symptomatic postural hypotension between 0.5 and 6 hours after the first dose necessitating termination of the study. In this study, 2 of the normotensive subjects experienced syncope. Subsequent trials in hypertensive patients always began doxazosin dosing at 1 mg/day resulting in a 4% incidence of postural side effects at 1 mg/day with no cases of syncope.

In multiple dose clinical trials in hypertension involving over 1500 hypertensive patients with dose titration every one to two weeks, syncope was reported in 0.7% of patients. None of these events occurred at the starting dose of 1 mg and 1.2% (8/664) occurred at 16 mg/day.

In placebo-controlled, clinical trials in BPH, 3 out of 665 patients (0.5%) taking doxazosin reported syncope. Two of the patients were taking 1 mg doxazosin, while one patient was taking 2 mg doxazosin when syncope occurred. In the open-label, long-term extension follow-up of approximately 450 BPH patients, there were 3 reports of syncope (0.7%). One patient was taking 2 mg, one patient was taking 8 mg and one patient was taking 12 mg when syncope occurred. In a clinical pharmacology study, one subject receiving 2 mg experienced syncope.

If syncope occurs, the patient should be placed in a recumbent position and treated supportively as necessary.

Priapism: Rarely (probably less frequently than once in every several thousand patients), $alpha_1$ antagonists such as doxazosin have been associated with priapism (painful penile erection, sustained for hours and unrelieved by sexual intercourse or masturbation). Because this condition can lead to permanent impotence if not promptly treated, patients must be advised about the seriousness of the condition (see **PRECAUTIONS: Information for Patients**).

PRECAUTIONS

General:

Prostate Cancer: Carcinoma of the prostate causes many of the symptoms associated with BPH and the two disorders frequently co-exist. Carcinoma of the prostate should therefore be ruled out prior to commencing therapy with CARDURA®.

Orthostatic Hypotension: While syncope is the most severe orthostatic effect of CARDURA®, other symptoms of lowered blood pressure, such as dizziness, lightheadedness, or vertigo can occur, especially at initiation of therapy or at the time of dose increases.

a) Hypertension

These symptoms were common in clinical trials in hypertension, occurring in up to 23% of all patients treated and causing discontinuation of therapy in about 2%.

In placebo-controlled titration trials in hypertension, orthostatic effects were minimized by beginning therapy at 1 mg per day and titrating every two weeks to 2, 4, or 8 mg per day. There was an increased frequency of orthostatic effects in patients given 8 mg or more, 10%, compared to 5% at 1–4 mg and 3% in the placebo group.

b) Benign Prostatic Hyperplasia

In placebo-controlled trials in BPH, the incidence of orthostatic hypotension with doxazosin was 0.3% and did not increase with increasing dosage (to 8 mg/day). The incidence of discontinuations due to hypotensive or orthostatic symptoms was 3.3% with doxazosin and 1% with placebo. The titration interval in these studies was one to two weeks.

Patients in occupations in which orthostatic hypotension could be dangerous should be treated with particular caution. As $alpha_1$ antagonists can cause orthostatic effects, it is important to evaluate standing blood pressure two minutes after standing and patients should be advised to exercise care when arising from a supine or sitting position.

If hypotension occurs, the patient should be placed in the supine position and, if this measure is inadequate, volume expansion with intravenous fluids or vasopressor therapy may be used. A transient hypotensive response is not a contraindication to further doses of CARDURA® (doxazosin mesylate).

Information for Patients (See Patient Package Insert): Patients should be made aware of the possibility of syncopal and orthostatic symptoms, especially at the initiation of therapy, and urged to avoid driving or hazardous tasks for 24 hours after the first dose, after a dosage increase, and after interruption of therapy when treatment is resumed. They should be cautioned to avoid situations where injury could result should syncope occur during initiation of doxazosin therapy. They should also be advised of the need to sit or lie down when symptoms of lowered blood pressure occur, although these symptoms are not always orthostatic, and to be careful when rising from a sitting or lying position. If dizziness, lightheadedness, or palpitations are bothersome they should be reported to the physician, so that dose adjustment can be considered. Patients should also be told that drowsiness or somnolence can occur with CARDURA® (doxazosin mesylate) or any selective $alpha_1$ adrenoceptor antagonist, requiring caution in people who must drive or operate heavy machinery.

Patients should be advised about the possibility of priapism as a result of treatment with $alpha_1$ antagonists. Patients should know that this adverse event is very rare. If they experience priapism, it should be brought to immediate medical attention for if not treated promptly it can lead to permanent erectile dysfunction (impotence).

Drug/Laboratory Test Interactions: CARDURA® does not affect the plasma concentration of prostate specific antigen in patients treated for up to 3 years. Both doxazosin, an $alpha_1$ inhibitor, and finasteride, a 5-alpha reductase inhibitor, are highly protein bound and hepatically metabolized. There is no definitive controlled clinical experience on the concomitant use of $alpha_1$ inhibitors and 5-alpha reductase inhibitors at this time.

Impaired Liver Function: CARDURA® should be administered with caution to patients with evidence of impaired hepatic function or to patients receiving drugs known to influence hepatic metabolism (see CLINICAL PHARMACOLOGY).

Leukopenia/Neutropenia: Analysis of hematologic data from hypertensive patients receiving CARDURA® in controlled hypertension clinical trials showed that the mean WBC (N=474) and mean neutrophil counts (N=419) were decreased by 2.4% and 1.0%, respectively, compared to placebo, a phenomenon seen with other alpha blocking drugs. In BPH patients the incidence of clinically significant WBC

Continued on next page

Cardura—Cont.

abnormalities was 0.4% (2/459) with CARDURA® and 0% (0/147) with placebo, with no statistically significant difference between the two treatment groups. A search through a data base of 2400 hypertensive patients and 665 BPH patients revealed 4 hypertensives in which drug-related neutropenia could not be ruled out and one BPH patient in which drug related leukopenia could not be ruled out. Two hypertensives had a single low value on the last day of treatment. Two hypertensives had stable, non-progressive neutrophil counts in the 1000/mm³ range over periods of 20 and 40 weeks. One BPH patient had a decrease from a WBC count of 4800/mm³ to 2700/mm³ at the end of the study; there was no evidence of clinical impairment. In cases where follow-up was available the WBCs and neutrophil counts returned to normal after discontinuation of CARDURA®. No patients became symptomatic as a result of the low WBC or neutrophil counts.

Drug Interactions: Most (98%) of plasma doxazosin is protein bound. *In vitro* data in human plasma indicate that CARDURA® has no effect on protein binding of digoxin, warfarin, phenytoin or indomethacin. There is no information on the effect of other highly plasma protein bound drugs on doxazosin binding. CARDURA® has been administered without any evidence of an adverse drug interaction to patients receiving thiazide diuretics, beta-blocking agents, and nonsteroidal anti-inflammatory drugs. In a placebo-controlled trial in normal volunteers, the administration of a single 1 mg dose of doxazosin on day 1 of a four-day regimen of oral cimetidine (400 mg twice daily) resulted in a 10% increase in mean AUC of doxazosin (p=0.006), and a slight but not statistically significant increase in mean C_{max} and mean half-life of doxazosin. The clinical significance of this increase in doxazosin AUC is unknown.

In clinical trials, CARDURA® tablets have been administered to patients on a variety of concomitant medications; while no formal interaction studies have been conducted, no interactions were observed. CARDURA® tablets have been used with the following drugs or drug classes: 1) analgesic/anti-inflammatory (e.g., acetaminophen, aspirin, codeine and codeine combinations, ibuprofen, indomethacin); 2) antibiotics (e.g., erythromycin, trimethoprim and sulfamethoxazole, amoxicillin); 3) antihistamines (e.g., chlorpheniramine); 4) cardiovascular agents (e.g., atenolol, hydrochlorothiazide, propranolol); 5) corticosteroids; 6) gastrointestinal agents (e.g., antacids); 7) hypoglycemics and endocrine drugs; 8) sedatives and tranquilizers (e.g., diazepam); 9) cold and flu remedies.

Cardiac Toxicity in Animals: An increased incidence of myocardial necrosis or fibrosis was displayed by Sprague-Dawley rats after 6 months of dietary administration at concentrations calculated to provide 80 mg doxazosin/kg/day and after 12 months of dietary administration at concentrations calculated to provide 40 mg doxazosin/kg/day (AUC exposure in rats 8 times the human AUC exposure with a 12 mg/day therapeutic dose). Myocardial fibrosis was observed in both rats and mice treated in the same manner with 40 mg doxazosin/kg/day for 18 months (exposure 8 times human AUC exposure in rats and somewhat equivalent to human C_{max} exposure in mice). No cardiotoxicity was observed at lower doses (up to 10 or 20 mg/kg/day, depending on the study) in either species. These lesions were not observed after 12 months of oral dosing in dogs at maximum doses of 20 mg/kg/day [maximum plasma concentrations (C_{max}) in dogs 14 times the C_{max} exposure in humans receiving a 12 mg/day therapeutic dose] and in Wistar rats at doses of 100 mg/kg/day (C_{max} exposures 15 times human C_{max} exposure with a 12 mg/day therapeutic dose). There is no evidence that similar lesions occur in humans.

Carcinogenesis, Mutagenesis, Impairment of Fertility: Chronic dietary administration (up to 24 months) of doxazosin mesylate at maximally tolerated doses of 40 mg/kg/day in rats and 120 mg/kg/day in mice revealed no evidence of carcinogenic potential. The highest doses evaluated in the rat and mouse studies are associated with AUCs (a measure of systemic exposure) that are 8 times and 4 times, respectively, the human AUC at a dose of 16 mg/day.

Mutagenicity studies revealed no drug- or metabolite-related effects at either chromosomal or subchromosomal levels.

Studies in rats showed reduced fertility in males treated with doxazosin at oral doses of 20 (but not 5 or 10) mg/kg/day, about 4 times the AUC exposures obtained with a 12 mg/day human dose. This effect was reversible within two weeks of drug withdrawal. There have been no reports of any effects of doxazosin on male infertility in humans.

Pregnancy: Teratogenic Effects, Pregnancy Category C. Studies in pregnant rabbits and rats at daily oral doses of up to 41 and 20 mg/kg, respectively (plasma drug concentrations 10 and 4 times human C_{max} and AUC exposures with a 12 mg/day therapeutic dose), have revealed no evidence of harm to the fetus. A dosage regimen of 82 mg/kg/day in the rabbit was associated with reduced fetal survival. There are no adequate and well-controlled studies in preg-

nant women. Because animal reproduction studies are not always predictive of human response, CARDURA® should be used during pregnancy only if clearly needed.

Radioactivity was found to cross the placenta following oral administration of labelled doxazosin to pregnant rats.

Nonteratogenic Effects. In peri-postnatal studies in rats, postnatal development at maternal doses of 40 or 50 mg/kg/day of doxazosin (8 times human AUC exposure with a 12 mg/day therapeutic dose) was delayed as evidenced by slower body weight gain and slightly later appearance of anatomical features and reflexes.

Nursing Mothers: Studies in lactating rats given a single oral dose of 1 mg/kg of [2-¹⁴C]-CARDURA® indicate that doxazosin accumulates in rat breast milk with a maximum concentration about 20 times greater than the maternal plasma concentration. It is not known whether this drug is excreted in human milk. Because many drugs are excreted in human milk, caution should be exercised when CARDURA® is administered to a nursing mother.

Pediatric Use: The safety and effectiveness of CARDURA® as an antihypertensive agent have not been established in children.

Use in Elderly: The safety and effectiveness profile of CARDURA® in BPH was similar in the elderly (age ≥65 years) and younger (age <65 years) patients.

ADVERSE REACTIONS

A. *Benign Prostatic Hyperplasia*

The incidence of adverse events has been ascertained from worldwide clinical trials in 965 BPH patients. The incidence rates presented below (Table 3) are based on combined data from seven placebo-controlled trials involving once daily administration of CARDURA® (doxazosin mesylate) in doses of 1–16 mg in hypertensives and 0.5–8 mg in normotensives. The adverse events when the incidence in the CARDURA® group was at least 1% are summarized in Table 3. No significant difference in the incidence of adverse events compared to placebo was seen except for dizziness, fatigue, hypotension, edema and dyspnea. Dizziness and dyspnea appeared to be dose-related.

TABLE 3
ADVERSE REACTIONS DURING
PLACEBO-CONTROLLED STUDIES
BENIGN PROSTATIC HYPERPLASIA

Body System	CARDURA® (N=665)	PLACEBO (N=300)
BODY AS A WHOLE		
Back pain	1.8%	2.0%
Chest pain	1.2%	0.7%
Fatigue	8.0%*	1.7%
Headache	9.9%	9.0%
Influenza-like symptoms	1.1%	1.0%
Pain	2.0%	1.0%
CARDIOVASCULAR SYSTEM		
Hypotension	1.7%*	0.0%
Palpitation	1.2%	0.3%
DIGESTIVE SYSTEM		
Abdominal Pain	2.4%	2.0%
Diarrhea	2.3%	2.0%
Dyspepsia	1.7%	1.7%
Nausea	1.5%	0.7%
METABOLIC AND NUTRITIONAL DISORDERS		
Edema	2.7%*	0.7%
NERVOUS SYSTEM		
Dizziness†	15.6%*	9.0%
Mouth Dry	1.4%	0.3%
Somnolence	3.0%	1.0%
RESPIRATORY SYSTEM		
Dyspnea	2.6%*	0.3%
Respiratory Disorder	1.1%	0.7%
SPECIAL SENSES		
Vision Abnormal	1.4%	0.7%
UROGENITAL SYSTEM		
Impotence	1.1%	1.0%
Urinary Tract Infection	1.4%	2.3%
SKIN & APPENDAGES		
Sweating Increased	1.1%	1.0%
PSYCHIATRIC DISORDERS		
Anxiety	1.1%	0.3%
Insomnia	1.2%	0.3%

*p ≤0.05 for treatment differences   †Includes vertigo

In these placebo-controlled studies of 665 CARDURA® (doxazosin mesylate) patients, treated for a mean of 85 days, additional adverse reactions have been reported. These are less than 1% and not distinguishable from those that occurred in the placebo group. Adverse reactions with an incidence of less than 1% but of clinical interest are (CARDURA® vs. placebo): *Cardiovascular System:* angina pectoris (0.6% vs. 0.7%), postural hypotension (0.3% vs. 0.3%), syncope (0.5% vs. 0.0%), tachycardia (0.9% vs. 0.0%); *Urogenital System:* dysuria (0.5% vs. 1.3%), and *Psychiatric Disorders:* libido decreased (0.8% vs. 0.3%). The safety profile in patients treated for up to three years was similar to that in the placebo-controlled studies.

The majority of adverse experiences with CARDURA® were mild.

B. *Hypertension*

CARDURA® (doxazosin mesylate) has been administered to approximately 4000 hypertensive patients, of whom 1679 were included in the hypertension clinical development program. In that program, minor adverse effects were frequent, but led to discontinuation of treatment in only 7% of patients. In placebo-controlled studies adverse effects occurred in 49% and 40% of patients in the doxazosin and placebo groups, respectively, and led to discontinuation in 2% of patients in each group. The major reasons for discontinuation were postural effects (2%), edema, malaise/fatigue, and some heart rate disturbance, each about 0.7%.

In controlled hypertension clinical trials directly comparing CARDURA® to placebo there was no significant difference in the incidence of side effects, except for dizziness (including postural), weight gain, somnolence and fatigue/malaise. Postural effects and edema appeared to be dose related. The prevalence rates presented below are based on combined data from placebo-controlled studies involving once daily administration of doxazosin at doses ranging from 1–16 mg. Table 4 summarizes those adverse experiences (possibly/probably related) reported for patients in these hypertension studies where the prevalence rate in the doxazosin group was at least 0.5% or where the reaction is of particular interest.

TABLE 4
ADVERSE REACTIONS DURING
PLACEBO-CONTROLLED STUDIES
HYPERTENSION

	DOXAZOSIN (N=339)	PLACEBO (N=336)
CARDIOVASCULAR SYSTEM		
Dizziness	19%	9%
Vertigo	2%	1%
Postural Hypotension	0.3%	0%
Edema	4%	3%
Palpitation	2%	3%
Arrhythmia	1%	0%
Hypotension	1%	0%
Tachycardia	0.3%	1%
Peripheral Ischemia	0.3%	0%
SKIN & APPENDAGES		
Rash	1%	1%
Pruritus	1%	1%
MUSCULOSKELETAL SYSTEM		
Arthralgia/Arthritis	1%	0%
Muscle Weakness	1%	0%
Myalgia	1%	0%
CENTRAL & PERIPHERAL N.S.		
Headache	14%	16%
Paresthesia	1%	1%
Kinetic Disorders	1%	0%
Ataxia	1%	0%
Hypertonia	1%	0%
Muscle Cramps	1%	0%
AUTONOMIC		
Mouth Dry	2%	2%
Flushing	1%	0%
SPECIAL SENSES		
Vision Abnormal	2%	1%
Conjunctivitis/Eye Pain	1%	1%
Tinnitus	1%	0.3%
PSYCHIATRIC		
Somnolence	5%	1%
Nervousness	2%	2%
Depression	1%	1%
Insomnia	1%	1%
Sexual Dysfunction	2%	1%

GASTROINTESTINAL

Nausea	3%	4%
Diarrhea	2%	3%
Constipation	1%	1%
Dyspepsia	1%	1%
Flatulence	1%	1%
Abdominal Pain	0%	2%
Vomiting	0%	1%

RESPIRATORY

Rhinitis	3%	1%
Dyspnea	1%	1%
Epistaxis	1%	0%

URINARY

Polyuria	2%	0%
Urinary Incontinence	1%	0%
Micturition Frequency	0%	2%

GENERAL

Fatigue/Malaise	12%	6%
Chest Pain	2%	2%
Asthenia	1%	1%
Face Edema	1%	0%
Pain	2%	2%

Additional adverse reactions have been reported, but these are, in general, not distinguishable from symptoms that might have occurred in the absence of exposure to doxazosin. The following adverse reactions occurred with a frequency of between 0.5% and 1%: syncope, hypoesthesia, increased sweating, agitation, increased weight. The following additional adverse reactions were reported by <0.5% of 3960 patients who received doxazosin in controlled or open, short- or long-term clinical studies, including international studies. *Cardiovascular System:* angina pectoris, myocardial infarction, cerebrovascular accident; *Autonomic Nervous System:* pallor; *Metabolic:* thirst, gout, hypokalemia; *Hematopoietic:* lymphadenopathy, purpura; *Reproductive System:* breast pain; *Skin Disorders:* alopecia, dry skin, eczema; *Central Nervous System:* paresis, tremor, twitching, confusion, migraine, impaired concentration; *Psychiatric:* paroniria, amnesia, emotional lability, abnormal thinking, depersonalization; *Special Senses:* parosmia, earache, taste perversion, photophobia, abnormal lacrimation; *Gastrointestinal System:* increased appetite, anorexia, fecal incontinence, gastroenteritis; *Respiratory System:* bronchospasm, sinusitis, coughing, pharyngitis; *Urinary System:* renal calculus; *General Body System:* hot flushes, back pain, infection, fever/rigors, decreased weight, influenza-like symptoms.

CARDURA® (doxazosin mesylate) has not been associated with any clinically significant changes in routine biochemical tests. No clinically relevant adverse effects were noted on serum potassium, serum glucose, uric acid, blood urea nitrogen, creatinine or liver function tests. CARDURA® has been associated with decreases in white blood cell counts (see PRECAUTIONS).

OVERDOSAGE

Experience with CARDURA® overdosage is limited. Two adolescents who each intentionally ingested 40 mg CARDURA® with diclofenac or paracetamol, were treated with gastric lavage with activated charcoal and made full recoveries. A two-year-old child who accidently ingested 4 mg CARDURA® was treated with gastric lavage and remained normotensive during the five-hour emergency room observation period. A six-month-old child accidentally received a crushed 1 mg tablet of CARDURA® and was reported to have been drowsy. A 32-year-old female with chronic renal failure, epilepsy and depression intentionally ingested 60 mg CARDURA® (blood level 0.9 µg/mL; normal values in hypertensives=0.02 µg/mL); death was attributed to a grand mal seizure resulting from hypotension. A 39-year-old female who ingested 70 mg CARDURA®, alcohol and Dalmane® (flurazepam) developed hypotension which responded to fluid therapy.

The oral LD_{50} of doxazosin is greater than 1000 mg/kg in mice and rats. The most likely manifestation of overdosage would be hypotension, for which the usual treatment would be intravenous infusion of fluid. As doxazosin is highly protein bound, dialysis would not be indicated.

DOSAGE AND ADMINISTRATION

DOSAGE MUST BE INDIVIDUALIZED. The initial dosage of CARDURA® in patients with hypertension and/or BPH is 1 mg given once daily in the a.m. or p.m. This starting dose is intended to minimize the frequency of postural hypotension and first dose syncope associated with CARDURA®. Postural effects are most likely to occur between 2 and 6 hours after a dose. Therefore blood pressure measurements should be taken during this time period after the first dose and with each increase in dose. If CARDURA® administration is discontinued for several days, therapy should be restarted using the initial dosing regimen.

A. *BENIGN PROSTATIC HYPERPLASIA 1-8 mg once daily.* The initial dosage of CARDURA® is 1 mg, given once daily in the a.m. or p.m. Depending on the individual patient's urodynamics and BPH symptomatology, dosage may then be increased to 2 mg and thereafter to 4 mg and 8 mg once daily, the maximum recommended dose for BPH. The recommended titration interval is 1-2 weeks. Blood pressure should be evaluated routinely in these patients.

B. *HYPERTENSION 1-16 mg once daily.* The initial dosage of CARDURA® is 1 mg given once daily. Depending on the individual patient's standing blood pressure response (based on measurements taken at 2-6 hours post-dose and 24 hours post-dose), dosage may then be increased to 2 mg and thereafter if necessary to 4 mg, 8 mg and 16 mg to achieve the desired reduction in blood pressure. **Increases in dose beyond 4 mg increase the likelihood of excessive postural effects including syncope, postural dizziness/vertigo and postural hypotension. At a titrated dose of 16 mg once daily the frequency of postural effects is about 12% compared to 3% for placebo.**

HOW SUPPLIED

CARDURA® (doxazosin mesylate) is available as colored tablets for oral administration. Each tablet contains doxazosin mesylate equivalent to 1 mg (white), 2 mg (yellow), 4 mg (orange) or 8 mg (green) of the active constituent, doxazosin.

CARDURA® TABLETS (doxazosin mesylate) are available as 1 mg (white), 2 mg (yellow), 4 mg (orange) and 8 mg (green) scored tablets.

Bottles of 100:	1 mg (NDC 0049-2750-66)
	2 mg (NDC 0049-2760-66)
	4 mg (NDC 0049-2770-66)
	8 mg (NDC 0049-2780-66)
Unit Dose Packages of 100:	1 mg (NDC 0049-2750-41)
	2 mg (NDC 0049-2760-41)
	4 mg (NDC 0049-2770-41)
	8 mg (NDC 0049-2780-41)

Recommended Storage: Store below 86°F (30°C).

CAUTION: Federal law prohibits dispensing without prescription.

©1997 PFIZER INC
70-4538-00-6 Revised June 1997

PATIENT INFORMATION ABOUT CARDURA®

Generic Name:
doxazosin mesylate
FOR BENIGN PROSTATIC HYPERPLASIA (BPH)

Read this leaflet:
• before you start taking CARDURA®
• each time you get a new prescription.
You and your doctor should discuss this treatment and your BPH symptoms before you start taking CARDURA® and at your regular checkups. This leaflet does NOT take the place of discussions with your doctor.

CARDURA® is used to treat both benign prostatic hyperplasia (BPH) and high blood pressure (hypertension). This leaflet describes CARDURA® as treatment for BPH (although you may be taking CARDURA® for both your BPH and high blood pressure).

What is BPH?
BPH is an enlargement of the prostate gland. This gland surrounds the tube that drains the urine from the bladder. The symptoms of BPH can be caused by a tensing of the enlarged muscle in the prostate gland which blocks the passage of urine. This can lead to such symptoms as:
• a weak or start-and-stop stream when urinating
• a feeling that the bladder is not completely emptied after urination
• a delay or difficulty in the beginning of urination
• a need to urinate often during the day and especially at night
• a feeling that you must urinate immediately.

Treatment Options for BPH
The four main treatment options for BPH are:
• If you are not bothered by your symptoms, you and your doctor may decide on a program of "watchful waiting." It is not an active treatment like taking medication or surgery but involves having regular checkups to see if your condition is getting worse or causing problems.
• Treatment with CARDURA® or other similar drugs. CARDURA® is the medication your doctor has prescribed for you. See "What CARDURA® Does," below.
• Treatment with the medication class of 5-alpha reductase inhibitors (e.g., Proscar®). It can cause the prostate to shrink. It may take 6 months or more for the full benefit of finasteride to be seen.
• Various surgical procedures. Your doctor can describe these procedures to you. The best procedure for you depends on your BPH symptoms and medical condition.

What CARDURA® Does
CARDURA® works on a specific type of muscle found in the prostate, causing it to relax. This in turn decreases the pressure within the prostate, thus improving the flow of urine and your symptoms.

• CARDURA® (doxazosin mesylate) helps relieve the symptoms of BPH (weak stream, start-and-stop stream, a feeling that your bladder is not completely empty, delay in beginning of urination, need to urinate often during the day and especially at night, and feeling that you must urinate immediately). It does not change the size of the prostate. The prostate may continue to grow; however, a larger prostate is not necessarily related to more symptoms or to worse symptoms. CARDURA® can decrease your symptoms and improve urinary flow, without decreasing the size of the prostate.
• If CARDURA® is helping you, you should notice an effect within 1 to 2 weeks after you start your medication. CARDURA® has been studied in over 900 patients for up to 2 years and the drug has been shown to continue to work during long-term treatment. Even though you take CARDURA® and it may help you, CARDURA® may not prevent the need for surgery in the future.
• CARDURA® does not affect PSA levels. PSA is the abbreviation for Prostate Specific Antigen. Your doctor may have done a blood test called PSA. You may want to ask your doctor more about this if you have had a PSA test done.

Other Important Facts
• You should see an improvement of your symptoms within 1 to 2 weeks. In addition to your other regular checkups you will need to continue seeing your doctor regularly to check your progress regarding your BPH and to monitor your blood pressure.
• CARDURA® (doxazosin mesylate) is not a treatment for prostate cancer. Your doctor has prescribed CARDURA® for your BPH and not for prostate cancer; however, a man can have BPH and prostate cancer at the same time. Doctors usually recommend that men be checked for prostate cancer once a year when they turn 50 (or 40 if a family member has had prostate cancer). A higher incidence of prostate cancer has been noted in men of African-American descent. These checks should continue even if you are taking CARDURA®.

How To Take CARDURA® and What You Should Know While Taking CARDURA® for BPH
CARDURA® Can Cause a Sudden Drop in Blood Pressure After the VERY FIRST DOSE. You may feel dizzy, faint or "light-headed," especially after you stand up from a lying or sitting position. This is more likely to occur after you've taken the first few doses or if you increase your dose, but can occur at any time while you are taking the drug. It can also occur if you stop taking the drug and then restart treatment. If you feel very dizzy, faint or "light-headed" you should contact your doctor. Your doctor will discuss with you how often you need to visit and how often your blood pressure should be checked.
Your blood pressure should be checked when you start taking CARDURA® even if you do not have high blood pressure (hypertension). Your doctor will discuss with you the details of how blood pressure is measured.
Blood Pressure Measurement: Whatever equipment is used, it is usual for your blood pressure to be measured in the following way: measure your blood pressure after lying quietly on your back for five minutes. Then, after standing for two minutes measure your blood pressure again. Your doctor will discuss with you what other times during the day your blood pressure should be taken, such as two to six hours after a dose, before bedtime or after waking up in the morning. Note that moderate to high-intensity exercise can, over a period of time, lower your average blood pressure.
You can take CARDURA® either in the morning or at bedtime and it will be equally effective. If you take CARDURA® at bedtime but need to get up from bed to go to the bathroom, get up slowly and cautiously until you are sure how the medication affects you. It is important to get up slowly from a chair or bed at any time until you learn how you react to CARDURA®. You should not drive or do any hazardous tasks until you are used to the effects of the medication. If you begin to feel dizzy, sit or lie down until you feel better.
• You will start with a 1 mg dose of CARDURA® once daily. Then the once daily dose will be increased as your body gets used to the effects of the medication. Follow your doctor's instructions about how to take CARDURA®. You must take it every day at the dose prescribed. Talk with your doctor if you don't take it for a few days for some reason; you may then need to restart the medication at a 1 mg dose, increase your dose gradually and again be cautious about possible dizziness. Do not share CARDURA® with anyone else; it was prescribed only for you.
• Other side effects you could have while taking CARDURA® (doxazosin mesylate), in addition to lowering of the blood pressure, include dizziness, fatigue (tiredness), swelling of the feet and shortness of breath. Most side effects are mild. However, you should discuss any unexpected effects you notice with your doctor.
• **WARNING:** Extremely rarely, CARDURA® and similar medications have caused painful erection of the penis,

Continued on next page

Cardura—Cont.

sustained for hours and unrelieved by sexual intercourse or masturbation. This condition is serious, and if untreated it can be followed by permanent inability to have an erection. If you have a prolonged abnormal erection, call your doctor or go to an emergency room as soon as possible.

• Keep CARDURA® and all medicines out of the reach of children.

FOR MORE INFORMATION ABOUT CARDURA® AND BPH TALK WITH YOUR DOCTOR, NURSE, PHARMACIST OR OTHER HEALTH CARE PROVIDER.

©1997 PFIZER INC
70-5039-00-1

Revised May 1997
Shown in Product Identification Guide, page 330

CEFOBID® ℞
[sĕf ′ō-bĭd]
(sterile cefoperazone sodium)
For Intravenous or Intramuscular Use

CEFOBID® ℞
(cefoperazone sodium injection USP)
in Galaxy® Plastic Container (PL 2040)
For Intravenous Use

DESCRIPTION

CEFOBID® (sterile cefoperazone sodium) and CEFOBID (cefoperazone sodium injection) in Galaxy® plastic container (PL 2040) contain cefoperazone as cefoperazone sodium. It is a semisynthetic, broad-spectrum, cephalosporin antibiotic. Chemically, cefoperazone sodium is sodium $(6R, 7R)$-7-[(R)-2-(4-ethyl-2,3-dioxo-1-piperazinecarboxamido)-2-(p-hydroxyphenyl)-acetamido)-3-[[(1-methyl- $1H$- tetrazol-5-yl)thio] methyl]-8-oxo-5-thia-1-azabicyclo[4.2.0]oct-2-ene-2-carboxylate. Its molecular formula is $C_{25}H_{26}N_9NaO_8S_2$ with a molecular weight of 667.65. The structural formula is given below:

CEFOBID (sterile cefoperazone sodium) contains 34 mg sodium (1.5 mEq) per gram. CEFOBID is a white powder which is freely soluble in water. The pH of a 25% (w/v) freshly reconstituted solution varies between 4.5–6.5 and the solution ranges from colorless to straw yellow depending on the concentration.

CEFOBID (sterile cefoperazone sodium) in crystalline form is supplied in vials containing 1 g or 2 g cefoperazone as cefoperazone sodium for intravenous or intramuscular administration.

CEFOBID (sterile cefoperazone sodium) is also supplied in Piggy Back Units for intravenous administration only.

CEFOBID (cefoperazone sodium injection) in Galaxy® plastic container (PL 2040) is a frozen, iso-osmotic, sterile, non-pyrogenic premixed 50 mL solution containing 1 g or 2 g of cefoperazone as cefoperazone sodium. Dextrose hydrous, USP, has been added to adjust the osmolality to approximately 300 mOsmol/kg (approximately 2.3 g and 1.8 g to the 1 g and 2 g dosages, respectively). The pH may have been adjusted with sodium hydroxide and/or hydrochloric acid. After thawing to room temperature, it is intended for intravenous use only.

The Galaxy® container is fabricated from a specially designed multilayer plastic (PL 2040). Solutions are in contact with the polyethylene layer of this container and can leach out certain chemical components of the plastic in very small amounts within the expiration dating period. The suitability of the plastic has been confirmed in test in animals according to the USP biological tests for plastic containers, as well as by tissue culture toxicity studies.

CLINICAL PHARMACOLOGY

High serum and bile levels of CEFOBID are attained after a single dose of the drug. Table 1 demonstrates the serum concentrations of CEFOBID in normal volunteers following either a single 15-minute constant rate intravenous infusion of 1, 2, 3 or 4 grams of the drug, or a single intramuscular injection of 1 or 2 grams of the drug.
[See table 1 at right]
The mean serum half-life of CEFOBID is approximately 2.0 hours, independent of the route of administration.
In vitro studies with human serum indicate that the degree of CEFOBID reversible protein binding varies with the serum concentration from 93% at 25 mcg/mL of CEFOBID to 90% at 250 mcg/mL and 82% at 500 mcg/mL.
CEFOBID achieves therapeutic concentrations in the following body tissues and fluids:

Tissue or Fluid	Dose		Concentration	
Ascitic Fluid	2	g	64	mcg/mL
Cerebrospinal Fluid	50	mg/kg	1.8	mcg/mL
(in patients with			to	
inflamed meninges)			8.0	mcg/mL
Urine	2	g	3,286	mcg/mL
Sputum	3	g	6.0	mcg/mL
Endometrium	2	g	74	mcg/g
Myometrium	2	g	54	mcg/g
Palatine Tonsil	1	g	8	mcg/g
Sinus Mucous Membrane	1	g	8	mcg/g
Umbilical Cord Blood	1	g	25	mcg/mL
Amniotic Fluid	1	g	4.8	mcg/mL
Lung	1	g	28	mcg/g
Bone	2	g	40	mcg/g

CEFOBID is excreted mainly in the bile. Maximum bile concentrations are generally obtained between one and three hours following drug administration and exceed concurrent serum concentrations by up to 100 times. Reported biliary concentrations of CEFOBID range from 66 mcg/mL at 30 minutes to as high as 6000 mcg/mL at 3 hours after an intravenous bolus injection of 2 grams.

Following a single intramuscular or intravenous dose, the urinary recovery of CEFOBID over a 12-hour period averages 20–30%. No significant quantity of metabolites has been found in the urine. Urinary concentrations greater than 2200 mcg/mL have been obtained following a 15-minute infusion of a 2 g dose. After an IM injection of 2 g, peak urine concentrations of almost 1000 mcg/mL have been obtained, and therapeutic levels are maintained for 12 hours. Repeated administration of CEFOBID at 12-hour intervals does not result in accumulation of the drug in normal subjects. Peak serum concentrations, areas under the curve (AUC's), and serum half-lives in patients with severe renal insufficiency are not significantly different from those in normal volunteers. In patients with hepatic dysfunction, the serum half-life is prolonged and urinary excretion is increased. In patients with combined renal and hepatic insufficiencies, CEFOBID may accumulate in the serum.

CEFOBID has been used in pediatrics, but the safety and effectiveness in children have not been established. The half-life of CEFOBID in serum is 6–10 hours in low birthweight neonates.

Microbiology

CEFOBID is active *in vitro* against a wide range of aerobic and anaerobic, gram-positive and gram-negative pathogens. The bactericidal action of CEFOBID results from the inhibition of bacterial cell wall synthesis. CEFOBID has a high degree of stability in the presence of beta-lactamases produced by most gram-negative pathogens. CEFOBID is usually active against organisms which are resistant to other beta-lactam antibiotics because of beta-lactamase production. CEFOBID is usually active against the following organisms *in vitro* and in clinical infections:

Gram-Positive Aerobes:
Staphylococcus aureus, penicillinase and non-penicillinase-producing strains
Staphylococcus epidermidis
Streptococcus pneumoniae (formerly *Diplococcus pneumoniae*)
Streptococcus pyogenes (Group A beta-hemolytic streptococci)
Streptococcus agalactiae (Group B beta-hemolytic streptococci)
Enterococcus (*Streptococcus faecalis, S. faecium* and *S. durans*)

Gram-Negative Aerobes:
Escherichia coli
Klebsiella species (including *K. pneumoniae*)
Enterobacter species
Citrobacter species
Haemophilus influenzae
Proteus mirabilis
Proteus vulgaris
Morganella morganii (formerly *Proteus morganii*)
Providencia stuartii
Providencia rettgeri (formerly *Proteus rettgeri*)
Serratia marcescens
Pseudomonas aeruginosa

Pseudomonas species
Some strains of *Acinetobacter calcoaceticus*
Neisseria gonorrhoeae

Anaerobic Organisms:
Gram-positive cocci (including *Peptococcus* and *Peptostreptococcus*)
Clostridium species
Bacteroides fragilis
Other *Bacteroides* species

CEFOBID is also active *in vitro* against a wide variety of other pathogens although the clinical significance is unknown. These organisms include: *Salmonella* and *Shigella* species, *Serratia liquefaciens, N. meningitidis, Bordetella pertussis, Yersinia enterocolitica, Clostridium difficile, Fusobacterium* species, *Eubacterium* species and beta-lactamase producing strains of *H. influenzae* and *N. gonorrhoeae*.

Susceptibility Testing:

Diffusion Technique. For the disk diffusion method of susceptibility testing, a 75 mcg CEFOBID diffusion disk should be used. Organisms should be tested with the CEFOBID 75 mcg disk since CEFOBID has been shown *in vitro* to be active against organisms which are found to be resistant to other beta-lactam antibiotics.
Tests should be interpreted by the following criteria:

Zone Diameter	Interpretation
Greater than or equal to 21 mm	Susceptible
16–20 mm	Moderately Susceptible
Less than or equal to 15 mm	Resistant

Quantitative procedures that require measurement of zone diameters give the most precise estimate of susceptibility. One such method which has been recommended for use with the CEFOBID 75 mcg disk is the NCCLS approved standard. (Performance Standards for Antimicrobial Disk Susceptibility Tests. Second Information Supplement Vol. 2 No. 2 pp. 49–69. Publisher—National Committee for Clinical Laboratory Standards, Villanova, Pennsylvania.)

A report of "susceptible" indicates that the infecting organism is likely to respond to CEFOBID therapy and a report of "resistant" indicates that the infecting organism is not likely to respond to therapy. A "moderately susceptible" report suggests that the infecting organism will be susceptible to CEFOBID if a higher than usual dosage is used or if the infection is confined to tissues and fluids (e.g., urine or bile) in which high antibiotic levels are attained.

Dilution Techniques. Broth or agar dilution methods may be used to determine the minimal inhibitory concentration (MIC) of CEFOBID. Serial twofold dilutions of CEFOBID should be prepared in either broth or agar. Broth should be inoculated to contain 5×10^5 organisms/mL and agar "spotted" with 10^4 organisms.

MIC test results should be interpreted in light of serum, tissue, and body fluid concentrations of CEFOBID. Organisms inhibited by CEFOBID at 16 mcg/mL or less are considered susceptible, while organisms with MIC's of 17–63 mcg/mL are moderately susceptible. Organisms inhibited at CEFOBID concentrations of greater than or equal to 64 mcg/mL are considered resistant, although clinical cures have been obtained in some patients infected by such organisms.

INDICATIONS AND USAGE

CEFOBID is indicated for the treatment of the following infections when caused by susceptible organisms:

Respiratory Tract Infections caused by *S. pneumoniae, H. influenzae, S. aureus* (penicillinase and non-penicillinase producing strains), *S. pyogenes** (Group A beta-hemolytic streptococci), *P. aeruginosa, Klebsiella pneumoniae, E. coli, Proteus mirabilis,* and *Enterobacter* species.

Peritonitis and Other Intra-abdominal Infections caused by *E. coli, P. aeruginosa,** and anaerobic gram-negative bacilli (including *Bacteroides fragilis*).

Bacterial Septicemia caused by *S. pneumoniae, S. agalactiae*, S. aureus, Pseudomonas aeruginosa*, E. coli, Klebsiella* spp.,* *Klebsiella pneumoniae** , *Proteus* species* (indole-positive and indole-negative), *Clostridium* spp.* and anaerobic gram-positive cocci.*

Infections of the Skin and Skin Structures caused by *S. aureus* (penicillinase and non-penicillinase producing strains), *S. pyogenes*,* and *P. aeruginosa.*

TABLE 1. Cefoperazone Serum Concentrations

Dose/Route	Mean Serum Concentrations (mcg/mL)						
	0*	0.5 hr	1 hr	2 hr	4 hr	8 hr	12 hr
1 g IV	153	114	73	38	16	4	0.5
2 g IV	252	153	114	70	32	8	2
3 g IV	340	210	142	89	41	9	2
4 g IV	506	325	251	161	71	19	6
1 g IM	32 **	52	65	57	33	7	1
2 g IM	40 **	69	93	97	58	14	4

* Hours post-administration, with 0 time being the end of the infusion.
** Values obtained 15 minutes post-injection.

Pelvic Inflammatory Disease, Endometritis, and Other Infections of the Female Genital Tract caused by *N. gonorrhoeae, S. epidermidis**, *S. agalactiae, E. coli, Clostridium* spp.,* *Bacteroides* species (including *Bacteroides fragilis*) and anaerobic gram-positive cocci.

Urinary Tract Infections caused by *Escherichia coli* and *Pseudomonas aeruginosa.*

Enterococcal Infections: Although cefoperazone has been shown to be clinically effective in the treatment of infections caused by enterococci in cases of **peritonitis and other intra-abdominal infections, infections of the skin and skin structures, pelvic inflammatory disease, endometritis and other infections of the female genital tract, and urinary tract infection,*** the majority of clinical isolates of enterococci tested are not susceptible to cefoperazone but fall just at or in the intermediate zone of susceptibilty, and are moderately resistant to cefoperazone. However, *in vitro* susceptibility testing may not correlate directly with *in vivo* results. Despite this, cefoperazone therapy has resulted in clinical cures of enterococcal infections, chiefly in polymicrobial infections. Cefoperazone should be used in enterococcal infections with care and at doses that achieve satisfactory serum levels of cefoperazone.

*Efficacy of this organism in this organ system was studied in fewer than 10 infections.

Susceptibility Testing

Before instituting treatment with CEFOBID, appropriate specimens should be obtained for isolation of the causative organism and for determination of its susceptibility to the drug. Treatment may be started before results of susceptibility testing are available.

Combination Therapy

Synergy between CEFOBID and aminoglycosides has been demonstrated with many gram-negative bacilli. However, such enhanced activity of these combinations is not predictable. If such therapy is considered, *in vitro* susceptibility tests should be performed to determine the activity of the drugs in combination, and renal function should be monitored carefully. (See PRECAUTIONS, and DOSAGE AND ADMINISTRATION sections).

CONTRAINDICATIONS

CEFOBID is contraindicated in patients with known allergy to the cephalosporin-class of antibiotics.

WARNINGS

BEFORE THERAPY WITH CEFOBID IS INSTITUTED, CAREFUL INQUIRY SHOULD BE MADE TO DETERMINE WHETHER THE PATIENT HAS HAD PREVIOUS HYPERSENSITIVITY REACTIONS TO CEPHALOSPORINS, PENICILLINS OR OTHER DRUGS. THIS PRODUCT SHOULD BE GIVEN CAUTIOUSLY TO PENICILLIN-SENSITIVE PATIENTS. ANTIBIOTICS SHOULD BE ADMINISTERED WITH CAUTION TO ANY PATIENT WHO HAS DEMONSTRATED SOME FORM OF ALLERGY, PARTICULARLY TO DRUGS. SERIOUS ACUTE HYPERSENSITIVITY REACTIONS MAY REQUIRE THE USE OF SUBCUTANEOUS EPINEPHRINE AND OTHER EMERGENCY MEASURES.

PSEUDOMEMBRANOUS COLITIS HAS BEEN REPORTED WITH THE USE OF CEPHALOSPORINS (AND OTHER BROAD-SPECTRUM ANTIBIOTICS); THEREFORE, IT IS IMPORTANT TO CONSIDER ITS DIAGNOSIS IN PATIENTS WHO DEVELOP DIARRHEA IN ASSOCIATION WITH ANTIBIOTIC USE.

Treatment with broad-spectrum antibiotics alters normal flora of the colon and may permit overgrowth of clostridia. Studies indicate a toxin produced by *Clostridium difficile* is one primary cause of antibiotic-associated colitis. Cholestyramine and colestipol resins have been shown to bind the toxin *in vitro.*

Mild cases of colitis may respond to drug discontinuance alone.

Moderate to severe cases should be managed with fluid, electrolyte, and protein supplementation as indicated.

When the colitis is not relieved by drug discontinuance or when it is severe, oral vancomycin is the treatment of choice for antibiotic-associated pseudomembranous colitis produced by *C. difficile.* Other causes of colitis should also be considered.

PRECAUTIONS

Although transient elevations of the BUN and serum creatinine have been observed, CEFOBID alone does not appear to cause significant nephrotoxicity. However, concomitant administration of aminoglycosides and other cephalosporins has caused nephrotoxicity.

CEFOBID is extensively excreted in bile. The serum half-life of CEFOBID is increased 2–4 fold in patients with hepatic disease and/or biliary obstruction. In general, total daily dosage above 4 g should not be necessary in such patients. If higher dosages are used, serum concentrations should be monitored.

Because renal excretion is not the main route of elimination of CEFOBID (see CLINICAL PHARMACOLOGY), patients with renal failure require no adjustment in dosage when usual doses are administered. When high doses of CEFOBID are used, concentrations of drug in the serum should be monitored periodically. If evidence of accumulation exists, dosage should be decreased accordingly.

The half-life of CEFOBID is reduced slightly during hemodialysis. Thus, dosing should be scheduled to follow a dialysis period. In patients with both hepatic dysfunction and significant renal disease, CEFOBID dosage should not exceed 1–2 g daily without close monitoring of serum concentrations.

As with other antibiotics, vitamin K deficiency has occurred rarely in patients treated with CEFOBID. The mechanism is most probably related to the suppression of gut flora which normally synthesize this vitamin. Those at risk include patients with a poor nutritional status, malabsorption states (e.g., cystic fibrosis), alcoholism, and patients on prolonged hyper-alimentation regimens (administered either intravenously or via a naso-gastric tube). Prothrombin time should be monitored in these patients and exogenous vitamin K administered as indicated.

A disulfiram-like reaction characterized by flushing, sweating, headache, and tachycardia has been reported when alcohol (beer, wine) was ingested within 72 hours after CEFOBID administration. Patients should be cautioned about the ingestion of alcoholic beverages following the administration of CEFOBID. A similar reaction has been reported with other cephalosporins.

Prolonged use of CEFOBID may result in the overgrowth of nonsusceptible organisms. Careful observation of the patient is essential. If superinfection occurs during therapy, appropriate measures should be taken.

CEFOBID should be prescribed with caution in individuals with a history of gastrointestinal disease, particularly colitis.

Drug Laboratory Test Interactions

A false-positive reaction for glucose in the urine may occur with Benedict's or Fehling's solution.

Carcinogenesis, Mutagenesis, Impairment of Fertility

Long term studies in animals have not been performed to evaluate carcinogenic potential. The maximum duration of CEFOBID animal toxicity studies is six months. In none of the *in vivo* or *in vitro* genetic toxicology studies did CEFOBID show any mutagenic potential at either the chromosomal or subchromosomal level. CEFOBID produced no impairment of fertility and had no effects on general reproductive performance or fetal development when administered subcutaneously at daily doses up to 500 to 1000 mg/kg prior to and during mating, and to pregnant female rats during gestation. These doses are 10 to 20 times the estimated usual single clinical dose. CEFOBID had adverse effects on the testes of prepubertal rats at all doses tested. Subcutaneous administration of 1000 mg/kg per day (approximately 16 times the average adult human dose) resulted in reduced testicular weight, arrested spermatogenesis, reduced germinal cell population and vacuolation of Sertoli cell cytoplasm. The severity of lesions was dose dependent in the 100 to 1000 mg/kg per day range; the low dose caused a minor decrease in spermatocytes. This effect has not been observed in adult rats. Histologically the lesions were reversible at all but the highest dosage levels. However, these studies did not evaluate subsequent development of reproductive function in the rats. The relationship of these findings to humans is unknown.

Usage in Pregnancy

Pregnancy Category B: Reproduction studies have been performed in mice, rats, and monkeys at doses up to 10 times the human dose and have revealed no evidence of impaired fertility or harm to the fetus due to CEFOBID. There are, however, no adequate and well controlled studies in pregnant women. Because animal reproduction studies are not always predictive of human response, this drug should be used during pregnancy only if clearly needed.

Usage in Nursing Mothers

Only low concentrations of CEFOBID are excreted in human milk. Although CEFOBID passes poorly into breast milk of nursing mothers, caution should be exercised when CEFOBID is administered to a nursing woman.

Pediatric Use

Safety and effectiveness in children have not been established. For information concerning testicular changes in prepubertal rats (see Carcinogenesis, Mutagenesis, Impairment of Fertility).

ADVERSE REACTIONS

In clinical studies the following adverse effects were observed and were considered to be related to CEFOBID therapy or of uncertain etiology:

Hypersensitivity: As with all cephalosporins, hypersensitivity manifested by skin reactions (1 patient in 45), drug fever (1 in 260), or a change in Coombs' test (1 in 60) has been reported. These reactions are more likely to occur in patients with a history of allergies, particularly to penicillin.

Hematology: As with other beta-lactam antibiotics, reversible neutropenia may occur with prolonged administration. Slight decreases in neutrophil count (1 patient in 50) have been reported. Decreased hemoglobins (1 in 20) or hematocrits (1 in 20) have been reported, which is consistent with published literature on other cephalosporins. Transient eosinophilia has occurred in 1 patient in 10.

Hepatic: Of 1285 patients treated with cefoperazone in clinical trials, one patient with a history of liver disease developed significantly elevated liver function enzymes during CEFOBID therapy. Clinical signs and symptoms of nonspecific hepatitis accompanied these increases. After CEFOBID therapy was discontinued, the patient's enzymes returned to pre-treatment levels and the symptomatology resolved. As with other antibiotics that achieve high bile levels, mild transient elevations of liver function enzymes have been observed in 5–10% of the patients receiving CEFOBID therapy. The relevance of these findings, which were not accompanied by overt signs or symptoms of hepatic dysfunction, has not been established.

Gastrointestinal: Diarrhea or loose stools has been reported in 1 in 30 patients. Most of these experiences have been mild or moderate in severity and self-limiting in nature. In all cases, these symptoms responded to symptomatic therapy or ceased when cefoperazone therapy was stopped. Nausea and vomiting have been reported rarely. Symptoms of pseudomembranous colitis can appear during or for several weeks subsequent to antibiotic therapy (see WARNINGS).

Renal Function Tests: Transient elevations of the BUN (1 in 16) and serum creatinine (1 in 48) have been noted.

Local Reactions: CEFOBID is well tolerated following intramuscular administration. Occasionally, transient pain (1 in 140) may follow administration by this route. When CEFOBID is administered by intravenous infusion some patients may develop phlebitis (1 in 120) at the infusion site.

DOSAGE AND ADMINISTRATION

The usual adult daily dose of CEFOBID is 2 to 4 grams per day administered in divided doses every 12 hours.

In severe infections or infections caused by less sensitive organisms, the total daily dose and/or frequency may be increased. Patients have been successfully treated with a total daily dosage of 6–12 grams divided into 2, 3 or 4 administrations ranging from 1.5 to 4 grams per dose.

In a pharmacokinetic study, a total daily dose of 16 grams was administered to severely immunocompromised patients by constant infusion without complications. Steady state serum concentrations were approximately 150 mcg/mL in these patients.

When treating infections caused by *Streptococcus pyogenes,* therapy should be continued for at least 10 days.

Solutions of CEFOBID and aminoglycoside should not be directly mixed, since there is a physical incompatibility between them. If combination therapy with CEFOBID and an aminoglycoside is contemplated (see INDICATIONS) this can be accomplished by sequential intermittent intravenous infusion provided that separate secondary intravenous tubing is used, and that the primary intravenous tubing is adequately irrigated with an approved diluent between doses. It is also suggested that CEFOBID be administered prior to the aminoglycoside. *In vitro* testing of the effectiveness of drug combination(s) is recommended.

RECONSTITUTION

The following solutions may be used for the initial reconstitution of CEFOBID (sterile cefoperazone sodium).

Table 1. Solutions for Initial Reconstitution.

5% Dextrose Injection (USP)
5% Dextrose and 0.9% Sodium Chloride Injection (USP)
5% Dextrose and 0.2% Sodium Chloride Injection (USP)
10% Dextrose Injection (USP)
Bacteriostatic Water for Injection [Benzyl Alcohol or Parabens] (USP)*†
0.9% Sodium Chloride Injection (USP)
Normosol® M and 5% Dextrose Injection
Normosol® R
Sterile Water for Injection*

---

* Not to be used as a vehicle for intravenous infusion

† Preparations containing Benzyl Alcohol should not be used in neonates.

General Reconstitution Procedures

CEFOBID (sterile cefoperazone sodium) for intravenous or intramuscular use may be initially reconstituted with any compatible solution mentioned above in Table 1. Solutions should be allowed to stand after reconstitution to allow any foaming to dissipate to permit visual inspection for complete solubilization. Vigorous and prolonged agitation may be necessary to solubilize CEFOBID in higher concentrations (above 333 mg cefoperazone/mL). The maximum solubility of CEFOBID (sterile cefoperazone sodium) is approximately 475 mg cefoperazone/mL of compatible diluent.

Continued on next page

Cefobid IV/IM—Cont.

Preparation For Intravenous Use

General. CEFOBID (sterile cefoperazone sodium) concentrations between 2 mg/mL and 50 mg/mL are recommended for intravenous administration.

Preparation of Vials. Vials of CEFOBID (sterile cefoperazone sodium) may be initially reconstituted with a minimum of 2.8 mL per gram of cefoperazone of any compatible reconstituting solution appropriate for intravenous administration listed above in Table 1. For ease of reconstitution the use of 5 mL of compatible solution per gram of CEFOBID is recommended. The entire quantity of the resulting solution should then be withdrawn for further dilution and administration using any of the following vehicles for intravenous infusion:

Table 2. Vehicles for Intravenous Infusion

5% Dextrose Injection (USP)
5% Dextrose and Lactated Ringer's Injection
5% Dextrose and 0.9% Sodium Chloride Injection (USP)
5% Dextrose and 0.2% Sodium Chloride Injection (USP)
10% Dextrose Injection (USP)
Lactated Ringer's Injection (USP)
0.9% Sodium Chloride Injection (USP)
Normosol® M and 5% Dextrose Injection
Normosol® R

Preparation of Piggy Back Units. CEFOBID (sterile cefoperazone sodium) in Piggy Back Units for intravenous use may be prepared by adding between 20 mL and 40 mL of any appropriate diluent listed in Table 2 per gram of cefoperazone. If 5% Dextrose and Lactated Ringer's Injection or Lactated Ringer's Injection (USP) is the chosen vehicle for administration the CEFOBID (sterile cefoperazone sodium) should initially be reconstituted using 2.8–5 mL per gram of any compatible reconstituting solution listed in Table 1 prior to the final dilution.

The resulting intravenous solution should be administered in one of the following manners:

Intermittent Infusion: Solutions of CEFOBID should be administered over a 15–30 minute time period.

Continuous Infusion: CEFOBID can be used for continuous infusion after dilution to a final concentration of between 2 and 25 mg cefoperazone per mL.

Preparation For Intramuscular Injection

Any suitable solution listed above may be used to prepare CEFOBID (sterile cefoperazone sodium) for intramuscular injection. When concentrations of 250 mg/mL or more are to be administered, a lidocaine solution should be used. These solutions should be prepared using a combination of Sterile Water for Injection and 2% Lidocaine Hydrochloride Injection (USP) that approximates a 0.5% Lidocaine Hydrochloride Solution. A two-step dilution process as follows is recommended: First, add the required amount of Sterile Water for Injection and agitate until CEFOBID powder is completely dissolved. Second, add the required amount of 2% lidocaine and mix.

[See first table below]

Storage and Stability: CEFOBID (sterile cefoperazone sodium) is to be stored at or below 25°C (77°F) and protected from light prior to reconstitution. After reconstitution, protection from light is not necessary.

The following parenteral diluents and approximate concentrations of CEFOBID provide stable solutions under the following conditions for the indicated time periods. (After the indicated time periods, unused portions of solutions should be discarded.)

	Final Cefoperazone Concentration	Step 1 Volume of Sterile Water	Step 2 Volume of 2% Lidocaine	Withdrawable Volume*†
1 g vial	333 mg/mL	2.0 mL	0.6 mL	3 mL
	250 mg/mL	2.8 mL	1.0 mL	4 mL
2 g vial	333 mg/mL	3.8 mL	1.2 mL	6 mL
	250 mg/mL	5.4 mL	1.8 mL	8 mL

When a diluent other than Lidocaine HCl Injection (USP) is used reconstitute as follows:

	Cefoperazone Concentration	Volume of Diluent to be Added	Withdrawable Volume*
1 g vial	333 mg/mL	2.6 mL	3 mL
	250 mg/mL	3.8 mL	4 mL
2 g vial	333 mg/mL	5.0 mL	6 mL
	250 mg/mL	7.2 mL	8 mL

* There is sufficient excess present to allow for withdrawal of the stated volume.
† Final lidocaine concentration will approximate that obtained if a 0.5% Lidocaine Hydrochloride Solution is used as diluent.

Room Temperature (15°–25°C/59°–77°F) 24 Hours	Approximate Concentrations
Bacteriostatic Water for Injection [Benzyl Alcohol or Parabens] (USP)	300 mg/mL
5% Dextrose Injection (USP)	2 mg to 50 mg/mL
5% Dextrose and Lactated Ringer's Injection	2 mg to 50 mg/mL
5% Dextrose and 0.9% Sodium Chloride Injection (USP)	2 mg to 50 mg/mL
5% Dextrose and 0.2% Sodium Chloride Injection (USP)	2 mg to 50 mg/mL
10% Dextrose Injection (USP)	2 mg to 50 mg/mL
Lactated Ringer's Injection (USP)	2 mg/mL
0.5% Lidocaine Hydrochloride Injection (USP)	300 mg/mL
0.9% Sodium Chloride Injection (USP)	2 mg to 300 mg/mL
Normosol® M and 5% Dextrose Injection	2 mg to 50 mg/mL
Normosol® R	2 mg to 50 mg/mL
Sterile Water for Injection	300 mg/mL

Reconstituted CEFOBID solutions may be stored in glass or plastic syringes, or in glass or flexible plastic parenteral solution containers.

Refrigerator Temperature (2°–8°C/36°–46°F) 5 Days	Approximate Concentrations
Bacteriostatic Water for Injection [Benzyl Alcohol or Parabens] (USP)	300 mg/mL
5% Dextrose Injection (USP)	2 mg to 50 mg/mL
5% Dextrose and 0.9% Sodium Chloride Injection (USP)	2 mg to 50 mg/mL
5% Dextrose and 0.2% Sodium Chloride Injection (USP)	2 mg to 50 mg/mL
Lactated Ringer's Injection (USP)	2 mg/mL
0.5% Lidocaine Hydrochloride Injection (USP)	300 mg/mL
0.9% Sodium Chloride Injection (USP)	2 mg to 300 mg/mL
Normosol® M and 5% Dextrose Injection	2 mg to 50 mg/mL
Normosol® R	2 mg to 50 mg/mL
Sterile Water for Injection	300 mg/mL

Reconstituted CEFOBID solutions may be stored in glass or plastic syringes, or in glass or flexible plastic parenteral solution containers.

Freezer Temperature (−20° to −10°C/−4° to 14°F) 3 Weeks	Approximate Concentrations
5% Dextrose Injection (USP)	50 mg/mL
5% Dextrose and 0.9% Sodium Chloride Injection (USP)	2 mg/mL
5% Dextrose and 0.2% Sodium Chloride Injection (USP)	2 mg/mL
5 Weeks	
0.9% Sodium Chloride Injection (USP)	300 mg/mL
Sterile Water for Injection	300 mg/mL

Reconstituted CEFOBID solutions may be stored in plastic syringes, or in flexible plastic parenteral solution containers.

[See second table below]

DIRECTIONS FOR USE OF CEFOBID® (cefoperazone sodium injection) IN GALAXY® PLASTIC CONTAINER (PL 2040)

CEFOBID in Galaxy® Container (PL 2040 Plastic) is to be administered either as a continuous or intermittent infusion.

Storage

Store in a freezer capable of maintaining a temperature of −20°C/−4°F.

Thawing of Plastic Container

Thaw frozen container at room temperature (25°C/77°F) or under refrigeration (5°C/41°F). [DO NOT FORCE THAW BY IMMERSION IN WATER BATHS OR BY MICROWAVE IRRADIATION.]

Check for minute leaks by squeezing container firmly. If leaks are detected, discard solution as sterility may be impaired.

DO NOT ADD SUPPLEMENTARY MEDICATION.

Preparation for Intravenous Administration (Use Aseptic Technique).

1. Suspend container from eyelet support
2. Remove protector from outlet port at bottom of container.
3. Attach administration set. Refer to complete directions accompanying set.

Caution: Do not use plastic containers in series connections. Such use could result in an embolism due to residual air being drawn from the primary container before administration of the fluid from the secondary container is complete.

HOW SUPPLIED

CEFOBID® (sterile cefoperazone sodium) is available in vials containing cefoperazone sodium equivalent to 1 g cefoperazone × 10 (NDC 0049-1201-83), and 2 g cefoperazone × 10 (NDC 0049-1202-83) for intramuscular and intravenous administration.

CEFOBID® (sterile cefoperazone sodium) is available in Piggy Back Units containing cefoperazone sodium equivalent to 1 g cefoperazone × 10 (NDC 0049-1211-83), and 2 g cefoperazone × 10 (NDC 0049-1212-83), and 10 g (NDC 0049-1219-28) Pharmacy Bulk Package for intravenous administration.

CEFOBID® (sterile cefoperazone sodium) is supplied as a frozen, iso-osmotic, pre-mixed solution in a single dose Galaxy® plastic container (PL 2040) as follows:

1 g/50 mL .... NDC 0049–1216–18
2 g/50 mL .... NDC 0049–1215–18

Store container(s) at or below −20°C/−4°F.

See DIRECTIONS FOR USE OF CEFOBID® (cefoperazone sodium injection) IN GALAXY® PLASTIC CONTAINER (PL 2040).

CEFOBID® (cefoperazone sodium injection) in Galaxy® plastic container (PL 2040) is manufactured for Roerig Division of Pfizer Pharmaceuticals by Baxter Healthcare Corporation, Deerfield, IL 60015.

CEFOBID® is a registered trademark of Pfizer Inc. Galaxy® is a registered trademark of Baxter International Inc.

©1996 PFIZER INC
70–4169–00–7   Revised October 1996

CEFOBID®   ℞

[sĕf 'ō-bĭd]
Sterile Cefoperazone Sodium, USP
PHARMACY BULK PACKAGE
NOT FOR DIRECT INFUSION

DESCRIPTION

CEFOBID (cefoperazone sodium) is a sterile, semisynthetic, broad-spectrum, parenteral cephalosporin antibiotic for intravenous or intramuscular administration. It is the sodium salt of 7-[(R)-2-(4-ethyl-2,3-dioxo-1-piperazinecarboxamido)-2-(p -hydroxyphenyl)acetamido-3-[[(1-methyl-H -tetrazol-5-yl)thio]methyl]-8-oxo-5-thia-1-azabicyclo[4.2.0]oct-2-ene-2-carboxylate. Its chemical formula is $C_{25}H_{26}N_9$-NaO_8S_2 with a molecular weight of 667.65. The structural formula is given below:

CEFOBID contains 34 mg sodium (1.5 mEq) per gram. CEFOBID is a white powder which is freely soluble in water. The pH of a 25% (w/v) freshly reconstituted solution varies between 4.5–6.5 and the solution ranges from colorless to straw yellow depending on the concentration.

CEFOBID in crystalline form is supplied in vials equivalent to 1 g or 2 g of cefoperazone and in Piggyback Units for in-

travenous administration equivalent to 1 g or 2 g cefoperazone. CEFOBID is also supplied premixed as a frozen, sterile, nonpyrogenic, iso-osmotic solution equivalent to 1 g or 2 g cefoperazone in plastic containers. After thawing, the solution is intended for intravenous use.
The plastic container is fabricated from specially formulated polyvinyl chloride. Solutions in contact with the plastic container can leach out certain of its chemical components in very small amounts within the expiration period, e.g., di 2-ethylhexyl phthalate (DEHP), up to 5 parts per million. However, the safety of the plastic has been confirmed in tests in animals according to the USP biological tests for plastic containers, as well as by tissue culture toxicity studies.
A pharmacy bulk package is a container of a sterile preparation for parenteral use that contains many single doses. This Pharmacy Bulk Package is for use in a pharmacy admixture service; it provides many single doses of cefoperazone for addition to suitable parenteral fluids in the preparation of admixtures for intravenous infusion. (See DOSAGE AND ADMINISTRATION, and DIRECTIONS FOR PROPER USE OF PHARMACY BULK PACKAGE).

CLINICAL PHARMACOLOGY

High serum and bile levels of CEFOBID are attained after a single dose of the drug. Table 1 demonstrates the serum concentrations of CEFOBID in normal volunteers following either a single 15-minute constant rate intravenous infusion of 1, 2, 3 or 4 grams of the drug, or a single intramuscular injection of 1 or 2 grams of the drug.
[See table 1 below]
The mean serum half-life of CEFOBID is approximately 2.0 hours, independent of the route of administration.
In vitro studies with human serum indicate that the degree of CEFOBID reversible protein binding varies with the serum concentration from 93% at 25 mcg/mL of CEFOBID to 90% at 250 mcg/mL and 82% at 500 mcg/mL.
CEFOBID achieves therapeutic concentrations in the following body tissues and fluids:

Tissue or Fluid	Dose	Concentration
Ascitic Fluid	2 g	64 mcg/mL
Cerebrospinal Fluid (in patients with inflamed meninges)	50 mg/kg	1.8 mcg/mL to 8.0 mcg/mL
Urine	2 g	3,286 mcg/mL
Sputum	3 g	6.0 mcg/mL
Endometrium	2 g	74 mcg/g
Myometrium	2 g	54 mcg/g
Palatine Tonsil	1 g	8 mcg/g
Sinus Mucous Membrane	1 g	8 mcg/g
Umbilical Cord Blood	1 g	25 mcg/mL
Amniotic Fluid	1 g	4.8 mcg/mL
Lung	1 g	28 mcg/g
Bone	2 g	40 mcg/g

CEFOBID is excreted mainly in the bile. Maximum bile concentrations are generally obtained between one and three hours following drug administration and exceed concurrent serum concentrations by up to 100 times. Reported biliary concentrations of CEFOBID range from 66 mcg/mL at 30 minutes to as high as 6000 mcg/mL at 3 hours after an intravenous bolus injection of 2 grams.
Following a single intramuscular or intravenous dose, the urinary recovery of CEFOBID over a 12-hour period averages 20–30%. No significant quantity of metabolites has been found in the urine. Urinary concentrations greater than 2200 mcg/mL have been obtained following a 15-minute infusion of a 2 g dose. After an IM injection of 2 g, peak urine concentrations of almost 1000 mcg/mL have been obtained, and therapeutic levels are maintained for 12 hours.
Repeated administration of CEFOBID at 12-hour intervals does not result in accumulation of the drug in normal subjects. Peak serum concentrations, areas under the curve (AUC's), and serum half-lives in patients with severe renal insufficiency are not significantly different from those in normal volunteers. In patients with hepatic dysfunction, the serum half-life is prolonged and urinary excretion is increased. In patients with combined renal and hepatic insufficiencies, CEFOBID may accumulate in the serum.
CEFOBID has been used in pediatrics, but the safety and effectiveness in children have not been established. The half-life of CEFOBID in serum is 6–10 hours in low birth-weight neonates.

Microbiology
CEFOBID is active *in vitro* against a wide range of aerobic and anaerobic, gram-positive and gram-negative pathogens. The bactericidal action of CEFOBID results from the inhibition of bacterial cell wall synthesis. CEFOBID has a high degree of stability in the presence of beta-lactamases produced by most gram-negative pathogens. CEFOBID is usually active against organisms which are resistant to other beta-lactam antibiotics because of beta-lactamase production. CEFOBID is usually active against the following organisms *in vitro* and in clinical infections:

Gram-Positive Aerobes:
Staphylococcus aureus, penicillinase and non-penicillinase-producing strains.
Staphylococcus epidermidis
Streptococcus pneumoniae (formerly *Diplococcus pneumoniae*)
Streptococcus pyogenes (Group A beta-hemolytic streptococci)
Streptococcus agalactiae (Group B beta-hemolytic streptococci)
Enterococcus (*Streptococcus faecalis, S. faecium* and *S. durans*)

Gram-Negative Aerobes:
Escherichia coli
Klebsiella species (including *K. pneumoniae*)
Enterobacter species
Citrobacter species
Haemophilus influenzae
Proteus mirabilis
Proteus vulgaris
Morganella morganii (formerly *Proteus morganii*)
Providencia stuartii
Providencia rettgeri (formerly *Proteus rettgeri*)
Serratia marcescens
Pseudomonas aeruginosa
Pseudomonas species
Some strains of *Acinetobacter calcoaceticus*
Neisseria gonorrhoeae

Anaerobic Organisms:
Gram-positive cocci (including *Peptococcus* and *Peptostreptococcus*)
Clostridium species
Bacteroides fragilis
Other *Bacteroides* species
CEFOBID is also active *in vitro* against a wide variety of other pathogens although the clinical significance is unknown. These organisms include: *Salmonella* and *Shigella* species, *Serratia liquefaciens, N. meningitidis, Bordetella pertussis, Yersinia enterocolitica, Clostridium difficile, Fusobacterium* species, *Eubacterium* species and beta-lactamase producing strains of *H. influenzae* and *N. gonorrhoeae.*

SUSCEPTIBILITY TESTING

Diffusion Technique. For the disk diffusion method of susceptibility testing, a 75 mcg CEFOBID diffusion disk should be used. Organisms should be tested with the CEFOBID 75 mcg disk since CEFOBID has been shown *in vitro* to be active against organisms which are found to be resistant to other beta-lactam antibiotics.
Tests should be interpreted by the following criteria:

Zone Diameter	Interpretation
Greater than or equal to 21 mm	Susceptible
16–20 mm	Moderately Susceptible
Less than or equal to 15 mm	Resistant

Quantitative procedures that require measurement of zone diameters give the most precise estimate of susceptibility. One such method which has been recommended for use with the CEFOBID 75 mcg disk is the NCCLS approved standard. (Performance Standards for Antimicrobic Disk Susceptibility Tests. Second Information Supplement Vol. 2 No. 2 pp. 49–69. Publisher—National Committee for Clinical Laboratory Standards, Villanova, Pennsylvania.)
A report of "susceptible" indicates that the infecting organism is likely to respond to CEFOBID therapy and a report of "resistant" indicates that the infecting organism is not likely to respond to therapy. A "moderately susceptible" report suggests that the infecting organism will be susceptible to CEFOBID if a higher than usual dosage is used or if the infection is confined to tissues and fluids (e.g., urine or bile) in which high antibiotic levels are attained.
Dilution Techniques. Broth or agar dilution methods may be used to determine the minimal inhibitory concentration (MIC) of CEFOBID. Serial twofold dilutions of CEFOBID should be prepared in either broth or agar. Broth should be inoculated to contain 5×10^5 organisms/mL and agar "spotted" with 10^4 organisms.
MIC test results should be interpreted in light of serum, tissue, and body fluid concentrations of CEFOBID. Organisms inhibited by CEFOBID at 16 mcg/mL or less are considered susceptible, while organisms with MIC's of 17–63 mcg/mL are moderately susceptible. Organisms inhibited at CEFOBID concentrations of greater than or equal to 64 mcg/mL are considered resistant, although clinical cures have been obtained in some patients infected by such organisms.

INDICATIONS AND USAGE

CEFOBID is indicated for the treatment of the following infections when caused by susceptible organisms:
Respiratory Tract Infections caused by *S. pneumoniae, H. influenzae, S. aureus* (penicillinase and non-penicillinase producing strains), *S. pyogenes** (Group A beta-hemolytic streptococci), *P. aeruginosa, Klebsiella pneumoniae, E. coli, Proteus mirabilis,* and *Enterobacter* species.
Peritonitis and Other Intra-abdominal Infections caused by *E. coli, P. aeruginosa,** and anaerobic gram-negative bacilli (including *Bacteroides fragilis*).
Bacterial Septicemia caused by *S. pneumoniae, S. agalactiae,** *S. aureus, Pseudomonas aeruginosa,** *E. coli, Klebsiella* spp.,* *Klebsiella pneumoniae,** *Proteus* species* (indole-positive and indole-negative), *Clostridium* spp.* and anaerobic gram-positive cocci.*
Infections of the Skin and Skin Structures caused by *S. aureus* (penicillinase and non-penicillinase producing strains), *S. pyogenes,** and *P. aeruginosa.*
Pelvic Inflammatory Disease, Endometritis, and Other Infections of the Female Genital Tract caused by *N. gonorrhoeae, S. epidermidis,** *S. agalactiae, E. coli, Clostridium* spp.,* *Bacteroides* species (including *Bacteroides fragilis*) and anaerobic gram-positive cocci.
Cefobid,® like other cephalosporins, has no activity against *Chlamydia trachomatis.* Therefore, when cephalosporins are used in the treatment of patients with pelvic inflammatory disease and *C. trachomatis* is one of the suspected pathogens, appropriate anti-chlamydial coverage should be added.
Urinary Tract Infections caused by *Escherichia coli* and *Pseudomonas aeruginosa.*
Enterococcal Infections: Although cefoperazone has been shown to be clinically effective in the treatment of infections caused by enterococci in cases of **peritonitis and other intra-abdominal infections, infections of the skin and skin structures, pelvic inflammatory disease, endometritis and other infections of the female genital tract, and urinary tract infections,*** the majority of clinical isolates of enterococci tested are not susceptible to cefoperazone but fall just at or in the intermediate zone of susceptibilty, and are moderately resistant to cefoperazone. However, *in vitro* susceptibility testing may not correlate directly with *in vivo* results. Despite this, cefoperazone therapy has resulted in clinical cures of enterococcal infections, chiefly in polymicrobial infections. Cefoperazone should be used in enterococcal infections with care and at doses that achieve satisfactory serum levels of cefoperazone.

*Efficacy of this organism in this organ system was studied in fewer than 10 infections.

Susceptibility Testing
Before instituting treatment with CEFOBID, appropriate specimens should be obtained for isolation of the causative organism and for determination of its susceptibility to the drug. Treatment may be started before results of susceptibility testing are available.
Combination Therapy
Synergy between CEFOBID and aminoglycosides has been demonstrated with many gram-negative bacilli. However, such enhanced activity of these combinations is not predictable. If such therapy is considered, *in vitro* susceptibility tests should be performed to determine the activity of the drugs in combination, and renal function should be monitored carefully. (See PRECAUTIONS, and DOSAGE AND ADMINISTRATION sections).

CONTRAINDICATIONS

CEFOBID is contraindicated in patients with known allergy to the cephalosporin-class of antibiotics.

TABLE 1. Cefoperazone Serum Concentrations

	Mean Serum Concentrations (mcg/mL)						
Dose/Route	0*	0.5 hr	1 hr	2 hr	4 hr	8 hr	12 hr
1 g IV	153	114	73	38	16	4	0.5
2 g IV	252	153	114	70	32	8	2
3 g IV	340	210	142	89	41	9	2
4 g IV	506	325	251	161	71	19	6
1 g IM	32**	52	65	57	33	7	1
2 g IM	40**	69	93	97	58	14	4

* Hours post-administration, with 0 time being the end of the infusion.
** Values obtained 15 minutes post-injection.

Continued on next page

Cefobid Pharmacy Bulk—Cont.

WARNINGS

BEFORE THERAPY WITH CEFOBID IS INSTITUTED, CAREFUL INQUIRY SHOULD BE MADE TO DETERMINE WHETHER THE PATIENT HAS HAD PREVIOUS HYPERSENSITIVITY REACTIONS TO CEPHALOSPORINS, PENICILLINS OR OTHER DRUGS. THIS PRODUCT SHOULD BE GIVEN CAUTIOUSLY TO PENICILLIN-SENSITIVE PATIENTS. ANTIBIOTICS SHOULD BE ADMINISTERED WITH CAUTION TO ANY PATIENT WHO HAS DEMONSTRATED SOME FORM OF ALLERGY, PARTICULARLY TO DRUGS. SERIOUS ACUTE HYPERSENSITIVITY REACTIONS MAY REQUIRE THE USE OF SUBCUTANEOUS EPINEPHRINE AND OTHER EMERGENCY MEASURES.

PSEUDOMEMBRANOUS COLITIS HAS BEEN REPORTED WITH THE USE OF CEPHALOSPORINS (AND OTHER BROAD-SPECTRUM ANTIBIOTICS); THEREFORE, IT IS IMPORTANT TO CONSIDER ITS DIAGNOSIS IN PATIENTS WHO DEVELOP DIARRHEA IN ASSOCIATION WITH ANTIBIOTIC USE.

Treatment with broad-spectrum antibiotics alters normal flora of the colon and may permit overgrowth of clostridia. Studies indicate a toxin produced by *Clostridium difficile* is one primary cause of antibiotic-associated colitis. Cholestyramine and colestipol resins have been shown to bind the toxin *in vitro*.

Mild cases of colitis may respond to drug discontinuance alone.

Moderate to severe cases should be managed with fluid, electrolyte, and protein supplementation as indicated.

When the colitis is not relieved by drug discontinuance or when it is severe, oral vancomycin is the treatment of choice for antibiotic-associated pseudomembranous colitis produced by *C. difficile*. Other causes of colitis should also be considered.

PRECAUTIONS

Although transient elevations of the BUN and serum creatinine have been observed, CEFOBID alone does not appear to cause significant nephrotoxicity. However, concomitant administration of aminoglycosides and other cephalosporins has caused nephrotoxicity.

CEFOBID is extensively excreted in bile. The serum half-life of CEFOBID is increased 2–4 fold in patients with hepatic disease and/or biliary obstruction. In general, total daily dosage above 4 g should not be necessary in such patients. If higher dosages are used, serum concentrations should be monitored.

Because renal excretion is not the main route of elimination of CEFOBID (see CLINICAL PHARMACOLOGY), patients with renal failure require no adjustment in dosage when usual doses are administered. When high doses of CEFOBID are used, concentrations of drug in the serum should be monitored periodically. If evidence of accumulation exists, dosage should be decreased accordingly.

The half-life of CEFOBID is reduced slightly during hemodialysis. Thus, dosing should be scheduled to follow a dialysis period. In patients with both hepatic dysfunction and significant renal disease, CEFOBID dosage should not exceed 1–2 g daily without close monitoring of serum concentrations.

As with other antibiotics, vitamin K deficiency has occurred rarely in patients treated with CEFOBID. The mechanism is most probably related to the suppression of gut flora which normally synthesize this vitamin. Those at risk include patients with a poor nutritional status, malabsorption states (e.g., cystic fibrosis), alcoholism, and patients on prolonged hyper-alimentation regimens (administered either intravenously or via a naso-gastric tube). Prothrombin time should be monitored in these patients and exogenous vitamin K administered as indicated.

A disulfiram-like reaction characterized by flushing, sweating, headache, and tachycardia has been reported when alcohol (beer, wine) was ingested within 72 hours after CEFOBID administration. Patients should be cautioned about the ingestion of alcoholic beverages following the administration of CEFOBID. A similar reaction has been reported with other cephalosporins.

Prolonged use of CEFOBID may result in the overgrowth of nonsusceptible organisms. Careful observation of the patient is essential. If superinfection occurs during therapy, appropriate measures should be taken.

CEFOBID should be prescribed with caution in individuals with a history of gastrointestinal disease, particularly colitis.

Drug Laboratory Test Interactions

A false-positive reaction for glucose in the urine may occur with Benedict's or Fehling's solution.

Carcinogenesis, Mutagenesis, Impairment of Fertility

Long-term studies in animals have not been performed to evaluate carcinogenic potential. The maximum duration of CEFOBID animal toxicity studies is six months. In none of the *in vivo* or *in vitro* genetic toxicology studies did CEFOBID show any mutagenic potential at either the chromosomal or subchromosomal level. CEFOBID produced no impairment of fertility and had no effects on general reproductive performance or fetal development when administered subcutaneously at daily doses up to 500 to 1000 mg/kg prior to and during mating, and to pregnant female rats during gestation. These doses are 10 to 20 times the estimated usual single clinical dose. CEFOBID had adverse effects on the testes of prepubertal rats at all doses tested. Subcutaneous administration of 1000 mg/kg per day (approximately 16 times the average adult human dose) resulted in reduced testicular weight, arrested spermatogenesis, reduced germinal cell population and vacuolation of Sertoli cell cytoplasm. The severity of lesions was dose dependent in the 100 to 1000 mg/kg per day range; the low dose caused a minor decrease in spermatocytes. This effect has not been observed in adult rats. Histologically the lesions were reversible at all but the highest dosage levels. However, these studies did not evaluate subsequent development of reproductive function in the rats. The relationship of these findings to humans is unknown.

Usage in Pregnancy

Pregnancy Category B: Reproduction studies have been performed in mice, rats, and monkeys at doses up to 10 times the human dose and have revealed no evidence of impaired fertility or harm to the fetus due to CEFOBID. There are, however, no adequate and well controlled studies in pregnant women. Because animal reproduction studies are not always predictive of human response, this drug should be used during pregnancy only if clearly needed.

Usage in Nursing Mothers

Only low concentrations of CEFOBID are excreted in human milk. Although CEFOBID passes poorly into breast milk of nursing mothers, caution should be exercised when CEFOBID is administered to a nursing woman.

Pediatric Use

Safety and effectiveness in children have not been established. For information concerning testicular changes in prepubertal rats, see Carcinogenesis, Mutagenesis, Impairment of Fertility.

ADVERSE REACTIONS

In clinical studies the following adverse effects were observed and were considered to be related to CEFOBID therapy or of uncertain etiology:

Hypersensitivity: As with all cephalosporins, hypersensitivity manifested by skin reactions (1 patient in 45), drug fever (1 in 260), or a change in Coombs' test (1 in 60) has been reported. These reactions are more likely to occur in patients with a history of allergies, particularly to penicillin.

Hematology: As with other beta-lactam antibiotics, reversible neutropenia may occur with prolonged administration. Slight decreases in neutrophil count (1 patient in 50) have been reported. Decreased hemoglobins (1 in 20) or hematocrits (1 in 20) have been reported, which is consistent with published literature on other cephalosporins. Transient eosinophilia has occurred in 1 patient in 10.

Hepatic: Of 1285 patients treated with cefoperazone in clinical trials, one patient with a history of liver disease developed significantly elevated liver function enzymes during CEFOBID therapy. Clinical signs and symptoms of nonspecific hepatitis accompanied these increases. After CEFOBID therapy was discontinued, the patient's enzymes returned to pre-treatment levels and the symptomatology resolved. As with other antibiotics that achieve high bile levels, mild transient elevations of liver function enzymes have been observed in 5–10% of the patients receiving CEFOBID therapy. The relevance of these findings, which were not accompanied by overt signs or symptoms of hepatic dysfunction, has not been established.

Gastrointestinal: Diarrhea or loose stools has been reported in 1 in 30 patients. Most of these experiences have been mild or moderate in severity and self-limiting in nature. In all cases, these symptoms responded to symptomatic therapy or ceased when cefoperazone therapy was stopped. Nausea and vomiting have been reported rarely. Symptoms of pseudomembranous colitis can appear during or for several weeks subsequent to antibiotic therapy (see WARNINGS).

Renal Function Tests: Transient elevations of the BUN (1 in 16) and serum creatinine (1 in 48) have been noted.

Local Reactions: CEFOBID is well tolerated following intramuscular administration. Occasionally, transient pain (1 in 140) may follow administration by this route. When CEFOBID is administered by intravenous infusion some patients may develop phlebitis (1 in 120) at the infusion site.

DOSAGE AND ADMINISTRATION

Sterile cefoperazone sodium can be administered by IM or IV injection (following dilution). However, the intent of this pharmacy bulk package is for the preparation of solutions for IV infusion only.

The usual adult daily dose of CEFOBID is 2 to 4 grams per day administered in equally divided doses every 12 hours. In severe infections or infections caused by less sensitive organisms, the total daily dose and/or frequency may be increased. Patients have been successfully treated with a total daily dosage of 6–12 grams divided into 2, 3 or 4 administrations ranging from 1.5 to 4 grams per dose.

When treating infections caused by *Streptococcus pyogenes*, therapy should be continued for at least 10 days.

If *C. trachomatis* is a suspected pathogen, appropriate anti-chlamydial coverage should be added, because cefoperazone has no activity against this organism.

Solutions of CEFOBID and aminoglycoside should not be directly mixed, since there is a physical incompatibility between them. If combination therapy with CEFOBID and an

Controlled Room Temperature (15°–25°C/59°–77°F) **24 Hours**	**Approximate Concentrations**
Bacteriostatic Water for Injection [Benzyl Alcohol or Parabens] (USP)	300 mg/mL
5% Dextrose Injection (USP)	2 mg to 50 mg/mL
5% Dextrose and Lactated Ringer's Injection	2 mg to 50 mg/mL
5% Dextrose and 0.9% Sodium Chloride Injection (USP)	2 mg to 50 mg/mL
5% Dextrose and 0.2% Sodium Chloride Injection (USP)	2 mg to 50 mg/mL
10% Dextrose Injection (USP)	2 mg to 50 mg/mL
Lactated Ringer's Injection (USP)	2 mg/mL
0.5% Lidocaine Hydrochloride Injection (USP)	300 mg/mL
0.9% Sodium Chloride Injection (USP)	2 mg to 300 mg/mL
Normosol® M and 5% Dextrose Injection	2 mg to 50 mg/mL
Normosol® R	2 mg to 50 mg/mL
Sterile Water for Injection	100 mg to 300 mg/mL

Reconstituted CEFOBID solutions may be stored in glass or plastic syringes, or in glass or flexible plastic parenteral solution containers.

Refrigerator Temperature (2°–8°C/36°–46°F) **5 Days**	**Approximate Concentrations**
Bacteriostatic Water for Injection [Benzyl Alcohol or Parabens] (USP)	300 mg/mL
5% Dextrose Injection (USP)	2 mg to 50 mg/mL
5% Dextrose and 0.9% Sodium Chloride Injection (USP)	2 mg to 50 mg/mL
5% Dextrose and 0.2% Sodium Chloride Injection (USP)	2 mg to 50 mg/mL
Lactated Ringer's Injection (USP)	2 mg/mL
0.5% Lidocaine Hydrochloride Injection (USP)	300 mg/mL
0.9% Sodium Chloride Injection (USP)	2 mg to 300 mg/mL
Normosol® M and 5% Dextrose Injection	2 mg to 50 mg/mL
Normosol® R	2 mg to 50 mg/mL
Sterile Water for Injection	100 mg to 300 mg/mL

Reconstituted CEFOBID solutions may be stored in glass or plastic syringes, or in glass or flexible plastic parenteral solution containers.

Freezer Temperature (−20° to −10°C/−4° to 14°F)	**Approximate Concentrations**
3 Weeks	
5% Dextrose Injection (USP)	50 mg/mL
5% Dextrose and 0.9% Sodium Chloride Injection (USP)	2 mg/mL
5% Dextrose and 0.2% Sodium Chloride Injection (USP)	2 mg/mL
5 Weeks	
0.9% Sodium Chloride Injection (USP)	300 mg/mL
Sterile Water for Injection	300 mg/mL

Reconstituted CEFOBID solutions may be stored in plastic syringes, or in flexible plastic parenteral solution containers.

Frozen samples should be thawed at room temperature before use. After thawing, unused portions should be discarded. Do not refreeze.

aminoglycoside is contemplated (see INDICATIONS) this can be accomplished by sequential intermittent intravenous infusion provided that separate secondary intravenous tubing is used, and that the primary intravenous tubing is adequately irrigated with an approved diluent between doses. It is also suggested that CEFOBID be administered prior to the aminoglycoside. *In vitro* testing of the effectiveness of drug combination(s) is recommended.

In a pharmacokinetic study, a total daily dose of 16 grams was administered to severely immunocompromised patients by constant infusion without complications. Steady state serum concentrations were approximately 150 mcg/mL in these patients.

RECONSTITUTION

The following solutions may be used for the initial reconstitution of CEFOBID sterile powder:

Table 1. Solutions for Initial Reconstitution

- 5% Dextrose Injection (USP)
- 5% Dextrose and 0.9% Sodium Chloride Injection (USP)
- 5% Dextrose and 0.2% Sodium Chloride Injection (USP)
- 10% Dextrose Injection (USP)
- Bacteriostatic Water for Injection [Benzyl Alcohol or Parabens] (USP)*†
- 0.9% Sodium Chloride Injection (USP)
- Normosol® M and 5% Dextrose Injection
- Normosol® R
- Sterile Water for Injection*

* Not to be used as a vehicle for intravenous infusion.

† Preparations containing Benzyl Alcohol should not be used in neonates.

General Reconstitution Procedures

CEFOBID sterile powder for intravenous or intramuscular use may be initially reconstituted with any compatible solution mentioned above in Table 1. Solutions should be allowed to stand after reconstitution to allow any foaming to dissipate to permit visual inspection for complete solubilization. Vigorous and prolonged agitation may be necessary to solubilize CEFOBID in higher concentrations (above 333 mg cefoperazone/mL). The maximum solubility of CEFOBID sterile powder is approximately 475 mg cefoperazone/mL of compatible diluent.

Preparation For Intravenous Use

General. CEFOBID concentrations between 2 mg/mL and 50 mg/mL are recommended for intravenous administration.

Table 2. Vehicles for Intravenous Infusion

- 5% Dextrose Injection (USP)
- 5% Dextrose and Lactated Ringer's Injection
- 5% Dextrose and 0.9% Sodium Chloride Injection (USP)
- 5% Dextrose and 0.2% Sodium Chloride Injection(USP)
- 10% Dextrose Injection (USP)
- Lactated Ringer's Injection (USP)
- 0.9% Sodium Chloride Injection (USP)
- Normosol® M and 5% Dextrose Injection
- Normosol® R

DIRECTIONS FOR PROPER USE OF PHARMACY BULK PACKAGE

The 10 gram vial should be reconstituted with 95 mL of sterile water for injection in two separate aliquots in a suitable work area such as a laminar flow hood. Add 45 mL of solution, shake to dissolve and add 50 mL, shake for final solution. The resulting solution will contain 100 mg/mL of cefoperazone. This closure may be penetrated only one time after reconstitution, if needed, using a suitable sterile transfer device or dispensing set which allows measured dispensing of the contents.

Discard unused solution within 24 hours of initial entry.

Reconstituted Bulk Solutions Should Not Be Used For Direct Infusion.

Although after reconstitution of the Pharmacy Bulk Package, no significant loss of potency occurs for 24 hours at room temperature and for 5 days if refrigerated, transfer individual dose to appropriate intravenous infusion solutions as soon as possible following reconstitution of the bulk package. Discard unused portions of solution held longer than these recommended periods at room temperature or under refrigeration. The stability of the solution which has been transferred into a container varies according to diluent and concentration. (See STORAGE AND STABILITY.)

The 10 gram vials may be further diluted with the parenteral diluents listed under **Table 2. Vehicles for Intravenous Infusion.** The parenteral diluents and approximate concentrations of CEFOBID that provide stable solutions are presented under STORAGE AND STABILITY.

Parenteral drug products should be inspected visually for particulate matter and discoloration prior to administration, whenever solution and container permit.

DIRECTIONS FOR USE OF CEFOBID (cefoperazone sodium) INJECTION IN PLASTIC CONTAINERS

CEFOBID supplied premixed as a frozen, sterile, iso-osmotic solution in plastic containers is to be administered either as continuous or intermittent infusion.

Thaw container at room temperature. After thawing, check for minute leaks by squeezing bag firmly. If leaks are found, discard solution as sterility may be impaired. Additives should not be introduced into this solution. Do not use if the solution is cloudy or precipitated or if the seal is not intact. After thawing, the solution is stable for 10 days if stored under refrigeration (5°C) and for 48 hours at room temperature. DO NOT REFREEZE. Use sterile equipment.

CAUTION: Do not use plastic container in series connections. Such use could result in air embolism due to residual air being drawn from the primary container before administration of the fluid from the secondary container is complete.

Preparation for Administration

1. Suspend container from eyelet support.
2. Remove plastic protector from outlet port at bottom of container.
3. Attach administration set. Refer to complete directions accompanying set.

STORAGE AND STABILITY

CEFOBID sterile powder is to be stored at or below 25°C (77°F) and protected from light prior to reconstitution. After reconstitution, protection from light is not necessary.

The following parenteral diluents and approximate concentrations of CEFOBID provide stable solutions under the following conditions for the indicated time periods. (After the indicated time periods, unused portions of solutions should be discarded.)

[See table at bottom of previous page]

HOW SUPPLIED

CEFOBID sterile powder is available in Pharmacy Bulk Package containing cefoperazone sodium equivalent to 10 g cefoperazone × 1 (NDC 0049-1219-28).

OTHER SIZE PACKAGES AVAILABLE

CEFOBID sterile powder is available in vials containing cefoperazone sodium equivalent to 1 g cefoperazone × 10 (NDC 0049-1201-83) and 2 g cefoperazone × 10 (NDC 0049-1202-83) for intramuscular and intravenous administration.

CEFOBID sterile powder is available in Piggyback Units containing cefoperazone sodium equivalent to 1 g cefoperazone × 10 (NDC 0049-1211-83), and 2 g cefoperazone × 10 (NDC 0049-1212-83).

CEFOBID (cefoperazone sodium) injection is supplied premixed as a frozen, sterile, nonpyrogenic, iso-osmotic solution in plastic containers. Each 50 mL unit contains cefoperazone sodium equivalent to 1 g cefoperazone with approximately 2.3 g dextrose hydrous USP added (NDC 0049-1216-18) or 2 g cefoperazone with approximately 1.8 g dextrose hydrous USP added (NDC 0049-1215-18). The solution is iso-osmotic (approximately 300 mOsmol/L), and solution pH may have been adjusted with sodium hydroxide and/or hydrochloric acid. Do not store above −20°C.

CEFOBID supplied as a frozen, sterile, nonpyrogenic, iso-osmotic solution in 50 ml plastic containers is manufactured for Roerig Division of Pfizer Pharmaceuticals by Baxter Healthcare Corporation, Deerfield, IL 60015.

70-4482-00-5 Revised April 1995

DIABINESE® ℞

[*dī-ab 'in-ees*]

(chlorpropamide)
Tablets, USP
For Oral Use

DESCRIPTION

DIABINESE® (chlorpropamide), is an oral blood-glucoselowering drug of the sulfonylurea class. Chlorpropamide is 1-[(p-Chlorophenyl) sulfonyl]-3-propylurea, $C_{10}H_{13}ClN_2O_3S$, and has the structural formula:

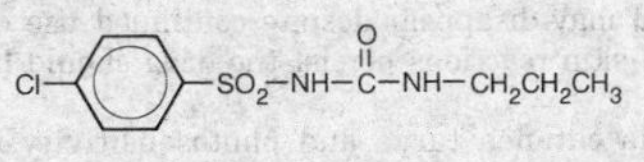
Cl
SO2–NH–C–NH–CH2CH2CH3
O

Chlorpropamide is a white crystalline powder, that has a slight odor. It is practically insoluble in water at pH 7.3 (solubility at pH 6 is 2.2 mg/ml). It is soluble in alcohol and moderately soluble in chloroform. The molecular weight of chlorpropamide is 276.74. DIABINESE is available as 100 mg and 250 mg tablets.

Inert ingredients are: alginic acid; Blue 1 Lake; hydroxypropyl cellulose; magnesium stearate; precipitated calcium carbonate; sodium lauryl sulfate; starch.

CLINICAL PHARMACOLOGY

DIABINESE appears to lower the blood glucose acutely by stimulating the release of insulin from the pancreas, an effect dependent upon functioning beta cells in the pancreatic islets. The mechanism by which DIABINESE lowers blood glucose during long-term administration has not been clearly established. Extra-pancreatic effects may play a part in the mechanism of action of oral sulfonylurea hypoglycemic drugs. While chlorpropamide is a sulfonamide derivative, it is devoid of antibacterial activity.

DIABINESE may also prove effective in controlling certain patients who have experienced primary or secondary failure to other sulfonylurea agents.

A method developed which permits easy measurement of the drug in blood is available on request.

Chlorpropamide does not interfere with the usual tests to detect albumin in the urine.

DIABINESE is absorbed rapidly from the gastrointestinal tract. Within one hour after a single oral dose, it is readily detectable in the blood, and the level reaches a maximum within two to four hours. It undergoes metabolism in humans and it is excreted in the urine as unchanged drug and as hydroxylated or hydrolyzed metabolites. The biological half-life of chlorpropamide averages about 36 hours. Within 96 hours, 80–90% of a single oral dose is excreted in the urine. However, long-term administration of therapeutic doses does not result in undue accumulation in the blood, since absorption and excretion rates become stabilized in about 5 to 7 days after the initiation of therapy.

DIABINESE exerts a hypoglycemic effect in normal humans within one hour, becoming maximal at 3 to 6 hours and persisting for at least 24 hours. The potency of chlorpropamide is approximately six times that of tolbutamide. Some experimental results suggest that its increased duration of action may be the result of slower excretion and absence of significant deactivation.

INDICATIONS AND USAGE

DIABINESE is indicated as an adjunct to diet to lower the blood glucose in patients with non-insulin-dependent diabetes mellitus (type II) whose hyperglycemia cannot be controlled by diet alone.

In initiating treatment for non-insulin-dependent diabetes, diet should be emphasized as the primary form of treatment. Caloric restriction and weight loss are essential in the obese diabetic patient. Proper dietary management alone may be effective in controlling the blood glucose and symptoms of hyperglycemia. The importance of regular physical activity should also be stressed, and cardiovascular risk factors should be identified and corrective measures taken where possible.

If this treatment program fails to reduce symptoms and/or blood glucose, the use of an oral sulfonylurea or insulin should be considered. Use of DIABINESE must be viewed by both the physician and patient as a treatment in addition to diet, and not as a substitute for diet or as a convenient mechanism for avoiding dietary restraint. Furthermore, loss of blood glucose control on diet alone may be transient, thus requiring only short-term administration of DIABINESE.

During maintenance programs, DIABINESE should be discontinued if satisfactory lowering of blood glucose is no longer achieved. Judgments should be based on regular clinical and laboratory evaluations.

In considering the use of DIABINESE in asymptomatic patients, it should be recognized that controlling the blood glucose in non-insulin-dependent diabetes, has not been definitely established to be effective in preventing the long-term cardiovascular or neural complications of diabetes.

CONTRAINDICATIONS

DIABINESE is contraindicated in patients with:

1. Known hypersensitivity to the drug.
2. Diabetic ketoacidosis, with or without coma. This condition should be treated with insulin.

WARNINGS

SPECIAL WARNING ON INCREASED RISK OF CARDIOVASCULAR MORTALITY

The administration of oral hypoglycemic drugs has been reported to be associated with increased cardiovascular mortality as compared to treatment with diet alone or diet plus insulin. This warning is based on the study conducted by the University Group Diabetes Program (UGDP), a long-term prospective clinical trial designed to evaluate the effectiveness of glucose-lowering drugs in preventing or delaying vascular complications in patients with non-insulin-dependent diabetes. The study involved 823 patients who were randomly assigned to one of four treatment groups (*Diabetes,* 19 (supp. 2): 747–830, 1970.)

UGDP reported that patients treated for 5 to 8 years with diet plus a fixed dose of tolbutamide (1.5 grams per day) had a rate of cardiovascular mortality approximately $2^1/_2$ times that of patients treated with diet alone. A significant increase in total mortality was not observed, but the use of tolbutamide was discontinued based on the increase in cardiovascular mortality, thus limiting the opportunity for the study to show an increase in over-all mortality. Despite controversy regarding the interpretation of these results, the findings of the UGDP study provide an adequate basis for this warning. The patient should be informed of the potential risks and advantages of DIABINESE and of alternative modes of therapy.

Although only one drug in the sulfonylurea class (tolbutamide) was included in this study, it is prudent from a safety

Continued on next page

Diabinese—Cont.

standpoint to consider that this warning may also apply to other oral hypoglycemic drugs in this class, in view of their close similarities in mode of action and chemical structure.

PRECAUTIONS

General

Hypoglycemia: All sulfonylurea drugs are capable of producing severe hypoglycemia. Proper patient selection, dosage, and instructions are important to avoid hypoglycemic episodes. Renal or hepatic insufficiency may cause elevated blood levels of DIABINESE and the latter may also diminish gluconeogenic capacity, both of which increase the risk of serious hypoglycemic reactions. Elderly, debilitated or malnourished patients, and those with adrenal or pituitary insufficiency are particularly susceptible to the hypoglycemic action of glucose-lowering drugs. Hypoglycemia may be difficult to recognize in the elderly, and in people who are taking beta-adrenergic blocking drugs. Hypoglycemia is more likely to occur when caloric intake is deficient, after severe or prolonged exercise, when alcohol is ingested, or when more than one glucose-lowering drug is used.

Because of the long half-life of chlorpropamide, patients who become hypoglycemic during therapy require careful supervision of the dose and frequent feedings for at least 3 to 5 days. Hospitalization and intravenous glucose may be necessary.

Loss of control of blood glucose: When a patient stabilized on any diabetic regimen is exposed to stress such as fever, trauma, infection, or surgery, a loss of control may occur. At such times, it may be necessary to discontinue DIABINESE and administer insulin.

The effectiveness of any oral hypoglycemic drug, including DIABINESE, in lowering blood glucose to a desired level decreases in many patients over a period of time, which may be due to progression of the severity of the diabetes or to diminished responsiveness to the drug. This phenomenon is known as secondary failure, to distinguish it from primary failure in which the drug is ineffective in an individual patient when first given.

INFORMATION FOR PATIENTS

Patients should be informed of the potential risks and advantages of DIABINESE and of alternative modes of therapy. They should also be informed about the importance of adherence to dietary instructions, of a regular exercise program, and of regular testing of urine and/or blood glucose.

The risks of hypoglycemia, its symptoms and treatment, and conditions that predispose to its development should be explained to patients and responsible family members. Primary and secondary failure should also be explained.

Patients should be instructed to contact their physician promptly if they experience symptoms of hypoglycemia or other adverse reactions.

LABORATORY TESTS

Blood and urine glucose should be monitored periodically. Measurement of glycosylated hemoglobin may be useful.

DRUG INTERACTIONS

The hypoglycemic action of sulfonylurea may be potentiated by certain drugs including nonsteroidal anti-inflammatory agents and other drugs that are highly protein bound, salicylates, sulfonamides, chloramphenicol, probenecid, coumarins, monoamine oxidase inhibitors, and beta adrenergic blocking agents. When such drugs are administered to a patient receiving DIABINESE, the patient should be observed closely for hypoglycemia. When such drugs are withdrawn from a patient receiving DIABINESE, the patient should be observed closely for loss of control.

Certain drugs tend to produce hyperglycemia and may lead to loss of control. These drugs include the thiazides and other diuretics, corticosteroids, phenothiazines, thyroid products, estrogens, oral contraceptives, phenytoin, nicotinic acid, sympathomimetics, calcium channel blocking drugs, and isoniazid. When such drugs are administered to a patient receiving DIABINESE, the patient should be closely observed for loss of control. When such drugs are withdrawn from a patient receiving DIABINESE, the patient should be observed closely for hypoglycemia.

Since animal studies suggest that the action of barbiturates may be prolonged by therapy with chlorpropamide, barbiturates should be employed with caution. In some patients, a disulfiram-like reaction may be produced by the ingestion of alcohol.

A potential interaction between oral miconazole and oral hypoglycemic agents leading to severe hypoglycemia has been reported. Whether this interaction also occurs with the intravenous, topical, or vaginal preparations of miconazole is not known.

Carcinogenesis, Mutagenesis, Impairment of Fertility: Chronic toxicity studies have been carried out in dogs and rats. Dogs treated for 6, 13, or 20 months with doses of DIABINESE greater than 20 times the human dose, have not shown any gross histological or pathological abnormalities.

Strength	Tablet Description	Tablet Code	NDC	Package Size
DIABINESE (chlorpropamide) 100 mg	Blue, D-shaped, scored	393	0663-3930-66 0069-3930-66	100's
			0663-3930-73 0069-3930-73	500's
			0663-3930-41 0069-3930-41	100 (10 × 10) unit dose
DIABINESE (chlorpropamide) 250 mg	Blue, D-shaped, scored	394	0663-3940-66 0069-3940-66	100's
			0663-3940-71 0069-3940-71	250's
			0663-3940-82 0069-3940-82	1000's
			0663-3940-41 0069-3940-41	100 (10 × 10) unit dose

After treatment with 100 mg/kg of DIABINESE for 20 months, a dog showed no histopathological liver changes. Rats treated with continuous DIABINESE therapy for 6 to 12 months showed varying degrees of suppression of spermatogenesis at higher dosage levels (up to 125 mg/kg). The extent of suppression seemed to follow that of growth retardation associated with chronic administration of high-dose DIABINESE in rats.

Pregnancy

Teratogenic Effects:

Pregnancy Category C. Animal reproductive studies have not been conducted with DIABINESE. It is also not known whether DIABINESE can cause fetal harm when administered to a pregnant woman or can affect reproduction capacity. DIABINESE should be given to a pregnant woman only if clearly needed.

Because recent information suggests that abnormal blood glucose levels during pregnancy are associated with a higher incidence of congenital abnormalities, many experts recommend that insulin be used during pregnancy to maintain blood glucose levels as close to normal as possible.

Nonteratogenic Effects:

Prolonged severe hypoglycemia (4 to 10 days) has been reported in neonates born to mothers who were receiving a sulfonylurea drug at the time of delivery. This has been reported more frequently with the use of agents with prolonged half-lives. If DIABINESE is used during pregnancy, it should be discontinued at least one month before the expected delivery date.

Nursing Mothers: An analysis of a composite of two samples of human breast milk, each taken five hours after ingestion of 500 mg of chlorpropamide by a patient, revealed a concentration of 5 mcg/ml. For reference, the normal peak blood level of chlorpropamide after a single 250 mg dose is 30 mcg/ml. Therefore, it is not recommended that a woman breast feed while taking this medication.

Use in Children: Safety and effectiveness in children have not been established.

ADVERSE REACTIONS

Hypoglycemia: See PRECAUTIONS and OVERDOSAGE sections.

Gastrointestinal Reactions: Cholestatic jaundice may occur rarely; DIABINESE should be discontinued if this occurs. Gastrointestinal disturbances are the most common reactions; nausea has been reported in less than 5% of patients, and diarrhea, vomiting, anorexia, and hunger in less than 2%. Other gastrointestinal disturbances have occurred in less than 1% of patients including proctocolitis. They tend to be dose related and may disappear when dosage is reduced.

Dermatologic Reactions: Pruritus has been reported in less than 3% of patients. Other allergic skin reactions, e.g., urticaria and maculopapular eruptions have been reported in approximately 1% or less of patients. These may be transient and may disappear despite continued use of DIABINESE; if skin reactions persist the drug should be discontinued.

Porphyria cutanea tarda and photosensitivity reactions have been reported with sulfonylureas.

Skin eruptions rarely progressing to erythema multiforme and exfoliative dermatitis have also been reported.

Hematologic Reactions: Leukopenia, agranulocytosis, thrombocytopenia, hemolytic anemia, aplastic anemia, pancytopenia, and eosinophilia have been reported with sulfonylureas.

Metabolic Reactions: Hepatic porphyria and disulfiram-like reactions have been reported with DIABINESE. See DRUG INTERACTIONS section.

Endocrine Reactions: On rare occasions, chlorpropamide has caused a reaction identical to the syndrome of inappropriate antidiuretic hormone (ADH) secretion. The features of this syndrome result from excessive water retention and include hyponatremia, low serum osmolality, and high urine osmolality. This reaction has also been reported for other sulfonylureas.

OVERDOSAGE

Overdosage of sulfonylureas including DIABINESE can produce hypoglycemia. Mild hypoglycemic symptoms without loss of consciousness or neurologic findings should be treated aggressively with oral glucose and adjustments in drug dosage and/or meal patterns. Close monitoring should continue until the physician is assured that the patient is out of danger. Severe hypoglycemic reactions with coma, seizure, or other neurological impairment occur infrequently, but constitute medical emergencies requiring immediate hospitalization. If hypoglycemic coma is diagnosed or suspected, the patient should be given a rapid intravenous injection of concentrated (50%) glucose solution. This should be followed by a continuous infusion of a more dilute (10%) glucose solution at a rate that will maintain the blood glucose at a level above 100 mg/dL. Patients should be closely monitored for a minimum of 24 to 48 hours since hypoglycemia may recur after apparent clinical recovery.

DOSAGE AND ADMINISTRATION

There is no fixed dosage regimen for the management of diabetes mellitus with DIABINESE or any other hypoglycemic agent. In addition to the usual monitoring of urinary glucose, the patient's blood glucose must also be monitored periodically to determine the minimum effective dose for the patient; to detect primary failure, i.e., inadequate lowering of blood glucose at the maximum recommended dose of medication; and to detect secondary failure, i.e., loss of an adequate blood glucose lowering response after an initial period of effectiveness. Glycosylated hemoglobin levels may also be of value in monitoring the patient's response to therapy.

Short-term administration of DIABINESE may be sufficient during periods of transient loss of control in patients usually controlled well on diet.

The total daily dosage is generally taken at a single time each morning with breakfast. Occasionally cases of gastrointestinal intolerance may be relieved by dividing the daily dosage. A LOADING OR PRIMING DOSE IS NOT NECESSARY AND SHOULD NOT BE USED.

Initial Therapy: 1. The mild to moderately severe, middle-aged, stable, non-insulin-dependent diabetic patient should be started on 250 mg daily. In elderly patients, debilitated or malnourished patients, and patients with impaired renal or hepatic function, the initial and maintenance dosing should be conservative to avoid hypoglycemic reactions (see PRECAUTIONS section). Older patients should be started on smaller amounts of DIABINESE, in the range of 100 to 125 mg daily.

2. No transition period is necessary when transferring patients from other oral hypoglycemic agents to DIABINESE. The other agent may be discontinued abruptly and chlorpropamide started at once. In prescribing chlorpropamide, due consideration must be given to its greater potency.

Many mild to moderately severe, middle-aged, stable non-insulin-dependent diabetic patients receiving insulin can be placed directly on the oral drug and their insulin abruptly discontinued. For patients requiring more than 40 units of insulin daily, therapy with DIABINESE may be initiated with a 50 per cent reduction in insulin for the first few days, with subsequent further reductions dependent upon the response.

During the initial period of therapy with chlorpropamide, hypoglycemic reactions may occasionally occur, particularly during the transition from insulin to the oral drug. Hypoglycemia within 24 hours after withdrawal of the intermediate or long-acting types of insulin will usually prove to be the result of insulin carry-over and not primarily due to the effect of chlorpropamide.

During the insulin withdrawal period, the patient should test his urine for sugar and ketone bodies at least three times daily and report the results frequently to his physician. If they are abnormal, the physician should be notified immediately. In some cases, it may be advisable to consider hospitalization during the transition period.

Five to seven days after the initial therapy, the blood level of chlorpropamide reaches a plateau. Dosage may subse-

quently be adjusted upward or downward by increments of not more than 50 to 125 mg at intervals of three to five days to obtain optimal control. More frequent adjustments are usually undesirable.

Maintenance Therapy: Most moderately severe, middle-aged, stable non-insulin-dependent diabetic patients are controlled by approximately 250 mg daily. Many investigators have found that some milder diabetics do well on daily doses of 100 mg or less. Many of the more severe diabetics may require 500 mg daily for adequate control. PATIENTS WHO DO NOT RESPOND COMPLETELY TO 500 MG DAILY WILL USUALLY NOT RESPOND TO HIGHER DOSES. MAINTENANCE DOSES ABOVE 750 mg DAILY SHOULD BE AVOIDED.

HOW SUPPLIED

[See table at top of previous page]

RECOMMENDED STORAGE

Store below 86°F (30°C).

CAUTION

Federal law prohibits dispensing without prescription.

69-2141-00-1 Revised April 1995

DIFLUCAN® ℞

(fluconazole tablets)
(fluconazole injection–
for intravenous infusion only)
(fluconazole for oral suspension)

DESCRIPTION

DIFLUCAN® (fluconazole), the first of a new subclass of synthetic triazole antifungal agents, is available as tablets for oral administration, as a powder for oral suspension and as a sterile solution for intravenous use in glass and in Viaflex® Plus plastic containers.

Fluconazole is designated chemically as 2,4-difluoro-α,α^1-bis(1H-1,2,4-triazol-1-ylmethyl) benzyl alcohol with an empirical formula of $C_{13}H_{12}F_2N_6O$ and molecular weight 306.3. The structural formula is:

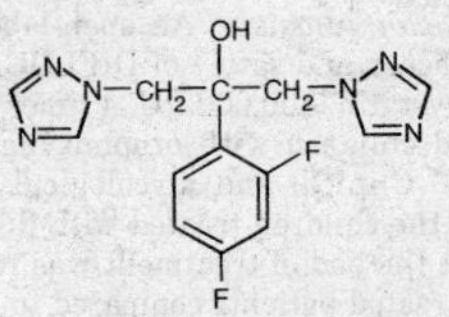

Fluconazole is a white crystalline solid which is slightly soluble in water and saline.

DIFLUCAN tablets contain 50, 100, 150, or 200 mg of fluconazole and the following inactive ingredients: microcrystalline cellulose, dibasic calcium phosphate anhydrous, povidone, croscarmellose sodium, FD&C Red No. 40 aluminum lake dye, and magnesium stearate.

DIFLUCAN for oral suspension contains 350 mg or 1400 mg of fluconazole and the following inactive ingredients: sucrose, sodium citrate dihydrate, citric acid anhydrous, sodium benzoate, titanium dioxide, colloidal silicon dioxide, xanthan gum and natural orange flavor. After reconstitution with 24 mL of distilled pure water or Purified Water (USP), each mL of reconstituted suspension contains 10 mg or 40 mg of fluconazole.

DIFLUCAN injection is an iso-osmotic, sterile, nonpyrogenic solution of fluconazole in a sodium chloride or dextrose diluent. Each mL contains 2 mg of fluconazole and 9 mg of sodium chloride or 56 mg of dextrose, hydrous. The pH ranges from 4.0 to 8.0 in the sodium chloride diluent and from 3.5 to 6.5 in the dextrose diluent. Injection volumes of 100 mL and 200 mL are packaged in glass and in Viaflex® Plus plastic containers.

The Viaflex® Plus plastic container is fabricated from a specially formulated polyvinyl chloride (PL 146® Plastic) (Viaflex and PL 146 are registered trademarks of Baxter International, Inc.). The amount of water that can permeate from inside the container into the overwrap is insufficient to affect the solution significantly. Solutions in contact with the plastic container can leach out certain of its chemical components in very small amounts within the expiration period, e.g. di-2-ethylhexylphthalate (DEHP), up to 5 parts per million. However, the suitability of the plastic has been confirmed in tests in animals according to USP biological tests for plastic containers as well as by tissue culture toxicity studies.

CLINICAL PHARMACOLOGY

Mode of Action

Fluconazole is a highly selective inhibitor of fungal cytochrome P-450 sterol C-14 alpha-demethylation. Mammalian cell demethylation is much less sensitive to fluconazole inhibition. The subsequent loss of normal sterols correlates with the accumulation of 14 alpha-methyl sterols in fungi and may be responsible for the fungistatic activity of fluconazole.

Age Studied	Dose (mg/kg)	Clearance (mL/min/kg)	Half-life (Hours)	Cmax (µg/mL)	Vdss (L/kg)
9 Months–13 years	Single-Oral 2 mg/kg	0.40 (38%) N=14	25.0	2.9 (22%) N=16	—
9 Months–13 years	Single-Oral 8 mg/kg	0.51 (60%) N=15	19.5	9.8 (20%) N=15	—
5–15 years	Multiple i.v. 2 mg/kg	0.49 (40%) N=4	17.4	5.5 (25%) N=5	0.722 (36%) N=4
5–15 years	Multiple i.v. 4 mg/kg	0.59 (64%) N=5	15.2	11.4 (44%) N=6	0.729 (33%) N=5
5–15 years	Multiple i.v. 8 mg/kg	0.66 (31%) N=7	17.6	14.1 (22%) N=8	1.069 (37%) N=7

Phamacokinetics and Metabolism

The pharmacokinetic properties of fluconazole are similar following administration by the intravenous or oral routes. In normal volunteers, the bioavailability of orally administered fluconazole is over 90% compared with intravenous administration. Bioequivalence was established between the 100 mg tablet and both suspension strengths when administered as a single 200 mg dose.

Peak plasma concentrations (Cmax) in fasted normal volunteers occur between 1 and 2 hours with a terminal plasma elimination half-life of approximately 30 hours (range 20–50 hours) after oral administration.

In fasted normal volunteers, administration of a single oral 400 mg dose of DIFLUCAN (fluconazole) leads to a mean Cmax of 6.72 µg/mL (range: 4.12 to 8.08 µg/mL) and after single oral doses of 50–400 mg, fluconazole plasma concentrations and AUC (area under the plasma concentration-time curve) are dose proportional.

Administration of a single oral 150 mg tablet of DIFLUCAN (fluconazole) to ten lactating women resulted in a mean Cmax of 2.61 µg/mL (range: 1.57 to 3.65 µg/mL).

Steady-state concentrations are reached within 5–10 days following oral doses of 50–400 mg given once daily. Administration of a loading dose (on day 1) of twice the usual daily dose results in plasma concentrations close to steady-state by the second day. The apparent volume of distribution of fluconazole approximates that of total body water. Plasma protein binding is low (11–12%). Following either single- or multiple-oral doses for up to 14 days, fluconazole penetrates into all body fluids studied (see table below). In normal volunteers, saliva concentrations of fluconazole were equal to or slightly greater than plasma concentrations regardless of dose, route, or duration of dosing. In patients with bronchiectasis, sputum concentrations of fluconazole following a single 150 mg oral dose were equal to plasma concentrations at both 4 and 24 hours post dose. In patients with fungal meningitis, fluconazole concentrations in the CSF are approximately 80% of the corresponding plasma concentrations.

A single oral 150 mg dose of fluconazole administered to 27 patients penetrated into vaginal tissue, resulting in tissue: plasma ratios ranging from 0.94 to 1.14 over the first 48 hours following dosing.

A single oral 150 mg dose of fluconazole administered to 14 patients penetrated into vaginal fluid, resulting in fluid: plasma ratios ranging from 0.36 to 0.71 over the first 72 hours following dosing.

Tissue or Fluid	Ratio of Fluconazole Tissue (Fluid)/ Plasma Concentration*
Cerebrospinal fluid†	.5–.9
Saliva	1
Sputum	1
Blister fluid	1
Urine	10
Normal skin	10
Nails	1
Blister skin	2
Vaginal tissue	1
Vaginal fluid	0.4–0.7

*Relative to concurrent concentrations in plasma in subjects with normal renal function.

†Independent of degree of meningeal inflammation.

In normal volunteers, fluconazole is cleared primarily by renal excretion, with approximately 80% of the administered dose appearing in the urine as unchanged drug. About 11% of the dose is excreted in the urine as metabolites.

The pharmacokinetics of fluconazole are markedly affected by reduction in renal function. There is an inverse relationship between the elimination half-life and creatinine clearance. The dose of DIFLUCAN may need to be reduced in patients with impaired renal function. (See DOSAGE AND ADMINISTRATION.) A 3-hour hemodialysis session decreases plasma concentrations by approximately 50%.

In normal volunteers, DIFLUCAN administration (doses ranging from 200 mg to 400 mg once daily for up to 14 days) was associated with small and inconsistent effects on testosterone concentrations, endogenous corticosteroid concentrations, and the ACTH-stimulated cortisol response.

Pharmacokinetics in Children

In children, the following pharmacokinetic data [MEAN(%cv)] have been reported:

[See table above]

Clearance corrected for body weight was not affected by age in these studies. Mean body clearance in adults is reported to be 0.23 (17%) mL/min/kg.

In premature newborns (gestational age 26 to 29 weeks), the mean (%cv) clearance within 36 hours of birth was 0.180 (35%, N=7) mL/min/kg, which increased with time to a mean of 0.218 (31%, N=9) mL/min/kg six days later and 0.333 (56%, N=4) mL/min/kg 12 days later. Similarly, the half-life was 73.6 hours, which decreased with time to a mean of 53.2 hours six days later and 46.6 hours 12 days later.

Drug Interaction Studies

Oral contraceptives: Oral contraceptives were administered as a single dose both before and after the oral administration of DIFLUCAN 50 mg once daily for 10 days in 10 healthy women. There was no significant difference in ethinyl estradiol or levonorgestrel AUC after the administration of 50 mg of DIFLUCAN. The mean increase in ethinyl estradiol AUC was 6% (range: –47 to 108%) and levonorgestrel AUC increased 17% (range: –33 to 141%).

Twenty-five normal females received daily doses of both 200 mg of DIFLUCAN tablets or placebo for two, ten-day periods. The treatment cycles were one month apart with all subjects receiving DIFLUCAN during one cycle and placebo during the other. The order of study treatment was random. Single doses of an oral contraceptive tablet containing levonorgestrel and ethinyl estradiol were administered on the final treatment day (day 10) of both cycles. Following administration of 200 mg of DIFLUCAN, the mean percentage increase of AUC for levonorgestrel compared to placebo was 25% (range: –12 to 82%) and the mean percentage increase for ethinyl estradiol compared to placebo was 38% (range: –11 to 101%). Both of these increases were statistically significantly different from placebo.

Cimetidine: DIFLUCAN 100 mg was administered as a single oral dose alone and two hours after a single dose of cimetidine 400 mg to six healthy male volunteers. After the administration of cimetidine, there was a significant decrease in fluconazole AUC and Cmax. There was a mean ± SD decrease in fluconazole AUC of 13% ± 11% (range: –3.4 to –31%) and Cmax decreased 19% ± 14% (range: –5 to –40%). However, the administration of cimetidine 600 mg to 900 mg intravenously over a four hour period (from one hour before to 3 hours after a single oral dose of DIFLUCAN 200 mg) did not affect the bioavailability or pharmacokinetics of fluconazole in 24 healthy male volunteers.

Antacid: Administration of Maalox® (20 mL) to 14 normal male volunteers immediately prior to a single dose of DIFLUCAN 100 mg had no effect on the absorption or elimination of fluconazole.

Hydrochlorothiazide: Concomitant oral administration of 100 mg DIFLUCAN and 50 mg hydrochlorothiazide for 10 days in 13 normal volunteers resulted in a significant increase in fluconazole AUC and Cmax compared to DIFLUCAN given alone. There was a mean ± SD increase in fluconazole AUC and Cmax of 45% ± 31% (range: 19 to 114%) and 43% ± 31% (range: 19 to 122%), respectively. These changes are attributed to a mean ± SD reduction in renal clearance of 30% ± 12% (range: –10 to –50%).

Rifampin: Administration of a single oral 200 mg dose of DIFLUCAN after 15 days of rifampin administered as 600 mg daily in eight healthy male volunteers resulted in a significant decrease in fluconazole AUC and a significant increase in apparent oral clearance of fluconazole. There was a mean ± SD reduction in fluconazole AUC of 23% ± 9% (range: –13 to –42%). Apparent oral clearance of fluconazole

Continued on next page

Diflucan—Cont.

increased 32% ± 17% (range: 16 to 72%). Fluconazole half-life decreased from 33.4 ± 4.4 hours to 26.8 ± 3.9 hours. (See PRECAUTIONS.)

Warfarin: There was a significant increase in prothrombin time response (area under the prothrombin time-time curve) following a single dose of warfarin (15 mg) administered to 13 normal male volunteers following oral DIFLUCAN 200 mg administered daily for 14 days as compared to the administration of warfarin alone. There was a mean ± SD increase in the prothrombin time response (area under the prothrombin time-time curve) of 7% ± 4% (range: −2 to 13%). (See PRECAUTIONS.) Mean is based on data from 12 subjects as one of 13 subjects experienced a 2-fold increase in his prothrombin time response.

Phenytoin: Phenytoin AUC was determined after 4 days of phenytoin dosing (200 mg daily, orally for 3 days followed by 250 mg intravenously for one dose) both with and without the administration of fluconazole (oral DIFLUCAN 200 mg daily for 16 days) in 10 normal male volunteers. There was a significant increase in phenytoin AUC. The mean ± SD increase in phenytoin AUC was 88% ± 68% (range: 16 to 247%). The absolute magnitude of this interaction is unknown because of the intrinsically nonlinear disposition of phenytoin. (See PRECAUTIONS.)

Cyclosporine: Cyclosporine AUC and Cmax were determined before and after the administration of fluconazole 200 mg daily for 14 days in eight renal transplant patients who had been on cyclosporine therapy for at least 6 months and on a stable cyclosporine dose for at least 6 weeks. There was a significant increase in cyclosporine AUC, Cmax, Cmin (24 hour concentration), and a significant reduction in apparent oral clearance following the administration of fluconazole. The mean ± SD increase in AUC was 92% ± 43% (range: 18 to 147%). The Cmax increased 60% ± 48% (range: −5 to 133%). The Cmin increased 157% ± 96% (range: 33 to 360%). The apparent oral clearance decreased 45% ± 15% (range: −15 to −60%). (See PRECAUTIONS.)

Zidovudine: Plasma zidovudine concentrations were determined on two occasions (before and following fluconazole 200 mg daily for 15 days) in 13 volunteers with AIDS or ARC who were on a stable zidovudine dose for at least two weeks. There was a significant increase in zidovudine AUC following the administration of fluconazole. The mean ± SD increase in AUC was 20% ± 32% (range: −27 to 104%). The metabolite, GZDV, to parent drug ratio significantly decreased after the administration of fluconazole, from 7.6 ± 3.6 to 5.7 ± 2.2.

Theophylline: The pharmacokinetics of theophylline were determined from a single intravenous dose of aminophylline (6 mg/kg) before and after the oral administration of fluconazole 200 mg daily for 14 days in 16 normal male volunteers. There were significant increases in theophylline AUC, Cmax, and half-life with a corresponding decrease in clearance. The mean ± SD theophylline AUC increased 21% ± 16% (range: −5 to 48%). The Cmax increased 13% ± 17% (range: −13 to 40%). Theophylline clearance decreased 16% ± 11% (range: −32 to 5%). The half-life of theophylline increased from 6.6 ± 1.7 hours to 7.9 ± 1.5 hours.

Terfenadine: Six healthy volunteers received terfenadine 60 mg BID for 15 days. Fluconazole 200 mg was administered daily from days 9 through 15. Fluconazole did not affect terfenadine plasma concentrations. Terfenadine acid metabolite AUC increased 36% ± 36% (range: 7 to 102%) from day 8 to day 15 with the concomitant administration of fluconazole. There was no change in cardiac repolarization as measured by Holter QTc intervals. (See PRECAUTIONS.)

Oral hypoglycemics: The effects of fluconazole on the pharmacokinetics of the sulfonylurea oral hypoglycemic agents tolbutamide, glipizide, and glyburide were evaluated in three placebo-controlled studies in normal volunteers. All subjects received the sulfonylurea alone as a single dose and again as a single dose following the administration of DIFLUCAN 100 mg daily for 7 days. In these three studies 22/46 (47.8%) of DIFLUCAN treated patients and 9/22 (40.1%) of placebo treated patients experienced symptoms consistent with hypoglycemia. (See PRECAUTIONS.)

Tolbutamide: In 13 normal male volunteers, there was significant increase in tolbutamide (500 mg single dose) AUC and Cmax following the administration of fluconazole. There was a mean ± SD increase in tolbutamide AUC of 26% ± 9% (range: 12 to 39%). Tolbutamide Cmax increased 11% ± 9% (range: −6 to 27%). (See PRECAUTIONS.)

Glipizide: The AUC and Cmax of glipizide (2.5 mg single dose) were significantly increased following the administration of fluconazole in 13 normal male volunteers. There was a mean ± SD increase in AUC of 49% ± 13% (range: 27 to 73%) and an increase in Cmax of 19% ± 23% (range: −11 to 79%). (See PRECAUTIONS.)

Glyburide: The AUC and Cmax of glyburide (5 mg single dose) were significantly increased following the administration of fluconazole in 20 normal male volunteers.

There was a mean ± SD increase in AUC of 44% ± 29% (range: −13 to 115%) and Cmax increased 19% ± 19% (range: −23 to 62%). Five subjects required oral glucose following the ingestion of glyburide after 7 days of fluconazole administration. (See PRECAUTIONS.)

Microbiology
Fluconazole exhibits *in vitro* activity against *Cryptococcus neoformans* and *Candida* spp. Fungistatic activity has also been demonstrated in normal and immunocompromised animal models for systemic and intracranial fungal infections due to *Cryptococcus neoformans* and for systemic infections due to *Candida albicans*.

In common with other azole antifungal agents, most fungi show a higher apparent sensitivity to fluconazole *in vivo* than *in vitro*. Fluconazole administered orally and/or intravenously was active in a variety of animal models of fungal infection using standard laboratory strains of fungi. Activity has been demonstrated against fungal infections caused by *Aspergillus flavus* and *Aspergillus fumigatus* in normal mice. Fluconazole has also been shown to be active in animal models of endemic mycoses, including one model of *Blastomyces dermatitidis* pulmonary infections in normal mice; one model of *Coccidioides immitis* intracranial infections in normal mice; and several models of *Histoplasma capsulatum* pulmonary infection in normal and immunosuppressed mice. The clinical significance of results obtained in these studies is unknown.

Oral fluconazole has been shown to be active in an animal model of vaginal candidiasis.

Concurrent administration of fluconazole and amphotericin B in infected normal and immunosuppressed mice showed the following results: a small additive antifungal effect in systemic infection with *C. albicans*, no interaction in intracranial infection with *Cr. neoformans*, and antagonism of the two drugs in systemic infection with *Asp. fumigatus*. The clinical significance of results obtained in these studies is unknown.

There have been reports of cases of superinfection with Candida species other than *C. albicans*, which are often inherently not susceptible to DIFLUCAN (e.g., *Candida krusei*). Such cases may require alternative antifungal therapy.

INDICATIONS AND USAGE
DIFLUCAN (fluconazole) is indicated for the treatment of:
1. Vaginal Candidiasis (vaginal yeast infections due to *Candida*).
2. Oropharyngeal and esophageal candidiasis. In open noncomparative studies of relatively small numbers of patients, DIFLUCAN was also effective for the treatment of Candida urinary tract infections, peritonitis, and systemic Candida infections including candidemia, disseminated candidiasis, and pneumonia.
3. Cryptococcal meningitis. Before prescribing DIFLUCAN (fluconazole) for AIDS patients with cryptococcal meningitis, please see CLINICAL STUDIES section. Studies comparing DIFLUCAN to amphotericin B in non-HIV infected patients have not been conducted.

Prophylaxis. DIFLUCAN is also indicated to decrease the incidence of candidiasis in patients undergoing bone marrow transplantation who receive cytotoxic chemotherapy and/or radiation therapy.

Specimens for fungal culture and other relevant laboratory studies (serology, histopathology) should be obtained prior to therapy to isolate and identify causative organisms. Therapy may be instituted before the results of the cultures and other laboratory studies are known; however, once these results become available, anti-infective therapy should be adjusted accordingly.

CLINICAL STUDIES
Cryptococcal meningitis: In a multicenter study comparing DIFLUCAN (200 mg/day) to amphotericin B (0.3 mg/kg/day) for treatment of cryptococcal meningitis in patients with AIDS, a multivariate analysis revealed three pretreatment factors that predicted death during the course of therapy: abnormal mental status, cerebrospinal fluid cryptococcal antigen titer greater than 1:1024, and cerebrospinal fluid white blood cell count of less than 20 cells/mm³. Mortality among high risk patients was 33% and 40% for amphotericin B and DIFLUCAN patients, respectively (p=0.58), with overall deaths 14% (9 of 63 subjects) and 18% (24 of 131 subjects) for the 2 arms of the study (p=0.48). Optimal doses and regimens for patients with acute cryptococcal meningitis and at high risk for treatment failure remain to be determined. (Saag, *et al.* N Engl J Med 1992; 326:83-9)

Vaginal candidiasis: Two adequate and well-controlled studies were conducted in the U.S. using the 150 mg tablet. In both, the results of the fluconazole regimen were comparable to the control regimen (clotrimazole or miconazole intravaginally for 7 days) both clinically and statistically at the one month post-treatment evaluation.

The therapeutic cure rate, defined as a complete resolution of signs and symptoms of vaginal candidiasis (clinical cure), along with a negative KOH examination and negative culture for *Candida* (microbiologic eradication), was 55% in both the fluconazole group and the vaginal products group.

	Fluconazole PO 150 mg tablet	Vaginal Product qhs × 7 days
Enrolled	448	422
Evaluable at		
Late Follow-up	347 (77%)	327 (77%)
Clinical cure	239/347 (69%)	235/327 (72%)
Mycologic erad.	213/347 (61%)	196/327 (60%)
Therapeutic cure	190/347 (55%)	179/327 (55%)

Approximately three-fourths of the enrolled patients had acute vaginitis (<4 episodes/12 months) and achieved 80% clinical cure, 67% mycologic eradication and 59% therapeutic cure when treated with a 150 mg DIFLUCAN tablet administered orally. These rates were comparable to control products. The remaining one-fourth of enrolled patients had recurrent vaginitis (≥4 episodes/12 months) and achieved 57% clinical cure, 47% mycologic eradication and 40% therapeutic cure. The numbers are too small to make meaningful clinical or statistical comparisons with vaginal products in the treatment of patients with recurrent vaginitis. Substantially more gastrointestinal events were reported in the fluconazole group compared to the vaginal product group. Most of the events were mild to moderate. Because fluconazole was given as a single dose, no discontinuations occurred.

Parameter	Fluconazole PO	Vaginal Products
Evaluable patients	448	422
With any adverse event	141 (31%)	112 (27%)
Nervous System	90 (20%)	69 (16%)
Gastrointestinal	73 (16%)	18 (4%)
With drug-related event	117 (26%)	67 (16%)
Nervous System	61 (14%)	29 (7%)
Headache	58 (13%)	28 (7%)
Gastrointestinal	68 (15%)	13 (3%)
Abdominal pain	25 (6%)	7 (2%)
Nausea	30 (7%)	3 (1%)
Diarrhea	12 (3%)	2 (<1%)
Application site event	0 (0%)	19 (5%)
Taste Perversion	6 (1%)	0 (0%)

Pediatric Studies
Oropharyngeal candidiasis: An open-label, comparative study of the efficacy and safety of DIFLUCAN (2–3 mg/kg/day) and oral nystatin (400,000 I.U. 4 times daily) in immunocompromised children with oropharyngeal candidiasis was conducted. Clinical and mycological response rates were higher in the children treated with fluconazole.

Clinical cure at the end of treatment was reported for 86% of fluconazole treated patients compared to 46% of nystatin treated patients. Mycologically, 76% of fluconazole treated patients had the infecting organism eradicated compared to 11% for nystatin treated patients.

	Fluconazole	Nystatin
Enrolled	96	90
Clinical Cure	76/88 (86%)	36/78 (46%)
Mycological eradication*	55/72 (76%)	6/54 (11%)

*Subjects without follow-up cultures for any reason were considered nonevaluable for mycological response.

The proportion of patients with clinical relapse 2 weeks after the end of treatment was 14% for subjects receiving DIFLUCAN and 16% for subjects receiving nystatin. At 4 weeks after the end of treatment the percentages of patients with clinical relapse were 22% for DIFLUCAN and 23% for nystatin.

CONTRAINDICATIONS
DIFLUCAN (fluconazole) is contraindicated in patients who have shown hypersensitivity to fluconazole or to any of its excipients. There is no information regarding cross hypersensitivity between fluconazole and other azole antifungal agents. Caution should be used in prescribing DIFLUCAN to patients with hypersensitivity to other azoles. Coadministration of terfenadine is contraindicated in patients receiving DIFLUCAN (fluconazole) at multiple doses of 400 mg or higher based upon results of a multiple dose interaction study. (See PRECAUTIONS.)

WARNINGS
(1) Hepatic injury: DIFLUCAN has been associated with rare cases of serious hepatic toxicity, including fatalities primarily in patients with serious underlying medical conditions. In cases of DIFLUCAN associated hepatotoxicity, no obvious relationship to total daily dose, duration of therapy, sex or age of the patient has been observed. DIFLUCAN hepatotoxicity has usually, but not always, been reversible on discontinuation of therapy. Patients who develop abnormal liver function tests during DIFLUCAN therapy should be monitored for the development of more severe hepatic injury. DIFLUCAN should be discontinued if clinical signs and symptoms consistent with liver disease develop that may be attributable to DIFLUCAN.

(2) Anaphylaxis: In rare cases, anaphylaxis has been reported.

(3) Dermatologic: Patients have rarely developed exfoliative skin disorders during treatment with DIFLUCAN. In patients with serious underlying diseases (predominantly AIDS and malignancy), these have rarely resulted in a fatal outcome. Patients who develop rashes during treatment with DIFLUCAN should be monitored closely and the drug discontinued if lesions progress.

(4) Cisapride: There have been reports of cardiac events including torsade de pointes in patients receiving concomitant administration of fluconazole with cisapride. Patients should be carefully monitored if fluconazole is to be coadministered with cisapride. (See PRECAUTIONS.)

PRECAUTIONS
General
Single Dose
The convenience and efficacy of the single dose oral tablet of fluconazole regimen for the treatment of vaginal yeast infections should be weighed against the acceptability of a higher incidence of drug related adverse events with DIFLUCAN (26%) versus intravaginal agents (16%) in U.S. comparative clinical studies. (See ADVERSE REACTIONS and CLINICAL STUDIES.)

Drug Interactions: (See CLINICAL PHARMACOLOGY and PRECAUTIONS—General)
Clinically or potentially significant drug interactions between DIFLUCAN and the following agents/classes have been observed. These are described in greater detail below.
Oral hypoglycemics
Coumarin-type anticoagulants
Phenytoin
Cyclosporine
Rifampin
Theophylline
Terfenadine
Cisapride
Astemizole

Oral hypoglycemics: Clinically significant hypoglycemia may be precipitated by the use of DIFLUCAN with oral hypoglycemic agents; one fatality has been reported from hypoglycemia in association with combined DIFLUCAN and glyburide use. DIFLUCAN reduces the metabolism of tolbutamide, glyburide, and glipizide and increases the plasma concentration of these agents. When DIFLUCAN is used concomitantly with these or other sulfonylurea oral hypoglycemic agents, blood glucose concentrations should be carefully monitored and the dose of the sulfonylurea should be adjusted as necessary.

Coumarin-type anticoagulants: Prothrombin time may be increased in patients receiving concomitant DIFLUCAN and coumarin-type anticoagulants. Careful monitoring of prothrombin time in patients receiving DIFLUCAN and coumarin-type anticoagulants is recommended.

Phenytoin: DIFLUCAN increases the plasma concentrations of phenytoin. Careful monitoring of phenytoin concentrations in patients receiving DIFLUCAN and phenytoin is recommended.

Cyclosporine: DIFLUCAN may significantly increase cyclosporine levels in renal transplant patients with or without renal impairment. Careful monitoring of cyclosporine concentrations and serum creatinine is recommended in patients receiving DIFLUCAN and cyclosporine.

Rifampin: Rifampin enhances the metabolism of concurrently administered DIFLUCAN. Depending on clinical circumstances, consideration should be given to increasing the dose of DIFLUCAN when it is administered with rifampin.

Theophylline: DIFLUCAN increases the serum concentrations of theophylline. Careful monitoring of serum theophylline concentrations in patients receiving DIFLUCAN and theophylline is recommended.

Terfenadine: Because of the occurrence of serious cardiac dysrhythmias secondary to prolongation of the QTc interval in patients receiving azole antifungals in conjunction with terfenadine, interaction studies have been performed. One study at a 200 mg daily dose of fluconazole failed to demonstrate a prolongation in QTc interval. Another study at a 400 mg and 800 mg daily dose of fluconazole demonstrated that DIFLUCAN taken in doses of 400 mg per day or greater significantly increases plasma levels of terfenadine when taken concomitantly. The combined use of fluconazole at doses of 400 mg or greater with terfenadine is contraindicated. (See CONTRAINDICATIONS, DRUG INTERACTION STUDIES.) The coadministration of fluconazole at doses lower than 400 mg/day with terfenadine should be carefully monitored.

Cisapride and Astemizole: There have been reports of cardiac events including torsade de pointes in patients to whom fluconazole and cisapride were coadministered. The use of fluconazole in patients concurrently taking cisapride, astemizole or other drugs metabolized by the cytochrome P450 system may be associated with elevations in serum levels of these drugs. In the absence of definitive information, caution should be used when coadministering fluconazole. Patients should be carefully monitored.
Fluconazole tablets coadministered with ethinyl estradiol-and levonorgestrel-containing oral contraceptives produced

an overall mean increase in ethinyl estradiol and levonorgestrel levels; however, in some patients there were decreases up to 47% and 33% of ethinyl estradiol and levonorgestrel levels. (See Drug Interaction Studies.) The data presently available indicate that the decreases in some individual ethinyl estradiol and levonorgestrel AUC values with fluconazole treatment are likely the result of random variation. While there is evidence that fluconazole can inhibit the metabolism of ethinyl estradiol and levonorgestrel, there is no evidence that fluconazole is a net inducer of ethinyl estradiol or levonorgestrel metabolism. The clinical significance of these effects is presently unknown.

Physicians should be aware that interaction studies with medications other than those listed in the CLINICAL PHARMACOLOGY section have not been conducted, but such interactions may occur.

Carcinogenesis, Mutagenesis and Impairment of Fertility
Fluconazole showed no evidence of carcinogenic potential in mice and rats treated orally for 24 months at doses of 2.5, 5 or 10 mg/kg/day (approximately 2–7× the recommended human dose). Male rats treated with 5 and 10 mg/kg/day had an increased incidence of hepatocellular adenomas.

Fluconazole, with or without metabolic activation, was negative in tests for mutagenicity in 4 strains of *S. typhimurium*, and in the mouse lymphoma L5178Y system. Cytogenetic studies *in vivo* (murine bone marrow cells, following oral administration of fluconazole) and *in vitro* (human lymphocytes exposed to fluconazole at 1000 µg/mL) showed no evidence of chromosomal mutations.

Fluconazole did not affect the fertility of male or female rats treated orally with daily doses of 5, 10 or 20 mg/kg or with parenteral doses of 5, 25 or 75 mg/kg, although the onset of parturition was slightly delayed at 20 mg/kg p.o. In an intravenous perinatal study in rats at 5, 20 and 40 mg/kg, dystocia and prolongation of parturition were observed in a few dams at 20 mg/kg (approximately 5–15× the recommended human dose) and 40 mg/kg, but not at 5 mg/kg. The disturbances in parturition were reflected by a slight increase in the number of still-born pups and decrease of neonatal survival at these dose levels. The effects on parturition in rats are consistent with the species specific estrogen-lowering property produced by high doses of fluconazole. Such a hormone change has not been observed in women treated with fluconazole (See CLINICAL PHARMACOLOGY.)

Pregnancy
Teratogenic Effects. Pregnancy Category C: Fluconazole was administered orally to pregnant rabbits during organogenesis in two studies, at 5, 10 and 20 mg/kg and at 5, 25, and 75 mg/kg, respectively. Maternal weight gain was impaired at all dose levels, and abortions occurred at 75 mg/kg (approximately 20–60× the recommended human dose); no adverse fetal effects were detected. In several studies in which pregnant rats were treated orally with fluconazole during organogenesis, maternal weight gain was impaired and placental weights were increased at 25 mg/kg. There were no fetal effects at 5 or 10 mg/kg; increases in fetal anatomical variants (supernumerary ribs, renal pelvis dilation) and delays in ossification were observed at 25 and 50 mg/kg and higher doses. At doses ranging from 80 mg/kg (approximately 20–60× the recommended human dose) to 320 mg/kg embryolethality in rats was increased and fetal abnormalities included wavy ribs, cleft palate and abnormal cranio-facial ossification. These effects are consistent with the inhibition of estrogen synthesis in rats and may be a result of known effects of lowered estrogen on pregnancy, organogenesis and parturition.

There are no adequate and well controlled studies in pregnant women. There have been reports of multiple congenital abnormalities in infants whose mothers were being treated for 3 or more months with high dose (400–800 mg/day) fluconazole therapy for coccidioidomycosis (an unindicated use). The relationship between fluconazole use and these events is unclear. DIFLUCAN should be used in pregnancy only if the potential benefit justifies the possible risk to the fetus.

Nursing Mothers
Fluconazole is secreted in human milk at concentrations similar to plasma. Therefore, the use of DIFLUCAN in nursing mothers is not recommended.

Pediatric Use
An open-label, randomized, controlled trial has shown DIFLUCAN to be effective in the treatment of oropharyngeal candidiasis in children 6 months to 13 years of age. (See CLINICAL STUDIES.)

The use of DIFLUCAN in children with cryptococcal meningitis, Candida esophagitis, or systemic Candida infections is supported by the efficacy shown for these indications in adults and by the results from several small noncomparative pediatric clinical studies. In addition, pharmacokinetic studies in children (see CLINICAL PHARMACOLOGY) have established a dose proportionality between children and adults. (See DOSAGE AND ADMINISTRATION.)

In a noncomparative study of children with serious systemic fungal infections, most of which were candidemia, the effectiveness of DIFLUCAN was similar to that reported for the

treatment of candidemia in adults. Of 17 subjects with culture-confirmed candidemia, 11 of 14 (79%) with baseline symptoms (3 were asymptomatic) had a clinical cure; 13/15 (87%) of evaluable patients had a mycologic cure at the end of treatment but two of these patients relapsed at 10 and 18 days, respectively, following cessation of therapy.

The efficacy of DIFLUCAN for the suppression of cryptococcal meningitis was successful in 4 of 5 children treated in a compassionate-use study of fluconazole for the treatment of life-threatening or serious mycosis. There is no information regarding the efficacy of fluconazole for primary treatment of cryptococcal meningitis in children.

The safety profile of DIFLUCAN in children has been studied in 577 children ages 1 day to 17 years who received doses ranging from 1 to 15 mg/kg/day for 1 to 1,616 days. (See ADVERSE REACTIONS.)

Efficacy of DIFLUCAN has not been established in infants less than 6 months of age. (See CLINICAL PHARMACOLOGY.) A small number of patients (29) ranging in age from 1 day to 6 months have been treated safely with DIFLUCAN.

ADVERSE REACTIONS
In Patients Receiving a Single Dose for Vaginal Candidiasis:
During comparative clinical studies conducted in the United States, 448 patients with vaginal candidiasis were treated with DIFLUCAN, 150 mg single dose. The overall incidence of side effects possibly related to DIFLUCAN was 26%. In 422 patients receiving active comparative agents, the incidence was 16%. The most common treatment-related adverse events reported in the patients who received 150 mg single dose fluconazole for vaginitis were headache (13%), nausea (7%), and abdominal pain (6%). Other side effects reported with an incidence equal to or greater than 1% included diarrhea (3%), dyspepsia (1%), dizziness (1%), and taste perversion (1%). Most of the reported side effects were mild to moderate in severity. Rarely, angioedema and anaphylactic reaction have been reported in marketing experience.

In Patients Receiving Multiple Doses for Other Infections:
Sixteen percent of over 4000 patients treated with DIFLUCAN (fluconazole) in clinical trials of 7 days or more experienced adverse events. Treatment was discontinued in 1.5% of patients due to adverse clinical events and in 1.3% of patients due to laboratory test abnormalities.

Clinical adverse events were reported more frequently in HIV infected patients (21%) than in non-HIV infected patients (13%); however, the patterns in HIV infected and non-HIV infected patients were similar. The proportions of patients discontinuing therapy due to clinical adverse events were similar in the two groups. (1.5%).

The following treatment-related clinical adverse events occurred at an incidence of 1% or greater in 4048 patients receiving DIFLUCAN for 7 or more days in clinical trials: nausea 3.7%, headache 1.9%, skin rash 1.8%, vomiting 1.7%, abdominal pain 1.7%, and diarrhea 1.5%.

The following adverse events have occurred under conditions where a causal association is probable:

Hepatobiliary: In combined clinical trials and marketing experience, there have been rare cases of serious hepatic reactions during treatment with DIFLUCAN. (See WARNINGS.) The spectrum of these hepatic reactions has ranged from mild transient elevations in transaminases to clinical hepatitis, cholestasis and fulminant hepatic failure, including fatalities. Instances of fatal hepatic reactions were noted to occur primarily in patients with serious underlying medical conditions (predominantly AIDS or malignancy) and often while taking concomitant medications. Transient hepatic reactions, including hepatitis and jaundice, have occurred among patients with no other identifiable risk factors. In each of these cases, liver function returned to baseline on discontinuation of DIFLUCAN.

In two comparative trials evaluating the efficacy of DIFLUCAN for the suppression of relapse of cryptococcal meningitis, a statistically significant increase was observed in median AST (SGOT) levels from a baseline value of 30 IU/L to 41 IU/L in one trial and 34 IU/L to 66 IU/L in the other. The overall rate of serum transaminase elevations of more than 8 times the upper limit of normal was approximately 1% in fluconazole-treated patients in clinical trials. These elevations occurred in patients with severe underlying disease, predominantly AIDS or malignancies, most of whom were receiving multiple concomitant medications, including many known to be hepatotoxic. The incidence of abnormally elevated serum transaminases was greater in patients taking DIFLUCAN concomitantly with one or more of the following medications: rifampin, phenytoin, isoniazid, valproic acid, or oral sulfonylurea hypoglycemic agents.

Immunologic: In rare cases, anaphylaxis has been reported.

The following adverse events have occurred under conditions where a causal association is uncertain.

Central Nervous System: seizures.

Dermatologic: Exfoliative skin disorders including Stevens-Johnson Syndrome and toxic epidermal necrolysis (see WARNINGS), alopecia.

Continued on next page

Diflucan—Cont.

Hematopoietic and *Lymphatic:* leukopenia, including neutropenia and agranulocytosis, thrombocytopenia.
Metabolic: hypercholesterolemia, hypertriglyceridemia, hypokalemia.

Adverse Reactions in Children:
In Phase 2/3 clinical trials conducted in the United States and in Europe, 577 pediatric patients, ages 1 day to 17 years were treated with DIFLUCAN at doses up to 15 mg/kg/day for up to 1,616 days. Thirteen percent of children experienced treatment related adverse events. The most commonly reported events were vomiting (5%), abdominal pain (3%), nausea (2%), and diarrhea (2%). Treatment was discontinued in 2.3% of patients due to adverse clinical events and in 1.4% of patients due to laboratory test abnormalities. The majority of treatment-related laboratory abnormalities were elevations of transaminases or alkaline phosphate.

Percentage of Patients With Treatment-Related Side Effects

	Fluconazole (N=577)	Comparative Agents (N=451)
With any side effect	13.0	9.3
Vomiting	5.4	5.1
Abdominal pain	2.8	1.6
Nausea	2.3	1.6
Diarrhea	2.1	2.2

OVERDOSAGE

There has been one reported case of overdosage with DIFLUCAN (fluconazole). A 42-year-old patient infected with human immunodeficiency virus developed hallucinations and exhibited paranoid behavior after reportedly ingesting 8200 mg of DIFLUCAN. The patient was admitted to the hospital, and his condition resolved within 48 hours.

In the event of overdose, symptomatic treatment (with supportive measures and gastric lavage if clinically indicated) should be instituted.

Fluconazole is largely excreted in urine. A three hour hemodialysis session decreases plasma levels by approximately 50%.

In mice and rats receiving very high doses of fluconazole, clinical effects in both species included decreased motility and respiration, ptosis, lacrimation, salivation, urinary incontinence, loss of righting reflex and cyanosis; death was sometimes preceded by clonic convulsions.

DOSAGE AND ADMINISTRATION

Dosage and Administration in Adults:
Single Dose

Vaginal candidiasis: The recommended dosage of DIFLUCAN for vaginal candidiasis is 150 mg as a single oral dose.

Multiple Dose

SINCE ORAL ABSORPTION IS RAPID AND ALMOST COMPLETE, THE DAILY DOSE OF DIFLUCAN (FLUCONAZOLE) IS THE SAME FOR ORAL (TABLETS AND SUSPENSION) AND INTRAVENOUS ADMINISTRATION. In general, a loading dose of twice the daily dose is recommended on the first day of therapy to result in plasma concentrations close to steady-state by the second day of therapy.

The daily dose of DIFLUCAN for the treatment of infections other than vaginal candidiasis should be based on the infecting organism and the patient's response to therapy. Treatment should be continued until clinical parameters or laboratory tests indicate that active fungal infection has subsided. An inadequate period of treatment may lead to recurrence of active infection. Patients with AIDS and cryptococcal meningitis or recurrent oropharyngeal candidiasis usually require maintenance therapy to prevent relapse.

Oropharyngeal candidiasis: The recommended dosage of DIFLUCAN for oropharyngeal candidiasis is 200 mg on the first day, followed by 100 mg once daily. Clinical evidence of oropharyngeal candidiasis generally resolves within several days, but treatment should be continued for at least 2 weeks to decrease the likelihood of relapse.

Esophageal candidiasis: The recommended dosage of DIFLUCAN for esophageal candidiasis is 200 mg on the first day, followed by 100 mg once daily. Doses up to 400 mg/day may be used, based on medical judgment of the patient's response to therapy. Patients with esophageal candidiasis should be treated for a minimum of three weeks and for at least two weeks following resolution of symptoms.

Systemic Candida infections: For systemic Candida infections including candidemia, disseminated candidiasis, and pneumonia, optimal therapeutic dosage and duration of therapy have not been established. In open, noncomparative studies of small numbers of patients, doses of up to 400 mg daily have been used.

Urinary tract infection and peritonitis: For the treatment of Candida urinary tract infections and peritonitis, daily doses of 50–200 mg have been used in open, noncomparative studies of small numbers of patients.

Cryptococcal meningitis: The recommended dosage for treatment of acute cryptococcal meningitis is 400 mg on the first day, followed by 200 mg once daily. A dosage of 400 mg once daily may be used, based on medical judgment of the patient's response to therapy. The recommended duration of treatment for initial therapy of cryptococcal meningitis is 10–12 weeks after the cerebrospinal fluid becomes culture negative. The recommended dosage of DIFLUCAN for suppression of relapse of cryptococcal meningitis in patients with AIDS is 200 mg once daily.

Prophylaxis in patients undergoing bone marrow transplantation: The recommended DIFLUCAN daily dosage for the prevention of candidiasis of patients undergoing bone marrow transplantation is 400 mg, once daily. Patients who are anticipated to have severe granulocytopenia (less than 500 neutrophils per cu mm) should start DIFLUCAN prophylaxis several days before the anticipated onset of neutropenia, and continue for 7 days after the neutrophil count rises above 1000 cells per cu mm.

Dosage and Administration in Children:
The following dose equivalency scheme should generally provide equivalent exposure in pediatric and adult patients:

Pediatric Patients	Adults
3 mg/kg	100 mg
6 mg/kg	200 mg
12* mg/kg	400 mg

*Some older children may have clearances similar to that of adults. Absolute doses exceeding 600 mg/day are not recommended.

Experience with DIFLUCAN in neonates is limited to pharmacokinetic studies in premature newborns. (See CLINICAL PHARMACOLOGY.) Based on the prolonged half-life seen in premature newborns (gestational age 26 to 29 weeks), these children, in the first two weeks of life, should receive the same dosage (mg/kg) as in older children, but administered every 72 hours. After the first two weeks, these children should be dosed once daily. No information regarding DIFLUCAN pharmacokinetics in full-term newborns is available.

Oropharyngeal candidiasis: The recommended dosage of DIFLUCAN for oropharyngeal candidiasis in children is 6 mg/kg on the first day, followed by 3 mg/kg once daily. Treatment should be administered for at least 2 weeks to decrease the likelihood of relapse.

Esophageal Candidiasis: For the treatment of esophageal candidiasis, the recommended dosage of DIFLUCAN in children is 6 mg/kg on the first day, followed by 3 mg/kg once daily. Doses up to 12 mg/kg/day may be used based on medical judgment of the patient's response to therapy. Patients with esophageal candidiasis should be treated for a minimum of three weeks and for at least 2 weeks following the resolution of symptoms.

Systemic Candida infections: For the treatment of candidemia and disseminated Candida infections, daily doses of 6–12 mg/kg/day have been used in an open, noncomparative study of a small number of children.

Cryptococcal meningitis: For the treatment of acute cryptococcal meningitis, the recommended dosage is 12 mg/kg on the first day, followed by 6 mg/kg once daily. A dosage of 12 mg/kg once daily may be used, based on medical judgment of the patient's response to therapy. The recommended duration of treatment for initial therapy of cryptococcal meningitis is 10–12 weeks after the cerebrospinal fluid becomes culture negative. For suppression of relapse of cryptococcal meningitis in children with AIDS, the recommended dose of DIFLUCAN is 6 mg/kg once daily.

Dosage in Patients With Impaired Renal Function:
Fluconazole is cleared primarily by renal excretion as unchanged drug. There is no need to adjust single dose therapy for vaginal candidiasis because of impaired renal function. In patients with impaired renal function who will receive multiple doses of DIFLUCAN, an initial loading dose of 50 to 400 mg should be given. After the loading dose, the daily dose (according to indication) should be based on the following table:

Creatinine Clearance (mL/min)	Percent of Recommended Dose
>50	100%
≤50 (no dialysis)	50%
Regular dialysis	100% after each dialysis

These are suggested dose adjustments based on pharmacokinetics following administration of multiple doses. Further adjustments may be needed depending upon clinical condition.

When serum creatinine is the only measure of renal function available, the following formula (based on sex, weight, and age of the patient) should be used to estimate the creatinine clearance in adults:

Males:
$$\frac{\text{Weight (kg)} \times (140-\text{age})}{72 \times \text{serum creatinine (mg/100 mL)}}$$

Females: $0.85 \times$ above value

Although the pharmacokinetics of fluconazole has not been studied in children with renal insufficiency, dosage reduction in children with renal insufficiency should parallel that recommended for adults. The following formula may be used to estimate creatinine clearance in children:

$$K \times \frac{\text{linear length or height (cm)}}{\text{serum creatinine (mg/100 mL)}}$$

(Where K=0.55 for children older than 1 year and 0.45 for infants.)

Administration

DIFLUCAN may be administered either orally or by intravenous infusion. DIFLUCAN injection has been used safely for up to fourteen days of intravenous therapy. The intravenous infusion of DIFLUCAN should be administered at a maximum rate of approximately 200 mg/hour, given as a continuous infusion.

DIFLUCAN injections in glass and Viaflex® Plus plastic containers are intended only for intravenous administration using sterile equipment.

Parenteral drug products should be inspected visually for particulate matter and discoloration prior to administration whenever solution and container permit.

Do not use if the solution is cloudy or precipitated or if the seal is not intact.

Directions for Mixing the Oral Suspension
Prepare a suspension at time of dispensing as follows: tap bottle until all the powder flows freely. To reconstitute, add 24 mL of distilled water or Purified Water (USP) to fluconazole bottle and shake vigorously to suspend powder. Each bottle will deliver 35 mL of suspension. The concentrations of the reconstituted suspensions are as follows:

Fluconazole Content per Bottle	Concentration of Reconstituted Suspension
350 mg	10 mg/mL
1400 mg	40 mg/mL

Note: Shake oral suspension well before using. Store reconstituted suspension between 86°F (30°C) and 41°F (5°C) and discard unused portion after 2 weeks. Protect from freezing.

Directions for IV Use of DIFLUCAN in Viaflex® Plus Plastic Containers
Do not remove unit from overwrap until ready for use. The overwrap is a moisture barrier. The inner bag maintains the sterility of the product.

CAUTION: Do not use plastic containers in series connections. Such use could result in air embolism due to residual air being drawn from the primary container before administration of the fluid from the secondary container is completed.

To Open
Tear overwrap down side at slit and remove solution container. Some opacity of the plastic due to moisture absorption during the sterilization process may be observed. This is normal and does not affect the solution quality or safety. The opacity will diminish gradually. After removing overwrap, check for minute leaks by squeezing the inner bag firmly. If leaks are found, discard solution as sterility may be impaired.

DO NOT ADD SUPPLEMENTARY MEDICATION.

Preparation for Administration:
1. Suspend container from eyelet support.
2. Remove plastic protector from outlet port at bottom of container.
3. Attach administration set. Refer to complete directions accompanying set.

HOW SUPPLIED

DIFLUCAN® Tablets: Pink trapezoidal tablets containing 50, 100 or 200 mg of fluconazole are packaged in bottles or unit dose blisters. The 150 mg fluconazole tablets are pink and oval shaped, packaged in a single dose unit blister.
DIFLUCAN® Tablets are supplied as follows:
DIFLUCAN® 50 mg Tablets: Engraved with DIFLUCAN® and 50 on the front and ROERIG on the back.
NDC 0049-3410-30 Bottles of 30
DIFLUCAN® 100 mg Tablets: Engraved with DIFLUCAN® and 100 on the front and ROERIG on the back.
NDC 0049-3420-30 Bottles of 30
NDC 0049-3420-41 Unit dose package of 100
DIFLUCAN® 150 mg Tablets: Engraved with DIFLUCAN® and 150 mg on the front and ROERIG on the back.
NDC 0049-3500-79 Unit dose package of 1
DIFLUCAN® 200 mg Tablets: Engraved with DIFLUCAN® and 200 on the front and ROERIG on the back.
NDC 0049-3430-30 Bottles of 30
NDC 0049-3430-41 Unit dose package of 100
Storage: Store tablets below 86°F (30°C).

DIFLUCAN® for Oral Suspension: DIFLUCAN® for oral suspension is supplied as an orange-flavored powder to provide 35 mL per bottle as follows:
NDC 0049-3440-19 Fluconazole 350 mg per bottle
NDC 0049-3450-19 Fluconazole 1400 mg per bottle
Storage: Store dry powder below 86°F (30°C). Store reconstituted suspension between 86°F (30°C) and 41°F (5°C) and discard unused portion after 2 weeks.
Protect from freezing.
DIFLUCAN® Injections: DIFLUCAN® injections for intravenous infusion administration are formulated as sterile iso-osmotic solutions containing 2 mg/mL of fluconazole. They are supplied in glass bottles or in Viaflex® Plus plastic containers containing volumes of 100 mL or 200 mL affording doses of 200 mg and 400 mg of fluconazole, respectively. DIFLUCAN® injections in Viaflex® Plus plastic containers are available in both sodium chloride and dextrose diluents.
DIFLUCAN® Injections in Glass Bottles:
NDC 0049-3371-26 Fluconazole in Sodium Chloride Diluent 200 mg/100 mL × 6
NDC 0049-3372-26 Fluconazole in Sodium Chloride Diluent 400 mg/200 mL × 6
Storage: Store between 86°F (30°C) and 41°F (5°C). Protect from freezing.
DIFLUCAN® Injections in Viaflex® Plus Plastic Containers:
NDC 0049-3435-26 Fluconazole in Sodium Chloride Diluent 200 mg/100 mL × 6
NDC 0049-3436-26 Fluconazole in Sodium Chloride Diluent 400 mg/200 mL × 6
NDC 0049-3437-26 Fluconazole in Dextrose Diluent 200 mg/100 mL × 6
NDC 0049-3438-26 Fluconazole in Dextrose Diluent 400 mg/200 mL × 6
Storage: Store between 77°F (25°C) and 41°F (5°C). Brief exposure up to 104°F (40°C) does not adversely affect the product. Protect from freezing.

70-4526-00-6 Revised February 1997

Shown in Product Identification Guide, page 330

FELDENE® ℞
[fĕl 'deen]
(piroxicam)
CAPSULES
For Oral Use

DESCRIPTION

FELDENE® (piroxicam) is 4-Hydroxy-2-methyl-*N* -2- pyridinyl-2*H* -1,2-benzothiazine-3-carboxamide 1,1-dioxide, an oxicam. Members of the oxicam family are not carboxylic acids, but they are acidic by virtue of the enolic 4-hydroxy substituent. FELDENE occurs as a white crystalline solid, sparingly soluble in water, dilute acid and most organic solvents. It is slightly soluble in alcohols and in aqueous alkaline solution. It exhibits a weakly acidic 4-hydroxy proton (pKa 5.1) and a weakly basic pyridyl nitrogen (pKa 1.8). It has the following structure:

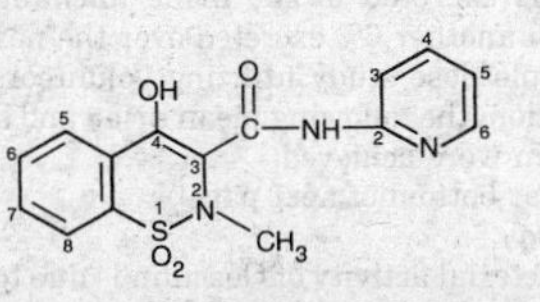

Molecular Formula: $C_{15}H_{13}N_3O_4S$
Molecular Weight 331.35

Inert ingredients in the formulations are: hard gelatin capsules (which may contain Blue 1, Red 3, and other inert ingredients); lactose; magnesium stearate; sodium lauryl sulfate; starch.

CLINICAL PHARMACOLOGY

FELDENE has shown anti-inflammatory, analgesic and antipyretic properties in animals. Edema, erythema, tissue proliferation, fever, and pain can all be inhibited in laboratory animals by the administration of FELDENE. It is effective regardless of the etiology of the inflammation. The mode of action of FELDENE is not fully established at this time. However, a common mechanism for the above effects may exist in the ability of FELDENE to inhibit the biosynthesis of prostaglandins, known mediators of inflammation. It is established that FELDENE does not act by stimulating the pituitary-adrenal axis.
FELDENE is well absorbed following oral administration. Drug plasma concentrations are proportional for 10 and 20 mg doses, generally peak within three to five hours after medication, and subsequently decline with a mean half-life of 50 hours (range of 30 to 86 hours, although values outside of this range have been encountered).
This prolonged half-life results in the maintenance of relatively stable plasma concentrations throughout the day on once daily doses and to significant drug accumulation upon multiple dosing. A single 20 mg dose generally produces peak piroxicam plasma levels of 1.5 to 2 mcg/mL, while maximum drug plasma concentrations, after repeated daily ingestion of 20 mg FELDENE, usually stabilize at 3–8 mcg/mL. Most patients approximate steady state plasma levels within 7 to 12 days. Higher levels, which approximate steady state at two to three weeks, have been observed in patients in whom longer plasma half-lives of piroxicam occurred.
FELDENE and its biotransformation products are excreted in urine and feces, with about twice as much appearing in the urine as the feces. Metabolism occurs by hydroxylation at the 5 position of the pyridyl side chain and conjugation of this product; by cyclodehydration; and by a sequence of reactions involving hydrolysis of the amide linkage, decarboxylation, ring contraction, and N-demethylation. Less than 5% of the daily dose is excreted unchanged.
Concurrent administration of aspirin (3900 mg/day) and FELDENE (20 mg/day), resulted in a reduction of plasma levels of piroxicam to about 80% of their normal values. The use of FELDENE in conjunction with aspirin is not recommended because data are inadequate to demonstrate that the combination produces greater improvement than that achieved with aspirin alone and the potential for adverse reactions is increased. Concomitant administration of antacids had no effect on FELDENE plasma levels. The effects of impaired renal function or hepatic disease on plasma levels have not been established.
FELDENE, like salicylates and other nonsteroidal anti-inflammatory agents, is associated with symptoms of gastrointestinal tract irritation (see ADVERSE REACTIONS). However, in a study utilizing ^{51}Cr-tagged red blood cells, 20 mg of FELDENE administered as a single dose for four days did not result in a significant increase in fecal blood loss and did not detectably affect the gastric mucosa. In the same study a total daily dose of 3900 mg of aspirin, i.e., 972 mg q.i.d., caused a significant increase in fecal blood loss and mucosal lesions as demonstrated by gastroscopy.
In controlled clinical trials, the effectiveness of FELDENE (piroxicam) has been established for both acute exacerbations and long-term management of rheumatoid arthritis and osteoarthritis.
The therapeutic effects of FELDENE are evident early in the treatment of both diseases with a progressive increase in response over several (8–12) weeks. Efficacy is seen in terms of pain relief and, when present, subsidence of inflammation.
Doses of 20 mg/day FELDENE display a therapeutic effect comparable to therapeutic doses of aspirin, with a lower incidence of minor gastrointestinal effects and tinnitus.
FELDENE has been administered concomitantly with fixed doses of gold and corticosteroids. The existence of a "steroid-sparing" effect has not been adequately studied to date.

INDICATIONS AND USAGE

FELDENE is indicated for acute or long-term use in the relief of signs and symptoms of the following:
1. osteoarthritis
2. rheumatoid arthritis

Dosage recommendations for use in children have not been established.

CONTRAINDICATIONS

FELDENE should not be used in patients who have previously exhibited hypersensitivity to it, or in individuals with the syndrome comprised of bronchospasm, nasal polyps, and angioedema precipitated by aspirin or other nonsteroidal anti-inflammatory drugs.

WARNINGS

Risk of GI Ulceration, Bleeding and Perforation with NSAID Therapy

Serious gastrointestinal toxicity such as bleeding, ulceration, and perforation can occur at any time, with or without warning symptoms, in patients treated chronically with NSAID therapy. Although minor upper gastrointestinal problems, such as dyspepsia, are common, usually developing early in therapy, physicians should remain alert for ulceration and bleeding in patients treated chronically with NSAIDs even in the absence of previous GI tract symptoms. In patients observed in clinical trials of several months to two years duration, symptomatic upper GI ulcers, gross bleeding or perforation appear to occur in approximately 1% of patients treated for 3–6 months, and in about 2–4% of patients treated for one year. Physicians should inform patients about the signs and/or symptoms of serious GI toxicity and what steps to take if they occur.
Studies to date have not identified any subset of patients not at risk of developing peptic ulceration and bleeding. Except for a prior history of serious GI events and other risk factors known to be associated with peptic ulcer disease, such as alcoholism, smoking, etc., no risk factors (e.g., age, sex) have been associated with increased risk. Elderly or debilitated patients seem to tolerate ulceration or bleeding less well than other individuals and most spontaneous reports of fatal GI events are in this population. Studies to date are inconclusive concerning the relative risk of various NSAIDs in causing such reactions. High doses of any NSAID probably carry a greater risk of these reactions, although controlled clinical trials showing this do not exist in most cases. In considering the use of relatively large doses (within the recommended dosage range), sufficient benefit should be anticipated to offset the potential increased risk of GI toxicity.

PRECAUTIONS

Renal Effects: As with other nonsteroidal anti-inflammatory drugs, long-term administration of piroxicam to animals has resulted in renal papillary necrosis and other abnormal renal pathology. In humans, there have been reports of acute interstitial nephritis with hematuria, proteinuria, and occasionally, nephrotic syndrome.
A second form of renal toxicity has been seen in patients with prerenal conditions leading to a reduction in renal blood flow or blood volume, where the renal prostaglandins have a supportive role in the maintenance of renal perfusion. In these patients administration of an NSAID may cause a dose-dependent reduction in prostaglandin formation and may precipitate overt renal decompensation. Patients at greatest risk of this reaction are those with impaired renal function, heart failure, liver dysfunction, those taking diuretics, and the elderly. Discontinuation of NSAID therapy is typically followed by recovery to the pretreatment state.
Because of extensive renal excretion of piroxicam and its biotransformation products (less than 5% of the daily dose excreted unchanged, see CLINICAL PHARMACOLOGY), lower doses of piroxicam should be anticipated in patients with impaired renal function, and they should be carefully monitored.
Although other nonsteroidal anti-inflammatory drugs do not have the same direct effects on platelets that aspirin does, all drugs inhibiting prostaglandin biosynthesis do interfere with platelet function to some degree; therefore, patients who may be adversely affected by such an action should be carefully observed when FELDENE is administered.
Because of reports of adverse eye findings with nonsteroidal anti-inflammatory agents, it is recommended that patients who develop visual complaints during treatment with FELDENE have ophthalmic evaluation.
As with other nonsteroidal anti-inflammatory drugs, borderline elevations of one or more liver tests may occur in up to 15% of patients. These abnormalities may progress, may remain essentially unchanged, or may be transient with continued therapy. The SGPT (ALT) test is probably the most sensitive indicator of liver dysfunction. Meaningful (3 times the upper limit of normal) elevations of SGPT or SGOT (AST) occurred in controlled clinical trials in less than 1% of patients. A patient with symptoms and/or signs suggesting liver dysfunction, or in whom an abnormal liver test has occurred, should be evaluated for evidence of the development of more severe hepatic reaction while on therapy with FELDENE. Severe hepatic reactions, including jaundice and cases of fatal hepatitis, have been reported with FELDENE. Although such reactions are rare, if abnormal liver tests persist or worsen, if clinical signs and symptoms consistent with liver disease develop, or if systemic manifestations occur (e.g. eosinophilia, rash, etc.), FELDENE should be discontinued. (See also ADVERSE REACTIONS.)
Although at the recommended dose of 20 mg/day of FELDENE increased fecal blood loss due to gastrointestinal irritation did not occur (see CLINICAL PHARMACOLOGY), in about 4% of the patients treated with FELDENE alone or concomitantly with aspirin, reductions in hemoglobin and hematocrit values were observed. Therefore, these values should be determined if signs or symptoms of anemia occur.
Peripheral edema has been observed in approximately 2% of the patients treated with FELDENE. Therefore, as with other nonsteroidal anti-inflammatory drugs, FELDENE should be used with caution in patients with heart failure, hypertension or other conditions predisposing to fluid retention, since its usage may be associated with a worsening of these conditions.
A combination of dermatological and/or allergic signs and symptoms suggestive of serum sickness have occasionally occurred in conjunction with the use of FELDENE. These include arthralgias, pruritus, fever, fatigue, and rash including vesiculo bullous reactions and exfoliative dermatitis.

Information for Patients

FELDENE, like other drugs of its class, is not free of side effects. The side effects of these drugs can cause discomfort and, rarely, there are more serious side effects, such as gastrointestinal bleeding, which may result in hospitalization and even fatal outcomes.
NSAIDs (Nonsteroidal Anti-Inflammatory Drugs) are often essential agents in the management of arthritis, but they also may be commonly employed for conditions which are less serious.

Continued on next page

Feldene—Cont.

Physicians may wish to discuss with their patients the potential risks (see WARNINGS, PRECAUTIONS, and ADVERSE REACTIONS sections) and likely benefits of NSAID treatment, particularly when the drugs are used for less serious conditions where treatment without NSAIDs may represent an acceptable alternative to both the patient and physician.

Laboratory Tests

Because serious GI tract ulceration and bleeding can occur without warning symptoms, physicians should follow chronically treated patients for the signs and symptoms of ulceration and bleeding and should inform them of the importance of this follow-up (see Risk of GI Ulceration, Bleeding and Perforation with NSAID Therapy).

Drug Interactions

FELDENE is highly protein bound, and, therefore, might be expected to displace other protein-bound drugs. Although this has not occurred in *in vitro* studies with coumarin-type anticoagulants, interactions with coumarin-type anticoagulants have been reported with FELDENE since marketing, therefore, physicians should closely monitor patients for a change in dosage requirements when administering FELDENE to patients on coumarin-type anticoagulants and other highly protein-bound drugs.

Plasma levels of piroxicam are depressed to approximately 80% of their normal values when FELDENE is administered in conjunction with aspirin (3900 mg/day), but concomitant administration of antacids has no effect on piroxicam plasma levels (see CLINICAL PHARMACOLOGY).

Nonsteroidal anti-inflammatory agents, including FELDENE, have been reported to increase steady state plasma lithium levels. It is recommended that plasma lithium levels be monitored when initiating, adjusting and discontinuing FELDENE.

Carcinogenesis, Chronic Animal Toxicity and Impairment of Fertility

Subacute and chronic toxicity studies have been carried out in rats, mice, dogs, and monkeys.

The pathology most often seen was that characteristically associated with the animal toxicology of anti-inflammatory agents: renal papillary necrosis (see PRECAUTIONS) and gastrointestinal lesions.

In classical studies in laboratory animals piroxicam did not show any teratogenic potential.

Reproductive studies revealed no impairment of fertility in animals.

Pregnancy and Nursing Mothers

Like other drugs which inhibit the synthesis and release of prostaglandins, piroxicam increased the incidence of dystocia and delayed parturition in pregnant animals when piroxicam administration was continued late into pregnancy. Gastrointestinal tract toxicity was increased in pregnant females in the last trimester of pregnancy compared to non-pregnant females or females in earlier trimesters of pregnancy.

FELDENE is not recommended for use in nursing mothers or in pregnant women because of the animal findings and since safety for such use has not been established in humans.

Use in Children

Dosage recommendations and indications for use in children have not been established.

ADVERSE REACTIONS

The incidence of adverse reactions to piroxicam is based on clinical trials involving approximately 2300 patients, about 400 of whom were treated for more than one year and 170 for more than two years. About 30% of all patients receiving daily doses of 20 mg of FELDENE experienced side effects. Gastrointestinal symptoms were the most prominent side effects—occurring in approximately 20% of the patients, which in most instances did not interfere with the course of therapy. Of the patients experiencing gastrointestinal side effects, approximately 5% discontinued therapy with an overall incidence of peptic ulceration of about 1%.

Other than the gastrointestinal symptoms, edema, dizziness, headache, changes in hematological parameters, and rash have been reported in a small percentage of patients. Routine ophthalmoscopy and slit-lamp examinations have revealed no evidence of ocular changes in 205 patients followed from 3 to 24 months while on therapy.

Incidence Greater Than 1% The following adverse reactions occurred more frequently than 1 in 100.

Gastrointestinal: stomatitis, anorexia, epigastric distress*, nausea*, constipation, abdominal discomfort, flatulence, diarrhea, abdominal pain, indigestion

Hematological: decreases in hemoglobin* and hematocrit* (see PRECAUTIONS), anemia, leucopenia, eosinophilia

Dermatologic: pruritus, rash

Central Nervous System: dizziness, somnolence, vertigo

Urogenital: BUN and creatinine elevations (see PRECAUTIONS)

Body as a Whole: headache, malaise

Special Senses: tinnitus

Cardiovascular/Respiratory: edema (see PRECAUTIONS)

*Reactions occurring in 3% to 9% of patients treated with FELDENE. Reactions occurring in 1–3% of patients are unmarked.

Incidence Less Than 1% (Causal Relationship Probable)

The following adverse reactions occurred less frequently than 1 in 100. The probability exists that there is a causal relationship between FELDENE and these reactions.

Gastrointestinal: liver function abnormalities, jaundice, hepatitis (see PRECAUTIONS), vomiting, hematemesis, melena, gastrointestinal bleeding, perforation and ulceration (see WARNINGS), dry mouth

Hematological: thrombocytopenia, petechial rash, ecchymosis, bone marrow depression including aplastic anemia, epistaxis

Dermatologic: sweating, erythema, bruising, desquamation, exfoliative dermatitis, erythema multiforme, toxic epidermal necrolysis, Stevens-Johnson syndrome, vesiculo bullous reaction, photoallergic skin reactions

Central Nervous System: depression, insomnia, nervousness

Urogenital: hematuria, proteinuria, interstitial nephritis, renal failure, hyperkalemia, glomerulitis, papillary necrosis, nephrotic syndrome (see PRECAUTIONS)

Body as a Whole: pain (colic), fever, flu-like syndrome (see PRECAUTIONS)

Special Senses: swollen eyes, blurred vision, eye irritations

Cardiovascular/Respiratory: hypertension, worsening of congestive heart failure (see PRECAUTIONS), exacerbation of angina

Metabolic: hypoglycemia, hyperglycemia, weight increase, weight decrease

Hypersensitivity: anaphylaxis, bronchospasm, urticaria/angioedema, vasculitis, "serum sickness" (see PRECAUTIONS)

Incidence Less Than 1% (Causal Relationship Unknown)

Other adverse reactions were reported with a frequency of less than 1 in 100, but a causal relationship between FELDENE and the reaction could not be determined.

Gastrointestinal: pancreatitis

Dermatologic: onycholysis, loss of hair

Central Nervous System: akathisia, hallucinations, mood alterations, dream abnormalities, mental confusion, paresthesias

Urogenital System: dysuria

Body as a Whole: weakness

Cardiovascular/Respiratory: palpitations, dyspnea

Hypersensitivity: positive ANA

Special Senses: transient hearing loss

Hematological: hemolytic anemia

OVERDOSAGE

In the event treatment for overdosage is required the long plasma half-life (see CLINICAL PHARMACOLOGY) of piroxicam should be considered. The absence of experience with acute overdosage precludes characterization of sequelae and recommendation of specific antidotal efficacy at this time. It is reasonable to assume, however, that the standard measures of gastric evacuation and general supportive therapy would apply. In addition to supportive measures, the use of activated charcoal may effectively reduce the absorption and reabsorption of piroxicam. Experiments in dogs have demonstrated that the use of multiple-dose treatments with activated charcoal could reduce the half-life of piroxicam elimination from 27 hours (without charcoal) to 11 hours and reduce the systemic bioavailability of piroxicam by as much as 37% when activated charcoal is given as late as 6 hours after administration of piroxicam.

ADMINISTRATION AND DOSAGE

Rheumatoid Arthritis, Osteoarthritis

It is recommended that FELDENE therapy be initiated and maintained at a single daily dose of 20 mg. If desired the daily dose may be divided. Because of the long half-life of FELDENE, steady-state blood levels are not reached for 7–12 days. Therefore although the therapeutic effects of FELDENE are evident early in treatment, there is a progressive increase in response over several weeks and the effect of therapy should not be assessed for two weeks.

Dosage recommendations and indications for use in children have not been established.

HOW SUPPLIED

FELDENE® Capsules for oral administration

Bottles of 100: 10 mg (NDC 0069-3220-66)
(NDC 0663-3220-66)
(NDC 59012-322-66) maroon and blue # 322
20 mg (NDC 0069-3230-66)
(NDC 59012-323-66) maroon #323
Bottles of 500: 20 mg (NDC 0069-3230-73)
(NDC 0663-3230-73)
(NDC 59012-323-73) maroon #323
Unit dose packages of 100: 20 mg (NDC 0069-3230-41)
(NDC 59012-323-41) maroon #323

©1982 PFIZER INC

69-4100-32-4 Rev. Oct. 1993

Shown in Product Identification Guide, page 330

GEOCILLIN® ℞

[*gē 'ō-sil-ĭn*]

(carbenicillin indanyl sodium)

TABLETS

For Oral Use

DESCRIPTION

Geocillin, a semisynthetic penicillin, is the sodium salt of the indanyl ester of Geopen® (carbenicillin disodium). The chemical name is:

1-(5-Indanyl)-N-(2-carboxy-3,3-dimethyl-7-oxo-4-thia-1-azabicyclo[3.2.0]hept-6-yl)-2-phenylmalonamate monosodium salt.

The structural formula is:

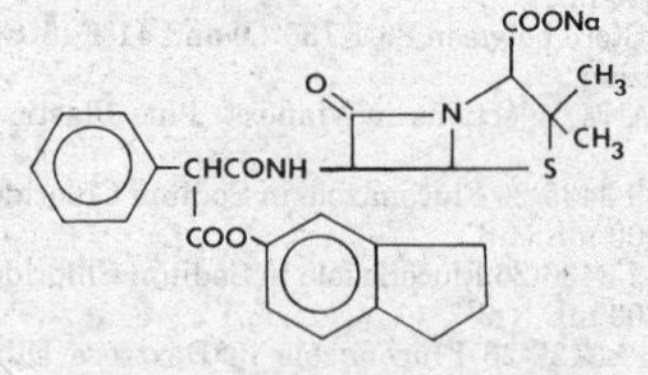

The empirical formula is: $C_{26}H_{25}N_2NaO_6S$ and mol. wt. is 516.55.

Geocillin tablets are yellow, capsule-shaped and film-coated, made of a white crystalline solid. Carbenicillin is freely soluble in water. Each Geocillin tablet contains 382 mg of carbenicillin, 118 mg of indanyl sodium ester. Each Geocillin tablet contains 23 mg of sodium.

Inert ingredients are: glycine; magnesium stearate and sodium lauryl sulfate. May also include the following: hydroxypropyl cellulose; hydroxypropyl methylcellulose; opaspray (which may include Blue 2 Lake, Yellow 6 Lake, Yellow 10 Lake, and other inert ingredients); opadry light yellow (which may contain D&C Yellow 10 Lake, FD&C Yellow 6 Lake and other inert ingredients); opadry clear (which may contain other inert ingredients).

CLINICAL PHARMACOLOGY

Free carbenicillin is the predominant pharmacologically active fraction of Geocillin. Carbenicillin exerts its antibacterial activity by interference with final cell wall synthesis of susceptible bacteria.

Geocillin is acid stable, and rapidly absorbed from the small intestine following oral administration. It provides relatively low plasma concentrations of antibiotic and is primarily excreted in the urine. After absorption, Geocillin is rapidly converted to carbenicillin by hydrolysis of the ester linkage. Following ingestion of a single 500 mg tablet of Geocillin, a peak carbenicillin plasma concentration of approximately 6.5 mcg/ml is reached in 1 hour. About 30% of this dose is excreted in the urine unchanged within 12 hours, with another 6% excreted over the next 12 hours.

In a multiple dose study utilizing volunteers with normal renal function, the following mean urine and serum levels of carbenicillin were achieved:

[See table at bottom of next page]

Microbiology

The antibacterial activity of Geocillin is due to its rapid conversion to carbenicillin by hydrolysis after absorption. Though Geocillin provides substantial *in vitro* activity against a variety of both gram-positive and gram-negative microorganisms, the most important aspect of its profile is in its antipseudomonal and antiproteal activity. Because of the high urine levels obtained following administration, Geocillin has demonstrated clinical efficacy in urinary infections due to susceptible strains of:

Escherichia coli
Proteus mirabilis
Proteus vulgaris
Morganella morganii (formerly *Proteus morganii*)
Pseudomonas species
Providencia rettgeri (formerly *Proteus rettgeri*)
Enterobacter species
Enterococci *(S. faecalis)*

In addition, *in vitro* data, not substantiated by clinical studies, indicate the following pathogens to be usually susceptible to Geocillin:

Staphylococcus species (nonpenicillinase producing)
Streptococcus species

Resistance

Most *Klebsiella* species are usually resistant to the action of Geocillin. Some strains of *Pseudomonas* species have developed resistance to carbenicillin.

Susceptibility Testing

Geopen (carbenicillin disodium) Susceptibility Powder or 100 ug Geopen Susceptibility Discs may be used to deter-

mine microbial susceptibility to Geocillin using one of the following standard methods recommended by the National Committee for Clinical Laboratory Standards:

M2-A3, "Performance Standards for Antimicrobial Disk Susceptibility Tests"

M7-A, "Methods for Dilution Antimicrobial Susceptibility Tests for Bacteria that Grow Aerobically"

M11-A, "Reference Agar Dilution Procedure for Antimicrobial Susceptibility Testing of Anaerobic Bacteria"

M17-P, "Alternative Methods for Antimicrobial Susceptibility Testing of Anaerobic Bacteria"

Tests should be interpreted by the following criteria:

Organisms	Disk Diffusion Zone diameter (mm) Suscept.	Intermed.	Resist.
Enterobacter	≥23	18–22	≤17
Pseudomonas sp.	≥17	14–16	≤13

Organisms	Dilution MIC (µ/ml) Suscept.	Moderately Suscept.	Resist.
Enterobacter	≤16	32	≥64
Pseudomonas sp.	≥128	—	≥156

Interpretations of susceptible, intermediate, and resistant correlate zone size diameters with MIC values. A laboratory report of "susceptible" indicates that the suspected causative microorganism most likely will respond to therapy with carbenicillin. A laboratory report of "resistant" indicates that the infecting microorganism most likely will not respond to therapy. A laboratory report of "moderately susceptible" indicates that the microorganism is most likely susceptible if a high dosage of carbenicillin is used, or if the infection is such that high levels of carbenicillin may be attained as in urine. A report of "intermediate" using the disk diffusion method may be considered an equivocal result, and dilution tests may be indicated.

INDICATIONS AND USAGE

Geocillin (carbenicillin indanyl sodium) is indicated in the treatment of acute and chronic infections of the upper and lower urinary tract and in asymptomatic bacteriuria due to susceptible strains of the following organisms:

Escherichia coli
Proteus mirabilis
Morganella morganii
  (formerly Proteus morganii)
Providencia rettgeri
  (formerly Proteus rettgeri)
Proteus vulgaris
Pseudomonas
Enterobacter
Enterococci

Geocillin is also indicated in the treatment of prostatitis due to susceptible strains of the following organisms:

Escherichia coli
  Enterococcus (S. faecalis)
Proteus mirabilis
Enterobacter sp.

WHEN HIGH AND RAPID BLOOD AND URINE LEVELS OF ANTIBIOTIC ARE INDICATED, THERAPY WITH GEOPEN (CARBENICILLIN DISODIUM) SHOULD BE INITIATED BY PARENTERAL ADMINISTRATION FOLLOWED, AT THE PHYSICIAN'S DISCRETION, BY ORAL THERAPY.

NOTE: Susceptibility testing should be performed prior to and during the course of therapy to detect the possible emergence of resistant organisms which may develop.

CONTRAINDICATIONS

Geocillin is ordinarily contraindicated in patients who have a known penicillin allergy.

WARNINGS

Serious and occasionally fatal hypersensitivity (anaphylactic) reactions have been reported in patients on oral penicillin therapy. Although anaphylaxis is more frequent following parenteral therapy, it has occurred in patients on oral penicillins. These reactions are more apt to occur in individuals with a history of penicillin hypersensitivity and/or a history of sensitivity to multiple allergens.

There have been reports of individuals with a history of penicillin hypersensitivity who have experienced severe hypersensitivity reactions when treated with a cephalosporin, and vice versa. Before initiating therapy with a penicillin, careful inquiry should be made concerning previous hypersensitivity reactions to penicillins, cephalosporins, or other allergens. If an allergic reaction occurs, the drug should be discontinued and the appropriate therapy instituted.

SERIOUS ANAPHYLACTOID REACTIONS REQUIRE IMMEDIATE EMERGENCY TREATMENT WITH EPINEPHRINE. OXYGEN, INTRAVENOUS STEROIDS AND AIRWAY MANAGEMENT, INCLUDING INTUBATION, SHOULD ALSO BE ADMINISTERED AS INDICATED.

PRECAUTIONS

General: As with any penicillin preparation, an allergic response, including anaphylaxis, may occur particularly in a hypersensitive individual.

Long term use of Geocillin may result in the overgrowth of nonsusceptible organisms. If superinfection occurs during therapy, appropriate measures should be taken.

Since carbenicillin is primarily excreted by the kidney, patients with severe renal impairment (creatinine clearance of less than 10 ml/min) will not achieve therapeutic urine levels of carbenicillin.

In patients with creatinine clearance of 10–20 ml/min it may be necessary to adjust dosage to prevent accumulation of drug.

Laboratory Tests: As with other penicillins, periodic assessment of organ system function including renal, hepatic, and hematopoietic systems is recommended during prolonged therapy.

Drug Interactions: Geocillin (carbenicillin indanyl sodium) blood levels may be increased and prolonged by concurrent administration of probenecid.

Carcinogenesis, Mutagenesis, Impairment of Fertility: There are no long-term animal or human studies to evaluate carcinogenic potential. Rats fed 250–1000 mg/kg/day for 18 months developed mild liver pathology (e.g., bile duct hyperplasia) at all dose levels, but there was no evidence of drug-related neoplasia. Geocillin administered at daily doses ranging to 1000 mg/kg had no apparent effect on the fertility or reproductive performance of rats.

Pregnancy Category B: Reproduction studies have been performed at dose levels of 1000 or 500 mg/kg in rats, 200 mg/kg in mice, and at 500 mg/kg in monkeys with no harm to fetus due to Geocillin. There are, however, no adequate and well controlled studies in pregnant women. Because animal reproduction studies are not always predictive of human response, this drug should be used during pregnancy only if clearly needed.

Labor and Delivery: It is not known whether the use of Geocillin in humans during labor or delivery has immediate or delayed adverse effects on the fetus, prolongs the duration of labor, or increases the likelihood that forceps delivery or other obstetrical intervention or resuscitation of the newborn will be necessary.

Nursing Mothers: Carbenicillin class antibiotics are excreted in milk although the amounts excreted are unknown; therefore, caution should be exercised if administered to a nursing woman.

Pediatric Use: Since only limited clinical data is available to date in children, the safety of Geocillin administration in this age group has not yet been established.

ADVERSE REACTIONS

The following adverse reactions have been reported as possibly related to Geocillin administration in controlled studies which include 344 patients receiving Geocillin.

Gastrointestinal: The most frequent adverse reactions associated with Geocillin therapy are related to the gastrointestinal tract. Nausea, bad taste, diarrhea, vomiting, flatulence, and glossitis were reported. Abdominal cramps, dry mouth, furry tongue, rectal bleeding, anorexia, and unspecified epigastric distress were rarely reported.

Dermatologic: Hypersensitivity reactions such as skin rash, urticaria, and less frequently pruritus.

Hematologic: As with other penicillins, anemia, thrombocytopenia, leukopenia, neutropenia, and eosinophilia have infrequently been observed. The clinical significance of these abnormalities is not known.

Miscellaneous: Other reactions rarely reported were hyperthermia, headache, itchy eyes, vaginitis, and loose stools.

Abnormalities of Hepatic Function Tests: Mild SGOT elevations have been observed following Geocillin administration.

OVERDOSAGE

Geocillin is generally nontoxic. Geocillin when taken in excessive amounts may produce mild gastrointestinal irritation. The drug is rapidly excreted in the urine and symptoms are transitory. The usual symptoms of anaphylaxis may occur in hypersensitive individuals.

Carbenicillin blood levels achievable with Geocillin are very low, and toxic reactions as a function of overdosage should not occur systematically. The oral LD_{50} in mice is 3,600 mg/kg, in rats 2,000 mg/kg, and in dogs is in excess of 500 mg/kg. The lethal human dose is not known.

Although never reported, the possibility of accumulation of indanyl should be considered when large amounts of Geocillin are ingested. Free indole, which is a phenol derivative, may be potentially toxic. In general 8–15 grams of phenol, and presumably a similar amount of indole, are required orally before toxicity (peripheral vascular collapse) may occur. The metabolic by-products of indole are nontoxic. In patients with hepatic failure it may be possible for unmetabolized indole to accumulate.

The metabolic by-products of Geocillin, indanyl sulfate and glucuronide, as well as free carbenicillin, are dialyzable.

DOSAGE AND ADMINISTRATION

Geocillin is available as a coated tablet to be administered orally.

Usual Adult Dose

URINARY TRACT INFECTIONS	
Escherichia coli, Proteus species, and Enterobacter	1–2 tablets 4 times daily
Pseudomonas and Enterococcus	2 tablets 4 times daily
PROSTATITIS	
Escherichia coli, Proteus mirabilis, Enterobacter and Enterococcus	2 tablets 4 times daily

HOW SUPPLIED

Geocillin is available as film-coated tablets in bottles of 100's (NDC 0049-1430-66), and unit-dose packages of 100 (10 × 10's) (NDC 0049-1430-41). Each tablet contains carbenicillin indanyl sodium equivalent to 382 mg of carbenicillin.

Revised Sept. 1991   69-1970-00-2

GLUCOTROL®   ℞

[glū 'kă-trōl]
(glipizide)
TABLETS
For Oral Use

DESCRIPTION

GLUCOTROL (glipizide) is an oral blood-glucose-lowering drug of the sulfonylurea class.

The Chemical Abstracts name of glipizide is 1-cyclohexyl-3-[[p- [2-(5-methylpyrazinecarboxamido)ethyl]phenyl] sulfonyl]urea. The molecular formula is $C_{21}H_{27}N_5O_4S$; the molecular weight is 445.55; the structural formula is shown below:

Glipizide is a whitish, odorless powder with a pKa of 5.9. It is insoluble in water and alcohols, but soluble in 0.1 N

Continued on next page

Mean Urine Concentration of Carbenicillin mcg/ml Hours After Initial Dose

DRUG	DOSE	0–3	3–6	6–24
Geocillin	1 tablet q.6 hr	1130	352	292
Geocillin	2 tablets q.6 hr	1428	789	809

Mean serum concentrations of carbenicillin in this study for these dosages are:

Mean Serum Concentration mcg/ml Hours After Initial Dose

DRUG	DOSE	1/2	1	2	4	6	24	25	26	28
Geocillin	1 tablet q.6 hr	5.1	6.5	3.2	1.9	0.0	0.4	8.8	5.4	0.4
Geocillin	2 tablets q.6 hr	6.1	9.6	7.9	2.6	0.4	0.8	13.2	12.8	3.8

Glucotrol—Cont.

NaOH; it is freely soluble in dimethylformamide. GLUCOTROL tablets for oral use are available in 5 and 10 mg strengths.
Inert ingredients are: colloidal silicon dioxide; lactose; microcrystalline cellulose; starch; stearic acid.

CLINICAL PHARMACOLOGY

Mechanism of Action: The primary mode of action of GLUCOTROL in experimental animals appears to be the stimulation of insulin secretion from the beta cells of pancreatic islet tissue and is thus dependent on functioning beta cells in the pancreatic islets. In humans GLUCOTROL appears to lower the blood glucose acutely by stimulating the release of insulin from the pancreas, an effect dependent upon functioning beta cells in the pancreatic islets. The mechanism by which GLUCOTROL lowers blood glucose during long-term administration has not been clearly established. In man, stimulation of insulin secretion by GLUCOTROL in response to a meal is undoubtedly of major importance. Fasting insulin levels are not elevated even on long-term GLUCOTROL administration, but the postprandial insulin response continues to be enhanced after at least 6 months of treatment. The insulinotropic response to a meal occurs within 30 minutes after an oral dose of GLUCOTROL in diabetic patients, but elevated insulin levels do not persist beyond the time of the meal challenge. Extrapancreatic effects may play a part in the mechanism of action of oral sulfonylurea hypoglycemic drugs.
Blood sugar control persists in some patients for up to 24 hours after a single dose of GLUCOTROL, even though plasma levels have declined to a small fraction of peak levels by that time (see Pharmacokinetics below).
Some patients fail to respond initially, or gradually lose their responsiveness to sulfonylurea drugs, including GLUCOTROL. Alternatively, GLUCOTROL may be effective in some patients who have not responded or have ceased to respond to other sulfonylureas.
Other Effects: It has been shown that GLUCOTROL therapy was effective in controlling blood sugar without deleterious changes in the plasma lipoprotein profiles of patients treated for NIDDM.
In a placebo-controlled, crossover study in normal volunteers, GLUCOTROL had no antidiuretic activity, and, in fact, led to a slight increase in free water clearance.
Pharmacokinetics: Gastrointestinal absorption of GLUCOTROL in man is uniform, rapid, and essentially complete. Peak plasma concentrations occur 1–3 hours after a single oral dose. The half-life of elimination ranges from 2–4 hours in normal subjects, whether given intravenously or orally. The metabolic and excretory patterns are similar with the two routes of administration, indicating that first-pass metabolism is not significant. GLUCOTROL does not accumulate in plasma on repeated oral administration. Total absorption and disposition of an oral dose was unaffected by food in normal volunteers, but absorption was delayed by about 40 minutes. Thus GLUCOTROL was more effective when administered about 30 minutes before, rather than with, a test meal in diabetic patients. Protein binding was studied in serum from volunteers who received either oral or intravenous GLUCOTROL and found to be 98–99% one hour after either route of administration. The apparent volume of distribution of GLUCOTROL after intravenous administration was 11 liters, indicative of localization within the extracellular fluid compartment. In mice no GLUCOTROL or metabolites were detectable autoradiographically in the brain or spinal cord of males or females, nor in the fetuses of pregnant females. In another study, however, very small amounts of radioactivity were detected in the fetuses of rats given labelled drug.
The metabolism of GLUCOTROL is extensive and occurs mainly in the liver. The primary metabolites are inactive hydroxylation products and polar conjugates and are excreted mainly in the urine. Less than 10% unchanged GLUCOTROL is found in the urine.

INDICATIONS AND USAGE

GLUCOTROL is indicated as an adjunct to diet for the control of hyperglycemia and its associated symptomatology in patients with non-insulin-dependent diabetes mellitus (NIDDM; type II), formerly known as maturity-onset diabetes, after an adequate trial of dietary therapy has proved unsatisfactory.
In initiating treatment for non-insulin-dependent diabetes, diet should be emphasized as the primary form of treatment. Caloric restriction and weight loss are essential in the obese diabetic patient. Proper dietary management alone may be effective in controlling the blood glucose and symptoms of hyperglycemia. The importance of regular physical activity should also be stressed, and cardiovascular risk factors should be identified, and corrective measures taken where possible.
If this treatment program fails to reduce symptoms and/or blood glucose, the use of an oral sulfonylurea or insulin should be considered. Use of GLUCOTROL must be viewed by both the physician and patient as a treatment in addition to diet, and not as a substitute for diet or as a convenient mechanism for avoiding dietary restraint. Furthermore, loss of blood glucose control on diet alone also may be transient, thus requiring only short-term administration of GLUCOTROL.
During maintenance programs, GLUCOTROL should be discontinued if satisfactory lowering of blood glucose is no longer achieved. Judgments should be based on regular clinical and laboratory evaluations.
In considering the use of GLUCOTROL in asymptomatic patients, it should be recognized that controlling blood glucose in non-insulin-dependent diabetes has not been definitely established to be effective in preventing the long-term cardiovascular or neural complications of diabetes.

CONTRAINDICATIONS

GLUCOTROL is contraindicated in patients with:
1. Known hypersensitivity to the drug.
2. Diabetic ketoacidosis, with or without coma. This condition should be treated with insulin.

WARNINGS

SPECIAL WARNING ON INCREASED RISK OF CARDIOVASCULAR MORTALITY: The administration of oral hypoglycemic drugs has been reported to be associated with increased cardiovascular mortality as compared to treatment with diet alone or diet plus insulin. This warning is based on the study conducted by the University Group Diabetes Program (UGDP), a long-term prospective clinical trial designed to evaluate the effectiveness of glucose-lowering drugs in preventing or delaying vascular complications in patients with non-insulin-dependent diabetes. The study involved 823 patients who were randomly assigned to one of four treatment groups (*Diabetes,* 19, supp. 2: 747–830, 1970). UGDP reported that patients treated for 5 to 8 years with diet plus a fixed dose of tolbutamide (1.5 grams per day) had a rate of cardiovascular mortality approximately $2^1/_2$ times that of patients treated with diet alone. A significant increase in total mortality was not observed, but the use of tolbutamide was discontinued based on the increase in cardiovascular mortality, thus limiting the opportunity for the study to show an increase in overall mortality. Despite controversy regarding the interpretation of these results, the findings of the UGDP study provide an adequate basis for this warning. The patient should be informed of the potential risks and advantages of GLUCOTROL and of alternative modes of therapy.

Although only one drug in the sulfonylurea class (tolbutamide) was included in this study, it is prudent from a safety standpoint to consider that this warning may also apply to other oral hypoglycemic drugs in this class, in view of their close similarities in mode of action and chemical structure.

PRECAUTIONS

General

Renal and Hepatic Disease: The metabolism and excretion of GLUCOTROL may be slowed in patients with impaired renal and/or hepatic function. If hypoglycemia should occur in such patients, it may be prolonged and appropriate management should be instituted.
Hypoglycemia: All sulfonylurea drugs are capable of producing severe hypoglycemia. Proper patient selection, dosage, and instructions are important to avoid hypoglycemic episodes. Renal or hepatic insufficiency may cause elevated blood levels of GLUCOTROL and the latter may also diminish gluconeogenic capacity, both of which increase the risk of serious hypoglycemic reactions. Elderly, debilitated or malnourished patients, and those with adrenal or pituitary insufficiency are particularly susceptible to the hypoglycemic action of glucose-lowering drugs. Hypoglycemia may be difficult to recognize in the elderly, and in people who are taking beta-adrenergic blocking drugs. Hypoglycemia is more likely to occur when caloric intake is deficient, after severe or prolonged exercise, when alcohol is ingested, or when more than one glucose-lowering drug is used.
Loss of Control of Blood Glucose: When a patient stabilized on any diabetic regimen is exposed to stress such as fever, trauma, infection, or surgery, a loss of control may occur. At such times, it may be necessary to discontinue GLUCOTROL and administer insulin.
The effectiveness of any oral hypoglycemic drug, including GLUCOTROL, in lowering blood glucose to a desired level decreases in many patients over a period of time, which may be due to progression of the severity of the diabetes or to diminished responsiveness to the drug. This phenomenon is known as secondary failure, to distinguish it from primary failure in which the drug is ineffective in an individual patient when first given.
Laboratory Tests: Blood and urine glucose should be monitored periodically. Measurement of glycosylated hemoglobin may be useful.
Information for Patients: Patients should be informed of the potential risks and advantages of GLUCOTROL and of alternative modes of therapy. They should also be informed about the importance of adhering to dietary instructions, of a regular exercise program, and of regular testing of urine and/or blood glucose.
The risks of hypoglycemia, its symptoms and treatment, and conditions that predispose to its development should be explained to patients and responsible family members. Primary and secondary failure should also be explained.
Drug Interactions: The hypoglycemic action of sulfonylureas may be potentiated by certain drugs including nonsteroidal anti-inflammatory agents, some azoles, and other drugs that are highly protein bound, salicylates, sulfonamides, chloramphenicol, probenecid, coumarins, monoamine oxidase inhibitors, and beta adrenergic blocking agents. When such drugs are administered to a patient receiving GLUCOTROL, the patient should be observed closely for hypoglycemia. When such drugs are withdrawn from a patient receiving GLUCOTROL, the patient should be observed closely for loss of control. *In vitro* binding studies with human serum proteins indicate that GLUCOTROL binds differently than tolbutamide and does not interact with salicylate or dicumarol. However, caution must be exercised in extrapolating these findings to the clinical situation and in the use of GLUCOTROL with these drugs.
Certain drugs tend to produce hyperglycemia and may lead to loss of control. These drugs include the thiazides and other diuretics, corticosteroids, phenothiazines, thyroid products, estrogens, oral contraceptives, phenytoin, nicotinic acid, sympathomimetics, calcium channel blocking drugs, and isoniazid. When such drugs are administered to a patient receiving GLUCOTROL, the patient should be closely observed for loss of control. When such drugs are withdrawn from a patient receiving GLUCOTROL, the patient should be observed closely for hypoglycemia.
A potential interaction between oral miconazole and oral hypoglycemic agents leading to severe hypoglycemia has been reported. Whether this interaction also occurs with the intravenous, topical, or vaginal preparations of miconazole is not known. The effect of concomitant administration of DIFLUCAN (fluconazole) and GLUCOTROL has been demonstrated in a placebo-controlled crossover study in normal volunteers. All subjects received GLUCOTROL alone and following treatment of 100 mg of DIFLUCAN as a single daily oral dose for 7 days. The mean percentage increase in the GLUCOTROL AUC after fluconazole administration was 56.9% (range: 35 to 81).
Carcinogenesis, Mutagenesis, Impairment of Fertility: A twenty month study in rats and an eighteen month study in mice at doses up to 75 times the maximum human dose revealed no evidence of drug-related carcinogenicity. Bacterial and *in vivo* mutagenicity tests were uniformly negative. Studies in rats of both sexes at doses up to 75 times the human dose showed no effects on fertility.
Pregnancy: Pregnancy Category C: GLUCOTROL (glipizide) was found to be mildly fetotoxic in rat reproductive studies at all dose levels (5–50 mg/kg). This fetotoxicity has been similarly noted with other sulfonylureas, such as tolbutamide and tolazamide. The effect is perinatal and believed to be directly related to the pharmacologic (hypoglycemic) action of GLUCOTROL. In studies in rats and rabbits no teratogenic effects were found. There are no adequate and well controlled studies in pregnant women. GLUCOTROL should be used during pregnancy only if the potential benefit justifies the potential risk to the fetus.
Because recent information suggests that abnormal blood glucose levels during pregnancy are associated with a higher incidence of congenital abnormalities, many experts recommend that insulin be used during pregnancy to maintain blood glucose levels as close to normal as possible.
Nonteratogenic Effects: Prolonged severe hypoglycemia (4 to 10 days) has been reported in neonates born to mothers who were receiving a sulfonylurea drug at the time of delivery. This has been reported more frequently with the use of agents with prolonged half-lives. If GLUCOTROL is used during pregnancy, it should be discontinued at least one month before the expected delivery date.
Nursing Mothers: Although it is not known whether GLUCOTROL is excreted in human milk, some sulfonylurea drugs are known to be excreted in human milk. Because the potential for hypoglycemia in nursing infants may exist, a decision should be made whether to discontinue nursing or to discontinue the drug, taking into account the importance of the drug to the mother. If the drug is discontinued and if diet alone is inadequate for controlling blood glucose, insulin therapy should be considered.
Pediatric Use: Safety and effectiveness in children have not been established.

ADVERSE REACTIONS

In U.S. and foreign controlled studies, the frequency of serious adverse reactions reported was very low. Of 702 patients, 11.8% reported adverse reactions and in only 1.5% was GLUCOTROL discontinued.
Hypoglycemia: See PRECAUTIONS and OVERDOSAGE sections.
Gastrointestinal: Gastrointestinal disturbances are the most common reactions. Gastrointestinal complaints were

reported with the following approximate incidence: nausea and diarrhea, one in seventy; constipation and gastralgia, one in one hundred. They appear to be dose-related and may disappear on division or reduction of dosage. Cholestatic jaundice may occur rarely with sulfonylureas: GLUCOTROL should be discontinued if this occurs.

Dermatologic: Allergic skin reactions including erythema, morbilliform or maculopapular eruptions, urticaria, pruritus, and eczema have been reported in about one in seventy patients. These may be transient and may disappear despite continued use of GLUCOTROL; if skin reactions persist, the drug should be discontinued. Porphyria cutanea tarda and photosensitivity reactions have been reported with sulfonylureas.

Hematologic: Leukopenia, agranulocytosis, thrombocytopenia, hemolytic anemia, aplastic anemia, and pancytopenia have been reported with sulfonylureas.

Metabolic: Hepatic porphyria and disulfiram-like reactions have been reported with sulfonylureas. In the mouse, GLUCOTROL pretreatment did not cause an accumulation of acetaldehyde after ethanol administration. Clinical experience to date has shown that GLUCOTROL has an extremely low incidence of disulfiram-like alcohol reactions.

Endocrine Reactions: Cases of hyponatremia and the syndrome of inappropriate antidiuretic hormone (SIADH) secretion have been reported with this and other sulfonylureas.

Miscellaneous: Dizziness, drowsiness, and headache have each been reported in about one in fifty patients treated with GLUCOTROL. They are usually transient and seldom require discontinuance of therapy.

Laboratory Tests: The pattern of laboratory test abnormalities observed with GLUCOTROL was similar to that for other sulfonylureas. Occasional mild to moderate elevations of SGOT, LDH, alkaline phosphatase, BUN and creatinine were noted. One case of jaundice was reported. The relationship of these abnormalities to GLUCOTROL is uncertain, and they have rarely been associated with clinical symptoms.

OVERDOSAGE

There is no well documented experience with GLUCOTROL overdosage. The acute oral toxicity was extremely low in all species tested (LD_{50} greater than 4 g/kg).

Overdosage of sulfonylureas including GLUCOTROL can produce hypoglycemia. Mild hypoglycemic symptoms without loss of consciousness or neurologic findings should be treated aggressively with oral glucose and adjustments in drug dosage and/or meal patterns. Close monitoring should continue until the physician is assured that the patient is out of danger. Severe hypoglycemic reactions with coma, seizure, or other neurological impairment occur infrequently, but constitute medical emergencies requiring immediate hospitalization. If hypoglycemic coma is diagnosed or suspected, the patient should be given a rapid intravenous injection of concentrated (50%) glucose solution. This should be followed by a continuous infusion of a more dilute (10%) glucose solution at a rate that will maintain the blood glucose at a level above 100 mg/dL. Patients should be closely monitored for a minimum of 24 to 48 hours since hypoglycemia may recur after apparent clinical recovery. Clearance of GLUCOTROL from plasma would be prolonged in persons with liver disease. Because of the extensive protein binding of GLUCOTROL, dialysis is unlikely to be of benefit.

DOSAGE AND ADMINISTRATION

There is no fixed dosage regimen for the management of diabetes mellitus with GLUCOTROL or any other hypoglycemic agent. In addition to the usual monitoring of urinary glucose, the patient's blood glucose must also be monitored periodically to determine the minimum effective dose for the patient; to detect primary failure, i.e., inadequate lowering of blood glucose at the maximum recommended dose of medication; and to detect secondary failure, i.e., loss of an adequate blood-glucose-lowering response after an initial period of effectiveness. Glycosylated hemoglobin levels may also be of value in monitoring the patient's response to therapy.

Short-term administration of GLUCOTROL may be sufficient during periods of transient loss of control in patients usually controlled well on diet.

In general, GLUCOTROL should be given approximately 30 minutes before a meal to achieve the greatest reduction in postprandial hyperglycemia.

Initial Dose: The recommended starting dose is 5 mg, given before breakfast. Geriatric patients or those with liver disease may be started on 2.5 mg.

Titration: Dosage adjustments should ordinarily be in increments of 2.5–5 mg, as determined by blood glucose response. At least several days should elapse between titration steps. If response to a single dose is not satisfactory, dividing that dose may prove effective. The maximum recommended once daily dose is 15 mg. Doses above 15 mg should ordinarily be divided and given before meals of adequate caloric content. The maximum recommended total daily dose is 40 mg.

Maintenance: Some patients may be effectively controlled on a once-a-day regimen, while others show better response with divided dosing. Total daily doses above 15 mg should ordinarily be divided. Total daily doses above 30 mg have been safely given on a b.i.d. basis to long-term patients.

In elderly patients, debilitated or malnourished patients, and patients with impaired renal or hepatic function, the initial and maintenance dosing should be conservative to avoid hypoglycemic reactions (see PRECAUTIONS section).

Patients Receiving Insulin: As with other sulfonylurea-class hypoglycemics, many stable non-insulin-dependent diabetic patients receiving insulin may be safely placed on GLUCOTROL. When transferring patients from insulin to GLUCOTROL, the following general guidelines should be considered:

For patients whose daily insulin requirement is 20 units or less, insulin may be discontinued and GLUCOTROL therapy may begin at usual dosages. Several days should elapse between GLUCOTROL titration steps.

For patients whose daily insulin requirement is greater than 20 units, the insulin dose should be reduced by 50% and GLUCOTROL therapy may begin at usual dosages. Subsequent reductions in insulin dosage should depend on individual patient response. Several days should elapse between GLUCOTROL titration steps.

During the insulin withdrawal period, the patient should test urine samples for sugar and ketone bodies at least three times daily. Patients should be instructed to contact the prescriber immediately if these tests are abnormal. In some cases, especially when patient has been receiving greater than 40 units of insulin daily, it may be advisable to consider hospitalization during the transition period.

Patients Receiving Other Oral Hypoglycemic Agents: As with other sulfonylurea-class hypoglycemics, no transition period is necessary when transferring patients to GLUCOTROL. Patients should be observed carefully (1–2 weeks) for hypoglycemia when being transferred from longer half-life sulfonylureas (e.g., chlorpropamide) to GLUCOTROL due to potential overlapping of drug effect.

HOW SUPPLIED

GLUCOTROL tablets are white, dye-free, scored, diamond-shaped, and imprinted as follows:

5 mg–Pfizer 411; 10 mg–Pfizer 412.

5 mg Bottles: 100's (NDC 0049-4110-66) (NDC 59012-411-66);

500's (NDC 0049-4110-73) (NDC 59012-411-73);

UNIT DOSE 100's (NDC 0049-4110-41) (NDC 59012-411-41).

10 mg Bottles: 100's (NDC 0049-4120-66) (NDC 59012-412-66);

500's (NDC 0049-4120-73) (NDC 59012-412-73);

UNIT DOSE 100's (NDC 0049-4120-41) (NDC 59012-412-41).

RECOMMENDED STORAGE: Store below 86°F (30°C).

CAUTION: Federal law prohibits dispensing without a prescription.

Rev. September 1993 69-4227-00-9

Shown in Product Identification Guide, page 330

GLUCOTROL XL® ℞

(glipizide)

Extended Release Tablets

For Oral Use

DESCRIPTION

Glipizide is an oral blood-glucose-lowering drug of the sulfonylurea class.

The Chemical Abstracts name of glipizide is 1-cyclohexyl-3-[[p-[2-(5-methylpyrazinecarboxamido)ethyl] phenyl]sulfonyl]urea. The molecular formula is $C_{21}H_{27}N_5O_4S$; the molecular weight is 445.55; the structural formula is shown below:

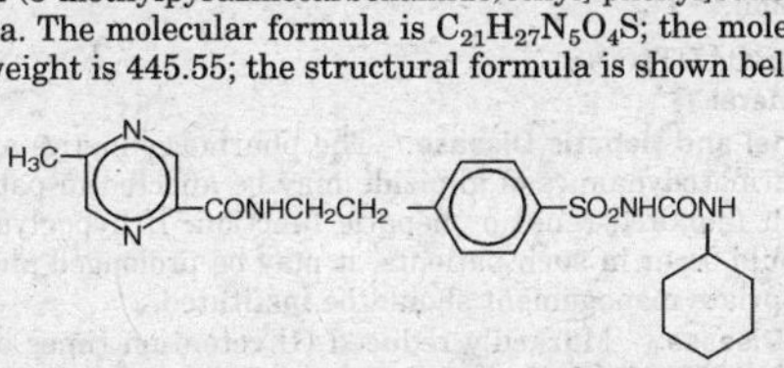

Glipizide is a whitish, odorless powder with a pKa of 5.9. It is insoluble in water and alcohols, but soluble in 0.1 *N* NaOH; it is freely soluble in dimethylformamide. GLUCOTROL XL® is a registered trademark for glipizide GITS. Glipizide GITS (Gastrointestinal Therapeutic System) is formulated as a once-a-day controlled release tablet for oral use and is designed to deliver 5 or 10 mg of glipizide. Inert ingredients in the formulations are: polyethylene oxide, hydroxypropyl methylcellulose, magnesium stearate, sodium chloride, red ferric oxide, cellulose acetate, polyethylene glycol, opadry white (YS-2-7063) and black ink (S-1-8106).

System Components and Performance

GLUCOTROL XL Extended Release Tablet is similar in appearance to a conventional tablet. It consists, however, of an osmotically active drug core surrounded by a semipermeable membrane. The core itself is divided into two layers: an "active" layer containing the drug, and a "push" layer containing pharmacologically inert (but osmotically active) components. The membrane surrounding the tablet is permeable to water but not to drug or osmotic excipients. As water from the gastrointestinal tract enters the tablet, pressure increases in the osmotic layer and "pushes" against the drug layer, resulting in the release of drug through a small, laser-drilled orifice in the membrane on the drug side of the tablet.

The GLUCOTROL XL Extended Release Tablet is designed to provide a controlled rate of delivery of glipizide into the gastrointestinal lumen which is independent of pH or gastrointestinal motility. The function of the GLUCOTROL XL Extended Release Tablet depends upon the existence of an osmotic gradient between the contents of the bi-layer core and fluid in the GI tract. Drug delivery is essentially constant as long as the osmotic gradient remains constant, and then gradually falls to zero. The biologically inert components of the tablet remain intact during GI transit and are eliminated in the feces as an insoluble shell.

CLINICAL PHARMACOLOGY

Mechanism of Action: Glipizide appears to lower blood glucose acutely by stimulating the release of insulin from the pancreas, an effect dependent upon functioning beta cells in the pancreatic islets. Extrapancreatic effects also may play a part in the mechanism of action of oral sulfonylurea hypoglycemic drugs. Two extrapancreatic effects shown to be important in the action of glipizide are an increase in insulin sensitivity and a decrease in hepatic glucose production. However, the mechanism by which glipizide lowers blood glucose during long-term administration has not been clearly established. Stimulation of insulin secretion by glipizide in response to a meal is of major importance. The insulinotropic response to a meal is enhanced with GLUCOTROL XL administration in diabetic patients. The postprandial insulin and C-peptide responses continue to be enhanced after at least 6 months of treatment. In 2 randomized, double-blind, dose-response studies comprising a total of 347 patients, there was no significant increase in fasting insulin in all GLUCOTROL XL-treated patients combined compared to placebo, although minor elevations were observed at some doses. There was no increase in fasting insulin over the long term.

Some patients fail to respond initially, or gradually lose their responsiveness to sulfonylurea drugs, including glipizide. Alternatively, glipizide may be effective in some patients who have not responded or have ceased to respond to other sulfonylureas.

Effects on Blood Glucose

The effectiveness of GLUCOTROL XL Extended Release Tablets in NIDDM at doses from 5-60 mg once daily has been evaluated in 4 therapeutic clinical trials each with long-term open extensions involving a total of 598 patients. Once daily administration of 5, 10 and 20 mg produced statistically significant reductions from placebo in hemoglobin A_{1C}, fasting plasma glucose and postprandial glucose in mild to severe NIDDM patients. In a pooled analysis of the patients treated with 5 mg and 20 mg, the relationship between dose and GLUCOTROL XL's effect of reducing hemoglobin A_{1C} was not established. However, in the case of fasting plasma glucose patients treated with 20 mg had a statistically significant reduction of fasting plasma glucose compared to the 5 mg-treated group.

The reductions in hemoglobin A_{1C} and fasting plasma glucose were similar in younger and older patients. Efficacy of GLUCOTROL XL was not affected by gender, race or weight (as assessed by body mass index). In long term extension trials, efficacy of GLUCOTROL XL was maintained in 81% of patients for up to 12 months.

In an open, two-way crossover study 132 patients were randomly assigned to either GLUCOTROL XL or Glucotrol® for 8 weeks and then crossed over to the other drug for an additional 8 weeks. GLUCOTROL XL administration resulted in significantly lower fasting plasma glucose levels and equivalent hemoglobin A_{1C} levels, as compared to Glucotrol.

Other Effects: It has been shown that GLUCOTROL XL therapy is effective in controlling blood glucose without deleterious changes in the plasma lipoprotein profiles of patients treated for NIDDM.

In a placebo-controlled, crossover study in normal volunteers, glipizide had no anti-diuretic activity, and, in fact, led to a slight increase in free water clearance.

Pharmacokinetics and Metabolism: Glipizide is rapidly and completely absorbed following oral administration in an immediate release dosage form. The absolute bioavailability of glipizide was 100% after single oral doses in patients with NIDDM. Beginning 2 to 3 hours after administration of GLUCOTROL XL Extended Release Tablets, plasma drug concentrations gradually rise reaching maximum concentrations within 6 to 12 hours after dosing. With subsequent once daily dosing of GLUCOTROL XL Extended Release

Continued on next page

Glucotrol XL—Cont.

Tablets, effective plasma glipizide concentrations are maintained throughout the 24 hour dosing interval with less peak to trough fluctuation than that observed with twice daily dosing of immediate release glipizide. The mean relative bioavailability of glipizide in 21 males with NIDDM after administration of 20 mg GLUCOTROL XL Extended Release Tablets, compared to immediate release Glucotrol (10 mg given twice daily), was 90% at steady-state. Steady-state plasma concentrations were achieved by at least the fifth day of dosing with GLUCOTROL XL Extended Release Tablets in 21 males with NIDDM and patients younger than 65 years. Approximately 1 to 2 days longer were required to reach steady-state in 24 elderly (≥65 years) males and females with NIDDM. No accumulation of drug was observed in patients with NIDDM during chronic dosing with GLUCOTROL XL Extended Release Tablets. Administration of GLUCOTROL XL with food has no effect on the 2 to 3 hour lag time in drug absorption. In a single dose, food effect study in 21 healthy male subjects, the administration of GLUCOTROL XL immediately before a high fat breakfast resulted in a 40% increase in the glipizide mean Cmax value, which was significant, but the effect on the AUC was not significant. There was no change in glucose response between the fed and fasting state. Markedly reduced GI retention times of the GLUCOTROL XL tablets over prolonged periods (e.g., short bowel syndrome) may influence the pharmacokinetic profile of the drug and potentially result in lower plasma concentrations. In a multiple dose study in 26 males with NIDDM, the pharmacokinetics of glipizide were linear over the dose range of 5 to 60 mg of GLUCOTROL XL in that the plasma drug concentrations increased proportionately with dose. In a single dose study in 24 healthy subjects, four 5 mg, two 10 mg, and one 20 mg GLUCOTROL XL Extended Release Tablets were bioequivalent.

Glipizide is eliminated primarily by hepatic biotransformation: less than 10% of a dose is excreted as unchanged drug in urine and feces; approximately 90% of a dose is excreted as biotransformation products in urine (80%) and feces (10%). The major metabolites of glipizide are products of aromatic hydroxylation and have no hypoglycemic activity. A minor metabolite which accounts for less than 2% of a dose, an acetylamino-ethyl benzene derivative, is reported to have 1/10 to 1/3 as much hypoglycemic activity as the parent compound. The mean total body clearance of glipizide was approximately 3 liters per hour after single intravenous doses in patients with NIDDM. The mean apparent volume of distribution was approximately 10 liters. Glipizide is 98–99% bound to serum proteins, primarily to albumin. The mean terminal elimination half-life of glipizide ranged from 2 to 5 hours after single or multiple doses in patients with NIDDM. There were no significant differences in the pharmacokinetics of glipizide after single dose administration to older diabetic subjects compared to younger healthy subjects. There is only limited information regarding the effects of renal impairment on the disposition of glipizide, and no information regarding the effects of hepatic disease. However, since glipizide is highly protein bound and hepatic biotransformation is the predominant route of elimination, the pharmacokinetics and/or pharmacodynamics of glipizide may be altered in patients with renal or hepatic impairment.

In mice no glipizide or metabolites were detectable autoradiographically in the brain or spinal cord of males or females, nor in the fetuses of pregnant females. In another study, however, very small amounts of radioactivity were detected in the fetuses of rats given labelled drug.

INDICATIONS AND USAGE

GLUCOTROL XL is indicated as an adjunct to diet for the control of hyperglycemia and its associated symptomatology in patients with non-insulin-dependent diabetes mellitus (NIDDM; type II), formerly known as maturity-onset diabetes, after an adequate trial of dietary therapy has proved unsatisfactory. GLUCOTROL XL is indicated when diet alone has been unsuccessful in correcting hyperglycemia, but even after the introduction of the drug in the patient's regimen, dietary measures should continue to be considered as important. In 12 week, well-controlled studies there was a maximal average net reduction in hemoglobin A_{1C} of 1.7% in absolute units between placebo-treated and GLUCOTROL XL-treated patients.

In initiating treatment for non-insulin-dependent diabetes, diet should be emphasized as the primary form of treatment. Caloric restriction and weight loss are essential in the obese diabetic patient. Proper dietary management alone may be effective in controlling blood glucose and symptoms of hyperglycemia. The importance of regular physical activity should also be stressed, cardiovascular risk factors should be identified, and corrective measures taken where possible.

If this treatment program fails to reduce symptoms and/or blood glucose, the use of an oral sulfonylurea should be considered. If additional reduction of symptoms and/or blood glucose is required, the addition of insulin to the treatment regimen should be considered. Use of GLUCOTROL XL must be viewed by both the physician and patient as a treatment in addition to diet, and not as a substitute for diet or as a convenient mechanism for avoiding dietary restraint. Furthermore, loss of blood glucose control on diet alone also may be transient, thus requiring only short-term administration of glipizide.

Some patients fail to respond initially or gradually lose their responsiveness to sulfonylurea drugs, including GLUCOTROL XL. In these cases, the addition of another oral blood glucose-lowering agent to GLUCOTROL XL therapy can be considered. Other approaches that can be considered include substitution of GLUCOTROL XL therapy with that of another oral blood glucose-lowering agent or insulin. GLUCOTROL XL should be discontinued if it no longer contributes to glucose lowering. Judgment of response to therapy should be based on regular clinical and laboratory evaluations.

In considering the use of GLUCOTROL XL in asymptomatic patients, it should be recognized that controlling blood glucose in non-insulin-dependent diabetes has not been definitely established to be effective in preventing the long-term cardiovascular or neural complications of diabetes. However, in insulin-dependent diabetes mellitus controlling blood glucose has been effective in slowing the progression of diabetic retinopathy, nephropathy, and neuropathy.

CONTRAINDICATIONS

Glipizide is contraindicated in patients with:

1. Known hypersensitivity to the drug.
2. Diabetic ketoacidosis, with or without coma. This condition should be treated with insulin.

WARNINGS

SPECIAL WARNING ON INCREASED RISK OF CARDIOVASCULAR MORTALITY: The administration of oral hypoglycemic drugs has been reported to be associated with increased cardiovascular mortality as compared to treatment with diet alone or diet plus insulin. This warning is based on the study conducted by the University Group Diabetes Program (UGDP), a long-term prospective clinical trial designed to evaluate the effectiveness of glucose-lowering drugs in preventing or delaying vascular complications in patients with non-insulin-dependent diabetes. The study involved 823 patients who were randomly assigned to one of four treatment groups (*Diabetes*, 19, SUPP. 2: 747-830, 1970).

UGDP reported that patients treated for 5 to 8 years with diet plus a fixed dose of tolbutamide (1.5 grams per day) had a rate of cardiovascular mortality approximately $2^1/_2$ times that of patients treated with diet alone. A significant increase in total mortality was not observed, but the use of tolbutamide was discontinued based on the increase in cardiovascular mortality, thus limiting the opportunity for the study to show an increase in overall mortality. Despite controversy regarding the interpretation of these results, the findings of the UGDP study provide an adequate basis for this warning. The patient should be informed of the potential risks and advantages of glipizide and of alternative modes of therapy.

Although only one drug in the sulfonylurea class (tolbutamide) was included in this study, it is prudent from a safety standpoint to consider that this warning may also apply to other oral hypoglycemic drugs in this class, in view of their close similarities in mode of action and chemical structure.

As with any other non-deformable material, caution should be used when administering GLUCOTROL XL Extended Release Tablets in patients with preexisting severe gastrointestinal narrowing (pathologic or iatrogenic). There have been rare reports of obstructive symptoms in patients with known strictures in association with the ingestion of another drug in this non-deformable sustained release formulation.

PRECAUTIONS

General

Renal and Hepatic Disease: The pharmacokinetics and/or pharmacodynamics of glipizide may be affected in patients with impaired renal or hepatic function. If hypoglycemia should occur in such patients, it may be prolonged and appropriate management should be instituted.

GI Disease: Markedly reduced GI retention times of the GLUCOTROL XL Extended Release Tablets may influence the pharmacokinetic profile and hence the clinical efficacy of the drug.

Hypoglycemia: All sulfonylurea drugs are capable of producing severe hypoglycemia. Proper patient selection, dosage, and instructions are important to avoid hypoglycemic episodes. Renal or hepatic insufficiency may affect the disposition of glipizide and the latter may also diminish gluconeogenic capacity, both of which increase the risk of serious hypoglycemic reactions. Elderly, debilitated or malnourished patients, and those with adrenal or pituitary insufficiency are particularly susceptible to the hypoglycemic action of glucose-lowering drugs. Hypoglycemia may be difficult to recognize in the elderly, and in people who are taking beta-adrenergic blocking drugs. Hypoglycemia is more likely to occur when caloric intake is deficient, after severe or prolonged exercise, when alcohol is ingested, or when more than one glucose-lowering drug is used. Therapy with a combination of glucose-lowering agents may increase the potential for hypoglycemia.

Loss of Control of Blood Glucose: When a patient stabilized on any diabetic regimen is exposed to stress such as fever, trauma, infection, or surgery, a loss of control may occur. At such times, it may be necessary to discontinue glipizide and administer insulin.

The effectiveness of any oral hypoglycemic drug, including glipizide, in lowering blood glucose to a desired level decreases in many patients over a period of time, which may be due to progression of the severity of the diabetes or to diminished responsiveness to the drug. This phenomenon is known as secondary failure, to distinguish it from primary failure in which the drug is ineffective in an individual patient when first given. Adequate adjustment of dose and adherence to diet should be assessed before classifying a patient as a secondary failure.

Laboratory Tests: Blood and urine glucose should be monitored periodically. Measurement of hemoglobin A_{1C} may be useful.

Information for Patients: Patients should be informed that GLUCOTROL XL Extended Release Tablets should be swallowed whole. Patients should not chew, divide or crush tablets. Patients should not be concerned if they occasionally notice in their stool something that looks like a tablet. In the GLUCOTROL XL Extended Release Tablet, the medication is contained within a nonabsorbable shell that has been specially designed to slowly release the drug so the body can absorb it. When this process is completed, the empty tablet is eliminated from the body.

Patients should be informed of the potential risks and advantages of GLUCOTROL XL and of alternative modes of therapy. They should also be informed about the importance of adhering to dietary instructions, of a regular exercise program, and of regular testing of urine and/or blood glucose. The risks of hypoglycemia, its symptoms and treatment, and conditions that predispose to its development should be explained to patients and responsible family members. Primary and secondary failure also should be explained.

Drug Interactions: The hypoglycemic action of sulfonylureas may be potentiated by certain drugs including nonsteroidal anti-inflammatory agents and other drugs that are highly protein bound, salicylates, sulfonamides, chloramphenicol, probenecid, coumarins, monoamine oxidase inhibitors, and beta-adrenergic blocking agents. When such drugs are administered to a patient receiving glipizide, the patient should be observed closely for hypoglycemia. When such drugs are withdrawn from a patient receiving glipizide, the patient should be observed closely for loss of control. *In vitro* binding studies with human serum proteins indicate that glipizide binds differently than tolbutamide and does not interact with salicylate or dicumarol. However, caution must be exercised in extrapolating these findings to the clinical situation and in the use of glipizide with these drugs.

Certain drugs tend to produce hyperglycemia and may lead to loss of control. These drugs include the thiazides and other diuretics, corticosteroids, phenothiazines, thyroid products, estrogens, oral contraceptives, phenytoin, nicotinic acid, sympathomimetics, calcium channel blocking drugs, and isoniazid. When such drugs are administered to a patient receiving glipizide, the patient should be closely observed for loss of control. When such drugs are withdrawn from a patient receiving glipizide, the patient should be observed closely for hypoglycemia.

A potential interaction between oral miconazole and oral hypoglycemic agents leading to severe hypoglycemia has been reported. Whether this interaction also occurs with the intravenous, topical, or vaginal preparations of miconazole is not known. The effect of concomitant administration of Diflucan® (fluconazole) and Glucotrol has been demonstrated in a placebo-controlled crossover study in normal volunteers. All subjects received Glucotrol alone and following treatment with 100 mg of Diflucan® as a single daily oral dose for 7 days. The mean percentage increase in the Glucotrol AUC after fluconazole administration was 56.9% (range: 35 to 81%).

Carcinogenesis, Mutagenesis, Impairment of Fertility: A twenty month study in rats and an eighteen month study in mice at doses up to 75 times the maximum human dose revealed no evidence of drug-related carcinogenicity. Bacterial and *in vivo* mutagenicity tests were uniformly negative. Studies in rats of both sexes at doses up to 75 times the human dose showed no effects on fertility.

Pregnancy: Pregnancy Category C: Glipizide was found to be mildly fetotoxic in rat reproductive studies at all dose levels (5-50 mg/kg). This fetotoxicity has been similarly noted with other sulfonylureas, such as tolbutamide and tolazamide. The effect is perinatal and believed to be directly related to the pharmacologic (hypoglycemic) action of glipizide. In studies in rats and rabbits no teratogenic effects were found. There are no adequate and well controlled studies in pregnant women. Glipizide should be used during

pregnancy only if the potential benefit justifies the potential risk to the fetus.

Because recent information suggests that abnormal blood glucose levels during pregnancy are associated with a higher incidence of congenital abnormalities, many experts recommend that insulin be used during pregnancy to maintain blood glucose levels as close to normal as possible.

Nonteratogenic Effects: Prolonged severe hypoglycemia (4 to 10 days) has been reported in neonates born to mothers who were receiving a sulfonylurea drug at the time of delivery. This has been reported more frequently with the use of agents with prolonged half-lives. If glipizide is used during pregnancy, it should be discontinued at least one month before the expected delivery date.

Nursing Mothers: Although it is not known whether glipizide is excreted in human milk, some sulfonylurea drugs are known to be excreted in human milk. Because the potential for hypoglycemia in nursing infants may exist, a decision should be made whether to discontinue nursing or to discontinue the drug, taking into account the importance of the drug to the mother. If the drug is discontinued and if diet alone is inadequate for controlling blood glucose, insulin therapy should be considered.

Pediatric Use: Safety and effectiveness in children have not been established.

Geriatric Use: Of the total number of patients in clinical studies of GLUCOTROL XL, 33 percent were 65 and over. No overall differences in effectiveness or safety were observed between these patients and younger patients, but greater sensitivity of some individuals cannot be ruled out. Approximately 1–2 days longer were required to reach steady-state in the elderly. (See CLINICAL PHARMACOLOGY and DOSAGE AND ADMINISTRATION).

ADVERSE REACTIONS

In U.S. controlled studies the frequency of serious adverse experiences reported was very low and causal relationship has not been established.

The 580 patients from 31 to 87 years of age who received GLUCOTROL XL Extended Release Tablets in doses from 5 mg to 60 mg in both controlled and open trials were included in the evaluation of adverse experiences. All adverse experiences reported were tabulated independently of their possible causal relation to medication.

Hypoglycemia: See PRECAUTIONS and OVERDOSAGE sections.

Only 3.4% of patients receiving GLUCOTROL XL Extended Release Tablets had hypoglycemia documented by a blood glucose measurement <60 mg/dL and/or symptoms believed to be associated with hypoglycemia. In a comparative efficacy study of GLUCOTROL XL and Glucotrol, hypoglycemia occurred rarely with an incidence of less than 1% with both drugs.

In double-blind, placebo-controlled studies the adverse experiences reported with an incidence of 3% or more in GLUCOTROL XL-treated patients include:

	GLUCOTROL XL (%) (N=278)	Placebo (%) (N=69)
Adverse Effect		
Asthenia	10.1	13.0
Headache	8.6	8.7
Dizziness	6.8	5.8
Nervousness	3.6	2.9
Tremor	3.6	0.0
Diarrhea	5.4	0.0
Flatulence	3.2	1.4

The following adverse experiences occurred with an incidence of less than 3% in GLUCOTROL XL-treated patients:

Body as a whole–pain

Nervous system–insomnia, paresthesia, anxiety, depression and hypesthesia

Gastrointestinal–nausea, dyspepsia, constipation and vomiting

Metabolic–hypoglycemia

Musculoskeletal –arthralgia, leg cramps and myalgia

Cardiovascular–syncope

Skin–sweating and pruritus

Respiratory–rhinitis

Special senses–blurred vision

Urogenital–polyuria

Other adverse experiences occurred with an incidence of less than 1% in GLUCOTROL XL-treated patients:

Body as a whole–chills

Nervous system–hypertonia, confusion, vertigo, somnolence, gait abnormality and decreased libido

Gastrointestinal–anorexia and trace blood in stool

Metabolic–thirst and edema

Cardiovascular–arrhythmia, migraine, flushing and hypertension

Skin–rash and urticaria

Respiratory–pharyngitis and dyspnea

Special senses–pain in the eye, conjunctivitis and retinal hemorrhage

Urogenital–dysuria

Although these adverse experiences occurred in patients treated with GLUCOTROL XL, a causal relationship to the medication has not been established in all cases.

There have been rare reports of gastrointestinal irritation and gastrointestinal bleeding with use of another drug in this non-deformable sustained release formulation, although causal relationship to the drug is uncertain.

The following are adverse experiences reported with immediate release glipizide and other sulfonylureas, but have not been observed with GLUCOTROL XL:

Hematologic: Leukopenia, agranulocytosis, thrombocytopenia, hemolytic anemia, aplastic anemia, and pancytopenia have been reported with sulfonylureas.

Metabolic: Hepatic porphyria and disulfiram-like reactions have been reported with sulfonylureas. In the mouse, glipizide pretreatment did not cause an accumulation of acetaldehyde after ethanol administration. Clinical experience to date has shown that glipizide has an extremely low incidence of disulfiram-like alcohol reactions.

Endocrine Reactions: Cases of hyponatremia and the syndrome of inappropriate antidiuretic hormone (SIADH) secretion have been reported with glipizide and other sulfonylureas.

Laboratory Tests: The pattern of laboratory test abnormalities observed with glipizide was similar to that for other sulfonylureas. Occasional mild to moderate elevations of SGOT, LDH, alkaline phosphatase, BUN and creatinine were noted. One case of jaundice was reported. The relationship of these abnormalities to glipizide is uncertain, and they have rarely been associated with clinical symptoms.

OVERDOSAGE

There is no well-documented experience with GLUCOTROL XL overdosage in humans. There have been no known suicide attempts associated with purposeful overdosing with GLUCOTROL XL. In nonclinical studies the acute oral toxicity of glipizide was extremely low in all species tested (LD_{50} greater than 4 g/kg). Overdosage of sulfonylureas including glipizide can produce hypoglycemia. Mild hypoglycemic symptoms without loss of consciousness or neurologic findings should be treated aggressively with oral glucose and adjustments in drug dosage and/or meal patterns. Close monitoring should continue until the physician is assured that the patient is out of danger. Severe hypoglycemic reactions with coma, seizure, or other neurological impairment occur infrequently, but constitute medical emergencies requiring immediate hospitalization. If hypoglycemic coma is diagnosed or suspected, the patient should be given rapid intravenous injection of concentrated (50%) glucose solution. This should be followed by a continuous infusion of a more dilute (10%) glucose solution at a rate that will maintain the blood glucose at a level above 100 mg/dL. Patients should be closely monitored for a minimum of 24 to 48 hours since hypoglycemia may recur after apparent clinical recovery. Clearance of glipizide from plasma may be prolonged in persons with liver disease. Because of the extensive protein binding of glipizide, dialysis is unlikely to be of benefit.

DOSAGE AND ADMINISTRATION

There is no fixed dosage regimen for the management of diabetes mellitus with GLUCOTROL XL Extended Release Tablet or any other hypoglycemic agent. Glycemic control should be monitored with hemoglobin A_{1C} and/or blood glucose levels to determine the minimum effective dose for the patient; to detect primary failure, i.e., inadequate lowering of blood glucose at the maximum recommended dose of medication; and to detect secondary failure, i.e., loss of an adequate blood-glucose-lowering response after an initial period of effectiveness. Home blood glucose monitoring may also provide useful information to the patient and physician. Short-term administration of GLUCOTROL XL Extended Release Tablet may be sufficient during periods of transient loss of control in patients usually controlled on diet.

In general, GLUCOTROL XL should be given with breakfast.

Recommended Dosing: The recommended starting dose of GLUCOTROL XL is 5 mg per day, given with breakfast. The recommended dose for geriatric patients is also 5 mg per day.

Dosage adjustment should be based on laboratory measures of glycemic control. While fasting blood glucose levels generally reach steady-state following initiation or change in GLUCOTROL XL dosage, a single fasting glucose determination may not accurately reflect the response to therapy. In most cases, hemoglobin A_{1C} level measured at three month intervals is the preferred means of monitoring response to therapy.

Hemoglobin A_{1C} should be measured as GLUCOTROL XL therapy is initiated at the 5 mg dose and repeated approximately three months later. If the result of this test suggests that glycemic control over the preceding three months was inadequate, the GLUCOTROL XL dose may be increased to 10 mg. Subsequent dosage adjustments should be made on the basis of hemoglobin A_{1C} levels measured at three month intervals. If no improvement is seen after three months of

therapy with a higher dose, the previous dose should be resumed. Decisions which utilize fasting blood glucose to adjust GLUCOTROL XL therapy should be based on at least two or more similar, consecutive values obtained seven days or more after the previous dose adjustment.

Most patients will be controlled with 5 mg or 10 mg taken once daily. However, some patients may require up to the maximum recommended daily dose of 20 mg. While the glycemic control of selected patients may improve with doses which exceed 10 mg, clinical studies conducted to date have not demonstrated an additional group average reduction of hemoglobin A_{1C} beyond what was achieved with the 10 mg dose.

Based on the results of a randomized crossover study, patients receiving immediate release glipizide may be switched safely to GLUCOTROL XL Extended Release Tablets once-a-day at the nearest equivalent total daily dose. Patients receiving immediate release Glucotrol may also be titrated to the appropriate dose of GLUCOTROL XL starting with 5 mg once daily. The decision to switch to the nearest equivalent dose or to titrate should be based on clinical judgment.

In elderly patients, debilitated or malnourished patients, and patients with impaired renal or hepatic function, the initial and maintenance dosing should be conservative to avoid hypoglycemic reactions (see PRECAUTIONS section). When GLUCOTROL XL is used in combination with other oral blood glucose-lowering agents, the second agent should be added at the lowest recommended dose and patients should be observed carefully. Titration of the added oral agent should be based on clinical judgment.

Patients Receiving Insulin: As with other sulfonylurea-class hypoglycemics, many stable non-insulin-dependent diabetic patients receiving insulin may be transferred safely to treatment with GLUCOTROL XL Extended Release Tablets. When transferring patients from insulin to GLUCOTROL XL, the following general guidelines should be considered:

For patients whose daily insulin requirement is 20 units or less, insulin may be discontinued and GLUCOTROL XL therapy may begin at usual dosages. Several days should elapse between titration steps.

For patients whose daily insulin requirement is greater than 20 units, the insulin dose should be reduced by 50% and GLUCOTROL XL therapy may begin at usual dosages. Subsequent reductions in insulin dosage should depend on individual patient response. Several days should elapse between titration steps.

During the insulin withdrawal period, the patient should test urine samples for sugar and ketone bodies at least three times daily. Patients should be instructed to contact the prescriber immediately if these tests are abnormal. In some cases, especially when the patient has been receiving greater than 40 units of insulin daily, it may be advisable to consider hospitalization during the transition period.

Patients Receiving Other Oral Hypoglycemic Agents: As with other sulfonylurea-class hypoglycemics, no transition period is necessary when transferring patients to GLUCOTROL XL Extended Release Tablets. Patients should be observed carefully (1–2 weeks) for hypoglycemia when being transferred from longer half-life sulfonylureas (e.g., chlorpropamide) to GLUCOTROL XL due to potential overlapping of drug effect.

HOW SUPPLIED

GLUCOTROL XL® Extended Release Tablets are supplied as 5 mg and 10 mg white, round, biconvex tablets and imprinted with black ink as follows:

5 mg tablets are imprinted with "GLUCOTROL XL 5" on one side.

    Bottles of 100: NDC 0049-1550-66
    Bottles of 500: NDC 0049-1550-73

10 mg tablets are imprinted with "GLUCOTROL XL 10" on one side.

    Bottles of 100: NDC 0049-1560-66
    Bottles of 500: NDC 0049-1560-73

Recommended Storage: The tablets should be protected from moisture and humidity and stored at controlled room temperature, 59° to 86°F (15° to 30°C).

CAUTION: Federal law prohibits dispensing without prescription.

©1998 PFIZER INC

69-4952-00-3
Revised Feb. 1998

Shown in Product Identification Guide, page 330

LIPITOR®
(Atorvastatin Calcium) Tablets

℞

DESCRIPTION

Lipitor® (atorvastatin calcium) is a synthetic lipid-lowering agent. Atorvastatin is an inhibitor of 3-hydroxy-3-methyl-

Continued on next page

Lipitor—Cont.

glutaryl-coenzyme A (HMG-CoA) reductase. This enzyme catalyzes the conversion of HMG-CoA to mevalonate, an early and rate-limiting step in cholesterol biosynthesis.
Atorvastatin calcium is [R-(R*, R*)]-2-(4-fluorophenyl)-β, δ-dihydroxy-5-(1-methylethyl)-3-phenyl-4-[(phenylamino)carbonyl]-1H-pyrrole-1-heptanoic acid, calcium salt (2:1) trihydrate. The empirical formula of atorvastatin calcium is $(C_{33}H_{34}FN_2O_5)_2Ca{\cdot}3H_2O$ and its molecular weight is 1209.42. Its structural formula is:

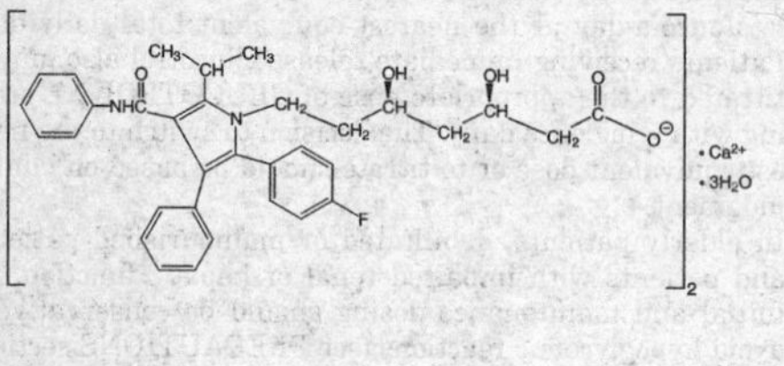

Atorvastatin calcium is a white to off-white crystalline powder that is insoluble in aqueous solutions of pH 4 and below. Atorvastatin calcium is very slightly soluble in distilled water, pH 7.4 phosphate buffer, and acetonitrile, slightly soluble in ethanol, and freely soluble in methanol.
Lipitor tablets for oral administration contain 10, 20, or 40 mg atorvastatin and the following inactive ingredients: calcium carbonate, USP; candelilla wax, FCC; croscarmellose sodium, NF; hydroxypropyl cellulose, NF; lactose monohydrate, NF; magnesium stearate, NF; microcrystalline cellulose, NF; Opadry White YS-1-7040 (hydroxypropylmethylcellulose, polyethylene glycol, talc, titanium dioxide); polysorbate 80, NF; simethicone emulsion.

CLINICAL PHARMACOLOGY

Mechanism of Action

Atorvastatin is a selective, competitive inhibitor of HMG-CoA reductase, the rate-limiting enzyme that converts 3-hydroxy-3-methyl-glutaryl-coenzyme A to mevalonate, a precursor of sterols, including cholesterol. Cholesterol and triglycerides circulate in the bloodstream as part of lipoprotein complexes. With ultracentrifugation, these complexes separate into HDL (high-density lipoprotein), IDL (intermediate-density lipoprotein), LDL (low-density lipoprotein), and VLDL (very-low-density lipoprotein) fractions. Triglycerides (TG) and cholesterol in the liver are incorporated into VLDL and released into the plasma for delivery to peripheral tissues. LDL is formed from VLDL and is catabolized primarily through the high-affinity LDL receptor. Clinical and pathologic studies show that elevated plasma levels of total cholesterol (total-C), LDL-cholesterol (LDL-C), and apolipoprotein B (apo B) promote human atherosclerosis and are risk factors for developing cardiovascular disease, while increased levels of HDL-C are associated with a decreased cardiovascular risk.
In animal models, Lipitor lowers plasma cholesterol and lipoprotein levels by inhibiting HMG-CoA reductase and cholesterol synthesis in the liver and by increasing the number of hepatic LDL receptors on the cell-surface to enhance uptake and catabolism of LDL; Lipitor also reduces LDL production and the number of LDL particles. Lipitor reduces LDL-C in some patients with homozygous familial hypercholesterolemia (FH), a population that rarely responds to other lipid-lowering medication(s).
A variety of clinical studies have demonstrated that elevated levels of total-C, LDL-C, and apo B (a membrane complex for LDL-C) promote human atherosclerosis. Similarly, decreased levels of HDL-C (and its transport complex, apo A) are associated with the development of atherosclerosis. Epidemiologic investigations have established that cardiovascular morbidity and mortality vary directly with the level of total-C and LDL-C, and inversely with the level of HDL-C.
Lipitor reduces total-C, LDL-C, and apo B in patients with homozygous and heterozygous FH, nonfamilial forms of hypercholesterolemia, and mixed dyslipidemia. Lipitor also reduces VLDL-C and TG and produces variable increases in HDL-C and apolipoprotein A-1. The effect of Lipitor on cardiovascular morbidity and mortality has not been determined.

Pharmacodynamics

Atorvastatin as well as some of its metabolites are pharmacologically active in humans. The liver is the primary site of action and the principal site of cholesterol synthesis and LDL clearance. Drug dosage rather than systemic drug concentration correlates better with LDL-C reduction. Individualization of drug dosage should be based on therapeutic response (see **DOSAGE AND ADMINISTRATION**).

TABLE 1. Dose-Response in Patients With Primary Hypercholesterolemia (Adjusted Mean % Change From Baseline)[a]

Dose	N	TC	LDL-C	Apo B	TG	HDL-C	Non-HDL-C/ HDL-C
Placebo	21	4	4	3	10	−3	7
10	22	−29	−39	−32	−19	6	−34
20	20	−33	−43	−35	−26	9	−41
40	21	−37	−50	−42	−29	6	−45
80	23	−45	−60	−50	−37	5	−53

[a] Results are pooled from 2 dose-response studies.

Pharmacokinetics and Drug Metabolism

Absorption: Atorvastatin is rapidly absorbed after oral administration; maximum plasma concentrations occur within 1 to 2 hours. Extent of absorption increases in proportion to atorvastatin dose. The absolute bioavailability of atorvastatin (parent drug) is approximately 12% and the systemic availability of HMG-CoA reductase inhibitory activity is approximately 30%. The low systemic availability is attributed to presystemic clearance in gastrointestinal mucosa and/or hepatic first-pass metabolism. Although food decreases the rate and extent of drug absorption by approximately 25% and 9%, respectively, as assessed by Cmax and AUC, LDL-C reduction is similar whether atorvastatin is given with or without food. Plasma atorvastatin concentrations are lower (approximately 30% for Cmax and AUC) following evening drug administration compared with morning. However, LDL-C reduction is the same regardless of the time of day of drug administration (see **DOSAGE AND ADMINISTRATION**).
Distribution: Mean volume of distribution of atorvastatin is approximately 565 liters. Atorvastatin is ≥98% bound to plasma proteins. A blood/plasma ratio of approximately 0.25 indicates poor drug penetration into red blood cells. Based on observations in rats, atorvastatin is likely to be secreted in human milk (see **CONTRAINDICATIONS, Pregnancy and Lactation**, and **PRECAUTIONS, Nursing Mothers**).
Metabolism: Atorvastatin is extensively metabolized to ortho- and parahydroxylated derivatives and various beta-oxidation products. *In vitro* inhibition of HMG-CoA reductase by ortho- and parahydroxylated metabolites is equivalent to that of atorvastatin. Approximately 70% of circulating inhibitory activity for HMG-CoA reductase is attributed to active metabolites. *In vitro* studies suggest the importance of atorvastatin metabolism by cytochrome P450 3A4, consistent with increased plasma concentrations of atorvastatin in humans following coadministration with erythromycin, a known inhibitor of this isoenzyme (see **PRECAUTIONS, Drug Interactions**). In animals, the ortho-hydroxy metabolite undergoes further glucuronidation.
Excretion: Atorvastatin and its metabolites are eliminated primarily in bile following hepatic and/or extrahepatic metabolism; however, the drug does not appear to undergo enterohepatic recirculation. Mean plasma elimination half-life of atorvastatin in humans is approximately 14 hours, but the half-life of inhibitory activity for HMG-CoA reductase is 20 to 30 hours due to the contribution of active metabolites. Less than 2% of a dose of atorvastatin is recovered in urine following oral administration.

Special Populations

Geriatric: Plasma concentrations of atorvastatin are higher (approximately 40% for Cmax and 30% for AUC) in healthy elderly subjects (age ≥65 years) than in young adults. LDL-C reduction is comparable to that seen in younger patient populations given equal doses of Lipitor.
Pediatric: Pharmacokinetic data in the pediatric population are not available.
Gender: Plasma concentrations of atorvastatin in women differ from those in men (approximately 20% higher for Cmax and 10% lower for AUC); however, there is no clinically significant difference in LDL-C reduction with Lipitor between men and women.
Renal Insufficiency: Renal disease has no influence on the plasma concentrations or LDL-C reduction of atorvastatin; thus, dose adjustment in patients with renal dysfunction is not necessary (see **DOSAGE AND ADMINISTRATION**).
Hemodialysis: While studies have not been conducted in patients with end-stage renal disease, hemodialysis is not expected to significantly enhance clearance of atorvastatin since the drug is extensively bound to plasma proteins.
Hepatic Insufficiency: In patients with chronic alcoholic liver disease, plasma concentrations of atorvastatin are markedly increased. Cmax and AUC are each 4-fold greater in patients with Childs-Pugh A disease. Cmax and AUC are approximately 16-fold and 11-fold increased, respectively, in patients with Childs-Pugh B disease (see **CONTRAINDICATIONS**).

Clinical Studies

Hypercholesterolemia (Heterozygous Familial and Nonfamilial) and Mixed Dyslipidemia (*Fredrickson* Types IIa and IIb)

Lipitor reduces total-C, LDL-C, VLDL-C, apo B, and TG, and increases HDL-C in patients with hypercholesterolemia and mixed dyslipidemia. Therapeutic response is seen within 2 weeks, and maximum response is usually achieved within 4 weeks and maintained during chronic therapy.
Lipitor is effective in a wide variety of patient populations with hypercholesterolemia, with and without hypertriglyceridemia, in men and women, and in the elderly. Experience in pediatric patients has been limited to patients with homozygous FH.
In two multicenter, placebo-controlled, dose-response studies in patients with hypercholesterolemia, Lipitor given as a single dose over 6 weeks significantly reduced total-C, LDL-C, apo B, and TG (Pooled results are provided in Table 1).
[See table 1 above]
In three multicenter, double-blind studies in patients with hypercholesterolemia, Lipitor was compared to other HMG-CoA reductase inhibitors. After randomization, patients were treated for 16 weeks with either Lipitor 10 mg per day or a fixed dose of the comparative agent (Table 2).
[See table 2 below]
The impact on clinical outcomes of the differences in lipid-altering effects between treatments shown in Table 2 is not known. Table 2 does not contain data comparing the effects of atorvastatin 10 mg and higher doses of lovastatin, pravastatin, and simvastatin. The drugs compared in the studies summarized in the table are not necessarily interchangeable.
In a large clinical study, the number of patients meeting their National Cholesterol Education Program-Adult Treatment Panel (NCEP-ATP) II target LDL-C levels on 10 mg of

TABLE 2. Mean Percent Change From Baseline at End Point (Double-Blind, Randomized, Active-Controlled Trials)

Treatment (Daily Dose)	N	Total-C	LDL-C	Apo B	TG	HDL-C	Non-HDL-C/ HDL-C
Study 1							
Atorvastatin 10 mg	707	−27[a]	−36[a]	−28[a]	−17[a]	+7	−37[a]
Lovastatin 20 mg	191	−19	−27	−20	− 6	+7	−28
95% CI for Diff[1]		−9.2, −6.5	−10.7, −7.1	−10.0, −6.5	−15.2, −7.1	−1.7, 2.0	−11.1, −7.1
Study 2							
Atorvastatin 10 mg	222	−25[b]	−35[b]	−27[b]	−17[b]	+6	−36[b]
Pravastatin 20 mg	77	−17	−23	−17	− 9	+8	−28
95% CI for Diff[1]		−10.8, −6.1	−14.5, −8.2	−13.4, −7.4	−14.1, −0.7	−4.9, 1.6	−11.5, −4.1
Study 3							
Atorvastatin 10 mg	132	−29[c]	−37[c]	−34[c]	−23[c]	+7	−39[c]
Simvastatin 10 mg	45	−24	−30	−30	−15	+7	−33
95% CI for Diff[1]		−8.7, −2.7	−10.1, −2.6	−8.0, −1.1	−15.1, −0.7	−4.3, 3.9	−9.6, −1.9

[1] A negative value for the 95% CI for the difference between treatments favors atorvastatin for all except HDL-C, for which a positive value favors atorvastatin. If the range does not include 0, this indicates a statistically significant difference.
[a] Significantly different from lovastatin, ANCOVA, p≤0.05
[b] Significantly different from pravastatin, ANCOVA, p≤0.05
[c] Significantly different from simvastatin, ANCOVA, p≤0.05

TABLE 3. NCEP Guidelines for Lipid Management

Definite Atherosclerotic Disease[a]	Two or More Other Risk Factors[b]	LDL-Cholesterol mg/dL (mmol/L) Initiation Level	Minimum Goal
No	No	≥190 (≥4.9)	<160 (<4.1)
No	Yes	≥160 (≥4.1)	<130 (<3.4)
Yes	Yes or No	≥130[c] (≥3.4)	≤100 (≤2.6)

[a] Coronary heart disease or peripheral vascular disease (including symptomatic carotid artery disease).
[b] Other risk factors for coronary heart disease (CHD) include: age (males: ≥45 years; females: ≥55 years or premature menopause without estrogen replacement therapy); family history of premature CHD; current cigarette smoking; hypertension; confirmed HDL-C <35 mg/dL (<0.91 mmol/L); and diabetes mellitus. Subtract 1 risk factor if HDL-C is ≥60 mg/dL (≥1.6 mmol/L).
[c] In CHD patients with LDL-C levels 100 to 129 mg/dL, the physician should exercise clinical judgment in deciding whether to initiate drug treatment.

Lipitor daily was assessed. After 16 weeks, 156/167 (93%) of patients with less than 2 risk factors for CHD and baseline LDL-C ≥190 mg/dL reached a target of ≤160 mg/dL; 141/218 (65%) of patients with 2 or more risk factors for CHD and LDL-C ≥160 mg/dL achieved a level of ≤130 mg/dL LDL-C, and 21/113 (19%) of patients with CHD and LDL-C ≥130 mg/dL reached a target level of ≤100 mg/dL LDL-C.

Homozygous Familial Hypercholesterolemia

In a study without a concurrent control group, 29 patients ages 6 to 37 years with homozygous FH received maximum daily doses of 20 to 80 mg of Lipitor. The mean LDL-C reduction in this study was 18%. Twenty-five patients with a reduction in LDL-C had a mean response of 20% (range of 7% to 53%, median of 24%); the remaining 4 patients had 7% to 24% increases in LDL-C. Five of the 29 patients had absent LDL-receptor function. Of these, 2 patients also had a portacaval shunt and had no significant reduction in LDL-C. The remaining 3 receptor-negative patients had a mean LDL-C reduction of 22%.

INDICATIONS AND USAGE

Lipitor is indicated as an adjunct to diet to reduce elevated total-C, LDL-C, apo B, and TG levels in patients with primary hypercholesterolemia (heterozygous familial and nonfamilial) and mixed dyslipidemia (*Fredrickson* Types IIa and IIb).

Lipitor is also indicated to reduce total-C and LDL-C in patients with homozygous familial hypercholesterolemia as an adjunct to other lipid-lowering treatments (e.g., LDL apheresis) or if such treatments are unavailable.

Therapy with lipid-altering agents should be a component of multiple-risk-factor intervention in individuals at increased risk for atherosclerotic vascular disease due to hypercholesterolemia. Lipid-altering agents should be used in addition to a diet restricted in saturated fat and cholesterol only when the response to diet and other nonpharmacological measures has been inadequate (see *National Cholesterol Education Program (NCEP) Guidelines*, summarized in Table 3).

[See table 3 above]

At the time of hospitalization for an acute coronary event, consideration can be given to initiating drug therapy at discharge if the LDL-C level is ≥130 mg/dL (NCEP-ATP II).

Prior to initiating therapy with Lipitor, secondary causes for hypercholesterolemia (e.g., poorly controlled diabetes mellitus, hypothyroidism, nephrotic syndrome, dysproteinemias, obstructive liver disease, other drug therapy, and alcoholism) should be excluded, and a lipid profile performed to measure total-C, LDL-C, HDL-C, and TG. For patients with TG <400 mg/dL (<4.5 mmol/L), LDL-C can be estimated using the following equation: LDL-C = total-C - (0.20 × [TG] + HDL-C). For TG levels >400 mg/dL (>4.5 mmol/L), this equation is less accurate and LDL-C concentrations should be determined by ultracentrifugation.

CONTRAINDICATIONS

Active liver disease or unexplained persistent elevations of serum transaminases.

Hypersensitivity to any component of this medication.

Pregnancy and Lactation

Atherosclerosis is a chronic process and discontinuation of lipid-lowering drugs during pregnancy should have little impact on the outcome of long-term therapy of primary hypercholesterolemia. Cholesterol and other products of cholesterol biosynthesis are essential components for fetal development (including synthesis of steroids and cell membranes). Since HMG-CoA reductase inhibitors decrease cholesterol synthesis and possibly the synthesis of other biologically active substances derived from cholesterol, they may cause fetal harm when administered to pregnant women. Therefore, HMG-CoA reductase inhibitors are contraindicated during pregnancy and in nursing mothers. ATORVASTATIN SHOULD BE ADMINISTERED TO WOMEN OF CHILDBEARING AGE ONLY WHEN SUCH PATIENTS ARE HIGHLY UNLIKELY TO CONCEIVE AND HAVE BEEN INFORMED OF THE POTENTIAL HAZARDS. If the patient becomes pregnant while taking this drug, therapy should be discontinued and the patient apprised of the potential hazard to the fetus.

WARNINGS

Liver Dysfunction

HMG-CoA reductase inhibitors, like some other lipid-lowering therapies, have been associated with biochemical abnormalities of liver function. **Persistent elevations (>3 times the upper limit of normal [ULN] occurring on 2 or more occasions) in serum transaminases occurred in 0.7% of patients who received atorvastatin in clinical trials. The incidence of these abnormalities was 0.2%, 0.2%, 0.6%, and 2.3% for 10, 20, 40, and 80 mg, respectively.**

One patient in clinical trials developed jaundice. Increases in liver function tests (LFT) in other patients were not associated with jaundice or other clinical signs or symptoms. Upon dose reduction, drug interruption, or discontinuation, transaminase levels returned to or near pretreatment levels without sequelae. Eighteen of 30 patients with persistent LFT elevations continued treatment with a reduced dose of atorvastatin.

It is recommended that liver function tests be performed before the initiation of treatment, at 6 and 12 weeks after initiation of therapy or elevation in dose, and periodically (e.g., semiannually) thereafter. Liver enzyme changes generally occur in the first 3 months of treatment with atorvastatin. Patients who develop increased transaminase levels should be monitored until the abnormalities resolve. Should an increase in ALT or AST of >3 times ULN persist, reduction of dose or withdrawal of atorvastatin is recommended.

Atorvastatin should be used with caution in patients who consume substantial quantities of alcohol and/or have a history of liver disease. Active liver disease or unexplained persistent transaminase elevations are contraindications to the use of atorvastatin (see **CONTRAINDICATIONS**).

Skeletal Muscle

Rhabdomyolysis with acute renal failure secondary to myoglobinuria has been reported with other drugs in this class.

Uncomplicated myalgia has been reported in atorvastatin-treated patients (see **ADVERSE REACTIONS**). Myopathy, defined as muscle aches or muscle weakness in conjunction with increases in creatine phosphokinase (CPK) values >10 times ULN, should be considered in any patient with diffuse myalgias, muscle tenderness or weakness, and/or marked elevation of CPK. Patients should be advised to report promptly unexplained muscle pain, tenderness or weakness, particularly if accompanied by malaise or fever. Atorvastatin therapy should be discontinued if markedly elevated CPK levels occur or myopathy is diagnosed or suspected.

The risk of myopathy during treatment with other drugs in this class is increased with concurrent administration of cyclosporine, fibric acid derivatives, erythromycin, niacin, or azole antifungals. Physicians considering combined therapy with atorvastatin and fibric acid derivatives, erythromycin, immunosuppressive drugs, azole antifungals, or lipid-lowering doses of niacin should carefully weight the potential benefits and risks and should carefully monitor patients for any signs or symptoms of muscle pain, tenderness, or weakness, particularly during the initial months of therapy and during any periods of upward dosage titration of either drug. Periodic creatine phosphokinase (CPK) determinations may be considered in such situations, but there is no assurance that such monitoring will prevent the occurrence of severe myopathy.

Atorvastatin therapy should be temporarily withheld or discontinued in any patient with an acute, serious condition suggestive of a myopathy or having a risk factor predisposing to the development of renal failure secondary to rhabdomyolysis (e.g., severe acute infection, hypotension, major surgery, trauma, severe metabolic, endocrine and electrolyte disorders, and uncontrolled seizures).

PRECAUTIONS

General

Before instituting therapy with atorvastatin, an attempt should be made to control hypercholesterolemia with appropriate diet, exercise, and weight reduction in obese patients, and to treat other underlying medical problems (see **INDICATIONS AND USAGE**).

Information for Patients

Patients should be advised to report promptly unexplained muscle pain, tenderness, or weakness, particularly if accompanied by malaise or fever.

Drug Interactions

The risk of myopathy during treatment with other drugs of this class is increased with concurrent administration of cyclosporine, fibric acid derivatives, niacin (nicotinic acid), erythromycin, azole antifungals (see **WARNINGS, Skeletal Muscle**).

Antacid: When atorvastatin and Maalox® TC suspension were coadministered, plasma concentrations of atorvastatin decreased approximately 35%. However, LDL-C reduction was not altered.

Antipyrine: Because atorvastatin does not affect the pharmacokinetics of antipyrine, interactions with other drugs metabolized via the same cytochrome isozymes are not expected.

Colestipol: Plasma concentrations of atorvastatin decreased approximately 25% when colestipol and atorvastatin were coadministered. However, LDL-C reduction was greater when atorvastatin and colestipol were coadministered than when either drug was given alone.

Cimetidine: Atorvastatin plasma concentrations and LDL-C reduction were not altered by coadministration of cimetidine.

Digoxin: When multiple doses of atorvastatin and digoxin were coadministered, steady-state plasma digoxin concentrations increased by approximately 20%. Patients taking digoxin should be monitored appropriately.

Erythromycin: In healthy individuals, plasma concentrations of atorvastatin increased approximately 40% with coadministration of atorvastatin and erythromycin, a known inhibitor of cytochrome P450 3A4 (see **WARNINGS, Skeletal Muscle**).

Oral Contraceptives: Coadministration of atorvastatin and an oral contraceptive increased AUC values for norethindrone and ethinyl estradiol by approximately 30% and 20%. These increases should be considered when selecting an oral contraceptive for a woman taking atorvastatin.

Warfarin: Atorvastatin had no clinically significant effect on prothrombin time when administered to patients receiving chronic warfarin treatment.

Endocrine Function

HMG-CoA reductase inhibitors interfere with cholesterol synthesis and theoretically might blunt adrenal and/or gonadal steroid production. Clinical studies have shown that atorvastatin does not reduce basal plasma cortisol concentration or impair adrenal reserve. The effects of HMG-CoA reductase inhibitors on male fertility have not been studied in adequate numbers of patients. The effects, if any, on the pituitary-gonadal axis in premenopausal women are unknown. Caution should be exercised if an HMG-CoA reductase inhibitor is administered concomitantly with drugs that may decrease the levels or activity of endogenous steroid hormones, such as ketoconazole, spironolactone, and cimetidine.

CNS Toxicity

Brain hemorrhage was seen in a female dog treated for 3 months at 120 mg/kg/day. Brain hemorrhage and optic nerve vacuolation were seen in another female dog that was sacrificed in moribund condition after 11 weeks of escalating doses up to 280 mg/kg/day. The 120 mg/kg dose resulted in a systemic exposure approximately 16 times the human plasma area-under-the curve (AUC, 0-24 hours) based on the maximum human dose of 80 mg/day. A single tonic convulsion was seen in each of 2 male dogs (one treated at 10 mg/kg/day and one at 120 mg/kg/day) in a 2-year study. No CNS lesions have been observed in mice after chronic treatment for up to 2 years at doses up to 400 mg/kg/day or in rats at doses up to 100 mg/kg/day. These doses were 6 to 11 times (mouse) and 8 to 16 times (rat) the human AUC (0-24) based on the maximum recommended human dose of 80 mg/day.

CNS vascular lesions, characterized by perivascular hemorrhages, edema, and mononuclear cell infiltration of perivascular spaces, have been observed in dogs treated with other members of this class. A chemically similar drug in this class produced optic nerve degeneration (Wallerian degeneration of retino-geniculate fibers) in clinically normal dogs in a dose-dependent fashion at a dose that produced plasma drug levels about 30 times higher than the mean drug level in humans taking the highest recommended dose.

Continued on next page

Lipitor—Cont.

Carcinogenesis, Mutagenesis, Impairment of Fertility

In a 2-year carcinogenicity study in rats at dose levels of 10, 30, and 100 mg/kg/day, 2 rare tumors were found in muscle in high-dose females: in one, there was a rhabdomyosarcoma and, in another, there was a fibrosarcoma. This dose represents a plasma AUC (0-24) value of approximately 16 times the mean human plasma drug exposure after an 80 mg oral dose.

A 2-year carcinogenicity study in mice given 100, 200, or 400 mg/kg/day resulted in a significant increase in liver adenomas in high-dose males and liver carcinomas in high-dose females. These findings occurred at plasma AUC (0-24) values of approximately 6 times the mean human plasma drug exposure after an 80 mg oral dose.

In vitro, atorvastatin was not mutagenic or clastogenic in the following tests with and without metabolic activation: the Ames test with *Salmonella typhimurium* and *Escherichia coli*, the HGPRT forward mutation assay in Chinese hamster lung cells, and the chromosomal aberration assay in Chinese hamster lung cells. Atorvastatin was negative in the *in vivo* mouse micronucleus test.

Studies in rats performed at doses up to 175 mg/kg (15 times the human exposure) produced no changes in fertility. There was aplasia and aspermia in the epididymis of 2 of 10 rats treated with 100 mg/kg/day of atorvastatin for 3 months (16 times the human AUC at the 80 mg dose); testis weights were significantly lower at 30 and 100 mg/kg and epididymal weight was lower at 100 mg/kg. Male rats given 100 mg/kg/day for 11 weeks prior to mating had decreased sperm motility, spermatid head concentration, and increased abnormal sperm. Atorvastatin caused no adverse effects on semen parameters, or reproductive organ histopathology in dogs given doses of 10, 40, or 120 mg/kg for two years.

Pregnancy

Pregnancy Category X

See CONTRAINDICATIONS

Safety in pregnant women has not been established. Atorvastatin crosses the rat placenta and reaches a level in fetal liver equivalent to that of maternal plasma. Atorvastatin was not teratogenic in rats at doses up to 300 mg/kg/day or in rabbits at doses up to 100 mg/kg/day. These doses resulted in multiples of about 30 times (rat) or 20 times (rabbit) the human exposure based on surface area (mg/m²).

In a study in rats given 20, 100, or 225 mg/kg/day, from gestation day 7 through to lactation day 21 (weaning), there was decreased pup survival at birth, neonate, weaning, and maturity in pups of mothers dosed with 225 mg/kg/day. Body weight was decreased on days 4 and 21 in pups of mothers dosed at 100 mg/kg/day; pup body weight was decreased at birth and at days 4, 21, and 91 at 225 mg/kg/day. Pup development was delayed (rotorod performance at 100 mg/kg/day and acoustic startle at 225 mg/kg/day; pinnae detachment and eye opening at 225 mg/kg/day). These doses correspond to 6 times (100 mg/kg) and 22 times (225 mg/kg) the human AUC at 80 mg/day.

Rare reports of congenital anomalies have been received following intrauterine exposure to HMG-CoA reductase inhibitors. There has been one report of severe congenital bony deformity, tracheo-esophageal fistula, and anal atresia (VATER association) in a baby born to a woman who took lovastatin with dextroamphetamine sulfate during the first trimester of pregnancy. Lipitor should be administered to women of child-bearing potential only when such patients are highly unlikely to conceive and have been informed of the potential hazards. If the woman becomes pregnant while taking Lipitor, it should be discontinued and the patient advised again as to the potential hazards to the fetus.

Nursing Mothers

Nursing rat pups had plasma and liver drug levels of 50% and 40%, respectively, of that in their mother's milk. Because of the potential for adverse reactions in nursing infants, women taking Lipitor should not breast-feed (see **CONTRAINDICATIONS**).

Pediatric Use

Treatment experience in a pediatric population is limited to doses of Lipitor up to 80 mg/day for 1 year in 8 patients with homozygous FH. No clinical or biochemical abnormalities were reported in these patients. None of these patients was below 9 years of age.

Geriatric Use

Treatment experience in adults age ≥70 years with doses of Lipitor up to 80 mg/day has been evaluated in 221 patients. The safety and efficacy of Lipitor in this population were similar to those of patients <70 years of age.

ADVERSE REACTIONS

Lipitor is generally well-tolerated. Adverse reactions have usually been mild and transient. In controlled clinical studies of 2502 patients, <2% of patients were discontinued due to adverse experiences attributable to atorvastatin. The most frequent adverse events thought to be related to atorvastatin were constipation, flatulence, dyspepsia, and abdominal pain.

Clinical Adverse Experiences

Adverse experiences reported in ≥2% of patients in placebo-controlled clinical studies of atorvastatin, regardless of causality assessment, are shown in Table 4.

[See table 4 below]

The following adverse events were reported, regardless of causality assessment in patients treated with atorvastatin in clinical trials. The events in italics occurred in ≥2% of patients and the events in plain type occurred in <2% of patients.

Body as a Whole: *Chest pain*, face edema, fever, neck rigidity, malaise, photosensitivity reaction, generalized edema.

Digestive System: *Nausea*, gastroenteritis, liver function tests abnormal, colitis, vomiting, gastritis, dry mouth, rectal hemorrhage, esophagitis, eructation, glossitis, mouth ulceration, anorexia, increased appetite, stomatitis, biliary pain, cheilitis, duodenal ulcer, dysphagia, enteritis, melena, gum hemorrhage, stomach ulcer, tenesmus, ulcerative stomatitis, hepatitis, pancreatitis, cholestatic jaundice.

Respiratory System: *Bronchitis, rhinitis*, pneumonia, dyspnea, asthma, epistaxis.

Nervous System: *Insomnia, dizziness*, paresthesia, somnolence, amnesia, abnormal dreams, libido decreased, emotional lability, incoordination, peripheral neuropathy, torticollis, facial paralysis, hyperkinesia, depression, hypesthesia, hypertonia.

Musculoskeletal System: *Arthritis*, leg cramps, bursitis, tenosynovitis, myasthenia, tendinous contracture, myositis.

Skin and Appendages: Pruritus, contact dermatitis, alopecia, dry skin, sweating, acne, urticaria, eczema, seborrhea, skin ulcer.

Urogenital System: *Urinary tract infection*, urinary frequency, cystitis, hematuria, impotence, dysuria, kidney calculus, nocturia, epididymitis, fibrocystic breast, vaginal hemorrhage, albuminuria, breast enlargement, metrorrhagia, nephritis, urinary incontinence, urinary retention, urinary urgency, abnormal ejaculation, uterine hemorrhage.

Special Senses: Amblyopia, tinnitus, dry eyes, refraction disorder, eye hemorrhage, deafness, glaucoma, parosmia, taste loss, taste perversion.

Cardiovascular System: Palpitation, vasodilation, syncope, migraine, postural hypotension, phlebitis, arrhythmia, angina pectoris, hypertension.

Metabolic and Nutritional Disorders: *Peripheral edema*, hyperglycemia, creatine phosphokinase increased, gout, weight gain, hypoglycemia.

Hemic and Lymphatic System: Ecchymosis, anemia, lymphadenopathy, thrombocytopenia, petechia.

Postintroduction Reports

Adverse events associated with Lipitor that have been received since market introduction, that are not listed above, and that may have no causal relationship to drug include the following: anaphylaxis, anginoneurotic edema and rhabdomyolysis.

OVERDOSAGE

There is no specific treatment for atorvastatin overdosage. In the event of an overdose, the patient should be treated symptomatically, and supportive measures instituted as required. Due to extensive drug binding to plasma proteins, hemodialysis is not expected to significantly enhance atorvastatin clearance.

DOSAGE AND ADMINISTRATION

The patient should be placed on a standard cholesterol-lowering diet before receiving Lipitor and should continue on this diet during treatment with Lipitor.

Hypercholesterolemia (Heterozygous Familial and Nonfamilial) and Mixed Dyslipidemia (*Fredrickson* Types IIa and IIb)

The recommended starting dose of Lipitor is 10 mg once daily. The dosage range is 10 to 80 mg once daily. Lipitor can be administered as a single dose at any time of the day, with or without food. Therapy should be individualized according to goal of therapy and response (see *NCEP Guidelines*, summarized in Table 3). After initiation and/or upon titration of Lipitor, lipid levels should be analyzed within 2 to 4 weeks and dosage adjusted accordingly.

Since the goal of treatment is to lower LDL-C, the NCEP recommends that LDL-C levels be used to initiate and assess treatment response. Only if LDL-C levels are not available, should total-C be used to monitor therapy.

Homozygous Familial Hypercholesterolemia

The dosage of Lipitor in patients with homozygous FH is 10 to 80 mg daily. Lipitor should be used as an adjunct to other lipid-lowering treatments (e.g., LDL apheresis) in these patients or if such treatments are unavailable.

Concomitant Therapy

Atorvastatin may be used in combination with a bile acid binding resin for additive effect. The combination of HMG-CoA reductase inhibitors and fibrates should generally be avoided (see **WARNINGS, Skeletal Muscle,** and **PRECAUTIONS, Drug Interactions** for other drug-drug interactions).

Dosage in Patients With Renal Insufficiency

Renal disease does not affect the plasma concentrations nor LDL-C reduction of atorvastatin; thus, dosage adjustment in patients with renal dysfunction is not necessary (see CLINICAL PHARMACOLOGY, Pharmacokinetics).

HOW SUPPLIED

Lipitor is supplied as white, elliptical, film-coated tablets of atorvastatin calcium containing 10, 20, and 40 mg of atorvastatin.

10 mg tablets: coded "PD 155" on one side and "10" on the other.
N0071-0155-23   bottles of 90
N0071-0155-34   bottles of 5000
N0071-0155-40 10 × 10 unit dose blisters

20 mg tablets: coded "PD 156" on one side and "20" on the other.
N0071-0156-23   bottles of 90
N0071-0156-40 10 × 10 unit dose blisters

40 mg tablets: coded "PD 157" on one side and "40" on the other.
N0071-0157-23   bottles of 90

Storage
Store at controlled room temperature 20°C to 25°C (68°F to 77°F) [see USP].

Rx only.
Revised April, 1998
Manufactured by:
Warner-Lambert Export, Ltd. ©1998
Dublin Ireland
Distributed by:
PARKE-DAVIS
Div of Warner-Lambert Co
Morris Plains, NJ 07950 USA
MADE IN GERMANY
Marketed by:
PARKE-DAVIS
Div of Warner-Lambert Co and
PFIZER Inc.
New York, NY 10017   0155G026
Shown in Product Identification Guide, page 331

TABLE 4. Adverse Events in Placebo-Controlled Studies (% of Patients)

BODY SYSTEM/ Adverse Event	Placebo N=270	Atorvastatin 10 mg N=863	Atorvastatin 20 mg N=36	Atorvastatin 40 mg N=79	Atorvastatin 80 mg N=94
BODY AS A WHOLE					
Infection	10.0	10.3	2.8	10.1	7.4
Headache	7.0	5.4	16.7	2.5	6.4
Accidental Injury	3.7	4.2	0.0	1.3	3.2
Flu Syndrome	1.9	2.2	0.0	2.5	3.2
Abdominal Pain	0.7	2.8	0.0	3.8	2.1
Back Pain	3.0	2.8	0.0	3.8	1.1
Allergic Reaction	2.6	0.9	2.8	1.3	0.0
Asthenia	1.9	2.2	0.0	3.8	0.0
DIGESTIVE SYSTEM					
Constipation	1.8	2.1	0.0	2.5	1.1
Diarrhea	1.5	2.7	0.0	3.8	5.3
Dyspepsia	4.1	2.3	2.8	1.3	2.1
Flatulence	3.3	2.1	2.8	1.3	1.1
RESPIRATORY SYSTSEM					
Sinusitis	2.6	2.8	0.0	2.5	6.4
Pharyngitis	1.5	2.5	0.0	1.3	2.1
SKIN AND APPENDAGES					
Rash	0.7	3.9	2.8	3.8	1.1
MUSCULOSKELETAL SYSTEM					
Arthralgia	1.5	2.0	0.0	5.1	0.0
Myalgia	1.1	3.2	5.6	1.3	0.0

MARAX®, MARAX® DF ℞

[*mă 'rax*]

(ephedrine sulfate, theophylline, hydroxyzine HCl)

TABLETS AND DF SYRUP

CONTENTS

	Each Tablet Contains:	Each Teaspoon (5 ml) Syrup Contains:
Ephedrine Sulfate	25 mg	6.25 mg
Theophylline	130 mg	32.50 mg
Atarax® (hydroxyzine HCl)	10 mg	2.5 mg
Alcohol (Ethyl Alcohol)		5% v/v.

Inert ingredients for tablets are: alginic acid; magnesium stearate; precipitated calcium carbonate; sodium lauryl sulfate.

Inert ingredients for syrup are: alcohol; cherry flavor; hydrochloric acid; sodium benzoate; special flavor compound; sucrose; water.

ACTIONS

The action of ephedrine as a vasoconstrictor is well known. It is therefore of significant benefit in symptomatic relief of the congestion occurring in bronchial asthma. As a bronchodilator, it has a slower onset but longer duration of action than does epinephrine, which, in contrast to ephedrine, is not effective upon oral administration.

The diverse actions of theophylline—bronchospasmolytic, cardiovascular, and diuretic—are well established, and make it a particularly useful drug in the treatment of bronchial asthma, both in the acute attack and in the prophylactic therapy of the disease.

Atarax (hydroxyzine HCl) modifies the central stimulatory action of ephedrine preventing excessive excitation in patients on Marax therapy.

In animal studies Atarax has demonstrated antiserotonin activity and antispasmodic potency of a nonspecific nature.

Marax-DF Syrup produces an expectorant action wherein the tenacity of the sputum is decreased and the ease of expectoration is increased.

INDICATIONS

Based on a review of this drug by the National Academy of Sciences-National Research Council and/or other information, FDA has classified the indications as follows:

"Possibly" Effective: For controlling bronchospastic disorders.

Final classification of the less than effective indication requires further investigation.

CONTRAINDICATIONS

Because of the ephedrine, Marax is contraindicated in cardiovascular disease, hyperthyroidism, and hypertension. This drug is contraindicated in individuals who have shown hypersensitivity to the drug or its components.

Hydroxyzine, when administered to the pregnant mouse, rat, and rabbit induced fetal abnormalities in the rat at doses substantially above the human therapeutic range. Clinical data in human beings are inadequate to establish safety in early pregnancy. Until such data are available, hydroxyzine is contraindicated in early pregnancy.

PRECAUTIONS

Because of the ephedrine component this drug should be used with caution in elderly males or those with known prostatic hypertrophy.

The potentiating action of hydroxyzine, although mild, must be taken into consideration when the drug is used in conjunction with central nervous system depressants; and when other central nervous system depressants are administered concomitantly with hydroxyzine their dosage should be reduced. Patients should be cautioned that hydroxyzine can increase the effect of alcohol.

Patients should be warned—because of the hydroxyzine component—of the possibility of drowsiness occurring and cautioned against driving a car or operating dangerous machinery while taking this drug.

ADVERSE REACTIONS

With large doses of ephedrine, excitation, tremulousness, insomnia, nervousness, palpitation, tachycardia, precordial pain, cardiac arrhythmias, vertigo, dryness of the nose and throat, headache, sweating, and warmth may occur. Because ephedrine is a sympathomimetic agent some patients may develop vesical sphincter spasm and resultant urinary hesitation, and occasionally acute urinary retention. This should be borne in mind when administering preparations containing ephedrine to elderly males or those with known prostatic hypertrophy. At the recommended dose for Marax, a side effect occasionally reported is palpitation, and this can be controlled with dosage adjustment, additional amounts of concurrently administered Atarax (hydroxyzine HCl), or discontinuation of the medication. When ephedrine is given three or more times daily patients may develop tolerance after several weeks of therapy.

Theophylline when given on an empty stomach frequently causes gastric irritation accompanied by upper abdominal discomfort, nausea, and vomiting. Administration of the medication after meals will serve to minimize this side effect. Theophylline may cause diuresis and cardiac stimulation. The amount of Atarax present in Marax has not resulted in disturbing side effects. When used alone specifically as a tranquilizer in the normal dosage range (25 to 50 mg three or four times a day), side effects are infrequent; even at these higher doses, no serious side effects have been reported and confirmed to date. Those which do occasionally occur when Atarax is used alone are drowsiness, xerostomia and, at extremely high doses, involuntary motor activity, unsteadiness of gait, neuromuscular weakness, all of which may be controlled by reduction of the dosage or discontinuation of the medication.

With the relatively low dose of Atarax in Marax, these effects are not likely to occur. In addition, the ataractic action of Atarax may modify the cardiac stimulatory action of ephedrine, and concurrently, increasing the amount of Atarax may control or abolish this undesirable effect of ephedrine.

DOSAGE AND ADMINISTRATION

The dosage of Marax should be adjusted according to the severity of complaints, and the patient's individual toleration.

Tablets: In general, an adult dose of 1 tablet, 2 to 4 times daily, should be sufficient. Some patients are controlled adequately with $^1/_2$ to 1 tablet at bedtime. The time interval between doses should not be shorter than four hours. The dosage for children over 5 years of age and for adults who are sensitive to ephedrine, is one-half the usual adult dose. Clinical experience to date has been confined to ages above 5 years.

Syrup: The dose for children over 5 years of age is 1 teaspoon (5 ml), 3 to 4 times daily. Dosage for children 2 to 5 years of age is $^1/_2$ to 1 teaspoon (2.5-5 ml), 3 to 4 times daily. Not recommended for children under 2 years of age.

HOW SUPPLIED

Marax Tablets are available as scored, dye free, m-shaped tablets in bottles of 100 (NDC 0049-2540-66) and 500 (NDC 0049-2540-73).

Marax-DF Syrup is available in pints (NDC 0049-2550-93) and gallons (NDC 0049-2550-54) as a colorless syrup, free of all coal tar dyes, and should be dispensed in tight, light-resistant containers (USP).

69-0928-32-7
66-2265-00-4

MINIPRESS® CAPSULES ℞

[*mĭn 'ē-prĕs*]

(prazosin hydrochloride)

For Oral Use

DESCRIPTION

MINIPRESS® (prazosin hydrochloride), a quinazoline derivative, is the first of a new chemical class of antihypertensives. It is the hydrochloride salt of 1-(4-amino-6,7-dimethoxy-2-quinazolinyl)-4-(2-furoyl) piperazine and its structural formula is:

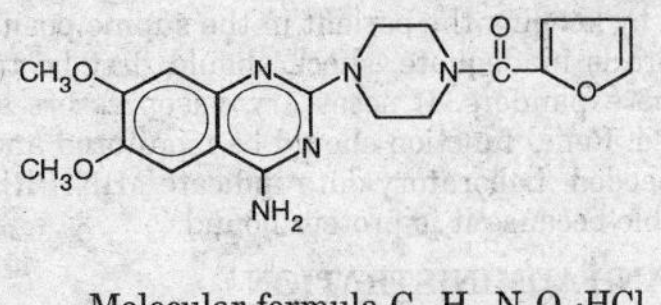

Molecular formula $C_{19}H_{21}N_5O_4 \cdot HCl$

It is a white, crystalline substance, slightly soluble in water and isotonic saline, and has a molecular weight of 419.87. Each 1 mg capsule of MINIPRESS for oral use contains drug equivalent to 1 mg free base.

Inert ingredients in the formulations are: hard gelatin capsules (which may contain Blue 1, Red 3, Red 28, Red 40, and other inert ingredients); magnesium stearate; sodium lauryl sulfate; starch; sucrose.

CLINICAL PHARMACOLOGY

The exact mechanism of the hypotensive action of prazosin is unknown. Prazosin causes a decrease in total peripheral resistance and was originally thought to have a direct relaxant action on vascular smooth muscle. Recent animal studies, however, have suggested that the vasodilator effect of prazosin is also related to blockade of postsynaptic *alpha*-adrenoceptors. The results of dog forelimb experiments demonstrate that the peripheral vasodilator effect of prazosin is confined mainly to the level of the resistance vessels (arterioles). Unlike conventional *alpha*-blockers, the antihypertensive action of prazosin is usually not accompanied by a reflex tachycardia. Tolerance has not been observed to develop in long term therapy.

Hemodynamic studies have been carried out in man following acute single dose administration and during the course of long term maintenance therapy. The results confirm that the therapeutic effect is a fall in blood pressure unaccompanied by a clinically significant change in cardiac output, heart rate, renal blood flow and glomerular filtration rate. There is no measurable negative chronotropic effect.

In clinical studies to date, MINIPRESS (prazosin hydrochloride) has not increased plasma renin activity.

In man, blood pressure is lowered in both the supine and standing positions. This effect is most pronounced on the diastolic blood pressure.

Following oral administration, human plasma concentrations reach a peak at about three hours with a plasma half-life of two to three hours. The drug is highly bound to plasma protein. Bioavailability studies have demonstrated that the total absorption relative to the drug in a 20% alcoholic solution is 90%, resulting in peak levels approximately 65% of that of the drug in solution. Animal studies indicate that MINIPRESS (prazosin hydrochloride) is extensively metabolized, primarily by demethylation and conjugation, and excreted mainly via bile and feces. Less extensive human studies suggest similar metabolism and excretion in man.

In clinical studies in which lipid profiles were followed, there were generally no adverse changes noted between pre- and post-treatment lipid levels.

INDICATIONS AND USAGE

MINIPRESS (prazosin hydrochloride) is indicated in the treatment of hypertension. It can be used alone or in combination with other antihypertensive drugs such as diuretics or beta-adrenergic blocking agents.

CONTRAINDICATIONS

None known.

WARNINGS

MINIPRESS (prazosin hydrochloride) may cause syncope with sudden loss of consciousness. In most cases this is believed to be due to an excessive postural hypotensive effect, although occasionally the syncopal episode has been preceded by a bout of severe tachycardia with heart rates of 120–160 beats per minute. Syncopal episodes have usually occurred within 30 to 90 minutes of the initial dose of the drug; occasionally they have been reported in association with rapid dosage increases or the introduction of another antihypertensive drug into the regimen of a patient taking high doses of MINIPRESS (prazosin hydrochloride). The incidence of syncopal episodes is approximately 1% in patients given an initial dose of 2 mg or greater. Clinical trials conducted during the investigational phase of this drug suggest that syncopal episodes can be minimized by limiting the initial dose of the drug to 1 mg, by subsequently increasing the dosage slowly, and by introducing any additional antihypertensive drugs into the patient's regimen with caution (see DOSAGE AND ADMINISTRATION). Hypotension may develop in patients given MINIPRESS who are also receiving a beta-blocker such as propranolol.

If syncope occurs, the patient should be placed in the recumbent position and treated supportively as necessary. This adverse effect is self-limiting and in most cases does not recur after the initial period of therapy or during subsequent dose titration.

Patients should always be started on the 1 mg capsules of MINIPRESS (prazosin hydrochloride). The 2 and 5 mg capsules are not indicated for initial therapy.

More common than loss of consciousness are the symptoms often associated with lowering of the blood pressure, namely, dizziness and lightheadedness. The patient should be cautioned about these possible adverse effects and advised what measures to take should they develop. The patient should also be cautioned to avoid situations where injury could result should syncope occur during the initiation of MINIPRESS (prazosin hydrochloride) therapy.

PRECAUTIONS

Information for Patients: Dizziness or drowsiness may occur after the first dose of this medicine. Avoid driving or performing hazardous tasks for the first 24 hours after taking this medicine or when the dose is increased. Dizziness, lightheadedness or fainting may occur, especially when rising from a lying or sitting position. Getting up slowly may help lessen the problem. These effects may also occur if you

Continued on next page

Minipress—Cont.

drink alcohol, stand for long periods of time, exercise, or if the weather is hot. While taking MINIPRESS, be careful in the amount of alcohol you drink. Also, use extra care during exercise or hot weather, or if standing for long periods. Check with your physician if you have any questions.

Drug Interactions

MINIPRESS (prazosin hydrochloride) has been administered without any adverse drug interaction in limited clinical experience to date with the following: (1) cardiac glycosides—digitalis and digoxin; (2) hypoglycemics—insulin, chlorpropamide, phenformin, tolazamide, and tolbutamide; (3) tranquilizers and sedatives—chlordiazepoxide, diazepam, and phenobarbital; (4) antigout—allopurinol, colchicine, and probenecid; (5) antiarrhythmics—procainamide, propranolol (see WARNINGS however), and quinidine; and (6) analgesics, antipyretics and anti-inflammatories—propoxyphene, aspirin, indomethacin, and phenylbutazone.

Addition of a diuretic or other antihypertensive agent to MINIPRESS has been shown to cause an additive hypotensive effect. This effect can be minimized by reducing the MINIPRESS dose to 1 to 2 mg three times a day, by introducing additional antihypertensive drugs cautiously and then by retitrating MINIPRESS based on clinical response.

Drug/Laboratory Test Interactions

In a study on five patients given from 12 to 24 mg of prazosin per day for 10 to 14 days, there was an average increase of 42% in the urinary metabolite of norepinephrine and an average increase in urinary VMA of 17%. Therefore, false positive results may occur in screening tests for pheochromocytoma in patients who are being treated with prazosin. If an elevated VMA is found, prazosin should be discontinued and the patient retested after a month.

Laboratory Tests

In clinical studies in which lipid profiles were followed, there were generally no adverse changes noted between pre- and post-treatment lipid levels.

Carcinogenesis, Mutagenesis, Impairment of Fertility: No carcinogenic potential was demonstrated in an 18 month study in rats with MINIPRESS at dose levels more than 225 times the usual maximum recommended human dose of 20 mg per day. MINIPRESS was not mutagenic in in vivo genetic toxicology studies. In a fertility and general reproductive performance study in rats, both males and females, treated with 75 mg/kg (225 times the usual maximum recommended human dose), demonstrated decreased fertility while those treated with 25 mg/kg (75 times the usual maximum recommended human dose) did not.

In chronic studies (one year or more) of MINIPRESS in rats and dogs, testicular changes consisting of atrophy and necrosis occurred at 25 mg/kg/day (75 times the usual maximum recommended human dose). No testicular changes were seen in rats or dogs at 10 mg/kg/day (30 times the usual maximum recommended human dose). In view of the testicular changes observed in animals, 105 patients on long term MINIPRESS therapy were monitored for 17-ketosteroid excretion and no changes indicating a drug effect were observed. In addition, 27 males on MINIPRESS for up to 51 months did not have changes in sperm morphology suggestive of drug effect.

Usage in Pregnancy: Pregnancy Category C. MINIPRESS has been shown to be associated with decreased litter size at birth, 1, 4, and 21 days of age in rats when given doses more than 225 times the usual maximum recommended human dose. No evidence of drug-related external, visceral, or skeletal fetal abnormalities were observed. No drug-related external, visceral, or skeletal abnormalities were observed in fetuses of pregnant rabbits and pregnant monkeys at doses more than 225 times and 12 times the usual maximum recommended human dose respectively.

The use of prazosin and a beta-blocker for the control of severe hypertension in 44 pregnant women revealed no drug-related fetal abnormalities or adverse effects. Therapy with prazosin was continued for as long as 14 weeks.[1]

Prazosin has also been used alone or in combination with other hypotensive agents in severe hypertension of pregnancy by other investigators. No fetal or neonatal abnormalities have been reported with the use of prazosin.[2]

There are no adequate and well controlled studies which establish the safety of MINIPRESS (prazosin HCl) in pregnant women. MINIPRESS should be used during pregnancy only if the potential benefit justifies the potential risk to the mother and fetus.

Nursing Mothers: MINIPRESS has been shown to be excreted in small amounts in human milk. Caution should be exercised when MINIPRESS is administered to a nursing woman.

Usage in Children: Safety and effectiveness in children have not been established.

ADVERSE REACTIONS

Clinical trials were conducted on more than 900 patients. During these trials and subsequent marketing experience, the most frequent reactions associated with MINIPRESS therapy are: dizziness 10.3%, headache 7.8%, drowsiness

Strength	Capsule Color	Capsule Code	NDC	Package Size
MINIPRESS® 1 mg	White	431	0069-4310-71	250's
			0069-4310-82	1000's
			0063-4310-82	
			0069-4310-41	100 (10×10)
			0663-4310-41	Unit Dose
MINIPRESS® 2 mg	Pink and White	437	0069-4370-71	250's
			0663-4370-71	
			0069-4370-82	1000's
			0663-4370-82	
			0069-4370-41	100 (10×10)
			0663-4370-41	Unit Dose
MINIPRESS® 5 mg	Blue and White	438	0069-4380-71	250's
			0663-4380-71	
			0069-4380-73	500's
			0663-4380-73	
			0069-4380-41	100 (10×10)
			0663-4380-41	Unit Dose

7.6%, lack of energy 6.9%, weakness 6.5%, palpitations 5.3%, and nausea 4.9%. In most instances side effects have disappeared with continued therapy or have been tolerated with no decrease in dose of drug.

Less frequent adverse reactions which are reported to occur in 1–4% of patients are:

Gastrointestinal: vomiting, diarrhea, constipation.
Cardiovascular: edema, orthostatic hypotension, dyspnea, syncope.
Central Nervous System: vertigo, depression, nervousness.
Dermatologic: rash.
Genitourinary: urinary frequency.
EENT: blurred vision, reddened sclera, epistaxis, dry mouth, nasal congestion.

In addition, fewer than 1% of patients have reported the following (in some instances, exact causal relationships have not been established):

Gastrointestinal: abdominal discomfort and/or pain, liver function abnormalities, pancreatitis.
Cardiovascular: tachycardia.
Central Nervous System: paresthesia, hallucinations.
Dermatologic: pruritus, alopecia, lichen planus.
Genitourinary: incontinence, impotence, priapism.
EENT: tinnitus.
Other: diaphoresis, fever, positive ANA titer, arthralgia.

Single reports of pigmentary mottling and serous retinopathy, and a few reports of cataract development or disappearance have been reported. In these instances, the exact causal relationship has not been established because the baseline observations were frequently inadequate.

In more specific slit-lamp and funduscopic studies, which included adequate baseline examinations, no drug-related abnormal ophthalmological findings have been reported.

Literature reports exist associating MINIPRESS therapy with a worsening of pre-existing narcolepsy. A causal relationship is uncertain in these cases.

OVERDOSAGE

Accidental ingestion of at least 50 mg of MINIPRESS (prazosin hydrochloride) in a two year old child resulted in profound drowsiness and depressed reflexes. No decrease in blood pressure was noted. Recovery was uneventful.

Should overdosage lead to hypotension, support of the cardiovascular system is of first importance. Restoration of blood pressure and normalization of heart rate may be accomplished by keeping the patient in the supine position. If this measure is inadequate, shock should first be treated with volume expanders. If necessary, vasopressors should then be used. Renal function should be monitored and supported as needed. Laboratory data indicate MINIPRESS is not dialysable because it is protein bound.

DOSAGE AND ADMINISTRATION

The dose of MINIPRESS should be adjusted according to the patient's individual blood pressure response. The following is a guide to its administration:

Initial Dose

1 mg two or three times a day. (See WARNINGS)

Maintenance Dose

Dosage may be slowly increased to a total daily dose of 20 mg given in divided doses. The therapeutic dosages most commonly employed have ranged from 6 mg to 15 mg daily given in divided doses. Doses higher than 20 mg usually do not increase efficacy, however a few patients may benefit from further increases up to a daily dose of 40 mg given in divided doses. After initial titration some patients can be maintained adequately on a twice daily dosage regimen.

Use With Other Drugs

When adding a diuretic or other antihypertensive agent, the dose of MINIPRESS should be reduced to 1 mg or 2 mg three times a day and retitration then carried out.

HOW SUPPLIED

[See table above]

References

1. Lubbe, WF, and Hodge, JV: *New Zealand Med J* **94** (691) 169–172, 1981.
2. Davey, DA, and Dommisse, J: *S.A. Med J,* Oct 4, 1980 (551–556).

©1996 Pfizer Inc
69-2318-00-3   Revised June 1996

MINIZIDE® CAPSULES   ℞
[mĭn 'ē-zīd]
(prazosin hydrochloride/polythiazide)
FOR ORAL ADMINISTRATION

> This fixed combination drug is not indicated for initial therapy of hypertension. Hypertension requires therapy titrated to the individual patient. If the fixed combination represents the dose so determined, its use may be more convenient in patient management. The treatment of hypertension is not static, but must be re-evaluated as conditions in each patient warrant.

DESCRIPTION

MINIZIDE® is a combination of MINIPRESS® (prazosin hydrochloride) plus RENESE® (polythiazide).

MINIPRESS (prazosin hydrochloride), a quinazoline derivative, is the first of that chemical class of antihypertensives. It is the hydrochloride salt of 1-(4-amino-6, 7-dimethoxy-2-quinazolinyl)-4-(2-furoyl) piperazine and its structural formula is:

It is a white, crystalline substance, slightly soluble in water and isotonic saline, and has a molecular weight of 419.87. Each 1 mg capsule of MINIPRESS (prazosin hydrochloride) contains drug equivalent to 1 mg free base.

RENESE (polythiazide) is an orally effective, nonmercurial diuretic, saluretic, and antihypertensive agent.

It is designated chemically as 2*H*-1,2,4-Benzothiadiazine-7-sulfonamide,6-chloro-3,4-dihydro -2- methyl -3-[[(2,2,2-trifluoroethyl) thio]methyl]-,1,1-dioxide, and has the following structural formula:

It is a white, crystalline substance insoluble in water, but readily soluble in alkaline solution.

Inert ingredients in the formulations are: hard gelatin capsules (which may contain Blue 1, Green 3, Red 3 and other inert ingredients); magnesium stearate; sodium lauryl sulfate; starch; sucrose.

CLINICAL PHARMACOLOGY

MINIZIDE (prazosin hydrochloride/polythiazide)

Minizide produces a more pronounced antihypertensive response than occurs after either prazosin hydrochloride or polythiazide alone in equivalent doses.

MINIPRESS (prazosin hydrochloride)

The exact mechanism of the hypotensive action of prazosin is unknown. Prazosin causes a decrease in total peripheral resistance and was originally thought to have a direct relaxant action on vascular smooth muscle. Recent animal studies, however, have suggested that the vasodilator effect of prazosin is also related to blockade of postsynaptic *alpha*-adrenoceptors. The results of dog forelimb experiments demonstrate that the peripheral vasodilator effect of prazosin is confined mainly to the level of the resistance vessels (arterioles). Unlike conventional *alpha*-blockers, the antihypertensive action of prazosin is usually not accompanied by a reflex tachycardia. Tolerance has not been observed to develop in long term therapy.

Hemodynamic studies have been carried out in man following acute single dose administration and during the course of long term maintenance therapy. The results confirm that the therapeutic effect is a fall in blood pressure unaccompanied by a clinically significant change in cardiac output, heart rate, renal blood flow, and glomerular filtration rate. There is no measurable negative chronotropic effect.

In clinical studies to date, MINIPRESS has not increased plasma renin activity.

In man, blood pressure is lowered in both the supine and standing positions. This effect is most pronounced on the diastolic blood pressure.

Following oral administration, human plasma concentrations reach a peak at about three hours with a plasma half-life of two to three hours. The drug is highly bound to plasma protein. Bioavailability studies have demonstrated that the total absorption relative to the drug in a 20% alcoholic solution is 90%, resulting in peak levels approximately 65% of that of the drug in solution. Animal studies indicate that MINIPRESS is extensively metabolized, primarily by demethylation and conjugation, and excreted mainly via bile and feces. Less extensive human studies suggest similar metabolism and excretion in man.

MINIPRESS has been administered without any adverse drug interaction in limited clinical experience to date with the following: (1) cardiac glycosides—digitalis and digoxin; (2) hypoglycemics—insulin, chlorpropamide, phenformin, tolazamide, and tolbutamide; (3) tranquilizers and sedatives—chlordiazepoxide, diazepam, and phenobarbital; (4) antigout—allopurinol, colchicine, and probenecid; (5) antiarrhythmics—procainamide, propranolol (see WARNINGS however), and quinidine; and (6) analgesics, antipyretics and anti-inflammatories—propoxyphene, aspirin, indomethacin, and phenylbutazone.

RENESE (polythiazide)

RENESE is a member of the benzothiadiazine (thiazide) family of diuretic/antihypertensive agents. Its mechanism of action results in an interference with the renal tubular mechanism of electrolyte reabsorption. At maximal therapeutic dosage all thiazides are approximately equal in their diuretic potency. The mechanism whereby thiazides function in the control of hypertension is unknown. Renese is well absorbed, giving peak human plasma concentrations about 5 hours after oral administration. Drug is removed slowly thereafter with a plasma elimination half-life of approximately 27 hours. One fifth of the drug is recovered unchanged in human urine; the remainder is cleared via feces and as metabolites. Animal studies indicate metabolism occurs by rupture of the thiadiazine ring and loss of the side chain.

INDICATIONS AND USAGE

MINIZIDE is indicated in the treatment of hypertension. (See box warning.)

CONTRAINDICATIONS

RENESE is contraindicated in patients with anuria, and in patients known to be sensitive to thiazides or to other sulfonamide derivatives.

WARNINGS

MINIPRESS (prazosin hydrochloride)

MINIPRESS may cause syncope with sudden loss of consciousness. In most cases this is believed to be due to an excessive postural hypotensive effect, although occasionally the syncopal episode has been preceded by a bout of severe tachycardia with heart rates of 120–160 beats per minute. Syncopal episodes have usually occurred within 30 to 90 minutes of the initial dose of the drug; occasionally they have been reported in association with rapid dosage increases or the introduction of another antihypertensive drug into the regimen of a patient taking high doses of MINIPRESS. The incidence of syncopal episodes is approximately 1% in patients given an initial dose of 2 mg or greater. Clinical trials

conducted during the investigational phase of this drug suggest that syncopal episodes can be minimized by limiting the initial dose of the drug to 1 mg, by subsequently increasing the dosage slowly, and by introducing any additional antihypertensive drugs into the patient's regimen with caution (see DOSAGE AND ADMINISTRATION). Hypotension may develop in patients given MINIPRESS who are also receiving a beta-blocker such as propranolol.

If syncope occurs, the patient should be placed in the recumbent position and treated supportively as necessary. This adverse effect is self-limiting and in most cases does not recur after the initial period of therapy or during subsequent dose titration.

Patients should always be started on the 1 mg capsules of MINIPRESS (prazosin hydrochloride). The 2 and 5 mg capsules are not indicated for initial therapy.

More common than loss of consciousness are the symptoms often associated with lowering of the blood pressure, namely, dizziness and lightheadedness. The patient should be cautioned about these possible adverse effects and advised what measures to take should they develop. The patient should also be cautioned to avoid situations where injury could result should syncope occur during the initiation of MINIPRESS therapy.

RENESE (polythiazide)

RENESE should be used with caution in severe renal disease. In patients with renal disease, thiazides may precipitate azotemia. Cumulative effects of the drug may develop in patients with impaired renal function.

Thiazides should be used with caution in patients with impaired hepatic function or progressive liver disease, since minor alterations of fluid and electrolyte balance may precipitate hepatic coma.

Sensitivity reactions may occur in patients with a history of allergy or bronchial asthma.

The possibility of exacerbation or activation of systemic lupus erythematosus has been reported.

Thiazides may be additive or potentiative of the action of other antihypertensive drugs.

Potentiation occurs with ganglionic or peripheral adrenergic blocking drugs.

Periodic determinations of serum electrolytes to detect possible electrolyte imbalance should be performed at appropriate intervals.

All patients receiving thiazide therapy should be observed for clinical signs of fluid or electrolyte imbalance, namely, hyponatremia, hypochloremic alkalosis, and hypokalemia. Serum and urine electrolyte determinations are particularly important when the patient is vomiting excessively or receiving parenteral fluids. Medications such as digitalis may also influence serum electrolytes. Warning signs, irrespective of cause, are: dryness of mouth, thirst, weakness, lethargy, drowsiness, restlessness, muscle pains or cramps, muscular fatigue, hypotension, oliguria, tachycardia, and gastrointestinal disturbances such as nausea and vomiting. Hypokalemia may develop with thiazides as with any potent diuretic, especially with brisk diuresis, when severe cirrhosis is present, or during concomitant use of corticosteroids or ACTH.

Interference with adequate oral electrolyte intake will also contribute to hypokalemia. Digitalis therapy may exaggerate the metabolic effects of hypokalemia, especially with reference to myocardial activity.

Any chloride deficit is generally mild and usually does not require specific treatment except under extraordinary circumstances (as in hepatic or renal disease). Dilutional hyponatremia may occur in edematous patients in hot weather; appropriate therapy is water restriction rather than administration of salt, except in rare instances when the hyponatremia is life-threatening. In actual salt depletion, appropriate replacement is the therapy of choice.

Hyperuricemia may occur or frank gout may be precipitated in certain patients receiving thiazide therapy.

Insulin requirements in diabetic patients may be either increased, decreased, or unchanged. Latent diabetes mellitus may become manifest during thiazide administration.

Thiazide drugs may increase responsiveness to tubocurarine.

The antihypertensive effects of the drug may be enhanced in the post-sympathectomy patient.

Thiazides may decrease arterial responsiveness to norepinephrine. This diminution is not sufficient to preclude effectiveness of the pressor agent for therapeutic use.

If progressive renal impairment becomes evident, as indicated by a rising nonprotein nitrogen or blood urea nitrogen, a careful reappraisal of therapy is necessary with consideration given to withholding or discontinuing diuretic therapy.

Thiazides may decrease serum protein-bound iodine levels without signs of thyroid disturbance.

PRECAUTIONS

Drug/Laboratory Test Interactions: In a study on five patients given from 12 to 24 mg of prazosin per day for 10 to 14 days, there was an average increase of 42% in the urinary metabolite of norepinephrine and an average increase in urinary VMA of 17%. Therefore, false positive results may occur in screening tests for pheochromocytoma in patients who are being treated with prazosin. If an elevated VMA is found, prazosin should be discontinued and the patient retested after a month.

Carcinogenesis, Mutagenesis, Impairment of Fertility: No carcinogenic or mutagenic studies have been conducted with MINIZIDE. However, no carcinogenic potential was demonstrated in 18 month studies in rats with either MINIPRESS or RENESE at dose levels more than 100 times the usual maximum human doses. MINIPRESS was not mutagenic in *in vivo* genetic toxicology studies.

MINIZIDE produced no impairment of fertility in male or female rats at 50 and 25 mg/kg/day of MINIPRESS and RENESE respectively. In chronic studies (one year or more) of MINIPRESS in rats and dogs, testicular changes consisting of atrophy and necrosis occurred at 25 mg/kg/day (60 times the usual maximum recommended human dose). No testicular changes were seen in rats or dogs at 10 mg/kg/day (24 times the usual maximum recommended human dose). In view of the testicular changes observed in animals, 105 patients on long term MINIPRESS therapy were monitored for 17-ketosteroid excretion and no changes indicating a drug effect were observed. In addition, 27 males on MINIPRESS alone for up to 51 months did not have changes in sperm morphology suggestive of drug effect.

Use in Pregnancy: Pregnancy Category C. MINIZIDE was not teratogenic in either rats or rabbits when administered in oral doses more than 100 times the usual maximum human dose. Studies in rats indicated that the combination of RENESE (40 times the usual maximum recommended human dose) and MINIPRESS (8 times the usual maximum recommended human dose) caused a greater number of stillbirths, a more prolonged gestation, and a decreased survival of pups to weaning than that caused by MINIPRESS alone. There are no adequate and well controlled studies in pregnant women. Therefore, MINIZIDE should be used in pregnancy only if the potential benefit justifies the potential risk to the fetus.

Nursing Mothers: It is not known whether MINIPRESS or RENESE is excreted in human milk. Thiazides appear in breast milk. Thus, if use of the drug is deemed essential the patient should stop nursing.

Pediatric Use: Safety and effectiveness in children has not been established.

ADVERSE REACTIONS

MINIPRESS (prazosin hydrochloride)

The most common reactions associated with MINIPRESS therapy are: dizziness 10.3%, headache 7.8%, drowsiness 7.6%, lack of energy 6.9%, weakness 6.5%, palpitations 5.3%, and nausea 4.9%. In most instances side effects have disappeared with continued therapy or have been tolerated with no decrease in dose of drug.

The following reactions have been associated with MINIPRESS, some of them rarely. (In some instances exact causal relationships have not been established.)

Continued on next page

STRENGTH	COMPONENTS	COLOR	CAPSULE CODE	PKG. SIZE
MINIZIDE® 1	1 mg prazosin + 0.5 mg polythiazide (NDC 0663-4300-66) (NDC 0069-4300-66)	Blue-Green	430	100's
MINIZIDE® 2	2 mg prazosin + 0.5 mg polythiazide (NDC 0663-4320-66) (NDC 0069-4320-66)	Blue-Green/Pink	432	100's
MINIZIDE® 5	5 mg prazosin + 0.5 mg polythiazide (NDC 0663-4360-66) (NDC 0069-4360-66)	Blue-Green/Blue	436	100's

Minizide—Cont.

Gastrointestinal: vomiting, diarrhea, constipation, abdominal discomfort and/or pain, liver function abnormalities, pancreatitis.
Cardiovascular: edema, dyspnea, syncope, tachycardia.
Central Nervous System: nervousness, vertigo, depression, paresthesia, hallucinations.
Dermatologic: rash, pruritus, alopecia, lichen planus.
Genitourinary: urinary frequency, incontinence, impotence, priapism.
EENT: blurred vision, reddened sclera, epistaxis, tinnitus, dry mouth, nasal congestion.
Other: diaphoresis, fever.

Single reports of pigmentary mottling and serous retinopathy, and a few reports of cataract development or disappearance have been reported. In these instances, the exact causal relationship has not been established because the baseline observations were frequently inadequate.
In more specific slit-lamp and funduscopic studies, which included adequate baseline examinations, no drug-related abnormal ophthalmological findings have been reported.
Literature reports exist associating MINIPRESS therapy with a worsening of pre-existing narcolepsy. A causal relationship is uncertain in these cases.

RENESE (polythiazide)
Gastrointestinal: anorexia, gastric irritation, nausea, vomiting, cramping, diarrhea, constipation, jaundice (intrahepatic cholestatic jaundice), pancreatitis.
Central Nervous System: dizziness, vertigo, paresthesia, headache, xanthopsia.
Hematologic: leukopenia, agranulocytosis, thrombocytopenia, aplastic anemia.
Dermatologic: purpura, photosensitivity, rash, urticaria, necrotizing angiitis, (vasculitis) (cutaneous vasculitis).
Cardiovascular: Orthostatic hypotension may occur and be aggravated by alcohol, barbiturates, or narcotics.
Other: hyperglycemia, glycosuria, hyperuricemia, muscle spasm, weakness, restlessness.

OVERDOSAGE

MINIPRESS (prazosin hydrochloride)
Accidental ingestion of at least 50 mg of MINIPRESS in a two year old child resulted in profound drowsiness and depressed reflexes. No decrease in blood pressure was noted. Recovery was uneventful.
Should overdosage lead to hypotension, support of the cardiovascular system is of first importance. Restoration of blood pressure and normalization of heart rate may be accomplished by keeping the patient in the supine position. If this measure is inadequate, shock should first be treated with volume expanders. If necessary, vasopressors should then be used. Renal function should be monitored and supported as needed. Laboratory data indicate that MINIPRESS is not dialyzable because it is protein bound.

RENESE (polythiazide)
Should overdosage with RENESE occur, electrolyte balance and adequate hydration should be maintained. Gastric lavage is recommended, followed by supportive treatment. Where necessary, this may include intravenous dextrose and saline with potassium and other electrolyte therapy, administered with caution as indicated by laboratory testing at appropriate intervals.

DOSAGE AND ADMINISTRATION

MINIZIDE (prazosin hydrochloride/polythiazide)
Dosage: as determined by individual titration of MINIPRESS (prazosin hydrochloride) and RENESE (polythiazide). (See box warning.)
Usual MINIZIDE dosage is one capsule two or three times daily, the strength depending upon individual requirement following titration.
The following is a general guide to the administration of the individual components of MINIZIDE:

MINIPRESS (prazosin hydrochloride)
Initial Dose: 1 mg two or three times a day. (See WARNINGS.)
Maintenance Dose: Dosage may be slowly increased to a total daily dose of 20 mg given in divided doses. The therapeutic dosages most commonly employed have ranged from 6 mg to 15 mg daily given in divided doses. Doses higher than 20 mg usually do not increase efficacy, however a few patients may benefit from further increases up to a daily dose of 40 mg given in divided doses. After initial titration some patients can be maintained adequately on a twice daily dosage regimen.
Use With Other Drugs: When adding a diuretic or other antihypertensive agent, the dose of MINIPRESS should be reduced to 1 mg or 2 mg three times a day and retitration then carried out.

RENESE (polythiazide)
The usual dose of RENESE for antihypertensive therapy is 2 to 4 mg daily.

HOW SUPPLIED

[See table at bottom of previous page]
#69-2463-00-7 Revised Oct. 1995

NAVANE® ℞
[nah 'vān]
(thiothixene) CAPSULES
NAVANE® ℞
(thiothixene hydrochloride) CONCENTRATE

DESCRIPTION

Navane® (thiothixene) is a thioxanthene derivative. Specifically, it is the *cis* isomer of N,N-dimethyl-9-[3-(4-methyl-1-piperazinyl)-propylidene] thioxanthene-2-sulfonamide.

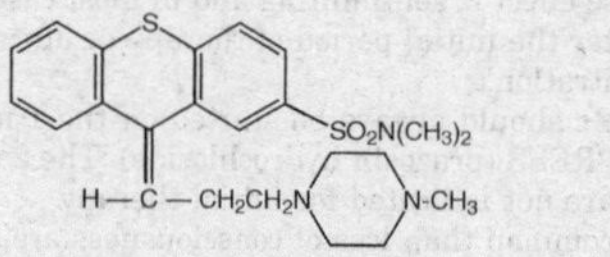

The thioxanthenes differ from the phenothiazines by the replacement of nitrogen in the central ring with a carbon-linked side chain fixed in space in a rigid structural configuration. An N,N-dimethyl sulfonamide functional group is bonded to the thioxanthene nucleus.
Inert ingredients for the capsule formulations are: hard gelatin capsules (which contain gelatin and titanium dioxide; may contain Yellow 10, Yellow 6, Blue 1, Green 3, Red 3, and other inert ingredients); lactose; magnesium stearate; sodium lauryl sulfate; starch.
Inert ingredients for the oral concentrate formulation are: alcohol; cherry flavor; dextrose; passion fruit flavor; sorbitol solution; water.

ACTIONS

Navane is a psychotropic agent of the thioxanthene series. Navane possesses certain chemical and pharmacological similarities to the piperazine phenothiazines and differences from the aliphatic group of phenothiazines.

INDICATIONS

Navane is effective in the management of manifestations of psychotic disorders. Navane has not been evaluated in the management of behavioral complications in patients with mental retardation.

CONTRADICTIONS

Navane is contraindicated in patients with circulatory collapse, comatose states, central nervous system depression due to any cause, and blood dycrasias. Navane is contraindicated in individuals who have shown hypersensitivity to the drug. It is not known whether there is a cross sensitivity between the thioxanthenes and the phenothiazine derivatives, but this possibility should be considered.

WARNINGS

Tardive Dyskinesia—Tardive dyskinesia, a syndrome consisting of potentially irreversible, involuntary, dyskinetic movements may develop in patients treated with neuroleptic (antipsychotic) drugs. Although the prevalence of the syndrome appears to be highest among the elderly, especially elderly women, it is impossible to rely upon prevalence estimates to predict, at the inception of neuroleptic treatment, which patients are likely to develop the syndrome. Whether neuroleptic drug products differ in their potential to cause tardive dyskinesia is unknown.
Both the risk of developing the syndrome and the likelihood that it will become irreversible are believed to increase as the duration of treatment and the total cumulative dose of neuroleptic drugs administered to the patient increase. However, the syndrome can develop, although much less commonly, after relatively brief treatment periods at low doses.
There is no known treatment for established cases of tardive dyskinesia, although the syndrome may remit, partially or completely, if neuroleptic treatment is withdrawn. Neuroleptic treatment, itself, however, may suppress (or partially suppress) the signs and symptoms of the syndrome and thereby may possibly mask the underlying disease process. The effect that symptomatic suppression has upon the long-term course of the syndrome is unknown.
Given these considerations, neuroleptics should be prescribed in a manner that is most likely to minimize the occurrence of tardive dyskinesia. Chronic neuroleptic treatment should generally be reserved for patients who suffer from a chronic illness that, 1) is known to respond to neuroleptic drugs, and, 2) for whom alternative, equally effective, but potentially less harmful treatments are not available or appropriate. In patients who do require chronic treatment, the smallest dose and the shortest duration of treatment producing a satisfactory clinical response should be sought. The need for continued treatment should be reassessed periodically.
If signs and symptoms of tardive dyskinesia appear in a patient on neuroleptics, drug discontinuation should be considered. However, some patients may require treatment despite the presence of the syndrome. (For further information about the description of tardive dyskinesia and its clinical detection, please refer to "Information for Patients" in the PRECAUTIONS section, and to the ADVERSE REACTIONS section.)

Neuroleptic Malignant Syndrome (NMS)—A potentially fatal symptom complex sometimes referred to as Neuroleptic Malignant Syndrome (NMS) has been reported in association with antipsychotic drugs. Clinical manifestations of NMS are hyperpyrexia, muscle rigidity, altered mental status and evidence of autonomic instability (irregular pulse or blood pressure, tachycardia, diaphoresis, and cardiac dysrhythmias).
The diagnostic evaluation of patients with this syndrome is complicated. In arriving at a diagnosis, it is important to identify cases where the clinical presentation includes both serious medical illness (e.g., pneumonia, systemic infection, etc.) and untreated or inadequately treated extrapyramidal signs and symptoms (EPS). Other important considerations in the differential diagnosis include central anticholinergic toxicity, heat stroke, drug fever and primary central nervous system (CNS) pathology.
The management of NMS should include 1) immediate discontinuation of antipsychotic drugs and other drugs not essential to concurrent therapy, 2) intensive symptomatic treatment and medical monitoring, and 3) treatment of any concomitant serious medical problems for which specific treatments are available. There is no general agreement about specific pharmacological treatment regimens for uncomplicated NMS.
If a patient requires antipsychotic drug treatment after recovery from NMS, the potential reintroduction of drug therapy should be carefully considered. The patient should be carefully monitored, since recurrences of NMS have been reported.
Usage in Pregnancy—Safe use of Navane during pregnancy has not been established. Therefore, this drug should be given to pregnant patients only when, in the judgment of the physician, the expected benefits from the treatment exceed the possible risks to mother and fetus. Animal reproduction studies and clinical experience to date have not demonstrated any teratogenic effects.
In the animal reproduction studies with Navane, there was some decrease in conception rate and litter size, and an increase in resorption rate in rats and rabbits. Similar findings have been reported with other psychotropic agents. After repeated oral administration of Navane to rats (5 to 15 mg/kg/day), rabbits (3 to 50 mg/kg/day), and monkeys (1 to 3 mg/kg/day) before and during gestation, no teratogenic effects were seen.
Usage in Children—The use of Navane in children under 12 years of age is not recommended because safe conditions for its use have not been established.
As is true with many CNS drugs, Navane may impair the mental and/or physical abilities required for the performance of potentially hazardous tasks such as driving a car or operating machinery, especially during the first few days of therapy. Therefore, the patient should be cautioned accordingly.
As in the case of other CNS-acting drugs, patients receiving Navane (thiothixene) should be cautioned about the possible additive effects (which may include hypotension) with CNS depressants and with alcohol.

PRECAUTIONS

An antiemetic effect was observed in animal studies with Navane; since this effect may also occur in man, it is possible that Navane may mask signs of overdosage of toxic drugs and may obscure conditions such as intestinal obstruction and brain tumor.
In consideration of the known capability of Navane and certain other psychotropic drugs to precipitate convulsions, extreme caution should be used in patients with a history of convulsive disorders or those in a state of alcohol withdrawal, since it may lower the convulsive threshold. Although Navane potentiates the actions of the barbiturates, the dosage of the anticonvulsant therapy should not be reduced when Navane is administered concurrently.
Though exhibiting rather weak anticholinergic properties, Navane should be used with caution in patients who might be exposed to extreme heat or who are receiving atropine or related drugs.
Use with caution in patients with cardiovascular disease.
Caution as well as careful adjustment of the dosages is indicated when Navane is used in conjunction with other CNS depressants.
Also, careful observation should be made for pigmentary retinopathy and lenticular pigmentation (fine lenticular pigmentation has been noted in a small number of patients treated with Navane for prolonged periods). Blood dyscrasias (agranulocytosis, pancytopenia, thrombocytopenic purpura), and liver damage (jaundice, biliary stasis) have been reported with related drugs.
Neuroleptic drugs elevate prolactin levels; the elevation persists during chronic administration. Tissue culture experiments indicate that approximately one-third of human breast cancers are prolactin dependent *in vitro*, a factor of potential importance if the prescription of these drugs is contemplated in a patient with a previously detected breast cancer. Although disturbances such as galactorrhea, amenorrhea, gynecomastia, and impotence have been reported,

the clinical significance of elevated serum prolactin levels is unknown for most patients. An increase in mammary neoplasms has been found in rodents after chronic administration of neuroleptic drugs. Neither clinical studies nor epidemiologic studies conducted to date, however, have shown an association between chronic administration of these drugs and mammary tumorigenesis; the available evidence is considered too limited to be conclusive at this time.

Information for Patients: Given the likelihood that some patients exposed chronically to neuroleptics will develop tardive dyskinesia, it is advised that all patients in whom chronic use is contemplated be given, if possible, full information about this risk. The decision to inform patients and/or their guardians must obviously take into account the clinical circumstances and the competency of the patient to understand the information provided.

ADVERSE REACTIONS

NOTE: Not all of the following adverse reactions have been reported with Navane. However, since Navane has certain chemical and pharmacologic similarities to the phenothiazines, all of the known side effects and toxicity associated with phenothiazine therapy should be borne in mind when Navane is used.

Cardiovascular Effects: Tachycardia, hypotension, lightheadedness, and syncope. In the event hypotension occurs, epinephrine should not be used as a pressor agent since a paradoxical further lowering of blood pressure may result. Nonspecific EKG changes have been observed in some patients receiving Navane. These changes are usually reversible and frequently disappear on continued Navane therapy. The incidence of these changes is lower than that observed with some phenothiazines. The clinical significance of these changes is not known.

CNS Effects: Drowsiness, usually mild, may occur although it usually subsides with continuation of Navane therapy. The incidence of sedation appears similar to that of the piperazine group of phenothiazines but less than that of certain aliphatic phenothiazines. Restlessness, agitation and insomnia have been noted with Navane. Seizures and paradoxical exacerbation of psychotic symptoms have occurred with Navane infrequently.

Hyperreflexia has been reported in infants delivered from mothers having received structurally related drugs.

In addition, phenothiazine derivatives have been associated with cerebral edema and cerebrospinal fluid abnormalities.

Extrapyramidal symptoms, such as pseudoparkinsonism, akathisia and dystonia have been reported. Management of these extrapyramidal symptoms depends upon the type and severity. Rapid relief of acute symptoms may require the use of an injectable antiparkinson agent. More slowly emerging symptoms may be managed by reducing the dosage of Navane and/or administering an oral antiparkinson agent.

Persistent Tardive Dyskinesia: As with all antipsychotic agents, tardive dyskinesia may appear in some patients on long-term therapy or may occur after drug therapy has been discontinued. The syndrome is characterized by rhythmical involuntary movements of the tongue, face, mouth or jaw (e.g., protrusion of tongue, puffing of cheeks, puckering of mouth, chewing movements). Sometimes these may be accompanied by involuntary movements of extremities.

Since early detection of tardive dyskinesia is important, patients should be monitored on an ongoing basis. It has been reported that fine vermicular movement of the tongue may be an early sign of the syndrome. If this or any other presentation of the syndrome is observed, the clinician should consider possible discontinuation of neuroleptic medication. (See WARNINGS section.)

Hepatic Effects: Elevations of serum transaminase and alkaline phosphatase, usually transient, have been infrequently observed in some patients. No clinically confirmed cases of jaundice attributable to Navane (thiothixene) have been reported.

Hematologic Effects: As is true with certain other psychotropic drugs, leukopenia and leucocytosis, which are usually transient, can occur occasionally with Navane. Other antipsychotic drugs have been associated with agranulocytosis, eosinophilia, hemolytic anemia, thrombocytopenia and pancytopenia.

Allergic Reactions: Rash, pruritus, urticaria, photosensitivity and rare cases of anaphylaxis have been reported with Navane. Undue exposure to sunlight should be avoided. Although not experienced with Navane, exfoliative dermatitis and contact dermatitis (in nursing personnel) have been reported with certain phenothiazines.

Endocrine Disorders: Lactation, moderate breast enlargement and amenorrhea have occurred in a small percentage of females receiving Navane. If persistent, this may necessitate a reduction in dosage or the discontinuation of therapy. Phenothiazines have been associated with false positive pregnancy tests, gynecomastia, hypoglycemia, hyperglycemia and glycosuria.

Autonomic Effects: Dry mouth, blurred vision, nasal congestion, constipation, increased sweating, increased salivation and impotence have occurred infrequently with Navane therapy. Phenothiazines have been associated with miosis, mydriasis, and adynamic ileus.

Other Adverse Reactions: Hyperpyrexia, anorexia, nausea, vomiting, diarrhea, increase in appetite and weight, weakness or fatigue, polydipsia, and peripheral edema.

Although not reported with Navane, evidence indicates there is a relationship between phenothiazine therapy and the occurrence of a systemic lupus erythematosus-like syndrome.

Neuroleptic Malignant Syndrome (NMS): Please refer to the text regarding NMS in the WARNINGS section.

NOTE: Sudden deaths have occasionally been reported in patients who have received certain phenothiazine derivatives. In some cases the cause of death was apparently cardiac arrest or asphyxia due to failure of the cough reflex. In others, the cause could not be determined nor could it be established that death was due to phenothiazine administration.

DOSAGE AND ADMINISTRATION

Dosage of Navane should be individually adjusted depending on the chronicity and severity of the condition. In general, small doses should be used initially and gradually increased to the optimal effective level, based on patient response.

Some patients have been successfully maintained on once-a-day Navane therapy.

The use of Navane in children under 12 years of age is not recommended because safe conditions for its use have not been established.

In milder conditions, an initial dose of 2 mg three times daily. If indicated, a subsequent increase to 15 mg/day total daily dose is often effective.

In more severe conditions, an initial dose of 5 mg twice daily.

The usual optimal dose is 20 to 30 mg daily. If indicated, an increase to 60 mg/day total daily dose is often effective. Exceeding a total daily dose of 60 mg rarely increases the beneficial response.

OVERDOSAGE

Manifestations include muscular twitching, drowsiness and dizziness. Symptoms of gross overdosage may include CNS depression, rigidity, weakness, torticollis, tremor, salivation, dysphagia, hypotension, disturbances of gait, or coma.

Treatment: Essentially symptomatic and supportive. Early gastric lavage is helpful. Keep patient under careful observation and maintain an open airway, since involvement of the extrapyramidal system may produce dysphagia and respiratory difficulty in severe overdosage. If hypotension occurs, the standard measures for managing circulatory shock should be used (I.V. fluids and/or vasoconstrictors).

If a vasoconstrictor is needed, levarterenol and phenylephrine are the most suitable drugs. Other pressor agents, including epinephrine, are not recommended, since phenothiazine derivatives may reverse the usual pressor action of these agents and cause further lowering of blood pressure.

If CNS depression is marked, symptomatic treatment is indicated. Extrapyramidal symptoms may be treated with antiparkinson drugs.

There are no data on the use of peritoneal or hemodialysis, but they are known to be of little value in phenothiazine intoxication.

HOW SUPPLIED

Navane® (thiothixene) Capsules

Bottles of 100's:	1 mg (NDC 0049-5710-66)
	2 mg (NDC 0049-5720-66)
	5 mg (NDC 0049-5730-66)
	10 mg (NDC 0049-5740-66)
	20 mg (NDC 0049-5770-66)
1000's:	2 mg (NDC 0049-5720-82)
	5 mg (NDC 0049-5730-82)
	10 mg (NDC 0049-5740-82)
500's:	20 mg (NDC 0049-5770-73).
Unit Doses of:	1 mg (NDC 0049-5710-41)
	2 mg (NDC 0049-5720-41)
	5 mg (NDC 0049-5730-41)
	10 mg (NDC 0049-5740-41)
	20 mg (NDC 0049-5770-41)

Navane® (thiothixene hydrochloride) Concentrate is available in 120 mL (4 oz) bottles (NDC 0049-5750-47), with an accompanying dropper calibrated at 2 mg, 3 mg, 4 mg, 5 mg, 6 mg, 8 mg, and 10 mg; in 30 mL (1 oz) bottles (NDC 0049-5750-51), with an accompanying dropper calibrated at 2 mg, 3 mg, 4 mg, and 5 mg. Each mL contains thiothixene hydrochloride equivalent to 5mg of thiothixene. Contains alcohol U.S.P. 7.0% v/v (small loss unavoidable).

©1997 PFIZER INC

69-1655-00-8 Revised January 1997

Shown in Product Identification Guide, page 331

NAVANE® ℞

[*nah 'vān*]

(thiothixene hydrochloride)
Intramuscular For Injection
STERILE

DESCRIPTION

Navane (thiothixene hydrochloride) is a thioxanthene derivative. Specifically, thiothixene is the *cis* isomer of N,N-dimethyl-9-[3-(4-methyl-1-piperazinyl)-propylidene] thioxanthene-2-sulfonamide.

The thioxanthenes differ from the phenothiazines by the replacement of nitrogen in the central ring with a carbon-linked side chain fixed in space in a rigid structural configuration. An N,N-dimethyl sulfonamide functional group is bonded to the thioxanthene nucleus.

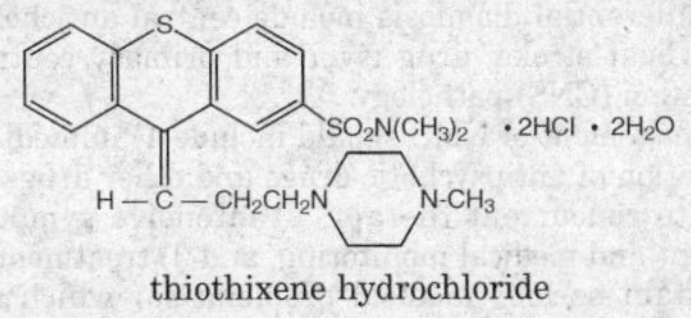

thiothixene hydrochloride

Inert ingredients for the intramuscular for injection formulation are: water; mannitol.

ACTIONS

Navane is a psychotropic agent of the thioxanthene series. Navane possesses certain chemical and pharmacological similarities to the piperazine phenothiazines and differences from the aliphatic group of phenothiazines. Navane's mode of action has not been clearly established.

INDICATIONS

Navane is effective in the management of manifestations of psychotic disorders. Navane has not been evaluated in the management of behavioral complications in patients with mental retardation.

CONTRAINDICATIONS

Navane is contraindicated in patients with circulatory collapse, comatose states, central nervous system depression due to any cause, and blood dyscrasias. Navane is contraindicated in individuals who have shown hypersensitivity to the drug. It is not known whether there is a cross sensitivity between the thioxanthenes and the phenothiazine derivatives, but this possibility should be considered.

WARNINGS

Tardive Dyskinesia—Tardive dyskinesia, a syndrome consisting of potentially irreversible, involuntary, dyskinetic movements may develop in patients treated with neuroleptic (antipsychotic) drugs. Although the prevalence of the syndrome appears to be highest among the elderly, especially elderly women, it is impossible to rely upon prevalence estimates to predict, at the inception of neuroleptic treatment, which patients are likely to develop the syndrome. Whether neuroleptic drug products differ in their potential to cause tardive dyskinesia is unknown.

Both the risk of developing the syndrome and the likelihood that it will become irreversible are believed to increase as the duration of treatment and the total cumulative dose of neuroleptic drugs administered to the patient increase. However, the syndrome can develop, although much less commonly, after relatively brief treatment periods at low doses.

There is no known treatment for established cases of tardive dyskinesia, although the syndrome may remit, partially or completely, if neuroleptic treatment is withdrawn. Neuroleptic treatment, itself, however, may suppress (or partially suppress) the signs and symptoms of the syndrome and thereby may possibly mask the underlying disease process. The effect that symptomatic suppression has upon the long-term course of the syndrome is unknown.

Given these considerations, neuroleptics should be prescribed in a manner that is most likely to minimize the occurrence of tardive dyskinesia. Chronic neuroleptic treatment should generally be reserved for patients who suffer from a chronic illness that, 1) is known to respond to neuroleptic drugs, and, 2) for whom alternative, equally effective, but potentially less harmful treatments are *not* available or appropriate. In patients who do require chronic treatment, the smallest dose and the shortest duration of treatment producing a satisfactory clinical response should be sought. The need for continued treatment should be reassessed periodically.

If signs and symptoms of tardive dyskinesia appear in a patient on neuroleptics, drug discontinuation should be considered. However, some patients may require treatment despite the presence of the syndrome.

(For further information about the description of tardive dyskinesia and its clinical detection, please refer to "Information for Patients" in the PRECAUTIONS section, and to the ADVERSE REACTIONS section.)

Continued on next page

Navane IM—Cont.

Neuroleptic Malignant Syndrome (NMS)—A potentially fatal symptom complex sometimes referred to as Neuroleptic Malignant Syndrome (NMS) has been reported in association with antipsychotic drugs. Clinical manifestations of NMS are hyperpyrexia, muscle rigidity, altered mental status and evidence of autonomic instability (irregular pulse or blood pressure, tachycardia, diaphoresis, and cardiac dysrhythmias).

The diagnostic evaluation of patients with this syndrome is complicated. In arriving at a diagnosis, it is important to identify cases where the clinical presentation includes both serious medical illness (e.g., pneumonia, systemic infection, etc.) and untreated or inadequately treated extrapyramidal signs and symptoms (EPS). Other important considerations in the differential diagnosis include central anticholinergic toxicity, heat stroke, drug fever and primary central nervous system (CNS) pathology.

The management of NMS should include 1) immediate discontinuation of antipsychotic drugs and other drugs not essential to concurrent therapy, 2) intensive symptomatic treatment and medical monitoring, and 3) treatment of any concomitant serious medical problems for which specific treatments are available. There is no general agreement about specific pharmacological treatment regimens for uncomplicated NMS.

If a patient requires antipsychotic drug treatment after recovery from NMS, the potential reintroduction of drug therapy should be carefully considered. The patient should be carefully monitored, since recurrences of NMS have been reported.

Usage in Pregnancy—Safe use of Navane during pregnancy has not been established. Therefore, this drug should be given to pregnant patients only when, in the judgment of the physician, the expected benefits from treatment exceed the possible risks to mother and fetus. Animal reproductive studies and clinical experience to date have not demonstrated any teratogenic effects.

In the animal reproduction studies with Navane, there was some decrease in conception rate and litter size, and an increase in resorption rate in rats and rabbits, changes which have been similarly reported with other psychotropic agents. After repeated oral administration of Navane to rats (5 to 15 mg/kg/day), rabbits (3 to 50 mg/kg/day), and monkeys (1 to 3 mg/kg/day) before and during gestation, no teratogenic effects were seen. (See Precautions)

Usage in Children—The use of Navane in children under 12 years of age is not recommended because safety and efficacy in the pediatric age group have not been established.

As is true with many CNS drugs, Navane may impair the mental and/or physical abilities required for the performance of potentially hazardous tasks such as driving a car or operating machinery, especially during the first few days of therapy. Therefore, the patient should be cautioned accordingly.

As in the case of other CNS-acting drugs, patients receiving Navane should be cautioned about the possible additive effects (which may include hypotension) with CNS depressants and with alcohol.

PRECAUTIONS

General: An antiemetic effect was observed in animal studies with Navane (thiothixene hydrochloride); since this effect may also occur in man, it is possible that Navane may mask signs of overdosage of toxic drugs and may obscure conditions such as intestinal obstruction and brain tumor.

In consideration of the known capability of Navane and certain other psychotropic drugs to precipitate convulsions, extreme caution should be used in patients with a history of convulsive disorders, or those in a state of alcohol withdrawal since it may lower the convulsive threshold. Although Navane potentiates the actions of the barbiturates, the dosage of the anticonvulsant therapy should not be reduced when Navane is administered concurrently.

Caution as well as careful adjustment of the dosage is indicated when Navane is used in conjunction with other CNS depressants other than anticonvulsant drugs.

Though exhibiting rather weak anticholinergic properties, Navane should be used with caution in patients who are known or suspected to have glaucoma, or who might be exposed to extreme heat, or who are receiving atropine or related drugs.

Use with caution in patients with cardiovascular disease.

Also, careful observation should be made for pigmentary retinopathy, and lenticular pigmentation (fine lenticular pigmentation has been noted in a small number of patients treated with Navane for prolonged periods). Blood dyscrasias (agranulocytosis, pancytopenia, thrombocytopenic purpura), and liver damage (jaundice, biliary stasis), have been reported with related drugs.

Undue exposure to sunlight should be avoided. Photosensitive reactions have been reported in patients on Navane.

As with all intramuscular preparations, Navane Intramuscular For Injection should be injected well within the body of a relatively large muscle. The preferred sites are the upper outer quadrant of the buttock (i.e., gluteus maximus) and the mid-lateral thigh.

The deltoid area should be used only if well developed such as in certain adults and older children, and then only with caution to avoid radial nerve injury. Intramuscular injections should not be made into the lower and mid-thirds of the upper arm. As with all intramuscular injections, aspiration is necessary to help avoid inadvertent injection into a blood vessel.

Neuroleptic drugs elevate prolactin levels; the elevation persists during chronic administration. Tissue culture experiments indicate that approximately one-third of human breast cancers are prolactin dependent *in vitro*, a factor of potential importance if the prescription of these drugs is contemplated in a patient with a previously detected breast cancer. Although disturbances such as galactorrhea, amenorrhea, gynecomastia, and impotence have been reported, the clinical significance of elevated serum prolactin levels is unknown for most patients. An increase in mammary neoplasms has been found in rodents after chronic administration of neuroleptic drugs. Neither clinical studies nor epidemiologic studies conducted to date, however, have shown an association between chronic administration of these drugs and mammary tumorigenesis; the available evidence is considered too limited to be conclusive at this time.

Information for Patients: Given the likelihood that some patients exposed chronically to neuroleptics will develop tardive dyskinesia, it is advised that all patients in whom chronic use is contemplated be given, if possible, full information about this risk. The decision to inform patients and/or their guardians must obviously take into account the clinical circumstances and the competency of the patient to understand the information provided.

ADVERSE REACTIONS

NOTE: Not all of the following adverse reactions have been reported with Navane. However, since Navane has certain chemical and pharmacologic similarities to the phenothiazines, all of the known side effects and toxicity associated with phenothiazine therapy should be borne in mind when Navane is used.

Cardiovascular Effects: Tachycardia, hypotension, lightheadedness, and syncope. In the event hypotension occurs, epinephrine should not be used as a pressor agent since a paradoxical further lowering of blood pressure may result. Nonspecific EKG changes have been observed in some patients receiving Navane. These changes are usually reversible and frequently disappear on continued Navane therapy. The clinical significance of these changes is not known.

CNS Effects: Drowsiness, usually mild, may occur although it usually subsides with continuation of Navane therapy. The incidence of sedation appears similar to that of the piperazine group of phenothiazines, but less than that of certain aliphatic phenothiazines. Restlessness, agitation and insomnia have been noted with Navane. Seizures and paradoxical exacerbation of psychotic symptoms have occurred with Navane infrequently.

Hyperreflexia has been reported in infants delivered from mothers having received structurally related drugs.

In addition, phenothiazine derivatives have been associated with cerebral edema and cerebrospinal fluid abnormalities. Extrapyramidal symptoms, such as pseudo-parkinsonism, akathisia, and dystonia have been reported. Management of these extrapyramidal symptoms depends upon the type and severity. Rapid relief of acute symptoms may require the use of an injectable antiparkinson agent. More slowly emerging symptoms may be managed by reducing the dosage of Navane and/or administering an oral antiparkinson agent.

Persistent Tardive Dyskinesia: As with all antipsychotic agents tardive dyskinesia may appear in some patients on long term therapy or may occur after drug therapy has been discontinued. The syndrome is characterized by rhythmical involuntary movements of the tongue, face, mouth or jaw (e.g., protrusion of tongue, puffing of cheeks, puckering of mouth, chewing movements). Sometimes these may be accompanied by involuntary movements of extremities.

Since early detection of tardive dyskinesia is important, patients should be monitored on an ongoing basis. It has been reported that fine vermicular movement of the tongue may be an early sign of the syndrome. If this or any other presentation of the syndrome is observed, the clinician should consider possible discontinuation of neuroleptic medication. (See WARNINGS section.)

Hepatic Effects: Elevations of serum transaminase and alkaline phosphatase, usually transient, have been infrequently observed in some patients. No clinically confirmed cases of jaundice attributable to Navane (thiothixene hydrochloride) have been reported.

Hematologic Effects: As is true with certain other psychotropic drugs, leukopenia and leucocytosis, which are usually transient, can occur occasionally with Navane. Other antipsychotic drugs have been associated with agranulocytosis, eosinophilia, hemolytic anemia, thrombocytopenia and pancytopenia.

Allergic Reactions: Rash, pruritus, urticaria, and rare cases of anaphylaxis have been reported with Navane. Undue exposure to sunlight should be avoided. Although not experienced with Navane, exfoliative dermatitis, contact dermatitis (in nursing personnel), have been reported with certain phenothiazines.

Endocrine Disorders: Lactation, moderate breast enlargement and amenorrhea have occurred in a small percentage of females receiving Navane. If persistent, this may necessitate a reduction in dosage or the discontinuation of therapy. Phenothiazines have been associated with false positive pregnancy tests, gynecomastia, hypoglycemia, hyperglycemia, and glycosuria.

Autonomic Effects: Dry mouth, blurred vision, nasal congestion, constipation, increased sweating, increased salivation, and impotence have occurred infrequently with Navane therapy. Phenothiazines have been associated with miosis, mydriasis, and adynamic ileus.

Other Adverse Reactions: Hyperpyrexia, anorexia, nausea, vomiting, diarrhea, increase in appetite and weight, weakness or fatigue, polydipsia and peripheral edema.

Although not reported with Navane, evidence indicates there is a relationship between phenothiazine therapy and the occurrence of a systemic lupus erythematosus-like syndrome.

Neuroleptic Malignant Syndrome (NMS): Please refer to the text regarding NMS in the WARNINGS section.

NOTE: Sudden deaths have occasionally been reported in patients who have received certain phenothiazine derivatives. In some cases the cause of death was apparently cardiac arrest or asphyxia due to failure of the cough reflex. In others, the cause could not be determined nor could it be established that death was due to phenothiazine administration.

DOSAGE AND ADMINISTRATION

Preparation

Navane (thiothixene hydrochloride) Intramuscular For Injection must be reconstituted with 2.2 ml of sterile water for injection.

For Intramuscular Use Only

Dosage of Navane should be individually adjusted depending on the chronicity and severity of the condition. In general, small doses should be used initially and gradually increased to the optimal effective level, based on patient response.

Usage in children under 12 years of age is not recommended.

Where more rapid control and treatment of acute behavior is desirable, the intramuscular form of Navane may be indicated. It is also of benefit where the very nature of the patient's symptomatology, whether acute or chronic, renders oral administration impractical or even impossible.

For treatment of acute symptomatology or in patients unable or unwilling to take oral medication, the usual dose is 4 mg of Navane Intramuscular For Injection administered 2 to 4 times daily. Dosage may be increased or decreased depending on response. Most patients are controlled on a total daily dosage of 16 to 20 mg. The maximum recommended dosage is 30 mg/day. An oral form should supplant the injectable form as soon as possible. It may be necessary to adjust the dosage when changing from the intramuscular to oral dosage forms. Dosage recommendations for Navane Capsules and Concentrate can be found in the Navane oral package insert.

OVERDOSAGE

Manifestations include muscular twitching, drowsiness, and dizziness. Symptoms of gross overdosage may include CNS depression, rigidity, weakness, torticollis, tremor, salivation, dysphagia, hypotension, disturbances of gait, or coma.

Treatment: Essentially symptomatic and supportive. Keep patient under careful observation and maintain an open airway, since involvement of the extrapyramidal system may produce dysphagia and respiratory difficulty in severe overdosage. If hypotension occurs, the standard measures for managing circulatory shock should be used (I.V. fluids and/or vasoconstrictors).

If a vasoconstrictor is needed, levarterenol and phenylephrine are the most suitable drugs. Other pressor agents, including epinephrine, are not recommended, since phenothiazine derivatives may reverse the usual pressor elevating action of these agents and cause further lowering of blood pressure.

If CNS depression is marked, symptomatic treatment is indicated. Extrapyramidal symptoms may be treated with antiparkinson drugs.

There are no data on the use of peritoneal or hemodialysis, but they are known to be of little value in phenothiazine intoxication.

HOW SUPPLIED

Navane (thiothixene hydrochloride) Intramuscular For Injection is available in amber glass vials in packages of 10 vials (NDC 0049-5765-83). When reconstituted with 2.2 ml of STERILE WATER FOR INJECTION, each ml contains

thiothixene hydrochloride equivalent to 5 mg of thiothixene, and 59.6 mg of mannitol. The reconstituted solution of Navane Intramuscular For Injection may be stored for 48 hours at room temperature before discarding.

70-4177-00-4
Revised January 1988

NORVASC® ℞

[*nor 'vask*]
(amlodipine besylate)
Tablets

DESCRIPTION

NORVASC® is the besylate salt of amlodipine, a long-acting calcium channel blocker.

NORVASC is chemically described as (R.S.) 3-ethyl-5-methyl-2-(2-amino-ethoxymethyl)-4-(2-chlorophenyl)-1,4-dihydro-6-methyl-3,5-pyridinedicarboxylate benzenesulphonate. Its empirical formula is $C_{20}H_{25}ClN_2O_5 \cdot C_6H_6O_3S$, and its structural formula is:

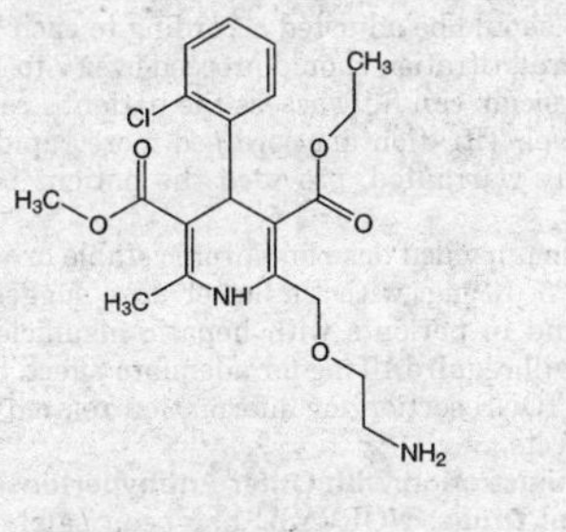

$C_6H_6O_3S$

Amlodipine besylate is a white crystalline powder with a molecular weight of 567.1. It is slightly soluble in water and sparingly soluble in ethanol. NORVASC (amlodipine besylate) tablets are formulated as white tablets equivalent to 2.5, 5 and 10 mg of amlodipine for oral administration. In addition to the active ingredient, amlodipine besylate, each tablet contains the following inactive ingredients: microcrystalline cellulose, dibasic calcium phosphate anhydrous, sodium starch glycolate, and magnesium stearate.

CLINICAL PHARMACOLOGY

Mechanism of Action: NORVASC is a dihydropyridine calcium antagonist (calcium ion antagonist or slow-channel blocker) that inhibits the transmembrane influx of calcium ions into vascular smooth muscle and cardiac muscle. Experimental data suggest that NORVASC binds to both dihydropyridine and nondihydropyridine binding sites. The contractile processes of cardiac muscle and vascular smooth muscle are dependent upon the movement of extracellular calcium ions into these cells through specific ion channels. NORVASC inhibits calcium ion influx across cell membranes selectively, with a greater effect on vascular smooth muscle cells than on cardiac muscle cells. Negative inotropic effects can be detected *in vitro* but such effects have not been seen in intact animals at therapeutic doses. Serum calcium concentration is not affected by NORVASC. Within the physiologic pH range, NORVASC is an ionized compound (pKa=8.6), and its kinetic interaction with the calcium channel receptor is characterized by a gradual rate of association and dissociation with the receptor binding site, resulting in a gradual onset of effect.

NORVASC is a peripheral arterial vasodilator that acts directly on vascular smooth muscle to cause a reduction in peripheral vascular resistance and reduction in blood pressure.

The precise mechanisms by which NORVASC relieves angina have not been fully delineated, but are thought to include the following:

Exertional Angina: In patients with exertional angina, NORVASC reduces the total peripheral resistance (afterload) against which the heart works and reduces the rate pressure product, and thus myocardial oxygen demand, at any given level of exercise.

Vasospastic Angina: NORVASC has been demonstrated to block constriction and restore blood flow in coronary arteries and arterioles in response to calcium, potassium epinephrine, serotonin, and thromboxane A_2 analog in experimental animal models and in human coronary vessels *in vitro*. This inhibition of coronary spasm is responsible for the effectiveness of NORVASC in vasospastic (Prinzmetal's or variant) angina.

Pharmacokinetics and Metabolism: After oral administration of therapeutic doses of NORVASC, absorption produces peak plasma concentrations between 6 and 12 hours. Absolute bioavailability has been estimated to be between 64 and 90%. The bioavailability of NORVASC is not altered by the presence of food.

NORVASC is extensively (about 90%) converted to inactive metabolites via hepatic metabolism with 10% of the parent compound and 60% of the metabolites excreted in the urine. *Ex vivo* studies have shown that approximately 93% of the circulating drug is bound to plasma proteins in hypertensive patients. Elimination from the plasma is biphasic with a terminal elimination half-life of about 30–50 hours. Steady-state plasma levels of NORVASC are reached after 7 to 8 days of consecutive daily dosing.

The pharmacokinetics of NORVASC are not significantly influenced by renal impairment. Patients with renal failure may therefore receive the usual initial dose.

Elderly patients and patients with hepatic insufficiency have decreased clearance of amlodipine with a resulting increase in AUC of approximately 40–60%, and a lower initial dose may be required. A similar increase in AUC was observed in patients with moderate to severe heart failure.

Pharmacodynamics: *Hemodynamics* Following administration of therapeutic doses to patients with hypertension, NORVASC produces vasodilation resulting in a reduction of supine and standing blood pessures. These decreases in blood pressure are not accompanied by a significant change in heart rate or plasma catecholamine levels with chronic dosing. Although the acute intravenous administration of amlodipine decreases arterial blood pressure and increases heart rate in hemodynamic studies of patients with chronic stable angina, chronic administration of oral amlodipine in clinical trials did not lead to clinically significant changes in heart rate or blood pressures in normotensive patients with angina.

With chronic once daily oral administration, antihypertensive effectiveness is maintained for at least 24 hours. Plasma concentrations correlate with effect in both young and elderly patients. The magnitude of reduction in blood pressure with NORVASC is also correlated with the height of pretreatment elevation; thus, individuals with moderate hypertension (diastolic pressure 105–114 mmHg) had about a 50% greater response than patients with mild hypertension (diastolic pressure 90–104 mmHg). Normotensive subjects experienced no clinically significant change in blood pressures (+1/ – 2 mmHg).

In hypertensive patients with normal renal function, therapeutic doses of NORVASC resulted in a decrease in renal vascular resistance and an increase in glomerular filtration rate and effective renal plasma flow without change in filtration fraction or proteinuria.

As with other calcium channel blockers, hemodynamic measurements of cardiac function at rest and during exercise (or pacing) in patients with normal ventricular function treated with NORVASC have generally demonstrated a small increase in cardiac index without significant influence on dP/dt or on left ventricular end diastolic pressure or volume. In hemodynamic studies, NORVASC has not been associated with a negative inotropic effect when administered in the therapeutic dose range to intact animals and man, even when co-administered with beta-blockers to man. Similar findings, however, have been observed in normals or well-compensated patients with heart failure with agents possessing significant negative inotropic effects.

Studies in Patients with Congestive Heart Failure: NORVASC has been compared to placebo in four 8–12 week studies of patients with NYHA class II/III heart failure, involving a total of 697 patients. In these studies, there was no evidence of worsened heart failure based on measures of exercise tolerance, NYHA classification, symptoms, or LVEF. In a long-term (follow-up at least 6 months, mean 13.8 months) placebo-controlled mortality/morbidity study of NORVASC 5–10 mg in 1153 patients with NYHA classes III (n=931) or IV (n=222) heart failure on stable doses of diuretics, digoxin, and ACE inhibitors, NORVASC had no effect on the primary endpoint of the study which was the combined endpoint of all-cause mortality and cardiac morbidity (as defined by life-threatening arrhythmia, acute myocardial infarction, or hospitalization for worsened heart failure), or on NYHA classification, or symptoms of heart failure. Total combined all-cause mortality and cardiac morbidity events were 222/571 (39%) for patients on NORVASC and 246/583 (42%) for patients on placebo; the cardiac morbid events represented about 25% of the endpoints in the study.

Electrophysiologic Effects: NORVASC does not change sinoatrial nodal function or atrioventricular conduction in intact animals or man. In patients with chronic stable angina, intravenous administration of 10 mg did not significantly alter A-H and H-V conduction and sinus node recovery time after pacing. Similar results were obtained in patients receiving NORVASC and concomitant beta blockers. In clinical studies in which NORVASC was administered in combination with beta-blockers to patients with either hypertension or angina, no adverse effects on electrocardiographic parameters were observed. In clinical trials with angina patients alone, NORVASC therapy did not alter electrocardiographic intervals or produce higher degrees of AV blocks.

Effects in Hypertension: The antihypertensive efficacy of NORVASC has been demonstrated in a total of 15 double-blind, placebo-controlled, randomized studies involving 800 patients on NORVASC and 538 on placebo. Once daily administration produced statistically significant placebo-corrected reductions in supine and standing blood pressures at 24 hours postdose, averaging about 12/6 mmHg in the standing position and 13/7 mmHg in the supine position in patients with mild to moderate hypertension. Maintenance of the blood pressure effect over the 24-hour dosing interval was observed, with little difference in peak and trough effect. Tolerance was not demonstrated in patients studied for up to 1 year. The 3 parallel, fixed dose, dose response studies showed that the reduction in supine and standing blood pressures was dose-related within the recommended dosing range. Effects on diastolic pressure were similar in young and older patients. The effect on systolic pressure was greater in older patients, perhaps because of greater baseline systolic pressure. Effects were similar in black patients and in white patients.

Effects in Chronic Stable Angina: The effectiveness of 5–10 mg/day of NORVASC in exercise-induced angina has been evaluated in 8 placebo-controlled, double-blind clinical trials of up to 6 weeks duration involving 1038 patients (684 NORVASC, 354 placebo) with chronic stable angina. In 5 of the 8 studies significant increases in exercise time (bicycle or treadmill) were seen with the 10 mg dose. Increases in symptom-limited exercise time averaged 12.8% (63 sec) for NORVASC 10 mg, and averaged 7.9% (38 sec) for NORVASC 5 mg. NORVASC 10 mg also increased time to 1 mm ST segment deviation in several studies and decreased angina attack rate. The sustained efficacy of NORVASC in angina patients has been demonstrated over long-term dosing. In patients with angina there were no clinically significant reductions in blood pressures (4/1 mmHg) or changes in heart rate (+0.3 bpm).

Effects in Vasospastic Angina: In a double-blind, placebo-controlled clinical trial of 4 weeks duration in 50 patients, NORVASC therapy decreased attacks by approximately 4/week compared with a placebo decrease of approximately 1/week ($p<0.01$). Two of 23 NORVASC and 7 of 27 placebo patients discontinued from the study due to lack of clinical improvement.

INDICATIONS AND USAGE

1. Hypertension

NORVASC is indicated for the treatment of hypertension. It may be used alone or in combination with other antihypertensive agents.

2. Chronic Stable Angina

NORVASC is indicated for the treatment of chronic stable angina. NORVASC may be used alone or in combination with other antianginal agents.

3. Vasospastic Angina (Prinzmetal's or Variant Angina)

NORVASC is indicated for the treatment of confirmed or suspected vasospastic angina. NORVASC may be used as monotherapy or in combination with other antianginal drugs.

CONTRAINDICATIONS

NORVASC is contraindicated in patients with known sensitivity to amlodipine.

WARNINGS

Increased Angina and/or Myocardial Infarction: Rarely, patients, particularly those with severe obstructive coronary artery disease, have developed documented increased frequency, duration and/or severity of angina or acute myocardial infarction on starting calcium channel blocker therapy or at the time of dosage increase. The mechanism of this effect has not been elucidated.

PRECAUTIONS

General: Since the vasodilation induced by NORVASC is gradual in onset, acute hypotension has rarely been reported after oral administration of NORVASC. Nonetheless, caution should be exercised when administering NORVASC as with any other peripheral vasodilator particularly in patients with severe aortic stenosis.

Use in Patients with Congestive Heart Failure: In general, calcium channel blockers should be used with caution in patients with heart failure. NORVASC (5–10 mg per day) has been studied in a placebo-controlled trial of 1153 patients with NYHA Class III or IV heart failure (see CLINICAL PHARMACOLOGY) on stable doses of ACE inhibitor, digoxin, and diuretics. Follow-up was at least 6 months, with a mean of about 14 months. There was no overall adverse effect on survival or cardiac morbidity (as defined by life-threatening arrhythmia, acute myocardial infarction, or hospitalization for worsened heart failure). NORVASC has been compared to placebo in four 8–12 week studies of patients with NYHA class II/III heart failure, involving a total of 697 patients. In these studies, there was no evidence of worsened heart failure based on measures of exercise tolerance, NYHA classification, symptoms, or LVEF.

Continued on next page

Norvasc—Cont.

Beta-Blocker Withdrawal: NORVASC is not a beta-blocker and therefore gives no protection against the dangers of abrupt beta-blocker withdrawal; any such withdrawal should be by gradual reduction of the dose of beta-blocker.

Patients with Hepatic Failure: Since NORVASC is extensively metabolized by the liver and the plasma elimination half-life (t 1/2) is 56 hours in patients with impaired hepatic function, caution should be exercised when administering NORVASC to patients with severe hepatic impairment.

Drug Interactions: *In vitro* data in human plasma indicate that NORVASC has no effect on the protein binding of drugs tested (digoxin, phenytoin, warfarin, and indomethacin). Special studies have indicated that the co-administration of NORVASC with digoxin did not change serum digoxin levels or digoxin renal clearance in normal volunteers; that co-administration with cimetidine did not alter the pharmacokinetics of amlodipine; and that co-administration with warfarin did not change the warfarin prothrombin response time.

In clinical trials, NORVASC has been safely administered with thiazide diuretics, beta-blockers, angiotensin-converting enzyme inhibitors, long-acting nitrates, sublingual nitroglycerin, digoxin, warfarin, non-steroidal anti-inflammatory drugs, antibiotics, and oral hypoglycemic drugs.

Drug/Laboratory Test Interactions: None known.

Carcinogenesis, Mutagenesis, Impairment of Fertility: Rats and mice treated with amlodipine in the diet for two years, at concentrations calculated to provide daily dosage levels of 0.5, 1.25, and 2.5 mg/kg/day showed no evidence of carcinogenicity. The highest dose (for mice, similar to, and for rats twice* the maximum recommended clinical dose of 10 mg on a mg/m^2 basis) was close to the maximum tolerated dose for mice but not for rats.

Mutagenicity studies revealed no drug related effects at either the gene or chromosome levels.

There was no effect on the fertility of rats treated with amlodipine (males for 64 days and females 14 days prior to mating) at doses up to 10 mg/kg/day (8 times* the maximum recommended human dose of 10 mg on a mg/m^2 basis).

Pregnancy Category C: No evidence of teratogenicity or other embryo/fetal toxicity was found when pregnant rats or rabbits were treated orally with up to 10 mg/kg amlodipine (respectively 8 times* and 23 times* the maximum recommended human dose of 10 mg on a mg/m^2 basis) during their respective periods of major organogenesis. However, litter size was significantly decreased (by about 50%) and the number of intrauterine deaths was significantly increased (about 5-fold) in rats administered 10 mg/kg amlodipine for 14 days before mating and throughout mating and gestation. Amlodipine has been shown to prolong both the gestation period and the duration of labor in rats at this dose. There are no adequate and well-controlled studies in pregnant women. Amlodipine should be used during pregnancy only if the potential benefit justifies the potential risk to the fetus.

Nursing Mothers: It is not known whether amlodipine is excreted in human milk. In the absence of this information, it is recommended that nursing be discontinued while NORVASC is administered.

Pediatric Use: Safety and effectiveness of NORVASC in children have not been established.

*Based on patient weight of 50 kg.

ADVERSE REACTIONS

NORVASC has been evaluated for safety in more than 11,000 patients in U.S. and foreign clinical trials. In general, treatment with NORVASC was well-tolerated at doses up to 10 mg daily. Most adverse reactions reported during therapy with NORVASC were of mild or moderate severity. In controlled clinical trials directly comparing NORVASC (N=1730) in doses up to 10 mg to placebo (N=1250), discontinuation of NORVASC due to adverse reactions was required in only about 1.5% of patients and was not significantly different from placebo (about 1%). The most common side effects are headache and edema. The incidence (%) of side effects which occurred in a dose related manner are as follows:

Adverse Event	2.5 mg N=275	5.0 mg N=296	10.0 mg N=268	Placebo N=520
Edema	1.8	3.0	10.8	0.6
Dizziness	1.1	3.4	3.4	1.5
Flushing	0.7	1.4	2.6	0.0
Palpitation	0.7	1.4	4.5	0.6

Other adverse experiences which were not clearly dose related but which were reported with an incidence greater than 1.0% in placebo-controlled clinical trials include the following:

Placebo-Controlled Studies

	NORVASC (%) (N=1730)	PLACEBO (%) (N=1250)
Headache	7.3	7.8
Fatigue	4.5	2.8
Nausea	2.9	1.9
Abdominal Pain	1.6	0.3
Somnolence	1.4	0.6

For several adverse experiences that appear to be drug and dose related, there was a greater incidence in women than men associated with amlodipine treatment as shown in the following table:

ADR	NORVASC M=% (N=1218)	NORVASC F=% (N=512)	PLACEBO M=% (N=914)	PLACEBO F=% (N=336)
Edema	5.6	14.6	1.4	5.1
Flushing	1.5	4.5	0.3	0.9
Palpitations	1.4	3.3	0.9	0.9
Somnolence	1.3	1.6	0.8	0.3

The following events occurred in ≤1% but >0.1% of patients in controlled clinical trials or under conditions of open trials or marketing experience where a causal relationship is uncertain; they are listed to alert the physician to a possible relationship:

Cardiovascular: arrhythmia (including ventricular tachycardia and atrial fibrillation), bradycardia, chest pain, hypotension, peripheral ischemia, syncope, tachycardia, postural dizziness, postural hypotension.

Central and Peripheral Nervous System: hypoesthesia, paresthesia, tremor, vertigo.

Gastrointestinal: anorexia, constipation, dyspepsia,** dysphagia, diarrhea, flatulence, vomiting, gingival hyperplasia.

General: asthenia,** back pain, hot flushes, malaise, pain, rigors, weight gain.

Musculoskeletal System: arthralgia, arthrosis, muscle cramps,** myalgia.

Psychiatric: sexual dysfunction (male** and female), insomnia, nervousness, depression, abnormal dreams, anxiety, depersonalization.

Respiratory System: dyspnea,** epistaxis.

Skin and Appendages: pruritus,** rash,** rash erythematous, rash maculopapular.

**These events occurred in less than 1% in placebo-controlled trials, but the incidence of these side effects was between 1% and 2% in all multiple dose studies.

Special Senses: abnormal vision, conjunctivitis, diplopia, eye pain, tinnitus.

Urinary System: micturition frequency, micturition disorder, nocturia.

Autonomic Nervous System: dry mouth, sweating increased.

Metabolic and Nutritional: thirst.

Hemopoietic: purpura.

The following events occurred in ≤0.1% of patients: cardiac failure, pulse irregularity, extrasystoles, skin discoloration, urticaria, skin dryness, alopecia, dermatitis, muscle weakness, twitching, ataxia, hypertonia, migraine, cold and clammy skin, apathy, agitation, amnesia, gastritis, increased appetite, loose stools, coughing, rhinitis, dysuria, polyuria, parosmia, taste perversion, abnormal visual accommodation, and xerophthalmia.

Other reactions occurred sporadically and cannot be distinguished from medications or concurrent disease states such as myocardial infarction and angina.

NORVASC therapy has not been associated with clinically significant changes in routine laboratory tests. No clinically relevant changes were noted in serum potassium, serum glucose, total triglycerides, total cholesterol, HDL cholesterol, uric acid, blood urea nitrogen, or creatinine.

The following postmarketing event has been reported infrequently where a causal relationship is uncertain: gynecomastia. In postmarketing experience, jaundice and hepatic enzyme elevations (mostly consistent with cholestasis) in some cases severe enough to require hospitalization have been reported in association with use of amlodipine.

NORVASC has been used safely in patients with chronic obstructive pulmonary disease, well-compensated congestive heart failure, peripheral vascular disease, diabetes mellitus, and abnormal lipid profiles.

OVERDOSAGE

Single oral doses of 40 mg/kg and 100 mg/kg in mice and rats, respectively, caused deaths. A single oral dose of 4 mg/kg or higher in dogs caused a marked peripheral vasodilation and hypotension.

Overdosage might be expected to cause excessive peripheral vasodilation with marked hypotension and possibly a reflex tachycardia. In humans, experience with intentional overdose of NORVASC is limited. Reports of intentional overdosage include a patient who ingested 250 mg and was asymptomatic and was not hospitalized; another (120 mg) was hospitalized, underwent gastric lavage and remained normotensive; the third (105 mg) was hospitalized and had hypotension (90/50 mmHg) which normalized following plasma expansion. A patient who took 70 mg amlodipine and an unknown quantity of benzodiazepine in a suicide attempt developed shock which was refractory to treatment and died the following day with abnormally high benzodiazepine plasma concentration. A case of accidental drug overdose has been documented in a 19-month-old male who ingested 30 mg amlodipine (about 2mg/kg). During the emergency room presentation, vital signs were stable with no evidence of hypotension, but a heart rate of 180 bpm. Ipecac was administered 3.5 hours after ingestion and on subsequent observation (overnight) no sequelae were noted.

If massive overdose should occur, active cardiac and respiratory monitoring should be instituted. Frequent blood pressure measurements are essential. Should hypotension occur, cardiovascular support including elevation of the extremities and the judicious administration of fluids should be initiated. If hypotension remains unresponsive to these conservative measures, administration of vasopressors (such as phenylephrine) should be considered with attention to circulating volume and urine output. Intravenous calcium gluconate may help to reverse the effects of calcium entry blockade. As NORVASC is highly protein bound, hemodialysis is not likely to be of benefit.

DOSAGE AND ADMINISTRATION

The usual initial antihypertensive oral dose of NORVASC is 5 mg once daily with a maximum dose of 10 mg once daily. Small, fragile, or elderly individuals, or patients with hepatic insufficiency may be started on 2.5 mg once daily and this dose may be used when adding NORVASC to other antihypertensive therapy.

Dosage should be adjusted according to each patient's need. In general, titration should proceed over 7 to 14 days so that the physician can fully assess the patient's response to each dose level. Titration may proceed more rapidly, however, if clinically warranted, provided the patient is assessed frequently.

The recommended dose for chronic stable or vasospastic angina is 5–10 mg, with the lower dose suggested in the elderly and in patients with hepatic insufficiency. Most patients will require 10 mg for adequate effect. See ADVERSE REACTIONS section for information related to dosage and side effects.

Co-administration with Other Antihypertensive and/or Antianginal Drugs: NORVASC has been safely administered with thiazides, ACE inhibitors, betablockers, long-acting nitrates, and/or sublingual nitroglycerin.

HOW SUPPLIED

NORVASC®–2.5 mg Tablets (amlodipine besylate equivalent to 2.5 mg of amlodipine per tablet) are supplied as white, diamond, flat-faced, beveled edged engraved with "NORVASC" on one side and "2.5" on the other side and supplied as follows:

NDC 0069-1520-68	Bottle of 90
NDC 0069-1520-66	Bottle of 100

NORVASC®–5 mg Tablets (amlodipine besylate equivalent to 5 mg of amlodipine per tablet) are white, elongated octagon, flat-faced, beveled edged engraved with both "NORVASC" and "5" on one side and plain on the other side and supplied as follows:

NDC 0069-1530-68	Bottle of 90
NDC 0069-1530-66	Bottle of 100
NDC 0069-1530-41	Unit Dose package of 100
NDC 0069-1530-72	Bottle of 300

NORVASC®–10 mg Tablets (amlodipine besylate equivalent to 10 mg of amlodipine per tablet) are white, round, flat-faced, beveled edged engraved with both "NORVASC" and "10" on one side and plain on the other side and supplied as follows:

NDC 0069-1540-68	Bottle of 90
NDC 0069-1540-66	Bottle of 100
NDC 0069-1540-41	Unit Dose package of 100

Store bottles at controlled room temperature, 59° to 86°F (15° to 30°C) and dispense in tight, light-resistant containers (USP).

© 1996 Pfizer Inc
Revised November 1996
Shown in Product Identification Guide, page 331

**Buffered
PFIZERPEN®
(penicillin G potassium)
for Injection**

℞

DESCRIPTION

Buffered Pfizerpen (penicillin G potassium) for Injection is a sterile, pyrogen-free powder for reconstitution. Buffered Pfizerpen for Injection is an antibacterial agent for intramuscular, continuous intravenous drip, intrapleural or other local infusion, and intrathecal administration.

Each million units contains approximately 6.8 milligrams of sodium (0.3 mEq) and 65.6 milligrams of potassium (1.68 mEq).

Chemically, Pfizerpen is monopotassium 3,3-dimethyl-7-oxo-6-(2-phenylacetamido)-4-thia-1-azabicyclo (3.2.0) heptane-2-carboxylate. It has a molecular weight of 372.48 and the following chemical structure.

[See chemical structure at top of next column]

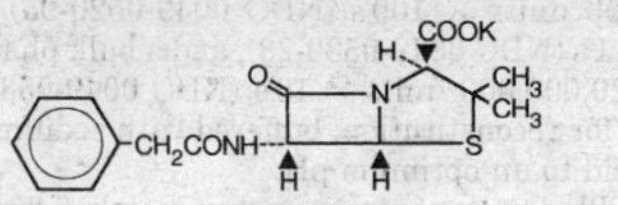

Formula
$C_{16}H_{17}KN_2O_4S$

Penicillin G potassium is a colorless or white crystal, or a white crystalline powder which is odorless, or practically so, and moderately hygroscopic. Penicillin G potassium is very soluble in water. The pH of the reconstituted product is between 6.0–8.5.

CLINICAL PHARMACOLOGY

Aqueous penicillin G is rapidly absorbed following both intramuscular and subcutaneous injection. Initial blood levels following parenteral administration are high but transient. Penicillins bind to serum proteins, mainly albumin. Therapeutic levels of the penicillins are easily achieved under normal circumstances in extracellular fluid and most other body tissues. Penicillins are distributed in varying degrees into pleural, pericardial, peritoneal, ascitic, synovial, and interstitial fluids. Penicillins are excreted in breast milk. Penetration into the cerebrospinal fluid, eyes, and prostate is poor. Penicillins are rapidly excreted in the urine by glomerular filtration and active tubular secretion, primarily as unchanged drug. Approximately 60 percent of the total dose of 300,000 units is excreted in the urine within this 5 hour period. For this reason high and frequent doses are required to maintain the elevated serum levels desirable in treating certain severe infections in individuals with normal kidney function. In neonates and young infants, and in individuals with impaired kidney function, excretion is considerably delayed.

Microbiology

Penicillin G exerts a bactericidal action against penicillin-susceptible microorganisms during the stage of active multiplication. It acts through the inhibition of biosynthesis of cell wall mucopeptide rendering the cell wall osmotically unstable. It is not active against the penicillinase-producing bacteria, which include many strains of staphylococci. While *in vitro* studies have demonstrated the susceptibility of most strains of the following organisms, clinical efficacy for infections other than those included in the INDICATIONS AND USAGE section has not been documented. Penicillin G exerts high *in vitro* activity against staphylococci (except penicillinase-producing strains), streptococci (groups A, C, G, H, L, and M), and pneumococci. Other organisms susceptible to penicillin G are *N. gonorrhoeae, Corynebacterium diphtheriae, Bacillus anthracis,* Clostridia, *Actinomyces bovis, Streptobacillus moniliformis, Listeria monocytogenes* and Leptospira. *Treponema pallidum* is extremely sensitive to the bactericidal action of penicillin G. Some species of gram-negative bacilli are sensitive to moderate to high concentrations of the drug obtained with intravenous administration. These include most strains of *Escherichia coli;* all strains of *Proteus mirabilis,* Salmonella and Shigella; and some strains of *Aerobacter aerogenes* and *Alcaligenes faecalis.*

Penicillin acts synergistically with gentamicin or tobramycin against many strains of enterococci.

Susceptibility Testing: Penicillin G Susceptibility Powder or 10 units Penicillin G Susceptibility Discs may be used to determine microbial susceptibility to penicillin G using one of the following standard methods recommended by the National Committee for Laboratory Standards:

M2-A3, "Performance Standards for Antimicrobial Disk Susceptibility Tests"

M7-A, "Methods for Dilution Antimicrobial Susceptibility Tests for Bacteria that Grow Aerobically"

M11-A, "Reference Agar Dilution Procedure for Antimicrobial Susceptibility Testing of Anaerobic Bacteria"

M17-P, "Alternative Methods for Antimicrobial Susceptibility Testing of Anaerobic Bacteria"

Tests should be interpreted by the following criteria:

	Zone Diameter, nearest whole mm		
	Susceptible	Moderately Susceptible	Resistant
Staphylococci	≥29	—	≤28
N. gonorrhoeae	≥20	—	≤19
Enterococci	—	≥15	≤14
Non-enterococcal streptococci and *L. monocytogenes*	≥28	20–27	≤19

	Approximate MIC Correlates	
	Susceptible	Resistant
Staphylococci	≤0.1 μg/mL	β-lactamase
N. gonorrhoeae	≤0.1 μg/mL	β-lactamase
Enterococci	—	≥16 μg/mL
Non-enterococcal streptococci and *L. monocytogenes*	≤0.12 μg/mL	≥4 μg/mL

Interpretations of susceptible, intermediate, and resistant correlate zone size diameters with MIC values. A laboratory report of "susceptible" indicates that the suspected causative microorganism most likely will respond to therapy with penicillin G. A laboratory report of "resistant" indicates that the infecting microorganism most likely will not respond to therapy. A laboratory report of "moderately susceptible" indicates that the microorganism is most likely susceptible if a high dosage of penicillin G is used, or if the infection is such that high levels of penicillin G may be attained, as in urine. A report of "intermediate" using the disk diffusion method may be considered an equivocal result, and dilution tests may be indicated.

Control organisms are recommended for susceptibility testing. Each time the test is performed the following organisms should be included. The range for zones of inhibition is shown below:

Control Organism	Zone of Inhibition Range
Staphylococcus aureus (ATCC 25923)	27–35

INDICATIONS AND USAGE

Aqueous penicillin G (parenteral) is indicated in the therapy of severe infections caused by penicillin G-susceptible microorganisms when rapid and high penicillin levels are required in the conditions listed below. Therapy should be guided by bacteriological studies (including susceptibility tests) and by clinical response.

The following infections will usually respond to adequate dosage of aqueous penicillin G (parenteral):

Streptococcal infections.

NOTE: Streptococci in groups A, C, H, G, L, and M are very sensitive to penicillin G. Some group D organisms are sensitive to the high serum levels obtained with aqueous penicillin G.

Aqueous penicillin G (parenteral) is the penicillin dosage form of choice for bacteremia, empyema, severe pneumonia, pericarditis, endocarditis, meningitis, and other severe infections caused by sensitive strains of the gram-positive species listed above.

Pneumococcal infections.

Staphylococcal infections—penicillin G sensitive.

Other infections:

Anthrax.

Actinomycosis.

Clostridial infections (including tetanus).

Diphtheria (to prevent carrier state).

Erysipeloid (*Erysipelothrix insidiosa*) endocarditis.

Fusospirochetal infections—severe infections of the oropharynx (Vincent's), lower respiratory tract and genital area due to *Fusobacterium fusiformisans* spirochetes.

Gram-negative bacillary infections (bacteremias)—(*E. coli, A. aerogenes, A. faecalis,* Salmonella, Shigella and *P. mirabilis*).

Listeria infections (*Listeria monocytogenes*).

Meningitis and endocarditis.

Pasteurella infections (*Pasteurella multocida*).

Bacteremia and meningitis.

Rat-bite fever (*Spirillum minus* or *Streptobacillus moniliformis*).

Gonorrheal endocarditis and arthritis (*N. gonorrhoeae*).

Syphilis (*T. pallidum*) including congenital syphilis.

Meningococcic meningitis.

Although no controlled clinical efficacy studies have been conducted, aqueous crystalline penicillin G for injection and penicillin G procaine suspension have been suggested by the American Heart Association and the American Dental Association for use as part of a combined parenteral-oral regimen for prophylaxis against bacterial endocarditis in patients with congenital heart disease or rheumatic, or other acquired valvular heart disease when they undergo dental procedures and surgical procedures of the upper respiratory tract.[1] Since it may happen that *alpha* hemolytic streptococci relatively resistant to penicillin may be found when patients are receiving continuous oral penicillin for secondary prevention of rheumatic fever, prophylactic agents other than penicillin may be chosen for these patients and prescribed in addition to their continuous rheumatic fever prophylactic regimen.

NOTE: When selecting antibiotics for the prevention of bacterial endocarditis the physician or dentist should read the full joint statement of the American Heart Association and the American Dental Association.[1]

CONTRAINDICATIONS

A history of a previous hypersensitivity reaction to any penicillin is a contraindication.

WARNINGS

Serious and occasionally fatal hypersensitivity (anaphylactoid) reactions have been reported in patients on penicillin therapy. These reactions are more likely to occur in individuals with a history of penicillin hypersensitivity and/or a history of sensitivity to multiple allergens. There have been reports of individuals with a history of penicillin hypersensitivity who have experienced severe reactions when treated with cephalosporins. Before initiating therapy with any penicillin, careful inquiry should be made concerning previous hypersensitivity reactions to penicillin, cephalosporins, or other allergens. If an allergic reaction occurs, the drug should be discontinued and the appropriate therapy instituted. Serious anaphylactoid reactions require immediate emergency treatment with epinephrine. Oxygen, intravenous steroids, and airway management including intubation, should also be administered as indicated.

PRECAUTIONS

General: Penicillin should be used with caution in individuals with histories of significant allergies and/or asthma.

Intramuscular Therapy: Care should be taken to avoid intravenous or accidental intraarterial administration, or injection into or near major peripheral nerves or blood vessels, since such injections may produce neurovascular damage. Particular care should be taken with IV administration because of the possibility of thrombophlebitis.

In streptococcal infections, therapy must be sufficient to eliminate the organism (10 days minimum) otherwise the sequelae of streptococcal disease may occur. Cultures should be taken following the completion of treatment to determine whether streptococci have been eradicated.

The use of antibiotics may result in overgrowth of nonsusceptible organisms. Constant observation of the patient is essential. If new infections due to bacteria or fungi appear during therapy, the drug should be discontinued and appropriate measures taken. Whenever allergic reactions occur, penicillin should be withdrawn unless, in the opinion of the physician, the condition being treated is life threatening and amenable only to penicillin therapy.

Aqueous penicillin G by the intravenous route in high doses (above 10 million units), should be administered slowly because of the adverse effects of electrolyte imbalance from either the potassium or sodium content of the penicillin. Potassium penicillin G contains 1.7 mEq potassium and 0.3 mEq sodium per million units. The patient's renal, cardiac, and vascular status should be evaluated and if impairment of function is suspected or known to exist a reduction in the total dosage should be considered. Frequent evaluation of electrolyte balance, renal and hematopoietic function is recommended during therapy when high doses of intravenous aqueous penicillin G are used.

Laboratory Tests: In prolonged therapy with penicillin, periodic evaluation of the renal, hepatic, and hematopoietic systems is recommended for organ system dysfunction. This is particularly important in prematures, neonates and other infants, and when high doses are used.

Positive Coomb's tests have been reported after large intravenous doses.

Monitor serum potassium and implement corrective measures when necessary.

When treating gonococcal infections in which primary and secondary syphilis are suspected, proper diagnostic procedures, including dark field examinations, should be done before receiving penicillin and monthly serological tests made for at least four months. All cases of penicillin treated syphilis should receive clinical and serological examinations every six months for two to three years.

In suspected staphylococcal infections, proper laboratory studies, including susceptibility tests, should be performed. In streptococcal infections, cultures should be taken following completion of treatment to determine whether streptococci have been eradicated. Therapy must be sufficient to eliminate the organism (a minimum of 10 days), otherwise the sequelae of streptococcal disease (e.g., endocarditis, rheumatic fever) may occur.

Drug Interactions: Concurrent administration of bacteriostatic antibiotics (e.g., erythromycin, tetracycline) may diminish the bactericidal effects of penicillins by slowing the rate of bacterial growth. Bactericidal agents work most effectively against the immature cell wall of rapidly proliferating microorganisms. This has been demonstrated *in vitro;* however, the clinical significance of this interaction is not well documented. There are few clinical situations in which the concurrent use of "static" and "cidal" antibiotics are indicated. However, in selected circumstances in which such therapy is appropriate, using adequate doses of antibacterial agents and beginning penicillin therapy first, should minimize the potential for interaction.

Penicillin blood levels may be prolonged by concurrent administration of probenecid which blocks the renal tubular secretion of penicillins.

Displacement of penicillin from plasma protein binding sites will elevate the level of free penicillin in the serum.

Carcinogenesis, Mutagenesis, Impairment of Fertility: No information on long-term studies are available on the carcinogenesis, mutagenesis, or the impairment of fertility with the use of penicillins.

Continued on next page

Pfizerpen—Cont.

Pregnancy Category B—*Teratogenic Effects:* Reproduction studies performed in the mouse, rat, and rabbit have revealed no evidence of impaired fertility or harm to the fetus due to penicillin G. Human experience with the penicillins during pregnancy has not shown any positive evidence of adverse effects on the fetus. There are, however, no adequate and well controlled studies in pregnant women showing conclusively that harmful effects of these drugs on the fetus can be excluded. Because animal reproduction studies are not always predictive of human response, this drug should be used during pregnancy only if clearly needed.

Nursing Mothers: Penicillins are excreted in human milk. Caution should be exercised when penicillin G is administered to a nursing woman.

Pediatric Use: Penicillins are excreted largely unchanged by the kidney. Because of incompletely developed renal function in infants, the rate of elimination will be slow. Use caution in administering to newborns and evaluate organ system function frequently.

ADVERSE REACTIONS

Penicillin is a substance of low toxicity but does have a significant index of sensitization. The following hypersensitivity reactions have been reported: skin rashes ranging from maculopapular eruptions to exfoliative dermatitis; urticaria; and reactions resembling serum sickness, including chills, fever, edema, arthralgia and prostration. Severe and occasionally fatal anaphylaxis has occurred (see WARNINGS).

Hemolytic anemia, leucopenia, thrombocytopenia, nephropathy, and neuropathy are rarely observed adverse reactions and are usually associated with high intravenous dosage.

Patients given continuous intravenous therapy with penicillin G potassium in high dosage (10 million to 100 million units daily) may suffer severe or even fatal potassium poisoning, particularly if renal insufficiency is present. Hyperreflexia, convulsions and coma may be indicative of this syndrome.

Cardiac arrhythmias and cardiac arrest may also occur. (High dosage of penicillin G sodium may result in congestive heart failure due to high sodium intake.)

The Jarisch-Herxheimer reaction has been reported in patients treated for syphilis.

OVERDOSAGE

Neurological adverse reactions, including convulsions, may occur with the attainment of high CSF levels of beta-lactams. In case of overdosage, discontinue medication, treat symptomatically, and institute supportive measures as required.

Penicillin G potassium is hemodialyzable.

DOSAGE AND ADMINISTRATION

Severe infections due to Susceptible Strains of Streptococci, Pneumococci and Staphylococci—bacteremia, pneumonia, endocarditis, pericarditis, empyema, meningitis, and other severe infections—a minimum of 5 million units daily.

Syphilis: —Aqueous penicillin G may be used in the treatment of acquired and congenital syphilis, but because of the necessity of frequent dosage, hospitalization is recommended. Dosage and duration of therapy will be determined by age of patient and stage of the disease.

Gonorrheal endocarditis —a minimum of 5 million units daily.

Meningococcic meningitis —1–2 million units intramuscularly every 2 hours, or continuous IV drip of 20–30 million units/day.

Actinomycosis —1–6 million units/day for cervicofacial cases; 10–20 million units/day for thoracic and abdominal disease.

Clostridial infections —20 million units/day; penicillin is adjunctive therapy to antitoxin.

Fusospirochetal infections —severe infections of oropharynx, lower respiratory tract and genital area—5–10 million units/day.

Rat-bite fever (*Spirillum minus* or *Streptobacillus moniliformis*)—12–15 million units/day for 3–4 weeks.

Listeria infections (*Listeria monocytogenes*)

Neonates—500,000 to 1 million units/day.

Adults with meningitis—15–20 million units/day for 2 weeks.

Adults with endocarditis—15–20 million units/day for 4 weeks.

Pasteurella infections (*Pasteurella multocida*)

Bacteremia and meningitis—4–6 million units/day for 2 weeks.

Erysipeloid (*Erysipelothrix insidiosa*)

Endocarditis—2–20 million units/day for 4–6 weeks.

Gram-negative bacillary infections (*E. coli, Enterobacter aerogenes, A. faecalis,* Salmonella, Shigella and *Proteus mirabilis*)

Bacteremia—20–80 million units/day.

Diphtheria (carrier state): 300,000–400,000 units of penicillin/day in divided doses for 10–12 days.

Anthrax —A minimum of 5 million units of penicillin/day in divided doses until cure is effected.

For prophylaxis against bacterial endocarditis[1] in patients with congenital heart disease or rheumatic or other acquired valvular heart disease, when undergoing dental procedures or surgical procedures of the upper respiratory tract, use a combined parenteral-oral regimen. One million units of aqueous crystalline penicillin G (30,000 units/kg in children) intramuscularly, mixed with 600,000 units procaine penicillin G (600,000 units for children) should be given one-half to one hour before the procedure. Oral penicillin V (phenoxymethyl penicillin), 500 mg for adults or 250 mg for children less than 60 lb, should be given every 6 hours for 8 doses. Doses for children should not exceed recommendations for adults for a single dose or for a 24 hour period.

Reconstitution

The following table shows the amount of solvent required for solution of various concentrations.

[See table below]

When the required volume of solvent is greater than the capacity of the vial, the penicillin can be dissolved by first injecting only a portion of the solvent into the vial, then withdrawing the resultant solution and combining it with the remainder of the solvent in a larger sterile container.

Buffered Pfizerpen (penicillin G potassium) for Injection is highly water soluble. It may be dissolved in small amounts of Water for Injection, or Sterile Isotonic Sodium Chloride Solution for Parenteral Use. All solutions should be stored in a refrigerator. When refrigerated, penicillin solutions may be stored for seven days without significant loss of potency.

Buffered Pfizerpen for Injection may be given intramuscularly or by continuous intravenous drip for dosages of 500,000, 1,000,000, or 5,000,000 units. It is also suitable for intrapleural, intraarticular, and other local instillations.

THE 20,000,000 UNIT DOSAGE MAY BE ADMINISTERED BY INTRAVENOUS INFUSION ONLY.

(1) Intramuscular Injection: Keep total volume of injection small. The intramuscular route is the preferred route of administration. Solutions containing up to 100,000 units of penicillin per ml of diluent may be used with a minimum of discomfort. Greater concentration of penicillin G per ml is physically possible and may be employed where therapy demands. When large dosages are required, it may be advisable to administer aqueous solutions of penicillin by means of continuous intravenous drip.

(2) Continuous Intravenous Drip: Determine the volume of fluid and rate of its administration required by the patient in a 24-hour period in the usual manner for fluid therapy, and add the appropriate daily dosage of penicillin to this fluid. For example, if an adult patient requires 2 liters of fluid in 24 hours and a daily dosage of 10 million units of penicillin, add 5 million units to 1 liter and adjust the rate of flow so that the liter will be infused in 12 hours.

(3) Intrapleural or Other Local Infusion: If fluid is aspirated, give infusion in a volume equal to $^1/_4$ or $^1/_2$ the amount of fluid aspirated, otherwise, prepare as for intramuscular injection.

(4) Intrathecal Use: The intrathecal use of penicillin in meningitis must be highly individualized. It should be employed only with full consideration of the possible irritating effects of penicillin when used by this route. The preferred route of therapy in bacterial meningitides is intravenous, supplemented by intramuscular injection.

Parenteral drug products should be inspected visually for particulate matter and discoloration prior to administration, whenever solution and container permit.

Sterile solution may be left in refrigerator for one week without significant loss of potency.

HOW SUPPLIED

Buffered Pfizerpen (penicillin G potassium) for Injection is available in vials containing respectively 1,000,000 units × 10's (NDC 0049-0510-83), 1,000,000 units × 100's (NDC 0049-0510-95), 5,000,000 units × 10's (NDC 0049-0520-83), 5,000,000 units × 100's (NDC 0049-0520-95), 20,000,000 units × 1's (NDC 0049-0530-28), and a bulk pharmacy package of 20,000,000 units × 10's (NDC 0049-0530-83) of dry powder for reconstitution; buffered with sodium citrate and citric acid to an optimum pH.

Each million units contains approximately 6.8 milligrams of sodium (0.3 mEq) and 65.6 milligrams of potassium (1.68 mEq).

Store the dry powder below 86°F (30°C).

Reference

1. American Heart Association. 1977. Prevention of bacterial endocarditis. Circulation. 56:139A–143A.

Revised April 1987 70-4209-00-5

Approx. Desired Concentration (units/ml)	Approx. Volume (ml) 1,000,000 units	Solvent for Vial of 5,000,000 units	Infusion Only 20,000,000 units
50,000	20.0	—	
100,000	10.0	—	—
250,000	4.0	18.2	75.0
500,000	1.8	8.2	33.0
750,000	—	4.8	—
1,000,000	—	3.2	11.5

PROCARDIA® ℞

[*pro-car 'dē-ă*]

nifedipine

CAPSULES

For Oral Use

DESCRIPTION

PROCARDIA® (nifedipine) is an antianginal drug belonging to a class of pharmacological agents, the calcium channel blockers. Nifedipine is 3,5-pyridinedicarboxylic acid, 1,4-dihydro-2, 6-dimethyl-4-(2-nitrophenyl)-, dimethyl ester, $C_{17}H_{18}N_2O_6$, and has the structural formula:

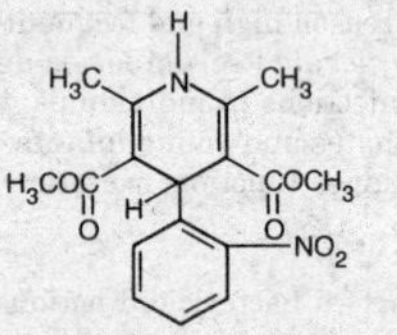

Nifedipine is a yellow crystalline substance, practically insoluble in water but soluble in ethanol. It has a molecular weight of 346.3. PROCARDIA capsules are formulated as soft gelatin capsules for oral administration each containing 10 mg or 20 mg nifedipine.

Inert ingredients in the formulations are: glycerin; peppermint oil; polyethylene glycol; soft gelatin capsules (which contain Yellow 6, and may contain Red Ferric Oxide and other inert ingredients), and water. The 10 mg capsules also contain saccharin sodium.

CLINICAL PHARMACOLOGY

PROCARDIA is a calcium ion influx inhibitor (slow-channel blocker or calcium ion antagonist) and inhibits the transmembrane influx of calcium ions into cardiac muscle and smooth muscle. The contractile processes of cardiac muscle and vascular smooth muscle are dependent upon the movement of extracellular calcium ions into these cells through specific ion channels. PROCARDIA selectively inhibits calcium ion influx across the cell membrane of cardiac muscle and vascular smooth muscle without changing serum calcium concentrations.

Mechanism of Action

The precise means by which this inhibition relieves angina has not been fully determined, but includes at least the following two mechanisms:

1) Relaxation and Prevention of Coronary Artery Spasm

PROCARDIA dilates the main coronary arteries and coronary arterioles, both in normal and ischemic regions, and is a potent inhibitor of coronary artery spasm, whether spontaneous or ergonovine-induced. This property increases myocardial oxygen delivery in patients with coronary artery spasm, and is responsible for the effectiveness of PROCARDIA in vasospastic (Prinzmetal's or variant) angina. Whether this effect plays any role in classical angina is not clear, but studies of exercise tolerance have not shown an increase in the maximum exercise rate-pressure product, a widely accepted measure of oxygen utilization. This suggests that, in general, relief of spasm or dilation of coronary arteries is not an important factor in classical angina.

2) Reduction of Oxygen Utilization

PROCARDIA regularly reduces arterial pressure at rest and at a given level of exercise by dilating peripheral arterioles and reducing the total peripheral resistance (afterload) against which the heart works. This unloading of the heart reduces myocardial energy consumption and oxygen requirements and probably accounts for the effectiveness of PROCARDIA in chronic stable angina.

Pharmacokinetics and Metabolism

PROCARDIA is rapidly and fully absorbed after oral administration. The drug is detectable in serum 10 minutes after oral administration, and peak blood levels occur in approximately 30 minutes. Bioavailability is proportional to dose from 10 to 30 mg; half-life does not change significantly with dose. There is little difference in relative bioavailability when PROCARDIA capsules are given orally and either

swallowed whole, bitten and swallowed, or, bitten and held sublingually. However, biting through the capsule prior to swallowing does result in slightly earlier plasma concentrations (27 ng/mL 10 minutes after 10 mg) than if capsules are swallowed intact. It is highly bound by serum proteins. PROCARDIA is extensively converted to inactive metabolites and approximately 80 percent of PROCARDIA and metabolites are eliminated via the kidneys. The half-life of nifedipine in plasma is approximately two hours. Since hepatic biotransformation is the predominant route for the disposition of nifedipine, the pharmacokinetics may be altered in patients with chronic liver disease. Patients with hepatic impairment (liver cirrhosis) have a longer disposition half-life and higher bioavailability of nifedipine than healthy volunteers. The degree of serum protein binding of nifedipine is high (92–98%). Protein binding may be greatly reduced in patients with renal or hepatic impairment.

Hemodynamics

Like other slow channel blockers, PROCARDIA exerts a negative inotropic effect on isolated myocardial tissue. This is rarely, if ever, seen in intact animals or man, probably because of reflex responses to its vasodilating effects. In man, PROCARDIA causes decreased peripheral vascular resistance and a fall in systolic and diastolic pressure, usually modest (5–10mm Hg systolic), but sometimes larger. There is usually a small increase in heart rate, a reflex response to vasodilation. Measurements of cardiac function in patients with normal ventricular function have generally found a small increase in cardiac index without major effects on ejection fraction, left ventricular end diastolic pressure (LVEDP) or volume (LVEDV). In patients with impaired ventricular function, most acute studies have shown some increase in ejection fraction and reduction in left ventricular filling pressure.

Electrophysiologic Effects

Although, like other members of its class, PROCARDIA decreases sinoatrial node function and atrioventricular conduction in isolated myocardial preparations, such effects have not been seen in studies in intact animals or in man. In formal electrophysiologic studies, predominantly in patients with normal conduction systems, PROCARDIA has had no tendency to prolong atrioventricular conduction, prolong sinus node recovery time, or slow sinus rate.

INDICATIONS AND USAGE

I. Vasospastic Angina

PROCARDIA (nifedipine) is indicated for the management of vasospastic angina confirmed by any of the following criteria: 1) classical pattern of angina at rest accompanied by ST segment elevation, 2) angina or coronary artery spasm provoked by ergonovine, or 3) angiographically demonstrated coronary artery spasm. In those patients who have had angiography, the presence of significant fixed obstructive disease is not incompatible with the diagnosis of vasospastic angina, provided that the above criteria are satisfied. PROCARDIA may also be used where the clinical presentation suggests a possible vasospastic component but where vasospasm has not been confirmed, e.g., where pain has a variable threshold on exertion or when angina is refractory to nitrates and/or adequate doses of beta blockers.

II. Chronic Stable Angina
(Classical Effort-Associated Angina)

PROCARDIA is indicated for the management of chronic stable angina (effort-associated angina) without evidence of vasospasm in patients who remain symptomatic despite adequate doses of beta blockers and/or organic nitrates or who cannot tolerate those agents.

In chronic stable angina (effort-associated angina) PROCARDIA has been effective in controlled trials of up to eight weeks duration in reducing angina frequency and increasing exercise tolerance, but confirmation of sustained effectiveness and evaluation of long term safety in these patients are incomplete.

Controlled studies in small numbers of patients suggest concomitant use of PROCARDIA and beta-blocking agents may be beneficial in patients with chronic stable angina, but available information is not sufficient to predict with confidence the effects of concurrent treatment, especially in patients with compromised left ventricular function or cardiac conduction abnormalities. When introducing such concomitant therapy, care must be taken to monitor blood pressure closely since severe hypotension can occur from the combined effects of the drugs. (See WARNINGS.)

CONTRAINDICATIONS

Known hypersensitivity reaction to PROCARDIA.

WARNINGS

Excessive Hypotension

Although in most patients, the hypotensive effect of PROCARDIA is modest and well tolerated, occasional patients have had excessive and poorly tolerated hypotension. These responses have usually occurred during initial titration or at the time of subsequent upward dosage adjustment. Although patients have rarely experienced excessive hypotension on PROCARDIA alone, this may be more common in patients on concomitant beta-blocker therapy. Although not approved for this purpose, PROCARDIA and

other immediate-release nifedipine capsules have been used (orally and sublingually) for acute reduction of blood pressure. Several well-documented reports describe cases of profound hypotension, myocardial infarction, and death when immediate-release nifedipine was used in this way. **PROCARDIA capsules should not be used for the acute reduction of blood pressure.**

PROCARDIA and other immediate-release nifedipine capsules have also been used for the long-term control of essential hypertension, although no properly-controlled studies have been conducted to define an appropriate dose or dose interval for such treatment. **PROCARDIA capsules should not be used for the control of essential hypertension.**

Several well-controlled, randomized trials studied the use of immediate-release nifedipine in patients who had just sustained myocardial infarctions. In none of these trials did immediate-release nifedipine appear to provide any benefit. In some of the trials, patients who received immediate-release nifedipine had significantly worse outcomes than patients who received placebo. **PROCARDIA capsules should not be administered within the first week or two after myocardial infarction, and they should also be avoided in the setting of acute coronary syndrome (when infarction may be imminent).**

Severe hypotension and/or increased fluid volume requirements have been reported in patients receiving PROCARDIA together with a beta blocking agent who underwent coronary artery bypass surgery using high dose fentanyl anesthesia. The interaction with high dose fentanyl appears to be due to the combination of PROCARDIA and a beta-blocker, but the possibility that it may occur with PROCARDIA alone, with low doses of fentanyl, in other surgical procedures, or with other narcotic analgesics cannot be ruled out. In PROCARDIA treated patients where surgery using high dose fentanyl anesthesia is contemplated, the physician should be aware of these potential problems and, if the patient's condition permits, sufficient time (at least 36 hours) should be allowed for PROCARDIA to be washed out of the body prior to surgery.

Increased Angina and/or Myocardial Infarction

Rarely, patients, particularly those who have severe obstructive coronary artery disease, have developed well documented increased frequency, duration and/or severity of angina or acute myocardial infarction on starting PROCARDIA or at the time of dosage increase. The mechanism of this effect is not established.

Beta Blocker Withdrawal

Patients recently withdrawn from beta blockers may develop a withdrawal syndrome with increased angina, probably related to increased sensitivity to catecholamines. Initiation of PROCARDIA treatment will not prevent this occurrence and might be expected to exacerbate it by provoking reflex catecholamine release. There have been occasional reports of increased angina in a setting of beta blocker withdrawal and PROCARDIA initiation. It is important to taper beta blockers if possible, rather than stopping them abruptly before beginning PROCARDIA.

Congestive Heart Failure

Rarely, patients, usually receiving a beta blocker, have developed heart failure after beginning PROCARDIA. Patients with tight aortic stenosis may be at greater risk for such an event, as the unloading effect of PROCARDIA would be expected to be of less benefit to these patients, owing to their fixed impedance to flow across the aortic valve.

PRECAUTIONS

General: Hypotension: Because PROCARDIA decreases peripheral vascular resistance, careful monitoring of blood pressure during the initial administration and titration of PROCARDIA is suggested. Close observation is especially recommended for patients already taking medications that are known to lower blood pressure. (See WARNINGS.)

Peripheral Edema: Mild to moderate peripheral edema, typically associated with arterial vasodilation and not due to left ventricular dysfunction, occurs in about one in ten patients treated with PROCARDIA (nifedipine). This edema occurs primarily in the lower extremities and usually responds to diuretic therapy. With patients whose angina is complicated by congestive heart failure, care should be taken to differentiate this peripheral edema from the effects of increasing left ventricular dysfunction.

Laboratory Tests: Rare, usually transient, but occasionally significant elevations of enzymes such as alkaline phosphatase, CPK, LDH, SGOT and SGPT have been noted. The relationship to PROCARDIA therapy is uncertain in most cases, but probable in some. These laboratory abnormalities have rarely been associated with clinical symptoms; however, cholestasis with or without jaundice has been reported. Rare instances of allergic hepatitis have been reported.

PROCARDIA, like other calcium channel blockers, decreases platelet aggregation *in vitro*. Limited clinical studies have demonstrated a moderate but statistically significant decrease in platelet aggregation and an increase in bleeding time in some PROCARDIA patients. This is

thought to be a function of inhibition of calcium transport across the platelet membrane. No clinical significance for these findings has been demonstrated.

Positive direct Coombs Test with/without hemolytic anemia has been reported but a causal relationship between PROCARDIA administration and positivity of this laboratory test, including hemolysis, could not be determined.

Although PROCARDIA has been used safely in patients with renal dysfunction and has been reported to exert a beneficial effect in certain cases, rare, reversible elevations in BUN and serum creatinine have been reported in patients with pre-existing chronic renal insufficiency. The relationship to PROCARDIA therapy is uncertain in most cases but probable in some.

Drug Interactions: Beta-adrenergic blocking agents: (See INDICATIONS AND USAGE and WARNINGS.) Experience in over 1400 patients in a non-comparative clinical trial has shown that concomitant administration of PROCARDIA and beta-blocking agents is usually well tolerated, but there have been occasional literature reports suggesting that the combination may increase the likelihood of congestive heart failure, severe hypotension or exacerbation of angina.

Long-acting nitrates: PROCARDIA may be safely co-administered with nitrates, but there have been no controlled studies to evaluate the antianginal effectiveness of this combination.

Digitalis: Since there have been isolated reports of patients with elevated digoxin levels, and there is a possible interaction between digoxin and nifedipine, it is recommended that digoxin levels be monitored when initiating, adjusting, and discontinuing nifedipine to avoid possible over- or under-digitalization.

Quinidine: There have been rare reports of an interaction between quinidine and nifedipine (with a decreased plasma level of quinidine).

Coumarin anticoagulants: There have been rare reports of increased prothrombin time in patients taking coumarin anticoagulants to whom PROCARDIA was administered. However, the relationship to PROCARDIA therapy is uncertain.

Cimetidine: A study in six healthy volunteers has shown a significant increase in peak nifedipine plasma levels (80%) and area-under-the-curve (74%) after a one week course of cimetidine at 1000 mg per day and nifedipine at 40 mg per day. Ranitidine produced smaller, non-significant increases. The effect may be mediated by the known inhibition of cimetidine on hepatic cytochrome P-450, the enzyme system probably responsible for the first-pass metabolism of nifedipine. If nifedipine therapy is initiated in a patient currently receiving cimetidine, cautious titration is advised.

Carcinogenesis, Mutagenesis, Impairment of Fertility: Nifedipine was administered orally to rats for two years and was not shown to be carcinogenic. When given to rats prior to mating, nifedipine caused reduced fertility at a dose approximately 30 times the maximum recommended human dose. There is a literature report of reversible reduction in the ability of human sperm obtained from a limited number of infertile men taking recommended doses of nifedipine to bind to and fertilize an ovum *in vitro*. *In vivo* mutagenicity studies were negative.

Pregnancy: Pregnancy Category C: Nifedipine has been shown to produce teratogenic findings in rats and rabbits, including digital anomalies similar to those reported for phenytoin. Digital anomalies have been reported to occur with other members of the dihydropyridine class and are possibly a result of compromised uterine blood flow. Nifedipine administration was associated with a variety of embryotoxic, placentotoxic, and fetotoxic effects, including stunted fetuses (rats, mice, rabbits), rib deformities (mice), cleft palate (mice), small placentas and underdeveloped chorionic villi (monkeys), embryonic and fetal deaths (rats, mice, rabbits), and prolonged pregnancy/decreased neonatal survivial (rats; not evaluated in other species). On a mg/kg basis, all of the doses associated with the teratogenic embryotoxic or fetotoxic effects in animals were higher (3.5 to 42 times) than the maximum recommended human dose of 120 mg/day. On a mg/m^2 basis, some doses were higher and some were lower than the maximum recommended human dose but all are within an order of magnitude of it. The doses associated with placentotoxic effects in monkeys were equivalent to or lower than the maximum recommended human dose on mg/m^2 basis.

There are no adequate and well-controlled studies in pregnant women. PROCARDIA should be used during pregnancy only if the potential benefit justifies the potential risk to the fetus.

Pediatric Use: Safety and effectiveness in pediatric patients have not been established. Use in pediatric population is not recommended.

ADVERSE REACTIONS

In multiple-dose U.S. and foreign controlled studies in which adverse reactions were reported spontaneously, adverse effects were frequent but generally not serious and

Continued on next page

Procardia—Cont.

rarely required discontinuation of therapy or dosage adjustment. Most were expected consequences of the vasodilator effects of PROCARDIA.

Adverse Effect	PROCARDIA CAPSULES (%) (N=226)	Placebo (%) (N=235)
Dizziness, lightheadedness, giddiness	27	15
Flushing, heat sensation	25	8
Headache	23	20
Weakness	12	10
Nausea, heartburn	11	8
Muscle cramps, tremor	8	3
Peripheral edema	7	1
Nervousness, mood changes	7	4
Palpitation	7	5
Dyspnea, cough, wheezing	6	3
Nasal congestion, sore throat	6	8

There is also a large uncontrolled experience in over 2100 patients in the United States. Most of the patients had vasospastic or resistant angina pectoris, and about half had concomitant treatment with beta-adrenergic blocking agents. The most common adverse events were:

Incidence Approximately 10%
Cardiovascular: peripheral edema
Central Nervous System: dizziness or lightheadedness
Gastrointestinal: nausea
Systemic: headache and flushing, weakness

Incidence Approximately 5%
Cardiovascular: transient hypotension

Incidence 2% or Less
Cardiovascular: palpitation
Respiratory: nasal and chest congestion, shortness of breath
Gastrointestinal: diarrhea, constipation, cramps, flatulence
Musculoskeletal: inflammation, joint stiffness, muscle cramps
Central Nervous System: shakiness, nervousness, jitteriness, sleep disturbances, blurred vision, difficulties in balance
Other: dermatitis, pruritus, urticaria, fever, sweating, chills, sexual difficulties

Incidence Approximately 0.5%
Cardiovascular: syncope (mostly with initial dosing and/or an increase in dose), erythromelalgia.

Incidence Less Than 0.5%
Hematologic: thrombocytopenia, anemia, leukopenia, purpura
Gastrointestinal: allergic hepatitis
Face and Throat: angioedema (mostly oropharyngeal edema with breathing difficulty in a few patients), gingival hyperplasia.
CNS: depression, paranoid syndrome
Special Senses: transient blindness at the peak of plasma level, tinnitus
Urogenital: nocturia, polyuria
Other: arthritis with ANA (+), exfoliative dermatitis, gynecomastia
Musculoskeletal: myalgia

Several of these side effects appear to be dose related. Peripheral edema occurred in about one in 25 patients at doses less than 60 mg per day and in about one patient in eight at 120 mg per day or more. Transient hypotension, generally of mild to moderate severity and seldom requiring discontinuation of therapy, occurred in one of 50 patients at less than 60 mg per day and in one of 20 patients at 120 mg per day or more.

Very rarely, introduction of PROCARDIA therapy was associated with an increase in anginal pain, possibly due to associated hypotension. Transient unilateral loss of vision has also occurred.

In addition, more serious adverse events were observed, not readily distinguishable from the natural history of the disease in these patients. It remains possible, however, that some or many of these events were drug related. Myocardial infarction occurred in about 4% of patients and congestive heart failure or pulmonary edema in about 2%. Ventricular arrhythmias or conduction disturbances each occurred in fewer than 0.5% of patients.

In a subgroup of over 1000 patients receiving PROCARDIA with concomitant beta blocker therapy, the pattern and incidence of adverse experiences was not different from that of the entire group of PROCARDIA (nifedipine) treated patients. (See PRECAUTIONS.)

In a subgroup of approximately 250 patients with a diagnosis of congestive heart failure as well as angina pectoris (about 10% of the total patient population), dizziness or lightheadedness, peripheral edema, headache or flushing each occurred in one in eight patients. Hypotension occurred in about one in 20 patients. Syncope occurred in approximately one patient in 250. Myocardial infarction or symptoms of congestive heart failure each occurred in about one patient in 15. Atrial or ventricular dysrhythmias each occurred in about one patient in 150.

In post-marketing experience, there have been rare reports of exfoliative dematitis caused by nifedipine.

There have been rare reports of exfoliative or bullous skin adverse events (such as exfoliative dermatitis, erythema mutiforme, Stevens-Johnson Syndrome, and toxic epidermal necrolysis) and photosensitivity reactions.

OVERDOSAGE

Experience with nifedipine overdosage is limited. Generally, overdosage with nifedipine leading to pronounced hypotension calls for active cardiovascular support including monitoring of cardiovascular and respiratory function, elevation of extremities, and judicious use of calcium infusion, pressor agents and fluids. Clearance of nifedipine would be expected to be prolonged in patients with impaired liver function. Since nifedipine is highly protein bound, dialysis is not likely to be of any benefit; however, plasmapheresis may be beneficial.

DOSAGE AND ADMINISTRATION

The dosage of PROCARDIA needed to suppress angina and that can be tolerated by the patient must be established by titration. Excessive doses can result in hypotension.

Therapy should be initiated with the 10 mg capsule. The starting dose is one 10 mg capsule, swallowed whole, 3 times/day. The usual effective dose range is 10–20 mg three times daily. Some patients, especially those with evidence of coronary artery spasm, respond only to higher doses, more frequent administration, or both. In such patients, doses of 20–30 mg three or four times daily may be effective. Doses above 120 mg daily are rarely necessary. More than 180 mg per day is not recommended.

In most cases, PROCARDIA titration should proceed over a 7–14 day period so that the physician can assess the response to each dose level and monitor the blood pressure before proceeding to higher doses.

If symptoms so warrant, titration may proceed more rapidly provided that the patient is assessed frequently. Based on the patient's physical activity level, attack frequency, and sublingual nitroglycerin consumption, the dose of PROCARDIA may be increased from 10 mg t.i.d. to 20 mg t.i.d. and then to 30 mg t.i.d. over a three-day period.

In hospitalized patients under close observation, the dose may be increased in 10 mg increments over four- to six-hour periods as required to control pain and arrhythmias due to ischemia. A single dose should rarely exceed 30 mg.

No "rebound effect" has been observed upon discontinuation of PROCARDIA. However, if discontinuation of PROCARDIA is necessary, sound clinical practice suggests that the dosage should be decreased gradually with close physician supervision.

Co-Administration with Other Antianginal Drugs

Sublingual nitroglycerin may be taken as required for the control of acute manifestations of angina, particularly during PROCARDIA titration. See **PRECAUTIONS, Drug Interactions**, for information on co-administration of PROCARDIA with beta blockers or long-acting nitrates.

HOW SUPPLIED

PROCARDIA® soft gelatin capsules are supplied in:

Bottles of 100:
10 mg (NDC 0069-2600-66) (NDC 59012-260-66) orange #260;
20 mg (NDC 0069-2610-66) (NDC 59012-261-66) orange and light brown #261

Bottles of 300:
10 mg (NDC 0069-2600-72) (NDC 59012-260-72) orange #260;
20 mg (NDC 0069-2610-72) (NDC 59012-261-72) orange and light brown #261

Unit dose packages of 100:
10 mg (NDC 0069-2600-41) (NDC 59012-260-41) orange #260;
20 mg (NDC 0069-2610-41) (NDC 59012-261-41) orange and light brown #261

The capsules should be protected from light and moisture and stored at controlled room temperature 59° to 77°F (15° to 25°C) in the manufacturer's original container.

Manufactured by Pfizer Inc. Encapsulated by R.P. Scherer, Clearwater, FL 33518
69-4990-00-9 Revised March 1997

Shown in Product Identification Guide, page 331

PROCARDIA XL® ℞

[pro-car ' dē-ă]
(nifedipine)
Extended Release Tablets
For Oral Use

DESCRIPTION

Nifedipine is a drug belonging to a class of pharmacological agents known as the calcium channel blockers. Nifedipine is 3,5-pyridinedicarboxylic acid, 1,4-dihydro-2,6-dimethyl-4-(2-nitrophenyl)-, dimethyl ester, $C_{17}H_{18}N_2O_6$, and has the structural formula:

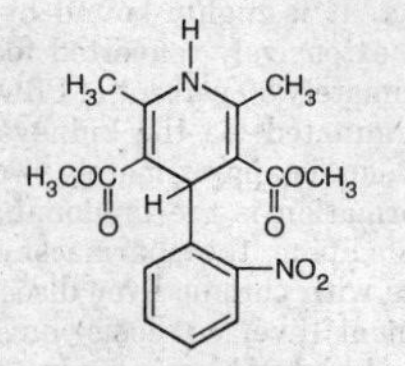

Nifedipine is a yellow crystalline substance, practically insoluble in water but soluble in ethanol. It has a molecular weight of 346.3. PROCARDIA XL is a registered trademark for Nifedipine GITS. Nifedipine GITS (Gastrointestinal Therapeutic System) Tablet is formulated as a once-a-day controlled-release tablet for oral administration designed to deliver 30, 60, or 90 mg of nifedipine.

Inert ingredients in the formulations are: cellulose acetate; hydroxypropyl cellulose; hydroxypropyl methylcellulose; magnesium stearate; polyethylene glycol; polyethylene oxide; red ferric oxide; sodium chloride; titanium dioxide.

System Components and Performance

PROCARDIA XL Extended Release Tablet is similar in appearance to a conventional tablet. It consists, however, of a semipermeable membrane surrounding an osmotically active drug core. The core itself is divided into two layers: an "active" layer containing the drug, and a "push" layer containing pharmacologically inert (but osmotically active) components. As water from the gastrointestinal tract enters the tablet, pressure increases in the osmotic layer and "pushes" against the drug layer, releasing drug through the precision laser-drilled tablet orifice in the active layer.

PROCARDIA XL Extended Release Tablet is designed to provide nifedipine at an approximately constant rate over 24 hours. This controlled rate of drug delivery into the gastrointestinal lumen is independent of pH or gastrointestinal motility. PROCARDIA XL depends for its action on the existence of an osmotic gradient between the contents of the bi-layer core and fluid in the GI tract. Drug delivery is essentially constant as long as the osmotic gradient remains constant, and then gradually falls to zero. Upon swallowing, the biologically inert components of the tablet remain intact during GI transit and are eliminated in the feces as an insoluble shell.

CLINICAL PHARMACOLOGY

Nifedipine is a calcium ion influx inhibitor (slow-channel blocker or calcium ion antagonist) and inhibits the transmembrane influx of calcium ions into cardiac muscle and smooth muscle. The contractile processes of cardiac muscle and vascular smooth muscle are dependent upon the movement of extracellular calcium ions into these cells through specific ion channels. Nifedipine selectively inhibits calcium ion influx across the cell membrane of cardiac muscle and vascular smooth muscle without altering serum calcium concentrations.

Mechanism of Action

A) Angina

The precise mechanisms by which inhibition of calcium influx relieves angina has not been fully determined, but includes at least the following two mechanisms:

1) Relaxation and Prevention of Coronary Artery Spasm

Nifedipine dilates the main coronary arteries and coronary arterioles, both in normal and ischemic regions, and is a potent inhibitor of coronary artery spasm, whether spontaneous or ergonovine-induced. This property increases myocardial oxygen delivery in patients with coronary artery spasm, and is responsible for the effectiveness of nifedipine in vasospastic (Prinzmetal's or variant) angina. Whether this effect plays any role in classical angina is not clear, but studies of exercise tolerance have not shown an increase in the maximum exercise rate-pressure product, a widely accepted measure of oxygen utilization. This suggests that, in general, relief of spasm or dilation of coronary arteries is not an important factor in classical angina.

2) Reduction of Oxygen Utilization

Nifedipine regularly reduces arterial pressure at rest and at a given level of exercise by dilating peripheral arterioles and reducing the total peripheral vascular resistance (afterload) against which the heart works. This unloading of the heart reduces myocardial energy consumption and oxygen requirements, and probably accounts for the effectiveness of nifedipine in chronic stable angina.

B) Hypertension

The mechanism by which nifedipine reduces arterial blood pressure involves peripheral arterial vasodilatation and the resulting reduction in peripheral vascular resistance. The increased peripheral vascular resistance that is an underlying cause of hypertension results from an increase in active tension in the vascular smooth muscle. Studies have demonstrated that the increase in active tension reflects an increase in cytosolic free calcium.

Nifedipine is a peripheral arterial vasodilator which acts directly on vascular smooth muscle. The binding of nifedipine to voltage-dependent and possibly receptor-operated channels in vascular smooth muscle results in an inhibition of calcium influx through these channels. Stores of intracellular calcium in vascular smooth muscle are limited and thus dependent upon the influx of extracellular calcium for contraction to occur. The reduction in calcium influx by nifedipine causes arterial vasodilation and decreased peripheral vascular resistance which results in reduced arterial blood pressure.

Pharmacokinetics and Metabolism
Nifedipine is completely absorbed after oral administration. Plasma drug concentrations rise at a gradual, controlled rate after a PROCARDIA XL Extended Release Tablet dose and reach a plateau at approximately six hours after the first dose. For subsequent doses, relatively constant plasma concentrations at this plateau are maintained with minimal fluctuations over the 24-hour dosing interval. About a four-fold higher fluctuation index (ratio of peak to trough plasma concentration) was observed with the conventional immediate-release Procardia® capsule at t.i.d. dosing than with once daily PROCARDIA XL Extended Release Tablet. At steady-state the bioavailability of the PROCARDIA XL Extended Release Tablet is 86% relative to Procardia capsules. Administration of the PROCARDIA XL Extended Release Tablet in the presence of food slightly alters the early rate of drug absorption, but does not influence the extent of drug bioavailability. Markedly reduced GI retention time over prolonged periods (i.e., short bowel syndrome), however, may influence the pharmacokinetic profile of the drug which could potentially result in lower plasma concentrations. Pharmacokinetics of PROCARDIA XL Extended Release Tablets are linear over the dose range of 30 to 180 mg in that plasma drug concentrations are proportional to dose administered. There was no evidence of dose dumping either in the presence or absence of food for over 150 subjects in pharmacokinetic studies.

Nifedipine is extensively metabolized to highly water-soluble, inactive metabolites accounting for 60 to 80% of the dose excreted in the urine. The elimination half-life of nifedipine is approximately two hours. Only traces (less than 0.1% of the dose) of unchanged form can be detected in the urine. The remainder is excreted in the feces in metabolized form, most likely as a result of biliary excretion. Thus, the pharmacokinetics of nifedipine are not significantly influenced by the degree of renal impairment. Patients in hemodialysis or chronic ambulatory peritoneal dialysis have not reported significantly altered pharmacokinetics of nifedipine. Since hepatic biotransformation is the predominant route for the disposition of nifedipine, the pharmacokinetics may be altered in patients with chronic liver disease. Patients with hepatic impairment (liver cirrhosis) have a longer disposition half-life and higher bioavailability of nifedipine than healthy volunteers. The degree of serum protein binding of nifedipine is high (92–98%). Protein binding may be greatly reduced in patients with renal or hepatic impairment.

Hemodynamics
Like other slow-channel blockers, nifedipine exerts a negative inotropic effect on isolated myocardial tissue. This is rarely, if ever, seen in intact animals or man, probably because of reflex responses to its vasodilating effects. In man, nifedipine decreases peripheral vascular resistance which leads to a fall in systolic and diastolic pressures, usually minimal in normotensive volunteers (less than 5–10 mm Hg systolic), but sometimes larger. With PROCARDIA XL Extended Release Tablets, these decreases in blood pressure are not accompanied by any significant change in heart rate. Hemodynamic studies in patients with normal ventricular function have generally found a small increase in cardiac index without major effects on ejection fraction, left ventricular end diastolic pressure (LVEDP) or volume (LVEDV). In patients with impaired ventricular function, most acute studies have shown some increase in ejection fraction and reduction in left ventricular filling pressure.

Electrophysiologic Effects
Although, like other members of its class, nifedipine causes a slight depression of sinoatrial node function and atrioventricular conduction in isolated myocardial preparations, such effects have not been seen in studies in intact animals or in man. In formal electrophysiologic studies, predominantly in patients with normal conduction systems, nifedipine has had no tendency to prolong atrioventricular conduction or sinus node recovery time, or to slow sinus rate.

INDICATIONS AND USAGE
I. Vasospastic Angina
PROCARDIA XL is indicated for the management of vasospastic angina confirmed by any of the following criteria: 1) classical pattern of angina at rest accompanied by ST segment elevation, 2) angina or coronary artery spasm provoked by ergonovine, or 3) angiographically demonstrated coronary artery spasm. In those patients who have had angiography, the presence of significant fixed obstructive disease is not incompatible with the diagnosis of vasospastic angina, provided that the above criteria are satisfied. PROCARDIA XL may also be used where the clinical presentation suggests a possible vasospastic component but where vasospasm has not been confirmed, e.g., where pain has a variable threshold on exertion or in unstable angina where electrocardiographic findings are compatible with intermittent vasospasm, or when angina is refractory to nitrates and/or adequate doses of beta blockers.

II. Chronic Stable Angina
(Classical Effort-Associated Angina)
PROCARDIA XL is indicated for the management of chronic stable angina (effort-associated angina) without evidence of vasospasm in patients who remain symptomatic despite adequate doses of beta blockers and/or organic nitrates or who cannot tolerate those agents.

In chronic stable angina (effort-associated angina) nifedipine has been effective in controlled trials of up to eight weeks duration in reducing angina frequency and increasing exercise tolerance, but confirmation of sustained effectiveness and evaluation of long-term safety in these patients is incomplete.

Controlled studies in small numbers of patients suggest concomitant use of nifedipine and beta-blocking agents may be beneficial in patients with chronic stable angina, but available information is not sufficient to predict with confidence the effects of concurrent treatment, especially in patients with compromised left ventricular function or cardiac conduction abnormalities. When introducing such concomitant therapy, care must be taken to monitor blood pressure closely since severe hypotension can occur from the combined effects of the drugs. (See WARNINGS.)

III. Hypertension
PROCARDIA XL is indicated for the treatment of hypertension. It may be used alone or in combination with other antihypertensive agents.

CONTRAINDICATIONS
Known hypersensitivity reaction to nifedipine.

WARNINGS
Excessive Hypotension
Although in most angina patients the hypotensive effect of nifedipine is modest and well tolerated, occasional patients have had excessive and poorly tolerated hypotension. These responses have usually occurred during initial titration or at the time of subsequent upward dosage adjustment, and may be more likely in patients on concomitant beta blockers.

Severe hypotension and/or increased fluid volume requirements have been reported in patients receiving nifedipine together with a beta-blocking agent who underwent coronary artery bypass surgery using high dose fentanyl anesthesia. The interaction with high dose fentanyl appears to be due to the combination of nifedipine and a beta blocker, but the possibility that it may occur with nifedipine alone, with low doses of fentanyl, in other surgical procedures, or with other narcotic analgesics cannot be ruled out. In nifedipine-treated patients where surgery using high dose fentanyl anesthesia is contemplated, the physician should be aware of these potential problems and if the patient's condition permits, sufficient time (at least 36 hours) should be allowed for nifedipine to be washed out of the body prior to surgery.

The following information should be taken into account in those patients who are being treated for hypertension as well as angina:

Increased Angina and/or Myocardial Infarction
Rarely, patients, particularly those who have severe obstructive coronary artery disease, have developed well documented increased frequency, duration and/or severity of angina or acute myocardial infarction on starting nifedipine or at the time of dosage increase. The mechanism of this effect is not established.

Beta Blocker Withdrawal
It is important to taper beta blockers if possible, rather than stopping them abruptly before beginning nifedipine. Patients recently withdrawn from beta blockers may develop a withdrawal syndrome with increased angina, probably related to increased sensitivity to catecholamines. Initiation of nifedipine treatment will not prevent this occurrence and on occasion has been reported to increase it.

Congestive Heart Failure
Rarely, patients, usually receiving a beta blocker, have developed heart failure after beginning nifedipine. Patients with tight aortic stenosis may be at greater risk for such an event, as the unloading effect of nifedipine would be expected to be of less benefit to those patients, owing to their fixed impedance to flow across the aortic valve.

PRECAUTIONS
General—Hypotension: Because nifedipine decreases peripheral vascular resistance, careful monitoring of blood pressure during the initial administration and titration of nifedipine is suggested. Close observation is especially recommended for patients already taking medications that are known to lower blood pressure. (See WARNINGS.)
Peripheral Edema: Mild to moderate peripheral edema occurs in a dose dependent manner with an incidence ranging from approximately 10% to about 30% at the highest dose studied (180 mg). It is a localized phenomenon thought to be associated with vasodilation of dependent arterioles and small blood vessels and not due to left ventricular dysfunction or generalized fluid retention. With patients whose angina or hypertension is complicated by congestive heart failure, care should be taken to differentiate this peripheral edema from the effects of increasing left ventricular dysfunction.

Other: As with any other non-deformable material, caution should be used when administering PROCARDIA XL in patients with preexisting severe gastrointestinal narrowing (pathologic or iatrogenic). There have been rare reports of obstructive symptoms in patients with known strictures in association with the ingestion of PROCARDIA XL.
Information for Patients: PROCARDIA XL Extended Release Tablets should be swallowed whole. Do not chew, divide or crush tablets. Do not be concerned if you occasionally notice in your stool something that looks like a tablet. In PROCARDIA XL, the medication is contained within a nonabsorbable shell that has been specially designed to slowly release the drug for your body to absorb. When this process is completed, the empty tablet is eliminated from your body.
Laboratory Tests: Rare, usually transient, but occasionally significant elevations of enzymes such as alkaline phosphatase, CPK, LDH, SGOT, and SGPT have been noted. The relationship to nifedipine therapy is uncertain in most cases, but probable in some. These laboratory abnormalities have rarely been associated with clinical symptoms; however, cholestasis with or without jaundice has been reported. A small (5.4%) increase in mean alkaline phosphatase was noted in patients treated with PROCARDIA XL. This was an isolated finding not associated with clinical symptoms and it rarely resulted in values which fell outside the normal range. Rare instances of allergic hepatitis have been reported. In controlled studies, PROCARDIA XL did not adversely affect serum uric acid, glucose, or cholesterol. Serum potassium was unchanged in patients receiving PROCARDIA XL in the absence of concomitant diuretic therapy, and slightly decreased in patients receiving concomitant diuretics.

Nifedipine, like other calcium channel blockers, decreases platelet aggregation in vitro. Limited clinical studies have demonstrated a moderate but statistically significant decrease in platelet aggregation and an increase in bleeding time in some nifedipine patients. This is thought to be a function of inhibition of calcium transport across the platelet membrane. No clinical significance for these findings has been demonstrated.

Positive direct Coombs test with/without hemolytic anemia has been reported but a causal relationship between nifedipine administration and positivity of this laboratory test, including hemolysis, could not be determined.

Although nifedipine has been used safely in patients with renal dysfunction and has been reported to exert a beneficial effect, in certain cases, rare, reversible elevations in BUN and serum creatinine have been reported in patients with pre-existing chronic renal insufficiency. The relationship to nifedipine therapy is uncertain in most cases but probable in some.

Drug Interactions: Beta-adrenergic blocking agents: (See INDICATIONS AND USAGE and WARNINGS.) Experience in over 1400 patients with Procardia capsules in a noncomparative clinical trial has shown that concomitant administration of nifedipine and beta-blocking agents is usually well tolerated, but there have been occasional literature reports suggesting that the combination may increase the likelihood of congestive heart failure, severe hypotension, or exacerbation of angina.

Long-acting Nitrates: Nifedipine may be safely co-administered with nitrates, but there have been no controlled studies to evaluate the antianginal effectiveness of this combination.

Digitalis: Administration of nifedipine with digoxin increased digoxin levels in nine of twelve normal volunteers. The average increase was 45%. Another investigator found no increase in digoxin levels in thirteen patients with coronary artery disease. In an uncontrolled study of over two hundred patients with congestive heart failure during which digoxin blood levels were not measured, digitalis toxicity was not observed. Since there have been isolated reports of patients with elevated digoxin levels, it is recommended that digoxin levels be monitored when initiating, adjusting, and discontinuing nifedipine to avoid possible over- or under-digitalization.

Coumarin Anticoagulants: There have been rare reports of increased prothrombin time in patients taking coumarin anticoagulants to whom nifedipine was administered. However, the relationship to nifedipine therapy is uncertain.

Cimetidine: A study in six healthy volunteers has shown a significant increase in peak nifedipine plasma levels (80%) and area-under-the-curve (74%), after a one week course of cimetidine at 1000 mg per day and nifedipine at 40 mg per day. Ranitidine produced smaller, non-significant increases.

Continued on next page

Procardia XL—Cont.

The effect may be mediated by the known inhibition of cimetidine on hepatic cytochrome P-450, the enzyme system probably responsible for the first-pass metabolism of nifedipine. If nifedipine therapy is initiated in a patient currently receiving cimetidine, cautious titration is advised.

Carcinogenesis, Mutagenesis, Impairment of Fertility: Nifedipine was administered orally to rats for two years and was not shown to be carcinogenic. When given to rats prior to mating, nifedipine caused reduced fertility at a dose approximately 30 times the maximum recommended human dose. There is a literature report of reversible reduction in the ability of human sperm obtained from a limited number of infertile men taking recommended doses of nifedipine to bind to and fertilize an ovum *in vitro*. *In vivo* mutagenicity studies were negative.

Pregnancy: Pregnancy Category C: Nifedipine has been shown to produce teratogenic findings in rats and rabbits, including digital anomalies similar to those reported for phenytoin. Digital anomalies have been reported to occur with other members of the dihydropyridine class and are possibly a result of compromised uterine blood flow. Nifedipine administration was associated with a variety of embryotoxic, placentotoxic, and fetotoxic effects, including stunted fetuses (rats, mice, rabbits), rib deformities (mice), cleft palate (mice), small placentas and underdeveloped chorionic villi (monkeys), embryonic and fetal deaths (rats, mice, rabbits), and prolonged pregnancy/decreased neonatal survival (rats; not evaluated in other species). On a mg/kg basis, all of the doses associated with the teratogenic embryotoxic or fetotoxic effects in animals were higher (3.5 to 42 times) than the maximum recommended human dose of 120 mg/day. On a mg/m^2 basis, some doses were higher and some were lower than the maximum recommended human dose but all are within an order of magnitude of it. The doses associated with placentotoxic effects in monkeys were equivalent to or lower than the maximum recommended human dose on a mg/m^2 basis.

There are no adequate and well-controlled studies in pregnant women. PROCARDIA XL Extended Release Tablets should be used during pregnancy only if the potential benefit justifies the potential risk to the fetus.

Pediatric Use: Safety and effectiveness in pediatric patients have not been established.

ADVERSE EXPERIENCES

Over 1000 patients from both controlled and open trials with PROCARDIA XL Extended Release Tablets in hypertension and angina were included in the evaluation of adverse experiences. All side effects reported during PROCARDIA XL Extended Release Tablet therapy were tabulated independent of their causal relation to medication. The most common side effect reported with PROCARDIA XL was edema which was dose related and ranged in frequency from approximately 10% to about 30% at the highest dose studied (180 mg). Other common adverse experiences reported in placebo-controlled trials include:

Adverse Effect	PROCARDIA XL (%) (N=707)	Placebo (%) (N=266)
Headache	15.8	9.8
Fatigue	5.9	4.1
Dizziness	4.1	4.5
Constipation	3.3	2.3
Nausea	3.3	1.9

Of these, only edema and headache were more common in PROCARDIA XL patients than placebo patients.

The following adverse reactions occurred with an incidence of less than 3.0%. With the exception of leg cramps, the incidence of these side effects was similar to that of placebo alone.

Body as a Whole/Systemic: asthenia, flushing, pain
Cardiovascular: palpitations
Central Nervous System: insomnia, nervousness, paresthesia, somnolence
Dermatologic: pruritus, rash
Gastrointestinal: abdominal pain, diarrhea, dry mouth, dyspepsia, flatulence
Musculoskeletal: arthralgia, leg cramps
Respiratory: chest pain (nonspecific), dyspnea
Urogenital: impotence, polyuria

Other adverse reactions were reported sporadically with an incidence of 1.0% or less. These include:

Body as a Whole/Systemic: face edema, fever, hot flashes, malaise, periorbital edema, rigors
Cardiovascular: arrhythmia, hypotension, increased angina, tachycardia, syncope
Central Nervous System: anxiety, ataxia, decreased libido, depression, hypertonia, hypoesthesia, migraine, paroniria, tremor, vertigo
Dermatologic: alopecia, increased sweating, urticaria, purpura
Gastrointestinal: eructation, gastroesophageal reflux, gum hyperplasia, melena, vomiting, weight increase
Musculoskeletal: back pain, gout, myalgias
Respiratory: coughing, epistaxis, upper respiratory tract infection, respiratory disorder, sinusitis
Special Senses: abnormal lacrimation, abnormal vision, taste perversion, tinnitus
Urogenital/Reproductive: breast pain, dysuria, hematuria, nocturia

Adverse experiences which occurred in less than 1 in 1000 patients cannot be distinguished from concurrent disease states or medications.

The following adverse experiences, reported in less than 1% of patients, occurred under conditions (e.g., open trials, marketing experience) where a causal relationship is uncertain: gastrointestinal irritation, gastrointestinal bleeding, gynecomastia.

In multiple-dose U.S. and foreign controlled studies with nifedipine capsules in which adverse reactions were reported spontaneously, adverse effects were frequent but generally not serious and rarely required discontinuation of therapy or dosage adjustment. Most were expected consequences of the vasodilator effects of nifedipine.

Adverse Effect	PROCARDIA CAPSULES (%) (N=226)	Placebo (%) (N=235)
Dizziness, lightheadedness, giddiness	27	15
Flushing, heat sensation	25	8
Headache	23	20
Weakness	12	10
Nausea, heartburn	11	8
Muscle cramps, tremor	8	3
Peripheral edema	7	1
Nervousness, mood changes	7	4
Palpitation	7	5
Dyspnea, cough, wheezing	6	3
Nasal congestion, sore throat	6	8

There is also a large uncontrolled experience in over 2100 patients in the United States. Most of the patients had vasospastic or resistant angina pectoris, and about half had concomitant treatment with beta-adrenergic blocking agents. The relatively common adverse events were similar in nature to those seen with PROCARDIA XL.

In addition, more serious adverse events were observed, not readily distinguishable from the natural history of the disease in these patients. It remains possible, however, that some or many of these events were drug related. Myocardial infarction occurred in about 4% of patients and congestive heart failure or pulmonary edema in about 2%. Ventricular arrhythmias or conduction disturbances each occurred in fewer than 0.5% of patients.

In a subgroup of over 1000 patients receiving PROCARDIA with concomitant beta blocker therapy, the pattern and incidence of adverse experiences was not different from that of the entire group of PROCARDIA (nifedipine) treated patients. (See PRECAUTIONS.)

In a subgroup of approximately 250 patients with a diagnosis of congestive heart failure as well as angina, dizziness, or lightheadedness, peripheral edema, headache or flushing each occurred in one in eight patients. Hypotension occurred in about one in 20 patients. Syncope occurred in approximately one patient in 250. Myocardial infarction or symptoms of congestive heart failure each occurred in about one patient in 15. Atrial or ventricular dysrhythmias each occurred in about one patient in 150.

In post-marketing experience, there have been rare reports of exfoliative dermatitis caused by nifedipine.

There have been rare reports of exfoliative or bullous skin adverse events (such as exfoliative dermatitis, erythema multiforme, Stevens-Johnson Syndrome, and toxic epidermal necrolysis) and photosensitivity reactions.

OVERDOSAGE

Experience with nifedipine overdosage is limited. Generally, overdosage with nifedipine leading to pronounced hypotension calls for active cardiovascular support including monitoring of extremities, cardiac and respiratory function, elevation of extremities, judicious use of calcium infusion, pressor agents and fluids. Clearance of nifedipine would be expected to be prolonged in patients with impaired liver function. Since nifedipine is highly protein-bound, dialysis is not likely to be of any benefit.

There has been one reported case of massive overdosage with PROCARDIA XL Extended Release Tablets. The main effects of ingestion of approximately 4800 mg of PROCARDIA XL in a young man attempting suicide as a result of cocaine-induced depression was initial dizziness, palpitations, flushing, and nervousness. Within several hours of ingestion, nausea, vomiting, and generalized edema developed. No significant hypotension was apparent at presentation, 18 hours post-ingestion. Electrolyte abnormalities consisted of a mild, transient elevation of serum creatinine, and modest elevations of LDH and CPK, but normal SGOT. Vital signs remained stable, no electrocardiographic abnormalities were noted and renal function returned to normal within 24 to 48 hours with routine supportive measures alone. No prolonged sequelae were observed.

The effect of a single 900 mg ingestion of Procardia capsules in a depressed anginal patient also on tricyclic antidepressants was loss of consciousness within 30 minutes of ingestion, and profound hypotension, which responded to calcium infusion, pressor agents, and fluid replacement. A variety of ECG abnormalities were seen in this patient with a history of bundle branch block, including sinus bradycardia and varying degrees of AV block. These dictated the prophylactic placement of a temporary ventricular pacemaker, but otherwise resolved spontaneously. Significant hyperglycemia was seen initially in this patient, but plasma glucose levels rapidly normalized without further treatment.

A young hypertensive patient with advanced renal failure ingested 280 mg of Procardia capsules at one time, with resulting marked hypotension responding to calcium infusion and fluids. No AV conduction abnormalities, arrhythmias, or pronounced changes in heart rate were noted, nor was there any further deterioration in renal function.

DOSAGE AND ADMINISTRATION

Dosage must be adjusted according to each patient's needs. Therapy for either hypertension or angina should be initiated with 30 or 60 mg once daily. PROCARDIA XL Extended Release Tablets should be swallowed whole and should not be bitten or divided. In general, titration should proceed over a 7–14 day period so that the physician can fully assess the response to each dose level and monitor blood pressure before proceeding to higher doses. Since steady-state plasma levels are achieved on the second day of dosing, if symptoms so warrant, titration may proceed more rapidly provided the patient is assessed frequently. Titration to doses above 120 mg are not recommended.

Angina patients controlled on Procardia capsules alone or in combination with other antianginal medications may be safely switched to PROCARDIA XL Extended Release Tablets at the nearest equivalent total daily dose (e.g., 30 mg t.i.d. of Procardia capsules may be changed to 90 mg once daily of PROCARDIA XL Extended Release Tablets). Subsequent titration to higher or lower doses may be necessary and should be initiated as clinically warranted. Experience with doses greater than 90 mg in patients with angina is limited. Therefore, doses greater than 90 mg should be used with caution and only when clinically warranted.

No "rebound effect" has been observed upon discontinuation of PROCARDIA XL Extended Release Tablets. However, if discontinuation of nifedipine is necessary, sound clinical practice suggests that the dosage should be decreased gradually with close physician supervision.

Care should be taken when dispensing PROCARDIA XL to assure that the extended release dosage form has been prescribed.

Co-Administration with Other Antianginal Drugs

Sublingual nitroglycerin may be taken as required for the control of acute manifestations of angina, particularly during nifedipine titration. See PRECAUTIONS, Drug Interactions, for information on co-administration of nifedipine with beta blockers or long-acting nitrates.

HOW SUPPLIED

PROCARDIA XL® Extended Release Tablets are supplied as 30 mg, 60 mg and 90 mg round, biconvex, rose-pink, film-coated tablets in:

Bottles of 100: 30 mg (NDC 0069-2650-66)
(NDC 59012-265-66)
60 mg (NDC 0069-2660-66)
(NDC 59012-266-66)
90 mg (NDC 0069-2670-66)
(NDC 59012-267-66)

Bottles of 300: 30 mg (NDC 0069-2650-72)
(NDC 59012-265-72)
60 mg (NDC 0069-2660-72)
(NDC 59012-266-72)

Bottles of 5000: 30 mg (NDC 0069-2650-94)
(NDC 59012-265-94)
60 mg (NDC 0069-2660-94)
(NDC 59012-266-94)

Unit dose packages of 100: 30 mg (NDC 0069-2650-41)
(NDC 59012-265-41)
60 mg (NDC 0069-2660-41)
(NDC 59012-266-41)
90 mg (NDC 0069-2670-41)
(NDC 59012-267-41)

Store below 86°F (30°C).
Protect from moisture and humidity.

© 1997 PFIZER INC

69-4467-00-6 Revised March 1997

Shown in Product Identification Guide, page 331

RENESE® ℞

[rĕ-nēs]
(polythiazide)
TABLETS
for Oral Administration

DESCRIPTION

Renese® is designated generically as polythiazide, and chemically as 2*H*-1,2,4-Benzothiadiazine-7-sulfonamide,

6-chloro-3,4-dihydro-2-methyl-3-[[(2,2,2-trifluoroethyl)thio]methyl]-, 1,1-dioxide. It is a white crystalline substance, insoluble in water but readily soluble in alkaline solution. Inert Ingredients: dibasic calcium phosphate; lactose; magnesium stearate; polyethylene glycol; sodium lauryl sulfate; starch; vanillin. The 2 mg tablets also contain: Yellow 6; Yellow 10.

ACTION

The mechanism of action results in an interference with the renal tubular mechanism of electrolyte reabsorption. At maximal therapeutic dosage all thiazides are approximately equal in their diuretic potency. The mechanism whereby thiazides function in the control of hypertension is unknown.

INDICATIONS

Renese is indicated as adjunctive therapy in edema associated with congestive heart failure, hepatic cirrhosis, and corticosteroid and estrogen therapy.

Renese has also been found useful in edema due to various forms of renal dysfunction as: Nephrotic syndrome; Acute glomerulonephritis; and Chronic renal failure.

Renese is indicated in the management of hypertension either as the sole therapeutic agent or to enhance the effectiveness of other antihypertensive drugs in the more severe forms of hypertension.

Usage in Pregnancy. The routine use of diuretics in an otherwise healthy woman is inappropriate and exposes mother and fetus to unnecessary hazard. Diuretics do not prevent development of toxemia of pregnancy, and there is no satisfactory evidence that they are useful in the treatment of developed toxemia.

Edema during pregnancy may arise from pathological causes or from the physiologic and mechanical consequences of pregnancy. Thiazides are indicated in pregnancy when edema is due to pathologic causes, just as they are in the absence of pregnancy (however, see Warnings, below). Dependent edema in pregnancy, resulting from restriction of venous return by the expanded uterus, is properly treated through elevation of the lower extremities and use of support hose; use of diuretics to lower intravascular volume in this case is illogical and unnecessary. There is hypervolemia during normal pregnancy which is harmful to neither the fetus nor the mother (in the absence of cardiovascular disease), but which is associated with edema, including generalized edema, in the majority of pregnant women. If this edema produces discomfort, increased recumbency will often provide relief. In rare instances, this edema may cause extreme discomfort which is not relieved by rest. In these cases, a short course of diuretics may provide relief and may be appropriate.

CONTRAINDICATIONS

Anuria. Hypersensitivity to this or other sulfonamide derived drugs.

WARNINGS

Thiazides should be used with caution in severe renal disease. In patients with renal disease, thiazides may precipitate azotemia. Cumulative effects of the drug may develop in patients with impaired renal function.

Thiazides should be used with caution in patients with impaired hepatic function or progressive liver disease, since minor alterations of fluid and electrolyte balance may precipitate hepatic coma.

Thiazides may add to or potentiate the action of other antihypertensive drugs. Potentiation occurs with ganglionic or peripheral adrenergic blocking drugs.

Sensitivity reactions may occur in patients with a history of allergy or bronchial asthma.

The possibility of exacerbation or activation of systemic lupus erythematosus has been reported.

Usage in Pregnancy. Thiazides cross the placental barrier and appear in cord blood. The use of thiazides in pregnant women requires that the anticipated benefit be weighed against possible hazards to the fetus. These hazards include fetal or neonatal jaundice, thrombocytopenia, and possibly other adverse reactions which have occurred in the adult.

Nursing Mothers. Thiazides appear in breast milk. If use of the drug is deemed essential, the patient should stop nursing.

PRECAUTIONS

Periodic determination of serum electrolytes to detect possible electrolyte imbalance should be performed at appropriate intervals.

All patients receiving thiazide therapy should be observed for clinical signs of fluid or electrolyte imbalance; namely, hyponatremia, hypochloremic alkalosis, and hypokalemia. Serum and urine electrolyte determinations are particularly important when the patient is vomiting excessively or receiving parenteral fluids. Medication such as digitalis may also influence serum electrolytes. Warning signs, irrespective of cause, are: dryness of mouth, thirst, weakness, lethargy, drowsiness, restlessness, muscle pains or cramps, muscular fatigue, hypotension, oliguria, tachycardia, and gastrointestinal disturbances such as nausea and vomiting.

Hypokalemia may develop with thiazides as with any other potent diuretic, especially with brisk diuresis, when severe cirrhosis is present, or during concomitant use of corticosteroids or ACTH.

Interference with adequate oral electrolyte intake will also contribute to hypokalemia. Digitalis therapy may exaggerate metabolic effects of hypokalemia especially with reference to myocardial activity.

Any chloride deficit is generally mild and usually does not require specific treatment except under extraordinary circumstances (as in liver disease or renal disease). Dilutional hyponatremia may occur in edematous patients in hot weather; appropriate therapy is water restriction, rather than administration of salt except in rare instances when the hyponatremia is life threatening. In actual salt depletion, appropriate replacement is the therapy of choice.

Hyperuricemia may occur or frank gout may be precipitated in certain patients receiving thiazide therapy.

Insulin requirements in diabetic patients may be increased, decreased, or unchanged. Latent diabetes mellitus may become manifest during thiazide administration.

Thiazide drugs may increase the responsiveness to tubocurarine.

The antihypertensive effects of the drug may be enhanced in the postsympathectomy patient.

Thiazides may decrease arterial responsiveness to norepinephrine. This diminution is not sufficient to preclude effectiveness of the pressor agent for therapeutic use.

If progressive renal impairment becomes evident, as indicated by a rising nonprotein nitrogen or blood urea nitrogen, a careful reappraisal of therapy is necessary with consideration given to withholding or discontinuing diuretic therapy.

Thiazides may decrease serum PBI levels without signs of thyroid disturbance.

Pediatric Use: Safety and effectiveness in pediatric patients have not been established.

ADVERSE REACTIONS

A. GASTROINTESTINAL SYSTEM REACTIONS

1. anorexia
2. gastric irritation
3. nausea
4. vomiting
5. cramping
6. diarrhea
7. constipation
8. jaundice (intrahepatic cholestatic jaundice)
9. pancreatitis

B. CENTRAL NERVOUS SYSTEM REACTIONS

1. dizziness
2. vertigo
3. paresthesias
4. headache
5. xanthopsia

C. HEMATOLOGIC REACTIONS

1. leukopenia
2. agranulocytosis
3. thrombocytopenia
4. aplastic anemia

D. DERMATOLOGIC—HYPERSENSITIVITY REACTIONS

1. purpura
2. photosensitivity
3. rash
4. urticaria
5. necrotizing angiitis
   (vasculitis)
   (cutaneous vasculitis)

E. CARDIOVASCULAR REACTION

Orthostatic hypotension may occur and may be aggravated by alcohol, barbiturates or narcotics.

F. OTHER

1. hyperglycemia
2. glycosuria
3. hyperuricemia
4. muscle spasm
5. weakness
6. restlessness

Whenever adverse reactions are moderate or severe, thiazide dosage should be reduced or therapy withdrawn.

DOSAGE AND ADMINISTRATION

Therapy should be individualized according to patient response. This therapy should be titrated to gain maximal therapeutic response as well as the minimal dose possible to maintain that therapeutic response. The usual dose of Renese tablets for diuretic therapy is 1 to 4 mg daily, and for antihypertensive therapy is 2 to 4 mg daily.

HOW SUPPLIED

RENESE® (polythiazide) Tablets are available as:

1 mg white, scored tablets in bottles of 100 (NDC 0069-3750-66).

2 mg yellow, scored tablets in bottles of 100 (NDC 0069-3760-66).

4 mg white, scored tablets in bottles of 100 (NDC 0069-3770-66).

Pfizer Labs
Division of Pfizer Inc, NY, NY 10017
69-1116-00-6   Revised April 1997

SINEQUAN®   ℞
[*sin 'a-kwon*]
(doxepin HCl)
Capsules
Oral Concentrate

DESCRIPTION

SINEQUAN® (doxepin hydrochloride) is one of a class of psychotherapeutic agents known as dibenzoxepin tricyclic compounds. The molecular formula of the compound is $C_{19}H_{21}NO \cdot HCl$ having a molecular weight of 316. It is a white crystalline solid readily soluble in water, lower alcohols and chloroform.

Inert ingredients for the capsule formulations are: hard gelatin capsules (which may contain Blue 1, Red 3, Red 40, Yellow 10, and other inert ingredients); magnesium stearate; sodium lauryl sulfate; starch.

Inert ingredients for the oral concentrate formulation are: glycerin; methylparaben; peppermint oil; propylparaben; water.

CHEMISTRY

SINEQUAN (doxepin HCl) is a dibenzoxepin derivative and is the first of a family of tricyclic psychotherapeutic agents. Specifically, it is an isomeric mixture of: 1-Propanamine, 3-dibenz[*b,e*]oxepin-11(6*H*)ylidene-*N,N*-dimethyl-, hydrochloride.

SINEQUAN (doxepin HCl)

ACTIONS

The mechanism of action of SINEQUAN (doxepin HCl) is not definitely known. It is not a central nervous system stimulant nor a monoamine oxidase inhibitor. The current hypothesis is that the clinical effects are due, at least in part, to influences on the adrenergic activity at the synapses so that deactivation of norepinephrine by reuptake into the nerve terminals is prevented. Animal studies suggest that doxepin HCl does not appreciably antagonize the antihypertensive action of guanethidine. In animal studies anticholinergic, antiserotonin and antihistamine effects on smooth muscle have been demonstrated. At higher than usual clinical doses, norepinephrine response was potentiated in animals. This effect was not demonstrated in humans.

At clinical dosages up to 150 mg per day, SINEQUAN can be given to man concomitantly with guanethidine and related compounds without blocking the antihypertensive effect. At dosages above 150 mg per day blocking of the antihypertensive effect of these compounds has been reported.

SINEQUAN is virtually devoid of euphoria as a side effect. Characteristic of this type of compound, SINEQUAN has not been demonstrated to produce the physical tolerance or psychological dependence associated with addictive compounds.

INDICATIONS

SINEQUAN is recommended for the treatment of:

1. Psychoneurotic patients with depression and/or anxiety.
2. Depression and/or anxiety associated with alcoholism (not to be taken concomitantly with alcohol).
3. Depression and/or anxiety associated with organic disease (the possibility of drug interaction should be considered if the patient is receiving other drugs concomitantly).
4. Psychotic depressive disorders with associated anxiety including involutional depression and manic-depressive disorders.

The target symptoms of psychoneurosis that respond particularly well to SINEQUAN include anxiety, tension, depression, somatic symptoms and concerns, sleep disturbances, guilt, lack of energy, fear, apprehension and worry.

Clinical experience has shown that SINEQUAN is safe and well tolerated even in the elderly patient. Owing to lack of clinical experience in the pediatric population, SINEQUAN is not recommended for use in children under 12 years of age.

CONTRAINDICATIONS

SINEQUAN is contraindicated in individuals who have shown hypersensitivity to the drug. Possibility of cross sensitivity with other dibenzoxepines should be kept in mind.

Continued on next page

Sinequan—Cont.

SINEQUAN is contraindicated in patients with glaucoma or a tendency to urinary retention. These disorders should be ruled out, particularly in older patients.

WARNINGS

The once-a-day dosage regimen of SINEQUAN in patients with intercurrent illness or patients taking other medications should be carefully adjusted. This is especially important in patients receiving other medications with anticholinergic effects.

Usage in Geriatrics: The use of SINEQUAN on a once-a-day dosage regimen in geriatric patients should be adjusted carefully based on the patient's condition.

Usage in Pregnancy: Reproduction studies have been performed in rats, rabbits, monkeys and dogs and there was no evidence of harm to the animal fetus. The relevance to humans is not known. Since there is no experience in pregnant women who have received this drug, safety in pregnancy has not been established. There has been a report of apnea and drowsiness occurring in a nursing infant whose mother was taking SINEQUAN.

Usage in Children: The use of SINEQUAN in children under 12 years of age is not recommended because safe conditions for its use have not been established.

PRECAUTIONS

Drug Interactions: *Drugs Metabolized by P450 2D6:* The biochemical activity of the drug metabolizing isozyme cytochrome P450 2D6 (debrisoquin hydroxylase) is reduced in a subset of the Caucasian population (about 7–10% of Caucasians are so-called "poor metabolizers"); reliable estimates of the prevalence of reduced P450 2D6 isozyme activity among Asian, African and other populations are not yet available. Poor metabolizers have higher than expected plasma concentrations of tricyclic antidepressants (TCAs) when given usual doses. Depending on the fraction of drug metabolized by P450 2D6, the increase in plasma concentration may be small, or quite large (8-fold increase in plasma AUC of the TCA).

In addition, certain drugs inhibit the activity of this isozyme and make normal metabolizers resemble poor metabolizers. An individual who is stable on a given dose of TCA may become abruptly toxic when given one of these inhibiting drugs as concomitant therapy. The drugs that inhibit cytochrome P450 2D6 include some that are not metabolized by the enzyme (quinidine; cimetidine) and many that are substrates for P450 2D6 (many other antidepressants, phenothiazines, and the Type 1C antiarrythmics propafenone and flecainide). While all the selective serotonin reuptake inhibitors (SSRIs), e.g., fluoxetine, sertraline, and paroxetine, inhibit P450 2D6, they may vary in the extent of inhibition. The extent to which SSRI-TCA interactions may pose clinical problems will depend on the degree of inhibition and the pharmacokinetics of the SSRI involved. Nevertheless, caution is indicated in the co-administration of TCAs with any of the SSRIs and also in switching from one class to the other. Of particular importance, sufficient time must elapse before initiating TCA treatment in a patient being withdrawn from fluoxetine, given the long half-life of the parent and active metabolite (at least 5 weeks may be necessary). Concomitant use of tricyclic antidepressants with drugs that can inhibit cytochrome P450 2D6 may require lower doses than usually prescribed for either the tricyclic antidepressant or the other drug. Furthermore, whenever one of these other drugs is withdrawn from co-therapy, an increased dose of tricyclic antidepressant may be required. It is desirable to monitor TCA plasma levels whenever a TCA is going to be coadministered with another drug known to be an inhibitor of P450 2D6.

MAO Inhibitors: Serious side effects and even death have been reported following the concomitant use of certain drugs with MAO inhibitors. Therefore, MAO inhibitors should be discontinued at least two weeks prior to the cautious initiation of therapy with SINEQUAN. The exact length of time may vary and is dependent upon the particular MAO inhibitor being used, the length of time it has been administered, and the dosage involved.

Cimetidine: Cimetidine has been reported to produce clinically significant fluctuations in steady-state serum concentrations of various tricyclic antidepressants. Serious anticholinergic symptoms (i.e., severe dry mouth, urinary retention and blurred vision) have been associated with elevations in the serum levels of tricyclic antidepressant when cimetidine therapy is initiated. Additionally, higher than expected tricyclic antidepressant levels have been observed when they are begun in patients already taking cimetidine. In patients who have been reported to be well controlled on tricyclic antidepressants receiving concurrent cimetidine therapy, discontinuation of cimetidine has been reported to decrease established steady-state serum tricyclic antidepressant levels and compromise their therapeutic effects.

Alcohol: It should be borne in mind that alcohol ingestion may increase the danger inherent in any intentional or unintentional SINEQUAN overdosage. This is especially important in patients who may use alcohol excessively.

Tolazamide: A case of severe hypoglycemia has been reported in a type II diabetic patient maintained on tolazamide (1 gm/day) 11 days after the addition of doxepin (75 mg/day).

Drowsiness: Since drowsiness may occur with the use of this drug, patients should be warned of the possibility and cautioned against driving a car or operating dangerous machinery while taking the drug. Patients should also be cautioned that their response to alcohol may be potentiated.

Suicide: Since suicide is an inherent risk in any depressed patient and may remain so until significant improvement has occurred, patients should be closely supervised during the early course of therapy. Prescriptions should be written for the smallest feasible amount.

Psychosis: Should increased symptoms of psychosis or shift to manic symptomatology occur, it may be necessary to reduce dosage or add a major tranquilizer to the dosage regimen.

ADVERSE REACTIONS

NOTE: Some of the adverse reactions noted below have not been specifically reported with SINEQUAN use. However, due to the close pharmacological similarities among the tricyclics, the reactions should be considered when prescribing SINEQUAN (doxepin HCl).

Anticholinergic Effects: Dry mouth, blurred vision, constipation, and urinary retention have been reported. If they do not subside with continued therapy, or become severe, it may be necessary to reduce the dosage.

Central Nervous System Effects: Drowsiness is the most commonly noticed side effect. This tends to disappear as therapy is continued. Other infrequently reported CNS side effects are confusion, disorientation, hallucinations, numbness, paresthesias, ataxia, extrapyramidal symptoms, seizures, tardive dyskinesia, and tremor.

Cardiovascular: Cardiovascular effects including hypotension, hypertension, and tachycardia have been reported occasionally.

Allergic: Skin rash, edema, photosensitization, and pruritus have occasionally occurred.

Hematologic: Eosinophilia has been reported in a few patients. There have been occasional reports of bone marrow depression manifesting as agranulocytosis, leukopenia, thrombocytopenia, and purpura.

Gastrointestinal: Nausea, vomiting, indigestion, taste disturbances, diarrhea, anorexia, and aphthous stomatitis have been reported. (See Anticholinergic Effects.)

Endocrine: Raised or lowered libido, testicular swelling, gynecomastia in males, enlargement of breasts and galactorrhea in the female, raising or lowering of blood sugar levels, and syndrome of inappropriate antidiuretic hormone secretion have been reported with tricyclic administration.

Other: Dizziness, tinnitus, weight gain, sweating, chills, fatigue, weakness, flushing, jaundice, alopecia, headache, exacerbation of asthma, and hyperpyrexia (in association with chlorpromazine) have been occasionally observed as adverse effects.

Withdrawal Symptoms: The possibility of development of withdrawal symptoms upon abrupt cessation of treatment after prolonged SINEQUAN administration should be borne in mind. These are not indicative of addiction and gradual withdrawal of medication should not cause these symptoms.

DOSAGE AND ADMINISTRATION

For most patients with illness of mild to moderate severity, a starting daily dose of 75 mg is recommended. Dosage may subsequently be increased or decreased at appropriate intervals and according to individual response. The usual optimum dose range is 75 mg/day to 150 mg/day.

In more severely ill patients higher doses may be required with subsequent gradual increase to 300 mg/day if necessary. Additional therapeutic effect is rarely to be obtained by exceeding a dose of 300 mg/day.

In patients with very mild symptomatology or emotional symptoms accompanying organic disease, lower doses may suffice. Some of these patients have been controlled on doses as low as 25-50 mg/day.

The total daily dosage of SINEQUAN may be given on a divided or once-a-day dosage schedule. If the once-a-day schedule is employed, the maximum recommended dose is 150 mg/day. This dose may be given at bedtime. **The 150 mg capsule strength is intended for maintenance therapy only and is not recommended for initiation of treatment.**

Anti-anxiety effect is apparent before the antidepressant effect. Optimal antidepressant effect may not be evident for two to three weeks.

OVERDOSAGE

Deaths may occur from overdosage with this class of drugs. Multiple drug ingestion (including alcohol) is common in deliberate tricyclic antidepressant overdose. As the management is complex and changing, it is recommended that the physician contact a poison control center for current information on treatment. Signs and symptoms of toxicity develop rapidly after tricyclic antidepressant overdose; therefore, hospital monitoring is required as soon as possible.

Manifestations: Critical manifestations of overdose include: cardiac dysrhythmias, severe hypotension, convulsions, and CNS depression, including coma. Changes in the electrocardiogram, particularly in QRS axis or width, are clinically significant indicators of tricyclic antidepressant toxicity.

Other signs of overdose may include: confusion, disturbed concentration, transient visual hallucinations, dilated pupils, agitation, hyperactive reflexes, stupor, drowsiness, muscle rigidity, vomiting, hypothermia, hyperpyrexia, or any of the symptoms listed under ADVERSE REACTIONS.

General Recommendations:

General: Obtain an ECG and immediately initiate cardiac monitoring. Protect the patient's airway, establish an intravenous line and initiate gastric decontamination. A minimum of six hours of observation with cardiac monitoring and observation for signs of CNS or respiratory depression, hypotension, cardiac dysrhythmias and/or conduction blocks, and seizures is strongly advised. If signs of toxicity occur at any time during this period, extended monitoring is recommended. There are case reports of patients succumbing to fatal dysrhythmias late after overdose; these patients had clinical evidence of significant poisoning prior to death and most received inadequate gastrointestinal decontamination. Monitoring of plasma drug levels should not guide management of the patient.

Gastrointestinal Decontamination: All patients suspected of tricyclic antidepressant overdose should receive gastrointestinal decontamination. This should include large volume gastric lavage followed by activated charcoal. If consciousness is impaired, the airway should be secured prior to lavage. Emesis is contraindicated.

Cardiovascular: A maximal limb-lead QRS duration of ≥0.10 seconds may be the best indication of the severity of the overdose. Intravenous sodium bicarbonate should be used to maintain the serum pH in the range of 7.45 to 7.55. If the pH response is inadequate, hyperventilation may also be used. Concomitant use of hyperventilation and sodium bicarbonate should be done with extreme caution, with frequent pH monitoring. A pH >7.60 or a pCO$_2$ <20 mm Hg is undesirable. Dysrhythmias unresponsive to sodium bicarbonate therapy/hyperventilation may respond to lidocaine, bretylium or phenytoin. Type 1A and 1C antiarrhythmics are generally contraindicated (e.g., quinidine, disopyramide, and procainamide).

In rare instances, hemoperfusion may be beneficial in acute refractory cardiovascular instability in patients with acute toxicity. However, hemodialysis, peritoneal dialysis, exchange tranfusions, and forced diuresis generally have been reported as ineffective in tricyclic antidepressant poisoning.

CNS: In patients with CNS depression, early intubation is advised because of the potential for abrupt deterioration. Seizures should be controlled with benzodiazepines, or if these are ineffective, other anticonvulsants (e.g., phenobarbital, phenytoin). Physostigmine is not recommended except to treat life-threatening symptoms that have been unresponsive to other therapies, and then only in consultation with a poison control center.

Psychiatric Follow-up: Since overdosage is often deliberate, patients may attempt suicide by other means during the recovery phase. Psychiatric referral may be appropriate.

Pediatric Management: The principles of management of child and adult overdosages are similar. It is strongly recommended that the physician contact the local poison control center for specific pediatric treatment.

HOW SUPPLIED

SINEQUAN® is available as capsules containing doxepin HCl equivalent to:

10 mg—100's (NDC 0049-5340-66) (NDC 0662-5340-66), 1000's (NDC 0049-5340-82) (NDC 0662-5340-82)
25 mg—100's (NDC 0049-5350-66) (NDC 0662-5350-66), 1000's (NDC 0049-5350-82) (NDC 0662-5350-82), 5000's (NDC 0049-5350-94) (NDC 0662-5350-94)
50 mg—100's (NDC 0049-5360-66) (NDC 0662-5360-66), 1000's (NDC 0049-5360-82) (NDC 0662-5360-82), 5000's (NDC 0049-5360-94) (NDC 0662-5360-94)
75 mg—100's (NDC 0049-5390-66) (NDC 0662-5390-66), 1000's (NDC 0049-5390-82) (NDC 0662-5390-82)
100 mg—100's (NDC 0049-5380-66) (NDC 0662-5380-66), 1000's (NDC 0049-5380-82) (NDC 0662-5380-82)
150 mg—50's (NDC 0049-5370-50) (NDC 0662-5370-50), 500's (NDC 0049-5370-73) (NDC 0062-5370-73)

SINEQUAN® Oral Concentrate is available in 120 mL bottles (NDC 0049-5100-47) (NDC 0662-5100-47) with an accompanying dropper calibrated at 5 mg, 10 mg, 15 mg, 20 mg, and 25 mg. Each mL contains doxepin HCl equivalent to 10 mg doxepin. Just prior to administration, SINEQUAN® Oral Concentrate should be diluted with approximately 120 mL of water, whole or skimmed milk, or orange, grapefruit, tomato, prune or pineapple juice. SINEQUAN® Oral Concentrate is not physically compatible with a number of carbonated beverages. For those patients requiring antidepressant therapy who are on methadone maintenance, SINEQUAN® Oral Concentrate and methadone syrup can be mixed together with Gatorade®,

lemonade, orange juice, sugar water, Tang®, or water; but not with grape juice. Preparation and storage of bulk dilutions is not recommended.

©1996 Pfizer Inc

69-2135-00-0 Revised May 1996

Shown in Product Identification Guide, page 331

SPECTROBID® ℞
[spek 'trō-bid]
(bacampicillin HCl)
TABLETS

DESCRIPTION

SPECTROBID® (bacampicillin HCl) is a member of the ampicillin class of semi-synthetic penicillins derived from the basic penicillin nucleus: 6-aminopenicillanic acid. SPECTROBID, as well as ampicillin and other ampicillin analogues, is acid resistant and suitable for oral administration.

SPECTROBID is the hydrochloride salt of 1-ethoxycarbonyloxyethyl ester of ampicillin and is available as a tablet. During the process of absorption from the gastrointestinal tract, SPECTROBID is hydrolyzed rapidly to ampicillin, a well characterized and effective antibacterial agent. Each 400 mg tablet of SPECTROBID is chemically equivalent to 280 mg of ampicillin.

Chemically, SPECTROBID is 1′-ethoxycarbonyloxyethyl - 6 - (D-α aminophenylacetamide) - penicillinate hydrochloride. It has a molecular weight of 501.96 and the following structural formula:

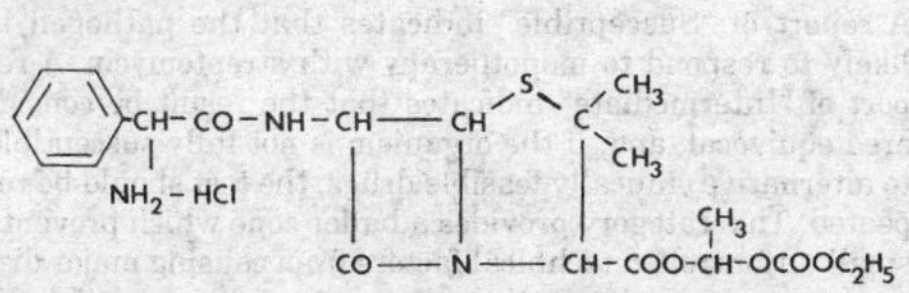

Inert ingredients for the tablets are: microcrystalline cellulose, lactose and magnesium stearate. May also include the following: hydroxypropyl methylcellulose; and opaspray white, opadry white and opadry clear (these components may contain other inert ingredients).

ACTIONS

Clinical Pharmacology

SPECTROBID is characterized by its more complete and more rapid absorption from the GI tract than ampicillin. SPECTROBID tablets of 400 mg, 800 mg, and 1600 mg have provided ampicillin peak serum concentrations of 7.9, 12.9, and 20.1 mcg/mL. These peak levels are approximately three times the levels obtained with administration of equivalent amounts of ampicillin. The areas-under-the-serum-concentration curves obtained during the first 6 hours were 24.8 and 12.9 mcg/mL/hr., when bacampicillin HCl 800 mg and ampicillin 500 mg were administered to adults. (See Graph.)

In fasting adult volunteers, a 400 mg dose of the tablet gave a peak serum ampicillin concentration of 7.2 mcg/mL. In fasting pediatric patients a 12.5 mg/kg dose provided a peak of 8.4 mcg/mL.

After oral administration of SPECTROBID tablet, ampicillin activity in serum peaks at 0.7–0.9 hours (compared to 1.5–2.0 hours after administration of ampicillin). Serum ampicillin half-life is 1.1 hours after either SPECTROBID or ampicillin administration.

Peak tissue and body fluid ampicillin concentrations also are higher after administration of SPECTROBID. Utilizing a special skin window technique to determine ampicillin levels, therapeutic levels in the interstitial fluid were higher and more prolonged after SPECTROBID than after ampicillin administration. SPECTROBID is stable in the presence of gastric acid. Food does not retard absorption of SPECTROBID tablets which may be given without regard to meals. SPECTROBID has been shown to be rapidly and well absorbed after oral administration, with about 75% of a given dose being recoverable in the urine as active ampicillin within 8 hours of administration. Urinary excretion can be delayed by concurrent administration of probenecid. The active moiety of SPECTROBID (i.e., ampicillin) diffuses readily into most body tissues and fluids. In serum, ampicillin is only 20% protein-bound, compared to 60–90% for other penicillins.

Microbiology

SPECTROBID per se has no *in vitro* antibacterial activity and owes its *in vivo* bactericidal activity to the parent compound, ampicillin. The ampicillin class of penicillins (including SPECTROBID) has a broad spectrum of activity against many gram-negative and gram-positive bacteria. Like other penicillins, the ampicillin class of penicillins inhibits the synthesis of cell wall mucopeptide.

Ampicillin class antibiotics are inactivated by β-lactamases produced by certain strains of *Enterobacter, Citrobacter, Haemophilus influenzae,* and *Escherichia coli,* and by most strains of staphylococci and indole-positive *Proteus* spp. Ampicillin class antibiotics are not active against *Pseudomonas, Klebsiella,* or *Serratia* spp.

SUSCEPTIBILITY TESTING

Elution Technique: For the automated method of susceptibility testing (i.e., Autobac™), gram-negative organisms should be tested with the 4.5 mcg ampicillin elution disk, while gram-positive organisms should be tested with the 0.22 mcg disk.

Diffusion Technique: For the Kirby-Bauer method of susceptibility testing, a 10 mcg ampicillin diffusion disk should be used. With this procedure, a laboratory report of "susceptible" indicates that the infecting organism is likely to respond to SPECTROBID therapy, and a report of "resistant" indicates that the infecting organism is not likely to respond to therapy. An "intermediate susceptibility" report suggests that the infecting organism would be susceptible to SPECTROBID if a high dosage is used or if the infection is confined to tissues and fluids (e.g., urine) in which high antibiotic levels are attained.

Dilution Techniques: Broth or agar dilution methods may be used to determine the minimal inhibitory concentration (MIC) value for susceptibility of bacterial isolates to SPECTROBID. Since SPECTROBID per se has no *in vitro* activity, ampicillin powder should be used in a twofold concentration series of the antibiotic prepared in either broth (in tubes) or agar (in petri plates). Tubes should be inoculated to contain 10^4 to 10^5 organisms/mL or plates "spotted" with 10^3 to 10^4 organisms.

INDICATIONS AND USAGE

SPECTROBID is indicated for the treatment of the following infections when caused by ampicillin-susceptible organisms:

1. Upper and Lower Respiratory Tract Infections (including acute exacerbations of chronic bronchitis) due to streptococci (β-hemolytic streptococci, *Streptococcus pyogenes*), pneumococci (*Streptococcus pneumoniae*), nonpenicillinase-producing staphylococci and *H. influenzae;*
2. Urinary Tract Infections due to *E. coli, Proteus mirabilis,* and *Streptococcus faecalis* (enterococci);
3. Skin and Skin Structure Infections due to streptococci and susceptible staphylococci;
4. Gonorrhea (acute uncomplicated urogenital infections) due to *Neisseria gonorrhoeae.*

Bacteriological studies to determine the causative organisms and their susceptibility to SPECTROBID (i.e., ampicillin) should be performed. Therapy may be instituted prior to obtaining results of susceptibility testing. Indicated surgical procedures should be performed.

CONTRAINDICATIONS

The use of ampicillin class antibiotics is contraindicated in individuals with a history of an allergic reaction to any of the penicillin antibiotics and/or cephalosporins.

WARNINGS

Serious and occasional fatal hypersensitivity (anaphylactic) reactions have been reported in patients on penicillin therapy. Although anaphylaxis is more frequent following parenteral therapy, it has occurred in patients on oral penicillins. These reactions are more apt to occur in individuals with a history of penicillin hypersensitivity and/or hypersensitivity to multiple allergens.

There have been reports of individuals with a history of penicillin hypersensitivity who have experienced severe reactions when treated with cephalosporins. Before therapy with a penicillin, careful inquiry should be made concerning previous hypersensitivity reactions to penicillins, cephalosporins, and other allergens.

IF AN ALLERGIC REACTION OCCURS, THE DRUG SHOULD BE DISCONTINUED AND THE APPROPRIATE THERAPY INSTITUTED. SERIOUS ANAPHYLACTOID REACTIONS REQUIRE IMMEDIATE EMERGENCY TREATMENT WITH EPINEPHRINE. OXYGEN, INTRAVENOUS STEROIDS, AND AIRWAY MANAGEMENT, INCLUDING INTUBATION, SHOULD ALSO BE ADMINISTERED AS INDICATED.

PRECAUTIONS

1. General: The possibility of superinfections with mycotic or bacterial pathogens should be kept in mind during therapy. If superinfections occur (usually involving *Aerobacter, Pseudomonas,* or *Candida*), the drug should be discontinued and appropriate therapy instituted.

As with any potent agent, it is advisable to check periodically for organ system dysfunction during prolonged therapy. This includes renal, hepatic, and hematopoietic systems and is particularly important in prematures, neonates, and patients with liver or renal impairments.

A high percentage of patients with mononucleosis who receive ampicillin develop a skin rash. Thus, ampicillin class antibiotics should not be administered to patients with mononucleosis.

2. Clinically Significant Drug Interactions: The concurrent administration of allopurinol and ampicillin increases substantially the incidence of rashes in patients receiving both drugs as compared to patients receiving ampicillin alone. It is not known whether this potentiation of ampicillin rashes is due to allopurinol or the hyperuricemia present in these patients. There are no data available on the incidence of rash in patients treated concurrently with SPECTROBID (bacampicillin HCl) and allopurinol. SPECTROBID should not be co-administered with Antabuse (disulfiram).

3. Drug and Laboratory Test Interactions: When testing for the presence of glucose in urine using Clinitest™, Benedict's Solution, or Fehling's Solution, high urine concentrations of ampicillin may result in false-positive reactions. Therefore, it is recommended that glucose tests based on enzymatic glucose oxidase reactions (such as Clinistix™ or Testape™) be used.

Following administration of ampicillin to pregnant women a transient decrease in plasma concentration of total conjugated estriol, estriol-glucuronide, conjugated estrone and estradiol, has been noted.

4. Pregnancy Category B: Reproduction studies have been performed in mice and rats at SPECTROBID doses of up to 750 mg/kg (more than 25 times the human dose) and have revealed no evidence of impaired fertility or harm to the fetus due to SPECTROBID. There are, however, no adequate and well controlled studies in pregnant women. Because animal reproduction studies are not always predictive of human response, this drug should be used during pregnancy only if clearly needed.

5. Carcinogenesis, Mutagenesis, Impairment of Fertility: No carcinogenicity or mutagenicity studies were conducted. No impairment of fertility and no significant effect on general reproductive performance was observed in rats administered oral doses of up to 750 mg/kg of bacampicillin HCl per day prior to and during mating and gestation. In addition, bacampicillin HCl caused no drug-related effects on the reproductive organs of rats or dogs receiving daily oral doses of up to 800 and 650 mg/kg respectively for 6 months.

6. Labor and Delivery: Oral ampicillin class antibiotics are generally poorly absorbed during labor. Studies in guinea pigs showed that intravenous administration of ampicillin decreased the uterine tone, frequency of contractions, height of contractions, and duration of contractions. However, it is not known whether use of SPECTROBID in humans during labor or delivery has immediate or delayed adverse effects on the fetus, prolongs the duration of labor, or increases the likelihood that forceps delivery or other obstetrical intervention or resuscitation of the newborn will be necessary.

7. Nursing Mothers: Ampicillin class antibiotics are excreted in milk; therefore, caution should be exercised when ampicillin class antibiotics are administered to a nursing woman.

8. Pediatric Use: SPECTROBID tablets are indicated for children weighing 25 kg or more.

ADVERSE REACTIONS

As with other penicillins, it may be expected that untoward reactions will be essentially limited to sensitivity phenomena. They are more likely to occur in individuals who have previously demonstrated hypersensitivity to penicillins and in those with a history of allergy, asthma, hay fever, or urticaria.

In well controlled clinical trials conducted in the U.S. the most frequent adverse reactions to SPECTROBID were epigastric upset (2%) and diarrhea (2%). Increased dosage may result in an increased incidence of diarrhea. In the same clinical trials the most frequent adverse effects for amoxicillin were diarrhea (4%) and nausea (2%).

The following adverse reactions have been reported for ampicillin.

Gastrointestinal: diarrhea, gastritis, stomatitis, nausea, vomiting, glossitis, black "hairy" tongue, enterocolitis, and pseudomembranous colitis.

Hypersensitivity Reactions: skin rashes, urticaria, erythema multiforme, and an occasional case of exfoliative dermatitis. These reactions may be controlled with antihistamines and, if necessary, systemic corticosteroids. Whenever such reactions occur, the drug should be discontinued, unless the opinion of the physician dictates otherwise.

Serious and occasional fatal hypersensitivity (anaphylactic) reactions can occur with oral penicillins. (See WARNINGS.)

Liver: A moderate rise in serum glutamic oxaloacetic transaminase (SGOT) has been noted in some ampicillin treated patients, but the significance of this finding is unknown. In well controlled clinical trials no difference was noted between ampicillin and SPECTROBID with regard to the incidence of liver function test abnormalities.

Hemic and Lymphatic Systems: Anemia, thrombocytopenia, thrombocytopenic purpura, eosinophilia, leukopenia, and agranulocytosis have been reported during therapy with penicillins. These reactions are usually reversible on discontinuation of therapy and are believed to be hypersensitivity phenomena.

Continued on next page

Spectrobid—Cont.

DOSAGE AND ADMINISTRATION

SPECTROBID tablets may be given without regard to meals.

UPPER RESPIRATORY TRACT INFECTIONS (including otitis media) due to streptococci, pneumococci, nonpenicillinase-producing staphylococci and *H. influenzae;*

URINARY TRACT INFECTIONS due to *E. coli, Proteus mirabilis,* and *Streptococcus faecalis;*

SKIN AND SKIN STRUCTURES INFECTIONS due to streptococci and susceptible staphylococci:

Usual Dosage

Adults: 1 × 400 mg tablet every 12 hours (for patients weighing 25 kg or more).

Children: (≥ 25kg) 25 mg/kg per day in 2 equally divided doses at 12 hour intervals.

IN SEVERE INFECTIONS OR THOSE CAUSED BY LESS SUSCEPTIBLE ORGANISMS:

Usual Dosage

Adults: 2 × 400 mg tablets every 12 hours (for patients weighing 25 kg or more).

Children: (≥ 25 kg) 50 mg/kg per day in 2 equally divided doses at 12 hour intervals.

LOWER RESPIRATORY TRACT INFECTIONS due to streptococci, pneumococci, nonpenicillinase-producing staphylococci, and *H. influenzae:*

Usual Dosage

Adults: 2 × 400 mg tablets every 12 hours (for patients weighing 25 kg or more).

Children: (≥ 25 kg) 50 mg/kg per day in 2 equally divided doses at 12 hour intervals.

GONORRHEA—acute uncomplicated urogenital infections due to *N. gonorrhoeae* (males and females):

1.6 grams (4 × 400 mg tablet plus 1 gram probenecid) as a single oral dose.

No pediatric dosage has been established.

Cases of gonorrhea with a suspected lesion of syphilis should have dark field examination before receiving SPECTROBID and monthly serological tests for a minimum of four months. Larger doses may be required for stubborn or severe infections.

It should be recognized that in the treatment of chronic urinary tract infections, frequent bacteriological and clinical appraisals are necessary. Smaller doses than those recommended above should not be used. In stubborn infections, therapy may be required for several weeks. It may be necessary to continue clinical and/or bacteriological follow-up for several months after cessation of therapy. Except for gonorrhea, treatment should be continued for a minimum of 48 to 72 hours beyond the time that the patient becomes asymptomatic or evidence of bacterial eradication has been obtained.

IT IS RECOMMENDED THAT THERE BE AT LEAST 10 DAYS' TREATMENT FOR ANY INFECTION CAUSED BY HEMOLYTIC STREPTOCOCCI TO PREVENT THE OCCURRENCE OF ACUTE RHEUMATIC FEVER OR GLOMERULONEPHRITIS.

HOW SUPPLIED

SPECTROBID® (bacampicillin HCl) Tablets

400 mg (NDC 0049-0350-66): white, film-coated, oblong, unscored are available in bottles of 100.

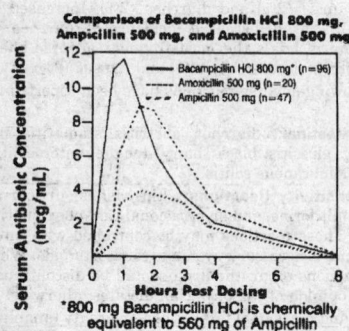

Comparison of Bacampicillin HCl 800 mg, Ampicillin 500 mg, and Amoxicillin 500 mg

*800 mg Bacampicillin HCl is chemically equivalent to 560 mg of Ampicillin

Rev. July 1992

© 1992, Pfizer Inc
69-4092-00-7

STREPTOMYCIN SULFATE Injection, USP ℞
1 g/2.5 mL Ampules
For Intramuscular Use Only

WARNING
THE RISK OF SEVERE NEUROTOXIC REACTIONS IS SHARPLY INCREASED IN PATIENTS WITH IMPAIRED RENAL FUNCTION OR PRE-RENAL AZOTEMIA. THESE INCLUDE DISTURBANCES OF VESTIBULAR AND COCHLEAR FUNCTION. OPTIC NERVE DYSFUNCTION, PERIPHERAL NEURITIS, ARACHNOIDITIS, AND ENCEPHALOPATHY MAY ALSO OCCUR. THE INCIDENCE OF CLINICALLY DETECTABLE, IRREVERSIBLE VESTIBULAR DAMAGE IS PARTICULARLY HIGH IN PATIENTS TREATED WITH STREPTOMYCIN.

RENAL FUNCTION SHOULD BE MONITORED CAREFULLY; PATIENTS WITH RENAL IMPAIRMENT AND/OR NITROGEN RETENTION SHOULD RECEIVE REDUCED DOSAGES. THE PEAK SERUM CONCENTRATION IN INDIVIDUALS WITH KIDNEY DAMAGE SHOULD NOT EXCEED 20 TO 25 MCG/ML. THE CONCURRENT OR SEQUENTIAL USE OF OTHER NEUROTOXIC AND/OR NEPHROTOXIC DRUGS WITH STREPTOMYCIN SULFATE, INCLUDING NEOMYCIN, KANAMYCIN, GENTAMICIN, CEPHALORIDINE, PAROMOMYCIN, VIOMYCIN, POLYMYXIN B, COLISTIN, TOBRAMYCIN AND CYCLOSPORINE SHOULD BE AVOIDED.

THE NEUROTOXICITY OF STREPTOMYCIN CAN RESULT IN RESPIRATORY PARALYSIS FROM NEUROMUSCULAR BLOCKAGE, ESPECIALLY WHEN THE DRUG IS GIVEN SOON AFTER THE USE OF ANESTHESIA OR OF MUSCLE RELAXANTS.

THE ADMINISTRATION OF STREPTOMYCIN IN PARENTERAL FORM SHOULD BE RESERVED FOR PATIENTS WHERE ADEQUATE LABORATORY AND AUDIOMETRIC TESTING FACILITIES ARE AVAILABLE DURING THERAPY.

DESCRIPTION

Streptomycin is a water-soluble aminoglycoside derived from *Streptomyces griseus.* It is marketed as the sulfate salt of streptomycin. The chemical name of streptomycin sulfate is D-Streptamine, *O*-2-deoxy-2-(methylamino)-α-L-glucopyranosyl-(1→2)-*O*-5-deoxy-3-*C*-formyl-α-L-lyxofuranosyl-(1⁻4)-*N,N* '-bis(aminoiminomethyl)-, sulfate (2:3) (salt). The empirical formula for Streptomycin Sulfate is $(C_{21}H_{39}N_7O_{12})_2.3H_2SO_4$ and the molecular weight is 1457.38. It has the following structure:

$$\cdot 3H_2SO_4$$

Streptomycin Sulfate Injection, 1 g/2.5 mL (400 mg/mL), is supplied as a sterile, nonpyrogenic solution for intramuscular use.

Each mL contains: Streptomycin sulfate equivalent to 400 mg of streptomycin, sodium citrate dihydrate 12 mg, phenol 0.25% w/v as preservative, sodium metabisulfite 2 mg in Water for Injection. pH range 5.0 to 8.0.

CLINICAL PHARMACOLOGY

Following intramuscular injection of 1 g of streptomycin, as the sulfate, a peak serum level of 25 to 50 mcg/mL is reached within 1 hour, diminishing slowly to about 50 percent after 5 to 6 hours.

Appreciable concentrations are found in all organ tissues except the brain. Significant amounts have been found in pleural fluid and tuberculous cavities. Streptomycin passes through the placenta with serum levels in the cord blood similar to maternal levels. Small amounts are excreted in milk, saliva, and sweat.

Streptomycin is excreted by glomerular filtration. In patients with normal kidney function, between 29% and 89% of a single 600 mg dose is excreted in the urine within 24 hours. Any reduction of glomerular function results in decreased excretion of the drug and concurrent rise in serum and tissue levels.

Microbiology

Streptomycin sulfate is a bactericidal antibiotic. It acts by interfering with normal protein synthesis.

Streptomycin has been shown to be active against most strains of the following organisms both *in vitro* and in clinical infection. (See INDICATIONS AND USAGE.):

Brucella (brucellosis),

Calymmatobacterium granulomatis (donovanosis, granuloma inguinale),

Escherichia coli, Proteus spp., Aerobacter aerogenes, Klebsiella pneumoniae, and *Enterococcus faecalis* in urinary tract infections,

Francisella tularensis,

Haemophilus ducreyi (chancroid),

Haemophilus influenzae (in respiratory, endocardial, and meningeal infections—concomitantly with another antibacterial agent),

Klebsiella pneumoniae pneumonia (concomitantly with another antibacterial agent),

Mycobacterium tuberculosis,

Pasteurella pestis

Streptococcus viridans, *Enterococcus faecalis* (in endocardial infections—concomitantly with penicillin).

SUSCEPTIBILITY TESTS: Diffusion Techniques

Quantitative methods that require measurement of zone diameters give the most precise estimate of the susceptibility of bacteria to antimicrobial agents. One such standard procedure[1] which has been recommended for use with disks to test susceptibility of organisms to streptomycin uses the 10 mcg streptomycin disk. Interpretation involves the correlation of the diameter obtained in the disk test with the minimum inhibitory concentration (MIC) for streptomycin.

Reports from the laboratory giving results of the standard single disk susceptibility test with a 10 mcg streptomycin disk should be interpreted according to the following criteria:

Zone Diameter (mm)	Interpretation
≥15	(S) Susceptible
11–12	(I) Intermediate
≤10	(R) Resistant

A report of "Susceptible" indicates that the pathogen is likely to respond to monotherapy with streptomycin. A report of "Intermediate" indicates that the result be considered equivocal, and, if the organism is not fully susceptible to alternative clinically feasible drugs, the test should be repeated. This category provides a buffer zone which prevents small uncontrolled technical factors from causing major discrepancies in interpretations. A report of "Resistant" indicates that achievable drug concentrations are unlikely to be inhibitory and other therapy should be selected.

Standardized procedures require the use of laboratory control organisms. The 10 mcg streptomycin disk should give the following zone diameter:

Organism	Zone diameter (mm)
E. coli ATCC 25922	12–20
S. aureus ATCC 25923	14–22

Methods Section:

Two standardized *in vitro* susceptibility methods are available for testing streptomycin against *Mycobacterium tuberculosis* organisms. The agar proportion method (CDC or NCCLS M24–P) utilizes middlebrook 7H10 medium impregnated with streptomycin at two final concentrations, 2.0 and 10.0 mcg/mL. MIC_{90} values are calculated by comparing the quantity of organisms growing in the medium containing drug to the control cultures. Mycobacterial growth in the presence of drug ≥ 1% of the control indicates resistance.

The radiometric broth method employs the BACTEC 460 machine to compare the growth index from untreated control cultures to cultures grown in the presence of 6.0 mcg/mL of streptomycin. Strict adherence to the manufacturer's instructions for sample processing and data interpretation is required for this assay.

Susceptibility test results obtained by these two different methods cannot be compared unless equivalent drug concentrations are evaluated.

The clinical relevance of *in vitro* susceptibility test results for mycobacterial species other than *M. tuberculosis* using either the BACTEC or the proportion method has not been determined.

INDICATIONS AND USAGE

Streptomycin is indicated for the treatment of individuals with moderate to severe infections caused by susceptible strains of microorganisms in the specific conditions listed below:

1. Mycobacterium tuberculosis: The Advisory Council for the Elimination of Tuberculosis, the American Thoracic Society, and the Center for Disease Control recommend that either streptomycin or ethambutol be added as a fourth drug in a regimen containing isoniazid (INH), rifampin and pyrazinamide for initial treatment of tuberculosis unless the likelihood of INH or rifampin resistance is very low. The need for a fourth drug should be reassessed when the results of susceptibility testing are known. In the past when the national rate of primary drug resistance to isoniazid was known to be less than 4% and was either stable or declining, therapy with two and three drug regimens was considered adequate. If community rates of INH resistance are currently less than 4%, an initial treatment regimen with less than four drugs may be considered.

Streptomycin is also indicated for therapy of tuberculosis when one or more of the above drugs is contraindicated because of toxicity or intolerance. The management of tuberculosis has become more complex as a consequence of increasing rates of drug resistance and concomitant HIV infection. Additional consultation from experts in the treatment of tuberculosis may be desirable in those settings.

2. Non-tuberculosis infections: The use of streptomycin should be limited to the treatment of infections caused by bacteria which have been shown to be susceptible to the antibacterial effects of streptomycin and which are not amenable to therapy with less potentially toxic agents.

a. *Pasteurella pestis* (plague),
b. *Francisella tularensis* (tularemia),
c. *Brucella,*
d. *Calymmatobacterium granulomatis* (donovanosis, granuloma inguinale),
e. *H. ducreyi* (chancroid),
f. *H. influenzae* (in respiratory, endocardial, and meningeal infections—concomitantly with another antibacterial agent),
g. *K. pneumoniae* pneumonia (concomitantly with another antibacterial agent),
h. *E. coli, Proteus, A. aerogenes, K. pneumoniae,* and *Enterococcus faecalis* in urinary tract infections,
i. *Streptococcus* viridans, *Enterococcus faecalis* (in endocardial infections—concomitantly with penicillin),
j. Gram-negative bacillary bacteremia (concomitantly with another antibacterial agent).

CONTRAINDICATIONS

A history of clinically significant hypersensitivity to streptomycin is a contraindication to its use. Clinically significant hypersensitivity to other aminoglycosides may contraindicate the use of streptomycin because of the known cross-sensitivity of patients to drugs in this class.

WARNINGS

Ototoxicity: Both vestibular and auditory dysfunction can follow the administration of streptomycin. The degree of impairment is directly proportional to the dose and duration of streptomycin administration, to the age of the patient, to the level of renal function and to the amount of underlying existing auditory dysfunction. The ototoxic effects of the aminoglycosides, including streptomycin, are potentiated by the co-administration of ethacrynic acid, mannitol, furosemide and possibly other diuretics.

The vestibulotoxic potential of streptomycin exceeds that of its capacity for cochlear toxicity. Vestibular damage is heralded by headache, nausea, vomiting and disequilibrium. Early cochlear injury is demonstrated by the loss of high frequency hearing. Appropriate monitoring and early discontinuation of the drug may permit recovery prior to irreversible damage to the sensorineural cells.

Sulfites: Streptomycin contains sodium metabisulfite, a sulfite that may cause allergic type reactions including anaphylactic symptoms and life-threatening or less severe asthmatic episodes in certain susceptible people. The overall prevalence of sulfite sensitivity in the general population is unknown and probably low. Sulfite sensitivity is seen more frequently in asthmatic than in non-asthmatic people.

Pregnancy: Streptomycin can cause fetal harm when administered to a pregnant woman. Because streptomycin readily crosses the placental barrier, caution in use of the drug is important to prevent ototoxicity in the fetus. If this drug is used during pregnancy, or if the patient becomes pregnant while taking this drug, the patient should be apprised of the potential hazard to the fetus.

PRECAUTIONS

General: Baseline and periodic caloric stimulation tests and audiometric tests are advisable with extended streptomycin therapy. Tinnitus, roaring noises, or a sense of fullness in the ears indicates need for audiometric examination or termination of streptomycin therapy or both.

Care should be taken by individuals handling streptomycin for injection to avoid skin sensitivity reactions. As with all intramuscular preparations, Streptomycin Sulfate Injection should be injected well within the body of a relatively large muscle and care should be taken to minimize the possibility of damage to peripheral nerves. (See DOSAGE AND ADMINISTRATION.)

Extreme caution must be exercised in selecting a dosage regimen in the presence of pre-existing renal insuffiency. In severely uremic patients a single dose may produce high blood levels for several days and the cumulative effect may produce ototoxic sequelae. When streptomycin must be given for prolonged periods of time alkalinization of the urine may minimize or prevent renal irritation.

A syndrome of apparent central nervous system depression, characterized by stupor and flaccidity, occasionally coma and deep respiratory depression, has been reported in very young infants in whom streptomycin dosage had exceeded the recommended limits. Thus, infants should not receive streptomycin in excess of the recommended dosage.

In the treatment of venereal infections such as granuloma inguinale, and chancroid, if concomitant syphilis is suspected, suitable laboratory procedures such as a dark field examination should be performed before the start of treatment, and monthly serologic tests should be done for at least four months.

As with other antibiotics, use of this drug may result in overgrowth of nonsusceptible organisms, including fungi. If superinfection occurs, appropriate therapy should be instituted.

Drug Interactions: The ototoxic effects of the aminoglycosides, including streptomycin, are potentiated by the co-administration of ethacrynic acid, furosemide, mannitol and possibly other diuretics.

Pregnancy: Category D: See WARNINGS section.

Nursing Mothers: Because of the potential for serious adverse reactions in nursing infants from streptomycin, a decision should be made whether to discontinue nursing or to discontinue the drug, taking into account the importance of the drug to the mother.

Pediatric Use: (See DOSAGE AND ADMINISTRATION.)

ADVERSE REACTIONS

The following reactions are common: vestibular ototoxicity (nausea, vomiting, and vertigo); paresthesia of face; rash; fever; urticaria; angioneurotic edema; and eosinophilia.

The following reactions are less frequent: cochlear ototoxicity (deafness); exfoliative dermatitis; anaphylaxis; azotemia; leucopenia; thrombocytopenia, pancytopenia; hemolytic anemia; muscular weakness; and amblyopia.

Vestibular dysfunction resulting from the parenteral administration of streptomycin is cumulatively related to the total daily dose. When 1.8 to 2 g/day are given, symptoms are likely to develop in the large percentage of patients—especially in the elderly or patients with impaired renal function—within four weeks. Therefore, it is recommended that caloric and audiometric tests be done prior to, during, and following intensive therapy with streptomycin in order to facilitate detection of any vestibular dysfunction and/or impairment of hearing which may occur.

Vestibular symptoms generally appear early and usually are reversible with early detection and cessation of streptomycin administration. Two to three months after stopping the drug, gross vestibular symptoms usually disappear, except for the relative inability to walk in total darkness or on very rough terrain.

Although streptomycin is the least nephrotoxic of the aminoglycosides, nephrotoxicity does occur rarely.

Clinical judgment as to termination of therapy must be exercised when side effects occur.

DOSAGE AND ADMINISTRATION

Intramuscular Route Only

Adults: The preferred site is the upper outer quadrant of the buttock, (*i.e.,* gluteus maximus), or the mid-lateral thigh.

Children: It is recommended that intramuscular injections be given preferably in the mid-lateral muscles of the thigh. In infants and small children the periphery of the upper outer quadrant of the gluteal region should be used only when necessary, such as in burn patients, in order to minimize the possibility of damage to the sciatic nerve.

The deltoid area should be used only if well developed such as in certain adults and older children, and then only with caution to avoid radial nerve injury. Intramuscular injections should not be made into the lower and mid-third of the upper arm. As with all intramuscular injections, aspiration is necessary to help avoid inadvertent injection into a blood vessel.

Injection sites should be alternated. As higher doses or more prolonged therapy with streptomycin may be indicated for more severe or fulminating infections (endocarditis, meningitis, etc.), the physician should always take adequate measures to be immediately aware of any toxic signs or symptoms occurring in the patient as a result of streptomycin therapy.

1. TUBERCULOSIS: The standard regimen for the treatment of drug susceptible tuberculosis has been two months of INH, rifampin and pyrazinamide followed by four months of INH and rifampin (patients with concomitant infection with tuberculosis and HIV may require treatment for a longer period). When streptomycin is added to this regimen because of suspected or proven drug resistance (see **INDICATIONS AND USAGE** section), the recommended dosing for streptomycin is as follows:

	Daily	*Twice Weekly*	*Thrice Weekly*
Children	20–40 mg/kg	25–30 mg/kg	25–30 mg/kg
	Max 1 g	Max 1.5 g	Max 1.5 g
Adults	15 mg/kg	25–30 mg/kg	25–30 mg/kg
	Max 1 g	Max 1.5 g	Max 1.5 g

Streptomycin is usually administered daily as a single intramuscular injection. A total dose of not more than 120 g over the course of therapy should be given unless there are no other therapeutic options. In patients older than 60 years of age the drug should be used at a reduced dosage due to the risk of increased toxicity. (See **BOXED WARNING**).

Therapy with streptomycin may be terminated when toxic symptoms have appeared, when impending toxicity is feared, when organisms become resistant, or when full treatment effect has been obtained. The total period of drug treatment of tuberculosis is a minimum of 1 year; however, indications for terminating therapy with streptomycin may occur at any time as noted above.

2. TULAREMIA: One to 2 g daily in divided doses for 7 to 14 days until the patient is afebrile for 5 to 7 days.
3. PLAGUE: Two grams of streptomycin daily in two divided doses should be administered intramuscularly. A minimum of 10 days of therapy is recommended.
4. BACTERIAL ENDOCARDITIS:

a. *Streptococcal endocarditis:* In penicillin-sensitive alpha and non-hemolytic streptococcal endocarditis (penicillin MIC≤0.1 mcg/mL), streptomycin may be used for 2-week treatment concomitantly with penicillin. The streptomycin regimen is 1 g b.i.d. for the first week, and 500 mg b.i.d. for the second week. If the patient is over 60 years of age, the dosage should be 500 mg b.i.d. for the entire 2-week period.

b. *Enterococcal endocarditis:* Streptomycin in doses of 1 g b.i.d. for 2 weeks and 500 mg b.i.d. for an additional 4 weeks is given in combination with penicillin. Ototoxicity may require termination of the streptomycin prior to completion of the 6-week course of treatment.

5. CONCOMITANT USE WITH OTHER AGENTS: For concomitant use with other agents to which the infecting organism is also sensitive: Streptomycin is considered a second-line agent for the treatment of gram-negative bacillary bacteremia, meningitis, and pneumonia; brucellosis; granuloma inguinale; chancroid, and urinary tract infection.

For adults: 1 to 2 grams in divided doses every six to twelve hours for moderate to severe infections. Doses should generally not exceed 2 grams per day.

For children: 20 to 40 mg/kg/day (8 to 20 mg/lb/day) in divided doses every 6 to 12 hours. (Particular care should be taken to avoid excessive dosage in children.)

Parenteral drug products should be inspected visually for particulate matter and discoloration prior to administration, whenever solution and container permit.

HOW SUPPLIED

Streptomycin Sulfate Injection, USP is supplied in packages of 10 ampules (NDC 0049-0620-33). Each ampule contains streptomycin sulfate equivalent to 1 g of streptomycin in 2.5 mL.

Store under refrigeration at 36° to 46°F (2° to 8°C).

REFERENCES

[1] National Committee for Clinical Laboratory Standards. Performance Standards for Antimicrobial Disk Susceptibility Tests—Fourth Edition. Approved Standard NCCLS Document M2-A4. Vol. 10, No. 7. NCCLS, Villanova, PA 1990.

© 1992 PFIZER INC.

70-4895-00-0 Issued April 1993

TAO® ℞
[*tā ′ō*]
(troleandomycin)
Capsules

DESCRIPTION

TAO (troleandomycin) is a synthetically derived acetylated ester of oleandomycin, an antibiotic elaborated by a species of *Streptomyces antibioticus.* It is a white crystalline compound, insoluble in water, but readily soluble and stable in the presence of gastric juice. The compound has a molecular weight of 814 and corresponds to the empirical formula $C_{41}H_{67}NO_{15}$.

Inert ingredients in the formulation are: hard gelatin capsules (which may contain inert ingredients); lactose; magnesium stearate; sodium lauryl sulfate; starch.

ACTIONS

TAO is an antibiotic shown to be active *in vitro* against the following gram-positive organisms:

Streptococcus pyogenes
Diplococcus pneumoniae

Susceptibility plate testing: If the Kirby-Bauer method of disc sensitivity is used, a 15 mcg. oleandomycin disc should give a zone of over 18 mm when tested against a troleandomycin sensitive bacterial strain.

INDICATIONS

Diplococcus pneumoniae
Pneumococcal pneumonia due to susceptible strains.
Streptococcus pyogenes

Continued on next page

Tao Capsules—Cont.

Group A beta-hemolytic streptococcal infections of the upper respiratory tract.
Injectable benzathine penicillin G is considered by the American Heart Association to be the drug of choice in the treatment and prevention of streptococcal pharyngitis and in long term prophylaxis of rheumatic fever.
Troleandomycin is generally effective in the eradication of streptococci from the nasopharynx. However, substantial data establishing the efficacy of TAO in the subsequent prevention of rheumatic fever are not available at present.

CONTRAINDICATIONS

Troleandomycin is contraindicated in patients with known hypersensitivity to this antibiotic.

WARNINGS

Usage in Pregnancy: Safety for use in pregnancy has not been established.
The administration of troleandomycin has been associated with an allergic type of cholestatic hepatitis. Some patients receiving troleandomycin for more than two weeks or in repeated courses have shown jaundice accompanied by right upper quadrant pain, fever, nausea, vomiting, eosinophilia, and leukocytosis. These changes have been reversible on discontinuance of the drug. Liver function tests should be monitored in patients on such dosage, and the drug discontinued if abnormalities develop. Reports in the literature have suggested that the concurrent use of ergotamine-containing drugs and troleandomycin may induce ischemic reactions. Therefore, the concurrent use of ergotamine-containing drugs and troleandomycin should be avoided. Troleandomycin should be administered with caution to patients concurrently receiving estrogen containing oral contraceptives.
Studies in chronic asthmatic patients have suggested that the concurrent use of theophylline and troleandomycin may result in elevated serum concentrations of theophylline. Therefore, it is recommended that patients receiving such concurrent therapy be observed for signs of theophylline toxicity, and that therapy be appropriately modified if such signs develop.

PRECAUTIONS

Troleandomycin is principally excreted by the liver.
Caution should be exercised in administering the antibiotic to patients with impaired hepatic function.

ADVERSE REACTIONS

The most frequent side effects of troleandomycin preparations are gastrointestinal, such as abdominal cramping and discomfort, and are dose related. Nausea, vomiting, and diarrhea occur infrequently with usual oral doses.
During prolonged or repeated therapy, there is a possibility of overgrowth of nonsusceptible bacteria or fungi. If such infections occur, the drug should be discontinued and appropriate therapy instituted.
Mild allergic reactions such as urticaria and other skin rashes have occurred. Serious allergic reactions, including anaphylaxis, have been reported.

DOSAGE AND ADMINISTRATION

Clinical judgment based on the type of infection and its severity should determine dosage within the below listed ranges.
Adults: 250 to 500 mg 4 times a day
Children: 125 to 250 mg (3-5 mg/lb or 6.6 to 11 mg/kg) every 6 hours
When used in streptococcal infection, therapy should be continued for ten days.

HOW SUPPLIED

TAO is supplied as:
Capsules 250 mg: Each capsule contains troleandomycin equivalent to 250 mg of oleandomycin; bottles of 100 (NDC 0049-1590-66).
Revised July 1995 69-1800-00-8

TERRA-CORTRIL® ℞

Terramycin® (oxytetracycline HCl)
—Cortril® (hydrocortisone acetate)
OPHTHALMIC SUSPENSION

DESCRIPTION

Terra-Cortril suspension combines the antibiotic, oxytetracycline HCl ($C_{22}H_{24}N_2O_9{\cdot}HCl$) and the adrenocorticoid, hydrocortisone acetate ($C_{23}H_{32}O_6$). **Each ml of Terra-Cortril contains Terramycin (oxytetracycline HCl) equivalent to 5 mg of oxytetracycline, and 15 mg of Cortril (hydrocortisone acetate) incorporated in mineral oil with aluminum tristearate.**

For Ophthalmic Use Only.

CLINICAL PHARMACOLOGY

Corticosteroids suppress the inflammatory response to a variety of agents and they probably delay or slow healing. Since corticoids may inhibit the body's defense mechanism against infection, a concomitant antimicrobial drug may be used when this inhibition is considered to be clinically significant in a particular case.
The anti-infective component in the combination is included to provide action against specific organisms susceptible to it.
Terramycin is considered active against the following microorganisms:
Rickettsiae (Rocky Mountain spotted fever, typhus fever and the typhus group, Q fever, rickettsialpox and tick fevers),
Mycoplasma pneumoniae (PPLO, Eaton Agent),
Agents of psittacosis and ornithosis,
Agents of lymphogranuloma venereum and granuloma inguinale,
The spirochetal agent of relapsing fever (*Borrelia recurrentis*).
The following gram-negative microorganisms:
Haemophilus ducreyi (chancroid),
Pasteurella pestis and *Pasteurella tularensis,*
Bartonella bacilliformis,
Bacteroides species,
Vibrio comma and *Vibrio fetus,*
Brucella species (in conjunction with streptomycin).
Because many strains of the following groups of microorganisms have been shown to be resistant to tetracyclines, culture and susceptibility testing are recommended.
Oxytetracycline is indicated for treatment of infections caused by the following gram-negative microorganisms, when bacteriologic testing indicates appropriate susceptibility to the drug:
Escherichia coli,
Enterobacter aerogenes (formerly *Aerobacter aerogenes*),
Shigella species,
Mima species and *Herellea* species,
Haemophilus influenzae (respiratory infections),
Klebsiella species (respiratory and urinary infections).
Oxytetracycline is indicated for treatment of infections caused by the following gram-positive microorganisms when bacteriologic testing indicates appropriate susceptibility to the drug:
Streptococcus species:
Up to 44 percent of strains of *Streptococcus pyogenes* and 74 percent of *Streptococcus faecalis* have been found to be resistant to tetracycline drugs. Therefore, tetracyclines should not be used for streptococcal disease unless the organism has been demonstrated to be sensitive.
For upper respiratory infections due to Group A beta-hemolytic streptococci, pencillin is the usual drug of choice, including prophylaxis of rheumatic fever.
Diplococcus pneumoniae,
Staphylococcus aureus, skin and soft tissue infections. Oxytetracycline is not the drug of choice in the treatment of any type of staphylococcal infections.
When penicillin is contraindicated, tetracyclines are alternative drugs in the treatment of infections due to:
Neisseria gonorrhoeae,
Treponema pallidum and *Treponema pertenue* (syphilis and yaws),
Listeria monocytogenes,
Clostridium species,
Bacillus anthracis,
Fusobacterium fusiforme (Vincent's infection),
Actinomyces species.
Tetracyclines are indicated in the treatment of trachoma, although the infectious agent is not always eliminated, as judged by immunofluorescence.
Inclusion conjunctivitis may be treated with oral tetracyclines or with a combination of oral and topical agents.
When a decision to administer both a corticoid and an antimicrobial is made, the administration of such drugs in combination has the advantage of greater patient compliance and convenience, with the added assurance that the appropriate dosage of both drugs is administered, plus assured compatibility of ingredients when both types of drug are in the same formulation and, particularly, that the correct volume of drug is delivered and retained.
The relative potency of corticosteroids depends on the molecular structure, concentration, and release from the vehicle.

INDICATIONS AND USAGE

For steroid-responsive inflammatory ocular conditions for which a corticosteroid is indicated and where bacterial infection or risk of bacterial ocular infection exists.
Ocular steroids are indicated in inflammatory conditions of the palpebral and bulbar conjunctiva, cornea, and anterior segment of the globe where the inherent risk of steroid use in certain infective conjunctivitides is accepted to obtain a diminution in edema and inflammation. They are also indicated in chronic anterior uveitis and corneal injury from chemical radiation, thermal burns, or penetration of foreign bodies.
The use of a combination drug with an anti-infective component is indicated where the risk of infection is high or where there is an expectation that potentially dangerous numbers of bacteria will be present in the eye.
The particular anti-infective drug in this product is active against the following common bacterial eye pathogens:
Staphylococcus aureus
Streptococci, including *Streptococcus pneumoniae*
Escherichia coli
Neisseria species
The product does not provide adequate coverage against:
Haemophilus influenzae
Klebsiella/Enterobacter species
Pseudomonas aeruginosa
Serratia marcescens

CONTRAINDICATIONS

Epithelial herpes simplex keratitis (dendritic keratitis), vaccinia, varicella, and many other viral diseases of the cornea and conjunctiva. Mycobacterial infection of the eye. Fungal diseases of ocular structures. Hypersensitivity to a component of the medication. (Hypersensitivity to the antibiotic component occurs at a higher rate than for other components.)
The use of these combinations is always contraindicated after uncomplicated removal of a corneal foreign body.

WARNINGS

Prolonged use may result in glaucoma, with damage to the optic nerve, defects in visual acuity and fields of vision, and posterior subcapsular cataract formation. Prolonged use may suppress the host response and thus increase the hazard of secondary ocular infections. In those diseases causing thinning of the cornea or sclera, perforations have been known to occur with the use of topical steroids. In acute purulent conditions of the eye, steroids may mask infection or enhance existing infection. If these products are used for 10 days or longer, intraocular pressure should be routinely monitored even though it may be difficult in children and uncooperative patients.
Employment of steroid medication in the treatment of herpes simplex requires great caution.

PRECAUTIONS

The initial prescription and renewal of the medication order beyond 20 milliliters should be made by a physician only after examination of the patient with the aid of magnification, such as slit lamp biomicroscopy and, where appropriate, fluorescein staining.
The possibility of persistent fungal infections of the cornea should be considered after prolonged steroid dosing.

ADVERSE REACTIONS

Adverse reactions have occurred with steroid/anti-infective combination drugs which can be attributed to the steroid component, the anti-infective component, or the combination. Exact incidence figures are not available since no denominator of treated patients is available.
Reactions occurring most often from the presence of the anti-infective ingredient are allergic sensitizations. The reactions due to the steroid component in decreasing order of frequency are: elevation of intraocular pressure (IOP) with possible development of glaucoma, and infrequent optic nerve damage; posterior subcapsular cataract formation; and delayed wound healing.
Secondary Infection: The development of secondary infection has occurred after use of combinations containing steroids and antimicrobials. Fungal infections of the cornea are particularly prone to develop coincidentally with long-term applications of steroid. The possibility of fungal invasion must be considered in any persistent corneal ulceration where steroid treatment has been used.
Secondary bacterial ocular infection following suppression of host responses also occurs.

DOSAGE AND ADMINISTRATION

Instill 1 or 2 drops of Terra-Cortril Ophthalmic Suspension into the affected eye three times daily.
Not more than 20 milliliters should be prescribed initially and the prescription should not be refilled without further evaluation as outlined in "Precautions" above.

HOW SUPPLIED

Terra-Cortril Ophthalmic Suspension (NDC 0049-0670-48) is supplied in 5 ml vials with separate sterile dropper.
Revised August 1987 60-2323-00-3

TERRAMYCIN® ℞

(oxytetracycline)
INTRAMUSCULAR SOLUTION*
FOR INTRAMUSCULAR USE ONLY
contains 2% lidocaine

DESCRIPTION

Oxytetracycline is a product of the metabolism of *Streptomyces rimosus* and is one of the family of tetracycline antibiotics.

Terramycin Intramuscular
contents per ml (m/v)

Ingredient	2 ml Single Dose Ampules		10 ml Vial Multidose
	100 mg/2 ml	250 mg/2 ml	50 mg/ml 10 ml (5 × 2 ml Doses)
oxytetracycline	50 mg	125 mg	50 mg
lidocaine	2.0%	2.0%	2.0%
magnesium chloride hexahydrate	2.5%	6.0%	2.5%
sodium formaldehyde sulfoxylate	0.5%	0.5%	0.3%
α-monothioglycerol			1.0%
monoethanolamine	approx. 1.7%	approx. 4.2%	approx. 2.6%
citric acid			1.0%
propyl gallate			0.02%
propylene glycol	75.2%	67.0%	74.1%
water	18.8%	16.8%	18.5%

Oxytetracycline diffuses readily through the placenta into the fetal circulation, into the pleural fluid and, under some circumstances, into the cerebrospinal fluid. It appears to be concentrated in the hepatic system and excreted in the bile, so that it appears in the feces, as well as in the urine, in a biologically active form.

COMPOSITION

[See table above]

ACTIONS

Oxytetracycline is primarily bacteriostatic and is thought to exert its antimicrobial effect by the inhibition of protein synthesis. Oxytetracycline is active against a wide range of gram-negative and gram-positive organisms.

The drugs in the tetracycline class have closely similar antimicrobial spectra, and cross resistance among them is common. Microorganisms may be considered susceptible if the M.I.C. (minimum inhibitory concentration) is not more than 4.0 mcg/ml and intermediate if the M.I.C. is 4.0 to 12.5 mcg/ml.

Susceptibility plate testing: A tetracycline disc may be used to determine microbial susceptibility to drugs in the tetracycline class. If the Kirby-Bauer method of disc susceptibility testing is used, a 30 mcg tetracycline disc should give a zone of at least 19 mm when tested against an oxytetracycline-susceptible bacterial strain.

Tetracyclines are readily absorbed and are bound to plasma proteins in varying degree. They are concentrated by the liver in the bile, and excreted in the urine and feces at high concentrations and in a biologically active form.

INDICATIONS

Oxytetracycline is indicated in infections caused by the following microorganisms:

Rickettsiae (Rocky Mountain spotted fever, typhus fever and the typhus group, Q fever, rickettsialpox and tick fevers),

Mycoplasma pneumoniae (PPLO, Eaton Agent),

Agents of psittacosis and ornithosis,

Agents of lymphogranuloma venereum and granuloma inguinale,

The spirochetal agent of relapsing fever *(Borrelia recurrentis).*

The following gram-negative microorganisms:

Haemophilus ducreyi (chancroid),

Pasteurella pestis, and *Pasteurella tularensis,*

Bartonella bacilliformis,

Bacteroides species,

Vibrio comma and *Vibrio fetus,*

Brucella species (in conjunction with streptomycin).

Because many strains of the following groups of microorganisms have been shown to be resistant to tetracyclines, culture and susceptibility testing are recommended.

Oxytetracycline is indicated for treatment of infections caused by the following gram-negative microorganisms, when bacteriologic testing indicates appropriate susceptibility to the drug:

Escherichia coli,

Enterobacter aerogenes (formerly *Aerobacter aerogenes*),

Shigella species,

Mima species and *Herellea* species,

Haemophilus influenzae (respiratory infections),

Klebsiella species (respiratory and urinary infections).

Oxytetracycline is indicated for treatment of infections caused by the following gram-positive microorganisms when bacteriologic testing indicates appropriate susceptibility to the drug:

Streptococcus species:

Up to 44 percent of strains of *Streptococcus pyogenes* and 74 percent of *Streptococcus faecalis* have been found to be resistant to tetracycline drugs. Therefore, tetracyclines should not be used for streptococcal disease unless the organism has been demonstrated to be sensitive.

For upper respiratory infections due to Group A beta-hemolytic streptococci, penicillin is the usual drug of choice, including prophylaxis of rheumatic fever.

Diplococcus pneumoniae,

Staphylococcus aureus, skin and soft tissue infections. Oxytetracycline is not the drug of choice in the treatment of any type of staphylococcal infections.

When penicillin is contraindicated, tetracyclines are alternative drugs in the treatment of infections due to:

Neisseria gonorrhoeae,

Treponema pallidum and *Treponema pertenue* (syphilis and yaws),

Listeria monocytogenes,

Clostridium species,

Bacillus anthracis,

Fusobacterium fusiforme (Vincent's infection),

Actinomyces species.

In acute intestinal amebiasis, the tetracyclines may be a useful adjunct to amebicides.

Tetracyclines are indicated in the treatment of trachoma, although the infectious agent is not always eliminated, as judged by immunofluorescence.

Inclusion conjunctivitis may be treated with oral tetracyclines or with a combination of oral and topical agents.

CONTRAINDICATIONS

This drug is contraindicated in persons who have shown hypersensitivity to any of the tetracyclines.

WARNINGS

THE USE OF TETRACYCLINES DURING TOOTH DEVELOPMENT (LAST HALF OF PREGNANCY, INFANCY, AND CHILDHOOD TO THE AGE OF 8 YEARS) MAY CAUSE PERMANENT DISCOLORATION OF THE TEETH (YELLOW-GRAY-BROWN). This adverse reaction is more common during long term use of the drugs but has been observed following repeated short term courses. Enamel hypoplasia has also been reported. *TETRACYCLINES, THEREFORE, SHOULD NOT BE USED IN THIS AGE GROUP UNLESS OTHER DRUGS ARE NOT LIKELY TO BE EFFECTIVE OR ARE CONTRAINDICATED.*

If renal impairment exists, even usual oral or parenteral doses may lead to excessive systemic accumulation of the drug and possible liver toxicity. Under such conditions, lower than usual total doses are indicated and, if therapy is prolonged, serum level determinations of the drug may be advisable. This hazard is of particular importance in the parenteral administration of tetracyclines to pregnant or postpartum patients with pyelonephritis. When used under these circumstances, the blood level should not exceed 15 mcg/ml and liver function tests should be made at frequent intervals. Other potentially hepatotoxic drugs should not be prescribed concomitantly.

(In the presence of renal dysfunction, particularly in pregnancy, intravenous tetracycline therapy in daily doses exceeding 2 grams has been associated with deaths due to liver failure.)

Photosensitivity manifested by an exaggerated sunburn reaction has been observed in some individuals taking tetracyclines. Patients apt to be exposed to direct sunlight or ultraviolet light should be advised that this reaction can occur with tetracycline drugs, and treatment should be discontinued at the first evidence of skin erythema.

The antianabolic action of the tetracyclines may cause an increase in BUN. While this is not a problem in those with normal renal function, in patients with significantly impaired function, higher serum levels of this drug may lead to azotemia, hyperphosphatemia, and acidosis.

The product contains sodium formaldehyde sulfoxylate which serves as an antioxidant. Upon oxidation, this compound can form a potential sulfiting agent. Sulfiting agents may cause allergic-type reactions including anaphylactic symptoms and life-threatening or less severe asthmatic epi-

sodes in certain susceptible people. The over-all prevalence of sulfite sensitivity in the general population is unknown and probably low. Sulfite sensitivity is seen more frequently in asthmatic than in nonasthmatic people.

Usage in pregnancy. (See above "Warnings" about use during tooth development.)

Results of animal studies indicate that tetracyclines cross the placenta, are found in fetal tissues and can have toxic effects on the developing fetus (often related to retardation of skeletal development). Evidence of embryotoxicity has also been noted in animals treated early in pregnancy.

Usage in newborns, infants, and children. (See above "Warnings" about use during tooth development).

All tetracyclines form a stable calcium complex in any bone-forming tissue. A decrease in the fibula growth rate has been observed in prematures given oral tetracycline in doses of 25 mg/kg every 6 hours. This reaction was shown to be reversible when the drug was discontinued.

Tetracyclines are present in the milk of lactating women who are taking a drug in this class.

PRECAUTIONS

As with all intramuscular preparations, Terramycin (oxytetracycline) Intramuscular Solution should be injected well within the body of a relatively large muscle. ADULTS: The preferred sites are the upper outer quadrant of the buttock, (i.e., gluteus maximus), and the mid-lateral thigh. CHILDREN: It is recommended that intramuscular injections be given preferably in the mid-lateral muscles of the thigh. In infants and small children the periphery of the upper outer quadrant of the gluteal region should be used only when necessary, such as in burn patients, in order to minimize the possibility of damage to the sciatic nerve.

The deltoid area should be used only if well developed such as in certain adults and older children, and then only with caution to avoid radial nerve injury. Intramuscular injections should not be made into the lower and mid-thirds of the upper arm. As with all intramuscular injections, aspiration is necessary to help avoid inadvertent injection into a blood vessel.

As with other antibiotic preparations, use of this drug may result in overgrowth of nonsusceptible organisms, including fungi. If superinfection occurs, the antibiotic should be discontinued and appropriate therapy instituted.

In venereal diseases when coexistent syphilis is suspected, a dark field examination should be done before treatment is started and the blood serology repeated monthly for at least 4 months.

Because tetracyclines have been shown to depress plasma prothrombin activity, patients who are on anticoagulant therapy may require downward adjustment of their anticoagulant dosage.

In long term therapy, periodic laboratory evaluation of organ systems, including hematopoietic, renal and hepatic studies should be performed.

All infections due to Group A beta-hemolytic streptococci should be treated for at least 10 days.

Since bacteriostatic drugs may interfere with the bactericidal action of penicillin, it is advisable to avoid giving tetracycline in conjunction with penicillin.

ADVERSE REACTIONS

Local irritation may be present after intramuscular injection. The injection should be deep, with care taken not to injure the sciatic nerve nor inject intravascularly.

Gastrointestinal: anorexia, nausea, vomiting, diarrhea, glossitis, dysphagia, enterocolitis, and inflammatory lesions (with monilial overgrowth) in the anogenital region. These reactions have been caused by both the oral and parenteral administration of tetracyclines.

Skin: maculopapular and erythematous rashes. Exfoliative dermatitis has been reported but is uncommon. Photosensitivity is discussed above. (See "Warnings").

Renal toxicity: Rise in BUN has been reported and is apparently dose related. (See "Warnings").

Hypersensitivity reactions: Urticaria, angioneurotic edema, anaphylaxis, anaphylactoid purpura, pericarditis, and exacerbation of systemic lupus erythematosus.

Bulging fontanels in infants and benign intracranial hypertension in adults have been reported in individuals receiving full therapeutic dosages. These conditions disappeared rapidly when the drug was discontinued.

Blood: Hemolytic anemia, thrombocytopenia, neutropenia, and eosinophilia have been reported.

When given over prolonged periods, tetracyclines have been reported to produce brown-black microscopic discoloration of thyroid glands. No abnormalities of thyroid function studies are known to occur.

DOSAGE AND ADMINISTRATION

Intramuscular Administration:

Adults: The usual daily dose is 250 mg administered once every 24 hours or 300 mg given in divided doses at 8 to 12 hour intervals.

For children above eight years of age: 15–25 mg/kg of body weight up to a maximum of 250 mg per single daily injection. Dosage may be divided and given at 8 to 12 hour intervals.

Continued on next page

Terramycin Solution—Cont.

Intramuscular therapy should be reserved for situations in which oral therapy is not feasible.

The intramuscular administration of oxytetracycline produces lower blood levels than oral administration in the recommended dosages. Patients placed on intramuscular oxytetracycline should be changed to the oral dosage form as soon as possible. If rapid, high blood levels are needed, oxytetracycline should be administered intravenously.

In patients with renal impairment: (See "Warnings") Total dosage should be decreased by reduction of recommended individual doses and/or by extending time intervals between doses.

HOW SUPPLIED

Terramycin (oxytetracycline) Intramuscular Solution is available as follows:

250 mg/2ml—in 2 ml pre-scored glass ampules, packages of 5 (NDC 0049-0770-09).

100 mg/2ml—in 2 ml pre-scored glass ampules, packages of 5 (NDC 0049-0760-09).

50 mg/ml—in 10 ml multiple dose vials, packages of 5 (NDC 0049-0750-77).

*U.S. Pat. Nos. 3,017,323 and 3,026,248
Revised March 1987   70-1051-00-2

TERRAMYCIN®
(oxytetracycline HCl with polymyxin B sulfate)
OPHTHALMIC OINTMENT
STERILE

DESCRIPTION

Each gram of sterile ointment contains oxytetracycline HCl equivalent to 5 mg oxytetracycline, 10,000 units of polymyxin B sulfate, white petrolatum, and liquid petrolatum.

ACTIONS

Terramycin® is a widely used antibiotic with clinically proved activity against gram-positive and gram-negative bacteria, rickettsiae, spirochetes, large viruses, and certain protozoa.

Polymyxin B Sulfate, one of a group of related antibiotics derived from *Bacillus polymyxa*, is rapidly bactericidal. This action is exclusively against gram-negative organisms. It is particularly effective against *Pseudomonas aeruginosa (B. pyocyaneus)* and Koch-Weeks bacillus, frequently found in local infections of the eye.

There is thus made available a particularly effective antimicrobial combination of the broad-spectrum antibiotic Terramycin as well as polymyxin B sulfate against primarily causative or secondarily infecting organisms.

INDICATIONS

The sterile preparation, Terramycin with Polymyxin B Sulfate Ophthalmic Ointment, is indicated for the treatment of superficial ocular infections involving the conjunctiva and/or cornea caused by Terramycin with Polymyxin B Sulfate-susceptible organisms.

It may be administered topically alone, or as an adjunct to systemic therapy.

It is effective in infections caused by susceptible strains of staphylococci, streptococci, pneumococci, *Hemophilus influenzae, Pseudomonas aeruginosa,* Koch-Weeks bacillus, and *Proteus.*

CONTRAINDICATIONS

This drug is contraindicated in individuals who have shown hypersensitivity to any of its components.

PRECAUTIONS

As with all antibiotic preparations, use of this drug may result in overgrowth of nonsusceptible organisms, including fungi. If superinfection occurs, the antibiotic should be discontinued and appropriate specific therapy should be instituted.

ADVERSE REACTIONS

Terramycin with Polymyxin B Sulfate Ophthalmic Ointment is well tolerated by the epithelial membranes and other tissues of the eye. Allergic or inflammatory reactions due to individual hypersensitivity are rare.

DOSAGE AND ADMINISTRATION

Approximately $\frac{1}{2}$ inch of the ointment is squeezed from the tube onto the lower lid of the affected eye two to four times daily.

The patient should be instructed to avoid contamination of the tip of the tube when applying the ointment.

HOW SUPPLIED

Terramycin with Polymyxin B Sulfate Ophthalmic Ointment is supplied in $\frac{1}{8}$ oz (3.5 g) tubes (NDC 0049-0801-08).

August 1987   60-2324-00-1

TROVAN™ Tablets   ℞
[trō-văn]
(trovafloxacin mesylate)

TROVAN™ I.V.   ℞
(alatrofloxacin mesylate injection)
For Intravenous Infusion

TROVAN™ is available as TROVAN Tablets (trovafloxacin mesylate) for oral administration and as TROVAN I.V. (alatrofloxacin mesylate injection), a prodrug of trovafloxacin, for intravenous administration.

DESCRIPTION

TROVAN Tablets

TROVAN Tablets contain trovafloxacin mesylate, a synthetic broad-spectrum antibacterial agent for oral administration. Chemically, trovafloxacin mesylate, a fluoronaphthyridone related to the fluoroquinolone antibacterials, is (1α, 5α, 6α)-7-(6-amino-3-azabicyclo[3.1.0]hex-3-yl)-1-(2,4-difluorophenyl)-6-fluoro-1,4-dihydro-4-oxo-1,8- naphthyridine-3-carboxylic acid, monomethanesulfonate. Trovafloxacin mesylate differs from other quinolone derivatives by having a 1,8-naphthyridine nucleus.

The chemical structure is:

Its empirical formula is $C_{20}H_{15}F_3N_4O_3 \bullet CH_3SO_3H$ and its molecular weight is 512.46.

Trovafloxacin mesylate is a white to off-white powder. Trovafloxacin mesylate is available in 100 mg and 200 mg (trovafloxacin equivalent) blue, film-coated tablets. TROVAN Tablets contain microcrystalline cellulose, crosslinked sodium carboxymethylcellulose and magnesium stearate. The tablet coating is a mixture of hydroxypropylcellulose, hydroxypropylmethylcellulose, titanium dioxide, polyethylene glycol and FD&C blue #2 aluminum lake.

TROVAN I.V.

TROVAN I.V. contains alatrofloxacin mesylate, the L-alanyl-L-alanyl prodrug of trovafloxacin mesylate. Chemically, alatrofloxacin mesylate is (1α, 5α, 6α)-L-alanyl-N-[3-[6-carboxy-8-(2,4-difluorophenyl)-3-fluoro-5,8-dihydro-5-oxo-1,8-naphthyridin-2-yl]-3-azabicyclo[3.1.0]hex-6-yl]-L-alaninamide, monomethanesulfonate. It is intended for administration by intravenous infusion.

Following intravenous administration, the alanine substituents in alatrofloxacin are rapidly hydrolyzed *in vivo* to yield trovafloxacin. (See **CLINICAL PHARMACOLOGY**.)

The chemical structure is:

Its empirical formula is $C_{26}H_{25}F_3N_6O_5 \bullet CH_3SO_3H$ and its molecular weight is 654.62.

Alatrofloxacin mesylate is a white to light yellow powder. TROVAN I.V. is available in 40 mL and 60 mL single use vials as a sterile, preservative-free aqueous concentrate of 5 mg trovafloxacin/mL as alatrofloxacin mesylate intended for dilution prior to intravenous administration of doses of 200 mg or 300 mg of trovafloxacin, respectively. (See **HOW SUPPLIED**.)

The formulation contains Water for Injection, and may contain sodium hydroxide or hydrochloric acid for pH adjustment. The pH range for the 5 mg/mL aqueous concentrate is 3.5 to 4.3.

CLINICAL PHARMACOLOGY

After intravenous administration, alatrofloxacin is rapidly converted to trovafloxacin. Plasma concentrations of alatrofloxacin are below quantifiable levels within 5 to 10 minutes of completion of a one hour infusion.

Absorption

Trovafloxacin is well-absorbed from the gastrointestinal tract after oral administration. The absolute bioavailability is approximately 88%. For comparable dosages, no dosage adjustment is necessary when switching from parenteral to oral administration (Figure 1). (See **DOSAGE AND ADMINISTRATION**.)

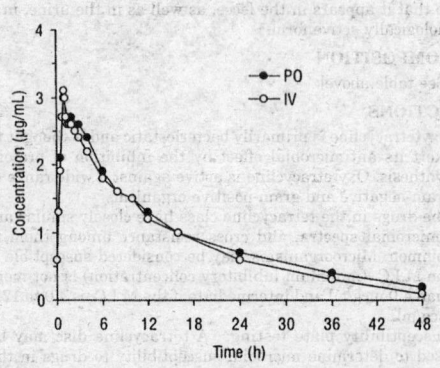

Figure 1. Mean trovafloxacin serum concentrations determined following 1 hour intravenous infusions of alatrofloxacin at daily doses of 200 mg (trovafloxacin equivalents) to healthy male volunteers and following daily oral administration of 200 mg trovafloxacin for seven days to six male and six female healthy young volunteers.

Pharmacokinetics

The mean pharmacokinetic parameters (±SD) of trovafloxacin after single and multiple 100 mg and 200 mg oral doses and one hour intravenous infusions of alatrofloxacin in doses of 200 and 300 mg (trovafloxacin equivalents) appear in the chart below.

[See table below]

Serum concentrations of trovafloxacin are dose-proportional after oral administration of trovafloxacin in the dose range of 30 to 1000 mg or after intravenous administration of alatrofloxacin in the dose range of 30 to 400 mg (trovafloxacin equivalents). Steady state concentrations are achieved by the third daily oral or intravenous dose of trovafloxacin with an accumulation factor of approximately 1.3 times the single dose concentrations.

Oral absorption of trovafloxacin is not altered by concomitant food intake; therefore, it can be administered without regard to food.

The systemic exposure to trovafloxacin ($AUC_{0-\infty}$) administered as crushed tablets via nasogastric tube into the stom-

---

TROVAFLOXACIN PHARMACOKINETIC PARAMETERS

	C_{max} (µg/mL)	T_{max} (hrs)	$AUC^{1,2}$ (µg·h/mL)	$T_{1/2}$ (hrs)	Vd_{ss} (L/Kg)	CL (mL/hr/Kg)	CL_r (mL/hr/Kg)
Trovafloxacin 100 mg							
Single dose	1.0±0.3	0.9±0.4	11.2±2.2	9.1	—	—	—
Multiple dose	1.1±0.2	1.0±0.5	11.8±1.8	10.5	—	—	—
Trovafloxacin 200 mg							
Single dose	2.1±0.5	1.8±0.9	26.7±7.5	9.6	—	—	—
Multiple dose	3.1±1.0	1.2±0.5	34.4±5.7	12.2	—	—	—
Alatrofloxacin 200 mg*							
Single dose	2.7±0.4	1.0±0.0	28.1±5.1	9.4	1.2±0.2	93.0±17.4	6.5±3.5
Multiple dose	3.1±0.6	1.0±0.0	32.2±7.3	11.7	1.3±0.1	81.7±17.8	8.6±2.4
Alatrofloxacin 300 mg*							
Single dose	3.6±0.6	1.3±0.4	46.1±5.2	11.2	1.2±0.1	84.6±6.0	6.9±0.5
Multiple dose	4.4±0.6	1.2±0.2	46.3±3.9	12.7	1.4±0.1	84.5±11.1	8.4±1.8

* trovafloxacin equivalents
[1,2] Single dose: AUC(−∞), multiple dose: AUC(0–24)
C_{max}= Maximum serum concentration; T_{max}=Time to C_{max}; AUC=Area under the concentration vs. time curve;
$T_{1/2}$=serum half-life; Vd_{ss}=Volume of distribution; Cl=Total clearance; Cl_r=Renal clearance

Fluid or Tissue	Tissue-Fluid/Serum Ratio* (Range)
Respiratory	
bronchial macrophages	
(multiple dose)	24.1 (9.6–41.8)
lung mucosa	1.1 (0.7–1.5)
lung epithelial lining fluid	
(multiple dose)	5.8 (1.1–17.5)
whole lung	2.1 (0.42–5.03)
Skin, Musculoskeletal	
skin	1.0 (0.20–1.88)
subcutaneous tissue	0.4 (0.15–0.68)
skin blister fluid	0.7–0.9 (blister/plasma)
skeletal muscle	1.5 (0.50–2.90)
bone	1.0 (0.55–1.67)
Gastrointestinal	
colonic tissue	0.7 (0.0–1.47)
peritoneal fluid	0.4 (0.0–1.25)
bile	15.4 (11.9–21.0)
Central Nervous System	
cerebrospinal fluid (CSF), adults	0.25 (0.03–0.33)
cerebrospinal fluid (CSF), children	0.28**
Reproductive	
prostatic tissue	1.0 (0.5–1.6)
cervix (multiple dose)	0.6 (0.5–0.7)
ovary	1.6 (0.3–2.2)
fallopian tube	0.7 (0.2–1.1)
myometrium (multiple dose)	0.6 (0.4–0.8)
uterus	0.6 (0.3–0.8)
vaginal fluid (multiple dose)	4.7 (0.8–20.8)

* Mean values in adults over 2–29 hours following drug administration, except individual lung tissues, which were single time points of 6 hours following drug administration
** Ratio of composite AUC(0–24) in CSF/composite AUC(0–24) in serum in 22 pediatric patients aged 1 to 12 years after 1 hour I.V. infusion in single dose alatrofloxacin (equivalent trovafloxacin dose range: 4.5–9.9 mg/kg)

ach was identical to that of orally administered intact tablets. Administration of concurrent enteral feeding solutions had no effect on the absorption of trovafloxacin given via nasogastric tube into the stomach. When trovafloxacin was administered as crushed tablets into the duodenum via nasogastric tube, the $AUC_{0-\infty}$ and peak serum concentration (C_{max}) were reduced by 30% relative to the orally administered intact tablets. Time to peak serum level (T_{max}) was also decreased from 1.7 hrs to 1.1 hrs.

Distribution
The mean plasma protein bound fraction is approximately 76%, and is concentration-independent. Trovafloxacin is widely distributed throughout the body. Rapid distribution of trovafloxacin into tissues results in significantly higher trovafloxacin concentrations in most target tissues than in plasma or serum.
[See table above]

Presence in Breast Milk
Trovafloxacin was found in measurable concentrations in the breast milk of three lactating subjects. The average measurable breast milk concentration was 0.8 µg/mL (range: 0.3–2.1 µg/mL) after single I.V. alatrofloxacin (300 mg trovafloxacin equivalents) and repeated oral trovafloxacin (200 mg) doses.

Metabolism
Trovafloxacin is metabolized by conjugation (the role of cytochrome P450 oxidative metabolism of trovafloxacin is minimal). Thirteen percent of the administered dose appears in the urine in the form of the ester glucuronide and 9% appears in the feces as the N-acetyl metabolite (2.5% of the dose is found in the serum as the active N-acetyl metabolite). Other minor metabolites (diacid, sulfamate, hydroxy-carboxylic acid) have been identified in both urine and feces in small amounts (<4% of the administered dose).

Excretion
Approximately 50% of an oral dose is excreted unchanged (43% in the feces and 6% in the urine).
After multiple 200 mg doses, to healthy subjects, mean (±SD) cumulative urinary trovafloxacin concentrations were 12.1±3.4 µg/mL. With these levels of trovafloxacin in urine, crystals of trovafloxacin have not been observed in the urine of human subjects.

Special Populations
Geriatric
In adult subjects, the pharmacokinetics of trovafloxacin are not affected by age (range 19–78 years).
Pediatric
Limited information is available in the pediatric population (see **Distribution**). The pharmacokinetics of trovafloxacin have not been fully characterized in pediatric populations less than 18 years of age.
Gender
There are no significant differences in trovafloxacin pharmacokinetics between males and females when differences in body weight are taken into account. After single 200 mg doses, trovafloxacin Cmax and AUC(0–∞) were 60% and 32% higher, respectively, in healthy females compared to healthy males. Following repeated daily administration of 200 mg for 7 days, the Cmax for trovafloxacin was 38% higher and AUC(0–24) was 16% higher in healthy females compared to healthy males. The clinical importance of the increases in serum levels of trovafloxacin in females has not been established. (See **PRECAUTIONS: Information for Patients.**)
Chronic Hepatic Disease
Following repeated administration of 100 mg for 7 days to patients with mild cirrhosis (Child-Pugh Class A), the AUC(0–24) for trovafloxacin was increased ~45% compared

to matched controls. Repeated administration of 200 mg for 7 days to patients with moderate cirrhosis (Child-Pugh Class B) resulted in an increase of ~50% in AUC(0–24) compared to matched controls. There appeared to be no significant effect on trovafloxacin Cmax for either group. The oral clearance of trovafloxacin was reduced ~30% in both cirrhosis groups, which corresponded to prolongation of half-life by 2–2.5 hours (25–30% increase) compared to controls. There are no data in patients with severe cirrhosis (Child-Pugh Class C). Dosage adjustment is recommended in patients with mild to moderate cirrhosis. (See **DOSAGE AND ADMINISTRATION**.)
Renal Insufficiency
The pharmacokinetics of trovafloxacin are not affected by renal impairment. Trovafloxacin serum concentrations are not significantly altered in subjects with severe renal insufficiency (creatinine clearance < 20 mL/min), including patients on hemodialysis.
Photosensitivity Potential
In a study of the skin response to ultraviolet and visible radiation conducted in 48 healthy volunteers (12 per group), the minimum erythematous dose (MED) was measured for ciprofloxacin, lomefloxacin, trovafloxacin and placebo before and after drug administration for 5 days. In this study, trovafloxacin (200 mg q.d.) was shown to have a lower potential for producing delayed photosensitivity skin reactions than ciprofloxacin (500 mg b.i.d.) or lomefloxacin (400 mg q.d.), although greater than placebo. (See **PRECAUTIONS: Information for Patients**.)
Drug-drug Interactions
The systemic availability of trovafloxacin following oral tablet administration is significantly reduced by the concomitant administration of antacids containing aluminum and magnesium salts, sucralfate, vitamins or minerals containing iron, and concomitant intravenous morphine administration.
Administration of trovafloxacin (300 mg p.o.) 30 minutes after administration of an antacid containing magnesium hydroxide and aluminum hydroxide resulted in reductions in systemic exposure to trovafloxacin (AUC) of 66% and peak serum concentration (Cmax) of 60%. (See **PRECAUTIONS: Drug Interactions, DOSAGE AND ADMINISTRATION**.)
Concomitant sucralfate administration (1g) with trovafloxacin 200 mg p.o. resulted in a 70% decrease in trovafloxacin systemic exposure (AUC) and a 77% reduction in peak serum concentration (Cmax). (See **PRECAUTIONS: Drug Interactions, DOSAGE AND ADMINISTRATION**.)
Concomitant administration of ferrous sulfate (120 mg elemental iron) with trovafloxacin 200 mg p.o. resulted in a 40% reduction in trovafloxacin systemic exposure (AUC) and a 48% decrease in trovafloxacin Cmax. (See **PRECAUTIONS: Drug Interactions, DOSAGE AND ADMINISTRATION**.)
Concomitant administration of intravenous morphine (0.15 mg/kg) with oral trovafloxacin (200 mg) resulted in a 36% reduction in trovafloxacin AUC and a 46% decrease in trovafloxacin Cmax. Trovafloxacin administration had no effect on the pharmacokinetics of morphine or its pharmacologically active metabolite, morphine-6-β-glucuronide. (See **PRECAUTIONS: Drug Interactions, DOSAGE AND ADMINISTRATION**.)
Minor pharmacokinetic interactions that are most likely without clinical significance include calcium carbonate, omeprazole and caffeine.
Concomitant administration of calcium carbonate (1000 mg) with trovafloxacin 200 mg p.o. resulted in a 20% reduction in trovafloxacin AUC and a 17% reduction in peak serum trovafloxacin concentration (Cmax).
A 40 mg dose of omeprazole given 2 hours prior to trovafloxacin (300 mg p.o.) resulted in a 17% reduction in trovafloxacin AUC and a 17% reduction in trovafloxacin peak serum concentration (Cmax).
Administration of trovafloxacin (200 mg) concomitantly with caffeine (200 mg) resulted in a 17% increase in caffeine AUC and a 15% increase in caffeine Cmax. These changes in caffeine exposure are not considered clinically significant.
No significant pharmacokinetic interactions include cimetidine, theophylline, digoxin, warfarin and cyclosporine. Cimetidine co-administration (400 mg twice daily for 5 days) with trovafloxacin (200 mg p.o. daily for 3 days) resulted in changes in trovafloxacin AUC and Cmax of less than 5%.
Trovafloxacin (200 mg p.o. daily for 7 days) co-administration with theophylline (300 mg twice daily for 14 days) resulted in no change in theophylline AUC and Cmax.
Trovafloxacin (200 mg p.o. daily for 10 days) co-administration with digoxin (0.25 mg daily for 20 days) did not significantly alter systemic exposure (AUC) to digoxin or the renal clearance of digoxin.
Trovafloxacin (200 mg p.o. daily for 7 days) does not interfere with the pharmacokinetics nor the pharmacody-

Continued on next page

Trovan Tabs/IV—Cont.

namics of warfarin (daily for 21 days). Concomitant oral administration of trovafloxacin did not affect the systemic exposure (AUC) or peak plasma concentrations (Cmax) of the S or R isomers of warfarin, nor did it influence prothrombin times.

Trovafloxacin (200 mg p.o. daily for 7 days) co-administration with cyclosporine (daily doses from 150–450 mg for 7 days) resulted in decreases of 10% or less in systemic exposure to cyclosporine (AUC) and in the peak blood concentrations of cyclosporine.

Microbiology

Trovafloxacin is a fluoronaphthyridone related to the fluoroquinolones with *in vitro* activity against a wide range of gram-negative and gram-positive aerobic, and anaerobic microorganisms. The bactericidal action of trovafloxacin results from inhibition of DNA gyrase and topoisomerase IV. DNA gyrase is an essential enzyme that is involved in the replication, transcription and repair of bacterial DNA. Topoisomerase IV is an enzyme known to play a key role in the partitioning of the chromosomal DNA during bacterial cell division. Mechanism of action of fluoroquinolones including trovafloxacin is different from that of penicillins, cephalosporins, aminoglycosides, macrolides, and tetracyclines. Therefore, fluoroquinolones may be active against pathogens that are resistant to these antibiotics. There is no cross-resistance between trovafloxacin and the mentioned classes of antibiotics. The overall results obtained from *in vitro* synergy studies, testing combinations of trovafloxacin with beta-lactams and aminoglycosides, indicate that synergy is strain specific and not commonly encountered. This agrees with results obtained previously with other fluoroquinolones. Resistance to trovafloxacin *in vitro* develops slowly via multiple-step mutation in a manner similar to other fluoroquinolones. Resistance to trovafloxacin *in vitro* occurs at a general frequency of between 1×10^{-7} to 10^{-10}. Although cross-resistance has been observed between trovafloxacin and some other fluoroquinolones, some microorganisms resistant to other fluoroquinolones may be susceptible to trovafloxacin.

Trovafloxacin has been shown to be active against most strains of the following microorganisms, both *in vitro* and in clinical infections as described in the **INDICATIONS AND USAGE** section:

Aerobic gram-positive microorganisms

Enterococcus faecalis (many strains are only moderately susceptible)
Staphylococcus aureus (methicillin-susceptible strains)
Staphylococcus epidermidis (methicillin-susceptible strains)
Streptococcus agalactiae
Streptococcus pneumoniae (penicillin-susceptible strains)
Streptococcus pyogenes
Viridans group streptococci

Aerobic gram-negative microorganisms

Escherichia coli
Gardnerella vaginalis
Haemophilus influenzae
Haemophilus parainfluenzae
Klebsiella pneumoniae
Moraxella catarrhalis
Neisseria gonorrhoeae
Proteus mirabilis
Pseudomonas aeruginosa

Anaerobic microorganisms

Bacteroides fragilis
Prevotella species
Peptostreptococcus species

Other microorganisms

Chlamydia pneumoniae
Chlamydia trachomatis
Legionella pneumophila
Mycoplasma pneumoniae
The following *in vitro* data are available, **but their clinical significance is unknown.**
Trovafloxacin exhibits *in vitro* minimum inhibitory concentrations (MICs) of ≤2 μg/mL against most (90%) strains of the following microorganisms; however, the safety and effectiveness of trovafloxacin in treating clinical infections due to these microorganisms have not been established in adequate and well-controlled clinical trials.

Aerobic gram-positive microorganisms

Streptococcus pneumoniae (penicillin-resistant strains)

Aerobic gram-negative microorganisms

Citrobacter freundii
Enterobacter aerogenes
Morganella morganii
Proteus vulgaris

Anaerobic microorganisms

Bacteroides distasonis
Clostridium perfringens
Bacteroides ovatus

Microorganism	MIC Range (μg/mL)
Escherichia coli ATCC 25922	0.004-0.016
Staphylococcus aureus ATCC 29213	0.008-0.03
Pseudomonas aeruginosa ATCC 27853	0.25-2.0
Enterococcus faecalis ATCC 29212	0.06-0.25
Haemophilus influenzae[e] ATCC 49247	0.004-0.016
Streptococcus pneumoniae[f] ATCC 49619	0.06-0.25
Neisseria gonorrhoeae[g] ATCC 49226	0.004-0.016

[e] This quality control range is applicable to only *H. influenzae* ATCC 49247 tested by a microdilution procedure using HTM[1].

[f] This quality control range is applicable to only *S. pneumoniae* ATCC 49619 tested by a microdilution procedure using cation-adjusted Mueller-Hinton broth with 2–5% lysed horse blood.

[g] This quality control range is applicable to only *N. gonorrhoeae* ATCC 49226 tested by agar dilution procedure using GC agar base with 1% defined growth supplement[1].

Other microorganisms

Mycoplasma hominis
Ureaplasma urealyticum
NOTE: *Mycobacterium tuberculosis* and *Mycobacterium avium-intracellulare* complex organisms are commonly resistant to trovafloxacin.

NOTE: The activity of trovafloxacin against *Treponema pallidum* has not been evaluated; however, other quinolones are not active against *Treponema pallidum*. (See **WARNINGS**.)

Susceptibility Tests:

Dilution Techniques: Quantitative methods are used to determine antimicrobial minimum inhibitory concentrations (MICs). These MICs provide estimates of the susceptibility of bacteria to antimicrobial compounds. The MICs should be determined using a standardized procedure. Standardized procedures are based on dilution methods[1] (broth or agar) or equivalent with standardized inoculum concentrations and standardized concentrations of trovafloxacin mesylate powder. The MIC values should be interpreted according to the following criteria:

For testing non-fastidious aerobic organisms:

MIC (μg/mL)	Interpretation
≤2.0	Susceptible (S)
4.0	Intermediate (I)
≥8.0	Resistant (R)

For testing *Haemophilus* spp.[a]:

MIC (μg/mL)	Interpretation[b]
≤1.0	Susceptible (S)

[a] This interpretive standard is applicable only to broth microdilution susceptibility tests with *Haemophilus* spp. using Haemophilus Test Medium (HTM)[1].
[b] The current absence of data on resistant strains precludes defining any results other than "Susceptible". Strains yielding MIC results suggestive of a "nonsusceptible" category should be submitted to a reference laboratory for further testing.

For testing *Streptococcus* spp. including *Streptococcus pneumoniae*[c]:

MIC (μg/mL)	Interpretation
≤1.0	Susceptible (S)
2.0	Intermediate (I)
≥4.0	Resistant (R)

[c] These interpretive standards are applicable only to broth microdilution susceptibility tests using cation-adjusted Mueller-Hinton broth with 2–5% lysed horse blood.

For testing *Neisseria gonorrhoeae*[d]:

MIC (μg/mL)	Interpretation
≤0.125	Susceptible (S)
0.25	Intermediate (I)
≥0.5	Resistant (R)

[d] These interpretive standards are applicable to agar dilution tests with GC agar base and 1% defined growth supplement[1].

A report of "Susceptible" indicates that the pathogen is likely to be inhibited if the antimicrobial compound in the blood reaches the concentration usually achievable. A report of "Intermediate" indicates that the result should be considered equivocal, and, if the microorganism is not fully susceptible to alternative, clinically feasible drugs, the test should be repeated. This category implies possible clinical applicability in body sites where the drug is physiologically concentrated or in situations where high dosage of drug can be used. This category also provides a buffer zone which prevents small uncontrolled technical factors from causing major discrepancies in interpretation. A report of "Resistant"

indicates that the pathogen is not likely to be inhibited if the antimicrobial compound in the blood reaches the concentration usually achievable; other therapy should be selected.

Standardized susceptibility test procedures require the use of laboratory control microorganisms to control the technical aspects of the laboratory procedures. Standard trovafloxacin mesylate powder should provide the following MIC values:

[See table above]

Diffusion Techniques: Quantitative methods that require measurement of zone diameters also provide reproducible estimates of the susceptibility of bacteria to antimicrobial compounds. One such standardized procedure[2] requires the use of standardized inoculum concentrations. This procedure uses paper disks impregnated with trovafloxacin mesylate equivalent to 10 μg trovafloxacin to test the susceptibility of microorganisms to trovafloxacin.

Reports from the laboratory providing results of the standard single-disk susceptibility test with a trovafloxacin mesylate disk (equivalent to 10 mg trovafloxacin) should be interpreted according to the following criteria:

The following zone diameter interpretive criteria should be used for testing non-fastidious aerobic organisms:

Zone Diameter (mm)	Interpretation
≥17	Susceptible (S)
14–16	Intermediate (I)
≤13	Resistant (R)

For testing *Haemophilus* spp.[h]:

Zone Diameter (mm)	Interpretation[i]
≥22	Susceptible (S)

[h] This zone diameter standard is applicable only to tests with *Haemophilus* spp. using HTM[2].
[i] The current absence of data on resistant strains precludes defining any results other than "Susceptible". Strains yielding MIC results suggestive of "nonsusceptible" category should be submitted to a reference laboratory for further testing.

For testing *Streptococcus* spp. including *Streptococcus pneumoniae*[j]:

Zone Diameter (mm)	Interpretation
≥19	Susceptible (S)
18–16	Intermediate (I)
≤15	Resistant (R)

[j] These zone diameter standards only apply to tests performed using Mueller-Hinton agar supplemented with 5% sheep blood incubated in 5% CO_2.

For testing *Neisseria gonorrhoeae*[k]:

Zone Diameter (mm)	Interpretation
≥37	Susceptible (S)
34–36	Intermediate (I)
≤33	Resistant (R)

[k] These interpretive standards are applicable to disk diffusion tests with GC agar base and 1% defined growth supplement[2] incubated in 5% CO_2.

Interpretation should be as stated above for results using dilution techniques. Interpretation involves correlation of the diameter obtained in the disk test with the MIC for trovafloxacin.

As with standardized dilution techniques, diffusion methods require the use of laboratory control microorganisms that are used to control the technical aspects of the laboratory procedures. For the diffusion technique, the trovafloxacin mesylate equivalent to 10-μg trovafloxacin disk should provide the following zone diameters in these laboratory quality control strains:

[See table at top of next page]

Microorganism	Zone Diameter Range (mm)
Escherichia coli ATCC 25922	29–36
Staphylococcus aureus ATCC 25923	29–35
Pseudomonas aeruginosa ATCC 27853	21–27
Haemophilus influenzae[l] ATCC 49247	32–39
Streptococcus pneumoniae[m] ATCC 49619	25–32
Neisseria gonorrhoeae[n] ATCC 49226	42–55

[l] This quality control limit applies to tests conducted with *Haemophilus influenzae* ATCC 49247 using HTM[2].
[m] This quality control range is applicable only to tests performed by disk diffusion using Mueller-Hinton agar supplemented with 5% defibrinated sheep blood.
[n] This quality control range is only applicable to tests performed by disk diffusion using GC agar base and 1% defined growth supplement[2].

Anaerobic Techniques: For anaerobic bacteria, the susceptibility to trovafloxacin as MICs can be determined by standardized test methods[3]. The MIC values obtained should be interpreted according to the following criteria:

MIC (μg/mL)	Interpretation
≤2.0	Susceptible (S)
4.0	Intermediate (I)
≥8.0	Resistant (R)

Interpretation is identical to that stated above for results using dilution techniques.
As with other susceptibility techniques, the use of laboratory control microorganisms is required to control the technical aspects of the laboratory standardized procedures. Standardized trovafloxacin mesylate powder should provide the following MIC values:
[See table below]

INDICATIONS AND USAGE

TROVAN is indicated for the treatment of infections caused by susceptible strains of the designated microorganisms in the conditions listed below. (See **DOSAGE AND ADMINISTRATION.**)

Nosocomial pneumonia caused by *Escherichia coli, Pseudomonas aeruginosa, Haemophilus influenzae*, or *Staphylococcus aureus*. As with other antimicrobials, where *Pseudomonas aeruginosa* is a documented or presumptive pathogen, combination therapy with either an aminoglycoside or aztreonam may be clinically indicated.

Community acquired pneumonia caused by *Streptococcus pneumoniae, Haemophilus influenzae, Klebsiella pneumoniae, Staphylococcus aureus, Mycoplasma pneumoniae, Moraxella catarrhalis, Legionella pneumophila*, or *Chlamydia pneumoniae*.

Acute bacterial exacerbation of chronic bronchitis caused by *Haemophilus influenzae, Moraxella catarrhalis, Streptococcus pneumoniae, Staphylococcus aureus*, or *Haemophilus parainfluenzae*.

Acute sinusitis caused by *Haemophilus influenzae, Moraxella catarrhalis*, or *Streptococcus pneumoniae*.

Complicated intra-abdominal infections, including post-surgical infections caused by *Escherichia coli, Bacteroides fragilis*, viridans group streptococci, *Pseudomonas aeruginosa, Klebsiella pneumoniae, Peptostreptococcus* species, or *Prevotella* species.

Gynecologic and pelvic infections including endomyometritis, parametritis, septic abortion and post-partum infections caused by *Escherichia coli, Bacteroides fragilis*, viridans group streptococci, *Enterococcus faecalis, Streptococcus agalactiae, Peptostreptococcus* species, *Prevotella* species, or *Gardnerella vaginalis*.

Prophylaxis of infection associated with elective colorectal surgery, vaginal and abdominal hysterectomy. Uncomplicated skin and skin structure infections caused by *Staphylococcus aureus, Streptococcus pyogenes*, or *Streptococcus agalactiae*.

Complicated skin and skin structure infections, including diabetic foot infections, caused by *Staphylococcus aureus, Streptococcus agalactiae, Pseudomonas aeruginosa, Enterococcus faecalis, Escherichia coli*, or *Proteus mirabilis*. **NOTE**: TROVAN has not been studied in the treatment of osteomyelitis. The safety and efficacy of TROVAN given for >4 weeks have not been studied. (See **PRECAUTIONS: General.**)

Uncomplicated urinary tract infections (cystitis) caused by *Escherichia coli*.

Chronic bacterial prostatitis caused by *Escherichia coli, Enterococcus faecalis*, or *Staphylococcus epidermidis*.

Uncomplicated urethral gonorrhea in males and endocervical and rectal gonorrhea in females caused by *Neisseria gonorrhoeae*. (See **WARNINGS.**)

Cervicitis due to *Chlamydia trachomatis*. **NOTE**: In males with nongonococcal urethritis TROVAN was somewhat less effective than doxycycline.

Pelvic inflammatory disease (mild to moderate) caused by *Neisseria gonorrhoeae* or *Chlamydia trachomatis*.

CONTRAINDICATIONS

TROVAN is contraindicated in persons with a history of hypersensitivity to trovafloxacin, alatrofloxacin, quinolone antimicrobial agents or any other components of these products.

WARNINGS

THE SAFETY AND EFFECTIVENESS OF TROVAFLOXACIN IN PEDIATRIC POPULATIONS LESS THAN 18 YEARS OF AGE, PREGNANT WOMEN, AND NURSING WOMEN HAVE NOT BEEN ESTABLISHED. (See **PRECAUTIONS: Pediatric Use, Pregnancy,** and **Nursing Mothers** subsections.)

As with other members of the quinolone class, trovafloxacin has caused arthropathy and/or chondrodysplasia in immature rats and dogs. The significance of these findings to humans is unknown. (See **ANIMAL PHARMACOLOGY.**)

Convulsions, increased intracranial pressure and psychosis have been reported in patients receiving quinolones. Quinolones may also cause central nervous system stimulation which may lead to tremors, restlessness, lightheadedness, confusion, hallucinations, paranoia, depression, nightmares and insomnia. These reactions may occur following the first dose. If these reactions occur in patients receiving trovafloxacin or alatrofloxacin, the drug should be discontinued and appropriate measures instituted. (See **PRECAUTIONS: General, Information for Patients, Drug Interactions** and **ADVERSE REACTIONS.**)

As with other quinolones, TROVAN should be used with caution in patients with known or suspected CNS disorders, such as severe cerebral atherosclerosis, epilepsy, and other factors that predispose to seizures. (See **ADVERSE REACTIONS.**)

Serious and occasionally fatal hypersensitivity and/or anaphylactic reactions have been reported in patients receiving therapy with quinolones. These reactions may occur following the first dose. Some reactions have been accompanied by cardiovascular collapse, hypotension/shock, seizure, loss of consciousness, tingling, angioedema (including tongue, laryngeal, throat or facial edema/swelling), airway obstruction (including bronchospasm, shortness of breath and acute respiratory distress), dyspnea, urticaria, itching and other serious skin reactions.

TROVAN should be discontinued at the first appearance of a skin rash or any other sign of hypersensitivity. Serious acute hypersensitivity reactions may require treatment with epinephrine and other resuscitative measures, including oxygen, intravenous fluids, antihistamines, corticosteroids, pressor amines and airway management, as clinically indicated. (See **PRECAUTIONS** and **ADVERSE REACTIONS.**)

Serious and sometimes fatal events, some due to hypersensitivity and some due to uncertain etiology, have been reported in patients receiving therapy with all antibiotics. These events may be severe and generally occur following the administration of multiple doses. Clinical manifestations may include one or more of the following: fever, rash or severe dermatologic reactions (e.g., toxic epidermal necrolysis, Stevens-Johnson Syndrome); vasculitis, arthralgia, myalgia, serum sickness; allergic pneumonitis, interstitial nephritis; acute renal insufficiency or failure; hepatitis, jaundice, acute hepatic necrosis or failure; anemia, including hemolytic and aplastic; thrombocytopenia, including thrombotic thrombocytopenic purpura; leukopenia; agranulocytosis; pancytopenia; and/or other hematologic abnormalities.

Pseudomembranous colitis has been reported with nearly all antibacterial agents, including TROVAN, and may range in severity from mild to life-threatening. Therefore, it is important to consider this diagnosis in patients who present with diarrhea subsequent to the administration of any antibacterial agent.

Microorganism	MIC[p] (μg/mL)
Bacteroides fragilis ATCC 25285	0.125–0.5
Bacteroides thetaiotaomicron ATCC 29741	0.25–1.0
Eubacterium lentum ATCC 43055	0.25–1.0

[p] These quality control ranges were derived from tests performed in the broth formulation of Wilkins-Chalgren agar.

Treatment with antibacterial agents alters the flora of the colon and may permit overgrowth of clostridia. Studies indicate that a toxin produced by *Clostridium difficile* is the primary cause of "antibiotic-associated colitis."

After the diagnosis of pseudomembranous colitis has been established, therapeutic measures should be initiated. Mild cases of pseudomembranous colitis usually respond to drug discontinuation alone. In moderate to severe cases, consideration should be given to management with fluids and electrolytes, protein supplementation, and treatment with an antibacterial drug clinically effective against *C. difficile* colitis. (See **ADVERSE REACTIONS.**)

Although not seen in TROVAN clinical trials, ruptures of the shoulder, hand, and Achilles tendons that required surgical repair or resulted in prolonged disability have been reported in patients receiving quinolones. TROVAN should be discontinued if the patient experiences pain, inflammation or rupture of a tendon. Patients should rest and refrain from exercise until the diagnosis of tendinitis or tendon rupture has been confidently excluded. Tendon rupture can occur during or after therapy with quinolones.

Trovafloxacin has not been shown to be effective in the treatment of syphilis. Antimicrobial agents used in high doses for short periods of time to treat gonorrhea may mask or delay the symptoms of incubating syphilis. All patients with gonorrhea should have a serologic test for syphilis at the time of diagnosis.

PRECAUTIONS

General:

Because TROVAN can cause elevations of liver function tests during or soon after prolonged therapy (i.e., ≥21 days), periodic assessment of hepatic function is advisable. The safety and efficacy of TROVAN given for >4 weeks have not been studied. (See **ADVERSE REACTIONS.**)

Moderate to severe phototoxicity reactions have been observed in patients who are exposed to direct sunlight while receiving some drugs in this class. Therapy should be discontinued if phototoxicity (e.g., a skin eruption, etc.) occurs.

The safety and efficacy of TROVAN in patients with severe cirrhosis (Child-Pugh Class C) have not been studied.

Information for Patients:

Patients should be advised:

- that TROVAN Tablets may be taken without regard to meals;
- that vitamins or minerals containing iron, aluminum- or magnesium-base antacids, antacids containing citric acid buffered with sodium citrate, or sucralfate should be taken at least two hours before or two hours after taking TROVAN Tablets. (See **Drug Interactions.**);
- that TROVAN may cause lightheadedness and/or dizziness. Dizziness and/or lightheadedness was the most common adverse reaction reported, and for females under 45 years, it was reported significantly more frequently than in other groups. The incidence of dizziness may be substantially reduced if TROVAN Tablets are taken at bedtime or with food. Patients should know how they react to trovafloxacin before they operate an automobile or machinery or engage in activities requiring mental alertness and coordination. (See **WARNINGS** and **ADVERSE REACTIONS.**);
- to discontinue treatment and inform their physician if they experience pain, inflammation or rupture of a tendon, and to rest and refrain from exercise until the diagnosis of tendinitis or tendon rupture has been confidently excluded;
- that TROVAN may be associated with hypersensitivity reactions, even following the first dose, and to discontinue the drug at the first sign of a skin rash, hives or other skin reactions, difficulty in swallowing or breathing, any swelling suggesting angioedema (e.g., swelling of the lips, tongue, face, tightness of the throat, hoarseness), or other symptoms of an allergic reaction. (See **WARNINGS** and **ADVERSE REACTIONS.**);
- to avoid excessive sunlight or artificial ultraviolet light (e.g., tanning beds) while taking TROVAN and to discontinue therapy if phototoxicity (e.g., sunburn-like reaction or skin eruption) occurs.

Drug Interactions:

No significant interactions with theophylline, cimetidine, digoxin, warfarin, or cyclosporine have been observed with TROVAN Tablets. (See **CLINICAL PHARMACOLOGY.**)

Minor pharmacokinetic interactions without clinical significance have been observed with co-administration of TROVAN Tablets with caffeine, omeprazole and calcium carbonate. (See **CLINICAL PHARMACOLOGY.**)

Antacids, Sucralfate, and Iron: The absorption of oral trovafloxacin is significantly reduced by the concomitant administration of some antacids containing magnesium or aluminum, citric acid/sodium citrate (Bicitra®), as well as sucralfate and iron (as ferrous ions). The above oral agents should be taken at least two hours before or two hours after oral trovafloxacin administration. (See **CLINICAL PHARMACOLOGY.**)

Continued on next page

Trovan Tabs/IV—Cont.

Morphine: Co-administration of intravenous morphine significantly reduces the absorption of oral trovafloxacin. Intravenous morphine should be administered at least 2 hours after oral TROVAN dosing in the fasted state and at least 4 hours after oral TROVAN is taken with food. Trovafloxacin administration had no effect on the pharmacokinetics of morphine or its metabolite, morphine-6-β-glucuronide. (See **CLINICAL PHARMACOLOGY**.)

Alatrofloxacin should not be co-administered with any solution containing multivalent cations, e.g., magnesium, through the same intravenous line. (See **DOSAGE AND ADMINISTRATION**.)

Laboratory Test Interactions: There are no reported laboratory test interactions.

Carcinogenesis, Mutagenesis, Impairment of Fertility:
Long term studies in animals to determine the carcinogenic potential of trovafloxacin or alatrofloxacin have not been conducted.

Trovafloxacin was not mutagenic in the Ames Salmonella reversion assay or CHO/HGPRT mammalian cell gene mutation assay and it was not clastogenic in mitogen-stimulated human lymphocytes or mouse bone marrow cells. A mouse micronucleus test conducted with alatrofloxacin was also negative. The positive response observed in the *E. coli* bacterial mutagenicity assay may be due to the inhibition of DNA gyrase by trovafloxacin.

Trovafloxacin and alatrofloxacin did not affect the fertility of male or female rats at oral and I.V. doses of 75 mg/kg/day and 50 mg/kg/day, respectively. These doses are 15 and 10 times the recommended maximum human dose based on mg/kg or approximately 2 times based on mg/m². However, oral doses of trovafloxacin at 200 mg/kg/day (40 times the recommended maximum human dose based on mg/kg or about 6 times based on mg/m²) were associated with increased preimplantation loss in rats.

Pregnancy: Teratogenic Effects. Pregnancy Category C:
An increase in skeletal variations was observed in rat fetuses after daily oral 75 mg/kg maternal doses of trovafloxacin (approximately 15 times the highest recommended human dose based on mg/kg or two times based upon body surface area) were administered during organogenesis. However, fetal skeletal variations were not observed in rats dosed orally with 15 mg/kg trovafloxacin. Evidence of fetotoxicity (increased perinatal mortality and decreased body weights) was also observed in rats at 75 mg/kg. Daily oral doses of trovafloxacin at 45 mg/kg (approximately 9 times the highest recommended human dose based on mg/kg or 2.7 times based upon body surface area) in the rabbit were not associated with an increased incidence of fetal skeletal variations or malformations.

An increase in skeletal variations and malformations was observed in rat fetuses after daily intravenous doses of alatrofloxacin at ≥20 mg/kg/day (approximately 4 times the highest recommended human dose based on mg/kg or 0.6 times based upon body surface area) were administered to dams during organogenesis. In the rabbit, an increase in fetal skeletal malformations was also observed when 20 mg/kg/day (approximately equal to the highest recommended human dose based upon body surface area) of alatrofloxacin was given intravenously during the period of organogenesis. Intravenous dosing of alatrofloxacin at 6.5 mg/kg in the rat or rabbit was not associated with an increased incidence of skeletal variations or malformations. Fetotoxicity and fetal skeletal malformations have been associated with other quinolones.

Oral doses of trovafloxacin >5mg/kg were associated with an increased gestation time in rats, and several dams at 75 mg/kg experienced uterine dystocia.

There are no adequate and well-controlled studies in pregnant women. TROVAN should be used during pregnancy only if the potential benefit justifies the potential risk to the fetus. (See **WARNINGS**.)

Nursing Mothers:
Trovafloxacin is excreted in human milk and was found in measurable concentrations in the breast milk of lactating subjects. (See **CLINICAL PHARMACOLOGY, Distribution**.)

Because of the potential for unknown effects from trovafloxacin in nursing infants from mothers taking trovafloxacin, a decision should be made either to discontinue nursing or to discontinue the drug, taking into account the importance of the drug to the mother.

Pediatric Use:
The safety and effectiveness of trovafloxacin in pediatric populations less than 18 years of age have not been established. Quinolones, including trovafloxacin, cause arthropathy and osteochondrosis in juvenile animals of several species. (See **WARNINGS**.)

Geriatric Use:
In multiple-dose clinical trials of trovafloxacin, 27% of patients were ≥65 years of age and 12% of patients were ≥75 years of age. The overall incidence of drug-related adverse reactions, including central nervous system and gastroin-

TROVAN Drug-Related Adverse Reactions (frequency ≥1%) in Multiple-Dose Clinical Trials

	100 mg oral qd (N=1536)	200 mg oral qd (N=3259)	200 mg I.V. 200 mg oral qd (N=634)	300 mg I.V. 200 mg oral qd (N=623)
Dizziness	3%	11%	2%	2%
Lightheadedness	2%	4%	2%	<1%
Nausea	4%	8%	5%	4%
Headache	4%	5%	5%	1%
Vomiting	<1%	3%	1%	3%
Diarrhea	2%	2%	2%	2%
Abdominal pain	<1%	1%	1%	0%
Application/injection/ insertion site reaction	n/a	n/a	5%	2%
Vaginitis	1%	1%	<1%	<1%
Pruritus	<1%	<1%	2%	2%
Rash	<1%	<1%	2%	2%

DOSAGE GUIDELINES

INFECTION*/LOCATION AND TYPE	DAILY UNIT DOSE AND ROUTE OF ADMINISTRATION	TOTAL DURATION
Nosocomial Pneumonia (See NOTE 1 below.)	300 mg I.V. followed by 200 mg oral	10–14 days
Community Acquired Pneumonia	200 mg oral or 200 mg I.V. followed by 200 mg oral	7–14 days
Acute Bacterial Exacerbation of Chronic Bronchitis	100 mg oral	7–10 days
Acute Sinusitis	200 mg oral	10 days
Complicated Intra-Abdominal Infections, including post-surgical infections	300 mg I.V. followed by 200 mg oral	7–14 days
Gynecological and Pelvic Infections	300 mg I.V. followed by 200 mg oral	7–14 days
Surgical Prophylaxis—Elective Colorectal Surgery (See NOTE 2 below.)	200 mg I.V. or oral	Single intravenous or oral dose within 30 min. to 4 hours before surgery
Surgical Prophylaxis—Elective Abdominal and Vaginal Hysterectomy (See NOTE 2 below.)	200 mg I.V. or oral	Single intravenous or oral dose within 30 min. to 4 hours before surgery
Skin and Skin Structure Infections, Uncomplicated	100 mg oral	7–10 days
Skin and Skin Structure Infections, Complicated, including diabetic foot infections	200 mg oral or 200 mg I.V. followed by 200 mg oral	10–14 days
Uncomplicated Urinary Tract Infections (cystitis)	100 mg oral	3 days
Chronic Bacterial Prostatitis	200 mg oral	28 days
Uncomplicated Urethral Gonorrhea in Males; Endocervical and Rectal Gonorrhea in Females	100 mg oral	Single dose
Cervicitis due to *Chlamydia trachomatis*	200 mg oral	5 days
Pelvic Inflammatory Disease (mild to moderate)	200 mg oral	14 days

*due to the designated pathogens (See INDICATIONS AND USAGE.)

testinal side effects, was less in the ≥65 year group than the other age groups.

ADVERSE REACTIONS

Over 6000 patients have been treated with TROVAN in multidose clinical efficacy trials worldwide.

In TROVAN studies the majority of adverse reactions were described as mild in nature (over 90% were described as mild or moderate). TROVAN was discontinued for adverse events thought related to drug in 5% of patients (dizziness 2.4%, nausea 1.9%, headache 1.1%, and vomiting 1.0%). [See first table above]

Dizziness/lightheadedness on TROVAN is generally mild, lasts for a few hours following a dose, and in most cases, resolves with continued dosing. The incidence of dizziness and lightheadedness in TROVAN patients over 65 years is 3.1% and 0.6%, respectively. (See **PRECAUTIONS: Information for Patients**.)

TROVAN appears to have a low potential for phototoxicity. In clinical trials with TROVAN, only mild, treatment-related phototoxicity was observed in less than 0.03% (2/7096) of patients.

Additional reported drug-related events in clinical trials (remotely, possibly, probably or unknown) that occurred in <1% of TROVAN-treated patients are:

APPLICATION/INJECTION/INSERTION SITE: Application/injection/insertion site device complications, inflammation, pain, edema

AUTONOMIC NERVOUS: flushing, increased sweating, dry mouth, cold clammy skin, increased saliva

CARDIOVASCULAR: peripheral edema, chest pain, thrombophlebitis, hypotension, palpitation, periorbital edema, hypertension, syncope, tachycardia, angina pectoris, bradycardia, peripheral ischemia, edema, dizziness postural.

CENTRAL & PERIPHERAL NERVOUS SYSTEM: confusion, paresthesia, vertigo, hypoesthesia, ataxia, convulsions, dysphonia, hypertonia, migraine, involuntary muscle contractions, speech disorder, encephalopathy, abnormal gait, hyperkinesia, hypokinesia, tongue paralysis, abnormal coordination, tremor, dyskinesia

GASTROINTESTINAL: abdominal pain, altered bowel habit, constipation, diarrhea-*Clostridium difficile*, dyspepsia, flatulence, loose stools, gastritis, dysphagia, increased appetite, gastroenteritis, rectal disorder, colitis, pseudomembranous colitis, enteritis, eructation, gastrointestinal disorder, melena, hiccup

ORAL CAVITY: gingivitis, stomatitis, altered saliva, tongue disorder, tongue edema, tooth disorder, chelitis, halitosis

GENERAL/OTHER: fever, fatigue, pain, asthenia, moniliasis, hot flushes, back pain, chills, infection (bacterial, fungal), malaise, sepsis, alcohol intolerance, allergic reaction, anaphylactoid reaction, drug (other) toxicity/reaction, weight increase, weight decrease

HEMATOPOIETIC: anemia, granulocytopenia, hemorrhage unspecified, leukopenia, prothrombin decreased, thrombocythemia, thrombocytopenia

LIVER/BILIARY: increased hepatic enzymes, hepatic function abnormal, bilirubinemia, discolored feces, jaundice

METABOLIC/NUTRITIONAL: hyperglycemia, thirst

MUSCULOSKELETAL: arthralgia, muscle cramps, myalgia, muscle weakness, skeletal pain, tendinitis, arthropathy

PSYCHIATRIC: anxiety, anorexia, agitation, nervousness, somnolence, insomnia, depression, amnesia, concentration impaired, depersonalization, dreaming abnormal, emotional lability, euphoria, hallucination, impotence, libido decreased-male, paroniria, thinking abnormal

REPRODUCTIVE: Female: leukorrhea, menstrual disorder; Male: balanoposthitis

RESPIRATORY: dyspnea, rhinitis, sinusitis, bronchospasm, coughing, epistaxis, respiratory insufficiency, upper respiratory tract infection, respiratory disorder, asthma, hemoptysis, hypoxia, stridor

SKIN/APPENDAGES: pruritus, pruritus ani, skin disorder, skin ulceration, angioedema, dermatitis, dermatitis fungal, photosensitivity skin reaction, seborrhea, skin exfoliation, urticaria

SPECIAL SENSES: taste perversion, eye pain, abnormal vision, conjunctivitis, photophobia, conjuctival hemorrhage, hyperacusis, scotoma, tinnitus, visual field defect, diplopia, xerophthalmia

URINARY SYSTEM: dysuria, face edema, micturition frequency, interstitial nephritis, renal failure acute, renal function abnormal, urinary incontinence

LABORATORY CHANGES: Changes in laboratory parameters, without regard to drug relationship, occurring in ≥1% of TROVAN-treated patients were: decreased hemoglobin and hematocrit; increased platelets; decreased and increased WBC; eosinophilia; increased ALT (SGPT), AST (SGOT), and alkaline phosphatase; decreased protein and albumin; increased BUN and creatinine; decreased sodium; and bicarbonate. It is not known whether these abnormalities were caused by the drug or the underlying condition being treated.

The incidence and magnitude of liver function abnormalities with TROVAN were the same as comparator agents except in the only study in which oral TROVAN was administered for 28 days. In this study (chronic bacterial prostatitis) nine percent (13/140) of TROVAN-treated patients experienced elevations of serum transaminases (AST and/or ALT) of ≥3 times the upper limit of normal. These liver function test abnormalities generally developed at the end of, or following completion of, the planned 28-day course of therapy, but were not associated with concurrent elevations of related laboratory measures of hepatic function (such as serum bilirubin, alkaline phosphatase, or lactate dehydrogenase). Patients were asymptomatic with these abnormalities, which generally returned to normal within 1–2 months after discontinuation of therapy. (See **PRECAUTIONS: General.**)

OVERDOSAGE

Trovafloxacin has a low order of acute toxicity. The minimum lethal oral dose in mice and rats was 2000 mg/kg or greater. The minimum lethal I.V. dose for the prodrug, alatrofloxacin, was 50–125 mg/kg for mice and greater than 75 mg/kg for rats. Clinical signs observed included decreased activity and respiration, ataxia, ptosis, tremors and convulsions.

In the event of acute oral overdosage, the stomach should be emptied by inducing vomiting or by gastric lavage. The patient should be carefully observed and given symptomatic and supportive treatment. Adequate hydration should be maintained. Trovafloxacin is not efficiently removed from the body by hemodialysis.

DOSAGE AND ADMINISTRATION

The recommended dosage for TROVAN Tablets or TROVAN I.V. for the treatment of infections is described in the table below. Doses of TROVAN are administered once every 24 hours.

Oral doses should be administered at least two hours before or two hours after antacids containing magnesium or aluminum, as well as sucralfate, citric acid buffered with sodium citrate (e.g., Bicitra®) and metal cations (e.g., ferrous sulfate).

Intravenous morphine should be administered at least 2 hours after oral TROVAN dosing in the fasted state and at least 4 hours after oral TROVAN is taken with food.

When switching from intravenous to oral dosage administration, for comparable dosages, no adjustment is necessary. Patients whose therapy is started with TROVAN I.V. may be switched to TROVAN Tablets when clinically indicated at the discretion of the physician.

TROVAN I.V. (alatrofloxacin mesylate injection) should only be administered by INTRAVENOUS infusion. It is not for intramuscular, intrathecal, intraperitoneal, or subcutaneous administration.

Single-use vials require dilution prior to administration. (See **PREPARATION OF ALATROFLOXACIN MESYLATE INJECTION FOR ADMINISTRATION.**)

[See second table at top of previous page]

NOTE 1: As with other antimicrobials, where *Pseudomonas aeruginosa* is a documented or presumptive pathogen, combination therapy with either an aminoglycoside or aztreonam may be clinically indicated.

NOTE 2: In patients where surgical prophylaxis with oral TROVAN is indicated, Bicitra® should not be given within 2 hours. (See **PRECAUTIONS: Drug Interactions.**)

The safety and efficacy of TROVAN use for >4 weeks have not been studied. (See **PRECAUTIONS.**)

IMPAIRED RENAL FUNCTION: No adjustment in the dosage of TROVAN is necessary in patients with impaired renal function. Trovafloxacin is eliminated primarily by biliary excretion. Trovafloxacin is not efficiently removed from the body by hemodialysis.

CHRONIC HEPATIC DISEASE (cirrhosis): The following table provides dosing guidelines for patients with mild or moderate cirrhosis (Child-Pugh Class A and B). There are no data in patients with severe cirrhosis (Child-Pugh Class C).

INDICATED DOSE (Normal hepatic function)	CHRONIC HEPATIC DISEASE DOSE
300 mg I.V.	200 mg I.V.
200 mg I.V. or oral	100 mg I.V. or oral
100 mg oral	100 mg oral

INTRAVENOUS ADMINISTRATION

AFTER DILUTION WITH AN APPROPRIATE DILUENT, TROVAN I.V. SHOULD BE ADMINISTERED BY INTRAVENOUS INFUSION OVER A PERIOD OF 60 MINUTES. CAUTION: RAPID OR BOLUS INTRAVENOUS INFUSION SHOULD BE AVOIDED.

TROVAN I.V. is supplied in single-use vials containing a concentrated solution of alatrofloxacin mesylate in Water for Injection (equivalent of 200 mg or 300 mg as trovafloxacin). Each mL contains alatrofloxacin mesylate equivalent to 5 mg trovafloxacin. (See **HOW SUPPLIED** for container sizes.) THESE TROVAN I.V. SINGLE-USE VIALS MUST BE FURTHER DILUTED WITH AN APPROPRIATE SOLUTION PRIOR TO INTRAVENOUS ADMINISTRATION.

This parenteral drug product should be inspected visually for discoloration and particulate matter prior to dilution and administration. Since no preservative or bacteriostatic agent is present in this product, aseptic technique must be used in preparation of the final parenteral solution.

PREPARATION OF ALATROFLOXACIN MESYLATE INJECTION FOR ADMINISTRATION

The intravenous dose should be prepared by aseptically withdrawing the appropriate volume of concentrate from the vials of TROVAN I.V. This should be diluted with a suitable intravenous solution to a final concentration of 1–2 mg/mL. (See **Compatible Intravenous Solutions.**) The resulting solution should be infused over a period of 60 minutes by direct infusion or through a Y-type intravenous infusion set which may already be in place.

Since the vials are for single use only, any unused portion should be discarded.

Since only limited data are available on the compatibility of alatrofloxacin intravenous injection with other intravenous substances, additives or other medications should not be added to TROVAN I.V. in single-use vials or infused simultaneously through the same intravenous line.

If the same intravenous line is used for sequential infusion of several different drugs, the line should be flushed before and after infusion of TROVAN I.V. with an infusion solution compatible with TROVAN I.V. and with any other drug(s) administered via this common line.

If TROVAN I.V. is to be given concomitantly with another drug, each drug should be given separately in accordance with the recommended dosage and route of administration for each drug.

The desired dosage of TROVAN I.V. may be prepared according to the following chart:

[See table above]

DOSAGE STRENGTH (mg) (trovafloxacin equivalent)	VOLUME TO WITHDRAW (mL)	DILUENT VOLUME (mL)	TOTAL VOLUME (mL)	INFUSION CONC (mg/mL)
100 mg	20	30	50	2
100 mg	20	80	100	1
200 mg	40	60	100	2
200 mg	40	160	200	1
300 mg	60	90	150	2
300 mg	60	240	300	1

For example, to prepare a 200 mg dose at an infusion concentration of 2 mg/mL (as trovafloxacin), 40 mL of TROVAN I.V. is withdrawn from a vial and diluted with 60 mL of a compatible intravenous fluid to produce a total infusion solution volume of 100 mL.

Compatible Intravenous Solutions:

5% Dextrose Injection, USP
0.45% Sodium Chloride Injection, USP
5% Dextrose and 0.45% Sodium Chloride Injection, USP
5% Dextrose and 0.2% Sodium Chloride Injection, USP
Lactated Ringer's and 5% Dextrose Injection, USP

Stability of TROVAN I.V. as Supplied:

When stored under recommended conditions, TROVAN I.V., as supplied in 40 mL or 60 mL vials, is stable through the expiration date printed on the label.

Stability of TROVAN I.V. Following Dilution:

TROVAN I.V., when diluted with the following intravenous solutions to concentrations of 0.5 to 2.0 mg/mL (as trovafloxacin), is physically and chemically stable for up to 7 days when refrigerated or up to 3 days at room temperature stored in glass bottles or plastic (PVC type) intravenous containers.

HOW SUPPLIED

Tablets

TROVAN™ (trovafloxacin mesylate) Tablets are available as blue, film-coated tablets. The 100 mg tablets are round and contain trovafloxacin mesylate equivalent to 100 mg trovafloxacin. The 200 mg tablets are modified oval-shaped and contain trovafloxacin mesylate equivalent to 200 mg trovafloxacin.

TROVAN Tablets are packaged and in unit dose blister strips in the following configurations:

100-mg tablets: color: blue; shape: round; debossing: "PFIZER" on one side and "378" on the other
Bottles of 30 (NDC 0049-3780-30)
Unit Dose/ 40 tablets (NDC 0049-3780-43)

200-mg tablets: color: blue; shape: modified oval; debossing: "PFIZER" on one side and "379" on the other
Bottles of 30 (NDC 0049-3790-30)
Unit Dose/ 40 tablets (NDC 0049-3790-43)

Storage

TROVAN Tablets should be stored at 15°C to 30°C (59°F to 86°F) in tight containers (USP).

Continued on next page

Trovan Tabs/IV—Cont.

Injection

TROVAN is also available for intravenous administration as the prodrug, TROVAN™ I.V. (alatrofloxacin mesylate injection), in the following configurations:

Single-use vials containing a clear, colorless to pale-yellow concentrated solution of alatrofloxacin mesylate equivalent to 5 mg trovafloxacin/mL.

   5 mg/mL, 40 mL, 200 mg
      Unit dose package (NDC 0049-3890-28)
   5 mg/mL, 60 mL, 300 mg
      Unit dose package (NDC 0049-3900-28)

Storage

TROVAN I.V. should be stored at 15°C to 30°C (59°F to 86°F). Protect From Light. Do Not Freeze.

ANIMAL PHARMACOLOGY

Quinolones have been shown to cause arthropathy in immature animals.

Arthropathy and chondrodysplasia were observed in immature animals given trovafloxacin. (See **WARNINGS**.)

At doses from 10 to 15 times the human dose based on mg/kg or approximately 3 to 5 times based on mg/m^2, trovafloxacin has been shown to cause arthropathy in immature rats and dogs. In addition, these drugs are associated with an increased incidence of chondrodysplasia in rats compared to controls. There is no evidence of arthropathies in fully mature rats and dogs at doses from 40 or 10 times the human dose based on mg/kg or approximately 5 times based on mg/m^2 for a 6 month exposure period.

Unlike some other members of the quinolone class, crystalluria and ocular toxicity were not observed in chronic safety studies with rats or dogs with either trovafloxacin or its prodrug, alatrofloxacin.

Quinolones have been reported to have proconvulsant activity that is exacerbated with concomitant use of non-steroidal antiinflammatory drugs (NSAIDS). Neither trovafloxacin administered orally at 500 mg/kg, nor alatrofloxacin administered intravenously at 75 mg/kg, showed an increase in measures of seizure activity in mice at doses when used in combination with the active metabolite of the NSAID, fenbufen.

As with other members of the quinolone class, trovafloxacin at doses 5 to 10 times the human dose based on mg/kg or 1 to 5 times the human dose based on mg/m^2 produces testicular degeneration in rats and dogs dosed for 6 months.

At a dose of trovafloxacin 10 times the highest human dose based on mg/kg or approximately 5 times based on mg/m^2, elevated liver enzyme levels which correlated with centrilobar hepatocellular vacuolar degeneration and necrosis were observed in dogs in a 6 month study. A subsequent study demonstrated reversibility of these effects when trovafloxacin was discontinued.

CLINICAL STUDIES

Acute Bacterial Exacerbation of Chronic Bronchitis

Patients with clinically documented acute bacterial exacerbation of chronic bronchitis participated in a randomized, double blind, multicenter trial comparing oral trovafloxacin (100 mg once daily) with oral clarithromycin (500 mg twice daily) for 7 days. The clinical success rate (cure + improvement, with no need for further antibiotic therapy) at the End of Treatment was 89% (181/203) and 85% (160/188) for trovafloxacin and clarithromycin, respectively. The clinical success rate at the End of Study (Day 28) was 80% (158/197) and 74% (131/178) for trovafloxacin and clarithromycin, respectively.

The following are the clinical success rates for the clinically evaluable groups by pathogen:

[See first table above]

Of the above patients with clinical failure at end of treatment or study, no trovafloxacin and 2 clarithromycin patients (both *H. influenzae*) had positive post treatment cultures for the baseline pathogen. There was no emergence of resistance in either treatment group. Fewer patients required hospitalization during study (Day 1–35) in the trovafloxacin group (3/210) than in the clarithromycin group (10/200), p=0.039.

Hospitalized Community Acquired Pneumonia

Adult patients with clinically and radiologically documented community acquired pneumonia, requiring hospitalization and initial intravenous therapy, participated in two randomized, multicenter, double-blind, double-dummy trials. The first trial compared intravenous alatrofloxacin (200 mg once daily for 2 to 7 days) followed by oral trovafloxacin (200 mg once daily) for a total of 7 to 14 days of therapy to intravenous ciprofloxacin (400 mg BID) plus ampicillin (500 mg QID) for 2 to 7 days followed by oral ciprofloxacin (500 mg BID) plus amoxicillin (500 mg TID) for a total of 7 to 14 days of therapy. The second study compared intravenous alatrofloxacin (200 mg once daily for 2 to 7 days) followed by oral trovafloxacin (200 mg once daily) for a total of 7 to 14 days of therapy to intravenous ceftriaxone (1000 mg once daily for 2 to 7 days) followed by oral cefpodoxime (400 mg BID) for 7 to 14 days of total therapy with optional blinded erythromycin added to the ceftriaxone/cefpodoxime arm if an atypical pneumonia was suspected. The clinical success rate (cure + improvement with no need for further antibiotic therapy) at the End of Treatment was 90% (311/346) and 90% (325/363) for TROVAN and the comparator agents, respectively. The clinical success rate at the End of Study (Day 30) was 86% (256/299) and 85% (283/334) for TROVAN and the comparator agents, respectively. All cause mortality (Day 1–35) was 2.45% (10/408) on TROVAN and 5.45% (23/422) on the comparator agents.

The following outcomes are the clinical success rates for the clinically evaluable patient groups by pathogen in these two studies:

[See second table above]

Of the above patients with clinical failure at end of treatment or study, only one alatrofloxacin patient (*H. influenzae* + *S. pneumoniae*) and one ceftriaxone + erythromycin patient (*Legionella*) had a microbiologically confirmed persistent pathogen at the time of failure with no emergence of resistance in either study.

Nosocomial Pneumonia

Adult patients with clinically and radiologically documented nosocomial pneumonia participated in a randomized, multicenter, double-blind, double-dummy trial comparing intravenous alatrofloxacin (300 mg once daily for 2 to 7 days) followed by oral trovafloxacin (200 mg once daily) for a total of 7 to 14 days of therapy to intravenous ciprofloxacin (400 mg BID) for 2 to 7 days followed by oral ciprofloxacin (750 mg BID) for a total of 7 to 14 days of therapy with optional blinded clindamycin or metronidazole added to the ciprofloxacin arm if an anaerobic pneumonia was suspected. In subjects with documented Pseudomonas infection or methicillin-resistant *S. aureus*, aztreonam or vancomycin, respectively, could have been added to either treatment regimen.

The clinical success rate (cure + improvement with no need for further antibiotic therapy) at the End of Treatment was 77% (68/88) and 78% (79/101) for TROVAN and ciprofloxacin, respectively. The clinical success rate at the End of Study (Day 30) was 69% (50/72) and 68% (54/79) for TROVAN and ciprofloxacin, respectively.

	End of Treatment		End of Study	
Pathogen	Trovafloxacin 100 mg	Clarithromycin 500 mg BID	Trovafloxacin 100 mg	Clarithromycin 500 mg BID
H. influenzae	92% (24/26)	89% (16/18)	92% (24/26)	44% (7/16)*
M. catarrhalis	78% (14/18)	80% (16/20)	71% (12/17)	74% (14/19)
S. pneumoniae	100% (7/7)	91% (10/11)	86% (6/7)	91% (10/11)
H. parainfluenzae	100% (6/6)	86% (6/7)	100% (6/6)	86% (6/7)
S. aureus	93% (13/14)	83% (10/12)	85% (11/13)	75% (9/12)

* p=0.001

	End of Treatment		End of Study	
Pathogen	TROVAN	Comparators	TROVAN	Comparators
S. pneumoniae	89% (63/71)	95% (62/65)	87% (55/63)	91% (50/55)
H. influenzae	97% (35/36)	94% (46/49)	90% (28/31)	94% (44/47)
M. catarrhalis	100% (8/8)	100% (4/4)	100% (6/6)	100% (4/4)
S. aureus	100% (8/8)	93% (13/14)	100% (6/6)	91% (10/11)
K. pneumoniae	100% (3/3)	89% (8/9)	100% (3/3)	86% (6/7)
L. pneumophila	77% (10/13)	86% (12/14)	75% (9/12)	86% (12/14)
M. pneumoniae	100% (20/20)	87% (13/15)	94% (17/18)	79% (11/14)
C. pneumoniae	75% (6/8)	100% (18/18)	67% (4/6)	94% (16/17)

	End of Treatment		End of Study	
Pathogen	TROVAN	Ciprofloxacin	TROVAN	Ciprofloxacin
P. aeruginosa	67% (10/15)	55% (6/11)	62% (8/13)	25% (2/8)
H. influenzae	88% (7/8)	89% (8/9)	83% (5/6)	86% (6/7)
E. coli	71% (5/7)	80% (4/5)	50% (3/6)	80% (4/5)
S. aureus	64% (7/11)	80% (8/10)	50% (4/8)	67% (4/6)

	End of Treatment		End of Study	
Pathogen	TROVAN	Imipenem/Cila Amox/Clav	TROVAN	Imipenem/Cila Amox/Clav
E. coli	94% (72/77)	90% (52/58)	86% (66/77)	86% (51/59)
Bacteroides fragilis	97% (30/31)	82% (28/34)	84% (26/31)	75% (27/36)
viridans group streptococci	90% (18/20)	83% (19/23)	90% (18/20)	78% (18/23)
Pseudomonas aeruginosa	94% (15/16)	82% (14/17)	88% (14/16)	83% (15/18)
Klebsiella pneumoniae	80% (12/15)	71% (10/14)	67% (10/15)	71% (10/14)
Peptostreptococcus spp.	86% (12/14)	88% (7/8)	79% (11/14)	75% (6/8)
Prevotella spp.	77% (10/13)	50% (2/4)	77% (10/13)	60% (3/5)

The following outcomes are the clinical success rates for the clinically evaluable patient groups by pathogen:
[See third table on previous page]
Of the above patients with clinical failure at end of treatment or study, two alatrofloxacin patients (*S. aureus, P. aeruginosa*) and 4 ciprofloxacin patients (all *P. aeruginosa*) had a microbiologically confirmed persistent pathogen at the time of failure. Three of the 4 ciprofloxacin patients with clinical failure and persistence had emergence of resistance with none on alatrofloxacin.

Complicated Intra-Abdominal Infections
Patients hospitalized with clinically-documented, complicated intra-abdominal infections, including post-surgical infections, participated in a randomized, double-blind, multicenter trial comparing intravenous alatrofloxacin (300 mg once daily) followed by oral trovafloxacin (200 mg once daily) to intravenous imipenem/cilastatin (1g q8h) followed by oral amoxicillin/clavulanic acid (500 mg TID) for a maximum of 14 days of therapy. The clinical success rate (cure + improvement) at the End of Treatment was 88% (136/155) and 86% (122/142) for alatrofloxacin→trovafloxacin and imipenem/cilastatin→amoxicillin/clavulanic acid, respectively. The clinical success rate at the End of Study (Day 30) was 83% (129/156) and 84% (127/152) for alatrofloxacin→trovafloxacin and imipenem/cilastatin→amoxicillin/clavulanic acid, respectively.
The following are the clinical success rates for the clinically evaluable patient groups by pathogen:
[See fourth table on previous page]
Of patients with a baseline pathogen and a clinical response of failure at the End of Study, 9 of 26 on TROVAN and 10 of 21 on imipenem/cilastatin had microbiologically-confirmed persistence of the baseline pathogen with no emergence of resistance in either group.

CAUTION: Federal (USA) law prohibits dispensing without a prescription.

REFERENCES:
1. National Committee for Clinical Laboratory Standards, Methods for Dilution Antimicrobial Susceptibility Tests for Bacteria That Grow Aerobically—Fourth Edition; Approved Standard, NCCLS Document M7-A4, Vol. 17, No. 2, NCCLS, Villanova, PA, January, 1997.
2. National Committee for Clinical Laboratory Standards. Performance Standards for Antimicrobial Disk Susceptibility Tests—Sixth Edition; Approved Standard, NCCLS Document M2-A6, Vol. 17, No. 1, NCCLS, Villanova, PA, January, 1997.
3. National Committee for Clinical Laboratory Standards. Methods for Antimicrobial Susceptibility Testing of Anaerobic Bacteria—Third Edition; Approved Standard, NCCLS Document M11-A3, Vol. 13, No. 26, NCCLS, Villanova, PA, December, 1993.

U.S. Patent No. 5,164,402 © 1997 Pfizer Inc
69-5328-00-0 Issued December 1997
Shown in Product Identification Guide, page 331

UNASYN® ℞
(ampicillin sodium/sulbactam sodium)

DESCRIPTION
UNASYN is an injectable antibacterial combination consisting of the semisynthetic antibiotic ampicillin sodium and the beta-lactamase inhibitor sulbactam sodium for intravenous and intramuscular administration.
Ampicillin sodium is derived from the penicillin nucleus, 6-aminopenicillanic acid. Chemically, it is monosodium (2S, 5R, 6R)-6-[(R)-2-amino-2-phenylacetamido]-3,3-dimethyl-7-oxo-4-thia-1-azabicyclo[3.2.0]heptane-2-carboxylate and has a molecular weight of 371.39. Its chemical formula is $C_{16}H_{18}N_3NaO_4S$. The structural formula is:

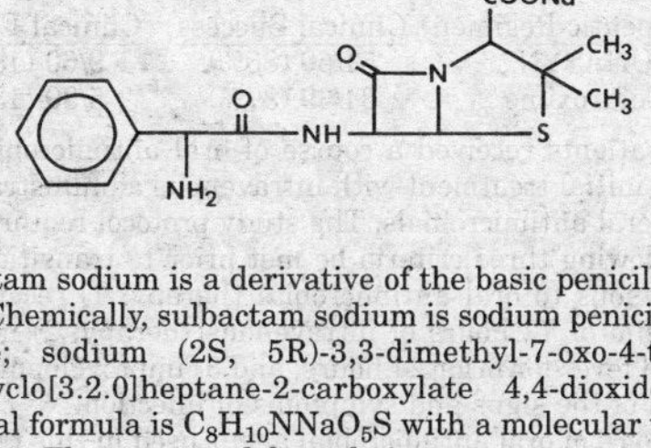

Sulbactam sodium is a derivative of the basic penicillin nucleus. Chemically, sulbactam sodium is sodium penicillinate sulfone; sodium (2S, 5R)-3,3-dimethyl-7-oxo-4-thia-1-azabicyclo[3.2.0]heptane-2-carboxylate 4,4-dioxide. Its chemical formula is $C_8H_{10}NNaO_5S$ with a molecular weight of 255.22. The structural formula is:

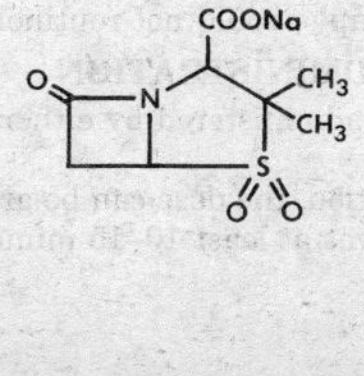

UNASYN, ampicillin sodium/sulbactam sodium parenteral combination, is available as a white to off-white dry powder for reconstitution. UNASYN dry powder is freely soluble in aqueous diluents to yield pale yellow to yellow solutions containing ampicillin sodium and sulbactam sodium equivalent to 250 mg ampicillin per mL and 125 mg sulbactam per mL. The pH of the solutions is between 8.0 and 10.0.
Dilute solutions (up to 30 mg ampicillin and 15 mg sulbactam per mL) are essentially colorless to pale yellow. The pH of dilute solutions remains the same.
1.5 g of UNASYN (1 g ampicillin as the sodium salt plus 0.5 g sulbactam as the sodium salt) parenteral contains approximately 115 mg (5 mEq) of sodium.
3 g of UNASYN (2 g ampicillin as the sodium salt plus 1 g sulbactam as the sodium salt) parenteral contains approximately 230 mg (10 mEq) of sodium.

CLINICAL PHARMACOLOGY
General: Immediately after completion of a 15-minute intravenous infusion of UNASYN, peak serum concentrations of ampicillin and sulbactam are attained. Ampicillin serum levels are similar to those produced by the administration of equivalent amounts of ampicillin alone. Peak ampicillin serum levels ranging from 109 to 150 mcg/mL are attained after administration of 2000 mg of ampicillin plus 1000 mg sulbactam and 40 to 71 mcg/mL after administration of 1000 mg ampicillin plus 500 mg sulbactam. The corresponding mean peak serum levels for sulbactam range from 48 to 88 mcg/mL and 21 to 40 mcg/mL, respectively. After an intramuscular injection of 1000 mg ampicillin plus 500 mg sulbactam, peak ampicillin serum levels ranging from 8 to 37 mcg/mL and peak sulbactam serum levels ranging from 6 to 24 mcg/mL are attained.
The mean serum half-life of both drugs is approximately 1 hour in healthy volunteers.
Approximately 75 to 85% of both ampicillin and sulbactam are excreted unchanged in the urine during the first 8 hours after administration of UNASYN to individuals with normal renal function. Somewhat higher and more prolonged serum levels of ampicillin and sulbactam can be achieved with the concurrent administration of probenecid.
In patients with impaired renal function the elimination kinetics of ampicillin and sulbactam are similarly affected, hence the ratio of one to the other will remain constant whatever the renal function. The dose of UNASYN in such patients should be administered less frequently in accordance with the usual practice for ampicillin (see Dosage and Administration).
Ampicillin has been found to be approximately 28% reversibly bound to human serum protein and sulbactam approximately 38% reversibly bound.
The following average levels of ampicillin and sulbactam were measured in the tissues and fluids listed:

TABLE A
Concentration of UNASYN in Various Body Tissues and Fluids

Fluid or Tissue	Dose (grams) Ampicillin/ Sulbactam	Concentration (mcg/mL or mcg/g) Ampicillin Sulbactam
Peritoneal Fluid	0.5/0.5 IV	7/14
Blister Fluid (Cantharides)	0.5/0.5 IV	8/20
Tissue Fluid	1/0.5 IV	8/4
Intestinal Mucosa	0.5/0.5 IV	11/18
Appendix	2/1 IV	3/40

Penetration of both ampicillin and sulbactam into cerebrospinal fluid in the presence of inflamed meninges has been demonstrated after IV administration of UNASYN.

MICROBIOLOGY
Ampicillin is similar to benzyl penicillin in its bactericidal action against susceptible organisms during the stage of active multiplication. It acts through the inhibition of cell wall mucopeptide biosynthesis. Ampicillin has a broad spectrum of bactericidal activity against many gram-positive and gram-negative aerobic and anaerobic bacteria. (Ampicillin is, however, degraded by beta-lactamases and therefore the spectrum of activity does not normally include organisms which produce these enzymes.)
A wide range of beta-lactamases found in microorganisms resistant to penicillins and cephalosporins have been shown in biochemical studies with cell free bacterial systems to be irreversibly inhibited by sulbactam. Although sulbactam alone possesses little useful antibacterial activity except against the *Neisseriaciae,* whole organism studies have shown that sulbactam restores ampicillin activity against beta-lactamase producing strains. In particular, sulbactam has good inhibitory activity against the clinically important plasmid mediated beta-lactamases most frequently responsible for transferred drug resistance. Sulbactam has no effect on the activity of ampicillin against ampicillin susceptible strains.
The presence of sulbactam in the UNASYN formulation effectively extends the antibiotic spectrum of ampicillin to include many bacteria normally resistant to it and to other beta-lactam antibiotics. Thus, UNASYN possesses the properties of a broad-spectrum antibiotic and a beta-lactamase inhibitor.
While *in vitro* studies have demonstrated the susceptibility of most strains of the following organisms, clinical efficacy for infections other than those included in the indications section has not been documented.
Gram-Positive Bacteria: *Staphylococcus aureus* (beta-lactamase and non-beta-lactamase producing), *Staphylococcus epidermidis* (beta-lactamase and non-beta-lactamase producing), *Staphylococcus saprophyticus* (beta-lactamase and non-beta-lactamase producing), *Streptococcus faecalis*† (Enterococcus), *Streptococcus pneumoniae*† (formerly *D. pneumoniae), Streptococcus pyogenes*†, *Streptococcus viridans*†.
Gram-Negative Bacteria: *Hemophilus influenzae* (beta-lactamase and non-beta-lactamase producing). *Moraxella (Branhamella) catarrhalis* (beta-lactamase and non-beta-lactamase producing). *Escherichia coli* (beta-lactamase and non-beta-lactamase producing). *Klebsiella* species (all known strains are beta-lactamase producing). *Proteus mirabilis* (beta-lactamase and non-beta-lactamase producing). *Proteus vulgaris, Providencia rettgeri, Providencia stuartii, Morganella morganii,* and *Neisseria gonorrhoeae* (beta-lactamase and non-beta-lactamase producing).
Anaerobes: *Clostridium* species†, *Peptococcus* species†, *Peptostreptococcus* species, *Bacteroides* species, including *B. fragilis*.
†These are not beta-lactamase producing strains and, therefore, are susceptible to ampicillin alone.

Susceptibility Testing
Diffusion Technique: For the Kirby-Bauer method of susceptibility testing, a 20 mcg (10 mcg ampicillin + 10 mcg sulbactam) diffusion disk should be used. The method is one outlined in the NCCLS publication M2-A4.[1] With this procedure, a report from the laboratory of "Susceptible" indicates that the infecting organism is likely to respond to UNASYN therapy and a report of "Resistant" indicates that the infecting organism is not likely to respond to therapy. An "Intermediate" susceptibility report suggests that the infecting organism would be susceptible to UNASYN if a higher dosage is used or if the infection is confined to tissues or fluids (e.g., urine) in which high antibiotic levels are attained.
Dilution Techniques: Broth or agar dilution methods may be used to determine the minimal inhibitory concentration (MIC) value for susceptibility of bacterial isolates to ampicillin/sulbactam. The method used is one outlined in the NCCLS publication M7-A2.[2] Tubes should be inoculated to contain 10^5 to 10^6 organisms/mL or plates "spotted" with 10^4 organisms.
The recommended dilution method employs a constant ampicillin/sulbactam ratio of 2:1 in all tubes with increasing concentrations of ampicillin. MIC's are reported in terms of ampicillin concentration in the presence of sulbactam at a constant 2 parts ampicillin to 1 part sulbactam.
[See table at top of next page]

INDICATIONS AND USAGE
UNASYN is indicated for the treatment of infections due to susceptible strains of the designated microorganisms in the conditions listed below.
Skin and Skin Structure Infections caused by beta-lactamase producing strains of *Staphylococcus aureus, Escherichia coli,* Klebsiella* spp.* (including *K. pneumoniae*), Proteus mirabilis,* Bacteroides fragilis,* Enterobacter* spp.,* and *Acinetobacter calcoaceticus.**
NOTE: For information on use in pediatric patients see PRECAUTIONS—Pediatric Use and CLINICAL STUDIES sections.
Intra-Abdominal Infections caused by beta-lactamase producing strains of *Escherichia coli, Klebsiella* spp. (including *K. pneumoniae*), Bacteroides* spp. (including *B. fragilis*), and *Enterobacter* spp.*
Gynecological Infections caused by beta-lactamase producing strains of *Escherichia coli,** and *Bacteroides* spp.* (including *B. fragilis**).
*Efficacy for this organism in this organ system was studied in fewer than 10 infections.
While UNASYN is indicated only for the conditions listed above, infections caused by ampicillin-susceptible organisms are also amenable to treatment with UNASYN due to its ampicillin content. Therefore, mixed infections caused by ampicillin-susceptible organisms and beta-lactamase producing organisms susceptible to UNASYN should not require the addition of another antibiotic.

Continued on next page

Unasyn—Cont.

Appropriate culture and susceptibility tests should be performed before treatment in order to isolate and identify the organisms causing infection and to determine their susceptibility to UNASYN.

Therapy may be instituted prior to obtaining the results from bacteriological and susceptibility studies, when there is reason to believe the infection may involve any of the beta-lactamase producing organisms listed above in the indicated organ systems. Once the results are known, therapy should be adjusted if appropriate.

CONTRAINDICATIONS

The use of UNASYN is contraindicated in individuals with a history of hypersensitivity reactions to any of the penicillins.

WARNINGS

SERIOUS AND OCCASIONALLY FATAL HYPERSENSITIVITY (ANAPHYLACTIC) REACTIONS HAVE BEEN REPORTED IN PATIENTS ON PENICILLIN THERAPY. THESE REACTIONS ARE MORE APT TO OCCUR IN INDIVIDUALS WITH A HISTORY OF PENICILLIN HYPERSENSITIVITY AND/OR HYPERSENSITIVITY REACTIONS TO MULTIPLE ALLERGENS. THERE HAVE BEEN REPORTS OF INDIVIDUALS WITH A HISTORY OF PENICILLIN HYPERSENSITIVITY WHO HAVE EXPERIENCED SEVERE REACTIONS WHEN TREATED WITH CEPHALOSPORINS. BEFORE THERAPY WITH A PENICILLIN, CAREFUL INQUIRY SHOULD BE MADE CONCERNING PREVIOUS HYPERSENSITIVITY REACTIONS TO PENICILLINS, CEPHALOSPORINS, AND OTHER ALLERGENS. IF AN ALLERGIC REACTION OCCURS, UNASYN SHOULD BE DISCONTINUED AND THE APPROPRIATE THERAPY INSTITUTED.

SERIOUS ANAPHYLACTOID REACTIONS REQUIRE IMMEDIATE EMERGENCY TREATMENT WITH EPINEPHRINE. OXYGEN, INTRAVENOUS STEROIDS, AND AIRWAY MANAGEMENT, INCLUDING INTUBATION, SHOULD ALSO BE ADMINISTERED AS INDICATED.

Pseudomembranous colitis has been reported with nearly all antibacterial agents, including UNASYN, and has ranged in severity from mild to life-threatening. Therefore, it is important to consider this diagnosis in patients who present with diarrhea subsequent to the administration of antibacterial agents.

Treatment with antibacterial agents alters the normal flora of the colon and may permit overgrowth of clostridia. Studies indicate that toxin produced by *Clostridium difficile* is one primary cause of "antibiotic-associated colitis."

Mild cases of pseudomembranous colitis usually respond to drug discontinuation alone. In moderate to severe cases, consideration should be given to management with fluids and electrolytes, protein supplementation and treatment with an antibacterial drug clinically effective against *C. difficile* colitis.

PRECAUTIONS

General: A high percentage of patients with mononucleosis who receive ampicillin develop a skin rash. Thus, ampicillin-class antibiotics should not be administered to patients with mononucleosis. In patients treated with UNASYN the possibility of superinfections with mycotic or bacterial pathogens should be kept in mind during therapy. If superinfections occur (usually involving *Pseudomonas* or *Candida*), the drug should be discontinued and/or appropriate therapy instituted.

Drug Interactions: Probenecid decreases the renal tubular secretion of ampicillin and sulbactam. Concurrent use of probenecid with UNASYN may result in increased and prolonged blood levels of ampicillin and sulbactam. The concurrent administration of allopurinol and ampicillin increases substantially the incidence of rashes in patients receiving both drugs as compared to patients receiving ampicillin alone. It is not known whether this potentiation of ampicillin rashes is due to allopurinol or the hyperuricemia present in these patients. There are no data with UNASYN and allopurinol administered concurrently. UNASYN and aminoglycosides should not be reconstituted together due to the *in vitro* inactivation of aminoglycosides by the ampicillin component of UNASYN.

Drug/Laboratory Test Interactions: Administration of UNASYN will result in high urine concentration of ampicillin. High urine concentrations of ampicillin may result in false positive reactions when testing for the presence of glucose in urine using Clinitest™, Benedict's Solution or Fehling's Solution. It is recommended that glucose tests based on enzymatic glucose oxidase reactions (such as Clinistix™ or Testape™) be used. Following administration of ampicillin to pregnant women, a transient decrease in plasma concentration of total conjugated estriol, estriol-glucuronide, conjugated estrone and estradiol has been noted. This effect may also occur with UNASYN.

Carcinogenesis, Mutagenesis, Impairment of Fertility: Long-term studies in animals have not been performed to evaluate carcinogenic or mutagenic potential.

Recommended ampicillin/sulbactam, Susceptibility Ranges [1,2,3]

	Resistant	Intermediate	Susceptible
Gram(−) and Staphylococcus			
Bauer/Kirby Zone Sizes	≤11 mm	12–13 mm	≥14 mm
MIC (mcg of ampicillin/mL)	≥32	16	≤ 8
Hemophilus influenzae			
Bauer/Kirby Zone Sizes	≤19	—	≥20
MIC (mcg of ampicillin/mL)	≥ 4	—	≤ 2

[1]The non-beta-lactamase producing organisms which are normally susceptible to ampicillin, such as *Streptococci,* will have similar zone sizes as for ampicillin disks.
[2]*Staphylococci* resistant to methicillin, oxacillin, or nafcillin must be considered resistant to UNASYN.
[3]The quality control cultures should have the following assigned daily ranges for ampicillin/sulbactam:

		Disks	Mode MIC (mcg/mL ampicillin/mcg/mL sulbactam)
E. coli	(ATCC 25922)	20–24 mm	2/1
S. aureus	(ATCC 25923)	29–37 mm	0.12/0.06
E. coli	(ATCC 35218)	13–19 mm	8/4

Pregnancy

Pregnancy Category B: Reproduction studies have been performed in mice, rats, and rabbits at doses up to ten (10) times the human dose and have revealed no evidence of impaired fertility or harm to the fetus due to UNASYN. There are, however, no adequate and well controlled studies in pregnant women. Because animal reproduction studies are not always predictive of human response, this drug should be used during pregnancy only if clearly needed. (See—Drug/Laboratory Test Interactions.)

Labor and Delivery: Studies in guinea pigs have shown that intravenous administration of ampicillin decreased the uterine tone, frequency of contractions, height of contractions, and duration of contractions. However, it is not known whether the use of UNASYN in humans during labor or delivery has immediate or delayed adverse effects on the fetus, prolongs the duration of labor, or increases the likelihood that forceps delivery or other obstetrical intervention or resuscitation of the newborn will be necessary.

Nursing Mothers: Low concentrations of ampicillin and sulbactam are excreted in the milk; therefore, caution should be exercised when UNASYN is administered to a nursing woman.

Pediatric Use: The safety and effectiveness of UNASYN have been established for pediatric patients one year of age and older for skin and skin structure infections as approved in adults. Use of UNASYN in pediatric patients is supported by evidence from adequate and well-controlled studies in adults with additional data from pediatric pharmacokinetic studies, a controlled clinical trial conducted in pediatric patients and post-marketing adverse events surveillance. (See **CLINICAL PHARMACOLOGY, INDICATIONS AND USAGE, ADVERSE REACTIONS, DOSAGE AND ADMINISTRATION**, and **CLINICAL STUDIES** sections.)

The safety and effectiveness of UNASYN have not been established for pediatric patients for intra-abdominal infections.

ADVERSE REACTIONS

UNASYN is generally well tolerated. The following adverse reactions have been reported.

Local Adverse Reactions

Pain at IM injection site—16%
Pain at IV injection site—3%
Thrombophlebitis—3%

Systemic Adverse Reactions

The most frequently reported adverse reactions were diarrhea in 3% of the patients and rash in less than 2% of the patients.

Additional systemic reactions reported in less than 1% of the patients were: itching, nausea, vomiting, candidiasis, fatigue, malaise, headache, chest pain, flatulence, abdominal distension, glossitis, urine retention, dysuria, edema, facial swelling, erythema, chills, tightness in throat, substernal pain, epistaxis and mucosal bleeding.

Pediatric Patients: Available safety data for pediatric patients treated with UNASYN demonstrate a similar adverse events profile to those observed in adult patients. Additionally, atypical lymphocytosis has been observed in one pediatric patient receiving UNASYN.

Adverse Laboratory Changes

Adverse laboratory changes without regard to drug relationship that were reported during clinical trials were:

Hepatic: Increased AST (SGOT), ALT (SGPT), alkaline phosphatase, and LDH.

Hematologic: Decreased hemoglobin, hematocrit, RBC, WBC, neutrophils, lymphocytes, platelets and increased lymphocytes, monocytes, basophils, eosinophils, and platelets.

Blood Chemistry: Decreased serum albumin and total proteins.

Renal: Increased BUN and creatinine.

Urinalysis: Presence of RBC's and hyaline casts in urine. The following adverse reactions have been reported with ampicillin-class antibiotics and can also occur with UNASYN.

Gastrointestinal: Gastritis, stomatitis, black "hairy" tongue, and enterocolitis. Onset of pseudomembranous colitis symptoms may occur during or after antibiotic treatment. (See WARNINGS.)

Hypersensitivity Reactions: Urticaria, erythema multiforme, and an occasional case of exfoliative dermatitis have been reported. These reactions may be controlled with antihistamines and, if necessary, systemic corticosteroids. Whenever such reactions occur, the drug should be discontinued, unless the opinion of the physician dictates otherwise. Serious and occasional fatal hypersensitivity (anaphylactic) reactions can occur with a penicillin. (See WARNINGS.)

Hematologic: In addition to the adverse laboratory changes listed above for UNASYN, agranulocytosis has been reported during therapy with penicillins. All of these reactions are usually reversible on discontinuation of therapy and are believed to be hypersensitivity phenomena. Some individuals have developed positive direct Coombs Tests during treatment with UNASYN, as with other beta-lactam antibiotics.

OVERDOSAGE

Neurological adverse reactions, including convulsions, may occur with the attainment of high CSF levels of beta-lactams. Ampicillin may be removed from circulation by hemodialysis. The molecular weight, degree of protein binding and pharmacokinetics profile of sulbactam suggest that this compound may also be removed by hemodialysis.

CLINICAL STUDIES

Skin and Skin Structure Infections in Pediatric Patients: Data from a controlled clinical trial conducted in pediatric patients provided evidence supporting the safety and efficacy of UNASYN for the treatment of skin and skin structure infections. Of 99 pediatric patients evaluable for clinical efficacy, 60 patients received a regimen containing intravenous UNASYN, and 39 patients received a regimen containing intravenous cefuroxime. This trial demonstrated similar outcomes (assessed at an appropriate interval after discontinuation of all antimicrobial therapy) for UNASYN- and cefuroxime-treated patients:

Therapeutic Regimen	Clinical Success	Clinical Failure
UNASYN	51/60 (85%)	9/60 (15%)
Cefuroxime	34/39 (87%)	5/39 (13%)

Most patients received a course of oral antimicrobials following initial treatment with intravenous administration of parenteral antimicrobials. The study protocol required that the following three criteria be met prior to transition from intravenous to oral antimicrobial therapy: 1) receipt of a minimum of 72 hours of intravenous therapy; 2) no documented fever for prior 24 hours; and 3) improvement or resolution of the signs and symptoms of infection.

The choice of oral antimicrobial agent used in this trial was determined by susceptibility testing of the original pathogen, if isolated, to oral agents available. The course of oral antimicrobial therapy should not routinely exceed 14 days.

DOSAGE AND ADMINISTRATION

UNASYN may be administered by either the IV or the IM routes.

For IV administration, the dose can be given by slow intravenous injection over at least 10–15 minutes or can also be

Diluent	Maximum Concentration (mg/mL) UNASYN (Ampicillin/Sulbactam)	Use Periods
Sterile Water for Injection	45 (30/15)	8 hrs @ 25°C
	45 (30/15)	48 hrs @ 4°C
	30 (20/10)	72 hrs @ 4°C
0.9% Sodium Chloride Injection	45 (30/15)	8 hrs @ 25°C
	45 (30/15)	48 hrs @ 4°C
	30 (20/10)	72 hrs @ 4°C
5% Dextrose Injection	30 (20/10)	2 hrs @ 25°C
	30 (20/10)	4 hrs @ 4°C
	3 (2/1)	4 hrs @ 25°C
Lactated Ringer's Injection	45 (30/15)	8 hrs @ 25°C
	45 (30/15)	24 hrs @ 4°C
M/6 Sodium Lactate Injection	45 (30/15)	8 hrs @ 25°C
	45 (30/15)	8 hrs @ 4°C
5% Dextrose in 0.45% Saline	3 (2/1)	4 hrs @ 25°C
	15 (10/5)	4 hrs @ 4°C
10% Invert Sugar	3 (2/1)	4 hrs @ 25°C
	30 (20/10)	3 hrs @ 4°C

delivered, in greater dilutions with 50–100 mL of a compatible diluent as an intravenous infusion over 15–30 minutes. UNASYN may be administered by deep intramuscular injection. (See Preparation for Intramuscular Injection.)

The recommended adult dosage of UNASYN is 1.5 g (1 g ampicillin as the sodium salt plus 0.5 g sulbactam as the sodium salt) to 3 g (2 g ampicillin as the sodium salt plus 1 g sulbactam as the sodium salt) every six hours. This 1.5 to 3 g range represents the total of ampicillin content plus the sulbactam content of UNASYN, and corresponds to a range of 1 g ampicillin/0.5 g sulbactam to 2 g ampicillin/1 g sulbactam. The total dose of sulbactam should not exceed 4 grams per day.

Impaired Renal Function
In patients with impairment of renal function the elimination kinetics of ampicillin and sulbactam are similarly affected, hence the ratio of one to the other will remain constant whatever the renal function. The dose of UNASYN in such patients should be administered less frequently in accordance with the usual practice for ampicillin and according to the following recommendations:

UNASYN Dosage Guide For Patients With Renal Impairment

Creatinine Clearance (mL/min/1.73m²)	Ampicillin/ Sulbactam Half-Life (Hours)	Recommended UNASYN Dosage
≥30	1	1.5–3.0 g q 6h–q 8h
15–29	5	1.5–3.0 g q 12h
5–14	9	1.5–3.0 g q 24h

When only serum creatinine is available, the following formula (based on sex, weight, and age of the patient) may be used to convert this value into creatinine clearance. The serum creatinine should represent a steady state of renal function.

$$\text{Males} \quad \frac{\text{weight (kg)} \times (140-\text{age})}{72 \times \text{serum creatinine}}$$

Females   0.85 × above value

COMPATABILITY, RECONSTITUTION AND STABILITY
UNASYN sterile powder is to be stored at or below 30°C (86°F) prior to reconstitution.

When concomitant therapy with aminoglycosides is indicated, UNASYN and aminoglycosides should be reconstituted and administered separately, due to the *in vitro* inactivation of aminoglycosides by any of the aminopenicillins.

DIRECTIONS FOR USE
General Dissolution Procedures: UNASYN sterile powder for intravenous and intramuscular use may be reconstituted with any of the compatible diluents described in this insert. Solutions should be allowed to stand after dissolution to allow any foaming to dissipate in order to permit visual inspection for complete solubilization.

Preparation for Intravenous Use
1.5 g and 3.0 g Bottles: UNASYN sterile powder in piggyback units may be reconstituted directly to the desired concentrations using any of the following parenteral diluents. Reconstitution of UNASYN, at the specified concentrations, with these diluents provide stable solutions for the time periods indicated in the following table: (After the indicated time periods, any unused portions of solutions should be discarded.)

[See table at top of page]

If piggyback bottles are unavailable, standard vials of UNASYN sterile powder may be used. Initially, the vials may be reconstituted with Sterile Water for Injection to yield solutions containing 375 mg UNASYN per mL (250 mg ampicillin/125 mg sulbactam per mL). An appropriate volume should then be immediately diluted with a suitable parenteral diluent to yield solutions containing 3 to 45 mg UNASYN per mL (2 to 30 mg ampicillin/1 to 15 mg sulbactam per mL).

1.5 g ADD-Vantage® Vials: UNASYN in the ADD-Vantage® system is intended as a single dose for intravenous administration after dilution with the ADD-Vantage® Flexible Diluent Container containing 50 mL, 100 mL or 250 mL of 0.9% Sodium Chloride Injection, USP.

3 g ADD-Vantage® Vials: UNASYN in the ADD-Vantage® system is intended as a single dose for intravenous administration after dilution with the ADD-Vantage® Flexible Diluent Container containing 100 mL or 250 mL of 0.9% Sodium Chloride Injection, USP.

UNASYN in the ADD-Vantage® system is to be reconstituted with 0.9% Sodium Chloride Injection, USP only. See INSTRUCTIONS FOR USE OF THE ADD-Vantage® VIAL. Reconstitution of UNASYN, at the specified concentration, with 0.9% Sodium Chloride Injection, USP provides stable solutions for the time period indicated below:

Diluent	Maximum Concentration (mg/mL) UNASYN (Ampicillin/ Sulbactam)	Use Period
0.9% Sodium Chloride Injection	30 (20/10)	8 hrs @ 25°C

In 0.9% Sodium Chloride Injection, USP
The final diluted solution of UNASYN should be completely administered *within 8 hours* in order to assure proper potency.

Preparation for Intramuscular Injection
1.5 g and 3.0 g Standard Vials: Vials for intramuscular use may be reconstituted with Sterile Water for Injection USP, 0.5% Lidocaine Hydrochloride Injection USP or 2% Lidocaine Hydrochloride Injection USP. Consult the following table for recommended volumes to be added to obtain solutions containing 375 mg UNASYN per mL (250 mg ampicillin/125 mg sulbactam per mL). Note: *Use only freshly prepared solutions and administer within one hour after preparation.*

UNASYN Vial Size	Volume of Diluent to be Added	Withdrawal Volume*
1.5 g	3.2 mL	4.0 mL
3.0 g	6.4 mL	8.0 mL

*There is sufficient excess present to allow withdrawal and administration of the stated volumes.

Animal Pharmacology: While reversible glycogenosis was observed in laboratory animals, this phenomenon was dose- and time-dependent and is not expected to develop at the therapeutic doses and corresponding plasma levels attained during the relatively short periods of combined ampicillin/sulbactam therapy in man.

HOW SUPPLIED
UNASYN (ampicillin sodium/sulbactam sodium) is supplied as a sterile off-white dry powder in glass vials and piggyback bottles. The following packages are available:

Vials containing 1.5 g (NDC 0049-0013-83) equivalent of UNASYN (1 g ampicillin as the sodium salt plus 0.5 g sulbactam as the sodium salt)

Vials containing 3 g (NDC 0049-0014-83) equivalent of UNASYN (2 g ampicillin as the sodium salt plus 1 g sulbactam as the sodium salt)

Bottles containing 1.5 g (NDC 0049-0022-83) equivalent of UNASYN (1 g ampicillin as the sodium salt plus 0.5 g sulbactam as the sodium salt)

Bottles containing 3 g (NDC 0049-0023-83) equivalent of UNASYN (2 g ampicillin as the sodium salt plus 1 g sulbactam as the sodium salt)

Pharmacy Bulk Package containing 15 g (NDC 0049-0024-28) equivalent of UNASYN (10 g ampicillin as the sodium salt plus 5 g sulbactam as the sodium salt)

ADD-Vantage® vials containing 1.5 g (NDC 0049-0031-83) equivalent of UNASYN (1 g ampicillin as the sodium salt plus 0.5 g sulbactam as the sodium salt) are distributed by Pfizer Inc.

ADD-Vantage® vials containing 3 g (NDC 0049-0032-83) equivalent of UNASYN (2 g ampicillin as the sodium salt plus 1 g sulbactum as the sodium salt) are distributed by Pfizer Inc.

The 1.5 g UNASYN ADD-Vantage® vials are only to be used with Abbott Laboratories' ADD-Vantage® Flexible Diluent Container containing 0.9% Sodium Chloride Injection, USP, 50 mL, 100 mL, or 250 mL sizes.

The 3 g UNASYN ADD-Vantage® vials are only to be used with Abbott Laboratories' ADD-Vantage® Flexible Diluent Container containing 0.9% Sodium Chloride Injection, USP, 100 mL or 250 mL sizes.

INSTRUCTIONS FOR USE OF THE ADD-Vantage® VIAL
To Open Diluent Container: Peel overwrap from the corner and remove container. Some opacity of the plastic due to moisture absorption during the sterilization process may be observed. This is normal and does not affect the solution quality or safety. The opacity will diminish gradually.

To Assemble Vial and Flexible Diluent Container: (Use Aseptic Technique)
1. Remove the protective covers from the top of the vial and the vial port on the diluent container as follows:
a. To remove the breakaway vial cap, swing the pull ring over the top of the vial and pull down far enough to start the opening (see Figure 1), pull the ring approximately half way around the cap and then pull straight up to remove the cap (see Figure 2).
NOTE: Do not access vial with syringe.

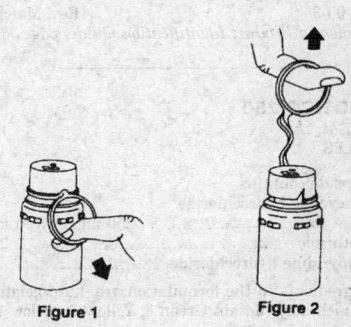

Figure 1   Figure 2

b. To remove the vial port cover, grasp the tab on the pull ring, pull up to break the three tie strings, then pull back to remove the cover. (See Figure 3.)
2. Screw the vial into the vial port until it will go no further. THE VIAL MUST BE SCREWED IN TIGHTLY TO ASSURE A SEAL. This occurs approximately 1/2 turn (180°) after the first audible click. (See Figure 4.) The clicking sound does not assure a seal, the vial must be turned as far as it will go.
NOTE: Once vial is sealed, do not attempt to remove. (See Figure 4.)
3. Recheck the vial to assure that it is tight by trying to turn it further in the direction of assembly.
4. Label appropriately.

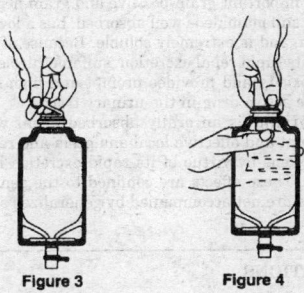

Figure 3   Figure 4

To Prepare Admixture
1. Squeeze the bottom of the diluent container gently to inflate the portion of the container surrounding the end of the drug vial.
2. With the other hand, push the drug vial down into the container telescoping the walls of the container. Grasp the inner cap of the vial through the walls of the container. (See Figure 5.)
3. Pull the inner cap from the drug vial. (See Figure 6.) Verify that the rubber stopper has been pulled out, allowing the drug and diluent to mix.
4. Mix container contents thoroughly and use within the specified time.
[See figures 5 & 6 at top of next column]

Continued on next page

Unasyn—Cont.

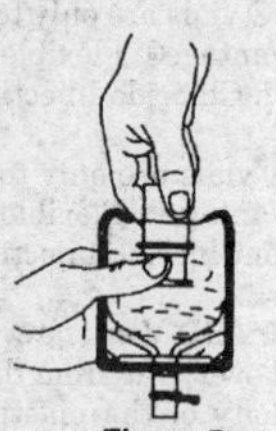

Figure 5

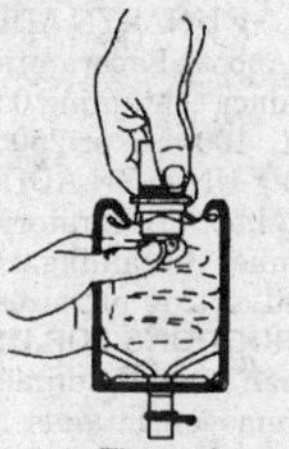

Figure 6

REFERENCES

1. National Committee for Clinical Laboratory Standards, *Performance Standards for Antimicrobial Disk Susceptibility Tests*—Fourth Edition. Approved Standard NCCLS Document M2-A4, Vol. 10, No. 7 NCCLS. Villanova, PA. April 1990.
2. National Committee for Clinical Laboratory Standards, *Methods for Dilution Antimicrobial Susceptibility Tests for Bacteria that Grow Aerobically.* Second Edition. Approved Standard NCCLS Document M7-A2. Vol. 10, No. 8 NCCLS. Villanova, PA. April 1990.

69-4361-00-3 Rev. March 1997

Shown in Product Identification Guide, page 331

UROBIOTIC®-250 ℞

[*u "rō-bī-ot 'ik*]
CAPSULES

Each capsule contains

Oxytetracycline hydrochloride equivalent to	250 mg. oxytetracycline
Sulfamethizole	250 mg
Phenazopyridine hydrochloride	50 mg

Inert ingredients in the formulation are: hard gelatin capsules (which may contain Green 3, Yellow 6, Yellow 10 and other inert ingredients); magnesium stearate; sodium lauryl sulfate; starch.

ACTIONS

Urobiotic-250 is a product designed for use specifically in urinary tract infections.

Terramycin® (oxytetracycline HCl) is a widely used antibiotic with clinically proved activity against gram-positive and gram-negative bacteria, rickettsiae, spirochetes, large viruses, and certain protozoa. Terramycin is well tolerated and well absorbed after oral administration. It diffuses readily through the placenta and is present in the fetal circulation. It diffuses into the pleural fluid, and under some circumstances, into the cerebrospinal fluid. Oxytetracycline HCl appears to be concentrated in the hepatic system and is excreted in the bile. It is excreted in the urine and in the feces, in high concentrations, in a biologically active form.

Sulfamethizole is a chemotherapeutic agent active against a number of important gram-positive and gram-negative bacteria. This sulfonamide is well absorbed, has a low degree of acetylation, and is extremely soluble. Because of these features and its rapid renal excretion, sulfamethizole has a low order of toxicity and provides prompt and high concentrations of the active drug in the urinary tract.

Phenazopyridine is an orally absorbed agent which produces prompt and effective local analgesia and relief of urinary symptoms by virtue of its rapid excretion in the urinary tract. These effects are confined to the genitourinary system and are not accompanied by generalized sedation or narcosis.

INDICATIONS

Based on a review of this drug by the National Academy of Sciences-National Research Council and/or other information, FDA has classified the indications as follows:

"Lacking substantial evidence of effectiveness as a fixed combination":

Urobiotic-250 is indicated in the therapy of a number of genitourinary infections caused by susceptible organisms. These infections include the following: pyelonephritis, pyelitis, ureteritis, cystitis, prostatitis, and urethritis.

Since both Terramycin and sulfamethizole provide effective levels in blood, tissue, and urine, Urobiotic-250 provides a multiple antimicrobial approach at the site of infection. Both antibacterial components are active against the most common urinary pathogens, including *Escherichia coli, Pseudomonas aeruginosa, Aerobacter aerogenes, Streptococcus faecalis, Streptococcus hemolyticus,* and *Micrococcus pyogenes.* Urobiotic-250 is particularly useful in the treatment of infections caused by bacteria more sensitive to the combination than to either component alone. The combination is also of value in those cases with mixed infections, and in those instances where the causative organism is unknown pending laboratory isolation. **Final classification of the less than effective indications requires further investigation. Clinical studies to substantiate the efficacy of Urobiotic-250 are ongoing. Completion of these ongoing studies will provide data for final classification of these indications.**

CONTRAINDICATIONS

This drug is contraindicated in individuals who have shown hypersensitivity to any of its components.

This drug, because of the sulfonamide component, should not be used in patients with a history of sulfonamide sensitivities, and in pregnant females at term.

WARNINGS

If renal impairment exists, even usual oral or parenteral doses may lead to excessive systemic accumulation of the drug and possible liver toxicity. Under such conditions, lower than usual doses are indicated and if therapy is prolonged, tetracycline serum level determinations may be advisable.

Oxytetracycline HCl, which is one of the ingredients of Urobiotic-250, may form a stable calcium complex in any bone-forming tissue with no serious harmful effects reported thus far in humans. However, use of oxytetracycline during tooth development (last trimester of pregnancy, neonatal period and early childhood) may cause discoloration of the teeth (yellow-grey-brownish). This effect occurs mostly during long term use of the drug but it also has been observed in usual short treatment courses.

Because of its sulfonamide content, this drug should be used only after critical appraisal in patients with liver damage, renal damage, urinary obstruction, or blood dyscrasias. Deaths have been reported from hypersensitivity reactions, agranulocytosis, aplastic anemia, and other blood dyscrasias associated with sulfonamide administration. When used intermittently, or for a prolonged period, blood counts and liver and kidney function tests should be performed.

Certain hypersensitive individuals may develop a photodynamic reaction precipitated by exposure to direct sunlight during the use of this drug. This reaction is usually of the photoallergic type which may also be produced by other tetracycline derivatives. Individuals with a history of photosensitivity reactions should be instructed to avoid exposure to direct sunlight while under treatment with this or other tetracycline drugs, and treatment should be discontinued at first evidence of skin discomfort.

NOTE: Reactions of a photoallergic nature are exceedingly rare with Terramycin (oxytetracycline HCl). Phototoxic reactions are not believed to occur with Terramycin.

PRECAUTIONS

As with all antibiotic preparations, use of this drug may result in overgrowth of nonsusceptible organisms, including fungi. If superinfection occurs, the antibiotic should be discontinued and appropriate specific therapy should be instituted. This drug should be used with caution in persons having histories of significant allergies and/or asthma.

ADVERSE REACTIONS

Glossitis, stomatitis, proctitis, nausea, diarrhea, vaginitis, and dermatitis, as well as reactions of an allergic nature, may occur during oxytetracycline HCl therapy, but are rare. If adverse reactions, individual idiosyncrasy, or allergy occur, discontinue medication. Rare instances of esophagitis and esophageal ulcerations have been reported in patients receiving capsule forms of drugs in the tetracycline class. Most of these patients took medications immediately before going to bed. (See Dosage and Administration.)

With oxytetracycline therapy bulging fontanels in infants and benign intracranial hypertension in adults have been reported in individuals receiving full therapeutic dosages. These conditions disappeared rapidly when the drug was discontinued.

As in all sulfonamide therapy, the following reactions may occur: nausea, vomiting, diarrhea, hepatitis, pancreatitis, blood dyscrasias, neuropathy, drug fever, skin rash, infection of the conjunctiva and sclera, petechiae, purpura, hematuria and crystalluria. The dosage should be decreased or the drug withdrawn, depending upon the severity of the reaction.

DOSAGE AND ADMINISTRATION

Urobiotic-250 is recommended in adults only. A dose of 1 capsule four times daily is suggested. In refractory cases 2 capsules four times a day may be used.

Therapy should be continued for a minimum of seven days or until bacteriologic cure in acute urinary tract infections. Administration of adequate amounts of fluid along with capsule forms of drugs in the tetracycline class is recommended to wash down the drugs and reduce the risk of esophageal irritation and ulceration. (See Adverse Reactions.)

To aid absorption of the drug, it should be given at least one hour before or two hours after eating. Aluminum hydroxide gel given with antibiotics has been shown to decrease their absorption and is contraindicated.

SUPPLY

Urobiotic-250 capsules: bottles of 50 (NDC 0049-0920-50), and unit dose packages of 100 (10 × 10's) (NDC 0049-0920-41).

LITERATURE AVAILABLE

Yes.

70-1636-00-9
Revised Dec. 1986

VIAGRA® ℞

[*vī agra*]
(sildenafil citrate)
Tablets

DESCRIPTION

VIAGRA®, an oral therapy for erectile dysfunction, is the citrate salt of sildenafil, a selective inhibitor of cyclic guanosine monophosphate (cGMP)-specific phosphodiesterase type 5 (PDE5).

Sildenafil citrate is designated chemically as 1-[[3-(6,7-dihydro-1-methyl-7-oxo-3-propyl-1*H*-pyrazolo[4,3-*d*]pyrimidin-5-yl)-4-ethoxyphenyl]sulfonyl]-4-methylpiperazine citrate and has the following structural formula:

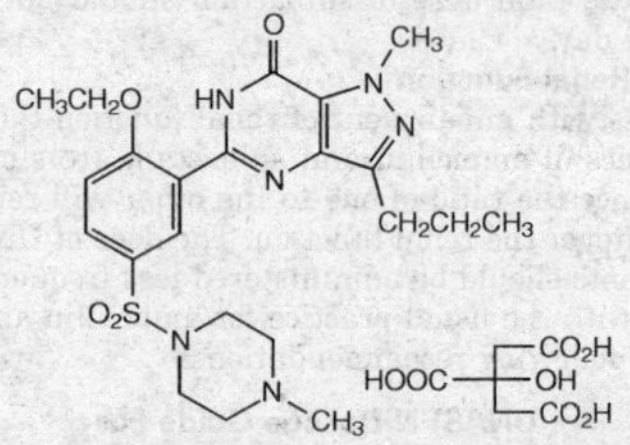

Sildenafil citrate is a white to off-white crystalline powder with a solubility of 3.5 mg/mL in water and a molecular weight of 666.7. VIAGRA (sildenafil citrate) is formulated as blue, film-coated rounded-diamond-shaped tablets equivalent to 25 mg, 50 mg and 100 mg of sildenafil for oral administration. In addition to the active ingredient, sildenafil citrate, each tablet contains the following inactive ingredients: microcrystalline cellulose, anhydrous dibasic calcium phosphate, croscarmellose sodium, magnesium stearate, hydroxypropyl methylcellulose, titanium dioxide, lactose, triacetin, and FD & C Blue #2 aluminum lake.

CLINICAL PHARMACOLOGY

Mechanism of Action

The physiologic mechanism of erection of the penis involves release of nitric oxide (NO) in the corpus cavernosum during sexual stimulation. NO then activates the enzyme guanylate cyclase, which results in increased levels of cyclic guanosine monophosphate (cGMP), producing smooth muscle relaxation in the corpus cavernosum and allowing inflow of blood. Sildenafil has no direct relaxant effect on isolated human corpus cavernosum, but enhances the effect of nitric oxide (NO) by inhibiting phosphodiesterase type 5 (PDE5), which is responsible for degradation of cGMP in the corpus cavernosum. When sexual stimulation causes local release of NO, inhibition of PDE5 by sildenafil causes increased levels of cGMP in the corpus cavernosum, resulting in smooth muscle relaxation and inflow of blood to the corpus cavernosum. Sildenafil at recommended doses has no effect in the absence of sexual stimulation.

Studies *in vitro* have shown that sildenafil is selective for PDE5. Its effect is more potent on PDE5 than on other known phosphodiesterases (>80-fold for PDE1, >1,000-fold for PDE2, PDE3, and PDE4). The approximately 4,000-fold selectivity for PDE5 versus PDE3 is important because that PDE is involved in control of cardiac contractility. Sildenafil is only about 10-fold as potent for PDE5 compared to PDE6, an enzyme found in the retina; this lower selectivity is thought to be the basis for abnormalities related to color vision observed with higher doses or plasma levels (see Pharmacodynamics).

Pharmacokinetics and Metabolism

VIAGRA is rapidly absorbed after oral administration, with absolute bioavailability of about 40%. Its pharmacokinetics are dose-proportional over the recommended dose range. It is eliminated predominantly by hepatic metabolism (mainly cytochrome P450 3A4) and is converted to an active metabolite with properties similar to the parent, sildenafil. Both sildenafil and the metabolite have terminal half lives of about 4 hours.

Absorption and Distribution: VIAGRA is rapidly absorbed. Maximum observed plasma concentrations are reached within 30 to 120 minutes (median 60 minutes) of oral dosing

in the fasted state. When VIAGRA is taken with a high fat meal, the rate of absorption is reduced, with a mean delay in T_{max} of 60 minutes and a mean reduction in C_{max} of 29%. The mean steady state volume of distribution (Vss) for sildenafil is 105 L, indicating distribution into the tissues. Sildenafil and its major circulating N-desmethyl metabolite are both approximately 96% bound to plasma proteins. Protein binding is independent of total drug concentrations. Based upon measurements of sildenafil in semen of healthy volunteers 90 minutes after dosing, less than 0.001% of the administered dose may appear in the semen of patients.

Metabolism and Excretion: Sildenafil is cleared predominantly by the CYP3A4 (major route) and CYP2C9 (minor route) hepatic microsomal isoenzymes. The major circulating metabolite results from N-desmethylation of sildenafil, and is itself further metabolized. This metabolite has a PDE selectivity profile similar to sildenafil and an *in vitro* potency for PDE5 approximately 50% of the parent drug. Plasma concentrations of this metabolite are approximately 40% of those seen for sildenafil, so that the metabolite accounts for about 20% of sildenafil's pharmacologic effects. After either oral or intravenous administration, sildenafil is excreted as metabolites predominantly in the feces (approximately 80% of administered oral dose) and to a lesser extent in the urine (approximately 13% of the administered oral dose). Similar values for pharmacokinetic parameters were seen in normal volunteers and in the patient population, using a population pharmacokinetic approach.

Pharmacokinetics in Special Populations

Geriatrics: Healthy elderly volunteers (65 years or over) had a reduced clearance of sildenafil, with free plasma concentrations approximately 40% greater than those seen in healthy younger volunteers (18–45 years).

Renal insufficiency: In volunteers with mild (CLcr = 50-80 mL/min) and moderate (CLcr = 30-49 mL/min) renal impairment, the pharmacokinetics of a single oral dose of VIAGRA (50 mg) were not altered. In volunteers with severe (CLcr = <30 mL/min) renal impairment, sildenafil clearance was reduced, resulting in approximately doubling of AUC and C_{max} compared to age-matched volunteers with no renal impairment.

Hepatic insufficiency: In volunteers with hepatic cirrhosis (Child-Pugh A and B), sildenafil clearance was reduced, resulting in increases in AUC (84%) and C_{max} (47%) compared to age-matched volunteers with no hepatic impairment.

Pharmacodynamics

In eight double-blind, placebo-controlled crossover studies of patients with either organic or psychogenic erectile dysfunction, sexual stimulation resulted in improved erections, as assessed by penile plethysmography, after VIAGRA administration compared with placebo. Most studies assessed the efficacy of VIAGRA approximately 60 minutes post dose. The erectile response, as assessed by penile plethysmography, generally increased with increasing sildenafil dose and plasma concentration. The time course of effect was examined in one study, showing an effect for up to 4 hours but the response was diminished compared to 2 hours.

Single oral doses of sildenafil up to 100 mg produced no clinically relevant changes in the ECGs of normal male volunteers. Single oral doses of sildenafil (100 mg) produced an average decrease of about 10 mmHg in normals, similar to the effect in patients with ischemic heart disease given 40 mg of sildenafil I.V. Larger but similarly transient effects on blood pressure were recorded among patients receiving concomitant nitrates (see CONTRAINDICATIONS). These effects are possibly related to PDE5 in vascular smooth muscle.

A comprehensive battery of visual function tests was conducted at doses up to twice the maximum recommended dose. Mild, transient, dose-related impairment of color discrimination (blue/green) was detected using the Farnsworth-Munsell 100-hue test, with peak effects near the time of peak plasma levels. This finding is consistent with the inhibition of PDE6, which is involved in phototransduction in the retina. In flexible titration studies of 4 to 26 weeks, 3% of patients on sildenafil reported visual disturbances, described as color tinge or light sensitivity, compared to no such findings in placebo-treated patients.

Clinical Studies

In clinical studies, VIAGRA was assessed for its effect on the ability of men with erectile dysfunction (ED) to engage in sexual activity and in many cases specifically on the ability to achieve and maintain an erection sufficient for satisfactory sexual activity. VIAGRA was evaluated primarily at doses of 25 mg, 50 mg and 100 mg in 21 randomized, double-blind, placebo-controlled trials of up to 6 months in duration, using a variety of study designs (fixed dose, titration, parallel, crossover). VIAGRA was administered to more than 3,000 patients aged 19 to 87 years, with ED of various etiologies (organic, psychogenic, mixed) with a mean duration of 5 years. VIAGRA demonstrated statistically significant improvement compared to placebo in all 21 studies.

The effectiveness of VIAGRA was evaluated in most studies using several assessment instruments. The primary measure in the principal studies was a sexual function questionnaire (the International Index of Erectile Function - IIEF)

administered during a 4-week treatment-free run-in period, at baseline, at follow-up visits, and at the end of double-blind, placebo-controlled, at-home treatment. Two of the questions from the IIEF served as primary study endpoints; categorical responses were elicited to questions about (1) the ability to achieve erections sufficient for sexual intercourse and (2) the maintenance of erections after penetration. Both questions were addressed by the patient at the final visit for the last 4 weeks of the study. The possible categorical responses to these questions were (0) no attempted intercourse, (1) never or almost never, (2) a few times, (3) sometimes, (4) most times, and (5) almost always or always. Also collected as part of the IIEF was information about other aspects of sexual function, including information on erectile function, orgasm, desire, satisfaction with intercourse, and overall sexual satisfaction. Sexual function data were also recorded by patients in a daily diary. In addition, patients were asked a global efficacy question and an optional partner questionnaire was administered.

The effect on one of the major endpoints, maintenance of erections after penetration, is shown in Figure 1, for the pooled results of 5 fixed dose, dose-response studies of greater than one month duration, showing response according to baseline function. Results with all doses have been pooled, but scores showed greater improvement at the 50 and 100 mg doses than at 25 mg. The pattern of responses was similar for the other principal question, the ability to achieve an erection sufficient for intercourse. The titration studies, in which most patients received 100 mg, showed similar results. Figure 1 shows that regardless of the baseline levels of function, subsequent function in patients treated with VIAGRA was better than that seen in patients treated with placebo. At the same time, on-treatment function was better in treated patients who were less impaired at baseline.

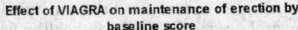

Effect of VIAGRA on maintenance of erection by baseline score

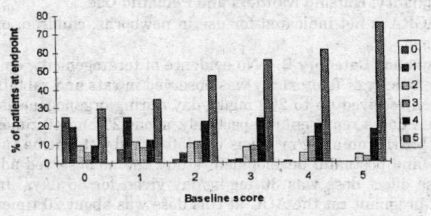

Effect of placebo on maintenance of erection by baseline score

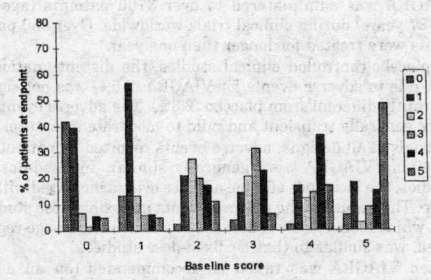

Figure 1. Effect of VIAGRA and placebo on maintenance of erection by baseline score.

The frequency of patients reporting improvement of erections in response to a global question in four of the randomized, double-blind, parallel, placebo-controlled fixed dose studies (1797 patients) of 12 to 24 weeks duration is shown in Figure 2. These patients had erectile dysfunction at baseline that was characterized by median categorical scores of 2 (a few times) on principal IIEF questions. Erectile dysfunction was attributed to organic (58%; generally not characterized, but including diabetes and excluding spinal cord injury), psychogenic (17%), or mixed (24%) etiologies. Sixty-three percent, 74%, and 82% of the patients on 25 mg, 50 mg and 100 mg of VIAGRA, respectively, reported an improvement in their erections, compared to 24% on placebo. In the titration studies (n=644) (with most patients eventually receiving 100 mg), results were similar.

[See figure 2 at top of next column]

The patients in studies had varying degrees of ED. One-third to one-half of the subjects in these studies reported successful intercourse at least once during a 4-week, treatment-free run-in period.

In many of the studies, of both fixed dose and titration designs, daily diaries were kept by patients. In these studies, involving about 1600 patients, analyses of patient diaries showed no effect of VIAGRA on rates of attempted inter-

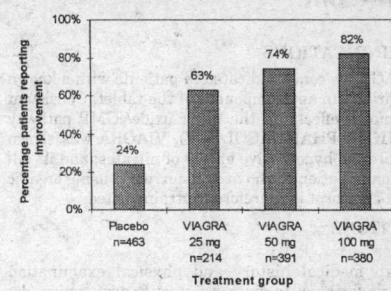

Figure 2. Percentage of Patients Reporting an Improvement in Erections.

course (about 2 per week), but there was clear treatment-related improvement in sexual function: per patient weekly success rates averaged 1.3 on 50–100 mg of VIAGRA vs 0.4 on placebo; similarly, group mean success rates (total successes divided by total attempts) were about 66% on VIAGRA vs about 20% on placebo.

During 3 to 6 months of double-blind treatment or longer-term (1 year), open-label studies, few patients withdrew from active treatment for any reason, including lack of effectiveness. At the end of the long-term study, 88% of patients reported that VIAGRA improved their erections.

Men with untreated ED had relatively low baseline scores for all aspects of sexual function measured (again using a 5-point scale) in the IIEF. VIAGRA improved these aspects of sexual function: frequency, firmness and maintenance of erections; frequency of orgasm; frequency and level of desire; frequency, satisfaction and enjoyment of intercourse; and overall relationship satisfaction.

One randomized, double-blind, flexible-dose, placebo-controlled study included only patients with erectile dysfunction attributed to complications of diabetes mellitus (n=268). As in the other titration studies, patients were started on 50 mg and allowed to adjust the dose up to 100 mg or down to 25 mg of VIAGRA; all patients, however, were receiving 50 mg or 100 mg at the end of the study. There were highly statistically significant improvements on the two principal IIEF questions (frequency of successful penetration during sexual activity and maintenance of erections after penetration) on VIAGRA compared to placebo. On a global improvement question, 57% of VIAGRA patients reported improved erections versus 10% on placebo. Diary data indicated that on VIAGRA, 48% of intercourse attempts were successful versus 12% on placebo.

One randomized, double-blind, placebo-controlled, crossover, flexible-dose (up to 100 mg) study of patients with erectile dysfunction resulting from spinal cord injury (n=178) was conducted. The changes from baseline in scoring on the two end point questions (frequency of successful penetration during sexual activity and maintenance of erections after penetration) were highly statistically significantly in favor of VIAGRA. On a global improvement question, 83% of patients reported improved erections on VIAGRA versus 12% on placebo. Diary data indicated that on VIAGRA, 59% of attempts at sexual intercourse were successful compared to 13% on placebo.

Across all trials, VIAGRA improved the erections of 43% of radical prostatectomy patients compared to 15% on placebo. Subgroup analyses of responses to a global improvement question in patients with psychogenic etiology in two fixed-dose studies (total n=179) and two titration studies (total n=149) showed 84% of VIAGRA patients reported improvement in erections compared with 26% of placebo. The changes from baseline in scoring on the two end point questions (frequency of successful penetration during sexual activity and maintenance of erections after penetration) were highly statistically significantly in favor of VIAGRA. Diary data in two of the studies (n=178) showed rates of successful intercourse per attempt of 70% for VIAGRA and 29% for placebo.

A review of population subgroups demonstrated efficacy regardless of baseline severity, etiology, race and age. VIAGRA was effective in a broad range of ED patients, including those with a history of coronary artery disease, hypertension, other cardiac disease, peripheral vascular disease, diabetes mellitus, depression, coronary artery bypass graft (CABG), radical prostatectomy, trans-urethral resection of the prostate (TURP) and spinal cord injury, and in patients taking anti-depressants/anti-psychotics and anti-hypertensives/diuretics.

INDICATION AND USAGE

VIAGRA is indicated for the treatment of erectile dysfunction. The studies that established benefit demonstrated improvements in success rates for sexual intercourse compared with placebo.

Continued on next page

Viagra—Cont.

CONTRAINDICATIONS

Use of VIAGRA is contraindicated in patients with a known hypersensitivity to any component of the tablet. Consistent with its known effects on the nitric oxide/cGMP pathway (see CLINICAL PHARMACOLOGY), VIAGRA was shown to potentiate the hypotensive effects of nitrates, and its administration to patients who are concurrently using organic nitrates in any form is therefore contraindicated.

PRECAUTIONS

General

A thorough medical history and physical examination should be undertaken to diagnose erectile dysfunction, determine potential underlying causes, and identify appropriate treatment.

There is a degree of cardiac risk associated with sexual activity; therefore, physicians may wish to consider the cardiovascular status of their patients prior to initiating any treatment for erectile dysfunction.

Agents for the treatment of erectile dysfunction should be used with caution in patients with anatomical deformation of the penis (such as angulation, cavernosal fibrosis or Peyronie's disease), or in patients who have conditions which may predispose them to priapism (such as sickle cell anemia, multiple myeloma, or leukemia).

The safety and efficacy of combinations of VIAGRA with other treatments for erectile dysfunction have not been studied. Therefore, the use of such combinations is not recommended.

VIAGRA has no effect on bleeding time when taken alone or with aspirin. In vitro studies with human platelets indicate that sildenafil potentiates the antiaggregatory effect of sodium nitroprusside (a nitric oxide donor). There is no safety information on the administration of VIAGRA to patients with bleeding disorders or active peptic ulceration. Therefore, VIAGRA should be administered with caution to these patients.

A minority of patients with the inherited condition retinitis pigmentosa have genetic disorders of retinal phosphodiesterases. There is no safety information on the administration of VIAGRA to patients with retinitis pigmentosa. Therefore, VIAGRA should be administered with caution to these patients.

Information for Patients

Physicians should discuss with patients the contraindication of VIAGRA with concurrent organic nitrates.

The use of VIAGRA offers no protection against sexually transmitted diseases. Counseling of patients about the protective measures necessary to guard against sexually transmitted diseases, including the Human Immunodeficiency Virus (HIV), may be considered.

Drug Interactions

Effects of Other Drugs on VIAGRA

In vitro studies: Sildenafil metabolism is principally mediated by the cytochrome P450 (CYP) isoforms 3A4 (major route) and 2C9 (minor route). Therefore, inhibitors of these isoenzymes may reduce sildenafil clearance.

In vivo studies: Cimetidine (800 mg), a non-specific CYP inhibitor, caused a 56% increase in plasma sildenafil concentrations when co-administered with VIAGRA (50 mg) to healthy volunteers.

When a single 100 mg dose of VIAGRA was administered with erythromycin, a specific CYP3A4 inhibitor, at steady state (500 mg bid for 5 days), there was a 182% increase in sildenafil systemic exposure (AUC). Stronger CYP3A4 inhibitors such as ketoconazole, itraconazole or mibefradil would be expected to have still greater effects, and population data from patients in clinical trials did indicate a reduction in sildenafil clearance when it was co-administered with CYP3A4 inhibitors (such as ketoconazole, erythromycin, or cimetidine). It can be expected that concomitant administration of CYP3A4 inducers, such as rifampin, will decrease plasma levels of sildenafil.

Single doses of antacid (magnesium hydroxide/aluminum hydroxide) did not affect the bioavailability of VIAGRA.

Pharmacokinetic data from patients in clinical trials showed no effect on sildenafil pharmacokinetics of CYP2C9 inhibitors (such as tolbutamide, warfarin), CYP2D6 inhibitors (such as selective serotonin reuptake inhibitors, tricyclic antidepressants), thiazide and related diuretics, ACE inhibitors, and calcium channel blockers. The AUC of the active metabolite, N-desmethyl sildenafil, was increased 62% by loop and potassium-sparing diuretics and 102% by non-specific beta-blockers. These effects on the metabolite are not expected to be of clinical consequence.

Effects of VIAGRA on Other Drugs

In vitro studies: Sildenafil is a weak inhibitor of the cytochrome P450 isoforms 1A2, 2C9, 2C19, 2D6, 2E1 and 3A4 (IC50 >150 μM). Given sildenafil peak plasma concentrations of approximately 1 μM after recommended doses, it is unlikely that VIAGRA will alter the clearance of substrates of these isoenzymes.

In vivo studies: No significant interactions were shown with tolbutamide (250 mg) or warfarin (40 mg), both of which are metabolized by CYP2C9.

VIAGRA (50 mg) did not potentiate the increase in bleeding time caused by aspirin (150 mg).

VIAGRA (50 mg) did not potentiate the hypotensive effect of alcohol in healthy volunteers with mean maximum blood alcohol levels of 0.08%.

No interaction was seen when VIAGRA (100 mg) was co-administered with amlodipine in hypertensive patients. The mean additional reduction on supine blood pressure (systolic, 8 mmHg; diastolic, 7 mmHg) was of a similar magnitude to that seen when VIAGRA was administered alone to healthy volunteers (see CLINICAL PHARMACOLOGY).

Analysis of the safety database showed no difference in the side effect profile in patients taking VIAGRA with and without anti-hypertensive medication.

Carcinogenesis, Mutagenesis, Impairment of Fertility

Sildenafil was not carcinogenic when administered to rats for 24 months at a dose resulting in total systemic drug exposure (AUCs) for unbound sildenafil and its major metabolite of 29- and 42-times, for male and female rats, respectively, the exposures observed in human males given the Maximum Recommended Human Dose (MRHD) of 100 mg. Sildenafil was not carcinogenic when administered to mice for 18–21 months at dosages up to the Maximum Tolerated Dose (MTD) of 10 mg/kg/day, approximately 0.6 times the MRHD on a mg/m² basis.

Sildenafil was negative in in vitro bacterial and Chinese hamster ovary cell assays to detect mutagenicity, and in vitro human lymphocytes and in vivo mouse micronucleus assays to detect clastogenicity.

There was no impairment of fertility in rats given sildenafil up to 60 mg/kg/day for 36 days to females and 102 days to males, a dose producing an AUC value of more than 25 times the human male AUC.

There was no effect on sperm motility or morphology after single 100 mg oral doses of VIAGRA in healthy volunteers.

Pregnancy, Nursing Mothers and Pediatric Use

VIAGRA is not indicated for use in newborns, children, or women.

Pregnancy Category B. No evidence of teratogenicity, embryotoxicity or fetotoxicity was observed in rats and rabbits which received up to 200 mg/kg/day during organogenesis. These doses represent, respectively, about 20 and 40 times the MRHD on a mg/m² basis in a 50 kg subject. In the rat pre- and postnatal development study, the no observed adverse effect dose was 30 mg/kg/day given for 36 days. In non-pregnant rat the AUC at this dose was about 20 times human AUC. There are no adequate and well-controlled studies of sildenafil in pregnant women.

ADVERSE REACTIONS

VIAGRA was administered to over 3700 patients (aged 19–87 years) during clinical trials worldwide. Over 550 patients were treated for longer than one year.

In placebo-controlled clinical studies, the discontinuation rate due to adverse events for VIAGRA (2.5%) was not significantly different from placebo (2.3%). The adverse events were generally transient and mild to moderate in nature.

In trials of all designs, adverse events reported by patients receiving VIAGRA were generally similar. In fixed-dose studies, the incidence of some adverse events increased with dose. The nature of the adverse events in flexible-dose studies, which more closely reflect the recommended dosage regimen, was similar to that for fixed-dose studies.

When VIAGRA was taken as recommended (on an as-needed basis) in flexible-dose, placebo-controlled clinical trials the following adverse events were reported:

TABLE 1. ADVERSE EVENTS REPORTED BY ≥2% OF PATIENTS TREATED WITH VIAGRA AND MORE FREQUENT ON DRUG THAN PLACEBO IN PRN FLEXIBLE-DOSE PHASE II/III STUDIES

Adverse Event	Percentage of Patients Reporting Event	
	VIAGRA N=734	PLACEBO N=725
Headache	16%	4%
Flushing	10%	1%
Dyspepsia	7%	2%
Nasal Congestion	4%	2%
Urinary Tract Infection	3%	2%
Abnormal Vision†	3%	0%
Diarrhea	3%	1%
Dizziness	2%	1%
Rash	2%	1%

†Abnormal Vision: Mild and transient, predominantly color tinge to vision, but also increased sensitivity to light or blurred vision. In these studies, only one patient discontinued due to abnormal vision.

Other adverse reactions occurred at a rate of >2%, but equally common on placebo: respiratory tract infection, back pain, flu syndrome, and arthralgia.

In fixed-dose studies, dyspepsia (17%) and abnormal vision (11%) were more common at 100 mg than at lower doses. At doses above the recommended dose range, adverse events were similar to those detailed above but generally were reported more frequently.

No cases of priapism were reported.

The following events occurred in < 2% of patients in controlled clinical trials; a causal relationship to VIAGRA is uncertain. Reported events include those with a plausible relation to drug use; omitted are minor events and reports too imprecise to be meaningful:

Body as a whole: face edema, photosensitivity reaction, shock, asthenia, pain, chills, accidental fall, abdominal pain, allergic reaction, chest pain, accidental injury.

Cardiovascular: angina pectoris, AV block, migraine, syncope, tachycardia, palpitation, hypotension, postural hypotension, myocardial ischemia, cerebral thrombosis, cardiac arrest, heart failure, abnormal electrocardiogram, cardiomyopathy.

Digestive: vomiting, glossitis, colitis, dysphagia, gastritis, gastroenteritis, esophagitis, stomatitis, dry mouth, liver function tests abnormal, rectal hemorrhage, gingivitis.

Hemic and Lymphatic: anemia and leukopenia.

Metabolic and Nutritional: thirst, edema, gout, unstable diabetes, hyperglycemia, peripheral edema, hyperuricemia, hypoglycemic reaction, hypernatremia.

Musculoskeletal: arthritis, arthrosis, myalgia, tendon rupture, tenosynovitis, bone pain, myasthenia, synovitis.

Nervous: ataxia, hypertonia, neuralgia, neuropathy, paresthesia, tremor, vertigo, depression, insomnia, somnolence, abnormal dreams, reflexes decreased, hypesthesia.

Respiratory: asthma, dyspnea, laryngitis, pharyngitis, sinusitis, bronchitis, sputum increased, cough increased.

Skin and appendages: urticaria, herpes simplex, pruritus, sweating, skin ulcer, contact dermatitis, exfoliative dermatitis.

Special senses: mydriasis, conjunctivitis, photophobia, tinnitus, eye pain, deafness, ear pain, eye hemorrhage, cataract, dry eyes.

Urogenital: cystitis, nocturia, urinary frequency, breast enlargement, urinary incontinence, abnormal ejaculation, genital edema and anorgasmia.

OVERDOSAGE

In studies with healthy volunteers of single doses up to 800 mg, adverse events were similar to those seen at lower doses but incidence rates were increased.

In cases of overdose, standard supportive measures should be adopted as required. Renal dialysis is not expected to accelerate clearance as sildenafil is highly bound to plasma proteins and it is not eliminated in the urine.

DOSAGE AND ADMINISTRATION

For most patients, the recommended dose is 50 mg taken, as needed, approximately 1 hour before sexual activity. However, VIAGRA may be taken anywhere from 4 hours to 0.5 hour before sexual activity. Based on effectiveness and toleration, the dose may be increased to a maximum recommended dose of 100 mg or decreased to 25 mg. The maximum recommended dosing frequency is once per day.

The following factors are associated with increased plasma levels of sildenafil: age >65 (40% increase in AUC), hepatic impairment (e.g., cirrhosis, 80%), severe renal impairment (creatinine clearance <30 mL/min, 100%), and concomitant use of potent cytochrome P450 3A4 inhibitors (erythromycin, ketoconazole, itraconazole, 200%). Since higher plasma levels may increase both the efficacy and incidence of adverse events, a starting dose of 25 mg should be considered in these patients.

VIAGRA was shown to potentiate the hypotensive effects of nitrates and its administration in patients who use nitric oxide donors or nitrates in any form is therefore contraindicated.

HOW SUPPLIED

VIAGRA® (sildenafil citrate) is supplied as blue, film-coated, rounded-diamond-shaped tablets containing sildenafil citrate equivalent to the nominally indicated amount of sildenafil as follows:

[See table below]

	25 mg	50 mg	100 mg
Obverse	VGR25	VGR50	VGR100
Reverse	PFIZER	PFIZER	PFIZER
Bottle of 30	NDC-0069-4200-30	NDC-0069-4210-30	NDC-0069-4220-30

Recommended Storage: Store at controlled room temperature, 15° to 30°C (59° to 86°F).

Rx only

© 1998 PFIZER INC

Distributed by
Pfizer Labs
Division of Pfizer Inc, NY, NY 10017
70-5485-00-1   Issued May 1998
Shown in Product Identification Guide, page 331

VIBRAMYCIN® Calcium   ℞
[vī-brə 'mīs-ᵊn]
doxycycline calcium
oral suspension
SYRUP

VIBRAMYCIN® Hyclate
[vī-brə 'mīs-ᵊn]
doxycycline hyclate
CAPSULES

VIBRAMYCIN® Monohydrate
[vī-brə 'mīs-ᵊn]
doxycycline monohydrate
for ORAL SUSPENSION

VIBRA–TABS®
[vī-brə 'mīs-ᵊn]
doxycycline hyclate
FILM COATED TABLETS

DESCRIPTION

Vibramycin is a broad-spectrum antibiotic synthetically derived from oxytetracycline, and is available as Vibramycin Monohydrate (doxycycline monohydrate); Vibramycin Hyclate and Vibra-Tabs (doxycycline hydrochloride hemiethanolate hemihydrate); and Vibramycin Calcium (doxycycline calcium) for oral administration.

The structural formula of doxycycline monohydrate is

with a molecular formula of $C_{22}H_{24}N_2O_8 \cdot H_2O$ and a molecular weight of 462.46. The chemical designation for doxycycline is 4-(Dimethylamino)-1, 4, 4a, 5, 5a, 6, 11, 12a-octahydro-3, 5, 10, 12, 12a-pentahydroxy-6-methyl-1, 11-dioxo-2-naphthacenecarboxamide monohydrate. The molecular formula for doxycycline hydrochloride hemiethanolate hemihydrate is $(C_{22}H_{24}N_2O_8 \cdot HCl)_2 \cdot C_2H_6O \cdot H_2O$ and the molecular weight is 1025.89. Doxycycline is a light-yellow crystalline powder. Doxycycline hyclate is soluble in water, while doxycycline monohydrate is very slightly soluble in water.

Doxycycline has a high degree of lipoid solubility and a low affinity for calcium binding. It is highly stable in normal human serum. Doxycycline will not degrade into an epianhydro form.

Inert ingredients in the syrup formulation are: apple flavor; butylparaben; calcium chloride; carmine; glycerin; hydrochloric acid; magnesium aluminum silicate; povidone; propylene glycol; propylparaben; raspberry flavor; simethicone emulsion; sodium hydroxide; sodium metabisulfite; sorbitol solution; water.

Inert ingredients in the capsule formulations are: hard gelatin capsules (which may contain Blue 1 and other inert ingredients); magnesium stearate; microcrystalline cellulose; sodium lauryl sulfate.

Inert ingredients for the oral suspension formulation are: carboxymethylcellulose sodium; Blue 1; methylparaben; microcrystalline cellulose; propylparaben; raspberry flavor; Red 28; simethicone emulsion; sucrose.

Inert ingredients for the tablet formulation are: ethylcellulose; hydroxypropyl methylcellulose; magnesium stearate; microcrystalline cellulose; propylene glycol; sodium lauryl sulfate; talc; titanium dioxide; Yellow 6 Lake.

CLINICAL PHARMACOLOGY

Tetracyclines are readily absorbed and are bound to plasma proteins in varying degree. They are concentrated by the liver in the bile, and excreted in the urine and feces at high concentrations and in a biologically active form. Doxycycline is virtually completely absorbed after oral administration. Following a 200 mg dose, normal adult volunteers averaged peak serum levels of 2.6 mcg/mL of doxycycline at 2 hours decreasing to 1.45 mcg/mL at 24 hours. Excretion of doxycycline by the kidney is about 40%/72 hours in individuals with normal function (creatinine clearance about 75 mL/min.). This percentage excretion may fall as low as 1–5%/72

hours in individuals with severe renal insufficiency (creatinine clearance below 10 mL/min.). Studies have shown no significant difference in serum half-life of doxycycline (range 18–22 hours) in individuals with normal and severely impaired renal function.

Hemodialysis does not alter serum half-life.

Results of animal studies indicate that tetracyclines cross the placenta and are found in fetal tissues.

Microbiology

The tetracyclines are primarily bacteriostatic and are thought to exert their antimicrobial effect by the inhibition of protein synthesis. The tetracyclines, including doxycycline, have a similar antimicrobial spectrum of activity against a wide range of gram-positive and gram-negative organisms. Cross-resistance of these organisms to tetracyclines is common.

Gram-Negative Bacteria
Neisseria gonorrhoeae
Calymmatobacterium granulomatis
Haemophilus ducreyi
Haemophilus influenzae
Yersinia pestis (formerly *Pasteurella pestis*)
Francisella tularensis (formerly *Pasteurella tularensis*)
Vibrio cholera (formerly *Vibrio comma*)
Bartonella bacilliformis
Brucella species

Because many strains of the following groups of gram-negative microorganisms have been shown to be resistant to tetracyclines, culture and susceptibility testing are recommended:
Escherichia coli
Klebsiella species
Enterobacter aerogenes
Shigella species
Acinetobacter species (formerly *Mima* species and *Herellea* species)
Bacteroides species

Gram-Positive Bacteria
Because many strains of the following groups of gram-positive microorganisms have been shown to be resistant to tetracycline, culture and susceptibility testing are recommended. Up to 44 percent of strains of *Streptococcus pyogenes* and 74 percent of *Streptococcus faecalis* have been found to be resistant to tetracycline drugs. Therefore, tetracycline should not be used for streptococcal disease unless the organism has been demonstrated to be susceptible.
Streptococcus pyogenes
Streptococcus pneumoniae
Enterococcus group (*Streptococcus faecalis* and *Streptococcus faecium*)
Alpha-hemolytic streptococci (viridans group)

Other Microorganisms
Rickettsiae
Chlamydia psittaci
Chlamydia trachomatis
Mycoplasma pneumoniae
Ureaplasma urealyticum
Borrelia recurrentis
Treponema pallidum
Treponema pertenue
Clostridium species
Fusobacterium fusiforme
Actinomyces species
Bacillus anthracis
Propionbacterium acnes
Entamoeba species
Balantidium coli
Plasmodium falciparum

Doxycycline has been found to be active against the asexual erythrocytic forms of *Plasmodium falciparum* but not against the gametocytes of *P. falciparum*. The precise mechanism of action of the drug is not known.

Susceptibility tests: Diffusion techniques: Quantitative methods that require measurement of zone diameters give the most precise estimate of the susceptibility of bacteria to antimicrobial agents. One such standard procedure[1] which has been recommended for use with disks to test susceptibility of organisms to doxycycline uses the 30-mcg tetracycline-class disk or the 30-mcg doxycycline disk. Interpretation involves the correlation of the diameter obtained in the disk test with the minimum inhibitory concentration (MIC) for tetracycline or doxycycline, respectively.

Reports from the laboratory giving results of the standard single-disk susceptibility test with a 30-mcg tetracycline-class disk or the 30-mcg doxycycline disk should be interpreted according to the following criteria:

Zone Diameter (mm)		Interpretation
tetracycline	doxycycline	
≥19	≥16	Susceptible
15–18	13–15	Intermediate
≤14	≤12	Resistant

A report of "Susceptible" indicates that the pathogen is likely to be inhibited by generally achievable blood levels. A report of "Intermediate" suggests that the organism would be susceptible if a high dosage is used or if the infection is

confined to tissues and fluids in which high antimicrobial levels are attained. A report of "Resistant" indicates that achievable concentrations are unlikely to be inhibitory, and other therapy should be selected.

Standardized procedures require the use of laboratory control organisms. The 30-mcg tetracycline-class disk or the 30-mcg doxycycline disk should give the following zone diameters:

Organism	Zone Diameter (mm)	
	tetracycline	doxycycline
E. coli ATCC 25922	18–25	18–24
S. aureus ATCC 25923	19–28	23–29

Dilution techniques: Use a standardized dilution method[2] (broth, agar, microdilution) or equivalent with tetracycline powder. The MIC values obtained should be interpreted according to the following criteria:

MIC (mcg/mL)	Interpretation
≤4	Susceptible
8	Intermediate
≥16	Resistant

As with standard diffusion techniques, dilution methods require the use of laboratory control organisms. Standard tetracycline powder should provide the following MIC values:

Organism	MIC (mcg/mL)
E. coli ATCC 25922	1.0–4.0
S. aureus ATCC 29213	0.25–1.0
E. faecalis ATCC 29212	8–32
P. aeruginosa ATCC 27853	8–32

INDICATIONS AND USAGE

Treatment:
Doxycycline is indicated for the treatment of the following infections:

Rocky mountain spotted fever, typhus fever and the typhus group, Q fever, rickettsialpox, and tick fevers caused by Rickettsiae.

Respiratory tract infections caused by *Mycoplasma pneumoniae*.

Lymphogranuloma venereum caused by *Chlamydia trachomatis*.

Psittacosis (ornithosis) caused by *Chlamydia psittaci*.

Trachoma caused by *Chlamydia trachomatis*, although the infectious agent is not always eliminated as judged by immunofluorescence.

Inclusion conjunctivitis caused by *Chlamydia trachomatis*.

Uncomplicated urethral, endocervical or rectal infections in adults caused by *Chlamydia trachomatis*.

Nongonococcal urethritis caused by *Ureaplasma urealyticum*.

Relapsing fever due to *Borrelia recurrentis*.

Doxycycline is also indicated for the treatment of infections caused by the following gram-negative microorganisms:

Chancroid caused by *Haemophilus ducreyi*.

Plague due to *Yersinia pestis* (formerly *Pasteurella pestis*).

Tularemia due to *Francisella tulerensis* (formerly *Pasteurella tulerensis*).

Cholera caused by *Vibrio cholerae* (formerly *Vibrio comma*).

Campylobacter fetus infections caused by *Campylobacter fetus* (formerly *Vibrio fetus*).

Brucellosis due to *Brucella* species (in conjunction with streptomycin).

Bartonellosis due to *Bartonella bacilliformis*.

Granuloma inguinale caused by *Calymmatobacterium granulomatis*.

Because many strains of the following groups of microorganisms have been shown to be resistant to doxycycline, culture and susceptibility testing are recommended.

Doxycycline is indicated for treatment of infections caused by the following gram-negative microorganisms, when bacteriologic testing indicates appropriate susceptibility to the drug:

Escherichia coli.

Enterobacter aerogenes (formerly *Aerobacter aerogenes*).

Shigella species.

Acinetobacter species (formerly *Mima* species and *Herellea* species).

Respiratory tract infections caused by *Haemophilus influenzae*.

Respiratory tract and urinary tract infections caused by *Klebsiella* species.

Doxycycline is indicated for treatment of infections caused by the following gram-positive microorganisms when bacteriologic testing indicates appropriate susceptibility to the drug:

Upper respiratory infections caused by *Streptococcus pneumoniae* (formerly *Diplococcus pneumoniae*).

When penicillin is contraindicated, doxycycline is an alternative drug in the treatment of the following infections:

Uncomplicated gonorrhea caused by *Neisseria gonorrhoeae*.

Syphilis caused by *Treponema pallidum*.

Yaws caused by *Treponema pertenue*.

Continued on next page

Vibramycin/Vibra-Tabs—Cont.

Listeriosis due to *Listeria monocytogenes*.
Anthrax due to *Bacillus anthracis*.
Vincent's infection caused by *Fusobacterium fusiforme*.
Actinomycosis caused by *Actinomyces israelii*.
Infections caused by *Clostridium* species.
In acute intestinal amebiasis, doxycycline may be a useful adjunct to amebicides.
In severe acne, doxycycline may be useful adjunctive therapy.

Prophylaxis:
Doxycycline is indicated for the prophylaxis of malaria due to *Plasmodium falciparum* in short-term travelers (<4 months) to areas with chloroquine and/or pyrimethamine-sulfadoxine resistant strains. See DOSAGE AND ADMINISTRATION section and Information for Patients subsection of the PRECAUTIONS section.

CONTRAINDICATIONS
This drug is contraindicated in persons who have shown hypersensitivity to any of the tetracyclines.

WARNINGS
THE USE OF DRUGS OF THE TETRACYCLINE CLASS DURING TOOTH DEVELOPMENT (LAST HALF OF PREGNANCY, INFANCY AND CHILDHOOD TO THE AGE OF 8 YEARS) MAY CAUSE PERMANENT DISCOLORATION OF THE TEETH (YELLOW-GRAY-BROWN). This adverse reaction is more common during long-term use of the drugs, but has been observed following repeated short-term courses. Enamel hypoplasia has also been reported. TETRACYCLINE DRUGS, THEREFORE, SHOULD NOT BE USED IN THIS AGE GROUP UNLESS OTHER DRUGS ARE NOT LIKELY TO BE EFFECTIVE OR ARE CONTRAINDICATED.

All tetracyclines form a stable calcium complex in any bone-forming tissue. A decrease in fibula growth rate has been observed in prematures given oral tetracycline in doses of 25 mg/kg every 6 hours. This reaction was shown to be reversible when the drug was discontinued.

Results of animal studies indicate that tetracyclines cross the placenta, are found in fetal tissues, and can have toxic effects on the developing fetus (often related to retardation of skeletal development). Evidence of embryotoxicity has also been noted in animals treated early in pregnancy. If any tetracycline is used during pregnancy or if the patient becomes pregnant while taking this drug, the patient should be apprised of the potential hazard to the fetus.

The antianabolic action of the tetracyclines may cause an increase in BUN. Studies to date indicate that this does not occur with the use of doxycycline in patients with impaired renal function.

Photosensitivity manifested by an exaggerated sunburn reaction has been observed in some individuals taking tetracyclines. Patients apt to be exposed to direct sunlight or ultraviolet light should be advised that this reaction can occur with tetracycline drugs, and treatment should be discontinued at the first evidence of skin erythema.

Vibramycin Syrup contains sodium metabisulfite, a sulfite that may cause allergic-type reactions including anaphylactic symptoms and life-threatening or less severe asthmatic episodes in certain susceptible people. The over-all prevalence of sulfite sensitivity in the general population is unknown and probably low. Sulfite sensitivity is seen more frequently in asthmatic than in non-asthmatic people.

PRECAUTIONS
General
As with other antibiotic preparations, use of this drug may result in overgrowth of nonsusceptible organisms, including fungi. If superinfection occurs, the antibiotic should be discontinued and appropriate therapy instituted.

Bulging fontanels in infants and benign intracranial hypertension in adults have been reported in individuals receiving tetracyclines. These conditions disappeared when the drug was discontinued.

Incision and drainage or other surgical procedures should be performed in conjunction with antibiotic therapy, when indicated.

Doxycycline offers substantial but not complete suppression of the asexual blood stages of *Plasmodium* strains.

Doxycycline does not suppress *P. falciparum*'s sexual blood stage gametocytes. Subjects completing this prophylactic regimen may still transmit the infection to mosquitoes outside endemic areas.

Information for Patients
Patients taking doxycycline for malaria prophylaxis should be advised:
—that no present-day antimalarial agent, including doxycycline, guarantees protection against malaria.
—to avoid being bitten by mosquitoes by using personal protective measures that help avoid contact with mosquitoes, especially from dusk to dawn (e.g., staying in well-screened areas, using mosquito nets, covering the body with clothing, and using an effective insect repellent.)

—that doxycycline prophylaxis:
—should begin 1–2 days before travel to the malarious area,
—should be continued daily while in the malarious area and after leaving the malarious area,
—should be continued for 4 further weeks to avoid development of malaria after returning from an endemic area,
—should not exceed 4 months.

All patients taking doxycycline should be advised:
—to avoid excessive sunlight or artificial ultraviolet light while receiving doxycycline and to discontinue therapy if phototoxicity (e.g., skin eruption, etc.) occurs. Sunscreen or sunblock should be considered. (See WARNINGS.)
—to drink fluids liberally along with doxycycline to reduce the risk of esophageal irritation and ulceration. (See ADVERSE REACTIONS.)
—that the absorption of tetracyclines is reduced when taken with foods, especially those which contain calcium. However, the absorption of doxycycline is not markedly influenced by simultaneous ingestion of food or milk. (See DRUG INTERACTIONS.)
—that the absorption of tetracyclines is reduced when taking bismuth subsalicylate. (See DRUG INTERACTIONS.)
—that the use of doxycycline might increase the incidence of vaginal candidiasis.

Laboratory Tests
In venereal disease, when co-existent syphilis is suspected, dark field examinations should be done before treatment is started and the blood serology repeated monthly for at least 4 months.

In long-term therapy, periodic laboratory evaluation of organ systems, including hematopoietic, renal, and hepatic studies, should be performed.

Drug Interactions
Because tetracyclines have been shown to depress plasma prothrombin activity, patients who are on anticoagulant therapy may require downward adjustment of their anticoagulant dosage.

Since bacteriostatic drugs may interfere with the bactericidal action of penicillin, it is advisable to avoid giving tetracyclines in conjunction with penicillin.

Absorption of tetracyclines is impaired by antacids containing aluminum, calcium, or magnesium, and iron-containing preparations.

Absorption of tetracyclines is impaired by bismuth subsalicylate.

Barbiturates, carbamazepine, and phenytoin decrease the half-life of doxycycline.

The concurrent use of tetracycline and Penthrane (methoxyflurane) has been reported to result in fatal renal toxicity.

Concurrent use of tetracycline may render oral contraceptives less effective.

Drug/Laboratory Test Interactions
False elevations of urinary catecholamine levels may occur due to interference with the fluorescence test.

Carcinogenesis, Mutagenesis, Impairment of Fertility
Long-term studies in animals to evaluate carcinogenic potential of doxycycline have not been conducted. However, there has been evidence of oncogenic activity in rats in studies with the related antibiotics, oxytetracycline (adrenal and pituitary tumors), and minocycline (thyroid tumors). Likewise, although mutagenicity studies of doxycycline have not been conducted, positive results in *in vitro* mammalian cell assays have been reported for related antibiotics (tetracycline, oxytetracycline).

Doxycycline administered orally at dosage levels as high as 250 mg/kg/day had no apparent effect on the fertility of female rats. Effect on male fertility has not been studied.

Pregnancy Category
Teratogenic effects: Category "D" — (See WARNINGS).
Nonteratogenic effects: (See WARNINGS).

Labor and Delivery
The effect of tetracyclines on labor and delivery is unknown.

Nursing Mothers
Tetracyclines are excreted in human milk. Because of the potential for serious adverse reactions in nursing infants from doxycycline, a decision should be made whether to discontinue nursing or to discontinue the drug, taking into account the importance of the drug to the mother. (See WARNINGS).

Pediatric Use
See WARNINGS and DOSAGE AND ADMINISTRATION.

ADVERSE REACTIONS
Due to oral doxycycline's virtually complete absorption, side effects of the lower bowel, particularly diarrhea, have been infrequent. The following adverse reactions have been observed in patients receiving tetracyclines:
Gastrointestinal: anorexia, nausea, vomiting, diarrhea, glossitis, dysphagia, enterocolitis, and inflammatory lesions (with monilial overgrowth) in the anogenital region. Hepatotoxicity has been reported rarely. These reactions have been caused by both the oral and parenteral administration of tetracyclines. Rare instances of esophagitis and esophageal ulcerations have been reported in patients receiving capsule and tablet forms of the drugs in the tetracycline

class. Most of these patients took medications immediately before going to bed. (See DOSAGE AND ADMINISTRATION.)
Skin: maculopapular and erythematous rashes. Exfoliative dermatitis has been reported but is uncommon. Photosensitivity is discussed above. (See WARNINGS.)
Renal toxicity: Rise in BUN has been reported and is apparently dose related. (See WARNINGS.)
Hypersensitivity reactions: urticaria, angioneurotic edema, anaphylaxis, anaphylactoid purpura, serum sickness, pericarditis, and exacerbation of systemic lupus erythematosus.
Blood: Hemolytic anemia, thrombocytopenia, neutropenia, and eosinophilia have been reported.
Other: bulging fontanels in infants and intracranial hypertension in adults. (See PRECAUTIONS—General.)
When given over prolonged periods, tetracyclines have been reported to produce brown-black microscopic discoloration of the thyroid gland. No abnormalities of thyroid function studies are known to occur.

OVERDOSAGE
In case of overdosage, discontinue medication, treat symptomatically and institute supportive measures. Dialysis does not alter serum half-life and thus would not be of benefit in treating cases of overdosage.

DOSAGE AND ADMINISTRATION
THE USUAL DOSAGE AND FREQUENCY OF ADMINISTRATION OF DOXYCYCLINE DIFFERS FROM THAT OF THE OTHER TETRACYCLINES. EXCEEDING THE RECOMMENDED DOSAGE MAY RESULT IN AN INCREASED INCIDENCE OF SIDE EFFECTS. Adults: The usual dose of oral doxycycline is 200 mg on the first day of treatment (administered 100 mg every 12 hours) followed by a maintenance dose of 100 mg/day. The maintenance dose may be administered as a single dose or as 50 mg every 12 hours.

In the management of more severe infections (particularly chronic infections of the urinary tract), 100 mg every 12 hours is recommended.

For children above eight years of age: The recommended dosage schedule for children weighing 100 pounds or less is 2 mg/lb of body weight divided into two doses on the first day of treatment, followed by 1 mg/lb of body weight given as a single daily dose or divided into two doses, on subsequent days. For more severe infections up to 2 mg/lb of body weight may be used. For children over 100 lb the usual adult dose should be used.

The therapeutic antibacterial serum activity will usually persist for 24 hours following recommended dosage.

When used in streptococcal infections, therapy should be continued for 10 days.

Administration of adequate amounts of fluid along with capsule and tablet forms of drugs in the tetracycline class is recommended to wash down the drugs and reduce the risk of esophageal irritation and ulceration. (See ADVERSE REACTIONS.)

If gastric irritation occurs, it is recommended that doxycycline be given with food or milk. The absorption of doxycycline is not markedly influenced by simultaneous ingestion of food or milk.

Studies to date have indicated that administration of doxycycline at the usual recommended doses does not lead to excessive accumulation of the antibiotic in patients with renal impairment.

Uncomplicated gonococcal infections in adults (except anorectal infections in men): 100 mg, by mouth, twice a day for 7 days. As an alternate single visit dose, administer 300 mg stat followed in one hour by a second 300 mg dose. The dose may be administered with food, including milk or carbonated beverage, as required.

Uncomplicated urethral, endocervical, or rectal infection in adults caused by *Chlamydia trachomatis*: 100 mg by mouth twice a day for 7 days.

Nongonococcal urethritis (NGU) caused by *C. trachomatis* or *U. urealyticum*: 100 mg by mouth twice a day for 7 days.

Syphilis—early: Patients who are allergic to penicillin should be treated with doxycycline 100 mg by mouth twice a day for 2 weeks.

Syphilis of more than one year's duration: Patients who are allergic to penicillin should be treated with doxycycline 100 mg by mouth twice a day for 4 weeks.

Acute epididymo-orchitis caused by *N. gonorrhoeae*: 100 mg, by mouth, twice a day for at least 10 days.

Acute epididymo-orchitis caused by *C. trachomatis*: 100 mg, by mouth, twice a day for at least 10 days.

For prophylaxis of malaria: For adults, the recommended dose is 100 mg daily. For children over 8 years of age, the recommended dose is 2 mg/kg given once daily up to the adult dose. Prophylaxis should begin 1–2 days before travel to the malarious area. Prophylaxis should be continued daily during travel in the malarious area and for 4 weeks after the traveler leaves the malarious area.

HOW SUPPLIED
Vibramycin Hyclate (doxycycline hyclate) is available in capsules containing doxycycline hyclate equivalent to:

<u>*50 mg doxycycline*</u>
bottles of 50 (NDC 0069-0940-50),
unit-dose pack of 100 (10 × 10's) (NDC 0069-0940-41).
The capsules are white and light blue and are imprinted with "VIBRA" on one half and "PFIZER 094" on the other half.
<u>*100 mg doxycycline*</u>
bottles of 50 (NDC 0069-0950-50) and 500 (NDC 0069-0950-73),
unit-dose pack of 100 (10 × 10's) (NDC 0069-0950-41).
The capsules are light blue and are imprinted with "VIBRA" on one half and "PFIZER 095" on the other half.
Vibra-Tabs (doxycycline hyclate) is available in salmon colored film-coated tablets containing doxycycline hyclate equivalent to:
<u>*100 mg doxycycline*</u>
bottles of 50 (NDC 0069-0990-50) and 500 (NDC 0069-0990-73),
The tablets are imprinted on one side with "VIBRA-TABS" and "PFIZER 099" on the other side.
Vibramycin Calcium Syrup (doxycycline calcium oral suspension) is available as a raspberry-apple flavored oral suspension. Each teaspoonful (5 mL) contains doxycycline calcium equivalent to 50 mg of doxycycline: bottles of 1 oz (30 mL) (NDC 0069-0971-51), and 1 pint (473 mL) (NDC 0069-0971-93).
Vibramycin Monohydrate (doxycycline monohydrate) for Oral Suspension is available as a raspberry-flavored, dry powder for oral suspension. When reconstituted, each teaspoonful (5 mL) contains doxycycline monohydrate equivalent to 25 mg of doxycycline: 2 oz (60 mL) bottles (NDC 0069-0970-65).
All products are to be stored below 86°F (30°C) and dispensed in tight, light-resistant containers (USP). The unit dose packs should also be stored in a dry place.

ANIMAL PHARMACOLOGY AND ANIMAL TOXICOLOGY

Hyperpigmentation of the thyroid has been produced by members of the tetracycline class in the following species: in rats by oxytetracycline, doxycycline, tetracycline PO_4, and methacycline; in minipigs by doxycycline, minocycline, tetracycline PO_4, and methacycline; in dogs by doxycycline and minocycline; in monkeys by minocycline.
Minocycline, tetracycline PO_4, methacycline, doxycycline, tetracycline base, oxytetracycline HCl, and tetracycline HCl were goitrogenic in rats fed a low iodine diet. This goitrogenic effect was accompanied by high radioactive iodine uptake. Administration of minocycline also produced a large goiter with high radioiodine uptake in rats fed a relatively high iodine diet.
Treatment of various animal species with this class of drugs has also resulted in the induction of thyroid hyperplasia in the following: in rats and dogs (minocycline); in chickens (chlortetracycline); and in rats and mice (oxytetracycline). Adrenal gland hyperplasia has been observed in goats and rats treated with oxytetracycline.

REFERENCES

1. National Committee for Clinical Laboratory Standards, *Performance Standards for Antimicrobial Disk Susceptibility Tests,* Fourth Edition. Approved Standard NCCLS Document M2-A4, Vol. 10, No. 7 NCCLS, Villanova, PA, April 1990.
2. National Committee for Clinical Laboratory Standards, *Methods for Dilution Antimicrobial Susceptibility Tests for Bacteria that Grow Aerobically,* Second Edition. Approved Standard NCCLS Document M7-A2, Vol. 10, No. 8 NCCLS, Villanova, PA, April 1990.

65-1680-00-5 Revised April 1993

VIBRAMYCIN® Hyclate ℞
[vī "bra-mī 'sin]
doxycycline hyclate for injection
INTRAVENOUS
For Intravenous Use Only

DESCRIPTION

Vibramycin (doxycycline hyclate for injection) Intravenous is a broad–spectrum antibiotic synthetically derived from oxytetracycline, and is available as Vibramycin Hyclate (doxycycline hydrochloride hemiethanolate hemihydrate). The chemical designation of this light-yellow crystalline powder is alpha-6-deoxy-5-oxytetracycline. Doxycycline has a high degree of lipoid solubility and a low affinity for calcium binding. It is highly stable in normal human serum.

ACTIONS

Doxycycline is primarily bacteriostatic and thought to exert its antimicrobial effect by the inhibition of protein synthesis. Doxycycline is active against a wide range of gram-positive and gram-negative organisms.
The drugs in the tetracycline class have closely similar antimicrobial spectra and cross resistance among them is common. Microorganisms may be considered susceptible to doxycycline (likely to respond to doxycycline therapy) if the minimum inhibitory concentration (M.I.C.) is not more than 4.0 mcg/mL. Microorganisms may be considered intermediate (harboring partial resistance) if the M.I.C. is 4.0 to 12.5 mcg/mL and resistant (not likely to respond to therapy) if the M.I.C. is greater than 12.5 mcg/mL.
Susceptibility plate testing: If the Kirby-Bauer method of disc susceptibility testing is used, a 30 mcg doxycycline disc should give a zone of at least 16 mm when tested against a doxycycline-susceptible bacterial strain. A tetracycline disc may be used to determine microbial susceptibility. If the Kirby-Bauer method of disc susceptibility testing is used, a 30 mcg tetracycline disc should give a zone of at least 19 mm when tested against a tetracycline-susceptible bacterial strain.
Tetracyclines are readily absorbed and are bound to plasma proteins in varying degree. They are concentrated by the liver in the bile, and excreted in the urine and feces at high concentrations and in a biologically active form.
Following a single 100 mg dose administered in a concentration of 0.4 mg/mL in a one-hour infusion, normal adult volunteers average a peak of 2.5 mcg/mL, while 200 mg of a concentration of 0.4 mg/mL administered over two hours averaged a peak of 3.6 mcg/mL.
Excretion of doxycycline by the kidney is about 40 percent/72 hours in individuals with normal function (creatinine clearance about 75 mL/min.). This percentage excretion may fall as low as 1-5 percent/72 hours in individuals with severe renal insufficiency (creatinine clearance below 10 mL/min.). Studies have shown no significant difference in serum half-life of doxycycline (range 18-22 hours) in individuals with normal and severely impaired renal function. Hemodialysis does not alter this serum half-life of doxycycline.

INDICATIONS

Doxycycline is indicated in infections caused by the following microorganisms:
- Rickettsiae (Rocky Mountain spotted fever, typhus fever, and the typhus group, Q fever, rickettsialpox and tick fevers).
- *Mycoplasma pneumoniae* (PPLO, Eaton Agent).
- Agents of psittacosis and ornithosis.
- Agents of lymphogranuloma venereum and granuloma inguinale.
- The spirochetal agent of relapsing fever (*Borrelia recurrentis).*

The following gram-negative microorganisms:
- *Haemophilus ducreyi* (chancroid),
- *Pasteurella pestis* and *Pasteurella tularensis,*
- *Bartonella bacilliformis,*
- *Bacteroides* species,
- *Vibrio comma* and *Vibrio fetus,*
- *Brucella* species (in conjunction with streptomycin).

Because many strains of the following groups of microorganisms have been shown to be resistant to tetracyclines, culture and susceptibility testing are recommended.
Doxycycline is indicated for treatment of infections caused by the following gram-negative microorganisms when bacteriologic testing indicates appropriate susceptibility to the drug:
- *Escherichia coli,*
- *Enterobacter aerogenes* (formerly *Aerobacter aerogenes),*
- *Shigella* species,
- *Mima* species and *Herellea* species,
- *Haemophilus influenzae* (respiratory infections),
- *Klebsiella* species (respiratory and urinary infections).

Doxycycline is indicated for treatment of infections caused by the following gram-positive microorganisms when bacteriologic testing indicates appropriate susceptibility to the drug:
Streptococcus species:
Up to 44 percent of strains of *Streptococcus pyogenes* and 74 percent of *Streptococcus faecalis* have been found to be resistant to tetracycline drugs. Therefore, tetracyclines should not be used for streptococcal disease unless the organism has been demonstrated to be sensitive.
For upper respiratory infections due to group A beta-hemolytic streptococci, penicillin is the usual drug of choice, including prophylaxis of rheumatic fever.
- *Diplococcus pneumoniae,*
- *Staphylococcus aureus,* respiratory, skin and soft tissue infections. Tetracyclines are not the drugs of choice in the treatment of any type of staphylococcal infections.

When penicillin is contraindicated, doxycycline is an alternative drug in the treatment of infections due to:
- *Neisseria gonorrhoeae* and *N. meningitidis,*
- *Treponema pallidum* and *Treponema pertenue* (syphilis and yaws),
- *Listeria monocytogenes,*
- *Clostridium* species,
- *Bacillus anthracis,*
- *Fusobacterium fusiforme* (Vincent's infection),
- *Actinomyces* species.

In acute intestinal amebiasis, doxycycline may be a useful adjunct to amebicides.
Doxycycline is indicated in the treatment of trachoma, although the infectious agent is not always eliminated, as judged by immunofluorescence.

CONTRAINDICATIONS

This drug is contraindicated in persons who have shown hypersensitivity to any of the tetracyclines.

WARNINGS

THE USE OF DRUGS OF THE TETRACYCLINE CLASS DURING TOOTH DEVELOPMENT (LAST HALF OF PREGNANCY, INFANCY AND CHILDHOOD TO THE AGE OF 8 YEARS) MAY CAUSE PERMANENT DISCOLORATION OF THE TEETH (YELLOW-GRAY-BROWN). This adverse reaction is more common during long-term use of the drugs but has been observed following repeated short-term courses. Enamel hypoplasia has also been reported. *TETRACYCLINE DRUGS, THEREFORE, SHOULD NOT BE USED IN THIS AGE GROUP UNLESS OTHER DRUGS ARE NOT LIKELY TO BE EFFECTIVE OR ARE CONTRAINDICATED.*
Photosensitivity manifested by an exaggerated sunburn reaction has been observed in some individuals taking tetracyclines. Patients apt to be exposed to direct sunlight or ultraviolet light should be advised that this reaction can occur with tetracycline drugs, and treatment should be discontinued at the first evidence of skin erythema.
The antianabolic action of the tetracyclines may cause an increase in BUN. Studies to date indicate that this does not occur with the use of doxycycline in patients with impaired renal function.

Usage in Pregnancy

(See above WARNINGS about use during tooth development.)
Vibramycin Intravenous has not been studied in pregnant patients. It should not be used in pregnant women unless, in the judgment of the physician, it is essential for the welfare of the patient.
Results of animal studies indicate that tetracyclines cross the placenta, are found in fetal tissues and can have toxic effects on the developing fetus (often related to retardation of skeletal development). Evidence of embryotoxicity has also been noted in animals treated early in pregnancy.

Usage in Children

The use of Vibramycin Intravenous in children under 8 years is not recommended because safe conditions for its use have not been established.
(See above WARNINGS about use during tooth development.)
As with other tetracyclines, doxycycline forms a stable calcium complex in any bone-forming tissue. A decrease in the fibula growth rate has been observed in prematures given oral tetracycline in doses of 25 mg/kg every 6 hours. This reaction was shown to be reversible when the drug was discontinued.
Tetracyclines are present in the milk of lactating women who are taking a drug in this class.

PRECAUTIONS

As with other antibiotic preparations, use of this drug may result in overgrowth of nonsusceptible organisms, including fungi. If superinfection occurs, the antibiotic should be discontinued and appropriate therapy instituted.
In venereal diseases when coexistent syphilis is suspected, a dark field examination should be done before treatment is started and the blood serology repeated monthly for at least 4 months.
Because tetracyclines have been shown to depress plasma prothrombin activity, patients who are on anticoagulant therapy may require downward adjustment of their anticoagulant dosage.
In long-term therapy, periodic laboratory evaluation of organ systems, including hematopoietic, renal, and hepatic studies should be performed.
All infections due to group A beta-hemolytic streptococci should be treated for at least 10 days.
Since bacteriostatic drugs may interfere with the bactericidal action of penicillin, it is advisable to avoid giving tetracycline in conjunction with penicillin.

ADVERSE REACTIONS

Gastrointestinal: anorexia, nausea, vomiting, diarrhea, glossitis, dysphagia, enterocolitis, and inflammatory lesions (with monilial overgrowth) in the anogenital region. Hepatotoxicity has been reported rarely. These reactions have been caused by both the oral and parenteral administration of tetracyclines.
Skin: maculopapular and erythematous rashes. Exfoliative dermatitis has been reported but is uncommon. Photosensitivity is discussed above. (See WARNINGS.)
Renal toxicity: Rise in BUN has been reported and is apparently dose related. (See WARNINGS.)
Hypersensitivity reactions: urticaria, angioneurotic edema, anaphylaxis, anaphylactoid purpura, pericarditis and exacerbation of systemic lupus erythematosus.

Continued on next page

Vibramycin Intravenous—Cont.

Bulging fontanels in infants and benign intracranial hypertension in adults have been reported in individuals receiving full therapeutic dosages. These conditions disappeared rapidly when the drug was discontinued.
Blood: Hemolytic anemia, thrombocytopenia, neutropenia and eosinophilia have been reported.
When given over prolonged periods, tetracyclines have been reported to produce brown-black microscopic discoloration of thyroid glands. No abnormalities of thyroid function studies are known to occur.

DOSAGE AND ADMINISTRATION

Note: Rapid administration is to be avoided. Parenteral therapy is indicated only when oral therapy is not indicated. Oral therapy should be instituted as soon as possible. If intravenous therapy is given over prolonged periods of time, thrombophlebitis may result.
THE USUAL DOSAGE AND FREQUENCY OF ADMINISTRATION OF VIBRAMYCIN I.V. (100-200 MG/DAY) DIFFERS FROM THAT OF THE OTHER TETRACYCLINES (1-2 G/DAY). EXCEEDING THE RECOMMENDED DOSAGE MAY RESULT IN AN INCREASED INCIDENCE OF SIDE EFFECTS.
Studies to date have indicated that Vibramycin at the usual recommended doses does not lead to excessive accumulation of the antibiotic in patients with renal impairment.
Adults: The usual dosage of Vibramycin I.V. is 200 mg on the first day of treatment administered in one or two infusions. Subsequent daily dosage is 100 to 200 mg depending upon the severity of infection, with 200 mg administered in one or two infusions.
In the treatment of primary and secondary syphilis, the recommended dosage is 300 mg daily for at least 10 days.
For children above eight years of age: The recommended dosage schedule for children weighing 100 pounds or less is 2 mg/lb of body weight on the first day of treatment, administered in one or two infusions. Subsequent daily dosage is 1 to 2 mg/lb of body weight given as one or two infusions, depending on the severity of the infection. For children over 100 pounds the usual adult dose should be used. (See WARNINGS Section for Usage in Children.)
General: The duration of infusion may vary with the dose (100 to 200 mg per day), but is usually one to four hours. A recommended minimum infusion time for 100 mg of a 0.5 mg/mL solution is one hour. Therapy should be continued for at least 24-48 hours after symptoms and fever have subsided. The therapeutic antibacterial serum activity will usually persist for 24 hours following recommended dosage.
Intravenous solutions should not be injected intramuscularly or subcutaneously. Caution should be taken to avoid the inadvertent introduction of the intravenous solution into the adjacent soft tissue.

PREPARATION OF SOLUTION

To prepare a solution containing 10 mg/mL, the contents of the vial should be reconstituted with 10 mL (for the 100 mg/vial container) or 20 mL (for the 200 mg/vial container) of Sterile Water for Injection or any of the ten intravenous infusion solutions listed below. Each 100 mg of Vibramycin (i.e., withdraw entire solution from the 100 mg vial) is further diluted with 100 mL to 1000 mL of the intravenous solutions listed below. Each 200 mg of Vibramycin (i.e., withdraw entire solution from the 200 mg vial) is further diluted with 200 mL to 2000 mL of the following intravenous solutions:

1. Sodium Chloride Injection, USP
2. 5% Dextrose Injection, USP
3. Ringer's Injection, USP
4. Invert Sugar, 10% in Water
5. Lactated Ringer's Injection, USP
6. Dextrose 5% in Lactated Ringer's
7. Normosol-M® in D5-W (Abbott)
8. Normosol-R® in D5-W (Abbott)
9. Plasma-Lyte® 56 in 5% Dextrose (Travenol)
10. Plasma-Lyte® 148 in 5% Dextrose (Travenol)

This will result in desired concentrations of 0.1 to 1.0 mg/mL. Concentrations lower than 0.1 mg/mL or higher than 1.0 mg/mL are not recommended.

Stability

Vibramycin IV is stable for 48 hours in solution when diluted with Sodium Chloride Injection, USP, or 5% Dextrose Injection, USP, to concentrations between 1.0 mg/mL and 0.1 mg/ mL and stored at 25°C. Vibramycin IV in these solutions is stable under fluorescent light for 48 hours, but must be protected from direct sunlight during storage and infusion. Reconstituted solutions (1.0 to 0.1 mg/mL) may be stored up to 72 hours prior to start of infusion if refrigerated and protected from sunlight and artificial light. Infusion must then be completed within 12 hours. Solutions must be used within these time periods or discarded.
Vibramycin IV, when diluted with Ringer's Injection, USP, or Invert Sugar, 10% in Water, or Normosol-M® in D5-W (Abbott), or Normosol-R®in D5-W (Abbott), or Plasma-Lyte® 56 in 5% Dextrose (Travenol), or Plasma-Lyte® 148 in 5% Dextrose (Travenol) to a concentration between 1.0 mg/mL and 0.1 mg/mL, must be completely infused within 12 hours after reconstitution to ensure adequate stability. During infusion, the solution must be protected from direct sunlight. Reconstituted solutions (1.0 to 0.1 mg/mL) may be stored up to 72 hours prior to start of infusion if refrigerated and protected from sunlight and artifical light. Infusion must then be completed within 12 hours. Solutions must be used within these time periods or discarded.
When diluted with Lactated Ringer's Injection, USP, or Dextrose 5% in Lactated Ringer's, infusion of the solution (ca. 1.0 mg/mL) or lower concentrations (not less than 0.1 mg/mL) must be completed within six hours after reconstitution to ensure adequate stability. During infusion, the solution must be protected from direct sunlight. Solutions must be used within this time period or discarded.
Solutions of Vibramycin (doxycycline hyclate for injection) at a concentration of 10 mg/mL in Sterile Water for Injection, when frozen immediately after reconstitution are stable for 8 weeks when stored at −20°C. If the product is warmed, care should be taken to avoid heating it after the thawing is complete. Once thawed the solution should not be refrozen.

HOW SUPPLIED

Vibramycin (doxycycline hyclate for injection) Intravenous is available as a sterile powder in a vial containing doxycycline hyclate equivalent to 100 mg of doxycycline with 480 mg of ascorbic acid, packages of 5 (NDC 0049-0960-77), and in individually packaged vials containing doxycycline hyclate equivalent to 200 mg of doxycycline with 960 mg of ascorbic acid (0049–0980–81).

65-1940-00-2

LITERATURE AVAILABLE

Yes.

Revised March 1991

VISTARIL® ℞

[*vĭs 'tăr-ĭl*]
(hydroxyzine pamoate)
Capsules and Oral Suspension

DESCRIPTION

Hydroxyzine pamoate is designated chemically as 1-(p-chlorobenzhydryl) 4- [2- (2-hydroxyethoxy) ethyl] diethylenediamine salt of 1,1'- methylene bis (2 hydroxy-3-naphthalene carboxylic acid).
Inert ingredients for the capsule formulations are: hard gelatin capsules (which may contain Yellow 10, Green 3, Yellow 6, Red 33, and other inert ingredients); magnesium stearate; sodium lauryl sulfate; starch; sucrose.
Inert ingredients for the oral suspension formulation are: carboxymethylcellulose sodium; lemon flavor; propylene glycol; sorbic acid; sorbitol solution; water.

CLINICAL PHARMACOLOGY

Vistaril® (hydroxyzine pamoate) is unrelated chemically to the phenothiazines, reserpine, meprobamate, or the benzodiazepines.
Vistaril is not a cortical depressant, but its action may be due to a suppression of activity in certain key regions of the subcortical area of the central nervous system. Primary skeletal muscle relaxation has been demonstrated experimentally. Bronchodilator activity, and antihistaminic and analgesic effects have been demonstrated experimentally and confirmed clinically. An antiemetic effect, both by the apomorphine test and the veriloid test, has been demonstrated. Pharmacological and clinical studies indicate that hydroxyzine in therapeutic dosage does not increase gastric secretion or acidity and in most cases has mild antisecretory activity. Hydroxyzine is rapidly absorbed from the gastrointestinal tract and Vistaril's clinical effects are usually noted within 15 to 30 minutes after oral administration.

INDICATIONS

For symptomatic relief of anxiety and tension associated with psychoneurosis and as an adjunct in organic disease states in which anxiety is manifested.
Useful in the management of pruritus due to allergic conditions such as chronic urticaria and atopic and contact dermatoses, and in histamine-mediated pruritus.
As a sedative when used as premedication and following general anesthesia, **Hydroxyzine may potentiate meperidine (Demerol®) and barbiturates,** so their use in pre-anesthetic adjunctive therapy should be modified on an individual basis. Atropine and other belladonna alkaloids are not affected by the drug. Hydroxyzine is not known to interfere with the action of digitalis in any way and it may be used concurrently with this agent.
The effectiveness of hydroxyzine as an antianxiety agent for long–term use, that is, more than 4 months, has not been assessed by systematic clinical studies. The physician should reassess periodically the usefulness of the drug for the individual patient.

CONTRAINDICATIONS

Hydroxyzine, when administered to the pregnant mouse, rat, and rabbit, induced fetal abnormalities in the rat and mouse at doses substantially above the human therapeutic range. Clinical data in human beings are inadequate to establish safety in early pregnancy. Until such data are available, hydroxyzine is contraindicated in early pregnancy.
Hydroxyzine pamoate is contraindicated for patients who have shown a previous hypersensitivity to it.

WARNINGS

Nursing Mothers: It is not known whether this drug is excreted in human milk. Since many drugs are so excreted, hydroxyzine should not be given to nursing mothers.

PRECAUTIONS

THE POTENTIATING ACTION OF HYDROXYZINE MUST BE CONSIDERED WHEN THE DRUG IS USED IN CONJUNCTION WITH CENTRAL NERVOUS SYSTEM DEPRESSANTS SUCH AS NARCOTICS, NON-NARCOTIC ANALGESICS AND BARBITURATES. Therefore, when central nervous system depressants are administered concomitantly with hydroxyzine, their dosage should be reduced. Since drowsiness may occur with use of the drug, patients should be warned of this possibility and cautioned against driving a car or operating dangerous machinery while taking Vistaril (hydroxyzine pamoate). Patients should be advised against the simultaneous use of other CNS depressant drugs, and cautioned that the effect of alcohol may be increased.

ADVERSE REACTIONS

Side effects reported with the administration of Vistaril are usually mild and transitory in nature.
Anticholinergic: Dry mouth.
Central Nervous System: Drowsiness is usually transitory and may disappear in a few days of continued therapy or upon reduction of the dose. Involuntary motor activity, including rare instances of tremor and convulsions, has been reported, usually with doses considerably higher than those recommended. Clinically significant respiratory depression has not been reported at recommended doses.

OVERDOSAGE

The most common manifestation of overdosage of Vistaril is hypersedation. As in the management of overdosage with any drug, it should be borne in mind that multiple agents may have been taken.
If vomiting has not occurred spontaneously, it should be induced. Immediate gastric lavage is also recommended. General supportive care, including frequent monitoring of the vital signs and close observation of the patient, is indicated. Hypotension, though unlikely, may be controlled with intravenous fluids and Levophed® (levarterenol) or Aramine® (metaraminol). Do not use epinephrine, as Vistaril counteracts its pressor action. Caffeine and Sodium Benzoate Injection, USP, may be used to counteract central nervous system depressant effects.
There is no specific antidote. It is doubtful that hemodialysis would be of any value in the treatment of overdosage with hydroxyzine. However, if other agents such as barbiturates have been ingested concomitantly, hemodialysis may be indicated. There is no practical method to quantitate hydroxyzine in body fluids or tissue after its ingestion or administration.

DOSAGE

For symptomatic relief of anxiety and tension associated with psychoneurosis and as an adjunct in organic disease states in which anxiety is manifested: in adults, 50–100 mg q.i.d.; children under 6 years, 50 mg daily in divided doses and over 6 years, 50–100 mg daily in divided doses.
For use in the management of pruritus due to allergic conditions such as chronic urticaria and atopic and contact dermatoses, and in histamine-mediated pruritus: in adults, 25 mg t.i.d. or q.i.d.; children under 6 years, 50 mg daily in divided doses and over 6 years, 50–100 mg daily in divided doses.
As a sedative when used as a premedication and following general anesthesia: 50–100 mg in adults, and 0.6 mg/kg in children.
When treatment is initiated by the intramuscular route of administration, subsequent doses may be administered orally.
As with all medications, the dosage should be adjusted according to the patient's response to therapy.

HOW SUPPLIED

Vistaril® Capsules (hydroxyzine pamoate equivalent to hydroxyzine hydrochloride)

25 mg: 100's (NDC 0069-5410-66), 500's (NDC 0069-5410-73), and Unit Dose (10 × 10's) (NDC 0069-5410-41) two-tone green capsules

50 mg: 100's (NDC 0069-5420-66), 500's (NDC 0069-5420-73), and Unit Dose (10 × 10's) (NDC 0069-5420-41) green and white capsules

100 mg: 100's (NDC 0069-5430-66), 500's (NDC 0069-5430-73), and Unit Dose (10 × 10's) (NDC 0069-5430-41) green and gray capsules

Vistaril® Oral Suspension (hydroxyzine pamoate equivalent to 25 mg hydroxyzine hydrochloride per teaspoonful-5 mL): 1 pint (473 mL) bottles (NDC 0069-5440-93) and 4 ounce (120 mL) bottles (NDC 0069-5440-97) in packages of 4.

Shake vigorously until product is completely resuspended.

BIBLIOGRAPHY

Available on request.

69-0846-00-1   Revised November 1994

VISTARIL®
hydroxyzine hydrochloride
Intramuscular Solution
For Intramuscular Use Only

℞

CHEMISTRY

Hydroxyzine hydrochloride is designated chemically as 1-(p-chlorobenzhydryl) 4-[2-(2-hydroxyethoxy) ethyl] piperazine dihydrochloride.

ACTIONS

VISTARIL (hydroxyzine hydrochloride) is unrelated chemically to phenothiazine, reserpine, and meprobamate. Hydroxyzine has demonstrated its clinical effectiveness in the chemotherapeutic aspect of the total management of neuroses and emotional disturbances manifested by anxiety, tension, agitation, apprehension or confusion.

Hydroxyzine has been shown clinically to be a rapid-acting true ataraxic with a wide margin of safety. It induces a calming effect in anxious, tense, psychoneurotic adults and also in anxious, hyperkinetic children without impairing mental alertness. It is not a cortical depressant, but its action may be due to a suppression of activity in certain key regions of the subcortical area of the central nervous system.

Primary skeletal muscle relaxation has been demonstrated experimentally.

Hydroxyzine has been shown experimentally to have antispasmodic properties, apparently mediated through interference with the mechanism that responds to spasmogenic agents such as serotonin, acetylcholine, and histamine.

Antihistaminic effects have been demonstrated experimentally and confirmed clinically.

An antiemetic effect, both by the apomorphine test and the veriloid test, has been demonstrated. Pharmacological and clinical studies indicate that hydroxyzine in therapeutic dosage does not increase gastric secretion or acidity and in most cases provides mild antisecretory benefits.

INDICATIONS

The total management of anxiety, tension, and psychomotor agitation in conditions of emotional stress requires in most instances a combined approach of psychotherapy and chemotherapy. Hydroxyzine has been found to be particularly useful for this latter phase of therapy in its ability to render the disturbed patient more amenable to psychotherapy in long term treatment of the psychoneurotic and psychotic, although it should not be used as the sole treatment of psychosis or of clearly demonstrated cases of depression. Hydroxyzine is also useful in alleviating the manifestations of anxiety and tension as in the preparation for dental procedures and in acute emotional problems. It has also been recommended for the management of anxiety associated with organic disturbances and as adjunctive therapy in alcoholism and allergic conditions with strong emotional overlay, such as in asthma, chronic urticaria, and pruritus.

VISTARIL (hydroxyzine hydrochloride) Intramuscular Solution is useful in treating the following types of patients when intramuscular administration is indicated:

1. The acutely disturbed or hysterical patient.
2. The acute or chronic alcoholic with anxiety withdrawal symptoms or delirium tremens.
3. As pre- and postoperative and pre- and postpartum adjunctive medication to permit reduction in narcotic dosage, allay anxiety and control emesis.

VISTARIL (hydroxyzine hydrochloride) has also demonstrated effectiveness in controlling nausea and vomiting, excluding nausea and vomiting of pregnancy. (See Contraindications.)

In prepartum states, the reduction in narcotic requirement effected by hydroxyzine is of particular benefit to both mother and neonate.

Hydroxyzine benefits the cardiac patient by its ability to allay the associated anxiety and apprehension attendant to certain types of heart disease. Hydroxyzine is not known to interfere with the action of digitalis in any way and may be used concurrently with this agent.

The effectiveness of hydroxyzine in long term use, that is, more than 4 months, has not been assessed by systematic clinical studies. The physician should reassess periodically the usefulness of the drug for the individual patient.

CONTRAINDICATIONS

Hydroxyzine hydrochloride intramuscular solution is intended only for intramuscular administration and should not, under any circumstances, be injected subcutaneously, intra-arterially, or intravenously.

This drug is contraindicated for patients who have shown a previous hypersensitivity to it.

Hydroxyzine, when administered to the pregnant mouse, rat, and rabbit, induced fetal abnormalities in the rat at doses substantially above the human therapeutic range. Clinical data in human beings are inadequate to establish safety in early pregnancy. Until such data are available, hydroxyzine is contraindicated in early pregnancy.

PRECAUTIONS

THE POTENTIATING ACTION OF HYDROXYZINE MUST BE CONSIDERED WHEN THE DRUG IS USED IN CONJUNCTION WITH CENTRAL NERVOUS SYSTEM DEPRESSANTS SUCH AS NARCOTICS, BARBITURATES, AND ALCOHOL. Rarely, cardiac arrests and death have been reported in association with the combined use of hydroxyzine hydrochloride IM and other CNS depressants. Therefore when central nervous system depressants are administered concomitantly with hydroxyzine their dosage should be reduced up to 50 per cent. The efficacy of hydroxyzine as adjunctive pre- and postoperative sedative medication has also been well established, especially as regards its ability to allay anxiety, control emesis, and reduce the amount of narcotic required.

HYDROXYZINE MAY POTENTIATE NARCOTICS AND BARBITURATES, so their use in preanesthetic adjunctive therapy should be modified on an individual basis. Atropine and other belladonna alkaloids are not affected by the drug. When hydroxyzine is used preoperatively or prepartum, narcotic requirements may be reduced as much as 50 per cent. Thus, when 50 mg of VISTARIL (hydroxyzine hydrochloride) Intramuscular Solution is employed, meperidine dosage may be reduced from 100 mg to 50 mg. The administration of meperidine may result in severe hypotension in the postoperative patient or any individual whose ability to maintain blood pressure has been compromised by a depleted blood volume. Meperidine should be used with great caution and in reduced dosage in patients who are receiving other pre- and/or postoperative medications and in whom there is a risk of respiratory depression, hypotension, and profound sedation or coma occurring. Before using any medications concomitant with hydroxyzine, the manufacturer's prescribing information should be read carefully.

Since drowsiness may occur with the use of this drug, patients should be warned of this possibility and cautioned against driving a car or operating dangerous machinery while taking this drug.

As with all intramuscular preparations, VISTARIL Intramuscular Solution should be injected well within the body of a relatively large muscle. Inadvertent subcutaneous injection may result in significant tissue damage.

ADULTS: The preferred site is the upper outer quadrant of the buttock, (i.e., gluteus maximus), or the mid-lateral thigh.

CHILDREN: It is recommended that intramuscular injections be given preferably in the mid-lateral muscles of the thigh. In infants and small children the periphery of the upper outer quadrant of the gluteal region should be used only when necessary, such as in burn patients, in order to minimize the possibility of damage to the sciatic nerve.

The deltoid area should be used only if well developed such as in certain adults and older children, and then only with caution to avoid radial nerve injury. Intramuscular injections should not be made into the lower and mid-third of the upper arm. As with all intramuscular injections, aspiration is necessary to help avoid inadvertent injection into a blood vessel.

ADVERSE REACTIONS

Therapeutic doses of hydroxyzine seldom produce impairment of mental alertness. However, drowsiness may occur; if so, it is usually transitory and may disappear in a few days of continued therapy or upon reduction of the dose. Dryness of the mouth may be encountered at higher doses. Extensive clinical use has substantiated the absence of toxic effects on the liver or bone marrow when administered in the recommended doses for over four years of uninterrupted therapy. The absence of adverse effects has been further demonstrated in experimental studies in which excessively high doses were administered.

Involuntary motor activity, including rare instances of tremor and convulsions, has been reported, usually with doses considerably higher than those recommended. Continuous therapy with over one gram per day has been employed in some patients without these effects having been encountered.

DOSAGE AND ADMINISTRATION

The recommended dosages for VISTARIL (hydroxyzine hydrochloride) Intramuscular Solution are:

For adult psychiatric and emotional emergencies, including acute alcoholism.	IM: 50–100 mg stat., and q. 4–6h., p.r.n.
Nausea and vomiting excluding nausea and vomiting of pregnancy.	Adults: 25–100 mg IM Children: 0.5 mg/lb body weight IM
Pre- and postoperative adjunctive medication.	Adults: 25–100 mg IM Children: 0.5 mg/lb body weight IM
Pre- and postpartum adjunctive therapy.	25–100 mg IM

As with all potent medications, the dosage should be adjusted according to the patient's response to therapy.

FOR ADDITIONAL INFORMATION OF THE ADMINISTRATION AND SITE OF SELECTION SEE PRECAUTIONS SECTION. NOTE: VISTARIL (hydroxyzine hydrochloride) Intramuscular Solution may be administered without further dilution.

Patients may be started on intramuscular therapy when indicated. They should be maintained on oral therapy whenever this route is practicable.

HOW SUPPLIED

VISTARIL (hydroxyzine hydrochloride) Intramuscular Solution
Multi-Dose Vials
25 mg/mL: 10 mL vials (NDC 0049-5450-74)
50 mg/mL: 10 mL vials (NDC 0049-5460-74)
Unit Dose Vials
50 mg/mL–1 mL fill: packages of 25 vials (NDC 0049-5462-76)
100 mg/2 mL–2 mL fill: packages of 25 vials (NDC 0049-5460-76)

STORAGE

Store below 86° F (30°C).
Protect from freezing.

FORMULA

Dosage Strength	25 mg/1 mL	50 mg/1 mL 100 mg/2 mL
Hydroxyzine hydrochloride	25 mg/mL	50 mg/mL
Benzyl Alcohol	0.9%	0.9%
Sodium hydroxide	to adjust to optimum pH	

70-0843-00-5
Revised May 1993

ZITHROMAX®
(azithromycin tablets)
(azithromycin capsules)
and
(azithromycin for oral suspension)

℞

DESCRIPTION

ZITHROMAX® (azithromycin tablets, azithromycin capsules and azithromycin for oral suspension) contain the active ingredient azithromycin, an azalide, a subclass of macrolide antibiotics, for oral administration. Azithromycin has the chemical name (2R,3S,4R,5R,8R,10R,11R,12S,13S,14R)-13-[(2,6-dideoxy-3-C-methyl- 3-O-methyl-α-L-ribo-hexopyranosyl)oxy]-2-ethyl-3,4,10-trihydroxy-3,5,6,8,10,12,14-heptamethyl-11-[[3,4,6-trideoxy-3-(dimethylamino)- β-D-xylo-hexopyranosyl]oxy]-1-oxa-6-azacyclopentadecan-15-one. Azithromycin is derived from erythromycin; however, it differs chemically from erythromycin in that a methyl-substituted nitrogen atom is incorporated into the lactone ring. Its molecular formula is $C_{38}H_{72}N_2O_{12}$, and its molecular weight is 749.00. Azithromycin has the following structural formula:

Continued on next page

Zithromax—Cont.

Azithromycin, as the dihydrate, is a white crystalline powder with a molecular formula of $C_{38}H_{72}N_2O_{12} \cdot 2H_2O$ and a molecular weight of 785.0.

ZITHROMAX® is supplied for oral administration as film-coated, modified capsular shaped tablets containing azithromycin dihydrate equivalent to 250 mg azithromycin and the following inactive ingredients: dibasic calcium phosphate anhydrous, pregelatinized starch, sodium croscarmellose, magnesium stearate, sodium lauryl sulfate, hydroxypropyl methylcellulose, lactose, titanium dioxide, triacetin and D&C Red #30 aluminum lake.

ZITHROMAX® capsules contain azithromycin dihydrate equivalent to 250 mg of azithromycin. The capsules are supplied in red opaque hard-gelatin capsules (containing FD&C Red #40). They also contain the following inactive ingredients: anhydrous lactose, corn starch, magnesium stearate, and sodium lauryl sulfate.

It is also supplied as a powder for oral suspension.

ZITHROMAX® for oral suspension is supplied in bottles containing azithromycin dihydrate powder equivalent to 300 mg, 600 mg, 900 mg, or 1200 mg azithromycin per bottle and the following inactive ingredients: sucrose; sodium phosphate, tribasic, anhydrous; hydroxypropyl cellulose; xanthan gum; FD&C Red #40; and spray dried artificial cherry, creme de vanilla and banana flavors. After constitution, each 5 mL of suspension contains 100 mg or 200 mg of azithromycin.

CLINICAL PHARMACOLOGY

Adult Pharmacokinetics: Following oral administration, azithromycin is rapidly absorbed and widely distributed throughout the body. Rapid distribution of azithromycin into tissues and high concentration within cells result in significantly higher azithromycin concentrations in tissues than in plasma or serum.

The pharmacokinetic parameters of azithromycin capsules in plasma after a loading dose of 500 mg (2–250 mg capsules) on day one followed by 250 mg (1–250 mg capsule) q.d. on days two through five in healthy young adults (age 18–40 years old) are portrayed in the following chart:

Pharmacokinetic Parameters
(Mean)

	Total n=12 Day 1	Day 5
C_{max} (µg/mL)	0.41	0.24
T_{max} (h)	2.5	3.2
AUC_{0-24} (µg·h/mL)	2.6	2.1
C_{min} (µg/mL)	0.05	0.05
Urinary Excret. (% dose)	4.5	6.5

In this study, there was no significant difference in the disposition of azithromycin between male and female subjects. Plasma concentrations of azithromycin following single 500 mg oral and i.v. doses declined in a polyphasic pattern resulting in an average terminal half-life of 68 hours. With a regimen of 500 mg on Day 1 and 250 mg/day on Days 2–5, C_{min} and C_{max} remained essentially unchanged from Day 2 through Day 5 of therapy. However, without a loading dose, azithromycin C_{min} levels required 5 to 7 days to reach steady-state.

In an open, randomized, two-way crossover study, pharmacokinetic parameters (AUC_{0-72}, C_{max}, T_{max}) determined from 36 fasted healthy male volunteers who received two 250-mg commercial capsules and two 250-mg tablets were:

	Capsule	Tablet	90% CI
AUC_{0-72} (µg·h/mL)	4.1 (1.2)	4.3 (1.2)	(99–113%)
C_{max} (µg/mL)	0.5 (0.2)	0.5 (0.2)	(96–121%)
T_{max} (hours)	2.1 (0.8)	2.2 (0.9)	

When azithromycin capsules were administered with food to 11 adult healthy male subjects, the rate of absorption (C_{max}) of azithromycin from the capsule formulation was reduced by 52% and the extent of absorption (AUC) by 43%. In an open label, randomized, two-way crossover study in 12 healthy subjects to assess the effect of a high fat standard meal on the serum concentrations of azithromycin resulting from the oral administration of two 250-mg film-coated tablets, it was shown that food increased C_{max} by 23% while there was no change in AUC.

When azithromycin suspension was administered with food to 28 adult healthy male subjects, the rate of absorption (C_{max}) was increased by 56% while the extent of absorption (AUC) was unchanged.

The AUC of azithromycin was unaffected by co-administration of an antacid containing aluminum and magnesium hydroxide with ZITHROMAX® capsules (azithromycin); however, the C_{max} was reduced by 24%. Administration of cimetidine (800 mg) two hours prior to azithromycin had no effect on azithromycin absorption.

When studied in healthy elderly subjects from age 65 to 85 years, the pharmacokinetic parameters of azithromycin in elderly men were similar to those in young adults; however, in elderly women, although higher peak concentrations (increased by 30 to 50%) were observed, no significant accumulation occurred.

The high values in adults for apparent steady-state volume of distribution (31.1 L/kg) and plasma clearance (630 mL/min) suggest that the prolonged half-life is due to extensive uptake and subsequent release of drug from tissues.

The serum protein binding of azithromycin is variable in the concentration range of approximating human exposure, decreasing from 51% at 0.02 µg/mL to 7% at 2 µg/mL.

Biliary excretion of azithromycin, predominantly as unchanged drug, is a major route of elimination. Over the course of a week, approximately 6% of the administered dose appears as unchanged drug in urine.

There are no pharmacokinetic data available from studies in hepatically- or renally-impaired individuals.

The effect of azithromycin on the plasma levels or pharmacokinetics of theophylline administered in multiple doses adequate to reach therapeutic steady-state plasma levels is not known. (See **PRECAUTIONS.**)

Selected tissue (or fluid) concentration and tissue (or fluid) to plasma/serum concentration ratios are shown in the following table:

AZITHROMYCIN CONCENTRATIONS FOLLOWING TWO-250 mg (500 mg) CAPSULES IN ADULTS

TISSUE OR FLUID	TIME AFTER DOSE (h)	TISSUE OR FLUID CONCENTRATION (µg/g or µg/mL)[1]
SKIN	72–96	0.4
LUNG	72–96	4.0
SPUTUM*	2–4	1.0
SPUTUM**	10–12	2.9
TONSIL***	9–18	4.5
TONSIL***	180	0.9
CERVIX****	19	2.8

TISSUE OR FLUID	CORRESPONDING PLASMA OR SERUM LEVEL (µg/mL)	TISSUE (FLUID) PLASMA (SERUM) RATIO[1]
SKIN	0.012	35
LUNG	0.012	>100
SPUTUM*	0.64	2
SPUTUM**	0.1	30
TONSIL***	0.03	>100
TONSIL***	0.006	>100
CERVIX****	0.04	70

[1] High tissue concentrations should not be interpreted to be quantitatively related to clinical efficacy. The antimicrobial activity of azithromycin is pH related. Azithromycin is concentrated in cell lysosomes which have a low intraorganelle pH, at which the drug's activity is reduced. However, the extensive distribution of drug to tissues may be relevant to clinical activity.

* Sample was obtained 2–4 hours after the first dose.

** Sample was obtained 10–12 hours after the first dose.

*** Dosing regimen of 2 doses of 250 mg each, separated by 12 hours.

**** Sample was obtained 19 hours after a single 500 mg dose.

The extensive tissue distribution was confirmed by examination of additional tissues and fluids (bone, ejaculum, prostate, ovary, uterus, salpinx, stomach, liver, and gallbladder). As there are no data from adequate and well-controlled studies of azithromycin treatment of infections in these additional body sites, the clinical significance of these tissue concentration data is unknown.

Following a regimen of 500 mg on the first day and 250 mg daily for 4 days, only very low concentrations were noted in cerebrospinal fluid (less than 0.01 µg/mL) in the presence of non-inflamed meninges.

Pediatric Pharmacokinetics:

In two clinical studies, azithromycin for oral suspension was dosed at 10 mg/kg on day 1, followed by 5 mg/kg on days 2 through 5 to two groups of children (aged 1–5 years and 5–15 years, respectively). The mean pharmacokinetic parameters at Day 5 were $C_{max} = 0.216$ µg/mL, $T_{max} = 1.9$ hours, and $AUC_{0-24} = 1.822$ µg·hr/mL for the 1- to 5-year-old group and were $C_{max} = 0.383$ µg/mL, $T_{max} = 2.4$ hours, and $AUC_{0-24} = 3.109$ µg·hr/mL for the 5- to 15-year-old group. There are no pharmacokinetic data on azithromycin suspension when administered at a dose of 12 mg/kg/day in the presence or absence of food. (For the pediatric pharyngitis/tonsillitis dose, see **DOSAGE AND ADMINISTRATION.**)

Microbiology: Azithromycin acts by binding to the 50S ribosomal subunit of susceptible microorganisms and, thus, interfering with microbial protein synthesis. Nucleic acid synthesis is not affected.

Azithromycin concentrates in phagocytes and fibroblasts as demonstrated by in vitro incubation techniques. Using such methodology, the ratio of intracellular to extracellular concentration was > 30 after one hour incubation. In vivo studies suggest that concentration in phagocytes may contribute to drug distribution to inflamed tissues.

Azithromycin has been shown to be active against most strains of the following microorganisms, both in vitro and in clinical infections as described in the **INDICATIONS AND USAGE** section.

Aerobic gram-positive microorganisms
Staphylococcus aureus
Streptococcus agalactiae
Streptococcus pneumoniae
Streptococcus pyogenes
NOTE: Azithromycin demonstrates cross-resistance with erythromycin-resistant gram-positive strains. Most strains of *Enterococcus faecalis* and methicillin-resistant staphylococci are resistant to azithromycin.

Aerobic gram-negative microorganisms
Haemophilus ducreyi
Haemophilus influenzae
Moraxella catarrhalis
Neisseria gonorrhoeae

"Other" microorganisms
Chlamydia pneumoniae
Chlamydia trachomatis
Mycoplasma pneumoniae
Beta-lactamase production should have no effect on azithromycin activity.

The following in vitro data are available, **but their clinical significance is unknown.**

Azithromycin exhibits in vitro minimum inhibitory concentrations (MIC's) of 0.5 µg/mL or less against most (≥90%) strains of streptococci and MIC's of 2.0 µg/mL or less against most (≥90%) strains of other listed microorganisms. However, the safety and effectiveness of azithromycin in treating clinical infections due to these microorganisms have not been established in adequate and well-controlled trials.

Aerobic gram-positive microorganisms
Streptococci (Groups C, F, G)
Viridans group streptococci

Anaerobic microorganisms
Peptostreptococcus species
Prevotella bivia

Aerobic gram-negative microorganisms
Bordetella pertussis
Legionella pneumophila

"Other" microorganisms
Ureaplasma urealyticum

Susceptibility Tests

Azithromycin can be solubilized for in vitro susceptibility testing using dilution techniques by dissolving in a minimum amount of 95% ethanol and diluting to the working stock concentration with broth. Further dilutions may be made in water.

Dilution Techniques:

Quantitative methods are used to determine antimicrobial minimum inhibitory concentrations (MIC's). These MIC's provide estimates of the susceptibility of bacteria to antimicrobial compounds. The MIC's should be determined using a standardized procedure. Standardized procedures are based on a dilution method[1] (broth or agar) or equivalent with standardized inoculum concentrations and standardized concentrations of azithromycin powder. The MIC values should be interpreted according to the following criteria:

For testing aerobic microorganisms other than *Haemophilus* species, *Neisseria gonorrhoeae*, and streptococci:

MIC (µg/mL)	Interpretation
≤2	Susceptible (S)
4	Intermediate (I)
≥8	Resistant (R)

For testing *Haemophilus* species:[a]

MIC (µg/mL)	Interpretation
≤4	Susceptible (S)

[a] These interpretive standards are applicable only to broth microdilution susceptibility testing with *Haemophilus* species using Haemophilus Test Medium.[1]

The current absence of data on resistant strains precludes defining any categories other than "Susceptible." Strains yielding MIC results suggestive of a "nonsusceptible" category should be submitted to a reference laboratory for further testing.

For testing Streptococci including *S. pneumoniae*:[b]

MIC (µg/mL)	Interpretation
≤0.5	Susceptible (S)
1	Intermediate (I)
≥2	Resistant (R)

[b] These interpretive standards are applicable only to broth microdilution susceptibility tests using cation-adjusted Mueller-Hinton broth with 2–5% lysed horse blood.

No interpretive criteria have been established for testing *Neisseria gonorrhoeae*. This species is not usually tested. A report of "Susceptible" indicates that the pathogen is likely to respond to monotherapy with azithromycin. A re-

port of "Intermediate" indicates that the result should be considered equivocal, and, if the microorganism is not fully susceptible to alternative, clinically feasible drugs, the test should be repeated. This category implies possible clinical applicability in body sites where the drug is physiologically concentrated or in situations where high dosage of drug can be used. This category also provides a buffer zone which prevents small uncontrolled technical factors from causing major discrepancies in interpretation. A report of "Resistant" indicates that achievable drug concentrations are unlikely to be inhibitory; other therapy should be selected.

Standardized susceptibility test procedures require the use of laboratory control microorganisms to control the technical aspects of the laboratory procedures. Standard azithromycin powder should provide the following MIC values:

Microorganism	MIC (μg/mL)
Haemophilus influenzae ATCC 49247[a]	1.0–4.0
Staphylococcus aureus ATCC 29213	0.5–2.0
Streptococcus pneumoniae ATCC 49619[b]	0.06–0.25

[a] This quality control range is applicable only to H. influenzae ATCC 49247 tested by a broth microdilution procedure using Haemophilus Test Medium (HTM).[1]
[b] This quality control range is applicable to only S. pneumoniae ATCC 49619 tested by a broth microdilution procedure using cation-adjusted Mueller-Hinton broth with 2–5% lysed horse blood.

No interpretive criteria have been established for testing Neisseria gonorrhoeae. This species is not usually tested.

Diffusion Techniques:
Quantitative methods that require measurement of zone diameters also provide reproducible estimates of the susceptibility of bacteria to antimicrobial compounds. One such standardized procedure[2] requires the use of standardized inoculum concentrations. This procedure uses paper disks impregnated with 15-μg azithromycin to test the susceptibility of microorganisms to azithromycin.

Reports from the laboratory providing results of the standard single-disk susceptibility test with a 15-μg azithromycin disk should be interpreted according to the following criteria:

For testing aerobic microorganisms (including streptococci)[a] except Haemophilus species and Neisseria gonorrhoeae:

Zone Diameter (mm)	Interpretation
≥18	Susceptible (S)
14–17	Intermediate (I)
≤13	Resistant (R)

[a] These zone diameter standards for streptococci apply only to tests performed using Mueller-Hinton agar supplemented with 5% sheep blood and incubated in 5% CO$_2$.

For testing Haemophilus species:[b]

Zone Diameter (mm)	Interpretation
≥12	Susceptible (S)

[b] These zone diameter standards apply only to tests with Haemophilus species using Haemophilus Test Medium (HTM).[2]

The current absence of data on resistant strains precludes defining any categories other than "Susceptible." Strains yielding zone diameter results suggestive of a "nonsusceptible" category should be submitted to a reference laboratory for further testing.

No interpretive criteria have been established for testing Neisseria gonorrhoeae. This species is not usually tested.

Interpretation should be as stated above for results using dilution techniques. Interpretation involves correlation of the diameter obtained in the disk test with the MIC for azithromycin.

As with standardized dilution techniques, diffusion methods require the use of laboratory control microorganisms that are used to control the technical aspects of the laboratory procedures. For the diffusion technique, the 15-μg azithromycin disk should provide the following zone diameters in these laboratory test quality control strains:

Microorganism	Zone Diameter (mm)
Haemophilus influenzae ATCC 49247[a]	13–21
Staphylococcus aureus ATCC 25923	21–26
Streptococcus pneumoniae ATCC 49619[b]	19–25

[a] These quality control limits apply only to tests conducted with H. influenzae ATCC 49247 using Haemophilus Test Medium (HTM).[2]
[b] These quality control limits apply only to tests conducted with S. pneumoniae ATCC 49619 using Mueller-Hinton agar supplemented with 5% sheep blood incubated in 5% CO$_2$.

INDICATIONS AND USAGE

ZITHROMAX® (azithromycin) is indicated for the treatment of patients with mild to moderate infections (pneumonia: see **WARNINGS**) caused by susceptible strains of the designated microorganisms in the specific conditions listed below. As recommended dosages, durations of therapy, and applicable patient populations vary among these infections, please see **DOSAGE AND ADMINISTRATION** for specific dosing recommendations.

Adults:

Acute bacterial exacerbations of chronic obstructive pulmonary disease due to Haemophilus influenzae, Moraxella catarrhalis, or Streptococcus pneumoniae.

Community-acquired pneumonia due to Chlamydia pneumoniae, Haemophilus influenzae, Mycoplasma pneumoniae, or Streptococcus pneumoniae in patients appropriate for oral therapy.

NOTE: Azithromycin should not be used in patients with pneumonia who are judged to be inappropriate for oral therapy because of moderate to severe illness or risk factors such as any of the following:

patients with cystic fibrosis,
patients with nosocomially acquired infections,
patients with known or suspected bacteremia,
patients requiring hospitalization,
elderly or debilitated patients, or
patients with significant underlying health problems that may compromise their ability to respond to their illness (including immunodeficiency or functional asplenia).

Pharyngitis/tonsillitis caused by Streptococcus pyogenes as an alternative to first-line therapy in individuals who cannot use first-line therapy.

NOTE: Penicillin by the intramuscular route is the usual drug of choice in the treatment of Streptococcus pyogenes infection and the prophylaxis of rheumatic fever. ZITHROMAX® is often effective in the eradication of susceptible strains of Streptococcus pyogenes from the nasopharynx. Because some strains are resistant to ZITHROMAX®, susceptibility tests should be performed when patients are treated with ZITHROMAX®. Data establishing efficacy of azithromycin in subsequent prevention of rheumatic fever are not available.

Uncomplicated skin and skin structure infections due to Staphylococcus aureus, Streptococcus pyogenes, or Streptococcus agalactiae. Abscesses usually require surgical drainage.

Urethritis and cervicitis due to Chlamydia trachomatis or Neisseria gonorrhoeae.

Genital ulcer disease in men due to Haemophilus ducreyi (chancroid). Due to the small number of women included in clinical trials, the efficacy of azithromycin in the treatment of chancroid in women has not been established.

ZITHROMAX®, at the recommended dose, should not be relied upon to treat syphilis. Antimicrobial agents used in high doses for short periods of time to treat non-gonococcal urethritis may mask or delay the symptoms of incubating syphilis. All patients with sexually-transmitted urethritis or cervicitis should have a serologic test for syphilis and appropriate cultures for gonorrhea performed at the time of diagnosis. Appropriate antimicrobial therapy and follow-up tests for these diseases should be initiated if infection is confirmed.

Appropriate culture and susceptibility tests should be performed before treatment to determine the causative organism and its susceptibility to azithromycin. Therapy with ZITHROMAX® may be initiated before results of these tests are known; once the results become available, antimicrobial therapy should be adjusted accordingly.

Children: (See **Pediatric Use** and **CLINICAL STUDIES IN PEDIATRIC PATIENTS.**)

Acute otitis media caused by Haemophilus influenzae, Moraxella catarrhalis, or Streptococcus pneumoniae. (For specific dosage recommendation, see **DOSAGE AND ADMINISTRATION.**)

Community-acquired pneumonia due to Chlamydia pneumoniae, Haemophilus influenzae, Mycoplasma pneumoniae, or Streptococcus pneumoniae in patients appropriate for oral therapy. (For specific dosage recommendation, see **DOSAGE AND ADMINISTRATION.**)

NOTE: Azithromycin should not be used in pediatric patients with pneumonia who are judged to be inappropriate for oral therapy because of moderate to severe illness or risk factors such as any of the following:

patients with cystic fibrosis,
patients with nosocomially acquired infections,
patients with known or suspected bacteremia,
patients requiring hospitalization, or
patients with significant underlying health problems that may compromise their ability to respond to their illness (including immunodeficiency or functional asplenia).

Pharyngitis/tonsillitis caused by Streptococcus pyogenes as an alternative to first-line therapy in individuals who cannot use first-line therapy. (For specific dosage recommendation, see **DOSAGE AND ADMINISTRATION.**)

NOTE: Penicillin by the intramuscular route is the usual drug of choice in the treatment of Streptococcus pyogenes infection and the prophylaxis of rheumatic fever. ZITHROMAX® is often effective in the eradication of susceptible strains of Streptococcus pyogenes from the nasopharynx. Because some strains are resistant to ZITHROMAX®, susceptibility tests should be performed when patients are treated with ZITHROMAX®. Data establishing efficacy of azithromycin in subsequent prevention of rheumatic fever are not available.

Appropriate culture and susceptibility tests should be performed before treatment to determine the causative organism and its susceptibility to azithromycin. Therapy with ZITHROMAX® may be initiated before results of these tests are known; once the results become available, antimicrobial therapy should be adjusted accordingly.

CONTRAINDICATIONS

ZITHROMAX® is contraindicated in patients with known hypersensitivity to azithromycin, erythromycin, or any macrolide antibiotic.

WARNINGS

Serious allergic reactions, including angioedema, anaphylaxis, and dermatologic reactions including Stevens Johnson Syndrome and toxic epidermal necrolysis have been reported rarely in patients on azithromycin therapy. Although rare, fatalities have been reported. (See **CONTRAINDICATIONS.**) Despite initially successful symptomatic treatment of the allergic symptoms, when symptomatic therapy was discontinued, the allergic symptoms **recurred soon thereafter in some patients without further azithromycin exposure.** These patients required prolonged periods of observation and symptomatic treatment. The relationship of these episodes to the long tissue half-life of azithromycin and subsequent prolonged exposure to antigen is unknown at present.

If an allergic reaction occurs, the drug should be discontinued and appropriate therapy should be instituted. Physicians should be aware that reappearance of the allergic symptoms may occur when symptomatic therapy is discontinued.

In the treatment of pneumonia, azithromycin has only been shown to be safe and effective in the treatment of community-acquired pneumonia due to Chlamydia pneumoniae, Haemophilus influenzae, Mycoplasma pneumoniae, or Streptococcus pneumoniae in patients appropriate for oral therapy. Azithromycin should not be used in patients with pneumonia who are judged to be inappropriate for oral therapy because of moderate to severe illness or risk factors such as any of the following: patients with cystic fibrosis, patients with nosocomially acquired infections, patients with known or suspected bacteremia, patients requiring hospitalization, elderly or debilitated patients, or patients with significant underlying health problems that may compromise their ability to respond to their illness (including immunodeficiency or functional asplenia).

Pseudomembranous colitis has been reported with nearly all antibacterial agents and may range in severity from mild to life-threatening. Therefore, it is important to consider this diagnosis in patients who present with diarrhea subsequent to the administration of antibacterial agents.

Treatment with antibacterial agents alters the normal flora of the colon and may permit overgrowth of clostridia. Studies indicate that a toxin produced by Clostridium difficile is a primary cause of "antibiotic-associated colitis."

After the diagnosis of pseudomembranous colitis has been established, therapeutic measures should be initiated. Mild cases of pseudomembranous colitis usually respond to discontinuation of the drug alone. In moderate to severe cases, consideration should be given to management with fluids and electrolytes, protein supplementation, and treatment with an antibacterial drug clinically effective against Clostridium difficile colitis.

PRECAUTIONS

General: Because azithromycin is principally eliminated via the liver, caution should be exercised when azithromycin is administered to patients with impaired hepatic function. There are no data regarding azithromycin usage in patients with renal impairment; thus, caution should be exercised when prescribing azithromycin in these patients.

The following adverse events have not been reported in clinical trials with azithromycin, an azalide; however, they have been reported with macrolide products: ventricular arrhythmias, including ventricular tachycardia and torsades de pointes, in individuals with prolonged QT intervals.

There has been a spontaneous report from the post-marketing experience of a patient with previous history of arrhythmias who experienced torsades de pointes and subsequent myocardial infarction following a course of azithromycin therapy.

Information for Patients:
Patients should be cautioned to take ZITHROMAX® capsules and ZITHROMAX® suspension at least one hour prior to a meal or at least two hours after a meal. These medications should not be taken with food.

Continued on next page

Zithromax—Cont.

ZITHROMAX® tablets can be taken with or without food. Patients should also be cautioned not to take aluminum- and magnesium-containing antacids and azithromycin simultaneously.

The patient should be directed to discontinue azithromycin immediately and contact a physician if any signs of an allergic reaction occur.

Drug Interactions: Aluminum- and magnesium-containing antacids reduce the peak serum levels (rate) but not the AUC (extent) of azithromycin absorption.

Administration of cimetidine (800 mg) two hours prior to azithromycin had no effect on azithromycin absorption.

Azithromycin did not affect the plasma levels or pharmacokinetics of theophylline administered as a single intravenous dose. The effect of azithromycin on the plasma levels or pharmacokinetics of theophylline administered in multiple doses resulting in therapeutic steady-state levels of theophylline is not known. However, concurrent use of macrolides and theophylline has been associated with increases in the serum concentrations of theophylline. Therefore, until further data are available, prudent medical practice dictates careful monitoring of plasma theophylline levels in patients receiving azithromycin and theophylline concomitantly.

Azithromycin did not affect the prothrombin time response to a single dose of warfarin. However, prudent medical practice dictates careful monitoring of prothrombin time in all patients treated with azithromycin and warfarin concomitantly. Concurrent use of macrolides and warfarin in clinical practice has been associated with increased anticoagulant effects.

The following drug interactions have not been reported in clinical trials with azithromycin; however, no specific drug interaction studies have been performed to evaluate potential drug-drug interaction. Nonetheless, they have been observed with macrolide products. Until further data are developed regarding drug interactions when azithromycin and these drugs are used concomitantly, careful monitoring of patients is advised:

Digoxin—elevated digoxin levels.

Ergotamine or dihydroergotamine—acute ergot toxicity characterized by severe peripheral vasospasm and dysesthesia.

Triazolam—decrease the clearance of triazolam and thus may increase the pharmacologic effect of triazolam.

Drugs metabolized by the cytochrome P^{450} system—elevations of serum carbamazepine, terfenadine, cyclosporine, hexobarbital, and phenytoin levels.

Laboratory Test Interactions: There are no reported laboratory test interactions.

Carcinogenesis, Mutagenesis, Impairment of Fertility: Long-term studies in animals have not been performed to evaluate carcinogenic potential. Azithromycin has shown no mutagenic potential in standard laboratory tests: mouse lymphoma assay, human lymphocyte clastogenic assay, and mouse bone marrow clastogenic assay. No evidence of impaired fertility due to azithromycin was found.

Pregnancy: Teratogenic Effects. Pregnancy Category B: Reproduction studies have been performed in rats and mice at doses up to moderately maternally toxic dose levels (i.e., 200 mg/kg/day). These doses, based on a mg/m^2 basis, are estimated to be 4 and 2 times, respectively, the human daily dose of 500 mg. In the animal studies, no evidence of harm to the fetus due to azithromycin was found. There are, however, no adequate and well-controlled studies in pregnant women. Because animal reproduction studies are not always predictive of human response, azithromycin should be used during pregnancy only if clearly needed.

Nursing Mothers: It is not known whether azithromycin is excreted in human milk. Because many drugs are excreted in human milk, caution should be exercised when azithromycin is administered to a nursing woman.

Pediatric Use: (See **CLINICAL PHARMACOLOGY, INDICATIONS AND USAGE,** and **DOSAGE AND ADMINISTRATION.**)

Acute Otitis Media (dosage regimen: 10 mg/kg on Day 1 followed by 5 mg/kg on Days 2–5): Safety and effectiveness in the treatment of children with otitis media under 6 months of age have not been established.

Community-Acquired Pneumonia (dosage regimen: 10 mg/kg on Day 1 followed by 5 mg/kg on Days 2–5): Safety and effectiveness in the treatment of children with community-acquired pneumonia under 6 months of age have not been established. Safety and effectiveness for pneumonia due to Chlamydia pneumoniae and Mycoplasma pneumoniae were documented in pediatric clinical trials. Safety and effectiveness for pneumonia due to Haemophilus influenzae and Streptococcus pneumoniae were not documented bacteriologically in the pediatric clinical trial due to difficulty in obtaining specimens. Use of azithromycin for these two microorganisms is supported, however, by evidence from adequate and well-controlled studies in adults.

Pharyngitis/Tonsillitis (dosage regimen: 12 mg/kg on Days 1–5): Safety and effectiveness in the treatment of children with pharyngitis/tonsillitis under 2 years of age have not been established.

Studies evaluating the use of repeated courses of therapy have not been conducted. (See CLINICAL PHARMACOLOGY and ANIMAL TOXICOLOGY.)

Geriatric Use: Pharmacokinetic parameters in older volunteers (65–85 years old) were similar to those in younger volunteers (18–40 years old) for the 5-day therapeutic regimen. Dosage adjustment does not appear to be necessary for older patients with normal renal and hepatic function receiving treatment with this dosage regimen. (See **CLINICAL PHARMACOLOGY.**)

ADVERSE REACTIONS

In clinical trials, most of the reported side effects were mild to moderate in severity and were reversible upon discontinuation of the drug. Approximately 0.7% of the patients (adults and children) from the multiple-dose clinical trials discontinued ZITHROMAX® (azithromycin) therapy because of treatment-related side effects. Most of the side effects leading to discontinuation were related to the gastrointestinal tract, e.g., nausea, vomiting, diarrhea, or abdominal pain. Potentially serious side effects of angioedema and cholestatic jaundice were reported rarely.

Clinical:

Adults:

Multiple-dose regimen: Overall, the most common side effects in adult patients receiving a multiple-dose regimen of ZITHROMAX® were related to the gastrointestinal system with diarrhea/loose stools (5%), nausea (3%), and abdominal pain (3%) being the most frequently reported.

No other side effects occurred in patients on the mutliple-dose regimen of ZITHROMAX® with a frequency greater than 1%. Side effects that occurred with a frequency of 1% or less included the following:

Cardiovascular: Palpitations, chest pain.

Gastrointestinal: Dyspepsia, flatulence, vomiting, melena, and cholestatic jaundice.

Genitourinary: Monilia, vaginitis, and nephritis.

Nervous System: Dizziness, headache, vertigo, and somnolence.

General: Fatigue.

Allergic: Rash, photosensitivity, and angioedema.

Single 1-gram dose regimen: Overall, the most common side effects in patients receiving a single-dose regimen of 1 gram of ZITHROMAX® were related to the gastrointestinal system and were more frequently reported than in patients receiving the multiple-dose regimen.

Side effects that occurred in patients on the single one-gram dosing regimen of ZITHROMAX® with a frequency of 1% or greater included diarrhea/loose stools (7%), nausea (5%), abdominal pain (5%), vomiting (2%), dyspepsia (1%), and vaginitis (1%).

Single 2-gram dose regimen: Overall, the most common side effects in patients receiving a single 2-gram dose of ZITHROMAX® were related to the gastrointestinal system. Side effects that occurred in patients in this study with a frequency of 1% or greater included nausea (18%), diarrhea/loose stools (14%), vomiting (7%), abdominal pain (7%), vaginitis (2%), dyspepsia (1%), and dizziness (1%). The majority of these complaints were mild in nature.

Children:

Multiple-dose regimens: The types of side effects in children were comparable to those seen in adults, with different incidence rates for the two dosage regimens recommended in children.

Acute Otitis Media: For the recommended dosage regimen of 10 mg/kg on Day 1 followed by 5 mg/kg on Days 2–5, the most frequent side effects attributed to treatment were diarrhea/loose stools (2%), abdominal pain (2%), vomiting (1%), and nausea (1%).

Community-Acquired Pneumonia: For the recommended dosage regimen of 10 mg/kg on Day 1 followed by 5 mg/kg on Days 2–5, the most frequent side effects attributed to treatment were diarrhea/loose stools (5.8%), abdominal pain, vomiting, and nausea (1.9% each), and rash (1.6%).

Pharyngitis/tonsillitis: For the recommended dosage regimen of 12 mg/kg on Days 1–5, the most frequent side effects attributed to treatment were diarrhea/loose stools (6%), vomiting (5%), abdominal pain (3%), nausea (2%), and headache (1%).

With either treatment regimen, no other side effects occurred in children treated with ZITHROMAX® with a frequency greater than 1%. Side effects that occurred with a frequency of 1% of less included the following:

Cardiovascular: Chest pain.

Gastrointestinal: Dyspepsia, constipation, anorexia, flatulence, and gastritis.

Nervous System: Headache (otitis media dosage), hyperkinesia, dizziness, agitation, nervousness, insomnia.

General: Fever, fatigue, malaise.

Allergic: Rash.

Skin and Appendages: Pruritus, urticaria.

Special Senses: Conjunctivitis.

Post-Marketing Experience:

Adverse events reported with azithromycin during the post-marketing period in adult and/or pediatric patients for which a causal relationship may not be established include:

Allergic: Arthralgia, edema, urticaria.

Cardiovascular: Arrhythmias including ventricular tachycardia.

Gastrointestinal: Anorexia, constipation, dyspepsia, flatulence, vomiting/diarrhea rarely resulting in dehydration.

General: Asthenia, paresthesia.

Genitourinary: Interstitial nephritis and acute renal failure.

Liver/Biliary: Abnormal liver function including hepatitis and cholestatic jaundice.

Nervous System: Convulsions.

Skin/Appendages: Rarely serious skin reactions including erythema multiforme, Stevens Johnson Syndrome, and toxic epidermal necrolysis.

Special Senses: Hearing disturbances including hearing loss, deafness, and/or tinnitus, rare reports of taste disturbances.

Laboratory Abnormalities:

Adults:

Significant abnormalities (irrespective of drug relationship) occurring during the clinical trials were reported as follows: with an incidence of 1–2%, elevated serum creatine phosphokinase, potassium, ALT (SGPT), GGT, and AST (SGOT); with an incidence of less than 1%, leukopenia, neutropenia, decreased platelet count, elevated serum alkaline phosphatase, bilirubin, BUN, creatinine, blood glucose, LDH, and phosphate.

When follow-up was provided, changes in laboratory tests appeared to be reversible.

In multiple-dose clinical trials involving more than 3000 patients, 3 patients discontinued therapy because of treatment-related liver enzyme abnormalities and 1 because of a renal function abnormality.

Children:

Significant abnormalities (irrespective of drug relationship) occurring during clinical trials were all reported at a frequency of less than 1%, but were similar in type to the adult pattern.

In multiple-dose clinical trials involving almost 3300 pediatric patients, no patients discontinued therapy because of treatment-related laboratory abnormalities

DOSAGE AND ADMINISTRATION

(See INDICATIONS AND USAGE and CLINICAL PHARMACOLOGY.)

Adults:

The recommended dose of ZITHROMAX® for the treatment of mild to moderate acute bacterial exacerbations of chronic obstructive pulmonary disease, community-acquired pneumonia of mild severity, pharyngitis/tonsillitis (as second-line therapy), and uncomplicated skin and skin structure infections due to the indicated organisms is: 500 mg as a single dose on the first day followed by 250 mg once daily on days 2 through 5.

ZITHROMAX® capsules should be given at least 1 hour before or 2 hours after a meal. ZITHROMAX® capsules should not be taken with food.

ZITHROMAX® tablets can be taken with or without food.

The recommended dose of ZITHROMAX® for the treatment of genital ulcer disease due to Haemophilus ducreyi (chancroid), non-gonococcal urethritis and cervicitis due to C. trachomatis is: a single 1 gram (1000 mg) dose of ZITHROMAX®.

The recommended dose of ZITHROMAX® for the treatment of urethritis and cervicitis due to Neisseria gonorrhoeae is a single 2 gram (2000 mg) dose of ZITHROMAX®.

Children:

Acute Otitis Media and Community-Acquired Pneumonia: The recommended dose of ZITHROMAX® for oral suspension for the treatment of children with acute otitis media and community-acquired pneumonia is 10 mg/kg as a single dose on the first day (not to exceed 500 mg/day) followed by 5 mg/kg on days 2 through 5 (not to exceed 250 mg/day). (See chart below.)

ZITHROMAX® for oral suspension should be given at least 1 hour before or 2 hours after a meal.

ZITHROMAX® for oral suspension should not be taken with food.

[See table at top right of next page]

Pharyngitis/Tonsillitis: The recommended dose for children with pharyngitis/tonsillitis is 12 mg/kg once a day for 5 days (not to exceed 500 mg/day). (See chart below.)

ZITHROMAX® for oral suspension should be given at least 1 hour before or 2 hours after a meal.

ZITHROMAX® for oral suspension should not be taken with food.

PEDIATRIC DOSAGE GUIDELINES FOR PHARYNGITIS/TONSILLITIS
(Age 2 years and above, see Pediatric Use.)
Based on Body Weight

PHARYNGITIS/TONSILLITIS

Dosing Calculated on 12 mg/kg once daily Days 1 to 5.

Weight Kg	lbs	200 mg/5 mL Suspension Day 1–5	Total mL per Treatment Course
8	18	2.5 mL (½ tsp)	12.5 mL
17	37	5 mL (1 tsp)	25 mL
25	55	7.5 mL (1½ tsp)	37.5 mL
33	73	10 mL (2 tsp)	50 mL
40	88	12.5 mL (2½ tsp)	62.5 mL

Constituting instructions for ZITHROMAX® Oral Suspension, 300, 600, 900, 1200 mg bottles. The table below indicates the volume of water to be used for constitution.

Amount of water to be added	Total volume after constitution (azithromycin content)	Azithromycin concentration after constitution
9 mL (300 mg)	15 mL (300 mg)	100 mg/5 mL
9 mL (600 mg)	15 mL (600 mg)	200 mg/5 mL
12 mL (900 mg)	22.5 mL (900 mg)	200 mg/5 mL
15 mL (1200 mg)	30 mL (1200 mg)	200 mg/5 mL

Shake well before each use. Oversized bottle provides shake space. Keep tightly closed.
After mixing, store at 5° to 30°C (41° to 86°F) and use within 10 days. Discard after full dosing is completed.

HOW SUPPLIED

ZITHROMAX® tablets are supplied as red modified capsular shaped, engraved, film-coated tablets containing azithromycin dihydrate equivalent to 250 mg of azithromycin. ZITHROMAX® tablets are engraved with "Pfizer" on one side and "306" on the other. These are packaged in bottles and blister cards of 6 tablets (Z-PAKS®) as follows:

Bottles of 30	NDC 0069-3060-30
Boxes of 3 (Z-PAKS® of 6)	NDC 0069-3060-75
Unit Dose package of 50	NDC 0069-3060-86

ZITHROMAX® tablets should be stored between 15° to 30°C (59° to 86°F).
ZITHROMAX® for oral suspension after constitution contains a flavored suspension. ZITHROMAX® for oral suspension is supplied in bottles with accompanying calibrated dropper as follows:

Azithromycin contents per bottle	NDC
300 mg	0069-3110-19
600 mg	0069-3120-19
900 mg	0069-3130-19
1200 mg	0069-3140-19

Storage: Store dry powder below 30°C (86°F). Store constituted suspension between 5° to 30°C (41° to 86°F) and discard when full dosing is completed.

CLINICAL STUDIES IN PEDIATRIC PATIENTS
(See INDICATIONS AND USAGE and Pediatric Use.)
From the perspective of evaluating pediatric clinical trials, Days 11–14 (6–9 days after completion of the five-day regimen) were considered on-therapy evaluations because of the extended half-life of azithromycin. Day 11–14 data are provided for clinical guidance. Day 30 evaluations were considered the primary test of cure endpoint.

Acute Otitis Media
Efficacy Protocol 1
In a double-blind, controlled clinical study of acute otitis media performed in the United States, azithromycin (10 mg/kg on Day 1 followed by 5 mg/kg on Days 2–5) was compared to an antimicrobial/beta-lactamase inhibitor. In this study, very strict evaluability criteria were used to determine clinical response and safety results were obtained. For the 553 patients who were evaluated for clinical efficacy, the clinical success rate (i.e., cure plus improvement) at the Day 11 visit was 88% for azithromycin and 88% for the control agent. For the 521 patients who were evaluated at the Day 30 visit, the clinical success rate was 73% for azithromycin and 71% for the control agent.
In the safety analysis of the above study, the incidence of adverse events, primarily gastrointestinal, in all patients

PEDIATRIC DOSAGE GUIDELINES FOR OTITIS MEDIA AND COMMUNITY-ACQUIRED PNEUMONIA
(Age 6 months and above, see Pediatric Use.)
Based on Body Weight

OTITIS MEDIA AND COMMUNITY-ACQUIRED PNEUMONIA

Dosing Calculated on 10 mg/kg on Day 1 dose, followed by 5 mg/kg on Days 2 to 5.

Weight Kg	lbs	100 mg/5mL Suspension Day 1	Days 2–5	200 mg/5 mL Suspension Day 1	Days 2–5	Total mL per Treatment Course
10	22	5 mL (1 tsp)	2.5 mL (½ tsp)			15 mL
20	44			5 mL (1 tsp)	2.5 mL (½ tsp)	15 mL
30	66			7.5 mL (1½ tsp)	3.75 mL (¾ tsp)	22.5 mL
40	88			10 mL (2 tsp)	5 mL (1 tsp)	30 mL

treated was 9% with azithromycin and 31% with the control agent. The most common side effects were diarrhea/loose stools (4% azithromycin vs. 20% control), vomiting (2% azithromycin vs. 7% control), and abdominal pain (2% azithromycin vs. 5% control).
Efficacy Protocol 2
In a noncomparative clinical and microbiologic trial performed in the United States, where significant rates of beta-lactamase producing organisms (35%) were found, 131 patients were evaluable for clinical efficacy. The combined clinical success rate (i.e., cure and improvement) at the Day 11 visit was 84% for azithromycin. For the 122 patients who were evaluated at the Day 30 visit, the clinical success rate was 70% for azithromycin.
Microbiologic determinations were made at the pre-treatment visit. Microbiology was not reassessed at later visits. The following presumptive bacterial/clinical cure outcomes (i.e., clinical success) were obtained from the evaluable group.
Bacteriologic Eradication:

	Day 11 Azithromycin	Day 30 Azithromycin
S. pneumoniae	61/74 (82%)	40/56 (71%)
H. influenzae	43/54 (80%)	30/47 (64%)
M. catarrhalis	28/35 (80%)	19/26 (73%)
S. pyogenes	11/11 (100%)	7/7
Overall	177/217 (82%)	97/137 (73%)

In the safety analysis of this study, the incidence of adverse events, primarily gastrointestinal, in all patients treated was 9%. The most common side effect was diarrhea (4%).
Efficacy Protocol 3
In another controlled comparative clinical and microbiologic study of otitis media performed in the United States, azithromcyin was compared to an antimicrobial/beta-lactamase inhibitor. This study utilized two of the same investigators as Efficacy Protocol 2 (above), and these two investigators enrolled 90% of the patients in Efficacy Protocol 3. For this reason, Efficacy Protocol 3 was not considered to be an independent study. Significant rates of beta-lactamase producing organisms (20%) were found. Ninety-two (92) patients were evaluable for clinical and microbiologic efficacy. The combined clinical success rate (i.e., cure and improvement) of those patients with a baseline pathogen at the Day 11 visit was 88% for azithromycin vs. 100% for control; at the Day 30 visit, the clinical success rate was 82% for azithromycin vs. 80% for control.
Microbiologic determinations were made at the pre-treatment visit. Microbiology was not reassessed at later visits. At the Day 11 and Day 30 visits, the following presumptive bacterial/clinical cure outcomes (i.e., clinical success) were obtained from the evaluable group:
[See table below]
In the safety analysis of the above study, the incidence of adverse events, primarily gastrointestinal, in all patients treated was 4% with azithromycin and 31% with the control agent. The most common side effect was diarrhea/loose stools (2% azithromycin vs. 29% control.)
Pharyngitis/Tonsillitis
In 3 double-blind controlled studies, conducted in the United States, azithromycin (12 mg/kg once a day for 5 days) was compared to penicillin V (250 mg three times a

day for 10 days) in the treatment of pharyngitis due to documented Group A β-hemolytic streptococci (GABHS or S. pyogenes). Azithromycin was clinically and microbiologically statistically superior to penicillin at Day 14 and Day 30 with the following clinical success (i.e., cure and improvement) and bacteriologic efficacy rates (for the combined evaluable patient with documented GABHS):

Three U.S. Streptococcal Pharyngitis Studies
Azithromycin vs. Penicillin V
EFFICACY RESULTS

	Day 14	Day 30
Bacteriologic Eradication:		
Azithromycin	323/340 (95%)	255/330 (77%)
Penicillin V	242/332 (73%)	206/325 (63%)
Clinical Success (Cure plus improvement):		
Azithromycin	336/343 (98%)	310/330 (94%)
Penicillin V	284/338 (84%)	241/325 (74%)

Approximately 1% of azithromycin-susceptible S. pyogenes isolates were resistant to azithromycin following therapy. The incidence of adverse events, primarily gastrointestinal, in all patients treated was 18% on azithromycin and 13% on penicillin. The most common side effects were diarrhea/loose stools (6% azithromycin vs. 2% penicillin), vomiting (6% azithromycin vs. 4% penicillin), and abdominal pain (3% azithromycin vs. 1% penicillin).

ANIMAL TOXICOLOGY

Phospholipidosis (intracellular phospholipid accumulation) has been observed in some tissues of mice, rats, and dogs given multiple doses of azithromycin. It has been demonstrated in numerous organ systems (e.g., eye, dorsal root ganglia, liver, gallbladder, kidney, spleen, and pancreas) in dogs treated with azithromycin at doses which, expressed on a mg/kg basis, are only 2 times greater than the recommended adult human dose and in rats at doses comparable to the recommended adult human dose. This effect has been reversible after cessation of azithromycin treatment. Phospholipidosis has been observed to a similar extent in the tissues of neonatal rats and dogs given daily doses of azithromycin ranging from 10 days to 30 days. Based on the pharmacokinetic data, phospholipidosis has been seen in the rat (30 mg/kg dose) at observed C_{max} value of 1.3 μg/mL (6 times greater than the observed C_{max} of 0.216 μg/mL at the pediatric dose of 10 mg/kg). Similarly, it has been shown in the dog (10 mg/kg dose) at observed C_{max} value of 1.5 μg/mL (7 times greater than the observed same C_{max} and drug dose in the studied pediatric population). On mg/m² basis, 30 mg/kg dose in the rat (135 mg/m²) and 10 mg/kg dose in the dog (79 mg/m²) are approximately 0.4 and 0.6 times, respectively, the recommended dose in the pediatric patients with an average body weight of 25 kg. This effect, similar to that seen in the adult animals, is reversible after cessation of azithromycin treatment. The significance of these findings for animals and for humans is unknown.

REFERENCES
1. National Committee for Clinical Laboratory Standards. Methods for Dilution Antimicrobial Susceptibility Tests for Bacteria that Grow Aerobically—Third Edition. Approved Standard NCCLS Document M7-A3, Vol. 13, No. 25, NCCLS, Villanova, PA, December 1993.

Continued on next page

Bacteriologic Eradication:

	Day 11 Azithromycin	Control	Day 30 Azithromycin	Control
S. pneumoniae	25/29 (86%)	26/26 (100%)	22/28 (79%)	18/22 (82%)
H. influenzae	9/11 (82%)	9/9	8/10 (80%)	6/8
M. catarrhalis	7/7	5/5	5/5	2/3
S. pyogenes	2/2	5/5	2/2	4/4
Overall	43/49 (88%)	45/45 (100%)	37/45 (82%)	30/37 (81%)

Zithromax—Cont.

2. National Committee for Clinical Laboratory Standards. Performance Standards for Antimicrobial Disk Susceptibility Tests—Fifth Edition. Approved Standard NCCLS Document M2-A5, Vol. 13, No. 24, NCCLS, Villanova, PA, December 1993.

Licensed from Pliva
70-5179-00-6

©1997 PFIZER INC
Revised April 1997

Shown in Product Identification Guide, page 331

ZITHROMAX® ℞
(azithromycin capsules)
(azithromycin tablets)
and
(azithromycin for oral suspension)

DESCRIPTION

ZITHROMAX® (azithromycin capsules, azithromycin tablets and azithromycin for oral suspension) contain the active ingredient azithromycin, an azalide, a subclass of macrolide antibiotics, for oral administration. Azithromycin has the chemical name (2R,3S,4R,5R,8R,10R,11R,12S,13S,14R)-13-[(2,6-dideoxy-3-C-methyl-3-O-methyl-α-L-ribo-hexopyranosyl)oxy]-2-ethyl-3,4,10-trihydroxy-3,5,6,8,10,12,14-heptamethyl-11-[[3,4,6-trideoxy-3-(dimethylamino)-β-D-xylo-hexopyranosyl]oxy]-1-oxa-6-azacyclopentadecan-15-one. Azithromycin is derived from erythromycin; however, it differs chemically from erythromycin in that a methyl-substituted nitrogen atom is incorporated into the lactone ring. Its molecular formula is $C_{38}H_{72}N_2O_{12}$, and its molecular weight is 749.0. Azithromycin has the following structural formula:

Azithromycin, as the dihydrate, is a white crystalline powder with a molecular formula of $C_{38}H_{72}N_2O_{12}\cdot2H_2O$ and a molecular weight of 785.0.

ZITHROMAX® capsules contain azithromycin dihydrate equivalent to 250 mg of azithromycin. The capsules are supplied in red opaque hard-gelatin capsules (containing FD&C Red #40). They also contain the following inactive ingredients: anhydrous lactose, corn starch, magnesium stearate, and sodium lauryl sulfate.

ZITHROMAX® tablets contain azithromycin dihydrate equivalent to 600 mg azithromycin. The tablets are supplied as white, modified oval-shaped, film-coated tablets. They also contain the following inactive ingredients: dibasic calcium phosphate anhydrous, pregelatinized starch, sodium croscarmellose, magnesium stearate, sodium lauryl sulfate, and an aqueous film coat consisting of hydroxypropyl methyl cellulose, titanium dioxide, lactose and triacetin.

ZITHROMAX® for oral suspension is supplied in a single dose packet containing azithromycin dihydrate equivalent to 1 g azithromycin. It also contains the following inactive ingredients: colloidal silicon dioxide, sodium phosphate tribasic, anhydrous; spray dried artificial banana flavor, spray dried artificial cherry flavor, and sucrose.

CLINICAL PHARMACOLOGY

Pharmacokinetics: Following oral administration, azithromycin is rapidly absorbed and widely distributed throughout the body. Rapid distribution of azithromycin into tissues and high concentration within cells result in significantly higher azithromycin concentrations in tissues than in plasma or serum. The 1 g single dose packet is bioequivalent to four 250 mg capsules.

The pharmacokinetic parameters of azithromycin in plasma after dosing as per labeled recommendations in healthy young adults (age 18–40 years old) are portrayed in the following chart:

[See table at top of page]

In these studies (500 mg Day 1, 250 mg Days 2–5), there was no significant difference in the disposition of azithromycin between male and female subjects. Plasma concentrations of azithromycin following single 500 mg oral and i.v. doses declined in a polyphasic pattern resulting in an average terminal half-life of 68 hours. With a regimen of 500 mg

MEAN (CV%) PK PARAMETER

DOSE/DOSAGE FORM	Subjects	Day No.	C_{max} μg/ml	T_{max} (hr)	C_{24} (μg/ml)	AUC (μg *hr/ ml)	$T_{1/2}$ (hr)	Urinary Excretion (% of dose)
500 mg/250 mg capsule	12	Day 1	0.41	2.5	0.05	2.6[a]	—	4.5
and 250 mg on Days 2–5	12	Day 5	0.24	3.2	0.05	2.1[a]	—	6.5
1200 mg/600 mg tablets	12	Day 1	0.66	2.5	0.074	6.8[b]	40	—
			(62%)	(79%)	(49%)	(64%)	(33%)	—

[a] 0–24 hr
[b] 0–last.

on Day 1 and 250 mg/day on Days 2–5, C_{min} and C_{max} remained essentially unchanged from Day 2 through Day 5 of therapy. However, without a loading dose, azithromycin C_{min} levels required 5 to 7 days to reach steady-state.

When azithromycin capsules were administered with food, the rate of absorption (C_{max}) of azithromycin was reduced by 52% and the extent of absorption (AUC) by 43%.

When the oral suspension of azithromycin was administered with food, the C_{max} increased by 46% and the AUC by 14%.

The absolute bioavailability of two 600 mg tablets was 34% (CV=56%). Administration of two 600 mg tablets with food increased C_{max} by 31% (CV=43%) while the extent of absorption (AUC) was unchanged (mean ratio of AUCs=1.00; CV=55%).

The AUC of azithromycin in 250 mg capsules was unaffected by coadministration of an antacid containing aluminum and magnesium hydroxide with ZITHROMAX® (azithromycin); however, the C_{max} was reduced by 24%. Administration of cimetidine (800 mg) two hours prior to azithromycin had no effect on azithromycin absorption.

When studied in healthy elderly subjects from age 65 to 85 years, the pharmacokinetic parameters of azithromycin (500 mg Day 1, 250 mg Days 2–5) in elderly men were similar to those in young adults; however, in elderly women, although higher peak concentrations (increased by 30 to 50%) were observed, no significant accumulation occurred. The high values in adults for apparent steady-state volume of distribution (31.1 L/kg) and plasma clearance (630 mL/min) suggest that the prolonged half-life is due to extensive uptake and subsequent release of drug from tissues. Selected tissue (or fluid) concentration and tissue (or fluid) to plasma/serum concentration ratios are shown in the following table:

AZITHROMYCIN CONCENTRATIONS FOLLOWING TWO 250 mg (500 mg) CAPSULES IN ADULTS

TISSUE OR FLUID	TIME AFTER DOSE (h)	TISSUE OR FLUID CONCENTRATION (μg/g or μg/mL)[1]
SKIN	72–96	0.4
LUNG	72–96	4.0
SPUTUM*	2–4	1.0
SPUTUM**	10–12	2.9
TONSIL***	9–18	4.5
TONSIL***	180	0.9
CERVIX****	19	2.8

TISSUE OR FLUID	CORRESPONDING PLASMA OR SERUM LEVEL (μg/mL)	TISSUE (FLUID) PLASMA (SERUM) RATIO[1]
SKIN	0.012	35
LUNG	0.012	>100
SPUTUM*	0.64	2
SPUTUM**	0.1	30
TONSIL***	0.03	>100
TONSIL***	0.006	>100
CERVIX****	0.04	70

[1] High tissue concentrations should not be interpreted to be quantitatively related to clinical efficacy. The antimicrobial activity of azithromycin is pH related. Azithromycin is concentrated in cell lysosomes which have a low intraorganelle pH, at which the drug's activity is reduced. However, the extensive distribution of drug to tissues may be relevant to clinical activity.
* Sample was obtained 2–4 hours after the first dose.
** Sample was obtained 10–12 hours after the first dose.
*** Dosing regimen of 2 doses of 250 mg each, separated by 12 hours.
**** Sample was obtained 19 hours after a single 500 mg dose.

The extensive tissue distribution was confirmed by examination of additional tissues and fluids (bone, ejaculum, prostate, ovary, uterus, salpinx, stomach, liver, and gallbladder). As there are no data from adequate and well-controlled studies of azithromycin treatment of infections in these additional body sites, the clinical significance of these tissue concentration data is unknown.

Following a regimen of 500 mg on the first day and 250 mg daily for 4 days, only very low concentrations were noted in cerebrospinal fluid (less than 0.01 μg/mL) in the presence of non-inflamed meninges.

Following oral administration of a single 1200 mg dose (two 600 mg tablets), the mean maximum concentration in peripheral leukocytes was 140 μg/mL. Concentrations remained above 32 μg/mL for approximately 60 hr. The mean half-lives for 6 males and 6 females were 34 hr and 57 hr, respectively. Leukocyte to plasma C_{max} ratios for males and females were 258 (±77%) and 175 (±60%), respectively, and the AUC ratios were 804 (±31%) and 541 (±28%), respectively. The clinical relevance of these findings is unknown. The serum protein binding of azithromycin is variable in the concentration range approximating human exposure, decreasing from 51% at 0.02 μg/mL to 7% at 2 μg/mL. Biliary excretion of azithromycin, predominantly as unchanged drug, is a major route of elimination. Over the course of a week, approximately 6% of the administered dose appears as unchanged drug in urine.

There are no pharmacokinetic data available from studies in hepatically- or renally-impaired individuals.

The effect of azithromycin on the plasma levels or pharmacokinetics of theophylline administered in multiple doses adequate to reach therapeutic steady-state plasma levels is not known. (See PRECAUTIONS.)

Mechanism of Action: Azithromycin acts by binding to the 50S ribosomal subunit of susceptible microorganisms and, thus, interfering with microbial protein synthesis. Nucleic acid synthesis is not affected.

Azithromycin concentrates in phagocytes and fibroblasts as demonstrated by *in vitro* incubation techniques. Using such methodology, the ratio of intracellular to extracellular concentration was >30 after one hour incubation. *In vivo* studies suggest that concentration in phagocytes may contribute to drug distribution to inflamed tissues.

Microbiology:

Azithromycin has been shown to be active against most strains of the following microorganisms, both *in vitro* and in clinical infections as described in the INDICATIONS AND USAGE section.

Aerobic Gram-Positive Microorganisms
Staphylococcus aureus
Streptococcus agalactiae
Streptococcus pneumoniae
Streptococcus pyogenes
NOTE: Azithromycin demonstrates cross-resistance with erythromycin-resistant gram-positive strains. Most strains of *Enterococcus faecalis* and methicillin-resistant staphylococci are resistant to azithromycin.

Aerobic Gram-Negative Microorganisms
Haemophilus influenzae
Moraxella catarrhalis

"Other" Microorganisms
Chlamydia trachomatis
Beta-lactamase production should have no effect on azithromycin activity.

Azithromycin has been shown to be active *in vitro* and in the prevention of disease caused by the following microorganisms:

Mycobacteria
Mycobacterium avium complex (MAC) consisting of:
Mycobacterium avium
Mycobacterium intracellulare.
The following *in vitro* data are available, *but their clinical significance is unknown.*

Azithromycin exhibits *in vitro* minimal inhibitory concentrations (MICs) of 2.0 μg/mL or less against most (≥90%) strains of the following microorganisms; however, the safety and effectiveness of azithromycin in treating clinical infections due to these microorganisms have not been established in adequate and well-controlled trials.

Aerobic Gram-Positive Microorganisms
Streptococci (Groups C, F, G)
Viridans group streptococci

Aerobic Gram-Negative Microorganisms
Bordetella pertussis
Campylobacter jejuni
Haemophilus ducreyi
Legionella pneumophila

Anaerobic Microorganisms
Bacteroides bivius
Clostridium perfringens
Peptostreptococcus species

"Other" Microorganisms

Borrelia burgdorferi
Mycoplasma pneumoniae
Treponema pallidum
Ureaplasma urealyticum

Susceptibility Testing of Bacteria Excluding Mycobacteria

The *in vitro* potency of azithromycin is markedly affected by the pH of the microbiological growth medium during incubation. Incubation in a $10\% \ CO_2$ atmosphere will result in lowering of media pH (7.2 to 6.6) within 18 hours and in an apparent reduction of the *in vitro* potency of azithromycin. Thus, the initial pH of the growth medium should be 7.2–7.4, and the CO_2 content of the incubation atmosphere should be as low as practical.

Azithromycin can be solubilized for *in vitro* susceptibility testing by dissolving in a minimum amount of 95% ethanol and diluting to working concentration with water.

Dilution Techniques:

Quantitative methods are used to determine minimal inhibitory concentrations that provide reproducible estimates of the susceptibility of bacteria to antimicrobial compounds. One such standardized procedure uses a standardized dilution method[1] (broth, agar or microdilution) or equivalent with azithromycin powder. The MIC values should be interpreted according to the following criteria:

MIC (µg/mL)	Interpretation
≤2	Susceptible (S)
4	Intermediate (I)
≥8	Resistant (R)

A report of "Susceptible" indicates that the pathogen is likely to respond to monotherapy with azithromycin. A report of "Intermediate" indicates that the result should be considered equivocal, and, if the microorganism is not fully susceptible to alternative, clinically feasible drugs, the test should be repeated. This category also provides a buffer zone which prevents small uncontrolled technical factors from causing major discrepancies in interpretation. A report of "Resistant" indicates that usually achievable drug concentrations are unlikely to be inhibitory and that other therapy should be selected.

Measurement of MIC or MBC and achieved antimicrobial compound concentrations may be appropriate to guide therapy in some infections. (See CLINICAL PHARMACOLOGY section for further information on drug concentrations achieved in infected body sites and other pharmacokinetic properties of this antimicrobial drug product.)

Standardized susceptibility test procedures require the use of laboratory control microorganisms. Standard azithromycin powder should provide the following MIC values:

Microorganism	MIC (µg/mL)
Escherichia coli ATCC 25922	2.0–8.0
Enterococcus faecalis ATCC 29212	1.0–4.0
Staphylococcus aureus ATCC 29213	0.25–1.0

Diffusion Techniques:

Quantitative methods that require measurement of zone diameters also provide reproducible estimates of the susceptibility of bacteria to antimicrobial compounds. One such standardized procedure[2] that has been recommended for use with disks to test the susceptibility of microorganisms to azithromycin uses the 15-µg azithromycin disk. Interpretation involves the correlation of the diameter obtained in the disk test with the minimal inhibitory concentration (MIC) for azithromycin.

Reports from the laboratory providing results of the standard single-disk susceptibility test with a 15 µg azithromycin disk should be interpreted according to the following criteria:

Zone Diameter (mm)	Interpretation
≥18	(S) Susceptible
14–17	(I) Intermediate
≤13	(R) Resistant

Interpretation should be as stated above for results using dilution techniques.

As with standardized dilution techniques, diffusion methods require the use of laboratory control microorganisms. The 15-µg azithromycin disk should provide the following zone diameters in these laboratory test quality control strains:

Microorganism	Zone Diameter (mm)
Staphylococcus aureus ATCC 25923	21–26

In Vitro Activity of Azithromycin Against Mycobacteria.

Azithromycin has demonstrated *in vitro* activity against *Mycobacterium avium* complex (MAC) organisms. While gene probe techniques may be used to distinguish *M. avium* species from *M. intracellulare*, many studies only report results on *M. avium* complex (MAC) isolates. Azithromycin has also been shown to be active against phagocytized *M. avium* complex (MAC) organisms in mouse and human macrophage cell cultures as well as in the beige mouse infection model.

Various *in vitro* methodologies employing broth or solid media at different pHs, with and without oleic acid-albumin

dextrose-catalase (OADC), have been used to determine azithromycin MIC values for *Mycobacterium avium* complex strains. In general, MIC values decreased 4 to 8 fold as the pH of middlebrook 7H11 agar media increased from 6.6 to 7.4. At pH 7.4, MIC values determined with Mueller-Hinton agar were 4 fold higher than that observed with middlebrook 7H12 media at the same pH. Utilization of oleic acid-albumin-dextrose-catalase (OADC) in these assays has been shown to further alter MIC values. The ability to correlate MIC values and plasma drug levels is difficult as azithromycin concentrates in macrophages and tissues.

A cross resistance relationship between azithromycin and clarithromycin has been observed with some *Mycobacterium avium* complex (MAC) isolates. The various mechanisms of cross resistance between azithromycin and clarithromycin for *M. avium* complex organisms have not been fully characterized. The clinical significance of azithromycin and clarithromycin cross resistance is unknown.

Susceptibility testing for *Mycobacterium avium* complex (MAC):

The disk diffusion techniques and dilution methods for susceptibility testing against gram-positive and gram-negative bacteria should not be used for determining azithromycin MIC values against mycobacteria. *In vitro* susceptibility testing methods and diagnostic products currently available for determining minimal inhibitory concentration (MIC) values against *Mycobacterium avium* complex (MAC) organisms have not been established or validated. Azithromycin MIC values will vary depending on the susceptibility testing method employed, composition and pH of media and the utilization of nutritional supplements. Breakpoints to determine whether clinical isolates of *M. avium* or *M. intracellulare* are susceptible to azithromycin have not been established.

INDICATIONS AND USAGE

ZITHROMAX® (azithromycin) is indicated for the treatment of patients with mild to moderate infections (pneumonia: see WARNINGS) caused by susceptible strains of the designated microorganisms in the specific conditions listed below.

Lower Respiratory Tract:

Acute bacterial exacerbations of chronic obstructive pulmonary disease due to *Haemophilus influenzae*, *Moraxella catarrhalis*, or *Streptococcus pneumoniae*.

Community-acquired pneumonia of mild severity due to *Streptococcus pneumoniae* or *Haemophilus influenzae* in patients appropriate for outpatient oral therapy.

NOTE: Azithromycin should not be used in patients with pneumonia who are judged to be inappropriate for outpatient oral therapy because of moderate to severe illness or risk factors such as any of the following:

    patients with nosocomially acquired infections,

    patients with known or suspected bacteremia,

    patients requiring hospitalization,

    elderly or debilitated patients, or

    patients with significant underlying health problems that may compromise their ability to respond to their illness (including immunodeficiency or functional asplenia).

Upper Respiratory Tract:

Streptococcal pharyngitis/tonsillitis—As an alternative to first line therapy of acute pharyngitis/tonsillitis due to *Streptococcus pyogenes* occurring in individuals who cannot use first line therapy.

NOTE: Penicillin is the usual drug of choice in the treatment of *Streptococcus pyogenes* infection and the prophylaxis of rheumatic fever. ZITHROMAX® is often effective in the eradication of susceptible strains of *Streptococcus pyogenes* from the nasopharynx. Data establishing efficacy of azithromycin in subsequent prevention of rheumatic fever are not available.

Skin and Skin Structure

Uncomplicated skin and skin structure infections due to *Staphylococcus aureus*, *Streptococcus pyogenes*, or *Streptococcus agalactiae*. Abscesses usually require surgical drainage.

Sexually Transmitted Diseases

Non-gonococcal urethritis and cervicitis due to *Chlamydia trachomatis*.

ZITHROMAX®, at the recommended dose, should not be relied upon to treat gonorrhea or syphilis. Anitmicrobial agents used in high doses for short periods of time to treat non-gonococcal urethritis may mask or delay the symptoms of incubating gonorrhea or syphilis. All patients with sexually-transmitted urethritis or cervicitis should have a serologic test for syphilis and appropriate cultures for gonorrhea performed at the time of diagnosis. Appropriate antimicrobial therapy and follow-up tests for these diseases should be initiated if infection is confirmed.

Appropriate culture and susceptibility tests should be performed before treatment to determine the causative organism and its susceptibility to azithromycin. Therapy with ZITHROMAX® may be initiated before results of these tests are known; once the results become available, antimicrobial therapy should be adjusted accordingly.

Disseminated *Mycobacterium Avium* Complex (MAC) Disease

ZITHROMAX®, taken alone or in combination with rifabutin at its approved dose, is indicated for the prevention of disseminated *Mycobacterium avium* complex (MAC) disease in persons with advanced HIV infection. (See Clinical Trials section.)

CONTRAINDICATIONS

ZITHROMAX® is contraindicated in patients with known hypersensitivity to azithromycin, erythromycin, or any macrolide antibiotic.

WARNINGS

Rare serious allergic reactions, including angioedema and anaphylaxis, have been reported rarely in patients on azithromycin therapy. (See CONTRAINDICATIONS.) Despite initially successful symptomatic treatment of the allergic symptoms, when symptomatic therapy was discontinued, the allergic symptoms **recurred soon thereafter in some patients without further azithromycin exposure.** These patients required prolonged periods of observation and symptomatic treatment. The relationship of these episodes to the long tissue half-life of azithromycin and subsequent prolonged exposure to antigen is unknown at present. If an allergic reaction occurs, the drug should be discontinued and appropriate therapy should be instituted. Physicians should be aware that reappearance of the allergic symptoms may occur when symptomatic therapy is discontinued.

In the treatment of pneumonia, azithromycin has only been shown to be safe and effective in the treatment of community-acquired pneumonia of mild severity due to *Streptococcus pneumoniae* or *Haemophilus influenzae* in patients appropriate for outpatient oral therapy. Azithromycin should not be used in patients with pneumonia who are judged to be inappropriate for outpatient oral therapy because of moderate to severe illness or risk factors such as any of the following: patients with nosocomially acquired infections, patients with known or suspected bacteremia, patients requiring hospitalization, elderly or debilitated patients, or patients with significant underlying health problems that may compromise their ability to respond to their illness (including immunodeficiency or functional asplenia). Pseudomembranous colitis has been reported with nearly all antibacterial agents and may range in severity from mild to life-threatening. Therefore, it is important to consider this diagnosis in patients who present with diarrhea subsequent to the administration of antibacterial agents.

Treatment with antibacterial agents alters the normal flora of the colon and may permit overgrowth of clostridia. Studies indicate that a toxin produced by *Clostridium difficile* is a primary cause of "antibiotic-associated colitis."

After the diagnosis of pseudomembranous colitis has been established, therapeutic measures should be initiated. Mild cases of pseudomembranous colitis usually respond to discontinuation of the drug alone. In moderate to severe cases, consideration should be given to management with fluids and electrolytes, protein supplementation, and treatment with an antibacterial drug clinically effective against *Clostridium difficile* colitis.

PRECAUTIONS

General: Because azithromycin is principally eliminated via the liver, caution should be exercised when azithromycin is administered to patients with impaired hepatic function. There are no data regarding azithromycin usage in patients with renal impairment; thus, caution should be exercised when prescribing azithromycin in these patients.

The following adverse events have not been reported in clinical trials with azithromycin, an azalide; however, they have been reported with macrolide products: ventricular arrhythmias, including ventricular tachycardia and *torsades de pointes*, in individuals with prolonged QT intervals.

Information for Patients:

Patients should be cautioned to take ZITHROMAX® capsules at least one hour prior to a meal or at least two hours after a meal. Azithromycin capsules should not be taken with food.

ZITHROMAX® tablets may be taken with or without food. However, increased tolerability has been observed when tablets are taken with food.

ZITHROMAX® for oral suspension in single 1 g packets can be taken with or without food after constitution.

Patients should also be cautioned not to take aluminum- and magnesium-containing antacids and azithromycin simultaneously.

The patient should be directed to discontinue azithromycin immediately and contact a physician if any signs of an allergic reaction occur.

Drug Interactions: Aluminum- and magnesium-containing antacids reduce the peak serum levels (rate) but not the AUC (extent) of azithromycin (500 mg) absorption.

Continued on next page

Zithromax—Cont.

Administration of cimetidine (800 mg) two hours prior to azithromycin had no effect on azithromycin (500 mg) absorption.

Azithromycin (500 mg Day 1, 250 mg Days 2–5) did not affect the plasma levels or pharmacokinetics of theophylline administered as a single intravenous dose. The effect of azithromycin on the plasma levels or pharmacokinetics of theophylline administered in multiple doses resulting in therapeutic steady-state levels of theophylline is not known. However, concurrent use of macrolides and theophylline has been associated with increases in the serum concentrations of theophylline. Therefore, until further data are available, prudent medical practice dictates careful monitoring of plasma theophylline levels in patients receiving azithromycin and theophylline concomitantly.

Azithromycin (500 mg Day 1, 250 mg Days 2–5) did not affect the prothrombin time response to a single dose of warfarin. However, prudent medical practice dictates careful monitoring of prothrombin time in all patients treated with azithromycin and warfarin concomitantly. Concurrent use of macrolides and warfarin in clinical practice has been associated with increased anticoagulant effects.

Dose adjustments are not indicated when azithromycin and zidovudine are coadministered. When zidovudine (100 mg q3h ×5) was coadministered with daily azithromycin (600 mg, n=5 or 1200 mg, n=7), mean C_{max}, AUC and Clr increased by 26% (CV 54%), 10% (CV 26%) and 38% (CV114%), respectively. The mean AUC of phosphorylated zidovudine increased by 75% (CV 95%), while zidovudine glucuronide C_{max} and AUC increased by less than 10%. In another study, addition of 1 gram azithromycin per week to a regimen of 10 mg/kg daily zidovudine resulted in 25% (CV 70%) and 13% (CV 37%) increases in zidovudine C_{max} and AUC, respectively. Zidovudine glucuronide mean C_{max} and AUC increased by 16% (CV 61%) and 8.0% (CV 32%), respectively.

Doses of 1200 mg/day azithromycin for 14 days in 6 subjects increased C_{max} of concurrently administered didanosine (200 mg *q.* 12h) by 44% (54% CV) and AUC by 14% (23% CV). However, none of these changes were significantly different from those produced in a parallel placebo control group of subjects.

Preliminary data suggest that coadministration of azithromycin and rifabutin did not markedly affect the mean serum concentrations of either drug. Administration of 250 mg azithromycin daily for 10 days (500 mg on the first day) produced mean concentrations of azithromycin 1 day after the last dose of 53 ng/ml when coadministered with 300 mg daily rifabutin and 49 mg/ml when coadministered with placebo. Mean concentrations 5 days after the last dose were 23 ng/ml and 21 ng/ml in the two groups of subjects. Administration of 300 mg rifabutin for 10 days produced mean concentrations of rifabutin one half day after the last dose of 60 mg/ml when coadministered with daily 250 mg azithromycin and 71 ng/ml when coadministered with placebo. Mean concentrations 5 days after the last dose were 8.1 ng/ml and 9.2 ng/ml in the two groups of subjects.

The following drug interactions have not been reported in clinical trials with azithromycin; however, no specific drug interaction studies have been performed to evaluate potential drug-drug interaction. Nonetheless, they have been observed with macrolide products. Until further data are developed regarding drug interactions when azithromycin and these drugs are used concomitantly, careful monitoring of patients is advised:

Digoxin—elevated digoxin levels.

Ergotamine or dihydroergotamine—acute ergot toxicity characterized by severe peripheral vasospasm and dysesthesia.

Triazolam—decrease the clearance of triazolam and thus may increase the pharmacologic effect of triazolam.

Drugs metabolized by the cytochrome P^{450} system—elevations of serum carbamazepine, cyclosporine, hexobarbital, and phenytoin levels.

Laboratory Test Interactions: There are no reported laboratory test interactions.

Carcinogenesis, Mutagenesis, Impairment of Fertility: Long-term studies in animals have not been performed to evaluate carcinogenic potential. Azithromycin has shown no mutagenic potential in standard laboratory tests: mouse lymphoma assay, human lymphocyte clastogenic assay, and mouse bone marrow clastogenic assay.

Pregnancy: Teratogenic Effects. Pregnancy Category B: Reproduction studies have been performed in rats and mice at doses up to moderately maternally toxic dose levels (i.e., 200 mg/kg/day). These doses, based on a mg/m² basis, are estimated to be 4 to 2 times, respectively, the human daily dose of 500 mg.

With regard to the MAC prophylaxis dose of 1200 mg weekly, on a mg/m²/day basis, the doses in rats and mice are approximately 2 and 1 times the human dose, respectively. No evidence of impaired fertility or harm to the fetus due to azithromycin was found. There are, however, no adequate

and well-controlled studies in pregnant women. Because animal reproduction studies are not always predictive of human response, azithromycin should be used during pregnancy only if clearly needed.

Nursing Mothers: It is not known whether azithromycin is excreted in human milk. Because many drugs are excreted in human milk, caution should be exercised when azithromycin is administered to a nursing woman.

Pediatric Use:
In controlled clinical studies, azithromycin has been administered to pediatric patients ranging in age from 6 months to 12 years. For information regarding the use of ZITHROMAX (azithromycin for oral suspension) in the treatment of pediatric patients, please refer to the INDICATIONS AND USAGE and DOSAGE AND ADMINISTRATION sections of the prescribing information for ZITHROMAX (azithromycin for oral suspension) 100 mg/5 mL and 200 mg/5 mL bottles. Prevention of Disseminated *Mycobacterium avium* complex (MAC) Disease: Safety and efficacy of azithromycin for the prevention of MAC in children have not been established. Limited safety data are available for 24 children 5 months to 14 years of age (mean 4.6 years) who received azithromycin for treatment of opportunistic infections. The mean duration of therapy was 186.7 days (range 13–710 days) at doses of <5 to 20 mg/kg/day. Three children were treated for 6 months or more and 4 children were treated for 1 month or more with a dose of >10 mg/kg/day. Adverse events were similar to those observed in the adult population, most of which involved the gastrointestinal tract. While none of these children prematurely discontinued treatment due to a side effect, one child discontinued due to a laboratory abnormality (eosinophilia). The protocols upon which these data are based specified a daily dose of 10–20 mg/kg/day of azithromycin.

Geriatric Use: Pharmacokinetic parameters in older volunteers (65–85 years old) were similar to those in younger volunteers (18–40 years old) for the 5-day therapeutic regimen. Dosage adjustment does not appear to be necessary for older patients with normal renal and hepatic function receiving treatment with this dosage regimen. (See CLINICAL PHARMACOLOGY.)

ADVERSE REACTIONS

In clinical trials, most of the reported side effects were mild to moderate in severity and were reversible upon discontinuation of the drug. Approximately 0.7% of the patients from the multiple-dose clinical trials discontinued ZITHROMAX® (azithromycin) therapy because of treatment-related side effects. Most of the side effects leading to discontinuation were related to the gastrointestinal tract, e.g., nausea, vomiting, diarrhea, or abdominal pain. Rarely but potentially serious side effects were angioedema and cholestatic jaundice.

Clinical:
Multiple-dose regimen:
Overall, the most common side effects in adult patients receiving a multiple-dose regimen of ZITHROMAX® were related to the gastrointestinal system with diarrhea/loose stools (5%), nausea (3%), and abdominal pain (3%) being the most frequently reported.

No other side effects occurred in patients on the multiple-dose regimen of ZITHROMAX® with a frequency greater than 1%. Side effects that occurred with a frequency of 1% or less included the following:

Cardiovascular: Palpitations, chest pain.

Gastrointestinal: Dyspepsia, flatulence, vomiting, melena, and cholestatic jaundice.

Genitourinary: Monilia, vaginitis, and nephritis.

Nervous System: Dizziness, headache, vertigo, and somnolence.

General: Fatigue.

Allergic: Rash, photosensitivity, and angioedema.

Chronic therapy with 1200 mg weekly regimen: The nature of side effects seen with the 1200 mg weekly dosing regimen for the prevention of *Mycobacterium avium* infection in severely immunocompromised HIV-infected patients were similar to those seen with short term dosing regimens. (See CLINICAL TRIALS.)

Single 1-gram dose regimen: Overall, the most common side effects in patients receiving a single-dose regimen of 1

gram of ZITHROMAX® were related to the gastrointestinal system and were more frequently reported than in patients receiving the multiple-dose regimen.

Side effects that occurred in patients on the single one-gram dosing regimen of ZITHROMAX® with a frequency of 1% or greater included diarrhea/loose stools (7%), nausea (5%), abdominal pain (5%), vomiting (2%), dyspepsia (1%), and vaginitis (1%).

Laboratory Abnormalities:
Significant abnormalities (irrespective of drug relationship) occurring during the clinical trials were reported as follows: With an incidence of 1–2%, elevated serum creatine phosphokinase, potassium, ALT (SGPT), GGT, and AST (SGOT). With an incidence of less than 1%, leukopenia, neutropenia, decreased platelet count, elevated serum alkaline phosphatase, bilirubin, BUN, creatinine, blood glucose, LDH, and phosphate.

When follow-up was provided, changes in laboratory tests appeared to be reversible.

In multiple-dose clinical trials involving more than 3000 patients, 3 patients discontinued therapy because of treatment-related liver enzyme abnormalities and 1 because of a renal function abnormality.

In a phase I drug interaction study performed in normal volunteers, 1 of 6 subjects given the combination of azithromycin and rifabutin, 1 of 7 given rifabutin alone and 0 of 6 given azithromycin alone developed a clinically significant neutropenia (<500 cells/mm³).

Laboratory abnormalities seen in clinical trials for the prevention of disseminated *Mycobacterium avium* disease in severely immunocompromised HIV-infected patients are presented in the CLINICAL TRIALS section.

DOSAGE AND ADMINISTRATION (See INDICATIONS AND USAGE.)

ZITHROMAX® capsules should be given at least 1 hour before or 2 hours after a meal. ZITHROMAX® capsules should not be mixed with or taken with food.

ZITHROMAX® for oral suspension (single dose 1 g packet) can be taken with or without food after constitution. Not for pediatric use. For pediatric suspension, please refer to the INDICATIONS AND USAGE and DOSAGE AND ADMINISTRATION sections of the prescribing information for ZITHROMAX (azithromycin for oral suspension) 100 mg/5 mL and 200 mg/5 mL bottles.

ZITHROMAX® tablets may be taken without regard to food. However, increased tolerability has been observed when tablets are taken with food.

The recommended dose of ZITHROMAX® for the treatment of individuals 16 years of age and older with mild to moderate acute bacterial exacerbations of chronic obstructive pulmonary disease, pneumonia, pharyngitis/tonsillitis (as second line therapy), and uncomplicated skin and skin structure infections due to the indicated organisms is: 500 mg as a single dose on the first day followed by 250 mg once daily on Days 2 through 5 for a total dose of 1.5 grams of ZITHROMAX®.

The recommended dose of ZITHROMAX® for the prevention of disseminated *Mycobacterium avium* complex (MAC) disease is: 1200 mg taken once weekly. This dose of ZITHROMAX® may be combined with the approved dosage regimen of rifabutin.

The recommended dose of ZITHROMAX® for the treatment of non-gonococcal urethritis and cervicitis due to *C. trachomatis* is: a single 1 gram (1000 mg) dose of ZITHROMAX®. This dose can be administered as four 250 mg capsules or as one single dose packet (1 g).

DIRECTIONS FOR ADMINISTRATION OF ZITHROMAX® for oral suspension in the single dose packet (1 g): The entire contents of the packet should be mixed thoroughly with two ounces (approximately 60 mL) of water. Drink the entire contents immediately; add an additional two ounces of water, mix, and drink to assure complete consumption of dosage. **The single dose packet should not be used to administer doses other than 1000 mg of azithromycin. This packet not for pediatric use.**

HOW SUPPLIED

ZITHROMAX® capsules (imprinted with "Pfizer 305") are supplied in red opaque hard-gelatin capsules containing

Cumulative Incidence Rate, %: Placebo (n=89)

Month	MAC Free and Alive	MAC	Adverse Experience	Lost to Follow-up
6	69.7	13.5	6.7	10.1
12	47.2	19.1	15.7	18.0
18	37.1	22.5	18.0	22.5

Cumulative Incidence Rate, %: Azithromycin (n=85)

Month	MAC Free and Alive	MAC	Adverse Experience	Lost to Follow-up
6	84.7	3.5	9.4	2.4
12	63.5	8.2	16.5	11.8
18	44.7	11.8	25.9	17.6

Cumulative Incidence Rate, %: Ritabutin (n=223)

Month	MAC Free and Alive	MAC	Adverse Experience	Lost to Follow-up
6	83.4	7.2	8.1	1.3
12	60.1	15.2	16.1	8.5
18	40.8	21.5	24.2	13.5

Cumulative Incidence Rate, %: Azithromycin (n=223)

Month	MAC Free and Alive	MAC	Adverse Experience	Lost to Follow-up
6	85.2	3.6	5.8	5.4
12	65.5	7.6	16.1	10.8
18	45.3	12.1	23.8	18.8

Cumulative Incidence Rate, %: Azithromycin/Rifabutin Combination (n=218)

Month	MAC Free and Alive	MAC	Adverse Experience	Lost to Follow-up
6	89.4	1.8	5.5	3.2
12	71.6	2.8	15.1	10.6
18	49.1	6.4	29.4	15.1

INCIDENCE OF ONE OR MORE TREATMENT RELATED* ADVERSE EVENTS** IN HIV INFECTED PATIENTS RECEIVING PROPHYLAXIS FOR DISSEMINATED MAC OVER APPROXIMATELY 1 YEAR

	Study 155		Study 174		
	Placebo (N=91)	Azithromycin 1200 mg weekly (N=89)	Azithromycin 1200 mg weekly (N=233)	Rifabutin 300 mg daily (N=236)	Azithromycin + Rifabutin (N=224)
Mean Duration of Therapy (days)	303.8	402.9	315	296.1	344.4
Discontinuation of Therapy	2.3	8.2	13.5	15.9	22.7
Autonomic Nervous System					
Mouth Dry	0	0	0	3.0	2.7
Central Nervous System					
Dizziness	0	1.1	3.9	1.7	0.4
Headache	0	0	3.0	5.5	4.5
Gastrointestinal					
Diarrhea	15.4	52.8	50.2	19.1	50.9
Loose Stools	6.6	19.1	12.9	3.0	9.4
Abdominal Pain	6.6	27	32.2	12.3	31.7
Dyspepsia	1.1	9	4.7	1.7	1.8
Flatulence	4.4	9	10.7	5.1	5.8
Nausea	11	32.6	27.0	16.5	28.1
Vomiting	1.1	6.7	9.0	3.8	5.8
General					
Fever	1.1	0	2.1	4.2	4.9
Fatigue	0	2.2	3.9	2.1	3.1
Malaise	0	1.1	0.4	0	2.2
Musculoskeletal					
Arthralgia	0	0	3.0	4.2	7.1
Psychiatric					
Anorexia	1.1	0	2.1	2.1	3.1
Skin & Appendages					
Pruritus	3.3	0	3.9	3.4	7.6
Rash	3.2	3.4	8.1	9.4	11.1
Skin discoloration	0	0	0	2.1	2.2
Special Senses					
Tinnitus	4.4	3.4	0.9	1.3	0.9
Hearing Decreased	2.2	1.1	0.9	0.4	0
Uveitis	0	0	0.4	1.3	1.8
Taste Perversion	0	0	1.3	2.5	1.3

* Includes those events considered possibly or probably related to study drug
** >2% adverse event rates for any group (except uveitis).

Prophylaxis Against Disseminated MAC Abnormal Laboratory Values*

		Placebo	Azithromycin 1200 mg weekly	Rifabutin 300 mg daily	Azithromycin & Rifabutin
Hemoglobin	<8 g/dl	1/51 2%	4/170 2%	4/114 4%	8/107 8%
Platelet Count	$<50 \times 10^3/mm^3$	1/71 1%	4/260 2%	2/182 1%	6/181 3%
WBC Count	$<1 \times 10^3/mm^3$	0/8 0%	2/70 3%	2/47 4%	0/43 0%
Neutrophils	<500/mm³	0/26 0%	4/106 4%	3/82 4%	2/78 3%
SGOT	$>5 \times ULN^a$	1/41 2%	8/158 5%	3/121 3%	6/114 5%
SGPT	$>5 \times ULN$	0/49 0%	8/166 5%	3/130 2%	5/117 4%
Alk Phos	$>5 \times ULN$	1/80 1%	4/247 2%	2/172 1%	3/164 2%

^{a}= Upper Limit of Normal
* excludes subjects outside of the relevant normal range at baseline

azithromycin dihydrate equivalent to 250 mg of azithromycin. These are packaged in bottles and blister cards of 6 capsules (Z-PAKS™) as follows:

Bottles of 50　　　　　　　　　　NDC 0069-3050-50
Boxes of 3 (Z-PAKS™ of 6)　　　NDC 0069-3050-34
Unit Dose package of 50　　　　　NDC 0069-3050-86

Store capsules below 30°C (86°F).

ZITHROMAX® 600 mg tablets (engraved on front with "PFIZER" and on back with "308") are supplied as white, modified oval-shaped, film-coated tablets containing azithromycin dihydrate equivalent to 600 mg azithromycin.

These are packaged in bottles of 30 tablets. ZITHROMAX® tablets are supplied as follows:
Bottles of 30　　　　　　　　　NDC 0069-3080-30
Tablets should be stored at or below 30° C (86°F).
ZITHROMAX® for oral suspension is supplied in single dose packets containing azithromycin dihydrate equivalent to 1 gram of azithromycin as follows:
Boxes of 10 Single Dose
Packets (1 g)　　　　　　　　　NDC 0069-3051-07
Boxes of 3 Single Dose
Packets (1 g)　　　　　　　　　NDC 0069-3051-75
Store single dose packets between 5° and 30°C (41° and 86°F).

CLINICAL STUDIES IN PATIENTS WITH ADVANCED HIV INFECTION FOR THE PREVENTION OF DISEASE DUE TO DISSEMINATED *MYCOBACTERIUM AVIUM* COMPLEX (MAC) (See INDICATIONS AND USAGE):
Two randomized, double blind clinical trials were performed in patients with CD4 counts <100 cells/μL. The first study (155) compared azithromycin (1200 mg once weekly) to placebo and enrolled 182 patients with a mean CD4 count of 35 cells/μL. The second study (174) randomized 723 patients to either azithromycin (1200 mg once weekly), rifabutin (300 mg daily) or the combination of both. The mean CD4 count was 51 cells/μL. The primary endpoint in these studies was disseminated MAC disease. Other endpoints included the incidence of clinically significant MAC disease and discontinuations from therapy for drug-related side effects.

MAC bacteremia
In trial 155, 85 patients randomized to receive azithromycin and 89 patients randomized to receive placebo met study entrance criteria. Cumulative incidences at 6, 12 and 18 months of the possible outcomes are in the following table:
[See table at bottom of previous page]
The difference in the one year cumulative incidence rates of disseminated MAC disease (placebo–azithromycin) is 10.9%. This difference is statistically significant (p=0.037) with a 95% confidence interval for this difference of (0.8%, 20.9%). The comparable number of patients experiencing adverse events and the fewer number of patients lost to follow-up on azithromycin should be taken into account when interpreting the significance of this difference.
In trial 174, 223 patients randomized to receive rifabutin, 223 patients randomized to receive azithromycin, and 218 patients randomized to receive both rifabutin and azithromycin met study entrance criteria. Cumulative incidences at 6, 12 and 18 months of the possible outcomes are recorded in the following table:
[See first table above]
Comparing the cumulative one year incidence rates, azithromycin monotherapy is at least as effective as rifabutin monotherapy. The difference (rifabutin–azithromycin) in the one year rates (7.6%) is statistically significant (p=0.022) with an adjusted 95% confidence interval (0.9%, 14.3%). Additionally, azithromycin/rifabutin combination therapy is more effective than rifabutin alone. The difference (rifabutin–azithromycin/rifabutin) in the cumulative one year incidence rates (12.5%) is statistically significant (p<0.001) with an adjusted 95% confidence interval of (6.6%, 18.4%). The comparable number of patients experiencing adverse events and the fewer number of patients lost to follow-up on rifabutin should be taken into account when interpreting the significance of this difference.
In Study 174, sensitivity testing* was performed on all available MAC isolates from subjects randomized to either azithromycin, rifabutin or the combination. The distribution of MIC values for azithromycin from susceptibility testing of the breakthrough isolates was similar between study arms. As the efficacy of azithromycin in the treatment of disseminated MAC has not been established, the clinical relevance of these *in vitro* MICs as an indicator of susceptibility or resistance is not known. (*Methodology per Inderlied CB, et al. Determination of *In Vitro* Susceptibility of *Mycobacterium avium* Complex Isolates to Antimicrobial Agents by Various Methods. Antimicrob. Agents Chemother 1987; 31: 1697–1702.)

Clinically Significant Disseminated MAC Disease
In association with the decreased incidence of bacteremia, patients in the groups randomized to either azithromycin alone or azithromycin in combination with rifabutin showed reductions in the signs and symptoms of disseminated MAC disease, including fever or night sweats, weight loss and anemia.

Discontinuations From Therapy For Drug-Related Side Effects
In Study 155, discontinuations for drug-related toxicity occurred in 8.2% of subjects treated with azithromycin and 2.3% of those given placebo (p=0.121). In Study 174, more subjects discontinued from the combination of azithromycin and rifabutin (22.7%) than from azithromycin alone (13.5%; p=0.026) or rifabutin alone (15.9%; p=0.209).

Safety
As these patients with advanced HIV disease were taking multiple concomitant medications and experienced a variety of intercurrent illnesses, it was often difficult to attribute adverse events to study medication. Overall, the nature of side effects seen on the weekly dosage regimen of

Continued on next page

Zithromax—Cont.

azithromycin over a period of approximately one year in patients with advanced HIV disease was similar to that previously reported for shorter course therapies.
[See second table on previous page]
Side effects related to the gastrointestinal tract were seen more frequently in patients receiving azithromycin than in those receiving placebo or rifabutin. In Study 174, 86% of diarrheal episodes were mild to moderate in nature with discontinuation of therapy for this reason occurring in only 9/233 (3.8%) of patients.

Changes in Laboratory Values

In these immunocompromised patients with advanced HIV infection, it was necessary to assess laboratory abnormalities developing on study with additional criteria if baseline values were outside the relevant normal range.
[See third table on previous page]

ANIMAL TOXICOLOGY

Phospholipidosis (intracellular phospholipid binding) has been observed in some tissues of mice, rats, and dogs given multiple doses of azithromycin. It has been demonstrated in numerous organ systems (e.g., eye, dorsal root ganglia, liver, gallbladder, kidney, spleen, and pancreas) in dogs administered doses which, based on pharmacokinetics, are as low as 2 times greater than the recommended adult human dose and in rats at doses comparable to the recommended adult human dose. This effect has been reversible after cessation of azithromycin treatment. The significance of these findings for humans is unknown.

REFERENCES

1. National Committee for Clinical Laboratory Standards. Methods for Dilution Antimicrobial Susceptibility Tests for Bacteria that Grow Aerobically—Third Edition. Approved Standard NCCLS Document M7-A3, Vol. 13, No. 25, NCCLS, Villanova, PA, December 1993.
2. National Committee for Clinical Laboratory Standards. Performance Standards for Antimicrobial Disk Susceptibility Tests—Fifth Edition. Approved Standard NCCLS Document M2-A5, Vol. 13, No. 24, NCCLS, Villanova, PA, December 1993.

Licensed from Pliva
©1996 PFIZER INC
Pfizer   **Printed in U.S.A.**
70-4763-00-2   Revised June 1996
Shown in Product Identification Guide, page 331

ZITHROMAX®
℞
(azithromycin for injection)
For IV infusion only

DESCRIPTION

ZITHROMAX® (azithromycin for injection) contains the active ingredient azithromycin, an azalide, a subclass of macrolide antibiotics, for intravenous injection. Azithromycin has the chemical name (2R,3S,4R,5R,8R,10R,11R,12S,13S,14R)-13-[(2,6-dideoxy-3-C-methyl-3-O-methyl-α-L-ribo-hexopyranosyl)oxy]-2-ethyl-3,4,10-trihydroxy-3,5,6,8,10,12,14-heptamethyl-11-[[3, 4, 6-trideoxy-3-(dimethylamino)-β-D-xylo-hexopyranosyl] oxy]-1-oxa-6-azacyclopentadecan-15-one. Azithromycin is derived from erythromycin; however, it differs chemically from erythromycin in that a methyl-substituted nitrogen atom is incorporated into the lactone ring. Its molecular formula is $C_{38}H_{72}N_2O_{12}$, and its molecular weight is 749.00. Azithromycin has the following structural formula:

Azithromycin, as the dihydrate, is a white crystalline powder with a molecular formula of $C_{38}H_{72}N_2O_{12} \cdot 2H_2O$ and a molecular weight of 785.0.
ZITHROMAX® (azithromycin for injection) consists of azithromycin dihydrate and the following inactive ingredients: citric acid and sodium hydroxide. ZITHROMAX® (azithromycin for injection) is supplied in lyophilized form in a 10-mL vial equivalent to 500 mg of azithromycin for intravenous administration. Reconstitution, according to label directions, results in approximately 5 mL of

---

Plasma concentrations (µg/mL ± S.D.) after the last daily intravenous infusion of 500 mg azithromycin

Infusion Concentration, Duration	Time after starting the infusion (hr)								
	0.5	1	2	3	4	6	8	12	24
2 mg/mL, 1 hr[a]	2.98 ±1.12	3.63 ±1.73	0.60 ±0.31	0.40 ±0.23	0.33 ±0.16	0.26 ±0.14	0.27 ±0.15	0.20 ±0.12	0.20 ±0.15
1 mg/mL, 3 hr[b]	0.91 ±0.13	1.02 ±0.11	1.14 ±0.13	1.13 ±0.16	0.32 ±0.05	0.28 ±0.04	0.27 ±0.03	0.22 ±0.02	0.18 ±0.02

[a]=500 mg (2 mg/mL) for 2–5 days in Community-acquired pneumonia patients.
[b]=500 mg (1 mg/mL) for 5 days in healthy subjects.

ZITHROMAX® for intravenous injection with each mL containing azithromycin dihydrate equivalent to 100 mg of azithromycin.

CLINICAL PHARMACOLOGY

In patients hospitalized with community-acquired pneumonia receiving single daily one-hour intravenous infusions for 2 to 5 days of 500 mg azithromycin at a concentration of 2 mg/mL, the mean Cmax ± S.D. achieved was 3.63 ± 1.60 µg/mL, while the 24-hour trough level was 0.20 ± 0.15 µg/mL, and the AUC₂₄ was 9.60 ± 4.80 µg·h/mL.
The mean Cmax, 24-hour trough and AUC₂₄ values were 1.14 ± 0.14 µg/mL, 0.18 ± 0.02 µg/mL, and 8.03 ±0.86 µg·h/mL, respectively, in normal volunteers receiving a 3-hour intravenous infusion of 500 mg azithromycin at a concentration of 1 mg/mL. Similar pharmacokinetic values were obtained in patients hospitalized with community-acquired pneumonia that received the same 3-hour dosage regimen for 2–5 days.
[See table above]
The average CL_t and V_d values were 10.18 mL/min/kg and 33.3 L/kg, respectively, in 18 normal volunteers receiving 1000 to 4000-mg doses given as 1 mg/mL over 2 hours.
Comparison of the plasma pharmacokinetic parameters following the 1st and 5th daily doses of 500 mg intravenous azithromycin showed only an 8% increase in C_{max} but a 61% increase in AUC₂₄ reflecting a threefold rise in C_{24} trough levels.
Following single oral doses of 500 mg azithromycin to 12 healthy volunteers, C_{max}, trough level, and AUC₂₄ were reported to be 0.41 µg/mL, 0.05 µg/mL, and 2.6 µg·h/mL, respectively. These oral values are approximately 38%, 83%, and 52% of the values observed following a single 500-mg I.V. 3-hour infusion (C_{max}: 1.08 µg/mL, trough: 0.06 µg/mL, and AUC²⁴: 5.0 µg·h/mL). Thus, plasma concentrations are higher following the intravenous regimen throughout the 24-hour interval. The pharmacokinetic parameters on day 5 of azithromycin 250-mg capsules following a 500-mg oral loading dose to healthy young adults (age 18–40 years old) were as follows: C_{max}: 0.24 µg/mL, AUC₂₄: 2.1 µg·h/mL. Tissue levels have not been obtained following intravenous infusions of azithromycin. Selected tissue (or fluid) concentration and tissue (or fluid) to plasma/serum concentration ratios following oral administration of azithromycin are shown in the following table:
[See table below]
Tissue levels were determined following a single oral dose of 500 mg azithromycin in 7 gynecological patients. Approximately 17 hours after dosing, azithromycin concentrations were 2.7 µg/g in ovarian tissue, 3.5 µg/g in uterine tissue, and 3.3 µg/g in salpinx. Tissue levels have not been obtained following intravenous infusion of azithromycin.
In a multiple-dose study in 12 normal volunteers utilizing a 500-mg (1 mg/mL) one-hour intravenous-dosage regimen for

five days, the amount of administered azithromycin dose excreted in urine in 24 hours was about 11% after the 1st dose and 14% after the 5th dose. These values are greater than the reported 6% excreted unchanged in urine after oral administration of azithromycin. Biliary excretion is a major route of elimination for unchanged drug, following oral administration.
The serum protein binding of azithromycin is variable in the concentration range approximating human exposure decreasing from 51% at 0.02 µg/mL to 7% at 2 µg/mL.
Microbiology: Azithromycin acts by binding to the 50S ribosomal subunit of susceptible microorganisms and, thus, interfering with microbial protein synthesis. Nucleic acid synthesis is not affected.
Azithromycin concentrates in phagocytes and fibroblasts as demonstrated by *in vitro* incubation techniques. Using such methodology, the ratio of intracellular to extracellular concentration was >30 after one hour incubation. *In vivo* studies suggest that concentration in phagocytes may contribute to drug distribution to inflamed tissues.
Azithromycin has been shown to be active against most strains of the following microorganisms, both in vitro and in clinical infections as described in the **INDICATIONS AND USAGE** section of the package insert for ZITHROMAX® (azithromycin for injection).

Aerobic gram-positive microorganisms
Staphylococcus aureus
Streptococcus pneumoniae
NOTE: Azithromycin demonstrates cross-resistance with erythromycin-resistant gram-positive strains. Most strains of *Enterococcus faecalis* and methicillin-resistant staphylococci are resistant to azithromycin.

Aerobic gram-negative microorganisms
Haemophilus influenzae
Moraxella catarrhalis
Neisseria gonorrhoeae

"Other" microorganisms
Chlamydia pneumoniae
Chlamydia trachomatis
Legionella pneumophila
Mycoplasma hominis
Mycoplasma pneumoniae

Beta-lactamase production should have no effect on azithromycin activity.
Azithromycin has been shown to be active against most strains of the following microorganisms, both *in vitro* and in clinical infections as described in the **INDICATIONS AND USAGE** section of the package insert for ZITHROMAX® (azithromycin tablets) and ZITHROMAX® (azithromycin for oral suspension).

AZITHROMYCIN CONCENTRATIONS FOLLOWING TWO - 250 mg (500 mg) CAPSULES IN ADULTS

TISSUE OR FLUID	TIME AFTER DOSE (h)	TISSUE OR FLUID CONCENTRATION (µg/g or µg/mL)[1]	CORRESPONDING PLASMA OR SERUM LEVEL (µg/mL)	TISSUE (FLUID) PLASMA (SERUM) RATIO[1]
SKIN	72–96	0.4	0.012	35
LUNG	72–96	4.0	0.012	>100
SPUTUM*	2–4	1.0	0.64	2
SPUTUM**	10–12	2.9	0.1	30
TONSIL***	9–18	4.5	0.03	>100
TONSIL***	180	0.9	0.006	>100
CERVIX****	19	2.8	0.04	70

[1] High tissue concentrations should not be interpreted to be quantitatively related to clinical efficacy. The antimicrobial activity of azithromycin is pH related. Azithromycin is concentrated in cell lysosomes which have a low intraorganelle pH, at which the drug's activity is reduced. However, the extensive distribution of drug to tissues may be relevant to clinical activity.

* Sample was obtained 2–4 hours after the first dose.
** Sample was obtained 10–12 hours after the first dose.
*** Dosing regimen of 2 doses of 250 mg each, separated by 12 hours.
**** Sample was obtained 19 hours after a single 500 mg dose.

Aerobic gram-positive microorganisms
Staphylococcus aureus
Streptococcus agalactiae
Streptococcus pneumoniae
Streptococcus pyogenes

Aerobic gram-negative microorganisms
Haemophilus ducreyi
Haemophilus influenzae
Moraxella catarrhalis
Neisseria gonorrhoeae

"Other" microorganisms
Chlamydia pneumoniae
Chlamydia trachomatis
Mycoplasma pneumoniae

The following *in vitro* data are available, **but their clinical significance is unknown.**

Azithromycin exhibits *in vitro* minimum inhibitory concentrations (MIC's) of 0.5 µg/mL or less against most (≥90%) strains of streptococci listed below and MIC's of 2.0 µg/mL or less against most (≥90%) strains of other listed microorganisms. However, the safety and effectiveness of azithromycin in treating clinical infections due to these microorganisms have not been established in adequate and well-controlled clinical trials.

Aerobic gram-positive microorganisms
Streptococci (Groups C, F, G)
Viridans group streptococci

Aerobic gram-negative microorganisms
Bordetella pertussis

Anaerobic microorganisms
Peptostreptococcus species
Prevotella bivia

"Other" microorganisms
Ureaplasma urealyticum

Susceptibility Tests

Azithromycin can be solubilized for *in vitro* susceptibility testing using dilution techniques by dissolving in a minimum amount of 95% ethanol and diluting to the working stock concentration with broth.

Dilution Techniques:

Quantitative methods are used to determine antimicrobial minimum inhibitory concentrations (MIC's). These MIC's provide estimates of the susceptibility of bacteria to antimicrobial compounds. The MIC's should be determined using a standardized procedure. Standardized procedures are based on a dilution method[1] (broth or agar) or equivalent with standardized inoculum concentrations and standardized concentrations of azithromycin powder. The MIC values should be interpreted according to the following criteria:

For testing aerobic microorganisms other than *Haemophilus* species, *Neisseria gonorrhoeae*, and streptococci:

MIC (µg/mL)	Interpretation
≤2	Susceptible (S)
4	Intermediate (I)
≥8	Resistant (R)

For testing *Haemophilus* species:[a]

MIC (µg/mL)	Interpretation
≤4	Susceptible (S)

[a] This interpretive standard is applicable only to broth microdilution susceptibility testing with *Haemophilus* species using *Haemophilus* Test Medium (HTM).[1]

The current absence of data on resistant strains precludes defining any categories other than "Susceptible". Strains yielding MIC results suggestive of a "nonsusceptible" category should be submitted to a reference laboratory for further testing.

For testing streptococci including *S. pneumoniae:* [b]

MIC (µg/mL)	Interpretation
≤0.5	Susceptible (S)
1	Intermediate (I)
≥2	Resistant (R)

[b] These interpretive standards are applicable only to broth microdilution susceptibility tests using cation-adjusted Mueller-Hinton broth with 2–5% lysed horse blood.[1]

No interpretive criteria have been established for testing *Neisseria gonorrhoeae*. This species is not usually tested.

A report of "Susceptible" indicates that the pathogen is likely to respond to monotherapy with azithromycin. A report of "Intermediate" indicates that the result should be considered equivocal, and, if the microorganism is not fully susceptible to alternative, clinically feasible drugs, the test should be repeated. This category implies possible clinical applicability in body sites where the drug is physiologically concentrated or in situations where high dosage of drug can be used. This category also provides a buffer zone which prevents small uncontrolled technical factors from causing major discrepancies in interpretation. A report of "Resistant" indicates that achievable drug concentrations are unlikely to be inhibitory; other therapy should be selected.

Standardized susceptibility test procedures require the use of laboratory control microorganisms to control the technical aspects of the laboratory procedures. Standard azithromycin powder should provide the following MIC values:

Microorganism	MIC (µg/mL)
Haemophilus influenzae ATCC 49247[a]	1.0–4.0
Staphylococcus aureus ATCC 29213	0.5–2.0
Streptococcus pneumoniae ATCC 49619[b]	0.06–0.25

[a] This quality control range is applicable to only *H. influenzae* ATCC 49247 tested by a broth microdilution procedure using *Haemophilus* Test Medium (HTM)[1].

[b] This quality control range is applicable to only *S. pneumoniae* ATCC 49619 tested by a broth microdilution procedure using cation-adjusted Mueller-Hinton broth with 2–5% lysed horse blood.[1]

Diffusion Techniques:

Quantitative methods that require measurement of zone diameters also provide reproducible estimates of the susceptibility of bacteria to antimicrobial compounds. One such standardized procedure[2] requires the use of standardized inoculum concentrations. This procedure uses paper disks impregnated with 15-µg azithromycin to test the susceptibility of microorganisms to azithromycin.

Reports from the laboratory providing results of the standard single-disk susceptibility test with a 15-µg azithromycin disk should be interpreted according to the following criteria:

For testing aerobic microorganisms (including streptococci)[a] except *Haemophilus* species and *Neisseria gonorrhoeae:*

Zone Diameter (mm)	Interpretation
≥18	Susceptible (S)
14–17	Intermediate (I)
≤13	Resistant (R)

[a] These zone diameter standards for streptococci apply only to tests performed using Mueller-Hinton agar supplemented with 5% sheep blood and incubated in 5% CO_2[2].

For testing *Haemophilus* species:[b]

Zone Diameter (mm)	Interpretation
≥12	Susceptible (S)

[b] This zone diameter standard is applicable only to tests with *Haemophilus* species using *Haemophilus* Test Medium (HTM)[2].

The current absence of data on resistant strains precludes defining any categories other than "Susceptible". Strains yielding zone diameter results suggestive of a "nonsusceptible" category should be submitted to a reference laboratory for further testing.

No interpretive criteria have been established for testing *Neisseria gonorrhoeae*. This species is not usually tested.

Interpretation should be as stated above for results using dilution techniques. Interpretation involves correlation of the diameter obtained in the disk test with the MIC for azithromycin.

As with standardized dilution techniques, diffusion methods require the use of laboratory control microorganisms that are used to control the technical aspects of the laboratory procedures. For the diffusion technique, the 15-µg azithromycin disk should provide the following zone diameters in these laboratory test quality control strains:

Microorganism	Zone Diameter (mm)
Haemophilus influenzae ATCC 49247[a]	13–21
Staphylococcus aureus ATCC 25923	21–26
Streptococcus pneumoniae ATCC 49619[b]	19–25

[a] These quality control limits are applicable only to tests conducted with *H. influenzae* ATCC 49247 using *Haemophilus* Test Medium (HTM)[2].

[b] These quality control limits are applicable only to tests conducted with *S. pneumoniae* ATCC 49619 using Mueller-Hinton agar supplemented with 5% sheep blood incubated in 5% CO_2[2].

INDICATIONS AND USAGE

ZITHROMAX® (azithromycin for injection) is indicated for the treatment of patients with infections caused by susceptible strains of the designated microorganisms in the conditions listed below. As recommended dosages, durations of therapy, and applicable patient populations vary among these infections, please see **DOSAGE AND ADMINISTRATION** for dosing recommendations.

Community-acquired pneumonia due to *Chlamydia pneumoniae, Haemophilus influenzae, Legionella pneumophila, Moraxella catarrhalis, Mycoplasma pneumoniae, Staphylococcus aureus,* or *Streptococcus pneumoniae* in patients who require initial intravenous therapy.

Pelvic inflammatory disease due to *Chlamydia trachomatis, Neisseria gonorrhoeae,* or *Mycoplasma hominis* in patients who require initial intravenous therapy. If anaerobic microorganisms are suspected of contributing to the infection, an antimicrobial agent with anaerobic activity should be administered in combination with ZITHROMAX®.

ZITHROMAX® (azithromycin for injection) should be followed by ZITHROMAX® by the oral route as required. (See **DOSAGE AND ADMINISTRATION.**)

Appropriate culture and susceptibility tests should be performed before treatment to determine the causative microorganism and its susceptibility to azithromycin. Therapy with ZITHROMAX® may be initiated before results of these tests are known; once the results become available, antimicrobial therapy should be adjusted accordingly.

CONTRAINDICATIONS

ZITHROMAX® is contraindicated in patients with known hypersensitivity to azithromycin, erythromycin, or any macrolide antibiotic.

WARNINGS

Serious allergic reactions, including angioedema, anaphylaxis, and dermatologic reactions including Stevens Johnson Syndrome and toxic epidermal necrolysis have been reported rarely in patients on azithromycin therapy. Although rare, fatalities have been reported. (See **CONTRAINDICATIONS.**) Despite initially successful symptomatic treatment of the allergic symptoms, when symptomatic therapy was discontinued, the allergic symptoms **recurred soon thereafter in some patients without further azithromycin exposure.** These patients required prolonged periods of observation and symptomatic treatment. The relationship of these episodes to the long tissue half-life of azithromycin and subsequent prolonged exposure to antigen is unknown at present.

If an allergic reaction occurs, the drug should be discontinued and appropriate therapy should be instituted. Physicians should be aware that reappearance of the allergic symptoms may occur when symptomatic therapy is discontinued.

Pseudomembranous colitis has been reported with nearly all antibacterial agents and may range in severity from mild to life-threatening. Therefore, it is important to consider this diagnosis in patients who present with diarrhea subsequent to the administration of antibacterial agents.

Treatment with antibacterial agents alters the normal flora of the colon and may permit overgrowth of clostridia. Studies indicate that a toxin produced by *Clostridium difficile* is a primary cause of "antibiotic-associated colitis."

After the diagnosis of pseudomembranous colitis has been established, therapeutic measures should be initiated. Mild cases of pseudomembranous colitis usually respond to discontinuation of the drug alone. In moderate to severe cases, consideration should be given to management with fluids and electrolytes, protein supplementation, and treatment with an antibacterial drug clinically effective against *Clostridium difficile* colitis.

PRECAUTIONS

General: Because azithromycin is principally eliminated via the liver, caution should be exercised when azithromycin is administered to patients with impaired hepatic function. There are no data regarding azithromycin usage in patients with renal impairment; therefore, caution should be exercised when prescribing azithromycin in these patients.

ZITHROMAX® (azithromycin for injection) should be reconstituted and diluted as directed and administered as an intravenous infusion over not less than 60 minutes. (See **DOSAGE AND ADMINISTRATION.**)

Local I.V. site reactions have been reported with the intravenous administration of azithromycin. The incidence and severity of these reactions were the same when 500 mg azithromycin were given over 1 hour (2 mg/mL as 250 mL infusion) or over 3 hours (1 mg/mL as 500 mL infusion). (See **ADVERSE REACTIONS.**) All volunteers who received infusate concentrations above 2.0 mg/mL experienced local I.V. site reactions and, therefore, higher concentrations should be avoided.

The following adverse events have not been reported in clinical trials with azithromycin; however, they have been reported with macrolide products: ventricular arrhythmias, including ventricular tachycardia, and *torsades de pointes*, in individuals with prolonged QT intervals. There has been a spontaneous report from the post-marketing experience of

Continued on next page

Zithromax IV—Cont.

a patient with previous history of arrhythmias who experienced *torsades de pointes* and subsequent myocardial infarction following a course of oral azithromycin therapy.

Information for Patients:
Patients should be cautioned not to take aluminum- and magnesium-containing antacids and azithromycin by the oral route simultaneously.

Patients should be directed to discontinue azithromycin and contact a physician if any signs of an allergic reaction occur.

Drug Interactions: Aluminum- and magnesium-containing antacids reduce the peak serum levels (rate) but not the AUC (extent) of orally administered azithromycin.

Administration of cimetidine (800 mg) two hours prior to orally administered azithromycin had no effect on azithromycin absorption.

Azithromycin given by the oral route did not affect the plasma levels or pharmacokinetics of theophylline administered as a single intravenous dose. The effect of azithromycin on the plasma levels or pharmacokinetics of theophylline administered in multiple doses resulting in therapeutic steady-state levels of theophylline is not known. However, concurrent use of macrolides and theophylline has been associated with increases in the serum concentrations of theophylline. Therefore, until further data are available, prudent medical practice dictates careful monitoring of plasma theophylline levels in patients receiving azithromycin and theophylline concomitantly.

Azithromycin given by the oral route did not affect the prothrombin time response to a single dose of warfarin. However, prudent medical practice dictates careful monitoring of prothrombin time in all patients treated with azithromycin and warfarin concomitantly. Concurrent use of macrolides and warfarin in clinical practice has been associated with increased anticoagulant effects.

The following drug interactions have not been reported in clinical trials with azithromycin; however, no specific drug interaction studies have been performed to evaluate potential drug-drug interaction. Nonetheless, they have been observed with macrolide products. Until further data are developed regarding drug interactions when azithromycin and these drugs are used concomitantly, careful monitoring of patients is advised:

Digoxin — elevated digoxin levels.

Ergotamine or dihydroergotamine — acute ergot toxicity characterized by severe peripheral vasospasm and dysesthesia.

Triazolam — Increased pharmacologic effect of triazolam by decreasing the clearance of triazolam.

Drugs metabolized by the cytochrome P450 system — elevations of serum carbamazepine, terfenadine, cyclosporine, hexobarbital, and phenytoin levels.

Laboratory Test Interactions: There are no reported laboratory test interactions.

Carcinogenesis, Mutagenesis, Impairment of Fertility: Long-term studies in animals have not been performed to evaluate carcinogenic potential. Azithromycin has shown no mutagenic potential in standard laboratory tests: mouse lymphoma assay, human lymphocyte clastogenic assay, and mouse bone marrow clastogenic assay. No evidence of impaired fertility due to azithromycin was found.

Pregnancy: Teratogenic Effects. Pregnancy Category B: Reproduction studies have been performed in rats and mice at doses up to moderately maternally toxic dose levels (i.e., 200 mg/kg/day by the oral route). These doses, based on a mg/m^2 basis, are estimated to be 4 and 2 times, respectively, the human daily dose of 500 mg by the oral route. In the animal studies, no evidence of harm to the fetus due to azithromycin was found. There are, however, no adequate and well-controlled studies in pregnant women. Because animal reproduction studies are not always predictive of human response, azithromycin should be used during pregnancy only if clearly needed.

Nursing Mothers: It is not known whether azithromycin is excreted in human milk. Because many drugs are excreted in human milk, caution should be exercised when azithromycin is administered to a nursing woman.

Pediatric Use: Safety and effectiveness of azithromycin for injection in children or adolescents under 16 years have not been established. In controlled clinical studies, azithromycin has been administered to pediatric patients (age 6 months to 16 years) by the oral route. For information regarding the use of ZITHROMAX® (azithromycin for oral suspension) in the treatment of pediatric patients, refer to the **INDICATIONS AND USAGE** and **DOSAGE AND ADMINISTRATION** sections of the prescribing information for ZITHROMAX® (azithromycin for oral suspension) 100 mg/5 mL and 200 mg/5 mL bottles.

Geriatric Use: Pharmacokinetic studies with intravenous azithromycin have not been performed in older volunteers. Pharmacokinetics of azithromycin following oral administration in older volunteers (65–85 years old) were similar to those in younger volunteers (18–40 years old) for the 5-day therapeutic regimen.

ADVERSE REACTIONS

In clinical trials of intravenous azithromycin for community-acquired pneumonia, in which 2–5 I.V. doses were given, most of the reported side effects were mild to moderate in severity and were reversible upon discontinuation of the drug. The majority of patients in these trials had one or more comorbid diseases and were receiving concomitant medications. Approximately 1.2% of the patients discontinued intravenous ZITHROMAX® therapy, and a total of 2.4% discontinued azithromycin therapy by either the intravenous or oral route because of clinical or laboratory side effects.

In clinical trials conducted in patients with pelvic inflammatory disease, in which 1–2 I.V. doses were given, 2% of women who received monotherapy with azithromycin and 4% who received azithromycin plus metronidazole discontinued therapy due to clinical side effects.

Clinical side effects leading to discontinuations from these studies were most commonly gastrointestinal (abdominal pain, nausea, vomiting, diarrhea), and rashes; laboratory side effects leading to discontinuation were increases in transaminase levels and/or alkaline phosphatase levels.

Clinical:
Overall, the most common side effects associated with treatment in adult patients who received I.V./P.O. ZITHROMAX® in studies of community-acquired pneumonia were related to the gastrointestinal system with diarrhea/loose stools (4.3%), nausea (3.9%), abdominal pain (2.7%), and vomiting (1.4%) being the most frequently reported. Approximately 12% of patients experienced a side effect related to the intravenous infusion; most common were pain at the injection site (6.5%) and local inflammation (3.1%).

The most common side effects associated with treatment in adult women who received I.V./P.O. ZITHROMAX® in studies of pelvic inflammatory disease were related to the gastrointestinal system. Diarrhea (8.5%) and nausea (6.6%) were most commonly reported, followed by vaginitis (2.8%), abdominal pain (1.9%), anorexia (1.9%), rash and pruritus (1.9%). When azithromycin was co-administered with metronidazole in these studies, a higher proportion of women experienced side effects of nausea (10.3%), abdominal pain (3.7%), vomiting (2.8%), application site reaction, stomatitis, dizziness, or dyspnea (all at 1.9%).

No other side effects occurred in patients on the multiple dose I.V./P.O. regimen of ZITHROMAX® in these studies with a frequency greater than 1%.

Side effects that occurred with a frequency of 1% or less included the following:

Gastrointestinal: dyspepsia, flatulence, mucositis, oral moniliasis, and gastritis

Nervous System: headache, somnolence

Allergic: bronchospasm

Special Senses: taste perversion

Post-Marketing Experience:
Adverse events reported with orally administered azithromycin during the post-marketing period in adult and/or pediatric patients for which a causal relationship could not be established include:

Allergic: arthralgia, edema, urticaria

Cardiovascular: arrhythmias, including ventricular tachycardia

Gastrointestinal: anorexia, constipation, dyspepsia, flatulence, vomiting/diarrhea rarely resulting in dehydration

General: asthenia, paresthesia

Genitourinary: interstitial nephritis and acute renal failure

Liver/Biliary: abnormal liver function including hepatitis and cholestatic jaundice

Nervous System: convulsions

Skin/Appendages: rarely, serious skin reactions including erythema multiforme, Stevens Johnson Syndrome, and toxic epidermal necrolysis

Special Senses: hearing disturbances including hearing loss, deafness, and/or tinnitus, rare reports of taste disturbances

Laboratory Abnormalities:
Significant abnormalities (irrespective of drug relationship) occurring during the clinical trials were reported as follows: with an incidence of 4–6%, elevated ALT (SGPT), AST (SGOT), creatinine with an incidence of 1–3%, elevated LDH, bilirubin with an incidence of less than 1%, leukopenia, neutropenia, decreased platelet count, and elevated serum alkaline phosphatase.

When follow-up was provided, changes in laboratory tests appeared to be reversible.

In multiple-dose clinical trials involving more than 750 patients treated with ZITHROMAX® (I.V./P.O.), less than 2% of patients discontinued azithromycin therapy because of treatment-related liver enzyme abnormalities.

DOSAGE AND ADMINISTRATION
(See INDICATIONS AND USAGE and CLINICAL PHARMACOLOGY.)

The recommended dose of ZITHROMAX® (azithromycin for injection) for the treatment of adult patients with community-acquired pneumonia due to the indicated organisms is: 500 mg as a single daily dose by the intravenous route for at least two days. Intravenous therapy should be followed by azithromycin by the oral route at a single, daily dose of 500 mg, administered as two 250-mg tablets to complete a 7- to 10-day course of therapy. The timing of the switch to oral therapy should be done at the discretion of the physician and in accordance with clinical response.

The recommended dose of ZITHROMAX® (azithromycin) for the treatment of adult patients with pelvic inflammatory disease due to the indicated organisms is: 500 mg as a single daily dose by the intravenous route for one or two days. Intravenous therapy should be followed by azithromycin by the oral route at a single, daily dose of 250 mg to complete a 7-day course of therapy. The timing of the switch to oral therapy should be done at the discretion of the physician and in accordance with clinical response. If anaerobic microorganisms are suspected of contributing to the infection, an antimicrobial agent with anaerobic activity should be administered in combination with ZITHROMAX®.

The infusate concentration and rate of infusion for ZITHROMAX® (azithromycin for injection) should be either 1 mg/mL over 3 hours or 2 mg/mL over 1 hour.

Preparation of the solution for intravenous administration is as follows:

Reconstitution
Prepare the initial solution of ZITHROMAX® (azithromycin for injection) by adding 4.8 mL of Sterile Water For Injection to the 500 mg vial and shaking the vial until all of the drug is dissolved. Each mL of reconstituted solution contains 100 mg azithromycin. Reconstituted solution is stable for 24 hours when stored below 30°C or 86°F.

Parenteral drug products should be inspected visually for particulate matter prior to administration. If particulate matter is evident in reconstituted fluids, the drug solution should be discarded.

Dilute this solution further prior to administration as instructed below.

Dilution
To provide azithromycin over a concentration range of 1.0–2.0 mg/mL, transfer 5 mL of the 100 mg/mL azithromycin solution into the appropriate amount of any of the diluents listed below:

Normal Saline (0.9% sodium chloride)
1/2 Normal Saline (0.45% sodium chloride)
5% Dextrose in Water
Lactated Ringer's Solution
5% Dextrose in 1/2 Normal Saline (0.45% sodium chloride) with 20 mEq KCl
5% Dextrose in Lactated Ringer's Solution
5% Dextrose in 1/3 Normal Saline (0.3% sodium chloride)
5% Dextrose in 1/2 Normal Saline (0.45% sodium chloride)
Normosol®-M in 5% Dextrose
Normosol®-R in 5% Dextrose

Final Infusion Solution Concentration (mg/mL)	Amount of Diluent (mL)
1.0 mg/mL	500 mL
2.0 mg/mL	250 mL

It is recommended that a 500-mg dose of ZITHROMAX® (azithromycin for injection), diluted as above, be infused over a period of not less than 60 minutes.

ZITHROMAX® (azithromycin for injection) should not be given as a bolus or as an intramuscular injection.

Storage
When diluted according to the instructions (1.0 mg/mL to 2.0 mg/mL), ZITHROMAX® (azithromycin for injection) is stable for 24 hours at or below room temperature (30°C or 86°F), or for 7 days if stored under refrigeration (5°C or 41°F).

HOW SUPPLIED

ZITHROMAX® (azithromycin for injection) is supplied in lyophilized form under a vacuum in a 10-mL vial equivalent to 500 mg of azithromycin for intravenous administration. Each vial also contains sodium hydroxide and 413.6 mg citric acid.

CAUTION: Federal (U.S.) law prohibits dispensing without prescription.

These are packaged as follows:
10 vials of 500 mg   NDC 0069-3150-83

CLINICAL STUDIES
Community-Acquired Pneumonia
In a controlled study of community-acquired pneumonia performed in the U.S., azithromycin (500 mg as a single

Evidence of Infection	Total	Cure	Improved	Cure + Improved
Mycoplasma pneumoniae	18	11 (61%)	5 (28%)	16 (89%)
Chlamydia pneumoniae	34	15 (44%)	13 (38%)	28 (82%)
Legionella pneumophila	16	5 (31%)	8 (50%)	13 (81%)

daily dose by the intravenous route for 2–5 days, followed by 500 mg/day by the oral route to complete 7–10 days therapy) was compared to cefuroxime (2250 mg/day in three divided doses by the intravenous route for 2–5 days followed by 1000 mg/day in two divided doses by the oral route to complete 7–10 days therapy), with or without erythromycin. For the 291 patients who were evaluable for clinical efficacy, the clinical outcome rates, i.e., cure, improved, and success (cure + improved) among the 277 patients seen at 10–14 days post-therapy were as follows:

Clinical Outcome	Azithromycin	Comparator
Cure	46%	44%
Improved	32%	30%
Success (Cure + Improved)	78%	74%

In a separate, uncontrolled clinical and microbiological trial performed in the U.S., 94 patients with community-acquired pneumonia who received azithromycin in the same regimen were evaluable for clinical efficacy. The clinical outcome rates, i.e., cure, improved, and success (cure + improved) among the 84 patients seen at 10–14 days post-therapy were as follows:

Clinical Outcome	Azithromycin
Cure	60%
Improved	29%
Success (Cure + Improved)	89%

Microbiological determinations in both trials were made at the pre-treatment visit and, where applicable, were reassessed at later visits. Serological testing was done on baseline and final visit specimens. The following combined presumptive bacteriological eradication rates were obtained from the evaluable groups:

Combined Bacteriological Eradication Rates for Azithromycin:

(at last completed visit)	Azithromycin
S. pneumoniae	64/67 (96%)[a]
H. influenzae	41/43 (95%)
M. catarrhalis	9/10
S. aureus	9/10

[a] Nineteen of twenty-four patients (79%) with positive blood cultures for *S. pneumoniae* were cured (intent to treat analysis) with eradication of the pathogen.

The presumed bacteriological outcomes at 10–14 days post-therapy for patients treated with azithromycin with evidence (serology and/or culture) of atypical pathogens for both trials were as follows:

[See table at bottom of previous page]

ANIMAL TOXICOLOGY

Phospholipidosis (intracellular phospholipid accumulation) has been observed in some tissues of mice, rats, and dogs given multiple doses of azithromycin. It has been demonstrated in numerous organ systems (e.g., eye, dorsal root ganglia, liver, gallbladder, kidney, spleen, and pancreas) in dogs treated with azithromycin at doses which, expressed on a mg/kg basis, are only 2 times greater than the recommended adult human dose and in rats at doses comparable to the recommended adult human dose. This effect has been reversible after cessation of azithromycin treatment. Phospholipidosis has been observed to a similar extent in the tissues of neonatal rats and dogs given daily doses of azithromycin ranging from 10 days to 30 days. Based on the pharmacokinetic data, phospholipidosis has been seen in the rat (30 mg/kg dose) at observed C_{max} value of 1.3 μg/mL (6 times greater than the observed C_{max} of 0.216 μg/mL at the pediatric dose of 10 mg/kg). Similarly, it has been shown in the dog (10 mg/kg dose) at observed C_{max} value of 1.5 μg/mL (7 times greater than the observed same C_{max} and drug dose in the studied pediatric population). On mg/m^2 basis, 30 mg/kg dose in the rat (135 mg/m^2) and 10 mg/kg dose in the dog (79 mg/m^2) are approximately 0.4 and 0.6 times, respectively, the recommended dose in the pediatric patients with an average body weight of 25 kg. This effect, similar to that seen in the adult animals, is reversible after cessation of azithromycin treatment. The significance of these findings for animals and for humans is unknown.

REFERENCES

1. National Committee for Clinical Laboratory Standards. Methods for Dilution Antimicrobial Susceptibility Tests for Bacteria that Grow Aerobically—Third Edition. Approved Standard NCCLS Document M7-A3, Vol. 13, No. 25, NCCLS, Villanova, PA, December, 1993.

2. National Committee for Clinical Laboratory Standards. Performance Standards for Antimicrobial Disk Susceptibility Tests — Fifth Edition. Approved Standard NCCLS Document M2-A5, Vol. 13, No. 24, NCCLS, Villanova, PA, December, 1993.

Licensed from Pliva ©1997 PFIZER INC

70-5191-00-1 Issued October 1997

Show in Product Information Guide, page 331

ZOLOFT® ℞
(sertraline hydrochloride)
Tablets

DESCRIPTION

ZOLOFT® (sertraline hydrochloride) is a selective serotonin reuptake inhibitor (SSRI) for oral administration. It is chemically unrelated to other SSRIs, tricyclic, tetracyclic, or other available antidepressant agents. It has a molecular weight of 342.7. Sertraline hydrochloride has the following chemical name: (1S-cis)-4-(3,4-dichlorophenyl)-1,2,3,4-tetrahydro-N-methyl-1-naphthalenamine hydrochloride. The empirical formula $C_{17}H_{17}NCl_2 \bullet HCl$ is represented by the following structural formula:

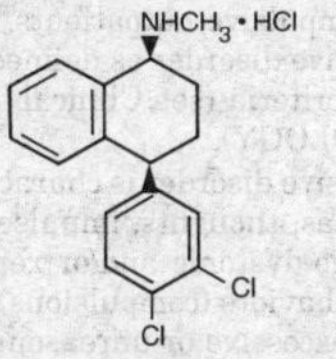

Sertraline hydrochloride is a white crystalline powder that is slightly soluble in water and isopropyl alcohol, and sparingly soluble in ethanol.

ZOLOFT is supplied for oral administration as scored tablets containing sertraline hydrochloride equivalent to 25, 50 and 100 mg of sertraline and the following inactive ingredients: dibasic calcium phosphate dihydrate, D & C Yellow #10 aluminum lake (in 25 mg tablet), FD & C Blue #1 aluminum lake (in 25 mg tablet), FD & C Red #40 aluminum lake (in 25 mg tablet), FD & C Blue #2 aluminum lake (in 50 mg tablet), hydroxypropyl cellulose, hydroxypropyl methylcellulose, magnesium stearate, microcrystalline cellulose, polyethylene glycol, polysorbate 80, sodium starch glycolate, synthetic yellow iron oxide (in 100 mg tablet), and titanium dioxide.

CLINICAL PHARMACOLOGY

Pharmacodynamics

The mechanism of action of sertraline is presumed to be linked to its inhibition of CNS neuronal uptake of serotonin (5HT). Studies at clinically relevant doses in man have demonstrated that sertraline blocks the uptake of serotonin into human platelets. *In vitro* studies in animals also suggest that sertraline is a potent and selective inhibitor of neuronal serotonin reuptake and has only very weak effects on norepinephrine and dopamine neuronal reuptake. *In vitro* studies have shown that sertraline has no significant affinity for adrenergic (alpha$_1$, alpha$_2$, beta), cholinergic, GABA, dopaminergic, histaminergic, serotonergic (5HT$_{1A}$, 5HT$_{1B}$, 5HT$_2$), or benzodiazepine receptors; antagonism of such receptors has been hypothesized to be associated with various anticholinergic, sedative, and cardiovascular effects for other psychotropic drugs. The chronic administration of sertraline was found in animals to downregulate brain norepinephrine receptors, as has been observed with other clinically effective antidepressants. Sertraline does not inhibit monoamine oxidase.

Pharmacokinetics

Systemic Bioavailability–In man, following oral once-daily dosing over the range of 50 to 200 mg for 14 days, mean peak plasma concentrations (Cmax) of sertraline occurred between 4.5 to 8.4 hours post-dosing. The average terminal elimination half-life of plasma sertraline is about 26 hours. Based on this pharmacokinetic parameter, steady-state sertraline plasma levels should be achieved after approximately one week of once-daily dosing. Linear dose-proportional pharmacokinetics were demonstrated in a single dose study in which the Cmax and area under the plasma concentration time curve (AUC) of sertraline were proportional to dose over a range of 50 to 200 mg. Consistent with the terminal elimination half-life, there is an approximately two-fold accumulation, compared to a single dose, of sertraline with repeated dosing over a 50 to 200 mg dose range. The single dose bioavailability of sertraline tablets is approximately equal to an equivalent dose of solution.

The effects of food on the bioavailability of sertraline were studied in subjects administered a single dose with and without food. AUC was slightly increased when drug was administered with food but the Cmax was 25% greater, while the time to reach peak plasma concentration decreased from 8 hours post-dosing to 5.5 hours.

Metabolism–Sertraline undergoes extensive first pass metabolism. The principal initial pathway of metabolism for sertraline is N-demethylation. N-desmethylsertraline has a plasma terminal elimination half-life of 62 to 104 hours. Both *in vitro* biochemical and *in vivo* pharmacological testing have shown N-desmethylsertraline to be substantially less active than sertraline. Both sertraline and N-desmethylsertraline undergo oxidative deamination and subsequent reduction, hydroxylation, and glucuronide conjugation. In a study of radiolabeled sertraline involving two healthy male subjects, sertraline accounted for less than 5% of the plasma radioactivity. About 40–45% of the administered radioactivity was recovered in urine in 9 days. Unchanged sertraline was not detectable in the urine. For the same period, about 40–45% of the administered radioactivity was accounted for in feces, including 12–14% unchanged sertraline.

Desmethylsertraline exhibits time-related, dose dependent increases in AUC (0–24 hour), Cmax and Cmin, with about a 5–9 fold increase in these pharmacokinetic parameters between day 1 and day 14.

Protein Binding–*In vitro* protein binding studies performed with radiolabeled ^{3}H-sertraline showed that sertraline is highly bound to serum proteins (98%) in the range of 20 to 500 ng/mL. However, at up to 300 and 200 ng/mL concentrations, respectively, sertraline and N-desmethylsertraline did not alter the plasma protein binding of two other highly protein bound drugs, viz., warfarin and propranolol (see PRECAUTIONS).

Pediatric Pharmacokinetics–Sertraline pharmacokinetics were evaluated in a group of 61 pediatric patients (29 aged 6–12 years, 32 aged 13–17 years) with a DSM-III-R diagnosis of depression or obsessive-compulsive disorder. Patients included both males (n=28) and females (n=33). During 42 days of chronic sertraline dosing, sertraline was titrated up to 200 mg/day and maintained at that dose for a minimum of 11 days. On the final day of sertraline 200 mg/day, the 6–12 year old group exhibited a mean sertraline AUC (0–24 hr) of 3107 ng-hr/mL, mean Cmax of 165 ng/mL, and mean half-life of 26.2 hr. The 13–17 year old group exhibited a mean sertraline AUC (0–24 hr) of 2296 ng-hr/mL, mean Cmax of 123 ng/mL, and mean half-life of 27.8 hr. Higher plasma levels in the 6–12 year old group were largely attributable to patients with lower body weights. No gender associated differences were observed. By comparison, a group of 22 separately studied adults between 18 and 45 years of age (11 male, 11 female) received 30 days of 200 mg/day sertraline and exhibited a mean sertraline AUC (0–24 hr) of 2570 ng-hr/mL, mean Cmax of 142 ng/mL, and mean half-life of 27.2 hr. Relative to the adults, both the 6–12 year olds and the 13–17 year olds showed about 22% lower AUC (0–24 hr) and Cmax values when plasma concentration was adjusted for weight. These data suggest that pediatric patients metabolize sertraline with slightly greater efficiency than adults. Nevertheless, lower doses may be advisable for pediatric patients given their lower body weights, especially in very young patients, in order to avoid excessive plasma levels (see DOSAGE AND ADMINISTRATION).

Age–Sertraline plasma clearance in a group of 16 (8 male, 8 female) elderly patients treated for 14 days at a dose of 100 mg/day was approximately 40% lower than in a similarly studied group of younger (25 to 32 y.o.) individuals. Steady-state, therefore, should be achieved after 2 to 3 weeks in older patients. The same study showed a decreased clearance of desmethylsertraline in older males, but not in older females.

Liver Disease–As might be predicted from its primary site of metabolism, liver impairment can affect the elimination of sertraline. The elimination half-life of sertraline was prolonged in a single dose study of patients with mild, stable cirrhosis, with a mean of 52 hours compared to 22 hours seen in subjects without liver disease. In hepatically impaired patients, it was observed that the Cmax and AUC were increased by 1.7 and 4.4 fold, respectively, compared to healthy subjects. This suggests that the use of sertraline in patients with liver disease must be approached with caution. If sertraline is administered to patients with liver disease, a lower or less frequent dose should be used (see PRECAUTIONS and DOSAGE AND ADMINISTRATION).

Renal Disease—The pharmacokinetics of sertraline in patients with significant renal dysfunction have not been determined.

Clinical Trials

Depression–The efficacy of ZOLOFT as a treatment for depression was established in two placebo-controlled studies in adult outpatients meeting DSM-III criteria for major depression. Study 1 was an 8-week study with flexible dosing of ZOLOFT in a range of 50 to 200 mg/day; the mean dose for completers was 145 mg/day. Study 2 was a 6-week fixed-dose study, including ZOLOFT doses of 50, 100, and 200 mg/day. Overall, these studies demonstrated ZOLOFT to be superior to placebo on the Hamilton Depression Rating Scale and the Clinical Global Impression Severity and Improvement scales. Study 2 was not readily interpretable regarding a dose response relationship for effectiveness.

Study 3 involved depressed outpatients who had responded by the end of an initial 8-week open treatment phase on ZOLOFT 50–200 mg/day. These patients (N=295) were randomized to continuation for 44 weeks on double-blind ZOLOFT 50–200 mg/day or placebo. A statistically significantly lower relapse rate was observed for patients taking ZOLOFT compared to those on placebo. The mean dose for completers was 70 mg/day.

Continued on next page

Zoloft—Cont.

Analyses for gender effects on outcome did not suggest any differential responsiveness on the basis of sex.

Obsessive-Compulsive Disorder (OCD)–The effectiveness of ZOLOFT in the treatment of OCD was demonstrated in three multicenter placebo-controlled studies of adult outpatients (Studies 1–3). Patients in all studies had moderate to severe OCD (DSM-III or DSM-III-R) with mean baseline ratings on the Yale Brown Obsessive-Compulsive Scale (YBOCS) total score ranging from 23 to 25.

Study 1 was an 8-week study with flexible dosing of ZOLOFT in a range of 50 to 200 mg/day; the mean dose for completers was 186 mg/day. Patients receiving ZOLOFT experienced a mean reduction of approximately 4 points on the YBOCS total score which was significantly greater than the mean reduction of 2 points in placebo-treated patients. Study 2 was a 12-week fixed-dose study, including ZOLOFT doses of 50, 100, and 200 mg/day. Patients receiving ZOLOFT doses of 50 and 200 mg/day experienced mean reductions of approximately 6 points on the YBOCS total score which were significantly greater than the approximately 3 point reduction in placebo-treated patients. Study 3 was a 12-week study with flexible dosing of ZOLOFT in a range of 50 to 200 mg/day; the mean dose for completers was 185 mg/day. Patients receiving ZOLOFT experienced a mean reduction of approximately 7 points on the YBOCS total score which was significantly greater than the mean reduction of approximately 4 points in placebo-treated patients.

Analyses for age and gender effects on outcome did not suggest any differential responsiveness on the basis of age or sex.

The effectiveness of ZOLOFT for the treatment of OCD was also demonstrated in a 12-week, multicenter, parallel group study in a pediatric outpatient population (children and adolescents, ages 6–17). Patients in this study were initiated at doses of either 25 mg/day (children, ages 6–12) or 50 mg/day (adolescents, ages 13–17), and then titrated over the next four weeks to a maximum dose of 200 mg/day, as tolerated. The mean dose for completers was 178 mg/day. Dosing was once a day in the morning or evening. Patients in this study had moderate to severe OCD (DSM-III-R) with mean baseline ratings on the Children's Yale-Brown Obsessive-Compulsive Scale (CYBOCS) total score of 22. Patients receiving sertraline experienced a mean reduction of approximately 7 units on the CYBOCS total score which was significantly greater than the 3 unit reduction for placebo patients. Analyses for age and gender effects on outcome did not suggest any differential responsiveness on the basis of age or sex.

Panic Disorder–The effectiveness of ZOLOFT in the treatment of panic disorder was demonstrated in three double-blind, placebo-controlled studies (Studies 1–3) of adult outpatients who had a primary diagnosis of panic disorder (DSM-III-R), with or without agoraphobia.

Studies 1 and 2 were 10-week flexible dose studies. ZOLOFT was initiated at 25 mg/day for the first week, and then patients were dosed in a range of 50–200 mg/day on the basis of clinical response and toleration. The mean ZOLOFT doses for completers to 10 weeks were 131 mg/day and 144 mg/day, respectively, for studies 1 and 2. In these studies, ZOLOFT was shown to be significantly more effective than placebo on change from baseline in panic attack frequency and on the Clinical Global Impression Severity of Illness and Global Improvement scores. The difference between ZOLOFT and placebo in reduction from baseline in the number of full panic attacks was approximately 2 panic attacks per week in both studies.

Study 3 was a 12-week fixed-dose study, including ZOLOFT doses of 50, 100, and 200 mg/day. Patients receiving ZOLOFT experienced a significantly greater reduction in panic attack frequency than patients receiving placebo. Study 3 was not readily interpretable regarding a dose response relationship for effectiveness.

Subgroup analyses did not indicate that there were any differences in treatment outcomes as a function of age, race, or gender.

INDICATIONS AND USAGE

Depression–ZOLOFT® (sertraline hydrochloride) is indicated for the treatment of depression.

The efficacy of ZOLOFT in the treatment of a major depressive episode was established in six to eight week controlled trials of outpatients whose diagnoses corresponded most closely to the DSM-III category of major depressive disorder (see Clinical Trials under CLINICAL PHARMACOLOGY). A major depressive episode implies a prominent and relatively persistent depressed or dysphoric mood that usually interferes with daily functioning (nearly every day for at least 2 weeks); it should include at least 4 of the following 8 symptoms: change in appetite, change in sleep, psychomotor agitation or retardation, loss of interest in usual activities or decrease in sexual drive, increased fatigue, feelings of guilt or worthlessness, slowed thinking or impaired concentration, and a suicide attempt or suicidal ideation.

The antidepressant action of ZOLOFT in hospitalized depressed patients has not been adequately studied.

The efficacy of ZOLOFT in maintaining an antidepressant response for up to 44 weeks following 8 weeks of open-label acute treatment (52 weeks total) was demonstrated in a placebo-controlled trial. The usefulness of the drug in patients receiving ZOLOFT for extended periods should be reevaluated periodically (see Clinical Trials under CLINICAL PHARMACOLOGY).

Obsessive-Compulsive Disorder–ZOLOFT is indicated for the treatment of obsessions and compulsions in patients with obsessive-compulsive disorder (OCD), as defined in the DSM-III-R; i.e., the obsessions or compulsions cause marked distress, are time-consuming, or significantly interfere with social or occupational functioning.

The efficacy of ZOLOFT was established in 12-week trials with obsessive-compulsive outpatients having diagnoses of obsessive-compulsive disorder as defined according to DSM-III or DSM-III-R criteria (see Clinical Trials under CLINICAL PHARMACOLOGY).

Obsessive-compulsive disorder is characterized by recurrent and persistent ideas, thoughts, impulses, or images (obsessions) that are ego-dystonic and/or repetitive, purposeful, and intentional behaviors (compulsions) that are recognized by the person as excessive or unreasonable.

The effectiveness of ZOLOFT in long-term use for OCD, i.e., for more than 12 weeks, has not been systematically evaluated in placebo-controlled trials. Therefore, the physician who elects to use ZOLOFT for extended periods should periodically reevaluate the long-term usefulness of the drug for the individual patient (see DOSAGE AND ADMINISTRATION).

Panic Disorder–ZOLOFT is indicated for the treatment of panic disorder, with or without agoraphobia, as defined in DSM-IV. Panic disorder is characterized by the occurrence of unexpected panic attacks and associated concern about having additional attacks, worry about the implications or consequences of the attacks, and/or a significant change in behavior related to the attacks.

The efficacy of ZOLOFT was established in three 10–12 week trials in panic disorder patients whose diagnoses corresponded to the DSM-III-R category of panic disorder (see Clinical Trials under CLINICAL PHARMACOLOGY).

Panic disorder (DSM-IV) is characterized by recurrent unexpected panic attacks, i.e., a discrete period of intense fear or discomfort in which four (or more) of the following symptoms develop abruptly and reach a peak within 10 minutes: (1) palpitations, pounding heart, or accelerated heart rate; (2) sweating; (3) trembling or shaking; (4) sensations of shortness of breath or smothering; (5) feeling of choking; (6) chest pain or discomfort; (7) nausea or abdominal distress; (8) feeling dizzy, unsteady, lightheaded, or faint; (9) derealization (feelings of unreality) or depersonalization (being detached from oneself); (10) fear of losing control; (11) fear of dying; (12) paresthesias (numbness or tingling sensations); (13) chills or hot flushes.

The effectiveness of ZOLOFT® (sertraline hydrochloride) in long-term use, that is, for more than 12 weeks, has not been systematically evaluated in controlled trials. Therefore, the physician who elects to use ZOLOFT for extended periods should periodically re-evaluate the long-term usefulness of the drug for the individual patient (See DOSAGE AND ADMINISTRATION).

CONTRAINDICATIONS

Concomitant use in patients taking monoamine oxidase inhibitors (MAOIs) is contraindicated (see WARNINGS).

WARNINGS

Cases of serious sometimes fatal reactions have been reported in patients receiving ZOLOFT® (sertraline hydrochloride), a selective serotonin reuptake inhibitor (SSRI), in combination with a monoamine oxidase inhibitor (MAOI). Symptoms of a drug interaction between an SSRI and an MAOI include: hyperthermia, rigidity, myoclonus, autonomic instability with possible rapid fluctuations of vital signs, mental status changes that include confusion, irritability, and extreme agitation progressing to delirium and coma. These reactions have also been reported in patients who have recently discontinued an SSRI and have been started on an MAOI. Some cases presented with features resembling neuroleptic malignant syndrome. Therefore, ZOLOFT should not be used in combination with an MAOI, or within 14 days of discontinuing treatment with an MAOI. Similarly, at least 14 days should be allowed after stopping ZOLOFT before starting an MAOI.

PRECAUTIONS

General

Activation of Mania/Hypomania–During premarketing testing, hypomania or mania occurred in approximately 0.4% of ZOLOFT® (sertraline hydrochloride) treated patients.

Weight Loss–Significant weight loss may be an undesirable result of treatment with sertraline for some patients, but on average, patients in controlled trials had minimal, 1 to 2 pound weight loss, versus smaller changes on placebo. Only rarely have sertraline patients been discontinued for weight loss.

Seizure–ZOLOFT has not been evaluated in patients with a seizure disorder. These patients were excluded from clinical studies during the product's premarket testing. No seizures were observed among approximately 3000 patients treated with ZOLOFT in the development program for depression. However, 4 patients out of approximately 1800 (220<18 years of age) exposed during the development program for obsessive-compulsive disorder experienced seizures, representing a crude incidence of 0.2%. Three of these patients were adolescents, two with a seizure disorder and one with a family history of seizure disorder, none of whom were receiving anticonvulsant medication. Accordingly, ZOLOFT should be introduced with care in patients with a seizure disorder.

Suicide–The possibility of a suicide attempt is inherent in depression and may persist until significant remission occurs. Close supervision of high risk patients should accompany initial drug therapy. Prescriptions for ZOLOFT should be written for the smallest quantity of tablets consistent with good patient management, in order to reduce the risk of overdose.

Because of the well-established comorbidity between both OCD and depression and panic disorder and depression, the same precautions observed when treating patients with depression should be observed when treating patients with OCD or panic disorder.

Weak Uricosuric Effect–ZOLOFT® (sertraline hydrochloride) is associated with a mean decrease in serum uric acid of approximately 7%. The clinical significance of this weak uricosuric effect is unknown, and there have been no reports of acute renal failure with ZOLOFT.

Use in Patients with Concomitant Illness–Clinical experience with ZOLOFT in patients with certain concomitant systemic illness is limited. Caution is advisable in using ZOLOFT in patients with diseases or conditions that could affect metabolism or hemodynamic responses.

ZOLOFT has not been evaluated or used to any appreciable extent in patients with a recent history of myocardial infarction or unstable heart disease. Patients with these diagnoses were excluded from clinical studies during the product's premarket testing. However, the electrocardiograms of 774 patients who received ZOLOFT in double-blind trials were evaluated and the data indicate that ZOLOFT is not associated with the development of significant ECG abnormalities.

ZOLOFT is extensively metabolized by the liver. In subjects with mild, stable cirrhosis of the liver, the clearance of sertraline was decreased, thus increasing the elimination half-life. A lower or less frequent dose should be used in patients with cirrhosis.

Since ZOLOFT is extensively metabolized, excretion of unchanged drug in urine is a minor route of elimination. However, until the pharmacokinetics of ZOLOFT have been studied in patients with renal impairment and until adequate numbers of patients with severe renal impairment have been evaluated during chronic treatment with ZOLOFT, it should be used with caution in such patients.

Interference with Cognitive and Motor Performance–In controlled studies, ZOLOFT did not cause sedation and did not interfere with psychomotor performance.

Hyponatremia–Several cases of hyponatremia have been reported and appeared to be reversible when ZOLOFT was discontinued. Some cases were possibly due to the syndrome of inappropriate antidiuretic hormone secretion. The majority of these occurrences have been in elderly individuals, some in patients taking diuretics or who were otherwise volume depleted.

Platelet Function–There have been rare reports of altered platelet function and/or abnormal results from laboratory studies in patients taking ZOLOFT. While there have been reports of abnormal bleeding or purpura in several patients taking ZOLOFT, it is unclear whether ZOLOFT had a causative role.

Information for Patients

Physicians are advised to discuss the following issues with patients for whom they prescribe ZOLOFT:

Patients should be told that although ZOLOFT has not been shown to impair the ability of normal subjects to perform tasks requiring complex motor and mental skills in laboratory experiments, drugs that act upon the central nervous system may affect some individuals adversely.

Patients should be told that although ZOLOFT has not been shown in experiments with normal subjects to increase the mental and motor skill impairments caused by alcohol, the concomitant use of ZOLOFT and alcohol is not advised.

Patients should be told that while no adverse interaction of ZOLOFT with over-the-counter (OTC) drug products is known to occur, the potential for interaction exists. Thus, the use of any OTC product should be initiated cautiously according to the directions of use given for the OTC product.

Patients should be advised to notify their physician if they become pregnant or intend to become pregnant during therapy.

Patients should be advised to notify their physician if they are breast feeding an infant.

Laboratory Tests
None.

Drug Interactions
Potential Effects of Coadministration of Drugs Highly Bound to Plasma Proteins–Because sertraline is tightly bound to plasma protein, the administration of ZOLOFT® (sertraline hydrochloride) to a patient taking another drug which is tightly bound to protein (e.g., warfarin, digitoxin) may cause a shift in plasma concentrations potentially resulting in an adverse effect.

Conversely, adverse effects may result from displacement of protein bound ZOLOFT by other tightly bound drugs.

In a study comparing prothrombin time AUC (0–120 hr) following dosing with warfarin (0.75 mg/kg) before and after 21 days of dosing with either ZOLOFT (50–200 mg/day) or placebo, there was a mean increase in prothrombin time of 8% relative to baseline for ZOLOFT compared to a 1% decrease for placebo (p<0.02). The normalization of prothrombin time for the ZOLOFT group was delayed compared to the placebo group. The clinical significance of this change is unknown. Accordingly, prothrombin time should be carefully monitored when ZOLOFT therapy is initiated or stopped.

Cimetidine–In a study assessing disposition of ZOLOFT (100 mg) on the second of 8 days of cimetidine administration (800 mg daily), there were significant increases in ZOLOFT mean AUC (50%), Cmax (24%) and half-life (26%) compared to the placebo group. The clinical significance of these changes is unknown.

CNS Active Drugs–In a study comparing the disposition of intravenously administered diazepam before and after 21 days of dosing with either ZOLOFT (50 to 200 mg/day escalating dose) or placebo, there was a 32% decrease relative to baseline in diazepam clearance for the ZOLOFT group compared to a 19% decrease relative to baseline for the placebo group (p<0.03). There was a 23% increase in Tmax for desmethyldiazepam in the ZOLOFT group compared to a 20% decrease in the placebo group (p<0.03). The clinical significance of these changes is unknown.

In a placebo-controlled trial in normal volunteers, the administration of two doses of ZOLOFT did not significantly alter steady-state lithium levels or the renal clearance of lithium.

Nonetheless, at this time, it is recommended that plasma lithium levels be monitored following initiation of ZOLOFT therapy with appropriate adjustments to the lithium dose. The risk of using ZOLOFT in combination with other CNS active drugs has not been systematically evaluated. Consequently, caution is advised if the concomitant administration of ZOLOFT and such drugs is required.

There is limited controlled experience regarding the optimal timing of switching from other antidepressants to ZOLOFT. Care and prudent medical judgment should be exercised when switching, particularly from long-acting agents. The duration of an appropriate washout period which should intervene before switching from one selective serotonin reuptake inhibitor (SSRI) to another has not been established.

Monoamine Oxidase Inhibitors–See CONTRAINDICATIONS and WARNINGS.

Drugs Metabolized by P450 3A4–In two separate in vivo interaction studies, sertraline was co-administered with cytochrome P450 3A4 substrates, terfenadine or carbamazepine, under steady-state conditions. The results of these studies demonstrated that sertraline co-administration did not increase plasma concentrations of terfenadine or carbamazepine. These data suggest that sertraline's extent of inhibition of P450 3A4 activity is not likely to be of clinical significance.

Drugs Metabolized by P450 2D6–Many antidepressants, e.g., the SSRIs, including sertraline, and most tricyclic antidepressants inhibit the biochemical activity of the drug metabolizing isozyme cytochrome P450 2D6 (debrisoquin hydroxylase); and, thus, may increase the plasma concentrations of co-administered drugs that are metabolized by P450 2D6. The drugs for which this potential interaction is of greatest concern are those metabolized primarily by 2D6 and which have a narrow therapeutic index, e.g., the tricyclic antidepressants and the Type 1C antiarrhythmics propafenone and flecainide. The extent to which this interaction is an important clinical problem depends on the extent of the inhibition of P450 2D6 by the antidepressant and the therapeutic index of the co-administered drug. There is variability among the antidepressants in the extent of clinically important 2D6 inhibition, and in fact sertraline at lower doses has a less prominent inhibitory effect on 2D6 than some others in the class. Nevertheless, even sertraline has the potential for clinically important 2D6 inhibition. Consequently, concomitant use of a drug metabolized by P450 2D6 with ZOLOFT may require lower doses than usually prescribed for the other drug. Furthermore, whenever ZOLOFT is withdrawn from co-therapy, an increased dose of

the co-administered drug may be required (see Tricyclic Antidepressants under PRECAUTIONS).

Tricyclic Antidepressants (TCAs)–The extent to which SSRI-TCA interactions may pose clinical problems will depend on the degree of inhibition and the pharmacokinetics of the SSRI involved. Nevertheless, caution is indicated in the co-administration of TCAs with ZOLOFT, because sertraline may inhibit TCA metabolism. Plasma TCA concentrations may need to be monitored, and the dose of TCA may need to be reduced, if a TCA is co-administered with ZOLOFT (see Drugs Metabolized by P450 2D6 under PRECAUTIONS).

Hypoglycemic Drugs–In a placebo-controlled trial in normal volunteers, administration of ZOLOFT for 22 days (including 200 mg/day for the final 13 days) caused a statistically significant 16% decrease from baseline in the clearance of tolbutamide following an intravenous 1000 mg dose. ZOLOFT administration did not noticeably change either the plasma protein binding or the apparent volume of distribution of tolbutamide, suggesting that the decreased clearance was due to a change in the metabolism of the drug. The clinical significance of this decrease in tolbutamide clearance is unknown.

Atenolol–ZOLOFT (100 mg) when administered to 10 healthy male subjects had no effect on the beta-adrenergic blocking ability of atenolol.

Digoxin–In a placebo-controlled trial in normal volunteers, administration of ZOLOFT for 17 days (including 200 mg/day for the last 10 days) did not change serum digoxin levels or digoxin renal clearance.

Microsomal Enzyme Induction–Preclinical studies have shown ZOLOFT to induce hepatic microsomal enzymes. In clinical studies, ZOLOFT was shown to induce hepatic enzymes minimally as determined by a small (5%) but statistically significant decrease in antipyrine half-life following administration of 200 mg/day for 21 days. This small change in antipyrine half-life reflects a clinically insignificant change in hepatic metabolism.

Electroconvulsive Therapy–There are no clinical studies establishing the risks or benefits of the combined use of electroconvulsive therapy (ECT) and ZOLOFT.

Alcohol–Although ZOLOFT did not potentiate the cognitive and psychomotor effects of alcohol in experiments with normal subjects, the concomitant use of ZOLOFT and alcohol is not recommended.

Carcinogenesis–Lifetime carcinogenicity studies were carried out in CD-1 mice and Long-Evans rats at doses up to 40 mg/kg/day. These doses correspond to 1 times (mice) and 2 times (rats) the maximum recommended human dose (MRHD) on a mg/m² basis. There was a dose-related increase of liver adenomas in male mice receiving sertraline

at 10–40 mg/kg (0.25–1.0 times the MRHD on a mg/m² basis). No increase was seen in female mice or in rats of either sex receiving the same treatments, nor was there an increase in hepatocellular carcinomas. Liver adenomas have a variable rate of spontaneous occurrence in the CD-1 mouse and are of unknown significance to humans. There was an increase in follicular adenomas of the thyroid in female rats receiving sertraline at 40 mg/kg (2 times the MRHD on a mg/m² basis); this was not accompanied by thyroid hyperplasia. While there was an increase in uterine adenocarcinomas in rats receiving sertraline at 10–40 mg/kg (0.5–2.0 times the MRHD on a mg/m² basis) compared to placebo controls, this effect was not clearly drug related.

Mutagenesis–Sertraline had no genotoxic effects, with or without metabolic activation, based on the following assays: bacterial mutation assay; mouse lymphoma mutation assay; and tests for cytogenetic aberrations in vivo in mouse bone marrow and in vitro in human lymphocytes.

Impairment of Fertility–A decrease in fertility was seen in one of two rat studies at a dose of 80 mg/kg (4 times the maximum recommended human dose on a mg/m₂ basis).

Pregnancy–Pregnancy Category C–Reproduction studies have been performed in rats and rabbits at doses up to 80 mg/kg/day and 40 mg/kg/day, respectively. These doses correspond to approximately 4 times the maximum recommended human dose (MRHD) on a mg/m² basis. There was no evidence of teratogenicity at any dose level. When pregnant rats and rabbits were given sertraline during the period of organogenesis, delayed ossification was observed in fetuses at doses of 10 mg/kg (0.5 times the MRHD on a mg/m² basis) in rats and 40 mg/kg (4 times the MRHD on a mg/m² basis) in rabbits. When female rats received sertraline during the last third of gestation and throughout lactation, there was an increase in the number of stillborn pups and in the number of pups dying during the first 4 days after birth. Pup body weights were also decreased during the first four days after birth. These effects occurred at a dose of 20 mg/kg (1 times the MRHD on a mg/m² basis). The no effect dose for rat pup mortality was 10 mg/kg (0.5 times the MRHD on a mg/m² basis). The decrease in pup survival was shown to be due to in utero exposure to sertraline. The clinical significance of these effects is unknown. There are no adequate and well-controlled studies in pregnant women. ZOLOFT® (sertraline hydrochloride) should be used during pregnancy only if the potential benefit justifies the potential risk to the fetus.

Labor and Delivery–The effect of ZOLOFT on labor and delivery in humans is unknown.

TABLE 1
MOST COMMON TREATMENT-EMERGENT ADVERSE EVENTS: INCIDENCE IN PLACEBO-CONTROLLED CLINICAL TRIALS

Body System/Adverse Event	Percentage of Patients Reporting Event					
	Depression/Other*		OCD		Panic Disorder	
	ZOLOFT (N=861)	Placebo (N=853)	ZOLOFT (N=533)	Placebo (N=373)	ZOLOFT (N=430)	Placebo (N=275)
Autonomic Nervous System Disorders						
Ejaculation Failure[1]	7	<1	17	2	19	1
Sweating Increased	8	3	6	1	5	1
Centr. & Periph. Nerv. System Disorders						
Somnolence	13	6	15	8	15	9
Tremor	11	3	8	1	5	1
Gastrointestinal Disorders						
Anorexia	3	2	11	2	7	2
Constipation	8	6	6	4	7	3
Diarrhea/Loose Stools	18	9	24	10	20	9
Dyspepsia	6	3	10	4	10	8
Nausea	26	12	30	11	29	18
Psychiatric Disorders						
Agitation	6	4	6	3	6	2
Insomnia	16	9	28	12	25	18
Libido Decreased	1	<1	11	2	7	1

[1]Primarily ejaculatory delay. Denominator used was for male patients only (N=271 ZOLOFT depression/other*; N=271 placebo depression/other*; N=296 ZOLOFT OCD; N=219 placebo OCD; N=216 ZOLOFT panic disorder; N=134 placebo panic disorder).

*Depression and other premarketing controlled trials.

Continued on next page

Zoloft—Cont.

Nursing Mothers—It is not known whether, and if so in what amount, sertraline or its metabolites are excreted in human milk. Because many drugs are excreted in human milk, caution should be exercised when ZOLOFT is administered to a nursing woman.

Pediatric Use—The efficacy of ZOLOFT for the treatment of obsessive-compulsive disorder was demonstrated in a 12-week, multicenter, placebo-controlled study with 187 outpatients ages 6–17 (see Clinical Trials under CLINICAL PHARMACOLOGY). The effectiveness of ZOLOFT in pediatric patients with depression or panic disorder has not been systematically evaluated.

Sertraline pharmacokinetics were evaluated in 61 pediatric patients between 6 and 17 years of age with depression or OCD and revealed similar drug exposures to those of adults when plasma concentration was adjusted for weight (see Pharmacokinetics under CLINICAL PHARMACOLOGY).

More than 250 patients with depression or OCD between 6 and 17 years of age have received ZOLOFT in clinical trials. The adverse event profile observed in these patients was generally similar to that observed in adult studies with ZOLOFT (see ADVERSE REACTIONS). As with other SSRIs, decreased appetite and weight loss have been observed in association with the use of ZOLOFT. Consequently, regular monitoring of weight and growth is recommended if treatment of a child with an SSRI is to be continued long term. Safety and effectiveness in pediatric patients below the age of 6 have not been established.

The risks, if any, that may be associated with sertraline's extended use in children and adolescents with OCD have not been systematically assessed. The prescriber should be mindful that the evidence relied upon to conclude that sertraline is safe for use in children and adolescents derives from relatively short-term clinical studies and from extrapolation of experience gained with adult patients. In particular, there are no studies that directly evaluate the effects of long-term sertraline use on the growth, development, and maturation of children and adolescents. Although there is no affirmative finding to suggest that sertraline possesses a capacity to adversely affect growth, development or maturation, the absence of such findings is not compelling evidence of the absence of the potential of sertraline to have adverse effects in chronic use.

Geriatric Use—Several hundred elderly patients have participated in clinical studies with ZOLOFT. The pattern of adverse reactions in the elderly was similar to that in younger patients.

ADVERSE REACTIONS

During its premarketing assessment, multiple doses of ZOLOFT were administered to approximately 3800 adult subjects as of June 30, 1995. The conditions and duration of exposure to ZOLOFT varied greatly, and included (in overlapping categories) clinical pharmacology studies, open and double-blind studies, uncontrolled and controlled studies, inpatient and outpatient studies, fixed-dose and titration studies, and studies for multiple indications, including depression, OCD, and panic disorder.

Untoward events associated with this exposure were recorded by clinical investigators using terminology of their own choosing. Consequently, it is not possible to provide a meaningful estimate of the proportion of individuals experiencing adverse events without first grouping similar types of untoward events into a smaller number of standardized event categories.

In the tabulations that follow, a World Health Organization dictionary of terminology has been used to classify reported adverse events. The frequencies presented, therefore, represent the proportion of the approximately 3800 adult individuals exposed to multiple doses of ZOLOFT who experienced a treatment-emergent adverse event of the type cited on at least one occasion while receiving ZOLOFT. An event was considered treatment-emergent if it occurred for the first time or worsened while receiving therapy following baseline evaluation. It is important to emphasize that events reported during therapy were not necessarily caused by it.

The prescriber should be aware that the figures in the tables and tabulations cannot be used to predict the incidence of side effects in the course of usual medical practice where patient characteristics and other factors differ from those that prevailed in the clinical trials. Similarly, the cited frequencies cannot be compared with figures obtained from other clinical investigations involving different treatments, uses, and investigators. The cited figures, however, do provide the prescribing physician with some basis for estimating the relative contribution of drug and nondrug factors to the side effect incidence rate in the population studied.

Incidence in Placebo-Controlled Trials—Table 1 enumerates the most common treatment-emergent adverse events associated with the use of ZOLOFT (incidence of at least 5% for ZOLOFT and at least twice that for placebo within at least one of the indications) for the treatment of adult patients with depression/other*, OCD, and panic disorder in placebo-controlled clinical trials. Most patients received doses of 50 to 200 mg/day. Table 2 enumerates treatment-emergent adverse events that occurred in 2% or more of patients treated with ZOLOFT and with incidence greater than placebo who participated in controlled clinical trials comparing ZOLOFT with placebo in the treatment of depression/other*, OCD, and panic disorder. Table 2 provides combined data for the pool of studies that are provided separately by indication in Table 1.

[See table 1 at top of previous page]
[See table 2 at left]

Associated with Discontinuation in Placebo-Controlled Clinical Trials

Table 3 lists the adverse events associated with discontinuation of ZOLOFT® (sertraline hydrochloride) treatment (incidence at least twice that for placebo and at least 1% for ZOLOFT in clinical trials) in depression/other*, OCD, and panic disorder.

[See table 3 at bottom of next page]

Other Adverse Events in Pediatric Patients—In approximately n=250 pediatric patients treated with ZOLOFT, the overall profile of adverse events was generally similar to that seen in adult studies, as shown in Tables 1 and 2. However, the following adverse events, not appearing in Tables 1 and 2, were reported at an incidence of at least 2% and occurred at a rate of at least twice the placebo rate in a controlled trial (n=187): hyperkinesia, twitching, fever, malaise, purpura, weight decrease, concentration impaired, manic reaction, emotional lability, thinking abnormal, and epistaxis.

Other Events Observed During the Premarketing Evaluation of ZOLOFT® (sertraline hydrochloride)—Following is a list of treatment-emergent adverse events reported during premarketing assessment of ZOLOFT in clinical trials (approximately 3800 adult subjects) except those already listed in the previous tables or elsewhere in labeling.

In the tabulations that follow, a World Health Organization dictionary of terminology has been used to classify reported adverse events. The frequencies presented, therefore, repre-

TABLE 2
TREATMENT-EMERGENT ADVERSE EVENTS: INCIDENCE IN
PLACEBO-CONTROLLED CLINICAL TRIALS

Body System/Adverse Event**	Percentage of Patients Reporting Event Depression/Other*, OCD, and Panic Disorder combined	
	ZOLOFT (N=1824)	Placebo (N=1501)
Autonomic Nervous System Disorders		
Ejaculation Failure[1]	14	1
Mouth Dry	15	9
Sweating Increased	7	2
Centr. & Periph. Nerv. System Disorders		
Somnolence	14	7
Dizziness	13	8
Headache	26	23
Paresthesia	3	2
Tremor	9	2
Disorders of Skin and Appendages		
Rash	3	2
Gastrointestinal Disorders		
Anorexia	6	2
Constipation	7	5
Diarrhea/Loose Stools	20	9
Dyspepsia	8	4
Flatulence	3	2
Nausea	28	13
Vomiting	4	2
General		
Fatigue	12	8
Hot Flushes	2	1
Psychiatric Disorders		
Agitation	6	4
Anxiety	4	3
Insomnia	22	11
Libido Decreased	5	1
Nervousness	6	4
Special Senses		
Vision Abnormal	4	2

[1]Primarily ejaculatory delay. Denominator used was for male patients only (N=783 ZOLOFT; N=624 placebo).
*Depression and other premarketing controlled trials.
**Included are events reported by at least 2% of patients taking ZOLOFT except the following events, which had an incidence on placebo greater than or equal to ZOLOFT: abdominal pain and pharyngitis.

sent the proportion of the approximately 3800 adult individuals exposed to multiple doses of ZOLOFT who experienced an event of the type cited on at least one occasion while receiving ZOLOFT. All events are included except those already listed in the previous tables or elsewhere in labeling and those reported in terms so general as to be uninformative and those for which a causal relationship to ZOLOFT treatment seemed remote. It is important to emphasize that although the events reported occurred during treatment with ZOLOFT, they were not necessarily caused by it.

Events are further categorized by body system and listed in order of decreasing frequency according to the following definitions: frequent adverse events are those occurring on one or more occasions in at least 1/100 patients; infrequent adverse events are those occurring in 1/100 to 1/1000 patients; rare events are those occurring in fewer than 1/1000 patients. Events of major clinical importance are also described in the PRECAUTIONS section.

Autonomic Nervous System Disorders–*Frequent:* impotence; *Infrequent:* flushing, increased saliva, cold clammy skin, mydriasis; *Rare:* pallor, glaucoma, priapism, vasodilation.

Body as a Whole–General Disorders–*Rare:* allergic reaction, allergy.

Cardiovascular–*Frequent:* palpitations, chest pain; *Infrequent:* hypertension, tachycardia, postural dizziness, postural hypotension, periorbital edema, peripheral edema, hypotension, peripheral ischemia, syncope, edema, dependent edema; *Rare:* precordial chest pain, substernal chest pain, aggravated hypertension, myocardial infarction, cerebrovascular disorder.

Central and Peripheral Nervous System Disorders–*Frequent:* hypertonia, hypoesthesia; *Infrequent:* twitching, confusion, hyperkinesia, vertigo, ataxia, migraine, abnormal coordination, hyperesthesia, leg cramps, abnormal gait, nystagmus, hypokinesia; *Rare:* dysphonia, coma, dyskinesia, hypotonia, ptosis, choreoathetosis, hyporeflexia.

Disorders of Skin and Appendages–*Infrequent:* pruritus, acne, urticaria, alopecia, dry skin, erythematous rash, photosensitivity reaction, maculopapular rash; *Rare:* follicular rash, eczema, dermatitis, contact dermatitis, bullous eruption, hypertrichosis, skin discoloration, pustular rash.

Endocrine Disorders–*Rare:* exophthalmos, gynecomastia.

Gastrointestinal Disorders–*Frequent:* appetite increased; *Infrequent:* dysphagia, tooth caries aggravated, eructation, esophagitis, gastroenteritis; *Rare:* melena, glossitis, gum hyperplasia, hiccup, stomatitis, tenesmus, colitis, diverticulitis, fecal incontinence, gastritis, rectum hemorrhage, hemorrhagic peptic ulcer, proctitis, ulcerative stomatitis, tongue edema, tongue ulceration.

General–*Frequent:* back pain, asthenia, malaise, weight increase; *Infrequent:* fever, rigors, generalized edema; *Rare:* face edema, aphthous stomatitis.

Hearing and Vestibular Disorders–*Rare:* hyperacusis, labyrinthine disorder.

Hematopoietic and Lymphatic–*Rare:* anemia, anterior chamber eye hemorrhage.

Liver and Biliary System Disorders–*Rare:* abnormal hepatic function.

Metabolic and Nutritional Disorders–*Infrequent:* thirst; *Rare:* hypoglycemia, hypoglycemic reaction.

Musculoskeletal System Disorders–*Frequent:* myalgia; *Infrequent:* arthralgia, dystonia, arthrosis, muscle cramps, muscle weakness.

Psychiatric Disorders–*Frequent:* yawning, other male sexual dysfunction, other female sexual dysfunction; *Infrequent:* depression, amnesia, paroniria, teeth-grinding, emotional lability, apathy, abnormal dreams, euphoria, paranoid reaction, hallucination, aggressive reaction, aggravated depression, delusions; *Rare:* withdrawal syndrome, suicide ideation, libido increased, somnambulism, illusion.

Reproductive–*Infrequent:* menstrual disorder, dysmenorrhea, intermenstrual bleeding, vaginal hemorrhage, amenorrhea, leukorrhea; *Rare:* female breast pain, menorrhagia, balanoposthitis, breast enlargement, atrophic vaginitis, acute female mastitis.

Respiratory System Disorders–*Frequent:* rhinitis; *Infrequent:* coughing, dyspnea, upper respiratory tract infection, epistaxis, bronchospasm, sinusitis; *Rare:* hyperventilation, bradypnea, stridor, apnea, bronchitis, hemoptysis, hypoventilation, laryngismus, laryngitis.

Special Senses–*Frequent:* tinnitus; *Infrequent:* conjunctivitis, earache, eye pain, abnormal accommodation; *Rare:* xerophthalmia, photophobia, diplopia, abnormal lacrimation, scotoma, visual field defect.

Urinary System Disorders–*Infrequent:* micturition frequency, polyuria, urinary retention, dysuria, nocturia, urinary incontinence; *Rare:* cystitis, oliguria, pyelonephritis, hematuria, renal pain, strangury.

Laboratory Tests–In man, asymptomatic elevations in serum transaminases (SGOT [or AST] and SGPT [or ALT]) have been reported infrequently (approximately 0.8%) in association with ZOLOFT® (sertraline hydrochloride) administration. These hepatic enzyme elevations usually occurred within the first 1 to 9 weeks of drug treatment and promptly diminished upon drug discontinuation.

ZOLOFT therapy was associated with small mean increases in total cholesterol (approximately 3%) and triglycerides (approximately 5%), and a small mean decrease in serum uric acid (approximately 7%) of no apparent clinical importance.

The safety profile observed with ZOLOFT treatment in patients with depression, OCD and panic disorder is similar.

Other Events Observed During the Postmarketing Evaluation of ZOLOFT–Reports of adverse events temporally associated with ZOLOFT that have been received since market introduction, that are not listed above and that may have no causal relationship with the drug include the following: increased coagulation times, bradycardia, AV block, atrial arrhythmias, hypothyroidism, leukopenia, thrombocytopenia, hyperglycemia, priapism, galactorrhea, hyperprolactinemia, neuroleptic malignant syndrome-like events, psychosis, severe skin reactions, which potentially can be fatal, such as Stevens-Johnson Syndrome, vasculitis, photosensitivity and other severe cutaneous disorders, rare reports of pancreatitis, and liver events–clinical features (which in the majority of cases appeared to be reversible with discontinuation of ZOLOFT) occurring in one or more patients include: elevated enzymes, increased bilirubin, hepatomegaly, hepatitis, jaundice, abdominal pain, vomiting, liver failure and death.

DRUG ABUSE AND DEPENDENCE

Controlled Substance Class–ZOLOFT® (sertraline hydrochloride) is not a controlled substance.

Physical and Psychological Dependence–In a placebo-controlled, double-blind, randomized study of the comparative abuse liability of ZOLOFT, alprazolam, and d-amphetamine in humans, ZOLOFT did not produce the positive subjective effects indicative of abuse potential, such as euphoria or drug liking, that were observed with the other two drugs. Premarketing clinical experience with ZOLOFT did not reveal any tendency for a withdrawal syndrome or any drug-seeking behavior. In animal studies ZOLOFT does not demonstrate stimulant or barbiturate-like (depressant) abuse potential. As with any CNS active drug, however, physicians should carefully evaluate patients for history of drug abuse and follow such patients closely, observing them for signs of ZOLOFT misuse or abuse (e.g., development of tolerance, incrementation of dose, drug-seeking behavior).

OVERDOSAGE

Human Experience–As of November 1992, there were 79 reports of non-fatal acute overdoses involving ZOLOFT, of which 28 were overdoses of ZOLOFT alone and the remainder involved a combination of other drugs and/or alcohol in addition to ZOLOFT. In those cases of overdose involving only ZOLOFT, the reported doses ranged from 500 mg to 6000 mg. In a subset of 18 of these patients in whom ZOLOFT blood levels were determined, plasma concentrations ranged from <5 ng/mL to 554 ng/mL. Symptoms of overdose with ZOLOFT alone included somnolence, nausea, vomiting, tachycardia, ECG changes, anxiety and dilated pupils. Treatment was primarily supportive and included monitoring and use of activated charcoal, gastric lavage or cathartics and hydration. Although there were no reports of death when ZOLOFT was taken alone, there were 4 deaths involving overdoses of ZOLOFT in combination with other drugs and/or alcohol. Therefore, any overdosage should be treated aggressively.

Management of Overdoses–Establish and maintain an airway, insure adequate oxygenation and ventilation. Activated charcoal, which may be used with sorbitol, may be as or more effective than emesis or lavage, and should be considered in treating overdose.

Cardiac and vital signs monitoring is recommended along with general symptomatic and supportive measures.

There are no specific antidotes for ZOLOFT.

Due to the large volume of distribution of ZOLOFT, forced diuresis, dialysis, hemoperfusion, and exchange transfusion are unlikely to be of benefit.

In managing overdosage, consider the possibility of multiple drug involvement. The physician should consider contacting a poison control center on the treatment of any overdose.

DOSAGE AND ADMINISTRATION

Initial Treatment

Dosage for Adults

Depression and Obsessive-Compulsive Disorder–ZOLOFT treatment should be administered at a dose of 50 mg once daily.

Panic Disorder–ZOLOFT treatment should be initiated with a dose of 25 mg once daily. After one week, the dose should be increased to 50 mg once daily.

While a relationship between dose and effect has not been established for depression, OCD, or panic disorder, patients were dosed in a range of 50–200 mg/day in the clinical trials

TABLE 3
MOST COMMON ADVERSE EVENTS ASSOCIATED WITH DISCONTINUATION IN PLACEBO-CONTROLLED CLINICAL TRIALS

Adverse Event	Depression/Other* OCD, and Panic Disorder combined (N=1824)	Depression/Other* (N=861)	OCD (N=533)	Panic Disorder (N=430)
Agitation	1%	1%	–	3%
Anorexia	–	–	–	1%
Anxiety	–	–	–	1%
Concentration Impaired	–	–	–	1%
Depersonalization	–	–	–	1%
Diarrhea	3%	2%	2%	4%
Dizziness	–	–	1%	2%
Dry Mouth	1%	1%	–	3%
Dyspepsia	–	–	–	3%
Ejaculation Failure[1]	1%	1%	1%	2%
Fatigue	1%	–	–	3%
Headache	2%	2%	–	5%
Insomnia	2%	1%	3%	4%
Nausea	4%	4%	3%	6%
Nervousness	1%	–	–	3%
Paresthesia	–	–	–	2%
Somnolence	2%	1%	2%	3%
Tremor	1%	2%	–	–
Vomiting	–	–	–	1%

[1] Primarily ejaculatory delay. Denominator used was for male patients only (N=271 depression/other*; N=296 OCD; N=216 panic disorder).
*Depression and other premarketing controlled trials.

Continued on next page

Zoloft—Cont.

demonstrating the effectiveness of ZOLOFT for these indications. Consequently, a dose of 50 mg, administered once daily, is recommended as the initial dose. Patients not responding to a 50 mg dose may benefit from dose increases up to a maximum of 200 mg/day. Given the 24 hour elimination half-life of ZOLOFT, dose changes should not occur at intervals of less than 1 week. ZOLOFT should be administered once daily, either in the morning or evening.

Dosage for Pediatric Population (Children and Adolescents)

Obsessive-Compulsive Disorder–ZOLOFT treatment should be initiated with a dose of 25 mg once daily in children (ages 6–12) and at a dose of 50 mg once daily in adolescents (ages 13–17).

While a relationship between dose and effect has not been established for OCD, patients were dosed in a range of 25–200 mg/day in the clinical trials demonstrating the effectiveness of ZOLOFT for pediatric patients (6–17 years) with OCD. Patients not responding to an initial dose of 25 or 50 mg/day may benefit from dose increases up to a maximum of 200 mg/day. For children with OCD, their generally lower body weights compared to adults should be taken into consideration in advancing the dose, in order to avoid excess dosing. Given the 24 hour elimination half-life of ZOLOFT, dose changes should not occur at intervals of less than 1 week.

ZOLOFT should be administered once daily, either in the morning or evening.

Dosage for Hepatically or Renally Impaired Patients

As indicated under PRECAUTIONS, a lower or less frequent dosage should be used in patients with hepatic impairment. In addition, particular care should be used in patients with renal impairment.

Maintenance/Continuation/Extended Treatment

Depression–It is generally agreed that acute episodes of depression require several months or longer of sustained pharmacologic therapy. Whether the dose of antidepressant needed to induce remission is identical to the dose needed to maintain and/or sustain euthymia is unknown. Systematic evaluation of ZOLOFT has shown that its antidepressant efficacy is maintained for periods of up to 44 weeks following 8 weeks of open-label acute treatment (52 weeks total) at a dose of 50–200 mg/day (mean dose of 70 mg/day) (see Clinical Trials under CLINICAL PHARMACOLOGY).

Obsessive-Compulsive Disorder and Panic Disorder–Although the efficacy of ZOLOFT beyond 10–12 weeks of dosing for OCD and panic disorder has not been documented in controlled trials, both are chronic conditions, and it is reasonable to consider continuation of a responding patient for either indication. Dosage adjustments may be needed to maintain the patient on the lowest effective dosage, and patients should be periodically reassessed to determine the need for continued treatment.

Switching Patients to or from a Monoamine Oxidase Inhibitor–At least 14 days should elapse between discontinuation of an MAOI and initiation of therapy with ZOLOFT. In addition, at least 14 days should be allowed after stopping ZOLOFT before starting an MAOI (see CONTRAINDICATIONS and WARNINGS).

HOW SUPPLIED

ZOLOFT® (sertraline hydrochloride) capsular-shaped scored tablets, containing sertraline hydrochloride equivalent to 25, 50 and 100 mg of sertraline, are packaged in bottles.

ZOLOFT® 25mg Tablets: light green film coated tablets engraved on one side with ZOLOFT and on the other side scored and engraved with 25 mg.

NDC 0049-4960-50	Bottles of 50

ZOLOFT® 50 mg Tablets: light blue film coated tablets engraved on one side with ZOLOFT and on the other side scored and engraved with 50 mg.

NDC 0049-4900-66	Bottles of 100
NDC 0049-4900-73	Bottles of 500
NDC 0049-4900-94	Bottles of 5000
NDC 0049-4900-41	Unit Dose Packages of 100

ZOLOFT® 100 mg Tablets: light yellow film coated tablets engraved on one side with ZOLOFT and on the other side scored and engraved with 100 mg.

NDC 0049-4910-66	Bottles of 100
NDC 0049-4910-73	Bottles of 500
NDC 0049-4910-94	Bottles of 5000
NDC 0049-4910-41	Unit Dose Packages of 100

Store at controlled room temperature, 59° to 86°F (15° to 30°C).

©1997 Pfizer Inc

69-4721-00-4 Revised October 1997

Shown in Product Identification Guide, page 331

ZYRTEC® ℞

(cetirizine hydrochloride)
Tablets and Syrup
For Oral Use

DESCRIPTION

Cetirizine hydrochloride, the active component of ZYRTEC® tablets and syrup, is an orally active and selective H_1-receptor antagonist. The chemical name is (±) - [2-[4- [(4-chlorophenyl)phenylmethyl] -1- piperazinyl] ethoxy] acetic acid, dihydrochloride. Cetirizine hydrochloride is a racemic compound with an empirical formula of $C_{21}H_{25}ClN_2O_3 \bullet 2HCl$. The molecular weight is 461.82 and the chemical structure is shown below:

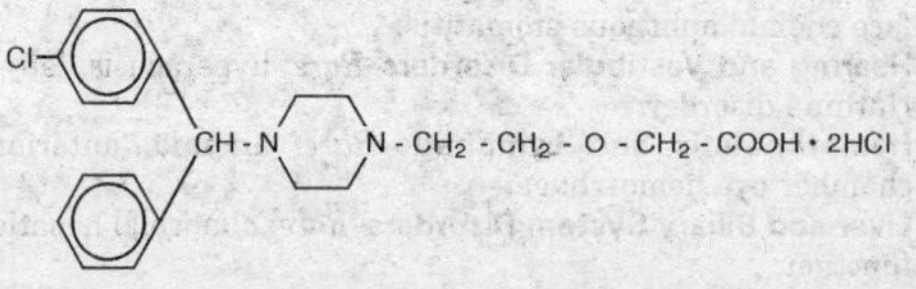

Cetirizine hydrochloride is a white, crystalline powder and is water soluble. ZYRTEC tablets are formulated as white, film-coated, rounded-off rectangular shaped tablets for oral administration and are available in 5 and 10 mg strengths. Inactive ingredients are: lactose; magnesium stearate; povidone; titanium dioxide; hydroxypropyl methylcellulose; polyethylene glycol; and corn starch.

ZYRTEC syrup is a colorless to slightly yellow syrup containing cetirizine hydrochloride at a concentration of 1 mg/mL (5 mg/5 mL) for oral administration. The pH is between 4 and 5. The inactive ingredients of the syrup are: banana flavor; glacial acetic acid; glycerin; grape flavor; methylparaben, propylene glycol; propylparaben; sodium acetate; sugar syrup; and water.

CLINICAL PHARMACOLOGY

Mechanism of Actions: Cetirizine, a human metabolite of hydroxyzine, is an antihistamine; its principal effects are mediated via selective inhibition of peripheral H_1 receptors. The antihistaminic activity of cetirizine has been clearly documented in a variety of animal and human models. *In vivo* and *ex vivo* animal models have shown negligible anticholinergic and antiserotonergic activity. In clinical studies, however, dry mouth was more common with cetirizine than with placebo. *In vitro* receptor binding studies have shown no measurable affinity for other than H_1 receptors. Autoradiographic studies with radiolabeled cetirizine in the rat have shown negligible penetration into the brain. *Ex vivo* experiments in the mouse have shown that systemically administered cetirizine does not significantly occupy cerebral H_1 receptors.

Pharmacokinetics:

Absorption: Cetirizine was rapidly absorbed with a time to maximum concentration (Tmax) of approximately 1 hour following oral administration of tablets or syrup in adults. Comparable bioavailability was found between the tablet and syrup dosage forms. When healthy volunteers were administered multiple doses of cetirizine (10 mg tablets once daily for 10 days), a mean peak plasma concentration (Cmax) of 311 ng/mL was observed. No accumulation was observed. Cetirizine pharmacokinetics were linear for oral doses ranging from 5 to 60 mg. Food had no effect on the extent of cetirizine exposure (AUC) but Tmax was delayed by 1.7 hours and Cmax was decreased by 23% in the presence of food.

Distribution: The mean plasma protein binding of cetirizine is 93%, independent of concentration in the range of 25–1000 ng/mL, which includes the therapeutic plasma levels observed.

Metabolism: A mass balance study in 6 healthy male volunteers indicated that 70% of the administered radioactivity was recovered in the urine and 10% in the feces. Approximately 50% of the radioactivity was identified in the urine as unchanged drug. Most of the rapid increase in peak plasma radioactivity was associated with parent drug, suggesting a low degree of first-pass metabolism. Cetirizine is metabolized to a limited extent by oxidative O-dealkylation to a metabolite with negligible antihistaminic activity. The enzyme or enzymes responsible for this metabolism have not been identified.

Elimination: The mean elimination half-life in 146 healthy volunteers across multiple pharmacokinetic studies was 8.3 hours and the apparent total body clearance for cetirizine was approximately 53 mL/min.

Interaction Studies

Pharmacokinetic interaction studies with cetirizine in adults were conducted with pseudoephedrine, antipyrine, ketoconazole, erythromycin and azithromycin. No interactions were observed. In a multiple dose study of theophylline (400 mg once daily for 3 days) and cetirizine (20 mg once daily for 3 days), a 16% decrease in the clearance of cetirizine was observed. The disposition of theophylline was not altered by concomitant cetirizine administration.

Special Populations

Pediatric Patients: When pediatric patients aged 7 to 12 years received a single, 5-mg oral cetirizine capsule, the mean Cmax was 275 ng/mL. Based on cross-study comparisons, the weight-normalized, apparent total body clearance was 33% greater and the elimination half-life was 33% shorter in this pediatric population than in adults. In pediatric patients aged 2 to 5 years who received 5 mg of cetirizine, the mean Cmax was 660 ng/mL. Based on cross-study comparisons, the weight-normalized apparent total body clearance was 81 to 111% greater and the elimination half-life was 33 to 41% shorter in this pediatric population than in adults.

Geriatric Patients: Following a single, 10-mg oral dose, the elimination half-life was prolonged by 50% and the apparent total body clearance was 40% lower in 16 geriatric subjects with a mean age of 77 years compared to 14 adult subjects with a mean age of 53 years. The decrease in cetirizine clearance in these elderly volunteers may be related to decreased renal function.

Effect of Gender: The effect of gender on cetirizine pharmacokinetics has not been adequately studied.

Effect of Race: No race-related differences in the kinetics of cetirizine have been observed.

Renal Impairment: The kinetics of cetirizine were studied following multiple, oral, 10-mg daily doses of cetirizine for 7 days in 7 normal volunteers (creatinine clearance 89–128 mL/min), 8 patients with mild renal function impairment (creatinine clearance 42–77 mL/min) and 7 patients with moderate renal function impairment (creatinine clearance 11–31 mL/min). The pharmacokinetics of cetirizine were similar in patients with mild impairment and normal volunteers. Moderately impaired patients had a 3-fold increase in half-life and a 70% decrease in clearance compared to normal volunteers.

Patients on hemodialysis (n=5) given a single, 10-mg dose of cetirizine had a 3-fold increase in half-life and a 70% decrease in clearance compared to normal volunteers. Less than 10% of the administered dose was removed during the single dialysis session.

Dosing adjustment is necessary in patients with moderate or severe renal impairment and in patients on dialysis (see **DOSAGE AND ADMINISTRATION**).

Hepatic Impairment: Sixteen patients with chronic liver diseases (hepatocellular, cholestatic, and biliary cirrhosis), given 10 to 20 mg of cetirizine as a single, oral dose had a 50% increase in half-life along with a corresponding 40% decrease in clearance compared to 16 healthy subjects.

Dosing adjustment may be necessary in patients with hepatic impairment (see **DOSAGE AND ADMINISTRATION**).

Pharmacodynamics: Studies in 69 adult normal volunteers (aged 20 to 61 years) showed that ZYRTEC at doses of 5 and 10 mg strongly inhibited the skin wheal and flare caused by the intradermal injection of histamine. The onset of this activity after a single 10-mg dose occurred within 20 minutes in 50% of subjects and within one hour in 95% of subjects; this activity persisted for at least 24 hours. ZYRTEC at doses of 5 and 10 mg also strongly inhibited the wheal and flare caused by intradermal injection of histamine in 19 pediatric volunteers (aged 5 to 12 years) and the activity persisted for at least 24 hours. In a 35-day study in children aged 5 to 12, no tolerance to the antihistaminic (suppression of wheal and flare response) effects of ZYRTEC was found. The effects of intradermal injection of various other mediators or histamine releasers were also inhibited by cetirizine, as was response to a cold challenge in patients with cold-induced urticaria. In mildly asthmatic subjects, ZYRTEC at 5 to 20 mg blocked bronchoconstriction due to nebulized histamine, with virtually total blockade after a 20-mg dose. In studies conducted for up to 12 hours following cutaneous antigen challenge, the late phase recruitment of eosinophils, neutrophils and basophils, components of the allergic inflammatory response, was inhibited by ZYRTEC at a dose of 20 mg.

In four clinical studies in healthy adult males, no clinically significant mean increases in QTc were observed in ZYRTEC treated subjects. In the first study, a placebo-controlled crossover trial, ZYRTEC was given at doses up to 60 mg per day, 6 times the maximum clinical dose, for 1 week, and no significant mean QTc prolongation occurred. In the second study, a crossover trial, ZYRTEC 20 mg and erythromycin (500 mg every 8 hours) were given alone and in combination. There was no significant effect on QTc with the combination or with ZYRTEC alone. In the third trial, also a crossover study, ZYRTEC 20 mg and ketoconazole (400 mg per day) were given alone and in combination. ZYRTEC caused a mean increase in QTc of 9.1 msec from baseline after 10 days of therapy. Ketoconazole also increased QTc by 8.3 msec. The combination caused an increase of 17.4 msec, equal to the sum of the individual effects. Thus, there was no significant drug interaction on QTc with the combination of ZYRTEC and ketoconazole. In the fourth study, a placebo-controlled parallel trial, ZYRTEC 20 mg was given alone or in combination with azithromycin (500 mg as a single dose on the first day followed by 250 mg once daily). There was no significant increase in OTc with ZYRTEC 20 mg alone or in combination with azithromycin.

In a four-week clinical trial in pediatric patients aged 6 to 11 years, results of randomly obtained ECG measurements

before treatment and after 2 weeks of treatment showed that ZYRTEC 5 or 10 mg did not significantly increase QTc versus placebo. The effects of ZYRTEC on the QTc interval at doses higher than the 10 mg dose have not been studied in children less than 12 years of age. The effect of ZYRTEC on the QTc interval in children less than 6 years of age has not been studied.

In a six-week, placebo-controlled study of 186 patients (aged 12 to 64 years) with allergic rhinitis and mild to moderate asthma, ZYRTEC 10 mg once daily improved rhinitis symptoms and did not alter pulmonary function. In a two-week, placebo-controlled clinical trial, a subset analysis of 65 pediatric (aged 6 to 11 years) allergic rhinitis patients with asthma showed ZYRTEC did not alter pulmonary function. These studies support the safety of administering ZYRTEC to pediatric and adult allergic rhinitis patients with mild to moderate asthma.

Clinical Studies: Nine multicenter, randomized, double-blind, clinical trials comparing cetirizine 5 to 20 mg to placebo in patients 12 years and older with seasonal or perennial allergic rhinitis were conducted in the United States. Five of these showed significant reductions in symptoms of allergic rhinitis, 3 in seasonal allergic rhinitis (1 to 4 weeks in duration) and 2 in perennial allergic rhinitis for up to 8 weeks in duration. Two 4-week multicenter, randomized, double-blind, clinical trials comparing cetirizine 5 to 20 mg to placebo in patients with chronic idiopathic urticaria were also conducted and showed significant improvement in symptoms of chronic idiopathic urticaria. In general, the 10-mg dose was more effective than the 5-mg dose and the 20-mg dose gave no added effect. Some of these trials included pediatric patients aged 12 to 16 years. In addition, four multicenter, randomized, placebo-controlled, double-blind 2–4 week trials in 534 pediatric patients aged 6 to 11 years with seasonal allergic rhinitis were conducted in the United States at doses up to 10 mg.

INDICATIONS AND USAGE

Seasonal Allergic Rhinitis: ZYRTEC is indicated for the relief of symptoms associated with seasonal allergic rhinitis due to allergens such as ragweed, grass and tree pollens in adults and children 2 years of age and older. Symptoms treated effectively include sneezing, rhinorrhea, nasal pruritus, ocular pruritus, tearing, and redness of the eyes.

Perennial Allergic Rhinitis: ZYRTEC is indicated for the relief of symptoms associated with perennial allergic rhinitis due to allergens such as dust mites, animal dander and molds in adults and children 2 years of age and older. Symptoms treated effectively include sneezing, rhinorrhea, postnasal discharge, nasal pruritus, ocular pruritus, and tearing.

Chronic Urticaria: ZYRTEC is indicated for the treatment of the uncomplicated skin manifestations of chronic idiopathic urticaria in adults and children 2 years of age and older. It significantly reduces the occurrence, severity, and duration of hives and significantly reduces pruritus.

CONTRAINDICATIONS

ZYRTEC is contraindicated in those patients with a known hypersensitivity to it or any of its ingredients or hydroxyzine.

PRECAUTIONS

Activities Requiring Mental Alertness: In clinical trials, the occurrence of somnolence has been reported in some patients taking ZYRTEC; due caution should therefore be exercised when driving a car or operating potentially dangerous machinery. Concurrent use of ZYRTEC with alcohol or other CNS depressants should be avoided because additional reductions in alertness and additional impairment of CNS performance may occur.

Drug-Drug Interactions: No clinically significant drug interactions have been found with theophylline at a low dose, azithromycin, pseudoephedrine, ketoconazole, or erythromycin. There was a small decrease in the clearance of cetirizine caused by a 400-mg dose of theophylline; it is possible that larger theophylline doses could have a greater effect.

Carcinogenesis, Mutagenesis and Impairment of Fertility: In a 2-year carcinogenicity study in rats, cetirizine was not carcinogenic at dietary doses up to 20 mg/kg (approximately 15 times the maximum recommended daily oral dose in adults on a mg/m^2 basis, or approximately 10 times the maximum recommended daily oral dose in children on a mg/m^2 basis). In a 2-year carcinogenicity study in mice, cetirizine caused an increased incidence of benign liver tumors in males at a dietary dose of 16 mg/kg (approximately 6 times the maximum recommended daily oral dose in adults on a mg/m^2 basis, or approximately 4 times the maximum recommended daily oral dose in children on a mg/m^2 basis). No increase in the incidence of liver tumors was observed in mice at a dietary dose of 4 mg/kg (approximately 2 times the maximum recommended daily oral dose in adults on a mg/m^2 basis, or approximately equal to the maximum recommended daily oral dose in children on a mg/m^2 basis).

The clinical significance of these findings during long-term use of ZYRTEC is not known.

Cetirizine was not mutagenic in the Ames test, and not clastogenic in the human lymphocyte assay, the mouse lymphoma assay, and *in vivo* micronucleus test in rats.

In a fertility and general reproductive performance study in mice, cetirizine did not impair fertility at an oral dose of 64 mg/kg (approximately 25 times the maximum recommended daily oral dose in adults on a mg/m^2 basis).

Pregnancy Category B: In mice, rats, and rabbits, cetirizine was not teratogenic at oral doses up to 96, 225, and 135 mg/kg, respectively (approximately 40, 180 and 220 times the maximum recommended daily oral dose in adults on a mg/m^2 basis). There are no adequate and well-controlled studies in pregnant women. Because animal studies are not always predictive of human response, ZYRTEC should be used in pregnancy only if clearly needed.

Nursing Mothers: In mice, cetirizine caused retarded pup weight gain during lactation at an oral dose in dams of 96 mg/kg (approximately 40 times the maximum recommended daily oral dose in adults on a mg/m^2 basis). Studies in beagle dogs indicated that approximately 3% of the dose was excreted in milk. Cetirizine has been reported to be excreted in human breast milk. Because many drugs are excreted in human milk, use of ZYRTEC in nursing mothers is not recommended.

Geriatric Use: In placebo-controlled trials, 186 patients aged 65 to 94 years received doses of 5 to 20 mg of ZYRTEC per day. Adverse events were similar in this group to patients under age 65. Subset analysis of efficacy in this group was not done.

Pediatric Use: The safety of ZYRTEC, at daily doses of 5 or 10 mg, has been demonstrated in 376 pediatric patients aged 6 to 11 years in placebo-controlled trials lasting up to four weeks and in 254 patients in a non-placebo-controlled 12-week trial. The safety of cetirizine has been demonstrated in 168 patients aged 2 to 5 years in placebo-controlled trials of up to 4 weeks duration. On a mg/kg basis, most of the 168 patients received between 0.2 and 0.4 mg/kg of cetirizine HCl.

The effectiveness of ZYRTEC for the treatment of seasonal and perennial allergic rhinitis and chronic idiopathic urticaria in pediatric patients aged 2 to 11 years is based on an extrapolation of the demonstrated efficacy of ZYRTEC in adults in these conditions and the likelihood that the disease course, pathophysiology and the drug's effect are substantially similar between these two populations. The recommended doses for the pediatric population are based on cross-study comparisons of the pharmacokinetics and pharmacodynamics of cetirizine in adult and pediatric subjects and on the safety profile of cetirizine in both adult and pediatric patients at doses equal to or higher than the recommended doses. The cetirizine AUC and Cmax in pediatric subjects aged 2 to 5 years who received a single dose of 5 mg of cetirizine syrup and in pediatric subjects aged 6 to 11 years who received a single dose of 10 mg of cetirizine syrup were estimated to be intermediate between that observed in adults who received a single dose of 10 mg of cetirizine tablets and those who received a single dose of 20 mg of cetirizine tablets.

The safety and effectiveness of cetirizine in pediatric patients under the age of 2 years have not yet been established.

ADVERSE REACTIONS

Controlled and uncontrolled clinical trials conducted in the United States and Canada included more than 6000 patients aged 12 years and older, with more than 3900 receiving ZYRTEC at doses of 5 to 20 mg per day. The duration of treatment ranged from 1 week to 6 months, with a mean exposure of 30 days.

Most adverse reactions reported during therapy with ZYRTEC were mild or moderate. In placebo-controlled trials, the incidence of discontinuations due to adverse reactions in patients receiving ZYRTEC 5 or 10 mg was not significantly different from placebo (2.9% vs. 2.4%, respectively).

The most common adverse reaction in patients aged 12 years and older that occurred more frequently on ZYRTEC than placebo was somnolence. The incidence of somnolence associated with ZYRTEC was dose related, 6% in placebo, 11% at 5 mg and 14% at 10 mg. Discontinuations due to somnolence for ZYRTEC was uncommon (1.0% on ZYRTEC vs. 0.6% on placebo). Fatigue and dry mouth also appeared to be treatment-related adverse reactions. There were no differences by age, race, gender or by body weight with regard to the incidence of adverse reactions.

Table 1 lists adverse experiences in patients aged 12 years and older which were reported for ZYRTEC 5 and 10 mg in controlled clinical trials in the United States and that were more common with ZYRTEC than placebo.

Table 1.
Adverse Experiences Reported in Patients Aged 12 Years and Older in Placebo-Controlled United States ZYRTEC Trials (Maximum Dose of 10 mg) at Rates of 2% or Greater (Percent Incidence)

Adverse Experience	ZYRTEC (N=2034)	Placebo (N=1612)
Somnolence	13.7	6.3
Fatigue	5.9	2.6
Dry Mouth	5.0	2.3
Pharyngitis	2.0	1.9
Dizziness	2.0	1.2

In addition, headache and nausea occurred in more than 2% of the patients, but were more common in placebo patients. Pediatric studies were also conducted with ZYRTEC. More than 1300 pediatric patients aged 6 to 11 years with more than 900 treated with ZYRTEC at doses of 1.25 to 10 mg per day were included in controlled and uncontrolled clinical trials conducted in the United States. The duration of treatment ranged from 2 to 12 weeks. Placebo-controlled trials up to 4 weeks duration included 168 pediatric patients aged 2 to 5 years who received cetirizine, the majority of whom received single daily doses of 5 mg.

The majority of adverse reactions reported in pediatric patients aged 2 to 11 years with ZYRTEC were mild or moderate. In placebo-controlled trials, the incidence of discontinuations due to adverse reactions in pediatric patients receiving up to 10 mg of ZYRTEC was uncommon (0.4% on ZYRTEC vs. 1.0% on placebo).

Table 2 lists adverse experiences which were reported for ZYRTEC 5 and 10 mg in pediatric patients aged 6 to 11 years in placebo-controlled clinical trials in the United States and were more common with ZYRTEC than placebo. Of these, abdominal pain was considered treatment-related and somnolence appeared to be dose-related, 1.3% in placebo, 1.9% at 5 mg and 4.2% at 10 mg. The adverse experiences reported in pediatric patients aged 2 to 5 years in placebo-controlled trials were qualitatively similar in nature and generally similar in frequency to those reported in trials with children aged 6 to 11 years.

Table 2.
Adverse Experiences Reported in Pediatric Patients Aged 6 to 11 Years in Placebo-Controlled United States ZYRTEC Trials (5 or 10 mg Dose) Which Occurred at a Frequency of ≥2% in Either the 5-mg or the 10-mg ZYRTEC Group, and More Frequently Than in the Placebo Group

Adverse Experiences	Placebo (N=309)	ZYRTEC 5 mg (N=161)	ZYRTEC 10 mg (N=215)
Headache	12.3%	11.0%	14.0%
Pharyngitis	2.9%	6.2%	2.8%
Abdominal pain	1.9%	4.4%	5.6%
Coughing	3.9%	4.4%	2.8%
Somnolence	1.3%	1.9%	4.2%
Diarrhea	1.3%	3.1%	1.9%
Epistaxis	2.9%	3.7%	1.9%
Bronchospasm	1.9%	3.1%	1.9%
Nausea	1.9%	1.9%	2.8%
Vomiting	1.0%	2.5%	2.3%

The following events were observed infrequently (less than 2%), in either 3982 adults and children 12 years and older or in 659 pediatric patients aged 6 to 11 years who received ZYRTEC in U.S. trials, including an open adult study of six months duration. A causal relationship of these infrequent events with ZYRTEC administration has not been established.

Autonomic Nervous System: anorexia, flushing, increased salivation, urinary retention.

Cardiovascular: cardiac failure, hypertension, palpitation, tachycardia.

Central and Peripheral Nervous Systems: abnormal coordination, ataxia, confusion, dysphonia, hyperesthesia, hyperkinesia, hypertonia, hypoesthesia, leg cramps, migraine,

Continued on next page

Zyrtec—Cont.

myelitis, paralysis, paresthesia, ptosis, syncope, tremor, twitching, vertigo, visual field defect.

Gastrointestinal: abnormal hepatic function, aggravated tooth caries, constipation, dyspepsia, eructation, flatulence, gastritis, hemorrhoids, increased appetite, melena, rectal hemorrhage, stomatitis including ulcerative stomatitis, tongue discoloration, tongue edema.

Genitourinary: cystitis, dysuria, hematuria, micturition frequency, polyuria, urinary incontinence, urinary tract infection.

Hearing and Vestibular: deafness, earache, ototoxicity, tinnitus.

Metabolic/Nutritional: dehydration, diabetes mellitus, thirst.

Musculoskeletal: arthralgia, arthritis, arthrosis, muscle weakness, myalgia.

Psychiatric: abnormal thinking, agitation, amnesia, anxiety, decreased libido, depersonalization, depression, emotional lability, euphoria, impaired concentration, insomnia, nervousness, paroniria, sleep disorder.

Respiratory System: bronchitis, dyspnea, hyperventilation, increased sputum, pneumonia, respiratory disorder, rhinitis, sinusitis, upper respiratory tract infection.

Reproductive: dysmenorrhea, female breast pain, intermenstrual bleeding, leukorrhea, menorrhagia, vaginitis.

Reticuloendothelial: lymphadenopathy.

Skin: acne, alopecia, angioedema, bullous eruption, dermatitis, dry skin, eczema, erythematous rash, furunculosis, hyperkeratosis, hypertrichosis, increased sweating, maculopapular rash, photosensitivity reaction, photosensitivity toxic reaction, pruritus, purpura, rash, seborrhea, skin disorder, skin nodule, urticaria.

Special Senses: parosmia, taste loss, taste perversion.

Vision: blindness, conjunctivitis, eye pain, glaucoma, loss of accommodation, ocular hemorrhage, xerophthalmia.

Body as a Whole: accidental injury, asthenia, back pain, chest pain, enlarged abdomen, face edema, fever, generalized edema, hot flashes, increased weight, leg edema, malaise, nasal polyp, pain, pallor, periorbital edema, peripheral edema, rigors.

Occasional instances of transient, reversible hepatic transaminase elevations have occurred during cetirizine therapy. Hepatitis with significant transaminase elevation and elevated bilirubin in association with the use of ZYRTEC has been reported.

In foreign marketing experience the following additional rare, but potentially severe adverse events have been reported: anaphylaxis, cholestasis, glomerulonephritis, hemolytic anemia, hepatitis, orofacial dyskinesia, severe hypotension, stillbirth, and thrombocytopenia.

DRUG ABUSE AND DEPENDENCE

There is no information to indicate that abuse or dependency occurs with ZYRTEC.

OVERDOSAGE

Overdosage has been reported with ZYRTEC. In one adult patient who took 150 mg of ZYRTEC, the patient was somnolent but did not display any other clinical signs or abnormal blood chemistry or hematology results. In an 18 month old pediatric patient who took an overdose of ZYRTEC (approximately 180 mg), restlessness and irritability were observed initially; this was followed by drowsiness. Should overdose occur, treatment should be symptomatic or supportive, taking into account any concomitantly ingested medications. There is no known specific antidote to ZYRTEC. ZYRTEC is not effectively removed by dialysis, and dialysis will be ineffective unless a dialyzable agent has been concomitantly ingested. The acute minimal lethal oral doses were 237 mg/kg in mice (approximately 95 times the maximum recommended daily oral dose in adults on a mg/m^2 basis, or approximately 55 times the maximum recommended daily oral dose in children on a mg/m^2 basis) and 562 mg/kg in rats (approximately 460 times the maximum recommended daily oral dose in adults on a mg/m^2 basis, or approximately 270 times the maximum recommended daily oral dose in children on a mg/m^2 basis). In rodents, the target of acute toxicity was the central nervous system, and the target of multiple-dose toxicity was the liver.

DOSAGE AND ADMINISTRATION

Adults and Children 12 Years and Older: The recommended initial dose of ZYRTEC is 5 or 10 mg per day in adults and children 12 years and older, depending on symptom severity. Most patients in clinical trials started at 10 mg. ZYRTEC is given as a single daily dose, with or without food. The time of administration may be varied to suit individual patient needs.

Children 6 to 11 Years: The recommended initial dose of ZYRTEC in children aged 6 to 11 years is 5 or 10 mg (1 or 2 teaspoons) once daily depending on symptom severity. The time of administration may be varied to suit individual patient needs.

Children 2 to 5 Years: The recommended initial dose of ZYRTEC syrup in children aged 2 to 5 years is 2.5 mg (½ teaspoon) once daily. The dosage in this age group can be increased to a maximum dose of 5 mg per day given as 1 teaspoon (5 mg) once daily, or as ½ teaspoon (2.5 mg) given every 12 hours, depending on symptom severity and patient response.

Dose Adjustment for Renal and Hepatic Impairment: In patients 12 years of age and older with decreased renal function (creatinine clearance 11–31 mL/min), patients on hemodialysis (creatinine clearance less than 7 mL/min), and in hepatically impaired patients, a dose of 5 mg once daily is recommended. Similarly, pediatric patients aged 6 to 11 years with impaired renal or hepatic function should use the lower recommended dose. Because of the difficulty in reliably administering doses of less than 2.5 mg (½ teaspoon) of ZYRTEC syrup and in the absence of pharmacokinetic and safety information for cetirizine in children below the age of 6 years with impaired renal or hepatic function, its use in this impaired patient population is not recommended.

HOW SUPPLIED

ZYRTEC® tablets are white, film-coated, rounded-off rectangular shaped containing 5 mg or 10 mg cetirizine hydrochloride.

5 mg tablets are engraved with "ZYRTEC" on one side and "5" on the other.

Bottles of 100: NDC 0069-5500-66

10 mg tablets are engraved with "ZYRTEC" on one side and "10" on the other.

Bottles of 100: NDC 0069-5510-66

STORAGE: Store at room temperature 59° to 86°F (15° to 30°C).

ZYRTEC® syrup is colorless to slightly yellow with a banana-grape flavor. Each teaspoonful (5 mL) contains 5 mg cetirizine hydrochloride. ZYRTEC® syrup is supplied as follows:

120 mL amber glass bottles   NDC 0069-5530-47
1 pint amber glass bottles   NDC 0069-5530-93

STORAGE: Store at 41° to 86°F (5° to 30°C).

Cetirizine is licensed from UCB Pharma, Inc.

©1998 PFIZER INC

Manufactured / Marketed by
Pfizer Labs
Division of Pfizer Inc, NY, NY 10017
Marketed by
UCB Pharma, Inc.
Smyrna, GA 30080
70-4573-00-3   Revised May 1998
Shown in Product Identification Guide, page 331

Pfizer Labs Division
See Pfizer Inc

Pharmaceutical Associates, Inc.
A Subsidiary of Beach Products, Inc.
201 DELAWARE STREET
GREENVILLE, SC 29605

Direct Inquiries to:
Clete Harmon, Director of Q.A.
PH: (800) 845-8210
     (864) 277-7282
FAX: (864) 277-8045

HOSPITAL UNIT DOSE / TRADE PACKAGE

NDC Prefix: 00121-

PRODUCT LISTING

ACETAMINOPHEN ORAL SOLUTION USP   OTC
(160 mg per 5 mL)
   Unit Dose 10.15 mL and 20.3 mL

ACETAMINOPHEN and CODEINE PHOSPHATE   ℂ℞
ORAL SOLUTION USP
(120 mg/12 mg per 5 mL)
   Unit Dose 5 mL, 10 mL, 12.5 mL, and 15 mL
   Bottles of 4 fl oz and 16 fl oz

ALUMINUM HYDROXIDE GEL USP   OTC
(320 mg per 5 mL)
   Unit Dose 30 mL
   Bottles of 12 fl oz and 16 fl oz

ALUMINUM HYDROXIDE GEL CONCENTRATE   OTC
(600 mg per 5 mL)
   Bottles of 12 fl oz

AMANTADINE HYDROCHLORIDE SYRUP USP   ℞
(50 mg per 5 mL)
   Unit Dose 10 mL and 20 mL
   Bottles of 16 fl oz

AROMATIC CASCARA FLUIDEXTRACT USP   OTC
   Unit Dose 5 mL

CHLORAL HYDRATE SYRUP USP   ℂⅣ℞
(500 mg per 5 mL)
   Unit Dose 5 mL
   Bottles of 4 fl oz

CIMETIDINE HYDROCHLORIDE ORAL SOLUTION   ℞
(300 mg per 5 mL)
   Bottles of 8 fl oz

DIPHENHYDRAMINE HYDROCHLORIDE ELIXIR USP   ℞
(12.5 mg per 5 mL)
   Unit Dose 5 mL, 10 mL, and 20 mL

DOCUSATE SODIUM LIQUID   OTC
(50 mg per 5 mL)
   Unit Dose 10 mL and 25 mL
   Bottles of 16 fl oz

DOCUSATE SODIUM SYRUP USP   OTC
(20 mg per 5 mL)
   Unit Dose 25 mL
   Bottles of 16 fl oz

DOCUSATE SODIUM with CASANTHRANOL   OTC
(20 mg/10 mg per 5 mL)
   Unit Dose 15 mL and 30 mL
   Bottles of 16 fl oz

FERROUS SULFATE LIQUID   OTC
(300 mg per 5 mL)
   Unit Dose 5 mL

FLUPHENAZINE HYDROCHLORIDE ELIXIR USP   ℞
(2.5 mg per 5 mL)
   Bottles of 60 mL and 16 fl oz

FLUPHENAZINE HYDROCHLORIDE ORAL SOLUTION   ℞
USP Concentrate
(5 mg per 1 mL)
   Bottles of 4 fl oz

GUAIFENESIN SYRUP USP   OTC
(100 mg per 5 mL)
   Unit Dose 5 mL, 10 mL, and 15 mL
   Bottles of 4 fl oz

GUAIFENESIN SYRUP with CODEINE   ℂⅤ OTC
(100 mg/10 mg per 5 mL)
   Unit Dose 5 mL and 10 mL
   Bottles of 4 fl oz and 16 fl oz

GUAIFENESIN SYRUP and DEXTROMETHORPHAN   OTC
(100 mg/10 mg per 5 mL)
   Unit Dose 5 mL and 10 mL
   Bottles of 4 fl oz

HALOPERIDOL ORAL SOLUTION USP   ℞
Concentrate
(2 mg per 1 mL)
   Unit Dose 5 mL and 10 mL
   Bottles of 4 fl oz

HYDROCODONE BITARTRATE and   ℂⅢ℞
ACETAMINOPHEN ELIXIR
(7.5 mg/500 mg per 15 mL)
   Unit Dose 15 mL
   Bottles of 4 fl oz and 16 fl oz

HYDROCODONE BITARTRATE and GUAIFENESIN   ℂⅢ℞
EXPECTORANT
(5 mg/100 mg per 5 mL)
   Unit Dose 5 mL and 10 mL
   Bottles of 16 fl oz

HYDROCODONE BITARTRATE/PHENYLEPHRINE   ℂⅢ℞
HYDROCHLORIDE/CHLORPHENIRAMINE MALEATE
SYRUP
(1.67 mg/5 mg/2 mg per 5 mL)
   Bottles of 16 fl oz

LACTULOSE SOLUTION USP   ℞
(10 g per 15 mL)
   Unit Dose 30 mL
   Bottles of 8 fl oz

METOCLOPRAMIDE ORAL SOLUTION USP   ℞
(5 mg per 5 mL)
   Unit Dose 10 mL
   Bottles of 16 fl oz

MILK OF MAGNESIA USP   OTC
(400 mg per 5 mL)
   Unit Dose 15 mL and 30 mL

MILK OF MAGNESIA CONCENTRATE   OTC
(2400 mg per 10 mL)
   Unit Dose 10 mL

MILK OF MAGNESIA CASCARA SUSPENSION   OTC
(2400 mg/5 mL per 30 mL)
   Unit Dose 15 mL and 30 mL
   Bottles of 4 fl oz

MINERAL OIL   OTC
   Unit Dose 30 mL

PHENOBARBITAL ELIXIR   ℂⅣ℞
(20 mg per 5 mL)
   Unit Dose 5 mL, 7.5 mL, and 15 mL

POTASSIUM CHLORIDE ORAL SOLUTION USP 10%   ℞
(20 mEq per 15 mL)
   Unit Dose 15 mL and 30 mL

POTASSIUM CHLORIDE ORAL SOLUTION USP 20% ℞
(40 mEq per 15 mL)
  Unit Dose 15 mL
POTASSIUM CITRATE and CITRIC ACID ℞
ORAL SOLUTION USP
(1100 mg/334 mg per 5 mL)
  Unit Dose 15 mL and 30 mL
  Bottles of 16 fl oz
PROMETHAZINE HYDROCHLORIDE and CODEINE Ⓥ℞
PHOSPHATE SYRUP
(6.25 mg/10 mg per 5 mL)
  Unit Dose 5 mL
PSEUDOEPHEDRINE HYDROCHLORIDE SYRUP USP OTC
(30 mg per 5 mL)
  Bottles of 4 fl oz
SODIUM CITRATE and CITRIC ACID ORAL ℞
SOLUTION USP
(500 mg/334 mg per 5 mL)
  Unit Dose 15 mL and 30 mL
  Bottles of 16 fl oz
SORBITOL SOLUTION USP OTC
(70% w/w)
  Unit Dose 30 mL
  Bottles of 16 fl oz
SORE THROAT SPRAY OTC
(Phenol 1.4%) Cherry and Menthol
  Bottles of 6 fl oz
THIORIDAZINE HYDROCHLORIDE ORAL ℞
SOLUTION USP Concentrate
(30 mg per 1 mL)
  Bottles of 4 fl oz
THIORIDAZINE HYDROCHLORIDE ORAL ℞
SOLUTION USP Concentrate
(100 mg per 1 mL)
  Bottles of 4 fl oz
TRICITRATES ORAL SOLUTION ℞
(550 mg/500 mg/334 mg per 5 mL)
  Unit Dose 15 mL and 30 mL
  Bottles of 16 fl oz
TRIHEXYPHENIDYL HYDROCHLORIDE ELIXIR USP ℞
(2 mg per 5 mL)
  Unit Dose 5 mL, 10 mL, and 12.5 mL
  Bottles of 16 fl oz

Pharmacia & Upjohn Company
Bridgewater, NJ 08807-1265

Direct Inquiries to:
1-888-768-5501

For Medical and Pharmaceutical Information, Including Emergencies, Contact:
(616) 833-8244

PRODUCT IDENTIFICATION
Prescription capsules and tablets manufactured by Pharmacia & Upjohn Company are imprinted with one or a combination of the following: (1) Product trademark, (2) Dosage strength, (3) "Adria," "Pharmacia," "Upjohn," "U," or the code "KP." That portion of the National Drug Code (NDC) number that indicates product and strength.
A list of oral solid dosage forms with NDC product identification numbers is provided below.

Code #	Product	Strength
01	**DOSTINEX®** Tablets (carbergoline tablets)	0.5 mg
02	**MIRAPEX®** Tablets (pramipexole dihydrochloride tablets)	0.125 mg
04	**MIRAPEX®** Tablets (pramipexole dihydrochloride tablets)	0.25 mg
06	**MIRAPEX®** Tablets (pramipexole dihydrochloride tablets)	1 mg
08	**MIRAPEX®** Tablets (pramipexole dihydrochloride tablets)	0.5 mg
10	**HALCION®** Tablets (triazolam tablets, USP) *See Product Identification Guide*	0.125 mg
12	**CORTEF®** Tablets (hydrocortisone tablets, USP)	5 mg
14	**HALOTESTIN®** Tablets (fluoxymesterone tablets, USP) *See Product Identification Guide*	2 mg
15	**CORTISONE ACETATE** Tablets, USP	5 mg
17	**HALCION®** Tablets (triazolam tablets, USP) *See Product Identification Guide*	0.25 mg

Code #	Product	Strength
18	**DIDREX®** Tablets (benzphetamine hydrochloride tablets) *See Product Identification Guide*	50 mg
19	**HALOTESTIN®** Tablets (fluoxymesterone tablets, USP) *See Product Identification Guide*	5 mg
23	**CORTISONE ACETATE** Tablets, USP *See Product Identification Guide*	10 mg
29	**XANAX®** Tablets (alprazolam tablets, USP) *See Product Identification Guide*	0.25 mg
31	**CORTEF®** Tablets (hydrocortisone tablets, USP)	10 mg
32	**DELTASONE®** Tablets (prednisone tablets, USP) *See Product Identification Guide*	2.5 mg
32	**EMCYT** Capsules (estramustine phosphate sodium)	140 mg
34	**CORTISONE ACETATE** Tablets, USP	25 mg
36	**HALOTESTIN®** Tablets (fluoxymesterone tablets, USP) *See Product Identification Guide*	10 mg
37	**MIRAPEX®** Tablets (pramipexole dihydrochloride tablets) *See Product Identification Guide*	1.5 mg
41	**DETROL®** Tablets (tolterodine tartrate tablets) *See Product Identification Guide*	2 mg
44	**CORTEF®** Tablets (hydrocortisone tablets, USP)	20 mg
45	**DELTASONE®** Tablets (prednisone tablets, USP) *See Product Identification Guide*	5 mg
49	**MEDROL®** Tablets (methylprednisolone tablets, USP)	2 mg
50	**PROVERA®** Tablets (medroxyprogesterone acetate tablets, USP) *See Product Identification Guide*	10 mg
55	**XANAX®** Tablets (alprazolam tablets, USP) *See Product Identification Guide*	0.5 mg
61	**RESCRIPTOR®** Tablets (delavirdine mesylate tablets) *See Product Identification Guide*	100 mg
64	**PROVERA®** Tablets (medroxyprogesterone acetate tablets, USP) *See Product Identification Guide*	2.5 mg
90	**XANAX®** Tablets (alprazolam tablets, USP) *See Product Identification Guide*	1 mg
94	**XANAX®** Tablets (alprazolam tablets, USP) *See Product Identification Guide*	2 mg
100	**ORINASE®** Tablets (tolbutamide tablets, USP)	500 mg
101	**ALBAMYCIN®** Capsules (novobiocin sodium capsules)	250 mg
101	**AZULFIDINE** Tablets (sulfasalazine)	500 mg
102	**AZULFIDINE EN-tabs** (sulfasalazine delayed release)	500 mg
105	**DIPENTUM** Capsules (olsalazine sodium)	250 mg
121	**LONITEN®** Tablets (minoxidil tablets, USP) *See Product Identification Guide*	2.5 mg
131	**MICRONASE®** Tablets (glyburide tablets) *See Product Identification Guide*	1.25 mg
137	**LONITEN®** Tablets (minoxidil tablets, USP) *See Product Identification Guide*	10 mg
141	**MICRONASE®** Tablets (glyburide tablets) *See Product Identification Guide*	2.5 mg
165	**DELTASONE®** Tablets (prednisone tablets, USP) *See Product Identification Guide*	20 mg
171	**MICRONASE®** Tablets (glyburide tablets) *See Product Identification Guide*	5 mg
193	**DELTASONE®** Tablets (prednisone tablets, USP) *See Product Identification Guide*	10 mg
225	**CLEOCIN HCl®** Capsules (clindamycin hydrochloride capsules, USP) *See Product Identification Guide*	150 mg
286	**PROVERA®** Tablets (medroxyprogesterone acetate tablets, USP) *See Product Information Guide*	5 mg

Code #	Product	Strength
301	**MYCOBUTIN** (rifabutin capsules)	150 mg
331	**CLEOCIN HCl®** Capsules (clindamycin hydrochloride capsules, USP) *See Product Identification Guide*	75 mg
341	**GLYNASE®** PresTab® Tablets (micronized glyburide tablets) *See Product Identification Guide*	1.5 mg
352	**GLYNASE®** PresTab® Tablets (micronized glyburide tablets) *See Product Identification Guide*	3 mg
388	**DELTASONE®** Tablets (prednisone tablets, USP) *See Product Identification Guide*	50 mg
395	**CLEOCIN HCl®** Capsules (clindamycin hydrochloride capsules, USP) *See Product Identification Guide*	300 mg
450	**COLESTID®** Tablets (micronized colestipol hydrochloride)	1 g
500	**LINCOCIN®** Capsules (lincomycin hydrochloride capsules, USP)	500 mg
617	**VANTIN®** Tablets (cefpodoxime proxetil tablets)	100 mg
618	**VANTIN®** Tablets (cefpodoxime proxetil tablets)	200 mg
3449	**GLYNASE®** PresTab Tablets (micronized glyburide tablets)	6 mg
3772	**OGEN®** Tablets (estropipate tablets, USP)	0.75 mg
3773	**OGEN®** Tablets (estropipate tablets, USP)	1.5 mg
3774	**OGEN®** Tablets (estropipate tablets, USP)	3 mg

ADRIAMYCIN RDF® ℞
[adrēē′ah-mī-cĭn]
doxorubicin hydrochloride
for injection, USP

ADRIAMYCIN PFS® ℞
doxorubicin hydrochloride
injection, USP
FOR INTRAVENOUS USE ONLY

WARNING
1. Severe local tissue necrosis will occur if there is extravasation during administration (See DOSAGE AND ADMINISTRATION). Doxorubicin must not be given by the intramuscular or subcutaneous route.
2. Myocardial toxicity manifested in its most severe form by potentially fatal congestive heart failure may occur either during therapy or months to years after termination of therapy. The probability of developing impaired myocardial function based on a combined index of signs, symptoms and decline in left ventricular ejection fraction (LVEF) is estimated to be 1 to 2% at a total cumulative dose of 300 mg/m^2 of doxorubicin, 3 to 5% at a dose of 400 mg/m^2, 5 to 8% at 450 mg/m^2 and 6 to 20% at 500 mg/m^2.* The risk of developing CHF increases rapidly with increasing total cumulative doses of doxorubicin in excess of 450 mg/m^2. This toxicity may occur at lower cumulative doses in patients with prior mediastinal irradiation or on concurrent cyclophosphamide therapy or with preexisting heart disease.
3. Dosage should be reduced in patients with impaired hepatic function.
4. Severe myelosuppression may occur.
5. Doxorubicin should be administered only under the supervision of a physician who is experienced in the use of cancer chemotherapeutic agents.

---

* Data on file at Pharmacia & Upjohn

DESCRIPTION
Doxorubicin is a cytotoxic anthracycline antibiotic isolated from cultures of *Streptomyces peucetius* var. *caesius*.
Doxorubicin consists of a naphthacenequinone nucleus linked through a glycosidic bond at ring atom 7 to an amino sugar, daunosamine.

Continued on next page

Information on these Pharmacia & Upjohn products is based on labeling in effect June 1, 1998. Further information concerning these and other Pharmacia & Upjohn products may be obtained by direct inquiry to Medical Information, Pharmacia & Upjohn, Kalamazoo, MI 49001.

Adriamycin—Cont.

Chemically, doxorubicin hydrochloride is:
5,12-Naphthacenedione, 10-[(3-amino-2,3,6-trideoxy-αL-*lyxo*-hexopyranosyl)oxy]-7,8,9,10-tetrahydro-6,8,11-trihydroxy-8-(hydroxylacetyl)-1-methoxy-, hydrochloride (8*S*-*cis*)-. The structural formula is as follows:

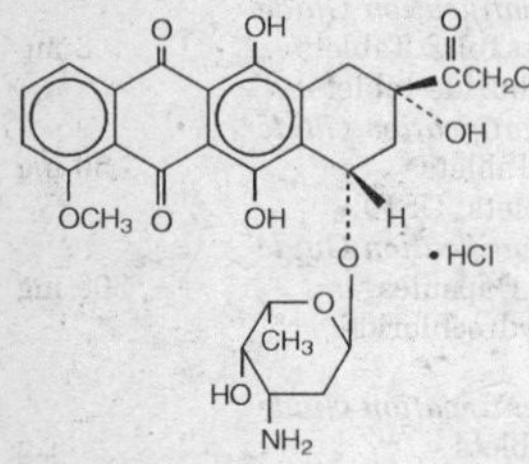

$C_{27}H_{29}NO_{11} \cdot HCl$
M.W.—579.99

Doxorubicin binds to nucleic acids, presumably by specific intercalation of the planar anthracycline nucleus with the DNA double helix. The anthracycline ring is lipophilic, but the saturated end of the ring system contains abundant hydroxyl groups adjacent to the amino sugar, producing a hydrophilic center. The molecule is amphoteric, containing acidic functions in the ring phenolic groups and a basic function in the sugar amino group. It binds to cell membranes as well as plasma proteins.

ADRIAMYCIN RDF® (doxorubicin hydrochloride for injection, USP) a sterile red-orange lyophilized powder for intravenous use only, is available in 10, 20 and 50 mg single dose vials and a 150 mg multidose vial.

Each 10 mg single dose vial contains 10 mg of doxorubicin HCl, USP, 50 mg of lactose, NF (hydrous) and 1 mg of methylparaben, NF (added to enhance dissolution) as a sterile red-orange lyophilized powder.

Each 20 mg single dose vial contains 20 mg of doxorubicin HCl, USP, 100 mg of lactose, NF (hydrous) and 2 mg of methylparaben, NF (added to enhance dissolution) as a sterile red-orange lyophilized powder.

Each 50 mg single dose vial contains 50 mg of doxorubicin HCl, USP, 250 mg of lactose, NF (hydrous) and 5 mg of methylparaben, NF (added to enhance dissolution) as a sterile red-orange lyophilized powder.

Each 150 mg multidose vial contains 150 mg of doxorubicin HCl, USP, 750 mg of lactose, NF (hydrous) and 15 mg of methylparaben, NF (added to enhance dissolution) as a sterile red-orange lyophilized powder.

ADRIAMYCIN PFS® (doxorubicin hydrochloride injection, USP) is a sterile parenteral, isotonic solution for intravenous use only, containing no preservative, available in 5 mL (10 mg), 10 mL (20 mg), 25 mL (50 mg), and 37.5 mL (75 mg) single dose vials and a 100 mL (200 mg) multidose vial.

Each mL contains doxorubicin HCl 2 mg, USP and the following inactive ingredients: sodium chloride 0.9% and water for injection q.s. Hydrochloric acid is used to adjust the pH to a target pH of 3.0.

CLINICAL PHARMACOLOGY

The cytotoxic effect of doxorubicin on malignant cells and its toxic effects on various organs are thought to be related to nucleotide base intercalation and cell membrane lipid binding activities of doxorubicin. Intercalation inhibits nucleotide replication and action of DNA and RNA polymerases. The interaction of doxorubicin with topoisomerase II to form DNA-cleavable complexes appears to be an important mechanism of doxorubicin cytocidal activity. Doxorubicin cellular membrane binding may effect a variety of cellular functions. Enzymatic electron reduction of doxorubicin by a variety of oxidases, reductases and dehydrogenases generate highly reactive species including the hydroxyl free radical OH•. Free radical formation has been implicated in doxorubicin cardiotoxicity by means of Cu (II) and Fe (III) reduction at the cellular level.

Animal studies have shown activity in a spectrum of experimental tumors, immunosuppression, carcinogenic properties in rodents, induction of a variety of toxic effects, including delayed and progressive cardiac toxicity, myelosuppression in all species and atrophy to testes in rats and dogs.

Pharmacokinetic studies, determined in patients with various types of tumors undergoing either single or multi-agent therapy have shown that doxorubicin follows a multiphasic disposition after intravenous injection. The initial distributive half-life of approximately 5.0 minutes suggests rapid tissue uptake of doxorubicin, while its slow elimination from tissues is reflected by a terminal half-life of 20 to 48 hours. Steady-state distribution volumes exceed 20 to 30 L/kg and are indicative of extensive drug uptake into tissues. Plasma clearance is in the range of 8 to 20 mL/min/kg and is predominately by metabolism and biliary excretion. Approximately 40% of the dose appears in the bile in 5 days, while only 5 to 12% of the drug and its metabolites appear in the urine during the same time period. Binding of doxorubicin and its major metabolite, doxorubicinol to plasma proteins is about 74 to 76% and is independent of plasma concentration of doxorubicin up to 2 μM. Enzymatic reduction at the 7 position and cleavage of the daunosamine sugar yields aglycones which are accompanied by free radical formation, the local production of which may contribute to the cardiotoxic activity of doxorubicin. Disposition of doxorubicinol (DOX-OL) in patients is formation rate limited. The terminal half-life of DOX-OL is similar to doxorubicin. The relative exposure of DOX-OL, compared to doxorubicin ranges between 0.4 to 0.6. In urine, <3% of the dose was recovered as DOX-OL over 7 days. The literature contains no information regarding gender related differences in the pharmacokinetics of doxorubicin and doxorubicinol.

In four patients, dose-independent pharmacokinetics have been shown for doxorubicin in the dose range of 30 to 70 mg/m². Systemic clearance of doxorubicin is significantly reduced in obese women with ideal body weight greater than 130%. There was a significant reduction in clearance without any change in volume of distribution in obese patients when compared with normal patients with less than 115% ideal body weight. The clearance of doxorubicin and doxorubicinol was also reduced in patients with impaired hepatic function. Doxorubicin was excreted in the milk of one lactating patient, with peak milk concentration at 24 hours after treatment being approximately 4.4 -fold greater than the corresponding plasma concentration. Doxorubicin was detectable in the milk up to 72 hours after therapy with 70 mg/m² of doxorubicin given as a 15 minute intravenous infusion and 100 mg/m² of cisplatin as a 26 hour intravenous infusion. The peak concentration of doxorubicinol in milk at 24 hours was 0.2 μM and AUC up to 24 hours was 16.5 μM.hr while the AUC for doxorubicin was 9.9 μM.hr. Doxorubicin does not cross the blood brain barrier.

INDICATIONS AND USAGE

ADRIAMYCIN PFS and ADRIAMYCIN RDF have been used successfully to produce regression in disseminated neoplastic conditions such as acute lymphoblastic leukemia, acute myeloblastic leukemia, Wilms' tumor, neuroblastoma, soft tissue and bone sarcomas, breast carcinoma, ovarian carcinoma, transitional cell bladder carcinoma, thyroid carcinoma, gastric carcinoma, Hodgkin's disease, malignant lymphoma and bronchogenic carcinoma in which the small cell histologic type is the most responsive compared to other cell types.

CONTRAINDICATIONS

Doxorubicin therapy should not be started in patients who have marked myelosuppression induced by previous treatment with other antitumor agents or by radiotherapy. Doxorubicin treatment is contraindicated in patients who received previous treatment with complete cumulative doses of doxorubicin, daunorubicin, idarubicin, and/or other anthracyclines and anthracenes.

WARNINGS

Special attention must be given to the cardiotoxicity induced by doxorubicin. Irreversible myocardial toxicity, manifested in its most severe form by life-threatening and potentially fatal congestive heart failure, may occur either during therapy or months to years after termination of therapy. The probability of developing impaired myocardial function, based on a combined index of signs, symptoms and decline in left ventricular ejection fraction (LVEF) is estimated to be 1 to 2% at a total cumulative dose of 300 mg/m² of doxorubicin, 3 to 5% at a dose of 400 mg/m², 5 to 8% at a dose of 450 mg/m² and 6 to 20% at a dose of 500 mg/m² given in a schedule of a bolus injection once every 3 weeks (data on file at Pharmacia & Upjohn). In a retrospective review by Von Hoff et al, the probability of developing congestive heart failure was reported to be 5/168 (3%) at a cumulative dose of 430 mg/m² of doxorubicin, 8/110 (7%) at 575 mg/m² and 3/14 (21%) at 728 mg/m². The cumulative incidence of CHF was 2.2%. In a prospective study of doxorubicin in combination with cyclophosphamide, fluorouracil and/or vincristine in patients with breast cancer or small cell lung cancer, the cumulative incidence of congestive heart failure was 5 to 6%. The probability of CHF at various cumulative doses of doxorubicin was 1.5% at 300 mg/m², 4.9% at 400 mg/m², 7.7% at 450 mg/m² and 20.5% at 500 mg/m².

Cardiotoxicity may occur at lower doses in patients with prior mediastinal irradiation, concurrent cyclophosphamide therapy and advanced age. Data also suggest that pre-existing heart disease is a co-factor for increased risk of doxorubicin cardiotoxicity. In such cases, cardiac toxicity may occur at doses lower than the respective recommended cumulative dose of doxorubicin. Studies have suggested that concomitant administration of doxorubicin and calcium channel entry blockers may increase the risk of doxorubicin cardiotoxicity. The total dose of doxorubicin administered to the individual patient should also take into account previous or concomitant therapy with related compounds such as daunorubicin, idarubicin and mitoxantrone. Cardiomyopathy and/or congestive heart failure may be encountered several months or years after discontinuation of doxorubicin therapy.

The risk of congestive heart failure and other acute manifestations of doxorubicin cardiotoxicity in children may be as much or lower than in adults. Children appear to be at particular risk for developing delayed cardiac toxicity in that doxorubicin induced cardiomyopathy impairs myocardial growth as children mature, subsequently leading to possible development of congestive heart failure during early adulthood. As many as 40% of children may have subclinical cardiac dysfunction and 5 to 10% of children may develop congestive heart failure on long term follow-up. This late cardiac toxicity may be related to the dose of doxorubicin. The longer the length of follow-up the greater the increase in the detection rate.

Treatment of doxorubicin induced congestive heart failure includes the use of digitalis, diuretics, after load reducers such as angiotensin I converting enzyme (ACE) inhibitors, low salt diet, and bed rest. Such intervention may relieve symptoms and improve the functional status of the patient.

Monitoring Cardiac Function

In adult patients severe cardiac toxicity may occur precipitously without antecedent ECG changes. Cardiomyopathy induced by anthracyclines is usually associated with very characteristic histopathologic changes on an endomyocardial biopsy (EM biopsy), and a decrease of left ventricular ejection fraction (LVEF), as measured by multi-gated radionuclide angiography (MUGA scans) and/or echocardiogram (ECHO), from pretreatment baseline values. However, it has not been demonstrated that monitoring of the ejection fraction will predict when individual patients are approaching their maximally tolerated cumulative dose of doxorubicin. Cardiac function should be carefully monitored during treatment to minimize the risk of cardiac toxicity. A baseline cardiac evaluation with an ECG, LVEF, and/or an echocardiogram (ECHO) is recommended especially in patients with risk factors for increased cardiac toxicity (pre-existing heart disease, mediastinal irradiation, or concurrent cyclophosphamide therapy). Subsequent evaluations should be obtained at a cumulative dose of doxorubicin of at least 400 mg/m² and periodically thereafter during the course of therapy. Children are at increased risk for developing delayed cardiotoxicity following doxorubicin administration and therefore a follow-up cardiac evaluation is recommended periodically to monitor for this delayed cardiotoxicity.

In adults, a 10% decline in LVEF to below the lower limit of normal or an absolute LVEF of 45%, or a 20% decline in LVEF at any level is indicative of deterioration in cardiac function. In children, deterioration in cardiac function during or after the completion of therapy with doxorubicin is indicated by a drop in fractional shortening (FS) by an absolute value of ≥10 percentile units or below 29%, and a decline in LVEF of 10 percentile units or an LVEF below 55%. In general, if test results indicate deterioration in cardiac function associated with doxorubicin, the benefit of continued therapy should be carefully evaluated against the risk of producing irreversible cardiac damage.

Acute life-threatening arrhythmias have been reported to occur during or within a few hours after doxorubicin administration.

There is a high incidence of bone marrow depression, primarily of leukocytes, requiring careful hematologic monitoring. With the recommended dose schedule, leukopenia is usually transient, reaching its nadir 10 to 14 days after treatment with recovery usually occurring by the 21st day. White blood counts as low as 1000/mm3 are to be expected during treatment with appropriate doses of doxorubicin. Red blood cell and platelet levels should also be monitored since they may also be depressed. Hematologic toxicity may require dose reduction or suspension or delay of doxorubicin therapy. Persistent severe myelosuppression may result in superinfection or hemorrhage.

Doxorubicin may potentiate the toxicity of other anticancer therapies. Exacerbation of cyclophosphamide induced hemorrhagic cystitis and enhancement of the hepatotoxicity of 6-mercaptopurine have been reported. Radiation induced toxicity to the myocardium, mucosae, skin and liver have been reported to be increased by the administration of doxorubicin.

Since metabolism and excretion of doxorubicin occurs predominantly by the hepatobiliary route, toxicity to recommended doses of doxorubicin can be enhanced by hepatic impairment; therefore, prior to the individual dosing, evaluation of hepatic function is recommended using conventional laboratory tests such as SGOT, SGPT, alkaline phosphatase and bilirubin (See DOSAGE AND ADMINISTRATION).

Necrotizing colitis manifested by typhlitis (cecal inflammation), bloody stools and severe and sometimes fatal infections have been associated with a combination of doxorubicin given by i.v. push daily for 3 days and cytarabine given by continuous infusion daily for 7 or more days.

On intravenous administration of doxorubicin, extravasation may occur with or without an accompanying stinging or burning sensation, even if blood returns well on aspiration of the infusion needle (See DOSAGE AND ADMINISTRATION). If any signs or symptoms of extravasation have occurred, the injection or infusion should be immediately terminated and restarted in another vein.

Pregnancy Category D—Safe use of doxorubicin in pregnancy has not been established. Doxorubicin is embryotoxic and teratogenic in rats and embryotoxic and abortifacient in rabbits. There are no adequate and well-controlled studies in pregnant women. If doxorubicin is to be used during pregnancy, or if the patient becomes pregnant during therapy, the patient should be apprised of the potential hazard to the fetus. Women of childbearing age should be advised to avoid becoming pregnant.

PRECAUTIONS
General
Doxorubicin is not an anti-microbial agent.
Information for Patients
ADRIAMYCIN PFS and ADRIAMYCIN RDF impart a red coloration to the urine for 1 to 2 days after administration, and patients should be advised to expect this during active therapy.
Drug Interactions
Literature contain the following drug interactions with doxorubicin in humans: cyclosporine (Sandimmune) may induce coma and/or seizures, phenobarbital increases the elimination of doxorubicin, phenytoin levels may be decreased by doxorubicin, streptozocin (Zanosar) may inhibit the hepatic metabolism, and administration of live vaccines to immunosuppressed patients, including those undergoing cytotoxic chemotherapy, may be hazardous. Information on other potential drug interactions may be found in the literature.
Laboratory Tests
Initial treatment with doxorubicin requires observation of the patient and periodic monitoring of complete blood counts, hepatic function tests, and radionuclide left ventricular ejection fraction (See WARNINGS section).
Like other cytotoxic drugs, doxorubicin may induce "tumor lysis syndrome" and hyperuricemia in patients with rapidly growing tumors. Appropriate supportive and pharmacologic measures may prevent or alleviate this complication.
Carcinogenesis, Mutagenesis, Impairment of Fertility
Formal long-term carcinogenicity studies have not been conducted with doxorubicin. Doxorubicin and related compounds have been shown to have mutagenic and carcinogenic properties when tested in experimental models (including bacterial systems, mammalian cells in culture, and female Sprague-Dawley rats).
The possible adverse effect on fertility in males and females in humans or experimental animals have not been adequately evaluated. Testicular atrophy was observed in rats and dogs.
A variant of chemotherapy-related acute non-lymphocytic leukemia has been reported to occur infrequently a few years after multiple drug treatment of some neoplasms, which sometimes included doxorubicin. The exact role of doxorubicin has not been elucidated.
Pregnancy Category D
(See WARNINGS section.)
Nursing Mothers:
Because of the potential for serious adverse reactions in nursing infants from doxorubicin, mothers should be advised to discontinue nursing during doxorubicin therapy.

ADVERSE REACTIONS
Dose limiting toxicities of therapy are myelosuppression and cardiotoxicity. Other reactions reported are:
Cardiotoxicity—(See WARNINGS section.)
Cutaneous—Reversible complete alopecia occurs in most cases. Hyperpigmentation of nailbeds and dermal crease, primarily in children, and onycholysis have been reported in a few cases. Recall of skin reaction due to prior radiotherapy has occurred with doxorubicin administration.
Gastrointestinal—Acute nausea and vomiting occurs frequently and may be severe. This may be alleviated by antiemetic therapy. Mucositis (stomatitis and esophagitis) may occur 5 to 10 days after administration. The effect may be severe leading to ulceration and represents a site of origin for severe infections. The dosage regimen consisting of administration of doxorubicin on three successive days results in greater incidence and severity of mucositis. Ulceration and necrosis of the colon, especially the cecum, may occur leading to bleeding or severe infections which can be fatal. This reaction has been reported in patients with acute non-lymphocytic leukemia treated with a 3-day course of doxorubicin combined with cytarabine. Anorexia and diarrhea have been occasionally reported.
Vascular—Phlebosclerosis has been reported especially when small veins are used or a single vein is used for repeated administration. Facial flushing may occur if the injection is given too rapidly.
Local—Severe cellulitis, vesication and tissue necrosis will occur if extravasation of doxorubicin occurs during administration. Erythematous streaking along the vein proximal to the site of injection had been reported (See DOSAGE AND ADMINISTRATION).
Hematologic—The occurrence of secondary acute myeloid leukemia with or without a preleukemic phase has been reported rarely in patients concurrently treated with doxorubicin in association with DNA-damaging antineoplastic agents. Such cases could have a short (1–3 years) latency period.
Hypersensitivity—Fever, chills and urticaria have been reported occasionally. Anaphylaxis may occur. A case of apparent cross sensitivity to lincomycin has been reported.
Other—Conjunctivitis and lacrimation occur rarely.

OVERDOSAGE
Acute overdosage with doxorubicin enhances the toxic effect of mucositis, leukopenia and thrombocytopenia. Treatment of acute overdosage consists of treatment of the severely myelosuppressed patient with hospitalization, antimicrobials, platelet transfusions and symptomatic treatment of mucositis. Use of hemopoietic growth factor (G-CSF, GM-CSF) may be considered.
The 150 mg ADRIAMYCIN RDF and the 100 mL (2 mg/mL) ADRIAMYCIN PFS vials are packaged as multiple dose vials and caution should be exercised to prevent inadvertent overdosage.
Cumulative dosage with doxorubicin increases the risk of cardiomyopathy and resultant congestive heart failure (See WARNINGS Section). Treatment consists of vigorous management of congestive heart failure with digitalis preparations, diuretics, and after-load reducers such as ACE inhibitors.

DOSAGE AND ADMINISTRATION
Care in the administration of ADRIAMYCIN PFS and ADRIAMYCIN RDF will reduce the chance of perivenous infiltration (See WARNINGS). It may also decrease the chance of local reactions such as urticaria and erythematous streaking. On intravenous administration of doxorubicin, extravasation may occur with or without an accompanying burning or stinging sensation, even if blood returns well on aspiration of the infusion needle. If any signs or symptoms of extravasation have occurred, the injection or infusion should be immediately terminated and restarted in another vein. If extravasation is suspected, intermittent application of ice to the site for 15 min. q.i.d. x 3 days may be useful. The benefit of local administration of drugs has not been clearly established. Because of the progressive nature of extravasation reactions, close observation and plastic surgery consultation is recommended. Blistering, ulceration and/or persistent pain are indications for wide excision surgery, followed by split-thickness skin grafting.[1]
The most commonly used dose schedule when used as a single agent is 60 to 75 mg/m^2 as a single intravenous injection administered at 21-day intervals. The lower dosage should be given to patients with inadequate marrow reserves due to old age, or prior therapy, or neoplastic marrow infiltration. ADRIAMYCIN PFS and ADRIAMYCIN RDF have been used concurrently with other approved chemotherapeutic agents. Evidence is available that in some types of neoplastic disease combination chemotherapy is superior to single agents. The benefits and risks of such therapy continue to be elucidated. When used in combination with other chemotherapy drugs, the most commonly used dosage of doxorubicin is 40 to 60 mg/m^2 given as a single intravenous injection every 21 to 28 days. Doxorubicin dosage must be reduced in case of hyperbilirubinemia as follows:

Plasma bilirubin concentration (mg/dL)	Dosage reduction (%)
1.2–3.0	50
3.1–5.0	75

Reconstitution Directions: ADRIAMYCIN RDF 10 mg, 20 mg, 50 mg, and 150 mg vials should be reconstituted with 5 mL, 10 mL, 25 mL, and 75 mL, respectively, of Sodium Chloride Injection, USP (0.9%), to give a final concentration of 2 mg/mL of doxorubicin hydrochloride. An appropriate volume of air should be withdrawn from the vial during reconstitution to avoid excessive pressure buildup. Bacteriostatic diluents are not recommended.
After adding the diluent, the vial should be shaken and the contents allowed to dissolve. The reconstituted solution is stable for 7 days at room temperature and under normal room light (100 foot-candles) and 15 days under refrigeration (2° to 8°C). It should be protected from exposure to sunlight. Discard any of the unused solution from the 10 mg, 20 mg, and 50 mg single dose vials. Unused solutions of the multiple dose vial remaining beyond the recommended storage times should be discarded.
It is recommended that ADRIAMYCIN PFS and ADRIAMYCIN RDF be slowly administered into the tubing of a freely running intravenous infusion of Sodium Chloride Injection, USP, or 5% Dextrose Injection, USP. The tubing should be attached to a Butterfly® needle inserted preferably into a large vein. If possible, avoid veins over joints or in extremities with compromised venous or lymphatic drainage. The rate of administration is dependent on the size of the vein, and the dosage. However, the dose should be administered in not less than 3 to 5 minutes. Local erythematous streaking along the vein as well as facial flushing may be indicative of too rapid an administration. A burning or stinging sensation may be indicative of perivenous infiltration and the infusion should be immediately terminated and restarted in another vein. Perivenous infiltration may occur painlessly.
Doxorubicin should not be mixed with heparin or fluorouracil since it has been reported that these drugs are incompatible to the extent that a precipitate may form. Until specific compatibility data are available, it is not recommended that doxorubicin be mixed with other drugs.
Parenteral drug products should be inspected visually for particulate matter and discoloration prior to administration, whenever solution and container permit.
Handling and Disposal: Skin reactions associated with doxorubicin have been reported. Skin accidentally exposed to doxorubicin should be rinsed copiously with soap and warm water, and if the eyes are involved, standard irrigation techniques should be used immediately. The use of goggles, gloves, and protective gowns is recommended during preparation and administration of the drug.
Procedures for proper handling and disposal of anti-cancer drugs should be considered. Several guidelines on this subject have been published.[2-8] There is no general agreement that all the procedures recommended in the guidelines are necessary or appropriate.

HOW SUPPLIED
ADRIAMYCIN RDF® Powder for Injection (doxorubicin hydrochloride for injection, USP) is available as follows:

NDC 0013-1086-91	10 mg single dose vial, 10 vial packs
NDC 0013-1096-91	20 mg single dose vial, 10 vial packs
NDC 0013-1106-79	50 mg single dose vial, single packs

Store at controlled room temperature, 15° to 30°C (59° to 86°F). Protect from light.
Retain in carton until time of use. Contains no preservative. Discard unused portion.
MULTIDOSE VIAL:
NDC 0013-1116-83   150 mg multidose vial, single packs
Store at controlled room temperature, 15° to 30°C (59° to 86°F). Protect from light.
Retain in carton until time of use.
RECONSTITUTED SOLUTION STABILITY:
After adding the diluent, the vial should be shaken and the contents allowed to dissolve. The reconstituted solution is stable for 7 days at room temperature and under normal room light (100 foot-candles) and 15 days under refrigeration (2° to 8°C). It should be protected from exposure to sunlight. Discard any unused solution from the 10 mg, 20 mg and 50 mg single dose vials. Unused solutions of the multiple dose vial remaining beyond the recommended storage times should be discarded.
MANUFACTURER:
Pharmacia & Upjohn S.p.A.
Milan, Italy

HOW SUPPLIED
ADRIAMYCIN PFS® Injection (doxorubicin hydrochloride injection, USP)

SINGLE DOSE VIALS:
Sterile single use only, contains no preservative.

NDC 0013-1136-91	10 mg vial, 2 mg/mL, 5 mL, 10 vial packs
NDC 0013-1146-91	20 mg vial, 2 mg/mL, 10 mL, 10 vial packs
NDC 0013-1156-79	50 mg vial, 2 mg/mL, 25 mL, single vial packs
NDC 0013-1176-87	75 mg vial, 2 mg/mL, 37.5 mL, single vial packs

Store under refrigeration, 2° to 8°C (36° to 46°F). Protect from light. Retain in carton until time of use.
Discard unused portion.

MULTIDOSE VIAL:
Sterile multidose vial, contains no preservative.
NDC 0013-1166-83   200 mg, 2 mg/mL, 100 mL, multidose vial, single vial packs

Store under refrigeration, 2° to 8°C (36° to 46°F). Protect from light. Retain in carton until contents are used.

Continued on next page

Information on these Pharmacia & Upjohn products is based on labeling in effect June 1, 1998. Further information concerning these and other Pharmacia & Upjohn products may be obtained by direct inquiry to Medical Information, Pharmacia & Upjohn, Kalamazoo, MI 49001.

Adriamycin—Cont.

MANUFACTURERS:
Pharmacia & Upjohn S.p.A.
Milan, Italy
SP Pharmaceuticals LLC
Albuquerque, NM 87109, USA
Rx only

REFERENCES
1. Rudolph R., Larson DL: Etiology and Treatment of Chemotherapeutic Agent Extravasation Injuries: A Review J. Clin Oncol 5:1116-1126, 1987.
2. Recommendations for the Safe Handling of Parenteral Antineoplastic Drugs. NIH Publication No. 83-2621. For sale by the Superintendent of Documents, US Government Printing Office, Washington, DC 20402.
3. AMA Council Report, Guidelines for Handling Parenteral Antineoplastics, JAMA. 1985; 253 (11): 1590-1592.
4. National Study Commission on Cytotoxic Exposure-Recommendations for Handling Cytotoxic Agents. Available from Louis P. Jeffrey, Sc.D., Chairman, National Study Commission on Cytotoxic Exposure, Massachusetts College of Pharmacy and Allied Health Sciences, 179 Longwood Avenue, Boston, Massachusetts 02115.
5. Clinical Oncological Society of Australia. Guidelines and Recommendations for Safe Handling of Antineoplastic Agents. Med J Australia. 1983; 1:426-428.
6. Jones RB, et al: Safe Handling of Chemotherapeutic Agents: A Report from the Mount Sinai Medical Center. CA - A Cancer Journal for Clinicians. 1983; (Sept/Oct) 258-263.
7. American Society of Hospital Pharmacists Technical Assistance Bulletin on Handling Cytotoxic and Hazardous Drugs. Am J Hosp Pharm. 1990; 47:1033-1049.
8. OSHA Work-Practice Guidelines for Personnel Dealing with Cytotoxic (Antineoplastic) Drugs. Am J Hosp Pharm. 1986; 43:1193-1204.

DISTRIBUTED BY:
Pharmacia & Upjohn Company
Kalamazoo, MI 49001, USA

817 336 000   March 1998

AZULFIDINE EN-tabs®
[azul ′ fidine]
sulfasalazine delayed release tablets, USP
Enteric-coated Tablets

DESCRIPTION
AZULFIDINE EN-tabs Tablets contain sulfasalazine, formulated in a delayed release tablet (enteric-coated), 500 mg, for oral administration.

AZULFIDINE EN-tabs Tablets are film coated with cellulose acetate phthalate to retard disintegration of the tablet in the stomach and reduce potential irritation of the gastric mucosa.

Therapeutic Classification: Anti-inflammatory agent and/or immunomodulatory agent.

Chemical Designation: 5-([p-(2-pyridylsulfamoyl)phenyl]azo) salicylic acid.

Chemical Structure:

Molecular Formula: $C_{18}H_{14}N_4O_5S$

HOW SUPPLIED
AZULFIDINE EN-tabs Tablets, 500 mg, are elliptical, gold-colored, film enteric-coated tablets, monogrammed "102" on one side and "KPh" on the other. They are available in the following package sizes:

Bottles of 100	NDC 0013–0102–01
Bottles of 300	NDC 0013–0102–20

Storage: Store at 25°C (77°F); excursions permitted to 15-30°C (59-86°F) [see USP controlled Room Temperature].
Rx only

Mfd for: Pharmacia & Upjohn Company
Kalamazoo, MI 49001, USA

By: Pharmacia & Upjohn AB
Stockholm, Sweden

801862101
Revised: May 1998
Shown in Product Identification Guide, page 331

CAMPTOSAR®
Injection   ℞
Irinotecan hydrochloride injection
For Intravenous Use Only

WARNINGS
1. CAMPTOSAR Injection should be administered only under the supervision of a physician who is experienced in the use of cancer chemotherapeutic agents. Appropriate management of complications is possible only when adequate diagnostic and treatment facilities are readily available.
2. CAMPTOSAR can induce both early and late forms of diarrhea that appear to be mediated by different mechanisms. Both forms of diarrhea may be severe. Early diarrhea (occurring during or within 24 hours of administration of CAMPTOSAR) may be preceded by complaints of diaphoresis and abdominal cramping and may be ameliorated by atropine. Late diarrhea (occurring more than 24 hours after administration of CAMPTOSAR) can be prolonged, may lead to dehydration and electrolyte imbalance, and can be life-threatening. Late diarrhea should be treated promptly with loperamide; patients with severe diarrhea should be carefully monitored and given fluid and electrolyte replacement if they become dehydrated (see WARNINGS section). Administration of CAMPTOSAR should be interrupted if severe diarrhea occurs.
3. Severe myelosuppression may occur (see WARNINGS section).

DESCRIPTION
CAMPTOSAR Injection (irinotecan hydrochloride injection) is an antineoplastic agent of the topoisomerase I inhibitor class. Irinotecan hydrochloride was clinically investigated as CPT-11.

CAMPTOSAR is supplied as a sterile, pale yellow, clear, aqueous solution. It is available in two single-dose sizes: 2 mL-fill vials contain 40 mg irinotecan hydrochloride and 5 mL-fill vials contain 100 mg irinotecan hydrochloride. Each milliliter of solution contains 20 mg of irinotecan hydrochloride (on the basis of the trihydrate salt), 45 mg of sorbitol NF powder, and 0.9 mg of lactic acid, USP. The pH of the solution is adjusted to 3.5 (range, 3.0 to 3.8) with sodium hydroxide or hydrochloric acid. CAMPTOSAR is intended for dilution with 5% Dextrose Injection, USP (D5W), or 0.9% Sodium Chloride Injection, USP, prior to intravenous infusion. The preferred diluent is 5% Dextrose Injection, USP.

Irinotecan hydrochloride is a semisynthetic derivative of camptothecin, an alkaloid extract from plants such as *Camptotheca acuminata*. The chemical name is (4S)-4,11-diethyl-4-hydroxy-9-[(4-piperidinopiperidino)carbonyloxy]-1H-pyrano[3′,4′:6,7] indolizino[1,2-b]quinoline-3,14(4H,12H)-dione hydrochloride. Its structural formula is as follows:

Irinotecan Hydrochloride

Irinotecan hydrochloride is a pale yellow to yellow crystalline powder, with the empirical formula $C_{33}H_{38}N_4O_6 \cdot HCl \cdot 3H_2O$ and a molecular weight of 677.19. It is slightly soluble in water and organic solvents.

CLINICAL PHARMACOLOGY
Irinotecan is a derivative of camptothecin. Camptothecins interact specifically with the enzyme topoisomerase I which relieves torsional strain in DNA by inducing reversible single-strand breaks. Irinotecan and its active metabolite SN-38 bind to the topoisomerase I - DNA complex and prevent religation of these single-strand breaks. Current re-

search suggests that the cytotoxicity of irinotecan is due to double-strand DNA damage produced during DNA synthesis when replication enzymes interact with the ternary complex formed by topoisomerase I, DNA, and either irinotecan or SN-38. Mammalian cells cannot efficiently repair these double-strand breaks.

Irinotecan serves as a water-soluble precursor of the lipophilic metabolite SN-38. SN-38 is formed from irinotecan by carboxylesterase-mediated cleavage of the carbamate bond between the camptothecin moiety and the dipiperidino side chain. SN-38 is approximately 1000 times as potent as irinotecan as an inhibitor of topoisomerase I purified from human and rodent tumor cell lines. In vitro cytotoxicity assays show that the potency of SN-38 relative to irinotecan varies from 2- to 2000-fold. However, the plasma area under the concentration versus time curve (AUC) values for SN-38 are 2% to 8% of irinotecan and SN-38 is 95% bound to plasma proteins compared to approximately 50% bound to plasma proteins for irinotecan (see Pharmacokinetics). The precise contribution of SN-38 to the activity of CAMPTOSAR is thus unknown. Both irinotecan and SN-38 exist in an active lactone form and an inactive hydroxy acid anion form. A pH-dependent equilibrium exists between the two forms such that an acid pH promotes the formation of the lactone, while a more basic pH favors the hydroxy acid anion form.

Administration of irinotecan has resulted in anti tumor activity in mice bearing cancers of rodent origin and in human carcinoma xenografts of various histological types.

Pharmacokinetics
After intravenous infusion of CAMPTOSAR in humans, irinotecan plasma concentrations decline in a multiexponential manner, with a mean terminal elimination half-life of about 6 hours. The mean terminal elimination half-life of the active metabolite SN-38 is about 10 hours. The half-lives of the lactone (active) forms of irinotecan and SN-38 are similar to those of total irinotecan and SN-38, as the lactone and hydroxy acid forms are in equilibrium.

Over the dose range of 50 to 350 mg/m², the AUC of irinotecan increases linearly with dose; the AUC of SN-38 increases less than proportionally with dose. Maximum concentrations of the active metabolite SN-38 are generally seen within 1 hour following the end of a 90-minute infusion of CAMPTOSAR.

Irinotecan exhibits moderate plasma protein binding (30% to 68% bound). SN-38 is highly bound to human plasma proteins (approximately 95% bound). The plasma protein to which irinotecan and SN-38 predominantly binds is albumin.

[See table below]

Metabolism and Excretion: The metabolic conversion of irinotecan to the active metabolite SN-38 is mediated by carboxylesterase enzymes and primarily occurs in the liver. SN-38 subsequently undergoes conjugation to form a glucuronide metabolite. SN-38 glucuronide had 1/50 to 1/100 the activity of SN-38 in cytotoxicity assays using two cell lines in vitro. The disposition of irinotecan has not been fully elucidated in humans. The urinary excretion of irinotecan is 11% to 20%; SN-38, <1%; and SN-38 glucuronide, 3%. The cumulative biliary and urinary excretion of irinotecan and its metabolites (SN-38 and SN-38 glucuronide) over a period of 48 hours following administration of CAMPTOSAR in two patients ranged from approximately 25% (100 mg/m²) to 50% (300 mg/m²).

Pharmacokinetics in Special Populations
Geriatric: The terminal half-life of irinotecan was 6.0 hours in patients who were 65 years or older and 5.5 hours in patients younger than 65 years. Dose-normalized AUC_{0-24} for SN-38 in patients who were at least 65 years of age was 11% higher than in patients younger than 65 years. No change in dosage and administration is recommended for geriatric patients.

Pediatric: The pharmacokinetics of irinotecan have not been studied in the pediatric population.

Gender: The pharmacokinetics of irinotecan do not appear to be influenced by gender.

Race: The influence of race on the pharmacokinetics of irinotecan has not been evaluated.

Hepatic Insufficiency: The influence of hepatic insufficiency on the pharmacokinetic characteristics of irinotecan and its

Summary of Mean (± Standard Deviation) Irinotecan and SN-38 Pharmacokinetic Parameters in Patients With Metastatic Carcinoma of the Colon and Rectum

Dose (mg/m²)	Irinotecan						SN-38		
	C_{max} (ng/mL)	AUC_{0-24} (ng·hr/mL)	$t_{1/2}$ (hr)	V_{area} (L/m²)	CL (L/hr/m²)		C_{max} (ng/mL)	AUC_{0-24} (ng·hr/mL)	$t_{1/2}$ (hr)
125 (N=64)	1,660± 797	10,200± 3,270	5.8± 0.7	110± 48.5	13.3± 6.01		26.3± 11.9	229± 108	10.4± 3.1

C_{max} - Maximum plasma concentration.
AUC_{0-24} - Area under the plasma concentration-time curve from time 0 to 24 hours after the end of the 90-minute infusion.
$t_{1/2}$ - Terminal elimination half-life.
V_{area} - Volume of distribution of terminal elimination phase.
CL - Total systemic clearance.

metabolites has not been formally studied. Among patients with known hepatic tumor involvement (a majority of patients), irinotecan and SN-38 AUC values were somewhat higher than values for patients without liver metastases. For patients having liver metastases without decreased hepatic function, no change in dosage and administration is recommended.

Renal Insufficiency: The influence of renal insufficiency on the pharmacokinetics of irinotecan has not been evaluated.

Drug-Drug Interactions

Possible pharmacokinetic interactions of CAMPTOSAR with other concomitantly administered medications have not been formally investigated.

CLINICAL STUDIES

In phase 1 studies of CAMPTOSAR Injection, the maximum-tolerated dose as a single agent in the treatment of patients with solid tumors was 120 to 150 mg/m² when administered once weekly for 4 weeks, followed by a 2-week rest period. The dose-limiting toxicities were diarrhea and neutropenia. In one study, use of granulocyte colony-stimulating factor (G-CSF) appeared to increase the tolerated dose from 120 to 145 mg/m².

Data from three open-label, phase 2, single-agent clinical studies, involving a total of 304 patients in 59 centers, support the use of CAMPTOSAR in the treatment of patients with metastatic cancer of the colon or rectum that has recurred or progressed following treatment with fluorouracil (5-FU)-based therapy. These studies were designed to evaluate tumor response rate and do not provide information on actual clinical benefit, such as effect on survival and disease-related symptoms. In each study, CAMPTOSAR was administered in repeated 6-week courses consisting of a 90-minute intravenous infusion once weekly for 4 weeks, followed by a 2-week rest period. Starting doses of CAMPTOSAR in these trials were 100, 125, or 150 mg/m², but the 150 mg/m² dose proved poorly tolerated (unacceptably high rates of grade 4 late diarrhea and febrile neutropenia). Study 1 enrolled 48 patients and was conducted under the auspices of a single investigator at several regional hospitals. Study 2 was a multicenter study conducted by the North Central Cancer Treatment Group. All 90 patients enrolled in Study 2 received a starting dose of 125 mg/m². Study 3 was a multicenter study that enrolled 166 patients from 30 institutions. The initial dose in Study 3 was 125 mg/m² but was reduced to 100 mg/m² because the toxicity seen at the 125 mg/m² dose was perceived to be greater than that seen in previous studies. All patients in these studies had metastatic colorectal cancer, and the majority had disease that recurred or progressed following a 5-FU-based regimen administered for metastatic disease.

The results of the individual studies are shown in the following table:

[See table above]

In the intent-to-treat analysis of the pooled data across all three studies, 193 of the 304 patients began therapy at the recommended starting dose of 125 mg/m². Among these 193 patients, 2 complete and 27 partial responses were observed, for an overall response rate of 15.0% (95% Confidence Interval [CI], 10.0% to 20.1%) at this starting dose. A considerably lower response rate was seen with a starting dose of 100 mg/m². The majority of responses were observed within the first two courses of therapy, and all but one of the responses were observed by the fourth course of therapy (one response was observed after the eighth course). The response duration (median) for patients beginning therapy at 125 mg/m² was 5.8 months (range, 2.6 to 15.1 months).

Response rates to CAMPTOSAR were similar in males and females and among patients older and younger than 65 years. Rates were also similar in patients with cancer of the colon or cancer of the rectum and in patients with single and multiple metastatic sites. Response rate was 18.5% in patients with a performance status of 0 and 7.6% in patients with a performance status of 1 or 2. Patients with a performance status of 3 or 4 have not been studied. Over half of the patients responding to CAMPTOSAR had not responded to prior 5-FU-based treatment given for metastatic disease. Patients who had received previous irradiation to the pelvis also responded to CAMPTOSAR at approximately the same rate as those who had not previously received irradiation.

INDICATIONS AND USAGE

CAMPTOSAR Injection is indicated for the treatment of patients with metastatic carcinoma of the colon or rectum whose disease has recurred or progressed following 5-FU-based therapy.

CONTRAINDICATIONS

CAMPTOSAR is contraindicated in patients with a known hypersensitivity to the drug.

WARNINGS

Diarrhea:

CAMPTOSAR Injection can induce both early and late forms of diarrhea that appear to be mediated by different mechanisms. Early diarrhea (occurring during or within 24 hours of administration of CAMPTOSAR) is cholinergic in nature. It can be severe but is usually transient. It may be

	Study			
	1	2	3	
Number of Patients	48	90	64	102
Dose (mg/m²/wk × 4)	125*	125	125	100
Male (%)	54	64	50	49
Age <65 yr (%)	54	54	64	54
Ethnic Origin (%)				
White	79.2	95.6	81.3	91.2
African American	12.5	4.4	10.9	4.9
Hispanic	8.3	0.0	7.8	2.0
Oriental/Asian	0.0	0.0	0.0	2.0
Performance Status 0 (%)	60	38	59	44
Performance Status 1 (%)	38	48	33	51
Performance Status 2 (%)	2	14	8	5
Prior 5-FU Therapy (%)				
For Metastatic Disease	81.3	65.5	73.4	67.7
≤6 months after Adjuvant	14.6	6.7	26.6	27.5
>6 months after Adjuvant	2.1	15.6	0.0	2.0
Classification Unknown	2.1	12.2	0.0	2.9
Primary Tumor (%)				
Colon	100	71	89	87
Rectum	0	29	11	8
Number of Courses of CAMPTOSAR (median)	3.5	3.0	3.0	3.0
Median Dose Intensity† (mg/m²/wk)	62	56	61	54
Objective Response Rate (%)‡ [95% CI]	20.8 [9.3, 32.3]	13.8 [6.3, 20.4]	14.1 [5.5, 22.6]	7.8 [2.6, 13.1]
Time to Response (median, months)	2.6	2.1	2.8	2.8
Response Duration (median, months)	6.4	5.9	5.6	6.2
Survival (median, months)	10.4	8.1	10.7	9.3

*Nine patients received 150 mg/m² as a starting dose; 2 (22.2%) responded to CAMPTOSAR.

†Total dose administered in a course ÷ 6 (number of weeks in a course).

‡There were 2/304 complete responses; the remainder were partial responses.

preceded by complaints of diaphoresis and abdominal cramping. Early diarrhea may be ameliorated by administration of atropine (see PRECAUTIONS, General, for dosing recommendations for atropine).

Late diarrhea (occurring more than 24 hours after administration of CAMPTOSAR) can be prolonged, may lead to dehydration and electrolyte imbalance, and can be life-threatening. Late diarrhea should be treated promptly with loperamide (see PRECAUTIONS, Information for Patients, for dosing recommendations for loperamide). Patients with severe diarrhea should be carefully monitored and given fluid and electrolyte replacement if they become dehydrated. National Cancer Institute (NCI) grade 3 diarrhea is defined as an increase of 7 to 9 stools daily, or incontinence, or severe cramping and NCI grade 4 diarrhea is defined as an increase of ≥10 stools daily, or grossly bloody stool, or need for parenteral support. If grade 3 or 4 late diarrhea occurs, administration of CAMPTOSAR should be delayed until the patient recovers and subsequent doses should be decreased (see DOSAGE AND ADMINISTRATION).

Myelosuppression:

Deaths due to sepsis following severe myelosuppression have been reported in patients treated with CAMPTOSAR. Therapy with CAMPTOSAR should be temporarily discontinued if neutropenic fever occurs or if the absolute neutrophil count drops below 500/mm³. The dose of CAMPTOSAR should be reduced if there is a clinically significant decrease in the total white blood cell count (<2000/mm³), neutrophil count (<1000/mm³), hemoglobin (<8 gm/dL), or platelet count (<100,000/mm³) (see DOSAGE AND ADMINISTRATION). Routine administration of a colony-stimulating factor (CSF) is not necessary, but physicians may wish to consider CSF use in individual patients experiencing significant neutropenia.

Pregnancy:

CAMPTOSAR may cause fetal harm when administered to a pregnant woman. Radioactivity related to ^{14}C-irinotecan crosses the placenta of rats following intravenous administration of 10 mg/kg (which in separate studies produced an irinotecan C_{max} and AUC about 3 and 0.5 times, respec-

tively, the corresponding values in patients administered 125 mg/m²). Administration of 6 mg/kg/day intravenous irinotecan to rats (which in separate studies produced an irinotecan C_{max} and AUC about 2 and 0.2 times, respectively, the corresponding values in patients administered 125 mg/m²) and rabbits (about one-half the recommended human dose on a mg/m² basis) during the period of organogenesis, is embryotoxic as characterized by increased postimplantation loss and decreased numbers of live fetuses. Irinotecan was teratogenic in rats at doses greater than 1.2 mg/kg/day (which in separate studies produced an irinotecan C_{max} and AUC about 2/3 and 1/40th, respectively, of the corresponding values in patients administered 125 mg/m²) and in rabbits at 6.0 mg/kg/day (about one-half the recommended weekly human dose on a mg/m² basis). Teratogenic effects included a variety of external, visceral, and skeletal abnormalities. Irinotecan administered to rat dams for the period following organogenesis through weaning at doses of 6 mg/kg/day caused decreased learning ability and decreased female body weights in the offspring. There are no adequate and well-controlled studies of irinotecan in pregnant women. If the drug is used during pregnancy, or if the patient becomes pregnant while receiving this drug, the patient should be apprised of the potential hazard to the fetus. Women of childbearing potential should be advised to avoid becoming pregnant while receiving treatment with CAMPTOSAR.

PRECAUTIONS

General

Care of Intravenous Site:

CAMPTOSAR is administered by intravenous infusion. Care should be taken to avoid extravasation, and the infu-

Continued on next page

Information on these Pharmacia & Upjohn products is based on labeling in effect June 1, 1998. Further information concerning these and other Pharmacia & Upjohn products may be obtained by direct inquiry to Medical Information, Pharmacia & Upjohn, Kalamazoo, MI 49001.

Consult 1999 PDR® supplements and future editions for revisions

Camptosar—Cont.

sion site should be monitored for signs of inflammation. Should extravasation occur, flushing the site with sterile water and application of ice are recommended.

Premedication with Antiemetics:

Irinotecan is emetigenic. It is recommended that patients receive premedication with antiemetic agents. In clinical studies, the majority of patients received 10 mg of dexamethasone given in conjunction with another type of antiemetic agent, such as a 5-HT_3 blocker (eg, ondansetron or granisetron). Antiemetic agents should be given on the day of treatment, starting at least 30 minutes before administration of CAMPTOSAR. Physicians should also consider providing patients with an antiemetic regimen (eg, prochlorperazine) for subsequent use as needed.

Treatment of Early Diarrhea:

Administration of 0.25 to 1 mg of intravenous atropine should be considered (unless clinically contraindicated) in patients experiencing diaphoresis, abdominal cramping, or early diarrhea (diarrhea occurring during or within 24 hours following administration of CAMPTOSAR).

Patients at Particular Risk:

Physicians should exercise particular caution in monitoring the effects of CAMPTOSAR in the elderly (≥65 years) and in patients who had previously received pelvic/abdominal irradiation (see ADVERSE REACTIONS).

The use of CAMPTOSAR in patients with significant hepatic dysfunction has not been established. In clinical trials, CAMPTOSAR was not administered to patients with serum bilirubin >2.0 mg/dL, or transaminase >3 times the upper limit of normal if no liver metastasis, or transaminase >5 times the upper limit of normal with liver metastasis.

However, patients with even modest elevations in total serum bilirubin levels (1.0 to 2.0 mg/dL) have had a significantly greater likelihood of experiencing first-course grade 3 or 4 neutropenia than those with bilirubin levels that were less than 1.0 mg/dL (50% versus 17.7%; $p<0.001$). Patients with abnormal glucoronidation of bilirubin, such as those with Gilbert's syndrome, may also be at greater risk of myleosuppression when receiving therapy with CAMPTOSAR. An association between bilirubin elevations and an increased risk of late diarrhea has not been observed.

Information for Patients

Patients and patients' caregivers should be informed of the expected toxic effects of CAMPTOSAR, particularly of its gastrointestinal manifestations, such as nausea, vomiting, and diarrhea. Each patient should be instructed to have loperamide readily available and to begin treatment for late diarrhea (occurring more than 24 hours after administration of CAMPTOSAR) at the first episode of poorly formed or loose stools or the earliest onset of bowel movements more frequent than normally expected for the patient. One dosage regimen for loperamide used in clinical trials consisted of the following (Note: This dosage regimen exceeds the usual dosage recommendations for loperamide.): 4 mg at the first onset of late diarrhea and then 2 mg every 2 hours until the patient is diarrhea-free for at least 12 hours. During the night, the patient may take 4 mg of loperamide every 4 hours. The patient should also be instructed to notify the physician if diarrhea occurs. Premedication with loperamide is not recommended.

The use of drugs with laxative properties should be avoided because of the potential for exacerbation of diarrhea. Patients should be advised to contact their physician to discuss any laxative use.

Patients should consult their physician if vomiting occurs, fever or evidence of infection develops, or if symptoms of dehydration, such as fainting, light-headedness, or dizziness, are noted following therapy with CAMPTOSAR.

Patients should be alerted to the possibility of alopecia.

Laboratory Tests

Careful monitoring of the white blood cell count with differential, hemoglobin, and platelet count is recommended before each dose of CAMPTOSAR.

Drug Interactions

The adverse effects of CAMPTOSAR, such as myelosuppression and diarrhea, would be expected to be exacerbated by other antineoplastic agents having similar adverse effects. Patients who have previously received pelvic/abdominal irradiation are at increased risk of severe myelosuppression following the administration of CAMPTOSAR. The concurrent administration of CAMPTOSAR with irradiation has not been adequately studied and is not recommended.

Lymphocytopenia has been reported in patients receiving CAMPTOSAR, and it is possible that the administration of dexamethasone as antiemetic prophylaxis may have enhanced the likelihood of this effect. However, serious opportunistic infections have not been observed, and no complications have specifically been attributed to lymphocytopenia.

Hyperglycemia has also been reported in patients receiving CAMPTOSAR. Usually, this has been observed in patients with a history of diabetes mellitus or evidence of glucose intolerance prior to administration of CAMPTOSAR. It is probable that dexamethasone, given as antiemetic prophylaxis, contributed to hyperglycemia in some patients.

The incidence of akathisia in clinical trials was greater (8.5%, 4/47 patients) when prochlorperazine was administered on the same day as CAMPTOSAR than when these drugs were given on separate days (1.3%, 1/80 patients). The 8.5% incidence of akathisia, however, is within the range reported for use of prochlorperazine when given as a premedication for other chemotherapies.

It would be expected that laxative use during therapy with CAMPTOSAR would worsen the incidence or severity of diarrhea, but this has not been studied.

In view of the potential risk of dehydration secondary to vomiting and/or diarrhea induced by CAMPTOSAR, the physician may wish to withhold diuretics during dosing with CAMPTOSAR and, certainly, during periods of active vomiting or diarrhea.

Drug-Laboratory Test Interactions

There are no known interactions between CAMPTOSAR and laboratory tests.

Carcinogenesis, Mutagenesis & Impairment of Fertility

Long-term carcinogenicity studies with irinotecan were not conducted. Rats were, however, administered intravenous doses of 2 mg/kg or 25 mg/kg irinotecan once per week for 13 weeks (in separate studies, the 25 mg/kg dose produced an irinotecan C_{max} and AUC that were about 7.0 times and 1.3 times the respective values in patients administered 125 mg/m^2) and were then allowed to recover for 91 weeks. Under these conditions, there was a significant linear trend with dose for the incidence of combined uterine horn endometrial stromal polyps and endometrial stromal sarcomas. Neither irinotecan or SN-38 was mutagenic in the in vitro Ames assay. Irinotecan was clastogenic both in vitro (chromosome aberrations in Chinese hamster ovary cells) and in vivo (micronucleus test in mice). No significant adverse effects on fertility and general reproductive performance were observed after intravenous administration of irinotecan in doses of up to 6 mg/kg/day to rats and rabbits. However, atrophy of male reproductive organs was observed after multiple daily irinotecan doses both in rodents at 20 mg/kg (which in separate studies produced an irinotecan C_{max} and AUC about 5 and 1 times, respectively, the corresponding values in patients administered 125 mg/m^2) and dogs at 0.4 mg/kg (which in separate studies produced an irinotecan C_{max} and AUC about one-half and 1/15th, respectively, the corresponding values in patients administered 125 mg/m^2).

Pregnancy

Pregnancy Category D—see WARNINGS.

Nursing Mothers

Radioactivity appeared in rat milk within 5 minutes of intravenous administration of radiolabeled irinotecan and was concentrated up to 65-fold at 4 hours after administration relative to plasma concentrations. Because many drugs are excreted in human milk and because of the potential for serious adverse reactions in nursing infants, it is recommended that nursing be discontinued when receiving therapy with CAMPTOSAR.

Pediatric Use

The safety and effectiveness of CAMPTOSAR in pediatric patients have not been established.

ADVERSE REACTIONS

US Clinical Trials

In three clinical studies, 304 patients with metastatic carcinoma of the colon or rectum that had recurred or progressed following 5-FU-based therapy were treated with CAMPTOSAR. Seventeen of the patients died within 30 days of the administration of CAMPTOSAR; in five cases (1.6%, 5/304), the deaths were potentially drug-related. These five patients experienced a constellation of medical events that included known effects of CAMPTOSAR. One of these patients died of neutropenic sepsis without fever. Neutropenic fever, defined as NCI grade 4 neutropenia and grade 2 or greater fever, occurred in nine (3.0%) other patients; these patients recovered with supportive care. One hundred and nineteen (39.1%) of the 304 patients were hospitalized a total of 156 times because of adverse events; 81 (26.6%) patients were hospitalized for events judged to be related to administration of irinotecan. The primary reasons for drug-related hospitalization were diarrhea, with or without nausea and/or vomiting (18.4%); neutropenia/leukopenia, with or without diarrhea and/or fever (8.2%); and nausea and/or vomiting (4.9%). Adjustments in the dose of CAMPTOSAR were made during the course of treatment and for subsequent courses based on individual patient tolerance. The first dose of at least one course of CAMPTOSAR was reduced for 67% of patients who began the studies at the 125 mg/m^2 starting dose. Within-course dose reductions were required for 32% of the courses initiated at the 125 mg/m^2 dose level. The most common reasons for dose reduction were late diarrhea, neutropenia, and leukopenia. Thirteen (4.3%) patients discontinued treatment with CAMPTOSAR because of adverse events. The adverse events in the following table are based on the experience of the 304 patients enrolled in the three studies described in the CLINICAL STUDIES section.

Adverse Events Occurring in >10% of 304 Previously Treated Patients with Metastatic Carcinoma of the Colon or Rectum

Body System & Event	% of Patients Reporting	
	NCI Grades 1–4	NCI Grades 3 & 4
GASTROINTESTINAL		
Diarrhea (late)*	87.8	30.6
7-9 stools/day (grade 3)	—	(16.4)
≥10 stools/day (grade 4)	—	(14.1)
Nausea	86.2	16.8
Vomiting	66.8	12.5
Anorexia	54.9	5.9
Diarrhea (early)†	50.7	7.9
Constipation	29.9	2.0
Flatulence	12.2	0
Stomatitis	11.8	0.7
Dyspepsia	10.5	0
HEMATOLOGIC		
Leukopenia	63.2	28.0
Anemia	60.5	6.9
Neutropenia	53.9	26.3
500 to <1000/mm^3 (grade 3)	—	(14.8)
<500/mm^3 (grade 4)	—	(11.5)
BODY AS A WHOLE		
Asthenia	75.7	12.2
Abdominal cramping/pain	56.9	16.4
Fever	45.4	0.7
Pain	23.7	2.3
Headache	16.8	0.7
Back pain	14.5	1.6
Chills	13.8	0.3
Minor Infection‡	14.5	0
Edema	10.2	1.3
Abdominal Enlargement	10.2	0.3
METABOLIC & NUTRITIONAL		
↓ Body weight	30.3	0.7
Dehydration	14.8	4.3
↑ Alkaline phosphatase	13.2	3.9
↑ SGOT	10.5	1.3
DERMATOLOGIC		
Alopecia	60.5	NA§
Sweating	16.4	0
Rash	12.8	0.7
RESPIRATORY		
Dyspnea	22.0	3.6
↑ Coughing	17.4	0.3
Rhinitis	15.5	0
NEUROLOGIC		
Insomnia	19.4	0
Dizziness	14.8	0
CARDIOVASCULAR		
Vasodilation (Flushing)	11.2	0

* Occurring >24 hours after administration of CAMPTOSAR.
† Occurring ≤24 hours after administration of CAMPTOSAR.
‡ Primarily upper respiratory infections.
§ Not applicable, complete hair loss = NCI grade 2.

First 6-Week Dosing Schedule for CAMPTOSAR for a Patient Experiencing No Toxicity Requiring Dosing Delays

Week (day)	1 (1)	2 (8)	3 (15)	4 (22)	5 (29)	6* (36)
Treatment (given on first day of weeks 1–4)	one 90-min IV infusion	one 90-min IV infusion	one 90-min IV infusion	one 90-min IV infusion	rest	rest

* The second 6-week course of treatment may begin week 7 (day 43).

Recommended Dose Modifications†

A new course of therapy should not begin until the granulocyte count has recovered to ≥1500/mm³, and the platelet count has recovered to ≥100,000mm³, and treatment-related diarrhea is fully resolved. Treatment should be delayed 1 to 2 weeks to allow for recovery from treatment-related toxicities. If the patient has not recovered after a 2-week delay, consideration should be given to discontinuing CAMPTOSAR.

Toxicity NCI Grade* Value)	During a Course of Therapy†	At the Start of the Next Courses of Therapy† (After Adequate Recovery), Compared to the Starting Dose in the Previous Course
No toxicity	Maintain dose level	↑ 25 mg/m² up to a maximum dose of 150 mg/m²
Neutropenia 1 (1500 to 1999/mm³) 2 (1000 to 1499/mm³) 3 (500 to 999/mm³) 4 (<500/mm³)	Maintain dose level ↓ 25 mg/m² Omit dose, then ↓ 25 mg/m² when resolved to ≤ grade 2 Omit dose, then ↓ 50 mg/m² when resolved to ≤ grade 2	Maintain dose level Maintain dose level ↓ 25 mg/m² ↓ 50 mg/m²
Neutropenia fever (grade 4 neutropenia & ≥ grade 2 fever)	Omit dose, then ↓ 50 mg/m² when resolved	↓ 50 mg/m²
Other hematologic toxicities	Dose modifications for leukopenia, thrombocytopenia, and anemia during a course of therapy and at the start of subsequent courses of therapy are also based on NCI toxicity criteria and are the same as recommended for neutropenia above.	
Diarrhea 1 (2–3 stools/day > pretx‡) 2 (4–6 stools/day > pretx) 3 (7–9 stools/day > pretx) 4 (≥ 10 stools/day > pretx)	Maintain dose level ↓ 25 mg/m² Omit dose, then ↓ 25 mg/m² when resolved to ≤ grade 2 Omit dose, then ↓ 50 mg/m² when resolved to ≤ grade 2	Maintain dose level Maintain, if the only grade 2 tox§ ↓ 25 mg/m², if the only grade 3 tox ↓ 50 mg/m²
Other nonhematologic toxicities 1 2 3 4	Maintain dose level ↓ 25 mg/m² Omit dose, then ↓ 25 mg/m² when resolved to ≤ grade 2 Omit dose, then ↓ 50 mg/m² when resolved to ≤ grade 2	Maintain dose level ↓ 25 mg/m² ↓ 50 mg/m² ↓ 50 mg/m²

*National Cancer Institute Common Toxicity Criteria.
†All dose modifications should be based on the worst preceding toxicity.
‡Pretreatment.
§Toxicity.

Gastrointestinal: Diarrhea, nausea, and vomiting were common adverse events following treatment with CAMPTOSAR and could be severe. These events occurred early (during or within 24 hours of administration of CAMPTOSAR) or late (more than 24 hours after administration of CAMPTOSAR). The median time to onset of late diarrhea was 11 days following administration of CAMPTOSAR. For patients starting treatment at the 125 mg/m² dose, the median duration of any grade of diarrhea was 3 days. Among those patients treated at the 125 mg/m² dose who experienced grade 3 or 4 diarrhea, the median duration of the entire episode of diarrhea was 7 days. The frequency of grade 3 or 4 late diarrhea was somewhat greater in patients starting treatment at 125 mg/m² than in patients given a 100 mg/m² starting dose (34% versus 24%). The frequency of grade 3 and 4 late diarrhea was significantly greater in patients ≥65 years than in patients <65 years of age (39.8% versus 23.4%; p = 0.0025). In Study 2, the frequency of grade 3 and 4 late diarrhea was significantly greater in male than in female patients (43.1% versus 15.6%; p = 0.01). However, there were no gender differences in the frequency of grade 3 and 4 late diarrhea in the other two studies. Colonic ulceration, sometimes with gastrointestinal bleeding, has been observed in association with administration of CAMPTOSAR.
Hematology: CAMPTOSAR commonly caused neutropenia, leukopenia (including lymphocytopenia), and anemia. Serious thrombocytopenia was uncommon. Neutropenic fever (concurrent NCI grade 4 neutropenia and fever of grade 2 or greater) occurred in 3.0% of the patients; 5.6% of patients received G-CSF for the treatment of neutropenia. NCI grade 3 or 4 anemia was noted in 6.9% of the patients. Blood transfusions were given to 9.9% of the patients. The frequency of grade 3 and 4 neutropenia was significantly higher in patients who received previous pelvic/abdominal irradiation than in those who had not received irradiation (48.1% versus 24.1%; p = 0.0356). Patients with total serum bilirubin levels of 1.0 mg/dL or more also have had a significantly greater likelihood of experiencing first-course grade 3 or 4 neutropenia than those with bilirubin levels that were less than 1.0 mg/dL (50% versus 17.7%; p<0.001). There were no significant differences in the frequency of grade 3 and 4 neutropenia by age or gender.
Body as a Whole: Asthenia, fever, and abdominal pain were the most common events of this type.

Hepatic: NCI grade 3 or 4 liver enzyme abnormalities were observed in fewer than 10% of patients. These events typically occurred in patients with known hepatic metastases.
Dermatologic: Alopecia was reported during treatment with CAMPTOSAR. Rashes have also been reported but did not result in discontinuation of treatment.
Respiratory: Severe pulmonary events were infrequent; NCI grade 3 or 4 dyspnea was reported in 3.6% of patients. Over half the patients with dyspnea had lung metastases; the extent to which malignant pulmonary involvement or other preexisting lung disease may have contributed to dyspnea in these patients is unknown.
Neurologic: Insomnia and dizziness were observed, but were not usually considered to be directly related to the administration of CAMPTOSAR. Dizziness may sometimes have represented symptomatic evidence of orthostatic hypotension in patients with dehydration.
Cardiovascular: Vasodilation (flushing) has been observed during administration of CAMPTOSAR but has not required intervention.

Non-US Clinical Trials

Irinotecan has been studied in over 1100 patients in Japan and in over 400 patients in France. Patients in these studies had a variety of tumor types, including cancer of the colon or rectum, and were treated with several different doses and schedules. In general, the types of toxicities observed were similar to those seen in US trials with CAMPTOSAR. There is some information from Japanese trials that patients with considerable ascites or pleural effusions were at increased risk for neutropenia or diarrhea. A potentially life-threatening pulmonary syndrome, consisting of dyspnea, fever, and a reticulonodular pattern on chest x-ray, was observed in a small percentage of patients in early Japanese studies. The contribution of irinotecan to these preliminary events was difficult to assess because these patients also had lung tumors and some had preexisting nonmalignant pulmonary disease. As a result of these observations, however, clinical studies in the United States have enrolled few patients with compromised pulmonary function, significant ascites, or pleural effusions.

OVERDOSAGE

In US phase 1 trials, single doses of up to 345 mg/m² of irinotecan injection were administered to patients with var-

ious cancers. Single doses of up to 750 mg/m² of irinotecan have been given in non-US trials. The adverse events in these patients were similar to those reported with the recommended dosage and regimen. There is no known antidote for overdosage of CAMPTOSAR. Maximum supportive care should be instituted to prevent dehydration due to diarrhea and to treat any infectious complications.
Lethality was observed after single intravenous irinotecan doses of approximately 111 mg/kg in mice and 73 mg/kg in rats (approximately 2.6 and 3.4 times the recommended human dose of 125 mg/m², respectively). Death was preceded by cyanosis, tremors, respiratory distress, and convulsions.

DOSAGE AND ADMINISTRATION
Starting Dose and Dose Modifications
The usual recommended starting dose of CAMPTOSAR Injection is 125 mg/m² (see First 6-week Dosing Schedule table). In patients with a combined history of prior pelvic/abdominal irradiation and modestly elevated total serum bilirubin levels (1.0 to 2.0 mg/dL) prior to treatment with CAMPTOSAR, there may be a substantially increased likelihood of grade 3 or 4 neutropenia. Consideration may be given to starting CAMPTOSAR at a lower dose (eg 100 mg/m²) in such patients (See PRECAUTIONS). Definite recommendations regarding the most appropriate starting doses in patients who have pretreatment total serum bilirubin elevations above 2.0 mg/dL are not yet available, but it is likely that lower starting doses will need to be considered in such patients.
After initiation of treatment with CAMPTOSAR, subsequent doses should be adjusted to as high as 150 mg/m² or to as low as 50 mg/m² in 25 to 50 mg/m² increments depending upon individual patient tolerance of treatment (see Recommended Dose Modifications table).
All doses should be administered as an intravenous infusion over 90 minutes (see Preparation of Infusion Solution). The recommended treatment regimen (one treatment course) is once weekly treatment for 4 weeks, followed by a 2-week rest period. The first treatment course is shown in the fol-

Continued on next page

Information on these Pharmacia & Upjohn products is based on labeling in effect June 1, 1998. Further information concerning these and other Pharmacia & Upjohn products may be obtained by direct inquiry to Medical Information, Pharmacia & Upjohn, Kalamazoo, MI 49001.

Camptosar–Cont.

lowing table. Thereafter, additional courses of treatment may be repeated every 6 weeks (4 weeks on therapy, followed by 2 weeks rest). Provided intolerable toxicity does not develop, treatment and additional courses of CAMPTOSAR may be continued indefinitely in patients who attain a response or in patients whose disease remains stable. Patients should be carefully monitored for toxicity.

[See table at bottom of page 2456]

The table below describes the recommended dose modifications during a course of therapy and at the start of each subsequent course of therapy. These recommendations are based on toxicities commonly observed with the administration of CAMPTOSAR. Therapy with CAMPTOSAR should be interrupted when grade 3 or 4 late diarrhea occurs (see PRECAUTIONS, Information for Patients) or when other intolerable toxicity is observed. Dose modifications for hematologic toxicities other than neutropenia (eg, leukopenia, anemia or thrombocytopenia, and platelets) during a course of therapy and at the start of a subsequent course of therapy are the same as recommended for neutropenia. Dose modifications for nonhematologic toxicities other than diarrhea (nausea, vomiting, etc) during a course of therapy are the same as those recommended for diarrhea. At the start of a subsequent course of therapy, the dose of CAMPTOSAR should be decreased by 25 mg/m^2, compared to the initial dose of the previous course, for other NCI grade 2 or by 50 mg/m^2 for other grade 3 or 4 nonhematologic toxicities. All dose modifications should be based on the worst preceding toxicity. A new course of therapy should not begin until the granulocyte count has recovered to $\geq$1500/mm^3 and the platelet count has recovered to $\geq$100,000/mm^3 and treatment-related diarrhea is fully resolved. Treatment should be delayed 1 to 2 weeks to allow for recovery from treatment-related toxicity. If the patient has not recovered after a 2-week delay, consideration should be given to discontinuing CAMPTOSAR.

It is recommended that patients receive premedication with antiemetic agents (see PRECAUTIONS, General).

[See table at top of previous page]

Preparation & Administration Precautions

As with other potentially toxic anticancer agents, care should be exercised in the handling and preparation of infusion solutions prepared from CAMPTOSAR Injection. The use of gloves is recommended. If a solution of CAMPTOSAR contacts the skin, wash the skin immediately and thoroughly with soap and water. If CAMPTOSAR contacts the mucous membranes, flush thoroughly with water. Several published guidelines for handling and disposal of anticancer agents are available.[1-7]

Preparation of Infusion Solution

Inspect vial contents for particulate matter and repeat inspection when drug product is withdrawn from vial into syringe.

CAMPTOSAR Injection must be diluted prior to infusion. CAMPTOSAR should be diluted in 5% Dextrose Injection, USP, (preferred) or 0.9% Sodium Chloride Injection, USP, to a final concentration range of 0.12 to 1.1 mg/mL. In most clinical trials, CAMPTOSAR was administered in 500 mL of 5% Dextrose Injection, USP.

The solution is physically and chemically stable for up to 24 hours at room temperature (approximately 25°C) and in ambient fluorescent lighting. Solutions diluted in 5% Dextrose Injection, USP, and stored at refrigerated temperatures (approximately 2° to 8°C), and protected from light are physically and chemically stable for 48 hours. Refrigeration of admixtures using 0.9% Sodium Chloride Injection, USP, is not recommended due to a low and sporadic incidence of visible particulates. **Freezing CAMPTOSAR and admixtures of CAMPTOSAR may result in precipitation of the drug and should be avoided.** Because of possible microbial contamination during dilution, it is advisable to use the admixture prepared with 5% Dextrose Injection, USP, within 24 hours if refrigerated (2° to 8°C, 36° to 46°F). In the case of admixtures prepared with 5% Dextrose Injection, USP, or Sodium Chloride Injection, USP, the solutions should be used within 6 hours if kept at room temperature (15° to 30°C, 59° to 86°F).

Other drugs should not be added to the infusion solution. Parenteral drug products should be inspected visually for particulate matter and discoloration prior to administration whenever solution and container permit.

HOW SUPPLIED

Each mL of CAMPTOSAR Injection contains 20 mg irinotecan (on the basis of the trihydrate salt); 45 mg sorbitol; and 0.9 mg lactic acid. When necessary, pH has been adjusted to 3.5 (range, 3.0 to 3.8) with sodium hydroxide or hydrochloric acid.

CAMPTOSAR Injection is available in single-dose amber glass vials in the following package sizes:

2 mL NDC 0009-7529-02
5 mL NDC 0009-7529-01

This is packaged in a backing/plastic blister to protect against inadvertent breakage and leakage. **The vial should be inspected for damage and visible signs of leaks before removing the backing/plastic blister. If damaged, incinerate the unopened package.**

Store at controlled room temperature 15° to 30°C (59° to 86°F). Protect from light. It is recommended that the vial (and backing/plastic blister) should remain in the carton until the time of use.

Caution: Federal law prohibits dispensing without prescription.

REFERENCES

1. Recommendations for the Safe Handling of Parenteral Antineoplastic Drugs. NIH Publication No. 83-2621. For sale by the Superintendent of Documents, US Government Printing Office, Washington, DC 20402.
2. AMA Council Report. Guidelines for handling parenteral antineoplastics. JAMA 1985; 253(11): 1590–2.
3. National Study Commission on Cytotoxic Exposure. Recommendations for handling cytotoxic agents. Available from Louis P. Jeffrey, ScD, Chairman, National Study Commission on Cytotoxic Exposure, Massachusetts College of Pharmacy and Allied Health Sciences, 179 Longwood Avenue, Boston, MA 02115.
4. Clinical Oncological Society of Australia. Guidelines and recommendations for safe handling of antineoplastic agents. Med J Australia 1983;1:426–8.
5. Jones RB, et. al. Safe handling of chemotherapeutic agents: a report from the Mount Sinai Medical Center. CA-A Cancer J for Clinicians, 1983;Sept./Oct., 258–63.
6. American Society of Hospital Pharmacists Technical Assistance Bulletin on handling cytotoxic and hazardous drugs. Am J Hosp Pharm 1990;47:1033–49.
7. OSHA work-practice guidelines for personnel dealing with cytotoxic (antineoplastic) drugs. Am J Hosp Pharm 1986;43:1193–1204.

Manufactured by Pharmacia & Upjohn Company, Kalamazoo, Michigan 49001, USA

Licensed from Yakult Honsha Co, LTD, Japan, and Daiichi Pharmaceutical Co, LTD, Japan

Revised December 1997 816 907 005
692053

CAVERJECT® Sterile Powder ℞
alprostadil for injection
For Intracavernosal Use

DESCRIPTION

CAVERJECT Sterile Powder contains alprostadil as the naturally occurring form of prostaglandin E_1 (PGE_1) and is designated chemically as (11α,13E,15S)-11,15-dihydroxy-9-oxoprost-13-en-1-oic acid. The molecular weight is 354.49.

Alprostadil is a white to off-white crystalline powder with a melting point between 115° and 116°C. Its solubility at 35°C is 8000 micrograms per 100 milliliter double distilled water.

CAVERJECT is available as a sterile freeze-dried powder for intracavernosal use in four sizes: 5, 10, 20 and 40 micrograms per vial—When reconstituted as directed with 1 milliliter of bacteriostatic water for injection or sterile water, both preserved with benzyl alcohol 0.945% w/v, gives 1.13 milliliters of reconstituted solution. Each milliliter of CAVERJECT contains 5.4, 10.5, 20.5 or 41.1 micrograms of alprostadil depending on vial strength, 172 milligrams of lactose, 47 micrograms of sodium citrate and 8.4 milligrams of benzyl alcohol. The deliverable amount of alprostadil is 5, 10, 20 or 40 micrograms per milliliter because approximately 0.4 microgram for the 5 microgram strength, 0.5 microgram for the 10 and 20 microgram strengths and 1.1 microgram for the 40 microgram strength is lost due to adsorption to the vial and syringe. When necessary, the pH of alprostadil for injection was adjusted with hydrochloric acid and/or sodium hydroxide before lyophilization.

The structural formula of alprostadil is represented below:

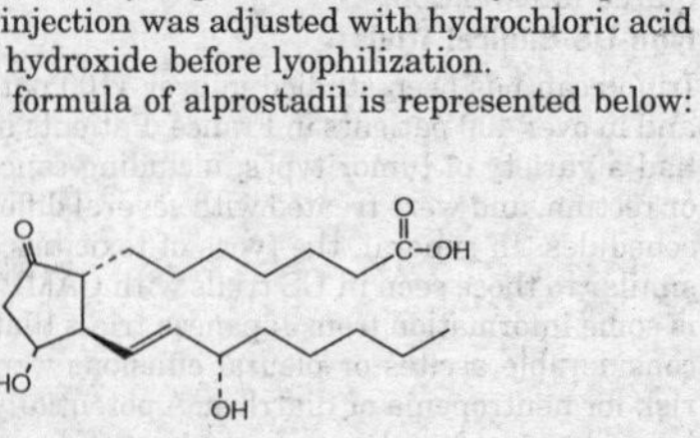

HOW SUPPLIED

CAVERJECT is a dry lyophilized powder and is supplied in vials containing 6.15, 11.9, 23.2 or 46.4 micrograms of alprostadil for intracavernosal administration. Store the 5, 10 and 20 microgram strengths at or below 25°C (77°F).

Store the 40 microgram strength at 2° to 8°C (36° to 46°F) until dispensed. After dispensing, the CAVERJECT 40 microgram strength may be stored at or below 25°C (77°F) for 3 months or until expiration date, whichever occurs first.

When reconstituted and used as directed, the deliverable amount of alprostadil is 5, 10, 20 or 40 micrograms, respectively. The reconstituted solution should be used immediately and not stored or frozen. Only the accompanying diluent or bacteriostatic water for injection with benzyl alcohol should be used when reconstituting CAVERJECT.

CAVERJECT is available in the following packages:

6–5 microgram vials with diluent syringes NDC 0009-7212-03
6–10 microgram vials with diluent syringes NDC 0009-3778-08
6–20 microgram vials with diluent syringes NDC 0009-3701-01

Other available packages:

6–10 microgram vials NDC 0009-3778-05
6–20 microgram vials NDC 0009-3701-05
6–40 microgram vials NDC 0009-7686-04

Pharmacia & Upjohn Company • Kalamazoo, MI 49001, USA

Revised October 1997 816 442 004
691811

Shown in Product Identification Guide, page 331

CLEOCIN HCl® ℞
clindamycin hydrochloride capsules, USP

WARNING

Pseudomembranous colitis has been reported with nearly all antibacterial agents, including clindamycin, and may range in severity from mild to life-threatening. Therefore, it is important to consider this diagnosis in patients who present with diarrhea subsequent to the administration of antibacterial agents.

Because clindamycin therapy has been associated with severe colitis which may end fatally, it should be reserved for serious infections where less toxic antimicrobial agents are inappropriate, as described in the **INDICATIONS AND USAGE** section. It should not be used in patients with nonbacterial infections such as most upper respiratory tract infections. Treatment with antibacterial agents alters the normal flora of the colon and may permit overgrowth of clostridia. Studies indicate that a toxin produced by *Clostridium difficile* is one primary cause of "antibiotic-associated colitis".

After the diagnosis of pseudomembranous colitis has been established, therapeutic measures should be initiated. Mild cases of pseudomembranous colitis usually respond to drug discontinuation alone. In moderate to severe cases, consideration should be given to management with fluids and electrolytes, protein supplementation, and treatment with an antibacterial drug clinically effective against *C. difficile* colitis.

Diarrhea, colitis, and pseudomembranous colitis have been observed to begin up to several weeks following cessation of therapy with clindamycin.

DESCRIPTION

Clindamycin hydrochloride is the hydrated hydrochloride salt of clindamycin. Clindamycin is a semisynthetic antibiotic produced by a 7(S)-chloro-substitution of the 7(R)-hydroxyl group of the parent compound lincomycin.

CLEOCIN HCl Capsules contain clindamycin hydrochloride equivalent to 75 mg, 150 mg or 300 mg of clindamycin.

Inactive ingredients: **75 mg**—corn starch, FD&C blue no. 1, FD&C yellow no. 5, gelatin, lactose, magnesium stearate and talc; **150 mg**—corn starch, FD&C blue no. 1, FD&C yellow no. 5, gelatin, lactose, magnesium stearate, talc and titanium dioxide; **300 mg**—corn starch, FD&C blue no. 1, gelatin, lactose, magnesium stearate, talc and titanium dioxide.

The structural formula is represented below:

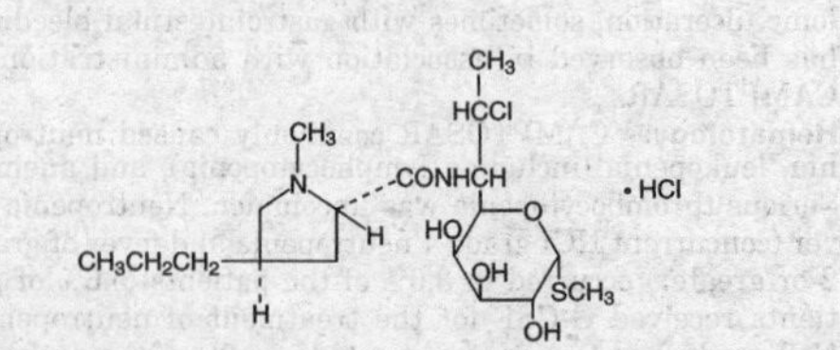

The chemical name for clindamycin hydrochloride is Methyl 7-chloro-6,7,8-trideoxy-6-(1-methyl-*trans*-4-propyl-L-2-pyrrolidinecarboxamido)-1-thio-L-*threo*-α-D-*galacto*-octopyranoside monohydrochloride.

CLINICAL PHARMACOLOGY

Microbiology: Clindamycin has been shown to have *in vitro* activity against isolates of the following organisms:

Aerobic gram-positive cocci, including:

Staphylococcus aureus
Staphylococcus epidermidis
(penicillinase and nonpenicillinase producing strains).

When tested by *in vitro* methods some staphylococcal strains originally resistant to erythromycin rapidly develop resistance to clindamycin.

Streptococci (except *Streptococcus faecalis*)

Pneumococci

Anaerobic gram-negative bacilli, including:

Bacteroides species (including *Bacteroides fragilis* group and *Bacteroides melaninogenicus* group)

Fusobacterium species

Anaerobic gram-positive nonsporeforming bacilli, including:

Propionibacterium

Eubacterium

Actinomyces species

Anaerobic and microaerophilic gram-positive cocci, including:

Peptococcus species

Peptostreptococcus species

Microaerophilic streptococci

Clostridia: Clostridia are more resistant than most anaerobes to clindamycin. Most *Clostridium perfringens* are susceptible, but other species, eg, *Clostridium sporogenes* and *Clostridium tertium* are frequently resistant to clindamycin. Susceptibility testing should be done.

Cross resistance has been demonstrated between clindamycin and lincomycin.

Antagonism has been demonstrated between clindamycin and erythromycin.

Human Pharmacology: Serum level studies with a 150 mg oral dose of clindamycin hydrochloride in 24 normal adult volunteers showed that clindamycin was rapidly absorbed after oral administration. An average peak serum level of 2.50 mcg/mL was reached in 45 minutes; serum levels averaged 1.51 mcg/mL at 3 hours and 0.70 mcg/mL at 6 hours. Absorption of an oral dose is virtually complete (90%), and the concomitant administration of food does not appreciably modify the serum concentrations; serum levels have been uniform and predictable from person to person and dose to dose. Serum level studies following multiple doses of CLEOCIN HCl for up to 14 days show no evidence of accumulation or altered metabolism of drug.

Serum half-life of clindamycin is increased slightly in patients with markedly reduced renal function. Hemodialysis and peritoneal dialysis are not effective in removing clindamycin from the serum.

Concentrations of clindamycin in the serum increased linearly with increased dose. Serum levels exceed the MIC (minimum inhibitory concentration) for most indicated organisms for at least six hours following administration of the usually recommended doses. Clindamycin is widely distributed in body fluids and tissues (including bones). The average biological half-life is 2.4 hours. Approximately 10% of the bioactivity is excreted in the urine and 3.6% in the feces; the remainder is excreted as bioinactive metabolites.

Doses of up to 2 grams of clindamycin per day for 14 days have been well tolerated by healthy volunteers, except that the incidence of gastrointestinal side effects is greater with the higher doses.

No significant levels of clindamycin are attained in the cerebrospinal fluid, even in the presence of inflamed meninges.

Pharmacokinetic studies in elderly volunteers (61–79 years) and younger adults (18–39 years) indicate that age alone does not alter clindamycin pharmacokinetics (clearance, elimination half-life, volume of distribution, and area under the serum concentration-time curve) after IV administration of clindamycin phosphate. After oral administration of clindamycin hydrochloride, elimination half-life is increased to approximately 4.0 hours (range 3.4–5.1 h) in the elderly compared to 3.2 hours (range 2.1–4.2 h) in younger adults. The extent of absorption, however, is not different between age groups and no dosage alteration is necessary for the elderly with normal hepatic function and normal (age-adjusted) renal function[1].

INDICATIONS AND USAGE

Clindamycin is indicated in the treatment of serious infections caused by susceptible anaerobic bacteria.

Clindamycin is also indicated in the treatment of serious infections due to susceptible strains of streptococci, pneumococci, and staphylococci. Its use should be reserved for penicillin-allergic patients or other patients for whom, in the judgment of the physician, a penicillin is inappropriate. Because of the risk of colitis, as described in the WARNING box, before selecting clindamycin the physician should consider the nature of the infection and the suitability of less toxic alternatives (eg, erythromycin).

Anaerobes: Serious respiratory tract infections such as empyema, anaerobic pneumonitis and lung abscess; serious skin and soft tissue infections; septicemia; intra-abdominal infections such as peritonitis and intra-abdominal abscess (typically resulting from anaerobic organisms resident in the normal gastrointestinal tract); infections of the female pelvis and genital tract such as endometritis, nongonococcal tubo-ovarian abscess, pelvic cellulitis and postsurgical vaginal cuff infection.

Streptococci: Serious respiratory tract infections; serious skin and soft tissue infections.

Staphylococci: Serious respiratory tract infections; serious skin and soft tissue infections.

Pneumococci: Serious respiratory tract infections.

Bacteriologic studies should be performed to determine the causative organisms and their susceptibility to clindamycin.

In Vitro **Susceptibility Testing:** A standardized disk testing procedure* is recommended for determining susceptibility of aerobic bacteria to clindamycin. A description is contained in the CLEOCIN® Susceptibility Disk insert. Using this method, the laboratory can designate isolates as resistant, intermediate, or susceptible. Tube or agar dilution methods may be used for both anaerobic and aerobic bacteria. When the directions in the CLEOCIN® Susceptibility Powder insert are followed, an MIC of 1.6 mcg/mL may be considered susceptible; MICs of 1.6 to 4.8 mcg/mL may be considered intermediate and MICs greater than 4.8 mcg/mL may be considered resistant.

*Bauer AW, Kirby WMM, Sherris JC, et al: Antibiotic susceptibility testing by a standardized single disc method. *Am J Clin Pathol* 45:493-496, 1966. Standardized disc susceptibility test. *Federal Register* 37:20527-29, 1972.

CLEOCIN Susceptibility Disks 2 mcg. See package insert for use.

CLEOCIN Susceptibility Powder 20 mg. See package insert for use.

For anaerobic bacteria the minimal inhibitory concentration (MIC) of clindamycin can be determined by agar dilution and broth dilution (including microdilution) techniques. If MICs are not determined routinely, the disk broth method is recommended for routine use. THE KIRBY-BAUER DISK DIFFUSION METHOD AND ITS INTERPRETIVE STANDARDS ARE NOT RECOMMENDED FOR ANAEROBES.

CONTRAINDICATIONS

CLEOCIN HCl is contraindicated in individuals with a history of hypersensitivity to preparations containing clindamycin or lincomycin.

WARNINGS

See WARNING box.

Pseudomembranous colitis has been reported with nearly all antibacterial agents, including clindamycin, and may range in severity from mild to life-threatening. Therefore, it is important to consider this diagnosis in patients who present with diarrhea subsequent to the administration of antibacterial agents.

Treatment with antibacterial agents alters the normal flora of the colon and may permit overgrowth of clostridia. Studies indicate that a toxin produced by *Clostridium difficile* is one primary cause of "antibiotic-associated colitis".

After the diagnosis of pseudomembranous colitis has been established, therapeutic measures should be initiated. Mild cases of pseudomembranous colitis usually respond to drug discontinuation alone. In moderate to severe cases, consideration should be given to management with fluids and electrolytes, protein supplementation, and treatment with an antibacterial drug clinically effective against *C. difficile* colitis.

A careful inquiry should be made concerning previous sensitivities to drugs and other allergens.

Usage in Meningitis—Since clindamycin does not diffuse adequately into the cerebrospinal fluid, the drug should not be used in the treatment of meningitis.

PRECAUTIONS

General

Review of experience to date suggests that a subgroup of older patients with associated severe illness may tolerate diarrhea less well. When clindamycin is indicated in these patients, they should be carefully monitored for change in bowel frequency.

CLEOCIN HCl should be prescribed with caution in individuals with a history of gastrointestinal disease, particularly colitis.

CLEOCIN HCl should be prescribed with caution in atopic individuals.

Indicated surgical procedures should be performed in conjunction with antibiotic therapy.

The use of CLEOCIN HCl occasionally results in overgrowth of nonsusceptible organisms—particularly yeasts. Should superinfections occur, appropriate measures should be taken as indicated by the clinical situation.

Clindamycin dosage modification may not be necessary in patients with renal disease. In patients with moderate to severe liver disease, prolongation of clindamycin half-life has been found. However, it was postulated from studies that when given every eight hours, accumulation should rarely occur. Therefore, dosage modification in patients with liver disease may not be necessary. However, periodic liver enzyme determinations should be made when treating patients with severe liver disease.

The 75 mg and 150 mg capsules contain FD&C yellow no. 5 (tartrazine) which may cause allergic-type reactions (including bronchial asthma) in certain susceptible individuals. Although the overall incidence of FD&C yellow no. 5

(tartrazine) sensitivity in the general population is low, it is frequently seen in patients who also have aspirin hypersensitivity.

Laboratory Tests

During prolonged therapy, periodic liver and kidney function tests and blood counts should be performed.

Drug Interactions

Clindamycin has been shown to have neuromuscular blocking properties that may enhance the action of other neuromuscular blocking agents. Therefore, it should be used with caution in patients receiving such agents.

Antagonism has been demonstrated between clindamycin and erythromycin *in vitro*. Because of possible clinical significance, these two drugs should not be administered concurrently.

Carcinogenesis, Mutagenesis, Impairment of Fertility

Long term studies in animals have not been performed with clindamycin to evaluate carcinogenic potential. Genotoxicity tests performed included a rat micronucleus test and an Ames Salmonella reversion test. Both tests were negative. Fertility studies in rats treated orally with up to 300 mg/kg/day (approximately 1.6 times the highest recommended adult human dose based on mg/m²) revealed no effects on fertility or mating ability.

Pregnancy: Teratogenic effects

Pregnancy category B

Reproduction studies performed in rats and mice using oral doses of clindamycin up to 600 mg/kg/day (3.2 and 1.6 times the highest recommended adult human dose based on mg/m², respectively) or subcutaneous doses of clindamycin up to 250 mg/kg/day (1.3 and 0.7 times the highest recommended adult human dose based on mg/m², respectively) revealed no evidence of teratogenicity.

There are, however, no adequate and well-controlled studies in pregnant women. Because animal reproduction studies are not always predictive of the human response, this drug should be used during pregnancy only if clearly needed.

Nursing Mothers

Clindamycin has been reported to appear in breast milk in the range of 0.7 to 3.8 mcg/mL.

Pediatric Use

When CLEOCIN HCl is administered to the pediatric population (birth to 16 years), appropriate monitoring of organ system functions is desirable.

Geriatric Use

Clinical studies of clindamycin did not include sufficient numbers of patients age 65 and over to determine whether they respond differently from younger patients. However, other reported clinical experience indicates that antibiotic-associated colitis and diarrhea (due to *Clostridium difficile*) seen in association with most antibiotics occur more frequently in the elderly (>60 years) and may be more severe. These patients should be carefully monitored for the development of diarrhea.

Pharmacokinetic studies with clindamycin have shown no clinically important differences between young and elderly subjects with normal hepatic function and normal (age-adjusted) renal function after oral or intravenous administration.

ADVERSE REACTIONS

The following reactions have been reported with the use of clindamycin.

Gastrointestinal: Abdominal pain, pseudomembranous colitis, esophagitis, nausea, vomiting and diarrhea (see **WARNING** box). The onset of pseudomembranous colitis symptoms may occur during or after antibacterial treatment (see **WARNINGS**).

Hypersensitivity Reactions: Generalized mild to moderate morbilliform-like (maculopapular) skin rashes are the most frequently reported adverse reactions. Vesiculobullous rashes, as well as urticaria, have been observed during drug therapy. Rare instances of erythema multiforme, some resembling Stevens-Johnson syndrome, and a few cases of anaphylactoid reactions have also been reported.

Skin and Mucous Membranes: Pruritus, vaginitis, and rare instances of exfoliative dermatitis have been reported. (See *Hypersensitivity Reactions.*)

Liver: Jaundice and abnormalities in liver function tests have been observed during clindamycin therapy.

Renal: Although no direct relationship of clindamycin to renal damage has been established, renal dysfunction as evidenced by azotemia, oliguria, and/or proteinuria has been observed in rare instances.

Hematopoietic: Transient neutropenia (leukopenia) and eosinophilia have been reported. Reports of agranulocytosis and thrombocytopenia have been made. No direct etiologic

Continued on next page

Information on these Pharmacia & Upjohn products is based on labeling in effect June 1, 1998. Further information concerning these and other Pharmacia & Upjohn products may be obtained by direct inquiry to Medical Information, Pharmacia & Upjohn, Kalamazoo, MI 49001.

Cleocin HCl–Cont.

relationship to concurrent clindamycin therapy could be made in any of the foregoing.

Musculoskeletal: Rare instances of polyarthritis have been reported.

OVERDOSAGE

Significant mortality was observed in mice at an intravenous dose of 855 mg/kg and in rats at an oral or subcutaneous dose of approximately 2618 mg/kg. In the mice, convulsions and depression were observed.

Hemodialysis and peritoneal dialysis are not effective in removing clindamycin from the serum.

ANIMAL TOXICOLOGY

One year oral toxicity studies in Spartan Sprague-Dawley rats and beagle dogs at dose levels up to 300 mg/kg/day (approximately 1.6 and 5.4 times the highest recommended adult human dose based on mg/m^2, respectively) have shown clindamycin to be well tolerated. No appreciable difference in pathological findings has been observed between groups of animals treated with clindamycin and comparable control groups. Rats receiving clindamycin hydrochloride at 600 mg/kg/day (approximately 3.2 times the highest recommended adult human dose based on mg/m^2) for 6 months tolerated the drug well; however, dogs dosed at this level (approximately 10.8 times the highest recommended adult human dose based on mg/m^2) vomited, would not eat, and lost weight.

DOSAGE AND ADMINISTRATION

If significant diarrhea occurs during therapy, this antibiotic should be discontinued (see **WARNING** box).

Adults: *Serious infections*—150 to 300 mg every 6 hours. *More severe infections*—300 to 450 mg every 6 hours. **Pediatric Patients:** *Serious infections*—8 to 16 mg/kg/day (4 to 8 mg/lb/day) divided into three or four equal doses. *More severe infections*—16 to 20 mg/kg/day (8 to 10 mg/lb/day) divided into three or four equal doses.

To avoid the possibility of esophageal irritation, CLEOCIN HCl Capsules should be taken with a full glass of water.

Serious infections due to anaerobic bacteria are usually treated with CLEOCIN PHOSPHATE® Sterile Solution. However, in clinically appropriate circumstances, the physician may elect to initiate treatment or continue treatment with CLEOCIN HCl Capsules.

In cases of β-hemolytic streptococcal infections, treatment should continue for at least 10 days.

HOW SUPPLIED

CLEOCIN HCl Capsules are available in the following strengths, colors and sizes:

75 mg Green
Bottles of 100   NDC 0009-0331-02
150 mg Light Blue and Green
Bottles of 16   NDC 0009-0225-01
Bottles of 100   NDC 0009-0225-02
Unit dose package of 100   NDC 0009-0225-03
300 mg Light Blue
Bottles of 16   NDC 0009-0395-13
Bottles of 100   NDC 0009-0395-14
Unit dose package of 100   NDC 0009-0395-02

Store at controlled room temperature 20° to 25° C (68° to 77° F) [see USP].

Rx only

REFERENCES

1. Smith RB, Phillips JP: Evaluation of CLEOCIN HCl and CLEOCIN Phosphate in an Aged Population. Upjohn TR 8147-82-9122-021, December 1982.

Made in Canada for
Pharmacia & Upjohn Company
Kalamazoo, MI 49001, USA
By Global Pharm Inc.
Don Mills, Ontario M3B 1Y5
Canada
Revised April 1998   810 570 624
     692166

CLEOCIN PHOSPHATE®   ℞
Sterile Solution
clindamycin phosphate injection, USP and clindamycin phosphate injection in 5% dextrose
Sterile Solution is for Intramuscular and Intravenous Use
CLEOCIN PHOSPHATE in the ADD-Vantage™ Vial is For Intravenous Use Only

patients who present with diarrhea subsequent to the administration of antibacterial agents.

Because clindamycin therapy has been associated with severe colitis which may end fatally, it should be reserved for serious infections where less toxic antimicrobial agents are inappropriate, as described in the **INDICATIONS AND USAGE** section. It should not be used in patients with nonbacterial infections such as most upper respiratory tract infections. Treatment with antibacterial agents alters the normal flora of the colon and may permit overgrowth of clostridia. Studies indicate that a toxin produced by *Clostridium difficile* is one primary cause of "antibiotic-associated colitis".

After the diagnosis of pseudomembranous colitis has been established, therapeutic measures should be initiated. Mild cases of pseudomembranous colitis usually respond to drug discontinuation alone. In moderate to severe cases, consideration should be given to management with fluids and electrolytes, protein supplementation, and treatment with an antibacterial drug clinically effective against *C. difficile* colitis.

Diarrhea, colitis, and pseudomembranous colitis have been observed to begin up to several weeks following cessation of therapy with clindamycin.

DESCRIPTION

CLEOCIN PHOSPHATE Sterile Solution in vials contains clindamycin phosphate, a water soluble ester of clindamycin and phosphoric acid. Each mL contains the equivalent of 150 mg clindamycin, 0.5 mg disodium edetate and 9.45 mg benzyl alcohol added as preservative in each mL. Clindamycin is a semisynthetic antibiotic produced by a 7(S)-chlorosubstitution of the 7(R)-hydroxyl group of the parent compound lincomycin.

The chemical name of clindamycin phosphate is L-*threo*-α-D-*galacto*-Octopyranoside, methyl 7-chloro-6,7,8-trideoxy-6-[[(1-methyl-4-propyl-2-pyrrolidinyl) carbonyl] amino]-1-thio-, 2-(dihydrogen phosphate), (2S-*trans*)-.

The molecular formula is $C_{18}H_{34}ClN_2O_8PS$ and the molecular weight is 504.96.

The structural formula is represented below:

CLEOCIN PHOSPHATE in the ADD-Vantage Vial is intended for intravenous use only after further dilution with appropriate volume of ADD-Vantage diluent base solution.

CLEOCIN PHOSPHATE IV Solution in the Galaxy® plastic container for intravenous use is composed of clindamycin phosphate equivalent to 300, 600 and 900 mg of clindamycin premixed with 5% dextrose as a sterile solution. Disodium edetate has been added at a concentration of 0.04 mg/mL. The pH has been adjusted with sodium hydroxide and/or hydrochloric acid.

The plastic container is fabricated from a specially designed multilayer plastic, PL 2501. Solutions in contact with the plastic container can leach out certain of its chemical components in very small amounts within the expiration period. The suitability of the plastic has been confirmed in tests in animals according to the USP biological tests for plastic containers, as well as by tissue culture toxicity studies.

CLINICAL PHARMACOLOGY

Biologically inactive clindamycin phosphate is rapidly converted to active clindamycin.

By the end of short-term intravenous infusion, peak serum levels of active clindamycin are reached. Biologically inactive clindamycin phosphate disappears rapidly from the serum; the average elimination half-life is 6 minutes; however, the serum elimination half-life of active clindamycin is about 3 hours in adults and 2½ hours in children.

After intramuscular injection of clindamycin phosphate, peak levels of active clindamycin are reached within 3 hours in adults and 1 hour in children. Serum level curves may be constructed from IV peak serum levels as given in Table 1 by application of elimination half-lives listed above.

Serum levels of clindamycin can be maintained above the *in vitro* minimum inhibitory concentrations for most indicated organisms by administration of clindamycin phosphate every 8 to 12 hours in adults and every 6 to 8 hours in children, or by continuous intravenous infusion. An equilibrium state is reached by the third dose.

The elimination half-life of clindamycin is increased slightly in patients with markedly reduced renal or hepatic function. Hemodialysis and peritoneal dialysis are not effective

in removing clindamycin from the serum. Dosage schedules need not be modified in the presence of mild or moderate renal or hepatic disease.

No significant levels of clindamycin are attained in the cerebrospinal fluid even in the presence of inflamed meninges. Pharmacokinetic studies in elderly volunteers (61–79 years) and younger adults (18–39 years) indicate that age alone does not alter clindamycin pharmacokinetics (clearance, elimination half-life, volume of distribution, and area under the serum concentration-time curve) after IV administration of clindamycin phosphate. After oral administration of clindamycin hydrochloride, elimination half-life is increased to approximately 4.0 hours (range 3.4–5.1 h) in the elderly compared to 3.2 hours (range 2.1–4.2 h) in younger adults. The extent of absorption, however, is not different between age groups and no dosage alteration is necessary for the elderly with normal hepatic function and normal (age-adjusted) renal function[1].

Serum assays for active clindamycin require an inhibitor to prevent *in vitro* hydrolysis of clindamycin phosphate.

Table 1. Average Peak and Trough Serum Concentrations of Active Clindamycin After Dosing With Clindamycin Phosphate

Dosage Regimen	Peak mcg/mL	Trough mcg/mL
Healthy Adult Males (Post equilibrium)		
600 mg IV in 30 min q6h	10.9	2.0
600 mg IV in 30 min q8h	10.8	1.1
900 mg IV in 30 min q8h	14.1	1.7
600 mg IM q12h*	9	
Children (first dose)*		
5–7 mg/kg IV in 1 hour	10	
5–7 mg/kg IM	8	
3–5 mg/kg IM	4	

*Data in this group from patients being treated for infection.

Microbiology: Although clindamycin phosphate is inactive *in vitro*, rapid *in vivo* hydrolysis converts this compound to the antibacterially active clindamycin.

Clindamycin has been shown to have *in vitro* activity against isolates of the following organisms:
Aerobic gram positive cocci, including:

Staphylococcus aureus   (penicillinase and non-penicillinase producing strains). When tested by *in vitro* methods, some staphylococcal strains originally resistant to erythromycin rapidly develop resistance to clindamycin.
Staphylococcus epidermidis

Streptococci (except *Enterococcus faecalis*)
Pneumococci
Anaerobic gram negative bacilli, including:
   Bacteroides species (including *Bacteroides fragilis* group and *Bacteroides melaninogenicus* group)
   Fusobacterium species
Anaerobic gram positive nonsporeforming bacilli, including:
   Propionibacterium
   Eubacterium
   Actinomyces species
Anaerobic and *microaerophilic gram positive cocci,* including
   Peptococcus species
   Peptostreptococcus species
   Microaerophilic streptococci
Clostridia: Clostridia are more resistant than most anaerobes to clindamycin. Most *Clostridium perfringens* are susceptible, but other species, e.g., *Clostridium sporogenes* and *Clostridium tertium* are frequently resistant to clindamycin. Susceptibility testing should be done.

Cross resistance has been demonstrated between clindamycin and lincomycin.

Antagonism has been demonstrated between clindamycin and erythromycin.

In vitro Susceptibility Testing:

Disk diffusion technique-Quantitative methods that require measurement of zone diameters give the most precise estimates of antibiotic susceptibility. One such procedure[2] has been recommended for use with disks to test susceptibility to clindamycin.

Reports from a laboratory using the standardized single-disk susceptibility test[1] with a 2 mcg clindamycin disk should be interpreted according to the following criteria:

Susceptible organisms produce zones of 17 mm or greater, indicating that the tested organism is likely to respond to therapy.

Organisms of intermediate susceptibility produce zones of 15–16 mm, indicating that the tested organism would be

susceptible if a high dosage is used or if the infection is confined to tissues and fluids (e.g., urine), in which high antibiotic levels are attained.

Resistant organisms produce zones of 14 mm or less, indicating that other therapy should be selected.

Standardized procedures require the use of control organisms. The 2 mcg clindamycin disk should give a zone diameter between 24 and 30 mm for *S. aureus* ATCC 25923.

Dilution techniques—A bacterial isolate may be considered susceptible if the minimum inhibitory concentration (MIC) for clindamycin is not more than 1.6 mcg/mL. Organisms are considered moderately susceptible if the MIC is greater than 1.6 mcg/mL and less than or equal to 4.8 mcg/mL. Organisms are considered resistant if the MIC is greater than 4.8 mcg per mL.

The range of MICs for the control strains are as follows:

S. aureus ATCC 29213, 0.06–0.25 mcg/mL.

E. faecalis ATCC 29212, 4.0–16 mcg/mL.

For anaerobic bacteria the minimum inhibitory concentration (MIC) of clindamycin can be determined by agar dilution and broth dilution (including microdilution) techniques.[3] If MICs are not determined routinely, the disk broth method is recommended for routine use. THE KIRBY-BAUER DISK DIFFUSION METHOD AND ITS INTERPRETIVE STANDARDS ARE NOT RECOMMENDED FOR ANAEROBES.

INDICATIONS AND USAGE

CLEOCIN PHOSPHATE products are indicated in the treatment of serious infections caused by susceptible anaerobic bacteria.

CLEOCIN PHOSPHATE products are also indicated in the treatment of serious infections due to susceptible strains of streptococci, pneumococci, and staphylococci. Its use should be reserved for penicillin-allergic patients or other patients for whom, in the judgment of the physician, a penicillin is inappropriate. Because of the risk of antibiotic-associated pseudomembranous colitis, as described in the WARNING box, before selecting clindamycin the physician should consider the nature of the infection and the suitability of less toxic alternatives (e.g., erythromycin).

Bacteriologic studies should be performed to determine the causative organisms and their susceptibility to clindamycin.

Indicated surgical procedures should be performed in conjunction with antibiotic therapy.

CLEOCIN PHOSPHATE is indicated in the treatment of serious infections caused by susceptible strains of the designated organisms in the conditions listed below:

Lower respiratory tract infections including pneumonia, empyema, and lung abscess caused by anaerobes, *Streptococcus pneumoniae*, other streptococci (except *E. faecalis*), and *Staphylococcus aureus*.

Skin and skin structure infections caused by *Streptococcus pyogenes*, *Staphylococcus aureus*, and anaerobes.

Gynecological infections including endometritis, nongonococcal tubo-ovarian abscess, pelvic cellulitis, and postsurgical vaginal cuff infection caused by susceptible anaerobes.

Intra-abdominal infections including peritonitis and intra-abdominal abscess caused by susceptible anaerobic organisms.

Septicemia caused by *Staphylococcus aureus*, streptococci (except *Enterococcus faecalis*), and susceptible anaerobes.

Bone and joint infections including acute hematogenous osteomyelitis caused by *Staphylococcus aureus* and as adjunctive therapy in the surgical treatment of chronic bone and joint infections due to susceptible organisms.

CONTRAINDICATIONS

This drug is contraindicated in individuals with a history of hypersensitivity to preparations containing clindamycin or lincomycin.

WARNINGS

See **WARNING** box.

Pseudomembranous colitis has been reported with nearly all antibacterial agents, including clindamycin, and may range in severity from mild to life-threatening. Therefore, it is important to consider this diagnosis in patients who present with diarrhea subsequent to the administration of antibacterial agents.

Treatment with antibacterial agents alters the normal flora of the colon and may permit overgrowth of clostridia. Studies indicate that a toxin produced by *clostridium difficile* is one primary cause of "antibiotic-associated colitis".

After the diagnosis of pseudomembranous colitis has been established, therapeutic measures should be initiated. Mild cases of pseudomembranous colitis usually respond to drug discontinuation alone. In moderate to severe cases, consideration should be given to management with fluids and electrolytes, protein supplementation, and treatment with an antibacterial drug clinically effective against *C. difficile* colitis.

A careful inquiry should be made concerning previous sensitivities to drugs and other allergens.

This product contains benzyl alcohol as a preservative. Benzyl alcohol has been associated with a fatal "Gasping Syndrome" in premature infants. (See **PRECAUTIONS—Pediatric Use.**)

Usage in Meningitis—Since clindamycin does not diffuse adequately into the cerebrospinal fluid, the drug should not be used in the treatment of meningitis.

SERIOUS ANAPHYLACTOID REACTIONS REQUIRE IMMEDIATE EMERGENCY TREATMENT WITH EPINEPHRINE. OXYGEN AND INTRAVENOUS CORTICOSTEROIDS SHOULD ALSO BE ADMINISTERED AS INDICATED.

PRECAUTIONS

General

Review of experience to date suggests that a subgroup of older patients with associated severe illness may tolerate diarrhea less well. When clindamycin is indicated in these patients, they should be carefully monitored for change in bowel frequency.

CLEOCIN PHOSPHATE products should be prescribed with caution in individuals with a history of gastrointestinal disease, particularly colitis.

CLEOCIN PHOSPHATE should be prescribed with caution in atopic individuals.

Certain infections may require incision and drainage or other indicated surgical procedures in addition to antibiotic therapy.

The use of CLEOCIN PHOSPHATE may result in overgrowth of nonsusceptible organisms—particularly yeasts. Should superinfections occur, appropriate measures should be taken as indicated by the clinical situation.

CLEOCIN PHOSPHATE should not be injected intravenously undiluted as a bolus, but should be infused over at least 10–60 minutes as directed in the DOSAGE AND ADMINISTRATION section.

Clindamycin dosage modification may not be necessary in patients with renal disease. In patients with moderate to severe liver disease, prolongation of clindamycin half-life has been found. However, it was postulated from studies that when given every eight hours, accumulation should rarely occur. Therefore, dosage modification in patients with liver disease may not be necessary. However, periodic liver enzyme deter minations should be made when treating patients with severe liver disease.

Laboratory Tests

During prolonged therapy periodic liver and kidney function tests and blood counts should be performed.

Drug Interactions

Clindamycin has been shown to have neuromuscular blocking properties that may enhance the action of other neuromuscular blocking agents. Therefore, it should be used with caution in patients receiving such agents.

Antagonism has been demonstrated between clindamycin and erythromycin *in vitro*. Because of possible clinical significance, the two drugs should not be administered concurrently.

Carcinogenesis, Mutagenesis, Impairment of Fertility

Long term studies in animals have not been performed with clindamycin to evaluate carcinogenic potential. Genotoxicity tests performed included a rat micronucleus test and an Ames Salmonella reversion test. Both tests were negative. Fertility studies in rats treated orally with up to 300 mg/kg/day (approximately 1.1 times the highest recommended adult human dose based on mg/m^2) revealed no effects on fertility or mating ability.

Pregnancy: Teratogenic effects

Pregnancy category B

Reproduction studies performed in rats and mice using oral doses of clindamycin up to 600 mg/kg/day (2.1 and 1.1 times the highest recommended adult human dose based on mg/m^2, respectively) or subcutaneous doses of clindamycin up to 250 mg/kg/day (0.9 and 0.5 times the highest recommended adult human dose based on mg/m^2, respectively) revealed no evidence of teratogenicity.

There are, however, no adequate and well-controlled studies in pregnant women. Because animal reproduction studies are not always predictive of the human response, this drug should be used during pregnancy only if clearly needed.

Nursing Mothers

Clindamycin has been reported to appear in breast milk in the range of 0.7 to 3.8 mcg/mL at dosages of 150 mg orally to 600 mg intravenously. Because of the potential for adverse reactions due to clindamycin in neonates (see **Pediatric Use**), the decision to discontinue the drug should be made, taking into account the importance of the drug to the mother.

Pediatric Use

When CLEOCIN PHOSPHATE Sterile Solution is administered to the pediatric population (birth to 16 years) appropriate monitoring of organ system functions is desirable.

Usage in Newborns and Infants

This product contains benzyl alcohol as a preservative. Benzyl alcohol has been associated with a fatal "Gasping Syndrome" in premature infants.

The potential for the toxic effect in the pediatric population from chemicals that may leach from the single dose premixed IV preparation in plastic has not been evaluated.

Geriatric Use

Clinical studies of clindamycin did not include sufficient numbers of patients age 65 and over to determine whether they respond differently from younger patients. However, other reported clinical experience indicates that antibiotic-associated colitis and diarrhea (due to *Clostridium difficile*) seen in association with most antibiotics occur more frequently in the elderly (>60 years) and may be more severe. These patients should be carefully monitored for the development of diarrhea.

Pharmacokinetic studies with clindamycin have shown no clinically important differences between young and elderly subjects with normal hepatic function and normal (age-adjusted) renal function after oral or intravenous administration.

ADVERSE REACTIONS

The following reactions have been reported with the use of clindamycin.

Gastrointestinal: Antibiotic-associated colitis (see **WARNINGS**), pseudomembranous colitis, abdominal pain, nausea, and vomiting. The onset of pseudomembranous colitis symptoms may occur during or after antibacterial treatment (see **WARNINGS**). An unpleasant or metallic taste occasionally has been reported after intravenous administration of the higher doses of clindamycin phosphate.

Hypersensitivity Reactions: Maculopapular rash and urticaria have been observed during drug therapy. Generalized mild to moderate morbilliform-like skin rashes are the most frequently reported of all adverse reactions. Rare instances of erythema multiforme, some resembling Stevens-Johnson syndrome, have been associated with clindamycin. A few cases of anaphylactoid reactions have been reported. If a hypersensitivity reaction occurs, the drug should be discontinued. The usual agents (epinephrine, corticosteroids, antihistamines) should be available for emergency treatment of serious reactions.

Skin and Mucous Membranes: Pruritus, vaginitis, and rare instances of exfoliative dermatitis have been reported (see *Hypersensitivity Reactions*).

Liver: Jaundice and abnormalities in liver function tests have been observed during clindamycin therapy.

Renal: Although no direct relationship of clindamycin to renal damage has been established, renal dysfunction as evidenced by azotemia, oliguria, and/or proteinuria has been observed in rare instances.

Hematopoietic: Transient neutropenia (leukopenia) and eosinophilia have been reported. Reports of agranulocytosis and thrombocytopenia have been made. No direct etiologic relationship to concurrent clindamycin therapy could be made in any of the foregoing.

Local Reactions: Pain, induration and sterile abscess have been reported after intramuscular injection and thrombophlebitis after intravenous infusion. Reactions can be minimized or avoided by giving deep intramuscular injections and avoiding prolonged use of indwelling intravenous catheters.

Musculoskeletal: Rare instances of polyarthritis have been reported.

Cardiovascular: Rare instances of cardiopulmonary arrest and hypotension have been reported following too rapid intravenous administration. (See **DOSAGE AND ADMINISTRATION** section.)

OVERDOSAGE

Significant mortality was observed in mice at an intravenous dose of 855 mg/kg and in rats at an oral or subcutaneous dose of approximately 2618 mg/kg. In the mice, convulsions and depression were observed.

Hemodialysis and peritoneal dialysis are not effective in removing clindamycin from the serum.

ANIMAL TOXICOLOGY

One year oral toxicity studies in Spartan Sprague-Dawley rats and beagle dogs at dose levels up to 300 mg/kg/day (approximately 1.1 and 3.6 times the highest recommended adult human dose based on mg/m^2, respectively) have shown clindamycin to be well tolerated. No appreciable difference in pathological findings has been observed between groups of animals treated with clindamycin and comparable control groups. Rats receiving clindamycin hydrochloride at 600 mg/kg/day (approximately 2.1 times the highest recommended adult human dose based on mg/m^2) for 6 months tolerated the drug well; however, dogs dosed at this level

Continued on next page

Information on these Pharmacia & Upjohn products is based on labeling in effect June 1, 1998. Further information concerning these and other Pharmacia & Upjohn products may be obtained by direct inquiry to Medical Information, Pharmacia & Upjohn, Kalamazoo, MI 49001.

Cleocin Phosphate—Cont.

(approximately 7 times the highest recommended adult human dose based in mg/m²) vomited, would not eat, and lost weight.

DOSAGE AND ADMINISTRATION

If diarrhea occurs during therapy, this antibiotic should be discontinued (see WARNING box).

Adults: Parenteral (IM or IV Administration): Serious infections due to aerobic gram-positive cocci and the more susceptible anaerobes (NOT generally including *Bacteroides fragilis*, *Peptococcus* species and *Clostridium* species other than *Clostridium perfringens*):

600–1200 mg/day in 2, 3 or 4 equal doses.

More serious infections, particularly those due to proven or suspected *Bacteroides fragilis*, *Peptococcus* species, or *Clostridium* species other than *Clostridium perfringens*:

1200–2700 mg/day in 2, 3 or 4 equal doses.

For more serious infections, these doses may have to be increased. In life-threatening situations due to either aerobes or anaerobes these doses may be increased. Doses of as much as 4800 mg daily have been given intravenously to adults. See Dilution and Infusion Rates section below.

Single intramuscular injections of greater than 600 mg are not recommended.

Alternatively, drug may be administered in the form of a single rapid infusion of the first dose followed by continuous IV infusion as follows:

[See table at bottom of page]

Neonates (less than 1 month):

15 to 20 mg/kg/day in 3 to 4 equal doses. The lower dosage may be adequate for small prematures.

Pediatric patients 1 month of age to 16 years: Parenteral (IM or IV) administration: 20 to 40 mg/kg/day in 3 or 4 equal doses. The higher doses would be used for more severe infections. As an alternative to dosing on a body weight basis, children may be dosed on the basis of square meters body surface: 350 mg/m²/day for serious infections and 450 mg/m²/day for more severe infections.

Parenteral therapy may be changed to oral CLEOCIN PEDIATRIC® Flavored Granules (clindamycin palmitate hydrochloride) or CLEOCIN HCl® Capsules (clindamycin hydrochloride) when the condition warrants and at the discretion of the physician.

In cases of β-hemolytic streptococcal infections, treatment should be continued for at least 10 days.

Dilution and Infusion Rates: Clindamycin phosphate must be diluted prior to IV administration. The concentration of clindamycin in diluent for infusion should not exceed 18 mg per mL. Infusion rates should not exceed 30 mg per minute. The usual infusion dilutions and rates are as follows:

Dose	Diluent	Time
300 mg	50 mL	10 min
600 mg	50 mL	20 min
900 mg	50–100 mL	30 min
1200 mg	100 mL	40 min

Administration of more than 1200 mg in a single 1-hour infusion is not recommended.

Parenteral drug products should be inspected visually for particulate matter and discoloration prior to administration, whenever solution and container permit.

Dilution and Compatibility: Physical and biological compatibility studies monitored for 24 hours at room temperature have demonstrated no inactivation or incompatibility with the use of CLEOCIN PHOSPHATE Sterile Solution (clindamycin phosphate) in IV solutions containing sodium chloride, glucose, calcium or potassium, and solutions containing vitamin B complex in concentrations usually used clinically. No incompatibility has been demonstrated with the antibiotics cephalothin, kanamycin, gentamicin, penicillin or carbenicillin.

The following drugs are physically incompatible with clindamycin phosphate: ampicillin sodium, phenytoin sodium, barbiturates, aminophylline, calcium gluconate, and magnesium sulfate.

The compatibility and duration of stability of drug admixtures will vary depending on concentration and other conditions. For current information regarding compatibilities of clindamycin phosphate under specific conditions, please contact the Medical and Drug Information Unit, Pharmacia & Upjohn Company.

To maintain serum clindamycin levels	Rapid infusion rate	Maintenance infusion rate
Above 4 mcg/mL	10 mg/min for 30 min	0.75 mg/min
Above 5 mcg/mL	15 mg/min for 30 min	1.00 mg/min
Above 6 mcg/mL	20 mg/min for 30 min	1.25 mg/min

Physico-Chemical Stability of diluted solutions of CLEOCIN PHOSPHATE

Room temperature: 6, 9 and 12 mg/mL (equivalent to clindamycin base) in dextrose injection 5%, sodium chloride injection 0.9%, or Lactated Ringers Injection in glass bottles or minibags, demonstrated physical and chemical stability for at least 16 days at 25°C. Also, 18 mg/mL (equivalent to clindamycin base) in dextrose injection 5%, in minibags, demonstrated physical and chemical stability for at least 16 days at 25°C.

Refrigeration: 6, 9 and 12 mg/mL (equivalent to clindamycin base) in dextrose injection 5%, sodium chloride injection 0.9%, or Lactated Ringers Injection in glass bottles or minibags, demonstrated physical and chemical stability for at least 32 days at 4°C.

IMPORTANT: This chemical stability information in no way indicates that it would be acceptable practice to use this product well after the preparation time. Good professional practice suggests that compounded admixtures should be administered as soon after preparation as is feasible.

Frozen: 6, 9 and 12 mg/mL (equivalent to clindamycin base) in dextrose injection 5%, sodium chloride injection 0.9%, or Lactated Ringers Injection in minibags demonstrated physical and chemical stability for at least eight weeks at -10°C. Frozen solutions should be thawed at room temperature and not refrozen.

DIRECTIONS FOR DISPENSING

Pharmacy Bulk Package—Not for Direct Infusion

The Pharmacy Bulk Package is for use in a Pharmacy Admixture Service only under a laminar flow hood. Entry into the vial should be made with a small diameter sterile transfer set or other small diameter sterile dispensing device, and contents dispensed in aliquots using aseptic technique. Multiple entries with a needle and syringe are not recommended. AFTER ENTRY USE ENTIRE CONTENTS OF VIAL PROMPTLY. ANY UNUSED PORTION MUST BE DISCARDED WITHIN 24 HOURS AFTER INITIAL ENTRY.

DIRECTIONS FOR USE

CLEOCIN PHOSPHATE IV Solution in Galaxy Plastic Container

Premixed CLEOCIN PHOSPHATE IV Solution is for intravenous administration using sterile equipment. Check for minute leaks prior to use by squeezing bag firmly. If leaks are found, discard solution as sterility may be impaired. Do not add supplementary medication. Parenteral drug products should be inspected visually for particulate matter and discoloration prior to administration whenever solution and container permit. Do not use unless solution is clear and seal is intact.

Caution: Do not use plastic containers in series connections. Such use could result in air embolism due to residual air being drawn from the primary container before administration of the fluid from the secondary container is complete.

Preparation for Administration:
1. Suspend container from eyelet support.
2. Remove protector from outlet port at bottom of container.
3. Attach administration set. Refer to complete directions accompanying set.

Preparation of CLEOCIN PHOSPHATE in ADD-Vantage System—For IV Use Only. CLEOCIN PHOSPHATE 600 mg and 900 mg may be reconstituted in 50 mL or 100 mL, respectively, of Dextrose Injection 5% or Sodium Chloride Injection 0.9% in the ADD-diluent container. Refer to separate instructions for ADD-Vantage‡ System.

HOW SUPPLIED

Each mL of CLEOCIN PHOSPHATE Sterile Solution contains clindamycin phosphate equivalent to 150 mg clindamycin; 0.5 mg disodium edetate; 9.45 mg benzyl alcohol added as preservative. When necessary, pH is adjusted with sodium hydroxide and/or hydrochloric acid. CLEOCIN PHOSPHATE is available in the following packages:

25–2 mL vials	NDC 0009-0870-21
25–4 mL vials	NDC 0009-0775-26
25–6 mL vials	NDC 0009-0902-11
1–60 mL Pharmacy Bulk Package	NDC 0009-0728-05

CLEOCIN PHOSPHATE is supplied in ADD-Vantage vials as follows:

NDC	Vial Size	Total Clindamycin Phosphate/ vial	Amount of Diluent
0009-3124-01	4 mL	600 mg	50 mL
0009-3447-01	6 mL	900 mg	100 mL

Store at controlled room temperature 20° to 25°C (68° to 77°F) [see USP].

CLEOCIN PHOSPHATE IV Solution in Galaxy plastic containers is a sterile solution of clindamycin phosphate with 5% dextrose. The single dose Galaxy plastic containers are available as follows:

24-300 mg/50 mL containers	NDC 0009-3381-01
24-600 mg/50 mL containers	NDC 0009-3375-01
24-900 mg/50 mL containers	NDC 0009-3382-01

Exposure of pharmaceutical products to heat should be minimized. It is recommended that Galaxy plastic containers be stored at room temperature (25°C).

Avoid temperatures above 30°C.

Caution: Federal law prohibits dispensing without prescription.

Pharmacia & Upjohn Company • Kalamazoo, MI 49001, USA

Revised December 1997

810 020 033
691273

REFERENCES

1. Smith RB, Phillips JP: Evaluation of CLEOCIN HCl and CLEOCIN Phosphate in an Aged Population. Upjohn TR 8147-82-9122-021, December 1982.
2. Bauer AW, Kirby WMM, Sherris JC, Turck M; Antibiotic susceptibility testing by a standardized single disk method. *Am. J. Clin. Path.*, **45**:493–496, 1966. Standardized Disk Susceptibility Test, *Federal Register*, 37:20527–29, 1972.
3. National Committee for Clinical Lab. Standards. Methods for Antimicrobial Susceptibility Testing of Anaerobic Bacteria—Second Edition; Tentative Standard. NCCLS publication M11-T2. Villanova, PA; NCCLS; 1988.

‡ADD-Vantage is a registered trademark of Abbott Laboratories.

CLEOCIN PHOSPHATE IV Solution in the Galaxy plastic containers is manufactured for Pharmacia & Upjohn Company by Baxter Healthcare Corporation, Deerfield, IL 60015.

Galaxy® is a registered trademark of Baxter International, Inc.

CLEOCIN®
Vaginal Cream
clindamycin phosphate vaginal cream, USP
FOR INTRAVAGINAL USE ONLY
NOT FOR OPHTHALMIC, DERMAL, OR ORAL USE

℞

DESCRIPTION

Clindamycin phosphate is a water soluble ester of the semi-synthetic antibiotic produced by a 7(S)-chloro-substitution of the 7(R)-hydroxyl group of the parent antibiotic lincomycin. The chemical name for clindamycin phosphate is methyl 7-chloro-6,7,8-trideoxy-6-(1-methyl-*trans*-4-propyl-L-2-pyrrolidinecarboxamido)-1-thio-L-*threo*-α-D-*galacto*-octopyranoside 2-(dihydrogen phosphate). It has a molecular weight of 504.96, and the molecular formula is $C_{18}H_{34}ClN_2O_8PS$. The structural formula is represented below:

Cleocin Vaginal Cream 2%, is a semi-solid, white cream, which contains 2% clindamycin phosphate, USP, at a concentration equivalent to 20 mg clindamycin per gram. The pH of the cream is between 3.0 and 6.0. The cream also contains benzyl alcohol, cetostearyl alcohol, cetyl palmitate, mineral oil, polysorbate 60, propylene glycol, purified water, sorbitan monostearate, and stearic acid.

Each applicatorful of 5 grams of vaginal cream contains approximately 100 mg of clindamycin phosphate.

CLINICAL PHARMACOLOGY

Following a once a day intra vaginal dose of 100 mg of clindamycin phosphate vaginal cream 2%, administered to 6 healthy female volunteers for 7 days, approximately 5% (range 0.6% to 11%) of the administered dose was absorbed systemically. The peak serum clindamycin concentration observed on the first day averaged 18 ng/mL (range 4 to 47 ng/mL) and on day 7 it averaged 25 ng/mL (range 6 to 61 ng/mL). These peak concentrations were attained approximately 10 hours post-dosing (range 4–24 hours).

Following a once a day intravaginal dose of 100 mg of clindamycin phosphate vaginal cream 2%, administered for 7 consecutive days to 5 women with bacterial vaginosis, absorption was slower and less variable than that observed in healthy females. Approximately 5% (range 2% to 8%) of the dose was absorbed systemically. The peak serum clindamycin concentration observed on the first day averaged 13 ng/mL (range 6 to 34 ng/mL) and on day 7 it averaged 16 ng/mL (range 7 to 26 ng/mL). These peak concentrations were attained approximately 14 hours post-dosing (range 4–24 hours).
There was little or no systemic accumulation of clindamycin after repeated vaginal dosing of clindamycin phosphate vaginal cream 2%. The systemic half-life was 1.5 to 2.6 hours.

MICROBIOLOGY

Clindamycin inhibits bacterial protein synthesis at the level of the bacterial ribosome. The antibiotic binds preferentially to the 50S ribosomal subunit and affects the process of peptide chain initiation. Although clindamycin phosphate is inactive *in vitro,* rapid *in vivo* hydrolysis converts this compound to the antibacterially active clindamycin.
Culture and sensitivity testing of bacteria are not routinely performed to establish the diagnosis of bacterial vaginosis. (See INDICATIONS AND USAGE.) Standard methodology for the susceptibility testing of the potential bacterial vaginosis pathogens, *Gardnerella vaginalis, Mobiluncus* spp., or *Mycoplasma hominis,* has not been defined. Nonetheless, clindamycin is an antimicrobial agent active *in vitro* against most strains of the following organisms that have been reported to be associated with bacterial vaginosis:
Bacteroides spp.
Gardnerella vaginalis
Mobiluncus spp.
Mycoplasma hominis
Peptostreptococcus spp.

INDICATIONS AND USAGE

CLEOCIN Vaginal Cream 2%, is indicated in the treatment of bacterial vaginosis (formerly referred to as *Haemophilus* vaginitis, *Gardnerella* vaginitis, nonspecific vaginitis, *Corynebacterium* vaginitis, or anaerobic vaginosis). CLEOCIN Vaginal Cream 2%, can be used to treat non-pregnant women and pregnant women during the second and third trimester. (See CLINICAL STUDIES.)
NOTE: For purposes of this indication, a clinical diagnosis of bacterial vaginosis is usually defined by the presence of a homogeneous vaginal discharge that (a) has a pH of greater than 4.5, (b) emits a "fishy" amine odor when mixed with a 10% KOH solution, and (c) contains clue cells on microscopic examination. Gram's stain results consistent with a diagnosis of bacterial vaginosis include (a) markedly reduced or absent *Lactobacillus* morphology, (b) predominance of *Gardnerella* morphotype, and (c) absent or few white blood cells. Other pathogens commonly associated with vulvovaginitis, eg, *Trichomonas vaginalis, Chlamydia trachomatis, N. gonorrhoeae, Candida albicans,* and *Herpes simplex* virus should be ruled out.

CONTRAINDICATIONS

CLEOCIN Vaginal Cream 2%, is contraindicated in individuals with a history of hypersensitivity to clindamycin, lincomycin, or any of the components of this vaginal cream. CLEOCIN Vaginal Cream 2%, is also contraindicated in individuals with a history of regional enteritis, ulcerative colitis, or a history of "antibiotic-associated" colitis.

WARNINGS

Pseudomembranous colitis has been reported with nearly all antibacterial agents, including clindamycin, and may range in severity from mild to life-threatening. Orally and parenterally administered clindamycin has been associated with severe colitis which may end fatally. Diarrhea, bloody diarrhea, and colitis (including pseudomembranous colitis) have been reported with the use of orally and parenterally administered clindamycin, as well as with topical (dermal) formulations of clindamycin. Therefore, it is important to consider this diagnosis in patients who present with diarrhea subsequent to the administration of clindamycin, even when administered by the vaginal route, because approximately 5% of the clindamycin dose is systemically absorbed from the vagina.
Treatment with antibacterial agents alters the normal flora of the colon and may permit overgrowth of clostridia. Studies indicate that a toxin produced by *Clostridium difficile* is a primary cause of "antibiotic-associated" colitis.
After the diagnosis of pseudomembranous colitis has been established, therapeutic measures should be initiated. Mild cases of pseudomembranous colitis usually respond to discontinuation of the drug alone. In moderate to severe cases, consideration should be given to management with fluids and electrolytes, protein supplementation, and treatment with an antibacterial drug clinically effective against *Clostridium difficile* colitis.
Onset of pseudomembranous colitis symptoms may occur during or after antimicrobial treatment.

PRECAUTIONS

General

CLEOCIN Vaginal Cream 2%, contains ingredients that will cause burning and irritation of the eye. In the event of accidental contact with the eye, rinse the eye with copious amounts of cool tap water.
The use of CLEOCIN Vaginal Cream 2% may result in the overgrowth of nonsusceptible organisms in the vagina. In clinical studies involving 600 non-pregnant women who received treatment for 3 days, *Candida albicans* was detected, either symptomatically or by culture, in 8.8% of patients. In 9% of the patients, vaginitis was recorded. In clinical studies involving 1325 non-pregnant women who received treatment for 7 days, *Candida albicans* was detected, either symptomatically or by culture, in 10.5% of patients. Vaginitis was recorded in 10.7% of the patients. In 180 pregnant women who received treatment for 7 days, *Candida albicans* was detected, either symptomatically or by culture, in 13.3% of patients. In 7.2% of the patients, vaginitis was recorded. *Candida albicans,* as reported here, includes the terms: vaginal moniliasis and moniliasis (body as a whole). Vaginitis includes the terms: vulvovaginal disorder, vulvovaginitis, vaginal discharge, trichomonal vaginitis, and vaginitis.

Information for the Patient:

The patient should be instructed not to engage in vaginal intercourse, or use other vaginal products (such as tampons or douches) during treatment with this product.
The patient should also be advised that this cream contains mineral oil that may weaken latex or rubber products such as condoms or vaginal contraceptive diaphragms. Therefore, use of such products within 72 hours following treatment with CLEOCIN Vaginal Cream 2%, is not recommended.

Drug Interactions

Clindamycin has been shown to have neuromuscular blocking properties that may enhance the action of other neuromuscular blocking agents. Therefore, it should be used with caution in patients receiving such agents.

Carcinogenesis, Mutagenesis, Impairment of Fertility

Long term studies in animals have not been performed with clindamycin to evaluate carcinogenic potential. Genotoxicity tests performed included a rat micronucleus test and an Ames test. Both tests were negative. Fertility studies in rats treated orally with up to 300 mg/kg/day (31 times the human exposure based on mg/m^2) revealed no effects on fertility or mating ability.

Pregnancy: Teratogenic effects

Pregnancy Category B
There are no adequate and well-controlled studies in pregnant women during the first trimester of pregnancy. This drug should be used during the first trimester of pregnancy only if clearly needed.
CLEOCIN Vaginal Cream 2% has been studied in pregnant women during the second trimester. In women treated for seven days, abnormal labor was reported in 1.1% of patients who received clindamycin vaginal cream 2% compared with 0.5% of patients who received placebo.
Reproduction studies have been performed in rats and mice using oral and parenteral doses of clindamycin up to 600 mg/kg/day (62 and 25 times, respectively, the maximum human exposure based on mg/m^2) and have revealed no evidence of harm to the fetus due to clindamycin. In one mouse strain, cleft palates were observed in treated fetuses; this outcome was not produced in other mouse strains or in other species and is, therefore, considered to be a strain specific effect.
See INDICATIONS AND USAGE; PRECAUTIONS, General; and ADVERSE REACTIONS.

Nursing Mothers

Clindamycin has been detected in human milk after oral or parenteral administration. It is not known if clindamycin is excreted in human milk following the use of vaginally administered clindamycin phosphate.
Because of the potential for serious adverse reactions in nursing infants from clindamycin phosphate, a decision should be made whether to discontinue nursing or to discontinue the drug, taking into account the importance of the drug to the mother.

Pediatric Use

Safety and effectiveness in pediatric patients have not been established.

ADVERSE REACTIONS

Clinical trials

Non-pregnant Women: In clinical trials involving non-pregnant women, 1.8% of 600 patients who received treatment with CLEOCIN Vaginal Cream 2% for 3 days and 2.7% of 1325 patients who received treatment for 7 days discontinued therapy due to drug-related adverse events. Medical events judged to be related, probably related, possibly related, or of unknown relationship to vaginally administered clindamycin phosphate vaginal cream 2%, were reported for 20.7% of the patients receiving treatment for 3 days and 21.3% of the patients receiving treatment for 7 days. Events occurring in ≥1% of patients receiving clindamycin phosphate vaginal cream 2% are shown in Table 1.

TABLE 1—Events Occurring in ≥1% of Non-pregnant Patients Receiving Clindamycin Phosphate Vaginal Cream 2%

	CLEOCIN Vaginal Cream	
Event	3 Day n=600	7 Day n=1325
Urogenital		
Vaginal moniliasis	7.7	10.4
Vulvovaginitis	6.0	4.4
Vulvovaginal disorder	3.2	5.3
Trichomonal vaginitis	0	1.3
Body as a Whole		
Moniliasis (body)	1.3	0.2

Other events occurring in <1% of the clindamycin vaginal cream 2% groups include:
Urogenital system: vaginal discharge, metrorrhagia, urinary tract infection, endometriosis, menstrual disorder, vaginitis/vaginal infection, and vaginal pain.
Body as a whole: localized abdominal pain, generalized abdominal pain, abdominal cramps, halitosis, headache, bacterial infection, inflammatory swelling, allergic reaction, and fungal infection.
Digestive system: nausea, vomiting, constipation, dyspepsia, flatulence, diarrhea, and gastrointestinal disorder.
Endocrine system: hyperthyroidism.
Central nervous system: dizziness and vertigo.
Respiratory system: epistaxis.
Skin: pruritus (non-application site), moniliasis, rash, maculopapular rash, erythema, and urticaria.
Special senses: taste perversion.
Pregnant Women: In a clinical trial involving pregnant women during the second trimester, 1.7% of 180 patients who received treatment for 7 days discontinued therapy due to drug-related adverse events. Medical events judged to be related, probably related, possibly related, or of unknown relationship to vaginally administered clindamycin phosphate vaginal cream 2%, were reported for 22.8% of pregnant patients. Events occurring in ≥ 1% of patients receiving either clindamycin phosphate vaginal cream 2% or placebo are shown in Table 2.

TABLE 2—Events Occurring in ≥1% of Pregnant Patients Receiving Clindamycin Phosphate Vaginal Cream 2% or Placebo

Event	CLEOCIN Vaginal Cream 7 Day n=180	Placebo 7 Day n=184
Urogenital		
Vaginal moniliasis	13.3	7.1
Vulvovaginal disorder	6.7	7.1
Abnormal labor	1.1	0.5
Body as a Whole		
Fungal infection	1.7	0
Skin		
Pruritus, non-application site	1.1	0

Other events occurring in <1% of the clindamycin vaginal cream 2% group include:
Urogenital system: dysuria, metrorrhagia, vaginal pain, and trichomonal vaginitis.
Body as a whole: upper respiratory infection.
Skin: pruritus (topical application site) and erythema.
Other clindamycin formulations: Clindamycin vaginal cream affords minimal peak serum levels and systemic exposure (AUCs) of clindamycin compared to 100 mg oral clindamycin dosing. Although these lower levels of exposure are less likely to produce the common reactions seen with oral clindamycin, the possibility of these and other reactions cannot be excluded presently. Data from well-controlled trials directly comparing clindamycin administered orally to clindamycin administered vaginally are not available.

Continued on next page

Information on these Pharmacia & Upjohn products is based on labeling in effect June 1, 1998. Further information concerning these and other Pharmacia & Upjohn products may be obtained by direct inquiry to Medical Information, Pharmacia & Upjohn, Kalamazoo, MI 49001.

Cleocin Vaginal Cream—Cont.

The following adverse reactions and altered laboratory tests have been reported with the **oral or parenteral** use of clindamycin:

Gastrointestinal: Abdominal pain, esophagitis, nausea, vomiting, and diarrhea. (See WARNINGS.)

Hematopoietic: Transient neutropenia (leukopenia), eosinophilia, agranulocytosis, and thrombocytopenia have been reported. No direct etiologic relationship to concurrent clindamycin therapy could be made in any of these reports.

Hypersensitivity Reactions: Maculopapular rash and urticaria have been observed during drug therapy. Generalized mild to moderate morbilliform-like skin rashes are the most frequently reported of all adverse reactions. Rare instances of erythema multiforme, some resembling Stevens-Johnson syndrome, have been associated with clindamycin. A few cases of anaphylactoid reactions have been reported. If a hypersensitivity reaction occurs, the drug should be discontinued.

Liver: Jaundice and abnormalities in liver function tests have been observed during clindamycin therapy.

Musculoskeletal: Rare instances of polyarthritis have been reported.

Renal: Although no direct relationship of clindamycin to renal damage has been established, renal dysfunction as evidenced by azotemia, oliguria, and/or proteinuria has been observed in rare instances.

OVERDOSAGE

Vaginally applied clindamycin phosphate vaginal cream 2% could be absorbed in sufficient amounts to produce systemic effects. (See WARNINGS.)

DOSAGE AND ADMINISTRATION

The recommended dose is one applicatorful of clindamycin phosphate vaginal cream 2%, (5 grams containing approximately 100 mg of clindamycin phosphate) intravaginally, preferably at bedtime, for 3 or 7 consecutive days in nonpregnant patients and for 7 consecutive days in pregnant patients. (See CLINICAL STUDIES.)

HOW SUPPLIED

CLEOCIN Vaginal Cream 2%, (clindamycin phosphate vaginal cream) is supplied as follows:

21 g tube
(with 3 disposable applicators)   NDC 0009-3448-04
40 g tube
(with 7 disposable applicators)   NDC 0009-3448-01
Store at controlled room temperature 20° to 25°C (68° to 77°F) [see USP]. Protect from freezing.

CLINICAL STUDIES

In two clinical studies involving 674 evaluable non-pregnant women with bacterial vaginosis comparing CLEOCIN Vaginal Cream 2% for 3 or 7 days, the clinical cure rates, determined at 1 month posttherapy, ranged from 72% to 81% for the 3-day treatment and 84% to 86% for the 7-day treatment.

	CLEOCIN 3 Day		CLEOCIN 7 Day	
US Study	94/131	72%	110/128	86%
European Study	161/199	81%	181/216	84%

In a clinical study involving 249 evaluable pregnant patients in the second and third trimester treated for 7 days, the clinical cure rate, determined at 1 month posttherapy, was 60% (77/129) in the clindamycin arm and 9% (11/120) for the vehicle arm. The determination of clinical cure was based on the absence of a "fishy" amine odor when the vaginal discharge was mixed with a 10% KOH solution and the absence of clue cells on microscopic examination.

Rx only

Pharmacia & Upjohn Company
Kalamazoo, Michigan 49001, USA
Revised March 1998
          815 255 405
          692116

DIRECTIONS FOR USE

Disposable plastic applicators are provided with this package. They are designed to allow proper vaginal administration of the cream.
Remove cap from cream tube. Screw a plastic applicator on the threaded end of the tube.
Rolling tube from the bottom, squeeze gently and force the medication into the applicator. The applicator is filled when the plunger reaches its predetermined stopping point.
Unscrew the applicator from the tube and replace the cap.

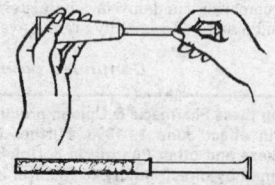

While lying on your back, firmly grasp the applicator barrel and insert into vagina as far as possible without causing discomfort.
Slowly push the plunger until it stops.
Carefully withdraw applicator from vagina, and discard applicator.

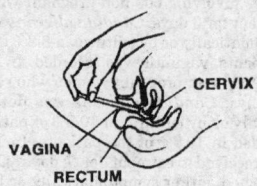

REMEMBER TO APPLY ONE APPLICATORFUL EACH NIGHT BEFORE BEDTIME, OR AS PRESCRIBED BY YOUR DOCTOR.

CLEOCIN T®   ℞
[klē̄o-sin]

Topical Solution, Topical Gel, Topical Lotion
clindamycin phosphate topical solution, USP, topical gel, and topical lotion
For External Use

DESCRIPTION

CLEOCIN T Topical Solution and CLEOCIN T Topical Lotion contain clindamycin phosphate, USP, at a concentration equivalent to 10 mg clindamycin per milliliter. CLEOCIN T Topical Gel contains clindamycin phosphate, USP, at a concentration equivalent to 10 mg clindamycin per gram. Each CLEOCIN T Topical Solution pledget applicator contains approximately 1 mL of topical solution.
Clindamycin phosphate is a water soluble ester of the semisynthetic antibiotic produced by a 7(S)-chloro-substitution of the 7(R)-hydroxyl group of the parent antibiotic lincomycin.
The solution contains isopropyl alcohol 50% v/v, propylene glycol, and water.
The gel contains allantoin, carbomer 934P, methylparaben, polyethylene glycol 400, propylene glycol, sodium hydroxide, and purified water.
The lotion contains cetostearyl alcohol (2.5%); glycerin; glyceryl stearate SE (with potassium monostearate); isostearyl alcohol (2.5%); methylparaben (0.3%); sodium lauroyl sarcosinate; stearic acid; and purified water.
The structural formula is represented below:

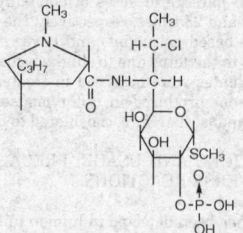

The chemical name for clindamycin phosphate is Methyl 7-chloro-6,7,8-trideoxy-6-(1-methyl-*trans*-4-propyl-L-2-pyrrolidinecarboxamido)-1-thio-L-*threo*-α-D-*galacto*-octopyranoside 2-(dihydrogen phosphate).

CLINICAL PHARMACOLOGY

Although clindamycin phosphate is inactive *in vitro*, rapid *in vivo* hydrolysis converts this compound to the antibacterially active clindamycin.
Cross resistance has been demonstrated between clindamycin and lincomycin.
Antagonism has been demonstrated between clindamycin and erythromycin.
Following multiple topical applications of clindamycin phosphate at a concentration equivalent to 10 mg clindamycin per mL in an isopropyl alcohol and water solution, very low levels of clindamycin are present in the serum (0–3 ng/mL) and less than 0.2% of the dose is recovered in urine as clindamycin.
Clindamycin activity has been demonstrated in comedones from acne patients. The mean concentration of antibiotic activity in extracted comedones after application of CLEOCIN T Topical Solution for 4 weeks was 597 mcg/g of comedonal material (range 0–1490). Clindamycin *in vitro* inhibits all

Propionibacterium acnes cultures tested (MICs 0.4 mcg/mL). Free fatty acids on the skin surface have been decreased from approximately 14% to 2% following application of clindamycin.

INDICATIONS AND USAGE

CLEOCIN T Topical Solution, CLEOCIN T Topical Gel and CLEOCIN T Topical Lotion are indicated in the treatment of acne vulgaris. In view of the potential for diarrhea, bloody diarrhea and pseudomembranous colitis, the physician should consider whether other agents are more appropriate. (See CONTRAINDICATIONS, WARNINGS and ADVERSE REACTIONS.)

CONTRAINDICATIONS

CLEOCIN T Topical Solution, CLEOCIN T Topical Gel and CLEOCIN T Topical Lotion are contraindicated in individuals with a history of hypersensitivity to preparations containing clindamycin or lincomycin, a history of regional enteritis or ulcerative colitis, or a history of antibiotic-associated colitis.

WARNINGS

Orally and parenterally administered clindamycin has been associated with severe colitis which may result in patient death. Use of the topical formulation of clindamycin results in absorption of the antibiotic from the skin surface. Diarrhea, bloody diarrhea, and colitis (including pseudomembranous colitis) have been reported with the use of topical and systemic clindamycin.

Studies indicate a toxin(s) produced by clostridia is one primary cause of antibiotic-associated colitis. The colitis is usually characterized by severe persistent diarrhea and severe abdominal cramps and may be associated with the passage of blood and mucus. Endoscopic examination may reveal pseudomembranous colitis. Stool culture for *Clostridium difficile* and stool assay for *C. difficile* toxin may be helpful diagnostically.

When significant diarrhea occurs, the drug should be discontinued. Large bowel endoscopy should be considered to establish a definitive diagnosis in cases of severe diarrhea.

Antiperistaltic agents such as opiates and diphenoxylate with atropine may prolong and/or worsen the condition. Vancomycin has been found to be effective in the treatment of antibiotic-associated pseudomembranous colitis produced by *Clostridium difficile*. The usual adult dosage is 500 milligrams to 2 grams of vancomycin orally per day in three to four divided doses administered for 7 to 10 days. Cholestyramine or colestipol resins bind vancomycin *in vitro*. If both a resin and vancomycin are to be administered concurrently, it may be advisable to separate the time of administration of each drug.

Diarrhea, colitis, and pseudomembranous colitis have been observed to begin up to several weeks following cessation of oral and parenteral therapy with clindamycin.

PRECAUTIONS

General
CLEOCIN T Topical Solution contains an alcohol base which will cause burning and irritation of the eye. In the event of accidental contact with sensitive surfaces (eye, abraded skin, mucous membranes), bathe with copious amounts of cool tap water. The solution has an unpleasant taste and caution should be exercised when applying medication around the mouth.
CLEOCIN T should be prescribed with caution in atopic individuals.

Drug Interactions
Clindamycin has been shown to have neuromuscular blocking properties that may enhance the action of other neuromuscular blocking agents. Therefore it should be used with caution in patients receiving such agents.

Pregnancy: Teratogenic effects—Pregnancy Category B
Reproduction studies have been performed in rats and mice using subcutaneous and oral doses of clindamycin ranging from 100 to 600 mg/kg/day and have revealed no evidence of impaired fertility or harm to the fetus due to clindamycin. There are, however, no adequate and well-controlled studies in pregnant women. Because animal reproduction studies are not always predictive of human response, this drug should be used during pregnancy only if clearly needed.

Nursing Mothers
It is not known whether clindamycin is excreted in human milk following use of CLEOCIN T. However, orally and parenterally administered clindamycin has been reported to appear in breast milk. Because of the potential for serious adverse reactions in nursing infants, a decision should be made whether to discontinue nursing or to discontinue the drug, taking into account the importance of the drug to the mother.

Pediatric Use
Safety and effectiveness in pediatric patients under the age of 12 have not been established.

ADVERSE REACTIONS

In 18 clinical studies of various formulations of CLEOCIN T using placebo vehicle and/or active comparator drugs as controls, patients experienced a number of treatment emergent adverse dermatologic events [see table below].

Number of Patients Reporting Events

Treatment Emergent Adverse Event	Solution n=553 (%)	Gel n=148 (%)	Lotion n=160 (%)
Burning	62 (11)	15 (10)	17 (11)
Itching	36 (7)	15 (10)	17 (11)
Burning/Itching	60 (11)	# (—)	# (—)
Dryness	105 (19)	34 (23)	29 (18)
Erythema	86 (16)	10 (7)	22 (14)
Oiliness/Oily Skin	8 (1)	26 (18)	12* (10)
Peeling	61 (11)	# (—)	11 (7)

not recorded
* of 126 subjects

Orally and parenterally administered clindamycin has been associated with severe colitis which may end fatally.
Cases of diarrhea, bloody diarrhea and colitis (including pseudomembranous colitis) have been reported as adverse reactions in patients treated with oral and parenteral formulations of clindamycin and rarely with topical clindamycin (see WARNINGS).
Abdominal pain and gastrointestinal disturbances as well as gram-negative folliculitis have also been reported in association with the use of topical formulations of clindamycin.

OVERDOSAGE

Topically applied CLEOCIN T can be absorbed in sufficient amounts to produce systemic effects. (See WARNINGS.)

DOSAGE AND ADMINISTRATION

Apply a thin film of CLEOCIN T Topical Solution, CLEOCIN T Topical Lotion, CLEOCIN T Topical Gel, or use a CLEOCIN T Topical Solution pledget for the application of CLEOCIN T twice daily to affected area. More than one pledget may be used. Each pledget should be used only once and then be discarded.
Lotion: Shake well immediately before using.
Pledget: Remove pledget from foil just before use. Do not use if the seal is broken. Discard after single use.
Keep all liquid dosage forms in containers tightly closed.

HOW SUPPLIED

CLEOCIN T Topical Solution containing clindamycin phosphate equivalent to 10 mg clindamycin per milliliter is available in the following sizes:
30 mL applicator bottle—NDC 0009-3116-01
60 mL applicator bottle—NDC 0009-3116-02
Carton of 60 single-use pledget applicators—NDC 0009-3116-14
CLEOCIN T Topical Gel containing clindamycin phosphate equivalent to 10 mg clindamycin per gram is available in the following sizes:
60 gram tube—NDC 0009-3331-01
30 gram tube—NDC 0009-3331-02
CLEOCIN T Topical Lotion containing clindamycin phosphate equivalent to 10 mg clindamycin per milliliter is available in the following size:
60 mL plastic squeeze bottle—NDC 0009-3329-01
Store at controlled room temperature 20° to 25° C (68° to 77° F) [see USP].
Protect from freezing.
CAUTION
Federal law prohibits dispensing without prescription.
Pharmacia & Upjohn Company, Kalamazoo, MI 49001, USA
Revised February 1998   811 373 428
                                     691223
Shown in Product Identification Guide, pages 331 and 332

COLESTID® ℞
[kō-less-tid]
micronized colestipol hydrochloride tablets

DESCRIPTION

The active ingredient in COLESTID Tablets is micronized colestipol hydrochloride, which is a lipid lowering agent for oral use. Colestipol is an insoluble, high molecular weight basic anion-exchange copolymer of diethylenetriamine and 1-chloro-2, 3-epoxypropane, with approximately 1 out of 5 amine nitrogens protonated (chloride form). It is a light yellow water-insoluble resin which is hygroscopic and swells when suspended in water or aqueous fluids.
Each COLESTID Tablet contains one gram of micronized colestipol hydrochloride. COLESTID Tablets are light yellow in color and are tasteless and odorless. Inactive ingredients: cellulose acetate phthalate, glyceryl triacetate, car-

nauba wax, hydroxypropyl methylcellulose, magnesium stearate, povidone, silicon dioxide. COLESTID Tablets contain no calories.

HOW SUPPLIED

COLESTID Tablets are yellow, elliptical, imprinted U, and are supplied as follows:
Bottles of 120   NDC 0009-0450-03
Bottles of 500   NDC 0009-0450-04
Each tablet contains 1 gram of colestipol hydrochloride.
Store at controlled room temperature 20° to 25° C (68° to 77° F) [see USP].
Caution: Federal law prohibits dispensing without prescription.
Pharmacia & Upjohn Company
Kalamazoo, MI 49001, USA
Revised November 1997   815 838 104
                                     692166

COLESTID® ℞
[kō-less-tid]
FLAVORED COLESTID®
colestipol hydrochloride for oral suspension

DESCRIPTION

COLESTID Granules and FLAVORED COLESTID Granules contain colestipol hydrochloride, which is a lipid lowering agent for oral use. Colestipol hydrochloride is an insoluble, high molecular weight basic anion-exchange copolymer of diethylenetriamine and 1-chloro-2, 3-epoxypropane, with approximately 1 out of 5 amine nitrogens protonated (chloride form). It is a light yellow water-insoluble resin which is hygroscopic and swells when suspended in water or aqueous fluids.
COLESTID is tasteless and odorless. Inactive ingredient: silicon dioxide. One dose (1 packet or 1 level teaspoon) of COLESTID contains 5 grams of colestipol hydrochloride.
FLAVORED COLESTID is orange flavored and light orange in color. One dose (1 packet or 1 level scoopful) of FLAVORED COLESTID is approximately 7.5 grams which contains 5 grams of colestipol hydrochloride. This product also contains the following inactive ingredients: aspartame, beta carotene, citric acid, flavor (natural and artificial), glycerine, maltol, mannitol, and methylcellulose.

CLINICAL PHARMACOLOGY

Cholesterol is the major, and probably the sole precursor of bile acids. During normal digestion, bile acids are secreted via the bile from the liver and gall bladder into the intestines. Bile acids emulsify the fat and lipid materials present in food, thus facilitating absorption. A major portion of the bile acids secreted is reabsorbed from the intestines and returned via the portal circulation to the liver, thus completing the enterohepatic cycle. Only very small amounts of bile acids are found in normal serum.
Colestipol hydrochloride binds bile acids in the intestine forming a complex that is excreted in the feces. This nonsystemic action results in a partial removal of the bile acids from the enterohepatic circulation, preventing their reabsorption. Since colestipol hydrochloride is an anion exchange resin, the chloride anions of the resin can be replaced by other anions, usually those with a greater affinity for the resin than chloride ion.
Colestipol hydrochloride is hydrophilic, but it is virtually water insoluble (99.75%) and it is not hydrolyzed by digestive enzymes. The high molecular weight polymer in colestipol hydrochloride apparently is not absorbed. In humans, less than 0.17% of a single ^{14}C-labeled colestipol hydrochloride dose is excreted in the urine when given following 60 days of chronic dosing of 20 grams of colestipol hydrochloride per day.
The increased fecal loss of bile acids due to colestipol hydrochloride administration leads to an increased oxidation of cholesterol to bile acids. This results in an increase in the number of low-density lipoprotein (LDL) receptors, increased hepatic uptake of LDL and a decrease in beta lipoprotein or low density lipoprotein serum levels, and a decrease in serum cholesterol levels. Although colestipol hydrochloride produces an increase in the hepatic synthesis of cholesterol in man, serum cholesterol levels fall.
There is evidence to show that this fall in cholesterol is secondary to an increased rate of clearance of cholesterol-rich lipoproteins (beta or low density lipoproteins) from the plasma. Serum triglyceride levels may increase or remain unchanged in colestipol hydrochloride treated patients.
The decline in serum cholesterol levels with colestipol hydrochloride treatment is usually evident by one month. When colestipol hydrochloride is discontinued, serum cholesterol levels usually return to baseline levels within one month. Periodic determinations of serum cholesterol levels

as outlined in the National Cholesterol Education Program (NCEP) guidelines should be done to confirm a favorable initial and long-term response[1].
In a large, placebo-controlled, multiclinic study, the LRC-CPPT,[2] hypercholesterolemic subjects treated with cholestyramine, a bile-acid sequestrant with a mechanism of action and an effect on serum cholesterol similar to that of colestipol hydrochloride, had reductions in total and low-density lipoprotein cholesterol (LDL-C). Over the seven-year study period the cholestyramine group experienced a 19% reduction (relative to the incidence in the placebo group) in the combined rate of coronary heart disease death plus non-fatal myocardial infarction (cumulative incidences of 7% cholestyramine and 8.6%, placebo). The subjects included in the study were middle-aged men (age 35–59) with serum cholesterol-levels above 265 mg/dL, LDL-C above 175 mg/dL on a moderate cholesterol-lowering diet, and no history of heart disease. It is not clear to what extent these findings can be extrapolated to other segments of the hypercholesterolemic population not studied.
Treatment with colestipol hydrochloride results in a significant increase in lipoprotein LpAI. Lipoprotein LpAI is one of the two major lipoprotein particles within the high-density lipoprotein (HDL) density range[3], and has been shown in cell culture to promote cholesterol efflux or removal from cells[4]. Although the significance of this finding has not been established in clinical studies, the elevation of the lipoprotein LpAI particle within the HDL fraction is consistent with an antiatherogenic effect of colestipol hydrochloride, even though little change is observed in HDL cholesterol.
In patients with heterozygous familial hypercholesterolemia who have not obtained an optimal response to colestipol hydrochloride alone in maximal doses, the combination of colestipol hydrochloride and nicotinic acid has been shown to further lower serum cholesterol, triglyceride, and LDL cholesterol (LDL-C) values. Simultaneously, HDL cholesterol (HDL-C) values increased significantly. In many such patients it is possible to normalize serum lipid values.[5-7]
Preliminary evidence suggests that the cholesterol-lowering effects of lovastatin and the bile acid sequestrant, colestipol hydrochloride, are additive.
The effect of intensive lipid-lowering therapy on coronary atherosclerosis has been assessed by arteriography in hyperlipidemic patients. In these randomized, controlled clinical trials, patients were treated for two to four years by either conventional measures (diet, placebo, or in some cases low-dose resin), or with intensive combination therapy using diet and COLESTID Granules plus either nicotinic acid or lovastatin. When compared to conventional measures, intensive lipid-lowering combination therapy significantly reduced the frequency of progression and increased the frequency of regression of coronary atherosclerotic lesions in patients with or at risk for coronary artery disease.[8-11]

INDICATIONS AND USAGE

Since no drug is innocuous, strict attention should be paid to the indications and contraindications, particularly when selecting drugs for chronic long-term use.
COLESTID Granules and FLAVORED COLESTID Granules are indicated as adjunctive therapy to diet for the reduction of elevated serum total and low-density lipoprotein (LDL) cholesterol in patients with primary hypercholesterolemia (elevated low density lipoproteins [LDL] cholesterol) who do not respond adequately to diet. Generally, COLESTID and FLAVORED COLESTID have no clinically significant effect on serum triglycerides, but with its use triglyceride levels may be raised in some patients.
Therapy with lipid-altering agents should be a component of multiple risk factor intervention in those individuals at significantly increased risk for atherosclerotic vascular disease due to hypercholesterolemia. Treatment should begin and continue with dietary therapy (see NCEP guidelines). A minimum of six months of intensive dietary therapy and counseling should be carried out prior to initiation of drug therapy. Shorter periods may be considered in patients with severe elevations of LDL-C or with definite CHD.
According to the NCEP guidelines, the goal of treatment is to lower LDL-C, and LDL-C is to be used to initiate and assess treatment response. Only if LDL-C levels are not available, should the Total-C be used to monitor therapy. The NCEP treatment guidelines are shown below.

Continued on next page

Information on these Pharmacia & Upjohn products is based on labeling in effect June 1, 1998. Further information concerning these and other Pharmacia & Upjohn products may be obtained by direct inquiry to Medical Information, Pharmacia & Upjohn, Kalamazoo, MI 49001.

Consult 1999 PDR® supplements and future editions for revisions

Colestid Granules—Cont.

		LDL-Cholesterol mg/dL (mmol/L)	
Definite Atherosclerotic Disease*	Two or More Other Risk Factors**	Initiation Level	Goal
No	No	≥190 (≥4.9)	<160 (<4.1)
No	Yes	≥160 (≥4.1)	<130 (<3.4)
Yes	Yes or No	≥130 (≥3.4)	≤100 (≤2.6)

*Coronary heart disease or peripheral vascular disease (including symptomatic carotid artery disease).

**Other risk factors for coronary heart disease (CHD) include: age (males: ≥45 years; females: ≥55 years or premature menopause without estrogen replacement therapy); family history of premature CHD; current cigarette smoking; hypertension; confirmed HDL-C <35 mg/dL (0.91 mmol/L); and diabetes mellitus. Subtract one risk factor if HDL-C is ≥60 mg/dL (1.6 mmol/L).

CONTRAINDICATIONS

COLESTID Granules and FLAVORED COLESTID Granules are contraindicated in those individuals who have shown hypersensitivity to any of its components.

WARNINGS

TO AVOID ACCIDENTAL INHALATION OR ESOPHAGEAL DISTRESS, *COLESTID GRANULES* AND *FLAVORED COLESTID GRANULES* SHOULD NOT BE TAKEN IN ITS DRY FORM. ALWAYS MIX *COLESTID* AND *FLAVORED COLESTID* WITH WATER OR OTHER FLUIDS BEFORE INGESTING.
PHENYLKETONURICS: *FLAVORED COLESTID* CONTAINS 18.2 MG PHENYLALANINE PER 7.5-GRAM DOSE.

PRECAUTIONS

Prior to initiating therapy with COLESTID Granules and FLAVORED COLESTID Granules, secondary causes of hypercholesterolemia (e.g., poorly controlled diabetes mellitus, hypothyroidism, nephrotic syndrome, dysproteinemias, obstructive liver disease, other drug therapy, alcoholism), should be excluded, and a lipid profile performed to assess Total cholesterol, HDL-C, and triglycerides (TG). For individuals with TG less than 400 mg/dL (<4.5 mmol/L), LDL-C can be estimated using the following equation:

LDL-C = Total cholesterol-[(Triglycerides/5)+HDL-C]

For TG levels >400 mg/dL, this equation is less accurate and LDL-C concentrations should be determined by ultracentrifugation. In hypertriglyceridemic patients, LDL-C may be low or normal despite elevated Total-C. In such cases COLESTID and FLAVORED COLESTID may not be indicated.

Because it sequesters bile acids, colestipol hydrochloride may interfere with normal fat absorption and thus may reduce absorption of folic acid and fat soluble vitamins such as A, D, and K.

Chronic use of colestipol hydrochloride may be associated with an increased bleeding tendency due to hypoprothrombinemia from vitamin K deficiency. This will usually respond promptly to parenteral vitamin K$_1$ and recurrences can be prevented by oral administration of vitamin K$_1$.

Serum cholesterol and triglyceride levels should be determined periodically based on NCEP guidelines to confirm a favorable initial and adequate long-term response.

COLESTID and FLAVORED COLESTID may produce or severely worsen pre-existing constipation. The dosage should be increased gradually in patients to minimize the risk of developing fecal impaction. In patients with pre-existing constipation, the starting dose should be 1 packet or 1 scoop once daily for 5–7 days, increasing to twice daily with monitoring of constipation and of serum lipoproteins, at least twice, 4–6 weeks apart. Increased fluid and fiber intake should be encouraged to alleviate constipation and a stool softener may occasionally be indicated. If the initial dose is well tolerated, the dose may be increased as needed by one dose/day (at monthly intervals) with periodic monitoring of serum lipoproteins. If constipation worsens or the desired therapeutic response is not achieved at one to six doses/day, combination therapy or alternate therapy should be considered. Particular effort should be made to avoid constipation in patients with symptomatic coronary artery disease. Constipation associated with COLESTID and FLAVORED COLESTID may aggravate hemorrhoids.

While there have been no reports of hypothyroidism induced in individuals with normal thyroid function, the theoretical possibility exists, particularly in patients with limited thyroid reserve.

Since colestipol hydrochloride is a chloride form of an anion exchange resin, there is a possibility that prolonged use may lead to the development of hyperchloremic acidosis.

Carcinogenesis, mutagenesis and impairment of fertility
In studies conducted in rats in which cholestyramine resin (a bile acid sequestering agent similar to colestipol hydrochloride) was used as a tool to investigate the role of various intestinal factors, such as fat, bile salts and microbial flora, in the development of intestinal tumors induced by potent carcinogens, the incidence of such tumors was observed to be greater in cholestyramine resin treated rats than in control rats.

The relevance of this laboratory observation from studies in rats with cholestyramine resin to the clinical use of colestipol hydrochloride is not known. In the LRC-CPPT study referred to above, the total incidence of fatal and non-fatal neoplasms was similar in both treatment groups. When the many different categories of tumors are examined, various alimentary system cancers were somewhat more prevalent in the cholestyramine group. The small numbers and the multiple categories prevent conclusions from being drawn. Further follow-up of the LRC-CPPT participants by the sponsors of that study is planned for cause-specific mortality and cancer morbidity.

When colestipol hydrochloride was administered in the diet to rats for 18 months, there was no evidence of any drug related intestinal tumor formation. In the Ames assay, colestipol hydrochloride was not mutagenic.

Use in Pregnancy
Since colestipol hydrochloride is essentially not absorbed systemically (less than 0.17% of the dose), it is not expected to cause fetal harm when administered during pregnancy in recommended dosages. There are no adequate and well controlled studies in pregnant women, and the known interference with absorption of fat soluble vitamins may be detrimental even in the presence of supplementation. The use of COLESTID or FLAVORED COLESTID in pregnancy or by women of childbearing potential requires that the potential benefits of drug therapy be weighed against possible hazards to the mother or child.

Nursing Mother
Caution should be exercised when COLESTID or FLAVORED COLESTID is administered to a nursing mother. The possible lack of proper vitamin absorption described in the "pregnancy" section may have an effect on nursing infants.

Pediatric Use
Safety and effectiveness in the pediatric population have not been established.

Drug Interactions
Since colestipol hydrochloride is an anion exchange resin, it may have a strong affinity for anions other than the bile acids. *In vitro* studies have indicated that colestipol hydrochloride binds a number of drugs. Therefore, COLESTID and FLAVORED COLESTID resin may delay or reduce the absorption of concomitant oral medication. The interval between the administration of COLESTID and FLAVORED COLESTID and any other medication should be as long as possible. Patients should take other drugs at least one hour before or four hours after COLESTID and FLAVORED COLESTID to avoid impeding their absorption.

Repeated doses of colestipol hydrochloride given prior to a single dose of propranolol in human trials have been reported to decrease propranolol absorption. However, in a follow-up study in normal subjects, single dose administration of colestipol hydrochloride and propranolol and twice-a-day administration for 5 days of both agents did not effect the extent of propranolol absorption, but had a small yet statistically significant effect on its rate of absorption; the time to reach maximum concentration was delayed 30 minutes. Effects on the absorption of other beta-blockers have not been determined. Therefore, patients on propranolol should be observed when COLESTID or FLAVORED COLESTID is either added or deleted from a therapeutic regimen.

Studies in humans show that the absorption of chlorothiazide as reflected in urinary excretion is markedly decreased even when administered one hour before colestipol hydrochloride. The absorption of tetracycline, furosemide, penicillin G, hydrochlorothiazide, and gemfibrozil was significantly decreased when given simultaneously with colestipol hydrochloride; these drugs were not tested to determine the effect of administration one hour before colestipol hydrochloride.

No depressant effect on blood levels in humans was noted when colestipol hydrochloride was administered with any of the following drugs: aspirin, clindamycin, clofibrate, methyldopa, nicotinic acid (niacin), tolbutamide, phenytoin or warfarin. Particular caution should be observed with digitalis preparations since there are conflicting results for the effect of colestipol hydrochloride on the availability of digoxin and digitoxin. The potential for binding of these drugs if given concomitantly is present. Discontinuing colestipol hydrochloride could pose a hazard to health if a potentially toxic drug that is significantly bound to the resin has been titrated to a maintenance level while the patient was taking colestipol hydrochloride.

Bile acid binding resins may also interfere with the absorption of oral phosphate supplements and hydrocortisone.

ADVERSE REACTIONS

Gastrointestinal
The most common adverse reactions are confined to the gastrointestinal tract. To achieve minimal GI disturbance with an optimal LDL-cholesterol lowering effect, a gradual increase of dosage starting with one dose/day is recommended. Constipation is the major single complaint and at times is severe. Most instances of constipation are mild, transient, and controlled with standard treatment. Increased fluid intake and inclusion of additional dietary fiber should be the first step; a stool softener may be added if needed. Some patients require decreased dosage or discontinuation of therapy. Hemorrhoids may be aggravated.

Other, less frequent gastrointestinal complaints consist of abdominal discomfort (abdominal pain and cramping), intestinal gas, (bloating and flatulence), indigestion and heartburn, diarrhea and loose stools, and nausea and vomiting. Bleeding hemorrhoids and blood in the stool have been infrequently reported. Peptic ulceration, cholecystitis, and cholelithiasis have been rarely reported in patients receiving colestipol hydrochloride granules, and are not necessarily drug related.

Transient and modest elevations of aspartate aminotransferase (AST, SGOT), alanine aminotransferase (ALT, SGPT) and alkaline phosphatase were observed on one or more occasions in various patients treated with colestipol hydrochloride.

The following non-gastrointestinal adverse reactions have been reported with generally equal frequency in patients receiving COLESTID Granules, FLAVORED COLESTID Granules, or placebo in clinical studies:

Cardiovascular
Chest pain, angina, and tachycardia have been infrequently reported.

Hypersensitivity
Rash has been infrequently reported. Urticaria and dermatitis have been rarely noted in patients receiving colestipol hydrochloride granules.

Musculoskeletal
Musculoskeletal pain, aches and pains in the extremities, joint pains, arthritis, and backache have been reported.

Neurologic
Headache, migraine headache and sinus headache have been reported. Other infrequently reported complaints include dizziness, light-headedness, and insomnia.

Miscellaneous
Anorexia, fatigue, weakness, shortness of breath, and swelling of the hands or feet, have been infrequently reported.

OVERDOSAGE

Overdosage of COLESTID Granules or FLAVORED COLESTID Granules has not been reported. Should overdosage occur, however, the chief potential harm would be obstruction of the gastrointestinal tract. The location of such potential obstruction, the degree of obstruction and the presence or absence of normal gut motility would determine treatment.

DOSAGE AND ADMINISTRATION

One dose (1 packet or 1 level teaspoon) of COLESTID Granules contains 5 grams of colestipol hydrochloride. One dose (1 packet or 1 level scoopful) of FLAVORED COLESTID Granules is approximately 7.5 grams which contains 5 grams of colestipol hydrochloride. The recommended daily adult dose is one to six packets or level scoopfuls given once or in divided doses. Treatment should be started with one dose once or twice daily with an increment of one dose/day at one- or two-month intervals. Appropriate use of lipid profiles as per NCEP guidelines including LDL-cholesterol and triglycerides is advised so that optimal, but not excessive doses are used to obtain the desired therapeutic effect on LDL-cholesterol level. If the desired therapeutic effect is not obtained at one to six doses/day with good compliance and acceptable side effects, combined therapy or alternate treatment should be considered.

To avoid accidental inhalation or esophageal distress, COLESTID and FLAVORED COLESTID should not be taken in its dry form. COLESTID and FLAVORED COLESTID should always be mixed with water or other fluids before ingesting. Patients should take other drugs at least one hour before or four hours after COLESTID or FLAVORED COLESTID to minimize possible interference with their absorption. (See PRECAUTIONS, Drug Interactions.)

Before COLESTID or FLAVORED COLESTID Administration
1. Define the type of hyperlipoproteinemia, as described in NCEP guidelines.
2. Institute a trial of diet and weight reduction.
3. Establish baseline serum total and LDL-cholesterol and triglyceride levels.

During COLESTID or FLAVORED COLESTID Administration

1. The patient should be carefully monitored clinically, including serum cholesterol and triglyceride levels. Periodic determinations of serum cholesterol levels as outlined in the NCEP guidelines should be done to confirm a favorable initial and longer-term response.

2. Failure of total or LDL-cholesterol to fall within the desired range should lead one to first examine dietary and drug compliance. If these are deemed acceptable, combined therapy or alternate treatment should be considered.

3. Significant rise in triglyceride level should be considered as indication for dose reduction, drug discontinuation, or combined or alternate therapy.

Mixing and Administration Guide

COLESTID and FLAVORED COLESTID should always be mixed in a liquid such as water or the beverage of your choice. It may also be taken in soups or with cereals or pulpy fruits. COLESTID or FLAVORED COLESTID *should never be taken in its dry form.*

FLAVORED COLESTID is an orange-flavored product. Although it may be mixed with a variety of liquids or foods, the selection should be based on patient preference.

With Beverages

1. Add the prescribed amount of COLESTID or FLAVORED COLESTID to a glassful (three ounces or more) of water or the beverage of your choice. A heavy or pulpy juice may minimize complaints relative to consistency.

2. Stir the mixture until the medication is completely mixed. (COLESTID and FLAVORED COLESTID will not dissolve in the liquid.) COLESTID and FLAVORED COLESTID may also be mixed with carbonated beverages, slowly stirred in a large glass; however, this mixture may be associated with GI complaints.

Rinse the glass with a small amount of additional beverage to make sure all the medication is taken.

With cereals, soups, and fruits

COLESTID and FLAVORED COLESTID may be taken mixed with milk in hot or regular breakfast cereals, or even mixed in soups that have a high fluid content. It may also be added to fruits that are pulpy such as crushed pineapple, pears, peaches, or fruit cocktail.

HOW SUPPLIED

COLESTID Granules are available as follows:
Cartons of 30 foil packets — NDC 0009-0260-01
Cartons of 90 foil packets — NDC 0009-0260-04
Bottles of 300 grams with scoop — NDC 0009-0260-17
Bottles of 500 grams with scoop — NDC 0009-0260-02
Each packet or level scoop supplies 5 grams of COLESTID.
FLAVORED COLESTID Granules are available as follows:
Cartons of 60 foil packets — NDC 0009-0370-03
Bottles of 450 grams (equivalent to approximately 60 doses) with scoop — NDC 0009-0370-05
Each packet or each level scoopful supplies approximately 7.5 grams of FLAVORED COLESTID containing 5 grams of colestipol hydrochloride.
Store at controlled room temperature 20° to 25°C (68° to 77°F) [see USP].

REFERENCES

1. Summary of the Second Report of the National Cholesterol Education Program (NCEP) Expert Panel on Detection, Evaluation, and Treatment of High Blood Cholesterol in Adults (Adult Treatment Panel II). *JAMA* 269(23):3015–3023, 1993.

2. Lipid Metabolism-Atherogenesis Branch, National Heart, Lung, and Blood Institute, Bethesda, MD: The Lipid Research Clinics Coronary Primary Prevention Trial Results. I. Reduction in Incidence of Coronary Heart Disease. *JAMA* 251:351–364, 1984.

3. Parra HJ, et al. Differential electroimmunoassay of human LpA-I lipoprotein particles on ready-to-use plates. *Clin. Chem.* 36(8):1431–1435, 1990.

4. Barbaras R, et al. Cholesterol efflux from cultured adipose cells is mediated by LpAI particles but not by LpAI:AII particles. *Biochem. Biophys. Res. Comm.* 142(1):63–69, 1987.

5. Kane JP, et al. Normalization of low-density-lipoprotein levels in heterozygous familial hypercholesterolemia with a combined drug regimen. *N Engl. J. Med.* 304:251–258, 1981.

6. Illingworth DR, et al. Colestipol plus nicotinic acid in treatment of heterozygous familial hypercholerolemia. *Lancet* 1:296–298, 1981.

7. Kuo PT, et al. Familial type II hyperlipoproteinemia with coronary heart disease: Effect of diet-colestipol-nicotinic acid treatment. *Chest* 79:286–291, 1981.

8. Blankenhorn DH, et al. Beneficial Effects of Combined Colestipol-Niacin Therapy on Coronary Atherosclerosis and Coronary Venous Bypass Grafts. *JAMA* 257(23):3233–3240, 1987.

9. Cashin-Hemphill L, et al. Beneficial Effects of Colestipol-Niacin on Coronary Atherosclerosis: A 4-Year Follow-up. *JAMA* 264:3013–3017, 1990.

10. Brown G, et al. Regression of Coronary Artery Disease as a Result of Intensive Lipid-Lowering Therapy in Men with High Levels of Apolipoprotein B. *N Engl, J. Med* 323:1289–1298, 1990.

11. Kane JP, et al. Regression of Coronary Atherosclerosis During Treatment of Familial Hypercholesterolemia with Combined Drug Regimens. *JAMA* 264:3007–3012, 1990.

Rx only
COLESTID Granules
Made by
Pharmacia & Upjohn Company
Kalamazoo, MI 49001, USA
FLAVORED COLESTID Granules
Made in Canada for
Pharmacia & Upjohn Company
Kalamazoo, MI 49001, USA
By Global Pharm Inc.
Don Mills, Ontario M3B 1Y5
Canada
Revised March 1998

816 577 105
691344

CORVERT®
Injection
[cŏr-vĕrt]
Ibutilide fumarate injection

℞

DESCRIPTION

CORVERT Injection (ibutilide fumarate injection) is an antiarrhythmic drug with predominantly class III (cardiac action potential prolongation) properties according to the Vaughan Williams Classification. Each milliliter of CORVERT Injection contains 0.1 mg of ibutilide fumarate (equivalent to 0.087 mg ibutilide free base), 0.189 mg sodium acetate trihydrate, 8.90 mg sodium chloride, hydrochloric acid to adjust pH to approximately 4.6, and Water for Injection.

CORVERT Injection is an isotonic, clear, colorless, sterile aqueous solution.

Ibutilide fumarate has one chiral center, and exists as a racemate of the (+) and (−) enantiomers.

The chemical name for ibutilide fumarate is Methanesulfonamide, N-{4-{4-(ethylheptylamino)-1-hydroxybutyl]phenyl}, (+) (−), (E)-2-butenedioate (1:0.5) (hemifumarate salt). Its molecular formula is $C_{22}H_{38}N_2O_5S$, and its molecular weight is 442.62.

Ibutilide fumarate is a white to off-white powder with an aqueous solubility of over 100 mg/mL at pH 7 or lower.

The structural formula is represented below:

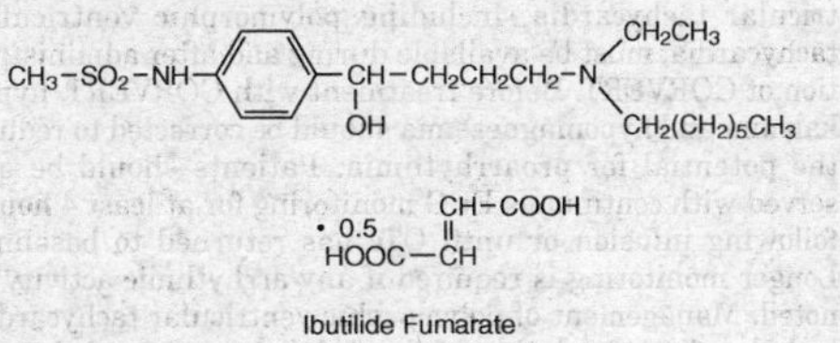

$$CH_3-SO_2-NH-\text{(benzene ring)}-\underset{OH}{CH}-CH_2CH_2CH_2-N\underset{CH_2(CH_2)_5CH_3}{\overset{CH_2CH_3}{}}$$

$$\cdot 0.5 \quad \underset{HOOC-CH}{\overset{CH-COOH}{\|}}$$

Ibutilide Fumarate

CLINICAL PHARMACOLOGY

Mechanism of Action: CORVERT Injection prolongs action potential duration in isolated adult cardiac myocytes and increases both atrial and ventricular refractoriness *in vivo,* ie, class III electrophysiologic effects. Voltage clamp studies indicate that CORVERT, at nanomolar concentrations, delays repolarization by activation of a slow, inward current (predominantly sodium), rather than by blocking outward potassium currents, which is the mechanism by which most other class III antiarrhythmics act. These effects lead to prolongation of atrial and ventricular action potential duration and refractoriness, the predominant electrophysiologic properties of CORVERT in humans that are thought to be the basis for its antiarrhythmic effect.

Electrophysiologic Effects: CORVERT produces mild slowing of the sinus rate and atrioventricular conduction. CORVERT produces no clinically significant effect on QRS duration at intravenous doses up to 0.03 mg/kg administered over a 10-minute period. Although there is no established relationship between plasma concentration and antiarrhythmic effect, CORVERT produces dose-related prolongation of the QT interval, which is thought to be associated with its antiarrhythmic activity. (See WARNINGS for relationship between QTc prolongation and torsades de pointes-type arrhythmias.) In a study in healthy volunteers, intravenous infusions of CORVERT resulted in prolongation of the QT interval that was directly correlated with ibutilide plasma concentration during and after 10-minute and 8-hour infusions. A steep ibutilide concentration/response (QT prolongation) relationship was shown. The maximum effect was a function of both the dose of CORVERT and the infusion rate.

Hemodynamic Effects: A study of hemodynamic function in patients with ejection fractions both above and below 35% showed no clinically significant effects on cardiac output, mean pulmonary arterial pressure, or pulmonary capillary wedge pressure at doses of CORVERT up to 0.03 mg/kg.

Pharmacokinetics: After intravenous infusion, ibutilide plasma concentrations rapidly decrease in a multiexponential fashion. The pharmacokinetics of ibutilide are highly variable among subjects. Ibutilide has a high systemic plasma clearance that approximates liver blood flow (about 29 mL/min/kg), a large steady-state volume of distribution (about 11 L/kg) in healthy volunteers, and minimal (about 40%) protein binding. Ibutilide is also cleared rapidly and highly distributed in patients being treated for atrial flutter or atrial fibrillation. The elimination half-life averages about 6 hours (range from 2 to 12 hours). The pharmacokinetics of ibutilide are linear with respect to the dose of CORVERT over the dose range of 0.01 mg/kg to 0.10 mg/kg. The enantiomers of ibutilide fumarate have pharmacokinetic properties similar to each other and to ibutilide fumarate. The pharmacokinetics of CORVERT Injection in patients with atrial flutter or atrial fibrillation are similar regardless of the type of arrhythmia, patient age, sex, or the concomitant use of digoxin, calcium channel blockers, or beta blockers.

Metabolism and elimination: In healthy male volunteers, about 82% of a 0.01 mg/kg dose of [^{14}C] ibutilide fumarate was excreted in the urine (about 7% of the dose as unchanged ibutilide) and the remainder (about 19%) was recovered in the feces.

Eight metabolites of ibutilide are detected in metabolic profiling of urine. These metabolites are thought to be formed primarily by ω-oxidation followed by sequential β-oxidation of the heptyl side chain of ibutilide. Of the eight metabolites, only the ω-hydroxy metabolite possesses class III electrophysiologic properties similar to that of ibutilide in an *in vitro* isolated rabbit myocardium model. The plasma concentrations of this active metabolite, however, are less than 10% of that of ibutilide.

Clinical Studies: Treatment with intravenous ibutilide fumarate for acute termination of recent onset atrial flutter/fibrillation was evaluated in 466 patients participating in two randomized, double-blind, placebo-controlled clinical trials. Patients had had their arrhythmias for 3 hours to 90 days, were anticoagulated for at least 2 weeks if atrial fibrillation was present more than 3 days, had serum potassium of at least 4.0 mEq/L and QTc below 440 msec, and were monitored by telemetry for at least 24 hours. Patients could not be on class I or other class III antiarrhythmics (these had to be discontinued at least 5 half-lives prior to infusion) but could be on calcium channel blockers, beta blockers, or digoxin. In one trial, single 10-minute infusions of 0.005 to 0.025 mg/kg were tested in parallel groups (0.3 to 1.5 mg in a 60 kg person). In the second trial, up to two infusions of ibutilide fumarate were evaluated—the first 1.0 mg, the second given 10 minutes after completion of the first infusion, either 0.5 or 1.0 mg. In a third double-blind study, 319 patients with atrial fibrillation or atrial flutter of 3 hours to 45 days duration were randomized to receive single, 10-minute intravenous infusions of either sotalol (1.5 mg/kg) or CORVERT (1 mg or 2 mg). Among patients with atrial flutter, 53% receiving 1 mg ibutilide fumarate and 70% receiving 2 mg ibutilide fumarate converted, compared to 18% of those receiving sotalol. In patients with atrial fibrillation, 22% receiving 1 mg ibutilide fumarate and 43% receiving 2 mg ibutilide fumarate converted compared to 10% of patients receiving sotalol.

Patients in clinical trials were hemodynamically stable. Patients with specific cardiovascular conditions such as symptomatic heart failure, recent acute myocardial infarction, and angina were excluded. About two thirds had cardiovascular symptoms, and the majority of patients had left atrial enlargement, decreased left ventricular ejection fraction, a history of valvular disease, or previous history of atrial fibrillation or flutter. Electrical cardioversion was allowed 90 minutes after the infusion was complete. Patients could be given other antiarrhythmic drugs 4 hours postinfusion.

Results of the first two studies are shown in the tables below. Conversion of atrial flutter/fibrillation usually (70% of those who converted) occurred within 30 minutes of the start of infusion and was dose related. The latest conversion seen was at 90 minutes after the start of the infusion. Most converted patients remained in normal sinus rhythm for 24 hours. Overall responses in these patients, defined as termination of arrhythmias for any length of time during or within 1 hour following completed infusion of randomized dose, were in the range of 43% to 48% at doses above 0.0125

Continued on next page

Information on these Pharmacia & Upjohn products is based on labeling in effect June 1, 1998. Further information concerning these and other Pharmacia & Upjohn products may be obtained by direct inquiry to Medical Information, Pharmacia & Upjohn, Kalamazoo, MI 49001.

Consult 1999 PDR® supplements and future editions for revisions

Corvert—Cont.

mg/kg (vs 2% for placebo). Twenty-four hour responses were similar. For these atrial arrhythmias, ibutilide was more effective in patients with flutter than fibrillation (≥48% vs ≤40%).

[See table at right]

[See table below]

The numbers of patients who remained in the converted rhythm at the end of 24 hours were slightly less than those patients who converted initially, but the difference between conversion rates for ibutilide compared to placebo was still statistically significant. In long-term follow-up, approximately 40% of all patients remained recurrence free, usually with chronic prophylactic treatment, 400 to 500 days after acute treatment, regardless of the method of conversion.

Patients with more recent onset of arrhythmia had a higher rate of conversion. Response rates were 42% and 50% for patients with onset of atrial fibrillation/flutter for less than 30 days in the two efficacy studies compared to 16% and 31% in those with more chronic arrhythmias.

Ibutilide was equally effective in patients below and above 65 years of age and in men and women. Female patients constituted about 20% of patients in controlled studies.

INDICATIONS AND USAGE

CORVERT Injection is indicated for the rapid conversion of atrial fibrillation or atrial flutter of recent onset to sinus rhythm. Patients with atrial arrhythmias of longer duration are less likely to respond to CORVERT. The effectiveness of ibutilide has not been determined in patients with arrhythmias of more than 90 days in duration.

LIFE-THREATENING ARRHYTHMIAS—APPROPRIATE TREATMENT ENVIRONMENT

CORVERT can cause potentially fatal arrhythmias, particularly sustained polymorphic ventricular tachycardia, usually in association with QT prolongation (torsades de pointes), but sometimes without documented QT prolongation. In clinical studies, these arrhythmias, which require cardioversion, occurred in 1.7% of treated patients during, or within a number of hours of, use of CORVERT. These arrhythmias can be reversed if treated promptly (see WARNINGS, Proarrhythmia). It is essential that CORVERT be administered in a setting of continuous ECG monitoring and by personnel trained in identification and treatment of acute ventricular arrhythmias, particularly polymorphic ventricular tachycardia. *Patients with atrial fibrillation of more than 2 to 3 days' duration must be adequately anticoagulated, generally for at least 2 weeks.*

CHOICE OF PATIENTS

Patients with chronic atrial fibrillation have a strong tendency to revert after conversion to sinus rhythm (see CLINICAL STUDIES) and treatments to maintain sinus rhythm carry risks. Patients to be treated with CORVERT, therefore, should be carefully selected such that the expected benefits of maintaining sinus rhythm outweigh the immediate risks of CORVERT, and the risks of maintenance therapy, and are likely to offer an advantage compared with alternative management.

CONTRAINDICATIONS

CORVERT Injection is contraindicated in patients who have previously demonstrated hypersensitivity to ibutilide fumarate or any of the other product components.

WARNINGS

Proarrhythmia: Like other antiarrhythmic agents, CORVERT Injection can induce or worsen ventricular arrhythmias in some patients. This may have potentially fatal consequences. Torsades de pointes, a polymorphic ventricular tachycardia that develops in the setting of a prolonged QT interval, may occur because of the effect CORVERT has on cardiac repolarization, but CORVERT can also cause polymorphic VT in the absence of excessive prolongation of the QT interval. In general, with drugs that prolong the QT interval, the risk of torsades de pointes is thought to increase progressively as the QT interval is prolonged and may be worsened with bradycardia, a varying heart rate, and hypokalemia. In clinical trials conducted in patients with atrial fibrillation and atrial flutter, those with QTc intervals >440 msec were not usually allowed to participate, and serum potassium had to be above 4.0 mEq/L. Although change in QTc was dose dependent for ibutilide, there was no clear relationship between risk of serious proarrhythmia and dose in clinical studies, possibly due to the small number of events. In clinical trials of intravenous ibutilide, patients with a history of congestive heart failure (CHF) or low left ventricular ejection fraction appeared to have a higher incidence of sustained polymorphic ventricular tachycardia (VT), than those without such underlying conditions; for sustained polymorphic VT the rate was 5.4% in patients with a history

of CHF and 0.8% without it. There was also a suggestion that women had a higher risk of proarrhythmia, but the sex difference was not observed in all studies and was most prominent for nonsustained ventricular tachycardia. The incidence of sustained ventricular arrhythmias was similar in male (1.8%) and female (1.5%) patients, possibly due to the small number of events. CORVERT is not recommended in patients who have previously demonstrated polymorphic ventricular tachycardia (eg, torsades de pointes).

During clinical trials, 1.7% of patients with atrial flutter or atrial fibrillation treated with CORVERT developed sustained polymorphic ventricular tachycardia requiring cardioversion. In these clinical trials, many initial episodes of polymorphic ventricular tachycardia occurred after the infusion of CORVERT was stopped but generally not more than 40 minutes after the start of the first infusion. There were, however, instances of recurrent polymorphic VT that occurred about 3 hours after the initial infusion. In two cases, the VT degenerated into ventricular fibrillation, requiring immediate defibrillation. Other cases were managed with cardiac pacing and magnesium sulfate infusions. Nonsustained polymorphic ventricular tachycardia occurred in 2.7% of patients and nonsustained monomorphic ventricular tachycardias occurred in 4.9% of the patients (see ADVERSE REACTIONS).

Proarrhythmic events must be anticipated. Skilled personnel and proper equipment, including cardiac monitoring equipment, intracardiac pacing facilities, a cardioverter/defibrillator, and medication for treatment of sustained ventricular tachycardia, including polymorphic ventricular tachycardia, must be available during and after administration of CORVERT. Before treatment with CORVERT, hypokalemia and hypomagnesemia should be corrected to reduce the potential for proarrhythmia. Patients should be observed with continuous ECG monitoring for at least 4 hours following infusion or until QTc has returned to baseline. Longer monitoring is required if any arrhythmic activity is noted. Management of polymorphic ventricular tachycardia includes discontinuation of ibutilide, correction of electrolyte abnormalities, especially potassium and magnesium, and overdrive cardiac pacing, electrical cardioversion, or defibrillation. Pharmacologic therapies include magnesium sulfate infusions. Treatment with antiarrhythmics should generally be avoided.

PRECAUTIONS

General

Antiarrhythmics: Class Ia antiarrhythmic drugs (Vaughan Williams Classification), such as disopyramide, quinidine, and procainamide, and other class III drugs, such as amiodarone and sotalol, should not be given concomitantly with

CORVERT Injection or within 4 hours postinfusion because of their potential to prolong refractoriness. In the clinical trials, class I or other class III antiarrhythmic agents were withheld for at least 5 half-lives prior to ibutilide infusion and for 4 hours after dosing, but thereafter were allowed at the physician's discretion.

Other drugs that prolong the QT interval: The potential for proarrhythmia may increase with the administration of CORVERT Injection to patients who are being treated with drugs that prolong the QT interval, such as phenothiazines, tricyclic antidepressants, tetracyclic antidepressants, and certain antihistamine drugs (H_1 receptor antagonists).

Heart block: Of the nine (1.5%) ibutilide-treated patients with reports of reversible heart block, five had first degree, three had second degree, and one had complete heart block.

Laboratory Test Interactions: None known.

Drug Interactions: No specific pharmacokinetic or other formal drug interaction studies were conducted.

Digoxin: Supraventricular arrhythmias may mask the cardiotoxicity associated with excessive digoxin levels. Therefore, it is advisable to be particularly cautious in patients whose plasma digoxin levels are above or suspected to be above the usual therapeutic range. Coadministration of digoxin did not have effects on either the safety or efficacy of ibutilide in the clinical trials.

Calcium channel blocking agents: Coadministration of calcium channel blockers did not have any effect on either the safety or efficacy of ibutilide in the clinical trials.

Beta-adrenergic blocking agents: Coadministration of beta-adrenergic blocking agents did not have any effect on either the safety or efficacy of ibutilide in the clinical trials.

Carcinogenesis, Mutagenesis, Impairment of Fertility: No animal studies have been conducted to determine the carcinogenic potential of CORVERT; however, it was not genotoxic in a battery of assays, (Ames assay, mammalian cell forward gene mutation assay, unscheduled DNA synthesis assay, and mouse micronucleus assay). Similarly, no drug-related effects on fertility or mating were noted in a reproductive study in rats in which ibutilide was administered orally to both sexes up to doses of 20 mg/kg/day. On a mg/m² basis, corrected for 3% bioavailability, the highest dose tested was approximately four times the maximum recommended human dose (MRHD).

Pregnancy: Pregnancy Category C. Ibutilide administered orally was teratogenic (abnormalities included adactyly, interventricular septal defects, and scoliosis) and embryocidal in reproduction studies in rats. On a mg/m² basis, corrected for the 3% oral bioavailability, the "no adverse effect dose" (5 mg/kg/day given orally) was approximately the same as the maximum recommended human dose (MRHD); the terato-

PERCENT OF PATIENTS WHO CONVERTED (First Trial)

		Placebo	Ibutilide			
			0.005 mg/kg	0.01 mg/kg	0.015 mg/kg	0.025 mg/kg
	n	41	41	40	38	40
Both	Initially*	2	12	33	45	48
	At 24 hours†	2	12	28	42	43
Atrial flutter	Initially*	0	14	30	58	55
	At 24 hours†	0	14	30	58	50
Atrial fibrillation	Initially*	5	10	35	32	40
	At 24 hours†	5	10	25	26	35

* Percent of patients who converted within 70 minutes after the start of infusion.
† Percent of patients who remained in sinus rhythm 24 hours after dosing.

PERCENT OF PATIENTS WHO CONVERTED (Second Trial)

		Placebo	Ibutilide	
			1.0 mg/0.5 mg	1.0 mg/1.0 mg
	n	86	86	94
Both	Initially*	2	43	44
	At 24 hours†	2	34	37
Atrial flutter	Initially*	2	48	63
	At 24 hours†	2	45	59
Atrial fibrillation	Initially*	2	38	25
	At 24 hours†	2	21	17

*Percent of patients who converted within 90 minutes after the start of infusion.
†Percent of patients who remained in sinus rhythm 24 hours after dosing.

genic dose (20 mg/kg/day given orally) was about four times the MRHD on a mg/m^2 basis, or 16 times the MRHD on a mg/kg basis. CORVERT should not be administered to a pregnant woman unless clinical benefit outweighs potential risk to the fetus.

Nursing Mothers: The excretion of ibutilide into breast milk has not been studied; accordingly, breastfeeding should be discouraged during therapy with CORVERT.

Pediatric Use: Clinical trials with CORVERT in patients with atrial fibrillation and atrial flutter did not include anyone under the age of 18. Safety and effectiveness of ibutilide in pediatric patients has not been established.

Geriatric Use: The mean age of patients in clinical trials was 65. No age-related differences were observed in pharmacokinetic, efficacy, or safety parameters for patients less than 65 compared to patients 65 years and older.

Use in Patients With Hepatic or Renal Dysfunction: The safety, effectiveness, and pharmacokinetics of CORVERT have not been established in patients with hepatic or renal dysfunction. However, it is unlikely that dosing adjustments would be necessary in patients with compromised renal or hepatic function based on the following considerations: (1) CORVERT is indicated for rapid intravenous therapy (duration ≤30 minutes) and is dosed to a known, well-defined pharmacologic action (termination of arrhythmia) or to a maximum of two 10-minute infusions; (2) less than 10% of the dose of CORVERT is excreted unchanged in the urine; and (3) drug distribution appears to be one of the primary mechanisms responsible for termination of the pharmacologic effect. Nonetheless, patients with abnormal liver function should be monitored by telemetry for more than the 4-hour period generally recommended.

In 285 patients with atrial fibrillation or atrial flutter who were treated with CORVERT, the clearance of ibutilide was independent of renal function, as assessed by creatinine clearance (range 21 to 140 mL/min).

ADVERSE REACTIONS

CORVERT Injection was generally well tolerated in clinical trials. Of the 586 patients with atrial fibrillation or atrial flutter who received CORVERT in phase II/III studies, 149 (25%) reported medical events related to the cardiovascular system, including sustained polymorphic ventricular tachycardia (1.7%) and nonsustained polymorphic ventricular tachy cardia (2.7%).

Other clinically important adverse events with an uncertain relationship to CORVERT include the following (0.2% represents one patient): sustained monomorphic ventricular tachycardia (0.2%), nonsustained monomorphic ventricular tachycardia (4.9%), AV block (1.5%), bundle branch block (1.9%), ventricular extrasystoles (5.1%), supraventricular extrasystoles (0.9%), hypotension/postural hypotension (2.0%), bradycardia/sinus bradycardia (1.2%), nodal arrhythmia (0.7%), congestive heart failure (0.5%), tachycardia/sinus tachycardia/supraventricular tachycardia (2.7%), idioventricular rhythm (0.2%), syncope (0.3%), and renal failure (0.3%). The incidence of these events, except for syncope, was greater in the group treated with CORVERT than in the placebo group.

Another adverse reaction that may be associated with the administration of CORVERT was nausea, which occurred with a frequency greater than 1% more in ibutilide-treated patients than those treated with placebo.

The medical events reported for more than 1% of the placebo- and ibutilide-treated patients are shown in the following Table.

Treatment-Emergent Medical Events With Frequency of More Than 1% and Higher Than That of Placebo

Event	Placebo N=127		All Ibutilide N=586	
	Patients		Patients	
	n	%	n	%
CARDIOVASCULAR				
Ventricular extrasystoles	1	0.8	30	5.1
Nonsustained monomorphic VT	1	0.8	29	4.9
Nonsustained polymorphic VT	—	—	16	2.7
Hypotension	2	1.6	12	2.0
Bundle branch block	—	—	11	1.9
Sustained polymorphic VT	—	—	10	1.7
AV block	1	0.8	9	1.5
Hypertension	—	—	7	1.2
QT segment prolonged	—	—	7	1.2
Bradycardia	1	0.8	7	1.2
Palpitation	1	0.8	6	1.0
Tachycardia	1	0.8	16	2.7
GASTROINTESTINAL				
Nausea	1	0.8	11	1.9
CENTRAL NERVOUS SYSTEM				
Headache	4	3.1	21	3.6

Recommended Dose of CORVERT Injection

Patient Weight	*Initial Infusion (over 10 minutes)*	*Second Infusion*
60 kg (132 lb) or more	*One vial (1 mg ibutilide fumarate)*	*If the arrhythmia does not terminate within 10 minutes after the end of the initial infusion, a second 10-minute infusion of equal strength may be administered 10 minutes after completion of the first infusion.*
Less than 60 kg (132 lb)	*0.1 mL/kg (0.01 mg/kg ibutilide fumarate)*	

OVERDOSAGE

Acute Experience in Animals: Acute overdose in animals results in CNS toxicity; notably, CNS depression, rapid gasping breathing, and convulsions. The intravenous median lethal dose in the rat was more than 50 mg/kg which is, on a mg/m^2 basis, at least 250 times the maximum recommended human dose.

Human Experience: In the clinical trials with CORVERT Injection, four patients were unintentionally overdosed. The largest dose was 3.4 mg administered over 15 minutes. One patient (0.025 mg/kg) developed increased ventricular ectopy and monomorphic ventricular tachycardia, another patient (0.032 mg/kg) developed AV block—3rd degree and nonsustained polymorphic VT, and two patients (0.038 and 0.020 mg/kg) had no medical event reports. Based on known pharmacology, the clinical effects of an overdosage with ibutilide could exaggerate the expected prolongation of repolarization seen at usual clinical doses. Medical events (eg, proarrhythmia, AV block) that occur after the overdosage should be treated with measures appropriate for that condition.

DOSAGE AND ADMINISTRATION

The recommended dose based on controlled trials (see CLINICAL STUDIES) is outlined in the Table below. Ibutilide infusion should be stopped as soon as the presenting arrhythmia is terminated or in the event of sustained or nonsustained ventricular tachycardia, or marked prolongation of QT or QTc.

[See table above]

In a trial comparing ibutilide and sotalol (see CLINICAL STUDIES), 2 mg ibutilide fumarate administered as a single infusion to patients weighing more than 60 kg was also effective in terminating atrial fibrillation or atrial flutter.

Patients should be observed with continuous ECG monitoring for at least 4 hours following infusion or until QTc has returned to baseline. Longer monitoring is required if any arrhythmic activity is noted. Skilled personnel and proper equipment (see WARNINGS, Proarrhythmia), such as a cardioverter/defibrillator, and medication for treatment of sustained ventricular tachycardia, including polymorphic ventricular tachycardia, must be available during administration of CORVERT and subsequent monitoring of the patient.

Dilution: CORVERT Injection may be administered undiluted or diluted in 50 mL of diluent. CORVERT may be added to 0.9% Sodium Chloride Injection or 5% Dextrose Injection before infusion. The contents of one 10 mL vial (0.1 mg/mL) may be added to a 50 mL infusion bag to form an admixture of approximately 0.017 mg/mL ibutilide fumarate. Parenteral drug products should be inspected visually for particulate matter and discoloration prior to administration whenever solution and container permit.

Compatibility and Stability: The following diluents are compatible with CORVERT Injection (0.1 mg/mL):

5% Dextrose Injection
0.9% Sodium Chloride Injection

The following intravenous solution containers are compatible with admixtures of CORVERT Injection (0.1 mg/mL):

polyvinyl chloride plastic bags
polyolefin bags

Admixtures of the product, with approved diluents, are chemically and physically stable for 24 hours at room temperature (15° to 30° C or 59° to 86° F) and for 48 hours at refrigerated temperatures (2° to 8°C or 36° to 46°F). Strict adherence to the use of aseptic technique during the preparation of the admixture is recommended in order to maintain sterility.

HOW SUPPLIED

CORVERT Injection (ibutilide fumarate injection) is supplied as an acetate-buffered isotonic solution at a concentration of 0.1 mg/mL that has been adjusted to approximately pH 4.6 in 10 mL clear glass, single-dose, flip-top vials.

Single-dose 10 mL vial,
1 mg/10 mL (0.1 mg/mL) NDC 0009-3794-01

Store at controlled room temperature 20° to 25°C (68° to 77°F) [see USP]. Store vial in carton until used.

Caution: Federal law prohibits dispensing without prescription.

Pharmacia & Upjohn Company • Kalamazoo, Michigan 49001, USA
Revised August 1997 816 418 002
691659

CYTOSAR-U® ℞

sterile cytarabine, USP
For Intravenous, Intrathecal and Subcutaneous Use Only

WARNING

Only physicians experienced in cancer chemotherapy should use CYTOSAR-U Sterile Powder.

For induction therapy patients should be treated in a facility with laboratory and supportive resources sufficient to monitor drug tolerance and protect and maintain a patient compromised by drug toxicity. The main toxic effect of CYTOSAR-U is bone marrow suppression with leukopenia, thrombocytopenia and anemia. Less serious toxicity includes nausea, vomiting, diarrhea and abdominal pain, oral ulceration, and hepatic dysfunction.

The physician must judge possible benefit to the patient against known toxic effects of this drug in considering the advisability of therapy with CYTOSAR-U. Before making this judgment or beginning treatment, the physician should be familiar with the following text.

DESCRIPTION

CYTOSAR-U (cytarabine) Sterile Powder, commonly known as ara-C, an antineoplastic, is a sterile lyophilized material for reconstitution and intravenous, intrathecal or subcutaneous administration. It is available in multi-dose vials containing 100 mg, 500 mg, 1 g or 2 g sterile cytarabine. The pH of CYTOSAR-U was adjusted, when necessary, with hydrochloric acid and/or sodium hydroxide.

Cytarabine is chemically 4-amino-1-β-D-arabinofuranosyl-2 (1H)-pyrimidinone. The structural formula is:

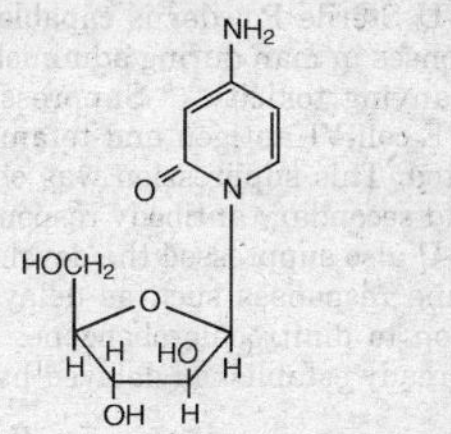

Cytarabine is an odorless, white to off-white, crystalline powder which is freely soluble in water and slightly soluble in alcohol and in chloroform.

PHARMACOLOGY

Cell Culture Studies

Cytarabine is cytotoxic to a wide variety of proliferating mammalian cells in culture. It exhibits cell phase specificity, primarily killing cells undergoing DNA synthesis (S-phase) and under certain conditions blocking the progression of cells from the G_1 phase to the S-phase. Although the mechanism of action is not completely understood, it appears that cytarabine acts through the inhibition of DNA polymerase. A limited, but significant, incorporation of cytarabine into both DNA and RNA has also been reported. Extensive chromosomal damage, including chromatoid breaks, have been produced by cytarabine and malignant transformation of rodent cells in culture has been reported. Deoxycytidine prevents or delays (but does not reverse) the cytotoxic activity.

Cell culture studies have shown an antiviral effect.[1] However, efficacy against herpes zoster or smallpox could not be demonstrated in controlled clinical trials.[2–4]

Cellular Resistance and Sensitivity

Cytarabine is metabolized by deoxycytidine kinase and other nucleotide kinases to the nucleotide triphosphate, an effective inhibitor of DNA polymerase; it is inactivated by a pyrimidine nucleoside deaminase, which converts it to the

Continued on next page

Information on these Pharmacia & Upjohn products is based on labeling in effect June 1, 1998. Further information concerning these and other Pharmacia & Upjohn products may be obtained by direct inquiry to Medical Information, Pharmacia & Upjohn, Kalamazoo, MI 49001.

Cytosar-U—Cont.

nontoxic uracil derivative. It appears that the balance of kinase and deaminase levels may be an important factor in determining sensitivity or resistance of the cell to cytarabine.

Animal Studies

In experimental studies with mouse tumors, cytarabine was most effective in those tumors with a high growth fraction. The effect was dependent on the treatment schedule; optimal effects were achieved when the schedule (multiple closely spaced doses or constant infusion) ensured contact of the drug with the tumor cells when the maximum number of cells were in the susceptible S-phase. The best results were obtained when courses of therapy were separated by intervals sufficient to permit adequate host recovery.

Human Pharmacology

Cytarabine is rapidly metabolized and is not effective orally; less than 20 percent of the orally administered dose is absorbed from the gastrointestinal tract.

Following rapid intravenous injection of cytarabine labeled with tritium, the disappearance from plasma is biphasic. There is an initial distributive phase with a half-life of about 10 minutes, followed by a second elimination phase with a half-life of about 1 to 3 hours. After the distributive phase, more than 80 percent of plasma radioactivity can be accounted for by the inactive metabolite 1-β-D-arabinofuranosyluracil (ara-U). Within 24 hours about 80 percent of the administered radioactivity can be recovered in the urine, approximately 90 percent of which is excreted as ara-U.

Relatively constant plasma levels can be achieved by continuous intravenous infusion.

After subcutaneous or intramuscular administration of cytarabine labeled with tritium, peak-plasma levels of radioactivity are achieved about 20 to 60 minutes after injection and are considerably lower than those after intravenous administration.

Cerebrospinal fluid levels of cytarabine are low in comparison to plasma levels after single intravenous injection. However, in one patient in whom cerebrospinal levels were examined after 2 hours of constant intravenous infusion, levels approached 40 percent of the steady state plasma level. With intrathecal administration, levels of cytarabine in the cerebrospinal fluid declined with a first order half-life of about 2 hours. Because cerebrospinal fluid levels of deaminase are low, little conversion to ara-U was observed.

Immunosuppressive Action

CYTOSAR-U Sterile Powder is capable of obliterating immune responses in man during administration with little or no accompanying toxicity.[5–6] Suppression of antibody responses to E-coli-VI antigen and tetanus toxoid have been demonstrated. This suppression was obtained during both primary and secondary antibody responses.

CYTOSAR-U also suppressed the development of cell-mediated immune responses such as delayed hypersensitivity skin reaction to dinitrochlorobenzene. However, it had no effect on already established delayed hypersensitivity reactions.

Following 5-day courses of intensive therapy with CYTOSAR-U the immune response was suppressed, as indicated by the following parameters: macrophage ingress into skin windows; circulating antibody response following primary antigenic stimulation; lymphocyte blastogenesis with phytohemagglutinin. A few days after termination of therapy there was a rapid return to normal.[7]

INDICATIONS AND USAGE

CYTOSAR-U in combination with other approved anticancer drugs is indicated for remission induction in acute nonlymphocytic leukemia of adults and pediatric patients. It has also been found useful in the treatment of acute lymphocytic leukemia and the blast phase of chronic myelocytic leukemia. Intrathecal administration of CYTOSAR-U is indicated in the prophylaxis and treatment of meningeal leukemia.

CONTRAINDICATIONS

CYTOSAR-U Sterile Powder is contraindicated in those patients who are hypersensitive to the drug.

WARNINGS (See boxed WARNING)

Cytarabine is a potent bone marrow suppressant. Therapy should be started cautiously in patients with pre-existing drug-induced bone marrow suppression. Patients receiving this drug must be under close medical supervision and, during induction therapy, should have leukocyte and platelet counts performed daily. Bone marrow examinations should be performed frequently after blasts have disappeared from the peripheral blood. Facilities should be available for management of complications, possibly fatal, of bone marrow suppression (infection resulting from granulocytopenia and other impaired body defenses, and hemorrhage secondary to thrombocytopenia). One case of anaphylaxis that resulted in acute cardiopulmonary arrest and required resuscitation has been reported. This occurred immediately after the intravenous administration of CYTOSAR-U Sterile Powder.

Severe and at times fatal CNS, GI and pulmonary toxicity (different from that seen with conventional therapy regimens of CYTOSAR-U) has been reported following some experimental dose schedules for CYTOSAR-U.[8–11] These reactions include reversible corneal toxicity, and hemorrhagic conjunctivitis, which may be prevented or diminished by prophylaxis with a local corticosteroid eye drop; cerebral and cerebellar dysfunction, including personality changes, somnolence and coma, usually reversible; severe gastrointestinal ulceration, including pneumatosis cystoides intestinalis leading to peritonitis; sepsis and liver abscess; pulmonary edema, liver damage with increased hyperbilirubinemia; bowel necrosis; and necrotizing colitis. Rarely, severe skin rash, leading to desquamation has been reported. Complete alopecia is more commonly seen with experimental high dose therapy than with standard treatment programs using CYTOSAR-U. If experimental high dose therapy is used, do not use a diluent containing benzyl alcohol.

Cases of cardiomyopathy with subsequent death have been reported following experimental high dose therapy with cytarabine in combination with cyclophosphamide when used for bone marrow transplant preparation.[12]

A syndrome of sudden respiratory distress, rapidly progressing to pulmonary edema and radiographically pronounced cardiomegaly has been reported following experimental high dose therapy with cytarabine used for the treatment of relapsed leukemia from one institution in 16/72 patients. The outcome of this syndrome can be fatal.[13]

Benzyl alcohol is contained in the diluent for this product. Benzyl alcohol has been reported to be associated with a fatal "Gasping Syndrome" in premature infants.

Two patients with childhood acute myelogenous leukemia who received intrathecal and intravenous CYTOSAR-U at conventional doses (in addition to a number of other concomitantly administered drugs) developed delayed progressive ascending paralysis resulting in death in one of the two patients.[14]

Use in Pregnancy (Category D)

CYTOSAR-U can cause fetal harm when administered to a pregnant woman. (See ANIMAL TOXICOLOGY). There are no adequate and well-controlled studies in pregnant women. If CYTOSAR-U is used during pregnancy, or if the patient becomes pregnant while taking CYTOSAR-U, the patient should be apprised of the potential hazard to the fetus. Women of childbearing potential should be advised to avoid becoming pregnant.

A review of the literature has shown 32 reported cases where CYTOSAR-U was given during pregnancy, either alone or in combination with other cytotoxic agents:

Eighteen normal infants were delivered. Four of these had first trimester exposure. Five infants were premature or of low birth weight. Twelve of the 18 normal infants were followed up at ages ranging from six weeks to seven years, and showed no abnormalities. One apparently normal infant died at 90 days of gastroenteritis.

Two cases of congenital abnormalities have been reported, one with upper and lower distal limb defects,[16] and the other with extremity and ear deformities.[17] Both of these cases had first trimester exposure.

There were seven infants with various problems in the neonatal period, including pancytopenia; transient depression of WBC, hematocrit or platelets; electrolyte abnormalities; transient eosinophilia; and one case of increased IgM levels and hyperpyrexia possibly due to sepsis. Six of the seven infants were also premature. The child with pancytopenia died at 21 days of sepsis.

Therapeutic abortions were done in five cases. Four fetuses were grossly normal, but one had an enlarged spleen and another showed Trisomy C chromosome abnormality in the chorionic tissue.

Because of the potential for abnormalities with cytotoxic therapy, particularly during the first trimester, a patient who is or who may become pregnant while on CYTOSAR-U should be apprised of the potential risk to the fetus and the advisability of pregnancy continuation. There is a definite, but considerably reduced risk if therapy is initiated during the second or third trimester. Although normal infants have been delivered to patients treated in all three trimesters of pregnancy, follow-up of such infants would be advisable.

PRECAUTIONS

1. General Precautions

Patients receiving CYTOSAR-U Sterile Powder must be monitored closely. Frequent platelet and leukocyte counts and bone marrow examinations are mandatory. Consider suspending or modifying therapy when drug-induced marrow depression has resulted in a platelet count under 50,000 or a polymorphonuclear granulocyte count under $1000/mm^3$. Counts of formed elements in the peripheral blood may continue to fall after the drug is stopped and reach lowest values after drug-free intervals of 12 to 24 days. When indicated, restart therapy when definite signs of marrow recovery appear (on successive bone marrow studies). Patients whose drug is withheld until "normal" peripheral blood values are attained may escape from control.

When large intravenous doses are given quickly, patients are frequently nauseated and may vomit for several hours postinjection. This problem tends to be less severe when the drug is infused.

The human liver apparently detoxifies a substantial fraction of an administered dose. In particular, patients with renal or hepatic function impairment may have a higher likelihood of CNS toxicity after high-dose CYTOSAR-U treatment.[46,47,49] Use the drug with caution and possibly at reduced dose in patients whose liver or kidney function is poor.

Periodic checks of bone marrow, liver and kidney functions should be performed in patients receiving CYTOSAR-U.

Like other cytotoxic drugs, CYTOSAR-U may induce hyperuricemia secondary to rapid lysis of neoplastic cells. The clinician should monitor the patient's blood uric acid level and be prepared to use such supportive and pharmacologic measures as might be necessary to control this problem.

Acute pancreatitis has been reported to occur in patients being treated with CYTOSAR-U who have had prior treatment with L-asparaginase.[15] There is evidence that this may be schedule dependent.[50]

2. Information for patient

Not applicable

3. Laboratory tests

See General Precautions

4. Drug Interactions

Reversible decreases in steady-state plasma digoxin concentrations and renal glycoside excretion were observed in patients receiving beta-acetyldigoxin and chemotherapy regimens containing cyclophosphamide, vincristine and prednisone with or without CYTOSAR-U or procarbazine.[39] Steady-state plasma digitoxin concentrations did not appear to change. Therefore, monitoring of plasma digoxin levels may be indicated in patients receiving similar combination chemotherapy regimens. The utilization of digitoxin for such patients may be considered as an alternative.

An *in vitro* interaction study between gentamicin and cytarabine showed a cytarabine related antagonism for the susceptibility of *K. pneumoniae* strains. This study suggests that in patients on cytarabine being treated with gentamicin for a *K. pneumoniae* infection, the lack of a prompt therapeutic response may indicate the need for reevaluation of antibacterial therapy.[40]

Clinical evidence in one patient showed possible inhibition of fluorocytosine efficacy during therapy with CYTOSAR-U.[41] This may be due to potential competitive inhibition of its uptake[42]

5. Carcinogenesis, mutagenesis, impairment of fertility

Extensive chromosomal damage, including chromatoid breaks have been produced by cytarabine and malignant transformation of rodent cells in culture has been reported.

6. Pregnancy

Pregnancy Category D. See WARNINGS.

7. Labor and delivery

Not applicable

8. Nursing mothers

It is not known whether this drug is excreted in human milk. Because many drugs are excreted in human milk and because of the potential for serious adverse reactions in nursing infants from cytarabine, a decision should be made whether to discontinue nursing or to discontinue the drug, taking into account the importance of the drug to the mother.

9. Pediatric use

See INDICATIONS AND USAGE

ADVERSE REACTIONS

Expected Reactions

Because cytarabine is a bone marrow suppressant, anemia, leukopenia, thrombocytopenia, megaloblastosis and reduced reticulocytes can be expected as a result of administration with CYTOSAR-U Sterile Powder. The severity of these reactions are dose and schedule dependent.[18] Cellular changes in the morphology of bone marrow and peripheral smears can be expected.[19]

Following 5-day constant infusions or acute injections of 50 mg/m^2 to 600 mg/m^2, white cell depression follows a biphasic course. Regardless of initial count, dosage level, or schedule, there is an initial fall starting the first 24 hours with a nadir at days 7–9. This is followed by a brief rise which peaks around the twelfth day. A second and deeper fall reaches nadir at days 15–24. Then there is rapid rise to above baseline in the next 10 days. Platelet depression is noticeable at 5 days with a peak depression occurring between days 12–15. Thereupon, a rapid rise to above baseline occurs in the next 10 days.[20]

Infectious Complications

Infection: Viral, bacterial, fungal, parasitic, or saprophytic infections, in any location in the body may be associated with the use of CYTOSAR-U alone or in combination with other immunosuppressive agents following immunosuppressant doses that affect cellular or humoral immunity. These infections may be mild, but can be severe and at times fatal.

The Cytarabine (Ara-C) Syndrome
A cytarabine syndrome has been described by Castleberry.[21] It is characterized by fever, myalgia, bone pain, occasionally chest pain, maculopapular rash, conjunctivitis and malaise. It usually occurs 6–12 hours following drug administration. Corticosteroids have been shown to be beneficial in treating or preventing this syndrome. If the symptoms of the syndrome are deemed treatable, corticosteroids should be contemplated as well as continuation of therapy with CYTOSAR-U.

Most Frequent Adverse Reactions
anorexia
nausea
vomiting
diarrhea
oral and anal inflammation or ulceration
hepatic dysfunction
fever
rash
thrombophlebitis
bleeding (all sites)

Nausea and vomiting are most frequent following rapid injection.

Less Frequent Adverse Reactions
sepsis
pneumonia
cellulitis at injection site
skin ulceration
urinary retention
renal dysfunction
neuritis
neural toxicity
sore throat
esophageal ulceration
esophagitis
chest pain
pericarditis
bowel necrosis
abdominal pain
pancreatitis
freckling
jaundice
conjunctivitis (may occur with rash)
dizziness
alopecia
anaphylaxis (See WARNINGS)
allergic edema
pruritus
shortness of breath
urticaria
headache

Experimental Doses
Severe and at times fatal CNS, GI and pulmonary toxicity (different from that seen with conventional therapy regimens of CYTOSAR-U) has been reported following some experimental dose schedules of CYTOSAR-U.[8-11] These reactions include reversible corneal toxicity and hemorrhagic conjunctivitis, which may be prevented or diminished by prophylaxis with a local corticosteroid eye drop; cerebral and cerebellar dysfunction, including personality changes, somnolence and coma, usually reversible; severe gastrointestinal ulceration, including pneumatosis cystoides intestinalis leading to peritonitis; sepsis and liver abscess; pulmonary edema, liver damage with increased hyperbilirubinemia; bowel necrosis; and necrotizing colitis. Rarely, severe skin rash, leading to desquamation has been reported. Complete alopecia is more commonly seen with experimental high dose therapy than with standard treatment programs using CYTOSAR-U. If experimental high dose therapy is used, do not use a diluent containing benzyl alcohol.

Cases of cardiomyopathy with subsequent death have been reported following experimental high dose therapy with cytarabine in combination with cyclophosphamide when used for bone marrow transplant preparation.[12] **This cardiac toxicity may be schedule dependent.**[45]

A syndrome of sudden respiratory distress, rapidly progressing to pulmonary edema and radiographically pronounced cardiomegaly has been reported following experimental high dose therapy with cytarabine used for the treatment of relapsed leukemia from one institution in 16/72 patients. The outcome of this syndrome can be fatal.[13]

Two patients with adult acute non-lymphocytic leukemia developed peripheral motor and sensory neuropathies after consolidation with high-dose CYTOSAR-U, daunorubicin, and asparaginase. Patients treated with high-dose CYTOSAR-U should be observed for neuropathy since dose schedule alterations may be needed to avoid irreversible neurologic disorders.[22]

Ten patients treated with experimental intermediate doses of CYTOSAR-U (1 g/m^2) with and without other chemotherapeutic agents (meta-AMSA, daunorubicin, etoposide) at various dose regimes developed a diffuse interstitial pneumonitis without clear cause that may have been related to the CYTOSAR-U.[43]

Two cases of pancreatitis have been reported following experimental doses of CYTOSAR-U and numerous other drugs. CYTOSAR-U could have been the causative agent.[44]

OVERDOSAGE

There is no antidote for overdosage of CYTOSAR-U. Doses of 4.5 g/m^2 by intravenous infusion over 1 hour every 12 hours for 12 doses has caused an unacceptable increase in irreversible CNS toxicity and death.[9]

Single doses as high as 3 g/m^2 have been administered by rapid intravenous infusion without apparent toxicity.[23]

DOSAGE AND ADMINISTRATION

CYTOSAR-U Sterile Powder is not active orally. The schedule and method of administration varies with the program of therapy to be used. CYTOSAR-U may be given by intravenous infusion or injection, subcutaneously, or intrathecally. Thrombophlebitis has occurred at the site of drug injection or infusion in some patients, and rarely patients have noted pain and inflammation at subcutaneous injection sites. In most instances, however, the drug has been well tolerated.

Patients can tolerate higher total doses when they receive the drug by rapid intravenous injection as compared with slow infusion. This phenomenon is related to the drug's rapid inactivation and brief exposure of susceptible normal and neoplastic cells to significant levels after rapid injection. Normal and neoplastic cells seem to respond in somewhat parallel fashion to these different modes of administration and no clear-cut clinical advantage has been demonstrated for either.

In the induction therapy of acute non-lymphocytic leukemia, the usual cytarabine dose in combination with other anti-cancer drugs is 100 mg/m^2 /day by continuous IV infusion (Days 1–7) or 100 mg/m^2 IV every 12 hours (Days 1–7). The literature should be consulted for the current recommendations for use in acute lymphocytic leukemia.

Intrathecal Use in Meningeal Leukemia
CYTOSAR-U has been used intrathecally in acute leukemia in doses ranging from 5 mg/m^2 to 75 mg/m^2 of body surface area. The frequency of administration varied from once a day for 4 days to once every 4 days. The most frequently used dose was 30 mg/m^2 every 4 days until cerebrospinal fluid findings were normal, followed by one additional treatment. [24-28] The dosage schedule is usually governed by the type and severity of central nervous system manifestations and the response to previous therapy.

If used intrathecally, do not use a diluent containing benzyl alcohol. Many clinicians reconstitute with autologous spinal fluid or preservative-free 0.9% Sodium Chloride, USP, for Injection and use immediately.

CYTOSAR-U given intrathecally may cause systemic toxicity and careful monitoring of the hemopoietic system is indicated. Modification of other anti-leukemia therapy may be necessary. Major toxicity is rare. The most frequently reported reactions after intrathecal administration were nausea, vomiting and fever; these reactions are mild and self-limiting. Paraplegia has been reported.[29] Necrotizing leukoencephalopathy occurred in 5 children; these patients had also been treated with intrathecal methotrexate and hydrocortisone, as well as by central nervous system radiation.[30] Isolated neurotoxicity has been reported.[31] Blindness occurred in two patients in remission whose treatment had consisted of combination systemic chemotherapy, prophylactic central nervous system radiation and intrathecal CYTOSAR-U.[32]

When CYTOSAR-U is administered both intrathecally and intravenously within a few days, there is an increased risk of spinal cord toxicity, however, in serious life-threatening disease, concurrent use of intravenous and intrathecal CYTOSAR-U is left to the discretion of the treating physician.[48]

Focal leukemic involvement of the central nervous system may not respond to intrathecal CYTOSAR-U and may better be treated with radiotherapy.

The 100 mg vial may be reconstituted with 5 mL of Bacteriostatic Water for Injection with Benzyl Alcohol 0.945% w/v added as preservative. The resulting solution contains 20 mg of cytarabine per mL. (Do not use Bacteriostatic Water for Injection with Benzyl Alcohol 0.945% w/v as a diluent for intrathecal use. See WARNINGS).

The 500 mg vial may be reconstituted with 10 mL Bacteriostatic Water for Injection with Benzyl Alcohol 0.945% w/v added as preservative. The resulting solution contains 50 mg of cytarabine per mL. (Do not use Bacteriostatic Water for Injection with Benzyl Alcohol 0.945% w/v as a diluent for intrathecal use. See WARNINGS).

The 1 gram vial may be reconstituted with 10 mL of Bacteriostatic Water for Injection with Benzyl Alcohol 0.945% w/v added as preservative. The resulting solution contains 100 mg of cytarabine per mL. (Do not use Bacteriostatic Water for Injection with Benzyl Alcohol 0.945% w/v as a diluent for intrathecal use. See WARNINGS).

The 2 gram vial may be reconstituted with 20 mL of Bacteriostatic Water for Injection with Benzyl Alcohol 0.945% w/v added as preservative. The resulting solution contains 100 mg of cytarabine per mL. (Do not use Bacteriostatic Water for Injection with Benzyl Alcohol 0.945% w/v as a diluent for intrathecal use. See WARNINGS).

If used intrathecally many clinicians reconstitute with preservative-free 0.9% Sodium Chloride for Injection and use immediately.

The pH of the reconstituted solutions is about 5. Solutions reconstituted with Bacteriostatic Water for Injection with Benzyl Alcohol 0.945% w/v may be stored at controlled room temperature, 20° to 25° C (68° to 77° F) for 48 hours. Discard any solutions in which a slight haze develops.

Solutions reconstituted without a preservative should be used immediately.

Chemical Stability of Infusion Solutions:
Chemical stability studies were performed by ultraviolet assay on CYTOSAR-U in infusion solutions. These studies showed that when reconstituted CYTOSAR-U was added to Water for Injection, 5% Dextrose in Water or Sodium Chloride Injection, 94 to 96 percent of the cytarabine was present after 192 hours storage at room temperature.

Parenteral drugs should be inspected visually for particulate matter and discoloration, prior to administration, whenever solution and container permit.

Procedures for proper handling and disposal of anticancer drugs should be considered. Several guidelines on this subject have been published.[33-38] There is no general agreement that all of the procedures recommended in the guidelines are necessary or appropriate.

HOW SUPPLIED

CYTOSAR-U Sterile Powder (sterile cytarabine) is available in multi-dose vials of four sizes:
100 mg vial, NDC 0009-0373-01
500 mg vial, NDC 0009-0473-01
1 g vial, NDC 0009-3295-01
2 g vial, NDC 0009-3296-01

Store the product at controlled room temperature 20° to 25° C (68° to 77° F) [see USP].

REFERENCES

1. Zaky DA, Betts RF, Douglas RG, et al: Varicella-Zoster Virus and Subcutaneous Cytarabine: Correlation of In Vitro Sensitivities to Blood Levels. *Antimicrob Agents Chemother* 1975; 7:229-232.
2. Davis CM, VanDersarl JV, Coltman CA Jr: Failure of Cytarabine in Varicella-Zoster Infections. *JAMA* 1973; *224*: 122-123.
3. Betts RF, Zaky DA, Douglas RG, et al: Ineffectiveness of Subcutaneous Cytosine Arabinoside in Localized Herpes Zoster. *Ann Intern Med* 1975; *82*:778-783.
4. Dennis DT, Doberstyn EB, Awoke S, et al: Failure of Cytosine Arabinoside in Treatment Smallpox; A Double-blind Study, *Lancet* 1974; *2*:377-379.
5. Gray GD: ARA-C and Derivatives as Examples of Immunosuppressive Nucleoside Analogs. *Ann NY Acad Sci* 1975; *255*:372-379.
6. Mitchell MS, Wade ME, DeConti RC, et al: Immunosuppressive Effects of Cytosine Arabinoside and Methotrexate in Man. *Ann Intern Med* 1969; *70*:535-547
7. Frei E, Ho DHW, Bodey GP, et al: Pharmacologic and Cytokinetic Studies of Arabinosyl Cytosine, In *Unifying Concepts of Leukemia. Bibl. Hematol.* No. 39. Karger, Basel 1973, pp 1085-1097.
8. Hopen G, Mondino BJ, Johnson BL, et al: Corneal Toxicity with Systemic Cytarabine. *Am J Ophthalmol* 1981; *91*:500-504.
9. Lazarus HM, Herzig RH, Herzig GP, et al: Central Nervous System Toxicity of High-Dose Systemic Cytosine Arabinoside. *Cancer* 1981; *48*:2577-2582.
10. Slavin RE, Dias MA, Soral R: Cytosine Arabinoside Induced Gastrointestinal Toxic Alterations in Sequential Chemotherapeutic Protocols—A Clinical Pathologic Study of 33 Patients. *Cancer* 1978; *42*:1747-1759.
11. Haupt HM, Hutchins GM, Moore GW: Ara-C Lung: Noncardiogenic Pulmonary Edema Complicating Cytosine Arabinoside Therapy of Leukemia. *Am J Med* 1981; *70*: 256-261.
12. Takvorian T, Anderson K, Ritz J: A Fatal Cardiomyopathy Associated with High Dosage Ara-C (HIDAC) and Cyclophosphamide (CTX) in Bone Marrow Transplantation (BMTx). (Abstract submitted for 1985 AACR Meetings in Houston, Texas.)

Continued on next page

Information on these Pharmacia & Upjohn products is based on labeling in effect June 1, 1998. Further information concerning these and other Pharmacia & Upjohn products may be obtained by direct inquiry to Medical Information, Pharmacia & Upjohn, Kalamazoo, MI 49001.

Cytosar-U—Cont.

13. Andersson BS, Cogan B, Keating MJ, Estey EH, et al: Subacute Pulmonary Failure Complicating Therapy with High-Dose Ara-C in Acute Leukemia. *Cancer* 1985; 56: 2181-2184.

14. Dunton SF, Ruprecht N, Spruce W, et al: Progressive Ascending Paralysis Following Administration of Intrathecal and Intravenous Cytosine Arabinoside. *Cancer* 1986; 57:1083-1088.

15. Altman AJ, Dinndorf P, Quinn JJ: Acute Pancreatitis in Association with Cytosine Arabinoside Therapy. *Cancer* 1982; 49:1384-1386.

16. Shafer AI: Teratogenic Effects of Antileukemic Chemotherapy. *Arch Intern Med* 1981; 141:514-515.

17. Wagner VM, et al: Congenital Abnormalities in Baby Born to Cytarabine Treated Mother. *Lancet* 1980; 2:98-99.

18. Frei E III, Bickers JN, Hewlett JS, et al: Dose Schedule and Antitumor Studies of Arabinosyl Cytosine (NSC 63878). *Cancer Res* 1969; 29:1325-1332.

19. Bell WR, Wang JJ, Carbone PP, et al: Cytogenetic and Morphologic Abnormalities in Human Bone Marrow Cells during Cytosine Arabinoside Therapy. *J Hematol* 1966; 27:771-781.

20. Burke PJ, Serpick AA, Carbone PP, et al: A Clinical Evaluation of Dose and Schedule of Administration of Cytosine Arabinoside (NSC 63878). *Cancer Res* 1968; 28: 274-279.

21. Castleberry RP, Crist WM, Holbrook T, et al: The Cytosine Arabinoside (Ara-C) Syndrome. *Med Pediatr Oncol* 1981; 9:257-264.

22. Powell BL, Capizzi RL, Lyerly EW, et al: Peripheral Neuropathy After High-Dose Cytosine Arabinoside, Daunorubicin, and Asparaginase Consolidation for Acute Nonlymphocytic Leukemia. *J Clin Oncol* 1986; 4 (1):95- 97.

23. Rudnick SA, et al: High Dose Cytosine Arabinoside (HDARAC) In Refractory Acute Leukemia. *Cancer* 1979; 44:1189-1193.

24. Proceedings of the Chemotherapy Conference on ARA-C: Development and Application (Cytosine Arabinoside Hydrochloride—NSC 63878), Oct. 10, 1969

25. Lay HN, Colebatch JH, Ekert H: Experiences with Cytosine Arabinoside in Childhood Leukaemia and Lymphoma. *Med J Aust* 1971; 2:187-192.

26. Halikowski B, Cyklis R, Armata J, et al: Cytosine Arabinoside Administered Intrathecally in Cerebromeningeal Leukemia, *Acta Paediat Scand* 1970; 59: 164-168.

27. Wang JJ, Pratt CB: Intrathecal Arabinosyl Cytosine in Meningeal Leukemia. *Cancer* 1970; 25:531-534.

28. Band PR, Holland JF, Bernard J, et al: Treatment of Central Nervous System Leukemia with Intrathecal Cytosine Arabinoside. *Cancer* 1973; 32:744-748.

29. Saiki JH, Thompson S, Smith F, et al: Paraplegia Following Intrathecal Chemotherapy. *Cancer* 1972; 29:370-374.

30. Rubinstein LJ, Herman MM, Long TF, et al: Disseminated Necrotizing Leukoencephalopathy: A Complication of Treated Central System Leukemia and Lymphoma. *Cancer* 1975; 35:291-305.

31. Marmont AM, Damasio EE: Neurotoxicity of Intrathecal Chemotherapy for Leukaemia. *Brit Med J* 1973; 4:47.

32. Margileth DA, Poplack DG, Pizzo PA, et al: Blindness During Remission in Two Patients with Acute Lymphoblastic Leukemia. *Cancer* 1977; 39:58-61

33. Recommendations for the Safe Handling of Parenteral Antineoplastic Drugs. NIH Publication No. 83-2621. For sale by the Superintendent of Documents, US Government Printing Office, Washington, DC 20402.

34. AMA Council Report, Guidelines for Handling Parenteral Antineoplastics. *JAMA*, March 15, 1985.

35. National Study Commission on Cytotoxic Exposure-Recommendations for Handling Cytotoxic Agents. Available from Louis P. Jeffrey, ScD, Director of Pharmacy Services, Rhode Island Hospital, 593 Eddy Street, Providence, Rhode Island 02902.

36. Clinical Oncological Society of Australia: Guidelines and recommendations for safe handling of antineoplastic agents. *Med J Australia* 1983; 1:426-428.

37. Jones, RB, et al: Safe handling of chemotherapeutic agents: A report from the Mount Sinai Medical Center CA-A *Cancer Journal for Clinicians* Sept/Oct., 1983, pp. 258-263.

38. American Society of Hospital Pharmacists Technical assistance bulletin on handling cytotoxic drugs in hospitals. *Am J Hosp Pharm* 1985; 42:131-137.

39. Kuhlman J: Inhibition of Digoxin Absorption but not of Digitoxin During Cytostatic Drug Therapy. *Arzneim Forsch* 1982; 32:698-704.

40. Moody MR, Morris JJ, Yang VM, et al: Effect of Two Cancer Chemotherapeutic Agents on the Antibacterial Activity of Three Antimicrobial Agents. *Antimicrob Agents Chemother* 1978; 14:737-742.

41. Holt RJ: Clinical Problems with 5-Fluorocytosine. *Mykosen* 1978; 21(11):363-369.

42. Polak A, Grenson M: Interference Between the Uptake of Pyrimidines and Purines in Yeasts. *Path Microbiol* 1973; 39:37-38.

43. Peters WG, Willemze R, Colly LP: Results of Induction and Consolidation Treatment with Intermediate and High-Dose Ara-C and m-AMSA Containing Regimens in Patients with Primarily Failed or Relapsed Acute Leukemia and Non-Hodgkin's Lymphoma. *Scan J Hemat* 1986; 36 (Suppl 44):7-16.

44. Siemers RF, Friedenberg WR, Norfleet RG: High-Dose Cytosine Arabinoside-Associated Pancreatitis. *Cancer* 1985; 56:1940-1942.

45. Paul S, et al: "High Dose Ara-C Does Not Increase the Cardiotoxicity of cyclophosphamide —Total Body Irradiation Conditioning Regimes for Bone Marrow Transplantation". *Proceeding of ASCO* 1989; 8:16, abstract 60.

46. Nand S, Messmore HL, Patel R, et al: Neurotoxicity Associated With Systemic High-Dose Cytosine Arabinoside. *J Clin Oncol* 1986; 4 (4):571-575.

47. Damon LE, Mass R, Linker CA: The Association Between High-Dose Cytarabine Neurotoxicity and Renal Insufficiency. *J Clin Oncol* 1989; 7 (10):1563-1568.

48. Watterson J, Toogood I, Nieder M, et al: Excessive Spinal Cord Toxicity from Intensive Central Nervous System-Directed Therapies. *Cancer* 1994; 74:3034-3041.

49. Smith GA, Damon LE, Rugo HS, et al: High-Dose Cytarabine Dose Modification Reduces the Incidence of Neurotoxicity in Patients with Renal Insufficiency. *J Clin Oncol* 1997; 15:833-839.

50. McBride CE, Yavorski RT, Moses FM, et al: Acute Pancreatitis Associated with Continuous Infusion Cytarabine Therapy: A Case Report. *Cancer* 1996; 77:2588-2591.

ANIMAL TOXICOLOGY

Toxicity of cytarabine in experimental animals, as well as activity, is markedly influenced by the schedule of administration. For example, in mice, the LD_{10} for single intraperitoneal administration is greater than 6000 mg/m². However, when administered as 8 doses, each separated by 3 hours, the LD_{10} is less than 750 mg/m² total dose. Similarly, although a total dose of 1920 mg/m² administered as 12 injections at 6-hour intervals was lethal to beagle dogs (severe bone marrow hypoplasia with evidence of liver and kidney damage), dogs receiving the same total dose administered in 8 injections (again at 6-hour intervals) over a 48-hour period survived with minimal signs of toxicity. The most consistent observation in surviving dogs was elevated transaminase levels. In all experimental species the primary limiting toxic effect is marrow suppression with leukopenia. In addition, cytarabine causes abnormal cerebellar development in the neonatal hamster and is teratogenic to the rat fetus.

Caution: Federal law prohibits dispensing without prescription.

Pharmacia & Upjohn Company • Kalamazoo, Michigan 49001, USA

Revised September 1997

810 126 322
691618

DEPO-MEDROL®   ℞

[depō' mĕ-drōl]
methylprednisolone acetate
sterile aqueous suspension
(sterile methylprednisolone acetate
suspension, USP)

Not For Intravenous Use

DESCRIPTION

DEPO-MEDROL Sterile Aqueous Suspension contains methylprednisolone acetate which is the 6-methyl derivative of prednisolone. Methylprednisolone acetate is a white or practically white, odorless, crystalline powder which melts at about 215° with some decomposition. It is soluble in dioxane, sparingly soluble in acetone, in alcohol, in chloroform, and in methanol, and slightly soluble in ether. It is practically insoluble in water. The chemical name for methylprednisolone acetate is pregna-1,4-diene-3,20-dione, 21-(acetyloxy)-11,17-dihydroxy-6-methyl-, (6α,11β)-and the molecular weight is 416.51. The structural formula is represented below:

DEPO-MEDROL is an anti-inflammatory glucocorticoid for intramuscular, intrasynovial, soft tissue or intralesional injection. It is available in three strengths: 20 mg/mL; 40 mg/mL; 80 mg/mL.

Each mL of these preparations contains:

Methylprednisolone acetate	20 mg	40 mg	80 mg
Polyethylene glycol 3350	29.5 mg	29.1 mg	28.2 mg
Polysorbate 80	1.97 mg	1.94 mg	1.88 mg
Monobasic sodium phosphate	6.9 mg	6.8 mg	6.59 mg
Dibasic sodium phosphate USP	1.44 mg	1.42 mg	1.37 mg
Benzyl alcohol added as a preservative	9.3 mg	9.16 mg	8.88 mg

Sodium Chloride was added to adjust tonicity.
When necessary, pH was adjusted with sodium hydroxide and/or hydrochloric acid.
The pH of the finished product remains within the USP specified range; ie, 3.5 to 7.0.

HOW SUPPLIED

DEPO-MEDROL Sterile Aqueous Suspension is available in the following strengths and package sizes:

20 mg per mL
    5 mL vials   NDC 0009-0274-01
40 mg per mL
    5 mL vials   NDC 0009-0280-02
    25 × 5 mL vials   NDC 0009-0280-51
    10 mL vials   NDC 0009-0280-03
    25 × 10 mL vials   NDC 0009-0280-52
80 mg per mL
    5 mL vials   NDC 0009-0306-02
    25 × 5 mL vials   NDC 0009-0306-12

Store at controlled room temperature 20° to 25° C (68° to 77° F) [see USP].

Caution: Federal law prohibits dispensing without prescription.

Pharmacia & Upjohn Company • Kalamazoo, Michigan 49001, USA

Revised November 1997

810 341 225
691211

DEPO-PROVERA®   ℞

[dep-ō-prō-vera]
Contraceptive Injection
medroxyprogesterone acetate injectable suspension,
USP

Patients should be counseled that this product does not protect against HIV infection (AIDS) and other sexually transmitted diseases.

DESCRIPTION

DEPO-PROVERA Contraceptive Injection contains medroxyprogesterone acetate, a derivative of progesterone, as its active ingredient. Medroxyprogesterone acetate is active by the parenteral and oral routes of administration. It is a white to off-white, odorless crystalline powder that is stable in air and that melts between 200° C and 210° C. It is freely soluble in chloroform, soluble in acetone and dioxane, sparingly soluble in alcohol and methanol, slightly soluble in ether, and insoluble in water.

The chemical name for medroxyprogesterone acetate is pregn-4-ene-3,20-dione, 17-(acetyloxy)-6-methyl-, (6α)-. The structural formula is as follows:

medroxyprogesterone acetate

DEPO-PROVERA Contraceptive Injection for intramuscular (IM) injection is available in vials and prefilled syringes, each containing 1 mL of medroxyprogesterone acetate sterile aqueous suspension 150 mg/mL.

Each mL contains:

Medroxyprogesterone acetate	150 mg
Polyethylene glycol 3350	28.9 mg
Polysorbate 80	2.41 mg
Sodium chloride	8.68 mg
Methylparaben	1.37 mg
Propylparaben	0.150 mg
Water for injection	qs

When necessary, pH is adjusted with sodium hydroxide or hydrochloric acid, or both.

CLINICAL PHARMACOLOGY

DEPO-PROVERA Contraceptive Injection (medroxyprogesterone acetate), when administered at the recommended dose to women every 3 months, inhibits the secretion of gonadotropins which, in turn, prevents follicular maturation and ovulation and results in endometrial thinning. These actions produce its contraceptive effect.

Following a single 150 mg IM dose of DEPO-PROVERA Contraceptive Injection, medroxyprogesterone acetate concentrations, measured by an extracted radioimmunoassay procedure, increase for approximately 3 weeks to reach peak plasma concentrations of 1 to 7 ng/mL. The levels then decrease exponentially until they become undetectable (<100 pg/mL) between 120 to 200 days following injection. Using an unextracted radioimmunoassay procedure for the assay of medroxyprogesterone acetate in serum, the apparent half-life for medroxyprogesterone acetate following IM administration of DEPO-PROVERA Contraceptive Injection is approximately 50 days.

Women with lower body weights conceive sooner than women with higher body weights after discontinuing DEPO-PROVERA Contraceptive Injection.

The effect of hepatic and/or renal disease on the pharmacokinetics of DEPO-PROVERA Contraceptive Injection is unknown.

INDICATIONS AND USAGE

DEPO-PROVERA Contraceptive Injection is indicated only for the prevention of pregnancy. To ensure that DEPO-PROVERA Contraceptive Injection is not administered inadvertently to a pregnant woman, the first injection must be given **ONLY** during the first 5 days of a normal menstrual period; **ONLY** within the first 5-days postpartum if not breast-feeding, and if exclusively breast-feeding, **ONLY** at the sixth postpartum week. The efficacy of DEPO-PROVERA Contraceptive Injection depends on adherence to the recommended dosage schedule (see DOSAGE AND ADMINISTRATION). It is a long-term injectable contraceptive in women when administered at 3-month (13-week) intervals. Dosage does not need to be adjusted for body weight.

In five clinical studies using DEPO-PROVERA Contraceptive Injection, the 12-month failure rate for the group of women treated with DEPO-PROVERA Contraceptive Injection was zero (no pregnancies reported) to 0.7 by Life-Table method. Pregnancy rates with contraceptive measures are typically reported for only the first year of use as shown in Table 1. Except for intrauterine devices (IUD), implants, sterilization, and DEPO-PROVERA Contraceptive Injection, the efficacy of these contraceptive measures depends in part on the reliability of use. The effectiveness of DEPO-PROVERA Contraceptive Injection is dependent on the patient returning every 3 months (13 weeks) for reinjection. [See table 1 above]

CONTRAINDICATIONS

1. Known or suspected pregnancy or as a diagnostic test for pregnancy.
2. Undiagnosed vaginal bleeding.
3. Known or suspected malignancy of breast.
4. Active thrombophlebitis, or current or past history of thromboembolic disorders, or cerebral vascular disease.
5. Liver dysfunction or disease.
6. Known hypersensitivity to DEPO-PROVERA Contraceptive Injection (medroxyprogesterone acetate or any of its other ingredients).

WARNINGS

1. Bleeding Irregularities

Most women using DEPO-PROVERA Contraceptive Injection experience disruption of menstrual bleeding patterns. Altered menstrual bleeding patterns include irregular or unpredictable bleeding or spotting, or rarely, heavy or continuous bleeding. If abnormal bleeding persists or is severe, appropriate investigation should be instituted to rule out the possibility of organic pathology, and appropriate treatment should be instituted when necessary.

As women continue using DEPO-PROVERA Contraceptive Injection, fewer experience irregular bleeding and more experience amenorrhea. By month 12 amenorrhea was reported by 55% of women, and by month 24 amenorrhea was reported by 68% of women using DEPO-PROVERA Contraceptive Injection.[2]

2. Bone Mineral Density Changes

Use of DEPO-PROVERA Contraceptive Injection may be considered among the risk factors for development of osteoporosis. The rate of bone loss is greatest in the early years of use and then subsequently approaches the normal rate of age related fall.

3. Cancer Risks

Long-term case-controlled surveillance of users of DEPO-PROVERA Contraceptive Injection found slight or no increased overall risk of breast cancer[3] and no overall increased risk of ovarian,[4] liver,[5] or cervical[6] cancer and a prolonged, protective effect of reducing the risk of endometrial[7] cancer in the population of users.

A pooled analysis[14] from two case-control studies, the World Health Organization Study[3] and the New Zealand Study[13],

Table 1
Lowest Expected and Typical Failure Rates*
Expressed as Percent of Women Experiencing an Accidental Pregnancy in the First Year of Continuous Use

Method	Lowest Expected	Typical
Injectable progestogen DEPO-PROVERA	0.3	0.3
Implants Norplant (6 capsules)	0.2†	0.2†
Female sterilization	0.2	0.4
Male sterilization	0.1	0.15
Pill		3
Combined	0.1	
Progestogen	0.5	
IUD		3
Progestasert	2	
Copper T 380A	0.8	
Condom	2	12
Diaphragm	6	18
Cap	6	18
Spermicides	3	21
Sponge		
Parous women	9	28
Nulliparous women	6	18
Periodic abstinence	1–9	20
Withdrawal	4	18
No method	85	85

Source: Trussell et al[1]

* Lowest expected - when used exactly as directed.
  Typical - includes those not following directions exactly.
† from Norplant® package insert.

reported the relative risk (RR) of breast cancer for women who had ever used DEPO-PROVERA Contraceptive Injection as 1.1 (95% confidence interval (CI) 0.97 to 1.4). Overall, there was no increase in risk with increasing duration of use of DEPO-PROVERA Contraceptive Injection. The RR of breast cancer for women of all ages who had initiated use of DEPO-PROVERA Contraceptive Injection within the previous 5 years was estimated to be 2.0 (95% CI 1.5 to 2.8).

The World Health Organization Study[3], a component of the pooled analysis[14] described above, showed an increased RR of 2.19 (95% CI 1.23 to 3.89) of breast cancer associated with use of DEPO-PROVERA Contraceptive Injection in women whose first exposure to drug was within the previous 4 years and who were under 35 years of age. However, the overall RR for ever-users of DEPO-PROVERA Contraceptive Injection was only 1.2 (95% CI 0.96 to 1.52).

[NOTE: A RR of 1.0 indicates neither an increased nor a decreased risk of cancer associated with the use of the drug, relative to no use of the drug. In the case of the subpopulation with a RR of 2.19, the 95% CI is fairly wide and does not include the value of 1.0, thus inferring an increased risk of breast cancer in the defined subgroup relative to nonusers. The value of 2.19 means that women whose first exposure to drug was within the previous 4 years and who are under 35 years of age have a 2.19-fold (95% CI 1.23 to 3.89-fold) increased risk of breast cancer relative to nonusers. The National Cancer Institute[8] reports an average annual incidence rate for breast cancer for US women, all races, age 30 to 34 years of 26.7 per 100,000. A RR of 2.19, thus, increases the possible risk from 26.7 to 58.5 cases per 100,000 women. The attributable risk, thus, is 31.8 per 100,000 women per year.]

A statistically insignificant increase in RR estimates of invasive squamous-cell cervical cancer has been associated with the use of DEPO-PROVERA Contraceptive Injection in women who were first exposed before the age of 35 years (RR 1.22 to 1.28 and 95% CI 0.93 to 1.70). The overall, nonsignificant relative risk of invasive squamous-cell cervical cancer in women who ever used DEPO-PROVERA Contraceptive Injection was estimated to be 1.11 (95% CI 0.96 to 1.29). No trends in risk with duration of use or times since initial or most recent exposure were observed.

4. Thromboembolic Disorders

The physician should be alert to the earliest manifestations of thrombotic disorders (thrombophlebitis, pulmonary embolism, cerebrovascular disorders, and retinal thrombosis). Should any of these occur or be suspected, the drug should not be readministered.

5. Ocular Disorders

Medication should not be readministered pending examination if there is a sudden partial or complete loss of vision or if there is a sudden onset of proptosis, diplopia, or migraine. If examination reveals papilledema or retinal vascular lesions, medication should not be readministered.

6. Unexpected Pregnancies

To ensure that DEPO-PROVERA Contraceptive Injection is not administered inadvertently to a pregnant woman, the first injection must be given **ONLY** during the first 5 days of a normal menstrual period; **ONLY** within the first 5-days postpartum if not breast-feeding, and if exclusively breast-feeding, **ONLY** at the sixth postpartum week (see DOSAGE AND ADMINISTRATION).

Neonates from unexpected pregnancies that occur 1 to 2 months after injection of DEPO-PROVERA Contraceptive Injection may be at an increased risk of low birth weight, which, in turn, is associated with an increased risk of neonatal death. The attributable risk is low because such pregnancies are uncommon.[9,10]

A significant increase in incidence of polysyndactyly and chromosomal anomalies was observed among infants of users of DEPO-PROVERA Contraceptive Injection, the former being most pronounced in women under 30 years of age. The unrelated nature of these defects, the lack of confirmation from other studies, the distant preconceptual exposure to DEPO-PROVERA Contraceptive Injection, and the chance effects due to multiple statistical comparisons, make a causal association unlikely.[11]

Neonates exposed to medroxyprogesterone acetate *in utero* and followed to adolescence, showed no evidence of any adverse effects on their health including their physical, intellectual, sexual, or social development.

Continued on next page

Information on these Pharmacia & Upjohn products is based on labeling in effect June 1, 1998. Further information concerning these and other Pharmacia & Upjohn products may be obtained by direct inquiry to Medical Information, Pharmacia & Upjohn, Kalamazoo, MI 49001.

Depo-Provera Injection—Cont.

Several reports suggest an association between intrauterine exposure to progestational drugs in the first trimester of pregnancy and genital abnormalities in male and female fetuses. The risk of hypospadias (five to eight per 1,000 male births in the general population) may be approximately doubled with exposure to these drugs. There are insufficient data to quantify the risk to exposed female fetuses, but because some of these drugs induce mild virilization of the external genitalia of the female fetus and because of the increased association of hypospadias in the male fetus, it is prudent to avoid the use of these drugs during the first trimester of pregnancy.
To ensure that DEPO-PROVERA Contraceptive Injection is not administered inadvertently to a pregnant woman, it is important that the first injection be given only during the first 5 days after the onset of a normal menstrual period within 5 days postpartum if not breast-feeding and if breast-feeding, at the sixth week postpartum (see DOSAGE AND ADMINISTRATION).
7. Ectopic Pregnancy
Health-care providers should be alert to the possibility of an ectopic pregnancy among women using DEPO-PROVERA Contraceptive Injection who become pregnant or complain of severe abdominal pain.
8. Lactation
Detectable amounts of drug have been identified in the milk of mothers receiving DEPO-PROVERA Contraceptive Injection. In nursing mothers treated with DEPO-PROVERA Contraceptive Injection, milk composition, quality, and amount are not adversely affected. Neonates and infants exposed to medroxyprogesterone from breast milk have been studied for developmental and behavioral effects through puberty. No adverse effects have been noted.
9. Anaphylaxis and Anaphylactoid Reaction
Anaphylaxis and anaphylactoid reaction have been reported with the use of DEPO-PROVERA Contraceptive Injection. If an anaphylactic reaction occurs appropriate therapy should be instituted. Serious anaphylactic reactions require emergency medical treatment.

PRECAUTIONS

GENERAL
1. Physical Examination
The pretreatment and annual history and physical examination should include special reference to breast and pelvic organs, as well as a Papanicolaou smear.
2. Fluid Retention
Because progestational drugs may cause some degree of fluid retention, conditions that might be influenced by this condition, such as epilepsy, migraine, asthma, and cardiac or renal dysfunction, require careful observation.
3. Weight Changes
There is a tendency for women to gain weight while on therapy with DEPO-PROVERA Contraceptive Injection. From an initial average body weight of 136 lb, women who completed 1 year of therapy with DEPO-PROVERA Contraceptive Injection gained an average of 5.4 lb. Women who completed 2 years of therapy gained an average of 8.1 lb.
Women who completed 4 years gained an average of 13.8 lb.
Women who completed 6 years gained an average of 16.5 lb.
Two percent of women withdrew from a large-scale clinical trial because of excessive weight gain.
4. Return of Fertility
DEPO-PROVERA Contraceptive Injection has a prolonged contraceptive effect. In a large US study of women who discontinued use of DEPO-PROVERA Contraceptive Injection to become pregnant, data are available for 61% of them. Based on Life-Table analysis of these data, it is expected that 68% of women who do become pregnant may conceive within 12 months, 83% may conceive within 15 months, and 93% may conceive within 18 months from the last injection. The median time to conception for those who do conceive is 10 months following the last injection with a range of 4 to 31 months, and is unrelated to the duration of use. No data are available for 39% of the patients who discontinued DEPO-PROVERA Contraceptive Injection to become pregnant and who were lost to follow-up or changed their mind.
5. CNS Disorders and Convulsions
Patients who have a history of psychic depression should be carefully observed and the drug not be readministered if the depression recurs.
There have been a few reported cases of convulsions in patients who were treated with DEPO-PROVERA Contraceptive Injection. Association with drug use or pre-existing conditions is not clear.
6. Carbohydrate Metabolism
A decrease in glucose tolerance has been observed in some patients on DEPO-PROVERA Contraceptive Injection treatment. The mechanism of this decrease is obscure. For this reason, diabetic patients should be carefully observed while receiving such therapy.
7. Liver Function
If jaundice develops, consideration should be given to not readministering the drug.
8. Protection Against Sexually Transmitted Diseases
Patients should be counseled that this product does not protect against HIV infection (AIDS) and other sexually transmitted diseases.

DRUG INTERACTIONS
Aminoglutethimide administered concomitantly with the DEPO-PROVERA Contraceptive Injection may significantly depress the serum concentrations of medroxyprogesterone acetate.[12] Users of DEPO-PROVERA Contraceptive Injection should be warned of the possibility of decreased efficacy with the use of this or any related drugs.

LABORATORY TEST INTERACTIONS
The pathologist should be advised of progestin therapy when relevant specimens are submitted.
The following laboratory tests may be affected by progestins including DEPO-PROVERA Contraceptive Injection:
(a) Plasma and urinary steroid levels are decreased (eg, progesterone, estradiol, pregnanediol, testosterone, cortisol).
(b) Gonadotropin levels are decreased.
(c) Sex-hormone-binding-globulin concentrations are decreased.
(d) Protein-bound iodine and butanol extractable protein-bound iodine may increase.
T_3-uptake values may decrease.
(e) Coagulation test values for prothrombin (Factor II), and Factors VII, VIII, IX, and X may increase.
(f) Sulfobromophthalein and other liver function test values may be increased.
(g) The effects of medroxyprogesterone acetate on lipid metabolism are inconsistent. Both increases and decreases in total cholesterol, triglycerides, low-density lipoprotein (LDL) cholesterol, and high-density lipoprotein (HDL) cholesterol have been observed in studies.

CARCINOGENESIS
See "WARNINGS" section 3.

PREGNANCY
Pregnancy Category X. See "WARNINGS" section 6.

NURSING MOTHERS
See "WARNINGS" section 8.

PEDIATRIC USE
Safety and effectiveness in pediatric patients have not been established. See "WARNINGS" section 6.

INFORMATION FOR THE PATIENT
See Patient Labeling.
Patient labeling is included with each single-dose vial and prefilled syringe of DEPO-PROVERA Contraceptive Injection to help describe its characteristics to the patient. It is recommended that prospective users be given this labeling and be informed about the risks and benefits associated with the use of DEPO-PROVERA Contraceptive Injection, as compared with other forms of contraception or with no contraception at all. It is recommended that physicians or other health-care providers responsible for those patients advise them at the beginning of treatment that their menstrual cycle may be disrupted and that irregular and unpredictable bleeding or spotting results, and that this usually decreases to the point of amenorrhea as treatment with DEPO-PROVERA Contraceptive Injection continues, without other therapy being required.

ADVERSE REACTIONS

In the largest clinical trial with DEPO-PROVERA Contraceptive Injection, over 3,900 women, who were treated for up to 7 years, reported the following adverse reactions, which may or may not be related to the use of DEPO-PROVERA Contraceptive Injection.
The following adverse reactions were reported by more than 5% of subjects:
Menstrual irregularities
(bleeding or amenorrhea, or both)
Weight changes
Headache
Nervousness
Abdominal pain or discomfort
Dizziness
Asthenia (weakness or fatigue)
Adverse reactions reported by 1% to 5% of subjects using DEPO-PROVERA Contraceptive Injection were:
Decreased libido or anorgasmia
Backache
Leg cramps
Depression
Nausea
Insomnia
Leukorrhea
Acne
Vaginitis
Pelvic pain
Breast pain
No hair growth or alopecia
Bloating
Rash
Edema
Hot flashes
Arthralgia
Events reported by fewer than 1% of subjects included: galactorrhea, melasma, chloasma, convulsions, changes in appetite, gastrointestinal disturbances, jaundice, genitourinary infections, vaginal cysts, dyspareunia, paresthesia, chest pain, pulmonary embolus, allergic reactions, anemia, drowsiness, syncope, dyspnea and asthma, tachycardia, fever, excessive sweating and body odor, dry skin, chills, increased libido, excessive thirst, hoarseness, pain at injection site, blood dyscrasia, rectal bleeding, changes in breast size, breast lumps or nipple bleeding, axillary swelling, breast cancer, prevention of lactation, sensation of pregnancy, lack of return to fertility, paralysis, facial palsy, scleroderma, osteoporosis, uterine hyperplasia, cervical cancer, varicose veins, dysmenorrhea, hirsutism, unexpected pregnancy, thrombophlebitis, deep vein thrombosis.
In addition, voluntary reports have been received of anaphylaxis and anaphylactoid reaction with use of DEPO-PROVERA Contraceptive Injection.

DOSAGE AND ADMINISTRATION

Both the 1 mL vial and the 1 mL prefilled syringe of DEPO-PROVERA Contraceptive Injection should be vigorously shaken just before use to ensure that the dose being administered represents a uniform suspension.
The recommended dose is 150 mg of DEPO-PROVERA Contraceptive Injection every 3 months (13 weeks) administered by deep, IM injection in the gluteal or deltoid muscle.
To ensure the patient is not pregnant at the time of the first injection, the first injection **MUST** be given **ONLY** during the first 5 days of a normal menstrual period; **ONLY** within the first 5-days postpartum if not breast-feeding; and if exclusively breast-feeding, **ONLY** at the sixth postpartum week.
If the time interval between injections is greater than 13 weeks, the physician should determine that the patient is not pregnant before administering the drug. The efficacy of DEPO-PROVERA Contraceptive Injection depends on adherence to the dosage schedule of administration.

HOW SUPPLIED

DEPO-PROVERA Contraceptive Injection (medroxyprogesterone acetate injectable suspension 150 mg/mL) is available as:

NDC 0009-0746-30	1 mL vial
NDC 0009-0746-34	5 × 1 mL vials
NDC 0009-0746-35	25 × 1 mL vials
NDC 0009-7376-01	1 mL prefilled syringe
NDC 0009-7376-02	6 × 1 mL prefilled syringes
NDC 0009-7376-03	24 × 1 mL prefilled syringes

Store at controlled room temperature 20° to 25° C (68° to 77° F) [see USP].

REFERENCES

1. Trussell J, Hatcher RA, Cates W Jr, Stewart FH, Kost K. A guide to interpreting contraceptive efficacy studies. Obstet Gynecol. 1990; *76*:558–567.
2. Schwallie PC, Assenzo JR. Contraceptive use-efficacy study utilizing medroxyprogesterone acetate administered as an intramuscular injection once every 90 days. Fertil Steril. 1973; *24*:331–339.
3. WHO Collaborative Study of Neoplasia and Steroid Contraceptives. Breast cancer and depot-medroxyprogesterone acetate: a multi-national study. Lancet. 1991; *338*:833–838.
4. WHO Collaborative Study of Neoplasia and Steroid Contraceptives. Depot-medroxyprogesterone acetate (DMPA) and risk of epithelial ovarian cancer. Int J Cancer. 1991; *49*:191–195
5. WHO Collaborative Study of Neoplasia and Steroid Contraceptives. Depot-medroxyprogesterone acetate (DMPA) and risk of liver cancer. Int J Cancer. 1991; *49*:182–185.
6. WHO Collaborative Study of Neoplasia and Steroid Contraceptives. Depot-medroxyprogesterone acetate (DMPA) and risk of invasive squamous-cell cervical cancer. Contraception. 1992; *45*:299–312.
7. WHO Collaborative Study of Neoplasia and Steroid Contraceptives. Depot-medroxyprogesterone acetate (DMPA) and risk of endometrial cancer. Int J Cancer. 1991; *49*:186–190.
8. Surveillance, Epidemiology, and End Results: Incidence and Mortality Data, 1973-1977. National Cancer Institute Monograph, 57: June 1981. (NIH publication No. 81-2330).
9. Gray RH, Pardthaisong T. *In Utero* exposure to steroid contraceptives and survival during infancy. Am J Epidemiol. 1991; *134*:804–811.
10. Pardthaisong T, Gray RH. *In Utero* exposure to steroid contraceptives and outcome of pregnancy. Am J Epidemiol. 1991; *134*:795–803.
11. Pardthaisong T, Gray RH, McDaniel EB, Chandacham A. Steroid contraceptive use and pregnancy outcome. Teratology. 1988; *38*:51–58.
12. Van Deijk WA, Blijham GH, Mellink WAM, Meulenberg PMM. Influence of aminoglutethimide on plasma levels of medroxyprogesterone acetate: its correlation with serum cortisol. Cancer Treatment Reports. 1985; *69*:1, 85–90.

13. Paul C, Skegg DCG, Spears GFS. Depot medroxyprogesterone (Depo-Provera) and risk of breast cancer. Br Med J. 1989; 299:759–762.

14. Skegg DCG, Noonan EA, Paul C, Spears GFS, Meirik O, Thomas DB. Depot Medroxyprogesterone Acetate and Breast Cancer: A Pooled Analysis from the World Health Organization and New Zealand Studies. JAMA. 1995; 273(10):799–804.

Caution: Federal law prohibits dispensing without prescription.

DEPO-PROVERA Contraceptive Injection 1 mL vials are manufactured by
Pharmacia & Upjohn Company, Kalamazoo, MI 49001, USA
DEPO-PROVERA Contraceptive Injection 1 mL prefilled syringes are manufactured by
Pharmacia & Upjohn N.V./S.A., Puurs, Belgium for Pharmacia & Upjohn Company, Kalamazoo, MI 49001, USA
Revised February 1998   815 459 311
                                         691400

DEPO-PROVERA®
Contraceptive Injection
medroxyprogesterone acetate
injectable suspension, USP

This product is intended to prevent pregnancy. It does not protect against HIV infection (AIDS) and other sexually transmitted diseases.

Patient Labeling
Introduction
Every woman who considers using DEPO-PROVERA Contraceptive Injection needs to understand the benefits and risks of this form of birth control and to discuss them with her health-care provider. This leaflet is intended to give you much of the information you will need in order to decide if DEPO-PROVERA Contraceptive Injection is the right choice for you. Your health-care provider will help you to compare DEPO-PROVERA Contraceptive Injection with other contraceptive methods and will answer any questions you have after you have read this information.

DEPO-PROVERA Contraceptive Injection is given as an intramuscular injection (a shot) in the buttock or upper arm once every 3 months (13 weeks). Promptly at the end of the 3-month interval, you will need to return to your health-care provider for your next injection in order to continue your contraceptive protection.

DEPO-PROVERA Contraceptive Injection contains medroxy progesterone acetate, a chemical similar to (but not the same as) the natural hormone progesterone that is produced by your ovaries during the second half of your menstrual cycle. DEPO-PROVERA Contraceptive Injection acts by preventing your egg cells from ripening. If an egg is not released from the ovaries during your menstrual cycle, it cannot become fertilized by sperm and result in pregnancy. DEPO-PROVERA Contraceptive Injection also causes changes in the lining of your uterus that make it less likely for pregnancy to occur.

Effectiveness of DEPO-PROVERA Contraceptive Injection
To ensure that DEPO-PROVERA Contraceptive Injection is not administered inadvertently to a pregnant woman, the first injection must be given **ONLY** during the first 5 days of a normal menstrual period; **ONLY** within the first 5-days postpartum if not breast-feeding, and if exclusively breast-feeding, **ONLY** at the sixth postpartum week (see **Administration of DEPO-PROVERA Contraceptive Injection**). The efficacy of DEPO-PROVERA Contraceptive Injection depends on adherence to the recommended dosage schedule.

DEPO-PROVERA Contraceptive Injection is over 99% effective, making it one of the most reliable methods of birth control available. This means that the average annual pregnancy rate is less than one for every 100 women who use DEPO-PROVERA Contraceptive Injection. The effectiveness of most contraceptive methods depends, in part, on how reliably each woman uses the method. The effectiveness of DEPO-PROVERA Contraceptive Injection depends only on the patient returning every 3 months (13 weeks) for her next injection.

The following table shows the percent of women who become pregnant while using different kinds of contraceptive methods. It gives both the lowest expected rate of pregnancy (the rate expected in women who use each method exactly as it should be used) and the typical rate of pregnancy (which includes women who became pregnant because they forgot to use their birth control or because they did not follow the directions exactly).

Percent of Women Experiencing an Accidental Pregnancy in the First Year of Continuous Use

Method	Lowest Expected	Typical
DEPO-PROVERA	0.3	0.3
Implants (Norplant)	0.2*	0.2*
Female sterilization	0.2	0.4
Male sterilization	0.1	0.15
Oral contraceptives (pill)	–	3
Combined	0.1	–
Progestogen only	0.5	–
IUD		
Progestasert	2	–
Copper T 380A	0.8	–
Condom (without spermicide)	2	12
Diaphragm (with spermicide)	6	18
Cervical cap	6	18
Withdrawal	4	18
Periodic abstinence	1–9	20
Spermicide alone	3	21
Vaginal sponge	–	–
used before childbirth	6	18
used after childbrith	9	28
No method	85	85

Source: Trussell et al: Obstet Gynecol 1990;76:558–567.

* From Norplant® package insert.

Who Should Not Use DEPO-PROVERA Contraceptive Injection
Certain women should not use DEPO-PROVERA Contraceptive Injection. You should not use DEPO-PROVERA Contraceptive Injection if you have any of the following conditions:
• if you think you might be pregnant
• if you have any vaginal bleeding without a known reason
• if you have had cancer of the breast
• if you have had a stroke
• if you have or have had blood clots (phlebitis) in your legs
• if you have problems with your liver or liver disease
• if you are allergic to DEPO-PROVERA Contraceptive Injection (medroxyprogesterone acetate or any of its other ingredients)

Other Things to Consider Before Choosing DEPO-PROVERA Contraceptive Injection
Before your doctor prescribes DEPO-PROVERA Contraceptive Injection, you will have a physical examination. It is important to tell your doctor or health-care provider if you have any of the following:
• a family history of cancer of the breast
• an abnormal mammogram (breast X-ray), fibrocystic breast disease, breast nodules or lumps, or bleeding from your nipples
• kidney disease
• irregular or scanty menstrual periods
• high blood pressure
• migraine headaches
• asthma
• epilepsy (convulsions or seizures)
• diabetes or a family history of diabetes
• a history of depression
• if you are taking any prescription or over-the-counter medications

This product is intended to prevent pregnancy. It does not protect against transmission of HIV (AIDS) and other sexually transmitted diseases such as chlamydia, genital herpes, genital warts, gonorrhea, hepatitis B, and syphilis.

Return of Fertility
Because DEPO-PROVERA Contraceptive Injection is a long-acting birth control method, it takes some time after your last injection for its effect to wear off. Based on the results from a large study done in the United States, of those women who stop using DEPO-PROVERA Contraceptive Injection in order to become pregnant, about half of those who become pregnant do so in about 10 months after their last injection; about two-thirds of those who become pregnant do so in about 12 months; about 83% of those who become pregnant do so in about 15 months, and about 93% of those who become pregnant do so in about 18 months after their last injection. The length of time you use DEPO-PROVERA Contraceptive Injection has no effect on how long it takes you to become pregnant after you stop using it.

Risks of Using DEPO-PROVERA Contraceptive Injection
1. Irregular Menstrual Bleeding
The side effect reported most frequently by women who use DEPO-PROVERA Contraceptive Injection for contraception is a change in their normal menstrual cycle. During the first year of using DEPO-PROVERA Contraceptive Injection, you might have one or more of the following changes:
• irregular or unpredictable bleeding or spotting,
• an increase or decrease in menstrual bleeding, or
• no bleeding at all.
Unusually heavy or continuous bleeding, however, is not a usual effect of DEPO-PROVERA Contraceptive Injection and if this happens you should see your health-care provider right away.
With continued use of DEPO-PROVERA Contraceptive Injection, bleeding usually decreases and many women stop having periods completely. In clinical studies of DEPO-PROVERA Contraceptive Injection, 55% of the women studied reported no menstrual bleeding (amenorrhea) after 1 year of use and 68% of the women studied reported no menstrual bleeding after 2 years of use.

The reason that your periods stop is because DEPO-PROVERA Contraceptive Injection causes a resting state in your ovaries. When your ovaries do not release an egg monthly, the regular monthly growth of the lining of your uterus does not occur and, therefore, the bleeding that comes with your normal menstruation does not take place. When you stop using DEPO-PROVERA Contraceptive Injection your menstrual period will usually, in time, return to its normal cycle.

2. Bone Mineral Changes
Use of DEPO-PROVERA Contraceptive Injection may be associated with a decrease in the amount of mineral stored in your bones. This could increase your risk of developing bone fractures. The rate of bone mineral loss is greatest in the early years of DEPO-PROVERA Contraceptive Injection use but, after that, it begins to resemble the normal rate of age-related bone mineral loss.

3. Cancer
Studies of women who have used different forms of contraception found that women who used DEPO-PROVERA Contraceptive Injection for contraception had no increased overall risk of developing cancer of the breast, ovary, uterus, cervix, or liver. However, women under 35 years of age whose first exposure to DEPO-PROVERA Contraceptive Injection was within the previous 4 to 5 years may have a slightly increased risk of developing breast cancer similar to that seen with oral contraceptives. You should discuss this with your health-care provider.

4. Unexpected Pregnancy
Because DEPO-PROVERA Contraceptive Injection is such an effective contraceptive method, the risk of unexpected pregnancy for women who get their shots regularly (every 3 months [13 weeks]) is very low. While there have been reports of an increased risk of low birth weight and neonatal infant death or other health problems in infants conceived close to the time of injection, such pregnancies are uncommon. If you think you may have become pregnant while using DEPO-PROVERA Contraceptive Injection for contraception, see your health-care provider as soon as possible.

5. Allergic Reactions
Severe allergic reactions known as anaphylaxis and anaphylactoid reactions have also been reported in some women using DEPO-PROVERA Contraceptive Injection.

6. Other Risks
Women who use hormone-based contraceptives may have an increased risk of blood clots or stroke. Also, if a contraceptive method fails, there is a possibility that the fertilized egg will begin to develop outside of the uterus (ectopic pregnancy). While these events are rare, you should tell your health-care provider if you have any of the Warning Signals listed in the next section.

Warning Signals
If any of these problems occur following an injection of DEPO-PROVERA Contraceptive Injection, call your health-care provider immediately:
• Sharp chest pain, coughing up of blood, or sudden shortness of breath (indicating a possible clot in the lung)
• Sudden severe headache or vomiting, dizziness or fainting, problems with your eyesight or speech, weakness, or numbness in an arm or leg (indicating a possible stroke)
• Severe pain or swelling in the calf (indicating a possible clot in the leg)
• Unusually heavy vaginal bleeding
• Severe pain or tenderness in the lower abdominal area
• Persistent pain, pus, or bleeding at the injection site

Side Effects of DEPO-PROVERA Contraceptive Injection
1. Weight Gain
You may experience a weight gain while you are using DEPO-PROVERA Contraceptive Injection. About two-thirds of the women who used DEPO-PROVERA Contraceptive Injection in the clinical trials reported a weight gain of about 5 pounds during the first year of use. You may continue to gain weight after the first year. Women in one large study who used DEPO-PROVERA Contraceptive Injection for 2 years gained an average total of 8.1 pounds over those 2 years, or approximately 4 pounds per year. Women who continued for 4 years gained an average total of 13.8 pounds over those 4 years, or approximately 3.5 pounds per year. Women who continued for 6 years gained an average total of 16.5 pounds over those 6 years, or approximately 2.75 pounds per year.

2. Other Side Effects
In a clinical study of over 3,900 women who used DEPO-PROVERA Contraceptive Injection for up to 7 years, some women reported the following effects that may or may not have been related to their use of DEPO-PROVERA Contraceptive Injection:

Continued on next page

Information on these Pharmacia & Upjohn products is based on labeling in effect June 1, 1998. Further information concerning these and other Pharmacia & Upjohn products may be obtained by direct inquiry to Medical Information, Pharmacia & Upjohn, Kalamazoo, MI 49001.

Consult 1999 PDR® supplements and future editions for revisions

Depo-Provera Injection—Cont.

- irregular menstrual bleeding
- amenorrhea
- headache
- nervousness
- abdominal cramps
- dizziness
- weakness or fatigue
- decreased sexual desire
- leg cramps
- nausea
- vaginal discharge or irritation
- breast swelling and tenderness
- bloating
- swelling of the hands or feet
- backache
- depression
- insomnia
- acne
- pelvic pain
- no hair growth or excessive hair loss
- rash
- hot flashes
- joint pain

Other problems were reported by very few of the women in the clinical trials, but some of these could be serious. These include: convulsions, jaundice, urinary tract infections, allergic reactions, fainting, paralysis, osteoporosis, lack of return to fertility, deep vein thrombosis, pulmonary embolus, breast cancer, or cervical cancer. If these or any other problems occur during your use of DEPO-PROVERA Contraceptive Injection, discuss them with your health-care provider.

General Precautions

1. Missed Periods

During the time you are using DEPO-PROVERA Contraceptive Injection for contraception, you may skip a period, or your periods may stop completely. If you have been receiving your injection of DEPO-PROVERA Contraceptive Injection regularly every 3 months (13 weeks), then you are probably not pregnant. However, if you think that you may be pregnant, see your health-care provider.

2. Laboratory Test Interactions

If you are scheduled for any laboratory tests, tell your health-care provider that you are using DEPO-PROVERA Contraceptive Injection for contraception. Certain blood tests are affected by hormones such as DEPO-PROVERA Contraceptive Injection.

3. Drug Interactions

Cytadren (aminoglutethimide) is an anticancer drug that may significantly decrease the effectiveness of DEPO-PROVERA Contraceptive Injection if the two drugs are given during the same time.

4. Nursing Mothers

Although DEPO-PROVERA Contraceptive Injection can be passed to the nursing infant in the breast milk, no harmful effects have been found in these children. DEPO-PROVERA Contraceptive Injection does not prevent the breasts from producing milk, so it can be used by nursing mothers. However, to minimize the amount of DEPO-PROVERA Contraceptive Injection that is passed to the infant in the first weeks after birth, you should wait until 6 weeks after childbirth before you start using DEPO-PROVERA Contraceptive Injection for contraception.

Administration of DEPO-PROVERA Contraceptive Injection

The recommended dose of DEPO-PROVERA Contraceptive Injection is 150 mg every 3 months (13 weeks) given in a single intramuscular injection in the buttock or upper arm. To ensure that you are not pregnant at the time of the first injection, it is essential that the injection be given **ONLY** during the first 5 days of a normal menstrual period. If used following the delivery of a child, the first injection of DEPO-PROVERA Contraceptive Injection **MUST** be given within 5 days after childbirth if you are not breast-feeding, or if you are exclusively breast-feeding, the injection **MUST** be given 6 weeks after childbirth. If you wait longer than 3 months (13 weeks) between injections, or longer than 6 weeks after delivery, your health-care provider should determine that you are not pregnant before giving you your injection of DEPO-PROVERA Contraceptive Injection.

Caution: Federal law prohibits dispensing without prescription.

Pharmacia & Upjohn Company
Kalamazoo, MI 49001, USA
Revised February 1998 815 459 311
691400

Shown in Product Identification Guide, page 332

DEPO-PROVERA® ℞
[dep-ō-prō-vera]
medroxyprogesterone acetate
injectable suspension, USP

DESCRIPTION

DEPO-PROVERA Sterile Aqueous Suspension contains medroxyprogesterone acetate, which is a derivative of progesterone and is active by the parenteral and oral routes of administration. It is a white to off-white, odorless crystalline powder, stable in air, melting between 200° and 210° C. It is freely soluble in chloroform, soluble in acetone and in dioxane, sparingly soluble in alcohol and methanol, slightly soluble in ether and insoluble in water.

The chemical name for medroxyprogesterone acetate is Pregn-4-ene-3,20-dione, 17-(acetyloxy)-6-methyl-, (6α)-. The structural formula is:

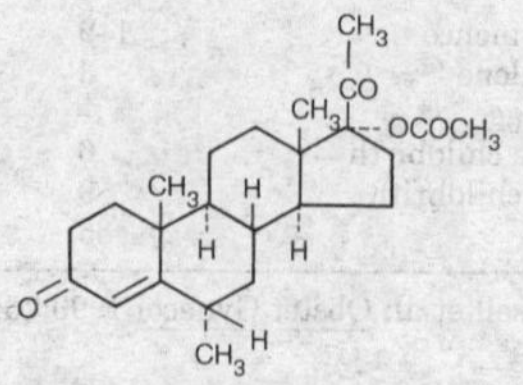

DEPO-PROVERA for intramuscular injection is available as 400 mg/mL medroxyprogesterone acetate. Each mL of the 400 mg/mL suspension contains:

Medroxyprogesterone acetate	400 mg
Polyethylene glycol 3350	20.3 mg
Sodium sulfate anhydrous	11 mg
with	
Myristyl-gamma-picolinium chloride	1.69 mg
added as preservative	

When necessary, pH was adjusted with sodium hydroxide and/or hydrochloric acid.

ACTIONS

Medroxyprogesterone acetate, administered parenterally in the recommended doses to women with adequate endogenous estrogen, transforms proliferative endometrium into secretory endometrium.

Medroxyprogesterone acetate inhibits (in the usual dose range) the secretion of pituitary gonadotropin which, in turn, prevents follicular maturation and ovulation.

Because of its prolonged action and the resulting difficulty in predicting the time of withdrawal bleeding following injection, medroxyprogesterone acetate is not recommended in secondary amenorrhea or dysfunctional uterine bleeding. In these conditions oral therapy is recommended.

INDICATIONS AND USES

Adjunctive therapy and palliative treatment of inoperable, recurrent, and metastatic endometrial or renal carcinoma.

CONTRAINDICATIONS

1. Known or suspected pregnancy or as a diagnostic test for pregnancy
2. Undiagnosed vaginal bleeding
3. Known or suspected malignancy of breast
4. Active thrombophlebitis, or current or past history of thromboembolic disorders, or cerebral vascular disease
5. Liver dysfunction or disease
6. Known sensitivity to DEPO-PROVERA (medroxyprogesterone acetate or any of its other ingredients).

WARNINGS

1. *Pregnancy* The use of progestational drugs during the first four months of pregnancy is not recommended. Progestational agents have been used beginning with the first trimester of pregnancy in attempts to prevent abortion but there is no evidence that such use is effective. Further more, the use of progestational agents, with their uterine-relaxant properties, in patients with fertilized defective ova may cause a delay in spontaneous abortion.

2. *Intrauterine Exposure* Several reports suggest an association between intrauterine exposure to progestational drugs in the first trimester of pregnancy and genital abnormalities in male and female fetuses. The risk of hypospadias (5 to 8 per 1,000 male births in the general population) may be approximately doubled with exposure to these drugs. There are insufficient data to quantify the risk to exposed female fetuses, but insofar as some of these drugs induce mild virilization of the external genitalia of the female fetus, and because of the increased association of hypospadias in the male fetus, it is prudent to avoid the use of these drugs during the first trimester of pregnancy.

If the patient is exposed to DEPO-PROVERA Sterile Aqueous Suspension during the first four months of pregnancy or if she becomes pregnant while taking this drug, she should be apprised of the potential risks to the fetus.

3. *Thromboembolic Disorders* The physician should be alert to the earliest manifestations of thrombotic disorder (thrombophlebitis, cerebrovascular disorder, pulmonary embolism, and retinal thrombosis). Should any of these occur or be suspected, the drug should be discontinued immediately.

4. *Ocular Disorders* Medication should be discontinued pending examination if there is a sudden partial or complete loss of vision, or if there is a sudden onset of proptosis, diplopia or migraine. If examination reveals papilledema or retinal vascular lesions, medication should be withdrawn.

5. *Lactation* Detectable amounts of drug have been identified in the milk of mothers receiving progestational drugs. The effect of this on the nursing infant has not been determined.

6. *Multi-dose Use* Multi-dose use of DEPO-PROVERA Sterile Aqueous Suspension from a single vial requires special care to avoid contamination. Although initially sterile, any multi-dose use of vials may lead to contamination unless strict aseptic technique is observed.

PRECAUTIONS

1. *Physical Examination* It is good medical practice for all women to have annual history and physical examinations, including women using DEPO-PROVERA Contraceptive Injection. The physical examination, however, may be deferred until after initiation of DEPO-PROVERA if requested by the woman and judged appropriate by the clinician. The physical examination should include special reference to blood pressure, breasts, abdomen and pelvic organs, including cervical cytology and relevant laboratory tests. In case of undiagnosed, persistent or recurrent abnormal vaginal bleeding, appropriate measures should be conducted to rule out malignancy. Women with a strong family history of breast cancer or who have breast nodules should be monitored with particular care.

2. *Fluid Retention* Because progestational drugs may cause some degree of fluid retention, conditions which might be influenced by this condition, such as epilepsy, migraine, asthma, cardiac or renal dysfunction, require careful observation.

3. *Vaginal Bleeding* In cases of breakthrough bleeding, as in all cases of irregular bleeding per vaginum, nonfunctional causes should be borne in mind and adequate diagnostic measures undertaken.

4. *Depression Patients* who have a history of psychic depression should be carefully observed and the drug discontinued if the depression recurs to a serious degree.

5. *Masking of Climacteric* The age of the patient constitutes no absolute limiting factor although treatment with progestin may mask the onset of the climacteric.

6. *Use with Estrogen* Studies of the addition of a progestin product to an estrogen replacement regimen for seven or more days of a cycle of estrogen administration have reported a lowered incidence of endometrial hyperplasia. Morphological and biochemical studies of endometria suggest that 10–13 days of a progestin are needed to provide maximal maturation of the endometrium and to eliminate any hyperplastic changes. Whether this will provide protection from endometrial carcinoma has not been clearly established.

There are possible risks which may be associated with the inclusion of progestin in estrogen replacement regimen, including adverse effects on carbohydrate and lipid metabolism. The dosage used may be important in minimizing these adverse effects.

A decrease in glucose tolerance has been observed in a small percentage of patients on estrogen-progestin combination treatment. The mechanism of this decrease is obscure. For this reason, diabetic patients should be carefully observed while receiving such therapy.

7. *Prolonged Use* The effect of prolonged use of DEPO-PROVERA Sterile Aqueous Suspension at the recommended doses on pituitary, ovarian, adrenal, hepatic, and uterine function is not known.

8. *Multi-dose Use* When multi-dose vials are used, special care to prevent contamination of the contents is essential. There is some evidence that benzalkonium chloride is not an adequate antiseptic for sterilizing DEPO-PROVERA Sterile Aqueous Suspension multi-dose vials. A povidone-iodine solution or similar product is recommended to cleanse the vial top prior to aspiration of contents. (See WARNINGS)

DRUG INTERACTIONS

Aminoglutethimide administered concomitantly with DEPO-PROVERA Sterile Aqueous Suspension may significantly depress the serum concentrations of medroxyprogesterone acetate. DEPO-PROVERA users should be warned of the possibility of decreased efficacy with the use of this or any related drugs.

LABORATORY TEST INTERACTIONS

The pathologist should be advised of progestin therapy when relevant specimens are submitted. The following laboratory tests may be affected by progestins including DEPO-PROVERA Sterile Aqueous Suspension:

a) Plasma and urinary steroid levels are decreased (e.g. progesterone, estradiol, pregnanediol, testosterone, cortisol).

b) Gonadotropin levels are decreased.

c) Sex-hormone binding globulin concentrations are decreased.

d) Protein bound iodine and butanol extractable protein bound iodine may increase. T_3 uptake values may decrease.

e) Coagulation test values for prothrombin (Factor II), and Factors VII, VIII, IX, and X may increase.

f) Sulfobromophthalein and other liver function test values may be increased.

g) The effects of medroxyprogesterone acetate on lipid metabolism are inconsistent. Both increases and decreases in total cholesterol, triglycerides, low-density lipoprotein (LDL) cholesterol, and high-density lipoprotein (HDL) cholesterol have been observed in studies.

CARCINOGENESIS, MUTAGENESIS, IMPAIRMENT OF FERTILITY

Long-term intramuscular administration of Medroxyprogesterone acetate (MPA) has been shown to produce mammary tumors in beagle dogs. There is no evidence of a carcinogenic effect associated with the oral administration of MPA to rats and mice. Medroxyprogesterone acetate was not mutagenic in a battery of *in vitro* or *in vivo* genetic toxicity assays.

Medroxyprogesterone acetate at high doses is an anti-fertility drug and high doses would be expected to impair fertility until the cessation of treatment.

INFORMATION FOR THE PATIENT

See Patient Information at end of insert.

ADVERSE REACTIONS

— (See WARNINGS for possible adverse effects on the fetus)
— breakthrough bleeding
— spotting
— change in menstrual flow
— amenorrhea
— headache
— nervousness
— dizziness
— edema
— change in weight (increase or decrease)
— changes in cervical erosion and cervical secretions
— cholestatic jaundice, including neonatal jaundice
— breast tenderness and galactorrhea
— skin sensitivity reactions consisting of urticaria, pruritus, edema and generalized rash
— acne, alopecia and hirsutism
— rash (allergic) with and without pruritis
— anaphylactoid reactions and anaphylaxis
— mental depression
— pyrexia
— fatigue
— insomnia
— nausea
— somnolence

In a few instances there have been undesirable sequelae at the site of injection, such as residual lump, change in color of skin, or sterile abscess.

A statistically significant association has been demonstrated between use of estrogen-progestin combination drugs and pulmonary embolism and cerebral thrombosis and embolism. For this reason patients on progestin therapy should be carefully observed. There is also evidence suggestive of an association with neuro-ocular lesions, e.g. retinal thrombosis and optic neuritis.

The following adverse reactions have been observed in patients receiving estrogen-progestin combination drugs:
— rise in blood pressure in susceptible individuals
— premenstrual syndrome
— changes in libido
— changes in appetite
— cystitis-like syndrome
— headache
— nervousness
— fatigue
— backache
— hirsutism
— loss of scalp hair
— erythema multiforma
— erythema nodosum
— hemorrhagic eruption
— itching
— dizziness

The following laboratory results may be altered by the use of estrogen-progestin combination drugs:
— increased sulfobromophthalein retention and other hepatic function tests
— coagulation tests: increase in prothrombin factors VII, VIII, IX, and X
— metyrapone test
— pregnanediol determinations
— thyroid function: increase in PBI, and butanol extractable protein bound iodine and decrease in T_3 uptake values

DOSAGE AND ADMINISTRATION

The suspension is intended for intramuscular administration only.

Endometrial or renal carcinoma—doses of 400 mg to 1000 mg of DEPO-PROVERA Sterile Aqueous Suspension per week are recommended initially. If improvement is noted within a few weeks or months and the disease appears stabilized, it may be possible to maintain improvement with as little as 400 mg per month. Medroxyprogesterone acetate is not recommended as primary therapy, but as adjunctive and palliative treatment in advanced inoperable cases including those with recurrent or metastatic disease.

When multi-dose vials are used, special care to prevent contamination of the contents is essential (See WARNINGS).

HOW SUPPLIED

DEPO-PROVERA Sterile Aqueous Suspension is available as 400 mg/mL in 2.5 and 10 mL vials.

The text of the patient insert for progestational drugs is set forth below.

PATIENT INFORMATION

DEPO-PROVERA Sterile Aqueous Suspension is a progestational drug. The information below is required by the U.S. Food and Drug Administration to be provided to all patients taking such products. This information relates only to the risk to the unborn child associated with use of progestational drugs during pregnancy. For further information on the use, side effects, and other risks associated with this product, ask your doctor.

WARNING FOR WOMEN

Progesterone or progesterone-like drugs have been used to prevent miscarriage in the first few months of pregnancy. No adequate evidence is available to show that they are effective for this purpose. Furthermore, most cases of early miscarriage are due to causes which could not be helped by these drugs.

There is an increased risk of minor birth defects in children whose mothers take this drug during the first 4 months of pregnancy. Several reports suggest an association between mothers who take these drugs in the first trimester of pregnancy and genital abnormalities in male and female babies. The risk to the male baby is the possibility of being born with a condition in which the opening of the penis is on the underside rather than the tip of the penis (hypospadias). Hypospadias occurs in about 5 to 8 per 1000 male births and is about doubled with exposure to these drugs. There is not enough information to quantify the risk to exposed female fetuses, but enlargement of the clitoris and fusion of the labia may occur, although rarely.

Therefore, since drugs of this type may induce mild masculinization of the external genitalia of the female fetus, as well as hypospadias in the male fetus, it is wise to avoid using the drug during the first trimester of pregnancy.

These drugs have been used as a test for pregnancy but such use is no longer considered safe because of possible damage to a developing baby. Also, more rapid methods for testing for pregnancy are now available.

If you take DEPO-PROVERA Sterile Aqueous Suspension and later find you were pregnant when you took it, be sure to discuss this with your doctor as soon as possible.

Rx only

Pharmacia & Upjohn Company
Kalamazoo, Michigan 49001, U.S.A.
Revised April 1998 810 597 212
692166

DETROL™ ℞

[*dĕ trōl*]

tolterodine tartrate tablets

DESCRIPTION

DETROL Tablets contain tolterodine tartrate. The active moiety, tolterodine, is a muscarinic receptor antagonist. The chemical name of tolterodine tartrate is (R)-N,N-diisopropyl-3-(2-hydroxy-5-methylphenyl)-3-phenylpropanamine L-hydrogen tartrate. The empirical formula of tolterodine tartrate is $C_{26}H_{37}NO_7$, and its molecular weight is 475.6. The structural formula of tolterodine tartrate is represented below:

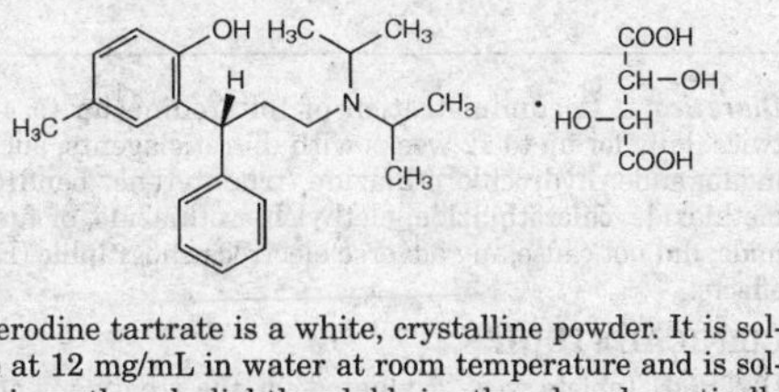

Tolterodine tartrate is a white, crystalline powder. It is soluble at 12 mg/mL in water at room temperature and is soluble in methanol, slightly soluble in ethanol, and practically insoluble in toluene.

DETROL Tablets for oral administration contain 1 or 2 mg of tolterodine tartrate. The inactive ingredients are colloidal anhydrous silica, calcium hydrogen phosphate dihydrate, cellulose microcrystalline, hydroxypropyl methylcellulose, magnesium stearate, sodium starch glycolate (pH 3.0 to 5.0), stearic acid, and titanium dioxide.

CLINICAL PHARMACOLOGY

Tolterodine is a competitive muscarinic receptor antagonist. Both urinary bladder contraction and salivation are mediated via cholinergic muscarinic receptors. In the anesthetized cat, tolterodine shows a selectivity for the urinary bladder over salivary glands; however, the clinical relevance of this finding has not been established.

After oral administration, tolterodine is metabolized in the liver, resulting in the formation of the 5-hydroxymethyl derivative, a major pharmacologically active metabolite. The 5-hydroxymethyl metabolite, which exhibits an antimuscarinic activity similar to that of tolterodine, contributes significantly to the therapeutic effect. Both tolterodine and the 5-hydroxymethyl metabolite exhibit a high specificity for muscarinic receptors, since both show negligible activity or affinity for other neurotransmitter receptors and other potential cellular targets, such as calcium channels.

Tolterodine has a pronounced effect on bladder function in healthy volunteers. The main effects following a 6.4-mg single dose of tolterodine were an increase in residual urine, reflecting an incomplete emptying of the bladder, and a decrease in detrusor pressure. These findings are consistent with a potent antimuscarinic action on the lower urinary tract.

Pharmacokinetics

Absorption: In a study of ^{14}C-tolterodine in healthy volunteers who received a 5-mg oral dose, at least 77% of the radiolabeled dose was absorbed. Tolterodine is rapidly absorbed, and maximum serum concentrations (C_{max}) typically occur within 1 to 2 hours after dose administration. The pharmacokinetics of tolterodine, based on C_{max} and area under the concentration-time curve (AUC) determinations, are dose-proportional over the range of 1 to 4 mg.

Effect of Food: Food intake increases the bioavailability of tolterodine (average increase 53%) and does not affect the levels of the 5-hydroxymethyl metabolite in extensive metabolizers. This change is not expected to be a safety concern and adjustment of dose is not needed.

Distribution: Tolterodine is highly bound to plasma proteins, primarily α_1-acid glycoprotein. Unbound concentrations of tolterodine average 3.7% ± 0.13% over the concentration range achieved in clinical studies. The 5-hydroxymethyl metabolite is not extensively protein bound, with unbound fraction concentrations averaging 36% ± 4.0%. The blood to serum ratio of tolterodine and the 5-hydroxymethyl metabolite averages 0.6 and 0.8, respectively, indicating that these compounds do not distribute extensively into erythrocytes. The volume of distribution of tolterodine following administration of a 1.28-mg intravenous dose is 113 ± 26.7 L.

Metabolism: Tolterodine is extensively metabolized by the liver following oral dosing. The primary metabolic route involves the oxidation of the 5-methyl group and is mediated by the cytochrome P450 2D6 and leads to the formation of a pharmacologically active 5-hydroxymethyl metabolite. Further metabolism leads to formation of the 5-carboxylic acid and N-dealkylated 5-carboxylic acid metabolites, which account for 51% ± 14% and 29% ± 6.3% of the metabolites recovered in the urine, respectively.

Variability in Metabolism: A subset (about 7%) of the population is devoid of cytochrome P450 2D6, the enzyme responsible for the formation of the 5-hydroxymethyl metabolite of tolterodine. The identified pathway of metabolism for these individuals, referred to as "poor metabolizers," is dealkylation via cytochrome P450 3A4 to N-dealkylated tolterodine. The remainder of the population is referred to as "extensive metabolizers." Pharmacokinetic studies revealed that tolterodine is metabolized at a slower rate in poor metabolizers than in extensive metabolizers; this results in significantly higher serum concentrations of tolterodine and in negligible concentrations of the 5-hydroxymethyl metabolite. Because of differences in the protein-binding characteristics of tolterodine and the 5-hydroxymethyl metabolite, the sum of unbound serum concentrations of tolterodine and the 5-hydroxymethyl metabolite is similar in extensive and poor metabolizers at steady state. Since tolterodine and the 5-hydroxymethyl metabolite have similar antimuscarinic effects, the net activity of DETROL Tablets is expected to be similar in extensive and poor metabolizers.

Excretion: Following administration of a 5-mg oral dose of ^{14}C-tolterodine to healthy volunteers, 77% of radioactivity was recovered in urine and 17% was recovered in feces. Less than 1% (<2.5% in poor metabolizers) of the dose was recovered as intact tolterodine, and 5% to 14% (<1% in poor metabolizers) was recovered as the active 5-hydroxymethyl metabolite. Most of the radioactivity was recovered within the first 24 hours, which is consistent with the apparent half-life of tolterodine: 1.9 to 3.7 hours in pharmacokinetic studies.

Continued on next page

Information on these Pharmacia & Upjohn products is based on labeling in effect June 1, 1998. Further information concerning these and other Pharmacia & Upjohn products may be obtained by direct inquiry to Medical Information, Pharmacia & Upjohn, Kalamazoo, MI 49001.

Detrol—Cont.

A summary of mean (± standard deviation) pharmacokinetic parameters of tolterodine and the 5-hydroxymethyl metabolite in extensive (EM) and poor (PM) metabolizers is provided in the following table. These data were obtained following single- and multiple-doses of tolterodine 4 mg administered twice daily to 16 healthy male subjects (8 EM, 8 PM).

[See first table above]

Pharmacokinetics in Special Populations

Age: In Phase 1, multiple-dose studies in which tolterodine 2 mg was administered twice daily, serum concentrations of tolterodine and of the 5-hydroxymethyl metabolite were similar in healthy elderly volunteers (aged 64 through 80 years) and healthy young volunteers (aged less than 40 years). In another Phase 1 study, elderly volunteers (aged 71 through 81 years) were given tolterodine 1 or 2 mg twice daily. Mean serum concentrations of tolterodine and the 5-hydroxymethyl metabolite in these elderly volunteers were approximately 20% and 50% higher, respectively, than reported in young healthy volunteers. However, no overall differences were observed in safety between older and younger patients in Phase 3, 12-week, controlled clinical studies; therefore, no dosage adjustment is recommended (see PRECAUTIONS, Geriatric Use).

Pediatric: The pharmacokinetics of tolterodine have not been established in pediatric patients.

Gender: The pharmacokinetics of tolterodine and the 5-hydroxymethyl metabolite are not influenced by gender. Mean C_{max} of tolterodine (1.6 µg/L in males versus 2.2 µg/L in females) and the active 5-hydroxymethyl metabolite (2.2 µg/L in males versus 2.5 µg/L in females) are similar in males and females who were administered tolterodine 2 mg. Mean AUC values of tolterodine (6.7 µg/L in males versus 7.8 µg/L in females) and the 5-hydroxymethyl metabolite (10 µg/L in males versus 11 µg/L in females) are also similar. The elimination half-life of tolterodine for both males and females is 2.4 hours, and the half-life of the 5-hydroxymethyl metabolite is 3.0 hours in females and 3.3 hours in males.

Race: Pharmacokinetic differences due to race have not been established.

Renal Insufficiency: The pharmacokinetics of tolterodine in patients with renal insufficiency have not been evaluated. The renal excretion of tolterodine and the 5-hydroxymethyl metabolite are negligible, and a decrease in total body clearance is not expected in patients with renal insufficiency. However, patients with renal impairment should be treated with caution.

Hepatic Insufficiency: Liver impairment can significantly alter the disposition of tolterodine. In a study conducted in cirrhotic patients, the elimination half-life of tolterodine was longer in cirrhotic patients (mean, 8.7 hours) than in healthy, young and elderly volunteers (mean, 2 to 4 hours). The clearance of orally administered tolterodine was substantially lower in cirrhotic patients (1.1 ± 1.7 L/h/kg) than in the healthy volunteers (5.7 ± 3.8 L/h/kg). Patients with significantly reduced hepatic function should not receive doses of DETROL greater than 1 mg twice daily (see PRECAUTIONS, General).

Drug-Drug Interactions

Fluoxetine: Fluoxetine is a selective serotonin reuptake inhibitor and a potent inhibitor of cytochrome P450 2D6 activity. In a study to assess the effect of fluoxetine on the pharmacokinetics of tolterodine and its metabolites, it was observed that fluoxetine significantly inhibited the metabolism of tolterodine in extensive metabolizers, resulting in a 4.8-fold increase in tolterodine AUC. There was a 52% decrease in C_{max} and a 20% decrease in AUC of the 5-hydroxymethyl metabolite. Fluoxetine thus alters the pharmacokinetics in patients who would otherwise be extensive metabolizers of tolterodine to resemble the pharmacokinetic profile in poor metabolizers. The sums of unbound serum concentrations of tolterodine and the 5-hydroxymethyl metabolite are only 25% higher during the interaction. No dose adjustment is required when DETROL and fluoxetine are coadministered.

Other Drugs Metabolized by Cytochrome P450 2D6: Tolterodine is not expected to influence the pharmacokinetics of drugs that are metabolized by cytochrome P450 2D6, such as flecainide, vinblastine, carbamazepine, and tricyclic antidepressants; however, the potential effect of tolterodine on the pharmacokinetics of these drugs has not been formally evaluated.

Warfarin: In healthy volunteers, coadministration of tolterodine 2 mg twice daily for 7 days and a single 25-mg dose of warfarin on day 4 had no effect on prothrombin time, Factor VII suppression, or on the pharmacokinetics of warfarin.

Oral Contraceptives: Tolterodine 2 mg twice daily had no effect on the pharmacokinetics of an oral contraceptive (ethinyl estradiol 30 µg/levonorgestrel 150 µg) as evidenced by the monitoring of ethinyl estradiol and levonorgestrel over a 2-month cycle in healthy female volunteers.

Phenotype (CYP2D6)	Tolterodine					5-Hydroxymethyl Metabolite			
	t_{max} (h)	C_{max}* (µg/L)	C_{avg}* (µg/L)	$t_{1/2}$ (h)	CL/F (L/h)	t_{max} (h)	C_{max}* (µg/L)	C_{avg}* (µg/L)	$t_{1/2}$ (h)
Single-dose									
EM	1.6±1.5	1.6±1.2	0.50±0.35	2.0±0.7	534±697	1.8±1.4	1.8±0.7	0.62±0.26	3.1±0.7
PM	1.4±0.5	10±4.9	8.3±4.3	6.5±1.6	17±7.3	—†	—	—	—
Multiple-dose									
EM	1.2±0.5	2.6±2.8	0.58±0.54	2.2±0.4	415±377	1.2±0.5	2.4±1.3	0.92±0.46	2.9±0.4
PM	1.9±1.0	19±7.5	12±5.1	9.6±1.5	11±4.2	—	—	—	—

*Parameter was dose-normalized from 4 mg to 2 mg.
C_{max} = Maximum plasma concentration; t_{max} = Time of occurrence of C_{max};
C_{avg} = Average plasma concentration; $t_{1/2}$ = Terminal elimination half-life; CL/F = Apparent oral clearance.
†— = not applicable.

95% Confidence Intervals for the Difference between DETROL (2 mg bid) and Placebo for the Median Change at Week 12 from Baseline

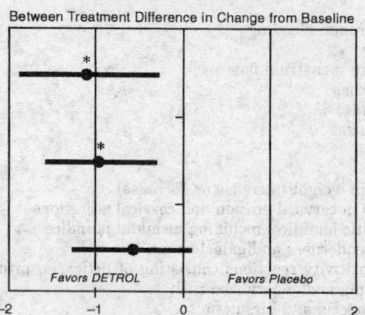

Number of Micturitions per 24 Hours

Study		DETROL	Placebo
008	number of patients	118	56
	median baseline	10.5	10.6
	median (SD) change from baseline	-2.2 (3.8)	-1.1 (3.6)
009	number of patients	128	64
	median baseline	10.4	10.4
	median (SD) change from baseline	-2.2 (2.1)	-1.2 (2.3)
010	number of patients	108	56
	median baseline	11.0	10.9
	median (SD) change from baseline	-1.6 (2.3)	-1.1 (2.8)

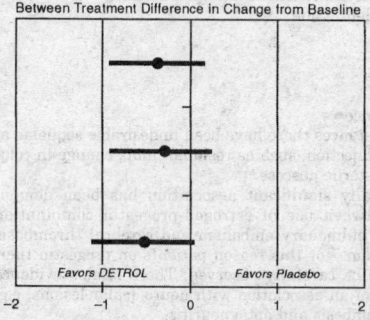

Number of Incontinence Episodes per 24 Hours

Study		DETROL	Placebo
008	number of patients	93	40
	median baseline	2.4	2.5
	median (SD) change from baseline	-1.2 (3.2)	-0.8 (1.5)
009	number of patients	116	55
	median baseline	2.5	3.2
	median (SD) change from baseline	-1.4 (2.5)	-1.1 (2.5)
010	number of patients	90	50
	median baseline	2.7	2.2
	median (SD) change from baseline	-1.5 (2.4)	-0.9 (2.1)

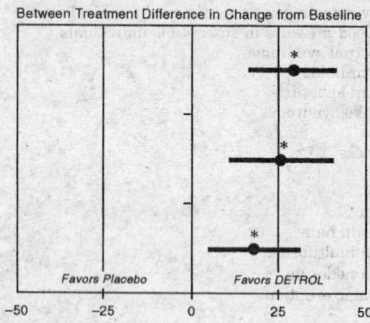

Volume Voided per Micturition (mL)

Study		DETROL	Placebo
008	number of patients	118	56
	median baseline	156	155
	median (SD) change from baseline	34 (54)	5 (42)
009	number of patients	128	64
	median baseline	149	157
	median (SD) change from baseline	34 (50)	8 (47)
010	number of patients	108	56
	median baseline	148	164
	median (SD) change from baseline	27 (45)	10 (52)

*The difference between DETROL and placebo was statistically significant.

Diuretics: Coadministration of tolterodine up to 4 mg twice daily for up to 12 weeks with diuretic agents, such as indapamide, hydrochlorothiazide, triamterene, bendroflumethiazide, chlorothiazide, methylchlorothiazide, or furosemide, did not cause any adverse electrocardiographic (ECG) effects.

CLINICAL STUDIES

DETROL Tablets were evaluated for the treatment of patients with an overactive bladder with symptoms of urinary frequency, urgency, or urge incontinence in three placebo-controlled, 12-week studies. A total of 339 patients received DETROL 2 mg twice daily and 177 patients received placebo. The majority of patients were Caucasian (95%) and female (75%), with a mean age of 60 years (range, 19 to 91 years). At study entry, nearly all patients perceived they had urgency (98%) and most patients had increased frequency of micturitions (89%) and urge incontinence (83%). These characteristics were well balanced across treatment groups for the three studies.

The efficacy endpoints included the change from baseline for:
- number of micturitions per 24 hours (averaged over 7 days)
- number of incontinence episodes per 24 hours (averaged over 7 days)
- volume of urine voided per micturition (averaged over 2 days)

Efficacy results for the three placebo-controlled, 12-week studies are presented in the following figures:
[See second table above]

INDICATIONS AND USAGE

DETROL Tablets are indicated for the treatment of patients with an overactive bladder with symptoms of urinary frequency, urgency, or urge incontinence.

CONTRAINDICATIONS

DETROL Tablets are contraindicated in patients with urinary retention, gastric retention, or uncontrolled narrow-angle glaucoma. DETROL is also contraindicated in pa-

tients who have demonstrated hypersensitivity to the drug or its ingredients.angle glaucoma.

PRECAUTIONS

General

Risk of Urinary Retention and Gastric Retention: DETROL should be administered with caution to patients with clinically significant bladder outflow obstruction because of the risk of urinary retention and to patients with gastrointestinal obstructive disorders, such as pyloric stenosis, because of the risk of gastric retention (see CONTRAINDICATIONS).

Controlled Narrow-Angle Glaucoma: DETROL should be used with caution in patients being treated for narrow-angle glaucoma.

Reduced Hepatic and Renal Function: Patients with significantly reduced hepatic function should not receive doses of DETROL greater than 1 mg twice daily. Patients with renal impairment should be treated with caution (see CLINICAL PHARMACOLOGY, Pharmacokinetics in Special Populations).

Information for Patients

Patients should be informed that antimuscarinic agents such as tolterodine may produce blurred vision.

Drug Interactions

Cytochrome P450 3A4 Inhibitors: Pharmacokinetic studies with patients concomitantly receiving cytochrome P450 3A4 inhibitors, such as macrolide antibiotics (erythromycin and clarithromycin) or antifungal agents (ketoconazole, itraconazole, and miconazole), have not been performed. Patients receiving cytochrome P450 3A4 inhibitors should not receive doses of DETROL greater than 1 mg twice daily.

Drug-Laboratory-Test Interactions

Interactions between tolterodine and laboratory tests have not been studied.

Carcinogenesis, Mutagenesis, Impairment of Fertility

Carcinogenicity studies with tolterodine were conducted in mice and rats. At the maximum tolerated dose in mice (30 mg/kg/day), female rats (20 mg/kg/day), and male rats (30 mg/kg/day), AUC values obtained for tolterodine were 355, 291, and 462 μg•h/L, respectively. In comparison, the human AUC value for a 2-mg dose administered twice daily is estimated at 34 μg•h/L. Thus, tolterodine exposure in the carcinogenicity studies was 9- to 14-fold higher than expected in humans. No increase in tumors was found in either mice or rats.

No mutagenic effects of tolterodine were detected in a battery of in vitro tests, including bacterial mutation assays (Ames test) in four strains of *Salmonella typhimurium* and in two strains of *Escherichia coli*, a gene mutation assay in L5178Y mouse lymphoma cells, and chromosomal aberration tests in human lymphocytes. Tolterodine was also negative in vivo in the bone marrow micronucleus test in the mouse.

In female mice treated for 2 weeks before mating and during gestation with 20 mg/kg/day (corresponding to AUC value of about 500 μg•h/L), neither effects on reproductive performance or fertility were seen. Based on AUC values, the systemic exposure was about 15-fold higher in animals than in humans. In male mice, a dose of 30 mg/kg/day did not induce any adverse effects on fertility.

Pregnancy

Pregnancy Category C. At oral doses of 20 mg/kg/day (approximately 14 times the human exposure), no anomalies or malformations were observed in mice. When given at doses of 30 to 40 mg/kg/day, tolterodine has been shown to cause embryolethality, reduce fetal weight, and increase the incidence of fetal abnormalities (cleft palate, digital abnormalities, intra-abdominal hemorrhage, and various skeletal abnormalities, primarily reduced ossification) in mice. At these doses, the AUC values were about 20- to 25-fold higher than in humans. Rabbits treated subcutaneously at a dose of 0.8 mg/kg/day achieved an AUC of 100 μg•h/L, which is about three-fold higher than that resulting from the human dose. This dose did not result in any embryotoxicity or teratogenicity. There are no studies of tolterodine in pregnant women. Therefore, DETROL should be used during pregnancy only if the potential benefit for the mother justifies the potential risk for the fetus.

Nursing Mothers

Tolterodine is excreted into the milk in mice. Offspring of female mice treated with tolterodine 20 mg/kg/day during the lactation period had slightly reduced body-weight gain. The offspring regained the weight during the maturation phase. It is not known whether tolterodine is excreted in human milk; therefore, administration of DETROL should be discontinued during nursing.

Pediatric Use

The safety and effectiveness of DETROL in pediatric patients have not been established.

Geriatric Use

Of the 1120 patients who were treated in the four, Phase 3, 12-week clinical studies of DETROL, 474 (42%) were 65 to 91 years of age. No overall differences in safety were observed between the older and younger patients (see CLINICAL PHARMACOLOGY, Pharmacokinetics in Special Populations).

Incidence (%) of Adverse Events Reported in ≥1% of Patients Treated with DETROL (2 mg bid) in 12-Week, Phase 3 Clinical Studies

Body System	Adverse Event*	DETROL 2 mg bid N=474	Placebo N=176
% Patients Reporting Adverse Events		75.5	77.8
% Patients Reporting Serious Adverse Events		3.7	3.4
% Patients Discontinuing due to Adverse Events		8.0	5.7
Autonomic Nervous	dry mouth	39.5	15.9
General	back pain	2.7	3.4
	chest pain	3.4	1.7
	fatigue	6.8	7.4
	headache	11.0	7.4
	influenza-like symptoms	4.4	6.3
	fall	1.3	0.6
Central/ Peripheral Nervous	paresthesia	1.1	0.6
	vertigo/dizziness	8.6	9.1
Gastrointestinal	abdominal pain	7.6	6.3
	constipation	6.5	4.5
	diarrhea	4.0	6.3
	dyspepsia	5.9	1.7
	flatulence	1.3	0.6
	nausea	4.2	5.7
	vomiting/nausea	1.7	0.6
Respiratory	bronchitis	2.1	0.6
	coughing	2.1	1.7
	pharyngitis	1.5	2.3
	rhinitis	1.1	1.1
	sinusitis	1.1	5.7
	URI	5.9	9.1
Urinary	dysuria	2.5	4.0
	micturition frequency	1.1	1.7
	urinary retention/mict dis	1.7	2.8
	UTI	5.5	7.4
Skin/ Appendages	pruritus	1.3	1.1
	rash/erythema	1.9	2.8
	skin dry	1.7	0.6
Musculoskeletal	arthralgia	2.3	2.8
Vision	vision abnormal (including accommodation)	4.7	4.0
	xerophthalmia	3.8	1.7
Psychiatric	nervousness	1.1	0.6
	somnolence	3.0	1.7
Metabolic/Nutritional	weight gain	1.5	1.1
Cardiovascular	hypertension	1.5	0.6
Resistance Mechanism	infection	2.1	1.1
	infection fungal	1.1	0.0

*Abbreviations: URI = upper respiratory infection, UTI = urinary tract infection, mict dis = micturition disorders.

ADVERSE REACTIONS

The Phase 2 and 3 clinical trial program for DETROL included 2049 patients who were treated with DETROL (N=1619) or placebo (N=430). No differences in the safety profile of tolterodine were identified based on age, gender, race, or metabolism. Four Phase 3, 12-week, controlled clinical studies form the basis for the main evaluation of safety, and the results are summarized below.

Adverse events considered to be treatment-related were dry mouth, dyspepsia, headache, constipation, and xerophthalmia. Dry mouth, constipation, abnormal vision (accommodation abnormalities), urinary retention, and xerophthalmia are expected side effects of antimuscarinic agents.

Dry mouth was the most frequently reported adverse event for patients treated with DETROL 2 mg twice daily in the Phase 3 clinical studies, occurring in 39.5% of patients treated with DETROL and 15.9% of placebo-treated patients; 0.8% of patients treated with DETROL discontinued treatment due to dry mouth.

The frequency of discontinuation due to adverse events was highest during the first 4 weeks of treatment. Eight percent of patients treated with DETROL 2 mg twice daily discontinued treatment due to adverse events; the most common adverse events leading to discontinuation were dizziness and headache.

The following table lists the adverse events reported in 1% or more of the patients treated with DETROL 2 mg twice daily in the 12-week studies. The adverse events are reported regardless of causality.

[See table above]

OVERDOSAGE

A 27-month-old child who ingested 5 to 7 tablets of DETROL 2 mg was treated with a suspension of activated charcoal and was hospitalized overnight with symptoms of dry mouth. The child fully recovered.

Management of Overdosage

Overdosage with DETROL can potentially result in severe central anticholinergic effects and should be treated accordingly.

ECG monitoring is recommended in the event of overdosage. In dogs, changes in the QT interval (slight prolongation of 10% to 20%) were observed at a suprapharmacologic dose of 4.5 mg/kg, which is about 68 times higher than the recommended human dose. In clinical trials of normal volunteers and patients, QT interval prolongation was not observed at doses up to 4 mg twice daily of tolterodine (higher doses were not evaluated).

DOSAGE AND ADMINISTRATION

The initial recommended dose is 2 mg twice daily. The dose may be lowered to 1 mg twice daily based on individual re-

Continued on next page

Information on these Pharmacia & Upjohn products is based on labeling in effect June 1, 1998. Further information concerning these and other Pharmacia & Upjohn products may be obtained by direct inquiry to Medical Information, Pharmacia & Upjohn, Kalamazoo, MI 49001.

Consult 1999 PDR® supplements and future editions for revisions

Detrol—Cont.

sponse and tolerability. For patients with significantly reduced hepatic function or who are currently taking drugs that are inhibitors of cytochrome P450 3A4, the recommended dose is 1 mg twice daily (see PRECAUTIONS, General).

HOW SUPPLIED

DETROL Tablets 1 mg (white, round, biconvex, film-coated tablets engraved with arcs above and below the letters "TO") and **DETROL Tablets 2 mg** (white, round, biconvex, film-coated tablets engraved with arcs above and below the letters "DT") are supplied as follows:

Bottles of 60
- 1 mg NDC 0009-4541-02
- 2 mg NDC 0009-4544-02

Bottles of 500
- 1 mg NDC 0009-4541-03
- 2 mg NDC 0009-4544-03

Unit Dose Pack of 140
- 1 mg NDC 0009-4541-01
- 2 mg NDC 0009-4544-01

Store at controlled room temperature 20° to 25°C (68° to 77°F) [see USP].

Rx only

US Patent No. 5,382,600

Manufactured by:
Pharmacia & Upjohn S.p.A.
Ascoli Piceno, Italy
For:
Pharmacia & Upjohn Company
Kalamazoo, MI 49001, USA
March 1998 817 413 000
692167

Shown in Product Identification Guide, page 332

DIPENTUM® ℞

[di-pent ' um]
(olsalazine sodium capsules)

DESCRIPTION

The active ingredient in DIPENTUM Capsules (olsalazine sodium) is a sodium salt of salicylate, disodium 3,3′-azobis (6-hydroxybenzoate) a compound that is effectively bioconverted to 5-aminosalicylic acid (5- ASA), which has anti-inflammatory activity in ulcerative colitis. Its empirical formula is $C_{14}H_8N_2Na_2O_6$ with a molecular weight of 346.21. The structural formula is:

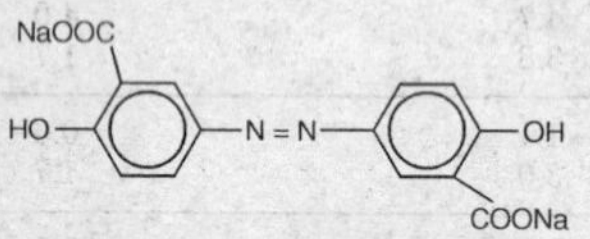
NaOOC
HO
N = N
OH
COONa

Olsalazine sodium is a yellow crystalline powder which melts with decomposition at 240°C. It is the sodium salt of a weak acid, soluble in water and DMSO, and practically insoluble in ethanol, chloroform and ether. Olsalazine sodium has acceptable stability under acidic or basic conditions.

DIPENTUM is supplied in hard gelatin capsules for oral administration. The inert ingredient in each 250 mg capsule of olsalazine sodium is magnesium stearate. The capsule shell has the following inactive ingredients: black iron oxide, caramel, gelatin, and titanium dioxide.

HOW SUPPLIED

Beige colored capsules, containing 250 mg olsalazine sodium imprinted with "DIPENTUM® 250 mg" on the capsule shell. Packaged in bottles of 100 (NDC 0013-0105-01) and 300 (NDC 0013-0105-20).

Storage

Store at 25°C (77°F). Excursions permitted to 15° to 30°C (59° to 86°F) [see USP Controlled Room Temperature].

Rx only

Manufactured for: Pharmacia & Upjohn Company, Kalamazoo, MI 49001, USA
by: Pharmacia & Upjohn AB, Stockholm, Sweden
Revised: February 1998 111010298

DOSTINEX ℞

[dŏs 'tinex]
brand of cabergoline tablets

DESCRIPTION

DOSTINEX Tablets contain cabergoline, a dopamine receptor agonist. The chemical name for cabergoline is 1-[(6-allylergolin-8β-yl)- carbonyl] -1- [3-(dimethylamino)propyl]-3-ethylurea. Its empirical formula is $C_{26}H_{37}N_5O_2$, and its molecular weight is 451.62. The structural formula is as follows:

[See chemical structure at top of next column]

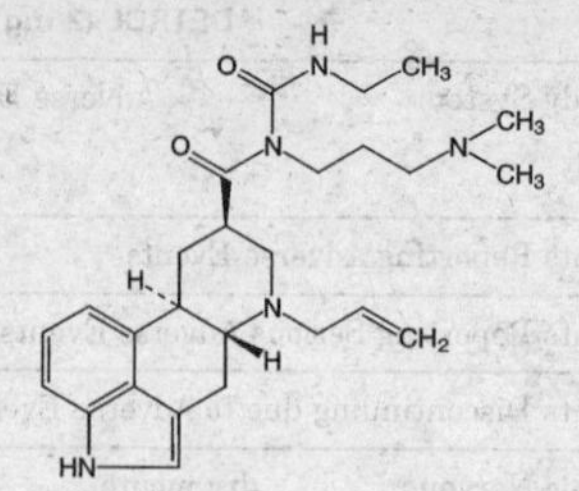
H
O
N
CH3
N
N
CH3
CH3
H
N
CH2
H
HN

Cabergoline is a white powder soluble in ethyl alcohol, chloroform, and N, N-dimethylformamide (DMF); slightly soluble in 0.1N hydrochloric acid; very slightly soluble in n-hexane; and insoluble in water.

DOSTINEX Tablets, for oral administration, contain 0.5 mg of cabergoline. Inactive ingredients consist of leucine, USP, and lactose, NF.

CLINICAL PHARMACOLOGY

Mechanism of Action: The secretion of prolactin by the anterior pituitary is mainly under hypothalamic inhibitory control, likely exerted through release of dopamine by tuberoinfundibular neurons. Cabergoline is a long-acting dopamine receptor agonist with a high affinity for D_2 receptors. Results of in vitro studies demonstrate that cabergoline exerts a direct inhibitory effect on the secretion of prolactin by rat pituitary lactotrophs. Cabergoline decreased serum prolactin levels in reserpinized rats. Receptor-binding studies indicate that cabergoline has low affinity for dopamine D_1, α_1- and α_2-adrenergic, and 5-HT_1- and 5-HT_2-serotonin receptors.

Clinical Studies: The prolactin-lowering efficacy of DOSTINEX was demonstrated in hyperprolactinemic women in two randomized, double-blind, comparative studies, one with placebo and the other with bromocriptine. In the placebo-controlled study (placebo n=20; cabergoline n=168), DOSTINEX produced a dose-related decrease in serum prolactin levels with prolactin normalized after 4 weeks of treatment in 29%, 76%, 74% and 95% of the patients receiving 0.125, 0.5, 0.75, and 1.0 mg twice weekly respectively.

In the 8-week, double-blind period of the comparative trial with bromocriptine (cabergoline n=223; bromocriptine n=236 in the intent-to-treat analysis), prolactin was normalized in 77% of the patients treated with DOSTINEX at 0.5 mg twice weekly compared with 59% of those treated with bromocriptine at 2.5 mg twice daily. Restoration of menses occurred in 77% of the women treated with DOSTINEX, compared with 70% of those treated with bromocriptine. Among patients with galactorrhea, this symptom disappeared in 73% of those treated with DOSTINEX compared with 56% of those treated with bromocriptine.

Pharmacokinetics

Absorption: Following single oral doses of 0.5 mg to 1.5 mg given to 12 healthy adult volunteers, mean peak plasma levels of 30 to 70 picograms (pg)/mL of cabergoline were observed within 2 to 3 hours. Over the 0.5-to-7 mg dose range, cabergoline plasma levels appeared to be dose-proportional in 12 healthy adult volunteers and nine adult parkinsonian patients. A repeat-dose study in 12 healthy volunteers suggests that steady-state levels following a once-weekly dosing schedule are expected to be twofold to threefold higher than after a single dose. The absolute bioavailability of cabergoline is unknown. A significant fraction of the administered dose undergoes a first-pass effect. The elimination half-life of cabergoline estimated from urinary data of 12 healthy subjects ranged between 63 to 69 hours. The prolonged prolactin-lowering effect of cabergoline may be related to its slow elimination and long half-life.

Distribution: In animals, based on total radioactivity, cabergoline (and/or its metabolites) has shown extensive tissue distribution. Radioactivity in the pituitary exceeded that in plasma by > 100-fold and was eliminated with a half-life of approximately 60 hours. This finding is consistent with the long-lasting prolactin-lowering effect of the drug. Whole body autoradiography studies in pregnant rats showed no fetal uptake but high levels in the uterine wall. Significant radioactivity (parent plus metabolites) detected in the milk of lactating rats suggests a potential for exposure to nursing infants. The drug is extensively distributed throughout the body. Cabergoline is moderately bound (40% to 42%) to human plasma proteins in a concentration-independent manner. Concomitant dosing of highly protein-bound drugs is unlikely to affect its disposition.

Metabolism: In both animals and humans, cabergoline is extensively metabolized, predominately via hydrolysis of the acylurea bond or the urea moiety. Cytochrome P-450 mediated metabolism appears to be minimal. Cabergoline does not cause enzyme induction and/or inhibition in the rat. Hydrolysis of the acylurea or urea moiety abolishes the prolactin-lowering effect of cabergoline, and major metabolites identified thus far do not contribute to the therapeutic effect.

Excretion: After oral dosing of radioactive cabergoline to five healthy volunteers, approximately 22% and 60% of the dose was excreted within 20 days in the urine and feces, respectively. Less than 4% of the dose was excreted unchanged in the urine. Nonrenal and renal clearances for cabergoline are about 3.2 L/min and 0.08 L/min, respectively. Urinary excretion in hyperprolactinemic patients was similar.

Special Populations

Renal Insufficiency: The pharmacokinetics of cabergoline were not altered in 12 patients with moderate-to-severe renal insufficiency as assessed by creatinine clearance.

Hepatic Insufficiency: In 12 patients with mild-to-moderate hepatic dysfunction (Child-Pugh score ≤ 10), no effect on mean cabergoline C_{max} or area under the plasma concentration curve (AUC) was observed. However, patients with severe insufficiency (Child-Pugh score > 10) show a substantial increase in the mean cabergoline C_{max} and AUC, and thus necessitate caution.

Elderly: Effect of age on the pharmacokinetics of cabergoline has not been studied.

Food-Drug Interaction

In 12 healthy adult volunteers, food did not alter cabergoline kinetics.

Pharmacodynamics

Dose response with inhibition of plasma prolactin, onset of maximal effect, and duration of effect has been documented following single cabergoline doses to healthy volunteers (0.05 to 1.5 mg) and hyperprolactinemic patients (0.3 to 1 mg). In volunteers, prolactin inhibition was evident at doses > 0.2 mg, while doses ≥ 0.5 mg caused maximal suppression in most subjects. Higher doses produce prolactin suppression in a greater proportion of subjects and with an earlier onset and longer duration of action. In 12 healthy volunteers, 0.5, 1, and 1.5 mg doses resulted in complete prolactin inhibition, with a maximum effect within 3 hours in 92% to 100% of subjects after the 1 and 1.5 mg doses compared with 50% of subjects after the 0.5 mg dose.

In hyperprolactinemic patients (N=51), the maximal prolactin decrease after a 0.6 mg single dose of cabergoline was comparable to 2.5 mg bromocriptine; however, the duration of effect was markedly longer (14 days vs 24 hours). The time to maximal effect was shorter for bromocriptine than cabergoline (6 hours vs 48 hours).

In 72 healthy volunteers, single or multiple doses (up to 2 mg) of cabergoline resulted in selective inhibition of prolactin with no apparent effect on other anterior pituitary hormones (GH, FSH, LH, ACTH, and TSH) or cortisol.

INDICATIONS AND USAGE

DOSTINEX Tablets are indicated for the treatment of hyperprolactinemic disorders, either idiopathic or due to pituitary adenomas.

CONTRAINDICATIONS

DOSTINEX Tablets are contraindicated in patients with uncontrolled hypertension or known hypersensitivity to ergot derivatives.

WARNINGS

Dopamine agonists in general should not be used in patients with pregnancy-induced hypertension, for example, preeclampsia and eclampsia, unless the potential benefit is judged to outweigh the possible risk.

PRECAUTIONS

General: Initial doses higher than 1.0 mg may produce orthostatic hypotension. Care should be exercised when administering DOSTINEX with other medications known to lower blood pressure.

Postpartum Lactation Inhibition or Suppression: DOSTINEX is not indicated for the inhibition or suppression of physiologic lactation. Use of bromocriptine, another dopamine agonist for this purpose, has been associated with cases of hypertension, stroke, and seizures.

Hepatic Impairment: Since cabergoline is extensively metabolized by the liver, caution should be used, and careful monitoring exercised, when administering DOSTINEX to patients with hepatic impairment.

Information for Patients: A patient should be instructed to notify her physician if she suspects she is pregnant, becomes pregnant, or intends to become pregnant during therapy. A pregnancy test should be done if there is any suspicion of pregnancy and continuation of treatment should be discussed with her physician.

Drug Interactions: DOSTINEX should not be administered concurrently with D_2-antagonists, such as phenothiazines, butyrophenones, thioxanthines, or metoclopramide.

Carcinogenesis, Mutagenesis, Impairment of Fertility: Carcinogenicity studies were conducted in mice and rats with cabergoline given by gavage at doses up to 0.98 mg/kg/day and 0.32 mg/kg/day, respectively. These doses are 7 times

and 4 times the maximum recommended human dose calculated on a body surface area basis using total mg/m^2/week in rodents and mg/m^2/week for a 50 kg human.

There was a slight increase in the incidence of cervical and uterine leiomyomas and uterine leiomyosarcomas in mice. In rats, there was a slight increase in malignant tumors of the cervix and uterus and interstitial cell adenomas. The occurrence of tumors in female rodents may be related to the prolonged suppression of prolactin secretion because prolactin is needed in rodents for the maintenance of the corpus luteum. In the absence of prolactin, the estrogen/progesterone ratio is increased, thereby increasing the risk for uterine tumors. In male rodents, the decrease in serum prolactin levels was associated with an increase in serum luteinizing hormone, which is thought to be a compensatory effect to maintain testicular steroid synthesis. Since these hormonal mechanisms are thought to be species-specific, the relevance of these tumors to humans is not known.

The mutagenic potential of cabergoline was evaluated and found to be negative in a battery of in vitro tests. These tests included the bacterial mutation (Ames) test with *Salmonella typhimurium*, the gene mutation assay with *Schizosaccharomyces pombe* P_1 and V79 Chinese hamster cells, DNA damage and repair in *Saccharomyces cerevisiae* D_4, and chromosomal aberrations in human lymphocytes. Cabergoline was also negative in the bone marrow micronucleus test in the mouse.

In female rats, a daily dose of 0.003 mg/kg for 2 weeks prior to mating and throughout the mating period inhibited conception. This dose represents approximately 1/28 the maximum recommended human dose calculated on a body surface area basis using total mg/m^2/week in rats and mg/m^2/week for a 50 kg human.

Pregnancy: Teratogenic Effects: Category B. Reproduction studies have been performed with cabergoline in mice, rats, and rabbits administered by gavage.

(Multiples of the maximum recommended human dose in this section are calculated on a body surface area basis using total mg/m^2/week for animals and mg/m^2/week for a 50 kg human.)

There were maternotoxic effects but no teratogenic effects in mice given cabergoline at doses up to 8 mg/kg/day (approximately 55 times the maximum recommended human dose) during the period of organogenesis.

A dose of 0.012 mg/kg/day (approximately 1/7 the maximum recommended human dose) during the period of organogenesis in rats caused an increase in post-implantation embryofetal losses. These losses could be due to the prolactin inhibitory properties of cabergoline in rats. At daily doses of 0.5 mg/kg/day (approximately 19 times the maximum recommended human dose) during the period of organogenesis in the rabbit, cabergoline caused maternotoxicity characterized by a loss of body weight and decreased food consumption. Doses of 4 mg/kg/day (approximately 150 times the maximum recommended human dose) during the period of organogenesis in the rabbit caused an increased occurrence of various malformations. However, in another study in rabbits, no treatment-related malformations or embryofetotoxicity were observed at doses up to 8 mg/kg/day (approximately 300 times the maximum recommended human dose).

In rats, doses higher than 0.003 mg/kg/day (approximately 1/28 the maximum recommended human dose) from 6 days before parturition and throughout the lactation period inhibited growth and caused death of offspring due to decreased milk secretion.

There are, however, no adequate and well-controlled studies in pregnant women. Because animal reproduction studies are not always predictive of human response, this drug should be used during pregnancy only if clearly needed.

Nursing Mothers: It is not known whether this drug is excreted in human milk. Because many drugs are excreted in human milk and because of the potential for serious adverse reactions in nursing infants from cabergoline, a decision should be made whether to discontinue nursing or to discontinue the drug, taking into account the importance of the drug to the mother. Use of DOSTINEX for the inhibition or suppression of physiologic lactation is not recommended (see PRECAUTIONS section).

The prolactin-lowering action of cabergoline suggests that it will interfere with lactation. Due to this interference with lactation, DOSTINEX should not be given to women postpartum who are breastfeeding or who are planning to breastfeed.

Pediatric Use: Safety and effectiveness of DOSTINEX in pediatric patients have not been established.

ADVERSE REACTIONS

The safety of DOSTINEX Tablets has been evaluated in more than 900 patients with hyperprolactinemic disorders. Most adverse events were mild or moderate in severity.

In a 4-week, double-blind, placebo-controlled study, treatment consisted of placebo or cabergoline at fixed doses of 0.125, 0.5, 0.75, or 1.0 mg twice weekly. Doses were halved during the first week. Since a possible dose-related effect was observed for nausea only, the four cabergoline treat-

ment groups have been combined. The incidence of the most common adverse events during the placebo-controlled study is presented in the following table.

Incidence of Reported Adverse Events During the 4-Week, Double-Blind, Placebo-Controlled Trial

Adverse Event*	Cabergoline (n=168) 0.125 to 1 mg two times a week	Placebo (n=20)
	Number (percent)	
Gastrointestinal		
Nausea	45 (27)	4 (20)
Constipation	16 (10)	0
Abdominal pain	9 (5)	1 (5)
Dyspepsia	4 (2)	0
Vomiting	4 (2)	0
Central and Peripheral Nervous System		
Headache	43 (26)	5 (25)
Dizziness	25 (15)	1 (5)
Paresthesia	2 (1)	0
Vertigo	2 (1)	0
Body As a Whole		
Asthenia	15 (9)	2 (10)
Fatigue	12 (7)	0
Hot flashes	2 (1)	1 (5)
Psychiatric		
Somnolence	9 (5)	1 (5)
Depression	5 (3)	1 (5)
Nervousness	4 (2)	0
Autonomic Nervous System		
Postural hypotension	6 (4)	0
Reproductive— Female		
Breast pain	2 (1)	0
Dysmenorrhea	2 (1)	0
Vision		
Abnormal vision	2 (1)	0

* Reported at ≥1% for cabergoline

In the 8-week, double-blind period of the comparative trial with bromocriptine, DOSTINEX (at a dose of 0.5 mg twice weekly) was discontinued because of an adverse event in 4 of 221 patients (2%) while bromocriptine (at a dose of 2.5 mg two times a day) was discontinued in 14 of 231 patients (6%). The most common reasons for discontinuation from DOSTINEX were headache, nausea and vomiting (3, 2 and 2 patients respectively); the most common reasons for discontinuation from bromocriptine were nausea, vomiting, headache, and dizziness or vertigo (10, 3, 3, and 3 patients respectively). The incidence of the most common adverse events during the double-blind portion of the comparative trial with bromocriptine is presented in the following table.

Incidence of Reported Adverse Events During the 8-Week, Double-Blind Period of the Comparative Trial With Bromocriptine

Adverse Event*	Cabergoline (n=221)	Bromocriptine (n=231)
	Number (percent)	
Gastrointestinal		
Nausea	63 (29)	100 (43)
Constipation	15 (7)	21 (9)
Abdominal pain	12 (5)	19 (8)
Dyspepsia	11 (5)	16 (7)
Vomiting	9 (4)	16 (7)
Dry mouth	5 (2)	2 (1)
Diarrhea	4 (2)	7 (3)
Flatulence	4 (2)	3 (1)
Throat irritation	2 (1)	0
Toothache	2 (1)	0
Centeral and Peripheral Nervous System		
Headache	58 (26)	62 (27)
Dizziness	38 (17)	42 (18)
Vertigo	9 (4)	10 (4)
Paresthesia	5 (2)	6 (3)

Body As a Whole		
Asthenia	13 (6)	15 (6)
Fatigue	10 (5)	18 (8)
Syncope	3 (1)	3 (1)
Influenza-like symptoms	2 (1)	0
Malaise	2 (1)	0
Periorbital edema	2 (1)	2 (1)
Peripheral edema	2 (1)	1
Psychiatric		
Depression	7 (3)	5 (2)
Somnolence	5 (2)	5 (2)
Anorexia	3 (1)	3 (1)
Anxiety	3 (1)	3 (1)
Insomnia	3 (1)	2 (1)
Impaired concentration	2 (1)	1
Nervousness	2 (1)	5 (2)
Cardiovascular		
Hot flashes	6 (3)	3 (1)
Hypotension	3 (1)	4 (2)
Dependent edema	2 (1)	1
Palpitation	2 (1)	5 (2)
Reproductive— Female		
Breast pain	5 (2)	8 (3)
Dysmenorrhea	2 (1)	1
Skin and Appendages		
Acne	3 (1)	0
Pruritus	2 (1)	1
Musculoskeletal		
Pain	4 (2)	6 (3)
Arthralgia	2 (1)	0
Respiratory		
Rhinitis	2 (1)	9 (4)
Vision		
Abnormal vision	2 (1)	2 (1)

* Reported at ≥1% for cabergoline

Other adverse events that were reported at an incidence of <1.0% in the overall clinical studies follow.

Body As a Whole: facial edema, influenza-like symptoms, malaise

Cardiovascular System: hypotension, syncope, palpitations

Digestive System: dry mouth, flatulence, diarrhea, anorexia

Metabolic and Nutritional System: weight loss, weight gain

Nervous System: somnolence, nervousness, paresthesia, insomnia, anxiety

Respiratory System: nasal stuffiness, epistaxis

Skin and Appendages: acne, pruritus

Special Senses: abnormal vision

Urogenital System: dysmenorrhea, increased libido

The safety of cabergoline has been evaluated in approximately 1,200 patients with Parkinson's disease in controlled and uncontrolled studies at dosages of up to 11.5 mg/day which greatly exceeds the maximum recommended dosage of cabergoline for hyperprolactinemic disorders. In addition to the adverse events that occurred in the patients with hyperprolactinemic disorders, the most common adverse events in patients with Parkinson's disease were dyskinesia, hallucinations, confusion, and peripheral edema. Heart failure, pleural effusion, pulmonary fibrosis, and gastric or duodenal ulcer occurred rarely. One case of constrictive pericarditis has been reported.

OVERDOSAGE

Overdosage might be expected to produce nasal congestion, syncope, or hallucinations. Measures to support blood pressure should be taken if necessary.

DOSAGE AND ADMINISTRATION

The recommended dosage of DOSTINEX Tablets for initiation of therapy is 0.25 mg twice a week. Dosage may be increased by 0.25 mg twice weekly up to a dosage of 1 mg twice a week according to the patient's serum prolactin level.

Dosage increases should not occur more rapidly than every 4 weeks, so that the physician can assess the patient's response to each dosage level. If the patient does not respond

Continued on next page

Information on these Pharmacia & Upjohn products is based on labeling in effect June 1, 1998. Further information concerning these and other Pharmacia & Upjohn products may be obtained by direct inquiry to Medical Information, Pharmacia & Upjohn, Kalamazoo, MI 49001.

Dostinex—Cont.

adequately, and no additional benefit is observed with higher doses, the lowest dose that achieved maximal response should be used and other therapeutic approaches considered.

After a normal serum prolactin level has been maintained for 6 months, DOSTINEX may be discontinued, with periodic monitoring of the serum prolactin level to determine whether or when treatment with DOSTINEX should be reinstituted. The durability of efficacy beyond 24 months of therapy with DOSTINEX has not been established.

HOW SUPPLIED

DOSTINEX Tablets are white, scored, capsule-shaped tablets containing 0.5 mg cabergoline. Each tablet is scored on one side and has the letter P and the letter U on either side of the breakline. The other side of the tablet is engraved with the number 700.

DOSTINEX is available as follows:

Bottles of 8 tablets   NDC 0013-7001-12

STORAGE

Store at controlled room temperature 20° to 25° C (68° to 77° F) [see USP].

Caution: Federal law prohibits dispensing without prescription.

Manufactured by: Pharmacia & Upjohn S.p.A.
      Milan, Italy

For: **Pharmacia & Upjohn Company**
      Kalamazoo, MI 49001, USA

816 989 000   N.808010530   December 1996

EMCYT®   ℞
(estramustine phosphate sodium)
capsules

DESCRIPTION

Estramustine phosphate sodium, an antineoplastic agent, is an off-white powder readily soluble in water. EMCYT Capsules are white and opaque, each containing estramustine phosphate sodium as the disodium salt monohydrate equivalent to 140 mg estramustine phosphate, for oral administration. Each capsule also contains magnesium stearate, silicon dioxide, sodium lauryl sulfate, and talc. Gelatin capsule shells contain the following pigment: titanium dioxide. Chemically, estramustine phosphate sodium is estra-1,3,5(10)-triene-3,17-diol(17β)-, 3-[bis(2-chloroethyl)carbamate] 17-(dihydrogen phosphate), disodium salt, monohydrate. It is also referred to as estradiol 3-[bis(2-chloroethyl)carbamate] 17-(dihydrogen phosphate), disodium salt, monohydrate.

Estramustine phosphate sodium has an empiric formula of $C_{23}H_{30}Cl_2NNa_2O_6P \cdot H_2O$, a calculated molecular weight of 582.4, and the following structural formula:

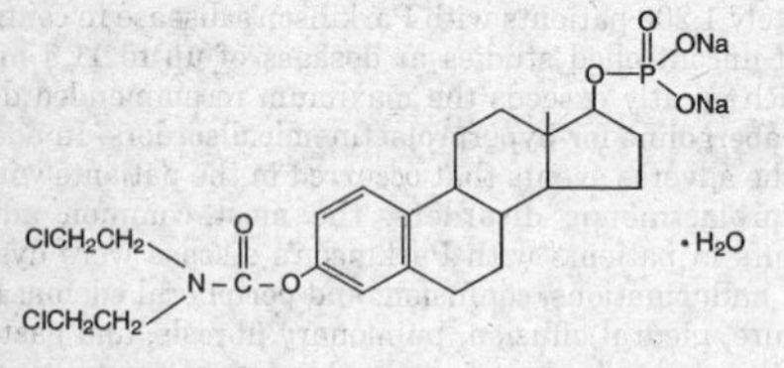

CLINICAL PHARMACOLOGY

Estramustine phosphate (Figure 1) is a molecule combining estradiol and nornitrogen mustard by a carbamate link. The molecule is phosphorylated to make it water soluble.

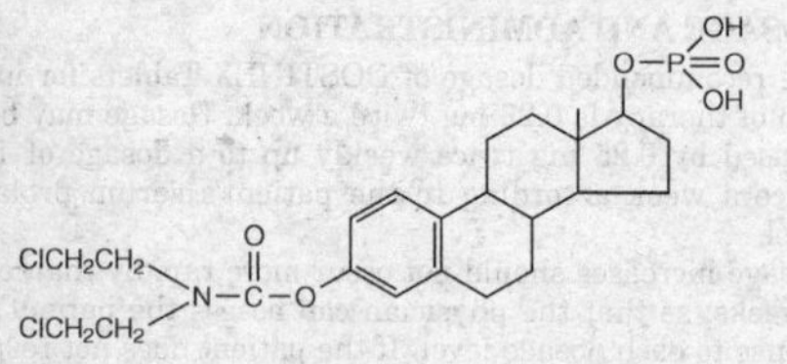

Figure 1. Estramustine Phosphate

Estramustine phosphate taken orally is readily dephosphorylated during absorption, and the major metabolites in plasma are estramustine (Figure 2), the estrone analog (Figure 3), estradiol, and estrone.
[See chemical structures at top of next column]
Prolonged treatment with estramustine phosphate produces elevated total plasma concentrations of estradiol that

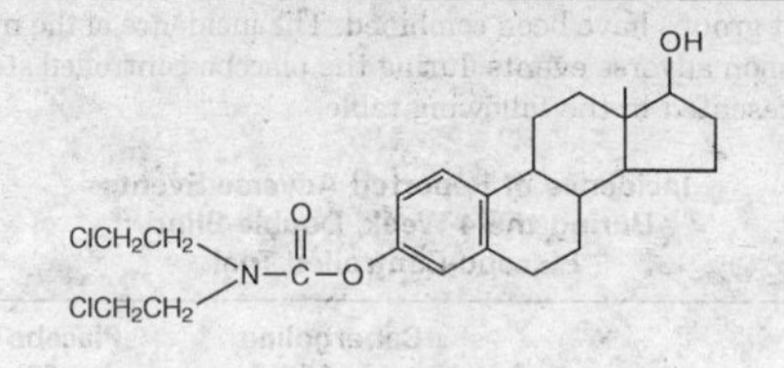

Figure 2. Estramustine

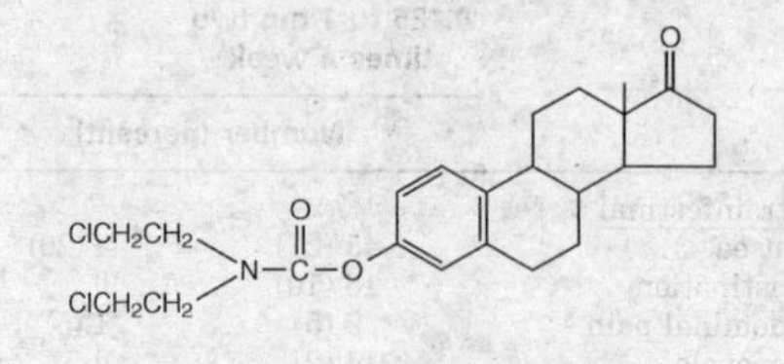

Figure 3. Estrone Analog of Estramustine

fall within ranges similar to the elevated estradiol levels found in prostatic cancer patients given conventional estradiol therapy. Estrogenic effects, as demonstrated by changes in circulating levels of steroids and pituitary hormones, are similar in patients treated with either estramustine phosphate or conventional estradiol.

The metabolic urinary patterns of the estradiol moiety of estramustine phosphate and estradiol itself are very similar, although the metabolites derived from estramustine phosphate are excreted at a slower rate.

INDICATIONS AND USAGE

EMCYT Capsules are indicated in the palliative treatment of patients with metastatic and/or progressive carcinoma of the prostate.

CONTRAINDICATIONS

EMCYT Capsules should not be used in patients with any of the following conditions:
1) Known hypersensitivity to either estradiol or to nitrogen mustard.
2) Active thrombophlebitis or thromboembolic disorders, except in those cases where the actual tumor mass is the cause of the thromboembolic phenomenon and the physician feels the benefits of therapy may outweigh the risks.

WARNINGS

It has been shown that there is an increased risk of thrombosis, including fatal and nonfatal myocardial infarction, in men receiving estrogens for prostatic cancer. EMCYT Capsules should be used with caution in patients with a history of thrombophlebitis, thrombosis, or thromboembolic disorders, especially if they were associated with estrogen therapy. Caution should also be used in patients with cerebral vascular or coronary artery disease.

Glucose Tolerance—Because glucose tolerance may be decreased, diabetic patients should be carefully observed while receiving EMCYT.

Elevated Blood Pressure—Because hypertension may occur, blood pressure should be monitored periodically.

PRECAUTIONS
General
Fluid Retention. Exacerbation of preexisting or incipient peripheral edema or congestive heart disease has been seen in some patients receiving therapy with EMCYT Capsules. Other conditions which might be influenced by fluid retention, such as epilepsy, migraine, or renal dysfunction, require careful observation.

EMCYT may be poorly metabolized in patients with impaired liver function and should be administered with caution in such patients.

Because EMCYT may influence the metabolism of calcium and phosphorus, it should be used with caution in patients with metabolic bone diseases that are associated with hypercalcemia or in patients with renal insufficiency.

Gynecomastia and impotence are known estrogenic effects. Allergic reactions and angioedema at times involving the airway have been reported.
Information for the Patient
Because of the possibility of mutagenic effects, patients should be advised to use contraceptive measures.
Laboratory Tests
Certain endocrine and liver function tests may be affected by estrogen-containing drugs. EMCYT may depress testosterone levels. Abnormalities of hepatic enzymes and of bilirubin have occurred in patients receiving EMCYT. Such tests should be done at appropriate intervals during therapy and repeated after the drug has been withdrawn for two months.
Food/Drug Interaction
Milk, milk products, and calcium-rich foods or drugs may impair the absorption of EMCYT.
Carcinogenesis, Mutagenesis, Impairment of Fertility
Long-term continuous administration of estrogens in certain animal species increases the frequency of carcinomas of

the breast and liver. Compounds structurally similar to EMCYT are carcinogenic in mice. Carcinogenic studies of EMCYT have not been conducted in man. Although testing by the Ames method failed to demonstrate mutagenicity for estramustine phosphate sodium, it is known that both estradiol and nitrogen mustard are mutagenic. For this reason and because some patients who had been impotent while on estrogen therapy have regained potency while taking EMCYT, the patient should be advised to use contraceptive measures.

ADVERSE REACTIONS

In a randomized, double-blind trial comparing therapy with EMCYT Capsules in 93 patients (11.5 to 15.9 mg/kg/day) or diethylstilbestrol (DES) in 93 patients (3.0 mg/day), the following adverse effects were reported:

	EMCYT n=93	DES n=93
CARDIOVASCULAR-RESPIRATORY		
Cardiac Arrest	0	2
Cerebrovascular Accident	2	0
Myocardial Infarction	3	1
Thrombophlebitis	3	7
Pulmonary Emboli	2	5
Congestive Heart Failure	3	2
Edema	19	17
Dyspnea	11	3
Leg Cramps	8	11
Upper Respiratory Discharge	1	1
Hoarseness	1	0
GASTROINTESTINAL		
Nausea	15	8
Diarrhea	12	11
Minor Gastrointestinal Upset	11	6
Anorexia	4	3
Flatulence	2	0
Vomiting	1	1
Gastrointestinal Bleeding	1	0
Burning Throat	1	0
Thirst	1	0
INTEGUMENTARY		
Rash	1	4
Pruritus	2	2
Dry Skin	2	0
Pigment Changes	0	3
Easy Bruising	3	0
Flushing	1	0
Night Sweats	0	1
Fingertip—Peeling Skin	1	0
Thinning Hair	1	1
BREAST CHANGES		
Tenderness	66	64
Enlargement		
Mild	60	54
Moderate	10	16
Marked	0	5
MISCELLANEOUS		
Lethargy Alone	4	3
Depression	0	2
Emotional Lability	2	0
Insomnia	3	0
Headache	1	1
Anxiety	1	0
Chest Pain	1	1
Hot Flashes	0	1
Pain in Eyes	0	1
Tearing of Eyes	1	1
Tinnitus	0	1
LABORATORY ABNORMALITIES		
Hematologic		
Leukopenia	4	2
Thrombopenia	1	2
Hepatic		
Bilirubin Alone	1	5
Bilirubin and LDH	0	1
Bilirubin and SGOT	2	1
Bilirubin, LDH and SGOT	2	0
LDH and/or SGOT	31	28
Miscellaneous		
Hypercalcemia—Transient	0	1

OVERDOSAGE

Although there has been no experience with overdosage to date, it is reasonable to expect that such episodes may produce pronounced manifestations of the known adverse reactions. In the event of overdosage, the gastric contents should be evacuated by gastric lavage and symptomatic therapy should be initiated. Hematologic and hepatic parameters should be monitored for at least 6 weeks after overdosage of EMCYT Capsules.

DOSAGE AND ADMINISTRATION

The recommended daily dose is 14 mg per kg of body weight (ie, one 140 mg capsule for each 10 kg or 22 lb of body

weight), given in 3 or 4 divided doses. Most patients in studies in the United States have been treated at a dosage range of 10 to 16 mg per kg per day.
Patients should be instructed to take EMCYT Capsules at least 1 hour before or 2 hours after meals. EMCYT should be swallowed with water. Milk, milk products, and calcium-rich foods or drugs (such as calcium-containing antacids) must not be taken simultaneously with EMCYT.
Patients should be treated for 30 to 90 days before the physician determines the possible benefits of continued therapy. Therapy should be continued as long as the favorable response lasts. Some patients have been maintained on therapy for more than 3 years at doses ranging from 10 to 16 mg per kg of body weight per day.
Procedures for proper handling and disposal of anticancer drugs should be considered. Several guidelines on this subject have been published.[1-7] There is no general agreement that all of the procedures recommended in the guidelines are necessary or appropriate.

HOW SUPPLIED

White opaque capsules, each containing estramustine phosphate sodium as the disodium salt monohydrate equivalent to 140 mg estramustine phosphate—bottle of 100 (NDC 0013-0132-02).

NOTE

EMCYT Capsules should be stored at 36° to 46°F (2° to 8°C). Federal law prohibits dispensing without prescription.

REFERENCES

1. Recommendations for the Safe Handling of Parenteral Antineoplastic Drugs. NIH Publication No. 83-2621. For sale by the Superintendent of Documents, U.S. Government Printing Office, Washington, DC, 20402.
2. AMA Council Report, Guidelines for Handling Parenteral Antineoplastics, *JAMA*. 1985; 253 (11):1590–1592.
3. National Study Commission on Cytotoxic Exposure-Recommendations for Handling Cytotoxic Agents. Available from Louis P. Jeffrey, Sc.D., Chairman, National Study Commission on Cytotoxic Exposure, Massachusetts College of Pharmacy and Allied Health Sciences, 179 Longwood Avenue, Boston, Massachusetts 02115.
4. Clinical Oncological Society of Australia. Guidelines and Recommendations for Safe Handling of Antineoplastic Agents. *Med J Australia*. 1983; 1:426–428.
5. Jones RB, et al. Safe Handling of Chemotherapeutic Agents: A Report from the Mount Sinai Medical Center. *CA-A Cancer Journal for Clinicians*. 1983; (Sept/Oct) 258–263.
6. American Society of Hospital Pharmacists Technical Assistance Bulletin on Handling Cytotoxic and Hazardous Drugs. *Am J Hosp Pharm*. 1990; 47:1033–1049.
7. OSHA Work-Practice Guidelines for Personnel Dealing with Cytotoxic (Antineoplastic) Drugs. *Am J Hosp Pharm*. 1986; 43:1193–1204.

Manufactured for: Pharmacia & Upjohn Company
Kalamazoo, MI 49001, USA
by: Hoffmann-La Roche Inc.
Nutley, N.J. 07110
108001297
25893310-1297 Revised: December 1997

ESTRING® ℞

Vaginal Ring
estradiol vaginal ring
2 mg

PHYSICIAN'S LEAFLET

1. ESTROGENS HAVE BEEN REPORTED TO INCREASE THE RISK OF ENDOMETRIAL CARCINOMA IN POSTMENOPAUSAL WOMEN.
Close clinical surveillance of all women taking estrogens is important. Adequate diagnostic measures, including endometrial sampling when indicated, should be undertaken to rule out malignancy in all cases of undiagnosed persistent or recurring abnormal vaginal bleeding. There is no evidence that "natural" estrogens are more or less hazardous than "synthetic" estrogens at equi-estrogenic doses.
2. ESTROGENS SHOULD NOT BE USED DURING PREGNANCY.
There is no indication for estrogen therapy during pregnancy or during immediate postpartum period. Estrogens are ineffective for the prevention or treatment of threatened or habitual abortion. Estrogens are not indicated for the prevention of postpartum breast engorgement.
Estrogen therapy during pregnancy is associated with an increased risk of congenital defects in the reproductive organs of the fetus, and possibly other birth defects. Studies of women who received diethylstilbestrol (DES) during pregnancy have shown that female offspring have an increased risk of vaginal adenosis, squamous cell dysplasia of the uterine cervix, and clear cell vaginal cancer later in life; male offspring have an increased risk of urogenital abnormalities and possibly testicular cancer later in life. The 1985 DES Task Force concluded that the use of DES during pregnancy is associated with a subsequent increased risk of breast cancer in the mothers, although a causal relationship remains unproven and the observed level of excess risk is similar to that for a number of other breast cancer risk factors.

DESCRIPTION

ESTRING (estradiol vaginal ring) is a slightly opaque ring with a whitish core containing a drug reservoir of 2 mg estradiol. Estradiol, silicone polymers and barium sulfate are combined to form the ring. When placed in the vagina, ESTRING releases estradiol, approximately 7.5 µg/24 hours, in a consistent stable manner over 90 days. ESTRING has the following dimensions: outer diameter 55 mm; cross-sectional diameter 9 mm; core diameter 2 mm. One ESTRING should be inserted into the upper third of the vaginal vault, to be worn continuously for three months.
Estradiol is chemically described as estra-1,3,5(10)-triene-3,17β-diol. The molecular formula of estradiol is $C_{18}H_{24}O_2$ and the structural formula is:

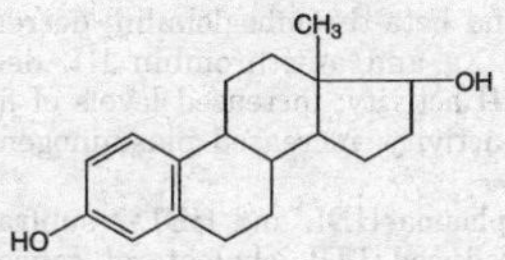

The molecular weight of estradiol is 272.39.

CLINICAL PHARMACOLOGY

Pharmacokinetics

ABSORPTION

Estrogens used in therapeutics are well absorbed through the skin, mucous membranes, and the gastrointestinal (GI) tract. The vaginal delivery of estrogens circumvents first-pass metabolism possibly reducing the induction of several other hepatic proteins.
In a Phase I study of 14 postmenopausal women, the insertion of ESTRING (estradiol vaginal ring) rapidly increased serum estradiol (E_2) levels attesting to the rapid absorption of estradiol via the vaginal mucosa. The time to attain peak serum estradiol levels (T_{max}) was 0.5 to 1 hour. Peak serum estradiol concentrations post-initial burst declined rapidly over the next 24 hours and were virtually indistinguishable from the baseline mean (range: 5 to 22 pg/mL). Serum levels of estradiol and estrone (E_1) over the following 12 weeks during which the ring was maintained in the vaginal vault remained relatively unchanged (see Table 1).
The initial estradiol peak post-application of the second ring in the same women resulted in ~ 38% lower C_{max}, apparently due to reduced systemic absorption via the revitalized vaginal epithelium. The relative systemic exposure from the initial peak of ESTRING accounted for approximately 4% of the total estradiol exposure over the 12 week period.
The constant and stable release of estradiol from ESTRING was demonstrated in a Phase II study of 166 – 222 postmenopausal women who inserted up to four rings consecutively at three month intervals. Low dose systemic delivery of estradiol from ESTRING resulted in mean steady state serum estradiol estimates of 7.8, 7.0, 7.0, 8.1 pg/mL at weeks 12, 24, 36, and 48, respectively. Similar reproducibility is also seen in levels of estrone. Lower systemic exposure to estradiol and estrone is further supported by serum levels measured during a pivotal Phase III study.
In post-menopausal women, mean dose of estradiol systemically absorbed unchanged from ESTRING is ~ 8% [95% CI: 2.8–12.8%] of the daily amount released locally. Low systemic exposure to estradiol and estrone resulting from ESTRING should elicit lower estrogen-dependent effects.

DISTRIBUTION

Circulating, unbound estrogens are known to modulate pharmacological response. Estrogens circulate in blood bound to sex-hormone binding globulin (SHBG) and albumin. A dynamic equilibrium exists between the conjugated and the unconjugated forms of estradiol and estrone, which undergo rapid interconversion.

METABOLISM

Exogenously delivered or endogenously derived estrogens are primarily metabolized in the liver to estrone and estriol, which are also found in the systemic circulation. Estrogen metabolites are primarily excreted in the urine as glucuronides and sulphates. Of the several estrogen metabolites, urinary estrone and estrone sulphate (E_1S), post-ESTRING use, are in the normal post-menopausal range.

EXCRETION

Mean percent dose excreted in the 24-hour urine as estradiol, 4 and 12 weeks post-application of ESTRING in a Phase I study was 5 and 8%, respectively, of the daily released amount.

Drug-Drug Interactions

No formal *drug-drug* interactions studies have been done with ESTRING. It is anticipated that lower exposure to systemic estrogens may reduce the potential for drug interactions thus maintaining the benefit to risk ratio of concomitant drugs.

TABLE 1: PHARMACOKINETIC MEAN ESTIMATES FOLLOWING ESTRING APPLICATION

Estrogen	C_{max} (pg/mL)	$C_{ss-48\ hr}$ (pg/mL)	C_{ss-4w} (pg/mL)	C_{ss-12w} (pg/mL)
Estradiol (E_2)	63.2[a]	11.2	9.5	8.0
Baseline-adjusted E_2[b]	55.6	3.6	2.0	0.4
Estrone (E_1)	66.3	52.5	43.8	47.0
Baseline-adjusted E_1	20.0	6.2	−2.4	0.8

[a] n=14
[b] Based on means

Pharmacodynamics

In-vivo, estrogens diffuse through cell membranes, distribute throughout the cell, bind to and activate the estrogen receptors, thereby eliciting their biological effects. Estrogen receptors have been identified in tissues of the reproductive tract, breast, pituitary, hypothalamus, liver and bone of women. ESTRING delivers estradiol constantly at a mean rate of ~ 7.5 µg/24 hours for a period of up to 90 days. Its use in post-menopausal patients in Phase I and II studies showed no apparent effects on systemic levels of hepatic protein SHBG, or FSH. Lowering of the pretreatment vaginal pH from a mean of 6.0 to a mean of 4.6 (as found in fertile women) over the 12 to 48 week treatment period, and improvements evident in the vaginal mucosal epithelium seen in all studies attest to the local dynamic effects of estrogens.

INDICATIONS AND USAGE

ESTRING (estradiol vaginal ring) is indicated for the treatment of urogenital symptoms associated with post-menopausal atrophy of the vagina (such as dryness, burning, pruritus and dyspareunia) and/or the lower urinary tract (urinary urgency and dysuria).

CLINICAL STUDIES

Two pivotal controlled studies have demonstrated the efficacy of ESTRING (estradiol vaginal ring) in the treatment of post-menopausal urogenital symptoms due to estrogen deficiency.
In a U.S. study where ESTRING was compared with conjugated estrogens vaginal cream, no difference in efficacy between the treatment groups was found with respect to improvement in the physician's global assessment of vaginal symptoms (83% and 82% of patients receiving ESTRING and cream, respectively) and in the patient's global assessment of vaginal symptoms (83% and 82% of patients receiving ESTRING and cream, respectively) after 12 weeks of treatment. In an Australian study, ESTRING was also compared with conjugated estrogens vaginal cream and no difference in the physician's assessment of improvement of vaginal mucosal atrophy (79% and 75% for ESTRING and cream, respectively) or in the patient's assessment of improvement in vaginal dryness (82% and 76% for ESTRING and cream, respectively) after 12 weeks of treatment.
In the U.S. study, symptoms of dysuria and urinary urgency improved in 74% and 65%, respectively, of patients receiving ESTRING as assessed by the patient. In the Australian study, symptoms of dysuria and urinary urgency improved in 90% and 71%, respectively, of patients receiving ESTRING as assessed by the patient.
In both studies, ESTRING and conjugated estrogens vaginal cream had a similar ability to reduce vaginal pH levels and to mature the vaginal mucosa (as measured cytologically using the maturation index and/or the maturation value) after 12 weeks of treatment. In supportive studies, ESTRING was also shown to have a similar significant treatment effect on the maturation of the urethral mucosa.

Continued on next page

Information on these Pharmacia & Upjohn products is based on labeling in effect June 1, 1998. Further information concerning these and other Pharmacia & Upjohn products may be obtained by direct inquiry to Medical Information, Pharmacia & Upjohn, Kalamazoo, MI 49001.

Estring—Cont.

Endometrial overstimulation, as evaluated in non-hysterectomized patients participating in the U.S. study by the progestogen challenge test and pelvic sonogram, was reported for none of the 58 (0%) patients receiving ESTRING and 4 of the 35 patients (11%) receiving conjugated estrogens vaginal cream.

Of the U.S. women who completed 12 weeks of treatment, 95% rated product comfort for ESTRING as excellent or very good compared with 65% of patients receiving conjugated estrogens vaginal cream, 95% of ESTRING patients judged the product to be very easy or easy to use compared with 88% of cream patients, and 82% gave ESTRING an overall rating of excellent or very good compared with 58% for the cream.

CONTRAINDICATIONS
1. Estrogens should not be used in women with any of the following conditions:
   a. Known or suspected pregnancy (see **BOXED WARNING**).
   b. Undiagnosed abnormal genital bleeding.
   c. Known or suspected cancer of the breast.
   d. Known or suspected estrogen-dependent neoplasia.
2. ESTRING (estradiol vaginal ring) should not be used in patients hypersensitive to any of its ingredients.

WARNINGS
1. **Breast cancer.**
   While the majority of studies have not shown an increased risk of breast cancer in women who have ever used estrogen replacement therapy, some have reported a moderately increased risk (relative risks of 1.3 to 2.0) in those taking higher doses or those taking lower doses for prolonged periods of time, especially in excess of ten years. Other studies have not shown this relationship.
2. **Other.**
   Congenital lesions with malignant potential, gallbladder disease, cardiovascular disease, elevated blood pressure and hypercalcemia have been associated with systemic estrogen treatment.

PRECAUTIONS
A. General
1. **Use of Progestins.**
   It is common practice with systemic administration of estrogen to add progestin for ten or more days during a cycle to lower the incidence of endometrial proliferation or hyperplasia. From the available clinical data, it seems unlikely that ESTRING would have adverse effects on the endometrium. Furthermore, addition of progestins to a patient being treated with ESTRING is not expected to result in vaginal bleeding.
2. **Physical Examination.**
   A complete medical and family history should be taken prior to the initiation of any estrogen therapy. The pretreatment and periodic physical examinations should include special reference to blood pressure, breasts, abdomen, and pelvic organs and should include a Papanicolaou smear. As a general rule, estrogen should not be prescribed for longer than one year without reexamining the patient.
3. **Uterine Bleeding and Mastodynia.**
   Although uncommon with ESTRING, certain patients may develop undesirable manifestations of estrogenic stimulation, such as abnormal uterine bleeding and mastodynia.
4. **Liver Disease.**
   ESTRING should be used with caution in patients with impaired liver function.
5. **Location of ESTRING.**
   Some women have experienced moving or gliding of ESTRING within the vagina. Instances of ESTRING being expelled from the vagina in connection with moving the bowels, strain, or constipation have been reported. If this occurs, ESTRING can be rinsed in lukewarm water and reinserted into the vagina by the patient.
6. **Vaginal Irritation.**
   ESTRING may not be suitable for women with narrow, short, or stenosed vaginas. Narrow vagina, vaginal stenosis, prolapse, and vaginal infections are conditions that make the vagina more susceptible to ESTRING-caused irritation or ulceration. Women with signs or symptoms of vaginal irritation should alert their physician.
7. **Vaginal Infection.**
   Vaginal infection is generally more common in postmenopausal women due to the lack of the normal flora of fertile women, especially lactobacillus, and the subsequent higher pH. Vaginal infections should be treated with appropriate antimicrobial therapy before initiation of ESTRING. If a vaginal infection develops during use of ESTRING, then ESTRING should be removed and reinserted only after the infection has been appropriately treated.

8. **Other.**
   Hypercoagulability and hyperlipidemia have been reported in women on other types of estrogen replacement therapy but, these have not been seen with ESTRING patients.
   Fluid retention is another known risk factor with estrogen therapy and may be harmful to patients with asthma, epilepsy, migraine and cardiac or renal dysfunction.
   ESTRING treatment has not been associated with any indication of increase in body weight up to 48 weeks of treatment.

B. Information for the Patient.
See text of **Information for Patients** which appears at the end of this insert.

C. Drug-Drug and Drug-Laboratory Interactions.
It is recommended that ESTRING be removed during treatment with other vaginally administered preparations.

Drug-drug and drug-laboratory interactions have been reported with estrogen administration overall, but were not observed in clinical trials with ESTRING. However, the possibility of the following interactions should be considered when treating patients with ESTRING.
1. Accelerated prothrombin time, partial thromboplastin time, and platelet aggregation time; increased platelet count; increased factors II, VII antigen, VIII antigen, VIII coagulant activity, IX, X, XII, VII-X complex, II-VII-X complex, and beta-thromboglobulin; decreased levels of anti-factor Xa and antithrombin III, decreased antithrombin III activity; increased levels of fibrinogen and fibrinogen activity; increased plasminogen antigen and activity.
2. Increased plasma HDL and HDL-2 subfraction concentrations, reduced LDL cholesterol concentration, increased triglycerides levels.

D. Carcinogenesis, Mutagenesis, and Impairment of Fertility.
Long term continuous administration of natural and synthetic estrogens in certain animal species increases the frequency of carcinomas of the breast, uterus, cervix, vagina, and liver (see **CONTRAINDICATIONS** and **BOXED WARNING**).

E. Pregnancy Category X.
Estrogens should not be used during pregnancy (see **CONTRAINDICATIONS** and **BOXED WARNING**).

F. Nursing Mothers.
This product is not intended for nursing mothers. As a general principle, the administration of any drug to nursing mothers should be done only when clearly necessary since many drugs are excreted in human milk. In addition, estrogen administration to nursing mothers has been shown to decrease the quantity and quality of the milk.

ADVERSE REACTIONS
The biological safety of the silicone elastomer has been studied in various *in vitro* and *in vivo* test models. The results show that the silicone elastomer is non-toxic, non-pyrogenic, non-irritating, and non-sensitizing. Long-term implantation induced encapsulation equal to or less than the negative control (polyethylene) used in the USP test. No toxic reaction or tumor formation was observed with the silicone elastomer.

In general, ESTRING (estradiol vaginal ring) was well tolerated. In the two pivotal controlled studies, discontinuation of treatment due to an adverse event was required by 5.4% of patients receiving ESTRING and 3.9% of patients receiving conjugated estrogens vaginal cream. The most common reasons for withdrawal from ESTRING treatment due to an adverse event were vaginal discomfort and gastrointestinal symptoms.

The adverse events reported with a frequency of 3% or greater in the two pivotal controlled studies by patients receiving ESTRING or conjugated estrogens vaginal cream are listed in Table 2.

Table 2: Adverse Events Reported by 3% or More of Patients Receiving Either ESTRING or Conjugated Estrogens Vaginal Cream in Two Pivotal Controlled Studies

ADVERSE EVENT	Estring (n=257) %	Conjugated Estrogens Vaginal Cream (n=129) %
Musculoskeletal		
Back Pain	6	8
Arthritis	4	2
Arthralgia	3	5
Skeletal Pain	2	4
CNS/Peripheral Nervous System		
Headache	13	16
Psychiatric		
Insomnia	4	0
Gastrointestinal		
Abdominal Pain	4	2
Nausea	3	2
Respiratory		
Upper Respiratory Tract Infection	5	6
Sinusitis	4	3
Pharyngitis	1	3
Urinary		
Urinary Tract Infection	2	7
Female Reproductive		
Leukorrhea	7	3
Vaginitis	5	2
Vaginal Discomfort/Pain	5	5
Vaginal Hemorrhage	4	5
Asymptomatic Genital Bacterial Growth	4	6
Breast Pain	1	7
Resistance Mechanisms		
Genital Moniliasis	6	7
Body as a Whole		
Flu-Like Symptoms	3	2
Hot Flushes	2	3
Allergy	1	4
Miscellaneous		
Family Stress	2	3

Other adverse events (listed alphabetically) occurring at a frequency of 1 to 3% in the two pivotal controlled studies by patients receiving ESTRING include: anxiety, bronchitis, chest pain, cystitis, dermatitis, diarrhea, dyspepsia, dysuria, flatulence, gastritis, genital eruption, genital pruritus, hemorrhoids, leg edema, migraine, otitis media, skin hypertrophy, syncope, toothache, tooth disorder, urinary incontinence.

The following additional adverse events were reported at least once by patients receiving ESTRING in the worldwide clinical program, which includes controlled and uncontrolled studies. A causal relationship with ESTRING has not been established.

Body as a Whole: allergic reaction
CNS/Peripheral Nervous System: dizziness
Gastrointestinal: enlarged abdomen, vomiting
Metabolic/Nutritional Disorders: weight decrease or increase
Psychiatric: depression, decreased libido, nervousness
Reproductive: breast engorgement, breast enlargement, intermenstrual bleeding, genital edema, vulval disorder
Skin/Appendages: pruritus, pruritus ani
Urinary: micturition frequency, urethral disorder
Vascular: thrombophlebitis
Vision: abnormal vision

OVERDOSAGE
Given the nature and design of ESTRING (estradiol vaginal ring), it is unlikely that overdosage will occur. However, should overdosage occur, it may manifest itself as nausea, vomiting, and/or vaginal bleeding. Serious ill effects have not been reported following acute ingestion of large doses of estrogen-containing oral contraceptives by young children.

DOSAGE AND ADMINISTRATION
One ESTRING (estradiol vaginal ring) is to be inserted as deeply as possible into the upper one-third of the vaginal vault. The ring is to remain in place continuously for three months, after which it is to be removed and, if appropriate, replaced by a new ring. The need to continue treatment should be assessed at 3 or 6 month intervals.

Should the ring be removed or fall out at any time during the 90-day treatment period, the ring should be rinsed in lukewarm water and re-inserted by the patient, or, if necessary, by a physician or nurse.

Retention of the ring for greater than 90 days does not represent overdosage but will result in progressively greater underdosage with the attendant risk of loss of efficacy and increasing risk of vaginal infections and/or erosions.

Instructions for Use
ESTRING (estradiol vaginal ring) insertion
The ring should be pressed into an oval and inserted into the upper third of the vaginal vault. The exact position is not critical. When ESTRING is in place, the patient should not feel anything. If the patient feels discomfort, ESTRING is probably not far enough inside. Gently push ESTRING further into the vagina.
ESTRING use
ESTRING should be left in place continuously for 90 days and then, if continuation of therapy is deemed appropriate, replaced by a new ESTRING.
The patient should not feel ESTRING when it is in place and it should not interfere with sexual intercourse. Straining at defecation may make ESTRING move down in the lower part of the vagina. If so, it may be pushed up again with a finger.
If ESTRING is expelled totally from the vagina, it should be rinsed in lukewarm water and reinserted by the patient (or doctor/nurse if necessary).

ESTRING removal
ESTRING may be removed by hooking a finger through the ring and pulling it out.

For patient instructions, see **Information for Patients**.

HOW SUPPLIED
Each ESTRING (estradiol vaginal ring) is individually packaged in a heat-sealed rectangular pouch consisting of three layers, from outside to inside: polyester, aluminum foil, and low density polyethylene, respectively. The pouch is provided with a tear-off notch on one side.

NDC 0013-2150-36 ESTRING (estradiol vaginal ring) 2 mg - available in single packs.

STORAGE - Store at controlled room temperature 15° to 30°C (59° to 86°F).

CAUTION: Federal law prohibits dispensing without prescription.

INFORMATION FOR PATIENTS
INTRODUCTION
This leaflet describes when and how to use ESTRING (estradiol vaginal ring), and the risks and benefits of estrogen treatment. Please read this information carefully before starting treatment.

Estrogens have important benefits but also some risks. You must decide, with your doctor, whether the risks to you of estrogen use are acceptable because of their benefits. If you use estrogens, check with your doctor to be sure you are using the dose that is appropriate for you, and that you don't use them longer than necessary. How long you need to use estrogens should be decided by you and your doctor.

1. **ESTROGENS INCREASE THE RISK OF CANCER OF THE UTERUS IN WOMEN WHO HAVE HAD THEIR MENOPAUSE ("CHANGE OF LIFE")**
If you use any estrogen-containing drug, it is important to visit your doctor regularly and report any unusual vaginal bleeding right away. Vaginal bleeding after menopause may be a warning sign of uterine cancer. Your doctor should evaluate any unusual vaginal bleeding to find out the cause.

2. **ESTROGENS SHOULD NOT BE USED DURING PREGNANCY**
Estrogens do not prevent miscarriage (spontaneous abortion) and are not needed in the days following childbirth. If you take estrogens during pregnancy, your unborn child has a greater than usual chance of having birth defects. The risk of developing these defects is small, but clearly larger than the risk in children whose mothers did not take estrogens during pregnancy. These birth defects may affect the baby's urinary system and sex organs. Daughters born to mothers who took DES (an estrogen drug) have a higher than usual chance of developing cancer of the vagina or cervix when they become teenagers or young adults. Sons may have a higher than usual chance of developing cancer of the testicles when they become teenagers or young adults.

USES OF ESTROGEN
Estrogens are hormones made by the ovaries of women during their reproductive years. Between ages 45 and 55, the ovaries normally stop making estrogens. This leads to a drop in body estrogen levels which causes the "change of life" or menopause (the end of monthly menstrual periods). If both ovaries are removed during an operation before natural menopause takes place, the sudden drop in estrogen levels results in what is known as "surgically induced menopause".

When the estrogen levels begin dropping, some women develop very uncomfortable symptoms, such as feelings of warmth in the face, neck, and chest, or sudden intense episodes of heat and sweating ("hot flashes" or "hot flushes"). Using estrogen drugs can help the body adjust to lower estrogen levels and reduce these symptoms. ESTRING (estradiol vaginal ring) DOES NOT PROVIDE ENOUGH ESTROGEN TO REDUCE THESE SYMPTOMS.

The declining estrogen levels associated with advancing age after menopause may also result in thinning and drying of the tissue in the urinary tract and vagina (urogenital atrophy). Vaginal symptoms of this condition include dryness in the vagina (atrophic vaginitis), genital itching and burning, and pain with intercourse. Urinary symptoms may include urinary urgency and pain on urination. Small amounts of estrogen delivered directly to the local tissue can be used to help reduce these symptoms.

USE OF ESTRING (estradiol vaginal ring)
ESTRING is a local estrogen therapy designed to relieve vaginal and urinary symptoms of postmenopausal estrogen deficiency for a full 90 days. ESTRING exerts its effect locally in the lower urogenital tract and has not been shown to have significant effects in other estrogen-sensitive organs or tissues of the body. Consequently, ESTRING PROVIDES RELIEF OF LOCAL SYMPTOMS OF MENOPAUSE ONLY.

DESCRIPTION
ESTRING (estradiol vaginal ring) contains a drug reservoir of 2 mg of the estrogen, estradiol, in its core. ESTRING releases estradiol into the vagina in a consistent, stable manner for 90 days. The soft, flexible ring is placed in the upper third of the vagina (by the physician or the patient) and worn continuously for 90 days, then removed and replaced if continuation of therapy is indicated.

WHO SHOULD NOT USE ESTRING (estradiol vaginal ring)
ESTRING should not be used:

During pregnancy (see **BOXED WARNING**).
Women who are definitely postmenopausal cannot become pregnant. Women who believe they are postmenopausal because their menstrual cycles have recently stopped should confirm that they are not pregnant before using any form of estrogen-containing drug. Using estrogens while pregnant may cause the unborn child to have birth defects. Estrogens do not prevent miscarriage.

In the presence of unusual vaginal bleeding which has not been evaluated by a doctor (see **BOXED WARNING**).
Unusual vaginal bleeding after menopause can be a warning sign of cancer of the uterus. Estrogens may increase the risk of cancer of the uterus in women who have had their menopause ("change of life"). If you use any estrogen-containing drug, it is important to visit your doctor regularly and report any unusual vaginal bleeding right away. Your doctor should evaluate any unusual vaginal bleeding to find out the cause.

If there is a history of certain types of cancer.
Estrogens may increase the risk of certain types of cancer. In general, ESTRING should not be used in women who have ever had cancer of the breast or uterus.

During treatment for vaginal infection with vaginal antimicrobial therapy.
It is recommended that ESTRING be discontinued while other vaginal medications are being used to treat a vaginal infection. Use of ESTRING can be resumed after termination of the other vaginal medication, and after first consulting with a physician.

After childbirth or when breastfeeding a baby.
ESTRING should not be used to try to stop the breasts from filling with milk after a baby is born. Women who are breast-feeding should avoid using any drugs because many drugs pass through to the baby in the milk. While nursing a baby, drugs should only be taken on the advice of your healthcare giver.

POSSIBLE RISKS FROM TREATMENT WITH ESTROGENS
The following risk factors apply to estrogens in general:

Cancer of the uterus.
Estrogens increase the risk of developing a condition (endometrial hyperplasia) that may lead to cancer of the lining of the uterus (endometrial cancer). The risk of endometrial cancer is greater in estrogen users than nonusers. Studies have shown that this increased risk depends on estrogen dose, duration of treatment, and treatment regimen. If the uterus has been removed (total hysterectomy), there is no danger of developing cancer of the uterus.

Cancer of the breast.
Most studies have not shown a higher risk of breast cancer in women who have ever used estrogens. However, some studies have reported that breast cancer developed more often (up to twice the usual rate) in women who used estrogens for long periods of time (especially more than 10 years), or who used higher doses for shorter time periods. Regular breast examinations by a health professional and monthly self-examination are recommended for all women.

Gallbladder disease and abnormal blood clotting.
Gallbladder disease and abnormal blood clotting are risk factors associated with medium to high doses of estrogen. Most studies of low dose estrogen usage by women do not show an increased risk of these complications, and to date have not been seen with ESTRING (estradiol vaginal ring) treatment.

SIDE EFFECTS
Like all medications, ESTRING (estradiol vaginal ring) may cause side effects. The most frequently reported side effect is increased vaginal secretions. Many of these vaginal secretions are like those that occur normally prior to menopause and indicate that ESTRING is working. Vaginal secretions that are associated with a bad odor, vaginal itching, or other signs of vaginal infection are NOT normal and may indicate a risk or a cause for concern. Other side effects may include vaginal discomfort, abdominal pain, or genital itching.

Estrogens in General
In addition to the risks listed above, the following side effects have been reported with estrogen use:
— Nausea and vomiting.
— Breast tenderness or enlargement.
— Enlargement of benign tumors ("fibroids") of the uterus.
— Retention of excess fluid. This may worsen some conditions, such as asthma, epilepsy, migraine, heart disease, or kidney disease.
— Spotty darkening of the skin, particularly on the face.

REDUCING RISK OF ESTROGEN USE
If you use estrogens, you may reduce your risks by doing these things:
See your doctor regularly.
While you are using estrogens, it is important to visit your doctor at least once a year for a check-up. If you develop vaginal bleeding while taking estrogens, call your doctor - you may need further evaluation. If members of your family have had breast cancer or if you have ever had breast lumps or an abnormal mammogram (breast X-ray), you may need to have more frequent breast examinations.
Reassess your need for estrogens.
You and your doctor should reevaluate whether or not you still need estrogens at least every 6 months.
Be alert for warning signs.
If any of these warning signals (or any other unusual symptoms) happen while you are using estrogens, call your doctor immediately:
— Abnormal bleeding from the vagina (possible uterine cancer).
— Pains in the calves or chest, sudden shortness of breath, or coughing blood (possible clot in the legs, heart, or lungs).
— Severe headache or vomiting, dizziness, faintness, changes in vision or speech, weakness or numbness of an arm or leg (possible clot in the brain or eye).
— Breast lumps (possible breast cancer; ask your doctor or health professional to show you how to examine your breasts monthly).
— Yellowing of skin or eyes (possible liver problem).
— Pain, swelling, or tenderness in the abdomen (possible gallbladder problem).

OTHER INFORMATION
1. Estrogens increase the risk of developing a condition (endometrial hyperplasia) that may lead to cancer of the lining of the uterus. Progestin, another hormone drug, is usually prescribed with higher-dose estrogen preparations to lower the risk of developing endometrial hyperplasia. Progestins are not usually needed for women using ESTRING (estradiol vaginal ring) alone.
2. Some women have experienced moving or sliding of ESTRING within the vagina. If this happens, ESTRING can be gently pushed back into position with a clean finger. Instances of ESTRING slipping out of the vagina have been infrequent and were usually associated with moving the bowels, straining, or constipation within the first few weeks of treatment. If this occurs, ESTRING can be washed with lukewarm (NOT hot) water and reinserted. If this happens repeatedly, you should consult with your doctor or healthcare giver and determine whether continued treatment is appropriate for you.
3. ESTRING may not be suitable for women with narrow, short, or stenosed (constricted) vaginas. A narrow vagina, vaginal stenosis (constriction), significant prolapse, and vaginal infections are conditions that make the vagina more susceptible to irritation or ulceration caused by ESTRING. Women with signs or symptoms of vaginal irritation should alert their doctor or healthcare giver.
4. Vaginal infection is generally more common in postmenopausal women. Vaginal infections should be treated with appropriate antimicrobial therapy before initiation of ESTRING. If a vaginal infection develops during use of ESTRING, then ESTRING should be removed and reinserted only after the infection has been appropriately treated. See your doctor or healthcare giver if you have vaginal discomfort or suspect you have a vaginal infection.
5. Your doctor has prescribed this drug for you and you alone. Do not give the drug to anyone else.
6. Keep this and all drugs out of the reach of children.
7. This leaflet provides a summary of important information about ESTRING. If you want more information, ask your doctor or pharmacist to show you the professional labeling. The professional labeling is also published in a book called the "Physicians' Desk Reference®," which is available in book stores and public libraries. Generic drugs carry virtually the same labeling information as their brand name versions.

HOW SUPPLIED
Each ESTRING (estradiol vaginal ring) is individually packaged in a heat-sealed rectangular pouch. The pouch is provided with a tear-off notch on one side.
NDC 0013-2150-36 ESTRING (estradiol vaginal ring) 2 mg available in single units.
Storage: Store at controlled room temperature 15° to 30° C (59° to 86°F).
Caution: Federal law prohibits dispensing without prescription.

Continued on next page

Information on these Pharmacia & Upjohn products is based on labeling in effect June 1, 1998. Further information concerning these and other Pharmacia & Upjohn products may be obtained by direct inquiry to Medical Information, Pharmacia & Upjohn, Kalamazoo, MI 49001.

Estring—Cont.

A Patient Guide to ESTRING
(estradiol vaginal ring) 2 mg
Insertion and Removal

FEMALE ANATOMY

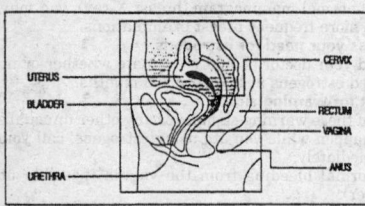

ESTRING INSERTION

ESTRING can be inserted and removed by you or your doctor. To insert ESTRING yourself, choose the position that is most comfortable for you: standing with one leg up, squatting, or lying down.

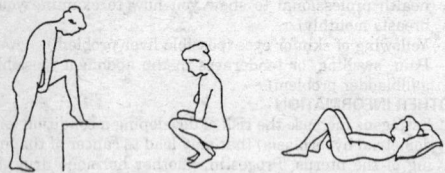

1. After washing and drying your hands, remove ESTRING from its pouch using the tear-off notch on the side. (Since the ring becomes slippery when wet, be sure your hands are dry before handling it.)
2. Hold ESTRING between your thumb and index finger and press the opposite sides of the ring together as shown.

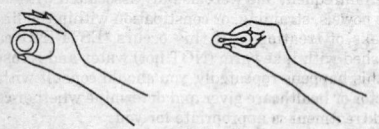

3. Gently push the compressed ring into your vagina as far as you can.

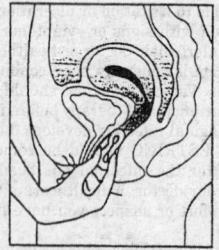

ESTRING PLACEMENT

The exact position of ESTRING is not critical, as long as it is placed in the upper third of the vagina.

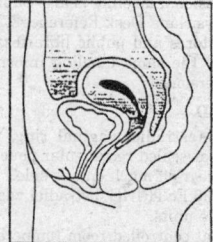

When ESTRING is in place, you should not feel anything. If you feel uncomfortable, ESTRING is probably not far enough inside. Use your finger to gently push ESTRING further into your vagina.
There is no danger of ESTRING being pushed too far up in the vagina or getting lost. ESTRING can only be inserted as far as the end of the vagina, where the cervix (the narrow, lower end of the uterus) will block ESTRING from going any further (see diagram of Female Anatomy).

ESTRING USE

Once inserted, ESTRING should remain in place in the vagina for 90 days.

Most women and their partners experience no discomfort with ESTRING in place during intercourse, so it is NOT necessary that the ring be removed. If ESTRING should cause you or your partner any discomfort, you may remove it prior to intercourse (see ESTRING Removal, below). Be sure to reinsert ESTRING as soon as possible afterwards. ESTRING may slide down into the lower part of the vagina as a result of the abdominal pressure or straining that sometimes accompanies constipation. If this should happen, gently guide ESTRING back into place with your finger. There have been rare reports of ESTRING falling out in some women following intense straining or coughing. If this should occur, simply wash ESTRING with lukewarm (NOT hot) water and reinsert it.

ESTRING DRUG DELIVERY

Once in the vagina, ESTRING begins to release estradiol immediately. ESTRING will continue to release a low, continuous dose of estradiol for the full 90 days it remains in place.

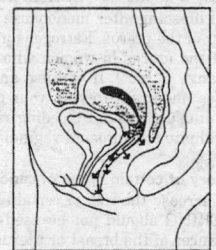

It will take about 2 to 3 weeks to restore the tissue of the vagina and urinary tract to a healthier condition and to feel the full effect of ESTRING in relieving vaginal and urinary symptoms. If your symptoms persist for more than a few weeks after beginning ESTRING therapy, contact your doctor.
One of the most frequently reported effects associated with the use of ESTRING is an increase in vaginal secretions. These secretions are like those that occur normally prior to menopause and indicate that ESTRING is working. However, if the secretions are associated with a bad odor or vaginal itching or discomfort, be sure to contact your doctor.

ESTRING REMOVAL

After 90 days there will no longer be enough estradiol in the ring to maintain its full effect in relieving your vaginal or urinary symptoms. ESTRING should be removed at that time and replaced with a new ESTRING, if your doctor determines that you need to continue your therapy.
To remove ESTRING:
1. Wash and dry your hands thoroughly.
2. Assume a comfortable position, either standing with one leg up, squatting, or lying down.
3. Loop your finger through the ring and gently pull it out.
4. Discard the used ring in a waste receptacle.
   (Do not flush ESTRING).

If you have any additional questions about removing ESTRING, contact your doctor or healthcare giver.
Manufactured for:
Pharmacia & Upjohn Company
Kalamazoo, MI 49001, USA
By:
Ferring AB
Malmö, Sweden
101021197
November 1997

FRAGMIN®   ℞
[frăg-mĭn]
dalteparin sodium injection
For *Subcutaneous* Use Only

> **SPINAL/EPIDURAL HEMATOMAS**
> When neuraxial anesthesia (epidural/spinal anesthesia) or spinal puncture is employed, patients anticoagulated or scheduled to be anticoagulated with low molecular weight heparins or heparinoids for prevention of thromboembolic complications are at risk of developing an epidural or spinal hematoma which can result in long-term or permanent paralysis.
> The risk of these events is increased by the use of indwelling epidural catheters for administration of analgesia or by the concomitant use of drugs affecting hemostasis such as nonsteroidal anti-inflammatory drugs, platelet inhibitors, or other anticoagulants. The risk also appears to be increased by traumatic or repeated epidural or spinal puncture.
> Patients should be frequently monitored for signs and symptoms of neurological impairment. If neurological compromise is noted, urgent treatment is necessary.
> The physician should consider the potential benefit versus risk before neuraxial intervention in patients anticoagulated or to be anticoagulated for thromboprophylaxis (also see WARNINGS, Hemorrhage and PRECAUTIONS, Drug Interactions).

DESCRIPTION

FRAGMIN Injection (dalteparin sodium injection) is a sterile, low molecular weight heparin. It is available in single-dose, prefilled syringes and a multiple-dose vial. With reference to the W.H.O. First International Low Molecular Weight Heparin Reference Standard, each syringe contains 2500 (16 mg dalteparin sodium) or 5000 (32 mg dalteparin sodium) anti-Factor Xa international units (IU) in 0.2 mL. Each 9.5 mL vial contains 10,000 (64 mg dalteparin sodium) anti-Factor Xa IU per 1 mL, for a total of 95,000 anti-Factor Xa IU per vial.
Each prefilled syringe also contains Water for Injection and sodium chloride, when required, to maintain physiologic ionic strength. The prefilled syringes are preservative free. Each multiple-dose vial also contains Water for Injection and 14 mg of benzyl alcohol per mL as a preservative. The pH of both formulations is 5.0 to 7.5.
Dalteparin sodium is produced through controlled nitrous acid depolymerization of sodium heparin from porcine intestinal mucosa followed by a chromatographic purification process. It is composed of strongly acidic sulphated polysaccharide chains (oligosaccharide, containing 2,5-anhydro-D-mannitol residues as end groups) with an average molecular weight of 5000 and about 90% of the material within the range 2000–9000. The molecular weight distribution is:

<3000 daltons	3.0–15.0%
3000 to 8000 daltons	65.0–78.0%
>8000 daltons	14.0–26.0%

Structural Formula

$$R = H \text{ or } SO_3Na$$
$$R_1 = COCH_3 \text{ or } SO_3Na$$
$$R_2 = H \text{ or } R_3 = COONa$$
$$\text{or}$$
$$R_2 = COONa \quad R_3 = H$$
$$n = 3\text{-}20$$

CLINICAL PHARMACOLOGY

Dalteparin is a low molecular weight heparin with antithrombotic properties. It acts by enhancing the inhibition of Factor Xa and thrombin by antithrombin. In man, dalteparin potentiates preferentially the inhibition of coagulation Factor Xa, while only slightly affecting clotting time, e.g., activated partial thromboplastin time (APTT).

Pharmacodynamics:
Doses of FRAGMIN Injection of up to 10,000 anti-Factor Xa IU administered subcutaneously as a single dose or two 5,000 IU doses 12 hours apart to healthy subjects do not produce a significant change in platelet aggregation, fibrinolysis, or global clotting tests such as prothrombin time (PT), thrombin time (TT) or APTT. Subcutaneous administration of doses of 5,000 IU b.i.d. of FRAGMIN for seven consecutive days to patients undergoing abdominal surgery did not markedly affect APTT, Platelet Factor 4 (PF4), or lipoprotein lipase.

Pharmacokinetics:
Mean peak levels of plasma anti-Factor Xa activity following single subcutaneous doses of 2,500, 5,000 and 10,000 IU were 0.19 ± 0.04, 0.41 ± 0.07 and 0.82 ± 0.10 IU/mL, respectively, and were attained in about 4 hours in most subjects. Absolute bioavailability in healthy volunteers, measured as the anti-Factor Xa activity, was $87 \pm 6\%$. Increasing the dose from 2,500 to 10,000 IU resulted in an overall increase in anti-Factor Xa AUC that was greater than proportional by about one-third.
Peak anti-Factor Xa activity increased more or less linearly with dose over the same dose range. There appeared to be no appreciable accumulation of anti-Factor Xa activity with twice-daily dosing of 100 IU/kg subcutaneously for up to 7 days.
The volume of distribution for dalteparin anti-Factor Xa activity was 40 to 60 mL/kg. The mean plasma clearances of

dalteparin anti-Factor Xa activity in normal volunteers following single intravenous bolus doses of 30 and 120 anti-Factor Xa IU/kg were 24.6 ± 5.4 and 15.6 ± 2.4 mL/hr/kg, respectively. The corresponding mean disposition half-lives are 1.47 ± 0.3 and 2.5 ± 0.3 hr.

Following intravenous doses of 40 and 60 IU/kg, mean terminal half-lives were 2.1 ± 0.3 and 2.3 ± 0.4 hrs, respectively. Longer apparent terminal half-lives (3 to 5 hrs) are observed following subcutaneous dosing, possibly due to delayed absorption. In patients with chronic renal insufficiency requiring hemodialysis, the mean terminal half-life of anti-Factor Xa activity following a single intravenous dose of 5,000 IU FRAGMIN was 5.7 ± 2.0 hrs, i.e. considerably longer than values observed in healthy volunteers, therefore, greater accumulation can be expected in these patients.

Clinical Trials

FRAGMIN Injection, administered once daily beginning prior to surgery and continuing for 5 to 10 days after surgery, has been shown to prevent deep vein thrombosis (DVT) in patients at risk for thromboembolic complications (see INDICATIONS and DOSAGE AND ADMINISTRATION). Data from two double-blind randomized controlled clinical trials performed in patients undergoing major abdominal surgery, summarized in the following tables, show that FRAGMIN 2500 IU was superior to placebo and similar to heparin in preventing DVT (see Tables 1 and 2).

Table 1
Abdominal Surgery

	Treatment Group	
	FRAGMIN	Placebo
Dosing Regimen	2500 IU qd	qd
Number of Patients Treated	102	102
Treatment Failures		
Total Thromboembolic Events (%)	4/91 (4.4)*	16/91 (17.6)
Proximal DVT (%)	0/91 (0)	5/91 (5.5)
Distal DVT (%)	4/91 (4.4)	11/91 (12.1)
PE (%)	0/91 (0)	2/91 (2.2)**

* P-value versus placebo = 0.008
** Both patients also had DVT, 1 proximal and 1 distal

Table 2
Abdominal Surgery

	Treatment Group	
	FRAGMIN	Heparin
Dosing Regimen	2500 IU qd	5000 IU bid
Number of Patients Treated	195	196
Treatment Failures		
Total Thromboembolic Events (%)	7/178 (3.9)*	7/174 (4.0)
Proximal DVT (%)	3/178 (1.7)	4/174 (2.3)
Distal DVT (%)	3/178 (1.7)	3/174 (1.7)
PE (%)	1/178 (0.6)	0/174 (0)

* P-value versus heparin = 0.74

Data from a double-blind randomized controlled clinical trial show that FRAGMIN 5000 IU once daily is more effective than FRAGMIN 2500 IU once daily in preventing DVT in patients undergoing abdominal surgery with malignancy (see Table 3).

Table 3
Abdominal Surgery
Patients With Malignancy

	Intent to Treat	
	FRAGMIN	FRAGMIN
Dosing Regimen	2500 IU qd	5000 IU qd
Number of Patients Treated	696	679
Treatment Failures		
Total Thromboembolic Events (%)	99/656 (15.1)*	60/645 (9.3)
Proximal DVT (%)	18/657 (2.7)	14/646 (2.2)
Distal DVT (%)	80/657 (12.2)	41/646 (6.3)
PE (%)		
Fatal	1/674 (0.1)	1/669 (0.1)
Non-fatal	2	4

* P-value = 0.001

INDICATIONS AND USAGE

FRAGMIN Injection is indicated for prophylaxis against deep vein thrombosis, which may lead to pulmonary embolism, in patients undergoing abdominal surgery who are at risk for thromboembolic complications.

Patients at risk include patients who are over 40 years of age, obese, undergoing surgery under general anesthesia

	FRAGMIN vs. Heparin*				FRAGMIN vs. Placebo		FRAGMIN vs. FRAGMIN	
	FRAGMIN 2500 IU/ 24 hr	Heparin 10000 IU/ 24 hr	FRAGMIN 5000 IU/ 24 hr	Heparin 10000 IU/ 24 hr	FRAGMIN 2500 IU/ 24 hr	Placebo	FRAGMIN 2500 IU/ 24 hr	FRAGMIN 5000 IU/ 24 hr
Post-Operational Transfusions	5.7% (n = 459)	7.9% (n = 454)	15.9% (n = 508)	12.7% (n = 498)	7.7% (n = 182)	7.1% (n = 182)	8.7% (n = 1025)	12.1% (n = 1033)
Wound Hematoma	3.4% (n = 467)	3.9% (n = 467)	2.4% (n = 508)	1.2% (n = 498)	2.5% (n = 79)	2.6% (n = 77)	0.1% (n = 1030)	0.4% (n = 1039)
Reoperation due to Bleeding	0.5% (n = 392)	0.8% (n = 392)	0.8% (n = 508)	0.4% (n = 498)	1.3% (n = 79)	1.3% (n = 78)	0.2% (n = 1030)	1.3% (n = 1038)
Injection Site Hematoma	0.2% (n = 466)	1.1% (n = 464)	7.1% (n = 506)	9.5% (n = 493)	4.7% (n = 172)	1.1% (n = 174)	3.5% (n = 1026)	5.5% (n = 1035)

*FRAGMIN administered once daily, heparin administered twice daily at a dose of 5000 IU.

lasting longer than 30 minutes or who have additional risk factors such as malignancy or a history of deep vein thrombosis or pulmonary embolism.

CONTRAINDICATIONS

FRAGMIN Injection is contraindicated in patients with known hypersensitivity to the drug, active major bleeding, or thrombocytopenia associated with positive in vitro tests for anti-platelet antibody in the presence of FRAGMIN. Patients with known hypersensitivity to heparin or pork products should not be treated with FRAGMIN.

WARNINGS

FRAGMIN Injection is not intended for intramuscular administration.

FRAGMIN cannot be used interchangeably (unit for unit) with unfractionated heparin or other low molecular weight heparins.

FRAGMIN should be used with extreme caution in patients with history of heparin-induced thrombocytopenia.

Hemorrhage:

FRAGMIN, like other anticoagulants, should be used with extreme caution in patients who have an increased risk of hemorrhage, such as those with severe uncontrolled hypertension, bacterial endocarditis, congenital or acquired bleeding disorders, active ulceration and angiodysplastic gastrointestinal disease, hemorrhagic stroke or shortly after brain, spinal or ophthalmological surgery.

Spinal or epidural hematomas can occur with the associated use of low molecular weight heparins or heparinoids and neuraxial (spinal/epidural) anesthesia or spinal puncture, which can result in long-term or permanent paralysis. The risk of these events is higher with the use of postoperative indwelling epidural catheters or concomitant use of additional drugs affecting hemostasis such as nonsteroidal anti-inflammatory drugs (see boxed WARNING).

As with other anticoagulants, bleeding can occur at any site during therapy with FRAGMIN. An unexpected drop in hematocrit or blood pressure should lead to a search for a bleeding site.

Thrombocytopenia:

In clinical trials, thrombocytopenia with platelet counts of <50,000/mm³ and <100,000/mm³ occurred in <1% and <1%, respectively, of patients undergoing abdominal surgery. In clinical practice, rare cases of thrombocytopenia with thrombosis have also been observed.

Thrombocytopenia of any degree should be monitored closely. Heparin-induced thrombocytopenia can occur with the administration of FRAGMIN. The incidence of this complication is unknown at present.

Miscellaneous:

The multiple-dose vial of FRAGMIN contains benzyl alcohol as a preservative. Benzyl alcohol has been reported to be associated with a fatal "Gasping Syndrome" in premature infants. Because benzyl alcohol may cross the placenta, FRAGMIN preserved with benzyl alcohol should not be used in pregnant women. (See PRECAUTIONS, Pregnancy Category B., Nonteratogenic Effects.)

PRECAUTIONS

General:

FRAGMIN Injection should not be mixed with other injections or infusions unless specific compatibility data are available that support such mixing.

FRAGMIN should be used with caution in patients with bleeding diathesis, thrombocytopenia or platelet defects; severe liver or kidney insufficiency, hypertensive or diabetic retinopathy, and recent gastrointestinal bleeding.

If a thromboembolic event should occur despite dalteparin prophylaxis, FRAGMIN should be discontinued and appropriate therapy initiated.

Drug Interactions:

FRAGMIN should be used with care in patients receiving oral anticoagulants and/or platelet inhibitors because of increased risk of bleeding.

Laboratory Tests:

Periodic routine complete blood counts, including platelet count, and stool occult blood tests are recommended during the course of treatment with FRAGMIN. No special monitoring of blood clotting times (e.g., APTT) is needed.

When administered at recommended prophylaxis doses, routine coagulation tests such as Prothrombin Time [PT] and Activated Partial Thromboplastin Time [APTT] are relatively insensitive measures of FRAGMIN activity and, therefore, unsuitable for monitoring.

Drug/Laboratory Test Interactions:
Elevations of Serum Transaminases

Asymptomatic increases in transaminase levels (SGOT/AST and SGPT/ALT) greater than three times the upper limit of normal of the laboratory reference range have been reported in 1.7 and 4.3%, respectively, of patients during treatment with FRAGMIN. Similar significant increases in transaminase levels have also been observed in patients treated with heparin and other low molecular weight heparins. Such elevations are fully reversible and are rarely associated with increases in bilirubin. Since transaminase determinations are important in the differential diagnosis of myocardial infarction, liver disease and pulmonary emboli, elevations that might be caused by drugs like FRAGMIN should be interpreted with caution.

Carcinogenicity, Mutagenesis, Impairment of Fertility:

Dalteparin sodium has not been tested for its carcinogenic potential in long-term animal studies. It was not mutagenic in the in vitro Ames Test, mouse lymphoma cell forward mutation test and human lymphocyte chromosomal aberration test and in the in vivo mouse micronucleus test. Dalteparin sodium at subcutaneous doses up to 1,200 IU/kg (7080 IU/m²) did not affect the fertility or reproductive performance of male and female rats.

Pregnancy: Pregnancy Category B.
Teratogenic Effects:

Reproduction studies with dalteparin sodium at intravenous doses up to 2400 IU/kg (14160 IU/m²) in pregnant rats and 4800 IU/kg (40800 IU/m²) in pregnant rabbits did not produce any evidence of impaired fertility or harm to the fetuses. There are, however, no adequate and well-controlled studies in pregnant women. Because animal reproduction studies are not always predictive of human response, this drug should be used during pregnancy only if clearly needed.

Nonteratogenic Effects:

Cases of "Gasping Syndrome" have occurred when large amounts of benzyl alcohol have been administered (99–404 mg/kg/day). The 9.5 mL multi-dose vial of FRAGMIN contains 14 mg/mL of benzyl alcohol.

Nursing Mothers:

It is not known whether dalteparin sodium is excreted in human milk. Because many drugs are excreted in human milk, caution should be exercised when FRAGMIN is administered to a nursing mother.

Pediatric Use:

Safety and effectiveness in pediatric patients have not been established.

ADVERSE REACTIONS

Hemorrhage:

The incidence of hemorrhagic complications during treatment with FRAGMIN Injection has been low. The most commonly reported side effect is hematoma at the injection site. The incidence of bleeding may increase with higher doses;

Continued on next page

Information on these Pharmacia & Upjohn products is based on labeling in effect June 1, 1998. Further information concerning these and other Pharmacia & Upjohn products may be obtained by direct inquiry to Medical Information, Pharmacia & Upjohn, Kalamazoo, MI 49001.

Fragmin—Cont.

however, in abdominal surgery patients with malignancy, no significant increase in bleeding was observed when comparing FRAGMIN 5000 IU to either FRAGMIN 2500 IU or low dose heparin.

In a study comparing FRAGMIN 5000 IU once daily to FRAGMIN 2500 IU once daily in patients undergoing surgery for malignancy, the incidence of bleeding events was 4.6% and 3.6%, respectively (n.s.). In a study comparing FRAGMIN 5000 IU once daily to heparin 5000 IU twice daily, the incidence of bleeding events was 3.2% and 2.7%, respectively (n.s.) in the malignancy subgroup.

The following table summarizes adverse bleeding events that occurred in clinical trials which studied FRAGMIN 2500 and 5000 IU administered once daily to abdominal surgery patients.

[See table at top of previous page]

Thrombocytopenia:

During clinical trials with FRAGMIN in thromboprophylaxis, thrombocytopenia, platelet counts of <50,000/mm^3 and <100,000/mm^3 were reported in <1% and <1%, respectively, of patients given FRAGMIN and <1% and 1% of patients given heparin. (See WARNINGS.)

Other:

Pain at injection site was seen in the following percentages of patients involved in clinical trials: 0% for FRAGMIN 2500 IU qd vs 0.4% for heparin 5000 IU bid; 4.5% for FRAGMIN 5000 IU qd vs 11.8% for heparin 5000 IU bid; 0% for FRAGMIN 2500 IU qd vs 0% for placebo and 1.1% for FRAGMIN 2500 IU qd vs 1.8% for FRAGMIN 5000 IU qd.

Allergic reactions (i.e., pruritus, rash, fever, injection site reaction, bulleous eruption) and skin necrosis have occurred rarely. A few cases of anaphylactoid reactions have been reported.

OVERDOSAGE

Symptoms/Treatment:

An excessive dosage of FRAGMIN Injection may lead to hemorrhagic complications. These may generally be stopped by the slow intravenous injection of protamine sulfate (1% solution), at a dose of 1 mg protamine for every 100 anti-Xa IU of FRAGMIN given. A second infusion of 0.5 mg protamine sulfate per 100 anti-Xa IU of FRAGMIN may be administered if the APTT measured 2 to 4 hours after the first infusion remains prolonged. Even with these additional doses of protamine, the APTT may remain more prolonged than would usually be found following administration of conventional heparin. In all cases, the anti-Factor Xa activity is never completely neutralized (maximum about 60 to 75%).

Particular care should be taken to avoid overdosage with protamine sulfate. Administration of protamine sulfate can cause severe hypotensive and anaphylactoid reactions. Because fatal reactions, often resembling anaphylaxis, have been reported with protamine sulfate, it should be given only when resuscitation techniques and treatment of anaphylactic shock are readily available. For additional information, consult the labeling of Protamine Sulfate Injection, USP, products. A single subcutaneous dose of 100,000 IU/kg of FRAGMIN to mice caused a mortality of 8% (1/12) whereas 50,000 IU/kg was a non-lethal dose. The observed sign was hematoma at the site of injection.

DOSAGE AND ADMINISTRATION

In patients undergoing abdominal surgery with a risk of thromboembolic complications, 2500 IU of FRAGMIN Injection should be administered subcutaneously only, each day, starting 1 to 2 hours prior to surgery and repeated once daily for 5 to 10 days postoperatively (See INDICATIONS).

In abdominal surgery associated with a high risk of thromboembolic complications, such as malignant disorder, 5000 IU should be administered subcutaneously only the evening before surgery and repeated once daily for 5 to 10 days postoperatively. Alternatively in patients with malignancy, the first 5000 IU dose can be administered as 2500 IU s.c. 1 to 2 hours prior to surgery with an additional 2500 IU s.c. dose 12 hours later and then 5000 IU once daily for 5 to 10 days.

Dosage adjustment and routine monitoring of coagulation parameters are not required if the dosage and administration recommendations specified above are followed.

Administration:

FRAGMIN is administered by subcutaneous injection. It must not be administered by intramuscular injection.

Subcutaneous injection technique: Patients should be sitting or lying down and FRAGMIN administered by deep subcutaneous injection. FRAGMIN may be injected in a U-shape area around the navel, the upper outer side of the thigh or the upper outer quadrangle of the buttock. The injection site should be varied daily. When the area around the navel or the thigh is used, using the thumb and forefinger, you must lift up a fold of skin while giving the injection. The entire length of the needle should be inserted at a 45 to 90 degree angle.

Parenteral drug products should be inspected visually for particulate matter and discoloration prior to administration, whenever solution and container permit.

HOW SUPPLIED

FRAGMIN Injection is available in the following strengths and package sizes:

0.2 mL single-dose prefilled syringe, affixed with a 27-gauge x 1/2 inch needle.

Package of 10:

2500 anti-Factor Xa IU	NDC 0013-2406-91
5000 anti-Factor Xa IU	NDC 0013-2426-91

9.5 mL multiple-dose vial:

10,000 anti-Factor Xa IU/mL (95,000 anti-Factor Xa IU/vial)	NDC 0013-2436-06

Storage

Store at controlled room temperature 20° to 25°C (68° to 77°F) [see USP].

Rx only

U.S. Patent 4,303,651

Manufactured for:
Pharmacia & Upjohn Company
Kalamazoo, MI 49001, USA

By: Vetter Pharma-Fertigung
Ravensburg, Germany
(prefilled syringes)

Pharmacia & Upjohn AB
Stockholm, Sweden
(multiple-dose vial)

132020398 Revised March 1998

GENOTROPIN™ ℞

[gen-ō″ trō-pĭn]

somatropin (rDNA origin) for injection

In a Two-Chamber Cartridge

DESCRIPTION

GENOTROPIN Lyophilized Powder contains somatropin [rDNA origin], which is a polypeptide hormone of recombinant DNA origin. It has 191 amino acid residues and a molecular weight of 22,124 daltons. The amino acid sequence of the product is identical to that of human growth hormone of pituitary origin (somatropin). GENOTROPIN is synthesized in a strain of *Escherichia coli* that has been modified by the addition of the gene for human growth hormone. GENOTROPIN is a sterile white lyophilized powder intended for subcutaneous injection.

GENOTROPIN 1.5 mg is dispensed in a two-chamber cartridge. The front chamber contains recombinant somatropin 1.5 mg (approximately 4.5 IU), glycine 27.6 mg, sodium dihydrogen phosphate anhydrous 0.3 mg, and disodium phosphate anhydrous 0.3 mg; the rear chamber contains 1.13 mL water for injection.

GENOTROPIN 5.8 mg is dispensed in a two-chamber cartridge. The front chamber contains recombinant somatropin 5.8 mg (approximately 17.4 IU), glycine 2.2 mg, mannitol 1.8 mg, sodium dihydrogen phosphate anhydrous 0.32 mg, and disodium phosphate anhydrous 0.31 mg; the rear chamber contains 0.3% m-Cresol (as a preservative) and mannitol 45 mg in 1.14 mL water for injection.

GENOTROPIN 13.8 mg is dispensed in a two-chamber cartridge. The front chamber contains recombinant somatropin 13.8 mg (approximately 41.4 IU), glycine 2.3 mg, mannitol 14.0 mg, sodium dihydrogen phosphate anhydrous 0.47 mg, and disodium phosphate anhydrous 0.46 mg; the rear chamber contains 0.3% m-Cresol (as a preservative) and mannitol 32 mg in 1.13 mL water for injection.

GENOTROPIN is a highly purified preparation. The reconstituted recombinant somatropin solution has a concentration of 1.3 mg/mL (approximately 4 IU/mL), for GENOTROPIN 1.5 mg, 5 mg/mL (approximately 15 IU/mL), for GENOTROPIN 5.8 mg, or 12 mg/mL (approximately 36 IU/mL) for GENOTROPIN 13.8 mg, an osmolality of approximately 300 mOsm/kg, and a pH of approximately 6.7.

HOW SUPPLIED

GENOTROPIN Lyophilized Powder is available in the following packages:

1.5 mg two-chamber cartridge (without preservative)
concentration of 1.3 mg/mL (approximately 4 IU/mL)

Preassembled in a GENOTROPIN INTRA-MIX™ Growth Hormone Reconstitution Device and packaged with a pressure release needle

Package of 5 NDC 0013-2606-94

5.8 mg two-chamber cartridge (with preservative)
concentration of 5 mg/mL (approximately 15 IU/mL)

For use with the GENOTROPIN PEN™ 5 Growth Hormone Delivery Device and/or the GENOTROPIN MIXER™ Growth Hormone Reconstitution Device

Package of 5 NDC 0013-2626-94
Package of 1 NDC 0013-2626-81

Preassembled in a GENOTROPIN INTRA-MIX™ Growth Hormone Reconstitution Device and packaged with a pressure release needle

Package of 5 NDC 0013-2616-94
Package of 1 NDC 0013-2616-81

13.8 mg two-chamber cartridge (with preservative)
concentration of 12 mg/mL (approximately 36 IU/mL)

For use with the GENOTROPIN PEN™ 12 Growth Hormone Delivery Device and/or the GENOTROPIN MIXER Growth Hormone Reconstitution Device

Package of 5 NDC 0013-2646-94
Package of 1 NDC 0013-2646-81

Please see accompanying directions for use of the reconstitution and/or delivery device.

Rx only

Manufactured for:
Pharmacia & Upjohn Company
Kalamazoo, MI 49001, USA
By:
Pharmacia & Upjohn AB
Stockholm, Sweden
Revised March 1998 439-169-1
121020398

Shown in Product Identification Guide, page 332

GLYNASE® PresTab® ℞

Tablets

micronized glyburide tablets; 1.5, 3, and 6 mg

DESCRIPTION

GLYNASE PresTab Tablets contain micronized (smaller particle size) glyburide, which is an oral blood-glucose-lowering drug of the sulfonylurea class. Glyburide is a white, crystalline compound, formulated as GLYNASE PresTab Tablets of 1.5, 3, and 6 mg strengths for oral administration. Inactive ingredients: colloidal silicon dioxide, corn starch, lactose, magnesium stearate. In addition, the **3 mg** strength contains FD&C Blue No. 1 Aluminum Lake, and the **6 mg** tablet contains D&C Yellow No. 10 Aluminum Lake. The chemical name for glyburide is 1-[[p-[2-(5-chloro-o-anisamido)ethyl]phenyl]-sulfonyl]-3-cyclohexylurea and the molecular weight is 493.99. The structural formula is represented below:

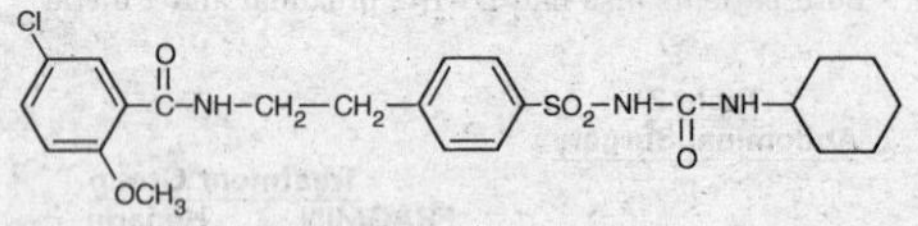

CLINICAL PHARMACOLOGY

Actions

Glyburide appears to lower the blood glucose acutely by stimulating the release of insulin from the pancreas, an effect dependent upon functioning beta cells in the pancreatic islets. The mechanism by which glyburide lowers blood glucose during long-term administration has not been clearly established. With chronic administration in Type II diabetic patients, the blood glucose lowering effect persists despite a gradual decline in the insulin secretory response to the drug. Extrapancreatic effects may be involved in the mechanism of action of oral sulfonylurea hypoglycemic drugs. The combination of glyburide and metformin may have a synergistic effect, since both agents act to improve glucose tolerance by different but complementary mechanisms.

Some patients who are initially responsive to oral hypoglycemic drugs, including glyburide, may become unresponsive or poorly responsive over time. Alternatively, glyburide may be effective in some patients who have become unresponsive to one or more other sulfonylurea drugs.

In addition to its blood glucose lowering actions, glyburide produces a mild diuresis by enhancement of renal free water clearance. Disulfiram-like reactions have very rarely been reported in patients treated with glyburide.

Pharmacokinetics

Single dose studies with GLYNASE PresTab Tablets in normal subjects demonstrate significant absorption of glyburide within one hour, peak drug levels at about two to three hours, and low but detectable levels at twenty-four hours.

Bioavailability studies have demonstrated that GLYNASE PresTab Tablets 3 mg provide serum glyburide concentrations that are not bioequivalent to those from MICRONASE® Tablets 5 mg. Therefore, the patient should be retitrated.

In a single-dose bioavailability study (see Figure A) in which subjects received GLYNASE PresTab Tablets 3 mg and MICRONASE Tablets 5 mg with breakfast, the peak of the mean serum glyburide concentration-time curve was 97.2 ng/mL for GLYNASE PresTab Tablets 3 mg and 87.5 ng/mL for MICRONASE Tablets 5 mg. The mean of the individual maximum serum concentration values of glyburide (C_{max}) from GLYNASE PresTab Tablets 3 mg was 106 ng/mL and that from MICRONASE Tablets 5 mg was 104 ng/mL. The mean glyburide area under the serum concentration-time curve (AUC) for this study was 568 ng x hr/mL

for GLYNASE PresTab Tablets 3 mg and 746 ng x hr/mL for MICRONASE Tablets 5 mg.

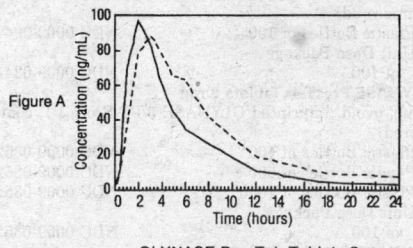

Figure A

```
GLYNASE PresTab Tablets 3 mg
--------- MICRONASE Tablets 5 mg
```

Mean serum levels of glyburide, as reflected by areas under the serum concentration-time curve, increase in proportion to corresponding increases in dose. Multiple dose studies with glyburide in diabetic patients demonstrate drug level concentration-time curves similar to single dose studies, indicating no buildup of drug in tissue depots.

In a steady-state study in diabetic patients receiving GLYNASE PresTab Tablets 6 mg once daily or GLYNASE PresTab Tablets 3 mg twice daily, no difference was seen between the two dosage regimens in average 24-hour glyburide concentrations following two weeks of dosing. The once-daily and twice-daily regimens provided equivalent glucose control as measured by fasting plasma glucose levels, 4-hour postprandial glucose AUC values, and 24-hour glucose AUC values. Insulin AUC response over the 24-hour period was not different for the two regimens. There were differences in insulin response between the regimens for the breakfast and supper 4-hour postprandial periods, but these did not translate into differences in glucose control.

The serum concentration of glyburide in normal subjects decreased with a half-life of about four hours.

In single dose studies in fasting normal subjects who were administered glyburide (MICRONASE Tablets) in doses ranging from 1.25 mg to 5 mg, the degree and duration of blood glucose lowering is proportional to the dose administered and to the area under the drug level concentration-time curve. The blood glucose lowering effect persists for 24 hours following single morning doses in nonfasting diabetic patients. Under conditions of repeated administration in diabetic patients, however, there is no reliable correlation between blood drug levels and fasting blood glucose levels. A one year study of diabetic patients treated with glyburide showed no reliable correlation between administered dose and serum drug level.

The major metabolite of glyburide is the 4-trans-hydroxy derivative. A second metabolite, the 3-cis-hydroxy derivative, also occurs. These metabolites probably contribute no significant hypoglycemic action in humans since they are only weakly active (1/400th and 1/40th as active, respectively, as glyburide) in rabbits.

Glyburide is excreted as metabolites in the bile and urine, approximately 50% by each route. This dual excretory pathway is qualitatively different from that of other sulfonylureas, which are excreted primarily in the urine.

Sulfonylurea drugs are extensively bound to serum proteins. Displacement from protein binding sites by other drugs may lead to enhanced hypoglycemic action. In vitro, the protein binding exhibited by glyburide is predominantly non-ionic, whereas that of other sulfonylureas (chlorpropamide, tolbutamide, tolazamide) is predominantly ionic. Acidic drugs such as phenylbutazone, warfarin, and salicylates displace the ionic-binding sulfonylureas from serum proteins to a far greater extent than the non-ionic binding glyburide. It has not been shown that this difference in protein binding will result in fewer drug-drug interactions with glyburide in clinical use.

INDICATIONS AND USAGE

GLYNASE PresTab Tablets are indicated as an adjunct to diet to lower the blood glucose in patients with non-insulin-dependent diabetes mellitus (Type II) whose hyperglycemia cannot be satisfactorily controlled by diet alone.

Glyburide may be used concomitantly with metformin when diet and glyburide or diet and metformin alone do not result in adequate glycemic control (see metformin insert).

In initiating treatment for non-insulin-dependent diabetes, diet should be emphasized as the primary form of treatment. Caloric restriction and weight loss are essential in the obese diabetic patient. Proper dietary management alone may be effective in controlling the blood glucose and symptoms of hyperglycemia. The importance of regular physical activity should also be stressed, and cardiovascular risk factors should be identified and corrective measures taken where possible. If this treatment program fails to reduce symptoms and/or blood glucose, the use of an oral sulfonylurea or insulin should be considered. Use of GLYNASE

PresTab must be viewed by both the physician and patient as a treatment in addition to diet and not as a substitution or as a convenient mechanism for avoiding dietary restraint. Furthermore, loss of blood glucose control on diet alone may be transient, thus requiring only short-term administration of GLYNASE PresTab.

During maintenance programs, GLYNASE PresTab should be discontinued if satisfactory lowering of blood glucose is no longer achieved. Judgment should be based on regular clinical and laboratory evaluations.

In considering the use of GLYNASE PresTab in asymptomatic patients, it should be recognized that controlling blood glucose in non-insulin-dependent diabetes has not been definitely established to be effective in preventing the long-term cardiovascular or neural complications of diabetes.

CONTRAINDICATIONS

GLYNASE PresTab Tablets are contraindicated in patients with:
1. Known hypersensitivity or allergy to the drug.
2. Diabetic ketoacidosis, with or without coma. This condition should be treated with insulin.
3. Type I diabetes mellitus, as sole therapy.

SPECIAL WARNING ON INCREASED RISK OF CARDIOVASCULAR MORTALITY

The administration of oral hypoglycemic drugs has been reported to be associated with increased cardiovascular mortality as compared to treatment with diet alone or diet plus insulin. This warning is based on the study conducted by the University Group Diabetes Program (UGDP), a long-term prospective clinical trial designed to evaluate the effectiveness of glucose-lowering drugs in preventing or delaying vascular complications in patients with non-insulin-dependent diabetes. The study involved 823 patients who were randomly assigned to one of four treatment groups (Diabetes, 19 (Suppl. 2):747-830, 1970).

UGDP reported that patients treated for 5 to 8 years with diet plus a fixed dose of tolbutamide (1.5 grams per day) had a rate of cardiovascular mortality approximately 2 1/2 times that of patients treated with diet alone. A significant increase in total mortality was not observed, but the use of tolbutamide was discontinued based on the increase in cardiovascular mortality, thus limiting the opportunity for the study to show an increase in overall mortality. Despite controversy regarding the interpretation of these results, the findings of the UGDP study provide an adequate basis for this warning. The patient should be informed of the potential risks and advantages of GLYNASE PresTab and of alternative modes of therapy.

Although only one drug in the sulfonylurea class (tolbutamide) was included in this study, it is prudent from a safety standpoint to consider that this warning may also apply to other oral hypoglycemic drugs in this class, in view of their close similarities in mode of action and chemical structure.

PRECAUTIONS

Bioavailability studies have demonstrated that GLYNASE PresTab Tablets 3 mg provide serum glyburide concentrations that are not bioequivalent to those from MICRONASE Tablets 5 mg. Therefore, patients should be retitrated when transferred from MICRONASE or Diabeta or other oral hypoglycemic agents.

General

Hypoglycemia: All sulfonylureas are capable of producing severe hypoglycemia. Proper patient selection and dosage and instructions are important to avoid hypoglycemic episodes. Renal or hepatic insufficiency may cause elevated drug levels of glyburide and the latter may also diminish gluconeogenic capacity, both of which increase the risk of serious hypoglycemic reactions. Elderly, debilitated or malnourished patients, and those with adrenal or pituitary insufficiency, are particularly susceptible to the hypoglycemic action of glucose-lowering drugs. Hypoglycemia may be difficult to recognize in the elderly and in people who are taking beta-adrenergic blocking drugs. Hypoglycemia is more likely to occur when caloric intake is deficient, after severe or prolonged exercise, when alcohol is ingested, or when more than one glucose lowering drug is used. The risk of hypoglycemia may be increased with combination therapy.

Loss of Control of Blood Glucose: When a patient stabilized on any diabetic regimen is exposed to stress such as fever, trauma, infection or surgery, a loss of control may occur. At such times it may be necessary to discontinue GLYNASE PresTab and administer insulin.

The effectiveness of any hypoglycemic drug, including GLYNASE PresTab, in lowering blood glucose to a desired level decreases in many patients over a period of time which may be due to progression of the severity of diabetes or to diminished responsiveness to the drug. This phenomenon is known as secondary failure, to distinguish it from primary failure in which the drug is ineffective in an individual patient when GLYNASE PresTab is first given. Adequate adjustment of dose and adherence to diet should be assessed before classifying a patient as a secondary failure.

Information for Patients: Patients should be informed of the potential risks and advantages of GLYNASE PresTab and of

alternative modes of therapy. They also should be informed about the importance of adherence to dietary instructions, of a regular exercise program, and of regular testing of urine and/or blood glucose.

The risks of hypoglycemia, its symptoms and treatment, and conditions that predispose to its development should be explained to patients and responsible family members. Primary and secondary failure also should be explained.

Laboratory Tests

Therapeutic response to GLYNASE PresTab Tablets should be monitored by frequent urine glucose tests and periodic blood glucose tests. Measurement of glycosylated hemoglobin levels may be helpful in some patients.

Drug Interactions

The hypoglycemic action of sulfonylureas may be potentiated by certain drugs including nonsteroidal anti-inflammatory agents and other drugs that are highly protein bound, salicylates, sulfonamides, chloramphenicol, probenecid, coumarins, monoamine oxidase inhibitors, and beta adrenergic blocking agents. When such drugs are administered to a patient receiving glyburide, the patient should be observed closely for hypoglycemia. When such drugs are withdrawn from a patient receiving glyburide, the patient should be observed closely for loss of control.

Certain drugs tend to produce hyperglycemia and may lead to loss of control. These drugs include the thiazides and other diuretics, corticosteroids, phenothiazines, thyroid products, estrogens, oral contraceptives, phenytoin, nicotinic acid, sympathomimetics, calcium channel blocking drugs, and isoniazid. When such drugs are administered to a patient receiving glyburide, the patient should be closely observed for loss of control. When such drugs are withdrawn from a patient receiving glyburide, the patient should be observed closely for hypoglycemia.

A possible interaction between glyburide and ciprofloxacin, a fluoroquinolone antibiotic, has been reported, resulting in a potentiation of the hypoglycemic action of glyburide. The mechanism of action for this interaction is not known.

A potential interaction between oral miconazole and oral hypoglycemic agents leading to severe hypoglycemia has been reported. Whether this interaction also occurs with the intravenous, topical or vaginal preparations of miconazole is not known.

Metformin: In a single-dose interaction study in NIDDM subjects, decreases in glyburide AUC and C_{max} were observed, but were highly variable. The single-dose nature of this study and the lack of correlation between glyburide blood levels and pharmacodynamic effects, makes the clinical significance of this inter action uncertain. Coadministration of glyburide and metformin did not result in any changes in either metformin pharmacokinetics or pharmacodynamics.

Carcinogenesis, Mutagenesis, and Impairment of Fertility

Studies in rats at doses up to 300 mg/kg/day for 18 months showed no carcinogenic effects. Glyburide is nonmutagenic when studied in the Salmonella microsome test (Ames test) and in the DNA damage/alkaline elution assay.

No drug-related effects were noted in any of the criteria evaluated in the two-year oncogenicity study of glyburide in mice.

Pregnancy

Teratogenic Effects: Pregnancy Category B

Reproduction studies have been performed in rats and rabbits at doses up to 500 times the human dose and have revealed no evidence of impaired fertility or harm to the fetus due to glyburide. There are, however, no adequate and well-controlled studies in pregnant women. Because animal reproduction studies are not always predictive of human response, this drug should be used during pregnancy only if clearly needed.

Because recent information suggests that abnormal blood glucose levels during pregnancy are associated with a higher incidence of congenital abnormalities, many experts recommend that insulin be used during pregnancy to maintain blood glucose as close to normal as possible.

Nonteratogenic Effects: Prolonged severe hypoglycemia (4 to 10 days) has been reported in neonates born to mothers who were receiving a sulfonylurea drug at the time of delivery. This has been reported more frequently with the use of agents with prolonged half-lives. If GLYNASE PresTab is used during pregnancy, it should be discontinued at least two weeks before the expected delivery date.

Nursing Mothers

Although it is not known whether glyburide is excreted in human milk, some sulfonylurea drugs are known to be excreted in human milk. Because the potential for hypoglyce-

Continued on next page

Information on these Pharmacia & Upjohn products is based on labeling in effect June 1, 1998. Further information concerning these and other Pharmacia & Upjohn products may be obtained by direct inquiry to Medical Information, Pharmacia & Upjohn, Kalamazoo, MI 49001.

Glynase PresTab—Cont.

mia in nursing infants may exist, a decision should be made whether to discontinue nursing or to discontinue the drug, taking into account the importance of the drug to the mother. If the drug is discontinued, and if diet alone is inadequate for controlling blood glucose, insulin therapy should be considered.

Pediatric Use

Safety and effectiveness in pediatric patients have not been established.

ADVERSE REACTIONS

Hypoglycemia: See PRECAUTIONS and OVERDOSAGE Sections.

Gastrointestinal Reactions: Cholestatic jaundice and hepatitis may occur rarely; GLYNASE PresTab Tablets should be discontinued if this occurs.

Liver function abnormalities, including isolated transaminase elevations, have been reported.

Gastrointestinal disturbances, *eg*, nausea, epigastric fullness, and heartburn are the most common reactions, having occurred in 1.8% of treated patients during clinical trials. They tend to be dose related and may disappear when dosage is reduced.

Dermatologic Reactions: Allergic skin reactions, *eg*, pruritus, erythema, urticaria, and morbilliform or maculopapular eruptions occurred in 1.5% of treated patients during clinical trials. These may be transient and may disappear despite continued use of glyburide. If skin reactions persist, the drug should be discontinued.

Porphyria cutanea tarda and photosensitivity reactions have been reported with sulfonylureas.

Hematologic Reactions: Leukopenia, agranulocytosis, thrombocytopenia, hemolytic anemia, aplastic anemia, and pancytopenia have been reported with sulfonylureas.

Metabolic Reactions: Hepatic porphyria and disulfiram-like reactions have been reported with sulfonylureas; however, hepatic porphyria has not been reported with glyburide and disulfiram-like reactions have been reported very rarely.

Cases of hyponatremia have been reported with glyburide and all other sulfonylureas, most often in patients who are on other medications or have medical conditions known to cause hyponatremia or increase release of antidiuretic hormone. The syndrome of inappropriate antidiuretic hormone (SIADH) secretion has been reported with certain other sulfonylureas, and it has been suggested that these sulfonylureas may augment the peripheral (antidiuretic) action of ADH and/or increase release of ADH.

Other Reactions: Changes in accommodation and/or blurred vision have been reported with glyburide and other sulfonylureas. These are thought to be related to fluctuation in glucose levels.

In addition to dermatologic reactions, allergic reactions such as angioedema, arthralgia, myalgia and vasculitis have been reported.

OVERDOSAGE

Overdosage of sulfonylureas, including glyburide, can produce hypoglycemia. Mild hypoglycemic symptoms, without loss of consciousness or neurological findings, should be treated aggressively with oral glucose and adjustments in drug dosage and/or meal patterns. Close monitoring should continue until the physician is assured that the patient is out of danger. Severe hypoglycemic reactions with coma, seizure, or other neurological impairment occur infrequently, but constitute medical emergencies requiring immediate hospitalization. If hypoglycemic coma is diagnosed or suspected, the patient should be given a rapid intravenous injection of concentrated (50%) glucose solution. This should be followed by a continuous infusion of a more dilute (10%) glucose solution at a rate which will maintain the blood glucose at a level above 100 mg/dL. Patients should be closely monitored for a minimum of 24 to 48 hours, since hypoglycemia may recur after apparent clinical recovery.

DOSAGE AND ADMINISTRATION

Patients should be retitrated when transferred from MICRONASE or Diabeta or other oral hypoglycemic agents.

There is no fixed dosage regimen for the management of diabetes mellitus with GLYNASE PresTab Tablets or any other hypoglycemic agent. In addition to the usual monitoring of urinary glucose, the patient's blood glucose must also be monitored periodically to determine the minimum effective dose for the patient; to detect primary failure, ie, inadequate lowering of blood glucose at the maximum recommended dose of medication; and to detect secondary failure, ie, loss of adequate blood glucose lowering response after an initial period of effectiveness. Glycosylated hemoglobin levels may also be of value in monitoring the patient's response to therapy.

Short-term administration of GLYNASE PresTab may be sufficient during periods of transient loss of control in patients usually controlled well on diet.

Usual Starting Dose

The suggested starting dose of GLYNASE PresTab is 1.5 to 3 mg daily, administered with breakfast or the first main meal. Those patients who may be more sensitive to hypoglycemic drugs should be started at 0.75 mg daily. (See PRECAUTIONS Section for patients at increased risk.) Failure to follow an appropriate dosage regimen may precipitate hypoglycemia. Patients who do not adhere to their prescribed dietary and drug regimen are more prone to exhibit unsatisfactory response to therapy.

Transfer From Other Hypoglycemic Therapy; Patients Receiving Other Oral Antidiabetic Therapy: Patients should be retitrated when transferred from MICRONASE or other oral hypoglycemic agents. The initial daily dose should be 1.5 to 3 mg. When transferring patients from oral hypoglycemic agents other than chlorpropamide to GLYNASE PresTab, no transition period and no initial or priming dose are necessary. When transferring patients from chlorpropamide, particular care should be exercised during the first two weeks because the prolonged retention of chlorpropamide in the body and subsequent overlapping drug effects may provoke hypoglycemia.

Patients Receiving Insulin: Some Type II diabetic patients being treated with insulin may respond satisfactorily to GLYNASE PresTab. If the insulin dose is less than 20 units daily, substitution of GLYNASE PresTab 1.5 to 3 mg as a single daily dose may be tried. If the insulin dose is between 20 and 40 units daily, the patient may be placed directly on GLYNASE PresTab Tablets 3 mg daily as a single dose. If the insulin dose is more than 40 units daily, a transition period is required for conversion to GLYNASE PresTab. In these patients, insulin dosage is decreased by 50% and GLYNASE PresTab Tablets 3 mg daily is started. Please refer to Titration to Maintenance Dose for further explanation.

Titration to Maintenance Dose

The usual maintenance dose is in the range of 0.75 to 12 mg daily, which may be given as a single dose or in divided doses (See Dosage Interval Section). Dosage increases should be made in increments of no more than 1.5 mg at weekly intervals based upon the patient's blood glucose response.

No exact dosage relationship exists between GLYNASE PresTab and the other oral hypoglycemic agents, including MICRONASE or Diabeta. Although patients may be transferred from the maximum dose of other sulfonylureas, the maximum starting dose of 3 mg of GLYNASE PresTab Tablets should be observed. A maintenance dose of 3 mg of GLYNASE PresTab Tablets provides approximately the same degree of blood glucose control as 250 to 375 mg chlorpropamide, 250 to 375 mg tolazamide, 5 mg of glyburide (nonmicronized tablets), 500 to 750 mg acetohexamide, or 1000 to 1500 mg tolbutamide.

When transferring patients receiving more than 40 units of insulin daily, they may be started on a daily dose of GLYNASE PresTab Tablets 3 mg concomitantly with a 50% reduction in insulin dose. Progressive withdrawal of insulin and increase of GLYNASE PresTab in increments of 0.75 to 1.5 mg every 2 to 10 days is then carried out. During this conversion period when both insulin and GLYNASE PresTab are being used, hypoglycemia may rarely occur. During insulin withdrawal, patients should test their urine for glucose and acetone at least three times daily and report results to their physician. The appearance of persistent acetonuria with glycosuria indicates that the patient is a Type I diabetic who requires insulin therapy.

Concomitant Glyburide and Metformin Therapy

GLYNASE PresTab Tablets should be added gradually to the dosing regimen of patients who have not responded to the maximum dose of metformin monotherapy after four weeks (see Usual Starting Dose and Titration to Maintenance Dose). Refer to metformin package insert.

With concomitant glyburide and metformin therapy, the desired control of blood glucose may be obtained by adjusting the dose of each drug. However, attempts should be made to identify the optimal dose of each drug needed to achieve this goal. With concomitant glyburide and metformin therapy, the risk of hypoglycemia associated with sulfonylurea therapy continues and may be increased. Appropriate precautions should be taken (see PRECAUTIONS Section).

Maximum Dose

Daily doses of more than 12 mg are not recommended.

Dosage Interval

Once-a-day therapy is usually satisfactory. Some patients, particularly those receiving more than 6 mg daily, may have a more satisfactory response with twice-a-day dosage.

Specific Patient Populations

GLYNASE PresTab Tablets are not recommended for use in pregnancy or for use in pediatric patients.

In elderly patients, debilitated or malnourished patients, and patients with impaired renal or hepatic function, the initial and maintenance dosing should be conservative to avoid hypoglycemic reactions. (See PRECAUTIONS Section.)

HOW SUPPLIED

GLYNASE PresTab Tablets are supplied as follows:

GLYNASE PresTab Tablets 1.5 mg

(white, ovoid, imprinted GLYNASE 1.5/PT Score PT, contour, scored)

Plastic Bottles of 100	NDC 0009-0341-01
Unit Dose Package of 100	NDC 0009-0341-02

GLYNASE PresTab Tablets 3 mg

(blue, ovoid, imprinted GLYNASE 3/PT Score PT, contour, scored)

Plastic Bottles of 100	NDC 0009-0352-01
Plastic Bottles of 500	NDC 0009-0352-03
Plastic Bottles of 1000	NDC 0009-0352-04
Unit Dose Package of 100	NDC 0009-0352-02

GLYNASE PresTab Tablets 6 mg

(yellow, ovoid, imprinted GLYNASE 6/PT Score PT, contour, scored)

Plastic Bottles of 100	NDC 0009-3449-01
Plastic Bottles of 500	NDC 0009-3449-03

The PresTab Tablet can be easily divided in half for a more flexible dosing regimen. Press gently on the score and the PresTab Tablet will split in even halves.

Caution: Federal law prohibits dispensing without prescription. Store at controlled room temperature 20° to 25° C (68° to 77° F) [see USP]. Dispensed in well closed containers with safety closures. Keep container tightly closed.

GLYNASE is a trademark of Pharmacia & Upjohn Company

PresTab is a trademark of Pharmacia & Upjohn Company

Diabeta is a trademark of
Hoechst-Roussel Pharmaceuticals, Inc.

Pharmacia & Upjohn Company
Kalamazoo, MI 49001, USA

Revised May 1997 814 930 108
691439

Shown in Product Identification Guide, page 332

HALCION® Ⓒ ℞
Tablets
triazolam tablets, USP

DESCRIPTION

HALCION Tablets contain triazolam, a triazolobenzodiazepine hypnotic agent.

Triazolam is a white crystalline powder, soluble in alcohol and poorly soluble in water. It has a molecular weight of 343.21.

The chemical name for triazolam is 8-chloro-6-(o-chlorophenyl)-1-methyl-4H-s-tria-zolo-[4,3-α][1,4] benzodiazepine.

The structural formula is represented below:

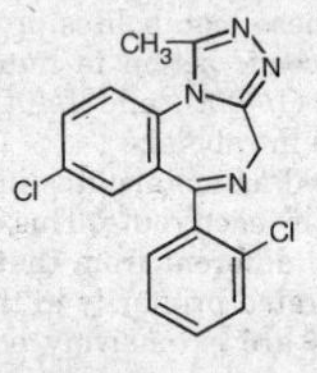

Each HALCION Tablet, for oral administration, contains 0.125 mg or 0.25 mg of triazolam. Inactive ingredients: **0.125 mg**—cellulose, corn starch, docusate sodium, lactose, magnesium stearate, silicon dioxide, sodium benzoate; **0.25 mg**—cellulose, corn starch, docusate sodium, FD&C Blue No. 2, lactose, magnesium stearate, silicon dioxide, sodium benzoate.

CLINICAL PHARMACOLOGY

Triazolam is a hypnotic with a short mean plasma half-life reported to be in the range of 1.5 to 5.5 hours. In normal subjects treated for 7 days with four times the recommended dosage, there was no evidence of altered systemic bioavailability, rate of elimination, or accumulation. Peak plasma levels are reached within 2 hours following oral administration. Following recommended doses of HALCION, triazolam peak plasma levels in the range of 1 to 6 ng/mL are seen. The plasma levels achieved are proportional to the dose given.

Triazolam and its metabolites, principally as conjugated glucuronides, which are presumably inactive, are excreted primarily in the urine. Only small amounts of unmetabolized triazolam appear in the urine. The two primary metabolites accounted for 79.9% of urinary excretion. Urinary excretion appeared to be biphasic in its time course.

HALCION Tablets 0.5 mg, in two separate studies, did not affect the prothrombin times or plasma warfarin levels in male volunteers administered sodium warfarin orally.

Extremely high concentrations of triazolam do not displace bilirubin bound to human serum albumin *in vitro*.

Triazolam ^{14}C was administered orally to pregnant mice. Drug-related material appeared uniformly distributed in the fetus with ^{14}C concentrations approximately the same as in the brain of the mother.

In sleep laboratory studies, HALCION Tablets significantly decreased sleep latency, increased the duration of sleep, and decreased the number of nocturnal awakenings. After 2 weeks of consecutive nightly administration, the drug's effect on total wake time is decreased, and the values recorded in the last third of the night approach baseline levels. On the first and/or second night after drug discontinuance (first or second post-drug night), total time asleep, percentage of time spent sleeping, and rapidity of falling asleep frequently were significantly less than on baseline (predrug) nights. This effect is often called "rebound" insomnia.

The type and duration of hypnotic effects and the profile of unwanted effects during administration of benzodiazepine drugs may be influenced by the biologic half-life of administered drug and any active metabolites formed. When half-lives are long, the drug or metabolites may accumulate during periods of nightly administration and be associated with impairments of cognitive and motor performance during waking hours; the possibility of interaction with other psychoactive drugs or alcohol will be enhanced. In contrast, if half-lives are short, the drug and metabolites will be cleared before the next dose is ingested, and carry-over effects related to excessive sedation or CNS depression should be minimal or absent. However, during nightly use for an extended period pharmacodynamic tolerance or adaptation to some effects of benzodiazepine hypnotics may develop. If the drug has a short half-life of elimination, it is possible that a relative deficiency of the drug or its active metabolites (ie, in relationship to the receptor site) may occur at some point in the interval between each night's use. This sequence of events may account for two clinical findings reported to occur after several weeks of nightly use of rapidly eliminated benzodiazepine hypnotics: 1) increased wakefulness during the last third of the night and 2) the appearance of increased daytime anxiety after 10 days of continuous treatment.

INDICATIONS AND USAGE

HALCION is indicated for the short-term treatment of insomnia (generally 7–10 days). Use for more than 2–3 weeks requires complete reevaluation of the patient (see WARNINGS).

Prescriptions for HALCION should be written for short-term use (7–10 days) and it should not be prescribed in quantities exceeding a 1-month supply.

CONTRAINDICATIONS

HALCION Tablets are contraindicated in patients with known hypersensitivity to this drug or other benzodiazepines.

Benzodiazepines may cause fetal damage when administered during pregnancy. An increased risk of congenital malformations associated with the use of diazepam and chlordiazepoxide during the first trimester of pregnancy has been suggested in several studies. Transplacental distribution has resulted in neonatal CNS depression following the ingestion of therapeutic doses of a benzodiazepine hypnotic during the last weeks of pregnancy.

HALCION is contraindicated in pregnant women. If there is a likelihood of the patient becoming pregnant while receiving HALCION, she should be warned of the potential risk to the fetus. Patients should be instructed to discontinue the drug prior to becoming pregnant. The possibility that a woman of childbearing potential may be pregnant at the time of institution of therapy should be considered.

HALCION is contraindicated with ketoconazole, itraconazole, and nefazodone, medications that significantly impair the oxidative metabolism mediated by cytochrome P450 3A (CYP 3A) (see WARNINGS and PRECAUTIONS–Drug Interactions).

WARNINGS

Sleep disturbance may be the presenting manifestation of a physical and/or psychiatric disorder. Consequently, a decision to initiate symptomatic treatment of insomnia should only be made after the patient has been carefully evaluated. The failure of insomnia to remit after 7–10 days of treatment may indicate the presence of a primary psychiatric and/or medical illness.

Worsening of insomnia or the emergence of new abnormalities of thinking or behavior may be the consequence of an unrecognized psychiatric or physical disorder. These have also been reported to occur in association with the use of HALCION.

Because some of the adverse effects of HALCION appear to be dose related (see PRECAUTIONS and DOSAGE AND ADMINISTRATION), it is important to use the smallest possible effective dose. Elderly patients are especially susceptible to dose related adverse effects.

An increase in daytime anxiety has been reported for HALCION after as few as 10 days of continuous use. In some patients this may be a manifestation of interdose with-drawal (see CLINICAL PHARMACOLOGY). If increased daytime anxiety is observed during treatment, discontinuation of treatment may be advisable.

A variety of abnormal thinking and behavior changes have been reported to occur in association with the use of benzodiazepine hypnotics including HALCION. Some of these changes may be characterized by decreased inhibition, eg, aggressiveness and extroversion that seem excessive, similar to that seen with alcohol and other CNS depressants (eg, sedative/hypnotics). Other kinds of behavioral changes have also been reported, for example, bizarre behavior, agitation, hallucinations, depersonalization. In primarily depressed patients, the worsening of depression, including suicidal thinking, has been reported in association with the use of benzodiazepines.

It can rarely be determined with certainty whether a particular instance of the abnormal behaviors listed above is drug induced, spontaneous in origin, or a result of an underlying psychiatric or physical disorder. Nonetheless, the emergence of any new behavioral sign or symptom of concern requires careful and immediate evaluation.

Because of its depressant CNS effects, patients receiving triazolam should be cautioned against engaging in hazardous occupations requiring complete mental alertness such as operating machinery or driving a motor vehicle. For the same reason, patients should be cautioned about the concomitant ingestion of alcohol and other CNS depressant drugs during treatment with HALCION Tablets.

As with some, but not all benzodiazepines, anterograde amnesia of varying severity and paradoxical reactions have been reported following therapeutic doses of HALCION. Data from several sources suggest that anterograde amnesia may occur at a higher rate with HALCION than with other benzodiazepine hypnotics.

Triazolam interaction with drugs that inhibit metabolism via cytochrome P450 3A:
The initial step in triazolam metabolism is hydroxylation catalyzed by cytochrome P450 3A (CYP 3A). Drugs that inhibit this metabolic pathway may have a profound effect on the clearance of triazolam. Consequently, triazolam should be avoided in patients receiving very potent inhibitors of CYP 3A. With drugs inhibiting CYP 3A to a lesser but still significant degree, triazolam should be used only with caution and consideration of appropriate dosage reduction. For some drugs, an interaction with triazolam has been quantified with clinical data; for other drugs, interactions are predicted from *in vitro* data and/or experience with similar drugs in the same pharmacologic class.

The following are examples of drugs known to inhibit the metabolism of triazolam and/or related benzodiazepines, presumably through inhibition of CYP 3A.

Potent CYP 3A inhibitors: Potent inhibitors of CYP 3A that should not be used concomitantly with triazolam include ketoconazole, itraconazole, and nefazodone. Although data concerning the effects of azole-type antifungal agents other than ketoconazole and itraconazole on triazolam metabolism are not available, they should be considered potent CYP 3A inhibitors, and their coadministration with triazolam is not recommended (see CONTRAINDICATIONS).

Drugs demonstrated to be CYP 3A inhibitors on the basis of clinical studies involving triazolam (caution and consideration of dose reduction are recommended during coadministration with triazolam):
Macrolide Antibiotics—Coadministration of erythromycin increased the maximum plasma concentration of triazolam by 46%, decreased clearance by 53%, and increased half-life by 35%; caution and consideration of appropriate triazolam dose reduction are recommended. Similar caution should be observed during coadministration with clarithromycin and other macrolide antibiotics.

Cimetidine—Coadministration of cimetidine increased the maximum plasma concentration of triazolam by 51%, decreased clearance by 55%, and increased half-life by 68%; caution and consideration of appropriate triazolam dose reduction are recommended.

Other drugs possibly affecting triazolam metabolism:
Other drugs possibly affecting triazolam metabolism by inhibition of CYP 3A are discussed in the PRECAUTIONS section (see PRECAUTIONS–Drug Interactions).

PRECAUTIONS

General: In elderly and/or debilitated patients it is recommended that treatment with HALCION Tablets be initiated at 0.125 mg to decrease the possibility of development of oversedation, dizziness, or impaired coordination.

Some side effects reported in association with the use of HALCION appear to be dose related. These include drowsiness, dizziness, light-headedness, and amnesia.

The relationship between dose and what may be more serious behavioral phenomena is less certain. Specifically, some evidence, based on spontaneous marketing reports, suggests that confusion, bizarre or abnormal behavior, agitation, and hallucinations may also be dose related, but this evidence is inconclusive. In accordance with good medical practice it is recommended that therapy be initiated at the lowest effective dose (see DOSAGE AND ADMINISTRATION).

Cases of "traveler's amnesia" have been reported by individuals who have taken HALCION to induce sleep while traveling, such as during an airplane flight. In some of these cases, insufficient time was allowed for the sleep period prior to awakening and before beginning activity. Also, the concomitant use of alcohol may have been a factor in some cases.

Caution should be exercised if HALCION is prescribed to patients with signs or symptoms of depression that could be intensified by hypnotic drugs. Suicidal tendencies may be present in such patients and protective measures may be required. Intentional overdosage is more common in these patients, and the least amount of drug that is feasible should be available to the patient at any one time.

The usual precautions should be observed in patients with impaired renal or hepatic function, chronic pulmonary insufficiency, and sleep apnea. In patients with compromised respiratory function, respiratory depression and apnea have been reported infrequently.

Information for patients: The text of a patient package insert is printed at the end of this insert. To assure safe and effective use of HALCION, the information and instructions provided in this patient package insert should be discussed with patients.

Laboratory tests: Laboratory tests are not ordinarily required in otherwise healthy patients.

Drug interactions: Both pharmacodynamic and pharmacokinetic interactions have been reported with benzodiazepines. In particular, triazolam produces additive CNS depressant effects when coadministered with other psychotropic medications, anticonvulsants, antihistamines, ethanol, and other drugs which themselves produce CNS depression.

Drugs that inhibit triazolam metabolism via cytochrome P450 3A: The initial step in triazolam metabolism is hydroxylation catalyzed by cytochrome P450 3A (CYP 3A). Drugs which inhibit this metabolic pathway may have a profound effect on the clearance of triazolam (see CONTRAINDICATIONS and WARNINGS for additional drugs of this type).

Drugs and other substances demonstrated to be CYP 3A inhibitors of possible clinical significance on the basis of clinical studies involving triazolam (caution is recommended during coadministration with triazolam):
Isoniazid—Coadministration of isoniazid increased the maximum plasma concentration of triazolam by 20%, decreased clearance by 42%, and increased half-life by 31%.
Oral contraceptives—Coadministration of oral contraceptives increased maximum plasma concentration by 6%, decreased clearance by 32%, and increased half-life by 16%.
Grapefruit juice—Coadministration of grapefruit juice increased the maximum plasma concentration of triazolam by 25%, increased the area under the concentration curve by 48%, and increased half-life by 18%.

Drugs demonstrated to be CYP 3A inhibitors on the basis of clinical studies involving benzodiazepines metabolized similarly to triazolam or on the basis of in vitro studies with triazolam or other benzodiazepines (caution is recommended during coadministration with triazolam): Available data from clinical studies of benzodiazepines other than triazolam suggest a possible drug interaction with triazolam for the following: fluvoxamine, diltiazem, and verapamil. Data from *in vitro* studies of triazolam suggest a possible drug interaction with triazolam for the following: sertraline and paroxetine. Data from *in vitro* studies of benzodiazepines other than triazolam suggest a possible drug interaction with triazolam for the following: ergotamine, cyclosporine, amiodarone, nicardipine, and nifedipine. Caution is recommended during coadministration of any of these drugs with triazolam (see WARNINGS).

Drugs that affect triazolam pharmacokinetics by other mechanisms:
Ranitidine—Coadministration of ranitidine increased the maximum plasma concentration of triazolam by 30%, increased the area under the concentration curve by 27%, and increased half-life by 3.3%. Caution is recommended during coadministration with triazolam.

Carcinogenesis, mutagenesis, impairment of fertility: No evidence of carcinogenic potential was observed in mice during a 24-month study with HALCION in doses up to 4,000 times the human dose.

Pregnancy:
1. Teratogenic effects: Pregnancy category X (see CONTRAINDICATIONS).
2. Non-teratogenic effects: It is to be considered that the child born of a mother who is on benzodiazepines may be at

Continued on next page

Information on these Pharmacia & Upjohn products is based on labeling in effect June 1, 1998. Further information concerning these and other Pharmacia & Upjohn products may be obtained by direct inquiry to Medical Information, Pharmacia & Upjohn, Kalamazoo, MI 49001.

Halcion—Cont.

some risk for withdrawal symptoms from the drug, during the postnatal period. Also, neonatal flaccidity has been reported in an infant born of a mother who had been receiving benzodiazepines.

Nursing mothers: Human studies have not been performed; however, studies in rats have indicated that HALCION and its metabolites are secreted in milk. Therefore, administration of HALCION to nursing mothers is not recommended.

Pediatric use: Safety and effectiveness of HALCION in individuals below 18 years of age have not been established.

ADVERSE REACTIONS

During placebo-controlled clinical studies in which 1,003 patients received HALCION Tablets, the most troublesome side effects were extensions of the pharmacologic activity of triazolam, eg, drowsiness, dizziness, or light-headedness. The figures cited below are estimates of untoward clinical event incidence among subjects who participated in the relatively short duration (ie, 1 to 42 days) placebo-controlled clinical trials of HALCION. The figures cannot be used to predict precisely the incidence of untoward events in the course of usual medical practice where patient characteristics and other factors often differ from those in clinical trials. These figures cannot be compared with those obtained from other clinical studies involving related drug products and placebo, as each group of drug trials is conducted under a different set of conditions.

Comparison of the cited figures, however, can provide the prescriber with some basis for estimating the relative contributions of drug and nondrug factors to the untoward event incidence rate in the population studied. Even this use must be approached cautiously, as a drug may relieve a symptom in one patient while inducing it in others. (For example, an anticholinergic, anxiolytic drug may relieve dry mouth [a sign of anxiety] in some subjects but induce it [an untoward event] in others.)

	HALCION	PLACEBO
Number of Patients	1003	997
% Patients Reporting:		
Central Nervous System		
Drowsiness	14.0	6.4
Headache	9.7	8.4
Dizziness	7.8	3.1
Nervousness	5.2	4.5
Light-headedness	4.9	0.9
Coordination disorders/ataxia	4.6	0.8
Gastrointestinal		
Nausea/vomiting	4.6	3.7

In addition to the relatively common (ie, 1% or greater) untoward events enumerated above, the following adverse events have been reported less frequently (ie, 0.9% to 0.5%): euphoria, tachycardia, tiredness, confusional states/memory impairment, cramps/pain, depression, visual disturbances.

Rare (ie, less than 0.5%) adverse reactions included constipation, taste alterations, diarrhea, dry mouth, dermatitis/allergy, dreaming/nightmares, insomnia, paresthesia, tinnitus, dysesthesia, weakness, congestion, death from hepatic failure in a patient also receiving diuretic drugs.

In addition to these untoward events for which estimates of incidence are available, the following adverse events have been reported in association with the use of HALCION and other benzodiazepines: amnestic symptoms (anterograde amnesia with appropriate or inappropriate behavior), confusional states (disorientation, derealization, depersonalization, and/or clouding of consciousness), dystonia, anorexia, fatigue, sedation, slurred speech, jaundice, pruritus, dysarthria, changes in libido, menstrual irregularities, incontinence, and urinary retention. Other factors may contribute to some of these reactions, eg, concomitant intake of alcohol or other drugs, sleep deprivation, an abnormal premorbid state, etc.

Other events reported include: paradoxical reactions such as stimulation, mania, an agitational state (restlessness, irritability, and excitation), increased muscle spasticity, sleep disturbances, hallucinations, delusions, aggressiveness, falling, somnambulism, syncope, inappropriate behavior and other adverse behavioral effects. Should these occur, use of the drug should be discontinued.

The following events have also been reported: chest pain, burning tongue/ glossitis/stomatitis.

Laboratory analyses were performed on all patients participating in the clinical program for HALCION. The following incidences of abnormalities were ob served in patients receiving HALCION and the corresponding placebo group. None of these changes were considered to be of physiological significance.

	HALCION		PLACEBO	
Number of Patients	380		361	
% of Patients Reporting:	Low	High	Low	High
Hematology				
Hematocrit	*	*	*	*
Hemoglobin	*	*	*	*
Total WBC count	1.7	2.1	*	1.3
Neutrophil count	1.5	1.5	3.3	1.0
Lymphocyte count	2.3	4.0	3.1	3.8
Monocyte count	3.6	*	4.4	1.5
Eosinophil count	10.2	3.2	9.8	3.4
Basophil count	1.7	2.1	*	1.8
Urinalysis				
Albumin	–	1.1	–	*
Sugar	–	*	–	*
RBC/HPF	–	2.9	–	2.9
WBC/HPF	–	11.7	–	7.9
Blood chemistry				
Creatinine	2.4	1.9	3.6	1.5
Bilirubin	*	1.5	1.0	*
SGOT	*	5.3	*	4.5
Alkaline phosphatase	*	2.2	*	2.6

* Less than 1%

When treatment with HALCION is protracted, periodic blood counts, urinalysis, and blood chemistry analyses are advisable.

Minor changes in EEG patterns, usually low-voltage fast activity, have been observed in patients during therapy with HALCION and are of no known significance.

DRUG ABUSE AND DEPENDENCE

Controlled Substance: Triazolam is a controlled substance under the Controlled Substance Act, and HALCION Tablets have been assigned to Schedule IV.

Abuse, Dependence and Withdrawal: Withdrawal symptoms, similar in character to those noted with barbiturates and alcohol (convulsions, tremor, abdominal and muscle cramps, vomiting, sweating, dysphoria, perceptual disturbances and insomnia), have occurred following abrupt discontinuance of benzodiazepines, including HALCION. The more severe symptoms are usually associated with higher dosages and longer usage, although patients at therapeutic dosages given for as few as 1–2 weeks can also have withdrawal symptoms and in some patients there may be withdrawal symptoms (daytime anxiety, agitation) between nightly doses (see CLINICAL PHARMACOLOGY). Consequently, abrupt discontinuation should be avoided and a gradual dosage tapering schedule is recommended in any patient taking more than the lowest dose for more than a few weeks. The recommendation for tapering is particularly important in any patient with a history of seizure.

The risk of dependence is increased in patients with a history of alcoholism, drug abuse, or in patients with marked personality disorders. Such dependence-prone individuals should be under careful surveillance when receiving HALCION. As with all hypnotics, repeat prescriptions should be limited to those who are under medical supervision.

OVERDOSAGE

Because of the potency of triazolam, some manifestations of overdosage may occur at 2 mg, four times the maximum recommended therapeutic dose (0.5 mg).

Manifestations of overdosage with HALCION Tablets include somnolence, confusion, impaired coordination, slurred speech, and, ultimately, coma. Respiratory depression and apnea have been reported with overdosages of HALCION. Seizures have occasionally been reported after overdosages. Death has been reported in association with overdoses of triazolam by itself, as it has with other benzodiazepines. In addition, fatalities have been reported in patients who have overdosed with a combination of a single benzodiazepine, including triazolam, and alcohol; benzodiazepine and alcohol levels seen in some of these cases have been lower than those usually associated with reports of fatality with either substance alone.

As in all cases of drug overdosage, respiration, pulse, and blood pressure should be monitored and supported by general measures when necessary. Immediate gastric lavage should be performed. An adequate airway should be maintained. Intravenous fluids may be administered.

Flumazenil, a specific benzodiazepine receptor antagonist, is indicated for the complete or partial reversal of the sedative effects of benzodiazepines and may be used in situations when an overdose with a benzodiazepine is known or suspected. Prior to the administration of flumazenil, necessary measures should be instituted to secure airway, ventilation and intravenous access. Flumazenil is intended as an adjunct to, not as a substitute for, proper management of benzodiazepine overdose. Patients treated with flumazenil should be monitored for re-sedation, respiratory depression, and other residual benzodiazepine effects for an appropriate period after treatment. The prescriber should be aware of a risk of seizure in association with flumazenil treatment, particularly in long-term benzodiazepine users and in cyclic antidepressant overdose. The complete flumazenil package insert including CONTRAINDICATIONS, WARNINGS and PRECAUTIONS should be consulted prior to use.

Experiments in animals have indicated that cardiopulmonary collapse can occur with massive intravenous doses of triazolam. This could be reversed with positive mechanical respiration and the intravenous infusion of norepinephrine bitartrate or metaraminol bitartrate. Hemodialysis and forced diuresis are probably of little value. As with the management of intentional overdosage with any drug, the physician should bear in mind that multiple agents may have been ingested by the patient.

The oral LD_{50} in mice is greater than 1,000 mg/kg and in rats is greater than 5,000 mg/kg.

DOSAGE AND ADMINISTRATION

It is important to individualize the dosage of HALCION Tablets for maximum beneficial effect and to help avoid significant adverse effects.

The recommended dose for most adults is 0.25 mg before retiring. A dose of 0.125 mg may be found to be sufficient for some patients (eg, low body weight). A dose of 0.5 mg should be used only for exceptional patients who do not respond adequately to a trial of a lower dose since the risk of several adverse reactions increases with the size of the dose administered. A dose of 0.5 mg should not be exceeded.

In geriatric and/or debilitated patients the recommended dosage range is 0.125 mg to 0.25 mg. Therapy should be initiated at 0.125 mg in this group and the 0.25 mg dose should be used only for exceptional patients who do not respond to a trial of the lower dose. A dose of 0.25 mg should not be exceeded in these patients.

As with all medications, the lowest effective dose should be used.

HOW SUPPLIED

HALCION Tablets are available in the following strengths and package sizes:

0.125 mg (white, elliptical, imprinted HALCION 0.125):
Reverse numbered

Unit Dose (100)	NDC 0009-0010-32
10–10 Tablet Bottles	NDC 0009-0010-38
Bottles of 500	NDC 0009-0010-11

0.25 mg (powder blue, elliptical, scored, imprinted HALCION 0.25):
Reverse numbered

Unit Dose (100)	NDC 0009-0017-55
10–10 Tablet Bottles	NDC 0009-0017-59
Bottles of 500	NDC 0009-0017-02

Store at controlled room temperature 20° to 25° C (68° to 77° F) [see USP].

Caution: Federal law prohibits dispensing without prescription.

The text of the patient insert for HALCION is set forth below.

PATIENT INFORMATION

INTRODUCTION

HALCION is intended to help you sleep. It is one of several benzodiazepine sleeping pills that have generally similar properties. Anyone who is considering using one of these medications should be aware of both their benefits and several important risks and limitations, including diminishing effectiveness with continued use and the possible development of dependence (addiction) and possibly mental changes particularly when the drugs are used for more than a few days to a week. This patient information statement is intended to provide you with knowledge about this class of medications in general and about HALCION in particular that will be useful to guide you in the safe use of this product, BUT IT SHOULD NOT REPLACE A DISCUSSION BETWEEN YOU AND YOUR PHYSICIAN ABOUT THE RISKS AND BENEFITS OF HALCION.

This leaflet will focus on the beneficial and adverse effects of all members of this class of medications, as well as some specific information about HALCION. There are some differences among these products, and your physician may wish to discuss any specific advantages and disadvantages of particular members of this drug class with you.

EFFECTIVENESS OF BENZODIAZEPINE SLEEPING PILLS

Benzodiazepine sleeping pills are effective medications and are relatively free of serious problems when they are used for short-term management of sleep problems (insomnia). Insomnia is not always the same. It may be reflected in difficulty in falling asleep, frequent awakening during the night, and/or early morning awakening. Insomnia is often transient in nature, responding to brief treatment with sleeping pills. Use for more than a short while requires discussion with your physician about the risks and benefits of prolonged use.

SIDE EFFECTS

Common Side Effects
The most common side effects of benzodiazepine sleeping pills are related to the ability of the medications to make you sleepy; drowsiness, dizziness, light-headedness, and dif-

ficulty with coordination. Users must be cautious about engaging in hazardous activities requiring complete mental alertness, eg, operating machinery or driving a motor vehicle. Do not take alcohol while using HALCION. Benzodiazepine sleeping pills should not be used with other medications or substances that may cause drowsiness, without discussing said use with your physician.

How sleepy you are the day after you use one of these sleep medications depends on your individual response and on how quickly the product is eliminated from your body. The larger the dose, the more likely an individual will experience next day residual effects such as drowsiness. For this reason, it is important to use the lowest effective dose for each individual patient. Benzodiazepines that are eliminated rapidly, eg, HALCION, tend to cause less next day drowsiness but may cause more withdrawal problems the day after use (see below).

Special Concerns

Memory Problems

All benzodiazepine sleeping pills can cause a special type of amnesia (memory loss) in which a person may not recall events occurring during some period of time, usually several hours, after taking a drug. This is ordinarily not a problem, because the person taking a sleeping pill intends to be asleep during this vulnerable period of time. It can be a problem when the drugs are taken to induce sleep while traveling, such as during an airplane flight, because the person may awake before the effect of the drug is gone. This has been called "traveler's amnesia". HALCION is more likely than other members of the class to cause this problem.

Tolerance/Withdrawal Phenomena

Some loss of effectiveness or adaptation to the sleep inducing effects of these medications may develop after nightly use for more than a few weeks and there may be a degree of dependence that develops. For the benzodiazepine sleeping pills that are eliminated quickly from the body, a relative deficiency of the drug may occur at some point in the interval between each night's use. This can lead to (1) increased wakefulness during the last third of the night, and (2) the appearance of increased signs of daytime anxiety or nervousness. These two events have been reported in particular for HALCION.

There can be more severe 'withdrawal' effects when a benzodiazepine sleeping pill is stopped. Such effects can occur after discontinuing these drugs following use for only a week or two, but may be more common and more severe after longer periods of continuous use. One type of withdrawal phenomenon is the occurrence of what is known as 'rebound insomnia'. That is, on the first few nights after the drug is stopped, insomnia is actually worse than before the sleeping pill was given. Other withdrawal phenomena following abrupt stopping of benzodiazepine sleeping pills range from mild unpleasant feelings to a major withdrawal syndrome which may include abdominal and muscle cramps, vomiting, sweating, tremor, and rarely, convulsions. These more severe withdrawal phenomena are uncommon.

Dependence/Abuse Phenomena

All benzodiazepine sleeping pills can cause dependence (addiction), especially when used regularly for more than a few weeks or at higher doses. Some people develop a need to continue taking these drugs, either at the prescribed dose or at increasing doses, not so much for continued therapeutic effect, but rather, to avoid withdrawal phenomena and/or to achieve nontherapeutic effects. Individuals who have been dependent on alcohol or other drugs may be at particular risk of becoming dependent on drugs in this class, but all people appear to be at some risk. This possibility must be considered before extending the use of these drugs for more than a few weeks.

Mental and Behavioral Changes

A variety of abnormal thinking and behavior changes have been reported to occur in association with the use of benzodiazepine sleeping pills. Some of these changes are like the release of inhibition seen in association with alcohol, eg, aggressiveness and extroversion that seem out of character. Others, however, can be more unusual and more extreme, such as confusion, bizarre behavior, agitation, hallucinations, depersonalization, and worsening of depression, including suicidal thinking. It is rarely clear whether such events are induced by the drug being taken, are caused by some underlying illness or are simply spontaneous happenings. In fact, worsened insomnia may in some cases be associated with illnesses that were present before the medication was used. In any event, the most important fact is to understand that regardless of the cause, users of these medications should promptly report any mental or behavioral changes to their doctor.

Effects on Pregnancy

Certain benzodiazepines have been linked to birth defects when administered during the early months of pregnancy. In addition, the administration of benzodiazepines during the last weeks of pregnancy has been associated with sedation of the fetus. Consequently, the use of this drug should be avoided at any time during pregnancy.

Interactions with Other Medications

HALCION should not be taken with ketoconazole, itraconazole and nefazodone. Taking HALCION with certain other medications may cause increased levels of the drug in the blood and result in an excessive effect. Always tell your doctor about all medications you are taking.

SAFE USE OF BENZODIAZEPINE SLEEPING PILLS

To assure the safe and effective use of HALCION, you should adhere to the following cautions:

1. HALCION is a prescription medication and, therefore, should be used only as directed by your doctor. Follow your doctor's advice about how to take it, when to take it, and how long to take it. As with other prescription medication, HALCION should be taken only by the individual for whom it is prescribed.
2. Do not extend your use of HALCION beyond 7–10 days without first consulting your physician.
3. If you develop any unusual and disturbing thoughts or behavior during treatment with HALCION, you should discuss such problems with your physician.
4. Inform your physician about any alcohol consumption and medicine you are taking now, including drugs you may buy without a prescription. Do not use alcohol while taking HALCION.
5. Do not take HALCION in circumstances where a full night's sleep and elimination of the drug from the body are not possible before you would again need to be active and functional, eg, an overnight flight of less than 7–8 hours, because amnestic episodes have been reported in such situations.
6. Do not increase the prescribed dose except on the advice of your physician.
7. Until you experience how this medication affects you, do not drive a car or operate potentially dangerous machinery, etc.
8. Be aware that you may experience an increase in sleep difficulties (rebound insomnia) on the first night or two after discontinuing HALCION.
9. Inform your physician if you are planning to become pregnant, if you are pregnant, or if you become pregnant while you are taking this medicine. The use of HALCION should be avoided at any time during pregnancy.
10. Always tell your doctor about all medications you are taking.

Pharmacia & Upjohn Company
Kalamazoo, Michigan 49001, USA
Revised August 1997 812 110 728
691439

Shown in Product Identification Guide, page 332

IDAMYCIN PFS ℞

[*eye-dă-mī-sin PFS*]

idarubicin hydrochloride injection

FOR INTRAVENOUS USE ONLY

WARNINGS

1. IDAMYCIN PFS Injection should be given slowly into a freely flowing intravenous infusion. It must *never* be given intramuscularly or subcutaneously. Severe local tissue necrosis can occur if there is extravasation during administration.
2. As is the case with other anthracyclines the use of IDAMYCIN PFS can cause myocardial toxicity leading to congestive heart failure. Cardiac toxicity is more common in patients who have received prior anthracyclines or who have pre-existing cardiac disease.
3. As is usual with antileukemic agents, severe myelosuppression occurs when IDAMYCIN PFS is used at effective therapeutic doses.
4. It is recommended that IDAMYCIN PFS be administered only under the supervision of a physician who is experienced in leukemia chemotherapy and in facilities with laboratory and supportive resources adequate to monitor drug tolerance and protect and maintain a patient compromised by drug toxicity. The physician and institution must be capable of responding rapidly and completely to severe hemorrhagic conditions and/or overwhelming infection.
5. Dosage should be reduced in patients with impaired hepatic or renal function. (See DOSAGE AND ADMINISTRATION.)

DESCRIPTION

IDAMYCIN PFS Injection contains idarubicin hydrochloride and is a sterile, semi-synthetic, preservative-free solution (PFS) antineoplastic anthracycline for intravenous use. Chemically, idarubicin hydrochloride is 5, 12-Naphthacenedione, 9-acetyl-7-[(3-amino-2,3,6-trideoxy-α-L-*lyxo*-hexopyranosyl)oxy]-7,8,9,10-tetrahydro-6,9,11-trihydroxyhydrochloride, (7S-*cis*). The structural formula is as follows:

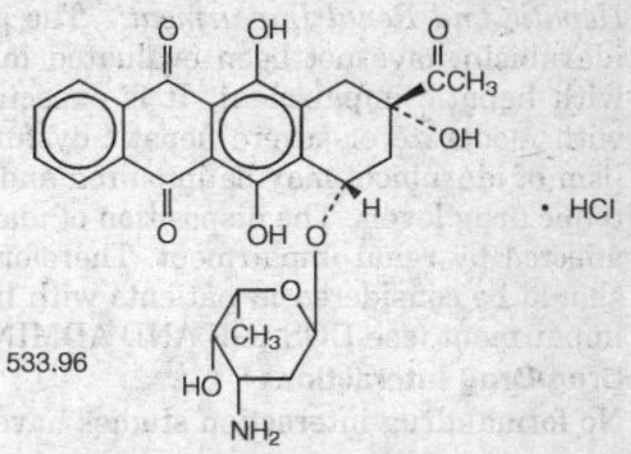

$C_{26}H_{27}NO_9.HCl$ M.W. 533.96

IDAMYCIN PFS is a sterile, red-orange, isotonic parenteral preservative-free solution, available in 5 mL (5 mg), 10 mL (10 mg) and 20 mL (20 mg) single use only vials.

Each mL contains Idarubicin HCl, USP 1 mg and the following inactive ingredients: Glycerin, USP 25 mg and Water for Injection, USP q.s. Hydrochloric Acid, NF is used to adjust the pH to a target of 3.5.

CLINICAL PHARMACOLOGY

Mechanism of Action

Idarubicin hydrochloride is a DNA-intercalating analog of daunorubicin which has an inhibitory effect on nucleic acid synthesis and interacts with the enzyme topoisomerase II. The absence of a methoxy group at position 4 of the anthracycline structure gives the compound a high lipophilicity which results in an increased rate of cellular uptake compared with other anthracyclines.

Pharmacokinetics

General Pharmacokinetics: Pharmacokinetic studies have been performed in adult leukemia patients with normal renal and hepatic function following intravenous administration of 10 to 12 mg/m^2 of idarubicin daily for 3 to 4 days as a single agent or combined with cytarabine. The plasma concentrations of idarubicin are best described by a two or three compartment open model. The elimination rate of idarubicin from plasma is slow with an estimated mean terminal half-life of 22 hours (range, 4 to 48 hours) when used as a single agent and 20 hours (range, 7 to 38 hours) when used in combination with cytarabine. The elimination of the primary active metabolite, idarubicinol, is considerably slower than that of the parent drug with an estimated mean terminal half-life that exceeds 45 hours; hence, its plasma levels are sustained for a period greater than 8 days.

Distribution: The disposition profile shows a rapid distributive phase with a very high volume of distribution presumably reflecting extensive tissue binding. Studies of cellular (nucleated blood and bone marrow cells) drug concentrations in leukemia patients have shown that peak cellular idarubicin concentrations are reached a few minutes after injection. Concentrations of idarubicin and idarubicinol in nucleated blood and bone marrow cells are more than a hundred times the plasma concentrations. Idarubicin disappearance rates in plasma and cells were comparable with a terminal half-life of about 15 hours. The terminal half-life of idarubicinol in cells was about 72 hours. The extent of drug and metabolite accumulation predicted in leukemia patients for Days 2 and 3 of dosing, based on the mean plasma levels and half-life obtained after the first dose, is 1.7- and 2.3-fold, respectively, and suggests no change in kinetics following a daily × 3 regimen. The percentages of idarubicin and idarubicinol bound to human plasma proteins averaged 97% and 94%, respectively, at concentrations similar to maximum plasma levels obtained in the pharmacokinetic studies. The binding is concentration independent. The plasma clearance is twice the expected hepatic plasma flow indicating extensive extrahepatic metabolism.

Metabolism: The primary active metabolite formed is idarubicinol. As idarubicinol has cytotoxic activity, it presumably contributes to the effects of idarubicin.

Elimination: The drug is eliminated predominately by biliary and to a lesser extent by renal excretion, mostly in the form of idarubicinol.

Pharmacokinetics in Special Populations

Pediatric Patients: Idarubicin studies in pediatric leukemia patients, at doses of 4.2 to 13.3 mg/m^2 /day × 3, suggest dose independent kinetics. There is no difference between the half-lives of the drug following daily × 3 or weekly × 3 administration. Cerebrospinal fluid (CSF) levels of idarubicin and idarubicinol were measured in pediatric leukemia patients treated intravenously. Idarubicin was detected in 2 of 21 CSF samples (0.14 and 1.57 ng/mL), while idarubicinol was detected in 20 of these 21 CSF samples obtained 18 to 30 hours after dosing (mean = 0.51 ng/mL; range, 0.22 to 1.05 ng/mL). The clinical relevance of these findings is unknown.

Continued on next page

Information on these Pharmacia & Upjohn products is based on labeling in effect June 1, 1998. Further information concerning these and other Pharmacia & Upjohn products may be obtained by direct inquiry to Medical Information, Pharmacia & Upjohn, Kalamazoo, MI 49001.

Idamycin PFS—Cont.

Hepatic and Renal Impairment: The pharmacokinetics of idarubicin have not been evaluated in leukemia patients with hepatic impairment. It is expected that in patients with moderate or severe hepatic dysfunction, the metabolism of idarubicin may be impaired and lead to higher systemic drug levels. The disposition of idarubicin may be also affected by renal impairment. Therefore, a dose reduction should be considered in patients with hepatic and/or renal impairment (see DOSAGE AND ADMINISTRATION).

Drug-Drug Interactions

No formal drug interaction studies have been performed.

CLINICAL STUDIES

Four prospective randomized studies, three U.S. and one Italian, have been conducted to compare the efficacy and safety of idarubicin (IDR) to that of daunorubicin (DNR), each in combination with cytarabine as induction therapy in previously untreated adult patients with acute myeloid leukemia (AML). These data are summarized in the following table and demonstrate significantly greater complete remission rates for the IDR regimen in two of the three U.S. studies and significantly longer overall survival for the IDR regimen in two of the three U.S. studies.

	Induction[a] Regimen Dose in mg/m²-Daily × 3 Days		Complete Remission Rate, All Pts Randomized		Median Survival (Days) All Pts Randomized	
	IDR	DNR	IDR	DNR	IDR	DNR
U.S. (IND Studies)						
1. MSKCC* (Age ≤ 60 years)	12[b]	50[b]	51/65† (78%)	38/65 (58%)	508†	435
2. SEG** (Age ≥ 15 years)	12[c]	45[c]	76/111† (69%)	65/119 (55%)	328	277
3. U.S. Multicenter (Age ≥ 18 years)	13[c]	45[c]	68/101 (67%)	66/113 (58%)	393†	281
Foreign (non-IND study)						
GIMEMA*** (Age ≥ 55 years)	12[c]	45[c]	49/124 (40%)	49/125 (39%)	87	169

*Memorial Sloan Kettering Cancer Center
**Southeastern Cancer Study Group
***Gruppo Italiano Malattie Ematologiche Maligne dell' Adulto
†Overall $p < 0.05$, unadjusted for prognostic factors or multiple endpoints.
[a]Patients who had persistent leukemia after the first induction course received a second course.
[b]Cytarabine 25 mg/m² bolus IV followed by 200 mg/m² daily × 5 days by continuous infusion
[c]Cytarabine 100 mg/m² daily × 7 days by continuous infusion.

[See table above]

There is no consensus regarding optional regimens to be used for consolidation; however, the following consolidation regimens were used in U.S. controlled trials. Patients received the same anthracycline for consolidation as was used for induction.

Studies 1 and 3 utilized 2 courses of consolidation therapy consisting of idarubicin 12 or 13 mg/m² daily for 2 days, respectively (or DNR 50 or 45 mg/m² daily for 2 days), and cytarabine, either 25 mg/m² by IV bolus followed by 200 mg/m² daily by continuous infusion for 4 days (Study 1), or 100 mg/m² daily for 5 days by continuous infusion (Study 3). A rest period of 4 to 6 weeks is recommended prior to initiation of consolidation and between the courses. Hematologic recovery is mandatory prior to initiation of each consolidation course.

Study 2 utilized 3 consolidation courses, administered at intervals of 21 days or upon hematologic recovery. Each course consisted of idarubicin 15 mg/m² IV for 1 dose (or DNR 50 mg/m² IV for 1 dose), cytarabine 100 mg/m² every 12 hours for 10 doses and 6-thioguanine 100 mg/m² orally for 10 doses. If severe myelosuppression occurred, subsequent courses were given with 25% reduction in the doses of all drugs. In addition, this study included 4 courses of maintenance therapy (2 days of the same anthracycline as was used in induction and 5 days of cytarabine).

Toxicities and duration of aplasia were similar during induction on the 2 arms in the U.S. studies except for an increase in mucositis on the IDR arm in one study. During consolidation, duration of aplasia on the IDR arm was longer in all three studies and mucositis was more frequent in two studies. During consolidation, transfusion requirements were higher on the IDR arm in the two studies in which they were tabulated, and patients on the IDR arm in Study 3 spent more days on IV antibiotics (Study 3 used a higher dose of idarubicin).

The benefit of consolidation and maintenance therapy in prolonging the duration of remission and survival is not proven.

Intensive maintenance with idarubicin is not recommended in view of the considerable toxicity (including deaths in remission) experienced by patients during the maintenance phase of Study 2.

A higher induction death rate was noted in patients on the IDR arm in the Italian trial. Since this was not noted in patients of similar age in the U.S. trials, one may speculate that it was due to a difference in the level of supportive care.

INDICATIONS AND USAGE

IDAMYCIN PFS Injection in combination with other approved antileukemic drugs is indicated for the treatment of acute myeloid leukemia (AML) in adults. This includes French-American-British (FAB) classifications M1 through M7.

WARNINGS

Idarubicin is intended for administration under the supervision of a physician who is experienced in leukemia chemotherapy.

Idarubicin is a potent bone marrow suppressant. Idarubicin should not be given to patients with pre-existing bone marrow suppression induced by previous drug therapy or radiotherapy unless the benefit warrants the risk.

Severe myelosuppression will occur in all patients given a therapeutic dose of this agent for induction, consolidation or maintenance. Careful hematologic monitoring is required. Deaths due to infection and/or bleeding have been reported during the period of severe myelosuppression. Facilities with laboratory and supportive resources adequate to monitor drug tolerability and protect and maintain a patient compromised by drug toxicity should be available. It must be possible to treat rapidly and completely a severe hemorrhagic condition and/or a severe infection.

Pre-existing heart disease and previous therapy with anthracyclines at high cumulative doses or other potentially cardiotoxic agents are co-factors for increased risk of idarubicin-induced cardiac toxicity and the benefit to risk ratio of idarubicin therapy in such patients should be weighed before starting treatment with idarubicin.

Myocardial toxicity as manifested by potentially fatal congestive heart failure, acute life-threatening arrhythmias or other cardiomyopathies may occur following therapy with idarubicin. Appropriate therapeutic measures for the management of congestive heart failure and/or arrhythmias are indicated.

Cardiac function should be carefully monitored during treatment in order to minimize the risk of cardiac toxicity of the type described for other anthracycline compounds. The risk of such myocardial toxicity may be higher following concomitant or previous radiation to the mediastinal-pericardial area or in patients with anemia, bone marrow depression, infections, leukemic pericarditis and/or myocarditis. While there are no reliable means for predicting congestive heart failure, cardiomyopathy induced by anthracyclines is usually associated with a decrease of the left ventricular ejection fraction (LVEF) from pretreatment baseline values.

Since hepatic and/or renal function impairment can affect the disposition of idarubicin, liver and kidney function should be evaluated with conventional clinical laboratory tests (using serum bilirubin and serum creatinine as indicators) prior to and during treatment. In a number of Phase III clinical trials, treatment was not given if bilirubin and/or creatinine serum levels exceeded 2 mg%. However, in one Phase III trial, patients with bilirubin levels between 2.6 and 5 mg% received the anthracycline with a 50% reduction in dose. Dose reduction of idarubicin should be considered if the bilirubin and/or creatinine levels are above the normal range. (See DOSAGE AND ADMINISTRATION.)

Pregnancy Category D—Idarubicin was embryotoxic and teratogenic in the rat at a dose of 1.2 mg/m²/day or one tenth the human dose, which was nontoxic to dams. Idarubicin was embryotoxic but not teratogenic in the rabbit even at a dose of 2.4 mg/m²/day or two tenths the human dose, which was toxic to dams. There is no conclusive information about idarubicin adversely affecting human fertility or causing teratogenesis. There has been one report of a fetal fatality after maternal exposure to idarubicin during the second trimester.

There are no adequate and well-controlled studies in pregnant women. If idarubicin is to be used during pregnancy, or if the patient becomes pregnant during therapy, the patient should be apprised of the potential hazard to the fetus. Women of childbearing potential should be advised to avoid pregnancy.

PRECAUTIONS

General

Therapy with idarubicin requires close observation of the patient and careful laboratory monitoring. Hyperuricemia secondary to rapid lysis of leukemic cells may be induced. Appropriate measures must be taken to prevent hyperuricemia and to control any systemic infection before beginning therapy.

Extravasation of idarubicin can cause severe local tissue necrosis. Extravasation may occur with or without an accompanying stinging or burning sensation even if blood returns well on aspiration of the infusion needle. If signs or symptoms of extravasation occur the injection or infusion should be terminated immediately and restarted in another vein. (See DOSAGE AND ADMINISTRATION.)

Laboratory Tests

Frequent complete blood counts and monitoring of hepatic and renal function tests are recommended.

Carcinogenesis, Mutagenesis, Impairment of Fertility

Formal long-term carcinogenicity studies have not been conducted with idarubicin. Idarubicin and related compounds have been shown to have mutagenic and carcinogenic properties when tested in experimental models (including bacterial systems, mammalian cells in culture and female Sprague-Dawley rats).

In male dogs given 1.8 mg/m²/day 3 times/week (about one seventh the weekly human dose on a mg/m² basis) for 13 weeks, or 3 times the human dose, testicular atrophy was observed with inhibition of spermatogenesis and sperm maturation with few or no mature sperm. These effects were not readily reversed after a recovery of 8 weeks.

Pregnancy Category D

(See WARNINGS.)

Nursing Mothers

It is not known whether this drug is excreted in human milk. Because many drugs are excreted in human milk and because of the potential for serious adverse reactions in nursing infants from idarubicin, mothers should discontinue nursing prior to taking this drug.

Pediatric Use

Safety and effectiveness in children have not been established.

ADVERSE REACTIONS

Approximately 550 patients with AML have received idarubicin in combination with cytarabine in controlled clinical trials worldwide. In addition, over 550 patients with acute leukemia have been treated in uncontrolled trials utilizing idarubicin as a single agent or in combination. The table below lists the adverse experiences reported in U.S. Study 2 (see CLINICAL STUDIES) and is representative of the experiences in other studies. These adverse experiences constitute all reported or observed experiences, including those not considered to be drug related. Patients undergoing induction therapy for AML are seriously ill due to their disease, are receiving multiple transfusions, and concomitant medications including potentially toxic antibiotics and antifungal agents. The contribution of the study drug to the adverse experience profile is difficult to establish.

Induction Phase	Percentage of Patients	
Adverse Experiences	IDR (N=110)	DNR (N=118)
Infection	95%	97%
Nausea & Vomiting	82%	80%
Hair Loss	77%	72%
Abdominal Cramps/Diarrhea	73%	68%
Hemorrhage	63%	65%
Mucositis	50%	55%
Dermatologic	46%	40%
Mental Status	41%	34%
Pulmonary-Clinical	39%	39%
Fever (not elsewhere classified)	26%	28%
Headache	20%	24%
Cardiac-Clinical	16%	24%
Neurologic-Peripheral Nerves	7%	9%
Pulmonary Allergy	2%	4%
Seizure	4%	5%
Cerebellar	4%	4%

The duration of aplasia and incidence of mucositis were greater on the IDR arm than the DNR arm, especially during consolidation in some U.S. controlled trials (see CLINICAL STUDIES).

The following information reflects experience based on U.S. controlled clinical trials.

Myelosuppression
Severe myelosuppression is the major toxicity associated with idarubicin therapy, but this effect of the drug is required in order to eradicate the leukemic clone. During the period of myelosuppression, patients are at risk of developing infection and bleeding which may be life-threatening or fatal.
Gastrointestinal
Nausea and/or vomiting, mucositis, abdominal pain and diarrhea were reported frequently, but were severe (equivalent to WHO Grade 4) in less than 5% of patients. Severe enterocolitis with perforation has been reported rarely. The risk of perforation may be increased by instrumental intervention. The possibility of perforation should be considered in patients who develop severe abdominal pain and appropriate steps for diagnosis and management should be taken.
Dermatologic
Alopecia was reported frequently and dermatologic reactions including generalized rash, urticaria and a bullous erythrodermatous rash of the palms and soles have occurred. The dermatologic reactions were usually attributed to concomitant antibiotic therapy. Local reactions including hives at the injection site have been reported. Recall of skin reaction due to prior radiotherapy has occurred with idarubicin administration.
Hepatic and Renal
Changes in hepatic and renal function tests have been observed. These changes were usually transient and occurred in the setting of sepsis and while patients were receiving potentially hepatotoxic and nephrotoxic antibiotics and antifungal agents. Severe changes in renal function (equivalent to WHO Grade 4) occurred in no more than 1% of patients, while severe changes in hepatic function (equivalent to WHO Grade 4) occurred in less than 5% of patients.
Cardiac
Congestive heart failure (frequently attributed to fluid overload), serious arrhythmias including atrial fibrillation, chest pain, myocardial infarction and asymptomatic declines in LVEF have been reported in patients undergoing induction therapy for AML. Myocardial insufficiency and arrhythmias were usually reversible and occurred in the setting of sepsis, anemia and aggressive intravenous fluid administration. The events were reported more frequently in patients over age 60 years and in those with pre-existing cardiac disease.

OVERDOSAGE

There is no known antidote to idarubicin. Two cases of fatal overdosage in patients receiving therapy for AML have been reported. The doses were 135 mg/m^2 over 3 days and 45 mg/m^2 of idarubicin and 90 mg/m^2 of daunorubicin over a three day period.
It is anticipated that overdosage with idarubicin will result in severe and prolonged myelosuppression and possibly in increased severity of gastrointestinal toxicity. Adequate supportive care including platelet transfusions, antibiotics and symptomatic treatment of mucositis is required. The effect of acute overdose on cardiac function is not fully known, but severe arrhythmia occurred in 1 of the 2 patients exposed. It is anticipated that very high doses of idarubicin may cause acute cardiac toxicity and may be associated with a higher incidence of delayed cardiac failure.
Disposition studies with idarubicin in patients undergoing dialysis have not been carried out. The profound multicompartment behavior, extensive extravascular distribution and tissue binding, coupled with the low unbound fraction available in the plasma pool make it unlikely that therapeutic efficacy or toxicity would be altered by conventional peritoneal or hemodialysis.

DOSAGE AND ADMINISTRATION (See WARNINGS)

For induction therapy in adult patients with AML the following dose schedule is recommended:
IDAMYCIN PFS Injection 12 mg/m^2 daily for 3 days by slow (10 to 15 min) intravenous injection in combination with cytarabine. The cytarabine may be given as 100 mg/m^2 daily by continuous infusion for 7 days or as cytarabine 25 mg/m^2 intravenous bolus followed by cytarabine 200 mg/m^2 daily for 5 days continuous infusion. In patients with unequivocal evidence of leukemia after the first induction course, a second course may be administered. Administration of the second course should be delayed in patients who experience severe mucositis, until recovery from this toxicity has occurred, and a dose reduction of 25% is recommended. In patients with hepatic and/or renal impairment, a dose reduction of IDAMYCIN PFS should be considered. IDAMYCIN PFS should not be administered if the bilirubin level exceeds 5 mg%. (See WARNINGS.)
The benefit of consolidation in prolonging the duration of remissions and survival is not proven. There is no consensus regarding optional regimens to be used for consolidation. (See CLINICAL STUDIES for doses used in U.S. Clinical studies.)
Preparation and Administration Precautions
Caution in handling the solution must be exercised as skin reactions associated with IDAMYCIN PFS may occur. Skin accidentally exposed to IDAMYCIN PFS should be washed thoroughly with soap and water and if the eyes are involved, standard irrigation techniques should be used immediately. The use of goggles, gloves, and protective gowns is recommended during preparation and administration of the drug.
Care in the administration of IDAMYCIN PFS will reduce the chance of perivenous infiltration. It may also decrease the chance of local reactions such as urticaria and erythematous streaking. During intravenous administration of IDAMYCIN PFS extravasation may occur with or without an accompanying stinging or burning sensation even if blood returns well on aspiration of the infusion needle. If any signs or symptoms of extravasation have occurred, the injection or infusion should be immediately terminated and restarted in another vein. If it is known or suspected that subcutaneous extravasation has occurred, it is recommended that intermittent ice packs (1/2 hour immediately, then 1/2 hour 4 times per day for 3 days) be placed over the area of extravasation and that the affected extremity be elevated. Because of the progressive nature of extravasation reactions, the area of injection should be frequently examined and plastic surgery consultation obtained early if there is any sign of a local reaction such as pain, erythema, edema or vesication. If ulceration begins or there is severe persistent pain at the site of extravasation, early wide excision of the involved area should be considered.[1]
IDAMYCIN PFS should be administered slowly (over 10 to 15 minutes) into the tubing of a freely running intravenous infusion of Sodium Chloride Injection, USP (0.9%) or 5% Dextrose Injection, USP. The tubing should be attached to a Butterfly needle or other suitable device and inserted preferably into a large vein.
Incompatibility
Unless specific compatibility data are available, IDAMYCIN PFS should not be mixed with other drugs. Precipitation occurs with heparin. Prolonged contact with any solution of an alkaline pH will result in degradation of the drug. Parenteral drug products should be inspected visually for particulate matter and discoloration prior to administration whenever solution and containers permit.
Handling and Disposal—Procedures for handling and disposal of anticancer drugs should be considered. Several guidelines on this subject have been published.[2–8] There is no general agreement that all of the procedures recommended in the guidelines are necessary or appropriate.

HOW SUPPLIED

IDAMYCIN PFS Injection (idarubicin hydrochloride injection)
Single Dose Vials: Sterile single use only, contains no preservative.
NDC 0013-2536-78 5 mg vial, 1 mg/mL, 5 mL, 5 vial packs.
NDC 0013-2546-86 10 mg vial, 1 mg/mL, 10 mL, single vials.
NDC 0013-2556-67 20 mg vial, 1 mg/mL, 20 mL, single vials.
Store under refrigeration 2° to 8°C (36° to 46°F), and protect from light. Retain in carton until time of use.
Rx only

Manufactured by:
Pharmacia & Upjohn S.p.A.
Milan, Italy

For:
Pharmacia & Upjohn Company
Kalamazoo, MI 49001, USA

REFERENCES

1. Rudolph R, Larson DL: Etiology and Treatment of Chemotherapeutic Agent Extravasation Injuries: A Review. J Clin Oncol 5: 1116-1126, 1987.
2. Recommendations for the Safe Handling of Parenteral Antineoplastic Drugs. NIH Publication No. 83-2621. For sale by the Superintendent of Documents, US Government Printing Office, Washington, DC 20402.
3. AMA Council Report, Guidelines for Handling Parenteral Antineoplastics, JAMA. 1985; 253 (11): 1590-1592.
4. National Study Commission on Cytotoxic Exposure-Recommendations for Handling Cytotoxic Agents. Available from Louis P. Jeffrey, Sc.D., Chairman, National Study Commission on Cytotoxic Exposure, Massachusetts College of Pharmacy and Allied Health Sciences, 179 Longwood Avenue, Boston, Massachusetts 02115.
5. Clinical Oncological Society of Australia. Guidelines and Recommendations for Safe Handling of Antineoplastic Agents. Med J Australia. 1983; 1:426-428.
6. Jones RB, et al: Safe Handling of Chemotherapeutic Agents: A Report from the Mount Sinai Medical Center. CA-A Cancer Journal for Clinicians. 1983; (Sept/Oct) 258-263.
7. American Society of Hospital Pharmacists Technical Assistance Bulletin on Handling Cytotoxic and Hazardous Drugs. Am J Hosp Pharm. 1990; 47:1033-1049.
8. OSHA Work-Practice Guidelines for Personnel Dealing with Cytotoxic (Antineoplastic) Drugs. Am J Hosp Pharm. 1986; 43:1193-1204.

817 166 002 March 1998
N.224295407.01.0

MEDROL® Tablets ℞

[*mĕ-drŏl*]
methylprednisolone tablets, USP

DESCRIPTION

MEDROL Tablets contain methylprednisolone which is a glucocorticoid. Glucocorticoids are adrenocortical steroids, both naturally occurring and synthetic, which are readily absorbed from the gastrointestinal tract. Methylprednisolone occurs as a white to practically white, odorless, crystalline powder. It is sparingly soluble in alcohol, in dioxane, and in methanol, slightly soluble in acetone, and in chloroform, and very slightly soluble in ether. It is practically insoluble in water.
The chemical name for methylprednisolone is pregna - 1,4 - diene - 3,20-dione, 11, 17, 21-trihydroxy-6-methyl-, (6α,11β)- and the molecular weight is 374.48. The structural formula is represented below:

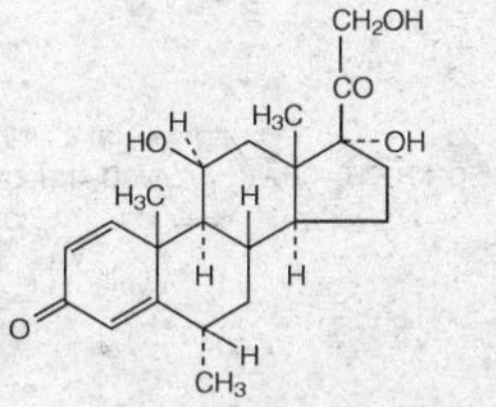

Each MEDROL Tablet for oral administration contains 2 mg, 4 mg, 8 mg, 16 mg, 24 mg or 32 mg of methylprednisolone.
Inactive ingredients:

2 mg	**4 and 16 mg**
Calcium Stearate	Calcium Stearate
Corn Starch	Corn Starch
Erythosine Sodium	Lactose
Lactose	Mineral Oil
Mineral Oil	Sorbic Acid
Sorbic Acid	Sucrose
Sucrose	

8 and 32 mg	**24 mg**
Calcium Stearate	Calcium Stearate
Corn Starch	Corn Starch
F D & C Yellow No. 6	F D & C Yellow No. 5
Lactose	Lactose
Mineral Oil	Mineral Oil
Sorbic Acid	Sorbic Acid
Sucrose	Sucrose

HOW SUPPLIED

MEDROL Tablets are available in the following strengths and packages sizes:
2 mg (pink, elliptical, scored, imprinted MEDROL 2)
Bottles of 100 NDC 0009-0049-02
4 mg (white, elliptical, scored, imprinted MEDROL 4)
Bottles of 100 NDC 0009-0056-02
Bottles of 500 NDC 0009-0056-03
Unit dose packages of 100 NDC 0009-0056-05
DOSEPAK™ Unit of Use (21 tablets) NDC 0009-0056-04
8 mg (peach, elliptical, scored, imprinted MEDROL 8)
Bottles of 25 NDC 0009-0022-01
16 mg (white, elliptical, scored, imprinted MEDROL 16)
Bottles of 50 NDC 0009-0073-01
24 mg (yellow, elliptical, scored, imprinted MEDROL 24)
Bottles of 25 NDC 0009-0155-01
32 mg (peach, elliptical, scored, imprinted MEDROL 32)
Bottles of 25 NDC 0009-0176-01
Store at controlled room temperature 20° to 25°C (68° to 77°F) [see USP].
Caution: Federal law prohibits dispensing without prescription.
Pharmacia & Upjohn Company
Kalamazoo, Michigan 49001, USA
Revised September 1997 810 487 722
692166

Continued on next page

Information on these Pharmacia & Upjohn products is based on labeling in effect June 1, 1998. Further information concerning these and other Pharmacia & Upjohn products may be obtained by direct inquiry to Medical Information, Pharmacia & Upjohn, Kalamazoo, MI 49001.

MICRONASE® Tablets ℞
[*mīk-run-aze*]
glyburide tablets
(1.25, 2.5, and 5 mg)

DESCRIPTION
MICRONASE Tablets contain glyburide, which is an oral blood-glucose-lowering drug of the sulfonyl urea class. Glyburide is a white, crystalline compound, formulated as MICRONASE Tablets of 1.25, 2.5, and 5 mg strengths for oral administration. Inactive ingredients: colloidal silicon dioxide, dibasic calcium phosphate, magnesium stearate, microcrystalline cellulose, sodium alginate, talc. In addition, the **2.5 mg** contains aluminum oxide and FD&C Red No. 40 and the **5 mg** contains aluminum oxide and FD&C Blue No. 1. The chemical name for glyburide is 1-[[p-[2-(5-chloro-o-anisamido)-ethyl]phenyl]-sulfonyl]-3-cyclohexylurea and the molecular weight is 493.99. The structural formula is represented below.

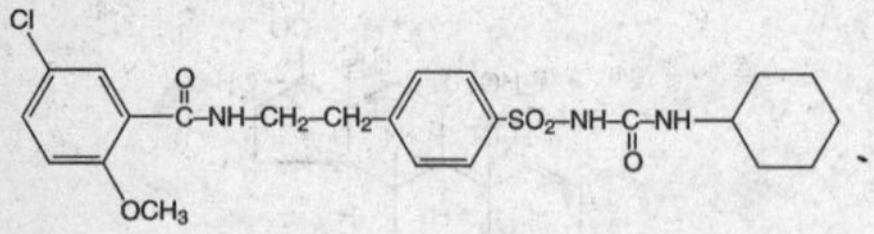

CLINICAL PHARMACOLOGY
Actions
Glyburide appears to lower the blood glucose acutely by stimulating the release of insulin from the pancreas, an effect dependent upon functioning beta cells in the pancreatic islets. The mechanism by which glyburide lowers blood glucose during long-term administration has not been clearly established. With chronic administration in Type II diabetic patients, the blood glucose lowering effect persists despite a gradual decline in the insulin secretory response to the drug. Extrapancreatic effects may be involved in the mechanism of action of oral sulfonylurea hypoglycemic drugs. The combination of glyburide and metformin may have a synergistic effect, since both agents act to improve glucose tolerance by different but complementary mechanisms.
Some patients who are initially responsive to oral hypoglycemic drugs, including MICRONASE, may become unresponsive or poorly responsive over time. Alternatively, MICRONASE Tablets may be effective in some patients who have become unresponsive to one or more other sulfonylurea drugs.
In addition to its blood glucose lowering actions, glyburide produces a mild diuresis by enhancement of renal free water clearance. Disulfiram-like reactions have very rarely been reported in patients treated with MICRONASE Tablets.
Pharmacokinetics
Single dose studies with MICRONASE Tablets in normal subjects demonstrate significant absorption of glyburide within one hour, peak drug levels at about four hours, and low but detectable levels at twenty-four hours. Mean serum levels of glyburide, as reflected by areas under the serum concentration-time curve, increase in proportion to corresponding increases in dose. Multiple dose studies with MICRONASE in diabetic patients demonstrate drug level concentration-time curves similar to single dose studies, indicating no buildup of drug in tissue depots. The decrease of glyburide in the serum of normal healthy individuals is biphasic; the terminal half-life is about 10 hours. In single dose studies in fasting normal subjects, the degree and duration of blood glucose lowering is proportional to the dose administered and to the area under the drug level concentration-time curve. The blood glucose lowering effect persists for 24 hours following single morning doses in nonfasting diabetic patients. Under conditions of repeated administration in diabetic patients, however, there is no reliable correlation between blood drug levels and fasting blood glucose levels. A one year study of diabetic patients treated with MICRONASE showed no reliable correlation between administered dose and serum drug level.
The major metabolite of glyburide is the 4-trans-hydroxy derivative. A second metabolite, the 3-cis-hydroxy derivative, also occurs. These metabolites probably contribute no significant hypoglycemic action in humans since they are only weakly active (1/400th and 1/40th as active, respectively, as glyburide) in rabbits.
Glyburide is excreted as metabolites in the bile and urine, approximately 50% by each route. This dual excretory pathway is qualitatively different from that of other sulfonylureas, which are excreted primarily in the urine.
Sulfonylurea drugs are extensively bound to serum proteins. Displacement from protein binding sites by other drugs may lead to enhanced hypoglycemic action. *In vitro*, the protein binding exhibited by glyburide is predominantly non-ionic, whereas that of other sulfonylureas (chlorpropamide, tolbutamide, tolazamide) is predominantly ionic. Acidic drugs such as phenylbutazone, warfarin, and salicylates displace the ionic-binding sulfonylureas from serum proteins to a far greater extent than the non-ionic binding glyburide. It has not been shown that this difference in protein binding will result in fewer drug-drug interactions with MICRONASE Tablets in clinical use.

INDICATIONS AND USAGE
MICRONASE Tablets are indicated as an adjunct to diet to lower the blood glucose in patients with non-insulin-dependent diabetes mellitus (Type II) whose hyperglycemia cannot be satisfactorily controlled by diet alone.
Glyburide may be used concomitantly with metformin when diet and glyburide or diet and metformin alone do not result in adequate glycemic control (see metformin insert).
In initiating treatment for non-insulin-dependent diabetes, diet should be emphasized as the primary form of treatment. Caloric restriction and weight loss are essential in the obese diabetic patient. Proper dietary management alone may be effective in controlling the blood glucose and symptoms of hyperglycemia. The importance of regular physical activity should also be stressed, and cardiovascular risk factors should be identified and corrective measures taken where possible. If this treatment program fails to reduce symptoms and/or blood glucose, the use of an oral sulfonylurea or insulin should be considered. Use of MICRONASE must be viewed by both the physician and patient as a treatment in addition to diet and not as a substitution or as a convenient mechanism for avoiding dietary restraint. Furthermore, loss of blood glucose control on diet alone may be transient, thus requiring only short-term administration of MICRONASE.
During maintenance programs, MICRONASE should be discontinued if satisfactory lowering of blood glucose is no longer achieved. Judgment should be based on regular clinical and laboratory evaluations.
In considering the use of MICRONASE in asymptomatic patients, it should be recognized that controlling blood glucose in non-insulin-dependent diabetes has not been definitely established to be effective in preventing the long-term cardiovascular or neural complications of diabetes.

CONTRAINDICATIONS
MICRONASE Tablets are contraindicated in patients with:
1. Known hypersensitivity or allergy to the drug.
2. Diabetic ketoacidosis, with or without coma. This condition should be treated with insulin.
3. Type I diabetes mellitus, as sole therapy.

SPECIAL WARNING ON INCREASED RISK OF CARDIOVASCULAR MORTALITY
The administration of oral hypoglycemic drugs has been reported to be associated with increased cardiovascular mortality as compared to treatment with diet alone or diet plus insulin. This warning is based on the study conducted by the University Group Diabetes Program (UGDP), a long-term prospective clinical trial designed to evaluate the effectiveness of glucose-lowering drugs in preventing or delaying vascular complications in patients with non-insulin-dependent diabetes. The study involved 823 patients who were randomly assigned to one of four treatment groups (*Diabetes,* 19 (Suppl. 2):747-830, 1970).
UGDP reported that patients treated for 5 to 8 years with diet plus a fixed dose of tolbutamide (1.5 grams per day) had a rate of cardiovascular mortality approximately 2½ times that of patients treated with diet alone. A significant increase in total mortality was not observed, but the use of tolbutamide was discontinued based on the increase in cardiovascular mortality, thus limiting the opportunity for the study to show an increase in overall mortality. Despite controversy regarding the interpretation of these results, the findings of the UGDP study provide an adequate basis for this warning. The patient should be informed of the potential risks and advantages of MICRONASE and of alternative modes of therapy.
Although only one drug in the sulfonylurea class (tolbutamide) was included in this study, it is prudent from a safety standpoint to consider that this warning may also apply to other oral hypoglycemic drugs in this class, in view of their close similarities in mode of action and chemical structure.

PRECAUTIONS
General
Hypoglycemia: All sulfonylureas are capable of producing severe hypoglycemia. Proper patient selection and dosage and instructions are important to avoid hypoglycemic episodes. Renal or hepatic insufficiency may cause elevated drug levels of glyburide and the latter may also diminish gluconeogenic capacity, both of which increase the risk of serious hypoglycemic reactions. Elderly, debilitated or malnourished patients, and those with adrenal or pituitary insufficiency, are particularly susceptible to the hypoglycemic action of glucose-lowering drugs. Hypoglycemia may be difficult to recognize in the elderly and in people who are taking beta-adrenergic blocking drugs. Hypoglycemia is more likely to occur when caloric intake is deficient, after severe or prolonged exercise, when alcohol is ingested, or when more than one glucose lowering drug is used. The risk of hypoglycemia may be increased with combination therapy.
Loss of Control of Blood Glucose: When a patient stabilized on any diabetic regimen is exposed to stress such as fever, trauma, infection or surgery, a loss of control may occur. At such times it may be necessary to discontinue MICRONASE and administer insulin.
The effectiveness of any hypoglycemic drug, including MICRONASE, in lowering blood glucose to a desired level decreases in many patients over a period of time which may be due to progression of the severity of diabetes or to diminished responsiveness to the drug. This phenomenon is known as secondary failure, to distinguish it from primary failure in which the drug is ineffective in an individual patient when MICRONASE is first given. Adequate adjustment of dose and adherence to diet should be assessed before classifying a patient as a secondary failure.
Information for Patients: Patients should be informed of the potential risks and advantages of MICRONASE and of alternative modes of therapy. They also should be informed about the importance of adherence to dietary instructions, of a regular exercise program, and of regular testing of urine and/or blood glucose.
The risks of hypoglycemia, its symptoms and treatment, and conditions that predispose to its development should be explained to patients and responsible family members. Primary and secondary failure also should be explained.
Laboratory Tests
Therapeutic response to MICRONASE Tablets should be monitored by frequent urine glucose tests and periodic blood glucose tests. Measurement of glycosylated hemoglobin levels may be helpful in some patients.
Drug Interactions
The hypoglycemic action of sulfonylureas may be potentiated by certain drugs including nonsteroidal anti-inflammatory agents and other drugs that are highly protein bound, salicylates, sulfonamides, chloramphenicol, probenecid, coumarins, monoamine oxidase inhibitors, and beta adrenergic blocking agents. When such drugs are administered to a patient receiving MICRONASE, the patient should be observed closely for hypoglycemia. When such drugs are withdrawn from a patient receiving MICRONASE, the patient should be observed closely for loss of control.
Certain drugs tend to produce hyperglycemia and may lead to loss of control. These drugs include the thiazides and other diuretics, corticosteroids, phenothiazines, thyroid products, estrogens, oral contraceptives, phenytoin, nicotinic acid, sympathomimetics, calcium channel blocking drugs, and isoniazid. When such drugs are administered to a patient receiving MICRONASE, the patient should be closely observed for loss of control. When such drugs are withdrawn from a patient receiving MICRONASE, the patient should be observed closely for hypoglycemia.
A possible interaction between glyburide and ciprofloxacin, a fluoroquinolone antibiotic, has been reported, resulting in a potentiation of the hypoglycemic action of glyburide. The mechanism for this interaction is not known.
A potential interaction between oral miconazole and oral hypoglycemic agents leading to severe hypoglycemia has been reported. Whether this interaction also occurs with the intravenous, topical or vaginal preparations of miconazole is not known.
Metformin: In a single-dose interaction study in NIDDM subjects, decreases in glyburide AUC and C_{max} were observed, but were highly variable. The single-dose nature of this study and the lack of correlation between glyburide blood levels and pharmacodynamic effects, makes the clinical significance of this interaction uncertain. Coadministration of glyburide and metformin did not result in any changes in either metformin pharmacokinetics or pharmacodynamics.
Carcinogenesis, Mutagenesis, and Impairment of Fertility
Studies in rats at doses up to 300 mg/kg/day for 18 months showed no carcinogenic effects. Glyburide is nonmutagenic when studied in the Salmonella microsome test (Ames test) and in the DNA damage/alkaline elution assay. No drug related effects were noted in any of the criteria evaluated in the two year oncogenicity study of glyburide in mice.
Pregnancy
Teratogenic Effects: Pregnancy Category B
Reproduction studies have been performed in rats and rabbits at doses up to 500 times the human dose and have revealed no evidence of impaired fertility or harm to the fetus due to glyburide. There are, however, no adequate and well controlled studies in pregnant women. Because animal reproduction studies are not always predictive of human response, this drug should be used during pregnancy only if clearly needed.
Because recent information suggests that abnormal blood glucose levels during pregnancy are associated with a higher incidence of congenital abnormalities, many experts recommend that insulin be used during pregnancy to maintain blood glucose as close to normal as possible.
Nonteratogenic Effects: Prolonged severe hypoglycemia (4 to 10 days) has been reported in neonates born to mothers

who were receiving a sulfonylurea drug at the time of delivery. This has been reported more frequently with the use of agents with prolonged half-lives. If MICRONASE is used during pregnancy, it should be discontinued at least two weeks before the expected delivery date.

Nursing Mothers

Although it is not known whether glyburide is excreted in human milk, some sulfonylurea drugs are known to be excreted in human milk. Because the potential for hypoglycemia in nursing infants may exist, a decision should be made whether to discontinue nursing or to discontinue the drug, taking into account the importance of the drug to the mother. If the drug is discontinued, and if diet alone is inadequate for controlling blood glucose, insulin therapy should be considered.

Pediatric Use

Safety and effectiveness in pediatric patients have not been established.

ADVERSE REACTIONS

Hypoglycemia: See Precautions and Overdosage Sections.

Gastrointestinal Reactions: Cholestatic jaundice and hepatitis may occur rarely; MICRONASE Tablets should be discontinued if this occurs.

Liver function abnormalities, including isolated transaminase elevations, have been reported.

Gastrointestinal disturbances, *eg,* nausea, epigastric fullness, and heartburn are the most common reactions, having occurred in 1.8% of treated patients during clinical trials. They tend to be dose related and may disappear when dosage is reduced.

Dermatologic Reactions: Allergic skin reactions, *eg,* pruritus, erythema, urticaria, and morbilliform or maculopapular eruptions occurred in 1.5% of treated patients during clinical trials. These may be transient and may disappear despite continued use of MICRONASE; if skin reactions persist, the drug should be discontinued.

Porphyria cutanea tarda and photosensitivity reactions have been reported with sulfonylureas.

Hematologic Reactions: Leukopenia, agranulocytosis, thrombocytopenia, hemolytic anemia, aplastic anemia, and pancytopenia have been reported with sulfonylureas.

Metabolic Reactions: Hepatic porphyria and disulfiram-like reactions have been reported with sulfonylureas; however, hepatic porphyria has not been reported with MICRONASE and disulfiram-like reactions have been reported very rarely.

Cases of hyponatremia have been reported with glyburide and all other sulfonylureas, most often in patients who are on other medications or have medical conditions known to cause hyponatremia or increase release of antidiuretic hormone. The syndrome of inappropriate antidiuretic hormone (SIADH) secretion has been reported with certain other sulfonylureas, and it has been suggested that these sulfonylureas may augment the peripheral (antidiuretic) action of ADH and/or increase release of ADH.

Other Reactions: Changes in accommodation and/or blurred vision have been reported with glyburide and other sulfonylureas. These are thought to be related to fluctuation in glucose levels.

In addition to dermatologic reactions, allergic reactions such as angioedema, arthralgia, myalgia and vasculitis have been reported.

OVERDOSAGE

Overdosage of sulfonylureas, including MICRONASE Tablets, can produce hypoglycemia. Mild hypoglycemic symptoms, without loss of consciousness or neurological findings, should be treated aggressively with oral glucose and adjustments in drug dosage and/or meal patterns. Close monitoring should continue until the physician is assured that the patient is out of danger. Severe hypoglycemic reactions with coma, seizure, or other neurological impairment occur infrequently, but constitute medical emergencies requiring immediate hospitalization. If hypoglycemic coma is diagnosed or suspected, the patient should be given a rapid intravenous injection of concentrated (50%) glucose solution. This should be followed by a continuous infusion of a more dilute (10%) glucose solution at a rate which will maintain the blood glucose at a level above 100 mg/dL. Patients should be closely monitored for a minimum of 24 to 48 hours, since hypoglycemia may recur after apparent clinical recovery.

DOSAGE AND ADMINISTRATION

There is no fixed dosage regimen for the management of diabetes mellitus with MICRONASE Tablets or any other hypoglycemic agent. In addition to the usual monitoring of urinary glucose, the patient's blood glucose must also be monitored periodically to determine the minimum effective dose for the patient; to detect primary failure, *ie,* inadequate lowering of blood glucose at the maximum recommended dose of medication; and to detect secondary failure, *ie,* loss of adequate blood glucose lowering response after an initial period of effectiveness. Glycosylated hemoglobin levels may also be of value in monitoring the patient's response to therapy.

Short-term administration of MICRONASE may be sufficient during periods of transient loss of control in patients usually controlled well on diet.

Usual Starting Dose

The usual starting dose of MICRONASE Tablets is 2.5 to 5 mg daily, administered with breakfast or the first main meal. Those patients who may be more sensitive to hypoglycemic drugs should be started at 1.25 mg daily. (See PRECAUTIONS section for patients at increased risk.) Failure to follow an appropriate dosage regimen may precipitate hypoglycemia. Patients who do not adhere to their prescribed dietary and drug regimen are more prone to exhibit unsatisfactory response to therapy.

Transfer From Other Hypoglycemic Therapy Patients Receiving Other Oral Antidiabetic Therapy: Transfer of patients from other oral antidiabetic regimens to MICRONASE should be done conservatively and the initial daily dose should be 2.5 to 5 mg. When transferring patients from oral hypoglycemic agents other than chlorpropamide to MICRONASE, no transition period and no initial or priming dose are necessary. When transferring patients from chlorpropamide, particular care should be exercised during the first two weeks because the prolonged retention of chlorpropamide in the body and subsequent overlapping drug effects may provoke hypoglycemia.

Patients Receiving Insulin: Some Type II diabetic patients being treated with insulin may respond satisfactorily to MICRONASE. If the insulin dose is less than 20 units daily, substitution of MICRONASE Tablets 2.5 to 5 mg as a single daily dose may be tried. If the insulin dose is between 20 and 40 units daily, the patient may be placed directly on MICRONASE Tablets 5 mg daily as a single dose. If the insulin dose is more than 40 units daily, a transition period is required for conversion to MICRONASE. In these patients, insulin dosage is decreased by 50% and MICRONASE Tablets 5 mg daily is started. Please refer to Titration to Maintenance Dose for further explanation.

Titration to Maintenance Dose

The usual maintenance dose is in the range of 1.25 to 20 mg daily, which may be given as a single dose or in divided doses (See Dosage Interval section). Dosage increases should be made in increments of no more than 2.5 mg at weekly intervals based upon the patient's blood glucose response.

No exact dosage relationship exists between MICRONASE and the other oral hypoglycemic agents. Although patients may be transferred from the maximum dose of other sulfonylureas, the maximum starting dose of 5 mg of MICRONASE Tablets should be observed. A maintenance dose of 5 mg of MICRONASE Tablets provides approximately the same degree of blood glucose control as 250 to 375 mg chlorpropamide, 250 to 375 mg tolazamide, 500 to 750 mg acetohexamide, or 1000 to 1500 mg tolbutamide.

When transferring patients receiving more than 40 units of insulin daily, they may be started on a daily dose of MICRONASE Tablets 5 mg concomitantly with a 50% reduction in insulin dose. Progressive withdrawal of insulin and increase of MICRONASE in increments of 1.25 to 2.5 mg every 2 to 10 days is then carried out. During this conversion period when both insulin and MICRONASE are being used, hypoglycemia may rarely occur. During insulin withdrawal, patients should test their urine for glucose and acetone at least three times daily and report results to their physician. The appearance of persistent acetonuria with glycosuria indicates that the patient is a Type I diabetic who requires insulin therapy.

Concomitant Glyburide and Metformin Therapy

MICRONASE Tablets should be added gradually to the dosing regimen of patients who have not responded to the maximum dose of metformin monotherapy after four weeks (see Usual Starting Dose and Titration to Maintenance Dose). Refer to metformin package insert.

With concomitant glyburide and metformin therapy, the desired control of blood glucose may be obtained by adjusting the dose of each drug. However, attempts should be made to identify the optimal dose of each drug needed to achieve this goal. With concomitant glyburide and metformin therapy, the risk of hypoglycemia associated with sulfonylurea therapy continues and may be increased. Appropriate precautions should be taken (see PRECAUTIONS section).

Maximum Dose

Daily doses of more than 20 mg are not recommended.

Dosage Interval

Once-a-day therapy is usually satisfactory. Some patients, particularly those receiving more than 10 mg daily, may have a more satisfactory response with twice-a-day dosage.

Specific Patient Populations

MICRONASE is not recommended for use in pregnancy or for use in pediatric patients.

In elderly patients, debilitated or malnourished patients, and patients with impaired renal or hepatic function, the initial and maintenance dosing should be conservative to avoid hypoglycemic reactions. (See PRECAUTIONS section.)

HOW SUPPLIED

MICRONASE Tablets are supplied as follows:

MICRONASE Tablets 1.25 mg (White, Round, Scored, imprinted MICRONASE 1.25)

Bottles of 100	NDC 0009-0131-01

MICRONASE Tablets 2.5 mg (Dark Pink, Round, Scored, imprinted MICRONASE 2.5)

Bottles of 100	NDC 0009-0141-01
Bottles of 500	NDC 0009-0141-11
Bottles of 1000	NDC 0009-0141-03
Unit Dose Pkg of 100	NDC 0009-0141-02

MICRONASE Tablets 5 mg (Blue, Round, Scored imprinted MICRONASE 5)

Bottles of 30	NDC 0009-0171-11
Bottles of 60	NDC 0009-0171-12
Bottles of 100	NDC 0009-0171-05
Bottles of 500	NDC 0009-0171-06
Bottles of 1000	NDC 0009-0171-07
Unit Dose Pkg of 100	NDC 0009-0171-03

Caution: Federal law prohibits dispensing without prescription. Store at controlled room temperature 20° to 25° C (68° to 77° F) [see USP]. Dispensed in well closed containers with safety closures. Keep container tightly closed.

Pharmacia & Upjohn Company
Kalamazoo, MI 49001, USA
Revised May 1997 811 985 420
691015

MIRAPEX® ℞
[*mĭr-ă-pex*]
pramipexole
dihydrochloride tablets

DESCRIPTION

MIRAPEX Tablets contain pramipexole, a dopamine agonist indicated for the treatment of the signs and symptoms of idiopathic Parkinson's disease. The chemical name of pramipexole dihydrochloride is (*S*)-2-amino-4,5,6,7-tetrahydro-6-(propylamino)benzothiazole dihydrochloride monohydrate. Its empirical formula is $C_{10}H_{17}N_3S$ • 2 HCl • H_2O, and its molecular weight is 302.27.

The structural formula is:

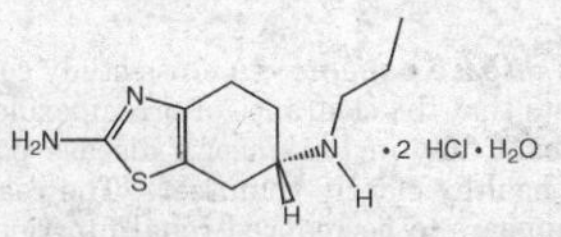

Pramipexole dihydrochloride is a white to off-white powder substance. Melting occurs in the range of 296° C to 301° C, with decomposition. Pramipexole dihydrochloride is more than 20% soluble in water, about 8% in methanol, about 0.5% in ethanol, and practically insoluble in dichloromethane.

MIRAPEX Tablets, for oral administration, contain 0.125 mg, 0.25 mg, 0.5 mg, 1.0 mg, or 1.5 mg of pramipexole dihydrochloride monohydrate. Inactive ingredients consist of mannitol, corn starch, colloidal silicon dioxide, povidone, and magnesium stearate.

CLINICAL PHARMACOLOGY

Pramipexole is a nonergot dopamine agonist with high relative in vitro specificity and full intrinsic activity at the D_2 subfamily of dopamine receptors, binding with higher affinity to D_3 than to D_2 or D_4 receptor subtypes. The relevance of D_3 receptor binding in Parkinson's disease is unknown.

The precise mechanism of action of pramipexole as a treatment for Parkinson's disease is unknown, although it is believed to be related to its ability to stimulate dopamine receptors in the striatum. This conclusion is supported by electrophysiologic studies in animals that have demonstrated that pramipexole influences striatal neuronal firing rates via activation of dopamine receptors in the striatum and the substantia nigra, the site of neurons that send projections to the striatum.

Pharmacokinetics

Pramipexole is rapidly absorbed, reaching peak concentrations in approximately 2 hours. The absolute bioavailability of pramipexole is greater than 90%, indicating that it is well absorbed and undergoes little presystemic metabolism. Food does not affect the extent of pramipexole absorption, although the time of maximum plasma concentration (T_{max}) is increased by about 1 hour when the drug is taken with a meal.

Continued on next page

Information on these Pharmacia & Upjohn products is based on labeling in effect June 1, 1998. Further information concerning these and other Pharmacia & Upjohn products may be obtained by direct inquiry to Medical Information, Pharmacia & Upjohn, Kalamazoo, MI 49001.

Mirapex—Cont.

Pramipexole is extensively distributed, having a volume of distribution of about 500 L (coefficient of variation [CV]=20%). It is about 15% bound to plasma proteins. Pramipexole distributes into red blood cells as indicated by an erythrocyte-to-plasma ratio of approximately 2.

Pramipexole displays linear pharmacokinetics over the clinical dosage range. Its terminal half-life is about 8 hours in young healthy volunteers and about 12 hours in elderly volunteers (see CLINICAL PHARMACOLOGY, Pharmacokinetics in Special Populations). Steady-state concentrations are achieved within 2 days of dosing.

Metabolism and elimination: Urinary excretion is the major route of pramipexole elimination, with 90% of a pramipexole dose recovered in urine, almost all as unchanged drug. Nonrenal routes may contribute to a small extent to pramipexole elimination, although no metabolites have been identified in plasma or urine. The renal clearance of pramipexole is approximately 400 mL/min (CV=25%), approximately three times higher than the glomerular filtration rate. Thus, pramipexole is secreted by the renal tubules, probably by the organic cation transport system.

Pharmacokinetics in Special Populations

Because therapy with pramipexole is initiated at a subtherapeutic dosage and gradually titrated upward according to clinical tolerability to obtain the optimum therapeutic effect, adjustment of the initial dose based on gender, weight, or age is not necessary. However, renal insufficiency, which can cause a large decrease in the ability to eliminate pramipexole, may necessitate dosage adjustment (see CLINICAL PHARMACOLOGY, Renal Insufficiency).

Gender: Pramipexole clearance is about 30% lower in women than in men, but most of this difference can be accounted for by differences in body weight. There is no difference in half-life between males and females.

Age: Pramipexole clearance decreases with age as the half-life and clearance are about 40% longer and 30% lower, respectively, in elderly (aged 65 years or older) compared with young healthy volunteers (aged less than 40 years). This difference is most likely due to the well-known reduction in renal function with age, since pramipexole clearance is correlated with renal function, as measured by creatinine clearance (see CLINICAL PHARMACOLOGY, Renal Insufficiency).

Parkinson's disease patients: A cross-study comparison of data suggests that the clearance of pramipexole may be reduced by about 30% in Parkinson's disease patients compared with healthy elderly volunteers. The reason for this difference appears to be reduced renal function in Parkinson's disease patients, which may be related to their poorer general health. The pharmacokinetics of pramipexole were comparable between early and advanced Parkinson's disease patients.

Pediatric: The pharmacokinetics of pramipexole in the pediatric population have not been evaluated.

Hepatic insufficiency: The influence of hepatic insufficiency on pramipexole pharmacokinetics has not been evaluated. Because approximately 90% of the recovered dose is excreted in the urine as unchanged drug, hepatic impairment would not be expected to have a significant effect on pramipexole elimination.

Renal insufficiency: The clearance of pramipexole was about 75% lower in patients with severe renal impairment (creatinine clearance approximately 20 mL/min) and about 60% lower in patients with moderate impairment (creatinine clearance approximately 40 mL/min) compared with healthy volunteers. A lower starting and maintenance dose is recommended in these patients (see PRECAUTIONS and DOSAGE AND ADMINISTRATION). In patients with varying degrees of renal impairment, pramipexole clearance correlates well with creatinine clearance. Therefore, creatinine clearance can be used as a predictor of the extent of decrease in pramipexole clearance. Pramipexole clearance is extremely low in dialysis patients, as a negligible amount of pramipexole is removed by dialysis. Caution should be exercised when administering pramipexole to patients with renal disease.

CLINICAL STUDIES

The effectiveness of MIRAPEX Tablets in the treatment of Parkinson's disease was evaluated in a multinational drug development program consisting of seven randomized, controlled trials. Three were conducted in patients with early Parkinson's disease who were not receiving concomitant levodopa, and four were conducted in patients with advanced Parkinson's disease who were receiving concomitant levodopa. Among these seven studies, three studies provide the most persuasive evidence of pramipexole's effectiveness in the management of patients with Parkinson's disease who were and were not receiving concomitant levodopa. Two of these three trials enrolled patients with early Parkinson's disease (not receiving levodopa), and one enrolled patients with advanced Parkinson's disease who were receiving maximally tolerated doses of levodopa.

In all studies, the Unified Parkinson's Disease Rating Scale (UPDRS), or one or more of its subparts, served as the primary outcome assessment measure. The UPDRS is a four-part multi-item rating scale intended to evaluate mentation (part I), activities of daily living (part II), motor performance (part III), and complications of therapy (part IV). Part II of the UPDRS contains 13 questions relating to activities of daily living (ADL), which are scored from 0 (normal) to 4 (maximal severity) for a maximum (worst) score of 52. Part III of the UPDRS contains 27 questions (for 14 items) and is scored as described for part II. It is designed to assess the severity of the cardinal motor findings in patients with Parkinson's disease (eg, tremor, rigidity, bradykinesia, postural instability, etc), scored for different body regions, and has a maximum (worst) score of 108.

Studies in Patients With Early Parkinson's Disease

Patients (N=599) in the two studies of early Parkinson's disease had a mean disease duration of 2 years, limited or no prior exposure to levodopa (generally none in the preceding 6 months), and were not experiencing the "on-off" phenomenon and dyskinesia characteristic of later stages of the disease.

One of the two early Parkinson's disease studies (N=335) was a double-blind, placebo-controlled, parallel trial consisting of a 7-week dose-escalation period and a 6-month maintenance period. Patients could be on selegiline, anticholinergics, or both, but could not be on levodopa products or amantadine. Patients were randomized to MIRAPEX or placebo. Patients treated with MIRAPEX had a starting daily dose of 0.375 mg and were titrated to a maximally tolerated dose, but no higher than 4.5 mg/day in three divided doses. At the end of the 6-month maintenance period, the mean improvement from baseline on the UPDRS part II (ADL) total score was 1.9 in the group receiving MIRAPEX and −0.4 in the placebo group, a difference that was statistically significant. The mean improvement from baseline on the UPDRS part III total score was 5.0 in the group receiving MIRAPEX and −0.8 in the placebo group, a difference that was also statistically significant. A statistically significant difference between groups in favor of MIRAPEX was seen beginning at week 2 of the UPDRS part II (maximum dose 0.75 mg/day) and at week 3 of the UPDRS part III (maximum dose 1.5 mg/day).

The second early Parkinson's disease study (N=264) was a double-blind, placebo-controlled, parallel trial consisting of a 6-week dose-escalation period and a 4-week maintenance period. Patients could be on selegiline, anticholinergics, amantadine, or any combination of these, but could not be on levodopa products. Patients were randomized to 1 of 4 fixed doses of MIRAPEX (1.5 mg, 3.0 mg, 4.5 mg, or 6.0 mg per day) or placebo. At the end of the 4-week maintenance period, the mean improvement from baseline on the UPDRS part II total score was 1.8 in the patients treated with MIRAPEX, regardless of assigned dose group, and 0.3 in placebo-treated patients. The mean improvement from baseline on the UPDRS part III total score was 4.2 in patients treated with MIRAPEX and 0.6 in placebo-treated patients. No dose-response relationship was demonstrated. The between-treatment differences on both parts of the UPDRS were statistically significant in favor of MIRAPEX for all doses.

No differences in effectiveness based on age or gender were detected. There were too few non-Caucasian patients to evaluate the effect of race. Patients receiving selegiline or anticholinergics had responses similar to patients not receiving these drugs.

Studies in Patients With Advanced Parkinson's Disease

In the advanced Parkinson's disease study, the primary assessments were the UPDRS and daily diaries that quantified amounts of "on" and "off" time.

Patients in the advanced Parkinson's disease study (N=360) had a mean disease duration of 9 years, had been exposed to levodopa for long periods of time (mean 8 years), used concomitant levodopa during the trial, and had "on-off" periods. The advanced Parkinson's disease study was a double-blind, placebo-controlled, parallel trial consisting of a 7-week dose-escalation period and a 6-month maintenance period. Patients were all treated with concomitant levodopa products and could additionally be on concomitant selegiline, anticholinergics, amantadine, or any combination. Patients treated with MIRAPEX had a starting dose of 0.375 mg/day and were titrated to a maximally tolerated dose, but no higher than 4.5 mg/day in three divided doses. At selected times during the 6-month maintenance period, patients were asked to record the amount of "off", "on", or "on with dyskinesia" time per day for several sequential days. At the end of the 6-month maintenance period, the mean improvement from baseline on the UPDRS part II total score was 2.7 in the group treated with MIRAPEX and 0.5 in the placebo group, a difference that was statistically significant. The mean improvement from baseline on the UPDRS part III total score was 5.6 in the group treated with MIRAPEX and 2.8 in the placebo group, a difference that was statistically significant. A statistically significant difference between groups in favor of MIRAPEX was seen at week 3 of the UPDRS part II (maximum dose 1.5 mg/day) and at week

2 of the UPDRS part III (maximum dose 0.75 mg/day). Dosage reduction of levodopa was allowed during this study if dyskinesia (or hallucinations) developed; levodopa dosage reduction occurred in 76% of patients treated with MIRAPEX versus 54% of placebo patients. On average, the levodopa dose was reduced 27%.

The mean number of "off" hours per day during baseline was 6 hours for both treatment groups. Throughout the trial, patients treated with MIRAPEX had a mean of 4 "off" hours per day, while placebo-treated patients continued to experience 6 "off" hours per day.

No differences in effectiveness based on age or gender were detected. There were too few non-Caucasian patients to evaluate the effect of race.

INDICATIONS AND USAGE

MIRAPEX Tablets are indicated for the treatment of the signs and symptoms of idiopathic Parkinson's disease.

The effectiveness of MIRAPEX was demonstrated in randomized, controlled trials in patients with early Parkinson's disease who were not receiving concomitant levodopa therapy as well as in patients with advanced disease on concomitant levodopa (see CLINICAL STUDIES).

CONTRAINDICATIONS

MIRAPEX Tablets are contraindicated in patients who have demonstrated hypersensitivity to the drug or its ingredients.

WARNINGS

Symptomatic Hypotension: Dopamine agonists, in clinical studies and clinical experience, appear to impair the systemic regulation of blood pressure, with resulting orthostatic hypotension, especially during dose escalation. Parkinson's disease patients, in addition, appear to have an impaired capacity to respond to an orthostatic challenge. For these reasons, Parkinson's disease patients being treated with dopaminergic agonists ordinarily require careful monitoring for signs and symptoms of orthostatic hypotension, especially during dose escalation, and should be informed of this risk (see PRECAUTIONS, Information for Patients).

In clinical trials of pramipexole, however, and despite clear orthostatic effects in normal volunteers, the reported incidence of clinically significant orthostatic hypotension was not greater among those assigned to MIRAPEX Tablets than among those assigned to placebo. This result is clearly unexpected in light of the previous experience with the risks of dopamine agonist therapy.

While this finding could reflect a unique property of pramipexole, it might also be explained by the conditions of the study and the nature of the population enrolled in the clinical trials. Patients were very carefully titrated, and patients with active cardiovascular disease or significant orthostatic hypotension at baseline were excluded.

Hallucinations: In the three double-blind, placebo-controlled trials in early Parkinson's disease, hallucinations were observed in 9% (35 of 388) of patients receiving MIRAPEX, compared with 2.6% (6 of 235) of patients receiving placebo. In the four double-blind, placebo-controlled trials in advanced Parkinson's disease, where patients received MIRAPEX and concomitant levodopa, hallucinations were observed in 16.5% (43 of 260) of patients receiving MIRAPEX compared with 3.8% (10 of 264) of patients receiving placebo. Hallucinations were of sufficient severity to cause discontinuation of treatment in 3.1% of the early Parkinson's disease patients and 2.7% of the advanced Parkinson's disease patients compared with about 0.4% of placebo patients in both populations.

Age appears to increase the risk of hallucinations attributable to pramipexole. In the early Parkinson's disease patients, the risk of hallucinations was 1.9 times greater than placebo in patients younger than 65 years and 6.8 times greater than placebo in patients older than 65 years. In the advanced Parkinson's disease patients, the risk of hallucinations was 3.5 times greater than placebo in patients younger than 65 years and 5.2 times greater than placebo in patients older than 65 years.

PRECAUTIONS

Rhabdomyolysis: A single case of rhabdomyolysis occurred in a 49-year-old male with advanced Parkinson's disease treated with MIRAPEX Tablets. The patient was hospitalized with an elevated CPK (10,631 IU/L). The symptoms resolved with discontinuation of the medication.

Renal: Since pramipexole is eliminated through the kidneys, caution should be exercised when prescribing MIRAPEX to patients with renal insufficiency (see DOSAGE AND ADMINISTRATION).

Dyskinesia: MIRAPEX may potentiate the dopaminergic side effects of levodopa and may cause or exacerbate preexisting dyskinesia. Decreasing the dose of levodopa may ameliorate this side effect.

Retinal pathology in albino rats: Pathologic changes (degeneration and loss of photoreceptor cells) were observed in the retina of albino rats in the 2-year carcinogenicity study. Evaluation of the retinas of albino mice, pigmented rats, monkeys, and minipigs did not reveal similar changes. The potential significance of this effect in humans has not been

established, but cannot be disregarded because disruption of a mechanism that is universally present in vertebrates (ie, disk shedding) may be involved (see ANIMAL TOXICOLOGY).

Events Reported With Dopaminergic Therapy
Although the events enumerated below have not been reported in association with the use of pramipexole in its development program, they are associated with the use of other dopaminergic drugs. The expected incidence of these events, however, is so low that even if pramipexole caused these events at rates similar to those attributable to other dopaminergic therapies, it would be unlikely that even a single case would have occurred in a cohort of the size exposed to pramipexole in studies to date.

Withdrawal-emergent hyperpyrexia and confusion: Although not reported with pramipexole in the clinical development program, a symptom complex resembling the neuroleptic malignant syndrome (characterized by elevated temperature, muscular rigidity, altered consciousness, and autonomic instability), with no other obvious etiology, has been reported in association with rapid dose reduction, withdrawal of, or changes in antiparkinsonian therapy.

Fibrotic complications: Although not reported with pramipexole in the clinical development program, cases of retroperitoneal fibrosis, pulmonary infiltrates, pleural effusion, and pleural thickening have been reported in some patients treated with ergot-derived dopaminergic agents. While these complications may resolve when the drug is discontinued, complete resolution does not always occur.

Although these adverse events are believed to be related to the ergoline structure of these compounds, whether other, nonergot derived dopamine agonists can cause them is unknown.

Information for Patients: Patients should be instructed to take MIRAPEX only as prescribed.

Patients should be informed that hallucinations can occur and that the elderly are at a higher risk than younger patients with Parkinson's disease.

Patients may develop postural (orthostatic) hypotension, with or without symptoms such as dizziness, nausea, fainting or blackouts, and sometimes, sweating. Hypotension may occur more frequently during initial therapy. Accordingly, patients should be cautioned against rising rapidly after sitting or lying down, especially if they have been doing so for prolonged periods and especially at the initiation of treatment with MIRAPEX.

Patients should be advised that MIRAPEX may cause somnolence and that they should neither drive a car nor operate other complex machinery until they have gained sufficient experience on MIRAPEX to gauge whether or not it affects their mental and/or motor performance adversely. Because of the possible additive sedative effects, caution should also be used when patients are taking other CNS depressants in combination with MIRAPEX.

Because the teratogenic potential of pramipexole has not been completely established in laboratory animals, and because experience in humans is limited, patients should be advised to notify their physicians if they become pregnant or intend to become pregnant during therapy (see PRECAUTIONS, Pregnancy).

Because of the possibility that pramipexole may be excreted in breast milk, patients should be advised to notify their physicians if they intend to breast-feed or are breast-feeding an infant.

If patients develop nausea, they should be advised that taking MIRAPEX with food may reduce the occurrence of nausea.

Laboratory Tests: During the development of MIRAPEX, no systematic abnormalities on routine laboratory testing were noted. Therefore, no specific guidance is offered regarding routine monitoring; the practitioner retains responsibility for determining how best to monitor the patient in his or her care.

Drug Interactions
Carbidopa/levodopa: Carbidopa/levodopa did not influence the pharmacokinetics of pramipexole in healthy volunteers (N=10). Pramipexole did not alter the extent of absorption (AUC) or the elimination of carbidopa/levodopa, although it caused an increase in levodopa C_{max} by about 40% and a decrease in T_{max} from 2.5 to 0.5 hours.

Selegiline: In healthy volunteers (N=11), selegiline did not influence the pharmacokinetics of pramipexole.

Amantadine: Population pharmacokinetic analysis suggests that amantadine is unlikely to alter the oral clearance of pramipexole (N=54).

Cimetidine: Cimetidine, a known inhibitor of renal tubular secretion of organic bases via the cationic transport system, caused a 50% increase in pramipexole AUC and a 40% increase in half-life (N=12).

Probenecid: Probenecid, a known inhibitor of renal tubular secretion of organic acids via the anionic transporter, did not noticeably influence pramipexole pharmacokinetics (N=12).

Other drugs eliminated via renal secretion: Population pharmacokinetic analysis suggests that coadministration of drugs that are secreted by the cationic transport system (eg,

cimetidine, ranitidine, diltiazem, triamterene, verapamil, quinidine, and quinine) decreases the oral clearance of pramipexole by about 20%, while those secreted by the anionic transport system (eg, cephalosporins, penicillins, indomethacin, hydrochlorothiazide, and chlorpropamide) are likely to have little effect on the oral clearance of pramipexole.

CYP interactions: Inhibitors of cytochrome P450 enzymes would not be expected to affect pramipexole elimination because pramipexole is not appreciably metabolized by these enzymes in vivo or in vitro. Pramipexole does not inhibit CYP enzymes CYP1A2, CYP2C9, CYP2C19, CYP2E1, and CYP3A4. Inhibition of CYP2D6 was observed with an apparent Ki of 30 μM, indicating that pramipexole will not inhibit CYP enzymes at plasma concentrations observed following the highest recommended clinical dose (1.5 mg tid).

Dopamine antagonists: Since pramipexole is a dopamine agonist, it is possible that dopamine antagonists, such as the neuroleptics (phenothiazines, butyrophenones, thio xanthenes) or metoclopramide, may diminish the effectiveness of MIRAPEX.

Drug/Laboratory Test Interactions: There are no known interactions between MIRAPEX and laboratory tests.

Carcinogenesis, Mutagenesis, Impairment of Fertility: Two-year carcinogenicity studies with pramipexole have been conducted in mice and rats. Pramipexole was administered in the diet to Chbb:NMRI mice at doses of 0.3, 2, and 10 mg/kg/day (0.3, 2.2, and 11 times the highest recommended clinical dose [1.5 mg tid] on a mg/m² basis). Pramipexole was administered in the diet to Wistar rats at 0.3, 2, and 8 mg/kg/day (plasma AUCs equal to 0.3, 2.5, and 12.5 times the AUC in humans receiving 1.5 mg tid). No significant increases in tumors occurred in either species.

Pramipexole was not mutagenic or clastogenic in a battery of assays, including the in vitro Ames assay, V79 gene mutation assay for HGPRT mutants, chromosomal aberration assay in Chinese hamster ovary cells, and in vivo mouse micronucleus assay.

In rat fertility studies, pramipexole at a dose of 2.5 mg/kg/day (5.4 times the highest clinical dose on a mg/m² basis), prolonged estrus cycles and inhibited implantation. These effects were associated with reductions in serum levels of prolactin, a hormone necessary for implantation and maintenance of early pregnancy in rats.

Pregnancy: Pregnancy Category C. When pramipexole was given to female rats throughout pregnancy, implantation was inhibited at a dose of 2.5 mg/kg/day (5.4 times the highest clinical dose on a mg/m² basis). Administration of 1.5 mg/kg/day of pramipexole to pregnant rats during the period of organogenesis (gestation days 7 through 16) resulted in a high incidence of total resorption of embryos. The plasma AUC in rats dosed at this level was 4.3 times the AUC in humans receiving 1.5 mg tid. These findings are thought to be due to the prolactin-lowering effect of pramipexole, since prolactin is necessary for implantation and maintenance of early pregnancy in rats (but not rabbits or humans). Because of pregnancy disruption and early embryonic loss in these studies, the teratogenic potential of pramipexole could not be adequately evaluated. There was no evidence of adverse effects on embryo-fetal development following administration of up to 10 mg/kg/day to pregnant rabbits during organogenesis (plasma AUC was 71 times that in humans receiving 1.5 mg tid). Postnatal growth was inhibited in the offspring of rats treated with 0.5 mg/kg/day (approximately equivalent to the highest clinical dose on a mg/m² basis) or greater during the latter part of pregnancy and throughout lactation.

There are no studies of pramipexole in human pregnancy. Because animal reproduction studies are not always predictive of human response, pramipexole should be used during pregnancy only if the potential benefit outweighs the potential risk to the fetus.

Nursing Mothers: A single-dose, radio-labeled study showed that drug-related materials were excreted into the breast milk of lactating rats. Concentrations of radioactivity in milk were three to six times higher than concentrations in plasma at equivalent time points.

Other studies have shown that pramipexole treatment resulted in an inhibition of prolactin secretion in humans and rats.

It is not known whether this drug is excreted in human milk. Because many drugs are excreted in human milk and because of the potential for serious adverse reactions in nursing infants from pramipexole, a decision should be made as to whether to discontinue nursing or to discontinue the drug, taking into account the importance of the drug to the mother.

Pediatric Use: The safety and efficacy of MIRAPEX in pediatric patients has not been established.

Geriatric Use: Pramipexole total oral clearance was approximately 30% lower in subjects older than 65 years compared with younger subjects, because of a decline in pramipexole renal clearance due to an age-related reduction in renal function. This resulted in an increase in elimination half-life from approximately 8.5 hours to 12 hours. In clinical studies, 38.7% of patients were older than 65 years.

There were no apparent differences in efficacy or safety between older and younger patients, except that the relative risk of hallucination associated with the use of MIRAPEX was increased in the elderly.

ADVERSE EVENTS
During the premarketing development of pramipexole, patients with either early or advanced Parkinson's disease were enrolled in clinical trials. Apart from the severity and duration of their disease, the two populations differed in their use of concomitant levodopa therapy. Patients with early disease did not receive concomitant levodopa therapy during treatment with pramipexole; those with advanced Parkinson's disease all received concomitant levodopa treatment. Because these two populations may have differential risks for various adverse events, this section will, in general, present adverse-event data for these two populations separately.

Because the controlled trials performed during premarketing development all used a titration design, with a resultant confounding of time and dose, it was impossible to adequately evaluate the effects of dose on the incidence of adverse events.

Early Parkinson's Disease
In the three double-blind, placebo-controlled trials of patients with early Parkinson's disease, the most commonly observed adverse events (>5%) that were numerically more frequent in the group treated with MIRAPEX Tablets were nausea, dizziness, somnolence, insomnia, constipation, asthenia, and hallucinations.

Approximately 12% of 388 patients with early Parkinson's disease and treated with MIRAPEX who participated in the double-blind, placebo-controlled trials discontinued treatment due to adverse events compared with 11% of 235 patients who received placebo. The adverse events most commonly causing discontinuation of treatment were related to the nervous system (hallucinations [3.1% on MIRAPEX vs 0.4% on placebo]; dizziness [2.1% on MIRAPEX vs 1% on placebo]; somnolence [1.6% on MIRAPEX vs 0% on placebo]; extrapyramidal syndrome [1.6% on MIRAPEX vs 6.4% on placebo]; headache and confusion [1.3% and 1.0%, respectively, on MIRAPEX vs 0% on placebo]); and gastrointestinal system (nausea [2.1% on MIRAPEX vs 0.4% on placebo]).

Adverse-event incidence in controlled clinical studies in early Parkinson's disease: Table 1 lists treatment-emergent adverse events that occurred in the double-blind, placebo-controlled studies in early Parkinson's disease that were reported by ≥1% of patients treated with MIRAPEX and were numerically more frequent than in the placebo group. In these studies, patients did not receive concomitant levodopa. Adverse events were usually mild or moderate in intensity.

The prescriber should be aware that these figures cannot be used to predict the incidence of adverse events in the course of usual medical practice where patient characteristics and other factors differ from those that prevailed in the clinical studies. Similarly, the cited frequencies cannot be compared with figures obtained from other clinical investigations involving different treatments, uses, and investigators. However, the cited figures do provide the prescribing physician with some basis for estimating the relative contribution of drug and nondrug factors to the adverse-event incidence rate in the population studied.

Table 1
Treatment-Emergent Adverse-Event* Incidence in Double-Blind, Placebo-Controlled Trials in Early Parkinson's Disease (Events ≥1% of Patients Treated With MIRAPEX and Numerically More Frequent Than in the Placebo Group)

Body System/ Adverse Event	MIRAPEX N=388	Placebo N=235
Body as a Whole		
Asthenia	14	12
General edema	5	3
Malaise	2	1
Reaction unevaluable	2	1
Fever	1	0
Digestive System		
Nausea	28	18
Constipation	14	6
Anorexia	4	2
Dysphagia	2	0

Continued on next page

Information on these Pharmacia & Upjohn products is based on labeling in effect June 1, 1998. Further information concerning these and other Pharmacia & Upjohn products may be obtained by direct inquiry to Medical Information, Pharmacia & Upjohn, Kalamazoo, MI 49001.

Consult 1999 PDR® supplements and future editions for revisions

Mirapex—Cont.

Metabolic & Nutritional System		
Peripheral edema	5	4
Decreased weight	2	0

Nervous System		
Dizziness	25	24
Somnolence	22	9
Insomnia	17	12
Hallucinations	9	3
Confusion	4	1
Amnesia	4	2
Hypesthesia	3	1
Dystonia	2	1
Akathisia	2	0
Thinking abnormalities	2	0
Decreased libido	1	0
Myoclonus	1	0

Special Senses		
Vision abnormalities	3	0

Urogenital System		
Impotence	2	1

*Patients may have reported multiple adverse experiences during the study or at discontinuation; thus, patients may be included in more than one category.

Other events reported by 1% or more of patients with early Parkinson's disease and treated with MIRAPEX but reported equally or more frequently in the placebo group were infection, accidental injury, headache, pain, tremor, back pain, syncope, postural hypotension, hypertonia, depression, abdominal pain, anxiety, dyspepsia, flatulence, diarrhea, rash, ataxia, dry mouth, extrapyramidal syndrome, leg cramps, twitching, pharyngitis, sinusitis, sweating, rhinitis, urinary tract infection, vasodilation, flu syndrome, increased saliva, tooth disease, dyspnea, increased cough, gait abnormalities, urinary frequency, vomiting, allergic reaction, hypertension, pruritis, hypokinesia, increased creatine PK, nervousness, dream abnormalities, chest pain, neck pain, paresthesia, tachycardia, vertigo, voice alteration, conjunctivitis, paralysis, accommodation abnormalities, tinnitus, diplopia, and taste perversions.

Advanced Parkinson's Disease

In the four double-blind, placebo-controlled trials of patients with advanced Parkinson's disease, the most commonly observed adverse events (>5%) that were numerically more frequent in the group treated with MIRAPEX and concomitant levodopa were postural (orthostatic) hypotension, dyskinesia, extrapyramidal syndrome, insomnia, dizziness, hallucinations, accidental injury, dream abnormalities, confusion, constipation, asthenia, somnolence, dystonia, gait abnormality, hypertonia, dry mouth, amnesia, and urinary frequency.

Approximately 12% of 260 patients with advanced Parkinson's disease who received MIRAPEX and concomitant levodopa in the double-blind, placebo-controlled trials discontinued treatment due to adverse events compared with 16% of 264 patients who received placebo and concomitant levodopa. The events most commonly causing discontinuation of treatment were related to the nervous system (hallucinations [2.7% on MIRAPEX vs 0.4% on placebo]; dyskinesia [1.9% on MIRAPEX vs 0.8% on placebo]; extrapyramidal syndrome [1.5% on MIRAPEX vs 4.9% on placebo]; dizziness [1.2% on MIRAPEX vs 1.5% on placebo]; confusion [1.2% on MIRAPEX vs 2.3% on placebo]); and cardiovascular system (postural [orthostatic] hypotension [2.3% on MIRAPEX vs 1.1% on placebo]).

Adverse-event incidence in controlled clinical studies in advanced Parkinson's disease:
Table 2 lists treatment-emergent adverse events that occurred in the double-blind, placebo-controlled studies in advanced Parkinson's disease that were reported by ≥1% of patients treated with MIRAPEX and were numerically more frequent than in the placebo group. In these studies, MIRAPEX or placebo was administered to patients who were also receiving concomitant levodopa. Adverse events were usually mild or moderate in intensity.

The prescriber should be aware that these figures cannot be used to predict the incidence of adverse events in the course of usual medical practice where patient characteristics and other factors differ from those that prevailed in the clinical studies. Similarly, the cited frequencies cannot be compared with figures obtained from other clinical investigations involving different treatments, uses, and investigators. However, the cited figures do provide the prescribing physician with some basis for estimating the relative contribution of drug and nondrug factors to the adverse-events incidence rate in the population studied.

Table 2
Treatment-Emergent Adverse-Event* Incidence in Double-Blind, Placebo-Controlled Trials in Advanced Parkinson's Disease (Events ≥ 1% of Patients Treated With MIRAPEX and Numerically More Frequent Than in the Placebo Group)

Body System/ Adverse Event	MIRAPEX† N=260	Placebo† N=264
Body as a Whole		
Accidental injury	17	15
Asthenia	10	8
General edema	4	3
Chest pain	3	2
Malaise	3	2
Cardiovascular System		
Postural hypotension	53	48
Digestive System		
Constipation	10	9
Dry mouth	7	3
Metabolic & Nutritional System		
Peripheral edema	2	1
Increased creatine PK	1	0
Musculoskeletal System		
Arthritis	3	1
Twitching	2	0
Bursitis	2	0
Myasthenia	1	0
Nervous System		
Dyskinesia	47	31
Extrapyramidal syndrome	28	26
Insomnia	27	22
Dizziness	26	25
Hallucinations	17	4
Dream abnormalities	11	10
Confusion	10	7
Somnolence	9	6
Dystonia	8	7
Gait abnormalities	7	5
Hypertonia	7	6
Amnesia	6	4
Akathisia	3	2
Thinking abnormalities	3	2
Paranoid reaction	2	0
Delusions	1	0
Sleep disorders	1	0
Respiratory System		
Dyspnea	4	3
Rhinitis	3	1
Pneumonia	2	0
Skin & Appendages		
Skin disorders	2	1
Special Senses		
Accommodation abnormalities	4	2
Vision abnormalities	3	1
Diplopia	1	0
Urogenital System		
Urinary frequency	6	3
Urinary tract infection	4	3
Urinary incontinence	2	1

*Patients may have reported multiple adverse experiences during the study or at discontinuation; thus, patients may be included in more than one category.
†Patients received concomitant levodopa.

Other events reported by 1% or more of patients with advanced Parkinson's disease and treated with MIRAPEX but reported equally or more frequently in the placebo group were nausea, pain, infection, headache, depression, tremor, hypokinesia, anorexia, back pain, dyspepsia, flatulence, ataxia, flu syndrome, sinusitis, diarrhea, myalgia, abdominal pain, anxiety, rash, paresthesia, hypertension, increased saliva, tooth disorder, apathy, hypotension, sweating, vasodilation, vomiting, increased cough, nervousness, pruritus, hypesthesia, neck pain, syncope, arthralgia, dysphagia, palpitations, pharyngitis, vertigo, leg cramps, conjunctivitis, and lacrimation disorders.

Adverse Events; Relationship to Age, Gender, and Race:
Among the treatment-emergent adverse events in patients treated with MIRAPEX, hallucination appeared to exhibit a positive relationship to age. No gender-related differences were observed. Only a small percentage (4%) of patients enrolled were non-Caucasian, therefore, an evaluation of adverse events related to race is not possible.

Other Adverse Events Observed During All Phase 2 and 3 Clinical Trials: MIRAPEX has been administered to 1,408 individuals during all clinical trials (Parkinson's disease and other patient populations), 648 of whom were in seven double-blind, placebo-controlled Parkinson's disease trials. During these trials, all adverse events were recorded by the clinical investigators using terminology of their own choosing. To provide a meaningful estimate of the proportion of individuals having adverse events, similar types of events were grouped into a smaller number of standardized categories using modified COSTART dictionary terminology. These categories are used in the listing below. The events listed below occurred in less than 1% of the 1,408 individuals exposed to MIRAPEX and occurred on at least two occasions (on one occasion if the event was serious). All reported events, except those already listed above, are included, without regard to determination of a causal relationship to MIRAPEX.

Events are listed within body-system categories in order of decreasing frequency.

Body as a whole: enlarged abdomen, death, fever, suicide attempt.
Cardiovascular system: peripheral vascular disease, myocardial infarction, angina pectoris, atrial fibrillation, heart failure, arrhythmia, atrial arrhythmia, pulmonary embolism.
Digestive system: thirst.
Musculoskeletal system: joint disorder, myasthenia.
Nervous system: agitation, CNS stimulation, hyperkinesia, psychosis, convulsions.
Respiratory system: pneumonia.
Special senses: cataract, eye disorder, glaucoma.
Urogenital system: dysuria, abnormal ejaculation, prostate cancer, hematuria, prostate disorder.

DRUG ABUSE AND DEPENDENCE

Pramipexole is not a controlled substance.
Pramipexole has not been systematically studied in animals or humans for its potential for abuse, tolerance, or physical dependence. However, in a rat model on cocaine self-administration, pramipexole had little or no effect.

OVERDOSAGE

There is no clinical experience with massive overdosage. One patient, with a 10-year history of schizophrenia, took 11 mg/day of pramipexole for 2 days; this is two to three times the protocol recommended daily dose. No adverse events were reported related to the increased dose. Blood pressure remained stable although pulse rate increased to between 100 and 120 beats/minute. The patient withdrew from the study at the end of week 2 due to lack of efficacy. There is no known antidote for overdosage of a dopamine agonist. If signs of central nervous system stimulation are present, a phenothiazine or other butyrophenone neuroleptic agent may be indicated; the efficacy of such drugs in reversing the effects of overdosage has not been assessed. Management of overdose may require general supportive measures along with gastric lavage, intravenous fluids, and electrocardiogram monitoring.

DOSAGE AND ADMINISTRATION

In all clinical studies, dosage was initiated at a subtherapeutic level to avoid intolerable adverse effects and orthostatic hypotension. MIRAPEX should be titrated gradually in all patients. The dosage should be increased to achieve a maximum therapeutic effect, balanced against the principal side effects of dyskinesia, hallucinations, somnolence, and dry mouth.

Dosing in Patients With Normal Renal Function Initial Treatment: Dosages should be increased gradually from a starting dose of 0.375 mg/day given in three divided doses and should not be increased more frequently than every 5 to 7 days. A suggested ascending dosage schedule that was used in clinical studies is shown in the following table:

Ascending Dosage Schedule of MIRAPEX

Week	Dosage (mg)	Total Daily Dose (mg)
1	0.125 tid	0.375
2	0.25 tid	0.75
3	0.5 tid	1.50
4	0.75 tid	2.25
5	1.0 tid	3.0
6	1.25 tid	3.75
7	1.5 tid	4.50

Maintenance Treatment: MIRAPEX Tablets were effective and well tolerated over a dosage range of 1.5 to 4.5 mg/day

administered in equally divided doses three times per day with or without concomitant levodopa (approximately 800 mg/day).

In a fixed-dose study in early Parkinson's disease patients, doses of 3 mg, 4.5 mg, and 6 mg per day of MIRAPEX were not shown to provide any significant benefit beyond that achieved at a daily dose of 1.5 mg/day.

When MIRAPEX is used in combination with levodopa, a reduction of the levodopa dosage should be considered. In a controlled study in advanced Parkinson's disease, the dosage of levodopa was reduced by an average of 27% from baseline.

Patients with Renal Impairment

Pramipexole Dosage in the Renally Impaired

Renal Status	Starting Dose (mg)	Maximum Dose (mg)
Normal to mild impairment (creatinine Cl > 60 mL/min)	0.125 tid	1.5 tid
Moderate impairment (creatinine Cl = 35 to 59 mL/min)	0.125 bid	1.5 bid
Severe impairment (creatinine Cl = 15 to 34 mL/min)	0.125 qd	1.5 qd
Very severe impairment (creatinine Cl < 15 mL/min and hemodialysis patients)	The use of MIRAPEX has not been adequately studied in this group of patients.	

Discontinuation of Treatment: It is recommended that MIRAPEX be discontinued over a period of 1 week; in some studies, however, abrupt discontinuation was uneventful.

HOW SUPPLIED

MIRAPEX Tablets are available as follows:

0.125 mg: white, round tablet with "U" on one side and "2" on the reverse side.

Bottles of 63 NDC 0009-0002-02

0.25 mg: white, oval, scored tablet with "U" twice on one side and "4" twice on the reverse side.

Bottles of 90 NDC 0009-0004-02
Unit dose packages of 100 NDC 0009-0004-06

0.5 mg: white, oval, scored tablet with "U" twice on one side and "8" twice on the reverse side.

Bottles of 90 NDC 0009-0008-02

1 mg: white, round, scored tablet with "U" twice on one side and "6" twice on the reverse side.

Bottles of 90 NDC 0009-0006-02
Unit dose packages of 100 NDC 0009-0006-06

1.5 mg: white, round, scored tablet with "U" twice on one side and "37" twice on the reverse side.

Bottles of 90 NDC 0009-0037-02
Unit dose packages of 100 NDC 0009-0037-06

Store at 25°C (77°F); excursions permitted to 15°–30°C (59°–86°F) [see USP Controlled Room Temperature]. Protect from light.

Rx only

ANIMAL TOXICOLOGY

Retinal Pathology in Albino Rats

Pathologic changes (degeneration and loss of photoreceptor cells) were observed in the retina of albino rats in the 2-year carcinogenicity study with pramipexole. These findings were first observed during week 76 and were dose dependent in animals receiving 2 or 8 mg/kg/day (plasma AUCs equal to 2.5 and 12.5 times the AUC in humans that received 1.5 mg tid). Similar findings were not present in rats receiving 0.3 mg/kg/day (plasma AUC equal to 0.3 times the AUC in humans that received 1.5 mg tid).

Investigative studies demonstrated that pramipexole reduced the rate of disk shedding from the photoreceptor rod cells of the retina in albino rats, which was associated with enhanced sensitivity to the damaging effects of light. In a comparative study, degeneration and loss of photoreceptor cells occurred in albino rats after 13 weeks of treatment with 25 mg/kg/day of pramipexole (54 times the highest clinical dose on a mg/m^2 basis) and constant light (100 lux) but not in pigmented rats exposed to the same dose and higher light intensities (500 lux). Thus, the retina of albino rats is considered to be uniquely sensitive to the damaging effects of pramipexole and light. Similar changes in the retina did not occur in a 2-year carcinogenicity study in albino mice treated with 0.3, 2, or 10 mg/kg/day (0.3, 2.2 and 11 times the highest clinical dose on a mg/m^2 basis). Evaluation of the retinas of monkeys given 0.1, 0.5, or 2.0 mg/kg/day of pramipexole (0.4, 2.2, and 8.6 times the highest clinical dose on a mg/m^2 basis) for 12 months and minipigs given 0.3, 1, or 5 mg/kg/day of pramipexole for 13 weeks also detected no changes.

The potential significance of this effect in humans has not been established, but cannot be disregarded because disruption of a mechanism that is universally present in vertebrates (ie, disk shedding) may be involved.

Fibro-osseous Proliferative Lesions in Mice

An increased incidence of fibro-osseous proliferative lesions occurred in the femurs of female mice treated for 2 years with 0.3, 2.0, or 10 mg/kg/day (0.3, 2.2, and 11 times the highest clinical dose on a mg/m^2 basis). Lesions occurred at a lower rate in control animals. Similar lesions were not observed in male mice or rats and monkeys of either sex that were treated chronically with pramipexole. The significance of this lesion to humans is not known.

Pharmacia & Upjohn Company
Kalamazoo, Michigan 49001, USA
Revised March 1998 817 017 004
691439

Shown in Product Identification Guide, page 332

MYCOBUTIN® ℞

(Rifabutin Capsules, USP)

DESCRIPTION

MYCOBUTIN® is the brand name for the antimycobacterial agent rifabutin. It is a semisynthetic ansamycin antibiotic derived from rifamycin S. MYCOBUTIN capsules for oral administration contain 150 mg of Rifabutin, USP per capsule, along with the inactive ingredients microcrystalline cellulose, magnesium stearate, red iron oxide, silica gel, sodium lauryl sulfate, titanium dioxide, and edible white ink.

The chemical name for rifabutin is 1′,4-didehydro-1-deoxy-1,4-dihydro-5′-(2-methylpropyl)-1-oxorifamycin XIV (Chemical Abstracts Service, 9th Collective Index) or (9*S*, 12*E*, 14*S*, 15*R*, 16*S*, 17*R*, 18*R*, 19*R*, 20*S*, 21*S*, 22*E*, 24*Z*)-6, 16, 18, 20-tetrahydroxy -1′- isobutyl -14- methoxy -7,9, 15,17,19,21,25 -heptamethyl-spiro [9,4-(epoxypentadeca[1, 11, 13]trienimino)-2*H*-furo[2′,3′:7,8]naphth[1,2-*d*]imidazole-2,4′-piperidine]-5,10,26-(3*H*,9*H*)-trione-16-acetate.

Rifabutin has a molecular formula of $C_{46}H_{62}N_4O_{11}$, a molecular weight of 847.02 and the following structure:

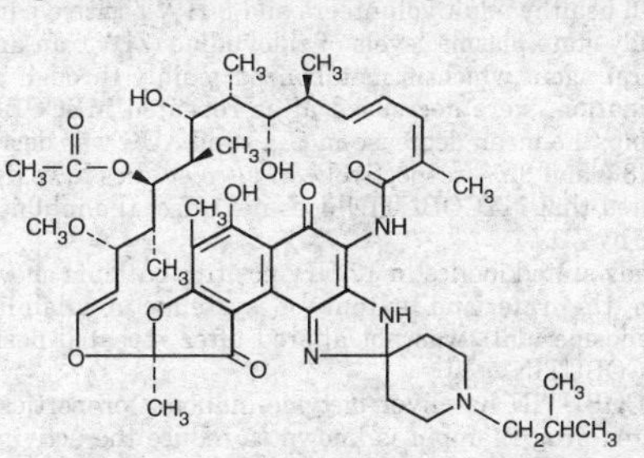

Rifabutin is a red-violet powder soluble in chloroform and methanol, sparingly soluble in ethanol, and very slightly soluble in water (0.19 mg/mL). Its log P value (the base 10 logarithm of the partition coefficient between n-octanol and water) is 3.2 (n-octanol/water).

CLINICAL PHARMACOLOGY

Pharmacokinetics

Following a single oral dose of 300 mg to nine healthy adult volunteers, MYCOBUTIN was readily absorbed from the gastrointestinal tract with mean (±SD) peak plasma levels (C_{max}) of 375 (±267) ng/mL (range: 141 to 1033 ng/mL) attained in 3.3 (±0.9) hours (T_{max} range: 2 to 4 hours). Plasma concentrations post -C_{max} declined in an apparent biphasic manner. Kinetic dose-proportionality has been established over the 300 to 600 mg dose range in nine healthy adult volunteers (crossover design) and in 16 early symptomatic human immunodeficiency virus (HIV)-positive patients over a 300 to 900 mg dose range. Rifabutin was slowly eliminated from plasma in seven healthy adult volunteers, presumably because of *distribution-limited elimination*, with a mean terminal half-life of 45 (±17) hours (range: 16 to 69 hours). Although the systemic levels of rifabutin following multiple dosing decreased by 38%, its terminal half-life remained unchanged. Rifabutin, due to its high lipophilicity, demonstrates a high propensity for distribution and intracellular tissue uptake. Estimates of apparent steady-state distribution volume (9.3 ± 1.5 L/kg) in five HIV-positive patients, following I.V. dosing, exceed total body water by approximately 15-fold. Substantially higher intracellular tissue levels than those seen in plasma have been observed in both rat and man. The lung to plasma concentration ratio, obtained at 12 hours, was found to be approximately 6.5 in four surgical patients administered an oral dose. Mean rifabutin steady-state trough levels ($C_{p,min}^{ss}$; 24-hour post-dose) ranged from 50 to 65 ng/mL in HIV-positive patients and in healthy adult volunteers. About 85% of the drug is bound in a concentration-independent manner to plasma proteins over a concentration range of 0.05 to 1 µg/mL. Binding does not appear to be influenced by renal or hepatic dysfunction.

Mean systemic clearance (CL_s/F) in healthy adult volunteers following a single oral dose was 0.69 (±0.32) L/hr/kg (range: 0.46 to 1.34 L/hr/kg). Renal and biliary clearance of unchanged drug each contribute approximately 5% to CL_s/F. About 30% of the dose is excreted in the feces. A mass-balance study in three healthy adult volunteers with ^{14}C-labeled drug has shown that 53% of the oral dose was excreted in the urine, primarily as metabolites. Of the five metabolites that have been identified, 25-O-desacetyl and 31-hydroxy are the most predominant, and show a plasma metabolite:parent area under the curve ratio of 0.10 and 0.07, respectively. The former has an activity equal to the parent drug and contributes up to 10% to the total antimicrobial activity.

Absolute bioavailability assessed in five HIV-positive patients, who received both oral and I.V. doses, averaged 20%. Total recovery of radioactivity in the urine indicates that at least 53% of the orally administered rifabutin dose is absorbed from the G.I. tract. The bioavailability of rifabutin from the capsule dosage form, relative to a solution, was 85% in 12 healthy adult volunteers. High-fat meals slow the rate without influencing the extent of absorption from the capsule dosage form. The overall pharmacokinetics of MYCOBUTIN are modified only slightly by alterations in hepatic function or age. MYCOBUTIN steady-state kinetics in early symptomatic HIV-positive patients are similar to healthy volunteers. Compared to healthy volunteers, steady-state kinetics of MYCOBUTIN are more variable in elderly patients (>70 years) and in symptomatic HIV-positive patients. Somewhat reduced drug distribution and faster elimination of rifabutin in patients with compromised renal function may result in decreased drug concentrations. The clinical implications of this are unknown.

No rifabutin disposition information is currently available in children or adolescents under 18 years of age.

Microbiology

Mechanism of Action

Rifabutin inhibits DNA-dependent RNA polymerase in susceptible strains of *Escherichia coli* and *Bacillus subtilis* but not in mammalian cells. In resistant strains of *E. coli*, rifabutin, like rifampin, did not inhibit this enzyme. It is not known whether rifabutin inhibits DNA-dependent RNA polymerase in *Mycobacterium avium* or in M. *intracellulare* which comprise *M. avium* complex (MAC).

Susceptibility Testing

In vitro susceptibility testing methods and diagnostic products used for determining minimum inhibitory concentration (MIC) values against *M. avium* complex (MAC) organisms have not been standardized. Breakpoints to determine whether clinical isolates of MAC and other mycobacterial species are susceptible or resistant to rifabutin have not been established.

In Vitro Studies

Rifabutin has demonstrated *in vitro* activity against *M. avium* complex (MAC) organisms isolated from both HIV-positive and HIV-negative people. While gene probe techniques may be used to identify these two organisms, many reported studies did not distinguish between these two species. The vast majority of isolates from MAC-infected, HIV-positive people are *M. avium*, whereas in HIV-negative people, about 40% of the MAC isolates are *M. intracellulare*.

Various *in vitro* methodologies employing broth or solid media, with and without polysorbate 80 (Tween 80), have been used to determine rifabutin MIC values for mycobacterial species. In general, MIC values determined in broth are several fold lower than that observed with methods employing solid media. Utilization of Tween 80 in these assays has been shown to further lower MIC values. However, MIC values were substantially higher for egg based compared to agar based solid media.

Rifabutin activity against 211 MAC isolates from HIV-positive people was evaluated *in vitro* utilizing a radiometric broth and an agar dilution method. Results showed that 78% and 82% of these isolates had MIC_{99} values of ≤0.25µg/mL and ≤1.0µg/mL, respectively, when evaluated by these two methods. Rifabutin was also shown to be active against phagocytized, *M avium* complex in a mouse macrophage cell culture model.

Continued on next page

Information on these Pharmacia & Upjohn products is based on labeling in effect June 1, 1998. Further information concerning these and other Pharmacia & Upjohn products may be obtained by direct inquiry to Medical Information, Pharmacia & Upjohn, Kalamazoo, MI 49001.

Mycobutin—Cont.

Rifabutin has *in vitro* activity against many strains of *Mycobacterium tuberculosis*. In one study, utilizing the radiometric broth method, each of 17 and 20 rifampin-naive clinical isolates tested from the United States and Taiwan, respectively, were shown to be susceptible to rifabutin concentrations of ≤0.125μg/mL.

Cross-resistance between rifampin and rifabutin is commonly observed with *M. tuberculosis* and *M. avium* complex isolates. Isolates of *M. tuberculosis* resistant to rifampin are likely to be resistant to rifabutin. Rifampicin and rifabutin MIC_{99} values against 523 isolates of *M. avium* complex were determined utilizing the agar dilution method (Ref. Heifets, Leonid B. and Iseman, Michael D. 1985. Determination of *in vitro* susceptibility of Mycobacteria to Ansamycin. Am. Rev. Respir. Dis. 132 (3):710-711).
[See table above]

SUSCEPTIBILITY OF *M. AVIUM* COMPLEX STRAINS TO RIFAMPIN AND RIFABUTIN

Susceptibility to Rifampin (μg/mL)	Number of Strains	% of Strains Susceptible/Resistant to Different Concentrations of Rifabutin (μg/mL)			
		Susceptible to 0.5	Resistant to 0.5 only	Resistant to 1.0	Resistant to 2.0
Susceptible to 1.0	30	100.0	0.0	0.0	0.0
Resistant to 1.0 only	163	88.3	11.7	0.0	0.0
Resistant to 5.0	105	38.0	57.1	2.9	2.0
Resistant to 10.0	225	20.0	50.2	19.6	10.2
TOTAL	523	49.5	36.7	9.0	4.8

Rifabutin *in vitro* MIC $_{99}$ values of ≤0.5 μg/mL, determined by the agar dilution method, for *M. kansasii, M. gordonae* and *M. marinum* have been reported; however, the clinical significance of these results is unknown.

INDICATIONS AND USAGE

MYCOBUTIN is indicated for the prevention of disseminated *Mycobacterium avium* complex (MAC) disease in patients with advanced HIV infection.

Clinical Studies

Two randomized, double-blind clinical trials (study 023 and study 027) compared MYCOBUTIN (300 mg/day) to placebo in patients with CDC-defined AIDS and CD4 counts ≤ 200 cells/μL. These studies accrued patients from 2/90 through 2/92. Study 023 enrolled 590 patients, with a median CD4 cell count at study entry of 42 cells/μL (mean 61). Study 027 enrolled 556 patients, with a median CD4 cell count at study entry of 40 cells/μL (mean 58).

Endpoints included the following:
(1) MAC bacteremia, defined as at least one blood culture positive for *M. avium* complex bacteria.
(2) Clinically significant disseminated MAC disease, defined as MAC bacteremia accompanied by signs or symptoms of serious MAC infection, including one or more of the following: fever, night sweats, rigors, weight loss, worsening anemia, and/or elevations in alkaline phosphatase.
(3) Survival

MAC bacteremia

Participants who received MYCOBUTIN were one-third to one-half as likely to develop MAC bacteremia as were participants who received placebo. These results were statistically significant (study 023: p<0.001; study 027: p = 0.002). In study 023, the one-year cumulative incidence of MAC bacteremia, on an intent to treat basis, was 9% for patients randomized to MYCOBUTIN and 22% for patients randomized to placebo. In study 027, these rates were 13% and 28% for MYCOBUTIN-treated and placebo-treated patients, respectively.

Most cases of MAC bacteremia (approximately 90% in these studies) occurred among participants whose CD4 count at study entry was ≤ 100 cells/μL. The median and mean CD4 counts at onset of MAC bacteremia were 13 cells/μL and 24 cells/μL, respectively. These studies did not investigate the optimal time to begin MAC prophylaxis.

Clinically significant disseminated MAC disease

In association with the decreased incidence of bacteremia, patients on MYCOBUTIN showed reductions in the signs and symptoms of disseminated MAC disease, including fever, night sweats, weight loss, fatigue, abdominal pain, anemia, and hepatic dysfunction.

Survival

The one year survival rates in study 023 were 77% for the MYCOBUTIN group and 77% for the placebo group. In study 027, the one year survival rates were 77% for the MYCOBUTIN group and 70% for the placebo group. These differences were not statistically significant.

CONTRAINDICATIONS

Rifabutin is contraindicated in patients who have had clinically significant hypersensitivity to this drug, or to any other rifamycins.

WARNINGS

MYCOBUTIN prophylaxis must not be administered to patients with active tuberculosis. Tuberculosis in HIV-positive patients is common and may present with atypical or extrapulmonary findings. Patients are likely to have a nonreactive purified protein derivative (PPD) despite active disease. In addition to chest X-ray and sputum culture, the following studies may be useful in the diagnosis of tuberculosis in the HIV-positive patient: blood culture, urine culture, or biopsy of a suspicious lymph node.

Patients who develop complaints consistent with active tuberculosis while on MYCOBUTIN prophylaxis should be evaluated immediately, so that those with active disease may be given an effective combination regimen of antituberculosis medications. Administration of single-agent MYCOBUTIN to patients with active tuberculosis is likely to lead to the development of tuberculosis that is resistant both to MYCOBUTIN and to rifampin.

There is no evidence that MYCOBUTIN is effective prophylaxis against *M. tuberculosis*. Patients requiring prophylaxis against both *M. tuberculosis* and *Mycobacterium avium* complex may be given isoniazid and MYCOBUTIN concurrently.

PRECAUTIONS

Because MYCOBUTIN may be associated with neutropenia, and more rarely thrombocytopenia, physicians should consider obtaining hematologic studies periodically in patients receiving MYCOBUTIN prophylaxis.

Information for Patients

Patients should be advised of the signs and symptoms of both MAC and tuberculosis, and should be instructed to consult their physicians if they develop new complaints consistent with either of these diseases. In addition, since MYCOBUTIN may rarely be associated with myositis and uveitis, patients should be advised to notify their physicians if they develop signs or symptoms suggesting either of these disorders.

Urine, feces, saliva, sputum, perspiration, tears, and skin may be colored brown-orange with rifabutin and some of its metabolites. Soft contact lenses may be permanently stained. Patients to be treated with MYCOBUTIN should be made aware of these possibilities.

Drug Interactions

In 10 healthy adult volunteers and 8 HIV-positive patients, steady-state plasma levels of zidovudine (ZDV), an antiretroviral agent which is metabolized mainly through glucuronidation, were decreased after repeated MYCOBUTIN dosing; the mean decrease in C_{max} and AUC was decreased by 48% and 32%, respectively. *In vitro* studies have demonstrated that MYCOBUTIN does not affect the inhibition of HIV by ZDV.

Steady-state kinetics in 12 HIV-positive patients show that both the rate and extent of systemic availability of didanosine (ddI), was not altered after repeated dosing of MYCOBUTIN.

MYCOBUTIN has liver enzyme-inducing properties. The related drug rifampin is known to reduce the activity of a number of other drugs, including dapsone, narcotics (including methadone), anticoagulants, corticosteroids, cyclosporine, cardiac glycoside preparations, quinidine, oral contraceptives, oral hypoglycemic agents (sulfonylureas), and analgesics. Rifampin has also been reported to decrease the effects of concurrently administered ketoconazole, barbiturates, diazepam, verapamil, beta-adrenergic blockers, clofibrate, progestins, disopyramide, mexiletine, theophylline, chloramphenicol, and anticonvulsants. Because of the structural similarity of rifabutin and rifampin, MYCOBUTIN may be expected to have some effect on these drugs as well. However, unlike rifampin, MYCOBUTIN appears not to affect the acetylation of isoniazid. When rifabutin was compared with rifampin in a study with 8 healthy normal volunteers, rifabutin appeared to be a less potent enzyme inducer than rifampin. The significance of this finding for clinical drug interactions is not known. Dosage adjustment of drugs listed above may be necessary if they are given concurrently with MYCOBUTIN. Patients using oral contraceptives should consider changing to nonhormonal methods of birth control.

Carcinogenesis, Mutagenesis, Impairment of Fertility:

Long term carcinogenicity studies were conducted with rifabutin in mice and in rats. Rifabutin was not carcinogenic in mice at doses up to 180 mg/kg/day, or approximately 36 times the recommended human daily dose. Rifabutin was not carcinogenic in the rat at doses up to 60 mg/kg/day, about 12 times the recommended human dose. Rifabutin was not mutagenic in the bacterial mutation assay (Ames Test) using both rifabutin-susceptible and resistant strains. Rifabutin was not mutagenic in *Schizosaccharomyces pombe P_1* and was not genotoxic in V-79 Chinese hamster cells, human lymphocytes *in vitro*, or mouse bone marrow cells *in vivo*.

Fertility was impaired in male rats given 160 mg/kg (32 times the recommended human daily dose).

Pregnancy:

Pregnancy Category B: Reproduction studies have been carried out in rats and rabbits given rifabutin using dose levels up to 200 mg/kg (40 times the recommended human daily dose). No teratogenicity was observed in either species. In rats, given 200 mg/kg/day, there was a decrease in fetal viability. In rats, at 40 mg/kg/day (8 times the recommended human daily dose), rifabutin caused an increase in fetal skeletal variants. In rabbits, at 80 mg/kg/day (16 times the recommended human daily dose), rifabutin caused maternotoxicity and increase in fetal skeletal anomalies. There are no adequate and well-controlled studies in pregnant women. Because animal reproduction studies are not always predictive of human response, rifabutin should be used in pregnant women only if the potential benefit justifies the potential risk to the fetus.

Nursing Mothers:

It is not known whether rifabutin is excreted in human milk. Because many drugs are excreted in human milk and because of the potential for serious adverse reactions in nursing infants, a decision should be made whether to discontinue nursing or discontinue the drug, taking into account the importance of the drug to the mother.

Pediatric Use:

Safety and effectiveness of rifabutin for prophylaxis of MAC in children have not been established. Limited safety data are available from treatment use in 22 HIV-positive children with MAC who received MYCOBUTIN in combination with at least two other antimycobacterials for periods from 1 to 183 weeks. Mean doses (mg/kg) for these children were: 18.5 (range 15.0 to 25.0) for infants one year of age; 8.6 (range 4.4 to 18.8) for children 2 to 10 years of age; and 4.0 (range 2.8 to 5.4) for adolescents 14 to 16 years of age. There is no evidence that doses greater than 5 mg/kg daily are useful. Adverse experiences were similar to those observed in the adult population, and included leukopenia, neutropenia and rash. Doses of MYCOBUTIN may be administered mixed with foods such as applesauce.

ADVERSE REACTIONS

MYCOBUTIN was generally well tolerated in the controlled clinical trials. Discontinuation of therapy due to an adverse event was required in 16% of patients receiving MYCOBUTIN compared to 8% of patients receiving placebo in these trials. Primary reasons for discontinuation of MYCOBUTIN were rash (4% of treated patients), gastrointestinal intolerance (3%), and neutropenia (2%).

The following table enumerates adverse experiences that occurred at a frequency of 1% or greater, among the patients treated with MYCOBUTIN in studies 023 and 027.

CLINICAL ADVERSE EXPERIENCES REPORTED IN ≥ 1% OF PATIENTS TREATED WITH MYCOBUTIN

ADVERSE EVENT	MYCOBUTIN (n=566) %	PLACEBO (n=580) %
BODY AS A WHOLE		
Abdominal Pain	4	3
Asthenia	1	1
Chest Pain	1	1
Fever	2	1
Headache	3	5
Pain	1	2
DIGESTIVE SYSTEM		
Anorexia	2	2
Diarrhea	3	3
Dyspepsia	3	1

Eructation	3	1
Flatulence	2	1
Nausea	6	5
Nausea and Vomiting	3	2
Vomiting	1	1
MUSCULOSKELETAL SYSTEM		
Myalgia	2	1
NERVOUS SYSTEM		
Insomnia	1	1
SKIN AND APPENDAGES		
Rash	11	8
SPECIAL SENSES		
Taste Perversion	3	1
UROGENITAL SYSTEM		
Discolored Urine	30	6

CLINICAL ADVERSE EVENTS REPORTED IN <1% OF PATIENTS WHO RECEIVED MYCOBUTIN

Considering data from the 023 and 027 pivotal trials, and from other clinical studies, MYCOBUTIN appears to be a likely cause of the following adverse events which occurred in less than 1% of treated patients: flu-like syndrome, hepatitis, hemolysis, arthralgia, myositis, chest pressure or pain with dyspnea, and skin discoloration.

The following adverse events have occurred in more than one patient receiving MYCOBUTIN, but an etiologic role has not been established: seizure, paresthesia, aphasia, confusion, and non-specific T wave changes on electrocardiogram.

When MYCOBUTIN was administered at doses from 1050 mg/day to 2400 mg/day, generalized arthralgia and uveitis were reported. These adverse experiences abated when MYCOBUTIN was discontinued.

The following table enumerates the changes in laboratory values that were considered as laboratory abnormalities in studies 023 and 027.

PERCENTAGE OF PATIENTS WITH LABORATORY ABNORMALITIES

LABORATORY ABNORMALITIES	MYCOBUTIN (n=566) %	PLACEBO (n=580) %
Chemistry:		
Increased Alkaline Phosphatase[1]	<1	3
Increased SGOT[2]	7	12
Increased SGPT[2]	9	11
Hematology:		
Anemia[3]	6	7
Eosinophilia	1	1
Leukopenia[4]	17	16
Neutropenia[5]	25	20
Thrombocytopenia[6]	5	4

INCLUDES GRADE 3 OR 4 TOXICITIES AS SPECIFIED:
1 all values >450 U/L
2 all values >150 U/L
3 all hemoglobin values <8.0 g/dL
4 all WBC values <1,500/mm^3
5 all ANC values <750/mm^3
6 all platelet count values <50,000/mm^3

The incidence of neutropenia in patients treated with MYCOBUTIN was significantly greater than in patients treated with placebo (p = 0.03). Although thrombocytopenia was not significantly more common among MYCOBUTIN treated patients in these trials, MYCOBUTIN has been clearly linked to thrombocytopenia in rare cases. One patient in study 023 developed thrombotic thrombocytopenic purpura, which was attributed to MYCOBUTIN.

Uveitis is rare when MYCOBUTIN is used as a single agent at 300 mg/day for prophylaxis of MAC in HIV-infected persons, even with the concomitant use of fluconazole and/or macrolide antibiotics. However, if higher doses of MYCOBUTIN are administered in combination with these agents, the incidence of uveitis is higher.

Patients who developed uveitis had mild to severe symptoms that resolved after treatment with corticosteroids and/or mydriatic eye drops; in some severe cases, however, resolution of symptoms occurred after several weeks.

When uveitis occurs, temporary discontinuance of MYCOBUTIN and ophthalmologic evaluation are recommended. In most mild cases, MYCOBUTIN may be restarted; however if signs or symptoms recur, use of MYCOBUTIN should be discontinued (Morbidity and Mortality Weekly Report, September 9, 1994).

ANIMAL TOXICOLOGY

Liver abnormalities, (increased bilirubin and liver weight), occurred in all species tested, in rats at doses 5 times, in monkeys at doses 8 times, and in mice at doses 6 times the recommended human daily dose. Testicular atrophy occurred in baboons at doses 4 times the recommended human dose, and in rats at doses 40 times the recommended human daily dose.

OVERDOSAGE

No information is available on accidental overdosage in humans.

Treatment

While there is no experience in the treatment of overdose with MYCOBUTIN, clinical experience with rifamycins suggest that gastric lavage to evacuate gastric contents (within a few hours of overdose), followed by instillation of an activated charcoal slurry into the stomach, may help absorb any remaining drug from the gastrointestinal tract.

Rifabutin is 85% protein bound and distributed extensively into tissues (Vss:8 to 9 L/kg). It is not primarily excreted via the urinary route (less than 10% as unchanged drug), therefore, neither hemodialysis nor forced diuresis is expected to enhance the systemic elimination of unchanged rifabutin from the body in a patient with MYCOBUTIN overdose.

DOSAGE AND ADMINISTRATION

It is recommended that 300 mg of MYCOBUTIN be administered once daily. For those patients with propensity to nausea, vomiting, or other gastrointestinal upset, administration of MYCOBUTIN at doses of 150 mg twice daily taken with food may be useful.

HOW SUPPLIED

MYCOBUTIN® (Rifabutin Capsules, USP) is supplied as hard gelatin capsules having an opaque red-brown cap and body, imprinted with MYCOBUTIN/PHARMACIA in white ink, each containing 150 mg of Rifabutin, USP.

MYCOBUTIN is available as follows:
NDC 0013-5301-17 Bottles of 100 capsules
Keep tightly closed and dispense in a tight container as defined in the USP. Store at controlled room temperature, 15° to 30°C (59° to 86°F).

CAUTION: Federal law prohibits dispensing without prescription.

Manufactured by:
PHARMACIA S.p.A.
ASCOLI PICENO, ITALY
057000496   Revised April 1, 1996
Shown in Product Identification Guide, page 332

OGEN®
brand of estropipate tablets, USP
℞

DESCRIPTION

OGEN (estropipate tablets), (formerly piperazine estrone sulfate), is a natural estrogenic substance prepared from purified crystalline estrone, solubilized as the sulfate and stabilized with piperazine. It is appreciably soluble in water and has almost no odor or taste — properties which are ideally suited for oral administration. The amount of piperazine in OGEN is not sufficient to exert a pharmacological action. Its addition ensures solubility, stability, and uniform potency of the estrone sulfate. Chemically estropipate, molecular weight: 436.56, is represented by estra-1,3,5(10)-trien-17–one, 3–(sulfooxy)-, compound with piperazine (1:1). The structural formula may be represented as follows:

OGEN is available as tablets for oral administration containing either 0.75 mg (OGEN .625), 1.5 mg (OGEN 1.25), or 3 mg (OGEN 2.5) estropipate (Calculated as sodium estrone sulfate 0.625 mg, 1.25 mg, and 2.5 mg, respectively).

Inactive Ingredients

Each tablet contains: Colloidal silicon dioxide, dibasic potassium phosphate, hydrogenated vegetable oil wax, hydroxypropyl cellulose, lactose, magnesium stearate, microcrystalline cellulose, sodium starch glycolate and tromethamine.

OGEN .625 also contains D&C Yellow No. 10 and FD&C Yellow No. 6.
OGEN 1.25 also contains: FD&C Yellow No. 6.
OGEN 2.5 also contains: FD&C Blue No. 2.

HOW SUPPLIED

OGEN (estropipate tablets, USP) is supplied as OGEN .625 (0.75 mg estropipate; calculated as sodium estrone sulfate 0.625 mg), yellow, scored tablets, imprinted U 3772, NDC 0009-3772-01; OGEN 1.25 (1.5 mg estropipate; calculated as sodium estrone sulfate 1.25 mg), peach-colored, scored tablets, imprinted U 3773, NDC 0009-3773-01; and OGEN 2.5 (3 mg estropipate; calculated as sodium estrone sulfate 2.5 mg), blue, scored tablets, imprinted U 3774, NDC 0009-3774-01. Tablets of all three dosage levels are standardized to provide uniform estrone activity and are scored to provide dosage flexibility. All tablet sizes of OGEN are available in bottles of 100.

Recommended storage: Store below 77°F (25°C).
Revised March 1994   816 035 002

PREPIDIL® Gel
brand of dinoprostone cervical gel
For Endocervical Use
℞

DESCRIPTION

PREPIDIL Gel contains dinoprostone as the naturally occurring form of prostaglandin E$_2$ (PGE$_2$) and is designated chemically as (5Z, 11α, 13E, 15S) - 11,15 - Dihydroxy-9-oxo-prosta-5, 13-dien-1-oic acid. The molecular formula is C$_{20}$H$_{32}$O$_5$ and the molecular weight is 352.5. Dinoprostone occurs as a white to off-white crystalline powder with a melting point within the range of 65° to 69°C. It is soluble in ethanol, in 25% ethanol in water, and in water to the extent of 130 mg/100 mL. The active constituent of PREPIDIL Gel is dinoprostone 0.5 mg/3 g (2.5 mL gel); other constituents are colloidal silicon dioxide NF (240 mg/3 g) and triacetin USP (2760 mg/3 g).

The structural formula is represented below:

CLINICAL PHARMACOLOGY

PREPIDIL Gel (dinoprostone) administered endocervically may stimulate the myometrium of the gravid uterus to contract in a manner similar to contractions seen in the term uterus during labor. Whether or not this action results from a direct effect of dinoprostone on the myometrium has not been determined.

Dinoprostone is also capable of stimulating smooth muscle of the gastrointestinal tract in humans. This activity may be responsible for the vomiting and/or diarrhea that is occasionally seen when dinoprostone is used for preinduction cervical ripening.

In laboratory animals, and also in humans, large doses of dinoprostone can lower blood pressure, probably as a result of its effect on smooth muscle of the vascular system. With the doses of dinoprostone used for cervical ripening this effect has not been seen. In laboratory animals, and also in humans, dinoprostone can elevate body temperature; however, with the dosing used for cervical ripening this effect has not been seen.

In addition to an oxytocic effect, there is evidence suggesting that this agent has a local cervical effect in initiating softening, effacement, and dilation. These changes, referred to as cervical ripening, occur spontaneously as the normal pregnancy progresses toward term and allow evacuation of uterine contents by decreasing cervical resistance at the same time that myometrial activity increases. While not completely understood, biochemical changes within the cervix during natural cervical ripening are similar to those following PGE$_2$-induced ripening. Further, it has been shown that these changes can take place independent of myometrial activity; however, it is quite likely that PGE$_2$ administered endocervically produces effacement and softening by combined contraction-inducing and cervical-ripening properties. There is evidence to suggest that the changes that take place within the cervix are due to collagen degradation resulting from collagenase secretion as a response, at least in part, to PGE$_2$.

Using an unvalidated assay, the following information was determined. When PREPIDIL Gel was administered endocervically to women undergoing preinduction ripening, results from measurement of plasma levels of the metabolite 13,14-dihydro-15-keto-PGE$_2$ (DHK-PGE$_2$) showed that PGE$_2$ was relatively rapidly absorbed and the T$_{max}$ was 0.5 to 0.75 hours. Plasma mean C$_{max}$ for gel-treated subjects

Continued on next page

Information on these Pharmacia & Upjohn products is based on labeling in effect June 1, 1998. Further information concerning these and other Pharmacia & Upjohn products may be obtained by direct inquiry to Medical Information, Pharmacia & Upjohn, Kalamazoo, MI 49001.

Prepidil—Cont.

was 433 ± 51 pg/mL versus 137 ± 24 pg/mL for untreated controls. In those subjects in which a clinical response was observed, mean C_{max} was 484 ± 57 pg/mL versus 213 ± 69 pg/mL in nonresponders and 219 ± 92 pg/mL in control subjects who had positive clinical progression toward normal labor. These elevated levels in gel-treated subjects appear to be largely a result of absorption of PGE_2 from the gel rather than from endogenous sources.

PGE_2 is completely metabolized in humans. PGE_2 is extensively metabolized in the lungs, and the resulting metabolites are further metabolized in the liver and kidney. The major route of elimination of the products of PGE_2 metabolism is the kidneys.

INDICATIONS AND USAGE

PREPIDIL Gel is indicated for ripening an unfavorable cervix in pregnant women at or near term with a medical or obstetrical need for labor induction.

CONTRAINDICATIONS

Endocervically administered PREPIDIL Gel is not recommended for the following:

a. Patients in whom oxytocic drugs are generally contraindicated or where prolonged contractions of the uterus are considered inappropriate, such as:
- cases with a history of cesarean section or major uterine surgery
- cases in which cephalopelvic disproportion is present
- cases in which there is a history of difficult labor and/or traumatic delivery
- grand multiparae with six or more previous term pregnancies
- cases with non-vertex presentation
- cases with hyperactive or hypertonic uterine patterns
- cases of fetal distress where delivery is not imminent
- in obstetric emergencies where the benefit-to-risk ratio for either the fetus or the mother favors surgical intervention

b. Patients with hypersensitivity to prostaglandins or constituents of the gel.

c. Patients with placenta previa or unexplained vaginal bleeding during this pregnancy.

d. Patients for whom vaginal delivery is not indicated, such as vasa previa or active herpes genitalia.

WARNINGS

FOR HOSPITAL USE ONLY

Dinoprostone, as with other potent oxytocic agents, should be used only with strict adherence to recommended dosages. Dinoprostone should be administered by physicians in a hospital that can provide immediate intensive care and acute surgical facilities.

PRECAUTIONS

1. General Precautions:

During use, uterine activity, fetal status, and character of the cervix (dilation and effacement) should be carefully monitored either by auscultation or electronic fetal monitoring to detect possible evidence of undesired responses, eg, hypertonus, sustained uterine contractility, or fetal distress. In cases where there is a history of hypertonic uterine contractility or tetanic uterine contractions, it is recommended that uterine activity and the state of the fetus should be continuously monitored. The possibility of uterine rupture should be borne in mind when high-tone myometrial contractions are sustained. Feto-pelvic relationships should be carefully evaluated before use of PREPIDIL Gel (see CONTRAINDICATIONS).

Caution should be exercised in administration of PREPIDIL Gel in patients with:
- asthma or history of asthma
- glaucoma or raised intraocular pressure

Caution should be taken so as not to administer PREPIDIL Gel above the level of the internal os. Careful vaginal examination will reveal the degree of effacement which will regulate the size of the shielded endocervical cathe-

ter to be used. That is, the 20 mm endocervical catheter should be used if no effacement is present, and the 10 mm catheter should be used if the cervix is 50% effaced. Placement of PREPIDIL Gel into the extra-amniotic space has been associated with uterine hyperstimulation.

As PREPIDIL Gel is extensively metabolized in the lung, liver, and kidney, and the major route of elimination is the kidney, PREPIDIL Gel should be used with caution in patients with renal and hepatic dysfunction.

2. Patients With Ruptured Membranes:

Caution should be exercised in the administration of PREPIDIL Gel in patients with ruptured membranes. The safety of use of PREPIDIL Gel in these patients has not been determined.

3. Drug Interactions:

PREPIDIL Gel may augment the activity of other oxytocic agents and their concomitant use is not recommended. For the sequential use of oxytocin following PREPIDIL Gel administration, a dosing interval of 6–12 hours is recommended.

4. Carcinogenesis, Mutagenesis, Impairment of Fertility:

Carcinogenic bioassay studies have not been conducted in animals with PREPIDIL Gel due to the limited indications for use and short duration of administration. No evidence of mutagenicity was observed in the Micronucleus Test or Ames Assay.

5. Pregnancy, Teratogenic Effects:

PREGNANCY CATEGORY C

Prostaglandin E_2 produced an increase in skeletal anomalies in rats and rabbits. No effect would be expected clinically, when used as indicated, since PREPIDIL Gel is administered after the period of organogenesis. PREPIDIL Gel has been shown to be embryotoxic in rats and rabbits, and any dose that produces sustained increased uterine tone could put the embryo or fetus at risk. See statements under General Precautions.

ADVERSE REACTIONS

PREPIDIL Gel is generally well-tolerated. In controlled trials, in which 1731 women were entered, the following events were reported at an occurrence of ≥1%:
[See table below]

In addition, in other trials amnionitis and intrauterine fetal sepsis have been associated with extra-amniotic intrauterine administration of PGE_2. Uterine rupture has been reported in association with the use of PREPIDIL Gel intracervically. Additional events reported in the literature, associated by the authors with the use of PREPIDIL Gel, included premature rupture of membranes, fetal depression (1 min Apgar<7), and fetal acidosis (umbilical artery pH<7.15).

DRUG ABUSE AND DEPENDENCE

No drug abuse or drug dependence has been seen with the use of PREPIDIL Gel.

OVERDOSAGE

Overdosage with PREPIDIL Gel may be expressed by uterine hypercontractility and uterine hypertonus. Because of the transient nature of PGE_2-induced myometrial hyperstimulation, nonspecific, conservative management was found to be effective in the vast majority of the cases; ie, maternal position change and administration of oxygen to the mother. β-adrenergic drugs may be used as a treatment of hyperstimulation following the administration of PGE_2 for cervical ripening.

DOSAGE AND ADMINISTRATION

NOTE: USE CAUTION IN HANDLING THIS PRODUCT TO PREVENT CONTACT WITH SKIN. WASH HANDS THOROUGHLY WITH SOAP AND WATER AFTER ADMINISTRATION.

PREPIDIL Gel should be brought to room temperature (59° to 86°F; 15° to 30°C) just prior to administration. Do not force the warming process by using a water bath or other source of external heat (eg, microwave oven).

To prepare the product for use, remove the peel-off seal from the end of the syringe. Then remove the protective end cap

(to serve as plunger extension) and insert the protective end cap into the plunger stopper assembly in the barrel of syringe. Choose the appropriate length shielded catheter (10 mm or 20 mm) and aseptically remove the sterile shielded catheter from the package. Careful vaginal examination will reveal the degree of effacement which will regulate the size of the shielded endocervical catheter to be used. That is, the 20 mm endocervical catheter should be used if no effacement is present, and the 10 mm catheter should be used if the cervix is 50% effaced. Firmly attach the catheter hub to the syringe tip as evidenced by a distinct click. Fill the catheter with sterile gel by pushing the plunger assembly to expel air from the catheter prior to administration to the patient. Proper assembly of the dosing apparatus is shown below.

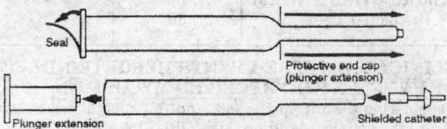

To properly administer the product, the patient should be in a dorsal position with the cervix visualized using a speculum. Using sterile technique, introduce the gel with the catheter provided into the cervical canal just below the level of the internal os. Administer the contents of the syringe by gentle expulsion and then remove the catheter. The gel is easily extrudable from the syringe. Use the contents of one syringe for one patient only. No attempt should be made to administer the small amount of gel remaining in the catheter. The syringe, catheter, and any unused package contents should be discarded after use. Following administration of PREPIDIL Gel, the patient should remain in the supine position for at least 15–30 minutes to minimize leakage from the cervical canal. If the desired response is obtained from PREPIDIL Gel, the recommended interval before giving intravenous oxytocin is 6–12 hours. If there is no cervical/uterine response to the initial dose of PREPIDIL Gel, repeat dosing may be given. The recommended repeat dose is 0.5 mg dinoprostone with a dosing interval of 6 hours. The need for additional dosing and the interval must be determined by the attending physician based on the course of clinical events. The maximum recommended cumulative dose for a 24-hour period is 1.5 mg of dinoprostone (7.5 mL PREPIDIL Gel).

HOW SUPPLIED

PREPIDIL Gel is available as a sterile semitranslucent viscous preparation for endocervical application: 0.5 mg PGE_2 per 3.0 g (2.5 mL) in syringe. In addition, each package contains two shielded catheters (10 mm and 20 mm tip) enclosed in sterile envelopes. The contents are not guaranteed sterile if envelopes are not intact.

Each 3-gram syringe applicator contains: dinoprostone, 0.5 mg; colloidal silicon dioxide, 240 mg; triacetin, 2760 mg.

| 3 gram syringe | NDC 0009-3359-01 |
| 5 × 3 gram syringes | NDC 0009-3359-02 |

PREPIDIL Gel has a shelf life of 24 months when stored under continuous refrigeration (36° to 46°F; 2° to 8°C).

Caution: Federal law prohibits dispensing without prescription.

Manufactured by N.V. Upjohn S.A.,
Puurs-Belgium for
Pharmacia & Upjohn Company
Kalamazoo, MI 49001, USA
Revised January 1995

815 040 004
5R2685/1

PROSTIN E2®
dinoprostone vaginal suppository

℞

DESCRIPTION

PROSTIN E2 Vaginal Suppository, an oxytocic, contains dinoprostone as the naturally occurring prostaglandin E2 (PGE2).

Its chemical name is (5Z,11α,13E,15S)-11,15-Dihydroxy-9-oxo-prosta-5,13-dien-1-oic acid and the structural formula is represented below:

The molecular formula is $C_{20}H_{32}O_5$. The molecular weight of dinoprostone is 352.5. Dinoprostone occurs as a white crystalline powder. It has a melting point within the range

Adverse Reaction	PGE$_2$ (N=884)		Control* (N=847)	
	N	(%)	N	(%)
Maternal				
Uterine contractile abnormality	58	(6.6)	34	(4.0)
Any gastrointestinal effect	50	(5.7)	22	(2.6)
Back pain	27	(3.1)	0	(0)
Warm feeling in vagina	13	(1.5)	0	(0)
Fever	12	(1.4)	10	(1.2)
Fetal				
Any fetal heart rate abnormality	150	(17.0)	123	(14.5)
Bradycardia	36	(4.1)	26	(3.1)
Deceleration				
Late	25	(2.8)	18	(2.1)
Variable	38	(4.3)	29	(3.4)
Unspecified	19	(2.1)	19	(2.2)

* placebo gel or no treatment

of 64° to 71° C. Dinoprostone is soluble in ethanol and in 25% ethanol in water. It is soluble in water to the extent of 130 mg/100 mL.

Each suppository contains 20 mg of dinoprostone in a mixture of glycerides of fatty acids.

CLINICAL PHARMACOLOGY

PROSTIN E2 Vaginal Suppository administered intravaginally stimulates the myometrium of the gravid uterus to contract in a manner that is similar to the contractions seen in the term uterus during labor. Whether or not this action results from a direct effect of dinoprostone on the myometrium has not been determined with certainty at this time. Nonetheless, the myometrial contractions induced by the vaginal administration of dinoprostone are sufficient to produce evacuation of the products of conception from the uterus in the majority of cases.

Dinoprostone is also capable of stimulating the smooth muscle of the gastrointestinal tract of man. This activity may be responsible for the vomiting and/or diarrhea that is not uncommon when dinoprostone is used to terminate pregnancy. In laboratory animals, and also in man, large doses of dinoprostone can lower blood pressure, probably as a consequence of its effect on the smooth muscle of the vascular system. With the doses of dinoprostone used for terminating pregnancy this effect has not been clinically significant. In laboratory animals, and also in man, dinoprostone can elevate body temperature. With the clinical doses of dinoprostone used for the termination of pregnancy some patients do exhibit temperature increases.

INDICATIONS AND USAGE

1. PROSTIN E2 Vaginal Suppository is indicated for the termination of pregnancy from the 12th through the 20th gestational week as calculated from the first day of the last normal menstrual period.
2. PROSTIN E2 is also indicated for evacuation of the uterine contents in the management of missed abortion or intrauterine fetal death up to 28 weeks of gestational age as calculated from the first day of the last normal menstrual period.
3. PROSTIN E2 is indicated in the management of nonmetastatic gestational trophoblastic disease (benign hydatidiform mole).

CONTRAINDICATIONS

1. Hypersensitivity to dinoprostone
2. Acute pelvic inflammatory disease
3. Patients with active cardiac, pulmonary, renal, or hepatic disease

> ### WARNINGS
> Dinoprostone, as with other potent oxytocic agents, should be used only with strict adherence to recommended dosages. Dinoprostone should be used by medically trained personnel in a hospital which can provide immediate intensive care and acute surgical facilities.

Dinoprostone does not appear to directly affect the fetoplacental unit. Therefore, the possibility does exist that the previable fetus aborted by dinoprostone could exhibit transient life signs. Dinoprostone is not indicated if the fetus in utero has reached the stage of viability. Dinoprostone should not be considered a feticidal agent.

Evidence from animal studies has suggested that certain prostaglandins may have some teratogenic potential. Therefore, any failed pregnancy termination with dinoprostone should be completed by some other means.

PROSTIN E2 Vaginal Suppository should not be used for extemporaneous preparation of any other dosage form.

Neither the PROSTIN E2 Vaginal Suppository, as dispensed nor any extemporaneous formulation made from the PROSTIN E2 Vaginal Suppository should be used for cervical ripening or other indication in the patient with term pregnancy.

PRECAUTIONS

1. **General precautions**

Animal studies lasting several weeks at high doses have shown that prostaglandins of the E and F series can induce proliferation of bone. Such effects have also been noted in newborn infants who have received prostaglandin E1 during prolonged treatment. There is no evidence that short term administration of PROSTIN E2 Vaginal Suppository can cause similar bone effects.

As in spontaneous abortion, where the process is sometimes incomplete, abortion induced by PROSTIN E2 may sometimes be incomplete. In such cases, other measures should be taken to assure complete abortion.

In patients with a history of asthma, hypo- or hypertension, cardiovascular disease, renal disease, hepatic disease, anemia, jaundice, diabetes or history of epilepsy, dinoprostone should be used with caution.

Dinoprostone administered by the vaginal route should be used with caution in the presence of cervicitis, infected endocervical lesions, or acute vaginitis.

As with any oxytocic agent, dinoprostone should be used with caution in patients with compromised (scarred) uteri.

Endometritis pyrexia

a. **Time of onset**: Typically, on third post-abortional day (38° C or higher).

b. **Duration**: Untreated pyrexia and infection continue and may give rise to other infective pelvic pathology.

c. **Retention**: Products of conception are often retained in the cervical os or uterine cavity.

d. **Histology**: Endometrium shows evidence of inflammatory lymphocytic infiltration with areas of necrotic hemorrhagic tissue.

e. **The uterus**: Often remains boggy and soft with tenderness over the fundus, and pain on moving the cervix, on bimanual examination.

f. **Discharge**: Often associated foul-smelling lochia and leukorrhea.

g. **Cervical culture**
The culture of pathological organisms from the cervix or uterine cavity after abortion does not, of itself, warrant the diagnosis of septic abortion in the absence of clinical evidence of sepsis. It is not uncommon to culture pathogens from cases of recent abortion *not* clinically infected. Persistent positive culture with clear clinical signs of infection are significant in the differential diagnosis.

h. **Blood count**
Leukocytosis and differential white cell counts are not of major clinical importance in distinguishing between the two conditions, since total WBC's may be increased as a result of infection and transient leukocytosis may also be drug induced.

PGE2 induced pyrexia

Within 15–45 minutes of suppository administration.

Elevations revert to pretreatment levels within 2–6 hours after discontinuation of therapy or removal of suppository from vagina without any other treatment.

Elevation occurs irrespective of any retained tissue.

Although the endometrial stroma may be edematous and vascular, there is relative absence of inflammatory reaction.

Normal uterine involution not tender.

Lochia normal.

Dinoprostone vaginal therapy is associated with transient pyrexia that may be due to its effect on hypothalamic thermoregulation. In the patients studied, temperature elevations in excess of 2° F (1.1° C) were observed in approximately one-half of the patients on the recommended dosage regimen. In all cases, temperature returned to normal on discontinuation of therapy. Differentiation of post-abortion endometritis from drug-induced temperature elevations is difficult, but with increasing clinical exposure and experience with PGE2 vaginal therapy the distinctions become more obviously apparent and are summarized below:
[See table above]

In the absence of clinical or bacteriological evidence of intrauterine infection, supportive therapy for drug induced fevers includes the forcing of fluids. As all PGE2-induced fevers have been found to be transient and self-limiting, it is doubtful if any simple empirical measures for temperature reduction are indicated.

2. **Laboratory tests**

When a pregnancy diagnosed as missed abortion is electively interrupted with intravaginal administration of dinoprostone, confirmation of intrauterine fetal death should be obtained in respect to a *negative pregnancy test* for chorionic gonadotropic activity (U.C.G. test or equivalent). When a pregnancy with late fetal intrauterine death is interrupted with intravaginal administration of dinoprostone, confirmation of intrauterine fetal death should be obtained prior to treatment.

3. **Drug interactions**

PROSTIN E2 may augment the activity of other oxytocic drugs. Concomitant use with other oxytocic agents is not recommended.

4. **Carcinogenesis, mutagenesis, impairment of fertility**

Carcinogenic bioassay studies have not been conducted in animals with PROSTIN E2 due to the limited indications for use and short duration of administration. No evidence of mutagenicity was observed in the Micronucleus Test or Ames Assay.

5. **Pregnancy:** Teratogenic Effects: Pregnancy Category C

Animal studies do not indicate that PROSTIN E2 is teratogenic, however, it has been shown to be embryotoxic in rats and rabbits and any dose which produces increased uterine tone could put the embryo or fetus at risk. See WARNINGS section.

6. **Pediatric use:** Safety and effectiveness in pediatric patients have not been established.

ADVERSE REACTIONS

The most frequent adverse reactions observed with the use of dinoprostone for abortion are related to its contractile effect on smooth muscle.

In the patients studied, approximately two-thirds experienced vomiting, one-half temperature elevations, two-fifths diarrhea, one-third some nausea, one-tenth headache, and one-tenth shivering and chills.

In addition, approximately one-tenth of the patients studied exhibited transient diastolic blood pressure decreases of greater than 20 mmHg.

Two cases of myocardial infarction following the use of dinoprostone have been reported in patients with a history of cardiovascular disease.

It is not known whether these events were related to the administration of dinoprostone.

Adverse effects in decreasing order of their frequency, observed with the use of dinoprostone, not all of which are clearly drug related include:

Vomiting	Nocturnal leg cramps
Diarrhea	Uterine rupture
Nausea	Breast tenderness
Fever	Blurred vision
Headache	Coughing
Chills or shivering	Rash
Backache	Myalgia
Joint inflammation or pain new or exacerbated	Stiff neck
	Dehydration
Flushing or hot flashes	Tremor
Dizziness	Paresthesia
Arthralgia	Hearing impairment
Vaginal pain	Urine retention
Chest pain	Pharyngitis
Dyspnea	Laryngitis
Endometritis	Diaphoresis
Syncope or fainting sensation	Eye pain
	Wheezing
Vaginitis or vulvitis	Cardiac arrhythmia
Weakness	Skin discoloration
Muscle cramp or pain	Vaginismus
Tightness in chest	Tension

DOSAGE AND ADMINISTRATION

STORE IN A FREEZER NOT ABOVE –20° C (–4° F) BUT BRING TO ROOM TEMPERATURE JUST PRIOR TO USE. REMOVE FOIL BEFORE USE.

A suppository containing 20 mg of dinoprostone should be inserted high into the vagina. The patient should remain in the supine position for ten minutes following insertion. Additional intravaginal administration of each subsequent suppository should be at 3- to 5-hour intervals until abortion occurs. Within the above recommended intervals administration time should be determined by abortifacient progress, uterine contractility response, and by patient tolerance. Continuous administration of the drug for more than 2 days is not recommended.

HOW SUPPLIED

PROSTIN E2 Vaginal Suppositories are available in foil strips of 5 individually sealed suppositories. Each suppository contains 20 mg of dinoprostone in a mixture of glycerides of fatty acids.

STORE IN A FREEZER NOT ABOVE –20° C (–4° F).

Rx only

Pharmacia & Upjohn Company
Kalamazoo, MI 49001, USA
Revised December 1997

810 994 413
692166

Continued on next page

Information on these Pharmacia & Upjohn products is based on labeling in effect June 1, 1998. Further information concerning these and other Pharmacia & Upjohn products may be obtained by direct inquiry to Medical Information, Pharmacia & Upjohn, Kalamazoo, MI 49001.

PROVERA®
[prō-vera]
medroxyprogesterone acetate tablets

R̲

WARNING

THE USE OF PROVERA (MEDROXYPROGESTER-ONE ACETATE) DURING THE FIRST FOUR MONTHS OF PREGNANCY IS NOT RECOMMENDED.

Progestational agents have been used beginning with the first trimester of pregnancy in an attempt to prevent habitual abortion. There is no adequate evidence that such use is effective when such drugs are given during the first four months of pregnancy. Furthermore, in the vast majority of women, the cause of abortion is a defective ovum, which progestational agents could not be expected to influence. In addition, the use of progestational agents, with their uterine-relaxant properties, in patients with fertilized defective ova may cause a delay in spontaneous abortion. Therefore, the use of such drugs during the first four months of pregnancy is not recommended.

Several reports suggest an association between intrauterine exposure to progestational drugs in the first trimester of pregnancy and genital abnormalities in male and female fetuses. The risk of hypospadias, 5 to 8 per 1,000 male births in the general population, may be approximately doubled with exposure to these drugs. There are insufficient data to quantify the risk to exposed female fetuses, but insofar as some of these drugs induce mild virilization of the external genitalia of the female fetus, and because of the increased association of hypospadias in the male fetus, it is prudent to avoid the use of these drugs during the first trimester of pregnancy.

If the patient is exposed to PROVERA Tablets (medroxyprogesterone acetate) during the first four months of pregnancy or if she becomes pregnant while taking this drug, she should be apprised of the potential risks to the fetus.

DESCRIPTION

PROVERA Tablets contain medroxyprogesterone acetate, which is a derivative of progesterone. It is a white to off-white, odorless crystalline powder, stable in air, melting between 200 and 210° C. It is freely soluble in chloroform, soluble in acetone and in dioxane, sparingly soluble in alcohol and in methanol, slightly soluble in ether, and insoluble in water.

The chemical name for medroxyprogesterone acetate is Pregn-4-ene-3,20-dione, 17-(acetyloxy)-6-methyl-, (6α)-. The structural formula is:

Each PROVERA tablet for oral administration contains 2.5 mg, 5 mg or 10 mg of medroxyprogesterone acetate. Inactive ingredients: calcium stearate, corn starch, lactose, mineral oil, sorbic acid, sucrose, talc. The 2.5 mg tablet contains FD&C Yellow no. 6.

ACTIONS

Medroxyprogesterone acetate, administered orally or parenterally in the recommended doses to women with adequate endogenous estrogen, transforms proliferative into secretory endometrium. Androgenic and anabolic effects have been noted, but the drug is apparently devoid of significant estrogenic activity. While parenterally administered medroxyprogesterone acetate inhibits gonadotropin production, which in turn prevents follicular maturation and ovulation, available data indicate that this does not occur when the usually recommended oral dosage is given as single daily doses.

INDICATIONS AND USAGE

Secondary amenorrhea; abnormal uterine bleeding due to hormonal imbalance in the absence of organic pathology, such as fibroids or uterine cancer.

CONTRAINDICATIONS

1. Thrombophlebitis, thromboembolic disorders, cerebral apoplexy or patients with a past history of these conditions.

2. Liver dysfunction or disease.
3. Known or suspected malignancy of breast or genital organs.
4. Undiagnosed vaginal bleeding.
5. Missed abortion.
6. As a diagnostic test for pregnancy.
7. Known sensitivity to PROVERA Tablets.

WARNINGS

1. The physician should be alert to the earliest manifestations of thrombotic disorders (thrombophlebitis, cerebrovascular disorders, pulmonary embolism, and retinal thrombosis). Should any of these occur or be suspected, the drug should be discontinued immediately.

2. Beagle dogs treated with medroxyprogesterone acetate developed mammary nodules some of which were malignant. Although nodules occasionally appeared in control animals, they were intermittent in nature, whereas the nodules in the drug-treated animals were larger, more numerous, persistent, and there were some breast malignancies with metastases. Their significance with respect to humans has not been established.

3. Discontinue medication pending examination if there is sudden partial or complete loss of vision, or if there is a sudden onset of proptosis, diplopia or migraine. If examination reveals papilledema or retinal vascular lesions, medication should be withdrawn.

4. Detectable amounts of progestin have been identified in the milk of mothers receiving the drug. The effect of this on the nursing neonate and infant has not been determined.

5. Usage in pregnancy is not recommended (See WARNING Box).

6. Retrospective studies of morbidity and mortality in Great Britain and studies of morbidity in the United States have shown a statistically significant association between thrombophlebitis, pulmonary embolism, and cerebral thrombosis and embolism and the use of oral contraceptives.[1-4] The estimate of the relative risk of thromboembolism in the study by Vessey and Doll[3] was about sevenfold, while Sartwell and associates[4] in the United States found a relative risk of 4.4, meaning that the users are several times as likely to undergo thromboembolic disease without evident cause as nonusers. The American study also indicated that the risk did not persist after discontinuation of administration, and that it was not enhanced by long continued administration. The American study was not designed to evaluate a difference between products.

PRECAUTIONS

1. The pretreatment physical examination should include special reference to breast and pelvic organs, as well as Papanicolaou smear.

2. Because progestogens may cause some degree of fluid retention, conditions which might be influenced by this factor, such as epilepsy, migraine, asthma, cardiac or renal dysfunction, require careful observation.

3. In cases of breakthrough bleeding, as in all cases of irregular bleeding per vaginum, nonfunctional causes should be borne in mind. In cases of undiagnosed vaginal bleeding, adequate diagnostic measures are indicated.

4. Patients who have a history of psychic depression should be carefully observed and the drug discontinued if the depression recurs to a serious degree.

5. Any possible influence of prolonged progestin therapy on pituitary, ovarian, adrenal, hepatic or uterine functions awaits further study.

6. A decrease in glucose tolerance has been observed in a small percentage of patients on estrogen-progestin combination drugs. The mechanism of this decrease is obscure. For this reason, diabetic patients should be carefully observed while receiving progestin therapy.

7. The age of the patient constitutes no absolute limiting factor although treatment with progestins may mask the onset of the climacteric.

8. The pathologist should be advised of progestin therapy when relevant specimens are submitted.

9. Because of the occasional occurrence of thrombotic disorders, (thrombophlebitis, pulmonary embolism, retinal thrombosis, and cerebrovascular disorders) in patients taking estrogen-progestin combinations and since the mechanism is obscure, the physician should be alert to the earliest manifestation of these disorders.

10. Studies of the addition of a progestin product to an estrogen replacement regimen for seven or more days of a cycle of estrogen administration have reported a lowered incidence of endometrial hyperplasia. Morphological and biochemical studies of endometrium suggest that 10–13 days of a progestin are needed to provide maximal maturation of the endometrium and to eliminate any hyperplastic changes. Whether this will provide protection from endometrial carcinoma has not been clearly established. There are possible additional risks which may be associated with the inclusion of progestin in estrogen replacement regimen. The potential

risks include adverse effects on carbohydrate and lipid metabolism. The dosage used may be important in minimizing these adverse effects.

11. Aminoglutethimide administered concomitantly with PROVERA may significantly depress the bioavailability of PROVERA.

12. Safety and effectiveness in pediatric patients below the age of 12 years have not been established.

Carcinogenesis, Mutagenesis, Impairment of Fertility.
Long-term intramuscular administration of PROVERA has been shown to produce mammary tumors in beagle dogs (see WARNINGS). There was no evidence of a carcinogenic effect associated with the oral administration of PROVERA to rats and mice. Medroxyprogesterone acetate was not mutagenic in a battery of *in vitro* or *in vivo* genetic toxicity assays.

Medroxyprogesterone acetate at high doses is an antifertility drug and high doses would be expected to impair fertility until the cessation of treatment.

Information for the Patient

See Patient Information at end of insert.

ADVERSE REACTIONS

Pregnancy—(See WARNING Box for possible adverse effects on the fetus).

Breast—Breast tenderness or galactorrhea has been reported rarely.

Skin—Sensitivity reactions consisting of urticaria, pruritus, edema and generalized rash have occurred in an occasional patient. Acne, alopecia and hirsutism have been reported in a few cases.

Thromboembolic Phenomena—Thromboembolic phenomena including thrombophlebitis and pulmonary embolism have been reported.

The following adverse reactions have been observed in women taking progestins including PROVERA Tablets:

    breakthrough bleeding
    spotting
    change in menstrual flow
    amenorrhea
    edema
    change in weight
      (increase or decrease)
    changes in cervical erosion and cervical secretions
    cholestatic jaundice
    anaphylactoid reactions and anaphylaxis rash (allergic)
      with and without pruritus
    mental depression
    pyrexia
    insomnia
    nausea
    somnolence

A statistically significant association has been demonstrated between use of estrogen-progestin combination drugs and the following serious adverse reactions: thrombophlebitis; pulmonary embolism and cerebral thrombosis and embolism. For this reason patients on progestin therapy should be carefully observed.

Although available evidence is suggestive of an association, such a relationship has been neither confirmed nor refuted for the following serious adverse reactions:

    neuro-ocular lesions, eg, retinal thrombosis and optic
      neuritis.

The following adverse reactions have been observed in patients receiving estrogen-progestin combination drugs:

    rise in blood pressure in susceptible individuals
    premenstrual-like syndrome
    changes in libido
    changes in appetite
    cystitis-like syndrome
    headache
    nervousness
    fatigue
    backache
    hirsutism
    loss of scalp hair
    erythema multiforme
    erythema nodosum
    hemorrhagic eruption
    itching
    dizziness

In view of these observations, patients on progestin therapy should be carefully observed.

The following laboratory results may be altered by the use of estrogen-progestin combination drugs:

Increased sulfobromophthalein retention and other hepatic function tests.

Coagulation tests: increase in prothrombin factors VII, VIII, IX and X.

Metyrapone test.

Pregnanediol determination.

Thyroid function: increase in PBI, and butanol extractable protein bound iodine and decrease in T^3 uptake values.

DOSAGE AND ADMINISTRATION

Secondary Amenorrhea—PROVERA Tablets may be given in dosages of 5 to 10 mg daily for 5 to 10 days. A dose for

inducing an optimum secretory transformation of an endometrium that has been adequately primed with either endogenous or exogenous estrogen is 10 mg of PROVERA daily for 10 days. In cases of secondary amenorrhea, therapy may be started at any time. Progestin withdrawal bleeding usually occurs within three to seven days after discontinuing PROVERA therapy.

Abnormal Uterine Bleeding Due to Hormonal Imbalance in the Absence of Organic Pathology—Beginning on the calculated 16th or 21st day of the menstrual cycle, 5 to 10 mg of medroxyprogesterone acetate may be given daily for 5 to 10 days. To produce an optimum secretory transformation of an endometrium that has been adequately primed with either endogenous or exogenous estrogen, 10 mg of medroxyprogesterone acetate daily for 10 days beginning on the 16th day of the cycle is suggested. Progestin withdrawal bleeding usually occurs within three to seven days after discontinuing therapy with PROVERA. Patients with a past history of recurrent episodes of abnormal uterine bleeding may benefit from planned menstrual cycling with PROVERA.

HOW SUPPLIED

PROVERA Tablets are available in the following strengths and package sizes:

2.5 mg (scored, round, orange)

Bottles of 30	NDC 0009-0064-06
Bottles of 100	NDC 0009-0064-04

5 mg (scored, hexagonal, white)

Bottles of 30	NDC 0009-0286-32
Bottles of 100	NDC 0009-0286-03

10 mg (scored, round, white)

Bottles of 30	NDC 0009-0050-09
Bottles of 100	NDC 0009-0050-02
Bottles of 500	NDC 0009-0050-11

Store at controlled room temperature 20° to 25° C (68° to 77° F) [see USP].

REFERENCES

1. Royal College of General Practitioners: Oral contraception and thromboembolic disease. J Coll Gen Pract **13**: 267-279, 1967.
2. Inman WHW, Vessey MP: Investigation of deaths from pulmonary, coronary, and cerebral thrombosis and embolism in women of child-bearing age. Br Med J **2**:193-199, 1968.
3. Vessey MP, Doll R: Investigation of relation between use of oral contraceptives and thromboembolic disease. A further report. Br Med J **2**:651-657, 1969.
4. Sartwell PE, Masi AT, Arthes FG, et al: Thromboembolism and oral contraceptives: An epidemiological case-control study. Am J Epidemiol **90**:365-380, 1969.

The text of the patient insert for progesterone and progesterone-like drugs is set forth below.

PATIENT INFORMATION

PROVERA Tablets contain medroxyprogesterone acetate, a progesterone. The information below is that which the U.S. Food and Drug Administration requires be provided for all patients taking progesterones. The information below relates only to the risk to the unborn child associated with use of progesterone during pregnancy. For further information on the use, side effects and other risks associated with this product, ask your doctor.

WARNING FOR WOMEN

Progesterone or progesterone-like drugs have been used to prevent miscarriage in the first few months of pregnancy. No adequate evidence is available to show that they are effective for this purpose. Furthermore, most cases of early miscarriage are due to causes which could not be helped by these drugs.

There is an increased risk of minor birth defects in children whose mothers take this drug during the first 4 months of pregnancy. Several reports suggest an association between mothers who take these drugs in the first trimester of pregnancy and genital abnormalities in male and female babies. The risk to the male baby is the possibility of being born with a condition in which the opening of the penis is on the underside rather than the tip of the penis (hypospadias). Hypospadias occurs in about 5 to 8 per 1,000 male births and is about doubled with exposure to these drugs. There is not enough information to quantify the risk to exposed female fetuses, but enlargement of the clitoris and fusion of the labia may occur, although rarely.

Therefore, since drugs of this type may induce mild masculinization of the external genitalia of the female fetus, as well as hypospadias in the male fetus, it is wise to avoid using the drug during the first trimester of pregnancy.

These drugs have been used as a test for pregnancy but such use is no longer considered safe because of possible damage to a developing baby. Also, more rapid methods for testing for pregnancy are now available.

If you take PROVERA and later find you were pregnant when you took it, be sure to discuss this with your doctor as soon as possible.

Rx only

Pharmacia & Upjohn Company
Kalamazoo, MI 49001, USA

Revised April 1998 812 584 511
691015

Shown in Product Identification Guide, page 332

RESCRIPTOR
Tablets ℞
delavirdine mesylate tablets

> **WARNING:** RESCRIPTOR Tablets are indicated for the treatment of HIV-1 infection in combination with appropriate antiretroviral agents when therapy is warranted. This indication is based on surrogate marker changes in clinical studies. Clinical benefit was not demonstrated for RESCRIPTOR based on survival or incidence of AIDS-defining clinical events in a completed trial comparing RESCRIPTOR plus didanosine with didanosine monotherapy (see DESCRIPTION OF CLINICAL STUDIES).
> Resistant virus emerges rapidly when RESCRIPTOR is administered as monotherapy. Therefore, RESCRIPTOR should always be administered in combination with appropriate antiretroviral therapy.

DESCRIPTION

RESCRIPTOR Tablets contain delavirdine mesylate, a synthetic non-nucleoside reverse transcriptase inhibitor of the human immunodeficiency virus type 1 (HIV-1). The chemical name of delavirdine mesylate is piperazine, 1-[3-[(1-methyl-ethyl)amino]-2-pyridinyl]-4-[[5-[(methylsulfonyl)-amino]-1*H*-indol-2-yl]carbonyl]-, monomethanesulfonate. Its molecular formula is $C_{22}H_{28}N_6O_3S \bullet CH_4O_3S$, and its molecular weight is 552.68. The structural formula is:

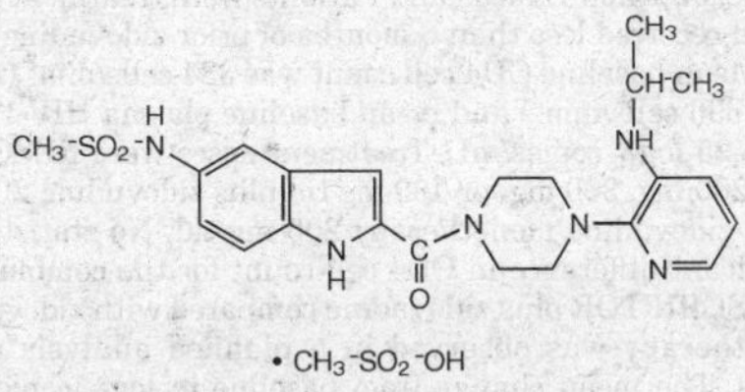

Delavirdine mesylate is an odorless white-to-tan crystalline powder. The aqueous solubility of delavirdine free base at 23°C is 2,942 µg/mL at pH 1.0, 295 µg/mL at pH 2.0, and 0.81 µg/mL at pH 7.4.

RESCRIPTOR Tablets, for oral administration, contain 100 mg of delavirdine mesylate (henceforth referred to as delavirdine). Inactive ingredients consist of lactose, microcrystalline cellulose, croscarmellose sodium, colloidal silicon dioxide, magnesium stearate, Opadry YS-1-7000-E White and carnauba wax.

MICROBIOLOGY

Mechanism of action: Delavirdine is a non-nucleoside reverse transcriptase inhibitor (NNRTI) of HIV-1. Delavirdine binds directly to reverse transcriptase (RT) and blocks RNA-dependent and DNA-dependent DNA polymerase activities. Delavirdine does not compete with template: primer or deoxynucleoside triphosphates. HIV-2 RT and human cellular DNA polymerases α, γ, or δ are not inhibited by delavirdine. In addition, HIV-1 group O, a group of highly divergent strains that are uncommon in North America, may not be inhibited by delavirdine.

In vitro HIV-1 susceptibility: In vitro anti–HIV-1 activity of delavirdine was assessed by infecting cell lines of lymphoblastic and monocytic origin and peripheral blood lymphocytes with laboratory and clinical isolates of HIV-1. IC_{50} and IC_{90} values (50% and 90% inhibitory concentrations) for laboratory isolates (N=5) ranged from 0.005 to 0.030 µM and 0.04 to 0.10 µM, respectively. Mean IC_{50} of clinical isolates (N=74) was 0.038 µM (range 0.001 to 0.69 µM); 73 of 74 clinical isolates had an $IC_{50} \leq 0.18$ µM. The IC_{90} of 24 of these clinical isolates ranged from 0.05 to 0.10 µM. In drug combination studies of delavirdine with zidovudine, didanosine, zalcitabine, lamivudine, interferon-α, and protease inhibitors, additive to synergistic anti–HIV-1 activity was observed in cell culture. The relationship between the in vitro susceptibility of HIV-1 RT inhibitors and the inhibition of HIV replication in humans has not been established.

Drug resistance: Phenotypic analyses of isolates from patients treated with delavirdine as monotherapy showed a 50-fold to 500-fold reduction in sensitivity in 14 of 15 patients by week 8 of therapy. Genotypic analyses of HIV-1 isolates from patients receiving delavirdine plus zidovudine combination therapy (N=19) showed mutations in 16 of 19 isolates by week 24 of therapy. Mutations occurred predominantly at position 103 and less frequently at positions 181 and 236. In a separate study, an average 86-fold increase in the zidovudine sensitivity of patient isolates (N=24) was observed after 24 weeks on delavirdine and zidovudine combination therapy. The clinical relevance of the phenotypic and the genotypic changes associated with delavirdine therapy has not been determined.

Cross-resistance: Rapid emergence of HIV strains that are cross-resistant to certain NNRTIs has been observed in vitro. Mutations at positions 103 and 181 have been associated with resistance to other NNRTIs. RESCRIPTOR may confer cross-resistance to other non-nucleoside reverse transcriptase inhibitors when used alone or in combination.

The potential for cross-resistance between delavirdine and protease inhibitors is low because of the different enzyme targets involved. The potential for cross-resistance between NNRTIs and nucleoside analogue RT inhibitors is low because of different sites of binding on the viral RT and distinct mechanisms of action.

CLINICAL PHARMACOLOGY

Pharmacokinetics

Absorption and Bioavailability: Delavirdine is rapidly absorbed following oral administration, with peak plasma concentrations occurring at approximately one hour. Following administration of delavirdine 400 mg tid (n=67, HIV-1–infected patients), the mean ± SD steady-state peak plasma concentration (C_{max}) was 35 ± 20 µM (range 2 to 100 µM), systemic exposure (AUC) was 180 ± 100 µM • hr (range 5 to 515 µM • hr) and trough concentration (C_{min}) was 15 ± 10 µM (range 0.1 to 45 µM). The single-dose bioavailability of delavirdine tablets relative to an oral solution was 85 ± 25% (n=16, non-HIV–infected subjects). The single-dose bioavailability of delavirdine tablets was increased by approximately 20% when a slurry of drug was prepared by allowing delavirdine tablets to disintegrate in water before administration (n=16, non-HIV–infected subjects).

Delavirdine may be administered with or without food. Following single-dose administration of delavirdine tablets with a high-fat meal (874 kcal, 57 g fat), mean C_{max} was decreased by 60% and mean AUC was decreased by 26%, relative to fasted administration (n=12, non-HIV–infected subjects). In a multiple-dose study, delavirdine was administered every eight hours with food or every eight hours, one hour before or two hours after a meal (n=13, HIV-1–infected patients). Patients remained on their typical diet throughout the study; meal content was not standardized. When multiple doses of delavirdine were administered with food, mean C_{max} was reduced by 22% but AUC and C_{min} were not altered.

Distribution: Delavirdine is extensively bound (approximately 98%) to plasma proteins, primarily albumin. The percentage of delavirdine that is protein bound is constant over a delavirdine concentration range of 0.5 to 196 µM. In five HIV-1–infected patients whose total daily dose of delavirdine ranged from 600 to 1200 mg, cerebrospinal fluid concentrations of delavirdine averaged 0.4% ± 0.07% of the corresponding plasma delavirdine concentrations; this represents about 20% of the fraction not bound to plasma proteins. Steady-state delavirdine concentrations in saliva (n=5, HIV-1–infected patients who received delavirdine 400 mg tid) and semen (n=5 healthy volunteers who received delavirdine 300 mg tid) were about 6% and 2%, respectively, of the corresponding plasma delavirdine concentrations collected at the end of a dosing interval.

Metabolism and Elimination: Delavirdine is extensively converted to several inactive metabolites. Delavirdine is primarily metabolized by cytochrome P450 3A (CYP3A), but in vitro data suggest that delavirdine may also be metabolized by CYP2D6. The major metabolic pathways for delavirdine are N-desalkylation and pyridine hydroxylation. Delavirdine exhibits nonlinear steady-state elimination pharmacokinetics, with apparent oral clearance decreasing by about 22-fold as the total daily dose of delavirdine increases from 60 to 1200 mg/day. In a study of ^{14}C-delavirdine in six healthy volunteers who received multiple doses of delavirdine tablets 300 mg tid, approximately 44% of the radio labeled dose was recovered in feces, and approximately 51% of the dose was excreted in urine. Less than 5% of the dose was recovered unchanged in urine. The apparent plasma half-life of delavirdine increases with dose; mean half-life following 400 mg tid is 5.8 hours, with a range of 2 to 11 hours.

In vitro and in vivo studies have shown that delavirdine reduces CYP3A activity and inhibits its own metabolism. In vitro studies have also shown that delavirdine reduces CYP2C9 and CYP2C19 activity. Inhibition of CYP3A by delavirdine is reversible within 1 week after discontinuation of drug.

Special Populations

Hepatic or Renal Impairment: The pharmacokinetics of delavirdine in patients with hepatic or renal impairment have not been investigated (see PRECAUTIONS).

Continued on next page

Information on these Pharmacia & Upjohn products is based on labeling in effect June 1, 1998. Further information concerning these and other Pharmacia & Upjohn products may be obtained by direct inquiry to Medical Information, Pharmacia & Upjohn, Kalamazoo, MI 49001.

Rescriptor—Cont.

Age: The pharmacokinetics of delavirdine have not been studied in patients <16 years or >65 years of age.

Gender: Following administration of delavirdine (400 mg every eight hours), median delavirdine AUC was 31% higher in female patients (n=12) than in male patients (n=55).

Race: No significant differences in the mean trough delavirdine concentrations were observed between different racial or ethnic groups.

Drug Interactions (see also PRECAUTIONS—Drug Interactions)

Antacids: In a single-dose study in twelve healthy volunteers, simultaneous administration of 300 mg delavirdine with alumina and magnesia oral suspension resulted in a 41 ± 19% reduction in delavirdine AUC (see PRECAUTIONS—Drug Interactions).

Clarithromycin: In a study in six HIV-1–infected patients, coadministration of clarithromycin (500 mg bid) with delavirdine (300 mg tid) resulted in a 44 ± 50% increase in delavirdine AUC. Compared to historical data, clarithromycin AUC was increased by approximately 100% and 14-hydroxyclarithromycin AUC was decreased by 75%.

Didanosine: In a study in nine HIV-1–infected patients, simultaneous administration of didanosine (125 mg or 250 mg bid) with delavirdine (400 mg tid) for two weeks resulted in an approximately 20% decrease in both didanosine AUC and delavirdine AUC, relative to when administration of delavirdine and didanosine was separated by at least one hour (see PRECAUTIONS—Drug Interactions).

Fluconazole: In a study in eight HIV-1–infected patients, coadministration of fluconazole (400 mg once daily) with delavirdine (300 mg tid) did not significantly alter the pharmacokinetics of delavirdine. Compared to historical data, fluconazole pharmacokinetics were not altered by delavirdine.

Fluoxetine: Population pharmacokinetic data available for 36 patients suggest that fluoxetine increases trough plasma delavirdine concentrations by about 50%.

Indinavir: Preliminary data (n=14) indicate that delavirdine inhibits the metabolism of indinavir such that coadministration of a 400 mg single dose of indinavir with delavirdine (400 mg tid) resulted in indinavir AUC values slightly less than those observed following administration of an 800 mg dose of indinavir alone. Also, coadministration of a 600 mg dose of indinavir with delavirdine (400 mg tid) resulted in indinavir AUC values approximately 40% greater than those observed following administration of an 800 mg dose of indinavir alone. Indinavir had no effect on delavirdine pharmacokinetics (see PRECAUTIONS—Drug Interactions).

Ketoconazole: Population pharmacokinetic data available for 26 patients suggest that ketoconazole increases trough plasma delavirdine concentrations by about 50%.

Phenytoin, Phenobarbital, and Carbamazepine: Population pharmacokinetic data available for eight patients suggest that coadministration of phenytoin, phenobarbital, or carbamazepine with delavirdine results in a substantial reduction in trough plasma delavirdine concentrations (see PRECAUTIONS—Drug Interactions).

Rifabutin: In a study in seven HIV-1–infected patients, coadministration of rifabutin (300 mg once daily) with delavirdine (400 mg tid) resulted in an 80 ± 10% decrease in delavirdine AUC. Compared to historical data, rifabutin AUC was increased by at least 100% (see PRECAUTIONS—Drug Interactions).

Rifampin: In a study in seven HIV-1–infected patients, coadministration of rifampin (600 mg once daily) with delavirdine (400 mg tid) resulted in a 96 ± 4% decrease in delavirdine AUC (see PRECAUTIONS—Drug Interactions).

Ritonavir: Preliminary data (n=13) indicate that coadministration of delavirdine (400 mg or 600 mg bid) with ritonavir (300 mg bid) did not alter ritonavir pharmacokinetics. Coadministration of ritonavir (300 mg bid) with delavirdine (400 mg bid) did not significantly alter delavirdine pharmacokinetics (n=9). The pharmacokinetic interaction between delavirdine and ritonavir at their recommended doses has not been studied (see PRECAUTIONS—Drug Interactions).

Saquinavir: In 13 healthy volunteers, coadministration of saquinavir (600 mg tid) with delavirdine (400 mg tid) resulted in a five-fold increase in saquinavir AUC. In seven healthy volunteers, coadministration of saquinavir (600 mg tid) with delavirdine (400 mg tid) resulted in a 15 ± 16% decrease in delavirdine AUC (see PRECAUTIONS—Drug Interactions).

Sulfamethoxazole and Trimethoprim/Sulfamethoxazole (TMP/SMX): Population pharmacokinetic data available for 311 patients suggest that the pharmacokinetics of delavirdine are not affected by sulfamethoxazole or TMP/SMX.

Zidovudine: Zidovudine and delavirdine do not alter one another's pharmacokinetics.

INDICATIONS AND USAGE

RESCRIPTOR Tablets are indicated for the treatment of HIV-1 infection in combination with appropriate antiretroviral agents when therapy is warranted. This indication is based on surrogate marker changes in clinical studies. Clinical benefit was not demonstrated for RESCRIPTOR based on survival or incidence of AIDS-defining clinical events in a completed trial comparing RESCRIPTOR plus didanosine with didanosine monotherapy (see DESCRIPTION OF CLINICAL STUDIES).

Resistant virus emerges rapidly when RESCRIPTOR is administered as monotherapy. Therefore, RESCRIPTOR should always be administered in combination with appropriate antiretroviral therapy.

DESCRIPTION OF CLINICAL STUDIES

In two of the clinical studies described below (Study 0021, Part 1 and Study 0017), an experimental HIV nucleic acid amplification assay was used to estimate the level of circulating HIV RNA in plasma. In the clinical study ACTG 261, also described below, an approved HIV nucleic acid amplification assay was used.

Figures 1-3 below present results for all patients with data available at the time points shown. The decrease in sample size reflects patients leaving the study, missed visits, and those who had not reached specified time points at data cutoff. In general, patients who left the study had lower CD4 cell counts and higher plasma HIV RNA values than patients remaining on study. Therefore, absolute changes from baseline are overstated in all treatment arms, increasingly so at later time points. However, the added effect of delavirdine treatment relative to the control arms does not appear to be significantly affected by patient dropout.

Study 0021, Part 1: RESCRIPTOR-Zidovudine Dual Therapy Trial

Study 0021, Part 1 was a randomized, double-blind trial comparing treatment with RESCRIPTOR plus zidovudine and zidovudine monotherapy in 718 HIV-1–infected patients (median age 34.3 years [range 17 to 70 years], 19% female, 32% non-Caucasian). Patients were treatment naive or had received less than 6 months of prior zidovudine therapy. Mean baseline CD4 cell count was 334 cells/mm^3 (range 75 to 696 cells/mm^3) and mean baseline plasma HIV-1 RNA was 5.25 $\log_{10}$ copies/mL. Treatment doses were RESCRIPTOR 200 mg, 300 mg, or 400 mg tid plus zidovudine 200 mg tid or zidovudine monotherapy 200 mg tid. No statistically significant difference in CD4 cell count for the combination of RESCRIPTOR plus zidovudine compared with zidovudine monotherapy was observed in a planned analysis at 24 weeks. The mean change from baseline in $\log_{10}$ copies/mL plasma HIV-1 RNA is summarized in Fig 1 for RESCRIPTOR 400 mg tid plus zidovudine and zidovudine monotherapy. All patients had not completed 52 weeks at the time of this analysis.

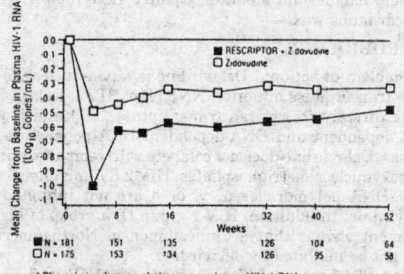

Fig 1: Mean Change From Baseline in Plasma HIV-1 RNA* Study 0021

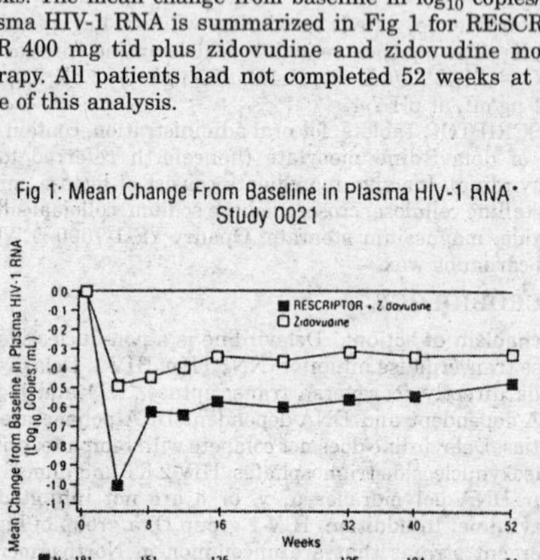

*Clinical significance of changes in plasma HIV-1 RNA levels has not been established.

Study 0017 RESCRIPTOR-Didanosine Dual Therapy Trial

Study 0017 was a randomized, double-blind trial comparing treatment with RESCRIPTOR plus didanosine versus didanosine monotherapy in 1,190 HIV-1–infected patients (median age 37.4 years [range 19 to 78 years], 13% female, 32% non-Caucasian). Patients had received up to 4 months prior didanosine therapy; there were no restrictions on prior zidovudine use. Mean baseline CD4 cell count was 142 cells/mm^3 (range 0 to 541 cells/mm^3) and mean baseline plasma HIV-1 RNA was 5.77 $\log_{10}$ copies/mL. Treatment doses were RESCRIPTOR 400 mg tid plus didanosine or didanosine monotherapy. The dose of didanosine was adjusted by body weight (<60 kg, 125 mg bid; >60 kg, 200 mg bid). Mean changes from baseline in CD4 cell count and $\log_{10}$ copies/mL plasma HIV-1 RNA are summarized in Figs 2 and 3, respectively. All patients had not completed 52 weeks at the time of this analysis.

[See figures 2 & 3 at top of next column]

An analysis of clinical efficacy end points (death, clinical progression defined as time to AIDS or death) was performed when all patients had completed at least 6 months in the trial. Comparable rates of deaths and AIDS progression between the didanosine monotherapy arm and the combination of RESCRIPTOR plus didanosine arm were observed. Refer to Fig 4.

Fig 2: Mean Change From Baseline in CD4 Cell Counts Study 0017

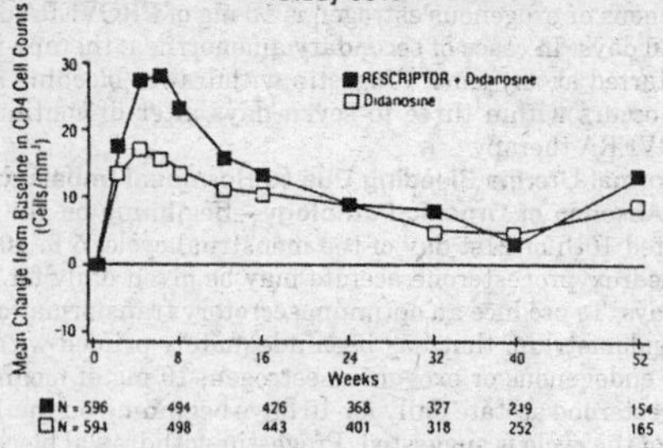

Fig 3: Mean Change From Baseline in Plasma HIV-1 RNA* Study 0017

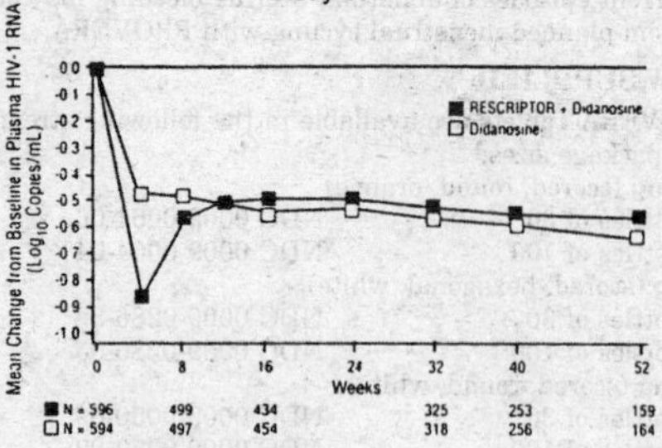

*Clinical significance of changes in plasma HIV-1 RNA levels has not been established.

Fig 4: Time to Clinical Progression or Death Study 0017

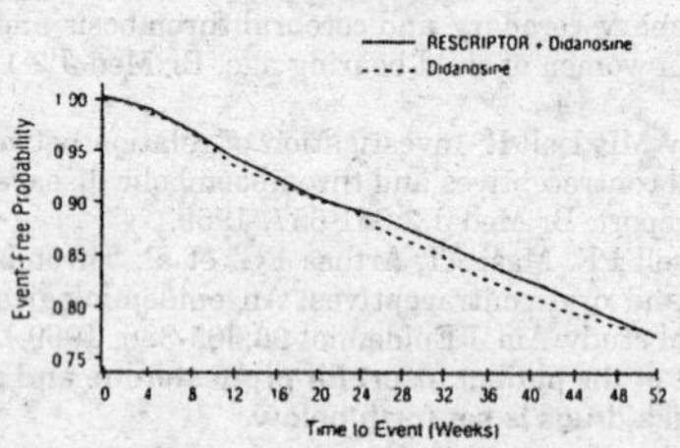

ACTG 261: RESCRIPTOR-Zidovudine-Didanosine Triple Therapy Trial

AIDS Clinical Trials Group (ACTG) Protocol 261 was a randomized trial comparing the following four treatment regimens: RESCRIPTOR plus didanosine, RESCRIPTOR plus zidovudine, RESCRIPTOR plus didanosine and zidovudine, and zidovudine plus didanosine. The study enrolled 544 HIV-1–infected patients (median age 35 years, 18% female and 44% non-Caucasian patients) who were either nucleoside treatment naive or had prior treatment with zidovudine or didanosine (not both) for less than 6 months. Thirty-seven percent reported previous antiretroviral therapy (194 patients with zidovudine and 6 with didanosine). Mean baseline CD4 cell count was 296 cells/mm^3 (range 55 to 640 cells/mm^3). Median baseline plasma HIV-1 RNA level (available for 229 patients) was 4.45 $\log_{10}$ copies/mL (28,260 copies/mL). Treatment doses were RESCRIPTOR 400 mg tid, zidovudine 200 mg tid, and didanosine dose adjusted by body weight (<60 kg, 125 mg bid; >60 kg, 200 mg bid).

Preliminary results showed no statistically significant difference in CD4 cell count for the three drug combination of RESCRIPTOR, zidovudine, and didanosine compared with the combination of zidovudine plus didanosine. No statistically significant difference in plasma HIV-1 RNA for the three-drug combination of RESCRIPTOR, zidovudine, and didanosine compared with the combination of zidovudine plus didanosine was observed. The mean change from baseline in CD4 cell count is shown in Fig 5. The mean change from baseline in plasma HIV-1 RNA is displayed through week 32 due to the small number of subjects having HIV-1 RNA determinations at week 48 and is shown in Fig 6.

[See figures 5 & 6 at top of next column]

CONTRAINDICATIONS

RESCRIPTOR Tablets are contraindicated in patients with previously demonstrated clinically significant hypersensitivity to any of the components of the formulation.

WARNINGS

Coadministration of RESCRIPTOR Tablets with certain nonsedating antihistamines, sedative hypnotics, antiarrhythmics, calcium channel blockers, ergot alkaloid preparations, amphetamines, and cisapride, may result in poten-

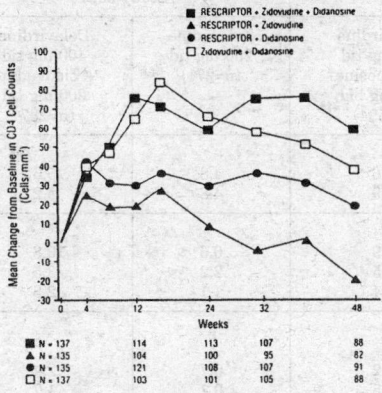

Fig 5: Mean Change From Baseline in CD4 Cell Counts ACTG 261

Symbol	N				
RESCRIPTOR + Zidovudine + Didanosine	N = 137	114	113	107	88
RESCRIPTOR + Zidovudine	N = 135	104	100	95	82
RESCRIPTOR + Didanosine	N = 135	121	108	107	91
Zidovudine + Didanosine	N = 137	103	101	105	88

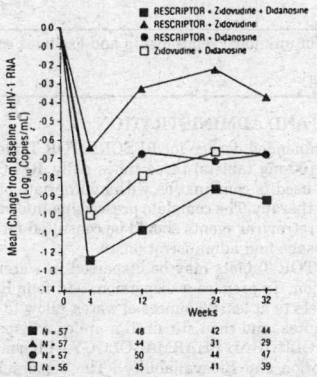

Fig 6: Mean Change From Baseline in Plasma HIV-1 RNA*, ACTG 261

Symbol	N				
RESCRIPTOR + Zidovudine + Didanosine	N = 57	48	42	44	
RESCRIPTOR + Zidovudine	N = 57	44	31	29	
RESCRIPTOR + Didanosine	N = 57	50	44	47	
Zidovudine + Didanosine	N = 56	45	41	39	

*Clinical significance of changes in plasma HIV-1 RNA levels has not been established.

tially serious and/or life-threatening adverse events due to possible effects of RESCRIPTOR on the hepatic metabolism of certain drugs (see PRECAUTIONS section).

PRECAUTIONS

General: Delavirdine is metabolized primarily by the liver. Therefore, caution should be exercised when administering RESCRIPTOR Tablets to patients with impaired hepatic function.

Resistance/Cross-Resistance: Non-nucleoside reverse transcriptase inhibitors, when used alone or in combination, may confer cross-resistance to other non-nucleoside reverse transcriptase inhibitors.

Skin Rash: Skin rash attributable to RESCRIPTOR has occurred in 18% of all patients in combination regimens in phase II and III controlled trials who received RESCRIPTOR 400 mg tid. Forty-two percent to 50% of patients treated with RESCRIPTOR 400 mg tid in Studies 0021 and 0017 experienced rash compared with 24% to 32% of patients receiving monotherapy with zidovudine or didanosine, respectively. In Studies 0021 and 0017, 4.3% of patients treated with RESCRIPTOR 400 mg tid discontinued treatment due to rash. Dose titration did not significantly reduce the incidence of rash. Rash was typically diffuse, maculopapular, erythematous, and often pruritic. Skin rash was more common in patients with lower CD4 cell counts and usually occurred within 1 to 3 weeks (median = 11 days) of treatment. Rash classified as severe was observed in 3.6% of patients in Studies 0021 and 0017. In most cases, the duration of the rash was less than 2 weeks and did not require dose reduction or discontinuation of RESCRIPTOR. Most patients were able to resume therapy after rechallenge with RESCRIPTOR following a treatment interruption due to rash. The distribution of the rash was mainly on the upper body and proximal arms, with decreasing intensity of the lesions on the neck and face, and progressively less on the rest of the trunk and limbs. Erythema multiforme and Stevens-Johnson syndrome were rarely seen and resolved after withdrawal of RESCRIPTOR. Any patient experiencing severe rash or rash accompanied by symptoms such as fever, blistering, oral lesions, conjunctivitis, swelling, muscle or joint aches should discontinue RESCRIPTOR and consult a physician. Occurrence of a delavirdine-related rash after 1 month of therapy is uncommon unless prolonged interruption of treatment with RESCRIPTOR occurs. Symptomatic relief has been obtained using diphenhydramine hydrochloride, hydroxyzine hydrochloride, and/or topical corticosteroids.

Information for Patients: Patients should be informed that RESCRIPTOR is not a cure for HIV-1 infection and that they may continue to acquire illnesses associated with HIV-1 infection, including opportunistic infections. Treatment with RESCRIPTOR has not been shown to reduce the incidence or frequency of such illnesses, and patients should be advised to remain under the care of a physician when using RESCRIPTOR.

Patients should be advised that the long-term effects of treatment with RESCRIPTOR are unknown at this time. They should be advised that the use of RESCRIPTOR has not been shown to reduce the risk of transmission of HIV-1. Patients should be instructed that the major toxicity of RESCRIPTOR is rash and should be advised to promptly notify their physician should rash occur. The majority of rashes associated with RESCRIPTOR occur within 1 to 3 weeks after initiating treatment with RESCRIPTOR. The rash normally resolves in 3 to 14 days and may be treated symptomatically while therapy with RESCRIPTOR is continued. Any patient experiencing severe rash or rash accompanied by symptoms such as fever, blistering, oral lesions, conjunctivitis, swelling, muscle or joint aches should discontinue medication and consult a physician.

Patients should be informed to take RESCRIPTOR every day as prescribed. Patients should not alter the dose of RESCRIPTOR without consulting their doctor. If a dose is missed, patients should take the next dose as soon as possible. However, if a dose is skipped, the patient should not double the next dose.

Patients with achlorhydria should take RESCRIPTOR with an acidic beverage (eg, orange or cranberry juice). However, the effect of an acidic beverage on the absorption of delavirdine in patients with achlorhydria has not been investigated.

Patients taking both RESCRIPTOR and antacids should be advised to take them at least one hour apart.

Because RESCRIPTOR may interact with certain drugs, patients should be advised to report to their doctor the use of any prescription or over-the-counter medications.

Drug Interactions (see also CLINICAL PHARMACOLOGY-Pharmacokinetics-Drug Interactions)

General: Coadministration of RESCRIPTOR with certain nonsedating antihistamines, sedative hypnotics, antiarrhythmics, calcium channel blockers, ergot alkaloid preparations, amphetamines, and cisapride, may result in potentially serious and/or life-threatening adverse events. Due to the inhibitory effect of delavirdine on CYP3A and CYP2C9, coadministration of RESCRIPTOR with drugs primarily metabolized by these liver enzymes may result in increased plasma concentrations. Higher plasma concentrations of these drugs could increase or prolong both therapeutic and adverse effects (Table 1). Therefore, appropriate dose adjustments may be necessary for these drugs. Drugs that induce CYP3A may also reduce plasma delavirdine concentrations (Table 2). Physicians should consider using alternatives to drugs that induce CYP3A while a patient is taking RESCRIPTOR.

Table 1. Selected Drugs that are Predicted to Have Plasma Concentrations Increased by Delavirdine*

HIV protease inhibitors: Indinavir, saquinavir
Antihistamines: terfenadine,† astemizole†
Antimicrobial agents: clarithromycin, dapsone, rifabutin
Anti-migraine agents: ergot derivatives
Benzodiazepines: alprazolam,† midazolam,† triazolam†
Calcium channel blockers: dihydropyridines, eg, nifedipine
GI motility agents: cisapride†
Other: quinidine, warfarin

*This table is not all inclusive.
†See WARNINGS.

Table 2. Selected Drugs that are Predicted to Decrease Plasma Delavirdine Concentrations‡§

Anticonvulsants: carbamazepine, phenobarbital, phenytoin
Antimycobacterial agents: rifabutin, rifampin

‡This table is not all inclusive.
§RESCRIPTOR may not be effective when administered concomitantly with these drugs.

Antacids: Doses of an antacid and RESCRIPTOR should be separated by at least one hour, because the absorption of delavirdine is reduced when coadministered with antacids.

Anticonvulsant Agents: *Phenytoin, phenobarbital, carbamazepine:* Coadministration with these agents is not recommended, because limited population pharmacokinetic data indicate that a substantial reduction in plasma delavirdine concentrations may result (see CLINICAL PHARMACOLOGY—Pharmacokinetics).

Antimycobacterial Agents:
Rifabutin: Coadministration of delavirdine and rifabutin is not recommended, because rifabutin substantially de-

creases plasma delavirdine concentrations and delavirdine increases plasma concentrations of rifabutin (see CLINICAL PHARMACOLOGY—Pharmacokinetics).
Rifampin: Delavirdine should not be coadministered with rifampin, because rifampin reduces delavirdine systemic exposure (AUC) by almost 100% (see CLINICAL PHARMACOLOGY—Pharmacokinetics).

H₂ Receptor Antagonists:
Cimetidine, famotidine, nizatidine, and ranitidine: These agents increase gastric pH and may reduce the absorption of delavirdine. Although the effect of these drugs on delavirdine absorption has not been evaluated, chronic use of these drugs with delavirdine is not recommended.

Nucleoside Analogue Reverse Transcriptase Inhibitors:
Didanosine: Administration of didanosine and delavirdine should be separated by at least one hour, because coadministration of didanosine and delavirdine resulted in reduced systemic exposure to both drugs by approximately 20% (see CLINICAL PHARMACOLOGY—Pharmacokinetics).

Protease Inhibitors (see CLINICAL PHARMACOLOGY—Pharmacokinetics):
Indinavir: Due to an increase in indinavir plasma concentrations (preliminary results), a dose reduction of indinavir to 600 mg tid should be considered when delavirdine and indinavir are coadministered. Currently, there are no safety and efficacy data available from the use of this combination.
Ritonavir: No studies have been conducted with combination therapy of delavirdine and ritonavir at their recommended doses. Preliminary results indicate there is no evidence of an interaction at doses of delavirdine 400 mg to 600 mg bid and ritonavir 300 mg bid. Currently, there are no safety and efficacy data available from the use of this combination.
Saquinavir: Saquinavir AUC increased 5-fold when delavirdine (400 mg tid) and saquinavir (600 mg tid) were administered in combination. Currently, there are limited safety and no efficacy data available from the use of this combination. In a small, preliminary study, hepatocellular enzyme elevations occurred in 13% of subjects during the first several weeks of the delavirdine and saquinavir combination (6% grade 3 or 4). Hepatocellular enzymes (ALT/AST) should be monitored frequently if this combination is prescribed.

Carcinogenesis, Mutagenesis and Impairment of Fertility: Long-term carcinogenicity studies with delavirdine in animals have not been completed. A battery of genetic toxicology tests was conducted with delavirdine, including the Ames assay, in vitro unscheduled DNA synthesis (UDS) assay, an in vitro cytogenetics (chromosome aberration) assay in human peripheral lymphocytes, a mammalian mutation assay in Chinese hamster ovary cells, and the micronucleus test in mice. The results were negative indicating delavirdine is not mutagenic.

Delavirdine at doses of 20, 100, and 200 mg/kg/day did not cause impairment of fertility in rats when males were treated for 70 days and females were treated for 14 days prior to mating.

Pregnancy: Pregnancy Category C: Delavirdine has been shown to be teratogenic in rats. Delavirdine caused ventricular septal defects in rats at doses of 50, 100, and 200 mg/kg/day when administered during the period of organogenesis. The lowest dose of delavirdine that caused malformations produced systemic exposures in pregnant rats equal to or lower than the expected human exposure to RESCRIPTOR ($C_{min} \approx 15$ μM) at the recommended dose. Exposure in rats approximately 5-fold higher than the expected human exposure resulted in marked maternal toxicity, embryotoxicity, fetal developmental delay, and reduced pup survival. Additionally, reduced pup survival on postpartum day 0 occurred at an exposure (mean C_{min}) approximately equal to the expected human exposure. Delavirdine was excreted in the milk of lactating rats at a concentration three to five times that of rat plasma.

Delavirdine at doses of 200 and 400 mg/kg/day administered during the period of organogenesis caused maternal toxicity, embryotoxicity and abortions in rabbits. The lowest dose of delavirdine that resulted in these toxic effects produced systemic exposures in pregnant rabbits approximately 6-fold higher than the expected human exposure to RESCRIPTOR ($C_{min} \approx 15$ μM) at the recommended dose. The no-observed-adverse-effect dose in the pregnant rabbit was 100 mg/kg/day. Various malformations were observed at this dose, but the incidence of such malformations was not statistically significantly different from those observed in the control group. Systemic exposures in pregnant rabbits at a dose of 100 mg/kg/day were lower than those expected in

Continued on next page

Information on these Pharmacia & Upjohn products is based on labeling in effect June 1, 1998. Further information concerning these and other Pharmacia & Upjohn products may be obtained by direct inquiry to Medical Information, Pharmacia & Upjohn, Kalamazoo, MI 49001.

Rescriptor—Cont.

humans at the recommended clinical dose. Malformations were not apparent at 200 and 400 mg/kg/day; however, only a limited number of fetuses were available for examination as a result of maternal and embryo death.

No adequate and well-controlled studies in pregnant women have been conducted. RESCRIPTOR should be used during pregnancy only if the potential benefit justifies the potential risk to the fetus. Of 7 unplanned pregnancies reported in premarketing clinical studies, 3 were ectopic pregnancies and 3 pregnancies resulted in healthy live births. One infant was born prematurely with a small muscular ventricular septal defect to a patient who received approximately six weeks of treatment with delavirdine and zidovudine early in the course of the pregnancy.

Nursing Mothers: The U.S. Public Health Services Centers for Disease Control and Prevention advises HIV-infected women not to breast-feed to avoid postnatal transmission of HIV to a child who may not yet be infected.

Pediatric Use: Safety and effectiveness of delavirdine in combination with other antiretroviral agents have not been established in HIV-1–infected individuals younger than 16 years of age.

ADVERSE REACTIONS

The safety of RESCRIPTOR Tablets alone and in combination with other therapies has been studied in 1,969 patients receiving RESCRIPTOR.

Adverse events of moderate or severe intensity reported in ≥ 2% of patients receiving RESCRIPTOR in combination with didanosine or zidovudine in Studies 0017 and 0021 are summarized in Table 3. The median duration of treatment in Studies 0017 and 0021 was 34 and 42 weeks (up to 107 weeks for both studies), respectively, at the time of the safety assessment. The most frequently reported drug-related medical event was rash (see PRECAUTIONS—Skin Rash).

[See table 3 above]

Medical events occurring in less than 2% of patients receiving RESCRIPTOR (in combination treatment) in all phase II and III studies, considered possibly related to treatment, and of at least ACTG grade 2 in intensity are listed below by body system.

Body as a Whole: Abdominal cramps, abdominal distention, abdominal pain (generalized or localized), allergic reaction, asthenia, back pain, chest pain, chills, edema (generalized or localized), epidermal cyst, fever, flank pain, flu syndrome, lethargy, lip edema, malaise, neck rigidity, pain (generalized or localized), sebaceous cyst, trauma, and upper respiratory infection.

Cardiovascular System: Bradycardia, migraine, pallor, palpitation, postural hypotension, syncope, tachycardia, and vasodilation.

Digestive System: Anorexia, aphthous stomatitis, bloody stool, colitis, constipation, decreased appetite, diarrhea (*Clostridium difficile*), diverticulitis, duodenitis, dry mouth, dyspepsia, dysphagia, enteritis, esophagitis, fecal incontinence, flatulence, gagging, gastritis, gastroesophageal reflux, gastrointestinal bleeding, gastrointestinal disorder, gingivitis, gum hemorrhage, increased appetite, increased saliva, increased thirst, mouth ulcer, nonspecific hepatitis, pancreatitis, rectal disorder, sialadenitis, stomatitis, and tongue edema or ulceration.

Hemic and Lymphatic System: Anemia, bruise, ecchymosis, eosinophilia, granulocytosis, neutropenia, pancytopenia, petechia, prolonged partial thromboplastin time, purpura, spleen disorder, and thrombocytopenia.

Metabolic and Nutritional Disorders: Alcohol intolerance, bilirubinemia, hyperkalemia, hyperuricemia, hypocalcemia, hyponatremia, hypophosphatemia, increased gamma glutamyl transpeptidase, increased lipase, increased serum alkaline phosphatase, increased serum amylase, increased serum creatine phosphokinase, increased serum creatinine, peripheral edema, and weight increase or decrease.

Musculoskeletal System: Arthralgia or arthritis of single and multiple joints, bone disorder, bone pain, leg cramps, muscular weakness, myalgia, tendon disorder, tenosynovitis, and tetany.

Nervous System: Abnormal coordination, agitation, amnesia, anxiety, change in dreams, cognitive impairment, confusion, decreased libido, depressive symptoms, disorientation, dizziness, emotional lability, hallucination, hyperesthesia, hyperreflexia, hypesthesia, impaired concentration, insomnia, manic symptoms, muscle cramp, nervousness, neuropathy, nightmares, nystagmus, paralysis, paranoid symptoms, paresthesia, restlessness, somnolence, tingling, tremor, vertigo, and weakness.

Respiratory System: Bronchitis, chest congestion, cough, dyspnea, epistaxis, laryngismus, pharyngitis, rhinitis, and sinusitis.

Skin and Appendages: Angioedema, dermal leukocytoclastic vasculitis, dermatitis, desquamation, diaphoresis, dry skin, erythema, erythema multiforme, folliculitis, fungal derma-

titis, hair loss, nail disorder, petechial rash, seborrhea, skin disorder, skin nodule, Stevens-Johnson syndrome, urticaria, and vesiculobullous rash.

Special Senses: Blepharitis, conjunctivitis, diplopia, dry eyes, ear pain, photophobia, taste perversion, and tinnitus.

Urogenital System: Breast enlargement, calculi of the kidney, epididymitis, hematuria, hemospermia, impotence, kidney pain, metrorrhagia, nocturia, polyuria, proteinuria, and vaginal moniliasis.

Laboratory Abnormalities: The frequency of clinically important laboratory abnormalities observed during therapy in Studies 0017 and 0021 is summarized in Table 4. There was no significant difference in ACTG grades 3 and 4 laboratory abnormalities between treatment groups except a two-fold reduction in neutropenia in the delavirdine plus zidovudine combination group compared with the zidovudine monotherapy group in Study 0021.

[See table 4 below]

OVERDOSAGE

No reports of overdose with RESCRIPTOR Tablets are available in humans. Several patients have received up to 850 mg tid for up to 6 months with no serious drug-related medical events.

Management of Overdosage: Treatment of overdosage with RESCRIPTOR should consist of general supportive measures, including monitoring of vital signs and observation of the patient's clinical status. There is no specific antidote for overdosage with RESCRIPTOR. If indicated, elimination of unabsorbed drug should be achieved by emesis or gastric lavage. Since delavirdine is extensively metabolized by the liver and is highly protein bound, dialysis is unlikely to be beneficial in significant removal of the drug.

DOSAGE AND ADMINISTRATION

The recommended dosage for RESCRIPTOR Tablets is 400 mg (four 100-mg tablets) three times daily. RESCRIPTOR should be used in combination with appropriate other antiretroviral therapy. The complete prescribing information for other antiretroviral agents should be consulted for information on dosage and administration.

RESCRIPTOR Tablets may be dispersed in water prior to consumption. To prepare a dispersion, add four RESCRIPTOR Tablets to at least 3 ounces of water, allow to stand for a few minutes, and then stir until a uniform dispersion occurs (see CLINICAL PHARMACOLOGY—Pharmacokinetics-Absorption and Bioavailability). The dispersion should be consumed promptly. The glass should be rinsed and the rinse swallowed to insure the entire dose is consumed.

RESCRIPTOR Tablets may be administered with or without food (see CLINICAL PHARMACOLOGY—Pharmacokinetics-Absorption and Bioavailability). Patients with achlorhydria should take RESCRIPTOR with an acidic beverage (eg, orange or cranberry juice). However, the effect of an acidic beverage on the absorption of delavirdine in patients with achlorhydria has not been investigated.

Patients taking both RESCRIPTOR and antacids should be advised to take them at least one hour apart.

HOW SUPPLIED

RESCRIPTOR Tablets are available as follows:
100 mg: white, capsule-shaped tablets marked with "U 3761".
Bottles of 360 tablets   NDC 0009-3761-03
Store at controlled room temperature 20° to 25°C (68° to 77°F) [see USP]. Keep container tightly closed. Protect from high humidity.

Table 3. — Adverse Events of Moderate or Severe Intensity in ≥2% of Patients Receiving RESCRIPTOR*

Body System/ Adverse Event	Study 0017		Study 0021	
	Didanosine† 200 mg bid (n=591)	Delavirdine 400 mg tid + Didanosine† 200 mg bid (n=594)	Zidovudine 200 mg tid (n=271)	Delavirdine 400 mg tid + Zidovudine 200 mg tid (n=287)
Body as a Whole				
Headache	4.7	5.6	4.8	5.6
Fatigue	2.7	2.9	4.8	5.2
Digestive				
Nausea	3.4	4.9	6.6	10.8
Diarrhea	4.4	4.5	2.2	3.5
Vomiting	1.2	2.4	1.1	2.8
Metabolic and Nutritional				
Increased ALT (SGPT)	3.6	5.2	0.7	2.4
Increased AST (SGOT)	3.0	4.5	0.7	1.7
Skin				
Rash	3.0	9.8	1.5	12.5
Maculopapular rash	2.0	6.6	1.1	4.5
Pruritus	1.7	2.2	1.5	3.1

*Includes those adverse events at least possibly related to study drug or of unknown relationship and excludes concurrent HIV conditions.
†Dose adjusted body weight < 60 kg = 125 mg bid; ≥ 60 kg = 200 mg bid.

Table 4. — Frequency (%)* of Clinically Important Laboratory Abnormalities

Laboratory Test	Study 0017		Study 0021	
	Didanosine† (n=591)	Delavirdine 400 mg tid + Didanosine† (n=594)	Zidovudine 200 mg tid (n=271)	Delavirdine 400 mg tid + Zidovudine 200 mg tid (n=287)
Neutropenia (ANC <750/mm^3)	6.7	5.7	7.7‡	3.5
Anemia (Hgb <7.0 g/dL)	0.2	0.7	1.1	1.0
Thrombocytopenia (platelets <50,000/mm^3)	1.4	1.5	0.0	0.0
ALT (>5.0 × ULN)	4.6	6.7	3.7	3.8
AST (>5.0 × ULN)	4.9	5.6	3.0	2.1
Bilirubin (>2.5 ULN)	0.7	0.5	0.4	1.0
Amylase (>2.0 ULN)	6.5	5.2	1.1	0.0

*Percentage was based on the number of patients for which data on that laboratory test was available.
†Dose adjusted by body weight <60 kg = 125 mg bid; ≥ 60 kg = 200 mg bid.
‡Significant (P <.05) delavirdine + zidovudine vs zidovudine.
ANC = Absolute neutrophil count; ULN = upper limit of normal.

Caution: Federal law prohibits dispensing without prescription.

ANIMAL TOXICOLOGY

Toxicities among various organs and organ systems in rats, mice, rabbits, dogs, and monkeys were observed following the administration of delavirdine. Necrotizing vasculitis was the most significant toxicity that occurred in dogs when mean nadir serum concentrations of delavirdine were at least 7-fold higher than the expected human exposure to RESCRIPTOR ($C_{min} \approx 15\ \mu M$) at the recommended dose. Vasculitis in dogs was not reversible during a 2.5-month recovery period; however, partial resolution of the vascular lesion characterized by reduced inflammation, diminished necrosis, and intimal thickening occurred during this period. Other major target organs included the gastrointestinal tract, endocrine organs, liver, kidneys, bone marrow, lymphoid tissue, lung, and reproductive organs.

Pharmacia & Upjohn Company
Kalamazoo, Michigan 49001, USA
Revised August 1997

816 885 002
692151

Shown in Product Identification Guide, page 332

SOLU-MEDROL®   ℞
[*sŏlū-medrŏl*]
Sterile Powder
methylprednisolone sodium succinate sterile powder
(methylprednisolone sodium succinate for injection, USP)
For Intravenous or Intramuscular Administration

DESCRIPTION

SOLU-MEDROL Sterile Powder contains methylprednisolone sodium succinate as the active ingredient. Methylprednisolone sodium succinate, USP, occurs as a white, or nearly white, odorless hygroscopic, amorphous solid. It is very soluble in water and in alcohol; it is insoluble in chloroform and is very slightly soluble in acetone.

The chemical name for methylprednisolone sodium succinate is pregna-1,4-diene-3,20-dione,21-(3-carboxy-1-oxopropoxy)-11,17-dihydroxy-6-methyl-monosodium salt, (6α, 11β), and the molecular weight is 496.53.

The structural formula is represented below:

Methylprednisolone sodium succinate is so extremely soluble in water that it may be administered in a small volume of diluent and is especially well suited for intravenous use in situations in which high blood levels of methylprednisolone are required rapidly.

SOLU-MEDROL is available in several strengths and packages for intravenous or intramuscular administration.

40 mg Act-O-Vial® System (Single-Dose Vial)—Each mL (when mixed) contains methylprednisolone sodium succinate equivalent to 40 mg methylprednisolone; also 1.6 mg monobasic sodium phosphate anhydrous; 17.46 mg dibasic sodium phosphate dried; 25 mg lactose hydrous; 8.8 mg benzyl alcohol added as preservative.

125 mg Act-O-Vial System (Single-Dose Vial)—Each 2 mL (when mixed) contains methylprednisolone sodium succinate equivalent to 125 mg methylprednisolone; also 1.6 mg monobasic sodium phosphate anhydrous; 17.4 mg dibasic sodium phosphate dried; 17.6 mg benzyl alcohol added as preservative.

500 mg Vial—Each 8 mL (when mixed as directed) contains methylprednisolone sodium succinate equivalent to 500 mg methylprednisolone; also 6.4 mg monobasic sodium phosphate anhydrous; 69.6 mg dibasic sodium phosphate dried.

500 mg Vial with Diluent—Each 8 mL (when mixed as directed) contains methylprednisolone sodium succinate equivalent to 500 mg methylprednisolone; also 6.4 mg monobasic sodium phosphate anhydrous; 69.6 mg dibasic sodium phosphate dried; 70.2 mg benzyl alcohol added as preservative.

500 mg Act-O-Vial System (Single-Dose Vial)—Each 4 mL (when mixed) contains methylprednisolone sodium succinate equivalent to 500 mg methylprednisolone; also 6.4 mg monobasic sodium phosphate anhydrous; 69.6 mg dibasic sodium phosphate dried; 33.7 mg benzyl alcohol added as preservative.

1 gram Vial—Each 16 mL (when mixed as directed) contains methylprednisolone sodium succinate equivalent to 1 gram methylprednisolone; also 12.8 mg monobasic sodium phosphate anhydrous; 139.2 mg dibasic sodium phosphate dried.

1 gram Act-O-Vial System (Single-Dose Vial)—Each 8 mL (when mixed) contains methylprednisolone sodium succinate equivalent to 1 gram methylprednisolone; also 12.8 mg monobasic sodium phosphate anhydrous; 139.2 mg dibasic sodium phosphate dried; 66.8 mg benzyl alcohol added as preservative.

2 gram Vial—Each 30.6 mL (when mixed as directed) contains methylprednisolone sodium succinate equivalent to 2 grams methylprednisolone; also 25.6 mg monobasic sodium phosphate anhydrous; 278 mg dibasic sodium phosphate dried.

2 gram Vial with Diluent—Each 30.6 mL (when mixed as directed) contains methylprednisolone sodium succinate equivalent to 2 grams methylprednisolone; also 25.6 mg monobasic sodium phosphate anhydrous; 278 mg dibasic sodium phosphate dried; 273 mg benzyl alcohol added as preservative.

When necessary, the pH of each formula was adjusted with sodium hydroxide so that the pH of the reconstituted solution is within the USP specified range of 7 to 8 and the tonicities are, for the 40 mg per mL solution, 0.50 osmolar; for the 125 mg per 2 mL, 500 mg per 8 mL and 1 gram per 16 mL solutions, 0.40 osmolar; for the 1 gram per 8 mL solution, 0.44 osmolar; for the 2 gram per 30.6 mL solutions, 0.42 osmolar. (Isotonic saline = 0.28 osmolar).

IMPORTANT—Use only the accompanying diluent or Bacteriostatic Water For Injection with Benzyl Alcohol when reconstituting SOLU-MEDROL. **Use within 48 hours after mixing.**

ACTIONS

Naturally occurring glucocorticoids (hydrocortisone and cortisone), which also have salt-retaining properties, are used as replacement therapy in adrenocortical deficiency states. Their synthetic analogs are primarily used for their potent anti-inflammatory effects in disorders of many organ systems.

Glucocorticoids cause profound and varied metabolic effects. In addition, they modify the body's immune responses to diverse stimuli.

Methylprednisolone is a potent anti-inflammatory steroid synthesized in the Research Laboratories of The Upjohn Company. It has a greater anti-inflammatory potency than prednisolone and even less tendency than prednisolone to induce sodium and water retention.

Methylprednisolone sodium succinate has the same metabolic and anti-inflammatory actions as methylprednisolone. When given parenterally and in equimolar quantities, the two compounds are equivalent in biologic activity. The relative potency of SOLU-MEDROL Sterile Powder and hydrocortisone sodium succinate, as indicated by depression of eosinophil count, following intravenous administration, is at least four to one. This is in good agreement with the relative oral potency of methylprednisolone and hydrocortisone.

INDICATIONS

When oral therapy is not feasible, and the strength, dosage form and route of administration of the drug reasonably lend the preparation to the treatment of the condition, SOLU-MEDROL Sterile Powder is indicated for intravenous or intramuscular use in the following conditions:

1. **Endocrine Disorders**
   Primary or secondary adrenocortical insufficiency (hydrocortisone or cortisone is the drug of choice; synthetic analogs may be used in conjunction with mineralocorticoids where applicable; in infancy, mineralocorticoid supplementation is of particular importance)
   Acute adrenocortical insufficiency (hydrocortisone or cortisone is the drug of choice; mineralocorticoid supplementation may be necessary, particularly when synthetic analogs are used)
   Preoperatively and in the event of serious trauma or illness, in patients with known adrenal insufficiency or when adrenocortical reserve is doubtful
   Shock unresponsive to conventional therapy if adrenocortical insufficiency exists or is suspected
   Congenital adrenal hyperplasia
   Hypercalcemia associated with cancer
   Nonsuppurative thyroiditis

2. **Rheumatic Disorders**
   As adjunctive therapy for short-term administration (to tide the patient over an acute episode or exacerbation) in:
   Post-traumatic osteoarthritis
   Synovitis of osteoarthritis
   Rheumatoid arthritis, including juvenile rheumatoid arthritis (selected cases may require low-dose maintenance therapy)
   Acute and subacute bursitis
   Epicondylitis
   Acute nonspecific tenosynovitis
   Acute gouty arthritis
   Psoriatic arthritis
   Ankylosing spondylitis

3. **Collagen Diseases**
   During an exacerbation or as maintenance therapy in selected cases of:

Systemic lupus erythematosus
Systemic dermatomyositis (polymyositis)
Acute rheumatic carditis

4. **Dermatologic Diseases**
   Pemphigus
   Severe erythema multiforme (Stevens-Johnson syndrome)
   Exfoliative dermatitis
   Bullous dermatitis herpetiformis
   Severe seborrheic dermatitis
   Severe psoriasis
   Mycosis fungoides

5. **Allergic States**
   Control of severe or incapacitating allergic conditions intractable to adequate trials of conventional treatment in:
   Bronchial asthma
   Contact dermatitis
   Atopic dermatitis
   Serum sickness
   Seasonal or perennial allergic rhinitis
   Drug hypersensitivity reactions
   Urticarial transfusion reactions
   Acute noninfectious laryngeal edema (epinephrine is the drug of first choice)

6. **Ophthalmic Diseases**
   Severe acute and chronic allergic and inflammatory processes involving the eye, such as:
   Herpes zoster ophthalmicus
   Iritis, iridocyclitis
   Chorioretinitis
   Diffuse posterior uveitis and choroiditis
   Optic neuritis
   Sympathetic ophthalmia
   Anterior segment inflammation
   Allergic conjunctivitis
   Allergic corneal marginal ulcers
   Keratitis

7. **Gastrointestinal Diseases**
   To tide the patient over a critical period of the disease in:
   Ulcerative colitis (systemic therapy)
   Regional enteritis (systemic therapy)

8. **Respiratory Diseases**
   Symptomatic sarcoidosis
   Berylliosis
   Fulminating or disseminated pulmonary tuberculosis when used concurrently with appropriate antituberculous chemotherapy
   Loeffler's syndrome not manageable by other means
   Aspiration pneumonitis

9. **Hematologic Disorders**
   Acquired (autoimmune) hemolytic anemia
   Idiopathic thrombocytopenic purpura in adults (IV only; IM administration is contraindicated)
   Secondary thrombocytopenia in adults
   Erythroblastopenia (RBC anemia)
   Congenital (erythroid) hypoplastic anemia

10. **Neoplastic Diseases**
    For palliative management of:
    Leukemias and lymphomas in adults
    Acute leukemia of childhood

11. **Edematous States**
    To induce diuresis or remission of proteinuria in the nephrotic syndrome, without uremia, of the idiopathic type or that due to lupus erythematosus

12. **Nervous System**
    Acute exacerbations of multiple sclerosis

13. **Miscellaneous**
    Tuberculous meningitis with subarachnoid block or impending block when used concurrently with appropriate antituberculous chemotherapy
    Trichinosis with neurologic or myocardial involvement

CONTRAINDICATIONS

The use of SOLU-MEDROL Sterile Powder is contraindicated in premature infants because the **40 mg Act-O-Vial**, the **125 mg Act-O-Vial**, the **500 mg Act-O-Vial**, the **1 gram Act-O-Vial** system, and the accompanying diluent for the 500 mg and 2 gram vials contain benzyl alcohol. Benzyl alcohol has been reported to be associated with a fatal "Gasping Syndrome" in premature infants. SOLU-MEDROL Sterile Powder is also contraindicated in systemic fungal infections and patients with known hypersensitivity to the product and its constituents.

WARNINGS

In patients on corticosteroid therapy subjected to any unusual stress, increased dosage of rapidly acting corticosteroids before, during, and after the stressful situation is indicated.

Continued on next page

Information on these Pharmacia & Upjohn products is based on labeling in effect June 1, 1998. Further information concerning these and other Pharmacia & Upjohn products may be obtained by direct inquiry to Medical Information, Pharmacia & Upjohn, Kalamazoo, MI 49001.

Solu-Medrol—Cont.

Corticosteroids may mask some signs of infection, and new infections may appear during their use. There may be decreased resistance and inability to localize infection when corticosteroids are used. Infections with any pathogen including viral, bacterial, fungal, protozoan or helminthic infections, in any location of the body, may be associated with the use of corticosteroids alone or in combination with other immunosuppressive agents that affect cellular immunity, humoral immunity, or neutrophil function.[1]

These infections may be mild, but can be severe and at times fatal. With increasing doses of corticosteroids, the rate of occurrence of infectious complications increases.[2]

A study has failed to establish the efficacy of SOLU-MEDROL in the treatment of sepsis syndrome and septic shock. The study also suggests that treatment of these conditions with SOLU-MEDROL may increase the risk of mortality in certain patients (ie, patients with elevated serum creatinine levels or patients who develop secondary infections after SOLU-MEDROL).

Prolonged use of corticosteroids may produce posterior subcapsular cataracts, glaucoma with possible damage to the optic nerves, and may enhance the establishment of secondary ocular infections due to fungi or viruses.

Usage in pregnancy. Since adequate human reproduction studies have not been done with corticosteroids, the use of these drugs in pregnancy, nursing mothers, or women of childbearing potential requires that the possible benefits of the drug be weighed against the potential hazards to the mother and embryo or fetus. Infants born of mothers who have received substantial doses of corticosteroids during pregnancy should be carefully observed for signs of hypoadrenalism.

Average and large doses of cortisone or hydrocortisone can cause elevation of blood pressure, salt and water retention, and increased excretion of potassium. These effects are less likely to occur with the synthetic derivatives except when used in large doses. Dietary salt restriction and potassium supplementation may be necessary. All corticosteroids increase calcium excretion.

Administration of live or live, attenuated vaccines is contraindicated in patients receiving immunosuppressive doses of corticosteroids. Killed or inactivated vaccines may be administered to patients receiving immunosuppressive doses of corticosteroids; however, the response to such vaccines may be diminished. Indicated immunization procedures may be undertaken in patients receiving nonimmunosuppressive doses of corticosteroids.

The use of SOLU-MEDROL Sterile Powder in active tuberculosis should be restricted to those cases of fulminating or disseminated tuberculosis in which the corticosteroid is used for the management of the disease in conjunction with appropriate antituberculous regimen.

If corticosteroids are indicated in patients with latent tuberculosis or tuberculin reactivity, close observation is necessary as reactivation of the disease may occur. During prolonged corticosteroid therapy, these patients should receive chemoprophylaxis.

Because rare instances of anaphylactic (eg, bronchospasm) reactions have occurred in patients receiving parenteral corticosteroid therapy, appropriate precautionary measures should be taken prior to administration, especially when the patient has a history of allergy to any drug.

There are reports of cardiac arrhythmias and/or circulatory collapse and/or cardiac arrest following the rapid administration of large IV doses of SOLU-MEDROL (greater than 0.5 gram administered over a period of less than 10 minutes). Bradycardia has been reported during or after the administration of large doses of methylprednisolone sodium succinate, and may be unrelated to the speed or duration of infusion.

Persons who are on drugs which suppress the immune system are more susceptible to infections than healthy individuals. Chicken pox and measles, for example, can have a more serious or even fatal course in non-immune children or adults on corticosteroids. In such children or adults who have not had these diseases, particular care should be taken to avoid exposure. How the dose, route and duration of corticosteroid administration affects the risk of developing a disseminated infection is not known. The contribution of the underlying disease and/or prior corticosteroid treatment to the risk is also not known. If exposed to chicken pox, prophylaxis with varicella zoster immune globulin (VZIG) may be indicated. If exposed to measles, prophylaxis with pooled intramuscular immunoglobulin (IG) may be indicated. (See the respective package inserts for complete VZIG and IG prescribing information.) If chicken pox develops, treatment with antiviral agents may be considered. Similarly, corticosteroids should be used with great care in patients with known or suspected Strongyloides (threadworm) infestation. In such patients, corticosteroid-induced immunosuppression may lead to Strongyloides hyperinfection and dissemination with widespread larval migration, often accompanied by severe enterocolitis and potentially fatal gramnegative septicemia.

PRECAUTIONS
General precautions
Drug-induced secondary adrenocortical insufficiency may be minimized by gradual reduction of dosage. This type of relative insufficiency may persist for months after discontinuation of therapy; therefore, in any situation of stress occurring during that period, hormone therapy should be reinstituted. Since mineralocorticoid secretion may be impaired, salt and/or a mineralocorticoid should be administered concurrently.

There is an enhanced effect of corticosteroids on patients with hypothyroidism and in those with cirrhosis.

Corticosteroids should be used cautiously in patients with ocular herpes simplex because of possible corneal perforation.

The lowest possible dose of corticosteroid should be used to control the condition under treatment, and when reduction in dosage is possible, the reduction should be gradual.

Psychic derangements may appear when corticosteroids are used, ranging from euphoria, insomnia, mood swings, personality changes, and severe depression, to frank psychotic manifestations. Also, existing emotional instability or psychotic tendencies may be aggravated by corticosteroids.

Steroids should be used with caution in nonspecific ulcerative colitis, if there is a probability of impending perforation, abscess or other pyogenic infection; diverticulitis; fresh intestinal anastomoses; active or latent peptic ulcer; renal insufficiency; hypertension; osteoporosis; and myasthenia gravis.

Growth and development of infants and children on prolonged corticosteroid therapy should be carefully observed. Kaposi's sarcoma has been reported to occur in patients receiving corticosteroid therapy. Discontinuation of corticosteroids may result in clinical remission.

Although controlled clinical trials have shown corticosteroids to be effective in speeding the resolution of acute exacerbations of multiple sclerosis, they do not show that corticosteroids affect the ultimate outcome or natural history of the disease. The studies do show that relatively high doses of corticosteroids are necessary to demonstrate a significant effect. (See DOSAGE AND ADMINISTRATION.)

An acute myopathy has been observed with the use of high doses of corticosteroids, most often occurring in patients with disorders of neuromuscular transmission (eg, myasthenia gravis), or in patients receiving concomitant therapy with neuromuscular blocking drugs (eg, pancuronium). This acute myopathy is generalized, may involve ocular and respiratory muscles, and may result in quadriparesis. Elevations of creatine kinase may occur. Clinical improvement or recovery after stopping corticosteroids may require weeks to years.

Since complications of treatment with glucocorticoids are dependent on the size of the dose and the duration of treatment, a risk/benefit decision must be made in each individual case as to dose and duration of treatment and as to whether daily or intermittent therapy should be used.

DRUG INTERACTIONS
The pharmacokinetic interactions listed below are potentially clinically important. Mutual inhibition of metabolism occurs with concurrent use of cyclosporin and methylprednisolone; therefore, it is possible that adverse events associated with the individual use of either drug may be more apt to occur. Convulsions have been reported with concurrent use of methylprednisolone and cyclosporin. Drugs that induce hepatic enzymes such as phenobarbital, phenytoin and rifampin may increase the clearance of methylprednisolone and may require increases in methylprednisolone dose to achieve the desired response. Drugs such as troleandomycin and ketoconazole may inhibit the metabolism of methylprednisolone and thus decrease its clearance. Therefore, the dose of methylprednisolone should be titrated to avoid steroid toxicity. Methylprednisolone may increase the clearance of chronic high dose aspirin. This could lead to decreased salicylate serum levels or increase the risk of salicylate toxicity when methylprednisolone is withdrawn. Aspirin should be used cautiously in conjunction with corticosteroids in patients suffering from hypoprothrombinemia. The effect of methylprednisolone on oral anticoagulants is variable. There are reports of enhanced as well as diminished effects of anticoagulant when given concurrently with corticosteroids. Therefore, coagulation indices should be monitored to maintain the desired anticoagulant effect.

Information for the Patient
Persons who are on immunosuppressant doses of corticosteroids should be warned to avoid exposure to chicken pox or measles. Patients should also be advised that if they are exposed, medical advice should be sought without delay.

ADVERSE REACTIONS
Fluid and Electrolyte Disturbances
Sodium retention
Fluid retention
Congestive heart failure in susceptible patients
Potassium loss
Hypokalemic alkalosis
Hypertension

Musculoskeletal
Muscle weakness
Steroid myopathy
Loss of muscle mass
Severe arthralgia
Vertebral compression fractures
Aseptic necrosis of femoral and humeral heads
Pathologic fracture of long bones
Osteoporosis
Tendon rupture, particularly of the Achilles tendon

Gastrointestinal
Peptic ulcer with possible perforation and hemorrhage
Pancreatitis
Abdominal distention
Ulcerative esophagitis
Increases in alanine transaminase (ALT, SGPT), aspartate transaminase (AST, SGOT), and alkaline phosphatase have been observed following corticosteroid treatment. These changes are usually small, not associated with any clinical syndrome and are reversible upon discontinuation.

Dermatologic
Impaired wound healing
Thin fragile skin
Petechiae and ecchymoses
Facial erythema
Increased sweating
May suppress reactions to skin tests

Neurological
Increased intracranial pressure with papilledema (pseudo-tumor cerebri) usually after treatment
Convulsions
Vertigo
Headache

Endocrine
Development of Cushingoid state
Suppression of growth in children
Secondary adrenocortical and pituitary unresponsiveness, particularly in times of stress, as in trauma, surgery or illness
Menstrual irregularities
Decreased carbohydrate tolerance
Manifestations of latent diabetes mellitus
Increased requirements for insulin or oral hypoglycemic agents in diabetics

Ophthalmic
Posterior subcapsular cataracts
Increased intraocular pressure
Glaucoma
Exophthalmos

Metabolic
Negative nitrogen balance due to protein catabolism
The following *additional* adverse reactions are related to parenteral corticosteroid therapy:
Hyperpigmentation or hypopigmentation
Subcutaneous and cutaneous atrophy
Sterile abscess
Anaphylactic reaction with or without circulatory collapse, cardiac arrest, bronchospasm
Urticaria
Nausea and vomiting
Cardiac arrhythmias; hypotension or hypertension

DOSAGE AND ADMINISTRATION
When high dose therapy is desired, the recommended dose of SOLU-MEDROL Sterile Powder is 30 mg/kg administered intravenously over at least 30 minutes. This dose may be repeated every 4 to 6 hours for 48 hours.

In general, high dose corticosteroid therapy should be continued only until the patient's condition has stabilized; usually not beyond 48 to 72 hours.

Although adverse effects associated with high dose short-term corticoid therapy are uncommon, peptic ulceration may occur. Prophylactic antacid therapy may be indicated.

In other indications initial dosage will vary from 10 to 40 mg of methylprednisolone depending on the clinical problem being treated. The larger doses may be required for short-term management of severe, acute conditions. The initial dose usually should be given intravenously over a period of several minutes. Subsequent doses may be given intravenously or intramuscularly at intervals dictated by the patient's response and clinical condition. Corticoid therapy is an adjunct to, and not replacement for conventional therapy.

Dosage may be reduced for infants and children but should be governed more by the severity of the condition and response of the patient than by age or size. It should not be less than 0.5 mg per kg every 24 hours.

Dosage must be decreased or discontinued gradually when the drug has been administered for more than a few days. If a period of spontaneous remission occurs in a chronic condition, treatment should be discontinued. Routine laboratory studies, such as urinalysis, two-hour postprandial blood sugar, determination of blood pressure and body weight, and a chest X-ray should be made at regular intervals during prolonged therapy. Upper GI X-rays are desirable in patients with an ulcer history or significant dyspepsia.

SOLU-MEDROL may be administered by intravenous or intramuscular injection or by intravenous infusion, the preferred method for initial emergency use being intravenous injection. To administer by intravenous (or intramuscular) injection, prepare solution as directed. The desired dose may be administered intravenously over a period of several minutes. If desired, the medication may be administered in diluted solutions by adding Water for Injection or other suitable diluent (see below) to the **Act-O-Vial** and withdrawing the indicated dose.

To prepare solutions for intravenous infusion, first prepare the solution for injection as directed. This solution may then be added to indicated amounts of 5% dextrose in water, isotonic saline solution or 5% dextrose in isotonic saline solution.

Multiple Sclerosis

In treatment of acute exacerbations of multiple sclerosis, daily doses of 200 mg of prednisolone for a week followed by 80 mg every other day for 1 month have been shown to be effective (4 mg of methylprednisolone is equivalent to 5 mg of prednisolone).

DIRECTIONS FOR USING THE ACT-O-VIAL SYSTEM

1. Press down on plastic activator to force diluent into the lower compartment.
2. Gently agitate to effect solution.
3. Remove plastic tab covering center of stopper.
4. Sterilize top of stopper with a suitable germicide.
5. Insert needle **squarely through center** of stopper until tip is just visible. Invert vial and withdraw dose.

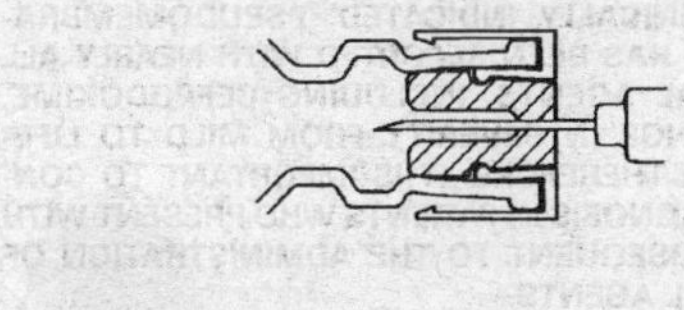

STORAGE CONDITIONS

Protect from light.

Store unreconstituted product at controlled room temperature 20° to 25° C (68° to 77° F) [see USP].

Store solution at controlled room temperature 20° to 25°C (68° to 77°F) [see USP].

Use solution within 48 hours after mixing.

HOW SUPPLIED

SOLU-MEDROL Sterile Powder is available in the following packages:

40 mg Act-O-Vial System (Single-Dose Vial)
1 mL NDC 0009-0113-12
25 × 1 mL NDC 0009-0113-19

125 mg Act-O-Vial System (Single-Dose Vial)
2 mL NDC 0009–0190–09
25 × 2 mL NDC 0009-0190-16
500 mg Vial NDC 0009-0758-01
500 mg Vial with Diluent NDC 0009-0887-01

500 mg Act-O-Vial System (Single-Dose Vial)
4 mL NDC 0009-0765-02

1 gram Vial NDC 0009-0698-01

1 gram Act-O-Vial System (Single-Dose Vial)
8 mL NDC 0009-3389-01

2 gram Vial NDC 0009-0988-01

2 gram Vial with Diluent NDC 0009-0796-01

REFERENCES

1. Fekety R. Infections associated with corticosteroids and immunosuppressive therapy. In: Gorbach SL, Bartlett JG, Blacklow NR, eds. *Infectious Diseases.* Philadelphia: WBSaunders Company 1992:1050-1.
2. Stuck AE, Minder CE, Frey FJ. Risk of infectious complications in patients taking glucocorticoids. *Rev Infect Dis* 1989:11(6):954-63.

Caution: Federal law prohibits dispensing without prescription.

Pharmacia & Upjohn Company • Kalamazoo, Michigan 49001, USA

Revised February 1997

810 431 032
691211

VANTIN® ℞

Tablets and Oral Suspension
cefpodoxime proxetil tablets and
cefpodoxime proxetil for oral suspension
For Oral Use Only

DESCRIPTION

Cefpodoxime proxetil is an orally administered, extended spectrum, semi-synthetic antibiotic of the cephalosporin class. The chemical name is (RS)-1(isopropoxycarbonyloxy) ethyl (+)-(6R,7R)-7-[2-(2-amino-4-thiazolyl)-2-{(Z)methoxyimino}acetamido]- 3- methoxymethyl-8-oxo- 5- thia - 1 - azabicyclo [4.2.0] oct-2-ene-2-carboxylate.

Its empirical formula is $C_{21}H_{27}N_5O_9S_2$ and its structural formula is represented below:

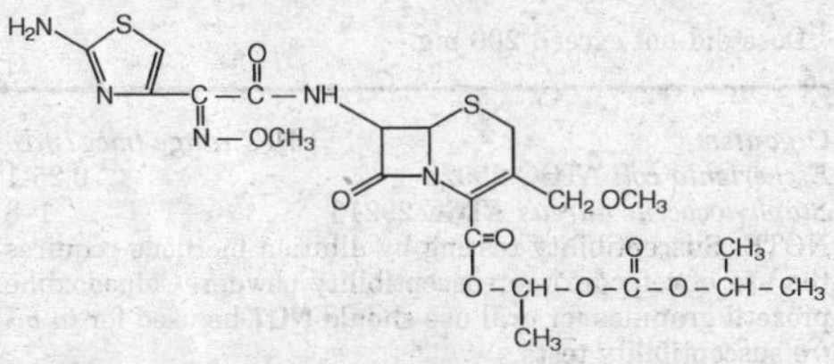

The molecular weight of cefpodoxime proxetil is 557,6.

Cefpodoxime proxetil is a prodrug; its active metabolite is cefpodoxime. All doses of cefpodoxime proxetil in this insert are expressed in terms of the active cefpodoxime moiety. The drug is supplied both as film-coated tablets and as flavored granules for oral suspension.

VANTIN Tablets contain cefpodoxime proxetil equivalent to 100 mg or 200 mg of cefpodoxime activity and the following inactive ingredients: carboxymethylcellulose calcium, carnauba wax, FD&C Yellow No. 6, hydroxypropylcellulose, hydroxypropylmethylcellulose, lactose hydrous, magnesium stearate, propylene glycol, sodium lauryl sulfate and titanium dioxide. In addition, the 100 mg film-coated tablets contain D&C Yellow No. 10 and the 200 mg film-coated tablets contain FD&C Red No. 40.

Each 5 mL of VANTIN for Oral Suspension contains cefpodoxime proxetil equivalent to 50 mg or 100 mg of cefpodoxime activity after constitution and the following inactive ingredients: artificial flavorings, butylated hydroxy anisole (BHA), carboxymethylcellulose sodium, microcrystalline cellulose, carrageenan, citric acid, colloidal silicon dioxide, croscarmellose sodium, hydroxypropylcellulose, lactose, maltodextrin, natural flavorings, propylene glycol alginate, sodium citrate, sodium benzoate, starch, sucrose, and vegetable oil.

CLINICAL PHARMACOLOGY

Absorption and Excretion:

Cefpodoxime proxetil is a prodrug that is absorbed from the gastrointestinal tract and de-esterified to its active metabolite, cefpodoxime. Following oral administration of 100 mg of cefpodoxime proxetil to fasting subjects, approximately 50% of the administered cefpodoxime dose was absorbed systemically. Over the recommended dosing range (100 to 400 mg), approximately 29 to 33% of the administered cefpodoxime dose was excreted unchanged in the urine in 12 hours. There is minimal metabolism of cefpodoxime *in vivo.*

Effects of Food:

The extent of absorption (mean AUC) and the mean peak plasma concentration increased when film-coated tablets were administered with food. Following a 200 mg tablet dose taken with food, the AUC was 21 to 33% higher than under fasting conditions, and the peak plasma concentration averaged 3.1 mcg/mL in fed subjects versus 2.6 mcg/mL in fasted subjects. Time to peak concentration was not significantly different between fed and fasted subjects.

When a 200 mg dose of the suspension was taken with food, the extent of absorption (mean AUC) and mean peak plasma concentration in fed subjects were not significantly different from fasted subjects, but the rate of absorption was slower with food (48% increase in T_{max}).

Pharmacokinetics of Cefpodoxime Proxetil Film-coated Tablets:

Over the recommended dosing range, (100 to 400 mg), the rate and extent of cefpodoxime absorption exhibited dose-dependency; dose-normalized C_{max} and AUC decreased by up to 32% with increasing dose. Over the recommended dosing range, the T_{max} was approximately 2 to 3 hours and the $T_{1/2}$ ranged from 2.09 to 2.84 hours. Mean C_{max} was 1.4 mcg/mL for the 100 mg dose, 2.3 mcg/mL for the 200 mg dose, and 3.9 mcg/mL for the 400 mg dose. In patients with normal renal function, neither accumulation nor significant changes in other pharmacokinetic parameters were noted following multiple oral doses of up to 400 mg Q 12 hours.

[See first table at top of next page]

Pharmacokinetics of Cefpodoxime Proxetil Suspension:

In adult subjects, a 100 mg dose of oral suspension produced an average peak cefpodoxime concentration of approximately 1.5 mcg/mL (range: 1.1 to 2.1 mcg/mL), which is equivalent to that reported following administration of the 100 mg tablet. Time to peak plasma concentration and area under the plasma concentration-time curve (AUC) for the oral suspension were also equivalent to those produced with film-coated tablets in adults following a 100 mg oral dose.

The pharmacokinetics of cefpodoxime were investigated in 29 patients aged 1 to 17 years. Each patient received a single, oral, 5 mg/kg dose of cefpodoxime oral suspension. Plasma and urine samples were collected for 12 hours after dosing. The plasma levels reported from this study are as follows:

[See second table at top of next page]

Distribution:

Protein binding of cefpodoxime ranges from 22 to 33% in serum and from 21 to 29% in plasma.

Skin Blister:

Following multiple-dose administration every 12 hours for 5 days of 200 mg or 400 mg cefpodoxime proxetil, the mean maximum cefpodoxime concentration in skin blister fluid averaged 1.6 and 2.8 mcg/mL, respectively. Skin blister fluid cefpodoxime levels at 12 hours after dosing averaged 0.2 and 0.4 mcg/mL for the 200 mg and 400 mg multiple-dose regimens, respectively.

Tonsil Tissue:

Following a single, oral 100 mg cefpodoxime proxetil film-coated tablet, the mean maximum cefpodoxime concentration in tonsil tissue averaged 0.24 mcg/g at 4 hours post-dosing and 0.09 mcg/g at 7 hours post-dosing. Equilibrium was achieved between plasma and tonsil tissue within 4 hours of dosing. No detection of cefpodoxime in tonsillar tissue was reported 12 hours after dosing. These results demonstrated that concentrations of cefpodoxime exceeded the MIC_{90} of *S. pyogenes* for at least 7 hours after dosing of 100 mg of cefpodoxime proxetil.

Lung Tissue:

Following a single, oral 200 mg cefpodoxime proxetil film-coated tablet, the mean maximum cefpodoxime concentration in lung tissue averaged 0.63 mcg/g at 3 hours post-dosing, 0.52 mcg/g at 6 hours post-dosing, and 0.19 mcg/g at 12 hours post-dosing. The results of this study indicated that cefpodoxime penetrated into lung tissue and produced sustained drug concentrations for at least 12 hours after dosing at levels that exceeded the MIC_{90} for *S. pneumoniae* and *H. influenzae.*

CSF:

Adequate data on CSF levels of cefpodoxime are not available.

Effects of Decreased Renal Function:

Elimination of cefpodoxime is reduced in patients with moderate to severe renal impairment (<50 mL/min creatinine clearance). (See **PRECAUTIONS** and **DOSAGE AND ADMINISTRATION.**) In subjects with mild impairment of renal function (50 to 80 mL/min creatinine clearance), the average plasma half-life of cefpodoxime was 3.5 hours. In subjects with moderate (30 to 49 mL/min creatinine clearance) or severe renal impairment (5 to 29 mL/min creatinine clearance), the half-life increased to 5.9 and 9.8 hours, respectively. Approximately 23% of the administered dose was cleared from the body during a standard 3-hour hemodialysis procedure.

Effect of Hepatic Impairment (cirrhosis):

Absorption was somewhat diminished and elimination unchanged in patients with cirrhosis. The mean cefpodoxime $T_{1/2}$ and renal clearance in cirrhotic patients were similar to those derived in studies of healthy subjects. Ascites did not appear to affect values in cirrhotic subjects. No dosage adjustment is recommended in this patient population.

Pharmacokinetics in Elderly Subjects:

Elderly subjects do not require dosage adjustments unless they have diminished renal function. (See **PRECAUTIONS.**) In healthy geriatric subjects, cefpodoxime half-life in plasma averaged 4.2 hours (vs 3.3 in younger subjects) and urinary recovery averaged 21% after a 400 mg dose was administered every 12 hours. Other pharmacokinetic parameters (C_{max}, AUC, and T_{max}) were unchanged relative to those observed in healthy young subjects.

Microbiology:

Cefpodoxime is active *in vitro* against a wide range of gram-positive and gram-negative bacteria. Cefpodoxime is highly stable in the presence of beta-lactamase enzymes. As a result, many organisms resistant to penicillins and some cephalosporins, due to the presence of beta-lactamases, may be susceptible to cefpodoxime.

The bactericidal activity of cefpodoxime results from its inhibition of cell wall synthesis. Cefpodoxime is usually active against the following organisms *in vitro* and in clinical infections. (See **INDICATIONS AND USAGE.**)

Continued on next page

Information on these Pharmacia & Upjohn products is based on labeling in effect June 1, 1998. Further information concerning these and other Pharmacia & Upjohn products may be obtained by direct inquiry to Medical Information, Pharmacia & Upjohn, Kalamazoo, MI 49001.

Vantin—Cont.

Gram-positive Aerobes:
Staphylococcus aureus (including penicillinase-producing strains)
NOTE: Cefpodoxime is inactive against methicillin-resistant staphylococci.
Staphylococcus saprophyticus
Streptococcus pneumoniae
Streptococcus pyogenes
Gram-negative Aerobes:
Escherichia coli
Haemophilus influenzae (including beta-lactamase-producing strains)
Klebsiella pneumoniae
Moraxella (Branhamella) catarrhalis
Neisseria gonorrhoeae (including penicillinase-producing strains)
Proteus mirabilis
The following *in vitro* data are available; *however, their clinical significance is unknown.*
Cefpodoxime exhibits *in vitro* minimum inhibitory concentrations of 2.0 mcg/mL or less against most strains of the following organisms. The safety and effectiveness of cefpodoxime proxetil in treating infections due to these organisms have not been established in adequate and well-controlled trials.
Gram-positive Aerobes:
Streptococcus agalactiae
Streptococcus spp. (Groups C, F, G)
NOTE: Cefpodoxime is inactive against most strains of *Enterococcus.*
Gram-negative Aerobes:
Citrobacter diversus
Haemophilus parainfluenzae
Klebsiella oxytoca
Proteus vulgaris
Providencia rettgeri
NOTE: Cefpodoxime is inactive against most strains of *Pseudomonas* and *Enterobacter.*
Anaerobes:
Peptostreptococcus magnus
SUSCEPTIBILITY TESTING
Diffusion Techniques: Quantitative methods that require measurement of zone diameters give the most precise estimate of the susceptibility of bacteria to antimicrobial agents. One such standardized procedure[1] recommended for use with the 10 mcg cefpodoxime disk is the National Committee for Clinical Laboratory Standards (NCCLS) approved procedure.
Interpretation involves correlation of the diameters obtained in the disk test with the minimum inhibitory concentration (MIC) for cefpodoxime.
Reports from the laboratory giving results of the standardized single disk susceptibility test using a 10 mcg cefpodoxime disk should be interpreted according to the following criteria:

Zone diameter (mm)	Interpretation
≥21	(S) Susceptible
18–20	(I) Intermediate
≤17	(R) Resistant

A report of "Susceptible" indicates that the pathogen is likely to be inhibited by generally achievable blood levels.
A report of "Intermediate" indicates that the result should be considered equivocal, and, if the organism is not fully susceptible to alternative, clinically feasible drugs, the test should be repeated. This category implies clinical applicability in body sites where the drug is physiologically concentrated or in situations where high dosage of drug can be used. This category provides a buffer zone that prevents small uncontrolled technical factors from causing major discrepancies in interpretation. A report of "Resistant" indicates that achievable concentrations of the antibiotic are unlikely to be inhibitory and other therapy should be selected.
Standardized procedures require the use of laboratory control organisms. The 10 mcg disk should give the following zone diameters:

Organism	Zone diameter (mm)
Escherichia coli ATCC 25922	23–28
Staphylococcus aureus ATCC 25923	19–25

Cephalosporin "class disks" should not be used to test for susceptibility to cefpodoxime.
Dilution Technique: Use a standardized dilution method[2] (broth, agar, microdilution) or equivalent with cefpodoxime susceptibility powder. The MIC values should be interpreted according to the following criteria:

MIC (mcg/mL)	Interpretation
≤2	(S) Susceptible
4	(I) Intermediate
≥8	(R) Resistant

As with standard diffusion methods, dilution procedures require the use of laboratory control organisms. Standard cefpodoxime susceptibility powder should give the following MIC values:

Organism	MIC range (mcg/mL)
Escherichia coli ATCC 25922	0.25–1
Staphylococcus aureus ATCC 29213	1–8

NOTE: Susceptibility testing by dilution methods requires the use of cefpodoxime susceptibility powder. Cefpodoxime proxetil granules for oral use should **NOT** be used for *in vitro* susceptibility tests.

INDICATIONS AND USAGE
Cefpodoxime proxetil is indicated for the treatment of patients with mild to moderate infections caused by susceptible strains of the designated microorganisms in the conditions listed below. **Recommended dosages, durations of therapy, and applicable patient populations vary among these infections. Please see DOSAGE AND ADMINISTRATION for specific recommendations.**
LOWER RESPIRATORY TRACT
Community-acquired pneumonia caused by *S. pneumoniae* or *H. influenzae* (including beta-lactamase-producing strains).
Acute bacterial exacerbation of chronic bronchitis caused by *S. pneumoniae, H. influenzae* (non-beta-lactamase-producing strains only), or *M. catarrhalis*. Data are insufficient at this time to establish efficacy in patients with acute bacterial exacerbations of chronic bronchitis caused by beta-lactamase-producing strains of *H. influenzae*.
SEXUALLY TRANSMITTED DISEASES
Acute, uncomplicated urethral and cervical gonorrhea caused by *Neisseria gonorrhoeae* (including penicillinase-producing strains)
Acute, uncomplicated ano-rectal infections in women due to *Neisseria gonorrhoeae* (including penicillinase-producing strains).
NOTE: The efficacy of cefpodoxime in treating male patients with rectal infections caused by *N. gonorrhoeae* has not been established. Data do not support the use of cefpodoxime proxetil in the treatment of pharyngeal infections due to *N. gonorrhoeae* in men or women.
SKIN AND SKIN STRUCTURES
Uncomplicated skin and skin structure infections caused by *Staphylococcus aureus* (including penicillinase-producing strains) or *Streptococcus pyogenes*. Abscesses should be surgically drained as clinically indicated.
NOTE: In clinical trials, successful treatment of uncomplicated skin and skin structure infections was dose-related. The effective therapeutic dose for skin infections was higher than those used in other recommended indications. (See **DOSAGE AND ADMINISTRATION**.)
UPPER RESPIRATORY TRACT
Acute otitis media caused by *Streptococcus pneumoniae, Haemophilus influenzae* (including beta-lactamase-producing strains), or *Moraxella (Branhamella) catarrhalis*.
Pharyngitis and/or tonsillitis caused by *Streptococcus pyogenes*.
NOTE: Only penicillin by the intramuscular route of administration has been shown to be effective in the prophylaxis of rheumatic fever. Cefpodoxime proxetil is generally effective in the eradication of streptococci from the oropharynx. However, data establishing the efficacy of cefpodoxime proxetil for the prophylaxis of subsequent rheumatic fever are not available.
URINARY TRACT
Uncomplicated urinary tract infections (cystitis) caused by *Escherichia coli, Klebsiella pneumoniae, Proteus mirabilis,* or *Staphylococcus saprophyticus*.
NOTE: In considering the use of cefpodoxime proxetil in the treatment of cystitis, cefpodoxime proxetil's lower bacterial eradication rates should be weighed against the increased eradication rates and different safety profiles of some other classes of approved agents. (See **CLINICAL STUDIES** section.)
Appropriate specimens for bacteriological examination should be obtained in order to isolate and identify causative organisms and to determine their susceptibility to cefpodoxime. Therapy may be instituted while awaiting the results of these studies. Once these results become available, antimicrobial therapy should be adjusted accordingly.

CEFPODOXIME PLASMA LEVELS (mcg/mL) IN FASTED ADULTS AFTER FILM-COATED TABLET ADMINISTRATION (Single Dose)

Dose (cefpodoxime equivalents)	Time after oral ingestion						
	1hr	2hr	3hr	4hr	6hr	8hr	12hr
100 mg	0.98	1.4	1.3	1.0	0.59	0.29	0.08
200 mg	1.5	2.2	2.2	1.8	1.2	0.62	0.18
400 mg	2.2	3.7	3.8	3.3	2.3	1.3	0.38

CEFPODOXIME PLASMA LEVELS (mcg/mL) IN FASTED PATIENTS (1 TO 17 YEARS OF AGE) AFTER SUSPENSION ADMINISTRATION

Dose (cefpodoxime equivalents)	Time after oral ingestion						
	1hr	2hr	3hr	4hr	6hr	8hr	12hr
5 mg/kg[1]	1.4	2.1	2.1	1.7	0.90	0.40	0.090

[1] Dose did not exceed 200 mg.

CONTRAINDICATIONS
Cefpodoxime proxetil is contraindicated in patients with a known allergy to cefpodoxime or to the cephalosporin group of antibiotics.

WARNINGS
BEFORE THERAPY WITH CEFPODOXIME PROXETIL IS INSTITUTED, CAREFUL INQUIRY SHOULD BE MADE TO DETERMINE WHETHER THE PATIENT HAS HAD PREVIOUS HYPERSENSITIVITY REACTIONS TO CEFPODOXIME, OTHER CEPHALOSPORINS, PENICILLINS, OR OTHER DRUGS. IF CEFPODOXIME IS TO BE ADMINISTERED TO PENICILLINSENSITIVE PATIENTS, CAUTION SHOULD BE EXERCISED BECAUSE CROSS HYPERSENSITIVITY AMONG BETA-LACTAM ANTIBIOTICS HAS BEEN CLEARLY DOCUMENTED AND MAY OCCUR IN UP TO 10% OF PATIENTS WITH A HISTORY OF PENICILLIN ALLERGY. IF AN ALLERGIC REACTION TO CEFPODOXIME PROXETIL OCCURS, DISCONTINUE THE DRUG. SERIOUS ACUTE HYPERSENSITIVITY REACTIONS MAY REQUIRE TREATMENT WITH EPINEPHRINE AND OTHER EMERGENCY MEASURES, INCLUDING OXYGEN, INTRAVENOUS FLUIDS, INTRAVENOUS ANTIHISTAMINE, AND AIRWAY MANAGEMENT, AS CLINICALLY INDICATED. PSEUDOMEMBRANOUS COLITIS HAS BEEN REPORTED WITH NEARLY ALL ANTIBACTERIAL AGENTS, INCLUDING CEFPODOXIME, AND MAY RANGE IN SEVERITY FROM MILD TO LIFE-THREATENING. THEREFORE, IT IS IMPORTANT TO CONSIDER THIS DIAGNOSIS IN PATIENTS WHO PRESENT WITH DIARRHEA SUBSEQUENT TO THE ADMINISTRATION OF ANTIBACTERIAL AGENTS.
Extreme caution should be observed when using this product in patients at increased risk for antibiotic-induced, pseudomembranous colitis because of exposure to institutional settings, such as nursing homes or hospitals with endemic *C. difficile.*
Treatment with broad-spectrum antibiotics, including cefpodoxime proxetil, alters the normal flora of the colon and may permit overgrowth of clostridia. Studies indicate a toxin produced by *Clostridium difficile* is the primary cause of "antibiotic-associated colitis".
After the diagnosis of pseudomembranous colitis has been established, therapeutic measures should be initiated. Mild cases of pseudomembranous colitis usually respond to drug discontinuation alone. In moderate to severe cases, consideration should be given to management with fluids and electrolytes, protein supplementation, and treatment with an oral antibacterial drug effective against *C. difficile.*
A concerted effort to monitor for *C. difficile* in cefpodoxime-treated patients with diarrhea was undertaken because of an increased incidence of diarrhea associated with *C. difficile* in early trials in normal subjects. *C. difficile* organisms or toxin was reported in 10% of the cefpodoxime-treated adult patients with diarrhea; however, no specific diagnosis of pseudomembranous colitis was made in these patients.
In post-marketing experience outside the United States, reports of pseudomembranous colitis associated with the use of cefpodoxime proxetil have been received.

PRECAUTIONS
General:
In patients with transient or persistent reduction in urinary output due to renal insufficiency, the total daily dose of cefpodoxime proxetil should be reduced because high and prolonged serum antibiotic concentrations can occur in such individuals following usual doses. Cefpodoxime, like other cephalosporins, should be administered with caution to patients receiving concurrent treatment with potent diuretics. (See **DOSAGE AND ADMINISTRATION**.)
As with other antibiotics, prolonged use of cefpodoxime proxetil may result in overgrowth of non-susceptible organisms. Repeated evaluation of the patient's condition is essential. If superinfection occurs during therapy, appropriate measures should be taken.
Drug Interactions:
Antacids: Concomitant administration of high doses of antacids (sodium bicarbonate and aluminum hydroxide) or H₂

blockers reduces peak plasma levels by 24% to 42% and the extent of absorption by 27% to 32%, respectively. The rate of absorption is not altered by these concomitant medications. Oral anti-cholinergics (e.g., propantheline) delay peak plasma levels (47% increase in T_{max}), but do not affect the extent of absorption (AUC).

Probenecid: As with other beta-lactam antibiotics, renal excretion of cefpodoxime was inhibited by probenecid and resulted in an approximately 31% increase in AUC and 20% increase in peak cefpodoxime plasma levels.

Nephrotoxic drugs: Although nephrotoxicity has not been noted when cefpodoxime proxetil was given alone, close monitoring of renal function is advised when cefpodoxime proxetil is administered concomitantly with compounds of known nephrotoxic potential.

Drug/Laboratory Test Interactions:
Cephalosporins, including cefpodoxime proxetil, are known to occasionally induce a positive direct Coombs' test.

Carcinogenesis, Mutagenesis, Impairment of Fertility:
Long-term animal carcinogenesis studies of cefpodoxime proxetil have not been performed. Mutagenesis studies of cefpodoxime, including the Ames test both with and without metabolic activation, the chromosome aberration test, the unscheduled DNA synthesis assay, mitotic recombination and gene conversion, the forward gene mutation assay and the *in vivo* micronucleus test, were all negative. No untoward effects on fertility or reproduction were noted when 100 mg/kg/day or less (2 times the human dose based on mg/m^2) was administered orally to rats.

Pregnancy — Teratogenic Effects:
Pregnancy Category B
Cefpodoxime proxetil was neither teratogenic nor embryocidal when administered to rats during organogenesis at doses up to 100 mg/kg/day (2 times the human dose based on mg/m^2) or to rabbits at doses up to 30 mg/kg/day (1–2 times the human dose based on mg/m^2).
There are, however, no adequate and well-controlled studies of cefpodoxime proxetil use in pregnant women. Because animal reproduction studies are not always predictive of human response, this drug should be used during pregnancy only if clearly needed.

Labor and Delivery:
Cefpodoxime proxetil has not been studied for use during labor and delivery. Treatment should only be given if clearly needed.

Nursing Mothers:
Cefpodoxime is excreted in human milk. In a study of 3 lactating women, levels of cefpodoxime in human milk were 0%, 2% and 6% of concomitant serum levels at 4 hours following a 200 mg oral dose of cefpodoxime proxetil. At 6 hours post-dosing, levels were 0%, 9% and 16% of concomitant serum levels. Because of the potential for serious reactions in nursing infants, a decision should be made whether to discontinue nursing or to discontinue the drug, taking into account the importance of the drug to the mother.

Pediatric Use:
Safety and efficacy in infants less than 5 months of age have not been established.

Geriatric Use:
Of the 3338 patients in multiple-dose clinical studies of cefpodoxime proxetil film-coated tablets, 521 (16%) were 65 and over, while 214 (6%) were 75 and over. No overall differences in effectiveness or safety were observed between the elderly and younger patients. In healthy geriatric subjects with normal renal function, cefpodoxime half-life in plasma averaged 4.2 hours and urinary recovery averaged 21% after a 400 mg dose was given every 12 hours for 15 days. Other pharmacokinetic parameters were unchanged relative to those observed in healthy younger subjects.
Dose adjustment in elderly patients with normal renal function is not necessary.

ADVERSE REACTIONS
Clinical Trials:
Film-coated Tablets (Multiple dose):
In clinical trials using multiple doses of cefpodoxime proxetil film-coated tablets, 3338 patients were treated with the recommended dosages of cefpodoxime (100 to 400 mg Q 12 hours). There were no deaths or permanent disabilities thought related to drug toxicity. Eighty-one (2.4%) patients discontinued medication due to adverse events thought possibly- or probably-related to drug toxicity. Sixty-six (66%) of the 100 patients who discontinued therapy (whether thought related to drug therapy or not) did so because of gastrointestinal disturbances, usually diarrhea. The percentage of cefpodoxime proxetil-treated patients who discontinued study drug because of adverse events was significantly greater at a dose of 800 mg daily than at a dose of 400 mg daily or at a dose of 200 mg daily. Adverse events thought possibly- or probably-related to cefpodoxime in multiple dose clinical trials (N=3338 cefpodoxime-treated patients) were:

Incidence Greater Than 1%:
Diarrhea   7.2%
Diarrhea or loose stools were dose related: decreasing from 10.6% of patients receiving 800 mg per day to 5.9% for those

Adults (age 13 years and older):

Type of Infection	Total Daily Dose	Dose Frequency	Duration
Acute community-acquired pneumonia	400 mg	200 mg Q 12 hours	14 days
Acute bacterial exacerbations of chronic bronchitis	400 mg	200 mg Q 12 hours	10 days
Uncomplicated gonorrhea (men and women) and rectal gonococcal infections (women)	200 mg	single dose	
Skin and skin structure	800 mg	400 mg Q 12 hours	7 to 14 days
Pharyngitis and/or tonsillitis	200 mg	100 mg Q 12 hours	5 to 10 days
Uncomplicated urinary tract infection	200 mg	100 mg Q 12 hours	7 days

Adults (age 13 years and older):

Type of Infection	Total Daily Dose	Dose Frequency	Duration
Acute community-acquired pneumonia	400 mg	200 mg Q 12 hours	14 days
Uncomplicated gonorrhea (men and women) and rectal gonococcal infections (women)	200 mg	single dose	
Skin and skin structure	800 mg	400 mg Q 12 hours	7 to 14 days
Pharyngitis and/or tonsillitis	200 mg	100 mg Q 12 hours	5 to 10 days
Uncomplicated urinary tract infection	200 mg	100 mg Q 12 hours	7 days

Children (age 5 months through 12 years):

Type of Infection	Total Daily Dose	Dose Frequency	Duration
Acute otitis media	10 mg/kg/day (Max 400 mg/day)	10 mg/kg Q 24 h (Max 400 mg/dose) or 5 mg/kg Q 12 h (Max 200 mg/dose)	10 days
Pharyngitis and/or tonsillitis	10 mg/kg/day (Max 200 mg/day)	5 mg/kg/dose Q 12 h (Max 100 mg/dose)	5 to 10 days

Constitution Directions For Oral Suspension		
Bottle Size	Final Concentration	Directions
100 mL	50 mg per 5 mL	Suspend in a total of 58 mL of water. Method: First, tap the bottle to loosen granules. Then add the water in two portions, shaking well after each aliquot of water.
75 mL	50 mg per 5 mL	Suspend in a total of 44 mL of water. Method: First, tap the bottle to loosen granules. Then add the water in two portions, shaking well after each aliquot of water.
50 mL	50 mg per 5 mL	Suspend in a total of 29 mL of water. Method: First, tap the bottle to loosen granules. Then add the water in two portions, shaking well after each aliquot of water.
100 mL	100 mg per 5 mL	Suspend in a total of 57 mL of water. Method: First, tap the bottle to loosen granules. Then add the water in two portions, shaking well after each aliquot of water.
75 mL	100 mg per 5 mL	Suspend in a total of 43 mL of water. Method: First, tap the bottle to loosen granules. Then add the water in two portions, shaking well after each aliquot of water.
50 mL	100 mg per 5 mL	Suspend in a total of 29 mL of water. Method: First, tap the bottle to loosen granules. Then add the water in two portions, shaking well after each aliquot of water.

receiving 200 mg per day. Of patients with diarrhea, 10% had *C. difficile* organism or toxin in the stool. (See **WARNINGS.**)

Nausea   3.8%
Vaginal Fungal Infections   3.1%
Abdominal Pain   1.6%
Rash   1.4%
Headache   1.1%
Vomiting   1.1%

Incidence Less Than 1%:
Cardiovascular: Chest pain, hypotension.
Dermatologic: Fungal skin infection, skin scaling/peeling.
Endocrine: Menstrual irregularity.
Genital: Pruritus.
Gastrointestinal: Flatulence, decreased salivation, candidiasis, pseudomembranous colitis.
Hypersensitivity: Anaphylactic shock.
Metabolic: Decreased appetite.
Miscellaneous: Malaise, fever.
Central Nervous System: Dizziness, fatigue, anxiety, insomnia, flushing, nightmares, weakness.
Respiratory: Cough, epistaxis.
Special Senses: Taste alteration, eye itching, tinnitus.
Granules for Oral Suspension (Multiple dose):
In clinical trials using multiple doses of cefpodoxime proxetil granules for oral suspension, 1586 pediatric patients

(90% of whom were less than 12 years of age) were treated with the recommended dosages of cefpodoxime (10 mg/kg/day Q 24 hours or divided Q 12 hours to a maximum equivalent adult dose).
There were no deaths or permanent disabilities in any of the patients in these studies. Twenty-three patients (1.5%) discontinued medication due to adverse events thought possibly- or probably-related to study drug. Primarily, these discontinuations were for gastrointestinal disturbances, usually diarrhea, vomiting, or diaper area rashes.
Adverse events thought possibly- or probably-related to cefpodoxime proxetil for oral suspension in multiple dose clinical trials (N=1586 cefpodoxime treated patients) were:
Incidence Greater Than 1%:
Diarrhea   5.7%
The incidence of diarrhea in infants and toddlers (age 6 months to 2 years) was 15.4%.

Continued on next page

Information on these Pharmacia & Upjohn products is based on labeling in effect June 1, 1998. Further information concerning these and other Pharmacia & Upjohn products may be obtained by direct inquiry to Medical Information, Pharmacia & Upjohn, Kalamazoo, MI 49001.

Vantin—Cont.

| Diaper Rash/Fungal Skin Rash | 2.3% |

The incidence of diaper rash in infants and toddlers was 12.1%.

| Other skin rashes | 1.8% |
| Vomiting | 2.1% |

Incidence Less Than 1%:
Central Nervous System: Headache, irritability.
Dermatologic: Exacerbation of acne, exfoliative dermatitis.
Genital: Pruritus or vaginitis.
Gastrointestinal: Nausea, abdominal pain, candidiasis, decreased salivation, pseudomembranous colitis.
Metabolic: Decreased appetite.
Miscellaneous: Fever.
Psychiatric: Hyperactivity/nervousness.
Respiratory: Epistaxis, rhinitis.

Film-coated Tablets (Single dose):
In clinical trials using a single dose of cefpodoxime proxetil film-coated tablets, 509 patients were treated with the recommended dosage of cefpodoxime (200 mg). There were no deaths or permanent disabilities thought related to drug toxicity in these studies.
Adverse events thought possibly- or probably-related to cefpodoxime in single dose clinical trials conducted in the United States were:

Incidence Greater Than 1%:
| Nausea | 1.4% |
| Diarrhea | 1.2% |

Incidence Less Than 1%:
Central Nervous System: Dizziness, headache, syncope.
Dermatologic: Rash.
Genital: Vaginitis.
Gastrointestinal: Abdominal pain.
Psychiatric: Anxiety.

Laboratory Changes (Adult patients):
Significant laboratory changes that have been reported in adult patients in clinical trials of cefpodoxime proxetil, without regard to drug relationship, were:
Hepatic: Transient increases in AST (SGOT), ALT (SGPT), GGT, alkaline phosphatase, bilirubin, and LDH.
Hematologic: Eosinophilia, leukocytosis, lymphocytosis, granulocytosis, basophilia, monocytosis, thrombocytosis, decreased hemoglobin, leukopenia, neutropenia, lymphocytopenia, thrombocytopenia, positive Coombs' test, and prolonged PT, and PTT.
Serum Chemistry: Increases in glucose, decreases in glucose, decreases in serum albumin, decreases in serum total protein.
Renal: Increases in BUN and creatinine.
Most of these abnormalities were transient and not clinically significant.

Laboratory Changes (Pediatric patients):
Significant laboratory changes that have been reported in pediatric patients in clinical trials of cefpodoxime proxetil, without regard to drug relationship, were:
Hematologic: Eosinophilia, decreased hemoglobin, decreased hematocrit.
Hepatic: Transiently increased ALT (SGPT)
Most of these abnormalities were transient and not clinically significant.

Post-marketing Experience:
The following serious adverse experiences have been reported: allergic reactions including Stevens-Johnson syndrome, toxic epidermal necrolysis, erythema multiforme and serum sickness-like reactions, pseudomembranous colitis, bloody diarrhea with abdominal pain, ulcerative colitis, rectorrhagia with hypotension, anaphylactic shock, acute liver injury, *in utero* exposure with miscarriage, purpuric nephritis, pulmonary infiltrate with eosinophilia, and eyelid dermatitis.
One death was attributed to pseudomembranous colitis and disseminated intravascular coagulation.

Cephalosporin Class Labeling:
In addition to the adverse reactions listed above which have been observed in patients treated with cefpodoxime proxetil, the following adverse reactions and altered laboratory tests have been reported for cephalosporin class antibiotics:
Adverse Reactions and Abnormal Laboratory Tests: Renal dysfunction, toxic nephropathy, hepatic dysfunction including cholestasis, aplastic anemia, hemolytic anemia, serum sickness-like reaction, hemorrhage, agranulocytosis, and pancytopenia.
Several cephalosporins have been implicated in triggering seizures, particularly in patients with renal impairment when the dosage was not reduced. (See **DOSAGE AND ADMINISTRATION** and **OVERDOSAGE**.) If seizures associated with drug therapy occur, the drug should be discontinued. Anticonvulsant therapy can be given if clinically indicated.

OVERDOSAGE

In acute rodent toxicity studies, a single 5 g/kg oral dose produced no adverse effects. In the event of serious toxic reaction from overdosage, hemodialysis or peritoneal dialysis may aid in the removal of cefpodoxime from the body, particularly if renal function is compromised.
The toxic symptoms following an overdose of beta-lactam antibiotics may include nausea, vomiting, epigastric distress, and diarrhea.

DOSAGE AND ADMINISTRATION

(See INDICATIONS AND USAGE for indicated pathogens.)
FILM-COATED TABLETS:
VANTIN Tablets should be administered orally with food to enhance absorption. (See **CLINICAL PHARMACOLOGY**.)
The recommended dosages, durations of treatment, and applicable patient population are as described in the following chart:
[See first table at top of previous page]
GRANULES FOR ORAL SUSPENSION:
VANTIN for Oral Suspension may be given without regard to food. The recommended dosages, durations of treatment, and applicable patient populations are as described in the following chart:
[See second table at top of previous page]
Patients with Renal Dysfunction:
For patients with severe renal impairment (<30 mL/min creatinine clearance), the dosing intervals should be increased to Q 24 hours. In patients maintained on hemodialysis, the dose frequency should be 3 times/week after hemodialysis.
When only the serum creatinine level is available, the following formula (based on sex, weight, and age of the patient) may be used to estimate creatinine clearance (mL/min). For this estimate to be valid, the serum creatinine level should represent a steady state of renal function.

Males:
(mL/min)
$$\frac{\text{Weight (kg)} \times (140 - \text{age})}{72 \times \text{serum creatinine (mg/100 mL)}}$$

Females: $0.85 \times$ above value
(mL/min)

Patients with Cirrhosis:
Cefpodoxime pharmacokinetics in cirrhotic patients (with or without ascites) are similar to those in healthy subjects. Dose adjustment is not necessary in this population.
Preparation of Suspension:
[See third table at top of previous page]
After mixing, the suspension should be stored in a refrigerator, 2° to 8°C (36° to 46°F). Shake well before using. Keep container tightly closed. The mixture may be used for 14 days. Discard unused portion after 14 days.

HOW SUPPLIED

VANTIN Tablets are available in the following strengths (cefpodoxime equivalents), colors, and sizes:
100 mg, (light orange, elliptical, debossed with U3617)
Bottles of 20	NDC 0009-3617-01
Bottles of 100	NDC 0009-3617-02
Unit dose packs of 100	NDC 0009-3617-03
200 mg, (coral red, elliptical, debossed with U3618)
Bottles of 20	NDC 0009-3618-01
Bottles of 100	NDC 0009-3618-02
Unit dose packs of 100	NDC 0009-3618-03
Store tablets at controlled room temperature 20° to 25°C (68° to 77°F) [see USP]. Replace cap securely after each opening. Protect unit dose packs from excessive moisture.
VANTIN for Oral Suspension is available in the following strengths (cefpodoxime equivalents when constituted according to directions), flavor, and size:
50 mg/5 mL, lemon creme
  flavor in 100 mL bottles NDC 0009-3531-01
50 mg/5 mL, lemon creme
  flavor in 75 mL bottles NDC 0009-3531-02
50 mg/5 mL, lemon creme
  flavor in 50 mL bottles NDC 0009-3531-03
100 mg/5 mL, lemon creme
  flavor in 100 mL bottles NDC 0009-3615-01
100 mg/5 mL, lemon creme
  flavor in 75 mL bottles NDC 0009-3615-02
100 mg/5 mL, lemon creme
  flavor in 50 mL bottles NDC 0009-3615-03
Store unsuspended granules at controlled room temperature 20° to 25°C (68° to 77°F) [see USP].
Directions for mixing are included on the label. After mixing, suspension should be stored in a refrigerator, 2° to 8°C (36° to 46°F). Shake well before using. Keep container tightly closed. The mixture may be used for 14 days. Discard unused portion after 14 days.

REFERENCES

1. National Committee for Clinical Laboratory Standards, Approved Standard: Performance Standards for Antimicrobial Disk Susceptibility Tests, 4th Edition, Vol. 10(7):M2-A4, Villanova, PA, April, 1990.
2. National Committee for Clinical Laboratory Standards, Approved Standard: Methods for Dilution Antimicrobial Susceptibility Tests for Bacteria That Grow Aerobically, 2nd Edition, Vol. 10(8):M7-A2, Villanova, PA, April, 1990.

CLINICAL TRIALS

Cystitis
In two double-blind, 2:1 randomized, comparative trials performed in adults in the United States, cefpodoxime proxetil was compared to other beta-lactam antibiotics. In these studies, the following bacterial eradication rates were obtained at 5 to 9 days after therapy:
[See first table above]
In these studies, clinical cure rates and bacterial eradication rates for cefpodoxime proxetil were comparable to the comparator agents; however, the clinical cure rates and bacteriologic eradication rates were lower than those observed with some other classes of approved agents for cystitis.
Acute Otitis Media Studies
In controlled studies of acute otitis media performed in the United States, where significant rates of beta-lactamase-producing organisms were found, cefpodoxime proxetil was compared to other oral antibiotics. In these studies, using very strict evaluability criteria and microbiologic and clinical response criteria at the 15-to-28 day post-therapy follow-up, the following presumptive bacterial eradication/clinical cure outcomes (ie, clinical success) were obtained.
[See second table above]
Rx only
U.S. Patent Nos. 4,486,425; 4,409,215.
Licensed from Sankyo Company, Ltd., Japan
Mfd by: Pharmacia & Upjohn N.V./S.A., Puurs - Belgium
For: Pharmacia & Upjohn Company, Kalamazoo, Michigan 49001, USA
Revised May 1998   815 267 013
Shown in Product Identification Guide, page 332

Pathogen	Cefpodoxime		Comparator	
E. coli	200/243 (82%)		99/123 (80%)	
Other pathogens	34/42 (81%)		23/28 (82%)	
K. pneumoniae				
P. mirabilis				
S. saprophyticus				
TOTAL	234/285 (82%)		122/151 (81%)	

Pathogen	Cefpodoxime Proxetil 5 mg/kg Q12h × 10 d	Comparator
H. influenzae	25/46 (54%)	18/36 (50%)
M. catarrhalis	20/42 (48%)	8/22 (36%)
S. pneumoniae	39/74 (53%)	19/37 (51%)

Pathogen	Cefpodoxime Proxetil 10 mg/kg Q24h × 10 d	Comparator
H. influenzae	36/56 (64%)	12/21 (57%)
M. catarrhalis	14/18 (78%)	8/12 (67%)
S. pneumoniae	56/89 (63%)	21/38 (55%)

XANAX®
Tablets
alprazolam tablets, USP

© IV ℞

DESCRIPTION

XANAX Tablets contain alprazolam which is a triazolo analog of the 1,4 benzodiazepine class of central nervous system-active compounds.
The chemical name of alprazolam is 8-Chloro-1-methyl-6-phenyl-4H-s-triazolo [4,3-α] [1,4] benzodiazepine.
The structural formula is represented below:
[See chemical structure at top of next column]
Alprazolam is a white crystalline powder, which is soluble in methanol or ethanol but which has no appreciable solubility in water at physiological pH.

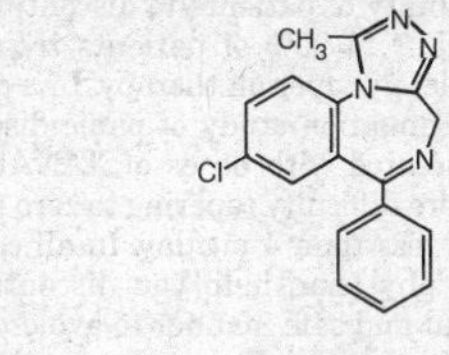

Each XANAX Tablet, for oral administration, contains 0.25, 0.5, 1 or 2 mg of alprazolam.
XANAX Tablets, 2 mg, are multi-scored and may be divided as shown below:

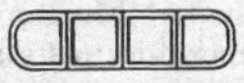

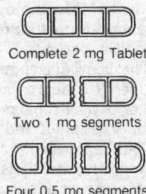

Complete 2 mg Tablet

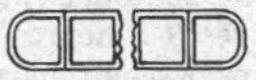

Two 1 mg segments

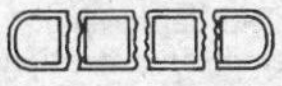

Four 0.5 mg segments

Inactive ingredients: Cellulose, corn starch, docusate sodium, lactose, magnesium stearate, silicon dioxide and sodium benzoate. In addition, the 0.5 mg tablet contains FD&C Yellow No. 6 and the 1 mg tablet contains FD&C Blue No. 2.

CLINICAL PHARMACOLOGY

CNS agents of the 1,4 benzodiazepine class presumably exert their effects by binding at stereo specific receptors at several sites within the central nervous system. Their exact mechanism of action is unknown. Clinically, all benzodiazepines cause a dose-related central nervous system depressant activity varying from mild impairment of task performance to hypnosis.
Following oral administration, alprazolam is readily absorbed. Peak concentrations in the plasma occur in one to two hours following administration. Plasma levels are proportionate to the dose given; over the dose range of 0.5 to 3.0 mg, peak levels of 8.0 to 37 ng/mL were observed. Using a specific assay methodology, the mean plasma elimination half-life of alprazolam has been found to be about 11.2 hours (range: 6.3–26.9 hours) in healthy adults.
The predominant metabolites are α-hydroxy-alprazolam and a benzophenone derived from alprazolam. The biological activity of α-hydroxy-alprazolam is approximately one-half that of alprazolam. The benzophenone metabolite is essentially inactive. Plasma levels of these metabolites are extremely low, thus precluding precise pharmacokinetic description. However, their half-lives appear to be of the same order of magnitude as that of alprazolam. Alprazolam and its metabolites are excreted primarily in the urine.
The ability of alprazolam to induce human hepatic enzyme systems has not yet been determined. However, this is not a property of benzodiazepines in general. Further, alprazolam did not affect the prothrombin or plasma warfarin levels in male volunteers administered sodium warfarin orally.
In vitro, alprazolam is bound (80 percent) to human serum protein.
Changes in the absorption, distribution, metabolism and excretion of benzodiazepines have been reported in a variety of disease states including alcoholism, impaired hepatic function and impaired renal function. Changes have also been demonstrated in geriatric patients. A mean half-life of alprazolam of 16.3 hours has been observed in healthy elderly subjects (range: 9.0–26.9 hours, n=16) compared to 11.0 hours (range: 6.3–15.8 hours, n=16) in healthy adult subjects. In patients with alcoholic liver disease the half-life of alprazolam ranged between 5.8 and 65.3 hours (mean: 19.7 hours, n=17) as compared to between 6.3 and 26.9 hours (mean=11.4 hours, n=17) in healthy subjects. In an obese group of subjects the half-life of alprazolam ranged between 9.9 and 40.4 hours (mean=21.8 hours, n=12) as compared to between 6.3 and 15.8 hours (mean=10.6 hours, n=12) in healthy subjects.
Because of its similarity to other benzodiazepines, it is assumed that alprazolam undergoes transplacental passage and that it is excreted in human milk.

INDICATIONS AND USAGE

XANAX Tablets (alprazolam) are indicated for the management of anxiety disorder (a condition corresponding most closely to the APA Diagnostic and Statistical Manual [DSM-III-R] diagnosis of generalized anxiety disorder) or the short-term relief of symptoms of anxiety. Anxiety or tension associated with the stress of everyday life usually does not require treatment with an anxiolytic.
Generalized anxiety disorder is characterized by unrealistic or excessive anxiety and worry (apprehensive expectation) about two or more life circumstances, for a period of six months or longer, during which the person has been bothered more days than not by these concerns. At least 6 of the following 18 symptoms are often present in these patients: *Motor Tension* (trembling, twitching, or feeling shaky; muscle tension, aches, or soreness; restlessness; easy fatigability); *Autonomic Hyperactivity* (shortness of breath or smothering sensations; palpitations or accelerated heart rate; sweating, or cold clammy hands; dry mouth; dizziness or light-headedness; nausea, diarrhea, or other abdominal distress; flushes or chills; frequent urination; trouble swallowing or 'lump in throat'); *Vigilance and Scanning* (feeling keyed up or on edge; exaggerated startle response; difficulty concentrating or 'mind going blank' because of anxiety; trouble falling or staying asleep; irritability). These symptoms must not be secondary to another psychiatric disorder or caused by some organic factor.
Anxiety associated with depression is responsive to XANAX.
XANAX is also indicated for the treatment of panic disorder, with or without agoraphobia.
Studies supporting this claim were conducted in patients whose diagnoses corresponded closely to the DSM-III-R criteria for panic disorder (see CLINICAL STUDIES).
Panic disorder is an illness characterized by recurrent panic attacks. The panic attacks, at least initially, are unexpected. Later in the course of this disturbance certain situations, eg, driving a car or being in a crowded place, may become associated with having a panic attack. These panic attacks are not triggered by situations in which the person is the focus of others' attention (as in social phobia). The diagnosis requires four such attacks within a four week period, or one or more attacks followed by at least a month of persistent fear of having another attack. The panic attacks must be characterized by at least four of the following symptoms: dyspnea or smothering sensations; dizziness, unsteady feelings, or faintness; palpitations or tachycardia; trembling or shaking; sweating; choking; nausea or abdominal distress; depersonalization or derealization; paresthesias; hot flashes or chills; chest pain or discomfort; fear of dying; fear of going crazy or of doing something uncontrolled. At least some of the panic attack symptoms must develop suddenly, and the panic attack symptoms must not be attributable to some known organic factors. Panic disorder is frequently associated with some symptoms of agoraphobia.
Demonstrations of the effectiveness of XANAX by systematic clinical study are limited to four months duration for anxiety disorder and four to ten weeks duration for panic disorder; however, patients with panic disorder have been treated on an open basis for up to eight months without apparent loss of benefit. The physician should periodically reassess the usefulness of the drug for the individual patient.

CONTRAINDICATIONS

XANAX Tablets are contraindicated in patients with known sensitivity to this drug or other benzodiazepines. XANAX may be used in patients with open angle glaucoma who are receiving appropriate therapy, but is contraindicated in patients with acute narrow angle glaucoma.
XANAX is contraindicated with ketoconazole and itraconazole, since these medications significantly impair the oxidative metabolism mediated by cytochrome P450 3A (CYP 3A) (see WARNINGS and PRECAUTIONS—Drug Interactions).

WARNINGS

Dependence and withdrawal reactions, including seizures:
Certain adverse clinical events, some life-threatening, are a direct consequence of physical dependence to XANAX. These include a spectrum of withdrawal symptoms; the most important is seizure (see DRUG ABUSE AND DEPENDENCE). Even after relatively short-term use at the doses recommended for the treatment of transient anxiety and anxiety disorder (ie, 0.75 to 4.0 mg per day), there is some risk of dependence. Spontaneous reporting system data suggest that the risk of dependence and its severity appear to be greater in patients treated with doses greater than 4 mg/day and for long periods (more than 12 weeks). However, in a controlled postmarketing discontinuation study of panic disorder patients, the duration of treatment (three months compared to six months) had no effect on the ability of patients to taper to zero dose. In contrast, patients treated with doses of XANAX greater than 4 mg/day had more difficulty tapering to zero dose than those treated with less than 4 mg/day.
The importance of dose and the risks of XANAX as a treatment for panic disorder:
Because the management of panic disorder often requires the use of average daily doses of XANAX above 4 mg, the risk of dependence among panic disorder patients may be higher than that among those treated for less severe anxiety. Experience in randomized placebo-controlled discontinuation studies of patients with panic disorder showed a high rate of rebound and withdrawal symptoms in patients treated with XANAX compared to placebo treated patients.
Relapse or return of illness was defined as a return of symptoms characteristic of panic disorder (primarily panic attacks) to levels approximately equal to those seen at baseline before active treatment was initiated. Rebound refers to a return of symptoms of panic disorder to a level substantially greater in frequency, or more severe in intensity than seen at baseline. Withdrawal symptoms were identified as those which were generally not characteristic of panic disorder and which occurred for the first time more frequently during discontinuation than at baseline.
In a controlled clinical trial in which 63 patients were randomized to XANAX and where withdrawal symptoms were specifically sought, the following were identified as symptoms of withdrawal: heightened sensory perception, impaired concentration, dysosmia, clouded sensorium, paresthesias, muscle cramps, muscle twitch, diarrhea, blurred vision, appetite decrease and weight loss. Other symptoms, such as anxiety and insomnia, were frequently seen during discontinuation, but it could not be determined if they were due to return of illness, rebound or withdrawal.
In a larger database comprised of both controlled and uncontrolled studies in which 641 patients received XANAX, discontinuation-emergent symptoms which occurred at a rate of over 5% in patients treated with XANAX and at a greater rate than the placebo treated group were as follows:
[See table above]

DISCONTINUATION-EMERGENT SYMPTOM INCIDENCE

Body System/Event	Percentage of 641 XANAX-Treated Panic Disorder Patients Reporting Events
Neurologic	
Insomnia	29.5
Light-headedness	19.3
Abnormal involuntary movement	17.3
Headache	17.0
Muscular twitching	6.9
Impaired coordination	6.6
Muscle tone disorders	5.9
Weakness	5.8
Psychiatric	
Anxiety	19.2
Fatigue and Tiredness	18.4
Irritability	10.5
Cognitive disorder	10.3
Memory impairment	5.5
Depression	5.1
Confusional state	5.0
Gastrointestinal	
Nausea/Vomiting	16.5
Diarrhea	13.6
Decreased salivation	10.6
Metabolic-Nutritional	
Weight loss	13.3
Decreased appetite	12.8
Dermatological	
Sweating	14.4
Cardiovascular	
Tachycardia	12.2
Special Senses	
Blurred vision	10.0

From the studies cited, it has not been determined whether these symptoms are clearly related to the dose and duration of therapy with XANAX in patients with panic disorder.
In two controlled trials of six to eight weeks duration where the ability of patients to discontinue medication was measured, 71%–93% of XANAX treated patients tapered completely off therapy compared to 89%–96% of placebo treated patients. In a controlled postmarketing discontinuation study of panic disorder patients, the duration of treatment (three months compared to six months) had no effect on the ability of patients to taper to zero dose.
Seizures attributable to XANAX were seen after drug discontinuance or dose reduction in 8 of 1980 patients with panic disorder or in patients participating in clinical trials

Continued on next page

Information on these Pharmacia & Upjohn products is based on labeling in effect June 1, 1998. Further information concerning these and other Pharmacia & Upjohn products may be obtained by direct inquiry to Medical Information, Pharmacia & Upjohn, Kalamazoo, MI 49001.

Xanax—Cont.

where doses of XANAX greater than 4 mg/day for over 3 months were permitted. Five of these cases clearly occurred during abrupt dose reduction, or discontinuation from daily doses of 2 to 10 mg. Three cases occurred in situations where there was not a clear relationship to abrupt dose reduction or discontinuation. In one instance, seizure occurred after discontinuation from a single dose of 1 mg after tapering at a rate of 1 mg every three days from 6 mg daily. In two other instances, the relationship to taper is indeterminate; in both of these cases the patients had been receiving doses of 3 mg daily prior to seizure. The duration of use in the above 8 cases ranged from 4 to 22 weeks. There have been occasional voluntary reports of patients developing seizures while apparently tapering gradually from XANAX. The risk of seizure seems to be greatest 24–72 hours after discontinuation (see DOSAGE AND ADMINISTRATION for recommended tapering and discontinuation schedule).

Status epilepticus and its treatment:

The medical event voluntary reporting system shows that withdrawal seizures have been reported in association with the discontinuation of XANAX. In most cases, only a single seizure was reported; however, multiple seizures and status epilepticus were reported as well. Ordinarily, the treatment of status epilepticus of any etiology involves use of intravenous benzodiazepines plus phenytoin or barbiturates, maintenance of a patent airway and adequate hydration. For additional details regarding therapy, consultation with an appropriate specialist may be considered.

Interdose Symptoms:

Early morning anxiety and emergence of anxiety symptoms between doses of XANAX have been reported in patients with panic disorder taking prescribed maintenance doses of XANAX. These symptoms may reflect the development of tolerance or a time interval between doses which is longer than the duration of clinical action of the administered dose. In either case, it is presumed that the prescribed dose is not sufficient to maintain plasma levels above those needed to prevent relapse, rebound or withdrawal symptoms over the entire course of the interdosing interval. In these situations, it is recommended that the same total daily dose be given divided as more frequent administrations (see DOSAGE AND ADMINISTRATION).

Risk of dose reduction:

Withdrawal reactions may occur when dosage reduction occurs for any reason. This includes purposeful tapering, but also inadvertent reduction of dose (eg, the patient forgets, the patient is admitted to a hospital, etc.). Therefore, the dosage of XANAX should be reduced or discontinued gradually (see DOSAGE AND ADMINISTRATION).

XANAX Tablets are not of value in the treatment of psychotic patients and should not be employed in lieu of appropriate treatment for psychosis. Because of its CNS depressant effects, patients receiving XANAX should be cautioned against engaging in hazardous occupations or activities requiring complete mental alertness such as operating machinery or driving a motor vehicle. For the same reason, patients should be cautioned about the simultaneous ingestion of alcohol and other CNS depressant drugs during treatment with XANAX.

Benzodiazepines can potentially cause fetal harm when administered to pregnant women. If XANAX is used during pregnancy, or if the patient becomes pregnant while taking this drug, the patient should be apprised of the potential hazard to the fetus. Because of experience with other members of the benzodiazepine class, XANAX is assumed to be capable of causing an increased risk of congenital abnormalities when administered to a pregnant woman during the first trimester. Because use of these drugs is rarely a matter of urgency, their use during the first trimester should almost always be avoided. The possibility that a woman of childbearing potential may be pregnant at the time of institution of therapy should be considered. Patients should be advised that if they become pregnant during therapy or intend to become pregnant they should communicate with their physicians about the desirability of discontinuing the drug.

Alprazolam interaction with drugs that inhibit metabolism via cytochrome P450 3A: The initial step in alprazolam metabolism is hydroxylation catalyzed by cytochrome P450 3A (CYP 3A). Drugs that inhibit this metabolic pathway may have a profound effect on the clearance of alprazolam. Consequently, alprazolam should be avoided in patients receiving very potent inhibitors of CYP 3A. With drugs inhibiting CYP 3A to a lesser but still significant degree, alprazolam should be used only with caution and consideration of appropriate dosage reduction. For some drugs, an interaction with alprazolam has been quantified with clinical data; for other drugs, interactions are predicted from *in vitro* data and/or experience with similar drugs in the same pharmacologic class.

The following are examples of drugs known to inhibit the metabolism of alprazolam and/or related benzodiazepines, presumably through inhibition of CYP 3A.

Potent CYP 3A inhibitors:

Azole antifungal agents—Although *in vivo* interaction data with alprazolam are not available, ketoconazole and itraconazole are potent CYP 3A inhibitors and the coadministration of alprazolam with them is not recommended. Other azole-type antifungal agents should also be considered potent CYP 3A inhibitors and the coadministration of alprazolam with them is not recommended (see CONTRAINDICATIONS).

Drugs demonstrated to be CYP 3A inhibitors on the basis of clinical studies involving alprazolam (caution and consideration of appropriate alprazolam dose reduction are recommended during coadministration with the following drugs):
Nefazodone—Coadministration of nefazodone increased alprazolam concentration two-fold.
Fluvoxamine—Coadministration of fluvoxamine approximately doubled the maximum plasma concentration of alprazolam, decreased clearance by 49%, increased half-life by 71%, and decreased measured psychomotor performance.
Cimetidine—Coadministration of cimetidine increased the maximum plasma concentration of alprazolam by 86%, decreased clearance by 42%, and increased half-life by 16%.

Other drugs possibly affecting alprazolam metabolism:
Other drugs possibly affecting alprazolam metabolism by inhibition of CYP 3A are discussed in the PRECAUTIONS section (see PRECAUTIONS—Drug Interactions).

PRECAUTIONS

General: If XANAX Tablets are to be combined with other psychotropic agents or anticonvulsant drugs, careful consideration should be given to the pharmacology of the agents to be employed, particularly with compounds which might potentiate the action of benzodiazepines (see DRUG INTERACTIONS).

As with other psychotropic medications, the usual precautions with respect to administration of the drug and size of the prescription are indicated for severely depressed patients or those in whom there is reason to expect concealed suicidal ideation or plans.

It is recommended that the dosage be limited to the smallest effective dose to preclude the development of ataxia or oversedation which may be a particular problem in elderly or debilitated patients. (See DOSAGE AND ADMINISTRATION.) The usual precautions in treating patients with impaired renal, hepatic or pulmonary function should be observed. There have been rare reports of death in patients with severe pulmonary disease shortly after the initiation of treatment with XANAX. A decreased systemic alprazolam elimination rate (eg, increased plasma half-life) has been observed in both alcoholic liver disease patients and obese patients receiving XANAX (see CLINICAL PHARMACOLOGY).

Episodes of hypomania and mania have been reported in association with the use of XANAX in patients with depression.

Alprazolam has a weak uricosuric effect. Although other medications with weak uricosuric effect have been reported to cause acute renal failure, there have been no reported instances of acute renal failure attributable to therapy with XANAX.

Information for Patients:
For all users of XANAX:
To assure safe and effective use of benzodiazepines, all patients prescribed XANAX should be provided with the following guidance. In addition, panic disorder patients, for whom doses greater than 4 mg/day are typically prescribed, should be advised about the risks associated with the use of higher doses.

1. Inform your physician about any alcohol consumption and medicine you are taking now, including medication you may buy without a prescription. Alcohol should generally not be used during treatment with benzodiazepines.

2. Not recommended for use in pregnancy. Therefore, inform your physician if you are pregnant, if you are planning to have a child, or if you become pregnant while you are taking this medication.

3. Inform your physician if you are nursing.

4. Until you experience how this medication affects you, do not drive a car or operate potentially dangerous machinery, etc.

5. Do not increase the dose even if you think the medication "does not work anymore" without consulting your physician. Benzodiazepines, even when used as recommended, may produce emotional and/or physical dependence.

6. Do not stop taking this medication abruptly or decrease the dose without consulting your physician, since withdrawal symptoms can occur.

Additional advice for panic disorder patients:
The use of XANAX at doses greater than 4 mg/day, often necessary to treat panic disorder, is accompanied by risks that you need to carefully consider. When used at doses greater than 4 mg/day, which may or may not be required for your treatment, XANAX has the potential to cause severe emotional and physical dependence in some patients and these patients may find it exceedingly difficult to terminate treatment. In two controlled trials of six to eight weeks

duration where the ability of patients to discontinue medication was measured, 7 to 29% of patients treated with XANAX did not completely taper off therapy. In a controlled postmarketing discontinuation study of panic disorder patients, the patients treated with doses of XANAX greater than 4 mg/day had more difficulty tapering to zero dose than patients treated with less than 4 mg/day. In all cases, it is important that your physician help you discontinue this medication in a careful and safe manner to avoid overly extended use of XANAX.

In addition, the extended use at doses greater than 4 mg/day appears to increase the incidence and severity of withdrawal reactions when XANAX is discontinued. These are generally minor but seizure can occur, especially if you reduce the dose too rapidly or discontinue the medication abruptly. Seizure can be life-threatening.

Laboratory Tests: Laboratory tests are not ordinarily required in otherwise healthy patients.

Drug Interactions: The benzodiazepines, including alprazolam, produce additive CNS depressant effects when coadministered with other psychotropic medications, anticonvulsants, antihistaminics, ethanol and other drugs which themselves produce CNS depression.

The steady state plasma concentrations of imipramine and desipramine have been reported to be increased an average of 31% and 20%, respectively, by the concomitant administration of XANAX Tablets in doses up to 4 mg/day. The clinical significance of these changes is unknown.

Drugs that inhibit alprazolam metabolism via cytochrome P450 3A: The initial step in alprazolam metabolism is hydroxylation catalyzed by cytochrome P450 3A (CYP 3A). Drugs which inhibit this metabolic pathway may have a profound effect on the clearance of alprazolam (see CONTRAINDICATIONS and WARNINGS for additional drugs of this type).

Drugs demonstrated to be CYP 3A inhibitors of possible clinical significance on the basis of clinical studies involving alprazolam (caution is recommended during coadministration with alprazolam):
Fluoxetine—Coadministration of fluoxetine with alprazolam increased the maximum plasma concentration of alprazolam by 46%, decreased clearance by 21%, increased half-life by 17%, and decreased measured psychomotor performance.
Propoxyphen—Coadministration of propoxyphene decreased the maximum plasma concentration of alprazolam by 6%, decreased clearance by 38%, and increased half-life by 58%.
Oral Contraceptives—Coadministration of oral contraceptives increased the maximum plasma concentration of alprazolam by 18%, decreased clearance by 22%, and increased half-life by 29%.

Drugs and other substances demonstrated to be CYP 3A inhibitors on the basis of clinical studies involving benzodiazepines metabolized similarly to alprazolam or on the basis of in vitro studies with alprazolam or other benzodiazepines (caution is recommended during coadministration with alprazolam): Available data from clinical studies of benzodiazepines other than alprazolam suggest a possible drug interaction with alprazolam for the following: diltiazem, isoniazid, macrolide antibiotics such as erythromycin and clarithromycin, and grapefruit juice. Data from *in vitro* studies of alprazolam suggest a possible drug interaction with alprazolam for the following: sertraline and paroxetine. Data from *in vitro* studies of benzodiazepines other than alprazolam suggest a possible drug interaction for the following: ergotamine, cyclosporine, amiodarone, nicardipine, and nifedipine. Caution is recommended during the coadministration of any of these with alprazolam (see WARNINGS).

Drug/Laboratory Test Interactions: Although interactions between benzodiazepines and commonly employed clinical laboratory tests have occasionally been reported, there is no consistent pattern for a specific drug or specific test.

Carcinogenesis, Mutagenesis, Impairment of Fertility: No evidence of carcinogenic potential was observed during 2-year bioassay studies of alprazolam in rats at doses up to 30 mg/kg/day (150 times the maximum recommended daily human dose of 10 mg/day) and in mice at doses up to 10 mg/kg/day (50 times the maximum recommended daily human dose).

Alprazolam was not mutagenic in the rat micronucleus test at doses up to 100 mg/kg, which is 500 times the maximum recommended daily human dose of 10 mg/day. Alprazolam also was not mutagenic *in vitro* in the DNA Damage/Alkaline Elution Assay or the Ames Assay.

Alprazolam produced no impairment of fertility in rats at doses up to 5 mg/kg/day, which is 25 times the maximum recommended daily human dose of 10 mg/day.

Pregnancy: Teratogenic Effects: Pregnancy Category D: (See WARNINGS Section).

Nonteratogenic Effects: It should be considered that the child born of a mother who is receiving benzodiazepines may be at some risk for withdrawal symptoms from the drug during the postnatal period. Also, neonatal flaccidity and respiratory problems have been reported in children

ANXIETY DISORDERS

	Treatment-Emergent Symptom Incidence†		Incidence of Intervention Because of Symptom
	XANAX	PLACEBO	XANAX
Number of Patients	565	505	565
% of Patients Reporting:			
Central Nervous System			
Drowsiness	41.0	21.6	15.1
Light-headedness	20.8	19.3	1.2
Depression	13.9	18.1	2.4
Headache	12.9	19.6	1.1
Confusion	9.9	10.0	0.9
Insomnia	8.9	18.4	1.3
Nervousness	4.1	10.3	1.1
Syncope	3.1	4.0	*
Dizziness	1.8	0.8	2.5
Akathisia	1.6	1.2	*
Tiredness/Sleepiness	*	*	1.8
Gastrointestinal			
Dry Mouth	14.7	13.3	0.7
Constipation	10.4	11.4	0.9
Diarrhea	10.1	10.3	1.2
Nausea/Vomiting	9.6	12.8	1.7
Increased Salivation	4.2	2.4	*
Cardiovascular			
Tachycardia/Palpitations	7.7	15.6	0.4
Hypotension	4.7	2.2	*
Sensory			
Blurred Vision	6.2	6.2	0.4
Musculoskeletal			
Rigidity	4.2	5.3	*
Tremor	4.0	8.8	0.4
Cutaneous			
Dermatitis/Allergy	3.8	3.1	0.6
Other			
Nasal Congestion	7.3	9.3	*
Weight Gain	2.7	2.7	*
Weight Loss	2.3	3.0	*

*None reported
†Events reported by 1% or more of XANAX patients are included.

born of mothers who have been receiving benzodiazepines.
Labor and Delivery: XANAX has no established use in labor or delivery.
Nursing Mothers: Benzodiazepines are known to be excreted in human milk. It should be assumed that alprazolam is as well. Chronic administration of diazepam to nursing mothers has been reported to cause their infants to become lethargic and to lose weight. As a general rule, nursing should not be undertaken by mothers who must use XANAX.
Pediatric Use: Safety and effectiveness of XANAX in individuals below 18 years of age have not been established.

ADVERSE REACTIONS

Side effects to XANAX Tablets, if they occur, are generally observed at the beginning of therapy and usually disappear upon continued medication. In the usual patient, the most frequent side effects are likely to be an extension of the pharmacological activity of alprazolam, eg, drowsiness or light-headedness.
The data cited in the two tables below are estimates of untoward clinical event incidence among patients who participated under the following clinical conditions: relatively short duration (ie, four weeks) placebo-controlled clinical studies with dosages up to 4 mg/day of XANAX (for the management of anxiety disorders or for the short-term relief of the symptoms of anxiety) and short-term (up to ten weeks) placebo-controlled clinical studies with dosages up to 10 mg/day of XANAX in patients with panic disorder, with or without agoraphobia.
These data cannot be used to predict precisely the incidence of untoward events in the course of usual medical practice where patient characteristics, and other factors often differ from those in clinical trials. These figures cannot be compared with those obtained from other clinical studies involving related drug products and placebo as each group of drug trials are conducted under a different set of conditions.
Comparison of the cited figures, however, can provide the prescriber with some basis for estimating the relative contributions of drug and non-drug factors to the untoward event incidence in the population studied. Even this use must be approached cautiously, as a drug may relieve a symptom in one patient but induce it in others. (For exam-

ple, an anxiolytic drug may relieve dry mouth [a symptom of anxiety] in some subjects but induce it [an untoward event] in others.)
Additionally, for anxiety disorders the cited figures can provide the prescriber with an indication as to the frequency with which physician intervention (eg, increased surveillance, decreased dosage or discontinuation of drug therapy) may be necessary because of the untoward clinical event. [See table above]
In addition to the relatively common (ie, greater than 1%) untoward events enumerated in the table above, the following adverse events have been reported in association with the use of benzodiazepines: dystonia, irritability, concentration difficulties, anorexia, transient amnesia or memory impairment, loss of coordination, fatigue, seizures, sedation, slurred speech, jaundice, musculoskeletal weakness, pruritus, diplopia, dysarthria, changes in libido, menstrual irregularities, incontinence and urinary retention.

PANIC DISORDER

	Treatment-Emergent Symptom Incidence*	
	XANAX	PLACEBO
Number of Patients	1388	1231
% of Patients Reporting:		
Central Nervous System		
Drowsiness	76.8	42.7
Fatigue and Tiredness	48.6	42.3
Impaired Coordination	40.1	17.9
Irritability	33.1	30.1
Memory Impairment	33.1	22.1
Light-headedness/Dizziness	29.8	36.9
Insomnia	29.4	41.8
Headache	29.2	35.6
Cognitive Disorder	28.8	20.5
Dysarthria	23.3	6.3
Anxiety	16.6	24.9
Abnormal Involuntary Movement	14.8	21.0
Decreased Libido	14.4	8.0
Depression	13.8	14.0
Confusional State	10.4	8.2

	XANAX	PLACEBO
Muscular Twitching	7.9	11.8
Increased Libido	7.7	4.1
Change in Libido (Not Specified)	7.1	5.6
Weakness	7.1	8.4
Muscle Tone Disorders	6.3	7.5
Syncope	3.8	4.8
Akathisia	3.0	4.3
Agitation	2.9	2.6
Disinhibition	2.7	1.5
Paresthesia	2.4	3.2
Talkativeness	2.2	1.0
Vasomotor Disturbances	2.0	2.6
Derealization	1.9	1.2
Dream Abnormalities	1.8	1.5
Fear	1.4	1.0
Feeling Warm	1.3	0.5
Gastrointestinal		
Decreased Salivation	32.8	34.2
Constipation	26.2	15.4
Nausea/Vomiting	22.0	31.8
Diarrhea	20.6	22.8
Abdominal Distress	18.3	21.5
Increased Salivation	5.6	4.4
Cardio-Respiratory		
Nasal Congestion	17.4	16.5
Tachycardia	15.4	26.8
Chest Pain	10.6	18.1
Hyperventilation	9.7	14.5
Upper Respiratory Infection	4.3	3.7
Sensory		
Blurred Vision	21.0	21.4
Tinnitus	6.6	10.4
Musculoskeletal		
Muscular Cramps	2.4	2.4
Muscle Stiffness	2.2	3.3
Cutaneous		
Sweating	15.1	23.5
Rash	10.8	8.1
Other		
Increased Appetite	32.7	22.8
Decreased Appetite	27.8	24.1
Weight Gain	27.2	17.9
Weight Loss	22.6	16.5
Micturition Difficulties	12.2	8.6
Menstrual Disorders	10.4	8.7
Sexual Dysfunction	7.4	3.7
Edema	4.9	5.6
Incontinence	1.5	0.6
Infection	1.3	1.7

*Events reported by 1% or more of XANAX patients are included.

In addition to the relatively common (ie, greater than 1%) untoward events enumerated in the table above, the following adverse events have been reported in association with the use of XANAX: seizures, hallucinations, depersonalization, taste alterations, diplopia, elevated bilirubin, elevated hepatic enzymes, and jaundice.
There have also been reports of withdrawal seizures upon rapid decrease or abrupt discontinuation of XANAX Tablets (see WARNINGS).
To discontinue treatment in patients taking XANAX, the dosage should be reduced slowly in keeping with good medical practice. It is suggested that the daily dosage of XANAX be decreased by no more than 0.5 mg every three days (see DOSAGE AND ADMINISTRATION). Some patients may benefit from an even slower dosage reduction. In a controlled postmarketing discontinuation study of panic disorder patients which compared this recommended taper schedule with a slower taper schedule, no difference was observed between the groups in the proportion of patients who tapered to zero dose; however, the slower schedule was associated with a reduction in symptoms associated with a withdrawal syndrome.
Panic disorder has been associated with primary and secondary major depressive disorders and increased reports of

Continued on next page

Information on these Pharmacia & Upjohn products is based on labeling in effect June 1, 1998. Further information concerning these and other Pharmacia & Upjohn products may be obtained by direct inquiry to Medical Information, Pharmacia & Upjohn, Kalamazoo, MI 49001.

Xanax—Cont.

suicide among untreated patients. Therefore, the same precaution must be exercised when using doses of XANAX greater than 4 mg/day in treating patients with panic disorders as is exercised with the use of any psychotropic drug in treating depressed patients or those in whom there is reason to expect concealed suicidal ideation or plans.

As with all benzodiazepines, paradoxical reactions such as stimulation, increased muscle spasticity, sleep disturbances, hallucinations and other adverse behavioral effects such as agitation, rage, irritability, and aggressive or hostile behavior have been reported rarely. In many of the spontaneous case reports of adverse behavioral effects, patients were receiving other CNS drugs concomitantly and/or were described as having underlying psychiatric conditions. Should any of the above events occur, alprazolam should be discontinued. Isolated published reports involving small numbers of patients have suggested that patients who have borderline personality disorder, a prior history of violent or aggressive behavior, or alcohol or substance abuse may be at risk for such events. Instances of irritability, hostility, and intrusive thoughts have been reported during discontinuation of alprazolam in patients with posttraumatic stress disorder.

Laboratory analyses were performed on patients participating in the clinical program for XANAX. The following incidences of abnormalities shown below were observed in patients receiving XANAX and in patients in the corresponding placebo group. Few of these abnormalities were considered to be of physiological significance.

	XANAX		PLACEBO	
	Low	High	Low	High
Hematology				
Hematocrit	*	*	*	*
Hemoglobin	*	*	*	*
Total WBC Count	1.4	2.3	1.0	2.0
Neutrophil Count	2.3	3.0	4.2	1.7
Lymphocyte Count	5.5	7.4	5.4	9.5
Monocyte Count	5.3	2.8	6.4	*
Eosinophil Count	3.2	9.5	3.3	7.2
Basophil Count	*	*	*	*
Urinalysis				
Albumin	—	*	—	*
Sugar	—	*	—	*
RBC/HPF	—	3.4	—	5.0
WBC/HPF	—	25.7	—	25.9
Blood Chemistry				
Creatinine	2.2	1.9	3.5	1.0
Bilirubin	*	1.6	*	*
SGOT	*	3.2	1.0	1.8
Alkaline Phosphatase	*	1.7	*	1.8

*Less than 1%

When treatment with XANAX is protracted, periodic blood counts, urinalysis and blood chemistry analyses are advisable.

Minor changes in EEG patterns, usually low-voltage fast activity have been observed in patients during therapy with XANAX and are of no known significance.

Post Introduction Reports: Various adverse drug reactions have been reported in association with the use of XANAX since market introduction. The majority of these reactions were reported through the medical event voluntary reporting system. Because of the spontaneous nature of the reporting of medical events and the lack of controls, a causal relationship to the use of XANAX cannot be readily determined. Reported events include: liver enzyme elevations, hepatitis, hepatic failure, Stevens-Johnson syndrome, hyperprolactinemia, gynecomastia and galactorrhea.

DRUG ABUSE AND DEPENDENCE

Physical and Psychological Dependence:
Withdrawal symptoms similar in character to those noted with sedative/hypnotics and alcohol have occurred following discontinuance of benzodiazepines, including XANAX. The symptoms can range from mild dysphoria and insomnia to a major syndrome that may include abdominal and muscle cramps, vomiting, sweating, tremors and convulsions. Distinguishing between withdrawal emergent signs and symptoms and the recurrence of illness is often difficult in patients undergoing dose reduction. The long term strategy for treatment of these phenomena will vary with their cause and the therapeutic goal. When necessary, immediate management of withdrawal symptoms requires re-institution of treatment at doses of XANAX sufficient to suppress symptoms. There have been reports of failure of other benzodiazepines to fully suppress these withdrawal symptoms. These failures have been attributed to incomplete cross-tolerance but may also reflect the use of an inadequate dosing regimen of the substituted benzodiazepine or the effects of concomitant medications.

While it is difficult to distinguish withdrawal and recurrence for certain patients, the time course and the nature of the symptoms may be helpful. A withdrawal syndrome typically includes the occurrence of new symptoms, tends to appear toward the end of taper or shortly after discontinuation, and will decrease with time. In recurring panic disorder, symptoms similar to those observed before treatment may recur either early or late, and they will persist.

While the severity and incidence of withdrawal phenomena appear to be related to dose and duration of treatment, withdrawal symptoms, including seizures, have been reported after only brief therapy with XANAX at doses within the recommended range for the treatment of anxiety (eg, 0.75 to 4 mg/day). Signs and symptoms of withdrawal are often more prominent after rapid decrease of dosage or abrupt discontinuance. The risk of withdrawal seizures may be increased at doses above 4 mg/day (see WARNINGS). Patients, especially individuals with a history of seizures or epilepsy, should not be abruptly discontinued from any CNS depressant agent, including XANAX. It is recommended that all patients on XANAX who require a dosage reduction be gradually tapered under close supervision (see WARNINGS and DOSAGE AND ADMINISTRATION).

Psychological dependence is a risk with all benzodiazepines, including XANAX. The risk of psychological dependence may also be increased at doses greater than 4 mg/day and with longer term use, and this risk is further increased in patients with a history of alcohol or drug abuse. Some patients have experienced considerable difficulty in tapering and discontinuing from XANAX, especially those receiving higher doses for extended periods. Addiction-prone individuals should be under careful surveillance when receiving XANAX. As with all anxiolytics, repeat prescriptions should be limited to those who are under medical supervision.

Controlled Substance Class: Alprazolam is a controlled substance under the Controlled Substance Act by the Drug Enforcement Administration and XANAX Tablets have been assigned to Schedule IV.

OVERDOSAGE

Manifestations of alprazolam overdosage include somnolence, confusion, impaired coordination, diminished reflexes and coma. Death has been reported in association with overdoses of alprazolam by itself, as it has with other benzodiazepines. In addition, fatalities have been reported in patients who have overdosed with a combination of a single benzodiazepine, including alprazolam, and alcohol; alcohol levels seen in some of these patients have been lower than those usually associated with alcohol-induced fatality.

The acute oral LD_{50} in rats is 331–2171 mg/kg. Other experiments in animals have indicated that cardiopulmonary collapse can occur following massive intravenous doses of alprazolam (over 195 mg/kg; 975 times the maximum recommended daily human dose of 10 mg/day). Animals could be resuscitated with positive mechanical ventilation and the intravenous infusion of norepinephrine bitartrate.

Animal experiments have suggested that forced diuresis or hemodialysis are probably of little value in treating overdosage.

General Treatment of Overdose: Overdosage reports with XANAX Tablets are limited. As in all cases of drug overdosage, respiration, pulse rate, and blood pressure should be monitored. General supportive measures should be employed, along with immediate gastric lavage. Intravenous fluids should be administered and an adequate airway maintained. If hypotension occurs, it may be combated by the use of vasopressors. Dialysis is of limited value. As with the management of intentional overdosing with any drug, it should be borne in mind that multiple agents may have been ingested.

Flumazenil, a specific benzodiazepine receptor antagonist, is indicated for the complete or partial reversal of the sedative effects of benzodiazepines and may be used in situations when an overdose with a benzodiazepine is known or suspected. Prior to the administration of flumazenil, necessary measures should be instituted to secure airway, ventilation and intravenous access. Flumazenil is intended as an adjunct to, not as a substitute for, proper management of benzodiazepine overdose. Patients treated with flumazenil should be monitored for re-sedation, respiratory depression, and other residual benzodiazepine effects for an appropriate period after treatment. **The prescriber should be aware of a risk of seizure in association with flumazenil treatment, particularly in long-term benzodiazepine users and in cyclic antidepressant overdose.** The complete flumazenil package insert including CONTRAINDICATIONS, WARNINGS and PRECAUTIONS should be consulted prior to use.

DOSAGE AND ADMINISTRATION

Dosage should be individualized for maximum beneficial effect. While the usual daily dosages given below will meet the needs of most patients, there will be some who require doses greater than 4 mg/day. In such cases, dosage should be increased cautiously to avoid adverse effects.

Anxiety disorders and transient symptoms of anxiety:
Treatment for patients with anxiety should be initiated with a dose of 0.25 to 0.5 mg given three times daily. The dose

may be increased to achieve a maximum therapeutic effect, at intervals of 3 to 4 days, to a maximum daily dose of 4 mg, given in divided doses. The lowest possible effective dose should be employed and the need for continued treatment reassessed frequently. The risk of dependence may increase with dose and duration of treatment.

In elderly patients, in patients with advanced liver disease or in patients with debilitating disease, the usual starting dose is 0.25 mg, given two or three times daily. This may be gradually increased if needed and tolerated. The elderly may be especially sensitive to the effects of benzodiazepines. If side effects occur at the recommended starting dose, the dose may be lowered.

In all patients, dosage should be reduced gradually when discontinuing therapy or when decreasing the daily dosage. Although there are no systematically collected data to support a specific discontinuation schedule, it is suggested that the daily dosage be decreased by no more than 0.5 mg every three days. Some patients may require an even slower dosage reduction.

Panic disorder:
The successful treatment of many panic disorder patients has required the use of XANAX at doses greater than 4 mg daily. In controlled trials conducted to establish the efficacy of XANAX in panic disorder, doses in the range of 1 to 10 mg daily were used. The mean dosage employed was approximately 5 to 6 mg daily. Among the approximately 1700 patients participating in the panic disorder development program, about 300 received XANAX in dosages of greater than 7 mg/day, including approximately 100 patients who received maximum dosages of greater than 9 mg/day. Occasional patients required as much as 10 mg a day to achieve a successful response.

Generally, therapy should be initiated at a low dose to minimize the risk of adverse responses in patients especially sensitive to the drug. Thereafter, the dose can be increased at intervals equal to at least 5 times the elimination half-life (about 11 hours in young patients, about 16 hours in elderly patients). Longer titration intervals should probably be used because the maximum therapeutic response may not occur until after the plasma levels achieve steady state. Dose should be advanced until an acceptable therapeutic response (ie, a substantial reduction in or total elimination of panic attacks) is achieved, intolerance occurs, or the maximum recommended dose is attained. For patients receiving doses greater than 4 mg/day, periodic reassessment and consideration of dosage reduction is advised. In a controlled postmarketing dose-response study, patients treated with doses of XANAX greater than 4 mg/day for three months were able to taper to 50% of their total maintenance dose without apparent loss of clinical benefit. Because of the danger of withdrawal, abrupt discontinuation of treatment should be avoided. (See WARNINGS, PRECAUTIONS, DRUG ABUSE AND DEPENDENCE).

The following regimen is one that follows the principles outlined above:

Treatment may be initiated with a dose of 0.5 mg three times daily. Depending on the response, the dose may be increased at intervals of 3 to 4 days in increments of no more than 1 mg per day. Slower titration to the dose levels greater than 4 mg/day may be advisable to allow full expression of the pharmacodynamic effect of XANAX. To lessen the possibility of interdose symptoms, the times of administration should be distributed as evenly as possible throughout the waking hours, that is, on a three or four times per day schedule.

The necessary duration of treatment for panic disorder patients responding to XANAX is unknown. After a period of extended freedom from attacks, a carefully supervised tapered discontinuation may be attempted, but there is evidence that this may often be difficult to accomplish without recurrence of symptoms and/or the manifestation of withdrawal phenomena.

In any case, reduction of dose must be undertaken under close supervision and must be gradual. If significant withdrawal symptoms develop, the previous dosing schedule should be reinstituted and, only after stabilization, should a less rapid schedule of discontinuation be attempted. In a controlled postmarketing discontinuation study of panic disorder patients which compared this recommended taper schedule with a slower taper schedule, no difference was observed between the groups in the proportion of patients who tapered to zero dose; however, the slower schedule was associated with a reduction in symptoms associated with a withdrawal syndrome. It is suggested that the dose be reduced by no more than 0.5 mg every three days, with the understanding that some patients may benefit from an even more gradual discontinuation. Some patients may prove resistant to all discontinuation regimens.

HOW SUPPLIED

XANAX Tablets are available as follows:
0.25 mg (white, oval, scored, imprinted "XANAX 0.25")

Bottles of 100	NDC 0009-0029-01
Reverse Numbered	
Unit Dose (100)	NDC 0009-0029-46
Bottles of 500	NDC 0009-0029-02
Bottles of 1000	NDC 0009-0029-14

0.5 mg (peach, oval, scored, imprinted "XANAX 0.5")

Bottles of 100	NDC 0009-0055-01
Reverse Numbered Unit Dose (100)	NDC 0009-0055-46
Bottles of 500	NDC 0009-0055-03
Bottles of 1000	NDC 0009-0055-15

1 mg (blue, oval, scored, imprinted "XANAX 1.0")

Bottles of 100	NDC 0009-0090-01
Bottles of 500	NDC 0009-0090-04
Bottles of 1000	NDC 0009-0090-13

2 mg (white, oblong, multi-scored, imprinted "XANAX" on one side and "2" on the reverse side)

Bottles of 100	NDC 0009-0094-01
Bottles of 500	NDC 0009-0094-03

Store at controlled room temperature 20° to 25° C (68° to 77° F) [see USP].

Caution: Federal law prohibits dispensing without prescription.

ANIMAL STUDIES

When rats were treated with alprazolam at 3, 10, and 30 mg/kg/day (15 to 150 times the maximum recommended human dose) orally for 2 years, a tendency for a dose related increase in the number of cataracts was observed in females and a tendency for a dose related increase in corneal vascularization was observed in males. These lesions did not appear until after 11 months of treatment.

CLINICAL STUDIES

Anxiety Disorders:

XANAX Tablets were compared to placebo in double blind clinical studies (doses up to 4 mg/day) in patients with a diagnosis of anxiety or anxiety with associated depressive symptomatology. XANAX was significantly better than placebo at each of the evaluation periods of these four week studies as judged by the following psychometric instruments: Physician's Global Impressions, Hamilton Anxiety Rating Scale, Target Symptoms, Patient's Global Impressions and Self-Rating Symptom Scale.

Panic Disorder:

Support for the effectiveness of XANAX in the treatment of panic disorder came from three short-term, placebo-controlled studies (up to 10 weeks) in patients with diagnoses closely corresponding to DSM-III-R criteria for panic disorder.

The average dose of XANAX was 5–6 mg/day in two of the studies, and the doses of XANAX were fixed at 2 and 6 mg/day in the third study. In all three studies, XANAX was superior to placebo on a variable defined as "the number of patients with zero panic attacks" (range, 37–83% met this criterion), as well as on a global improvement score. In two of the three studies, XANAX was superior to placebo on a variable defined as "change from baseline on the number of panic attacks per week" (range, 3.3–5.2), and also on a phobia rating scale. A subgroup of patients who were improved on XANAX during short-term treatment in one of these trials was continued on an open basis up to eight months, without apparent loss of benefit.

Pharmacia & Upjohn Company
Kalamazoo, Michigan 49001, USA 811 557 826
Revised May 1997 691439

Shown in Product Identification Guide, page 332

ZANOSAR® ℞
streptozocin sterile powder

WARNING

ZANOSAR Sterile Powder should be administered under the supervision of a physician experienced in the use of cancer chemotherapeutic agents.

A patient need not be hospitalized but should have access to a facility with laboratory and supportive resources sufficient to monitor drug tolerance and to protect and maintain a patient compromised by drug toxicity. Renal toxicity is dose-related and cumulative and may be severe or fatal. Other major toxicities are nausea and vomiting which may be severe and at times treatment-limiting. In addition, liver dysfunction, diarrhea, and hematological changes have been observed in some patients. Streptozocin is mutagenic. When administered parenterally, it has been found to be tumorigenic or carcinogenic in some rodents.

The physician must judge the possible benefit to his patient against the known toxic effects of this drug in considering the advisability of therapy with ZANOSAR. He should be familiar with the following text before making his judgment and beginning treatment.

DESCRIPTION

Each vial of ZANOSAR Sterile Powder contains 1 g of the active ingredient streptozocin 2 - deoxy - 2 -[[(methylnitrosoamino)carbonyl]amino] - α(and β) - D - glucopyranose and 220 mg citric acid anhydrous. ZANOSAR is available as a sterile, pale yellow, freeze-dried preparation for intravenous administration. The pH was adjusted with sodium hydroxide. When reconstituted as directed, the pH of the solution will be between 3.5 and 4.5. Streptozocin is a synthetic antineoplastic agent that is chemically related to other nitrosoureas used in cancer chemotherapy. Streptozocin is an ivory-colored crystalline powder with a molecular weight of 265.2. It is very soluble in water or physiological saline and is soluble in alcohol.

The structural formula is represented below:

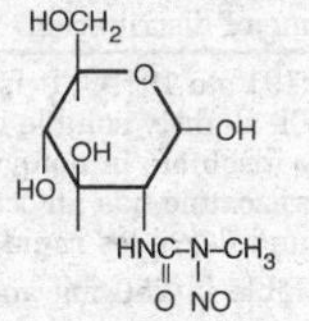

CLINICAL PHARMACOLOGY

Streptozocin inhibits DNA synthesis in bacterial and mammalian cells. In bacterial cells, a specific interaction with cytosine moieties leads to degradation of DNA. The biochemical mechanism leading to mammalian cell death has not been definitely established; streptozocin inhibits cell proliferation at a considerably lower level than that needed to inhibit precursor incorporation into DNA or to inhibit several of the enzymes involved in DNA synthesis. Although streptozocin inhibits the progression of cells into mitosis, no specific phase of the cell cycle is particularly sensitive to its lethal effects.

Streptozocin is active in the L1210 leukemic mouse over a fairly wide range of parenteral dosage schedules. In experiments in many animal species, streptozocin induced a diabetes that resembles human hyperglycemic nonketotic diabetes mellitus. This phenomenon, which has been extensively studied, appears to be mediated through a lowering of beta cell nicotinamide adenine dinucleotide (NAD) and consequent histopathologic alteration of pancreatic islet beta cells.

The metabolism and the chemical dissociation of streptozocin that occurs under physiologic conditions has not been extensively studied. When administered intravenously to a variety of experimental animals, streptozocin disappears from the blood very rapidly. In all species tested, it was found to concentrate in the liver and kidney. As much as 20% of the drug (or metabolites containing an N-nitrosourea group) is metabolized and/or excreted by the kidney. Metabolic products have not yet been identified.

INDICATIONS AND USAGE

ZANOSAR Sterile Powder is indicated in the treatment of metastatic islet cell carcinoma of the pancreas. Responses have been obtained with both functional and nonfunctional carcinomas. Because of its inherent renal toxicity, therapy with this drug should be limited to patients with symptomatic or progressive metastatic disease.

WARNINGS

Renal Toxicity

Many patients treated with ZANOSAR Sterile Powder have experienced renal toxicity, as evidenced by azotemia, anuria hypophosphatemia, glycosuria and renal tubular acidosis. **Such toxicity is dose-related and cumulative and may be severe or fatal.** Renal function must be monitored before and after each course of therapy. Serial urinalysis, blood urea nitrogen, plasma creatinine, serum electrolytes and creatinine clearance should be obtained prior to, at least weekly during, and for four weeks after drug administration. Serial urinalysis is particularly important for the early detection of proteinuria and should be quantitated with a 24 hour collection when proteinuria is detected. Mild proteinuria is one of the first signs of renal toxicity and may herald further deterioration of renal function. Reduction of the dose of ZANOSAR or discontinuation of treatment is suggested in the presence of significant renal toxicity.

Use of ZANOSAR in patients with preexisting renal disease requires a judgment by the physician of potential benefit as opposed to the known risk of serious renal damage.

This drug should not be used in combination with or concomitantly with other potential nephrotoxins.

When exposed dermally, some rats developed benign tumors at the site of application of streptozocin. Consequently, streptozocin may pose a carcinogenic hazard following topical exposure if not properly handled (see DOSAGE AND ADMINISTRATION).

See additional warnings at the beginning of this insert.

PRECAUTIONS

Laboratory Tests: Patients who are treated with ZANOSAR Sterile Powder must be monitored closely, particularly for evidence of renal, hepatic, and hematopoietic toxicity. Renal function tests are described in the WARNINGS section. Patients should also be monitored closely for evidence of hematopoietic and hepatic toxicities. Complete blood counts and liver function tests should be done at least weekly. Dosage adjustments or discontinuance of the drug may be indicated, depending upon the degree of toxicity noted.

Mutagenesis, Carcinogenesis, Impairment of Fertility: Streptozocin is mutagenic in bacteria, plants, and mammalian cells. When administered parenterally, it has been shown to induce renal tumors in rats and to induce liver tumors and other tumors in hamsters. Stomach and pancreatic tumors were observed in rats treated orally with streptozocin. Streptozocin has also been shown to be carcinogenic in mice.

Streptozocin adversely affected fertility when administered to male and female rats.

Pregnancy Category C: Reproduction studies revealed that streptozocin is teratogenic in the rat and has abortifacient effects in rabbits. When administered intravenously to pregnant monkeys, it appears rapidly in the fetal circulation. There are no studies in pregnant women. ZANOSAR should be used during pregnancy only if the potential benefit justifies the potential risk to the fetus.

Nursing Mothers: It is not known whether streptozocin is excreted in human milk. Because many drugs are excreted in human milk and because of the potential for serious adverse reactions in nursing infants, nursing should be discontinued in patients receiving ZANOSAR.

ADVERSE REACTIONS

Renal: See WARNINGS.

Gastrointestinal: Most patients treated with ZANOSAR Sterile Powder have experienced severe nausea and vomiting, occasionally requiring discontinuation of drug therapy. Some patients experienced diarrhea. A number of patients have experienced hepatic toxicity, as characterized by elevated liver enzyme (SGOT and LDH) levels and hypoalbuminemia.

Hematological: Hematological toxicity has been rare, most often involving mild decreases in hematocrit values. However, **fatal hematological toxicity with substantial reductions in leukocyte and platelet count** has been observed.

Metabolic: Mild to moderate abnormalities of glucose tolerance have been noted in some patients treated with ZANOSAR. These have generally been reversible, but insulin shock with hypoglycemia has been observed.

Genitourinary: Two cases of nephrogenic diabetes insipidus following therapy with ZANOSAR have been reported. One had spontaneous recovery and the second responded to indomethacin.

Post-marketing experience: Spontaneous reports have been received of local inflammation (i.e., edema, erythema, burning, tenderness) following extravasation of the product. In most cases, these events resolved the same day or within a few days.

OVERDOSAGE

No specific antidote for ZANOSAR is known.

DOSAGE AND ADMINISTRATION

ZANOSAR Sterile Powder should be administered intravenously. It is not active orally. Although it has been administered intra-arterially, this is not recommended pending further evaluation of the possibility that adverse renal effects may be evoked more rapidly by this route of administration. Two different dosage schedules have been employed successfully with ZANOSAR.

Daily Schedule—The recommended dose for daily intravenous administration is 500 mg/m^2 of body surface area for five consecutive days every six weeks until maximum benefit or until treatment-limiting toxicity is observed. Dose escalation on this schedule is not recommended.

Weekly Schedule—The recommended initial dose for weekly intravenous administration is 1000 mg/m^2 of body surface area at weekly intervals for the first two courses (weeks). In subsequent courses, drug doses may be escalated in patients who have not achieved a therapeutic response and who have not experienced significant toxicity with the previous course of treatment. However, A SINGLE DOSE OF 1500 mg/m^2 BODY SURFACE AREA SHOULD NOT BE EXCEEDED as a greater dose may cause azotemia. When administered on this schedule, the median time to onset of response is about 17 days and the median time to maximum response is about 35 days. The median **total** dose to onset of response is about 2000 mg/m^2 body surface area and the median **total** dose to maximum response is about 4000 mg/m^2 body surface area.

Continued on next page

Information on these Pharmacia & Upjohn products is based on labeling in effect June 1, 1998. Further information concerning these and other Pharmacia & Upjohn products may be obtained by direct inquiry to Medical Information, Pharmacia & Upjohn, Kalamazoo, MI 49001.

Zanosar—Cont.

The ideal duration of maintenance therapy with ZANOSAR has not yet been clearly established for either of the above schedules.

For patients with functional tumors, serial monitoring of fasting insulin levels allows a determination of biochemical response to therapy. For patients with either functional or nonfunctional tumors, response to therapy can be determined by measurable reductions of tumor size (reduction of organomegaly, masses, or lymph nodes).

Reconstitute ZANOSAR with 9.5 mL of Dextrose Injection USP, or 0.9% Sodium Chloride Injection USP. The resulting pale-gold solution will contain 100 mg of streptozocin and 22 mg of citric acid per mL. Where more dilute infusion solutions are desirable, further dilution in the above vehicles is recommended. The total storage time for streptozocin after it has been placed in solution should not exceed 12 hours. This product contains no preservatives and is not intended as a multiple-dose vial.

Caution in the handling and preparation of the powder and solution should be exercised, and the use of gloves is recommended. If ZANOSAR Sterile Powder or a solution prepared from ZANOSAR contacts the skin or mucosae, immediately wash the affected area with soap and water.

Procedures for proper handling and disposal of anticancer drugs should be considered. Several guidelines on this subject have been published.[4–9] There is no general agreement that all of the procedures recommended in the guidelines are necessary or appropriate.

HOW SUPPLIED

ZANOSAR Sterile Powder is supplied in 1 gram vials (NDC 0009-0844-01). Unopened vials of ZANOSAR should be stored at refrigeration temperatures (2° to 8° C) and protected from light (preferably stored in carton).

REFERENCES

1. Broder LE and Carter SK: *Ann Int Med,* 79:101–118, 1972.
2. Schein PS, O'Connell MJ, Blom J, Hubbard S, Magrath It, Bergevin P, Wiernik PH, Ziegler TL, and DeVita VT: *Cancer,* 34:993–1000, 1974.
3. Moertel CG, *et al: Cancer Chemother Rep,* 55:303–307, 1972.
4. Recommendations for the Safe Handling of Parenteral Antineoplastic Drugs. NIH Publication No. 83–2621. For sale by the Superintendent of Documents, US Government Printing Office, Washington, DC 20402.
5. AMA Council Report. Guidelines for Handling Parenteral Antineoplastics. JAMA, March 15, 1985.
6. National Study Commission on Cytotoxic Exposure-Recommendations for Handling Cytotoxic Agents. Available from Louis P. Jeffrey, ScD, Director of Pharmacy Services. Rhode Island Hospital. 593 Eddy Street. Providence. Rhode Island 02902.
7. Clinical Oncological Society of Australia: Guidelines and recommendations for safe handling of antineoplastic agents. *Med J Australia* 1:426–428, 1983.
8. Jones RB, et al, Safe handling of chemotherapeutic agents: A report from the Mount Sinai Medical Center CA-A Cancer Journal for Clinicians Sept./Oct., 1983, pp. 258–263.
9. American Society of Hospital Pharmacists Technical assistance bulletin on handling cytotoxic drugs in hospitals. *Am J Hosp Pharm* 42:131–137, 1985.

Caution: Federal law prohibits dispensing without prescription.

Pharmacia & Upjohn Company • Kalamazoo, Michigan 49001, USA

Revised November 1997 812 350 207
691272

ZINECARD® ℞

[zĭn "ă card ']

(dexrazoxane for injection)

DESCRIPTION

ZINECARD® (dexrazoxane for injection) is a sterile, pyrogen-free lyophilizate intended for intravenous administration. It is a cardioprotective agent for use in conjunction with doxorubicin.

Chemically, dexrazoxane is (S)-4,4'-(1-methyl-1,2-ethanediyl)bis-2,6-piperazinedione. The structural formula is as follows:

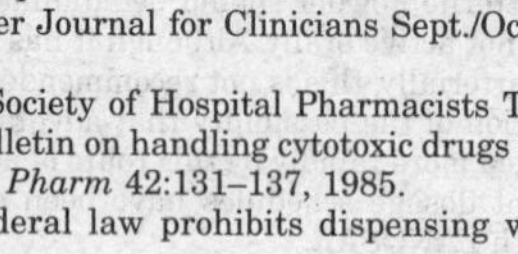

CH3
H
HN
N – CH2
C
N
NH

$C_{11}H_{16}N_4O_4$ M.W. 268.28

Dexrazoxane, a potent intracellular chelating agent is a derivative of EDTA. Dexrazoxane is a whitish crystalline powder which melts at 191° to 197°C. It is sparingly soluble in water and 0.1 N HCl, slightly soluble in ethanol and methanol and practically insoluble in nonpolar organic solvents. The pK_a is 2.1. Dexrazoxane has an octanol/water partition coefficient of 0.025 and degrades rapidly above a pH of 7.0.

ZINECARD is available in 250 mg and 500 mg single use only vials.

Each **250 mg vial** contains dexrazoxane hydrochloride equivalent to 250 mg dexrazoxane. Hydrochloric Acid, NF is added for pH adjustment. When reconstituted as directed with the 25 mL vial of 0.167 Molar (M/6) Sodium Lactate Injection, USP diluent provided, each mL contains: 10 mg dexrazoxane. The pH of the resultant solution is 3.5 to 5.5.

Each **500 mg vial** contains dexrazoxane hydrochloride equivalent to 500 mg dexrazoxane. Hydrochloric Acid, NF is added for pH adjustment. When reconstituted as directed with the 50 mL vial of 0.167 Molar (M/6) Sodium Lactate Injection, USP diluent provided, each mL contains: 10 mg dexrazoxane. The pH of the resultant solution is 3.5 to 5.5.

SUMMARY OF MEAN (%CV[a]) DEXRAZOXANE PHARMACOKINETIC PARAMETERS AT A DOSAGE RATIO OF 10:1 OF ZINECARD: DOXORUBICIN

Dose Doxorubicin (mg/m^2)	Dose Zinecard (mg/m^2)	Number of Subjects	Elimination Half-Life (h)	Plasma Clearance ($L/h/m^2$)	Renal Clearance ($L/h/m^2$)	[b]Volume of Distribution (L/m^2)
50	500	10	2.5 (16)	7.88 (18)	3.35 (36)	22.4 (22)
60	600	5	2.1 (29)	6.25 (31)	—	22.0 (55)

[a] Coefficient of variation
[b] Steady-state volume of distribution

CLINICAL PHARMACOLOGY

Mechanism of Action: The mechanism by which ZINECARD exerts its cardioprotective activity is not fully understood. Dexrazoxane is a cyclic derivative of EDTA that readily penetrates cell membranes. Results of laboratory studies suggest that dexrazoxane is converted intracellularly to a ring-opened chelating agent that interferes with iron-mediated free radical generation thought to be responsible, in part, for anthracycline-induced cardiomyopathy.

Pharmacokinetics: The pharmacokinetics of dexrazoxane have been studied in advanced cancer patients with normal renal and hepatic function. Generally, the pharmacokinetics of dexrazoxane can be adequately described by a two-compartment open model with first-order elimination. Dexrazoxane has been administered as a 15 minute infusion over a dose-range of 60 to 900 mg/m^2 with 60 mg/m^2 of doxorubicin, and at a fixed dose of 500 mg/m^2 with 50 mg/m^2 doxorubicin. The disposition kinetics of dexrazoxane are dose-independent, as shown by linear relationship between the area under plasma concentration-time curves and administered doses ranging from 60 to 900 mg/m^2. The mean peak plasma concentration of dexrazoxane was 36.5 µg/mL at the end of the 15 minute infusion of a 500 mg/m^2 dose of Zinecard administered 15 to 30 minutes prior to the 50 mg/m^2 doxorubicin dose. The important pharmacokinetic parameters of dexrazoxane are summarized in the following table. [See table above]

Following a rapid distributive phase (.2 to 0.3 hours), dexrazoxane reaches post-distributive equilibrium within two to four hours. The estimated steady-state volume of distribution of dexrazoxane suggests its distribution primarily in the total body water (25 L/m^2). The mean systemic clearance and steady-state volume of distribution of dexrazoxane in two Asian female patients at 500 mg/m^2 dexrazoxane along with 50 mg/m^2 doxorubicin were 15.15 $L/h/m^2$ and 36.27 L/m^2, respectively, but their elimination half-life and renal clearance of dexrazoxane were similar to those of the ten Caucasian patients from the same study. Qualitative metabolism studies with Zinecard have confirmed the presence of unchanged drug, a diacid-diamide cleavage product, and two monoacid-monoamide ring products in the urine of animals and man. The metabolite levels were not measured in the pharmacokinetic studies.

Urinary excretion plays an important role in the elimination of dexrazoxane. Forty-two percent of the 500 mg/m^2 dose of Zinecard was excreted in the urine.

Protein Binding: *In vitro* studies have shown that Zinecard is not bound to plasma proteins.

Special Populations: The pharmacokinetics of Zinecard have not been evaluated in pediatric populations nor in hepatic or renal insufficiency patients.

Drug Interactions: There was no significant change in the pharmacokinetics of doxorubicin (50 mg/m^2) and its predominant metabolite, doxorubicinol, in the presence of dexrazoxane (500 mg/m^2) in a crossover study in cancer patients.

Clinical Studies: The ability of ZINECARD to prevent/reduce the incidence and severity of doxorubicin-induced cardiomyopathy was demonstrated in three prospectively randomized placebo-controlled studies. In these studies, patients were treated with a doxorubicin-containing regimen and either ZINECARD or placebo starting with the first course of chemotherapy. There was no restriction on the cumulative dose of doxorubicin. Cardiac function was assessed by measurement of the left ventricular ejection fraction (LVEF), utilizing resting multigated nuclear medicine (MUGA) scans, and by clinical evaluations. Patients receiving ZINECARD had significantly smaller mean decreases from baseline in LVEF and lower incidences of congestive heart failure than the control group. The difference in decline from baseline in LVEF was evident beginning with a cumulative doxorubicin dose of 150 mg/m^2 and reached statistical significance in patients who received ≥400 mg/m^2 of doxorubicin. In addition to evaluating the effect of ZINECARD on cardiac function, the studies also assessed the effect of the addition of ZINECARD on the antitumor efficacy of the chemotherapy regimens. In one study (the largest of three breast cancer studies) patients with advanced breast cancer receiving fluorouracil, doxorubicin and cyclophosphamide (FAC) with ZINECARD had a lower response rate (48% vs 63%; p=0.007) and a shorter time to progression than patients who received FAC + placebo, although the survival of patients who did or did not receive ZINECARD with FAC was similar.

Two of the randomized breast cancer studies evaluating the efficacy and safety of FAC with either ZINECARD or placebo were amended to allow patients on the placebo arm who had attained a cumulative dose of doxorubicin of 300 mg/m^2 (six courses of FAC) to receive FAC with open-label ZINECARD for each subsequent course. This change in design allowed examination of whether there was a cardioprotective effect of Zinecard even when it was started after substantial exposure to doxorubicin.

Retrospective historical analyses were then performed to compare the likelihood of heart failure in patients to whom ZINECARD was added to the FAC regimen after they had received six (6) courses of FAC (and who then continued treatment with FAC therapy) with the heart failure rate in patients who had received six (6) courses of FAC and continued to receive this regimen without added ZINECARD. These analyses showed that the risk of experiencing a cardiac event (see Table 1 for definition) at a given cumulative dose of doxorubicin above 300 mg/m^2 was substantially greater in the 99 patients who did *not* receive ZINECARD beginning with their seventh course of FAC than in the 102 patients who did receive Zinecard (See Figure 1).

Table 1

The development of cardiac events is shown by:

1. Development of congestive heart failure, defined as having two or more of the following:
   a. Cardiomegaly by X-ray
   b. Basilar Rales
   c. S_3 Gallop
   d. Paroxysmal nocturnal dyspnea and/or orthopnea and/or significant dyspnea on exertion.
2. Decline from baseline in LVEF by ≥10% and to below the lower limit of normal for the institution.
3. Decline in LVEF by ≥20% from baseline value.
4. Decline in LVEF to ≥5% below lower limit of normal for the institution.

Figure 1 displays the risk of developing congestive heart failure by cumulative dose of doxorubicin in patients who received ZINECARD starting with their seventh course of FAC compared to patients who did not. Patients unprotected by ZINECARD had a 13 times greater risk of developing congestive heart failure. Overall, 3% of patients treated with ZINECARD developed CHF compared with 22% of patients not receiving ZINECARD.

Figure 1
DOX Dose at Congestive Heart Failure (CHF)
FAC vs. FAC/Zinecard Patients
Patients Receiving At Least Seven Courses of Treatment

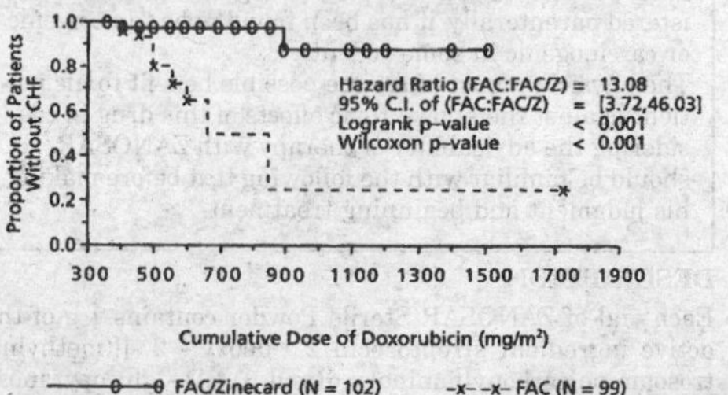

Proportion of Patients Without CHF
1.0
0.8
0.6
0.4
0.2
0.0
300
500
700
900
1100
1300
1500
1700
1900
Hazard Ratio (FAC:FAC/Z) = 13.08
95% C.I. of (FAC:FAC/Z) = [3.72,46.03]
Logrank p–value < 0.001
Wilcoxon p–value < 0.001
Cumulative Dose of Doxorubicin (mg/m²)
FAC/Zinecard (N = 102)
-x- -x- FAC (N = 99)

Because of its cardioprotective effect, ZINECARD permitted a greater percentage of patients to be treated with extended doxorubicin therapy. Figure 2 shows the number of patients still on treatment at increasing cumulative doses.

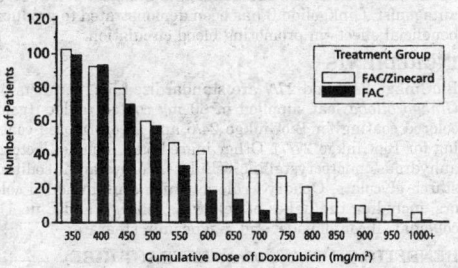

Figure 2
Cumulative Number of Patients On Treatment
FAC vs. FAC/Zinecard Patients
Patients Receiving at Least Seven Courses of Treatment

In addition to evaluating the cardioprotective efficacy of ZINECARD in this setting, the time to tumor progression and survival of these two groups of patients were also compared. There was a similar time to progression in the two groups and survival was at least as long for the group of patients that received ZINECARD starting with their seventh course, i.e., starting after a cumulative dose of doxorubicin of 300 mg/m² These time to progression and survival data should be interpreted with caution, however, because they are based on comparisons of groups entered sequentially in the studies and are not comparisons of prospectively randomized patients.

INDICATIONS AND USAGE

ZINECARD is indicated for reducing the incidence and severity of cardiomyopathy associated with doxorubicin administration in women with metastatic breast cancer who have received a cumulative doxorubicin dose of 300 mg/m² and who, in their physician's opinion, would benefit from continuing therapy with doxorubicin. It is not recommended for use with the initiation of doxorubicin therapy (see **WARNINGS**).

CONTRAINDICATIONS

ZINECARD should not be used with chemotherapy regimens that do not contain an anthracycline.

WARNINGS

ZINECARD may add to the myelosuppression caused by chemotherapeutic agents.

There is some evidence that the use of dexrazoxane concurrently with the initiation of fluorouracil, doxorubicin and cyclophosphamide (FAC) therapy interferes with the antitumor efficacy of the regimen, and this use is not recommended. In the largest of three breast cancer trials, patients who received dexrazoxane starting with their first cycle of FAC therapy had a lower response rate (48% vs 63%; p=0.007) and shorter time to progression than patients who did not receive dexrazoxane (see **Clinical Studies** section of **CLINICAL PHARMACOLOGY**). Therefore, ZINECARD should only be used in those patients who have received a cumulative doxorubicin dose of 300 mg/m² and are continuing with doxorubicin therapy.

Although clinical studies have shown that patients receiving FAC with ZINECARD may receive a higher cumulative dose of doxorubicin before experiencing cardiac toxicity than patients receiving FAC without ZINECARD, the use of ZINECARD in patients who have already received a cumulative dose of doxorubicin of 300 mg/m² without ZINECARD, does not eliminate the potential for anthracycline induced cardiac toxicity. Therefore, cardiac function should be carefully monitored.

Secondary malignancies (primarily acute myeloid leukemia) have been reported in patients treated chronically with oral razoxane. Razoxane is the racemic mixture, of which dexrazoxane is the S(+)-enantiomer. In these patients, the total cumulative dose of razoxane ranged from 26 to 480 grams and the duration of treatment was from 42 to 319 weeks. One case of T-cell lymphoma, a case of B-cell lymphoma and six to eight cases of cutaneous basal cell or squamous cell carcinoma have also been reported in patients treated with razoxane.

PRECAUTIONS
General

Doxorubicin should not be given prior to the intravenous injection of ZINECARD. ZINECARD should be given by slow I.V. push or rapid drip intravenous infusion from a bag. Doxorubicin should be given within 30 minutes after beginning the infusion with ZINECARD. (See **DOSAGE AND ADMINISTRATION**.)

As ZINECARD will always be used with cytotoxic drugs, patients should be monitored closely. While the myelosuppressive effects of ZINECARD at the recommended dose are mild, additive effects upon the myelosuppressive activity of chemotherapeutic agents may occur.

Laboratory tests
As ZINECARD may add to the myelosuppressive effects of cytotoxic drugs, frequent complete blood counts are recommended. (See **ADVERSE REACTIONS**).

Drug Interactions
ZINECARD does not influence the pharmacokinetics of doxorubicin.

Carcinogenesis, Mutagenesis, Impairment of Fertility (see **WARNINGS** section for information on human carcinogenicity) – No long-term carcinogenicity studies have been carried out with dexrazoxane in animals. Dexrazoxane was not mutagenic in the Ames test but was found to be clastogenic to human lymphocytes in vitro and to mouse bone marrow erythrocytes in vivo (micronucleus test).

The possible adverse effects of Zinecard on the fertility of humans and experimental animals, male or female, have not been adequately studied. Testicular atrophy was seen with dexrazoxane administration at doses as low as 30 mg/kg weekly for 6 weeks in rats (1/3 the human dose on a mg/m² basis) and as low as 20 mg/kg weekly for 13 weeks in dogs (approximately equal to the human dose on a mg/m² basis).

Pregnancy – *Pregnancy Category C* – Dexrazoxane was maternotoxic at doses of 2 mg/kg (1/40 the human dose on a mg/m² basis) and embryotoxic and teratogenic at 8 mg/kg (approximately 1/10 the human dose on a mg/m² basis) when given daily to pregnant rats during the period of organogenesis. Teratogenic effects in the rat included imperforate anus, microphthalmia, and anophthalmia. In offspring allowed to develop to maturity, fertility was impaired in the male and female rats treated in utero during organogenesis at 8 mg/kg. In rabbits, doses of 5 mg/kg (approximately 1/10 the human dose on a mg/m² basis) daily during the period of organogenesis were maternotoxic and dosages of 20 mg/kg (1/2 the human dose on a mg/m² basis) were embryotoxic and teratogenic. Teratogenic effects in the rabbit included several skeletal malformations such as short tail, rib and thoracic malformations, and soft tissue variations including subcutaneous, eye and cardiac hemorrhagic areas, as well as agenesis of the gallbladder and of the intermediate lobe of the lung. There are no adequate and well-controlled studies in pregnant women. ZINECARD should be used during pregnancy only if the potential benefit justifies the potential risk to the fetus.

Nursing Mothers – It is not known whether dexrazoxane is excreted in human milk. Because many drugs are excreted in human milk and because of the potential for serious adverse reactions in nursing infants exposed to dexrazoxane, mothers should be advised to discontinue nursing during dexrazoxane therapy.

Pediatric Use – Safety and effectiveness of dexrazoxane in children have not been established.

ADVERSE REACTIONS

ZINECARD at a dose of 500 mg/m² has been administered in combination with FAC in randomized, placebo-controlled, double-blind studies to patients with metastatic breast cancer. The dose of doxorubicin was 50 mg/m² in each of the trials. Courses were repeated every three weeks, provided recovery from toxicity had occurred. Table 2 below lists the incidence of adverse experiences for patients receiving FAC with either ZINECARD or placebo in the breast cancer studies. Adverse experiences occurring during courses 1 through 6 are displayed for patients receiving ZINECARD or placebo with FAC beginning with their first course of therapy (column 1 & 3, respectively). Adverse experiences occurring at course 7 and beyond for patients who received placebo with FAC during the first six courses and who then received either ZINECARD or placebo with FAC are also displayed (column 2 & 4, respectively).

[See table 2 above]

The adverse experiences listed above are likely attributable to the FAC regimen with the exception of pain on injection that was observed mainly on the ZINECARD arm.

Myelosuppression

Patients receiving FAC with ZINECARD experienced more severe leucopenia, granulocytopenia and thrombocytopenia

TABLE 2

PERCENTAGE (%) OF BREAST CANCER PATIENTS WITH ADVERSE EXPERIENCE

ADVERSE EXPERIENCE	FAC + ZINECARD Courses 1–6 N=413	FAC + ZINECARD Courses ≥7 N=102	FAC + PLACEBO Courses 1–6 N=458	FAC + PLACEBO Course ≥7 N=99
Alopecia	94	100	97	98
Nausea	77	51	84	60
Vomiting	59	42	72	49
Fatigue/Malaise	61	48	58	55
Anorexia	42	27	47	38
Stomatitis	34	26	41	28
Fever	34	22	29	18
Infection	23	19	18	21
Diarrhea	21	14	24	7
Pain on Injection	12	13	3	0
Sepsis	17	12	14	9
Neurotoxicity	17	10	13	5
Streaking/Erythema	5	4	4	2
Phlebitis	6	3	3	5
Esophagitis	6	3	7	4
Dysphagia	8	0	10	5
Hemorrhage	2	3	2	1
Extravasation	1	3	1	2
Urticaria	2	2	2	0
Recall Skin Reaction	1	1	2	0

Continued on next page

Information on these Pharmacia & Upjohn products is based on labeling in effect June 1, 1998. Further information concerning these and other Pharmacia & Upjohn products may be obtained by direct inquiry to Medical Information, Pharmacia & Upjohn, Kalamazoo, MI 49001.

Zinecard—Cont.

at nadir than patients receiving FAC without ZINECARD, but recovery counts were similar for the two groups of patients.

Hepatic and Renal

Some patients receiving FAC + ZINECARD or FAC + placebo experienced marked abnormalities in hepatic or renal function tests, but the frequency and severity of abnormalities in bilirubin, alkaline phosphatase, BUN, and creatinine were similar for patients receiving FAC with or without ZINECARD.

OVERDOSAGE

There have been no instances of drug overdose in the clinical studies sponsored by either Pharmacia Inc. or the National Cancer Institute. The maximum dose administered during the cardioprotective trials was 1000 mg/m^2 every three weeks.

Disposition studies with ZINECARD have not been conducted in cancer patients undergoing dialysis, but retention of a significant dose fraction (>0.4) of the unchanged drug in the plasma pool, minimal tissue partitioning or binding, and availability of greater than 90% of the systemic drug levels in the unbound form suggest that it could be removed using conventional peritoneal or hemodialysis.

There is no known antidote for dexrazoxane. Instances of suspected overdose should be managed with good supportive care until resolution of myelosuppression and related conditions is complete. Management of overdose should include treatment of infections, fluid regulation, and maintenance of nutritional requirements.

DOSAGE AND ADMINISTRATION

The recommended dosage ratio of ZINECARD:DOX is 10:1 (eg, 500 mg/m^2 ZINECARD:50 mg/m^2 DOX). ZINECARD must be reconstituted with 0.167 Molar (M/6) Sodium Lactate Injection, USP, to give a concentration of 10 mg ZINECARD for each mL of sodium lactate. The reconstituted solution should be given by slow I.V. push or rapid drip intravenous infusion from a bag. After completing the infusion of ZINECARD, and prior to a total elapsed time of 30 minutes (from the beginning of the ZINECARD infusion), the intravenous injection of doxorubicin should be given.

Reconstituted ZINECARD, when transferred to an empty infusion bag, is stable for 6 hours from the time of reconstitution when stored at controlled room temperature, 15° to 30°C (59° to 86°F) or under refrigeration, 2° to 8°C (36° to 46°F). DISCARD UNUSED SOLUTIONS.

The reconstituted ZINECARD solution may be diluted with either 0.9% Sodium Chloride Injection, USP or 5.0% Dextrose Injection, USP to a concentration range of 1.3 to 5.0 mg/mL in intravenous infusion bags. The resultant solutions are stable for 6 hours when stored at controlled room temperature, 15° to 30°C (59° to 86°F) or under refrigeration, 2° to 8°C (36° to 46°F). DISCARD UNUSED SOLUTIONS.

Incompatibility

ZINECARD should not be mixed with other drugs.

Parenteral drug products should be inspected visually for particulate matter and discoloration prior to administration, whenever solution and container permit.

Handling and Disposal: Caution in the handling and preparation of the reconstituted solution must be exercised and the use of gloves is recommended. If ZINECARD powder or solutions contact the skin or mucosae, immediately wash thoroughly with soap and water.

Procedures normally used for proper handling and disposal of anticancer drugs should be considered for use with ZINECARD. Several guidelines on this subject have been published.[1–7] There is no general agreement that all of the procedures recommended in the guidelines are necessary or appropriate.

HOW SUPPLIED

ZINECARD® (dexrazoxane for injection) is available in the following strengths as sterile, pyrogen-free lyophilizates.

NDC 0013-8715-62 250 mg single dose vial with a red flip-top seal, packaged in single vial packs.

(This package also contains a 25 mL vial of 0.167 Molar (M/6) Sodium Lactate Injection, USP.)

NDC 0013-8725-89 500 mg single dose vial with a blue flip-top seal, packaged in single vial packs.

(This package also contains a 50 mL vial of 0.167 Molar (M/6) Sodium Lactate Injection, USP.)

Store at controlled room temperature, 15° to 30°C (59° to 86°F). Reconstituted solutions of ZINECARD are stable for 6 hours at controlled room temperature or under refrigeration, 2° to 8°C (36° to 46°F). DISCARD UNUSED SOLUTIONS.

CAUTION: Federal law prohibits dispensing without prescription.

REFERENCES

1. Recommendations for the Safe Handling of Parenteral Antineoplastic Drugs. NIH Publication No. 83-2621. For sale by the Superintendent of Documents, U.S. Government Printing Office, Washington, DC 20402.
2. AMA Council Report. Guidelines for Handling Parenteral Antineoplastics JAMA. 1985 March 15.
3. National Study Commission on Cytotoxic Exposure-Recommendations for Handling Cytotoxic Agents. Available from Louis P. Jeffrey, Sc.D., Chairman, National Study Commission on Cytotoxic Exposure, Massachusetts College of Pharmacy and Allied Health Sciences, 179 Longwood Avenue, Boston, Massachusetts 02115.
4. Clinical Oncological Society of Australia. Guidelines and Recommendations for Safe Handling of Antineoplastic Agents. Med J Australia. 1983; 1:426–428.
5. Jones RB. et al. Safe handling of Chemotherapeutic Agents: A report from the Mount Sinai Medical Center. CA – A Cancer Journal for Clinicians. 1983; (Sept/Oct) 258–263.
6. American Society of Hospital Pharmacists Technical Assistance Bulletin on Handling Cytotoxic and Hazardous Drugs. Am J Hosp Pharm. 1990; 47:1033–1049.
7. OSHA Work-Practice Guidelines for Personnel Dealing with Cytotoxic (Antineoplastic) Drugs. Am J Hosp Pharm. 1986; 43:1193–1204.

770000496 April 1, 1996

Pharmanex, Inc.

625 COCHRAN STREET
SIMI VALLEY, CA 93065-1939

Direct Inquiries to:
Michael Chang, Ph.D or
Joseph Chang, Ph.D
(800) 999–6229
FAX: (805) 582-9301

Medical Emergency Contact:
Michael Chang, Ph.D.
(800) 999–6229
FAX: (805) 582-9301

Pharmanex is a science-based, natural healthcare company that develops and markets a line of proprietary natural healthcare products (listed below) as well as over 30 Premium Quality Self-care Botanical Extracts—ranging from Astragalus, Bilberry, CoQ10 and Echinacea, to Kava, Saw Palmetto, Valerian, etc. Each highly concentrated, scientifically standardized extract is formulated to provide clinically supported dosages that guarantee optimal levels of the key health promoting compounds in their proper ratios. For a full list of dietary supplement products and scientific support documents call toll free: **1-800-999-6229**.

BIO GINKGO 27/7™ Extra Strength and BIO GINKGO 24/6™

[bī 'ō-gĭng 'ko]
***Ginkgo biloba* leaf Extract**
60 mg tablets
Dietary Supplement

DESCRIPTION

BioGinkgo is an all-natural, standardized extract of the leaves of *Ginkgo biloba* trees for use as a dietary supplement to improve blood circulation to the brain and extremities, improve cognitive functions and conserve mental sharpness, and protect the body from oxidative cellular damage caused by free radicals.* *Ginkgo biloba* extract (GBE) is primarily used to affect the age-related relatively slow decline in cognitive functions.* There have been several controlled clinical trials designed to test the effectiveness of GBE in mitigating symptoms such as: difficulties of concentration and memory, absent mindedness, confusion, lack of energy, tiredness and decreased physical performance.*

GBE is one of the most widely used botanicals in the world and the focus of extensive scientific research, including over 300 published studies and reports to its credit. Twenty years of research led to the development of a standardized, concentrated extract from the leaves—with a scientifically-supported composition of 22 to 27% flavonoid glycoside content and 5 to 7% terpene lactone content as specified by European health authority standards for phytomedicines.

BioGinkgo is available in two scientifically-supported formulations: (1) BioGinkgo 27/7 Extra Strength (27% ginkgo flavone glycosides and 7% terpene lactones) contains significantly greater levels of the identified active constituents than the standard strength formulation listed below. In a bioavailability study in rabbits published in *Planta Medica* (Li C.L. and Wong Y.Y., December, 1997) comparing BioGinkgo 27/7 to another commercially available GBE, BioGinkgo 27/7 reached higher levels of plasma concentration of anti-PAF components, and manifested a faster onset and longer duration of action of anti-PAF activity over a 12-hour period. (2) BioGinkgo 24/6 (24% ginkgo flavone glycosides and 6% terpene lactones).

BioGinkgo formulations are specifically enriched to provide higher levels of ginkgolide B than other standardized GBE products. Ginkgolides are potent Platelet Activating Factor (PAF) antagonists, and ginkgolide B is the most potent PAF antagonist. Ginkgolide B has been demonstrated to produce beneficial effects in promoting blood circulation.*

INGREDIENTS

BioGinkgo 24/6 and 27/7 are standardized 50:1 extracts of *Ginkgo biloba* leaf supplied in 60 mg coated tablets (gold colored coating for BioGinkgo 24/6 and green colored coating for BioGinkgo 27/7). Other ingredients include: lactose anhydrous, microcrystalline cellulose, corn starch, sodium starch glycolate, Opadry® colors (which contain added colors, including the Lakes of Yellow 5, Yellow 6 and Blue 1), colloidal silicon dioxide, and magnesium stearate.

BENEFITS OF *Ginkgo biloba* EXTRACT (GBE)

GBE promotes healthy blood flow: A meta-analysis of several controlled clinical studies shows that GBE helps to maintain normal blood circulation in the body, including the brain and the extremities (arms, legs, eyes, inner ear, etc.) without a "borrowing" effect on adjacent areas of normal flow.* GBE promotes efficient circulation by helping to maintain the elasticity of arteries and capillaries.* Terpene lactones specific to GBE inhibit PAF, which may contribute to circulation blockage.* Ginkgolide B binds to PAF receptors.*

GBE improves memory and enhances cognitive function: GBE increases the rate at which information is transmitted between nerve cells by increasing blood flow to the brain and the Central Nervous System (CNS).* Also, by inhibiting PAF-induced platelet aggregation and reducing the resulting viscosity or "stickiness" of the blood, the ginkgolides increase cerebral blood flow and contribute to the improvement in cognitive function seen after GBE treatment.*

GBE promotes eye health: The macular area of the retina is responsible for fine reading, and is particularly sensitive to damage by lipid free radicals.* GBE may promote eye health in the elderly through its protective antioxidant properties.*

RECOMMENDED USE

As a dietary supplement, take one 60 mg tablet bid. Allow from 2 weeks up to 12 weeks for optimum benefits.

SAFETY

GBE appears to be well tolerated at prescribed doses. Adverse reactions include mild gastrointestinal discomfort, and rare reports of allergic skin reactions. Some people may experience a mild, transient headache for the first two or three days of use.

WARNINGS

BioGinkgo has not been evaluated in children and should only be used by adults. Pregnant or breast feeding mothers should consult a physician prior to use. Consult a physician if using concurrently with anticoagulant or NSAID medications.

HOW SUPPLIED

BioGinkgo 27/7 and 24/6 tablets of 60 mg each are supplied in packages of 40, 60 and 80 count, and can be purchased at major drug, grocery, discount and healthfood stores in the vitamin/dietary supplement section.

Shown in Product Identification Guide, page 332

BIO ST. JOHN'S™

[bī'ō-sānt jŏnz]
Enhanced St. John's wort (Hypericum) Extract
Dietary Supplement

DESCRIPTION

Bio St. John's [Patent Pending] is a dietary supplement that may help people cope with the daily stresses of our modern lifestyles—and may be particularly beneficial for individuals with a physically and mentally stressful lifestyle.* It consists of a complementary combination of a standardized extract of the herb St. John's wort *(Hypericum perforatum)*, together with a proprietary strain of the *Cordyceps sinensis* mushroom (CordyMax Cs-4™). St. John's wort is highly regarded and widely used in Europe as a safe, effective mood-promoting supplement.* Numerous clinical studies suggest that St. John's wort influences mood and helps people to maintain a positive mental outlook.* CordyMax helps to reduce symptoms of fatigue and increase stamina and resistance to stress while providing important protective and stabilizing benefits for numerous bodily systems, including the cardiovascular, respiratory, hepatic and nervous systems.*

INGREDIENTS

Bio St. John's [Patent Pending], at the recommended 4 capsules/day, contains clinically supported dosages of CordyMax Cs-4 mycelium (1500 mg/day) standardized to adenosine and mannitol content, and St. John's wort (900 mg/day) standardized to 0.3% hypericin within a complex or other natural compounds.

SCIENTIFIC SUPPORT

One of the essential active components of Bio St. John's is a standardized extract of St. John's wort. Animal and *in vitro* studies with St. John's wort extract have shown that it positively effects modulation of the functions and availability of serotonin and other neurotransmitters at nerve synapses and regulation of the expression of neurotransmitter receptors.* Its mechanism of action is incompletely understood—it is a weak MAOI and has not been demonstrated to act as an MAOI *in vivo*. In clinical studies, St. John's wort extract:

- Stabilizes mood and promotes a positive mental outlook*
- Improves sleep patterns in older individuals*
- Moderates seasonal mood changes*
- Is well-tolerated by most people

A systematic meta-analysis of 23 randomized clinical trials (including a total of 1757 outpatients) concluded that St. John's wort (Hypericum) preparations were 2.67 times more effective in the placebo controlled trials. Dropouts due to side effects were rare in the Hypericum treated group (0.8%). (Linde K. et al., 1996, *British Medical Journal*, 313: 253–8)

The other complementary ingredient in Bio St. John's, *Cordyceps sinensis* (Berk.) Sacc., a traditional Chinese mushroom, has been demonstrated in pre-clinical and clinical studies to act as a general tonic to:

- Improve energy, vitality and endurance*
- Elevate energy states (ATP) in organs*
- Have calming and stress-relieving effects*
- Optimize cardiac, respiratory, immune, liver and kidney functions*
- Optimize blood lipid metabolism and promote healthy blood lipid profiles*
- Provide a positive benefit for sexuality*

(See CordyMax Cs-4 section for additional information)

RECOMMENDED USE

As a dietary supplement, the recommended, clinically supported dosage is 2 capsules, 2 times per day with food and drink. It typically takes 4 to 6 weeks to achieve optimal results.

SAFETY

Toxicological studies in animals indicate that the toxicity of St. John's wort extracts is quite low. No mutagenic activity has been found. A potential for erythema exists for fair-skinned patients taking doses greater than 1800 mg/day of St. John's wort extract who are exposed to UV-A or UV-B. The most common side effects of St. John's wort extract reported in an open study of 3250 patients were gastrointestinal symptoms (0.6%), allergic reactions (0.5%) and fatigue (0.4%). (Woelk, H et al., 1994, *Journal of Geriatric Psychiatry Neurology*, 7:S34–38) No negative influences on performance or ability to drive have been reported. (See CordyMax Cs-4 section for safety information regarding this ingredient.)

WARNINGS

Patients on prescription medications for clinical depression should consult a physician before using St. John's wort extract as a dietary supplement. Pregnant and breast-feeding mothers should consult a physician prior to use. St. John's wort extract has been reported to significantly prolong narcotic-induced sleeping times and to antagonize the effects of reserpine. Hypericin causes a reduction in barbiturate-induced sleeping times. (See CordyMax Cs-4 section for warnings regarding this ingredient.)

HOW SUPPLIED

Bio St. John's capsules (600 mg each) are supplied in 64 count boxes and 90 count bottles, and can be purchased at major drug, grocery, health and discount stores in the vitamin/dietary supplement section. Clear gelatin capsules are USP quality and are designed to disintegrate within 30 minutes after ingestion.

CHOLESTIN™

[kō lĕs 'tĭn]

Monascus purpureus **Went (Red Yeast)**
600 mg capsules
Dietary Supplement

DESCRIPTION

Dietary supplementation with Cholestin (Patent Pending) is recommended for healthy adult males and postmenopausal women concerned about maintaining healthy blood cholesterol levels, and who—in consultation with their physicians—have determined that dietary supplementation rather than medical treatment is appropriate for cholesterol control.* Cholestin is intended for use as part of a cholesterol maintenance program that includes a healthy diet restricted in saturated fat and cholesterol, and other appropriate measures including regular exercise. **Cholestin is not recommended for treating a disease, and this product should not be substituted for prescribed medications.**

Cholestin has been rigorously evaluated in terms of its pharmacology and toxicity, and in clinical studies to confirm its safety and beneficial effects. It naturally contains HMG-CoA reductase inhibitors, including mevinolin, and unsaturated fatty acids. Thirty-three clinical trials in China and two in the U.S., including one at UCLA School of Medicine confirm its efficacy and safety; 17 were controlled, 18 were open label. In one major randomized multicenter clinical trial involving 446 hyperlipidemic patients with baseline total serum cholesterol levels >230 mg/dL, after 8 weeks of treatment, Monascus was found to promote the health of all lipid levels.* In total, more than 1,000 men and women with elevated lipid levels were given the proprietary ingredient in Cholestin at daily doses of 0.6 to 2.4 g/day for 8 weeks, and was found to promote healthy lipid levels in those patients.* For clinical results, refer to the following references listed below or call Pharmanex at 1-800-999-6229 for free reprints.

- Wang J, et al., "Multicenter Clinical Trial of the Serum Lipid-lowering Effects of a *Monascus purpureus* (Red Yeast) rice preparation from traditional Chinese medicine," *Current Therapeutic Research*, 1997; 58(12):964–978.
- Heber D, et al., "Cholesterol-lowering effects of a proprietary Chinese red yeast rice dietary supplement," *FASEB Journal*, 1998; 12(4):A206.

INGREDIENTS

Each capsule of Cholestin (Patent Pending) contains 600 mg of scientifically-standardized *Monascus purpureus* Went yeast fermented on premium rice. Among the key constituents found in Cholestin is a mixture of natural metabolites which resemble well-characterized HMG-CoA reductase inhibitors, including mevinolin, as well as significant levels of unsaturated fatty acids. Yeast in final product is inactive.

RECOMMENDED USE

As a dietary supplement, take two 600 mg capsules bid, or take all 4 capsules after dinner; take with food to minimize the risk of digestive tract discomfort. **Do not take more than four capsules in any 24-hour period, unless recommended by a physician. Immediately discontinue use if you experience any unexplained muscle pain, tenderness, or weakness, especially if accompanied by flu symptoms.**

SAFETY

Based on foreign and U.S. clinical studies involving thousands of subjects, only a small number of individuals reported slight discomfort in the digestive tract; otherwise, no adverse effects were observed during eight week study periods. Additionally, there were no clinically significant changes in laboratory tests for liver and kidney functions or in routine blood tests. Cholestin was also shown to be safe in acute and long-term animal toxicity studies where there were no adverse reactions at doses up to 50 times the normal human dose over 3 to 4 months.

WARNINGS

Keep out of reach of children.

- **Do not use if you are pregnant, can become pregnant, or are breast feeding.** Not to be used by anyone under 20 years of age. Consult with a physician if you are taking any medication or if you are under physician supervision for cholesterol control.
- One of the natural constituents in Cholestin (mevinolin) in much higher doses has been associated with some rare but serious side effects. Do not take Cholestin if: you are at risk for liver disease, have active liver disease or any history of liver disease; you consume more than 2 drinks of alcohol per day; you have a serious infection; you have undergone an organ transplantation; you have a serious disease or physical disorder or have recently undergone major surgery.

HOW SUPPLIED

Cholestin capsules of 600 mg each are supplied in packages of 48, 60, 80 or 120 count, and can be purchased at major drug, grocery, healthfood and discount stores in the vitamin/dietary supplement section.

Shown in Product Identification Guide, page 332

CORDYMAX Cs-4™

Cordyceps sinensis **mushroom mycelia**

[kord 'ə-măk sē ĕs fŏr, kord' ə-seps sĭ-nĕn-sĭs]

525 mg capsules
Dietary Supplement

DESCRIPTION

CordyMax Cs-4 (Patent Pending) is a dietary supplement used to reduce symptoms of fatigue, and to promote vitality and overall well-being.* It is an exclusive fermentation product derived from the mycelia of the principal fungal strain (*Paecilomyces hepiali* Chen Cs-4) isolated from the renown *Cordyceps sinensis* mushroom. CordyMax has been profiled extensively by chemical and pharmacological methods, and is recognized as having activity most similar to wild *Cordyceps sinensis*. For over two-thousand years, *Cordyceps sinensis* has remained the premier agent in the pharmacopoeia of traditional Chinese medicine to restore vitality and energy, and to serve as a potent tonic conducive to general health and aging concerns.* In humans and animals, CordyMax substantially increases the serum levels of the enzyme superoxide dismutase (SOD). This enhancement of the enzyme's proven ability to scavenge the free radicals associated with age-related oxidative cellular damage may explain the traditional use of the mushroom as a dietary supplement to improve vitality, energy, and quality of life.* Scientific studies also indicate that supplementation with CordyMax may:

(1) Reduce oxidative stress by scavenging oxygen-free radicals in mitochondria;*
(2) Promote efficient utilization of oxygen and enhance lung function;*
(3) Elevate energy states (ATP) in organs;*
(4) Redistribute blood flow to essential organs;*
(5) Improve liver and kidney functions through metabolizing and excreting toxic substances;*
(6) Provide a positive benefit for sexuality.*

INGREDIENTS

Each capsule of CordyMax Cs-4 contains 525 mg of the fermentation product of mycelia (*Paecilomyces hepiali* Chen, Cs-4) isolated from the mushroom *Cordyceps sinensis* (Berk.) Sacc., and is scientifically standardized by HPLC method to contain a minimum of 0.14% adenosine and no less than 5% mannitol (an indicator of polysaccharide content).

RECOMMENDED USE

As a dietary supplement, take two 525 mg capsules bid or tid with water or food. Optimal results typically take 3 to 6 weeks.

SAFETY

With the exception of one case of allergic skin reaction, no other adverse reactions have been reported. During clinical trials in China, some subjects noted a mild sensation of thirst, and one subject noted slight nausea. All subjects considered these effects quite tolerable. No cases of CNS effects have been reported. No contraindications were identified based on Chinese human studies. CordyMax is non-mutagenic and non-teratogenic.

WARNINGS

CordyMax has not been evaluated in children and should only be used by adults. Pregnant and breast feeding mothers should consult a physician prior to use. Consult a physician prior to use if taking a prescription medication.

HOW SUPPLIED

CordyMax capsules of 525 mg each are supplied in packages of 60, 64, 112, 120 count and can be purchased at major drug, grocery, discount and healthfood stores in the vitamin/dietary supplement section.

ESTROCARE™

[ĕs' trə-kâr]

Enhanced Black Cohosh Extract
Dietary Supplement

DESCRIPTION

EstroCare [Patent Pending] is a dietary supplement that addresses the challenges experienced by women during their post-reproductive years.* It consists of a complementary formulation that combines the tonic, energizing actions of CordyMax Cs-4, a proprietary strain of the *Cordyceps sinensis* mushroom, with the proven benefits of Black cohosh (*Cimicifuga racemosa*) root extract, a Native American herb which has been shown in extensive clinical trials to effectively and gently relieve the physical and psychological changes associated with menopause.* EstroCare provides complementary benefits for women experiencing menopause, as well as for younger women experiencing similar symptoms due to hormonal deficits.* Black cohosh extract and CordyMax have proven safety records and are well-tolerated. In combination, these herbs may help women to maintain energy, vitality and optimal health during the menopausal phase of life.*

INGREDIENTS

Estrocare [Patent Pending], at the recommended 3 capsules/day, contains clinically supported dosages of CordyMax Cs-4 mycelium (1500 mg/day) standardized to adeno-

Continued on next page

Estrocare—Cont.

sine and mannitol content, and Black cohosh root extract (81 mg/day) standardized to contain 2.5% triterpene glycosides, calculated as 27-deoxyactein.

SCIENTIFIC SUPPORT

The essential component of EstroCare is Black cohosh root extract. The primary application of Black cohosh extract is as a complement to hormonal (estrogen) therapy to help women manage normal menopausal changes.* Standardized extracts of Black cohosh are used in European phytotherapy and extensive clinical and pre-clinical investigations have shown that it:
• Has estrogen-like activity*
• Inhibits Luteinizing Hormone (LH) release from the pituitary
• Corrects and stabilizes hormonal imbalances associated with menopause*
• Has a calming effect and promotes a healthy hormonal balance*

In a study carried out by 131 general practitioners on 629 female patients with menopausal concerns, after receiving a standardized Black cohosh root extract twice a day for 6 to 8 weeks, 80% of patients experienced clear improvements in normal menopausal changes after four weeks. After 6 to 8 weeks, all menopausal changes experienced were abolished in approximately 40 to 50% of the patients, and were markedly reduced or improved in an additional 30 to 40% of patients. Overall, improvement ranged from 76% to 93% of patients. This dosage regime lacked side effects or had only minor side effects in 93% of the patients. (Stolze H, 1982, *Gyne*, 3:14–16)

The other complementary ingredient in EstroCare, *Cordyceps sinensis* (Berk.) Sacc., a traditional Chinese mushroom, has been demonstrated in pre-clinical and clinical studies to act as a general tonic to:
• Improve energy, vitality and endurance*
• Elevate energy states (ATP) in organs*
• Have calming and stress-relieving effects*
• Optimize cardiac, respiratory, immune, liver and kidney functions*
• Optimize blood lipid metabolism and promote healthy blood lipid profiles*
• Provide a positive benefit for sexuality*
(See CordyMax Cs-4 section for additional information about this ingredient)

RECOMMENDED USE

As a dietary supplement, the recommended, clinically supported dosage for adults is 3 capsules per day, 1 capsule in the morning and 2 capsules in the evening, taken with food or drink. Take for at least 8 weeks for optimal health benefits.

SAFETY

No contraindications or drug interactions have been identified. The action of standardized Black cohosh extract has been interpreted as "estriol-like"; however, individuals with estrogen-dependent tumors should consult their physician prior to use. Standardized Black cohosh extracts have been used in conjunction with estrogen replacement therapy with no adverse interactions. Black cohosh is not considered toxic. Overdoses may produce nausea, vomiting and dizziness; may reduce pulse and induce perspiration. (See CordyMax Cs-4 section for safety information regarding this ingredient.)

WARNINGS

Black cohosh should be avoided in pregnancy, as it may cause premature labor. No information is available on its safety for nursing mothers or breast-fed infants; as with any dietary supplement, a physician should be notified prior to use. A physician should be consulted before taking EstroCare if an individual is taking any physician prescribed medication. Consult a physician every 6 months to determine if further use is warranted.

HOW SUPPLIED

EstroCare capsules (527 mg each) are supplied in boxes of 60 count or 90 count bottles, and can be purchased at major drug, grocery, healthfood and discount stores in the vitamin/dietary supplement section. Clear gelatin capsules are USP quality and are designed to disintegrate within 30 minutes after ingestion.

TĒGREEN 97™
[tē 'grēn 97]
Green tea polyphenol extract
250 mg capsules
Dietary Supplement

DESCRIPTION

Tegreen 97 is a standardized, caffeine-free polyphenol extract of the fresh leaves of the tea plant *Camellia sinensis*.

The major components of Tegreen are polyphenols, which have proven free radical scavenging and antioxidant properties.* The polyphenols with the most active antioxidant activity are the catechins, specifically epigallocatechin gallate (EGCg) and epigallocatechin (EGC).* Using the Ames test, researchers at Kansas University found the EGCg component of Tegreen to be approximately 80 times more effective than Vitamin C, 10 times more effective than Vitamin E and twice as effective as the antioxidant compound in red wine at protecting cells from DNA degradation. The dietary supplement use of green tea polyphenols (especially the catechin EGCg) may help: (1) block the formation of toxic compounds, including nitrosamines* (2) suppress the activation of free radicals* (3) detoxify or trap free radicals* (4) inhibit spontaneous and photo-enhanced lipid peroxidation* (5) inhibit the enzyme urokinase.*

INGREDIENTS

Tēgreen Polyphenolic Profile

Total polyphenols	≥97%
Catechins fraction	≥65%
L-EGCg	≥38% (-)-epigallocatechin gallate
ECG	≥15% Epicatechin gallate
L-EGC	≥6% (-)-epigallocatechin

Caffeine-free formula, containing less than 3% caffeine or 6–8 mg, which is less than the caffeine in 1 ounce of a 5 minute brew green tea.

SCIENTIFIC SUPPORT

The ingestion of green tea polyphenols promotes general well-being by affecting a very broad spectrum of functions. In large-scale epidemiological studies in Asia (totaling more than 100,000 people for study periods up to 10 years), daily consumption of 4 or more cups of a green tea beverage was associated with significant overall health benefits, even after adjustments were made for potential confounding factors including age, tobacco and alcohol use, and body weight.

In addition to providing direct protection from the oxidative effects of toxic free radicals, green tea polyphenols may also enhance the body's natural resistance to environmental toxins and stresses by increasing the activity of certain antioxidant and detoxifying enzymes, including glutathione peroxidase, glutathione reductase, glutathione S-transferase, catalase, and quinone reductase in some cells and tissues.*

RECOMMENDED USE

As a dietary supplement, take one 250 mg capsule qd with food. Each capsule provides the green tea polyphenols typically found in about 4 cups of high-quality brewed green tea, but with only minimal amounts of caffeine.

SAFETY

Not known to be associated with any significant side effects or toxicity. Since Tegreen contains only minimal amounts of caffeine (approximately 6–8 mg), it should not produce the stimulant effect in some people caused by the consumption of caffeine-containing beverages.

WARNINGS

Tegreen has not been evaluated in children and should only be used by adults. Pregnant or breast feeding mothers should consult a physician prior to use.

HOW SUPPLIED

Tegreen capsules are supplied in packages of 30 and 60 count, and can be purchased at major drug, grocery, healthfood and discount stores in the vitamin/dietary supplement section.

STORAGE/SHELF LIFE

For all Pharmanex dietary supplements:
Storage: Store in a dry, cool place. Avoid excessive heat. Protect from light.
Shelf Life: Expiration date is imprinted on bottom of box and each foil blister pack.

---

*These statements have not been evaluated by the Food and Drug Administration. These products are not intended to diagnose, treat, cure or prevent any disease.

EDUCATIONAL MATERIALS

For more information and scientific support papers for Pharmanex Natural Healthcare Products: Call toll free 800-999-6229 or FAX 805-582-9301, Monday – Friday, 8 am to 5 pm, Pacific Time. Website: www.pharmanex.com

PolyMedica Pharmaceuticals (U.S.A.), Inc.
11 STATE STREET
WOBURN, MA 01801

For Medical Information Contact:
In Emergencies:
Peter Etzel or Arthur Siciliano
(781) 933-2020
FAX: (781) 933-7992

ANESTACON®   ℞
(lidocaine hydrochloride jelly, USP) 2%

DESCRIPTION

Each mL contains: Active: Lidocaine Hydrochloride 20 mg/ml (2%). Vehicle: Hydroxypropyl Methylcellulose 10 mg (1%). Preservative: Benzalkonium Chloride 0.1 mg (0.01%). Inactive: Sodium Chloride, Hydrochloric Acid and/or Sodium Hydroxide (to adjust pH to 6.0–7.0), Purified Water. The resulting mixture maximizes contact with mucosa and provides lubrication for instrumentation.

HOW SUPPLIED

In 15 ml. unit-dose for **SINGLE PATIENT USE.**

B & O SUPPRETTES®   ℂ ℞
No. 15A and No. 16A
(Belladonna and Opium) Rectal Suppositories

DESCRIPTION

Each B&O SUPPRETTE® contains (in the water-soluble NEOCERA® Suppository Base for rectal administration):
B&O No. 15A: Powdered opium* 30 mg (0.46 gr) and Powdered Belladonna Extract 16.2 mg (equivalent to 0.21 mg or 0.0032 gr belladonna alkaloids).
B&O No. 16A: Powdered opium* 60 mg (0.92 gr) and Powdered Belladonna Extract 16.2 mg (equivalent to 0.21 mg or 0.0032 gr belladonna alkaloids).
Store at room temperature. DO NOT REFRIGERATE.

HOW SUPPLIED

In strip packaged units of 12 and 144.

CYSTOSPAZ®   ℞
(hyoscyamine) Tablets

CYSTOSPAZ–M®   ℞
(hyoscyamine sulfate) Timed-Release Capsules

DESCRIPTION

CYSTOSPAZ® is a pale blue uncoated compressed tablet for oral administration. It contains the parasympatholytic agent hyoscyamine as the free base. Each tablet contains: hyoscyamine 0.15 mg.
CYSTOSPAZ-M® is a light blue timed-release capsule containing hyoscyamine sulfate 0.375 mg.

CLINICAL PHARMACOLOGY

Through its parasympatholytic action, hyoscyamine relaxes smooth muscle spasm resulting from parasympathetic stimulation. It inhibits gastrointestinal propulsive motility and decreases gastric acid secretion. It also controls excessive pharyngeal, tracheal and bronchial secretions. It is theλ-isomer of atropine and therefore exhibits the same clinical effects as atropine. It is, however, approximately twice as active peripherally as atropine, since the latter is the racemic (dλ) form of hyoscyamine and d-hyoscyamine possesses only a very weak anti-cholinergic action. Since only one-half the atropine dose is required for λ-hyoscyamine, it has only one-half the unwanted central effects of atropine.

INDICATIONS AND USAGE

In the management of disorders of the lower urinary tract associated with hypermotility. Although specific therapy is often required to remove the underlying cause of spasm, CYSTOSPAZ Tablets and CYSTOSPAZ-M Capsules are offered as antispasmodic agent dosage forms which may be combined with other forms of therapy where indicated. CYSTOSPAZ Tablets and CYSTOSPAZ-M capsules are effective as adjunctive therapy in the treatment of peptic ulcer and irritable bowel syndrome (irritable colon, spastic colon, mucous colitis), acute entercolitis and other functional gastrointestinal disorders.
CYSTOSPAZ Tablets and CYSTOSPAZ-M Capsules can also be used to control gastric secretion, visceral spasm and hypermotility in cystitis, pylorospasm and associated abdomi-

nal cramps. May be used in functional intestinal disorders to reduce symptoms such as those seen in mild dysenteries and diverticulitis. They are indicated (along with appropriate analgesics) in symptomatic relief of biliary and renal colic.

CONTRAINDICATIONS

Glaucoma, obstructive uropathy (for example, bladder neck obstruction due to prostatic hypertrophy); obstructive disease of the gastrointestinal tract (as in achalasia, pyloroduodenal stenosis); paralytic ileus, intestinal atony of elderly or debilitated patients; unstable cardiovascular status in acute hemorrhage; severe ulcerative colitis; toxic megacolon complicating ulcerative colitis; myasthenia gravis. Hypersensitivity to any of the ingredients.

WARNINGS

In the presence of high environmental temperature, heat prostration can occur with drug use (fever and heat stroke due to decreased sweating). Diarrhea may be an early symptom of incomplete intestinal obstruction, especially in patients with ileostomy or colostomy. In this instance, treatment with this drug would be inappropriate and possibly harmful. Like other anticholinergic agents, these products may produce drowsiness or blurred vision. In this event, the patient should be warned not to engage in activities requiring mental alertness such as operating a motor vehicle or other machinery or to perform hazardous work while taking this drug.

PRECAUTIONS

General: Use with caution in patients with autonomic neuropathy, hyperthyroidism, coronary heart disease, congestive heart failure, cardiac arrhythmias, and hypertension. Investigate any tachycardia before giving any anticholinergic drug since they may increase the heart rate. Use with caution in patients with hiatal hernia associated with reflux esophagitis.

Information for Patients: CYSTOSPAZ Tablets and CYSTOSPAZ-M Capsules may cause drowsiness, dizziness or blurred vision; patients should observe caution before driving, using machinery or performing other tasks requiring mental alertness. Use of CYSTOSPAZ Tablets or CYSTOSPAZ-M Capsules may decrease sweating resulting in heat prostration, fever or heat stroke; febrile patients or those who may be exposed to elevated environmental temperatures should use caution. Prolonged use of CYSTOSPAZ Tablets or CYSTOSPAZ-M Capsules may decrease or inhibit salivary flow, thus contributing to the development of caries, periodontal disease, oral candidiasis, and discomfort.

DRUG INTERACTIONS

Additive adverse effects resulting from cholinergic blockade may occur when CYSTOSPAZ® Tablets or CYSTOSPAZ-M Capsules are administered concomitantly with other antimuscarinics, amanatadine, haloperidol, phenothiazines, monoamine oxidase (MAO) inhibitors, tricyclic antidepressants or some antihistamines. Antacids may interfere with the absorption of CYSTOSPAZ Tablets or CYSTOSPAZ-M Capsules; take CYSTOSPAZ Tablets or CYSTOSPAZ-M Capsules before meals and antacids after meals.

Carcinogenesis, Mutagenesis, Impairment Of Fertility: No long term studies in animals have been performed to determine the carcinogenic, mutagenic or impairment of fertility potential of CYSTOSPAZ Tablets or CYSTOSPAZ-M Capsules.

Pregnancy Category C—Animal reproduction studies have not been conducted with CYSTOSPAZ Tablets or CYSTOSPAZ-M Capsules. It is also not known whether CYSTOSPAZ Tablets or CYSTOSPAZ-M Capsules can cause fetal harm when administered to a pregnant woman or can affect reproduction capacity. CYSTOSPAZ Tablets or CYSTOSPAZ-M Capsules should be taken by a pregnant woman only if clearly needed.

Nursing Mothers—Hyoscyamine is excreted in human milk. Caution should be exercised when CYSTOSPAZ Tablets or CYSTOSPAZ-M Capsules are administered to a nursing woman.

ADVERSE REACTIONS

Adverse reactions may include dryness of the mouth; urinary hesitancy and retention; blurred vision; tachycardia; palpitations; mydriasis; cycloplegia; increased ocular tension; headache; nervousness; drowsiness; weakness; suppression of lactation; allergic reactions or drug idiosyncrasies; urticaria and other dermal manifestations; and decreased sweating. **Note:** Slight dryness of the mouth is an indication that parasympathetic blockage is effective.

DRUG ABUSE AND DEPENDENCE

A dependence on the use of CYSTOSPAZ Tablets or CYSTOSPAZ-M Capsules has not been reported and due to the nature of their ingredients, abuse of CYSTOSPAZ Tablets or CYSTOSPAZ-M Capsules is not expected.

OVERDOSAGE

Symptoms of overdosage include severe dryness of the mouth, nose, throat, and hot dry flushed skin, hyperpyrexia (especially in children), difficulty or inability to swallow, difficult speech, dilated pupils until iris almost disappears, restlessness and garrulity indicating an irritability of the brain, marked tremors, convulsions, respiratory failure, death. In adults, symptoms of overdosage may begin in the range of ingestion of 0.6 to 1 mg with doses exceeding 1–2 mg eliciting more profound toxicity. Measures to be taken are immediate lavage of the stomach and injection of physostigmine 0.5 to 2 mg intravenously and repeated as necessary up to a total of 5 mg. Fever may be treated symptomatically (tepid water sponge baths, hypothermic blanket). Excitement to a degree which demands attention may be managed with sodium thiopental 2% solution given slowly intravenously or chloral hydrate (100–200 ml. of a 2% solution) by rectal infusion.

DOSAGE AND ADMINISTRATION

Adults: CYSTOSPAZ Tablets—One or two tablets four times daily or fewer if needed. CYSTOSPAZ-M Capsules—One capsule every twelve hours.

Children (12 and under): Reduce dosage in proportion to age and weight.

HOW SUPPLIED

CYSTOSPAZ Tablets— Bottles of 100 light blue tablets. Tablets are imprinted with a "**W** 2225". CYSTOSPAZ-M Capsules—Bottles of 100 light blue timed-release capsules. Capsules are identified with "**W** 2260" printed in black.

URISED® ℞

DESCRIPTION

URISED® is a dark blue, round, tablet for oral administration. It is a combination of antiseptics (Methenamine, Methylene Blue, Phenyl Salicylate, Benzoic Acid) and parasympatholytics (Atropine Sulfate, Hyoscyamine).

Each tablet contains: Methenamine 40.8 mg, Phenyl Salicylate 18.1 mg, Methylene Blue 5.4 mg, Benzoic Acid 4.5 mg, Atropine Sulfate 0.03 mg and Hyoscyamine (as the sulfate) 0.03 mg.

CLINICAL PHARMACOLOGY

Methenamine itself does not have antiseptic, irritant, or toxic properties in the urine. Methenamine, in an acid urine (pH 6 or below), hydrolyzes into formaldehyde within the urinary tract providing mild antiseptic activity. When given as directed and the daily urine volume is 1000 to 1500 mL, a daily dose of 2 grams will yield a urinary concentration of 18–60 mcg/mL of free formaldehyde in the urine. This is more than the minimal inhibitory dose of formaldehyde which must be available for most urinary tract pathogens. Methenamine is readily absorbed from the gastrointestinal tract and is rapidly excreted almost entirely in the urine. Methylene Blue and Benzoic Acid are mild but effective antiseptics which contribute to the antiseptic properties of Methenamine. Phenyl Salicylate is a mild analgesic and antipyretic with weak antiseptic activity. All of these compounds are readily absorbed from the gastrointestinal tract and excreted in the urine. Through parasympatholytic action, atropine and hyoscyamine relax smooth muscle spasms resulting from parasympathetic stimulation.

INDICATIONS AND USAGE

URISED is indicated for the relief of discomfort of the lower urinary tract caused by hypermotility resulting from inflammation or diagnostic procedures and in the treatment of cystitis, urethritis, and trigonitis when caused by organisms which maintain or produce an acid urine and are susceptible to formaldehyde.

CONTRAINDICATIONS

Glaucoma, urinary bladder neck obstruction, pyloric or duodenal obstruction, or cardiospasm. Hypersensitivity to any of the ingredients.

WARNINGS

Do not exceed recommended dose. Methenamine may combine with sulfonamides in the urine to give mutual antagonism and should not be used with sulfonamides.

PRECAUTIONS

Administer with caution to persons with known idiosyncrasy to atropine-like compounds and to patients suffering from cardiac disease. Bacteriological studies of the urine may be helpful in following the patient response. Methylene Blue interferes with the analysis for some urinary components such as free formaldehyde. Drugs and/or foods which produce an alkaline urine should be restricted.

Patient should be advised that the urine may become blue to blue-green and the feces may be discolored as a result of excretion of Methylene Blue, so care should be taken to avoid staining clothing or other items. Methenamine preparations should not be given to patients taking sulfonamides since insoluble precipitates may form with formaldehyde in the urine. No known long-term animal studies have been performed to evaluate carcinogenic potential. The precautions related to drug interaction, diagnostic interference, medical problems and side effects to use of belladonna alkaloids, should be observed.

Pregnancy Category C. Animal reproduction studies have not been conducted with URISED® tablets. It is also not known whether URISED tablets can cause fetal harm when administered to a pregnant woman or can affect reproduction capacity. URISED tablets should be given to a pregnant woman only if clearly needed.

Nursing Mothers: It is not known whether this drug is excreted in human milk. Because many drugs are excreted in human milk, caution should be exercised when URISED tablets are administered to a nursing woman.

Prolonged Use: There have been no studies to establish the safety of prolonged use in humans.

ADVERSE REACTIONS

Prolonged use may result in a generalized skin rash, pronounced dryness of the mouth, flushing, difficulty in initiating micturition, rapid pulse, dizziness or blurring of vision. If any of these reactions occurs, discontinue use immediately. Acute urinary retention may be precipitated in prostatic hypertrophy. See "OVERDOSAGE."

DRUG ABUSE AND DEPENDENCE

A dependence on the use of URISED has not been reported and due to the nature of its ingredients, abuse of URISED is not expected.

OVERDOSAGE

By exceeding the recommended dosage of URISED, symptomology related to the overdose of its individual active ingredients may be expected as follows:

Atropine Sulfate, Hyoscyamine: Symptoms associated with an overdosage of URISED will most probably be manifested in the symptoms related to overdosage of the alkaloids Atropine Sulfate and Hyoscyamine. Such symptoms as dryness of mucous membranes; dilatation of pupils; hot, dry, flushed skin; hyperpyrexia; tachycardia; palpitations; elevated blood pressure; coma; circulatory collapse and death from respiratory failure can occur due to overdosage of these alkaloids.

Methenamine: If large amounts of the drug (2–8 gm daily) are used over extended periods (3–4 weeks), bladder and gastrointestinal irritation, painful and frequent micturition, albuminuria and gross hematuria may be expected.

Methylene Blue: Symptoms of Methylene Blue overdosage associated with the overdosage of URISED are not expected to be discernible from those associated with the other active ingredients in URISED.

Benzoic Acid: Symptoms of Benzoic Acid overdosage associated with the overdosage of URISED are not expected to be discernible from those associated with the other active ingredients in URISED.

Phenyl Salicylate: Symptoms of Phenyl Salicylate overdosage include burning pain in throat and mouth, white necrotic lesions in the mouth, abdominal pain, vomiting, bloody diarrhea, pallor, sweating, weakness, headache, dizziness and tinnitus. The symptoms, however, are not expected to be discernible from those associated with the other active ingredients in URISED.

DOSAGE AND ADMINISTRATION

Adults: Two tablets four times daily. See "PRECAUTIONS."

Usual pediatric dosage: Children up to 6 years of age—Use is not recommended. Children 6 years of age and older—Dosage must be individualized by physician.

HOW SUPPLIED

Bottles of 100 and 500 tablets. Tablets are imprinted "**W** 2183".

Pratt Pharmaceuticals Division

see Pfizer Inc

For information on over-the-counter drugs, consult **PDR For Nonprescription Drugs.**

Procter & Gamble
P.O. BOX 5516
CINCINNATI, OH 45201

Direct Inquiries to:
Charles Lambert
(800) 358-8707

For Medical Emergencies:
Call Collect: (513) 558-4422

CHILDREN'S VICKS® NYQUIL®   OTC
COLD/COUGH RELIEF
Antihistamine/Nasal Decongestant/Cough Suppressant

(See PDR For Nonprescription Drugs.)

HEAD & SHOULDERS®
DANDRUFF SHAMPOO   OTC

Head & Shoulders Dandruff Shampoo for Normal hair offers effective control of persistent dandruff, and beautiful hair from a pleasant-to-use formula. Double-blind and expert-graded testing have proven that Head & Shoulders Dandruff Shampoo reduces dandruff. It is also gentle enough to use every day for clean, manageable hair.

ACTIVE INGREDIENT

1% pyrithione zinc suspended in a mild surfactant base. Shampoo also includes mild conditioning agents.

INDICATIONS

For effective control of dandruff of the scalp.

ACTIONS

Head & Shoulders reduces the flaking and itching caused by dandruff. The pyrithione zinc active helps kill the microscopic fungus associated with dandruff.

WARNINGS

For external use only. Avoid contact with eyes. If contact occurs, rinse eyes thoroughly with water. If condition worsens or does not improve after regular use of this product as directed, consult a doctor. Keep this and all drugs out of the reach of children.

DOSAGE AND ADMINISTRATION

For best results, use Head & Shoulders at least twice a week or as directed by a doctor. It is gentle enough to use for every shampoo.

INGREDIENTS

Pyrithione zinc in a shampoo base of water, ammonium laureth sulfate, ammonium lauryl sulfate, sodium lauroyl sarcosinate, glycol distearate, sodium sulfate, dimethicone, fragrance, DMDM hydantoin, disodium phosphate, sodium phosphate, lauryl alcohol, PEG-12, sodium chloride, polyquaternium-10 and FD&C Blue No. 1.

HOW SUPPLIED

Head & Shoulders Dandruff Shampoo is available in 2 FL OZ, 6.8 FL OZ, 15 FL OZ unbreakable plastic bottles.

HEAD & SHOULDERS®   OTC
DANDRUFF SHAMPOO DRY SCALP

Head & Shoulders Dandruff Shampoo for Normal hair offers effective control of persistent dandruff, and beautiful hair from a pleasant-to-use formula. Double-blind and expert-graded testing have proven that Head & Shoulders Dandruff Shampoo reduces dandruff. It is also gentle enough to use every day for clean, manageable hair.

ACTIVE INGREDIENT

1% pyrithione zinc suspended in a mild surfactant base. Shampoo also includes mild conditioning agents.

INDICATIONS

For effective control of dandruff of the scalp.

ACTIONS

Head & Shoulders reduces the flaking and itching caused by dandruff. The pyrithione zinc active helps kill the microscopic fungus associated with dandruff.

WARNINGS

For external use only. Avoid contact with eyes. If contact occurs, rinse eyes thoroughly with water. If condition worsens or does not improve after regular use of this product as directed, consult a doctor. Keep this and all drugs out of the reach of children.

DOSAGE AND ADMINISTRATION

For best results, use Head & Shoulders at least twice a week or as directed by a doctor. It is gentle enough to use for every shampoo.

INGREDIENTS

Pyrithione zinc in a shampoo base of water, ammonium laureth sulfate, ammonium lauryl sulfate, sodium lauroyl sarcosinate, glycol distearate, sodium sulfate, dimethicone, fragrance, DMDM hydantoin, disodium phosphate, sodium phosphate, lauryl alcohol, PEG-12, sodium chloride polyquaternium-10 and FD&C Blue No. 1.

HOW SUPPLIED

Head & Shoulders Dandruff Shampoo is available in 2 FL OZ, 6.8 FL OZ, 15 FL OZ unbreakable plastic bottles.

HEAD & SHOULDERS® INTENSIVE
TREATMENT DANDRUFF AND
SEBORRHEIC DERMATITIS SHAMPOO   OTC

Head & Shoulders Intensive Treatment Dandruff and Seborrheic Dermatitis Shampoo offers effective control of persistent dandruff, and beautiful hair from a pleasant-to-use formula. Double-blind and expert-graded testing have proven that Intensive Treatment Dandruff and Seborrheic Dermatitis Shampoo reduces persistent dandruff. It is also gentle enough to use every day for clean, manageable hair.

Active Ingredient 1% selenium sulfide suspended in a mild surfactant base. Shampoo also includes mild conditioning agents.

INDICATIONS

For effective control of seborrheic dermatitis and dandruff of the scalp.

ACTIONS

Selenium sulfide is substantive to the scalp and remains after rinsing. Its mechanism is believed to be antiproliferative, and to also control the microorganisms associated with persistent dandruff flaking and itching.

WARNINGS

For external use only. Avoid contact with the eyes. If contact occurs, rinse eyes thoroughly with water. If condition worsens or does not improve after regular use of this product as directed, consult a doctor. Keep this and all drugs out of the reach of children.

CAUTION

If used on bleached, tinted, grey, or permed hair, rinse for 5 minutes.

DOSAGE AND ADMINISTRATION

For best results, use at least twice a week or as directed by a doctor. It is gentle enough to use for every shampoo.

INGREDIENTS

Selenium sulfide in a shampoo base of water, ammonium laureth sulfate, ammonium lauryl sulfate, cocamide MEA, glycol distearate, ammonium xylenesulfonate, dimethicone, fragrance, tricetylmonium chloride, cetyl alcohol, DMDM hydantoin, sodium chloride, stearyl alcohol, hydroxypropyl methylcellulose, FD&C Red No. 4.

HOW SUPPLIED

Intensive Treatment Dandruff and Seborrheic Dermatitis Shampoo is available in 15 FL OZ unbreakable plastic bottles.

METAMUCIL®   OTC
[met uh-mū sil]
(psyllium husk fiber)

DESCRIPTION

Metamucil contains a bulk forming natural therapeutic fiber for restoring and maintaining regularity as recommended by a physician. It contains psyllium husk, a highly efficient fiber from the plant Plantago ovata. Metamucil contains no chemical stimulants and does not disrupt normal bowel function. Each dose contains approximately 3.4 grams of psyllium husk. Inactive ingredients, sodium, potassium, calories, carbohydrate, fat and phenylalanine content are shown in Table 1 for all forms and flavors. Phenylketonurics should be aware that phenylalanine is present in Metamucil products that contain aspartame. Metamucil Sugar-Free Regular Flavor contains no sugar and no artificial sweetners.
Metamucil in powdered forms is gluten-free. Wafers contain gluten: Apple Crisp contains 0.7g/dose, Cinnamon Spice contains 0.5g/dose.

ACTIONS

The active ingredient in Metamucil is psyllium husk, a natural fiber which promotes elimination due to its bulking ef-

---

fect in the colon. This bulking effect is due to both the water-holding capacity of undigested fiber and the increased bacterial mass following partial fiber digestion. These actions result in enlargement of the lumen of the colon, and softer stool, thereby decreasing intraluminal pressure and straining, and speeding colonic transit in constipated patients.

INDICATIONS

Metamucil is indicated in the management of chronic constipation, irritable bowel syndrome, as adjunctive therapy in the constipation of diverticular disease, the bowel management of patients with hemorrhoids, for constipation associated with convalescence and senility and for occasional constipation during pregnancy when under the care of a physician. Pregnancy: Category B.

CONTRAINDICATIONS

Intestinal obstruction, fecal impaction. Known allergy to any component.

WARNINGS

Patients are advised they should not use the product without consulting a doctor when abdominal pain, nausea, or vomiting are present or if they have noticed a sudden change in bowel habits that persists over a period of two weeks, or rectal bleeding. Patients are advised to consult a physician if constipation persists for longer than one week, as this may be a sign of a serious medical condition. **PATIENTS ARE CAUTIONED THAT TAKING THIS PRODUCT WITHOUT ADEQUATE FLUID MAY CAUSE IT TO SWELL AND BLOCK THE THROAT OR ESOPHAGUS AND MAY CAUSE CHOKING. THEY SHOULD NOT TAKE THE PRODUCT IF THEY HAVE DIFFICULTY IN SWALLOWING. IF THEY EXPERIENCE CHEST PAIN, VOMITING, OR DIFFICULTY IN SWALLOWING OR BREATHING AFTER TAKING THIS PRODUCT, THEY ARE ADVISED TO SEEK IMMEDIATE MEDICAL ATTENTION.** Psyllium products may cause allergic reaction in people sensitive to inhaled or ingested psyllium. Keep this and all medications out of the reach of children.

PRECAUTION

Notice to Health Care Professionals: To minimize the potential for allergic reaction, health care professionals who frequently dispense powdered psyllium products should avoid inhaling airborne dust while dispensing these products. Handling and Dispensing: To minimize generating airborne dust, spoon product from the canister into a glass according to label directions.

DOSAGE AND ADMINISTRATION

The usual adult dosage is 1 rounded teaspoonful or 1 rounded tablespoonful depending on product form. Some forms are available in packets. The appropriate dose should be mixed with 8 oz. of liquid (e.g., cool water, fruit juice, milk) following the labeled instructions. Metamucil wafers should be consumed with 8 oz. of liquid. **THE PRODUCT (CHILD OR ADULT DOSE) SHOULD BE TAKEN WITH AT LEAST 8 OZ (A FULL GLASS) OF WATER OR OTHER FLUID. TAKING THIS PRODUCT WITHOUT ENOUGH LIQUID MAY CAUSE CHOKING (SEE WARNINGS).** Metamucil can be taken orally one to three times a day, depending on the need and response. It may require continued use for 2 to 3 days to provide optimal benefit. Generally produces effect in 12–72 hours. For children (6 to 12 years old), use 1/2 the adult dose in/with 8 oz. of liquid, 1 to 3 times daily. Children under 6 consult a doctor.

LABEL STATEMENTS

• NEW USERS: Start with 1 dose daily. If minor bloating occurs when you increase doses, try slightly reducing the amount you are taking.
• Laxatives, including bulk fibers, may affect how well other medicines work. If you are taking a prescription medicine by mouth, take this product at least 2 hours before or 2 hours after the prescribed medicine.

HOW SUPPLIED

Powder: canisters (OTC) and cartons of single-dose packets (OTC). Wafers: cartons of single-dose packets (OTC). (See Table 1).
[See table at top of next page]

OIL OF OLAY®—Daily UV Protectant   OTC
SPF 15 Beauty Fluid—Regular &
Fragrance Free
Procter & Gamble

(See PDR For Nonprescription Drugs.)

OIL OF OLAY®—Daily UV Protectant   OTC
SPF 15
Cream—Regular & Fragrance Free
Procter & Gamble

(See PDR For Nonprescription Drugs.)

TABLE 1

METAMUCIL®

Dosage 1–3 Times Daily. Each Dose Contains 3.4 g Psyllium

Forms/ Flavors	Inactive Ingredients	Sodium mg/Dose	Potassium mg/Dose	Calories per dose	Carbohydrate g/Dose	Fat g/Dose	Phenylalanine mg/Dose	Husk Fiber	How Supplied
Smooth Texture Orange Flavor **METAMUCIL** Powder	Citric acid, Flavoring, Sucrose, Yellow 6, Yellow 10	5	32	50	12	—	—	1 rounded tablespoonful ~12 g	Canisters: 20.3, 30.4 and 48.2 ozs. (Doses: 48, 72 and 114); Cartons: 30 single-dose packets (OTC)
Smooth Texture Sugar-Free Orange Flavor **METAMUCIL** Powder	Aspartame, Citric acid, Flavoring, Maltodextrin, Yellow 6	5	31	20	5	—	25	1 rounded teaspoonful ~5.8 g	Canisters: 10, 15, 23.3 ozs. and 36.8 ozs. (Doses: 48, 72, 114 and 180); Cartons: 30 single-dose packets (OTC),
Smooth Texture Sugar-Free Regular Flavor **METAMUCIL** Powder	Citric Acid (less than 5%), Maltodextrin	<5	33	20	5	—	—	1 slightly rounded teaspoonful ~5.4 g	Canisters: 10, 15 and 23.3 ozs. (Doses: 48, 72 and 114)
Original Texture Regular Flavor **METAMUCIL** Powder	Sucrose	<5	29	25	6	—	—	1 rounded teaspoonful ~7 g	Canisters: 13, 19 and 29 ozs. (Doses: 48, 72 and 114)
Original Texture Orange Flavor **METAMUCIL** Powder	Citric acid, Flavoring, Sucrose, Yellow 6	5	30	45	10	—	—	1 rounded tablespoonful ~11 g	Canisters: 19, 29 and 44.2 ozs. (Doses: 48, 72 and 114)
Apple Crisp **METAMUCIL** Wafers	Ascorbic acid, Brown sugar, Cinnamon, Corn oil, Flavors, Fructose, Lecithin, Modified food starch, Molasses, Oat hull fiber, Sodium bicarbonate, Sucrose, Water, Wheat flour	21	63	121	18	5	—	2 wafers 25 g	Cartons: 12 doses
Cinnamon Spice **METAMUCIL** Wafers	Ascorbic acid, Cinnamon, Corn oil, Flavors, Fructose, Lecithin, Modified food starch, Molasses, Nutmeg, Oat hull fiber, Oats, Sodium bicarbonate, Sucrose, Water, Wheat flour	20	64	121	18	5	—	2 wafers 25 g	Cartons: 12 doses

---

PEDIATRIC VICKS® 44e   OTC
COUGH & CHEST CONGESTION RELIEF
Cough Suppressant/Expectorant

(See PDR For Nonprescription Drugs.)

PEDIATRIC VICKS® 44m   OTC
COUGH & COLD RELIEF
Cough Suppressant/Nasal Decongestant/Antihistamine

(See PDR For Nonprescription Drugs.)

PEPTO-BISMOL®   OTC
ORIGINAL LIQUID, ORIGINAL AND CHERRY TABLETS AND EASY-TO-SWALLOW CAPLETS
For upset stomach, indigestion, diarrhea, heartburn and nausea.

Multi-symptom Pepto-Bismol contains bismuth subsalicylate and is the only leading OTC stomach remedy clinically proven effective for both upper and lower GI symptoms. Pepto-Bismol is in more households than any other stomach remedy, making it a convenient recommendation with a name your patients will know. It has been clinically proven in double-blind placebo-controlled trials for relief of upset stomach symptoms and diarrhea.

DESCRIPTION
Each tablespoon (15 ml) of Pepto-Bismol Liquid contains 262 mg bismuth subsalicylate. Each tablespoonful of liquid contains a total of 130 mg non-aspirin salicylate. Pepto-Bismol liquid contains no sugar and is low in sodium (less than 5 mg/tablespoonful). Inactive ingredients: benzoic acid, D&C Red No. 22, D&C Red No. 28, flavor, magnesium aluminum silicate, methylcellulose, saccharin sodium, salicylic acid, sodium salicylate, sorbic acid and water.

Each Pepto-Bismol Tablet contains 262 mg bismuth subsalicylate. Each tablet contains a total of 102 mg non-aspirin salicylate (99 mg non-aspirin salicylate for Cherry). Pepto-Bismol tablets contain no sugar and are very low in sodium (less than 2 mg/tablet). Inactive ingredients include: adipic acid (in Cherry only), calcium carbonate, D&C Red No. 27, FD&C Red No. 40 (in Cherry only), flavors, magnesium stearate, mannitol, povidone, saccharin sodium and talc.
Each Pepto-Bismol Caplet contains 262 mg bismuth subsalicylate. Each caplet contains a total of 99 mg non-aspirin salicylate. Caplets contain no sugar and are low in sodium (less than 3 mg/caplet). Inactive ingredients include: calcium carbonate, D&C Red No. 27, magnesium stearate, mannitol, microcrystalline cellulose, polysorbate 80, povidone, silicon dioxide, and sodium starch glycolate.

INDICATIONS
Pepto-Bismol controls diarrhea within 24 hours, relieving associated abdominal cramps; soothes heartburn and indigestion without constipating; and relieves nausea and upset stomach.

ACTIONS
For upset stomach symptoms (i.e., indigestion, heartburn, nausea and fullness caused by over-indulgence), the active ingredient is believed to work via a topical effect on the stomach mucosa. For diarrhea, it is believed to work by several mechanisms in the gastrointestinal tract, including: 1) normalizing fluid movement via an antisecretory mechanism, 2) binding bacterial toxins and 3) antimicrobial activity.

WARNINGS
Children and teenagers who have or are recovering from chicken pox or flu should not use this medicine to treat nausea or vomiting. If nausea or vomiting is present, patients are advised to consult a doctor because this could be an early sign of Reye syndrome, a rare but serious illness.
This product contains non-aspirin salicylates. If taken with aspirin and ringing in the ears occurs, discontinue use. This product does not contain aspirin, but should not be admin-

istered to those patients who have a known allergy to aspirin or non-aspirin salicylates as an adverse reaction may occur. Caution is advised in the administration to patients taking medication for anticoagulation, diabetes and gout.
If diarrhea is accompanied by a high fever or continues more than 2 days, patients are advised to consult a physician. As with any drug, caution is advised in the administration to pregnant or nursing women.
Keep all medicine out of the reach of children.
Note: This medication may cause a temporary and harmless darkening of the tongue and/or stool. Stool darkening should not be confused with melena.

OVERDOSAGE
In case of overdose, patients are advised to contact a physician or Poison Control Center. Emesis induced by ipecac syrup is indicated in large ingestions provided ipecac can be administered within one hour of ingestion. Activated charcoal should be administered after gastric emptying. Patients should be evaluated for signs and symptoms of salicylate toxicity.

DOSAGE AND ADMINISTRATION
Liquid: Shake well before using.
Adults—   2 tablespoonsful
       (1 dose cup, 30 ml)
Children (according to age)—
9–12 yrs.   1 tablespoonful
       ($\frac{1}{2}$ dose cup, 15 ml)
6–9 yrs.   2 teaspoonsful
       ($\frac{1}{3}$ dose cup, 10 ml)
3–6 yrs.   1 teaspoonful
       ($\frac{1}{6}$ dose cup, 5 ml)

Repeat dosage every $\frac{1}{2}$ to 1 hour, if needed, to a maximum of 8 doses in a 24-hour period. Drink plenty of clear fluids to help prevent dehydration which may accompany diarrhea. For children under 3 years of age, consult a physician.

Continued on next page

Pepto-Bismol Original—Cont.

Tablets:
Adults—Two tablets
Children (according to age)—

9–12 yrs.	1 tablet
6–9 yrs.	$2/3$ tablet
3–6 yrs.	$1/3$ tablet

Chew or dissolve in mouth. Repeat every $1/2$ to 1 hour as needed, to a maximum of 8 doses in a 24-hour period. Drink plenty of clear fluids to help prevent dehydration, which may accompany diarrhea. For children under 3 years of age, consult a physician.

Caplets:
Adults—Two caplets
Children (according to age)—

9–12 yrs.	1 caplet
6–9 yrs.	$2/3$ caplet
3–6 yrs.	$1/3$ caplet

Swallow caplet(s) with water, do not chew. Repeat every $1/2$ to 1 hour as needed, to a maximum of 8 doses in a 24-hour period. Drink plenty of clear fluids to help prevent dehydration, which may accompany diarrhea. For children under 3 years of age, consult a physician.

HOW SUPPLIED

Pepto-Bismol Liquid is available in: 4, 8, 12, and 16 FL OZ bottles. Pepto-Bismol Tablets are pink, round, chewable tablets imprinted with a debossed triangle and "Pepto-Bismol" on one side. Tablets are available in: boxes of 30 and 48. Caplets are available in bottles of 24 and 40. Caplets are imprinted with "Pepto-Bismol" on one side.

PEPTO-BISMOL®   OTC
MAXIMUM STRENGTH LIQUID
For upset stomach, indigestion, diarrhea, heartburn and nausea.

Multi-symptom Pepto-Bismol contains bismuth subsalicylate and is the only leading OTC stomach remedy clinically proven effective for both upper and lower GI symptoms. Pepto-Bismol is in more households than any other stomach remedy, making it a convenient recommendation with a name your patients will know. It has been clinically-proven in double-blind placebo-controlled trials for relief of upset stomach symptoms and diarrhea.

DESCRIPTION

Each tablespoonful (15 ml) of Maximum Strength Pepto-Bismol Liquid contains 525 mg bismuth subsalicylate (236 mg non-aspirin salicylate). Maximum Strength Pepto-Bismol Liquid contains no sugar and is low in sodium (less than 5 mg/tablespoonful). Inactive ingredients include: benzoic acid, D&C Red No. 22, D&C Red No. 28, flavor, magnesium aluminum silicate, methylcellulose, saccharin sodium, salicylic acid, sodium salicylate, sorbic acid and water.

INDICATIONS

Maximum Strength Pepto-Bismol soothes upset stomach and indigestion without constipating; controls diarrhea within 24 hours, relieving associated abdominal cramps; and relieves heartburn and nausea.

ACTIONS

For upset stomach symptoms (i.e. indigestion, heartburn, nausea and fullness caused by over-indulgence), the active ingredient is believed to work via a topical effect on the stomach mucosa. For diarrhea, it is believed to work by several mechanisms in the gastrointestinal tract, including: 1) normalizing fluid movement via an antisecretory mechanism, 2) binding bacterial toxins, and 3) antimicrobial activity.

WARNINGS

Children and teenagers who have or are recovering from chicken pox or flu should not use this medicine to treat nausea or vomiting. If nausea or vomiting is present, patients are advised to consult a doctor because this could be an early sign of Reye syndrome, a rare but serious illness.
This product contains non-aspirin salicylates. If taken with aspirin and ringing in the ears occurs, discontinue use. This product does not contain aspirin, but should not be administered to those patients who have a known allergy to aspirin or other non-aspirin salicylates as an adverse reaction may occur. Caution is advised in the administration to patients taking medication for anticoagulation, diabetes and gout.
If diarrhea is accompanied by a high fever or continues more than 2 days, patients are advised to consult a physician. As with any drug, caution is advised in the administration to pregnant or nursing women.
Keep all medicine out of the reach of children.

Note: This medication may cause a temporary and harmless darkening of the tongue and/or stool. Stool darkening should not be confused with melena.

OVERDOSAGE

In case of overdose, patients are advised to contact a physician or Poison Control Center. Emesis induced by ipecac syrup is indicated in large ingestions provided ipecac can be administered within one hour of ingestion. Activated charcoal should be administered after gastric emptying. Patients should be evaluated for signs and symptoms of salicylate toxicity.

DOSAGE AND ADMINISTRATION

Shake well before using.

Adults—	2 tablespoonsful (1 dose cup, 30 ml)

Children (according to age)—

9–12 yrs.	1 tablespoonful ($1/2$ dose cup, 15 ml)
6–9 yrs.	2 teaspoonsful ($1/3$ dose cup, 10 ml)
3–6 yrs.	1 teaspoonful ($1/6$ dose cup, 5 ml)

Repeat dosage every hour, if needed, to a maximum of 4 doses in a 24-hour period. Drink plenty of clear fluids to help prevent dehydration, which may accompany diarrhea.

HOW SUPPLIED

Maximum Strength Pepto-Bismol is available in: 4, 8, and 12 FL OZ bottles.

ORIGINAL VICKS® COUGH DROPS   OTC
Menthol Cough Suppressant/Oral Anesthetic
Cherry Flavor

(See PDR For Nonprescription Drugs.)

ORIGINAL VICKS® CHLORASEPTIC®   OTC
COUGH & THROAT DROPS
Menthol Cough Suppressant/Oral Anesthetic
Cherry, Menthol & Honey Lemon Flavors

(See PDR For Nonprescription Drugs.)

VICKS® CHLORASEPTIC®   OTC
SORE THROAT SPRAY
Phenol/oral anesthetic
Cherry and Menthol Flavors

(See PDR For Nonprescription Drugs.)

VICKS® CHLORASEPTIC® SORE   OTC
THROAT LOZENGES
Cherry and Menthol Flavors
Menthol/Benzocaine
Oral Anesthetic

(See PDR For Nonprescription Drugs.)

VICKS® COUGH DROPS   OTC
Menthol Cough Suppressant/Oral Anesthetic
Menthol Flavor

(See PDR For Nonprescription Drugs.)

VICKS® DAYQUIL®   OTC
VICKS® DAYQUIL® LIQUICAPS®   OTC
MULTI-SYMPTOM COLD/FLU RELIEF
Nasal Decongestant/Pain Reliever
Cough Suppressant/Fever Reducer

(See PDR For Nonprescription Drugs.)

VICKS® DAYQUIL®   OTC
SINUS PRESSURE & PAIN RELIEF
WITH IBUPROFEN
Nasal Decongestant/Pain Reliever

(See PDR For Nonprescription Drugs.)

VICKS® 44   OTC
COUGH RELIEF
Dextromethorphan Hydrobromide
Cough Suppressant

(See PDR For Nonprescription Drugs.)

VICKS® 44D   OTC
COUGH & HEAD CONGESTION RELIEF
Cough Suppressant/Nasal Decongestant

(See PDR For Nonprescription Drugs.)

VICKS® 44E   OTC
COUGH & CHEST CONGESTION RELIEF
Cough Suppressant/Expectorant

(See PDR For Nonprescription Drugs.)

VICKS® 44M   OTC
COUGH, COLD & FLU RELIEF
Cough Suppressant/Nasal Decongestant/Antihistamine/Pain Reliever-Fever Reducer

(See PDR For Nonprescription Drugs.)

VICKS® NYQUIL® HOT THERAPY®   OTC
VICKS® NYQUIL® LIQUID
VICKS® NYQUIL® LIQUICAPS®
[nī quǐl]
Multi-Symptom Cold/Flu Relief
Antihistamine/Cough Suppressant/Pain Reliever/Nasal Decongestant/Fever Reducer

(See PDR For Nonprescription Drugs.)

VICKS® SINEX®   OTC
[sī 'něx]
NASAL SPRAY AND
ULTRA FINE MIST FOR SINUS RELIEF
Phenylephrine HCI Decongestant

(See PDR For Nonprescription Drugs.)

VICKS® SINEX® 12 HOUR   OTC
[sī 'něx]
NASAL SPRAY AND ULTRA FINE MIST
FOR SINUS RELIEF
Oxymetazoline HCI Nasal Decongestant

(See PDR For Nonprescription Drugs.)

VICKS® VAPOR INHALER   OTC
I-Desoxyephedrine/Nasal Decongestant

(See PDR For Nonprescription Drugs.)

VICKS® VAPORUB®   OTC
(cream) (ointment)
[vā 'pō-rub]
Nasal Decongestant/Cough Suppresssant/Topical Analgesic

(See PDR For Nonprescription Drugs.)

VICKS® VAPOSTEAM®   OTC
[vā 'pō "stēm]
Liquid Medication for Hot Steam Vaporizers.
Camphor/Cough Suppressant

(See PDR For Nonprescription Drugs.)

For EMERGENCY telephone numbers, consult the **Manufacturers' Index**.

Procter & Gamble
Pharmaceuticals, Inc.
SHARON WOODS TECHNICAL CENTER
11520 REED HARTMAN HIGHWAY
CINCINNATI, OH 45241

Direct Inquiries to:
Customer Service
(800) 448-4878

For Medical Information Contact:
Medical Communications
(800) 836-0658
Fax: (800) 438-0138
or write
Procter & Gamble Pharmaceuticals
Medical Communications Department
11450 Grooms Road
Cincinnati, OH 45242-9694

In Emergencies:
Medical Communications
(800) 836-0658

Information on these Procter & Gamble Pharmaceuticals products is based on labeling in effect July, 1998. Further information on these and other Procter & Gamble Pharmaceuticals products may be obtained by direct inquiry to Procter & Gamble Pharmaceuticals, Medical Communications Department, 11450 Grooms Rd. Cincinnati, OH 45242-9694, or phone 800-836-0658/FAX 800-438-0138.

ACTONEL™ ℞
[ac 'tŏn-ĕl]
(risedronate sodium tablets)

DESCRIPTION
ACTONEL Tablets (risedronate sodium tablets) inhibit osteoclast-mediated bone resorption and modulate bone metabolism. Each ACTONEL tablet for oral administration contains the equivalent of 30 mg of anhydrous risedronate sodium in the form of the hemi-pentahydrate. The empirical formula for risedronate sodium hemi-pentahydrate is $C_7H_{10}NO_7P_2Na \cdot 2.5\ H_2O$. The chemical name of risedronate sodium is [1-hydroxy-2-(3-pyridinyl)ethylidene]bis[phosphonic acid] mono-sodium salt and the chemical structure of risedronate sodium hemi-pentahydrate is the following:

Molecular Weight:
Anhydrous: 305.10
Hemi-pentahydrate: 350.13
Risedronate sodium is a fine, white to off-white, odorless, crystalline powder. It is soluble in water and in aqueous solutions, and essentially insoluble in common organic solvents.
Inactive Ingredients: Crospovidone, hydroxypropyl cellulose, hydroxypropyl methylcellulose, lactose monohydrate, magnesium stearate, microcrystalline cellulose, polyethylene glycol, silicon dioxide, titanium dioxide.

CLINICAL PHARMACOLOGY
Mechanism of Action: ACTONEL is a pyridinyl bisphosphonate that binds to bone hydroxyapatite. At the cellular level, ACTONEL inhibits osteoclasts. The osteoclasts adhere normally to the bone surface, but show evidence of reduced active resorption (e.g., lack of ruffled border). Histomorphometry in rats and dogs showed that ACTONEL treatment reduces bone turnover (activation frequency, i.e., the number of sites at which bone is remodeled) and bone resorption at remodeling sites.
Pharmacokinetics:
Absorption: Absorption after an oral dose is relatively rapid (t_{max} ~1 hour) and occurs throughout the upper gastrointestinal tract. Absorption is independent of dose over the range studied (2.5 to 30 mg). Mean oral bioavailability of the tablet is 0.63% (90% CI: 0.54% to 0.75%) and is decreased when risedronate is administered with food. Dosing either 0.5 hours prior to breakfast or 2 hours after dinner reduces extent of absorption by 55% as compared to dosing in the fasting state (no food or drink for 10 hours prior or 4 hours after dosing). Dosing 1 hour prior to breakfast reduces extent of absorption by 30% as compared to dosing in

the fasting state. ACTONEL is effective when administered at least 30 minutes before breakfast.
Distribution: Preclinical studies in rats and dogs dosed intravenously with single doses of [^{14}C] risedronate indicate that approximately 60% of the dose is distributed to bone. The remainder of the dose is excreted in the urine. The mean steady state volume of distribution is 6.3 L/kg in humans. Human plasma protein binding of drug is about 24%. After multiple oral dosing in rats, the uptake of risedronate in soft tissues was in the range of 0.001% to 0.01%.
Metabolism: Like other bisphosphonates, there is no evidence in support of systemic metabolism of risedronate.
Elimination: Approximately half of the absorbed dose is excreted in urine within 24 hours, and 85% of an intravenous dose is recovered in the urine over 28 days. Mean renal clearance is 105 mL/min (CV = 34%) and mean total clearance is 122 mL/min (CV = 19%), with the difference primarily reflecting nonrenal clearance or clearance due to adsorption to bone. The renal clearance is not concentration dependent, and there is a linear relationship between renal clearance and creatinine clearance. Unabsorbed drug is eliminated unchanged in feces. Once risedronate is absorbed, the serum concentration-time profile is multi-phasic with an initial half-life of about 1.5 hours and a terminal exponential half-life of 220 hours. Although the elimination rate from human bone is unknown, the 220 hour half-life is hypothesized to represent the dissociation of risedronate from the surface of bone.

Special Populations:
Pediatric: Risedronate pharmacokinetics have not been studied in patients < 18 years of age.
Gender: Bioavailability and pharmacokinetics following oral administration were similar in men and women.
Geriatric: Bioavailability and disposition were similar in elderly (> 60 years of age) and younger subjects. No dosage adjustment is necessary.
Race: Pharmacokinetic differences due to race have not been studied.
Renal Insufficiency: Risedronate is excreted unchanged primarily via the kidney. As compared to persons with normal renal function, the renal clearance of risedronate was decreased by about 70% in patients with creatinine clearance of approximately 30 mL/min. ACTONEL is not recommended for use in patients with severe renal impairment (creatinine clearance < 30 mL/min) because of lack of clinical experience. No dosage adjustment is necessary in patients with a creatinine clearance ≥ 30 mL/min.
Hepatic Insufficiency: No studies have been performed to assess risedronate's safety or efficacy in patients with hepatic impairment. Risedronate is not metabolized in rat, dog, and human liver preparations. Insignificant amounts (< 0.1% of intravenous dose) of drug are excreted in the bile in rats. Therefore, dosage adjustment is unlikely to be needed in patients with hepatic impairment.
Pharmacodynamics:
Paget's Disease: Paget's disease of bone is a chronic, focal skeletal disorder characterized by greatly increased and disordered bone remodeling. Excessive osteoclastic bone resorption is followed by osteoblastic new bone formation, leading to the replacement of the normal bone architecture by disorganized, enlarged, and weakened bone structure. Clinical manifestations of Paget's disease range from no symptoms to severe bone pain, bone deformity, pathological fractures, and neurological disorders. Serum alkaline phosphatase, the most frequently used biochemical marker of disease activity, provides an objective measure of disease severity and response to therapy.
In pagetic patients treated with ACTONEL 30 mg/day for 2 months, bone turnover returned to normal in a majority of patients as evidenced by significant reductions in serum alkaline phosphatase, a marker of bone formation, and in urinary hydroxyproline/creatinine and deoxypyridinoline/creatinine, markers of bone resorption. Radiographic structural changes of bone lesions, especially improvement of a majority of lesions with an osteolytic front in weight-bearing bones, were also observed after ACTONEL treatment.

In addition, histomorphometric data provide further support that ACTONEL can lead to a more normal bone structure in these patients.
Radiographs taken at baseline and after 6 months from patients treated with ACTONEL 30 mg daily demonstrate that ACTONEL decreases the extent of osteolysis in both the appendicular and axial skeleton. Osteolytic lesions in the lower extremities improved or were unchanged in 15/16 (94%) of assessed patients; 9/16 (56%) patients showed clear improvement in osteolytic lesions. No evidence of new fractures was observed.

CLINICAL STUDIES
The efficacy of ACTONEL was demonstrated in two clinical studies involving 120 male and 65 female patients. In a double-blind, active-controlled study of patients with moderate-to-severe Paget's disease (serum alkaline phosphatase levels of at least two times the upper limit of normal), patients were treated with risedronate 30 mg daily for 2 months or Didronel® (etidronate disodium) 400 mg/day for 6 months. Figure 1 shows that at Day 180, 77% (43/56) of risedronate-treated patients achieved normalization of serum alkaline phosphatase levels compared to 10.5% (6/57) of patients treated with Didronel (p < 0.001). At Day 540, 16 months after discontinuation of therapy, 53% (17/32) of risedronate-treated patients and 14% (4/29) of Didronel-treated patients with available data remained in biochemical remission.

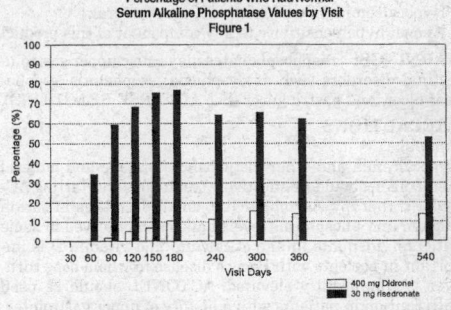

Percentage of Patients Who Had Normal
Serum Alkaline Phosphatase Values by Visit
Figure 1

During the first 180 days of the active-controlled study, 85% (51/60) of risedronate-treated patients demonstrated a ≥ 75% reduction from baseline in serum alkaline phosphatase excess (difference between measured level and midpoint of the normal range) with 2 months of treatment compared to 20% (12/60) in the Didronel-treated group with 6 months of treatment (p < 0.001). Changes in serum alkaline phosphatase excess over time (shown in Figure 2) are significant following only 30 days of treatment, with a 36% reduction in serum alkaline phosphatase excess at that time compared to only 6% seen with Didronel treatment at the same time point(p < 0.01).

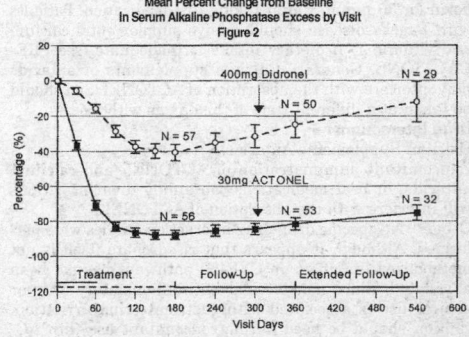

Mean Percent Change from Baseline
In Serum Alkaline Phosphatase Excess by Visit
Figure 2

Table 1
Mean Percent Reduction From Baseline at Day 180 in
Total Serum Alkaline Phosphatase Excess by Disease Severity

Subgroup: Baseline Disease Severity (AP)	30 mg ACTONEL			400 mg DIDRONEL		
	N	Baseline Serum AP (U/L)*	Mean % Reduction	N	Baseline Serum AP (U/L)*	Mean % Reduction
>2, <3×ULN	32	271.6 ± 5.3	−88.1	22	277.9 ± 7.45	−44.6
≥3, < 7×ULN	14	475.3 ± 28.8	−87.5	25	480.5 ± 26.44	−35.0
≥ 7×ULN	8	1336.5 ± 134.19	−81.8	6	1331.5 ± 167.58	−47.2

* Values shown are mean ± SEM; ULN = upper limit of normal

Continued on next page

Actonel—Cont.

Response to ACTONEL therapy was similar in patients with mild to very severe Paget's disease. Table 1 shows the mean percent reduction from baseline at Day 180 in excess serum alkaline phosphatase in patients with mild, moderate, or severe disease

[See table 1 at top of previous page]

Response to ACTONEL was similar between patients who had previously received anti-pagetic therapy and those who had not. In the active-controlled study, four patients previously non-responsive to one or more courses of anti-pagetic therapy (calcitonin, Didronel) responded to treatment with ACTONEL 30 mg daily (defined by at least a 30% change from baseline). Each of these patients achieved at least 90% reduction from baseline in serum alkaline phosphatase excess with three patients achieving normalization of serum alkaline phosphatase levels.

Histomorphometry of the bone was studied in 14 patients with bone biopsies: nine patients had biopsies from pagetic bone lesions and five patients from non-pagetic bone. Bone biopsy results in non-pagetic bone did not reveal osteomalacia, impairment of bone remodeling, or induction of a significant decline in bone turnover in patients treated with ACTONEL.

ANIMAL PHARMACOLOGY AND/OR TOXICOLOGY:

The potential for risedronate to induce osteomalacia was investigated in the Schenk rat assay. This assay is based on histologic examination of the epiphyses of growing rats after drug treatment. ACTONEL did not interfere with bone mineralization even at the highest dose tested (5 mg/kg/day, subcutaneously), which was > 3000 times the lowest antiresorptive dose (1.5 µg/kg/day). These data indicate that ACTONEL administered at therapeutic doses is unlikely to induce osteomalacia.

INDICATIONS AND USAGE

ACTONEL is indicated for treatment of Paget's disease of bone (osteitis deformans).

Treatment is indicated in patients with Paget's disease of bone (1) who have a level of serum alkaline phosphatase (SAP) at least two times the upper limit of normal, or (2) who are symptomatic, or (3) who are at risk for future complications from their disease, to induce remission (normalization of serum alkaline phosphatase).

CONTRAINDICATIONS

• Hypocalcemia (See PRECAUTIONS, General.)
• Known hypersensitivity to any component of this product

WARNINGS: Bisphosphonates may cause upper gastrointestinal disorders such as dysphagia, esophagitis, esophageal ulcer, and gastric ulcer (See ADVERSE REACTIONS).

PRECAUTIONS

General:

Hypocalcemia and other disturbances of bone and mineral metabolism should be effectively treated before starting ACTONEL therapy. Asymptomatic, small decreases in serum calcium and phosphorus levels have been observed in some patients. Adequate intake of calcium and vitamin D is important in patients with Paget's disease in whom bone turnover is significantly elevated. ACTONEL should be used with caution in patients with a history of upper gastrointestinal disorders. ACTONEL is not recommended for use in patients with severe renal impairment (creatinine clearance < 30 mL/min).

Information for Patients: The patient should be informed to pay particular attention to the dosing instructions as clinical benefits may be compromised by failure to take the drug according to instructions. Specifically, ACTONEL should be taken at least 30 minutes before the first food or drink of the day other than water.

In order to facilitate delivery to the stomach and minimize the possibility of gastrointestinal adverse effects, patients should take ACTONEL while in an upright position with a full glass (6 to 8 oz) of plain water and should avoid lying down for 30 minutes after taking this medication. Patients with Paget's disease should receive supplemental calcium and vitamin D if dietary intake is inadequate (see PRECAUTIONS, General). Calcium supplements or antacids may interfere with the absorption of ACTONEL and should be taken at a different time of the day as with food.

Drug Interactions:

Calcium Supplements/Antacids:

Concomitant administration of ACTONEL and calcium, antacids, or oral medications containing divalent cations will interfere with the absorption of ACTONEL.

Other: No specific drug-drug interaction studies were performed. Although it appears that risedronate itself is not metabolized, its affect on CYP450 pathways has not been elucidated. Since nonsteroidal anti-inflammatory drug or aspirin use is associated with gastrointestinal irritation, caution should be used during concomitant use with ACTONEL (See ADVERSE REACTIONS).

Drug/Laboratory Test Interactions: Bisphosphonates are known to interfere with the use of bone-imaging agents.

Specific studies with ACTONEL have not been performed.

Carcinogenesis, Mutagenesis, Impairment of Fertility:

Carcinogenesis: Long-term studies in animals to evaluate the carcinogenic potential of ACTONEL have not been completed.

Mutagenesis: Risedronate did not exhibit genetic toxicity in the following assays: *In vitro* bacterial mutagenesis in *Salmonella* and *E. coli* (Ames assay), mammalian cell mutagenesis in CHO/HGPRT assay, unscheduled DNA synthesis in rat hepatocytes and an assessment of chromosomal aberrations *in vivo* in rat bone marrow. Risedronate was positive in a chromosomal aberration assay in CHO cells at highly cytotoxic concentrations (> 675 mcg/mL, survival of 6% to 7%). When the assay was repeated at doses exhibiting appropriate cell survival (29%), there was no evidence of chromosomal damage.

Impairment of Fertility: In female rats, ovulation was inhibited at an oral dose of 16 mg/kg/day (approximately 5 times the human 30-mg dose based on surface area, mg/m²). Decreased implantation was noted in female rats treated with 7 and 16 mg/kg/day (2 and 5 times the human 30-mg dose based on surface area, mg/m²). In male rats, testicular and epididymal atrophy and inflammation were noted at 40 mg/kg/day (13 times the human 30-mg dose based on surface area, mg/m²). There was moderate to severe spermatid maturation block after 13 weeks in male dogs at a dose of 8 mg/kg/day (approximately 8 times the human 30-mg dose based on surface area, mg/m²). Testicular atrophy was noted in rats after 13 weeks of treatment at 16 mg/kg/day (5 times the human 30-mg dose based on surface area, mg/m²). These findings tended to increase in severity with increased dose and exposure time.

Pregnancy: Pregnancy Category C: Survival of neonates was decreased in rats treated during gestation with 16 and 80 mg/kg/day (5 and 27 times the human 30-mg dose based on surface area, mg/m²). Body weight was increased in neonates from dams treated with 7.1 and 16 mg/kg (2 and 5 times the human 30-mg dose based on surface area, mg/m²), but decreased in neonates from dams treated with 80 mg/kg (27 times the human 30-mg dose based on surface area, mg/m²). In rats treated during gestation, the number of fetuses exhibiting incomplete ossification of sternebrae or skull was statistically significantly decreased at 3.2 mg/kg/day, but increased at 7.1 mg/kg/day (1 and 2 times the human 30-mg dose based on surface area, mg/m²). The number of fetuses exhibiting unossified fetal sternebrae was statistically significantly decreased in rats at these same doses. Both incomplete ossification and unossified sternebrae were increased in rats treated with 16 and 80 mg/kg/day (5 and 27 times the human 30-mg dose based on surface area, mg/m²). A low incidence of cleft palate was observed in fetuses from female rats treated with 3.2 and 7.1 mg/kg/day (1 and 2 times the human 30-mg dose based on surface area, mg/m²). The relevance of this finding to human use of ACTONEL is unclear. No significant fetal ossification effects were seen in rabbits treated with up to 10 mg/kg/day during gestation (7 times the human 30-mg dose based on surface area, mg/m²). However, in rabbits treated with 10 mg/kg/day, 1 of 14 litters were aborted and 1 of 14 litters were delivered prematurely.

Similar to other bisphosphonates, treatment during mating and gestation with doses as low as 3.2 mg/kg/day (1 time the human 30-mg dose based on surface area, mg/m²) has resulted in periparturient hypocalcemia and mortality in pregnant rats allowed to deliver.

There are no adequate and well-controlled studies of ACTONEL in pregnant women. ACTONEL should be used during pregnancy only if the potential benefit justifies the potential risk to the mother and fetus.

Nursing Women: Risedronate was detected in feeding pups exposed to lactating rats for a 24-hour period postdosing, indicating a small degree of lacteal transfer. It is not known whether risedronate is excreted in human milk. Because many drugs are excreted in human milk and because of the potential for serious adverse reactions in nursing infants from bisphosphonates, a decision should be made whether to discontinue nursing or to discontinue the drug, taking into account the importance of the drug to the mother.

Pediatric Use: Safety and effectiveness in pediatric patients have not been established.

ADVERSE REACTIONS

ACTONEL has been studied in 392 patients with Paget's disease of bone. The adverse experiences reported have usually been mild or moderate and generally have not required discontinuation of treatment. The occurrence of adverse events does not appear to be related to patient age, gender, or race.

In a double-blind, active-controlled study, the adverse event profile was similar for ACTONEL and Didronel® (etidronate disodium): 6.6% (4/61) of patients treated with ACTONEL 30 mg/day for 2 months discontinued treatment due to adverse events, compared with 8.2% (5/61) of patients treated with Didronel 400 mg/day for 6 months. Adverse events reported in ≥ 2% of ACTONEL-treated patients in the Phase 3 study are shown in Table 2.

Table 2
Adverse Events Reported in ≥ 2% of ACTONEL-Treated Patients*

Body System	30 mg/day × 2 months ACTONEL % (N = 61)	400 mg/day × 6 months Didronel % (N = 61)
Body as a Whole		
Flu Syndrome	9.8	1.6
Chest Pain	6.6	3.3
Asthenia	4.9	0
Neoplasm	3.3	1.6
Gastrointestinal		
Diarrhea	19.7	14.8
Abdominal Pain	11.5	8.2
Nausea	9.8	9.8
Constipation	6.6	8.2
Belching	3.3	1.6
Colitis	3.3	3.3
Metabolic & Nutritional		
Peripheral Edema	8.2	6.6
Musculoskeletal		
Arthralgia	32.8	29.5
Bone Pain	4.9	4.9
Leg Cramps	3.3	3.3
Myasthenia	3.3	0
Nervous		
Headache	18.0	16.4
Dizziness	6.6	4.9
Respiratory		
Bronchitis	3.3	4.9
Sinusitis	4.9	1.6
Skin		
Rash	11.5	8.2
Special Senses		
Amblyopia	3.3	3.3
Tinnitus	3.3	3.3
Dry Eye	3.3	0

*Considered to be possibly or probably causally related in at least one patient

In the Phase 3 comparative study versus Didronel, patients with a history of upper gastrointestinal (GI) disease or abnormalities were not excluded. Patients were also not excluded based on nonsteroidal anti-inflammatory drug (NSAID) or aspirin use. The proportion of risedronate-treated patients with mild or moderate upper GI adverse events was similar to that in the Didronel-treated group, with no severe upper GI adverse events observed in either treatment group.

As expected, the incidence of GI adverse events in patients who took concomitant NSAIDs or aspirin was, in general, higher than in non-users. However, in these patients, the incidence of GI adverse events was similar in the Didronel- and risedronate-treated groups.

In one of the supportive studies, three patients receiving ACTONEL 30 mg/day were reported to have experienced acute iritis. One case resolved during ACTONEL therapy and did not recur with retreatment. In the second case, iritis initially resolved, but later recurred during ongoing ACTONEL therapy. This patient experienced a third episode of iritis after receiving pamidronate. In the third patient, iritis did not completely resolve until ACTONEL treatment was completed. In all cases, treatment with topical steroids was effective. Iritis has not been observed in other clinical studies, including the active-controlled study in which routine slit-lamp eye examinations were performed.

Laboratory Test Findings: Changes in bone metabolism parameters can be observed with ACTONEL therapy. These are usually asymptomatic and not associated with clinical signs. (See PRECAUTIONS, General.)

OVERDOSAGE

Decreases in serum calcium following substantial overdose may be expected in some patients. Signs and symptoms of hypocalcemia may also occur in some of these patients.

Gastric lavage may remove unabsorbed drug. Administration of milk or antacids to chelate ACTONEL may be helpful. Standard procedures that are effective for treating hypocalcemia, including the administration of calcium intravenously, would be expected to restore physiologic amounts of ionized calcium and to relieve signs and symptoms of hypocalcemia.

Lethality after single oral doses was seen in female rats at 903 mg/kg and male rats at 1703 mg/kg. The minimum lethal dose in mice and rabbits was 4000 mg/kg and 1000 mg/kg. These values represent 320 to 620 times the 30-mg human dose based on surface area (mg/m²).

DOSAGE AND ADMINISTRATION

The recommended treatment regimen is 30 mg once daily for 2 months.

Retreatment may be considered (following post-treatment observation of at least 2 months) if relapse occurs, or if treatment fails to normalize serum alkaline phosphatase. For retreatment, the dose and duration of therapy are the same as for initial treatment. No data are available on more than one course of retreatment.

ACTONEL should be taken at least 30 minutes before the first food or drink of the day other than water. In order to facilitate delivery to the stomach and minimize the possibility of gastrointestinal side effects, patients should take ACTONEL while in an upright position with a full glass (6 to 8 oz) of plain water and should avoid lying down for 30 minutes after taking this medication. Patients with Paget's disease should receive supplemental calcium and vitamin D if dietary intake is inadequate (see PRECAUTIONS, General). Calcium supplements and aluminum- and magnesium-containing antacids may interfere with the absorption of ACTONEL and should be taken at a different time of the day as with food. ACTONEL is not recommended for use in patients with severe renal impairment (creatinine clearance < 30 mL/min). No dosage adjustment is necessary in patients with a creatinine clearance ≥ 30 mL/min.

HOW SUPPLIED

ACTONEL is supplied as 30-mg film-coated, oval, white tablets with RSN on one face and 30 mg on the other.

NDC 0149-0470-01 Bottle of 30

Store at controlled room temperature 20°-25°C (68°-77°F) [See USP].

Rx Only

Sold Under U.S. Patent No. 5,583,122

Mfg. and Dist. by:

Proctor & Gamble Pharmaceuticals, TM Owner

Cincinnati, Ohio 45202

Co-Mkt. with:

Hoechst Marion Roussel, Inc.

Kansas City, Missouri 64137

MARCH 1998

Shown in Product Identification Guide, page 332

ALORA™ ℞

estradiol transdermal system

Continuous Delivery for Twice Weekly Dosing

PRESCRIBING INFORMATION

1. ESTROGENS HAVE BEEN REPORTED TO INCREASE THE RISK OF ENDOMETRIAL CARCINOMA IN POSTMENOPAUSAL WOMEN.

Close clinical surveillance of all women taking estrogens is important. Adequate diagnostic measures, including endometrial sampling when indicated, should be undertaken to rule out malignancy in all cases of undiagnosed persistent or recurring abnormal vaginal bleeding. There is currently no evidence that "natural" estrogens are more or less hazardous than "synthetic" estrogens at equi-estrogenic doses.

2. ESTROGENS SHOULD NOT BE USED DURING PREGNANCY.

There is no indication for estrogen therapy during pregnancy or during the immediate postpartum period. Estrogens are ineffective for the prevention or treatment of threatened or habitual abortion. Estrogens are not indicated for the prevention of postpartum breast engorgement.

Estrogen therapy during pregnancy is associated with an increased risk of congenital defects in the reproductive organs of the fetus, and possibly other birth defects. Studies of women who received diethylstilbestrol (DES) during pregnancy have shown that female offspring have an increased risk of vaginal adenosis, squamous cell dysplasia of the uterine cervix, and clear cell vaginal cancer later in life; male offspring have an increased risk of urogenital abnormalities and possibly testicular cancer later in life. The 1985 DES Task Force concluded that use of DES during pregnancy is associated with a subsequent increased risk of breast cancer in the mothers, although a causal relationship remains unproven and the observed level of excess risk is similar to that for a number of other breast cancer risk factors.

DESCRIPTION

Alora estradiol transdermal system is designed to deliver 17β-estradiol continuously and consistently over a 3 or 4-day interval upon application to intact skin. Three strengths of **Alora** systems are available, having nominal *in vivo* delivery of 0.05, 0.075, and 0.1 mg estradiol per day through skin of average permeability (inter-individual variation in skin permeability is approximately 20%). **Alora** systems have contact surface areas of 18, 27, and 36 cm^2 and contain 1.5, 2.3, and 3.0 mg of estradiol, USP, respectively. The composition of the systems per unit active surface area is identical. Estradiol, USP (17β-estradiol) is a white, crystalline powder that is chemically described as estra-1,3,5(10)-triene-3,17β-diol, has an empirical formula of $C_{18}H_{24}O_2$ and has molecular weight of 272.37. The structural formula is:

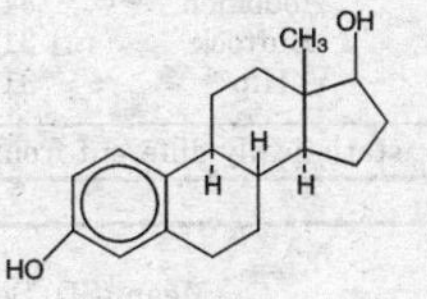

Estradiol

The **Alora** system consists of three layers. Proceeding from the polyethylene backing film as shown in the cross-sectional view below, the adhesive matrix drug reservoir that is in contact with the skin consists of estradiol, USP and sorbitan monooleate dissolved in an acrylic adhesive matrix. The polyester overlapped release liner protects the adhesive matrix during storage and is removed prior to application of the system to the skin.

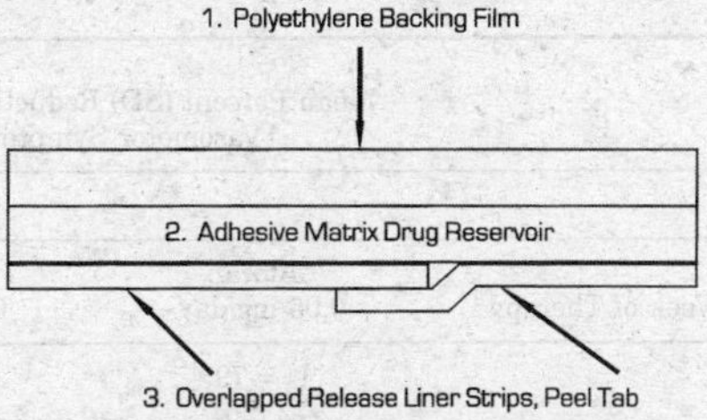

CLINICAL PHARMACOLOGY

Alora provides systemic estrogen replacement therapy by delivering estradiol, the major estrogenic hormone secreted by the human ovary, through the area of intact skin covered by the system. Estrogens are important in the development and maintenance of the female reproductive system and secondary sex characteristics. By a direct action, they cause growth and development of the uterus, Fallopian tubes, and vagina. With other hormones, such as pituitary hormones and progesterone, they cause enlargement of the breasts through promotion of ductal growth, stromal development, and the accretion of fat. They also contribute to the shaping of skeleton, maintenance of tone and elasticity of urogenital structures, changes in the epiphyses of the long bones that allow for the pubertal growth spurt and its termination, and pigmentation of the nipples and genitals.

Circulating estrogen concentration modulates the pituitary secretion of the gonadotrophins luteinizing hormone (LH) and follicle stimulating hormone (FSH) through a negative feedback mechanism and estrogen replacement therapy acts to reduce the elevated levels of these hormones seen in the postmenopausal woman. In a multiple dose study in 22 postmenopausal women, **Alora** 0.1 mg/day reduced circulating concentrations of LH and FSH by 34% and 45%, respectively, by the end of the third dose.

Estrogens occur naturally in several forms. The primary source of estrogen in normally cycling adult women is the ovarian follicle, which secretes 70 to 500 micrograms of estradiol daily, depending on the phase of the menstrual cycle. This is converted primarily to estrone, which circulates in roughly equal proportion to estradiol, and to a small amount of estriol. After menopause, most endogenous estrogen is produced by conversion of androstenedione, secreted by the adrenal cortex, to estrone by peripheral tissues. Thus, estrone (especially in its sulfate ester form) is the most abundant circulating estrogen in postmenopausal women. Although circulating estrogens exist in a dynamic equilibrium of metabolic interconversions, estradiol is the principal intracellular human estrogen and is substantially more potent than estrone or estriol at the receptor level.

Estrogen drug products act by regulating the transcription of a limited number of genes. Estrogens diffuse through cell membranes, distribute themselves throughout the cell, and bind to, and activate the nuclear estrogen receptor, a DNA-binding protein which is found in estrogen-responsive tissues. The activated estrogen receptor binds to specific DNA sequences, or hormone-response elements, which enhance the transcription of adjacent genes and in turn leads to the observed effects. Estrogen receptors have been identified in tissues of the reproductive tract, breast, pituitary, hypothalamus, liver, and in bone of women.

Estrogens used in therapy are well absorbed through the skin, mucous membranes, and gastrointestinal tract. When applied for a local action, absorption is usually sufficient to cause systemic effects. When conjugated with aryl and alkyl groups for parenteral administration, the rate of systemic absorption of injected oily preparations is slowed with a prolonged duration of action, such that a single intramuscular injection of estradiol valerate or estradiol cypionate is absorbed over several weeks.

Administered estrogens and their esters are handled within the body essentially the same as the endogenous hormones. Metabolic conversion of estrogens occurs primarily in the liver (first pass effect), but also at local target tissue sites. Complex metabolic processes result in a dynamic equilibrium of circulating conjugated and unconjugated estrogenic forms which are continually interconverted, especially between estrone and estradiol and between esterified and non-esterified forms. Although naturally-occurring estrogens circulate in the blood largely bound to sex hormone-binding globulin and albumin, only unbound estrogens enter target tissue cells. A significant proportion of the circulating estrogen exists as sulfate conjugates, especially estrone sulfate, which serves as a circulating reservoir for the formation of more active estrogenic species. A certain proportion of the estrogen is excreted into the bile and then reabsorbed from the intestine. During this enterohepatic recirculation, estrogens are desulfated and resulfated and undergo degradation through conversion to less active estrogens (estriol and other estrogens), oxidation to non-estrogenic substances (catecholestrogens, which interact with catecholamine metabolism, especially in the central nervous system), and conjugation with glucuronic acids (which are then rapidly excreted in the urine).

Loss of ovarian estradiol secretion after menopause can result in instability of thermoregulation, causing hot flushes associated with sleep disturbance and excessive sweating, and urogenital atrophy, causing dyspareunia and urinary incontinence. Estradiol replacement therapy alleviates many of these symptoms of estradiol deficiency in the menopausal woman.

Pharmacokinetics

Transdermal administration of **Alora** produces mean serum concentrations of estradiol comparable to those produced by premenopausal women in the early follicular phase of the ovulatory cycle. The pharmacokinetics and metabolism of transdermally administered estradiol using **Alora** have been evaluated in a total of 123 healthy postmenopausal women in three dose-range finding studies and in three definitive studies.

Absorption

Estradiol is transported across intact skin and into the systemic circulation by a passive diffusion process, the rate of diffusion across the stratum corneum being the principal factor. **Alora** presents sufficient concentration of estradiol to the surface of the skin to maintain continuous transport over the 3 to 4 day dosing interval.

Direct measurement of total absorbed dose of estradiol through analysis of residual estradiol content of systems worn over a continuous four day interval during 251 separate occasions in 123 postmenopausal women demonstrated that the average daily dose absorbed from **Alora** was 0.003 ± 0.001 mg estradiol per cm^2 active surface area. The nominal mean *in vivo* daily delivery rates of estradiol calculated from these data are 0.054 mg/day, 0.081 mg/day, and 0.11 mg/day for the 18 cm^2, 27 cm^2, and 36 cm^2 **Alora** systems, respectively.

In one multiple dose study, 22 postmenopausal women were treated with three consecutive **Alora** 0.1 mg/day systems on abdominal sites of application in a twice weekly dosing regimen and 3 consecutive Estraderm®[1] 0.1 estradiol transdermal systems in the same dosing regimen. During the third **Alora** dose, serum concentrations of estradiol increased above steady state baseline within 4 hours, achieved mean maximum concentration of 133 pg/ml within 18–24 hours, and remained relatively constant between 70 and 100 pg/ml until system removal at 96 hours. In contrast, Estraderm 0.1 mg/day produced higher fluctuations in estradiol serum concentrations, achieving and maintaining serum concentrations greater than 70 pg/ml only during the first 36 hours of the dosing period. Thereafter, serum estradiol concentrations declined steadily to a mean level of 22 pg/ml at system removal at 96 hours of the third dosing interval. The mean steady state estradiol serum concentration profiles for **Alora** 0.1 mg/day and Estraderm 0.1 mg/day are shown in Figure 1.

[See figure 1 at top of next column]

In another study, 20 women also were treated with three consecutive doses of **Alora** 0.05 mg/day, **Alora** 0.075 mg/day and **Alora** 0.1 mg/day on abdominal application sites. Mean steady state estradiol serum concentrations observed over the dosing interval are shown in Figure 2.

[See figure 2 in next column]

In a single dose randomized crossover study conducted to compare the effect of site of **Alora** application, 31 postmenopausal women wore single **Alora** 0.05 mg/day for four day periods on the lower abdomen, upper quadrant of the but-

Continued on next page

Alora—Cont.

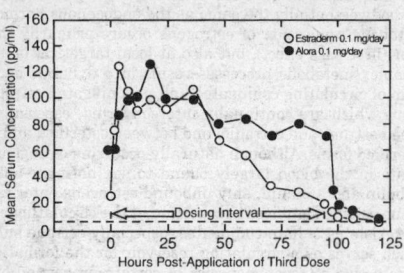

Figure 1
Mean steady state estradiol serum concentration during the third twice weekly dose of Alora 0.1 mg/day compared to Estraderm 0.1 mg/day in 22 postmenopausal women.

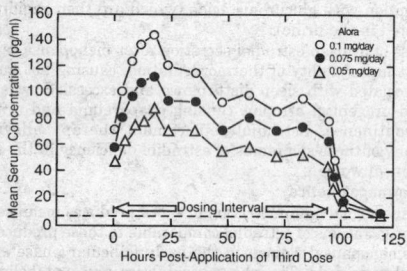

Figure 2
Mean steady state estradiol serum concentration during the third twice weekly dose of Alora 0.1 mg/day, Alora 0.075 mg/day, and Alora 0.05 mg/day in 20 postmenopausal women

tocks, and outside aspect of the hip. The estradiol serum concentration profiles are shown in Figure 3.

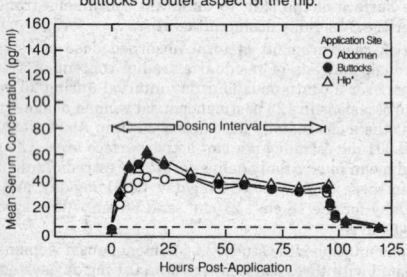

Figure 3
Mean estradiol serum concentration during a single 4 day wearing of Alora 0.05 mg/day applied by 31 postmenopausal women to the lower abdomen, upper quadrant of the buttocks or outer aspect of the hip.

*C_{max} and C_{avg} statistically different from abdomen.

Table I provides a summary of the estradiol pharmacokinetic parameters studied during biopharmaceutic evaluation of Alora.
[See table 1 above]

Distribution
No specific investigation of the tissue distribution of estradiol absorbed from Alora in humans has been conducted. However, a significant body of literature exists that indicates that estradiol is widely distributed in the body and is generally found in higher concentrations in the sex hormone target organs. Estradiol in blood is distributed between free estradiol, albumin bound estradiol, and sex hormone binding globulin (SHBG) bound estradiol. Serum concentrations reported here are expressed as total estradiol concentrations.

Metabolism
Since transdermally absorbed estradiol is not subject to first pass liver metabolism, the ratio of serum concentrations of estradiol to either of its major metabolites, estrone or estrone sulfate, is significantly greater than that seen for the oral route of administration. The clinical relevance of the estradiol to estrone ratio is presently unknown.

In controlled clinical trials using Alora compared to orally administered conjugated equine estrogens (CEE), the serum concentrations of estradiol and its metabolites were measured after 12 weeks therapy and are given in Table 2. The overall mean (SD) ratio of estradiol to estrone was 1.26 (0.80) for Alora and was 0.30 (0.39) for CEE.

Table 1
Mean (SD) Pharmacokinetic Profile of Alora Over an 84 Hour Dosing Interval

Alora (mg/day)	Application Site	N	Dosing	C_{max} (pg/ml)	C_{min} (pg/ml)	C_{avg} (pg/ml)	CL (L/hr)
0.05	Abdomen	20	Multiple	92 (33)	43 (12)	64 (19)	54 (18)
0.075	Abdomen	20	Multiple	120 (60)	53 (23)	86 (40)	53 (12)
0.1	Abdomen	42	Multiple	144 (57)	58 (20)	98 (38)	61 (18)
0.05	Abdomen	31	Single	53 (23)	—	41 (18)	69 (22)
	Buttock	31	Single	67 (45)	—	45 (21)	66 (23)
	Hip*	31	Single	69 (30)	—	48 (17)	62 (18)

* C_{max} and C_{avg} statistically different from abdomen

Table 2
Mean (SD) Serum Concentration of Estradiol and its Metabolites After 12 Weeks Therapy with Alora or CEE

	Concentrations after 12 Weeks Therapy			
	Alora 0.05 mg/day	CEE 0.625 mg/day	Alora 0.1 mg/day	CEE 1.25 mg/day
Estradiol (pg/ml)	49 (52)	25 (32)	105 (89)	52 (66)
Estrone (pg/ml)	43 (23)	89 (42)	69 (37)	232 (210)
Estrone Sulfate (pg/ml)	765 (710)	1714 (1112)	1243 (960)	2741 (2655)

Table 3
Mean Percent (SD) Reduction in Frequency of Moderate-to-Severe Vasomotor Symptoms for Alora Compared to CEE

	Mean Percent Reduction (SD)			
Week of Therapy	Alora 0.05 mg/day	CEE 0.625 mg/day	Alora 0.1 mg/day	CEE 1.25 mg/day
	N = 79	N = 78	N = 79	N = 78
4*	72 (26)	78 (30)	83 (28)	86 (20)
8*	81 (24)	88 (21)	91 (22)	92 (18)
12	87 (20)	91 (18)	92 (20)	96 (11)

Analysis includes all randomized patients who received at least one dose of study drug and who had a post-baseline measurement of efficacy. At weeks 4 and 8, * indicates statistically significant differences ($p < 0.05$) between Alora 0.05 mg/day and CEE 0.625 mg/day.

[See table 2 above]
Elimination
No specific studies of elimination of estradiol have been performed using Alora. However, elimination of estradiol is known to be primarily through liver metabolism and conjugation to more hydrophilic compounds such as sulfates and glucuronides which are then cleared through renal elimination. Because estradiol has a short half-life, transdermal administration of estradiol allows for rapid decline in blood levels after Alora is removed. The apparent mean (SD) serum half-life of estradiol determined from biopharmaceutic studies conducted with Alora is 1.75 ± 2.87 hours.
Special Populations
Alora has been studied only in postmenopausal women.

CONTROLLED CLINICAL STUDIES
Efficacy and safety of Alora have been studied in two double blind/double dummy, randomized, parallel group trials involving a total of 594 postmenopausal women over a 12 week dosing period. In both studies, measures of efficacy included reduction in weekly number of moderate-to-severe vasomotor symptoms when compared to a weekly baseline average determined during a 2-week pre-dosing screening period. Only women having estradiol and FSH serum concentrations in the postmenopausal range and who exhibited a weekly average of at least 60 moderate-to-severe hot flushes during the screening period were enrolled in the studies.

In a positive control study, each patient received unopposed estrogen for a duration of 12 weeks in the form of Alora 0.05 mg/day, Alora 0.1 mg/day, administered twice weekly; or once daily oral administration of conjugated equine estrogens (CEE) 0.625 mg, or CEE 1.25 mg. In this study, the population was primarily caucasian (88%), had a mean age of 50.4 years (range 29–75 years), and had undergone either natural menopause (46%) or surgical menopause (54%) at an average age of 42.5 years (range 19–62 years). Mean baseline frequency of moderate-to-severe vasomotor symptoms was 95 per week in the overall population studied. Mean percent reduction in frequency of moderate-to-severe hot flushes is shown in Table 3.
[See table 3 above]
In a placebo-controlled study, each patient received either Alora 0.05 mg/day, Alora 0.1 mg/day, or matching placebo unopposed and dosed twice weekly over a 12 week duration. In this study, the population was also primarily caucasian (88%), had a mean age of 50.9 years (range 31–70 years), and had undergone either natural menopause (44%) or sur-

gical menopause (56%) at an average age of 43.0 years (range 16–58 years). Mean baseline frequency of moderate-to-severe vasomotor symptoms was 89 per week in the overall population studied. Mean percent reduction in frequency of moderate-to-severe hot flushes is shown in Table 4.

Table 4
Mean Percent (SD) Reduction in Frequency of Moderate-to-Severe Vasomotor Symptoms for Alora Compared to Placebo

	Mean Percent Reduction (SD)		
Week of Therapy	Alora 0.05 mg/day N = 87	Alora 0.1 mg/day N = 91	Placebo N = 90
4*	67 (36)	81 (32)	50 (41)
8*	77 (42)	89 (27)	55 (42)
12*	80 (40)	90 (25)	60 (43)

Analysis includes all randomized patients who received at least one dose of study drug and who had a post-baseline measurement of efficacy. At weeks 4, 8, and 12, * indicates statistically significant differences ($p < 0.05$) between both strengths of Alora and placebo.

In the two clinical trials, vaginal cytology was obtained predosing and at last visit in a total of 103 women treated with Alora 0.05 mg/day, in 88 women treated with Alora 0.1 mg/day and in 46 women in the placebo group. Superficial cells increased by a mean of 15.4%, 26.6% and 8.1% for the Alora 0.05 mg/day, Alora 0.1 mg/day, and placebo groups, respectively. Corresponding reductions in basal/parabasal and intermediate cells were also observed.

INDICATIONS AND USAGE

Alora is indicated in:
1. Treatment of moderate-to-severe vasomotor symptoms associated with the menopause. There is no adequate evidence that estrogens are effective for nervous symptoms or depression which might occur during menopause and they should not be used to treat these conditions.
2. Treatment of vulval and vaginal atrophy.
3. Treatment of hypoestrogenism due to hypogonadism, castration or primary ovarian failure.

CONTRAINDICATIONS

Estrogens should not be used in individuals with any of the following conditions:

1. Known or suspected pregnancy (see Boxed Warning): Estrogens may cause fetal harm when administered to a pregnant woman.
2. Undiagnosed abnormal genital bleeding;
3. Known or suspected cancer of the breast;
4. Known or suspected estrogen-dependent neoplasia;
5. Active thrombophlebitis, or thromboembolic disorders.
6. Known hypersensitivity to any of the components of **Alora**.

WARNINGS

1. Induction of malignant neoplasms.

Endometrial cancer. The reported endometrial cancer risk among unopposed estrogen users is about 2 to 12 fold greater than in non-users, and appears dependent on duration of treatment and on estrogen dose. Most studies show no significant increased risk associated with use of estrogens for less than one year. The greatest risk appears associated with prolonged use—with increased risks of 15 to 24-fold for five to ten years or more. In three studies, persistence of risk was demonstrated for 8 to over 15 years after cessation of estrogen treatment. In one study a significant decrease in the incidence of endometrial cancer occurred six months after estrogen withdrawal. Concurrent progestin therapy may offset this risk but the overall health impact in postmenopausal women is not known (see PRECAUTIONS).

Breast cancer. Some studies have suggested a possible increased incidence of breast cancer in those women taking estrogen therapy at higher doses or for prolonged periods of time. While the majority of studies have not shown an increased risk of breast cancer in women who have ever used estrogen replacement therapy, some have reported a moderately increased risk (relative risks of 1.3–2.0) in those taking higher doses or those taking lower doses for prolonged periods of time, especially in excess of 10 years. On the other hand, other studies have not shown this relationship.

Congenital lesions with malignant potential. Estrogen therapy during pregnancy is associated with an increased risk of fetal congenital reproductive tract disorders, and possibly other birth defects. Studies of women who received DES during pregnancy have shown that female offspring have an increased risk of vaginal adenosis, squamous cell dysplasia of the uterine cervix, and clear cell vaginal cancer later in life; male offspring have an increased risk of urogenital abnormalities and possibly testicular cancer later in life. Although some of these changes are benign, others are precursors of malignancy.

2. Gallbladder disease. Two studies have reported a 2- to 4-fold increase in the risk of gallbladder disease requiring surgery in women receiving oral estrogen replacement therapy, similar to the 2-fold increase previously noted in users of oral contraceptives.
3. Cardiovascular disease: Large doses of estrogen (5 mg conjugated estrogens per day), comparable to those used to treat cancer of the prostate and breast, have been shown in a large prospective clinical trial in men to increase the risk of nonfatal myocardial infarction, pulmonary embolism, and thrombophlebitis. These risks cannot necessarily be extrapolated from men to women. However, to avoid the theoretical cardiovascular risk to women caused by high estrogen doses, the dose for estrogen replacement therapy should not exceed the lowest effective dose.
4. Elevated blood pressure: Occasional blood pressure increases during estrogen replacement therapy have been attributed to idiosyncratic reactions to estrogens. More often, blood pressure has remained the same or has dropped. One study showed that postmenopausal estrogen users have higher blood pressure than nonusers. Two other studies showed slightly lower blood pressure among estrogen users compared to nonusers. Postmenopausal estrogen use does not increase the risk of stroke. Nonetheless, blood pressure should be monitored at regular intervals during estrogen use.
5. Hypercalcemia: Administration of estrogens may lead to severe hypercalcemia in patients with breast cancer and bone metastases. If hypercalcemia occurs, use of the drug should be stopped and appropriate measures should be taken to reduce the serum calcium level.

PRECAUTIONS

A. General

1. Addition of a progestin. Studies of the addition of a progestin for 10 or more days of a cycle of estrogen administration have reported a lowered incidence of endometrial hyperplasia than would be induced by estrogen treatment alone. Morphologic and biochemical studies of endometrium suggest that 10 to 14 days of progestin are needed to provide maximal maturation of the endometrium and to reduce the likelihood of hyperplastic changes.

There are, however, possible risks which may be associated with the use of progestins in estrogen replacement regimens. These include:

(1) adverse effects on lipoprotein metabolism (lowering HDL and raising LDL) which could diminish the purported cardioprotective effect of estrogen therapy (see PRECAUTIONS below).
(2) impairment of glucose tolerance; and
(3) possible enhancement of mitotic activity in breast epithelial tissue, although few epidemiological data are available to address this point (see PRECAUTIONS below).

The choice of progestin, its dose, and its regimen may be important in minimizing these adverse effects, but these issues will require further study before they are clarified.

2. Cardiovascular risk. A causal relationship between estrogen replacement therapy and reduction of cardiovascular disease in postmenopausal women has not been proven. Furthermore, the effect of added progestins on this putative benefit is not yet known. In recent years, many published studies have suggested that there may be a cause-effect relationship between postmenopausal oral estrogen replacement therapy without added progestins and a decrease in cardiovascular disease in women. Although most of the observational studies which assess this statistical association have reported a 20% to 50% reduction in coronary heart disease risk and associated mortality in estrogen users, the following should be considered when interpreting these reports:

(1) Because only one of these studies was randomized and it was too small to yield statistically significant results, all relevant studies were subject to selection bias. Thus, the apparently reduced risk of coronary disease cannot be attributed with certainty to estrogen replacement therapy. It may instead have been caused by life-style and medical characteristics of the women studied with the results that healthier women were selected for estrogen therapy. In general, treated women were of higher socioeconomic and educational status, more slender, more physically active, more likely to have undergone surgical menopause, and less likely to have diabetes than the untreated women. Although some studies attempted to control for these selection factors, it is common for properly designed randomized trials to fail to confirm benefits suggested by less rigorous study designs. Thus, ongoing and future large-scale randomized trials may fail to confirm this apparent benefit.
(2) Current medical practice often includes the use of concomitant progestin therapy in women with intact uteri. (See PRECAUTIONS and WARNINGS.) While the effects of added progestins on the risk of ischemic heart disease are not known, all available progestins reverse at least some of the favorable effects of estrogens on HDL and LDL levels.
(3) While effects of added progestins on the risk of breast cancer are also unknown, available epidemiological evidence suggests that progestins do not reduce, and may enhance, the moderately increased breast cancer incidence that has been reported with prolonged estrogen replacement therapy (see WARNINGS above).

Because relatively long-term use of estrogens by a woman with a uterus has been shown to increase the risk of endometrial cancer, physicians often recommend that women who are deemed candidates for hormone replacement should take progestins as well as estrogens. When considering prescribing concomitant estrogens and progestins for hormone replacement therapy, physicians and patients are advised to carefully weigh the potential benefits and risks of the added progestin. Large-scale randomized, placebo-controlled, prospective clinical trials are required to clarify these issues.

3. Physical Examination. A complete medical and family history should be taken before initiation of any estrogen therapy. The pre-treatment and periodic physical examinations should include special reference to blood pressure, breasts, abdomen and pelvic organs, as well as a cervical Papanicolaou test. As a general rule, estrogen should be prescribed for no longer than 1 year without another physical examination being performed.
4. Hypercoagulability. Some studies have shown that women taking estrogen replacement therapy have hypercoagulability, primarily related to decreased antithrombin activity. This effect appears dose-and duration-dependent and is less pronounced than that associated with oral contraceptive use. Also, postmenopausal women tend to have increased coagulation parameters at baseline compared to premenopausal women. There is some suggestion that low dose postmenopausal mestranol may increase the risk of thromboembolism, although the majority of studies (primarily of oral conjugated estrogen users) report no such increase. There is insufficient information on hypercoagulability in women who have had previous thromboembolic disease.
5. Familial hyperlipoproteinemia. Estrogen therapy may be associated with massive elevations of plasma triglycerides leading to pancreatitis and other complications in patients with familial defects of lipoprotein metabolism.
6. Fluid retention. Because estrogens may cause some degree of fluid retention, careful observation is required when conditions that might be influenced by this factor are present (e.g., asthma, epilepsy, migraine, and cardiac or renal dysfunction).

7. Uterine bleeding and mastodynia. Certain patients may develop undesirable manifestations of estrogenic stimulation, such as abnormal uterine bleeding and mastodynia.
8. Impaired liver function. Estrogens may be poorly metabolized in patients with impaired liver function and should be administered with caution in such patients.

B. Information for the Patient

See Patient Package Insert printed below.

C. Laboratory Tests

Estrogen administration should generally be guided by clinical response at the smallest dose, rather than laboratory monitoring, for relief of symptoms for those indications in which symptoms are observable.

D. Drug/Laboratory Test Interactions

1. Accelerated prothrombin time, partial thromboplastin time, and platelet aggregation time; increased platelet count; increased factors II, VII antigen, VIII antigen, VIII coagulant activity; IX, X, XII, VII-X complex, and beta-thromboglobulin; decreased levels of anti-factor Xa and antithrombin III, decreased antithrombin III activity; increased levels of fibrinogen and fibrinogen activity; increased plasminogen antigen and activity.
2. Increased thyroid-binding globulin (TBG) leading to increased circulating total thyroid hormone, as measured by protein-bound iodine (PBI), T4 levels (by column or by radioimmunoassay) or T3 levels by radioimmunoassay. T3 resin uptake is decreased, reflecting the elevated TBG. Free T4 and free T3 concentrations are unaltered.
3. Other binding proteins may be elevated in serum, i.e., corticosteroid binding globulin (CBG), sex hormone- binding globulin (SHBG), leading to increased circulating corticosteroids and sex steroids, respectively. Free or biologically active hormone concentrations are unchanged. Other plasma proteins may be increased (angiotensinogen/renin substrate, alpha-1-antitrypsin, ceruloplasmin).
4. Increased plasma HDL and HDL-2 subfraction concentrations, reduced LDL cholesterol concentration, increased triglycerides levels.
5. Impaired glucose tolerance.
6. Reduced response to the metapyrone test.
7. Reduced serum folate concentration.

E. Carcinogenesis, Mutagenesis, Impairment of Fertility

Long-term continuous administration of natural and synthetic estrogens in certain animal species increases the frequency of carcinomas of the breast, uterus, cervix, vagina, testis, and liver (see CONTRAINDICATIONS and WARNINGS).

F. Pregnancy Category X

Estrogens should not be used during pregnancy (see CONTRAINDICATIONS and Boxed Warnings).

G. Nursing Mothers

As a general principle, the administration of any drug to nursing mothers should be done only when clearly necessary since many drugs are excreted in human milk. In addition, estrogen administration to nursing mothers has been shown to decrease the quantity and quality of the milk.

ADVERSE REACTIONS

Alora has been studied in two well-controlled clinical trials. One study compared twice weekly dosing of **Alora** at 0.05 mg/day and 0.1 mg/day to once daily dosing of 0.625 mg and 1.25 mg of orally administered conjugated equine estrogens (CEE) in the intent-to-treat population of 321 postmenopausal women. In addition, the same **Alora** doses were studied in a placebo-controlled study in an intent-to-treat population of 273 postmenopausal women. Incidence of adverse experiences > 5% of each treatment group is given below in Table 5.

Table 5
Incidence of Adverse Events > 5% in
a Placebo-Controlled Study of **Alora** Data are
Expressed as % of Treatment Group

Adverse Event	Alora 0.05 mg/day N = 88	Alora 0.1 mg/day N = 94	Placebo N = 91
Infection	17.0	18.1	16.5
Headache	12.5	21.3	23.1
Sinusitis	6.8	10.6	6.6
Pain	6.8	5.3	5.5
Arthralgia	6.8	1.1	4.4
Abdominal Pain	5.7	3.2	3.3
Vaginal Discharge	4.5	5.3	0.0
Breast Pain	4.5	5.3	0.0
Nausea	4.5	4.3	11.0
Vagina Bleeding	3.4	20.2	4.4
Back Pain	3.4	7.4	3.3
Vaginitis	3.4	3.2	9.9
Accidental Injury	2.3	6.4	4.4
Flatulence	2.3	5.3	1.1
Fibrocystic Breast	1.1	5.3	1.1
Pelvic Pain	0.0	5.3	2.2

Continued on next page

Alora—Cont.

Vaginal Bleeding

Overall in these two studies, 232 of the 594 patients enrolled possessed a partially or fully intact uterus. Fifty five (24%) of these women experienced at least one instance of vaginal bleeding during treatment. Of those patients receiving placebo, 12.9% of patients experienced at least one vaginal bleeding episode. The incidence of vaginal bleeding among estrogen treated patients increased with increasing dose of all estrogen treatments: 8.7% of those receiving **Alora** 0.05 mg/day, 20.0% of those receiving CEE 0.625 mg/day, 33.3% of those receiving CEE 1.25 mg/day, and 33.3% of those receiving **Alora** 0.1 mg/day.

Skin Irritation

In the total population of 594 postmenopausal women exposed to either placebo and/or **Alora** systems in these studies, a total of 46 (7.7%) patients reported cases of skin reaction at the site of transdermal system application. The majority of these cases were mild and resolved spontaneously. Overall, therapy was discontinued by 13 (2.2%) patients due to system application site reaction, 8 (2.3%) of those receiving both placebo and **Alora** and 5 (2.0%) of those receiving only placebo systems.

The following additional adverse reactions have been reported with estrogen therapy (see WARNINGS regarding induction of neoplasia, adverse effects on the fetus, increased incidence of gallbladder disease, cardiovascular disease, elevated blood pressure, and hypercalcemia).

1. Genitourinary System. Changes in vaginal bleeding pattern and abnormal withdrawal bleeding or flow; breakthrough bleeding, spotting. Increase in size of uterine leiomyomata; vaginal candidiasis; change in amount of cervical secretion.
2. Breasts. Tenderness, enlargement.
3. Gastrointestinal. Nausea, vomiting, abdominal cramps, bloating; cholestatic jaundice; increased incidence of gallbladder disease.
4. Skin. Chloasma or melasma that may persist when the drug is discontinued, erythema multiforme, erythema nodosum, hemorrhagic eruption, loss of scalp hair, hirsutism.
5. Eyes. Steepening of corneal curvature; intolerance to contact lenses.
6. Central Nervous System. Headache, migraine, dizziness, mental depression, chorea.
7. Miscellaneous. Increase or decrease in weight, reduced carbohydrate tolerance, aggravation of porphyria, edema, changes in libido.

OVERDOSAGE

Serious ill effects have not been reported following acute ingestion of large doses of estrogen containing oral contraceptives by young children. Overdosage of estrogen may cause nausea and vomiting, and withdrawal bleeding may occur in females.

DOSAGE AND ADMINISTRATION

Alora should be administered twice weekly, as instructed. The adhesive side of the **Alora** system should be placed on a clean, dry area of skin. The recommended application site is the lower abdomen. In addition, the upper quadrant of the buttocks or outer aspect of the hip may be used. ***Alora should not be applied to the breasts.*** The sites of application should be rotated, with an interval of at least 1 week allowed between applications to a particular site. The area selected should not be oily, damaged, or irritated. The waistline should be avoided, since tight clothing may rub the system off. The system should be applied immediately after opening the pouch and removing the protective liner. The system should be pressed firmly in place with the palm of the hand for about 10 seconds, making sure there is good contact, especially around the edges.

In the event that a system should fall off, the same system may be reapplied. If necessary, a new system may be applied. In either case, the original treatment schedule should be maintained.

Initiation of Therapy

Three **Alora** strengths having nominal estradiol *in vivo* delivery rates of 0.05 mg/day, 0.075 mg/day, and 0.1 mg/day (differentiated by the physical size of **Alora**) are available for treatment of moderate-to-severe vasomotor symptoms, vulval and vaginal atrophy associated with the menopause, hypogonadism, castration, or primary ovarian failure. Treatment is usually initiated with **Alora** 0.05 mg/day applied to the skin twice weekly. The dose should be adjusted as necessary and the lowest dose required to control symptoms should be used. Attempts to discontinue or taper medication should be made at 3-month to 6-month intervals.

In women who are not currently taking oral estrogens or in women switching from topical therapy or another transdermal estradiol therapy, treatment with **Alora** can be initiated at once. In women who are currently taking oral estrogens, treatment with **Alora** should be initiated 1 week after withdrawal of oral therapy or sooner if menopausal symptoms reappear in less than 1 week.

Therapeutic Regimen

Alora may be administered in a continuous regimen in patients who do not possess an intact uterus. In those patients with an intact uterus who are not using concomitant progestin therapy, **Alora** can be administered on a cyclic schedule (e.g. 3 weeks of therapy followed by 1 week without).

HOW SUPPLIED

Alora 0.05 mg/day (estradiol transdermal system). Each 18 cm^2 system contains 1.5 mg of estradiol USP for nominal delivery of 0.05 mg of estradiol per day when dosed in a twice weekly regimen.

NDC 0149-0491-01 Patient Calendar Pack of 8 Systems
NDC 0149-0491-03 Patient Calendar Pack of 24 Systems

Alora 0.075 mg/day (estradiol transdermal system). Each 27 cm^2 system contains 2.3 mg of estradiol USP for nominal delivery of 0.075 mg of estradiol per day when dosed in a twice weekly regimen.

NDC 0149-0492-01 Patient Calendar Pack of 8 Systems
NDC 0149-0492-03 Patient Calendar Pack of 24 Systems

Alora 0.1 mg/day (estradiol transdermal system). Each 36 cm^2 system contains 3.0 mg of estradiol USP for nominal delivery of 0.1 mg of estradiol per day when dosed in a twice weekly regimen.

NDC 0149-0493-01 Patient Calendar Pack of 8 Systems
NDC 0149-0493-03 Patient Calendar Pack of 24 Systems

Store at 15°–30°C (59°–86°F).

Do not store unpouched. Apply immediately upon removal from the protective pouch.

Discard used **Alora** in household trash in a manner that prevents accidental application or ingestion by children, pets, or others.

CAUTION: Federal law prohibits dispensing without prescription.

Developed and Manufactured by: **Thera Tech Inc.**, Salt Lake City, Utah 84108

For **Procter & Gamble Pharmaceuticals**, Cincinnati, Ohio 45202

Date: December 20, 1996

1. Registered trademark of Ciba-Geigy

PATIENT PACKAGE INSERT

Getting the Best Results with Alora—This Booklet Can Help

This booklet describes the correct way to apply and use the **Alora** patch—the key to getting the best results with **Alora**. It also talks about the risks and side effects of estrogen use. If you want to know more after you read it, ask your doctor, pharmacist, or other health care professional.

How to Use the Alora Patch

Alora is a thin, clear, plastic patch that sticks to the skin. Each patch is sealed in a pouch, which protects it until you're ready to put it on (figure 1). Don't open a pouch or remove a patch until just before you apply it.

What You Need to Do

1. Put on a new patch twice a week. Use one of the schedules on the inside flap of the Alora box (figure 2).

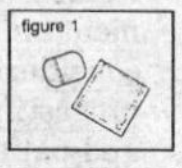
figure 1

For instance, if you apply your firstpatch on Sunday, take that patch off on Wednesday and put on a new one.

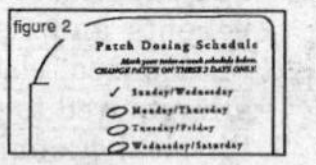

figure 2

Stick with this schedule as long as you use **Alora**. To help remind you, mark the schedule on the inside flap of the **Alora** box. Put a check next to the first day you apply the patch.

2. When you first start using Alora, apply the patch to the lower abdomen (below the panty line) (figure 3). As you gain more experience applying **Alora**, you may want to try the hips or buttocks to see which area works best for you. Do not apply Alora to your breasts or any other parts of the body.

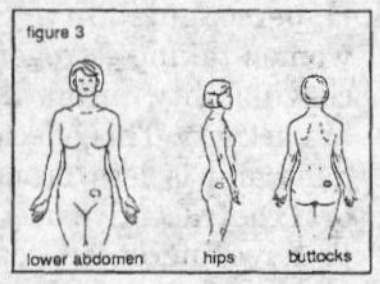

figure 3

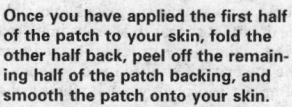

To help the patch stay in place:

- Try not to disturb the patch while putting on and removing clothes. It may help to place the patch where your underwear will cover it at all times.
- Try to avoid rubbing the patch while changing clothes, washing or drying off.
- Try different sites to see what works well with your body and your clothing.

When you change your patch, don't put the new one in the same place. For instance, if you had **Alora** on one side of the abdomen, put the new patch on the other side. Wait at least one week before you reuse any spot to help reduce the chance of skin redness or irritation.

3. Apply the patch with care—here's how.

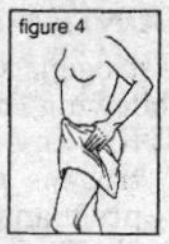
figure 4

- **Choose a spot for the patch and make sure the skin is clean. For best results the skin should be:**
  - **freshly washed;**
  - **free of body powder or lotion;**
  - **dry (figure 4) and cool (wait a few minutes after taking a hot shower);**
  - **free of cuts, rashes, or any other skin problem.**
- **Open the pouch by tearing along one of the outer edges (figure 5). Don't cut the pouch with scissors, which might damage the patch inside.**

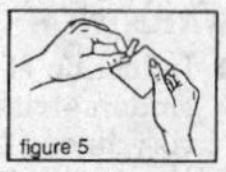
figure 5

- **Pull the patch out.**
- **Peel off one half of the backing which covers the sticky surface of the patch (figure 6).**

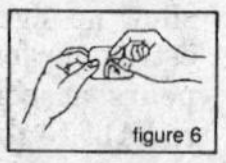
figure 6

Without touching the sticky surface, press that half of the patch onto yourskin (figure 7). (If you touch the sticky surface, the patch may not stay on as well.)

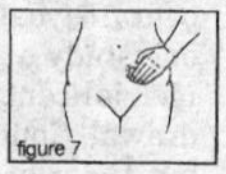
figure 7

- **Once you have applied the first half of the patch to your skin, fold the other half back, peel off the remaining half of the patch backing, and smooth the patch onto your skin.**

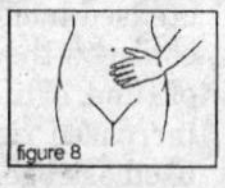
figure 8

- Press the entire patch firmly onto the skin with the palm of your hand for about 10 seconds (figure 8). Be sure all of the patch is touching your skin, even around the edges.
- Take off the old patch. Fold it in half and throw it away out of the reach of children and pets.

The skin under the old patch may look pink, but the color should fade away soon. In some cases, the skin may itch or look red; this may last from a couple of hours to a couple of days. Most of the time the problem is minor. But if it bothers you a lot or lasts longer than a few days, call your doctor.

Questions You May Have

Q. Should I take the patch off when I swim or bathe?

A. No. Wear each patch all the time until you put on a new one. Baths, showers, or swimming should not affect the **Alora** patch as long as you don't rub the patch as you wash. Avoid soaking in a hot tub for a long time, though, which can make the patch come off.

Wearing the patch while spending time in the sun should be no problem. Just be sure you put the patch on a spot your clothing or bathing suit covers.

Q. What should I do if the patch comes off?

A. Most women find that the **Alora** patch seldom comes off. But if it does, try putting the same patch back on the same spot. If it sticks firmly all over, leave it on. If not, take it off and put a new patch on a new spot. No matter what day this happens, stick to your twice-a-week schedule for the next patch.

Q. What should I do if I forget to change the patch on the day it's due?

A. Remove the old patch and apply a new one to a new spot as soon as you remember. No matter what day this happens, stick to your twice-a-week schedule for the next patch.

Q. How long should I keep using **Alora**?

A. The answer will be different for each woman. Talk to your doctor every 6 months about how you are feeling and whether you still need estrogen.

For Best Results, Stick with Your Patch Program

- **Replace your patch twice each week, on the two days you have chosen.** Until it becomes a habit, try:
  - Marking your schedule on the inside flap of the **Alora** carton;
  - Marking the days on your calendar;
  - Linking the days you change your patch to other things that always happen on those days (e.g., an exercise class, meetings, etc.)

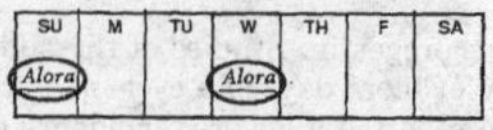

- **Handle each patch with care.**
  - Make sure the skin is clean, dry, and free of lotion and powder.
  - Try to avoid touching the sticky surface when applying the patch.
  - Avoid rubbing the patch while changing clothes, washing or drying off.

- **Keep working with your doctor, pharmacist, or other health care professional.** Ask questions. If you have concerns, talk them over- don't just stop using the patch on your own.
- **Get your refills of the Alora patch before your supply runs out.** For best results, replace your **Alora** patches on schedule.

If you would like more information on the **Alora** patch, please call toll free **1-888-ALORA-4-U** (1-888-256-7248).

INFORMATION FOR THE PATIENT

INTRODUCTION

This leaflet describes when and how to use estrogens, and the risks and benefits of estrogen treatment. Your doctor has prescribed the **Alora** estradiol transdermal system for the treatment of your menopausal symptoms. Estradiol is the same hormone that your ovaries produce abundantly before menopause. During menopause, production of estrogen hormones by your body decreases well below the amounts normally produced during your fertile years. In many women this decrease in estrogen production causes uncomfortable symptoms, most noticeably hot flashes and sleep disturbances. Estrogens can be given to reduce or eliminate these symptoms.

Estrogens have important benefits but also some risks. You must decide, with your doctor, whether the benefits of estrogen use outweigh the risks. If you use estrogens, check with your doctor to be sure you are using the lowest possible dose that works and that you don't use them longer than necessary. How long you need to use estrogens will depend on the reason for use.

1. ESTROGENS INCREASE THE RISK OF CANCER OF THE UTERUS IN WOMEN WHO HAVE HAD THEIR MENOPAUSE ("CHANGE OF LIFE")
If you use any estrogen-containing drug, it is important to visit your doctor regularly and report any unusual vaginal bleeding right away. Vaginal bleeding after menopause may be a warning sign of uterine cancer. Your doctor should evaluate any unusual vaginal bleeding to find out the cause.
2. ESTROGENS SHOULD NOT BE USED DURING PREGNANCY
Estrogens do not prevent miscarriage (spontaneous abortion) and are not needed in the days following childbirth. If you take estrogens during pregnancy, your unborn child has a greater than usual chance of having birth defects. The risk of developing these defects is small, but clearly larger than the risk in children whose mothers did not take estrogens during pregnancy. These birth defects may affect the baby's urinary system and sex organs. Daughters born to mothers who took DES (an estrogen drug) have a higher than usual chance of developing cancer of the vagina or cervix when they become teenagers or young adults. Sons may have a higher than usual chance of developing cancer of the testicles when they become teenagers or young adults.

INFORMATION ABOUT ALORA

How Alora Works

The **Alora** estradiol transdermal system that your doctor has prescribed for you, releases small amounts of estradiol through the skin and into the blood stream in a continuous way. The dose of estradiol you require will depend upon your individual response. The dose is adjusted by the size of the **Alora** estradiol transdermal system. **Alora** is available in three sizes.

Benefits of Treatment with Alora

Regular twice weekly use of **Alora** offers relief from moderate-to-severe symptoms of menopause, hot flashes and vaginal dryness. Small quantities of the naturally occurring hormone estradiol are absorbed through the skin from the **Alora** estradiol transdermal system, ensuring a continuous supply of circulating hormone in the body.

When estradiol is administered through the skin, the hormone does not undergo the rapid chemical changes in the liver and stomach that would occur if you were taking it in tablet or capsule form by mouth.

USES OF ESTROGEN

(Not every estrogen drug is approved for every use listed in this section. If you want to know which of these possible uses are approved for the medicine prescribed for you, ask your doctor or pharmacist to show you the professional labeling. You can also look up the specific estrogen product in a book called the "Physician's Desk Reference", which is available in many book stores and public libraries. Generic drugs carry virtually the same labeling information as their brand name versions.)

- **To reduce moderate or severe menopausal symptoms.**
Estrogens are hormones made by the ovaries of women. Between ages 45 and 55, the ovaries normally stop making estrogens. This drop in body estrogen levels causes the "change of life" or menopause (the end of monthly menstrual periods). Sometimes, both ovaries are removed during an operation before natural menopause takes place and the sudden drop in estrogen levels causes "surgical menopause."
When estrogen levels begin dropping, some women develop very uncomfortable symptoms, such as feelings of warmth in the face, neck, and chest, or sudden intense episodes of heat and sweating ("hot flashes" or "hot flushes"). Using estrogen drugs can help the body adjust to lower estrogen levels and reduce these symptoms. Some women have only mild menopausal symptoms, or none at all, and do not need estrogen therapy for these symptoms. Other women may need estrogens for a few months while their bodies adjust to lower estrogen levels. For the treatment of menopausal symptoms, the majority of women need estrogen replacement therapy for no longer than 6 months. Since every woman is different, you and your doctor should periodically reevaluate your need for continued estrogen use.
- **To treat vulval and vaginal atrophy** (itching, burning, dryness in or around the vagina, difficulty or burning on urination) associated with menopause.
- **To treat certain conditions in which a young woman's ovaries do not produce enough estrogen naturally.**
- **To treat certain types of abnormal vaginal bleeding due to hormonal imbalance when your doctor has found no serious cause of the bleeding.**
- **To treat certain cancers in special situations, in men and women.**
- **To prevent thinning of bones.**
Osteoporosis is a thinning of the bones that makes them weaker and allows them to break more easily. The bones of the spine, wrists, and hips break most often in osteoporosis. Both men and women start to lose bone mass after about age 40, but women lose bone mass faster after menopause. Using estrogens after menopause slows down bone thinning and may prevent bones from breaking. Lifelong adequate calcium intake, either in the diet (such as dairy products) or by calcium supplements (to reach a total daily intake of 1000 milligrams before menopause or 1500 milligrams after menopause) may help to prevent osteoporosis. Regular weight-bearing exercise (like walking or running for an hour, two or three times a week) may also help to prevent osteoporosis. Before you change your calcium intake or exercise habits, it is important to discuss these lifestyle changes with your doctor to find out if they are safe for you.
Since estrogen use has some risks, only women who are likely to develop osteoporosis should use estrogens to prevent this condition. Women who are likely to develop osteoporosis often have the following characteristics: white or Asian race, slim, cigarette smokers, and a family history of osteoporosis in a mother, sister, or aunt. Women who have relatively early menopause, often because their ovaries were surgically removed, are more likely to develop osteoporosis than women whose menopause happens at the average age (about 45 to 55 years).

WHO SHOULD NOT USE ESTROGENS

Estrogens should not be used:

- **During pregnancy (see Boxed Warning).**
If you think you may be pregnant, do not use any form of estrogen-containing drug. Using estrogens while you are pregnant may cause your unborn child to have birth defects. Estrogens do not prevent miscarriage.
- **If you have unusual vaginal bleeding which has not been evaluated by your doctor (see Boxed Warning).**
Unusual vaginal bleeding can be a warning sign of cancer of the uterus, especially if it happens after menopause. Your doctor must find out the cause of the bleeding so that he or she can recommend the proper treatment. Taking estrogens without visiting your doctor can cause you serious harm if your vaginal bleeding is caused by cancer of the uterus.
- **If you have had cancer.**
Since estrogens increase the risk of certain types of cancer, you should not use estrogens if you have ever had cancer of the breast or uterus, unless your doctor recommends that the drug may help in the cancer treatment. (For certain patients with breast or prostate cancer, estrogens may help.)
- **If you have any circulation problems.**
Estrogen therapy should not be used except in unusually special situations and only after consultation with your doctor and only in recommended doses. Patients with a tendency for abnormal blood clotting should avoid estrogen use (see DANGERS OF ESTROGENS, below).
- **When they do not work.**
During menopause, some women develop nervous symptoms or depression. Estrogens do not relieve these symptoms. You may have heard that taking estrogens for years after menopause will keep your skin soft and supple and keep you feeling young. There is no evidence for these claims and such long-term estrogen use may have serious risks.
- **After childbirth or when breast-feeding a baby.**
Estrogens should not be used to try to stop the breasts from filling with milk after a baby is born. Such treatment may increase the risk of developing blood clots (see DANGERS OF ESTROGENS, below).
If you are breast-feeding, you should avoid using any drugs because many drugs pass through to the baby in the milk. While nursing a baby, you should take drugs only on the advice of your health care provider.

DANGERS OF ESTROGENS

- **Cancer of the uterus.**
The risk of developing cancer of the uterus gets higher the longer estrogens are used and when larger doses are taken. One study showed that when estrogens are discontinued, this increased risk of cancer seems to fall off quickly. Three other studies showed that the risk for uterine cancer stayed high for 8 to more than 15 years after stopping estrogen treatment. Because of this risk, **IT IS IMPORTANT TO TAKE THE LOWEST DOSE THAT WORKS AND TO TAKE IT ONLY AS LONG AS YOU NEED IT.**
Using progestin therapy together with estrogen therapy may reduce the higher risk of uterine cancer related to estrogen use (see OTHER INFORMATION, below.)
If you have had your uterus removed (total hysterectomy), there is no danger of developing cancer of the uterus.
- **Cancer of the breast.**
Most studies have shown no association between the usual doses used for estrogen replacement therapy and breast cancer. However, some studies have reported that breast cancer developed more often (up to twice the usual rate) in women who used estrogens for long periods of time (especially longer than 10 years), or who used higher doses for shorter periods of time.
Regular breast examinations by a health professional and monthly self-examination are recommended for women receiving estrogen therapy, as they are for all women.
- **Gallbladder disease.**
Women who use estrogens after menopause are more likely to develop gallbladder disease needing surgery than women who do not use estrogens.
- **Abnormal blood clotting.**
Taking estrogens may increase the risk of blood clots. These changes allow the blood to clot more easily, possibly allowing clots to form in your bloodstream. If blood clots do form in your bloodstream, they can cut off the blood supply to vital organs, causing serious problems. These clots can cause a stroke (by cutting off blood to the brain), heart attack (by cutting off blood to the heart), a pulmonary embolus (by cutting off blood to the lungs), or other problems. Any of these conditions may be fatal or cause serious long-term disability. However, most studies of low-dose estrogen usage by women do not show an increased risk of these complications.

SIDE EFFECTS

In addition to the risks listed above, the following side effects have been reported with estrogen use:

- Nausea and vomiting.
- Breast tenderness or enlargement.
- Enlargement of benign tumors ("fibroids") of the uterus.
- Retention of excess fluid. This may make some conditions worsen, such as asthma, epilepsy, migraine, heart disease, or kidney disease.
- A spotty darkening of the skin, particularly on the face.
- Skin irritation, redness, or rash may occur at the site of application.

REDUCING RISK OF ESTROGEN USE

If you use estrogens, you can reduce your risks by doing these things:

- **See your doctor regularly.**
While you are using estrogens, it is important to visit your doctor at least once a year for a check-up. If you develop vaginal bleeding while taking estrogens, you may need further evaluation. If members of your family have had breast cancer or if you have ever had breast lumps or an abnormal mammogram (breast x-ray), you may need to have more frequent breast examinations.
- **Reassess your need for estrogens.**
You and your doctor should reevaluate whether or not you still need estrogens at least every six months.
- **Be alert for signs of trouble.**
If any of these warning signals (or any other unusual symptoms) happen while you are using estrogens, call your doctor immediately:
  - Abnormal bleeding from the vagina (possible uterine cancer).
  - Pains in the calves or chest, sudden shortness of breath, or coughing blood (possible clots in the legs, heart or lungs).
  - Severe headache or vomiting, dizziness, faintness, changes in vision or speech, weakness or numbness of an arm or leg (possible clot in the brain or eye).

Continued on next page

Alora—Cont.

- Breast lumps (possible breast cancer; ask your doctor or health professional to show you how to examine your breasts monthly).
- Yellowing of the skin or eyes (possible liver problem).
- Pain, swelling or tenderness in the abdomen (possible gallbladder problem).

OTHER INFORMATION

1. Estrogens increase the risk of developing a condition (endometrial hyperplasia) that may lead to cancer of the lining of the uterus. If your uterus has not been removed, your doctor may choose to prescribe a progestin, a different hormone drug to be used in association with estrogen treatment. Progestin lowers the risk of developing endometrial hyperplasia, a possible precancerous condition of the uterine lining, which may occur while using estrogen. There may be additional risks associated with the use of progestin together with estrogen treatment. The possible risks include:
   - unfavorable effects on blood fats (especially the lowering of HDL blood cholesterol, the "good" cholesterol which protects against heart disease);
   - unhealthy effects on blood sugar (which might make a diabetic condition worse); and
   - a possible further increase in breast cancer risk which may be associated with long-term estrogen use.

   Some research has suggested that estrogen taken without progestin may protect women against developing heart disease. However, this effect of estrogen is not certain because the estrogen-treated women had characteristics known to protect against heart disease; they were slimmer, more physically active, and less likely to have diabetes.

   You are cautioned to discuss very carefully with your doctor or healthcare provider all the possible risks and benefits of long-term estrogen and progestin treatment, as they affect you personally.
2. Your doctor has prescribed this drug for you and you alone. Do not give the drug to anyone else.
3. If you will be taking calcium supplements as part of the treatment to help prevent osteoporosis, check with your doctor about how much to take.
4. Keep this and all drugs out of the reach of children. In case of overdose, remove the system and call your doctor, hospital, or poison control center immediately. Dispose of used **Alora** estradiol transdermal systems in a manner that prevents accidental application or ingestion by children, pets, or others.

This leaflet provides a summary of the most important information about estrogens. If you want more information, ask your doctor or pharmacist to show you the professional labeling.

HOW SUPPLIED

Alora estradiol transdermal system 0.05 mg/day
Patient Calendar Pack of 8 Systems (**NDC** 0149-0491-01)
Patient Calendar Pack of 24 Systems (**NDC** 0149-0491-03)
Alora estradiol transdermal system 0.075 mg/day
Patient Calendar Pack of 8 Systems (**NDC** 0149-0492-01)
Patient Calendar Pack of 24 Systems (**NDC** 0149-0492-03)
Alora estradiol transdermal system 0.1 mg/day
Patient Calendar Pack of 8 Systems (**NDC** 0149-0493-01)
Patient Calendar Pack of 24 Systems (**NDC** 0149-0493-03)
Store at 15°- 30°C (59°- 86°F).
Do not store unpouched.
Apply immediately upon removal from the protective pouch.
Manufactured by: **TheraTech, Inc.**, Salt Lake City, Utah 84108
For: **Procter & Gamble Pharmaceuticals**, Cincinnati, Ohio 45202
Date: December 20, 1996 200178-01

Shown in Product Identification Guide, page 332

ASACOL® ℞

[*āce 'ah-kol*]
(mesalamine)
Delayed-Release Tablets

DESCRIPTION

Each **Asacol** delayed-release tablet for oral administration contains 400 mg of mesalamine, an anti-inflammatory drug. The **Asacol** delayed-release tablets are coated with acrylic based resin, Eudragit S (methacrylic acid copolymer B, NF), which dissolves at pH 7 or greater, releasing mesalamine in the terminal ileum and beyond for topical anti-inflammatory action in the colon. Mesalamine has the chemical name 5-amino-2-hydroxybenzoic acid; its structural formula is:
[See chemical structure at top of next column]

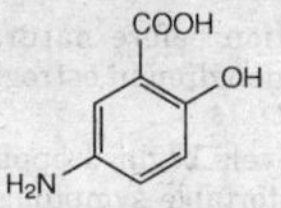

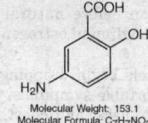

Molecular Weight: 153.1
Molecular Formula: $C_7H_7NO_3$

Inactive Ingredients: Each tablet contains colloidal silicon dioxide, dibutyl phthalate, edible black ink, iron oxide red, iron oxide yellow, lactose, magnesium stearate, methacrylic acid copolymer B (Eudragit S), polyethylene glycol, povidone, sodium starch glycolate, and talc.

CLINICAL PHARMACOLOGY

Mesalamine is thought to be the major therapeutically active part of the sulfasalazine molecule in the treatment of ulcerative colitis. Sulfasalazine is converted to equimolar amounts of sulfapyridine and mesalamine by bacterial action in the colon. The usual oral dose of sulfasalazine for active ulcerative colitis is 3 to 4 grams daily in divided doses, which provides 1.2 to 1.6 grams of mesalamine to the colon.
The mechanism of action of mesalamine (and sulfasalazine) is unknown, but appears to be topical rather than systemic. Mucosal production of arachidonic acid (AA) metabolites, both through the cyclooxygenase pathways, i.e., prostanoids, and through the lipoxygenase pathways, i.e., leukotrienes (LTs) and hydroxyeicosatetraenoic acids (HETEs), is increased in patients with chronic inflammatory bowel disease, and it is possible that mesalamine diminishes inflammation by blocking cyclooxygenase and inhibiting prostaglandin (PG) production in the colon.
Pharmacokinetics: **Asacol** tablets are coated with an acrylic-based resin that delays release of mesalamine until it reaches the terminal ileum and beyond. This has been demonstrated in human studies conducted with radiological and serum markers. Approximately 28% of the mesalamine in **Asacol** tablets is absorbed after oral ingestion, leaving the remainder available for topical action and excretion in the feces. Absorption of mesalamine is similar in fasted and fed subjects. The absorbed mesalamine is rapidly acetylated in the gut mucosal wall and by the liver. It is excreted mainly by the kidney as N-acetyl-5-aminosalicylic acid.
Mesalamine from orally administered **Asacol** tablets appears to be more extensively absorbed than the mesalamine released from sulfasalazine. Maximum plasma levels of mesalamine and N-acetyl-5-aminosalicylic acid following multiple **Asacol** doses are about 1.5 to 2 times higher than those following an equivalent dose of mesalamine in the form of sulfasalazine. Combined mesalamine and N-acetyl-5-aminosalicylic acid AUC's and urine drug dose recoveries following multiple doses of **Asacol** tablets are about 1.3 to 1.5 times higher than those following an equivalent dose of mesalamine in the form of sulfasalazine.
The t_{max} for mesalamine and its metabolite, N-acetyl-5-aminosalicylic acid, is usually delayed, reflecting the delayed release, and ranges from 4 to 12 hours. The half-lives of elimination ($t1/2_{elm}$) for mesalamine and N-acetyl-5-aminosalicylic acid are usually about 12 hours, but are variable, ranging from 2 to 15 hours. There is a large intersubject variability in the plasma concentrations of mesalamine and N-acetyl-5-aminosalicylic acid and in their elimination half-lives following administration of **Asacol** tablets.

Clinical Studies:

Mildly to moderately active ulcerative colitis: Two placebo-controlled studies have demonstrated the efficacy of **Asacol** tablets in patients with mildly to moderately active ulcerative colitis. In one randomized, double-blind, multi-center trial of 158 patients, **Asacol** doses of 1.6 g/day and 2.4 g/day were compared to placebo. At the dose of 2.4 g/day, **Asacol** tablets reduced the disease activity, with 21 of 43 (49%) **Asacol** patients showing improvement in sigmoidoscopic appearance of the bowel compared to 12 of 44 (27%) placebo patients (p = 0.048). In addition, significantly more patients in the **Asacol** 2.4 g/day group showed improvement in rectal bleeding and stool frequency. The 1.6 g/day dose did not produce consistent evidence of effectiveness.
In a second randomized, double-blind, placebo-controlled clinical trial of 6 weeks duration in 87 ulcerative colitis patients, **Asacol** tablets, at a dose of 4.8 g/day, gave sigmoidoscopic improvement in 28 of 38 (74%) patients compared to 10 of 38 (26%) placebo patients ($p < 0.001$). Also, more patients in the **Asacol** 4.8 g/day group showed improvement in overall symptoms.
Maintenance of remission of ulcerative colitis: A 6-month, randomized, double-blind, placebo-controlled, multi-center study involved 264 patients treated with **Asacol** 0.8 g/day (n = 90), 1.6 g/day (n = 87), or placebo (n = 87). The proportion of patients treated with 0.8 g/day who maintained endoscopic remission was not statistically significant compared to placebo. In the intention to treat (ITT) analysis of all 174 patients treated with **Asacol** 1.6 g/day or placebo, **Asacol** maintained endoscopic remission of ulcerative colitis in 61 of 87 (70.1%) of patients, compared to 42 of 87 (48.3%) of placebo recipients (p = 0.005).
A pooled efficacy analysis of 4 maintenance trials compared **Asacol**, at doses of 0.8 g/day to 2.8 g/day, with sulfasalazine, at doses of 2 g/day to 4 g/day (n = 200). Treatment success was 59 of 98 (59%) for **Asacol** and 70 of 102 (69%) for sulfasalazine, a non-significant difference.
Study to assess the effect on male fertility: The effect of **Asacol** (mesalamine) on sulfasalazine-induced impairment of male fertility was examined in an open-label study. Nine patients (age < 40 years) with chronic ulcerative colitis in clinical remission on sulfasalazine 2 g/day to 3 g/day were crossed over to an equivalent **Asacol** dose (0.8 g/day to 1.2 g/day) for 3 months. Improvement in sperm count ($p < 0.02$) and morphology ($p < 0.02$) occurred in all cases. Improvement in sperm motility ($p < 0.001$) occurred in 8 of the 9 patients.

INDICATIONS AND USAGE

Asacol tablets are indicated for the treatment of mildly to moderately active ulcerative colitis and for the maintenance of remission of ulcerative colitis.

CONTRAINDICATIONS

Asacol tablets are contraindicated in patients with hypersensitivity to salicylates or to any of the components of the **Asacol** tablet.

PRECAUTIONS

General: Patients with pyloric stenosis may have prolonged gastric retention of **Asacol** tablets which could delay release of mesalamine in the colon.
Exacerbation of the symptoms of colitis has been reported in 3% of **Asacol**-treated patients in controlled clinical trials. This acute reaction, characterized by cramping, abdominal pain, bloody diarrhea, and occasionally by fever, headache, malaise, pruritus, rash, and conjunctivitis, has been reported after the initiation of **Asacol** tablets as well as other mesalamine products. Symptoms usually abate when **Asacol** tablets are discontinued.
Some patients who have experienced a hypersensitivity reaction to sulfasalazine may have a similar reaction to **Asacol** tablets or to other compounds which contain or are converted to mesalamine.
Renal: Renal impairment, including minimal change nephropathy, and acute and chronic interstitial nephritis, has been reported in patients taking **Asacol** tablets as well as other compounds which contain or are converted to mesalamine. In animal studies (rats, dogs), the kidney is the principal target organ for toxicity. At doses of approximately 750 mg/kg to 1000 mg/kg [15 to 20 times the administered recommended human dose (based on a 50 kg person) on a mg/kg basis and 3 to 4 times on a mg/m^2 basis], mesalamine causes renal papillary necrosis. **Therefore, caution should be exercised when using Asacol (or other compounds which contain or are converted to mesalamine or its metabolites) in patients with known renal dysfunction or history of renal disease. It is recommended that all patients have an evaluation of renal function prior to initiation of Asacol tablets and periodically while on Asacol therapy.**
Information for Patients: Patients should be instructed to swallow the **Asacol** tablets whole, taking care not to break the outer coating. The outer coating is designed to remain intact to protect the active ingredient and thus ensure mesalamine availability for action in the colon. In 2% to 3% of patients in clinical studies, intact or partially intact tablets have been reported in the stool. If this occurs repeatedly, patients should contact their physician.
Patients with ulcerative colitis should be made aware that ulcerative colitis rarely remits completely, and that the risk of relapse can be substantially reduced by continued administration of **Asacol** at a maintenance dosage.
Drug Interactions: There are no known drug interactions.
Carcinogenesis, Mutagenesis, Impairment of Fertility: Dietary mesalamine was not carcinogenic in rats at doses as high as 480 mg/kg/day, or in mice at 2000 mg/kg/day. These doses are 2.4 and 5.1 times the maximum recommended human maintenance dose of **Asacol** of 1.6 g/day (32 mg/kg/day if 50 kg body weight assumed or 1184 mg/m^2), respectively, based on body surface area. Mesalamine was negative in the Ames assay for mutagenesis, negative for induction of sister chromatid exchanges (SCE) and chromosomal aberrations in Chinese hamster ovary cells *in vitro*, and negative for induction of micronuclei (MN) in mouse bone marrow polychromatic erythrocytes. Mesalamine, at oral doses up to 480 mg/kg/day, had no adverse effect on fertility or reproductive performance of male and female rats.
Pregnancy: Teratogenic Effects: Pregnancy Category B: Reproduction studies in rats and rabbits at oral doses up to 480 mg/kg/day have revealed no evidence of teratogenic effects or fetal toxicity due to mesalamine. There are, however, no adequate and well-controlled studies in pregnant women. Because animal reproduction studies are not always predictive of human response, this drug should be used during pregnancy only if clearly needed.
Nursing Mothers: Low concentrations of mesalamine and higher concentrations of its N-acetyl metabolite have been detected in human breast milk. While the clinical significance of this has not been determined, caution should be exercised when mesalamine is administered to a nursing woman.

Pediatric Use: Safety and effectiveness of **Asacol** tablets in pediatric patients have not been established.

ADVERSE REACTIONS

Asacol tablets have been evaluated in 3685 inflammatory bowel disease patients (most patients with ulcerative colitis) in controlled and open-label studies. Adverse events seen in clinical trials with **Asacol** tablets have generally been mild and reversible. Adverse events presented in the following sections may occur regardless of length of therapy and similar events have been reported in short- and long-term studies and in the post-marketing setting.

In two short-term (6 weeks) placebo-controlled clinical studies involving 245 patients, 155 of whom were randomized to **Asacol** tablets, five (3.2%) of the **Asacol** patients discontinued **Asacol** therapy because of adverse events as compared to two (2.2%) of the placebo patients. Adverse reactions leading to withdrawal from **Asacol** tablets included (each in one patient): diarrhea and colitis flare; dizziness, nausea, joint pain, and headache; rash, lethargy and constipation; dry mouth, malaise, lower back discomfort, mild disorientation, mild indigestion and cramping; headache, nausea, malaise, aching, vomiting, muscle cramps, a stuffy head, plugged ears, and fever.

Adverse events occurring in **Asacol**-treated patients at a frequency of 2% or greater in the two short-term, double-blind, placebo-controlled trials mentioned above are listed in Table 1 below. Overall, the incidence of adverse events seen with **Asacol** tablets was similar to placebo.

Table 1
Frequency (%) of Common Adverse Events Reported in Ulcerative Colitis Patients Treated with **Asacol** Tablets or Placebo in Short-Term (6-Week) Double-Blind Controlled Studies

Event	Percent of Patients with Adverse Events: Placebo (n = 87)	Asacol tablets (n = 152)
Headache	36	35
Abdominal pain	14	18
Eructation	15	16
Pain	8	14
Nausea	15	13
Pharyngitis	9	11
Dizziness	8	8
Asthenia	15	7
Diarrhea	9	7
Back pain	5	7
Fever	8	6
Rash	3	6
Dyspepsia	1	6
Rhinitis	5	5
Arthralgia	3	5
Hypertonia	5	5
Vomiting	2	5
Constipation	1	5
Flatulence	7	3
Dysmenorrhea	3	3
Chest pain	2	3
Chills	2	3
Flu syndrome	2	3
Peripheral edema	2	3
Myalgia	1	3
Sweating	1	3
Colitis exacerbation	0	3
Pruritus	0	3
Acne	1	2
Increased cough	1	2
Malaise	1	2
Arthritis	0	2
Conjunctivitis	0	2
Insomnia	0	2

Of these adverse events, only rash showed a consistently higher frequency with increasing **Asacol** dose in these studies.

In a 6-month placebo-controlled maintenance trial involving 264 patients, 177 of whom were randomized to **Asacol** tablets, six (3.4%) of the **Asacol** patients discontinued **Asacol** therapy because of adverse events, as compared to four (4.6%) of the placebo patients. Adverse reactions leading to withdrawal from **Asacol** tablets included (each in one patient): anxiety; headache; pruritus; decreased libido; rheumatoid arthritis; and stomatitis and asthenia.

In the 6-month placebo-controlled maintenance trial, the incidence of adverse events seen with **Asacol** tablets was similar to that seen with placebo. In addition to events listed in Table 1, the following adverse events occurred in **Asacol**-treated patients at a frequency of 2% or greater in this study: abdominal enlargement, anxiety, bronchitis, ear disorder, ear pain, gastroenteritis, gastrointestinal hemorrhage, infection, joint disorder, migraine, nervousness, paresthesia, rectal disorder, rectal hemorrhage, sinusitis, stool abnormalities, tenesmus, urinary frequency, vasodilation, and vision abnormalities.

In 3342 patients in uncontrolled clinical studies, the following adverse events occurred at a frequency of 5% or greater and appeared to increase in frequency with increasing dose: asthenia, fever, flu syndrome, pain, abdominal pain, back pain, flatulence, gastrointestinal bleeding, arthralgia, and rhinitis.

In addition to the adverse events listed above, the following events have been reported with **Asacol** use:

Body as a Whole: Neck pain, facial edema, edema.

Cardiovascular: Pericarditis (rare), myocarditis (rare).

Digestive: Anorexia, hepatitis (rare), pancreatitis, gastritis, increased appetite, cholecystitis, dry mouth, oral ulcers, perforated peptic ulcer (rare), bloody diarrhea.

Hematologic: Agranulocytosis (rare), aplastic anemia (rare), thrombocytopenia, eosinophilia, leukopenia, anemia, lymphadenopathy.

Musculoskeletal: Gout.

Nervous: Depression, somnolence, emotional lability, hyperesthesia, vertigo, confusion, tremor, peripheral neuropathy (rare), transverse myelitis (rare), Guillain-Barré syndrome (rare).

Respiratory/Pulmonary: Eosinophilic pneumonia, interstitial pneumonitis, asthma exacerbation.

Skin: Alopecia, psoriasis (rare), pyoderma gangrenosum (rare), dry skin, erythema nodosum, urticaria.

Special Senses: Eye pain, taste perversion, blurred vision, tinnitus.

Urogenital: Interstitial nephritis (See also Renal subsection in PRECAUTIONS), minimal change nephropathy (See also Renal subsection in PRECAUTIONS), dysuria, urinary urgency, hematuria, epididymitis, menorrhagia.

Laboratory Abnormalities: Elevated AST (SGOT) or ALT (SGPT), elevated alkaline phosphatase, elevated serum creatinine and BUN.

Hepatitis has been reported to occur rarely with **Asacol** tablets. More commonly, asymptomatic elevations of liver enzymes have occurred which usually resolve during continued use or with discontinuation of the drug.

DRUG ABUSE AND DEPENDENCY

Abuse: None reported.

Dependency: Drug dependence has not been reported with chronic administration of mesalamine.

OVERDOSAGE

Two cases of pediatric overdosage have been reported. A 3-year-old male who ingested 2 grams of **Asacol** tablets was treated with ipecac and activated charcoal; no adverse events occurred. Another 3-year-old male, approximately 16 kg, ingested an unknown amount of a maximum of 24 grams of **Asacol** crushed in solution (i.e., uncoated mesalamine); he was treated with orange juice and activated charcoal, and experienced no adverse events. In dogs, single doses of 6 grams of delayed-release **Asacol** tablets resulted in renal papillary necrosis but were not fatal. This was approximately 12.5 times the recommended human dose (based on a dose of 2.4 g/day in a 50 kg person). Single oral doses of uncoated mesalamine in mice and rats of 5000 mg/kg and 4595 mg/kg, respectively, or of 3000 mg/kg in cynomolgus monkeys, caused significant lethality.

DOSAGE AND ADMINISTRATION

For the treatment of mildly to moderately active ulcerative colitis: The usual dosage in adults is two 400-mg tablets to be taken three times a day for a total daily dose of 2.4 grams for a duration of 6 weeks.

For the maintenance of remission of ulcerative colitis: The recommended dosage in adults is 1.6 grams daily, in divided doses. Treatment duration in the prospective, well-controlled trial was 6 months.

HOW SUPPLIED

Asacol tablets are available as red-brown, capsule-shaped tablets containing 400 mg mesalamine and imprinted "Asacol NE" in black.

NDC 0149-0752-02 Bottle of 100

Store at controlled room temperature 20°–25°C (68°–77°F) [See USP].

CAUTION: Federal law prohibits dispensing without prescription.

Procter & Gamble Pharmaceuticals
Cincinnati, Ohio 45202
under license from Tillotts Pharma AG,
the registered trademark owner.
Made in Germany, D-64331 Weiterstadt
U.S. Patents Nos. 5,541,170 and 5,541,171
REVISED OCTOBER 1997 44003585

Shown in Product Identification Guide, page 332

DANTRIUM® capsules ℞

[*dan 'trē-um*]
(dantrolene sodium)

Dantrium (dantrolene sodium) has a potential for hepatotoxicity, and should not be used in conditions other than those recommended. Symptomatic hepatitis (fatal and non-fatal) has been reported at various dose levels of the drug. The incidence reported in patients taking up to 400 mg/day is much lower than in those taking doses of 800 mg or more per day. Even sporadic short courses of these higher dose levels within a treatment regimen markedly increased the risk of serious hepatic injury. Liver dysfunction as evidenced by blood chemical abnormalities alone (liver enzyme elevations) has been observed in patients exposed to **Dantrium** for varying periods of time. Overt hepatitis has occurred at varying intervals after initiation of therapy, but has been most frequently observed between the third and twelfth month of therapy. The risk of hepatic injury appears to be greater in females, in patients over 35 years of age, and in patients taking other medication(s) in addition to **Dantrium** (dantrolene sodium). **Dantrium** should be used only in conjunction with appropriate monitoring of hepatic function including frequent determination of SGOT or SGPT. If no observable benefit is derived from the administration of **Dantrium** after a total of 45 days, therapy should be discontinued. The lowest possible effective dose for the individual patient should be prescribed.

DESCRIPTION

The chemical formula of Dantrium (dantrolene sodium) is hydrated 1-[[[5-(4-nitrophenyl)-2-furanyl]methylene]amino]-2, 4-imidazolidinedione sodium salt. It is an orange powder, slightly soluble in water, but due to its slightly acidic nature the solubility increases somewhat in alkaline solution. The anhydrous salt has a molecular weight of 336. The hydrated salt contains approximately 15% water (3-1/2 moles) and has a molecular weight of 399. The structural formula for the hydrated salt is:

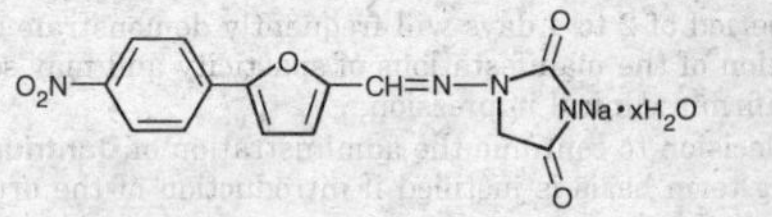

Dantrium is supplied in capsules of 25 mg, 50 mg, and 100 mg.

Inactive Ingredients: Each capsule contains edible black ink, FD&C Yellow No. 6, gelatin, lactose, magnesium stearate, starch, synthetic iron oxide red, synthetic iron oxide yellow, talc, and titanium dioxide.

CLINICAL PHARMACOLOGY

In isolated nerve-muscle preparation, **Dantrium** has been shown to produce relaxation by affecting the contractile response of the skeletal muscle at a site beyond the myoneural junction, directly on the muscle itself. In skeletal muscle, Dantrium dissociates the excitation-contraction coupling, probably by interfering with the release of Ca++ from the sarcoplasmic reticulum. This effect appears to be more pronounced in fast muscle fibers as compared to slow ones, but generally affects both. A central nervous system effect occurs, with drowsiness, dizziness, and generalized weakness occasionally present. Although **Dantrium** does not appear to directly affect the CNS, the extent of its indirect effect is unknown. The absorption of **Dantrium** after oral administration in humans is incomplete and slow but consistent, and dose-related blood levels are obtained. The duration and intensity of skeletal muscle relaxation is related to the dosage and blood levels. The mean biologic half-life of **Dantrium** in adults is 8.7 hours after a 100-mg dose. Specific metabolic pathways in the degradation and elimination of **Dantrium** in human subjects have been established. Metabolic patterns are similar in adults and pediatric patients. In addition to the parent compound, dantrolene, which is found in measurable amounts in blood and urine, the major metabolites noted in body fluids are the 5-hydroxy analog and the acetamido analog. Since **Dantrium** is probably metabolized by hepatic microsomal enzymes, enhancement of its metabolism by other drugs is possible. However, neither phenobarbital nor diazepam appears to affect **Dantrium** metabolism.

Clinical experience in the management of fulminant human malignant hyperthermia, as well as experiments conducted in malignant hyperthermia susceptible swine, have revealed that the administration of intravenous dantrolene, combined with indicated supportive measures, is effective in reversing the hypermetabolic process of malignant hyperthermia. Known differences between human and swine ma-

Continued on next page

Dantrium Capsules—Cont.

lignant hyperthermia are minor. The prophylactic administration of oral or intravenous dantrolene to malignant hyperthermia susceptible swine will attenuate or prevent the development of signs of malignant hyperthermia in a manner dependent upon the dosage of dantrolene administered and the intensity of the malignant hyperthermia triggering stimulus. Limited clinical experience with the administration of oral dantrolene to patients judged malignant hyperthermia susceptible, when combined with clinical experience in the use of intravenous dantrolene for the treatment of malignant hyperthermia and data derived from the above cited animal model experiments, suggests that oral dantrolene will also attenuate or prevent the development of signs of human malignant hyperthermia, provided that currently accepted practices in the management of such patients are adhered to (see INDICATIONS AND USAGE); intravenous dantrolene should also be available for use should the signs of malignant hyperthermia appear.

INDICATIONS AND USAGE

In Chronic Spasticity:

Dantrium is indicated in controlling the manifestations of clinical spasticity resulting from upper motor neuron disorders (e.g., spinal cord injury, stroke, cerebral palsy, or multiple sclerosis). It is of particular benefit to the patient whose functional rehabilitation has been retarded by the sequelae of spasticity. Such patients must have presumably reversible spasticity where relief of spasticity will aid in restoring residual function. **Dantrium** is not indicated in the treatment of skeletal muscle spasm resulting from rheumatic disorders.

If improvement occurs, it will ordinarily occur within the dosage titration (see DOSAGE AND ADMINISTRATION), and will be manifested by a decrease in the severity of spasticity and the ability to resume a daily function not quite attainable without **Dantrium**.

Occasionally, subtle but meaningful improvement in spasticity may occur with **Dantrium** therapy. In such instances, information regarding improvement should be solicited from the patient and those who are in constant daily contact and attendance with him. Brief withdrawal of **Dantrium** for a period of 2 to 4 days will frequently demonstrate exacerbation of the manifestations of spasticity and may serve to confirm a clinical impression.

A decision to continue the administration of **Dantrium** on a long-term basis is justified if introduction of the drug into the patient's regimen:

> produces a significant reduction in painful and/or disabling spasticity such as clonus, or
>
> permits a significant reduction in the intensity and/or degree of nursing care required, or
>
> rids the patient of any annoying manifestation of spasticity considered important by the patient himself.

In Malignant Hyperthermia:

Oral **Dantrium** is also indicated preoperatively to prevent or attenuate the development of signs of malignant hyperthermia in known, or strongly suspect, malignant hyperthermia susceptible patients who require anesthesia and/or surgery. Currently accepted clinical practices in the management of such patients must still be adhered to (careful monitoring for early signs of malignant hyperthermia, minimizing exposure to triggering mechanisms and prompt use of intravenous dantrolene sodium and indicated supportive measures should signs of malignant hyperthermia appear); see also the package insert for **Dantrium®** (dantrolene sodium) **Intravenous**.

Oral **Dantrium** should be administered following a malignant hyperthermic crisis to prevent recurrence of the signs of malignant hyperthermia.

CONTRAINDICATIONS

Active hepatic disease, such as hepatitis and cirrhosis, is a contraindication for use of **Dantrium**. **Dantrium** is contraindicated where spasticity is utilized to sustain upright posture and balance in locomotion or whenever spasticity is utilized to obtain or maintain increased function.

WARNINGS

It is important to recognize that fatal and non-fatal liver disorders of an idiosyncratic or hypersensitivity type may occur with **Dantrium** therapy.

At the start of **Dantrium** therapy, it is desirable to do liver function studies (SGOT, SGPT, alkaline phosphatase, total bilirubin) for a baseline or to establish whether there is pre-existing liver disease. If baseline liver abnormalities exist and are confirmed, there is a clear possibility that the potential for **Dantrium** hepatotoxicity could be enhanced, although such a possibility has not yet been established.

Liver function studies (e.g., SGOT or SGPT) should be performed at appropriate intervals during **Dantrium** therapy. If such studies reveal abnormal values, therapy should generally be discontinued. Only where benefits of the drug have been of major importance to the patient, should reinitiation

or continuation of therapy be considered. Some patients have revealed a return to normal laboratory values in the face of continued therapy while others have not.

If symptoms compatible with hepatitis, accompanied by abnormalities in liver function tests or jaundice appear, **Dantrium** should be discontinued. If caused by Dantrium and detected early, the abnormalities in liver function characteristically have reverted to normal when the drug was discontinued.

Dantrium therapy has been reinstituted in a few patients who have developed clinical and/or laboratory evidence of hepatocellular injury. If such reinstitution of therapy is done, it should be attempted only in patients who clearly need **Dantrium** and only after previous symptoms and laboratory abnormalities have cleared. The patient should be hospitalized and the drug should be restarted in very small and gradually increasing doses. Laboratory monitoring should be frequent and the drug should be withdrawn immediately if there is any indication of recurrent liver involvement. Some patients have reacted with unmistakable signs of liver abnormality upon administration of a challenge dose, while others have not.

Dantrium should be used with particular caution in females and in patients over 35 years of age in view of apparent greater likelihood of drug-induced, potentially fatal, hepatocellular disease in these groups.

Long-term safety of **Dantrium** in humans has not been established. Chronic studies in rats, dogs, and monkeys at dosages greater than 30 mg/kg/day showed growth or weight depression and signs of hepatopathy and possible occlusion nephropathy, all of which were reversible upon cessation of treatment. Sprague-Dawley female rats fed dantrolene sodium for 18 months at dosage levels of 15, 30, and 60 mg/kg/day showed an increased incidence of benign and malignant mammary tumors compared with concurrent controls. At the highest dose level, there was an increase in the incidence of benign hepatic lymphatic neoplasms. In a 30-month study at the same dose levels also in Sprague-Dawley rats, dantrolene sodium produced a decrease in the time of onset of mammary neoplasms. Female rats at the highest dose level showed an increased incidence of hepatic lymphangiomas and hepatic angiosarcomas.

The only drug-related effect seen in a 30-month study in Fischer-344 rats was a dose-related reduction in the time of onset of mammary and testicular tumors. A 24-month study in HaM/ICR mice revealed no evidence of carcinogenic activity. Carcinogenicity in humans cannot be fully excluded, so that this possible risk of chronic administration must be weighed against the benefits of the drug (i.e., after a brief trial) for the individual patient.

USAGE IN PREGNANCY

The safety of Dantrium for use in women who are or who may become pregnant has not been established. **Dantrium** should not be used in nursing mothers.

Usage in Pediatric Patients: The long-term safety of **Dantrium** in pediatric patients under the age of 5 years has not been established. Because of the possibility that adverse effects of the drug could become apparent only after many years, a benefit-risk consideration of the long-term use of **Dantrium** is particularly important in pediatric patients.

Drug Interactions:

Drowsiness may occur with Dantrium therapy, and the concomitant administration of CNS depressants such as sedatives and tranquilizing agents may result in further drowsiness.

While a definite drug interaction with estrogen therapy has not yet been established, caution should be observed if the two drugs are to be given concomitantly. Hepatotoxicity has occurred more often in women over 35 years of age receiving concomitant estrogen therapy.

Cardiovascular collapse in patients treated simultaneously with verapamil and dantrolene sodium is rare. The combination of therapeutic doses of intravenous dantrolene sodium and verapamil in halothane/α-chloralose anesthetized swine has resulted in ventricular fibrillation and cardiovascular collapse in association with marked hyperkalemia. Until the relevance of these findings to humans is established, the combination of dantrolene sodium and calcium channel blockers is not recommended during the management of malignant hyperthermia.

Administration of **Dantrium** may potentiate vecuronium-induced neuromuscular block.

PRECAUTIONS

Dantrium should be used with caution in patients with impaired pulmonary function, particularly those with obstructive pulmonary disease, and in patients with severely impaired cardiac function due to myocardial disease. It should be used with caution in patients with a history of previous liver disease or dysfunction (see WARNINGS).

Patients should be cautioned against driving a motor vehicle or participating in hazardous occupations while taking **Dantrium**. Caution should be exercised in the concomitant administration of tranquilizing agents.

Dantrium might possibly evoke a photosensitivity reaction; patients should be cautioned about exposure to sunlight while taking it.

ADVERSE REACTIONS

The most frequently occurring side effects of **Dantrium** have been drowsiness, dizziness, weakness, general malaise, fatigue, and diarrhea. These are generally transient, occurring early in treatment, and can often be obviated by beginning with a low dose and increasing dosage gradually until an optimal regimen is established. Diarrhea may be severe and may necessitate temporary withdrawal of **Dantrium** therapy. If diarrhea recurs upon readministration of **Dantrium**, therapy should probably be withdrawn permanently.

Other less frequent side effects, listed according to system, are:

Gastrointestinal: Constipation, rarely progressing to signs of intestinal obstruction, GI bleeding, anorexia, swallowing difficulty, gastric irritation, abdominal cramps, nausea and/or vomiting.

Hepatobiliary: Hepatitis (see WARNINGS).

Neurologic: Speech disturbance, seizure, headache, light-headedness, visual disturbance, diplopia, alteration of taste, insomnia, drooling.

Cardiovascular: Tachycardia, erratic blood pressure, phlebitis, heart failure.

Hematologic: Aplastic anemia, leukopenia, lymphocytic lymphoma, thrombocytopenia.

Psychiatric: Mental depression, mental confusion, increased nervousness.

Urogenital: Increased urinary frequency, crystalluria, hematuria, difficult erection, urinary incontinence and/or nocturia, difficult urination and/or urinary retention.

Integumentary: Abnormal hair growth, acne-like rash, pruritus, urticaria, eczematoid eruption, sweating.

Musculoskeletal: Myalgia, backache.

Respiratory: Feeling of suffocation, respiratory depression.

Special Senses: Excessive tearing.

Hypersensitivity: Pleural effusion with pericarditis, anaphylaxis.

Other: Chills and fever.

The published literature has included some reports of **Dantrium** use in patients with Neuroleptic Malignant Syndrome (NMS). **Dantrium** capsules are not indicated for the treatment of NMS and patients may expire despite treatment with **Dantrium** capsules.

DOSAGE AND ADMINISTRATION

For Use in Chronic Spasticity:

Prior to the administration of **Dantrium**, consideration should be given to the potential response to treatment. A decrease in spasticity sufficient to allow a daily function not otherwise attainable should be the therapeutic goal of treatment with **Dantrium**. Refer to INDICATIONS AND USAGE section for description of response to be anticipated.

It is important to establish a therapeutic goal (regain and maintain a specific function such as therapeutic exercise program, utilization of braces, transfer maneuvers, etc.) before beginning **Dantrium** therapy. Dosage should be increased until the maximum performance compatible with the dysfunction due to underlying disease is achieved. No further increase in dosage is then indicated.

Usual Dosage: It is important that the dosage be titrated and individualized for maximum effect. The lowest dose compatible with optimal response is recommended.

In view of the potential for liver damage in long-term **Dantrium** *use, therapy should be stopped if benefits are not evident within 45 days.*

Adults: The following gradual titration schedule is suggested. Some patients will not respond until higher daily dosage is achieved. Each dosage level should be maintained for seven days to determine the patient's response. If no further benefit is observed at the next higher dose, dosage should be decreased to the previous lower dose.

> 25 mg once daily for seven days, then
> 25 mg t.i.d. for seven days
> 50 mg t.i.d. for seven days
> 100 mg t.i.d.

Therapy with a dose four times daily may be necessary for some individuals. Doses higher than 100 mg four times daily should not be used. (See Box Warning.)

Pediatric Patients: The following gradual titration schedule is suggested. Some patients will not respond until higher daily dosage is achieved. Each dosage level should be maintained for seven days to determine the patient's response. If no further benefit is observed at the next higher dose, dosage should be decreased to the previous lower dose.

> 0.5 mg/kg once daily for seven days, then
> 0.5 mg/kg t.i.d. for seven days
> 1 mg/kg t.i.d. for seven days
> 2 mg/kg t.i.d.

Therapy with a dose four times daily may be necessary for some individuals. Doses higher than 100 mg four times daily should not be used. (See Box Warning.)

For Malignant Hyperthermia:

Preoperatively: Administer 4 to 8 mg/kg/day of oral **Dantrium** in 3 or 4 divided doses for one or two days prior to surgery, with the last dose being given approximately 3 to 4 hours before scheduled surgery with a minimum of water. This dosage will usually be associated with skeletal muscle weakness and sedation (sleepiness or drowsiness); adjustment can usually be made within the recommended dosage range to avoid incapacitation or excessive gastrointestinal irritation (including nausea and/or vomiting).

Post Crisis Follow-up:

Oral **Dantrium** should also be administered following a malignant hyperthermia crisis, in doses of 4 to 8 mg/kg per day in four divided doses, for a one to three day period to prevent recurrence of the manifestations of malignant hyperthermia.

OVERDOSAGE

Symptoms which may occur in case of overdose include, but are not limited to, muscular weakness and alterations in the state of consciousness (e.g. lethargy, coma), vomiting, diarrhea, and crystalluria. For acute overdosage, general supportive measures should be employed along with immediate gastric lavage.

Intravenous fluids should be administered in fairly large quantities to avert the possibility of crystalluria. An adequate airway should be maintained and artificial resuscitation equipment should be at hand. Electrocardiographic monitoring should be instituted, and the patient carefully observed. To date, no experience has been reported with dialysis and its value in Dantrium overdosage is not known.

HOW SUPPLIED

Dantrium (dantrolene sodium) is available in

25-mg opaque, orange and tan capsules:

NDC 0149-0030-05 bottle of 100

NDC 0149-0030-66 bottle of 500

NDC 0149-0030-77 hospital unit-dose strips in boxes of 100

50-mg opaque, orange and tan capsules:

NDC 0149-0031-05 bottle of 100

100-mg opaque, orange and tan capsules:

NDC 0149-0033-05 bottle of 100

NDC 0149-0033-77 hospital unit-dose strips in boxes of 100

Avoid excessive heat (over 104°F or 40°C).

Address medical inquiries to Procter & Gamble Pharmaceuticals, Medical Communications Department, 11450 Grooms Rd, Cincinnati, Ohio 45242.

CAUTION: Federal law prohibits dispensing without prescription.

Procter & Gamble Pharmaceuticals
Cincinnati, Ohio 45202
REVISED FEBRUARY 1997 03001-U7

DANTRIUM® INTRAVENOUS ℞
(dantrolene sodium for injection)

DESCRIPTION

Dantrium Intravenous is a sterile, non-pyrogenic, lyophilized formulation of dantrolene sodium for injection. **Dantrium Intravenous** is supplied in 70 mL vials containing 20 mg dantrolene sodium, 3000 mg mannitol, and sufficient sodium hydroxide to yield a pH of approximately 9.5 when reconstituted with 60 mL sterile water for injection USP (without a bacteriostatic agent).

Dantrium is classified as a direct-acting skeletal muscle relaxant. Chemically, **Dantrium** is hydrated 1-[[[5-(4-nitrophenyl)-2-furanyl]methylene]amino]-2,4-imidazolidinedione sodium salt. The structural formula for the hydrated salt is:

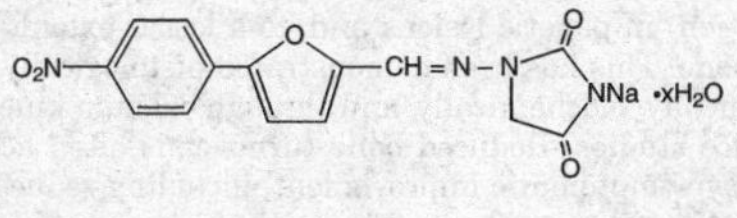

The hydrated salt contains approximately 15% water (3-1/2 moles) and has a molecular weight of 399. The anhydrous salt (dantrolene) has a molecular weight of 336.

CLINICAL PHARMACOLOGY

In isolated nerve-muscle preparation, **Dantrium** produces skeletal muscle relaxation by directly affecting the contractile response of the muscle at a site beyond the myoneural junction. In skeletal muscle, **Dantrium** dissociates excitation-contraction coupling, probably by interfering with the release of Ca^{++} from the sarcoplasmic reticulum. The administration of intravenous **Dantrium** to human volunteers is associated with loss of grip strength and weakness in the legs, as well as subjective CNS complaints (see also PRECAUTIONS, Information for Patients). Information concerning the passage of **Dantrium** across the blood-brain barrier is not available.

In the anesthetic-induced malignant hyperthermia syndrome, evidence points to an intrinsic abnormality of skeletal muscle tissue. In affected humans, it has been postulated that "triggering agents" (e.g., general anesthetics and depolarizing neuromuscular blocking agents) produce a change within the cell which results in an elevated myoplasmic calcium. This elevated myoplasmic calcium activates acute cellular catabolic processes that cascade to the malignant hyperthermia crisis.

It is hypothesized that addition of **Dantrium** to the "triggered" malignant hyperthermic muscle cell reestablishes a normal level of ionized calcium in the myoplasm. Inhibition of calcium release from the sarcoplasmic reticulum by **Dantrium** reestablishes the myoplasmic calcium equilibrium, increasing the percentage of bound calcium. In this way, physiologic, metabolic, and biochemical changes associated with the malignant hyperthermia crisis may be reversed or attenuated. Experimental results in malignant hyperthermia susceptible swine show that prophylactic administration of intravenous or oral dantrolene prevents or attenuates the development of vital sign and blood gas changes characteristic of malignant hyperthermia in a dose related manner. The efficacy of intravenous dantrolene in the treatment of human and porcine malignant hyperthermia crisis, when considered along with prophylactic experiments in malignant hyperthermia susceptible swine, lends support to prophylactic use of oral or intravenous dantrolene in malignant hyperthermia susceptible humans. When prophylactic intravenous dantrolene is administered as directed, whole blood concentrations remain at a near steady state level for 3 or more hours after the infusion is completed. Clinical experience has shown that early vital sign and/or blood gas changes characteristic of malignant hyperthermia may appear during or after anesthesia and surgery despite the prophylactic use of dantrolene and adherence to currently accepted patient management practices. These signs are compatible with attenuated malignant hyperthermia and respond to the administration of additional i.v. dantrolene (see DOSAGE AND ADMINISTRATION). The administration of the recommended prophylactic dose of intravenous dantrolene to healthy volunteers was not associated with clinically significant cardiorespiratory changes.

Specific metabolic pathways for the degradation and elimination of **Dantrium** in humans have been established. Dantrolene is found in measurable amounts in blood and urine. Its major metabolites in body fluids are 5-hydroxy dantrolene and an acetylamino metabolite of dantrolene. Another metabolite with an unknown structure appears related to the latter. **Dantrium** may also undergo hydrolysis and subsequent oxidation forming nitrophenylfuroic acid.

The mean biologic half-life of **Dantrium** after intravenous administration is variable, between 4 to 8 hours under most experimental conditions. Based on assays of whole blood and plasma, slightly greater amounts of dantrolene are associated with red blood cells than with the plasma fraction of blood. Significant amounts of dantrolene are bound to plasma proteins, mostly albumin, and this binding is readily reversible.

Cardiopulmonary depression has not been observed in malignant hyperthermia susceptible swine following the administration of up to 7.5 mg/kg i.v. dantrolene. This is twice the amount needed to maximally diminish twitch response to single supramaximal peripheral nerve stimulation (95% inhibition). A transient, inconsistent, depressant effect on gastrointestinal smooth muscles has been observed at high doses.

INDICATIONS AND USAGE

Dantrium Intravenous is indicated, along with appropriate supportive measures, for the management of the fulminant hypermetabolism of skeletal muscle characteristic of malignant hyperthermia crises in patients of all ages. **Dantrium Intravenous** should be administered by continuous rapid intravenous push as soon as the malignant hyperthermia reaction is recognized (i.e., tachycardia, tachypnea, central venous desaturation, hypercarbia, metabolic acidosis, skeletal muscle rigidity, increased utilization of anesthesia circuit carbon dioxide absorber, cyanosis and mottling of the skin, and, in many cases, fever).

Dantrium Intravenous is also indicated preoperatively, and sometimes postoperatively, to prevent or attenuate the development of clinical and laboratory signs of malignant hyperthermia in individuals judged to be malignant hyperthermia susceptible.

CONTRAINDICATIONS

None.

WARNINGS

The use of **Dantrium Intravenous** *in the management of malignant hyperthermia crisis is not a substitute for previously known supportive measures. These measures must be individualized, but it will usually be necessary to discontinue the suspect triggering agents, attend to increased oxygen requirements, manage the metabolic acidosis, institute cooling when necessary, monitor urinary output, and monitor for electrolyte imbalance.*

Since the effect of disease state and other drugs on the consequences of **Dantrium** related skeletal muscle weakness, including possible respiratory depression, cannot be predicted, patients who receive i.v. **Dantrium** preoperatively should have vital signs monitored.

If patients judged malignant hyperthermia susceptible are administered intravenous or oral **Dantrium** preoperatively, anesthetic preparation must still follow a standard malignant hyperthermia susceptible regimen, including the avoidance of known triggering agents. Monitoring for early clinical and metabolic signs of malignant hyperthermia is indicated because attenuation of malignant hyperthermia, rather than prevention, is possible. These signs usually call for the administration of additional i.v. dantrolene.

PRECAUTIONS

General: Care must be taken to prevent extravasation of **Dantrium** solution into the surrounding tissues due to the high pH of the intravenous formulation.

When mannitol is used for prevention or treatment of late renal complications of malignant hyperthermia, the 3 g of mannitol needed to dissolve each 20 mg vial of i.v. **Dantrium** should be taken into consideration.

Information for Patients: Based upon data in human volunteers, it will sometimes be appropriate to tell patients who receive **Dantrium Intravenous** that decrease in grip strength and weakness of leg muscles, especially walking down stairs, can be expected postoperatively. In addition, symptoms such as "lightheadedness" may be noted. Since some of these symptoms may persist for up to 48 hours, patients must not operate an automobile or engage in other hazardous activity during this time. Caution is also indicated at meals on the day of administration because difficulty swallowing and choking has been reported. Caution should be exercised in the concomitant administration of tranquilizing agents.

Hepatotoxicity seen with **Dantrium Capsules: Dantrium** (dantrolene sodium) has a potential for hepatotoxicity, and should not be used in conditions other than those recommended. Symptomatic hepatitis (fatal and non-fatal) has been reported at various dose levels of the drug. The incidence reported in patients taking up to 400 mg/day is much lower than in those taking doses of 800 mg or more per day. Even sporadic short courses of these higher dose levels within a treatment regimen markedly increased the risk of serious hepatic injury. Liver dysfunction as evidenced by blood chemical abnormalities alone (liver enzyme elevations) has been observed in patients exposed to **Dantrium** for varying periods of time. Overt hepatitis has occurred at varying intervals after initiation of therapy, but has been most frequently observed between the third and twelfth month of therapy. The risk of hepatic injury appears to be greater in females, in patients over 35 years of age, and in patients taking other medication(s) in addition to **Dantrium** (dantrolene sodium). **Dantrium** should be used only in conjunction with appropriate monitoring of hepatic function including frequent determination of SGOT or SGPT.

Fatal and non-fatal liver disorders of an idiosyncratic or hypersensitivity type may occur with **Dantrium** therapy.

Drug Interactions: **Dantrium** is metabolized by the liver, and it is theoretically possible that its metabolism may be enhanced by drugs known to induce hepatic microsomal enzymes. However, neither phenobarbital nor diazepam appears to affect **Dantrium** metabolism. Binding to plasma protein is not significantly altered by diazepam, diphenylhydantoin, or phenylbutazone. Binding to plasma proteins is reduced by warfarin and clofibrate and increased by tolbutamide.

Cardiovascular collapse in patients treated simultaneously with verapamil and dantrolene sodium is rare. The combination of therapeutic doses of intravenous dantrolene sodium and verapamil in halothane/α-chloralose anesthetized swine has resulted in ventricular fibrillation and cardiovascular collapse in association with marked hyperkalemia. It is recommended that the combination of intravenous dantrolene sodium and calcium channel blockers, such as verapamil, not be used together during the management of malignant hyperthermia crisis until the relevance of these findings to humans is established.

Administration of dantrolene may potentiate vecuronium-induced neuromuscular block.

Carcinogenesis, Mutagenesis, and Impairment of Fertility: Sprague-Dawley female rats fed **Dantrium** for 18 months at dosage levels of 15, 30, and 60 mg/kg/day showed an increased incidence of benign and malignant mammary tumors compared with concurrent controls. At the highest dose levels, there was an increase in the incidence of benign hepatic lymphatic neoplasms. In a 30-month study at the same dose levels also in Sprague-Dawley rats, dantrolene sodium produced a decrease in the time of onset of mammary neoplasms. Female rats at the highest dose level

Continued on next page

Dantrium Intravenous—Cont.

showed an increased incidence of hepatic lymphangiomas and hepatic angiosarcomas.
The only drug-related effect seen in a 30-month study in Fischer-344 rats was a dose-related reduction in the time of onset of mammary and testicular tumors. A 24-month study in HaM/ICR mice revealed no evidence of carcinogenic activity.
The significance of carcinogenicity data relative to use of **Dantrium** in humans is unknown.
Dantrolene sodium has produced positive results in the Ames *S. Typhimurium* bacterial mutagenesis assay in the presence and absence of a liver activating system.
Dantrolene sodium administered to male and female rats at dose levels up to 45 mg/kg/day showed no adverse effects on fertility or general reproductive performance.
Usage in Pregnancy: Pregnancy Category C: **Dantrium** has been shown to be embryocidal in the rabbit and has been shown to decrease pup survival in the rat when given at doses seven times the human oral dose. There are no adequate and well-controlled studies in pregnant women. **Dantrium Intravenous** should be used during pregnancy only if the potential benefit justifies the potential risk to the fetus.
Labor and Delivery: In one uncontrolled study, 100 mg per day of prophylactic oral **Dantrium** was administered to term pregnant patients awaiting labor and delivery. Dantrolene readily crossed the placenta, with maternal and fetal whole blood levels approximately equal at delivery; neonatal levels then fell approximately 50% per day for 2 days before declining sharply. No neonatal respiratory and neuromuscular side effects were detected at low dose. More data, at higher doses, are needed before more definitive conclusions can be made.

ADVERSE REACTIONS

There have been occasional reports of death following malignant hyperthermia crisis even when treated with intravenous dantrolene; incidence figures are not available (the pre-dantrolene mortality of malignant hyperthermia crisis was approximately 50%). Most of these deaths can be accounted for by late recognition, delayed treatment, inadequate dosage, lack of supportive therapy, intercurrent disease and/or the development of delayed complications such as renal failure or disseminated intravascular coagulopathy. In some cases there are insufficient data to completely rule out therapeutic failure of dantrolene.
There are rare reports of fatality in malignant hyperthermia crisis, despite initial satisfactory response to i.v. dantrolene, which involve patients who could not be weaned from dantrolene after initial treatment.
The administration of intravenous **Dantrium** to human volunteers is associated with loss of grip strength and weakness in the legs, as well as drowsiness and dizziness.
The following adverse reactions are in approximate order of severity:

There are rare reports of pulmonary edema developing during the treatment of malignant hyperthermia crisis in which the diluent volume and mannitol needed to deliver i.v. dantrolene possibly contributed.

There have been reports of thrombophlebitis following administration of intravenous dantrolene; actual incidence figures are not available.

There have been rare reports of urticaria and erythema possibly associated with the administration of i.v. **Dantrium**. There has been one case of anaphylaxis.

None of the serious reactions occasionally reported with long-term oral **Dantrium** use, such as hepatitis, seizures, and pleural effusion with pericarditis, have been reasonably associated with short-term **Dantrium Intravenous** therapy.
The following events have been reported in patients receiving oral dantrolene: aplastic anemia, leukopenia, lymphocytic lymphoma, and heart failure. (See package insert for **Dantrium** (dantrolene sodium) **Capsules** for a complete listing of adverse reactions.)
The published literature has included some reports of **Dantrium** use in patients with Neuroleptic Malignant Syndrome (NMS). **Dantrium Intravenous** is not indicated for the treatment of NMS and patients may expire despite treatment with **Dantrium Intravenous.**

OVERDOSAGE

Because **Dantrium Intravenous** must be administered at a low concentration in a large volume of fluid, acute toxicity of **Dantrium** could not be assessed in animals. In 14-day (subacute) studies, the intravenous formulation of **Dantrium** was relatively non-toxic to rats at doses of 10 mg/kg/day and 20 mg/kg/day. While 10 mg/kg/day in dogs for 14 days evoked little toxicity, 20 mg/kg/day for 14 days caused hepatic changes of questionable biologic significance.
Symptoms which may occur in case of overdose include, but are not limited to, muscular weakness and alterations in the state of consciousness (e.g. lethargy, coma), vomiting, diarrhea, and crystalluria.
For acute overdosage, general supportive measures should be employed.
Intravenous fluids should be administered in fairly large quantities to avert the possibility of crystalluria. An adequate airway should be maintained and artificial resuscitation equipment should be at hand. Electrocardiographic monitoring should be instituted, and the patient carefully observed. The value of dialysis in **Dantrium** overdose is not known.

DOSAGE AND ADMINISTRATION

As soon as the malignant hyperthermia reaction is recognized, all anesthetic agents should be discontinued; the administration of 100% oxygen is recommended. **Dantrium Intravenous** should be administered by continuous rapid intravenous push beginning at a minimum dose of 1 mg/kg, and continuing until symptoms subside or the maximum cumulative dose of 10 mg/kg has been reached.
If the physiologic and metabolic abnormalities reappear, the regimen may be repeated. It is important to note that administration of **Dantrium Intravenous** should be continuous until symptoms subside. The effective dose to reverse the crisis is directly dependent upon the individual's degree of susceptibility to malignant hyperthermia, the amount and time of exposure to the triggering agent, and the time elapsed between onset of the crisis and initiation of treatment.
Pediatric Dose: Experience to date indicates that the dose of **Dantrium Intravenous** for pediatric patients is the same as for adults.
Preoperatively: Dantrium Intravenous and/or **Dantrium Capsules** may be administered preoperatively to patients judged malignant hyperthermia susceptible as part of the overall patient management to prevent or attenuate the development of clinical and laboratory signs of malignant hyperthermia.

Dantrium Intravenous: The recommended prophylactic dose of **Dantrium Intravenous** is 2.5 mg/kg, starting approximately 1-1/4 hours before anticipated anesthesia and infused over approximately 1 hour. This dose should prevent or attenuate the development of clinical and laboratory signs of malignant hyperthermia provided that the usual precautions, such as avoidance of established malignant hyperthermia triggering agents, are followed. Additional **Dantrium Intravenous** may be indicated during anesthesia and surgery because of the appearance of early clinical and/or blood gas signs of malignant hyperthermia or because of prolonged surgery (see also CLINICAL PHARMACOLOGY, WARNINGS, and PRECAUTIONS). Additional doses must be individualized.

Oral administration of Dantrium Capsules: Administer 4 to 8 mg/kg/day of oral **Dantrium** in three or four divided doses for 1 or 2 days prior to surgery, with the last dose being given with a minimum of water approximately 3 to 4 hours before scheduled surgery. Adjustment can usually be made within the recommended dosage range to avoid incapacitation (weakness, drowsiness, etc.) or excessive gastrointestinal irritation (nausea and/or vomiting). See also the package insert for **Dantrium Capsules**.

Post Crisis Follow-up: Dantrium Capsules, 4 to 8 mg/kg/day, in four divided doses should be administered for 1 to 3 days following a malignant hyperthermia crisis to prevent recurrence of the manifestations of malignant hyperthermia.
Intravenous **Dantrium** may be used postoperatively to prevent or attenuate the recurrence of signs of malignant hyperthermia when oral **Dantrium** administration is not practical. The i.v. dose of **Dantrium** in the postoperative period must be individualized, starting with 1 mg/kg or more as the clinical situation dictates.

PREPARATION:

Each vial of **Dantrium Intravenous** should be reconstituted by adding 60 mL of *sterile water for injection USP (without a bacteriostatic agent), and the vial shaken until the solution is clear.* 5% Dextrose Injection USP, 0.9% Sodium Chloride Injection USP, and other acidic solutions are not compatible with **Dantrium Intravenous** and should not be used. The contents of the vial must be *protected from direct light* and *used within 6 hours* after reconstitution. Store reconstituted solutions at controlled room temperature (59°F to 86°F or 15°C to 30°C).
Reconstituted **Dantrium Intravenous** should *not* be transferred to large glass bottles for prophylactic infusion due to precipitate formation observed with the use of some glass bottles as reservoirs.
For prophylactic infusion, the required number of individual vials of **Dantrium Intravenous** should be reconstituted as outlined above. The contents of individual vials are then transferred to a larger volume sterile intravenous plastic bag. Stability data on file at Procter & Gamble Pharmaceuticals indicate commercially available sterile plastic bags are acceptable drug delivery devices. However, it is recommended that the prepared infusion be inspected carefully for cloudiness and/or precipitation prior to dispensing and administration. Such solutions should not be used. While stable for 6 hours, it is recommended that the infusion be prepared immediately prior to the anticipated dosage administration time.
Parenteral drug products should be inspected visually for particulate matter and discoloration prior to administration.

HOW SUPPLIED

Dantrium Intravenous (**NDC** 0149-0734-02) is available in vials containing a sterile lyophilized mixture of 20 mg dantrolene sodium, 3000 mg mannitol, and sufficient sodium hydroxide to yield a pH of approximately 9.5 when reconstituted with 60 mL sterile water for injection USP (without a bacteriostatic agent).
Store unreconstituted product at controlled room temperature (59°F to 86°F or 15°C to 30°C) and avoid prolonged exposure to light.
Address medical inquiries to Procter & Gamble Pharmaceuticals, Medical Communications Department, 11450 Grooms Rd, Cincinnati, Ohio 45242.
CAUTION: Rx only
Procter & Gamble Pharmaceuticals
Cincinnati, Ohio 45202
REVISED FEBRUARY 1997 73402–P2

DIDRONEL® ℞

[*dī 'drō-nel*]
(etidronate disodium)

DESCRIPTION

Didronel tablets contain either 200 mg or 400 mg of etidronate disodium, the disodium salt of (1-hydroxyethylidene) diphosphonic acid, for oral administration. This compound, also known as EHDP, regulates bone metabolism. It is a white powder, highly soluble in water, with a molecular weight of 250 and the following structural formula:

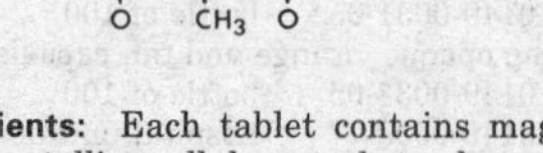

Inactive Ingredients: Each tablet contains magnesium stearate, microcrystalline cellulose, and starch.

CLINICAL PHARMACOLOGY

Didronel acts primarily on bone. It can inhibit the formation, growth, and dissolution of hydroxyapatite crystals and their amorphous precursors by chemisorption to calcium phosphate surfaces. Inhibition of crystal resorption occurs at lower doses than are required to inhibit crystal growth. Both effects increase as the dose increases.
Didronel is not metabolized. The amount of drug absorbed after an oral dose is approximately 3%. In normal subjects, plasma half-life ($t^1/_2$) of etidronate, based on non-compartmental pharmacokinetics is 1 to 6 hours. Within 24 hours, approximately half the absorbed dose is excreted in urine; the remainder is distributed to bone compartments from which it is slowly eliminated. Animal studies have yielded bone clearance estimates up to 165 days. In humans, the residence time on bone may vary due to such factors as specific metabolic condition and bone type. Unabsorbed drug is excreted intact in the feces. Preclinical studies indicate etidronate disodium does not cross the blood-brain barrier. **Didronel** therapy does not adversely affect serum levels of parathyroid hormone or calcium.
Paget's Disease: Paget's disease of bone (osteitis deformans) is an idiopathic, progressive disease characterized by abnormal and accelerated bone metabolism in one or more bones. Signs and symptoms may include bone pain and/or deformity, neurologic disorders, elevated cardiac output and other vascular disorders, and increased serum alkaline phosphatase and/or urinary hydroxyproline levels. Bone fractures are common in patients with Paget's disease.
Didronel slows accelerated bone turnover (resorption and accretion) in pagetic lesions and, to a lesser extent, in normal bone. This has been demonstrated histologically, scintigraphically, biochemically, and through calcium kinetic and balance studies. Reduced bone turnover is often accompanied by symptomatic improvement, including reduced bone pain. Also, the incidence of pagetic fractures may be reduced, and elevated cardiac output and other vascular disorders may be improved by **Didronel** therapy.
Heterotopic Ossification: Heterotopic ossification, also referred to as myositis ossificans (circumscripta, progressiva or traumatica), ectopic calcification, periarticular ossification, or paraosteoarthropathy, is characterized by metaplastic osteogenesis. It usually presents with signs of localized inflammation or pain, elevated skin temperature, and redness. When tissues near joints are involved, functional loss may also be present.
Heterotopic ossification may occur for no known reason as in myositis ossificans progressiva or may follow a wide variety of surgical, occupational, and sports trauma (eg, hip arthroplasty, spinal cord injury, head injury, burns, and severe thigh bruises). Heterotopic ossification has also been

observed in non-traumatic conditions (eg, infections of the central nervous system, peripheral neuropathy, tetanus, biliary cirrhosis, Peyronie's disease, as well as in association with a variety of benign and malignant neoplasms).

Clinical trials have demonstrated the efficacy of **Didronel** in heterotopic ossification following total hip replacement, or due to spinal cord injury.

— *Heterotopic ossification complicating total hip replacement* typically develops radiographically 3 to 8 weeks postoperatively in the pericapsular area of the affected hip joint. The overall incidence is about 50%; about one-third of these cases are clinically significant.

— *Heterotopic ossification due to spinal cord injury* typically develops radiographically 1 to 4 months after injury. It occurs below the level of injury, usually at major joints. The overall incidence is about 40%; about one-half of these cases are clinically significant.

Didronel chemisorbs to calcium hydroxyapatite crystals and their amorphous precursors, blocking the aggregation, growth, and mineralization of these crystals. This is thought to be the mechanism by which **Didronel** prevents or retards heterotopic ossification. There is no evidence **Didronel** affects mature heterotopic bone.

INDICATIONS AND USAGE

Didronel is indicated for the treatment of symptomatic Paget's disease of bone and in the prevention and treatment of heterotopic ossification following total hip replacement or due to spinal cord injury. **Didronel** is not approved for the treatment of osteoporosis.

Paget's Disease: **Didronel** is indicated for the treatment of symptomatic Paget's disease of bone. **Didronel** therapy usually arrests or significantly impedes the disease process as evidenced by:

— Symptomatic relief, including decreased pain and/or increased mobility (experienced by 3 out of 5 patients).

— Reductions in serum alkaline phosphatase and urinary hydroxy-proline levels (30% or more in 4 out of 5 patients).

— Histomorphometry showing reduced numbers of osteoclasts and osteoblasts, and more lamellar bone formation.

— Bone scans showing reduced radionuclide uptake at pagetic lesions.

In addition, reductions in pagetically elevated cardiac output and skin temperature have been observed in some patients.

In many patients, the disease process will be suppressed for a period of at least 1 year following cessation of therapy. The upper limit of this period has not been determined.

The effects of the **Didronel** treatment in patients with asymptomatic Paget's disease have not been studied. However, **Didronel** treatment of such patients may be warranted if extensive involvement threatens irreversible neurologic damage, major joints, or major weight-bearing bones.

Heterotopic Ossification: **Didronel** is indicated in the prevention and treatment of heterotopic ossification following total hip replacement or due to spinal cord injury.

Didronel reduces the incidence of clinically important heterotopic bone by about two-thirds. Among those patients who form heterotopic bone, **Didronel** retards the progression of immature lesions and reduces the severity by at least half. Follow-up data (at least 9 months posttherapy) suggest these benefits persist.

In total hip replacement patients, **Didronel** does not promote loosening of the prosthesis or impede trochanteric reattachment.

In spinal cord injury patients, **Didronel** does not inhibit fracture healing or stabilization of the spine.

CONTRAINDICATIONS

Didronel tablets are contraindicated in patients with known hypersensitivity to etidronate disodium or in patients with clinically overt osteomalacia.

WARNINGS

Paget's Disease: In Paget's patients the response to therapy may be of slow onset and continue for months after **Didronel** therapy is discontinued. Dosage should not be increased prematurely. A 90-day drug-free interval should be provided between courses of therapy.

Heterotopic Ossification: No specific warnings.

PRECAUTIONS

General: Patients should maintain an adequate nutritional status, particularly an adequate intake of calcium and vitamin D.

Therapy has been withheld from some patients with enterocolitis since diarrhea may be experienced, particularly at higher doses.

Didronel is not metabolized and is excreted intact via the kidney. Hyperphosphatemia may occur at doses of 10 to 20 mg/kg/day, apparently as a result of drug-related increases in tubular reabsorption of phosphate. Serum phosphate levels generally return to normal 2 to 4 weeks posttherapy. There is no experience to specifically guide treatment in patients with impaired renal function. **Didronel** dosage should be reduced when reductions in glomerular filtration rates are present. Patients with renal impairment should be closely monitored. In approximately 10% of patients in clinical trials of **Didronel® I. V. Infusion** (etidronate disodium) for hypercalcemia of malignancy, occasional, mild-to-moderate abnormalities in renal function (increases of >0.5 mg/dl serum creatinine) were observed during or immediately after treatment.

Didronel suppresses bone turnover, and may retard mineralization of osteoid laid down during the bone accretion process. These effects are dose and time dependent. Osteoid, which may accumulate noticeably at doses of 10 to 20 mg/kg/day, mineralizes normally posttherapy. In patients with fractures, especially of long bones, it may be advisable to delay or interrupt treatment until callus is evident.

Paget's Disease: In Paget's patients, treatment regimens exceeding the recommended (see DOSAGE AND ADMINISTRATION) daily maximum dose of 20 mg/kg or continuous administration of medication for periods greater than 6 months may be associated with osteomalacia and an increased risk of fracture.

Long bones predominantly affected by lytic lesions, particularly in those patients unresponsive to **Didronel** therapy, may be especially prone to fracture. Patients with predominantly lytic lesions should be monitored radiographically and biochemically to permit termination of **Didronel** in those patients unresponsive to treatment.

Drug Interactions: There have been isolated reports of patients experiencing increases in their prothrombin times when etidronate was added to warfarin therapy. The majority of these reports concerned variable elevations in prothrombin times without clinically significant sequelae. Although the relevance of these reports and any mechanism of coagulation alterations is unclear, patients on warfarin should have their prothrombin time monitored.

Carcinogenesis: Long-term studies in rats have indicated that **Didronel** is not carcinogenic.

Pregnancy: Teratogenic Effects: Pregnancy Category C. In teratology and developmental toxicity studies conducted in rats and rabbits treated with dosages of up to 100 mg/kg (5 to 20 times the clinical dose), no adverse or teratogenic effects have been observed in the offspring. Etidronate disodium has been shown to cause skeletal abnormalities in rats when given at oral dose levels of 300 mg/kg (15 to 60 times the human dose). Other effects on the offspring (including decreased live births) are at dosages that cause significant toxicity in the parent generation and are 25 to 200 times the human dose. The skeletal effects are thought to be the result of the pharmacological effects of the drug on bone.

There are no adequate and well-controlled studies in pregnant women, **Didronel** (etidronate disodium) should be used during pregnancy only if the potential benefit justifies the potential risk to the fetus.

Nursing Mothers: It is not known whether this drug is excreted in human milk. Because many drugs are excreted in human milk, caution should be exercised when **Didronel** is administered to a nursing woman.

Pediatric Use: Safety and effectiveness in pediatric patients have not been established. Pediatric patients have been treated with **Didronel**, at doses recommended for adults, to prevent heterotopic ossifications or soft tissue calcifications. A rachitic syndrome has been reported infrequently at doses of 10 mg/kg/day and more for prolonged periods approaching or exceeding a year. The epiphyseal radiologic changes associated with retarded mineralization of new osteoid and cartilage, and occasional symptoms reported, have been reversible when medication is discontinued.

ADVERSE REACTIONS

The incidence of gastrointestinal complaints (diarrhea, nausea) is the same for **Didronel** at 5 mg/kg/day as for placebo, about 1 patient in 15. At 10 to 20 mg/kg/day the incidence may increase to 2 or 3 in 10. These complaints are often alleviated by dividing the total daily dose.

Paget's Disease: In Paget's patients, increased or recurrent bone pain at pagetic sites, and/or the onset of pain at previously asymptomatic sites has been reported. At 5 mg/kg/day about 1 patient in 10 (versus 1 in 15 in the placebo group) report these phenomena. At higher doses the incidence rises to about 2 in 10. When therapy continues, pain resolves in some patients but persists in others.

Heterotopic Ossification: No specific adverse reactions.

Worldwide Postmarketing Experience: The worldwide postmarketing experience for etidronate disodium reflects its use in the following approved indications: Paget's disease, heterotopic ossification, and hypercalcemia of malignancy. It also reflects the use of etidronate disodium for osteoporosis where approved in countries outside the US. Other adverse events that have been reported and were thought to be possibly related to etidronate disodium include the following: alopecia; arthropathies, including arthralgia and arthritis; bone fracture; esophagitis; glossitis; hypersensitivity reactions, including angioedema, follicular eruption, macular rash, maculopapular rash, pruritus, a single case of Stevens-Johnson syndrome, and urticaria; osteomalacia; neuropsychiatric events, including amnesia, confusion, depression, and hallucination; and paresthesias. In patients receiving etidronate disodium, there have been rare reports of agranulocytosis, pancytopenia, and a report of leukopenia with recurrence on rechallenge. In addition, there have been rare reports of exacerbation of asthma. Exacerbation of existing peptic ulcer disease has been reported in a few patients. In one patient, perforation also occurred.

OVERDOSAGE

Clinical experience with acute **Didronel** overdosage is extremely limited. Decreases in serum calcium following substantial overdosage may be expected in some patients. Signs and symptoms of hypocalcemia also may occur in some of these patients. Some patients may develop vomiting. In one event, an 18-year-old female who ingested an estimated single dose of 4000 to 6000 mg (67 to 100 mg/kg) of **Didronel** was reported to be mildly hypocalcemic (7.52 mg/dl) and experienced paresthesia of the fingers. Hypocalcemia resolved 6 hours after lavage and treatment with intravenous calcium gluconate. A 92-year-old female who accidentally received 1600 mg of etidronate disodium per day for 3.5 days experienced marked diarrhea and required treatment for electrolyte imbalance. Orally administered etidronate disodium may cause hematologic abnormalities in some patients (see ADVERSE REACTIONS).

Etidronate disodium suppresses bone turnover and may retard mineralization of osteoid laid down during the bone accretion process. These effects are dose and time dependent. Osteoid which may accumulate noticeably at doses of 10 to 20 mg/kg/day of chronic, continuous dosing mineralizes normally posttherapy.

Prolonged continuous treatment (chronic overdosage) has been reported to cause nephrotic syndrome and fracture.

Gastric lavage may remove unabsorbed drug. Standard procedures for treating hypocalcemia, including the administration of Ca^{++} intravenously, would be expected to restore physiologic amounts of ionized calcium and relieve signs and symptoms of hypocalcemia. Such treatment has been effective.

DOSAGE AND ADMINISTRATION

Didronel should be taken as a single, oral dose. However, should gastrointestinal discomfort occur, the dose may be divided. To maximize absorption, patients should avoid taking the following items within two hours of dosing:

— Food, especially food high in calcium, such as milk or milk products.

— Vitamins with mineral supplements or antacids which are high in metals such as calcium, iron, magnesium, or aluminum.

***Paget's Disease:* Initial Treatment Regimens:** 5 to 10 mg/kg/day, not to exceed 6 months, or 11 to 20 mg/kg/day, not to exceed 3 months.

The recommended initial dose is 5 mg/kg/day for a period not to exceed 6 months. Doses above 10 mg/kg/day should be reserved for when 1) lower doses are ineffective or 2) there is an overriding need to suppress rapid bone turnover (especially when irreversible neurologic damage is possible) or reduce elevated cardiac output. Doses in excess of 20 mg/kg/day are not recommended.

Retreatment Guidelines: Retreatment should be initiated only after 1) a **Didronel**-free period of at least 90 days and 2) there is biochemical, symptomatic or other evidence of active disease process. It is advisable to monitor patients every 3 to 6 months although some patients may go drug free for extended periods. Retreatment regimens are the same as for initial treatment. For most patients the original dose will be adequate for retreatment. If not, consideration should be given to increasing the dose within the recommended guidelines.

Heterotopic Ossification: The following treatment regimens have been shown to be effective:

— Total Hip Replacement Patients: 20 mg/kg/day for 1 month before and 3 months after surgery (4 months total).

— Spinal Cord Injured Patients: 20 mg/kg/day for 2 weeks followed by 10 mg/kg/day for 10 weeks (12 weeks total). **Didronel** therapy should begin as soon as medically feasible following the injury, preferably prior to evidence of heterotopic ossification.

Retreatment has not been studied.

HOW SUPPLIED

Didronel is available as 200-mg, white, rectangular tablets with "P & G" on one face and "402" on the other.

NDC 0149-0405-60 bottle of 60

400-mg, white, scored, capsule-shaped tablets with "N E" on one face and "406" on the other.

NDC 0149-0406-60 bottle of 60

Avoid excessive heat (over 104°F or 40°C).

CAUTION: Federal law prohibits dispensing without prescription.

Procter & Gamble Pharmaceuticals
Cincinnati, Ohio 45202

Continued on next page

Didronel—Cont.

REVISED APRIL 1996 40560-P7

Shown in Product Identification Guide, page 332

HELIDAC® Therapy ℞

Pharmacist Information & Counseling Aid and Packaging Insert

PHARMACIST INFORMATION & COUNSELING AID
Not intended for distribution to Patient

- This Counseling Aid contains concise information for the Pharmacist and is meant to aid in counseling; please refer to the attached Package Insert for complete prescribing information.
- There is a detailed PATIENT INFORMATION BOOKLET contained in this package which should be read by the Patient prior to initiating therapy.
- Instructions for opening the enclosed dosing blister cards can be found on the top of this package.

For Your Information

- *Helicobacter pylori* infection has been found to play a primary role in the pathogenesis of duodenal ulcers, and is considered the causative organism in 80% to 95% of patients with duodenal ulcers.
- The components of HELIDAC Therapy [bismuth subsalicylate (BSS), metronidazole (MTZ), and tetracycline hydrochloride (TCN)] are indicated for the treatment of patients with an active duodenal ulcer associated with *Helicobacter pylori* infection. The eradication of *H. pylori* has been demonstrated to reduce the risk of duodenal ulcer recurrence. Appropriate doses of an H_2 antagonist indicated for the treatment of active duodenal ulcer should be prescribed for ulcer healing.
- HELIDAC Therapy is a combination of three antimicrobial agents: bismuth subsalicylate, metronidazole, and tetracycline hydrochloride. Clinical trials using this combination have demonstrated *H. pylori* eradication in up to 82% of patients with a duodenal ulcer. Please note: bismuth subsalicylate is used in this combination for its antimicrobial properties and not for symptomatic relief of upset stomach.
- Clinical data show that eradication of *H. pylori* is directly related to compliance. This therapy has been designed to enhance compliance and contains 14 blister cards, one for each day of the 14-day treatment plan, with each card divided into the 4 daily doses. The therapy also contains a patient-oriented information booklet and patient reminders.

Information To Share With Your Patient

- Scientists have discovered that most ulcers are caused by an infection from a specific germ called *H. pylori*.
- The medicines in this therapy have been demonstrated to treat the infection in the majority of cases when taken correctly. Treating the infection is important to reduce the risk of the ulcer coming back.
- Each pill of every dose is important. Studies have shown that taking all this medicine is very important to eradicate all the ulcer-causing germs. If doses are skipped or treatment is stopped early, some of these germs may not be eradicated and another ulcer can develop.

Dosing and Administration

It may be useful to open the therapy and explain dosing while showing the patient one of the dosing blister cards.

- Each dose includes 4 pills: 2 pink round chewable tablets (bismuth subsalicylate), 1 white round tablet (metronidazole), and 1 orange & white capsule (tetracycline hydrochloride).
- Take 1 dose (all 4 pills) 4 times a day - at mealtimes and bedtime.
- Chew and swallow the 2 pink tablets.
  Then swallow the white tablet and orange and white capsule whole with a full glass of water (8 ounces).
  Remember: Chew-Chew-Swallow-Swallow = 1 dose.
- All 4 daily doses are contained on an individual blister card.
- This therapy contains 14 blister cards, one card for each day of the 14-day treatment plan.
- If you miss a dose, do not take a double dose. Instead, make up any missed doses by continuing your normal dosing schedule until the medication is gone. (Please contact prescriber if more than 4 doses are missed.)
- Each dose should be taken with a full glass of water (8 ounces), especially the bedtime dose.*
- Concomitantly prescribed H_2 antagonist therapy should be taken as directed.

* To reduce risk of esophageal irritation and ulceration due to tetracycline

OTHER IMPORTANT INFORMATION TO GUIDE YOUR DISCUSSION WITH THE PATIENT

Contraindications:
HELIDAC Therapy is contraindicated in the following patient populations:

- Pregnant or nursing women
- Pediatric patients
- Patients with renal or hepatic impairment
- Patients with known hypersensitivity to bismuth subsalicylate, metronidazole or other nitroimidazole derivatives, or any of the tetracyclines; this product does not contain aspirin, but should not be administered to those patients who have a known allergy to aspirin or salicylates.

Warnings and Precautions (also see Contraindications):
The following is a partial list. Please refer to the Package Insert for more complete information.

- Patients should avoid:
  — Alcohol during therapy and at least 1 day after completion of all doses due to potential metronidazole effects
  — Sun lamps or sun because of possible photosensitivity secondary to tetracycline
  — Other medications without first consulting with your pharmacist or prescriber (See **Drug Interactions**.)
- Administer with caution in patients with central nervous system diseases.
- Administer with caution in elderly patients who may suffer from asymptomatic renal and hepatic dysfunction.
- Bismuth subsalicylate may cause a temporary and harmless darkening of the tongue and/or black stool. This should not be confused with melena (blood in the stool).

Adverse Reactions:
Adverse reactions associated with the individual components of HELIDAC Therapy have been well described and are included in the Package Insert. The most common adverse reactions (≥1%) reported in clinical trials where all three components were given concomitantly and where most patients were on concomitant acid suppression therapy, are as follows: nausea (10.2%), diarrhea (5.1%), abdominal pain (3%), melena (2.5%), anal discomfort (1.5%), anorexia (1.5%), dizziness (1.5%), paresthesia (1.5%), vomiting (1.5%), asthenia (1%), constipation (1%), insomnia (1%), pain (1%), and upper respiratory infection (1%). The majority of the events were related to the gastrointestinal tract, were reversible, and usually did not lead to discontinuation of therapy.

Some other possible adverse reactions include:

- Temporary and harmless darkening of the tongue and/or black stool
- Metallic taste in the mouth
- Temporary darkening of the urine (rare)
- Sore mouth
- Yeast infections in women

As with most medications, rare but serious side effects have been reported with the use of the components contained in HELIDAC Therapy. (See Package Insert.) Patients should be instructed to report any unusual symptoms to their pharmacist or prescriber.

Drug Interactions: See Package Insert for more complete information.

Alcohol: There is a potential for a disulfiram-like interaction with metronidazole. Patients should be warned not to drink alcoholic beverages or alcohol-containing products during therapy and for at least 1 day after the therapy is completed.

Antacids containing aluminum, calcium, or magnesium, and preparations containing iron, zinc, or sodium bicarbonate; or milk or dairy products: Absorption of tetracycline may be impaired when co-administered.

Anticoagulants: Individual components of HELIDAC Therapy have the potential to interact with anticoagulants. Monitoring anticoagulant therapy with appropriate adjustment of the anticoagulant dosage may be warranted if concurrent therapy is instituted. (See Package Insert.)

Antidiabetics: There is a possible enhanced hypoglycemic effect when given with salicylates.

Cimetidine: The simultaneous administration of drugs that decrease microsomal liver enzyme activity, such as cimetidine, may prolong the half-life and decrease plasma clearance of metronidazole.

Oral Contraceptives: As with many antibacterial preparations, concomitant use of HELIDAC Therapy may reduce the effectiveness of estrogen-containing oral contraceptives; breakthrough bleeding may occur. Patients should be advised to use an additional or different form of contraception. **Women who become pregnant while taking HELIDAC Therapy should be advised to notify their prescriber immediately.**

See the Package Insert regarding the following possible, suspected, or confirmed interactions: aspirin, probenecid, sulfinpyrazone, methoxyflurane, penicillin, disulfiram (within 2 weeks), lithium, and microsomal liver enzyme inducers, such as phenytoin or phenobarbital.

In patients stabilized on relatively high doses of lithium, short-term metronidazole therapy has been associated with elevation of serum lithium and, in a few cases, signs of lithium toxicity. Serum lithium and serum creatinine should be obtained several days after beginning metronidazole to detect any increase that may precede clinical symptoms of lithium toxicity.

Although there is an anticipated reduction in tetracycline systemic absorption due to an interaction with bismuth and/or bismuth subsalicylate tablet excipients (calcium carbonate), the relative contribution of systemic versus local antimicrobial activity against *H. pylori* for these agents has not been established.

PACKAGE INSERT

THESE PRODUCTS ARE INTENDED ONLY FOR USE AS DESCRIBED. The individual products contained in this package should not be used alone or in combination for other purposes. The information described in this labeling concerns only the use of these products as indicated in this combination package. For information on use of the individual components when dispensed as individual medications outside this combined use for treating *Helicobacter pylori*, please see the package inserts for each individual product.

WARNING
Metronizadole has been shown to be carcinogenic in mice and rats. (See **PRECAUTIONS**.) Unnecessary use of the drug should be avoided. Its use should be reserved for the conditions described in the **INDICATIONS AND USAGE** section below.

DESCRIPTION

HELIDAC Therapy consists of 112 bismuth subsalicylate 262.4-mg chewable tablets, 56 metronidazole 250-mg tablets, USP, and 56 tetracycline hydrochloride 500-mg capsules, USP, for oral administration.

Bismuth subsalicylate chewable tablets: Each pink round tablet contains 262.4 mg bismuth subsalicylate (102 mg salicylate) for oral administration.

Bismuth subsalicylate is a fine, white, odorless, and tasteless powder that is stable and non-hygroscopic. It is a highly insoluble salt of trivalent bismuth and salicylic acid.

Bismuth subsalicylate is 2-Hydroxybenzoic acid bismuth (3+) salt with the following structural formula:

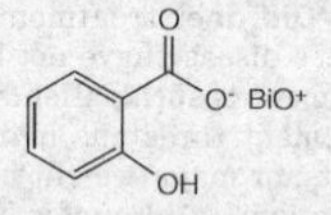

Molecular weight: 362.11

Inactive Ingredients: Each bismuth subsalicylate chewable tablet contains calcium carbonate, D&C Red No. 27 aluminum lake, flavor, magnesium stearate, mannitol, povidone, saccharin sodium, and talc.

Metronidazole tablets, USP: Each white round tablet contains 250 mg metronidazole. Metronidazole is 2-Methyl-5-nitroimidazole-1-ethanol, with the following structural formula:

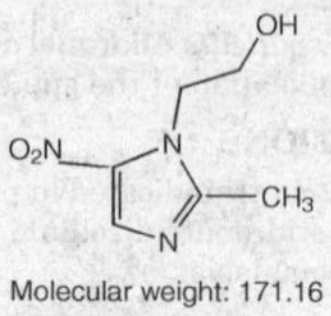

Molecular weight: 171.16

Inactive Ingredients: Each metronidazole tablet contains lactose monohydrate, magnesium stearate, microcrystalline cellulose, povidone, sodium starch glycolate, and stearic acid.

Tetracycline hydrochloride capsules, USP: Each pink and white capsule contains 500 mg tetracycline hydrochloride, causing it to appear pale orange and white in color when filled. Tetracycline is a yellow, odorless, crystalline powder. Tetracycline is stable in air but exposure to strong sunlight causes it to darken. Its potency is affected in solutions of pH below 2 and is rapidly destroyed by alkali hydroxide solutions. Tetracycline is very slightly soluble in water, freely soluble in dilute acid and in alkali hydroxide solutions, sparingly soluble in alcohol, and practically insoluble in chloroform and ether.

Tetracycline hydrochloride is (4S,4aS,5aS,6S,12aS)-4-(Dimethylamino)-1,4,4a,5,5a,6,11,12a-octahydro-3,6,10,12,12a-pentahydroxy-6-methyl-1,11-dioxo-2-naphthacenecarboxamide monohydrochloride, with the following structural formula:

[See chemical structure at top of next column]

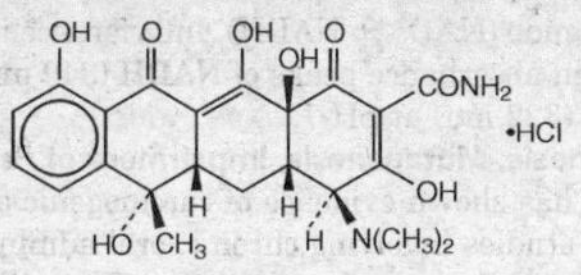

Molecular weight: 480.90

Inactive Ingredients: Each tetracycline hydrochloride capsule contains colloidal silicon dioxide, white ink, FD&C Red No. 40, gelatin, pregelatinized starch, stearic acid, and titanium dioxide.

CLINICAL PHARMACOLOGY

Pharmacokinetics: Pharmacokinetics for the HELIDAC Therapy components (bismuth subsalicylate chewable tablets, metronidazole tablets, and tetracycline hydrochloride capsules) when coadministered has not been studied. There is no information about the gastric mucosal concentrations of bismuth, metronidazole, and tetracycline after administration of these agents concomitantly or in combination with an acid suppressive agent. The systemic pharmacokinetic information presented below is based on studies in which each product was administered alone.

Bismuth Subsalicylate: Upon oral administration, bismuth subsalicylate is almost completely hydrolyzed in the gastrointestinal tract to bismuth and salicylic acid. Thus, the pharmacokinetics of bismuth subsalicylate following oral administration can be described by the individual pharmacokinetics of bismuth and salicylic acid.

Bismuth: Less than 1% of bismuth from oral doses of bismuth subsalicylate is absorbed from the gastrointestinal tract into the systemic circulation. Absorbed bismuth is distributed throughout the body. Bismuth is highly bound to plasma proteins (>90%). Bismuth has multiple disposition half-lives with an intermediate half-life of 5 to 11 days and a terminal half-life of 21 to 72 days. Elimination of bismuth is primarily through urinary and biliary routes with a renal clearance of 50 ± 18 mL/min. The mean trough blood bismuth concentration after 2 weeks oral administration of 787 mg bismuth subsalicylate (3 chewable tablets) four times daily under fasted condition was 5.1 ± 3.1 ng/mL. In another study, the mean trough blood bismuth concentration after 2 weeks oral administration of 525 mg bismuth subsalicylate (as PEPTO-BISMOL® liquid suspension) four times daily was 5 ng/mL with the highest value being 32 ng/mL.

Salicylic Acid: More than 80% of the salicylic acid is absorbed from oral doses of bismuth subsalicylate chewable tablets. Salicylic acid is about 90% plasma protein bound. The volume of distribution is about 170 mL/kg of body weight. Salicylic acid is extensively metabolized and about 10% is excreted unchanged in the urine. The metabolic clearance of salicylic acid is saturable; accordingly, nonlinear pharmacokinetics is observed at bismuth subsalicylate doses above 525 mg. Salicylic acid metabolic clearance is lower in females than in males. The terminal half-life of salicylic acid upon a single oral dose of 525 mg bismuth subsalicylate is between 2 to 5 hours. After a single oral dose of 525 mg bismuth subsalicylate (2 chewable tablets), the mean peak plasma salicylic acid concentration was 13.1 ± 3.4 µg/mL under fasted condition. The mean steady-state serum total salicylate concentration after 2 weeks oral administration of 525 mg bismuth subsalicylate (as PEPTO-BISMOL liquid suspension) four times daily was 24 µg/mL with the highest value being 70 µg/mL.

Metronidazole: Following oral administration, metronidazole is well absorbed, with peak plasma concentrations occurring between 1 and 2 hours after administration. Plasma concentrations of metronidazole are proportional to the administered dose, with oral administration of 250 mg producing a peak plasma concentration of 6 µg/mL. Studies reveal no significant bioavailability differences between males and females; however because of weight differences, the resulting plasma levels in males are generally lower.

Metronidazole is the major component appearing in the plasma, with lesser quantities of the 2-hydroxymethyl metabolite also being present. Less than 20% of the circulating metronidazole is bound to plasma proteins. Metronidazole also appears in cerebrospinal fluid, saliva, and human milk in concentrations similar to those found in plasma.

The average elimination half-life in normal volunteers is 8 hours. The major route of elimination of metronidazole and its metabolites is via the urine (60% to 80% of the dose), with fecal excretion accounting for 6% to 15% of the dose. The metabolites that appear in the urine result primarily from side-chain oxidation [1-(β-hydroxyethyl)-2-hydroxymethyl-5-nitroimidazole and 2-methyl-5-nitroimidazole-1-yl-acetic acid] and glucuronide conjugation, with unchanged metronidazole accounting for approximately 20% of the total. Renal clearance of metronidazole is approximately 10 mL/min/1.73 m^2.

Decreased renal function does not alter the single-dose pharmacokinetics of metronidazole. In patients with decreased liver function, plasma clearance of metronidazole is decreased.

Tetracycline Hydrochloride: Tetracyclines are readily absorbed and are bound to plasma proteins in varying degrees. They are concentrated by the liver in the bile and excreted in the urine and feces at high concentrations in a biologically active form.

The relative contribution of systemic versus local antimicrobial activity against *H. pylori* for agents used in eradication therapy has not been established.

Microbiology: Bismuth subsalicylate, metronidazole, and tetracycline individually have demonstrated *in vitro* activity against most susceptible strains of *Helicobacter pylori*.

Helicobacter: *Helicobacter pylori*: Metronidazole resistance has been increasing in the U.S. and mostly occurs in patients previously treated with metronidazole. Some *H. pylori* strains isolated from patients treated with bismuth, metronidazole, and tetracycline demonstrate an increase in metronidazole MIC's, indicating decreasing susceptibility and increasing resistance.

In the clinical studies, pretreatment and emerging resistance were not assessed for bismuth subsalicylate, metronidazole, or tetracycline, because susceptibility testing was not performed. No adequate data were collected during the clinical studies to indicate that bismuth subsalicylate can either decrease or increase metronidazole resistance.

It is recommended that all patients not eradicated of *H. pylori* following bismuth subsalicylate, metronidazole, and tetracycline treatment be considered to have *H. pylori* resistant to metronidazole. Patients who fail therapy should not be retreated with a regimen containing metronidazole.

***In vitro* Activity of Bismuth Subsalicylate, Metronidazole, and Tetracycline Hydrochloride against *Helicobacter pylori*:** Bismuth subsalicylate, metronidazole, and tetracycline individually have demonstrated *in vitro* activity against most susceptible strains of *Helicobacter pylori* isolated from patients with duodenal ulcers.

In vitro susceptibility testing methods (broth microdilution, agar dilution, E-test, and disk diffusion) and diagnostic products currently available for determining minimum inhibitory concentrations (MIC's) and zone sizes have not been standardized, validated, or approved for testing *H. pylori*. MIC values and zone sizes will vary depending on the susceptibility testing methodology employed, media, growth additives, inoculum concentration tested, growth phase, incubation atmosphere, and time.

INDICATIONS AND USAGE

The components of the HELIDAC Therapy (bismuth subsalicylate, metronidazole, and tetracycline hydrochloride), in combination with an H_2 antagonist are indicated for the treatment of patients with an active duodenal ulcer associated with *Helicobacter pylori* infection. The eradication of *H. pylori* has been demonstrated to reduce the risk of duodenal ulcer recurrence. Appropriate doses of H_2 antagonists for the treatment of active duodenal ulcers should be prescribed for ulcer healing. (See **DOSAGE AND ADMINISTRATION**.)

It is recommended that all patients not eradicated of *Helicobacter pylori* following HELIDAC Therapy plus an H_2 antagonist should be considered to have *Helicobacter pylori* resistant to metronidazole. Patients who fail therapy should not be retreated with a regimen containing metronidazole. (See **Microbiology** subsection.)

CLINICAL STUDIES

Investigators in the U.S. (Graham et al., 1991, 1992, and Cutler et al., 1993) and Germany (Labenz et al., 1993) studied the effect of therapy on the eradication of *H. pylori* using bismuth subsalicylate, metronidazole, and tetracycline hydrochloride. The patient population in these studies consisted predominantly of duodenal ulcer patients with active disease. In addition to bismuth subsalicylate, metronidazole, tetracycline hydrochloride triple therapy, most patients were also prescribed antisecretory therapy at doses recommended for ulcer healing, with the majority receiving ranitidine. The primary efficacy variable used in these studies to determine effectiveness of therapy was *H. pylori* eradication, or cure of infection. Use of cure of infection as a surrogate for reduced ulcer recurrence is based on an extensive review of the literature (Hopkins RJ, Girardi LS, Turney EA. The relationship between *H. pylori* eradication and reduced duodenal and gastric ulcer recurrence: A review. Gastroenterol 1996; 110:1244-52). Eradication rates are derived from results of the randomized, controlled study of Graham et al. and the uncontrolled, nonrandomized study of Cutler et al. *H. pylori* eradication was defined as no positive test (culture, histology, rapid urease, or ^{13}C breath test) at least 4 weeks following the end of treatment. In the analysis performed, dropouts and patients with missing *H. pylori* tests post-treatment were excluded. HELIDAC Therapy (bismuth subsalicylate, metronidazole, and tetracycline hydrochloride) was effective in eradicating *H. pylori*.

***Helicobacter pylori* Eradication Rates in Patients with Duodenal Ulcer**

Investigator	Eradication Rate in Duodenal Ulcer Patients†	95% Confidence Intervals
Graham[1,2]	77% (n=39)	61%–89%
Culter[3]	82% (n=51)	70%–92%

† Evaluable patients were defined as having a confirmed duodenal ulcer within 2 years prior to treatment and having taken 14 days of bismuth subsalicylate, metronidazole, and tetracycline (range 11 to 17 days). Eradication was defined as no evidence of *H. pylori* infection by culture, histology, rapid urease test and/or urea breath test from at least 4 weeks post-treatment up to 1 year post-treatment.

Graham et al. 1992 (2) studied long-term outcome in patients treated for active duodenal ulcer by frequently monitoring for ulcer recurrence for up to 1 year after therapy. This study compared patients who received bismuth subsalicylate (BSS), metronidazole (MTZ), and tetracycline hydrochloride (TCN) for 2 weeks with ranitidine to those who received ranitidine alone. The ulcer recurrence rates at 6 months and 1 year regardless of post-treatment eradication status are summarized below for duodenal ulcer patients who were *H. pylori* positive at baseline.

Duodenal Ulcer Recurrence Rates at 6 Months†

Therapy	All Patients	*H. pylori* Negative Patients Post-Treatment
BSS/MTZ/TCN + Ranitidine	4% (1/25)	6% (1/18)
Ranitidine	85% (17/20)	100% (1/1)

Duodenal Ulcer Recurrence Rates at 1 Year†

Therapy	All Patients	*H. pylori* Negative Patients Post-Treatment
BSS/MTZ/TCN + Ranitidine	9% (2/22)	13% (2/16)
Ranitidine	95% (18/19)	100% (1/1)

† Includes all patients randomized to therapy who were *H. pylori* positive at baseline (by culture, histology, and/or urea breath test) who had ulcer healing and 24 or 48 weeks of endoscopic follow-up data.

CONTRAINDICATIONS

This therapy is contraindicated in pregnant or nursing women, pediatric patients, in patients with renal or hepatic impairment, and in those with known hypersensitivity to bismuth subsalicylate, metronidazole or other nitroimidazole derivatives, or any of the tetracyclines. (See **WARNINGS** and **PRECAUTIONS**.) This product does not contain aspirin but should not be administered to those patients who have a known allergy to aspirin or salicylates.

WARNINGS

Bismuth Subsalicylate

Children and teenagers who have or who are recovering from chicken pox or flu should NOT use this medicine to treat nausea or vomiting. If nausea or vomiting is present, patients are advised to consult a doctor because this could be an early sign of Reye's syndrome, a rare but serious illness.

There have been rare reports of neurotoxicity associated with excessive doses of bismuth subsalicylate. Effects have been reversible with discontinuation of therapy.

Metronidazole

Central Nervous System Effects: Convulsive seizures and peripheral neuropathy, the latter characterized mainly by numbness or paresthesia of an extremity, have been reported in patients treated with metronidazole. The prevalence and severity of the neuropathy are directly related to the cumulative dose and duration of therapy, being most prevalent in patients taking high doses for prolonged treatment periods. The appearance of abnormal neurologic signs demands the prompt discontinuation of metronidazole therapy. Metronidazole should be administered with caution to patients with central nervous system diseases.

Pregnancy: Teratogenic Effects. Metronidazole crosses the placental barrier and its effects on the human fetal or-

Continued on next page

Helidac Therapy—Cont.

ganogenesis are not known. No fetotoxicity was observed when metronidazole was administered orally to pregnant mice at 20 mg/kg/day approximately one and a half times the most frequently recommended human dose (750 mg/day) based on mg/kg body weight; however, in a single small study where the drug was administered intraperitoneally, some intrauterine deaths were observed. The relationship of these findings to the drug is unknown.

Tetracycline

THE USE OF DRUGS OF THE TETRACYCLINE CLASS DURING TOOTH DEVELOPMENT (LAST HALF OF PREGNANCY, INFANCY, AND CHILDHOOD TO THE AGE OF 8 YEARS) MAY CAUSE PERMANENT DISCOLORATION OF THE TEETH (YELLOW-GRAY-BROWN). This adverse reaction is more common during long-term use of the drugs but has been observed following repeated short-term courses. Enamel hypoplasia has also been reported. TETRACYCLINE HYDROCHLORIDE IS A COMPONENT OF THE HELIDAC THERAPY, THEREFORE, HELIDAC THERAPY SHOULD NOT BE USED IN THESE PATIENT POPULATIONS. (See **CONTRAINDICATIONS**.)

Tetracycline hydrochloride, as a component of the HELIDAC Therapy, should not be used during pregnancy. Results of animal studies indicate that tetracyclines cross the placenta, are found in fetal tissues, and can have toxic effects on the developing fetus (often related to retardation of skeletal development). Evidence of embryotoxicity has also been noted in animals treated early in pregnancy. If this drug is used during pregnancy or if the patient becomes pregnant while taking this drug, the patient should be apprised of the potential hazard to the fetus.

Photosensitivity manifested by an exaggerated sunburn reaction has been observed in some individuals taking tetracyclines. Patients apt to be exposed to direct sunlight or ultraviolet light should be advised that this reaction can occur with tetracycline drugs. Treatment should be discontinued at the first evidence of skin erythema.

The antianabolic action of the tetracyclines may cause an increase in blood urea nitrogen (BUN). While this is not a problem in those with normal renal function, in patients with significantly impaired renal function, higher serum levels of tetracycline may lead to azotemia, hyperphosphatemia, and acidosis.

PRECAUTIONS

General:

Bismuth Subsalicylate

Bismuth subsalicylate may cause a temporary and harmless darkening of the tongue and/or black stool. Stool darkening should not be confused with melena.

Metronidazole

Patients with severe hepatic disease metabolize metronidazole slowly, with resultant accumulation of metronidazole and its metabolites in plasma. (See **CONTRAINDICATIONS**.) Metronidazole is a nitroimidazole and should be used with caution in patients with evidence of, or history of, blood dyscrasia. A mild leukopenia has been observed; however, no persistent hematologic abnormalities attributable to metronidazole have been observed.

Known or previously unrecognized candidiasis may present more prominent symptoms during therapy with metronidazole and requires treatment with a candicidal agent.

Tetracycline

As with other antibiotics, use of tetracycline hydrochloride may result in overgrowth of nonsusceptible organisms, including fungi. If superinfection occurs, tetracycline should be discontinued and appropriate therapy should be instituted.

Pseudotumor cerebri (benign intracranial hypertension) in adults has been associated with the use of tetracyclines. The usual clinical manifestations are headache and blurred vision. While this condition and related symptoms usually resolve soon after discontinuation of the tetracycline, the possibility for permanent sequelae exists.

Information for Patients: Each dose includes 4 pills: 2 pink round chewable tablets (bismuth subsalicylate), 1 white round tablet (metronidazole), and 1 orange and white capsule (tetracycline hydrochloride). Each dose (all 4 pills) should be taken 4 times a day, at mealtimes and bedtime. Patients should be instructed to chew and swallow the pink round tablets (bismuth subsalicylate tablets) and to swallow the white round tablet (metronidazole tablet) and the pale orange and white capsule (tetracycline hydrochloride capsule) whole with a full glass of water (8 ounces). Concomitantly prescribed H_2 antagonist therapy should be taken as directed.

Administration of adequate amounts of fluid, particularly with the bedtime dose of tetracycline hydrochloride, is recommended to reduce the risk of esophageal irritation and ulceration. (See **ADVERSE REACTIONS**.)

Missed doses can be made up by continuing the normal dosing schedule until the medication is gone. Patients should not take double doses. (If more than 4 doses are missed, the prescriber should be contacted.)

This treatment regimen includes salicylates. If taken with aspirin and ringing in the ears occurs, the prescriber should be consulted concerning discontinuation of the aspirin therapy until the HELIDAC Therapy is completed.

Concurrent use of tetracyclines may render oral contraceptives less effective. Patients should be advised to use a different or additional form of contraception. Breakthrough bleeding has been reported. Women who become pregnant while taking components of the HELIDAC Therapy should be advised to notify their prescriber immediately. (See **CONTRAINDICATIONS** and **WARNINGS**.)

Alcoholic beverages should be avoided while taking metronidazole and for at least 1 day afterward. (See **Drug Interactions**.)

Patients taking tetracycline hydrochloride should be cautioned to avoid exposure to sun or sun lamps. (See **WARNINGS**.)

Bismuth subsalicylate may cause temporary and harmless darkening of the tongue and/or black stool. Stool darkening should not be confused with melena (blood in the stool).

Drug Interactions: Individual components of the HELIDAC Therapy have a potential interaction with anticoagulants. Tetracycline has been shown to depress plasma prothrombin activity. Metronidazole has been reported to potentiate the anticoagulant effect of warfarin and other oral coumarin anticoagulants, resulting in a prolongation of prothrombin time. Salicylates may cause an increased risk of bleeding when administered with anticoagulant therapy. Therefore, monitoring anticoagulant therapy with appropriate adjustment of the anticoagulant dosage may be warranted if concurrent therapy is instituted.

Caution is advised in the administration of bismuth subsalicylate to patients taking medication for diabetes (possible enhanced hypoglycemic effect when given with salicylates) or patients taking aspirin, probenecid, or sulfinpyrazone.

Absorption of tetracyclines is impaired by antacids containing aluminum, calcium, or magnesium; preparations containing iron, zinc, or sodium bicarbonate; or milk or dairy products.

There is an anticipated reduction in tetracycline systemic absorption due to an interaction with bismuth and/or calcium carbonate, an excipient of bismuth subsalicylate tablets. The clinical significance of this is unknown as the relative contribution of systemic versus local antimicrobial activity against *H. pylori* for these agents has not been established.

Since bacteriostatic drugs, such as the tetracycline class of antibiotics, may interfere with the bactericidal action of penicillin, it is not advisable to administer these drugs concomitantly.

The concurrent use of tetracycline and methoxyflurane has been reported to result in fatal renal toxicity.

Concurrent use of tetracycline may render oral contraceptives less effective. Patients should be advised to use a different or additional form of contraception. Breakthrough bleeding has been reported. Women who become pregnant while on the HELIDAC Therapy should be advised to notify their prescriber immediately.

The simultaneous administration of drugs that decrease microsomal liver enzyme activity, such as cimetidine, may prolong the half-life and decrease plasma clearance of metronidazole.

The simultaneous administration of drugs that induce microsomal liver enzymes, such as phenytoin or phenobarbital, may accelerate the elimination of metronidazole, resulting in reduced plasma levels; impaired clearance of phenytoin has also been reported.

In patients stabilized on relatively high doses of lithium, short-term metronidazole therapy has been associated with elevation of serum lithium and, in a few cases, signs of lithium toxicity. Serum lithium and serum creatinine should be obtained several days after beginning metronidazole to detect any increase that may precede clinical symptoms of lithium intoxication.

Alcoholic beverages should not be consumed during metronidazole therapy and for at least 1 day afterward because abdominal cramps, nausea, vomiting, headaches, and flushing may occur.

Psychotic reactions have been reported in alcoholic patients who are using metronidazole and disulfiram concurrently. Metronidazole should not be given to patients who have taken disulfiram within the last 2 weeks.

Drug/Laboratory Test Interactions: Bismuth absorbs x-rays and may interfere with x-ray diagnostic procedures of the gastrointestinal tract.

Bismuth subsalicylate may cause a temporary and harmless darkening of the stool. However, this does not interfere with standard tests for occult blood.

Metronidazole may interfere with certain types of determinations of serum chemistry values, such as aspartate aminotransferase (AST, SGOT), alanine aminotransferase (ALT, SGPT), lactate dehydrogenase (LDH), triglycerides, and hexokinase glucose. Values of zero may be observed. All of the assays in which interference has been reported involve enzymatic coupling of the assay to oxidation-reduction of nicotinamide ($NAD^+ \Leftrightarrow NADH$). Interference is due to the similarity in absorbance peaks of NADH (340 nm) and metronidazole (322 nm) at pH 7.

Carcinogenesis, Mutagenesis, Impairment of Fertility: Metronidazole has shown evidence of carcinogenic activity in a number of studies involving chronic, oral administration in mice and rats. Prominent among the effects in the mouse was an increased incidence of pulmonary tumorigenesis. This has been observed in all six reported studies in that species, including one study in which the animals were dosed on an intermittent schedule (administration during every fourth week only). At very high dose levels, (approximately 500 mg/kg/day, which is approximately 33 times the most frequently recommended human dose for a 50 kg adult based on mg/kg body weight), there was a statistically significant increase in the incidence of malignant liver tumors in male mice. Also, the published results of one of the mouse studies indicate an increase in the incidence of malignant lymphomas as well as pulmonary neoplasms associated with lifetime feeding of the drug. All these effects are statistically significant. Long-term, oral-dosing studies in the rat showed statistically significant increases in the incidence of various neoplasms, particularly in mammary and hepatic tumors, among female rats administered metronidazole over those noted in the concurrent female control groups. Two lifetime tumorigenicity studies in hamsters have been performed and reported to be negative.

There has been no evidence of carcinogenicity for tetracycline hydrochloride in studies conducted with rats and mice. Some related antibiotics (oxytetracycline, minocycline) have shown evidence of oncogenic activity in rats.

No long-term toxicity studies have been conducted with bismuth subsalicylate.

No long-term studies have been performed to evaluate the effect of the combined use of bismuth subsalicylate, metronidazole, and tetracycline on carcinogenesis, mutagenesis, or impairment of fertility.

Although metronidazole has shown mutagenic activity in a number of *in vitro* assay systems, studies in mammals (*in vivo*) have failed to demonstrate a potential for genetic damage.

In two *in vitro* mammalian cell assay systems (L51784y mouse lymphoma and Chinese hamster lung cells), there was evidence of mutagenicity by tetracycline hydrochloride at concentrations of 60 and 10 μg/mL, respectively.

Bismuth did not show mutagenic potential in the NTP salmonella plate assay.

No reproductive toxicity studies have been conducted with bismuth subsalicylate.

Tetracycline hydrochloride had no effect on fertility when administered in the diet to male and female rats at a daily intake of 25 times the human dose.

Metronidazole, at doses up to 400 mg/kg/day (approximately 3.5 times the recommended maximum human dose based on mg/m^2) for 28 days, failed to produce any adverse effects on fertility and testicular function in male rats. Fertility studies have been performed in mice at doses up to six times the maximum recommended human dose based on mg/m^2 and have revealed no evidence of impaired fertility.

Pregnancy: Teratogenic Effects. Pregnancy Category D: Category D is based on the pregnancy category for tetracycline hydrochloride. (See **CONTRAINDICATIONS** and **WARNINGS**, **Tetracycline** and **Metronidazole** subsections.)

Non-teratogenic Effects: (See **WARNINGS**.)

Pregnant women with renal disease may be more prone to develop tetracycline-associated liver failure.

Labor and Delivery: The effect of this therapy on labor and delivery is unknown.

Nursing Mothers: Metronidazole and tetracycline are both secreted into human milk. Because of the potential for tumorigenicity shown for metronidazole in mouse and rat studies, and because of the potential for serious adverse reactions in nursing infants from tetracyclines, a decision should be made whether to discontinue nursing or to discontinue therapy, taking into account the importance of the therapy to the mother. Metronidazole is secreted in human milk in concentrations similar to those found in plasma. (See **CONTRAINDICATIONS**.)

Pediatric Use: Safety and effectiveness in pediatric patients infected with *H. pylori* have not been established. (See **CONTRAINDICATIONS** and **WARNINGS**.)

Geriatric Use: Elderly patients may suffer from asymptomatic renal and hepatic dysfunction. Care should be taken when administering this therapy to this patient population.

ADVERSE REACTIONS

The most common adverse reactions (≥1%) reported in clinical trials when all three components of this therapy were given concomitantly are listed in the table below. The majority of the adverse reactions were related to the gastrointestinal tract, were reversible, and infrequently led to discontinuation of therapy.

Incidence of Adverse Reactions Reported in Clinical Trials (≥1.0%)†

	BSS/MTZ/TCN‡ (n = 197)	Ranitidine (n = 73)
Adverse Reactions	**% Pts**	**% Pts**
Nausea	10.2%	1.4%
Diarrhea	5.1%	0.0%
Abdominal Pain	3.0%	0.0%
Melena	2.5%	0.0%
Anal Discomfort	1.5%	0.0%
Anorexia	1.5%	0.0%
Dizziness	1.5%	0.0%
Paresthesia	1.5%	0.0%
Vomiting	1.5%	0.0%
Asthenia	1.0%	0.0%
Constipation	1.0%	0.0%
Insomnia	1.0%	0.0%
Pain	1.0%	0.0%
Upper Respiratory Infection	1.0%	0.0%

†Includes reactions reported at ≥1.0% in patients taking BSS/MTZ/TCN
‡Most patients were on concomitant acid suppression therapy

The additional adverse reactions (<1%) reported in clinical trials when all three components of this therapy were given concomitantly are listed below and divided by body system:
Gastrointestinal: dry mouth, dyspepsia, dysphagia, flatulence, gastrointestinal hemorrhage, glossitis, stomatitis
Skin: photosensitivity reaction (see **WARNINGS**), rash
Cardiovascular: hypertension, myocardial infarction
CNS: nervousness
Musculoskeletal: rheumatoid arthritis
Other: malaise, syncope
The following adverse reactions from the labeling for bismuth subsalicylate are provided for information.
Gastrointestinal: black stools
Mouth: temporary and harmless darkening of the tongue
The following adverse reactions from the labeling for metronidazole are provided for information.
Gastrointestinal: The most common adverse reactions reported have been referable to the gastrointestinal tract, particularly nausea reported by about 12% of patients, sometimes accompanied by headache, anorexia, and occasionally vomiting, diarrhea, epigastric distress, and abdominal cramping. Constipation has also been reported.
Mouth: A sharp, unpleasant metallic taste is not unusual. Furry tongue, glossitis, stomatitis have occurred; these may be associated with a sudden overgrowth of *Candida* which may occur during therapy.
Blood: Reversible neutropenia (leukopenia); rarely, reversible thrombocytopenia.
Cardiovascular: Flattening of the T-wave may be seen in electrocardiographic tracings.
CNS: Convulsive seizures, peripheral neuropathy, dizziness, vertigo, incoordination, ataxia, confusion, irritability, depression, weakness, and insomnia. Two serious adverse reactions reported in patients treated with metronidazole have been convulsive seizures and peripheral neuropathy, the latter characterized mainly by numbness or paresthesia of an extremity. Since persistent peripheral neuropathy has been reported in some patients receiving prolonged administration of metronidazole, patients should be specifically warned about these reactions and should be told to stop the drug and report immediately to their physicians if any neurologic symptoms occur.
Hypersensitivity: urticaria, erythematous rash, flushing, nasal congestion, dryness of mouth (or vagina or vulva), and fever
Renal: Dysuria, cystitis, polyuria, incontinence, and a sense of pelvic pressure. Instances of darkened urine have been reported by approximately one patient in 100,000. Although the pigment which is probably responsible for this phenomenon has not been positively identified, it is almost certainly a metabolite of metronidazole and seems to have no clinical significance.
Other: Proliferation of *Candida* in the vagina, dyspareunia, decrease of libido, proctitis, and fleeting joint pains sometimes resembling "serum sickness." If patients receiving metronidazole drink alcoholic beverages, they may experience abdominal distress, nausea, vomiting, flushing, or headache. A modification of the taste of alcoholic beverages has also been reported. Crohn's disease patients are known to have an increased incidence of gastrointestinal and certain extraintestinal cancers. There have been some reports in the medical literature of breast and colon cancer in Crohn's disease patients who have been treated with metronidazole at high doses for extended periods of time. A cause and effect relationship has not been established. Rare cases of pancreatitis, which abated on withdrawal of the drug, have been reported.

The following adverse reactions from the labeling for tetracycline hydrochloride are provided for information.
Gastrointestinal: Anorexia, nausea, epigastric distress, vomiting, diarrhea, glossitis, black hairy tongue, dysphagia, enterocolitis, and inflammatory lesions (with monilial overgrowth) in the anogenital region. Rare instances of esophagitis and esophageal ulceration have been reported in patients taking the tetracycline-class antibiotics in capsule and tablet form. Most of the patients who experienced esophageal irritation took the medication immediately before going to bed. (See **DOSAGE AND ADMINISTRATION**.)
Liver: Hepatotoxicity and liver failure have been observed in patients receiving large doses of tetracycline and in tetracycline-treated patients with renal impairment. Increases in liver enzymes and hepatic toxicity have been reported rarely.
Teeth: Permanent discoloration of teeth may be caused during tooth development. Enamel hypoplasia has also been reported. (See **WARNINGS**.)
Blood: hemolytic anemia, thrombocytopenia, thrombocytopenic purpura, neutropenia, and eosinophilia
CNS: Pseudotumor cerebri (benign intracranial hypertension) in adults and bulging fontanels in infants. (See **PRECAUTIONS: Tetracycline**.) Dizziness, tinnitus, and visual disturbances have been reported. Myasthenic syndrome has been reported rarely.
Hypersensitivity: urticaria, angioneurotic edema, anaphylaxis, anaphylactoid purpura, pericarditis, exacerbation of systemic lupus erythematosus and serum sickness-like reactions, as fever, rash, and arthralgia
Renal: Rise in BUN has been reported and is apparently dose related. (See **WARNINGS**.)
Skin: Maculopapular and erythematous rashes have been reported. Exfoliative dermatitis has been rarely reported. Photosensitivity (see **WARNINGS**), onycholysis, and discoloration of the nails have been reported rarely.
Other: When given over prolonged periods, tetracyclines have been reported to produce brown-black microscopic discoloration of thyroid glands. No abnormalities of thyroid function studies are known to occur.

OVERDOSAGE

In case of an overdose, patients should contact a physician, poison control center, or emergency room. If all three components of this therapy are involved in an overdose, acute treatment should focus on the salicylate intoxication. There is neither a pharmacologic basis nor data suggesting an increased toxicity of the combination compared to individual components.
Bismuth Subsalicylate: The main concern of an acute bismuth subsalicylate (BSS) overdose focuses on the salicylate burden and not on bismuth, since less than 1% of the bismuth is normally absorbed. Each 262.4-mg tablet of BSS contains an amount of salicylate comparable to approximately 130 mg aspirin. Acute ingestion of less than 150 mg/kg of aspirin (i.e., less than one tablet of bismuth subsalicylate per kilogram of body weight) is not expected to lead to toxicity. Mild to moderate toxicity may result from the ingestion of 150 to 300 mg/kg, while severe toxicity may occur from ingestions over 300 mg/kg. Salicylate intoxication is well described in the literature and presents a complex clinical picture. Multiple respiratory and metabolic effects result in fluid, electrolyte, glucose, and acid-base disturbances. Initial symptoms of salicylate toxicity include hyperpnea, nausea, vomiting, tinnitus, hyperpyrexia, lethargy, tachycardia, and confusion. In severe cases, these symptoms may progress to severe hyperpnea, convulsions, pulmonary or cerebral edema, respiratory failure, cardiovascular collapse, coma, and death.
Treatment: There is no specific antidote for salicylate poisoning. If there are no contraindications, vomiting should be induced as soon as possible with syrup of ipecac, or gastric lavage should be instituted, provided that no more than one hour has elapsed since ingestion. Activated charcoal and a cathartic may be administered as primary decontamination therapy in those cases where greater than one hour has elapsed since ingestion, or to further decontaminate the gastrointestinal tract in those who have already received ipecac or gastric lavage. Plasma salicylate levels may be useful; a common nomogram can be used to help predict the severity of intoxication. Supportive and symptomatic treatment should be provided, with emphasis on correcting fluid, electrolyte, blood glucose, and acid-base disturbances. (Note: An acidotic blood pH increases the un-ionized salicylate form, allowing more to reach the central nervous system.) Elimination may be enhanced by urinary alkalinization, hemodialysis, or hemoperfusion. Since hemodialysis aids in correcting acid-base disturbances, this method may be preferred over hemoperfusion.
Metronidazole: Single oral doses of metronidazole, up to 19.5 g in adults, have been reported without resultant serious toxicity in suicide attempts and accidental overdoses. Symptoms reported include nausea, vomiting, and ataxia. Neurotoxic effects, including seizures and peripheral neuropathy, have been reported after 5 to 7 days of doses of 6 to 10.4 g every other day.
Treatment: There is no specific antidote for metronidazole overdose. Management of the patient should consist of symptomatic and supportive therapy. Metronidazole is dialyzable.
Tetracycline: The acute toxicity of tetracycline in overdose is not well established in the literature. Therapeutic and overdose quantities of tetracycline can cause gastrointestinal symptoms such as nausea, vomiting, and diarrhea.
Treatment: There is no specific antidote for tetracycline overdose. Management of the patient should consist of symptomatic and supportive therapy. Tetracycline is not dialyzable.

DOSAGE AND ADMINISTRATION

Adults: The recommended dosages are: bismuth subsalicylate, 525 mg (two 262.4 mg-chewable tablets), metronidazole, 250 mg (one 250-mg tablet), and tetracycline hydrochloride, 500 mg (one 500-mg capsule) taken four times daily (q.i.d.) for 14 days plus an H_2 antagonist approved for the treatment of acute duodenal ulcer. Patients should be instructed to take the medicines at mealtimes and at bedtime. The bismuth subsalicylate tablets should be chewed and swallowed. The metronidazole tablet and tetracycline hydrochloride capsule should be swallowed whole with a full glass of water (8 ounces). Concomitantly prescribed H_2 antagonist therapy should be taken as directed.
Ingestion of adequate amounts of fluid, particularly with the bedtime dose of tetracycline hydrochloride, is recommended to reduce the risk of esophageal irritation and ulceration. (See **ADVERSE REACTIONS**.)
Missed doses can be made up by continuing the normal dosing schedule until the medication is gone. Patients should not take double doses. If more than 4 doses are missed, the prescriber should be contacted.

HOW SUPPLIED

The HELIDAC Therapy is supplied in a carton containing patient instructions, patient reminders, and 14 blister cards, each card containing the following daily dosage:

8 bismuth subsalicylate 262.4-mg chewable tablets, each pink round tablet engraved "PG 11"

4 metronidazole 250-mg tablets, each white round tablet engraved "PG" on the upper half and "10" on the lower half of the tablet

4 tetracycline hydrochloride 500-mg capsules, each pale orange and white capsule printed "PG 12" in white ink

NDC 0149-0495-01 carton containing 14 days of therapy
Store at controlled room temperature 20°–25°C (68°–77°F) [See USP].

REFERENCES

1. Graham DY, Lew GM, Evans DG, Evans DJ Jr, Klein PD. Effect of triple therapy (antibiotics plus bismuth) on duodenal ulcer healing. Ann Intern Med 1991; 115:266-69.
2. Graham DY, Lew GM, Klein PD, Evans DG, Evans DJ Jr, Saeed ZA, Malaty HM. Effect of treatment of *Helicobacter pylori* infection on the long-term recurrence of gastric or duodenal ulcer. Ann Int Med 1992; 116:705-08.
3. Cutler AF, Schubert TT. Long-term *Helicobacter pylori* recurrence after successful eradication with triple therapy. Am J Gastroenterol 1993; 88:1359-61.

CAUTION: Federal law prohibits dispensing without prescription.

Sold Under U.S. Patent No. 5,256,684

PEPTO-BISMOL is the registered trademark of The Procter & Gamble Company.

Bismuth subsalicylate tablets are manufactured by Procter & Gamble Pharmaceuticals. Metronidazole 250-mg tablets, USP and tetracycline hydrochloride 500-mg capsules, USP are manufactured by Zenith Laboratories, Inc., Northvale, New Jersey 07647 for

Procter & Gamble Pharmaceuticals
Cincinnati, Ohio 45202

REVISED AUGUST 1997 44003435

Shown in Product Identification Guide, page 332

MACROBID® ℞

[mak 'rō bid]
(nitrofurantoin monohydrate/macrocrystals)
Capsules

DESCRIPTION

Nitrofurantoin is an antibacterial agent specific for urinary tract infections. The **Macrobid®** brand of nitrofurantoin is a hard gelatin capsule shell containing the equivalent of 100 mg of nitrofurantoin in the form of 25 mg of nitrofurantoin macrocrystals and 75 mg of nitrofurantoin monohydrate. The chemical name of nitrofurantoin macrocrystals is 1-[[[5-nitro-2-furanyl]methylene]amino]-2,4- imidazolidinedione. The chemical structure is the following:
[See chemical structure at top of next column]

Continued on next page

Macrobid—Cont.

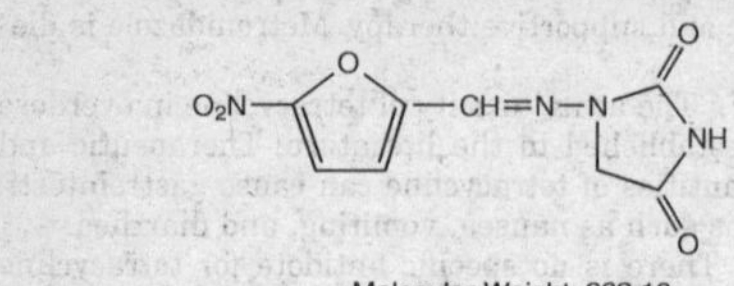

Molecular Weight: 238.16

The chemical name of nitrofurantoin monohydrate is 1-[[[5-nitro-2-furanyl]methylene]amino]-2,4- imidazolidinedione monohydrate. The chemical structure is the following:

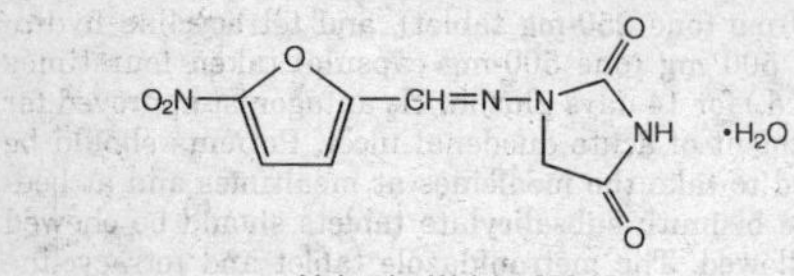

Molecular Weight: 256.17

Inactive Ingredients: Each capsule contains carbomer 934P, corn starch, compressible sugar, D&C Yellow No. 10, edible gray ink, FD&C Blue No. 1, FD&C Red No. 40, gelatin, lactose, magnesium stearate, povidone, talc, and titanium dioxide.

CLINICAL PHARMACOLOGY

Each **Macrobid** capsule contains two forms of nitrofurantoin. Twenty-five percent is macrocrystalline nitrofurantoin, which has slower dissolution and absorption than nitrofurantoin monohydrate. The remaining 75% is nitrofurantoin monohydrate contained in a powder blend which, upon exposure to gastric and intestinal fluids, forms a gel matrix that releases nitrofurantoin over time. Based on urinary pharmacokinetic data, the extent and rate of urinary excretion of nitrofurantoin from the 100-mg **Macrobid** capsule are similar to those of the 50-mg or 100-mg **Macrodantin®** (nitrofurantoin macrocrystals) capsule. Approximately 20–25% of a single dose of nitrofurantoin is recovered from the urine unchanged over 24 hours. Plasma nitrofurantoin concentrations after a single oral dose of the 100-mg **Macrobid** capsule are low, with peak levels usually less than 1 mcg/mL. Nitrofurantoin is highly soluble in urine, to which it may impart a brown color. When **Macrobid** is administered with food, the bioavailability of nitrofurantoin is increased by approximately 40%.

Microbiology: Nitrofurantoin is bactericidal in urine at therapeutic doses. The mechanism of the antimicrobial action of nitrofurantoin is unusual among antibacterials. Nitrofurantoin is reduced by bacterial flavoproteins to reactive intermediates which inactivate or alter bacterial ribosomal proteins and other macromolecules. As a result of such inactivations, the vital biochemical processes of protein synthesis, aerobic energy metabolism, DNA synthesis, RNA synthesis, and cell wall synthesis are inhibited. The broad-based nature of this mode of action may explain the lack of acquired bacterial resistance to nitrofurantoin, as the necessary multiple and simultaneous mutations of the target macromolecules would likely be lethal to the bacteria. Development of resistance to nitrofurantoin has not been a significant problem since its introduction in 1953. Cross-resistance with antibiotics and sulfonamides has not been observed, and transferable resistance is, at most, a very rare phenomenon. Nitrofurantoin, in the form of **Macrobid**, has been shown to be active against most strains of the following bacteria both *in vitro* and in clinical infections: (See **INDICATIONS AND USAGE.**)

Gram-Positive Aerobes
Staphylococcus saprophyticus

Gram-Negative Aerobes
Escherichia coli

Nitrofurantoin also demonstrates *in vitro* activity against the following microorganisms, although the clinical significance of these data with respect to treatment with **Macrobid** is unknown:

Gram-Positive Aerobes
Coagulase-negative staphylococci (including *Staphylococcus epidermidis*)
Enterococcus faecalis
Staphylococcus aureus
Streptococcus agalactiae
Group D streptococci
Viridans group streptococci

Gram-Negative Aerobes
Citrobacter amalonaticus
Citrobacter diversus
Citrobacter freundii
Klebsiella oxytoca
Klebsiella ozaenae

Nitrofurantoin is not active against most strains of *Proteus* species or *Serratia* species. It has no activity against *Pseudomonas* species. Antagonism has been demonstrated *in vitro* between nitrofurantoin and quinolone antimicrobials. The clinical significance of this finding is unknown.

Susceptibility Tests:
Dilution techniques:
Quantitative methods are used to determine antimicrobial minimal inhibitory concentrations (MIC's). These MIC's provide estimates of the susceptibility of bacteria to antimicrobial compounds. The MIC's should be determined using a standardized procedure. Standardized procedures are based on a dilution method[1] (broth or agar) or equivalent with standardized inoculum concentrations and standardized concentrations of nitrofurantoin powder. The MIC values should be interpreted according to the following criteria:

MIC (μg/mL)	Interpretation
≤ 32	Susceptible (S)
64	Intermediate (I)
≥ 128	Resistant (R)

A report of "Susceptible" indicates that the pathogen is likely to be inhibited if the antimicrobial compound in the urine reaches the concentrations usually achievable. A report of "Intermediate" indicates that the result should be considered equivocal, and, if the microorganism is not fully susceptible to alternative, clinically feasible drugs, the test should be repeated. This category implies possible clinical applicability in body sites where the drug is physiologically concentrated or in situations where high dosage of drug can be used. This category also provides a buffer zone which prevents small uncontrolled technical factors from causing major discrepancies in interpretation. A report of "Resistant" indicates that the pathogen is not likely to be inhibited if the antimicrobial compound in the urine reaches the concentrations usually achievable; other therapy should be selected. Standardized susceptibility test procedures require the use of laboratory control microorganisms to control the technical aspects of the laboratory procedures. Standard nitrofurantoin powder should provide the following MIC values:

Microorganism	MIC (μg/mL)
E. coli ATCC 25922	4–16
S. aureus ATCC 29213	8–32
E. faecalis ATCC 29212	4–16

Diffusion techniques:
Quantitative methods that require measurement of zone diameters also provide reproducible estimates of the susceptibility of bacteria to antimicrobial compounds. One such standardized procedure[2] requires the use of standardized inoculum concentrations. This procedure uses paper disks impregnated with 300-μg nitrofurantoin to test the susceptibility of microorganisms to nitrofurantoin.

Reports from the laboratory providing results of the standard single-disk susceptibility test with a 300-μg nitrofurantoin disk should be interpreted according to the following criteria:

Zone Diameter (mm)	Interpretation
≥ 17	Susceptible (S)
15–16	Intermediate (I)
≤ 14	Resistant (R)

Interpretation should be as stated above for results using dilution techniques. Interpretation involves correlation of the diameter obtained in the disk test with the MIC for nitrofurantoin.

As with standardized dilution techniques, diffusion methods require the use of laboratory control microorganisms that are used to control the technical aspects of the laboratory procedures. For the diffusion technique, the 300-μg nitrofurantoin disk should provide the following zone diameters in these laboratory test quality control strains:

Microorganism	Zone Diameter (mm)
E. coli ATCC 25922	20–25
S. aureus ATCC 25923	18–22

INDICATIONS AND USAGE

Macrobid is indicated only for the treatment of acute uncomplicated urinary tract infections (acute cystitis) caused by susceptible strains of *Escherichia coli* or *Staphylococcus saprophyticus*.

Nitrofurantoin is not indicated for the treatment of pyelonephritis or perinephric abscesses. Nitrofurantoins lack the broader tissue distribution of other therapeutic agents approved for urinary tract infections. Consequently, many patients who are treated with **Macrobid** are predisposed to persistence or reappearance of bacteriuria. (See **CLINICAL STUDIES**.) Urine specimens for culture and susceptibility testing should be obtained before and after completion of therapy. If persistence or reappearance of bacteriuria occurs after treatment with **Macrobid**, other therapeutic agents with broader tissue distribution should be selected. In considering the use of **Macrobid**, lower eradication rates should be balanced against the increased potential for systemic toxicity and for the development of antimicrobial resistance when agents with broader tissue distribution are utilized.

CONTRAINDICATIONS

Anuria, oliguria, or significant impairment of renal function (creatinine clearance under 60 mL per minute or clinically significant elevated serum creatinine) are contraindications. Treatment of this type of patient carries an increased risk of toxicity because of impaired excretion of the drug.

Because of the possibility of hemolytic anemia due to immature erythrocyte enzyme systems (glutathione instability), the drug is contraindicated in pregnant patients at term (38–42 weeks gestation), during labor and delivery, or when the onset of labor is imminent. For the same reason, the drug is contraindicated in neonates under one month of age. **Macrobid** is also contraindicated in those patients with known hypersensitivity to nitrofurantoin.

WARNINGS

ACUTE, SUBACUTE, OR CHRONIC PULMONARY REACTIONS HAVE BEEN OBSERVED IN PATIENTS TREATED WITH NITROFURANTOIN. IF THESE REACTIONS OCCUR, MACROBID SHOULD BE DISCONTINUED AND APPROPRIATE MEASURES TAKEN. REPORTS HAVE CITED PULMONARY REACTIONS AS A CONTRIBUTING CAUSE OF DEATH.

CHRONIC PULMONARY REACTIONS (DIFFUSE INTERSTITIAL PNEUMONITIS OR PULMONARY FIBROSIS, OR BOTH) CAN DEVELOP INSIDIOUSLY. THESE REACTIONS OCCUR RARELY AND GENERALLY IN PATIENTS RECEIVING THERAPY FOR SIX MONTHS OR LONGER. CLOSE MONITORING OF THE PULMONARY CONDITION OF PATIENTS RECEIVING LONG-TERM THERAPY IS WARRANTED AND REQUIRES THAT THE BENEFITS OF THERAPY BE WEIGHED AGAINST POTENTIAL RISKS. (SEE RESPIRATORY REACTIONS.)

Hepatic reactions, including hepatitis, cholestatic jaundice, chronic active hepatitis, and hepatic necrosis, occur rarely. Fatalities have been reported. The onset of chronic active hepatitis may be insidious, and patients should be monitored periodically for changes in biochemical tests that would indicate liver injury. If hepatitis occurs, the drug should be withdrawn immediately and appropriate measures should be taken.

Peripheral neuropathy, which may become severe or irreversible, has occurred. Fatalities have been reported. Conditions such as renal impairment (creatinine clearance under 60 mL per minute or clinically significant elevated serum creatinine), anemia, diabetes mellitus, electrolyte imbalance, vitamin B deficiency, and debilitating disease may enhance the occurrence of peripheral neuropathy. Patients receiving long-term therapy should be monitored periodically for changes in renal function.

Optic neuritis has been reported rarely in postmarketing experience with nitrofurantoin formulations.

Cases of hemolytic anemia of the primaquine-sensitivity type have been induced by nitrofurantoin. Hemolysis appears to be linked to a glucose-6-phosphate dehydrogenase deficiency in the red blood cells of the affected patients. This deficiency is found in 10 percent of Blacks and a small percentage of ethnic groups of Mediterranean and Near-Eastern origin. Hemolysis is an indication for discontinuing **Macrobid**; hemolysis ceases when the drug is withdrawn.

Pseudomembranous colitis has been reported with nearly all antibacterial agents, including nitrofurantoin, and may range from mild to life threatening. Therefore, it is important to consider this diagnosis in patients with diarrhea subsequent to the administration of antibacterial agents.

Treatment with antibacterial agents alters the normal flora of the colon and may permit overgrowth of clostridia. Studies indicate that a toxin produced by *Clostridium difficile* is one primary cause of antibiotic-associated colitis.

After the diagnosis of pseudomembranous colitis has been established, appropriate therapeutic measures should be initiated. Mild cases of pseudomembranous colitis usually respond to drug discontinuation alone. In moderate to severe cases, consideration should be given to management with fluids and electrolytes, protein supplementation, and treatment with an antibacterial drug clinically effective against *Clostridium difficile* colitis.

PRECAUTIONS

Information for Patients: Patients should be advised to take **Macrobid** with food (ideally breakfast and dinner) to further enhance tolerance and improve drug absorption. Patients should be instructed to complete the full course of therapy; however, they should be advised to contact their physician if any unusual symptoms occur during therapy.

Patients should be advised not to use antacid preparations containing magnesium trisilicate while taking **Macrobid**.

Drug Interactions: Antacids containing magnesium trisilicate, when administered concomitantly with nitrofurantoin, reduce both the rate and extent of absorption. The mechanism for this interaction probably is adsorption of nitrofurantoin onto the surface of magnesium trisilicate.

Uricosuric drugs, such as probenecid and sulfinpyrazone, can inhibit renal tubular secretion of nitrofurantoin. The re-

sulting increase in nitrofurantoin serum levels may increase toxicity, and the decreased urinary levels could lessen its efficacy as a urinary tract antibacterial.

Drug/Laboratory Test Interactions: As a result of the presence of nitrofurantoin, a false-positive reaction for glucose in the urine may occur. This has been observed with Benedict's and Fehling's solutions but not with the glucose enzymatic test.

Carcinogenesis, Mutagenesis, Impairment of Fertility: Nitrofurantoin was not carcinogenic when fed to female Holtzman rats for 44.5 weeks or to female Sprague-Dawley rats for 75 weeks. Two chronic rodent bioassays utilizing male and female Sprague-Dawley rats and two chronic bioassays in Swiss mice and in BDF_1 mice revealed no evidence of carcinogenicity. Nitrofurantoin presented evidence of carcinogenic activity in female $B6C3F_1$ mice as shown by increased incidences of tubular adenomas, benign mixed tumors, and granulosa cell tumors of the ovary. In male F344/N rats, there were increased incidences of uncommon kidney tubular cell neoplasms, osteosarcomas of the bone, and neoplasms of the subcutaneous tissue. In one study involving subcutaneous administration of 75 mg/kg nitrofurantoin to pregnant female mice, lung papillary adenomas of unknown significance were observed in the F1 generation. Nitrofurantoin has been shown to induce point mutations in certain strains of *Salmonella typhimurium* and forward mutations in L5178Y mouse lymphoma cells. Nitrofurantoin induced increased numbers of sister chromatid exchanges and chromosomal aberrations in Chinese hamster ovary cells but not in human cells in culture. Results of the sex-linked recessive lethal assay in Drosophila were negative after administration of nitrofurantoin by feeding or by injection. Nitrofurantoin did not induce heritable mutation in the rodent models examined.

The significance of the carcinogenicity and mutagenicity findings relative to the therapeutic use of nitrofurantoin in humans is unknown. The administration of high doses of nitrofurantoin to rats causes temporary spermatogenic arrest; this is reversible on discontinuing the drug. Doses of 10 mg/kg/day or greater in healthy human males may, in certain unpredictable instances, produce a slight to moderate spermatogenic arrest with a decrease in sperm count.

Pregnancy:

Teratogenic effects: Pregnancy Category B. Several reproduction studies have been performed in rabbits and rats at doses up to six times the human dose and have revealed no evidence of impaired fertility or harm to the fetus due to nitrofurantoin. In a single published study conducted in mice at 68 times the human dose (based on mg/kg administered to the dam), growth retardation and a low incidence of minor and common malformations were observed. However, at 25 times the human dose, fetal malformations were not observed; the relevance of these findings to humans is uncertain. There are, however, no adequate and well-controlled studies in pregnant women. Because animal reproduction studies are not always predictive of human response, this drug should be used during pregnancy only if clearly needed.

Non-teratogenic effects: Nitrofurantoin has been shown in one published transplacental carcinogenicity study to induce lung papillary adenomas in the F1 generation mice at doses 19 times the human dose on a mg/kg basis. The relationship of this finding to potential human carcinogenesis is presently unknown. Because of the uncertainty regarding the human implications of these animal data, this drug should be used during pregnancy only if clearly needed.

Labor and Delivery: **See CONTRAINDICATIONS.**

Nursing Mothers: Nitrofurantoin has been detected in human breast milk in trace amounts. Because of the potential for serious adverse reactions from nitrofurantoin in nursing infants under one month of age, a decision should be made whether to discontinue nursing or to discontinue the drug, taking into account the importance of the drug to the mother. (See **CONTRAINDICATIONS**.)

Pediatric Use: **Macrobid** is contraindicated in infants below the age of one month. (See **CONTRAINDICATIONS**.) Safety and effectiveness in pediatric patients below the age of twelve years have not been established.

ADVERSE REACTIONS

In clinical trials of **Macrobid**, the most frequent clinical adverse events that were reported as possibly or probably drug-related were nausea (8%), headache (6%), and flatulence (1.5%). Additional clinical adverse events reported as possibly or probably drug-related occurred in less than 1% of patients studied and are listed below within each body system in order of decreasing frequency:

Gastrointestinal: Diarrhea, dyspepsia, abdominal pain, constipation, emesis

Neurologic: Dizziness, drowsiness, amblyopia

Respiratory: Acute pulmonary hypersensitivity reaction (see **WARNINGS**)

Allergic: Pruritus, urticaria

Dermatologic: Alopecia

Miscellaneous: Fever, chills, malaise

The following additional clinical adverse events have been reported with the use of nitrofurantoin:

Gastrointestinal: Sialadenitis, pancreatitis. There have been sporadic reports of pseudomembranous colitis with the use of nitrofurantoin. The onset of pseudomembranous colitis symptoms may occur during or after antimicrobial treatment. (See **WARNINGS**.)

Neurologic: Peripheral neuropathy, which may become severe or irreversible, has occurred. Fatalities have been reported. Conditions such as renal impairment (creatinine clearance under 60 mL per minute or clinically significant elevated serum creatinine), anemia, diabetes mellitus, electrolyte imbalance, vitamin B deficiency, and debilitating diseases may increase the possibility of peripheral neuropathy. (See **WARNINGS**.)

Asthenia, vertigo, and nystagmus also have been reported with the use of nitrofurantoin. Benign intracranial hypertension (pseudotumor cerebri), confusion, depression, optic neuritis, and psychotic reactions have been reported rarely. Bulging fontanels, as a sign of benign intracranial hypertension in infants, have been reported rarely.

Respiratory:

CHRONIC, SUBACUTE, OR ACUTE PULMONARY HYPERSENSITIVITY REACTIONS MAY OCCUR WITH THE USE OF NITROFURANTOIN.

CHRONIC PULMONARY REACTIONS GENERALLY OCCUR IN PATIENTS WHO HAVE RECEIVED CONTINUOUS TREATMENT FOR SIX MONTHS OR LONGER. MALAISE, DYSPNEA ON EXERTION, COUGH, AND ALTERED PULMONARY FUNCTION ARE COMMON MANIFESTATIONS WHICH CAN OCCUR INSIDIOUSLY. RADIOLOGIC AND HISTOLOGIC FINDINGS OF DIFFUSE INTERSTITIAL PNEUMONITIS OR FIBROSIS, OR BOTH, ARE ALSO COMMON MANIFESTATIONS OF THE CHRONIC PULMONARY REACTION. FEVER IS RARELY PROMINENT.

THE SEVERITY OF CHRONIC PULMONARY REACTIONS AND THEIR DEGREE OF RESOLUTION APPEAR TO BE RELATED TO THE DURATION OF THERAPY AFTER THE FIRST CLINICAL SIGNS APPEAR. PULMONARY FUNCTION MAY BE IMPAIRED PERMANENTLY, EVEN AFTER CESSATION OF THERAPY. THE RISK IS GREATER WHEN CHRONIC PULMONARY REACTIONS ARE NOT RECOGNIZED EARLY.

In subacute pulmonary reactions, fever and eosinophilia occur less often than in the acute form. Upon cessation of therapy, recovery may require several months. If the symptoms are not recognized as being drug-related and nitrofurantoin therapy is not stopped, the symptoms may become more severe. Acute pulmonary reactions are commonly manifested by fever, chills, cough, chest pain, dyspnea, pulmonary infiltration with consolidation or pleural effusion on x-ray, and eosinophilia. Acute reactions usually occur within the first week of treatment and are reversible with cessation of therapy. Resolution often is dramatic. (See **WARNINGS**.)

Changes in EKG (e.g., non-specific ST/T wave changes, bundle branch block) have been reported in association with pulmonary reactions. Cyanosis has been reported rarely.

Hepatic: Hepatic reactions, including hepatitis, cholestatic jaundice, chronic active hepatitis, and hepatic necrosis, occur rarely. (See **WARNINGS**.)

Allergic: Lupus-like syndrome associated with pulmonary reaction to nitrofurantoin has been reported. Also, angioedema; maculopapular, erythematous, or eczematous eruptions; anaphylaxis; arthralgia; myalgia; drug fever; and chills have been reported. Hypersensitivity reactions represent the most frequent spontaneously-reported adverse events in worldwide postmarketing experience with nitrofurantoin formulations.

Dermatologic: Exfoliative dermatitis and erythema multiforme (including Stevens-Johnson syndrome) have been reported rarely.

Hematologic: Cyanosis secondary to methemoglobinemia has been reported rarely.

Miscellaneous: As with other antimicrobial agents, superinfections caused by resistant organisms, e.g., *Pseudomonas* species or *Candida* species, can occur.

In clinical trials of **Macrobid**, the most frequent laboratory adverse events (1–5%), without regard to drug relationship, were as follows: eosinophilia, increased AST (SGOT), increased ALT (SGPT), decreased hemoglobin, increased serum phosphorus. The following laboratory adverse events also have been reported with the use of nitrofurantoin: glucose-6-phosphate dehydrogenase deficiency anemia (see **WARNINGS**), agranulocytosis, leukopenia, granulocytopenia, hemolytic anemia, thrombocytopenia, megaloblastic anemia. In most cases, these hematologic abnormalities resolved following cessation of therapy. Aplastic anemia has been reported rarely.

OVERDOSAGE

Occasional incidents of acute overdosage of nitrofurantoin have not resulted in any specific symptoms other than vomiting. Induction of emesis is recommended. There is no specific antidote, but a high fluid intake should be maintained to promote urinary excretion of the drug. Nitrofurantoin is dialyzable.

DOSAGE AND ADMINISTRATION

Macrobid capsules should be taken with food.

Adults and Pediatric Patients Over 12 Years: One 100-mg capsule every 12 hours for seven days.

HOW SUPPLIED

Macrobid is available as 100-mg opaque black and yellow capsules imprinted "Macrobid" on one half and "Norwich Eaton" on the other.

NDC 0149-0710-01 bottle of 100

Store at controlled room temperature (59° to 86°F or 15° to 30°C).

Rx Only

REFERENCES

1. National Committee for Clinical Laboratory Standards. Methods for Dilution Antimicrobial Susceptibility Tests for Bacteria that Grow Aerobically—Third Edition. Approved Standard NCCLS Document M7-A3, Vol. 13, No. 25, NCCLS, Villanova, PA, December 1993.
2. National Committee for Clinical Laboratory Standards. Performance Standards for Antimicrobial Disk Susceptibility Tests—Fifth Edition. Approved Standard NCCLS Document M2-A5, Vol. 13, No. 24, NCCLS, Villanova, PA, December 1993.

CLINICAL STUDIES

Controlled clinical trials comparing **Macrobid** 100 mg p.o. q12h and **Macrodantin** 50 mg p.o. q6h in the treatment of acute uncomplicated urinary tract infections demonstrated approximately 75% microbiologic eradication of susceptible pathogens in each treatment group.

Procter & Gamble Pharmaceuticals
Cincinnati, Ohio 45202
REVISED FEBRUARY 1998

Shown in Product Identification Guide, page 332

MACRODANTIN® ℞

[*mak " rō-dan' tin*]
(nitrofurantoin macrocrystals)

DESCRIPTION

Macrodantin (nitrofurantoin macrocrystals) is a synthetic chemical of controlled crystal size. It is a stable, yellow, crystalline compound. **Macrodantin** is an antibacterial agent for specific urinary tract infections. It is available in 25-mg, 50-mg, and 100-mg capsules for oral administration.

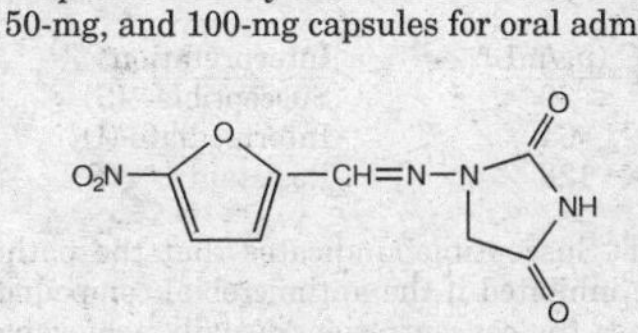

1-[[(5-NITRO-2-FURANYL)METHYLENE]AMINO]-2, 4-IMIDAZOLIDINEDIONE

Inactive Ingredients: Each capsule contains edible black ink, gelatin, lactose, starch, talc, titanium dioxide, and may contain FD&C Yellow No. 6 and D&C Yellow No. 10.

CLINICAL PHARMACOLOGY

Macrodantin is a larger crystal form of **Furadantin®** (nitrofurantoin). The absorption of **Macrodantin** is slower and its excretion somewhat less when compared to **Furadantin**. Blood concentrations at therapeutic dosage are usually low. It is highly soluble in urine, to which it may impart a brown color.

Following a dose regimen of 100 mg q.i.d. for 7 days, average urinary drug recoveries (0-24 hours) on day 1 and day 7 were 37.9% and 35.0%.

Unlike many drugs, the presence of food or agents delaying gastric emptying can increase the bioavailability of **Macrodantin**, presumably by allowing better dissolution in gastric juices.

Microbiology: Nitrofurantoin is bactericidal in urine at therapeutic doses. The mechanism of the antimicrobial action of nitrofurantoin is unusual among antibacterials. Nitrofurantoin is reduced by bacterial flavoproteins to reactive intermediates which inactivate or alter bacterial ribosomal proteins and other macromolecules. As a result of such inactivations, the vital biochemical processes of protein synthesis, aerobic energy metabolism, DNA synthesis, RNA synthesis, and cell wall synthesis are inhibited. The broad-based nature of this mode of action may explain the lack of acquired bacterial resistance to nitrofurantoin, as the necessary multiple and simultaneous mutations of the target macromolecules would likely be lethal to the bacteria. Development of resistance to nitrofurantoin has not been a significant problem since its introduction in 1953. Cross-resistance with antibiotics and sulfonamides has not been observed, and transferable resistance is, at most, a very rare phenomenon.

Continued on next page

Macrodantin—Cont.

Nitrofurantoin, in the form of **Macrodantin**, has been shown to be active against most strains of the following bacteria both *in vitro* and in clinical infections: (See **INDICATIONS AND USAGE**.)

Gram-Positive Aerobes
 Staphylococcus aureus
 Enterococci (e.g., *Enterococcus faecalis*)
Gram-Negative Aerobes
 Escherichia coli
NOTE: Some strains of *Enterobacter* species and *Klebsiella* species are resistant to nitrofurantoin.

Nitrofurantoin also demonstrates in vitro activity against the following microorganisms, although the clinical significance of these data with respect to treatment with **Macrodantin** is unknown:

Gram-Positive Aerobes
 Coagulase-negative staphylococci
 (including *Staphylococcus epidermidis* and *Staphylococcus saprophyticus*)
 Streptococcus agalactiae
 Group D streptococci
 Viridans group streptococci
Gram-Negative Aerobes
 Citrobacter amalonaticus
 Citrobacter diversus
 Citrobacter freundii
 Klebsiella oxytoca
 Klebsiella ozaenae
Nitrofurantoin is not active against most strains of *Proteus* species or *Serratia* species. It has no activity against *Pseudomonas species*.

Antagonism has been demonstrated *in vitro* between nitrofurantoin and quinolone antimicrobial agents. The clinical significance of this finding is unknown.

Susceptibility Tests:

Dilution techniques:
Quantitative methods are used to determine antimicrobial minimal inhibitory concentrations (MIC's). These MIC's provide estimates of the susceptibility of bacteria to antimicrobial compounds. The MIC's should be determined using a standardized procedure. Standardized procedures are based on a dilution method[1] (broth or agar) or equivalent with standardized inoculum concentrations and standardized concentrations of nitrofurantoin powder. The MIC values should be interpreted according to the following criteria:

MIC (µg/mL)	Interpretation
≤ 32	Susceptible (S)
64	Intermediate (I)
≥ 128	Resistant (R)

A report of "Susceptible" indicates that the pathogen is likely to be inhibited if the antimicrobial compound in the urine reaches the concentrations usually achievable. A report of "Intermediate" indicates that the result should be considered equivocal, and, if the microorganism is not fully susceptible to alternative, clinically feasible drugs, the test should be repeated. This category implies possible clinical applicability in body sites where the drug is physiologically concentrated or in situations where high dosage of drug can be used. This category also provides a buffer zone which prevents small uncontrolled technical factors from causing major discrepancies in interpretation. A report of "Resistant" indicates that the pathogen is not likely to be inhibited if the antimicrobial compound in the urine reaches the concentrations usually achievable; other therapy should be selected.

Standardized susceptibility test procedures require the use of laboratory control microorganisms to control the technical aspects of the laboratory procedures. Standard nitrofurantoin powder should provide the following MIC values:

Microorganism	MIC (µg/mL)
E. coli ATCC 25922	4–16
S. aureus ATCC 29213	8–32
E. faecalis ATCC 29212	4–16

Diffusion techniques:
Quantitative methods that require measurement of zone diameters also provide reproducible estimates of the susceptibility of bacteria to antimicrobial compounds. One such standardized procedure[2] requires the use of standardized inoculum concentrations. This procedure uses paper disks impregnated with 300-µg nitrofurantoin to test the susceptibility of microorganisms to nitrofurantoin.

Reports from the laboratory providing results of the standard single-disk susceptibility test with a 300-µg nitrofurantoin disk should be interpreted according to the following criteria:

Zone Diameter (mm)	Interpretation
≥ 17	Susceptible (S)
15-16	Intermediate (I)
≤ 14	Resistant (R)

Interpretation should be as stated above for results using dilution techniques. Interpretation involves correlation of the diameter obtained in the disk test with the MIC for nitrofurantoin.

As with standardized dilution techniques, diffusion methods require the use of laboratory control microorganisms that are used to control the technical aspects of the laboratory procedures. For the diffusion technique, the 300-æg nitrofurantoin disk should provide the following zone diameters in these laboratory test quality control strains:

Microorganism	Zone Diameter (mm)
E. coli ATCC 25922	20–25
S. aureus ATCC 25923	18–22

INDICATIONS AND USAGE

Macrodantin is specifically indicated for the treatment of urinary tract infections when due to susceptible strains of *Escherichia coli*, enterococci, *Staphylococcus aureus*, and certain susceptible strains of *Klebsiella* and *Enterobacter* species.

Nitrofurantoin is not indicated for the treatment of pyelonephritis or perinephric abscesses.

Nitrofurantoins lack the broader tissue distribution of other therapeutic agents approved for urinary tract infections. Consequently, many patients who are treated with **Macrodantin** are predisposed to persistence or reappearance of bacteriuria. Urine specimens for culture and susceptibility testing should be obtained before and after completion of therapy. If persistence or reappearance of bacteriuria occurs after treatment with **Macrodantin**, other therapeutic agents with broader tissue distribution should be selected. In considering the use of **Macrodantin**, lower eradication rates should be balanced against the increased potential for systemic toxicity and for the development of antimicrobial resistance when agents with broader tissue distribution are utilized.

CONTRAINDICATIONS

Anuria, oliguria, or significant impairment of renal function (creatinine clearance under 60 mL per minute or clinically significant elevated serum creatinine) are contraindications. Treatment of this type of patient carries an increased risk of toxicity because of impaired excretion of the drug.

Because of the possibility of hemolytic anemia due to immature erythrocyte enzyme systems (glutathione instability), the drug is contraindicated in pregnant patients at term (38-42 weeks gestation), during labor and delivery, or when the onset of labor is imminent. For the same reason, the drug is contraindicated in neonates under one month of age. **Macrodantin** is also contraindicated in those patients with known hypersensitivity to nitrofurantoin.

WARNINGS

ACUTE, SUBACUTE, OR CHRONIC PULMONARY REACTIONS HAVE BEEN OBSERVED IN PATIENTS TREATED WITH NITROFURANTOIN. IF THESE REACTIONS OCCUR, MACRODANTIN SHOULD BE DISCONTINUED AND APPROPRIATE MEASURES TAKEN. REPORTS HAVE CITED PULMONARY REACTIONS AS A CONTRIBUTING CAUSE OF DEATH.

CHRONIC PULMONARY REACTIONS (DIFFUSE INTERSTITIAL PNEUMONITIS OR PULMONARY FIBROSIS, OR BOTH) CAN DEVELOP INSIDI-OUSLY. THESE REACTIONS OCCUR RARELY AND GENERALLY IN PATIENTS RECEIVING THERAPY FOR SIX MONTHS OR LONGER. CLOSE MONITORING OF THE PULMONARY CONDITION OF PATIENTS RECEIVING LONG-TERM THERAPY IS WARRANTED AND REQUIRES THAT THE BENEFITS OF THERAPY BE WEIGHED AGAINST POTENTIAL RISKS. (SEE RESPIRATORY REACTIONS.)

Hepatic reactions, including hepatitis, cholestatic jaundice, chronic active hepatitis, and hepatic necrosis, occur rarely. Fatalities have been reported. The onset of chronic active hepatitis may be insidious, and patients should be monitored periodically for changes in biochemical tests that would indicate liver injury. If hepatitis occurs, the drug should be withdrawn immediately and appropriate measures should be taken.

Peripheral neuropathy, which may become severe or irreversible, has occurred. Fatalities have been reported. Conditions such as renal impairment (creatinine clearance under 60 mL per minute or clinically significant elevated serum creatinine), anemia, diabetes mellitus, electrolyte imbalance, vitamin B deficiency, and debilitating disease may enhance the occurrence of peripheral neuropathy. Patients receiving long-term therapy should be monitored periodically for changes in renal function.

Optic neuritis has been reported rarely in postmarketing experience with nitrofurantoin formulations.

Cases of hemolytic anemia of the primaquine-sensitivity type have been induced by nitrofurantoin. Hemolysis appears to be linked to a glucose-6-phosphate dehydrogenase deficiency in the red blood cells of the affected patients. This deficiency is found in 10 percent of Blacks and a small percentage of ethnic groups of Mediterranean and Near-East-

ern origin. Hemolysis is an indication for discontinuing **Macrodantin**; hemolysis ceases when the drug is withdrawn.

Pseudomembranous colitis has been reported with nearly all antibacterial agents, including nitrofurantoin, and may range from mild to life threatening. Therefore, it is important to consider this diagnosis in patients with diarrhea subsequent to the administration of antibacterial agents. Treatment with antibacterial agents alters the normal flora of the colon and may permit overgrowth of clostridia. Studies indicate that a toxin produced by *Clostridium difficile* is one primary cause of antibiotic-associated colitis.

After the diagnosis of pseudomembranous colitis has been established, appropriate therapeutic measures should be initiated. Mild cases of pseudomembranous colitis usually respond to drug discontinuation alone. In moderate to severe cases, consideration should be given to management with fluids and electrolytes, protein supplementation, and treatment with an antibacterial drug clinically effective against *Clostridium difficile* colitis.

PRECAUTIONS

Information for Patients: Patients should be advised to take **Macrodantin** with food to further enhance tolerance and improve drug absorption. Patients should be instructed to complete the full course of therapy; however, they should be advised to contact their physician if any unusual symptoms occur during therapy.

Many patients who cannot tolerate microcrystalline nitrofurantoin are able to take **Macrodantin** without nausea.

Patients should be advised not to use antacid preparations containing magnesium trisilicate while taking **Macrodantin**.

Drug Interactions: Antacids containing magnesium trisilicate, when administered concomitantly with nitrofurantoin, reduce both the rate and extent of absorption. The mechanism for this interaction probably is adsorption of nitrofurantoin onto the surface of magnesium trisilicate.

Uricosuric drugs, such as probenecid and sulfinpyrazone, can inhibit renal tubular secretion of nitrofurantoin. The resulting increase in nitrofurantoin serum levels may increase toxicity, and the decreased urinary levels could lessen its efficacy as a urinary tract antibacterial.

Drug/Laboratory Test Interactions: As a result of the presence of nitrofurantoin, a false-positive reaction for glucose in the urine may occur. This has been observed with Benedict's and Fehling's solutions but not with the glucose enzymatic test.

Carcinogenesis, Mutagenesis, Impairment of Fertility: Nitrofurantoin was not carcinogenic when fed to female Holtzman rats for 44.5 weeks or to female Sprague-Dawley rats for 75 weeks. Two chronic rodent bioassays utilizing male and female Sprague-Dawley rats and two chronic bioassays in Swiss mice and in BDF₁ mice revealed no evidence of carcinogenicity.

Nitrofurantoin presented evidence of carcinogenic activity in female B6C3F₁ mice as shown by increased incidences of tubular adenomas, benign mixed tumors, and granulosa cell tumors of the ovary. In male F344/N rats, there were increased incidences of uncommon kidney tubular cell neoplasms, osteosarcomas of the bone, and neoplasms of the subcutaneous tissue. In one study involving subcutaneous administration of 75 mg/kg nitrofurantoin to pregnant female mice, lung papillary adenomas of unknown significance were observed in the F1 generation.

Nitrofurantoin has been shown to induce point mutations in certain strains of *Salmonella typhimurium* and forward mutations in L5178Y mouse lymphoma cells. Nitrofurantoin induced increased numbers of sister chromatid exchanges and chromosomal aberrations in Chinese hamster ovary cells but not in human cells in culture. Results of the sex-linked recessive lethal assay in Drosophila were negative after administration of nitrofurantoin by feeding or by injection. Nitrofurantoin did not induce heritable mutation in the rodent models examined.

The significance of the carcinogenicity and mutagenicity findings relative to the therapeutic use of nitrofurantoin in humans is unknown.

The administration of high doses of nitrofurantoin to rats causes temporary spermatogenic arrest; this is reversible on discontinuing the drug. Doses of 10 mg/kg/day or greater in healthy human males may, in certain unpredictable instances, produce a slight to moderate spermatogenic arrest with a decrease in sperm count.

Pregnancy:

Teratogenic effects: Pregnancy Category B. Several reproduction studies have been performed in rabbits and rats at doses up to six times the human dose and have revealed no evidence of impaired fertility or harm to the fetus due to nitrofurantoin. In a single published study conducted in mice at 68 times the human dose (based on mg/kg administered to the dam), growth retardation and a low incidence of minor and common malformations were observed. However, at 25 times the human dose, fetal malformations were not observed; the relevance of these findings to humans is uncertain. There are, however, no adequate and well-con-

trolled studies in pregnant women. Because animal reproduction studies are not always predictive of human response, this drug should be used during pregnancy only if clearly needed.

Non-teratogenic effects: Nitrofurantoin has been shown in one published transplacental carcino-genicity study to induce lung papillary adenomas in the F1 generation mice at doses 19 times the human dose on a mg/kg basis. The relationship of this finding to potential human carcinogenesis is presently unknown. Because of the uncertainty regarding the human implications of these animal data, this drug should be used during pregnancy only if clearly needed.

Labor and Delivery: See **CONTRAINDICATIONS.**

Nursing Mothers: Nitrofurantoin has been detected in human breast milk in trace amounts. Because of the potential for serious adverse reactions from nitrofurantoin in nursing infants under one month of age, a decision should be made whether to discontinue nursing or to discontinue the drug, taking into account the importance of the drug to the mother. (See **CONTRAINDICATIONS.**)

Pediatric Use: **Macrodantin** is contraindicated in infants below the age of one month. (See **CONTRAINDICATIONS.**)

ADVERSE REACTIONS

Respiratory:
CHRONIC, SUBACUTE, OR ACUTE PULMONARY HYPERSENSITIVITY REACTIONS MAY OCCUR.
CHRONIC PULMONARY REACTIONS OCCUR GENERALLY IN PATIENTS WHO HAVE RECEIVED CONTINUOUS TREATMENT FOR SIX MONTHS OR LONGER. MALAISE, DYSPNEA ON EXERTION, COUGH, AND ALTERED PULMONARY FUNCTION ARE COMMON MANIFESTATIONS WHICH CAN OCCUR INSIDIOUSLY. RADIOLOGIC AND HISTOLOGIC FINDINGS OF DIFFUSE INTERSTITIAL PNEUMONITIS OR FIBROSIS, OR BOTH, ARE ALSO COMMON MANIFESTATIONS OF THE CHRONIC PULMONARY REACTION. FEVER IS RARELY PROMINENT.
THE SEVERITY OF CHRONIC PULMONARY REACTIONS AND THEIR DEGREE OF RESOLUTION APPEAR TO BE RELATED TO THE DURATION OF THERAPY AFTER THE FIRST CLINICAL SIGNS APPEAR. PULMONARY FUNCTION MAY BE IMPAIRED PERMANENTLY, EVEN AFTER CESSATION OF THERAPY. THE RISK IS GREATER WHEN CHRONIC PULMONARY REACTIONS ARE NOT RECOGNIZED EARLY.

In subacute pulmonary reactions, fever and eosinophilia occur less often than in the acute form. Upon cessation of therapy, recovery may require several months. If the symptoms are not recog-nized as being drug-related and nitrofurantoin therapy is not stopped, the symptoms may become more severe.

Acute pulmonary reactions are commonly manifested by fever, chills, cough, chest pain, dyspnea, pulmonary infiltration with consolidation or pleural effusion on x-ray, and eosinophilia. Acute reactions usually occur within the first week of treatment and are reversible with cessation of therapy. Resolution often is dramatic. (See **WARNINGS.**)

Changes in EKG (e.g., non-specific ST/T wave changes, bundle branch block) have been reported in association with pulmonary reactions.

Cyanosis has been reported rarely.

Hepatic: Hepatic reactions, including hepatitis, cholestatic jaundice, chronic active hepatitis, and hepatic necrosis, occur rarely. (See **WARNINGS.**)

Neurologic: Peripheral neuropathy, which may become severe or irreversible, has occurred. Fatalities have been reported. Conditions such as renal impairment (creatinine clearance under 60 mL per minute or clinically significant elevated serum creatinine), anemia, diabetes mellitus, electrolyte imbalance, vitamin B deficiency, and debilitating diseases may increase the possibility of peripheral neuropathy. (See **WARNINGS.**)

Asthenia, vertigo, nystagmus, dizziness, headache, and drowsiness also have been reported with the use of nitrofurantoin.

Benign intracranial hypertension (pseudotumor cerebri), confusion, depression, optic neuritis, and psychotic reactions have been reported rarely. Bulging fontanels, as a sign of benign intracranial hypertension in infants, have been reported rarely.

Dermatologic: Exfoliative dermatitis and erythema multiforme (including Stevens-Johnson syndrome) have been reported rarely. Transient alopecia also has been reported.

Allergic: A lupus-like syndrome associated with pulmonary reactions to nitrofurantoin has been reported. Also, angioedema; maculopapular, erythematous, or eczematous eruptions; pruritus; urticaria; anaphylaxis; arthralgia; myalgia; drug fever; and chills have been reported. Hyper sensitivity reactions represent the most frequent spontaneously-reported adverse events in worldwide postmarketing experience with nitrofurantoin formulations.

Gastrointestinal: Nausea, emesis, and anorexia occur most often. Abdominal pain and diarrhea are less common gastrointestinal reactions. These dose-related reactions can be minimized by reduction of dosage. Sialadenitis and pancreatitis have been reported. There have been sporadic re-

ports of pseudomembranous colitis with the use of nitrofurantoin. The onset of pseudomembranous colitis symptoms may occur during or after antimicrobial treatment. (See **WARNINGS.**)

Hematologic: Cyanosis secondary to methemoglobinemia has been reported rarely.

Miscellaneous: As with other antimicrobial agents, super-infections caused by resistant organisms, e.g., *Pseudomonas* species or *Candida* species, can occur.

Laboratory Adverse Events: The following laboratory adverse events have been reported with the use of nitrofurantoin: increased AST (SGOT), increased ALT (SGPT), decreased hemoglobin, increased serum phosphorus, eosinophilia, glucose-6-phosphate dehydrogenase deficiency anemia (see **WARNINGS**), agranulocytosis, leukopenia, granulo-cytopenia, hemolytic anemia, thrombocytopenia, megaloblastic anemia. In most cases, these hematologic abnormalities resolved following cessation of therapy. Aplastic anemia has been reported rarely.

OVERDOSAGE

Occasional incidents of acute overdosage of **Macrodantin** have not resulted in any specific symptoms other than vomiting. Induction of emesis is recommended. There is no specific antidote, but a high fluid intake should be maintained to promote urinary excretion of the drug. It is dialyzable.

DOSAGE AND ADMINISTRATION

Macrodantin should be given with food to improve drug absorption and, in some patients, tolerance.

Adults: 50–100 mg four times a day — the lower dosage level is recommended for uncomplicated urinary tract infections.

Pediatric Patients: 5–7 mg/kg of body weight per 24 hours, given in four divided doses (contraindicated under one month of age).

Therapy should be continued for one week or for at least 3 days after sterility of the urine is obtained. Continued infection indicates the need for reevaluation.

For long-term suppressive therapy in adults, a reduction of dosage to 50-100 mg at bedtime may be adequate. For long-term suppressive therapy in pediatric patients, doses as low as 1 mg/kg per 24 hours, given in a single dose or in two divided doses, may be adequate. **SEE WARNINGS SECTION REGARDING RISKS ASSOCIATED WITH LONG-TERM THERAPY.**

HOW SUPPLIED

Macrodantin is available as follows:
25-mg opaque, white capsule imprinted with one black line encircling the capsule and coded "MACRODANTIN 25 mg" and "0149-0007".*

NDC 0149-0007-05	bottle of 100

50-mg opaque, yellow and white capsule imprinted with two black lines encircling the capsule and coded "MACRODANTIN 50 mg" and "0149-0008".*

NDC 0149-0008-05	bottle of 100
NDC 0149-0008-66	bottle of 500
NDC 0149-0008-67	bottle of 1000
NDC 0149-0008-77	hospital unit-dose strips in box of 100

100-mg opaque, yellow capsule imprinted with three black lines encircling the capsule and coded "MACRODANTIN 100 mg" and "0149-0009".*

NDC 0149-0009-05	bottle of 100
NDC 0149-0009-66	bottle of 500
NDC 0149-0009-67	bottle of 1000
NDC 0149-0009-77	hospital unit-dose strips in box of 100

---

*Capsule design, registered trademark of Procter & Gamble Pharmaceuticals.

Rx Only

REFERENCES
1. National Committee for Clinical Laboratory Standards. Methods for Dilution Antimicrobial Susceptibility Tests for Bacteria that Grow Aerobically -- Third Edition. Approved Standard NCCLS Document M7-A3, Vol. 13, No. 25, NCCLS, Villanova, PA, December 1993.
2. National Committee for Clinical Laboratory Standards. Performance Standards for Antimicrobial Disk Susceptibility Tests -- Fifth Edition. Approved Standard NCCLS Document M2-A5, Vol. 13, No. 24, NCCLS, Villanova, PA, December 1993.

Procter & Gamble Pharmaceuticals
Cincinnati, Ohio 45202
REVISED FEBRUARY 1998
Shown in Product Identification Guide, page 332

EDUCATIONAL MATERIAL

Procter & Gamble Pharmaceuticals offers a wide range of educational services to the medical profession. Please write

to Manager, Professional Meetings & Conventions, Procter & Gamble Pharmaceuticals, Sharon Woods Technical Center, 11520 Reed Hartman Highway, Cincinnati, OH 45241 for further information.
• **Sponsorship of Educational Seminars**
• **Patient Education Booklets**
• **Resident/Fellow Conferences**
• **Newsletters**

The Purdue Frederick Company
100 CONNECTICUT AVENUE
NORWALK, CT 06850-3590

For Medical Information Contact:
Medical Department
(203) 853-0123

OxyContin® 10 mg Tablets
OxyContin® 20 mg Tablets
OxyContin® 40 mg Tablets
OxyContin® 80 mg Tablets
see listing under Purdue Pharma L.P., page 2569

OxyIR® Capsules—see listing under Purdue Pharma L.P., page 2574

BETADINE® BRAND PLUS   OTC
First Aid Antibiotics + Pain Reliever
Ointment
[bā 'tăh-dīn"]

ACTIONS
Topical broad-spectrum antibiotics plus topical anesthetic in a cholesterolized ointment* (moisturizer) base to help prevent infection and temporarily relieve pain; active ingredients per gram: polymyxin B sulfate (10,000 IU), bacitracin zinc (500 IU), and pramoxine HCl 10 mg.

INDICATIONS
Help prevent infection and provide temporary pain relief in minor cuts, scrapes and burns.

ADMINISTRATION
Clean affected area. Apply small amount of this product (an amount equal to the surface area of the tip of the finger) on the area 1 to 3 times daily. May be covered with a sterile bandage. **Children under 2 years of age: Consult a doctor.**

WARNINGS
For External Use Only. Do not use in the eyes or apply over large areas of the body. In case of deep or puncture wounds, animal bites, or serious burns, consult a physician. Stop use and consult a physician if the condition persists or gets worse. Do not use longer than 1 week unless directed by a physician. Keep this and all medications out of the reach of children. In case of accidental ingestion, seek professional assistance or contact a Poison Control Center immediately.

HOW SUPPLIED
1/2 oz. plastic tube with an applicator tip, and 1/32 oz. packettes.

---

*Formulated with Aquaphor®—a registered trademark of Beiersdorf AG.
Copyright 1998, The Purdue Frederick Company.

BETADINE® FIRST AID CREAM   OTC
[bā 'tăh-dīn"]
(povidone-iodine, 5%)

ACTION AND USES
BETADINE First Aid Cream is a topical antiseptic containing 5% povidone-iodine (PVP-I) in an oil-in-water emulsion. It is virtually nonirritating, nonstinging and nonburning when applied to minor cuts, burns or scrapes. It kills most bacteria and other pathogens virtually on contact. It enhances healing of minor wounds and has a very broad spectrum of microbicidal activity.
BETADINE First Aid Cream is easy to apply and remove. It is preservative-free.

ADMINISTRATION
Apply directly to affected area as needed. May be bandaged.

Continued on next page

Betadine Cream—Cont.

WARNINGS

For External Use Only. In case of deep or puncture wounds or serious burns, consult physician. If redness, irritation, swelling or pain persists or increases, or if infection occurs, discontinue use and consult physician. Keep out of reach of children.

SUPPLIED

$^1/_2$ oz. plastic tube, with an applicator tip for easy and economical application.
Copyright 1991, 1998. The Purdue Frederick Company

BETADINE®   OTC
BRAND First Aid Antibiotics + Moisturizer Ointment
[Bā 'tăh-dīn"]
Each gram contains: Polymyxin B Sulfate (10,000 IU) and Bacitracin Zinc (500 IU) in a cholesterolized ointment base.

ACTION AND USES

BETADINE Brand First Aid Antibiotics + Moisturizer Ointment is a topical antibiotic in a cholesterolized ointment base. It is formulated to help prevent infection in minor cuts, scrapes and burns.

ADVANTAGES

Its unique formula of two broad-spectrum antibiotics plus moisturizer helps prevent infection while helping to heal damaged skin.

ADMINISTRATION

Clean affected area. Apply small amount (an amount equal to the surface area of the tip of the finger) on the area 1 to 3 times daily. May be covered with a sterile bandage.

WARNINGS

For External Use Only. Do not use in the eyes or apply over large areas of the body. In case of deep or puncture wounds, animal bites, or serious burns, consult a physician. Stop use and consult a physician if the condition persists or gets worse or if a rash or other allergic reaction develops. Do not use this product if you are allergic to any of the ingredients. Do not use longer than 1 week unless directed by a physician. Keep this and all medications out of the reach of children. In case of accidental ingestion, seek professional assistance or contact a Poison Control Center immediately.

SUPPLIED

$^1/_2$ oz. plastic tubes, with an applicator-tip for easy and economical application, and $^1/_{32}$ oz. packettes.
Copyright 1996, 1998, The Purdue Frederick Company

BETADINE® MEDICATED DOUCHE   OTC
CONCENTRATE
[bā 'tăh-dīn"]
(povidone-iodine, 10%)

A pleasantly scented solution, BETADINE Medicated Douche is indicated for the prompt symptomatic relief of minor vaginal irritation, itching and soreness. May be used as a cleansing douche.

ADVANTAGES

Low surface tension, with uniform wetting action to assist penetration into vaginal crypts and crevices. Microbicidal activity is retained in the presence of moderate quantities of blood, pus, mucosal secretions and soap and water. Virtually nonirritating to vaginal mucosa. Will not stain skin or natural fabrics.

DIRECTIONS FOR USE

Directions for prompt symptomatic relief of minor vaginal irritation and itching: Fill 2 capfuls (2 tablespoonfuls) with douche. Mix with a quart of lukewarm water. Repeat procedure each day and use once daily for five days. Continue use for the full five days, even if symptoms are relieved earlier. Directions For Deodorizing and Cleansing Douche: Two (2) tablespoonfuls of BETADINE Douche Concentrate to a quart of lukewarm water once or twice per week.

When Not to Douche: Douching does not prevent pregnancy, nor should it be used for self-treatment or prevention of a sexually transmitted disease (STD). Do not use during pregnancy, while breast-feeding, or when symptoms of Pelvic Inflammatory Disease (PID) or an STD are present, except with the approval of your physician. Women with iodine sensitivity should not use this product.

When to Stop Use: If symptoms persist after five days of use, or redness, swelling or pain develops, discontinue use and consult a physician.

WARNINGS

Douching is reported to be associated with Pelvic Inflammatory Disease, a serious infection of the reproductive system which can lead to infertility and/or tubal (ectopic) pregnancy. Symptoms of PID and STD pain or tenderness in the lower part of the abdomen and pelvis; vaginal discharge and/or bleeding; nausea or fever; frequent urination; genital sores, and genital ulcers. If you suspect you have a STD or PID, stop using this product and see a physician immediately. Read and save the leaflet, *Important Information for Women*, which accompanies each package.

HOW SUPPLIED

8 oz. plastic bottles. Disposable $^1/_2$ oz. (1 tablespoonful) packets. Also available: BETADINE Medicated Disposable Douche (twin-pack) and BETADINE Pre-Mixed Medicated Disposable Douche, which requires no measuring or mixing (twin-pack).
Copyright 1991, 1998. The Purdue Frederick Company
Norwalk, CT 06850-3590

BETADINE® OINTMENT   OTC
[bā 'tăh-dīn"]
(povidone-iodine, 10%)

ACTION

Betadine ointment, in a water-soluble base, is a topical microbicide active against organisms commonly encountered in skin and wound infections.

INDICATIONS

Therapeutically, It may be used as an adjunct to systemic therapy where indicated; for primary or secondary topical infections, infected surgical incisions, infected decubitus or stasis ulcers, pyodermas, secondarily infected dermatoses, and infected traumatic lesions.
Prophylactically, It may be used to prevent microbial contamination in burns, incisions and other topical lesions; for degerming skin in hyperalimentation and catheter care. Its use for abrasions, minor cuts and wounds may prevent the development of infections and permit wound healing.

ADMINISTRATION

Apply directly to affected area as needed. Nonocclusion allows air to reach the wound. May be bandaged.

WARNINGS

For External Use Only. In case of deep or puncture wounds or serious burns, consult physician. If redness, irritation, swelling or pain persists or increases, or if infection occurs, discontinue use and consult physician. Keep out of reach of children.

SUPPLIED

$^1/_{32}$ oz. and $^1/_8$ oz. packettes; 1 oz. tubes.
Copyright 1991, 1998. The Purdue Frederick Company

BETADINE® SKIN CLEANSER   OTC
[bā 'tăh-dīn"]
(povidone-iodine, 7.5%)

BETADINE Skin Cleanser, a sudsing, antiseptic bactericidal, virucidal liquid cleanser, forms a rich, golden lather.

INDICATIONS

Helps prevent infection in cuts, scrapes and minor burns; used routinely for general hygiene; virtually nonirritating, nonstaining to skin.

DIRECTIONS FOR USE

Wet the skin, apply a sufficient amount to work up a rich golden lather. Allow lather to remain about 3 minutes and rinse off. Repeat 2–3 times a day or as directed by physician.

WARNINGS

For External Use Only. In case of deep or puncture wounds or serious burns, consult physician. If redness, irritation, swelling or pain persists or increases, or if infection occurs, discontinue use and consult physician. Keep out of reach of children. Avoid storing at excessive heat.

HOW SUPPLIED

4 fl. oz. plastic bottles.

NOTE

Blue stains on starched linen will wash off with soap and water.
Copyright 1991, 1998. The Purdue Frederick Company

BETADINE® SOLUTION   OTC
[bā 'tăh-dīn"]
(povidone-iodine,10%)
Topical Antiseptic Bactericide/Virucide

INDICATIONS

For preoperative prepping of operative site, including the vagina, and as a general topical bactericide/virucide for: dis-

infection of wounds; emergency treatment of lacerations and abrasions; second- and third-degree burns; as a prophylactic anti-infective agent in hospital and office procedures, including postoperative application to incisions to help prevent infection; oral moniliasis (thrush); bacterial and mycotic skin infections; decubitus and stasis ulcers; as a preoperative swab in the mouth and throat.

ADMINISTRATION

Apply full strength as often as needed as a paint, spray, or wet soak. May be bandaged.

WARNINGS

For External Use Only. In preoperative prepping, avoid "pooling" beneath the patient. Prolonged exposure to wet solution may cause irritation or rarely, severe skin reactions. In rare instance of local irritation or sensitivity, discontinue use. Do not heat prior to application.

HOW SUPPLIED

$^1/_2$ oz., 4 oz., 8 oz., 16 oz. (1 pt.), 32 oz. (1 qt.) and 1 gal. plastic bottles.

ALSO AVAILABLE

BETADINE® Solution Swab Aid® Pads for degerming small areas of skin or mucous membranes prior to injections, aspirations, catheterization and surgery; boxes of 100 packettes. Also: disposable BETADINE® Solution Swabsticks, in packettes of 1's and 3's. BETADINE® Aerosol Spray in 3 oz. bottles.
Copyright 1991, 1998. The Purdue Frederick Company

BETADINE® SURGICAL SCRUB   OTC
[bā 'tăh-dīn"]
(povidone-iodine, 7.5%)
Topical Antiseptic Bactericide/Virucide

INDICATIONS

A broad-spectrum antiseptic, bactericidal, virucidal sudsing skin cleanser for pre- and postoperative scrubbing or washing by hospital operating room personnel; for preoperative use on patients; and general use as an antiseptic microbicide in physician's office. Forms rich, golden lather.

DIRECTIONS FOR USE

A. For Preoperative Washing by Operating Personnel
1. Wet hands and forearms with water. Pour about 5 cc. (1 teaspoonful) of BETADINE Surgical Scrub on the palm of the hand and spread over both hands and forearms. Without adding more water, rub the Scrub thoroughly over all areas for about five minutes. Use a brush if desired. Clean thoroughly under fingernails. Add a little water and develop copious suds. Rinse thoroughly under running water.
2. Complete the wash by scrubbing with another 5 cc. of BETADINE Surgical Scrub in the same way.
B. For Preoperative Use on Patients
After the skin area is shaved, wet it with water. Apply BETADINE Surgical Scrub (1 cc. is sufficient to cover an area of 20-30 square inches), develop lather and scrub thoroughly for about five minutes. Rinse off by aid of sterile gauze saturated with water. The area may then be painted with BETADINE Solution or sprayed with BETADINE Aerosol Spray and allowed to dry.
C. For Use in the Physician's Office
Use for washing whenever a germicidal soap is required. For maximum degerming of the hands proceed as under (A). To prepare the patient's skin proceed as under (B).
Note: Blue stains on starched linen will wash off with soap and water.

WARNINGS

For External Use Only. Do not heat prior to application. In rare instances of local irritation or sensitivity, discontinue use. Keep out of reach of children.

SUPPLIED

4 oz. plastic bottle, 16 oz. (1 pint) plastic bottle with and without pump, 32 oz. (1 quart) and 1 gal. plastic bottles.
Copyright 1991, 1998. The Purdue Frederick Company
Norwalk, CT 06850-3590

BETASEPT® Surgical Scrub 4%   OTC
[bā 'tăh-sĕp-t"]
(chlorhexidine gluconate)

ACTION AND USES

BETASEPT Surgical Scrub (chlorhexidine gluconate) is an antiseptic/antimicrobial skin cleanser for hand scrubbing or washing by operating room personnel, for hand-washing by medical personnel, for pre-operative skin preparation, and for skin wound and general skin cleansing.

BETASEPT Surgical Scrub provides rapid bactericidal action and has a persistent antimicrobial effect against a wide range of microorganisms.

ADVANTAGES

BETASEPT Surgical Scrub is uniquely kind to hands,—a feature that encourages hospital personnel to follow correct hand-washing procedures.

BETASEPT Surgical Scrub is formulated in a highly viscous base which can help reduce waste and per-use cost during prepping and hand-washing. No unnecessary pink tint has been added.

DIRECTIONS FOR USE

Surgical Hand Scrub:

Wet hands and forearms with water. Scrub for 3 minutes with about 5 mL of BETASEPT Surgical Scrub and a wet brush, paying particular attention to the nails, cuticles and interdigital spaces. A separate nail cleaner may be used. Rinse thoroughly. Wash for an additional 3 minutes with 5 mL of BETASEPT Surgical Scrub and rinse under running water. Dry thoroughly.

Personnel Hand Wash:

Wet hands with water. Dispense about 5 mL of BETASEPT Surgical Scrub into cupped hands and wash in a vigorous manner for 15 seconds. Rinse and dry thoroughly.

Pre-Operative Skin Preparation:

Apply BETASEPT Surgical Scrub liberally to surgical site and swab for at least 2 minutes. Dry with a sterile towel. Repeat procedure for an additional 2 minutes and again dry with a sterile towel.

Skin Wound and General Skin Cleansing:

Wounds which involve more than the superficial layers of the skin should not be routinely treated with BETASEPT Surgical Scrub. BETASEPT Surgical Scrub should not be used for repeated general skin cleansing of large body areas except in those patients whose underlying condition makes it necessary to reduce the bacterial population of the skin. To use, thoroughly rinse the area to be cleansed with water. Apply the minimum amount of BETASEPT Surgical Scrub necessary to cover the skin or wound area and wash gently. Rinse again thoroughly.

WARNINGS

FOR EXTERNAL USE ONLY. KEEP OUT OF EYES, EARS AND MOUTH, BETASEPT SURGICAL SCRUB SHOULD NOT BE USED AS A PRE-OPERATIVE SKIN PREPARATION OF THE FACE OR HEAD, MISUSE OF PRODUCTS CONTAINING CHLORHEXIDINE GLUCONATE HAS BEEN REPORTED TO CAUSE SERIOUS AND PERMANENT EYE INJURY WHEN IT HAS BEEN PERMITTED TO ENTER AND REMAIN IN THE EYE DURING SURGICAL PROCEDURES. IF BETASEPT SURGICAL SCRUB SHOULD CONTACT THESE AREAS, RINSE OUT PROMPTLY AND THOROUGHLY WITH WATER.

Avoid contact with meninges. Betasept Surgical Scrub should not be used by persons who have sensitivity to it or its components. Chlorhexidine gluconate has been reported to cause deafness when instilled in the middle ear through perforated ear drums. Irritation, sensitization and generalized allergic reactions have been reported with chlorhexldine-containing products, especially in the genital areas. If adverse reactions occur, discontinue use immediately and if severe, contact a physician. Keep this and all drugs out of the reach of children. In case of accidental ingestion, seek professional assistance or contact a Poison Control Center immediately.

Avoid excessive heat (above 104°F).

HOW SUPPLIED

BETASEPT Surgical Scrub 4% is packaged in 1 gallon, 32 oz., 32 oz. with pump, 16 oz., 8 oz., and 4 oz. plastic bottles.

Copyright 1993, 1998, The Purdue Frederick Company, Norwalk, CT 06850-3590

CARDIOQUIN® ℞

(quinidine polygalacturonate)
tablets

DESCRIPTION

Quinidine is an antimalarial schizonticide and an antiarrhythmic agent with class 1a activity; it is the d-isomer of quinine, and its molecular weight is 324.43. Quinidine polygalacturonate is a polymer of quinidine and galacturonic acid; its structural formula is

[See chemical structure at top of next column]

and its empirical formula is

$(C_{20}H_{24}N_2O_2 \bullet C_6H_{10}O_7 \bullet H_2O)_n$. The molecular weight of the monomer is 536.58, of which 60.46% is quinidine base.

Quinidine polygalacturonate is a creamy white, amorphous powder, sparingly soluble in water but freely soluble in hot 40% ethanol. Each CARDIOQUIN tablet contains 275 mg of quinidine polygalacturonate (166 mg of quinidine base); the inactive ingredients include corn starch, lactose, magnesium stearate, povidone, and talc.

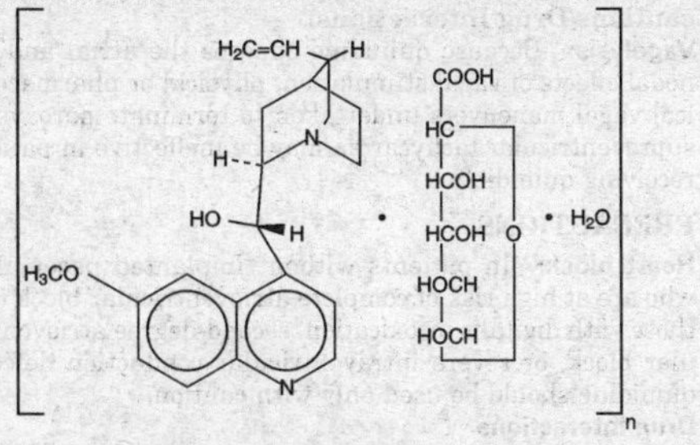

CLINICAL PHARMACOLOGY

Pharmacokinetics and Metabolism The absolute bioavailability of orally-administered CARDIOQUIN is about 70%, but this varies widely (45–100%) between patients. The less-than-complete bioavailability is the result of first-pass metabolism in the liver. Peak serum levels generally appear about 2 hours after dosing; absorption is delayed, but not changed in extent, when the drug is taken with food.

The **volume of distribution** of quinidine is 2–3 L/kg in healthy young adults, but this may be reduced to as little as 0.5 L/kg in patients with congestive heart failure, or increased to 3–5 L/kg in patients with cirrhosis of the liver. At concentrations of 2–5 mg/L (6.5–16.2 μmol/L), the fraction of quinidine bound to plasma proteins (mainly to α_1-acid glycoprotein and to albumin) is 80–88% in adults and older children, but it is lower in pregnant women, and in infants and neonates it may be as low as 50–70%. Because α_1-acid glycoprotein levels are increased in response to stress, serum levels of total quinidine may be greatly increased in settings such as acute myocardial infarction, even though the serum content of unbound (active) drug may remain normal. Protein binding is also increased in chronic renal failure, but binding abruptly descends toward or below normal when heparin is administered for hemodialysis.

Quinidine **clearance** typically proceeds at 3–5 mL/min/kg in adults, but clearance in children may be twice or three times as rapid. The elimination half-life is about 6–8 hours in adults and 3–4 hours in children. Quinidine clearance is unaffected by hepatic cirrhosis, so the increased volume of distribution seen in cirrhosis leads to a proportionate increase in the elimination half-life.

Most quinidine is eliminated hepatically via the action of cytochrome P450IIIA4; there are several different hydroxylated metabolites, and some of these have antiarrhythmic activity.

The most important of quinidine's metabolites is 3-hydroxyquinidine (3HQ), serum levels of which can approach those of quinidine in patients receiving conventional doses of CARDIOQUIN. The volume of distribution of 3HQ appears to be larger than that of quinidine, and the elimination half-life of 3HQ is about 12 hours.

As measured by antiarrhythmic effects in animals, by QT_c prolongation in human volunteers, or by various *in vitro* techniques, 3HQ has at least half the antiarrhythmic activity of the parent compound, so it may be responsible for a substantial fraction of the effect of CARDIOQUIN in chronic use.

When the urine pH is less than 7, about 20% of administered quinidine appears unchanged in the urine, but this fraction drops to as little as 5% when the urine is more alkaline. Renal clearance involves both glomerular filtration and active tubular secretion, moderated by (pH-dependent) tubular reabsorption. The net renal clearance is about 1 mL/min/kg in healthy adults.

When renal function is taken into account, quinidine clearance is apparently independent of patient age.

Assays of serum quinidine levels are widely available, but the results of modern assays may not be consistent with results cited in the older medical literature. The serum levels of quinidine cited in this package insert are those derived from specific assays, using either benzene extraction or (preferably) reverse-phase high-pressure liquid chromatography. In matched samples, older assays might unpredictably have given results that were as much as two or three times higher. A typical "therapeutic" concentration range is 2–6 mg/L (6.2–18.5 μmol/L).

Mechanisms of action In patients with malaria, quinidine acts primarily as an intra-erythrocytic schizonticide, with little effect upon sporozoites or upon pre-erythrocytic parasites. Quinidine is gametocidal to *Plasmodium vivax* and *P. malariae*, but not to *P. falciparum*.

In cardiac muscle and in Purkinje fibers, quinidine depresses the rapid inward depolarizing sodium current, thereby slowing phase-O depolarization and reducing the amplitude of the action potential without affecting the resting potential. In normal Purkinje fibers, it reduces the slope of phase-4 depolarization, shifting the threshold voltage upward toward zero. The result is slowed conduction and reduced automaticity in all parts of the heart, with increase of the effective refractory period relative to the duration of the action potential in the atria, ventricles, and Purkinje tissues. Quinidine also raises the fibrillation thresholds of the atria and ventricles, and it raises the ventricular defibrillation threshold as well. Quinidine's actions fall into class 1a in the Vaughn-Williams classification.

By slowing conduction and prolonging the effective refractory period, quinidine can interrupt or prevent reentrant arrhythmias and arrhythmias due to increased automaticity, including atrial flutter, atrial fibrillation, and paroxysmal supraventricular tachycardia.

In patients with the sick sinus syndrome, quinidine can cause marked sinus node depression and bradycardia. In most patients, however, quinidine is associated with an increase in sinus rate.

Quinidine prolongs the QT interval in a dose-related fashion. This may lead to increased ventricular automaticity and polymorphic ventricular tachycardias, including *torsades de pointes* (see **Warnings**).

In addition, quinidine has anticholinergic activity, it has negative inotropic activity, and it acts peripherally as an α-adrenergic antagonist (that is, as a vasodilator).

Clinical effects

Maintenance of sinus rhythm after conversion from atrial fibrillation: In six trials (published between 1970 and 1984) with a total of 808 patients, quinidine (418 patients) was compared to nontreatment (258 patients) or placebo (132 patients) for the maintenance of sinus rhythm after cardioversion from chronic atrial fibrillation. Quinidine was consistently more efficacious in maintaining sinus rhythm, but a meta-analysis found that mortality in the quinidine-exposed patients (2.9%) was significantly greater than mortality in the patients who had not been treated with active drug (0.8%). Suppression of atrial fibrillation with quinidine has theoretical patient benefits (*e.g.,* improved exercise tolerance; reduction in hospitalization for cardioversion; lack of arrhythmia-related palpitations, dyspnea, and chest pain; reduced incidence of systemic embolism and/or stroke), but these benefits have never been demonstrated in clinical trials. Some of these benefits (*e.g.,* reduction in stroke incidence) may be achievable by other means (anticoagulation).

By slowing the rate of atrial flutter/fibrillation, quinidine can decrease the degree of atrioventricular block and cause an increase, sometimes marked, in the rate at which supraventricular impulses are successfully conducted by the atrioventricular node, with a resultant paradoxical increase in ventricular rate (see **Warnings**).

Non-life-threatening ventricular arrhythmias: In studies of patients with a variety of ventricular arrhythmias (mainly frequent ventricular premature beats and non-sustained ventricular tachycardia), quinidine (total N=502) has been compared to flecainide (N=141), mexiletine (N=246), propafenone (N=53), and tocainide (N=67). In each of these studies, the mortality in the quinidine group was numerically greater than the mortality in the comparator group. When the studies were combined in a meta-analysis, quinidine was associated with a statistically significant threefold relative risk of death.

At therapeutic doses, quinidine's only consistent effect upon the surface electrocardiogram is an increase in the QT interval. This prolongation can be monitored as a guide to safety, and it may provide better guidance than serum drug levels (see **Warnings**).

INDICATIONS AND USAGE

Conversion of atrial fibrillation/flutter: In patients with symptomatic atrial fibrillation/flutter whose symptoms are not adequately controlled by measures that reduce the rate of ventricular response, CARDIOQUIN is indicated as a means of restoring normal sinus rhythm. If this use of CARDIOQUIN does not restore sinus rhythm within a reasonable time (see **Dosage and Administration**), then CARDIOQUIN should be discontinued.

Reduction of frequency of relapse into atrial fibrillation/flutter: Chronic therapy with CARDIOQUIN is indicated for some patients at high risk of symptomatic atrial fibrillation/flutter, generally patients who have had previous episodes of atrial fibrillation/flutter that were so frequent and poorly tolerated as to outweigh, in the judgment of the physician and the patient, the risks of prophylactic therapy with CARDIOQUIN. The increased risk of death should specifically be considered. CARDIOQUIN should be used only after alternative measures (*e.g.,* use of other drugs to control the ventricular rate) have been found to be inadequate.

In patients with histories of frequent symptomatic episodes of atrial fibrillation/flutter, the goal of therapy should be an increase in the average time between episodes. In most patients, the tachyarrhythmia *will recur* during therapy, and a single recurrence should not be interpreted as therapeutic failure.

Continued on next page

Cardioquin—Cont.

Suppression of ventricular arrhythmias: CARDIOQUIN is also indicated for the suppression of recurrent documented ventricular arrhythmias, such as sustained ventricular tachycardia, that in the judgment of the physician are life-threatening. Because of the proarrhythmic effects of quinidine, its use with ventricular arrhythmias of lesser severity is generally not recommended, and treatment of patients with asymptomatic ventricular premature contractions should be avoided. Where possible, therapy should be guided by the results of programmed electrical stimulation and/or Holter monitoring with exercise.

Antiarrhythmic drugs (including CARDIOQUIN) have not been shown to enhance survival in patients with ventricular arrhythmias.

CONTRAINDICATIONS

Quinidine is contraindicated in patients who are known to be allergic to it, or who have developed thrombocytopenic purpura during prior therapy with quinidine or quinine.

In the absence of a functioning artificial pacemaker, quinidine is also contraindicated in any patient whose cardiac rhythm is dependent upon a junctional or idioventricular pacemaker, including patients in complete atrioventricular block.

Quinidine is also contraindicated in patients who, like those with myasthenia gravis, might be adversely affected by an anticholinergic agent.

WARNINGS
Mortality:

In many trials of antiarrhythmic therapy for non-life-threatening arrhythmias, active antiarrhythmic therapy has resulted in increased mortality; the risk of active therapy is probably greatest in patients with structural heart disease.

In the case of quinidine used to prevent or defer recurrence of atrial flutter/fibrillation, the best available data come from a meta-analysis described under Clinical Pharmacology/Clinical Effects above. In the patients studied in the trials there analyzed, the mortality associated with the use of quinidine was more than three times as great as the mortality associated with the use of placebo.

Another meta-analysis, also described under Clinical Pharmacology/Clinical Effects, showed that in patients with various non-life-threatening ventricular arrhythmias, the mortality associated with the use of quinidine was consistently greater than that associated with the use of any of a variety of alternative antiarrhythmics.

Proarrhythmic effects: Like many other drugs (including all other class 1a antiarrhythmics), quinidine prolongs the QT_c interval, and this can lead to *torsades de pointes*, a life-threatening ventricular arrhythmia (see **Overdosage**). The risk of *torsades* is increased by any of: bradycardia, hypokalemia, hypomagnesemia, and high serum levels of quinidine, but it may appear in the absence of any of these risk factors. The best predictor of this arrhythmia appears to be the length of the QT_c interval, and quinidine should be used with extreme care in patients who have preexisting long-QT syndromes, who have histories of *torsades de pointes* of any cause, or who have previously responded to quinidine (or other drugs that prolong ventricular repolarization) with marked lengthening of the QT_c interval. Estimation of the incidence of *torsades* in patients with therapeutic levels of quinidine is not possible from the available data.

Other ventricular arrhythmias that have been reported with quinidine include frequent extrasystoles, ventricular tachycardia, ventricular flutter, and ventricular fibrillation.

Paradoxical increase in ventricular rate in atrial flutter/fibrillation: When quinidine is administered to patients with atrial flutter/fibrillation, the desired pharmacologic reversion to sinus rhythm may (rarely) be preceded by a slowing of the atrial rate with a consequent increase in the rate of beats conducted to the ventricles. The resulting ventricular rate may be very high (greater than 200 beats per minute) and poorly tolerated. This hazard may be decreased if partial atrioventricular block is achieved prior to initiation of quinidine therapy, using conduction-reducing drugs such as digitalis, verapamil, diltiazem, or a β-receptor blocking agent.

Exacerbated bradycardia in sick sinus syndrome: In patients with the sick sinus syndrome, quinidine has been associated with marked sinus node depression and bradycardia.

Pharmacokinetic considerations: Renal or hepatic dysfunction causes the elimination of quinidine to be slowed, while congestive heart failure causes a reduction in quinidine's apparent volume of distribution. Any of these conditions can lead to quinidine toxicity if dosage is not appropriately reduced. In addition, interactions with coadministered drugs can alter the serum concentration and activity of

quinidine, leading either to toxicity or to lack of efficacy if the dose of quinidine is not appropriately modified (see **Precautions/Drug Interactions**).

Vagolysis: Because quinidine opposes the atrial and A-V nodal effects of vagal stimulation, physical or pharmacological vagal maneuvers undertaken to terminate paroxysmal supraventricular tachycardia may be ineffective in patients receiving quinidine.

PRECAUTIONS

Heart block: In patients without implanted pacemakers who are at high risk of complete atrioventricular block (*e.g.*, those with digitalis intoxication, second-degree atrioventricular block, or severe intraventricular conduction defects), quinidine should be used only with caution.

Drug Interactions

Altered pharmacokinetics of quinidine: Drugs that alkalinize the urine (**carbonic-anhydrase inhibitors, sodium bicarbonate, thiazide diuretics**) reduce renal elimination of quinidine.

By pharmacokinetic mechanisms that are not well understood, quinidine levels are increased by coadministration of **amiodarone** or **cimetidine**. Very rarely, and again by mechanisms not understood, quinidine levels are decreased by coadministration of **nifedipine**.

Hepatic elimination of quinidine may be accelerated by coadministration of drugs (**phenobarbital, phenytoin, rifampin**) that induce production of cytochrome P450IIIA4. Perhaps because of competition for the P450IIIA4 metabolic pathway, quinidine levels rise when **ketoconazole** is coadministered.

Coadministration of propranolol usually does not affect quinidine pharmacokinetics, but in some studies the β-blocker appeared to cause increases in the peak serum levels of quinidine, decreases in quinidine's volume of distribution, and decreases in total quinidine clearance. The effects (if any) of coadministration of **other β-blockers** on quinidine pharmacokinetics have not been adequately studied.

Hepatic clearance of quinidine is significantly reduced during coadministration of **verapamil**, with corresponding increases in serum levels and half-life.

Altered pharmacokinetics of other drugs: Quinidine slows the elimination of **digoxin** and simultaneously reduces digoxin's apparent volume of distribution. As a result, serum digoxin levels may be as much as doubled. When quinidine and digoxin are coadministered, digoxin doses usually need to be reduced. Serum levels of **digitoxin** are also raised when quinidine is coadministered, although the effect appears to be smaller.

By a mechanism that is not understood, quinidine potentiates the anticoagulatory action of **warfarin**, and the anticoagulant dosage may need to be reduced.

Cytochrome P450IID6 is an enzyme critical to the metabolism of many drugs, notably including **mexiletine**, some **phenothiazines**, and most **polycyclic antidepressants**. Constitutional deficiency of cytochrome P450IID6 is found in less than 1% of Orientals, in about 2% of American blacks, and in some 8% of American whites.

Testing with debrisoquine is sometimes used to distinguish the P450IID6-deficient "poor metabolizers" from the majority-phenotype "extensive metabolizers."

When drugs whose metabolism is P450IID6-dependent are given to poor metabolizers, the serum levels achieved are higher, sometimes much higher, than the serum levels achieved when identical doses are given to extensive metabolizers. To obtain similar clinical benefit without toxicity, doses given to poor metabolizers may need to be greatly reduced. In the cases of prodrugs whose actions are actually mediated by P450IID6-produced metabolites (for example, **codeine** and **hydrocodone**, whose analgesic and antitussive effects appear to be mediated by morphine and hydromorphone, respectively), it may not be possible to achieve the desired clinical benefits in poor metabolizers.

Quinidine is not metabolized by cytochrome P450IID6, but therapeutic serum levels of quinidine inhibit the action of cytochrome P450IID6, effectively converting extensive metabolizers into poor metabolizers. Caution must be exercised whenever quinidine is prescribed together with drugs metabolized by cytochrome P450IID6.

Perhaps by competing for pathways of renal clearance, coadministration of quinidine causes an increase in serum levels of **procainamide**.

Serum levels of **haloperidol** are increased when quinidine is coadministered.

Presumably because both drugs are metabolized by cytochrome P450IIIA4, coadministration of quinidine causes variable slowing of the metabolism of **nifedipine**. Interactions with other dihydropyridine calcium-channel blockers have not been reported, but these agents (including **felodipine, nicardipine, and nimodipine**) are all dependent upon P450IIIA4 for metabolism, so similar interactions with quinidine should be anticipated.

Altered pharmacodynamics of other drugs: Quinidine's anticholinergic, vasodilating, and negative inotropic actions may be additive to those of other drugs with these effects,

and antagonistic to those of drugs with cholinergic, vasoconstricting, and positive inotropic effects. For example, when quinidine and **verapamil** are coadministered in doses that are each well tolerated as monotherapy, hypotension attributable to additive peripheral α-blockade is sometimes reported.

Quinidine potentiates the actions of depolarizing (succinylcholine, decamethonium) and nondepolarizing (*d*-tubocurarine, pancuronium) **neuromuscular blocking agents**. These phenomena are not well understood, but they are observed in animal models as well as in humans. In addition, *in vitro* addition of quinidine to the serum of pregnant women reduces the activity of pseudo-cholinesterase, an enzyme that is essential to the metabolism of succinylcholine.

Non-interaction of quinidine with other drugs: Quinidine has no clinically significant effect on the pharmacokinetics of **diltiazem, flecainide, mephenytoin, metoprolol, propafenone, propranolol, quinine, timolol, or tocainide.** Conversely, the pharmacokinetics of quinidine are not significantly affected by **caffeine, ciprofloxacin, digoxin, diltiazem, felodipine, omeprazole, or quinine.** Quinidine's pharmacokinetics are also unaffected by cigarette smoking.

Information for patients: Before prescribing CARDIOQUIN as prophylaxis against recurrence of atrial fibrillation, the physician should inform the patient of the risks and benefits to be expected (see **Clinical Pharmacology**). Discussion should include the facts:

• that the goal of therapy will be a reduction (probably not to zero) in the frequency of episodes of atrial fibrillation; and

• that reduced frequency of fibrillatory episodes may be expected, if achieved, to bring symptomatic benefits; but

• that no data are available to show that reduced frequency of fibrillatory episodes will reduce the risks of irreversible harm through stroke or death; and in fact

• that such data as are available suggest that treatment with CARDIOQUIN is likely to increase the patient's risk of death.

Carcinogenesis, mutagenesis, impairment of fertility Animal studies to evaluate quinidine's carcinogenic or mutagenic potential have not been performed. Similarly, there are no animal data as to quinidine's potential to impair fertility.

Pregnancy

Pregnancy Category C. Animal reproductive studies have not been conducted with quinidine. There are no adequate and well-controlled studies in pregnant women. Quinidine should be given to a pregnant woman only if clearly needed. In one neonate whose mother had received quinidine throughout her pregnancy, the serum level of quinidine was equal to that of the mother, with no apparent ill effect. The level of quinidine in amniotic fluid was about three times higher than that found in serum.

Labor and delivery Quinine is known to be oxytocic in humans, but there are no adequate data as to quinidine's effects (if any) on human labor and delivery.

Nursing mothers Quinidine is present in human milk at levels slightly lower than those in maternal serum; a human infant ingesting such milk should (scaling directly by weight) be expected to develop serum quinidine levels at least an order of magnitude lower than those of the mother. On the other hand, the pharmacokinetics and pharmacodynamics of quinidine in human infants have not been adequately studied, and neonates' reduced protein binding of quinidine may increase their risk of toxicity at low total serum levels. Administration of quinidine should (if possible) be avoided in lactating women who continue to nurse.

Geriatric use

Safety and efficacy of quinidine in elderly patients has not been systematically studied.

Pediatric use

In antimalarial trials, quinidine was as safe and effective in pediatric patients as in adults. Notwithstanding the known pharmacokinetic differences between children and adults (see **Pharmacokinetics and Metabolism**), children in these trials received the same doses (on a mg/kg basis) as adults. Safety and effectiveness of antiarrhythmic use in children have not been established.

ADVERSE REACTIONS

Quinidine preparations have been used for many years, but there are only sparse data from which to estimate the incidence of various adverse reactions. The adverse reactions most frequently reported have consistently been gastrointestinal, including diarrhea, nausea, vomiting, and heartburn/esophagitis. In one study of 245 adult outpatients who received quinidine to suppress premature ventricular contractions, the incidences of reported adverse experiences were as shown in the table below. The most serious quinidine-associated adverse reactions are described above under **Warnings.**

Adverse Experiences in a 245-Patient PVC Trial		
	Incidence	(%)
diarrhea	85	(35)
"upper gastrointestinal distress"	55	(22)
lightheadedness	37	(15)
headache	18	(7)
fatigue	17	(7)
palpitations	16	(7)
angina-like pain	14	(6)
weakness	13	(5)
rash	11	(5)
visual problems	8	(3)
change in sleep habits	7	(3)
tremor	6	(2)
nervousness	5	(2)
discoordination	3	(1)

Vomiting and diarrhea can occur as isolated reactions to therapeutic levels of quinidine, but they may also be the first signs of **cinchonism**, a syndrome that may also include tinnitus, reversible high-frequency hearing loss, deafness, vertigo, blurred vision, diplopia, photophobia, headache, confusion, and delirium. Cinchonism is most often a sign of chronic quinidine toxicity, but it may appear in sensitive patients after a single moderate dose.

A few cases of **hepatotoxicity**, including granulomatous hepatitis, have been reported in patients receiving quinidine. All of these have appeared during the first few weeks of therapy, and most (not all) have remitted once quinidine was withdrawn.

Autoimmune and inflammatory syndromes associated with quinidine therapy have included fever, urticaria, flushing, exfoliative rash, bronchospasm, psoriaform rash, pruritus and lymphadenopathy, hemolytic anemia, vasculitis, thrombocytopenic purpura, uveitis, angioedema, agranulocytosis, the sicca syndrome, arthralgia, myalgia, elevation in serum levels of skeletal-muscle enzymes, a disorder resembling systemic lupus erythematosus, and pneumonitis.

Convulsions, apprehension, and ataxia have been reported, but it is not clear that these were not simply the results of hypotension and consequent cerebral hypoperfusion. There are many reports of syncope. Acute psychotic reactions have been reported to follow the first dose of quinidine, but these reactions appear to be extremely rare.

Other adverse reactions occasionally reported include depression, mydriasis, disturbed color perception, night blindness, scotomata, optic neuritis, visual field loss, photosensitivity, and abnormalities of pigmentation.

OVERDOSAGE

Overdoses with various oral formulations of quinidine have been well described. Death has been described after a 5-gram ingestion by a toddler, while an adolescent was reported to survive after ingesting 8 grams of quinidine.

The most important ill effects of acute quinidine overdoses are ventricular arrhythmias and hypotension. Other signs and symptoms of overdose may include vomiting, diarrhea, tinnitus, high frequency hearing loss, vertigo, blurred vision, diplopia, photophobia, headache, confusion, and delirium.

Arrhythmias: Serum quinidine levels can be conveniently assayed and monitored, but the electrocardiographic QT_c interval is a better predictor of quinidine-induced ventricular arrhythmias.

The necessary treatment of hemodynamically unstable polymorphic ventricular tachycardia (including *torsades de pointes*) is withdrawal of treatment with quinidine and either immediate cardioversion or, if a cardiac pacemaker is in place or immediately available, immediate overdrive pacing. After pacing or cardioversion, further treatment must be guided by the length of the QT_c interval.

Quinidine-associated ventricular tachyarrhythmias with normal underlying QT_c intervals have not been adequately studied. Because of the theoretical possibility of QT-prolonging effects that might be additive to those of quinidine, other antiarrhythmics with Class I (disopyramide, procainamide) or Class III activities should (if possible) be avoided. Similarly, although the use of bretylium in quinidine overdose has not been reported, it is reasonable to expect that the α-blocking properties of bretylium might be additive to those of quinidine, resulting in problematic hypotension. If the post-cardioversion QT_c interval is prolonged, then the pre-cardioversion polymorphic ventricular tachyarrhythmia was (by definition) *torsades de pointes*. In this case, lidocaine and bretylium are unlikely to be of value, and other Class I antiarrhythmics (disopyramide, procainamide) are likely to exacerbate the situation. Factors contributing to QT_c prolongation (especially hypokalemia and hypomagnesemia) should be sought out and (if possible) aggressively corrected. Prevention of recurrent *torsades* may require sustained overdrive pacing or the cautious administration of isoproterenol (30–150 ng/kg/min).

Hypotension: Quinidine-induced hypotension that is not due to an arrhythmia is likely to be a consequence of quin-idine-related α-blockade and vasorelaxation. Simple repletion of central volume (Trendelenburg positioning, saline infusion) may be sufficient therapy; other interventions reported to have been beneficial in this setting are those that increase peripheral vascular resistance, including α-agonist catecholamines (norepinephrine, metaraminol) and the Military Anti-Shock Trousers.

Treatment: To obtain up-to-date information about the treatment of overdose, a good resource is your certified Regional Poison Control Center. Telephone numbers of certified poison control centers are listed in the *Physicians' Desk Reference (PDR)*. In managing overdose, consider the possibilities of multiple-drug overdoses, drug-drug interactions, and unusual drug kinetics in your patient.

Accelerated removal: Adequate studies of orally administered activated charcoal in human overdoses of quinidine have not been reported, but there are animal data showing significant enhancement of systemic elimination following this intervention, and there is at least one human case report in which the elimination half-life of quinidine in the serum was apparently shortened by repeated gastric lavage. Activated charcoal should be avoided if an ileus is present; the conventional dose is 1 gram/kg, administered every 2–6 hours as a slurry with 8 mL/kg of tap water.

Although renal elimination of quinidine might theoretically be accelerated by maneuvers to acidify the urine, such maneuvers are potentially hazardous and of no demonstrated benefit.

Quinidine is not usefully removed from the circulation by dialysis.

Following quinidine overdose, drugs that delay elimination of quinidine (cimetidine, carbonic-anhydrase inhibitors, thiazide diuretics) should be withdrawn unless absolutely required.

DOSAGE AND ADMINISTRATION

The dosage of quinidine varies considerably depending upon the general condition and the cardiovascular state of the patient.

Conversion of atrial fibrillation/flutter to sinus rhythm Especially in patients with known structural heart disease or other risk factors for toxicity, initiation or dose-adjustment of treatment with CARDIOQUIN should generally be performed in a setting where facilities and personnel for monitoring and resuscitation are continuously available. Patients with symptomatic atrial fibrillation/flutter should be treated with CARDIOQUIN only after ventricular rate control (*e.g.*, with digitalis or β-blockers) has failed to provide satisfactory control of symptoms.

Adequate trials have not identified an optimal regimen of CARDIOQUIN for conversion of atrial fibrillation/flutter to sinus rhythm. In one reported regimen, the patient first receives two tablets (550 mg; 333 mg of quinidine base) of CARDIOQUIN every six hours. If this regimen has not resulted in conversion after 4 or 5 doses, then the dose is cautiously increased. If, at any point during administration, the QRS complex widens to 130% of its pre-treatment duration; the QT_c interval widens to 130% of its pre-treatment duration and is then longer than 500 ms; P waves disappear; or the patient develops significant tachycardia, symptomatic bradycardia, or hypotension, then CARDIOQUIN is discontinued and other means of conversion (e.g., direct-current cardioversion) are considered.

Reduction of frequency of relapse into atrial fibrillation/flutter
In a patient with a history of frequent symptomatic episodes of atrial fibrillation/flutter, the goal of therapy with CARDIOQUIN should be an increase in the average time between episodes. In most patients, the tachyarrhythmia *will recur* during therapy with CARDIOQUIN, and a single recurrence should not be interpreted as therapeutic failure. Especially in patients with known structural heart disease or other risk factors for toxicity, initiation or dose-adjustment of treatment with CARDIOQUIN should generally be performed in a setting where facilities and personnel for monitoring and resuscitation are continuously available. Monitoring should be continued for two or three days after initiation of the regimen on which the patient will be discharged.

Therapy with CARDIOQUIN should begin with one tablet (275 mg; 166 mg of quinidine base) every six to eight hours. If this regimen is well tolerated, if the serum quinidine level is still well within the laboratory's therapeutic range, and if the average time between arrhythmic episodes has not been satisfactorily increased, then the dose may be cautiously raised. The total daily dosage should be reduced if the QRS complex widens to 130% of its pre-treatment duration; the QT_c interval widens to 130% of its pre-treatment duration and is longer than 500 ms: P waves disappear; or the patient develops significant tachycardia, symptomatic bradycardia, or hypotension.

Suppression of ventricular arrhythmias
Dosing regimens for the use of quinidine polygalacturonate in suppressing life-threatening ventricular arrhythmias have not been adequately studied. Described regimens have generally been similar to the regimen described just above

for the prophylaxis of symptomatic atrial fibrillation/flutter. Where possible, therapy should be guided by the results of programmed electrical stimulation and/or Holter monitoring with exercise.

HOW SUPPLIED

CARDIOQUIN is supplied as 275-mg, white, round, scored, uncoated tablets embossed **PF** on one side and **C275** on the other. The tablets are available in opaque white plastic bottles containing 100 tablets (NDC #0034-5470-80) and 500 tablets (NDC #0034-5470-90).
Store tablets at controlled room temperature (15–30°C; 59–86°F).
CAUTION: Federal (USA) law prohibits dispensing without prescription.
The Purdue Frederick Company
Norwalk, CT 06850-3590
Copyright© 1990, 1995
The Purdue Frederick Company
August 2, 1995   O8038

CERUMENEX® EARDROPS   ℞
[sĕ-rū 'mĕn-ĕx″]
(triethanolamine polypeptide oleate-condensate)

DESCRIPTION

CERUMENEX Eardrops contain Triethanolamine Polypeptide Oleate-Condensate (10%). Inactive Ingredients: Chlorobutanol 0.5%, Propylene Glycol and Water. Triethanolamine Polypeptide Oleate is a hygroscopic-miscible solution with low surface tension and optimal viscosity of 50–90 cps. It also has a slightly acid pH range (5.0–6.0) to approximate the surface of a normal ear canal.

CLINICAL PHARMACOLOGY

CERUMENEX Eardrops emulsify and disperse excess or impacted earwax. The triethanolamine polypeptide oleate, a surfactant, in a hygroscopic vehicle lyses cerumen to facilitate removal by subsequent water irrigation.

INDICATIONS AND USAGE

For removal of impacted cerumen prior to ear examination, otologic therapy and/or audiometry.

CONTRAINDICATIONS

Perforated tympanic membrane or otitis media is considered a contraindication to the use of this medication in the external ear canal.
A history of hypersensitivity to CERUMENEX Eardrops or to any of its components is also a contraindication to the use of this medication.

WARNINGS

Discontinue promptly if sensitization or irritation occurs.

PRECAUTIONS
General
It is recommended that the following precautions be observed in prescribing and administration of this agent:
1. Extreme caution is indicated in patients with demonstrable dermatologic idiosyncrasies or with history of allergic reactions in general.
2. Exposure of the ear canal to the CERUMENEX Eardrops should be limited to 15–30 minutes.
3. When administering CERUMENEX Eardrops, care must be taken to avoid undue exposure of the skin outside the ear during the instillation and the flushing out of the medication. If the medication comes in contact with the skin, the area should be washed with soap and water. Use of proper technique (see Dosage and Administration) will help avoid such undue exposure.
4. CERUMENEX Eardrops should be used only with caution in external otitis.

Information for Patients
1. Patients should be cautioned to avoid placing the applicator tip into the ear canal.
2. Patients should be cautioned to gently flush the ear with lukewarm water.
3. Patients should be warned to use CERUMENEX Eardrops in ears only. Surrounding skin should be promptly rinsed of any excess drops.
4. Patients should be instructed not to leave CERUMENEX Eardrops in the ear for longer than 30 minutes. A second application may be made, if needed, but more frequent use must be indicated by the physician.
5. Patients must be instructed not to exceed the time of exposure, nor to use the medication more frequently than directed by the physician.
6. Patients should be advised to discontinue the use of the medication in case of a possible reaction and to consult their physician promptly.

Carcinogenesis, Mutagenesis, Impairment of Fertility
Long-term animal studies have not been performed to evaluate the carcinogenic potential or the effect on fertility of CERUMENEX Eardrops.
Pregnancy
Teratogenic Effects: Pregnancy Category C. Animal reproduction studies have not yet been conducted with

Continued on next page

Cerumenex—Cont.

CERUMENEX Eardrops. It is also not known whether CERUMENEX Eardrops can cause fetal harm when administered to a pregnant woman or can affect reproduction capacity. CERUMENEX Eardrops should be given to a pregnant woman only if clearly needed.

Nursing Mothers

It is not known whether this drug is excreted in human milk. Because many drugs are excreted in human milk, caution should be exercised when CERUMENEX Eardrops are administered to a nursing mother.

Pediatric Use

Safety and effectiveness in children have not been established.

ADVERSE REACTIONS

Clinical Reactions of Possible Allergic Origin

Localized dermatitis reactions were reported in about 1% of 2,700 patients treated, ranging from a very mild erythema and pruritus of the external canal to a severe eczematoid reaction involving the external ear and periauricular tissue, generally with duration of 2–10 days. Other reactions which have been reported in connection with the use of CERUMENEX Eardrops include allergic contact dermatitis, skin ulcerations, burning and pain at the application site and skin rash.

DOSAGE AND ADMINISTRATION

1. Fill ear canal with CERUMENEX Eardrops with the patient's head tilted at a 45° angle.
2. Insert cotton plug and allow to remain 15–30 minutes.
3. Then gently flush with lukewarm water, using a soft rubber syringe (avoid excessive pressure). Exposure of skin outside the ear to the drug should be avoided. The procedure may be repeated if the first application fails to clear the impaction.

CAUTION: Federal Law Prohibits Dispensing Without a Prescription.

FOR EXTERNAL USE IN THE EAR ONLY

HOW SUPPLIED

CERUMENEX Eardrops (triethanolamine polypeptide oleate-condensate) are supplied in 6 ml (NDC 0034-5490-06) and 12 ml (NDC 0034-5490-12) bottles with a cellophane wrapped dropper.

Store at Controlled Room Temperature 15–30°C (59–86°F).

Copyright 1991, The Purdue Frederick Company

Norwalk, CT 06850-3590

May 15, 1991 L8037

MS CONTIN® 15 mg Tablets Ⓒ
MS CONTIN® 30 mg Tablets Ⓒ
MS CONTIN® 60 mg Tablets Ⓒ
MS CONTIN® 100 mg Tablets Ⓒ

MS CONTIN® 200 mg Tablets* Ⓒ
(For use in opioid tolerant patients only.)

[em es "kŏn "tĕn]

Morphine Sulfate Controlled-Release

WARNING: May be habit forming.

DESCRIPTION

Chemically, morphine sulfate is 7,8-didehydro-4,5α-epoxy-17- methylmorphinan-3,6 α-diol sulfate (2:1) (salt) pentahydrate and has the following structural formula:

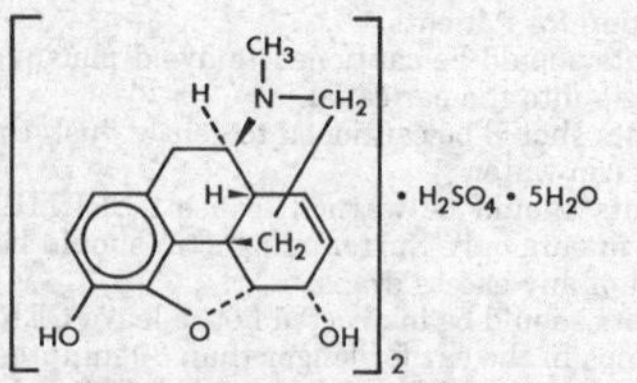

Each MS CONTIN 15 mg Controlled-Release Tablet contains: 15 mg Morphine sulfate U.S.P. Inactive ingredients: Cetostearyl alcohol, FD&C Blue No. 2, Hydroxyethyl cellulose, Hydroxypropyl methylcellulose, Lactose, Magnesium stearate, Talc, Titanium dioxide and other ingredients.

Each MS CONTIN 30 mg Controlled-Release Tablet contains: 30 mg Morphine sulfate U.S.P. Inactive ingredients: Cetostearyl alcohol, D&C Red No. 7, FD&C Blue No. 1, Hydroxyethyl cellulose, Hydroxypropyl methylcellulose, Lactose, Magnesium stearate, Talc, Titanium dioxide and other ingredients.

Each MS CONTIN 60 mg Controlled-Release Tablet contains: 60 mg Morphine sulfate U.S.P. Inactive ingredients: Cetostearyl alcohol, D&C Red No. 30, D&C Yellow No. 10, Hydroxyethyl cellulose, Hydroxypropyl methylcellulose, Lactose, Magnesium stearate, Talc, Titanium dioxide and other ingredients.

Each MS CONTIN 100 mg Controlled-Release Tablet contains: 100 mg Morphine sulfate U.S.P. Inactive ingredients: Cetostearyl alcohol, Hydroxyethyl cellulose, Hydroxypropyl methylcellulose, Magnesium stearate, Synthetic black iron oxide, Talc, Titanium dioxide and other ingredients.

MS CONTIN 200 mg Tablets*

(For use in opioid tolerant patients only.)

Each MS CONTIN 200 mg Controlled-Release Tablet* contains: 200 mg Morphine sulfate U.S.P. Inactive ingredients: Cetostearyl alcohol, D&C Yellow No. 10, FD&C Blue No. 1, Hydroxyethyl cellulose, Hydroxypropyl cellulose, Hydroxypropyl methylcellulose, Magnesium stearate, Polyethylene glycol, Talc, Titanium dioxide.

***FOR USE IN OPIOID TOLERANT PATIENTS ONLY.**

CLINICAL PHARMACOLOGY

Metabolism and Pharmacokinetics

MS CONTIN is a controlled-release tablet containing morphine sulfate. Following oral administration of a given dose of morphine, the amount ultimately absorbed is essentially the same whether the source is MS CONTIN or a conventional formulation. Morphine is released from MS CONTIN somewhat more slowly than from conventional oral preparations. Because of pre-systemic elimination (i.e., metabolism in the gut wall and liver) only about 40% of the administered dose reaches the central compartment.

Once absorbed, morphine is distributed to skeletal muscle, kidneys, liver, intestinal tract, lungs, spleen and brain. Morphine also crosses the placental membranes and has been found in breast milk.

Although a small fraction (less than 5%) of morphine is demethylated, for all practical purposes, virtually all morphine is converted to glucuronide metabolites; among these, morphine-3-glucuronide is present in the highest plasma concentration following oral administration.

The glucuronide system has a very high capacity and is not easily saturated even in disease. Therefore, rate of delivery of morphine to the gut and liver should not influence the total and, probably, the relative quantities of the various metabolites formed. Moreover, even if rate affected the relative amounts of each metabolite formed, it should be unimportant clinically because morphine's metabolites are ordinarily inactive.

The following pharmacokinetic parameters show considerable inter-subject variation but are representative of average values reported in the literature. The volume of distribution (Vd) for morphine is 4 liters per kilogram, and its terminal elimination half-life is normally 2 to 4 hours.

Following the administration of conventional oral morphine products, approximately fifty percent of the morphine that will reach the central compartment intact reaches it within 30 minutes. Following the administration of an equal amount of MS CONTIN to normal volunteers, however, this extent of absorption occurs, on average, after 1.5 hours.

The possible effect of food upon the systemic bioavailability of MS CONTIN has not been systematically evaluated for all strengths. Data from at least one study suggests that concurrent administration of MS CONTIN with a fatty meal may cause a slight decrease in peak plasma concentration.

Variation in the physical/mechanical properties of a formulation of an oral morphine drug product can affect both its absolute bioavailability and its absorption rate constant (k_a). The formulation employed in MS CONTIN has not been shown to affect morphine's oral bioavailability, but does decrease its apparent k_a. Other basic pharmacokinetic parameters (e.g., volume of distribution [Vd], elimination rate constant [k_e], clearance [Cl]), are unchanged as they are fundamental properties of morphine in the organism. However, in chronic use, the possibility that shifts in metabolite to parent drug ratios may occur cannot be excluded.

When immediate-release oral morphine or MS CONTIN is given on a fixed dosing regimen, steady state is achieved in about a day.

For a given dose and dosing interval, the AUC and average blood concentration of morphine at steady state (Css) will be independent of the specific type of oral formulation administered so long as the formulations have the same absolute bioavailability. The absorption rate of a formulation will, however, affect the maximum (Cmax) and minimum (Cmin) blood levels and the times of their occurrence.

PHARMACODYNAMICS

The effects described below are common to all morphine-containing products.

Central Nervous System

The principal actions of therapeutic value of morphine are analgesia and sedation (i.e., sleepiness and anxiolysis).

The precise mechanism of the analgesic action is unknown. However, specific CNS opiate receptors and endogenous compounds with morphine-like activity have been identified throughout the brain and spinal cord and are likely to play a role in the expression of analgesic effects.

Morphine produces respiratory depression by direct action on brain stem respiratory centers. The mechanism of respiratory depression involves a reduction in the responsiveness of the brain stem respiratory centers to increases in carbon dioxide tension, and to electrical stimulation.

Morphine depresses the cough reflex by direct effect on the cough center in the medulla. Antitussive effects may occur with doses lower than those usually required for analgesia.

Morphine causes miosis, even in total darkness. Pinpoint pupils are a sign of narcotic overdose but are not pathognomonic (e.g., pontine lesions of hemorrhagic or ischemic origins may produce similar findings). Marked mydriasis rather than miosis may be seen with worsening hypoxia.

Gastrointestinal Tract and Other Smooth Muscle

Gastric, biliary and pancreatic secretions are decreased by morphine. Morphine causes a reduction in motility associated with an increase in tone in the antrum of the stomach and duodenum. Digestion of food in the small intestine is delayed and propulsive contractions are decreased. Propulsive peristaltic waves in the colon are decreased, while tone is increased to the point of spasm. The end result is constipation. Morphine can cause a marked increase in biliary tract pressure as a result of spasm of sphincter of Oddi.

Cardiovascular System

Morphine produces peripheral vasodilation which may result in orthostatic hypotension. Release of histamine can occur and may contribute to narcotic-induced hypotension. Manifestations of histamine release and/or peripheral vasodilation may include pruritus, flushing, red eyes and sweating.

Plasma Level- Analgesia Relationships

In any particular patient, both analgesic effects and plasma morphine concentrations are related to the morphine dose. In non-tolerant individuals, plasma morphine concentration-efficacy relationships have been demonstrated and suggest that opiate receptors occupy effector compartments, leading to a lag-time, or hysteresis, between rapid changes in plasma morphine concentrations and effects of such changes. The most direct and predictable concentration-effect relationships can, therefore, be expected at distribution equilibrium and/or steady state conditions. In general, the minimum effective analgesic concentration in the plasma of non tolerant patients ranges from approximately 5 to 20ng/ml.

While plasma morphine-efficacy relationships can be demonstrated in non-tolerant individuals, they are influenced by a wide variety of factors and are not generally useful as a guide to the clinical use of morphine. The effective dose in opioid-tolerant patients may be 10–50 times as great (or greater) than the appropriate dose for opioid-naive individuals. Dosages of morphine should be chosen and must be titrated on the bases of clinical evaluation of the patient and the balance between therapeutic and adverse effects.

For any fixed dose and dosing interval, MS CONTIN will have at steady state, a lower Cmax and a higher Cmin than conventional morphine. This is a potential advantage; a reduced fluctuation in morphine concentration during the dosing interval should keep morphine blood levels more centered within the theoretical "therapeutic window." (Fluctuation for a dosing interval is defined as [Cmax-Cmin]/[Css-average].) On the other hand, the degree of fluctuation in serum morphine concentration might conceivably affect other phenomena. For example, reduced fluctuations in blood morphine concentrations might influence the rate of tolerance induction.

The elimination of morphine occurs primarily as renal excretion of 3-morphine glucuronide. A small amount of the glucuronide conjugate is excreted in the bile, and there is some minor enterohepatic recycling. Because morphine is primarily metabolized to inactive metabolites, the effects of renal disease on morphine's elimination are not likely to be pronounced. However, as with any drug, caution should be taken to guard against unanticipated accumulation if renal and/or hepatic function is seriously impaired.

INDICATIONS AND USAGE

MS CONTIN is a controlled-release oral morphine formulation indicated for the relief of moderate to severe pain. It is intended for use in patients who require repeated dosing with potent opioid analgesics over periods of more than a few days.

The MS CONTIN 200 mg Tablet strength is a high dose, controlled-release, oral morphine formulation indicated for the relief of pain in opioid tolerant patients only.

CONTRAINDICATIONS

MS CONTIN is contraindicated in patients with known hypersensitivity to the drug, in patients with respiratory depression in the absence of resuscitative equipment, and in patients with acute or severe bronchial asthma.

MS CONTIN is contraindicated in any patient who has or is suspected of having a paralytic ileus.

WARNINGS

(See also: CLINICAL PHARMACOLOGY)

Impaired Respiration

Respiratory depression is the chief hazard of all morphine preparations. Respiratory depression occurs most frequently in the elderly and debilitated patients, as well as in

those suffering from conditions accompanied by hypoxia or hypercapnia when even moderate therapeutic doses may dangerously decrease pulmonary ventilation.

Morphine should be used with extreme caution in patients with chronic obstructive pulmonary disease or cor pulmonale, and in patients having a substantially decreased respiratory reserve, hypoxia, hypercapnia, or preexisting respiratory depression. In such patients, even usual therapeutic doses of morphine may decrease respiratory drive while simultaneously increasing airway resistance to the point of apnea.

Head Injury and Increased Intracranial Pressure

The respiratory depressant effects of morphine with carbon dioxide retention and secondary elevation of cerebrospinal fluid pressure may be markedly exaggerated in the presence of head injury, other intracranial lesions, or preexisting increase in intracranial pressure. Morphine produces effects which may obscure neurologic signs of further increases in pressure in patients with head injuries.

Hypotensive Effect

MS CONTIN, like all opioid analgesics, may cause severe hypotension in an individual whose ability to maintain his blood pressure has already been compromised by a depleted blood volume, or a concurrent administration of drugs such as phenothiazines or general anesthetics. (See also: PRECAUTIONS: Drug Interactions.) MS CONTIN may produce orthostatic hypotension in ambulatory patients.

MS CONTIN, like all opioid analgesics, should be administered with caution to patients in circulatory shock, since vasodilation produced by the drug may further reduce cardiac output and blood pressure.

Interactions with other CNS Depressants

MS CONTIN, like all opioid analgesics, should be used with great caution and in reduced dosage in patients who are concurrently receiving other central nervous system depressants including sedatives or hypnotics, general anesthetics, phenothiazines, other tranquilizers and alcohol because respiratory depression, hypotension and profound sedation or coma may result.

Interactions with Mixed Agonist/Antagonist Opioid Analgesics

From a theoretical perspective, agonist/antagonist analgesics (i.e., pentazocine, nalbuphine, butorphanol and buprenorphine) should NOT be administered to a patient who has received or is receiving a course of therapy with a pure opioid agonist analgesic. In these patients, mixed agonist/antagonist analgesics may reduce the analgesic effect or may precipitate withdrawal symptoms.

Drug Dependence

Morphine can produce drug dependence and has a potential for being abused. Tolerance as well as psychological and physical dependence may develop upon repeated administration. Physical dependence, however, is not of paramount importance in the management of terminally ill patients or any patients in severe pain. Abrupt cessation or a sudden reduction in dose after prolonged use may result in withdrawal symptoms. After prolonged exposure to opioid analgesics, if withdrawal is necessary, it must be undertaken gradually. (See DRUG ABUSE AND DEPENDENCE.)

Infants born to mothers physically dependent on opioid analgesics may also be physically dependent and exhibit respiratory depression and withdrawal symptoms. (See DRUG ABUSE AND DEPENDENCE.)

PRECAUTIONS

(See also: CLINICAL PHARMACOLOGY)

Special precautions regarding MS CONTIN 200 mg Tablets

MS CONTIN 200 mg Tablets are for use only in opioid tolerant patients requiring daily morphine equivalent dosages of 400 mg or more. Care should be taken in its prescription and patients should be instructed against use by individuals other than the patient for whom it was prescribed, as this may have severe medical consequences for that individual.

General

MS CONTIN is intended for use in patients who require more than several days continuous treatment with a potent opioid analgesic. The controlled-release nature of the formulation allows it to be administered on a more convenient schedule than conventional immediate-release oral morphine products. (See CLINICAL PHARMACOLOGY: "Metabolism and Pharmacokinetics".) However, MS CONTIN does not release morphine continuously over the course of a dosing interval. The administration of single doses of MS CONTIN on a q12 hour dosing schedule will result in higher peak and lower trough plasma levels than those that occur when an identical daily dose of morphine is administered using conventional oral formulations on a q4h regimen. The clinical significance of greater fluctuations in morphine plasma level has not been systematically evaluated. (See DOSAGE AND ADMINISTRATION)

As with any potent opioid, it is critical to adjust the dosing regimen for each patient individually, taking into account the patient's prior analgesic treatment experience. Although it is clearly impossible to enumerate every consideration that is important to the selection of the initial dose and dos-

ing interval of MS CONTIN, attention should be given to 1) the daily dose, potency, and characteristics of the opioid the patient has been taking previously (e.g., whether it is a pure agonist or mixed agonist/antagonist), 2) the reliability of the relative potency estimate used to calculate the dose of morphine needed [N.B. potency estimates may vary with the route of administration], 3) the degree of opioid tolerance, if any, and 4) the general condition and medical status of the patient.

Selection of patients for treatment with MS CONTIN should be governed by the same principles that apply to the use of morphine or other potent opioid analgesics. Specifically, the increased risks associated with its use in the following populations should be considered: the elderly or debilitated and those with severe impairment of hepatic, pulmonary or renal function; myxedema or hypothyroidism; adrenocortical insufficiency (e.g., Addison's Disease); CNS depression or coma; toxic psychosis; prostatic hypertrophy or urethral stricture; acute alcoholism; delirium tremens; kyphoscoliosis, or inability to swallow.

The administration of morphine, like all opioid analgesics, may obscure the diagnosis or clinical course in patients with acute abdominal conditions.

Morphine may aggravate preexisting convulsions in patients with convulsive disorders. Morphine should be used with caution in patients about to undergo surgery of the biliary tract since it may cause spasm of the sphincter of Oddi. Similarly, morphine should be used with caution in patients with acute pancreatitis secondary to biliary tract disease.

Information for Patients

If clinically advisable, patients receiving MS CONTIN should be given the following instructions by the physician:

1. Appropriate pain management requires changes in the dose to maintain best pain control. Patients should be advised of the need to contact their physician if pain control is inadequate, but not to change the dose of MS CONTIN without consulting their physician.

2. Morphine may impair mental and/or physical ability required for the performance of potentially hazardous tasks (e.g., driving, operating machinery). Patients started on MS CONTIN or whose dose has been changed should refrain from dangerous activity until it is established that they are not adversely affected.

3. Morphine should not be taken with alcohol or other CNS depressants (sleep aids, tranquilizers) because additive effects including CNS depression may occur. A physician should be consulted if other prescription medications are currently being used or are prescribed for future use.

4. For women of childbearing potential who become or are planning to become pregnant, a physician should be consulted regarding analgesics and other drug use.

5. Upon completion of therapy, it may be appropriate to taper the morphine dose, rather than abruptly discontinue it.

6. While psychological dependence ("addiction") to morphine used in the treatment of pain is very rare, morphine is one of a class of drugs known to be abused and should be handled accordingly.

7. The MS CONTIN 200 mg Tablet is for use only in opioid tolerant patients requiring daily morphine equivalent dosages of 400 mg or more. Special care must be taken to avoid accidental ingestion or the use by individuals (including children) other than the patient for whom it was originally prescribed, as such unsupervised use may have severe, even fatal, consequences.

Drug Interactions (See WARNINGS)

The concomitant use of other central nervous system depressants including sedatives or hypnotics, general anesthetics, phenothiazines, tranquilizers and alcohol may produce additive depressant effects. Respiratory depression, hypotension and profound sedation or coma may occur. When such combined therapy is contemplated, the dose of one or both agents should be reduced. Opioid analgesics, including MS CONTIN, may enhance the neuromuscular blocking action of skeletal muscle relaxants and produce an increased degree of respiratory depression.

Carcinogenicity/Mutagenicity/Impairment of Fertility

Studies of morphine sulfate in animals to evaluate the drug's carcinogenic and mutagenic potential or the effect on fertility have not been conducted.

Pregnancy

Teratogenic effects—CATEGORY C: Adequate animal studies on reproduction have not been performed to determine whether morphine affects fertility in males or females. There are no well-controlled studies in women, but marketing experience does not include any evidence of adverse effects on the fetus following routine (short-term) clinical use of morphine sulfate products. Although there is no clearly defined risk, such experience cannot exclude the possibility of infrequent or subtle damage to the human fetus. MS CONTIN should be used in pregnant women only when clearly needed. (See also: PRECAUTIONS: Labor and Delivery, and DRUG ABUSE AND DEPENDENCE.)

Nonteratogenic effects: Infants born from mothers who have been taking morphine chronically may exhibit withdrawal symptoms.

Labor and Delivery

MS CONTIN is not recommended for use in women during and immediately prior to labor. Occasionally, opioid analgesics may prolong labor through actions which temporarily reduce the strength, duration and frequency of uterine contractions. However, this effect is not consistent and may be offset by an increased rate of cervical dilatation which tends to shorten labor.

Neonates whose mothers received opioid analgesics during labor should be observed closely for signs of respiratory depression. A specific narcotic antagonist, naloxone, should be available for reversal of narcotic-induced respiratory depression in the neonate.

Nursing Mothers

Low levels of *morphine* have been detected in the breast milk. Withdrawal symptoms can occur in breast-feeding infants when maternal administration of morphine sulfate is stopped. Ordinarily, nursing should not be undertaken while a patient is receiving MS CONTIN since morphine may be excreted in the milk.

Pediatric Use

Use of MS CONTIN has not been evaluated systematically in children.

ADVERSE REACTIONS

The adverse reactions caused by morphine are essentially those observed with other opioid analgesics. They include the following major hazards: respiratory depression, apnea, and to a lesser degree, circulatory depression; respiratory arrest, shock and cardiac arrest.

Most Frequently Observed

Constipation, lightheadedness, dizziness, sedation, nausea, vomiting, sweating, dysphoria and euphoria.

Some of these effects seem to be more prominent in ambulatory patients and in those not experiencing severe pain. Some adverse reactions in ambulatory patients may be alleviated if the patient lies down.

Less Frequently Observed Reactions

Central Nervous System: Weakness, headache, agitation, tremor, uncoordinated muscle movements, seizure, alterations of mood (nervousness, apprehension, depression, floating feelings), dreams, muscle rigidity, transient hallucinations and disorientation, visual disturbances, insomnia and increased intracranial pressure.

Gastrointestinal: Dry mouth, constipation, biliary tract spasm, laryngospasm, anorexia, diarrhea, cramps and taste alterations.

Cardiovascular: Flushing of the face, chills, tachycardia, bradycardia, palpitation, faintness, syncope, hypotension and hypertension.

Genitourinary: Urine retention or hesitance, reduced libido and/or potency.

Dermatologic: Pruritus, urticaria, other skin rashes, edema and diaphoresis.

Other: Antidiuretic effect, paresthesia, muscle tremor, blurred vision, nystagmus, diplopia and miosis.

DRUG ABUSE AND DEPENDENCE

Opioid analgesics may cause psychological and physical dependence (see WARNINGS). Physical dependence results in withdrawal symptoms in patients who abruptly discontinue the drug or may be precipitated through the administration of drugs with narcotic antagonist activity, e.g., naloxone or mixed agonist/antagonist analgesics (pentazocine, etc.; See also OVERDOSAGE). Physical dependence usually does not occur to a clinically significant degree until after several weeks of continued narcotic usage. Tolerance, in which increasingly large doses are required in order to produce the same degree of analgesia, is initially manifested by a shortened duration of analgesic effect, and, subsequently, by decreases in the intensity of analgesia.

In chronic pain patients, and in narcotic-tolerant cancer patients, the administration of MS CONTIN should be guided by the degree of tolerance manifested. Physical dependence, per se, is not ordinarily a concern when one is dealing with opioid-tolerant patients whose pain and suffering is associated with an irreversible illness.

If MS CONTIN is abruptly discontinued, a moderate to severe abstinence syndrome may occur. The opioid agonist abstinence syndrome is characterized by some or all of the following: restlessness, lacrimation, rhinorrhea, yawning, perspiration, gooseflesh, restless sleep or "yen" and mydriasis during the first 24 hours. These symptoms often increase in severity and over the next 72 hours may be accompanied by increasing irritability, anxiety, weakness, twitching and spasms of muscles; kicking movements; severe backache, abdominal and leg pains; abdominal and muscle cramps; hot and cold flashes, insomnia; nausea, anorexia, vomiting, intestinal spasm, diarrhea; coryza and repetitive sneezing; increase in body temperature, blood pressure, respiratory rate and heart rate. Because of excessive loss of fluids through sweating, vomiting and diarrhea, there is usually marked weight loss, dehydration, ketosis, and disturbances in acid-base balance. Cardiovascular collapse can occur.

Continued on next page

MS Contin—Cont.

Without treatment most observable symptoms disappear in 5–14 days; however, there appears to be a phase of secondary or chronic abstinence which may last for 2–6 months characterized by insomnia, irritability, and muscular aches. If treatment of physical dependence of patients on MS CONTIN is necessary, the patient may be detoxified by gradual reduction of the dosage. Gastrointestinal disturbances or dehydration should be treated accordingly.

OVERDOSAGE

Acute overdosage with morphine is manifested by respiratory depression, somnolence progressing to stupor or coma, skeletal muscle flaccidity, cold and clammy skin, constricted pupils, and, sometimes, bradycardia and hypotension.

In the treatment of overdosage, primary attention should be given to the re-establishment of a patent airway and institution of assisted or controlled ventilation. The pure opioid antagonist, naloxone, is a specific antidote against respiratory depression which results from opioid overdose. Naloxone (usually 0.4 to 2.0 mg) should be administered intravenously; however, because its duration of action is relatively short, the patient must be carefully monitored until spontaneous respiration is reliably re-established. If the response to naloxone is suboptimal or not sustained, additional naloxone may be re-administered, as needed, or given by continuous infusion to maintain alertness and respiratory function; however, there is no information available about the cumulative dose of naloxone that may be safely administered.

Naloxone should not be administered in the absence of clinically significant respiratory or circulatory depression secondary to morphine overdose. Naloxone should be administered cautiously to persons who are known, or suspected to be physically dependent on MS CONTIN. In such cases, an abrupt or complete reversal of narcotic effects may precipitate an acute abstinence syndrome.

Note: In an individual physically dependent on opioids, administration of the usual dose of the antagonist will precipitate an acute withdrawal syndrome. The severity of the withdrawal syndrome produced will depend on the degree of physical dependence and the dose of the antagonist administered. Use of a narcotic antagonist in such a person should be avoided. If necessary to treat serious respiratory depression in the physically dependent patient, the antagonist should be administered with care and by titration with smaller than usual doses of the antagonist.

Supportive measures (including oxygen, vasopressors) should be employed in the management of circulatory shock and pulmonary edema accompanying overdose as indicated. Cardiac arrest or arrhythmias may require cardiac massage or defibrillation.

DOSAGE AND ADMINISTRATION

(See also: CLINICAL PHARMACOLOGY, WARNINGS AND PRECAUTIONS sections)

MS CONTIN TABLETS ARE TO BE TAKEN WHOLE, AND ARE NOT TO BE BROKEN, CHEWED OR CRUSHED.

TAKING BROKEN, CHEWED OR CRUSHED MS CONTIN TABLETS COULD LEAD TO THE RAPID RELEASE AND ABSORPTION OF A POTENTIALLY TOXIC DOSE OF MORPHINE.

MS CONTIN is intended for use in patients who require more than several days continuous treatment with a potent opioid analgesic. The controlled-release nature of the formulation allows it to be administered on a more convenient schedule than conventional immediate-release oral morphine products. (See CLINICAL PHARMACOLOGY: "Metabolism and Pharmacokinetics".) However, MS CONTIN does not release morphine continuously over the course of a dosing interval. The administration of single doses of MS CONTIN on a q12h dosing schedule will result in higher peak and lower trough plasma levels than those that occur when an identical daily dose of morphine is administered using conventional oral formulations on a q4h regimen. The clinical significance of greater fluctuations in morphine plasma level has not been systematically evaluated.

As with any potent opioid drug product, it is critical to adjust the dosing regimen for each patient individually, taking into account the patient's prior analgesic treatment experience. Although it is clearly impossible to enumerate every consideration that is important to the selection of initial dose and dosing interval of MS CONTIN, attention should be given to 1) the daily dose, potency and precise characteristics of the opioid the patient has been taking previously (e.g., whether it is a pure agonist or mixed agonist/antagonist), 2) the reliability of the relative potency estimate used to calculate the dose of morphine needed [N.B. potency estimates may vary with the route of administration], 3) the degree of opioid tolerance, if any, and 4) the general condition and medical status of the patient.

The following dosing recommendations, therefore, can only be considered suggested approaches to what is actually a series of clinical decisions in the management of the pain of an individual patient.

Conversion from Conventional Oral Morphine to MS CONTIN

A patient's daily morphine requirement is established using immediate-release oral morphine (dosing every 4 to 6 hours). The patient is then converted to MS CONTIN in either of two ways: 1) by administering one-half of the patient's 24-hour requirement as MS CONTIN on an every 12-hour schedule; or, 2) by administering one-third of the patient's daily requirement as MS CONTIN on an every eight hour schedule. With either method, dose and dosing interval is then adjusted as needed (see discussion below). The 15 mg tablet should be used for initial conversion for patients whose total daily requirement is expected to be less than 60 mg. The 30 mg tablet strength is recommended for patients with a daily morphine requirement of 60 to 120 mg. When the total daily dose is expected to be greater than 120 mg, the appropriate combination of tablet strengths should be employed.

Conversion from Parenteral Morphine or Other Opioids (Parenteral or Oral) to MS CONTIN

MS CONTIN can be administered as the initial oral morphine drug product; in this case, however, particular care must be exercised in the conversion process. Because of uncertainty about, and intersubject variation in, relative estimates of opioid potency and cross tolerance, initial dosing regimens should be conservative; that is, an underestimation of the 24-hour oral morphine requirement is preferred to an overestimate. To this end, initial individual doses of MS CONTIN should be estimated conservatively. In patients whose daily morphine requirements are expected to be less than or equal to 120 mg per day, the 30 mg tablet strength is recommended for the initial titration period. Once a stable dose regimen is reached, the patient can be converted to the 60 mg or 100 mg tablet strength, or appropriate combination of tablet strengths, if desired.

Estimates of the relative potency of opioids are only approximate and are influenced by route of administration, individual patient differences, and, possibly, by an individual's medical condition. Consequently, it is difficult to recommend any fixed rule for converting a patient to MS CONTIN directly. The following general points should be considered, however.

1. *Parenteral to oral morphine ratio:* Estimates of the oral to parenteral potency of morphine vary. Some authorities suggest that a dose of oral morphine only three times the daily parenteral morphine requirement may be sufficient in chronic use settings.

2. *Other parenteral or oral opioids to oral morphine:* Because there is lack of systemic evidence bearing on these types of analgesic substitutions, specific recommendations are not possible.

Physicians are advised to refer to published relative potency data, keeping in mind that such ratios are only approximate. In general, it is safer to underestimate the daily dose of MS CONTIN required and rely upon ad hoc supplementation to deal with inadequate analgesia. (See discussion which follows.)

Use of MS CONTIN as the first opioid analgesic

There has been no systematic evaluation of MS CONTIN as an initial opioid analgesic in the management of pain. Because it may be more difficult to titrate a patient using a controlled-release morphine, it is ordinarily advisable to begin treatment using an immediate-release formulation.

Considerations in the Adjustment of Dosing Regimens

Whatever the approach, if signs of excessive opioid effects are observed early in a dosing interval, the next dose should be reduced. If this adjustment leads to inadequate analgesia, that is, "breakthrough" pain occurs late in the dosing interval, the dosing interval should be shortened. Alternatively, a supplemental dose of a short-acting analgesic may be given. As experience is gained, adjustments can be made to obtain an appropriate balance between pain relief, opioid side effects, and the convenience of the dosing schedule.

In adjusting dosing requirements, it is recommended that the dosing interval never be extended beyond 12 hours because the administration of very large single doses may lead to acute overdose. (N.B. MS CONTIN is a controlled-release formulation; it does not release morphine continuously over the dosing interval.)

For patients with low daily morphine requirements, the 15 mg tablet should be used.

Special Instructions for MS CONTIN 200 mg Tablets (For use in opioid tolerant patients only.)

The MS CONTIN 200 mg tablet is for use only in opioid tolerant patients requiring daily morphine equivalent dosages of 400 mg or more. It is recommended that this strength be reserved for patients that have already been titrated to a stable analgesic regimen using lower strengths of MS CONTIN or other opioid.

Conversion from MS CONTIN to parenteral opioids:

When converting a patient from MS CONTIN to parenteral opioids, it is best to assume that the parenteral to oral potency is high. NOTE THAT THIS IS THE CONVERSE OF THE STRATEGY USED WHEN THE DIRECTION OF CONVERSION IS FROM THE PARENTERAL TO ORAL FORMULATIONS. IN BOTH CASES, HOWEVER, THE

AIM IS TO ESTIMATE THE NEW DOSE CONSERVATIVELY. For example, to estimate the required 24-hour dose of morphine for IM use, one could employ a conversion of 1 mg of morphine IM for every 6 mg of morphine as MS CONTIN. Of course, the IM 24-hour dose would have to be divided by six and administered on a q4h regimen. This approach is recommended because it is least likely to cause overdose.

Safety and Handling

MS CONTIN TABLETS ARE TO BE TAKEN WHOLE, AND ARE NOT TO BE BROKEN, CHEWED, OR CRUSHED. TAKING BROKEN, CHEWED, OR CRUSHED MS CONTIN TABLETS COULD LEAD TO THE RAPID RELEASE AND ABSORPTION OF A POTENTIALLY TOXIC DOSE OF MORPHINE.

The MS CONTIN 200 mg Tablet strength is for use only in opioid tolerant patients requiring daily morphine equivalent dosages of 400 mg or more. This strength is potentially toxic if accidentally ingested and patients and their families should be instructed to take special care to avoid accidental or intentional ingestion by individuals other than those for whom the medication was originally prescribed.

HOW SUPPLIED

NDC 0034-0514-10: MS CONTIN (morphine sulfate controlled-release tablets) 15 mg are supplied in opaque plastic bottles containing 100 tablets.

NDC 0034-0514-90: MS CONTIN (morphine sulfate controlled-release tablets) 15 mg are supplied in opaque plastic bottles containing 500 tablets.

NDC 0034-0514-25: MS CONTIN (morphine sulfate controlled-release tablets) 15 mg are supplied in unit dose packaging with 25 individually numbered tablets per card; one card per tuck end carton.

NDC 0034-0515-50: MS CONTIN (morphine sulfate controlled-release tablets) 30 mg are supplied in opaque plastic bottles containing 50 tablets.

NDC 0034-0515-10: MS CONTIN (morphine sulfate controlled-release tablets) 30 mg are supplied in opaque plastic bottles containing 100 tablets.

NDC 0034-0515-45: MS CONTIN (morphine sulfate controlled-release tablets) 30 mg are supplied in opaque plastic bottles containing 250 tablets.

NDC 0034-0515-90: MS CONTIN (morphine sulfate controlled-release tablets) 30 mg are supplied in opaque plastic bottles containing 500 tablets.

NDC 0034-0515-25: MS CONTIN (morphine sulfate controlled-release tablets) 30 mg are supplied in unit dose packaging with 25 individually numbered tablets per card; one card per tuck end carton.

NDC 0034-0516-10: MS CONTIN (morphine sulfate controlled-release tablets) 60 mg are supplied in opaque plastic bottles containing 100 tablets.

NDC 0034-0516-90: MS CONTIN (morphine sulfate controlled-release tablets) 60 mg are supplied in opaque plastic bottles containing 500 tablets.

NDC 0034-0516-25: MS CONTIN (morphine sulfate controlled-release tablets) 60 mg are supplied in unit dose packaging with 25 individually numbered tablets per card; one card per tuck end carton.

NDC 0034-0517-10: MS CONTIN (morphine sulfate controlled-release tablets) 100 mg are supplied in opaque plastic bottles containing 100 tablets.

NDC 0034-0517-90: MS CONTIN (morphine sulfate controlled-release tablets) 100 mg are supplied in opaque plastic bottles containing 500 tablets.

NDC 0034-0517-25: MS CONTIN (morphine sulfate controlled-release tablets) 100 mg are supplied in unit dose packaging with 25 individually numbered tablets per card; one card per tuck end carton.

NDC 0034-0513-10: MS CONTIN (morphine sulfate controlled-release tablets) 200 mg are supplied in opaque plastic bottles containing 100 tablets.

NDC 0034-0513-25: MS CONTIN (morphine sulfate controlled-release tablets) 200 mg are supplied in unit dose packaging with 25 individually numbered tablets per card; one card per tuck end carton.

15 mg: Each round, blue-colored tablet bears the symbol PF on one side and M15 on the other side.

30 mg: Each round, lavender-colored tablet bears the symbol PF on one side and M30 on the other side.

60 mg: Each round, orange-colored tablet bears the symbol PF on one side and M60 on the other side.

100 mg: Each round, gray-colored tablet bears the symbol PF on one side and M100 on the other side.

200 mg: Each capsule-shaped, green-colored tablet bears the symbol PF on one side and 200 on the other side.

Store tablets at controlled room temperature 15°–30°C (59°–86°F).

Dispense in tight, light-resistant container.

CAUTION

DEA Order Form Required.

Federal law prohibits dispensing without prescription.

THE PURDUE FREDERICK COMPANY

Norwalk, CT 06850-3590

Copyright © 1987, 1994, The Purdue Frederick Company

U.S. Patent Numbers 4235870 and 4366310
January 28, 1994 **G3220**
Shown in Product Identification Guide, page 332

MSIR® CII
Oral Solution
[*em 'es ī "ahr*]
(morphine sulfate)
MSIR® CII
Oral Solution Concentrate*
(morphine sulfate)
MSIR® CII
Immediate-Release Oral Tablets
(morphine sulfate)
MSIR® CII
Immediate-Release Oral Capsules
(morphine sulfate)

*This product contains dry natural rubber

DESCRIPTION

Chemically, morphine sulfate is 7,8 didehydro-4,5 α-epoxy-17-methylmorphinan-3,6 α-diol sulfate (2:1) (salt) pentahydrate and has the following structural formula:

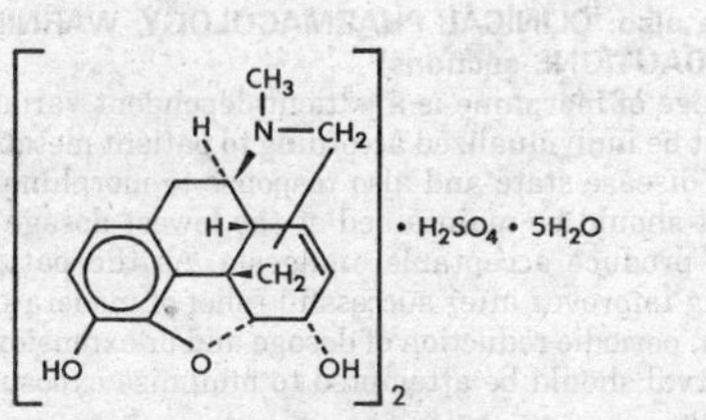

MSIR Oral Solution
Each 5 mL of MSIR Oral Solution contains:
Morphine Sulfate .... 10 or 20 mg
Inactive Ingredients: Edetate disodium, FD&C Red. No. 40, Glycerin, Invert Sugar, Sodium benzoate, Sodium chloride, Sucrose, Artificial & Natural Flavors, and other ingredients.
MSIR Oral Solution Concentrate
Each 1 mL of MSIR Oral Solution Concentrate contains:
Morphine Sulfate .... 20 mg
Inactive Ingredients: Edetate disodium, Sodium benzoate, and other ingredients.
MSIR Tablets
Each MSIR Tablet for oral administration contains:
Morphine Sulfate .... 15 or 30 mg
Inactive Ingredients: Croscarmellose sodium, Lactose, Magnesium stearate, Microcrystalline cellulose, and Talc.
MSIR Capsules
Each MSIR Capsule for oral administration contains:
Morphine Sulfate .... 15 or 30 mg
Inactive Ingredients: FD&C Blue No. 1, FD&C Blue No. 2, FD&C Red No. 40, FD&C Yellow No. 6, Gelatin, Hydroxypropyl methylcellulose, Lactose, Polyethylene glycol, Polysorbate 80, Polyvinylpyrrolidone, Starch, Sucrose, Titanium dioxide, and other ingredients. In addition, the 30 mg capsule contains Black iron oxide and D&C Red No. 28.

CLINICAL PHARMACOLOGY

Metabolism and Pharmacokinetics

MSIR Solutions, Tablets and Capsules containing morphine sulfate are for oral administration and are conventional immediate release products. Only about 40% of the administered dose reaches the central compartment because of presystemic elimination (i.e., metabolism in the gut wall and liver).

Once absorbed, morphine is distributed to skeletal muscle, kidneys, liver, intestinal tract, lungs, spleen and brain. Morphine also crosses the placental membranes and has been found in breast milk.

Although a small fraction (less than 5%) of morphine is demethylated, for all practical purposes, virtually all morphine is converted to glucuronide metabolites; among these, morphine-3-glucuronide is present in the highest plasma concentration following oral administration.

The glucuronide system has a very high capacity and is not easily saturated even in disease. Therefore, rate of delivery of morphine to the gut and liver should not influence the total and, probably, the relative quantities of the various metabolites formed. Moreover, even if rate affected the relative amounts of each metabolite formed, it should be unimportant clinically because morphine's metabolites are ordinarily inactive.

The following pharmacokinetic parameters show considerable intersubject variation but are representative of average values reported in the literature. The volume of distribution (Vd) for morphine is 4 liters per kilogram, and its terminal elimination half-life is approximately 2 to 4 hours. Following the administration of conventional oral morphine products, approximately fifty percent of the morphine that will reach the central compartment intact, reaches it within 30 minutes.

Variation in the physical/mechanical properties of a formulation of an oral morphine drug product can affect both its absolute bioavailability and its absorption rate constant (k_a). The basic pharmacokinetic parameters (e.g., volume of distribution [Vd], elimination rate constant [k_e], clearance [Cl]) are fundamental properties of morphine in the organism. However, in chronic use, the possibility that shifts in metabolite to parent drug ratios may occur cannot be excluded.

When immediate-release oral morphine is given on a fixed dosing regimen, steady state is achieved in about a day.

For a given dose and dosing interval, the AUC and average blood concentration of morphine at steady state (Css) will be independent of the specific type of oral formulation administered so long as the formulations have the same absolute bioavailability. The absorption rate of a formulation will, however, affect the maximum (Cmax) and minimum (Cmin) blood levels and the times of their occurrence.

While there is no predictable relationship between morphine blood levels and analgesic response, effective analgesia will not occur below some minimum blood level in a given patient. The minimum effective blood level for analgesia will vary among patients, especially among patients who have been previously treated with potent mu (μ) agonist opioids. Similarly, there is no predictable relationship between blood morphine concentration and untoward clinical responses; again, however, higher concentrations are more likely to be toxic than lower ones.

The elimination of morphine occurs primarily as renal excretion of 3-morphine glucuronide. A small amount of the glucuronide conjugate is excreted in the bile, and there is some minor enterohepatic recycling.

The elimination half-life of morphine is reported to vary between 2 and 4 hours. Thus, steady-state is probably achieved on most regimens within a day. Because morphine is primarily metabolized to inactive metabolites, the effects of renal disease on morphine's elimination are not likely to be pronounced. However, as with any drug, caution should be taken to guard against unanticipated accumulation if renal and/or hepatic function is seriously impaired.

Individual differences in the metabolism of morphine suggest that MSIR Oral Solutions, Tablets and Capsules be dosed conservatively according to the dosing initiation and titration recommendations in the Dosage and Administration section.

PHARMACODYNAMICS

The effects described below are common to all morphine-containing products.

Central Nervous System

The principal actions of therapeutic value of morphine are analgesia and sedation (i.e., sleepiness and anxiolysis).

The precise mechanism of analgesic action is unknown. However, specific CNS opiate receptors and endogenous compounds with morphine-like activity have been identified throughout the brain and spinal cord and are likely to play a role in the expression of analgesic effects.

Morphine produces respiratory depression by direct action on brain stem respiratory centers. The mechanism of respiratory depression involves a reduction in the responsiveness of the brain stem respiratory centers to increases in carbon dioxide tension, and to electrical stimulation.

Morphine depresses the cough reflex by direct effect on the cough center in the medulla. Antitussive effects may occur with doses lower than those usually required for analgesia.

Morphine causes miosis, even in total darkness. Pinpoint pupils are a sign of narcotic overdose but are not pathognomonic (e.g., pontine lesions of hemorrhagic or ischemic origins may produce similar findings). Marked mydriasis rather than miosis may be seen with worsening hypoxia.

Gastrointestinal Tract and Other Smooth Muscle

Gastric, biliary and pancreatic secretions are decreased by morphine. Morphine causes a reduction in motility associated with an increase in tone in the antrum of the stomach and duodenum. Digestion of food in the small intestine is delayed and propulsive contractions are decreased. In addition, propulsive peristaltic waves in the colon are decreased, while tone is increased to the point of spasm. The end result is constipation. Morphine can cause a marked increase in biliary tract pressure as a result of spasm of the sphincter of Oddi.

Cardiovascular System

Morphine produces peripheral vasodilation which may result in orthostatic hypotension. Release of histamine can occur and may contribute to narcotic-induced hypotension. Manifestations of histamine release and/or peripheral vasodilation may include pruritus, flushing, red eyes and sweating.

INDICATIONS AND USAGE

MSIR Oral Solutions, Tablets and Capsules are indicated for the relief of moderate to severe pain.

CONTRAINDICATIONS

MSIR Oral Solutions, Tablets and Capsules are contraindicated in patients with known hypersensitivity to the drug, in patients with respiratory depression in the absence of resuscitative equipment, and in patients with acute or severe bronchial asthma.

MSIR Oral Solutions, Tablets and Capsules are contraindicated in any patient who has or is suspected of having a paralytic ileus.

WARNINGS (See also: CLINICAL PHARMACOLOGY)

Impaired Respiration

Respiratory depression is the chief hazard of all morphine preparations.

Respiratory depression occurs most frequently in elderly and debilitated patients, and those suffering from conditions accompanied by hypoxia or hypercapnia when even moderate therapeutic doses may dangerously decrease pulmonary ventilation.

Morphine should be used with extreme caution in patients with chronic obstructive pulmonary disease or cor pulmonale, and in patients having a substantially decreased respiratory reserve, hypoxia, hypercapnia, or preexisting respiratory depression. In such patients, even usual therapeutic doses of morphine may decrease respiratory drive while simultaneously increasing airway resistance to the point of apnea.

Head Injury and Increased Intracranial Pressure

The respiratory depressant effects of morphine with carbon dioxide retention and secondary elevation of cerebrospinal fluid pressure may be markedly exaggerated in the presence of head injury, other intracranial lesions, or preexisting increase in intracranial pressure. Morphine produces effects which may obscure neurologic signs of further increase in pressure in patients with head injuries.

Hypotensive Effects

MSIR Oral Solutions, Tablets and Capsules, like all opioid analgesics, may cause severe hypotension in an individual whose ability to maintain his blood pressure has already been compromised by a depleted blood volume, or a concurrent administration of drugs such as phenothiazines, or general anesthetics. (See also: PRECAUTIONS: Drug Interactions.) MSIR Oral Solutions, Tablets and Capsules may produce orthostatic hypotension in ambulatory patients.

MSIR Oral Solutions, Tablets and Capsules, like all opioid analgesics, should be administered with caution to patients in circulatory shock, since vasodilation produced by the drug may further reduce cardiac output and blood pressure.

Interactions with Other CNS Depressants

MSIR Oral Solutions, Tablets and Capsules, like all opioid analgesics, should be used with great caution and in reduced dosage in patients who are concurrently receiving other central nervous system depressants including sedatives or hypnotics, general anesthetics, phenothiazines, other tranquilizers and alcohol, because respiratory depression, hypotension and profound sedation or coma may result.

Interactions with Mixed Agonist/Antagonist Opioid Analgesics

From a theoretical perspective, agonist/antagonist analgesics (i.e., pentazocine, nalbuphine, butorphanol and buprenorphine) should NOT be administered to a patient who has received or is receiving a course of therapy with a pure agonist opioid analgesic. In these patients, mixed agonist-antagonist analgesics may reduce the analgesic effect or may precipitate withdrawal symptoms.

Drug Dependence

Morphine can produce drug dependence and has a potential for being abused. Tolerance and psychological and physical dependence may develop upon repeated administration. Physical dependence, however, is not of paramount importance in the management of terminally ill patients or any patient in severe pain. Abrupt cessation or a sudden reduction in dose after prolonged use may result in withdrawal symptoms. After prolonged exposure to opioid analgesics, if withdrawal is necessary, it must be undertaken gradually. (See DRUG ABUSE AND DEPENDENCE.)

Infants born to mothers physically dependent on opioid analgesics may also be physically dependent and exhibit respiratory depression and withdrawal symptoms. (See DRUG ABUSE AND DEPENDENCE.)

PRECAUTIONS (See also: CLINICAL PHARMACOLOGY)

General

MSIR Oral Solutions, Tablets and Capsules are intended for use in patients who require a potent opioid analgesic for relief of moderate to severe pain.

Selection of patients for treatment with MSIR Oral Solutions, Tablets and Capsules should be governed by the same principles that apply to the use of morphine and other potent opioid analgesics. Specifically, the increased risks associated with its use in the following populations should be considered: the elderly or debilitated and those with severe

Continued on next page

MSIR—Cont.

impairment of hepatic, pulmonary or renal function; myxedema or hypothyroidism; adrenocortical insufficiency (e.g., Addison's Disease); CNS depression or coma; toxic psychoses; prostatic hypertrophy or urethral stricture; acute alcoholism; delirium tremens; kyphoscoliosis or inability to swallow.

The administration of morphine, like all opioid analgesics, may obscure the diagnosis or clinical course in patients with acute abdominal conditions.

Morphine may aggravate preexisting convulsions in patients with convulsive disorders.

Morphine should be used with caution in patients about to undergo surgery of the biliary tract, since it may cause spasm of the sphincter of Oddi. Similarly, morphine should be used with caution in patients with acute pancreatitis secondary to biliary tract disease.

Information for Patients

If clinically advisable, patients receiving MSIR Oral Solutions, Tablets and Capsules should be given the following instructions by the physician.

1. Morphine may produce physical and/or psychological dependence. For this reason, the dose of the drug should not be adjusted without consulting a physician.
2. Morphine may impair mental and/or physical ability required for the performance of potentially hazardous tasks (e.g., driving, operating machinery).
3. Morphine should not be taken with alcohol or other CNS depressants (sleep aids, tranquilizers) because additive effects including CNS depression may occur. A physician should be consulted if other prescription medications are currently being used or are prescribed for future use.
4. For women of childbearing potential who become or are planning to become pregnant, a physician should be consulted regarding analgesics and other drug use.

Drug Interactions (See also WARNINGS)

The concomitant use of other central nervous system depressants including sedatives or hypnotics, general anesthetics, phenothiazines, tranquilizers and alcohol may produce additive depressant effects. Respiratory depression, hypotension and profound sedation or coma may occur. When such combined therapy is contemplated, the dose of one or both agents should be reduced. Opioid analgesics, including MSIR Oral Solutions, Tablets and Capsules, may enhance the neuromuscular blocking action of skeletal muscle relaxants and produce an increased degree of respiratory depression.

Carcinogenicity/Mutagenicity/Impairment of Fertility

Studies of morphine sulfate in animals to evaluate the drug's carcinogenic and mutagenic potential or the effect on fertility have not been conducted.

Pregnancy

Teratogenic effects—CATEGORY C: Adequate animal studies on reproduction have not been performed to determine whether morphine affects fertility in males or females. There are no well-controlled studies in women, but marketing experience does not include any evidence of adverse effects on the fetus following routine (short-term) clinical use of morphine sulfate products. Although there is no clearly defined risk, such experience cannot exclude the possibility of infrequent or subtle damage to the human fetus. MSIR Oral Solutions, Tablets and Capsules should be used in pregnant women only when clearly needed. (See also: PRECAUTIONS: Labor and Delivery, and DRUG ABUSE AND DEPENDENCE.)

Nonteratogenic effects: Infants born from mothers who have been taking morphine chronically may exhibit withdrawal symptoms.

Labor and Delivery

MSIR Oral Solutions, Tablets and Capsules are not recommended for use in women during and immediately prior to labor. Occasionally, opioid analgesics may prolong labor through actions which temporarily reduce the strength, duration and frequency of uterine contractions. However, this effect is not consistent and may be offset by an increased rate of cervical dilatation which tends to shorten labor. Neonates whose mothers received opioid analgesics during labor should be observed closely for signs of respiratory depression. A specific narcotic antagonist, naloxone, should be available for reversal of narcotic-induced respiratory depression in the neonate.

Nursing Mothers

Low levels of morphine have been detected in human milk. Withdrawal symptoms can occur in breast-feeding infants when maternal administration of morphine sulfate is stopped. Nursing should not be undertaken while a patient is receiving MSIR Oral Solutions, Tablets and Capsules since morphine may be excreted in the milk.

Pediatric Use

MSIR Oral Solutions, Tablets and Capsules have not been evaluated systematically in children.

ADVERSE REACTIONS

The adverse reactions caused by morphine are essentially the same as those observed with other opioid analgesics.

They include the following major hazards: respiratory depression, apnea, and to a lesser degree, circulatory depression; respiratory arrest, shock, and cardiac arrest.

Most Frequently Observed

Constipation, lightheadedness, dizziness, sedation, nausea, vomiting, sweating, dysphoria and euphoria.

Some of these effects seem to be more prominent in ambulatory patients and in those not experiencing severe pain. Some adverse reactions in ambulatory patients may be alleviated if the patient lies down.

Less Frequently Observed Reactions

Central Nervous System: Weakness, headache, agitation, tremor, uncoordinated muscle movements, seizure, alterations of mood (nervousness, apprehension, depression, floating feelings), dreams, muscle rigidity, transient hallucinations and disorientation, visual disturbances, insomnia and increased intracranial pressure.

Gastrointestinal: Dry mouth, biliary tract spasm, laryngospasm, anorexia, diarrhea, cramps and taste alterations.

Cardiovascular: Flushing of the face, chills, tachycardia, bradycardia, palpitation, faintness, syncope, hypotension and hypertension.

Genitourinary: Urinary retention or hesitance, reduced libido, and/or potency.

Dermatologic: Pruritus, urticaria, other skin rashes, edema and diaphoresis.

Other: Antidiuretic effect, paresthesia, muscle tremor, blurred vision, nystagmus, diplopia and miosis.

DRUG ABUSE AND DEPENDENCE

Opioid analgesics may cause psychological and physical dependence. (See WARNINGS.) Physical dependence results in withdrawal symptoms in patients who abruptly discontinue the drug or may be precipitated through the administration of drugs with narcotic antagonist activity, e.g., naloxone or mixed agonist/antagonist analgesics (pentazocine, etc.: see also OVERDOSE). Physical dependence usually does not occur to a clinically significant degree until after several weeks of continued narcotic usage. Tolerance, in which increasingly large doses are required in order to produce the same degree of analgesia, is initially manifested by a shortened duration of analgesic effect, and, subsequently, by decreases in the intensity of analgesia.

In chronic-pain patients and in narcotic-tolerant cancer patients, the administration of MSIR Oral Solutions, Tablets and Capsules should be guided by the degree of tolerance manifested. Physical dependence, per se, is not ordinarily a concern when one is dealing with opioid-tolerant patients whose pain and suffering is associated with an irreversible illness.

If MSIR Oral Solutions, Tablets and Capsules are abruptly discontinued, a moderate to severe abstinence syndrome may occur. The opioid agonist abstinence syndrome is characterized by some or all of the following: restlessness, lacrimation, rhinorrhea, yawning, perspiration, cutis anserina, restless sleep known as the "yen" and mydriasis during the first 24 hours. These symptoms often increase in severity and over the next 72 hours may be accompanied by increasing irritability, anxiety, weakness, twitching and spasms of muscles; kicking movements; severe backache, abdominal and leg pains; abdominal and muscle cramps; hot and cold flashes; insomnia; nausea, anorexia, vomiting, intestinal spasm, diarrhea; coryza and repetitive sneezing; and increase in body temperature, blood pressure, respiratory rate and heart rate. Because of excessive loss of fluids through sweating, vomiting and diarrhea, there is usually marked weight loss, dehydration, ketosis, and disturbances in acid-base balance. Cardiovascular collapse can occur. Without treatment, most observable symptoms disappear in 5–14 days; however, there appears to be a phase of secondary or chronic abstinence which may last for 2–6 months, characterized by insomnia, irritability, and muscular aches.

If treatment of physical dependence on MSIR Oral Solutions, Tablets and Capsules is necessary, the patient may be detoxified by gradual reduction of the dosage. Gastrointestinal disturbances or dehydration should be treated accordingly.

OVERDOSE

Acute overdosage with morphine is manifested by respiratory depression, somnolence progressing to stupor or coma, skeletal muscle flaccidity, cold and clammy skin, constricted pupils, and, sometimes, bradycardia and hypotension.

In the treatment of overdosage, primary attention should be given to the re-establishment of a patent airway and institution of assisted or controlled ventilation. The pure opioid antagonist, naloxone, is a specific antidote against respiratory depression which results from opioid overdose. Naloxone (usually 0.4 to 2.0 mg) should be administered intravenously; however, because its duration of action is relatively short, the patient must be carefully monitored until spontaneous respiration is reliably reestablished. If the response to naloxone is suboptimal or not sustained, additional naloxone may be re-administered, as needed, or given by continuous infusion to maintain alertness and respiratory function; however, there is no information available about the cumulative dose of naloxone that may be safely administered.

Naloxone should not be administered in the absence of clinically significant respiratory or circulatory depression secondary to morphine overdose. Naloxone should be administered cautiously to persons who are known or suspected to be physically dependent on morphine. In such cases, an abrupt or complete reversal of narcotic effects may precipitate an acute abstinence syndrome.

Note: In an individual physically dependent on opioids, administration of the usual dose of the antagonist will precipitate an acute withdrawal syndrome. The severity of the withdrawal syndrome produced will depend on the degree of physical dependence and the dose of the antagonist administered. Use of a narcotic antagonist in such a person should be avoided. If necessary to treat serious respiratory depression in the physically dependent patient the antagonist should be administered with extreme care and by titration with smaller than usual doses of the antagonist.

Supportive measures (including oxygen, vasopressors) should be employed in the management of circulatory shock and pulmonary edema accompanying overdose as indicated. Cardiac arrest or arrhythmias may require cardiac massage or defibrillation.

DOSAGE AND ADMINISTRATION

(See also: CLINICAL PHARMACOLOGY, WARNINGS AND PRECAUTIONS sections)

Dosage of morphine is a patient-dependent variable, which must be individualized according to patient metabolism, age and disease state and also response to morphine. Each patient should be maintained at the lowest dosage level that will produce acceptable analgesia. As the patient's well-being improves after successful relief of moderate to severe pain, periodic reduction of dosage and/or extension of dosing interval should be attempted to minimize exposure to morphine.

Usual Adult Oral Dose: 5 to 30 mg every four (4) hours or as directed by physician, administered either as MSIR Oral Solutions, MSIR Oral Tablets or MSIR Oral Capsules. For control of pain in terminal illness, it is recommended that the appropriate dose of MSIR Oral Solutions, MSIR Oral Tablets or MSIR Oral Capsules be given on a regularly scheduled basis every four hours at the minimum dose to achieve acceptable analgesia. If converting a patient from another narcotic to morphine sulfate on the basis of standard equivalence tables, a 1 to 3 ratio of parenteral to oral morphine equivalence is suggested. This ratio is conservative and may underestimate the amount of morphine required. If this is the case, the dose of MSIR Oral Solutions, MSIR Oral Tablets or MSIR Oral Capsules should be gradually increased to achieve acceptable analgesia and tolerable side effects.

Sprinkling Contents of Capsule on Food or Liquids: MSIR Oral Capsules may be carefully opened and the entire beaded contents added to a small amount of cool, soft food, such as applesauce or pudding, or a liquid, such as water or orange juice. The bead-food mixture should be swallowed immediately and not stored for future use.

HOW SUPPLIED

MSIR (morphine sulfate) Oral Solution: (pleasantly flavored)

10 mg per 5 mL.
NDC 0034-0521-02: high density polyethylene plastic bottle of 120 mL with child-resistant closure.

20 mg per 5 mL.
NDC 0034-0522-02: high density polyethylene plastic bottle of 120 mL with child-resistant closure.

MSIR (morphine sulfate) Oral Solution Concentrate: (unflavored)

20 mg per 1 mL.
NDC 0034-0523-01: high density polyethylene plastic, child-resistant closure bottle with child-resistant dropper in 30 mL size.

NDC 0034-0523-02: high density polyethylene plastic, child-resistant closure bottle with child-resistant dropper in 120 mL size.

Discard opened bottle of Oral Solution after 90 days. Protect from light.

MSIR (morphine sulfate) Tablets:

15 mg round, white scored tablets
NDC 0034-0518-10: opaque plastic bottle containing 100 tablets. Each tablet bears the symbol *PF* on the scored side and *MI 15* on the other side.

30 mg capsule-shaped, white scored tablets
NDC 0034-0519-10: opaque plastic bottle containing 100 tablets. Each tablet bears the symbol *PF* on the scored side and *MI 30* on the other side.

MSIR (morphine sulfate) Capsules:

15 mg capsules, white opaque capsule body with blue cap
NDC 0034-1025-10: opaque plastic bottle containing 100 capsules. Each capsule bears the symbols "*PF MSIR 15*" and "*THIS END UP.*"

30 mg capsules, gray opaque capsule body with lavender cap
NDC 0034-1026-10: opaque plastic bottle containing 100 capsules. Each capsule bears the symbols *"PF MSIR 30"* and *"THIS END UP."*

Store MSIR Oral Solutions, Tablets and Capsules at controlled room temperature 15° to 30°C (59°–86°F).
CAUTION: DEA Order Form Required.
Rx Only
THE PURDUE FREDERICK COMPANY
Norwalk, CT 06850-3590
Copyright© 1985, 1998
The Purdue Frederick Company
June 5, 1998   I3154
Shown in Product Identification Guide, page 332

SENOKOT® CHILDREN'S SYRUP   OTC
[sĕn 'ō-kŏt]
(extract of senna concentrate)*

ACTION AND USES
To relieve functional constipation in children from two to under 12 years of age, Senokot Children's Syrup generally produces bowel movement in 6 to 12 hours. Taken at bedtime, it works gently overnight.

DESCRIPTION
Each teaspoon of Senokot Children's Syrup contains 8.8 mg sennosides. Active Ingredient: Extract of Senna Concentrate. Inactive Ingredients: Methylparaben, Potassium sorbate, Propylparaben, Sucrose, Water, Natural and artificial chocolate flavor, and other ingredients.

ADMINISTRATION AND DOSAGE
Recommended Dosage (or as directed by a doctor):
Take preferably at bedtime.

AGE	STARTING	MAXIMUM
6 to under 12 years of age	1-1¹/₂ tsp. once/day	1¹/₂ tsp. twice/day
2 to under 6 years of age	¹/₂-³/₄ tsp. once/day	³/₄ tsp. twice/day
Under 2 years	Consult a physician	

SENOKOT Children's Syrup is packaged with a free measuring cup to help assure accurate dosing. Formulated without alcohol, Senokot Children's Syrup has an appealing chocolaty flavor. It may be given with ice cream or stirred into milk. Its natural active ingredient is concentrated, making it effective with smaller doses than other children's laxatives.

WARNINGS
Do not use laxative products when abdominal pain, nausea, or vomiting are present unless directed by a doctor. If there has been a sudden change in the child's bowel movements that persists over a period of 2 weeks, consult a doctor before using a laxative. Laxative products should not be used for a period longer than 1 week unless directed by a doctor. Rectal bleeding or failure to have a bowel movement after use of a laxative may indicate a serious condition. Discontinue use and consult a doctor. As with any drug, if the user is pregnant or nursing a baby, seek the advice of a health professional before taking this product. In case of accidental overdose, seek professional assistance or contact a Poison Control Center immediately. Keep out of children's reach.

HOW SUPPLIED
2.5 fl. oz. plastic bottles; packaged with measuring cup.
Copyright 1996, 1998, The Purdue Frederick Company, Norwalk, CT 06850-3590

SENOKOT® TABLETS/GRANULES   OTC
[sen 'ō-kŏt]

SenokotXTRA® Tablets   OTC
(standardized senna concentrate)

SENOKOT-S® Tablets   OTC
(standardized senna concentrate and docusate sodium)
Natural Vegetable Laxative/Stool Softener Combination

INDICATIONS
SENOKOT Tablets/Granules and Double-Strength SenokotXTRA Tablets contain a natural vegetable derivative, standardized for uniform action. Each Double-Strength SenokotXTRA Tablet contains twice the active ingredient in one SENOKOT Tablet; patients may take one Double-Strength SenokotXTRA Tablet instead of two SENOKOT Tablets.
Senokot Laxatives provide a virtually colon-specific action which is gentle, effective and predictable, generally producing bowel movement in 6 to 12 hours. SENOKOT has been found to be effective even in many previously intractable cases of functional constipation. SENOKOT preparations may aid in rehabilitation of the constipated patient by facilitating regular elimination. At proper dosage levels, SENOKOT preparations are virtually free of adverse reactions (such as loose stools or abdominal discomfort) and enjoy high patient acceptance. Numerous and extensive clinical studies show their high degree of effectiveness in several types of functional constipation: geriatric and postpartum, drug-induced, pediatric, as well as in functional constipation concurrent with heart disease or anorectal surgery.
SENOKOT-S Tablets are designed to relieve both aspects of functional constipation—bowel inertia and hard, dry stools. They provide a natural neuroperistaltic stimulant combined with a classic stool softener, standardized senna concentrate gently stimulates the colon while docusate sodium softens the stool for smoother and easier evacuation. This coordinated dual action of the two ingredients results in colon-specific, predictable laxative effect, generally producing bowel movement in 6 to 12 hours. Flexibility of dosage permits fine adjustment to individual requirements. SENOKOT-S Tablets are highly suitable for relief of post-surgical and postpartum constipation, and effectively counter-act drug-induced constipation.

DESCRIPTION
SENOKOT Tablets: Each tablet contains 8.6 mg sennosides.
Active Ingredient: Standardized Senna Concentrate.
Inactive Ingredients: Corn starch, Glycerin, Lactose, Magnesium Stearate, Talc and other ingredients.
SENOKOT Granules: (cocoa-flavored): Each teaspoonful contains 15 mg sennosides.
Active Ingredient: Standardized Senna Concentrate.
Inactive Ingredients: Cocoa, Malt extract, Sodium lauryl sulfate, Sucrose, Vanillin and other ingredients.
SenokotXTRA Tablets: Each tablet contains 17 mg sennosides.
Active Ingredient: Standardized Senna Concentrate.
Inactive Ingredients: Corn Starch, Glycerin, Lactose, Magnesium stearate, Talc and other ingredients.
SENOKOT-S Tablets: Each tablet contains 8.6 mg sennosides and 50 mg of docusate sodium. Active Ingredients: Docusate Sodium and Standardized Senna Concentrate.
Inactive Ingredients: Cellulosic polymers, Corn starch, FD&C Yellow No. 10, FD&C Yellow No. 6 (Sunset Yellow), Guar Gum, Lactose, Polyethylene glycol, Talc, Titanium dioxide, and other ingredients.

RECOMMENDED DOSAGE
(or as directed by a doctor): Take preferably at bedtime. For older, debilitated, and OB/GYN patients, the physician may consider prescribing ¹/₂ the initial dose.
Senokot Tablets and Granules are available for children under 6 years of age. For children under 2 years of age, consult a physician.
SENOKOT Tablets and SENOKOT-S Tablets:
Recommended Dosage (or as directed by a doctor):
Take preferably at bedtime.

AGE	STARTING	MAXIMUM
Adults and children 12 years of age and over	2 tablets once a day	4 tablets twice a day
6 to under 12 years of age	1 tablet once a day	2 tablets twice a day
2 to under 6 years of age	¹/₂ tablet once a day	1 tablet twice a day
Under 2 years	Consult a physician.	

Double-Strength SenokotXTRA Tablets:
Recommended Dosage (or as directed by a doctor): Take preferably at bedtime.

AGE	STARTING	MAXIMUM
Adults and children 12 years of age and over	1 tablet once a day	2 tablets twice a day
6 to under 12 years of age	¹/₂ tablet once a day	1 tablet twice a day

SENOKOT Granules (May be eaten plain, mixed with liquids such as milk to make a delicious drink, or sprinkled on foods.):

AGE	STARTING	MAXIMUM
Adults and children 12 years of age and over	1 teaspoon once a day	2 teaspoons twice a day
6 to under 12 years of age	¹/₂ teaspoon once a day	1 teaspoon twice a day
2 to under 6 years of age	¹/₄ teaspoon once a day	¹/₂ teaspoon twice a day
Under 2 years	Consult a physician.	

WARNINGS
Do not use laxative products when abdominal pain, nausea or vomiting are present unless directed by a doctor. If you have noticed a sudden change in bowel movements that persists over a period of 2 weeks, consult a doctor before using a laxative. Laxative products should not be used for a period longer than 1 week unless directed by a doctor. Rectal bleeding or failure to have a bowel movement after use of a laxative may indicate a serious condition. Discontinue use and consult your doctor. As with any drug, if you are pregnant or nursing a baby, seek the advice of a health professional before using this product. In case of accidental overdose, seek professional assistance or contact a Poison Control Center immediately. Keep out of children's reach.

HOW SUPPLIED
Tablets: Boxes of 10 and 20; bottles of 50, 100 and 1000. Unit Strip Packs in boxes of 100 tablets: each tablet individually sealed. Double-Strength SenokotXTRA Tablets: Boxes of 12 and 36.
Senokot-S Tablets are supplied in packages of 10, bottles of 30, 60, and 1000 tablets, and Unit Strip Boxes of 100 tablets.
Granules: 2, 6, and 12 oz. plastic containers.
ALSO AVAILABLE
SENOKOT Syrup (extract of senna concentrate) in bottles of 2 and 8 fl. oz. Each teaspoon of SENOKOT Syrup contains 8.8 mg sennosides.
Active Ingredient: Extract of Senna Concentrate.
Inactive Ingredients: Alcohol 7% by volume, Methyl paraben, Potassium sorbate, Propylparaben, Sodium lauryl sulfate, Sucrose, Water, Natural and artificial flavors and other ingredients.
Copyright 1991, 1998. The Purdue Frederick Company

TRILISATE® TABLETS/LIQUID   Rx
[trĭl 'ĭ-sāt]
(choline magnesium trisalicylate)
500 mg, 750 mg, or 1000 mg
salicylate content

DESCRIPTION
TRILISATE Tablets/Liquid are nonsteroidal, anti-inflammatory preparations containing choline magnesium trisalicylate which is freely soluble in water. The absolute structure of choline magnesium trisalicylate is not known at this time. Choline magnesium trisalicylate has a molecular formula of $C_{26}H_{29}O_{10}NMg$, a molecular weight of 539.8, and it may be represented in the solid form as:

This substance when dissolved in water would appear to form 5 ions (1 choline ion, 1 magnesium ion and 3 salicylate ions) which may be represented as:

TRILISATE Tablets/Liquid are available in scored, salmon-colored, film-coated 500 mg tablets; in scored, white, film-coated 750 mg tablets, and in scored, red, film-coated 1000 mg tablets. TRILISATE Liquid is a cherry cordial-flavored liquid providing 500 mg salicylate content per teaspoonful (5 ml) for oral administration.
Each 500 mg tablet contains 293 mg of choline salicylate combined with 362 mg of magnesium salicylate to provide 500 mg salicylate content. Each 750 mg tablet contains 440 mg of choline salicylate combined with 544 mg of magnesium salicylate to provide 750 mg salicylate content. Each 1000 mg tablet contains 587 mg of choline salicylate com-

Continued on next page

Trilisate—Cont.

bined with 725 mg magnesium salicylate to provide 1000 mg salicylate content. TRILISATE Liquid contains 293 mg of choline salicylate combined with 362 mg of magnesium salicylate to provide 500 mg salicylate per teaspoonful (5 ml) in a clear amber, cherry cordial-flavored vehicle.

Inactive Ingredients: Each 500 mg tablet contains Carboxymethylcellulose sodium, Edetate disodium, FD&C Yellow No. 6, Polyethylene glycol, Polysorbate 20, Polysorbate 80, Stearic acid, Talc, and other ingredients.

Each 750 mg tablet contains Carboxymethylcellulose sodium, Edetate disodium, Hydroxypropyl methylcellulose, Polyethylene glycol, Polysorbate 20, Stearic acid, Talc, Titanium dioxide, and other ingredients.

Each 1000 mg tablet contains Carboxymethylcellulose sodium, Edetate disodium, FD&C Red No. 40, FD&C Yellow No. 6, FD&C Blue No. 2, Hydroxypropyl methylcellulose, Polyethylene glycol, Polysorbate 20, Polysorbate 80, Stearic acid, Talc, Titanium dioxide and other ingredients.

Each teaspoonful (5 ml) of Liquid contains: Caramel, Carboxymethylcellulose sodium, Edetate disodium, FD&C Yellow No. 6, Glycerin, High fructose corn syrup, Potassium sorbate, Water, and Artificial flavors.

CLINICAL PHARMACOLOGY

TRILISATE Tablets/Liquid contain salicylate with anti-inflammatory, analgesic and antipyretic action. On ingestion of TRILISATE Tablets/Liquid, the salicylate moiety is absorbed rapidly and reaches peak blood levels within an average of one to two hours after single doses of the tablets or liquid. The primary route of excretion is renal: the excretion products are chiefly the glycine and glucuronide conjugates. At higher serum salicylate concentrations, the glycine conjugation pathway becomes rapidly saturated. Thus, the slower glucuronide conjugation pathway becomes the rate limiting step for salicylate excretion. In addition, salicylate excreted in the bile as glucuronide conjugate may be reabsorbed. These factors account for the prolongation of salicylate half-life and the nonlinear increase in plasma salicylate level as the salicylate dose is increased. The serum concentration of salicylate is increased by conditions that decrease glomerular filtration rate or proximal tubular secretion.

The bioequivalence of TRILISATE Liquid and Tablets 500 mg/750 mg/1000 mg has been established. With the tablets, a steady-state condition is usually reached after 4 to 5 doses, and the half-life of elimination, on repeated administration of tablets, is 9 to 17 hours. This permits a maintenance dosage schedule of once or twice daily. Unlike aspirin and certain other non-steroidal anti-inflammatory agents, such as arylpropionic acid derivatives and arylacetic acid derivatives, choline magnesium trisalicylate, at therapeutic dosage levels, does not affect platelet aggregation, as shown by in-vitro and in-vivo studies.

INDICATIONS AND USAGE

Osteoarthritis, Rheumatoid Arthritis and Acute Painful Shoulder: Salicylates are considered the base therapy of choice in the arthritides; and TRILISATE preparations are indicated for the relief of the signs and symptoms of rheumatoid arthritis, osteoarthritis and other arthritides. TRILISATE Tablets or Liquid are indicated in the long-term management of these diseases and especially in the acute flare of rheumatoid arthritis. TRILISATE Tablets or Liquid are also indicated for the treatment of acute painful shoulder.

TRILISATE preparations are effective and generally well tolerated, and are logical choices whenever salicylate treatment is indicated. They are particularly suitable when a once-a-day or b.i.d. dosage regimen is important to patient compliance; when gastrointestinal intolerance to aspirin is encountered; when gastrointestinal microbleeding or hematologic effects of aspirin are considered a patient hazard; and when interference (or the risk of interference) with normal platelet function by aspirin or by propionic acid derivatives is considered to be clinically undesirable. Use of TRILISATE Liquid is appropriate when a liquid dosage form is preferred, as in the elderly patient.

The efficacy of TRILISATE preparations has not been studied in those patients who are designated by the American Rheumatism Association as belonging in Functional Class IV (incapacitated, largely or wholly bedridden or confined to a wheelchair, with little or no self-care). Analgesic and Antipyretic Action: TRILISATE Tablets/Liquid are also indicated for the relief of mild to moderate pain and for antipyresis.

Pediatric Use: **In children**, TRILISATE preparations are indicated for conditions requiring anti-inflammatory or analgesic action—such as juvenile rheumatoid arthritis and other appropriate conditions. In a four-week open label pilot study of patients with juvenile rheumatoid arthritis, children from 6 to 16 years of age previously on aspirin received weight adjusted doses (50–60 mg/kg) of TRILISATE 500 mg tablets on a divided b.i.d. schedule with subsequent dose titration to achieve therapeutic serum salicylate levels. Eighty-three percent (83%) of the patients rated the thera-

peutic effect of TRILISATE as good or excellent. Tinnitus, was reported by one patient and elevated SGOT levels at Week 1, which decreased during the trial, were detected in two patients. (See WARNINGS section).

CONTRAINDICATIONS

Patients who are hypersensitive to non-acetylated salicylates should not take TRILISATE Tablets or Liquid.

WARNINGS

Reye Syndrome is a rare but serious disease which may develop in children and teenagers who have chicken pox, influenza, or flu symptoms. While the cause of Reye Syndrome is unknown, some studies suggest a possible association between the development of Reye Syndrome and the use of medicines containing acetylated salicylates or aspirin. TRILISATE Tablets and Liquid are a combination of choline salicylate and magnesium salicylate which are nonacetylated salicylates, and there have been no reported cases associating TRILISATE with Reye Syndrome. Nevertheless, TRILISATE, as a salicylate-containing product, is not recommended for use in children and teenagers with chicken pox, influenza or flu symptoms.

PRECAUTIONS

General Precautions: As with other salicylates and non-steroidal anti-inflammatory drugs, TRILISATE preparations should be used with caution in patients with acute or chronic renal insufficiency, with acute or chronic hepatic dysfunction, or with gastritis or peptic ulcer disease.

Although reports exist of cross reactivity, including bronchospasm, with the use of non-acetylated salicylate products in aspirin-sensitive patients, TRILISATE preparations were found to be well tolerated with regard to pulmonary function and respiratory symptoms when these parameters were monitored in a group of documented aspirin-sensitive asthmatics dosed with TRILISATE in both controlled and open label studies.[1]

Concurrent use of other salicylate-containing products and TRILISATE preparations can lead to an increase in plasma salicylate concentration and may result in potentially toxic salicylate levels.

Laboratory Tests: Plasma salicylate levels can be periodically assessed during treatment with TRILISATE preparations to determine whether a therapeutically effective anti-inflammatory concentration of 15 to 30 mg/100 ml (150–300 micrograms/ml) is being maintained. Manifestations of systemic salicylate intoxication are usually not seen until the concentration exceeds 30 mg/100 ml. However, such tests rarely differentiate between the active free and inactive protein bound salicylate components. Since protein binding of salicylate is affected by age, nutritional status, competitive binding of other drugs, and underlying disease (e.g. rheumatoid arthritis), plasma salicylate level determinations may not always accurately reflect efficacious or toxic levels of active free salicylate. Acidification of the urine can significantly diminish the renal clearance of salicylate and increase plasma salicylate concentrations.

Drug Interactions: Foods and drugs that alter urine pH may affect renal clearance of salicylate and plasma salicylate concentrations. Raising urine pH, as with chronic antacid use, can enhance renal salicylate clearance and diminish plasma salicylate concentration; urine acidification can decrease urinary salicylate excretion and increase plasma levels.

When salicylate drug products are concurrently dosed with other plasma protein bound drug products, adverse effects may result. Although TRILISATE preparations are a rational choice for anti-inflammatory and analgesic therapy in patients on oral anticoagulants due to their demonstrated lack of effect in vivo and in vitro on platelet aggregation, bleeding time, platelet count, prothrombin time, and serum thromboxane B2 generation[1–7], the potential exists for increased levels of unbound warfarin with their concurrent use. Prothrombin time should be closely monitored and warfarin dose appropriately adjusted when therapy with TRILISATE preparations is initiated. The effect of TRILISATE on blood prothrombin levels has not been established. Salicylates may increase the therapeutic as well as toxic effects of methotrexate, particularly when administered in chemotherapeutic doses, by inhibition of renal methotrexate excretion and by displacement of plasma protein bound methotrexate. Caution should be exercised in administering TRILISATE to rheumatoid arthritis patients on methotrexate. When sulfonylurea oral hypoglycemic agents are co-administered with salicylates, the hypoglycemic effect may be enhanced via increased insulin secretion or by displacement of sulfonylurea agents from binding sites. Insulin-treated diabetics on high doses of salicylates should also be closely monitored for a similar hypoglycemic response. Other drugs with which salicylate competes for protein binding sites, and whose plasma concentration or free fraction may be altered by concurrent salicylate administration, include the following: phenytoin, valproic acid, and carbonic anhydrase inhibitors.

The efficacy of uricosuric agents may be decreased when administered with salicylate products. Although low doses of

salicylate (1 to 2 grams per day) have been reported to decrease urate excretion and elevate plasma urate concentrations, intermediate doses (2 to 3 grams per day) usually do not alter urate excretion. Larger salicylate doses (over 5 grams per day) can induce uricosuria and lower plasma urate levels.

Corticosteroids can reduce plasma salicylate levels by increasing renal elimination and perhaps by also stimulating hepatic metabolism of salicylates. By monitoring plasma salicylate levels, salicylate dosage may be titrated to accommodate changes in corticosteroid dose or to avoid salicylate toxicity during corticosteroid taper.

Drug/Laboratory Test Interactions: Free T4 values may be increased in patients on salicylate drug products due to competitive plasma protein binding; a concurrent decrease in total plasma T4 may be observed. Thyroid function is not affected.

Carcinogenesis: No long-term animal studies have been performed with TRILISATE to evaluate its carcinogenic potential.

Use in Pregnancy: Pregnancy Category C. Animal reproduction studies have not been conducted with TRILISATE preparations. It is also not known whether TRILISATE can cause fetal harm when administered to a pregnant woman or can affect reproduction capacity. TRILISATE should be given to a pregnant woman only if clearly needed. Because of the known effects of other salicylate drug products on the fetal cardiovascular system (closure of ductus arteriosus), use during late pregnancy should be avoided.

Labor and Delivery: The effects of TRILISATE on labor and delivery in pregnant women are unknown. Since prolonged gestation and prolonged labor due to prostaglandin inhibition have been reported with the use of other salicylate products, the use of TRILISATE preparations near term is not recommended. Other salicylate products have also been associated with alterations in maternal and neonatal hemostasis mechanisms and with perinatal mortality.

Nursing Mothers: Salicylate is excreted in human milk. Peak milk salicylate levels are delayed, occurring as long as 9 to 12 hours post dose, and the milk:plasma ratio has been reported to be as high as 0.34. Because of the potential for significant salicylate absorption by the nursing infant, caution should be exercised when TRILISATE is administered to a nursing woman.

Geriatric Use: The elderly may be prone to more side effects from salicylates than younger patients due to an age-related decline in renal clearance and/or increased use of concomitant medication. The elderly are more likely than younger patients to be taking a number of medications, some of which may affect the plasma protein binding of salicylate and thus increase the amount of free salicylate.

ADVERSE REACTIONS

The most frequent adverse reactions observed with TRILISATE preparations in clinical trials[7–12] are tinnitus and gastrointestinal complaints (including nausea, vomiting, gastric upset, indigestion, heartburn, diarrhea, constipation and epigastric pain). These occur in less than twenty percent (20%) of patients. Should tinnitus develop, reduction of daily dosage is recommended until the tinnitus is resolved. Less frequent adverse reactions, occurring in less than two percent (2%) of patients, are: hearing impairment, headache, lightheadedness, dizziness, drowsiness, and lethargy. Adverse reactions occurring in less than one percent (1%) of patients are: gastric ulceration, positive fecal occult blood, elevation in serum BUN and creatinine, rash, pruritus, anorexia, weight gain, edema, epistaxis and dysgeusia. Spontaneous reporting has yielded isolated or rare reports of the following adverse experiences: duodenal ulceration, elevated hepatic transaminases, hepatitis, esophagitis, asthma, erythema multiforme, urticaria, ecchymoses, irreversible hearing loss and/or tinnitus, mental confusion, hallucinations.

DRUG ABUSE AND DEPENDENCE

Drug abuse and dependence have not been reported with TRILISATE preparations.

OVERDOSAGE

Death in adults has been reported following ingestion of doses from 10 to 30 grams of salicylate; however, larger doses have been taken without resulting fatality.

Symptoms: Salicylate intoxication, known as salicylism, may occur with large doses or extended therapy. Common symptoms of salicylism include headache, dizziness, tinnitus, hearing impairment, confusion, drowsiness, sweating, vomiting, diarrhea, and hyperventilation. A more severe degree of salicylate intoxication can lead to CNS disturbances, alteration in electrolyte balance, respiratory and metabolic acidosis, hyperthermia, and dehydration.

Treatment: Reduction of further absorption of salicylate from the gastrointestinal tract can be achieved via emesis, gastric lavage, use of activated charcoal, or a combination of the above. Appropriate I.V. fluids should be administered to correct dehydration, electrolyte imbalance, and acidosis and to maintain adequate renal function. To accelerate salicylate excretion, forced diuresis with alkalinizing solution is

recommended. In extreme cases, peritoneal dialysis or hemodialysis should be considered for effective salicylate removal.

DOSAGE AND ADMINISTRATION

ADULTS: In rheumatoid arthritis, osteoarthritis, the more severe arthritides, and acute painful shoulder, the recommended starting dosage is 1500 mg given b.i.d. Some patients may be treated with 3000 mg given once per day (h.s.) In the elderly patient, a daily dosage of 2250 mg given as 750 mg t.i.d. may be efficacious and well tolerated. Dosage should be adjusted in accordance with the patient's response. In patients with renal dysfunction, monitor salicylate levels and adjust dose accordingly.

ELDERLY: In the elderly patients, a daily dosage of 2250 mg given as 750 mg t.i.d. may be efficacious and well tolerated. Dosage should be adjusted in accordance with the patient's response. In patients with renal dysfunction, monitor salicylate levels and adjust dose accordingly.

For mild to moderate pain or for antipyresis, the usual dosage is 2000 mg to 3000 mg daily in divided doses (b.i.d.). Based on patient response or salicylate blood levels, dosage may be adjusted to achieve optimum therapeutic effect. Salicylate blood levels should be in the range of 15 to 30 mg/100 ml for anti-inflammatory effect and 5 to 15 mg/100 ml for analgesia and antipyresis.

Each 500 mg tablet or teaspoonful is equivalent in salicylate content to 10 gr of aspirin; each 750 mg tablet, to 15 gr of aspirin; and each 1000 mg tablet, to 20 gr of aspirin.

If the physician prefers, the recommended daily dosage may be administered on a t.i.d. schedule.

As with other therapeutic agents, individual dosage adjustment is advisable, and a number of patients may require higher or lower dosages than those recommended. Certain patients require 2 to 3 weeks of therapy for optimal effect.

CHILDREN: Usual daily dose for children for anti-inflammatory or analgesic action:
TRILISATE 500 mg Tablets/Liquid and TRILISATE 750 mg and 1000 mg Tablets, 50 mg/kg/day.

Weight (kg)	Total daily dose
12–13	500 mg
14–17	750 mg
18–22	1000 mg
23–27	1250 mg
28–32	1500 mg
33–37	1750 mg

Total daily doses should be administered in divided doses (b.i.d.). Doses of TRILISATE preparations are calculated as the total daily dose of 50 mg/kg/day for children of 37 kg body weight or less and 2250 mg/day for heavier children. TRILISATE Liquid is available for greater convenience in treating younger patients and those adult patients unable to swallow a solid dosage form.

CAUTION
Federal law prohibits dispensing without a prescription.

HOW SUPPLIED

NDC 0034-0500-80: TRILISATE 500 mg Tablets (scored, salmon-colored, film-coated) supplied in bottles of 100 tablets.

NDC 0034-0500-50: TRILISATE 500 mg Tablets (scored, salmon-colored, film-coated) supplied in bottles of 500 tablets.

NDC 0034-0500-10: TRILISATE 500 mg Tablets (scored, salmon-colored, film-coated) supplied in unit dose packaging with 10 tablets per card. Ten cards are packed in each carton; 10 cartons are packed in each shipper.

NDC 0034-0505-80: TRILISATE 750 mg Tablets (scored, white, film-coated) in bottles of 100 tablets.

NDC 0034-0505-50: TRILISATE 750 mg Tablets (scored, white, film-coated) in bottles of 500 tablets.

NDC 0034-0505-10: TRILISATE 750 mg Tablets (scored, white, film-coated) supplied in unit dose packaging with 10 tablets per card. Ten cards are packed in each carton; 10 cartons are packed in each shipper.

NDC 0034-0510-80: TRILISATE 1000 mg Tablets (scored, red, film-coated) in bottles of 100 tablets.

NDC 0034-0520-80: TRILISATE Liquid in bottles of 8 fl. oz. (237 ml).

Store at controlled room temperature 59° to 86°F (15° to 30°C).

REFERENCES

1. Szczeklik, A et al; Choline magnesium trisalicylate in patients with aspirin-induced asthma; *Eur Respir J*; 3:535–539, 1990.
2. Zucker, MB and Rothwell KB; Differential influences of salicylate compounds on platelet aggregation and serotonin release; *Current Therapeutic Research*; 23(2), Feb 1987.
3. Stuart, JJ and Pisko, EJ; Choline magnesium trisalicylate does not impair platelet aggregation; *Pharma-therapeutica*; 2(8):547, 1981.
4. Danesh, BJZ, Saniabadi, AR, Russell, RI et al; Therapeutic potential of choline magnesium trisalicylate as an alternative to aspirin for patients with bleeding tendencies; *Scottish Medical Journal*; 32:167–168, 1987.
5. Danesh, BJZ, McLaren, M. Russell, RI et al; Does non-acetylated salicylate inhibit thromboxane biosynthesis in human platelets? *Scottish Medical Journal*; 33: 315–316, 1988.
6. Danesh, BJZ, McLaren, M, Russell, RI et al; Comparison of the effect of aspirin and choline magnesium trisalicylate on thromboxane biosynthesis in human platelets: role of the acetyl moiety; *Haemostasis*; 19: 169–173, 1989.
7. Data on file. Medical Department. The Purdue Frederick Company, 1989.
8. Blechman, WJ, and Lechner, BL; Clinical comparative evaluation of choline magnesium trisalicylate and acetylsalicylic acid in rheumatoid arthritis; *Rheumatology and Rehabilitation*; 18:119–124, 1979.
9. McLaughlin, G; Choline magnesium trisalicylate vs. naproxen in rheumatoid arthritis; *Current Therapeutic Research*; 32(4):579–585, 1982.
10. Ehrlich, GE; Miller, SB; and Zeiders, RS; Choline magnesium trisalicylate vs. ibuprofen in rheumatoid arthritis; *Rheumatology and Rehabilitation*; 19:30–41, 1980.
11. Goldenberg, A; Rudnicki, RD, and Koonce, ML; Clinical comparison of efficacy and safety of choline magnesium trisalicylate and indomethacin in treating osteoarthritis; *Current Therapeutic Research*; 24(3):245–260, 1978.
12. Guerin, BK and Burnstein, SL; Conservative therapy of acute painful shoulder; *Orthopedic Review*; XI(7):29–37, 1982.

The Purdue Frederick Company, Norwalk, CT 06850-3590
Copyright © 1982, 1995, The Purdue Frederick Company
U.S. Patent Number 4067974
December 7, 1995   R145

Shown in Product Identification Guide, page 333

UNIPHYL®   ℞
[ū 'nĭ-fĭl]
400 mg and 600 mg Tablets
(theophylline)
UNICONTIN® Controlled-Release System

DESCRIPTION

Uniphyl® (theophylline, anhydrous) Tablets in a controlled-release system allows a 24-hour dosing interval for appropriate patients.

Theophylline is structurally classified as a methylxanthine. It occurs as a white, odorless, crystalline powder with a bitter taste. Anhydrous theophylline has the chemical name 1H-Purine-2,6-dione,3,7-dihydro-1,3-dimethyl-, and is represented by the following structural formula:

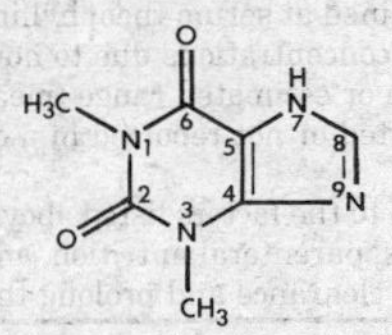

The molecular formula of anhydrous theophylline is $C_7H_8N_4O_2$ with a molecular weight of 180.17.

Each controlled-release tablet for oral administration, contains 400 or 600 mg of anhydrous theophylline per tablet.
Inactive Ingredients: Cetostearyl alcohol, Hydroxymethyl cellulose, Magnesium stearate, Povidone and Talc.

CLINICAL PHARMACOLOGY

Mechanism of Action: Theophylline has two distinct actions in the airways of patients with reversible obstruction; smooth muscle relaxation (i.e., bronchodilation) and suppression of the response of the airways to stimuli (i.e., non-bronchodilator prophylactic effects). While the mechanisms of action of theophylline are not known with certainty, studies in animals suggest that bronchodilatation is mediated by the inhibition of two isozymes of phosphodiesterase (PDE III and, to a lesser extent, PDE IV) while non-bronchodilator prophylactic actions are probably mediated through one or more different molecular mechanisms, that do not involve inhibition of PDE III or antagonism of adenosine receptors. Some of the adverse effects associated with theophylline appear to be mediated by inhibition of PDE III (e.g., hypotension, tachycardia, headache, and emesis) and adenosine receptor antagonism (e.g., alterations in cerebral blood flow). Theophylline increases the force of contraction of diaphragmatic muscles. This action appears to be due to enhancement of calcium uptake through an adenosine-mediated channel.

Serum Concentration-Effect Relationship: Bronchodilation occurs over the serum theophylline concentration range of 5–20 mcg/mL. Clinically important improvement in symptom control has been found in most studies to require peak serum theophylline concentrations >10 mcg/mL, but patients with mild disease may benefit from lower concentrations. At serum theophylline concentrations >20 mcg/mL, both the frequency and severity of adverse reactions increase. In general, maintaining peak serum theophylline concentrations between 10 and 15 mcg/mL will achieve most of the drug's potential therapeutic benefit while minimizing the risk of serious adverse events.

Pharmacokinetics:

Overview Theophylline is rapidly and completely absorbed after oral administration in solution or immediate-release solid oral dosage form. Theophylline does not undergo any appreciable pre-systemic elimination, distributes freely into fat-free tissues and is extensively metabolized in the liver. The pharmacokinetics of theophylline vary widely among similar patients and cannot be predicted by age, sex, body weight or other demographic characteristics. In addition, certain concurrent illnesses and alterations in normal physiology (see Table I) and co-administration of other drugs (see Table II) can significantly alter the pharmacokinetic characteristics of theophylline. Within-subject variability in metabolism has also been reported in some studies, especially in acutely ill patients. It is, therefore, recommended that serum theophylline concentrations be measured frequently in acutely ill patients (e.g., at 24-hr intervals) and periodically in patients receiving long-term therapy, e.g., at 6–12 month intervals. More frequent measurements should be made in the presence of any condition that may significantly alter theophylline clearance (see PRECAUTIONS, Laboratory tests).

[See table at top of next page]

Absorption Uniphyl® administered in the fed state is completely absorbed after oral administration.

In a single-dose crossover study, two 400 mg Uniphyl® Tablets were administered to 19 normal volunteers in the morning or evening immediately following the same standardized meal (769 calories consisting of 97 grams carbohydrates, 33 grams protein and 27 grams fat). There was no evidence of dose dumping nor were there any significant differences in pharmacokinetic parameters attributable to time of drug administration. On the morning arm, the pharmacokinetic parameters were AUC=241.9±83.0 mcg hr/mL, Cmax=9.3±2.0 mcg/mL, Tmax=12.8±4.2 hours. On the evening arm, the pharmacokinetic parameters were AUC=219.7±83.0 mcg hr/mL, Cmax=9.2±2.0 mcg/mL, Tmax=12.5±4.2 hours.

A study in which Uniphyl® 400 mg tablets were administered to 17 fed adult asthmatics produced similar theophylline level-time curves when administered in the morning or evening. Serum levels were generally higher in the evening regimen but there were no statistically significant differences between the two regimens.

	MORNING	**EVENING**
AUC (0–24 hrs)		
(mcg hr/mL)	236.0±76.7	256.0±80.4
Cmax (mcg/mL)	14.5±4.1	16.3±4.5
Cmin (mcg/mL)	5.5±2.9	5.0±2.5
Tmax (hours)	8.1±3.7	10.1±4.1

A single-dose study in 15 normal fasting male volunteers whose theophylline inherent mean elimination half-life was verified by a liquid theophylline product to be 6.9±2.5 (S.D.) hours were administered two or three 400 mg Uniphyl® Tablets. The relative bioavailability of Uniphyl® given in the fasting state in comparison to an immediate-release product was 59%. Peak serum theophylline levels occurred at 6.9±5.2 (S.D.) hours, with a normalized (to 800 mg) peak level being 6.2±2.1 (S.D.). The apparent elimination half-life for the 400 mg Uniphyl® Tablets was 17.2±5.8 (S.D.) hours.

Steady-state pharmacokinetics were determined in a study in 12 fasted patients with chronic reversible obstructive pulmonary disease. All were dosed with two 400 mg Uniphyl® Tablets given once daily in the morning and a reference controlled-release BID product administered as two 200 mg tablets given 12 hours apart. The pharmacokinetic parameters obtained for Uniphyl® Tablets given at doses of 800 mg once daily in the morning were virtually identical to the corresponding parameters for the reference drug when given as 400 mg BID. In particular, the AUC, Cmax and Cmin values obtained in this study were as follows:

	Uniphyl® Tablets 800 mg Q24h±S.D.	**Reference Drug 400 mg Q12h±S.D.**
AUC, (0–24 hours),		
mcg hr/mL	288.9±21.5	283.5±38.4
Cmax, mcg/mL	15.7±2.8	15.2±2.1
Cmin, mcg/mL	7.9±1.6	7.8±1.7
Cmax-Cmin diff.	7.7±1.5	7.4±1.5

Single-dose studies in which subjects were fasted for twelve (12) hours prior to and an additional four (4) hours following

Continued on next page

Uniphyl—Cont.

dosing, demonstrated reduced bioavailability as compared to dosing with food. One single-dose study in 20 normal volunteers dosed with two (2) 400 mg tablets in the morning, compared dosing under these fasting conditions with dosing immediately prior to a standardized breakfast (769 calories, consisting of 97 grams carbohydrates, 33 grams protein and 27 grams fat). Under fed conditions, the pharmacokinetic parameters were: AUC=231.7±92.4 mcg hr/mL, Cmax=8.4±2.6 mcg/mL, Tmax=17.3±6.7 hours. Under fasting conditions, these parameters were AUC=141.2±6.53 mcg hr/mL, Cmax=5.5±1.5 mcg/mL, Tmax=6.5±2.1 hours. Another single-dose study in 21 normal male volunteers, dosed in the evening, compared fasting to a standardized high calorie, high fat meal (870–1,020 calories, consisting of 33 grams protein, 55–75 grams fat, 58 grams carbohydrates). In the fasting arm subjects received one Uniphyl® 400 mg Tablet at 8 p.m. after an eight hour fast followed by a further four hour fast. In the fed arm, subjects were again dosed with one 400 mg Uniphyl® Tablet, but at 8 p.m. immediately after the high fat content standardized meal cited above. The pharmacokinetic parameters (normalized to 800 mg) fed were AUC=221.8±40.9 mcg hr/mL, Cmax=10.9±1.7 mcg/mL, Tmax=11.8±2.2 hours. In the fasting arm, the pharmacokinetic parameters (normalized to 800 mg) were AUC=146.4±40.9 mcg hr/mL, Cmax=6.7±1.7 mcg/mL, Tmax=7.3±2.2 hours.

Thus, administration of single Uniphyl® doses to healthy normal volunteers, under prolonged fasted conditions (at least 10 hour overnight fast before dosing followed by an additional four (4) hour fast after dosing) results in decreased bioavailability. However, there was no failure of this delivery system leading to a sudden and unexpected release of a large quantity of theophylline with Uniphyl® Tablets even when they are administered with a high fat, high calorie meal.

Similar studies were conducted with the 600 mg Uniphyl® Tablet. A single-dose study in 24 subjects with an established theophylline clearance of ≤ 4 L/hr, compared the pharmacokinetic evaluation of one 600 mg Uniphyl® Tablet and one and one-half 400 mg Uniphyl® Tablets under fed (using a standard high fat diet) and fasted conditions. The results of this 4-way randomized crossover study demonstrate the bioequivalence of the 400 mg and 600 mg Uniphyl® Tablets. Under fed conditions, the pharmacokinetic results for the one and one-half 400 mg Tablets were AUC=214.64±55.88 mcg hr/mL, Cmax=10.58±2.21 mcg/mL and Tmax=9.00±2.64 hours, and for the 600 mg Tablet were AUC=207.85±48.9 mcg hr/mL, Cmax=10.39±1.91 mcg/mL and Tmax=9.58 ±1.86 hours. Under fasted conditions the pharmacokinetic results for the one and one-half 400 mg Tablets were AUC=191.85±51.1 mcg hr/mL, Cmax=7.37±1.83 mcg/mL and Tmax=8.08±4.39 hours, and for the 600 mg Tablet were AUC=199.39±70.27 mcg hr/mL, Cmax=7.66±2.09 mcg/mL and Tmax=9.67±4.89 hours.

In this study the mean fed/fasted ratios for the one and one-half 400 mg Tablets and the 600 mg Tablet were about 112% and 104%, respectively.

In another study, the bioavailability of the 600 mg Uniphyl® Tablet was examined with morning and evening administration. This single-dose, crossover study in 22 healthy males was conducted under fed (standard high fat diet) conditions. The results demonstrated no clinically significant difference in the bioavailability of the 600 mg Uniphyl® Tablet administered in the morning or in the evening. The results were: AUC=233.6±45.1 mcg hr/mL, Cmax=10.6±1.3 mcg/mL and Tmax=12.5±3.2 hours with morning dosing; AUC=209.8±46.2 mcg hr/mL, Cmax=9.7±1.4 mcg/mL and Tmax=13.7±3.3 hours with evening dosing. The PM/AM ratio was 89.3%.

The absorption characteristics of Uniphyl® Tablets (theophylline, anhydrous) have been extensively studied. A steady-state crossover bioavailability study in 22 normal males compared two Uniphyl® 400 mg Tablets administered q24h at 8 a.m. immediately after breakfast with a reference controlled-release theophylline product administered BID in fed subjects at 8 a.m. immediately after breakfast and 8 p.m. immediately after dinner (769 calories, consisting of 97 grams carbohydrates, 33 grams protein and 27 grams fat).

The pharmacokinetic parameters for Uniphyl® 400 mg Tablets under these steady-state conditions were AUC=203.3±87.1 mcg hr/mL, Cmax=12.1±3.8 mcg/mL, Cmin=4.50±3.6, Tmax=8.8±4.6 hours. For the reference BID product, the pharmacokinetic parameters were AUC=219.2±88.4 mcg hr/mL, Cmax=11.0±4.1 mcg/mL, Cmin=7.28±3.5, Tmax=6.9±3.4 hours. The mean percent fluctuation [(Cmax-Cmin/Cmin) × 100] = 169% for the once-daily regimen and 51% for the reference product BID regimen.

The bioavailability of the 600 mg Uniphyl® tablet was further evaluated in a multiple dose, steady-state study in 26 healthy males comparing the 600 mg Tablet to one and one-half 400 mg Uniphyl® tablets. All subjects had previously

Table I. Mean and range of total body clearance and half-life of theophylline related to age and altered physiological states.¶

Population Characteristics	Total body clearance* mean (range)‡ (mL/kg/min)	Half-life mean (range)‡ (hr)
Age		
Premature neonates		
postnatal age 3–15 days	0.29 (0.09–0.49)	30 (17–43)
postnatal age 25–57 days	0.64 (0.04–1.2)	20 (9.4–30.6)
Term infants		
postnatal age 1–2 days	NR†	25.7 (25–26.5)
postnatal age 3–30 weeks	NR†	11 (6–29)
Children		
1–4 years	1.7 (0.5–2.9)	3.4 (1.2–5.6)
4–12 years	1.6 (0.8–2.4)	NR†
13–15 years	0.9 (0.48–1.3)	NR†
6–17 years	1.4 (0.2–2.6)	3.7 (1.5–5.9)
Adults (16–60 years)		
otherwise healthy		
non-smoking asthmatics	0.65 (0.27–1.03)	8.7 (6.1–12.8)
Elderly (>60 years)		
non-smokers with normal cardiac,		
liver, and renal function	0.41 (0.21–0.61)	9.8 (1.6–18)
Concurrent illness or altered physiological state		
Acute pulmonary edema	0.33** (0.07–2.45)	19** (3.1–82)
COPD->60 years, stable		
non-smoker >1 year	0.54 (0.44–0.64)	11 (9.4–12.6)
COPD with cor pulmonale	0.48 (0.08–0.88)	NR†
Cystic fibrosis (14–28 years)	1.25 (0.31–2.2)	6.0 (1.8–10.2)
Fever associated with		
acute viral respiratory illness		
(children 9–15 years)	NR†	7.0 (1.0–13)
Liver disease		
cirrhosis	0.31 ** (0.1–0.7)	32** (10–56)
acute hepatitis	0.35 (0.25–0.45)	19.2 (16.6–21.8)
cholestasis	0.65 (0.25–1.45)	14.4 (5.7–31.8)
Pregnancy		
1st trimester	NR†	8.5 (3.1–13.9)
2nd trimester	NR†	8.8 (3.8–13.8)
3rd trimester	NR†	13.0 (8.4–17.6)
Sepsis with multi-organ failure	0.47 (0.19–1.9)	18.8 (6.3–24.1)
Thyroid disease		
hypothyroid	0.38 (0.13–0.57)	11.6 (8.2–25)
hyperthyroid	0.8 (0.68–0.97)	4.5 (3.7–5.6)

¶ For various North American patient populations from literature reports. Different rates of elimination and consequent dosage requirements have been observed among other peoples.
* Clearance represents the volume of blood completely cleared of theophylline by the liver in one minute. Values listed were generally determined at serum theophylline concentrations <20 mcg/mL; clearance may decrease and half-life may increase at higher serum concentrations due to non-linear pharmacokinetics.
‡ Reported range or estimated range (mean ± 2 SD) where actual range not reported.
† NR = not reported or not reported in a comparable format.
** Median
Note: In addition to the factors listed above, theophylline clearance is increased and half-life decreased by low carbohydrate/high protein diets, parenteral nutrition, and daily consumption of charcoal-broiled beef. A high carbohydrate/low protein diet can decrease the clearance and prolong the half-life of theophylline.

established theophylline clearances of ≤ 4L/hr and were dosed once-daily for 6 days under fed conditions. The results showed no clinically significant difference between the 600 mg and one and one-half 400 mg Uniphyl® tablet regimens. Steady-state results were:

	600 MG TABLET FED	600 MG (ONE + ONE-HALF 400 MG TABLETS) FED
AUC 0–24hrs (mcg hr/mL)	209.77±51.04	212.32±56.29
Cmax (mcg/mL)	12.91±2.46	13.17±3.11
Cmin (mcg/mL)	5.52±1.79	5.39±1.95
Tmax (hours)	8.62±3.21	7.23±2.35
Percent Fluctuation	183.73±54.02	179.72±28.86

The bioavailability ratio for the 600/400 mg tablets was 98.8%. Thus, under all study conditions the 600 mg tablet is bioequivalent to one and one-half 400 mg tablets.
Studies demonstrate that as long as subjects were either consistently fed or consistently fasted, there is similar bioavailability with once-daily administration of Uniphyl® tablets whether dosed in the morning or evening.

Distribution Once theophylline enters the systemic circulation, about 40% is bound to plasma protein, primarily albumin. Unbound theophylline distributes throughout body water, but distributes poorly into body fat. The apparent volume of distribution of theophylline is approximately 0.45 L/kg (range 0.3–0.7 L/kg) based on ideal body weight. Theophylline passes freely across the placenta, into breast milk and into the cerebrospinal fluid (CSF). Saliva theophylline

concentrations approximate unbound serum concentrations, but are not reliable for routine or therapeutic monitoring unless special techniques are used. An increase in the volume of distribution of theophylline, primarily due to reduction in plasma protein binding, occurs in premature neonates, patients with hepatic cirrhosis, uncorrected acidemia, the elderly and in women during the third trimester of pregnancy. In such cases, the patient may show signs of toxicity at total (bound + unbound) serum concentrations of theophylline in the therapeutic range (10–20 mcg/mL) due to elevated concentrations of the pharmacologically active unbound drug. Similarly, a patient with decreased theophylline binding may have a sub-therapeutic total drug concentration while the pharmacologically active unbound concentration is in the therapeutic range. If only total serum theophylline concentration is measured, this may lead to an unnecessary and potentially dangerous dose increase. In patients with reduced protein binding, measurement of unbound serum theophylline concentration provides a more reliable means of dosage adjustment than measurement of total serum theophylline concentration. Generally, concentrations of unbound theophylline should be maintained in the range of 6–12 mcg/mL

Metabolism Following oral dosing, theophylline does not undergo any measurable first-pass elimination. In adults and children beyond one year of age, approximately 90% of the dose is metabolized in the liver. Biotransformation takes place through demethylation to 1-methylxanthine and 3-methylxanthine and hydroxylation to 1,3-dimethyluric acid. 1-methylxanthine is further hydroxylated, by xanthine oxidase, to 1-methyluric acid. About 6% of a theophylline dose is N-methylated to caffeine. Theophylline demethylation to 3-methylxanthine is catalyzed by cytochrome P-450 1A2, while cytochromes P-450 2E1 and P-450 3A3 catalyze the hydroxylation to 1,3-dimethyluric acid. Demethylation

to 1-methylxanthine appears to be catalyzed either by cytochrome P-450 1A2 or a closely related cytochrome. In neonates, the N-demethylation pathway is absent while the function of the hydroxylation pathway is markedly deficient. The activity of these pathways slowly increases to maximal levels by one year of age.

Caffeine and 3-methylxanthine are the only theophylline metabolites with pharmacologic activity. 3-methylxanthine has approximately one tenth the pharmacologic activity of theophylline and serum concentrations in adults with normal renal function are <1 mcg/mL. In patients with end-stage renal disease, 3-methylxanthine may accumulate to concentrations that approximate the unmetabolized theophylline concentration. Caffeine concentrations are usually undetectable in adults regardless of renal function. In neonates, caffeine may accumulate to concentrations that approximate the unmetabolized theophylline concentration and thus, exert a pharmacologic effect.

Both the N-demethylation and hydroxylation pathways of theophylline biotransformation are capacity-limited. Due to the wide intersubject variability of the rate of theophylline metabolism, non-linearity of elimination may begin in some patients at serum theophylline concentrations <10 mcg/mL. Since this non-linearity results in more than proportional changes in serum theophylline concentrations with changes in dose, it is advisable to make increases or decreases in dose in small increments in order to achieve desired changes in serum theophylline concentrations (see DOSAGE AND ADMINISTRATION, Table VI). Accurate prediction of dose-dependency of theophylline metabolism in patients *a priori* is not possible, but patients with very high initial clearance rates (i.e., low steady-state serum theophylline concentrations at above average doses) have the greatest likelihood of experiencing large changes in serum theophylline concentration in response to dosage changes.

Excretion In neonates, approximately 50% of the theophylline dose is excreted unchanged in the urine. Beyond the first three months of life, approximately 10% of the theophylline dose is excreted unchanged in the urine. The remainder is excreted in the urine mainly as 1,3-dimethyluric acid (35–40%), 1-methyluric acid (20–25%) and 3-methylxanthine (15–20%). Since little theophylline is excreted unchanged in the urine and since active metabolites of theophylline (i.e., caffeine, 3-methylxanthine) do not accumulate to clinically significant levels even in the face of end-stage renal disease, no dosage adjustment for renal insufficiency is necessary in adults and children >3 months of age. In contrast, the large fraction of the theophylline dose excreted in the urine as unchanged theophylline and caffeine in neonates requires careful attention to dose reduction and frequent monitoring of serum theophylline concentrations in neonates with reduced renal function (See WARNINGS).

Serum Concentrations at Steady State After multiple doses of theophylline, steady state is reached in 30–65 hours (average 40 hours) in adults. At steady state, on a dosage regimen with 24-hour intervals, the expected mean trough concentration is approximately 50% of the mean peak concentration, assuming a mean theophylline half-life of 8 hours. The difference between peak and trough concentrations is larger in patients with more rapid theophylline clearance. In these patients administration of Uniphyl® may be required more frequently (every 12 hours).

Special Populations (See Table I for mean clearance and half-life values)

Geriatric The clearance of theophylline is decreased by an average of 30% in healthy elderly adults (>60 yrs) compared to healthy young adults. Careful attention to dose reduction and frequent monitoring of serum theophylline concentrations are required in elderly patients (see WARNINGS).

Pediatrics The clearance of theophylline is very low in neonates (see WARNINGS). Theophylline clearance reaches maximal values by one year of age, remains relatively constant until about 9 years of age and then slowly decreases by approximately 50% to adult values at about age 16. Renal excretion of unchanged theophylline in neonates amounts to about 50% of the dose, compared to about 10% in children older than three months and in adults. Careful attention to dosage selection and monitoring of serum theophylline concentrations are required in pediatric patients (see WARNINGS and DOSAGE AND ADMINISTRATION).

Gender Gender differences in theophylline clearance are relatively small and unlikely to be of clinical significance. Significant reduction in theophylline clearance, however, has been reported in women on the 20th day of the menstrual cycle and during the third trimester of pregnancy.

Race Pharmacokinetic differences in theophylline clearance due to race have not been studied.

Renal insufficiency Only a small fraction, e.g., about 10%, of the administered theophylline dose is excreted unchanged in the urine of children greater than three months of age and adults. Since little theophylline is excreted unchanged in the urine and since active metabolites of theophylline (i.e., caffeine, 3-methylxanthine) do not accumulate to clinically significant levels even in the face of end-stage renal disease, no dosage adjustment for renal insufficiency is necessary in adults and children >3 months of age. In contrast,

approximately 50% of the administered theophylline dose is excreted unchanged in the urine in neonates. Careful attention to dose reduction and frequent monitoring of serum theophylline concentrations are required in neonates with decreased renal function (see WARNINGS).

Hepatic Insufficiency Theophylline clearance is decreased by 50% or more in patients with hepatic insufficiency (e.g., cirrhosis, acute hepatitis, cholestasis). Careful attention to dose reduction and frequent monitoring of serum theophylline concentrations are required in patients with reduced hepatic function (see WARNINGS).

Congestive Heart Failure (CHF) Theophylline clearance is decreased by 50% or more in patients with CHF. The extent of reduction in theophylline clearance in patients with CHF appears to be directly correlated to the severity of the cardiac disease. Since theophylline clearance is independent of liver blood flow, the reduction in clearance appears to be due to impaired hepatocyte function rather than reduced perfusion. Careful attention to dose reduction and frequent monitoring of serum theophylline concentrations are required in patients with CHF (see WARNINGS).

Smokers Tobacco and marijuana smoking appears to increase the clearance of theophylline by induction of metabolic pathways. Theophylline clearance has been shown to increase by approximately 50% in young adult tobacco smokers and by approximately 80% in elderly tobacco smokers compared to non-smoking subjects. Passive smoke exposure has also been shown to increase theophylline clearance by up to 50%. Abstinence from tobacco smoking for one week causes a reduction of approximately 40% in theophylline clearance. Careful attention to dose reduction and frequent monitoring of serum theophylline concentrations are required in patients who stop smoking (see WARNINGS). Use of nicotine gum has been shown to have no effect on theophylline clearance.

Fever Fever, regardless of its underlying cause, can decrease the clearance of theophylline. The magnitude and duration of the fever appear to be directly correlated to the degree of decrease of theophylline clearance. Precise data are lacking, but a temperature of 39°C (102°F) for at least 24 hours is probably required to produce a clinically significant increase in serum theophylline concentrations. Children with rapid rates of theophylline clearance (i.e., those who require a dose that is substantially larger than average [e.g., >22 mg/kg/day] to achieve a therapeutic peak serum theophylline concentration when afebrile) may be at greater risk of toxic effects from decreased clearance during sustained fever. Careful attention to dose reduction and frequent monitoring of serum theophylline concentrations are required in patients with sustained fever (see WARNINGS).

Miscellaneous Other factors associated with decreased theophylline clearance include the third trimester of pregnancy, sepsis with multiple organ failure, and hypothyroidism. Careful attention to dose reduction and frequent monitoring of serum theophylline concentrations are required in patients with any of these conditions (see WARNINGS). Other factors associated with increased theophylline clearance include hyperthyroidism and cystic fibrosis.

Clinical Studies: In patients with chronic asthma, including patients with severe asthma requiring inhaled corticosteroids or alternate-day oral corticosteroids, many clinical studies have shown that theophylline decreases the frequency and severity of symptoms, including nocturnal exacerbations, and decreases the "as needed" use of inhaled beta-2 agonists. Theophylline has also been shown to reduce the need for short courses of daily oral prednisone to relieve exacerbations of airway obstruction that are unresponsive to bronchodilators in asthmatics.

In patients with chronic obstructive pulmonary disease (COPD), clinical studies have shown that theophylline decreases dyspnea, air trapping, the work of breathing, and improves contractility of diaphragmatic muscles with little or no improvement in pulmonary function measurements.

INDICATIONS AND USAGE

Theophylline is indicated for the treatment of the symptoms and reversible airflow obstruction associated with chronic asthma and other chronic lung diseases, e.g., emphysema and chronic bronchitis.

CONTRAINDICATIONS

Uniphyl® is contraindicated in patients with a history of hypersensitivity to theophylline or other components in the product.

WARNINGS

Concurrent Illness: Theophylline should be used with extreme caution in patients with the following clinical conditions due to the increased risk of exacerbation of the concurrent condition:

Active peptic ulcer disease
Seizure disorders
Cardiac arrhythmias (not including bradyarrhythmias)

Conditions That Reduce Theophylline Clearance: There are several readily identifiable causes of reduced theophylline clearance. *If the total daily dose is not appropriately reduced in the presence of these risk factors, severe and*

potentially fatal theophylline toxicity can occur. Careful consideration must be given to the benefits and risks of theophylline use and the need for more intensive monitoring of serum theophylline concentrations in patients with the following risk factors:

Age
Neonates (term and premature)
Children <1 year
Elderly (>60 years)

Concurrent Diseases
Acute pulmonary edema
Congestive heart failure
Cor-pulmonale
Fever; ≥102° for 24 hours or more; or lesser temperature elevations for longer periods
Hypothyroidism
Liver disease, cirrhosis, acute hepatitis
Reduced renal function in infants <3 months of age
Sepsis with multi-organ failure
Shock

Cessation of Smoking

Drug Interactions
Adding a drug that inhibits theophylline metabolism (e.g., cimetidine, erythromycin, tacrine) or stopping a concurrently administered drug that enhances theophylline metabolism (e.g., carbamazepine, rifampin). (See PRECAUTIONS, Drug Interactions, Table II).

When Signs or Symptoms of Theophylline Toxicity Are Present:

Whenever a patient receiving theophylline develops nausea or vomiting, particularly repetitive vomiting, or other signs or symptoms consistent with theophylline toxicity (even if another cause may be suspected), additional doses of theophylline should be withheld and a serum theophylline concentration measured immediately. Patients should be instructed not to continue any dosage that causes adverse effects and to withhold subsequent doses until the symptoms have resolved, at which time the clinician may instruct the patient to resume the drug at a lower dosage (see DOSAGE AND ADMINISTRATION, Dosing Guidelines, Table VI).

Dosage Increases: Increases in the dose of theophylline should not be made in response to an acute exacerbation of symptoms of chronic lung disease since theophylline provides little added benefit to inhaled beta-2-selective agonists and systemically administered corticosteroids in this circumstance and increases the risk of adverse effects. A peak steady-state serum theophylline concentration should be measured before increasing the dose in response to persistent chronic symptoms to ascertain whether an increase in dose is safe. Before increasing the theophylline dose on the basis of a low serum concentration, the clinician should consider whether the blood sample was obtained at an appropriate time in relationship to the dose and whether the patient has adhered to the prescribed regimen (see PRECAUTIONS, Laboratory Tests).

As the rate of theophylline clearance may be dose-dependent (i.e., steady-state serum concentrations may increase disproportionately to the increase in dose), an increase in dose based upon a sub-therapeutic serum concentration measurement should be conservative. In general, limiting dose increases to about 25% of the previous total daily dose will reduce the risk of unintended excessive increases in serum theophylline concentration (see DOSAGE AND ADMINISTRATION, Table VI).

PRECAUTIONS

General: Careful consideration of the various interacting drugs and physiologic conditions that can alter theophylline clearance and require dosage adjustment should occur prior to initiation of theophylline therapy, prior to increases in theophylline dose, and during follow up (see WARNINGS). The dose of theophylline selected for initiation of therapy should be low and, *if tolerated,* increased slowly over a period of a week or longer with the final dose guided by monitoring serum theophylline concentrations and the patient's clinical response (see DOSAGE AND ADMINISTRATION, Table V).

Monitoring Serum Theophylline Concentrations: Serum theophylline concentration measurements are readily available and should be used to determine whether the dosage is appropriate. Specifically, the serum theophylline concentration should be measured as follows:

1. When initiating therapy to guide final dosage adjustment after titration.

2. Before making a dose increase to determine whether the serum concentration is sub-therapeutic in a patient who continues to be symptomatic.

3. Whenever signs or symptoms of theophylline toxicity are present.

4. Whenever there is a new illness, worsening of a chronic illness or a change in the patient's treatment regimen

Continued on next page

Uniphyl—Cont.

that may alter theophylline clearance (e.g., fever >102°F sustained for ≥24 hours, hepatitis, or drugs listed in Table II are added or discontinued).

To guide a dose increase, the blood sample should be obtained at the time of the expected peak serum theophylline concentration; 12 hours after an evening dose or 9 hours after a morning dose at steady-state. For most patients, steady-state will be reached after 3 days of dosing when no doses have been missed, no extra doses have been added, and none of the doses have been taken at unequal intervals. A trough concentration (i.e., at the end of the dosing interval) provides no additional useful information and may lead to an inappropriate dose increase since the peak serum theophylline concentration can be two or more times greater than the trough concentration with an immediate-release formulation. If the serum sample is drawn more than 12 hours after the evening dose, or more than 9 hours after a morning dose, the results must be interpreted with caution since the concentration may not be reflective of the peak concentration. In contrast, when signs or symptoms of theophylline toxicity are present, a serum sample should be obtained as soon as possible, analyzed immediately, and the result reported to the clinician without delay. In patients in whom decreased serum protein binding is suspected (e.g., cirrhosis, women during the third trimester of pregnancy), the concentration of unbound theophylline should be measured and the dosage adjusted to achieve an unbound concentration of 6–12 mcg/mL.

Saliva concentrations of theophylline cannot be used reliably to adjust dosage without special techniques.

Effects on Laboratory Tests: As a result of its pharmacological effects, theophylline at serum concentrations within the 10–20 mcg/mL range modestly increases plasma glucose (from a mean of 88 mg% to 98 mg%), uric acid (from a mean of 4 mg/dl to 6 mg/dl), free fatty acids (from a mean of 451 μEq/l to 800 μEq/l, total cholesterol (from a mean of 140 vs 160 mg/dl), HDL (from a mean of 36 to 50 mg/dl), HDL/LDL ratio (from a mean of 0.5 to 0.7), and urinary free cortisol excretion (from a mean of 44 to 63 mcg/24 hr). Theophylline at serum concentrations within the 10–20 mcg/mL range may also transiently decrease serum concentrations of triiodothyronine (144 before, 131 after one week and 142 ng/dL after 4 weeks of theophylline). The clinical importance of these changes should be weighed against the potential therapeutic benefit of theophylline in individual patients.

Information for Patients: The patient (or parent/care giver) should be instructed to seek medical advice whenever nausea, vomiting, persistent headache, insomnia or rapid heart beat occurs during treatment with theophylline, even if another cause is suspected. The patient should be instructed to contact their clinician if they develop a new illness, especially if accompanied by a persistent fever, if they experience worsening of a chronic illness, if they start or stop smoking cigarettes or marijuana, or if another clinician adds a new medication or discontinues a previously prescribed medication. Patients should be instructed to inform all clinicians involved in their care that they are taking theophylline, especially when a medication is being added or deleted from their treatment. Patients should be instructed to not alter the dose, timing of the dose, or frequency of administration without first consulting their clinician. If a dose is missed, the patient should be instructed to take the next dose at the usually scheduled time and to not attempt to make up for the missed dose.

Uniphyl® tablets can be taken once a day in the morning or evening. It is recommended that Uniphyl® be taken with meals. Patients should be advised that if they choose to take Uniphyl® with food it should be taken consistently with food and if they take it in a fasted condition it should routinely be taken fasted. It is important that the product whenever dosed be dosed consistently with or without food. Uniphyl® tablets are not to be chewed or crushed. The scored tablet may be split. Patients receiving Uniphyl® tablets may pass an intact matrix tablet in the stool or via colostomy. These matrix tablets usually contain little or no residual theophylline.

Drug Interactions: Theophylline interacts with a wide variety of drugs. The interaction may be pharmacodynamic, i.e., alterations in the therapeutic response to theophylline or another drug or occurrence of adverse effects without a change in serum theophylline concentration. More frequently, however, the interaction is pharmacokinetic, i.e., the rate of theophylline clearance is altered by another drug resulting in increased or decreased serum theophylline concentrations. Theophylline only rarely alters the pharmacokinetics of other drugs.

The drugs listed in Table II have the potential to produce clinically significant pharmacodynamic or pharmacokinetic interactions with theophylline. The information in the "Effect" column of Table II assumes that the interacting drug is being added to a steady-state theophylline regimen. If theophylline is being initiated in a patient who is already taking a drug that inhibits theophylline clearance (e.g., cimeti-

Table II. Clinically significant drug interactions with theophylline*

Drug	Type of Interaction	Effect**
Adenosine	Theophylline blocks adenosine receptors.	Higher doses of adenosine may be required to achieve desired effect.
Alcohol	A single large dose of alcohol (3 mL/kg of whiskey) decreases theophylline clearance for up to 24 hours.	30% increase
Allopurinol	Decreases theophylline clearance at allopurinol doses ≥600 mg/day.	25% increase
Aminoglutethimide	Increases theophylline clearance by induction of microsomal enzyme activity.	25% decrease
Carbamazepine	Similar to aminoglutethimide.	30% decrease
Cimetidine	Decreases theophylline clearance by inhibiting cytochrome P450 1A2.	70% increase
Ciprofloxacin	Similar to cimetidine.	40% increase
Clarithromycin	Similar to erythromycin.	25% increase
Diazepam	Benzodiazepines increase CNS concentrations of adenosine, a potent CNS depressant, while theophylline blocks adenosine receptors.	Larger diazepam doses may be required to produce desired level of sedation. Discontinuation of theophylline without reduction of diazepam dose may result in respiratory depression.
Disulfiram	Decreases theophylline clearance by inhibiting hydroxylation and demethylation.	50% increase
Enoxacin	Similar to cimetidine.	300% increase
Ephedrine	Synergistic CNS effects	Increased frequency of nausea, nervousness, and insomnia.
Erythromycin	Erythromycin metabolite decreases theophylline clearance by inhibiting cytochrome P450 3A3.	35% increase. Erythromycin steady-state serum concentrations decrease by a similar amount.
Estrogen	Estrogen containing oral contraceptives decrease theophylline clearance in a dose-dependent fashion. The effect of progesterone on theophylline clearance is unknown.	30% increase
Flurazepam	Similar to diazepam.	Similar to diazepam.
Fluvoxamine	Similar to cimetidine	Similar to cimetidine.
Halothane	Halothane sensitizes the myocardium to catecholamines, theophylline increases release of endogenous catecholamines.	Increased risk of ventricular arrhythmias.
Interferon, human recombinant alpha-A	Decreases theophylline clearance.	100% increase
Isoproterenol (IV)	Increases theophylline clearance.	20% decrease
Ketamine	Pharmacologic	May lower theophylline seizure threshold.
Lithium	Theophylline increases renal lithium clearance.	Lithium dose required to achieve a therapeutic serum concentration increased an average of 60%.
Lorazepam	Similar to diazepam.	Similar to diazepam.
Methotrexate (MTX)	Decreases theophylline clearance.	20% increase after low dose MTX, higher dose MTX may have a greater effect.
Mexiletine	Similar to disulfiram.	80% increase
Midazolam	Similar to diazepam.	Similar to diazepam.
Moricizine	Increases theophylline clearance.	25% decrease
Pancuronium	Theophylline may antagonize non-depolarizing neuromuscular blocking effects; possibly due to phosphodiesterase inhibition.	Larger dose of pancuronium may be required to achieve neuromuscular blockade.
Pentoxifylline	Decreases theophylline clearance.	30% increase
Phenobarbital (PB)	Similar to aminoglutethimide.	25% decrease after two weeks of concurrent PB.
Phenytoin	Phenytoin increases theophylline clearance by increasing microsomal enzyme activity. Theophylline decreases phenytoin absorption.	Serum theophylline and phenytoin concentrations decrease about 40%.
Propafenone	Decreases theophylline clearance and pharmacologic interaction.	40% increase. Beta-2 blocking effect may decrease efficacy of theophylline.
Propranolol	Similar to cimetidine and pharmacologic interaction.	100% increase. Beta-2 blocking effect may decrease efficacy of theophylline.
Rifampin	Increases theophylline clearance by increasing cytochrome P450 1A2 and 3A3 activity.	20–40% decrease
Sulfinpyrazone	Increases theophylline clearance by increasing demethylation and hydroxylation. Decreases renal clearance of theophylline.	20% decrease
Tacrine	Similar to cimetidine, also increases renal clearance of theophylline.	90% increase
Thiabendazole	Decreases theophylline clearance.	190% increase
Ticlopidine	Decreases theophylline clearance.	60% increase
Troleandomycin	Similar to erythromycin.	33–100% increase depending on troleandomycin dose.
Verapamil	Similar to disulfiram.	20% increase

* Refer to PRECAUTIONS, Drug Interactions for further information regarding table.
** Average effect on steady-state theophylline concentration or other clinical effect for pharmacologic interactions. Individual patients may experience larger changes in serum theophylline concentration than the value listed.

dine, erythromycin), the dose of theophylline required to achieve a therapeutic serum theophylline concentration will be smaller. Conversely, if theophylline is being initiated in a patient who is already taking a drug that enhances theophylline clearance (e.g., rifampin), the dose of theophylline required to achieve a therapeutic serum theophylline concentration will be larger. Discontinuation of a concomitant drug that increases theophylline clearance will result in accumulation of theophylline to potentially toxic levels, unless the theophylline dose is appropriately reduced. Discontinuation of a concomitant drug that inhibits theophylline clearance will result in decreased serum theophylline concentrations, unless the theophylline dose is appropriately increased.

The drugs listed in Table III have either been documented not to interact with theophylline or do not produce a clinically significant interaction (i.e., <15% change in theophylline clearance).

The listing of drugs in Tables II and III are current as of February 9, 1995. New interactions are continuously being reported for theophylline, especially with new chemical entities. **The clinician should not assume that a drug does not interact with theophylline if it is not listed in Table II.** Before addition of a newly available drug in a patient receiving theophylline, the package insert of the new drug and/or the medical literature should be consulted to determine if an interaction between the new drug and theophylline has been reported.

[See table II at top of previous page]

Table III. Drugs that have been documented not to interact with theophylline or drugs that produce no clinically significant interaction with theophylline.*

albuterol, systemic and inhaled	mebendazole
amoxicillin	medroxyprogesterone
ampicillin, with or without sulbactam	methylprednisolone
atenolol	metronidazole
azithromycin	metoprolol
caffeine, dietary ingestion	nadolol
cefaclor	nifedipine
co-trimoxazole (trimethoprim and sulfamethoxazole)	nizatidine
diltiazem	norfloxacin
dirithromycin	ofloxacin
enflurane	omeprazole
famotidine	prednisone, prednisolone
felodipine	ranitidine
finasteride	rifabutin
hydrocortisone	roxithromycin
isoflurane	sorbitol (purgative doses do not inhibit theophylline absorption)
isoniazid	sucralfate
isradipine	terbutaline, systemic
influenza vaccine	terfenadine
ketoconazole	tetracycline
lomefloxacin	tocainide

*** Refer to PRECAUTIONS, Drug Interactions for information regarding table.**

Drug-Food Interactions: The bioavailability of Uniphyl® tablets (theophylline, anhydrous) has been studied with coadministration of food. In three single-dose studies, subjects given Uniphyl® 400 mg or 600 mg tablets with a standardized high-fat meal were compared to fasted conditions. Under fed conditions, the peak plasma concentration and bioavailability were increased; however, a precipitous increase in the rate and extent of absorption was not evident (**See Pharmacokinetics-Absorption**). The increased peak and extent of absorption under fed conditions suggests that dosing should be ideally administered consistently either with or without food.

The Effect of Other Drugs on Theophylline Serum Concentration Measurements: Most serum theophylline assays in clinical use are immunoassays which are specific for theophylline. Other xanthines such as caffeine, dyphylline, and pentoxifylline are not detected by these assays. Some drugs (e.g., cefazolin, cephalothin), however, may interfere with certain HPLC techniques. Caffeine and xanthine metabolites in neonates or patients with renal dysfunction may cause the reading from some dry reagent office methods to be higher than the actual serum theophylline concentration.

Carcinogenesis, Mutagenesis, and Impairment of Fertility: Long term carcinogenicity studies have been carried out in mice (oral doses 30–150 mg/kg) and rats (oral doses 5–75 mg/kg). Results are pending.

Theophylline has been studied in Ames salmonella, *in vivo* and *in vitro* cytogenetics, micronucleus and Chinese hamster ovary test systems and has not been shown to be genotoxic.

In a 14 week continuous breeding study, theophylline, administered to mating pairs of $B6C3F_1$ mice at oral doses of 120, 270 and 500 mg/kg (approximately 1.0–3.0 times the human dose on a mg/m^2 basis) impaired fertility, as evidenced by decreases in the number of live pups per litter, decreases in the mean number of litters per fertile pair, and increases in the gestation period at the high dose as well as decreases in the proportion of pups born alive at the mid and high dose. In 13 week toxicity studies, theophylline was administered to F344 rats and $B6C3F_1$ mice at oral doses of 40–300 mg/kg (approximately 2.0 times the human dose on a mg/m^2 basis). At the high dose, systemic toxicity was observed in both species including decreases in testicular weight.

Pregnancy: CATEGORY C: There are no adequate and well controlled studies in pregnant women. Additionally, there are no teratogenicity studies in non-rodents (e.g., rabbits). Theophylline was not shown to be teratogenic in CD-1 mice at oral doses up to 400 mg/kg, approximately 2.0 times the human dose on a mg/m^2 basis or in CD-1 rats at oral doses up to 260 mg/kg, approximately 3.0 times the recommended human dose on a mg/m^2 basis. At a dose of 220 mg/kg, embryotoxicity was observed in rats in the absence of maternal toxicity.

Nursing Mothers: Theophylline is excreted into breast milk and may cause irritability or other signs of mild toxicity in nursing human infants. The concentration of theophylline in breast milk is about equivalent to the maternal serum concentration. An infant ingesting a liter of breast milk containing 10–20 mcg/mL of theophylline per day is likely to receive 10–20 mg of theophylline per day. Serious adverse effects in the infant are unlikely unless the mother has toxic serum theophylline concentrations.

Pediatric Use: Theophylline is safe and effective for the approved indications in pediatric patients. The maintenance dose of theophylline must be selected with caution in pediatric patients since the rate of theophylline clearance is highly variable across the pediatric age range (see CLINICAL PHARMACOLOGY, Table I, WARNINGS, and DOSAGE AND ADMINISTRATION, Table V).

Geriatric Use: Elderly patients are at significantly greater risk of experiencing serious toxicity from theophylline than younger patients due to pharmacokinetic and pharmacodynamic changes associated with aging. Theophylline clearance is reduced in patients greater than 60 years of age, resulting in increased serum theophylline concentrations in response to a given theophylline dose. Protein binding may be decreased in the elderly resulting in a larger proportion of the total serum theophylline concentration in the pharmacologically active unbound form. For these reasons, the maximum daily dose of theophylline in patients greater than 60 years of age ordinarily should not exceed 400 mg/day unless the patient continues to be symptomatic and the peak steady-state serum theophylline concentration is <10 mcg/mL (see DOSAGE AND ADMINISTRATION). Theophylline doses greater than 400 mg/d should be prescribed with caution in elderly patients.

ADVERSE REACTIONS

Adverse reactions associated with theophylline are generally mild when peak serum theophylline concentrations are <20 mcg/mL and mainly consist of transient caffeine-like adverse effects such as nausea, vomiting, headache, and insomnia. When peak serum theophylline concentrations exceed 20 mcg/mL, however, theophylline produces a wide range of adverse reactions including persistent vomiting, cardiac arrhythmias, and intractable seizures which can be lethal (see OVERDOSAGE). The transient caffeine-like adverse reactions occur in about 50% of patients when theophylline therapy is initiated at doses higher than recommended initial doses (e.g., >300 mg/day in adults and >12 mg/kg/day in children beyond >1 year of age). During the initiation of theophylline therapy, caffeine-like adverse effects may transiently alter patient behavior, especially in school age children, but this response rarely persists. Initiation of theophylline therapy at a low dose with subsequent slow titration to a predetermined age-related maximum dose will significantly reduce the frequency of these transient adverse effects (see DOSAGE AND ADMINISTRATION, Table V). In a small percentage of patients (<3% of children and <10% of adults) the caffeine-like adverse effects persist during maintenance therapy, even at peak serum theophylline concentrations within the therapeutic range (i.e., 10–20 mcg/mL). Dosage reduction may alleviate the caffeine-like adverse effects in these patients, however, persistent adverse effects should result in a reevaluation of the need for continued theophylline therapy and the potential therapeutic benefit of alternative treatment.

Other adverse reactions that have been reported at serum theophylline concentrations <20 mcg/mL include diarrhea, irritability, restlessness, fine skeletal muscle tremors, and transient diuresis. In patients with hypoxia secondary to COPD, multifocal atrial tachycardia and flutter have been reported at serum theophylline concentrations ≥15 mcg/mL. There have been a few isolated reports of seizures at serum theophylline concentrations <20 mcg/mL in patients with an underlying neurological disease or in elderly patients. The occurrence of seizures in elderly patients with serum theophylline concentrations <20 mcg/mL may be secondary to decreased protein binding resulting in a larger proportion of the total serum theophylline concentration in the pharmacologically active unbound form. The clinical characteristics of the seizures reported in patients with serum theophylline concentrations <20 mcg/mL have generally been milder than seizures associated with excessive serum theophylline concentrations resulting from an overdose (i.e. they have generally been transient, often stopped without anticonvulsant therapy, and did not result in neurological residua).

Table IV. Manifestations of theophylline toxicity.*

	Percentage of patients reported with sign or symptom			
	Acute Overdose (Large Single Ingestion)		Chronic Overdosage (Multiple Excessive Doses)	
Sign/Symptom	Study 1 (n=157)	Study 2 (n=14)	Study 1 (n=92)	Study 2 (n=102)
Asymptomatic	NR**	0	NR**	6
Gastrointestinal				
Vomiting	73	93	30	61
Abdominal Pain	NR**	21	NR**	12
Diarrhea	NR**	0	NR**	14
Hematemesis	NR**	0	NR**	2
Metabolic/Other				
Hypokalemia	85	79	44	43
Hyperglycemia	98	NR**	18	NR**
Acid/base disturbance	34	21	9	5
Rhabdomyolysis	NR**	7	NR**	0
Cardiovascular				
Sinus tachycardia	100	86	100	62
Other supraventricular tachycardias	2	21	12	14
Ventricular premature beats	3	21	10	19
Atrial fibrillation or flutter	1	NR**	12	NR**
Multifocal atrial tachycardia	0	NR**	2	NR**
Ventricular arrhythmias with hemodynamic instability	7	14	40	0
Hypotension/shock	NR**	21	NR**	8
Neurologic				
Nervousness	NR**	64	NR**	21
Tremors	38	29	16	14
Disorientation	NR**	7	NR**	11
Seizures	5	14	14	5
Death	3	21	10	4

* These data are derived from two studies in patients with serum theophylline concentrations >30 mcg/mL. In the first study (Study #1—Shanon, *Ann Intern Med* 1993; 119:1161–67), data were prospectively collected from 249 consecutive cases of theophylline toxicity referred to a regional poison center for consultation. In the second study (Study #2—Sessler, *Am J Med* 1990;88:567–76), data were retrospectively collected from 116 cases with serum theophylline concentrations >30 mcg/mL among 6000 blood samples obtained for measurement of serum theophylline concentrations in three emergency departments. Differences in the incidence of manifestations of theophylline toxicity between the two studies may reflect sample selection as a result of study design (e.g., in Study #1, 48% of the patients had acute intoxications versus only 10% in Study #2) and different methods of reporting results.

**NR=Not reported in a comparable manner.

OVERDOSAGE

General: The chronicity and pattern of theophylline overdosage significantly influences clinical manifestations of toxicity, management and outcome. There are two common presentations: (1) *acute overdose,* i.e., ingestion of a single large excessive dose (>10 mg/kg), as occurs in the context of an attempted suicide or isolated medication error, and (2) *chronic overdosage,* i.e., ingestion of repeated doses that are excessive for the patient's rate of theophylline clearance. The most common causes of chronic theophylline overdosage include patient or care giver error in dosing, clinician prescribing of an excessive dose or a normal dose in the presence of factors known to decrease the rate of theophylline clearance, and increasing the dose in response to an exacerbation of symptoms without first measuring the serum theophylline concentration to determine whether a dose increase is safe.

Severe toxicity from theophylline overdose is a relatively rare event. In one health maintenance organization, the fre-

Continued on next page

Uniphyl—Cont.

quency of hospital admissions for chronic overdosage of theophylline was about 1 per 1000 person-years exposure. In another study, among 6000 blood samples obtained for measurement of serum theophylline concentration, for any reason, from patients treated in an emergency department, 7% were in the 20–30 mcg/mL range and 3% were >30 mcg/mL. Approximately two-thirds of the patients with serum theophylline concentrations in the 20–30 mcg/mL range had one or more manifestations of toxicity while >90% of patients with serum theophylline concentrations >30 mcg/mL were clinically intoxicated. Similarly, in other reports, serious toxicity from theophylline is seen principally at serum concentrations >30 mcg/mL.

Several studies have described the clinical manifestations of theophylline overdose and attempted to determine the factors that predict life-threatening toxicity. In general, patients who experience an acute overdose are less likely to experience seizures than patients who have experienced a chronic overdosage, unless the peak serum theophylline concentration is >100 mcg/mL. After a chronic overdosage, generalized seizures, life-threatening cardiac arrhythmias, and death may occur at serum theophylline concentrations >30 mcg/mL. The severity of toxicity after chronic overdosage is more strongly correlated with the patient's age than the peak serum theophylline concentration; patients >60 years are at the greatest risk for severe toxicity and mortality after a chronic overdosage. Pre-existing or concurrent disease may also significantly increase the susceptibility of a patient to a particular toxic manifestation, e.g., patients with neurologic disorders have an increased risk of seizures and patients with cardiac disease have an increased risk of cardiac arrhythmias for a given serum theophylline concentration compared to patients without the underlying disease.

The frequency of various reported manifestations of theophylline overdose according to the mode of overdose are listed in Table IV.

Other manifestations of theophylline toxicity include increases in serum calcium, creatine kinase, myoglobin and leukocyte count, decreases in serum phosphate and magnesium, acute myocardial infarction, and urinary retention in men with obstructive uropathy.

Seizures associated with serum theophylline concentrations >30 mcg/mL are often resistant to anticonvulsant therapy and may result in irreversible brain injury if not rapidly controlled. Death from theophylline toxicity is most often secondary to cardiorespiratory arrest and/or hypoxic encephalopathy following prolonged generalized seizures or intractable cardiac arrhythmias causing hemodynamic compromise.

Overdose Management: General Recommendations for Patients with Symptoms of Theophylline Overdose or Serum Theophylline Concentrations >30 mcg/mL (Note: Serum theophylline concentrations may continue to increase after presentation of the patient for medical care.)

1. While simultaneously instituting treatment, contact a regional poison center to obtain updated information and advice on individualizing the recommendations that follow.
2. Institute supportive care, including establishment of intravenous access, maintenance of the airway, and electrocardiographic monitoring.
3. Treatment of seizures Because of the high morbidity and mortality associated with theophylline-induced seizures, treatment should be rapid and aggressive. Anticonvulsant therapy should be initiated with an intravenous benzodiazepine, e.g., diazepam, in increments of 0.1–0.2 mg/kg every 1–3 minutes until seizures are terminated. Repetitive seizures should be treated with a loading dose of phenobarbital (20 mg/kg infused over 30–60 minutes). Case reports of theophylline overdose in humans and animal studies suggest that phenytoin is ineffective in terminating theophylline-induced seizures. The doses of benzodiazepines and phenobarbital required to terminate theophylline-induced seizures are close to the doses that may cause severe respiratory depression or respiratory arrest; the clinician should therefore be prepared to provide assisted ventilation. Elderly patients and patients with COPD may be more susceptible to the respiratory depressant effects of anticonvulsants. Barbiturate-induced coma or administration of general anesthesia may be required to terminate repetitive seizures or status epilepticus. General anesthesia should be used with caution in patients with theophylline overdose because fluorinated volatile anesthetics may sensitize the myocardium to endogenous catecholamines released by theophylline. Enflurane appears less likely to be associated with this effect than halothane and may, therefore, be safer. Neuromuscular blocking agents alone should not be used to terminate seizures since they abolish the musculoskeletal manifestations without terminating seizure activity in the brain.

4. Anticipate Need for Anticonvulsants in patients with theophylline overdose who are at high risk for theophylline-induced seizures, e.g., patients with acute overdoses and serum theophylline concentrations >100 mcg/mL or chronic overdosage in patients >60 years of age with serum theophylline concentrations >30 mcg/mL, the need for anticonvulsant therapy should be anticipated. A benzodiazepine such as diazepam should be drawn into a syringe and kept at the patient's bedside and medical personnel qualified to treat seizures should be immediately available. In selected patients at high risk for theophylline-induced seizures, consideration should be given to the administration of prophylactic anticonvulsant therapy. Situations where prophylactic anticonvulsant therapy should be considered in high risk patients include anticipated delays in instituting methods for extracorporeal removal of theophylline (e.g., transfer of a high risk patient from one health care facility to another for extracorporeal removal) and clinical circumstances that significantly interfere with efforts to enhance theophylline clearance (e.g., a neonate where dialysis may not be technically feasible or a patient with vomiting unresponsive to antiemetics who is unable to tolerate multiple-dose oral activated charcoal). In animal studies, prophylactic administration of phenobarbital, but not phenytoin, has been shown to delay the onset of theophylline-induced generalized seizures and to increase the dose of theophylline required to induce seizures (i.e., markedly increases the LD_{50}). Although there are no controlled studies in humans, a loading dose of intravenous phenobarbital (20 mg/kg infused over 60 minutes) may delay or prevent life-threatening seizures in high risk patients while efforts to enhance theophylline clearance are continued. Phenobarbital may cause respiratory depression, particularly in elderly patients and patients with COPD.

5. Treatment of cardiac arrhythmias Sinus tachycardia and simple ventricular premature beats are not harbingers of life-threatening arrhythmias, they do not require treatment in the absence of hemodynamic compromise, and they resolve with declining serum theophylline concentrations. Other arrhythmias, especially those associated with hemodynamic compromise, should be treated with antiarrhythmic therapy appropriate for the type of arrhythmia.

6. Gastrointestinal decontamination Oral activated charcoal (0.5 g/kg up to 20 g and repeat at least once 1–2 hours after the first dose) is extremely effective in blocking the absorption of theophylline throughout the gastrointestinal tract, even when administered several hours after ingestion. If the patient is vomiting, the charcoal should be administered through a nasogastric tube or after administration of an antiemetic. Phenothiazine antiemetics such as prochlorperazine or perphenazine should be avoided since they can lower the seizure threshold and frequently cause dystonic reactions. A single dose of sorbitol may be used to promote stooling to facilitate removal of theophylline bound to charcoal from the gastrointestinal tract. Sorbitol, however, should be dosed with caution since it is a potent purgative which can cause profound fluid and electrolyte abnormalities, particularly after multiple doses. Commercially available fixed combinations of liquid charcoal and sorbitol should be avoided in young children and after the first dose in adolescents and adults since they do not allow for individualization of charcoal and sorbitol dosing. Ipecac syrup should be avoided in theophylline overdoses. Although ipecac induces emesis, it does not reduce the absorption of theophylline unless administered within 5 minutes of ingestion and even then is less effective than oral activated charcoal. Moreover, ipecac induced emesis may persist for several hours after a single dose and significantly decrease the retention and the effectiveness of oral activated charcoal.

7. Serum Theophylline Concentration Monitoring The serum theophylline concentration should be measured immediately upon presentation, 2–4 hours later, and then at sufficient intervals, e.g., every 4 hours, to guide treatment decisions and to assess the effectiveness of therapy. Serum theophylline concentrations may continue to increase after presentation of the patient for medical care as a result of continued absorption of theophylline from the gastrointestinal tract. Serial monitoring of serum theophylline serum concentrations should be continued until it is clear that the concentration is no longer rising and has returned to non-toxic levels.

8. General Monitoring Procedures Electrocardiographic monitoring should be initiated on presentation and continued until the serum theophylline level has returned to a non-toxic level. Serum electrolytes and glucose should be measured on presentation and at appropriate intervals indicated by clinical circumstances. Fluid and electrolyte abnormalities should be promptly corrected. **Monitoring and treatment should be continued until the serum concentration decreases below 20 mcg/mL.**

9. Enhance clearance of theophylline Multiple-dose oral activated charcoal (e.g., 0.5 mg/kg up to 20 g, every two

hours) increases the clearance of theophylline at least twofold by adsorption of theophylline secreted into gastrointestinal fluids. Charcoal must be retained in, and pass through, the gastrointestinal tract to be effective; emesis should therefore be controlled by administration of appropriate antiemetics. Alternatively, the charcoal can be administered continuously through a nasogastric tube in conjunction with appropriate antiemetics. A single dose of sorbitol may be administered with the activated charcoal to promote stooling to facilitate clearance of the adsorbed theophylline from the gastrointestinal tract. Sorbitol alone does not enhance clearance of theophylline and should be dosed with caution to prevent excessive stooling which can result in severe fluid and electrolyte imbalances. Commercially available fixed combinations of liquid charcoal and sorbitol should be avoided in young children and after the first dose in adolescents and adults since they do not allow for individualization of charcoal and sorbitol dosing. In patients with intractable vomiting, extracorporeal methods of theophylline removal should be instituted (see OVERDOSAGE, Extracorporeal Removal).

Specific Recommendations:
Acute Overdose
A. Serum Concentration >20 <30 mcg/mL
1. Administer a single dose of oral activated charcoal.
2. Monitor the patient and obtain a serum theophylline concentration in 2–4 hours to insure that the concentration is not increasing.
B. Serum Concentration >30 <100 mcg/mL
1. Administer multiple dose oral activated charcoal and measures to control emesis.
2. Monitor the patient and obtain serial theophylline concentrations every 2–4 hours to gauge the effectiveness of therapy and to guide further treatment decisions.
3. Institute extracorporeal removal if emesis, seizures, or cardiac arrhythmias cannot be adequately controlled (see OVERDOSAGE, Extracorporeal Removal).
C. Serum Concentration >100 mcg/mL
1. Consider prophylactic anticonvulsant therapy.
2. Administer multiple-dose oral activated charcoal and measures to control emesis.
3. Consider extracorporeal removal, even if the patient has not experienced a seizure (see OVERDOSAGE, Extracorporeal Removal).
4. Monitor the patient and obtain serial theophylline concentrations every 2–4 hours to gauge the effectiveness of therapy and to guide further treatment decisions.

Chronic Overdosage
A. Serum Concentration >20 <30 mcg/mL (with manifestations of theophylline toxicity)
1. Administer a single dose of oral activated charcoal.
2. Monitor the patient and obtain a serum theophylline concentration in 2–4 hours to insure that the concentration is not increasing.
B. Serum Concentration >30 mcg/mL in patients <60 years of age
1. Administer multiple-dose oral activated charcoal and measures to control emesis.
2. Monitor the patient and obtain serial theophylline concentrations every 2–4 hours to gauge the effectiveness of therapy and to guide further treatment decisions.
3. Institute extracorporeal removal if emesis, seizures, or cardiac arrhythmias cannot be adequately controlled (see OVERDOSAGE, Extracorporeal Removal).
C. Serum Concentration >30 mcg/mL in patients ≥60 years of age
1. Consider prophylactic anticonvulsant therapy.
2. Administer multiple-dose oral activated charcoal and measures to control emesis.
3. Consider extracorporeal removal even if the patient has not experienced a seizure (see OVERDOSAGE, Extracorporeal Removal).
4. Monitor the patient and obtain serial theophylline concentrations every 2–4 hours to gauge the effectiveness of therapy and to guide further treatment decisions.

Extracorporeal Removal: Increasing the rate of theophylline clearance by extracorporeal methods may rapidly decrease serum concentrations, but the risks of the procedure must be weighed against the potential benefit. Charcoal hemoperfusion is the most effective method of extracorporeal removal, increasing theophylline clearance up to six fold, but serious complications, including hypotension, hypocalcemia, platelet consumption and bleeding diatheses may occur. Hemodialysis is about as efficient as multiple-dose oral activated charcoal and has a lower risk of serious complications than charcoal hemoperfusion. Hemodialysis should be considered as an alternative when charcoal hemoperfusion is not feasible and multiple-dose oral charcoal is ineffective because of intractable emesis. Serum theophylline concentrations may rebound 5–10 mcg/mL after discontinuation of charcoal hemoperfusion or hemodialysis due to redistribution of theophylline from the tissue compartment. Perito-

neal dialysis is ineffective for theophylline removal; exchange transfusions in neonates have been minimally effective.

DOSAGE AND ADMINISTRATION

Uniphyl® 400 or 600 mg Tablets can be taken once a day in the morning or evening. It is recommended that Uniphyl be taken with meals. Patients should be advised that if they choose to take Uniphyl® with food it should be taken consistently with food and if they take it in a fasted condition it should routinely be taken fasted. It is important that the product whenever dosed be dosed consistently with or without food.

Uniphyl® Tablets are not to be chewed or crushed. The scored tablet may be split. Infrequently, patients receiving Uniphyl® 400 or 600 mg Tablets may pass an intact matrix tablet in the stool or via colostomy. These matrix tablets usually contain little or no residual theophylline.

Stabilized patients, 12 years of age or older, who are taking an immediate-release or controlled-release theophylline product may be transferred to once-daily administration of 400 mg or 600 mg Uniphyl® Tablets on a mg-for-mg basis. It must be recognized that the peak and trough serum theophylline levels produced by the once-daily dosing may vary from those produced by the previous product and/or regimen.

General Considerations: The steady-state peak serum theophylline concentration is a function of the dose, the dosing interval, and the rate of theophylline absorption and clearance in the individual patient. Because of marked individual differences in the rate of theophylline clearance, the dose required to achieve a peak serum theophylline concentration in the 10–20 mcg/mL range varies fourfold among otherwise similar patients in the absence of factors known to alter theophylline clearance (e.g., 400–1600 mg/day in adults <60 years old and 10–36 mg/kg/day in children 1–9 years old). For a given population there is no single theophylline dose that will provide both safe and effective serum concentrations for all patients. Administration of the median theophylline dose required to achieve a therapeutic serum theophylline concentration in a given population may result in either sub-therapeutic or potentially toxic serum theophylline concentrations in individual patients. For example, at a dose of 900 mg/d in adults <60 years or 22 mg/kg/d in children 1–9 years, the steady-state peak serum theophylline concentration will be <10 mcg/mL in about 30% of patients, 10–20 mcg/mL in about 50% and 20–30 mcg/mL in about 20% of patients. **The dose of theophylline must be individualized on the basis of peak serum theophylline concentration measurements in order to achieve a dose that will provide maximum potential benefit with minimal risk of adverse effects.**

Transient caffeine-like adverse effects and excessive serum concentrations in slow metabolizers can be avoided in most patients by starting with a sufficiently low dose and slowly increasing the dose, if judged to be clinically indicated, in small increments (See Table V). Dose increases should only be made if the previous dosage is well tolerated and at intervals of no less than 3 days to allow serum theophylline concentrations to reach the new steady-state. Dosage adjustment should be guided by serum theophylline concentration measurement (see PRECAUTIONS, Laboratory Tests and DOSAGE AND ADMINISTRATION, Table VI). Health care providers should instruct patients and care givers to discontinue any dosage that causes adverse effects, to withhold the medication until these symptoms are gone and to then resume therapy at a lower, previously tolerated dosage (see WARNINGS).

If the patient's symptoms are well controlled, there are no apparent adverse effects, and no intervening factors that might alter dosage requirements (see WARNINGS and PRECAUTIONS), serum theophylline concentrations should be monitored at 6 month intervals for rapidly growing children and at yearly intervals for all others. In acutely ill patients, serum theophylline concentrations should be monitored at frequent intervals, e.g., every 24 hours.

Theophylline distributes poorly into body fat, therefore, mg/kg dose should be calculated on the basis of ideal body weight.

Table V contains theophylline dosing titration schema recommended for patients in various age groups and clinical circumstances. Table VI contains recommendations for theophylline dosage adjustment based upon serum theophylline concentrations. **Application of these general dosing recommendations to individual patients must take into account the unique clinical characteristics of each patient. In general, these recommendations should serve as the upper limit for dosage adjustments in order to decrease the risk of potentially serious adverse events associated with unexpected large increases in serum theophylline concentration.**

Table V. Dosing initiation and titration (as anhydrous theophylline).*
A. Children (12–15 years) and adults (16–60 years) without risk factors for impaired clearance.

Titration Step	Children ≤ 45 kg	Children > 45 kg and adults
1. Starting Dosage	12–14 mg/kg/day up to a maximum of 300 mg/day admin. QD*	300–400 mg/day† admin. QD*
2. After 3 days, if tolerated, increase dose to:	16 mg/kg/day up to a maximum of 400 mg/day admin. QD*	400–600 mg/day† admin. QD*
3. After 3 more days, if tolerated and if needed increase dose to:	20 mg/kg/day up to a maximum of 600 mg/day admin. QD*	As with all theophylline products, doses greater than 600 mg should be titrated according to blood level (See Table VI)

†If caffeine-like adverse effects occur, then consideration should be given to a lower dose and titrating the dose more slowly (see ADVERSE REACTIONS).

B. Patients With Risk Factors For Impaired Clearance, The Elderly (>60 Years), And Those In Whom It Is Not Feasible To Monitor Serum Theophylline Concentrations:

In children 12–15 years of age, the theophylline dose should not exceed 16 mg/kg/day up to a maximum of 400 mg/day in the presence of risk factors for reduced theophylline clearance (see WARNINGS) or if it is not feasible to monitor serum theophylline concentrations.

In adolescents ≥16 years and adults, including the elderly, the theophylline dose should not exceed 400 mg/day in the presence of risk factors for reduced theophylline clearance (see WARNINGS) or if it is not feasible to monitor serum theophylline concentrations.

*Patients with more rapid metabolism clinically identified by higher than average dose requirements, should receive a smaller dose more frequently (every 12 hours) to prevent breakthrough symptoms resulting from low trough concentrations before the next dose.

Table VI. Dosage adjustment guided by serum theophylline concentration.

Peak Serum Concentration	Dosage Adjustment
<9.9 mcg/mL	If symptoms are not controlled and current dosage is tolerated, increase dose about 25%. Recheck serum concentration after three days for further dosage adjustment.
10–14.9 mcg/mL	If symptoms are controlled and current dosage is tolerated, maintain dose and recheck serum concentration at 6–12 month intervals.¶ If symptoms are not controlled and current dosage is tolerated consider adding additional medication(s) to treatment regimen.
15–19.9 mcg/mL	Consider 10% decrease in dose to provide greater margin of safety even if current dosage is tolerated.¶
20–24.9 mcg/mL	Decrease dose by 25% even if no adverse effects are present. Recheck serum concentration after 3 days to guide further dosage adjustment.
25–30 mcg/mL	Skip next dose and decrease subsequent doses at least 25% even if no adverse effects are present. Recheck serum concentration after 3 days to guide further dosage adjustment. If symptomatic, consider whether overdose treatment is indicated (see recommendations for chronic overdosage).
>30 mcg/mL	Treat overdose as indicated (see recommendations for chronic overdosage). If theophylline is subsequently resumed, decrease dose by at least 50% and recheck serum concentration after 3 days to guide further dosage adjustment.

¶ Dose reduction and/or serum theophylline concentration measurement is indicated whenever adverse effects are present, physiologic abnormalities that can reduce theophylline clearance occur (e.g., sustained fever), or a drug that interacts with theophylline is added or discontinued (see WARNINGS).

HOW SUPPLIED

Uniphyl® (theophylline, anhydrous) 400 mg Controlled-Release Tablets are supplied in white-opaque plastic bottles containing 100 tablets (NDC 0034-7004-80) or 500 tablets (NDC 0034-7004-70).

Each round, white, scored 400 mg tablet bears the symbol PF on one side and is marked U400 on the other side.

Uniphyl® (theophylline, anhydrous) 600 mg Controlled-Release Tablets are supplied in white-opaque plastic bottles containing 100 tablets (NDC 0034-7006-80).

Each rectangular, concave, white 600 mg scored tablet bears the symbol PF on one side and is marked U600 on the other side.

Store at controlled room temperature 15°–30°C (59°–86°F). Dispense in tight, light-resistant container.

CAUTION: Federal law prohibits dispensing without prescription.

The Purdue Frederick Company
Norwalk, CT 06850-3590
Copyright ©1996 The Purdue Frederick Company
U.S. Patent Numbers 4,235,870 and 4,366,310
June 12, 1996   R1374
Shown in Product Identification Guide, page 333

EDUCATIONAL MATERIAL

Laxative Protocol Sheets (PS77) 1 page (pad of 25)
Available to physicians, nurses and pharmacists

Purdue Pharma L.P.
100 CONNECTICUT AVENUE
NORWALK, CT 06850-3590

DHCplus® Capsules

MS Contin® Tablets—see listing under The Purdue Frederick Company, page 2556

MSIR® Capsules—see listing under The Purdue Frederick Company, page 2559

MSIR® Tablets—see listing under The Purdue Frederick Company, page 2559

MSIR® Liquid—see listing under The Purdue Frederick Company, page 2559

OXYCONTIN®   Ⓒ ℞
(OXYCODONE HCL CONTROLLED-RELEASE) TABLETS

Warning-May be habit forming.
10mg 20mg 40mg 80mg*

---

*80 mg For use in opioid tolerant patients only.

DESCRIPTION

OxyContin® (oxycodone hydrochloride controlled-release) tablets are an opioid analgesic supplied in 10 mg, 20 mg, 40 mg, and 80 mg tablet strengths for oral administration. The tablet strengths describe the amount of oxycodone per tablet as the hydrochloride salt. The structural formula for oxycodone hydrochloride is as follows:

$C_{18}H_{21}NO_4 \cdot HCl$ MW 351.83

The chemical formula is 4, 5-epoxy-14-hydroxy-3-methoxy-17-methylmorphinan-6-one hydrochloride.

Oxycodone is a white, odorless crystalline powder derived from the opium alkaloid, thebaine. Oxycodone hydrochloride dissolves in water (1 g in 6 to 7 mL). It is slightly soluble in alcohol (octanol water partition coefficient 0.7). The tablets contain the following inactive ingredients: ammonio

Continued on next page

OxyContin—Cont.

methacrylate copolymer, hydroxypropyl methylcellulose, lactose, magnesium stearate, povidone, red iron oxide (20 mg strength tablet only), stearyl alcohol, talc, titanium dioxide, triacetin, yellow iron oxide (40 mg strength tablet only), yellow iron oxide with FD&C blue No. 2 (80 mg strength tablet only), and other ingredients.

OxyContin® 80 mg Tablets ARE FOR USE IN OPIOID TOLERANT PATIENTS ONLY.

CLINICAL PHARMACOLOGY
Central Nervous System
Oxycodone is a pure agonist opioid whose principal therapeutic action is analgesia. Other therapeutic effects of oxycodone include anxiolysis, euphoria and feelings of relaxation. Like all pure opioid agonists, there is no ceiling effect to analgesia, such as is seen with partial agonists or non-opioid analgesics.

The precise mechanism of the analgesic action is unknown. However, specific CNS opioid receptors for endogenous compounds with opioid-like activity have been identified throughout the brain and spinal cord and play a role in the analgesic effects of this drug.

Oxycodone produces respiratory depression by direct action on brain stem respiratory centers. The respiratory depression involves both a reduction in the responsiveness of the brain stem respiratory centers to increases in carbon dioxide tension and to electrical stimulation.

Oxycodone depresses the cough reflex by direct effect on the cough center in the medulla. Antitussive effects may occur with doses lower than those usually required for analgesia. Oxycodone causes miosis, even in total darkness. Pinpoint pupils are a sign of opioid overdose but are not pathognomonic. Marked mydriasis rather than miosis may be seen due to hypoxia in overdose situations.

Gastrointestinal Tract and Other Smooth Muscle
Oxycodone causes a reduction in motility associated with an increase in smooth muscle tone in the antrum of the stomach and duodenum. Digestion of food in the small intestine is delayed and propulsive contractions are decreased. Propulsive peristaltic waves in the colon are decreased, while tone may be increased to the point of spasm resulting in constipation. Other opioid-induced effects may include a reduction in gastric, biliary and pancreatic secretions, spasm of sphincter of Oddi, and transient elevations in serum amylase.

Cardiovascular System
Oxycodone may produce release of histamine with or without associated peripheral vasodilation. Manifestations of histamine release and/or peripheral vasodilation may include pruritus, flushing, red eyes, sweating, and/or orthostatic hypotension.

Concentration—Efficacy Relationships (Pharmacodynamics)
Studies in normal volunteers and patients reveal predictable relationships between oxycodone dosage and plasma oxycodone concentrations, as well as between concentration and certain expected opioid effects. In normal volunteers these include pupillary constriction, sedation and overall "drug effect" and in patients, analgesia and feelings of "relaxation." In non-tolerant patients, analgesia is not usually seen at a plasma oxycodone concentration of less than 5–10 ng/mL.

As with all opioids, the minimum effective plasma concentration for analgesia will vary widely among patients, especially among patients who have been previously treated with potent agonist opioids. As a result, patients need to be treated with individualized titration of dosage to the desired effect. The minimum effective analgesic concentration of oxycodone for any individual patient may increase with repeated dosing due to an increase in pain and/or the development of tolerance.

Concentration—Adverse Experience Relationships
OxyContin tablets are associated with typical opioid-related adverse experiences similar to those seen with immediate-release oxycodone and all opioids. There is a general relationship between increasing oxycodone plasma concentration and increasing frequency of dose-related opioid adverse experiences such as nausea, vomiting, CNS effects and respiratory depression. In opioid-tolerant patients, the situation is altered by the development of tolerance to opioid-related side effects, and the relationship is poorly understood.

As with all opioids, the dose must be individualized (see DOSAGE AND ADMINISTRATION), because the effective analgesic dose for some patients will be too high to be tolerated by other patients.

PHARMACOKINETICS AND METABOLISM

The activity of OxyContin® (oxycodone hydrochloride controlled-release) tablets is primarily due to the parent drug oxycodone. OxyContin tablets are designed to provide controlled delivery of oxycodone over 12 hours. Oxycodone is well absorbed from OxyContin tablets with an oral bioavailability of from 60% to 87%. The relative oral bioavailability of OxyContin to immediate-release oral dosage forms is 100%. Upon repeated dosing in normal volunteers, steady-state levels were achieved within 24–36 hours. Dose proportionality has been established for the 10 mg, 20 mg, 40 mg, and 80 mg tablet strengths for both peak plasma levels (C_{max}) and extent of absorption (AUC). Oxycodone is extensively metabolized and eliminated primarily in the urine as both conjugated and unconjugated metabolites. The apparent elimination half-life of oxycodone following the administration of OxyContin was 4.5 hours compared to 3.2 hours for immediate-release oxycodone.

Absorption
About 60% to 87% of an oral dose of oxycodone reaches the central compartment in comparison to a parenteral dose. This high oral bioavailability is due to low pre-systemic and/or first-pass metabolism. In normal volunteers the $t^1/_2$ of absorption is 0.4 hours for immediate-release oral oxycodone. In contrast, OxyContin tablets exhibit a biphasic absorption pattern with two apparent absorption half-times of 0.6 and 6.9 hours, which describes the initial release of oxycodone from the tablet followed by a prolonged release.

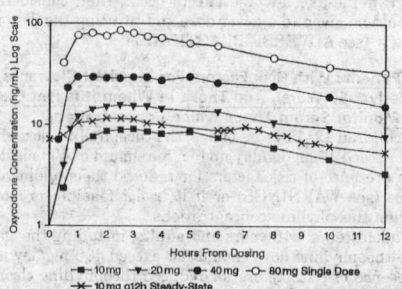

Plasma Oxycodone By Time

Dose proportionality has been established for the 10 mg, 20 mg, 40 mg, and 80 mg tablet strengths for both peak plasma concentrations (C_{max}) and extent of absorption (AUC) (see Table 1 below). Given the short half-life of elimination of oxycodone from OxyContin, steady-state plasma concentrations of oxycodone are achieved within 24–36 hours of initiation of dosing with OxyContin tablets. In a study comparing 10 mg of OxyContin every 12 hours to 5 mg of immediate-release oxycodone every 6 hours the two treatments were found to be equivalent for AUC and C_{max}, and similar for C_{min} (trough) concentrations. There was less fluctuation in plasma concentrations for the OxyContin tablets than for the immediate-release formulation.

[See table 1 below]

Food Effects
In contrast to immediate-release formulations, food has no significant effect on the absorption of oxycodone from OxyContin. Oxycodone release from OxyContin tablets is pH independent.

Distribution
Following intravenous administration, the volume of distribution (Vss) for oxycodone was 2.6L/kg. Oxycodone binding to plasma protein at 37°C and a pH of 7.4 was about 45%. Once absorbed, oxycodone is distributed to skeletal muscle, liver, intestinal tract, lungs, spleen and brain. Oxycodone has been found in breast milk (see PRECAUTIONS).

Metabolism
Oxycodone hydrochloride is extensively metabolized to noroxycodone, oxymorphone, and their glucuronides. The major circulating metabolite is noroxycodone with an AUC ratio of 0.6 relative to that of oxycodone. Noroxycodone is reported to be a considerably weaker analgesic than oxycodone. Oxymorphone, although possessing analgesic activity, is present in the plasma only in low concentrations. The correlation between oxymorphone concentrations and opioid effects was much less than that seen with oxycodone plasma concentrations. The analgesic activity profile of other metabolites is not known at present.

The formation of oxymorphone, but not noroxycodone, is mediated by CYP2D6 and as such its formation can, in theory, be affected by other drugs (see Drug-Drug Interactions).

Excretion
Oxycodone and its metabolites are excreted primarily via the kidney. The amounts measured in the urine have been reported as follows: free oxycodone up to 19%; conjugated oxycodone up to 50%; free oxymorphone 0%; conjugated oxymorphone ≤ 14%; both free and conjugated noroxycodone have been found in the urine but not quantified. The total plasma clearance was 0.8 L/min for adults.

Special Populations
Elderly
The plasma concentrations of oxycodone are only nominally affected by age, being 15% greater in elderly as compared to young subjects. There were no differences in adverse event reporting between young and elderly subjects.

Gender
Female subjects have, on average, plasma oxycodone concentrations up to 25% higher than males on a body weight adjusted basis. The reason for this difference is unknown.

Renal Impairment
Preliminary data from a study involving patients with mild to severe renal dysfunction (creatinine clearance <60 mL/min) show peak plasma oxycodone and noroxycodone concentrations 50% and 20% higher, respectively and AUC values for oxycodone, noroxycodone and oxymorphone 60%, 50% and 40% higher than normal subjects, respectively. This is accompanied by an increase in sedation but not by differences in respiratory rate, pupillary constriction, or several other measures of drug effect. There was an increase in $t^1/_2$ of elimination for oxycodone of only 1 hour (see PRECAUTIONS).

Hepatic Impairment
Preliminary data from a study involving patients with mild to moderate hepatic dysfunction show peak plasma oxycodone and noroxycodone concentrations 50% and 20% higher, respectively, than normal subjects. AUC values are 95% and 65% higher, respectively. Oxymorphone peak plasma concentrations and AUC values are lower by 30% and 40%. These differences are accompanied by increases in some, but not other, drug effects. The $t^1/_2$ elimination for oxycodone increased by 2.3 hours (see PRECAUTIONS).

Rectal Administration
Rectal administration of OxyContin tablets is not recommended. Preliminary data from a study involving 21 normal volunteers, show OxyContin tablets administered per rectum resulted in an AUC 39% greater and a C_{max} 9% higher than tablets administered by mouth (see PRECAUTIONS).

Drug-Drug Interactions (see PRECAUTIONS)
Oxycodone is metabolized in part via CYP2D6 to oxymorphone which represents less than 15% of the total administered dose. This route of elimination can be blocked by a variety of drugs (e.g., certain cardiovascular drugs and antidepressants). Patients receiving such drugs concomitantly with OxyContin do not appear to present different therapeutic profiles than other patients.

CLINICAL TRIALS

OxyContin® (oxycodone hydrochloride controlled-release) tablets were evaluated in studies involving 713 patients with either cancer or non-cancer pain. All patients receiving OxyContin were dosed q12h. Efficacy comparable to other forms of oral oxycodone was demonstrated in clinical studies using pharmacokinetic, pharmacodynamic and efficacy outcomes. The outcome of these trials indicated: (1) a positive relationship between dose and plasma oxycodone concentration, (2) a positive relationship between plasma oxy-

Table 1
Mean [% coefficient variation]

Regimen/Dosage Form	AUC (ng·hr/mL)†	C_{max} (ng/mL)	T_{max} (hrs)	Trough Conc. (ng/mL)
Single Dose				
10 mg OxyContin	100.7 [26.6]	10.6 [20.1]	2.7 [44.1]	n.a.
20 mg OxyContin	207.5 [35.9]	21.4 [36.6]	3.2 [57.9]	n.a.
40 mg OxyContin	423.1 [33.3]	39.3 [34.0]	3.1 [77.4]	n.a.
80 mg OxyContin*	1085.5 [32.3]	98.5 [32.1]	2.1 [52.3]	n.a.
Multiple Dose				
10 mg OxyContin Tablets q12h	103.6 [38.6]	15.1 [31.0]	3.2 [69.5]	7.2 [48.1]
5 mg immediate-release q6h	99.0 [36.2]	15.5 [28.8]	1.6 [49.7]	7.4 [50.9]

† for single-dose AUC=$AUC_{0\text{-inf}}$; for multiple-dose AUC=$AUC_{0\text{-T}}$
* data obtained while volunteers received naltexone which can enhance absorption.

codone concentration and analgesia, and (3) an observed peak to trough variation in plasma concentration with OxyContin lying within the observed range established with qid dosing of immediate-release oxycodone in clinical populations at the same total daily dose.

In clinical trials, OxyContin tablets were substituted for a wide variety of analgesics, including acetaminophen (APAP), aspirin (ASA), other non-steroidal anti-inflammatory drugs (NSAIDs), opioid combination products and single-entity opioids, primarily morphine. In cancer patients receiving adequate opioid therapy at baseline, pain intensity scores and acceptability of therapy remained unchanged by transfer to OxyContin. For non-cancer pain patients who had moderate to severe pain at baseline on prn opioid therapy, pain control and acceptability of therapy improved with the introduction of fixed-interval therapy with OxyContin.

Use in Cancer Pain

OxyContin was studied in three double-blind, controlled clinical trials involving 341 cancer patients and several open-label trials with therapy durations of over 10 months. Two, double-blind, controlled clinical studies indicated that OxyContin dosed q12h produced analgesic efficacy equivalent to immediate-release oxycodone dosed qid at the same total daily dose. Peak and trough plasma concentrations attained were similar to those attained with immediate-release oxycodone at equivalent total daily doses. With titration to analgesic effect and proper use of rescue medication, nearly every patient achieved adequate pain control with OxyContin.

In the third study, a double-blind, active-controlled, crossover trial, OxyContin dosed q12h was shown to be equivalent in efficacy and safety to immediate-release oxycodone dosed qid at the same total daily dose. Patients were able to be titrated to an acceptable analgesic effect with either OxyContin or immediate-release oxycodone with both treatments providing stable pain control within 2 days in most patients.

In patients with cancer pain, the total daily OxyContin doses tested ranged from 20 mg to 640 mg per day. The average total daily dose was approximately 105 mg per day.

Studies in Non-Cancer Pain

A double-blind, placebo-controlled, fixed-dose, parallel group study was conducted in 133 patients with moderate to severe osteoarthritis pain, who were judged as having inadequate pain control with prn opioids and maximal non-steroidal anti-inflammatory therapy. In this study, 20 mg OxyContin q12h significantly decreased pain and improved quality of life, mood and sleep, relative to placebo. Both dose-concentration and concentration-effect relationships were noted with a minimum effective plasma oxycodone concentration of approximately 5–10 ng/mL.

In a double-blind, active-controlled, crossover study involving 57 patients with low-back pain inadequately controlled with prn opioids and non-opioid therapy, OxyContin administered q12h provided analgesia equivalent to immediate-release oxycodone administered qid. Patients could be titrated to an acceptable analgesic effect with either OxyContin or immediate-release forms of oxycodone.

Single-Dose Comparison with Standard Therapy

A single-dose, double-blind, placebo-controlled, post-operative study of 182 patients was conducted utilizing graded doses of OxyContin (10, 20 and 30 mg). Twenty and 30 mg of OxyContin gave equivalent peak analgesic effect compared to two oxycodone 5 mg /acetaminophen 325 mg tablets and to 15 mg immediate-release oxycodone, while the 10 mg dose of OxyContin was intermediate between both the immediate-release and combination products and placebo. The onset of analgesic action with OxyContin occurred within 1 hour in most patients following oral administration.

OxyContin is not recommended pre-operatively (preemptive analgesia) or for the management of pain in the immediate post-operative period (the first 12 to 24 hours following surgery) because the safety or appropriateness of fixed-dose, long-acting opioids in this setting has not been established.

Other Clinical Trials

In open-label trials involving approximately 200 patients with cancer-related and non-cancer pain, dosed according to the package insert recommendations, appropriate analgesic effectiveness was noted without regard to age, gender, race, or disease state. There were no unusual drug interactions observed in patients receiving a wide range of medications common in these populations.

For opioid-naive patients, the average total daily dose of OxyContin was approximately 40 mg per day. There was no evidence of oxycodone and metabolite accumulation during 8 months of therapy. For cancer pain patients the average total daily dose was 105 mg (range 20 to 720 mg) per day. There was a significant decrease in acute opioid-related side effects, except for constipation, during the first several weeks of therapy. Development of significant tolerance to analgesia was uncommon.

A cohort of patients have been treated with OxyContin 80 mg tablets. There were no differences in the efficacy or safety profiles than seen with the other tablet strengths.

INDICATIONS AND USAGE

OxyContin® tablets are a controlled-release oral formulation of oxycodone hydrochloride indicated for the management of moderate to severe pain where use of an opioid analgesic is appropriate for more than a few days. (See: CLINICAL PHARMACOLOGY; CLINICAL TRIALS).

CONTRAINDICATIONS

OxyContin® is contraindicated in patients with known hypersensitivity to oxycodone, or in any situation where opioids are contraindicated. This includes patients with significant respiratory depression (in unmonitored settings or the absence of resuscitative equipment), and patients with acute or severe bronchial asthma or hypercarbia. OxyContin is contraindicated in any patient who has or is suspected of having paralytic ileus.

WARNINGS

OxyContin® (oxycodone hydrochloride controlled-release) TABLETS ARE TO BE SWALLOWED WHOLE, AND ARE NOT TO BE BROKEN, CHEWED OR CRUSHED. TAKING BROKEN, CHEWED OR CRUSHED OxyContin TABLETS COULD LEAD TO THE RAPID RELEASE AND ABSORPTION OF A POTENTIALLY TOXIC DOSE OF OXYCODONE.

Respiratory Depression

Respiratory depression is the chief hazard from all opioid agonist preparations. Respiratory depression occurs most frequently in elderly or debilitated patients, usually following large initial doses in non-tolerant patients, or when opioids are given in conjunction with other agents that depress respiration.

Oxycodone should be used with extreme caution in patients with significant chronic obstructive pulmonary disease or cor pulmonale, and in patients having a substantially decreased respiratory reserve, hypoxia, hypercapnia, or preexisting respiratory depression. In such patients, even usual therapeutic doses of oxycodone may decrease respiratory drive to the point of apnea. In these patients alternative non-opioid analgesics should be considered, and opioids should be employed only under careful medical supervision at the lowest effective dose.

Head Injury

The respiratory depressant effects of opioids include carbon dioxide retention and secondary elevation of cerebrospinal fluid pressure, and may be markedly exaggerated in the presence of head injury, intracranial lesions, or other sources of preexisting increased intracranial pressure. Oxycodone produces effects on pupillary response and consciousness which may obscure neurologic signs of further increases in intracranial pressure in patients with head injuries.

Hypotensive Effect

OxyContin®, like all opioid analgesics, may cause severe hypotension in an individual whose ability to maintain blood pressure has been compromised by a depleted blood volume, or after concurrent administration with drugs such as phenothiazines or other agents which compromise vasomotor tone. OxyContin may produce orthostatic hypotension in ambulatory patients. OxyContin, like all opioid analgesics, should be administered with caution to patients in circulatory shock, since vasodilation produced by the drug may further reduce cardiac output and blood pressure.

PRECAUTIONS

Special precautions regarding OxyContin® 80 mg Tablets

OxyContin® 80 mg Tablets are for use only in opioid tolerant patients requiring daily oxycodone equivalent dosages of 160 mg or more. Care should be taken in the prescription of this tablet strength. Patients should be instructed against use by individuals other than the patient for whom it was prescribed, as such inappropriate use may have severe medical consequences.

General

OxyContin® (oxycodone hydrochloride controlled-release) tablets are intended for use in patients who require oral pain therapy with an opioid agonist of more than a few days duration. As with any opioid analgesic, it is critical to adjust the dosing regimen individually for each patient (see DOSAGE AND ADMINISTRATION).

Selection of patients for treatment with OxyContin should be governed by the same principles that apply to the use of similar controlled-release opioid analgesics (see INDICATIONS AND USAGE). Opioid analgesics given on a fixed-dosage schedule have a narrow therapeutic index in certain patient populations, especially when combined with other drugs, and should be reserved for cases where the benefits of opioid analgesia outweigh the known risks of respiratory depression, altered mental state, and postural hypotension. Physicians should individualize treatment in every case, using non-opioid analgesics, prn opioids and/or combination products, and chronic opioid therapy with drugs such as OxyContin in a progressive plan of pain management such as outlined by the World Health Organization, the Agency for Health Care Policy and Research, and the American Pain Society.

Use of OxyContin is associated with increased potential risks and should be used only with caution in the following conditions: acute alcoholism; adrenocortical insufficiency (e.g., Addison's disease); CNS depression or coma; delirium tremens; debilitated patients; kyphoscoliosis associated with respiratory depression; myxedema or hypothyroidism; prostatic hypertrophy or urethral stricture; severe impairment of hepatic, pulmonary or renal function; and toxic psychosis.

The administration of oxycodone, like all opioid analgesics, may obscure the diagnosis or clinical course in patients with acute abdominal conditions. Oxycodone may aggravate convulsions in patients with convulsive disorders, and all opioids may induce or aggravate seizures in some clinical settings.

Interactions with other CNS Depressants

OxyContin, like all opioid analgesics, should be used with caution and started in a reduced dosage ($^1/_3$ to $^1/_2$ of the usual dosage) in patients who are concurrently receiving other central nervous system depressants including sedatives or hypnotics, general anesthetics, phenothiazines, other tranquilizers and alcohol. Interactive effects resulting in respiratory depression, hypotension, profound sedation or coma may result if these drugs are taken in combination with the usual doses of OxyContin.

Interactions with Mixed Agonist/Antagonist Opioid Analgesics

Agonist/antagonist analgesics (i.e., pentazocine, nalbuphine, butorphanol and buprenorphine) should be administered with caution to a patient who has received or is receiving a course of therapy with a pure opioid agonist analgesic such as oxycodone. In this situation, mixed agonist/antagonist analgesics may reduce the analgesic effect of oxycodone and/or may precipitate withdrawal symptoms in these patients.

Ambulatory Surgery

OxyContin is not recommended pre-operatively (preemptive analgesia) or for the management of pain in the immediate post-operative period (the first 12 to 24 hours following surgery) for patients not previously taking the drug, because its safety in this setting has not been established.

Patients who are already receiving OxyContin tablets as part of ongoing analgesic therapy may be safely continued on the drug if appropriate dosage adjustments are made considering the procedure, other drugs given and the temporary changes in physiology caused by the surgical intervention (see PRECAUTIONS: Drug-Drug Interactions, and DOSAGE AND ADMINISTRATION).

Post-Operative Use

Morphine and other opioids have been shown to decrease bowel motility. Ileus is a common post-operative complication, especially after intra-abdominal surgery with opioid analgesia. Caution should be taken to monitor for decreased bowel motility in post-operative patients receiving opioids. Standard supportive therapy should be implemented.

Use in Pancreatic/Biliary Tract Disease

Oxycodone may cause spasm of the sphincter of Oddi and should be used with caution in patients with biliary tract disease, including acute pancreatitis. Opioids like oxycodone may cause increases in the serum amylase level.

Tolerance and Physical Dependence

Tolerance is the need for increasing doses of opioids to maintain a defined effect such as analgesia (in the absence of disease progression or other external factors). Physical dependence is the occurrence of withdrawal symptoms after abrupt discontinuation of a drug or upon administration of an antagonist. Physical dependence and tolerance are not unusual during chronic opioid therapy.

Significant tolerance should not occur in most of the patients treated with the lowest doses of oxycodone. It should be expected, however, that a fraction of cancer patients will develop some degree of tolerance and require progressively higher dosages of OxyContin to maintain pain control during chronic treatment. Regardless of whether this occurs as a result of increased pain secondary to disease progression or pharmacological tolerance, dosages can usually be increased safely by adjusting the patient's dose to maintain an acceptable balance between pain relief and side effects. The dosage should be selected according to the patient's individual analgesic response and ability to tolerate side effects. Tolerance to the analgesic effect of opioids is usually paralleled by tolerance to side effects, except for constipation.

Physical dependence results in withdrawal symptoms in patients who abruptly discontinue the drug or may be precipitated through the administration of drugs with opioid antagonist activity (see OVERDOSAGE). If OxyContin is abruptly discontinued in a physically dependent patient, an abstinence syndrome may occur. This is characterized by some or all of the following: restlessness, lacrimation, rhinorrhea, yawning, perspiration, chills, myalgia and mydriasis. Other symptoms also may develop, including: irritability, anxiety, backache, joint pain, weakness, abdominal cramps, insomnia, nausea, anorexia, vomiting, diarrhea, or increased blood pressure, respiratory rate or heart rate.

If signs and symptoms of withdrawal occur, patients should be treated by reinstitution of opioid therapy followed by a

Continued on next page

OxyContin—Cont.

gradual, tapered dose reduction of OxyContin combined with symptomatic support (see DOSAGE AND ADMINISTRATION: Cessation of Therapy).

Information for Patients/Caregivers

If clinically advisable, patients receiving OxyContin (oxycodone hydrochloride controlled-release) tablets or their caregivers should be given the following information by the physician, nurse, pharmacist or caregiver:

1. Patients should be advised that OxyContin tablets were designed to work properly only if swallowed whole. They may release all their contents at once if broken, chewed or crushed, resulting in a risk of overdose.
2. Patients should be advised to report episodes of breakthrough pain and adverse experiences occurring during therapy. Individualization of dosage is essential to make optimal use of this medication.
3. Patients should be advised not to adjust the dose of OxyContin without consulting the prescribing professional.
4. Patients should be advised that OxyContin may impair mental and/or physical ability required for the performance of potentially hazardous tasks (e.g., driving, operating heavy machinery).
5. Patients should not combine OxyContin with alcohol or other central nervous system depressants (sleep aids, tranquilizers) except by the orders of the prescribing physician, because additive effects may occur.
6. Women of childbearing potential who become, or are planning to become, pregnant should be advised to consult their physician regarding the effects of analgesics and other drug use during pregnancy on themselves and their unborn child.
7. Patients should be advised that OxyContin is a potential drug of abuse. They should protect it from theft, and it should never be given to anyone other than the individual for whom it was prescribed.
8. Patients should be advised that they may pass empty matrix "ghosts" (tablets) via colostomy or in the stool, and that this is of no concern since the active medication has already been absorbed.
9. Patients should be advised that if they have been receiving treatment with OxyContin for more than a few weeks and cessation of therapy is indicated, it may be appropriate to taper the OxyContin dose, rather than abruptly discontinue it, due to the risk of precipitating withdrawal symptoms. Their physician can provide a dose schedule to accomplish a gradual discontinuation of the medication.

Laboratory Monitoring

Due to the broad range of plasma concentrations seen in clinical populations, the varying degrees of pain, and the development of tolerance, plasma oxycodone measurements are usually not helpful in clinical management. Plasma concentrations of the active drug substance may be of value in selected, unusual or complex cases.

Interactions with Alcohol and Drugs of Abuse

Oxycodone may be expected to have additive effects when used in conjunction with alcohol, other opioids or illicit drugs which cause central nervous system depression.

Use in Drug and Alcohol Addiction

OxyContin is an opioid with no approved use in the management of addictive disorders. Its proper usage in individuals with drug or alcohol dependence, either active or in remission, is for the management of pain requiring opioid analgesia.

Drug-Drug Interactions

Opioid analgesics, including OxyContin, may enhance the neuromuscular blocking action of skeletal muscle relaxants and produce an increased degree of respiratory depression. Oxycodone is metabolized in part to oxymorphone via CYP2D6. While this pathway may be blocked by a variety of drugs (e.g., certain cardiovascular drugs and antidepressants), such blockade has not yet been shown to be of clinical significance with this agent. Clinicians should be aware of this possible interaction, however.

Use with CNS Depressants

OxyContin, like all opioid analgesics, should be started at $1/3$ to $1/2$ of the usual dosage in patients who are concurrently receiving other central nervous system depressants including sedatives or hypnotics, general anesthetics, phenothiazines, centrally acting anti-emetics, tranquilizers and alcohol because respiratory depression, hypotension and profound sedation or coma may result. No specific interaction between oxycodone and monoamine oxidase inhibitors has been observed, but caution in the use of any opioid in patients taking this class of drugs is appropriate.

Mutagenicity/Carcinogenicity

Oxycodone was not mutagenic in the following assays: Ames Salmonella and E. Coli test with and without metabolic activation at doses of up to 5000 μg, chromosomal aberration test in human lymphocytes (in the absence of metabolic activation and with activation after 48 hours of exposure) at doses of up to 1500 μg/ml, and in the in vivo bone marrow micronucleus assay in mice (at plasma levels of up to 48 μg/ml). Mutagenic results occurred in the presence of metabolic activation in the human chromosomal aberration test (at greater than or equal to 1250 μg/ml) at 24 but not 48 hours of exposure and in the mouse lymphoma assay at doses of 50 μg/ml or greater with metabolic activation and at 400 μg/ml or greater without metabolic activation. The data from these tests indicate that the genotoxic risk to humans may be considered low.

Studies of oxycodone in animals to evaluate its carcinogenic potential have not been conducted owing to the length of clinical experience with the drug substance.

Pregnancy

Teratogenic Effects—Category B: Reproduction studies have been performed in rats and rabbits by oral administration at doses up to 8 mg/kg (48 mg/m²) and 125 mg/kg (1375 mg/m²), respectively. These doses are 4 and 60 times a human dose of 120 mg/day (74 mg/m²), based on mg/kg of a 60 kg adult (0.7 and 19 times this human dose based upon mg/m²). The results did not reveal evidence of harm to the fetus due to oxycodone. There are, however, no adequate and well-controlled studies in pregnant women. Because animal reproduction studies are not always predictive of human response, this drug should be used during pregnancy only if clearly needed.

Nonteratogenic Effects—Neonates whose mothers have been taking oxycodone chronically may exhibit respiratory depression and/or withdrawal symptoms, either at birth and/or in the nursery.

Labor and Delivery

OxyContin is not recommended for use in women during and immediately prior to labor and delivery because oral opioids may cause respiratory depression in the newborn.

Nursing Mothers

Low concentrations of oxycodone have been detected in breast milk. Withdrawal symptoms can occur in breast-feeding infants when maternal administration of an opioid analgesic is stopped. Ordinarily, nursing should not be undertaken while a patient is receiving OxyContin since oxycodone may be excreted in the milk.

Pediatric Use

Safety and effectiveness in pediatric patients below the age of 18 have not been established with this dosage form of oxycodone. However, oxycodone has been used extensively in the pediatric population in other dosage forms, as have the excipients used in this formulation. No specific increased risk is expected from the use of this form of oxycodone in pediatric patients old enough to safely take tablets if dosing is adjusted for the patient's weight (see DOSAGE AND ADMINISTRATION. **It must be remembered that OxyContin tablets cannot be crushed or divided for administration.**

Geriatric Use

In controlled pharmacokinetic studies in elderly subjects (greater than 65 years) the clearance of oxycodone appeared to be slightly reduced. Compared to young adults, the plasma concentrations of oxycodone were increased approximately 15%. In clinical trials with appropriate initiation of therapy and dose titration, no untoward or unexpected side effects were seen based on age, and the usual doses and dosing intervals are appropriate for the geriatric patient. As with all opioids, the starting dose should be reduced to $1/3$ to $1/2$ of the usual dosage in debilitated, non-tolerant patients.

Hepatic Impairment

A study of OxyContin in patients with hepatic impairment indicates greater plasma concentrations than those with normal function. The initiation of therapy at $1/3$ to $1/2$ the usual doses and careful dose titration is warranted.

Renal Impairment

In patients with renal impairment, as evidenced by decreased creatinine clearance (<60 mL/min.), the concentrations of oxycodone in the plasma are approximately 50% higher than in subjects with normal renal function. Dose initiation should follow a conservative approach. Dosages should be adjusted according to the clinical situation.

Gender Differences

In pharmacokinetic studies, opioid-naive females demonstrate up to 25% higher average plasma concentrations and greater frequency of typical opioid adverse events than males, even after adjustment for body weight. The clinical relevance of a difference of this magnitude is low for a drug intended for chronic usage at individualized dosages, and there was no male/female difference detected for efficacy or adverse events in clinical trials.

Rectal Administration

OxyContin® Tablets are not recommended for administration per rectum. A study in normal volunteers showed a significantly greater AUC and higher C_{max} during this route of administration (see PHARMACOKINETICS AND METABOLISM).

ADVERSE REACTIONS

Serious adverse reactions which may be associated with OxyContin® (oxycodone hydrochloride controlled-release) tablet therapy in clinical use are those observed with other opioid analgesics, including: respiratory depression, apnea, respiratory arrest, and (to an even lesser degree) circulatory depression, hypotension or shock (see OVERDOSE).

The non-serious adverse events seen on initiation of therapy with OxyContin are typical opioid side effects. These events are dose-dependent, and their frequency depends upon the dose, the clinical setting, the patient's level of opioid tolerance, and host factors specific to the individual. They should be expected and managed as a part of opioid analgesia. The most frequent (>5%) include constipation, nausea, somnolence, dizziness, vomiting, pruritus, headache, dry mouth, sweating and asthenia.

In many cases the frequency of these events during initiation of therapy may be minimized by careful individualization of starting dosage, slow titration, and the avoidance of large swings in the plasma concentrations of the opioid. Many of these adverse events will cease or decrease in intensity as OxyContin therapy is continued and some degree of tolerance is developed.

In clinical trials comparing OxyContin with immediate-release oxycodone and placebo, the most common adverse events (>5%) reported by patients (pts) at least once during therapy were:

Table 2

	OxyContin (n=227) #Pts (%)		Immediate-Release (n=225) #Pts (%)		Placebo (n=45) #Pts (%)	
Constipation	52	(23)	58	(26)	3	(7)
Nausea	52	(23)	60	(27)	5	(11)
Somnolence	52	(23)	55	(24)	2	(4)
Dizziness	29	(13)	35	(16)	4	(9)
Pruritus	29	(13)	28	(12)	1	(2)
Vomiting	27	(12)	31	(14)	3	(7)
Headache	17	(7)	19	(8)	3	(7)
Dry Mouth	13	(6)	15	(7)	1	(2)
Asthenia	13	(6)	16	(7)	—	—
Sweating	12	(5)	13	(6)	1	(2)

The following adverse experiences were reported in OxyContin treated patients with an incidence between 1% and 5%. In descending order of frequency they were anorexia, nervousness, insomnia, fever, confusion, diarrhea, abdominal pain, dyspepsia, rash, anxiety, euphoria, dyspnea, postural hypotension, chills, twitching, gastritis, abnormal dreams, thought abnormalities, and hiccups.

The following adverse reactions occurred in less than 1% of patients involved in clinical trials:

General: accidental injury, chest pain, facial edema, malaise, neck pain, pain

Cardiovascular: migraine, syncope, vasodilation, ST depression

Digestive: dysphagia, eructation, flatulence, gastrointestinal disorder, increased appetite, nausea and vomiting, stomatitis, ileus

Hemic and Lymphatic: lymphadenopathy

Metabolic and Nutritional: dehydration, edema, hyponatremia, peripheral edema, syndrome of inappropriate antidiuretic hormone secretion, thirst

Nervous: abnormal gait, agitation, amnesia, depersonalization, depression, emotional lability, hallucination, hyperkinesia, hypesthesia, hypotonia, malaise, paresthesia, seizures, speech disorder, stupor, tinnitus, tremor, vertigo, withdrawal syndrome with or without seizures

Respiratory: cough increased, pharyngitis, voice alteration

Skin: dry skin, exfoliative dermatitis, urticaria

Special Senses: abnormal vision, taste perversion

Urogenital: dysuria, hematuria, impotence, polyuria, urinary retention, urination impaired

DRUG ABUSE AND DEPENDENCE (Addiction)

OxyContin® is a mu-agonist opioid with an abuse liability similar to morphine and is a Schedule II controlled substance. Oxycodone products are common targets for both drug abusers and drug addicts. Delayed absorption, as provided by OxyContin tablets, is believed to reduce the abuse liability of a drug.

Drug addiction (drug dependence, psychological dependence) is characterized by a preoccupation with the procurement, hoarding, and abuse of drugs for non-medicinal purposes. Drug dependence is treatable, utilizing a multi-disciplinary approach, but relapse is common. Iatrogenic "addiction" to opioids legitimately used in the management of pain is very rare. "Drug seeking" behavior is very common to addicts. Tolerance and physical dependence in pain patients are *not* signs of psychological dependence. Preoccupation with achieving adequate pain relief can be appropriate behavior in a patient with poor pain control. Most chronic pain patients limit their intake of opioids to achieve a balance between the benefits of the drug and dose-limiting side effects.

Physicians should be aware that psychological dependence may not be accompanied by concurrent tolerance and symptoms of physical dependence in all addicts. In addition, abuse of opioids can occur in the absence of true psycholog-

ical dependence and is characterized by misuse for non-medical purposes, often in combination with other psycho-active substances.

OxyContin consists of a dual-polymer matrix, intended for oral use only. Parenteral venous injection of the tablet constituents, especially talc, can be expected to result in local tissue necrosis and pulmonary granulomas.

OVERDOSAGE

Acute overdosage with oxycodone can be manifested by respiratory depression, somnolence progressing to stupor or coma, skeletal muscle flaccidity, cold and clammy skin, constricted pupils, bradycardia, hypotension, and death.

In the treatment of oxycodone overdosage, primary attention should be given to the re-establishment of a patent airway and institution of assisted or controlled ventilation. Supportive measures (including oxygen and vasopressors) should be employed in the management of circulatory shock and pulmonary edema accompanying overdose as indicated. Cardiac arrest or arrhythmias may require cardiac massage or defibrillation.

The pure opioid antagonists such as naloxone or nalmefene are specific antidotes against respiratory depression from opioid overdose. Opioid antagonists should not be administered in the absence of clinically significant respiratory or circulatory depression secondary to oxycodone overdose. They should be administered cautiously to persons who are known, or suspected to be, physically dependent on any opioid agonist including OxyContin®. In such cases, an abrupt or complete reversal of opioid effects may precipitate an acute abstinence syndrome. The severity of the withdrawal syndrome produced will depend on the degree of physical dependence and the dose of the antagonist administered. Please see the prescribing information for the specific opioid antagonist for details of their proper use.

DOSAGE AND ADMINISTRATION

General Principles

OxyContin® (oxycodone hydrochloride controlled-release) TABLETS ARE TO BE SWALLOWED WHOLE, AND ARE NOT TO BE BROKEN, CHEWED OR CRUSHED. TAKING BROKEN, CHEWED OR CRUSHED OxyContin TABLETS COULD LEAD TO THE RAPID RELEASE AND ABSORPTION OF A POTENTIALLY TOXIC DOSE OF OXYCODONE.

In treating pain it is vital to assess the patient regularly and systematically. Therapy should also be regularly reviewed and adjusted based upon the patient's own reports of pain and side effects and the health professional's clinical judgment.

OxyContin is intended for the management of moderate to severe pain in patients who require treatment with an oral opioid analgesic for more than a few days. The controlled-release nature of the formulation allows it to be effectively administered every 12 hours. (See CLINICAL PHARMACOLOGY; PHARMACOKINETICS AND METABOLISM.) While symmetric (same dose AM and PM), around-the-clock, q12h dosing is appropriate for the majority of patients, some patients may benefit from asymmetric (different dose given in AM than in PM) dosing, tailored to their pain pattern. It is usually appropriate to treat a patient with only one opioid for around-the-clock therapy.

Initiation of Therapy

It is critical to initiate the dosing regimen for each patient individually, taking into account the patient's prior opioid and non-opioid analgesic treatment. Attention should be given to:

(1) the general condition and medical status of the patient
(2) the daily dose, potency and kind of the analgesic(s) the patient has been taking
(3) the reliability of the conversion estimate used to calculate the dose of oxycodone
(4) the patient's opioid exposure and opioid tolerance (if any)
(5) the balance between pain control and adverse experiences

Care should be taken to use low initial doses of OxyContin in patients who are not already opioid tolerant, especially those who are receiving concurrent treatment with muscle relaxants, sedatives, or other CNS active medications (see PRECAUTIONS: Drug-Drug Interactions).

Patients Not Already Taking Opioids (opioid naive)

Clinical trials have shown that patients may initiate analgesic therapy with OxyContin. A reasonable starting dose for most patients who are opioid naive is 10 mg q12h. If a non-opioid analgesic [aspirin (ASA), acetaminophen (APAP) or a non-steroidal anti-inflammatory (NSAID)] is being provided, it may be continued. If the current non-opioid is discontinued, early upward dose titration may be necessary.

Conversion from Fixed-Ratio Opioid/APAP, ASA, or NSAID Combination Drugs

Patients who are taking 1 to 5 tablets/capsules/caplets per day of a regular strength fixed-combination opioid/non-opioid should be started on 10 to 20 mg OxyContin q12h. For patients taking 6 to 9 tablets/capsules/ caplets, a starting dose of 20 to 30 mg q12h is suggested. For those taking 10 to 12 tablets, caplets or capsules a day, 30 to 40 mg q12h should be considered. The non-opioid may be continued as a separate drug. Alternatively, a different non-opioid analge-

sic may be selected. If the decision is made to discontinue the non-opioid analgesic, consideration should be given to early upward titration.

Patients Currently on Opioid Therapy

If a patient has been receiving opioid-containing medications prior to OxyContin therapy, the total daily (24-hour) dose of the other opioids should be determined.

1. Using standard conversion ratio estimates (see Table 3 below), multiply the mg/day of the previous opioids by the appropriate multiplication factors to obtain the equivalent total daily dose of oral oxycodone.
2. Divide this 24-hour oxycodone dose in half to obtain the twice a day (q12h) dose of OxyContin.
3. Round down to a dose which is appropriate for the tablet strengths available (10, 20, 40, and 80 mg tablets).
4. Discontinue all other around-the-clock opioid drugs when OxyContin therapy is initiated.

No fixed conversion ratio is likely to be satisfactory in all patients, especially patients receiving large opioid doses. The recommended doses shown in Table 3 are only a starting point, and close observation and frequent titration are indicated until patients are stable on the new therapy.

Table 3

Multiplication Factors for Converting the Daily Dose of Prior Opioids to the Daily Dose of Oral Oxycodone*
(Mg/Day Prior Opioid × Factor=Mg/Day Oral Oxycodone)

	Oral Prior Opioid	Parenteral Prior Opioid
Oxycodone	1	—
Codeine	0.15	—
Fentanyl TTS	SEE BELOW	SEE BELOW
Hydrocodone	0.9	—
Hydromorphone	4	20
Levorphanol	7.5	15
Meperidine	0.1	0.4
Methadone	1.5	3
Morphine	0.5	3

* **To be used only for conversion to oral oxycodone**. For patients receiving high-dose parenteral opioids, a more conservative conversion is warranted. For example, for high-dose parenteral morphine, use 1.5 instead of 3 as a multiplication factor.

In all cases, supplemental analgesia (see below) should be made available in the form of immediate-release oral oxycodone or another suitable short-acting analgesic.

OxyContin can be safely used concomitantly with usual doses of non-opioid analgesics and analgesic adjuvants, provided care is taken to select a proper initial dose (see PRECAUTIONS).

Conversion from Transdermal Fentanyl to OxyContin

Eighteen hours following the removal of the transdermal fentanyl patch, OxyContin treatment can be initiated. Although there has been no systematic assessment of such conversion, a conservative oxycodone dose, approximately 10 mg q12h of OxyContin, should be initially substituted for each 25 µg/hr fentanyl transdermal patch. The patient should be followed closely for early titration as there is very limited clinical experience with this conversion.

Managing Expected Opioid Adverse Experiences

Most patients receiving opioids, especially those who are opioid naive, will experience side effects. Frequently the side effects from OxyContin are transient, but may require evaluation and management. Adverse events such as constipation should be anticipated and treated aggressively and prophylactically with a stimulant laxative and/or stool softener. Patients do not usually become tolerant to the constipating effects of opioids.

Other opioid-related side effects such as sedation and nausea are usually self-limited and often do not persist beyond the first few days. If nausea persists and is unacceptable to the patient, treatment with anti-emetics or other modalities may relieve these symptoms and should be considered.

Patients receiving OxyContin may pass an intact matrix "ghost" in the stool or via colostomy. These ghosts contain little or no residual oxycodone and are of no clinical consequence.

Individualization of Dosage

Once therapy is initiated, pain relief and other opioid effects should be frequently assessed. Patients should be titrated to adequate effect (generally mild or no pain with the regular use of no more than two doses of supplemental analgesia per 24 hours). Rescue medication should be available (see: Supplemental Analgesia). Because steady-state plasma concentrations are approximated within 24 to 36 hours, dosage adjustment may be carried out every 1 to 2 days. It is most appropriate to increase the q12h dose, not the dosing frequency. There is no clinical information on dosing intervals shorter than q12h. As a guideline, except for the increase from 10 mg to 20 mg q12h, the total daily oxycodone dose usually can be increased by 25% to 50% of the current dose at each increase.

If signs of excessive opioid-related adverse experiences are observed, the next dose may be reduced. If this adjustment

leads to inadequate analgesia, a supplemental dose of immediate-release oxycodone may be given. Alternatively, non-opioid analgesic adjuvants may be employed. Dose adjustments should be made to obtain an appropriate balance between pain relief and opioid-related adverse experiences.

If significant adverse events occur before the therapeutic goal of mild or no pain is achieved, the events should be treated aggressively. Once adverse events are under control, upward titration should continue to an acceptable level of pain control.

During periods of changing analgesic requirements, including initial titration, frequent contact is recommended between physician, other members of the health-care team, the patient and the caregiver/family.

Special Instructions for OxyContin® 80 mg Tablets
(For use in opioid tolerant patients only.)

OxyContin® 80 mg Tablets are for use only in opioid tolerant patients requiring daily oxycodone equivalent dosages of 160 mg or more. Care should be taken in the prescription of this tablet strength. Patients should be instructed against use by individuals other than the patient for whom it was prescribed, as such inappropriate use may have severe medical consequences.

Supplemental Analgesia

Most cancer patients given around-the-clock therapy with controlled-release opioids will need to have immediate-release medication available for "rescue" from breakthrough pain or to prevent pain that occurs predictably during certain patient activities (incident pain).

Rescue medication can be immediate-release oxycodone, either alone or in combination with acetaminophen, aspirin or other NSAIDs as a supplemental analgesic. The supplemental analgesic should be prescribed at $1/4$ to $1/3$ of the 12-hour OxyContin dose as shown in Table 4. The rescue medication is dosed as needed for breakthrough pain and administered one hour before anticipated incident pain. If more than two doses of rescue medication are needed within 24 hours, the dose of OxyContin should be titrated upward. Caregivers and patients using prn rescue analgesia in combination with around-the-clock opioids should be advised to report incidents of breakthrough pain to the physician managing the patient's analgesia (see Information for Patients/Caregivers).

Table 4

Table of Appropriate Supplemental Analgesia

OxyContin q12h Dose (mg)	prn Rescue Dose immediate-release oxycodone (mg)
10 (1×10 mg)	5
20 (2×10 mg)	5
30 (3×10 mg)	10
40 (2×20 mg)	10
60 (3×20 mg)	15
80 (2×40 mg)	20
120 (3×40 mg)	30
160 (2×80 mg)	40
240 (3×80 mg)	60

Maintenance of Therapy

The intent of the titration period is to establish a patient-specific q12h dose that will maintain adequate analgesia with acceptable side effects for as long as pain relief is necessary. Should pain recur then the dose can be incrementally increased to re-establish pain control. The method of therapy adjustment outlined above should be employed to re-establish pain control.

During chronic therapy, especially for non-cancer pain syndromes, the continued need for around-the-clock opioid therapy should be reassessed periodically (e.g., every 6 to 12 months) as appropriate.

Cessation of Therapy

When the patient no longer requires therapy with OxyContin tablets, patients receiving doses of 20–60 mg/day can usually have the therapy stopped abruptly without incident. However, higher doses should be tapered over several days to prevent signs and symptoms of withdrawal in the physically dependent patient. The daily dose should be reduced by approximately 50% for the first two days and then reduced by 25% every two days thereafter until the total dose reaches the dose recommended for opioid naive patients (10 or 20 mg q12h). Therapy can then be discontinued.

If signs of withdrawal appear, tapering should be stopped. The dose should be slightly increased until the signs and symptoms of opioid withdrawal disappear. Tapering should then begin again but with longer periods of time between each dose reduction.

Conversion from OxyContin to Parenteral Opioids

To avoid overdose, conservative dose conversion ratios should be followed. Initiate treatment with about 50% of the estimated equianalgesic daily dose of parenteral opioid divided into suitable individual doses based on the appropriate dosing interval, and titrate based upon the patient's response.

Continued on next page

OxyContin—Cont.

SAFETY AND HANDLING

OxyContin® (oxycodone hydrochloride controlled-release) tablets are solid dosage forms that pose no known health risk to health-care providers beyond that of any controlled substance. As with all such drugs, care should be taken to prevent diversion or abuse by proper handling.

HOW SUPPLIED

OxyContin® (oxycodone hydrochloride controlled-release) 10 mg tablets are round, unscored, white-colored, convex tablets bearing the symbol OC on one side and 10 on the other. They are supplied as follows:

NDC 59011-100-10: child-resistant closure, opaque plastic bottles of 100

NDC 59011-100-25: unit dose packaging with 25 individually numbered tablets per card; one card per glue end carton

OxyContin® (oxycodone hydrochloride controlled-release) 20 mg tablets are round, unscored, pink-colored, convex tablets bearing the symbol OC on one side and 20 on the other. They are supplied as follows:

NDC 59011-103-10: child-resistant closure, opaque plastic bottles of 100

NDC 59011-103-25: unit dose packaging with 25 individually numbered tablets per card; one card per glue end carton

OxyContin® (oxycodone hydrochloride controlled-release) 40 mg tablets are round, unscored, yellow-colored, convex tablets bearing the symbol OC on one side and 40 on the other. They are supplied as follows:

NDC 59011-105-10: child-resistant closure, opaque plastic bottles of 100

NDC 59011-105-25: unit dose packaging with 25 individually numbered tablets per card; one card per glue end carton

OxyContin® (oxycodone hydrochloride controlled-release) 80 mg tablets are round, unscored, green-colored, convex tablets bearing the symbol OC on one side and 80 on the other. They are supplied as follows:

NDC 59011-107-10: child-resistant closure, opaque plastic bottles of 100.

NDC 59011-107-25: unit dose packaging with 25 individually numbered tablets per card: one card per glue end carton

Store tablets at controlled room temperature 15–30°C (59–86°F).

Dispense in tight, light-resistant container.

CAUTION

DEA Order Form Required.

Federal law prohibits dispensing without prescription.

Manufactured by The PF Laboratories, Inc.
Totowa, N.J. 07512
Distributed by Purdue Pharma L.P.
Norwalk, CT 06850-3590
Copyright© 1995, 1997 Purdue Pharma L.P.
U.S. Patent Numbers 4,861,598; 4,970,075; 5,266,331; 5,508,042; 5,549,912.
Other Patents Pending
July 29, 1997
F4909-811

Shown in Product Identification Guide, page 333

OXYIR® CII ℞

(oxycodone hydrochloride)
Immediate-Release Oral Capsules
5 mg

OXYFAST™ CII ℞

(oxycodone hydrochloride)
Immediate-Release
Oral CONCENTRATE Solution*
20 mg/1mL

***This product contains dry natural rubber**

DESCRIPTION

Oxycodone is 14-hydroxydihydrocodeinone, a white odorless crystalline powder which is derived from the opium alkaloid, thebaine, and may be represented by the following structural formula:

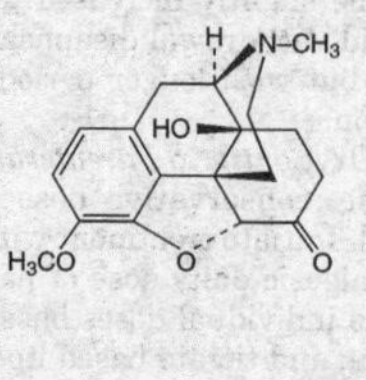

OxyIR Oral Capsules

Each 5 mg of OxyIR Capsules contains:

Oxycodone hydrochloride .... 5 mg

Inactive ingredients: Hydroxypropyl methycellulose, Maize starch, Polyethylene glycol, Polysorbate 80, Sucrose, Synthetic red iron oxide E172, Synthetic yellow iron oxide E172, Titanium dioxide E171.

OxyFAST Oral CONCENTRATE Solution

Each 1 mL of OxyFAST **Concentrate** Solution contains:

Oxycodone hydrochloride .... 20 mg

Inactive ingredients: Citric acid, FD&C Yellow #10, Sodium benzoate, Sodium citrate, Sodium saccharine and water.

ACTIONS

The analgesic ingredient, oxycodone, is a semisynthetic narcotic with multiple actions qualitatively similar to those of morphine; the most prominent of these involve the central nervous system and organs composed of smooth muscle. The principal actions of therapeutic value of oxycodone are analgesia and sedation.

CLINICAL PHARMACOLOGY

Central Nervous System: Oxycodone is a pure agonist opioid whose principal therapeutic action is analgesia. Other therapeutic effects of oxycodone include anxiolysis, euphoria and feelings of relaxation. Like all pure opioid agonists, there is no ceiling effect to analgesia, such as is seen with partial agonists or non-opioid analgesics.

The precise mechanism of the analgesic action is unknown. However, specific CNS opioid receptors for endogenous compounds with opioid-like activity have been identified throughout the brain and spinal cord and play a role in the analgesic effects of this drug.

Oxycodone produces respiratory depression by direct action on brain stem respiratory centers. The respiratory depression involves both a reduction in the responsiveness of the brain stem respiratory centers to increases in carbon dioxide tension and to electrical stimulation.

Oxycodone depresses the cough reflex by direct effect on the cough center in the medulla. Antitussive effects may occur with doses lower than those usually required for analgesia.

Oxycodone causes miosis, even in total darkness. Pinpoint pupils are a sign of opioid overdose but are not pathognomonic. Marked mydriasis rather than miosis may be seen due to hypoxia in overdose situations.

Gastrointestinal Tract and Other Smooth Muscle: Oxycodone causes a reduction in motility associated with an increase in smooth muscle tone in the antrum of the stomach and duodenum. Digestion of food in the small intestine is delayed and propulsive contractions are decreased. Propulsive peristaltic waves in the colon are decreased, while tone may be increased to the point of spasm resulting in constipation. Other opioid-induced effects may include a reduction in gastric, biliary and pancreatic secretions, spasm of sphincter of Oddi, and transient elevations in serum amylase.

Cardiovascular System: Oxycodone may produce release of histamine with or without associated peripheral vasodilation. Manifestations of histamine release and/or peripheral vasodilation may include pruritus, flushing, red eyes, sweating, and/or orthostatic hypotension.

Concentration—Efficacy Relationships (Pharmacodynamics): Studies in normal volunteers and patients reveal predictable relationships between oxycodone dosage and plasma oxycodone concentrations, as well as between concentration and certain expected opioid effects. In normal volunteers these include pupillary constriction, sedation and overall "drug effect" and in patients, analgesia and feelings of "relaxation." In nontolerant patients, analgesia is not usually seen at a plasma oxycodone concentration of less than 5–10 ng/mL.

As with all opioids, the minimum effective plasma concentration for analgesia will vary widely among patients, especially among patients who have been previously treated with potent agonist opioids. As a result, patients need to be treated with individualized titration of dosage to the desired effect. The minimum effective analgesic concentration of oxycodone for any individual patient may increase with repeated dosing due to an increase in pain and/or the development of tolerance.

Concentration—Adverse Experience Relationships: OxyIR Capsules and OxyFAST CONCENTRATE Solution are associated with typical opioid-related adverse experiences similar to those seen with all opioids. There is a general relationship between increasing oxycodone plasma concentration and increasing frequency of dose-related opioid adverse experiences such as nausea, vomiting, CNS effects and respiratory depression. In opioid-tolerant patients, the situation is altered by the development of tolerance to opioid-related side effects, and the relationship is poorly understood.

As with all opioids, the dose must be individualized (see DOSAGE AND ADMINISTRATION), because the effective analgesic dose for some patients will be too high to be tolerated by other patients.

INDICATIONS AND USAGE

For the relief of moderate to moderately severe pain.

CONTRAINDICATIONS

OxyIR and OxyFAST is contraindicated in patients with known hypersensitivity to oxycodone, or in any situation where opioids are contraindicated. This includes patients with significant respiratory depression (in unmonitored settings or the absence of resuscitative equipment), and patients with acute or severe bronchial asthma or hypercarbia. OxyIR and OxyFAST are contraindicated in any patient who has or is suspected of having paralytic ileus.

WARNINGS

Respiratory Depression: Respiratory depression is the chief hazard from all opioid agonist preparations. Respiratory depression occurs most frequently in elderly or debilitated patients, usually following large initial doses in non-tolerant patients, or when opioids are given in conjunction with other agents that depress respiration.

Oxycodone should be used with extreme caution in patients with significant chronic obstructive pulmonary disease or cor pulmonale, and in patients having a substantially decreased respiratory reserve, hypoxia, hypercapnia, or preexisting respiratory depression. In such patients, even usual therapeutic doses of oxycodone may decrease respiratory drive to the point of apnea. In these patients alternative non-opioid analgesics should be considered, and opioids should be employed only under careful medical supervision at the lowest effective dose.

Hypotensive Effect: OxyIR and OxyFAST, like all opioid analgesics, may cause severe hypotension in an individual whose ability to maintain blood pressure has been compromised by a depleted blood volume, or after concurrent administration with drugs such as phenothiazines or other agents which compromise vasomotor tone. OxyIR and OxyFAST may produce orthostatic hypotension in ambulatory patients. OxyIR and OxyFAST, like all opioid analgesics, should be administered with caution to patients in circulatory shock, since vasodilation produced by the drug may further reduce cardiac output and blood pressure.

Drug Dependence: Oxycodone can produce drug dependence of the morphine type, and therefore, has the potential for being abused. Psychic dependence, physical dependence and tolerance may develop upon repeated administration of this drug, and it should be prescribed and administered with the same degree of caution appropriate to the use of other oral narcotic-containing medications. Like other narcotic-containing medications, this drug is subject to the Federal Controlled Substances Act.

Usage in Ambulatory Patients: Oxycodone may impair the mental and/or physical abilities required for the performance of potential hazardous tasks such as driving a car or operating machinery. The patient using this drug should be cautioned accordingly.

Interaction with Other Central Nervous System Depressants: Patients receiving other narcotic analgesics, general anesthetics, phenothiazines, other tranquilizers, sedative-hypnotics or other CNS depressants (including alcohol) concomitantly with oxycodone hydrochloride may exhibit an additive CNS depression. When such combined therapy is contemplated, the dose of one or both agents should be reduced.

Usage in Pregnancy: Safe use in pregnancy has not been established relative to possible adverse effects on fetal development. Therefore, this drug should not be used in pregnant women unless, in the judgment of the physician, the potential benefits outweigh the possible hazards.

Usage in Children: This drug should not be administered to children.

PRECAUTIONS

Speical Precautions Regarding OxyFAST Oral CONCENTRATE 20 mg/1 mL Solution

OxyFAST 20 mg/1mL solution is a highly concentrated solution. Care should be taken in the prescription and dispensing of this solution strength. Patients should be instructed against use by individuals other than the patient, as inappropriate use may cause acute overdosage.

General

Opioid analgesics given on a fixed-dosage schedule have a narrow therapeutic index in certain patient populations, especially when combined with other drugs, and should be reserved for cases where the benefits of opioid analgesia outweigh the known risks of respiratory depression, altered mental state, and postural hypotension.

Use of OxyIR and OxyFAST is associated with increased potential risks and should be used only with caution in the following conditions: acute alcoholism; adrenocortical insufficiency (e.g., Addison's disease); CNS depression or coma; delirium tremens; debilitated patients; kyphoscoliosis associated with respiratory depression; myxedema or hypothyroidism; prostatic hypertrophy or urethral stricture; severe impairment of hepatic, pulmonary or renal function; and toxic psychosis.

The administration of oxycodone, like all opioid analgesics, may obscure the diagnosis or clinical course in patients with acute abdominal conditions. Oxycodone may aggravate con-

vulsions in patients with convulsive disorders, and all opioids may induce or aggravate seizures in some clinical settings.

Interactions with Mixed Agonist/ Antagonist Opioid Analgesics: Agonist/antagonist anagelsics (i.e., pentazocine, nalbuphine, butorphanol and buprenorphine) should be administered with caution to a patient who has received or is receiving a course of therapy with a pure opioid agonist analgesic such as oxycodone. In this situation, mixed agonist/antagonist analgesics may reduce the analgesic effect of oxycodone and/or may precipitate withdrawal symptoms in these patients.

Use in Pancreatic/Biliary Tract Disease: Oxycodone may cause spasm of the sphincter of Oddi and should be used with caution in patients with biliary tract disease, including acute pancreatitis. Opioids like oxycodone may cause increases in the serum amylase level.

Head Injury and Increased Intracranial Pressure: The respiratory depressant effects of narcotics and their capacity to elevate cerebrospinal fluid pressure may be markedly exaggerated in the presence of head injury, other intracranial lesions or a pre-existing increase in intracranial pressure. Furthermore, narcotics produce adverse reactions which may obscure the clinical course of patients with head injuries.

Acute Abdominal Conditions: The administration of this drug or other narcotics may obscure the diagnosis or clinical course in patients with acute abdominal conditions.

Information for Patients/Caregivers: If clinically advisable, patients receiving OxyIR (immediate-release) Capsules or OxyFAST CONCENTRATE Solution or their caregivers should be given the following information by the physician, nurse, pharmacist or caregiver:

1. Patients should be advised not to adjust the dose of this drug without consulting the prescribing professional.
2. Patients should be advised that this drug may impair mental and/or physical ability required for the performance of potentially hazardous tasks (e.g., driving, operating heavy machinery).
3. Patients should not combine this drug with alcohol or other central nervous system depressants (sleep aids, tranquilizers) except by the orders of the prescribing physician, because additive effects may occur.
4. Women of childbearing potential who become, or are planning to become, pregnant should be advised to consult their physician regarding the effects of analgesics and other drug use during pregnancy on themselves and their unborn child.
5. Patients should be advised that this drug is a potential drug of abuse. They should protect it from theft, and it should never be given to anyone other than the individual for whom it was prescribed.
6. Patients should be advised that if they have been receiving treatment with this drug for more than a few weeks and cessation of therapy is indicated, it may be appropriate to taper this drug dose, rather than abruptly discontinue it, due to the risk of precipitating withdrawal symptoms. Their physician can provide a dose schedule to accomplish a gradual discontinuation of the medication.

Laboratory Monitoring: Due to the broad range of plasma concentrations seen in clinical populations, the varying degrees of pain, and the development of tolerance, plasma oxycodone measurements are usually not helpful in clinical management. Plasma concentrations of the active drug substance may be of value in selected, unusual or complex cases.

Use in Drug and Alcohol Addiction: OxyIR and OxyFAST are opioids with no approved use in the management of addictive disorders. The proper usage of these drugs in individuals with drug or alcohol dependence, either active or in remission, is for the management of pain requiring opioid analgesia.

Drug-Drug Interactions: The CNS depressant effects of oxycodone hydrochloride may be additive with that of other CNS depressants. See WARNINGS.

Opioid analgesics, including OxyIR and OxyFAST, may enhance the neuromuscular blocking action of skeletal muscle relaxants and produce an increased degree of respiratory depression.

Oxycodone is metabolized in part to oxymorphone via CYP2D6. While this pathway may be blocked by a variety of drugs (e.g., certain cardiovascular drugs and antidepressants), such blockade has not yet been shown to be of clinical significance with this agent. Clinicians should be aware of this possible interaction, however.

Mutagenicity/Carcinogenicity: Oxycodone was not mutagenic in the following assays: Ames Salmonella and E. Coli test with and without metabolic activation at doses of up to 5000 μg, chromosomal aberration test in human lymphocytes (in the absence of metabolic activation and with activation after 48 hours of exposure) at doses of up to 1500 μg/ml, and in the in vivo bone marrow micronucleus assay in mice (at plasma levels of up to 48 μg/ml). Mutagenic results occurred in the presence of metabolic activation in the human chromosomal aberration test (at greater than or equal to 1250 μg/ml) at 24 but not 48 hours of exposure and in the mouse lymphoma assay at doses of 50 μg/ml or greater with metabolic activation and at 400 μg/ml or greater without metabolic activation. The data from these tests indicate that the genotoxic risk to humans may be considered low.

Studies of oxycodone in animals to evaluate its carcinogenic and mutagenic potential have not been conducted owing to the length of clinical experience with the drug substance.

Pregnancy: Teratogenic Effects—Category B: Reproduction studies have been performed in rats and rabbits by oral administration at doses up to 8 mg/kg (48 mg/m^2) and 125 mg/kg (1375 mg/m^2), respectively. These doses are 4 and 60 times a human dose of 120 mg/day (74 mg/m^2), based on mg/kg of a 60 kg adult (0.7 and 19 times this human dose based upon mg/m^2). The results did not reveal evidence of harm to the fetus due to oxycodone. There are, however, no adequate and well-controlled studies in pregnant women. Because animal reproduction studies are not always predictive of human response, this drug should be used during pregnancy only if clearly needed.

Nonteratogenic Effects—Neonates whose mothers have been taking oxycodone chronically may exhibit respiratory depression and/or withdrawal symptoms, either at birth and/or in the nursery.

Labor and Delivery: OxyIR and OxyFAST are not recommended for use in women during and immediately prior to labor and delivery because oral opioids may cause respiratory depression in the newborn.

Nursing Mothers: Low concentrations of oxycodone have been detected in breast milk. Withdrawal symptoms can occur in breast-feeding infants when maternal administration of an opioid analgesic is stopped. Ordinarily, nursing should not be undertaken while a patient is receiving OxyIR or OxyFAST since oxycodone may be excreted in the milk.

Pediatric Use: Safety and effectiveness in pediatric patients have not been established.

Special Risk Patients: This drug should be given with caution to certain patients such as the elderly, or debilitated, and those with severe impairment of hepatic or renal function, hypothyroidism, Addison's disease and prostatic hypertrophy or urethral stricture.

ADVERSE REACTIONS

The most frequently observed reactions include light-headedness, dizziness, sedation, nausea and vomiting. These effects seem to be more prominent in ambulatory than in non-ambulatory patients, and some of these adverse reactions may be alleviated if the patient lies down.

Other adverse reactions include euphoria, dysphoria, constipation, skin rash and pruritus.

DRUG ABUSE AND DEPENDENCE (Addiction)

Oxycodone products are common targets for both drug abusers and drug addicts.

Drug addiction (drug dependence, psychological dependence) is characterized by a preoccupation with the procurement, hoarding, and abuse of drugs for non-medicinal purposes. Drug dependence is treatable, utilizing a multi-disciplinary approach, but relapse is common. Iatrogenic "addiction" to opioids legitimately used in the management of pain is very rare. "Drug seeking" behavior is very common to addicts. Tolerance and physical dependence in pain patients are not signs of psychological dependence. Preoccupation with achieving adequate pain relief can be appropriate behavior in a patient with poor pain control. Most chronic pain patients limit their intake of opioids to achieve a balance between the benefits of the drug and dose-limiting side effects. Physicians should be aware that psychological dependence may not be accompanied by concurrent tolerance and symptoms of physical dependence in all addicts. In addition, abuse of opioids can occur in the absence of true psychological dependence and is characterized by misuse for non-medical purposes, often in combination with other psychoactive substances.

MANAGEMENT OF OVERDOSAGE

Signs and Symptoms: Serious overdose of oxycodone hydrochloride is characterized by respiratory depression (a decrease in respiratory rate and/or tidal volume, Cheyne-Stokes respiration, cyanosis), extreme somnolence progressing to stupor or coma, skeletal muscle flaccidity, cold and clammy skin, and sometimes bradycardia and hypotension. In severe overdosage, apnea, circulatory collapse, cardiac arrest and death may occur.

Treatment: Primary attention should be given to the reestablishment of adequate respiratory exchange through provision of a patent airway and the institution of assisted or controlled ventilation. The narcotic antagonist naloxone is a specific antidote against respiratory depression which may result from overdosage or unusual sensitivity to narcotics, including oxycodone.

Therefore, an appropriate dose of naloxone (usual initial adult dose: 0.4 mg) should be administered, preferably by the intravenous route, simultaneously with efforts at respiratory resuscitation. Since the duration of action of oxycodone may exceed that of the antagonist, the patient should be kept under continued surveillance and repeated doses of the antagonist should be administered as needed to maintain adequate respiration. An antagonist should not be administered in the absence of clinically significant respiratory or cardiovascular depression.

Oxygen, intravenous fluids, vasopressors and other supportive measures should be employed as indicated.

Gastric emptying may be useful in removing unabsorbed drug.

DOSAGE AND ADMINISTRATION

Special Precautions Regarding OxyFAST Oral CONCENTRATE 20 mg/1 mL Solution

OxyFAST 20 mg/1mL solution is a highly concentrated solution. Care should be taken in the prescription and dispensing of this solution strength. Patients should be instructed against use by individuals other than the patient, as inappropriate use may cause acute overdosage.

Dosage should be adjusted to the severity of the pain and the response of the patient. It may occasionally be necessary to exceed the usual dosage recommended below in cases of more severe pain or in those patients who have become tolerant to the analgesic effects of narcotics. This drug is given orally. The usual adult dosage is one 5 mg capsule every 6 hours as needed for pain.

HOW SUPPLIED

OxyIR (oxycodone hydrochloride) Capsules:
5 mg capsules, Cap: Beige Imprinted with O-IR; Body: Orange Imprinted with PF5mg.
NDC 59011-201-10: Opaque plastic bottle containing 100 capsules

OxyFAST (oxycodone hydrochloride)
Oral CONCENTRATE Solution
20 mg per 1 mL.
NDC 59011-225-20; High density polyethylene plastic, with child-resistant closure bottle with child-resistant dropper in 30 mL size.

Discard opened bottle of oral solution after 90 days. Protect from light.

Store OxyFAST oral **CONCENTRATE** solutions and capsules at controlled room temperature 15° to 30°C (59°–86°F).

Caution
DEA Order Form Required.
Rx Only
Purdue Pharma L.P., Norwalk, CT 06850-3590
Copyright ©1995, 1998
July 14, 1998
E4597

Shown in Product Identification Guide, page 333

R&D Laboratories, Inc.

4640 ADMIRALTY WAY, SUITE 710
MARINA DEL REY, CA 90292

Direct Inquiries to:
Rhoda Makoff, PhD
(310) 305-8053
(800) 338-9066
FAX (310) 305-9229

For Medical Emergencies:
Dwight Makoff, M.D.
(310) 652-9162

AMIN-AID® INSTANT DRINK OTC
Essential Amino Acid and Calorie Supplement

DESCRIPTION

Amin-Aid® is recommended for management of patients with distinctive nutritional requirements resulting from acute or chronic renal failure including essential amino acid deficiencies.

HOW SUPPLIED

Amin-Aid® Instant Drink is packaged 12 packages per carton, 2 cartons per case (24 packages per case).

Flavor	NDC No.
Orange	54391-6100-24
Strawberry	54391-6103-24
Berry	54391-6104-24

Manufactured by McGaw, Inc. For R&D Laboratories, Inc.

CALCI-CHEW® OTC

1.25 gm USP grade calcium carbonate chewable tablets—500 mg elemental calcium. Packaged as three separate flavors—cherry, lemon, orange.

Continued on next page

Calci-Chew—Cont.

DESCRIPTION
Tablets supplying 1.25 gm USP grade calcium carbonate. Contains no dyes and no sodium.

INDICATIONS
For use as calcium supplementation and in the treatment of hypocalcemia.

DOSAGE
For hypocalcemia, use as necessary to restore calcium to normal levels. For patients with impaired calcium absorption or on a calcium restricted diet, give under a physician's guidance.

HOW SUPPLIED
Plastic bottles of 100 tablets.

FLAVOR	NDC No.
CHERRY	54391-0025-2
LEMON	54391-0225-2
ORANGE	54391-0325-2

CALCI–MIX®　　　　　　　　　　OTC
1.25 gm USP grade calcium carbonate powdered in pull apart capsules. Contains 500 mg of elemental calcium. Can be swallowed or pulled apart and sprinkled on food or in drink.

DESCRIPTION
Gelatin capsules containing 1.25 gm USP grade calcium carbonate. Contains no sodium and no dyes.

INDICATIONS
For use as calcium supplementation and in the treatment of hypocalcemia.

DOSAGE
For hypocalcemia, use as necessary to restore calcium to normal levels. For patients with impaired calcium absorption or on a calcium restricted diet, give under a physician's guidance.

SUPPLIED
Plastic bottles of 100 capsules. NDC 54391-0027-3.

L-CARNITINE　　　　　　　　　　OTC
250 mg capsules.
Plastic bottles of 60 capsules
NDC 54391-0050-9

MAG-CARB™　　　　　　　　　　OTC
[măg-kărb]
A Nutritional Supplement

DESCRIPTION
A 250 mg magnesium carbonate supplement packaged in a gel capsule, delivering 70 mg of elemental magnesium. Used as a general supplement and especially suitable for the transplant recipient on cyclosporin therapy who is at risk for magnesium deficiency.

INGREDIENTS
Magnesium carbonate, magnesium stearate, cellulose, and gelatin.

DOSAGE
As needed or prescribed.

HOW SUPPLIED
Clear gelatin capsules in plastic bottles of 100. Store tightly in a cool, dry place.
NDC #54391-0031-03

NEPHRO–CALCI®　　　　　　　　　OTC
1.5 gm USP grade calcium carbonate tablets—600 mg elemental calcium.

DESCRIPTION
Tablets supplying 1.5 gm of (USP grade) calcium carbonate. Contains no dyes.

INDICATIONS
For use as calcium supplementation and in the treatment of hypocalcemia.

DOSAGE
For hypocalcemia, use as necessary to restore calcium to normal levels. For patients with impaired calcium absorption and patients on a calcium restricted diet, give under a physician's guidance.

SUPPLIED
Plastic bottles of 100 tablets. NDC 54391-0026-3.

NEPHRO–FER®　　　　　　　　　　OTC
Ferrous fumarate preparation for oral iron supplementation.

DESCRIPTION
Each tablet supplies 350 mg of ferrous fumarate—115 mg of elemental iron. Contains no dyes.

INDICATIONS
Patients taking EPO requiring oral iron supplementation—particularly patients who experience gastric problems with ferrous sulfate. Appropriate for any iron supplementation. (See Nephro-Fer® Rx for side effects.)

DOSAGE
One to three tablets daily as required, under the supervision of a physician.

SUPPLIED
Brown oval tablets marked RD13.
Tablets in unit dose blister packs of 30. NDC 54391-0013-8.

NEPHRO-FER® Rx　　　　　　　　　℞
Iron Supplement With Folic Acid

Oral iron supplement. For any patient needing iron supplementation for documented iron deficiency. Suitable for certain patients undergoing therapy with erythropoietin.

DESCRIPTION
Each tablet contains 324 mg ferrous fumarate—106.9 mg elemental iron—and 1 mg folic acid. Ferrous fumarate may be better tolerated than ferrous sulfate in some patients.

INDICATIONS
Renal failure patients and patients who have documented iron deficiency. Patients undergoing erythropoietin therapy who risk iron deficiency.

DOSAGE
One to three tablets daily between meals as required to correct iron deficiency, or as prescribed by physician.

SIDE EFFECTS
Transient bloating, flatulence, constipation, and diarrhea. Ingestion of greater than 400 mg per day of elemental iron can result in nausea and vomiting.

PRECAUTION
See folic acid precaution under NEPHRO-VITE® + FE

SUPPLIED
Brown, oval tablets marked RD33.
Tablets in unit dose blister packs of 30. NDC 54391-1313-8.
For use under medical supervision.

NEPHRAMINE®　　　　　　　　　　℞
5.4% Essential Amino Acid Injection

DESCRIPTION
5.4% NephrAmine® (Essential Amino Acid Injection) is a sterile, nonpyrogenic solution containing crystalline essential amino acids plus histidine. Each 250 mL unit provides Rose's recommended daily intake of essential amino acids[1] plus 625 mg of histidine, considered essential for uremics. The total nitrogen content of a 250 mL unit is approximately 1.6 grams (10 g of protein equivalent) in 14 grams of amino acids. All amino acids designated USP are the "L" isomer.
Each 100 mL contains:

Histidine USP*	0.25 g
Isoleucine USP	0.56 g
Leucine USP	0.88 g
Lysine	0.64 g
(added as Lysine Acetate USP	0.90 g)
Methionine USP	0.88 g
Phenylalanine USP	0.88 g
Threonine USP	0.40 g
Tryptophan USP	0.20 g
Valine USP	0.64 g
Cysteine	<0.014 g
(as Cysteine HCl·H₂O USP	<0.020 g)
Sodium Bisulfite (as an antioxidant)	<0.05 g
Water for Injection USP	qs

pH adjusted with Sodium Hydroxide NF as required
pH: 6.5 (6.0–7.0): Calculated Osmolarity: 435 mOsmol/liter
Total Nitrogen: Approx. 0.65 g/100 mL
Concentration of Electrolytes (mEq/liter): Sodium 5
Chloride <3, Acetate Approx. 44

*Histidine is considered an essential amino acid in uremic patients
[1] Rose WC: The sequence of events leading to the establishment of the amino acid needs of man **Am J Public Health: 1968; 58(11):** 2020–2027

CLINICAL PHARMACOLOGY
NephrAmine® provides an intravenously compatible mixture of essential amino acids which, when infused with hypertonic dextrose as a source of calories, plus electrolytes, minerals, and vitamins provides in a small volume of fluid all ingredients (with the exception of essential fatty acids) needed for total parenteral nutrition in patients with renal disease.
Infusion of NephrAmine® and hypertonic dextrose provides essential amino acids and calories for protein synthesis to promote improved cellular metabolic balance. Infusion of these components can decrease the rate of rise of blood urea nitrogen (bun) and minimize deterioration of serum potassium, magnesium and phosphorus balance in patients with impaired renal function. The extent to which essential amino acids and calories promote incorporation of waste urea nitrogen into newly synthesized amino acids in man, as it does in experimental animals, is, so far, not established.
The accelerated decrease in serum creatinine levels seen in patients with limited extra-renal complications suggests that treatment with NephrAmine® and hypertonic dextrose leads to earlier return of renal function in patients with potentially reversible acute renal failure. By providing nutritional support and promoting biochemical improvement as well as earlier return of renal function, NephrAmine® and hypertonic dextrose decrease morbidity associated with acute renal failure.
It is thought that acetate from lysine acetate, under the condition of parenteral nutrition, does not impact net acid-base balance when renal and respiratory functions are normal. Clinical evidence seems to support this thinking; however, confirmatory experimental evidence is not available.
The amounts of sodium and chloride present are not of clinical significance.

INDICATIONS AND USAGE
5.4% NephrAmine® (Essential Amino Acid Injection) is indicated for adult and pediatric use, in conjunction with other measures, to provide nutritional support for uremic patients, particularly when oral nutrition is infeasible or impractical. See *Special Precautions in Pediatric Patients* for additional information.

CONTRAINDICATIONS
NephrAmine® is contraindicated in patients with severe, uncorrected electrolyte and acid-base imbalance, hyperammonemia, decreased (subcritical) circulating blood volume, inborn errors of amino acid metabolism, or hypersensitivity to one or more amino acids present in the solution.

WARNINGS
This product contains sodium bisulfite, a sulfite that may cause allergic-type reactions including anaphylactic symptoms and life-threatening or less severe asthmatic episodes in certain susceptible people. The overall prevalence of sulfite sensitivity in the general population is unknown and probably low. Sulfite sensitivity is seen more frequently in asthmatic than in nonasthmatic people.
Safe and effective use of central venous nutrition requires a knowledge of nutrition as well as clinical expertise in recognition and treatment of the complications which can occur. **Frequent clinical evaluation and laboratory determinations are necessary for proper monitoring of central venous nutrition.** Studies should include blood sugar, serum proteins, kidney and liver function tests, electrolytes, hemogram, carbon dioxide combining power, serum osmolarity, blood cultures, blood ammonia levels, and circulating blood volume. NephrAmine® does not replace dialysis and conventional supportive therapy in patients with renal failure.
Administration of NephrAmine® to children or low birthweight infants, especially in high doses, may result in hyperammonemia.
Clinically significant hypokalemia, hypophosphatemia, or hypomagnesemia may occur as a result of therapy with NephrAmine® and hypertonic dextrose and replacement therapy may become necessary.
Administration of nitrogen in any form to patients with marked hepatic insufficiency or hepatic coma may result in plasma amino acid imbalances, hyperammonemia, or central nervous system deterioration. NephrAmine® should, therefore, be used with caution in such patients.
The intravenous administration of these solutions can cause fluid and/or solute overload resulting in dilution of serum electrolyte concentrations, overhydration, congested states

or pulmonary edema. The risk of dilutional states is inversely proportional to the solute concentration of the solution infused. The risk of solute overload causing congested states with peripheral and pulmonary edema is directly proportional to the concentration of the solution.

Conservative doses of amino acids should be given, dictated by the nutritional status of the patient.

PRECAUTIONS
General
Clinical evaluation and periodic laboratory determinations are necessary to monitor changes in fluid balance, electrolyte concentrations, and acid-base balance during prolonged parenteral therapy or whenever the condition of the patient warrants such evaluation. Significant deviations from normal concentrations may require the use of additional electrolyte supplements.

In order to promote urea nitrogen reutilization in patients with renal failure, it is essential to provide adequate calories with minimal amounts of the essential amino acids, and to severely restrict the intake of nonessential nitrogen. Hypertonic dextrose solutions are a convenient and metabolically effective source of concentrated calories.

Fluid balance must be carefully monitored in patients with renal failure and care should be taken to avoid circulatory overload, particularly in association with cardiac insufficiency.

In patients with myocardial infarct, infusion of amino acids should always be accompanied by dextrose, since in anoxia, free fatty acids cannot be utilized by the myocardium, and energy must be produced anaerobically from glycogen or glucose.

Strongly hypertonic nutrient solutions should be administered through an indwelling intravenous catheter with the tip located in the superior vena cava.

Special care must be taken when giving hypertonic dextrose to glucose-intolerant patients such as diabetic or prediabetic and uremic patients; especially when the latter are receiving peritoneal dialysis. To prevent severe hyperglycemia in such patients, insulin may be required.

Administration of glucose at a rate exceeding the patient's utilization may lead to hyperglycemia, coma, and death.

Administration of amino acids without carbohydrates may result in the accumulation of ketone bodies in the blood. Correction of this ketonemia may be achieved by the administration of carbohydrates. Abrupt cessation of hypertonic dextrose infusion may result in rebound hypoglycemia.

When 5.4% NephrAmine® (Essential Amino Acid Injection) is subjected to changes in temperature, there is a chance that some transient crystallization of amino acids may occur. Thorough shaking of the bottle for about one minute should redissolve the amino acids. If the amino acids do not completely redissolve, the bottle must be rejected.

To minimize the risk of possible incompatibilities arising from mixing this solution with other additives that may be prescribed, the final infusate should be inspected for cloudiness or precipitation immediately after mixing, prior to administration, and periodically during administration.

Use only if solution is clear and vacuum is present.

Usage in Pregnancy
Pregnancy Category C. Animal reproduction studies have not been conducted with 5.4% NephrAmine® (Essential Amino Acid Injection). It is also not known whether NephrAmine® can cause fetal harm when administered to a pregnant woman or can affect reproduction capacity. NephrAmine® should be given to a pregnant woman only if clearly needed.

Special Precautions for Central Venous Nutrition
Administration by central venous catheter should be used only by those familiar with this technique and its complications.

Central venous nutrition may be associated with complications which can be prevented or minimized by careful attention to all aspects of the procedure including solution preparation, administration, and patient monitoring. **It is essential that a carefully prepared protocol, based on current medical practices, be followed, preferably by an experienced team.**

SEE PACKAGE INSERT FOR ADDITIONAL INFORMATION ON CENTRAL VENOUS ADMINISTRATION.

Special Precautions in Patients with Renal Insufficiency
Frequent laboratory studies are necessary in patients with renal insufficiency due to underlying metabolic abnormalities. Hyperglycemia, a frequent complication, may not be reflected by glycosuria in renal failure. Blood glucose, therefore, must be determined frequently, often every six hours to guide dosage of dextrose and insulin if required.

Serum concentrations of potassium, phosphorus, and magnesium may dramatically decline with successful treatment, individually or together; these substances should be supplemented as required. Special care must be taken to avoid hypokalemia in digitalized patients, or those with cardiac arrhythmias.

Special Precautions in Pediatric Patients
5.4% NephrAmine® (Essential Amino Acid Injection) should be used with special caution in pediatric patients, especially low birth-weight infants, due to limited clinical experience.

Laboratory and clinical monitoring of pediatric patients, especially when nutritionally depleted, must be extensive and frequent. Initial total daily dose should be low, and increased slowly. Dosage of NephrAmine® above one gram of essential amino acids per kilogram body weight per day is not recommended.

Frequent monitoring of blood glucose is required in low birth-weight or septic infants as infusion of hypertonic dextrose carries a greater risk of hyperglycemia in such patients.

The absence of arginine in NephrAmine® may accentuate the risk of hyperammonemia in infants.

ADVERSE REACTIONS
See **WARNINGS** and *Special Precautions for Central Venous Nutrition.*

Reactions which may occur because of the solution or the technique of administration include febrile response, infection at the site of injection, venous thrombosis, and hypervolemia.

Symptoms may result from an excess or deficit of one or more of the ions present in the solution infused, therefore, frequent monitoring of electrolyte levels is essential.

Infrequent instances of hyperammonemia have been reported following administration of essential amino acid solutions to patients with massive gastrointestinal hemorrhage, nonuremic infants and children or following administration of higher than recommended doses to adult or pediatric patients. Serum ammonia levels and clinical symptoms may subside when the infusions are discontinued.

Phosphorus deficiency may lead to impaired tissue oxygenation and acute hemolytic anemia. Relative to calcium, excessive phosphorus intake can precipitate hypocalcemia with cramps, tetany and muscular hyperexcitability.

If an adverse reaction does occur, discontinue the infusion, evaluate the patient, institute appropriate therapeutic countermeasures and save the remainder of the fluid for examination if deemed necessary.

OVERDOSAGE
In the event of a fluid or solute overload during parenteral therapy, reevaluate the patient's condition, and institute appropriate corrective treatment.

DOSAGE AND ADMINISTRATION
The objective of nutritional management of renal decompensation is the provision of sufficient amino acid and caloric support for protein synthesis without greatly exceeding the renal capacity to excrete metabolic wastes.

Three grams of nitrogen per day provided as essential amino acids with adequate calories produce nitrogen equilibrium in many stable patients with chronic uremia. Although nitrogen requirements may be higher in stressed or acutely uremic patients, or those on dialysis, provision of additional nitrogen may not be possible due to fluid intake limits or glucose intolerance.

The usual methods of determining individual patient requirements for amino acids such as nitrogen balance or daily body weight are difficult to perform or interpret in the uremic patient. Therefore, dosage is guided by the patient's fluid intake limits and glucose and nitrogen tolerances, as well as metabolic and clinical response. Rate of rise of blood urea nitrogen generally diminishes with infusion of essential amino acids. However, excessive intake of dietary protein or increased protein catabolism may alter this response.

Adults: Generally, 250 to 500 mL of 5.4% NephrAmine® (Essential Amino Acid Injection), containing approximately 1.6 to 3.2 grams of nitrogen (in 13.4 to 26.8 grams of essential amino acids), are given daily. Adequate calories should be provided simultaneously. Each 250 mL of NephrAmine® is typically mixed aseptically with 500 mL of 70% dextrose to yield a solution of 1.8% NephrAmine® in 47% dextrose. This mixture provides a calorie-to-nitrogen ratio of 744.1.

Children: Initial total daily dose should be low and increased slowly. Dosage of NephrAmine® above one gram of essential amino acids per kg of body weight per day is not recommended. See *Special Precautions in Pediatric Patients* for additional information.

Fat emulsion coadministration should be considered when prolonged (more than 5 days) parenteral nutrition is required in order to prevent essential fatty acid deficiency (E.F.A.D.). Serum lipids should be monitored for evidence of E.F.A.D. in patients maintained on fat free TPN.

Electrolyte supplementation may be required. Undiluted NephrAmine® contains 5 mEq/liter of sodium. Elevated serum potassium, phosphorus, and magnesium levels generally decrease during treatment with NephrAmine®. Although these effects are beneficial, especially in acute renal failure, in some instances the reduction may be so great that supplementation of these electrolytes is required, especially in the presence of cardiac arrhythmias or digitalis toxicity. During periods of anuria or oliguria, electrolyte supplementation should be done with caution, even if serum levels are in the low normal range.

Compatibility of electrolyte additives to the 5.4% NephrAmine® (Essential Amino Acid Injection)/hypertonic dextrose mixture must be considered, and potentially incompatible ions such as calcium and phosphate may be added to alternate infusion bottles to avoid precipitation. In patients with hyperchloremic or other metabolic acidosis, sodium and potassium may be added as acetate or lactate salts to provide bicarbonate precursor. The electrolyte content of NephrAmine® must be considered when calculating daily electrolyte intake. Serum electrolytes, including magnesium and phosphorus, should be monitored frequently.

If a patient's nutritional intake is primarily parenteral, water soluble vitamins should also be provided.

Hypertonic mixtures of essential amino acids and dextrose may be safely administered by continuous infusion through a central venous catheter with the tip located in the superior vena cava. Initial infusion rates should be slow, generally 20–30 mL/hour. Increases by increments of 10 mL/hour each 24 hours are recommended to a maximum of 60–100 mL/hour. If administration rate should fall behind schedule, no attempt to "catch up" to planned intake should be made. Administration rate is governed by the patient's nitrogen, fluid, and glucose tolerance. Uremic patients are frequently glucose intolerant, especially in association with peritoneal dialysis, and may require the administration of exogenous insulin to prevent hyperglycemia. Blood glucose levels must be determined frequently. To prevent rebound hypoglycemia, a solution containing 5% dextrose should be administered when hypertonic dextrose infusions are abruptly discontinued.

Parenteral drug products should be inspected visually for particulate matter and discoloration prior to administration, whenever solution and container permit.

Care must be taken to avoid incompatible admixtures. Consult with pharmacist.

HOW SUPPLIED
5.4% NephrAmine® (Essential Amino Acid Injection) is supplied sterile and nonpyrogenic in glass containers packaged 12 per case.

NDC No.: 54391-1909-55   Size: 250 mL

Exposure of pharmaceutical products to heat should be minimized. Avoid excessive heat. Protect from freezing. It is recommended that the product be stored at room temperature (25°C); however, brief exposure up to 40°C does not adversely affect the product. Protect from light until use.

Manufactured By McGaw, Inc. For R&D Laboratories, Inc.
For Medical Emergencies:
McGaw Stat Line
(800) 854-6851

NEPHRO–VITE®Rx   ℞
Vitamin Formulation For Renal Patients

DESCRIPTION
The process of dialysis causes vitamin losses necessitating the regular replacement of the water soluble vitamins. It is important not to over supplement some vitamins. Vitamin A should not be supplemented and vitamin C supplementation should be limited to 60 mg per day to avoid the risk of increased oxalate formation.

Each tablet provides:

	Nephro-Vite®Rx	Nephro-Vite®
Vitamin C	60mg	60mg
Vitamin B_1	1.5mg	1.5mg
Vitamin B_2	1.7mg	1.7mg
Niacinamide	20mg	20mg
Vitamin B_6	10mg	10mg
Vitamin B_{12}	6mcg	6mcg
Folic Acid	1mg	.8mg
Pantothenic Acid	10mg	10mg
Biotin	300mcg	300mcg

INDICATIONS
Dialysis patients; Azotemic patients not on dialysis who eat poorly.

PRECAUTION
See Folic Acid Precaution under Nephro-Vite® +Fe

DOSAGE
One tablet daily, or as prescribed by physician.

SUPPLIED
Film coated, round yellow tablets, marked RD 12.
Plastic bottles of 100. NDC 54391-1002-1.
For use under medical supervision.

Continued on next page

NEPHRO–VITE®   OTC
Vitamin Formulation For Renal Patients

Renal vitamin replacement formulation—see table under Nephro-Vite® Rx for description. Same dosage as Nephro-Vite® Rx.
Film coated, round yellow tablets marked RD 02.
Supplied in plastic bottles of 100. NDC 54391-0002-1.

NEPHRO–VITE® +Fe   ℞
Vitamin Formulation For Renal Patients With Iron

COMPOSITION
Same as Nephro-Vite® Rx with the addition of 304 mg of ferrous fumarate—100 mg of elemental iron.

INDICATIONS
For any patient needing vitamin and iron supplementation for documented iron deficiency. Suitable for pre-dialysis and end stage renal disease patients.

PRECAUTION
Folic acid may partially correct the hematological damage due to vitamin B_{12} deficiency of pernicious anemia while the associated neurological damage progresses.

ADVERSE REACTIONS
Allergic sensitization has been reported following administration of folic acid. Iron sensitivity to low doses of iron has been reported and high doses result in iron toxicity. Transient bloating, flatulence, constipation and diarrhea. Ingestion of greater than 400 mg/day of iron can result in nausea and vomiting.

DOSAGE
One tablet daily between meals or as prescribed by a physician.

HOW SUPPLIED
Film coated, oval tablets marked RD23. Tablets in unit dose blister packs of 30.
NDC 54391-2213-8
For use under medical supervision.

REGAIN® MEDICAL NUTRITION BAR   OTC
[rē·gain]

DESCRIPTION
An effective oral nutrition supplement formulated for the malnourished renal failure patient. High nutritional value with no increase in fluid intake. Lower in sodium, potassium, phosphorus, and magnesium. Low in dextrose and sucrose.

DOSAGE
One bar daily or as prescribed by a medical professional.

HOW SUPPLIED
3 oz. bar; packaged in cases of 24, available in 3 flavors (vanilla, strawberry, malt) each with cocoa coating. Store in a cool place, 24°C (75°F) or less.
NDC: 54391-0240-05 vanilla; 54391-0140-05 malt; 54391-0040-05 strawberry

---

Reckitt & Colman Pharmaceuticals Inc.
**1909 HUGUENOT ROAD
RICHMOND, VA 23235**

Direct Inquiries to:
Professional Services
(804) 379-1090
FAX: (804) 379-1215

For Medical Information Contact:
In Emergencies
Medical Department
(804) 379-1090
FAX: (804) 379-1215

BUPRENEX®   ⓒ ℞
[būp´rĕn-ex]
**(buprenorphine hydrochloride)
INJECTABLE**

DESCRIPTION
Buprenex (buprenorphine hydrochloride) is a narcotic under the Controlled Substances Act due to its chemical derivation from thebaine. Chemically, it is 17-(cyclopropylmethyl)-α-(1,1-dimethylethyl)-4, 5-epoxy-18, 19-dihydro-3-hydroxy-6-methoxy-α-methyl-6, 14-ethenomorphinan-7-methanol, hydrochloride [5α, 7α(S)]. Buprenorphine hydrochloride is a white powder, weakly acidic and with limited solubility in water. Buprenex is a clear, sterile, injectable agonist-antagonist analgesic intended for intravenous or intramuscular administration. Each ml of Buprenex contains 0.324 mg buprenorphine hydrochloride (equivalent to 0.3 mg buprenorphine), 50 mg anhydrous dextrose, water for injection and HCl to adjust pH. Buprenorphine hydrochloride has the molecular formula, $C_{29}H_{41}NO_4\cdot HCl$, and the following structure:

Molecular weight: 504.09

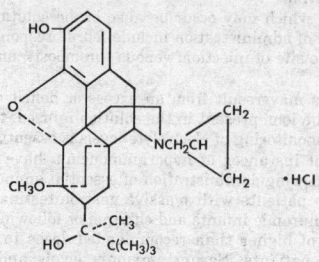

CLINICAL PHARMACOLOGY
Buprenex is a parenteral opioid analgesic with 0.3 mg Buprenex being approximately equivalent to 10 mg morphine sulfate in analgesic and respiratory depressant effects in adults. Pharmacological effects occur as soon as 15 minutes after intramuscular injection and persist for 6 hours or longer. Peak pharmacologic effects usually are observed at 1 hour. When used intravenously, the times to onset and peak effect are shortened.
The limits of sensitivity of available analytical methodology precluded demonstration of bioequivalence between intramuscular and intravenous routes of administration. In postoperative adults, pharmacokinetic studies have shown elimination half-lives ranging from 1.2–7.2 hours (mean 2.2 hours) after intravenous administration of 0.3 mg of buprenorphine. A single, ten-patient, pharmacokinetic study of doses of 3 µg/kg in children (age 5-7 years) showed a high inter-patient variability, but suggests that the clearance of the drug may be higher in children than in adults. This is supported by at least one repeat-dose study in postoperative pain that showed an optimal inter-dose interval of 4–5 hours in pediatric patients as opposed to the recommended 6–8 hours in adults.
Buprenorphine, in common with morphine and other phenolic opioid analgesics, is metabolized by the liver and its clearance is related to hepatic blood flow. Studies in patients anesthetized with 0.5% halothane have shown that this anesthetic decreases hepatic blood flow by about 30%.
Mechanism of Analgesic Action: Buprenex exerts its analgesic effect via high affinity binding to µ subclass opiate receptors in the central nervous system. Although Buprenex may be classified as a partial agonist, under the conditions of recommended use it behaves very much like classical µ agonists such as morphine. One unusual property of Buprenex observed in *in vitro* studies is its very slow rate of dissociation from its receptor. This could account for its longer duration of action than morphine, the unpredictability of its reversal by opioid antagonists, and its low level of manifest physical dependence.
Narcotic Antagonist Activity: Buprenorphine demonstrates narcotic antagonist activity and has been shown to be equipotent with naloxone as an antagonist of morphine in the mouse tail flick test.
Cardiovascular Effects: Buprenex may cause a decrease or, rarely, an increase in pulse rate and blood pressure in some patients.
Effects on Respiration: Under usual conditions of use in adults, both Buprenex and morphine show similar dose-related respiratory depressant effects. At adult therapeutic doses, Buprenex (0.3 mg buprenorphine) can decrease respiratory rate in an equivalent manner to an equianalgesic dose of morphine (10 mg). (See WARNINGS.)

INDICATIONS AND USAGE
Buprenex is indicated for the relief of moderate to severe pain.

CONTRAINDICATIONS
Buprenex should not be administered to patients who have been shown to be hypersensitive to the drug.

WARNINGS
Impaired Respiration: As with other potent opioids, clinically significant respiratory depression may occur within the recommended dose range in patients receiving therapeutic doses of buprenorphine. Buprenex should be used with caution in patients with compromised respiratory function (e.g., chronic obstructive pulmonary disease, cor pulmonale, decreased respiratory reserve, hypoxia, hypercapnia, or preexisting respiratory depression). Particular caution is advised if Buprenex is administered to patients taking or recently receiving drugs with CNS/respiratory depressant effects. In patients with the physical and/or pharmacological risk factors above, the dose should be reduced by approximately one-half.
NALOXONE MAY NOT BE EFFECTIVE IN REVERSING THE RESPIRATORY DEPRESSION PRODUCED BY BUPRENEX. THEREFORE, AS WITH OTHER POTENT OPIOIDS, THE PRIMARY MANAGEMENT OF OVERDOSE SHOULD BE THE REESTABLISHMENT OF ADEQUATE VENTILATION WITH MECHANICAL ASSISTANCE OF RESPIRATION, IF REQUIRED.
Interaction with Other Central Nervous System Depressants: Patients receiving Buprenex in the presence of other narcotic analgesics, general anesthetics, antihistamines, benzodiazepines, phenothiazines, other tranquilizers, sedative/hypnotics or other CNS depressants (including alcohol) may exhibit increased CNS depression. When such combined therapy is contemplated, it is particularly important that the dose of one or both agents be reduced.
Head Injury and Increased Intracranial Pressure: Buprenex, like other potent analgesics, may itself elevate cerebrospinal fluid pressure and should be used with caution in head injury, intracranial lesions and other circumstances where cerebrospinal pressure may be increased. Buprenex can produce miosis and changes in the level of consciousness which may interfere with patient evaluation.
Use in Ambulatory Patients: Buprenex may impair the mental or physical abilities required for the performance of potentially dangerous tasks such as driving a car or operating machinery. Therefore, Buprenex should be administered with caution to ambulatory patients who should be warned to avoid such hazards.
Use in Narcotic-Dependent Patients: Because of the narcotic antagonist activity of Buprenex, use in the physically dependent individual may result in withdrawal effects.

PRECAUTIONS
General: Buprenex should be administered with caution in the elderly, debilitated patients, in children and those with severe impairment of hepatic, pulmonary, or renal function; myxedema or hypothyroidism; adrenal cortical insufficiency (e.g., Addison's disease); CNS depression or coma; toxic psychoses; prostatic hypertrophy or urethral stricture; acute alcoholism, delirium tremens; or kyphoscoliosis.
Because Buprenex is metabolized by the liver, the activity of Buprenex may be increased and/or extended in those individuals with impaired hepatic function or those receiving other agents known to decrease hepatic clearance.
Buprenex has been shown to increase intracholedochal pressure to a similar degree as other opioid analgesics, and thus should be administered with caution to patients with dysfunction of the biliary tract.
Information for Patients: The effects of Buprenex, particularly drowsiness, may be potentiated by other centrally acting agents such as alcohol or benzodiazepines. It is particularly important that in these circumstances patients must not drive or operate machinery. Buprenex has some pharmacologic effects similar to morphine which in susceptible patients may lead to self-administration of the drug when pain no longer exists. Patients must not exceed the dosage of Buprenex prescribed by their physician. Patients should be urged to consult their physician if other prescription medications are currently being used or are prescribed for future use.
Drug Interactions: Drug interactions common to other potent opioid analgesics also may occur with Buprenex. Particular care should be taken when Buprenex is used in combination with central nervous system depressant drugs (see WARNINGS). Although specific information is not presently available, caution should be exercised when Buprenex is used in combination with MAO inhibitors. There have been reports of respiratory and cardiovascular collapse in patients who received therapeutic doses of diazepam and Buprenex. A suspected interaction between Buprenex and phenprocoumon resulting in purpura has been reported.
Carcinogenesis, Mutagenesis, Impairment of Fertility: The effects of Buprenex on fertility and gestation indices were investigated in rats by the subcutaneous and intramuscular routes at doses 10 to 1,000 times the proposed human doses. Dystocia was noted in dams treated with 1,000 times the human dose. No effects on fertility or gestation were noted in these Segment 1 studies.
Pregnancy: Pregnancy Category C. Reproduction studies have been performed in the rat at doses which ranged from 10 to 1,000 times the proposed human dose by the subcutaneous and intramuscular routes and 160 times the proposed human dose by the intravenous route. By the intramuscular route, Buprenex produced mild but statistically significant ($p < 0.05$) post-implantation losses and early fetal deaths at 10 and 100 but not 1,000 times the proposed human dose. No fetal malformations were noted in rats at any dose when Buprenex was administered by subcutaneous, intramuscu-

lar, or intravenous routes. In rabbits, intramuscularly administered Buprenex produced a dose-related trend for extra rib formation which attained statistical significance (p < 0.01) at 1,000 times the proposed human dose. By the intravenous route, doses in rats of 40 and 160 times the proposed human dose of Buprenex caused a slight increase in post-implantation losses that may have been treatment-related. No major fetal malformations were noted in drug treated groups when administered by intramuscular or intravenous routes.

There are no adequate and well-controlled studies in pregnant women. Buprenex should be used during pregnancy only if the potential benefit justifies the potential risk to the fetus.

Labor and Delivery: The safety of Buprenex given during labor and delivery has not been established.

Nursing Mothers: An apparent lack of milk production during general reproduction studies with Buprenex in rats caused decreased viability and lactation indices. It is unknown at this time whether or not Buprenex is excreted in human milk. Despite the lack of specific knowledge on this issue, it is reasonable to assume that Buprenex will enter human milk and caution should be exercised in the use of Buprenex when it is administered to nursing mothers.

Pediatric Use: The safety and effectiveness of Buprenex have been established for children between 2 and 12 years of age. Use of Buprenex in children is supported by evidence from adequate and well controlled trials of Buprenex in adults, with additional data from studies of 960 children ranging in age from 9 months to 18 years of age. Data is available from a pharmacokinetic study, several controlled clinical trials, and several large post-marketing studies and case series. The available information provides reasonable evidence that Buprenex may be used safely in children ranging from 2–12 years of age, and that it is of similar effectiveness in children as in adults.

ADVERSE REACTIONS

The most frequent side effect in clinical studies involving 1,133 patients was sedation which occurred in approximately two-thirds of the patients. Although sedated, these patients could easily be aroused to an alert state.

Other less frequent adverse reactions occurring in 5–10% of the patients were:

Nausea	Dizziness/Vertigo

Occurring in 1–5% of the patients:

Sweating	Headache
Hypotension	Nausea/Vomiting
Vomiting	Hypoventilation
Miosis	

The following adverse reactions were reported to have occurred in less than 1% of the patients:

CNS Effect: confusion, blurred vision, euphoria, weakness/fatigue, dry mouth, nervousness, depression, slurred speech, paresthesia.

Cardiovascular: hypertension, tachycardia, bradycardia.

Gastrointestinal: constipation.

Respiratory: dyspnea, cyanosis.

Dermatological: pruritus.

Ophthalmological: diplopia, visual abnormalities.

Miscellaneous: injection site reaction, urinary retention, dreaming, flushing/warmth, chills/cold, tinnitus, conjunctivitis, Wenckebach block, and psychosis.

Other effects observed infrequently include malaise, hallucinations, depersonalization, coma, dyspepsia, flatulence, apnea, rash, amblyopia, tremor, and pallor.

The following reactions have been reported to occur rarely: loss of appetite, dysphoria/agitation, diarrhea, urticaria, and convulsions/lack of muscle coordination.

In the United Kingdom, buprenorphine hydrochloride was made available under monitored release regulation during the first year of sale, and yielded data from 1,736 physicians on 9,123 patients (17,120 administrations). Data on 240 children under the age of 18 years were included in this monitored release program. No important new adverse effects attributable to buprenorphine hydrochloride were observed.

DRUG ABUSE AND DEPENDENCE

Buprenorphine hydrochloride is a partial agonist of the morphine type: i.e., it has certain opioid properties which may lead to psychic dependence of the morphine type due to an opiate-like euphoric component of the drug. Direct dependence studies have shown little physical dependence upon withdrawal of the drug. However, caution should be used in prescribing to individuals who are known to be drug abusers or ex-narcotic addicts. The drug may not substitute in acutely dependent narcotic addicts due to its antagonist component and may induce withdrawal symptoms.

OVERDOSAGE

Manifestations: Clinical experience with Buprenex overdosage has been insufficient to define the signs of this condition at this time. Although the antagonist activity of buprenorphine may become manifest at doses somewhat above the recommended therapeutic range, doses in the recom-

mended therapeutic range may produce clinically significant respiratory depression in certain circumstances. (See WARNINGS.)

Treatment: The respiratory and cardiac status of the patients should be monitored carefully. Primary attention should be given to the reestablishment of adequate respiratory exchange through provision of a patent airway and institution of assisted or controlled ventilation. Oxygen, intravenous fluids, vasopressors, and other supportive measures should be employed as indicated. Doxapram, a respiratory stimulant, may be used. **NALOXONE MAY NOT BE EFFECTIVE IN REVERSING THE RESPIRATORY DEPRESSION PRODUCED BY BUPRENEX. THEREFORE, AS WITH OTHER POTENT OPIOIDS, THE PRIMARY MANAGEMENT OF OVERDOSE SHOULD BE THE REESTABLISHMENT OF ADEQUATE VENTILATION WITH MECHANICAL ASSISTANCE OF RESPIRATION, IF REQUIRED.**

DOSAGE AND ADMINISTRATION

Adults: The usual dosage for persons 13 years of age and over is 1 ml Buprenex (0.3 mg buprenorphine) given by deep intramuscular or slow (over at least 2 minutes) intravenous injection at up to 6-hour intervals, as needed. Repeat once (up to 0.3 mg) if required, 30 to 60 minutes after initial dosage, giving consideration to previous dose pharmacokinetics, and thereafter only as needed. In high-risk patients (e.g., elderly, debilitated, presence of respiratory disease, etc.) and/or in patients where other CNS depressants are present, such as in the immediate postoperative period, the dose should be reduced by approximately one-half. Extra caution should be exercised with the intravenous route of administration, particularly with the initial dose.

Occasionally, it may be necessary to administer single doses of up to 0.6 mg to adults depending on the severity of the pain and the response of the patient. This dose should only be given I.M. and only to adult patients who are not in a high risk category (see WARNINGS and PRECAUTIONS). At this time, there are insufficient data to recommend single doses greater than 0.6 mg for long-term use.

Children: Buprenex has been used in children 2–12 years of age at doses between 2–6 micrograms/kg of body weight given every 4–6 hours. There is insufficient experience to recommend use in infants below the age of two years, single doses greater than 6 micrograms/kg of body weight, or the use of a repeat or second dose at 30–60 minutes (such as is used in adults). Since there is some evidence that not all children clear buprenorphine faster than adults, fixed interval or "round-the-clock" dosing should not be undertaken until the proper inter-dose interval has been established by clinical observation of the child. Physicians should recognize that, as with adults, some pediatric patients may not need to be remedicated for 6–8 hours.

Safety and Handling: Buprenex is supplied in sealed ampuls and poses no known environmental risk to health care providers. Accidental dermal exposure should be treated by removal of any contaminated clothing and rinsing the affected area with water.

Buprenex is a potent narcotic, and like all drugs of this class has been associated with abuse and dependence among health care providers. To control the risk of diversion, it is recommended that measures appropriate to the health care setting be taken to provide rigid accounting, control of wastage, and restriction of access.

Parenteral drug products should be inspected visually for particulate matter and discoloration prior to administration, whenever solution and container permit.

HOW SUPPLIED

Buprenex (buprenorphine hydrochloride) is supplied in clear glass snap-ampuls of 1 ml (0.3 mg buprenorphine).

NDC 12496-0757-1

Avoid excessive heat (over 104°F or 40°C). Protect from prolonged exposure to light.

Manufactured by:
Reckitt & Colman Products,
Hull, England HU8 7DS.

Distributed by:
Reckitt & Colman Pharmaceuticals Inc.,
Richmond, VA 23235.
Buprenex® is a trademark of Reckitt & Colman (Overseas) Limited.
REVISED JANUARY 1993

912801

Shown in Product Identification Guide, page 333

Check the **PINK** section
to find a particular **BRAND**.

Respa Pharmaceuticals, Inc.

P.O. BOX 88222
CAROL STREAM, IL 60188

Direct Inquiries to:
(630) 307-9920
FAX: (630) 307-2418

RESPA-DM TABLETS
DYE FREE/SUGAR FREE   ℞

Each tablet contain 30 mg Dextromethorphan and 600 mg Guaifenesin

DOSAGE

12 yr. and older 1 or 2 tab. B.I.D. 6 to 12 1 tab. B.I.D.

RESPA-GF TABLETS
DYE FREE/SUGAR FREE   ℞

Each tablet contain 600 mg Guaifenesin

DOSAGE

12 yr. and older 1 or 2 tab. B.I.D. 6 to 12 1 tab. B.I.D.

RESPA-1ST TABLETS
DYE FREE/SUGAR FREE   ℞

Each tab. contain 60 mg Pseudoephedrine and 600 mg Guaifenesin

DOSAGE

12 yr. and older 1 or 2 tab. B.I.D. 6 to 12 1 tab. B.I.D.

RESPAHIST CAPSULES
DYE FREE   ℞

Each capsule contain 6 mg Brompheniramine and 60 mg Pseudoephedrine

DOSAGE

12 yr. and older 1 or 2 capsules B.I.D. 6 to 12 1 Capsule B.I.D.

RESPA-A.R.M. Tablets
DYE FREE/SUGAR FREE   ℞

Each tablet contains: 25 mg Phenylephrine HCL, 50 mg Phenylpropanolamine HCL, 8 mg Chlorpheniramine MAL, Belladonna Alkaloids (Hyoscyamine Sulfate, Atropine Sulfate and Scopolamine Hydrobromide)

DOSAGE

Adults and Children over 12 years of age 1 tab B.I.D.

TRIKOF-D TABLETS
Dye Free/Sugar Free   ℞

Each tablet contain 600mg Guaifenesin, 30mg Dextromethorphan, 37.5mg Phenylpropanolamine

DOSAGE

12yr. and older 1 or 2 tab. B.I.D. 6 to 12 1 tab. B.I.D.

Rhône-Poulenc Rorer
Pharmaceuticals Inc.

500 ARCOLA ROAD
COLLEGEVILLE, PA 19426-0107

Direct Inquiries to:
QUALITY ASSURANCE QUESTIONS:
John Chiles, Manager, Quality Control
(610) 454-3130
REGULATORY AFFAIRS QUESTIONS:
Ron Panner, Group Director, Worldwide Regulatory Affairs
(610) 454-3026
For Medical Information Contact:
PRODUCT INFORMATION/ADVERSE DRUG EXPERIENCES/EMERGENCIES:
Medical Information and Education
1-800-340-7502
(610) 454-8110

Continued on next page

Following is a list of Rhône-Poulenc Rorer Pharmaceuticals Inc. products. Full prescribing information is provided on the following pages for those products indicated by an asterisk. For further information, please call Rhône-Poulenc Rorer Medical Information and Education at 1-800-340-7502 or (610) 454-8110.

H.P. ACTHAR® GEL ℞
80 USP Units/mL
Repository corticotropin injection available in 80 USP Units per mL.

*AZMACORT® Oral Inhaler ℞
Each metered-dose inhaler contains 60 mg triamcinolone acetonide. Each oral inhaler unit delivers 240 actuations of approximately 100 mcg of triamcinolone acetonide.
Pictured in Product Identification Guide, page 333

CALCIMAR® Injection, Synthetic ℞
Each 2-mL vial contains 400 I.U. (200 I.U. per mL) calcitonin-salmon as a sterile solution for subcutaneous or intramuscular injection.

*DDAVP® Injection ℞
Each mL of sterile, aqueous solution for injection provides 4 µg/mL desmopressin acetate.
Pictured in Product Identification Guide, page 333

*DDAVP® Injection 15 µg/mL ℞
Each mL of sterile, aqueous solution for injection provides 15 µg desmopressin acetate.
Pictured in Product Identification Guide, page 333

*DDAVP® Nasal Spray 5 mL ℞
Each mL of aqueous solution for intranasal use provides 0.1 mg desmopressin acetate.
Pictured in Product Identification Guide, page 333

DDAVP® Rhinal Tube 2.5 mL ℞
Each mL of aqueous solution for intranasal use provides 0.1 mg desmopressin acetate.

*DDAVP® Tablets ℞
Each tablet contains either 0.1 or 0.2 mg desmopressin acetate.
Pictured in Product Identification Guide, page 333

*GLIADEL® Wafer ℞
Each wafer implant contains the copolymer, polifeprosan 20, and 7.7 mg of carmustine.
Pictured in Product Identification Guide, page 333

HYGROTON® Tablets ℞
25 mg and 50 mg
Each tablet contains 25 mg or 50 mg chlorthalidone, USP.

*INTAL® Inhaler ℞
Each metered-dose aerosol unit delivers at least 112 (8.1 g canister) or at least 200 (14.2 g canister) inhalations containing 800 mcg cromolyn sodium.
Pictured in Product Identification Guide, page 333

*INTAL® Nebulizer Solution ℞
Each 2-mL ampule contains 20 mg cromolyn sodium inhalation solution, USP, in purified water.
Pictured in Product Identification Guide, page 333

*LOVENOX® Injection ℞
Prefilled syringes contain enoxaparin sodium in Water for Injection. Available in 30 mg, 40 mg, 60 mg, 80 mg, and 100 mg strengths. Each syringe contains 10 mg enoxaparin sodium per 0.1 mL Water for Injection. Also available in an ampule containing 30 mg enoxaparin sodium in 0.3 mL Water for Injection.
Pictured in Product Identification Guide, page 333

LOZOL® Tablets ℞
Each tablet contains 1.25 mg or 2.5 mg indapamide.

*NASACORT® AQ Nasal Spray ℞
Metered-dose pump spray unit delivers 120 actuations of 55 mcg aqueous triamcinolone acetonide.
Pictured in Product Identification Guide, page 333

*NASACORT® Nasal Inhaler ℞
This metered-dose aerosol unit delivers 100 actuations of 55 mcg of triamcinolone acetonide.
Pictured in Product Identification Guide, page 333

*NITROLINGUAL® SPRAY ℞
A 200-dose metered sublingual aerosol delivering 0.4 mg of nitroglycerin per actuation.
Pictured in Product Identification Guide, page 333

*ONCASPAR® ℞
Each 5-mL vial contains pegaspargase 750 IU/mL in a clear, colorless, phosphate buffered saline solution.

PAREPECTOLIN® Suspension
Each tablespoon contains 600 mg attapulgite in a pleasant-tasting suspension. (OTC)

*PENETREX™ Tablets ℞
Each 200-mg and 400-mg film-coated tablet contains enoxacin sesquihydrate equivalent to 200 mg and 400 mg of anhydrous enoxacin, respectively.
Pictured in Product Identification Guide, page 333

*RILUTEK® Tablets ℞
Each film-coated tablet contains 50 mg riluzole.
Pictured in Product Identification Guide, page 333

*SLO-BID™ Gyrocaps® ℞
50 mg, 75 mg, 100 mg, 125 mg, 200 mg, and 300 mg
Each extended-release capsule contains theophylline, anhydrous, USP.

SLO-PHYLLIN® Tablets ℞
100 mg and 200 mg
Each tablet contains 100 mg or 200 mg theophylline, anhydrous, USP.

SLO-PHYLLIN® Syrup ℞
Each 15 mL contains 80 mg theophylline, anhydrous, USP.

SLO-PHYLLIN® GG Capsules, Syrup ℞
Each capsule or 15 mL of syrup contains 150 mg of theophylline, anhydrous, and 90 mg of guaifenesin.

*TAXOTERE® for Injection Concentrate ℞
Single-dose vials contain either Taxotere (docetaxel) 80 mg Concentrate for Infusion or Taxotere (docetaxel) 20 mg Concentrate for Infusion with accompanying diluent. Taxotere Concentrate for Infusion contains polysorbate 80.
Pictured in Product Identification Guide, page 333

*TILADE® Inhaler ℞
Metered-dose aerosol unit delivers at least 104 metered inhalations of 1.75 mg nedocromil sodium from the mouthpiece.
Pictured in Product Identification Guide, page 334

TUSSAR® DM Syrup
Each 5 mL contains 15 mg dextromethorphan hydrobromide, USP; 2 mg chlorpheniramine maleate, USP; and 30 mg psuedoephedrine HCl, USP.

TUSSAR®–2 Syrup ℂ
Each 5 mL contains 10 mg codeine phosphate, USP; 30 mg pseudoephedrine HCl, USP; 100 mg guaifenesin, USP; and 2.5% alcohol.
(Warning: May be habit-forming.)

TUSSAR® SF Syrup ℂ
(Sugar Free)
Formulation identical to Tussar–2, except Tussar SF contains saccharin-sorbitol base for patients who must limit sugar intake. Alcohol content 2.5%.
(Warning: May be habit-forming.)

*ZAGAM® Tablets ℞
Each tablet contains 200 mg sparfloxacin.
Pictured in Product Identification Guide, page 334

*Please see full prescribing information on the following pages.

AZMACORT® ℞
[ăz 'ma-kort]
(triamcinolone acetonide)
Inhalation Aerosol

For Oral Inhalation Only
Shake Well Before Using

DESCRIPTION
Triamcinolone acetonide, USP, the active ingredient in **Azmacort®** Inhalation Aerosol, is a corticosteroid with a molecular weight of 434.5 and with the chemical designation 9-Fluoro-11β,16α,17,21-tetrahydroxypregna-1,4-diene-3,20-dione cyclic 16,17-acetal with acetone. ($C_{24}H_{31}FO_6$).

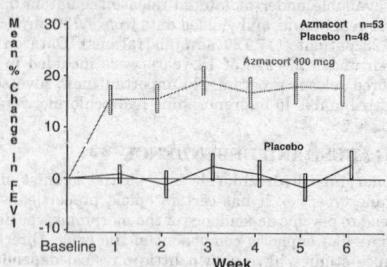

Azmacort Inhalation Aerosol is a metered-dose aerosol unit containing a microcrystalline suspension of triamcinolone acetonide in the propellant dichlorodifluoromethane and dehydrated alcohol USP 1% w/w. Each canister contains 60 mg triamcinolone acetonide. Each actuation delivers 200 mcg triamcinolone acetonide from the valve and 100 mcg from the spacer-mouthpiece under defined *in vitro* test conditions. There are at least 240 actuations in one **Azmacort** Inhalation Aerosol canister. **After 240 actuations, the amount delivered per actuation may not be consistent and the unit should be discarded.**

CLINICAL PHARMACOLOGY
Triamcinolone acetonide is a more potent derivative of triamcinolone. Although triamcinolone itself is approximately one to two times as potent as prednisone in animal models of inflammation, triamcinolone acetonide is approximately 8 times more potent than prednisone.
The precise mechanism of the action of glucocorticoids in asthma is unknown. However, the inhaled route makes it possible to provide effective local anti-inflammatory activity with reduced systemic corticosteroid effects. Though highly effective for asthma, glucocorticoids do not affect asthma symptoms immediately. While improvement in asthma may occur as soon as one week after initiation of **Azmacort** Inhalation Aerosol therapy, maximum improvement may not be achieved for 2 weeks or longer.
Based upon intravenous dosing of triamcinolone acetonide phosphate ester, the half-life of triamcinolone acetonide was reported to be 88 minutes. The volume of distribution (Vd) reported was 99.5 L (SD ± 27.5) and clearance was 45.2 L/hour (SD ± 9.1) for triamcinolone acetonide. The plasma half-life of glucocorticoids does not correlate well with the biologic half-life.
The pharmacokinetics of radiolabeled triamcinolone acetonide [14C] were evaluated following a single oral dose of 800 mcg to healthy male volunteers. Radiolabeled triamcinolone acetonide was found to undergo relatively rapid absorption following oral administration with maximum plasma triamcinolone acetonide and [14C]-derived radioactivity occurring between 1.5 and 2 hours. Plasma protein binding of triamcinolone acetonide appears to be relatively low and consistent over a wide plasma triamcinolone acetonide concentration range as a function of time. The overall mean percent fraction bound was approximately 68%.
The metabolism and excretion of triamcinolone acetonide were both rapid and extensive with no parent compound being detected in the plasma after 24 hours post-dose and a low ratio (10.6%) of parent compound $AUC_{0-\infty}$ to total [14C] radioactivity $AUC_{0-\infty}$. Greater than 90% of the oral [14C]-radioactive dose was recovered within 5 days after administration in 5 out of the 6 subjects in the study. Of the recovered [14C]-radioactivity, approximately 40% and 60% were found in the urine and feces, respectively.
Three metabolites of triamcinolone acetonide have been identified. They are 6β-hydroxytriamcinolone acetonide, 21-carboxytriamcinolone acetonide and 21-carboxy-6β-hydroxytriamcinolone acetonide. All three metabolites are expected to be substantially less active than the parent compound due to (a) the dependence of anti-inflammatory activity on the presence of a 21-hydroxyl group, (b) the decreased activity observed upon 6-hydroxylation, and (c) the markedly increased water solubility favoring rapid elimination. There appeared to be some quantitative differences in the metabolites among species. No differences were detected in metabolic pattern as a function of route of administration.

CLINICAL TRIALS
Double-blind, placebo controlled efficacy and safety studies have been conducted in asthma patients with a range of asthma severities, from those patients with mild disease to those with severe disease requiring oral steroid therapy.
The efficacy and safety of **Azmacort** Inhalation Aerosol given twice daily was demonstrated in two placebo-controlled clinical trials. In two separate studies, 222 asthmatic patients were randomized to receive either **Azmacort** Inhalation Aerosol 400 mcg twice daily or matching placebo for a treatment period of 6 weeks. Patients were adult asthmatics who were using inhaled beta$_2$-agonists on more than an occasional basis (at least three times weekly), either without or with inhaled corticosteroids, for control of their asthma symptoms. For the combined studies, 48% (52/109) patients randomized to placebo and 41% (46/113) patients randomized to **Azmacort** treatment were previously treated with inhaled corticosteroids.
Results of weekly lung function tests (FEV$_1$) from one of these trials is presented graphically below. Results of the second study are presented in tabular form as the changes in asthma measures from baseline to the end of the treatment period.

Mean Changes in Asthma Measures from Baseline to Endpoint[a]
All-Treated Patients
Results from a Placebo-Controlled, 6 Week Study

Asthma Measure	Placebo (N=61)	Azmacort 400 mcg bid (N=60)
Percent Change in FEV$_1$(%)	2.8%	17.5%
Increase in Morning Peak Flow Rate (L/min)	6.7	45.9

Decrease in Albuterol Use (puffs/day)	0.6	3.4
Decrease in Daily Asthma Symptom Score (units/day)[b]	0.5	2.3

[a] Endpoint Results are obtained from the last evaluable data, regardless of whether the patient completed 6 weeks of treatment.

[b] Scale (0–6) with 0 = no symptom: Maximum Score (AM + PM) = 12

In both studies, treatment with **Azmacort** Inhalation Aerosol (400 mcg twice daily) resulted in significant improvements in all clinical asthma measures (lung functions, asthma symptoms, use of as-needed $beta_2$-agonist medications) when compared to placebo.

INDICATIONS

Azmacort Inhalation Aerosol is indicated in the maintenance treatment of asthma as prophylactic therapy. **Azmacort** Inhalation Aerosol is also indicated for asthma patients who require systemic corticosteroid administration, where adding Azmacort may reduce or eliminate the need for the systemic corticosteroids.

Azmacort Inhalation Aerosol is NOT indicated for the relief of acute bronchospasm.

CONTRAINDICATIONS

Azmacort Inhalation Aerosol is contraindicated in the primary treatment of status asthmaticus or other acute episodes of asthma where intensive measures are required.

Hypersensitivity to triamcinolone acetonide or any of the other ingredients in this preparation contraindicates its use.

WARNINGS

Particular care is needed in patients who are transferred from systemically active corticosteroids to **Azmacort** Inhalation Aerosol because deaths due to adrenal insufficiency have occurred in asthmatic patients during and after transfer from systemic corticosteroids to aerosolized steroids in recommended doses.

After withdrawal from systemic corticosteroids, a number of months is usually required for recovery of hypothalamic-pituitary-adrenal (HPA) function. For some patients who have received large doses of oral steroids for long periods of time before therapy with **Azmacort** Inhalation Aerosol is initiated, recovery may be delayed for one year or longer. During this period of HPA suppression, patients may exhibit signs and symptoms of adrenal insufficiency when exposed to trauma, surgery, or infections, particularly gastroenteritis or other conditions with acute electrolyte loss. Although **Azmacort** Inhalation Aerosol may provide control of asthmatic symptoms during these episodes, in recommended doses it supplies only normal physiological amounts of corticosteroid systemically and does NOT provide the increased systemic steroid which is necessary for coping with these emergencies.

During periods of stress or a severe asthmatic attack, patients who have been recently withdrawn from systemic corticosteroids should be instructed to resume systemic steroids (in large doses) immediately and to contact their physician for further instruction. These patients should also be instructed to carry a warning card indicating that they may need supplementary systemic steroids during periods of stress or a severe asthma attack.

Localized infections with *Candida albicans* have occurred infrequently in the mouth and pharynx. These areas should be examined by the treating physician at each patient visit. The percentage of positive mouth and throat cultures for *Candida albicans* did not change during a year of continuous therapy. The incidence of clinically apparent infection is low (2.5%). These infections may disappear spontaneously or may require treatment with appropriate antifungal therapy or discontinuance of treatment with **Azmacort** Inhalation Aerosol.

Children who are on immunosuppressant drugs are more susceptible to infections than healthy children. Chickenpox and measles, for example, can have a more serious or even fatal course in children on immunosuppressant doses of corticosteroids. In such children, or in adults who have not had these diseases, particular care should be taken to avoid exposure. If exposed, therapy with varicella zoster immune globulin (VZIG) or pooled intravenous immunoglobulin (IVIG), as appropriate, may be indicated. If chickenpox develops, treatment with antiviral agents may be considered.

Azmacort Inhalation Aerosol is not to be regarded as a bronchodilator and is not indicated for rapid relief of bronchospasm.

As with other inhaled asthma medications, bronchospasm may occur with an immediate increase in wheezing following dosing. If bronchospasm occurs following use of **Azmacort** Inhalation Aerosol, it should be treated immediately with a fast-acting inhaled bronchodilator. Treatment with **Azmacort** Inhalation Aerosol should be discontinued and alternative treatment should be instituted.

Adverse Events Occurring at an Incidence of Greater Than 3% and Greater than Placebo

Adverse Event	Azmacort Dose 200 mcg bid (n=57)	Azmacort Dose 400 mcg bid (n=170)	Azmacort Dose 800 mcg bid (n=57)	Placebo (n=167)	Adverse Event	Azmacort Dose 200 mcg bid (n=57)	Azmacort Dose 400 mcg bid (n=170)	Azmacort Dose 800 mcg bid (n=57)	Placebo (n=167)
Sinusitis	5 (9%)	7 (4%)	1 (2%)	6 (4%)	Flu Syndrome	2 (4%)	8 (5%)	1 (2%)	5 (3%)
Pharyngitis	4 (7%)	42 (25%)	10 (18%)	19 (11%)	Back Pain	2 (4%)	3 (2%)	2 (4%)	3 (2%)
Headache	4 (7%)	35 (21%)	7 (12%)	24 (14%)					

Patients should be instructed to contact their physician immediately when episodes of asthma which are not responsive to bronchodilators occur during the course of treatment with **Azmacort** Inhalation Aerosol. During such episodes, patients may require therapy with systemic corticosteroids.

The use of **Azmacort** Inhalation Aerosol with systemic prednisone, dosed either daily or on alternate-days, could increase the likelihood of HPA suppression compared to a therapeutic dose of either one alone. Therefore, **Azmacort** Inhalation Aerosol should be used with caution in patients already receiving prednisone treatment for any disease.

Transfer of patients from systemic steroid therapy to **Azmacort** Inhalation Aerosol may unmask allergic conditions previously suppressed by the systemic steroid therapy, *e.g.,* rhinitis, conjunctivitis, and eczema.

PRECAUTIONS

During withdrawal from oral steroids, some patients may experience symptoms of systemically active steroid withdrawal, *e.g.,* joint and/or muscular pain, lassitude, and depression, despite maintenance or even improvement of respiratory function. (See **DOSAGE AND ADMINISTRATION**.) Although steroid withdrawal effects are usually transient and not severe, severe and even fatal exacerbation of asthma can occur if the previous daily oral corticosteroid requirement had significantly exceeded 10 mg/day of prednisone or equivalent.

In responsive patients, inhaled corticosteroids will often permit control of asthmatic symptoms with less suppression of HPA function than therapeutically equivalent oral doses of prednisone. Since triamcinolone acetonide is absorbed into the circulation and can be systemically active, the beneficial effects of **Azmacort** Inhalation Aerosol in minimizing or preventing HPA dysfunction may be expected only when recommended dosages are not exceeded.

Suppression of HPA function has been reported in volunteers who received 4000 mcg daily of triamcinolone acetonide by oral inhalation. In addition, suppression of HPA function has been reported in some patients who have received recommended doses for as little as 6 to 12 weeks. Since the response of HPA function to inhaled corticosteroids is highly individualized, the physician should consider this information when treating patients.

When used at excessive doses or at recommended doses in a small number of susceptible individuals, systemic corticosteroid effects such as hypercorticoidism and adrenal suppression may appear. If such changes occur, **Azmacort** Inhalation Aerosol should be discontinued slowly, consistent with accepted procedures for reducing systemic steroid therapy and for management of asthma symptoms.

Azmacort Inhalation Aerosol should be used with caution, if at all, in patients with active or quiescent tuberculosis infection of the respiratory tract; untreated systemic fungal, bacterial, parasitic, or viral infections; or ocular herpes simplex.

The long-term local and systemic effects of **Azmacort** Inhalation Aerosol in human subjects are still not fully known. While there has been no clinical evidence of adverse experiences, the effects resulting from chronic use of **Azmacort** Inhalation Aerosol on developmental or immunologic processes in the mouth, pharynx, trachea, and lung are unknown.

Because of the possibility of systemic absorption of inhaled corticosteroids, patients treated with these drugs should be observed carefully for any evidence of systemic corticosteroid effects including suppression of growth in children. Particular care should be taken in observing patients postoperatively or during periods of stress for evidence of a decrease in adrenal function.

Information for Patients: Patients being treated with **Azmacort** Inhalation Aerosol should receive the following information and instructions. This information is intended to aid them in the safe and effective use of this medication. It is not a complete disclosure of all possible adverse or intended effects.

Patients should use **Azmacort** Inhalation Aerosol at regular intervals as directed. Results of clinical trials indicate that significant improvement in asthma may occur by 1 week, but maximum benefit may not be achieved for 2 weeks or more. The patient should not increase the prescribed dosage but should contact the physician if symptoms do not improve or if the condition worsens.

In clinical studies and post-marketing experience with **Azmacort** Inhalation Aerosol, local infections of the oropharynx with *Candida albicans* have occurred. When such an infection develops, it should be treated with appropriate local or systemic (*i.e.,* oral antifungal) therapy while remaining on treatment with **Azmacort** Inhalation Aerosol. However, at times therapy with **Azmacort** Inhalation Aerosol may need to be interrupted.

Patients should be instructed to track their use of **Azmacort** Inhalation Aerosol and to dispose of the canister after 240 actuations since reliable dose delivery cannot be assured after 240 doses.

Patients who are on immunosuppressant doses of corticosteroids should be warned to avoid exposure to chickenpox or measles and, if exposed, to obtain medical advice.

Carcinogenesis, Mutagenesis, Impairment of Fertility: No evidence of treatment-related carcinogenicity was demonstrated after two years of once daily gavage of triamcinolone acetonide at doses of 0.05, 0.2, and 1.0 mcg/kg (approximately 0.02, 0.07, and 0.4% of the maximum recommended human daily inhalation dose on a mcg/m^2 basis) in the rat and 0.1, 0.6, and 3.0 mcg/kg (approximately 0.02, 0.1, and 0.6% of the maximum recommended human daily inhalation dose on a mcg/m^2 basis) in a mouse.

Mutagenesis studies with triamcinolone acetonide have not been carried out.

No evidence of impaired fertility was manifested when oral doses of up to 15.0 mcg/kg (8% of the maximum recommended human daily inhalation dose on a mcg/m^2 basis) were administered to female and male rats. However, triamcinolone acetonide at oral doses of 8 mcg/kg (approximately 4% of the maximum recommended human daily inhalation dose on a mcg/m^2 basis) caused dystocia and prolonged delivery and at oral doses of 5.0 mcg/kg (approximately 2.5% of the maximum recommended human daily inhalation dose on a mcg/m^2 basis) and above caused increases in fetal resorptions and stillbirths and decreases in pup body weight and survival. At a lower dose of 1.0 mcg/kg (approximately 0.5% of the maximum recommended human daily inhalation dose on a mcg/m^2 basis) it did not induce the above mentioned effects.

Pregnancy: Pregnancy Category C. Triamcinolone acetonide has been shown to be teratogenic at inhalational doses of 20, 40, and 80 mcg/kg in rats (approximately 0.1, 0.2, and 0.4 times the maximum recommended human daily inhalation dose on a mcg/m^2 basis, respectively), in rabbits at the same doses (approximately 0.2, 0.4, and 0.8 times the maximum recommended human daily inhalation dose on a mcg/m^2 basis, respectively) and in monkeys, at an inhalational dose of 500 mcg/kg (approximately 5 times the maximum recommended human daily inhalation dose on a mcg/m^2 basis). Dose related teratogenic effects in rats and rabbits included cleft palate and/or internal hydrocephaly and axial skeletal defects whereas the teratogenic effects observed in the monkey were CNS and/or cranial malformations. There are no adequate and well controlled studies in pregnant women. Triamcinolone acetonide should be used during pregnancy only if the potential benefit justifies the potential risk to the fetus.

Experience with oral glucocorticoids since their introduction in pharmacologic as opposed to physiologic doses suggests that rodents are more prone to teratogenic effects from glucocorticoids than humans. In addition, because there is a natural increase in glucocorticoid production during pregnancy, most women will require a lower exogenous steroid dose and many will not need glucocorticoid treatment during pregnancy.

Nonteratogenic Effects: Hypoadrenalism may occur in infants born of mothers receiving corticosteroids during pregnancy. Such infants should be carefully observed.

Nursing Mothers: It is not known whether triamcinolone acetonide is excreted in human milk. Because other corticosteroids are excreted in human milk, caution should be exercised when **Azmacort** Inhalation Aerosol is administered to nursing women.

Pediatric Use: Safety and effectiveness have not been established in pediatric patients below the age of 6. Oral corticosteroids have been shown to cause growth suppression

Continued on next page

Azmacort—Cont.

in children and teenagers, particularly with higher doses over extended periods. If a child or teenager on any corticosteroid appears to have growth suppression, the possibility that they are particularly sensitive to this effect of steroids should be considered.

ADVERSE REACTIONS

The table below describes the incidence of common adverse experiences based upon three placebo-controlled, multicenter US clinical trials of 507 patients (297 female and 210 male adults (age range 18-64)). These trials included asthma patients who had previously received inhaled beta$_2$-agonists alone, as well as those who previously required inhaled corticosteroid therapy for the control of their asthma. The patients were treated with **Azmacort** Inhalation Aerosol (including doses ranging from 200 to 800 mcg twice daily for 6 weeks) or placebo.

[See table at top of previous page]

Adverse events that occurred at an incidence of 1-3% in the overall **Azmacort** Inhalation Aerosol treatment group and greater than placebo included:

Body as a whole:	facial edema, pain, abdominal pain, photosensitivity
Digestive system:	diarrhea, oral monilia, toothache, vomiting
Metabolic and Nutrition:	weight gain
Musculoskeletal system:	bursitis, myalgia, tenosynovitis
Nervous system:	dry mouth
Organs of special sense:	rash
Respiratory system:	chest congestion, voice alteration
Urogenital system:	cystitis, urinary tract infection, vaginal monilia

In older controlled clinical trials of steroid dependent asthmatics, urticaria was reported rarely. Anaphylaxis was not reported in these controlled trials. Typical steroid withdrawal effects including muscle aches, joint aches, and fatigue were noted in clinical trials when patients were transferred from oral steroid therapy to **Azmacort** Inhalation Aerosol. Easy bruisability was also noted in these trials. Hoarseness, dry throat, irritated throat, dry mouth, facial edema, increased wheezing, and cough have been reported. These adverse effects have generally been mild and transient. Cases of oral candidiasis occurring with clinical use have been reported. (See **WARNINGS**.) Anaphylaxis has also been reported from post-marketing surveillance.

OVERDOSAGE

There are no data available on the effects of acute or chronic overdose. However, acute overdosing with **Azmacort** Inhalation Aerosol is unlikely in view of the total amount of active ingredient present and the route of administration. The maximum total daily dose (1600 mcg) has been well tolerated when administered as a single dose of 16 consecutive inhalations to adult asthmatics in a controlled clinical trial. Chronic overdosage may result in signs/symptoms of hypercorticoidism. (See **PRECAUTIONS**.) The risk of candidiasis could also be increased.

DOSAGE AND ADMINISTRATION

Adults: The usual recommended dosage is two inhalations (200 mcg) given three to four times a day or four inhalations (400 mcg) given twice daily. The maximal daily intake should not exceed 16 inhalations (1600 mcg) in adults. Higher initial doses (12 to 16 inhalations per day) may be considered in patients with more severe asthma.

Children 6 to 12 Years of Age: The usual recommended dosage is one or two inhalations (100 to 200 mcg) given three to four times a day or two to four inhalations (200 to 400 mcg) given twice daily. The maximal daily intake should not exceed 12 inhalations (1200 mcg) in children 6 to 12 years of age. Insufficient clinical data exist with respect to the safety and efficacy of the administration of **Azmacort** Inhalation Aerosol to children below the age of 6. The long-term effects of inhaled steroids, including **Azmacort** Inhalation Aerosol, on growth are still not fully known. Rinsing the mouth after inhalation is advised.

Different considerations must be given to the following groups of patients in order to obtain the full therapeutic benefit of **Azmacort** Inhalation Aerosol:

Note: In all patients, it is desirable to titrate to the lowest effective dose once asthma stability has been achieved.

Patients Not Receiving Systemic Corticosteroids: Patients who require maintenance therapy of their asthma may benefit from treatment with **Azmacort** Inhalation Aerosol at the doses recommended above. In patients who respond to **Azmacort** Inhalation Aerosol, improvement in pulmonary function is usually apparent within one to two weeks after the initiation of therapy.

Patients Maintained on Systemic Corticosteroids: Clinical studies have shown that **Azmacort** Inhalation Aerosol may be effective in the management of asthmatics dependent or maintained on systemic corticosteroids and may permit replacement or significant reduction in the dosage of systemic corticosteroids.

The patient's asthma should be reasonably stable before treatment with **Azmacort** Inhalation Aerosol is started. Initially, **Azmacort** Inhalation Aerosol should be used concurrently with the patient's usual maintenance dose of systemic corticosteroid. After approximately one week, gradual withdrawal of the systemic corticosteroid is started by reducing the daily or alternate daily dose. Reductions may be made after an interval of one or two weeks, depending on the response of the patient. A slow rate of withdrawal is strongly recommended. Generally, these decrements should not exceed 2.5 mg of prednisone or its equivalent. During withdrawal, some patients may experience symptoms of systemic corticosteroid withdrawal, e.g., joint and/or muscular pain, lassitude, and depression, despite maintenance or even improvement in pulmonary function. Such patients should be encouraged to continue with the inhaler but should be monitored for objective signs of adrenal insufficiency. If evidence of adrenal insufficiency occurs, the systemic corticosteroid doses should be increased temporarily and thereafter withdrawal should continue more slowly. Inhaled corticosteroids should be used with caution when used chronically in patients receiving prednisone regimens, either daily or alternate day. (See **WARNINGS**.)

During periods of stress or a severe asthma attack, transfer patients may require supplementary treatment with systemic corticosteroids.

Directions for Use: An illustrated leaflet of patient instructions for proper use accompanies each package of **Azmacort** Inhalation Aerosol.

HOW SUPPLIED

Azmacort Inhalation Aerosol contains 60 mg triamcinolone acetonide in a 20 gram package which delivers at least 240 actuations. It is supplied with a white plastic actuator, a white plastic spacer-mouthpiece and patient's leaflet of instructions: box of one. NDC 0075-0060-37. Each actuation delivers 200 mcg triamcinolone acetonide from the valve and 100 mcg from the spacer-mouthpiece under defined *in vitro* test conditions.

Avoid spraying in eyes.

For best results, the canister should be at room temperature before use.

Shake well before using.

CONTENTS UNDER PRESSURE. Do not puncture. Do not use or store near heat or open flame. Exposure to temperatures above 120°F may cause bursting. Never throw canister into fire or incinerator. Keep out of reach of children unless otherwise prescribed. STORE AT ROOM TEMPERATURE

Note: The indented statement below is required by the Federal government's Clean Air Act for all products containing or manufactured with chlorofluorocarbons (CFCs):

> WARNING: Contains CFC-12, a substance which harms public health and the environment by destroying ozone in the upper atmosphere.

A notice similar to the above WARNING has been placed in the "Information For The Patient" portion of this package insert under the Environmental Protection Agency's (EPA's) regulations. The patient's warning states that the patient should consult his or her physician if there are questions about alternatives.

Caution: Federal law prohibits dispensing without prescription.

Marketed by

RHÔNE-POULENC RORER PHARMACEUTICALS INC.
500 ARCOLA ROAD
COLLEGEVILLE, PA 19426
Rev. 6/97   IN-0367J

Shown in Product Identification Guide, page 333

DDAVP®
Injection 4 µg/mL   ℞
(desmopressin acetate)

DESCRIPTION

DDAVP® Injection 4 µg/mL (desmopressin acetate) is a synthetic analogue of the natural pituitary hormone 8-arginine vasopressin (ADH), an antidiuretic hormone affecting renal water conservation. It is chemically defined as follows:

Mol. Wt. 1183.34

Empirical Formula: $C_{46}H_{64}N_{14}O_{12}S_2 \cdot C_2H_4O_2 \cdot 3H_2O$

```
           O
           ‖
SCH₂CH₂C-Tyr-Phe-Gln-Asn-Cys-Pro-D-Arg-Gly-NH₂ • CH₃COOH • 3H₂O
 1       2   3   4   5   6   7   8   9
```

1-(3-mercaptopropionic acid)-8-D-arginine vasopressin monoacetate (salt) trihydrate.

DDAVP Injection 4 µg/mL is provided as a sterile, aqueous solution for injection.

Each mL provides:

Desmopressin acetate	4.0 µg
Sodium chloride	9.0 mg
Hydrochloric acid to adjust pH to 4	

The 10 mL vial contains chlorobutanol as a preservative (5.0 mg/mL).

CLINICAL PHARMACOLOGY

DDAVP Injection 4 µg/mL contains as active substance, desmopressin acetate, a synthetic analogue of the natural hormone arginine vasopressin. One mL (4 µg) of DDAVP (desmopressin acetate) solution has an antidiuretic activity of about 16 IU; 1 µg of DDAVP is equivalent to 4 IU.

DDAVP has been shown to be more potent than arginine vasopressin in increasing plasma levels of factor VIII activity in patients with hemophilia and von Willebrand's disease Type I.

Dose-response studies were performed in healthy persons, using doses of 0.1 to 0.4 µg/kg body weight, infused over a 10-minute period. Maximal dose response occurred at 0.3 to 0.4 µg/kg. The response to DDAVP of factor VIII activity and plasminogen activator is dose-related, with maximal plasma levels of 300 to 400 percent of initial concentrations obtained after infusion of 0.4 µg/kg body weight. The increase is rapid and evident within 30 minutes, reaching a maximum at a point ranging from 90 minutes to two hours. The factor VIII related antigen and ristocetin cofactor activity were also increased to a smaller degree, but still are dose-dependent.

1. The biphasic half-lives of DDAVP were 7.8 and 75.5 minutes for the fast and slow phases, respectively, compared with 2.5 and 14.5 minutes for lysine vasopressin, another form of the hormone. As a result, DDAVP provides a prompt onset of antidiuretic action with a long duration after each administration.

2. The change in structure of arginine vasopressin to DDAVP has resulted in a decreased vasopressor action and decreased actions on visceral smooth muscle relative to the enhanced antidiuretic activity, so that clinically effective antidiuretic doses are usually below threshold levels for effects on vascular or visceral smooth muscle.

3. When administered by injection, DDAVP has an antidiuretic effect about ten times that of an equivalent dose administered intranasally.

4. The bioavailability of the subcutaneous route of administration was determined qualitatively using urine output data. The exact fraction of drug absorbed by that route of administration has not been quantitatively determined.

5. The percentage increase of factor VIII levels in patients with mild hemophilia A and von Willebrand's disease was not significantly different from that observed in normal healthy individuals when treated with 0.3 µg/kg of DDAVP infused over 10 minutes.

6. Plasminogen activator activity increases rapidly after DDAVP infusion, but there has been no clinically significant fibrinolysis in patients treated with DDAVP.

7. The effect of repeated DDAVP administration when doses were given every 12 to 24 hours has generally shown a gradual diminution of the factor VIII activity increase noted with a single dose. The initial response is reproducible in any particular patient if there are 2 or 3 days between administrations.

INDICATIONS AND USAGE

Hemophilia A: DDAVP Injection 4 µg/mL is indicated for patients with hemophilia A with factor VIII coagulant activity levels greater than 5%.

DDAVP will often maintain hemostasis in patients with hemophilia A during surgical procedures and postoperatively when administered 30 minutes prior to scheduled procedure.

DDAVP will also stop bleeding in hemophilia A patients with episodes of spontaneous or trauma-induced injuries such as hemarthroses, intramuscular hematomas or mucosal bleeding.

DDAVP is not indicated for the treatment of hemophilia A with factor VIII coagulant activity levels equal to or less than 5%, or for the treatment of hemophilia B, or in patients who have factor VIII antibodies.

In certain clinical situations, it may be justified to try DDAVP in patients with factor VIII levels between 2% to 5%; however, these patients should be carefully monitored.

von Willebrand's Disease (Type I): DDAVP Injection 4 µg/mL is indicated for patients with mild to moderate classic von Willebrand's disease (Type I) with factor VIII levels greater than 5%. DDAVP will often maintain hemostasis in patients with mild to moderate von Willebrand's disease during surgical procedures and postoperatively when administered 30 minutes prior to the scheduled procedure.

DDAVP will usually stop bleeding in mild to moderate von Willebrand's patients with episodes of spontaneous or trauma-induced injuries such as hemarthroses, intramuscular hematomas or mucosal bleeding.

Those von Willebrand's disease patients who are least likely to respond are those with severe homozygous von Willebrand's disease with factor VIII coagulant activity and factor VIII von Willebrand factor antigen levels less

than 1%. Other patients may respond in a variable fashion depending on the type of molecular defect they have. Bleeding time and factor VIII coagulant activity, ristocetin cofactor activity, and von Willebrand factor antigen should be checked during administration of DDAVP to ensure that adequate levels are being achieved.

DDAVP is not indicated for the treatment of severe classic von Willebrand's disease (Type I) and when there is evidence of an abnormal molecular form of factor VIII antigen. (See **WARNINGS**.)

Diabetes Insipidus: DDAVP Injection 4 μg/mL is indicated as antidiuretic replacement therapy in the management of central (cranial) diabetes insipidus and for the management of the temporary polyuria and polydipsia following head trauma or surgery in the pituitary region. DDAVP is ineffective for the treatment of nephrogenic diabetes insipidus. DDAVP is also available as an intranasal preparation. However, this means of delivery can be compromised by a variety of factors that can make nasal insufflation ineffective or inappropriate. These include poor intranasal absorption, nasal congestion and blockage, nasal discharge, atrophy of nasal mucosa, and severe atrophic rhinitis. Intranasal delivery may be inappropriate where there is an impaired level of consciousness. In addition, cranial surgical procedures, such as transsphenoidal hypophysectomy, create situations where an alternative route of administration is needed as in cases of nasal packing or recovery from surgery.

CONTRAINDICATIONS

DDAVP Injection 4 μg/mL is contraindicated in individuals with known hypersensitivity to desmopressin acetate or any of the components of **DDAVP Injection 4 μg/mL.**

WARNINGS

Patients who do not have need of antidiuretic hormone for its antidiuretic effect, in particular those who are young or elderly, should be cautioned to ingest only enough fluid to satisfy thirst, in order to decrease the potential occurrence of water intoxication and hyponatremia.

Fluid intake should be adjusted downward, particularly in very young and elderly patients, in order to decrease the potential occurrence of water intoxication and hyponatremia. Particular attention should be paid to the possibility of the rare occurrence of an extreme decrease in plasma osmolality that may result in seizures which could lead to coma.

DDAVP should not be used to treat patients with Type IIB von Willebrand's disease since platelet aggregation may be induced.

PRECAUTIONS

General: For injection use only.

DDAVP® Injection 4 μg/mL (desmopressin acetate) has infrequently produced changes in blood pressure causing either a slight elevation in blood pressure or a transient fall in blood pressure and a compensatory increase in heart rate. The drug should be used with caution in patients with coronary artery insufficiency and/or hypertensive cardiovascular disease.

DDAVP (desmopressin acetate) should be used with caution in patients with conditions associated with fluid and electrolyte imbalance, such as cystic fibrosis, because these patients are prone to hyponatremia.

There have been rare reports of thrombotic events following **DDAVP Injection 4 μg/mL** in patients predisposed to thrombus formation. No causality has been determined, however, the drug should be used with caution in these patients.

Severe allergic reactions have been reported rarely. Fatal anaphylaxis has been reported in one patient who received intravenous DDAVP. It is not known whether antibodies to **DDAVP Injection 4 μg/mL** are produced after repeated injections.

Hemophilia A: Laboratory tests for assessing patient status include levels of factor VIII coagulant, factor VIII antigen and factor VIII ristocetin cofactor (von Willebrand factor) as well as activated partial thromboplastin time. Factor VIII coagulant activity should be determined before giving DDAVP for hemostasis. If factor VIII coagulant activity is present at less than 5% of normal, DDAVP should not be relied on.

von Willebrand's Disease: Laboratory tests for assessing patient status include levels of factor VIII coagulant activity, factor VIII ristocetin cofactor activity, and factor VIII von Willebrand factor antigen. The skin bleeding time may be helpful in following these patients.

Diabetes Insipidus: Laboratory tests for monitoring the patient include urine volume and osmolality. In some cases, plasma osmolality may be required.

Drug Interactions: Although the pressor activity of DDAVP is very low compared with the antidiuretic activity, use of doses as large as 0.3 μg/kg of DDAVP with other pressor agents should be done only with careful patient monitoring. DDAVP has been used with epsilon aminocaproic acid without adverse effects.

Carcinogenicity, Mutagenicity, Impairment of Fertility: Studies with DDAVP have not been performed to evaluate carcinogenic potential, mutagenic potential or effects on fertility.

Pregnancy Category B: Fertility studies have not been done. Teratology studies in rats and rabbits at doses from 0.05 to 10 μg/kg/day (approximately 0.1 times the maximum systemic human exposure in rats and up to 38 times the maximum systemic human exposure in rabbits based on surface area, mg/m²) revealed no harm to the fetus due to DDAVP. There are, however, no adequate and well controlled studies in pregnant women. Because animal reproduction studies are not always predictive of human response, this drug should be used during pregnancy only if clearly needed.

Several publications of desmopressin acetate's use in the management of diabetes insipidus during pregnancy are available; these include a few anecdotal reports of congenital anomalies and low birth weight babies. However, no causal connection between these events and desmopressin acetate has been established. A fifteen year, Swedish epidemiologic study of the use of desmopressin acetate in pregnant women with diabetes insipidus found the rate of birth defects to be no greater than that in the general population; however, the statistical power of this study is low. As opposed to preparations containing natural hormones, desmopressin acetate in antidiuretic doses has no uterotonic action and the physician will have to weigh the therapeutic advantages against the possible risks in each case.

Nursing Mothers: There have been no controlled studies in nursing women. A single study in postpartum women demonstrated a marked change in plasma, but little if any change in assayable DDAVP in breast milk following an intranasal dose of 10 μg. It is not known whether this drug is excreted in human milk. Because many drugs are excreted in human milk, caution should be exercised when DDAVP is administered to a nursing woman.

Pediatric Use: Use in infants and pediatric patients will require careful fluid intake restriction to prevent possible hyponatremia and water intoxication. **DDAVP Injection 4 μg/mL** *should not be used in infants less than three months of age* in the treatment of hemophilia A or von Willebrand's disease; safety and effectiveness in pediatric patients under 12 years of age with diabetes insipidus have not been established.

ADVERSE REACTIONS

Infrequently, DDAVP has produced transient headache, nausea, mild abdominal cramps and vulval pain. These symptoms disappeared with reduction in dosage. Occasionally, injection of DDAVP has produced local erythema, swelling or burning pain. Occasional facial flushing has been reported with the administration of DDAVP. **DDAVP Injection** has infrequently produced changes in blood pressure causing either a slight elevation or a transient fall and a compensatory increase in heart rate. Severe allergic reactions including anaphylaxis have been reported rarely with **DDAVP Injection.**

See **WARNINGS** for the possibility of water intoxication and hyponatremia.

There have been rare reports of thrombotic events (acute cerebrovascular thrombosis, acute myocardial infarction) following **DDAVP Injection** in patients predisposed to thrombus formation.

OVERDOSAGE

(See **ADVERSE REACTIONS**.) In case of overdosage, the dosage should be reduced, frequency of administration decreased, or the drug withdrawn according to the severity of the condition.

There is no known specific antidote for desmopressin acetate or **DDAVP Injection 4 μg/mL.**

An oral LD₅₀ has not been established. An intravenous dose of 2 mg/kg in mice demonstrated no effect.

DOSAGE AND ADMINISTRATION

Hemophilia A and von Willebrand's Disease (Type I): DDAVP Injection 4 μg/mL is administered as an intravenous infusion at a dose of 0.3 μg DDAVP/kg body weight diluted in sterile physiological saline and infused slowly over 15 to 30 minutes. In adults and children weighing more than 10 kg, 50 mL of diluent is recommended; in children weighing 10 kg or less, 10 mL of diluent is recommended. Blood pressure and pulse should be monitored during infusion. If **DDAVP Injection 4 μg/mL** is used preoperatively, it should be administered 30 minutes prior to the scheduled procedure.

The necessity for repeat administration of DDAVP or use of any blood products for hemostasis should be determined by laboratory response as well as the clinical condition of the patient. The tendency toward tachyphylaxis (lessening of response) with repeated administration given more frequently than every 48 hours should be considered in treating each patient.

Diabetes Insipidus: This formulation is administered subcutaneously or by direct intravenous injection. **DDAVP Injection 4 μg/mL** dosage must be determined for each patient and adjusted according to the pattern of response. Response should be estimated by two parameters: adequate duration of sleep and adequate, not excessive, water turnover.

The usual dosage range in adults is 0.5 mL (2.0 μg) to 1 mL (4.0 μg) daily, administered intravenously or subcutaneously, usually in two divided doses. The morning and evening doses should be separately adjusted for an adequate diurnal rhythm of water turnover. For patients who have been controlled on intranasal DDAVP and who must be switched to the injection form, either because of poor intranasal absorption or because of the need for surgery, the comparable antidiuretic dose of the injection is about one-tenth the intranasal dose.

Parenteral drug products should be inspected visually for particulate matter and discoloration prior to administration whenever solution and container permit.

HOW SUPPLIED

DDAVP Injection 4 μg/mL is available as a sterile solution in cartons of ten 1 mL single-dose ampules (NDC 0075-2451-01) and in 10 mL multiple-dose vials (NDC 0075-2451-53), each containing 4.0 μg DDAVP per mL.

Store refrigerated 2 to 8°C (36 to 46°F).

Caution: Federal law prohibits dispensing without prescription.

Keep out of the reach of children.

Military: 4 μg/mL—10 × 1 mL (NSN 6505-01-224-7450).

Rev. 9/97   IN-4708K

Manufactured for

RHÔNE-POULENC RORER PHARMACEUTICALS INC.
Collegeville, PA, U.S.A. 19426-0107
By Ferring Pharmaceuticals, Malmö, Sweden
Shown in Product Identification Guide, page 333

DDAVP®
Injection 15 μg/mL
(desmopressin acetate)   ℞

DESCRIPTION

DDAVP® Injection 15 μg/mL (desmopressin acetate) is a synthetic analogue of the natural pituitary hormone 8-arginine vasopressin (ADH), an antidiuretic hormone affecting renal water conservation. It is chemically defined as follows:
Mol. Wt. 1183.34
Empirical Formula: $C_{46}H_{64}N_{14}O_{12}S_2 \cdot C_2H_4O_2 \cdot 3H_2O$

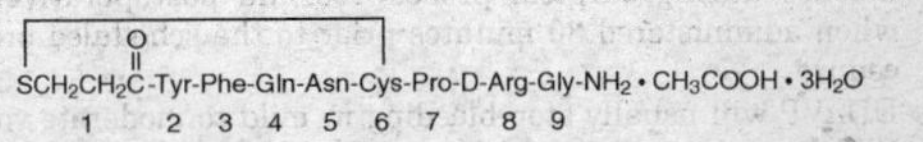

SCH₂CH₂C-Tyr-Phe-Gln-Asn-Cys-Pro-D-Arg-Gly-NH₂ • CH₃COOH • 3H₂O
1   2   3   4   5   6   7   8   9

1-(3-mercaptopropionic acid)-8-D-arginine vasopressin monoacetate (salt) trihydrate.

DDAVP Injection 15 μg/mL is provided as a sterile, aqueous solution for injection.
Each mL provides:
Desmopressin acetate .... 15.0 μg
Sodium chloride .... 9.0 mg
Hydrochloric acid to adjust pH to 4
The ampules contain either 1 mL (15 μg) or 2 mL (30 μg).

CLINICAL PHARMACOLOGY

DDAVP Injection 15 μg/mL contains as active substance, desmopressin acetate, a synthetic analogue of the natural hormone arginine vasopressin. One mL (15 μg) of DDAVP (desmopressin acetate) solution has an antidiuretic activity of about 60 IU; 1 μg of DDAVP is equivalent to 4 IU.

DDAVP has been shown to be more potent than arginine vasopressin in increasing plasma levels of factor VIII activity in patients with hemophilia and von Willebrand's disease Type I.

Dose-response studies were performed in healthy persons, using doses of 0.1 to 0.4 μg/kg body weight, infused over a 10-minute period. Maximal dose response occurred at 0.3 to 0.4 μg/kg. The response to DDAVP of factor VIII activity and plasminogen activator is dose-related, with maximal plasma levels of 300 to 400 percent of initial concentrations obtained after infusion of 0.4 μg/kg body weight. The increase is rapid and evident within 30 minutes, reaching a maximum at a point ranging from 90 minutes to two hours. The factor VIII related antigen and ristocetin cofactor activity were also increased to a smaller degree, but still are dose-dependent.

1. The biphasic half-lives of DDAVP were 7.8 and 75.5 minutes for the fast and slow phases, respectively, compared with 2.5 and 14.5 minutes for lysine vasopressin, another form of the hormone. As a result, DDAVP provides a prompt onset of antidiuretic action with a long duration after each administration.

2. The change in structure of arginine vasopressin to DDAVP has resulted in a decreased vasopressor action and decreased actions on visceral smooth muscle relative to the enhanced antidiuretic activity, so that clinically effective antidiuretic doses are usually below threshold levels for effects on vascular or visceral smooth muscle.

Continued on next page

DDAVP Injection 15 mcg/ml—Cont.

3. When administered by injection, DDAVP has an antidiuretic effect about ten times that of an equivalent dose administered intranasally.
4. The percentage increase of factor VIII levels in patients with mild hemophilia A and von Willebrand's disease was not significantly different from that observed in normal healthy individuals when treated with 0.3 µg/kg of DDAVP infused over 10 minutes.
5. Plasminogen activator activity increases rapidly after DDAVP infusion, but there has been no clinically significant fibrinolysis in patients treated with DDAVP.
6. The effect of repeated DDAVP administration when doses were given every 12 to 24 hours has generally shown a gradual diminution of the factor VIII activity increase noted with a single dose. The initial response is reproducible in any particular patient if there are 2 or 3 days between administrations.

INDICATIONS AND USAGE

Hemophilia A: DDAVP Injection 15 µg/mL is indicated for patients with hemophilia A with factor VIII coagulant activity levels greater than 5%.

DDAVP will often maintain hemostasis in patients with hemophilia A during surgical procedures and postoperatively when administered 30 minutes prior to scheduled procedure.

DDAVP will also stop bleeding in hemophilia A patients with episodes of spontaneous or trauma-induced injuries such as hemarthroses, intramuscular hematomas or mucosal bleeding.

DDAVP is not indicated for the treatment of hemophilia A with factor VIII coagulant activity levels equal to or less than 5%, or for the treatment of hemophilia B, or in patients who have factor VIII antibodies.

In certain clinical situations, it may be justified to try DDAVP in patients with factor VIII levels between 2% to 5%; however, these patients should be carefully monitored.

von Willebrand's Disease (Type I): DDAVP Injection 15 µg/mL is indicated for patients with mild to moderate classic von Willebrand's disease (Type I) with factor VIII levels greater than 5%. DDAVP will often maintain hemostasis in patients with mild to moderate von Willebrand's disease during surgical procedures and postoperatively when administered 30 minutes prior to the scheduled procedure.

DDAVP will usually stop bleeding in mild to moderate von Willebrand's patients with episodes of spontaneous or trauma-induced injuries such as hemarthroses, intramuscular hematomas or mucosal bleeding.

Those von Willebrand's disease patients who are least likely to respond are those with severe homozygous von Willebrand's disease with factor VIII coagulant activity and factor VIII von Willebrand factor antigen levels less than 1%. Other patients may respond in a variable fashion depending on the type of molecular defect they have. Bleeding time and factor VIII coagulant activity, ristocetin cofactor activity, and von Willebrand factor antigen should be checked during administration of DDAVP to ensure that adequate levels are being achieved.

DDAVP is not indicated for the treatment of severe classic von Willebrand's disease (Type I) and when there is evidence of an abnormal molecular form of factor VIII antigen. (See **WARNINGS**.)

CONTRAINDICATIONS

DDAVP Injection 15 µg/mL is contraindicated in individuals with known hypersensitivity to desmopressin acetate or to any of the components of **DDAVP Injection 15 µg/mL**.

WARNINGS

Patients who do not have need of antidiuretic hormone for its antidiuretic effect, in particular those who are young or elderly, should be cautioned to ingest only enough fluid to satisfy thirst, in order to decrease the potential occurrence of water intoxication and hyponatremia.

Fluid intake should be adjusted downward, particularly in very young and elderly patients, in order to decrease the potential occurrence of water intoxication and hyponatremia. Particular attention should be paid to the possibility of the rare occurrence of an extreme decrease in plasma osmolality that may result in seizures which could lead to coma.

DDAVP should not be used to treat patients with Type IIB von Willebrand's disease since platelet aggregation may be induced.

PRECAUTIONS

General: For injection use only.

DDAVP Injection 15 µg/mL has infrequently produced changes in blood pressure causing either a slight elevation in blood pressure or a transient fall in blood pressure and a compensatory increase in heart rate. The drug should be used with caution in patients with coronary artery insufficiency and/or hypertensive cardiovascular disease.

DDAVP (desmopressin acetate) should be used with caution in patients with conditions associated with fluid and electrolyte imbalance, such as cystic fibrosis, because these patients are prone to hyponatremia.

There have been rare reports of thrombotic events following **DDAVP® Injection 15 µg/mL** (desmopressin acetate) in patients predisposed to thrombus formation. No causality has been determined, however, the drug should be used with caution in these patients.

Severe allergic reactions have been reported rarely. Fatal anaphylaxis has been reported in one patient who received intravenous DDAVP. It is not known whether antibodies to **DDAVP Injection 15 µg/mL** are produced after repeated injections.

Hemophilia A: Laboratory tests for assessing patient status include levels of factor VIII coagulant, factor VIII antigen and factor VIII ristocetin cofactor (von Willebrand factor) as well as activated partial thromboplastin time. Factor VIII coagulant activity should be determined before giving DDAVP for hemostasis. If factor VIII coagulant activity is present at less than 5% of normal, DDAVP should not be relied on.

von Willebrand's Disease: Laboratory tests for assessing patient status include levels of factor VIII coagulant activity, factor VIII ristocetin cofactor activity, and factor VIII von Willebrand factor antigen. The skin bleeding time may be helpful in following these patients.

Drug Interactions: Although the pressor activity of DDAVP is very low compared with the antidiuretic activity, use of doses as large as 0.3 µg/kg of DDAVP with other pressor agents should be done only with careful patient monitoring. DDAVP has been used with epsilon aminocaproic acid without adverse effects.

Carcinogenicity, Mutagenicity, Impairment of Fertility: Studies with DDAVP have not been performed to evaluate carcinogenic potential, mutagenic potential or effects on fertility.

Pregnancy Category B: Fertility studies have not been done. Teratology studies in rats and rabbits at doses from 0.05 to 10 µg/kg/day (approximately 0.1 times the maximum systemic human exposure in rats and up to 38 times the maximum systemic human exposure in rabbits based on surface area, mg/m^2) revealed no harm to the fetus due to DDAVP. There are, however, no adequate and well controlled studies in pregnant women. Because animal reproduction studies are not always predictive of human response, this drug should be used during pregnancy only if clearly needed.

Several publications of desmopressin acetate's use in the management of diabetes insipidus during pregnancy are available; these include a few anecdotal reports of congenital anomalies and low birth weight babies. However, no causal connection between these events and desmopressin acetate has been established. A fifteen year, Swedish epidemiologic study of the use of desmopressin acetate in pregnant women with diabetes insipidus found the rate of birth defects to be no greater than that in the general population; however the statistical power of this study is low. As opposed to preparations containing natural hormones, desmopressin acetate in antidiuretic doses has no uterotonic action and the physician will have to weigh the therapeutic advantages against the possible risks in each case.

Nursing Mothers: There have been no controlled studies in nursing mothers. A single study in postpartum women demonstrated a marked change in plasma, but little if any change in assayable DDAVP in breast milk following an intranasal dose of 10 µg. It is not known whether this drug is excreted in human milk. Because many drugs are excreted in human milk, caution should be exercised when DDAVP is administered to a nursing woman.

Pediatric Use: Use in infants and pediatric patients will require careful fluid intake restriction to prevent possible hyponatremia and water intoxication. **DDAVP Injection 15 µg/mL** *should not be used in infants less than three months of age* in the treatment of hemophilia A or von Willebrand's disease.

ADVERSE REACTIONS

Infrequently, DDAVP has produced transient headache, nausea, mild abdominal cramps and vulval pain. These symptoms disappeared with reduction in dosage. Occasionally, injection of DDAVP has produced local erythema, swelling or burning pain. Occasional facial flushing has been reported with the administration of DDAVP. **DDAVP Injection** has infrequently produced changes in blood pressure causing either a slight elevation or a transient fall and a compensatory increase in heart rate. Severe allergic reactions including anaphylaxis have been reported rarely with **DDAVP Injection**.

See **WARNINGS** for the possibility of water intoxication and hyponatremia.

There have been rare reports of thrombotic events (acute cerebrovascular thrombosis, acute myocardial infarction) following **DDAVP Injection** in patients predisposed to thrombus formation.

OVERDOSAGE

(See **ADVERSE REACTIONS**.) In case of overdosage, the dosage should be reduced, frequency of administration decreased, or the drug withdrawn according to the severity of the condition.

There is no known specific antidote for desmopressin acetate or **DDAVP Injection 15 µg/mL.**

An oral LD_{50} has not been established. An intravenous dose of 2 mg/kg in mice demonstrated no effect.

DOSAGE AND ADMINISTRATION

Hemophilia A and von Willebrand's Disease (Type I): DDAVP Injection 15 µg/mL is administered as an intravenous infusion at a dose of 0.3 µg DDAVP/kg body weight diluted in sterile physiological saline and infused slowly over 15 to 30 minutes. In adults and children weighing more than 10 kg, 50 mL of diluent is recommended; in children weighing 10 kg or less, 10 mL of diluent is recommended. Blood pressure and pulse should be monitored during infusion. If **DDAVP Injection 15 µg/mL** is used preoperatively, it should be administered 30 minutes prior to the scheduled procedure.

The necessity for repeat administration of DDAVP or use of any blood products for hemostasis should be determined by laboratory response as well as the clinical condition of the patient. The tendency toward tachyphylaxis (lessening of response) with repeated administration given more frequently than every 48 hours should be considered in treating each patient.

Parenteral drug products should be inspected visually for particulate matter and discoloration prior to administration whenever solution and container permit.

See directions for use of One Point Cut (OPC) ampules for **DDAVP Injection** on back of carton.

HOW SUPPLIED

DDAVP Injection 15 µg/mL is available as a sterile solution in cartons of five 1 mL ampules (NDC 0075-0945-01) and five 2 mL ampules (NDC 0075-0945-02). Each vial is marked with two red rings and contains 15 µg DDAVP per mL.

Store refrigerated 2 to 8°C (36 to 46°F).

Caution: Federal law prohibits dispensing without prescription.

Keep out of the reach of children.

Manufactured for
RHÔNE-POULENC RORER PHARMACEUTICALS INC.
Collegeville, PA, U.S.A. 19426-0107
By Ferring Pharmaceuticals, Malmö, Sweden
Rev. 11/97 IN-6531C

Shown in Product Identification Guide, page 333

DDAVP® Nasal Spray ℞
(desmopressin acetate)

DESCRIPTION

DDAVP® Nasal Spray (desmopressin acetate) is a synthetic analogue of the natural pituitary hormone 8-arginine vasopressin (ADH), an antidiuretic hormone affecting renal water conservation. It is chemically defined as follows:

Mol. wt. 1183.34

Empirical formula: $C_{46}H_{64}N_{14}O_{12}S_2 \bullet C_2H_4O_2 \bullet 3H_2O$

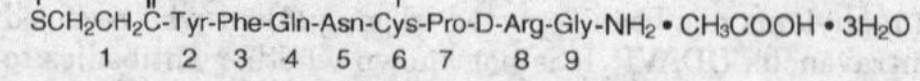
SCH2CH2C-Tyr-Phe-Gln-Asn-Cys-Pro-D-Arg-Gly-NH2 • CH3COOH • 3H2O
1 2 3 4 5 6 7 8 9

1-(3-mercaptopropionic acid)-8-D-arginine vasopressin monoacetate (salt) trihydrate.

DDAVP Nasal Spray is provided as an aqueous solution for intranasal use.

Each mL contains:

Desmopressin acetate	0.1 mg
Sodium Chloride	7.5 mg
Citric acid monohydrate	1.7 mg
Disodium phosphate dihydrate	3.0 mg
Benzalkonium chloride solution (50%)	0.2 mg

The **DDAVP Nasal Spray** compression pump delivers 0.1 mL (10 µg) of DDAVP (desmopressin acetate) per spray.

CLINICAL PHARMACOLOGY

DDAVP contains as active substance desmopressin acetate, a synthetic analogue of the natural hormone arginine vasopressin. One mL (0.1 mg) of intranasal DDAVP has an antidiuretic activity of about 400 IU; 10 µg of desmopressin acetate is equivalent to 40 IU.

1. The biphasic half-lives for intranasal DDAVP were 7.8 and 75.5 minutes for the fast and slow phases, compared with 2.5 and 14.5 minutes for lysine vasopressin, another form of the hormone used in this condition. As a result, intranasal DDAVP provides a prompt onset of antidiuretic action with a long duration after each administration.
2. The change in structure of arginine vasopressin to DDAVP has resulted in a decreased vasopressor action

and decreased actions on visceral smooth muscle relative to the enhanced antidiuretic activity, so that clinically effective antidiuretic doses are usually below threshold levels for effects on vascular or visceral smooth muscle.

3. DDAVP administered intranasally has an antidiuretic effect about one-tenth that of an equivalent dose administered by injection.

INDICATIONS AND USAGE

Primary Nocturnal Enuresis: DDAVP Nasal Spray is indicated for the management of primary nocturnal enuresis. It may be used alone or adjunctive to behavioral conditioning or other nonpharmacological intervention. It has been shown to be effective in some cases that are refractory to conventional therapies.

Central Cranial Diabetes Insipidus: DDAVP Nasal Spray is indicated as antidiuretic replacement therapy in the management of central cranial diabetes insipidus and for management of the temporary polyuria and polydipsia following head trauma or surgery in the pituitary region. It is ineffective for the treatment of nephrogenic diabetes insipidus.

The use of **DDAVP Nasal Spray** in patients with an established diagnosis will result in a reduction in urinary output with increase in urine osmolality and a decrease in plasma osmolality. This will allow the resumption of a more normal life-style with a decrease in urinary frequency and nocturia. There are reports of an occasional change in response with time, usually greater than 6 months. Some patients may show a decreased responsiveness, others a shortened duration of effect. There is no evidence this effect is due to the development of binding antibodies but may be due to a local inactivation of the peptide.

Patients are selected for therapy by establishing the diagnosis by means of the water deprivation test, the hypertonic saline infusion test, and/or the response to antidiuretic hormone. Continued response to intranasal DDAVP can be monitored by urine volume and osmolality.

DDAVP is also available as a solution for injection when the intranasal route may be compromised. These situations include nasal congestion and blockage, nasal discharge, atrophy of nasal mucosa, and severe atrophic rhinitis. Intranasal delivery may also be inappropriate where there is an impaired level of consciousness. In addition, cranial surgical procedures, such as transphenoidal hypophysectomy create situations where an alternative route of administration is needed as in cases of nasal packing or recovery from surgery.

CONTRAINDICATIONS

DDAVP Nasal Spray is contraindicated in individuals with known hypersensitivity to desmopressin acetate or to any of the components of **DDAVP Nasal Spray**.

WARNINGS

1. For intranasal use only.
2. In very young and elderly patients in particular, fluid intake should be adjusted downward in order to decrease the potential occurrence of water intoxication and hyponatremia. Particular attention should be paid to the possibility of the rare occurrence of an extreme decrease in plasma osmolality that may result in seizures which could lead to coma.

PRECAUTIONS

General: Intranasal DDAVP at high dosage has infrequently produced a slight elevation of blood pressure, which disappeared with a reduction in dosage. The drug should be used with caution in patients with coronary artery insufficiency and/or hypertensive cardiovascular disease because of possible rise in blood pressure.

DDAVP should be used with caution in patients with conditions associated with fluid and electrolyte imbalance, such as cystic fibrosis, because these patients are prone to hyponatremia.

Rare severe allergic reactions have been reported with DDAVP. Anaphylaxis has been reported with intravenous administration of DDAVP Injection, but not with DDAVP intranasal.

Central Cranial Diabetes Insipidus: Since DDAVP is used intranasally, changes in the nasal mucosa such as scarring, edema, or other disease may cause erratic, unreliable absorption in which case intranasal DDAVP should not be used. For such situations, DDAVP Injection should be considered.

Primary Nocturnal Enuresis: If changes in the nasal mucosa have occurred, unreliable absorption may result. **DDAVP Nasal Spray** should be discontinued until the nasal problems resolve.

Information for Patients: Patients should be informed that the **DDAVP Nasal Spray** bottle accurately delivers 50 doses of 10 µg each. Any solution remaining after 50 doses should be discarded since the amount delivered thereafter may be substantially less than 10 µg of drug. No attempt should be made to transfer remaining solution to another bottle. Patients should be instructed to read accompanying directions on use of the spray pump carefully before use.

Laboratory Tests: Laboratory tests for following the patient with central cranial diabetes insipidus or post-surgical or head trauma-related polyuria and polydipsia include urine volume and osmolality. In some cases plasma osmolality measurements may be required. For the healthy patient with primary nocturnal enuresis, serum electrolytes should be checked at least once if therapy is continued beyond 7 days.

Drug Interactions: Although the pressor activity of DDAVP is very low compared to the antidiuretic activity, use of large doses of intranasal DDAVP with other pressor agents should only be done with careful patient monitoring.

Carcinogenesis, Mutagenesis, Impairment of Fertility: Studies with DDAVP have not been performed to evaluate carcinogenic potential, mutagenic potential or effects on fertility.

Pregnancy: *Category B:* Fertility studies have not been done. Teratology studies in rats and rabbits at doses from 0.05 to 10 µg/kg/day (approximately 0.1 times the maximum systemic human exposure in rats and up to 38 times the maximum systemic human exposure in rabbits based on surface area, mg/m²) revealed no harm to the fetus due to DDAVP (desmopressin acetate). There are, however, no adequate and well controlled studies in pregnant women. Because animal reproduction studies are not always predictive of human response, this drug should be used during pregnancy only if clearly needed.

Several publications of desmopressin acetate's use in the management of diabetes insipidus during pregnancy are available; these include a few anecdotal reports of congenital anomalies and low birth weight babies. However, no causal connection between these events and desmopressin acetate has been established. A fifteen year Swedish epidemiologic study of the use of desmopressin acetate in pregnant women with diabetes insipidus found the rate of birth defects to be no greater than that in the general population; however, the statistical power of this study is low. As opposed to preparations containing natural hormones, desmopressin acetate in antidiuretic doses has no uterotonic action and the physician will have to weigh the therapeutic advantages against the possible risks in each case.

Nursing Mothers: There have been no controlled studies in nursing mothers. A single study in a post-partum woman demonstrated a marked change in plasma, but little if any change in assayable DDAVP in breast milk following an intranasal dose of 10 µg. It is not known whether this drug is excreted in human milk. Because many drugs are excreted in human milk, caution should be exercised when DDAVP is administered to a nursing woman.

Pediatric Use: *Primary Nocturnal Enuresis:*
DDAVP Nasal Spray (desmopressin acetate) has been used in childhood nocturnal enuresis. Short-term (4–8 weeks) **DDAVP Nasal Spray** administration has been shown to be safe and modestly effective in pediatric patients aged 6 years or older with severe childhood nocturnal enuresis. Adequately controlled studies with intranasal DDAVP in primary nocturnal enuresis have not been conducted beyond 4–8 weeks. The dose should be individually adjusted to achieve the best results.

Central Cranial Diabetes Insipidus: DDAVP Nasal Spray has been used in children with diabetes insipidus. Use in infants and children will require careful fluid intake restriction to prevent possible hyponatremia and water intoxication. The dose must be individually adjusted to the patient with attention in the very young to the danger of an extreme decrease in plasma osmolality with resulting convulsions. Dose should start at 0.05 mL or less.

Since the spray cannot deliver less than 0.1 mL (10 µg), smaller doses should be administered using the rhinal tube delivery system. Do not use the nasal spray in pediatric patients requiring less than 0.1 mL (10 µg) per dose.

There are reports of an occasional change in response with time, usually greater than 6 months. Some patients may show a decreased responsiveness, others a shortened duration of effect. There is no evidence this effect is due to the development of binding antibodies but may be due to a local inactivation of the peptide.

ADVERSE REACTIONS

Infrequently, high dosages of intranasal DDAVP have produced transient headache and nausea. Nasal congestion, rhinitis and flushing have also been reported occasionally along with mild abdominal cramps. These symptoms disappeared with reduction in dosage. Nosebleed, sore throat, cough and upper respiratory infections have also been reported.

The following table lists the percentage of patients having adverse experiences without regard to relationship to study drug from the pooled pivotal study data for nocturnal enuresis.

ADVERSE REACTION	PLACEBO (N=59) %	DDAVP 20 µg (N=60) %	DDAVP 40 µg (N=61) %
BODY AS A WHOLE			
Abdominal Pain	0	2	2
Asthenia	0	0	2
Chills	0	0	2
Headache	0	2	5
Throat Pain	2	0	0
NERVOUS SYSTEM			
Depression	2	0	0
Dizziness	0	0	3
RESPIRATORY SYSTEM			
Epistaxis	2	3	0
Nostril Pain	0	2	0
Respiratory Infection	2	0	0
Rhinitis	2	8	3
CARDIOVASCULAR SYSTEM			
Vasodilation	2	0	0
DIGESTIVE SYSTEM			
Gastrointestinal Disorder	0	2	0
Nausea	0	0	2
SKIN & APPENDAGES			
Leg Rash	2	0	0
Rash	2	0	0
SPECIAL SENSES			
Conjunctivitis	0	2	0
Edema Eyes	0	2	0
Lachrymation Disorder	0	0	2

See **WARNINGS** for the possibility of water intoxication and hyponatremia.

OVERDOSAGE

(See **ADVERSE REACTIONS**.) In case of overdosage, the dose should be reduced, frequency of administration decreased, or the drug withdrawn according to the severity of the condition. There is no known specific antidote for desmopressin acetate or **DDAVP Nasal Spray**.

An oral LD_{50} has not been established. An intravenous dose of 2 mg/kg in mice demonstrated no effect.

DOSAGE AND ADMINISTRATION

Primary Nocturnal Enuresis: Dosage should be adjusted according to the individual. The recommended initial dose for those 6 years of age and older is 20 µg or 0.2 mL solution intranasally at bedtime. Adjustment up to 40 µg is suggested if the patient does not respond.

Some patients may respond to 10 µg and adjustment to that lower dose may be done if the patient has shown a response to 20 µg. It is recommended that one-half of the dose be administered per nostril. Adequately controlled studies with intranasal DDAVP in primary nocturnal enuresis have not been conducted beyond 4–8 weeks.

Central Cranial Diabetes Insipidus: DDAVP Nasal Spray dosage must be determined for each individual patient and adjusted according to the diurnal pattern of response. Response should be estimated by two parameters: adequate duration of sleep and adequate, not excessive, water turnover. Patients with nasal congestion and blockage have often responded well to intranasal DDAVP. The usual dosage range in adults is 0.1 to 0.4 mL daily, either as a single dose or divided into two or three doses. Most adults require 0.2 mL daily in two divided doses. The morning and evening doses should be separately adjusted for an adequate diurnal rhythm of water turnover. For children aged 3 months to 12 years, the usual dosage range is 0.05 to 0.3 mL daily, either as a single dose or divided into two doses. About $^{1}/_{4}$ to $^{1}/_{3}$ of patients can be controlled by a single daily dose of DDAVP administered intranasally.

The nasal spray pump can only deliver doses of 0.1 mL (10 µg) or multiples of 0.1 mL. If doses other than these are required, the rhinal tube delivery system may be used.

The spray pump must be primed prior to the first use. To prime pump, press down four times. The bottle will now deliver 10 µg of drug per spray. Discard **DDAVP Nasal Spray** after 50 sprays since the amount delivered thereafter per spray may be substantially less than 10 µg of drug.

HOW SUPPLIED

DDAVP Nasal Spray is available in a 5-mL bottle with spray pump delivering 50 sprays of 10 µg (NDC 0075-2452-01). Desmopressin acetate is also available as DDAVP Rhinal Tube, a refrigerated product with 2.5 mL per vial, packaged with two rhinal tube applicators per carton (NDC 0075-2450-01).

Store at Controlled Room Temperature 20 to 25°C (68 to 77°F) [see USP]. STORE BOTTLE IN UPRIGHT POSITION.

Caution: Federal law prohibits dispensing without prescription.

Keep out of the reach of children.

Military: DDAVP Nasal Spray, 1 × 5.0 mL (NSN 6505-01–320-5579).

Rev. 2/97   IN-5534B

Manufactured for:

RHÔNE-POULENC RORER PHARMACEUTICALS INC.
Collegeville, PA, U.S.A. 19426-0107

By: Ferring Pharmaceuticals, Malmö, Sweden

Shown in Product Identification Guide, page 333

Continued on next page

DDAVP® Tablets ℞
(desmopressin acetate)

DESCRIPTION

DDAVP® Tablets (desmopressin acetate) are a synthetic analogue of the natural pituitary hormone 8-arginine vasopressin (ADH), an antidiuretic hormone affecting renal water conservation. It is chemically defined as follows:
Mol. Wt. 1183.34 Empirical Formula:
$C_{46}H_{64}N_{14}O_{12}S_2 \bullet C_2H_4O_2 \bullet 3H_2O$

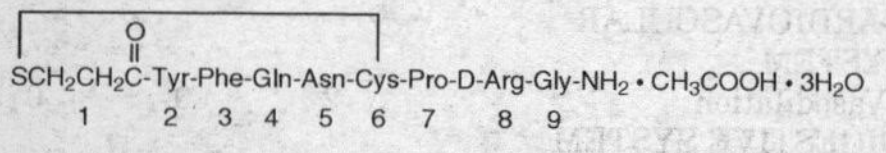
O
SCH2CH2C-Tyr-Phe-Gln-Asn-Cys-Pro-D-Arg-Gly-NH2 • CH3COOH • 3H2O
1 2 3 4 5 6 7 8 9

1-(3-mercaptopropionic acid)-8-D-arginine vasopressin monoacetate (salt) trihydrate.
DDAVP Tablets contain either 0.1 or 0.2 mg desmopressin acetate. Inactive ingredients include: lactose, potato starch, magnesium stearate and povidone.

CLINICAL PHARMACOLOGY

DDAVP Tablets contain as active substance, desmopressin acetate, a synthetic analogue of the natural hormone arginine vasopressin.
Central Diabetes Insipidus: Dose response studies in patients with diabetes insipidus have demonstrated that oral doses of 0.025 mg to 0.4 mg produced clinically significant antidiuretic effects. In most patients, doses of 0.1 mg to 0.2 mg produced optimal antidiuretic effects lasting up to eight hours. With doses of 0.4 mg, antidiuretic effects were observed for up to 12 hours; measurements beyond 12 hours were not recorded. Increasing oral doses produced dose dependent increases in the plasma levels of DDAVP (desmopressin acetate).
The plasma half-life of DDAVP followed a monoexponential time course with $t_{1/2}$ values of 1.5 to 2.5 hours which was independent of dose.
The bioavailability of DDAVP oral tablets is about 5% compared to intranasal DDAVP, and about 0.16% compared to intravenous DDAVP. The time to reach maximum plasma DDAVP levels ranged from 0.9 to 1.5 hours following oral or intranasal administration, respectively. Following administration of **DDAVP Tablets**, the onset of antidiuretic effect occurs at around 1 hour, and it reaches a maximum at about 4 to 7 hours based on the measurement of increased urine osmolality.
The use of **DDAVP Tablets** in patients with an established diagnosis will result in a reduction in urinary output with an accompanying increase in urine osmolality. These effects usually will allow resumption of a more normal life style, with a decrease in urinary frequency and nocturia.
There are reports of an occasional change in response to the intranasal formulations of DDAVP (DDAVP Nasal Spray and DDAVP Rhinal Tube). Usually, the change occurred over a period of time greater than six months. This change may be due to decreased responsiveness, or to shortened duration of effect. There is no evidence that this effect is due to the development of binding antibodies, but may be due to a local inactivation of the peptide. No lessening of effect was observed in the 46 patients who were treated with **DDAVP Tablets** for 12 to 44 months and no serum antibodies to desmopressin were detected.
The change in structure of arginine vasopressin to desmopressin acetate resulted in less vasopressor activity and decreased action on visceral smooth muscle relative to enhanced antidiuretic activity. Consequently, clinically effective antidiuretic doses are usually below the threshold for effects on vascular or visceral smooth muscle. In the four long-term studies of **DDAVP Tablets**, no increases in blood pressure in 46 patients receiving **DDAVP Tablets** for periods of 12 to 44 months were reported.
In one study, the pharmacodynamic characteristics of **DDAVP Tablets** and intranasal formulation were compared during an 8-hour dosing interval at steady state. The doses administered to 36 hydrated (water loaded) healthy male adult volunteers every 8 hours were 0.1, 0.2, 0.4 mg orally and 0.01 mg intranasally by rhinal tube. The results are shown in the following table:

Mean Changes from Baseline (SE) in Pharmacodynamic Parameters in Normal Healthy Adult Volunteers

Treatment	Total Urine Volume in mL	Maximum Urine Osmolality in mOsm/kg
0.1 mg PO q8h	−3689.3 (149.6)	514.8 (21.9)
0.2 mg PO q8h	−4429.9 (149.6)	686.3 (21.9)
0.4 mg PO q8h	−4998.8 (149.6)	769.3 (21.9)
0.01 mg IN q8h	−4844.9 (149.6)	754.1 (21.9)

(SE) = Standard error of the mean

With respect to the mean values of total urine volume decrease and maximum urine osmolality increase from baseline, the 90% confidence limits estimated that the 0.4 mg and 0.2 mg oral dose produced between 95% and 110% and 84% to 99% of pharmacodynamic activity, respectively, when compared to the 0.01 mg intranasal dose.
While both the 0.2 mg and 0.4 mg oral doses are considered pharmacodynamically similar to the 0.01 mg intranasal dose, the pharmacodynamic data on an inter-subject basis was highly variable and, therefore, individual dosing is recommended.
In another study in diabetes insipidus patients, the pharmacodynamic characteristics of **DDAVP Tablets** and intranasal formulations were compared over a 12-hour period. Ten fluid-controlled patients under age 18 were administered tablet doses of 0.2 mg and 0.4 mg, and intranasal doses of 0.01 mg and 0.02 mg.

Mean Peak Pharmacodynamic Parameters (SD) in Pediatric and Adolescent Diabetes Insipidus Patients

Treatment	Urine Volume in mL/min	Maximum Urine Osmolality in mOsm/kg
0.01 mg IN	0.3 (0.15)	717.0 (224.63)
0.02 mg IN	0.3 (0.25)	761.8 (298.82)
0.2 mg PO	0.3 (0.12)	678.3 (147.91)
0.4 mg PO	0.2 (0.15)	787.2 (73.34)

(SD) = Standard Deviation

All four dose formulations (0.01 mg IN, 0.02 mg IN, 0.2 mg PO and 0.4 mg PO) have a similar, pronounced pharmacodynamic effect on urine volume and urine osmolality. At two hours after study drug administration, mean urine volume was 4 mL/min and urine osmolality was >500 mOsm/kg. Mean plasma osmolality remained relatively constant over the time course recorded (0 to 12 hours). A statistical separation from baseline did not occur at any dose or time point. In these patients, the 0.2 mg tablets and the 0.01 mg intranasal spray exhibited similar pharmacodynamic profiles as did the 0.4 mg tablets and the 0.02 mg intranasal spray formulation. In another study of adult diabetes insipidus patients previously controlled on DDAVP intranasal spray, after one week of self-titration from spray to tablets, patients' diuresis was controlled with 0.1 mg **DDAVP Tablets** three times a day.
Primary Nocturnal Enuresis: Two double-blind, randomized, placebo-controlled studies were conducted in 340 patients with primary nocturnal enuresis. Patients were 5–17 years old, and 72% were males. A total of 329 patients were evaluated for efficacy. Patients were evaluated over a two-week baseline period in which the average number of wet nights was 10 (range 4–14). Patients were then randomized to receive 0.2, 0.4, or 0.6 mg of DDAVP or placebo. The pooled results after two weeks are shown in the following table:
[See table below]
Patients treated with DDAVP Tablets showed a statistically significant reduction in the number of wet nights compared to placebo-treated patients. A greater response was observed with increasing doses up to 0.6 mg.
In a six month, open-label extension study, patients completing the placebo-controlled studies were started on 0.2 mg/day DDAVP, and the dose was progressively increased until the optimal response was achieved (maximum dose 0.6 mg/day). A total of 230 patients were evaluated for efficacy; the average number of wet nights/2 weeks during the untreated baseline period was 10 (range 4–14), and the average duration (SD) of treatment was 4.2 (1.8) months. Twenty-five (25) patients (11%) achieved a complete or near complete response (≤2 wet nights/2 weeks) and did not require titration to the 0.6 mg/day dose. The majority of patients (198 of 230, 86%) were titrated to the highest dose. When all dose groups were combined, 128 (56%) showed at least a 50% reduction from baseline in the number of wet nights/2 weeks, while 87 (38%) patients achieved a complete or near complete response.

Response to DDAVP and Placebo at Two Weeks of Treatment
Mean (SE) Number of Wet Nights/2 Weeks

	Placebo (n = 85)	0.2 mg/day (n = 79)	0.4 mg/day (n = 82)	0.6 mg/day (n = 83)
Baseline	10 (0.3)	11 (0.3)	10 (0.3)	10 (0.3)
Reduction from Baseline	1 (0.3)	3 (0.4)	3 (0.4)	4 (0.4)
Percent Reduction from Baseline	10%	27%	30%	40%
p-value vs placebo	—	<0.05	<0.05	<0.05

INDICATIONS AND USAGE

Central Diabetes Insipidus: DDAVP Tablets are indicated as antidiuretic replacement therapy in the management of central diabetes insipidus and for the management of the temporary polyuria and polydipsia following head trauma or surgery in the pituitary region. DDAVP is ineffective for the treatment of nephrogenic diabetes insipidus.
Patients were selected for therapy based on the diagnosis by means of the water deprivation test, the hypertonic saline infusion test, and/or response to antidiuretic hormone. Continued response to DDAVP can be monitored by measuring urine volume and osmolality.
Primary Nocturnal Enuresis: DDAVP® Tablets (desmopressin acetate) are indicated for the management of primary nocturnal enuresis. DDAVP may be used alone or as an adjunct to behavioral conditioning or other non-pharmacologic intervention.

CONTRAINDICATIONS

DDAVP Tablets are contraindicated in individuals with known hypersensitivity to desmopressin acetate or to any of the components of **DDAVP Tablets.**

WARNINGS

In very young and elderly patients, in particular, fluid intake should be adjusted downward to decrease the potential occurrence of water intoxication and hyponatremia. Particular attention should be paid to the possibility of the rare occurrence of an extreme decrease in plasma osmolality that may result in seizures which could lead to coma.

PRECAUTIONS

General: Intranasal formulations of DDAVP at high doses and DDAVP Injection have infrequently produced a slight elevation of blood pressure which disappears with a reduction of dosage. Although this effect has not been observed when single oral doses up to 0.6 mg have been administered, the drug should be used with caution in patients with coronary artery insufficiency and/or hypertensive cardiovascular disease, because of a possible rise in blood pressure.
DDAVP should be used with caution in patients with conditions associated with fluid and electrolyte imbalance, such as cystic fibrosis, since these patients may develop hyponatremia.
Rare severe allergic reactions have been reported with DDAVP. Anaphylaxis has been reported with intravenous administration of DDAVP Injection, but not with **DDAVP Tablets.**
Laboratory Tests: *Central Diabetes Insipidus:* Laboratory tests for monitoring the patient with central diabetes insipidus or post-surgical or head trauma-related polyuria and polydipsia include urine volume and osmolality. In some cases, measurements of plasma osmolality may be useful.
Drug Interactions: Although the pressor activity of DDAVP is very low compared to its antidiuretic activity, large doses of **DDAVP Tablets** should be used with other pressor agents only with careful patient monitoring.
Carcinogenicity, Mutagenicity, Impairment of Fertility: Studies with DDAVP have not been performed to evaluate carcinogenic potential, mutagenic potential or effects on fertility.
Pregnancy: *Category B:* Fertility studies have not been done. Teratology studies in rats and rabbits at doses from 0.05 to 10 μg/kg/day (approximately 0.1 times the maximum systemic human exposure in rats and up to 38 times the maximum systemic human exposure in rabbits based on surface area, mg/m^2) revealed no harm to the fetus due to DDAVP (desmopressin acetate). There are, however, no adequate and well-controlled studies in pregnant women. Because animal studies are not always predictive of human response, this drug should be used during pregnancy only if clearly needed.
Several publications where desmopressin acetate was used in the management of diabetes insipidus during pregnancy are available; these include a few anecdotal reports of congenital anomalies and low birth weight babies. However, no causal connection between these events and desmopressin acetate has been established. A fifteen year Swedish epidemiologic study of the use of desmopressin acetate in pregnant women with diabetes insipidus found the rate of birth defects to be no greater than that in the general population; however, the statistical power of this study is low. As opposed to preparations containing natural hormones, desmo-

pressin acetate in antidiuretic doses has no uterotonic action and the physician will have to weigh the possible therapeutic advantages against the possible risks in each case.

Nursing Mothers: There have been no controlled studies in nursing mothers. A single study in postpartum women demonstrated a marked change in plasma, but little if any change in assayable DDAVP in breast milk following an intranasal dose of 0.01 mg.

It is not known whether the drug is excreted in human milk. Because many drugs are excreted in human milk, caution should be exercised when DDAVP is administered to nursing mothers.

Pediatric Use: *Central Diabetes Insipidus:* **DDAVP Tablets** have been used safely in pediatric patients, age 4 years and older, with diabetes insipidus for periods up to 44 months. In younger pediatric patients the dose must be individually adjusted in order to prevent an excessive decrease in plasma osmolality leading to hyponatremia and possible convulsions; dosing should start at 0.05 mg (1/2 of the 0.1 mg tablet). Use of **DDAVP Tablets** in pediatric patients requires careful fluid intake restrictions to prevent possible hyponatremia and water intoxication.

Primary Nocturnal Enuresis: DDAVP Tablets have been safely used in pediatric patients age 6 years and older with primary nocturnal enuresis for up to 6 months. Some patients respond to a dose of 0.2 mg; however, increasing responses are seen at doses of 0.4 mg and 0.6 mg. No increase in the frequency or severity of adverse reactions or decrease in efficacy was seen with an increased dose or duration. The dose should be individually adjusted to achieve the best results.

ADVERSE REACTIONS

Infrequently, large doses of the intranasal formulations of DDAVP and DDAVP Injection have produced transient headache, nausea, flushing and mild abdominal cramps. These symptoms have disappeared with reduction in dosage.

Central Diabetes Insipidus: In long-term clinical studies in which patients with diabetes insipidus were followed for periods up to 44 months of **DDAVP Tablet** therapy, transient increases in AST (SGOT) no higher than 1.5 times the upper limit of normal were occasionally observed. Elevated AST (SGOT) returned to the normal range despite continued use of **DDAVP Tablets**.

Primary Nocturnal Enuresis: The only adverse event occurring in ≥3% of patients in controlled clinical trials with DDAVP tablets that was probably, possibly, or remotely related to study drug was headache (4% DDAVP, 3% placebo).

Other: The following adverse events have been reported; however their relationship to DDAVP has not been established: abnormal thinking, diarrhea, and edema-weight gain.

See **WARNINGS** for the possibility of water intoxication and hyponatremia.

OVERDOSAGE

(See **ADVERSE REACTIONS**.) In case of overdose, the dose should be reduced, frequency of administration decreased, or the drug withdrawn according to the severity of the condition. There is no known specific antidote for DDAVP. The patient should be observed and treated with appropriate symptomatic therapy.

An oral LD_{50} has not been established. Oral doses up to 0.2 mg/kg/day have been administered to dogs and rats for 6 months without any significant drug-related toxicities reported. An intravenous dose of 2 mg/kg in mice demonstrated no effect.

DOSAGE AND ADMINISTRATION

Central Diabetes Insipidus: The dosage of **DDAVP Tablets** must be determined for each individual patient and adjusted according to the diurnal pattern of response. Response should be estimated by two parameters: adequate duration of sleep and adequate, not excessive, water turnover. Patients previously on intranasal DDAVP therapy should begin tablet therapy twelve hours after the last intranasal dose. During the initial dose titration period, patients should be observed closely and appropriate safety parameters measured to assure adequate response. Patients should be monitored at regular intervals during the course of **DDAVP Tablet** therapy to assure adequate antidiuretic response. Modifications in dosage regimen should be implemented as necessary to assure adequate water turnover.

Adults and Children: It is recommended that patients be started on doses of 0.05 mg (1/2 of the 0.1 mg tablet) two times a day and individually adjusted to their optimum therapeutic dose. Most patients in clinical trials found that the optimal dosage range is 0.1 mg to 0.8 mg daily, administered in divided doses. Each dose should be separately adjusted for an adequate diurnal rhythm of water turnover. Total daily dosage should be increased or decreased in the range of 0.1 mg to 1.2 mg divided into two or three daily doses as needed to obtain adequate antidiuresis. See **Pediatric Use** subsection for special considerations when administering desmopressin acetate to pediatric diabetes insipidus patients.

Primary Nocturnal Enuresis: The dosage of **DDAVP Tablets** must be determined for each individual patient and adjusted according to response. Patients previously on intranasal DDAVP therapy can begin tablet therapy the night following (24 hours after) the last intranasal dose. The recommended initial dose for patients age 6 years and older is 0.2 mg at bedtime. The dose may be titrated up to 0.6 mg to achieve the desired response.

HOW SUPPLIED

Strength	Size	NDC 0075-	Color	Markings
0.1 mg	Bottle of 100	0016-00	White	
0.2 mg	Bottle of 100	0026-00	White	

Store at Controlled Room Temperature 20 to 25°C (68 to 77°F) [see USP]. Avoid exposure to excessive heat or light.

Caution: Federal law prohibits dispensing without prescription.

Keep out of the reach of children.

Manufactured for
RHÔNE-POULENC RORER PHARMACEUTICALS INC.
COLLEGEVILLE, PA 19426

Rev. 3/98

By Ferring Pharmaceuticals, Malmö, Sweden   IN-5547C
Shown in Product Identification Guide, page 333

GLIADEL® Wafer
(polifeprosan 20 with carmustine implant)   ℞

DESCRIPTION

GLIADEL® Wafer (polifeprosan 20 with carmustine implant) is a sterile, off-white to pale yellow wafer approximately 1.45 cm in diameter and 1 mm thick. Each wafer contains 192.3 mg of a biodegradable polyanhydride copolymer and 7.7 mg of carmustine [1,3-bis (2-chloroethyl)-1-nitrosourea, or BCNU]. Carmustine is a nitrosourea oncolytic agent. The copolymer, polifeprosan 20, consists of poly[bis(p-carboxyphenoxy) propane: sebacic acid] in a 20:80 molar ratio and is used to control the local delivery of carmustine. Carmustine is homogeneously distributed in the copolymer matrix.

The structural formula for polifeprosan 20 is:

The structural formula for carmustine is:

CLINICAL PHARMACOLOGY

GLIADEL is designed to deliver carmustine directly into the surgical cavity created when a brain tumor is resected. On exposure to the aqueous environment of the resection cavity, the anhydride bonds in the copolymer are hydrolyzed, releasing carmustine, carboxyphenoxypropane, and sebacic acid. The carmustine released from GLIADEL diffuses into the surrounding brain tissue and produces an antineoplastic effect by alkylating DNA and RNA.

Carmustine has been shown to degrade both spontaneously and metabolically. The production of an alkylating moiety, hypothesized to be chloroethyl carbonium ion, leads to the formation of DNA cross-links.

The tumoricidal activity of GLIADEL is dependent on release of carmustine to the tumor cavity in concentrations sufficient for effective cytotoxicity.

More than 70% of the copolymer degrades by three weeks. The metabolic disposition and excretion of the monomers differ. Carboxyphenoxypropane is eliminated by the kidney and sebacic acid, an endogenous fatty acid, is metabolized by the liver and expired as CO_2 in animals.

The absorption, distribution, metabolism, and excretion of the copolymer in humans is unknown. Carmustine concentrations delivered by GLIADEL in human brain tissue have not been determined. Plasma levels of carmustine after

GLIADEL wafer implant were not determined. In rabbits implanted with wafers containing 3.85% carmustine, no detectible levels of carmustine were found in the plasma or cerebrospinal fluid.

Following an intravenous infusion of carmustine at doses ranging from 30 to 170 mg/m², the average terminal half-life, clearance, and steady-state volume of distribution were 22 minutes, 56 mL/min/kg, and 3.25 L/kg, respectively. Approximately 60% of the intravenous 200 mg/m² dose of ^{14}C-carmustine was excreted in the urine over 96 hours and 6% was expired as CO_2.

GLIADEL wafers are biodegradable in human brain when implanted into the cavity after tumor resection. The rate of biodegradation is variable from patient to patient. During the biodegradation process, a wafer remnant may be observed on brain imaging scans or at re-operation even though extensive degradation of all components has occurred. Data obtained from review of CT scans obtained 49 days after implantation of GLIADEL demonstrated that images consistent with wafers were visible to varying degrees in the scans of 11 of 18 patients. Data obtained at re-operation and autopsies have demonstrated wafer remnants up to 232 days after GLIADEL implantation.

Wafer remnants removed at re-operation from two patients with recurrent malignant glioma, one at 64 days and the second at 92 days after implantation, were analyzed for content. The following table presents the results of analyses completed on these remnants.

COMPOSITION OF WAFER REMNANTS REMOVED FROM TWO PATIENTS ON RE-OPERATION

Component	Patient A	Patient B
Days After GLIADEL Implantation	64	92
Anhydride Bonds	None detected	None detected
Water Content (% of wafer remnant weight)	95–97%	74–86%
Carmustine Content (% of initial)	<0.0004%	0.034%
Carboxyphenoxypropane Content (% of initial)	9%	14%
Sebacic Acid Content (% of initial)	4%	3%

The wafer remnants consisted mostly of water and monomeric components with minimal detectable carmustine present.

CLINICAL STUDIES

In a randomized, double-blind, placebo-controlled clinical trial in adults with recurrent malignant glioma, GLIADEL prolonged survival in patients with glioblastoma multiforme (GBM). Ninety-five percent of the patients treated with GLIADEL had 7–8 wafers implanted.

In 222 patients with recurrent malignant glioma who had failed initial surgery and radiation therapy, the six-month survival rate after surgery increased from 47% (53/112) for patients receiving placebo to 60% (66/110) for patients treated with GLIADEL. Median survival increased by 33%, from 24 weeks with placebo to 32 weeks with GLIADEL treatment. In patients with GBM, the six-month survival rate increased from 36% (26/73) with placebo to 56% (40/72) with GLIADEL treatment. Median survival of GBM patients increased by 41% from 20 weeks with placebo to 28 weeks with GLIADEL treatment. In patients with pathologic diagnoses other than GBM at the time of surgery for tumor recurrence, GLIADEL produced no survival prolongation.

6-MONTH KAPLAN-MEIER SURVIVAL CURVES FOR PATIENTS UNDERGOING SURGERY FOR RECURRENT GBM

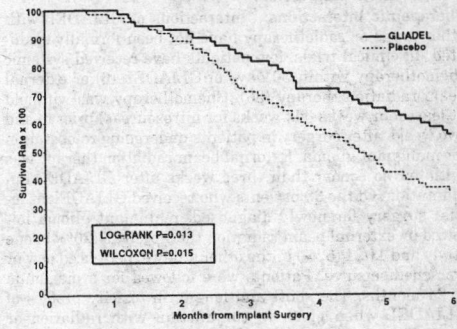

LOG-RANK P=0.013
WILCOXON P=0.015

[See figure at top of next column]

Continued on next page

Gliadel Wafer—Cont.

OVERALL KAPLAN-MEIER SURVIVAL CURVES FOR PATIENTS UNDERGOING SURGERY FOR RECURRENT GBM

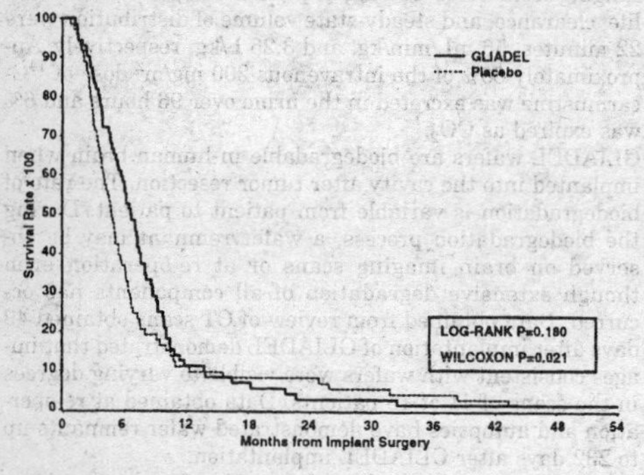
GLIADEL
Placebo
LOG-RANK P=0.180
WILCOXON P=0.021
Survival Rate x 100
Months from Implant Surgery
0
6
12
18
24
30
36
42
48
54
10
20
30
40
50
60
70
80
90
100

INDICATIONS AND USAGE

GLIADEL is indicated for use as an adjunct to surgery to prolong survival in patients with recurrent glioblastoma multiforme for whom surgical resection is indicated.

CONTRAINDICATIONS

GLIADEL contains carmustine. GLIADEL should not be given to individuals who have demonstrated a previous hypersensitivity to carmustine or any of the components of GLIADEL.

WARNINGS

Patients undergoing craniotomy for malignant glioma and implantation of GLIADEL should be monitored closely for known complications of craniotomy, including seizures, intracranial infections, abnormal wound healing, and brain edema. Cases of intracerebral mass effect unresponsive to corticosteroids have been described in patients treated with GLIADEL, including one case leading to brain herniation.

Pregnancy: There are no studies assessing the reproductive toxicity of GLIADEL. Carmustine, the active component of GLIADEL, can cause fetal harm when administered to a pregnant woman. Carmustine has been shown to be embryotoxic and teratogenic in rats at i.p. doses of 0.5, 1, 2, 4, or 8 mg/kg/day when given on gestation days 6 through 15. Carmustine caused fetal malformations (anophthalmia, micrognathia, omphalocele) at 1.0 mg/kg/day (about 1/6 the recommended human dose (eight wafers of 7.7 mg carmustine/wafer) on a mg/m^2 basis). Carmustine was embryotoxic in rabbits at i.v. doses of 4.0 mg/kg/day (about 1.2 times the recommended human dose on a mg/m^2 basis). Embryotoxicity was characterized by increased embryo-fetal deaths, reduced numbers of litters, and reduced litter sizes.

There are no studies of GLIADEL in pregnant women. If GLIADEL is used during pregnancy, or if the patient becomes pregnant after GLIADEL implantation, the patient must be warned of the potential hazard to the fetus.

PRECAUTIONS

General: Communication between the surgical resection cavity and the ventricular system should be avoided to prevent the wafers from migrating into the ventricular system and causing obstructive hydrocephalus. If a communication exists, it should be closed prior to wafer implantation.

Imaging Studies: Computed tomography and magnetic resonance imaging of the head may demonstrate enhancement in the brain tissue surrounding the resection cavity after implantation of GLIADEL wafers. This enhancement may represent edema and inflammation caused by GLIADEL or tumor progression.

Therapeutic Interactions: Interactions of GLIADEL with other drugs or radiotherapy have not been formally evaluated. In clinical trials, few patients have received systemic chemotherapy within 30 days of GLIADEL (6) or external beam radiation therapy (36). Chemotherapy was withheld at least four weeks (six weeks for nitrosoureas) prior to and two weeks after surgery in patients undergoing re-operation for malignant glioma. External beam radiation therapy was initiated no sooner than three weeks after GLIADEL implantation. Of the 36 patients who received GLIADEL at initial surgery for newly diagnosed, malignant glioma followed by external beam radiation therapy, 3/15 (20%) in one study and 11/21 (52%) in the other study experienced new or worsened seizures. Patients were followed for a maximum of 24 months. The short and long-term toxicity profiles of GLIADEL when given in conjunction with radiation or chemotherapy have not been fully explored.

Carcinogenesis, Mutagenesis, Impairment of Fertility: No carcinogenicity, mutagenicity or impairment of fertility studies have been conducted with GLIADEL. Carcinogenicity, mutagenicity and impairment of fertility studies have been conducted with carmustine, the active component of GLIADEL. Carmustine was given three times a week for six months, followed by 12 months observation, to Swiss mice at i.p. doses of 2.5 and 5.0 mg/kg (about 1/5 and 1/3 the recommended human dose (eight wafers of 7.7 mg carmustine/wafer) on a mg/m^2 basis) and to SD rats at i.p. dose of 1.5 mg/kg (about 1/4 the recommended human dose on a mg/m^2 basis.) There were increases in tumor incidence in all treated animals, predominantly subcutaneous and lung neoplasms.

Mutagenesis: Carmustine was mutagenic *in vitro* (Ames assay, human lymphoblast HGPRT assay) and clastogenic both *in vitro* (V79 hamster cell micronucleus assay) and *in vivo* (SCE assay in rodent brain tumors, mouse bone marrow micronucleus assay). *Impairment of Fertility:* Carmustine caused testicular degeneration at i.p. doses of 8 mg/kg/week for eight weeks (about 1.3 times the recommended human dose on a mg/m^2 basis) in male rats.

Pregnancy: Pregnancy Category D: see **WARNINGS**.

Nursing Mothers: It is not known if either carmustine, carboxyphenoxypropane, or sebacic acid is excreted in human milk. Because many drugs are excreted in human milk and because of the potential for serious adverse reactions from carmustine in nursing infants, it is recommended that patients receiving GLIADEL discontinue nursing.

Pediatric Use: The safety and effectiveness of GLIADEL in pediatric patients have not been established.

ADVERSE REACTIONS

Data in the following table are based on the experience of 222 patients with recurrent malignant glioma randomized to GLIADEL or placebo (wafer without carmustine).

The spectrum of adverse events observed in patients who received GLIADEL or placebo in clinical studies was consistent with that encountered in patients undergoing craniotomy for malignant gliomas.

GLIADEL was not reported to be the cause of death in any of the GLIADEL clinical trials.

The following post-operative adverse events were observed in 4% or more of the patients receiving GLIADEL in the placebo-controlled clinical trial. Except for nervous system effects, where there is a possibility that the placebo wafers could have been responsible, only events more common in the GLIADEL group are listed. These adverse events were either not present pre-operatively or worsened post-operatively during the follow-up period. The follow-up period in the randomized trial was up to 71 months.

COMMON ADVERSE EVENTS OBSERVED IN ≥4% OF PATIENTS IN THE RANDOMIZED TRIAL

Body System Adverse Event	GLIADEL Wafer with Carmustine [N=110] n (%)	PLACEBO Wafer without Carmustine [N=112] n (%)
Body as a Whole		
Fever	13 (12)	9 (8)
Pain*	8 (7)	1(1)
Digestive System		
Nausea and Vomiting	9 (8)	7 (6)
Metabolic and Nutritional Disorders		
Healing Abnormal*	15 (14)	6 (5)
Nervous System		
Aphasia	10 (9)	12 (11)
Brain Edema	4 (4)	1 (1)
Confusion	11(10)	9 (8)
Convulsion	21(19)	21 (19)
Headache	16 (15)	14 (13)
Hemiplegia	21(19)	22 (20)
Intracranial Hypertension	4 (4)	7 (6)
Meningitis or Abscess	4 (4)	1(1)
Somnolence	15 (14)	12 (11)
Stupor	7 (6)	7 (6)
Skin and Appendages		
Rash	6 (5)	4 (4)
Urogenital System		
Urinary Tract Infection	23 (21)	19 (17)

* $p < 0.05$ for comparison of GLIADEL versus placebo groups in the randomized trial (two-sided Fisher's Exact Test)

The following adverse events were also reported in 4–9% of GLIADEL patients but were at least as frequent in the placebo group as in GLIADEL-treated patients: infection, deep thrombophlebitis, pulmonary embolism, nausea, oral moniliasis, anemia, hyponatremia, pneumonia.

The following four categories of adverse events are possibly related to treatment with GLIADEL. The frequency with which they occurred in the randomized trial along with descriptive detail are provided below.

1. Seizures: In the randomized study, the majority of seizures in the placebo and GLIADEL groups were mild or moderate in severity. The incidence of new or worsened seizures was 19% in patients treated with GLIADEL and 19% in patients receiving placebo. Of the patients with new or worsened seizures post-operatively, 12/22 (54%) of patients treated with GLIADEL and 2/22 (9%) of placebo patients experienced the first new or worsened seizure within the first five post-operative days. The median time to onset of the first new or worsened post-operative seizure was 3.5 days in patients treated with GLIADEL and 61 days in placebo patients. The occurrence of seizures did not reduce the survival benefit of GLIADEL.

2. Brain Edema: In the randomized trial, brain edema was noted in 4% of patients treated with GLIADEL and in 1% of patients treated with placebo. Development of brain edema with mass effect (due to tumor recurrence, intracranial infection, or necrosis) may necessitate re-operation and, in some cases, removal of wafer or its remnants.

3. Healing Abnormalities: The majority of these events were mild to moderate in severity. Healing abnormalities occurred in 14% of GLIADEL-treated patients compared to 5% of placebo recipients. These events included cerebrospinal fluid leaks, subdural fluid collections, subgaleal or wound effusions, and wound breakdown.

4. Intracranial Infection: In the randomized trial, intracranial infection (meningitis or abscess) occurred in 4% of patients treated with GLIADEL and in 1% of patients receiving placebo. In GLIADEL-treated patients, there were two cases of bacterial meningitis, one case of chemical meningitis, and one case of meningitis which was not further specified. A brain abscess developed in one placebo-treated patient. The rate of deep wound infection (infection of subgaleal space, bone, meninges, or neural parenchyma) was 6% in both GLIADEL and placebo treated patients.

The following adverse events, not listed in the table above, were reported in less than 4% but at least 1% of patients treated with GLIADEL in all studies (n=273). The events listed were either not present pre-operatively or worsened post-operatively. Whether GLIADEL caused these events cannot be determined.

Body as a Whole: peripheral edema (2%); neck pain (2%); accidental injury (1%); back pain (1%); allergic reaction (1%); asthenia (1%); chest pain (1%); sepsis (1%)

Cardiovascular System: hypertension (3%); hypotension (1%)

Digestive System: diarrhea (2%); constipation (2%); dysphagia (1%); gastrointestinal hemorrhage (1%); fecal incontinence (1%)

Hemic and Lymphatic System: thrombocytopenia (1%); leukocytosis (1%)

Metabolic and Nutritional Disorders: hyponatremia (3%); hyperglycemia (3%); hypokalemia (1%)

Musculoskeletal System: infection (1%)

Nervous System: hydrocephalus (3%); depression (3%); abnormal thinking (2%); ataxia (2%); dizziness (2%); insomnia (2%); monoplegia (2%); coma (1%); amnesia (1%); diplopia (1%); paranoid reaction (1%). In addition, cerebral hemorrhage and cerebral infarct were each reported in less than 1% of patients treated with GLIADEL.

Respiratory System: infection (2%); aspiration pneumonia (1%)

Skin and Appendages: rash (2%)

Special Senses: visual field defect (2%); eye pain (1%)

Urogenital System: urinary incontinence (2%)

OVERDOSAGE

There is no clinical experience with use of more than eight GLIADEL wafers per surgical procedure.

DOSAGE AND ADMINISTRATION

Each GLIADEL wafer contains 7.7 mg of carmustine, resulting in a dose of 61.6 mg when eight wafers are implanted. It is recommended that eight wafers be placed in the resection cavity if the size and shape of it allows. Should the size and shape not accommodate eight wafers, the maximum number of wafers as allowed should be placed. Since there is no clinical experience, no more than eight wafers should be used per surgical procedure.

Handling and Disposal[1–7]: Wafers should only be handled by personnel wearing surgical gloves because exposure to carmustine can cause severe burning and hyperpigmentation of the skin. Use of double gloves is recommended and the outer gloves should be discarded into a biohazard waste container after use. A surgical instrument dedicated to the handling of the wafers should be used for wafer implantation. If repeat neurosurgical intervention is indicated, any wafer or wafer remnant should be handled as a potentially cytotoxic agent.

GLIADEL wafers should be handled with care. The aluminum foil laminate pouches containing GLIADEL should be delivered to the operating room and remain unopened until ready to implant the wafers. **The outside surface of the outer foil pouch is not sterile.**

Instructions for Opening Pouch Containing GLIADEL

Figure 1: To remove the sterile inner pouch from the outer pouch, locate the folded corner and slowly pull in an outward motion.

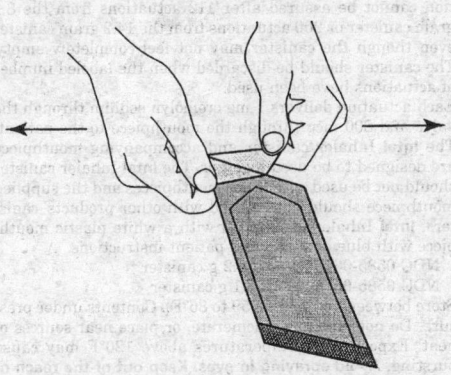

Figure 2: Do NOT pull in a downward motion rolling knuckles over the pouch. This may exert pressure on the wafer and cause it to break.

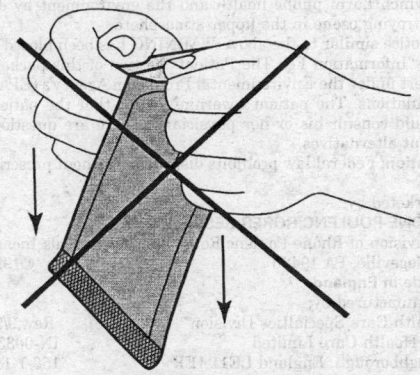

Figure 3: Remove the inner pouch by grabbing hold of the **crimped** edge and pulling upward.

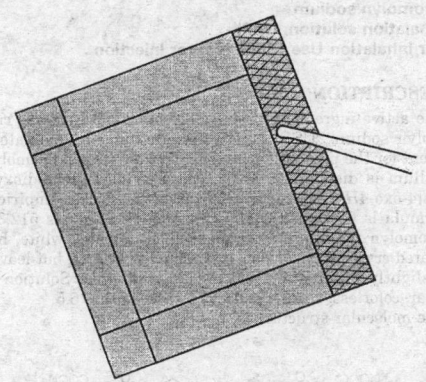

Figure 4: To open the inner pouch, gently hold the crimped edge and cut in an arc-like fashion around the wafer.

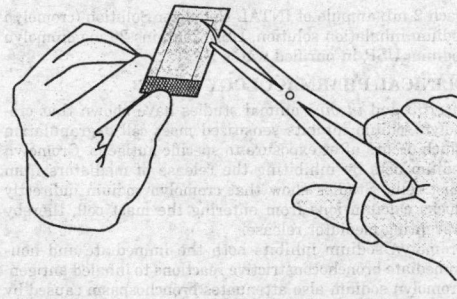

Figure 5: To remove the GLIADEL wafer, gently grasp the wafer with the aid of forceps and place it onto a designated sterile field.

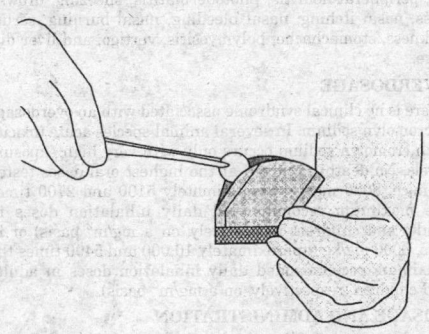

Once the tumor is resected, tumor pathology is confirmed, and hemostasis is obtained, up to eight GLIADEL® Wafers (polifeprosan 20 with carmustine implant) may be placed to cover as much of the resection cavity as possible. Slight overlapping of the wafers is acceptable. Wafers broken in half may be used, but wafers broken in more than two pieces should be discarded in a biohazard container. Oxidized regenerated cellulose (Surgicel®) may be placed over the wafers to secure them against the cavity surface. After placement of the wafers, the resection cavity should be irrigated and the dura closed in a water tight fashion.
Unopened foil pouches may be kept at ambient room temperature for a maximum of six hours at a time.

HOW SUPPLIED
GLIADEL is available in a single dose treatment box containing eight individually pouched wafers. Each wafer contains 7.7 mg of carmustine and is packaged in two aluminum foil laminate pouches. The inner pouch is sterile and is designed to maintain product sterility and protect the product from moisture. The outer pouch is a peelable overwrap. **The outside surface of the outer pouch is not sterile.**
GLIADEL must be stored at or below −20°C (−4°F).

REFERENCES
1. Recommendations for the Safe Handling of Parenteral Antineoplastic Drugs, NIH Publication No. 83-2621. For sale by the Superintendent of Documents, U.S. Government Printing Office, Washington, DC 20402.
2. AMA Council Report, Guidelines for Handling Parenteral Antineoplastics. JAMA, 1985; 253(11):1590-1592.
3. National Study Commission on Cytotoxic Exposure — Recommendations for Handling Cytotoxic Agents. Available from Louis P. Jeffrey, ScD., Chairman, National Study Commission on Cytotoxic Exposure, Massachusetts College of Pharmacy and Allied Health Sciences, 179 Longwood Avenue, Boston, Massachusetts 02115.
4. Clinical Oncological Society of Australia, Guidelines and Recommendations for Safe Handling of Antineoplastic Agents. Med J Australia, 1983; 1:426-428.
5. Jones RB, et al: Safe Handling of Chemotherapeutic Agents: A Report from the Mount Sinai Medical Center. CA — A Cancer Journal for Clinicians, 1983; (Sept/Oct) 258-263.
6. American Society of Hospital Pharmacists Technical Assistance Bulletin on Handling Cytotoxic and Hazardous Drugs. Am J. Hosp Pharm, 1990; 47:1033-1049.
7. OSHA Work-Practice Guidelines for Personnel Dealing with Cytotoxic (Antineoplastic) Drugs. Am J Hosp Pharm, 1986; 43:1193-1204.
NDC: 0075-9995-08
CAUTION: FEDERAL LAW PROHIBITS DISPENSING WITHOUT PRESCRIPTION.
U.S. Patent Nos. 4,789,724 and 5,179,189.
Manufactured for
RHÔNE-POULENC RORER PHARMACEUTICALS INC.
Collegeville, PA, U.S.A. 19426-0107
By
Guilford Pharmaceuticals Inc.
Baltimore, MD 21224
Rev. 10/96   IN-2250
Shown in Product Identification Guide, page 333

INTAL® INHALER
[ĭn ′tăl]
(cromolyn sodium inhalation aerosol)
For Oral Inhalation Only

DESCRIPTION
The active ingredient of **Intal** Inhaler is cromolyn sodium, USP. It is an inhaled anti-inflammatory agent for the preventive management of asthma. Cromolyn sodium is disodium 5,5′-[(2-hydroxytrimethylene)dioxy]bis[4-oxo-4H-1-benzopyran-2-carboxylate]. The empirical formula is $C_{23}H_{14}Na_2O_{11}$; the molecular weight is 512.34. Cromolyn sodium is a water soluble, odorless, white, hydrated crystal-line powder. It is tasteless at first, but leaves a slightly bitter aftertaste. The molecular structure of cromolyn sodium is:

Intal Inhaler (cromolyn sodium inhalation aerosol) is a metered dose aerosol unit for oral inhalation containing micronized cromolyn sodium, sorbitan trioleate with dichlorotetrafluoroethane and dichlorodifluoromethane as propellants. Each actuation delivers approximately 1 mg cromolyn sodium from the valve and 800 mcg cromolyn sodium through the mouthpiece to the patient. Each 8.1 g canister delivers at least 112 metered inhalations (56 doses); each 14.2 g canister delivers at least 200 metered inhalations (100 doses).

CLINICAL PHARMACOLOGY
In vitro and *in vivo* animal studies have shown that cromolyn sodium inhibits sensitized mast cell degranulation which occurs after exposure to specific antigens. Cromolyn sodium acts by inhibiting the release of mediators from mast cells. Studies show that cromolyn sodium indirectly blocks calcium ions from entering the mast cell, thereby preventing mediator release.
Cromolyn sodium inhibits both the immediate and non-immediate bronchoconstrictive reactions to inhaled antigen. Cromolyn sodium also attenuates bronchospasm caused by exercise, toluene diisocyanate, aspirin, cold air, sulfur dioxide, and environmental pollutants, at least in some patients.
Cromolyn sodium has no intrinsic bronchodilator or antihistamine activity.
After administration of cromolyn sodium capsules by inhalation, approximately 8% of the total dose administered is absorbed and rapidly excreted unchanged, approximately equally divided between urine and bile. The remainder of the dose is either exhaled or deposited in the oropharynx, swallowed, and excreted via the alimentary tract.

INDICATIONS AND USAGE
Intal Inhaler is a prophylactic agent indicated in the management of patients with bronchial asthma.
In patients whose symptoms are sufficiently frequent to require a continuous program of medication, **Intal** Inhaler is given by inhalation on a regular daily basis. (See **DOSAGE AND ADMINISTRATION**.) The effect of **Intal** Inhaler is usually evident after several weeks of treatment, although some patients show an almost immediate response.
If improvement occurs, it will ordinarily occur within the first 4 weeks of administration as manifested by a decrease in the severity of clinical symptoms of asthma, or in the need for concomitant therapy, or both.
In patients who develop acute bronchoconstriction in response to exposure to exercise, toluene diisocyanate, environmental pollutants, known antigens, etc., **Intal** Inhaler should be used shortly before exposure to the precipitating factor, *i.e.*, within 10 to 15 minutes but not more than 60 minutes. (See **DOSAGE AND ADMINISTRATION**.) **Intal** Inhaler may be effective in relieving bronchospasm in some, but not all, patients with exercise induced bronchospasm.

CONTRAINDICATIONS
Intal Inhaler is contraindicated in those patients who have shown hypersensitivity to cromolyn sodium or other ingredients in this preparation.

WARNINGS
Intal Inhaler has no role in the treatment of an acute attack of asthma, especially status asthmaticus. Severe anaphylactic reactions can occur after cromolyn sodium administration. The recommended dosage should be decreased in patients with decreased renal or hepatic function. Intal Inhaler should be discontinued if the patient develops eosinophilic pneumonia (or pulmonary infiltrates with eosinophilia). Because of the propellants in this preparation, it should be used with caution in patients with coronary artery disease or a history of cardiac arrhythmias.

PRECAUTIONS
General: In view of the biliary and renal routes of excretion for cromolyn sodium, consideration should be given to decreasing the dosage or discontinuing the administration of the drug in patients with impaired renal or hepatic function.
Occasionally, patients may experience cough and/or bronchospasm following cromolyn sodium inhalation. At times, patients who develop bronchospasm may not be able to continue administration despite prior bronchodilator administration. Rarely, very severe bronchospasm has been encountered.

Continued on next page

Intal Inhaler—Cont.

Carcinogenesis, Mutagenesis, and Impairment of Fertility: Long-term studies of cromolyn sodium in mice (12 months intraperitoneal administration at doses up to 150 mg/kg/day three days per week), hamsters (intraperitoneal administration at doses up to 53 mg/kg/day three days per week for 15 weeks followed by 17.5 mg/kg/day three days per week for 37 weeks), and rats (18 months subcutaneous treatment at doses up to 75 mg/kg/day six days per week) showed no neoplastic effects. These doses in mice, hamsters, and rats correspond to approximately 40, 10, and 80 times, respectively, the maximum recommended daily inhalation dose in adults on a mg/m^2 basis, or, approximately 20, 5, and 40 times, respectively, the maximum recommended daily inhalation dose in children on a mg/m^2 basis.

Cromolyn sodium showed no mutagenic potential in Ames Salmonella/microsome plate assays, mitotic gene conversion in *Saccharomyces cerevisiae*, and in an *in vitro* cytogenetic study in human peripheral lymphocytes.

No evidence of impaired fertility was shown in laboratory reproduction studies conducted subcutaneously in rats at the highest doses tested, 175 mg/kg/day in males and 100 mg/kg/day in females. These doses are approximately 220 and 130 times, respectively, the maximum recommended daily inhalation dose in adults on a mg/m^2 basis.

Pregnancy: *Pregnancy Category B:* Reproduction studies with cromolyn sodium administered subcutaneously to pregnant mice and rats at maximum daily doses of 540 mg/kg/day and 160 mg/kg/day, respectively, and intravenously to rabbits at a maximum daily dose of 485 mg/kg/day produced no evidence of fetal malformations. These doses represent approximately 340, 210, and 1,200 times, respectively, the maximum recommended daily inhalation dose in adults on a mg/m^2 basis. Adverse fetal effects (increased resorption and decreased fetal weight) were noted only at the very high parenteral doses that produced maternal toxicity. There are, however, no adequate and well-controlled studies in pregnant women.

Because animal reproduction studies are not always predictive of human response, **Intal** Inhaler should be used during pregnancy only if clearly needed.

Drug Interaction During Pregnancy: Cromolyn sodium and isoproterenol were studied following subcutaneous injections in pregnant mice. Cromolyn sodium alone in doses up to 540 mg/kg/day (approximately 340 times the maximum recommended daily inhalation dose in adults on a mg/m^2 basis) did not cause significant increases in resorptions or major malformations. Isoproterenol alone at a dose of 2.7 mg/kg/day (approximately 7 times the maximum recommended daily inhalation dose in adults on a mg/m^2 basis) increased both resorptions and malformations. The addition of 540 mg/kg/day of cromolyn sodium (approximately 340 times the maximum recommended daily inhalation dose in adults on a mg/m^2 basis) to 2.7 mg/kg/day of isoproterenol (approximately 7 times the maximum recommended daily inhalation dose in adults on a mg/m^2 basis) appears to have increased the incidence of both resorptions and malformations.

Nursing Mothers: It is not known whether this drug is excreted in human milk, therefore, caution should be exercised when **Intal** Inhaler is administered to a nursing woman and the attending physician must make a benefit/risk assessment in regard to its use in this situation.

Pediatric Use: Safety and effectiveness in pediatric patients below the age of 5 years have not been established. For young pediatric patients unable to utilize the Inhaler, **Intal** Nebulizer Solution (cromolyn sodium inhalation solution, USP) is recommended. Because of the possibility that adverse effects of this drug could become apparent only after many years, a benefit/risk consideration of the long-term use of **Intal** Inhaler is particularly important in pediatric patients.

ADVERSE REACTIONS

In controlled clinical studies of **Intal** Inhaler, the most frequently reported adverse reactions attributed to cromolyn sodium treatment were:

Throat irritation or dryness
Bad taste
Cough
Wheeze
Nausea

The most frequently reported adverse reactions attributed to other forms of cromolyn sodium (on the basis of reoccurrence following readministration) involve the respiratory tract and are: bronchospasm [sometimes severe, associated with a precipitous fall in pulmonary function (FEV_1)], cough, laryngeal edema (rare), nasal congestion (sometimes severe), pharyngeal irritation, and wheezing.

Adverse reactions which occur infrequently and are associated with administration of the drug are: anaphylaxis, angioedema, dizziness, dysuria and urinary frequency, joint swelling and pain, lacrimation, nausea and headache, rash, swollen parotid gland, urticaria, pulmonary infiltrates with eosinophilia, substernal burning, and myopathy.

The following adverse reactions have been reported as rare events and it is unclear whether they are attributable to the drug: anemia, exfoliative dermatitis, hemoptysis, hoarseness, myalgia, nephrosis, periarteritic vasculitis, pericarditis, peripheral neuritis, photodermatitis, sneezing, drowsiness, nasal itching, nasal bleeding, nasal burning, serum sickness, stomachache, polymyositis, vertigo, and liver disease.

OVERDOSAGE

There is no clinical syndrome associated with an overdosage of cromolyn sodium. In several animal species acute toxicity with cromolyn sodium occurs only with very high exposure levels. No deaths occurred at the highest oral doses tested in mice, 8000 mg/kg (approximately 5100 and 2700 times the maximum recommended daily inhalation doses in adults and children, respectively, on a mg/m^2 basis) or in rats, 8000 mg/kg (approximately 10,000 and 5400 times the maximum recommended daily inhalation doses in adults and children, respectively, on a mg/m^2 basis).

DOSAGE AND ADMINISTRATION

For management of bronchial asthma in adults and pediatric patients (5 years of age and over) who are able to use the Inhaler, the usual starting dosage is two metered inhalations four times daily at regular intervals. This dose should not be exceeded. Not all patients will respond to the recommended dose and there is evidence to suggest, at least in younger patients, that a lower dose may provide efficacy.

Patients with chronic asthma should be advised that the effect of **Intal** Inhaler therapy is dependent upon its administration at regular intervals, as directed. **Intal** Inhaler should be introduced into the patient's therapeutic regimen when the acute episode has been controlled, the airway has been cleared, and the patient is able to inhale adequately.

For the prevention of acute bronchospasm which follows exercise, exposure to cold, dry air, or environmental agents, the usual dose is two metered inhalations shortly before exposure to the precipitating factor, *i.e.*, within 10 to 15 minutes but not more than 60 minutes.

Intal Inhaler Therapy in Relation to Other Treatments for Asthma: *Non-steroidal agents:* **Intal** Inhaler should be *added* to the patient's existing treatment regimen (*e.g.*, bronchodilators). When a clinical response to **Intal** Inhaler is evident, usually within two to four weeks, and if the asthma is under good control, an attempt may be made to decrease concomitant medication usage gradually.

If concomitant medications are eliminated or required on no more than a prn basis, the frequency of administration of **Intal** Inhaler may be titrated downward to the lowest level consistent with the desired effect. The usual decrease is from two metered inhalations four times daily to three times daily to twice daily. It is important that the dosage be reduced gradually to avoid exacerbation of asthma. It is emphasized that in patients whose dosage has been titrated to fewer than four inhalations per day, an increase in the dosage of **Intal** Inhaler and the introduction of, or increase in, symptomatic medications may be needed if the patient's clinical condition deteriorates.

Corticosteroids: In patients chronically receiving corticosteroids for the management of bronchial asthma, the dosage should be maintained following the introduction of **Intal** Inhaler. If the patient improves, an attempt to decrease corticosteroids should be made. Even if the corticosteroid-dependent patient fails to show symptomatic improvement following **Intal** Inhaler administration, the potential to reduce corticosteroids may nonetheless be present. Thus, gradual tapering of corticosteroid dosage may be attempted. It is important that the dose be reduced slowly, maintaining close supervision of the patient to avoid an exacerbation of asthma.

It should be borne in mind that prolonged corticosteroid therapy frequently causes an impairment in the activity of the hypothalamic-pituitary-adrenal axis and a reduction in the size of the adrenal cortex. A potentially critical degree of impairment or insufficiency may persist asymptomatically for some time even after gradual discontinuation of adrenocortical steroids. Therefore, if a patient is subjected to significant stress, such as a severe asthmatic attack, surgery, trauma, or severe illness while being treated or within one year (occasionally up to two years) after corticosteroid treatment has been terminated, consideration should be given to reinstituting corticosteroid therapy. When respiratory function is impaired, as may occur in severe exacerbation of asthma, a temporary increase in the amount of corticosteroids may be required to regain control of the patient's asthma.

It is particularly important that great care be exercised if for any reason cromolyn sodium is withdrawn in cases where its use has permitted a reduction in the maintenance dose of corticosteroids. In such cases, continued close supervision of the patient is essential since there may be sudden reappearance of severe manifestations of asthma which will require immediate therapy and possible reintroduction of corticosteroids.

For best results, the canister should be at room temperature before use.

HOW SUPPLIED

Intal Inhaler is supplied as an aerosol canister which provides 112 metered dose actuations from the 8.1 gram inhaler and 200 metered dose actuations from the 14.2 gram inhaler. The correct amount of medication in each inhalation cannot be assured after 112 actuations from the 8.1 gram canister or 200 actuations from the 14.2 gram canister even though the canister may not feel completely empty. The canister should be discarded when the labeled number of actuations have been used.

Each actuation delivers 1 mg cromolyn sodium through the valve and 800 mcg through the mouthpiece to the patient. The **Intal** Inhaler canister and accompanying mouthpiece are designed to be used together. The **Intal** Inhaler canister should not be used with other mouthpieces and the supplied mouthpiece should not be used with other products' canisters. **Intal** Inhaler is supplied with a white plastic mouthpiece with blue dust cap and patient instructions.

NDC 0585-0675-01 14.2 g canister
NDC 0585-0675-02 8.1 g canister

Store between 15 to 30°C (59 to 86°F). Contents under pressure. Do not puncture, incinerate, or place near sources of heat. Exposure to temperatures above 120°F may cause bursting. **Avoid spraying in eyes. Keep out of the reach of children.**

Note: The indented statement below is required by the Federal government's Clean Air Act for all products containing or manufactured with chlorofluorocarbons (CFCs).

WARNING: Contains CFC-12 (dichlorodifluoromethane) and CFC-114 (dichlorotetrafluoroethane), substances which harm public health and the environment by destroying ozone in the upper atmosphere.

A notice similar to the above WARNING has been placed in the "Information For The Patient" portion of this package insert under the Environmental Protection Agency's (EPA's) regulations. The patient's warning states that the patient should consult his or her physician if there are questions about alternatives.

Caution: Federal law prohibits dispensing without prescription.

Marketed by:
RHÔNE-POULENC RORER RESPIRATORY
A division of Rhône-Poulenc Rorer Pharmaceuticals Inc.
Collegeville, PA 19426 ©1997
Made in England
Manufactured by:
Health Care Specialties Division Rev. 9/97
3M Health Care Limited IN-0033A
Loughborough, England LE11 1EP 156-1-140

Shown in Product Identification Guide, page 333

INTAL® Nebulizer Solution ℞

(cromolyn sodium inhalation solution, USP)
For Inhalation Use Only—Not for Injection

DESCRIPTION

The active ingredient of INTAL Nebulizer Solution is cromolyn sodium, USP. It is an inhaled anti-inflammatory agent for the preventive management of asthma. Cromolyn sodium is disodium 5,5'-[(2-hydroxytrimethylene)dioxy]-bis[4-oxo-4*H*-1-benzopyran-2-carboxylate]. The empirical formula is $C_{23}H_{14}Na_2O_{11}$; the molecular weight is 512.34. Cromolyn sodium is a water soluble, odorless, white, hydrated crystalline powder. It is tasteless at first, but leaves a slightly bitter aftertaste. INTAL Nebulizer Solution is clear, colorless, sterile, and has a target pH of 5.5.

The molecular structure is:

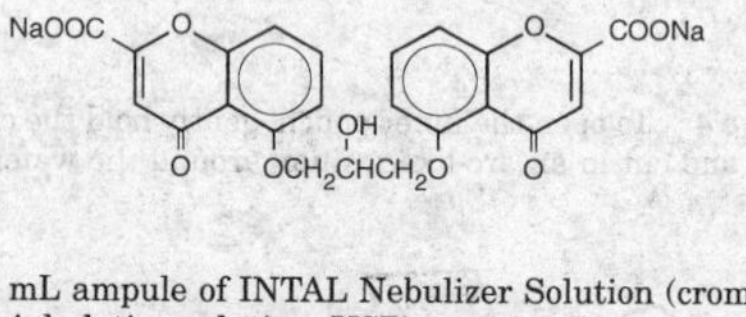

Each 2 mL ampule of INTAL Nebulizer Solution (cromolyn sodium inhalation solution, USP) contains 20 mg cromolyn sodium, USP, in purified water.

CLINICAL PHARMACOLOGY

In vitro and *in vivo* animal studies have shown that cromolyn sodium inhibits sensitized mast cell degranulation which occurs after exposure to specific antigens. Cromolyn sodium acts by inhibiting the release of mediators from mast cells. Studies show that cromolyn sodium indirectly blocks calcium ions from entering the mast cell, thereby preventing mediator release.

Cromolyn sodium inhibits both the immediate and non-immediate bronchoconstrictive reactions to inhaled antigen. Cromolyn sodium also attenuates bronchospasm caused by exercise, toluene diisocyanate, aspirin, cold air, sulfur dioxide, and environmental pollutants.

Cromolyn sodium has no intrinsic bronchodilator or antihistamine activity.

After administration by inhalation, approximately 8% of the total cromolyn sodium dose administered is absorbed and rapidly excreted unchanged, approximately equally divided between urine and bile. The remainder of the dose is either exhaled or deposited in the oropharynx, swallowed and excreted via the alimentary tract.

INDICATIONS AND USAGE

INTAL is a prophylactic agent indicated in the management of patients with bronchial asthma.

In patients whose symptoms are sufficiently frequent to require a continuous program of medication, INTAL is given by inhalation on a regular daily basis (see **DOSAGE AND ADMINISTRATION**). The effect of INTAL is usually evident after several weeks of treatment, although some patients show an almost immediate response.

In patients who develop acute bronchoconstriction in response to exposure to exercise, toluene diisocyanate, environmental pollutants, etc., INTAL should be given shortly before exposure to the precipitating factor (see **DOSAGE AND ADMINISTRATION**).

CONTRAINDICATIONS

INTAL is contraindicated in those patients who have shown hypersensitivity to cromolyn sodium.

WARNINGS

INTAL has no role in the treatment of status asthmaticus. Anaphylactic reactions with cromolyn sodium administration have been reported rarely.

PRECAUTIONS

General: Occasionally, patients may experience cough and/or bronchospasm following INTAL inhalation. At times, patients who develop bronchospasm may not be able to continue INTAL administration despite prior bronchodilator administration. Rarely, very severe bronchospasm has been encountered.

Symptoms of asthma may recur if INTAL is reduced below the recommended dosage or discontinued.

Information for Patients: INTAL is to be taken as directed by the physician. Because it is preventive medication, it may take up to four weeks before the patient experiences maximum benefit.

INTAL Nebulizer Solution should be used in a power-driven nebulizer with an adequate airflow rate equipped with a suitable face mask or mouthpiece.

Drug stability and safety of INTAL Nebulizer Solution when mixed with other drugs in a nebulizer have not been established.

For additional information, see the accompanying leaflet entitled *Living a Full Life with Asthma.*

Carcinogenesis, Mutagenesis, and Impairment of Fertility: Long term studies of cromolyn sodium in mice (12 months intraperitoneal administration at doses up to 150 mg/kg three days per week), hamsters (intraperitoneal administration at doses up to 52.6 mg/kg three days per week for 15 weeks followed by 17.5 mg/kg three days per week for 37 weeks), and rats (18 months subcutaneous administration at doses up to 75 mg/kg six days per week) showed no neoplastic effects. The average daily maximum dose levels administered in these studies were 192.9 mg/m^2 for mice, 47.2 mg/m^2 for hamsters and 385.8 mg/m^2 for rats. These doses correspond to approximately 330%, 80%, and 650% of the maximum daily human dose of 59.2 mg/m^2.

Cromolyn sodium showed no mutagenic potential in Ames Salmonella/microsome plate assays, mitotic gene conversion in *Saccharomyces cerevisiae* and in an *in vitro* cytogenetic study in human peripheral lymphocytes.

No evidence of impaired fertility was shown in laboratory reproduction studies conducted subcutaneously in rats at the highest doses tested, 175 mg/kg/day (1050 mg/m^2) in males and 100 mg/kg/day (600 mg/m^2) in females. These doses are approximately 18 and 10 times the maximum daily human dose, respectively, based on mg/m^2.

Pregnancy: Pregnancy Category B. Reproduction studies with cromolyn sodium administered subcutaneously to pregnant mice and rats at maximum daily doses of 540 mg/kg (1620 mg/m^2) and 164 mg/kg (984 mg/m^2), respectively, and intravenously to rabbits at a maximum daily dose of 485 mg/kg (5820 mg/m^2) produced no evidence of fetal malformations. These doses represent approximately 27, 16, and 98 times the maximum daily human dose, respectively, on a mg/m^2 basis. Adverse fetal effects (increased resorptions and decreased fetal weight) were noted only at the very high parenteral doses that produced maternal toxicity. There are, however, no adequate and well-controlled studies in pregnant women.

Because animal reproduction studies are not always predictive of human response, this drug should be used during pregnancy only if clearly needed.

Drug Interaction During Pregnancy: Cromolyn sodium and isoproterenol were studied following subcutaneous injections in pregnant mice. Cromolyn sodium alone in doses of 60 to 540 mg/kg (38 to 338 times the human dose) did not cause significant increases in resorptions or major malfor-

mations. Isoproterenol alone at a dose of 2.7 mg/kg (90 times the human dose) increased both resorptions and malformations. The addition of cromolyn sodium (338 times the human dose) to isoproterenol (90 times the human dose) appears to have increased the incidence of both resorptions and malformations.

Nursing Mothers: It is not known whether this drug is excreted in human milk. Because many drugs are excreted in human milk, caution should be exercised when INTAL is administered to a nursing woman.

Pediatric Use: Safety and effectiveness in pediatric patients below the age of 2 years have not been established.

ADVERSE REACTIONS

Clinical experience with the use of INTAL suggests that adverse reactions are rare events. The following adverse reactions have been associated with INTAL Nebulizer Solution: cough, nasal congestion, nausea, sneezing, and wheezing. Other reactions have been reported in clinical trials; however, a causal relationship could not be established: drowsiness, nasal itching, nose bleed, nose burning, serum sickness, and stomachache.

In addition, adverse reactions have been reported with INTAL Capsules (cromolyn sodium for inhalation, USP). The most common side effects are associated with inhalation of the powder and include transient cough (1 in 5 patients) and mild wheezing (1 in 25 patients). These effects rarely require treatment or discontinuation of the drug.

Information on the incidence of adverse reactions to INTAL Capsules has been derived from U.S. postmarketing surveillance experience. The following adverse reactions attributed to INTAL, based upon recurrence following readministration, have been reported in less than 1 in 10,000 patients: laryngeal edema, swollen parotid gland, angioedema, bronchospasm, joint swelling and pain, dizziness, dysuria and urinary frequency, nausea, cough, wheezing, headache, nasal congestion, rash, urticaria, and lacrimation.

Other adverse reactions have been reported in less than 1 in 100,000 patients, and it is unclear whether these are attributable to the drug: anaphylaxis, nephrosis, periarteritic vasculitis, pericarditis, peripheral neuritis, pulmonary infiltrates with eosinophilia, polymyositis, exfoliative dermatitis, hemoptysis, anemia, myalgia, hoarseness, photodermatitis, and vertigo.

OVERDOSAGE

There is no clinical syndrome associated with an overdosage of cromolyn sodium. Acute toxicity testing in a wide variety of species has demonstrated an extremely low order of toxicity for cromolyn sodium, regardless of whether administration was parenteral, oral or by inhalation. Parenteral administration in mice, rats, guinea pigs, hamsters, and rabbits demonstrated an LD$_{50}$ in the region of 4000 mg/kg. Intravenous administration in monkeys also indicated a similar order of toxicity. The highest dose administered by the oral route in rats and mice was 8000 mg/kg, and at this dose level no deaths occurred. By inhalation, even in long term studies, it proved impossible to achieve toxic dose levels of cromolyn sodium in a range of mammalian species.

DOSAGE AND ADMINISTRATION

For management of bronchial asthma in adults and pediatric patients (two years of age and over), the usual starting dosage is the contents of one ampule administered by nebulization four times a day at regular intervals.

Drug stability and safety of INTAL Nebulizer Solution when mixed with other drugs in a nebulizer have not been established.

Patients with chronic asthma should be advised that the effect of INTAL therapy is dependent upon its administration at regular intervals, as directed. INTAL should be introduced into the patient's therapeutic regimen when the acute episode has been controlled, the airway has been cleared and the patient is able to inhale adequately.

For the prevention of acute bronchospasm which follows exercise or exposure to cold dry air, environmental agents (e.g., animal danders, toluene diisocyanate, pollutants), etc., the usual dose is the contents of one ampule administered by nebulization shortly before exposure to the precipitating factor.

It should be emphasized to the patient that the drug is poorly absorbed when swallowed and is not effective by this route of administration.

INTAL Therapy in Relation to Other Treatments for Asthma: Non-steroidal agents: INTAL should be *added* to the patient's existing treatment regimen (e.g., bronchodilators). When a clinical response to INTAL is evident, usually within two to four weeks, and if the asthma is under good control, an attempt may be made to decrease concomitant medication usage gradually.

If concomitant medications are eliminated or required on no more than a prn basis, the frequency of administration of INTAL may be titrated downward to the lowest level consistent with the desired effect. The usual decrease is from four to three ampules per day. It is important that the dosage be reduced gradually to avoid exacerbation of asthma. It

is emphasized that in patients whose dosage has been titrated to fewer than four ampules per day, an increase in the dose of INTAL and the introduction of, or increase in, symptomatic medications may be needed if the patient's clinical condition deteriorates.

Corticosteroids: In patients chronically receiving corticosteroids for the management of bronchial asthma, the dosage should be maintained following the introduction of INTAL. If the patient improves, an attempt to decrease corticosteroids should be made. Even if the corticosteroid-dependent patient fails to show symptomatic improvement following INTAL administration, the potential to reduce corticosteroids may nonetheless be present. Thus, gradual tapering of corticosteroid dosage may be attempted. It is important that the dose be reduced slowly, maintaining close supervision of the patient to avoid an exacerbation of asthma.

It should be borne in mind that prolonged corticosteroid therapy frequently causes an impairment in the activity of the hypothalamic-pituitary-adrenal axis and a reduction in the size of the adrenal cortex. A potentially critical degree of impairment or insufficiency may persist asymptomatically for some time even after gradual discontinuation of adrenocortical steroids. Therefore, if a patient is subjected to significant stress, such as a severe asthmatic attack, surgery, trauma or severe illness while being treated or within one year (occasionally up to two years) after corticosteroid treatment has been terminated, consideration should be given to reinstituting corticosteroid therapy. When respiratory function is impaired, as may occur in severe exacerbation of asthma, a temporary increase in the amount of corticosteroids may be required to regain control of the patient's asthma.

It is particularly important that great care be exercised if, for any reason, INTAL is withdrawn in cases where its use has permitted a reduction in the maintenance dose of corticosteroids. In such cases, continued close supervision of the patient is essential since there may be sudden reappearance of severe manifestations of asthma which will require immediate therapy and possible reintroduction of corticosteroids.

HOW SUPPLIED

INTAL Nebulizer Solution is a colorless solution supplied in a low density polyethylene plastic unit dose ampule with 12 ampules per foil pouch. Each 2 mL ampule contains 20 mg cromolyn sodium, USP, in purified water.

NDC 0585-0673-02   60 ampules × 2 mL
NDC 0585-0673-03   120 ampules × 2 mL

Store at Controlled Room Temperature 20 to 25°C (68 to 77°F) [see USP]. Protect from light. Do not use if it contains a precipitate or becomes discolored. Keep out of the reach of children.

Store ampules in foil pouch until ready for use.

CAUTION: Federal law prohibits dispensing without prescription.

Manufactured by:
Automatic Liquid Packaging, Inc.
Woodstock, IL 60098

Rev. 11/96
IN-0030A

Shown in Product Identification Guide, page 333

LOVENOX®   ℞
(enoxaparin sodium)
Injection

SPINAL/EPIDURAL HEMATOMAS

When neuraxial anesthesia (epidural/spinal anesthesia) or spinal puncture is employed, patients anticoagulated or scheduled to be anticoagulated with low molecular weight heparins or heparinoids for prevention of thromboembolic complications are at risk of developing an epidural or spinal hematoma which can result in long-term or permanent paralysis.

The risk of these events is increased by the use of indwelling epidural catheters for administration of analgesia or by the concomitant use of drugs affecting hemostasis such as non steroidal anti-inflammatory drugs (NSAIDs), platelet inhibitors, or other anticoagulants. The risk also appears to be increased by traumatic or repeated epidural or spinal puncture.

Patients should be frequently monitored for signs and symptoms of neurological impairment. If neurologic compromise is noted, urgent treatment is necessary.

The physician should consider the potential benefit versus risk before neuraxial intervention in patients anticoagulated or to be anticoagulated for thromboprophy-

---

Continued on next page

Lovenox—Cont.

laxis (see also **WARNINGS, Hemorrhage**, and **PRE-CAUTIONS, Drug Interactions**).

DESCRIPTION

Lovenox Injection is a sterile solution for injection containing enoxaparin sodium, a low molecular weight heparin. It is available in: prefilled syringes (30 and 40 mg), graduated prefilled syringes (60, 80, and 100 mg), and ampules (30 mg). Each dosage unit contains 10 mg enoxaparin sodium per 0.1 mL Water for Injection. The solution is preservative-free and intended for use only as a single-dose injection. (See **DOSAGE AND ADMINISTRATION** and **HOW SUPPLIED** for dosage unit descriptions.)

The pH of the injection is 5.5 to 7.5, with an approximate anti-Factor Xa activity per dosage unit of 1000 IU per every 10 mg of enoxaparin sodium (with reference to the W.H.O. First International Low Molecular Weight Heparin Reference Standard). Nitrogen is used in the headspace to inhibit oxidation.

Enoxaparin is obtained by alkaline degradation of heparin benzyl ester derived from porcine intestinal mucosa. Its structure is characterized by a 2-O-sulfo-4-enepyranosuronic acid group at the non-reducing end and a 2-N,6-O-disulfo-D-glucosamine at the reducing end of the chain. The substance is the sodium salt. The average molecular weight is about 4500 daltons. The molecular weight distribution is:

<2000 daltons   ≤20%
2000 to 8000 daltons ≥68%
>8000 daltons   ≤15%

STRUCTURAL FORMULA

CLINICAL PHARMACOLOGY

Enoxaparin is a low molecular weight heparin which has antithrombotic properties. In humans, enoxaparin given at a dose of 1.5 mg/kg subcutaneously (s.c.) is characterized by a higher ratio of anti-Factor Xa to anti-Factor IIa activity (mean±SD, 14.0±3.1) (based on areas under anti-Factor activity versus time curves) compared to the ratios observed for heparin (mean±SD, 1.22±0.13). Increases of up to 1.5 times the control values were seen in the thrombin time (TT) and the activated partial thromboplastin time (aPTT). Following the administration of a single s.c. dose of up to 90 mg of enoxaparin to healthy subjects, no appreciable change was observed in fibrinogen level, other parameters of fibrinolysis, platelet aggregation, or prothrombin time (PT). Enoxaparin at 1 mg/kg dose, administered s.c. every 12h to patients in a large clinical trial produced minimal increases in aPTT (<45 seconds) in the majority of patients (n = 1607).

Pharmacodynamics: Maximum anti-Factor Xa and antithrombin (anti-Factor IIa) activities occur 3 to 5 hours after s.c. injection of enoxaparin. Mean peak anti-Factor Xa activity was 0.16 IU/mL (1.58 µg/mL) and 0.38 IU/mL (3.83 µg/mL) after the 20 mg and the 40 mg clinically tested doses, respectively. Mean (n = 46) peak anti-Factor Xa activity was 1.1 IU/mL at steady state in patients with unstable angina receiving 1.0 mg/kg every 12 hours for 14 days. Mean absolute bioavailability of enoxaparin based on anti-Factor Xa activity is 92% in healthy volunteers. The volume of distribution of anti-Factor Xa activity is about 6 L. Following intravenous (i.v.) dosing, the total body clearance of enoxaparin is 25 mL/min. After i.v. dosing of enoxaparin labeled with the gamma-emitter, ^{99m}Tc, 40% of radioactivity and 8 to 20% of anti-Factor Xa activity were recovered in urine in 24 hours. Elimination half-life based on anti-Factor Xa activity was 4.5 hours after s.c. administration. Following a 40 mg once daily dose, significant anti-Factor Xa activity persists in plasma for about 12 hours.

Clearance and C_{max} derived from anti-Factor Xa values following single and multiple s.c. dosing in elderly subjects and subjects with mild to moderate renal failure (creatinine clearance 30 to 80 mL/min) were close to those observed in healthy subjects. Following once daily dosing of 40 mg enoxaparin in elderly, healthy subjects, the Day 10 mean area under anti-Factor Xa activity versus time curve (AUC) was 25% greater than the mean AUC value obtained after the first dose. The kinetics of anti-Factor Xa activity in anuric patients undergoing dialysis are similar to those (in other studies) in healthy subjects receiving a comparable dose of 0.5 mg/kg given intravenously.

Efficacy of Lovenox in Hip Replacement Surgery

Indication	Lovenox Dosing Regimen		
	10 mg q.d. s.c. n (%)	30 mg q12h s.c. n (%)	40 mg q.d. s.c. n (%)
All Treated Hip Replacement Patients	161 (100)	208 (100)	199 (100)
Treatment Failures Total DVT (%)	40 (25)	22 (11)[1]	27 (14)
Proximal DVT (%)	17 (11)	8 (4)[2]	9 (5)

[1] p value versus Lovenox 10 mg q.d. = 0.0008
[2] p value versus Lovenox 10 mg q.d. = 0.0168

Efficacy of Lovenox with Extended Prophylaxis Following Hip Replacement Surgery

Indication (Post-discharge)	Post-Discharge Dosing Regimen	
	Lovenox 40 mg q.d. s.c. n (%)	Placebo q.d. s.c. n (%)
All Treated Extended Prophylaxis Patients	90 (100)	89 (100)
Treatment Failures Total DVT (%)	6 (7)[1] (95% CI: 3 to 14)	18 (20) (95% CI: 12 to 30)
Proximal DVT (%)	5 (6)[2] (95% CI: 2 to 13)	7 (8) (95% CI: 3 to 16)

[1] p value versus placebo = 0.008
[2] p value versus placebo = 0.537

Efficacy of Lovenox in Knee Replacement Surgery

Indication	Dosing Regimen	
	Lovenox 30 mg q12h s.c. n (%)	Placebo q12h s.c. n (%)
All Treated Knee Replacement Patients	47 (100)	52 (100)
Treatment Failures Total DVT (%)	5 (11)[1] (95% CI: 1 to 21)	32 (62) (95% CI: 47 to 76)
Proximal DVT (%)	0 (0)[2] (95% Upper CL: 5)	7 (13) (95% CI: 3 to 24)

[1] p value versus placebo = 0.0001
CI = Confidence Interval
[2] p value versus placebo = 0.013
CL = Confidence Limit

CLINICAL TRIALS

Hip or Knee Replacement Surgery: Lovenox has been shown to prevent post-operative deep vein thrombosis (DVT) following hip or knee replacement surgery.

In a double-blind study, Lovenox 30 mg every 12h s.c. was compared to placebo in patients with hip replacement. After hemostasis was established, treatment was initiated 12 to 24 hours after surgery and was continued for 10 to 14 days after surgery. The data are provided below.

Efficacy of Lovenox in Hip Replacement Surgery

Indication	Dosing Regimen	
	Lovenox 30 mg q12h s.c. n (%)	Placebo q12h s.c. n (%)
All Treated Hip Replacement Patients	50 (100)	50 (100)
Treatment Failures Total DVT (%)	5 (10)[1]	23 (46)
Proximal DVT (%)	1 (2)[2]	11 (22)

[1] p value versus placebo = 0.0002
[2] p value versus placebo = 0.0134

A double-blind, multicenter study compared three dosing regimens of Lovenox in patients with hip replacement. Treatment was initiated within two days after surgery and was continued for 7 to 11 days after surgery. The data are provided below.
[See first table at top of page]
There was no significant difference between the 30 mg every 12h and 40 mg once-a-day regimens.

Extended Prophylaxis in Hip Replacement Surgery: In a study of extended prophylaxis for patients undergoing hip replacement surgery, patients were treated, while hospitalized, with enoxaparin 40 mg s.c., initiated up to 12 hours prior to surgery for the prevention of post-operative deep vein thrombosis. At the end of the peri-operative period, all patients underwent bilateral venography. In a double-blind design, those patients with no venous thromboembolic disease were randomized to a post-discharge regimen of either enoxaparin 40 mg (n = 90) once daily s.c. or to placebo (n = 89) for 3 weeks. In this population of patients, the incidence of deep vein thrombosis during extended prophylaxis was significantly lower for enoxaparin compared to placebo. The data are provided below.
[See second table above]

In a second study, patients undergoing hip replacement surgery were treated, while hospitalized, with enoxaparin 40 mg s.c., initiated up to 12 hours prior to surgery. All patients were examined for clinical signs and symptoms of venous thromboembolic disease. In a double-blind design, patients without clinical signs and symptoms of venous thromboembolic disease were randomized to a post-discharge regimen of either enoxaparin 40 mg (n = 131) once daily s.c. or to placebo (n = 131) for 3 weeks. Similar to the first study the incidence of deep vein thrombosis during extended prophylaxis was significantly lower for enoxaparin compared to placebo, with a statistically significant difference in both total DVT (enoxaparin 21 [16%] versus placebo 45 [34%]; p = 0.001) and proximal DVT (enoxaparin 8 [6%] versus placebo 28 [21%]; p = <0.001).

In a double-blind study, Lovenox 30 mg every 12h s.c. was compared to placebo in 99 patients undergoing knee replacement surgery. After hemostasis was established, treatment was initiated 12 to 24 hours after surgery and was continued up to 15 days after surgery. The incidence of proximal and total deep vein thrombosis after surgery was significantly lower for enoxaparin compared to placebo. The data are provided below.

[See third table from top on previous page]
Additionally, in an open-label, parallel group, randomized clinical study, Lovenox 30 mg every 12h s.c. in patients undergoing elective knee replacement surgery was compared to heparin 5000 U every 8h s.c. Treatment was initiated after surgery and continued up to 14 days. The incidence of deep vein thrombosis was significantly lower for enoxaparin compared to heparin.

Abdominal Surgery: In a double-blind, parallel group study of 1115 patients undergoing elective cancer surgery of the gastrointestinal, urological, or gynecological tract, Lovenox 40 mg s.c., administered once daily, beginning 2 hours prior to surgery and continuing for a maximum of 12 days after surgery, was comparable to heparin 5000 U every 8h s.c. in preventing deep vein thrombosis (DVT). The data are provided below.
[See first table at right]
In a second double-blind, parallel group study, Lovenox 40 mg s.c. once daily was compared to heparin 5000 U every 8h s.c. in 1347 patients undergoing colorectal surgery (one-third with cancer). Treatment was initiated approximately 2 hours prior to surgery and continued for approximately 7 to 10 days after surgery. The data are provided below.
[See second table at right]

Unstable Angina and Non-Q-Wave Myocardial Infarction: In a multicenter, double-blind, parallel group study, 3171 patients who recently experienced unstable angina or non-Q-wave myocardial infarction were randomized to either Lovenox 1 mg/kg every 12h s.c. or heparin i.v. bolus (5000 U) followed by a continuous infusion (adjusted to achieve an aPTT of 55 to 85 seconds). **All** patients were also treated with aspirin 100 to 325 mg per day. Treatment was initiated within 24 hours of the event and continued until clinical stabilization, revascularization procedures, or hospital discharge, with a maximal duration of 8 days of therapy. The combined incidence of the triple endpoint of death, myocardial infarction, or recurrent angina was lower for Lovenox compared with heparin therapy at 14 days after initiation of treatment. The lower incidence of the triple endpoint was sustained up to 30 days after initiation of treatment. These results were observed in an analysis of both all-randomized and all-treated patients.
Urgent revascularization procedures were performed less frequently in the Lovenox group as compared to the heparin group, 6.3% compared to 8.2% at 30 days (p = 0.047).
[See third table at right]
The combined incidence of death or myocardial infarction at all time points was lower for Lovenox® (enoxaparin sodium) Injection compared to standard heparin therapy, but did not achieve statistical significance. The data are provided below.
[See fourth table at right]

INDICATIONS AND USAGE
- Lovenox Injection is indicated for the prevention of deep vein thrombosis, which may lead to pulmonary embolism:
  - in patients undergoing hip replacement surgery, during and following hospitalization;
  - in patients undergoing knee replacement surgery;
  - in patients undergoing abdominal surgery who are at risk for thromboembolic complications. Patients at risk include patients who are over 40 years of age, obese, undergoing surgery under general anesthesia lasting longer than 30 minutes or who have additional risk factors such as malignancy or a history of deep vein thrombosis or pulmonary embolism.
- Lovenox Injection is indicated for the prevention of ischemic complications of unstable angina and non-Q-wave myocardial infarction, when concurrently administered with aspirin.

See **DOSAGE AND ADMINISTRATION: Adult Dosage** for appropriate dosage regimens.

CONTRAINDICATIONS
Lovenox Injection is contraindicated in patients with active major bleeding, in patients with thrombocytopenia associated with a positive *in vitro* test for anti-platelet antibody in the presence of enoxaparin sodium, or in patients with hypersensitivity to enoxaparin sodium.
Patients with known hypersensitivity to heparin or pork products should not be treated with Lovenox Injection.

WARNINGS
Lovenox Injection is not intended for intramuscular administration.
Lovenox cannot be used interchangeably (unit for unit) with heparin or other low molecular weight heparins as they differ in manufacturing process, molecular weight distribution, anti-Xa and anti-IIa activities, units, and dosage. Each of these medicines has its own instructions for use.
Lovenox should be used with extreme caution in patients with a history of heparin-induced thrombocytopenia.
Hemorrhage: Lovenox Injection, like other anticoagulants, should be used with extreme caution in conditions with increased risk of hemorrhage, such as bacterial endocarditis, congenital or acquired bleeding disorders, active

ulcerative and angiodysplastic gastrointestinal disease, hemorrhagic stroke, or shortly after brain, spinal, or ophthalmological surgery, or in patients treated concomitantly with platelet inhibitors.
Cases of epidural or spinal hematomas have been reported with the associated use of enoxaparin and spinal/epidural anesthesia or spinal puncture resulting in long-term or permanent paralysis. The risk of these events is higher with the use of post-operative indwelling epidural catheters or by the concomitant use of additional drugs affecting hemo-

stasis such as NSAIDs (see boxed WARNING; ADVERSE REACTIONS, Ongoing Safety Surveillance; and PRECAUTIONS, Drug Interactions).
Bleeding can occur at any site during therapy with enoxaparin. An unexplained fall in hematocrit or blood pressure should lead to a search for a bleeding site.
Thrombocytopenia: Thrombocytopenia can occur with the administration of Lovenox.

Continued on next page

Efficacy of Lovenox in Abdominal Surgery Patients with Cancer

Indication	Dosing Regimen	
	Lovenox 40 mg q.d. s.c. n (%)	Heparin 5000 U q8h s.c. n (%)
All Treated Abdominal Surgery Patients	555 (100)	560 (100)
Treatment Failures Total VTE[1] (%)	56 (10.1) (95% CI[2]: 8 to 13)	63 (11.3) (95% CI: 9 to 14)
DVT Only (%)	54 (9.7) (95% CI: 7 to 12)	61 (10.9) (95% CI: 8 to 13)

[1]VTE = Venous thromboembolic events which included DVT, PE, and death considered to be thromboembolic in origin.
[2]CI = Confidence Interval

Efficacy of Lovenox in Colorectal Surgery

Indication	Dosing Regimen	
	Lovenox 40 mg q.d. s.c. n (%)	Heparin 5000 U q8h s.c. n (%)
All Treated Colorectal Surgery Patients	673 (100)	674 (100)
Treatment Failures Total VTE[1] (%)	48 (7.1) (95% CI[2]: 5 to 9)	45 (6.7) (95% CI: 5 to 9)
DVT Only (%)	47 (7.0) (95% CI: 5 to 9)	44 (6.5) (95% CI: 5 to 8)

[1]VTE = Venous thromboembolic events which included DVT, PE, and death considered to be thromboembolic in origin.
[2]CI = Confidence Interval

Efficacy of Lovenox in Unstable Angina and Non-Q-Wave Myocardial Infarction (Combined Endpoint of Death, Myocardial Infarction, or Recurrent Angina)

Indication	Dosing Regimen[1]		Reduction (%)	p Value
	Lovenox 1 mg/kg q12h s.c. n (%)	Heparin aPTT Adjusted i.v. Therapy n (%)		
All Randomized Unstable Angina and Non-Q-Wave MI Patients	1607 (100)	1564 (100)		
Timepoint[2]				
48 Hours	99 (6.2)	115 (7.4)	1.2	0.178
14 Days	266 (16.6)	309 (19.8)	3.2	0.019
30 Days	318 (19.8)	364 (23.3)	3.5	0.016

[1]All patients were also treated with aspirin 100 to 325 mg per day.
[2]Evaluation timepoints are after initiation of treatment. Therapy continued for up to 8 days (median duration of 2.6 days).

Efficacy of Lovenox in Unstable Angina and Non-Q-Wave Myocardial Infarction (Combined Endpoint of Death or Myocardial Infarction)

Indication	Dosing Regimen[1]		Reduction (%)	p Value
	Lovenox 1 mg/kg q12h s.c. n (%)	Heparin aPTT Adjusted i.v. Therapy n (%)		
All Randomized Unstable Angina and Non-Q-Wave MI Patients	1607 (100)	1564 (100)		
Timepoint[2]				
48 Hours	18 (1.1)	21 (1.3)	0.2	0.119
14 Days	79 (4.9)	96 (6.1)	1.2	0.132
30 Days	99 (6.2)	121 (7.7)	1.5	0.081

[1]All patients were also treated with aspirin 100 to 325 mg per day.
[2]Evaluation timepoints are after initiation of treatment. Therapy continued for up to 8 days (median duration of 2.6 days).

Lovenox—Cont.

Hip and Knee Replacement Surgery: During clinical trials in patients following hip and knee replacement surgery, moderate thrombocytopenia (platelet counts between 100,000/mm³ and 50,000/mm³) occurred at a rate of 1.5% in patients given Lovenox, 2.0% in patients given heparin, and 0.6% in patients given placebo.

Platelet counts less than 50,000/mm³ occurred at a rate of 0.05% in patients given Lovenox, 0.5% in patients given heparin, and 0% in patients given placebo in the same trials.

Abdominal Surgery: During clinical trials in patients following abdominal surgery, moderate thrombocytopenia (platelet counts between 100,000/mm³ and 50,000/mm³) occurred at a rate of 2% in patients given Lovenox, and 1.5% in patients given heparin.

Platelet counts less than 50,000/mm³ occurred at a rate of 0.08% in patients given Lovenox and in 0.3% of patients given heparin in the same trials.

Unstable Angina: During a clinical trial in patients with unstable angina or non-Q-wave myocardial infarctions, moderate thrombocytopenia (platelet counts between 100,000/mm³ and 50,000/mm³) occurred at a rate of 0.4% in patients given Lovenox as well as in patients given heparin.

Platelet counts less than 50,000/mm³ occurred at a rate of 0.1% in patients given Lovenox and in 0% of patients given heparin in the same trial.

Thrombocytopenia of any degree should be monitored closely. If the platelet count falls below 100,000/mm³, enoxaparin should be discontinued. Rare cases of thrombocytopenia with thrombosis have also been observed in clinical practice. The rate of incidence of this complication in usual medical practice is unknown at present.

PRECAUTIONS

General: Lovenox Injection should not be mixed with other injections or infusions.

Lovenox Injection should be used with care in patients with a bleeding diathesis, uncontrolled arterial hypertension or a history of recent gastrointestinal ulceration, diabetic retinopathy, and hemorrhage. Elderly patients and patients with renal insufficiency may show delayed elimination of enoxaparin. Enoxaparin should be used with care in these patients.

If thromboembolic events occur despite enoxaparin prophylaxis, Lovenox should be discontinued and appropriate therapy initiated.

Laboratory Tests: Periodic complete blood counts, including platelet count, and stool occult blood tests are recommended during the course of treatment with Lovenox Injection. When administered at recommended prophylaxis doses, routine coagulation tests such as Prothrombin Time (PT) and Activated Partial Thromboplastin Time (aPTT) are relatively insensitive measures of Lovenox activity and, therefore, unsuitable for monitoring. Anti-Factor Xa may be used to monitor the anticoagulant effect of Lovenox in patients with significant renal impairment. If during Lovenox therapy abnormal coagulation parameters or bleeding should occur, anti-Factor Xa levels may be used to monitor the anticoagulant effects of Lovenox (see **CLINICAL PHARMACOLOGY: Pharmacodynamics**).

Drug Interactions: Unless really needed, agents which may enhance the risk of hemorrhage should be discontinued prior to initiation of Lovenox therapy. These agents include medications such as: anticoagulants, platelet inhibitors including acetylsalicylic acid, salicylates, NSAIDs (including ketorolac tromethamine), dipyridamole, or sulfinpyrazone. If co-administration is essential, conduct close clinical and laboratory monitoring (see **PRECAUTIONS: Laboratory Tests**).

Carcinogenesis, Mutagenesis, Impairment of Fertility: No long-term studies in animals have been performed to evaluate the carcinogenic potential of enoxaparin. Enoxaparin was not mutagenic in *in vitro* tests, including the Ames test, mouse lymphoma cell forward mutation test, and human lymphocyte chromosomal aberration test, and the *in vivo* rat bone marrow chromosomal aberration test. Enoxaparin was found to have no effect on fertility or reproductive performance of male and female rats at s.c. doses up to 20 mg/kg/day or 141 mg/m²/day. The maximum human dose in clinical trials was 2.0 mg/kg/day or 78 mg/m²/day (for an average body weight of 70 kg, height of 170 cm, and body surface area of 1.8 m²).

Pregnancy: *Teratogenic Effects: Pregnancy Category B:* Teratology studies have been conducted in pregnant rats and rabbits at s.c. doses of enoxaparin up to 30 mg/kg/day or 211 mg/m²/day and 410 mg/m²/day, respectively. There was no evidence of teratogenic effects or fetotoxicity due to enoxaparin. There are, however, no adequate and well-controlled studies in pregnant women. Because animal reproduction studies are not always predictive of human response, this drug should be used during pregnancy only if clearly needed.

Non-teratogenic Effects: There have been a few spontaneous post-marketing reports of fetal death when pregnant

women received enoxaparin. Causality of the cases has not been determined. In one case, placental hemorrhage and detachment were found in association with the fetal death. If enoxaparin is used during pregnancy, or if the patient becomes pregnant while taking this drug, the patient should be apprised of the potential hazard to the fetus.

Nursing Mothers: It is not known whether this drug is excreted in human milk. Because many drugs are excreted in human milk, caution should be exercised when enoxaparin is administered to nursing women.

Pediatric Use: Safety and effectiveness of enoxaparin in pediatric patients have not been established.

ADVERSE REACTIONS

Hemorrhage: The incidence of major hemorrhagic complications during Lovenox Injection treatment has been low. The following rates of major bleeding events have been reported during clinical trials.

[See first table above]

NOTE: At no time point were the 40 mg q.d. pre-operative and the 30 mg q12h post-operative hip replacement surgery prophylactic regimens compared in clinical trials.

Injection site hematomas during the extended prophylaxis period after hip replacement surgery occurred in 9% of the enoxaparin patients versus 1.8% of the placebo patients.

Major Bleeding Episodes in Hip or Knee Replacement Surgery[1]

	Dosing Regimen		
Indications	**Lovenox** 40 mg q.d. s.c.	**Lovenox** 30 mg q12h s.c.	**Heparin** 15,000 U/24h s.c.
Hip Replacement Surgery Without Extended Prophylaxis[2]		n = 786 31 (4%)	n = 541 32 (6%)
Hip Replacement Surgery With Extended Prophylaxis Peri-operative Period[3]	n = 288 4 (2%)		
Extended Prophylaxis Period[4]	n = 221 0 (0%)		
Knee Replacement Surgery Without Extended Prophylaxis[2]		n = 294 3 (1%)	n = 225 3 (1%)

[1] Bleeding complications were considered major: (1) if the hemorrhage caused a significant clinical event, or (2) if accompanied by a hemoglobin decrease ≥2g/dL or transfusion of 2 or more units of blood products. Retroperitoneal and intracranial hemorrhages were always considered major. In the knee replacement surgery trials, intraocular hemorrhages were also considered major hemorrhages.
[2] Enoxaparin sodium 30 mg q12h s.c. initiated 12 to 24 hours after surgery and continued for up to 14 days after surgery.
[3] Enoxaparin sodium 40 mg s.c. q.d. initiated up to 12 hours prior to surgery and continued for up to 7 days after surgery.
[4] Enoxaparin sodium 40 mg s.c. q.d. for up to 21 days after discharge.

Adverse Events Occurring at ≥2% Incidence in Enoxaparin Treated Patients[1] Undergoing Hip or Knee Replacement Surgery

	Dosing Regimen							
	Lovenox 40 mg q.d. s.c.				**Lovenox** 30 mg q12h s.c.		**Heparin** 15,000 U/24h s.c.		**Placebo** q12h s.c.	
	Peri-operative Period n = 288[2]		Extended Prophylaxis Period n = 131[3]		n = 1080		n = 766		n = 115	
Adverse Event	Severe	Total	Severe	Total	Severe	Total	Severe	Total	Severe	Total
Fever	0%	8%	0%	0%	<1%	5%	<1%	4%	0%	3%
Hemorrhage	<1%	13%	0%	5%	<1%	4%	1%	4%	0%	3%
Nausea					<1%	3%	<1%	2%	0%	2%
Anemia	0%	16%	0%	<2%	<1%	2%	2%	5%	<1%	7%
Edema					<1%	2%	<1%	2%	0%	2%
Peripheral edema	0%	6%	0%	0%	<1%	3%	<1%	4%	0%	3%

[1] Excluding unrelated adverse events.
[2] Data represents enoxaparin sodium 40 mg s.c. q.d. initiated up to 12 hours prior to surgery in 288 hip replacement surgery patients who received enoxaparin perio-operatively in an unblinded fashion in one clinical trial.
[3] Data represents enoxaparin sodium 40 mg s.c. q.d. given in a blinded fashion as extended prophylaxis at the end of the peri-operative period in 131 of the original 288 hip replacement surgery patients for up to 21 days in one clinical trial.

Major Bleeding Episodes in Abdominal & Colorectal Surgery[1]

	Dosing Regimen	
Indications	**Lovenox** 40 mg q.d. s.c.	**Heparin** 5000 U q8h s.c.
Abdominal Surgery	n = 555 23 (4%)	n = 560 16 (3%)
Colorectal Surgery	n = 673 28 (4%)	n = 674 21 (3%)

[1] Bleeding complications were considered major: (1) if the hemorrhage caused a significant clinical event, or (2) if accompanied by a hemoglobin decrease ≥2g/dL or transfusion of 2 or more units of blood products. Retroperitoneal, intraocular, and intracranial hemorrhages were always considered major.

Major Bleeding Episodes in Unstable Angina and Non-Q-Wave Myocardial Infarction

	Dosing Regimen	
Indication	**Lovenox**[1] 1 mg/kg q12h s.c.	**Heparin**[1] aPTT Adjusted i.v. Therapy
Unstable Angina and Non-Q-Wave MI[2,3]	n = 1578 17 (1%)	n = 1529 18 (1%)

[1] The rates represent major bleeding on study medication up to 12 hours after dose.
[2] Aspirin therapy was administered concurrently (100 to 325 mg per day).
[3] Bleeding complications were considered major: (1) if the hemorrhage caused a significant clinical event, or (2) if accompanied by a hemoglobin decrease ≥3g/dL or transfusion of 2 or more units of blood products were required. Intraocular, retroperitoneal, and intracranial hemorrhages were always considered major.

Thrombocytopenia: see **WARNINGS: Thrombocytopenia.**
Elevations of Serum Aminotransferases: Asymptomatic increases in aspartate (AST [SGOT]) and alanine (ALT [SGPT]) aminotransferase levels greater than three times the upper limit of normal of the laboratory reference range have been reported in up to 3.9% and 5.5% of patients, respectively, during treatment with Lovenox® (enoxaparin sodium) Injection. Similar significant increases in aminotransferase levels have also been observed in patients and healthy volunteers treated with heparin and other low molecular weight heparins. Such elevations are fully reversible and are rarely associated with increases in bilirubin.

Since aminotransferase determinations are important in the differential diagnosis of myocardial infarction, liver disease, and pulmonary emboli, elevations that might be caused by drugs like Lovenox should be interpreted with caution.

Local Reactions: Mild local irritation, pain, hematoma, ecchymosis and erythema may follow s.c. injection of Lovenox Injection.

Other: Other adverse effects that were thought to be possibly or probably related to treatment with Lovenox Injection, heparin, or placebo in clinical trials with patients undergoing hip or knee replacement surgery, or abdominal or colorectal surgery, and that occurred at a rate of at least 2% in the enoxaparin group, are provided below.
[See second table at top of previous page]
[See first table at right]

Adverse Events in Enoxaparin Treated Patients With Unstable Angina or Non-Q-Wave Myocardial Infarction: Nonhemorrhagic clinical events reported to be related to enoxaparin therapy occurred at an incidence of ≤1%.
Non-major hemorrhagic episodes, primarily injection site ecchymoses and hematomas, were more frequently reported in patients treated with s.c. enoxaparin than in patients treated with i.v. heparin.
Serious adverse events with Lovenox® (enoxaparin sodium) Injection or heparin in a clinical trial in patients with unstable angina or non-q-wave myocardial infarction that occurred at a rate of at least 0.5% in the enoxaparin group, are provided below (irrespective of relationship to drug therapy).
[See scond table at right]

Ongoing Safety Surveillance: Since 1993, there have been more than 40 reports of epidural or spinal hematoma formation with concurrent use of enoxaparin and spinal/epidural anesthesia or spinal puncture. The majority of patients had a post-operative indwelling epidural catheter placed for analgesia or received additional drugs affecting hemostasis such as NSAIDs. Many of the epidural or spinal hematomas caused neurologic injury, including long-term or permanent paralysis. Because these events were reported voluntarily from a population of unknown size, estimates of frequency cannot be made.

Other reports include: local reactions at the injection site (*i.e.*, skin necrosis, nodules, inflammation, oozing), systemic allergic reactions (*i.e.*, pruritus, urticaria), vesiculobullous rash, purpura, and thrombocytosis.

OVERDOSAGE

Symptoms/Treatment: Accidental overdosage following administration of Lovenox Injection may lead to hemorrhagic complications. Injected Lovenox may be largely neutralized by the slow i.v. injection of protamine sulfate (1% solution). The dose of protamine sulfate should be equal to the dose of Lovenox® (enoxaparin sodium) Injection injected: 1 mg protamine sulfate should be administered to neutralize 1 mg Lovenox Injection. A second infusion of 0.5 mg protamine sulfate per 1 mg of Lovenox Injection may be administered if the aPTT measured 2 to 4 hours after the first infusion remains prolonged. However, even with higher doses of protamine, the aPTT may remain more prolonged than under normal conditions found following administration of heparin. In all cases, the anti-Factor Xa activity is never completely neutralized (maximum about 60%). Particular care should be taken to avoid overdosage with protamine sulfate. Administration of protamine sulfate can cause severe hypotensive and anaphylactoid reactions. Because fatal reactions, often resembling anaphylaxis, have been reported with protamine sulfate, it should be given only when resuscitation techniques and treatment of anaphylactic shock are readily available. For additional information consult the labeling of Protamine Sulfate Injection, USP, products.

A single s.c. dose of 46.4 mg/kg enoxaparin was lethal to rats. The symptoms of acute toxicity were ataxia, decreased motility, dyspnea, cyanosis, and coma.

DOSAGE AND ADMINISTRATION

All patients should be evaluated for a bleeding disorder before prophylactic administration of Lovenox. Since coagulation parameters are unsuitable for monitoring Lovenox activity, routine monitoring of coagulation parameters is not required (see **PRECAUTIONS, Laboratory Tests**).
Adult Dosage: *Hip or Knee Replacement Surgery:* In patients undergoing hip or knee replacement surgery, the rec-

Adverse Events Occurring at ≥2% Incidence in Enoxaparin Treated Patients[1]
Undergoing Abdominal or Colorectal Surgery

Adverse Event	Dosing Regimen			
	Lovenox 40 mg q.d. s.c. n = 1228		Heparin 5000 U q8h s.c. n = 1234	
	Severe	Total	Severe	Total
Hemorrhage	<1%	7%	<1%	6%
Anemia	<1%	3%	<1%	3%
Ecchymosis	0%	3%	0%	3%

[1]Excluding unrelated adverse events.

Serious Adverse Events Occurring at ≥0.5% Incidence in Enoxaparin Treated Patients
With Unstable Angina or Non-Q-Wave Myocardial Infarction

Adverse Event	Dosing Regimen	
	Lovenox 1 mg/kg q12h s.c. n = 1578 n (%)	Heparin aPTT Adjusted i.v. Therapy n = 1529 n (%)
Atrial fibrillation	11 (0.70)	3 (0.20)
Heart failure	15 (0.95)	11 (0.72)
Lung edema	11 (0.70)	11 (0.72)
Pneumonia	13 (0.82)	9 (0.59)

Dosage Unit	Strength[1]	Package Size (per carton)	Anti-Xa Activity[2]	NDC # 0075-
Ampules	30 mg / 0.3 mL	10 ampules	3000 IU	0624-03
Prefilled Syringes[3]	30 mg / 0.3 mL	10 syringes	3000 IU	0624-30
	40 mg / 0.4 mL	10 syringes	4000 IU	0620-40
Graduated Prefilled Syringes[3]	60 mg / 0.6 mL	10 syringes	6000 IU	0621-60
	80 mg / 0.8 mL	10 syringes	8000 IU	0622-80
	100 mg / 1.0 mL	10 syringes	10 000 IU	0623-00

[1] Strength represents the number of milligrams of enoxaparin sodium in Water for Injection. Lovenox ampules and prefilled syringes contain 10 mg enoxaparin sodium per 0.1 mL Water for Injection.
[2] Approximate anti-Factor Xa activity based on reference to the W.H.O. First International Low Molecular Weight Heparin Reference Standard.
[3] Each Lovenox syringe is affixed with a 27 gauge × 1/2 inch needle.

ommended dose of Lovenox Injection is **30 mg every 12 hours** administered by s.c. injection. Provided that hemostasis has been established, the initial dose should be given 12 to 24 hours post-operatively. Up to 14 days administration (average duration 7 to 10 days) of Lovenox 30 mg every 12 hours has been well tolerated in controlled clinical trials. For hip replacement surgery, a dose of **40 mg** once daily s.c., given initially 12 (±3) hours prior to surgery, may be considered. Following the initial phase of thromboprophylaxis in hip replacement surgery patients (Lovenox 30 mg every 12 hours or 40 mg once daily), continued prophylaxis with Lovenox Injection 40 mg once daily administered by s.c. injection for 3 weeks is recommended.

Abdominal Surgery: In patients undergoing abdominal surgery who are at risk for thromboembolic complications, the recommended dose of Lovenox Injection is **40 mg once daily** administered by s.c. injection with the initial dose given 2 hours prior to surgery. The usual duration of administration is 7 to 10 days; up to 12 days administration has been well tolerated in clinical trials.

Unstable Angina and Non-Q-Wave Myocardial Infarction: In patients with unstable angina or non-q-wave myocardial infarction, the recommended dose of Lovenox Injection is **1 mg/kg** administered subcutaneously **every 12 hours** in conjunction with oral aspirin therapy (100 to 325 mg once daily). Treatment with Lovenox Injection should be prescribed for a minimum of 2 days and continued until clinical stabilization. The usual duration of treatment is 2 to 8 days. To minimize the risk of bleeding following vascular instrumentation during the treatment of unstable angina, adhere precisely to the intervals recommended between Lovenox doses. The vascular access sheath for instrumentation should remain in place for 6 to 8 hours following a dose of Lovenox. The next scheduled dose should be given no sooner than 6 to 8 hours after sheath removal. The site of the procedure should be observed for signs of bleeding or hematoma formation.

Administration: Enoxaparin injection is a clear, colorless to pale yellow sterile solution, and as with other parenteral

drug products, should be inspected visually for particulate matter and discoloration prior to administration.

When using Lovenox ampules, to assure withdrawal of the appropriate volume of drug, the use of a tuberculin syringe or equivalent is recommended.

Lovenox Injection is administered by s.c. injection. It must not be administered by intramuscular injection.

Subcutaneous Injection Technique: Patients should be lying down and Lovenox Injection administered by deep s.c. injection. To avoid the loss of drug when using the prefilled syringes, do not expel the air bubble from the syringe before the injection. Administration should be alternated between the left and right anterolateral and left and right posterolateral abdominal wall. The whole length of the needle should be introduced into a skin fold held between the thumb and forefinger; the skin fold should be held throughout the injection. To minimize bruising, do not rub the injection site after completion of the injection. An automatic injector, Lovenox EasyInjector™, is available for patients to administer Lovenox Injection packaged in 30 mg and 40 mg prefilled syringes. Please see directions accompanying the Lovenox EasyInjector™ automatic injection device.

HOW SUPPLIED

Lovenox (enoxaparin sodium) Injection is available in:
[See third table above]
Store at Controlled Room Temperature, 15–25°C (59–77°F) [see USP].

Keep out of the reach of children.

Caution: Federal law prohibits dispensing without prescription.

Lovenox prefilled and graduated prefilled syringes manufactured in France.

Lovenox ampules manufactured in England.

Continued on next page

Lovenox—Cont.

RHÔNE-POULENC RORER PHARMACEUTICALS INC.
COLLEGEVILLE, PA 19426 ©1998
IN-1107Q Rev. 3/98
Shown in Product Identification Guide, page 333

NASACORT® ℞

[na 'za · cort]
(triamcinolone acetonide)
Nasal Inhaler
For Intranasal Use Only
Shake Well Before Using

DESCRIPTION

Triamcinolone acetonide, USP, the active ingredient in **Nasacort®** Nasal Inhaler, is a glucocorticosteroid with a molecular weight of 434.5 and with the chemical designation 9-Fluoro-11β,16α,17, 21-tetrahydroxypregna-1, 4-diene-3, 20-dione cyclic 16,17-acetal with acetone. ($C_{24}H_{31}FO_6$).

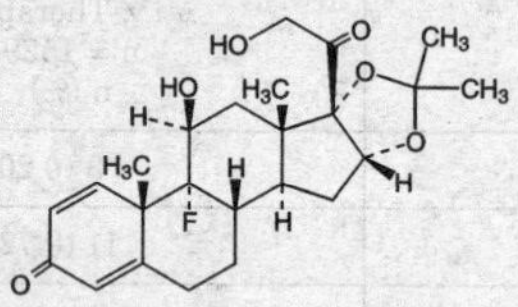

Nasacort Nasal Inhaler is a metered-dose aerosol unit containing a microcrystalline suspension of triamcinolone acetonide in dichlorodifluoromethane and dehydrated alcohol USP 0.7% w/w. Each canister contains 15 mg triamcinolone acetonide. Each actuation delivers 55 mcg triamcinolone acetonide from the nasal actuator to the patient (estimated from *in vitro* testing). There are at least 100 actuations in one **Nasacort** Nasal Inhaler canister. **After 100 actuations, the amount delivered per actuation may not be consistent and the unit should be discarded.** Patients are provided with a check-off card to track usage as part of the Information for Patients tear-off sheet.

CLINICAL PHARMACOLOGY

Triamcinolone acetonide is a more potent derivative of triamcinolone. Although triamcinolone itself is approximately one to two times as potent as prednisone in animal models of inflammation, triamcinolone acetonide is approximately 8 times more potent than prednisone.

Although the precise mechanism of corticosteroid antiallergic action is unknown, corticosteroids are very effective. However, they do not have an immediate effect on allergic signs and symptoms. When allergic symptoms are very severe, local treatment with recommended doses (microgram) of any available topical corticosteroids are not as effective as treatment with larger doses (milligram) of oral or parenteral formulations. When corticosteroids are prematurely discontinued, symptoms may not recur for several days.

Based upon intravenous dosing of triamcinolone acetonide phosphate ester, the half-life of triamcinolone acetonide was reported to be 88 minutes. The volume of distribution (Vd) reported was 99.5 L (SD ± 27.5) and clearance was 45.2 L/hour (SD ± 9.1) for triamcinolone acetonide. The plasma half-life of corticosteroids does not correlate well with the biologic half-life.

When administered intranasally to man at 440 mcg/day dose, the peak plasma concentration was <1 ng/mL and occurred on average at 3.4 hours (range 0.5 to 8.0 hours) postdosing. The apparent half-life was 4.0 hours (range 1.0 to 7.0 hours); however, this value probably reflects lingering absorption. Intranasal doses below 440 mcg/day gave sparse data and did not allow for the calculation of meaningful pharmacokinetic parameters.

In animal studies using rats and dogs, three metabolites of triamcinolone acetonide have been identified. They are 6β-hydroxytriamcinolone acetonide, 21-carboxytriamcinolone acetonide and 21-carboxy-6β-hydroxytriamcinolone acetonide. All three metabolites are expected to be substantially less active than the parent compound due to (a) the dependence of anti-inflammatory activity on the presence of a 21-hydroxyl group, (b) the decreased activity observed upon 6-hydroxylation, and (c) the markedly increased water solubility favoring rapid elimination. There appeared to be some quantitative differences in the metabolites among species. No differences were detected in metabolic pattern as a function of route of administration.

CLINICAL TRIALS

In double-blind, parallel, placebo-controlled clinical trials of seasonal and perennial allergic rhinitis, in adults and adolescents in fixed total daily doses of 110, 220 and 440 mcg per day, the responses to aerosolized triamcinolone acetonide demonstrated a statistically significant improvement over placebo. In open label trials where the doses were sometimes adjusted according to patients' signs and symptoms, the daily doses and regimens varied. The most commonly used dose was 110 mcg per day.

Nasacort Nasal Inhaler, at a dose of 220 mcg once daily, has also been studied in two double-blind, placebo-controlled trials of two and four weeks duration in children ages 6 through 11 years with seasonal and perennial allergic rhinitis. These trials included 162 males and 91 females. **Nasacort** administered at a fixed dose of 220 mcg once daily resulted in consistent and statistically significant reductions of allergic rhinitis symptoms over vehicle placebo.

In attempting to determine if systemic absorption played a role in the response to **Nasacort**, a clinical study comparing intranasal and depot intramuscular triamcinolone acetonide was conducted. The doses used were based on bioavailability studies of each formulation. The final doses of **Nasacort** 440 mcg once a day and Kenalog®-40, 4 mg intramuscularly once a week, were chosen to deliver comparable total amounts of weekly triamcinolone acetonide. However, the weekly injection yielded sustained plasma levels throughout the dosing interval while the daily **Nasacort** application resulted in daily peak and trough concentrations, the mean of which was 3.5 times below the Kenalog plasma levels. Both topical **Nasacort** and intramuscular Kenalog-40 were clinically effective. In addition, in some studies there was evidence of improvement of eye symptoms. This suggests that **Nasacort**, at least to some degree is acting by a systemic mechanism.

In order to evaluate the effects of systemic absorption on the Hypothalamic-Pituitary-Adrenal (HPA) axis, **Nasacort** administered to adults in doses of 440 mcg once a day was compared to placebo and 42 days of a single morning dose of prednisone 10 mg. Adrenal response to a six-hour cosyntropin stimulation test suggests that intranasal **Nasacort** 440 mcg/day for six weeks did not measurably affect adrenal activity. Conversely, oral prednisone at 10 mg/day significantly reduced the response to ACTH.

No evidence of adrenal axis suppression was observed in 26 pediatric patients exposed for 6 weeks to systemic levels of triamcinolone acetonide higher than the systemic levels observed following administration of the maximum recommended dose of **Nasacort** Nasal Inhaler.

INDIVIDUALIZATION OF DOSAGE

Individual patients will experience a variable time to onset and degree of symptom relief when using **Nasacort**. It is recommended that dosing be started at 220 mcg once a day and the effect be assessed in four to seven days.

Adults and Children 12 years of age and older: Some relief can be expected in approximately two-thirds of patients within four to seven days. If greater effect is desired an increase of dose to 440 mcg once a day can be tried. If adequate relief has not been obtained by the third week of **Nasacort** treatment, alternate forms of treatment should be considered.

A dose-response between 110 mcg/day (one spray/nostril/day) and 440 mcg/day (four sprays/nostril/day) is not clearly discernible. In general, in the clinical trials the highest dose tended to provide relief sooner. This suggests an alternative approach to starting therapy with **Nasacort**, *e.g.,* starting treatment with 440 mcg (four sprays/nostril/day) and then, depending on the patient's response, decreasing the dose by one spray per day every four to seven days. Although **Nasacort** may be used at 220 mcg/day or 440 mcg/day divided into two or four times a day, the degree of relief does not seem to be significantly different compared to once-a-day dosing. As with other nasal corticosteroids, the vehicle used to deliver the corticosteroid, may cause symptoms that are difficult to distinguish from the patient's rhinitis symptoms. Thus, depending upon the balance between these vehicle side effects and the benefits of treatment, in determining the optimal dose for the relief of symptoms, individual patients may need to have a trial of high and low doses.

Children 6 through 11 years of age: In children 6 through 11 years of age, it is recommended that dosing be started at 220 mcg given as two sprays (55 mcg/spray) in each nostril once a day. In clinical trials, significant relief of rhinitis symptoms in children was observed as early as the fourth day of treatment and generally, it took one to two weeks to achieve maximum benefit. If adequate relief has not been obtained by the third week of **Nasacort** treatment, alternate forms of treatment should be considered.

In general, it is always desirable to titrate an individual patient to the minimum effective dose to reduce the possibility of side effects. In clinical trials, after symptoms have been brought under control at the recommended starting doses, reducing the daily dose to 110 mcg (one spray in each nostril once per day) has been shown to be effective in controlling symptoms in approximately one-half of adult patients being treated long-term for allergic rhinitis. (See **PRECAUTIONS**, **WARNINGS**, **Information for Patients** and **ADVERSE REACTIONS** sections).

INDICATIONS AND USAGE

Nasacort Nasal Inhaler is indicated for the nasal treatment of seasonal and perennial allergic rhinitis symptoms in adults and children 6 years of age and older.

CONTRAINDICATIONS

Hypersensitivity to any of the ingredients of this preparation contraindicates its use.

WARNINGS

The replacement of a systemic corticosteroid with a topical corticoid can be accompanied by signs of adrenal insufficiency and, in addition, some patients may experience symptoms of withdrawal, *e.g.,* joint and/or muscular pain, lassitude and depression. Patients previously treated for prolonged periods with systemic corticosteroids and transferred to topical corticoids should be carefully monitored for acute adrenal insufficiency in response to stress. In those patients who have asthma or other clinical conditions requiring long-term systemic corticosteroid treatment, too rapid a decrease in systemic corticosteroids may cause a severe exacerbation of their symptoms.

Children who are on immunosuppressant drugs are more susceptible to infections than healthy children. Chickenpox and measles, for example, can have a more serious or even fatal course in children on immunosuppressant doses of corticosteroids. In such children, or in adults who have not had these diseases, particular care should be taken to avoid exposure. If exposed, therapy with varicella-zoster immune globulin (VZIG) or pooled intravenous immunoglobulin (IVIG), as appropriate, may be indicated. If chickenpox develops, treatment with antiviral agents may be considered.

The use of **Nasacort** Nasal Inhaler with alternate-day systemic prednisone could increase the likelihood of hypothalamic-pituitary-adrenal (HPA) suppression compared to a therapeutic dose of either one alone. Therefore, **Nasacort** Nasal Inhaler should be used with caution in patients already receiving alternate-day prednisone treatment for any disease.

PRECAUTIONS

General: In clinical studies with triamcinolone acetonide administered intranasally, the development of localized infections of the nose and pharynx with *Candida albicans* has rarely occurred. When such an infection develops, it may require treatment with appropriate local therapy and discontinuance of treatment with **Nasacort** Nasal Inhaler.

Triamcinolone acetonide administered intranasally has been shown to be absorbed into the systemic circulation in humans. Patients with active rhinitis showed absorption similar to that found in normal volunteers. **Nasacort** at 440 mcg/day for 42 days did not measurably affect adrenal response to a six hour cosyntropin test. In the same study, prednisone 10 mg/day significantly reduced adrenal response to ACTH over the same period (see **CLINICAL TRIALS** section).

Nasacort Nasal Inhaler should be used with caution, if at all, in patients with active or quiescent tuberculous infections of the respiratory tract or in patients with untreated fungal, bacterial, or systemic viral infections or ocular herpes simplex.

Because of the inhibitory effect of corticosteroids on wound healing in patients who have experienced recent nasal septal ulcers, nasal surgery or trauma, a corticosteroid should be used with caution until healing has occurred. As with other nasally inhaled corticosteroids, nasal septal perforations have been reported in rare instances.

When used at excessive doses, systemic corticosteroid effects such as hypercorticism and adrenal suppression may appear. If such changes occur, **Nasacort** Nasal Inhaler should be discontinued slowly, consistent with accepted procedures for discontinuing oral steroid therapy.

Information for Patients: Patients being treated with **Nasacort** Nasal Inhaler should receive the following information and instructions.

Patients who are on immunosuppressant doses of corticosteroids should be warned to avoid exposure to chickenpox or measles and, if exposed, to obtain medical advice.

Patients should use **Nasacort** Nasal Inhaler at regular intervals since its effectiveness depends on its regular use. A decrease in symptoms may occur as soon as 12 hours after starting steroid therapy and generally can be expected to occur within a few days of initiating therapy in allergic rhinitis. The patient should take the medication as directed and should not exceed the prescribed dosage. The patient should contact the physician if symptoms do not improve after three weeks, or if the condition worsens. Nasal irritation and/or burning or stinging after use of the spray occur only rarely with this product. The patient should contact the physician if they occur.

For the proper use of this unit and to attain maximum improvement, the patient should read and follow the accompanying patient instructions carefully. Spraying triamcinolone acetonide directly onto the nasal septum should be avoided. Because the amount dispensed per puff may not be consistent, it is important to shake the canister well. Also, the canister should be discarded after 100 actuations.

Carcinogenesis, Mutagenesis: No evidence of treatment-related carcinogenicity was demonstrated after 2 years of once daily gavage administration of triamcinolone acetonide at doses of 0.05, 0.2 and 1.0 mcg/kg (approximately 0.1, 0.4 and 1.8% of the recommended clinical dose on a mcg/m^2 basis) in the rat and 0.1, 0.6 and 3.0 mcg/kg (approximately 0.1, 0.6 and 3.0% of the recommended clinical dose on a mcg/m^2 basis) in the mouse.
Mutagenesis studies with triamcinolone acetonide have not been conducted.
Impairment of Fertility: No evidence of impaired fertility was demonstrated when oral doses up to 15 mcg/kg (approximately 28% of the recommended clinical dose on a mcg/m^2 basis) were administered to female and male rats. However, triamcinolone acetonide at oral doses of 8.0 mcg/kg (approximately 15.0% of the recommended clinical dose on a mcg/m^2 basis) caused dystocia and prolonged delivery and at oral doses of 5.0 mcg/kg (approximately 9.0% of the recommended clinical dose on a mcg/m^2 basis) and above produced increases in fetal resorptions and stillbirths as well as decreases in pup body weight and survival. At an oral dose of 1.0 mcg/kg (approximately 2.0% of the recommended clinical dose on a mcg/m^2 basis), it did not manifest the above mentioned effects.
Pregnancy: Pregnancy Category C. Triamcinolone acetonide was teratogenic at inhalational doses of 20, 40 and 80 mcg/kg in rats (approximately 0.4, 0.75 and 1.5 times the recommended clinical dose on a mcg/m^2 basis, respectively) and rabbits (approximately 0.75, 1.5 and 3.0 times the recommended dose on a mcg/m^2 basis, respectively). Triamcinolone acetonide was also teratogenic at an inhalational dose of 500 mcg/kg in monkeys (approximately 18 times the recommended clinical dose on a mcg/m^2 basis). Dose-related teratogenic effects in rats and rabbits included cleft palate, internal hydrocephaly, and axial skeletal defects. Teratogenic effects observed in the monkey were CNS and cranial malformations. There are no adequate and well-controlled studies in pregnant women. Triamcinolone acetonide should be used during pregnancy only if the potential benefits justify the potential risk to the fetus.
Experience with oral corticoids since their introduction in pharmacologic as opposed to physiologic doses suggests that rodents are more prone to teratogenic effects from corticoids than humans. In addition, because there is a natural increase in glucocorticoid production during pregnancy, most women will require a lower exogenous steroid dose and many will not need corticoid treatment during pregnancy.
Nonteratogenic Effects: Hypoadrenalism may occur in infants born of mothers receiving corticosteroids during pregnancy. Such infants should be carefully observed.
Nursing Mothers: It is not known whether triamcinolone acetonide is excreted in human milk. Because other corticosteroids are excreted in human milk, caution should be exercised when **Nasacort** Nasal Inhaler is administered to nursing women.
Pediatric Use: Safety and effectiveness in pediatric patients below the age of 6 have not been established. Oral corticosteroids have been shown to cause growth suppression in children and teenagers, particularly with higher doses over extended periods. If a child or teenager on any corticosteroid appears to have growth suppression, the possibility that they are particularly sensitive to this effect of steroids should be considered.

ADVERSE REACTIONS

Adults and Children 12 years of age and older: In controlled and uncontrolled studies, 1257 adult and adolescent patients received treatment with intranasal triamcinolone acetonide. Adverse reactions are based on the 567 patients who received a product similar to the marketed **Nasacort** canister.
These patients were treated for an average of 48 days (range 1 to 117 days). The 145 patients enrolled in uncontrolled studies received treatment from 1 to 820 days (average 332 days). The most prevalent adverse experience was headache, being reported by approximately 18% of the patients who received **Nasacort**. Nasal irritation was reported by 2.8% of the patients receiving **Nasacort**. Other nasopharyngeal side effects were reported by fewer than 5% of the patients who received **Nasacort** and included: dry mucous membranes, naso-sinus congestion, throat discomfort, sneezing, and epistaxis. The complaints do not usually interfere with treatment and in the controlled and uncontrolled studies approximately 1% of patients have discontinued because of these nasal adverse effects. In the event of accidental overdose, an increased potential for these adverse experiences may be expected, but systemic adverse experiences are unlikely (see **OVERDOSAGE** section).
Children 6 through 11 years of age: Adverse event data in children 6 through 11 years of age are derived from two controlled clinical trials of two and four weeks duration. In these trials, 127 patients received fixed doses of 220 mcg/day of triamcinolone acetonide for an average of 22 days (range 8 to 33 days).
Adverse events occurring at an incidence of 3% or greater and more common among children treated with 220 mcg triamcinolone acetonide daily than vehicle placebo were:

Adverse Events	220 mcg of triamcinolone acetonide daily (n=127)	Vehicle placebo (n=322)
Epistaxis	11.0%	9.3%
Cough	9.4%	9.3%
Fever	7.9%	5.6%
Nausea	6.3%	3.1%
Throat discomfort	5.5%	5.3%
Otitis	4.7%	3.7%
Dyspepsia	4.7%	2.2%

Adverse events occurring at a rate of 3% or greater that were more common in the placebo group were upper respiratory tract infection, headache and concurrent infection. Only 1.6% of patients discontinued due to adverse experiences. No patient discontinued due to a serious adverse event related to **Nasacort** therapy.
Though not observed in controlled clinical trials of **Nasacort** Nasal Inhaler in children, cases of nasal septum perforation among pediatric users have been reported in post-marketing surveillance of this product.

DOSAGE AND ADMINISTRATION

A decrease in symptoms may occur as soon as 12 hours after starting steroid therapy and generally can be expected to occur within a few days of initiating therapy in allergic rhinitis.
If improvement is not evident after 2 to 3 weeks, the patient should be re-evaluated. (See **INDIVIDUALIZATION OF DOSAGE** section).
Adults and Children 12 years of age and older: The recommended starting dose of **Nasacort** Nasal Inhaler is 220 mcg per day given as two sprays (55 mcg/spray) in each nostril once a day. If needed, the dose may be increased to 440 mcg per day (55 mcg/spray) either as once-a-day dosage or divided up to four times a day, *i.e.,* twice a day (two sprays/nostril), or four times a day (one spray/nostril). After the desired effect is obtained, some patients may be maintained on a dose of as little as one spray (55 mcg) in each nostril once a day (total daily dose 110 mcg per day).
Children 6 through 11 years of age: The recommended starting dose of **Nasacort** Nasal Inhaler is 220 mcg per day given as two sprays (55 mcg/spray) in each nostril once a day. Once the maximal effect has been achieved, it is always desirable to titrate the patient to the minimum effective dose.
Nasacort Nasal Inhaler is not recommended for children below 6 years of age since adequate numbers of patients have not been studied in this age group.
Directions for Use: Illustrated Patient's Instructions for use accompany each package of **Nasacort** Nasal Inhaler.

OVERDOSAGE

Acute overdosage with this dosage form is unlikely. The acute topical application of the entire 15 mg of the canister would most likely cause nasal irritation and headache. It would be unlikely to see acute systemic adverse effects even if the entire 15 mg of triamcinolone acetonide was administered intranasally all at once.

HOW SUPPLIED

Nasacort Nasal Inhaler is supplied as an aerosol canister which will provide 100 metered dose actuations. Each actuation delivers 55 mcg triamcinolone acetonide through the nasal actuator. The **Nasacort** Nasal Inhaler canister and accompanying nasal actuator are designed to be used together. The **Nasacort** Nasal Inhaler canister should not be used with other nasal actuators and the supplied nasal actuator should not be used with other products' canisters.
Nasacort Nasal Inhaler is supplied with a white plastic nasal actuator and patient instructions. Net weight of the canister contents is 10 grams.
NDC 0075-1505-43.
CONTENTS UNDER PRESSURE
Avoid spraying in eyes.
Do not puncture. Do not use or store near heat or open flame. Exposure to temperatures above 120°F may cause bursting. Never throw container into fire or incinerator. Keep out of reach of children. Store at Controlled Room Temperature 20 to 25°C (68 to 77°F) [see USP].
Note: The indented statement below is required by the Federal government's Clean Air Act for all products containing or manufactured with chlorofluorocarbons (CFC's):

> WARNING: Contains CFC-12, a substance which harms public health and the environment by destroying ozone in the upper atmosphere.

A notice similar to the above WARNING has been placed in the "Information For The Patient" portion of this package insert under the Environmental Protection Agency's (EPA's) regulations. The patient's warning states that the patient should consult his or her physician if there are questions about alternatives.
Caution: Federal (U.S.A.) law prohibits dispensing without prescription.
U.S. Pat. No. 4,767,612
Rev. 11/96
IN-0479J

Military and Veterans Administration: 1 ×10 gm (NSN 6505-01-345-2880).
Marketed by
RHÔNE-POULENC RORER PHARMACEUTICALS INC.
Collegeville, PA, U.S.A. 19426-0107
Shown in Product Identification Guide, page 333

NASACORT® AQ ℞

[na 'za · cort]
(triamcinolone acetonide)
For intranasal use only.
Shake Well Before Using

DESCRIPTION

Triamcinolone acetonide, USP, the active ingredient in **Nasacort® AQ** Nasal Spray, is a corticosteroid with a molecular weight of 434.51 and with the chemical designation 9-Fluoro-11β,16α,17,21-tetrahydroxypregna-1,4-diene-3,20-dione cyclic 16,17-acetal with acetone ($C_{24}H_{31}FO_6$).

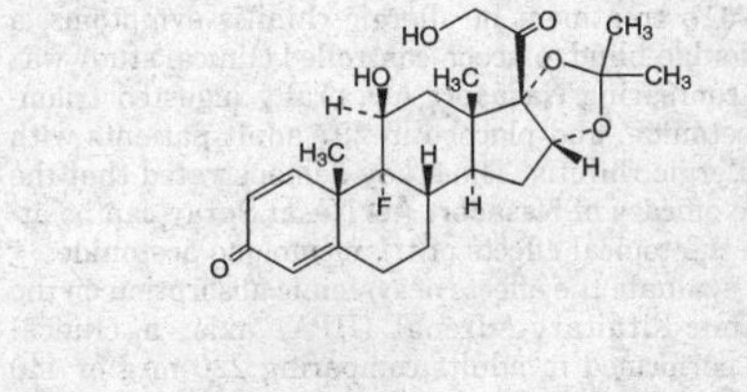

Nasacort AQ Nasal Spray is an unscented, thixotropic, water-based metered-dose pump spray formulation unit containing a microcrystalline suspension of triamcinolone acetonide in an aqueous medium. Microcrystalline cellulose, carboxymethylcellulose sodium, polysorbate 80, dextrose, benzalkonium chloride, and edetate disodium are contained in this aqueous medium; hydrochloric acid or sodium hydroxide may be added to adjust the pH to a target of 5.0 within a range of 4.5 and 6.0.
Each actuation delivers 55 mcg triamcinolone acetonide from the nasal actuator after an initial priming of 5 sprays. It will remain adequately primed for 2 weeks. If the product is not used for more than 2 weeks, then it can be adequately reprimed with one spray. The contents of one 6.5 gram sample bottle provide 30 actuations, and the contents of one 16.5 gram bottle provide 120 actuations. **After either 30 actuations or 120 actuations, the amount of triamcinolone acetonide delivered per actuation may not be consistent and the unit should be discarded.** Each 30 actuation sample bottle contains 3.575 mg of triamcinolone acetonide and each 120 actuation bottle contains 9.075 mg of triamcinolone acetonide.
In the Information for Patients tear-off sheet, patients are provided with a check-off form to track usage.

CLINICAL PHARMACOLOGY

Triamcinolone acetonide is a more potent derivative of triamcinolone. Although triamcinolone itself is approximately one to two times as potent as prednisone in animal models of inflammation, triamcinolone acetonide is approximately 8 times more potent than prednisone.
Although the precise mechanism of corticosteroid antiallergic action is unknown, corticosteroids are very effective. However, when allergic symptoms are very severe, local treatment with recommended doses (microgram) of any available topical corticosteroid are not as effective as treatment with larger doses (milligram) of oral or parenteral formulations.
Based upon intravenous dosing of triamcinolone acetonide phosphate ester in adults, the half-life of triamcinolone acetonide was reported to be 88 minutes. The volume of distribution (Vd) reported was 99.5 L (SD ± 27.5) and clearance was 45.2 L/hour (SD ± 9.1) for triamcinolone acetonide. The plasma half-life of corticosteroids does not correlate well with the biologic half-life.
Pharmacokinetic characterization of the **Nasacort AQ** Nasal Spray formulation was determined in both normal adult subjects and patients with allergic rhinitis. Single dose intranasal administration of 220 mcg of **Nasacort AQ** Nasal Spray in normal adult subjects and patients demonstrated minimal absorption of triamcinolone acetonide. The mean peak plasma concentration was approximately 0.5 ng/mL (range: 0.1 to 1.0 ng/mL) and occurred at 1.5 hours post dose. The mean plasma drug concentration was less than 0.06 ng/mL at 12 hours, and below the assay detection limit at 24 hours. The average terminal half-life was 3.1 hours. The range of mean $AUC_{0-\infty}$ values was 1.4 ng•hr/mL to 4.7 ng•hr/mL between doses of 110 mcg to 440 mcg in both patients and healthy volunteers. Dose proportionality was

Continued on next page

Nasacort AQ—Cont.

demonstrated in both normal adult subjects and in allergic rhinitis patients following single intranasal doses of 110 mcg or 220 mcg **Nasacort AQ** Nasal Spray. The C_{max} and AUC of the 440 mcg dose increased less than proportionally when compared to 110 and 220 mcg doses. Following multiple doses in pediatric patients receiving 440 mcg/day, plasma drug concentrations, AUC, C_{max} and T_{max} were similar to those values observed in adult patients.

In animal studies using rats and dogs, three metabolites of triamcinolone acetonide have been identified. They are 6β-hydroxytriamcinolone acetonide, 21-carboxytriamcinolone acetonide and 21-carboxy-6β-hydroxytriamcinolone acetonide. All three metabolites are expected to be substantially less active than the parent compound due to (a) the dependence of anti-inflammatory activity on the presence of a 21-hydroxyl group, (b) the decreased activity observed upon 6-hydroxylation, and (c) the markedly increased water solubility favoring rapid elimination. There appeared to be some quantitative differences in the metabolites among species. No differences were detected in metabolic pattern as a function of route of administration.

In order to determine if systemic absorption plays a role in **Nasacort AQ's** treatment of allergic rhinitis symptoms, a two week double-blind, placebo-controlled clinical study was conducted comparing **Nasacort AQ**, orally ingested triamcinolone acetonide, and placebo in 297 adult patients with seasonal allergic rhinitis. The study demonstrated that the therapeutic efficacy of **Nasacort AQ** Nasal Spray can be attributed to the topical effects of triamcinolone acetonide.

In order to evaluate the effects of systemic absorption on the Hypothalamic-Pituitary-Adrenal (HPA) axis, a clinical study was performed in adults comparing 220 mcg or 440 mcg **Nasacort AQ** per day, or 10 mg prednisone per day with placebo for 42 days. Adrenal response to a six-hour cosyntropin stimulation test showed that **Nasacort AQ** administered at doses of 220 mcg and 440 mcg had no statistically significant effect on HPA activity versus placebo. Conversely, oral prednisone at 10 mg/day significantly reduced the response to ACTH.

A study evaluating plasma cortisol response thirty and sixty minutes after cosyntropin stimulation in 80 pediatric patients who received 220 mcg or 440 mcg (twice the maximum recommended daily dose) daily for six weeks was conducted. No abnormal response to cosyntropin infusion (peak serum cortisol <18 mcg/dL) was observed in any pediatric patient after six weeks of dosing with **Nasacort AQ** at 440 mcg per day.

CLINICAL TRIALS

The safety and efficacy of **Nasacort AQ** Nasal Spray have been evaluated in 10 double-blind, placebo-controlled clinical trials of two- to four-weeks duration in adults and children 12 years and older with seasonal or perennial allergic rhinitis. The number of patients treated with **Nasacort AQ** Nasal Spray in these studies was 1266; of these patients, 675 were males and 591 were females.

Overall, the results of these clinical trials in adults and children 12 years and older demonstrated that **Nasacort AQ** Nasal Spray 220 mcg once daily (2 sprays in each nostril), when compared to placebo, provides statistically significant relief of nasal symptoms of seasonal or perennial allergic rhinitis including sneezing, stuffiness, discharge, and itching.

The safety and efficacy of **Nasacort AQ** Nasal Spray, at doses of 110 mcg or 220 mcg once daily, have also been adequately studied in two double-blind, placebo-controlled trials of two- and twelve-weeks duration in children ages 6 through 12 years with seasonal and perennial allergic rhinitis. These trials included 341 males and 177 females. **Nasacort AQ** administered at either dose resulted in statistically significant reductions in the severity of nasal symptoms of allergic rhinitis.

INDICATIONS AND USAGE

Nasacort AQ Nasal Spray is indicated for the treatment of the nasal symptoms of seasonal and perennial allergic rhinitis in adults and children 6 years of age and older.

CONTRAINDICATIONS

Hypersensitivity to any of the ingredients of this preparation contraindicates its use.

WARNINGS

The replacement of a systemic corticosteroid with a topical corticosteroid can be accompanied by signs of adrenal insufficiency and, in addition, some patients may experience symptoms of withdrawal; *e.g.*, joint and/or muscular pain, lassitude and depression. Patients previously treated for prolonged periods with systemic corticosteroids and transferred to topical corticosteroids should be carefully monitored for acute adrenal insufficiency in response to stress. In those patients who have asthma or other clinical conditions requiring long-term systemic corticosteroid treatment, too rapid a decrease in systemic corticosteroids may cause a severe exacerbation of their symptoms.

Adverse Events	Patients treated with 220 mcg triamcinolone acetonide (n=857) %	Vehicle Placebo (n=962) %
Pharyngitis	5.1	3.6
Epistaxis	2.7	0.8
Increase in cough	2.1	1.5

Children who are on immunosuppressant drugs are more susceptible to infections than healthy children. Chickenpox and measles, for example, can have a more serious or even fatal course in children on immunosuppressant doses of corticosteroids. In such children, or in adults who have not had these diseases, particular care should be taken to avoid exposure. If exposed, therapy with varicella-zoster immune globulin (VZIG) or pooled intravenous immunoglobulin (IVIG), as appropriate, may be indicated. If chickenpox develops, treatment with antiviral agents may be considered.

PRECAUTIONS

General: In clinical studies with triamcinolone acetonide nasal spray, the development of localized infections of the nose and pharynx with *Candida albicans* has rarely occurred. When such an infection develops it may require treatment with appropriate local or systemic therapy and discontinuance of treatment with **Nasacort AQ** Nasal Spray. **Nasacort AQ** Nasal Spray should be used with caution, if at all, in patients with active or quiescent tuberculous infection of the respiratory tract or in patients with untreated fungal, bacterial, or systemic viral infections or ocular herpes simplex.

Because of the inhibitory effect of corticosteroids, in patients who have experienced recent nasal septal ulcers, nasal surgery, or trauma, a corticosteroid should be used with caution until healing has occurred. As with other nasally inhaled corticosteroids, nasal septal perforations have been reported in rare instances.

When used at excessive doses, systemic corticosteroid effects such as hypercorticism and adrenal suppression may appear. If such changes occur, **Nasacort AQ** Nasal Spray should be discontinued slowly, consistent with accepted procedures for discontinuing oral steroid therapy.

Information for Patients: Patients being treated with **Nasacort AQ** Nasal Spray should receive the following information and instructions. Patients who are on immunosuppressant doses of corticosteroids should be warned to avoid exposure to chickenpox or measles and, if exposed, to obtain medical advice.

Patients should use **Nasacort AQ** Nasal Spray at regular intervals since its effectiveness depends on its regular use. (See **DOSAGE AND ADMINISTRATION**.)

An improvement in some patient symptoms may be seen within the first day of treatment, and generally, it takes one week of treatment to reach maximum benefit. Initial assessment for response should be made during this time frame and periodically until the patient's symptoms are stabilized. The patient should take the medication as directed and should not exceed the prescribed dosage. The patient should contact the physician if symptoms do not improve after three weeks, or if the condition worsens. Patients who experience recurrent episodes of epistaxis (nose bleeds) or nasal septum discomfort while taking this medication should contact their physician. For the proper use of this unit and to attain maximum improvement, the patient should read and follow the accompanying patient instructions carefully. It is important to shake the bottle well before each use. **Also, the bottle should be discarded after 120 actuations since the amount of triamcinolone acetonide delivered thereafter per actuation may be substantially less than 55 mcg of drug.** Do not transfer any remaining suspension to another bottle.

Carcinogenesis, Mutagenesis, and Impairment of Fertility: In a two-year study in rats, triamcinolone acetonide caused no treatment-related carcinogenicity at oral doses up to 1.0 mcg/kg (approximately 1/30 and 1/50 of the maximum recommended daily intranasal dose in adults and children on a mcg/m² basis, respectively). In a two-year study in mice, triamcinolone acetonide caused no treatment-related carcinogenicity at oral doses up to 3.0 mcg/kg (approximately 1/12 and 1/30 of the maximum recommended daily intranasal dose in adults and children on a mcg/m² basis, respectively). No mutagenicity studies with triamcinolone acetonide have been performed.

In male and female rats, triamcinolone acetonide caused no change in pregnancy rate at oral doses up to 15.0 mcg/kg (approximately 1/2 of the maximum recommended daily intranasal dose in adults on a mcg/m² basis). Triamcinolone acetonide caused increased fetal resorptions and stillbirths and decreases in pup weight and survival at doses of 5.0 mcg/kg and above (approximately 1/5 of the maximum recommended daily intranasal dose in adults on a mcg/m² basis). At 1.0 mcg/kg (approximately 1/30 of the maximum recommended daily intranasal dose in adults on a mcg/m² basis), it did not induce the above mentioned effects.

Pregnancy: *Teratogenic Effects: Pregnancy Category C.* Triamcinolone acetonide was teratogenic in rats, rabbits, and

monkeys. In rats, triamcinolone acetonide was teratogenic at inhalation doses of 20 mcg/kg and above (approximately 7/10 of the maximum recommended daily intranasal dose in adults on a mcg/m² basis). In rabbits, triamcinolone acetonide was teratogenic at inhalation doses of 20 mcg/kg and above (approximately 2 times the maximum recommended daily intranasal dose in adults on a mcg/m² basis). In monkeys, triamcinolone acetonide was teratogenic at an inhalation dose of 500 mcg/kg (approximately 37 times the maximum recommended daily intranasal dose in adults on a mcg/m² basis). Dose-related teratogenic effects in rats and rabbits included cleft palate and/or internal hydrocephaly and axial skeletal defects, whereas the effects observed in the monkey were cranial malformations.

There are no adequate and well-controlled studies in pregnant women. Therefore, triamcinolone acetonide should be used in pregnancy only if the potential benefit justifies the potential risk to the fetus. Since their introduction, experience with oral corticosteroids in pharmacologic as opposed to physiologic doses suggests that rodents are more prone to teratogenic effects from corticosteroids than humans. In addition, because there is a natural increase in glucocorticoid production during pregnancy, most women will require a lower exogenous corticosteroid dose and many will not need corticosteroid treatment during pregnancy.

Nonteratogenic Effects: Hypoadrenalism may occur in infants born of mothers receiving corticosteroids during pregnancy. Such infants should be carefully observed.

Nursing Mothers: It is not known whether triamcinolone acetonide is excreted in human milk. Because other corticosteroids are excreted in human milk, caution should be exercised when **Nasacort AQ** Nasal Spray is administered to nursing women.

Pediatric Use: Safety and effectiveness in pediatric patients below the age of 6 years have not been established. Corticosteroids have been shown to cause growth suppression in children and teenagers, particularly with higher doses over extended periods. If a child or teenager on any corticosteroid appears to have growth suppression, the possibility that they are particularly sensitive to this effect of corticosteroids should be considered.

ADVERSE REACTIONS

In placebo-controlled, double-blind, and open-label clinical studies, 1483 adults and children 12 years and older received treatment with triamcinolone acetonide aqueous nasal spray. These patients were treated for an average duration of 51 days. In the controlled trials (2–5 weeks duration) from which the following adverse reaction data are derived, 1394 patients were treated with **Nasacort AQ** Nasal Spray for an average of 19 days. In a long-term, open-label study, 172 patients received treatment for an average duration of 286 days.

Adverse events occurring at an incidence of 2% or greater and more common among **Nasacort AQ**-treated patients than placebo-treated patients in controlled adult clinical trials were:

[See table above]

A total of 602 children 6 to 12 years of age were studied in 3 double-blind, placebo-controlled clinical trials. Of these, 172 received 110 mcg/day and 207 received 220 mcg/day of **Nasacort AQ** Nasal Spray for two, six, or twelve weeks. The longest average durations of treatment for patients receiving 110 mcg/day and 220 mcg/day were 76 days and 80 days, respectively. Only 1% of those patients treated with **Nasacort AQ** were discontinued due to adverse experiences. No patient receiving 110 mcg/day discontinued due to a serious adverse event and one patient receiving 220 mcg/day discontinued due to a serious event that was considered not drug related. Overall, these studies found the adverse experience profile for **Nasacort AQ** to be similar to placebo. A similar adverse event profile was observed in pediatric patients 6–12 years of age as compared to older children and adults with the exception of epistaxis which occurred in less than 2% of the pediatric patients studied.

Adverse events occurring at an incidence of 2% or greater and more common among adult patients treated with placebo than **Nasacort AQ** were: headache, and rhinitis. In children aged 6 to 12 years these events included: asthma, epistaxis, headache, infection, otitis media, sinusitis, and vomiting.

In clinical trials, nasal septum perforation was reported in one adult patient although relationship to **Nasacort AQ** Nasal Spray has not been established.

In the event of accidental overdose, an increased potential for these adverse experiences may be expected, but acute systemic adverse experiences are unlikely. (See **OVERDOSAGE**.)

DOSAGE AND ADMINISTRATION

Recommended Doses: *Adults and children 12 years of age and older:* The recommended starting and maximum dose is 220 mcg per day as two sprays in each nostril once daily. *Children 6 to 12 years of age:* The recommended starting dose is 110 mcg per day given as one spray in each nostril once daily. The maximum recommended dose is 220 mcg per day as two sprays per nostril once daily.

Nasacort AQ Nasal Spray is not recommended for children under 6 years of age since adequate numbers of patients have not been studied in this age group.

Individualization of Dosage: It is always desirable to titrate an individual patient to the minimum effective dose to reduce the possibility of side effects. In adults, when the maximum benefit has been achieved and symptoms have been controlled, reducing the dose to 110 mcg per day (one spray in each nostril once a day) has been shown to be effective in maintaining control of the allergic rhinitis symptoms in patients who were initially controlled at 220 mcg/day.

In children six to twelve years of age, the recommended starting dose is 110 mcg per day given as one spray in each nostril once daily. The maximum recommended daily dose in children 6 to 12 years of age is 220 mcg per day (two sprays in each nostril once daily). Some patients who do not achieve maximum symptom control at a dose of 110 mcg per day may benefit from a dose of 220 mcg given as two sprays in each nostril once daily. The minimum effective dose should be used to ensure continued control of symptoms. Once symptoms are controlled, pediatric patients may be able to be maintained on 110 mcg per day (1 spray in each nostril once daily).

An improvement in some patient symptoms may be seen within the first day of treatment, and generally, it takes one week of treatment to reach maximum benefit. Initial assessment for response should be made during this time frame and periodically until the patient's symptoms are stabilized. If adequate relief of symptoms has not been obtained after 3 weeks of treatment, **Nasacort AQ** Nasal Spray should be discontinued. (See **WARNINGS, PRECAUTIONS, Information for Patients,** and **ADVERSE REACTIONS.**)

Directions For Use: Illustrated Patient's Instructions for use accompany each package of **Nasacort AQ** Nasal Spray.

OVERDOSAGE

Like any other nasally administered corticosteroid, acute overdosing is unlikely in view of the total amount of active ingredient present. In the event that the entire contents of the bottle were administered all at once, via either oral or nasal application, clinically significant systemic adverse events would most likely not result. The patient may experience some gastrointestinal upset.

HOW SUPPLIED

Nasacort AQ Nasal Spray is a nonchlorofluorocarbon (non-CFC) containing metered-dose pump spray. The contents of one 6.5 gram sample bottle provide 30 actuations, and the contents of one 16.5 gram bottle provide 120 actuations. The bottle should be discarded when the labeled number of actuations have been reached even though the bottle is not completely empty.

It is supplied in a white high-density polyethylene container with a metered-dose pump unit, white nasal adapter, and patient instructions.

NDC 0075-1506-16

Caution: Federal law prohibits dispensing without prescription.

Keep out of reach of children.

Store at Controlled Room Temperature, 20 to 25°C (68 to 77°F) [see USP].

Manufactured by Rhône-Poulenc Rorer Puerto Rico Inc.
Manati, Puerto Rico

RHÔNE-POULENC RORER PHARMACEUTICALS INC.
500 ARCOLA ROAD
COLLEGEVILLE, PA 19426
Patent Pending

Rev. 10/97
IN-6361B

Shown in Product Identification Guide, page 333

NITROLINGUAL® SPRAY   ℞
(nitroglycerin lingual aerosol)
0.4 mg/metered dose

DESCRIPTION

Nitroglycerin, an organic nitrate, is a vasodilator which has effects on both arteries and veins. The chemical name for nitroglycerin is 1,2,3-propanetriol trinitrate ($C_3H_5N_3O_9$). The compound has a molecular weight of 227.09. The chemical structure is:

[See chemical structure at top of next column]

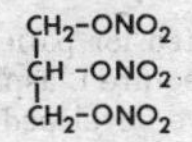

Nitrolingual® Spray (nitroglycerin lingual aerosol 0.4 mg) is a metered dose aerosol containing nitroglycerin in propellants (dichlorodifluoromethane and dichlorotetrafluoroethane). Each metered dose of Nitrolingual Spray delivers

$$CH_2-ONO_2$$
$$CH -ONO_2$$
$$CH_2-ONO_2$$

0.4 mg of nitroglycerin per spray emission. This product delivers nitroglycerin in the form of spray droplets onto or under the tongue. Inactive ingredients: caprylic/capric/diglyceryl succinate, ether, flavors.

CLINICAL PHARMACOLOGY

The principal pharmacological action of nitroglycerin is relaxation of vascular smooth muscle, producing a vasodilator effect on both peripheral arteries and veins with more prominent effects on the latter. Dilation of the post-capillary vessels, including large veins, promotes peripheral pooling of blood and decreases venous return to the heart, thereby reducing left ventricular end-diastolic pressure (pre-load). Arteriolar relaxation reduces systemic vascular resistance and arterial pressure (after-load).

The mechanism by which nitroglycerin relieves angina pectoris is not fully understood. Myocardial oxygen consumption or demand (as measured by the pressure-rate product, tension-time index, and stroke-work index) is decreased by both the arterial and venous effects of nitroglycerin and presumably, a more favorable supply-demand ratio is achieved. While the large epicardial coronary arteries are also dilated by nitroglycerin, the extent to which this action contributes to relief of exertional angina is unclear.

Nitroglycerin is rapidly metabolized *in vivo*, with a liver reductase enzyme having primary importance in the formation of glycerol nitrate metabolites and inorganic nitrate. Two active major metabolites, 1,2- and 1,3-dinitroglycerols, the products of hydrolysis, although less potent as vasodilators, have longer plasma half-lives than the parent compound. The dinitrates are further metabolized to mononitrates (considered biologically inactive with respect to cardiovascular effects) and ultimately glycerol and carbon dioxide.

Therapeutic doses of nitroglycerin may reduce systolic, diastolic and mean arterial blood pressure. Effective coronary perfusion pressure is usually maintained, but can be compromised if blood pressure falls excessively or increased heart rate decreases diastolic filling time.

Elevated central venous and pulmonary capillary wedge pressures, pulmonary vascular resistance and systemic vascular resistance are also reduced by nitroglycerin therapy. Heart rate is usually slightly increased, presumably a reflex response to the fall in blood pressure. Cardiac index may be increased, decreased, or unchanged. Patients with elevated left ventricular filling pressure and systemic vascular resistance values in conjunction with a depressed cardiac index are likely to experience an improvement in cardiac index. On the other hand, when filling pressures and cardiac index are normal, cardiac index may be slightly reduced.

A pharmacokinetic study in 13 healthy men showed no statistically significant differences between the mean values for maximum plasma concentration and time to achieve maximum plasma level with equal doses (0.8 mg) of Nitrolingual Spray and sublingual nitroglycerin tablets. Peak plasma concentration after 0.8 mg of Nitrolingual occurred within 4 minutes and the apparent plasma half-life was approximately 5 minutes. In a randomized, double-blind study in patients with exertional angina pectoris dose-related increases in exercise tolerance were seen following doses of 0.2, 0.4, and 0.8 mg delivered by metered spray.

INDICATIONS AND USAGE

Nitrolingual Spray is indicated for acute relief of an attack or prophylaxis of angina pectoris due to coronary artery disease.

CONTRAINDICATIONS

Nitrolingual Spray is contraindicated in patients who have shown purported hypersensitivity or idiosyncrasy to it or other nitrates or nitrites.

WARNINGS

The use of any form of nitroglycerin during the early days of acute myocardial infarction requires particular attention to hemodynamic monitoring and clinical status.

PRECAUTIONS: (General)

Severe hypotension, particularly with upright posture, may occur even with small doses of nitroglycerin. The drug, therefore, should be used with caution in subjects who may have volume depletion from diuretic therapy or in patients who have low systolic blood pressure (*e.g.,* below 90 mm Hg). Paradoxical bradycardia and increased angina pectoris may accompany nitroglycerin-induced hypotension.

Nitrate therapy may aggravate the angina caused by hypertrophic cardiomyopathy.

Tolerance to this drug and cross-tolerance to other nitrates and nitrites may occur. Tolerance to the vascular and antianginal effects of nitrates has been demonstrated in clinical trials, experience through occupational exposure, and in isolated tissue experiments in the laboratory.

In industrial workers continuously exposed to nitroglycerin, tolerance clearly occurs. Moreover, physical dependence also occurs since chest pain, acute myocardial infarction, and even sudden death have occurred during temporary withdrawal of nitroglycerin from the workers. In various clinical trials in angina patients, there are reports of anginal attacks being more easily provoked and of rebound in the hemodynamic effects soon after nitrate withdrawal. The relative importance of these observations to the routine, clinical use of nitroglycerin is not known.

DRUG INTERACTIONS: Alcohol may enhance sensitivity to the hypotensive effects of nitrates. Nitroglycerin acts directly on vascular muscle. Therefore, any other agents that depend on vascular smooth muscle as the final common path can be expected to have decreased or increased effect depending upon the agent.

Marked symptomatic orthostatic hypotension has been reported when calcium channel blockers and oral controlled-release nitroglycerin were used in combination. Dose adjustments of either class of agents may be necessary.

CARCINOGENESIS, MUTAGENESIS, IMPAIRMENT OF FERTILITY: Animal carcinogenesis studies with sublingual nitroglycerin have not been performed.

Rats receiving up to 434 mg/kg/day of dietary nitroglycerin for 2 years developed dose-related fibrotic and neoplastic changes in liver, including carcinomas, and interstitial cell tumors in testes. At high dose, the incidences of hepatocellular carcinomas in both sexes were 52% *vs.* 0% in controls, and incidences of testicular tumors were 52% *vs.* 8% in controls. Lifetime dietary administration of up to 1058 mg/kg/day of nitroglycerin was not tumorigenic in mice.

Nitroglycerin was weakly mutagenic in Ames tests performed in two different laboratories. Nevertheless, there was no evidence of mutagenicity in an *in vivo* dominant lethal assay with male rats treated with doses up to about 363 mg/kg/day, p.o., or in *in vitro* cytogenic tests in rat and dog tissues.

In a three-generation reproduction study, rats received dietary nitroglycerin at doses up to about 434 mg/kg/day for six months prior to mating of the F_0 generation with treatment continuing through successive F_1 and F_2 generations. The high-dose was associated with decreased feed intake and body weight gain in both sexes at all matings. No specific effect on the fertility of the F_0 generation was seen. Infertility noted in subsequent generations, however, was attributed to increased interstitial cell tissue and aspermatogenesis in the high-dose males. In this three-generation study there was no clear evidence of teratogenicity.

PREGNANCY: Pregnancy Category C – Animal teratology studies have not been conducted with nitroglycerin spray. Teratology studies in rats and rabbits, however, were conducted with topically applied nitroglycerin ointment at doses up to 80 mg/kg/day and 240 mg/kg/day, respectively. No toxic effects on dams or fetuses were seen at any dose tested. There are no adequate and well-controlled studies in pregnant women. Nitroglycerin should be given to pregnant women only if clearly needed.

NURSING MOTHERS: It is not known whether nitroglycerin is excreted in human milk. Because many drugs are excreted in human milk, caution should be exercised when Nitrolingual Spray is administered to a nursing woman.

PEDIATRIC USE: The safety and effectiveness of nitroglycerin in pediatric patients have not been established.

ADVERSE REACTIONS

Adverse reaction to Nitrolingual Spray, particularly headache and hypotension, is generally dose-related. In clinical trials at various doses of nitroglycerin, the following adverse effects have been observed:

Headache, which may be severe and persistent, is the most commonly reported side effect of nitroglycerin with an incidence on the order of about 50% in some studies. Cutaneous vasodilation with flushing may occur. Transient episodes of dizziness and weakness, as well as other signs of cerebral ischemia associated with postural hypotension, may occasionally develop. An occasional individual may exhibit marked sensitivity to the hypotensive effects of nitrates and severe responses (nausea, vomiting, weakness, restlessness, pallor, perspiration and collapse) may occur even with therapeutic doses. Drug rash and/or exfoliative dermatitis have been reported in patients receiving nitrate therapy. Nausea and vomiting appear to be uncommon.

OVERDOSAGE

Signs and Symptoms:

Nitrate overdosage may result in: severe hypotension, persistent throbbing headache, vertigo, palpitation, visual disturbance, flushing and perspiring skin (later becoming cold and cyanotic), nausea and vomiting (possibly with colic and even bloody diarrhea), syncope (especially in the upright posture), methemoglobinemia with cyanosis and anorexia, initial hypernea, dyspnea and slow breathing, slow pulse (dicrotic and intermittent), heart block, increased intracra-

Continued on next page

Nitrolingual—Cont.

nial pressure with cerebral symptoms of confusion and moderate fever, paralysis and coma followed by clonic convulsions, and possibly death due to circulatory collapse.
Treatment of Overdosage:
Keep the patient recumbent in a shock position and comfortably warm. Gastric lavage may be of use if the medication has only recently been swallowed. Passive movement of the extremities may aid venous return. Administer oxygen and artificial ventilation, if necessary. If methemoglobinemia is present, administration of methylene blue (1% solution), 1–2 mg per kilogram of body weight intravenously, may be required.
Methemoglobinemia:
Case reports of clinically significant methemoglobinemia are rare at conventional doses of organic nitrates. The formation of methemoglobin is dose-related and in the case of genetic abnormalities of hemoglobin that favor methemoglobin formation, even conventional doses of organic nitrates could produce harmful concentrations of methemoglobin.

WARNING

Epinephrine is ineffective in reversing the severe hypotensive events associated with overdosage. It and related compounds are contraindicated in this situation.

DOSAGE AND ADMINISTRATION

At the onset of an attack, one or two metered doses should be sprayed onto or under the tongue. No more than three metered doses are recommended within a 15-minute period. If the chest pain persists, prompt medical attention is recommended. Nitrolingual Spray may be used prophylactically five to ten minutes prior to engaging in activities which might precipitate an acute attack.
During application the patient should rest, ideally in the sitting position. The canister should be held vertically with the valve head uppermost and the spray orifice as close to the mouth as possible. The dose should preferably be sprayed onto the tongue by pressing the button firmly and the mouth should be closed immediately after each dose. THE SPRAY SHOULD NOT BE INHALED. Patients should be instructed to familiarize themselves with the position of the spray orifice, which can be identified by the finger rest on top of the valve, in order to facilitate orientation for administration at night.

HOW SUPPLIED

Nitrolingual Spray, 14.49 g (Net Contents) containing 200 metered doses, box of one. (NDC 0075-0850-84)
Note: The indented statement below is required by the Federal government's Clean Air Act for all products containing or manufactured with chlorofluorocarbons (CFCs):

WARNING: Contains CFC-11 and CFC-12, substances which harm public health and environment by destroying ozone in the upper atmosphere.

A notice similar to the above WARNING has been placed in the "Information For The Patient" portion of this package insert pursuant to EPA regulations.
STORE AT ROOM TEMPERATURE. Do not expose to temperatures exceeding 50°C (122°F).
Keep out of the reach of children.
CAUTION: Federal law prohibits dispensing without prescription.
Military and Veterans Administration: 0.4 mg–14.49 gm (NSN 6505-01-246-3781).
Rev. 7/97 IN-2997L
Manufactured by
G. Pohl-Boskamp GmbH & Co.
D-25551 Hohenlockstedt
Germany
Distributed by
RHÔNE-POULENC RORER PHARMACEUTICALS INC.
Collegeville, PA, U.S.A. 19426-0107
Shown in Product Identification Guide, page 333

ONCASPAR® ℞

[ən ′-cə-spər]
(pegaspargase)

PRODUCT OVERVIEW

KEY FACTS

ONCASPAR® (pegaspargase) is a modified version of the enzyme L-asparaginase. It is an oncolytic agent used in combination chemotherapy for the treatment of patients with acute lymphoblastic leukemia who are hypersensitive to native forms of L-asparaginase. Oncaspar was clinically researched as PEG-L-asparaginase. As a component of selected multiple agent regimens, the recommended dose of **ONCASPAR®** is 2,500 IU/m^2 every 14 days by either the intramuscular or intravenous route of administration. When a remission is obtained, appropriate maintenance therapy may be instituted. **ONCASPAR®** may be used as part of a maintenance regimen.

MAJOR USES

ONCASPAR® is indicated for patients with acute lymphoblastic leukemia who require L-asparaginase in their treatment regimen, but have developed hypersensitivity to the native forms of L-asparaginase. **ONCASPAR®**, like native L-asparaginase, is generally used in combination with other chemotherapeutic agents, such as vincristine, methotrexate, cytarabine, daunorubicin, and doxorubicin.[1,5] Use of **ONCASPAR®** as a single agent should only be undertaken when multi-agent chemotherapy is judged to be inappropriate for the patient.

SAFETY INFORMATION

ONCASPAR® is contraindicated in patients with pancreatitis or a history of pancreatitis. **ONCASPAR®** is contraindicated in patients who have had significant hemorrhagic events associated with prior L-asparaginase therapy. **ONCASPAR®** is also contraindicated in patients who have had previous serious allergic reactions, such as generalized urticaria, bronchospasm, laryngeal edema, hypotension, or other unacceptable adverse reactions to **ONCASPAR®**.

PRESCRIBING INFORMATION

ONCASPAR® ℞

[ən ′-cə-spər]
(pegaspargase)

DESCRIPTION

ONCASPAR®, the ENZON trademark for pegaspargase, is a modified version of the enzyme L-asparaginase. It is an oncolytic agent used in combination chemotherapy for the treatment of patients with acute lymphoblastic leukemia who are hypersensitive to native forms of L-asparaginase (as described in **CLINICAL PHARMACOLOGY**).
The generic name for **ONCASPAR®** is **pegaspargase**. The chemical name is monomethoxypolyethylene glycol succinimidyl L-asparaginase. L-asparaginase is modified by covalently conjugating units of monomethoxypolyethylene glycol (PEG), molecular weight of 5,000, to the enzyme, forming the active ingredient PEG-L-asparaginase. The L-asparaginase (L-asparagine amidohydrolase, type EC-2, EC 3.5.1.1) used in the manufacture of **ONCASPAR®** is derived from *Escherichia coli*. ENZON purchases the enzyme L-asparaginase in bulk from Merck, Sharp and Dohme, Division of Merck & Co., Inc., West Point, PA 19486, U.S. License Number 2. Merck & Co., Inc. supplies bulk L-asparaginase as a licensed intermediate for further manufacture by ENZON into PEG-L-asparaginase. Merck & Co., Inc. can only assume responsibility for the bulk intermediate supplied to ENZON.
ONCASPAR® is supplied as an isotonic sterile solution in phosphate buffered saline, pH 7.3, for intramuscular or intravenous administration only. The solution is clear, colorless and contains no preservatives. It is supplied in 5 mL single-dose vials.
ONCASPAR® activity is expressed in International Units (IU) according to the recommendation of the International Union of Biochemistry. One IU of L-asparaginase is defined as that amount of enzyme required to generate 1 μmol of ammonia per minute at pH 7.3 and 37°C.
Each milliliter of **ONCASPAR®** contains:

PEG-L-asparaginase	750 IU ± 20%
Monobasic sodium phosphate, USP	1.20 mg ± 5%
Dibasic sodium phosphate, USP	5.58 mg ± 5%
Sodium chloride, USP	8.50 mg ± 5%
Water for injection, USP	qs to 1.0 mL

The specific activity of **ONCASPAR®** is at least 85 IU per milligram protein.

CLINICAL PHARMACOLOGY

Leukemic cells are unable to synthesize asparagine due to a lack of asparagine synthetase and are dependent on an exogenous source of asparagine for survival. Rapid depletion of asparagine which results from treatment with the enzyme L-asparaginase, kills the leukemic cells. Normal cells, however, are less affected by the rapid depletion due to their ability to synthesize asparagine. This is an approach to therapy based on a specific metabolic defect in some leukemic cells which do not produce asparagine synthetase.[1]
In a study in predominately L-asparaginase naive adult patients with leukemia and lymphoma, initial plasma levels of L-asparaginase following intravenous administration were determined. Plasma half-life did not appear to be influenced by dose levels, and it could not be correlated with age, sex, surface area, renal or hepatic function, diagnosis or extent of disease. Apparent volume of distribution was equal to estimated plasma volume. L-asparaginase was measurable for at least 15 days following the initial treatment with **ONCASPAR®**. The enzyme could not be detected in the urine.[2]
In a study of newly diagnosed pediatric patients with acute lymphoblastic leukemia (ALL) who received either a single intramuscular injection of **ONCASPAR®** (2,500 IU/m^2), *E. coli* L-asparaginase (25,000 IU/m^2), or *Erwinia* L-asparaginase (25,000 IU/m^2), the plasma half-lives for the three forms of L-asparaginase were:[3]

PLASMA HALF-LIVES OF THREE FORMS OF L-ASPARAGINASE

TREATMENT GROUP	NO. OF PATIENTS	MEAN (DAYS)	STANDARD DEVIATION
ONCASPAR®	10	5.73	3.24
E. coli L-asparaginase	17	1.24	0.17
Erwinia L-asparaginase	10	0.65	0.13

In this same study of newly diagnosed pediatric ALL patients, the *in vivo* early leukemic cell kill after a single intramuscular injection of native *E. coli* L-asparaginase (25,000 IU/m^2), *Erwinia* L-asparaginase (25,000 IU/m^2), and **ONCASPAR®** (2,500 IU/m^2) during a five day "investigational window" was studied.[4] Bone marrow aspirates were taken before and five days after a single dose of one of the three different forms of L-asparaginase. Rhodamine-123 (RH-123), a selectively incorporated fluorescent mitochondrial dye, was used in an *in vitro* assay on the bone marrow aspirates to ascertain cell viability. The percent reduction of viable lymphoblasts at day five for each group is presented in the following table:[4]

RHODAMINE-123 (*IN VIVO* CELL KILL)

TREATMENT GROUP	NO. OF PATIENTS	PERCENT REDUCTION OF VIABLE LYMPHOBLASTS AT DAY 5 MEAN ± S.D.
ONCASPAR®	21	55.7 ± 10.2
E. coli L-asparaginase	28	57.8 ± 10.1
Erwinia L-asparaginase	19	57.9 ± 13.8

In three pharmacokinetic studies, 37 relapsed ALL patients received **ONCASPAR®** at 2,500 IU/m^2 every two weeks. The plasma half-life of **ONCASPAR®** was 3.24 ± 1.83 days in nine patients who were previously hypersensitive to native L-asparaginase and 5.69 ± 3.25 days in 28 non-hypersensitive patients. The area under the curve was 9.50 ± 3.95 IU/mL/day in the previously hypersensitive patients, and 9.83 ± 5.94 IU/mL/day in the non-hypersensitive patients.

Hypersensitivity Reactions

Hypersensitivity reactions to *E. coli* L-asparaginase have been reported in the literature in 3% to 73% of patients.[1] Patients in **ONCASPAR®** clinical studies were considered to be previously hypersensitive if they experienced a systemic rash, urticaria, bronchospasm, laryngeal edema, or hypotension following administration of any form of native L-asparaginase. Patients were also considered to be previously hypersensitive if they experienced local erythema, urticaria, or swelling, greater than two centimeters, for at least ten minutes following administration of any form of native L-asparaginase. The National Cancer Institute Common Toxicity Criteria (CTC) were used to classify the severity of the hypersensitivity reactions. These are: grade 1 — transient rash (mild); grade 2 — mild bronchospasm (moderate); grade 3 — moderate bronchospasm and/or serum sickness (severe); grade 4 — hypotension and/or anaphylaxis (life-threatening). Additionally, most transient local urticaria were considered grade 2 hypersensitivity reactions, while most sustained urticaria distant from the injection site were considered grade 3 hypersensitivity reactions. In general, the moderate to life-threatening hypersensitivity reactions were considered dose-limiting; that is, they required L-asparaginase treatment to be discontinued.
In separate studies, **ONCASPAR®** was administered intravenously to 48 patients and intramuscularly to 126 patients. The incidence of hypersensitivity reactions when **ONCASPAR®** was administered intramuscularly was 30% in patients who were previously hypersensitive to native L-asparaginase and 11% in non-hypersensitive patients (p-value of 0.007). The incidence of hypersensitivity reactions when **ONCASPAR®** was administered intravenously was 60% in patients who were previously hypersensitive to native L-asparaginase and 12% in non-hypersensitive patients. Since only five previously hypersensitive patients received **ONCASPAR®** intravenously, no meaningful analysis of the incidence of hypersensitivity reactions was possible between either the previously hypersensitive and non-hypersensitive patients, or between the intravenous and intramuscular routes of administration.
The overall incidence of hypersensitivity reactions in 174 patients who received **ONCASPAR®** in five clinical studies is shown in the table below:

INCIDENCE OF ONCASPAR® HYPERSENSITIVITY REACTIONS

PATIENT STATUS	N	CTC GRADE OF HYPERSENSITIVITY REACTION 1	2	3	4	TOTAL
Previously Hypersensitive Patients	62	7	8	4	1	20 (32%)

Non-Hypersensitive Patients	112	5	4	1	1	11 (10%)
Total Patients	174	12	12	5	2	31 (18%)

The probability of a previously hypersensitive or non-hypersensitive patient completing 8 doses of **ONCASPAR®** therapy without developing a dose-limiting hypersensitivity reaction was 77% and 95%, respectively.
All of the 62 hypersensitive patients treated with **ONCASPAR®** in five clinical studies had previous hypersensitivity reactions to one or more of the native forms of L-asparaginase. Of the 35 patients who had previous hypersensitivity reactions to *E. coli* L-asparaginase only, 5 (14%) had **ONCASPAR®** dose-limiting hypersensitivity reactions. Of the 27 patients who had hypersensitivity reactions to both *E. coli* and *Erwinia* L-asparaginase, 7 (26%) had **ONCASPAR®** dose-limiting hypersensitivity reactions. The overall incidence of dose-limiting hypersensitivity reactions in 174 patients treated with **ONCASPAR®** was 9% (19% in 62 hypersensitive and 3% in 112 non-hypersensitive patients). Of the total of 9% dose-limiting hypersensitivity reactions, 1% were anaphylactic (CTC grade 4) and the other 8% were ≤ CTC grade 3.

Clinical Activity

ONCASPAR® was evaluated as part of combination therapy in four open label studies comprising 42 multiply-relapsed, previously hypersensitive acute leukemia patients [39 (93%) with ALL] at a dose of 2,000 or 2,500 IU/m^2 administered intramuscularly or intravenously every 14 days during induction combination chemotherapy. The reinduction response rate was 50% (36% complete remissions and 14% partial remissions), with a 95% confidence interval of 35% to 65%. This response rate is comparable to that reported in the literature for relapsed patients treated with native L-asparaginase as part of combination chemotherapy.[1]
ONCASPAR® was also shown to have some activity as a single agent in multiply-relapsed hypersensitive ALL patients, the majority of whom were pediatric. Treatment with **ONCASPAR®** resulted in three responses (one complete remission and two partial remissions) in nine previously hypersensitive patients who would not have been able to receive any further L-asparaginase treatment.
ONCASPAR® was also studied in non-hypersensitive, relapsed ALL patients who were randomized to receive two doses of **ONCASPAR®** at 2,500 IU/m^2 every 14 days or twelve doses of *E. coli* L-asparaginase at 10,000 IU/m^2 three times a week during a 28 day induction combination chemotherapy regimen (which included vincristine and prednisone). Although the enrollment in this study was too small to be conclusive, the data showed that for 20 patients there was no significant difference between the overall response rates of 60% and 50%, respectively, or the complete remission rates of 50% and 50%, respectively.
ONCASPAR® was administered during maintenance therapy regimens to 33 previously hypersensitive patients. The average number of doses received during maintenance therapy was 5.8 (range of 1 to 24) and the average duration of maintenance therapy was 126 (range of 1 to 513) days for this patient population.

INDICATIONS AND USAGE

ONCASPAR® is indicated for patients with acute lymphoblastic leukemia who require L-asparaginase in their treatment regimen, but have developed hypersensitivity to the native forms of L-asparaginase **(SEE CLINICAL PHARMACOLOGY)**. **ONCASPAR®**, like native L-asparaginase, is generally used in combination with other chemotherapeutic agents, such as vincristine, methotrexate, cytarabine, daunorubicin, and doxorubicin.[1,5] Use of **ONCASPAR®** as a single agent should only be undertaken when multi-agent chemotherapy is judged to be inappropriate for the patient.

CONTRAINDICATIONS

ONCASPAR® is contraindicated in patients with pancreatitis or a history of pancreatitis. **ONCASPAR®** is contraindicated in patients who have had significant hemorrhagic events associated with prior L-asparaginase therapy. **ONCASPAR®** is also contraindicated in patients who have had previous serious allergic reactions, such as generalized urticaria, bronchospasm, laryngeal edema, hypotension, or other unacceptable adverse reactions to **ONCASPAR®**.

WARNINGS

It is recommended that **ONCASPAR®** be given under the supervision of an individual who is qualified by training and experience to administer cancer chemotherapeutic agents. Especially in patients with known hypersensitivity to the other forms of L-asparaginase, hypersensitivity reactions to **ONCASPAR®**, including life-threatening anaphylaxis, may occur during therapy. As a routine precaution, patients should be kept under observation for one hour with resuscitation equipment and other agents necessary to treat anaphylaxis (epinephrine, oxygen, intravenous steroids, etc.) available.

PRECAUTIONS

General

This drug may be a contact irritant, and the solution must be handled and administered with care. Gloves are recommended. Inhalation of vapors and contact with skin or mucous membranes, especially those of the eyes, must be avoided. In case of contact, wash with copious amounts of water for at least 15 minutes. Anaphylactic reactions require the immediate use of epinephrine, oxygen, intravenous steroids, and antihistamines. Patients taking **ONCASPAR®** are at higher than usual risk for bleeding problems, especially with simultaneous use of other drugs that have anticoagulant properties, such as aspirin, and non-steroidal anti-inflammatories **(SEE DRUG INTERACTIONS)**. **ONCASPAR®** may have immunosuppressive activity. Therefore, it is possible that use of the drug in patients may predispose the patient to infection. Severe hepatic and central nervous system toxicity following multi-agent chemotherapy that includes **ONCASPAR®** may occur. Caution appears warranted when treating patients with **ONCASPAR®** given in combination with hepatotoxic agents, particularly when liver dysfunction is present.
Patients undergoing **ONCASPAR®** therapy must be carefully monitored and the therapeutic regimen adjusted according to response and toxicity. Physicians using a given treatment regimen incorporating **ONCASPAR®** should be thoroughly familiar with its benefits and risks.

Information For Patients

Patients should be informed of the possibility of hypersensitivity reactions, including immediate anaphylaxis, to **ONCASPAR®**. Patients taking **ONCASPAR®** are at higher than usual risk for bleeding problems. Patients should be instructed that the simultaneous use of **ONCASPAR®** with other drugs that may increase the risk of bleeding should be avoided **(SEE DRUG INTERACTIONS)**. **ONCASPAR®** may affect the ability of the liver to function normally in some patients. Therapy with **ONCASPAR®** may increase the toxicity of other medications **(SEE DRUG INTERACTIONS)**. **ONCASPAR®** may have immunosuppressive activity. Therefore, it is possible that use of the drug in patients may predispose the patient to infection. Patients should notify their physicians of any adverse reactions that occur.

Laboratory Tests

A fall in circulating lymphoblasts is often noted after initiating therapy. This may be accompanied by a marked rise in serum uric acid. As a guide to the effects of therapy, the patient's peripheral blood count and bone marrow should be monitored.
Frequent serum amylase determinations should be obtained to detect early evidence of pancreatitis **(SEE CONTRAINDICATIONS)**. Blood sugar should be monitored during therapy with **ONCASPAR®** because hyperglycemia may occur. When using **ONCASPAR®** in conjunction with hepatotoxic chemotherapy, patients should be monitored for liver dysfunction.
ONCASPAR® may affect a number of plasma proteins; therefore, monitoring of fibrinogen, PT, and PTT may be indicated.

Drug Interactions

Unfavorable interactions of L-asparaginase with some antitumor agents have been demonstrated.[1] It is recommended, therefore, that **ONCASPAR®** be used in combination regimens only by physicians familiar with the benefits and risks of a given regimen. Depletion of serum proteins by **ONCASPAR®** may increase the toxicity of other drugs which are protein bound. Additionally, during the period of its inhibition of protein synthesis and cell replication, **ONCASPAR®** may interfere with the action of drugs such as methotrexate, which require cell replication for their lethal effects. **ONCASPAR®** may interfere with the enzymatic detoxification of other drugs, particularly in the liver. Physicians using a given treatment regimen should be thoroughly familiar with its benefits and risks.
Imbalances in coagulation factors have been noted with the use of **ONCASPAR®** predisposing to bleeding and/or thrombosis. Caution should be used when administering any concurrent anticoagulant therapy, such as coumadin, heparin, dipyridamole, aspirin, or non-steroidal anti-inflammatories.

Carcinogenesis, Mutagenesis, Impairment of Fertility

Long-term carcinogenic studies in animals have not been performed with **ONCASPAR®** nor have studies been performed on impairment of fertility. **ONCASPAR®** did not exhibit a mutagenic effect when tested against *Salmonella typhimurium* strains in the Ames assay.

Pregnancy

Pregnancy Category C. Animal reproduction studies have not been conducted with **ONCASPAR®**. It is also not known whether **ONCASPAR®** can cause fetal harm when administered to a pregnant woman or can affect reproduction capacity. **ONCASPAR®** should be given to a pregnant woman only if clearly needed.

Nursing Mothers

It is not known whether **ONCASPAR®** is excreted in human milk. Because many drugs are excreted in human milk and because of the potential for serious adverse reactions due to **ONCASPAR®** in nursing infants, a decision should be made to discontinue nursing or discontinue the drug, taking into account the importance of the drug to the mother.

ONCASPAR® ADVERSE REACTIONS

Adverse reactions have been reported in adults and pediatric patients. Overall, the adult patients treated with **ONCASPAR®** had a somewhat higher incidence of known L-asparaginase toxicities, except for hypersensitivity reactions, than the pediatric patients treated with **ONCASPAR®**.
Excluding hypersensitivity reactions, the most frequently occurring known L-asparaginase related toxicities and adverse experiences reported for the 174 patients in clinical studies were chemical hepatotoxicities and coagulopathies, the majority of which did not result in any significant clinical events. The incidence of significant clinical events included clinical pancreatitis (1%), hyperglycemia requiring insulin therapy (3%), and thrombosis (4%).
The following adverse reactions related to **ONCASPAR®** were reported for 174 patients in five clinical studies.
The adverse reactions reported most frequently (greater than 5%) were allergic reactions (which may have included rash, erythema, edema, pain, fever, chills, urticaria, dyspnea, or bronchospasm), SGPT increase, nausea and/or vomiting, fever, and malaise.
The adverse reactions reported occasionally (greater than 1% but less than 5%) were anaphylactic reactions, dyspnea, injection site hypersensitivity, lip edema, rash, urticaria, abdominal pain, chills, pain in the extremities, hypotension, tachycardia, thrombosis, anorexia, diarrhea, jaundice, abnormal liver function test, decreased anticoagulant effect, disseminated intravascular coagulation, decreased fibrinogen, hemolytic anemia, leukopenia, pancytopenia, thrombocytopenia, increased thromboplastin, injection site pain, injection site reaction, bilirubinemia, hyperglycemia, hyperuricemia, hypoglycemia, hypoproteinemia, peripheral edema, increased SGOT, arthralgia, myalgia, convulsion, headache, night sweats, and paresthesia.
The adverse reactions reported rarely (less than 1%) were bronchospasm, petechial rash, face edema, lesional edema, sepsis, septic shock, chest pain, endocarditis, hypertension, constipation, flatulence, gastrointestinal pain, hepatomegaly, increased appetite, liver fatty deposits, coagulation disorder, increased coagulation time, decreased platelet count, purpura, increased amylase, edema, excessive thirst, hyperammonemia, hyponatremia, weight loss, bone pain, joint disorder, confusion, dizziness, emotional lability, somnolence, increased cough, epistaxis, upper respiratory infection, erythema simplex, pruritus, hematuria, increased urinary frequency, and abnormal kidney function.
The following **ONCASPAR®** related adverse reactions have been observed in patients with hematologic malignancies, primarily acute lymphoblastic leukemia (approximately 75%), non-Hodgkins lymphoma (approximately 13%), acute myelogenous leukemia (approximately 3%), and a variety of solid tumors (approximately 9%):
HYPERSENSITIVITY REACTIONS: a variety of hypersensitivity reactions have occurred. These reactions may be acute or delayed, and include acute anaphylaxis, bronchospasm, dyspnea, urticaria, arthralgia, erythema, induration, edema, pain, tenderness, hives, swelling, lip edema, chills, fever, and skin rashes **(SEE WARNINGS AND CONTRAINDICATIONS)**.
PANCREATIC FUNCTION: pancreatitis, sometimes fulminant and fatal, has occurred. Increased serum amylase and lipase have also occurred.
LIVER FUNCTION: a variety of liver function abnormalities have been observed, including elevations of SGOT, SGPT, and bilirubin (direct and indirect). Jaundice, ascites, and hypoalbuminemia, which may be associated with peripheral edema, have been observed. These abnormalities usually are reversible on discontinuance of therapy, and some reversal may occur during the course of therapy. Fatty changes in the liver and liver failure have occurred.
HEMATOLOGIC: hypofibrinogenemia, prolonged prothrombin times, prolonged partial thromboplastin times, and decreased antithrombin III have been observed. Superficial and deep venous thrombosis, sagittal sinus thrombosis, venous catheter thrombosis, and atrial thrombosis have occurred. Leukopenia, agranulocytosis, pancytopenia, thrombocytopenia, disseminated intravascular coagulation, severe hemolytic anemia, and anemia have been observed. Clinical hemorrhage, which may be fatal; easy bruisability, and ecchymosis have also been observed.
METABOLIC: mild to severe hyperglycemia has been observed in low incidence, and usually responds to discontinuation of **ONCASPAR®** and the judicious use of intravenous fluid and insulin. Hypoglycemia, increased thirst and hyponatremia, uric acid nephropathy, hyperuricemia, hypoproteinemia, and peripheral edema have also been observed. Hypoalbuminemia, proteinuria, weight loss, and metabolic acidosis have occurred. Therapy with **ONCASPAR®** is associated with an increase in blood ammonia during the conversion of L-asparagine to aspartic acid by the enzyme.
NEUROLOGIC: status epilepticus and temporal lobe seizures, somnolence, coma, malaise, mental status changes, dizziness, emotional lability, headache, lip numbness, finger

Continued on next page

Oncaspar—Cont.

paresthesia, mood changes, night sweats, and a Parkinson-like syndrome have occurred. Mild to severe confusion, disorientation, and paresthesia have also occurred. These side effects usually have reversed spontaneously after treatment was stopped.

RENAL: increased BUN, increased creatinine, increased urinary frequency, hematuria due to thrombopenia, severe hemorrhagic cystitis, renal dysfunction, and renal failure have been observed.

CARDIOVASCULAR: chest pain, subacute bacterial endocarditis, hypertension, severe hypotension, and tachycardia have occurred.

DIGESTIVE: anorexia, constipation, decreased appetite, diarrhea, indigestion, flatulence, gas, gastrointestinal pain, mucositis, hepatomegaly, elevated gamma-glutamyltranspeptidase, increased appetite, mouth tenderness, severe colitis, and nausea and/or vomiting have been observed.

MUSCULOSKELETAL: diffuse and local musculoskeletal pain, arthralgia, joint stiffness, and cramps have occurred.

RESPIRATORY: cough, epistaxis, severe bronchospasm, and upper respiratory infection have been observed.

SKIN/APPENDAGES: itching, alopecia, fever blister, purpura, hand whiteness and fungal changes, nail whiteness and ridging, erythema simplex, jaundice, and petechial rash have occurred.

GENERAL: localized edema, injection site reactions (including pain, swelling, or redness), malaise, infection, sepsis, fatigue, and septic shock may occur.

OVERDOSAGE

Three patients received 10,000 IU/m² of **ONCASPAR®** as an intravenous infusion. One patient experienced a slight increase in liver enzymes. A second patient developed a rash ten minutes after the start of the infusion, which was controlled with the administration of an antihistamine and by slowing down the infusion rate. A third patient did not experience any adverse reactions.

DOSAGE AND ADMINISTRATION

As a component of selected multiple agent regimens, the recommended dose of **ONCASPAR®** is 2,500 IU/m² every 14 days by either the intramuscular or intravenous route of administration.

The preferred route of administration, however, is the intramuscular route because of the lower incidence of hepatotoxicity, coagulopathy, and gastrointestinal and renal disorders compared to the intravenous route of administration.

The safety and effectiveness of **ONCASPAR®** have been established in patients with known previous hypersensitivity to L-asparaginase whose ages ranged from 1 to 21 years old. The recommended dose of **ONCASPAR®** for children with a body surface area ≥0.6 m² is 2,500 IU/m² administered every 14 days. The recommended dose of **ONCASPAR®** for children with a body surface area <0.6 m² is 82.5 IU/kg administered every 14 days.

Do not administer ONCASPAR® if there is any indication that the drug has been frozen. Although there may not be an apparent change in the appearance of the drug, ONCASPAR®'s activity is destroyed after freezing.

When administering **ONCASPAR®** intramuscularly, the volume at a single injection site should be limited to 2 mL. If the volume to be administered is greater than 2 mL, multiple injection sites should be used.

When administered intravenously, **ONCASPAR®** should be given over a period of 1 to 2 hours in 100 mL of sodium chloride or dextrose injection 5%, through an infusion that is already running.

Anaphylactic reactions require the immediate use of antihistamines, epinephrine, oxygen, and intravenous steroids.

Use of **ONCASPAR®** as the sole induction agent should be undertaken only in an unusual situation when a combined regimen, which uses other chemotherapeutic agents such as vincristine, methotrexate, cytarabine, daunorubicin, or doxorubicin, is inappropriate because of toxicity or other specific patient-related factors, or in patients refractory to other therapy. When **ONCASPAR®** is to be used as the sole induction agent, the recommended dosage regimen is also 2,500 IU/m² every 14 days.

When a remission is obtained, appropriate maintenance therapy may be instituted. **ONCASPAR®** may be used as part of a maintenance regimen.

Parenteral drug products should be inspected visually for particulate matter, cloudiness or discoloration prior to administration, whenever solution and container permit.

HOW SUPPLIED

Dosage Form

ONCASPAR®: Use only one dose per vial; do not re-enter the vial. Discard unused portions. Do not save unused drug for later administration.

Sterile solution for injection in ready to use single-use vials. Preservative free.

Quantity per Individual Container

5 mL per vial containing 750 IU/mL **ONCASPAR®** in a clear, colorless, phosphate buffered saline solution, pH 7.3. Each vial contains 3,750 IU of **ONCASPAR®**.

Handling and Storage

Avoid excessive agitation. DO NOT SHAKE.

Keep refrigerated at +2°C to +8°C (36°F to 46°F).

Do not use if cloudy or if precipitate is present.

Do not use if stored at room temperature for more than 48 hours.

DO NOT FREEZE. Do not use product if it is known to have been frozen. Freezing destroys activity, which cannot be detected visually.

NDC 0075-0640-05

U.S. Patent 4,179,337 and pat. pending

40 Kingsbridge Road
Piscataway, NJ 08854-3998 USA

01/21/94

REFERENCES

1. Capizzi, RL and Holcenberg, JS. Asparaginase. In: Holland and Frei (eds). *Cancer Med* third edition, Lea and Febiger, Phila. PA, 1993.
2. Ho, DH, et al. Clinical pharmacology of polyethylene glycol-L-asparaginase. *Drug Metab Dispos* 14 (3): 349–352, 1986.
3. Asselin, BL, et al. Comparative Pharmacokinetic Studies of Three L-asparaginase Preparations. *J Clin Oncology* (11): 1780–1786, 1993.
4. Data on File at ENZON.
5. Clavell, LA, et al. Four-agent induction and intensive asparaginase therapy for treatment of childhood acute lymphoblastic leukemia. *N Engl J Med* 315 (11): 657–663, 1986.

IN-1724 Rev. 2/94

Mfg. by: Enzon, Inc.
Piscataway, NJ 08854 USA
License No. 1171

Dist. by: Rhône-Poulenc Rorer Pharmaceuticals Inc.
Collegeville, PA, U.S.A. 19426-0107

PENETREX™ ℞

(enoxacin) Tablets

DESCRIPTION

Penetrex™ (enoxacin) is a broad-spectrum azafluoroquinolone antibacterial agent for oral administration. Enoxacin is 1-ethyl-6-fluoro-1,4-dihydro-4-oxo-7-(1-piperazinyl)-1,8-naphthyridine-3-carboxylic acid sesquihydrate. The chemical structure of enoxacin is:

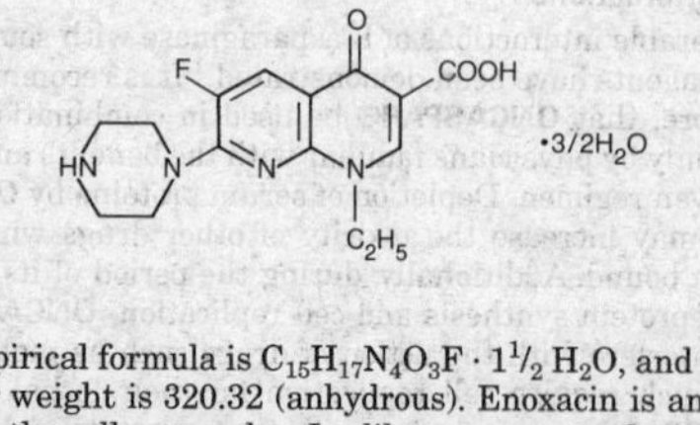

Its empirical formula is $C_{15}H_{17}N_4O_3F \cdot 1^1/_2\ H_2O$, and its molecular weight is 320.32 (anhydrous). Enoxacin is an ivory-to-slightly yellow powder. In dilute aqueous solution, it is unstable in strong sunlight.

Penetrex is available in 200 mg and 400 mg film-coated tablets. Each "200" and "400" Penetrex tablet contains enoxacin sesquihydrate equivalent to 200 mg and 400 mg of anhydrous enoxacin, respectively. Each Penetrex 200 mg and 400 mg tablet contains the following inactive ingredients: cellulose microcrystalline NF, colloidal silicon dioxide NF, croscarmellose sodium NF, FD&C Blue No. 2 aluminum lake, hydroxypropyl cellulose NF, hydroxypropyl methylcellulose, magnesium stearate USP, polyethylene glycol, simethicone, sorbic acid, stearate emulsifiers, and titanium dioxide.

CLINICAL PHARMACOLOGY

Following oral administration to healthy subjects, peak plasma enoxacin concentrations were achieved within 1 to 3 hours. Absolute oral bioavailability of enoxacin is approximately 90%. Maximum plasma concentrations of enoxacin average 0.93 μg/mL and 2.0 μg/mL after single 200 mg and 400 mg doses, respectively. Enoxacin plasma half-life is 3 to 6 hours. Enoxacin is excreted primarily via the kidney. After a single dose, greater than 40% was recovered in urine by 48 hours as unchanged drug. In elderly patients, the mean peak enoxacin plasma concentration was 50% higher than that in young adult volunteers receiving comparable single doses of enoxacin. This appears to correspond to age-associated reduction of renal function in the elderly population. Five metabolites of enoxacin have been identified in human urine and account for 15% to 20% of the administered dose.

Enoxacin diffuses into cervix, fallopian tube, and myometrium at levels approximately 1–2 times those achieved in plasma, and into kidney and prostate at levels approximately 2–4 times those achieved in plasma. Studies have not been conducted to assess the penetration of enoxacin into human cerebrospinal fluid.

Enoxacin is approximately 40% bound to plasma proteins in healthy subjects and is approximately 14% bound to plasma proteins in patients with impaired renal function.

The effect of food on the absorption of enoxacin from the tablet formulation has not been studied.

Some isozymes of the cytochrome P-450 hepatic microsomal enzyme system are inhibited by enoxacin. This inhibition results in significant drug/drug interactions with theophylline and caffeine. Enoxacin interferes with the metabolism of theophylline, resulting in a dose-related decrease in theophylline clearance. Elevated serum theophylline concentrations may increase the risk of theophylline-related adverse reactions. (See **PRECAUTIONS: Drug Interactions.**)

Clearance of enoxacin is reduced in patients with impaired renal function (creatinine clearance ≤30 mL/min/1.73 m²), and dosage adjustment is necessary. (See **DOSAGE AND ADMINISTRATION.)**

MICROBIOLOGY

Enoxacin is an inhibitor of the bacterial enzyme DNA gyrase and is a bactericidal agent. Enoxacin may be active against pathogens resistant to drugs that act by different mechanisms.

Enoxacin has been shown to be active against most strains of the following organisms both *in vitro* and in clinical infections: (See **INDICATIONS AND USAGE.)**

Gram-positive aerobes: *Staphylococcus epidermidis, Staphylococcus saprophyticus.*

Gram-negative aerobes: *Enterobacter cloacae, Escherichia coli, Klebsiella pneumoniae, Neisseria gonorrhoeae, Proteus mirabilis, Pseudomonas aeruginosa.*

The following *in vitro* data are available but their clinical significance is unknown.

In addition, enoxacin exhibits *in vitro* minimum inhibitory concentrations (MICs) of 2.0 μg/mL or less against most strains of the following organisms; however, the safety and effectiveness of enoxacin in treating clinical infections due to these organisms have not been established in adequate and well-controlled trials.

Gram-negative aerobes: *Aeromonas hydrophila, Citrobacter diversus, Citrobacter freundii, Citrobacter koseri, Enterobacter aerogenes, Haemophilus ducreyi, Klebsiella oxytoca, Klebsiella ozaenae, Morganella morganii, Proteus vulgaris, Providencia stuartii, Providencia alcalifaciens, Serratia marcescens, Serratia proteomaculans* (formerly *S. liquefaciens*)

Many strains of *Streptococcus* species and anaerobes are usually resistant to enoxacin.

The activity of enoxacin against *Treponema pallidum* has not been evaluated; however, other quinolones are not active against *T. pallidum.* (See **WARNINGS.)**

Cross-resistance with other quinolones has been demonstrated.

The addition of human serum has no effect on the *in vitro* MIC values; however, enoxacin activity is decreased in acidic (pH 5.5) environments.

Susceptibility Testing

Diffusion Techniques: Quantitative methods that require measurement of zone diameters give the most precise estimate of susceptibility of bacteria to antimicrobial agents. One such standardized procedure[1] that has been recommended for use with disks to test susceptibility of organisms to enoxacin uses the 10-μg enoxacin disk.

Interpretation involves the correlation of the diameter obtained in the disk test with the minimum inhibitory concentration (MIC) for enoxacin.

Reports from the laboratory giving results of the standard single-disk susceptibility test with a 10-μg enoxacin disk should be interpreted according to the following criteria:

Zone Diameter (mm)	Interpretation
≥18	(S) Susceptible
15–17	(MS) Moderately susceptible
≤14	(R) Resistant

A report of "Susceptible" indicates that the pathogen is likely to be inhibited by generally achievable blood concentrations. A report of "Moderately susceptible" suggests that the organism would be susceptible if high dosage is used or if the infection is confined to tissues or fluids in which high antimicrobial levels are attained. A report of "Resistant" indicates that achievable drug concentrations are unlikely to be inhibitory, and other therapy should be selected.

Standardized susceptibility test procedures require the use of laboratory control organisms. The 10-μg enoxacin disk should give the following zone diameters:

Organism	Zone Diameter (mm)
Escherichia coli (ATCC 25922)	28–36
Neisseria gonorrhoeae (ATCC 49226)	43–51
Pseudomonas aeruginosa (ATCC 27853)	22–28
Staphylococcus aureus (ATCC 25923)	22–28

Other quinolone antibacterial disks should not be substituted when performing susceptibility tests for enoxacin because of spectrum differences. The 10-µg enoxacin disk should be used for all *in vitro* testing of isolates for enoxacin susceptibility using diffusion techniques.
Dilution Techniques: Use a standardized dilution method[2] (broth, agar, or microdilution) or equivalent with enoxacin powder. The MIC values obtained should be interpreted according to the following criteria:

MIC (µg/mL)	Interpretation
≤2	(S) Susceptible
4	(MS) Moderately susceptible
≥8	(R) Resistant

As with standard diffusion methods, dilution procedures require the use of laboratory control organisms. Standard enoxacin powder should give the following MIC values:

Organism	MIC (µg/mL)
Enterococcus faecalis (ATCC 29212)	2–16
Escherichia coli (ATCC 25922)	0.06–0.25
Neisseria gonorrhoeae (ATCC 49226)	0.015–0.06
Pseudomonas aeruginosa (ATCC 27853)	2–8
Staphylococcus aureus (ATCC 29213)	0.5–2

INDICATIONS AND USAGE

Penetrex™ (enoxacin) is indicated for the treatment of adults (≥18 years of age) with the following infections caused by susceptible strains of the designated microorganisms:
Sexually Transmitted Diseases (See **WARNINGS.**)
Uncomplicated urethral or cervical gonorrhea due to *Neisseria gonorrhoeae*.
Urinary Tract
Uncomplicated urinary tract infections (cystitis) due to *Escherichia coli*, *Staphylococcus epidermidis**, or *Staphylococcus saprophyticus**.
Complicated urinary tract infections due to *Escherichia coli*, *Klebsiella pneumoniae*, *Proteus mirabilis*, *Pseudomonas aeruginosa*, *Staphylococcus epidermidis*, or *Enterobacter cloacae**.
*Efficacy for this organism in this organ system at the recommended dose was studied in fewer than ten infections. The dosage regimens for complicated and uncomplicated urinary tract infections are different. (See **DOSAGE AND ADMINISTRATION.**)
Penicillinase production should have no effect on enoxacin activity.
Appropriate culture and susceptibility tests should be performed before treatment in order to isolate and identify organisms causing the infection and to determine their susceptibility to enoxacin. Therapy with enoxacin may be initiated while awaiting the results of these studies; therapy should be adjusted if necessary once the results are known. Culture and susceptibility testing performed periodically during therapy will provide information not only on the therapeutic effect of the antimicrobial agent but also on the possible emergence of bacterial resistance.

CONTRAINDICATIONS

Penetrex is contraindicated in persons with a history of hypersensitivity, tendinitis, or tendon rupture associated with the use of enoxacin or any member of the quinolone group of antimicrobial agents.

WARNINGS

THE SAFETY AND EFFECTIVENESS OF ENOXACIN IN CHILDREN, ADOLESCENTS (UNDER THE AGE OF 18 YEARS), PREGNANT WOMEN, AND LACTATING WOMEN HAVE NOT BEEN ESTABLISHED. (See PRECAUTIONS: Pregnancy, Nursing Mothers, and Pediatric Use.) Enoxacin has been shown to cause arthropathy in immature rats and dogs when given in oral doses approximately 1.5 and 3.8 times, respectively, the highest human clinical dose based on a mg/m^2 basis after a four-week dosage regimen. Gross and histopathological examination of the weight-bearing joints of the dogs revealed lesions of the cartilage. Other quinolones also produce erosions of cartilage of weight-bearing joints and other signs of arthropathy in immature animals of various species. (See **ANIMAL PHARMACOLOGY.**)

Convulsions and abnormal electroencephalograms have been reported in some patients receiving enoxacin. Increased intracranial pressure, and toxic psychoses have been reported in patients receiving drugs in this class. Quinolones may also cause central nervous system stimulation which may lead to: tremors, restlessness/agitation, nervousness/anxiety, lightheadedness, confusion, hallucinations, paranoia, depression, nightmares, insomnia, and, rarely, suicidal thoughts or acts. These reactions may occur following the first dose. If these reactions occur in patients receiving enoxacin, the drug should be discontinued and appropriate measures instituted. As with all quinolones, enoxacin should be used with caution in patients with known or suspected CNS disorder that may predispose to seizures or lower the seizure threshold (*e.g.*, severe cerebral arteriosclerosis, epilepsy) or in the presence of other risk factors that may predispose to seizures or lower the seizure threshold (*e.g.*, certain drug therapy, renal dysfunction). (See **PRECAUTIONS: General, Information for Patients, Drug Interactions** and **ADVERSE REACTIONS.**)
Enoxacin is a potent inhibitor of the hepatic microsomal enzyme system, resulting in significant drug/drug interactions with theophylline and caffeine. (See **PRECAUTIONS: Drug Interactions.**)
Serious and occasionally fatal hypersensitivity (anaphylactoid or anaphylactic) reactions, some following the first dose, have been reported in patients receiving quinolone therapy. Some reactions were accompanied by cardiovascular collapse, loss of consciousness, tingling, pharyngeal or facial edema, dyspnea, urticaria, or itching. Only a few patients had a history of previous hypersensitivity reactions. Serious hypersensitivity reactions have also been reported following treatment with enoxacin. If an allergic reaction to enoxacin occurs, discontinue the drug. Serious acute hypersensitivity reactions may require immediate treatment with epinephrine. Oxygen, intravenous fluids, antihistamines, corticosteroids, pressor amines, and airway management, including intubation, should be administered as indicated.
Pseudomembranous colitis has been reported with nearly all antibacterial agents, including enoxacin, and may range in severity from mild to life-threatening. Therefore, it is important to consider this diagnosis in patients who present with diarrhea subsequent to the administration of antibacterial agents.
Treatment with broad-spectrum antibacterial agents alters the normal flora of the colon and may permit overgrowth of clostridia. Studies indicate that a toxin produced by *Clostridium difficile* is a primary cause of "antibiotic-associated colitis."
After the diagnosis of pseudomembranous colitis has been established, therapeutic measures should be initiated.
Mild cases of pseudomembranous colitis usually respond to discontinuation of the drug alone. In moderate to severe cases, consideration should be given to management with fluids and electrolytes, protein supplementation, and treatment with an antibacterial drug clinically effective against *C. difficile* colitis.
Ruptures of the shoulder, hand and Achilles tendons that required surgical repair or resulted in prolonged disability have been reported with fluoroquinolone antimicrobials. Enoxacin should be discontinued if the patient experiences pain, inflammation or rupture of a tendon. Patients should rest and refrain from exercise until the diagnosis of tendinitis or tendon rupture has been confidently excluded. Tendon rupture can occur at anytime during or after therapy with enoxacin.
Enoxacin has not been shown to be effective in the treatment of syphilis. Antimicrobial agents used in high doses for short periods of time to treat gonorrhea may mask or delay the symptoms of incubating syphilis. All patients with gonorrhea should have a serologic test for syphilis at the time of diagnosis. Patients treated with enoxacin should have a follow-up serologic test for syphilis after 3 months.

PRECAUTIONS

General: Alteration of the dosage regimen is necessary for patients with impaired renal function (creatinine clearance ≤30 mL/min/1.73 m^2). (See **DOSAGE AND ADMINISTRATION.**)
As with other quinolones, enoxacin should be used with caution in patients with a known or suspected CNS disorder that may predispose to seizures or lower the seizure threshold (*e.g.*, severe cerebral arteriosclerosis, epilepsy) or in the presence of other risk factors that may predispose to seizures or lower the seizure threshold (*e.g.*, certain drug therapy, renal dysfunction). (See **WARNINGS** and **PRECAUTIONS: Drug Interactions.**)
Moderate-to-severe phototoxicity reactions have been observed in patients exposed to direct sunlight while receiving enoxacin or some other drugs in this class. Excessive sunlight should be avoided. Therapy should be discontinued if phototoxicity occurs.
Ophthalmologic abnormalities, including cataracts and multiple punctate lenticular opacities, have been noted in patients undergoing treatment with enoxacin, as well as with some other quinolones, but have also been observed in

patients receiving placebo in comparative trials. In clinical trials using multiple-dose therapy, ophthalmic tissue levels of enoxacin and other quinolones were significantly higher than respective plasma concentrations. The causal relationship, if any, of quinolones to lenticular abnormalities has not been established.
Decreased spermatogenesis and subsequent decreased fertility were noted in rats and dogs treated with doses of enoxacin that produced plasma levels in the animals three times higher than those produced in humans at the recommended therapeutic dosage. The potential for enoxacin to affect spermatogenesis in male patients is unknown.
Information for Patients:
Patients should be advised:
• not to take magnesium-, aluminum-, or calcium-containing antacids, bismuth subsalicylate, products containing iron, or multivitamins containing zinc for 8 hours prior to enoxacin or for 2 hours after enoxacin administration (see **PRECAUTIONS: Drug Interactions**);
• to drink fluids liberally;
• to avoid consumption of caffeine-containing products (certain drugs, coffee, tea, chocolate, certain carbonated beverages) during enoxacin therapy (see **PRECAUTIONS: Drug Interactions**);
• that convulsions have been reported in patients taking quinolones, including enoxacin, and to notify their physicians before taking this drug if there is a history of this condition;
• to discontinue treatment and inform their physician if they experience pain, inflammation, or rupture of a tendon, and to rest and refrain from exercise until the diagnosis of tendinitis or tendon rupture has been confidently excluded;
• that enoxacin may cause dizziness and lightheadedness and, therefore, patients should know how they react to enoxacin before they operate an automobile or machinery or engage in activities requiring mental alertness and coordination;
• that enoxacin may be associated with hypersensitivity reaction, even following the first dose, and to discontinue the drug at the first sign of a skin rash or other allergic reaction;
• to avoid undue exposure to excessive sunlight while receiving enoxacin and to discontinue therapy if phototoxicity occurs.
Drug Interactions:
Bismuth: Bismuth subsalicylate, given concomitantly with enoxacin or 60 minutes following enoxacin administration, decreased enoxacin bioavailability by approximately 25%. Thus, concomitant administration of enoxacin and bismuth subsalicylate should be avoided.
Caffeine: Enoxacin is a potent inhibitor of the cytochrome P-450 isozymes responsible for the metabolism of methylxanthines. In a multiple-dose study, enoxacin caused a dose-related increase in the mean elimination half-life of caffeine, thereby decreasing the clearance of caffeine by up to 80% and leading to a five-fold increase in the AUC and the half-life of caffeine. Trough plasma enoxacin levels were also 20% higher when caffeine and enoxacin were administered concomitantly. Caffeine-related adverse effects have occurred in patients consuming caffeine while on therapy with enoxacin. (See **WARNINGS.**)
Cyclosporine: Elevated serum levels of cyclosporine have been reported with concomitant use of cyclosporine with other members of the quinolone class.
Digoxin: Enoxacin may raise serum digoxin levels in some individuals. If signs and symptoms suggestive of digoxin toxicity occur when enoxacin and digoxin are given concomitantly, physicians are advised to obtain serum digoxin levels and adjust digoxin doses appropriately.
Non-steroidal anti-inflammatory agents: Seizures have been reported in patients taking enoxacin concomitantly with the nonsteroidal anti-inflammatory drug fenbufen. Animal studies also suggest an increased potential for seizures when these two drugs are given concomitantly. Fenbufen is not approved in the United States at this time.
Sucralfate and antacids: Quinolones form chelates with metal cations. Therefore, administration of quinolones with antacids containing calcium, magnesium, or aluminum; with sucralfate; with divalent or trivalent cations such as iron; or with multivitamins containing zinc may substantially interfere with drug absorption and result in insufficient plasma and tissue quinolone concentrations. Antacids containing aluminum hydroxide and magnesium hydroxide reduce the oral absorption of enoxacin by 75%. The oral bioavailability of enoxacin is reduced by 60% with coadministration of ranitidine. These agents should not be taken for 8 hours before or for 2 hours after enoxacin administration.
Theophylline: Enoxacin is a potent inhibitor of the cytochrome P-450 isozymes responsible for the metabolism of methylxanthines. Enoxacin interferes with the metabolism of theophylline resulting in a 42% to 74% dose-related decrease in theophylline clearance and a subsequent 260% to 350% increase in serum theophylline levels. Theophylline-

Continued on next page

Penetrex—Cont.

related adverse effects have occurred in patients when theophylline and enoxacin were coadministered. (See **WARNINGS**.)

Warfarin: Quinolones, including enoxacin, decrease the clearance of R-warfarin, the less active isomer of racemic warfarin. Enoxacin does not affect the clearance of the active S-isomer, and changes in clotting time have not been observed when enoxacin and warfarin were coadministered. Nevertheless, the prothrombin time or other suitable coagulation test should be monitored when warfarin or its derivatives and enoxacin are given concomitantly.

Carcinogenesis, Mutagenesis, Impairment of Fertility: Long-term studies in animals to determine the carcinogenic potential of enoxacin have not been conducted.

Genetic toxicology tests included *in vitro* mutagenicity and cytogenetic assays and *in vivo* cytogenetic and micronucleus tests. Enoxacin did not induce point mutations in bacterial cells or mitotic gene conversion in yeast cells, with or without metabolic activation. Enoxacin did not induce sister chromatid exchanges or structural chromosomal aberrations in mammalian cells *in vitro*, with or without metabolic activation. In addition, enoxacin did not induce chromosomal aberrations in mice.

There was a minimal, dose-related, statistically significant increase in micronuclei at high doses in mice. The significance of these findings, in the absence of effects in other test systems, is not established.

Enoxacin produced no consistent effects on fertility and reproductive parameters in female rats given oral doses of enoxacin at levels up to 1000 mg/kg. Decreased spermatogenesis and subsequent impaired fertility was noted in male rats given oral doses of 1000 mg/kg. This dose is approximately 13-fold greater than the highest human clinical daily oral dose of 16 mg/kg, assuming a 50 kg person and based on a mg/m² basis.

Pregnancy: *Teratogenic effects.* Pregnancy Category C. Studies with enoxacin given orally to mice and rats have shown no evidence of teratogenic potential. The intravenous infusion of enoxacin into pregnant rabbits at doses of 10 to 50 mg/kg caused dose-related maternal toxicity (venous irritation, body weight loss, and reduced food intake) and, at 50 mg/kg, fetal toxicity (increased post-implantation loss and stunted fetuses).

At 50 mg/kg, the incidence of fetal malformations was significantly increased in the presence of overt maternal and fetal toxicity. There are no adequate and well-controlled studies in pregnant women. Enoxacin should be used during pregnancy only if the potential benefit justifies the potential risk to the fetus. (See **WARNINGS**.)

Nursing Mothers: It is not known whether enoxacin is excreted in human milk. Enoxacin is excreted in the milk of lactating rats. Because drugs of this class are excreted in human milk and because of the potential for serious adverse reactions from enoxacin in nursing infants, a decision should be made whether to discontinue nursing or to discontinue the drug, taking into account the importance of the drug to the mother.

Pediatric Use: Safety and effectiveness in pediatric patients and adolescents below the age of 18 years have not been established. Enoxacin causes arthropathy in juvenile animals. (See **WARNINGS** and **ANIMAL PHARMACOLOGY**.)

Geriatric Use: In multiple-dose clinical trials of enoxacin, elderly patients (≥65 years of age) experienced significantly more overall adverse events than patients under 65 years of age. However, the incidence of drug-related adverse reactions was comparable between age groups.

ADVERSE REACTIONS

Single-Dose Studies

During clinical trials, approximately 9% of patients treated with a single dose of 400 mg of enoxacin for uncomplicated urethral or endocervical gonorrhea reported adverse events. The most frequently reported events in single-dose trials, without regard to drug relationship, were nausea and vomiting (2%). Events that occurred in less than 1% of patients are listed below.

CENTRAL NERVOUS SYSTEM: headache, dizziness, somnolence; GASTROINTESTINAL: abdominal pain; GYNECOLOGIC: vaginal moniliasis; SKIN/HYPERSENSITIVITY: rash; LABORATORY ABNORMALITIES: increased AST (SGOT), decreased hemoglobin, decreased hematocrit, eosinophilia, leukocytosis, leukopenia,

thrombocytosis, increased urinary protein, increased alkaline phosphatase, increased ALT (SGPT), increased bilirubin, hyperkalemia.

Multiple-Dose Studies

The incidence of adverse events reported by patients in multiple-dose clinical trials, without regard to drug relationship, was 23%. The incidence of drug-related adverse reactions in multiple-dose clinical trials was 16%. Among patients receiving multiple-dose therapy, enoxacin was discontinued because of an adverse event in 3.8% of patients.

The following events were considered likely to be drug-related in patients receiving multiple doses of enoxacin in clinical trials: nausea and/or vomiting 6%, dizziness 2%, headache 1%, abdominal pain 1%, diarrhea 1%, dyspepsia 1%.

The most frequently reported events in all multiple-dose clinical trials, without regard to drug relationship, were as follows: nausea and/or vomiting 8%, dizziness and/or vertigo 3%, headache 2%, diarrhea 2%, abdominal pain 2%, insomnia 1%, dyspepsia 1%, rash 1%, nervousness and/or anxiety 1%, unusual taste 1%, pruritus 1%.

Additional events that occurred in less than 1% of patients but >0.1% of patients are listed below.

BODY AS A WHOLE: asthenia, fatigue, fever, malaise, back pain, chest pain, edema, chills; GASTROINTESTINAL: flatulence, constipation, dry mouth/throat, stomatitis, anorexia, gastritis, bloody stools; CENTRAL NERVOUS SYSTEM: somnolence, tremor, convulsions, paresthesia, confusion, agitation, depression, syncope, myoclonus, depersonalization, hypertonia; SKIN/HYPERSENSITIVITY: photosensitivity reaction, urticaria, hyperhidrosis, mycotic infection, erythema multiforme, toxic epidermal necrolysis, Stevens-Johnson syndrome; SPECIAL SENSES: tinnitus, conjunctivitis, visual disturbances including amblyopia; MUSCULOSKELETAL: myalgia, arthralgia; CARDIOVASCULAR: palpitations, tachycardia, vasodilation; RESPIRATORY: dyspnea, cough, epistaxis; HEMIC AND LYMPHATIC: purpura; UROGENITAL: vaginal moniliasis, vaginitis, urinary incontinence, renal failure.

The following adverse events occurred in less than 0.1% of patients in multiple-dose clinical trials but were considered significant: pseudomembranous colitis, hyperkinesia, amnesia, ataxia, hypotonia, psychosis, emotional lability, hallucination, schizophrenic reaction.

LABORATORY CHANGES: The following laboratory abnormalities appeared in ≥1.0% of patients receiving multiple doses of enoxacin: elevated AST (SGOT), elevated ALT (SGPT). It is not known whether these abnormalities were caused by the drug or the underlying conditions.

Worldwide Post-Marketing Experience

The most frequent spontaneously-reported adverse events in the worldwide post-marketing experience with multiple- and single-dose enoxacin use have been rashes, seizures/convulsions, and photosensitivity reactions; however, there is no evidence that the incidences of these events were larger than those observed in the clinical trials population.

Quinolone-class adverse reactions: Although not reported in completed clinical studies with enoxacin, a variety of adverse events have been reported with other quinolones. Clinical adverse events include: erythema nodosum, hepatic necrosis, possible exacerbation of myasthenia gravis, nystagmus, intestinal perforation, hyperpigmentation, interstitial nephritis, polyuria, urinary retention, renal calculi, cardiopulmonary arrest, cerebral thrombosis, and laryngeal or pulmonary edema.

Laboratory adverse events include: agranulocytosis, elevation of serum triglycerides and/or serum cholesterol, prolongation of the prothrombin time, candiduria, and crystalluria.

OVERDOSAGE

In the event of acute overdosage, the stomach should be emptied by inducing vomiting or by gastric lavage and the patient carefully observed and given supportive treatment. Enoxacin is poorly removed (<5% over 4 hours) by hemodialysis.

DOSAGE AND ADMINISTRATION

Penetrex™ (enoxacin) should be taken at least one hour before or at least two hours after a meal.

See **INDICATIONS AND USAGE** for information on appropriate pathogens and patient populations.

Sexually Transmitted Diseases

Uncomplicated urethral or cervical gonorrhea: 400 mg single dose

Urinary Tract Infections

Uncomplicated urinary tract infections: 200 mg q12h for 7 days

Complicated urinary tract infections: 400 mg q12h for 14 days

Dosage Adjustment for Renal Impairment: Dosage should be adjusted in patients with a creatinine clearance value of 30 mL/min/1.73 m² or less. After a normal initial dose, the dosing interval should be adjusted as follows:

Creatinine Clearance	Dosage Adjustment	Dosage Interval
>30 mL/min/1.73 m²	None	12 hours
≤30 mL/min/1.73 m²	½ recommended dose	12 hours

When only the serum creatinine is known, the following formula may be used to estimate creatinine clearance.

Men:
$$\frac{\text{creatinine}}{\text{clearance (mL/min)}} = \frac{\text{Weight (kg)} \times (140-\text{age})}{72 \times \text{serum creatinine (mg/dL)}}$$
Women: $0.85 \times$ the value calculated for men.

The serum creatinine should represent a steady state of renal function.

Dosage adjustment is not necessary in elderly patients with normal renal function, but dose should be adjusted according to the previous guidelines in elderly patients with compromised renal function.

HOW SUPPLIED

[See table below]

Store at controlled room temperature, 15° to 30°C (59° to 86°F).

This product should be dispensed in a container with a child-resistant cap.

Keep out of the reach of children.

ANIMAL PHARMACOLOGY

Enoxacin and other members of the quinolone class have been shown to cause arthropathy in immature animals of most species tested. (See **WARNINGS**.)

REFERENCES

1. National Committee for Clinical Laboratory Standards, Performance Standards for Antimicrobial Disk Susceptibility Tests—Fourth Edition. Approved Standard NCCLS Document M2-A4, Vol. 10, No. 7, NCCLS, Villanova, PA, 1990.
2. National Committee for Clinical Laboratory Standards, Methods for Dilution Antimicrobial Susceptibility Tests for Bacteria that Grow Aerobically—Second Edition. Approved Standard NCCLS Document M7-A2, Vol. 10, No. 8, NCCLS, Villanova, PA, 1990.

Caution: Federal law prohibits dispensing without a prescription.

Rev. 12/97   IN-5391C

RHONE-POULENC RORER PHARMACEUTICALS INC.
Collegeville, PA, U.S.A. 19426-0107

Shown in Product Identification Guide, page 333

RILUTEK®   ℞
(riluzole) Tablets
[*rĭl-ū-tĕk*]

DESCRIPTION

RILUTEK® (riluzole) is a member of the benzothiazole class. Chemically, riluzole is 2-amino-6-(trifluoromethoxy) benzothiazole. Its molecular formula is $C_8H_5F_3N_2OS$ and its molecular weight is 234.2. Its structural formula is as follows:

Riluzole is a white to slightly yellow powder that is very soluble in dimethylformamide, dimethylsulfoxide and methanol, freely soluble in dichloromethane, sparingly soluble in 0.1 N HCl and very slightly soluble in water and in 0.1 N NaOH. RILUTEK is available as a capsule-shaped, white, film-coated tablet for oral administration containing 50 mg of riluzole. Each tablet is engraved with "RPR 202" on one side.

Inactive Ingredients: Core: anhydrous dibasic calcium phosphate, USP; microcrystalline cellulose, NF; anhydrous

Strength	Size	NDC 0075-	Color	Markings
200 mg	Bottles of 50	5100-50	light blue	(℞) 5100
400 mg	Bottles of 50	5140-50	dark blue	(℞) 5140

colloidal silica, NF; magnesium stearate, NF; croscarmellose sodium, NF. **Film coating:** hydroxypropyl methylcellulose, USP; polyethylene glycol 6000; titanium dioxide, USP.

CLINICAL PHARMACOLOGY
Mechanism of Action
The etiology and pathogenesis of amyotrophic lateral sclerosis (ALS) are not known, although a number of hypotheses have been advanced. One hypothesis is that motor neurons, made vulnerable through either genetic predisposition or environmental factors, are injured by glutamate. In some cases of familial ALS the enzyme superoxide dismutase has been found to be defective.

The mode of action of RILUTEK is unknown. Its pharmacological properties include the following, some of which may be related to its effect: 1) an inhibitory effect on glutamate release, 2) inactivation of voltage-dependent sodium channels, and 3) ability to interfere with intracellular events that follow transmitter binding at excitatory amino acid receptors.

Riluzole has also been shown, in a single study, to delay median time to death in a transgenic mouse model of ALS. These mice express human superoxide dismutase bearing one of the mutations found in one of the familial forms of human ALS.

It is also neuroprotective in various *in vivo* experimental models of neuronal injury involving excitotoxic mechanisms. In *in vitro* tests, riluzole protected cultured rat motor neurons from the excitotoxic effects of glutamic acid and prevented the death of cortical neurons induced by anoxia. Due to its blockade of glutamatergic neurotransmission, riluzole also exhibits myorelaxant and sedative properties in animal models at doses of 30 mg/kg (about 20 times the recommended human daily dose) and anticonvulsant properties at a dose of 2.5 mg/kg (about 2 times the recommended human daily dose).

Pharmacokinetics
Riluzole is well-absorbed (approximately 90%), with average absolute oral bioavailability of about 60% (CV=30%). Pharmacokinetics are linear over a dose range of 25–100 mg given every 12 hours. A high fat meal decreases absorption, reducing AUC by about 20% and peak blood levels by about 45%. The mean elimination half-life of riluzole is 12 hours (CV=35%) after repeated doses. With multiple-dose administration, riluzole accumulates in plasma by about 2 fold and steady-state is reached in less than 5 days. Riluzole is 96% bound to plasma proteins, mainly to albumin and lipoproteins over the clinical concentration range.

The 50 mg market tablet was equivalent, with respect to AUC, to the tablet used in the dose ranging clinical trials, while the C_{max} was approximately 30% higher. Both tablets have been used in clinical trials. However, if doses greater than those recommended are given, it is likely that higher plasma levels will be achieved, the safety of which has not been established (see DOSAGE AND ADMINISTRATION).

Metabolism and Elimination
Riluzole is extensively metabolized to six major and a number of minor metabolites, not all of which have been identified. Some metabolites appear pharmacologically active in *in vitro* assays. The metabolism of riluzole is mostly hepatic and consists of cytochrome P450-dependent hydroxylation and glucuronidation.

There is marked inter-individual variability in the clearance of riluzole, probably attributable to variability of CYP 1A2 activity, the principal isozyme involved in N-hydroxylation.

In vitro studies using liver microsomes show that hydroxylation of the primary amine group producing N-hydroxyriluzole is the main metabolic pathway in human, monkey, dog and rabbit. In humans, cytochrome P450 1A2 is the principal isozyme involved in N-hydroxylation. *In vitro* studies predict that CYP 2D6, CYP 2C19, CYP 3A4 and CYP 2E1 are unlikely to contribute significantly to riluzole metabolism in humans. Whereas direct glucuroconjugation of riluzole (involving the glucurotransferase isoform UGT-HP4) is very slow in human liver microsomes, N-hydroxyriluzole is readily conjugated at the hydroxylamine group resulting in the formation of O- (>90%) and N-glucuronides.

Following a single 150 mg dose of ^{14}C-riluzole to 6 healthy males, 90% and 5% of the radioactivity was recovered in the urine and feces respectively over a period of 7 days. Glucuronides accounted for more than 85% of the metabolites in urine. Only 2% of a riluzole dose was recovered in the urine as unchanged drug.

Special Populations
The pharmacokinetics of riluzole have not been studied in renally and hepatically impaired subjects, nor is there information about the effects of smoking, age and gender on the pharmacokinetics of riluzole but certain differences in population subsets should be anticipated (see PRECAUTIONS).

Hepatic and Renal Disease: Since riluzole is extensively metabolized and subsequently excreted in the urine, it is likely that functional hepatic and renal impairment will reduce the clearance of riluzole and its metabolites and give higher plasma levels (see PRECAUTIONS and WARNINGS).

Age: Age-related decreased renal function would be expected to give higher plasma levels of riluzole and metabolites. However, in controlled clinical trials, in which approximately 30% of patients were over 65, there were no differences in adverse events between younger and older patients (see PRECAUTIONS).

Gender: CYP 1A2 activity has been reported to be lower in women than in men. Therefore, a gender effect on riluzole kinetics may be expected in women, resulting in higher blood concentrations of riluzole and its metabolites (see PRECAUTIONS). No gender effect on favorable or adverse effects of riluzole was seen in controlled trials, however.

Smoking: Cigarette smoking is known to induce CYP 1A2. Patients who smoke cigarettes would be expected to eliminate riluzole faster. There is no information, however, on the effect of, or need for, dosage adjustment in these patients.

Race: Clearance of riluzole in Japanese subjects native to Japan was found to be 50% lower as compared to Caucasians after normalizing for body weight. Although it is not clear if this difference is due to genetic or environmental factors (*e.g.*, smoking, alcohol, coffee, and dietary preferences), it is possible that Japanese subjects may possess a lower capacity (oxidative and/or conjugative) for metabolizing riluzole. There are no studies, however, of lower doses in Japanese subjects (see PRECAUTIONS).

Clinical Trials
The efficacy of RILUTEK as a treatment of ALS was established in two adequate and well-controlled trials in which the time to tracheostomy or death was longer for patients randomized to RILUTEK than for those randomized to placebo.

These studies admitted patients with either familial or sporadic ALS, a disease duration of less than 5 years, and a baseline forced vital capacity greater than or equal to 60%. In one study, performed in France and Belgium, 155 ALS patients were followed for at least 13 months (maximum duration 18 months) after being randomized to either 100 mg/day (given 50 mg BID) of RILUTEK or placebo.

Figure 1, which follows, displays the survival curves for time to death or tracheostomy. The vertical axis represents the proportion of individuals alive without tracheostomy at various times following treatment initiation (horizontal axis). Although these survival curves were not statistically significantly different when evaluated by the analysis specified in the study protocol (Logrank test p=0.12), the difference was found to be significant by another appropriate analysis (Wilcoxon test p=0.05). As seen, the study showed an early increase in survival in patients given riluzole. Among the patients in whom treatment failed during the study (tracheostomy or death) there was a difference between the treatment groups in median survival of approximately 90 days. There was no statistically significant difference in mortality at the end of the study.

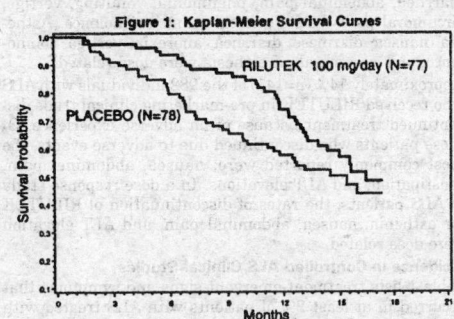

Figure 1: Kaplan-Meier Survival Curves

In the second study, performed in both Europe and North America, 959 ALS patients were followed for at least 1 year (North American centers) and up to 18 months (European centers) after being randomized to either 50, 100, 200 mg/day of RILUTEK or placebo.

Figure 2, which follows, displays the survival curves for time to death or tracheostomy for patients randomized to either 100 mg/day of RILUTEK or placebo. Although these survival curves were not statistically significantly different when evaluated by the analysis specified in the study protocol (Logrank test p = 0.076), the difference was found to be significant by another appropriate analysis (Wilcoxon test p = 0.05). Not displayed in Figure 2 are the results of 50 mg/day of RILUTEK which could not be statistically distinguished from placebo and the results of 200 mg/day which are essentially identical to 100 mg/day. As seen, the study showed an early increase in survival in patients given riluzole. Among the patients in whom treatment failed during the study (tracheostomy or death) there was a difference between the treatment groups in median survival of approximately 60 days. There was no statistically significant difference in mortality at the end of the study.

[See figure 2 at top of next column]

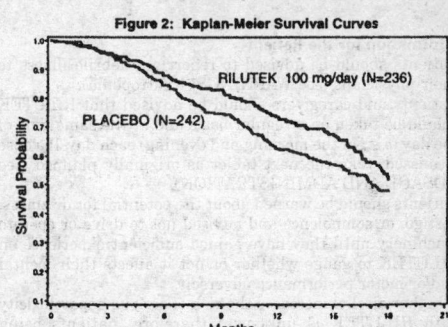

Figure 2: Kaplan-Meier Survival Curves

Although riluzole improved early survival in both studies, measures of muscle strength and neurological function did not show a benefit.

INDICATIONS AND USAGE
RILUTEK is indicated for the treatment of patients with amyotrophic lateral sclerosis (ALS). Riluzole extends survival and/or time to tracheostomy.

CONTRAINDICATIONS
RILUTEK is contraindicated in patients who have a history of severe hypersensitivity reactions to riluzole or any of the tablet components.

WARNINGS
Liver Injury/Monitoring Liver Chemistries
RILUTEK should be prescribed with care in patients with current evidence or history of abnormal liver function indicated by significant abnormalities in serum transaminase (ALT/SGPT; AST/SGOT), bilirubin, and/or gamma-glutamate transferase (GGT) levels (see PRECAUTIONS and DOSAGE AND ADMINISTRATION SECTIONS). Baseline elevations of several LFTs (especially elevated bilirubin) should preclude the use of RILUTEK.

RILUTEK, even in patients without a prior history of liver disease, causes serum aminotransferase elevations. Experience in almost 800 ALS patients indicates that about 50% of riluzole-treated patients will experience at least one ALT/SGPT level above the upper limit of normal, about 8% will have elevations > 3 × ULN, and about 2% of patients will have elevations > 5 × ULN. A single non-ALS patient with epilepsy treated with concomitant carbamazepine and phenobarbital experienced marked, rapid elevations of liver enzymes with jaundice (ALT 26 × ULN, AST 17 × ULN, and bilirubin 11 × ULN) four months after starting RILUTEK; these returned to normal 7 weeks after treatment discontinuation.

Maximum increases in serum ALT usually occurred within 3 months after the start of riluzole therapy and were usually transient when < 5 times ULN. In trials, if ALT levels were <5 times ULN, treatment continued and ALT levels usually returned to below 2 times ULN within 2 to 6 months. Treatment in studies was discontinued, however, if ALT levels exceeded 5 × ULN, so that there is no experience with continued treatment of ALS patients once ALT values exceed 5 times ULN (see PRECAUTIONS: Laboratory Tests). There were rare instances of jaundice.

Liver chemistries should be monitored (see PRECAUTIONS).

Neutropenia
Among approximately 4000 patients given riluzole for ALS, there were three cases of marked neutropenia (absolute neutrophil count less than 500/mm³), all seen within the first 2 months of riluzole treatment. In one case, neutrophil counts rose on continued treatment. In a second case, counts rose after therapy was stopped. A third case was more complex, with marked anemia as well as neutropenia and the etiology of both is uncertain. Patients should be warned to report any febrile illness to their physicians. The report of a febrile illness should prompt treating physicians to check white blood cell counts.

PRECAUTIONS
Use in Patients with Concomitant Disease
RILUTEK should be used with caution in patients with concomitant liver and/or renal insufficiency (see WARNINGS, CLINICAL PHARMACOLOGY). In particular, in cases of RILUTEK-induced hepatic injury manifested by elevated liver enzymes, the effect of the hepatic injury on RILUTEK metabolism is unknown.

Special Populations
Riluzole should be used with caution in elderly patients whose hepatic or renal functions may be compromised due to age. Also, females and Japanese patients may possess a lower metabolic capacity to eliminate riluzole compared to males and Caucasian subjects, respectively (see CLINICAL PHARMACOLOGY: Special Populations).

Continued on next page

Rilutek—Cont.

Information for the Patient

Patients should be advised to report any febrile illness to their physicians (see WARNINGS: Neutropenia).

Patients and caregivers should be advised that RILUTEK should be taken on a regular basis and at the same time of the day (*e.g.,* in the morning and evening) each day. If a dose is missed, take the next tablet as originally planned (see DOSAGE AND ADMINISTRATION).

Patients should be warned about the potential for dizziness, vertigo, or somnolence and advised not to drive or operate machinery until they have gained sufficient experience on RILUTEK to gauge whether or not it affects their mental and/or motor performance adversely.

Whether alcohol increases the risk of serious hepatotoxicity with RILUTEK is unknown; therefore, patients being treated with RILUTEK should be discouraged from drinking excessive amounts of alcohol.

Patients should also be made aware that RILUTEK should be stored at temperatures between 20°–25°C (68°–77°F) and protected from bright light.

RILUTEK must be kept out of the reach of children.

Laboratory Tests

It is recommended that serum aminotransferases including ALT levels be measured before and during riluzole therapy. Serum ALT levels should be evaluated every month during the first 3 months of treatment, every 3 months during the remainder of the first year, and periodically thereafter. Serum ALT levels should be evaluated more frequently in patients who develop elevations (see WARNINGS).

As noted in the WARNINGS Section, there is no experience with continued treatment of patients once ALT exceeds 5 × ULN. If a decision is made to continue to treat these patients, frequent monitoring (at least weekly) of complete liver function is recommended. Treatment should be discontinued if ALT exceeds 10 × ULN or if clinical jaundice develops. Because there is no experience with rechallenge of patients who have had RILUTEK discontinued for ALT > 5 × ULN, no recommendations about restarting RILUTEK can be made.

In the two controlled trials in patients with ALS, the frequency with which values for hemoglobin, hematocrit, and erythrocyte counts fell below the lower limit of normal was greater in RILUTEK-treated patients than in placebo-treated patients; however, these changes were mild and transient. The proportions of patients observed with abnormally low values for these parameters showed a dose-response relationship. Only one patient was discontinued from treatment because of severe anemia. The significance of this finding is unknown.

Drug Interactions

There have been no clinical studies designed to evaluate the interaction of riluzole with other drugs.

As with all drugs, the potential for interaction by a variety of mechanisms is a possibility.

Hepatotoxic Drugs: The clinical trials in ALS excluded patients on concomitant medications which were potentially hepatotoxic, (*e.g.,* allopurinol, methyldopa, sulfasalazine). Accordingly, there is no information about the safety of administering RILUTEK in conjunction with such medications. If the practitioner chooses to prescribe such a combination, caution should be exercised.

Drugs Highly Bound To Plasma Proteins: Riluzole is highly bound (96%) to plasma proteins, binding mainly to serum albumin and to lipoproteins. The effect of riluzole (up to 5 mcg/mL) on warfarin (5 mcg/mL) binding did not show any displacement of warfarin. Conversely, riluzole binding was unaffected by the addition of warfarin, digoxin, imipramine and quinine at high therapeutic concentrations.

Effect of Other Drugs On Riluzole Metabolism: *In vitro* studies using human liver microsomal preparations suggest that CYP 1A2 is the principal isozyme involved in the initial oxidative metabolism of riluzole and, therefore, potential interactions may occur when riluzole is given concurrently with agents that affect CYP 1A2 activity. Potential inhibitors of CYP 1A2 (*e.g.,* caffeine, phenacetin, theophylline, amitriptyline, and quinolones) could decrease the rate of riluzole elimination, while inducers of CYP 1A2 (*e.g.,* cigarette smoke, charcoal-broiled food, rifampicin, and omeprazole) could increase the rate of riluzole elimination.

Effect of Riluzole On the Metabolism of Other Drugs: CYP 1A2 is the principal isoenzyme involved in the initial oxidative metabolism of riluzole; potential interactions may occur when riluzole is given concurrently with other agents which are also metabolized primarily by CYP 1A2 (*e.g.,* theophylline, caffeine and tacrine). Currently, it is not known whether riluzole has any potential for enzyme induction in humans.

Drug Laboratory Test Interactions: None known

Carcinogenesis, Mutagenesis, Impairment of Fertility

Long-term studies to determine the carcinogenic potential of riluzole have not yet been completed.

The genotoxic potential of riluzole was evaluated in the bacterial mutagenicity (Ames) test, the mouse lymphoma mutation assay in L5178Y cells, the *in vitro* chromosomal aberration assay in human lymphocytes and the *in vivo* rat cytogenetic assay and *in vivo* mouse micronucleus assay in bone marrow. There was no evidence of mutagenic or clastogenic potential in the Ames test, the mouse lymphoma assay, or the *in vivo* assays in the mouse and rat. There was an equivocal clastogenic response in the *in vitro* lymphocyte chromosomal aberration assay.

Riluzole impaired fertility when administered to male and female rats prior to and during mating at an oral dose of 15 mg/kg or 1.5 times the maximum daily dose on a mg/m^2 basis (see PRECAUTIONS: "Pregnancy" for effects on fertility).

Pregnancy

Pregnancy category C:

Oral administration of riluzole to pregnant animals during the period of organogenesis caused embryotoxicity in rats and rabbits at doses of 27 mg/kg and 60 mg/kg, respectively, or 2.6 and 11.5 times, respectively, the recommended maximum human daily dose on a mg/m^2 basis. Evidence of maternal toxicity was also observed at these doses.

When administered to rats prior to and during mating (males and females) and throughout gestation and lactation (females), riluzole produced adverse effects on pregnancy (decreased implantations, increased intrauterine death) and offspring viability and growth at an oral dose of 15 mg/kg or 1.5 times the maximum daily dose on a mg/m^2 basis.

There are no adequate and well-controlled studies in pregnant women. Riluzole should be used during pregnancy only if the potential benefit justifies the potential risk to the fetus.

Nursing Women

In rat studies, ^{14}C-riluzole was detected in maternal milk. It is not known whether riluzole is excreted in human breast milk. Because many drugs are excreted in human milk, and because the potential for serious adverse reactions in nursing infants from RILUTEK® is unknown, women should be advised not to breast-feed during treatment with RILUTEK.

Use in the Elderly

Age-related compromised renal and hepatic function may cause a decrease in clearance of riluzole (see CLINICAL PHARMACOLOGY: Special Populations). In controlled clinical trials, about 30% of patients were over 65. There were no differences in adverse effects between younger and older patients.

Pediatric Use

The safety and the effectiveness of RILUTEK in pediatric patients have not been established.

ADVERSE REACTIONS

The most commonly observed AEs associated with the use of RILUTEK more frequently than placebo treated patients, were: asthenia, nausea, dizziness, decreased lung function, diarrhea, abdominal pain, pneumonia, vomiting, vertigo, circumoral paresthesia, anorexia, and somnolence. Asthenia, nausea, dizziness, diarrhea, anorexia, vertigo, somnolence, and circumoral paresthesia were dose related.

Approximately 14% (n=141) of the 982 individuals with ALS who received RILUTEK in pre-marketing clinical trials discontinued treatment because of an adverse experience. Of those patients who discontinued due to adverse events, the most commonly reported were: nausea, abdominal pain, constipation, and ALT elevations. In a dose response study in ALS patients, the rates of discontinuation of RILUTEK for asthenia, nausea, abdominal pain, and ALT elevation were dose related.

Incidence in Controlled ALS Clinical Studies

Table 1 lists treatment-emergent signs and symptoms that occurred in at least 2% of patients with ALS treated with RILUTEK (n=794) participating in placebo-controlled trials and were numerically greater in the patients treated with RILUTEK 100 mg/day than with placebo or for which a dose response relationship is suggested.

The prescriber should be aware that these figures cannot be used to predict the frequency of adverse experiences in the course of usual medical practice where patient characteristics and other factors may differ from those prevailing during clinical studies. Inspection of these frequencies, however, does provide the prescriber with one basis to estimate the relative contribution of drug and non-drug factors to the AE incidences in the population studied.

Table 1
Adverse Events Occurring in Placebo-Controlled Clinical Trials

Percentage of patients reporting events*

Body System/ Adverse Event*	Riluzole 50 mg/day (N=237)	Riluzole 100 mg/day (N=313)	Riluzole 200 mg/day (N=244)	Placebo (N=320)
Body as a Whole				
Asthenia	14.8	19.2	20.1	12.2
Headache	8.0	7.3	7.0	6.6
Abdominal pain	6.8	5.1	7.8	3.8
Back pain	1.7	3.2	4.1	2.5
Aggravation reaction	0.4	1.3	2.0	0.9
Malaise	0.4	0.6	1.2	0.0
Digestive				
Nausea	12.2	16.3	20.5	10.6
Vomiting	4.2	4.2	4.5	1.6
Dyspepsia	2.5	3.8	6.1	5.0
Anorexia	3.8	3.2	8.6	3.8
Diarrhea	5.5	2.9	9.0	3.1
Flatulence	2.5	2.6	2.0	1.9
Stomatitis	0.8	1.0	1.2	0.0
Tooth disorder	0.0	1.0	1.2	0.3
Oral Moniliasis	0.4	0.6	1.2	0.3
Nervous				
Hypertonia	5.9	6.1	5.3	5.9
Depression	4.2	4.5	6.1	5.0
Dizziness	5.1	3.8	12.7	2.5
Dry mouth	3.0	3.5	2.0	3.4
Insomnia	2.1	3.5	2.9	3.4
Somnolence	0.8	1.9	4.1	1.3
Vertigo	2.5	1.9	4.5	0.9
Circumoral paresthesia	1.3	1.6	3.3	0.0
Skin and Appendages				
Pruritus	3.8	3.8	2.5	3.1
Eczema	0.8	1.6	1.6	0.6
Alopecia	0.0	1.0	1.2	0.6
Exfoliative dermatitis	0.0	0.6	1.2	0.0
Respiratory				
Decreased lung function	13.1	10.2	16.0	9.4
Rhinitis	8.9	6.4	7.8	6.3
Increased cough	2.1	2.6	3.7	1.6
Sinusitis	0.4	1.0	1.6	0.9
Cardiovascular				
Hypertension	6.8	5.1	3.3	4.1
Tachycardia	1.3	2.6	2.0	1.3
Phlebitis	0.4	1.0	0.8	0.3
Palpitation	0.4	0.6	1.2	0.9
Postural hypotension	0.8	0.0	1.6	0.6
Metabolic and Nutritional Disorders				
Weight loss	4.6	4.8	3.7	4.7
Peripheral edema	4.2	2.9	3.3	2.2
Musculoskeletal System				
Arthralgia	5.1	3.5	1.6	3.4
Urogenital System				
Urinary tract infection	2.5	2.6	4.5	2.2
Dysuria	0.0	1.0	1.2	0.3

Other Adverse Events Observed

Other events which occurred in more than 2% of patients treated with RILUTEK 100 mg/day but equally or more frequently in the placebo group included: accidental injury, apnea, bronchitis, constipation, death, dysphagia, dyspnea, flu syndrome, heart arrest, increased sputum, pneumonia, and respiratory disorder.

The overall adverse event profile for RILUTEK was similar between females and males, and was independent of age. Because the largest non-white racial subgroup was only 2% of patients exposed to RILUTEK (18/794) in placebo-controlled trials, there are insufficient data to support a statement regarding the distribution of adverse experience reports by race. In ALS studies, dizziness did occur more commonly in females (11%) than in males (4%). There was not a difference between females and males in the rates of discontinuation of RILUTEK for individual adverse experiences.

Other Adverse Events Observed During All Clinical Trials

RILUTEK has been administered to 1713 individuals during all clinical trials, some of which were placebo-controlled. During these trials, all adverse events were recorded by the clinical investigators using terminology of their own choosing. To provide a meaningful estimate of the proportion of individuals having adverse events, similar types of events were grouped into a smaller number of standardized categories using modified COSTART dictionary terminology. The frequencies presented represent the proportion of the 1713 individuals exposed to RILUTEK who experienced an event of the type cited on at least one occasion while receiving RILUTEK. All reported events are included except those

already listed in the previous table, those too general to be informative, and those not reasonably associated with the use of the drug.

Events are further classified within body system categories and enumerated in order of decreasing frequency using the following definitions: *frequent* adverse events are defined as those occurring in at least 1/100 patients; *infrequent* adverse events are those occurring in 1/100 to 1/1000 patients; *rare* adverse events are those occurring in fewer than 1/1000 patients.

***=AE frequency ≤to placebo**

Body as a Whole: *Frequent:* Hostility*. *Infrequent:* Abscess*, sepsis*, photosensitivity reaction*, cellulitis, face edema*, hernia, peritonitis, attempted suicide, injection site reaction, chills*, flu syndrome, intentional injury, enlarged abdomen, neoplasm. *Rare:* Acrodynia, hypothermia, moniliasis*, rheumatoid arthritis.

Digestive System: *Infrequent:* Increased appetite, intestinal obstruction*, fecal impaction, gastrointestinal hemorrhage, gastrointestinal ulceration, gastritis*, fecal incontinence, jaundice, hepatitis, glossitis, gum hemorrhage*, pancreatitis, tenesmus, esophageal stenosis. *Rare:* Cheilitis*, cholecystitis, hematemesis, melena*, biliary pain, proctitis, pseudomembranous enterocolitis, enlarged salivary gland, tongue discoloration, tooth caries.

Nervous System: *Frequent:* Agitation*, tremor. *Infrequent:* Hallucinations, personality disorder*, abnormal thinking*, coma, paranoid reaction*, manic reaction, ataxia, extrapyramidal syndrome, hypokinesia, urinary retention, emotional lability, delusions, apathy, hypesthesia, incoordination, confusion*, convulsion, leg cramps, amnesia, dysarthria, increased libido, stupor, subdural hematoma, abnormal gait, delirium, depersonalization, facial paralysis, hemiplegia, decreased libido, myoclonus. *Rare:* Abnormal dreams, acute brain syndrome, CNS depression, dementia, cerebral embolism, euphoria*, hypotonia, ileus*, peripheral neuritis, psychosis*, psychotic depression, schizophrenic reaction, trismus, wristdrop.

Skin and Appendages: *Infrequent:* Skin ulceration, urticaria, psoriasis, seborrhea*, skin disorder, fungal dermatitis*. *Rare:* Angioedema, contact dermatitis, erythema multiforme, furunculosis*, skin moniliasis, skin granuloma, skin nodule.

Respiratory System: *Infrequent:* Hiccup, pleural disorder*, asthma, epistaxis, hemoptysis, yawn, hyperventilation*, lung edema*, hypoventilation*, lung carcinoma, hypoxia, laryngitis, pleural effusion, pneumothorax*, respiratory moniliasis, stridor.

Cardiovascular System: *Infrequent:* Syncope*, hypotension, heart failure, migraine, peripheral vascular disease, angina pectoris*, myocardial infarction*, ventricular extrasystoles, cerebral hemorrhage, atrial fibrillation*, bundle branch block, congestive heart failure, pericarditis, lower extremity embolus, myocardial ischemia*, shock*. *Rare:* Bradycardia, cerebral ischemia, hemorrhage, mesenteric artery occlusion, subarachnoid hemorrhage, supraventricular tachycardia*, thrombosis, ventricular fibrillation, ventricular tachycardia.

Metabolic and Nutritional Disorders: *Infrequent:* Gout*, respiratory acidosis, edema, thirst*, hypokalemia, hyponatremia, weight gain*. *Rare:* Generalized edema, hypercalcemia, hypercholesteremia.

Endocrine System: *Infrequent:* Diabetes mellitus, thyroid neoplasia. *Rare:* Diabetes insipidus, parathyroid disorder.

Hemic and Lymphatic System: *Infrequent:* Anemia*, leukocytosis, leukopenia, ecchymosis. *Rare:* Neutropenia, aplastic anemia, cyanosis, hypochromic anemia, iron deficiency anemia, lymphadenopathy, petechiae*, purpura.

Musculoskeletal System: *Infrequent:* Arthrosis, myasthenia*, bone neoplasm. *Rare:* Bone necrosis, osteoporosis, tetany.

Special Senses: *Infrequent:* Amblyopia, ophthalmitis. *Rare:* Blepharitis, cataract, deafness, diplopia*, ear pain, glaucoma, hyperacusis, photophobia, taste loss, vestibular disorder.

Urogenital System: *Infrequent:* Urinary urgency, urine abnormality, urinary incontinence, kidney calculus, hematuria, impotence, prostate carcinoma, kidney pain, metrorrhagia, priapism. *Rare:* Amenorrhea, breast abscess, breast pain, nephritis*, nocturia, pyelonephritis, enlarged uterine fibroids, uterine hemorrhage, vaginal moniliasis.

Laboratory Tests: *Infrequent:* Increased gamma glutamyl transferase, abnormal liver function/tests, increased alkaline phosphatase, positive direct Coombs test, increased gamma globulins. *Rare:* increased lactic dehydrogenase.

OVERDOSAGE

There have been no reports of overdose with RILUTEK. No specific antidote or information on treatment of overdosage with RILUTEK is available. In the event of overdose, RILUTEK therapy should be discontinued immediately. Treatment should be supportive and directed toward alleviating symptoms.

The estimated oral median lethal dose is 94 mg/kg and 39 mg/kg for male mice and rats, respectively.

DOSAGE AND ADMINISTRATION

The recommended dose for RILUTEK is 50 mg every 12 hours. No increased benefit can be expected from higher daily doses, but adverse events are increased.

RILUTEK tablets should be taken at least an hour before, or two hours after, a meal to avoid a food-related decrease in bioavailability.

Special Populations

Patients with Impaired Renal or Hepatic Function: Studies have not yet been completed in these populations (see WARNINGS, PRECAUTIONS, CLINICAL PHARMACOLOGY).

HOW SUPPLIED

RILUTEK 50 mg tablets are white, film-coated, capsule-shaped and engraved with "RPR 202" on one side. RILUTEK is supplied in bottles of 60 tablets, NDC 0075-7700-60. These bottles are designed with a special dispensing flip cap to aid dispensing with minimum effort.

STORE AT CONTROLLED ROOM TEMPERATURE 20°–25°C (68°–77°F) AND PROTECT FROM BRIGHT LIGHT.

KEEP OUT OF THE REACH OF CHILDREN.

Caution: Federal law prohibits dispensing without prescription.

Manufactured in Ireland

RHÔNE-POULENC RORER PHARMACEUTICALS INC.

Collegeville, PA, U.S.A. 19426-0107

IN-5336A Rev. 1/96

Shown in Product Identification Guide, page 333

SLO-BID™ ℞

[*slō 'bid"*]

(Theophylline, Extended-release Capsules, USP)

50 mg, 75 mg, 100 mg, 125 mg, 200 mg, and 300 mg Gyrocaps®

DESCRIPTION

Slo-bid™ Gyrocaps® contain 50 mg, 75 mg, 100 mg, 125 mg, 200 mg, or 300 mg theophylline, anhydrous in the form of long-acting beads within a dye-free hard gelatin capsule and are intended for oral administration. Theophylline is a bronchodilator structurally classified as a xanthine derivative.

Slo-bid Gyrocaps can be administered with a 12-hour dosing interval for a majority of patients and a 24-hour dosing interval for selected patients (see DOSAGE AND ADMINISTRATION section for description of appropriate patient population).

Theophylline is 1*H*-Purine-2,6-dione,3,7-dihydro-1,3-dimethyl represented by the following structural formula:

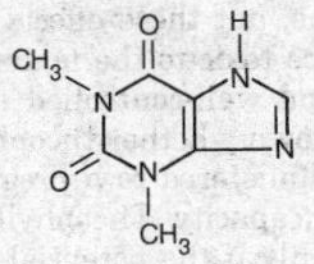

Theophylline is a white, odorless, crystalline powder having a bitter taste.

CLINICAL PHARMACOLOGY

Theophylline directly relaxes the smooth muscle of the bronchial airways and pulmonary blood vessels, thus acting as a bronchodilator and smooth muscle relaxant. It has also been demonstrated that aminophylline has a potent effect on diaphragmatic contractility in normal persons and may then be capable of reducing fatigability and thereby improve contractility in patients with chronic obstructive airways disease. The exact mode of action remains unsettled. Although theophylline does cause inhibition of phosphodiesterase with a resultant increase in intracellular cyclic AMP, other agents similarly inhibit the enzyme producing a rise of cyclic AMP but are unassociated with any demonstrable bronchodilation. Other mechanisms proposed include an effect on translocation of intracellular calcium; prostaglandin antagonism; stimulation of catecholamines endogenously; inhibition of cyclic guanosine monophosphate metabolism and adenosine receptor antagonism. None of these mechanisms has been proved, however.

In vitro, theophylline has been shown to act synergistically with beta agonists, and there are now available data that do demonstrate an additive effect *in vivo* with combined use.

Pharmacokinetics:

The half-life of theophylline is influenced by a number of known variables. It may be prolonged in chronic alcoholics, particularly those with liver disease (cirrhosis or alcoholic liver disease), in patients with congestive heart failure and in those patients taking certain other drugs (See PRECAUTIONS, Drug Interactions).

Newborns and neonates have extremely slow clearance rates compared to older infants and children, i.e., those over one year. Older children have rapid clearance rates while most nonsmoking adults have clearance rates between these two extremes. In premature neonates the decreased clearance is related to oxidative pathways that have yet to be established.

Theophylline Elimination Characteristics
Half-life (in hours)

	Range	Mean
Children	1–9	3.7
Adults	3–15	7.7

In cigarette smokers (1–2 packs/day) the mean half-life is 4–5 hours, much shorter than in nonsmokers. The increase in clearance associated with smoking is presumably due to stimulation of the hepatic metabolic pathway by components of cigarette smoke. The duration of this effect after cessation of smoking is unknown but may require 6 months to 2 years before the rate approaches that of the nonsmoker.

In a single-dose bioavailability study in 18 normal subjects, 300 mg extended-release Slo-bid Gyrocaps produced mean peak serum concentrations of 3.5 ± 0.7 µg/mL at a mean time of 7.8 ± 1.8 hours after dosing. Subjects fasted overnight before dosing and four hours after the dose. When compared to a syrup dosage form, relative bioavailability of Slo-bid Gyrocaps was about 91%. At steady state in a multiple-dose bioavailability study in 18 normal subjects with q12h dosing (600–1000 mg/day), the mean peak-trough variation was 3.5 ± 0.9 µg/mL. The mean C_{max} and C_{min} were 12.9 ± 3.0 and 9.4 ± 2.5 µg/mL, respectively. The mean percent fluctuation $[((C_{max}-C_{min})/C_{min})\times 100]$ was 40 ± 15%. Subjects fasted 12 hours before the dose and 4 hours after the dose was administered on the days that the blood samples were drawn. A multiple-dose bioequivalence study with 15 asthmatic children, ages 9–16, comparing Slo-bid Gyrocaps administered as intact capsules and as the beaded contents sprinkled on applesauce with b.i.d. dosing (150–600 mg/dose) indicated no significant differences in maximum and minimum theophylline concentrations, time to achieve peak concentration, and peak-trough differences. The bioavailability as measured by comparing area under the curves ($AUC_{0-12\ hours}$ granules/$AUC_{0-12\ hours}$ capsules) was 0.990 ± 0.214.

Taking Slo-bid immediately after a high-fat content meal may result in a decrease in the rate of absorption (lower C_{max} and later T_{max}) but with no significant difference in the extent of absorption (see PRECAUTIONS, Drug-Food Interactions). In a single-dose bioavailability study, 24 normal adult nonsmoking subjects were given 900 mg extended-release Slo-bid Gyrocaps with food and under fasting conditions. Results (mean ± S.D.) showed:

	Food	Fasting
AUC 0 → ∞ (µg-hr/mL)	260.5±60.6	280.5±68.7
C_{max} (µg/mL)	10.57±2.00	12.49±2.15
T_{max} (hr)	9.8±2.1	7.0±1.4

Steady-state pharmacokinetics were determined in 26 normal male volunteers (with theophylline clearance rates less than or equal to 5.0 L/hr and/or a theophylline elimination half-life of 6 to 12 hours) who received 900 mg of theophylline per day for five days. Twenty-six were dosed with three 300 mg extended-release Slo-bid Gyrocaps administered 24 hours apart immediately after the consumption of breakfast, and seventeen were dosed with one 300 mg, one 100 mg, and one 50 mg Slo-bid Gyrocap administered 12 hours apart (immediately after consuming breakfast and two hours after the consumption of dinner).

The pharmacokinetic parameters obtained for the extended-release Slo-bid Gyrocaps given as 900 mg once daily in the morning after a high-fat content breakfast were essentially the same as those parameters obtained after Slo-bid Gyrocaps administered in the widely-acceptable, approved manner of twice-daily. In particular, the area-under-the-curve values were 238 ± 27 (S.D.) and 251 ± 29 µg-hr/mL for the products administered q24h and q12h, respectively. Mean C_{max} values of 13.2 ± 2.0 µg/mL and 12.2 ± 2.2 µg/mL and C_{min} values of 5.9 ± 1.0 µg/mL and 8.6 ± 1.1 µg/mL were obtained after q24h and q12h administration, respectively. The mean percent fluctuation $[((C_{max}-C_{min})/C_{min})\times 100]$ was 140 ± 66% (S.D.) and 40 ± 15% (S.D.) when Slo-bid was given once- or twice-daily, respectively.

INDICATIONS AND USAGE

For relief and/or prevention of symptoms from asthma and reversible bronchospasm associated with chronic bronchitis and emphysema.

CONTRAINDICATIONS

Slo-bid is contraindicated in individuals who have shown hypersensitivity to any of the components of this product or to xanthine derivatives. It is also contraindicated in pa-

Continued on next page

Slo-Bid—Cont.

tients with active peptic ulcer disease and in individuals with underlying seizure disorders (unless receiving appropriate anticonvulsant medication).

WARNINGS

Serum levels above 20 µg/mL are rarely found after appropriate administration of the recommended doses. However, in individuals in whom theophylline plasma clearance is reduced *for any reason,* even conventional doses may result in increased serum levels and potential toxicity. Reduced theophylline clearance has been documented in the following readily identifiable groups: 1) patients with impaired renal or liver function; 2) patients over 55 years of age, particularly males and those with chronic lung disease; 3) those with cardiac failure from any cause; 4) patients with sustained high fever; 5) neonates and infants under 1 year of age; and 6) those patients taking certain drugs (see PRECAUTIONS, Drug Interactions). Frequently, such patients have markedly prolonged theophylline serum levels following discontinuation of the drug.

Decreased clearance of theophylline may be associated with either influenza immunization or active influenza, and with other viral infections.

It is important to consider reduction of dosage and measurement of serum theophylline levels in the above individuals. Serious side effects such as ventricular arrhythmias, convulsions or even death may appear as the first sign of toxicity without any previous warning. Less serious signs of theophylline toxicity (i.e., nausea and restlessness) may occur frequently when initiating therapy but are usually transient; when such signs are persistent during maintenance therapy, they are often associated with serum concentrations above 20 µg/mL. Stated differently, *serious toxicity is not reliably preceded by less severe side effects.* A serum concentration measurement is the only reliable method of identifying a potential for life-threatening toxicity.

Many patients who require theophylline exhibit tachycardia due to their underlying disease process, so the cause/effect relationship to elevated serum theophylline concentrations may not be appreciated.

Theophylline products may cause or worsen arrhythmias and any significant change in rate and/or rhythm warrants monitoring and further investigation.

Studies in laboratory animals (minipigs, rodents and dogs) recorded the occurrence of cardiac arrhythmias and sudden death (with histologic evidence of myocardial necrosis) when beta agonists and methylxanthines were administered concurrently. The significance of these findings when applied to humans is currently unknown.

PRECAUTIONS

General: On the average, theophylline half-life is shorter in cigarette and marijuana smokers than in nonsmokers, but smokers can have half-lives as long as nonsmokers. Theophylline should not be administered concurrently with other xanthine preparations. Use with caution in patients with hypoxemia, hypertension or with a history of peptic ulcer. Theophylline may occasionally act as a local irritant to the GI tract, although GI symptoms are more commonly centrally mediated and associated with serum drug concentrations over 20 µg/mL.

Xanthines can potentiate hypokalemia resulting from beta$_2$ agonist therapy, steroids, diuretics, other xanthines and hypoxia. Particular caution is advised in severe asthma. It is recommended that serum potassium levels be monitored in such situations.

Information for Patients:
The physician should reinforce the importance of taking only the prescribed dose at the prescribed time intervals. The patient should alert the physician if symptoms occur repeatedly, especially near the end of a dosing interval. When prescribing administration by the sprinkle method, details of the proper technique should be explained to the patient.

Laboratory Test: Serum levels should be monitored periodically to determine the theophylline levels associated with observed clinical response and to identify the potential for toxicity. For such measurements, the serum sample should be obtained at the time of peak concentration, approximately 5–9 hours after the morning dose. It is important that the patient has not missed or taken additional doses during the previous 48 hours and that dosing intervals have been reasonably equally spaced.

DOSE ADJUSTMENT BASED ON SERUM THEOPHYLLINE MEASUREMENTS WHEN THESE INSTRUCTIONS HAVE NOT BEEN FOLLOWED MAY RESULT IN RECOMMENDATIONS THAT PRESENT RISK OF TOXICITY TO THE PATIENT.

Drug Interactions:
Drug-Drug: Toxic synergism with ephedrine has been documented and may occur with some other sympathomimetic bronchodilators. In addition, the following drug interactions have been demonstrated:

Drug	Effect
Theophylline with:	
Allopurinol (high dose)	Increased serum theophylline levels
Cimetidine	Increased serum theophylline levels
Ciprofloxacin	Increased serum theophylline levels
Erythromycin, Troleandomycin	Increased serum theophylline levels
Lithium carbonate	Increased renal excretion of lithium
Oral contraceptives	Increased serum theophylline levels
Propranolol	Increased serum theophylline levels
Phenytoin	Decreased theophylline and phenytoin serum levels
Rifampin	Decreased serum theophylline levels

Drug-Food: Taking Slo-bid immediately after a high-fat content meal such as 8 ounces whole milk, 2 fried eggs, 2 strips bacon, one bran muffin with butter, 2 ounces hash brown potatoes (about 789 calories, including approximately 49 g of fat) may result in a decrease in the rate of absorption, but with no significant difference in the extent of absorption (see CLINICAL PHARMACOLOGY, Pharmacokinetics). The influence of the type and amount of other foods, as well as the time interval between drug and food, has not been studied.

Drug/Laboratory Test Interactions: Currently available analytic methods, including high-pressure liquid chromatography and immunoassay techniques, for measuring serum theophylline levels are specific. Metabolites and other drugs generally do not affect the results. Other new analytic methods are also now in use. The physician should be aware of the laboratory method used and whether other drugs will interfere with the assay for theophylline.

Carcinogenesis, Mutagenesis, Impairment of Fertility: Long-term carcinogenicity studies have not been performed with theophylline.

Chromosome-breaking activity was detected in human cell cultures at concentrations of theophylline up to 50 times the therapeutic serum concentrations in humans. Theophylline was not mutagenic in the dominant lethal assay in male mice given theophylline intraperitoneally in doses up to 30 times the maximum daily human oral dose.

Studies to determine the effect on fertility have not been performed with theophylline.

Pregnancy: Pregnancy Category C—Reproduction studies performed in mice and rats at oral doses from 7 to 17 times the human dose (maximum human dose for adults assumed to be 13 mg/kg/day) have indicated that theophylline may cause malformations, but these effects only occurred at or near doses that were toxic to the maternal animals. There are no adequate and well-controlled studies in pregnant women. It is not known whether theophylline can cause fetal harm when administered to a pregnant woman or can affect reproduction capacity. Theophylline should be used during pregnancy only if the potential benefit justifies the potential risk to the fetus.

Nursing Mothers: Theophylline is distributed into breast milk and may cause irritability or other signs of toxicity in nursing infants. Because of the potential for serious adverse reactions in nursing infants from theophylline, a decision should be made whether to discontinue nursing or to discontinue the drug, taking into account the importance of the drug to the mother.

Pediatric Use:
Safety and effectiveness of Slo-bid Gyrocaps adminstered:
1. Every 24 hours in children under 12 years of age, have not been established.
2. Every 12 hours in children under 6 years of age, have not been established.

ADVERSE REACTIONS

The following adverse reactions have been observed, but there has not been enough systematic collection of data to support an estimate of their frequency. The most consistent adverse reactions are usually due to overdosage.

Gastrointestinal: nausea, vomiting, epigastric pain, hematemesis, diarrhea.
Central Nervous System: headaches, irritability, restlessness, insomnia, reflex hyperexcitability, muscle twitching, clonic and tonic generalized convulsions.
Cardiovascular: palpitation, tachycardia, extrasystoles, flushing, hypotension, circulatory failure, ventricular arrhythmias.
Respiratory: tachypnea.
Renal: potentiation of diuresis.
Other: alopecia, hyperglycemia, inappropriate ADH syndrome, rash.

OVERDOSAGE

Management: It is suggested that the management principles (consistent with the clinical status of the patient when first seen) outlined below be instituted and that simultaneous contact with a Regional Poison Control Center be established. In this way both updated information and individualization regarding therapy may be provided.

1. When potential oral overdose is established and seizure has not occurred:
   a) If patient is alert and seen soon after ingestion, induction of emesis may be of value. Gastric lavage has been demonstrated to be of no value in influencing outcome in patients who present more than 1 hour after ingestion.
   b) Administer a cathartic. Sorbitol solution is reported to be of value.
   c) Administer repeated doses of activated charcoal and monitor theophylline serum levels.
   d) Prophylactic administration of phenobarbital has been shown to increase the seizure threshold in laboratory animals, and administration of this drug may be of value.
   e) Monitor serum potassium.
2. If patient presents with a seizure:
   a) Establish an airway.
   b) Administer oxygen.
   c) Treat the seizure with intravenous diazepam 0.1 to 0.3 mg/kg up to 10 mg. If seizures cannot be controlled, the use of general anesthesia should be considered.
   d) Monitor vital signs, maintain blood pressure and provide adequate hydration.
3. Postseizure Coma:
   a) Maintain airway and oxygenation.
   b) If a result of oral medication, follow above recommendations to prevent absorption of drug, but intubation and lavage will have to be performed instead of inducing emesis and the cathartic and charcoal will need to be introduced via a large-bore gastric lavage tube.
   c) Continue to provide full supportive care and adequate hydration until the drug is metabolized. In general, drug metabolism is sufficiently rapid so as not to warrant dialysis. If repeated oral activated charcoal is ineffective (as noted by stable or rising serum levels), charcoal hemoperfusion may be indicated.

DOSAGE AND ADMINISTRATION

Taking Slo-bid immediately after a high-fat content meal may alter its rate of absorption (see CLINICAL PHARMACOLOGY and PRECAUTIONS, Drug-Food Interactions). However, the differences are usually small and Slo-bid may normally be administered without regard to meals.

Effective use of theophylline (i.e., the concentration of drug in the serum associated with optimal benefit and minimal risk of toxicity) is considered to occur when the theophylline concentration is maintained from 10 to 20 µg/mL. The early studies from which these levels were derived were carried out in patients immediately or shortly after recovery from acute exacerbations of their disease (some hospitalized with status asthmaticus).

Although the 20 µg/mL level remains appropriate as a critical value (above which toxicity is more likely to occur) for safety purposes, additional data are now available that indicate that the serum theophylline concentrations required to produce maximum physiologic benefit may, in fact, fluctuate with the degree of bronchospasm present and are variable. Therefore, the physician should individualize the range appropriate to the patient's requirements, based on both symptomatic response and improvement in pulmonary function. It should be stressed that serum theophylline concentrations maintained at the upper level of the 10 to 20 µg/mL range may be associated with potential toxicity when factors known to reduce theophylline clearance are operative. (See WARNINGS.)

If it is not possible to obtain serum level determinations, restriction of the daily dose (in otherwise healthy adults) to not greater than 13 mg/kg/day, to a maximum of 900 mg, in divided doses will result in relatively few patients exceeding serum levels of 20 µg/mL and the resultant greater risk of toxicity.

Caution should be exercised for younger children who cannot complain of minor side effects. Older adults, those with cor pulmonale, congestive heart failure, and/or liver disease may have unusually low dosage requirements and thus may experience toxicity at the maximal dosage recommended below.

Theophylline does not distribute into fatty tissue. Dosage should be calculated on the basis of lean (ideal) body weight where mg/kg doses are presented.

Frequency of Dosing: When immediate-release products with rapid absorption are used, dosing to maintain serum levels generally requires administration every 6 hours. This is particularly true in children, but dosing intervals up to 8 hours may be satisfactory in adults since they eliminate the drug at a slower rate. Some children, and adults requiring higher than average doses (those having rapid rates of clearance, e.g., half-lives of under 6 hours) may benefit and be more effectively controlled during chronic therapy when given products with extended-release characteristics since these provide longer dosing intervals and/or less fluctuation

in serum concentration between dosing. Those extended-release products which provide flexibility in dosage through formulations of varying strengths are also helpful in controlling serum levels. Dosage guidelines are approximations only and the wide range of theophylline clearance between individuals (particularly those with concomitant disease) make indiscriminate usage hazardous.

Dosage Guidelines:

I. Acute Symptoms

NOTE: Status asthmaticus should be considered a medical emergency and is defined as that degree of bronchospasm that is not rapidly responsive to usual doses of conventional bronchodilators. Optimal therapy for such patients frequently requires both *additional medication* parenterally administered, and *close monitoring,* preferably in an intensive care setting.

Slo-bid is not intended for patients experiencing an acute episode of bronchospasm (associated with asthma, chronic bronchitis, or emphysema). Such patients require *rapid* relief of symptoms and should be treated with an immediate-release or intravenous theophylline preparation (or other bronchodilators) and not with extended-release products.

II. Chronic Therapy

A. Initiating Therapy with an Immediate-Release Product

It is recommended that the appropriate dosage be established using an immediate-release preparation. A dosage form that allows small incremental doses is desirable for initiating therapy. A liquid preparation should be considered for children to permit easier and more accurate dosage adjustment. Slow clinical titration is generally preferred to help assure acceptance and safety of the medication and to allow the patient to develop tolerance to transient caffeine-like side effects. Then, if the total 24-hour dose can be given by use of the available strengths of this product, the patient can usually be switched to Slo-bid, giving one third of the daily dose at 8-hour intervals or one half the daily dose at 12-hour intervals. Patients who metabolize theophylline rapidly, such as the young, smokers, and some non-smoking adults are the most likely candidates for dosing at 8-hour intervals. Such patients can generally be identified as having trough serum concentrations lower than desired or repeatedly exhibiting symptoms near the end of a dosing interval.

B. Initiating Therapy with Slo-bid Gyrocaps

Alternatively, therapy can be initiated with Slo-bid Gyrocaps since they are available in dosage strengths that permit titration and adjustments of dosage (in adults and older children). Children weighing less than 25 kg should have their daily dosage requirements established with Slo-Phyllin® 80 mg Syrup to permit small dosage increments.

Initial Dose: 16 mg/kg/24 hours or 400 mg/24 hours (whichever is less) of anhydrous theophylline in 2 or 3 divided doses at 8- or 12-hour intervals.

Increasing Dose: The above dosage may be increased in approximately 25-percent increments at 3-day intervals so long as the drug is tolerated. Following each adjustment, if the clinical response is satisfactory and serum levels can be measured, then such measurements should be obtained as directed under section IV (below). If serum levels cannot be obtained, then that dosage level should be maintained. Dosage increases may be made in this manner until the maximum dose indicated in section III (below) is reached. It is important that no patient be maintained on any dosage that is not tolerated. When instructing patients to increase dosage according to the schedule above, they should be told not to take a subsequent dose if apparent side effects occur and to resume therapy at a lower dose once adverse effects have disappeared.

C. Sprinkling Contents on Food

Slo-bid Gyrocaps may be administered by carefully opening the capsule and sprinkling the beaded contents on a spoonful of soft food such as applesauce or pudding; the soft food should be swallowed immediately without chewing and followed with a glass of cool water or juice to ensure complete swallowing of the beads. It is recommended that the food used should not be hot and should be soft enough to be swallowed without chewing. Any bead/food mixture should be used immediately and not stored for future use. SUBDIVIDING THE CONTENTS OF A CAPSULE IS NOT RECOMMENDED.

D. Once-Daily Dosing

The slow absorption rate of this preparation may allow once-daily administration in adult nonsmokers with appropriate total body clearance and other patients with low dosage requirements. Once-daily dosing should be considered only after the patient has been gradually and satisfactorily titrated to therapeutic levels with q12h dosing. Once-daily dosing should be based on twice the q12h dose and should be initiated at the end of the last q12h dosing interval. The trough concentration

		Dose per 8 hours	Dose per 12 hours
Age 6–under 9 years	24 mg/kg/day	8.0 mg/kg	12.0 mg/kg
Age 9–under 12 years	20 mg/kg/day	6.7 mg/kg	10.0 mg/kg
Age 12–under 16 years	18 mg/kg/day	6.0 mg/kg	9.0 mg/kg
Age over 16 years	13 mg/kg/day	4.3 mg/kg	6.5 mg/kg

OR 900 mg
(WHICHEVER IS LESS)

Strength	Size	NDC 0075-	Color	Markings
50 mg	Bottles of 100	0057-00	Opaque white capsule	50 printed in red
	Unit Dose 100	0057-62		
75 mg	Bottles of 100	1075-00	Opaque white capsule	75 printed in red
	Unit Dose 100	1075-62		
100 mg	Bottles of 100	0100-00	Opaque white capsule	100 printed in red
	Bottles of 1000	0100-99		
	Unit Dose 100	0100-62		
125 mg	Bottles of 100	1125-00	Opaque white capsule	125 print in red
	Unit Dose 100	1125-62		
200 mg	Bottles of 100	0200-00	Opaque white capsule	200 printed in red
	Bottles of 1000	0200-99		
	Unit Dose 100	0200-62		
300 mg	Bottles of 100	0300-00	Opaque white capsule	300 printed in red
	Bottles of 1000	0300-99		
	Unit Dose 100	0300-62		

(C_{min}) obtained following conversion to once-daily dosing may be lower (especially in high clearance patients) and the peak concentration (C_{max}) may be higher (especially in low clearance patients) than that obtained with q12h dosing. If symptoms recur, or signs of toxicity appear during the once-daily dosing interval, dosing on the q12h basis should be reinstituted.

It is essential that serum theophylline concentrations be monitored before and after transfer to once-daily dosing. Food and posture, along with changes associated with circadian rhythm, may influence the rate of absorption and/or clearance rates of theophylline from extended-release dosage forms administered at night. The exact relationship of these and other factors to night-time serum concentrations and the clinical significance of such findings require additional study. Therefore, it is not recommended that Slo-bid, when used as a once-a-day product, be administered at night.

III. Maximum Dose of Theophylline Where the Serum Concentration is Not Measured

WARNING: DO NOT ATTEMPT TO MAINTAIN ANY DOSE THAT IS NOT TOLERATED.

Not to exceed the following:

[See first table above]

IV. Measurement of Serum Theophylline Concentrations During Chronic Therapy

If the above maximum doses are to be maintained or exceeded, serum theophylline measurement is essential (See PRECAUTIONS, Laboratory Tests for guidance).

V. Final Adjustment of Dosage

Dosage adjustment after serum theophylline measurement

If serum theophylline is:		Directions:
Within desired range		Maintain dosage if tolerated.
Too high	20 to 25 µg/mL	Decrease doses by about 10% and recheck serum level after 3 days.
	25 to 30 µg/mL	Skip next dose and decrease subsequent doses by about 25%. Recheck serum level after 3 days.
	Over 30 µg/mL	Skip next 2 doses and decrease subsequent doses by 50%. Recheck serum level after 3 days.
Too low		Increase dosage by 25% at 3-day intervals until either the desired serum concentration and/or clinical response is achieved. The total daily dose may need to be administered at more frequent intervals if symptoms occur repeatedly at the end of a dosing interval.

The serum concentration may be rechecked at appropriate intervals, but at least at the end of any adjustment period. When the patient's condition is otherwise clinically stable and none of the recognized factors which alter elimination are present, measurement of serum levels need be repeated only every 6 to 12 months.

STORAGE CONDITIONS

Store at room temperature. Protect from excessive heat, light and moisture.

CAUTION

Federal (U.S.A.) law prohibits dispensing without prescription. Keep this and all medications out of the reach of children.

HOW SUPPLIED

[See second table above]

RHÔNE-POULENC RORER PHARMACEUTICALS INC.
Collegeville, PA, U.S.A. 19426-0107
Rev. 12/96   IN-0221F

TAXOTERE®   ℞
[tax-ō-tēr]
(docetaxel)
for Injection Concentrate

Rx only

WARNING

TAXOTERE® (docetaxel) for Injection Concentrate should be administered under the supervision of a qualified physician experienced in the use of antineoplastic agents. Appropriate management of complications is possible only when adequate diagnostic and treatment facilities are readily available.

The incidence of treatment-related mortality associated with TAXOTERE therapy is increased in patients with abnormal liver function and in patients receiving higher doses (see **WARNINGS**).

TAXOTERE should generally not be given to patients with bilirubin > upper limit of normal (ULN), or to patients with SGOT and/or SGPT >1.5 × ULN concomitant with alkaline phosphatase > 2.5 × ULN. Patients with elevations of bilirubin or abnormalities of transaminase concurrent with alkaline phosphatase are at increased risk for the development of grade 4 neutropenia,

Continued on next page

Taxotere—Cont.

febrile neutropenia, infections, severe thrombocytopenia, severe stomatitis, severe skin toxicity, and toxic death. Patients with isolated elevations of transaminase > 1.5 × ULN also had a higher rate of febrile neutropenia grade 4 but did not have an increased incidence of toxic death. Bilirubin, SGOT or SGPT, and alkaline phosphatase values should be obtained prior to each cycle of TAXOTERE therapy and reviewed by the treating physician.

TAXOTERE therapy should not be given to patients with neutrophil counts of < 1500 cells/mm³. In order to monitor the occurrence of neutropenia, which may be severe and result in infection, frequent blood cell counts should be performed on all patients receiving TAXOTERE.

Severe hypersensitivity reactions characterized by hypotension and/or bronchospasm, or generalized rash/erythema occurred in 2.2% (2/92) of patients who received the recommended 3-day dexamethasone premedication. Hypersensitivity reactions requiring discontinuation of the TAXOTERE infusion were reported in five patients who did not receive premedication. These reactions resolved after discontinuation of the infusion and the administration of appropriate therapy. TAXOTERE must not be given to patients who have a history of severe hypersensitivity reactions to TAXOTERE or to other drugs formulated with polysorbate 80 (see **WARNINGS**).

Severe fluid retention occurred in 6.5% (6/92) of patients despite use of a 3-day dexamethasone premedication regimen. It was characterized by one or more of the following events: poorly tolerated peripheral edema, generalized edema, pleural effusion requiring urgent drainage, dyspnea at rest, cardiac tamponade, or pronounced abdominal distention (due to ascites) (see **PRECAUTIONS**).

DESCRIPTION

Docetaxel is an antineoplastic agent belonging to the taxoid family. It is prepared by semisynthesis beginning with a precursor extracted from the renewable needle biomass of yew plants. The chemical name for docetaxel is (2R,3S)-N-carboxy-3-phenylisoserine,N-tert-butyl ester, 13-ester with 5β-20-epoxy-$1,2\alpha,4,7\beta,10\beta,13\alpha$-hexahydroxytax-11-en-9-one 4-acetate 2-benzoate, trihydrate. Docetaxel has the following structural formula:

Docetaxel is a white to almost-white powder with an empirical formula of $C_{43}H_{53}NO_{14} \cdot 3H_2O$, and a molecular weight of 861.9. It is highly lipophilic and practically insoluble in water. TAXOTERE (docetaxel) for Injection Concentrate is a clear yellow to brownish-yellow viscous solution. TAXOTERE is sterile, non-pyrogenic, and is available in single-dose vials containing 20 mg (0.5 mL) or 80 mg (2.0 mL) docetaxel (anhydrous). Each mL contains 40 mg docetaxel (anhydrous) and 1040 mg polysorbate 80.

TAXOTERE for Injection Concentrate requires dilution prior to use. A sterile, non-pyrogenic, single-dose diluent is supplied for that purpose. The diluent for TAXOTERE contains 13% ethanol in Water for Injection, and is supplied in 1.5 mL (to be used with 20 mg TAXOTERE for Injection Concentrate) and 6.0 mL (to be used with 80 mg TAXOTERE for Injection Concentrate) vials.

CLINICAL PHARMACOLOGY

Docetaxel is an antineoplastic agent that acts by disrupting the microtubular network in cells that is essential for mitotic and interphase cellular functions. Docetaxel binds to free tubulin and promotes the assembly of tubulin into stable microtubules while simultaneously inhibiting their disassembly. This leads to the production of microtubule bundles without normal function and to the stabilization of microtubules, which results in the inhibition of mitosis in cells. Docetaxel's binding to microtubules does not alter the number of protofilaments in the bound microtubules, a feature which differs from most spindle poisons currently in clinical use.

HUMAN PHARMACOKINETICS

The pharmacokinetics of docetaxel have been evaluated in cancer patients after administration of 20-115 mg/m² in

Efficacy of TAXOTERE in the Treatment of Breast Cancer Patients Previously Treated with an Anthracycline-Containing Regimen (Intent-to-Treat Analysis)

Efficacy Parameter	Docetaxel (N=203)	Mitomycin/ Vinblastine (N=189)	p-value
Median Survival	11.4 months	8.7 months	
Risk Ratio*, Mortality (Docetaxel:Control)	0.73		p=0.01 Log Rank
95% CI (Risk Ratio)	0.58–0.93		
Median Time to Progression	4.3 months	2.5 months	
Risk Ratio*, Progression (Docetaxel:Control)	0.75		p=0.01 Log Rank
95% CI (Risk Ratio)	0.61–0.94		
Overall Response Rate	28.1%	9.5%	p<0.0001
Complete Response Rate	3.4%	1.6%	Chi Square

*For the risk ratio, a value less than 1.00 favors docetaxel.

Efficacy of TAXOTERE in the Treatment of Breast Cancer Patients Previously Treated with an Alkylating-Containing Regimen (Intent-to-Treat Analysis)

Efficacy Parameter	Docetaxel (N=161)	Doxorubicin (165)	p-value
Median Survival	14.7 months	14.3 months	
Risk Ratio*, Mortality (Docetaxel:Control)	0.89		p=0.39 Log Rank
95% CI (Risk Ratio)	0.68–1.16		
Median Time to Progression	6.5 months	5.3 months	
Risk Ratio*, Progression (Docetaxel:Control)	0.93		p=0.45 Log Rank
95% CI (Risk Ratio)	0.71–1.16		
Overall Response Rate	45.3%	29.7%	p=0.004
Complete Response Rate	6.8%	4.2%	Chi Square

*For the risk ratio, a value less than 1.00 favors docetaxel.

phase I studies. The area under the curve (AUC) was dose proportional following doses of 70-115 mg/m² with infusion times of 1 to 2 hours. Docetaxel's pharmacokinetic profile is consistent with a three-compartment pharmacokinetic model, with half-lives for the α, β, and γ phases of 4 min, 36 min, and 11.1 hr, respectively. The initial rapid decline represents distribution to the peripheral compartments and the late (terminal) phase is due, in part, to a relatively slow efflux of docetaxel from the peripheral compartment. Mean values for total body clearance and steady state volume of distribution were 21 L/h/m² and 113 L, respectively. Mean total body clearance for Japanese patients dosed at the range of 10–90 mg/m² was similar to that of European/American populations dosed at 100 mg/m², suggesting no significant difference in the elimination of docetaxel in the two populations.

A study of ¹⁴C-docetaxel was conducted in three cancer patients. Docetaxel was eliminated in both the urine and feces following oxidative metabolism of the tert-butyl ester group, but fecal excretion was the main elimination route. Within 7 days, urinary and fecal excretion accounted for approximately 6% and 75% of the administered radioactivity, respectively. About 80% of the radioactivity recovered in feces is excreted during the first 48 hours as 1 major and 3 minor metabolites with very small amounts (less than 8%) of unchanged drug. Based on in vitro studies, isoenzymes of the cytochrome P45 03A (CYP 3A) subfamily appear to be involved in docetaxel metabolism.

A population pharmacokinetic analysis was carried out after TAXOTERE treatment of 535 patients dosed at 100 mg/m². Pharmacokinetic parameters estimated by this analysis were very close to those estimated from phase I studies. The pharmacokinetics of docetaxel were not influenced by age or gender and docetaxel total body clearance was not modified by pretreatment with dexamethasone. In patients with clinical chemistry data suggestive of mild to moderate liver function impairment (SGOT and/or SGPT >1.5 times the upper limit of normal [ULN] concomitant with alkaline phosphatase >2.5 times ULN), total body clearance was lowered by an average of 27%, resulting in a 38% increase in systemic exposure (AUC). This average,

however, includes a substantial range and there is, at present, no measurement that would allow recommendation for dose adjustment in such patients. Patients with combined abnormalities of transaminase and alkaline phosphatase should, in general, not be treated with TAXOTERE.

In vitro studies showed that docetaxel is about 94% protein bound, mainly to α_1-acid glycoprotein, albumin, and lipoproteins. In three cancer patients, the in vitro binding to plasma proteins was found to be approximately 97%. Dexamethasone does not affect the protein binding of docetaxel.

CLINICAL STUDIES

The efficacy and safety of TAXOTERE have been evaluated in locally advanced or metastatic breast cancer after failure of previous chemotherapy (alkylating agent-containing regimens or anthracycline-containing regimens), primarily at a dose of 100 mg/m² given as a 1-hour infusion every 3 weeks, but with some experience at 60 mg/m², in two large randomized trials and a number of smaller single arm studies.

Randomized Trials: In one randomized trial, patients with a history of prior treatment with an anthracycline-containing regimen were assigned to treatment with TAXOTERE or the combination of mitomycin (12 mg/m² every 6 weeks) and vinblastine (6 mg/m² every 3 weeks). 203 patients were randomized to TAXOTERE and 189 to the comparator arm. Most patients had received prior chemotherapy for metastatic disease; only 27 patients on the TAXOTERE arm and 33 patients on the comparator arm entered the study following relapse after adjuvant therapy. Three-quarters of patients had measurable, visceral metastases. The primary endpoint was time to progression. The following table summarizes the study results:

[See first table above]

In a second randomized trial, patients previously treated with an alkylating-containing regimen were assigned to treatment with TAXOTERE or doxorubicin (75 mg/m² every 3 weeks). 161 patients were randomized to TAXOTERE and 165 patients to doxorubicin. Approximately one-half of patients had received prior chemotherapy for metastatic disease, and one-half entered the study following relapse after adjuvant therapy. Three-quarters of patients had measurable, visceral metastases. The primary endpoint was time to progression. The study results are summarized below:

**Hematologic Adverse Events in Breast Cancer Patients
Previously Treated with Chemotherapy
Treated at TAXOTERE 100 mg/m² with Normal or Elevated Liver
Function Tests or 60 mg/m² with Normal Liver Function Tests**

| | TAXOTERE 100 mg/m² | | TAXOTERE 60 mg/m² |
| | Normal LFTs* | Elevated LFTs** | Normal LFTs* |
Adverse Event	n=730 %	n=18 %	n=174 %
Neutropenia			
Any <2000 cells/mm³	98.4	100	95.4
Grade 4 <500 cells/mm³	84.4	93.8	74.9
Thrombocytopenia			
Any <100,000 cells/mm³	10.8	44.4	14.4
Grade 4 <20,000 cells/mm³	0.6	16.7	1.1
Anemia <11 g/dL	94.6	94.4	64.9
Infection***			
Any	22.5	38.9	1.1
Grade 3 and 4	7.1	33.3	0
Febrile Neutropenia****			
By Patient	11.8	33.3	0
By Course	2.4	8.6	0
Septic Death	1.5	5.6	1.1
Non-Septic Death	1.1	11.1	0

* Normal Baseline LFTs: Transaminases ≤ 1.5 times ULN or alkaline phosphatase ≤ 2.5 times ULN or isolated elevations of transaminases or alkaline phosphatase up to 5 times ULN

** Elevated Baseline LFTs: SGOT and/or SGPT >1.5 times ULN concurrent with alkaline phosphatase >2.5 times ULN

*** Incidence of infection requiring hospitalization and/or intravenous antibiotics was 8.5% (n=62) among the 730 patients with normal LFTs at baseline; 7 patients had concurrent grade 3 neutropenia, and 46 patients had grade 4 neutropenia.

**** Febrile Neutropenia: For 100 mg/m², ANC grade 4 and fever > 38° C with IV antibiotics and/or hospitalization; for 60 mg/m², ANC grade 3/4 and fever > 38.1° C

**Non-Hematologic Adverse Events in Breast Cancer Patients
Previously Treated with Chemotherapy
Treated at TAXOTERE 100 mg/m² with Normal or Elevated Liver
Function Tests or 60 mg/m² with Normal Liver Function Tests**

| | TAXOTERE 100 mg/m² | | TAXOTERE 60 mg/m² |
| | Normal LFTs* | Elevated LFTs** | Normal LFTs* |
Adverse Event	n=730 %	n=18 %	n=174 %
Acute Hypersensitivity Reaction			
Regardless of Premedication			
Any	13.0	5.6	0.6
Severe	1.2	0	0
Fluid Retention***			
Regardless of Premedication			
Any	56.2	61.1	12.6
Severe	7.9	16.7	0
Neurosensory			
Any	56.8	50	19.5
Severe	5.8	0	0
Myalgia	22.7	33.3	3.4
Cutaneous			
Any	44.8	61.1	30.5
Severe	4.8	16.7	0
Asthenia			
Any	65.2	44.4	65.5
Severe	16.6	22.2	0
Diarrhea			
Any	42.2	27.8	NA
Severe	6.3	11.1	
Stomatitis			
Any	53.3	66.7	19.0
Severe	7.8	38.9	0.6

* Normal Baseline LFTs: Transaminases ≤ 1.5 times ULN or alkaline phosphatase ≤ 2.5 times ULN or isolated elevations of transaminases or alkaline phosphatase up to 5 times ULN

** Elevated Baseline Liver Function: SGOT and/or SGPT >1.5 times ULN concurrent with alkaline phosphatase >2.5 times ULN

*** Fluid Retention Includes (by COSTART): edema (peripheral, localized, generalized, lymphedema, pulmonary edema, and edema otherwise not specified) and effusion (pleural, pericardial, and ascites); no premedication given with the 60 mg/m² dose

NA = not available

[See second table at top of previous page]
Single Arm Studies: TAXOTERE at a dose of 100 mg/m² was studied in six single arm studies involving a total of 309 patients with metastatic breast cancer in whom previous chemotherapy had failed. Among these, 190 patients had anthracycline-resistant breast cancer, defined as progression during an anthracycline-containing chemotherapy regimen for metastatic disease, or relapse during an anthracycline-containing adjuvant regimen. In anthracycline-resistant patients, the overall response rate was 37.9% (72/190; 95% C.I.: 31.0-44.8) and the complete response rate was 2.1%.

TAXOTERE was also studied in three single arm Japanese studies at a dose of 60 mg/m², in 174 patients who had received prior chemotherapy for locally advanced or metastatic breast cancer. Among 26 patients whose best response to an anthracycline had been progression, the response rate was 34.6% (95% C.I.: 17.2-55.7), similar to the response rate in single arm studies of 100 mg/m².

Hematologic and Other Toxicity: Relation to dose and baseline liver chemistry abnormalities. Hematologic and other toxicity is increased at higher doses and in patients with elevated baseline liver function tests (LFTs). In the following tables, adverse drug reactions are compared for three populations: 730 patients with normal LFTs given TAXOTERE at 100 mg/m² in the randomized and single arm studies of metastatic breast cancer after failure of previous chemotherapy; 18 patients in these studies who had abnormal baseline LFTs (defined as SGOT and/or SGPT > 1.5 times ULN concurrent with alkaline phosphatase > 2.5 times ULN); and 174 patients in Japanese studies given TAXOTERE at 60 mg/m² who had normal LFTs.

[See first table at left]
[See second table at left]

INDICATIONS AND USAGE

TAXOTERE (docetaxel) for Injection Concentrate is indicated for the treatment of patients with locally advanced or metastatic breast cancer after failure of prior chemotherapy.

CONTRAINDICATIONS

TAXOTERE is contraindicated in patients who have a history of severe hypersensitivity reactions to docetaxel or to other drugs formulated with polysorbate 80.
TAXOTERE should not be used in patients with neutrophil counts of <1500 cells/mm³.

WARNINGS

TAXOTERE (docetaxel) for Injection Concentrate should be administered under the supervision of a qualified physician experienced in the use of antineoplastic agents. Appropriate management of complications is possible only when adequate diagnostic and treatment facilities are readily available.

Toxic Deaths: TAXOTERE administered at 100 mg/m² was associated with deaths considered possibly or probably related to treatment in 2.0% (19/965) of metastatic breast cancer patients, both previously treated and untreated, with normal baseline liver function and in 11.5% (7/61) of patients with various tumor types who had abnormal baseline liver function (SGOT and/or SGPT > 1.5 times ULN together with AP > 2.5 times ULN). Among patients dosed at 60 mg/m², mortality related to treatment occurred in 0.6% (3/481) of patients with normal liver function, and in 3 of 7 patients with abnormal liver function. Approximately half of these deaths occurred during the first cycle. Sepsis accounted for the majority of the deaths.

Premedication Regimen: All patients should be premedicated with oral corticosteroids such as dexamethasone 16 mg per day (*e.g.*, 8 mg BID) for 3 days starting 1 day prior to TAXOTERE to reduce the severity of fluid retention and hypersensitivity reactions (see **DOSAGE AND ADMINISTRATION** section). This regimen was evaluated in 92 patients with metastatic breast cancer previously treated with chemotherapy given TAXOTERE at a dose of 100 mg/m² every 3 weeks.

Hypersensitivity Reactions: Patients should be observed closely for hypersensitivity reactions, especially during the first and second infusions. Severe hypersensitivity reactions characterized by hypotension and/or bronchospasm, or generalized rash/erythema occurred in 2.2% of the 92 patients premedicated with 3-day corticosteroids. Hypersensitivity reactions requiring discontinuation of the TAXOTERE infusion were reported in 5 out of 1260 patients with various tumor types who did not receive premedication, but in 0/92 patients premedicated with 3-day corticosteroids. Patients with a history of severe hypersensitivity reactions should not be rechallenged with TAXOTERE.

Hematologic Effects: Neutropenia (< 2000 neutrophils/mm³) occurs in virtually all patients given 60–100 mg/m² of TAXOTERE and grade 4 neutropenia (< 500 cells/mm³) occurs in 85% of patients given 100 mg/m² and 75% of patients given 60 mg/m². Frequent monitoring of blood counts is, therefore, essential so that dose can be adjusted. TAXOTERE should not be administered to patients with neutrophils < 1500 cells/mm³.

Febrile neutropenia occurred in about 12% of patients given 100 mg/m² but was very uncommon in patients given 60 mg/m². Hematologic responses, febrile reactions and infections, and rates of septic death for different regimens are dose related and are described in **CLINICAL STUDIES**.

Three breast cancer patients with severe liver impairment (bilirubin > 1.7 times ULN) developed fatal gastrointestinal bleeding associated with severe drug-induced thrombocytopenia.

Continued on next page

Taxotere—Cont.

Hepatic Impairment: (see BOXED WARNING).

Fluid Retention: (see BOXED WARNING).

Pregnancy: TAXOTERE can cause fetal harm when administered to pregnant women. Studies in both rats and rabbits at doses ≥ 0.3 and 0.03 mg/kg/day, respectively (about $\frac{1}{50}$ and $\frac{1}{300}$ the daily maximum recommended human dose on a mg/m^2 basis), administered during the period of organogenesis, have shown that TAXOTERE is embryotoxic and fetotoxic (characterized by intrauterine mortality, increased resorption, reduced fetal weight, and fetal ossification delay). The doses indicated above also caused maternal toxicity.

There are no adequate and well-controlled studies in pregnant women using TAXOTERE. If TAXOTERE is used during pregnancy, or if the patient becomes pregnant while receiving this drug, the patient should be apprised of the potential hazard to the fetus or potential risk for loss of the pregnancy. Women of childbearing potential should be advised to avoid becoming pregnant during therapy with TAXOTERE.

PRECAUTIONS

General: Responding patients may not experience an improvement in performance status on therapy and may experience worsening. The relationship between changes in performance status, response to therapy, and treatment-related side effects has not been established.

Hematologic Effects: In order to monitor the occurrence of myelotoxicity, it is recommended that frequent peripheral blood cell counts be performed on all patients receiving TAXOTERE. Patients should not be retreated with subsequent cycles of TAXOTERE until neutrophils recover to a level > 1500 cells/mm^3 and platelets recover to a level > 100,000 cells/mm^3.

A 25% reduction in the dose of TAXOTERE is recommended during subsequent cycles following severe neutropenia (< 500 cells/mm^3) lasting 7 days or more, febrile neutropenia, or a grade 4 infection in a TAXOTERE® (docetaxel) for Injection Concentrate cycle (see DOSAGE AND ADMINISTRATION section).

Hypersensitivity Reactions: Hypersensitivity reactions may occur within a few minutes following initiation of a TAXOTERE infusion. If minor reactions such as flushing or localized skin reactions occur, interruption of therapy is not required. More severe reactions, however, require the immediate discontinuation of TAXOTERE and aggressive therapy. All patients should be premedicated with an oral corticosteroid prior to the initiation of the infusion of TAXOTERE (see BOXED WARNING and WARNINGS: Premedication Regimen).

Cutaneous: Localized erythema of the extremities with edema followed by desquamation has been observed. In case of severe skin toxicity, an adjustment in dosage is recommended (see DOSAGE AND ADMINISTRATION section). The discontinuation rate due to skin toxicity was 1.6% (15/965) for metastatic breast cancer patients. Among 92 breast cancer patients premedicated with 3-day corticosteroids, there were no cases of severe skin toxicity reported and no patient discontinued TAXOTERE due to skin toxicity.

Fluid Retention: Severe fluid retention has been reported following TAXOTERE therapy (see BOXED WARNING and WARNINGS: Premedication Regimen). Patients should be premedicated with oral corticosteroids prior to each TAXOTERE administration to reduce the incidence and severity of fluid retention (see DOSAGE AND ADMINISTRATION section). Patients with pre-existing effusions should be closely monitored from the first dose for the possible exacerbation of the effusions.

When fluid retention occurs, peripheral edema usually starts in the lower extremities and may become generalized with a median weight gain of 2 kg.

Among 92 breast cancer patients premedicated with 3-day corticosteroids, moderate fluid retention occurred in 27.2% and severe fluid retention in 6.5%. The median cumulative dose to onset of moderate or severe fluid retention was 819 mg/m^2. 9.8% (9/92) of patients discontinued treatment due to fluid retention: 4 patients discontinued with severe fluid retention; the remaining 5 had mild or moderate fluid retention. The median cumulative dose to treatment discontinuation due to fluid retention was 1021 mg/m^2. Fluid retention was completely, but sometimes slowly, reversible with a median of 16 weeks from the last infusion of TAXOTERE to resolution (range: 0 to 42+ weeks). Patients developing peripheral edema may be treated with standard measures, e.g., salt restriction, oral diuretic(s).

Neurologic: Severe neurosensory symptoms (paresthesia, dysesthesia, pain) were observed in 5.5% (53/965) of metastatic breast cancer patients, and resulted in treatment discontinuation in 6.1%. When these symptoms occur, dosage must be adjusted. If symptoms persist, treatment should be discontinued (see DOSAGE AND ADMINISTRATION section). Patients who experienced neurotoxicity in clinical trials and for whom follow-up information on the complete resolution of the event was available had spontaneous re-

versal of symptoms with a median of 9 weeks from onset (range: 0 to 106 weeks). Severe peripheral motor neuropathy mainly manifested as distal extremity weakness occurred in 4.4% (42/965).

Asthenia: Severe asthenia has been reported in 14.9% (144/965) of metastatic breast cancer patients but has led to treatment discontinuation in only 1.8%. Symptoms of fatigue and weakness may last a few days up to several weeks and may be associated with deterioration of performance status in patients with progressive disease.

Information for Patients: For additional information, see the accompanying Patient Information Leaflet.

Drug Interactions: There have been no formal clinical studies to evaluate the drug interactions of TAXOTERE with other medications. *In vitro* studies have shown that the metabolism of docetaxel may be modified by the concomitant administration of compounds that induce, inhibit, or are metabolized by cytochrome P450 3A4, such as cyclosporine, terfenadine, ketoconazole, erythromycin, and troleandomycin. Caution should be exercised with these drugs when treating patients receiving TAXOTERE as there is a potential for a significant interaction.

Carcinogenicity, Mutagenicity, Impairment of Fertility: No studies have been conducted to assess the carcinogenic potential of TAXOTERE. TAXOTERE has been shown to be clastogenic in the *in vitro* chromosome aberration test in CHO-K$_1$ cells and in the *in vivo* micronucleus test in the mouse, but it did not induce mutagenicity in the Ames test or the CHO/HGPRT gene mutation assays. TAXOTERE produced no impairment of fertility in rats when administered in multiple IV doses of up to 0.3 mg/kg (about $\frac{1}{50}$ the recommended human dose on a mg/m^2 basis), but decreased testicular weights were reported. This correlates with findings of a 10-cycle toxicity study (dosing once every 21 days for 6 months) in rats and dogs in which testicular atrophy or degeneration was observed at IV doses of 5 mg/kg in rats and 0.375 mg/kg in dogs (about $\frac{1}{3}$ and $\frac{1}{15}$ the recommended human dose on a mg/m^2 basis, respectively). An increased frequency of dosing in rats produced similar effects at lower dose levels.

Pregnancy: Pregnancy Category D (see WARNINGS section).

Nursing Mothers: It is not known whether TAXOTERE is excreted in human milk. Because many drugs are excreted in human milk, and because of the potential for serious adverse reactions in nursing infants from TAXOTERE, mothers should discontinue nursing prior to taking the drug.

Pediatric Use: The safety and effectiveness of TAXOTERE in pediatric patients have not been established.

ADVERSE REACTIONS

Adverse drug reactions occurring in at least 5% of patients are compared for three populations who received TAXOTERE administered at 100 mg/m^2 as a 1-hour infusion every 3 weeks: 2045 patients with various tumor types and normal baseline liver function tests; the subset of 965 patients with locally advanced or metastatic breast cancer, both previously treated and untreated with chemotherapy, who had normal baseline liver function tests; and an additional 61 patients with various tumor types who had abnormal liver function tests at baseline. These reactions were considered possibly or probably related to TAXOTERE. At least 95% of these patients did not receive hematopoietic support. The safety profile is generally similar in patients receiving TAXOTERE for the treatment of breast carcinoma and in patients with other tumor types.

[See table at top of next page]

Hematologic: (see WARNINGS). Reversible marrow suppression was the major dose-limiting toxicity of TAXOTERE. The median time to nadir was 7 days, while the median duration of severe neutropenia (<500 cells/mm^3) was 7 days. Among 2045 patients with solid tumors and normal baseline LFTs, severe neutropenia occurred in 75.4% and lasted for more than 7 days in 2.9% of cycles.

Febrile neutropenia (<500 cells/mm^3 with fever > 38° C with IV antibiotics and/or hospitalization) occurred in 11% of patients with solid tumors, in 12.3% of patients with metastatic breast cancer, and in 9.8% of 92 breast cancer patients premedicated with 3-day corticosteroids.

Severe infectious episodes occurred in 6.1% of patients with solid tumors, in 6.4% of patients with metastatic breast cancer, and in 5.4% of 92 breast cancer patients premedicated with 3-day corticosteroids.

Thrombocytopenia (<100,000 cells/mm^3) associated with fatal gastrointestinal hemorrhage has been reported.

Hypersensitivity Reactions: Severe hypersensitivity reactions are discussed in the BOXED WARNING, WARNINGS, and PRECAUTIONS sections. Minor events, including flushing, rash with or without pruritus, chest tightness, back pain, dyspnea, drug fever, or chills, have been reported and resolved after discontinuing the infusion and appropriate therapy.

Fluid Retention: (see BOXED WARNING, WARNINGS: Premedication Regimen, and PRECAUTIONS sections).

Cutaneous: Severe skin toxicity is discussed in PRECAUTIONS. Reversible cutaneous reactions characterized by a rash including localized eruptions, mainly on the feet and/or hands, but also on the arms, face, or thorax, usually associated with pruritus, have been observed. Eruptions generally occurred within 1 week after TAXOTERE infusion, recovered before the next infusion, and were not disabling. Severe nail disorders were characterized by hypo- or hyperpigmentation, and occasionally by onycholysis (in 0.8% of patients with solid tumors) and pain.

Neurologic: (see PRECAUTIONS).

Gastrointestinal: Gastrointestinal reactions (nausea and/or vomiting and/or diarrhea) were generally mild to moderate. Severe reactions occurred in 3–5% of patients with solid tumors and to a similar extent among metastatic breast cancer patients. The incidence of severe reactions was 1% or less for the 92 breast cancer patients premedicated with 3-day corticosteroids.

Severe stomatitis occurred in 5.5% of patients with solid tumors, in 7.4% of patients with metastatic breast cancer, and in 1.1% of the 92 breast cancer patients premedicated with 3-day corticosteroids.

Cardiovascular: Hypotension occurred in 2.8% of patients with solid tumors; 1.2% required treatment. Clinically meaningful events such as heart failure, sinus tachycardia, atrial flutter, dysrhythmia, unstable angina, pulmonary edema, and hypertension occurred rarely. 8.1% (7/86) of metastatic breast cancer patients receiving TAXOTERE 100 mg/m^2 in a randomized trial and who had serial left ventricular ejection fractions assessed developed deterioration of LVEF by $\geq 1.0\%$ associated with a drop below the institutional lower limit of normal.

Infusion Site Reactions: Infusion site reactions were generally mild and consisted of hyperpigmentation, inflammation, redness or dryness of the skin, phlebitis, extravasation, or swelling of the vein.

Hepatic: In patients with normal LFTs at baseline, bilirubin values greater than the ULN occurred in 8.9% of patients. Increases in SGOT or SGPT > 1.5 times the ULN, or alkaline phosphatase > 2.5 times ULN, were observed in 18.9% and 7.3% of patients, respectively. While on TAXOTERE, increases in SGOT and/or SGPT > 1.5 times ULN concomitant with alkaline phosphatase > 2.5 times ULN occurred in 4.3% of patients with normal LFTs at baseline. (Whether these changes were related to the drug or underlying disease has not been established.)

Ongoing Evaluation: The following serious adverse events of uncertain relationship to TAXOTERE have been reported:

Body as a whole: abdominal pain, diffuse pain, chest pain, radiation recall phenomenon

Cardiovascular: atrial fibrillation, deep vein thrombosis, ECG abnormalities, thrombophlebitis, pulmonary embolism, syncope, tachycardia, myocardial infarction

Digestive: constipation, duodenal ulcer, esophagitis, gastrointestinal hemorrhage, intestinal obstruction, ileus, gastrointestinal perforation, neutropenic enterocolitis, dehydration in relation to digestive disorders

Nervous: confusion, seizures

Respiratory: dyspnea, acute pulmonary edema, acute respiratory distress syndrome, interstitial pneumonia

Urogenital: renal insufficiency

OVERDOSAGE

There is no known antidote for TAXOTERE overdosage. In case of overdosage, the patient should be kept in a specialized unit where vital functions can be closely monitored. Anticipated complications of overdosage include: bone marrow suppression, peripheral neurotoxicity, and mucositis.

There were two reports of overdose. One patient received 150 mg/m^2 and the other received 200 mg/m^2 as 1-hour infusions. Both patients experienced severe neutropenia, mild asthenia, cutaneous reactions, and mild paresthesia, and recovered without incident.

In mice, lethality was observed following single IV doses that were ≥ 154 mg/kg (about 4.5 times the recommended human dose on a mg/m^2 basis); neurotoxicity associated with paralysis, non-extension of hind limbs, and myelin degeneration was observed in mice at 48 mg/kg (about 1.5 times the recommended human dose on a mg/m^2 basis). In male and female rats, lethality was observed at a dose of 20 mg/kg (comparable to the recommended human dose on a mg/m^2 basis) and was associated with abnormal mitosis and necrosis of multiple organs.

DOSAGE AND ADMINISTRATION

The recommended dose of TAXOTERE is 60–100 mg/m^2 administered intravenously over 1 hour every 3 weeks.

Premedication Regimen: All patients should be premedicated with oral corticosteroids such as dexamethasone 16 mg per day (e.g., 8 mg BID) for 3 days starting 1 day prior to TAXOTERE administration in order to reduce the

Summary of Adverse Events in Patients Receiving TAXOTERE at 100 mg/m²

Adverse Event	All Tumor Types Normal LFTs* n=2045 %	All Tumor Types Elevated LFTs** n=61 %	Breast Cancer Normal LFTs* n=965 %
Hematologic			
Neutropenia			
<2000 cells/mm³	95.5	96.4	98.5
<500 cells/mm³	75.4	87.5	85.9
Leukopenia			
<4000 cells/mm³	95.6	98.3	98.6
<1000 cells/mm³	31.6	46.6	43.7
Thrombocytopenia			
<100,000 cells/mm³	8.0	24.6	9.2
Anemia			
<11 g/dL	90.4	91.8	93.6
<8 g/dL	8.8	31.1	7.7
Febrile Neutropenia***	11.0	26.2	12.3
Septic Death	1.6	4.9	1.4
Non-Septic Death	0.6	6.6	0.6
Infections			
Any	21.6	32.8	22.2
Severe	6.1	16.4	6.4
Fever in Absence of Infection			
Any	31.2	41.0	35.1
Severe	2.1	8.2	2.2
Hypersensitivity Reactions			
Regardless of Premedication			
Any	21.0	19.7	17.6
Severe	4.2	9.8	2.6
With 3-day Premedication	n=92	n=3	n=92
Any	15.2	33.3	15.2
Severe	2.2	0	2.2
Fluid Retention			
Regardless of Premedication			
Any	47.0	39.3	59.7
Severe	6.9	8.2	8.9
With 3-day Premedication	n=92	n=3	n=92
Any	64.1	66.7	64.1
Severe	6.5	33.3	6.5
Neurosensory			
Any	49.3	34.4	58.3
Severe	4.3	0	5.5
Cutaneous			
Any	47.6	54.1	47.0
Severe	4.8	9.8	5.2
Nail Changes			
Any	30.6	23.0	40.5
Severe	2.5	4.9	3.7
Gastrointestinal			
Nausea	38.8	37.7	42.1
Vomiting	22.3	23.0	23.4
Diarrhea	38.7	32.8	42.6
Severe	4.7	4.9	5.5
Stomatitis			
Any	41.7	49.2	51.7
Severe	5.5	13.0	7.4
Alopecia	75.8	62.3	74.2
Asthenia			
Any	61.8	52.5	66.3
Severe	12.8	24.6	14.9
Myalgia			
Any	18.9	16.4	21.1
Severe	1.5	1.6	1.8
Arthralgia	9.2	6.6	8.2
Infusion Site Reactions	4.4	3.3	4.0

* **Normal Baseline LFTs:** Transaminases ≤ 1.5 times ULN or alkaline phosphatase ≤ 2.5 times ULN or isolated elevations of transaminases or alkaline phosphatase up to 5 times ULN

** **Elevated Baseline LFTs:** SGOT and/or SGPT >1.5 times ULN concurrent with alkaline phosphatase >2.5 times ULN

*** **Febrile Neutropenia:** ANC grade 4 with fever > 38°C with IV antibiotics and/or hospitalization

incidence and severity of fluid retention as well as the severity of hypersensitivity reactions (see **BOXED WARNING**, **WARNINGS**, and **PRECAUTIONS** sections).

Dosage Adjustments During Treatment: Patients who are dosed initially at 100 mg/m² and who experience either febrile neutropenia, neutrophils < 500 cells/mm³ for more than 1 week, severe or cumulative cutaneous reactions, or severe peripheral neuropathy during TAXOTERE therapy should have the dosage adjusted from 100 mg/m² to 75 mg/m². If the patient continues to experience these reactions, the dosage should either be decreased from 75 mg/m² to 55 mg/m² or the treatment should be discontinued. Conversely, patients who are dosed initially at 60 mg/m² and who do not experience febrile neutropenia, neutrophils <500 cells/mm³ for more than 1 week, severe or cumulative cutaneous reactions, or severe peripheral neuropathy during TAXOTERE therapy may tolerate higher doses.

Special Populations:

Hepatic Impairment: Patients with bilirubin > ULN should generally not receive TAXOTERE. Also, patients with SGOT and/or SGPT > 1.5 × ULN concomitant with alkaline phosphatase > 2.5 × ULN should generally not receive TAXOTERE.

Children: The safety and effectiveness of docetaxel in pediatric patients below the age of 16 years have not been established.

Elderly: No dosage adjustments are required for use in elderly.

PREPARATION AND ADMINISTRATION PRECAUTIONS

TAXOTERE is a cytotoxic anticancer drug and, as with other potentially toxic compounds, caution should be exercised when handling and preparing TAXOTERE solutions. The use of gloves is recommended. Please refer to **Handling and Disposal** section.

If TAXOTERE concentrate, premix solution, or infusion solution should come into contact with the skin, immediately and thoroughly wash with soap and water. If TAXOTERE concentrate, premix solution, or infusion solution should come into contact with mucosa, immediately and thoroughly wash with water.

TAXOTERE for Injection Concentrate requires dilution prior to administration. Please follow the preparation instructions provided below. Note: Both the TAXOTERE for Injection Concentrate and the diluent vials contain an overfill.

A. Preparation of the Premix Solution

1. Remove the appropriate number of vials of TAXOTERE for Injection Concentrate and diluent from the refrigerator. Allow the vials to stand at room temperature for approximately 5 minutes.
2. Aseptically withdraw the entire contents of the diluent vial into a syringe and transfer it to the vial of TAXOTERE for Injection Concentrate.

Information regarding fill volumes is listed below:

Strength	Vial Content	Diluent Vial
TAXOTERE 20 mg	23.6 mg/0.59 mL	1.83 mL
TAXOTERE 80 mg	94.4 mg/2.36 mL	7.33 mL

This will assure a final premix concentration of 10 mg docetaxel/mL

3. Gently rotate each premix solution vial for approximately 15 seconds to assure full mixture of the concentrate and diluent.
4. The TAXOTERE premix solution (10 mg docetaxel/mL) should be clear; however, there may be some foam on top of the solution due to the polysorbate 80. Allow the premix solution to stand for a few minutes to allow any foam to dissipate. It is not required that all foam dissipate prior to continuing the preparation process.

B. Preparation of the Infusion Solution

1. Aseptically withdraw the required amount of TAXOTERE premix solution (10 mg docetaxel/mL) with a calibrated syringe and inject the required volume of premix solution into a 250 mL infusion bag or bottle of either 0.9% Sodium Chloride solution or 5% Dextrose solution to produce a final concentration of 0.3 to 0.9 mg/mL.

If a dose greater than 240 mg of TAXOTERE is required, use a larger volume of the infusion vehicle so that a concentration of 0.9 mg/mL TAXOTERE is not exceeded.

2. Thoroughly mix the infusion by manual rotation.
3. As with all parenteral products, TAXOTERE should be inspected visually for particulate matter or discoloration prior to administration whenever the solution and container permit. If the TAXOTERE for Injection premix solution or infusion solution is not clear or appears to have precipitation, the solution should be discarded.

TAXOTERE infusion solution should be administered intravenously as a 1-hour infusion under ambient room temperature and lighting conditions.

Contact of the undiluted concentrate with plasticized PVC equipment or devices used to prepare solutions for infusion is not recommended. In order to minimize patient exposure to the plasticizer DEHP (di-2-ethylhexyl phthalate), which may be leached from PVC infusion bags or sets, diluted

Continued on next page

Taxotere—Cont.

TAXOTERE solution should be stored in bottles (glass, polypropylene) or plastic bags (polypropylene, polyolefin) and administered through polyethylene-lined administration sets.

Stability: Unopened vials of TAXOTERE are stable until the expiration date indicated on the package when stored refrigerated, 2° to 8° C (36° to 46° F), and protected from bright light. Freezing does not adversely affect the product.

HOW SUPPLIED

TAXOTERE for Injection Concentrate is supplied in a single-dose vial as a sterile, pyrogen-free, non-aqueous, viscous solution with an accompanying sterile, non-pyrogenic, diluent (13% ethanol in Water for Injection) vial. The following strengths are available:

TAXOTERE 80 MG   **(NDC 0075-8001-80)**
TAXOTERE (docetaxel) 80 mg Concentrate for Infusion: 80 mg docetaxel in 2 mL polysorbate 80 (Fill: 94.4 mg docetaxel in 2.36 mL polysorbate 80) and diluent for TAXOTERE 80 mg. 13% (w/w) ethanol in Water for Injection (Fill: 7.33 mL). Both items are in a blister pack in one carton.

TAXOTERE 20 MG   **(NDC 0075-8001-20)**
TAXOTERE (docetaxel) 20 mg Concentrate for Infusion: 20 mg docetaxel in 0.5 mL polysorbate 80 (Fill: 23.6 mg docetaxel in 0.59 mL polysorbate 80) and diluent for TAXOTERE 20 mg. 13% (w/w) ethanol in Water for Injection (Fill: 1.83 mL). Both items are in a blister pack in one carton.

Storage: Store refrigerated, 2° to 8° C (36° to 46° F). Retain in the original package to protect from bright light.

TAXOTERE premix solution (10 mg TAXOTERE/mL) and fully prepared TAXOTERE infusion solution (in either 0.9% Sodium Chloride solution or 5% Dextrose solution) should be used as soon as possible after preparation. However, the premix solution is stable for 8 hours either at room temperature, 15° to 25° C (59° to 77° F), or stored refrigerated, 2° to 8° C (36° to 46° F).

Handling and Disposal: Procedures for proper handling and disposal of anticancer drugs should be considered. Several guidelines on this subject have been published[1-8]. There is no general agreement that all of the procedures recommended in the guidelines are necessary or appropriate.

REFERENCES

1. OSHA Work-Practice Guidelines for Personnel Dealing with Cytotoxic (Antineoplastic) Drugs. *Am J Hosp Pharm.* 1986; 43(5): 1193-1204.
2. American Society of Hospital Pharmacists Technical Assistance Bulletin on Handling Cytotoxic and Hazardous Drugs. *Am J Hosp Pharm.* 1990; 47(95): 1033-1049.
3. AMA Council Report. Guidelines for Handling Parenteral Antineoplastics. *JAMA* 1985; 253 (11): 1590-1592.
4. Oncology Nursing Society Clinical Practice Committee. Cancer Chemotherapy Guidelines. Module II - Recommendations of Nursing Practice in the Acute Care Setting. *ONS* 1988; 2-14.
5. Recommendations for the Safe Handling of Parenteral Antineoplastic Drugs. NIH Publication No. 83-2621. For sale by the Superintendent of Documents, US Government Printing Office, Washington, DC 20402.
6. National Study Commission on Cytotoxic Exposure - Recommendations for Handling Cytotoxic Agents. Available from Louis P. Jeffry, Chairman, National Study Commission on Cytotoxic Exposure. Massachusetts College of Pharmacy and Allied Health Sciences, 179 Longwood Avenue, Boston, MA 02115.
7. Clinical Oncological Society of Australia. Guidelines and Recommendations for Safe Handling of Antineoplastic Agents. *Med J Austr.* 1983; 426-428.
8. Jones, RB, et al. Safe Handling of Chemotherapeutic Agents: A Report from the Mt. Sinai Medical Center. *CA-A Cancer Journal for Clinicians* 1983; Sept/Oct: 258-263.

RHÔNE-POULENC RORER PHARMACEUTICALS INC.
COLLEGEVILLE, PA 19426
IN-5493D   Rev. 7/98
Shown in Product Identification Guide, page 333

TILADE® INHALER   ℞
[tī lādĕ]
(NEDOCROMIL SODIUM INHALATION AEROSOL)

DESCRIPTION

Tilade (nedocromil sodium) is an inhaled anti-inflammatory agent for the preventive management of asthma. Nedocromil sodium is a pyranoquinoline with the chemical name 4H-Pyrano[3,2-g]quinoline-2,8-dicarboxylic acid, 9-ethyl-6,9-dihydro-4,6-dioxo-10-propyl-, disodium salt, and it has a

molecular weight of 415.3. The empirical formula is $C_{19}H_{15}NNa_2O_7$. Nedocromil sodium, a yellow powder, is soluble in water.

The molecular structure of nedocromil sodium is:

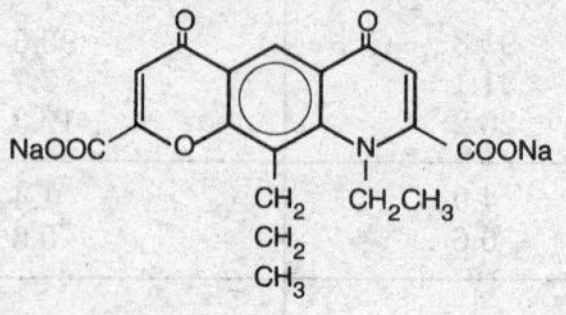

$NaOOC$ ... $COONa$
CH_2
CH_2CH_3
CH_2
CH_3

Chemical Class: Pyranoquinoline

Tilade Inhaler (nedocromil sodium inhalation aerosol) is a pressurized metered-dose aerosol suspension for oral inhalation containing micronized nedocromil sodium and sorbitan trioleate, as well as dichlorotetrafluoroethane and dichlorodifluoromethane as propellants. Each **Tilade** canister contains 210 mg nedocromil sodium. Each actuation meters 2.00 mg nedocromil sodium from the valve and delivers 1.75 mg nedocromil sodium from the mouthpiece. Each 16.2 g canister provides at least 104 metered actuations. **After 104 metered actuations, the amount delivered per actuation may not be consistent and the unit should be discarded.** Each **Tilade** Inhaler canister must be primed with 3 actuations prior to the first use. If a canister remains unused for more than 7 days, then it should be reprimed with 3 actuations.

CLINICAL PHARMACOLOGY

General: Nedocromil sodium has been shown to inhibit the *in vitro* activation of, and mediator release from, a variety of inflammatory cell types associated with asthma, including eosinophils, neutrophils, macrophages, mast cells, monocytes, and platelets. *In vitro* studies on cells obtained by bronchoalveolar lavage from antigen-sensitized macaque monkeys show that nedocromil sodium inhibits the release of mediators including histamine, leukotriene C_4, and prostaglandin D_2. Similar studies with human bronchoalveolar cells showed inhibition of histamine release from mast cells and beta-glucuronidase release from macrophages.

Nedocromil sodium has been tested in experimental models of asthma using allergic animals and shown to inhibit the development of early and late bronchoconstriction responses to inhaled antigen. The development of airway hyper-responsiveness to nonspecific bronchoconstrictors was also inhibited. Nedocromil sodium reduced antigen-induced increases in airway microvasculature leakage when administered intravenously in a model system.

In humans, nedocromil sodium has been shown to inhibit acutely the bronchoconstrictor response to several kinds of challenge. Pretreatment with single doses of nedocromil sodium inhibited the bronchoconstriction caused by sulfur dioxide, inhaled neurokinin A, various antigens, exercise, cold air, fog, and adenosine monophosphate.

Nedocromil sodium has no bronchodilator, antihistamine, or corticosteroid activity.

Nedocromil sodium, when delivered by inhalation at the recommended dose, has no known systemic activity.

Pharmacokinetics and Bioavailability: Systemic bioavailability of nedocromil sodium administered as an inhaled aerosol is low. In a single dose study involving 20 healthy adult subjects who were administered a 3.5 mg dose of nedocromil sodium (2 actuations of 1.75 mg each), the mean AUC was 5.0 ng-hr/mL and the mean C_{max} was 1.6 ng/mL attained about 28 minutes after dosing. The mean half-life was 3.3 hours. Urinary excretion over 12 hours averaged 3.4% of the administered dose, of which approximately 75% was excreted in the first six hours of dosing.

In a multiple dose study, six healthy adult volunteers (3 males and 3 females) received a 3.5 mg single dose followed by 3.5 mg four times a day for seven consecutive days. Accumulation of the drug was not observed. Following single and multiple dose inhalations, urinary excretion of nedocromil accounted for 5.6% and 12% of the drug administered, respectively. After intravenous administration to healthy adults, urinary excretion of nedocromil was approximately 70%. The absolute bioavailability of nedocromil was thus 8% (5.6/70) for single and 17% (12/70) for multiple inhaled doses.

Similarly, in a multiple dose study of 12 asthmatic adult patients, each given a 3.5 mg single dose followed by 3.5 mg four times a day for one month, both single dose and multiple dose inhalations gave a mean high plasma concentration of 2.8 ng/mL between 5 and 90 minutes, mean AUC of 5.6 ng-hr/mL, and a mean terminal half-life of 1.5 hours. The mean 24-hour urinary excretion after either single or multiple dose administration represented approximately 5% of the administered dose.

Studies involving very high oral doses of nedocromil (600 mg single dose, and subsequently 200 mg three times a day for seven days) showed an absolute bioavailability of less than 2%. In a radiolabeled (^{14}C) nedocromil intravenous study involving two healthy adult males, urinary excretion accounted for 64% of the dose, fecal excretion for 36%.

Although minimal pharmacokinetic data are available in children between the ages of 6 and 11 years, the nedocromil sodium levels obtained at 1 hour after chronic dosing in this age group appear to be similar to those observed in adults.

Protein Binding: Nedocromil is approximately 89% protein bound in human plasma over a concentration range of 0.5 to 50 µg/mL. This binding is reversible.

Metabolism: Nedocromil is not metabolized after IV administration and is excreted unchanged.

CLINICAL STUDIES

The worldwide clinical trial experience with **Tilade** comprises 6,469 patients, including 993 pediatric patients 6 through 11 years of age. Studies have been conducted both at twice daily and at four times daily dosage regimens. Evidence from these studies indicates that the four times daily regimen has been more effective than the twice daily regimen. Less frequent administration can be considered in patients under good control on the four times daily regimen. (See **DOSAGE AND ADMINISTRATION**.)

Adult Studies: *Tilade vs. Placebo:* The effectiveness of **Tilade** given four times daily was examined in a 14-week, double-blind, placebo-controlled, parallel-group trial in five centers in 120 patients (60/treatment). To be eligible for entry, the asthmatic patients had to be controlled using only sustained-release theophylline (SRT) and beta$_2$-agonists. Two weeks after the test therapies were begun the SRT was discontinued and four weeks after that oral beta$_2$-agonists were stopped. Beta$_2$-agonist metered dose inhalers could still be used after 6 weeks. Efficacy was assessed by symptom scores recorded on diary cards completed on a daily basis by the patients. Each morning the patient recorded nighttime asthma on a 0-2 scale, (0=slept well, no asthma; 1=woke once because of asthma; 2=woke more than once because of asthma). Before bedtime the patients recorded daytime asthma and cough on a 0-5 scale (0=no symptoms of asthma/cough today; 5=asthma/cough symptoms were noticed most of the day and caused a lot of trouble). At the end of the treatment phase, patients and clinicians were asked for their opinions on the effectiveness of the treatment based on a five point scale (1=very effective; 5=made condition worse). The results of these evaluations are shown in Table 1; **Tilade** was significantly superior to placebo for all measurements.

[See table 1 above]

The FEV$_1$ percentage change relative to baseline is shown in Figure 1; these also favored **Tilade** over placebo throughout the study, with an effect seen first at the two week measurement.

Table 1

Variable	Time Period	Tilade Mean	Placebo Mean
Daytime Asthma[1]	Weeks 7–14	1.26	2.08
Nighttime Asthma[2]	Weeks 7–14	0.67	0.96
Cough[1]	Weeks 7–14	0.68	1.49
Patient's Opinion[2]	Week 14	2.27	3.55
Clinician's Opinion[2]	Week 14	2.13	3.48
FEV$_1$[2] (liters)	Week 2	2.69	2.18
FEV$_1$[2] (liters)	Week 6	2.65	2.15
FEV$_1$[2] (liters)	Week 10	2.55	2.15
FEV$_1$[2] (liters)	Week 14	2.59	2.10

[1]**Tilade** significantly better than Placebo, $p<0.05$.
[2]**Tilade** significantly better than Placebo, $p<0.01$.

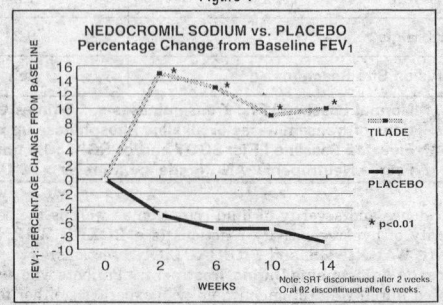

Figure 1

NEDOCROMIL SODIUM vs. PLACEBO
Percentage Change from Baseline FEV$_1$

TILADE
PLACEBO
* p<0.01

WEEKS

Note: SRT discontinued after 2 weeks.
Oral B2 discontinued after 6 weeks.

This study shows that **Tilade** improves symptom control and pulmonary function when it is added to an as-needed inhaled beta$_2$-adrenergic bronchodilator regimen and that a beneficial effect could be detected within two weeks.

Tilade vs. Cromolyn Sodium vs. Placebo: The effectiveness of **Tilade** was compared to cromolyn sodium and placebo in an eight-week, double-blind, parallel-group, 12-center trial during which medication was given four times daily. Three hundred and six patients were randomized to treatment (103/**Tilade**; 104/cromolyn sodium; 99/placebo). All patients were SRT dependent and this drug was stopped prior to starting the test treatment. Efficacy was assessed on the basis of diary card symptom scores and FEV$_1$. The diary scores were the same as used in the 14-week study except that nighttime symptoms were recorded on a 0–3 scale. The primary efficacy variable was a summary symptom score derived by averaging the scores for daytime asthma, nighttime asthma, and cough. The results of the study are shown in Table 2.

[See table 2 above]

This study corroborates the findings of the 14-week study, showing that **Tilade** is effective in the management of symptoms and pulmonary function in primarily atopic mild to moderate asthmatics. Both active treatments were statistically significantly better than placebo for the primary efficacy variable (summary symptom score); **Tilade** and cromolyn sodium were not significantly different for this parameter. A statistically significant difference favoring cromolyn sodium was, however, seen for nighttime asthma and FEV$_1$.

In allergic asthmatics who are well controlled on cromolyn sodium, there is no evidence that the substitution of **Tilade** for cromolyn sodium would confer additional benefit to the patient.

Available data on the relative efficacy of **Tilade** and cromolyn sodium are inconclusive and efficacy with one agent is not known to be predictive of efficacy with the other.

Pediatric Studies: *Tilade vs. Placebo in Pediatric Patients:* The effectiveness of **Tilade** in minimizing the anticipated seasonal increase in asthmatic symptoms in pediatric patients 6 through 11 years of age with mild seasonal ragweed-induced asthma was examined in an eight-week, double-blind, placebo-controlled, parallel-group trial in nine centers in 146 patients (75/**Tilade**; 71/placebo). These patients had a mean baseline FEV$_1$ that was 85% of predicted normal and a mean baseline beta$_2$-agonist requirement of less than 2 inhalations of albuterol from a metered dose inhaler per day. Study medication was given four times a day. Efficacy was assessed on the basis of diary card symptom scores (daytime asthma, sleep disturbance, daytime cough, and morning asthma, all rated on a six point scale: 0=no symptoms; 5=severe symptoms) and as-needed bronchodilator use. The primary efficacy variable was based on both the summary symptom score (total of daytime asthma, daytime cough, and sleep disturbance) and as-needed bronchodilator usage. At the end of the treatment phase, parents and clinicians assessed treatment effectiveness on a five point scale: 1=very effective; 5=made condition worse. After a two week baseline, patients were randomized to eight weeks of double-blind treatment. The results of these evaluations are shown in Table 3.

[See table 3 above]

The percentage change from baseline in summary symptom score by week is shown in Figure 2.

Table 2

Variable	Time Period	Tilade Mean	Placebo Mean	Cromolyn Sodium Mean
Summary Score[1]	Weeks 3–8	1.30	1.76	1.13
Daytime Asthma[1]	Weeks 3–8	1.59	2.05	1.41
Nighttime Asthma[2]	Weeks 3–8	0.91	1.23	0.77
Cough[3]	Weeks 3–8	1.11	1.58	0.93
FEV$_1$[2]	Weeks 3–8	2.46	2.23	2.56
Patient's Opinion[1]	Week 8	2.54	3.39	2.22
Clinician's Opinion[1]	Week 8	2.60	3.43	2.39

[1] **Tilade** significantly better than Placebo, $p<0.001$
[2] **Tilade** significantly better than Placebo, $p<0.01$, cromolyn sodium significantly better than **Tilade**, $p<0.05$
[3] **Tilade** significantly better than Placebo, $p<0.05$

Table 3
Comparison of Scores for Tilade and Placebo During the Primary Time Period of Evaluation

Variable	Time Period	Tilade Mean	Vehicle Placebo Mean
Summary Symptom Score[1,3,4]	Weeks 3–8	1.38	1.99
Bronchodilator Use[2,3,4]	Weeks 3–8	0.43	0.84
Parent's Opinion[4]	Week 8	2.13	2.75
Clinician's Opinion[4]	Week 8	2.16	2.74

[1] Daytime asthma, daytime cough, and sleep disturbance due to asthma (0–15)
[2] One unit for every two inhalations
[3] Adjusted for baseline
[4] **Tilade** significantly better than Placebo, $p<0.05$

ADVERSE EVENT (AE)	% Experiencing AE		% Withdrawing	
	Tilade (N=2632)	Placebo (N=2402)	Tilade	Placebo
Special Senses				
Unpleasant Taste*	11.6%	3.1%	1.6%	0.0%
Respiratory System Disorders				
Coughing	8.9%	10.2%	1.1%	1.2%
Pharyngitis	7.6%	7.5%	0.5%	0.4%
Rhinitis*	7.3%	6.0%	0.1%	0.1%
Upper Respiratory Infection	6.7%	6.3%	0.1%	0.2%
Sputum Increased	1.5%	1.4%	0.1%	0.2%
Bronchitis	1.1%	1.5%	0.1%	0.1%
Dyspnea	2.5%	3.3%	0.8%	1.0%
Bronchospasm**	8.4%	11.8%	1.4%	2.0%
Sinusitis	3.3%	4.1%	1.1%	0.0%
Respiratory Disorder	0.8%	1.1%	0.0%	0.0%
Gastrointestinal Tract				
Nausea*	3.9%	2.3%	1.1%	0.5%
Vomiting*	2.5%	1.6%	0.2%	0.3%
Dyspepsia	1.5%	1.1%	0.1%	0.1%
Diarrhea	1.3%	1.2%	0.1%	0.0%
Abdominal Pain*	1.9%	1.3%	0.2%	0.1%
Central and Peripheral Nervous System				
Dizziness	0.8%	1.3%	0.1%	0.2%
Body as a Whole				
Headache	8.1%	7.5%	0.4%	0.2%
Chest Pain	3.6%	3.8%	0.7%	0.5%
Fatigue	1.0%	0.8%	0.2%	0.0%
Fever	3.1%	3.7%	0.1%	0.1%
Resistance Mechanism Disorders				
Infection Viral	2.4%	3.2%	0.1%	0.1%
Vision Disorders				
Conjunctivitis	1.1%	0.7%	0.0%	0.1%
Skin and Appendages Disorders				
Rash**	0.5%	1.2%	0.1%	0.0%

* Statistically significant higher frequency on **Tilade**, $p<0.05$
**Statistically significant higher frequency on Placebo, $p<0.05$

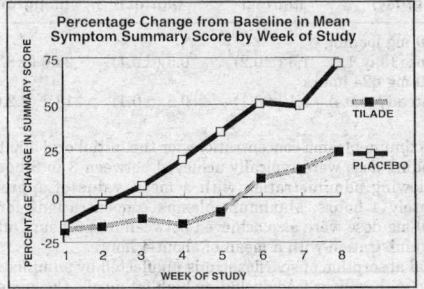

Figure 2

Percentage Change from Baseline in Mean Symptom Summary Score by Week of Study

TILADE
PLACEBO

(y-axis: PERCENTAGE CHANGE IN SUMMARY SCORE; x-axis: WEEK OF STUDY)

This study shows that **Tilade**, when used prophylactically in asthmatics with known seasonal exacerbations, can attenuate an increase in symptoms of asthma and reduce the need for rescue bronchodilator treatment.

INDICATIONS AND USAGE

Tilade Inhaler is indicated for maintenance therapy in the management of adult and pediatric patients 6 years and older with mild to moderate asthma.

Tilade is not indicated for the reversal of acute bronchospasm.

CONTRAINDICATIONS

Tilade Inhaler is contraindicated in patients who have shown hypersensitivity to nedocromil sodium or other ingredients in this preparation.

WARNINGS

Tilade® Inhaler (nedocromil sodium inhalation aerosol) is not a bronchodilator and, therefore, should not be used for the reversal of acute bronchospasm, particularly status asthmaticus. **Tilade** should ordinarily be continued during acute exacerbations, unless the patient becomes intolerant to the use of inhaled dosage forms.

As with other inhaled asthma medications, bronchospasm, which can be life-threatening, may occur immediately after administration. If this occurs, **Tilade** should be discontinued and alternative therapy instituted.

PRECAUTIONS

General: The role of **Tilade** as a corticosteroid-sparing agent in patients receiving oral or inhaled corticosteroids remains to be defined. If systemic or inhaled corticosteroid therapy is reduced in patients receiving **Tilade**, careful monitoring is necessary.

Information for Patients:
Patients should be told that:

- **Tilade** must be taken regularly to achieve benefit, even during symptom-free periods.
- **Tilade** is not meant to relieve acute asthma symptoms. If symptoms do not improve or the patient's condition worsens, the patient should not increase the dosage but should notify the physician immediately.
- They should not decrease the dose without the physician's knowledge. The recommended dose should not be exceeded.
- The full therapeutic effect of **Tilade** may not be obtained for 1 week or longer after initiating treatment.
- Because the therapeutic effect depends upon local delivery to the lungs, it is essential that patients be properly instructed in the correct method of use (see Patient Instructions for Use).
- An illustrated leaflet for the patient is included in each **Tilade** Inhaler pack.

Drug Interactions: In clinical studies, **Tilade** has been co-administered with other anti-asthma medications, including inhaled and oral bronchodilators, and inhaled corticosteroids, with no evidence of increased frequency of adverse events or laboratory abnormalities. No formal drug-drug interaction studies, however, have been conducted.

Continued on next page

Tilade—Cont.

Carcinogenesis, Mutagenesis, Impairment of Fertility: A two-year inhalation carcinogenicity study of nedocromil sodium at a dose of 24 mg/kg/day (approximately 8 times the maximum recommended human daily inhalation dose on a mg/m^2 basis) in Wistar rats showed no carcinogenic potential. A 21-month oral dietary carcinogenicity study of nedocromil sodium performed in B6C3F1 mice with doses up to 180 mg/kg/day (approximately 30 times the maximum recommended human daily inhalation dose on a mg/m^2 basis) showed no carcinogenic potential.
Nedocromil sodium showed no mutagenic potential in the Ames Salmonella/microsome plate assay, mitotic gene conversion in *Saccharomyces cerevisiae*, mouse lymphoma forward mutation, and mouse micronucleus assays.
Reproduction and fertility studies in mice and rats showed no effects on male and female fertility at a subcutaneous dose of 100 mg/kg/day (approximately 30 times and 60 times respectively, the maximum recommended human daily inhalation dose on a mg/m^2 basis).
Pregnancy: *Pregnancy Category B*. Reproduction studies performed in mice, rats, and rabbits using a subcutaneous dose of 100 mg/kg/day (approximately 30 times, 60 times, and 116 times, respectively, the maximum recommended human daily inhalation dose on a mg/m^2 basis) revealed no evidence of teratogenicity or harm to the fetus due to nedocromil sodium. There are, however, no adequate and well-controlled studies in pregnant women. Because animal reproduction studies are not always predictive of human response, this drug should be used during pregnancy only if clearly needed.
Nursing Mothers: It is not known whether this drug is excreted in human milk. Because many drugs are excreted in human milk, caution should be exercised when **Tilade** is administered to a nursing woman.
Pediatric Use: Safety data in normal volunteers and asthmatic patients between the ages of 6 and 11 years are available on a total of 311 children from U.S. clinical trials and 192 children from foreign clinical trials (total = 503) of 4–12 weeks duration. An additional 225 children received **Tilade** for 40 weeks and 24 received **Tilade** for 52 weeks.
The safety and effectiveness of **Tilade** in children ages 6 through 11 have been established in adequate and well-controlled clinical trials. (See **CLINICAL STUDIES**: **Pediatric Studies**.) Use of **Tilade** in children ages 6 through 11 years is also supported by evidence from adequate and well-controlled studies of **Tilade** in adults.
The safety and effectiveness of **Tilade** in patients below the age of 6 years have not been established.

ADVERSE REACTIONS

Tilade is generally well tolerated. Adverse event information was derived from 6,469 patients receiving **Tilade** in controlled and open-label clinical trials of 1–52 weeks in duration. A total of 4,400 patients received two inhalations four times a day. An additional 2,069 patients received two inhalations twice daily or another dose regimen. Seventy-seven percent of patients were treated with **Tilade** for eight weeks or longer.
Of the 4,400 patients who received two inhalations of **Tilade** four times a day, 2,632 were in placebo-controlled, parallel trials and of these 6.0% withdrew from the trials due to adverse events, compared to 5.7% of the 2,446 patients who received placebo.
The reasons for withdrawal were generally similar in the **Tilade** and placebo-treated groups, except that patients withdrew due to bad taste statistically more frequently on **Tilade** than on placebo. Headache reported as severe or very severe, some with nausea and ill feeling, was experienced by 1.0% of **Tilade** patients and 0.7% of placebo patients.
The events reported with a frequency of 1% or greater across all placebo-controlled studies are displayed for all patients ages 6 years and older who received **Tilade** or placebo at two inhalations four times daily.
The adverse event profile observed in children ages 6 through 11 was similar to that observed in adults.
[See third table from top on previous page]
Other adverse events present at less than the 1% level of occurrence, but that might be related to **Tilade** administration, include arthritis, tremor, and a sensation of warmth.
In clinical trials with 2,632 patients receiving **Tilade**, 2 patients (0.08%) developed neutropenia and 3 patients (0.11%) developed leukopenia. Although it is unclear if these reactions were caused by **Tilade**, in several cases these abnormal laboratory tests returned to normal when **Tilade** was discontinued.
There have been reports of clinically significant elevation of hepatic transaminases (ALT and AST greater than 10 times the upper limit of the normal reference range in one patient) associated with the administration of **Tilade**. It is unclear if these abnormal laboratory tests in asymptomatic patients were caused by **Tilade**.
Cases of bronchospasm immediately following dosing with **Tilade** have been reported from postmarketing experience. (See **WARNINGS**.) Isolated cases of pneumonitis with eosinophilia (PIE syndrome) and anaphylaxis have also been reported in which a relationship to drug is undetermined.

OVERDOSAGE

There is no experience to date with overdose of **Tilade** in humans. There were no deaths in rodents at an oral dose of 4,000 mg/kg (approximately 690 times [for mice] and 1,370 times [for rats] the maximum recommended human daily inhalation dose on a mg/m^2 basis). The subcutaneous or intravenous lethal dose in rats was between 2,000 and 4,000 mg/kg (approximately 690 and 1,370 times, respectively, the maximum recommended human daily inhalation dose on a mg/m^2 basis). No deaths occurred in mice at a subcutaneous dose of 4,000 mg/kg (approximately 690 times the maximum recommended human daily inhalation dose on a mg/m^2 basis), and the intravenous lethal dose in mice was between 2,000 and 4,000 mg/kg (approximately 345 and 690 times, respectively, the maximum recommended human daily inhalation dose on a mg/m^2 basis). An intravenous dose of 240 mg/kg (approximately 110 times the maximum recommended human daily inhalation dose on a mg/m^2 basis) did not produce any deaths in cats. Head shaking/tremor and salivation were observed in beagle dogs following daily inhalation doses of 5 mg/kg (approximately 6 times the maximum recommended human daily inhalation dose on a mg/m^2 basis) and transient hypotension was detected following daily subcutaneous doses of 8 mg/kg (approximately 9 times the maximum recommended human daily inhalation dose on a mg/m^2 basis). In addition, clonic convulsions were observed in dogs following daily inhalation doses of 20 mg/kg plus subcutaneous doses of 20 mg/kg giving peak plasma nedocromil levels of 7.6 µg/mL, some three orders of magnitude greater than peak plasma levels (2.5 ng/mL) of the maximum recommended human daily inhalation dose. Specific tests designed to evaluate CNS activity demonstrated no effects due to nedocromil sodium, and nedocromil sodium does not pass the blood brain barrier. Therefore, overdosage is unlikely to result in clinical manifestations requiring more than observation and discontinuation of the drug where appropriate.

DOSAGE AND ADMINISTRATION

The recommended dosage for adult and pediatric patients 6 years of age and older is two inhalations four times a day at regular intervals, which provides a dose of 14 mg per day. In patients whose asthma is well controlled on this dosage (*e.g.*, patients who only need occasional inhaled or oral $beta_2$-agonists and who are not experiencing serious exacerbations), less frequent administration may be effective.
Each **Tilade** Inhaler canister must be primed with 3 actuations prior to the first use. If a canister remains unused for more than 7 days, then it should be reprimed with 3 actuations.
Tilade Inhaler may be added to the patient's existing treatment regimen (*e.g.*, bronchodilators). When a clinical response to **Tilade** Inhaler is evident and if the patient's asthma is under good control, an attempt may be made to decrease concomitant medication usage gradually.
Proper inhalational technique is essential (see Patient Instructions for Use).
Patients should be advised that the optimal effect of **Tilade** therapy depends upon its administration at regular intervals, even during symptom-free periods.

HOW SUPPLIED

Tilade Inhaler is available in 16.2 g canisters providing at least 104 metered inhalations. Each **Tilade** canister contains 210 mg nedocromil sodium. Each pack is supplied with patient instructions, a tan-colored rubber valve cover, and white plastic mouthpiece and cover, bearing the **Tilade** logo. The **Tilade** mouthpiece should not be used with other aerosol medications and the **Tilade** canister should not be used with other mouthpieces. Each actuation meters 2.00 mg nedocromil sodium from the valve and delivers 1.75 mg nedocromil sodium from the mouthpiece.

NDC 0585-0685-02 One 16.2 g Canister (104 Metered Inhalations)

The canister should be discarded after the labeled number of actuations have been used. The amount of medication in each actuation cannot be assured after this point.
Store between 2 to 30°C (36 to 86°F). Do not freeze. **Avoid spraying in eyes.** Contents under pressure. Do not puncture, incinerate, place near sources of heat, or use with other mouthpieces. Exposure to temperatures above 120°F may cause bursting. Never throw canister into fire or incinerator. **Keep out of the reach of children.** For best results, the canister should be at room temperature before use. Shake well before using.
Note: The indented statement below is required by the Federal government's Clean Air Act for all products containing or manufactured with chlorofluorocarbons (CFCs).

> WARNING: Contains CFC-12 and CFC-114, substances which harm public health and the environment by destroying ozone in the upper atmosphere.

A notice similar to the above WARNING has been placed in the "Patient Instructions for Use" portion of this package insert under the Environmental Protection Agency's (EPA's) regulations. The patient's warning states that the patient should consult his or her physician if there are questions about alternatives.
Caution: Federal law prohibits dispensing without prescription.

RHÔNE-POULENC RORER RESPIRATORY
A division of Rhône-Poulenc Rorer Pharmaceuticals Inc.
Collegeville, PA 19426
© 1998
Made in England
Rev. 4/98
IN-0032B
Shown in Product Identification Guide, page 334

ZAGAM® ℞
(sparfloxacin) Tablets

DESCRIPTION

Zagam® (sparfloxacin) tablets contain sparfloxacin, a synthetic broad-spectrum antimicrobial agent for oral administration. Sparfloxacin, an aminodifluoroquinolone, is 5-Amino-1-cyclopropyl-7-(*cis*-3,5-dimethyl-1-piperazinyl)-6,8-difluoro-1,4-dihydro-4-oxo-3-quinolinecarboxylic acid. Its empirical formula is $C_{19}H_{22}F_2N_4O_3$ and it has the following chemical structure:

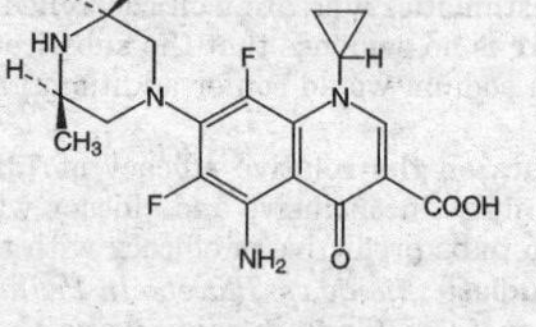

Sparfloxacin has a molecular weight of 392.41. It occurs as a yellow crystalline powder. It is sparingly soluble in glacial acetic acid or chloroform, very slightly soluble in ethanol (95%), and practically insoluble in water and ether. It dissolves in dilute acetic acid or 0.1 N sodium hydroxide.
Zagam is available as a 200-mg round, white film-coated tablet. Each 200-mg tablet contains the following inactive ingredients: microcrystalline cellulose NF, corn starch NF, L-hydroxypropylcellulose NF, magnesium stearate NF, and colloidal silicone dioxide NF. The film coating contains: methylhydroxypropylcellulose USP, polyethylene glycol 6000, and titanium dioxide USP.

CLINICAL PHARMACOLOGY

Absorption: Sparfloxacin is well absorbed following oral administration with an absolute oral bioavailability of 92%. The mean maximum plasma sparfloxacin concentration following a single 400-mg oral dose was approximately 1.3 (±0.2) µg/mL. The area under the curve (mean $AUC_{0\to\infty}$) following a single 400-mg oral dose was approximately 34 (±6.8) µg•hr/mL.
Steady-state plasma concentration was achieved on the first day by giving a loading dose that was double the daily dose. Mean (±SD) pharmacokinetic parameters observed for the 24-hour dosing interval with the recommended dosing regimen are shown below:

Dosing Regimen (mg/day)	Peak Cmax (µg/mL)	Trough C_{24} (µg/mL)	AUC $_{0\to24}$ hr. µg/mL
400 mg loading dose (day 1)	1.3 (±0.2)	0.5 (±0.1)	20.6 (±3.1)
200 mg q24 hours (steady-state)	1.1 (±0.1)	0.5 (±0.1)	18.7 (±2.6)

Maximum plasma concentrations for the initial oral 400-mg loading dose were typically achieved between 3 to 6 hours following administration with a mean value of approximately 4 hours. Maximum plasma concentrations for a 200-mg dose were also achieved between 3 to 6 hours after administration with a mean of about 4 hours.
Oral absorption of sparfloxacin is unaffected by administration with milk or food, including high fat meals. Concurrent administration of antacids containing magnesium hydroxide and aluminum hydroxide reduces the oral bioavailability of sparfloxacin by as much as 50%. (See **PRECAUTIONS, Information for Patients**, and **Drug Interactions**.)
Distribution: Upon reaching general circulation, sparfloxacin distributes well into the body, as reflected by the large mean steady-state volume of distribution (Vd_{ss}) of 3.9 (±0.8) L/kg. Sparfloxacin exhibits low plasma protein binding in serum at about 45%.
Sparfloxacin penetrates well into body fluids and tissues. Results of tissue and body fluid distribution studies demonstrated that oral administration of sparfloxacin produces sustained concentrations and that sparfloxacin concentra-

tions in lower respiratory tract tissues and fluids generally exceed the corresponding plasma concentrations. The concentration of sparfloxacin in respiratory tissues (pulmonary parenchyma, bronchial wall, and bronchial mucosa) at 2 to 6 hours following standard oral dosing was approximately 3 to 6 times greater than the corresponding concentration in plasma. Concentrations in these respiratory tissues increase at up to 24 hours following dosing. Sparfloxacin is also highly concentrated into alveolar macrophages compared to plasma. Tissue or fluid to plasma sparfloxacin concentration ratios for respiratory tissues and fluids are:
[See table at right]

Mean pleural effusion to plasma concentration ratios were 0.34 and 0.69 at 4 and 20 hours postdose, respectively.

Metabolism: Sparfloxacin is metabolized by the liver, primarily by phase II glucuronidation, to form a glucuronide conjugate. Its metabolism does not utilize or interfere with cytochrome-mediated oxidation, in particular cytochrome P450.

Excretion: The total body clearance and renal clearance of sparfloxacin were 11.4 (±3.5) and 1.5 (±0.5) L/hr, respectively. Sparfloxacin is excreted in both the feces (50%) and urine (50%). Approximately 10% of an orally administered dose is excreted in the urine as unchanged drug in patients with normal renal function. Following a 400-mg loading dose of sparfloxacin, the mean urine concentration 4 hours postdose was in excess of 12.0 μg/mL, and measurable concentrations of active drug persisted through six days for subjects with normal renal function.

The terminal elimination phase half-life ($t_{1/2}$) of sparfloxacin in plasma generally varies between 16 and 30 hours, with a mean $t_{1/2}$ of approximately 20 hours. The $t_{1/2}$ is independent of the administered dose, suggesting that sparfloxacin elimination kinetics are linear.

Special Populations

Geriatric: The pharmacokinetics of sparfloxacin are not altered in the elderly with normal renal function.

Pediatric: The pharmacokinetics of sparfloxacin in pediatric subjects have not been studied.

Gender: There are no gender differences in the pharmacokinetics of sparfloxacin.

Renal insufficiency: In patients with renal impairment (creatinine clearance <50 mL/min), the terminal elimination half-life of sparfloxacin is lengthened. Single or multiple doses of sparfloxacin in patients with varying degrees of renal impairment typically produce plasma concentrations that are twice those observed in subjects with normal renal function. (See **PRECAUTIONS: General** and **DOSAGE AND ADMINISTRATION.**)

Hepatic insufficiency: The pharmacokinetics of sparfloxacin are not altered in patients with mild or moderate hepatic impairment without cholestasis.

MICROBIOLOGY

Sparfloxacin has *in vitro* activity against a wide range of gram-negative and gram-positive microorganisms. Sparfloxacin exerts its antibacterial activity by inhibiting DNA gyrase, a bacterial topoisomerase. DNA gyrase is an essential enzyme which controls DNA topology and assists in DNA replication, repair, deactivation, and transcription. Quinolones differ in chemical structure and mode of action from β-lactam antibiotics. Quinolones may, therefore, be active against bacteria resistant to β-lactam antibiotics.

Although cross-resistance has been observed between sparfloxacin and other fluoroquinolones, some microorganisms resistant to other fluoroquinolones may be susceptible to sparfloxacin.

In vitro tests show that the combination of sparfloxacin and rifampin is antagonistic against *Staphylococcus aureus*.

Sparfloxacin has been shown to be active against most strains of the following microorganisms, both *in vitro* and in clinical infections as described in the **INDICATIONS AND USAGE** section:

Aerobic gram-positive microorganisms
Staphylococcus aureus
Streptococcus pneumoniae (penicillin-susceptible strains)
Aerobic gram-negative microorganisms
Enterobacter cloacae
Haemophilus influenzae
Haemophilus parainfluenzae
Klebsiella pneumoniae
Moraxella catarrhalis
Other microorganisms
Chlamydia pneumoniae
Mycoplasma pneumoniae
The following *in vitro* data are available, **but their clinical significance is unknown:**

Sparfloxacin exhibits *in vitro* minimal inhibitory concentrations (MIC's) of 1 μg/mL or less against most (≥90%) strains of the following microorganisms; however, the safety and effectiveness of sparfloxacin in treating clinical infections due to these microorganisms have not been established in adequate and well-controlled clinical trials.

Aerobic gram-positive microorganisms
Streptococcus agalactiae
Streptococcus pneumoniae (penicillin-resistant strains)

Respiratory tissues and fluids	n** value	Tissue to Plasma Sparfloxacin Concentration Mean Ratio (%CV)*	
		Time of Collection Postdose	
		2 to 6 hour	12 to 24 hour
alveolar macrophage	6/5	51.8 (88.7%)	68.1 (47.9%)
epithelial lining fluid	10/10	12.3 (26.7%)	17.6 (35.3%)
pulmonary parenchyma	8/7	5.9 (15.0%)	15.8 (32.0%)
bronchial wall	8/7	2.8 (16.0%)	5.7 (25.0%)
bronchial mucosa	6/5	2.7 (11.5%)	3.1 (11.6%)

* % CV (percent coefficient of variation)
** For tissues with two values, the first n is for 2 to 6 hours and the second n is for 12 to 24 hours.

Streptococcus pyogenes
Viridans group streptococci
Aerobic gram-negative microorganisms
Acinetobacter anitratus
Acinetobacter lwoffi
Citrobacter diversus
Enterobacter aerogenes
Klebsiella oxytoca
Legionella pneumophila
Morganella morganii
Proteus mirabilis
Proteus vulgaris

SUSCEPTIBILITY TESTS

Dilution techniques: Quantitative methods are used to determine antimicrobial minimal inhibitory concentrations (MIC's). These MIC's provide estimates of the susceptibility of bacteria to antimicrobial compounds. The MIC's should be determined using a standardized procedure. Standardized procedures are based on a dilution method[1] (broth or agar) or equivalent with standardized inoculum concentrations and standardized concentrations of sparfloxacin powder. The MIC values should be interpreted according to the following criteria:

For testing aerobic microorganisms other than *Haemophilus influenzae*, *Haemophilus parainfluenzae*, and *Streptococcus pneumoniae*:

MIC (μg/mL)	Interpretation
≤1	Susceptible (S)
2	Intermediate (I)
≥4	Resistant (R)

For testing *Haemophilus influenzae* and *Haemophilus parainfluenzae*:[a]

MIC (μg/mL)	Interpretation
≤0.25	Susceptible (S)

[a] These interpretive standards are applicable only to broth microdilution susceptibility testing with *Haemophilus influenzae* and *Haemophilus parainfluenzae* using Haemophilus Test Medium[1].

The current absence of data on resistant strains precludes defining any categories other than "Susceptible." Strains yielding MIC results suggestive of a "nonsusceptible" category should be submitted to a reference laboratory for further testing.

For testing *Streptococcus pneumoniae*:[b]

MIC (μg/mL)	Interpretation
≤0.5	Susceptible (S)

[b] These interpretive standards are applicable only to broth microdilution susceptibility tests using cation-adjusted Mueller-Hinton broth with 2–5% lysed horse blood.

The current absence of data on resistant strains precludes defining any categories other than "Susceptible." Strains yielding MIC results suggestive of a "nonsusceptible" category should be submitted to a reference laboratory for further testing.

A report of "Susceptible" indicates that the pathogen is likely to be inhibited if the antimicrobial compound in the blood reaches the concentration usually achievable. A report of "Intermediate" indicates that the result should be considered equivocal, and, if the microorganism is not fully susceptible to alternative, clinically feasible drugs, the test should be repeated. This category implies possible clinical applicability in body sites where the drug is physiologically concentrated or in situations where a high dosage of drug can be used. This category also provides a buffer zone which prevents small uncontrolled technical factors from causing major discrepancies in interpretation. A report of "Resistant" indicates that the pathogen is not likely to be inhibited if the antimicrobial compound in the blood reaches the concentration usually achievable; other therapy should be selected.

Standardized susceptibility test procedures require the use of laboratory control microorganisms to control the techni-

cal aspects of the laboratory procedures. Standard sparfloxacin powder should provide the following MIC values:

Microorganism	MIC Range (μg/mL)
Enterococcus faecalis ATCC 29212	0.12–0.5
Escherichia coli ATCC 25922	0.004–0.016
Haemophilus influenzae ATCC 49247[a]	0.004–0.016
Staphylococcus aureus ATCC 29213	0.03–0.12
Streptococcus pneumoniae ATCC 49619[b]	0.12–0.5

[a] This quality control range is applicable to only *H. influenzae* ATCC 49247 tested by a broth microdilution procedure using Haemophilus Test Medium (HTM)[1].

[b] This quality control range is applicable to only *S. pneumoniae* ATCC 49619 tested by a broth microdilution procedure using cation-adjusted Mueller-Hinton broth with 2–5% lysed horse blood.

Diffusion techniques: Quantitative methods that require measurement of zone diameters also provide reproducible estimates of the susceptibility of bacteria to antimicrobial compounds. One such standardized procedure[2] requires the use of standardized inoculum concentrations. This procedure uses paper disks impregnated with 5-μg sparfloxacin to test the susceptibility of microorganisms to sparfloxacin. Reports from the laboratory providing results of the standard single-disk susceptibility test with a 5-μg sparfloxacin disk should be interpreted according to the following criteria:

For aerobic microorganisms other than *Haemophilus influenzae*, *Haemophilus parainfluenzae*, and *Streptococcus pneumoniae*:

Zone Diameter (mm)	Interpretation
≥19	Susceptible (S)
16–18	Intermediate (I)
≤15	Resistant (R)

Haemophilus influenzae and *Haemophilus parainfluenzae* should not be tested by diffusion techniques. An MIC should be determined for these isolates.

For *Streptococcus pneumoniae*:[a]

Zone Diameter (mm)	Interpretation
≥19	Susceptible (S)

[a] These zone diameter standards for *Streptococcus pneumoniae* apply only to tests performed using Mueller-Hinton agar supplemented with 5% sheep blood and incubated in 5% CO_2.

The current absence of data on resistant strains precludes any category other than "Susceptible." Strains yielding zone diameter results suggestive of a "nonsusceptible" category should be submitted to a reference laboratory for further testing.

Interpretation should be as stated above for results using dilution techniques. Interpretation involves correlation of the diameter obtained in the disk test with the MIC for sparfloxacin.

As with standard dilution techniques, diffusion methods require the use of laboratory control microorganisms that are used to control the technical aspects of the laboratory procedures. For the diffusion technique, the 5-μg sparfloxacin disk should provide the following zone diameters in these laboratory quality control strains:

Continued on next page

Zagam—Cont.

Microorganism	Zone Diameter (mm)
Escherichia coli	
ATCC 25922	30–38
Staphylococcus aureus	
ATCC 25923	27–33
Streptococcus pneumoniae	
ATCC 49619[a]	21–27

[a] These quality control limits apply to tests conducted with *S. pneumoniae* ATCC 49619 using Mueller-Hinton agar supplemented with 5% sheep blood incubated in 5% CO_2.

INDICATIONS AND USAGE

Zagam (sparfloxacin) is indicated for the treatment of adults ($\geq$ 18 years of age) with the following infections caused by susceptible strains of the designated microorganisms:

Community-acquired pneumonia caused by *Chlamydia pneumoniae, Haemophilus influenzae, Haemophilus parainfluenzae, Moraxella catarrhalis, Mycoplasma pneumoniae,* or *Streptococcus pneumoniae*
Acute bacterial exacerbations of chronic bronchitis caused by *Chlamydia pneumoniae, Enterobacter cloacae, Haemophilus influenzae, Haemophilus parainfluenzae, Klebsiella pneumoniae, Moraxella catarrhalis, Staphylococcus aureus,* or *Streptococcus pneumoniae*

Appropriate culture and susceptibility tests should be performed before treatment in order to isolate and identify organisms causing the infection and to determine their susceptibility to sparfloxacin. Therapy with sparfloxacin may be initiated before results of these tests are known; once results become available, appropriate therapy should be selected. Culture and susceptibility testing performed periodically during therapy will provide information on the continued susceptibility of the pathogen to the antimicrobial agent and also on the possible emergence of bacterial resistance.

CONTRAINDICATIONS

Sparfloxacin is contraindicated for individuals with a history of hypersensitivity or photosensitivity reactions.
Torsade de pointes has been reported in patients receiving sparfloxacin concomitantly with disopyramide and amiodarone. Consequently, sparfloxacin is contraindicated for individuals receiving these drugs as well as other QT_c-prolonging antiarrhythmic drugs reported to cause torsade de pointes, such as class Ia antiarrhythmic agents (e.g., quinidine, procainamide), class III antiarrhythmic agents (e.g., sotalol), and bepridil. Sparfloxacin is contraindicated in patients with known QT_c prolongation or in patients being treated concomitantly with medications known to produce an increase in the QT_c interval and/or torsade de pointes (e.g., terfenadine). (See **WARNINGS** and **PRECAUTIONS.**)
It is essential to avoid exposure to the sun, bright natural light, and UV rays throughout the entire duration of treatment and for 5 days after treatment is stopped. Sparfloxacin is contraindicated in patients whose life-style or employment will not permit compliance with required safety precautions concerning phototoxicity. (See **WARNINGS** and **PRECAUTIONS.**)

WARNINGS

MODERATE TO SEVERE PHOTOTOXIC REACTIONS HAVE OCCURRED IN PATIENTS EXPOSED TO DIRECT OR INDIRECT SUNLIGHT OR TO ARTIFICIAL ULTRAVIOLET LIGHT (e.g., SUNLAMPS) DURING OR FOLLOWING TREATMENT. THESE REACTIONS HAVE ALSO OCCURRED IN PATIENTS EXPOSED TO SHADED OR DIFFUSE LIGHT, INCLUDING EXPOSURE THROUGH GLASS OR DURING CLOUDY WEATHER. PATIENTS SHOULD BE ADVISED TO DISCONTINUE SPARFLOXACIN THERAPY AT THE FIRST SIGNS OR SYMPTOMS OF A PHOTOTOXICITY REACTION SUCH AS A SENSATION OF SKIN BURNING, REDNESS, SWELLING, BLISTERS, RASH, ITCHING, OR DERMATITIS.
The overall incidence of drug related phototoxicity in the 1585 patients who received sparfloxacin during clinical trials with recommended dosage was 7.9% (n=126). Phototoxicity ranged from mild 4.1% (n=65) to moderate 3.3% (n=52) to severe 0.6% (n=9), with severe defined as involving at least significant curtailment of normal daily activity. The frequency of phototoxicity reactions characterized by blister formation was 0.8% (n=13) of which 3 were severe. The discontinuation rate due to phototoxicity independent of drug relationship was 1.1% (n=17).
As with some other types of phototoxicity, there is the potential for exacerbation of the reaction on re-exposure to sunlight or artificial ultraviolet light prior to complete recovery from the reaction. In a few cases, recovery from phototoxicity reactions was prolonged for several weeks. In rare cases, reactions have recurred up to several weeks after stopping sparfloxacin therapy.

EXPOSURE TO DIRECT AND INDIRECT SUNLIGHT (EVEN WHEN USING SUNSCREENS OR SUNBLOCKS) SHOULD BE AVOIDED WHILE TAKING SPARFLOXACIN AND FOR FIVE DAYS FOLLOWING THERAPY. SPARFLOXACIN THERAPY SHOULD BE DISCONTINUED IMMEDIATELY AT THE FIRST SIGNS OR SYMPTOMS OF PHOTOTOXICITY.
These phototoxic reactions have occurred with and without the use of sunscreens or sunblocks and have been associated with a single dose of sparfloxacin. However, a study in healthy volunteers has demonstrated that some sunscreen products, specifically those active in blocking UVA spectrum wavelengths (those containing the active ingredients octocrylene or Parsol® 1789), can moderate the photosensitizing effect of sparfloxacin. However, many over-the-counter sunscreens do not provide adequate UVA protection.
Increases in the QT_c interval have been observed in healthy volunteers treated with sparfloxacin. After a single loading dose of 400 mg, a mean increase in QT_c interval of 11 msec (2.9%) is seen; at steady-state the mean increase is 7 msec (1.9%). The magnitude of the QT_c effect does not increase with repeated administration, and the QT_c returns to baseline within 48 hours of the last dose. In clinical trials involving 1489 patients with a baseline QT_c measurement, the mean prolongation at steady-state was 10 msec (2.5%); 0.7% of patients had a QT_c interval greater than 500 msec; however, no arrhythmic effects were seen.
THE SAFETY AND EFFECTIVENESS OF SPARFLOXACIN IN CHILDREN, ADOLESCENTS (UNDER THE AGE OF 18 YEARS), PREGNANT WOMEN, AND LACTATING WOMEN HAVE NOT BEEN ESTABLISHED. (See PRECAUTIONS—Pregnancy, Nursing Mothers; and Pediatric Use.)
Sparfloxacin has been shown to cause arthropathy in immature dogs when given in oral doses of 25 mg/kg/day (approximately 1.9 times the highest human dose on a mg/m^2 basis) for seven consecutive days. Examination of the weight-bearing joints of the dogs revealed small erosive lesions of the cartilage. Other quinolones also produce erosions of cartilage of weight-bearing joints and other signs of arthropathy in immature animals of various species.
Convulsions and toxic psychoses have been reported in patients receiving quinolones, including sparfloxacin. Quinolones may also cause increased intracranial pressure and central nervous system stimulation which may lead to tremors, restlessness/agitation, anxiety/nervousness, lightheadedness, confusion, hallucinations, paranoia, depression, nightmares, insomnia, and, rarely, suicidal thoughts or acts. These reactions may occur following the first dose. If these reactions occur in patients receiving sparfloxacin, the drug should be discontinued and appropriate measures instituted. As with other quinolones, sparfloxacin should be used with caution in patients with a known or suspected CNS disorder that may predispose to seizures or lower the seizure threshold (e.g., severe cerebral arteriosclerosis, epilepsy) or in the presence of other risk factors that may predispose to seizures or lower the seizure threshold (e.g., certain drug therapy, renal dysfunction). Cases of seizure associated with hypoglycemia have been reported. (See **PRECAUTIONS: General Information for Patients, Drug Interactions** and **ADVERSE REACTIONS.**)
Serious and occasionally fatal hypersensitivity (including anaphylactoid or anaphylactic) reactions, some following the first dose, have been reported in patients receiving quinolones. Some reactions were accompanied by cardiovascular collapse, hypotension/shock, seizure, loss of consciousness, tingling, angioedema (including tongue, laryngeal, throat, or facial edema), airway obstruction (including bronchospasm, shortness of breath, and acute respiratory distress), dyspnea, urticaria, and/or itching. Only a few patients had a history of previous hypersensitivity reactions. If an allergic reaction to sparfloxacin occurs, the drug should be discontinued immediately. Serious acute hypersensitivity reactions may require immediate treatment with epinephrine, and other resuscitative measures including oxygen, intravenous fluids, antihistamines, corticosteroids, pressor amines, and airway management, including intubation, as clinically indicated.
Serious and sometimes fatal events, some due to hypersensitivity, and some due to uncertain etiology, have been reported rarely in patients receiving therapy with quinolones. These events may be severe and generally occur following the administration of multiple doses. Clinical manifestations may include one or more of the following: fever, rash or severe dermatologic reactions (e.g., toxic epidermal necrolysis, Stevens-Johnson Syndrome); vasculitis; arthralgia; myalgia; serum sickness; allergic pneumonitis; interstitial nephritis; acute renal insufficiency or failure; hepatitis; jaundice; acute hepatic necrosis or failure; anemia, including hemolytic and aplastic; thrombocytopenia, including thrombotic thrombocytopenic purpura; leukopenia; agranulocytosis; pancytopenia; and/or other hematologic abnormalities.

The drug should be discontinued immediately at the first appearance of a skin rash or any other sign of hypersensitivity and supportive measures instituted. (See **PRECAUTIONS: Information for Patients** and **ADVERSE REACTIONS.**)
Pseudomembranous colitis has been reported with nearly all antibacterial agents, including sparfloxacin, and may range in severity from mild to life-threatening. Therefore, it is important to consider this diagnosis in patients who present with diarrhea subsequent to the administration of antibacterial agents.
Treatment with antibacterial agents alters the normal flora of the colon and may permit overgrowth of clostridia. Studies indicate that a toxin produced by *Clostridium difficile* is one primary cause of "antibiotic-associated colitis."
After the diagnosis of pseudomembranous colitis has been established, therapeutic measures should be initiated. Mild cases of pseudomembranous colitis usually respond to drug discontinuation alone. In moderate to severe cases, consideration should be given to management with fluids and electrolytes, protein supplementation, and treatment with an antibacterial drug clinically effective against *C. difficile* colitis.
Ruptures of the shoulder, hand, and Achilles tendons that required surgical repair or resulted in prolonged disability have been reported with sparfloxacin and other quinolones. Sparfloxacin should be discontinued if the patient experiences pain, inflammation, or rupture of a tendon. Patients should rest and refrain from exercise until the diagnosis of tendonitis or tendon rupture has been confidently excluded. Tendon rupture can occur at any time during or after therapy with sparfloxacin.

PRECAUTIONS

General: Adequate hydration of patients receiving sparfloxacin should be maintained to prevent the formation of a highly concentrated urine.
Administer sparfloxacin with caution in the presence of renal insufficiency. Careful clinical observation and appropriate laboratory studies should be performed prior to and during therapy since elimination of sparfloxacin may be reduced. Adjustment of the dosage regimen is necessary for patients with impaired renal function-creatinine clearance <50 mL/min. (See **CLINICAL PHARMACOLOGY** and **DOSAGE AND ADMINISTRATION.**)
Avoid the concomitant prescription of medications known to prolong the QT_c interval, e.g., erythromycin, terfenadine, astemizole, cisapride, pentamidine, tricyclic antidepressants, some antipsychotics including phenothiazines. (See **CONTRAINDICATIONS.**) Sparfloxacin is not recommended for use in patients with pro-arrhythmic conditions (e.g., hypokalemia, significant bradycardia, congestive heart failure, myocardial ischemia, and atrial fibrillation).
Moderate to severe phototoxicity reactions have been observed in patients exposed to direct sunlight while receiving drugs in this class. Excessive exposure to sunlight should be avoided. In clinical trials with sparfloxacin, phototoxicity was observed in approximately 7% of patients. Therapy should be discontinued if phototoxicity (e.g., a skin eruption) occurs.
As with other quinolones, sparfloxacin should be used with caution in any patient with a known or suspected CNS disorder that may predispose to seizures or lower the seizure threshold (e.g., severe cerebral arteriosclerosis, epilepsy) or in the presence of other risk factors that may predispose to seizures or lower the seizure threshold (e.g., certain drug therapy, renal dysfunction). (See **WARNINGS** and **Drug Interactions.**)
Information for Patients:
Patients should be advised:
* to avoid exposure to direct or indirect sunlight (including through glass, while using sunscreens and sunblocks, reflected sunlight, and cloudy weather) and exposure to artificial ultraviolet light (e.g., sunlamps) during treatment with sparfloxacin and for five days after therapy. If brief exposure to the sun cannot be avoided, patients should cover as much of their skin as possible with clothing;
* to discontinue sparfloxacin therapy at the first sign or symptom of phototoxicity reaction such as a sensation of skin burning, redness, swelling, blisters, rash, itching or dermatitis;
* that a patient who has experienced a phototoxic reaction with sparfloxacin should also be advised to avoid further exposure to sunlight and artificial ultraviolet light until the phototoxicity reaction has resolved and he or she has completely recovered from the reaction or for five days whichever is longer. In rare cases, reactions have recurred up to several weeks after stopping sparfloxacin therapy;
* that sparfloxacin may cause neurologic adverse effects (e.g., dizziness, lightheadedness) and that patients should know how they react to sparfloxacin before they operate an automobile or machinery or engage in other activities requiring mental alertness and coordination (see **WARNINGS** and **ADVERSE REACTIONS**);
* to discontinue treatment and inform their physician if they experience pain, inflammation, or rupture of a tendon, and to rest and refrain from exercise until the diagnosis of tendonitis or tendon rupture has been confidently excluded;

- that sparfloxacin can be taken with food or milk or caffeine-containing products;
- that mineral supplements or vitamins with iron, or zinc, or calcium may be taken 4 hours after sparfloxacin administration;
- that sucralfate or magnesium- and aluminum-containing antacids may be taken 4 hours after sparfloxacin administration (see **PRECAUTIONS—Drug Interactions**);
- that sparfloxacin may be associated with hypersensitivity reactions, even following the first dose, and to discontinue the drug at the first sign of a skin rash or other allergic reaction;
- to drink fluids liberally.

Drug Interactions:

Digoxin: Sparfloxacin has no effect on the pharmacokinetics of digoxin.

Methylxanthines: Sparfloxacin does not increase plasma theophylline concentrations. Since there is no interaction with theophylline, interaction with other methylxanthines such as caffeine is unlikely.

Warfarin: Sparfloxacin does not increase the anti-coagulant effect of warfarin.

Cimetidine: Cimetidine does not affect the pharmacokinetics of sparfloxacin.

Antacids and Sucralfate: Aluminum and magnesium cations in antacids and sucralfate form chelation complexes with sparfloxacin. The oral bioavailability of sparfloxacin is reduced when an aluminum-magnesium suspension is administered between 2 hours before and 2 hours after sparfloxacin administration. The oral bioavailability of sparfloxacin is not reduced when the aluminum-magnesium suspension is administered 4 hours following sparfloxacin administration.

Zinc/iron salts: Absorption of quinolones is reduced significantly by these preparations. These products may be taken 4 hours after sparfloxacin administration.

Probenecid: Probenecid does not alter the pharmacokinetics of sparfloxacin.

Drug/Laboratory Test Interactions:

Sparfloxacin therapy may produce false-negative culture results for *Mycobacterium tuberculosis* by suppression of mycobacterial growth.

Carcinogenesis, Mutagenesis, Impairment of Fertility:

Carcinogenesis: Sparfloxacin was not carcinogenic in mice or rats when administered for 104 weeks at daily oral doses 3.5–6.2 times greater than the maximum human dose (400 mg), respectively, based upon mg/m². These doses corresponded to plasma concentrations approximately equal to (mice) and 2.2 times greater than (rats) maximum human plasma concentrations.

Mutagenesis: Sparfloxacin was not mutagenic in *Salmonella typhimurium* TA98, TA100, TA1535, or TA1537, in *Escherichia coli* strain WP2 uvrA, nor in Chinese hamster lung cells. Sparfloxacin and other quinolones have been shown to be mutagenic in *Salmonella typhimurium* strain TA102 and to induce DNA repair in *Escherichia coli*, perhaps due to their inhibitory effect on bacterial DNA gyrase. Sparfloxacin induced chromosomal aberrations in Chinese hamster lung cells *in vitro* at cytotoxic concentrations; however, no increase in chromosomal aberrations or micronuclei in bone marrow cells was observed after sparfloxacin was administered orally to mice.

Impairment of Fertility: Sparfloxacin had no effect on the fertility or reproductive performance of male or female rats at oral doses up to 15.4 times the maximum human dose (400 mg) based upon mg/m² (equivalent to approximately 12 times the maximum human plasma concentration).

Pregnancy: Teratogenic effects: Pregnancy Category C Reproduction studies performed in rats, rabbits, and monkeys at oral doses 6.2, 4.4, and 2.6 times higher than the maximum human dose, respectively, based upon mg/m² (corresponding to plasma concentrations 4.5- and 6.5-fold higher than in humans in the monkey and rat, respectively) did not reveal any evidence of teratogenic effects. At these doses, sparfloxacin was clearly maternally toxic to the rabbit and monkey with evidence of slight maternal toxicity observed in the rat. When administered to pregnant rats at clearly maternally toxic doses (≥9.3 times the maximum human dose based upon mg/m²), sparfloxacin induced a dose-dependent increase in the incidence of fetuses with ventricular septal defects. Among the three species tested, this effect was specific to the rat. There are, however, no adequate and well-controlled studies in pregnant women. Sparfloxacin should be used during pregnancy only if the potential benefit justifies the potential risk to the fetus. (See **WARNINGS.**)

Nursing mothers: Sparfloxacin is excreted in human milk. Because of the potential for serious adverse reactions in infants nursing from mothers taking sparfloxacin, a decision should be made whether to discontinue nursing or to discontinue the drug, taking into account the importance of the drug to the mother. (See **WARNINGS.**)

Pediatric use: Safety and effectiveness have not been established in patients below the age of 18 years. Quinolones,

Organism	Sparfloxacin	Erythromycin*	Cefaclor
C. pneumoniae	19/22 (86.4%)	3/4 (75%)	5/5 (100%)
H. influenzae	20/24 (83.3%)	0	25/31 (80.6%)
H. parainfluenzae	61/63 (96.8%)	4/4 (100%)	31/41 (75.6%)
M. catarrhalis	7/8 (87.5%)	4/4 (100%)	5/6 (83.3%)
M. pneumoniae	36/39 (92.3%)	15/15 (100%)	20/24 (83.3%)
S. pneumoniae	39/41 (95.1%)	10/11 (90%)	16/17 (94.1%)

* Pathogen numbers were smaller since many of the strains were intrinsically resistant to erythromycin.

Event	Sparfloxacin n=387	Erythromycin n=209	Cefaclor n=162
Abdominal Pain	6 (1.6%)	18 (8.6%)	2 (1.2%)
Photosensitivity Reaction	16 (4.1%)	0	1 (0.6%)
QT Interval Prolonged	8 (2.1%)	2 (1.0%)	1 (0.6%)
Sinus Bradycardia	2 (0.5%)	6 (2.9%)	0
Diarrhea	15 (3.9%)	33 (15.8%)	7 (4.3%)
Flatulence	0	5 (2.4%)	0
Nausea	11 (2.8%)	32 (15.3%)	4 (2.5%)
Vomiting	10 (2.6%)	15 (7.2%)	1 (0.6%)
Insomnia	6 (1.6%)	5 (2.4%)	0

Organism	Sparfloxacin	Ofloxacin
H. parainfluenzae	104/109 (95.4%)	90/95 (94.7%)
H. influenzae	51/57 (89.5%)	61/65 (93.8%)
C. pneumoniae	37/45 (82.2%)	36/40 (90%)
M. catarrhalis	36/38 (94.7%)	33/34 (97.1%)
S. pneumoniae	30/34 (88.2%)	20/22 (90.9%)
S. aureus	16/19 (84.2%)	13/14 (92.9%)
K. pneumoniae	17/17 (100%)	15/17 (88.2%)
E. cloacae	12/13 (92.3%)	12/15 (80%)

including sparfloxacin, cause arthropathy and osteochondrosis in juvenile animals of several species. (See **WARNINGS.**)

ADVERSE REACTIONS

In clinical trials, most of the adverse events were mild to moderate in severity and transient in nature. During clinical investigations with the recommended dosage, 1585 patients received sparfloxacin and 1331 patients received a comparator. The discontinuation rate due to adverse events was 6.6% for sparfloxacin versus 5.6% for cefaclor, 14.8% for erythromycin, 8.9% for ciprofloxacin, 7.4% for ofloxacin, and 8.3% for clarithromycin.

The most frequently reported events (remotely, possibly, or probably drug related with an incidence of ≥1%) among sparfloxacin treated patients in the US phase 3 clinical trials with the recommended dosage were: photosensitivity reaction (7.9%), diarrhea (4.6%), nausea (4.3%), headache (4.2%), dyspepsia (2.3%), dizziness (2.0%), insomnia (1.9%), abdominal pain (1.8%), pruritus (1.8%), taste perversion (1.4%), and QT_c interval prolongation (1.3%), vomiting (1.3%), flatulence (1.1%) and vasodilatation (1.0%).

In US phase 3 clinical trials of shorter treatment duration than the recommended dosage, the most frequently reported events (incidence ≥1%, remotely, possibly, or probably drug related) were: headache (8.1%), nausea (7.6%), dizziness (3.8%), photosensitivity reaction (3.6%), pruritus (3.3%), diarrhea (3.2%), vaginal moniliasis (2.8%), abdominal pain (2.4%), asthenia (1.7%), dyspepsia (1.6%), somnolence (1.5%), dry mouth (1.4%), and rash (1.1%).

Additional possibly or probably related events that occurred in less than 1% of all patients enrolled in US phase 3 clinical trials are listed below:

BODY AS A WHOLE: fever, chest pain, generalized pain, allergic reaction, cellulitis, back pain, chills, face edema, malaise, accidental injury, anaphylactoid reaction, infection, mucous membrane disorder, neck pain, rheumatoid arthritis;

CARDIOVASCULAR: palpitation, electrocardiogram abnormal, hypertension, tachycardia, sinus bradycardia, PR interval shortened, angina pectoris, arrhythmia, atrial fibrillation, atrial flutter, complete AV block, first degree AV block, second degree AV block, cardiovascular disorder, hemorrhage, migraine, peripheral vascular disorder, supraventricular extrasystoles, ventricular extrasystoles, postural hypotension;

GASTROINTESTINAL: constipation, anorexia, gingivitis, oral moniliasis, stomatitis, tongue disorder, tooth disorder, gastroenteritis, increased appetite, mouth ulceration, flatulence, vomiting;

HEMATOLOGIC: cyanosis, ecchymosis, lymphadenopathy;

METABOLISM: gout, peripheral edema, thirst;

MUSCULOSKELETAL: arthralgia, arthritis, joint disorder, myalgia;

CENTRAL NERVOUS SYSTEM: paresthesia, hypesthesia, nervousness, somnolence, abnormal dreams, dry mouth, depression, tremor, anxiety, confusion, hallucinations, hyperesthesia, hyperkinesia, sleep disorder, hypokinesia, vertigo, abnormal gait, agitation, lightheadedness, emotional lability, euphoria, abnormal thinking, amnesia, twitching;

RESPIRATORY: asthma, epistaxis, pneumonia, rhinitis, pharyngitis, bronchitis, hemoptysis, sinusitis, cough increased, dyspnea, laryngismus, lung disorder, pleural disorder;

SKIN/HYPERSENSITIVITY: rash, maculopapular rash, dry skin, herpes simplex, sweating, urticaria, vesiculobullous rash, exfoliative dermatitis, acne, alopecia, angioedema, contact dermatitis, fungal dermatitis, furunculosis, pustular rash, skin discoloration, herpes zoster, petechial rash;

SPECIAL SENSES: ear pain, amblyopia, photophobia, tinnitus, conjunctivitis, diplopia, abnormality of accommodation, blepharitis, ear disorder, eye pain, lacrimation disorder, otitis media;

UROGENITAL: vaginitis, dysuria, breast pain, dysmenorrhea, hematuria, menorrhagia, nocturia, polyuria, urinary tract infection, kidney pain, leukorrhea, metrorrhagia, vulvovaginal disorder.

LABORATORY CHANGES: In the US phase 3 clinical trials, with the recommended dosage, the most frequently (incidence ≥1%) reported changes in laboratory parameters listed as adverse events, regardless of relationship to drug, were: elevated ALT (SGPT) (2.0%), AST (SGOT) (2.3%) and white blood cells (1.1%).

Increases for the following laboratory tests were reported in less than 1% of all patients enrolled in clinical trials: alkaline phosphatase, serum amylase, aPTT, blood urea nitrogen, calcium, creatinine, eosinophils, serum lipase, monocytes, neutrophils, total bilirubin, urine glucose, urine protein, urine red blood cells, and urine white blood cells.

Decreases for the following laboratory tests were reported in less than 1% of all patients enrolled in clinical trials: albumin, creatinine clearance, hematocrit, hemoglobin, lymphocytes, phosphorus, red blood cells, and sodium.

Increases and decreases for the following laboratory tests were reported in less than 1% of all patients in clinical trials: blood glucose, platelets, potassium, and white blood cells.

Postmarketing Adverse Events: The following are additional adverse events (regardless of relationship to drug) reported from worldwide postmarketing experience with sparfloxacin or other quinolones: acidosis, acute renal failure, agranulocytosis, albuminuria, anaphylactic shock, angioedema, anosmia, ataxia, bullous eruption, candiduria, cardiopulmonary arrest, cerebral thrombosis, convulsions, crystalluria, dysgeusia, dysphasia, ebrious feeling, embolism, erythema nodosum, exacerbation of myasthenia gravis, gastralgia, hemolytic anemia, hepatic necrosis, hepatitis, hiccough, hyperpigmentation, interstitial nephritis, interstitial pneumonia, intestinal perforation, jaundice, laryngeal or

Continued on next page

Zagam—Cont.

pulmonary edema, manic reaction, numbness, nystagmus, painful oral mucosa, pancreatitis, phobia, prolongation of prothrombin time, pseudomembranous colitis, Quincke's edema, renal calculi, rhabdomyolysis, sensory disturbance, Stevens-Johnson syndrome, squamous cell carcinoma, tendonitis, tendon rupture, tremor, thrombocytopenia, thrombocytopenia purpura, toxic epidermal necrolysis, toxic psychosis, urinary retention, uveitis, vaginal candidiasis, vasculitis.

Laboratory changes: elevation of serum triglycerides, serum cholesterol, blood glucose, serum potassium, decrease in WBC counts, RBC counts, hemoglobin level, hematocrit level, thrombocyte counts, elevation in GOT, GPT, ALP, LDH, γ-GTP, total bilirubin.

OVERDOSAGE

In case of overdosage, the patient should be monitored in a suitably equipped medical facility and advised to avoid sun exposure for five days. ECG monitoring is recommended due to the possible prolongation of the QT_c interval. There is no known antidote for sparfloxacin overdosage.

It is not known whether sparfloxacin is dialyzable.

Single doses of sparfloxacin were relatively non-toxic via the oral route of administration in mice, rats, and dogs. No deaths occurred within a 14-day post-treatment observation period at the highest oral doses tested, up to 5000 mg/kg in either rodent species, or up to 600 mg/kg in the dog. Clinical signs observed included inactivity in mice and dogs, diarrhea in both rodent species, and vomiting, salivation, and tremors in dogs.

DOSAGE AND ADMINISTRATION

Zagam (sparfloxacin) can be taken with or without food.

The recommended daily dose of Zagam in patients with normal renal function is two 200-mg tablets taken on the first day as a loading dose. Thereafter, one 200-mg tablet should be taken every 24 hours for a total of 10 days of therapy (11 tablets).

The recommended daily dose of Zagam in patients with renal impairment (creatinine clearance <50 mL/min) is two 200-mg tablets taken on the first day as a loading dose. Thereafter, one 200-mg tablet should be taken every 48 hours for a total of 9 days of therapy (6 tablets).

CLINICAL STUDIES

Community-Acquired Pneumonia Studies

In two controlled clinical studies of community-acquired pneumonia conducted in the United States, sparfloxacin was compared to erythromycin and cefaclor. The patient clinical success and pathogen eradication rates for sparfloxacin were equivalent to those of the comparators. In these studies, the following pathogen eradication rates/presumed pathogen eradication rates were obtained:

[See first table at top of previous page]

Safety

The following table lists possibly and probably drug-related adverse events that occurred in these studies at an incidence of ≥2%:

[See second table at top of previous page]

Acute Bacterial Exacerbations of Chronic Bronchitis Study

In a controlled clinical study of acute bacterial exacerbations of chronic bronchitis conducted in the United States, sparfloxacin was compared to ofloxacin. In this study, the following pathogen eradication rates were obtained:

[See third table at top of previous page]

Safety

The following table lists possibly and probably drug-related adverse events that occurred in the study at an incidence of ≥2% for either compound.

Event	Sparfloxacin (n=395)		Ofloxacin (n=403)	
Headache	11	(2.8%)	6	(1.5%)
Photosensitivity Reaction	29	(7.3%)	3	(0.7%)
Diarrhea	6	(1.5%)	9	(2.2%)
Dyspepsia	8	(2.0%)	14	(3.5%)
Nausea	16	(4.1%)	29	(7.2%)
Dizziness	12	(3.0%)	10	(2.5%)
Insomnia	4	(1.0%)	46	(11.4%)
Taste Perversion	10	(2.5%)	10	(2.5%)

HOW SUPPLIED

Strength	Size	NDC 0075-	Description	Markings
200 mg	Blister Pack of 11 (RespiPac™)	5410-11	round, white tablet	RPR 201
	Bottle of 55	5410-55		

Store at Controlled Room Temperature 20 to 25°C (68 to 77°F) [see USP].

Caution: Federal law prohibits dispensing without a prescription.

Keep out of the reach of children.

ANIMAL PHARMACOLOGY

Sparfloxacin and other quinolones have been shown to cause arthropathy in juvenile animals of most species tested. (See **WARNINGS**.)

Sparfloxacin had no convulsive activity in mice when administered alone or in combination with the nonsteroidal anti-inflammatory agents ketoprofen, or naproxen.

References:

1. National Committee for Clinical Laboratory Standards. Methods for Dilution Antimicrobial Susceptibility Tests for Bacteria that Grow Aerobically—Third Edition. Approved Standard NCCLS Document M7-A3, Vol. 13, No. 25, NCCLS, Villanova, PA, December, 1993.

2. National Committee for Clinical Laboratory Standards. Performance Standards for Antimicrobial Disk Susceptibility Tests—Fifth Edition. Approved Standard NCCLS Document M2-A5, Vol. 13, No. 24, NCCLS, Villanova, PA, December 1993.

RHÔNE-POULENC RORER PHARMACEUTICALS INC.
Collegeville, PA, U.S.A. 19426-0107

IN-0010　　　　　　　　　　　　　　　　　　Rev. 3/97

Shown in Product Identification Guide, page 334

Richwood Pharmaceutical Company Inc.

7900 TANNER'S GATE DRIVE, SUITE 200 FLORENCE, KENTUCKY 41042
(For product information see Shire Richwood Inc.)

Roberts Pharmaceutical Corp.

4 INDUSTRIAL WAY WEST EATONTOWN, NJ 07724

Direct Inquiries to:
Customer Service
(732) 389-1182
(800) 828-2088
FAX: (732) 389-1014

For Medical Information Contact:
(800) 992-9306

AGRYLIN™　　　　　　　　　　　　　　　　　Rx

[ăg 'rä-lĭn]

(anagrelide hydrochloride)

Capsules

DESCRIPTION

Name: AGRYLIN™ (anagrelide hydrochloride)

Dosage Form: 0.5 mg and 1 mg capsules for oral administration

Active Ingredient: AGRYLIN™ Capsules contain either 0.5 mg or 1 mg of anagrelide base (as anagrelide hydrochloride).

Inactive Ingredients: Povidone USP, Anhydrous Lactose NF, Lactose Monohydrate NF, Microcrystalline Cellulose NF, Crospovidone NF, Magnesium Stearate NF.

Pharmacological Classification: Platelet-reducing agent.

Chemical Name: 6,7-dichloro-1,5-dihydroimidazo[2,1-b]quinazolin-2(3H)-one monohydrochloride monohydrate.

Molecular formula: $C_{10}H_7Cl_2N_3O \cdot HCl \cdot H_2O$

Molecular weight: 310.55

Structural formula:

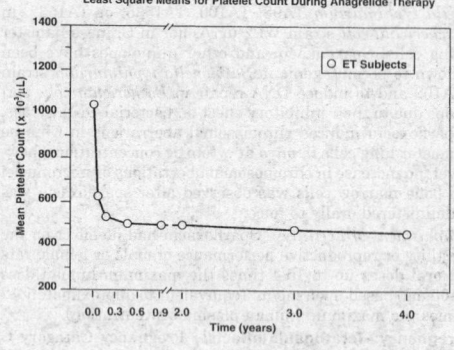

Appearance: Off-white powder.

Solubility:　Water .... Very slightly soluble

Dimethyl Sulfoxide .... Sparingly soluble

Dimethylformamide .... Sparingly soluble

CLINICAL PHARMACOLOGY

The mechanism by which anagrelide reduces blood platelet count is still under investigation. Studies in patients support a hypothesis of dose-related reduction in platelet production resulting from a decrease in megakaryocyte hypermaturation. In blood withdrawn from normal volunteers treated with anagrelide, a disruption was found in the post-

mitotic phase of megakaryocyte development and a reduction in megakaryocyte size and ploidy. At therapeutic doses, anagrelide does not produce significant changes in white cell counts or coagulation parameters, and may have a small, but clinically insignificant effect on red cell parameters. Platelet aggregation is inhibited in people at doses higher than those required to reduce platelet count. Anagrelide inhibits cyclic AMP phosphodiesterase, as well as ADP- and collagen-induced platelet aggregation.

Following oral administration of ^{14}C-anagrelide in people, more than 70% of radioactivity was recovered in urine. Based on limited data, there appears to be a trend toward dose linearity between doses of 0.5 mg and 2.0 mg. At fasting and at a dose of 0.5 mg of anagrelide, the plasma half-life is 1.3 hours. The available plasma concentration time data at steady state in patients showed that anagrelide does not accumulate in plasma after repeated administration. The drug is extensively metabolized; less than 1% is recovered in the urine as anagrelide.

When a 0.5 mg dose of anagrelide was taken after food, its bioavailability (based on AUC values) was modestly reduced by an average of 13.8% and its plasma half-life slightly increased (to 1.8 hours), when compared with drug administered to the same subjects in the fasted state. The peak plasma level was lowered by an average of 45% and delayed by 2 hours.

CLINICAL STUDIES

A total of 551 patients with Essential Thrombocythemia (ET) were treated with anagrelide in three clinical trials. Patients with ET were diagnosed based on the following criteria:

• Platelet count ≥900,000/μL on two determinations
• Profound megakaryocytic hyperplasia in bone marrow
• Absence of Philadelphia chromosome
• Normal red cell mass
• Normal serum iron and ferritin, and normal marrow iron stores.

The mean duration of anagrelide therapy for study patients was 65 weeks; 23% of patients received treatment for 2 years. In one unblinded, historically-controlled study, 276 ET patients were treated with anagrelide starting at doses of 0.5–2.0 mg every 6 hours. The dose was increased if the platelet count was still high, but to no more than 12 mg each day. Efficacy was defined as reduction of platelet count to or near physiologic levels (150,000–400,000/μL). The criteria for defining subjects as "responders" were reduction in platelets for at least 4 weeks to ≤600,000/μL, or by at least 50% from baseline value. Subjects treated for less than 4 weeks were not considered evaluable. The results are depicted graphically below:

Least Square Means for Platelet Count During Anagrelide Therapy

[Figure: graph of Mean Platelet Count (× 10³/μL) vs Time (years), ET Subjects]

		Time on Treatment						
		Weeks				**Years**		
	Baseline	4	12	24	48	2	3	4
Mean*	1045	627	537	506	508	501	474	464
N	274**	265	245	206	179	139	76	11

*× 10³/μL

**Two hundred seventy-six ET subjects were enrolled in this study. There is no anagrelide information available for two of those subjects. Therefore, 274 subjects represent the intent-to-treat population who received anagrelide therapy.

A second historically-controlled, unblinded study in 35 patients with ET treated with anagrelide showed similar decreases in platelet count over time. For 139 patients who had baseline symptoms thought to be secondary to thrombocythemia (e.g., headache, dizziness, neurological or visual symptoms) and who were treated for at least one year with anagrelide, there was a significant reduction in frequency of symptoms at one year compared with the first month of treatment.

INDICATIONS AND USAGE

AGRYLIN™ Capsules are indicated for the treatment of patients with Essential Thrombocythemia to reduce the elevated platelet count and the risk of thrombosis and to ameliorate associated symptoms (see CLINICAL STUDIES, DOSAGE and ADMINISTRATION).

WARNINGS

Cardiovascular

Anagrelide should be used with caution in patients with known or suspected heart disease, and only if the potential benefits of therapy outweigh the potential risks. Because of the positive inotropic effects and side-effects of anagrelide, a pre-treatment cardiovascular examination is recommended along with careful monitoring during treatment. In humans, therapeutic doses of anagrelide may cause cardiovascular effects, including vasodilation, tachycardia, palpitations, and congestive heart failure.

Renal

It is recommended that patients with renal insufficiency (creatinine $\geq$ 2 mg/dL) receive anagrelide when, in the physician's judgment, the potential benefits of therapy outweigh the potential risks. These patients should be monitored closely for signs of renal toxicity while receiving anagrelide (see ADVERSE REACTIONS, Urogenital System).

Hepatic

It is recommended that patients with evidence of hepatic dysfunction (bilirubin, SGOT, or measures of liver function > 1.5 times the upper limit of normal) receive anagrelide when, in the physician's judgment, the potential benefits of therapy outweigh the potential risks. These patients should be monitored closely for signs of hepatic toxicity while receiving anagrelide (see ADVERSE REACTIONS, Hepatic System).

PRECAUTIONS

Laboratory Tests: Anagrelide therapy requires close clinical supervision of the patient. While the platelet count is being lowered (usually during the first two weeks of treatment), blood counts (hemoglobin, white blood cells), liver function (SGOT, SGPT) and renal function (serum creatinine, BUN) should be monitored.

In 9 subjects receiving a single 5 mg dose of anagrelide, standing blood pressure fell an average of 22/15 mm Hg, usually accompanied by dizziness. Only minimal changes in blood pressure were observed following a dose of 2 mg.

Cessation of AGRYLIN™ Treatment: In general, interruption of anagrelide treatment is followed by an increase in platelet count. After sudden stoppage of anagrelide therapy, the increase in platelet count can be observed within four days.

Drug Interactions: Bioavailability studies evaluating possible interactions between anagrelide and other drugs have not been conducted. The most common medications used concomitantly with anagrelide have been aspirin, acetaminophen, furosemide, iron, ranitidine, hydroxyurea, and allopurinol. The most frequently used concomitant cardiac medication has been digoxin. Although drug-to-drug interaction studies have not been conducted, there is no clinical evidence to suggest that anagrelide interacts with any of these compounds.

There is a single case report which suggests that sucralfate may interfere with anagrelide absorption.

Food has no clinically significant effect on the bioavailability of anagrelide.

Carcinogenesis, Mutagenesis, Impairment of Fertility: No long-term studies in animals have been performed to evaluate carcinogenic potential of anagrelide hydrochloride. Anagrelide hydrochloride was not genotoxic in the Ames test, the mouse lymphoma cell (L5178Y, TK$^{+/-}$) forward mutation test, the human lymphocyte chromosome aberration test, or the mouse micronucleus test. Anagrelide hydrochloride at oral doses up to 240 mg/kg/day (1,440 mg/m²/day, 195 times the recommended maximum human dose based on body surface area) was found to have no effect on fertility and reproductive performance of male rats. However, in female rats, at oral doses of 60 mg/kg/day (360 mg/m²/day, 49 times the recommended maximum human dose based on body surface area) or higher, it disrupted implantation when administered in early pregnancy and retarded or blocked parturition when administered in late pregnancy.

Pregnancy: Pregnancy Category C.

i) Teratogenic Effects

Teratology studies have been performed in pregnant rats at oral doses up to 900 mg/kg/day (5,400 mg/m²/day, 730 times the recommended maximum human dose based on body surface area) and in pregnant rabbits at oral doses up to 20 mg/kg/day (240 mg/m²/day, 32 times the recommended maximum human dose based on body surface area) and have revealed no evidence of impaired fertility or harm to the fetus due to anagrelide hydrochloride.

ii) Nonteratogenic Effects

A fertility and reproductive performance study performed in female rats revealed that anagrelide hydrochloride at oral doses of 60 mg/kg/day (360 mg/m²/day, 49 times the recommended maximum human dose based on body surface area) or higher disrupted implantation and exerted adverse effect on embryo/fetal survival.

A perinatal and postnatal study performed in female rats revealed that anagrelide hydrochloride at oral doses of 60 mg/kg/day (360 mg/m²/day, 49 times the recommended maximum human dose based on body surface area) or higher produced delay or blockage of parturition, deaths of nondelivering pregnant dams and their fully developed fetuses, and increased mortality in the pups born.

Five women became pregnant while on anagrelide treatment at doses of 1 to 4 mg/day. Treatment was stopped as soon as it was realized that they were pregnant. All delivered normal, healthy babies. There are no adequate and well-controlled studies in pregnant women. Anagrelide hydrochloride should be used during pregnancy only if the potential benefit justifies the potential risk to the fetus.

Anagrelide is not recommended in women who are or may become pregnant. If this drug is used during pregnancy, or if the patient becomes pregnant while taking this drug, the patient should be apprised of the potential harm to the fetus. Women of child-bearing potential should be instructed that they must not be pregnant and that they should use contraception while taking anagrelide. Anagrelide may cause fetal harm when administered to a pregnant woman.

Nursing Mothers: It is not known whether this drug is excreted in human milk. Because many drugs are excreted in human milk and because of the potential for serious adverse reaction in nursing infants from anagrelide hydrochloride, a decision should be made whether to discontinue nursing or to discontinue the drug, taking into account the importance of the drug to the mother.

Pediatric Use: The safety and efficacy of anagrelide in patients under the age of 16 years have not been established. Anagrelide has been used successfully in eight pediatric patients (age range 8 to 17 years), including three patients with essential thrombocythemia, who were treated at a dose of 1 to 4 mg/day.

ADVERSE REACTIONS

While most reported adverse events during anagrelide therapy have been mild in intensity and have decreased in frequency with continued treatment, serious adverse events reported in patients with ET and/or in patients with thrombocythemias of other etiologies include: congestive heart failure, myocardial infarction, cardiomyopathy, cardiomegaly, complete heart block, atrial fibrillation, cerebrovascular accident, pericarditis, pulmonary infiltrates, pulmonary fibrosis, pulmonary hypertension, pancreatitis, gastric/duodenal ulceration, and seizure.

Of the 551 ET patients treated with anagrelide for a mean duration of 65 weeks, 82 (15%) were discontinued from the study because of adverse events or abnormal laboratory test results. The most common adverse events for treatment discontinuation were headache, diarrhea, edema, palpitation, and abdominal pain. Overall, the occurrence rate of all adverse events was 17.9 per 1,000 treatment days. The occurrence rate of adverse events increased at higher dosages of anagrelide.

The most frequently reported adverse reactions to anagrelide (in 5% or greater of 551 patients with ET) in clinical trials were:

Headache	44.5%
Palpitations	27.2%
Diarrhea	24.3%
Asthenia	22.1%
Edema, other	19.8%
Abdominal Pain	17.4%
Nausea	15.1%
Pain, other	14.7%
Dizziness	14.5%
Dyspnea	10.5%
Flatulence	10.5%
Chest Pain	7.8%
Rash, including urticaria	7.8%
Vomiting	7.4%
Paresthesia	7.3%
Tachycardia	7.3%
Peripheral Edema	7.1%
Dyspepsia	6.4%
Back Pain	6.4%
Anorexia	5.8%
Malaise	5.8%

Adverse events with an incidence of 1% to < 5% included:

Body as a Whole System: Fever, flu symptoms, chills, neck pain, photosensitivity.

Cardiovascular System: Arrhythmia, hemorrhage, cardiovascular disease, cerebrovascular accident, angina pectoris, heart failure, postural hypotension, vasodilatation, migraine, syncope.

Digestive System: Constipation, GI distress, GI hemorrhage, gastritis, melena, aphthous stomatitis, eructation, nausea, vomiting.

Hemic & Lymphatic System: Anemia, thrombocytopenia, ecchymosis, lymphadenoma.

Platelet counts below 100,000/µL occurred in 35 patients and reduction below 50,000/µL occurred in 7 of the 551 ET patients while on anagrelide therapy. Thrombocytopenia promptly recovered upon discontinuation of anagrelide.

Hepatic System: Elevated liver enzymes were observed in 2 of 551 patients during anagrelide therapy.

Musculoskeletal System: Arthralgia, myalgia, leg cramps.

Nervous System: Depression, somnolence, confusion, insomnia, hypertension, nervousness, amnesia.

Nutritional Disorders: Dehydration.

Respiratory System: Rhinitis, epistaxis, respiratory disease, sinusitis, pneumonia, bronchitis, asthma.

Skin and Appendages System: Pruritus, skin disease, alopecia.

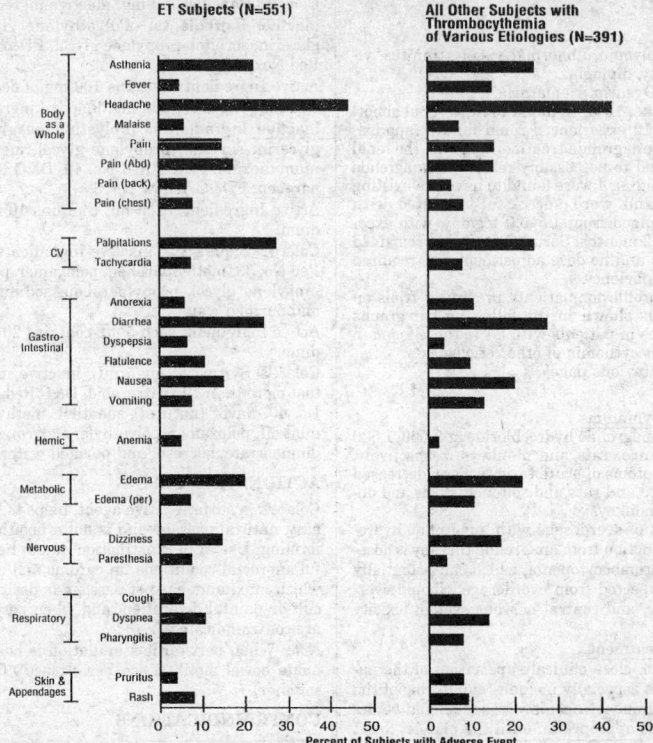

Continued on next page

Agrylin—Cont.

Special Senses: Amblyopia, abnormal vision, tinnitus, visual field abnormality, diplopia.
Urogenital System: Dysuria, Hematuria.
Of the 551 ET patients, 10 were found to have renal abnormalities. Six of the 10 experienced renal failure (approximately 1%) while on anagrelide treatment; in two, the renal failure was considered to be possibly related to anagrelide treatment. The remaining 4 were found to have pre-existing renal impairment and were successfully treated with anagrelide. Doses ranged from 1.5–6.0 mg/day, with exposure periods of 2 to 12 months. Serum creatinines remained within normal limits and no dose adjustment was required because of renal insufficiency.
The adverse event profile for patients in clinical trials on anagrelide therapy is shown in the following bar graphs comparing the profiles in patients with ET to those found in patients with thrombocythemia of other etiologies.
[See table at top of previous page]

OVERDOSAGE

Acute Toxicity and Symptoms
Single oral doses of anagrelide hydrochloride at 2,500, 1,500 and 200 mg/kg in mice, rats and monkeys, respectively, were not lethal. Symptoms of acute toxicity were: decreased motor activity in mice and rats and softened stools and decreased appetite in monkeys.
There are no reports of overdosage with anagrelide hydrochloride. Platelet reduction from anagrelide therapy is dose-related; therefore, thrombocytopenia, which can potentially cause bleeding, is expected from overdosage. Should overdosage occur, cardiac, and central nervous system toxicity can also be expected.
Management and Treatment
In case of overdosage, close clinical supervision of the patient is required; this especially includes monitoring of the platelet count for thrombocytopenia. Dosage should be decreased or stopped, as appropriate, until the platelet count returns to within the normal range.

DOSAGE AND ADMINISTRATION

Treatment with **AGRYLIN™** Capsules should be initiated under close medical supervision. The recommended starting dosage of **AGRYLIN™** is 0.5 mg qid or 1 mg bid, which should be maintained for at least one week. Dosage should then be adjusted to the lowest effective dosage required to reduce and maintain platelet count below 600,000/μL, and ideally to the normal range. The dosage should be increased by not more than 0.5 mg/day in any one week. Dosage should not exceed 10 mg/day or 2.5 mg in a single dose (see PRECAUTIONS). The decision to treat asymptomatic young adults with essential thrombocythemia should be individualized.
To monitor the effect of anagrelide and prevent the occurrence of thrombocytopenia, platelet counts should be performed every two days during the first week of treatment and at least weekly thereafter until the maintenance dosage is reached.
Typically, platelet count begins to respond within 7 to 14 days at the proper dosage. Most patients will experience an adequate response at a dose of 1.5 to 3.0 mg/day. Patients with known or suspected heart disease, renal insufficiency, or hepatic dysfunction should be monitored closely.

HOW SUPPLIED

AGRYLIN™ is available as:
0.5 mg, opaque, white capsules imprinted "ROBERTS 063" in black ink:
NDC 54092-063-01 = bottle of 100
1 mg, opaque, gray capsules imprinted "ROBERTS 064" in black ink:
NDC 54092-064-01 = bottle of 100
Store from 15° to 25°C (59° to 77°F), in a light-resistant container.
CAUTION: Federal law prohibits dispensing without prescription.
ROBERTS® PHARMACEUTICALS
Manufactured for
Roberts Laboratories Inc.
a subsidiary of
ROBERTS PHARMACEUTICAL CORP.
Eatontown, NJ 07724-2274, USA
by MALLINCKRODT INC.
Hobart, NY 13788
Copyright © 1998 Roberts Laboratories Inc.
Shown in Product Identification Guide, page 334

COLACE®   OTC
[*kō̄lās*]
docusate sodium,
capsules • syrup • liquid (drops)

DESCRIPTION

Colace® (docusate sodium) is a stool softener.
Active Ingredient: contains 50 mg of docusate sodium.

Colace® Capsules, 50 mg, inactive ingredients:
Inactive Ingredients: Polyethylene glycol 400, gelatin, glycerin, sorbitol, propylene glycol, FD&C Red No. 40, D&C Red No. 33.
Active Ingredient: contains 100 mg of docusate sodium.
Colace® Capsules, 100 mg, inactive ingredients:
Inactive Ingredients: Polyethylene glycol 400, gelatin, glycerin, sorbitol, propylene glycol, methylparaben, titanium dioxide, FD&C Red No. 40, D&C Red No. 33, propylparaben, FD&C Yellow No. 6.
Active Ingredient: each mL contains 10 mg of docusate sodium.
Colace® Liquid, 1%, inactive ingredients: citric acid, D&C Red No. 33, methylparaben, poloxamer, polyethylene glycol, propylene glycol, propylparaben, sodium citrate, vanillin, and purified water.
Active Ingredient: each 5 mL contains 20 mg of docusate sodium.
Colace® Syrup, 20 mg/5 mL, inactive ingredients: alcohol (not more than 1%), citric acid, D&C Red No. 33, FD&C Red No. 40, flavor (natural), menthol, methylparaben, peppermint oil, poloxamer, polyethylene glycol, propylparaben, sodium citrate, sucrose, and purified water.

ACTIONS AND USES

Colace®, a surface-active agent, helps to keep stools soft for easy, natural passage and is not a laxative, thus, not habit forming. Useful in constipation due to hard stools, in painful anorectal conditions, in cardiac and other conditions in which maximum ease of passage is desirable to avoid difficult or painful defecation, and when peristaltic stimulants are contraindicated.
Note: When peristaltic stimulation is needed due to inadequate bowel motility, see Peri-Colace® (laxative and stool softener).

CONTRAINDICATIONS

There are no known contraindications to Colace®.

WARNING

As with any drug, pregnant or nursing women should seek the advice of a health professional before using this product.

SIDE EFFECTS

The incidence of side effects—none of a serious nature—is exceedingly small. Bitter taste, throat irritation, and nausea (primarily associated with the use of the syrup and liquid) are the main side effects reported. Rash has occurred.

ADMINISTRATION AND DOSAGE

Orally —Suggested daily Dosage: *Adults and older children:* 50 to 200 mg *Children 6 to 12:* 40 to 120 mg Liquid.
Infants and children under 3 years of age: As prescribed by physician.
Children 3 to 6 years of age: 2mL one to three times daily
For retention or flushing enemas: Add 5 to 10mL (1 to 2 tsp) of COLACE® liquid to the enema fluid.
The higher doses are recommended for initial therapy. Dosage should be adjusted to individual response. The effect on stools is usually apparent 1 to 3 days after the first dose. Colace® liquid or syrup must be given in a 6 oz. to 8 oz. glass of milk or fruit juice or in infant's formula to prevent throat irritation. *In enemas*—Add 5 to 10 mL Colace® liquid) to a retention or flushing enema.

HOW SUPPLIED

Colace® capsules, 50 mg
  NDC 54092-052-30 Bottles of 30
  NDC 54092-052-60 Bottles of 60
  NDC 54092-052-52 Cartons of 100
    single unit packs
  NDC 54092-052-11 Blister Pack of 10
Colace® capsules, 100 mg
  NDC 54092-053-30 Bottles of 30
  NDC 54092-053-60 Bottles of 60
  NDC 54092-053-02 Bottles of 250
  NDC 54092-053-10 Bottles of 1000
  NDC 54092-053-52 Cartons of 100
    single unit packs
  NDC 54092-053-11 Blister Pack of 10
Note: Colace® capsules should be stored at controlled room temperature (59°–86°F or 15°–30°C)
Colace® liquid, 1% solution; 10 mg/mL (with calibrated dropper)
  NDC 54092-414-16 Bottles of 16 fl oz
  NDC 54092-414-30 Bottles of 30 mL
Colace® syrup, 20 mg/5-mL teaspoon; contains not more than 1% alcohol
  NDC 54092-415-08 Bottles of 8 fl oz
  NDC 54092-415-16 Bottles of 16 fl oz
Manufactured for:
Roberts Laboratories Inc., a subsidiary of
ROBERTS PHARMACEUTICAL CORPORATION
Eatontown, NJ 07724 USA

COLACE MICROENEMA   OTC
[*kō̄ lās*]
(docusate sodium)
(for rectal use only)

DESCRIPTION

Active ingredient: Each 5 mL contains 200 mg of docusate sodium.
Inactive ingredients: citric acid, sodium benzoate, hydroxypropyl methylcellulose, apricot kernel oil, PEG-6 esters, PEG-6 and PEG-32 and glycol stearate, glycerin 96%, and purified water.
Indications: For relief of occasional constipation (irregularity).
Directions for use: Adults and children 3 years of age and older: Express a drop of the mixture to lubricate the tip if necessary. Slowly insert the full length (half length for children 3 to 12 years old) of the nozzle into the rectum. Squeeze out the entire contents of the tube. Remove the nozzle completely before releasing grip on the tube, otherwise the contents may flow back into the tube.
Do not use in children under 3 years of age, except under the advise of a physician.
This product generally produces bowel movement in 2 to 15 minutes.

WARNINGS

Do not use laxative products when abdominal pain, nausea, or vomiting are present, unless directed by a doctor. If you have noticed a sudden change in bowel habits that persists over a period of 2 weeks, consult a doctor before using a laxative. Laxative products should not be used for a period longer than 1 week unless directed by a doctor. Rectal bleeding or failure to have a bowel movement after use of a laxative may indicate a serious condition. Discontinue use and consult your doctor.
Keep this and all medication out of the reach of children.
Store from 15°C to 30°C.

HOW SUPPLIED

200 mg
3 × 5 mL Microenemas
NDC 54092-491-70
Manufactured for
Roberts Laboratories Inc., a subsidiary of
ROBERTS PHARMACEUTICAL CORP.
Eatontown, NJ 07724, USA
Copyright ©1995 Roberts Laboratories Inc.
491 7004 001   10/95

EMINASE®   ℞
[*em-in-āz*]
brand of ANISTREPLASE

DESCRIPTION

Eminase® (anistreplase) is the p-anisoylated derivative of the Lys-Plasminogen-Streptokinase activator complex prepared *in vitro* by acylating human plasma-derived, purified, heat-treated, Lys-Plasminogen and purified Streptokinase from group C β-hemolytic streptococci. *Eminase* ® has a molecular weight of about 131,000. Each vial of *Eminase* ® is supplied as a sterile, lyophilized, white to off-white powder containing 30 units of Anistreplase, <3 mg dimethylsulfoxide, <0.2 mg sodium hydroxide and the following buffers and stabilizers: 150 μg p-amidinophenyl-p'-anisate (acylating agent), 100 mg mannitol, 46 mg L-lysine, 30 mg Albumin (Human), <2 mg glycerol, and 1.3 mg *ε* -aminocaproic acid. *Eminase* ® is intended only for intravenous (I.V.) injection after reconstitution with **Sterile Water for Injection, USP.** The preparation contains no preservatives and is intended to be used as a single dose. Potency is expressed in units of Anistreplase by using a reference standard which is specific for *Eminase* ® and is not comparable with units used for other fibrinolytics.
The Lys-Plasminogen and the Streptokinase used in the manufacture of *Eminase* ® are prepared under U.S. license by Oesterreichisches Institut fuer Haemoderivate GmbH and Behringwerke AG, respectively, under shared manufacturing arrangements.

CLINICAL PHARMACOLOGY

Eminase ® is an inactive derivative of a fibrinolytic enzyme with the catalytic center of the activator complex temporarily blocked by an anisoyl group. The anisoyl group does not decrease the high fibrin-binding ability of the complex. *Eminase* ® is made *in vitro* from Lys-Plasminogen and Streptokinase. *Eminase* ® differs from the complex initially formed *in vivo* upon administration of Streptokinase; the latter complex contains predominately glu-plasminogen. Activation of *Eminase* ® occurs with release of the anisoyl group by deacylation, a non-enzymatic first-order process with a half-life *in vitro* in human blood of about 2 hours. In solution, deacylation of *Eminase* ® starts immediately and the enzymatically active Lys-Plasminogen-Streptokinase acti-

vator complex is progressively formed. The production of plasmin from plasminogen by deacylated *Eminase®* can take place in the bloodstream or within the thrombus; the latter process is catalytically more efficient but both may contribute to thrombolysis. The half-life of fibrinolytic activity of the circulating *Eminase®* is 70 to 120 minutes (mean 94 minutes).

A number of controlled clinical studies have been performed with *Eminase®* to demonstrate benefit. Heparin anticoagulation was administered to all patients routinely following (about 4 to 6 hours) dosing with *Eminase®*.

Randomized, controlled studies have demonstrated that *Eminase®* reduces mortality when administered within 6 hours of the onset of the symptoms of acute myocardial infarction (AMI). The benefit of mortality reduction occurs acutely and is maintained for at least 1 year.

In a study of 1258 patients (AIMS trial), mortality at 30 days postinfarction was decreased (47.2%, p = 0.0001) in patients receiving *Eminase®* as compared with placebo. At 1 year, the reduction in mortality was maintained (38%, p = 0.001). The incidence of heart failure was less in patients treated with *Eminase®* (17.9%) compared with patients who received placebo (23.3%).[1,2] Similar mortality results were obtained from a smaller, randomized, controlled trial.[1,3]

In a double-blind, randomized trial of *Eminase®* compared with heparin bolus, left ventricular function was improved and infarction size reduced. There was significantly (p<0.01, two sample t-test) higher left ventricular ejection fraction (LVEF) for the *Eminase®* treatment group (53%) compared with the heparin treatment group (47.5%) when measured 4 days after treatment (intent-to-treat analysis). This difference was maintained when patients were reexamined by radionuclide ventriculography at day 19, even when patients who experienced successful angioplasty were excluded from the analysis (p = 0.04). About 3 weeks after treatment, mean infarct size was 24% lower in the patients treated with *Eminase®* compared with those treated with heparin (n = 188, p = 0.02).[1,4] Similarly, if those patients who experienced successful angioplasty were excluded from the analysis, the mean infarct size in patients treated with *Eminase®* was significantly less than that of heparin-treated patients (p <0.01).

In randomized, comparative studies reperfusion rates of between 50% and 68% have been reported in patients receiving *Eminase®* within 6 hours of symptom onset. However, for maximum rates of reperfusion, treatment should be initiated as soon as possible after onset of symptoms.

In two studies,[1,5,6] *Eminase®* and intracoronary (IC) Streptokinase were compared in patients with angiographically proven coronary artery occlusion. Reperfusion occurred about 45 minutes after the start of therapy for both treatment groups. When therapy was initiated within 4 hours of onset of AMI symptoms reperfusion rates of 59% (n = 87) and 68% (n = 41) were observed for *Eminase®* compared with 59% (n = 85) and 70% (n = 43) for IC Streptokinase. Of those patients who had coronary artery reperfusion, angiographically demonstrated reocclusion occurred within 24 hours in 3% to 4% of those treated with *Eminase®* and in 7% to 12% of those treated with Streptokinase.[1,5,6]

In a well-controlled, randomized study, a patency rate of 72% was obtained with *Eminase®* compared with 53% for I.V. Streptokinase. Patency for the 107 patients was determined by posttreatment angiography.[1,7]

Eminase® was also found to have a favorable risk/benefit profile in elderly patients (>65 years, n = 940) who participated in clinical trials. Use of *Eminase®* in patients over 75 years old has not been adequately studied.

INDICATIONS AND USAGE

Eminase® is indicated for use in the management of acute myocardial infarction (AMI) in adults, for the lysis of thrombi obstructing coronary arteries, the reduction of infarct size, the improvement of ventricular function following AMI, and the reduction of mortality associated with AMI. Treatment should be initiated as soon as possible after the onset of AMI symptoms (**see CLINICAL PHARMACOLOGY**).

CONTRAINDICATIONS

Because thrombolytic therapy increases the risk of bleeding, *Eminase®* is contraindicated in the following situations:
- active internal bleeding
- history of cerebrovascular accident
- recent (within 2 months) intracranial or intraspinal surgery or trauma (**see WARNINGS**)
- intracranial neoplasm, arteriovenous malformation, or aneurysm
- known bleeding diathesis
- severe, uncontrolled hypertension

Eminase® should not be administered to patients having experienced severe allergic reactions to either this product or Streptokinase.

WARNINGS

Bleeding: (**See ADVERSE REACTIONS**) The most common complication associated with *Eminase®* therapy is bleeding. The types of bleeding associated with thrombolytic therapy can be divided into two broad categories:
1. Internal bleeding involving the gastrointestinal tract, genitourinary tract, retroperitoneal, ocular, or intracranial sites.

2. Superficial or surface bleeding, observed mainly at invaded or disturbed sites (e.g., venous cutdowns, arterial punctures, sites of recent surgical intervention).

The concomitant use of heparin anticoagulation may contribute to the bleeding. Some of the hemorrhagic episodes occurred 1 or more days after the effects of *Eminase®* had dissipated, but while heparin therapy was continuing.

As fibrin is lysed during *Eminase®* therapy, bleeding from recent puncture sites may occur. Therefore, thrombolytic therapy requires careful attention to all potential bleeding sites (including catheter insertion sites, arterial and venous puncture sites, cutdown sites, and needle puncture sites). Intramuscular injections and nonessential handling of the patient should be avoided during treatment with *Eminase®*. Venipunctures should be performed carefully and only as required.

Should an arterial puncture be necessary following administration of *Eminase®*, it is preferable to use an upper-extremity vessel that is accessible to manual compression. A pressure dressing should be applied, and the puncture site should be checked frequently for evidence of bleeding.

Each patient being considered for therapy with *Eminase®* should be carefully evaluated and anticipated benefits should be weighed against potential risks associated with therapy.

In the following conditions, the risks of *Eminase®* therapy may be increased and should be weighed against the anticipated benefits:
- recent (within 10 days) major surgery (e.g., coronary artery bypass graft, obstetrical delivery, organ biopsy, previous puncture of noncompressible vessels)
- cerebrovascular disease
- recent gastrointestinal or genitourinary bleeding (within 10 days)
- recent trauma (within 10 days) including cardiopulmonary resuscitation
- hypertension: systolic BP ≥180 mmHg and/or diastolic BP ≥110 mmHg
- high likelihood of left heart thrombus (e.g., mitral stenosis with atrial fibrillation)
- subacute bacterial endocarditis
- acute pericarditis
- hemostatic defects including those secondary to severe hepatic or renal disease
- pregnancy
- age >75 years (Use of *Eminase®* in patients over 75 years old has not been adequately studied.)

diabetic hemorrhagic retinopathy or other hemorrhagic ophthalmic conditions

septic thrombophlebitis or occluded AV cannula at seriously infected site

patients currently receiving oral anticoagulants (e.g., warfarin sodium)

any other condition in which bleeding constitutes a significant hazard or would be particularly difficult to manage because of its location

Arrhythmias: Coronary thrombolysis may result in arrhythmias associated with reperfusion. These arrhythmias (such as sinus bradycardia, accelerated idioventricular rhythm, ventricular premature depolarizations, ventricular tachycardia, ventricular fibrillation) are not different from those often seen in the ordinary course of acute myocardial infarction and may be managed with standard antiarrhythmic measures. It is recommended that antiarrhythmic therapy for bradycardia and/or ventricular irritability be available when injections of *Eminase®* are administered.

Hypotension: Hypotension, sometimes severe, not secondary to bleeding or anaphylaxis, has occasionally been observed soon after intravenous *Eminase®* administration. Patients should be monitored closely and, should symptomatic or alarming hypotension occur, appropriate symptomatic treatment should be administered.

PRECAUTIONS

General: Standard management of myocardial infarction should be implemented concomitantly with *Eminase®* treatment. Invasive procedures should be minimized (**see WARNINGS**). Anaphylactoid reactions have rarely been reported in patients who received *Eminase®*. Accordingly, adequate treatment provisions such as epinephrine should be available for immediate use.

Readministration: Because of the increased likelihood of resistance due to antistreptokinase antibody, Eminase® (anistreplase) may not be as effective if administered more than 5 days after prior *Eminase®* or Streptokinase therapy, particularly between 5 days and 12 months. Increased antistreptokinase antibody levels after *Eminase®* or Streptokinase may also increase the risk of allergic reactions following readministration.

Repeated administration of *Eminase®* within 1 week of the initial dose has occurred in a small number of patients treated for AMI and non-AMI conditions. The incidence of hematomas/bruising was somewhat greater in those patients who received repeat doses of *Eminase®* but otherwise the adverse event profile was similar to those who received 1 dose.

Laboratory Tests: Intravenous administration of Eminase® will cause marked decreases in plasminogen and fibrinogen and increases in thrombin time (TT), activated partial thromboplastin time (APTT), and prothrombin time (PT).

Results of coagulation tests and/or measures of fibrinolytic activity performed during *Eminase®* therapy may be unreliable unless specific precautions are taken to prevent *in vitro* artifacts. *Eminase®* when present in blood in pharmacologic concentrations, remains active under *in vitro* conditions. This can lead to degradation of fibrinogen in blood samples removed for analysis. Collection of blood samples in the presence of aprotinin (2000 to 3000 KIU/mL) can, to some extent, mitigate this phenomenon.

Drug Interactions: The interaction of *Eminase®* (anistreplase) with other cardioactive drugs has not been studied. In addition to bleeding associated with heparin and vitamin K antagonists, drugs that alter platelet function (such as aspirin and dipyridamole) may increase the risk of bleeding if administered prior to *Eminase®* therapy.

Use of Anticoagulants: *Eminase®* alone or in combination with antiplatelet agents and anticoagulants may cause bleeding complications. Therefore, careful monitoring is advised, especially at arterial puncture sites. In clinical studies, a majority of patients treated received anticoagulant therapy postdosing with *Eminase®* during their hospital stay and a minority received heparin pretreatment with *Eminase®*. The use of antiplatelet agents increased the incidence of bleeding events similarly in patients treated with *Eminase®* or nonthrombolytic therapy. There was no evidence of a synergistic effect of combined *Eminase®* and antiplatelet agents on bleeding events. In addition, there was no difference in the incidence of hemorrhagic CVAs in *Eminase®*-treated patients who did or did not receive aspirin.

Carcinogenesis, Mutagenesis, Impairment of Fertility: Long-term studies in animals have not been performed to evaluate the carcinogenic potential or the effect on fertility. Studies to determine mutagenicity and chromosomal aberration assays in human lymphocytes were negative at all concentrations tested.

Pregnancy (Category C): Animal reproduction studies have not been conducted with *Eminase®*. It is also not known whether *Eminase®* can cause fetal harm when administered to a pregnant woman or can affect reproduction capacity. *Eminase®* should be given to a pregnant woman only if clearly needed.

Nursing Mothers: It is not known whether *Eminase®* is excreted in human milk. Because many drugs are excreted in human milk, the physician should decide whether the patient should discontinue nursing or not receive *Eminase®*.

Pediatric Use: Safety and effectiveness of Eminase® (anistreplase) in children have not been established.

ADVERSE REACTIONS

Bleeding: The incidence of bleeding (major or minor) varied widely from study to study and may depend on the use of arterial catheterization and other invasive procedures, patient population, and/or concomitant therapy. The overall incidence of bleeding in patients treated with *Eminase®* in clinical trials (n = 5275) was 14.6%, with nonpuncture-site bleeding occurring in 10.2%, and puncture-site bleeding occurring in 5.7%, of these patients. Bleeding at the puncture site occurred more frequently in clinical trials in which the patients underwent immediate coronary catheterization (13.3%, n = 637) compared with those who did not (3.0%, n = 2023). The incidence of presumed intracranial bleeding within 7 days postdosing with *Eminase®* was 0.57% (n = 5275); 0.34% etiology confirmed hemorrhagic; 0.23% etiology not confirmed) compared to 0.16% (n = 1249) after nonthrombolytic therapy.

In the AIMS trial the overall incidence of bleeding in patients treated with *Eminase®* was 14.8% compared with 3.8% for placebo. The incidence of specific bleeding events was:

Type of Bleeding	EMINASE® (n=500)	Placebo (n=501)
Puncture site	4.6%	<1%
Nonpuncture site hematoma	2.8%	<1%
Hematuria/Genitourinary	2.4%	<1%
Hemoptysis	2.2%	<1%
Gastrointestinal hemorrhage	2.0%	1.4%
Intracranial	1.0%	<1%
Gum/Mouth hemorrhage	1.0%	0
Epistaxis	<1%	<1%
Anemia	<1%	<1%
Eye hemorrhage	<1%	<1%
Hemorrhage (unspecified)	<1%	0

In this study there was no difference between *Eminase®* and placebo in the incidence of major bleeding events.

Should serious bleeding (not controlled by local pressure) occur in a critical location (intracranial, gastrointestinal, retroperitoneal, pericardial), any concomitant heparin should be terminated immediately and the administration

Continued on next page

Eminase—Cont.

of protamine to reverse heparinization should be considered. If necessary, the bleeding tendency can be reversed with appropriate replacement therapy.

Minor bleeding can be anticipated mainly at invaded or disturbed sites. If such bleeding occurs, local measures should be taken to control the bleeding **(see WARNINGS)**.

Cardiovascular: The most frequently reported adverse experiences in *Eminase* ® clinical trials (n = 5275) were arrhythmia/conduction disorders which were reported in 38% of patients treated with *Eminase* ® and 46% of nonthrombolytic control patients. Hypotension occurred in 10.4% of patients treated with *Eminase* ® compared to 7.9% for patients who received nonthrombolytic treatment **(see WARNINGS)**.

Allergic-type Reactions: Anaphylactic and anaphylactoid reactions have been observed rarely (0.2%) in patients treated with *Eminase* ® and are similar in incidence to Streptokinase (0.1% anaphylactic shock in 1 study). These included symptoms such as bronchospasm or angioedema. Other milder or delayed effects such as urticaria, itching, flushing, rashes and eosinophilia have been occasionally observed. A delayed purpuric rash appearing 1 to 2 weeks after treatment has been reported in 0.3% of patients. The rash may also be associated with arthralgia, ankle edema, gastrointestinal symptoms, mild hematuria, mild proteinuria and vasculitis. This syndrome was self-limiting and without long-term sequelae.

Risk of Viral Transmission: Six batches of *Eminase* ® (five different batches of Lys-Plasminogen) were used in clinical trials designed specifically to monitor possible hepatitis non-A, non-B transmission. No case of hepatitis was diagnosed in patients receiving *Eminase*®. Lys-Plasminogen is derived from human plasma obtained from FDA approved sources and tested for absence of viral contamination, including human immunodeficiency virus type-1 (HIV-1) and hepatitis B surface antigen. The manufacturing process includes a vapor-heat treatment step for inactivation of viruses. The entire manufacturing process has also been validated to yield a cumulative reduction of $\geq 10^{21}$ fold HIV-1 infectious particles, i.e., $\geq 10^{6}$ infectious particles removed by vapor-heat treatment and a cumulative total of $\geq 10^{15}$ infectious particles removed by the various steps in the purification process.

Causal Relationship Unknown: Since the following experiences may also be associated with AMI or other therapy, the causal relationship to *Eminase* ® administration is unknown. The following adverse experiences were infrequently (<10%) reported in clinical trials: **Body as a Whole**—chills, fever, headache, shock; **Cardiovascular**—cardiac rupture, chest pain, emboli; **Dermatology**—purpura, sweating; **Gastrointestinal**—nausea and/or vomiting; **Hemic and Lymphatic**—thrombocytopenia; **Metabolic and Nutritional**—elevated transaminase levels; **Musculoskeletal**—arthralgia; **Nervous**—agitation, dizziness, paresthesia, tremor, vertigo; **Respiratory**—dyspnea, lung edema. The following adverse experiences were rarely (less than one in a thousand) reported with use of commercially distributed *Eminase*®: **Nervous**—Guillain Barré syndrome; **Respiratory**—adult respiratory distress syndrome.

DOSAGE AND ADMINISTRATION

Administer *Eminase* ®as soon as possible after the onset of symptoms. The recommended dose is 30 units of *Eminase* ® administered only by intravenous injection over 2 to 5 minutes into an intravenous line or vein.

Reconstitution:

1. Slowly add 5 mL of **Sterile Water for Injection, USP**, by directing the stream of fluid against the side of the vial.
2. Gently roll the vial, mixing the dry powder and fluid. **Do not shake.** Try to minimize foaming.
3. The reconstituted preparation is a colorless to pale yellow transparent solution. Before administration, the product should be visually inspected for particulate matter and discoloration.
4. Withdraw the entire contents of the vial.
5. The reconstituted solution should not be further diluted before administration or added to any infusion fluids. No other medications should be added to the vial or syringe containing *Eminase*®.
6. If *Eminase* ® is not administered within 30 minutes of reconstitution, it should be discarded.

HOW SUPPLIED

Eminase ® is supplied as a sterile, lyophilized powder in 30-unit vials. NDC 54092-543-30.

Storage: Store lyophilized *Eminase* ® between 2° and 8°C (36° to 46°F).

Do not use beyond the expiration date printed on the vial.

REFERENCES

1. Data on File. SmithKline Beecham Pharmaceuticals, Philadelphia.
2. AIMS Trial Study Group. Effect of intravenous APSAC on mortality after acute myocardial infarction: preliminary report of a placebo-controlled clinical trial. Lancet 1988; 1:545–9.
3. Meinertz T, Kasper W, Schumacher M, Just H for the APSAC multicenter trial group. The German multicenter trial of anisoylated plasminogen streptokinase activator complex versus heparin for acute myocardial infarction. Am J Cardiol 1988; 62:347–51.
4. Bassand JP, Machecourt J, Cassagnes J, et al. Multicenter trial of intravenous anisoylated plasminogen streptokinase activator complex (APSAC) in acute myocardial infarction: effects on infarct size and left ventricular function. J Am Coll Cardiol 1989; 13:988–97.
5. Anderson JL, Rothbard RL, Hackworthy RA, et al. Multicenter reperfusion trial of intravenous anisoylated plasminogen streptokinase activator complex (APSAC) in acute myocardial infarction: controlled comparison with intracoronary streptokinase. J Am Coll Cardiol 1988; 11: 1153–63.
6. Bonnier HJRM, Visser RF, Klomps HC, Hoffmann HJML and the Dutch Invasive Reperfusion Study Group. Comparison of intravenous anisoylated plasminogen streptokinase activator complex and intracoronary streptokinase in acute myocardial infarction. Am J Cardiol 1988; 62:25–30.
7. Brochier ML, Quilliet L, Kulbertus H, et al. Intravenous anisoylated plasminogen streptokinase activator complex versus intravenous streptokinase in evolving myocardial infarction: preliminary data from a randomized multicentre study. Drugs 1987; 33(Suppl 3):140–5.

Manufactured by:
WÜLFING PHARMA GmbH
Gronau, Germany
U.S. License No. 1208

Distributed by:
Roberts Laboratories Inc.
a subsidiary of
ROBERTS PHARMACEUTICAL CORP.
Eatontown, NJ 07724, USA

Veterans Administration/Military/PHS—Vial, 30 mL, 6505-01-314-7922. EM:L3

ETHMOZINE® ℞
(moricizine hydrochloride)
TABLETS

DESCRIPTION

ETHMOZINE® (moricizine hydrochloride) is an orally active antiarrhythmic drug available for administration in tablets containing 200 mg, 250 mg and 300 mg of moricizine hydrochloride. The chemical name of moricizine hydrochloride is 10-(3-morpholinopropionyl) phenothiazine-2-carbamic acid ethyl ester hydrochloride and the structural formula is represented as follows:

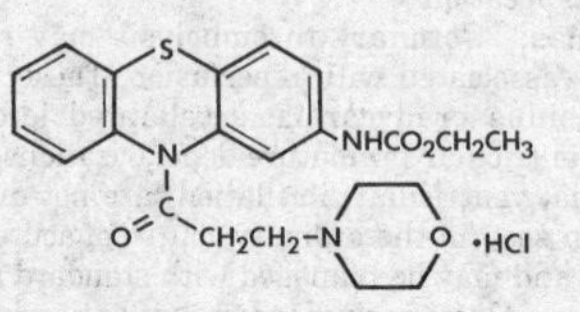

MW=464

Moricizine hydrochloride is a white to tan crystalline powder, freely soluble in water and has a pKa of 6.4 (weak acid). ETHMOZINE® tablets contain: lactose, microcrystalline cellulose, sodium starch glycolate, magnesium stearate, and dyes (FD&C Blue 1, D&C Yellow 10 and FD&C Yellow 6 [200 mg tablet]; FD&C Yellow 6 and FD&C Red 40 [250 mg tablet]; FD&C Blue 1 [300 mg tablet]).

CLINICAL PHARMACOLOGY

Mechanism of Action

ETHMOZINE® is a Class I antiarrhythmic agent with potent local anesthetic activity and myocardial membrane stabilizing effects. ETHMOZINE® reduces the fast inward current carried by sodium ions.

In isolated dog Purkinje fibers, ETHMOZINE® shortens Phase II and III repolarization, resulting in a decreased action potential duration and effective refractory period. A dose-related decrease in the maximum rate of Phase 0 depolarization (V_{max}) occurs without effect on maximum diastolic potential or action potential amplitude. The sinus node and atrial tissue of the dog are not affected.

Electrophysiology

Electrophysiology studies in patients with ventricular tachycardia have shown that ETHMOZINE®, at daily doses of 750 mg and 900 mg, prolongs atrioventricular conduction. Both AV nodal conduction time (AH interval) and His-Purkinje conduction time (HV interval) are prolonged by 10–13% and 21–26%, respectively. The PR interval is prolonged by 16–20% and the QRS by 7–18%. Prolongations of 2–5% in the corrected QT interval result from widening of the QRS interval, but there is shortening of the JT interval, indicating an absence of significant effect on ventricular repolarization. Intra-atrial conduction or atrial effective refractory periods are not consistently affected. In patients without sinus node dysfunction, ETHMOZINE® has minimal effects on sinus cycle length and sinus node recovery time. These effects may be significant in patients with sinus node dysfunction (see PRECAUTIONS: Electrocardiographic Changes/Conduction Abnormalities).

Hemodynamics

In patients with impaired left ventricular function, ETHMOZINE® has minimal effects on measurements of cardiac performance such as cardiac index, stroke volume index, pulmonary capillary wedge pressure, systemic or pulmonary vascular resistance or ejection fraction, either at rest or during exercise. ETHMOZINE® is associated with a small, but consistent increase in resting blood pressure and heart rate. Exercise tolerence in patients with ventricular arrhythmias is unaffected. In patients with a history of congestive heart failure or angina pectoris, exercise duration and rate-pressure product at maximal exercise are unchanged during ETHMOZINE® administration. Nonetheless, in some cases worsened heart failure in patients with severe underlying heart disease has been attributed to ETHMOZINE®.

Other Pharmacologic Effects

Although ETHMOZINE® is chemically related to the neuroleptic phenothiazines, it has no demonstrated central or peripheral dopaminergic activity in animals. Moreover, in patients on chronic ETHMOZINE®, serum prolactin levels did not increase.

Pharmacokinetics/Pharmacodynamics

The antiarrhythmic and electrophysiologic effects of ETHMOZINE® are not related in time course or intensity to plasma moricizine concentrations or to the concentrations of any identified metabolite, all of which have short (2–3 hours) half-lives. Following single doses of ETHMOZINE®, there is a prompt prolongation of the PR interval, which becomes normal within 2 hours, consistent with the rapid fall of plasma moricizine. JT interval shortening, however, peaks at about 6 hours and persists for at least 10 hours. Although an effect on VPD rates is seen within 2 hours after dosing, the full effect is seen after 10–14 hours and persists in full, when therapy is terminated, for more than 10 hours, after which the effect decays slowly, and is still substantial at 24 hours. This suggests either an unidentified, active, long half-life metabolite or a structural or functional "deep compartment" with slow entry from, and release to, the plasma. The following description of parent compound pharmacokinetics is therefore of uncertain relevance to clinical actions.

Following oral administration, ETHMOZINE® undergoes significant first-pass metabolism resulting in an absolute bioavailability of approximately 38%. Peak plasma concentrations of ETHMOZINE® are usually reached within 0.5–2 hours. Administration 30 minutes after a meal delays the rate of absorption, resulting in lower peak plasma concentrations, but the extent of absorption is not altered. ETHMOZINE® plasma levels are proportional to dose over the recommended therapeutic dose range.

The apparent volume of distribution after oral administration is very large (≥300L) and is not significantly related to body weight. ETHMOZINE® is approximately 95% bound to human plasma proteins. This binding interaction is independent of ETHMOZINE® plasma concentration.

ETHMOZINE® undergoes extensive biotransformation. Less than 1% of orally administered ETHMOZINE® is excreted unchanged in the urine. There are at least 26 metabolites, but no single metabolite has been found to represent as much as 1% of the administered dose, and as stated above, antiarrhythmic response has relatively slow onset and offset. Two metabolites are pharmacologically active in at least one animal model: moricizine sulfoxide and phenothiazine-2-carbamic acid ethyl ester sulfoxide. Each of these metabolites represents a small percentage of the administered dose (<0.6%), is present in lower concentrations in the plasma than the parent drug, and has a plasma elimination half-life of approximately three hours.

ETHMOZINE® has been shown to induce its own metabolism. Average ETHMOZINE® plasma concentrations in patients decrease with multiple dosing. This decrease in plasma levels of parent drug does not appear to affect clinical outcome for patients receiving chronic ETHMOZINE® therapy.

The plasma half-life of ETHMOZINE® is 1.5–3.5 hours (most values about 2 hours) following single or multiple oral doses in patients with ventricular ectopy. Approximately 56% of the administered dose is execreted in the feces and 39% is excreted in the urine. Some ETHMOZINE® is also recycled through enterohepatic circulation.

CLINICAL ACTIONS

ETHMOZINE® at daily doses of 600–900 mg produces a dose- related reduction in the occurrence of frequent ventricular premature depolarizations (VPDs) and reduces the incidence of nonsustained and sustained ventricular tachycardia (VT). In controlled clinical trials, ETHMOZINE® has

been shown to have antiarrhythmic activity that is generally similar to that of disopyramide, propranolol, and quinidine at the doses studied. In controlled and compassionate use programmed electrical stimulation studies (PES), ETHMOZINE® prevented the induction of sustained ventricular tachycardia in approximately 25% (19/75) of patients. In a post-marketing randomized comparative PES study, ETHMOZINE® had a response rate of approximately 12% (7/59). Activity of ETHMOZINE® is maintained during long-term use.

ETHMOZINE® is effective in treating ventricular arrhythmias in patients with and without organic heart disease. ETHMOZINE® may be effective in patients in whom other antiarrhythmic agents are ineffective, not tolerated and/or contraindicated.

Arrhythmia exacerbation or "rebound" is not noted following discontinuation of ETHMOZINE® therapy.

INDICATIONS AND USAGE

ETHMOZINE® is indicated for the treatment of documented ventricular arrhythmias, such as sustained ventricular tachycardia, that, in the judgement of the physician are life- threatening. Because of the proarrhythmic effects of ETHMOZINE®, its use with lesser arrhythmias is generally not recommended. Treatment of patients with asymptomatic ventricular premature contractions should be avoided.

Initiation of ETHMOZINE® treatment, as with other antiarrhythmic agents used to treat life-threatening arrhythmias, should be carried out in the hospital.

Antiarrhythmic drugs have not been shown to enhance survival in patients with ventricular arrhythmias.

CONTRAINDICATIONS

ETHMOZINE® (moricizine hydrochloride) is contraindicated in patients with pre-existing second- or third-degree AV block and in patients with right bundle branch block when associated with left hemiblock (bifascicular block) unless a pacemaker is present. ETHMOZINE® is also contraindicated in the presence of cardiogenic shock or known hypersensitivity to the drug.

WARNINGS

Mortality

Ethmozine® was one of the three antiarrhythmic drugs included in the National Heart Lung and Blood Institute's (NHLBI) Cardiac Arrhythmia Suppression Trial (CAST I), a long-term, multi-center, randomized, double-blind study in patients with asymptomatic non-life-threatening ventricular arrhythmias who had had a myocardial infarction more than six days, but less than two years previously. An excessive mortality or non-fatal cardiac arrest rate was seen in patients treated with both of the Class IC agents included in the trial, which led to discontinuation of those two arms of the trial. The average duration of treatment with these agents was 10 months. The Ethmozine® and placebo arms of the trial were continued in the NHLBI-sponsored CAST II. In this randomized, double-blind trial, patients with asymptomatic, non-life-threatening ventricular arrhythmias who had had a myocardial infarction within 4 to 90 days and left ventricular ejection fraction ≤0.40 prior to enrollment were evaluated. The average duration of treatment with Ethmozine® in this study was 18 months. The study was discontinued because of the unlikely possibility of demonstrating a benefit toward improved survival with Ethmozine® and because of an evolving adverse trend after long-term treatment, although there was no statistical significance versus placebo.

The applicability of the CAST results to other populations (e.g. those without recent myocardial infarction) is uncertain. Considering the known proarrhythmic properties of Ethmozine® and the lack of evidence of improved survival for any antiarrhythmic drug in patients without life-threatening arrhythmias, the use of Ethmozine®, as well as other antiarrhythmic agents, should be reserved for patients with life-threatening ventricular arrhythmias.

Proarrhythmia

Like other antiarrhythmic drugs, ETHMOZINE® can provoke new rhythm disturbances or make existing arrhythmias worse. These proarrhythmic effects can range from an increase in the frequency of VPDs to the development of new or more severe ventricular tachycardia, e.g., tachycardia that is more sustained or more resistant to conversion to sinus rhythm, with potentially fatal consequences. It is often not possible to distinguish a proarrhythmic effect from the patient's underlying rhythm disorder, so that the occurrence rates given below must be considered approximations. Note also that drug-induced arrhythmias can generally be identified only when they occur early after starting the drug and when the rhythm can be identified, usually because the patient is being monitored. It is clear from the NIH sponsored CAST (Cardiac Arrhythmia Suppression Trial) that some antiarrhythmic drugs can cause increased sudden death mortality, presumably due to new arrhythmias or asystole that do not appear early after treatment but that represent a sustained increased risk.

Domestic pre-marketing trials included 1072 patients given ETHMOZINE®; 397 had baseline lethal arrhythmias (sustained VT or VF and non-sustained VT with hemodynamic symptoms) and 576 had potentially lethal arrhythmias (increased VPDs or NSVT in patients with known structural heart disease, active ischemia, congestive heart failure or an LVEF<40% and/or CI<2.0 l/min/m^2). In this population there were 40 (3.7%) identified proarrhythmic events, 26 (2.5%) of which were serious, either fatal (6), new hemodynamically significant sustained VT or VF (4), new sustained VT that was not hemodynamically significant (11) or sustained VT that became syncopal/presyncopal when it had not been before (5). Proarrhythmic effects described as incessant ventricular tachycardia were observed in the post-marketing PES study and in post-marketing adverse event reports.

In general, serious proarrhythmic effects in the domestic pre-marketing trials were equally common in patients with more and less severe arrhythmias, 2.5% in the patients with baseline lethal arrhythmias vs. 2.8% in patients with potentially lethal arrhythmias, although the patients with serious effects were more likely to have a history of sustained VT (38% vs. 23%). In the post-marketing comparative PES study, patients treated with ETHMOZINE® (250–300 mg TID) had a proarrhythmia rate of 14% (8/59).

Five of the six fatal proarrhythmic events were in patients with baseline lethal arrhythmias; four had prior cardiac arrests. Rates and severity of proarrhythmic events were similar in patients given 600–900 mg of ETHMOZINE® per day and those given higher doses. Patients with proarrhythmic events were more likely than the overall population to have coronary artery disease (85% vs. 67%), history of acute myocardial infarction (75% vs. 53%), congestive heart failure (60% vs. 43%), and cardiomegaly (55% vs. 33%). All of the six proarrhythmic deaths were in patients with coronary artery disease; 5/6 each had documented acute myocardial infarction, congestive heart failure, and cardiomegaly.

Electrolyte Disturbances

Hypokalemia, hyperkalemia, or hypomagnesemia may alter the effects of Class I antiarrhythmic drugs. Electrolyte imbalances should be corrected before administration of ETHMOZINE®.

Sick Sinus Syndrome

ETHMOZINE® should be used only with extreme caution in patients with sick sinus syndrome, as it may cause sinus bradycardia, sinus pause or sinus arrest.

PRECAUTIONS

General:

Electrocardiographic Changes/Conduction Abnormalities

ETHMOZINE® slows AV nodal and intraventricular conduction, producing dose-related increases in the PR and QRS intervals. In clinical trials, the average increase in the PR interval was 12% and the QRS interval was 14%. Although the QTC interval is increased, this is wholly because of QRS prolongation; the JT interval is shortened, indicating the absence of significant slowing of ventricular repolarization. The degree of lengthening of PR and QRS intervals does not predict efficacy.

In controlled clinical trials and in open studies, the overall incidence of delayed ventricular conduction, including new bundle branch block pattern, was approximately 9.4%. In patients without baseline conduction abnormalities, the frequency of second-degree AV block was 0.2% and third-degree AV block did not occur. In patients with baseline conduction abnormalities, the frequencies of second-degree AV block and third-degree AV block were 0.9% and 1.4%, respectively.

ETHMOZINE® therapy was discontinued in 1.6% of patients due to electrocardiographic changes (0.6% due to sinus pause or asystole, 0.2% to AV block, 0.2% to junctional rhythm, 0.4% to intraventricular conduction delay, and 0.2% to wide QRS and/or PR interval).

In patients with pre-existing conduction abnormalities, ETHMOZINE® therapy should be initiated cautiously. If second- or third-degree AV block occurs, ETHMOZINE® therapy should be discontinued unless a ventricular pacemaker is in place. When changing the dose of ETHMOZINE® or adding concomitant medications which may also affect cardiac conduction, patients should be monitored electrocardiographically.

Hepatic Impairment

Patients with significant liver dysfunction have reduced plasma clearance and an increased half-life of ETHMOZINE®. Although the precise relationship of ETHMOZINE® levels to effect is not clear, patients with hepatic disease should be treated with lower doses and closely monitored for excessive pharmacological effects, including effects on ECG intervals, before dosage adjustment. Patients with severe liver disease should be administered ETHMOZINE® with particular care, if at all (See DOSAGE AND ADMINISTRATION).

Renal Impairment

Plasma levels of intact ETHMOZINE® are unchanged in hemodialysis patients, but a significant portion (39%) of ETHMOZINE® is metabolized and excreted in the urine. Although no identified active metabolite is known to increase in people with renal failure, metabolites of unrecognized importance could be affected. For this reason, ETHMOZINE® should be administered cautiously in patients with impaired renal function. Patients with significant renal dysfunction should be started on lower doses and monitored for excessive pharmacologic effects, including ECG intervals, before dosage adjustment (See DOSAGE AND ADMINISTRATION).

Congestive Heart Failure

Most patients with congestive heart failure have tolerated the recommended ETHMOZINE® daily doses without unusual toxicity or change in effect. Pharmacokinetic differences between ETHMOZINE® patients with and without congestive heart failure were not apparent (See Hepatic Impairment above). In some cases, worsened heart failure has been attributed to ETHMOZINE®. Patients with pre-existing heart failure should be monitored carefully when ETHMOZINE® is initiated.

Effects on Pacemaker Threshold

The effect of ETHMOZINE® on the sensing and pacing thresholds of artificial pacemakers has not been sufficiently studied. In such patients, pacing parameters must be monitored, if ETHMOZINE® is used.

Drug Interactions

No significant changes in serum digoxin levels or pharmacokinetics have been observed in patients or healthy subjects receiving concomitant ETHMOZINE® therapy. Concomitant use was associated with additive prolongation of the PR interval, but not with a significant increase in the rate of second- or third-degree AV block.

Concomitant administration of cimetidine resulted in a decrease in ETHMOZINE® clearance of 49% and a 1.4 fold increase in plasma levels in healthy subjects. During clinical trials, no significant changes in the efficacy or tolerance of ETHMOZINE® have been observed in patients receiving concomitant cimetidine therapy. Patients on cimetidine should have ETHMOZINE® therapy initiated at relatively low doses, not more than 600 mg/day. Patients should be monitored when concomitant cimetidine therapy is instituted or discontinued or when the ETHMOZINE® dose is changed.

Concomitant administration of beta blocker therapy did not reveal significant changes in overall electrocardiographic intervals in patients. In one controlled study, ETHMOZINE® (moricizine hydrochloride) and propranolol administered concomitantly produced a small additive increase in the PR interval.

Theophylline clearance and plasma half-life were significantly affected by multiple dose ETHMOZINE® administration when both conventional and sustained release theophylline were given to healthy subjects (clearance increased 44–66% and plasma half-life decreased 19–33%). Plasma theophylline levels should be monitored when concomitant ETHMOZINE® is initiated or discontinued.

Because of possible additive pharmocologic effects, caution is indicated when ETHMOZINE® is used with any drug that affects cardiac electrophysiology. Uncontrolled experience in patients indicates no serious adverse interaction during the concomitant use of ETHMOZINE® and diuretics, vasodilators, antihypertensive drugs, calcium channel blockers, beta-blockers, angiotensin-converting enzyme inhibitors, or warfarin. Plasma warfarin levels, warfarin pharmacokinetics, and prothrombin times were unaffected during multiple dose ETHMOZINE® administration to young, healthy, male subjects in a controlled study. However, there are isolated reports of the need to either increase or decrease warfarin doses after initiation of ETHMOZINE®. Some patients who were taking warfarin with a stable prothrombin time experienced excessive prolongation of the prothrombin time following the initiation of ETHMOZINE®. In some cases, liver enzymes also were elevated. Bleeding or bruising may occur. When ETHMOZINE® is started or stopped in a patient stabilized on warfarin, more frequent prothrombin time monitoring is advisable.

Results from *in vitro* studies do not suggest alterations in ETHMOZINE plasma protein binding in the presence of other highly plasma protein bound drugs.

CARCINOGENESIS, MUTAGENESIS, IMPAIRMENT OF FERTILITY

In a 24-month mouse study in which ETHMOZINE® was administered in the feed at concentrations calculated to provide doses ranging up to 320 mg/kg/day, ovarian tubular adenomas and granulosa cell tumors were limited in occurrence to ETHMOZINE® treated animals. Although the findings were of borderline statistical significance, or not statistically significant, historical control data indicate that both of these tumors are uncommon in the strain of mouse studied.

Continued on next page

Ethmozine—Cont.

In a 24-month study in which ETHMOZINE® was administered by gavage to rats at doses of 25, 50 and 100 mg/kg/day, Zymbal's Gland Carcinoma was observed in one mid-dose and two high-dose males. This tumor appears to be uncommon in the strain of rat studied. Rats of both sexes showed a dose-related increase in hepatocellular cholangioma (also described as bile ductile cystadenoma or cystic hyperplasia) along with fatty metamorphosis, possibly due to disruption of hepatic choline utilization for phospholipid biosynthesis. The rat is known to be uniquely sensitive to alteration in choline metabolism.

ETHMOZINE® was not mutagenic when assayed for genotoxicity in *in vitro* bacterial (Ames test) and mammalian (Chinese hamster ovary/hypoxanthine-guanine phosphoribosyl transferase and sister chromatid exchange) cell systems or in *in vivo* mammalian systems (rat bone cytogenicity and mouse micronucleus).

A general reproduction and fertility study was conducted in rats at dose levels up to 6.7 times the maximum recommended human dose of 900 mg/day (based upon 50 kg human body weight) and revealed no evidence of impaired male or female fertility.

Pregnancy—Teratogenic Effects:

Pregnancy Category B

Teratology studies have been performed with ETHMOZINE® in rats and in rabbits at doses up to 6.7 and 4.7 times the maximum recommended human daily dose, respectively, and have revealed no evidence of harm to the fetus. There are, however, no adequate and well-controlled studies in pregnant women. Because animal reproduction studies are not always predictive of human response, ETHMOZINE® should be used during pregnancy only if clearly needed.

Pregnancy—Nonteratogenic Effects:

In a study in which rats were dosed with ETHMOZINE® prior to mating, during mating and throughout gestation and lactation, dose levels 3.4 and 6.7 times the maximum recommended human daily dose produced a dose-related decrease in pup and maternal weight gain, possibly related to a larger litter size. In a study in which dosing was begun on Day 15 of gestation, ETHMOZINE®, at a level 6.7 times the maximum recommended human daily dose, produced a retardation in maternal weight gain but no effect on pup growth.

Nursing Mothers

ETHMOZINE® is secreted in the milk of laboratory animals and has been reported to be present in human milk. Because of the potential for serious adverse reactions in nursing infants from ETHMOZINE®, a decision should be made whether to discontinue the drug, taking into account the importance of the drug to the mother.

Pediatric Use

The safety and effectiveness of ETHMOZINE® in children less than 18 years of age have not been established.

ADVERSE REACTIONS

The most serious adverse reaction reported for ETHMOZINE® is proarrhythmia (see WARNINGS). This occurred in 3.7% of 1072 patients with ventricular arrhythmias who received a wide range of doses under a variety of circumstances.

In addition to discontinuations because of proarrhythmias, in controlled clinical trials and in open studies, adverse reactions led to discontinuation of ETHMOZINE® in 7% of 1105 patients with ventricular and supraventricular arrhythmias, including 3.2% due to nausea, 1.6% due to ECG abnormalities (principally conduction defects, sinus pause, junctional rhythm, or AV block), 1% due to congestive heart failure and 0.3–0.4% due to dizziness, anxiety, drug fever, urinary retention, blurred vision, gastrointestinal upset, rash, and laboratory abnormalities.

The most frequently occurring adverse reactions in the 1072 patients (including all adverse experiences whether or not considered ETHMOZINE®-related by the investigator) were dizziness (15.1%), nausea (9.6%), headache (8.0%), fatigue (5.9%), palpitations (5.8%) and dyspnea (5.7%). Dizziness appears to be related to the size of each dose. In a comparison of 900 mg/day given at 450 mg b.i.d. or 300 mg t.i.d., more than 20% of patients experienced dizziness on the b.i.d. regimen vs. 12% on the t.i.d. regimen.

Adverse reactions reported by less than 5%, but in 2% or greater of the patients were: sustained ventricular tachycardia, hypesthesias, abdominal pain, dyspepsia, vomiting, sweating, cardiac chest pain, asthenia, nervousness, paresthesias, congestive heart failure, musculoskeletal pain, diarrhea, dry mouth, cardiac death, sleep disorders and blurred vision.

Adverse reactions infrequently reported (in less than 2% of the patients) were:

Cardiovascular—hypotension, hypertension, syncope, supraventricular arrhythmias (including atrial fibrillation/flutter), cardiac arrest, bradycardia, pulmonary embolism, myocardial infarction, vasodilation, cerebrovascular events, thrombophlebitis;

INCIDENCE (%) OF THE MOST COMMON ADVERSE REACTIONS (THERAPY DURATION = 1–14 DAYS)

Adverse Reactions	>2% Moricizine No.	%	>2% Placebo No.	%	>2% Quinidine No.	%	>5% Disopyramide No.	%	>5% Propranolol No.	%
Total No. of Patients	1072		618		110		31		24	
Dizziness	121	11.3	33	5.3	8	7.3	—		2	8.3
Nausea	74	6.9	18	2.9	7	6.4	3	9.7	—	
Headache	62	5.8	27	4.4	—		—		4	16.7
Pain	41	3.8	31	5.0	6	5.5	2	6.5	—	
Dyspnea	41	3.8	22	3.6	—		—		—	
Hypesthesia	40	3.7	—		3	2.7	—		—	
Fatigue	33	3.1	16	2.6	6	5.5	2	6.5	3	12.5
Vomiting	22	2.1	—		—		—		—	
Dry Mouth	—		—		—		11	35.5	—	
Nervousness	—		—		—		3	9.7	—	
Blurred vision	—		—		3	2.7	2	6.5	3	12.5
Diarrhea	—		—		25	22.7	—		—	
Constipation	—		—		—		2	6.5	—	
Somnolence	—		—		—		—		2	8.3
Urinary Retention	—		—		—		4	12.9	—	

Nervous System—tremor, anxiety, depression, euphoria, confusion, somnolence, agitation, seizure, coma, abnormal gait, hallucinations, nystagmus, diplopia, speech disorder, akathisia, loss of memory, ataxia, abnormal coordination, dyskinesia, vertigo, tinnitus;

Genitourinary—urinary retention or frequency, dysuria, urinary incontinence, kidney pain, impotence, decreased libido;

Respiratory—hyperventilation, apnea, asthma, pharyngitis, cough, sinusitus;

Gastrointestinal—anorexia, bitter taste, dysphagia, flatulence, ileus;

Other—drug fever, hypothermia, temperature intolerence, eye pain, rash, pruritus, dry skin, urticaria, swelling of the lips and tongue, periorbital edema.

During ETHMOZINE® therapy, two patients developed thrombocytopenia that may have been drug-related. Clinically significant elevations in liver function tests (bilirubin, serum transaminases) and jaundice consistent with hepatitis were rarely reported. Although a cause and effect relationship has not been established, caution is advised in patients who develop unexplained signs of hepatic dysfunction, and consideration should be given to discontinuing therapy.

Three patients developed rechallenge-confirmed drug fever, with one patient experiencing an elevation above 103°F (to 105°F. with rigors). Fevers occurred at about 2 weeks in 2 cases, and after 21 weeks in the third. Fevers resolved within 48 hours of discontinuation of moricizine.

Adverse reactions were generally similar in patients over 65 (n=375) and under 65 (n=697), although discontinuation of therapy for reasons other than proarrhythmia was more common in older patients (13.9% vs. 7.7%). Overall mortality was greater in older patients (9.3% vs. 3.9%), but those were not deaths attributed to treatment and the older patients had more serious underlying heart disease.

The following table compares the most common (occurrence in more than 2% of the patients) non-cardiac adverse reactions (i.e., drug-related or of unknown relationship) in controlled clinical trials during the first one to two weeks of therapy with ETHMOZINE®, quinidine, placebo, disopyramide, or propranolol in patients with ventricular arrhythmias.

[See table above]

OVERDOSAGE

Deaths have occurred after accidental or intentional overdosages of 2,250 and 10,000 mg of ETHMOZINE® (moricizine hydrochloride), respectively.

Signs, Symptoms and Laboratory Findings Associated with an Overdosage of Drug

Overdosage with ETHMOZINE® may produce emesis, lethargy, coma, syncope, hypotension, conduction disturbances, exacerbation of congestive heart failure, myocardial infarction, sinus arrest, arrhythmias (including junctional bradycardia, ventricular tachycardia, ventricular fibrillation and asystole), and respiratory failure.

Lethal Dose in Animals

Oral doses of ETHMOZINE® of about 200 mg/kg in dogs, 250 mg/kg in monkeys, 420 mg/kg in mice and 905 mg/kg in rats were lethal to about one-half of the animals exposed. Death was usually preceded by tremors, convulsions and respiratory depression.

Recommended General Treatment Procedures

A specific antidote for ETHMOZINE® has not been identified. In the event of overdosage, treatment should be supportive. Patients should be hospitalized and monitored for cardiac, respiratory and CNS changes. Advanced life support systems, including an intracardiac pacing catheter, should be provided where necessary. Acute overdosage should be treated with appropriate gastric evacuation, and with special care to avoid aspiration. Accidental introduction of ETHMOZINE® into the lungs of monkeys resulted in rapid arrhythmic death.

DOSAGE AND ADMINISTRATION

The dosage of ETHMOZINE® must be individualized on the basis of antiarrhythmic response and tolerance. Clinical, cardiac rhythm monitoring, electrocardiogram intervals, exercise testing, and/or programmed electrical stimulation testing may be used to guide antiarrhythmic response and dosage adjustment. In general, the patients will be at high risk and should be hospitalized for the initiation of therapy (see INDICATIONS AND USAGE).

The usual adult dosage is between 600 and 900 mg per day, given every 8 hours in three equally divided doses. Within this range, the dosage can be adjusted as tolerated, in increments of 150 mg/day at 3-day intervals, until the desired effect is obtained. Patients with life-threatening arrhythmias who exhibit a beneficial response as judged by objective criteria (Holter monitoring, programmed electrical stimulation, exercise testing, etc.) can be maintained on chronic ETHMOZINE® therapy. As the antiarrhythmic effect of ETHMOZINE® persists for more than 12 hours, some patients whose arrhythmias are well-controlled on a Q8H regimen may be given the same total daily dose in a Q12H regimen to increase convenience and help assure compliance. When higher doses are used, patients may experience more dizziness and nausea on the Q12 hour regimen.

Patients with Hepatic Impairment

Patients with hepatic disease should be started at 600 mg/day or lower and monitored closely, including measurement of ECG intervals, before dosage adjustment.

Patients with Renal Impairment

Patients with significant renal dysfunction should be started at 600mg/day or lower and monitored closely, including measurement of ECG intervals, before dosage adjustment.

Transfer to ETHMOZINE®

Recommendations for transferring patients from another antiarrhythmic to ETHMOZINE® can be given based on theoretical considerations. Previous antiarrhythmic therapy should be withdrawn for 1–2 plasma half-lives before starting ETHMOZINE® at the recommended dosages. In patients in whom withdrawal of a previous antiarrhythmic is likely to produce life-threatening arrhythmias, hospitalization is recommended.

Transferred From	Start ETHMOZINE®
Quinidine, Disopyramide	6–12 hours after last dose
Procainamide	3–6 hours after last dose
Encainide, Propafenone, Tocainide, or Mexiletine	8–12 hours after last dose
Flecainide	12–24 hours after last dose

HOW SUPPLIED

ETHMOZINE® (moricizine hydrochloride) is available as oval, convex, film-coated tablets as follows:

200 mg (light green):	Bottles of 100 (NDC 54092-046-01)
	Hospital Unit Dose Carton of 100 (NDC 54092-046-52)
250 mg (light orange):	Bottles of 100 (NDC 54092-047-01)
	Hospital Unit Dose Carton of 100 (NDC 54092-047-52)
300 mg (light blue)	Bottles of 100 (NDC 54092-048-01)
	Hospital Unit Dose Carton of 100 (NDC 54092-048-52)

Store from 15°–30°C (59°–86°F) in a tightly-closed, light resistant container. Protect from light.

Manufactured for:
Roberts Laboratories Inc.
a wholly owned subsidiary of
Roberts Pharmaceutical Corporation
Eatontown, New Jersey 07724
US Patent 3,864,487

FUROXONE® ℞
[fewr-ox 'ōne]
(furazolidone)
Tablets and Liquid

DESCRIPTION

Furoxone (furazolidone) is one of the synthetic antimicrobial nitrofurans. It is a stable, yellow, crystalline compound with the following structure:

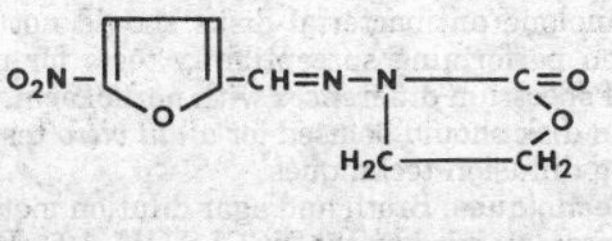

3-(5-nitrofurfurylideneamino)-2-oxazolidinone

Inactive Ingredients: Furoxone tablets contain calcium pyrophosphate, FD&C Blue #2, magnesium stearate, starch, and sucrose. Furoxone liquid contains carboxymethylcellulose sodium, flavors, glycerin, magnesium aluminum silicate, methylparaben, propylparaben, purified water, and saccharin sodium.

ACTION

Furoxone has a broad antibacterial spectrum covering the majority of gastrointestinal tract pathogens including *E. coli*, staphylococci, *Salmonella, Shigella, Proteus, Aerobacter aerogenes, Vibrio cholerae*[9,10,11] and *Giardia lamblia.*[5,6] Its bactericidal activity is based upon its interference with several bacterial enzyme systems; this antimicrobial action minimizes the development of resistant organisms. It neither significantly alters the normal bowel flora nor results in fungal overgrowth. The brown color found in the urine with adequate dosage is of no clinical significance.

INDICATIONS

Indicated in the specific and symptomatic treatment of bacterial or protozoal diarrhea and enteritis caused by susceptible organisms. Furoxone products are well tolerated, have a very low incidence of adverse reactions.

CONTRAINDICATIONS

1. To obviate an Antabuse® (disulfiram)-like reaction which may occur in some patients, the ingestion of alcohol should be avoided during or within four days after Furoxone therapy (see ADVERSE REACTIONS).
2. IN GENERAL MAOI DRUGS, TYRAMINE-CONTAINING FOODS AND INDIRECTLY-ACTING SYMPATHOMIMETIC AMINES ARE CONTRAINDICATED OR SHOULD BE USED WITH CAUTION IN PATIENTS RECEIVING FUROXONE (SEE PRECAUTIONS).
3. INFANTS UNDER 1 MONTH SHOULD NOT RECEIVE FUROXONE (SEE ADVERSE REACTIONS AND DOSAGE FOR CHILDREN).[4] THE FUROXONE CONCENTRATION IN THE BREAST MILK OF LACTATING WOMEN HAS NOT BEEN DETERMINED. THEREFORE THE SAFETY IN THIS CIRCUMSTANCE HAS NOT BEEN ESTABLISHED.
4. Prior sensitivity to Furoxone is a contraindication.

WARNINGS

(See CONTRAINDICATIONS listed above.)

Use In Pregnancy: The safety of Furoxone during the childbearing age has not been established; as with any potent antibacterial, Furoxone must be administered with caution during the childbearing age. However, animal breeding studies have revealed no evidence of teratogenicity following the administration of Furoxone for long periods of time and at doses far in excess of those recommended for the human. There have been no clinical reports regarding this possible adverse effect on the fetus or the newborn infant.

PRECAUTIONS

Monoamine Oxidase Inhibition:[7] Effective inhibition of monoamine oxidase by furazolidone has been demonstrated experimentally in man by the enhancement of tyramine and amphetamine sensitivity and by the directly measured monoamine oxidase inhibition.

A period of five days of furazolidone administration in the recommended doses in these patients was required to give an enhancement of the tyramine and amphetamine sensitivities by two to threefold. Administration of furazolidone in the recommended dose of 400 mg/day for a period of five days should not subject the adult patient to an undue hazard of hypertensive crisis due to monoamine oxidase inhibition. Hypertensive crises have never been reported even after the peroral administration of larger doses and/or for doses given over longer periods of time. Controlled studies reveal no signs or symptoms of hypertensive crisis even after the peroral administration of Furoxone in doses of 400 mg/day in excess of 48 consecutive months.[8]

If administered in doses larger than recommended or in excess of five days, the indications must be weighed against the possible hazards of hypertensive crisis related to the accumulation of monoamine oxidase inhibition. If indications are sufficient, the patients should be informed of drugs and foods which predispose to hypertensive crises:

(A) Other known MAOI drugs; however, when indicated they should be prescribed with caution and at a reduced dosage.
(B) Tyramine-containing foods such as broad beans, yeast extracts, strong unpasteurized cheeses, beer, wine, pickled herring, chicken livers, and fermented products are contraindicated.
(C) Indirectly-acting sympathomimetic amines such as those found in nasal decongestants (phenylephrine, ephedrine) and anorectics (amphetamines) are contraindicated.
(D) Likewise, sedatives, antihistamines, tranquilizers, and narcotics should be used in reduced dosages and with caution.

Orthostatic hypotension and hypoglycemia may occur.

Carcinogenesis, Mutagenesis, Impairment of Fertility: Furazolidone has shown evidence of tumorigenic activity in several studies involving chronic, high-dose oral administration to rodents. Promotion of the development of mammary neoplasia has been demonstrated in rats of two strains. Prominent among the findings in mice was that furazolidone caused significant increases in malignant lung tumors. The relevance of these animal findings, particularly in relationship to short-term therapy in humans, is not established.

ADVERSE REACTIONS

A few hypersensitivity reactions to Furoxone have been reported including a fall in blood pressure, urticaria, fever, arthralgia, and a vesicular morbilliform rash. These reactions subsided following withdrawal of the drug.

Nausea, emesis, headache, or malaise occur occasionally and may be minimized or eliminated by reduction in dosage or withdrawal of the drug.

Rarely, individuals receiving Furoxone have exhibited an Antabuse® (disulfiram)-like reaction to alcohol characterized by flushing, slight temperature elevation, dyspnea, and in some instances, a sense of constriction within the chest. All symptomatology disappeared within 24 hours with no lasting ill effects. During nine years of clinical use and approximately 3.5 million courses of therapy (in the U.S.A. alone) in the published literature and documented case reports 43 cases have been reported—of which 14 were produced under experimental conditions with planned doses of the compound in excess of those recommended.

Three of these experienced a fall in blood pressure necessitating active therapy. Indications are that levarterenol (Levophed®) may be used to combat such hypotensive episodes since human studies show that this drug is not potentiated in patients treated with Furoxone. (Indirectly acting pressor agents should be avoided.) The ingestion of alcohol in any form should be avoided during Furoxone therapy and for four days thereafter to prevent this reaction.

Furoxone may cause mild reversible intravascular hemolysis in certain ethnic groups of Mediterranean and Near-Eastern origin, and Negroes.[1,3] This is due to an intrinsic defect of red blood cell metabolism in a small percentage of these ethnic groups, making them unusually susceptible to hemolysis by numerous compounds.[2] It is necessary to observe such patients closely while receiving Furoxone and to discontinue its use if there is any indication of hemolysis.

Should not be administered to infants under 1 month of age because of the possibility of producing a hemolytic anemia due to immature enzyme systems (glutathione instability) in the early neonatal period.[4]

Colitis, proctitis, anal pruritus, staphylococcic enteritis and renal or hepatic toxicity have not been a significant problem with Furoxone.

DOSAGE AND ADMINISTRATION

FUROXONE TABLETS, 100 mg each, are green and scored to facilitate adjustment of dosage.

Average Adult Dosage: One 100 mg tablet four times daily.

Average Dosage for Children: Those 5 years of age or older should receive 25 to 50 mg (1/4 to 1/2 tablet) four times daily. The tablet dosage may be crushed and given in a spoonful of corn syrup.

FUROXONE LIQUID composition: each 15 ml tablespoonful contains Furoxone 50 mg per 15 ml (3.33 mg per ml) in a light-yellow aqueous vehicle. Suitable flavoring, suspending and preservative agents complete the formulation. (See Inactive Ingredients.) It is stable in storage. Prior to administering Furoxone Liquid shake the bottle vigorously. It should be dispensed in amber bottles.

Average Adult Dosage: Two tablespoonfuls four times daily.

Average Dosage for Children:

5 years or older—1/2 to 1 tablespoonful four times daily (7.5–15.0 ml)

1 to 4 years old—1 to 1 1/2 teaspoonfuls four times daily (5.0–7.5 ml)

1 month to 1 year—1/2 to 1 teaspoonful four times daily (2.5–5.0 ml)

This dosage is based on an average dose of 5 mg of Furoxone per Kg (2.3 mg per lb) of body weight given in four equally divided doses during 24 hours. The maximal dose of 8.8 mg of Furoxone per Kg (4 mg per lb) of body weight per 24 hours should probably not be exceeded because of the possibility of producing nausea or emesis. If these are severe, the dosage should be reduced.

The average case of diarrhea treated with Furoxone will respond within 2 to 5 days of therapy. Occasional patients may require a longer term of therapy. If satisfactory clinical response is not obtained within 7 days it indicates that the pathogen is refractory to Furoxone and the drug should be discontinued. Adjunctive therapy with other antibacterial agents or bismuth salts is not contraindicated. (N.B. Refer to WARNINGS.)

In order to administer furazolidone in doses larger than recommended or in excess of five days the indications must be weighed against the possible hazards of hypertensive crisis related to the accumulation of monoamine oxidase inhibition. If indications are sufficient, the patient should be informed of drugs and foods which predispose to hypertensive crises. (See PRECAUTIONS.)

HOW SUPPLIED

Furoxone Tablets, 100mg each, coded "Roberts 130", are supplied in amber bottles containing 20 tablets NDC 54092–130–20 and 100 tablets NDC 54092–130–01. (Should be dispensed in amber bottles.)

Furoxone Liquid is supplied in amber bottles containing 60 ml NDC 54092–430–60 and 473 ml NDC 54092–430–16. (Should be dispensed in amber bottles.)

REFERENCES

1. Kellermeyer, R.S., Tarlov, A.R., Schrier, S.L., and Alving, A.S.J. Lab. Clin. Med. 52:827–828 (Nov) 1958.
2. Tarlov et al. Arch. Int. Med. 109:209–234, 1962.
3. Kellermeyer et al. J.A.M.A. 180: No. 5, 388–394, 1962.
4. Zinkham, Pediatrics 23:18–32, 1959; Gross & Hurwitz, Pediatrics 22:453, 1958.
5. Fallas Vargas, M Un Nuevo Tratamiento para la Giardiasis (A New Treatment for Giardiasis). Rev. Med. Costa Rica 19:269–284 (July) 1962.
6. Webster, B. H. Furazolidone in the Treatment of Giardiasis. Amer. J. Dig. Diseases 5:618–622 (July) 1960.
7. Oates, J.A., Pettinger, W.A. Inhibition of Monoamine Oxidase by Furazolidone in Man. Data on file: Office of the Medical Director, Roberts Pharmaceutical Corp. Available upon request.
8. Kirsner, Joseph B., M.D., Ph.D. Data on file: Office of the Medical Director, Roberts Pharmaceutical Corp. Available upon request.
9. Neogy, K.N., et al. Furazolidone in Cholera, Journ. Indian Med. Assoc. 48:137, 1967.
10. Chaudhuri, R.N. et al. Furazolidone in Cholera. Lancet 2:909 (Oct 30) 1965.
11. Curlin, G. Comparison of Antibiotic Regimens in Cholera. Abstracts of papers, Epidemiological Intelligence Service Conference, Atlanta, Ga., April 11–14, 1967, p. 11.

FUROXONE (FURAZOLIDONE) SENSI-DISCS for laboratory determination of bacterial sensitivity are available from BBL, division of BioQuest.

CAUTION

Federal law prohibits dispensing without prescription.
Store at controlled room temperature: 15°–30°C (59°–86°F).
Do not refrigerate.

Manufactured for
Roberts Laboratories Inc.
a subsidiary of
Roberts Pharmaceutical Corporation
Eatontown, New Jersey 07724 USA

NOROXIN® Tablets ℞
(Norfloxacin), U.S.P.

DESCRIPTION

NOROXIN+ (Norfloxacin) is a synthetic, broad-spectrum antibacterial agent for oral administration. Norfloxacin, a fluoroquinolone, is 1-ethyl-6-fluoro-1,4-dihydro-4-oxo-7-(1-piperazinyl)-3-quinolinecarboxylic acid. Its empirical formula is $C_{16}H_{18}FN_3O_3$ and the structural formula is:

[See chemical structure at top of next column]

Continued on next page

Noroxin—Cont.

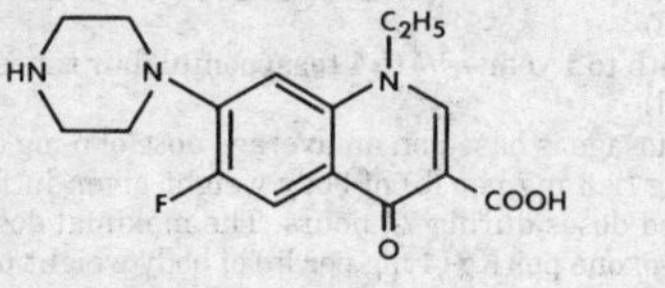

Norfloxacin is a white to pale yellow crystalline powder with a molecular weight of 319.34 and a melting point of about 221°C. It is freely soluble in glacial acetic acid, and very slightly soluble in ethanol, methanol and water.

NOROXIN is available in 400-mg tablets. Each tablet contains the following inactive ingredients: cellulose, croscarmellose sodium, hydroxypropyl cellulose, hydroxypropyl methylcellulose, iron oxide, magnesium stearate, and titanium dioxide.

Norfloxacin, a fluoroquinolone, differs from non-fluorinated quinolones by having a fluorine atom at the 6 position and a piperazine moiety at the 7 position.

+ Registered trademark of MERCK & CO., INC.

CLINICAL PHARMACOLOGY

In fasting healthy volunteers, at least 30–40% of an oral dose of NOROXIN is absorbed. Absorption is rapid following single doses of 200 mg, 400 mg and 800 mg. At the respective doses, mean peak serum and plasma concentrations of 0.8, 1.5 and 2.4 µg/mL are attained approximately one hour after dosing. The presence of food may decrease absorption. The effective half-life of norfloxacin in serum and plasma is 3–4 hours. Steady-state concentrations of norfloxacin will be attained within two days of dosing.

In healthy elderly volunteers (65–75 years of age with normal renal function for their age), norfloxacin is eliminated more slowly because of their slightly decreased renal function. Drug absorption appears unaffected. However, the effective half-life of norfloxacin in these elderly subjects is 4 hours.

The disposition of norfloxacin in patients with creatinine clearance rates greater than 30 mL/min/1.73m^2 is similar to that in healthy volunteers. In patients with creatinine clearance rates equal to or less than 30 mL/min/1.73m^2, the renal elimination of norfloxacin decreases so that the effective serum half-life is 6.5 hours. In these patients, alteration of dosage is necessary (see DOSAGE AND ADMINISTRATION). Drug absorption appears unaffected by decreasing renal function.

Norfloxacin is eliminated through metabolism, biliary excretion, and renal excretion. After a single 400-mg dose of NOROXIN, mean antimicrobial activities equivalent to 278, 773, and 82 µg of norfloxacin/g of feces were obtained at 12, 24, and 48 hours, respectively. Renal excretion occurs by both glomerular filtration and tubular secretion as evidenced by the high rate of renal clearance (approximately 275 mL/min). Within 24 hours of drug administration, 26 to 32% of the administered dose is recovered in the urine as norfloxacin with an additional 5–8% being recovered in the urine as six active metabolites of lesser antimicrobial potency. Only a small percentage (less than 1%) of the dose is recovered thereafter. Fecal recovery accounts for another 30% of the administered dose.

Two to three hours after a single 400-mg dose, urinary concentrations of 200 µg/mL or more are attained in the urine. In healthy volunteers, mean urinary concentrations of norfloxacin remain above 30 µg/mL for at least 12 hours following a 400-mg dose. The urinary pH may affect the solubility of norfloxacin. Norfloxacin is least soluble at urinary pH of 7.5 with greater solubility occurring at pHs above and below this value. The serum protein binding of norfloxacin is between 10 and 15%.

The following are mean concentrations of norfloxacin in various fluids and tissues measured 1 to 4 hours post-dose after two 400-mg doses, unless otherwise indicated:

Renal Parenchyma	7.3 µg/g
Prostate	2.5 µg/g
Seminal Fluid	2.7 µg/mL
Testicle	1.6 µg/g
Uterus/Cervix	3.0 µg/g
Vagina	4.3 µg/g
Fallopian Tube	1.9 µg/g
Bile	6.9 µg/mL (after two 200-mg doses)

Microbiology

Norfloxacin has *in vitro* activity against a broad range of gram-positive and gram-negative aerobic bacteria. The fluorine atom at the 6 position provides increased potency against gram-negative organisms, and the piperazine moiety at the 7 position is responsible for anti-pseudomonal activity.

Norfloxacin inhibits bacterial deoxyribonucleic acid synthesis and is bactericidal. At the molecular level, three specific events are attributed to norfloxacin in *E. coli* cells:

1) inhibition of the ATP-dependent DNA supercoiling reaction catalyzed by DNA gyrase,
2) inhibition of the relaxation of supercoiled DNA,
3) promotion of double-stranded DNA breakage.

Resistance to norfloxacin due to spontaneous mutation *in vitro* is a rare occurrence (range: 10^{-9} to 10^{-12} cells). Resistant organisms have emerged during therapy with norfloxacin in less than 1% of patients treated. Organisms in which development of resistance is greatest are the following:

Pseudomonas aeruginosa
Klebsiella pneumoniae
Acinetobacter species
Enterococcus species

For this reason, when there is a lack of satisfactory clinical response, repeat culture and susceptibility testing should be done. Nalidixic acid-resistant organisms are generally susceptible to norfloxacin *in vitro;* however, these organisms may have higher MICs to norfloxacin than nalidixic acid-susceptible strains. There is generally no cross-resistance between norfloxacin and other classes of antibacterial agents. Therefore, norfloxacin may demonstrate activity against indicated organisms resistant to some other antimicrobial agents including the aminoglycosides, penicillins, cephalosporins, tetracyclines, macrolides, and sulfonamides, including combinations of sulfamethoxazole and trimethoprim. Antagonism has been demonstrated *in vitro* between norfloxacin and nitrofurantoin.

Norfloxacin has been shown to be active against most strains of the following organisms both *in vitro* and in clinical infections (see INDICATIONS AND USAGE):

Gram-positive aerobes:
Enterococcus faecalis
Staphylococcus aureus
Staphylococcus epidermidis
Staphylococcus saprophyticus
Streptococcus agalactiae

Gram-negative aerobes:
Citrobacter freundii
Enterobacter aerogenes
Enterobacter cloacae
Escherichia coli
Klebsiella pneumoniae
Neisseria gonorrhoeae
Proteus mirabilis
Proteus vulgaris
Pseudomonas aeruginosa
Serratia marcescens

Norfloxacin has been shown to be active *in vitro* against most strains of the following organisms; however, the clinical significance of these data is unknown.

Gram-positive aerobes:
Bacillus cereus

Gram-negative aerobes:
Acinetobacter calcoaceticus
Aeromonas species
Alcaligenes species
Campylobacter species
Citrobacter diversus
Edwardsiella tarda
Flavobacterium species
Hafnia alvei
Klebsiella oxytoca
Klebsiella rhinoscleromatis
Morganella morganii
Providencia alcalifaciens
Providencia rettgeri
Providencia stuartii
Salmonella species
Shigella species
Vibrio cholerae
Vibrio parahemolyticus
Yersinia enterocolitica

Other:
Ureaplasma urealyticum

NOROXIN is not generally active against obligate anaerobes.

Norfloxacin has not been shown to be active against *Treponema pallidum.* (See WARNINGS.)

Susceptibility Tests

Diffusion Techniques: Quantitative methods that require measurement of zone diameters give the most precise estimate of the susceptibility of bacteria to antimicrobial agents. One such procedure is the National Committee for Clinical Laboratory Standards (NCCLS) approved procedure (M2-A4–Performance Standards for Antimicrobial Disk Susceptibility Tests 1990). This method has been recommended for use with the 10-µg norfloxacin disk to test susceptibility to norfloxacin. Interpretation involves correlation of the diameters obtained in the disk test with minimum inhibitory concentration (MIC) for norfloxacin. Reports from the laboratory giving results of the standard single-disk susceptibility test with a 10-µg norfloxacin disk should be interpreted according to the following criteria **(these criteria apply to isolates from urinary tract or prostatic infections):**

Zone diameter (mm)	Interpretation
≥17	(S) Susceptible
13–16	(I) Intermediate
≤12	(R) Resistant

A report of "Susceptible" indicates that the pathogen is likely to be inhibited by generally achievable urine/prostatic tissue levels. A report of "Intermediate" indicates that the test results be considered equivocal or indeterminate. A report of "Resistant" indicates that achievable concentrations of the antibiotic are unlikely to be inhibitory and other therapy should be selected.

Standardized procedures require the use of laboratory control organisms. The 10-µg norfloxacin disk should give the following zone diameter:

Organism	Zone diameter (mm)
E. coli ATCC 25922	28–35
P. aeruginosa ATCC 27853	22–29
S. aureus ATCC 25923	17–28

Other quinolone antibacterial disks should not be substituted when performing susceptibility tests for norfloxacin because of spectrum differences with norfloxacin. The 10-µg norfloxacin disk should be used for all *in vitro* testing of isolates using diffusion techniques.

Dilution Techniques: Broth and agar dilution methods, such as those recommended by the NCCLS (M7-A2—Methods for Dilution Antimicrobial Susceptibility Tests for Bacteria that Grow Aerobically 1990), may be used to determine the minimum inhibitory concentration (MIC) of norfloxacin. MIC test results should be interpreted according to the following criteria **(these criteria apply to isolates from urinary tract or prostatic infections):**

MIC (µg/mL)	Interpretation
≤4	(S) Susceptible
8	(I) Intermediate
≥16	(R) Resistant

As with standard diffusion methods, dilution procedures require the use of laboratory control organisms. Standard norfloxacin powder should give the following MIC values:

Organism	MIC range (µg/mL)
E. coli ATCC 25922	0.03–0.12
E. faecalis ATCC 29212	2.0–8.0
P. aeruginosa ATCC 27853	1.0–4.0
S. aureus ATCC 29213	0.05–2.0

INDICATIONS AND USAGE

NOROXIN is indicated for the treatment of adults with the following infections caused by susceptible strains of the designated microorganisms:

Urinary tract infections:
Uncomplicated urinary tract infections (including cystitis) due to *Enterococcus faecalis, Escherichia coli, Klebsiella pneumoniae, Proteus mirabilis, Pseudomonas aeruginosa, Staphylococcus epidermidis, Staphylococcus saprophyticus, Citrobacter freundii*, Enterobacter aerogenes*, Enterobacter cloacae*, Proteus vulgaris*, Staphylococcus aureus**, or *Streptococcus agalactiae**.

Complicated urinary tract infections due to *Enterococcus faecalis, Escherichia coli, Klebsiella pneumoniae, Proteus mirabilis, Pseudomonas aeruginosa,* or *Serratia marcescens**.

Sexually transmitted diseases (See WARNINGS.):
Uncomplicated urethral and cervical gonorrhea due to *Neisseria gonorrhoeae.*

Prostatitis:
Prostatitis due to *Escherichia coli.*

(See DOSAGE AND ADMINISTRATION for appropriate dosing instructions.)

Penicillinase production should have no effect on norfloxacin activity.

Appropriate culture and susceptibility tests should be performed before treatment in order to isolate and identify organisms causing the infection and to determine their susceptibility to norfloxacin. Therapy with norfloxacin may be initiated before results of these tests are known; once results become available, appropriate therapy should be given. Repeat culture and susceptibility testing performed periodically during therapy will provide information not only on the therapeutic effect of the antimicrobial agents but also on the possible emergence of bacterial resistance.

*Efficacy for this organism in this organ system was studied in fewer than 10 infections.

CONTRAINDICATIONS

NOROXIN (norfloxacin) is contraindicated in persons with a history of hypersensitivity, tendinitis, or tendon rupture associated with the use of norfloxacin or any member of the quinolone group of antimicrobial agents.

WARNINGS

THE SAFETY AND EFFICACY OF ORAL NORFLOXACIN IN CHILDREN, ADOLESCENTS (UNDER THE AGE OF 18), PREGNANT WOMEN, AND NURSING MOTHERS HAVE NOT BEEN ESTABLISHED. (See PRECAUTIONS-*Pregnancy,*

Nursing Mothers **and** ***Pediatric Use.***) The oral administration of single doses of norfloxacin, 6 times** the recommended human clinical dose (on a mg/kg basis), caused lameness in immature dogs. Histologic examination of the weight-bearing joints of these dogs revealed permanent lesions of the cartilage. Other quinolones also produced erosions of the cartilage in weight-bearing joints and other signs of arthropathy in immature animals of various species. (See ANIMAL PHARMACOLOGY.)

Convulsions have been reported in patients receiving norfloxacin. Convulsions, increased intracranial pressure, and toxic psychoses have been reported in patients receiving drugs in this class. Quinolones may also cause central nervous system (CNS) stimulation which may lead to tremors, restlessness, lightheadedness, confusion, and hallucinations. If these reactions occur in patients receiving norfloxacin, the drug should be discontinued and appropriate measures instituted.

The effects of norfloxacin on brain function or on the electrical activity of the brain have not been tested. Therefore, until more information becomes available, norfloxacin, like all other quinolones, should be used with caution in patients with known or suspected CNS disorders, such as severe cerebral arteriosclerosis, epilepsy, and other factors which predispose to seizures. (See ADVERSE REACTIONS.)

Serious and occasionally fatal hypersensitivity (anaphylactoid or anaphylactic) reactions, some following the first dose, have been reported in patients receiving quinolone therapy. Some reactions were accompanied by cardiovascular collapse, loss of consciousness, tingling, pharyngeal or facial edema, dyspnea, urticaria and itching. Only a few patients had a history of hypersensitivity reactions. If an allergic reaction to norfloxacin occurs, discontinue the drug. Serious acute hypersensitivity reactions may require immediate emergency treatment with epinephrine. Oxygen, intravenous fluids, antihistamines, corticosteroids, pressor amines, and airway management, including intubation, should be administered as indicated.

Pseudomembranous colitis has been reported with nearly all antibacterial agents, including norfloxacin, and may range in severity from mild to life-threatening. Therefore, it is important to consider this diagnosis in patients who present with diarrhea subsequent to the administration of antibacterial agents.

Treatment with antibacterial agents alters the normal flora of the colon and may permit overgrowth of clostridia. Studies indicate that a toxin produced by *Clostridium difficile* is one primary cause of "antibiotic-associated colitis".

After the diagnosis of pseudomembranous colitis has been established, therapeutic measures should be initiated. Mild cases of pseudomembranous colitis usually respond to drug discontinuation alone. In moderate to severe cases, consideration should be given to management with fluids and electrolytes, protein supplementation, and treatment with an antibacterial drug clinically effective against *C. difficile* colitis.

Ruptures of the shoulder, hand, and Achilles tendons that required surgical repair or resulted in prolonged disability have been reported with norfloxacin. Norfloxacin should be discontinued if the patient experiences pain, inflammation, or rupture of a tendon. Patients should rest and refrain from exercise until the diagnosis of tendinitis or tendon rupture has been confidently excluded. Tendon rupture can occur at any time during or after therapy with norfloxacin.

Norfloxacin has not been shown to be effective in the treatment of syphilis. Antimicrobial agents used in high doses for short periods of time to treat gonorrhea may mask or delay the symptoms of incubating syphilis. All patients with gonorrhea should have a serologic test for syphilis at the time of diagnosis. Patients treated with norfloxacin should have a follow-up serologic test for syphilis after three months.

**Based on a patient weight of 50 kg.

PRECAUTIONS

General:

Needle-shaped crystals were found in the urine of some volunteers who received either placebo, 800 mg norfloxacin, or 1600 mg norfloxacin (at or twice the recommended daily dose, respectively) while participating in a double-blind, crossover study comparing single doses of norfloxacin with placebo. While crystalluria is not expected to occur under usual conditions with a dosage regimen of 400 mg b.i.d., as a precaution, the daily recommended dosage should not be exceeded and the patient should drink sufficient fluids to ensure a proper state of hydration and adequate urinary output.

Alteration in dosage regimen is necessary for patients with impaired renal function (see DOSAGE AND ADMINISTRATION).

Moderate to severe phototoxicity reactions have been observed in patients who are exposed to excessive sunlight while receiving some members of this drug class. Excessive sunlight should be avoided. Therapy should be discontinued if phototoxicity occurs.

Infection	Description	Unit Dose	Frequency	Duration	Daily Dose
Urinary Tract	Uncomplicated UTI's (cystitis) due to *E. coli, K. pneumoniae, or P. mirabilis*	400 mg	q12h	3 days	800 mg
	Uncomplicated UTI's due to other indicated organisms	400 mg	q12h	7–10 days	800 mg
	Complicated UTI's	400 mg	q12h	10–21 days	800 mg
Sexually Transmitted Diseases	Uncomplicated Gonorrhea	800 mg	single dose	1 day	800 mg
Prostatitis	Acute or Chronic	400 mg	q12h	28 days	800 mg

Rarely, hemolytic reactions have been reported in patients with latent or actual defects in glucose-6-phosphate dehydrogenase activity who take quinolone antibacterial agents, including norfloxacin. (See ADVERSE REACTIONS.)

Information for Patients

Patients should be advised:
— to drink fluids liberally.
— that norfloxacin should be taken at least one hour before or at least two hours after a meal or milk ingestion.
— that multivitamins or other products containing iron or zinc, or antacids should not be taken within the two-hour period before or within the two-hour period after taking norfloxacin. (See *Drug Interactions.*)
— that norfloxacin can cause dizziness and lightheadedness and, therefore, patients should know how they react to norfloxacin before they operate an automobile or machinery or engage in activities requiring mental alertness and coordination.
— to discontinue treatment and inform their physician if they experience pain, inflammation, or rupture of a tendon, and to rest and refrain from exercise until the diagnosis of tendinitis or tendon rupture has been confidently excluded.
— that norfloxacin may be associated with hypersensitivity reactions, even following the first dose, and to discontinue the drug at the first sign of a skin rash or other allergic reaction.
— to avoid undue exposure to excessive sunlight while receiving norfloxacin and to discontinue therapy if phototoxicity occurs.
— that some quinolones may increase the effects of theophylline and/or caffeine. (See *Drug Interactions.*)

Laboratory Tests

As with any potent antibacterial agent, periodic assessment of organ system functions, including renal, hepatic, and hematopoietic, is advisable during prolonged therapy.

Drug Interactions

Elevated plasma levels of theophylline have been reported with concomitant quinolone use. There have been reports of theophylline-related side effects in patients on concomitant therapy with norfloxacin and theophylline. Therefore, monitoring of theophylline plasma levels should be considered and dosage of theophylline adjusted as required.

Elevated serum levels of cyclosporine have been reported with concomitant use of cyclosporine with norfloxacin. Therefore cyclosporine serum levels should be monitored and appropriate cyclosporine dosage adjustments made when these drugs are used concomitantly.

Quinolones, including norfloxacin, may enhance the effects of the oral anticoagulant warfarin or its derivatives. When these products are administered concomitantly, prothrombin time or other suitable coagulation tests should be closely monitored.

Diminished urinary excretion of norfloxacin has been reported during the concomitant administration of probenecid and norfloxacin.

The concomitant use of nitrofurantoin is not recommended since nitrofurantoin may antagonize the antibacterial effect of NOROXIN in the urinary tract.

Multivitamins, or other products containing iron or zinc, antacids or sucralfate should not be administered concomitantly with, or within 2 hours of, the administration of norfloxacin, because they may interfere with absorption resulting in lower serum and urine levels of norfloxacin.

Some quinolones have also been shown to interfere with the metabolism of caffeine. This may lead to reduced clearance of caffeine and a prolongation of its plasma half-life.

Carcinogenesis, Mutagenesis, Impairment of Fertility

No increase in neoplastic changes was observed with norfloxacin as compared to controls in a study in rats, lasting up to 96 weeks at doses 8–9 times** the usual human dose (on a mg/kg basis).

Norfloxacin was tested for mutagenic activity in a number of *in vivo* and *in vitro* tests. Norfloxacin had no mutagenic effect in the dominant lethal test in mice and did not cause chromosomal aberrations in hamsters or rats at doses 30–60 times** the usual human dose (on a mg/kg basis). Norfloxacin had no mutagenic activity *in vitro* in the Ames microbial mutagen test, Chinese hamster fibroblasts and V-79 mammalian cell assay. Although norfloxacin was weakly positive in the Rec-assay for DNA repair, all other mutagenic assays were negative including a more sensitive test (V-79).

Norfloxacin did not adversely affect the fertility of male and female mice at oral doses up to 30 times** the usual human dose (on a mg/kg basis).

Pregnancy

Teratogenic Effects. Pregnancy Category C. Norfloxacin has been shown to produce embryonic loss in monkeys when given in doses 10 times** the maximum daily total human dose (on a mg/kg basis). At this dose, peak plasma levels obtained in monkeys were approximately 2 times those obtained in humans. There has been no evidence of a teratogenic effect in any of the animal species tested (rat, rabbit, mouse, monkey) at 6–50 times** the maximum daily human dose (on a mg/kg basis). There are, however, no adequate and well controlled studies in pregnant women. Norfloxacin should be used during pregnancy only if the potential benefit justifies the potential risk to the fetus.

Nursing Mothers

It is not known whether norfloxacin is excreted in human milk.

When a 200-mg dose of NOROXIN was administered to nursing mothers, norfloxacin was not detected in human milk. However, because the dose studied was low, because other drugs in this class are secreted in human milk, and because of the potential for serious adverse reactions from norfloxacin in nursing infants, a decision should be made to discontinue nursing or to discontinue the drug, taking into account the importance of the drug to the mother.

Pediatric Use

The safety and effectiveness of oral norfloxacin in children and adolescents below the age of 18 years have not been established. Norfloxacin causes arthropathy in juvenile animals of several animal species. (See WARNINGS and ANIMAL PHARMACOLOGY.)

**Based on a patient weight of 50 kg.

ADVERSE REACTIONS

Single-Dose Studies

In clinical trials involving 82 healthy subjects and 228 patients with gonorrhea, treated with a single dose of norfloxacin, 6.5% reported drug-related adverse experiences. However, the following incidence figures were calculated without reference to drug relationship.

The most common adverse experiences (>1.0%) were: dizziness (2.6%), nausea (2.6%), headache (2.0%), and abdominal cramping (1.6%).

Additional reactions (0.3%–1.0%) were: anorexia, diarrhea, hyperhidrosis, asthenia, anal/rectal pain, constipation, dyspepsia, flatulence, tingling of the fingers, and vomiting.

Laboratory adverse changes considered drug-related were reported in 4.5% of patients/subjects. These laboratory changes were: increased AST (SGOT) (1.6%), decreased WBC (1.3%), decreased platelet count (1.0%), increased urine protein (1.0%), decreased hematocrit and hemoglobin (0.6%), and increased eosinophils (0.6%).

Multiple-Dose Studies

In clinical trials involving 52 healthy subjects and 1980 patients with urinary tract infections or prostatitis, treated

Continued on next page

Noroxin—Cont.

with multiple doses of norfloxacin, 3.6% reported drug-related adverse experiences. However, the incidence figures below were calculated without reference to drug relationship.
The most common adverse experiences (>1.0%) were: nausea (4.2%), headache (2.8%), dizziness (1.7%), and asthenia (1.3%).
Additional reactions (0.3%–1.0%) were: abdominal pain, back pain, constipation, diarrhea, dry mouth, dyspepsia/heartburn, fever, flatulence, hyperhidrosis, loose stools, pruritus, rash, somnolence, and vomiting.
Less frequent reactions (0.1%–0.2%) included: abdominal swelling, allergies, anorexia, anxiety, bitter taste, blurred vision, bursitis, chest pain, chills, depression, dysmenorrhea, edema, erythema, foot or hand swelling, insomnia, mouth ulcer, myocardial infarction, palpitation, pruritus ani, renal colic, sleep disturbances, and urticaria.
Abnormal laboratory values observed in these patients/subjects were: eosinophilia (1.5%), elevation of ALT (SGPT) (1.4%), decreased WBC and/or neutrophil count (1.4%), elevation of AST (SGOT) (1.4%), and increased alkaline phosphatase (1.1%). Those occurring less frequently included increased BUN, increased LDH, increased serum creatinine, decreased hematocrit, and glycosuria.
Post Marketing
The most frequently reported adverse reaction in post-marketing experience is rash.
CNS effects characterized as generalized seizures and myoclonus have been reported with NOROXIN®. A causal relationship to NOROXIN® has not been established (see WARNINGS). Visual disturbances have been reported with drugs in this class.
The following additional adverse reactions have been reported since the drug was marketed:
Hypersensitivity Reactions
Hypersensitivity reactions have been reported including anaphylactoid reactions, angioedema, dyspnea, vasculitis, urticaria, arthritis, arthralgia and myalgia (see WARNINGS).
Skin
Toxic epidermal necrolysis, Stevens-Johnson syndrome and erythema multiforme, exfoliative dermatitis, photosensitivity
Gastrointestinal
Pseudomembranous colitis, hepatitis, jaundice including cholestatic jaundice, pancreatitis (rare), stomatitis. The onset of pseudomembranous colitis symptoms may occur during or after antibacterial treatment. (See WARNINGS.)
Renal
Interstitial nephritis, renal failure
Nervous System/Psychiatric
Peripheral neuropathy, Guillain-Barré syndrome, ataxia, paresthesia; psychic disturbances including psychotic reactions and confusion
Musculoskeletal
Tendinitis, tendon rupture, possible exacerbation of myasthenia gravis
Hematologic
Neutropenia, leukopenia, hemolytic anemia, sometimes associated with glucose-6-phosphate dehydrogenase deficiency; thrombocytopenia
Special Senses
Transient hearing loss (rare), tinnitus, diplopia
Other adverse events reported with quinolones include: agranulocytosis, albuminuria, candiduria, crystalluria, cylindruria, dysphagia, elevation of blood glucose, elevation of serum cholesterol, elevation of serum potassium, elevation of serum triglycerides, hematuria, hepatic necrosis, symptomatic hypoglycemia, nystagmus, postural hypotension, prolongation of prothrombin time, and vaginal candidiasis.

OVERDOSAGE

No significant lethality was observed in male and female mice and rats at single oral doses up to 4 g/kg.
In the event of acute overdosage, the stomach should be emptied by inducing vomiting or by gastric lavage, and the patient carefully observed and given symptomatic and supportive treatment. Adequate hydration must be maintained.

DOSAGE AND ADMINISTRATION

Tablets NOROXIN should be taken at least one hour before or at least two hours after a meal or milk ingestion. Tablets NOROXIN should be taken with a glass of water. Patients receiving NOROXIN should be well hydrated (see PRECAUTIONS).
Normal Renal Function
The recommended daily dose of NOROXIN is as described in the following chart:
[See table at top of previous page]
Renal Impairment
NOROXIN may be used for the treatment of urinary tract infections in patients with renal insufficiency. In patients with a creatinine clearance rate of 30 mL/min/1.73m^2 or less, the recommended dosage is one 400-mg tablet once daily for the duration given above. At this dosage, the urinary concentration exceeds the MICs for most urinary pathogens susceptible to norfloxacin, even when the creatinine clearance is less than 10 mL/min/1.73m^2.
When only the serum creatinine level is available, the following formula (based on sex, weight, and age of the patient) may be used to convert this value into creatinine clearance. The serum creatinine should represent a steady state of renal function.

$$\text{Males: } \frac{(\text{weight in kg}) \times (140 - \text{age})}{(72) \times \text{serum creatinine (mg/100 mL)}}$$

$$\text{Females: } (0.85) \times (\text{above value})$$

Elderly
Elderly patients being treated for urinary tract infections who have a creatinine clearance of greater than 30 mL/min/1.73m^2 should receive the dosages recommended under *Normal Renal Function.*
Elderly patients being treated for urinary tract infections who have a creatinine clearance of 30 mL/min/1.73m^2 or less should receive 400 mg once daily as recommended under *Renal Impairment.*

HOW SUPPLIED

Tablets NOROXIN 400 mg are dark pink, oval shaped, film-coated tablets, coded MSD 705 on one side and NOROXIN on the other. They are supplied as follows:
NDC 54092-097-01 bottles of 100.
(6505-01-258-9542 100's)
NDC 54092-097-20 unit of use bottles of 20
NDC 54092-097-52 unit dose packages of 100.
Storage
Tablets NOROXIN should be stored in a tightly-closed container. Avoid storage at temperatures above 40°C (104°F).

ANIMAL PHARMACOLOGY

Norfloxacin and related drugs have been shown to cause arthropathy in immature animals of most species tested (see WARNINGS).
Crystalluria has occurred in laboratory animals tested with norfloxacin. In dogs, needle-shaped drug crystals were seen in the urine at doses of 50 mg/kg/day. In rats, crystals were reported following doses of 200 mg/kg/day.
Embryo lethality and slight maternotoxicity (vomiting and anorexia) were observed in cynomolgus monkeys at doses of 150 mg/kg/day or higher.
Ocular toxicity, seen with some related drugs, was not observed in any norfloxacin-treated animals.
COPYRIGHT © MERCK & CO., INC., 1986, 1989
All rights reserved
Manufactured by:
Merck & Co., Inc.
West Point, PA 19486, USA
Distributed by:
Roberts Laboratories, Inc. a subsidiary of
Roberts Pharmaceutical Corp.
Eatontown, NJ 07724, USA
Shown in Product Identification Guide, page 334

PENTASA® ℞
(mesalamine)
Controlled-Release Capsules 250 mg

Prescribing information as of December 1995

DESCRIPTION

PENTASA (mesalamine) for oral administration is a controlled-release formulation of mesalamine, an aminosalicylate anti-inflammatory agent for gastrointestinal use.
Chemically, mesalamine is 5-amino-2-hydroxybenzoic acid. It has a molecular weight of 153.14.
The structural formula is:

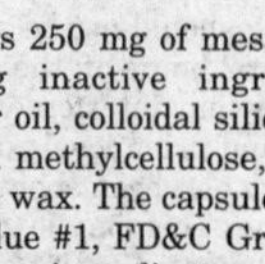

Each capsule contains 250 mg of mesalamine. It also contains the following inactive ingredients: acetylated monoglyceride, castor oil, colloidal silicon dioxide, ethylcellulose, hydroxypropyl methylcellulose, starch, stearic acid, sugar, talc, and white wax. The capsule shell contains D&C Yellow #10, FD&C Blue #1, FD&C Green #3, gelatin, titanium dioxide, and other ingredients.

CLINICAL PHARMACOLOGY

Sulfasalazine is split by bacterial action in the colon into sulfapyridine (SP) and mesalamine (5-ASA). It is thought that the mesalamine component is therapeutically active in ulcerative colitis. The usual oral dose of sulfasalazine for active ulcerative colitis in adults is 2 to 4 g per day in divided doses. Four grams of sulfasalazine provide 1.6 g of free mesalamine to the colon.
The mechanism of action of mesalamine (and sulfasalazine) is unknown, but appears to be topical rather than systemic. Mucosal production of arachidonic acid (AA) metabolites, both through the cyclooxygenase pathways, ie, prostanoids, and through the lipoxygenase pathways, ie, leukotrienes (LTs) and hydroxyeicosatetraenoic acids (HETEs), is increased in patients with chronic inflammatory bowel disease, and it is possible that mesalamine diminishes inflammation by blocking cyclooxygenase and inhibiting prostaglandin (PG) production in the colon.

Human Pharmacokinetics and Metabolism

Absorption. PENTASA is an ethylcellulose-coated controlled-release formulation of mesalamine designed to release therapeutic quantities of mesalamine throughout the gastrointestinal tract. Based on urinary excretion data, 20% to 30% of the mesalamine in PENTASA is absorbed. In contrast, when mesalamine is administered orally as an unformulated 1-g aqueous suspension, mesalamine is approximately 80% absorbed.
Plasma mesalamine concentration peaked at approximately 1 µg/mL 3 hours following a 1-g PENTASA dose and declined in a biphasic manner. The literature describes a mean terminal half-life of 42 minutes for mesalamine following intravenous administration. Because of the continuous release and absorption of mesalamine from PENTASA throughout the gastrointestinal tract, the true elimination half-life cannot be determined after oral administration. N-acetylmesalamine, the major metabolite of mesalamine, peaked at approximately 3 hours at 1.8 µg/mL, and its concentration followed a biphasic decline. Pharmacological activities of N-acetylmesalamine are unknown, and other metabolites have not been identified.
Oral mesalamine pharmacokinetics were nonlinear when PENTASA capsules were dosed from 250 mg to 1 g four times daily, with steady-state mesalamine plasma concentrations increasing about nine times, from 0.14 µg/mL to 1.21 µg/mL, suggesting saturable first-pass metabolism. N-acetylmesalamine pharmacokinetics were linear.
Elimination. About 130 mg free mesalamine was recovered in the feces following a single 1-g PENTASA dose, which was comparable to the 140 mg of mesalamine recovered from the molar equivalent sulfasalazine tablet dose of 2.5 g. Elimination of free mesalamine and salicylates in feces increased proportionately with PENTASA dose. N-acetylmesalamine was the primary compound excreted in the urine (19% to 30%) following PENTASA dosing.

CLINICAL TRIALS

In two randomized, double-blind, placebo-controlled, dose-response trials (UC-1 and UC-2) of 625 patients with active mild to moderate ulcerative colitis, PENTASA, at an oral dose of 4 g/day given 1 g four times daily, produced consistent improvement in prospectively identified primary efficacy parameters, PGA, Tx F, and Sl as shown in the table below.
The 4-g dose of PENTASA also gave consistent improvement in secondary efficacy parameters, namely the frequency of trips to the toilet, stool consistency, rectal bleeding, abdominal/rectal pain, and urgency. The 4-g dose of PENTASA induced remission as assessed by endoscopic and symptomatic endpoints.
In some patients, the 2-g dose of PENTASA was observed to improve efficacy parameters measured. However, the 2-g dose gave inconsistent results in primary efficacy parameters across the two adequate and well-controlled trials.
[See table at top of next page]

INDICATIONS AND USAGE

PENTASA is indicated for the induction of remission and for the treatment of patients with mildly to moderately active ulcerative colitis.

CONTRAINDICATIONS

PENTASA is contraindicated in patients who have demonstrated hypersensitivity to mesalamine, any other components of this medication, or salicylates.

PRECAUTIONS

General

Caution should be exercised if PENTASA is administered to patients with impaired hepatic function.
Mesalamine has been associated with an acute intolerance syndrome that may be difficult to distinguish from a flare of inflammatory bowel disease. Although the exact frequency of occurrence cannot be ascertained, it has occurred in 3% of patients in controlled clinical trials of mesalamine or sulfasalazine. Symptoms include cramping, acute abdominal pain and bloody diarrhea, sometimes fever, headache, and rash. If acute intolerance syndrome is suspected, prompt withdrawal is required. If a rechallenge is performed later in order to validate the hypersensitivity, it should be carried out under close medical supervision at reduced dose and only if clearly needed.

Renal

Caution should be exercised if PENTASA is administered to patients with impaired renal function. Single reports of nephrotic syndrome and interstitial nephritis associated with mesalamine therapy have been described in the foreign lit-

erature. There have been rare reports of interstitial nephritis in patients receiving PENTASA. In animal studies, a 13-week oral toxicity study in mice and 13-week and 52-week oral toxicity studies in rats and cynomolgus monkeys have shown the kidney to be the major target organ of mesalamine toxicity. Oral daily doses of 2400 mg/kg in mice and 1150 mg/kg in rats produced renal lesions including granular and hyaline casts, tubular degeneration, tubular dilation, renal infarct, papillary necrosis, tubular necrosis, and interstitial nephritis. In cynomolgus monkeys, oral daily doses of 250 mg/kg or higher produced nephrosis, papillary edema, and interstitial fibrosis. Patients with preexisting renal disease, increased BUN or serum creatinine, or proteinuria should be carefully monitored.

Carcinogenesis, Mutagenesis, Impairment of Fertility

Long-term studies of the carcinogenic potential of mesalamine in mice and rats are ongoing. No evidence of mutagenicity was observed in an in vitro Ames test and in an in vivo mouse micronucleus test. No effects on fertility or reproductive performance were observed in male or female rats at doses up to 400 mg/kg/day (2360 mg/M^2). For a 50-kg person (1.3 M^2 body surface area), this represents five times the recommended clinical dose (80 mg/kg/day) on a mg/kg basis and 0.8 times the clinical dose (2960 mg/M^2) on a body surface area basis.

Semen abnormalities and infertility in men, which have been reported in association with sulfasalazine have not been seen with PENTASA capsules during controlled clinical trials.

Pregnancy

Category B. Reproduction studies have been performed in rats at doses up to 1000 mg/kg/day (5900 mg/M^2) and rabbits at doses of 800 mg/kg/day (6856 mg/M^2) and have revealed no evidence of teratogenic effects or harm to the fetus due to mesalamine. There are, however, no adequate and well-controlled studies in pregnant women. Because animal reproduction studies are not always predictive of human response, PENTASA should be used during pregnancy only if clearly needed.

Mesalamine is known to cross the placental barrier.

Nursing Mothers

Minute quantities of mesalamine were distributed to breast milk and amniotic fluid of pregnant women following sulfasalazine therapy. When treated with sulfasalazine at a dose equivalent to 1.25 g/day of mesalamine, 0.02 µg/mL to 0.08 µg/mL and trace amounts of mesalamine were measured in amniotic fluid and breast milk, respectively. N-acetylmesalamine, in quantities of 0.07 µg/mL to 0.77 µg/mL and 1.13 µg/mL to 3.44 µg/mL, was identified in the same fluids, respectively.

Caution should be exercised when PENTASA is administered to a nursing woman.

Pediatric Use

Safety and efficacy of PENTASA in pediatric patients have not been established.

ADVERSE REACTIONS

In combined domestic and foreign clinical trials, more than 2100 patients with ulcerative colitis or Crohn's disease received PENTASA therapy. Generally, PENTASA therapy was well tolerated. The most common events (ie, greater than or equal to 1%) were diarrhea (3.4%), headache (2.0%), nausea (1.8%), abdominal pain (1.7%), dyspepsia (1.6%), vomiting (1.5%), and rash (1.0%).

In two domestic placebo-controlled trials involving over 600 ulcerative colitis patients, adverse events were fewer in PENTASA-treated patients than in the placebo group (PENTASA 14% vs placebo 18%) and were not dose-related. Events occurring at 1% or more are shown in the table below. Of these, only nausea and vomiting were more frequent in the PENTASA group. Withdrawal from therapy due to adverse events was more common on placebo than PENTASA (7% vs 4%).

[See table 1 above]

Clinical laboratory measurements showed no significant abnormal trends for any test, including measurement of hematologic, liver, and kidney function.

The following adverse events, presented by body system, were reported infrequently (ie, less than 1%) during domestic ulcerative colitis and Crohn's disease trials. In many cases, the relationship to PENTASA has not been established.

Gastrointestinal: abdominal distention, anorexia, constipation, duodenal ulcer, dysphagia, eructation, esophageal ulcer, fecal incontinence, GGTP increase, GI bleeding, increased alkaline phosphatase, LDH increase, mouth ulcer, oral moniliases, pancreatitis, rectal bleeding, SGOT increase, SGPT increase, stool abnormalities (color or texture change), thirst

Dermatological: acne, alopecia, dry skin, eczema, erythema nodosum, nail disorder, photosensitivity, pruritus, sweating, urticaria

Nervous System: depression, dizziness, insomnia, somnolence, paresthesia

Cardiovascular: palpitations, pericarditis, vasodilation

	Clinical Trial UC-1			**Clinical Trial UC-2**		
		PENTASA			**PENTASA**	
Parameter Evaluated	PL (n=90)	4 g/day (n=95)	2 g/day (n=97)	PL (n=83)	4 g/day (n=85)	2 g/day (n=83)
PGA	36%	59%*	57%*	31%	55%*	41%
Tx F	22%	9%*	18%	31%	9%*	17%*
SI	−2.5	−5.0*	−4.3*	−1.6	−3.8*	−2.6
Remission†	12%	26%*	24%*	12%	27%*	12%

* p <0.05 vs placebo.
PGA: Physician Global Assessment: proportion of patients with complete or marked improvement.
Tx F: Treatment Failure: proportion of patients developing severe or fulminant UC requiring steroid therapy or hospitalization or worsening of the disease at 7 days of therapy, or lack of significant improvement by 14 days of therapy.
SI: Sigmoidoscopic Index: an objective measure of disease activity rated by a standard (15-point) scale that includes mucosal vascular pattern, erythema, friability, granularity/ulcerations, and mucopus: improvement over baseline.
† Defined as complete resolution of symptoms plus improvement of endoscopic endpoints. To be considered in remission, patients had a "1" score for one of the endoscopic components (mucosal vascular pattern, erythema, granularity, for friability) and "0" for the others.

Table 1. Adverse Events Occurring in More Than 1% of Either Placebo or PENTASA Patients in Domestic Placebo-controlled Ulcerative Colitis Trials. (PENTASA Comparison to Placebo)

Event	PENTASA n=451	Placebo n=173
Diarrhea	16 (3.5%)	13 (7.5%)
Headache	10 (2.2%)	6 (3.5%)
Nausea	14 (3.1%)	—
Abdominal Pain	5 (1.1%)	7 (4.0%)
Melena (Bloody Diarrhea)	4 (0.9%)	6 (3.5%)
Rash	6 (1.3%)	2 (1.2%)
Anorexia	5 (1.1%)	2 (1.2%)
Fever	4 (0.9%)	2 (1.2%)
Rectal Urgency	1 (0.2%)	4 (2.3%)
Nausea and Vomiting	5 (1.1%)	—
Worsening of Ulcerative Colitis	2 (0.4%)	2 (1.2%)
Acne	1 (0.2%)	2 (1.2%)

Other: albuminuria, amenorrhea, amylase increase, arthralgia, asthenia, breast pain, conjunctivitis, ecchymosis, edema, fever, hematuria, hypomenorrhea, Kawasaki-like syndrome, leg cramps, lichen planus, lipase increase, malaise, menorrhagia, metrorrhagia, myalgia, pulmonary infiltrates, thrombocythemia, thrombocytopenia, urinary frequency

One week after completion of an 8-week ulcerative colitis study, a 72-year-old male, with no previous history of pulmonary problems, developed dyspnea. The patient was subsequently diagnosed with interstitial pulmonary fibrosis without eosinophilia by one physician and bronchiolitis obliterans with organizing pneumonitis by a second physician. A causal relationship between this event and mesalamine therapy has not been established.

Published case reports and/or spontaneous postmarketing surveillance have described infrequent instances of pericarditis, fatal myocarditis, chest pain and T-wave abnormalities, hypersensitivity pneumonitis, pancreatitis, nephrotic syndrome, interstitial nephritis, hepatitis, aplastic anemia, pancytopenia, leukopenia, or anemia while receiving mesalamine therapy. Anemia can be a part of the clinical presentation of inflammatory bowel disease.

OVERDOSAGE

Single oral doses of mesalamine up to 5 g/kg in pigs or a single intravenous dose of mesalamine at 920 mg/kg in rats were not lethal.

There is no clinical experience with PENTASA overdosage. PENTASA is an aminosalicylate, and symptoms of salicylate toxicity may be possible, such as: tinnitus, vertigo, headache, confusion, drowsiness, sweating, hyperventilation, vomiting, and diarrhea. Severe intoxication with salicylates can lead to disruption of electrolyte balance and blood pH, hyperthermia, and dehydration.

Treatment of Overdosage. Since PENTASA is an aminosalicylate, conventional therapy for salicylate toxicity may be beneficial in the event of acute overdosage. This includes prevention of further gastrointestinal tract absorption by emesis and, if necessary, by gastric lavage. Fluid and electrolyte imbalance should be corrected by the administration of appropriate intravenous therapy. Adequate renal function should be maintained.

DOSAGE AND ADMINISTRATION

The recommended dosage for the induction of remission and the symptomatic treatment of mildly to moderately active ulcerative colitis is 1 g (4 PENTASA capsules) four times a day for a total daily dose of 4 g. Treatment duration in controlled trials was up to 8 weeks.

HOW SUPPLIED

PENTASA controlled-release capsules are supplied in bottles of 240 capsules (NDC 54092-189-81); and blister packs of 80 capsules (NDC 54092-189-80). Each green and blue capsule contains 250 mg of mesalamine in controlled-release beads. PENTASA controlled-release capsules are identified with a pentagonal starburst logo and the number 2010 on the green portion and PENTASA 250 mg on the blue portion of the capsules.

Store at controlled room temperature 59° to 86°F (15° to 30°C).

Manufactured for
Roberts Laboratories Inc., a subsidiary of
ROBERTS PHARMACEUTICAL CORPORATION,
Eatontown, NJ 07724, USA
Prescribing Information as of December 1995
Licensed U.S. Patent Nos. B1 4,496,553 and 4,980,173
189 0117 001   50011416
Shown in Product Identification Guide, page 334

PERI-COLACE® capsules • syrup   OTC
(casanthranol and docusate sodium)

DESCRIPTION

Peri-Colace® is a combination of the mild stimulant laxative casanthranol, and the stool-softener Colace® (docusate sodium). Each capsule contains 30 mg of casanthranol and 100 mg of Colace®; the syrup contains 30 mg of casanthranol and 60 mg of Colace® per 15-mL tablespoon (10 mg of casanthranol and 20 mg of Colace® per 5-mL teaspoon) and 10% alcohol.

Peri-Colace® Capsules contain the following inactive ingredients: Polyethylene glycol 400, gelatin, glycerin, sorbitol, propylene glycol, titanium dioxide, methylparaben, FD&C Red No. 40, propylparaben, FD&C Blue No. 1.

Peri-Colace® Syrup contains the following inactive ingredients: alcohol (10% v/v), citric acid, flavors, methyl salicylate, methylparaben, poloxamer, polyethylene glycol, propylparaben, sodium citrate, sorbitol solution, sucrose, and purified water.

ACTION AND USES

Peri-Colace® provides gentle peristaltic stimulation and helps to keep stools soft for easier passage. Bowel movement is induced gently—usually overnight or in 8 to 12

Continued on next page

Peri-Colace—Cont.

hours. Nausea, griping, abnormally loose stools, and constipation rebound are minimized. Useful in management of chronic or temporary constipation.

Note: To prevent hard stools when laxative stimulation is not needed or undesirable, see Colace® (stool softener).

WARNINGS

Do not use when abdominal pain, nausea, or vomiting is present. Frequent or prolonged use of this preparation may result in dependence on laxatives.

As with any drug, pregnant or nursing women should seek the advice of a health professional before using this product.

SIDE EFFECTS

The incidence of side effects—none of a serious nature—is exceedingly small. Nausea, abdominal cramping or discomfort, diarrhea, and rash are the main side effects reported.

ADMINISTRATION AND DOSAGE

Adults—1 or 2 capsules, or 1 or 2 tablespoons syrup at bedtime, or as indicated. In severe cases, dosage may be increased to 2 capsules or 2 tablespoons twice daily, or 3 capsules at bedtime. *Children*—1 to 3 teaspoons of syrup at bedtime, or as indicated. Peri-Colace® syrup must be given in a 6 oz. to 8 oz. glass of milk or fruit juice or in infant's formula to prevent throat irritation.

OVERDOSAGE

In addition to symptomatic treatment, gastric lavage, if timely, is recommended in cases of large overdosage.

HOW SUPPLIED

Peri-Colace® Capsules
 NDC 54092-054-30 Bottles of 30
 NDC 54092-054-60 Bottles of 60
 NDC 54092-054-02 Bottles of 250
 NDC 54092-054-10 Bottles of 1000
 NDC 54092-054-52 Cartons of 100 single unit packs
Note: Peri-Colace® capsules should be stored at controlled room temperatures (59°–86°F or 15°–30°C).
Peri-Colace® Syrup
 NDC 54092-418-08 Bottles of 8 fl oz
 NDC 54092-418-16 Bottles of 16 fl oz
Peri-Colace®
 NDC 54092-054-11 Blister Pack of 10
Manufactured for:
Roberts Laboratories Inc., a subsidiary of
ROBERTS PHARMACEUTICAL CORPORATION
Eatontown, NJ 07724 USA

PROAMATINE®   ℞
(midodrine hydrochloride)
Tablets of 2.5 mg and 5 mg

> **WARNING: Because ProAmatine can cause marked elevation of supine blood pressure, it should be used in patients whose lives are considerably impaired despite standard clinical care. The indication for use of ProAmatine in the treatment of symptomatic orthostatic hypotension is based primarily on a change in a surrogate marker of effectiveness, an increase in systolic blood pressure measured one minute after standing, a surrogate marker considered likely to correspond to a clinical benefit. At present, however, clinical benefits of ProAmatine, principally improved ability to carry out activities of daily living, have not been verified.**

DESCRIPTION

Name: ProAmatine® (midodrine hydrochloride) Tablets
Dosage Form: 2.5-mg and 5-mg tablets for oral administration
Active Ingredient: Midodrine hydrochloride, 2.5 mg or 5 mg
Inactive Ingredients: Microcrystalline Cellulose NF, Colloidal Silicone Dioxide NF, Magnesium Stearate NF, Corn Starch NF, Talc USP, FD&C Yellow No. 6 Lake (5-mg tablet)
Pharmacological Classification: Vasopressor/Antihypotensive
Chemical Names (USAN: Midodrine Hydrochloride): (1) Acetamide, 2-amino-*N*-[2-(2,5-dimethoxyphenyl)-2-hydroxyethyl]-monohydrochloride,(±)-; (2) (±) -2-amino-*N*-(β-hydroxy-2,5-dimethoxyphenethyl)acetamide monohydrochloride BAN, INN, JAN: Midodrine
Structural Formula:
[See chemical structure at top of next column]
Molecular Formula: $C_{12}H_{18}N_2O_4HCl$; **Molecular Weight:** 290.7

Organoleptic Properties: Odorless, white, crystalline powder

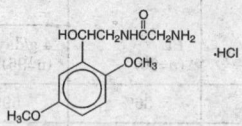

Solubility:	Water:	Soluble
	Methanol:	Sparingly soluble

pKa: 7.8 (0.3% aqueous solution)
pH: 3.5 to 5.5 (5% aqueous solution)
Melting Range: 200 to 203°C

CLINICAL PHARMACOLOGY

Mechanism of Action: ProAmatine forms an active metabolite, desglymidodrine, that is an alpha₁-agonist, and exerts its actions via activation of the alpha-adrenergic receptors of the arteriolar and venous vasculature, producing an increase in vascular tone and elevation of blood pressure. Desglymidodrine does not stimulate cardiac beta-adrenergic receptors. Desglymidodrine diffuses poorly across the blood-brain barrier, and is therefore not associated with effects on the central nervous system. Administration of ProAmatine results in a rise in standing, sitting, and supine systolic and diastolic blood pressure in patients with orthostatic hypotension of various etiologies. Standing systolic blood pressure is elevated by approximately 15 to 30 mmHg at 1 hour after a 10-mg dose of midodrine, with some effect persisting for 2 to 3 hours. ProAmatine has no clinically significant effect on standing or supine pulse rates in patients with autonomic failure.

Pharmacokinetics: ProAmatine is a prodrug, i.e., the therapeutic effect of orally administered midodrine is due to the major metabolite desglymidodrine, formed by deglycination of midodrine. After oral administration, ProAmatine is rapidly absorbed. The plasma levels of the prodrug peak after about half an hour, and decline with a half-life of approximately 25 minutes, while the metabolite reaches peak blood concentrations about 1 to 2 hours after a dose of midodrine and has a half-life of about 3 to 4 hours. The absolute bioavailability of midodrine (measured as desglymidodrine) is 93%. The bioavailability of desglymidodrine is not affected by food. Approximately the same amount of desglymidodrine is formed after intravenous and oral administration of midodrine. Neither midodrine nor desglymidodrine is bound to plasma proteins to any significant extent.

Metabolism and Excretion: Thorough metabolic studies have not been conducted, but it appears that deglycination of midodrine to desglymidodrine takes place in many tissues, and both compounds are metabolized in part by the liver. Neither midodrine nor desglymidodrine is a substrate for monoamine oxidase.

Renal elimination of midodrine is insignificant. The renal clearance of desglymidodrine is of the order of 385 mL/minute, most, about 80%, by active renal secretion. The actual mechanism of active secretion has not been studied, but it is possible that it occurs by the base-secreting pathway responsible for the secretion of several other drugs that are bases (see also **Potential for Drug Interactions**).

Clinical Studies

Midodrine has been studied in 3 principal controlled trials, one of 3-weeks duration and 2 of 1 to 2 days duration. All studies were randomized, double-blind and paralled-design trials in patients with orthostatic hypotension of any etiology and supine-to-standing fall of systolic blood pressure of at least 15 mmHg accompanied by at least moderate dizziness/lightheadedness. Patients with pre-existing sustained supine hypertension above 180/110 mmHg were routinely excluded. In a 3-week study in 170 patients, most previously untreated with midodrine, the midodrine-treated patients (10 mg t.i.d., with the last dose not later than 6 P.M.) had significantly higher (by about 20 mmHg) 1-minute standing systolic pressure 1 hour after dosing (blood pressures were not measured at other times) for all 3 weeks. After week 1, midodrine-treated patients had small improvements in dizziness/lightheadedness/unsteadiness scores and global evaluations, but these effects were made difficult to interpret by a high early drop-out rate (about 25% vs 5% on placebo). Supine and sitting blood pressure rose 16/8 and 20/10 mmHg, respectively, on average.

In a 2-day study, after open-label midodrine, known midodrine responders received midodrine 10 mg or placebo at 0, 3, and 6 hours. One-minute standing systolic blood pressures were increased 1 hour after each dose by about 15 mmHg and 3 hours after each dose by about 12 mmHg; 3-minute standing pressures were increased also at 1, but not 3, hours after dosing. There were increases in standing time seen intermittently 1 hour after dosing, but not at 3 hours.

In a 1-day, dose-response trial, single doses of 0, 2.5, 10, and 20 mg of midodrine were given to 25 patients. The 10- and 20-mg doses produced increases in standing 1-minute systolic pressure of about 30 mmHg at 1 hour; the increase was sustained in part for 2 hours after 10 mg and 4 hours after 20 mg. Supine systolic pressure was ≥200 mmHg in 22% of patients on 10 mg and 45% of patients on 20 mg; elevated pressures often lasted 6 hours or more.

INDICATIONS AND USAGE

ProAmatine is indicated for the treatment of symptomatic orthostatic hypotension (OH). Because ProAmatine can cause marked elevation of supine blood pressure (BP > 200 mmHg systolic), it should be used in patients whose lives are considerably impaired despite standard clinical care, including non-pharmacologic treatment (such as support stockings), fluid expansion, and lifestyle alterations. The indication is based on ProAmatine's effect on increases in 1-minute standing systolic blood pressure, a surrogate marker considered likely to correspond to a clinical benefit. At present, however, clinical benefits of ProAmatine, principally improved ability to perform life activities, have not been established. Further clinical trials are underway to verify and describe the clinical benefits of ProAmatine. After initiation of treatment, ProAmatine should be continued only for patients who report significant symptomatic improvement.

CONTRAINDICATIONS

ProAmatine is contraindicated in patients with severe organic heart disease, acute renal disease, urinary retention, pheochromocytoma or thyrotoxicosis. ProAmatine should not be used in patients with persistent and excessive supine hypertension.

WARNINGS

Supine Hypertension: The most potentially serious adverse reaction associated with ProAmatine therapy is marked elevation of supine arterial blood pressure (supine hypertension). Systolic pressure of about 200 mmHg were seen overall in about 13.4% of patients given 10 mg of ProAmatine. Systolic elevations of this degree were most likely to be observed in patients with relatively elevated pretreatment systolic blood pressures (mean 170 mmHg). There is no experience in patients with initial supine systolic pressure above 180 mmHg, as those patients were excluded from the clinical trials. Use of ProAmatine in such patients is not recommended. Sitting blood pressures were also elevated by ProAmatine therapy. It is essential to monitor supine and sitting blood pressures in patients maintained on ProAmatine.

PRECAUTIONS

General: The potential for supine and sitting hypertension should be evaluated at the beginning of ProAmatine therapy. Supine hypertension can often be controlled by preventing the patient from becoming fully supine, i.e., sleeping with the head of the bed elevated. The patient should be cautioned to report symptoms of supine hypertension immediately. Symptoms may include cardiac awareness, pounding in the ears, headache, blurred vision, etc. The patient should be advised to discontinue the medication immediately if supine hypertension persists. Blood pressure should be monitored carefully when ProAmatine is used concomitantly with other agents that cause vasoconstriction, such as phenylephrine, ephedrine, dihydroergotamine, phenylpropanolamine, or pseudoephedrine.

A slight slowing of the heart rate may occur after administration of ProAmatine, primarily due to vagal reflex. Caution should be exercised when ProAmatine is used concomitantly with cardiac glycosides (such as digitalis), psychopharmacologic agents, beta blockers or other agents that directly or indirectly reduce heart rate. Patients who experience any signs or symptoms suggesting bradycardia (pulse slowing, increased dizziness, syncope, cardiac awareness) should be advised to discontinue ProAmatine and should be re-evaluated.

ProAmatine should be used cautiously in patients with urinary retention problems, as desglymidodrine acts on the alpha-adrenergic receptors of the bladder neck.

ProAmatine should be used with caution in orthostatic hypotensive patients who are also diabetic, as well as those with a history of visual problems who are also taking fludrocortisone acetate, which is known to cause an increase in intraocular pressure and glaucoma.

ProAmatine use has not been studied in patients with renal impairment. Because desglymidodrine is eliminated via the kidneys, and higher blood levels would be expected in such patients. ProAmatine should be used with caution in patients with renal impairment, with a starting dose of 2.5 mg (see **DOSAGE AND ADMINISTRATION**). Renal function should be assessed prior to initial use of ProAmatine.

ProAmatine use has not been studied in patients with hepatic impairment. ProAmatine should be used with caution in patients with hepatic impairment, as the liver has a role in the metabolism of midodrine.

Information for Patients: Patients should be told that certain agents in over-the-counter products, such as cold remedies and diet aids, can elevate blood pressure, and therefore, should be used cautiously with ProAmatine, as they

may enhance or potentiate the pressor effects of ProAmatine (see **Drug Interactions**). Patients should also be made aware of the possibility of supine hypertension. They should be told to avoid taking their dose if they are to be supine for any length of time, i.e., they should take their last daily dose of ProAmatine 3 to 4 hours before bedtime to minimize nighttime supine hypertension.

Laboratory Tests: Since desglymidodrine is eliminated by the kidneys and the liver has a role in its metabolism, evaluation of the patient should include assessment of renal and hepatic function prior to initiating therapy and subsequently, as appropriate.

Drug Interactions: When administered concomitantly with ProAmatine, cardiac glycosides may enhance or precipitate bradycardia, A.V. block or arrhythmia.

The use of drugs that stimulate alpha-adrenergic receptors (e.g., phenylephrine, pseudoephedrine, ephedrine, phenylpropanolamine or dihydroergotamine) may enhance or potentiate the pressor effects of ProAmatine. Therefore, caution should be used when ProAmatine is administered concomitantly with agents that cause vasoconstriction.

ProAmatine has been used in patients concomitantly treated with salt-retaining steroid therapy (i.e., fludrocortisone acetate), with or without salt supplementation. The potential for supine hypertension should be carefully monitored in these patients and may be minimized by either reducing the dose of fludrocortisone acetate or decreasing the salt intake prior to initiation of treatment with ProAmatine. Alpha-adrenergic blocking agents, such as prazosin, terazosin, and doxazosin, can antagonize the effects of ProAmatine.

Potential for Drug Interactions: It appears possible, although there is no supporting experimental evidence, that the high renal clearance of desglymidodrine (a base) is due to active tubular secretion by the base-secreting system also responsible for the secretion of such drugs as metformin, cimetidine, ranitidine, procainamide, triamterene, flecainide, and quinidine. Thus there may be a potential for drug-drug interactions with these drugs.

Carcinogenesis, Mutagenesis, Impairment of Fertility: Long-term studies have been conducted in rats and mice at dosages of 3 to 4 times the maximum recommended daily human dose on a mg/m^2 basis, with no indication of carcinogenic effects related to ProAmatine. Studies investigating the mutagenic potential of ProAmatine revealed no evidence of mutagenicity. Other than the dominant lethal assay in male mice, where no impairment of fertility was observed, there have been no studies on the effects of ProAmatine on fertility.

Pregnancy: *Pregnancy Category C.* ProAmatine increased the rate of embryo resorption, reduced fetal body weight in rats and rabbits, and decreased fetal survival in rabbits when given in doses 13 (rat) and 7 (rabbit) times the maximum human dose based on body surface area (mg/m^2). There are no adequate and well-controlled studies in pregnant women. ProAmatine should be used during pregnancy only if the potential benefit justifies the potential risk to the fetus. No teratogenic effects have been observed in studies in rats and rabbits.

Nursing Mothers: It is not known whether this drug is excreted in human milk. Because many drugs are excreted in human milk, caution should be exercised when ProAmatine is administered to a nursing woman.

Pediatric Use: Safety and effectiveness in pediatric patients have not been established.

ADVERSE REACTIONS

The most frequent adverse reactions seen in controlled trials were supine and sitting hypertension; paresthesia and pruritus, mainly of the scalp; goosebumps; chills; urinary urge; urinary retention and urinary frequency.

The frequency of these events in a 3-week placebo-controlled trial is shown in the following table:

Adverse Events

Event	Placebo n=88 #of reports	Placebo n=88 % of patients	Midodrine n=82 #of reports	Midodrine n=82 % of patients
Total # of reports	22		77	
Paresthesia[1]	4	4.5	15	18.3
Piloerection	0	0	11	13.4
Dysuria[2]	0	0	11	13.4
Pruritus[3]	2	2.3	10	12.2
Supine hypertension[4]	0	0	6	7.3
Chills	0	0	4	4.9
Pain[5]	0	0	4	4.9
Rash	1	1.1	2	2.4

[1] Includes hyperesthesia and scalp paresthesia
[2] Includes dysuria (1), increased urinary frequency (2), impaired urination (1), urinary retention (5), urinary urgency (2)
[3] Includes scalp pruritis
[4] Includes patients who experienced an increase in supine hypertension
[5] Includes abdominal pain and pain increase

Less frequent adverse reactions were headache; feeling of pressure/fullness in the head; vasodilation/flushing face; confusion/thinking abnormality; dry mouth; nervousness/anxiety and rash. Other adverse reactions that occurred rarely were visual field defect; dizziness; skin hyperesthesia; insomnia; somnolence; erythema multiforme; canker sore; dry skin; dysuria; impaired urination; asthenia; backache; pyrosis; nausea; gastrointestinal distress; flatulence and leg cramps.

The most potentially serious adverse reaction associated with ProAmatine therapy is supine hypertension. The feelings of paresthesia, pruritus, piloerection and chills are pilomotor reactions associated with the action of midodrine on the alpha-adrenergic receptors of the hair follicles. Feelings of urinary urgency, retention and frequency are associated with the action of midodrine on the alpha-receptors of the bladder neck.

OVERDOSAGE

Symptoms of overdose could include hypertension, piloerection (goosebumps), a sensation of coldness and urinary retention. There are 2 reported cases of overdosage with ProAmatine, both in young males. One patient ingested ProAmatine drops, 250 mg, experienced systolic blood pressure of greater than 200 mmHg, was treated with an IV injection of 20 mg of phentolamine, and was discharged the same night without any complaints. The other patient ingested 205 mg of ProAmatine (41 5-mg tablets), and was found lethargic and unable to talk, unresponsive to voice but responsive to painful stimuli, hypertensive and bradycardic. Gastric lavage was performed, and the patient recovered fully by the next day without sequelae.

The single doses that would be associated with symptoms of overdosage or would be potentially life-threatening are unknown. The oral LD$_{50}$ is approximately 30 to 50 mg/kg in rats, 675 mg/kg in mice, and 125 to 160 mg/kg in dogs. Desglymidodrine is dialyzable.

Recommended general treatment, based on the pharmacology of the drug, includes induced emesis and administration of alpha-sympatholytic drugs (e.g., phentolamine).

DOSAGE AND ADMINISTRATION

The recommended dose of ProAmatine is 10 mg, 3 times daily. Dosing should take place during the daytime hours when the patient needs to be upright, pursuing the activities of daily life. A suggested dosing schedule of approximately 4-hour intervals is as follows: shortly before or upon arising in the morning, midday, and late afternoon (not later than 6 P.M.). Doses may be given in 3-hour intervals, if required, to control symptoms, but not more frequently. Single doses as high as 20 mg have been given to patients, but severe and persistent systolic supine hypertension occur at a high rate (about 45%) at this dose. In order to reduce the potential for supine hypertension during sleep, ProAmatine should not be given after the evening meal or less than 4 hours before bedtime. Total daily doses greater than 30 mg have been tolerated by some patients, but their safety and usefulness have not been studied systematically or established. Because of the risk of supine hypertension, ProAmatine should be continued only in patients who appear to attain symptomatic improvement during initial treatment.

The supine and standing blood pressure should be monitored regularly, and the administration of ProAmatine should be stopped if supine blood pressure increases excessively.

Because desglymidodrine is excreted renally, dosing in patients with abnormal renal function should be cautious; although this has not been systematically studied, it is recommended that treatment of these patients be initiated using 2.5-mg doses.

Dosing in children has not been adequately studied.

Blood levels of midodrine and desglymidodrine were similar when comparing levels in patients 65 or older vs. younger than 65 and when comparing males vs. females, suggesting dose modifications for these groups are not necessary.

HOW SUPPLIED

ProAmatine is supplied as 2.5-mg and 5-mg tablets for oral administration. The 2.5-mg tablet is white, round, and biplanar, with a bevelled edge, and is scored on 1 side with "RPC" above and "2.5" below the score, and "003" on the other side. The 5-mg tablet is orange, round, and biplanar, with a bevelled edge, and is scored on 1 side with "RPC" above and "5" below the score, and "004" on the other side.

2.5-milligram
  Tablets: NDC 54092-003-01   Bottle of 100
5-milligram
  Tablets: NDC 54092-004-01   Bottle of 100

Store from 15°C to 25°C (59°F to 77°F).

CAUTION: Keep this and all medication out of the reach of children.

ROBERTS® PHARMACEUTICALS
Manufactured by NYCOMED Austria GmbH
for Roberts Laboratories Inc.,
a subsidiary of **ROBERTS PHARMACEUTICAL CORPORATION,** Eatontown, NJ 07724-2274, USA
Copyright© 1997 Roberts Laboratories Inc.
Rev. 3/97   003 0107 003
Shown in Product Identification Guide, page 334

SLOW-MAG®   OTC
MAGNESIUM CHLORIDE

DESCRIPTION

SLOW-MAG® is enteric coated magnesium chloride available in tablet form in a dosage unit of 64mg magnesium per tablet. Magnesium is an essential mineral of a healthy diet and may help to maintain the functions of the heart, muscles and nervous system.
SLOW-MAG® is a dietary supplement that provides a magnesium chloride formulation that is enteric coated to avoid the stomach upset and diarrhea commonly associated with oral magnesium supplements.

INGREDIENTS

Each tablet contains magnesium chloride hexahydrate, calcium carbonate, povidone, talc, magnesium stearate, cellulose acetate phthalate, diethyl phthalate, titanium dioxide, hydroxypropyl cellulose, FD&C Blue No. 2 Lake.

DIRECTIONS FOR USE

As a dietary supplement, take 2 tablets daily or as directed by a physician. Two 64mg tablets contain 32% of the recommended daily allowance for magnesium.

HOW SUPPLIED

Bottles of 60 tablets.
Do not use if the inner seal or protective band around the cap is broken or missing.

TIGAN®   ℞
[tī 'găn]
brand of trimethobenzamide hydrochloride
CAPSULES
SUPPOSITORIES
INJECTABLE

DESCRIPTION

Chemically, trimethobenzamide HCl is N-[p-[2-(dimethylamino)-ethoxy] benzyl]-3,4,5-trimethoxybenzamide hydrochloride. It has a molecular weight of 424.93 and the following structural formula:

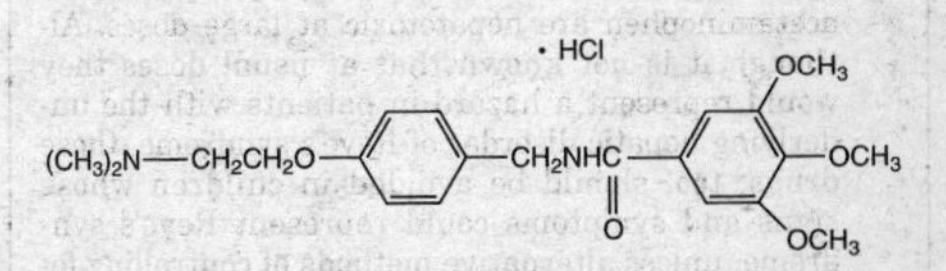

Capsules: Each 100 mg *Tigan®* capsule for oral use, with opaque blue cap and opaque white body, contains trimethobenzamide hydrochloride equivalent to 100 mg. Each 250 mg *Tigan®* capsule for oral use, with opaque blue cap and body, contains trimethobenzamide hydrochloride equivalent to 250 mg. Both caps and bodies of the 100 and 250 mg capsules are imprinted with TIGAN® 100 mg and TIGAN® 250 mg, respectively.
Inactive Ingredients: FD&C Blue No. 1, FD&C Red No. 3, lactose, magnesium stearate, starch and titanium dioxide.
Suppositories (200 mg): Each suppository contains 200 mg trimethobenzamide hydrochloride and 2% benzocaine in a base compounded with polysorbate 80, white beeswax and propylene glycol monostearate.
Suppositories, Pediatric (100 mg): Each suppository contains 100 mg trimethobenzamide hydrochloride and 2% benzocaine in a base compounded with polysorbate 80, white beeswax and propylene glycol monostearate.
Ampuls: Each 2 mL ampul contains 200 mg trimethobenzamide hydrochloride compounded with 0.2% parabens (methyl and propyl) as preservatives, 1 mg sodium citrate and 0.4 mg citric acid as buffers and pH adjusted to approximately 5.0 with sodium hydroxide.
Multi-Dose Vials: Each mL contains 100 mg trimethobenzamide hydrochloride compounded with 0.45% phenol as preservative, 0.5 mg sodium citrate and 0.2 mg citric acid as buffers and pH adjusted to approximately 5.0 with sodium hydroxide.
Thera-Ject® (Disposable Syringes): Each 2 mL contains 200 mg trimethobenzamide hydrochloride compounded with

Continued on next page

Tigan—Cont.

0.45% phenol as preservative, 1 mg sodium citrate and 0.4 mg citric acid as buffers, 0.2 mg disodium edetate as stabilizer and pH adjusted to approximately 5.0 with sodium hydroxide.

ACTIONS

The mechanism of action of *Tigan®* as determined in animals is obscure, but may be the chemoreceptor trigger zone (CTZ), an area in the medulla oblongata through which emetic impulses are conveyed to the vomiting center; direct impulses to the vomiting center apparently are not similarly inhibited. In dogs pretreated with trimethobenzamide HCl, the emetic response to apomorphine is inhibited, while little or no protection is afforded against emesis induced by intragastric copper sulfate.

INDICATIONS

Tigan® is indicated for the control of nausea and vomiting.

CONTRAINDICATIONS

The injectable form of *Tigan®* in children, the suppositories in premature or newborn infants, and use in patients with known hypersensitivity to trimethobenzamide are contraindicated. Since the suppositories contain benzocaine they should not be used in patients known to be sensitive to this or similar local anesthetics.

WARNINGS

Caution should be exercised when administering *Tigan®* to children for the treatment of vomiting. Antiemetics are not recommended for treatment of uncomplicated vomiting in children and their use should be limited to prolonged vomiting of known etiology. There are three principal reasons for caution:

1. There has been some suspicion that centrally acting antiemetics may contribute, in combination with viral illnesses (a possible cause of vomiting in children), to development of Reye's syndrome, a potentially fatal acute childhood encephalopathy with visceral fatty degeneration, especially involving the liver. Although there is no confirmation of this suspicion, caution is nevertheless recommended.

2. The extrapyramidal symptoms which can occur secondary to *Tigan®* may be confused with the central nervous system signs of an undiagnosed primary disease responsible for the vomiting, e.g., Reye's syndrome or other encephalopathy.

3. It has been suspected that drugs with hepatotoxic potential, such as *Tigan®*, may unfavorably alter the course of Reye's syndrome. Such drugs should therefore be avoided in children whose signs and symptoms (vomiting) could represent Reye's syndrome. It should also be noted that salicylates and acetaminophen are hepatotoxic at large doses. Although it is not known that at usual doses they would represent a hazard in patients with the underlying hepatic disorder of Reye's syndrome, these drugs, too, should be avoided in children whose signs and symptoms could represent Reye's syndrome, unless alternative methods of controlling fever are not successful.

Tigan® may produce drowsiness. Patients should not operate motor vehicles or other dangerous machinery until their individual responses have been determined. Reye's syndrome has been associated with the use of *Tigan®* and other drugs, including antiemetics, although their contribution, if any, to the cause and course of the disease has not been established. This syndrome is characterized by an abrupt onset shortly following a nonspecific febrile illness, with persistent, severe vomiting, lethargy, irrational behavior, progressive encephalopathy leading to coma, convulsions and death.

Usage in Pregnancy: Trimethobenzamide hydrochloride was studied in reproduction experiments in rats and rabbits and no teratogenicity was suggested. The only effects observed were an increased percentage of embryonic resorptions or stillborn pups in rats administered 20 mg and 100 mg/kg and increased resorptions in rabbits receiving 100 mg/kg. In each study these adverse effects were attributed to one or two dams. The relevance to humans is not known. Since there is no adequate experience in pregnant or lactating women who have received this drug, safety in pregnancy or in nursing mothers has not been established.

Usage with Alcohol: Concomitant use of alcohol with *Tigan®* may result in an adverse drug interaction.

PRECAUTIONS

During the course of acute febrile illness, encephalitides, gastroenteritis, dehydration and electrolyte imbalance, especially in children and the elderly or debilitated, CNS reactions such as opisthotonos, convulsions, coma and extrapyramidal symptoms have been reported with and with-

out use of *Tigan®* (trimethobenzamide hydrochloride) or other antiemetic agents. In such disorders caution should be exercised in administering *Tigan®* particularly to patients who have recently received other CNS-acting agents (phenothiazines, barbiturates, belladonna derivatives). It is recommended that severe emesis should not be treated with an antiemetic drug alone; where possible the cause of vomiting should be established. Primary emphasis should be directed toward the restoration of body fluids and electrolyte balance, the relief of fever and relief of the causative disease process. Overhydration should be avoided since it may result in cerebral edema.

The antiemetic effects of *Tigan®* may render diagnosis more difficult in such conditions as appendicitis and obscure signs of toxicity due to overdosage of other drugs.

ADVERSE REACTIONS

There have been reports of hypersensitivity reactions and Parkinson-like symptoms. There have been instances of hypotension reported following parenteral administration to surgical patients. There have been reports of blood dyscrasias, blurring of vision, coma, convulsions, depression of mood, diarrhea, disorientation, dizziness, drowsiness, headache, jaundice, muscle cramps and opisthotonos. If these occur, the administration of the drug should be discontinued. Allergic-type skin reactions have been observed; therefore, the drug should be discontinued at the first sign of sensitization. While these symptoms will usually disappear spontaneously, symptomatic treatment may be indicated in some cases.

DOSAGE AND ADMINISTRATION

(See WARNINGS and PRECAUTIONS.)
Dosage should be adjusted according to the indication for therapy, severity of symptoms and the response of the patient.

CAPSULES, 250 mg and 100 mg
Usual Adult Dosage
One 250 mg capsule t.i.d. or q.i.d.
Usual Children's Dosage
30 to 90 lbs: One or two 100 mg capsules t.i.d. or q.i.d.
SUPPOSITORIES, 200 mg (not to be used in premature or newborn infants)
Usual Adult Dosage
One suppository (200 mg) t.i.d. or q.i.d.
Usual Children's Dosage
Under 30 lbs: One-half suppository (100 mg) t.i.d. or q.i.d.
30 to 90 lbs: One-half to one suppository (100 to 200 mg) t.i.d. or q.i.d.
SUPPOSITORIES, PEDIATRIC, 100 mg (not to be used in premature or newborn infants)
Usual Children's Dosage
Under 30 lbs: One suppository (100 mg) t.i.d. or q.i.d.
30 to 90 lbs: One to two suppositories (100 to 200 mg) t.i.d. or q.i.d.
INJECTABLE, 100 mg/mL (not for use in children)
Usual Adult Dosage
2 mL (200 mg) t.i.d. or q.i.d. intramuscularly.
NOTE: The injectable form is intended for intramuscular administration only; it is not recommended for intravenous use.
Intramuscular administration may cause pain, stinging, burning, redness and swelling at the site of injection. Such effects may be minimized by deep injection into the upper outer quadrant of the gluteal region, and by avoiding the escape of solution along the route.

CAUTION

Federal law prohibits dispensing without prescription.

STORAGE

Store *Tigan®* from 15° to 30°C (59° to 86°F).

HOW SUPPLIED

Capsules, 100 mg trimethobenzamide hydrochloride each, bottles of 100; 250 mg trimethobenzamide hydrochloride each, bottles of 100 and 500
NDC 54092-186-01 100 mg 100's
NDC 54092-187-01 250 mg 100's
NDC 54092-187-05 250 mg 500's
Suppositories, Pediatric, 100 mg, boxes of 10
Suppositories, 200 mg, boxes of 10 and 50
NDC 54092-503-10 100 mg (box of 10)
NDC 54092-504-10 200 mg (box of 10)
NDC 54092-504-50 200 mg (box of 50)
Ampuls, 2 mL, boxes of 10
NDC 54092-540-02 100 mg/mL in 2 mL ampul
Multi-Dose Vials, 20 mL
NDC 54092-541-20 100 mg/mL in 20 mL Multi-Dose Vials
Thera-Ject® (Disposable Syringes), 2 mL, boxes of 25
NDC 54092-542-02 100 mg/mL in 2 mL Thera-Ject® Disposable Syringes
Manufactured for
Roberts Laboratories Inc.,
a subsidiary of
ROBERTS PHARMACEUTICAL CORP.
Eatontown, NJ 07724, USA

Veterans Administration/Military/PHS—Capsules, 250 mg, 100's. 6505-01-333-7733; 250 mg, 500's, 6505-00-965-2319; Suppositories, 100 mg, 10's, 6505-01-153-3395; 200 mg, 10's, 6505-01-234-4444; 200 mg, 50's, 6505-00-890-1819; Vials, 100 mg/mL, 2 mL, 1's, 6505-00-949-1410; 100 mg/mL, 20 mL, 1's, 6505-00-951-4759; Thera-Ject®, 2 mL, 1's, 6505-01-048-0827.
TN: L1

Shown in Product Identification Guide, page 334

A. H. Robins Company
1407 CUMMINGS DRIVE
RICHMOND, VA 23220

Direct General Inquiries to:
(610) 688-4400

For Emergency Medical Information Contact:
Day: (800) 934-5556 8:30 AM to 4:30 PM (Eastern Standard Time), Weekdays only
Night: (610) 688-4400 (Emergencies only; non-emergencies should wait until the next day)
For Medical/Pharmacy Inquiries on Marketed Products Call:
Medical Affairs, (800) 934-5556 8:30 AM to 4:30 PM (Eastern Standard Time), Weekdays only

A.H. Robins Products

The following is a list of products listed under A.H. Robins. All oral solid dosage forms are listed with their corresponding National Drug Code (NDC) numbers. All numbers are preceded by 0031.
[See table at bottom of next page]

DIMETANE®–DX ℞
[dĭ 'mĕ-tān]
COUGH SYRUP
SUGAR-FREE

DESCRIPTION

Dimetane-DX Cough Syrup is a light-red syrup with a butterscotch flavor.
Each 5 mL (1 teaspoonful) contains:
Brompheniramine Maleate, USP .... 2 mg
Pseudoephedrine Hydrochloride, USP .... 30 mg
Dextromethorphan Hydrobromide, USP .... 10 mg
Alcohol 0.95 percent
In a palatable, aromatic vehicle.
Inactive Ingredients: Citric Acid, FD&C Red 40, FD&C Yellow 6, Flavors, Glycerin, Saccharin Sodium, Sodium Benzoate, Sorbitol, Water.
Antihistamine/Nasal Decongestant/Antitussive syrup for oral administration.

CLINICAL PHARMACOLOGY

Brompheniramine maleate is a histamine antagonist, specifically an H_1-receptor-blocking agent belonging to the alkylamine class of antihistamines. Antihistamines appear to compete with histamine for receptor sites on effector cells. Brompheniramine also has anticholinergic (drying) and sedative effects. Among the antihistaminic effects, it antagonizes the allergic response (vasodilatation, increased vascular permeability, increased mucus secretion) of nasal tissue. Brompheniramine is well absorbed from the gastrointestinal tract, with peak plasma concentration after single, oral dose of 4 mg reached in 5 hours; urinary excretion is the major route of elimination, mostly as products of biodegradation; the liver is assumed to be the main site of metabolic transformation.
Pseudoephedrine acts on sympathetic nerve endings and also on smooth muscle, making it useful as a nasal decongestant. The nasal decongestant effect is mediated by the action of pseudoephedrine on α-sympathetic receptors, producing vasoconstriction of the dilated nasal arterioles. Following oral administration, effects are noted within 30 minutes with peak activity occurring at approximately one hour.
Dextromethorphan acts centrally to elevate the threshold for coughing. It has no analgesic or addictive properties. The onset of antitussive action occurs in 15 to 30 minutes after administration and is of long duration.

INDICATIONS AND USAGE

For relief of coughs and upper respiratory symptoms, including nasal congestion, associated with allergy or the common cold.

CONTRAINDICATIONS

Hypersensitivity to any of the ingredients. Do not use in the newborn, in premature infants, in nursing mothers, in pa-

tients with severe hypertension or severe coronary artery disease. Do not use dextromethorphan in patients receiving monoamine oxidase (MAO) inhibitors (see "DRUG INTERACTIONS").

Antihistamines should not be used to treat lower respiratory tract conditions including asthma.

WARNINGS

Especially in infants and small children, antihistamines in overdosage may cause hallucinations, convulsions, and death.

Antihistamines may diminish mental alertness. In the young child, they may produce excitation.

PRECAUTIONS
General

Because of its antihistamine component, Dimetane-DX Cough Syrup should be used with caution in patients with a history of bronchial asthma, narrow angle glaucoma, gastrointestinal obstruction, or urinary bladder neck obstruction. Because of its sympathomimetic component, Dimetane-DX Cough Syrup should be used with caution in patients with diabetes, hypertension, heart disease, or thyroid disease.

Information for Patients

Patients should be warned about engaging in activities requiring mental alertness, such as driving a car or operating dangerous machinery.

Drug Interactions

Monoamine oxidase (MAO) inhibitors—Hyperpyrexia, hypotension, and death have been reported coincident with the co-administration of MAO inhibitors and products containing dextromethorphan. In addition, MAO inhibitors prolong and intensify the anticholinergic (drying) effects of antihistamines and may enhance the effect of pseudoephedrine. Concomitant administration of Dimetane-DX and MAO inhibitors should be avoided (see "Contraindications").

Central nervous system (CNS) depressants—Antihistamines have additive effects with alcohol and other CNS depressants (hypnotics, sedatives, tranquilizers, antianxiety agents, etc).

Antihypertensive drugs—Sympathomimetics may reduce the effects of antihypertensive drugs.

Carcinogenesis, Mutagenesis, Impairment of Fertility

Animal studies of Dimetane-DX Cough Syrup to assess the carcinogenic and mutagenic potential or the effect on fertility have not been performed.

Pregnancy
Teratogenic Effects—Pregnancy Category C

Animal reproduction studies have not been conducted with Dimetane-DX Cough Syrup. It is also not known whether Dimetane-DX Cough Syrup can cause fetal harm when administered to a pregnant woman or can affect reproduction capacity. Dimetane-DX Cough Syrup should be given to a pregnant woman only if clearly needed.

Reproduction studies of brompheniramine maleate (a component of Dimetane-DX Cough Syrup) in rats and mice at doses up to 16 times the maximum human dose have revealed no evidence of impaired fertility or harm to the fetus.

Nursing Mothers

Because of the higher risk of intolerance of antihistamines in small infants generally, and in newborns and prematures in particular, Dimetane-DX Cough Syrup is contraindicated in nursing mothers.

Pediatric Use

Safety and effectiveness in pediatric patients below the age of 6 months have not been established (see "DOSAGE AND ADMINISTRATION").

ADVERSE REACTIONS

The most frequent adverse reactions to Dimetane-DX Cough Syrup are: sedation; dryness of mouth, nose and throat; thickening of bronchial secretions; dizziness. Other adverse reactions may include:

Dermatologic: Urticaria, drug rash, photosensitivity, pruritus.

Cardiovascular System: Hypotension, hypertension, cardiac arrhythmias, palpitation.

CNS: Disturbed coordination, tremor, irritability, insomnia, visual disturbances, weakness, nervousness, convulsions, headache, euphoria, and dysphoria.

G.U. System: Urinary frequency, difficult urination.

G.I. System: Epigastric discomfort, anorexia, nausea, vomiting, diarrhea, constipation.

Respiratory System: Tightness of chest and wheezing, shortness of breath.

Hematologic System: Hemolytic anemia, thrombocytopenia, agranulocytosis.

OVERDOSAGE
Signs and Symptoms

Central nervous system effects from overdosage of brompheniramine may vary from depression to stimulation, especially in children. Anticholinergic effects may be noted. Toxic doses of pseudoephedrine may result in CNS stimulation, tachycardia, hypertension, and cardiac arrhythmias; signs of CNS depression may occasionally be seen. Dextromethorphan in toxic doses will cause drowsiness, ataxia, nystagmus, opisthotonos, and convulsive seizures.

Toxic Doses

Data suggest that individuals may respond in an unexpected manner to apparently small amounts of a particular drug. A $2^1/_2$-year-old child survived the ingestion of 21 mg/kg of dextromethorphan exhibiting only ataxia, drowsiness, and fever, but seizures have been reported in 2 children following the ingestion of 13–17 mg/kg. Another $2^1/_2$-year-old child survived a dose of 300–900 mg of brompheniramine. The toxic dose of pseudoephedrine should be less than that of ephedrine, which is estimated to be 50 mg/kg.

Treatment

Induce emesis if patient is alert and is seen prior to 6 hours following ingestion. Precautions against aspiration must be taken, especially in infants and small children. Gastric lavage may be carried out, although in some instances tracheostomy may be necessary prior to lavage. Naloxone hydrochloride 0.005 mg/kg intravenously may be of value in reversing the CNS depression that may occur from an overdose of dextromethorphan. CNS stimulants may counter CNS depression. Should CNS hyperactivity or convulsive seizures occur, intravenous short-acting barbiturates may be indicated. Hypertensive responses and/or tachycardia should be treated appropriately. Oxygen, intravenous fluids, and other supportive measures should be employed as indicated.

DOSAGE AND ADMINISTRATION

Adults and pediatric patients 12 years of age and over: 2 teaspoonfuls every 4 hours. Children 6 to under 12 years: 1 teaspoonful every 4 hours. Children 2 to under 6 years: $^1/_2$ teaspoonful every 4 hours. Infants 6 months to under 2 years: Dosage to be established by physician.
Do not exceed 6 doses during a 24-hour period.

HOW SUPPLIED

Dimetane®-DX Cough Syrup is a light-red syrup containing in each 5 mL (1 teaspoonful) brompheniramine maleate 2 mg, pseudoephedrine hydrochloride 30 mg and dextromethorphan hydrobromide 10 mg, available in pints (NDC 0031-1836-25).

Store at controlled room temperature, between 20°C and 25°C (68°F and 77°F).

Dispense in tight, light-resistant container.

Manufactured by:
Pharmaceutical Division
A.H. Robins Company
Richmond, VA 23220

Continued on next page

NDC Number	Product
–	DIMETANE®-DX Cough Syrup (each teaspoonful [5 mL] contains 2 mg brompheniramine maleate, 30 mg pseudoephedrine HCl and 10 mg dextromethorphan hydrobromide)
1535	MITROLAN® (calcium polycarbophil) Tablets
4207	DONNATAL® Capsules (each capsule contains 16.2 mg phenobarbital, 0.1037 mg hyoscyamine sulfate, 0.0194 mg atropine sulfate and 0.0065 mg scopolamine hydrobromide)
–	DONNATAL® Elixir (each teaspoonful [5 mL] contains 16.2 mg phenobarbital, 0.1037 mg hyoscyamine sulfate, 0.0194 mg atropine sulfate and 0.0065 mg scopolamine hydrobromide)
4235	DONNATAL® EXTENTABS® (each Extentab tablet contains 48.6 mg phenobarbital, 0.311 mg hyoscyamine sulfate, 0.0582 mg atropine sulfate and 0.0195 mg scopolamine hydrobromide)
4250	DONNATAL® Tablets (each tablet contains 16.2 mg phenobarbital, 0.1037 mg hyoscyamine sulfate, 0.0194 mg atropine sulfate and 0.0065 mg scopolamine hydrobromide)
4650	DONNAZYME® Tablets (each tablet contains 500 mg pancreatin)
5720	MICRO-K EXTENCAPS® 600 mg (8 mEq K) (potassium chloride) extended-release capsules, USP
5730	MICRO-K 10 EXTENCAPS® 750 mg (10 mEq K) (potassium chloride) extended-release capsules, USP
6257	PHENAPHEN® with Codeine ⒸⅢ (acetaminophen and codeine phosphate) No. 3 Capsules, (325 mg/30 mg)
6274	PHENAPHEN® with Codeine ⒸⅢ (acetaminophen and codeine phosphate) No. 4 Capsules, (325 mg/60 mg)
6649	QUINIDEX EXTENTABS® (quinidine sulfate extended-release tablets, USP), 300 mg
–	REGLAN® (metoclopramide HCl) Syrup, 5 mg/5 mL
6701	REGLAN® (metoclopramide HCl) Tablets, 10 mg
6705	REGLAN® (metoclopramide HCl) Tablets, 5 mg
7429	ROBAXIN® (methocarbamol tablets, USP) Tablets, 500 mg
7449	ROBAXIN®-750 (methocarbamol tablets, USP) Tablets, 750 mg
7469	ROBAXISAL® Tablets (each tablet contains 400 mg methocarbamol and 325 mg aspirin)
7824	ROBINUL® (glycopyrrolate tablets, USP) Tablets, 1 mg
7840	ROBINUL® Forte (glycopyrrolate tablets, USP) Tablets, 2 mg
–	ROBITUSSIN A-C® Syrup ⒸⅤ (each teaspoonful [5 mL] contains 100 mg guaifenesin and 10 mg codeine phosphate)
–	ROBITUSSIN®-DAC Syrup ⒸⅤ (each teaspoonful [5 mL] contains 100 mg guaifenesin, 30 mg pseudoephedrine hydrochloride, and 10 mg codeine phosphate)
8901	TENEX® (guanfacine HCl) Tablets, 1 mg
8903	TENEX® (guanfacine HCl) Tablets, 2 mg

DONNATAL® TABLETS ℞
DONNATAL® CAPSULES ℞
DONNATAL® ELIXIR ℞
[don 'nă-tal]

DESCRIPTION
Each Donnatal tablet, capsule or 5 mL (teaspoonful) of elixir (23% alcohol) contains:

Phenobarbital, USP	16.2 mg
(Warning: May be habit forming)	
Hyoscyamine Sulfate, USP	0.1037 mg
Atropine Sulfate, USP	0.0194 mg
Scopolamine Hydrobromide, USP	0.0065 mg

INACTIVE INGREDIENTS:
Tablets: Dibasic Calcium Phosphate, Magnesium Stearate, Microcrystalline Cellulose, Silicon Dioxide, Sodium Starch Glycolate, Stearic Acid, Sucrose. May contain Corn Starch, Dextrose, or Invert Sugar.
Capsules: Corn Starch, Edible Ink, D&C Yellow 10 and FD&C Green 3 or FD&C Blue 1 and FD&C Yellow 6, FD&C Blue 2 Aluminum Lake, Gelatin, Lactose, Sucrose. May contain FD&C Red 40 and Yellow 6 Aluminum Lakes.
Elixir: D&C Yellow 10, FD&C Blue 1, FD&C Yellow 6, Flavors, Glucose, Saccharin Sodium, Water.

ACTIONS
This drug combination provides natural belladonna alkaloids in a specific, fixed ratio combined with phenobarbital to provide peripheral anticholinergic/antispasmodic action and mild sedation.

INDICATIONS
Based on a review of this drug by the National Academy of Sciences—National Research Council and/or other information, FDA has classified the following indications as "possibly" effective:
For use as adjunctive therapy in the treatment of irritable bowel syndrome (irritable colon, spastic colon, mucous colitis) and acute enterocolitis.
May also be useful as adjunctive therapy in the treatment of duodenal ulcer. IT HAS NOT BEEN SHOWN CONCLUSIVELY WHETHER ANTICHOLINERGIC/ ANTISPASMODIC DRUGS AID IN THE HEALING OF A DUODENAL ULCER, DECREASE THE RATE OF RECURRENCES OR PREVENT COMPLICATIONS.

CONTRAINDICATIONS
Glaucoma, obstructive uropathy (for example, bladder neck obstruction due to prostatic hypertrophy); obstructive disease of the gastrointestinal tract (as in achalasia, pyloroduodenal stenosis, etc.); paralytic ileus, intestinal atony of the elderly or debilitated patient; unstable cardiovascular status in acute hemorrhage; severe ulcerative colitis especially if complicated by toxic megacolon; myasthenia gravis; hiatal hernia associated with reflux esophagitis.
Donnatal is contraindicated in patients with known hypersensitivity to any of the ingredients. Phenobarbital is contraindicated in acute intermittent porphyria and in those patients in whom phenobarbital produces restlessness and/or excitement.

WARNINGS
In the presence of a high environmental temperature, heat prostration can occur with belladonna alkaloids (fever and heatstroke due to decreased sweating).
Diarrhea may be an early symptom of incomplete intestinal obstruction, especially in patients with ileostomy or colostomy. In this instance treatment with this drug would be inappropriate and possibly harmful.
Donnatal may produce drowsiness or blurred vision. The patient should be warned, should these occur, not to engage in activities requiring mental alertness, such as operating a motor vehicle or other machinery, and not to perform hazardous work.
Phenobarbital may decrease the effect of anticoagulants and necessitate larger doses of the anticoagulant for optimal effect. When the phenobarbital is discontinued, the dose of the anticoagulant may have to be decreased.
Phenobarbital may be habit forming and should not be administered to individuals known to be addiction prone or to those with a history of physical and/or psychological dependence upon drugs.
Since barbiturates are metabolized in the liver, they should be used with caution and initial doses should be small in patients with hepatic dysfunction.

PRECAUTIONS
Use with caution in patients with: autonomic neuropathy, hepatic or renal disease, hyperthyroidism, coronary heart disease, congestive heart failure, cardiac arrhythmias, tachycardia, and hypertension.
Belladonna alkaloids may produce a delay in gastric emptying (antral stasis) which would complicate the management of gastric ulcer.
Theoretically, with overdosage, a curare-like action may occur.
CARCINOGENESIS, MUTAGENESIS. Long-term studies in animals have not been performed to evaluate carcinogenic potential.
PREGNANCY CATEGORY C. Animal reproduction studies have not been conducted with Donnatal. It is not known whether Donnatal can cause fetal harm when administered to a pregnant woman or can affect reproduction capacity. Donnatal should be given to a pregnant woman only if clearly needed.
NURSING MOTHERS. It is not known whether this drug is excreted in human milk. Because many drugs are excreted in human milk, caution should be exercised when Donnatal is administered to a nursing mother.

ADVERSE REACTIONS
Adverse reactions may include xerostomia; urinary hesitancy and retention; blurred vision; tachycardia; palpitation; mydriasis; cycloplegia; increased ocular tension; loss of taste sense; headache; nervousness; drowsiness; weakness; dizziness; insomnia; nausea; vomiting; impotence; suppression of lactation; constipation; bloated feeling; musculoskeletal pain; severe allergic reaction or drug idiosyncrasies, including anaphylaxis, urticaria and other dermal manifestations; and decreased sweating. Elderly patients may react with symptoms of excitement, agitation, drowsiness, and other untoward manifestations to even small doses of the drug.
Phenobarbital may produce excitement in some patients, rather than a sedative effect. In patients habituated to barbiturates, abrupt withdrawal may produce delirium or convulsions.

DOSAGE AND ADMINISTRATION
The dosage of Donnatal should be adjusted to the needs of the individual patient to assure symptomatic control with a minimum of adverse effects.
Donnatal Tablets or Capsules. Adults: One or two Donnatal tablets or capsules three or four times a day according to condition and severity of symptoms.
Donnatal Elixir. Adults: One or two teaspoonfuls of elixir three or four times a day according to conditions and severity of symptoms.
Children (Elixir)—may be dosed every 4 or 6 hours.:

	Starting Dosage	
Body Weight	q4h	q6h
10 lb (4.5 kg)	0.5 mL	0.75 mL
20 lb (9.1 kg)	1.0 mL	1.5 mL
30 lb (13.6 kg)	1.5 mL	2.0 mL
50 lb (22.7 kg)	1/2 tsp	3/4 tsp
75 lb (34.0 kg)	3/4 tsp	1 tsp
100 lb (45.4 kg)	1 tsp	1 1/2 tsp

OVERDOSAGE
The signs and symptoms of overdose are headache, nausea, vomiting, blurred vision, dilated pupils, hot and dry skin, dizziness, dryness of the mouth, difficulty in swallowing, CNS stimulation. Treatment should consist of gastric lavage, emetics, and activated charcoal. If indicated, parenteral cholinergic agents such as physostigmine or bethanechol chloride, should be added.

HOW SUPPLIED
Donnatal® Tablets. White, compressed, scored and embossed "R"; in bottles of 100 (NDC 0031-4250-63), 1000 (NDC 0031-4250-74) and Dis-Co® Unit Dose Packs of 100 (NDC 0031-4250-64).
Donnatal® Capsules. Green and white, monogrammed "AHR" and "4207"; in bottles of 100 (NDC 0031-4207-63).
Donnatal® Elixir. Green, citrus flavored, in 4 fl. oz. (NDC 0031-4221-12), pints (NDC 0031-4221-25), gallons (NDC 0031-4221-29) and 5 mL Dis-Co® Unit Dose Packs (4 × 25s) (NDC 0031-4221-13).
Store at controlled room temperature, between 20°C and 25°C (68°F and 77°F).
Dispense in tight, light-resistant container.

Manufactured by:
Pharmaceutical Division
A.H. Robins Company
Richmond, VA 23220
Shown in Product Identification Guide, page 334

DONNATAL EXTENTABS® ℞
[don 'nă-tal ĕks "tĕn 'tabs]

DESCRIPTION
Each Donnatal Extentabs tablet contains:

Phenobarbital, USP (3/4 gr)	48.6 mg
(Warning: May be habit forming)	
Hyoscyamine Sulfate, USP	0.3111 mg
Atropine Sulfate, USP	0.0582 mg
Scopolamine Hydrobromide, USP	0.0195 mg

Each Donnatal Extentabs tablet contains the equivalent of three Donnatal tablets. Extentabs are designed to release the ingredients gradually to provide effects for up to twelve (12) hours.
Inactive Ingredients: Acacia, Acetylated Monoglycerides, Calcium Sulfate, Carnauba Wax, D&C Yellow 10, Edible Ink, FD&C Blue 1, FD&C Blue 2 Aluminum Lake, FD&C Yellow 6, Gelatin, Guar Gum, Magnesium Stearate, Polysorbates, Shellac, Sodium Phosphate, Sucrose, Titanium Dioxide, Wheat Flour, White Wax and other ingredients, one of which is a corn derivative. May include FD&C Red 40 and Yellow 6 Aluminum Lakes.

ACTIONS
This drug combination provides natural belladonna alkaloids in a specific, fixed ratio combined with phenobarbital to provide peripheral anticholinergic/antispasmodic action and mild sedation.

INDICATIONS
Based on a review of this drug by the National Academy of Sciences—National Research Council and/or other information, FDA has classified the following indications as "possibly" effective:
For use as adjunctive therapy in the treatment of irritable bowel syndrome (irritable colon, spastic colon, mucous colitis) and acute enterocolitis.
May also be useful as adjunctive therapy in the treatment of duodenal ulcer. IT HAS NOT BEEN SHOWN CONCLUSIVELY WHETHER ANTICHOLINERGIC/ ANTISPASMODIC DRUGS AID IN THE HEALING OF A DUODENAL ULCER, DECREASE THE RATE OF RECURRENCES OR PREVENT COMPLICATIONS.

CONTRAINDICATIONS
Glaucoma, obstructive uropathy (for example, bladder neck obstruction due to prostatic hypertrophy); obstructive disease of the gastrointestinal tract (as in achalasia, pyloroduodenal stenosis, etc.); paralytic ileus, intestinal atony of the elderly or debilitated patient; unstable cardiovascular status in acute hemorrhage; severe ulcerative colitis especially if complicated by toxic megacolon; myasthenia gravis, hiatal hernia associated with reflux esophagitis.
Donnatal is contraindicated in patients with known hypersensitivity to any of the ingredients. Phenobarbital is contraindicated in acute intermittent porphyria and in those patients in whom phenobarbital produces restlessness and/or excitement.

WARNINGS
In the presence of a high environmental temperature, heat prostration can occur with belladonna alkaloids (fever and heatstroke due to decreased sweating).
Diarrhea may be an early symptom of incomplete intestinal obstruction, especially in patients with ileostomy or colostomy. In this instance treatment with this drug would be inappropriate and possibly harmful.
Donnatal may produce drowsiness or blurred vision. The patient should be warned, should these occur, not to engage in activities requiring mental alertness, such as operating a motor vehicle or other machinery, and not to perform hazardous work.
Phenobarbital may decrease the effect of anticoagulants and necessitate larger doses of the anticoagulant for optimal effect. When the phenobarbital is discontinued, the dose of the anticoagulant may have to be decreased.
Phenobarbital may be habit forming and should not be administered to individuals known to be addiction prone or to those with a history of physical and/or psychological dependence upon drugs.
Since barbiturates are metabolized in the liver, they should be used with caution and initial doses should be small in patients with hepatic dysfunction.

PRECAUTIONS
Use with caution in patients with: autonomic neuropathy, hepatic or renal disease, hyperthyroidism, coronary heart disease, congestive heart failure, cardiac arrhythmias, tachycardia, and hypertension.
Belladonna alkaloids may produce a delay in gastric emptying (antral stasis) which would complicate the management of gastric ulcer.
Theoretically, with overdosage, a curare-like action may occur.
Carcinogenesis, mutagenesis. Long-term studies in animals have not been performed to evaluate carcinogenic potential.
Pregnancy Category C. Animal reproduction studies have not been conducted with Donnatal. It is not known whether Donnatal can cause fetal harm when administered to a pregnant woman or can affect reproduction capacity. Donnatal should be given to a pregnant woman only if clearly needed.

Nursing mothers. It is not known whether this drug is excreted in human milk. Because many drugs are excreted in human milk, caution should be exercised when Donnatal is administered to a nursing mother.

ADVERSE REACTIONS

Adverse reactions may include xerostomia; urinary hesitancy and retention; blurred vision; tachycardia; palpitation; mydriasis; cycloplegia; increased ocular tension; loss of taste sense; headache; nervousness; drowsiness; weakness; dizziness; insomnia; nausea; vomiting; impotence; suppression of lactation; constipation; bloated feeling; musculoskeletal pain; severe allergic reaction or drug idiosyncrasies, including anaphylaxis, urticaria and other dermal manifestations; and decreased sweating. Elderly patients may react with symptoms of excitement, agitation, drowsiness, and other untoward manifestations to even small doses of the drug.

Phenobarbital may produce excitement in some patients, rather than a sedative effect. In patients habituated to barbiturates, abrupt withdrawal may produce delirium or convulsions.

DOSAGE AND ADMINISTRATION

The dosage of Donnatal Extentabs should be adjusted to the needs of the individual patient to assure symptomatic control with a minimum of adverse reactions. The usual dose is one tablet every twelve (12) hours. If indicated, one tablet every eight (8) hours may be given.

OVERDOSAGE

The signs and symptoms of overdose are headache, nausea, vomiting, blurred vision, dilated pupils; hot and dry skin, dizziness, dryness of the mouth, difficulty in swallowing, CNS stimulation. Treatment should consist of gastric lavage, emetics, and activated charcoal. If indicated, parenteral cholinergic agents such as physostigmine or bethanechol chloride should be added.

HOW SUPPLIED

Pale green, coated tablets, monogrammed AHR and Donnatal Extentab in bottles of 100 (NDC 0031-4235-63) and 500 (NDC 0031-4235-70); and Dis-Co® Unit Dose Packs of 100 (NDC 0031-4235-64).

Store at controlled room temperature, between 20°C and 25°C (68°F and 77°F).

Dispense in well-closed, light-resistant container.

Manufactured by:
Pharmaceutical Division
A.H. Robins Company
Richmond, VA 23220

Shown in Product Identification Guide, page 334

DONNAZYME® Tablets ℞

[don 'nă " zīm]

Pancreatic Enzyme Replacement

DESCRIPTION

Donnazyme tablets are available for oral administration.

Each tablet contains:

Pancreatin, USP equivalent .... 500 mg

which provides not less than the following enzymatic activity—

Lipase	1,000 USP Units
Protease	12,500 USP Units
Amylase	12,500 USP Units

Inactive Ingredients: Acacia, Acetylated Monoglycerides, Calcium Sulfate, Carnauba Wax, Cellulose Acetate Phthalate, Corn Starch, D&C Yellow 10 Aluminum Lake, Diethyl Phthalate, Edible Ink, FD&C Blue 1 Aluminum Lake, FD&C Yellow 6 Aluminum Lake, Gelatin, Methylparaben, Microcrystalline Cellulose, Polysorbates, Povidone, Propylparaben, Shellac, Sodium Benzoate, Stearic Acid, Sucrose, Titanium Dioxide, Wheat Flour, White Wax. May contain Docusate Sodium.

CLINICAL PHARMACOLOGY

The outer layer of Donnazyme tablets is gastric-soluble. The core of the tablet contains pancreatin. It is designed to disintegrate in the alkaline medium of the duodenum where it releases the active enzyme components of pancreatin (trypsin, amylase and lipase). Trypsin breaks down larger protein fractions into peptides; amylase converts starch into maltose; lipase splits fat into fatty acids and glycerin.

INDICATIONS AND USAGE

Donnazyme is indicated for the treatment of exocrine pancreatic insufficiency.

CONTRAINDICATIONS

Donnazyme is contraindicated in patients with known hypersensitivity to the drug.

WARNINGS

Do not take this product if you are allergic to pork.

Do not take this product unless directed by a physician.

Do not exceed the labeled dose unless directed by a physician.

Do not chew tablets.

Swallow tablets quickly to lessen potential for mouth irritation.

PRECAUTIONS

Carcinogenesis, mutagenesis: Long-term studies in animals have not been performed to evaluate carcinogenic potential.

Pregnancy Category C. Animal reproduction studies have not been conducted with Donnazyme. It is not known whether Donnazyme can cause fetal harm when administered to a pregnant woman or can affect reproduction capacity. Donnazyme should be given to a pregnant woman only if clearly needed.

Nursing mothers: It is not known whether this drug is excreted in human milk. Because many drugs are excreted in human milk, caution should be exercised when Donnazyme is administered to a nursing mother.

Pediatric Use: Safety and effectiveness in children have not been established.

ADVERSE REACTIONS

Skin rash is the most frequently reported adverse reaction to Donnazyme and appears to be associated with hypersensitivity to pork protein in the pancreatin. At high doses, a laxative effect may occur.

OVERDOSAGE

Excessive dosage may produce a laxative effect. Systemic toxicity does not occur.

DOSAGE AND ADMINISTRATION

Two tablets with each meal and 2 tablets taken with food eaten between meals or as directed by a physician. Donnazyme tablets should be swallowed whole and not crushed or chewed.

HOW SUPPLIED

Kelly green tablets in bottles of 100 (NDC 0031-4650-63). Store at controlled room temperature, between 20°C and 25°C (68°F and 77°F). Dispense in tight container.

Manufactured by:
Pharamaceutical Division
A.H. Robins Company
Richmond, VA 23220

Shown in Product Identification Guide, page 334

DOPRAM® INJECTABLE ℞

[do 'pram]

brand of Doxapram Hydrochloride Injection, USP

DESCRIPTION

Dopram Injectable (Doxapram Hydrochloride Injection, USP) is a clear, colorless, sterile, non-pyrogenic, aqueous solution with pH 3.5—5.0, for intravenous administration.

Each 1 mL contains:

Doxapram Hydrochloride, USP	20 mg
Benzyl Alcohol, NF (as preservative)	0.9%
Water for Injection, USP	q.s.

Due to its benzyl alcohol content, Dopram Injectable should not be used in newborns.

Dopram Injectable is a respiratory stimulant.

Doxapram hydrochloride is a white to off-white, crystalline powder, sparingly soluble in water, alcohol and chloroform. It has the following chemical name:

1-ethyl-4-[2-(4-morpholinyl)ethyl]-3,3-diphenyl-2-pyrrolidinone monohydrochloride, monohydrate.

CLINICAL PHARMACOLOGY

Doxapram hydrochloride produces respiratory stimulation mediated through the peripheral carotid chemoreceptors. As the dosage level is increased, the central respiratory centers in the medulla are stimulated with progressive stimulation of other parts of the brain and spinal cord.

The onset of respiratory stimulation following the recommended single intravenous injection of doxapram hydrochloride usually occurs in 20–40 seconds with peak effect at 1–2 minutes. The duration of effect may vary from 5–12 minutes.

The respiratory stimulant action is manifested by an increase in tidal volume associated with a slight increase in respiratory rate.

A pressor response may result following doxapram administration. Provided there is no impairment of cardiac function, the pressor effect is more marked in hypovolemic than in normovolemic states. The pressor response is due to the improved cardiac output rather than peripheral vasoconstriction. Following doxapram administration, an increased release of catecholamines has been noted.

Although opiate induced respiratory depression is antagonized by doxapram, the analgesic effect is not affected.

INDICATIONS

1. ***Postanesthesia.***
   a. When the possibility of airway obstruction and/or hypoxia have been eliminated, doxapram may be used to stimulate respiration in patients with drug-induced postanesthesia respiratory depression or apnea other than that due to muscle relaxant drugs.
   b. To pharmacologically stimulate deep breathing in the so-called "stir-up" regimen in the postoperative patient. (Simultaneous administration of oxygen is desirable.)
2. ***Drug-induced central nervous system depression.***
   Exercising care to prevent vomiting and aspiration, doxapram may be used to stimulate respiration, hasten arousal, and to encourage the return of laryngopharyngeal reflexes in patients with mild to moderate respiratory and CNS depression due to drug overdosage.
3. ***Chronic pulmonary disease associated with acute hypercapnia.***
   Doxapram is indicated as a temporary measure in hospitalized patients with acute respiratory insufficiency superimposed on chronic obstructive pulmonary disease. Its use should be for a short period of time (approximately 2 hours) as an aid in the prevention of elevation of arterial CO_2 tension during the administration of oxygen. It should not be used in conjuction with mechanical ventilation.

CONTRAINDICATIONS

Due to its benzyl alcohol content, Dopram Injectable should not be used in newborns.

Doxapram should not be used in patients with epilepsy or other convulsive disorders.

Doxapram is contraindicated in patients with mechanical disorders of ventilation such as mechanical obstruction, muscle paresis, flail chest, pneumothorax, acute bronchial asthma, pulmonary fibrosis or other conditions resulting in restriction of chest wall, muscles of respiration or alveolar expansion.

Doxapram is contraindicated in patients with evidence of head injury or cerebral vascular accident and in those with significant cardiovascular impairment, severe hypertension, or known hypersensitivity to the drug.

WARNINGS

1. ***In postanesthetic use.***
   a. Doxapram is neither an antagonist to muscle relaxant drugs nor a specific narcotic antagonist. Adequacy of airway and oxygenation must be assured prior to doxapram administration.
   b. Doxapram should be administered with great care and only under careful supervision to patients with hypermetabolic states such as hyperthyroidism or pheochromocytoma.
   c. Since narcosis may recur after stimulation with doxapram, care should be taken to maintain close observation until the patient has been fully alert for $^1/_2$ to 1 hour.
2. ***In drug-induced CNS and respiratory depression.***
   Doxapram alone may not stimulate adequate spontaneous breathing or provide sufficient arousal in patients who are ***severely*** depressed either due to respiratory failure or to CNS depressant drugs, but should be used as an adjunct to established supportive measures and resuscitative techniques.
3. ***In chronic obstructive pulmonary disease.***
   a. Because of the associated increased work of breathing, do not increase the rate of infusion of doxapram in severely ill patients in an attempt to lower pCO_2.
   b. Doxapram should not be used in conjunction with mechanical ventilation.

PRECAUTIONS

1. ***General.***
   a. An adequate airway is essential.
   b. Recommended dosages of doxapram should be employed and maximum total dosages should not be exceeded. In order to avoid side effects, it is advisable to use the minimum effective dosage.
   c. Monitoring of the blood pressure and deep tendon reflexes is recommended to prevent overdosage.
   d. Vascular extravasation or use of a single injection site over an extended period should be avoided since either may lead to thrombophlebitis or local skin irritation.
   e. Rapid infusion may result in hemolysis.
   f. Lowered pCO_2 induced by hyperventilation produces cerebral vasoconstriction and slowing of the cerebral circulation. This should be taken into consideration on an individual basis.
   g. Intravenous short-acting barbiturates, oxygen and resuscitative equipment should be readily available to manage overdosage manifested by excessive central nervous system stimulation. Slow administration of the drug, and careful observation of the patient during administration and for some time subsequently are ad-

Continued on next page

Dopram—Cont.

visable. These precautions are to assure that the protective reflexes have been restored and to prevent possible post-hyperventilation hypoventilation.

h. Doxapram should be administered cautiously to patients receiving sympathomimetic or monoamine oxidase inhibiting drugs, since an additive pressor effect may occur.

i. Blood pressure increases are generally modest but significant increases have been noted in some patients. Because of this doxapram is not recommended for use in severe hypertension (see Contraindications).

j. If sudden hypotension or dyspnea develops, doxapram should be stopped.

2. *In postanesthetic use.*
   a. The same consideration to pre-existing disease states should be exercised as in non-anesthetized individuals. See Contraindications and Warnings covering use in hypertension, asthma, disturbances of respiratory mechanics including airway obstruction, CNS disorders including increased cerebrospinal fluid pressure, convulsive disorders, acute agitation, and profound metabolic disorders.
   b. See Drug Interactions.

3. *In chronic obstructive pulmonary disease.*
   a. Arrhythmias seen in some patients in acute respiratory failure secondary to chronic obstructive pulmonary disease are probably the result of hypoxia. Doxapram should be used with caution in these patients.
   b. Arterial blood gases should be drawn prior to the initiation of doxapram infusion and oxygen administration, then at least every $\frac{1}{2}$ hour. Doxapram administration does not diminish the need for careful monitoring of the patient or the need for supplemental oxygen in patients with acute respiratory failure. Doxapram should be stopped if the arterial blood gases deteriorate, and mechanical ventilation initiated.

Drug Interactions: Administration of doxapram to patients who are receiving sympathomimetic or monoamine oxidase inhibiting drugs may result in an additive pressor effect. (See Precautions).

In patients who have received muscle relaxants, doxapram may temporarily mask the residual effects of muscle relaxant drugs.

In patients who have received anesthetics known to sensitize the myocardium to catecholamines, such as halothane, cyclopropane and enflurane, initiation of doxapram therapy should be delayed for at least 10 minutes following discontinuance of anesthesia, since an increase in epinephrine release has been noted with doxapram.

Carcinogenesis, mutagenesis, impairment of fertility. No carcinogenic or mutagenic studies have been performed using doxapram. Doxapram did not adversely affect the breeding performance of rats.

Pregnancy Category B. Reproduction studies have been performed in rats at doses up to 1.6 times the human dose and have revealed no evidence of impaired fertility or harm to the fetus due to doxapram. There are, however, no adequate and well-controlled studies in pregnant women. Since the animals in the reproduction studies were dosed by the IM and oral routes and animal reproduction studies, in general, are not always predictive of human response, this drug should be used during pregnancy only if clearly needed.

Nursing mothers. It is not known whether this drug is excreted in human milk. Because many drugs are excreted in human milk, caution should be exercised when doxapram hydrochloride is administered to a nursing mother.

Pediatric use. The use of the preservative benzyl alcohol in the newborn has been associated with metabolic, CNS, respiratory, circulatory, and renal dysfunction. Safety and effectiveness in children below the age of 12 years have not been established.

ADVERSE REACTIONS

The following adverse reactions have been reported:

1. *Central and autonomic nervous systems.*
   Pyrexia, flushing, sweating; pruritus and paresthesia, such as a feeling of warmth, burning, or hot sensation, especially in the area of genitalia and perineum; apprehension, disorientation, pupillary dilatation, headache, dizziness, hyperactivity, involuntary movements, muscle spasticity, increased deep tendon reflexes, clonus, bilateral Babinski, and convulsions.

2. *Respiratory.*
   Dyspnea, cough, tachypnea, laryngospasm, bronchospasm, hiccough, and rebound hypoventilation.

3. *Cardiovascular.*
   Phlebitis, variations in heart rate, lowered T-waves, arrhythmias, chest pain, tightness in chest. A mild to moderate increase in blood pressure is commonly noted and may be of concern in patients with severe cardiovascular diseases.

4. *Gastrointestinal.*
   Nausea, vomiting, diarrhea, desire to defecate.

Table I. Dosage for postanesthetic use—I.V.

I.V. Administration	Recommended dosage		Maximum dose per single injection		Maximum total dose	
	mg/kg	mg/lb	mg/kg	mg/lb	mg/kg	mg/lb
Single Injection	0.5–1.0	0.25–0.5	1.5	0.70	1.5	0.70
Repeat Injections (5 min. intervals)	0.5–1.0	0.25–0.5	1.5	0.70	2.0	1.0
Infusion	0.5–1.0	0.25–0.5	—	—	4.0	2.0

Table II. Dosage for drug-induced CNS depression

Level of Depression	METHOD ONE Priming dose single/repeat i.v. injection		METHOD TWO Rate of intermittent i.v. infusion	
	mg/kg	mg/lb	mg/kg/hr	mg/lb/hr
Mild*	1.0	0.5	1.0–2.0	0.5–1.0
Moderate†	2.0	1.0	2.0–3.0	1.0–1.5

*Mild Depression
Class 0: Asleep, but can be aroused and can answer questions.
Class 1: Comatose, will withdraw from painful stimuli, reflexes intact.
†Moderate Depression
Class 2: Comatose, will not withdraw from painful stimuli, reflexes intact.
Class 3: Comatose, reflexes absent, no depression of circulation or respiration.

5. *Genitourinary.*
   Stimulation of urinary bladder with spontaneous voiding; urinary retention.

6. *Laboratory determinations.*
   A decrease in hemoglobin, hematocrit, or red blood cell count has been observed in postoperative patients. In the presence of pre-existing leukopenia, a further decrease in WBC has been observed following anesthesia and treatment with doxapram hydrochloride. Elevation of BUN and albuminuria have also been observed. As some of the patients cited above had received multiple drugs concomitantly, a cause and effect relationship could not be determined.

OVERDOSAGE

Signs and Symptoms. Symptoms of overdosage are extensions of the pharmacologic effects of the drug. Excessive pressor effect, tachycardia, skeletal muscle hyperactivity, and enhanced deep tendon reflexes may be early signs of overdosage. Therefore, the blood pressure, pulse rate and deep tendon reflexes should be evaluated periodically and the dosage or infusion rate adjusted accordingly.

Convulsive seizures are unlikely at recommended dosages. In unanesthetized animals, the convulsant dose is 70 times greater than the respiratory stimulant dose. Intravenous LD_{50} values in the mouse and rat were approximately 75 mg/kg and in the cat and dog were 40–80 mg/kg.

Except for management of chronic obstructive pulmonary disease associated with acute hypercapnia, the maximum recommended dosage is 3 GRAMS/24 HOURS. (See Dosage and Administration.)

Management. There is no specific antidote for doxapram. Management should be symptomatic. Short-acting intravenous barbiturates, oxygen and resuscitative equipment should be used as needed for supportive treatment.

There is no evidence that doxapram is dialyzable; further, the half-life of doxapram makes it unlikely that dialysis would be appropriate in managing overdose with this drug.

DOSAGE AND ADMINISTRATION

1. Doxapram hydrochloride is compatible with 5% and 10% dextrose in water or normal saline. ADMIXTURE OF DOXAPRAM WITH ALKALINE SOLUTIONS SUCH AS 2.5% THIOPENTAL SODIUM, BICARBONATE, OR AMINOPHYLLINE WILL RESULT IN PRECIPITATION OR GAS FORMATION.

2. *In postanesthetic use.*
   a. By i.v. injection (see Table I. Dosage for postanesthetic use—I.V.) Slow administration of the drug and careful observation of the patient during administration and for some time subsequently are advisable.
   [See table I above]
   b. By infusion. The solution is prepared by adding 250 mg of doxapram (12.5 mL) to 250 mL of dextrose or saline solution. The infusion is initiated at a rate of approximately 5 mg/minute until a satisfactory respiratory response is observed, and maintained at a rate of 1–3 mg/minute. The rate of infusion should be adjusted to sustain the desired level of respiratory stimulation with a minimum of side effects. The recommended total dosage by infusion is 4 mg/kg (2.0 mg/lb), or approximately 300 mg for the average adult.

3. *In the management of drug-induced CNS depression.*
   (See Table II. Dosage for drug-induced CNS depression.)
   [See table II above]
   METHOD ONE
   Using Single and/or Repeat Single I.V. *Injections.*
   a. Give priming dose of 1.0 mg/lb (2.0 mg/kg) body weight and repeat in 5 minutes.
   b. Repeat same dose q1–2h until patient wakens. Watch for relapse into unconsciousness or development of respiratory depression, since Dopram does not affect the metabolism of CNS-depressant drugs.
   c. If relapse occurs, resume injections q1–2h until arousal is sustained, or total maximum daily dose (3 grams) is given. Allow patients to sleep until 24 hours have elapsed from first injection of Dopram, using assisted or automatic respiration if necessary.
   d. Repeat procedure the following day until patient breathes spontaneously and sustains desired level of consciousness, or until maximum dose (3 grams) is given.
   e. Repetitive doses should be administered only to patients who have shown response to the initial dose.
   f. Failure to respond appropriately indicates the need for neurologic evaluation for a possible central nervous system source of sustained coma.
   METHOD TWO
   By Intermittent I.V. *Infusion.*
   a. Give priming dose as in Method One.
   b. If patient wakens, watch for relapse; if no response, continue general supportive treatment for 1–2 hours and repeat Dopram. If some respiratory stimulation occurs, prepare I.V. infusion by adding 250 mg of Dopram (12.5 mL) to 250 mL of saline or dextrose solution. Deliver at rate of 1–3 mg/min (60–180 mL/hr) according to size of patient and depth of coma. Discontinue Dopram if patient begins to waken or at end of 2 hours.
   c. Continue supportive treatment for $\frac{1}{2}$ to 2 hours and repeat Step b.
   d. Do not exceed 3 grams/day.

4. *Chronic obstructive pulmonary disease associated with acute hypercapnia.*
   a. One vial of doxapram (400 mg) should be mixed with 180 mL of dextrose or saline solution (concentration of 2.0 mg/mL). The infusion should be started at 1–2 mg/minute ($\frac{1}{2}$–1 mL/minute); if indicated, increase to a maximum of 3 mg/minute. Arterial blood gases should be determined prior to the onset of doxapram's administration and at least every half hour during the two hours of infusion to insure against the insidious development of CO_2-RETENTION AND ACIDOSIS. Alteration of oxygen concentration or flow rate may necessitate adjustment in the rate of doxapram infusion.
   b. Predictable blood gas patterns are more readily established with a continuous infusion of doxapram. If the blood gases show evidence of deterioration, the infusion of doxapram should be discontinued.
   c. ADDITIONAL INFUSIONS BEYOND THE SINGLE MAXIMUM TWO HOUR ADMINISTRATION PERIOD ARE NOT RECOMMENDED.

Parenteral drug products should be inspected visually for particulate matter and discoloration prior to administration, whenever solution and container permit.

HOW SUPPLIED

Dopram Injectable (Doxapram Hydrochloride Injection) is available in 20 mL multiple dose vials containing 20 mg of doxapram hydrochloride per mL. with benzyl alcohol 0.9% as the preservative (NDC 0031-4849-83).

Store at Controlled Room Temperature, Between 15°C and 30°C (59°F and 86°F).

Manufactured for Pharmaceutical Division
A. H. Robins Co.
Richmond, Virginia 23220
by Elkins-Sinn, Inc., Cherry Hill, New Jersey 08003-4099.

MICRO–K EXTENCAPS® ℞
[mi´cro˝ K ĕks˝tĕn´caps]

MICRO–K 10 EXTENCAPS® ℞
(Potassium Chloride Extended-Release Capsules, USP)

DESCRIPTION

Micro-K Extencaps capsules and Micro-K 10 Extencaps capsules are oral dosage forms of microencapsulated potassium chloride containing 600 and 750 mg, respectively, of potassium chloride USP equivalent to 8 and 10 mEq of potassium.

Dispersibility of potassium chloride (KCl) is accomplished by microencapsulation and a dispersing agent. The resultant flow characteristics of the KCl microcapsules and the controlled release of K+ ions by the microcapsular membrane are intended to avoid the possibility that excessive amounts of KCl can be localized at any point on the mucosa of the gastrointestinal tract.

Each crystal of KCl is microencapsulated by a patented process with an insoluble polymeric coating which functions as a semi-permeable membrane; it allows for the controlled release of potassium and chloride ions over an eight- to ten-hour period. Fluids pass through the membrane and gradually dissolve the potassium chloride within the microcapsules. The resulting potassium chloride solution slowly diffuses outward through the membrane. Micro-K and Micro-K 10 are electrolyte replenishers. The chemical name of the active ingredient is potassium chloride and the structural formula is KCl. Potassium chloride USP occurs as a white, granular powder or as colorless crystals. It is odorless and has a saline taste. Its solutions are neutral to litmus. It is freely soluble in water and insoluble in alcohol. The inactive ingredients present are edible ink, ethylcellulose, FD&C Blue 2 Aluminum Lake, FD&C Yellow 6, gelatin, magnesium stearate, sodium lauryl sulfate, titanium dioxide. May contain FD&C Red 40 and Yellow 6 Aluminum Lakes.

CLINICAL PHARMACOLOGY

Potassium ion is the principal intracellular cation of most body tissues. Potassium ions participate in a number of essential physiological processes, including the maintenance of intracellular tonicity, the transmission of nerve impulses, the contraction of cardiac, skeletal, and smooth muscle, and the maintenance of normal renal function.

The intracellullar concentration of potassium is approximately 150 to 160 mEq per liter. The normal adult plasma concentration is 3.5 to 5 mEq per liter. An active ion transport system maintains this gradient across the plasma membrane.

Potassium is a normal dietary constituent and under steady-state conditions the amount of potassium absorbed from the gastrointestinal tract is equal to the amount excreted in the urine. The usual dietary intake of potassium is 50 to 100 mEq per day.

Potassium depletion will occur whenever the rate of potassium loss through renal excretion and/or loss from the gastrointestinal tract exceeds the rate of potassium intake. Such depletion usually develops slowly as a consequence of therapy with diuretics, primary or secondary hyperaldosteronism, diabetic ketoacidosis, or inadequate replacement of potassium in patients on prolonged parenteral nutrition. Depletion can develop rapidly with severe diarrhea, especially if associated with vomiting. Potassium depletion due to these causes is usually accompanied by a concomitant loss of chloride and is manifested by hypokalemia and metabolic alkalosis. Potassium depletion may produce weakness, fatigue, disturbances of cardiac rhythm (primarily ectopic beats), prominent U-waves in the electrocardiogram, and in advanced cases, flaccid paralysis and/or impaired ability to concentrate urine.

If potassium depletion associated with metabolic alkalosis cannot be managed by correcting the fundamental cause of the deficiency, e.g., where the patient requires long-term diuretic therapy, supplemental potassium in the form of high potassium food or potassium chloride may be able to restore normal potassium levels.

In rare circumstances (e.g., patients with renal tubular acidosis) potassium depletion may be associated with metabolic acidosis and hyperchloremia. In such patients potassium replacement should be accomplished with potassium salts other than the chloride, such as potassium bicarbonate, potassium citrate, potassium acetate, or potassium gluconate.

INDICATIONS AND USAGE

BECAUSE OF REPORTS OF INTESTINAL AND GASTRIC ULCERATION AND BLEEDING WITH CONTROLLED-RELEASE POTASSIUM CHLORIDE PREPARATIONS, THESE DRUGS SHOULD BE RESERVED FOR THOSE PATIENTS WHO CANNOT TOLERATE OR REFUSE TO TAKE LIQUID OR EFFERVESCENT POTASSIUM PREPARATIONS OR FOR PATIENTS IN WHOM THERE IS A PROBLEM OF COMPLIANCE WITH THESE PREPARATIONS.

1. For the treatment of patients with hypokalemia with or without metabolic alkalosis; in digitalis intoxication, and in patients with hypokalemic familial periodic paralysis. If hypokalemia is the result of diuretic therapy, consideration should be given to the use of a lower dose of diuretic, which may be sufficient without leading to hypokalemia.

2. For the prevention of hypokalemia in patients who would be at particular risk if hypokalemia were to develop, e.g., digitalized patients or patients with significant cardiac arrhythmias, hepatic cirrhosis with ascites, states of aldosterone excess with normal renal function, potassium-losing nephropathy, and certain diarrheal states.

The use of potassium salts in patients receiving diuretics for uncomplicated essential hypertension is often unnecessary when such patients have a normal dietary pattern and when low doses of the diuretic are used. Serum potassium should be checked periodically, however, and if hypokalemia occurs, dietary supplementation with potassium-containing foods may be adequate to control milder cases. In more severe cases, and if dose adjustment of the diuretic is ineffective or unwarranted, supplementation with potassium salts may be indicated.

CONTRAINDICATIONS

Potassium supplements are contraindicated in patients with hyperkalemia since a further increase in serum potassium concentration in such patients can produce cardiac arrest. Hyperkalemia may complicate any of the following conditions: chronic renal failure, systemic acidosis such as diabetic acidosis, acute dehydration, extensive tissue breakdown as in severe burns, adrenal insufficiency, or the administration of a potassium-sparing diuretic (e.g., spironolactone, triamterene, amiloride) (see **OVERDOSAGE**).

Controlled-release formulations of potassium chloride have produced esophageal ulceration in certain cardiac patients with esophageal compression due to an enlarged left atrium. Potassium supplementation, when indicated in such patients, should be given as a liquid preparation.

All solid oral dosage forms of potassium chloride are contraindicated in any patient in whom there is structural, pathological (e.g., diabetic gastroparesis), or pharmacologic (use of anticholinergic agents or other agents with anticholinergic properties at sufficient doses to exert anticholinergic effects) cause for arrest or delay in capsule passage through the gastrointestinal tract.

WARNINGS

Hyperkalemia (see **OVERDOSAGE**)

In patients with impaired mechanisms for excreting potassium, the administration of potassium salts can produce hyperkalemia and cardiac arrest. This occurs most commonly in patients given potassium by the intravenous route but may also occur in patients given potassium orally. Potentially fatal hyperkalemia can develop rapidly and be asymptomatic.

The use of potassium salts in patients with chronic renal disease, or any other condition which impairs potassium excretion, requires particularly careful monitoring of the serum potassium concentration and appropriate dosage adjustments.

Interaction with Potassium-Sparing Diuretics

Hypokalemia should not be treated by the concomitant administration of potassium salts and a potassium-sparing diuretic (e.g., spironolactone, triamterene, or amiloride), since the simultaneous administration of these agents can produce severe hyperkalemia.

Interaction with Angiotensin Converting Enzyme Inhibitors

Angiotensin converting enzyme (ACE) inhibitors (e.g., captopril, enalapril) will produce some potassium retention by inhibiting aldosterone production. Potassium supplements should be given to patients receiving ACE inhibitors only with close monitoring.

Gastrointestinal Lesions

Solid oral dosage forms of potassium chloride can produce ulcerative and/or stenotic lesions of the gastrointestinal tract. Based on spontaneous adverse reaction reports, enteric coated preparations of potassium chloride are associated with an increased frequency of small bowel lesions (45–50 per 100,000 patient years) compared to sustained-release wax matrix formulations (less than one per 100,000 patient years). Because of the lack of extensive marketing experience with microencapsulated products, a comparison between such products and wax matrix or enteric coated products is not available. Micro-K Extencaps and Micro-K 10 Extencaps are microencapsulated capsules formulated to provide a controlled rate of release of microencapsulated potassium chloride and thus to minimize the possibility of a high local concentration of potassium near the gastrointestinal wall.

Prospective trials have been conducted in normal human volunteers in which the upper gastrointestinal tract was evaluated by endoscopic inspection before and after one week of solid oral potassium chloride therapy. The ability of this model to predict events occurring in usual clinical practice is unknown. Trials which approximated usual clinical practice did not reveal any clear differences between the wax matrix and microencapsulated dosage forms. In contrast, there was a higher incidence of gastric and duodenal lesions in subjects receiving a high dose of a wax matrix controlled-release formulation under conditions which did not resemble usual or recommended clinical practice (i.e., 96 mEq per day in divided doses of potassium chloride administered to fasted patients, in the presence of an anticholinergic drug to delay gastric emptying). The upper gastrointestinal lesions observed by endoscopy were asymptomatic and were not accompanied by evidence of bleeding (hemoccult testing). The relevance of these findings to the usual conditions (i.e., non-fasting, no anticholinergic agent, smaller doses) under which controlled-release potassium chloride products are used is uncertain; epidemiologic studies have not identified an elevated risk, compared to microencapsulated products, for upper gastrointestinal lesions in patients receiving wax matrix formulations. Micro-K® Extencaps® and Micro-K 10® Extencaps® should be discontinued immediately and the possibility of ulceration, obstruction or perforation considered if severe vomiting, abdominal pain, distention, or gastrointestinal bleeding occur.

Metabolic Acidosis

Hypokalemia in patients with metabolic acidosis should be treated with an alkalinizing potassium salt such as potassium bicarbonate, potassium citrate, potassium acetate, or potassium gluconate.

PRECAUTIONS

General

The diagnosis of potassium depletion is ordinarily made by demonstrating hypokalemia in a patient with a clinical history suggesting some cause for potassium depletion. In interpreting the serum potassium level, the physician should bear in mind that acute alkalosis per se can produce hypokalemia in the absence of a deficit in total body potassium, while acute acidosis per se can increase the serum potassium concentration into the normal range even in the presence of a reduced total body potassium. The treatment of potassium depletion, particularly in the presence of cardiac disease, renal disease, or acidosis, requires careful attention to acid-base balance and appropriate monitoring of serum electrolytes, the electrocardiogram, and the clinical status of the patient.

Information for Patients

Physicians should consider reminding the patient of the following:

To take each dose with meals and with a full glass of water or other suitable liquid.

To take each dose without crushing, chewing, or sucking the capsule.

To take this medicine following the frequency and amount prescribed by the physician. This is especially important if the patient is also taking diuretics and/or digitalis preparations.

To check with the physician if there is trouble swallowing capsules or if the capsules seem to stick in the throat.

To check with the physician at once if tarry stools or other evidence of gastrointestinal bleeding is noticed.

Laboratory Tests

Regular serum potassium determinations are recommended, especially in patients with renal insufficiency or diabetic nephropathy.

When blood is drawn for analysis of plasma potassium it is important to recognize that artifactual elevations can occur after improper venipuncture technique or as a result of in vitro hemolysis of the sample.

Drug Interactions

Potassium-sparing diuretic, angiotensin converting enzyme inhibitors (see **WARNINGS**).

Carcinogenesis, Mutagenesis, Impairment of Fertility

Carcinogenicity, mutagenicity and fertility studies in animals have not been performed. Potassium is a normal dietary constituent.

Pregnancy Category C

Animal reproduction studies have not been conducted with Micro-K. It is unlikely that potassium supplementation that does not lead to hyperkalemia would have an adverse effect on the fetus or would affect reproductive capacity.

Nursing Mothers

The normal potassium ion content of human milk is about 13 mEq per liter. Since oral potassium becomes part of the

Continued on next page

Micro-K—Cont.

body potassium pool, so long as body potassium is not excessive, the contribution of potassium chloride supplementation should have little or no effect on the level in human milk.

Pediatric Use

Safety and effectiveness in pediatric patients have not been established.

ADVERSE REACTIONS

One of the most severe adverse effects is hyperkalemia (see **CONTRAINDICATIONS**, **WARNINGS**, and **OVERDOSAGE**).

Gastrointestinal bleeding and ulceration have been reported in patients treated with Micro-K Extencaps (see **CONTRAINDICATIONS** and **WARNINGS**). In addition to gastrointestinal bleeding and ulceration, perforation and obstruction have been reported in patients treated with other solid KCl dosage forms, and may occur with Micro-K Extencaps.

The most common adverse reactions to the oral potassium salts are nausea, vomiting, flatulence, abdominal discomfort, and diarrhea. These symptoms are due to irritation of the gastrointestinal tract and are best managed by taking the dose with meals or reducing the amount taken at one time.

Skin rash has been reported rarely with potassium preparations.

OVERDOSAGE

The administration of oral potassium salts to persons with normal excretory mechanisms for potassium rarely causes serious hyperkalemia. However, if excretory mechanisms are impaired or if potassium is administered too rapidly intravenously, potentially fatal hyperkalemia can result (see **CONTRAINDICATIONS** and **WARNINGS**). It is important to recognize that hyperkalemia is usually asymptomatic and may be manifested only by an increased serum potassium concentration (6.5–8.0 mEq/L) and characteristic electrocardiogram changes (peaking of T-waves, loss of P-wave, depression of ST segment, and prolongation of the QT interval). Late manifestations include muscle paralysis and cardiovascular collapse from cardiac arrest (9–12 mEq/L).

Treatment measures for hyperkalemia include the following: (1) elimination of foods and medications containing potassium and of any agents with potassium-sparing properties; (2) intravenous administration of 300 to 500 ml/hr of 10% dextrose solution containing 10 to 20 units of crystalline insulin per 1,000 ml; (3) correction of acidosis, if present, with intravenous sodium bicarbonate; (4) use of exchange resins, hemodialysis, or peritoneal dialysis.

In treating hyperkalemia, it should be recalled that in patients who have been stabilized on digitalis, too rapid a lowering of the serum potassium concentration can produce digitalis toxicity.

DOSAGE AND ADMINISTRATION

The usual dietary intake of potassium by the average adult is 50 to 100 mEq per day. Potassium depletion sufficient to cause hypokalemia usually requires the loss of 200 or more mEq of potassium from the total body store.

Dosage must be adjusted to the individual needs of each patient. The dose for the prevention of hypokalemia is typically in the range of 20 mEq per day. Doses of 40 to 100 mEq per day or more are used for the treatment of potassium depletion. Dosage should be divided if more than 20 mEq per day is given such that no more than 20 mEq is given in a single dose.

Because of the potential for gastric irritation (see **WARNINGS**), Micro-K Extencaps should be taken with meals and with a full glass of water or other liquid.

Patients who have difficulty swallowing capsules may sprinkle the contents of the capsule onto a spoonful of soft food. The soft food, such as applesauce or pudding, should be swallowed immediately without chewing and followed with a glass of cool water or juice to ensure complete swallowing of the microcapsules. The food used should not be hot and should be soft enough to be swallowed without chewing. Any microcapsule/food mixture should be used immediately and not stored for future use.

HOW SUPPLIED

Micro-K Extencaps® are pale orange capsules monogrammed Micro-K and AHR/5720, each containing 600 mg microencapsulated potassium chloride (equivalent to 8 mEq K) in bottles of 100 (NDC 0031-5720-63), 500 (NDC 0031-5720-70) and Dis-Co® unit dose packs of 100 (NDC 0031-5720-64).

Micro-K 10 Extencaps® are pale orange and opaque white capsules monogrammed Micro-K 10 and AHR/5730, each containing 750 mg microencapsulated potassium chloride (equivalent to 10 mEq K), in bottles of 100 (NDC 0031-5730-63), 100 Unit-of-Use (NDC 0031-5730-68), 500 (NDC 0031-5730-70) and Dis-Co® unit dose packs of 100 (NDC 0031-5730-64).

Store at controlled room temperature, 20°–25°C (68°–77°F).
Dispense in tight container.

Caution: Federal law prohibits dispensing without a prescription.

Manufactured by:
Pharmaceutical Division
A.H. Robins Company
Richmond, VA 23220

Shown in Product Identification Guide, page 334

PHENAPHEN® WITH CODEINE Ⓒ℞

[*fen 'ah-fen "*]

(Acetaminophen and Codeine Phosphate Capsules)

DESCRIPTION

Each Phenaphen® with Codeine No. 3 capsule contains:

Acetaminophen, USP	325 mg
Codeine Phosphate, USP	30 mg
(Warning: May be habit forming)	

Inactive Ingredients: D&C Yellow 10, Edible Ink, FD&C Blue 1, (FD&C Green 3 and Red 40), FD&C Yellow 6, Gelatin, Magnesium Stearate, Sodium Starch Glycolate, Stearic Acid.

Each Phenaphen® with Codeine No. 4 capsule contains:

Acetaminophen, USP	325 mg
Codeine Phosphate, USP	60 mg
(Warning: May be habit forming)	

Inactive Ingredients: Corn Starch, D&C Yellow 10, Edible Ink, FD&C Green 3 or Blue 1, FD&C Yellow 6, Gelatin, Lactose, Magnesium Stearate, Sodium Starch Glycolate, Stearic Acid.

Acetaminophen, 4′-hydroxyacetanilide, is a non-opiate, non-salicylate analgesic and antipyretic which occurs as a white, odorless, crystalline powder, possessing a slightly bitter taste.

Codeine is an alkaloid, obtained from opium or prepared from morphine by methylation. Codeine phosphate occurs as fine, white, needle-shaped crystals, or white, crystalline powder. It is affected by light. Its chemical name is: 7,8-didehydro-4, 5α-epoxy-3-methoxy-17-methylmorphinan-6α-ol phosphate (1:1) (salt) hemihydrate.

HOW SUPPLIED

Phenaphen with Codeine No. 3, black and green capsules in bottles of 100 (NDC 0031-6257-63) and 500 (NDC 0031-6257-70).

Phenaphen with Codeine No. 4, green and white capsules in bottles of 100 (NDC 0031-6274-63).

Store at controlled room temperature, between 20°– 25°C (68°–77°F).

Dispense capsules in tight, light-resistant container.

Manufactured by:
Pharmaceutical Division
A.H. Robins Company
Richmond, VA 23220

For prescribing information write to Professional Service, Wyeth-Ayerst Laboratories, P.O. Box 8299, Philadelphia, PA 19101, or contact your local Wyeth-Ayerst representative.

QUINIDEX EXTENTABS® Tablets ℞

[*kwĭn 'ĭ "deks ĕks "tĕn 'tabs*]

(quinidine sulfate extended-release tablets, USP)

DESCRIPTION

Quinidine is an antimalarial schizonticide and an antiarrhythmic agent with Class la activity; it is the d-isomer of quinine, and its molecular weight is 324.43. Quinidine sulfate is the sulfate salt of quinidine; its chemical name is cinchonan-9-ol, 6′-methoxy-, (9S)-, sulfate(2:1) dihydrate; its structural formula is

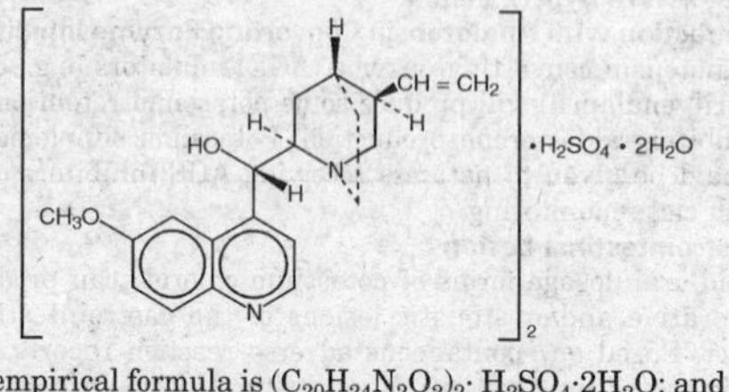

its empirical formula is $(C_{20}H_{24}N_2O_2)_2 \cdot H_2SO_4 \cdot 2H_2O$; and its molecular weight is 782.95, of which 82.9% is quinidine base.

Each Quinidex Extentabs® tablet contains 300 mg of quinidine sulfate (249 mg of quinidine base) in a formulation to provide extended release; the inactive ingredients are acacia, acetylated monoglycerides, calcium sulfate, carnauba wax, edible ink, FD&C Blue 2, gelatin, guar gum, magnesium oxide, magnesium stearate, polysorbates, shellac, sucrose, titanium dioxide, white wax, and other ingredients, one of which is a corn derivative. Tablets may also contain FD&C Red 40 and FD&C Yellow 6 Aluminum Lakes.

CLINICAL PHARMACOLOGY

PHARMACOKINETICS

The absolute bioavailability of quinidine from Quinidex is about 70%, but this varies widely (45–100%) between patients. The less-than-complete bioavailability is the result of first-pass metabolism in the liver. Peak serum levels generally appear about 6 hours after dosing.

Although the effect of food upon Quinidex absorption has not been studied, peak serum quinidine levels obtained from immediate-release quinidine sulfate are known to be delayed by nearly an hour (without change in total absorption) when these products are taken with food.

The **volume of distribution** of quinidine is 2 to 3 L/kg in healthy young adults, but this may be reduced to as little as 0.5 L/kg in patients with congestive heart failure, or increased to 3 to 5 L/kg in patients with cirrhosis of the liver. At concentrations of 2 to 5 mg/L (6.5 to 16.2 μmol/L), the fraction of quinidine bound to plasma proteins (mainly to α_1-acid glycoprotein and to albumin) is 80 to 88% in adults and older children, but it is lower in pregnant women, and in infants and neonates it may be as low as 50 to 70%. Because α_1-acid glycoprotein levels are increased in response to stress, serum levels of total quinidine may be greatly increased in settings such as acute myocardial infarction, even though the serum content of unbound (active) drug may remain normal. Protein binding is also increased in chronic renal failure, but binding abruptly descends toward or below normal when heparin is administered for hemodialysis.

Quinidine **clearance** typically proceeds at 3 to 5 mL/min/kg in adults, but clearance in children may be twice or three times as rapid. The elimination half-life is 6 to 8 hours in adults and 3 to 4 hours in children. Quinidine clearance is unaffected by hepatic cirrhosis, so the increased volume of distribution seen in cirrhosis leads to a proportionate increase in the elimination half-life.

Most quinidine is eliminated hepatically via the action of cytochrome $P_{450}IIIA_4$; there are several different hydroxylated metabolites, and some of these have antiarrhythmic activity.

The most important of quinidine's metabolites is 3-hydroxyquinidine (3HQ), serum levels of which can approach those of quinidine in patients receiving conventional doses of Quinidex. The volume of distribution of 3HQ appears to be larger than that of quinidine, and the elimination half-life of 3HQ is about 12 hours.

As measured by antiarrhythmic effects in animals, by QT_c prolongation in human volunteers, or by various *in vitro* techniques, 3HQ has at least half the antiarrhythmic activity of the parent compound, so it may be responsible for a substantial fraction of the effect of Quinidex in chronic use.

When the urine pH is less than 7, about 20% of administered quinidine appears unchanged in the urine, but this fraction drops to as little as 5% when the urine is more alkaline. Renal clearance involves both glomerular filtration and active tubular secretion, moderated by (pH-dependent) tubular reabsorption. The new renal clearance is about 1 mL/min/kg in healthy adults.

When renal function is taken into account, quinidine clearance is apparently independent of patient age.

Assays of serum quinidine levels are widely available, but the results of modern assays may not be consistent with results cited in the older medical literature. The serum levels of quinidine cited in this package insert are those derived from specific assays, using either benzene extraction or (preferably) reverse-phase high-pressure liquid chromatography. In matched samples, older assays might unpredictably have given results that were as much as two or three times higher. A typical "therapeutic" concentration range is 2 to 6 mg/L (6.2 to 18.5 μmol/L).

MECHANISMS OF ACTION

In patients with malaria, quinidine acts primarily as an intra-erythrocytic schizonticide, with little effect upon sporozites or upon pre-erythrocytic parasites. Quinidine is gametocidal to *Plasmodium vivax* and *P. malariae,* but not to *P. falciparum.*

In cardiac muscle and in Purkinje fibers, quinidine depresses the rapid inward depolarizing sodium current, thereby slowing phase-0 depolarization and reducing the amplitude of the action potential without affecting the resting potential. In normal Purkinje fibers, it reduces the slope of phase-4 depolarization, shifting the threshold voltage upward toward zero. The result is slow conduction and reduced automaticity in all parts of the heart, with increase of the effective refractory period relative to the duration of the action potential in the atria, ventricles, and Purkinje tissues. Quinidine also raises the fibrillation thresholds of the atria and ventricles, and it raises the ventricular *de* fibrillation threshold as well. Quinidine's actions fall into Class la in the Vaughan-Williams classification.

By slowing conduction and prolonging the effective refractory period, quinidine can interrupt or prevent reentrant arrhythmias and arrhythmias due to increased automaticity, including atrial flutter, atrial fibrillation, and paroxysmal supraventricular tachycardia.

In patients with the sick sinus syndrome, quinidine can cause marked sinus node depression and bradycardia. In most patients, however, use of quinidine is associated with an increase in the sinus rate.

Quinidine prolongs the QT interval in a dose-related fashion. This may lead to increased ventricular automaticity and polymorphic ventricular tachycardias, including *torsades de pointes* (see **WARNINGS**).

In addition, quinidine has anticholinergic activity, it has negative inotropic activity, and it acts peripherally as an α-adrenergic antagonist (that is, as a vasodilator).

CLINICAL EFFECTS

Maintenance of sinus rhythm after conversion from atrial fibrillation: In six clinical trials (published between 1970 and 1984) with a total of 808 patients, quinidine (418 patients) was compared to nontreatment (258 patients) or placebo (132 patients) for the maintenance of sinus rhythm after cardioversion from chronic atrial fibrillation. Quinidine was consistently more efficacious in maintaining sinus rhythm, but a meta-analysis found that mortality in the quinidine-exposed patients (2.9%) was significantly greater than mortality in the patients who had not been treated with active drug (0.8%). Suppression of atrial fibrillation with quinidine has theoretical patient benefits (e.g., improved exercise tolerance; reduction in hospitalization for cadioversion; lack of arrhythmia-related palpitations, dyspnea, and chest pain; reduced incidence of systemic embolism and/or stroke), but these benefits have never been demonstrated in clinical trials. Some of these benefits (e.g., reduction in stroke incidence) may be achievable by other means (anticoagulation).

By slowing the rate of atrial flutter/fibrillation, quinidine can decrease the degree of atrioventricular block and cause an increase, sometimes marked, in the rate at which supraventricular impulses are successfully conducted by the atrioventricular node, with a resultant paradoxical increase in ventricular rate (see **WARNINGS**).

Non-life-threatening ventricular arrhythmias: In studies of patients with a variety of ventricular arrhythmias (mainly frequent ventricular premature beats and non-sustained ventricular tachycardia), quinidine (total N=502) has been compared to flecainide (N=141), mexiletine (N=246), propafenone (N=53), and tocainide (N=67). In each of these studies, the mortality in the quinidine group was numerically greater than the mortality in the comparator group. When the studies were combined in a meta-analysis, quinidine was associated with a statistically significant threefold relative risk of death.

At therapeutic doses, quinidine's only consistent effect upon the surface electrocardiogram is an increase in the QT interval. This prolongation can be monitored as a guide to safety, and it may provide better guidance than serum drug levels (see **WARNINGS**).

INDICATIONS AND USAGE

CONVERSION OF ATRIAL FIBRILLATION/FLUTTER

In patients with symptomatic atrial fibrillation/flutter whose symptoms are not adequately controlled by measures that reduce the rate of ventricular response, Quinidex is indicated as a means of restoring normal sinus rhythm. If this use of Quinidex does not restore sinus rhythm within a reasonable time (see **DOSAGE AND ADMINISTRATION**), then Quinidex should be discontinued.

REDUCTION OF FREQUENCY OF RELAPSE INTO ATRIAL FIBRILLATION/FLUTTER

Chronic therapy with Quinidex is indicated for some patients at high risk of symptomatic atrial fibrillation/flutter; generally patients who have had previous episodes of atrial fibrillation/flutter that were so frequent and poorly tolerated as to outweigh, in the judgment of the physician and the patient, the risks of prophylactic therapy with Quinidex. The increased risk of death should specifically be considered. Quinidex should be used only after alternative measures (e.g., use of other drugs to control ventricular rate) have been found to be inadequate.

In patients with histories of frequent symptomatic episodes of atrial fibrillation/flutter, the goal of therapy should be an increase in the average time between episodes. In most patients, the tachyarrhythmia *will recur* during therapy, and a single recurrence should not be interpreted as therapeutic failure.

SUPPRESSION OF VENTRICULAR ARRHYTHMIAS

Quinidex is also indicated for the suppression of recurrent documented ventricular arrhythmias, such as sustained ventricular tachycardia, that in the judgment of the physician are life-threatening. Because of the proarrhythmic effects of quinidine, its use with ventricular arrhythmias of lesser severity is generally not recommended, and treatment of patients with asymptomatic ventricular premature contractions should be avoided. Where possible, therapy should be guided by the results of programmed electrical stimulation and/or Holter monitoring with exercise.

Antiarrhythmic drugs (including Quinidex) have not been shown to enhance survival in patients with ventricular arrhythmias.

CONTRAINDICATIONS

Quinidine is contraindicated in patients who are known to be allergic to it, or who have developed thrombocytopenic purpura during prior therapy with quinidine or quinine.

In the absence of a functioning artificial pacemaker, quinidine is also contraindicated in any patient whose cardiac rhythm is dependent upon a junctional or idioventricular pacemaker, including patients in complete atrioventricular block.

Quinidine is also contraindicated in patients who, like those will myasthenia gravis, might be adversely affected by an anticholinergic agent.

WARNINGS

MORTALITY

In many trials of antiarrhythmic therapy for non-life-threatening arrhythmias, active antiarrhythmic therapy has resulted in increased mortality; the risk of active therapy is probably greatest in patients with structural heart disease.

In the case of quinidine used to prevent or defer recurrence of atrial flutter/fibrillation, the best available data come from a meta-analysis described under Clinical Pharmacology—CLINICAL EFFECTS above. In the patients studied in the trials there analyzed, the mortality associated with the use of quinidine was more than three times as great as the mortality associated with the use of placebo.

Another meta-analysis, also described under Clinical Pharmacology—CLINICAL EFFECTS, showed that in patients with various non-life-threatening ventricular arrhythmias, the mortality associated with the use of quinidine was consistently greater than that associated with the use of any of a variety of alternative antiarrhythmics.

PROARRHYTHMIC EFFECTS

Like many other drugs (including all other Class la antiarrhythmics), quinidine prolongs the QT_c interval, and this can lead to *torsades de pointes*, a life-threatening ventricular arrhythmia (see **OVERDOSAGE**). The risk of *torsades* is increased by bradycardia, hypokalemia, hypomagnesemia, or high serum levels of quinidine, but it may appear in the absence of any of these risk factors. The best predictor of this arrhythmia appears to be the length of the QT_c interval, and quinidine should be used with extreme care in patients who have preexisting long-QT syndromes, who have histories of *torsades de pointes* of any cause, or who have previously responded to quinidine (or other drugs that prolong ventricular repolarization) with marked lengthening of the QT_c interval. Estimation of the incidence of *torsades* in patients with therapeutic levels of quinidine is not possible from the available data.

Other ventricular arrhythmias that have been reported with quinidine include frequent extrasystoles, ventricular tachycardia, ventricular flutter, and ventricular fibrillation.

PARADOXICAL INCREASE IN VENTRICULAR RATE IN ATRIAL FLUTTER/FIBRILLATION

When quinidine is administered to patients with atrial flutter/fibrillation the desired pharmacologic reversion to sinus rhythm may (rarely) be preceded by a showing of the atrial rate with a consequent increase in the rate of beats conducted to the ventricles. The resulting ventricular rate may be very high (greater than 200 beats per minute) and poorly tolerated. This hazard may be decreased if partial atrioventricular block is achieved prior to initiation of quinidine therapy, using conduction-reducing drugs such as digitalis, verapamil, diltiazem, or a β-receptor blocking agent.

EXACERBATED BRADYCARDIA IN SICK SINUS SYNDROME

In patients with the sick sinus syndrome, quinidine has been associated with marked sinus node depression and bradycardia.

PHARMACOKINETIC CONSIDERATIONS

Renal or hepatic dysfunction causes the elimination of quinidine to be slowed, while congestive heart failure causes a reduction in quinidine's apparent volume of distribution. Any of these conditions can lead to quinidine toxicity if dosage is not appropriately reduced. In addition, interactions with coadministered drugs can alter the serum concentration and activity of quinidine, leading either to toxicity or to lack of efficacy if the dose of quinidine is not appropriately modified. (See **PRECAUTIONS**—DRUG INTERACTIONS.)

VAGOLYSIS

Because quinidine opposes the atrial and A-V nodal effects of vagal stimulation, physical or pharmacological vagal maneuvers undertaken to terminate paroxysmal supraventricular tachycardia may be ineffective in patients receiving quinidine.

PRECAUTIONS

GENERAL

All the precautions applying to regular quinidine therapy apply to this product. Hypersensitivity or anaphylactoid reactions to quinidine, although rare, should be considered, especially during the first weeks of therapy. Hospitalization for close clinical observation, electrocardiographic monitoring, and determination of serum quinidine levels are indicated when large doses of quinidine are used or with patients who present an increased risk.

LABORATORY TESTS

Periodic blood counts and liver and kidney function tests should be performed during long-term therapy; the drug should be discontinued if blood dyscrasias or evidence of hepatic or renal dysfunction occurs.

HEART BLOCK

In patients without implanted pacemakers who are at high risk of complete atrioventricular block (e.g., those with digitalis intoxication, second-degree atrioventricular block, or severe intraventricular conduction defects), quinidine should be used only with caution.

DRUG INTERACTIONS

Altered pharmacokinetics of quinidine: Drugs that alkalinize the urine (**carbonic-anhydrase inhibitors, sodium bicarbonate, thiazide diuretics**) reduce renal elimination of quinidine.

By pharmacokinetic mechanisms that are not well understood, quinidine levels are increased by coadministration of **amiodarone** or **cimetidine**. Very rarely, and again by mechanisms not understood, quinidine levels are decreased by coadministration of **nifedipine**.

Hepatic elimination of quinidine may be accelerated by coadministration of drugs (**phenobarbital, phenytoin, rifampin**) that induce production of cytochrome $P_{450}IIIA_4$.

Perhaps because of competition for the $P_{450}IIIA_4$ metabolic pathway, quinidine levels rise when **ketaconazole** is coadministered.

Coadministration of **propranolol** usually does not affect quinidine pharmacokinetics, but in some studies the β-blocker appeared to cause increases in the peak serum levels of quinidine, decreases in quinidine's volume of distribution, and decreases in total quinidine clearance. The effects (if any) of coadministration of **other β-blockers** on quinidine pharmacokinetics have not been adequately studied.

Hepatic clearance of quinidine is significantly reduced during coadministration of **verapamil**, with corresponding increases in serum levels and half-life.

Altered pharmacokinetics of other drugs: Quinidine slows the elimination of **digoxin** and simultaneously reduces digoxin's apparent volume of distribution. As a result, serum digoxin levels may be as much as doubled. When quinidine and digoxin are coadministered, digoxin doses usually need to be reduced. Serum levels of **digitoxin** are also raised when quinidine is coadministered, although the effect appears to be smaller.

By a mechanism that is not understood, quinidine potentiates the anticoagulatory action of **warfarin**, and the anticoagulant dosage may need to be reduced.

Cytochrome $P_{450}IID_6$ is an enzyme critical to the metabolism of many drugs, notably including **mexiletine**, some **phenothiazines**, and most **polycyclic antidepressants**. Constitutional deficiency of cytochrome $P_{450}IID_6$ is found in less than 1% of Orientals, in about 2% of American blacks, and in about 8% of American whites. Testing with debrisoquine is sometimes used to distinguish the $P_{450}IID_6$-deficient "poor metabolizers" from the majority-phenotype "extensive metabolizers."

When drugs whose metabolism is $P_{450}IID_6$-dependent are given to poor metabolizers, the serum levels achieved are higher, sometimes much higher, than the serum levels achieved when identical doses are given to extensive metabolizers. To obtain similar clinical benefit without toxicity, doses given to poor metabolizers may need to be greatly reduced. In the cases of prodrugs whose actions are actually mediated by $P_{450}IID_6$-produced metabolites (for example, **codeine** and **hydrocodone**, whose analgesic and antitussive effects appear to be mediated by morphine and hydromorphone, respectively), it may not be possible to achieve the desired clinical benefits in poor metabolizers.

Quinidine is not metabolized by cytochrome $P_{450}IID_6$, but therapeutic serum levels of quinidine inhibit the action of cytochrome $P_{450}IID_6$, effectively converting extensive metabolizers into poor metabolizers. Caution must be exercised whenever quinidine is prescribed together with drugs metabolized by cytochrome $P_{450}IID_6$.

Perhaps by competing for pathways of renal clearance, coadministration of quinidine causes an increase in serum levels of **procainamide.**

Serum levels of **haloperidol** are increased when quinidine is coadministered.

Presumably because both drugs are metabolized by cytochrome $P_{450}IIIA_4$, coadministration of quinidine causes variable slowing of the metabolism of **nifedipine**. Interac-

Continued on next page

Quinidex—Cont.

tions with other dihydropyridine calcium-channel blockers have not been reported, but these agents (including **felodipine, nicardipine,** and **nimodipine**) are all dependent upon $P_{450}IIIA_4$ for metabolism, so similar interactions with quinidine should be anticipated.

Altered pharmacodynamics of other drugs: Quinidine's anticholinergic, vasodilating, and negative inotropic actions may be additive to those of other drugs with these effects, and antagonistic to those of drugs with cholinergic, vasoconstricting, and positive inotropic effects. For example, when quinidine and **verapamil** are coadministered in doses that are each well tolerated as monotherapy, hypotension attributable to additive peripheral α-blockade is sometimes reported.

Quinidine potentiates the actions of depolarizing (succinylcholine, decamethonium) and nondepolarizing (d-tubocurarine, pancuronium) **neuromuscular blocking agents**. These phenomena are not well understood, but they are observed in animals models as well as in humans. In addition, *in vitro* addition of quinidine to the serum of pregnant women reduces the activity of pseudocholinesterase, an enzyme that is essential to the metabolism of succinylcholine.

Non-interactions of quinidine with other drugs: Quinidine has no clinically significant effect on the pharmacokinetics of **diltiazem, flecainide, mephenytoin, metoprolol, propafenone, propranolol, quinine, timolol,** or **tocainide**.

Conversely, the pharmacokinetics of quinidine are not significantly affected by **caffeine, ciprofloxacin, digoxin, diltiazem, felodipine, omeprazole,** or **quinine**. Quinidine's pharmacokinetics are also unaffected by cigarette smoking.

INFORMATION FOR PATIENTS

Before prescribing Quinidex Extentabs® as prophylaxis against recurrence of atrial fibrillation, the physician should inform the patient of the risks and benefits to be expected (see **CLINICAL PHARMACOLOGY**).

Discussion should include the facts

- that the goal of therapy will be a reduction (probably not to zero) in the frequency of episodes of atrial fibrillation; and
- that reduced frequency of fibrillatory episodes may be expected, if achieved, to bring symptomatic benefit; but
- that no data are available to show that reduced frequency of fibrillatory episodes will reduce the risks of irreversible harm through stroke or death; and in fact
- that such data as are available suggest that treatment with Quinidex is likely to increase the patient's risk of death.

CARCINOGENESIS, MUTAGENESIS, IMPAIRMENT OF FERTILITY

Animal studies to evaluate quinidine's carcinogenic or mutagenic potential have not been performed. Similarly, there are no animal data as to quinidine's potential to impair fertility.

PREGNANCY

Pregnancy Category C: Animal reproductive studies have not been conducted with quinidine. There are no adequate and well-controlled studies in pregnant women. Quinidine should be given to a pregnant woman only if clearly needed. In one neonate whose mother had received quinidine throughout her pregnancy, the serum level of quinidine was equal to that of the mother, with no apparent ill effect. The level of quinidine in amniotic fluid was about three times higher than that found in serum.

LABOR AND DELIVERY

Quinine is said to be oxytocic in humans, but there are no adequate data as to quinidine's effects (if any) on human labor and delivery.

NURSING MOTHERS

Quinidine is present in human milk at levels slightly lower than those in maternal serum; a human infant ingesting such milk should (scaling directly by weight) be expected to develop serum quinidine levels at least an order of magnitude lower than those of the mother. On the other hand, the pharmacokinetics and pharmacodynamics of quinidine in human infants have not been adequately studied, and neonates' reduced protein binding of quinidine may increase their risk of toxicity at low total serum levels. Administration of quinidine should (if possible) be avoided in lactating women who continue to nurse.

GERIATRIC USE

Safety and efficacy of quinidine in elderly patients have not been systematically studied.

PEDIATRIC USE

In antimalarial trials, quinidine was as safe and effective in pediatric patients as in adults. Notwithstanding the known pharmacokinetic differences between the pediatric population and adults (see **CLINICAL PHARMACOLOGY—PHARMACOKINETICS**), pediatric patients in these trials received the same doses (on a mg/kg basis) as adults.

Safety and effectiveness of the antiarrhythmic use of quinidine in pediatric patients have not been established in well-controlled clinical trials.

ADVERSE REACTIONS

Quinidine preparations have been used for many years, but there are only sparse data from which to estimate the incidence of various adverse reactions. The adverse reactions most frequently reported have consistently been gastrointestinal, including diarrhea, nausea, vomiting, and heartburn/esophagitis. In one study of 245 adult outpatients who received quinidine to suppress premature ventricular contractions, the incidences of reported adverse experiences were as shown in the table below. The most serious quinidine-associated adverse reactions are described above under **WARNINGS**.

Adverse Experiences in a 245-Patient PVC Trial

	Incidence (%)
diarrhea	85 (35)
"upper gastrointestinal distress"	55 (22)
light-headedness	37 (15)
headache	18 (7)
fatigue	17 (7)
palpitations	16 (7)
angina-like pain	14 (6)
weakness	13 (5)
rash	11 (5)
visual problems	8 (3)
change in sleep habits	7 (3)
tremor	6 (2)
nervousness	5 (2)
discoordination	3 (1)

Vomiting and diarrhea can occur as isolated reactions to therapeutic levels of quinidine, but they also may be the first signs of **cinchonism**, a syndrome that also may include tinnitus, reversible high-frequency hearing loss, deafness, vertigo, blurred vision, diplopia, photophobia, headache, confusion, and delirium. Cinchonism is most often a sign of chronic quinidine toxicity, but it may appear in sensitive patients after a single moderate dose.

A few cases of **hepatotoxicity**, including granulomatous hepatitis, have been reported in patients receiving quinidine. All of these have appeared during the first few weeks of therapy, and most (not all) have remitted once quinidine was withdrawn.

Autoimmune and inflammatory syndromes associated with quinidine therapy have included pneumonitis, fever, urticaria, flushing, exfoliative rash, bronchospasm, psoriasiform rash, pruritus and lymphadenopathy, hemolytic anemia, vasculitis, thrombocytopenic purpura, uveitis, angioedema, agranulocytosis, the sicca syndrome, arthralgia, myalgia, elevation in serum levels of skeletal-muscle enzymes, and a disorder resembling systemic lupus erythematosus.

Convulsions, apprehension, and ataxia have been reported, but it is not clear that these were not simply the results of hypotension and consequent cerebral hypoperfusion. There are many reports of syncope. Acute psychotic reactions have been reported to follow the first dose of quinidine, but these reactions appear to be extremely rare.

Other adverse reactions occasionally reported include depression, mydriasis, disturbed color perception, night blindness, scotomata, optic neuritis, visual field loss, photosensitivity, and abnormalities of pigmentation.

OVERDOSAGE

Overdoses with various oral formulations of quinidine have been well described. Death has been described after a 5-gram ingestion by a toddler, while an adolescent was reported to survive after ingesting 8 grams of quinidine.

The most important ill effects of acute quinidine overdoses are ventricular arrhythmias and hypotension. Other signs and symptoms of overdose may include vomiting, diarrhea, tinnitus, high-frequency hearing loss, vertigo, blurred vision, diplopia, photophobia, headache, confusion, and delirium.

ARRHYTHMIAS

Serum quinidine levels can be conveniently assayed and monitored, but the electrocardiographic QT_c interval is a better predictor of quinidine-induced ventricular arrhythmias.

The necessary treatment of hemodynamically unstable polymorphic ventricular tachycardia (including *torsades de pointes*) is withdrawal of treatment with quinidine and either immediate cardioversion or, if a cardiac pacemaker is in place or immediately available, immediate overdrive pacing. After pacing or cardioversion, further management must be guided by the length of the QT_c interval.

Quinidine-associated ventricular tachyarrhythmias with normal underlying QT_c intervals have not been adequately studied. Because of the theoretical possibility of QT-prolonging effects that might be additive to those of quinidine, other antiarrhythmics with Class I (disopyramide, procainamide) or Class III activities should (if possible) be avoided. Similarly, although the use of bretylium in quinidine overdose has not been reported, it is reasonable to expect that the α-blocking properties of bretylium might be additive to those of quinidine, resulting in problematic hypotension.

If the post-cardioversion QT_c interval is prolonged, then the pre-cardioversion polymorphic ventricular tachyarrhythmia was (by definition) *torsades de pointes*. In this case, lidocaine and bretylium are unlikely to be of value, and other Class I antiarrhythmics (disopyramide, procainamide) are likely to exacerbate the situation. Factors contributing to QT_c prolongation (especially hypokalemia and hypomagnesemia) should be sought out and (if possible) aggressively corrected. Prevention of recurrent *torsades* may require sustained overdrive pacing or the cautious administration of isoproterenol (30 to 150 ng/kg/min).

HYPOTENSION

Quinidine-induced hypotension that is not due to an arrhythmia is likely to be a consequence of quinidine-related α-blockade and vasorelaxation. Simple repletion of central volume (Trendelenburg positioning, saline infusion) may be sufficient therapy; other interventions reported to have been beneficial in this setting are those that increase peripheral vascular resistance, including α-agonist catecholamines (norepinephrine, metaraminol) and the Military Anti-Shock Trousers.

TREATMENT

Adequate studies of orally-administered activated charcoal in human overdoses of quinidine have not been reported, but there are animal data showing significant enhancement of systemic elimination following this intervention, and there is at least one human case report in which the elimination half-life of quinidine in the serum was apparently shortened by repeated gastric lavage. Activated charcoal should be avoided if an ileus is present; the conventional dose is 1 gram/kg, administered every 2 to 6 hours as a slurry with 8 mL/kg of tap water. Although renal elimination of quinidine might theoretically be accelerated by maneuvers to acidify the urine, such maneuvers are potentially hazardous and of no demonstrated benefit.

Quinidine is not usefully removed from the circulation by dialysis. Following quinidine overdose, drugs that delay elimination of quinidine (cimetidine, carbonic-anhydrase inhibitors, thiazide diuretics) should be withdrawn unless absolutely required.

In managing overdose, consider the possibilities of multiple-drug overdoses, drug-drug interactions, and unusual drug kinetics in your patient.

DOSAGE AND ADMINISTRATION

CONVERSION OF ATRIAL FIBRILLATION/FLUTTER TO SINUS RHYTHM

Especially in patients with known structural heart disease or other risk factors for toxicity, initiation or dose-adjustment of treatment with Quinidex should generally be performed in a setting where facilities and personnel for monitoring and resuscitation are continuously available.

Patients with symptomatic atrial fibrillation/flutter should be treated with Quinidex only after ventricular rate control (e.g., with digitalis or β-blockers) has failed to provide satisfactory control of symptoms. Adequate trials have not identified an optimal regimen of Quinidex for conversion of atrial fibrillation/flutter to sinus rhythm. Therapy with Quinidex should begin with one tablet (300 mg; 249 mg of quinidine base) every 8 to 12 hours. If this regimen is well tolerated, if the serum quinidine level is still well within the laboratory's therapeutic range, and if this regimen has not resulted in conversion, then the dose may be cautiously raised. If, at any point during administration, the QRS complex widens to 130% of its pre-treatment duration; the QT_c interval widens to 130% of its pre-treatment duration and is then longer than 500 ms; P waves disappear; or the patient develops significant tachycardia, symptomatic bradycardia, or hypotension, then Quinidex is discontinued, and other means of conversion (e.g., direct-current cardioversion) are considered.

REDUCTION OF FREQUENCY OF RELAPSE INTO ATRIAL FIBRILLATION/FLUTTER

In a patient with a history of frequent symptomatic episodes of atrial fibrillation/flutter, the goal of therapy with Quinidex should be an increase in the average time between episodes. In most patients, the tachyarrhythmia *will recur* during therapy with Quinidex, and a single recurrence should not be interpreted as therapeutic failure.

Especially in patients with known structural heart disease or other risk factors for toxicity, initiation or dose-adjustment of treatment with Quinidex should generally be performed in a setting where facilities and personnel for monitoring and resuscitation are continously available.

Monitoring should be continued for two or three days after initiation of the regimen on which the patient will be discharged.

Therapy with Quinidex should begin with one tablet (300 mg; 249 mg of quinidine base) every eight to twelve hours. If this regimen is well tolerated, if the serum quinidine level is still well within the laboratory's therapeutic range, and if the average time between arrhythmic episodes has not been satisfactorily increased, then the dose may be cautiously raised. The total daily dosage should be reduced if the QRS complex widens to 130% of its pre-treatment duration; the QT_c interval widens to 130% of its pre-treatment duration and is then longer than 500 ms; P waves disappear; or the patient develops significant tachycardia, symptomatic bradycardia, or hypotension.

SUPPRESSION OF VENTRICULAR ARRHYTHMIAS
Dosing regimens for the use of quinidine sulfate in suppressing life-threatening ventricular arrhythmias have not been adequately studied.
Described regimens have generally been similar to the regimen described just above for the prophylaxis of symptomatic atrial fibrillation/flutter. Where possible, therapy should be guided by the results of programmed electrical stimulation and/or Holter monitoring with exercise.

HOW SUPPLIED

Quinidex Extentabs® Tablets (quinidine sulfate extended-release tablets, USP) are 300 mg, white, sugar-coated, round tablets marked with "QUINIDEX" and "AHR". The tablets are available in bottles and in DIS-CO® unit-dose packages as follows:

bottle of 100	NDC 0031-6649-63
bottle of 250	NDC 0031-6649-67
unit-dose pack of 100	NDC 0031-6649-64

Store tablets at controlled room temperature, 20°–25°C (68°–77°F).
Dispense in well-closed, light-resistant container.
Caution: Federal law prohibits dispensing without prescription.
Manufactured by:
Pharmaceutical Division
A.H. Robins Company
Richmond, VA 23220
Shown in Product Identification Guide, page 334

REGLAN® Tablets ℞
[rĕg 'lan]
(Metoclopramide Tablets, USP)

REGLAN® Syrup
(Metoclopramide Oral Solution, USP)

REGLAN® Injectable
(Metoclopramide Injection, USP)

DESCRIPTION

For oral administration, Reglan Tablets (Metoclopramide Tablets, USP) 10 mg are white. scored, capsule-shaped tablets engraved Reglan on one side and AHR 10 on the opposite side.
Each tablet contains:
Metoclopramide base 10 mg
(as the monohydrochloride monohydrate)
INACTIVE INGREDIENTS: Magnesium Stearate, Mannitol, Microcrystalline Cellulose, Stearic Acid.
Reglan Tablets (Metoclopramide Tablets, USP) 5 mg are green, elliptical-shaped tablets engraved Reglan 5 on one side and AHR on the opposite side.
Each tablet contains:
Metoclopramide base 5 mg
(as the monohydrochloride monohydrate)
INACTIVE INGREDIENTS: Corn Starch, D&C Yellow 10 Lake, FD&C Blue 1 Aluminum Lake, Lactose, Microcrystalline Cellulose, Silicon Dioxide, Stearic Acid.
Reglan Syrup (Metoclopramide Oral Solution, USP) is an orange-colored, palatable, aromatic, sugar-free liquid.
Each 5 mL (1 teaspoonful) contains:
Metoclopramide base 5 mg
(as the monohydrochloride monohydrate)
INACTIVE INGREDIENTS: Citric Acid, FD&C Yellow 6, Flavors, Glycerin, Methylparaben, Propylparaben, Sorbitol, Water.
For parenteral administration, Reglan Injectable (Metoclopramide Injection, USP) is a clear, colorless, sterile solution with a pH of 4.5–6.5 for intravenous or intramuscular administration.
CONTAINS NO PRESERVATIVE.
2 mL and 10 mL single dose vials; 2 mL single dose ampuls; 30 mL single dose vial
Each 1 mL contains:
Metoclopramide base 5 mg
(as the monohydrochloride monohydrate)
Sodium Chloride, USP 8.5 mg, Water for Injection, USP q.s. pH adjusted, when necessary, with hydrochloric acid and/or sodium hydroxide.
Metoclopramide hydrochloride is a white crystalline, odorless substance, freely soluble in water. Chemically, it is 4-amino-5-chloro-N-[2-(diethylamino)ethyl]-2-methoxy benzamide monohydrochloride monohydrate. Molecular weight: 354.3.

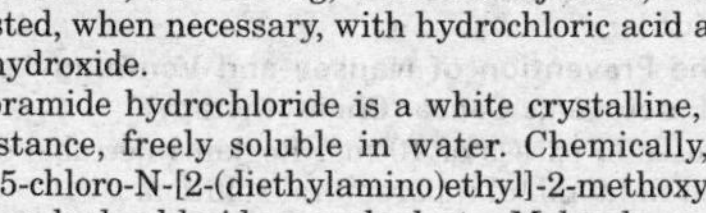

CLINICAL PHARMACOLOGY

Metoclopramide stimulates motility of the upper gastrointestinal tract without stimulating gastric, biliary, or pancreatic secretions. Its mode of action is unclear. It seems to sensitize tissues to the action of acetylcholine. The effect of metoclopramide on motility is not dependent on intact vagal innervation, but it can be abolished by anticholinergic drugs.
Metoclopramide increases the tone and amplitude of gastric (especially antral) contractions, relaxes the pyloric sphincter and the duodenal bulb, and increases peristalsis of the duodenum and jejunum resulting in accelerated gastric emptying and intestinal transit. It increases the resting tone of the lower esophageal sphincter. It has little, if any effect on the motility of the colon or gallbladder.
In patients with gastroesophageal reflux and low LESP (lower esophageal sphincter pressure), single oral doses of metoclopramide produce dose-related increases in LESP. Effects begin at about 5 mg and increase through 20 mg (the largest dose tested). The increase in LESP from a 5 mg dose lasts about 45 minutes and that of 20 mg lasts between 2 and 3 hours. Increased rate of stomach emptying has been observed with single oral doses of 10 mg.
The antiemetic properties of metoclopramide appear to be a result of its antagonism of central and peripheral dopamine receptors. Dopamine produces nausea and vomiting by stimulation of the medullary chemoreceptor trigger zone (CTZ), and metoclopramide blocks stimulation of the CTZ by agents like l-dopa or apomorphine which are known to increase dopamine levels or to possess dopamine-like effects. Metoclopramide also abolishes the slowing of gastric emptying caused by apomorphine.
Like the phenothiazines and related drugs, which are also dopamine antagonists, metoclopramide produces sedation and may produce extrapyramidal reactions, although these are comparatively rare (see **Warnings**). Metoclopramide inhibits the central and peripheral effects of apomorphine, induces release of prolactin and causes a transient increase in circulating aldosterone levels, which may be associated with transient fluid retention.
The onset of pharmacological action of metoclopramide is 1 to 3 minutes following an intravenous dose, 10 to 15 minutes following intramuscular administration, and 30 to 60 minutes following an oral dose; pharmacological effects persist for 1 to 2 hours.

Pharmacokinetics
Metoclopramide is rapidly and well absorbed. Relative to an intravenous dose of 20 mg, the absolute oral bioavailability of metoclopramide is 80% ± 15.5% as demonstrated in a crossover study of 18 subjects. Peak plasma concentrations occur at about 1–2 hr after a single oral dose. Similar time to peak is observed after individual doses at steady state.
In a single dose study of 12 subjects the area under the drug concentration-time curve increases linearly with doses from 20 to 100 mg. Peak concentrations increase linearly with dose; time to peak concentrations remains the same; whole body clearance is unchanged; and the elimination rate remains the same. The average elimination half-life in individuals with normal renal function is 5–6 hr. Linear kinetic processes adequately describe the absorption and elimination of metoclopramide.
Approximately 85% of the radioactivity of an orally administered dose appears in the urine within 72 hr. Of the 85% eliminated in the urine, about half is present as free or conjugated metoclopramide.
The drug is not extensively bound to plasma proteins (about 30%). The whole body volume of distribution is high (about 3.5 L/kg) which suggests extensive distribution of drug to the tissues.
Renal impairment affects the clearance of metoclopramide. In a study with patients with varying degrees of renal impairment, a reduction in creatinine clearance was correlated with a reduction in plasma clearance, renal clearance, non-renal clearance, and increase in elimination half-life. The kinetics of metoclopramide in the presence of renal impairment remained linear however. The reduction in clearance as a result of renal impairment suggests that adjustment downward of maintenance dosage should be done to avoid drug cumulation.

INDICATIONS AND USAGE

Symptomatic Gastroesophageal Reflux
Reglan Tablets and Syrup are indicated as short-term (4 to 12 weeks) therapy for adults with symptomatic, documented gastroesophageal reflux who fail to respond to conventional therapy.
The principal effect of metoclopramide is on symptoms of postprandial and daytime heartburn with less observed effect on nocturnal symptoms. If symptoms are confined to particular situations, such as following the evening meal, use of metoclopramide as single doses prior to the provocative situation should be considered, rather than using the drug throughout the day. Healing of esophageal ulcers and erosions has been endoscopically demonstrated at the end of a 12-week trial using doses of 15 mg q.i.d. As there is no documented correlation between symptoms and healing of esophageal lesions, patients with documented lesions should be monitored endoscopically.

Diabetic Gastroparesis (Diabetic Gastric Stasis)
Reglan (Metoclopramide Hydrochloride, USP) is indicated for the relief of symptoms associated with acute and recurrent diabetic gastric stasis. The usual manifestations of delayed gastric emptying (e.g., nausea, vomiting, heartburn, persistent fullness after meals and anorexia) appear to respond to Reglan within different time intervals. Significant relief of nausea occurs early and continues to improve over a three-week period. Relief of vomiting and anorexia may precede the relief of abdominal fullness by one week or more.

The Prevention of Nausea and Vomiting Associated with Emetogenic Cancer Chemotherapy
Reglan Injectable is indicated for the prophylaxis of vomiting associated with emetogenic cancer chemotherapy.

The Prevention of Postoperative Nausea and Vomiting
Reglan Injectable is indicated for the prophylaxis of postoperative nausea and vomiting in those circumstances where nasogastric suction is undesirable.

Small Bowel Intubation
Reglan Injectable may be used to facilitate small bowel intubation in adults and children in whom the tube does not pass the pylorus with conventional maneuvers.

Radiological Examination
Reglan Injectable may be used to stimulate gastric emptying and intestinal transit of barium in cases where delayed emptying interferes with radiological examination of the stomach and/or small intestine.

CONTRAINDICATIONS

Metoclopramide should not be used whenever stimulation of gastrointestinal motility might be dangerous, e.g., in the presence of gastrointestinal hemorrhage, mechanical obstruction, or perforation.
Metoclopramide is contraindicated in patients with pheochromocytoma because the drug may cause a hypertensive crisis, probably due to release of catecholamines from the tumor. Such hypertensive crises may be controlled by phentolamine.
Metoclopramide is contraindicated in patients with known sensitivity or intolerance to the drug.
Metoclopramide should not be used in epileptics or patients receiving other drugs which are likely to cause extrapyramidal reactions, since the frequency and severity of seizures or extrapyramidal reactions may be increased.

WARNINGS

Mental depression has occurred in patients with and without prior history of depression. Symptoms have ranged from mild to severe and have included suicidal ideation and suicide. Metoclopramide should be given to patients with a prior history of depression only if the expected benefits outweigh the potential risks.
Extrapyramidal symptoms, manifested primarily as acute dystonic reactions, occur in approximately 1 in 500 patients treated with the usual adult dosages of 30–40 mg/day of metoclopramide. These usually are seen during the first 24–48 hours of treatment with metoclopramide, occur more frequently in pediatric patients and young adults, and are even more frequent at the higher doses used in prophylaxis of vomiting due to cancer chemotherapy. These symptoms may include involuntary movements of limbs and facial grimacing, torticollis, oculogyric crisis, rhythmic protrusion of tongue, bulbar type of speech, trismus, or dystonic reactions resembling tetanus. Rarely, dystonic reactions may present as stridor and dyspnea, possibly due to laryngospasm. If these symptoms should occur, inject 50 mg Benadryl® (diphenhydramine hydrochloride) intramuscularly, and they usually will subside. Cogentin® (benztropine mesylate), 1 to 2 mg intramuscularly, may also be used to reverse these reactions.
Parkinsonian-like symptoms have occurred, more commonly within the first 6 months after beginning treatment with metoclopramide, but occasionally after longer periods. These symptoms generally subside within 2–3 months following discontinuance of metoclopramide. Patients with preexisting Parkinson's disease should be given metoclopramide cautiously, if at all, since such patients may experience exacerbation of parkinsonian symptoms when taking metoclopramide.

Tardive Dyskinesia
Tardive dyskinesia, a syndrome consisting of potentially irreversible, involuntary, dyskinetic movements may develop in patients treated with metoclopramide. Although the prevalence of the syndrome appears to be highest among the elderly, especially elderly women, it is impossible to predict which patients are likely to develop the syndrome. Both the risk of developing the syndrome and the likelihood that it will become irreversible are believed to increase with the duration of treatment and the total cumulative dose.

Continued on next page

Reglan—Cont.

Less commonly, the syndrome can develop after relatively brief treatment periods at low doses; in these cases, symptoms appear more likely to be reversible.

There is no known treatment for established cases of tardive dyskinesia although the syndrome may remit, partially or completely, within several weeks-to-months after metoclopramide is withdrawn. Metoclopramide itself, however, may suppress (or partially suppress) the signs of tardive dyskinesia, thereby masking the underlying disease process. The effect of this symptomatic suppression upon the long-term course of the syndrome is unknown. Therefore, the use of metoclopramide for the symptomatic control of tardive dyskenesia is not recommended.

PRECAUTIONS

General

In one study in hypertensive patients, intravenously administered metoclopramide was shown to release catecholamines; hence, caution should be exercised when metoclopramide is used in patients with hypertension.

Intravenous injections of undiluted metoclopramide should be made slowly allowing 1 to 2 minutes for 10 mg since a transient but intense feeling of anxiety and restlessness, followed by drowsiness, may occur with rapid administration.

Intravenous administration of Reglan Injectable diluted in a parenteral solution should be made slowly over a period of not less than 15 minutes.

Giving a promotility drug such as metoclopramide theoretically could put increased pressure on suture lines following a gut anastomosis or closure. Although adverse events related to this possibility have not been reported to date, the possibility should be considered and weighed when deciding whether to use metoclopramide or nasogastric suction in the prevention of postoperative nausea and vomiting.

Information for Patients

Metoclopramide may impair the mental and/or physical abilities required for the performance of hazardous tasks such as operating machinery or driving a motor vehicle. The ambulatory patient should be cautioned accordingly.

Drug Interactions

The effects of metoclopramide on gastrointestinal motility are antagonized by anticholinergic drugs and narcotic analgesics. Additive sedative effects can occur when metoclopramide is given with alcohol, sedatives, hypnotics, narcotics or tranquilizers.

The finding that metoclopramide releases catecholamines in patients with essential hypertension suggests that it should be used cautiously, if at all, in patients receiving monoamine oxidase inhibitors.

Absorption of drugs from the stomach may be diminished (e.g., digoxin) by metoclopramide, whereas the rate and/or extent of absorption of drugs from the small bowel may be increased (e.g., acetaminophen, tetracycline, levodopa, ethanol, cyclosporine).

Gastroparesis (gastric stasis) may be responsible for poor diabetic control in some patients. Exogenously administered insulin may begin to act before food has left the stomach and lead to hypoglycemia. Because the action of metoclopramide will influence the delivery of food to the intestines and thus the rate of absorption, insulin dosage or timing of dosage may require adjustment.

Carcinogenesis, Mutagenesis, Impairment of Fertility

A 77-week study was conducted in rats with oral doses up to about 40 times the maximum recommended human daily dose. Metoclopramide elevates prolactin levels and the elevation persists during chronic administration. Tissue culture experiments indicate that approximately one-third of human breast cancers are prolactin-dependent *in vitro*, a factor of potential importance if the prescription of metoclopramide is contemplated in a patient with previously detected breast cancer. Although disturbances such as galactorrhea, amenorrhea, gynecomastia, and impotence have been reported with prolactin-elevating drugs, the clinical significance of elevated serum prolactin levels is unknown for most patients. An increase in mammary neoplasms has been found in rodents after chronic administration of prolactin-stimulating neuroleptic drugs and metoclopramide. Neither clinical studies nor epidemiologic studies conducted to date, however, have shown an association between chronic administration of these drugs and mammary tumorigenesis; the available evidence is too limited to be conclusive at this time.

An Ames mutagenicity test performed on metoclopramide was negative.

Pregnancy Category B

Reproduction studies performed in rats, mice, and rabbits by the I.V., I.M., S.C. and oral routes at maximum levels ranging from 12 to 250 times the human dose have demonstrated no impairment of fertility or significant harm to the fetus due to metoclopramide. There are, however, no adequate and well-controlled studies in pregnant women. Because animal reproduction studies are not always predictive of human response, this drug should be used during pregnancy only if clearly needed.

Nursing Mothers

Metoclopramide is excreted in human milk. Caution should be exercised when metoclopramide is administered to a nursing mother.

Pediatric Use

There are insufficient data to support efficacy or make dosage recommendations for metoclopramide in patients less than 18 years of age except as stated to facilitate small bowel intubation (see **Overdosage** and **Dosage and Administration**).

ADVERSE REACTIONS

In general, the incidence of adverse reactions correlates with the dose and duration of metoclopramide administration. The following reactions have been reported, although in most instances, data do not permit an estimate of frequency:

CNS Effects

Restlessness, drowsiness, fatigue and lassitude occur in approximately 10% of patients receiving the most commonly prescribed dosage of 10 mg q.i.d. (see **Precautions**). Insomnia, headache, confusion, dizziness or mental depression with suicidal ideation (see **Warnings**) occur less frequently. In cancer chemotherapy patients being treated with 1–2 mg/kg per dose, incidence of drowsiness is about 70%. There are isolated reports of convulsive seizures without clearcut relationship to metoclopramide. Rarely, hallucinations have been reported.

Extrapyramidal Reactions (EPS)

Acute dystonic reactions, the most common type of EPS associated with metoclopramide, occur in approximately 0.2% of patients (1 in 500) treated with 30 to 40 mg of metoclopramide per day. In cancer chemotherapy patients receiving 1–2 mg/kg per dose, the incidence is 2% in patients over the ages of 30–35, and 25% or higher in pediatric patients and young adults who have not had prophylactic administration of diphenhydramine. Symptoms include involuntary movements of limbs, facial grimacing, torticollis, oculogyric crisis, rhythmic protrusion of tongue, bulbar type of speech, trismus, opisthotonus (tetanus-like reactions) and rarely, stridor and dyspnea, possibly due to laryngospasm; ordinarily these symptoms are readily reversed by diphenhydramine (see **Warnings**).

Parkinsonian-like symptoms may include bradykinesia, tremor, cogwheel rigidity, mask-like facies (see **Warnings**). Tardive dyskinesia most frequently is characterized by involuntary movements of the tongue, face, mouth or jaw, and sometimes by involuntary movements of the trunk and/or extremities; movements may be choreoathetotic in appearance (see **Warnings**).

Motor restlessness (akathisia) may consist of feelings of anxiety, agitation, jitteriness, and insomnia, as well as inability to sit still, pacing, foot tapping. These symptoms may disappear spontaneously or respond to a reduction in dosage.

Endocrine Disturbances

Galactorrhea, amenorrhea, gynecomastia, impotence secondary to hyperprolactinemia (see **Precautions**). Fluid retention secondary to transient elevation of aldosterone (see **Clinical Pharmacology**).

Cardiovascular

Hypotension, hypertension, supraventricular tachycardia, bradycardia and possible AV block (see **Contraindications** and **Precautions**).

Gastrointestinal

Nausea and bowel disturbances, primarily diarrhea.

Hepatic

Rarely, cases of hepatotoxicity, characterized by such findings as jaundice and altered liver function tests, when metoclopramide was administered with other drugs with known hepatotoxic potential.

Renal

Urinary frequency and incontinence.

Hematologic

A few cases of neutropenia, leukopenia, or agranulocytosis, generally without clearcut relationship to metoclopramide. Methemoglobinemia, especially with overdosage in neonates (see **Overdosage**).

Allergic Reactions

A few cases of rash, urticaria, or bronchospasm, especially in patients with a history of asthma. Rarely, angioneurotic edema, including glossal or laryngeal edema.

Miscellaneous

Visual disturbances. Porphyria. Rare occurrences of neuroleptic malignant syndrome (NMS) have been reported. This potentially fatal syndrome is comprised of the symptom complex of hyperthermia, altered consciousness, muscular rigidity and autonomic dysfunction.

Transient flushing of the face and upper body, without alterations in vital signs, following high doses intravenously.

OVERDOSAGE

Symptoms of overdosage may include drowsiness, disorientation and extrapyramidal reactions. Anticholinergic or antiparkinson drugs or antihistamines with anticholinergic properties may be helpful in controlling the extrapyramidal reactions. Symptoms are self-limiting and usually disappear within 24 hours.

Hemodialysis removes relatively little metoclopramide, probably because of the small amount of the drug in blood relative to tissues. Similarly, continuous ambulatory peritoneal dialysis does not remove significant amounts of drug. It is unlikely that dosage would need to be adjusted to compensate for losses through dialysis. Dialysis is not likely to be an effective method of drug removal in overdose situations.

Unintentional overdose due to misadministration has been reported in patients between the age of 2 months and 7 years with the use of Reglan syrup. While there was no consistent pattern to the reports associated with these overdoses, events included seizures, extrapyramidal reactions, and lethargy.

Methemoglobinemia has occurred in premature and full-term neonates who were given overdoses of metoclopramide (1–4 mg/kg/day orally, intramuscularly or intravenously for 1–3 or more days). Methemoglobinemia has not been reported in neonates treated with 0.5 mg/kg/day in divided doses. Methemoglobinemia can be reversed by the intravenous administration of methylene blue.

DOSAGE AND ADMINISTRATION

For the Relief of Symptomatic Gastroesophageal Reflux

Administer from 10 mg to 15 mg Reglan (Metoclopramide Hydrochloride, USP) orally up to q.i.d. 30 minutes before each meal and at bedtime, depending upon symptoms being treated and clinical response (see **Clinical Pharmacology** and **Indications and Usage**). If symptoms occur only intermittently or at specific times of the day, use of metoclopramide in single doses up to 20 mg prior to the provoking situation may be preferred rather than continuous treatment. Occasionally, patients (such as elderly patients) who are more sensitive to the therapeutic or adverse effects of metoclopramide will require only 5 mg per dose.

Experience with esophageal erosions and ulcerations is limited, but healing has thus far been documented in one controlled trial using q.i.d. therapy at 15 mg/dose, and this regimen should be used when lesions are present, so long as it is tolerated (see **Adverse Reactions**). Because of the poor correlation between symptoms and endoscopic appearance of the esophagus, therapy directed at esophageal lesions is best guided by endoscopic evaluation.

Therapy longer than 12 weeks has not been evaluated and cannot be recommended.

For the Relief of Symptoms Associated with Diabetic Gastroparesis (Diabetic Gastric Stasis)

Administer 10 mg of metoclopramide 30 minutes before each meal and at bedtime for two to eight weeks, depending upon response and the likelihood of continued well-being upon drug discontinuation.

The initial route of administration should be determined by the severity of the presenting symptoms. If only the earliest manifestations of diabetic gastric stasis are present, oral administration of Reglan may be initiated. However, if severe symptoms are present, therapy should begin with Reglan Injectable (I.M. or I.V.). Doses of 10 mg may be administered slowly by the intravenous route over a 1- to 2-minute period.

Administration of Reglan Injectable (Metoclopramide Injection, USP) up to 10 days may be required before symptoms subside, at which time oral administration may be instituted. Since diabetic gastric stasis is frequently recurrent, Reglan therapy should be reinstituted at the earliest manifestation.

For the Prevention of Nausea and Vomiting Associated with Emetogenic Cancer Chemotherapy

For doses in excess of 10 mg, Reglan Injectable should be diluted in 50 mL of a parenteral solution.

Container	Total Contents #	Concentration #	Administration
2 mL single dose vial/ampul	10 mg	5 mg/mL	FOR IV or IM ADMINISTRATION
10 mL single dose vial	50 mg	5 mg/mL	FOR IV INFUSION ONLY; DILUTE BEFORE USING
30 mL single dose vial	150 mg	5 mg/mL	FOR IV INFUSION ONLY; DILUTE BEFORE USING

Metoclopramide base (as the monohydrochloride monohydrate)

The preferred parenteral solution is Sodium Chloride Injection (normal saline), which when combined with Reglan Injectable, can be stored frozen for up to 4 weeks. Reglan Injectable is degraded when admixed and frozen with Dextrose-5% in Water. Reglan Injectable diluted in Sodium Chloride Injection, Dextrose-5% in Water, Dextrose-5% in 0.45% Sodium Chloride, Ringer's Injection or Lactated Ringer's Injection may be stored up to 48 hours (without freezing) after preparation if protected from light. All dilutions may be stored unprotected from light under normal light conditions up to 24 hours after preparation.

Intravenous infusions should be made slowly over a period of not less than 15 minutes, 30 minutes before beginning cancer chemotherapy and repeated every 2 hours for two doses, then every 3 hours for three doses.

The initial two doses should be 2 mg/kg if highly emetogenic drugs such as cisplatin or dacarbazine are used alone or in combination. For less emetogenic regimens, 1 mg/kg per dose may be adequate.

If extrapyramidal symptoms should occur, inject 50 mg Benadryl® (diphenhydramine hydrochloride) intramuscularly, and EPS usually will subside.

For the Prevention of Postoperative Nausea and Vomiting
Reglan Injectable should be given intramuscularly near the end of surgery. The usual adult dose is 10 mg; however, doses of 20 mg may be used.

To Facilitate Small Bowel Intubation
If the tube has not passed the pylorus with conventional maneuvers in 10 minutes, a single dose (undiluted) may be administered slowly by the intravenous route over a 1- to 2-minute period.

The recommended single dose is: Adults—10 mg metoclopramide base. Pediatric patients (6–14 years of age)—2.5 to 5 mg metoclopramide base; (under 6 years of age)—0.1 mg/kg metoclopramide base.

To Aid in Radiological Examinations
In patients where delayed gastric emptying interferes with radiological examination of the stomach and/or small intestine, a single dose may be administered slowly by the intravenous route over a 1- to 2-minute period.

For dosage, see intubation above.

Use in Patients with Renal or Hepatic Impairment
Since metoclopramide is excreted principally through the kidneys, in those patients whose creatinine clearance is below 40 mL/min, therapy should be initiated at approximately one-half the recommended dosage. Depending upon clinical efficacy and safety considerations, the dosage may be increased or decreased as appropriate.

See **Overdosage** section for information regarding dialysis.

Metoclopramide undergoes minimal hepatic metabolism, except for simple conjugation. Its safe use has been described in patients with advanced liver disease whose renal function was normal.

NOTE: Parenteral drug products should be inspected visually for particulate matter and discoloration prior to administration, whenever solution and container permit.

Admixture Compatibilities
Reglan Injectable (Metoclopramide Injection, USP) is compatible for mixing and injection with the following dosage forms to the extent indicated below:

PHYSICALLY AND CHEMICALLY COMPATIBLE UP TO 48 HOURS
Cimetidine Hydrochloride (SK&F), Mannitol, USP (Abbott), Potassium Acetate, USP (Invenex), Potassium Phosphate, USP (Invenex).

PHYSICALLY COMPATIBLE UP TO 48 HOURS
Ascorbic Acid, USP (Abbott), Benztropine Mesylate, USP (MS&D), Cytarabine, USP (Upjohn), Dexamethasone Sodium Phosphate, USP (ESI, MS&D), Diphenhydramine Hydrochloride, USP (Parke-Davis), Doxorubicin Hydrochloride, USP (Adria), Heparin Sodium, USP (ESI), Hydrocortisone Sodium Phosphate (MS&D), Lidocaine Hydrochloride, USP (ESI), Multi-Vitamin Infusion (must be refrigerated-USV), Vitamin B Complex with Ascorbic Acid (Roche).

PHYSICALLY COMPATIBLE UP TO 24 HOURS *(Do not use if precipitation occurs)*
Clindamycin Phosphate, USP (Upjohn), Cyclophosphamide, USP (Mead-Johnson), Insulin, USP (Lilly)

CONDITIONALLY COMPATIBLE *(Use within one hour after mixing or may be infused directly into the same running IV line)*
Ampicillin Sodium, USP (Bristol), Cisplatin (Bristol), Erythromycin Lactobionate, USP (Abbott), Methotrexate Sodium, USP (Lederle), Penicillin G Potassium, USP (Squibb), Tetracycline Hydrochloride, USP (Lederle).

INCOMPATIBLE *(Do Not Mix)*
Cephalothin Sodium, USP (Lilly), Chloramphenicol Sodium, USP (Parke-Davis), Sodium Bicarbonate, USP (Abbott).

HOW SUPPLIED

Each white, capsule-shaped, scored Reglan® Tablet contains 10 mg metoclopramide base (as the monohydrochloride monohydrate). Available in bottles of 100 (NDC 0031-6701-63), and 500 tablets (NDC 0031-6701-70) and Dis-Co® Unit Dose Packs of 100 tablets (NDC 0031-6701-64).

Each green, elliptical-shaped Reglan® Tablet contains 5 mg metoclopramide base (as the monohydrochloride monohydrate). Available in bottles of 100 (NDC 0031-6705-63) and Dis-Co® Unit Dose Packs of 100 tablets (NDC 0031-6705-64). Dispense tablets in tight, light-resistant container.

Reglan® Syrup, 5 mg metoclopramide base (as the monohydrochloride monohydrate) per 5 mL, available in pints (NDC 0031-6706-25). Dispense syrup in tight, light-resistant container.

Preservative-free:
Reglan® Injectable, 5 mg metoclopramide base (as the monohydrochloride monohydrate) per mL; available in 2 mL single dose vials in cartons of 25 (NDC 0031-6709-72), 10 mL single dose vials in cartons of 25 (NDC 0031-6709-78); and 30 mL single dose vials in cartons of 25 (NDC 0031-6709-24); 2 mL ampuls in cartons of 25 (NDC 0031-6709-95).

[See table at bottom of previous page]

Store vials and ampuls in carton until used. Do not store open single dose vials or ampuls for later use, as they contain no preservative.

Dilutions may be stored unprotected from light under normal light conditions up to 24 hours after preparation.

Tablets, Syrup and Injectable should be stored at controlled room temperature between 20°C and 25°C (68°F and 77°F).

Reglan Injectable is manufactured for Pharmaceutical Division, A. H. Robins Company, Richmond, Virginia 23220 by Elkins-Sinn, Cherry Hill, NJ 08003, a division of A.H. Robins

Shown in Product Identification Guide, page 334

ROBAXIN® INJECTABLE ℞

[ro "baks 'in]
brand of Methocarbamol Injection, USP

DESCRIPTION

Methocarbamol has the following structural formula:

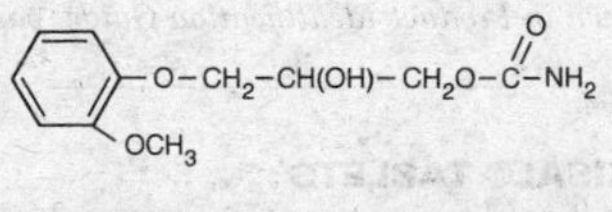

3-(2-methoxyphenoxy)-1,2-propanediol
1-carbamate, or methocarbamol

Robaxin Injectable is a parenteral dosage form.

Each mL contains:
Methocarbamol, USP **100 mg**; Polyethylene Glycol 300, NF 0.5 mL; Water for Injection, USP q.s. pH adjusted, when necessary, with hydrochloric acid and/or sodium hydroxide.

AFTER MIXING WITH I.V. INFUSION FLUIDS, **DO NOT REFRIGERATE.**

ACTIONS

The mechanism of action of methocarbamol in humans has not been established, but may be due to general central nervous system depression. It has no direct action on the contractile mechanism of striated muscle, the motor end plate or the nerve fiber.

INDICATIONS

The injectable form of methocarbamol is indicated as an adjunct to rest, physical therapy, and other measures for the relief of discomfort associated with acute, painful musculoskeletal conditions. The mode of action of this drug has not been clearly identified, but may be related to its sedative properties. Methocarbamol does not directly relax tense skeletal muscles in man.

CONTRAINDICATIONS

Robaxin Injectable should not be administered to patients with known or suspected renal pathology. This caution is necessary because of the presence of polyethylene glycol 300 in the vehicle.

A much larger amount of polyethylene glycol 300 than is present in recommended doses of Robaxin Injectable is known to have increased pre-existing acidosis and urea retention in patients with renal impairment. Although the amount present in this preparation is well within the limits of safety, caution dictates this contraindication.

Robaxin Injectable is contraindicated in patients hypersensitive to any of the ingredients.

WARNINGS

Since methocarbamol may possess a general central nervous system depressant effect, patients receiving Robaxin Injectable (methocarbamol injection) should be cautioned about combined effects with alcohol and other CNS depressants.

Safe use of Robaxin Injectable has not been established with regard to possible adverse effects upon fetal development. Therefore, Robaxin Injectable should not be used in women who are or may become pregnant and particularly during early pregnancy unless in the judgment of the physician the potential benefits outweigh the possible hazards.

PRECAUTIONS

As with other agents administered either intravenously or intramuscularly, careful supervision of dose and rate of injection should be observed. Rate of injection should not exceed 3 mL per minute—i.e., one 10 mL vial in approximately three minutes. Since Robaxin Injectable is hypertonic, vascular extravasation must be avoided. A recumbent position will reduce the likelihood of side reactions.

Blood aspirated into the syringe does not mix with the hypertonic solution. This phenomenon occurs with many other intravenous preparations. The blood may be safely injected with the methocarbamol, or the injection may be stopped when the plunger reaches the blood, whichever the physician prefers.

The total dosage should not exceed 30 mL (three vials) a day for more than three consecutive days except in the treatment of tetanus.

Caution should be observed in using the injectable form in suspected or known epileptic patients.

Safety and effectiveness in children below the age of 12 years have not been established except in tetanus. See special directions for use in tetanus.

It is not known whether this drug is secreted in human milk. As a general rule, nursing should not be undertaken while a patient is on a drug since many drugs are excreted in human milk.

Methocarbamol may cause a color interference in certain screening tests for 5-hydroxyindoleacetic acid (5-HIAA) and vanillylmandelic acid (VMA).

ADVERSE REACTIONS

Dizziness, lightheadedness, drowsiness, vertigo, fainting, syncope, hypotension, gastrointestinal upset, metallic taste, thrombophlebitis, sloughing at the site of injection, pain at the site of injection, anaphylactic reaction, urticaria, pruritus, rash, conjunctivitis with nasal congestion, flushing, nystagmus, diplopia, mild muscular incoordination, bradycardia, blurred vision, headache, fever. In most cases of syncope there was spontaneous recovery. In others, epinephrine, injectable steroids and/or injectable antihistamines were employed to hasten recovery. Certain of these complaints may have been due to any overly rapid rate of intravenous injection.

The onset of convulsive seizures during intravenous administration has been reported, including instances in known epileptics. The psychic trauma of the procedure may have been a contributing factor. Although several observers have reported success in terminating epileptiform seizures with Robaxin Injectable, its administration to patients with epilepsy is not recommended.

DOSAGE AND ADMINISTRATION

For Intravenous and Intramuscular Use Only. Total adult dosage should not exceed 30 mL (3 vials) a day for more than 3 consecutive days except in the treatment of tetanus. A like course may be repeated after a lapse of 48 hours if the condition persists. Dosage and frequency of injection should be based on the severity of the condition being treated and therapeutic response noted.

For the relief of symptoms of moderate degree, 10 mL (one vial) may be adequate. Ordinarily this injection need not be repeated, as the administration of the oral form will usually sustain the relief initiated by the injection. For the severest cases or in postoperative conditions in which oral administration is not feasible, 20 to 30 mL (two to three vials) may be required.

Directions for Intravenous Use. Robaxin Injectable may be administered undiluted directly into the vein at a ***maximum rate of three mL per minute.*** It may also be added to an intravenous drip of Sodium Chloride Injection (Sterile Isotonic Sodium Chloride Solution for Parenteral Use) or five per cent Dextrose Injection (Sterile 5 per cent Dextrose Solution); one vial given as a single dose should not be diluted to more than 250 mL for I. V. infusion. Care should be exercised to avoid vascular extravasation of this hypertonic solution which may result in thrombophlebitis. It is preferable that the patient be in a recumbent position during and for at least 10 to 15 minutes following the injection.

Directions for Intramuscular Use. When the intramuscular route is indicated, not more than five mL (one-half vial) should be injected into each gluteal region. The injections may be repeated at eight hour intervals, if necessary. When satisfactory relief of symptoms is achieved, it can usually be maintained with tablets.

Not Recommended for Subcutaneous Administration.

Special Directions for Use in Tetanus: There is clinical evidence which suggests that methocarbamol may have a beneficial effect in the control of the neuromuscular manifestations of tetanus. It does not, however, replace the usual procedure of debridement, tetanus antitoxin, penicillin,

Continued on next page

Robaxin Injectable—Cont.

tracheotomy, attention to fluid balance, and supportive care. Robaxin Injectable should be added to the regimen as soon as possible.

For adults: Inject one or two vials directly into the tubing of a previously inserted indwelling needle. An additional 10 mL or 20 mL may be added to the infusion bottle so that a total of up to 30 mL (three vials) is given as the initial dose (note Precautions). This procedure should be repeated every six hours until conditions allow for the insertion of a naso-gastric tube. Crushed Robaxin (methocarbamol) tablets suspended in water or saline may then be given through this tube. Total daily oral doses up to 24 grams may be required as judged by patient response.

For children: A minimum initial dose of 15 mg/kg is recommended. This dosage may be repeated every six hours as indicated. The maintenance dosage may be given by injection into the tubing or by I.V. infusion with an appropriate quantity of fluid. See directions for I.V. use.

HOW SUPPLIED

Robaxin Injectable—10 mL single dose vials in packages of 5 (NDC 0031-7409-87) and 25 (NDC 0031-7409-94). Manufactured for Pharmaceutical Division, A. H. ROBINS CO., Richmond, VA 23220, by ELKINS-SINN, INC., Cherry Hill, NJ 08034, a subsidiary of A.H. Robins.
Shown in Product Identification Guide, page 334

ROBAXIN®   ℞
[ro "baks 'ĭn]
brand of Methocarbamol Tablets, USP
500 mg per tablet
ROBAXIN®–750 brand of Methocarbamol Tablets,
USP   ℞
750 mg per tablet

DESCRIPTION

Inactive Ingredients: ROBAXIN—Corn Starch, FD&C Yellow 6 Aluminum Lake, Hydroxypropyl Cellulose, Hydroxypropyl Methylcellulose, Magnesium Stearate, Polysorbate 20, Povidone, Propylene Glycol, Saccharin Sodium, Sodium Lauryl Sulfate, Sodium Starch Glycolate, Stearic Acid, Titanium Dioxide.
ROBAXIN-750—Corn Starch, D&C Yellow 10 Aluminum Lake, FD&C Yellow 6 Aluminum Lake, Hydroxypropyl Cellulose, Hydroxypropyl Methylcellulose, Magnesium Stearate, Polysorbate 20, Povidone, Propylene Glycol, Saccharin Sodium, Sodium Lauryl Sulfate, Sodium Starch Glycolate, Stearic Acid, Titanium Dioxide.
Methocarbamol has the following structural formula:

O-CH$_2$-CH(OH)-CH$_2$-O-C-NH$_2$
OCH$_3$

1,2-Propanediol, 3-(2-methoxyphenoxy)-,
1-carbamate, (±)-.

ACTIONS

The mechanism of action of methocarbamol in humans has not been established, but may be due to general central nervous system depression. It has no direct action on the contractile mechanism of striated muscle, the motor end plate or the nerve fiber.

INDICATIONS

Robaxin (methocarbamol) is indicated as an adjunct to rest, physical therapy, and other measures for the relief of discomforts associated with acute, painful musculoskeletal conditions. The mode of action of this drug has not been clearly identified, but may be related to its sedative properties. Methocarbamol does not directly relax tense skeletal muscles in man.

CONTRAINDICATIONS

Robaxin is contraindicated in patients hypersensitive to any of the ingredients.

WARNINGS

Since methocarbamol may possess a general central nervous system depressant effect, patients receiving Robaxin/Robaxin-750 (methocarbamol tablets) should be cautioned about combined effects with alcohol and other CNS depressants.
Safe use of methocarbamol has not been established with regard to possible adverse effects upon fetal development. Therefore, methocarbamol tablets should not be used in women who are or may become pregnant and particularly during early pregnancy unless in the judgment of the physician the potential benefits outweigh the possible hazards.

PRECAUTIONS

Safety and effectiveness in children below the age of 12 years have not been established.

It is not known whether this drug is secreted in human milk. As a general rule, nursing should not be undertaken while a patient is on a drug since many drugs are excreted in human milk.
Methocarbamol may cause a color interference in certain screening tests for 5-hydroxyindoleacetic acid (5-HIAA) and vanillylmandelic acid (VMA).

ADVERSE REACTIONS

Lightheadedness, dizziness, drowsiness, nausea, allergic manifestations such as urticaria, pruritus, rash, conjunctivitis with nasal congestion, blurred vision, headache, fever.

DOSAGE AND ADMINISTRATION

Robaxin (methocarbamol), 500 mg—Adults: initial dosage, 3 tablets q.i.d.; maintenance dosage, 2 tablets q.i.d.
Robaxin-750 (methocarbamol), 750 mg — Adults: initial dosage, 2 tablets q.i.d.; maintenance dosage, 1 tablet q.4h. or 2 tablets t.i.d.
Six grams a day are recommended for the first 48 to 72 hours of treatment. (For severe conditions 8 grams a day may be administered.) Thereafter, the dosage can usually be reduced to approximately 4 grams a day.

HOW SUPPLIED

Robaxin—light orange, round, film-coated tablets monogrammed Robaxin and AHR in bottles of 100 (NDC 0031-7429-63), and 500 (NDC 0031-7429-70).
Robaxin-750—orange, capsule-shaped, film-coated tablets monogrammed Robaxin-750 and AHR in bottles of 100 (NDC 0031-7449-63), 500 (NDC 0031-7449-70), and Dis-Co® unit dose packs of 100 (NDC 0031-7449-64).
Store at Controlled Room Temperature, between 20°C and 25°C (68°F and 77°F).
Dispense in tight container.
Also available in the injectable form, 1 g methocarbamol in each 10 ml vial (NDC 0031-7409).
Manufactured by:
Pharmaceutical Division
A.H. Robins Company
Richmond, VA 23220
Shown in Product Identification Guide, page 334

ROBAXISAL® TABLETS   ℞
[ro "baks 'ĭ-sal "]

DESCRIPTION

For oral administration, Robaxisal is available as a pink and white laminated tablet containing:
Methocarbamol, USP .... 400 mg
Aspirin, USP .... 325 mg
Inactive Ingredients: Corn Starch, FD&C Red 3, Magnesium Stearate, Povidone, Sodium Lauryl Sulfate, Sodium Starch Glycolate, Stearic Acid.
Methocarbamol has the following structural formula and chemical name:

O-CH$_2$-CH(OH)-CH$_2$-O-C-NH$_2$
OCH$_3$

3-(2-Methoxyphenoxy)-1,2-propanediol
1-Carbamate

ACTIONS

Robaxisal provides a double approach to the management of discomforts associated with musculoskeletal disorders.
METHOCARBAMOL
The mechanism of action of methocarbamol in humans has not been established, but may be due to general central nervous system depression. It has no direct action on the contractile mechanism of striated muscle, the motor end plate or the nerve fiber.
ASPIRIN
Aspirin is a mild analgesic with anti-inflammatory and antipyretic activity.

INDICATIONS

Robaxisal is indicated as an adjunct to rest, physical therapy, and other measures for the relief of discomfort associated with acute, painful musculoskeletal conditions. The mode of action of methocarbamol has not been clearly identified but may be related to its sedative properties. Methocarbamol does not directly relax tense skeletal muscles in man.

CONTRAINDICATIONS

Hypersensitivity to methocarbamol or aspirin.

WARNINGS

Since methocarbamol may possess a general central nervous system depressant effect, patients receiving Robaxisal should be cautioned about combined effects with alcohol and other CNS depressants.

PRECAUTIONS

Products containing aspirin should be administered with caution to patients with gastritis or peptic ulceration, or those receiving hypoprothrombinemic anticoagulants.
Methocarbamol may cause a color interference in certain screening tests for 5-hydroxyindoleacetic acid (5-HIAA) and vanillylmandelic acid (VMA).
PREGNANCY
Safe use of Robaxisal has not been established with regard to possible adverse effects upon fetal development. Therefore, Robaxisal should not be used in women who are or may become pregnant and particularly during early pregnancy unless in the judgment of the physician the potential benefits outweigh the possible hazards.
NURSING MOTHERS
It is not known whether methocarbamol is secreted in human milk; however, aspirin does appear in human milk in moderate amounts. It can produce a bleeding tendency either by interfering with the function of the infant's platelets or by decreasing the amount of prothrombin in the blood. The risk is minimal if the mother takes the aspirin just after nursing and if the infant has an adequate store of vitamin K. As a general rule, nursing should not be undertaken while a patient is on a drug.
PEDIATRIC USE
Safety and effectiveness in children 12 years of age and below have not been established.
USE IN ACTIVITIES REQUIRING MENTAL ALERTNESS
Robaxisal may rarely cause drowsiness. Until the patient's response has been determined, he should be cautioned against the operation of motor vehicles or dangerous machinery.

ADVERSE REACTIONS

The most frequent adverse reaction to methocarbamol is dizziness or lightheadedness and nausea. This occurs in about one in 20–25 patients. Less frequent reactions are drowsiness, blurred vision, headache, fever, allergic manifestations such as urticaria, pruritus, and rash.
Adverse reactions that have been associated with the use of aspirin include: nausea and other gastrointestinal discomfort, gastritis, gastric erosion, vomiting, constipation, diarrhea, angio-edema, asthma, rash, pruritus, urticaria. Gastrointestinal discomfort may be minimized by taking Robaxisal with food.

DOSAGE AND ADMINISTRATION

Adults and children over 12 years of age: Two tablets four times daily. Three tablets four times daily may be used in severe conditions for one to three days in patients who are able to tolerate salicylates. These dosage recommendations provide respectively 3.2 and 4.8 grams of methocarbamol per day.

OVERDOSAGE

Toxicity due to overdosage of methocarbamol is unlikely; however, acute overdosage of aspirin may cause symptoms of salicylate intoxication.
TREATMENT OF OVERDOSAGE
Supportive therapy for 24 hours, as methocarbamol is excreted within that time. If salicylate intoxication occurs, especially in children, the hyperpnea may be controlled with sodium bicarbonate. Judicious use of 5% CO_2 with 95% O_2 may be of benefit. Abnormal electrolyte patterns should be corrected with appropriate fluid therapy.

HOW SUPPLIED

Robaxisal® is supplied as pink and white laminated, compressed tablets in bottles of 100 (NDC 0031-7469-63) and 500 (NDC 0031-7469-70).
Store at controlled room temperature, between 20° and 25°C (68° and 77°F).
Dispense in well-closed container.
Manufactured by:
Pharmaceutical Division
A.H. Robins Company
Richmond, VA 23220
Shown in Product Identification Guide, page 334

ROBINUL® TABLETS   ℞
[ro 'bĭ-nul]
ROBINUL® FORTE TABLETS   ℞
brand of Glycopyrrolate Tablets, USP

DESCRIPTION

Robinul® and Robinul® Forte tablets contain the synthetic anticholinergic, glycopyrrolate. Glycopyrrolate is a quaternary ammonium compound with the following chemical name: 3-[(cyclopentylhydroxyphenylacetyl)oxy]-1,1-dimethylpyrrolidinium bromide.
Robinul tablets are scored, compressed white tablets engraved AHR. Each tablet contains:
Glycopyrrolate, USP .... 1 mg
Robinul Forte tablets are scored, compressed white tablets engraved AHR. Each tablet contains:
Glycopyrrolate, USP .... 2 mg

Inactive Ingredients: Dibasic Calcium Phosphate, Lactose, Magnesium Stearate, Povidone, Sodium Starch Glycolate.

ACTIONS

Glycopyrrolate, like other anticholinergic (antimuscarinic) agents, inhibits the action of acetylcholine on structures innervated by postganglionic cholinergic nerves and on smooth muscles that respond to acetylcholine but lack cholinergic innervation. These peripheral cholinergic receptors are present in the autonomic effector cells of smooth muscle, cardiac muscle, the sino-atrial node, the atrioventricular node, exocrine glands and, to a limited degree, in the autonomic ganglia. Thus, it diminishes the volume and free acidity of gastric secretions and controls excessive pharyngeal, tracheal, and bronchial secretions.

Glycopyrrolate antagonizes muscarinic symptoms (e.g., bronchorrhea, bronchospasm, bradycardia, and intestinal hypermotility) induced by cholinergic drugs such as the anticholinesterases.

The highly polar quaternary ammonium group of glycopyrrolate limits its passage across lipid membranes, such as the blood-brain barrier, in contrast to atropine sulfate and scopolamine hydrobromide, which are non-polar tertiary amines which penetrate lipid barriers easily.

INDICATIONS

For use as adjunctive therapy in the treatment of peptic ulcer.

CONTRAINDICATIONS

Glaucoma; obstructive uropathy (for example, bladder neck obstruction due to prostatic hypertrophy); obstructive disease of the gastrointestinal tract (as in achalasia, pyloroduodenal stenosis, etc.); paralytic ileus; intestinal atony of the elderly or debilitated patient; unstable cardiovascular status in acute hemorrhage; severe ulcerative colitis; toxic megacolon complicating ulcerative colitis; myasthenia gravis. Robinul (glycopyrrolate) tablets are contraindicated in those patients with a hypersensitivity to glycopyrrolate.

WARNINGS

In the presence of a high environmental temperature, heat prostration (fever and heat stroke due to decreased sweating) can occur with use of Robinul.

Diarrhea may be an early symptom of incomplete intestinal obstruction, especially in patients with ileostomy or colostomy. In this instance treatment with this drug would be inappropriate and possibly harmful.

Robinul (glycopyrrolate) may produce drowsiness or blurred vision. In this event, the patient should be warned not to engage in activities requiring mental alertness such as operating a motor vehicle or other machinery, or performing hazardous work while taking this drug.

Theoretically, with overdosage, a curare-like action may occur, i.e., neuromuscular blockade leading to muscular weakness and possible paralysis.

PREGNANCY

The safety of this drug during pregnancy has not been established. The use of any drug during pregnancy requires that the potential benefits of the drug be weighed against possible hazards to mother and child. Reproduction studies in rats revealed no teratogenic effects from glycopyrrolate; however, the potent anticholinergic action of this agent resulted in diminished rates of conception and of survival at weaning, in a dose-related manner. Other studies in dogs suggest that this may be due to diminished seminal secretion which is evident at high doses of glycopyrrolate. Information on possible adverse effects in the pregnant female is limited to uncontrolled data derived from marketing experience. Such experience has revealed no reports of teratogenic or other fetus-damaging potential. No controlled studies to establish the safety of the drug in pregnancy have been performed.

NURSING MOTHERS

It is not known whether this drug is secreted in human milk. As a general rule, nursing should not be undertaken while a patient is on a drug since many drugs are excreted in human milk.

PEDIATRIC USE

Since there is no adequate experience in pediatric patients who have received this drug, safety and efficacy in pediatric patients have not been established.

PRECAUTIONS

Use Robinul with caution in the elderly and in all patients with:
- Autonomic neuropathy.
- Hepatic or renal disease.
- Ulcerative colitis—large doses may suppress intestinal motility to the point of producing a paralytic ileus and for this reason may precipitate or aggravate "toxic megacolon," a serious complication of the disease.
- Hyperthyroidism, coronary heart disease, congestive heart failure, cardiac tachyarrhythmias, tachycardia, hypertension and prostatic hypertrophy.
- Hiatal hernia associated with reflux esophagitis, since anticholinergic drugs may aggravate this condition.

ADVERSE REACTIONS

Anticholinergics produce certain effects, most of which are extensions of their fundamental pharmacological actions. Adverse reactions to anticholinergics in general may include xerostomia; decreased sweating; urinary hesitancy and retention; blurred vision; tachycardia; palpitations; dilatation of the pupil; cycloplegia; increased ocular tension; loss of taste; headaches; nervousness; mental confusion; drowsiness; weakness; dizziness; insomnia; nausea; vomiting; constipation; bloated feeling; impotence; suppression of lactation; severe allergic reaction or drug idiosyncrasies including anaphylaxis, urticaria and other dermal manifestations.

Robinul (glycopyrrolate) is chemically a quaternary ammonium compound; hence, its passage across lipid membranes, such as the blood-brain barrier, is limited in contrast to atropine sulfate and scopolamine hydrobromide. For this reason the occurrence of CNS related side effects is lower, in comparison to their incidence following administration of anticholinergics which are chemically tertiary amines that can cross this barrier readily.

OVERDOSAGE

The symptoms of overdosage of glycopyrrolate are peripheral in nature rather than central.

1. To guard against further absorption of the drug—use gastric lavage, cathartics and/or enemas.

2. To combat peripheral anticholinergic effects (residual mydriasis, dry mouth, etc.)—utilize a quaternary ammonium anticholinesterase, such as neostigmine methylsulfate.

3. To combat hypotension—use pressor amines (norepinephrine, metaraminol) i.v.; and supportive care.

4. To combat respiratory depression—administer oxygen; utilize a respiratory stimulant such as Dopram® i.v.; artificial respiration.

DOSAGE AND ADMINISTRATION

The dosage of Robinul or Robinul Forte should be adjusted to the needs of the individual patient to assure symptomatic control with a minimum of adverse reactions. The presently recommended maximum daily dosage of glycopyrrolate is 8 mg.

Robinul (glycopyrrolate, 1 mg) tablets. The recommended initial dosage of Robinul for adults is one tablet three times daily (in the morning, early afternoon, and at bedtime). Some patients may require two tablets at bedtime to assure overnight control of symptoms. For maintenance, a dosage of one tablet twice a day is frequently adequate.

Robinul Forte (glycopyrrolate, 2 mg) tablets. The recommended dosage of Robinul Forte for adults is one tablet two or three times daily at equally spaced intervals.

Robinul tablets are not recommended for use in children under the age of 12 years.

DRUG INTERACTIONS

There are no known drug interactions.

HOW SUPPLIED

Robinul® (glycopyrrolate, 1 mg) tablets in bottles of 100 (NDC 0031-7824-63).

Robinul® Forte (glycopyrrolate, 2 mg) tablets in bottles of 100 (NDC 0031-7840-63).

Store at controlled room temperature, 20°-25°C (68°-77°F). Dispense in tight container.

Manufactured by:
Pharmaceutical Division
A.H. Robins Company
Richmond, VA 23220

Shown in Product Identification Guide, page 334

ROBINUL® INJECTABLE ℞
[ro 'bĭ-nul]
(Glycopyrrolate Injection, USP)

DESCRIPTION

Robinul (glycopyrrolate) is a synthetic anticholinergic agent. Each 1 mL contains:

Glycopyrrolate, USP .... 0.2 mg
Water for Injection, USP .... q.s.
Benzyl Alcohol, NF (preservative) 0.9%
pH adjusted, when necessary, with hydrochloric acid and/or sodium hydroxide.

For Intramuscular or Intravenous administration.

Glycopyrrolate is a quaternary ammonium compound with the following chemical name:

3[(cyclopentylhydroxyphenylacetyl)oxy]-1,1-dimethyl pyrrolidinium bromide.

Unlike atropine, glycopyrrolate is completely ionized at physiological pH values.

Robinul Injectable is a clear, colorless, sterile liquid; pH 2.0–3.0.

CLINICAL PHARMACOLOGY

Glycopyrrolate, like other anticholinergic (antimuscarinic) agents, inhibits the action of acetylcholine on structures innervated by postganglionic cholinergic nerves and on smooth muscles that respond to acetylcholine but lack cholinergic innervation. These peripheral cholinergic receptors are present in the autonomic effector cells of smooth muscle, cardiac muscle, the sinoatrial node, the atrioventricular node, exocrine glands, and, to a limited degree, in the autonomic ganglia. Thus, it diminishes the volume and free acidity of gastric secretions and controls excessive pharyngeal, tracheal, and bronchial secretions.

Glycopyrrolate antagonizes muscarinic symptoms (e.g., bronchorrhea, bronchospasm, bradycardia, and intestinal hypermotility) induced by cholinergic drugs such as the anticholinesterases.

The highly polar quaternary ammonium group of glycopyrrolate limits its passage across lipid membranes, such as the blood-brain barrier, in contrast to atropine sulfate and scopolamine hydrobromide, which are non-polar tertiary amines which penetrate lipid barriers easily.

Peak effects occur approximately 30 to 45 minutes after intramuscular administration. The vagal blocking effects persist for 2 to 3 hours and the antisialagogue effects persist up to 7 hours, periods longer than for atropine. With intravenous injection, the onset of action is generally evident within one minute.

INDICATIONS AND USAGE

In Anesthesia: Robinul (glycopyrrolate) Injectable is indicated for use as a preoperative antimuscarinic to reduce salivary, tracheobronchial, and pharyngeal secretions; to reduce the volume and free acidity of gastric secretions; and, to block cardiac vagal inhibitory reflexes during induction of anesthesia and intubation. When indicated, Robinul Injectable may be used intraoperatively to counteract drug-induced or vagal traction reflexes with the associated arrhythmias. Glycopyrrolate protects against the peripheral muscarinic effects (e.g., bradycardia and excessive secretions) of cholinergic agents such as neostigmine and pyridostigmine given to reverse the neuromuscular blockade due to nondepolarizing muscle relaxants.

In Peptic Ulcer: For use in adults as adjunctive therapy for the treatment of peptic ulcer when rapid anticholinergic effect is desired or when oral medication is not tolerated.

CONTRAINDICATIONS

Known hypersensitivity to glycopyrrolate.

Due to its benzyl alcohol content, Robinul Injectable should not be used in newborns (children less than 1 month of age). In addition, in the management of *peptic ulcer* patients, because of the longer duration of therapy, Robinul Injectable may be contraindicated in patients with concurrent glaucoma; obstructive uropathy (for example, bladder neck obstruction due to prostatic hypertrophy); obstructive disease of the gastrointestinal tract (as in achalasia, pyloroduodenal stenosis, etc.); paralytic ileus; intestinal atony of the elderly or debilitated patient; unstable cardiovascular status in acute hemorrhage; severe ulcerative colitis; toxic megacolon complicating ulcerative colitis; myasthenia gravis.

WARNINGS

This drug should be used with great caution, if at all, in patients with glaucoma or asthma.

In the ambulatory patient. Robinul (glycopyrrolate) may produce drowsiness or blurred vision. The patient should be cautioned regarding activities requiring mental alertness such as operating a motor vehicle or other machinery or performing hazardous work while taking this drug.

In addition, in the presence of a high environmental temperature, heat prostration (fever and heat stroke due to decreased sweating) can occur with use of Robinul (glycopyrrolate).

Diarrhea may be an early symptom of incomplete intestinal obstruction, especially in patients with ileostomy or colostomy. In this instance treatment with Robinul (glycopyrrolate) would be inappropriate and possibly harmful.

PRECAUTIONS

General

Investigate any tachycardia before giving glycopyrrolate since an increase in the heart rate may occur.

Use with caution in patients with: coronary artery disease; congestive heart failure; cardiac arrhythmias; hypertension; hyperthyroidism.

In managing ulcer patients, use Robinul with caution in the elderly and in all patients with autonomic neuropathy, hepatic or renal disease, ulcerative colitis or hiatal hernia, since anticholinergic drugs may aggravate these conditions. With overdosage, a curare-like action may occur.

Drug Interactions

The intravenous administration of any anticholinergic in the presence of cyclopropane anesthesia can result in ventricular arrhythmias; therefore, caution should be observed if Robinul (glycopyrrolate) Injectable is used during cyclo-

Continued on next page

Robinul Injectable—Cont.

propane anesthesia. If the drug is given in small incremental doses of 0.1 mg or less, the likelihood of producing ventricular arrhythmias is reduced.

Carcinogenesis, Mutagenesis, Impairment of Fertility

Long-term studies in animals have not been performed to evaluate carcinogenic potential. In the teratology studies, diminished rates of conception and of survival at weaning were observed in rats, in a dose-related manner. Studies in dogs suggest that this may be due to diminished seminal secretion which is evident at high doses of glycopyrrolate.

Pregnancy Category B

Reproduction studies have been performed in rats and rabbits up to 1000 times the human dose and have revealed no teratogenic effects from glycopyrrolate. There are, however, no adequate and well-controlled studies in pregnant women. Because animal reproduction studies are not always predictive of human response, this drug should be used during pregnancy only if clearly needed.

Nursing Mothers

It is not known whether this drug is excreted in human milk. Because many drugs are excreted in human milk, caution should be exercised when Robinul is administered to a nursing woman.

Pediatric Use

Safety and effectiveness in children below the age of 12 years have not been established for the management of peptic ulcer.

ADVERSE REACTIONS

Anticholinergics produce certain effects, most of which are extensions of their pharmacologic actions. Adverse reactions to anticholinergics in general may include dry mouth; urinary hesitancy and retention; blurred vision due to mydriasis; increased ocular tension; tachycardia; palpitation; decreased sweating; loss of taste; headache; nervousness; drowsiness; weakness; dizziness; insomnia; nausea; vomiting; impotence; suppression of lactation; constipation; bloated feeling; severe allergic reaction or drug idiosyncrasies including anaphylaxis; urticaria and other dermal manifestations; some degree of mental confusion and/or excitement, especially in elderly persons.

Robinul is chemically a quaternary ammonium compound; hence, its passage across lipid membranes, such as the blood-brain barrier is limited in contrast to atropine sulfate and scopolamine hydrobromide. For this reason the occurrence of CNS related side effects is lower, in comparison to their incidence following administration of anticholinergics which are chemically tertiary amines that can cross this barrier readily.

OVERDOSAGE

To combat peripheral anticholinergic effects, a quaternary ammonium anticholinesterase such as neostigmine methylsulfate (which does not cross the blood-brain barrier) may be given intravenously in increments of 0.25 mg in adults. This dosage may be repeated every five to ten minutes until anticholinergic overactivity is reversed or up to a maximum of 2.5 mg. Proportionately smaller doses should be used in children. Indication for repetitive doses of neostigmine should be based on close monitoring of the decrease in heart rate and the return of bowel sounds.

In the unlikely event that CNS symptoms (excitement, restlessness, convulsions, psychotic behavior) occur, physostigmine (which does cross the blood-brain barrier) should be used. Physostigmine 0.5 to 2 mg should be slowly administered intravenously and repeated as necessary up to a total of 5 mg in adults. Proportionately smaller doses should be used in children.

Fever should be treated symptomatically. In the event of a curare-like effect on respiratory muscles, artificial respiration should be instituted and maintained until effective respiratory action returns.

DOSAGE AND ADMINISTRATION

Robinul (glycopyrrolate) Injectable may be administered intramuscularly, or intravenously, without dilution, in the following indications:

Adults: *Preanesthetic Medication.* The recommended dose of Robinul (glycopyrrolate) Injectable is 0.002 mg (0.01 mL) per pound of body weight by intramuscular injection, given 30 to 60 minutes prior to the anticipated time of induction of anesthesia or at the time the preanesthetic narcotic and/or sedative are administered.

Intraoperative Medication. Robinul (glycopyrrolate) Injectable may be used during surgery to counteract drug induced or vagal traction reflexes with the associated arrhythmias (e.g., bradycardia). It should be administered intravenously as single doses of 0.1 mg (0.5 mL) and repeated, as needed, at intervals of 2–3 minutes. The usual attempts should be made to determine the etiology of the arrhythmia, and the surgical or anesthetic manipulations necessary to correct parasympathetic imbalance should be performed.

Reversal of Neuromuscular Blockade. The recommended dose of Robinul (glycopyrrolate) Injectable is 0.2 mg (1.0 mL) for each 1.0 mg of neostigmine or 5.0 mg of pyridostigmine. In order to minimize the appearance of cardiac side effects, the drugs may be administered simultaneously by intravenous injection and may be mixed in the same syringe.

Children: (Read Contraindications). *Preanesthetic Medication.* The recommended dose of Robinul (glycopyrrolate) Injectable in children 1 month to 12 years of age is 0.002 mg (0.01 mL) per pound of body weight intramuscularly, given 30 to 60 minutes prior to the anticipated time of induction of anesthesia or at the time the preanesthetic narcotic and/or sedative are administered.

Children 1 month to 2 years of age may require up to 0.004 mg (0.02 mL) per pound of body weight.

Intraoperative Medication. Because of the long duration of action of Robinul (glycopyrrolate) if used as preanesthetic medication, additional Robinul (glycopyrrolate) Injectable for anticholinergic effect intraoperatively is rarely needed; in the event it is required the recommended pediatric dose is 0.002 mg (0.01 mL) per pound of body weight intravenously, not to exceed 0.1 mg (0.5 mL) in a single dose which may be repeated, as needed, at intervals of 2–3 minutes. The usual attempts should be made to determine the etiology of the arrhythmia, and the surgical or anesthetic manipulations necessary to correct parasympathetic imbalance should be performed.

Reversal of Neuromuscular Blockade. The recommended pediatric dose of Robinul (glycopyrrolate) Injectable is 0.2 mg (1.0 mL) for each 1.0 mg of neostigmine or 5.0 mg of pyridostigmine. In order to minimize the appearance of cardiac side effects, the drugs may be administered simultaneously by intravenous injection and may be mixed in the same syringe.

Adults: *Peptic Ulcer.* The usual recommended dose of Robinul Injectable is 0.1 mg (0.5 mL) administered at 4-hour intervals, 3 or 4 times daily intravenously or intramuscularly. Where more profound effect is required, 0.2 mg (1.0 mL) may be given. Some patients may need only a single dose, and frequency of administration should be dictated by patient response up to a maximum of four times daily.

Robinul Injectable is not recommended for peptic ulcers in children under 12 years of age. (See Precautions.)

NOTE: Parenteral drug products should be inspected visually for particulate matter and discoloration prior to administration whenever solution and container permit.

Admixture Compatibilities. Robinul (glycopyrrolate) Injectable is compatible for mixing and injection with the following injectable dosage forms: 5% and 10% glucose in water or saline; atropine sulfate, USP; Antilirium® (physostigmine salicylate); Benadryl® (diphenhydramine HCl); codeine phosphate, USP; Emete-Con® (benzquinamide HCl); hydromorphone HCl, USP; Inapsine® (droperidol); Innovar® (droperidol and fentanyl citrate); Largon® (propiomazine HCl); Levo-Dromoran® (levorphanol tartrate); lidocaine, USP; Mepergan® (meperidine and promethazine HCls); meperidine HCl, USP; Mestinon® /Regonol® (pyridostigmine bromide); morphine sulfate, USP; Nisentil® (alphaprodine HCl); Nubain® (nalbuphine HCl); Numorphan® (oxymorphone HCl); Pantopon® (opium alkaloids HCls); procaine HCl, USP; promethazine HCl, USP; Prostigmin® (neostigmine methylsulfate, USP); scopolamine HBr, USP; Sparine® (promazine HCl); Stadol® (butorphanol tartrate); Sublimaze® (fentanyl citrate); Talwin® (pentazocine lactate); Tigan® (trimethobenzamide HCl); Vesprin® (triflupromazine HCl); and Vistaril® (hydroxyzine HCl). Robinul Injectable may be administered via the tubing of a running infusion of physiological saline or lactated Ringer's solution. Since the stability of glycopyrrolate is questionable above a pH of 6.0, do *not* combine Robinul Injectable in the same syringe with Brevital® (methohexital Na); Chloromycetin® (chloramphenicol Na succinate); Dramamine® (dimenhydrinate); Nembutal® (pentobarbital Na); Pentothal® (thiopental Na); Seconal® (secobarbital Na); sodium bicarbonate (Abbott); or Valium® (diazepam). A gas will evolve or a precipitate may form. Mixing with Decadron® (dexamethasone Na phosphate) or a buffered solution of lactated Ringer's solution will result in a pH higher than 6.0. Mixing chlorpromazine HCl, USP, or Compazine® (prochlorperazine) with other agents in a syringe is not recommended by the manufacturer, although the mixture with Robinul Injectable is physically compatible.

HOW SUPPLIED

Robinul (glycopyrrolate) Injectable, 0.2 mg/mL, is available in 1 mL single dose vials packaged in 25's (NDC 0031-7890-11), 2 mL single dose vials packaged in 25's (NDC 0031-7890-95), 5 mL multiple dose vials packaged in 25's (NDC 0031-7890-06), and 20 mL (NDC 0031-7890-83) multiple dose vials.

Store at controlled room temperature, between 20°C and 25°C (68°F and 77°F).

Manufactured by:
Pharmaceutical Division
A. H. Robins Company
Richmond, VA 23220

Shown in Product Identification Guide, page 334

ROBITUSSIN A–C® Ⓒ

[ro "bĭ-tuss 'ĭn]

Expectorant
Cough Suppressant
Sugar-Free

Robitussin and Codeine

Each 5 mL (1 teaspoonful) contains:

Guaifenesin, USP	100 mg
Codeine Phosphate, USP	10 mg
(Warning: May be habit forming)	

Alcohol 3.5 percent

In a palatable, aromatic syrup

Inactive Ingredients: Caramel, Citric Acid, FD&C Red 40, Flavors, Glycerin, Saccharin Sodium, Sodium Benzoate, Sorbitol, Water.

ACTIONS

Robitussin A-C combines the expectorant, guaifenesin, with the cough suppressant, codeine. Guaifenesin enhances the output of lower respiratory tract fluid. The enhanced flow of less viscid secretions promotes and facilitates the removal of mucus. Codeine is a centrally acting agent which elevates the threshold for cough.

As a result, dry, unproductive coughs become more productive and less frequent.

Under Federal law, Robitussin A-C is available without a prescription. Certain state laws may differ. The container label contains the following indications, warnings and drug interaction precaution statements and directions:

INDICATIONS

Temporarily controls cough due to minor throat and bronchial irritation as may occur with the common cold or inhaled irritants. Helps loosen phlegm (mucus) and thin bronchial secretions to make coughs more productive.

WARNINGS

A persistent cough may be a sign of a serious condition. If cough persists for more than 1 week, tends to recur, or is accompanied by fever, rash, or persistent headache, consult a doctor. Do not take this product for persistent or chronic cough such as occurs with smoking, asthma, chronic bronchitis, emphysema, or if cough is accompanied by excessive phlegm (mucus) unless directed by a doctor. Adults and children who have a chronic pulmonary disease or shortness of breath, or children who are taking other drugs, should not take this product unless directed by a doctor. May cause or aggravate constipation. As with any drug, if you are pregnant or nursing a baby, seek the advice of a health professional before using this product.

PROFESSIONAL NOTE: Guaifenesin has been shown to produce a color interference with certain clinical laboratory determinations of 5-hydroxyindoleacetic acid (5-HIAA) and vanillylmandelic acid (VMA).

DRUG INTERACTION PRECAUTION

Caution should be used when taking this product with sedatives, tranquilizers and drugs used for depression, especially monoamine oxidase inhibitors (MAOIs). These combinations may cause greater sedation (drowsiness) than is caused by the products used alone.

DIRECTIONS

Take orally as stated below or use as directed by a doctor. Adults and children 12 years of age and over: 2 teaspoonfuls every 4 hours, not to exceed 12 teaspoonfuls in a 24-hour period; children 6 to under 12 years: 1 teaspoonful every 4 hours, not to exceed 6 teaspoonfuls in a 24-hour period; children under 6 years: consult a doctor. A special measuring device should be used to give an accurate dose of this product to children under 6 years of age. Giving a higher dose than recommended by a doctor could result in serious side effects for a child. Use of codeine-containing preparations is not recommended for children under 2 years of age. Do not exceed recommended dosage.

HOW SUPPLIED

Bottles of 4 fl. oz. (NDC 0031-8674-12), pints (NDC 0031-8674-25), and gallons (NDC 0031-8674-29).

Manufactured by:
Pharmaceutical Division
A.H. Robins Company
Richmond, VA 23220

ROBITUSSIN® –DAC Ⓒ

[ro "bĭ-tuss 'ĭn]

Expectorant
Nasal Decongestant
Cough-Suppressant
Sugar-Free

Each 5 mL (1 teaspoonful) contains:

Guaifenesin, USP	100 mg
Pseudoephedrine Hydrochloride, USP	30 mg
Codeine Phosphate, USP	10 mg
(Warning: May be habit forming)	

In a palatable, aromatic syrup
Alcohol 1.9 percent
Inactive Ingredients: Caramel, Citric Acid, FD&C Red 40, Flavors, Glycerin, Saccharin Sodium, Sodium Benzoate, Sorbitol, Water.

ACTIONS

Robitussin-DAC combines the expectorant, guaifenesin, the nasal decongestant, pseudoephedrine, and the cough suppressant, codeine. Guaifenesin enhances the output of lower respiratory tract fluid. The enhanced flow of less viscid secretions promotes and facilitates the removal of mucus. Codeine is a centrally acting agent which elevates the threshold for cough. As a result, dry, unproductive coughs become more productive and less frequent. The nasal decongestant, pseudoephedrine, reduces the swelling of nasal passages.
Under Federal law, Robitussin-DAC is available without a prescription. Certain state laws may differ. The container label contains the following indications, warnings and drug interaction precaution statements and directions:

INDICATIONS

Temporarily relieves nasal congestion and controls cough due to minor throat and bronchial irritation as may occur with the common cold or inhaled irritants. Temporarily restores freer breathing through the nose. Helps loosen phlegm (mucus) and thin bronchial secretions to make coughs more productive.

WARNINGS

A persistent cough may be a sign of a serious condition. If cough persists for more than 1 week, tends to recur, or is accompanied by fever, rash, or persistent headache, consult a doctor. Do not take this product for persistent or chronic cough such as occurs with smoking, asthma, chronic bronchitis, emphysema, or if cough is accompanied by excessive phlegm (mucus) unless directed by a doctor. Adults and children who have a chronic pulmonary disease or shortness of breath, or children who are taking other drugs, should not take this product unless directed by a doctor. Do not take this product if you have high blood pressure, heart disease, diabetes or thyroid disease, except under the advice and supervision of a doctor. Do not exceed recommended dosage because at higher doses nervousness, dizziness or sleeplessness may occur. May cause or aggravate constipation. As with any drug, if you are pregnant or nursing a baby, seek the advice of a health professional before using this product.
PROFESSIONAL NOTE: Guaifenesin has been shown to produce a color interference with certain clinical laboratory determinations of 5-hydroxyindoleacetic acid (5-HIAA) and vanillylmandelic acid (VMA).

DRUG INTERACTION PRECAUTION

Do not take this product if you are presently taking a prescription drug for high blood pressure or depression, especially monoamine oxidase inhibitors (MAOIs), without first consulting your doctor.

DIRECTIONS

Take orally as stated below or use as directed by a doctor.
Adults and children 12 years of age and over: 2 teaspoonfuls every 4 hours, not to exceed 8 teaspoonfuls in a 24-hour period; children 6 to under 12 years: 1 teaspoonful every 4 hours, not to exceed 4 teaspoonfuls in a 24-hour period; children under 6 years: consult a doctor. A special measuring device should be used to give an accurate dose of this product to children under 6 years of age. Giving a higher dose than recommended by a doctor could result in serious side effects for a child. Use of codeine-containing preparations is not recommended for children under 2 years of age. Do not exceed recommended dosage.

HOW SUPPLIED

Bottles of 4 fl. oz. (NDC 0031-8680-12) and one pint (NDC 0031-8680-25).
Manufactured by:
Pharmaceutical Division
A.H. Robins Company
Richmond, VA 23220

TENEX® ℞
[ten 'ex]
(Guanfacine Hydrochloride)
Tablets

DESCRIPTION

Tenex (guanfacine hydrochloride) is a centrally acting antihypertensive with α_2-adrenoceptor agonist properties in tablet form for oral administration.
The chemical name of Tenex (guanfacine hydrochloride) is N-amidino-2-(2,6-dichlorophenyl) acetamide hydrochloride and its molecular weight is 282.56.
Guanfacine hydrochloride is a white to off-white powder; sparingly soluble in water and alcohol and slightly soluble in acetone. The tablets contain the following inactive ingredients:

Mean Changes (mm Hg) from Baseline in Seated Systolic and Diastolic Blood Pressure for Patients Completing 4 to 8 Weeks of Treatment with Guanfacine Monotherapy

Mean Change S/D* Seated	n = (range)	Placebo	0.5 mg	1 mg	2 mg	3 mg	5 mg
White Patients	11–30	–1/–5	–6/–8	–8/–9	–12/–11	–15/–12	–18/–16
Black Patients	8–28	–3/–5	0/–2	–3/–5	–7/–7	–8/–9	–19/–15

* S/D = Systolic/diastolic blood pressure.

Mean Decreases (mm Hg) in Seated and Standing Blood Pressure for Patients Treated with Guanfacine in Combination with Chlorthalidone

Mean Change	n =	Placebo 63	0.5 mg 63	1 mg 64	2 mg 58	3 mg 59
S/D* Seated		–5/–7	–5/–6	–14/–13	–12/–13	–16/–13
S/D* Standing		–3/–5	–5/–4	–11/–9	–9/–10	–15/–12

* S/D = Systolic/diastolic blood pressure

1 mg—FD&C Red 40 aluminum lake, lactose, microcrystalline cellulose, povidone, stearic acid.
2 mg—D&C Yellow 10 aluminum lake, lactose, microcrystalline cellulose, povidone, stearic acid.

CLINICAL PHARMACOLOGY

Tenex (guanfacine hydrochloride) is an orally active antihypertensive agent whose principal mechanism of action appears to be stimulation of central α_2-adrenergic receptors. By stimulating these receptors, guanfacine reduces sympathetic nerve impulses from the vasomotor center to the heart and blood vessels. This results in a decrease in peripheral vascular resistance and a reduction in heart rate.
The dose-response relationship for blood pressure and adverse effects of guanfacine given once a day as monotherapy has been evaluated in patients with mild to moderate hypertension. In this study patients were randomized to placebo or to 0.5 mg, 1 mg, 2 mg, 3 mg, or 5 mg of Tenex. Results are shown in the following table. A useful effect was not observed overall until doses of 2 mg were reached, although responses in white patients were seen at 1 mg; 24 hour effectiveness of 1 mg to 3 mg doses was documented using 24 hour ambulatory monitoring. While the 5 mg dose added an increment of effectiveness, it caused an unacceptable increase in adverse reactions.
[See first table above]
Controlled clinical trials in patients with mild to moderate hypertension who were receiving a thiazide-type diuretic have defined the dose-response relationship for blood pressure response and adverse reactions of guanfacine given at bedtime and have shown that the blood pressure response to guanfacine can persist for 24 hours after a single dose. In the 12-week, placebo-controlled dose-response study, patients were randomized to placebo or to doses of 0.5, 1, 2, and 3 mg of guanfacine, in addition to 25 mg chlorthalidone, each given at bedtime. The observed mean changes from baseline, tabulated below, indicate the similarity of response for placebo and the 0.5 mg dose. Doses of 1, 2, and 3 mg resulted in decreased blood pressure in the sitting position with no real differences among the three doses. In the standing position there was some increase in response with dose.
[See second table above]
While most of the effectiveness of guanfacine in combination (and as monotherapy in white patients) was present at 1 mg, adverse reactions at this dose were not clearly distinguishable from those associated with placebo. Adverse reactions were clearly present at 2 and 3 mg (see **Adverse Reactions**).
In a second 12-week, placebo-controlled study of 1, 2 or 3 mg of Tenex (guanfacine hydrochloride) administered with 25 mg of chlorthalidone once daily, a significant decrease in blood pressure was maintained for a full 24 hours after dosing. While there was no significant difference between the 12 and 24 hour blood pressure readings, the fall in blood pressure at 24 hours was numerically smaller, suggesting possible escape of blood pressure in some patients and the need for individualization of therapy.
In a double-blind, randomized trial, either guanfacine or clonidine was given at recommended doses with 25 mg chlorthalidone for 24 weeks and then abruptly discontinued. Results showed equal degrees of blood pressure reduction with the two drugs and there was no tendency for blood pressures to increase despite maintenance of the same daily dose of the two drugs. Signs and symptoms of rebound phenomena were infrequent upon discontinuation of either drug. Abrupt withdrawal of clonidine produced a rapid return of diastolic and especially, systolic blood pressure to approximately pretreatment levels, with occasional values significantly greater than baseline, whereas guanfacine withdrawal produced a more gradual increase to pretreatment levels, but also with occasional values significantly greater than baseline.

PHARMACODYNAMICS
Hemodynamic studies in man showed that the decrease in blood pressure observed after single-dose or long-term oral treatment with guanfacine was accompanied by a significant decrease in peripheral resistance and a slight reduction in heart rate (5 beats/min). Cardiac output under conditions of rest or exercise was not altered by guanfacine.
Tenex (guanfacine hydrochloride) lowered elevated plasma renin activity and plasma catecholamine levels in hypertensive patients, but this does not correlate with individual blood-pressure responses.
Growth hormone secretion was stimulated with single oral doses of 2 and 4 mg of guanfacine. Long-term use of Tenex had no effect on growth hormone levels.
Guanfacine had no effect on plasma aldosterone. A slight but insignificant decrease in plasma volume occurred after one month of guanfacine therapy. There were no changes in mean body weight or electrolytes.
PHARMACOKINETICS
Relative to an intravenous dose of 3 mg, the absolute oral bioavailability of guanfacine is about 80%. Peak plasma concentrations occur from 1 to 4 hours with an average of 2.6 hours after single oral doses or at steady state.
The area under the concentration-time curve (AUC) increases linearly with the dose.
In individuals with normal renal function, the average elimination half-life is approximately 17 hr (range 10–30 hr). Younger patients tend to have shorter elimination half-lives (13–14 hr) while older patients tend to have half-lives at the upper end of the range. Steady state blood levels were attained within 4 days in most subjects.
In individuals with normal renal function, guanfacine and its metabolites are excreted primarily in the urine. Approximately 50% (40–75%) of the dose is eliminated in the urine as unchanged drug; the remainder is eliminated mostly as conjugates of metabolites produced by oxidative metabolism of the aromatic ring.
The guanfacine-to-creatinine clearance ratio is greater than 1.0, which would suggest that tubular secretion of drug occurs.
The drug is approximately 70% bound to plasma proteins, independent of drug concentration.
The whole body volume of distribution is high (a mean of 6.3 L/kg), which suggests a high distribution of drug to the tissues.
The clearance of guanfacine in patients with varying degrees of renal insufficiency is reduced, but plasma levels of drug are only slightly increased compared to patients with normal renal function. When prescribing for patients with renal impairment, the low end of the dosing range should be used. Patients on dialysis also can be given usual doses of guanfacine hydrochloride as the drug is poorly dialyzed.

INDICATIONS AND USAGE

Tenex (guanfacine hydrochloride) is indicated in the management of hypertension. Tenex may be given alone or in combination with other antihypertensive agents, especially thiazide-type diuretics.

CONTRAINDICATIONS

Tenex is contraindicated in patients with known hypersensitivity to guanfacine hydrochloride.

PRECAUTIONS

GENERAL
Like other antihypertensive agents, Tenex (guanfacine hydrochloride) should be used with caution in patients with severe coronary insufficiency, recent myocardial infarction, cerebrovascular disease or chronic renal or hepatic failure.
SEDATION
Tenex, like other orally active central α-2-adrenergic agonists, causes sedation or drowsiness, especially when beginning therapy. These symptoms are dose-related (see Ad-

Continued on next page

Tenex—Cont.

Adverse Reaction	Placebo n=73		0.5 mg n=72		1 mg n=72		2 mg n=72		3 mg n=72	
Dry Mouth	5	(7%)	4	(5%)	6	(8%)	8	(11%)	20	(28%)
Somnolence	1	(1%)	3	(4%)	0	(0%)	1	(1%)	10	(14%)
Asthenia	0	(0%)	2	(3%)	0	(0%)	2	(2%)	7	(10%)
Dizziness	2	(2%)	1	(1%)	3	(4%)	6	(8%)	3	(4%)
Headache	3	(4%)	4	(3%)	3	(4%)	1	(1%)	2	(2%)
Impotence	1	(1%)	1	(0%)	0	(0%)	1	(1%)	3	(4%)
Constipation	0	(0%)	0	(0%)	0	(0%)	1	(1%)	1	(1%)
Fatigue	3	(3%)	2	(3%)	2	(3%)	5	(6%)	3	(4%)

verse Reactions). When Tenex is used with other centrally active depressants (such as phenothiazines, barbiturates, or benzodiazepines), the potential for additive sedative effects should be considered.

REBOUND
Abrupt cessation of therapy with orally active central α-2 adrenergic agonists may be associated with increases (from depressed on-therapy levels) in plasma and urinary catecholamines, symptoms of "nervousness and anxiety" and, less commonly, increases in blood pressure to levels significantly greater than those prior to therapy.

INFORMATION FOR PATIENTS
Patients who receive Tenex should be advised to exercise caution when operating dangerous machinery or driving motor vehicles until it is determined that they do not become drowsy or dizzy from the medication. Patients should be warned that their tolerance for alcohol and other CNS depressants may be diminished. Patients should be advised not to discontinue therapy abruptly.

LABORATORY TESTS
In clinical trials, no clinically relevant laboratory test abnormalities were identified as causally related to drug during short-term treatment with Tenex (guanfacine hydrochloride).

DRUG INTERACTIONS
The potential for increased sedation when Tenex is given with other CNS-depressant drugs should be appreciated.
The administration of guanfacine concomitantly with a known microsomal enzyme inducer (phenobarbital or phenytoin) to two patients with renal impairment reportedly resulted in significant reductions in elimination half-life and plasma concentration. In such cases, therefore, more frequent dosing may be required to achieve or maintain the desired hypotensive response. Further, if guanfacine is to be discontinued in such patients, careful tapering of the dosage may be necessary in order to avoid rebound phenomena (see Rebound above).

ANTICOAGULANTS
Ten patients who were stabilized on oral anticoagulants were given guanfacine, 1–2 mg/day, for 4 weeks. No changes were observed in the degree of anticoagulation.
In several well-controlled studies, guanfacine was administered together with diuretics with no drug interactions reported. In the long-term safety studies, Tenex was given concomitantly with many drugs without evidence of any interactions. The principal drugs given (number of patients in parentheses) were: cardiac glycosides (115), sedatives and hypnotics (103), coronary vasodilators (52), oral hypoglycemics (45), cough and cold preparations (45), NSAIDs (38), antihyperlipidemics (29), antigout drugs (24), oral contraceptives (18), bronchodilators (13), insulin (10), and beta blockers (10).

DRUG/LABORATORY TEST INTERACTIONS
No laboratory test abnormalities related to the use of Tenex (guanfacine hydrochloride) have been identified.

CARCINOGENESIS, MUTAGENESIS, IMPAIRMENT OF FERTILITY
No carcinogenic effect was observed in studies of 78 weeks in mice at doses more than 150 times the maximum recommended human dose and 102 weeks in rats at doses more than 100 times the maximum recommended human dose. In a variety of test models, guanfacine was not mutagenic.
No adverse effects were observed in fertility studies in male and female rats.

PREGNANCY CATEGORY B
Administration of guanfacine to rats at 70 times the maximum recommended human dose and to rabbits at 20 times the maximum recommended human dose resulted in no evidence of harm to the fetus. Higher doses (100 and 200 times the maximum recommended human dose in rabbits and rats respectively) were associated with reduced fetal survival and maternal toxicity. Rat experiments have shown that guanfacine crosses the placenta.
There are, however, no adequate and well-controlled studies in pregnant women. Because animal reproduction studies are not always predictive of human response, this drug should be used during pregnancy only if clearly needed.

LABOR AND DELIVERY
Tenex (guanfacine hydrochloride) is not recommended in the treatment of acute hypertension associated with toxemia of pregnancy. There is no information available on the effects of guanfacine on the course of labor and delivery.

NURSING MOTHERS
It is not known whether Tenex (guanfacine hydrochloride) is excreted in human milk. Because many drugs are excreted in human milk, caution should be exercised when Tenex is administered to a nursing woman. Experiments with rats have shown that guanfacine is excreted in the milk.

PEDIATRIC USE
Safety and effectiveness in children under 12 years of age have not been demonstrated. Therefore, the use of Tenex in this age group is not recommended.

ADVERSE REACTIONS
Adverse reactions noted with Tenex (guanfacine hydrochloride) are similar to those of other drugs of the central α–2 adrenoreceptor agonist class: dry mouth, sedation (somnolence), weakness (asthenia), dizziness, constipation, and impotence. While the reactions are common, most are mild and tend to disappear on continued dosing.
Skin rash with exfoliation has been reported in a few cases; although clear cause and effect relationships to Tenex could not be established, should a rash occur, Tenex should be discontinued and the patient monitored appropriately.
In the dose-response monotherapy study described under **Clinical Pharmacology**, the frequency of the most commonly observed adverse reactions showed a dose relationship from 0.5 to 3 mg as follows:
[See table at bottom of page]
The percent of patients who dropped out because of adverse reactions are shown below for each dosage group.

	Placebo	0.5 mg	1 mg	2 mg	3 mg
Percent dropouts	0%	2.0%	5.0%	13%	32%

The most common reasons for dropouts among patients who received guanfacine were dry mouth, somnolence, dizziness, fatigue, weakness, and constipation.
In the 12-week, placebo-controlled, dose-response study of guanfacine administered with 25 mg chlorthalidone at bedtime, the frequency of the most commonly observed adverse reactions showed a clear dose relationship from 0.5 to 3 mg as follows:
[See table at top of page]
There were 41 premature terminations because of adverse reactions in this study. The percent of patients who dropped out and the dose at which the dropout occurred were as follows:

Dose:	Placebo	0.5 mg	1 mg	2 mg	3 mg
Percent dropouts	6.9%	4.2%	3.2%	6.9%	8.3%

Reasons for dropouts among patients who received guanfacine were: somnolence, headache, weakness, dry mouth, dizziness, impotence, insomnia, constipation, syncope, urinary incontinence, conjunctivitis, paresthesia, and dermatitis.
In a second 12-week placebo-controlled combination therapy study in which the dose could be adjusted upward to 3 mg per day in 1-mg increments at 3-week intervals, i.e., a setting more similar to ordinary clinical use, the most commonly recorded adverse reactions were: dry mouth, 47%; constipation, 16%; fatigue, 12%; somnolence, 10%; asthenia, 6%; dizziness, 6%; headache, 4%; and insomnia, 4%.
Reasons for dropouts among patients who received guanfacine were: somnolence, dry mouth, dizziness, impotence, constipation, confusion, depression, and palpitations.

In the clonidine/guanfacine comparison described in Clinical Pharmacology, the most common adverse reactions noted were as follows:

Adverse Reactions	Guanfacine (n = 279)	Clonidine (n = 278)
Dry mouth	30%	37%
Somnolence	21%	35%
Dizziness	11%	8%
Constipation	10%	5%
Fatigue	9%	8%
Headache	4%	4%
Insomnia	4%	3%

Adverse reactions occurring in 3% or less of patients in the three controlled trials of Tenex with a diuretic were:

Cardiovascular—	bradycardia, palpitations, substernal pain
Gastrointestinal—	abdominal pain, diarrhea, dyspepsia, dysphagia, nausea
CNS—	amnesia, confusion, depression, insomnia, libido decrease
ENT disorders—	rhinitis, taste perversion, tinnitus
Eye disorders—	conjunctivitis, iritis, vision disturbance
Musculoskeletal—	leg cramps, hypokinesia
Respiratory—	dyspnea
Dermatologic—	dermatitis, pruritus, purpura, sweating
Urogenital—	testicular disorder, urinary incontinence
Other—	malaise, paresthesia, paresis

Adverse reaction reports tend to decrease over time. In an open-label trial of one year's duration, 580 hypertensive subjects were given guanfacine, titrated to achieve goal blood pressure, alone (51%), with diuretic (38%), with beta blocker (3%), with diuretic plus beta blocker (6%), or with diuretic plus vasodilator (2%). The mean daily dose of guanfacine reached was 4.7 mg.

Adverse Reaction	Incidence of adverse reactions at any time during the study	Incidence of adverse reactions at the end of one year
	n=580	n=580
Dry mouth	60%	15%
Drowsiness	33%	6%
Dizziness	15%	1%
Constipation	14%	3%
Weakness	5%	1%
Headache	4%	0.2%
Insomnia	5%	0%

There were 52 (8.9%) dropouts due to adverse effects in this 1-year trial. The causes were: dry mouth (n = 20), weakness (n = 12), constipation (n = 7), somnolence (n = 3), nausea (n = 3), orthostatic hypotension (n = 2), insomnia (n = 1), rash (n = 1), nightmares (n = 1), headache (n = 1), and depression (n = 1).

POSTMARKETING EXPERIENCE
An open-label postmarketing study involving 21,718 patients was conducted to assess the safety of Tenex (guanfacine hydrochloride) 1 mg/day given at bedtime for 28 days. Tenex was administered with or without other antihypertensive agents. Adverse events reported in the postmarketing study at an incidence greater than 1% included dry mouth, dizziness, somnolence, fatigue, headache and nausea. The most commonly reported adverse events in this study were the same as those observed in controlled clinical trials.
Less frequent, possibly Tenex-related events observed in the postmarketing study and/or reported spontaneously include:

Adverse Reaction	Placebo n=59	0.5 mg n=60	1 mg n=61	2 mg n=60	3 mg n=59
Dry Mouth	0%	10%	10%	42%	54%
Somnolence	8%	5%	10%	13%	39%
Asthenia	0%	2%	3%	7%	3%
Dizziness	8%	12%	2%	8%	15%
Headache	8%	13%	7%	5%	3%
Impotence	0%	0%	0%	7%	3%
Constipation	0%	2%	0%	5%	15%
Fatigue	2%	2%	5%	8%	10%

BODY AS A WHOLE	asthenia, chest pain, edema, malaise, tremor
CARDIOVASCULAR	bradycardia, palpitations, syncope, tachycardia
CENTRAL NERVOUS SYSTEM	paresthesias, vertigo
EYE DISORDERS	blurred vision
GASTROINTESTINAL SYSTEM	abdominal pain, constipation, diarrhea, dyspepsia
LIVER AND BILIARY SYSTEM	abnormal liver function tests
MUSCULO-SKELETAL SYSTEM	arthralgia, leg cramps, leg pain, myalgia
PSYCHIATRIC	agitation, anxiety, confusion, depression, insomnia, nervousness
REPRODUCTIVE SYSTEM, MALE	impotence
RESPIRATORY SYSTEM	dyspnea
SKIN AND APPENDAGES	alopecia, dermatitis, exfoliative dermatitis, pruritus, rash
SPECIAL SENSES	alterations in taste
URINARY SYSTEM	nocturia, urinary frequency

Rare, serious disorders with no definitive cause and effect relationship to Tenex have been reported spontaneously and/or in the postmarketing study. These events include acute renal failure, cardiac fibrillation, cerebrovascular accident, congestive heart failure, heart block, and myocardial infarction.

Drug Abuse and Dependence
No reported abuse or dependence has been associated with the administration of Tenex (guanfacine hydrochloride).

OVERDOSAGE
SIGNS AND SYMPTOMS
Drowsiness, lethargy, bradycardia and hypotension have been observed following overdose with guanfacine.
A 25-year-old female intentionally ingested 60 mg. She presented with severe drowsiness and bradycardia of 45 beats/minute. Gastric lavage was performed and an infusion of isoproterenol (0.8 mg in 12 hours) was administered. She recovered quickly and without sequelae.
A 28-year-old female who ingested 30–40 mg developed only lethargy, was treated with activated charcoal and a cathartic, was monitored for 24 hours, and was discharged in good health.
A 2-year-old male weighing 12 kg, who ingested up to 4 mg of guanfacine, developed lethargy. Gastric lavage (followed by activated charcoal and sorbitol slurry via NG tube) removed some tablet fragments within 2 hours after ingestion, and vital signs were normal. During 24-hour observation in ICU, systolic pressure was 58 and heart rate 70 at 16 hours post-ingestion. No intervention was required, and the child was discharged fully recovered the next day.
TREATMENT OF OVERDOSAGE
Gastric lavage and supportive therapy as appropriate. Guanfacine is not dialyzable in clinically significant amounts (2.4%).

DOSAGE AND ADMINISTRATION
The recommended initial dose of Tenex (guanfacine hydrochloride) when given alone or in combination with another antihypertensive drug is 1 mg daily given at bedtime to minimize somnolence. If after 3 to 4 weeks of therapy, 1 mg does not give a satisfactory result, a dose of 2 mg may be given, although most of the effect of Tenex is seen at 1 mg (see **Clinical Pharmacology**). Higher daily doses have been used, but adverse reactions increase significantly with doses above 3 mg/day.
The frequency of rebound hypertension is low, but it can occur. When rebound occurs, it does so after 2–4 days, which is delayed compared with clonidine hydrochloride. This is consistent with the longer half-life of guanfacine. In most cases, after abrupt withdrawal of guanfacine, blood pressure returns to pretreatment levels slowly (within 2–4 days) without ill effects.

HOW SUPPLIED
Tenex® (guanfacine hydrochloride) Tablets are available in the following dosing stengths (expressed in equivalent amounts of guanfacine):
1 mg—light pink, diamond-shaped tablet embossed with a 1 and engraved AHR on one side and engraved TENEX on the other side in bottles of 100 (NDC 0031-8901-63) and 500 (NDC 0031-8901-70) and Dis-Co® Unit Dose Packs of 100 (NDC 0031-8901-64).
2 mg—yellow, diamond-shaped tablet, one side engraved TENEX, other side engraved 2 with AHR below it in bottles of 100 (NDC 0031-8903-63).
Store at controlled room temperature, between 20°C and 25°C (68°F and 77°F).
Dispense in tight, light-resistant container.

Manufactured by:
Pharmaceutical Division
A.H. Robins Company
Richmond, VA 23220
Shown in Product Identification Guide, page 334

Roche Pharmaceuticals

Roche Laboratories Inc.
340 Kingsland Street
Nutley, NJ 07110-1199

For Medical Information:
Write: Professional Product Information
Call: (800) 526-6367
In Emergencies: 24-hour service
Routine Inquiries: Press 1
Adverse Drug Events: Press 2
Product Complaints: Press 3
Medical Needs Program: Press 4

ACCUTANE®   ℞
[acc 'u-tane]
(isotretinoin)
CAPSULES

Avoid Pregnancy

The following text is complete product information based on official labeling in effect June 1998.

CONTRAINDICATION AND WARNING: Accutane must not be used by females who are pregnant or who may become pregnant while undergoing treatment. Although not every fetus exposed to Accutane has resulted in a deformed child, there is an extremely high risk that a deformed infant can result if pregnancy occurs while taking Accutane in any amount even for short periods of time. Potentially any fetus exposed during pregnancy can be affected. Presently, there is no accurate means of determining after Accutane exposure which fetus has been affected and which fetus has not been affected.

Accutane is contraindicated in females of childbearing potential unless the <u>patient meets all of the following conditions</u>:

- **has severe disfiguring nodular acne that is recalcitrant to standard therapies (see INDICATIONS AND USAGE section for definition)**
- **is reliable in understanding and carrying out instructions**
- **is capable of complying with the mandatory contraceptive measures**
- **has received both oral and written warnings of the hazards of taking Accutane during pregnancy and exposing a fetus to the drug**
- **has received both oral and written warnings of the risk of possible contraception failure and of the need to use two reliable forms of contraception simultaneously, unless abstinence is the chosen method, or the patient has undergone a hysterectomy and has acknowledged in writing her understanding of these warnings and of the need for using dual contraceptive methods**
- **has had a negative serum or urine pregnancy test with a sensitivity of at least 50 mIU/mL within 1 week prior to beginning therapy**
- **will begin therapy only on the second or third day of the next normal menstrual period**

It is also recommended that a prescription for Accutane should not be issued by the physician until a report of a negative pregnancy test has been obtained and the patient has begun her menstrual period. It is also recommended that pregnancy testing and contraception counseling be repeated on a monthly basis. To encourage compliance with this recommendation, the physician should prescribe no more than a 1 month supply of the drug.

Major human fetal abnormalities related to Accutane administration have been documented: CNS abnormalities (including cerebral abnormalities, cerebellar malformation, hydrocephalus, microcephaly, cranial nerve deficit); skull abnormality; external ear abnormalities

(including anotia, micropinna, small or absent external auditory canals); eye abnormalities (including microphthalmia); cardiovascular abnormalities; facial dysmorphia; cleft palate; thymus gland abnormality; parathyroid hormone deficiency. In some cases death has occurred with certain of the abnormalities previously noted. Cases of IQ scores less than 85 with or without obvious CNS abnormalities have also been reported. There is an increased risk of spontaneous abortion. In addition, premature births have been reported.

Effective contraception must be used for at least 1 month before beginning Accutane therapy, during therapy and for 1 month following discontinuation of therapy even where there has been a history of infertility, unless due to hysterectomy. It is recommended that two reliable forms of contraception be used simultaneously unless abstinence is the chosen method.

If pregnancy does occur during treatment, the physician and patient should discuss the desirability of continuing the pregnancy.

Accutane should be prescribed only by physicians who have special competence in the diagnosis and treatment of severe recalcitrant nodular acne, are experienced in the use of systemic retinoids and understand the risk of teratogenicity if Accutane is used during pregnancy.

DESCRIPTION
Accutane (isotretinoin), a retinoid which inhibits sebaceous gland function and keratinization, is available in 10-mg, 20-mg and 40-mg soft gelatin capsules for oral administration. Each capsule also contains beeswax, butylated hydroxyanisole, edetate disodium, hydrogenated soybean oil flakes, hydrogenated vegetable oil and soybean oil. Gelatin capsules contain glycerin and parabens (methyl and propyl), with the following dye systems: 10 mg — iron oxide (red) and titanium dioxide; 20 mg — FD&C Red No. 3, FD&C Blue No. 1 and titanium dioxide; 40 mg — FD&C Yellow No. 6, D&C Yellow No. 10 and titanium dioxide. Chemically, isotretinoin is 13-*cis*-retinoic acid and is related to both retinoic acid and retinol (vitamin A). It is a yellow-orange to orange crystalline powder with a molecular weight of 300.44.

CLINICAL PHARMACOLOGY
The exact mechanism of action of Accutane is unknown.
Nodular Acne: Clinical improvement in nodular acne patients occurs in association with a reduction in sebum secretion. The decrease in sebum secretion is temporary and is related to the dose and duration of treatment with Accutane, and reflects a reduction in sebaceous gland size and an inhibition of sebaceous gland differentiation.[1]
Clinical Pharmacokinetics: The pharmacokinetic profile of isotretinoin is predictable and can be described using linear pharmacokinetic theory.
After oral administration of 80 mg (two 40-mg capsules), peak blood concentrations ranged from 167 to 459 ng/mL (mean 256 ng/mL) and mean time to peak was 3.2 hours in normal volunteers, while in acne patients peak concentrations ranged from 98 to 535 ng/mL (mean 262 ng/mL) with a mean time to peak of 2.9 hours. The drug is 99.9% bound in human plasma almost exclusively to albumin. The terminal elimination half-life of isotretinoin ranged from 10 to 20 hours in volunteers and patients. Following an 80-mg liquid suspension oral dose of ^{14}C-isotretinoin, ^{14}C-activity in blood declined with a half-life of 90 hours. Relatively equal amounts of radioactivity were recovered in the urine and feces with 65% to 83% of the dose recovered.
The major identified metabolite in blood is 4-*oxo*-isotretinoin. The mean elimination half-life of this metabolite is 25 hours (range 17–50 hours). Tretinoin and 4-*oxo*-tretinoin were also observed. After two 40-mg capsules of isotretinoin, maximum concentrations of the metabolite of 87 to 399 ng/mL occurred at 6 to 20 hours. The blood concentration of the major metabolite generally exceeded that of isotretinoin after 6 hours.
When taken with food or milk, the oral absorption of isotretinoin is increased.
The mean ± SD minimum steady-state blood concentration of isotretinoin was 160 ± 19 ng/mL in ten patients receiving 40-mg bid doses. After single and multiple doses, the mean ratio of areas under the blood concentration:time curves of 4-*oxo*-isotretinoin to isotretinoin was 3 to 3.5.
Tissue Distribution in Animals: Tissue distribution of ^{14}C-isotretinoin in rats after oral dosing revealed high concentrations of radioactivity in many tissues after 15 minutes, with a maximum in 1 hour, and declining to nondetectable levels by 24 hours in most tissues. After 7 days, however, low levels of radioactivity were detected in the liver, ureter, adrenal, ovary and lacrimal gland.

INDICATIONS AND USAGE
Severe recalcitrant nodular acne: Accutane is indicated for the treatment of severe recalcitrant nodular acne. Nod-

Continued on next page

Accutane—Cont.

ules are inflammatory lesions with a diameter of 5 mm or greater. The nodules may become suppurative or hemorrhagic. "Severe," by definition,[2] means "many" as opposed to "few or several" nodules. Because of significant adverse effects associated with its use, Accutane should be reserved for patients with severe nodular acne who are unresponsive to conventional therapy, including systemic antibiotics.

A single course of therapy has been shown to result in complete and prolonged remission of disease in many patients.[1,3,4] If a second course of therapy is needed, it should not be initiated until at least 8 weeks after completion of the first course, because experience has shown that patients may continue to improve while off Accutane.

CONTRAINDICATIONS

Pregnancy: Category X. See boxed CONTRAINDICATION AND WARNING.

Accutane should not be given to patients who are sensitive to parabens, which are used as preservatives in the gelatin capsule.

WARNINGS

Psychiatric Disorders: **Accutane may cause depression, psychosis and, rarely, suicidal ideation, suicide attempts and suicide. Discontinuation of Accutane therapy may be insufficient; further evaluation may be necessary. No mechanism of action has been established for these events (see ADVERSE REACTIONS).**

Pseudotumor Cerebri: **Accutane use has been associated with a number of cases of pseudotumor cerebri (benign intracranial hypertension). Early signs and symptoms of pseudotumor cerebri include papilledema, headache, nausea and vomiting, and visual disturbances. Patients with these symptoms should be screened for papilledema and, if present, they should be told to discontinue Accutane immediately and be referred to a neurologist for further diagnosis and care.**

Decreased Night Vision: A number of cases of decreased night vision have occurred during Accutane therapy. Because the onset in some patients was sudden, patients should be advised of this potential problem and warned to be cautious when driving or operating any vehicle at night. Visual problems should be carefully monitored.

Corneal Opacities: Corneal opacities have occurred in patients receiving Accutane for acne and more frequently when higher drug dosages were used in patients with disorders of keratinization. All Accutane patients experiencing visual difficulties should discontinue the drug and have an ophthalmological examination. The corneal opacities that have been observed in patients treated with Accutane have either completely resolved or were resolving at follow-up 6 to 7 weeks after discontinuation of the drug (see ADVERSE REACTIONS).

Inflammatory Bowel Disease: Accutane has been temporally associated with inflammatory bowel disease (including regional ileitis) in patients without a prior history of intestinal disorders. Patients experiencing abdominal pain, rectal bleeding or severe diarrhea should discontinue Accutane immediately.

Lipids: Blood lipid determinations should be performed before Accutane is given and then at intervals until the lipid response to Accutane is established, which usually occurs within 4 weeks (see PRECAUTIONS).

Approximately 25% of patients receiving Accutane experienced an elevation in plasma triglycerides. Approximately 15% developed a decrease in high density lipoproteins and about 7% showed an increase in cholesterol levels. These effects on triglycerides, HDL and cholesterol were reversible upon cessation of Accutane therapy.

Patients with increased tendency to develop hypertriglyceridemia include those with diabetes mellitus, obesity, increased alcohol intake and familial history.

The cardiovascular consequences of hypertriglyceridemia are not well understood, but may increase the patient's risk status. In addition, acute pancreatitis, sometimes associated with elevation of serum triglycerides in excess of 800 mg/dL, has been reported. Therefore, every attempt should be made to control significant triglyceride elevation.

Some patients have been able to reverse triglyceride elevation by reduction in weight, restriction of dietary fat and alcohol, and reduction in dose while continuing Accutane.[5]

An obese male patient with Darier's disease developed elevated triglycerides and subsequent eruptive xanthomas.[6]

Hyperostosis: In clinical trials of disorders of keratinization with a mean dose of 2.24 mg/kg/day, a high prevalence of skeletal hyperostosis was noted. Two children showed x-ray findings suggestive of premature closure of the epiphysis. Additionally, skeletal hyperostosis was noted in 6 of 8 patients in a prospective study of disorders of keratinization.[7] Minimal skeletal hyperostosis has also been observed by x-rays in prospective studies of nodular acne patients treated with a single course of therapy at recommended doses.

Hepatotoxicity: Several cases of clinical hepatitis have been noted which are considered to be possibly or probably related to Accutane therapy. Additionally, mild to moderate elevations of liver enzymes have been observed in approximately 15% of individuals treated during clinical trials, some of which normalized with dosage reduction or continued administration of the drug. If normalization does not readily occur or if hepatitis is suspected during treatment with Accutane, the drug should be discontinued and the etiology further investigated.

Animal Studies: In rats given 32 or 8 mg/kg/day of isotretinoin for 18 months or longer, the incidences of focal calcification, fibrosis and inflammation of the myocardium, calcification of coronary, pulmonary and mesenteric arteries and metastatic calcification of the gastric mucosa were greater than in control rats of similar age. Focal endocardial and myocardial calcifications associated with calcification of the coronary arteries were observed in two dogs after approximately 6 to 7 months of treatment with isotretinoin at a dosage of 60 to 120 mg/kg/day.

In dogs given isotretinoin chronically at a dosage of 60 mg/kg/day, corneal ulcers and corneal opacities were encountered at a higher incidence than in control dogs. In general, these ocular changes tended to revert toward normal when treatment with isotretinoin was stopped, but did not completely clear during the observation period.

In rats given isotretinoin at a dosage of 32 mg/kg/day for approximately 15 weeks, long bone fracture has been observed.

PRECAUTIONS

Information for Patients: **Females of childbearing potential should be instructed that they must not be pregnant when Accutane therapy is initiated, and that they should use effective contraception while taking Accutane and for 1 month after Accutane has been stopped. They should also sign a consent form prior to beginning Accutane therapy (see boxed CONTRAINDICATION AND WARNING).**

Because of the relationship of Accutane to vitamin A, patients should be advised against taking vitamin supplements containing vitamin A to avoid additive toxic effects. Patients should be informed that transient exacerbation of acne has been seen, generally during the initial period of therapy.

Patients should be informed that they may experience decreased tolerance to contact lenses during and after therapy.

It is recommended that patients not donate blood during therapy and for 1 month following discontinuance of the drug.

Laboratory Tests: The incidence of hypertriglyceridemia is 1 patient in 4 on Accutane therapy. Pretreatment and follow-up blood lipids should be obtained under fasting conditions. After consumption of alcohol, at least 36 hours should elapse before these determinations are made. It is recommended that these tests be performed at weekly or biweekly intervals until the lipid response to Accutane is established. Since elevations of liver enzymes have been observed during clinical trials, pretreatment and follow-up liver function tests should be performed at weekly or biweekly intervals until the response to Accutane has been established.

Certain patients receiving Accutane have experienced problems in the control of their blood sugar. In addition, new cases of diabetes have been diagnosed during Accutane therapy, although no causal relationship has been established. Some patients undergoing vigorous physical activity while on Accutane therapy have experienced elevated CPK levels; however, the clinical significance is unknown.

Carcinogenesis, Mutagenesis and Impairment of Fertility: In Fischer 344 rats given oral isotretinoin at dosages of 8 or 32 mg/kg/day for greater than 18 months, there was an increased incidence of pheochromocytoma; the incidence of adrenal medullary hyperplasia was also increased at the higher dosage. The relatively high level of spontaneous pheochromocytomas occurring in the Fischer 344 rat makes it a poor model for study of this tumor. The increase in adrenal medullary proliferative lesions following chronic treatment with relatively high dosages of oral isotretinoin may be an accentuation of a genetic predisposition in the Fischer 344 rat; therefore, the relevance of this tumor to the human population is uncertain. In addition, decreased incidences of liver adenomas, liver angiomas and leukemia were noted at dosage levels of 8 and 32 mg/kg/day.

The Ames test was conducted with isotretinoin in two laboratories. The results of the tests in one laboratory were negative while in the second laboratory a weakly positive response (less than 1.6 × background) was noted in *S. typhimurium* TA100 when the assay was conducted with metabolic activation. No dose-response effect was seen and all other strains were negative. Additionally, other tests designed to assess genotoxicity (Chinese hamster cell assay, mouse micronucleus test, *S. cerevisiae* D7 assay, in vitro clastogenesis assay with human-derived lymphocytes and unscheduled DNA synthesis assay) were all negative.

No adverse effects on gonadal function, fertility, conception rate, gestation or parturition were observed in rats at oral dosages of isotretinoin of 2, 8 or 32 mg/kg/day.

In dogs, testicular atrophy was noted after treatment with oral isotretinoin for approximately 30 weeks at dosages of 20 or 60 mg/kg/day. In general, there was microscopic evidence for appreciable depression of spermatogenesis but some sperm were observed in all testes examined and in no instance were completely atrophic tubules seen. In studies of 66 men, 30 of whom were patients with nodular acne under treatment with oral isotretinoin, no significant changes were noted in the count or motility of spermatozoa in the ejaculate. In a study of 50 men (ages 17 to 32 years) receiving Accutane (isotretinoin) therapy for nodular acne, no significant effects were seen on ejaculate volume, sperm count, total sperm motility, morphology or seminal plasma fructose.

Pregnancy: **Category X. See boxed CONTRAINDICATION AND WARNING.**

Nursing Mothers: It is not known whether this drug is excreted in human milk. Because of the potential for adverse effects, nursing mothers should not receive Accutane.

ADVERSE REACTIONS

Clinical: Many of the side effects and adverse reactions seen or expected in patients receiving Accutane are similar to those described in patients taking high doses of vitamin A.

The percentages of adverse reactions listed below reflect the total experience in Accutane studies, including investigational studies of disorders of keratinization, with the exception of those pertaining to dry skin and mucous membranes. These latter reflect the experience only in patients with nodular acne because reactions relating to dryness are more commonly recognized as adverse reactions in this disease. Included in this category are dry skin, skin fragility, pruritus, epistaxis, dry nose and dry mouth, which may be seen in up to 80% of nodular acne patients.

The most frequent adverse reaction to Accutane is cheilitis, which occurs in over 90% of patients. A less frequent reaction was conjunctivitis (about 2 patients in 5).

Skeletal hyperostosis has been observed on x-rays of patients treated with Accutane (see WARNINGS). Other types of bone abnormalities have also been reported; however, no causal relationship has been established.

In the post-marketing period, a number of patients treated with Accutane have reported depression, psychosis and, rarely, suicidal ideation, suicide attempts and suicide. Of the patients reporting depression, some reported that the depression subsided with discontinuation of therapy and recurred with reinstitution of therapy (see WARNINGS).

Approximately 16% of patients treated with Accutane developed musculoskeletal symptoms (including arthralgia) during treatment. In general, these were mild to moderate and have occasionally required discontinuation of drug. Less frequently, transient pain in the chest has also been reported. These symptoms generally cleared rapidly after discontinuation of Accutane but in rare cases have persisted.

Less than 1 patient in 10 experienced rash (including erythema, seborrhea and eczema); thinning of hair, which in rare cases has persisted.

Approximately 1 patient in 20 experienced peeling of palms and soles, skin infections, nonspecific urogenital findings, nonspecific gastrointestinal symptoms, fatigue, headache and increased susceptibility to sunburn.

Accutane has been associated with a number of cases of pseudotumor cerebri, some of which involved concomitant use of tetracyclines (see WARNINGS).

The following CNS reactions have been reported and may bear no relationship to therapy — seizures, emotional instability, dizziness, nervousness, drowsiness, malaise, weakness, insomnia, lethargy and paresthesias.

The following reactions have been reported in less than 1% of patients and may bear no relationship to therapy — changes in skin pigment (hypo- and hyperpigmentation), flushing, urticaria, bruising, disseminated herpes simplex, edema, hair problems (other than thinning), hirsutism, respiratory infections, weight loss, erythema nodosum, paronychia, nail dystrophy, bleeding and inflammation of the gums, abnormal menses, optic neuritis, photophobia, eye lid inflammation, arthritis, anemia, palpitation, tachycardia, lymphadenopathy, sweating, tinnitus and voice alteration. Reports of acne fulminans and vasculitis, including Wegener's granulomatosis, have been received, but no causal relationship to Accutane therapy has been established.

In Accutane studies to date, of 72 patients who had normal pretreatment ophthalmological examinations, 5 developed corneal opacities while on Accutane (all 5 patients had a disorder of keratinization). Corneal opacities have also been reported in nodular acne patients treated with Accutane (see WARNINGS). Dry eyes and decrease in night vision have been reported and in rare instances have persisted (see WARNINGS). Cataracts, keratitis and visual disturbances have also been reported.

Accutane has been temporally associated with inflammatory bowel disease (see WARNINGS).

Delayed wound healing has been reported. As may be seen with healing inflammatory acne lesions, an occasional exaggerated healing response, manifested by exuberant granu-

ACCUTANE DOSING BY BODY WEIGHT

Body Weight			Total Mg/Day	
kilograms	pounds	0.5 mg/kg	1 mg/kg	2 mg/kg
40	88	20	40	80
50	110	25	50	100
60	132	30	60	120
70	154	35	70	140
80	176	40	80	160
90	198	45	90	180
100	220	50	100	200

lation tissue with crusting, has been reported in patients receiving therapy with Accutane. Pyogenic granuloma has also been diagnosed in a number of cases.

Laboratory: Accutane therapy induces change in serum lipids in a significant number of treated subjects. Approximately 25% of patients had elevation of plasma triglycerides. Five out of 135 patients treated for nodular acne and 32 out of 298 total subjects treated for all diagnoses showed an elevation of triglycerides above 500 mg percent. About 16% of patients showed a mild to moderate decrease in serum high density lipoprotein (HDL) levels while receiving treatment with Accutane, and about 7% of patients experienced minimal elevations of serum cholesterol during treatment. Abnormalities of serum triglycerides, HDL and cholesterol were reversible upon cessation of Accutane therapy. Approximately 40% of patients receiving Accutane developed elevated sedimentation rates, often from elevated baseline values.

From 1 in 10 to 1 in 5 patients showed decreases in red blood cell parameters and white blood cell counts, elevated platelet counts, white cells in the urine, increased alkaline phosphatase, SGOT, SGPT, GGTP or LDH (see WARNINGS: Hepatotoxicity).

Less than 1 in 10 patients showed proteinuria, microscopic or gross hematuria, elevated fasting blood sugar, elevated CPK, hyperuricemia or thrombocytopenia.

Dose Relationship and Duration: Cheilitis and hypertriglyceridemia are usually dose-related.

Most adverse reactions were reversible when therapy was discontinued; however, some have persisted after cessation of therapy (see WARNINGS and ADVERSE REACTIONS).

Overdosage: The oral LD$_{50}$ of isotretinoin is greater than 4000 mg/kg in rats and mice and is approximately 1960 mg/kg in rabbits. Overdose has been associated with vomiting, facial flushing, cheilosis, abdominal pain, headache, dizziness and ataxia. All symptoms quickly resolved without apparent residual effects.

DOSAGE AND ADMINISTRATION

The recommended dosage range for Accutane is 0.5 to 2 mg/kg given in 2 divided doses daily for 15 to 20 weeks. In studies comparing 0.1, 0.5 and 1 mg/kg/day,[8] it was found that all dosages provided initial clearing of disease, but there was a greater need for retreatment with the lower dosages.

It is recommended that for most patients the initial dosage of Accutane be 0.5 to 1 mg/kg/day. Patients whose disease is very severe or is primarily manifested on the body may require up to the maximum recommended dosage, 2 mg/kg/day. During treatment, the dose may be adjusted according to response of the disease and/or the appearance of clinical side effects — some of which may be dose-related.

If the total nodule count has been reduced by more than 70% prior to completing 15 to 20 weeks of treatment, the drug may be discontinued. After a period of 2 months or more off therapy, and if warranted by persistent or recurring severe nodular acne, a second course of therapy may be initiated. Contraceptive measures must be followed for any subsequent course of therapy.

Accutane should be administered with food.

[See table above]

HOW SUPPLIED

Soft gelatin capsules, 10 mg (light pink), imprinted ACCUTANE 10 ROCHE. Boxes of 100 containing 10 Prescription Paks of 10 capsules (NDC 0004-0155-49).

Soft gelatin capsules, 20 mg (maroon), imprinted ACCUTANE 20 ROCHE. Boxes of 100 containing 10 Prescription Paks of 10 capsules (NDC 0004-0169-49).

Soft gelatin capsules, 40 mg (yellow), imprinted ACCUTANE 40 ROCHE. Boxes of 100 containing 10 Prescription Paks of 10 capsules (NDC 0004-0156-49).

Store at 59° to 86°F (15° to 30°C). Protect from light.

REFERENCES

1. Peck GL, Olsen TG, Yoder FW, Strauss JS, Downing DT, Pandya M, Butkus D, Arnaud-Battandier J: Prolonged remissions of cystic and conglobate acne with 13-*cis*-retinoic acid. *N Engl J Med* 300:329-333, 1979. 2. Pochi PE, Shalita AR, Strauss JS, Webster SB: Report of the consensus conference on acne classification. *J Am Acad Dermatol* 24:495-500, 1991. 3. Farrell LN, Strauss JS, Stranieri AM: The treatment of severe cystic acne with 13-*cis*-retinoic acid:

evaluation of sebum production and the clinical response in a multiple-dose trial. *J Am Acad Dermatol* 3:602-611, 1980.
4. Jones H, Blanc D, Cunliffe WJ: 13-*cis*-retinoic acid and acne. *Lancet* 2:1048-1049, 1980. 5. Katz RA, Jorgensen H, Nigra TP: Elevation of serum triglyceride levels from oral isotretinoin in disorders of keratinization. *Arch Dermatol* 116:1369-1372, 1980. 6. Dicken CH, Connolly SM: Eruptive xanthomas associated with isotretinoin (13-*cis*-retinoic acid). *Arch Dermatol* 116:951-952, 1980. 7. Ellis CN, Madison KC, Pennes DR, Martel W, Voorhees JJ: Isotretinoin therapy is associated with early skeletal radiographic changes. *J Am Acad Dermatol* 10:1024-1029, 1984. 8. Strauss JS, Rapini RP, Shalita AR, Konecky E, Pochi PE, Comite H, Exner JH: Isotretinoin therapy for acne: results of a multicenter dose-response study. *J Am Acad Dermatol* 10:490-496, 1984.

PATIENT INFORMATION/CONSENT:

Accutane must not be used by females who are pregnant or who may become pregnant while undergoing treatment.

IMPORTANT INFORMATION AND WARNING: Accutane can cause severe birth defects if it is taken when a female is pregnant. There is an extremely high risk that you will have a severely deformed baby if:

• you are pregnant when you start taking Accutane,
• you become pregnant while you are taking Accutane,
• you do not wait 1 month after you stop taking Accutane before becoming pregnant.

It is recommended that you and your doctor schedule an appointment every month to repeat the pregnancy test and check your body's response to Accutane. For your health and well-being, be sure to keep your appointments as scheduled.

THE CONSENT:
My treatment with Accutane has been personally explained to me by Dr. _____. The following points of information, among others, have been specifically discussed and made clear:

1. I, _____,

(Patient's Name)

understand that Accutane is a very powerful medicine used to treat severe nodular acne that did not get better with other treatments including oral antibiotics.

INITIALS: _____

2. I understand that I must not take Accutane if I am pregnant or may become pregnant during treatment.

INITIALS: _____

3. I understand that severe birth defects have occurred in babies of females who took Accutane during pregnancy. I have been warned by my doctor that there is an extremely high risk of severe damage to my unborn baby if I am pregnant or become pregnant while taking Accutane.

INITIALS: _____

4. I have been told by my doctor that effective birth control (contraception) must be used for at least 1 month before starting Accutane, all during Accutane therapy and for 1 month after Accutane treatment has stopped. My doctor has told me that I must either abstain from sexual intercourse or use two reliable kinds of birth control at the same time. I have also been told that any method of birth control can fail. I must use two forms of reliable birth control simultaneously even if I think I cannot become pregnant, unless I abstain from sexual intercourse or have had a hysterectomy.

INITIALS: _____

5. I know that I must have a blood or urine test done by my doctor that shows I am not pregnant within 1 week before starting Accutane, and I understand that I must wait until the second or third day of my next normal menstrual period before starting Accutane.

INITIALS: _____

6. My doctor has told me that I can participate in the "Patient Referral" program for an initial free pregnancy test and birth control counseling session by a consulting physician.

INITIALS: _____

7. I also know that I must immediately stop taking Accutane if I become pregnant while taking the drug and immediately contact my doctor to discuss the desir-

ability of continuing the pregnancy. I also know that I must immediately contact my doctor if I become pregnant during the month after stopping Accutane.

INITIALS: _____

8. I have carefully read the Accutane patient brochure, "Important information concerning your treatment with Accutane," given to me by my doctor. I understand all of its contents and have talked over any questions I have with my doctor.

INITIALS: _____

9. I am not now pregnant, nor do I plan to become pregnant for 1 month after I have completely finished taking Accutane.

INITIALS: _____

10. My doctor has told me that I can participate in a survey concerning Accutane use in females by completing an additional form.

INITIALS: _____

I now authorize Dr. _____
to begin my treatment with Accutane.

_____
Patient, Parent or Guardian   Date

_____
Address

_____

_____
Telephone Number

I have fully explained to the patient, _____, the nature and purpose of the treatment described above and the risks to females of childbearing potential. I have asked the patient if she has any questions regarding her treatment with Accutane and have answered those questions to the best of my ability.

_____
Physician   Date

Revised: February 1998
Shown in Product Identification Guide, page 334

BACTRIM™ ℞

[bac 'trim]
brand of trimethoprim and sulfamethoxazole
IV INFUSION

The following text is complete prescribing information based on official labeling in effect June 1998.

DESCRIPTION

Bactrim (trimethoprim and sulfamethoxazole) IV Infusion, a sterile solution for intravenous infusion only, is a synthetic antibacterial combination product. Each 5 mL contains 80 mg trimethoprim (16 mg/mL) and 400 mg sulfamethoxazole (80 mg/mL) compounded with 40% propylene glycol, 10% ethyl alcohol and 0.3% diethanolamine; 1% benzyl alcohol and 0.1% sodium metabisulfite added as preservatives, water for injection, and pH adjusted to approximately 10 with sodium hydroxide.

Trimethoprim is 2,4-diamino-5-(3,4,5-trimethoxybenzyl)pyrimidine. It is a white to light yellow, odorless, bitter compound with a molecular weight of 290.3.

Sulfamethoxazole is N^1-(5-methyl-3-isoxazolyl)sulfanilamide. It is an almost white, odorless, tasteless compound with a molecular weight of 253.28.

CLINICAL PHARMACOLOGY

Following a 1-hour intravenous infusion of a single dose of 160 mg trimethoprim and 800 mg sulfamethoxazole to 11 patients whose weight ranged from 105 lbs to 165 lbs (mean, 143 lbs), the peak plasma concentrations of trimethoprim and sulfamethoxazole were 3.4 ± 0.3 µg/mL and 46.3 ± 2.7 µg/mL, respectively. Following repeated intravenous administration of the same dose at 8-hour intervals, the mean plasma concentrations just prior to and immediately after each infusion at steady state were 5.6 ± 0.6 µg/mL and 8.8 ± 0.9 µg/mL for trimethoprim and 70.6 ± 7.3 µg/mL and 105.6 ± 10.9 µg/mL for sulfamethoxazole. The mean plasma half-life was 11.3 ± 0.7 hours for trimethoprim and 12.8 ± 1.8 hours for sulfamethoxazole. All of these 11 patients had normal renal function, and their ages ranged from 17 to 78 years (median, 60 years).[1]

Pharmacokinetic studies in children and adults suggest an age-dependent half-life of trimethoprim, as indicated in the following table.[2]

Age (years)	No. of Patients	Mean TMP Half-life (hours)
<1	2	7.67
1–10	9	5.49
10–20	5	8.19
20–63	6	12.82

Continued on next page

Bactrim IV Infusion—Cont.

Patients with severely impaired renal function exhibit an increase in the half-lives of both components, requiring dosage regimen adjustment (See DOSAGE AND ADMINISTRATION section).

Both trimethoprim and sulfamethoxazole exist in the blood as unbound, protein-bound and metabolized forms; sulfamethaxazole also exists as the conjugated form. The metabolism of sulfamethoxazole occurs predominately by N_4-acetylation, although the glucuronide conjugate has been identified. The principal metabolites of trimethoprim are the 1- and 3-oxides and the 3'- and 4'-hydroxy derivatives. The free forms of trimethoprim and sulfamethoxazole are considered to be the therapeutically active forms. Approximately 44% of trimethoprim and 70% of sulfamethoxazole are bound to plasma proteins. The presence of 10 mg percent sulfamethoxazole in plasma decreases the protein binding of trimethoprim by an insignificant degree; trimethoprim does not influence the protein binding of sulfamethoxazole.

Excretion of trimethoprim and sulfamethoxazole is primarily by the kidneys through both glomerular filtration and tubular secretion. Urine concentrations of both trimethoprim and sulfamethoxazole are considerably higher than are the concentrations in the blood. The percent of dose excreted in urine over a 12-hour period following the intravenous administration of the first dose of 240 mg of trimethoprim and 1200 mg of sulfamethoxazole on day 1 ranged from 17% to 42.4% as free trimethoprim; 7% to 12.7% as free sulfamethoxazole; and 36.7% to 56% as total (free plus the N_4-acetylated metabolite) sulfamethoxazole. When administered together as Bactrim, neither trimethoprim nor sulfamethoxazole affects the urinary excretion pattern of the other. Both trimethoprim and sulfamethoxazole distribute to sputum and vaginal fluid; trimethoprim also distributes to bronchial secretions, and both pass the placental barrier and are excreted in breast milk.

Microbiology: Sulfamethoxazole inhibits bacterial synthesis of dihydrofolic acid by competing with para -aminobenzoic acid (PABA). Trimethoprim blocks the production of tetrahydrofolic acid from dihydrofolic acid by binding to and reversibly inhibiting the required enzyme, dihydrofolate reductase. Thus, Bactrim blocks two consecutive steps in the biosynthesis of nucleic acids and proteins essential to many bacteria.

In vitro studies have shown that bacterial resistance develops more slowly with Bactrim than with either trimethoprim or sulfamethoxazole alone.

In vitro serial dilution tests have shown that the spectrum of antibacterial activity of Bactrim includes common bacterial pathogens with the exception of *Pseudomonas aeruginosa*. The following organisms are usually susceptible: *Escherichia coli, Klebsiella* species, *Enterobacter* species, *Morganella morganii, Proteus mirabilis*, indole-positive *Proteus* species including *Proteus vulgaris, Haemophilus influenzae* (including ampicillin-resistant strains), *Streptococcus pneumoniae, Shigella flexneri* and *Shigella sonnei*. It should be noted, however, that there are little clinical data on the use of Bactrim IV Infusion in serious systemic infections due to *Haemophilus influenzae* and *Streptococcus pneumoniae.*

[See table below]

The recommended quantitative disc susceptibility method may be used for estimating the susceptibility of bacteria to Bactrim.[3,4] With this procedure, a report from the laboratory of "Susceptible to trimethoprim and sulfamethoxazole" indicates that the infection is likely to respond to therapy with Bactrim. If the infection is confined to the urine, a report of "Intermediate susceptibility to trimethoprim and sulfamethoxazole" also indicates that the infection is likely

to respond. A report of "Resistant to trimethoprim and sulfamethoxazole" indicates that the infection is unlikely to respond to therapy with Bactrim.

INDICATIONS AND USAGE

Pneumocystis Carinii Pneumonia: Bactrim IV Infusion is indicated in the treatment of *Pneumocystis carinii* pneumonia in children and adults.

Shigellosis: Bactrim IV Infusion is indicated in the treatment of enteritis caused by susceptible strains of *Shigella flexneri* and *Shigella sonnei* in children and adults.

Urinary Tract Infections: Bactrim IV Infusion is indicated in the treatment of severe or complicated urinary tract infections due to susceptible strains of *Escherichia coli, Klebsiella* species, *Enterobacter* species, *Morganella morganii* and *Proteus* species when oral administration of Bactrim is not feasible and when the organism is not susceptible to single-agent antibacterials effective in the urinary tract.

Although appropriate culture and susceptibility studies should be performed, therapy may be started while awaiting the results of these studies.

CONTRAINDICATIONS

Bactrim is contraindicated in patients with a known hypersensitivity to trimethoprim or sulfonamides and in patients with documented megaloblastic anemia due to folate deficiency. Bactrim is also contraindicated in pregnant patients and nursing mothers, because sulfonamides pass the placenta and are excreted in the milk and may cause kernicterus. Bactrim is contraindicated in infants less than 2 months of age.

WARNINGS

FATALITIES ASSOCIATED WITH THE ADMINISTRATION OF SULFONAMIDES, ALTHOUGH RARE, HAVE OCCURRED DUE TO SEVERE REACTIONS, INCLUDING STEVENS-JOHNSON SYNDROME, TOXIC EPIDERMAL NECROLYSIS, FULMINANT HEPATIC NECROSIS, AGRANULOCYTOSIS, APLASTIC ANEMIA AND OTHER BLOOD DYSCRASIAS.

BACTRIM SHOULD BE DISCONTINUED AT THE FIRST APPEARANCE OF SKIN RASH OR ANY SIGN OF ADVERSE REACTION. Clinical signs, such as rash, sore throat, fever, arthralgia, cough, shortness of breath, pallor, purpura or jaundice may be early indications of serious reactions. In rare instances a skin rash may be followed by more severe reactions, such as Stevens-Johnson syndrome, toxic epidermal necrolysis, hepatic necrosis or serious blood disorder. Complete blood counts should be done frequently in patients receiving sulfonamides.

BACTRIM SHOULD NOT BE USED IN THE TREATMENT OF STREPTOCOCCAL PHARYNGITIS. Clinical studies have documented that patients with group A β-hemolytic streptococcal tonsillopharyngitis have a greater incidence of bacteriologic failure when treated with Bactrim than do those patients treated with penicillin, as evidenced by failure to eradicate this organism from the tonsillopharyngeal area.

Bactrim IV Infusion contains sodium metabisulfite, a sulfite that may cause allergic-type reactions, including anaphylactic symptoms and life-threatening or less severe asthmatic episodes in certain susceptible people. The overall prevalence of sulfite sensitivity in the general population is unknown and probably low. Sulfite sensitivity is seen more frequently in asthmatic than in nonasthmatic people.

PRECAUTIONS

General: Bactrim should be given with caution to patients with impaired renal or hepatic function, to those with possible folate deficiency (eg, the elderly, chronic alcoholics, patients receiving anticonvulsant therapy, patients with malabsorption syndrome, and patients in malnutrition states) and to those with severe allergies or bronchial asthma. In

glucose-6-phosphate dehydrogenase deficient individuals, hemolysis may occur. This reaction is frequently dose-related.

Local irritation and inflammation due to extravascular infiltration of the infusion have been observed with Bactrim IV Infusion. If these occur the infusion should be discontinued and restarted at another site.

Use in the Elderly: There may be an increased risk of severe adverse reactions in elderly patients, particularly when complicating conditions exist, eg, impaired kidney and/or liver function, or concomitant use of other drugs. Severe skin reactions, generalized bone marrow suppression (see WARNINGS and ADVERSE REACTIONS sections) or a specific decrease in platelets (with or without purpura) are the most frequently reported severe adverse reactions in elderly patients. In those concurrently receiving certain diuretics, primarily thiazides, an increased incidence of thrombocytopenia with purpura has been reported. Appropriate dosage adjustments should be made for patients with impaired kidney function (see DOSAGE AND ADMINISTRATION section).

Use in the Treatment of Pneumocystis Carinii Pneumonia in Patients with Acquired Immunodeficiency Syndrome (AIDS): AIDS patients may not tolerate or respond to Bactrim in the same manner as non-AIDS patients. The incidence of side effects, particularly rash, fever, leukopenia, and elevated aminotransferase (transaminase) values, with Bactrim therapy in AIDS patients who are being treated for *Pneumocystis carinii* pneumonia has been reported to be greatly increased compared with the incidence normally associated with the use of Bactrim in non-AIDS patients.

Laboratory Tests: Appropriate culture and susceptibility studies should be performed before and throughout treatment. Complete blood counts should be done frequently in patients receiving Bactrim; if a significant reduction in the count of any formed blood element is noted, Bactrim should be discontinued. Urinalyses with careful microscopic examination and renal function tests should be performed during therapy, particularly for those patients with impaired renal function.

Drug Interactions: In elderly patients concurrently receiving certain diuretics, primarily thiazides, an increased incidence of thrombocytopenia with purpura has been reported. It has been reported that Bactrim may prolong the prothrombin time in patients who are receiving the anticoagulant warfarin. This interaction should be kept in mind when Bactrim is given to patients already on anticoagulant therapy, and the coagulation time should be reassessed.

Bactrim may inhibit the hepatic metabolism of phenytoin. Bactrim, given at a common clinical dosage, increased the phenytoin half-life by 39% and decreased the phenytoin metabolic clearance rate by 27%. When administering these drugs concurrently, one should be alert for possible excessive phenytoin effect.

Sulfonamides can also displace methotrexate from plasma protein binding sites, thus increasing free methotrexate concentrations.

Drug/Laboratory Test Interactions: Bactrim, specifically the trimethoprim component, can interfere with a serum methotrexate assay as determined by the competitive binding protein technique (CBPA) when a bacterial dihydrofolate reductase is used as the binding protein. No interference occurs, however, if methotrexate is measured by a radioimmunoassay (RIA).

The presence of trimethoprim and sulfamethoxazole may also interfere with the Jaffé alkaline picrate reaction assay for creatinine, resulting in overestimations of about 10% in the range of normal values.

Carcinogenesis, Mutagenesis, Impairment of Fertility:
Carcinogenesis: Long-term studies in animals to evaluate carcinogenic potential have not been conducted with Bactrim IV Infusion.

Mutagenesis: Bacterial mutagenic studies have not been performed with sulfamethoxazole and trimethoprim in combination. Trimethoprim was demonstrated to be nonmutagenic in the Ames assay. No chromosomal damage was observed in human leukocytes cultured in vitro with sulfamethoxazole and trimethoprim alone or in combination; the concentrations used exceeded blood levels of these compounds following therapy with Bactrim. Observations of leukocytes obtained from patients treated with Bactrim revealed no chromosomal abnormalities.

Impairment of Fertility: Bactrim IV Infusion has not been studied in animals for evidence of impairment of fertility. However, studies in rats at oral dosages as high as 70 mg/kg trimethoprim plus 350 mg/kg sulfamethoxazole daily showed no adverse effects on fertility or general reproductive performance.

Pregnancy: Teratogenic Effects: Pregnancy Category C. In rats, oral doses of 533 mg/kg sulfamethoxazole or 200 mg/kg trimethoprim produced teratological effects manifested mainly as cleft palates.

The highest dose which did not cause cleft palates in rats was 512 mg/kg sulfamethoxazole or 192 mg/kg trimethoprim when administered separately. In two studies in rats, no teratology was observed when 512 mg/kg of sulfamethoxazole was used in combination with 128 mg/kg of trimethoprim. In one study, however, cleft palates were observed in one litter out of 9 when 355 mg/kg of sulfamethoxazole was used in combination with 88 mg/kg of trimethoprim.

REPRESENTATIVE MINIMUM INHIBITORY CONCENTRATION VALUES FOR BACTRIM-SUSCEPTIBLE ORGANISMS (MIC—µg/mL)

Bacteria	TMP alone	SMX alone	TMP/SMX(1:20) TMP	SMX		
Escherichia coli	0.05–1.5		1.0–245	0.05–0.5	0.95	–9.5
Proteus species (indole positive)	0.5–5.0		7.35–300	0.05–1.5	0.95	–28.5
Morganella morganii	0.5–5.0		7.35–300	0.05–1.5	0.95	–28.5
Proteus mirabilis	0.5–1.5		7.35–30	0.05–0.15	0.95	–2.85
Klebsiella species	0.15–5.0		2.45–245	0.05–1.5	0.95	–28.5
Enterobacter species	0.15–5.0		2.45–245	0.05–1.5	0.95	–28.5
Haemophilus influenzae	0.15–1.5		2.85–95	0.015–0.15	0.285	–2.85
Streptococcus pneumoniae	0.15–1.5		7.35–24.5	0.05–0.15	0.95	–2.85
*Shigella flexneri**	<0.01–0.04		<0.16–>320	<0.002–0.03	0.04	–0.625
*Shigella sonnei**	0.02–0.08		0.625–>320	0.004–0.06	0.08	–1.25

TMP = trimethoprim
SMX = sulfamethoxazole

* Rudoy RC, Nelson JD, Haltalin KC. *Antimicrob Agents Chemother.* May 1974;5:439–443.

In some rabbit studies, an overall increase in fetal loss (dead and resorbed and malformed conceptuses) was associated with doses of trimethoprim six times the human therapeutic dose.
While there are no large, well-controlled studies on the use of trimethoprim and sulfamethoxazole in pregnant women, Brumfitt and Pursell,[5] in a retrospective study, reported the outcome of 186 pregnancies during which the mother received either placebo or oral trimethoprim and sulfamethoxazole. The incidence of congenital abnormalities was 4.5% (3 of 66) in those who received placebo and 3.3% (4 of 120) in those receiving trimethoprim and sulfamethoxazole. There were no abnormalities in the 10 children whose mothers received the drug during the first trimester. In a separate survey, Brumfitt and Pursell also found no congenital abnormalities in 35 children whose mothers had received oral trimethoprim and sulfamethoxazole at the time of conception or shortly thereafter.
Because trimethoprim and sulfamethoxazole may interfere with folic acid metabolism, Bactrim IV Infusion should be used during pregnancy only if the potential benefit justifies the potential risk to the fetus.
Nonteratogenic Effects: See CONTRAINDICATIONS section.
Nursing Mothers: See CONTRAINDICATIONS section.
Pediatric Use: Bactrim IV Infusion is not recommended for infants younger than two months of age (see CONTRAINDICATIONS section).

ADVERSE REACTIONS

The most common adverse effects are gastrointestinal disturbances (nausea, vomiting, anorexia) and allergic skin reactions (such as rash and urticaria). **FATALITIES ASSOCIATED WITH THE ADMINISTRATION OF SULFONAMIDES, ALTHOUGH RARE, HAVE OCCURRED DUE TO SEVERE REACTIONS, INCLUDING STEVENS-JOHNSON SYNDROME, TOXIC EPIDERMAL NECROLYSIS, FULMINANT HEPATIC NECROSIS, AGRANULOCYTOSIS, APLASTIC ANEMIA AND OTHER BLOOD DYSCRASIAS (SEE WARNINGS SECTION).** Local reaction, pain and slight irritation on IV administration are infrequent. Thrombophlebitis has rarely been observed.
Hematologic: Agranulocytosis, aplastic anemia, thrombocytopenia, leukopenia, neutropenia, hemolytic anemia, megaloblastic anemia, hypoprothrombinemia, methemoglobinemia, eosinophilia.
Allergic Reactions: Stevens-Johnson syndrome, toxic epidermal necrolysis, anaphylaxis, allergic myocarditis, erythema multiforme, exfoliative dermatitis, angioedema, drug fever, chills, Henoch-Schoenlein purpura, serum sickness-like syndrome, generalized allergic reactions, generalized skin eruptions, conjunctival and scleral injection, photosensitivity, pruritus, urticaria and rash. In addition, periarteritis nodosa and systemic lupus erythematosus have been reported.
Gastrointestinal: Hepatitis (including cholestatic jaundice and hepatic necrosis), elevation of serum transaminase and bilirubin, pseudomembraneous enterocolitis, pancreatitis, stomatitis, glossitis, nausea, emesis, abdominal pain, diarrhea, anorexia.
Genitourinary: Renal failure, interstitial nephritis, BUN and serum creatinine elevation, toxic nephrosis with oliguria and anuria, and crystalluria.
Neurologic: Aseptic meningitis, convulsions, peripheral neuritis, ataxia, vertigo, tinnitus, headache.
Psychiatric: Hallucinations, depression, apathy, nervousness.
Endocrine: The sulfonamides bear certain chemical similarities to some goitrogens, diuretics (acetazolamide and the thiazides) and oral hypoglycemic agents. Cross-sensitivity may exist with these agents. Diuresis and hypoglycemia have occurred rarely in patients receiving sulfonamides.
Musculoskeletal: Arthralgia and myalgia.
Respiratory: Pulmonary infiltrates.
Miscellaneous: Weakness, fatigue, insomnia.

OVERDOSAGE

Acute: Since there has been no extensive experience in humans with single doses of Bactrim IV Infusion in excess of 25 mL (400 mg trimethoprim and 2000 mg sulfamethoxazole), the maximum tolerated dose in humans is unknown. Signs and symptoms of overdosage reported with sulfonamides include anorexia, colic, nausea, vomiting, dizziness, headache, drowsiness and unconsciousness. Pyrexia, hematuria and crystalluria may be noted. Blood dyscrasias and jaundice are potential late manifestations of overdosage.
Signs of acute overdosage with trimethoprim include nausea, vomiting, dizziness, headache, mental depression, confusion and bone marrow depression.
General principles of treatment include the administration of intraveneous fluids if urine output is low and renal function is normal. Acidification of the urine will increase renal elimination of trimethoprim. The patient should be monitored with blood counts and appropriate blood chemistries, including electrolytes. If a significant blood dyscrasia or jaundice occurs, specific therapy should be instituted for these complications. Peritoneal dialysis is not effective and hemodialysis is only moderately effective in eliminating trimethoprim and sulfamethoxazole.
Chronic: Use of Bactrim IV Infusion at high doses and/or for extended periods of time may cause bone marrow depression manifested as thrombocytopenia, leukopenia and/or megaloblastic anemia. If signs of bone marrow depression occur, the patient should be given leucovorin 5 to 15 mg daily until normal hematopoiesis is restored.
Animal Toxicity: The LD_{50} of Bactrim IV Infusion in mice is 700 mg/kg or 7.3 mL/kg; in rats and rabbits the LD_{50} is >500 mg/kg or >5.2 mL/kg. The vehicle produced the same LD_{50} in each of these species as the active drug.
The signs and symptoms noted in mice, rats and rabbits with Bactrim IV Infusion or its vehicle at the high IV doses used in acute toxicity studies included ataxia, decreased motor activity, loss of righting reflex, tremors or convulsions, and/or respiratory depression.

DOSAGE AND ADMINISTRATION

CONTRAINDICATED IN INFANTS LESS THAN 2 MONTHS OF AGE. CAUTION—BACTRIM IV INFUSION MUST BE DILUTED IN 5% DEXTROSE IN WATER SOLUTION PRIOR TO ADMINISTRATION. DO NOT MIX BACTRIM IV INFUSION WITH OTHER DRUGS OR SOLUTIONS. RAPID INFUSION OR BOLUS INJECTION MUST BE AVOIDED.
Dosage:
CHILDREN AND ADULTS:
Pneumocystis Carinii Pneumonia: Total daily dose is 15 to 20 mg/kg (based on the trimethoprim component) given in 3 or 4 equally divided doses every 6 to 8 hours for up to 14 days. One investigator noted that a total daily dose of 10 to 15 mg/kg was sufficient in 10 adult patients with normal renal function.[6]
Severe Urinary Tract Infections and Shigellosis: Total daily dose is 8 to 10 mg/kg (based on the trimethoprim component) given in 2 or 4 equally divided doses every 6, 8 or 12 hours for up to 14 days for severe urinary tract infections and 5 days for shigellosis. The maximum recommended daily dose is 60 mL per day.
For Patients with Impaired Renal Function: When renal function is impaired, a reduced dosage should be employed using the following table:

Creatinine Clearance (mL/min)	Recommended Dosage Regimen
Above 30	Usual standard regimen
15–30	$^1/_2$ the usual regimen
Below 15	Use not recommended

Method of Preparation: Bactrim IV Infusion must be diluted. EACH 5 ML SHOULD BE ADDED TO 125 ML OF 5% DEXTROSE IN WATER. After diluting with 5% dextrose in water the solution should not be refrigerated and should be used within 6 hours. If a dilution of 5 mL per 100 mL of 5% dextrose in water is desired, it should be used within 4 hours. If upon visual inspection there is cloudiness or evidence of crystallization after mixing, the solution should be discarded and a fresh solution prepared.
Multidose Vials: After initial entry into the vial, the remaining contents must be used within 48 hours.
The following infusion systems have been tested and found satisfactory: unit-dose glass containers; unit-dose polyvinyl chloride and polyolefin containers. No other systems have been tested and therefore no others can be recommended.
Dilution: EACH 5 ML OF BACTRIM IV INFUSION SHOULD BE ADDED TO 125 ML OF 5% DEXTROSE IN WATER.
Note: In those instances where fluid restriction is desirable, each 5 mL may be added to 75 mL of 5% dextrose in water. Under these circumstances the solution should be mixed just prior to use and should be administered within 2 hours. If upon visual inspection there is cloudiness or evidence of crystallization after mixing, the solution should be discarded and a fresh solution prepared.
DO NOT MIX BACTRIM IV INFUSION–5% DEXTROSE IN WATER WITH DRUGS OR SOLUTIONS IN THE SAME CONTAINER.
Administration: The solution should be given by intravenous infusion over a period of 60 to 90 minutes. Rapid infusion or bolus injection must be avoided. Bactrim IV Infusion should not be given intramuscularly.

HOW SUPPLIED

10-mL *Vials,* containing 160 mg trimethoprim (16 mg/mL) and 800 mg sulfamethoxazole (80 mg/mL) for infusion with 5% dextrose in water. Boxes of 10 (NDC 0004-1955-01).
30-mL *Multidose Vials,* each 5 mL containing 80 mg trimethoprim (16 mg/mL) and 400 mg sulfamethoxazole (80 mg/mL) for infusion with 5% dextrose in water. Boxes of 1 (NDC 0004-1958-01).
STORE AT ROOM TEMPERATURE (15°–30°C or 59°–86°F). DO NOT REFRIGERATE.
Bactrim is also available as *DS (double strength) Tablets* (white, notched, capsule shaped), containing 160 mg trimethoprim and 800 mg sulfamethoxazole—bottles of 100 (NDC 0004-0117-01), 250 (NDC 0004-0117-04) and 500 (NDC 0004-0117-14). Imprint on tablets: (front) BACTRIM-DS; (back) ROCHE.
Tablets (light green, scored, capsule shaped), containing 80 mg trimethoprim and 400 mg sulfamethoxazole—bottles of 100 (NDC 0004-0050-01). Imprint on tablets: (front) BACTRIM; (back) ROCHE.
Pediatric Suspension (pink, cherry flavored), containing 40 mg trimethoprim and 200 mg sulfamethoxazole per teaspoonful (5 mL)—bottles of 16 oz (1 pint) (NDC 0004-1033-28).

REFERENCES

1. Grose WE, Bodey GP, Loo TL. Clinical Pharmacology of Intravenously Administered Trimethoprim-Sulfamethoxazole. *Antimicrob Agents Chemother.* Mar 1979;15:447-451. 2. Siber GR, Gorham C, Durbin W, Lesko L, Levin MJ. Pharmacology of Intravenous Trimethoprim-Sulfamethoxazole in Children and Adults. *Current Chemotherapy and Infectious Diseases.* American Society for Microbiology, Washington, D.C., 1980, Vol. 1, pp. 691-692. 3. Bauer AW, Kirby WMM, Sherris JC, Turck M. Antibiotic Susceptibility Testing by a Standardized Single Disk Method. *Am J Clin Pathol.* Apr 1966;45:493-496.4. National Committee for Clinical Laboratory Standards. *Performance Standards for Antimicrobial Disc Susceptibility Test.* 771 East Lancaster Avenue, Villanova, Pennsylvania 19085: Approved Standard ASM-2. 5. Brumfitt W, Pursell R. Trimethoprim/Sulfamethoxazole in the Treatment of Bacteriuria in Women. *J Infect Dis.* Nov 1973;128 (Suppl):S657-S663. 6. Winston DJ, Lau WK, Gale RP, Young LS. Trimethoprim-Sulfamethoxazole for the Treatment of *Pneumocystis carinii* pneumonia. *Ann Intern Med.* June 1980;92:762-769.

Revised: March 1994

BACTRIM™ ℞

[bac 'trim]
brand of trimethoprim and sulfamethoxazole
DS (double strength) Tablets,
Tablets
and
Pediatric Suspension

The following text is complete prescribing information based on official labeling in effect June 1998.

DESCRIPTION

Bactrim (trimethoprim and sulfamethoxazole) is a synthetic antibacterial combination product available in DS (double strength) tablets, tablets and pediatric suspension for oral administration. Each DS tablet contains 160 mg trimethoprim and 800 mg sulfamethoxazole plus magnesium stearate, pregelatinized starch and sodium starch glycolate. Each tablet contains 80 mg trimethoprim and 400 mg sulfamethoxazole plus magnesium stearate, pregelatinized starch, sodium starch glycolate, FD&C Blue No. 1 lake, FD&C Yellow No. 6 lake and D&C Yellow No. 10 lake. Each teaspoonful (5 mL) of the pediatric suspension contains 40 mg trimethoprim and 200 mg sulfamethoxazole in a vehicle containing 0.3 percent alcohol, edetate disodium, glycerin, microcrystalline cellulose, parabens (methyl and propyl), polysorbate 80, saccharin sodium, simethicone, sorbitol, sucrose, FD&C Yellow No. 6, FD&C Red No. 40, flavors and water.
Trimethoprim is 2,4-diamino-5-(3,4,5-trimethoxybenzyl)pyrimidine. It is a white to light yellow, odorless, bitter compound with a molecular weight of 290.3.
Sulfamethoxazole is N^1-(5-methyl-3-isoxazolyl)sulfanilamide. It is almost white, odorless, tasteless compound with a molecular weight of 253.28.

CLINICAL PHARMACOLOGY

Bactrim is rapidly absorbed following oral administration. Both sulfamethoxazole and trimethoprim exist in the blood as unbound, protein-bound and metabolized forms; sulfamethoxazole also exists as the conjugated form. The metabolism of sulfamethoxazole occurs predominately by N_4-acetylation, although the glucuronide conjugate has been identified. The principal metabolites of trimethoprim are the 1- and 3-oxides and the 3′- and 4′- hydroxy derivatives. The free forms of sulfamethoxazole and trimethoprim are considered to be the therapeutically active forms. Approximately 44% of trimethoprim and 70% of sulfamethoxazole are bound to plasma proteins. The presence of 10 mg percent sulfamethoxazole in plasma decreases the protein binding of trimethoprim by an insignificant degree; trimethoprim does not influence the protein binding of sulfamethoxazole.
Peak blood levels for the individual components occur 1 to 4 hours after oral administration. The mean serum half-lives of sulfamethoxazole and trimethoprim are 10 and 8 to 10 hours, respectively. However, patients with severely impaired renal function exhibit an increase in the half-lives of

Continued on next page

Bactrim Tablets/Ped. Susp.—Cont.

both components, requiring dosage regimen adjustment (see DOSAGE AND ADMINISTRATION section). Detectable amounts of trimethoprim and sulfamethoxazole are present in the blood 24 hours after drug administration. During administration of 160 mg trimethoprim and 800 mg sulfamethoxazole bid, the mean steady-state plasma concentration of trimethoprim was 1.72 µg/mL. The steady-state mean plasma levels of free and total sulfamethoxazole were 57.4 µg/mL and 68.0 µg/mL, respectively. These steady-state levels were achieved after three days of drug administration.[1]

Excretion of sulfamethoxazole and trimethoprim is primarily by the kidneys through both glomerular filtration and tubular secretion. Urine concentrations of both sulfamethoxazole and trimethoprim are considerably higher than are the concentrations in the blood. The average percentage of the dose recovered in urine from 0 to 72 hours after a single oral dose of Bactrim is 84.5% for total sulfonamide and 66.8% for free trimethoprim. Thirty percent of the total sulfonamide is excreted as free sulfamethoxazole, with the remaining as N_4-acetylated metabolite.[2] When administered together as Bactrim, neither sulfamethoxazole nor trimethoprim affects the urinary excretion pattern of the other.

Both trimethoprim and sulfamethoxazole distribute to sputum, vaginal fluid and middle ear fluid; trimethoprim also distributes to bronchial secretion, and both pass the placental barrier and are excreted in breast milk.

Microbiology: Sulfamethoxazole inhibits bacterial synthesis of dihydrofolic acid by competing with *para* -aminobenzoic acid (PABA). Trimethoprim blocks the production of tetrahydrofolic acid from dihydrofolic acid by binding to and reversibly inhibiting the required enzyme, dihydrofolate reductase. Thus, Bactrim blocks two consecutive steps in the biosynthesis of nucleic acids and proteins essential to many bacteria.

In vitro studies have shown that bacterial resistance develops more slowly with Bactrim than with either trimethoprim or sulfamethoxazole alone.

In vitro serial dilution tests have shown that the spectrum of antibacterial activity of Bactrim includes the common urinary tract pathogens with the exception of *Pseudomonas aeruginosa.* The following organisms are usually susceptible: *Escherichia coli, Klebsiella* species, *Enterobacter* species, *Morganella morganii, Proteus mirabilis,* and indole-positive *Proteus* species including *Proteus vulgaris.* The usual spectrum of antimicrobial activity of Bactrim includes the following bacterial pathogens isolated from middle ear exudate and from bronchial secretions: *Haemophilus influenzae,* including ampicillin-resistant strains, and *Streptococcus pneumoniae. Shigella flexneri* and *Shigella sonnei* are usually susceptible. The usual spectrum also includes enterotoxigenic strains of *Escherichia coli* (ETEC) causing bacterial gastroenteritis.

[See table below]

The recommended quantitative disc susceptibility method may be used for estimating the susceptibility of bacteria to Bactrim.[3,4] With this procedure, a report from the laboratory of "Susceptible to trimethoprim and sulfamethoxazole" indicates that the infection is likely to respond to therapy with Bactrim. If the infection is confined to the urine, a report of "Intermediate susceptibility to trimethoprim and sulfamethoxazole" also indicates that the infection is likely to respond. A report of "Resistant to trimethoprim and sulfamethoxazole" indicates that the infection is unlikely to respond to therapy with Bactrim.

INDICATIONS AND USAGE

Urinary Tract Infections: For the treatment of urinary tract infections due to susceptible strains of the following organisms: *Escherichia coli, Klebsiella* species, *Enterobacter* species, *Morganella morganii, Proteus mirabilis* and *Proteus vulgaris.* It is recommended that initial episodes of uncomplicated urinary tract infections be treated with a single effective antibacterial agent rather than the combination.

Acute Otitis Media: For the treatment of acute otitis media in children due to susceptible strains of *Streptococcus pneumoniae* or *Haemophilus influenzae* when in the judgment of the physician Bactrim offers some advantage over the use of other antimicrobial agents. To date, there are limited data on the safety of repeated use of Bactrim in children under two years of age. Bactrim is not indicated for prophylactic or prolonged administration in otitis media at any age.

Acute Exacerbations of Chronic Bronchitis in Adults: For the treatment of acute exacerbations of chronic bronchitis due to susceptible strains of *Streptococcus pneumoniae* or *Haemophilus influenzae* when in the judgment of the physician Bactrim offers some advantage over the use of a single antimicrobial agent.

Shigellosis: For the treatment of enteritis caused by susceptible strains of *Shigella flexneri* and *Shigella sonnei* when antibacterial therapy is indicated.

Pneumocystis Carinii Pneumonia: For the treatment of documented *Pneumocystis carinii* pneumonia. For prophylaxis against *Pneumocystis carinii* pneumonia in individuals who are immunosuppressed and considered to be at an increased risk of developing *Pneumocystis carinii* pneumonia.

Travelers' Diarrhea in Adults: For the treatment of travelers' diarrhea due to susceptible strains of enterotoxigenic *E. coli.*

CONTRAINDICATIONS

Bactrim is contraindicated in patients with a known hypersensitivity to trimethoprim or sulfonamides and in patients with documented megaloblastic anemia due to folate deficiency. Bactrim is also contraindicated in pregnant patients and nursing mothers, because sulfonamides pass the placenta and are excreted in the milk and may cause kernicterus. Bactrim is contraindicated in infants less than 2 months of age.

WARNINGS: FATALITIES ASSOCIATED WITH THE ADMINISTRATION OF SULFONAMIDES, ALTHOUGH RARE, HAVE OCCURRED DUE TO SEVERE REACTIONS, INCLUDING STEVENS-JOHNSON SYNDROME, TOXIC EPIDERMAL NECROLYSIS, FULMINANT HEPATIC NECROSIS, AGRANULOCYTOSIS, APLASTIC ANEMIA AND OTHER BLOOD DYSCRASIAS.

BACTRIM SHOULD BE DISCONTINUED AT THE FIRST APPEARANCE OF SKIN RASH OR ANY SIGN OF ADVERSE REACTION. Clinical signs, such as rash, sore throat, fever, arthralgia, cough, shortness of breath, pallor, purpura or jaundice may be early indications of serious reactions. In rare instances a skin rash may be followed by more severe reactions, such as Stevens-Johnson syndrome, toxic epidermal necrolysis, hepatic necrosis or serious blood disorder. Complete blood counts should be done frequently in patients receiving sulfonamides.

BACTRIM SHOULD NOT BE USED IN THE TREATMENT OF STREPTOCOCCAL PHARYNGITIS. Clinical studies have documented that patients with group A β-hemolytic streptococcal tonsillopharyngitis have a greater incidence of bacteriologic failure when treated with Bactrim than do those patients treated with penicillin, as evidenced by failure to eradicate this organism from the tonsillopharyngeal area.

REPRESENTATIVE MINIMUM INHIBITORY CONCENTRATION VALUES FOR BACTRIM-SUSCEPTIBLE ORGANISMS
(MIC—µg/mL)

Bacteria	TMP alone	SMX alone	TMP/SMX(1:20) TMP	TMP/SMX(1:20) SMX
Escherichia coli	0.05–1.5	1.0–245	0.05–0.5	0.95–9.5
Escherichia coli (enterotoxigenic strains)	0.015–0.15	0.285–>950	0.005–0.15	0.095–2.85
Proteus species (indole positive)	0.5–5.0	7.35–300	0.05–1.5	0.95–28.5
Morganella morganii	0.5–5.0	7.35–300	0.05–1.5	0.95–28.5
Proteus mirabilis	0.5–1.5	7.35–30	0.05–0.15	0.95–2.85
Klebsiella species	0.15–5.0	2.45–245	0.05–1.5	0.95–28.5
Enterobacter species	0.15–5.0	2.45–245	0.05–1.5	0.95–28.5
Haemophilus influenzae	0.15–1.5	2.85–95	0.015–0.15	0.285–2.85
Streptococcus pneumoniae	0.15–1.5	7.35–24.5	0.05–0.15	0.95–2.85
*Shigella flexneri**	<0.01–0.04	<0.16–>320	<0.002–0.03	0.04–0.625
*Shigella sonnei**	0.02–0.08	0.625–>320	0.004–0.06	0.08–1.25

TMP = trimethoprim SMX = sulfamethoxazole

*Rudoy RC, Nelson JD, Haltalin KC. *Antimicrob Agents Chemother.* May 1974;5:439–443.

PRECAUTIONS

General: Bactrim should be given with caution to patients with impaired renal or hepatic function, to those with possible folate deficiency (eg, the elderly, chronic alcoholics, patients receiving anticonvulsant therapy, patients with malabsorption syndrome, and patients in malnutrition states) and to those with severe allergies or bronchial asthma. In glucose-6-phosphate dehydrogenase deficient individuals, hemolysis may occur. This reaction is frequently dose-related.

Use in the Elderly: There may be an increased risk of severe adverse reactions in elderly patients, particularly when complicating conditions exist, eg, impaired kidney and/or liver function, or concomitant use of other drugs. Severe skin reactions, generalized bone marrow suppression (see WARNINGS and ADVERSE REACTIONS sections) or a specific decrease in platelets (with or without purpura) are the most frequently reported severe adverse reactions in elderly patients. In those concurrently receiving certain diuretics, primarily thiazides, an increased incidence of thrombocytopenia with purpura has been reported. Appropriate dosage adjustments should be made for patients with impaired kidney function (see DOSAGE AND ADMINISTRATION section).

Use in the Treatment of and Prophylaxis for Pneumocystis Carinii Pneumonia in Patients with Acquired Immunodeficiency Syndrome (AIDS): AIDS patients may not tolerate or respond to Bactrim in the same manner as non-AIDS patients. The incidence of side effects, particularly rash, fever, leukopenia and elevated aminotransferase (transaminase) values, with Bactrim therapy in AIDS patients who are being treated for *Pneumocystis carinii* pneumonia has been reported to be greatly increased compared with the incidence normally associated with the use of Bactrim in non-AIDS patients. Adverse effects are generally less severe in patients receiving Bactrim for prophylaxis. A history of mild intolerance to Bactrim in AIDS patients does not appear to predict intolerance of subsequent secondary prophylaxis.[5] However, if a patient develops skin rash or any sign of adverse reaction, therapy with Bactrim should be reevaluated (see WARNINGS).

Information for Patients: Patients should be instructed to maintain an adequate fluid intake in order to prevent crystalluria and stone formation.

Laboratory Tests: Complete blood counts should be done frequently in patients receiving Bactrim; if a significant reduction in the count of any formed blood element is noted, Bactrim should be discontinued. Urinalyses with careful microscopic examination and renal function tests should be performed during therapy, particularly for those patients with impaired renal function.

Drug Interactions: In elderly patients concurrently receiving certain diuretics, primarily thiazides, an increased incidence of thrombocytopenia with purpura has been reported. It has been reported that Bactrim may prolong the prothrombin time in patients who are receiving the anticoagulant warfarin. This interaction should be kept in mind when Bactrim is given to patients already on anticoagulant therapy, and the coagulation time should be reassessed.

Bactrim may inhibit the hepatic metabolism of phenytoin. Bactrim, given at a common clinical dosage, increased the phenytoin half-life by 39% and decreased the phenytoin metabolic clearance rate by 27%. When administering these drugs concurrently, one should be alert for possible excessive phenytoin effect.

Sulfonamides can also displace methotrexate from plasma protein binding sites, thus increasing free methotrexate concentrations.

Drug/Laboratory Test Interactions: Bactrim, specifically the trimethoprim component, can interfere with a serum methotrexate assay as determined by the competitive binding protein technique (CBPA) when a bacterial dihydrofolate reductase is used as the binding protein. No interference occurs, however, if methotrexate is measured by a radioimmunoassay (RIA).

The presence of trimethoprim and sulfamethoxazole may also interfere with the Jaffé alkaline picrate reaction assay for creatinine, resulting in overestimations of about 10% in the range of normal values.

Carcinogenesis, Mutagenesis, Impairment of Fertility:

Carcinogenesis: Long-term studies in animals to evaluate carcinogenic potential have not been conducted with Bactrim.

Mutagenesis: Bacterial mutagenic studies have not been performed with sulfamethoxazole and trimethoprim in combination. Trimethoprim was demonstrated to be nonmutagenic in the Ames assay. No chromosomal damage was observed in human leukocytes in vitro with sulfamethoxazole and trimethoprim alone or in combination; the concentrations used exceeded blood levels of these compounds following therapy with Bactrim. Observations of leukocytes obtained from patients treated with Bactrim revealed no chromosomal abnormalities.

Impairment of Fertility: No adverse effects on fertility or general reproductive performance were observed in rats given oral dosages as high as 70 mg/kg/day trimethoprim plus 350 mg/kg/day sulfamethoxazole.

Pregnancy: Teratogenic Effects: Pregnancy Category C. In rats, oral doses of 533 mg/kg sulfamethoxazole or 200 mg/kg trimethoprim produced teratologic effects manifested mainly as cleft palates.

The highest dose which did not cause cleft palates in rats was 512 mg/kg sulfamethoxazole or 192 mg/kg trimethoprim when administered separately. In two studies in rats, no teratology was observed when 512 mg/kg of sulfamethoxazole was used in combination with 128 mg/kg of trimethoprim. In one study, however, cleft palates were observed in one litter out of 9 when 355 mg/kg of sulfamethoxazole was used in combination with 88 mg/kg of trimethoprim.

In some rabbit studies, an overall increase in fetal loss (dead and resorbed and malformed conceptuses) was associated with doses of trimethoprim 6 times the human therapeutic dose.

While there are no large, well-controlled studies on the use of trimethoprim and sulfamethoxazole in pregnant women, Brumfitt and Pursell,[6] in a retrospective study, reported the outcome of 186 pregnancies during which the mother received either placebo or trimethoprim and sulfamethoxazole. The incidence of congenital abnormalities was 4.5% (3 of 66) in those who received placebo and 3.3% (4 of 120) in those receiving trimethoprim and sulfamethoxazole. There were no abnormalities in the 10 children whose mothers received the drug during the first trimester. In a separate survey, Brumfitt and Pursell also found no congenital abnormalities in 35 children whose mothers had received oral trimethoprim and sulfamethoxazole at the time of conception or shortly thereafter.

Because trimethoprim and sulfamethoxazole may interfere with folic acid metabolism, Bactrim should be used during pregnancy only if the potential benefit justifies the potential risk to the fetus.

Nonteratogenic Effects: See CONTRAINDICATIONS section.

Nursing Mothers: See CONTRAINDICATIONS section.

Pediatric Use: Bactrim is not recommended for infants younger than 2 months of age (see INDICATIONS and CONTRAINDICATIONS sections).

ADVERSE REACTIONS

The most common adverse effects are gastrointestinal disturbances (nausea, vomiting, anorexia) and allergic skin reactions (such as rash and urticaria). **FATALITIES ASSOCIATED WITH THE ADMINISTRATION OF SULFONAMIDES, ALTHOUGH RARE, HAVE OCCURRED DUE TO SEVERE REACTIONS, INCLUDING STEVENS-JOHNSON SYNDROME, TOXIC EPIDERMAL NECROLYSIS, FULMINANT HEPATIC NECROSIS, AGRANULOCYTOSIS, APLASTIC ANEMIA AND OTHER BLOOD DYSCRASIAS (SEE WARNINGS SECTION).**

Hematologic: Agranulocytosis, aplastic anemia, thrombocytopenia, leukopenia, neutropenia, hemolytic anemia, megaloblastic anemia, hypoprothrombinemia, methemoglobinemia, eosinophilia.

Allergic Reactions: Stevens-Johnson syndrome, toxic epidermal necrolysis, anaphylaxis, allergic myocarditis, erythema multiforme, exfoliative dermatitis, angioedema, drug fever, chills, Henoch-Schoenlein purpura, serum sickness-like syndrome, generalized allergic reactions, generalized skin eruptions, photosensitivity, conjunctival and scleral injection, pruritus, urticaria and rash. In addition, periarteritis nodosa and systemic lupus erythematosus have been reported.

Gastrointestinal: Hepatitis (including cholestatic jaundice and hepatic necrosis), elevation of serum transaminase and bilirubin, pseudomembranous enterocolitis, pancreatitis, stomatitis, glossitis, nausea, emesis, abdominal pain, diarrhea, anorexia.

Genitourinary: Renal failure, interstitial nephritis, BUN and serum creatinine elevation, toxic nephrosis with oliguria and anuria, and crystalluria.

Neurologic: Aseptic meningitis, convulsions, peripheral neuritis, ataxia, vertigo, tinnitus, headache.

Psychiatric: Hallucinations, depression, apathy, nervousness.

Endocrine: The sulfonamides bear certain chemical similarities to some goitrogens, diuretics (acetazolamide and the thiazides) and oral hypoglycemic agents. Cross-sensitivity may exist with these agents. Diuresis and hypoglycemia have occurred rarely in patients receiving sulfonamides.

Musculoskeletal: Arthralgia and myalgia.

Respiratory: Pulmonary infiltrates.

Miscellaneous: Weakness, fatigue, insomnia.

OVERDOSAGE

Acute: The amount of a single dose of Bactrim that is either associated with symptoms of overdosage or is likely to be life-threatening has not been reported. Signs and symptoms of overdosage reported with sulfonamides include anorexia, colic, nausea, vomiting, dizziness, headache, drowsiness and unconsciousness. Pyrexia, hematuria and crystalluria may be noted. Blood dyscrasias and jaundice are potential late manifestations of overdosage.

Signs of acute overdosage with trimethoprim include nausea, vomiting, dizziness, headache, mental depression, confusion and bone marrow depression.

General principles of treatment include the institution of gastric lavage or emesis, forcing oral fluids, and the administration of intravenous fluids if urine output is low and renal function is normal. Acidification of the urine will increase renal elimination of trimethoprim. The patient should be monitored with blood counts and appropriate blood chemistries, including electrolytes. If a significant blood dyscrasia or jaundice occurs, specific therapy should be instituted for these complications. Peritoneal dialysis is not effective and hemodialysis is only moderately effective in eliminating trimethoprim and sulfamethoxazole.

Chronic: Use of Bactrim at high doses and/or for extended periods of time may cause bone marrow depression manifested as thrombocytopenia, leukopenia and/or megaloblastic anemia. If signs of bone marrow depression occur, the patient should be given leucovorin 5 to 15 mg daily until normal hematopoiesis is restored.

DOSAGE AND ADMINISTRATION
Not recommended for use in infants less than 2 months of age.

Urinary Tract Infections and Shigellosis in Adults and Children, and Acute Otitis Media in Children:

Adults: The usual adult dosage in the treatment of urinary tract infections is 1 Bactrim DS (double strength) tablet, 2 Bactrim tablets or 4 teaspoonfuls (20 mL) of Bactrim Pediatric Suspension every 12 hours for 10 to 14 days. An identical daily dosage is used for 5 days in the treatment of shigellosis.

Children: The recommended dose for children with urinary tract infections or acute otitis media is 8 mg/kg trimethoprim and 40 mg/kg sulfamethoxazole per 24 hours, given in two divided doses every 12 hours for 10 days. An identical daily dosage is used for 5 days in the treatment of shigellosis. The following table is a guideline for the attainment of this dosage:

Children 2 months of age or older:

Weight		Dose—every 12 hours	
lb	kg	Teaspoonfuls	Tablets
22	10	1 (5 mL)	—
44	20	2 (10 mL)	1
66	30	3 (15 mL)	1½
88	40	4 (20 mL)	2 or 1 DS tablet

For Patients with Impaired Renal Function: When renal function is impaired, a reduced dosage should be employed using the following table:

Creatinine Clearance (mL/min)	Recommended Dosage Regimen
Above 30	Usual standard regimen
15–30	½ the usual regimen
Below 15	Use not recommended

Acute Exacerbations of Chronic Bronchitis in Adults:
The usual adult dosage in the treatment of acute exacerbations of chronic bronchitis is 1 Bactrim DS (double strength) tablet, 2 Bactrim tablets or 4 teaspoonfuls (20 mL) of Bactrim Pediatric Suspension every 12 hours for 14 days.

Pneumocystis Carinii Pneumonia:
Treatment: Adults and Children:
The recommended dosage for patients with documented *Pneumocystis carinii* pneumonia is 15 to 20 mg/kg trimethoprim and 75 to 100 mg/kg sulfamethoxazole per 24 hours given in equally divided doses every 6 hours for 14 to 21 days.[7] The following table is a guideline for the upper limit of this dosage:

Weight		Dose—every 6 hours	
lb	kg	Teaspoonfuls	Tablets
18	8	1 (5 mL)	—
35	16	2 (10 mL)	1
53	24	3 (15 mL)	1½
70	32	4 (20 mL)	2 or 1 DS tablet
88	40	5 (25 mL)	2½
106	48	6 (30 mL)	3 or 1½ DS tablets
141	64	8 (40 mL)	4 or 2 DS tablets
176	80	10 (50 mL)	5 or 2½ DS Tablets

For the lower limit dose (15 mg/kg trimethoprim and 75 mg/kg sulfamethoxazole per 24 hours) administer 75% of the dose in the above table.

Prophylaxis:
Adults:
The recommended dosage for prophylaxis in adults is 1 Bactrim DS (double strength) tablet daily.[8]

Children:
For children, the recommended dose is 150 mg/m²/day trimethoprim with 750 mg/m²/day sulfamethoxazole given orally in equally divided doses twice a day, on 3 consecutive days per week. The total daily dose should not exceed 320 mg trimethoprim and 1600 mg sulfamethoxazole.[9] The following table is a guideline for the attainment of this dosage in children:

Body Surface Area	Dose—every 12 hours	
(m²)	Teaspoonfuls	Tablets
0.26	½ (2.5 mL)	—
0.53	1 (5 mL)	½
1.06	2 (10 mL)	1

Travelers' Diarrhea in Adults:
For the treatment of travelers' diarrhea, the usual adult dosage is 1 Bactrim DS (double strength) tablet; 2 Bactrim tablets or 4 teaspoonfuls (20 mL) of Pediatric Suspension every 12 hours for 5 days.

HOW SUPPLIED

DS (double strength) Tablets (white, notched, capsule shaped), containing 160 mg trimethoprim and 800 mg sulfamethoxazole—bottles of 100 (NDC 0004-0117-01), 250 (NDC 0004-0117-04) and 500 (NDC 0004-0117-14). Imprint on tablets: (front) BACTRIM-DS; (back) ROCHE.

Tablets (light green, scored, capsule shaped), containing 80 mg trimethoprim and 400 mg sulfamethoxazole—bottles of 100 (NDC 0004-0050-01). Imprint on tablets: (front) BACTRIM; (back) ROCHE.

Pediatric Suspension (pink, cherry flavored), containing 40 mg trimethoprim and 200 mg sulfamethoxazole per teaspoonful (5 mL)—bottles of 16 oz (1 pint) (NDC 0004-1033-28).

TABLETS SHOULD BE STORED AT 15°–30°C (59°–86°F) IN A DRY PLACE AND PROTECTED FROM LIGHT.

SUSPENSION SHOULD BE STORED AT 15°–30°C (59°–86°F) AND PROTECTED FROM LIGHT.

REFERENCES
1. Kremers P, Duvivier J, Heusghem C. Pharmacokinetic Studies of Co-Trimoxazole in Man after Single and Repeated Doses. *J Clin Pharmacol.* Feb-Mar 1974; 14:112–117. 2. Kaplan SA, et al. Pharmacokinetic Profile of Trimethoprim-Sulfamethoxazole in Man. *J Infect Dis.* Nov 1973; 128 (Suppl): S547–S555. 3. *Federal Register.* 1972; 37:20527–20529, 4. Bauer AW, Kirby WMM, Sherris JC, Turck M. Antibiotic Susceptibility Testing by a Standardized Single Disk Method. *Am J Clin Path.* Apr 1966; 45: 493–496. 5. Hardy DW, et al. A controlled trial of trimethoprim-sulfamethoxazole or aerosolized pentamidine for secondary prophylaxis of *Pneumocystis carinii* pneumonia in patients with the acquired immunodeficiency syndrome. *N Engl J Med.* 1992; 327: 1842–1848. 6. Brumfitt W, Pursell R. Trimethoprim/Sulfamethoxazole in the Treatment of Bacteriuria in Women. *J Infect Dis.* Nov 1973; 128 (Suppl): S657–S663. 7. Masur H. Prevention and treatment of *Pneumocystis* pneumonia. *N Engl J Med.* 1992;327:1853–1880. 8. Recommendations for prophylaxis against *Pneumocystis carinii* pneumonia for adults and adolescents infected with human immunodeficiency virus. *MMWR,* 1992; 41(RR-4):1–11. 9. CDC Guidelines for prophylaxis against *Pneumocystis carinii* pneumonia for children infected with human immunodeficiency virus. *MMWR.* 1991;40(RR-2);1–13.

Revised: January 1994
Shown in Product Identification Guide, page 334

CELLCEPT®   ℞
[sel 'sep]
(mycophenolate mofetil capsules)
(mycophenolate mofetil tablets)

The following text is complete prescribing information based on official labeling in effect June 1998.

> **WARNING:** Increased susceptibility to infection and the possible development of lymphoma may result from immunosuppression. Only physicians experienced in immunosuppressive therapy and management of renal or cardiac transplant patients should use CellCept. Patients receiving the drug should be managed in facilities equipped and staffed with adequate laboratory and supportive medical resources. The physician responsible for maintenance therapy should have complete information requisite for the follow-up of the patient.

Continued on next page

Cellcept—Cont.

DESCRIPTION

CellCept (mycophenolate mofetil) is the 2-morpholinoethyl ester of mycophenolic acid (MPA), an immunosuppressive agent.

The chemical name for mycophenolate mofetil is 2-morpholinoethyl (E)-6-(1,3-dihydro-4-hydroxy-6-methoxy-7-methyl-3-oxo-5-isobenzofuranyl)-4-methyl-4-hexenoate. It has an empirical formula of $C_{23}H_{31}NO_7$, a molecular weight of 433.50.

CellCept is available for oral administration as capsules containing 250 mg of mycophenolate mofetil and tablets containing 500 mg of mycophenolate mofetil. Inactive ingredients in CellCept 250 mg capsules include croscarmellose sodium, magnesium stearate, povidone (K-90) and pregelatinized starch. The capsule shells contain black iron oxide, FD&C blue #2, gelatin, red iron oxide, silicon dioxide, sodium lauryl sulfate, titanium dioxide and yellow iron oxide. Inactive ingredients in CellCept 500 mg tablets include black iron oxide, croscarmellose sodium, FD&C blue #2 aluminum lake, hydroxypropyl cellulose, hydroxypropyl methylcellulose, magnesium stearate, microcrystalline cellulose, polyethylene glycol 400, povidone (K-90), red iron oxide, talc and titanium dioxide; may also contain ammonium hydroxide, ethyl alcohol, methyl alcohol, n-butyl alcohol, propylene glycol and shellac.

Mycophenolate mofetil is a white to off-white crystalline powder. It is slightly soluble in water (43 μg/mL at pH 7.4); the solubility increases in acidic medium (4.27 mg/mL at pH 3.6). It is freely soluble in acetone, soluble in methanol, and sparingly soluble in ethanol. The apparent partition coefficient in 1-octanol/water (pH 7.4) buffer solution is 238. The pKa values for mycophenolate mofetil are 5.6 for the morpholino group and 8.5 for the phenolic group.

CLINICAL PHARMACOLOGY

Mechanism of Action: Mycophenolate mofetil has been demonstrated in experimental animal models to prolong the survival of allogeneic transplants (kidney, heart, liver, intestine, limb, small bowel, pancreatic islets and bone marrow). Mycophenolate mofetil has also been shown to reverse ongoing acute rejection in the canine renal and rat cardiac allograft models. Mycophenolate mofetil also inhibited proliferative arteriopathy in experimental models of aortic and heart allografts in rats, as well as in primate cardiac xenografts. Mycophenolate mofetil was used alone or in combination with other immunosuppressive agents in these studies. Mycophenolate mofetil has been demonstrated to inhibit immunologically-mediated inflammatory responses in animal models and to inhibit tumor development and prolong survival in murine tumor transplant models.

Mycophenolate mofetil is rapidly absorbed following oral administration and hydrolyzed to form MPA, which is the active metabolite. MPA is a potent, selective, uncompetitive and reversible inhibitor of inosine monophosphate dehydrogenase (IMPDH), and therefore inhibits the de novo pathway of guanosine nucleotide synthesis without incorporation into DNA. Because T- and B-lymphocytes are critically dependent for their proliferation on de novo synthesis of purines whereas other cell types can utilize salvage pathways, MPA has potent cytostatic effects on lymphocytes. MPA inhibits proliferative responses of T- and B-lymphocytes to both mitogenic and allospecific stimulation. Addition of guanosine or deoxyguanosine reverses the cytostatic effects of MPA on lymphocytes. MPA also suppresses antibody formation by B-lymphocytes. MPA prevents the glycosylation of lymphocyte and monocyte glycoproteins that are involved in intercellular adhesion to endothelial cells and may inhibit recruitment of leukocytes into sites of inflammation and graft rejection. Mycophenolate mofetil did not inhibit early events in the activation of human peripheral blood mononuclear cells, such as the production of interleukin-1 (IL-1) and interleukin-2 (IL-2), but did block the coupling of these events to DNA synthesis and proliferation.

Pharmacokinetics: Following oral administration, mycophenolate mofetil undergoes rapid and extensive absorption and complete presystemic metabolism to MPA, the active metabolite. MPA is metabolized to form the phenolic glucuronide of MPA (MPAG) which is not pharmacologically active. Mycophenolate mofetil is not measurable systemically in plasma following oral administration.

Absorption: In 12 healthy volunteers, the mean absolute bioavailability of oral mycophenolate mofetil relative to IV mycophenolate mofetil (based on MPA AUC) was 94%. The area under the plasma-concentration time curve (AUC) for MPA appears to increase in a dose-proportional fashion in renal transplant patients receiving multiple doses of mycophenolate mofetil up to a daily dose of 3 g (see table below on pharmacokinetic parameters in renal and cardiac transplant patients).

The C_{max} and AUC of MPA in early transplant patients (<40 days posttransplant) are approximately 45% to 50% and 20% to 30% lower, respectively, as compared to healthy volunteers or to stable renal and cardiac transplant patients.

Pharmacokinetic Parameters for MPA [mean (±SD)] Following Administration of Mycophenolate Mofetil to Healthy Volunteers (Single Dose), Renal and Cardiac Transplant Patients (Multiple Doses)

	Dose	T_{max} (h)	C_{max} (μg/mL)	Total AUC (μg·h/mL)
Healthy Volunteers	1 g	0.80 (±0.36) (n=129)	24.5 (±9.5) (n=129)	63.9 (±16.2) (n=117)
Time After Renal Transplantation	**Dose**	T_{max} (h)	C_{max} (μg/mL)	Interdosing Interval AUC_{0-12} (μg·h/mL)
Early (<40 days)	1 g bid	1.31 (±0.76) (n=25)	8.16 (±4.50) (n=25)	27.3 (±10.9) (n=25)
Early (<40 days)	1.5 g bid	1.21 (±0.81) (n=27)	13.5 (±8.18) (n=27)	38.4 (±15.4) (n=27)
Late (>3 months)	1.5 g bid	0.90 (±0.24) (n=23)	24.1 (±12.1) (n=23)	65.3 (±35.4) (n=23)
Time After Cardiac Transplantation	**Dose**	T_{max} (h)	C_{max} (μg/mL)	Interdosing Interval AUC_{8-12} (μg·h/mL)
Early (Day before discharge)	1.5 g bid	1.8 (±1.3) (n=11)	11.5 (±6.8) (n=11)	43.3 (±20.8) (n=9)
Late (>6 months)	1.5 g bid	1.1 (±0.7) (n=52)	20.0 (±9.4) (n=52)	54.1* (±20.4) (n=49)

*AUC_{0-12} values quoted are extrapolated from data from samples collected over 4 hours.

Pharmacokinetic Parameters for MPA [mean (±SD)] Following Single Doses of Mycophenolate Mofetil in Chronic Renal and Hepatic Impairment

Renal Impairment (no. of patients)	Dose	T_{max} (h)	C_{max} (μg/mL)	AUC_{0-96} (μg·h/mL)
Healthy Volunteers GFR >80 mL/min/1.73m^2(n=6)	1 g	0.75 (±0.27)	25.3 (±7.99)	45.0 (±22.6)
Mild Renal Impairment GFR 50 to 80 mL/min/1.73m^2 (n=6)	1 g	0.75 (±0.27)	26.0 (±3.82)	59.9 (±12.9)
Moderate Renal Impairment GFR 25 to 49 mL/min/1.73m^2 (n=6)	1 g	0.75 (±0.27)	19.0 (±13.2)	52.9 (±25.5)
Severe Renal Impairment GFR <25 mL/min/1.73m^2 (n=7)	1 g	1.00 (±0.41)	16.3 (±10.8)	78.6 (±46.4)
Hepatic Impairment (no. of patients)	**Dose**	T_{max} (h)	C_{max} (μg/mL)	AUC_{0-48} (μg·h/mL)
Healthy Volunteers (n=6)	1 g	0.63 (±0.14)	24.3 (±5.73)	29.0 (±5.78)
Alcoholic cirrhosis (n=18)	1 g	0.85 (±0.58)	22.4 (±10.1)	29.8 (±10.7)

Food (27 g fat, 650 calories) had no effect on the extent of absorption (MPA AUC) of mycophenolate mofetil when administered at doses of 1.5 g bid to renal transplant patients. However, MPA C_{max} was decreased by 40% in the presence of food (see DOSAGE AND ADMINISTRATION).

Distribution: The mean (±SD) apparent volume of distribution of MPA in twelve healthy volunteers is approximately 3.6 (±1.5) and 4.0 (±1.2) L/kg following IV and oral administration, respectively. MPA, at clinically relevant concentrations, is 97% bound to plasma albumin. MPAG is 82% bound to plasma albumin at MPAG concentration ranges that are normally seen in stable renal transplant patients; however, at higher MPAG concentrations (observed in patients with renal impairment or delayed graft function), the binding of MPA may be reduced as a result of competition between MPAG and MPA for protein binding. Mean blood to plasma ratio of radioactivity concentrations was approximately 0.6 indicating that MPA and MPAG do not extensively distribute into the cellular fractions of blood.

In vitro studies to evaluate the effect of other agents on the binding of MPA to human serum albumin (HSA) or plasma proteins showed that salicylate (at 25 mg/dL with HSA) and MPAG (at ≥460 μg/mL with plasma proteins) increased the free fraction of MPA. At concentrations that exceeded what is encountered clinically, cyclosporine, digoxin, naproxen, prednisone, propranolol, tacrolimus, theophylline, tolbutamide and warfarin did not increase the free fraction of MPA. MPA at concentrations as high as 100 μg/mL had little effect on the binding of warfarin, digoxin or propranolol, but decreased the binding of theophylline from 53% to 45% and phenytoin from 90% to 87%.

Metabolism: Mycophenolate mofetil undergoes complete presystemic metabolism to MPA, the active metabolite. MPA is metabolized principally by glucuronyl transferase to form the phenolic glucuronide of MPA (MPAG) which is not pharmacologically active. The following metabolites of the 2-hydroxyethyl-morpholino moiety are also recovered in the urine following oral administration of mycophenolate mofetil to healthy subjects: N-(2-carboxymethyl)-morpholine, N-(2-hydroxyethyl)-morpholine, and the N-oxide of N-(2-hydroxyethyl)-morpholine.

Secondary peaks in the plasma MPA concentration-time profile are usually observed 6 to 12 hours postdose. The coadministration of cholestyramine (4 g tid) resulted in approximately a 40% decrease in the MPA AUC (largely as a consequence of lower concentrations in the terminal portion of the profile). These observations suggest that enterohepatic recirculation contributes to MPA plasma concentrations.

Increased plasma concentrations of mycophenolate mofetil metabolites (MPA 50% increase and MPAG about three- to six-fold increase) are observed in patients with renal insufficiency (see CLINICAL PHARMACOLOGY: Special Populations).

Excretion: Negligible amount of drug is excreted as MPA (<1% of dose) in the urine. Orally administered radiola-

beled mycophenolate mofetil resulted in complete recovery of the administered dose, with 93% of the administered dose recovered in the urine and 6% recovered in feces. Most (about 87%) of the administered dose is excreted in the urine as MPAG. MPA and MPAG are usually not removed by hemodialysis. However, at high MPAG plasma concentrations (>100 µg/mL), small amounts of MPAG are removed.

Mean ($\pm$SD) apparent half-life and plasma clearance of MPA are 17.9 ($\pm$6.5) hours and 193 ($\pm$48) mL/min following oral administration and 16.6 ($\pm$5.8) hours and 177 ($\pm$31) mL/min following IV administration, respectively.

Pharmacokinetics in Healthy Volunteers, Renal and Cardiac Transplant Patients: Shown below are the mean ($\pm$SD) pharmacokinetic parameters for MPA following the administration of oral mycophenolate mofetil given as single doses to healthy volunteers and multiple doses to renal and cardiac transplant patients. The C_{max} and AUC of MPA in early transplant patients (<40 days posttransplant) are approximately 45% to 50% and 20% to 30% lower, respectively, as compared to healthy volunteers or to stable renal and cardiac transplant patients.

[See first table at top of previous page]

Two 500 mg tablets have been shown to be bioequivalent to four 250 mg capsules.

Special Populations: Shown below are the mean ($\pm$SD) pharmacokinetic parameters for MPA following the administration of oral mycophenolate mofetil given as single doses to subjects with renal and hepatic impairment.

[See second table at top of previous page]

Renal Insufficiency: In a single-dose study (6 volunteers per group), plasma MPA AUCs observed in volunteers with severe chronic renal impairment [glomerular filtration rate (GFR) <25 mL/min/1.73 m²] were about 75% higher relative to those observed in healthy volunteers (GFR >80 mL/min/1.73 m²). In addition, the single-dose plasma MPAG AUC was three- to six-fold higher in volunteers with severe renal impairment than in volunteers with mild renal impairment or healthy volunteers, consistent with the known renal elimination of MPAG. Multiple dosing of mycophenolate mofetil in patients with severe chronic renal impairment has not been studied. No data are available on the safety of long-term exposure to this level of MPAG (see PRECAUTIONS: *General* and DOSAGE AND ADMINISTRATION). In patients with delayed renal graft function posttransplant, mean MPA AUC_{0-12} was comparable to that seen in posttransplant patients without delayed graft function. Mean plasma MPAG AUC_{0-12} was two- to three-fold higher than in posttransplant patients without delayed graft function (see PRECAUTIONS: *General* and DOSAGE AND ADMINISTRATION).

The pharmacokinetics of mycophenolate mofetil are not altered by hemodialysis. Hemodialysis usually does not remove MPA or MPAG. At high concentrations of MPAG (>100 µg/mL), hemodialysis removes only small amounts of MPAG.

Hepatic Insufficiency: In a single-dose (1 g) study of 18 volunteers with alcoholic cirrhosis and 6 healthy volunteers, hepatic MPA glucuronidation processes appeared to be relatively unaffected by hepatic parenchymal disease when pharmacokinetic parameters of healthy volunteers and alcoholic cirrhosis patients within this study were compared. However, it should be noted that for unexplained reasons, the healthy volunteers in this study had about a 50% lower AUC as compared to healthy volunteers in other studies, thus making comparisons between volunteers with alcoholic cirrhosis and healthy volunteers difficult. Effects of hepatic disease on this process probably depend on the particular disease. Hepatic disease with other etiologies may show a different effect.

Pediatrics: Very limited pharmacokinetic data are available for pediatric renal transplant recipients. Data on these patients collected on day 21 posttransplant are presented in the table below:

[See first table above]

Gender: Data obtained from several studies were pooled to look at any gender-related differences in the pharmacokinetics of MPA (data were adjusted to 1 g dose). Mean ($\pm$SD) MPA AUC_{0-12} for males (n=79) was 32.0 ($\pm$14.5) and for females (n=41) was 36.5 ($\pm$18.8) µg·h/mL while mean ($\pm$SD) MPA C_{max} was 9.96 ($\pm$6.19) in the males and 10.6 ($\pm$5.64) µg/mL in the females. These differences are not of clinical significance.

CLINICAL STUDIES

The safety and efficacy of CellCept in combination with corticosteroids and cyclosporine for the prevention of organ rejection were assessed in renal transplant patients in three randomized, double-blind, multicenter trials and in cardiac patients in one randomized double-blind, multicenter trial.

Renal Transplant: These three studies compared two dose levels of CellCept (1 g bid and 1.5 g bid) with azathioprine (2 studies) or placebo (1 study) when administered in combination with cyclosporine (Sandimmune®) and corticosteroids to prevent acute rejection episodes. One study also included antithymocyte globulin (ATGAM®) induction therapy. These studies are described by geographic location of

the investigational sites. One study was conducted in the USA at 14 sites, one study was conducted in Europe at 20 sites, and one study was conducted in Europe, Canada, and Australia at a total of 21 sites.

The primary efficacy endpoint was the proportion of patients in each treatment group who experienced treatment failure within the first six months after transplantation (defined as biopsy-proven acute rejection on treatment or the occurrence of death, graft loss or early termination from the study for any reason without prior biopsy-proven rejection). CellCept, when administered with antithymocyte globulin (ATGAM®) induction (one study) and with cyclosporine and corticosteroids (all three studies), was compared to the following three therapeutic regimens: (1) antithymocyte globulin (ATGAM®) induction/ azathioprine/ cyclosporine/corticosteroids, (2) azathioprine/cyclosporine/corticosteroids, and (3) cyclosporine/corticosteroids.

CellCept, in combination with corticosteroids and cyclosporine reduced (statistically significant at the <0.05 level) the incidence of treatment failure within the first 6 months following transplantation. The following tables summarize the results of these studies. These tables show (1) the proportion of patients experiencing treatment failure, (2) the proportion of patients who experienced biopsy-proven acute rejection on treatment, and (3) early termination, for any reason other than graft loss or death, without a prior biopsy-proven acute rejection episode. Patients who prematurely discontinued treatment were followed for the occurrence of death or graft loss, and the cumulative incidence of graft loss and patient death are summarized separately. Patients who prematurely discontinued treatment were not followed for the occurrence of acute rejection after termination. More patients discontinued receiving CellCept (without prior biopsy-proven rejection, death or graft loss) than discontinued in the control groups, with the highest rate in the CellCept 3 g/day group. Therefore, the acute rejection rates may be underestimates, particularly in the CellCept 3 g/day group. [See second table above]

Cumulative incidence of twelve-month graft loss and patient death are presented below. No advantage of CellCept with respect to graft loss and patient death was established. Numerically, patients receiving CellCept 2 g/day and 3 g/day experienced a better outcome than controls in all

Pharmacokinetic Parameters for MPA [mean ± (SD)] Following Multiple Oral Doses of Mycophenolate Mofetil in Pediatric Renal Transplant Patients

Age Range	Dose	T_{max} (h)	C_{max} (µg/mL)	AUC_{0-12} (µg·h/mL)
$\geq$ 3 mo to < 6 yr (Mean = 2.75) (n=4)	15 mg/kg bid	1.25 ($\pm$0.87)	3.70 ($\pm$2.08)	13.6 ($\pm$8.69)
$\geq$ 6 yr to < 12 yr (Mean = 9.0) (n=4)	15 mg/kg bid	0.50 ($\pm$0.00)	13.5 ($\pm$4.48)	23.4 ($\pm$2.84)
$\geq$ 12 yr to 18 yr (Mean = 15.6) (n=5)	15 mg/kg bid	0.50 ($\pm$0.00)	13.2 ($\pm$6.86)	30.0 ($\pm$8.34)
$\geq$ 12 yr to 18 yr (Mean = 14.0) (n=7)	23 mg/kg bid	1.14 ($\pm$0.80)	10.6 ($\pm$9.59)	28.3 ($\pm$12.8)

Renal Transplant Studies
Incidence of Treatment Failure (Biopsy-proven Rejection of Early Termination for Any Reason)

USA Study (N=499 patients)	CellCept 2 g/day (n=167 patients)	CellCept 3 g/day (n=166 patients)	Azathioprine 1 to 2 mg/kg/day (n=166 patients)
All treatment failures	31.1%	31.3%	47.6%
Early termination without prior acute rejection*	9.6%	12.7%	6.0%
Biopsy-proven rejection episode on treatment	19.8%	17.5%	38.0%
Europe/Canada/Australia Study (N=503 patients)	**CellCept 2 g/day (n=173 patients)**	**CellCept 3 g/day (n=164 patients)**	**Azathioprine 100 to 150 mg/day (n=166 patients)**
All treatment failures	38.2%	34.8%	50.0%
Early termination without prior acute rejection*	13.9%	15.2%	10.2%
Biopsy-proven rejection episode on treatment	19.7%	15.9%	35.5%
Europe Study (N=491 patients)	**CellCept 2 g/day (n=165 patients)**	**CellCept 3 g/day (n=160 patients)**	**Placebo (n=166 patients)**
All treatment failures	30.3%	38.8%	56.0%
Early termination without prior acute rejection*	11.5%	22.5%	7.2%
Biopsy-proven rejection episode on treatment	17.0%	13.8%	46.4%

*Does not include death and graft loss as reason for early termination.

Renal Transplant Studies
Cumulative Incidence of Combined Graft Loss and Patient Death at 12 Months

Study	CellCept 2 g/day	CellCept 3 g/day	Control (Azathioprine or Placebo)
USA	8.5%	11.5%	12.2%
Europe/Canada/Australia	11.7%	11.0%	13.6%
Europe	8.5%	10.0%	11.5%

Continued on next page

Cellcept—Cont.

three studies; patients receiving CellCept 2 g/day experienced a better outcome than CellCept 3 g/day in two of the three studies. Patients in all treatment groups who terminated treatment early were found to have a poor outcome with respect to graft loss and patient death at one year.
[See third table from top on previous page]

Cardiac Transplant: A double-blind, randomized, comparative, parallel-group, multicenter study in primary cardiac transplant recipients was performed at 20 centers in the United States, one in Canada, five in Europe and two in Australia. The total number of patients enrolled was 650; 72 never received study drug and 578 received study drug. Patients received CellCept 1.5 g bid (n=289) or azathioprine 1.5 to 3 mg/kg/day (n=289), in combination with cyclosporine (Sandimmune® or Neoral®) and corticosteroids as maintenance immunosuppressive therapy. The two primary efficacy endpoints were: (1) the proportion of patients who, after transplantation, had at least one endomyocardial biopsy-proven rejection with hemodynamic compromise, or were retransplanted or died, within the first 6 months, and (2) the proportion of patients who died or were transplanted during the first 12 months following transplantation. Patients who prematurely discontinued treatment were followed for the occurrence of allograft rejection for up to 6 months and for the occurrence of death for 1 year.

(1) Rejection: No difference was established between CellCept and azathioprine (AZA) with respect to biopsy-proven rejection with hemodynamic compromise, as presented below.
[See first table above]

(2) Survival: CellCept was shown to be at least as effective as AZA in preventing death or retransplantation at 1 year, as presented below.
[See second table above]

Rejection at 6 Months

	All Patients		Treated Patients	
	AZA N=323	CellCept N=327	AZA N=289	CellCept N=289
Biopsy-proven rejection with hemodynamic compromise*	121 (38%)	120 (37%)	100 (35%)	92 (32%)

* Hemodynamic compromise occurred if any of the following criteria were met: pulmonary capillary wedge pressure ≥20 mm or a 25% increase; cardiac index <2.0 l/min/m^2 or a 25% decrease; ejection fraction ≤30%; pulmonary artery oxygen saturation ≤60% or a 25% decrease; presence of new S_3 gallop; fractional shortening was ≤20% or a 25% decrease; inotropic support required to manage the clinical condition.

Death or Retransplantation at 1 year

	All Patients		Treated Patients	
	AZA N=323	CellCept N=327	AZA N=289	CellCept N=289
Death or Retransplantation	49 (15.2%)	42 (12.8%)	33 (11.4%)	18 (6.2%)

INDICATIONS AND USAGE

Renal and Cardiac Transplant: CellCept is indicated for the prophylaxis of organ rejection in patients receiving allogeneic renal transplants and in patients receiving allogeneic cardiac transplants. CellCept should be used concomitantly with cyclosporine and corticosteroids.

CONTRAINDICATIONS

Allergic reactions to CellCept have been observed; therefore, CellCept is contraindicated in patients with a hypersensitivity to mycophenolate mofetil, mycophenolic acid or any component of the drug product.

WARNINGS (See boxed WARNING):

Patients receiving immunosuppressive regimens involving combinations of drugs, including CellCept, as part of an immunosuppressive regimen are at increased risk of developing lymphomas and other malignancies, particularly of the skin. The risk appears to be related to the intensity and duration of immunosuppression rather than to the use of any specific agent. Oversuppression of the immune system can also increase susceptibility to infection.

As usual for patients with increased risk for skin cancer, exposure to sunlight and UV light should be limited by wearing protective clothing and using a sunscreen with a high protection factor.

CellCept has been administered in combination with the following agents in clinical trials: antithymocyte globulin (ATGAM®), OKT3 (Orthoclone OKT® 3), cyclosporine (Sandimmune®, Neoral®), and corticosteroids. The efficacy and safety of the use of CellCept in combination with other immunosuppressive agents have not been determined.

Lymphoproliferative disease or lymphoma developed in approximately 1% of patients receiving CellCept (2 g or 3 g) with other immunosuppressive agents in controlled clinical trials of renal and cardiac transplant patients (see ADVERSE REACTIONS).

Adverse effects on fetal development (including malformations) occurred when pregnant rats and rabbits were dosed during organogenesis. These responses occurred at doses lower than those associated with maternal toxicity, and at doses below the recommended clinical dose for renal or cardiac transplantation. There are no adequate and well-controlled studies in pregnant women. However, as CellCept has been shown to have teratogenic effects in animals, it may cause fetal harm when administered to a pregnant woman. Therefore, CellCept should not be used in pregnant women unless the potential benefit justifies the potential risk to the fetus.

Women of childbearing potential should have a negative serum or urine pregnancy test with a sensitivity of at least 50 mIU/mL within 1 week prior to beginning therapy. It is recommended that CellCept therapy should not be initiated by the physician until a report of a negative pregnancy test has been obtained.

Effective contraception must be used before beginning CellCept therapy, during therapy, and for 6 weeks following discontinuation of therapy, even where there has been a history of infertility, unless due to hysterectomy. Two reliable forms of contraception must be used simultaneously unless abstinence is the chosen method. If pregnancy does occur during treatment, the physician and patient should discuss the desirability of continuing the pregnancy (see PRECAUTIONS: *Pregnancy* and *Information for Patients*).

In controlled studies for prevention of renal or cardiac rejection, similar rates of fatal infection/sepsis (<2%) occurred in patients receiving CellCept (2 g or 3 g) (see ADVERSE REACTIONS).

Severe neutropenia [absolute neutrophil count (ANC) <0.5 × 10^3/µL] developed in up to 2.0% of renal transplant patients and up to 2.8% of cardiac transplant patients receiving CellCept (see ADVERSE REACTIONS). Patients receiving CellCept should be monitored for neutropenia (see PRECAUTIONS: *Laboratory Tests*). The development of neutropenia may be related to CellCept itself, concomitant medications, viral infections, or some combination of these causes. If neutropenia develops (ANC <1.3 x 10^3/µL), dosing with CellCept should be interrupted or the dose reduced, appropriate diagnostic tests performed, and the patient managed appropriately (see DOSAGE AND ADMINISTRATION). Neutropenia has been observed most frequently in the period from 31 to 180 days posttransplant in patients treated for prevention of renal and cardiac rejection.

Patients receiving CellCept should be instructed to report immediately any evidence of infection, unexpected bruising, bleeding or any other manifestation of bone marrow depression.

PRECAUTIONS

General: Gastrointestinal hemorrhage has been observed in approximately 3% of renal transplant patients and in 2.8% of cardiac transplant patients treated with CellCept 3 g daily. Gastrointestinal perforations have rarely been observed. Most patients receiving CellCept were also receiving other drugs known to be associated with these complications. Patients with active peptic ulcer disease were excluded from enrollment in studies with mycophenolate mofetil. Because CellCept has been associated with an increased incidence of digestive system adverse events, including infrequent cases of gastrointestinal tract ulceration, hemorrhage, and perforation, CellCept should be administered with caution in patients with active serious digestive system disease.

Subjects with severe chronic renal impairment (GFR <25 mL/min/1.73 m^2) who have received single doses of CellCept showed higher plasma MPA and MPAG AUCs relative to subjects with lesser degrees of renal impairment or normal healthy volunteers. No data are available on the safety of long-term exposure to these levels of MPAG. Doses of CellCept greater than 1 g administered twice a day to renal transplant patients should be avoided and they should be carefully observed (see CLINICAL PHARMACOLOGY: *Pharmacokinetics* and DOSAGE AND ADMINISTRATION). No data are available for cardiac transplant patients with severe chronic renal impairment. CellCept may be used for cardiac transplant patients with severe chronic renal impairment if the potential benefits outweigh the potential risks.

In patients with delayed renal graft function posttransplant, mean MPA AUC_{0-12} was comparable, but MPAG AUC_{0-12} was two- to three-fold higher, compared to that seen in posttransplant patients without delayed renal graft function. In the three controlled studies of prevention of renal rejection, there were 298 of 1483 patients (20%) with delayed graft function. Although patients with delayed graft function have a higher incidence of certain adverse events (anemia, thrombocytopenia, hyperkalemia) than patients without delayed graft function, these events were not more frequent in patients receiving CellCept than azathioprine or placebo. No dose adjustment is recommended for these patients; however, they should be carefully observed (see CLINICAL PHARMACOLOGY: *Pharmacokinetics* and DOSAGE AND ADMINISTRATION).

It is recommended that CellCept not be administered concomitantly with azathioprine because such concomitant administration has not been studied clinically.

In view of the significant reduction in the AUC of MPA by cholestyramine, caution should be used in the concomitant administration of CellCept with drugs that interfere with enterohepatic recirculation because of the potential to reduce the efficacy of CellCept (see PRECAUTIONS: *Drug Interactions*).

Information for Patients: Patients should be informed of the need for repeated appropriate laboratory tests while they are receiving CellCept. Patients should be given complete dosage instructions and informed of the increased risk of lymphoproliferative disease and certain other malignancies. Women of childbearing potential should be instructed of the potential risks during pregnancy, and that they should use effective contraception before beginning CellCept therapy, during therapy and for 6 weeks after CellCept has been stopped (see WARNINGS and PRECAUTIONS: *Pregnancy*).

Laboratory Tests: Complete blood counts should be performed weekly during the first month, twice monthly for the second and third months of treatment, then monthly through the first year (see WARNINGS, ADVERSE REACTIONS, and DOSAGE AND ADMINISTRATION).

Drug Interactions: Drug interaction studies with mycophenolate mofetil have been conducted with acyclovir, antacids, cholestyramine, cyclosporine, ganciclovir, oral contraceptives, and trimethoprim/sulfamethoxazole. Drug interaction studies have not been conducted with other drugs that may be commonly administered to renal or cardiac transplant patients. CellCept has not been administered concomitantly with azathioprine.

Acyclovir: Coadministration of mycophenolate mofetil (1 g) and acyclovir (800 mg) to twelve healthy volunteers resulted in no significant change in MPA AUC and C_{max}. However, MPAG and acyclovir plasma AUCs were increased 10.6% and 21.9%, respectively. Because MPAG plasma concentrations are increased in the presence of renal impairment, as are acyclovir concentrations, the potential exists for the two drugs to compete for tubular secretion, further increasing the concentrations of both drugs.

Antacids with Magnesium and Aluminum Hydroxides: Absorption of a single dose of mycophenolate mofetil (2 g) was decreased when administered to ten rheumatoid arthritis patients also taking Maalox® TC (10 mL qid). The C_{max} and AUC_{0-24} for MPA were 33% and 17% lower, respectively, than when mycophenolate mofetil was administered alone under fasting conditions. CellCept may be administered to patients who are also taking antacids containing magnesium and aluminum hydroxides; however, it is recommended that CellCept and the antacid not be administered simultaneously.

Cholestyramine: Following single-dose administration of 1.5 g mycophenolate mofetil to twelve healthy volunteers pretreated with 4 g tid of cholestyramine for 4 days, MPA AUC decreased approximately 40%. This decrease is consistent with interruption of enterohepatic recirculation which may be due to binding of recirculating MPAG with cholestyramine in the intestine. CellCept is not recommended to be given with cholestyramine or other agents that may interfere with enterohepatic recirculation.

Cyclosporine: Cyclosporine (Sandimmune®) pharmacokinetics (at doses of 275 to 415 mg/day) were unaffected by single and multiple doses of 1.5 g bid of mycophenolate mofetil in ten stable renal transplant patients. The mean (±SD) AUC_{0-12} and C_{max} of cyclosporine after 14 days of multiple doses of mycophenolate mofetil were 3290 (±822) ng·h/mL and 753 (±161) ng/mL, respectively, compared to 3245 (±1088) ng·h/mL and 700 (±246) ng/mL, respectively, one week before administration of mycophenolate mofetil. The effect of cyclosporine on mycophenolate mofetil phar-

Adverse Events in Controlled Studies in Prevention of Renal Allograft Rejection
USA Study Combined with Europe/Canada/Australia Study

	CellCept 2 g/day (n=336)	CellCept 3 g/day (n=330)	Azathioprine 1 to 2 mg/kg/day or 100 to 150 mg/day (n=326)
Body as a Whole			
Pain	33.0%	31.2%	32.2%
Abdominal pain	24.7	27.6	23.0
Fever	21.4	23.3	23.3
Headache	21.1	16.1	21.2
Infection	18.2	20.9	19.9
Sepsis	17.6	19.7	15.6
Asthenia	13.7	16.1	19.9
Chest pain	13.4	13.3	14.7
Back pain	11.6	12.1	14.1
Hemic and Lymphatic			
Anemia	25.6	25.8	23.6
Leukopenia	23.2	34.5	24.8
Thrombocytopenia	10.1	8.2	13.2
Hypochromic anemia	7.4	11.5	9.2
Leukocytosis	7.1	10.9	7.4
Urogenital			
Urinary tract infection	37.2	37.0	33.7
Hematuria	14.0	12.1	11.3
Kidney tubular necrosis	6.3	10.0	5.8
Cardiovascular			
Hypertension	32.4	28.2	32.2
Metabolic and Nutritional			
Peripheral edema	28.6	27.0	28.2
Hypercholesteremia	12.8	8.5	11.3
Hypophosphatemia	12.5	15.8	11.7
Edema	12.2	11.8	13.5
Hypokalemia	10.1	10.0	8.3
Hyperkalemia	8.9	10.3	16.9
Hyperglycemia	8.6	12.4	15.0
Digestive			
Diarrhea	31.0	36.1	20.9
Constipation	22.9	18.5	22.4
Nausea	19.9	23.6	24.5
Dyspepsia	17.6	13.6	13.8
Vomiting	12.5	13.6	9.2
Nausea and vomiting	10.4	9.7	10.7
Oral moniliasis	10.1	12.1	11.3
Respiratory			
Infection	22.0	23.9	19.6
Dyspnea	15.5	17.3	16.6
Cough Increased	15.5	13.3	15.0
Pharyngitis	9.5	11.2	8.0
Skin and Appendages			
Acne	10.1	9.7	6.4
Rash	7.7	6.4	10.4
Nervous System			
Tremor	11.0	11.8	12.3
Insomnia	8.9	11.8	10.4
Dizziness	5.7	11.2	11.0

Europe Study

	CellCept 2 g/day (n=165)	CellCept 3 g/day (n=160)	Placebo (n=166)
Body as a Whole			
Sepsis	21.8%	17.5%	13.9%
Infection	12.7	15.6	13.3
Abdominal pain	12.1	11.9	11.4
Hemic and Lymphatic			
Leukopenia	11.5	16.3	4.2
Urogenital			
Urinary tract infection	45.5	44.4	37.3
Urinary tract disorder	6.7	10.6	4.2
Cardiovascular			
Hypertension	17.6	16.9	19.3
Digestive			
Diarrhea	16.4	18.8	13.9
Respiratory			
Infection	15.8	13.1	9.0
Bronchitis	8.5	11.9	8.4
Pneumonia	3.6	10.6	10.8

macokinetics could not be evaluated in this study; however, plasma concentrations of MPA were similar to that for healthy volunteers.

Ganciclovir: Following single-dose administration to twelve stable renal transplant patients, no pharmacokinetic interaction was observed between mycophenolate mofetil (1.5 g) and IV ganciclovir (5 mg/kg). Mean ($\pm$SD) ganciclovir AUC and C_{max} (n=10) were 54.3 ($\pm$19.0) μg·h/mL and 11.5 ($\pm$1.8) μg/mL, respectively, after coadministration of the two drugs, compared to 51.0 ($\pm$17.0) μg·h/mL and 10.6 ($\pm$2.0) μg/mL, respectively, after administration of IV ganciclovir alone. The mean ($\pm$SD) AUC and C_{max} of MPA (n=12) after coadministration were 80.9 ($\pm$21.6) μg·h/mL and 27.8 ($\pm$13.9) μg/mL, respectively, compared to values of 80.3 ($\pm$16.4) μg·h/mL and 30.9 ($\pm$11.2) μg/mL, respectively, after administration of mycophenolate mofetil alone. Because MPAG plasma concentrations are increased in the presence of renal impairment, as are ganciclovir concentrations, the

potential exists for the two drugs to compete for tubular secretion and thus further increases in concentrations of both drugs may occur.

Oral Contraceptives: Following single-dose administration to fifteen healthy women, no pharmacokinetic interaction was observed between mycophenolate mofetil (1 g) and two tablets of Ortho-Novum® 7/7/7 (1 mg norethindrone [NET] and 35 μg estradiol ethinyl [EE]). This single-dose study suggests the lack of a gross pharmacokinetic interaction, but cannot exclude the possibility of changes in the pharmacokinetics of the oral contraceptive under long-term dosing conditions with CellCept, which might adversely affect the efficacy of the oral contraceptive.

Trimethoprim/sulfamethoxazole: Following single-dose administration of mycophenolate mofetil (1.5 g) to twelve healthy male volunteers on day 8 of a 10 day course of Bactrim™ DS (trimethoprim 160 mg/sulfamethoxazole 800 mg) administered bid, no effect on the bioavailability of MPA

was observed. The mean ($\pm$SD) AUC and C_{max} of MPA after concomitant administration were 75.2 ($\pm$19.8) μg·h/mL and 34.0 ($\pm$6.6) μg/mL, respectively, compared to 79.2 ($\pm$27.9) and 34.2 ($\pm$10.7), respectively, after administration of mycophenolate mofetil alone.

Other Interactions: The measured value for renal clearance of MPAG indicates removal occurs by renal tubular secretion as well as glomerular filtration. Consistent with this, coadministration of probenecid, a known inhibitor of tubular secretion, with mycophenolate mofetil in monkeys results in a three-fold increase in plasma MPAG AUC and a two-fold increase in plasma MPA AUC. Thus, other drugs known to undergo renal tubular secretion may compete with MPAG and thereby raise plasma concentrations of MPAG or the other drug undergoing tubular secretion.

Drugs that alter the gastrointestinal flora may interact with mycophenolate mofetil by disrupting enterohepatic recirculation. Interference of MPAG hydrolysis may lead to less MPA available for absorption.

Carcinogenesis, Mutagenesis, Impairment of Fertility: In a 104-week oral carcinogenicity study in mice, mycophenolate mofetil in daily doses up to 180 mg/kg was not tumorigenic. The highest dose tested was 0.5 times the recommended clinical dose (2 g/day) in renal transplant patients and 0.3 times the recommended clinical dose (3 g/day) in cardiac transplant patients when corrected for differences in body surface area (BSA). In a 104-week oral carcinogenicity study in rats, mycophenolate mofetil in daily doses up to 15 mg/kg was not tumorigenic. The highest dose was 0.08 times the recommended clinical dose in renal transplant patients and 0.05 times the recommended clinical dose in cardiac transplant patients when corrected for BSA. While these animal doses were lower than those given to patients, they were maximal in those species and were considered adequate to evaluate the potential for human risk (see WARNINGS).

Mycophenolate mofetil was not genotoxic, with or without metabolic activation, in several assays: the bacterial mutation assay, the yeast mitotic gene conversion assay, the mouse micronucleus aberration assay, or the Chinese hamster ovary cell (CHO) chromosomal aberration assay.

Mycophenolate mofetil had no effect on fertility of male rats at oral doses up to 20 mg/kg/day. This dose represents 0.1 times the recommended clinical dose in renal transplant patients and 0.07 times the recommended clinical dose in cardiac transplant patients when corrected for BSA. In a female fertility and reproduction study conducted in rats, oral doses of 4.5 mg/kg/day caused malformations (principally of the head and eyes) in the first generation offspring in the absence of maternal toxicity. This dose was 0.02 times the recommended clinical dose in renal transplant patients and 0.01 times the recommended clinical dose in cardiac transplant patients when corrected for BSA. No effects on fertility or reproductive parameters were evident in the dams or in the subsequent generation.

Pregnancy: *Category C.* In teratology studies in rats and rabbits, fetal resorptions and malformations occurred in rats at 6 mg/kg/day and in rabbits at 90 mg/kg/day, in the absence of maternal toxicity. These levels are equivalent to 0.03 to 0.92 times the recommended clinical dose in renal transplant patients and 0.02 to 0.61 times the recommended clinical dose in cardiac transplant patients on a BSA basis. In a female fertility and reproduction study conducted in rats, oral doses of 4.5 mg/kg/day caused malformations (principally of the head and eyes) in the first generation offspring in the absence of maternal toxicity. This dose was 0.02 times the recommended clinical dose in renal transplant patients and 0.01 times the recommended clinical dose in cardiac transplant patients when corrected for BSA.

There are no adequate and well-controlled studies in pregnant women. CellCept should not be used in pregnant women unless the potential benefit justifies the potential risk to the fetus. Effective contraception must be used before beginning CellCept therapy, during therapy and for 6 weeks after CellCept has been stopped (see WARNINGS, PRECAUTIONS: *Information for Patients*).

Nursing Mothers: Studies in rats treated with mycophenolate mofetil have shown mycophenolic acid to be excreted in milk. It is not known whether this drug is excreted in human milk. Because many drugs are excreted in human milk and because of the potential for serious adverse reactions in nursing infants from mycophenolate mofetil, a decision should be made whether to discontinue nursing or to discontinue the drug, taking into account the importance of the drug to the mother.

Pediatric Patients: Safety and effectiveness in pediatric patients have not been established. Very limited pharmacokinetic data are available in pediatric patients (see CLINICAL PHARMACOLOGY: *Pharmacokinetics*).

ADVERSE REACTIONS

The principal adverse reactions associated with the administration of CellCept include diarrhea, leukopenia, sepsis and vomiting, and there is evidence of a higher frequency of certain types of infections.

Continued on next page

Adverse Events in the Controlled Study in Prevention of Cardiac Allograft Rejection

	CellCept 3 g/day (n=289)	Azathioprine 1.5 to 3 mg/kg/day (n=289)
Body as a Whole		
Pain	75.8%	74.7%
Abdominal pain	33.9	33.2
Fever	47.4	46.4
Headache	54.3	51.9
Infection	25.6	19.4
Sepsis	18.7	18.7
Asthenia	43.3	36.3
Chest pain	26.3	26.0
Back pain	34.6	28.4
Accidental injury	19.0	14.9
Chills	11.4	11.4
Hemic and Lymphatic		
Anemia	42.9	43.9
Leukopenia	30.4	39.1
Thrombocytopenia	23.5	27.0
Hypochromic anemia	24.6	23.5
Leukocytosis	40.5	35.6
Ecchymosis	16.6	8.0
Urogenital		
Urinary tract infection	13.1	11.8
Kidney function abnormal	21.8	26.3
Oliguria	14.2	12.8
Cardiovascular		
Hypertension	77.5	72.3
Hypotension	32.5	36.0
Cardiovascular disorder	25.6	24.2
Tachycardia	20.1	18.0
Arrhythmia	19.0	18.7
Bradycardia	17.3	17.3
Pericardial effusion	15.9	13.5
Heart failure	11.8	8.7
Metabolic and Nutritional		
Peripheral edema	64.0	53.3
Hypercholesteremia	41.2	38.4
Edema	26.6	25.6
Hypokalemia	31.8	25.6
Hyperkalemia	14.5	19.7
Hyperglycemia	46.7	52.6
Creatinine increased	39.4	36.0
BUN increased	34.6	32.5
Lactic dehydrogenase increased	23.2	17.0
Bilirubinemia	18.0	21.8
Hypervolemia	16.6	22.8
Generalized edema	18.0	20.1
Hyperuricemia	16.3	17.6
SGOT increased	17.3	15.6
Hypomagnesemia	18.3	12.8
Acidosis	14.2	16.6
Weight gain	15.6	15.2
SGPT increased	15.6	12.5
Hyponatremia	11.4	11.8
Hyperlipemia	10.7	9.3
Digestive		
Diarrhea	45.3	34.3
Constipation	41.2	37.7
Nausea	54.0	54.3
Dyspepsia	18.7	19.4
Vomiting	33.9	28.4
Nausea and vomiting	11.1	7.6
Oral moniliasis	11.4	11.8
Flatulence	13.8	15.6
Respiratory		
Infection	37.0	35.3
Dyspnea	36.7	36.3
Cough increased	31.1	25.6
Pharyngitis	18.3	13.5
Lung disorder	30.1	29.1
Sinusitis	26.0	19.0
Rhinitis	19.0	15.6
Pleural effusion	17.0	13.8
Asthma	11.1	11.4
Pneumonia	10.7	10.4
Skin and Appendages		
Acne	12.1	9.3
Rash	22.1	18.0
Skin disorder	12.5	8.7
Nervous System		
Tremor	24.2	23.9
Insomnia	40.8	37.7
Dizziness	28.7	27.7
Anxiety	28.4	23.9
Paresthesia	20.8	18.0
Hypertonia	15.6	14.5
Depression	15.6	12.5
Agitation	13.1	12.8
Somnolence	11.1	10.4
Confusion	13.5	7.6
Nervousness	11.4	9.0

Continued

The incidence of adverse events for CellCept was determined in three randomized, comparative, double-blind trials in prevention of rejection in renal transplant patients, and in one randomized, comparative, double-blind trial in cardiac transplant patients.

Safety data are summarized below for all renal transplant patients in the double-blind prevention studies; approximately 53% of these patients have been treated for more than 1 year. Adverse events that were reported in ≥10% of patients in either CellCept treatment group are presented below for the two active-controlled studies combined (USA and Europe/Canada/Australia) and for the one European placebo-controlled study. Because of the lower overall reporting of events in the European placebo-controlled study, these data were not combined with the other two active-controlled prevention trials, but are instead presented separately.

[See table at top of previous page]

In the randomized, double-blind, comparative trial in cardiac transplant recipients, approximately 65% of patients have been treated for more than 1 year. Adverse events reported in ≥10% of patients in the group treated with CellCept are provided below.

[See table at left and at top of next page]

The above data demonstrate that in three controlled trials for prevention of renal rejection, patients receiving 2 g/day of CellCept had an overall better safety profile than did patients receiving 3 g/day of CellCept. Sepsis, which was generally CMV viremia, was slightly more common in those renal patients treated with CellCept, with an incidence of 18 to 22%, compared to 16% in patients receiving azathioprine and 14% in patients receiving placebo. In the controlled cardiac transplant study, there was no difference in the incidence of sepsis (18.7%) between patients treated with CellCept and control patients. In the digestive system, diarrhea was increased in renal and cardiac patients receiving CellCept, with an incidence of up to 36%, compared to 21% for patients receiving azathioprine and 14% for patients receiving placebo in the renal transplant studies. In the controlled cardiac transplant study, an incidence of diarrhea up to 45.3% in the patients treated with CellCept was reported compared to 34.3% for patients receiving azathioprine. The types of adverse events in the cardiac transplant patients studied in the multicenter controlled trial were qualitatively similar to those observed in renal transplant patients.

The incidence of malignancies among the 1483 patients treated in controlled trials for the prevention of renal allograft rejection who were followed for ≥1 year was similar to the incidence reported in the literature for renal allograft recipients. Lymphoproliferative disease or lymphoma developed in approximately 1% of patients receiving CellCept (2 g or 3 g) with other immunosuppressive agents in controlled clinical trials of renal and cardiac transplant patients (see WARNINGS). The following table summarizes the incidence of malignancies observed in the controlled renal and cardiac trials.

[See second table at top of next page]

Up to 2.0% of patients receiving CellCept 3 g daily for prevention of renal rejection developed severe neutropenia [absolute neutrophil count (ANC) <0.5 x 10^3/μL]. Up to 2.8% of cardiac transplant patients receiving CellCept 3 g daily developed severe neutropenia (see WARNINGS, PRECAUTIONS: *Laboratory Tests* and DOSAGE AND ADMINISTRATION).

The following tables show the incidence of opportunistic infections that occurred in the renal and cardiac transplant populations in the controlled prevention trials:

[See third table at top of next page]

[See fourth table at top of next page]

In controlled studies for prevention of renal or cardiac rejection, similar rates of fatal infection/sepsis (<2%) occurred in patients receiving CellCept (2 g or 3 g) (see WARNINGS). In cardiac transplant patients, the overall incidence of opportunistic infections was approximately 10% higher in patients treated with CellCept than in those receiving azathioprine, but this difference was not associated with excess mortality due to infection/sepsis among patients treated with CellCept.

The following adverse events, not mentioned in any of the tables above, were reported with ≥3% incidence in both renal and cardiac transplant patients treated with CellCept, in combination with cyclosporine and corticosteroids.

Body as a Whole: abdomen enlarged, chills occurring with fever, cyst, face edema, flu syndrome, hemorrhage, pelvic pain, malaise

Urogenital: dysuria, impotence, urinary frequency

Cardiovascular: angina pectoris, atrial fibrillation, palpitation, peripheral vascular disorder, postural hypotension

Metabolic and Nutritional: alkaline phosphatase increased, dehydration, hypervolemia, hypocalcemia, hypoglycemia, hypoproteinemia

Digestive: anorexia, esophagitis, gastritis, gastroenteritis, gingivitis, gum hyperplasia, infection, liver function tests abnormal, rectal disorder

Respiratory: lung edema

Skin and Appendages: fungal dermatitis, pruritus, skin benign neoplasm, skin hypertrophy, skin ulcer, sweating
Endocrine: diabetes mellitus
Musculoskeletal: arthralgia, joint disorder
Special Senses: conjunctivitis

The following adverse events, not mentioned in any of the tables above were reported with ≥3% incidence in renal transplant patients only treated with CellCept, in combination with other immunosuppressive agents:
Body as a Whole: accidental injury, hernia
Hemic and Lymphatic: ecchymosis, polycythemia
Urogenital: albuminuria, hydronephrosis, pain, pyelonephritis, urinary tract disorder
Cardiovascular: cardiovascular disorder, hypotension, tachycardia, thrombosis, vasodilatation
Metabolic and Nutritional: acidosis, creatinine increased, gamma glutamyl transpeptidase increased, hypercalcemia, hyperlipemia, hyperuricemia, lactic dehydrogenase increased, SGOT increased, SGPT increased, weight gain
Digestive: flatulence, gastrointestinal hemorrhage, gastrointestinal moniliasis, hepatitis, ileus, mouth ulceration
Respiratory: asthma, lung disorder, pleural effusion, rhinitis, sinusitis
Skin and Appendages: alopecia, hirsutism, rash, skin disorder
Nervous: anxiety, depression, hypertonia, paresthesia, somnolence
Endocrine: parathyroid disorder
Musculoskeletal: leg cramps, myalgia, myasthenia
Special Senses: amblyopia, cataract (not specified)

The following adverse events, not mentioned in any of the tables above, were reported with ≥3% incidence in cardiac transplant patients only treated with CellCept, in combination with other immunosuppressive agents:
Body as a Whole: neck pain, cellulitis
Hemic and Lymphatic: prothrombin increased, thromboplastin decreased, petechia
Urogenital: nocturia, kidney failure, urine abnormality, hematuria, urinary incontinence, prostatic disorder, urinary retention
Cardiovascular: ventricular extrasystole, congestive heart failure, supraventricular tachycardia, ventricular tachycardia, atrial flutter, pulmonary hypertension, heart arrest, venous pressure increased, syncope, supraventricular extrasystoles, extrasystoles, pallor, vasospasm
Metabolic and Nutritional: hypoxia, hypophosphatemia, gout, abnormal healing, alkalosis, weight loss, hypochloremia, thirst, respiratory acidosis
Digestive: gastrointestinal disorder, melena, liver damage, dysphagia, jaundice, stomatitis
Respiratory: atelectasis, hiccup, pneumothorax, sputum increased, respiratory disorder, epistaxis, apnea, voice alteration, pain, hemoptysis, neoplasm
Skin and Appendages: hemorrhage, skin carcinoma
Nervous: emotional lability, neuropathy, convulsion, hallucinations, thinking abnormal, vertigo
Endocrine: Cushing's syndrome, hypothyroidism
Special Senses: ear pain, deafness, ear disorder, tinnitus, abnormal vision, lacrimation disorder, eye hemorrhage

Postmarketing Experience

Digestive: colitis (sometimes caused by cytomegalovirus), pancreatitis
Resistance Mechanism Disorders: Serious life-threatening infections such as meningitis and infectious endocarditis have been reported occasionally and there is evidence of a higher frequency of certain types of serious infections such as tuberculosis and atypical mycobacterial infection.

OVERDOSAGE

There has been no reported experience of overdosage of mycophenolate mofetil in humans. The highest dose administered to renal transplant patients in clinical trials has been 4 g/day. In limited experience with cardiac and hepatic transplant patients in clinical trials, the highest doses used were 4 g/day or 5 g/day. At doses of 4 g/day or 5 g/day, there appears to be a higher rate, compared to the use of 3 g/day or less, of gastrointestinal intolerance (nausea, vomiting, and/or diarrhea), and occasional hematologic abnormalities, principally neutropenia, leading to a need to reduce or discontinue dosing.

In acute oral toxicity studies, no deaths occurred in adult mice at doses up to 4000 mg/kg or in adult monkeys at doses up to 1000 mg/kg; these were the highest doses of mycophenolate mofetil tested in these species. These doses represent 11 times the recommended clinical dose in renal transplant patients and approximately 7 times the recommended clinical dose in cardiac transplant patients when corrected for BSA. In adult rats, deaths occurred after single oral doses of 500 mg/kg of mycophenolate mofetil. The dose represents approximately 3 times the recommended clinical dose in cardiac transplant patients when corrected for BSA.

MPA and MPAG are usually not removed by hemodialysis. However, at high MPAG plasma concentrations (>100 µg/mL), small amounts of MPAG are removed. By increasing excretion of the drug, MPA can be removed by bile acid sequestrants, such as cholestyramine.

Adverse Events in the Controlled Study in Prevention of Cardiac Allograft Rejection -- (Continued)

	CellCept 3 g/day (n=289)	Azathioprine 1.5 to 3 mg/kg/day (n=289)
Musculoskeletal System		
Leg Cramps	16.6	15.6
Myasthenia	12.5	9.7
Myalgia	12.5	9.3
Special Senses		
Ambylopia	14.9	6.6
Endocrine System	12.1	12.8

Malignancies Observed in Renal and Cardiac Transplant Trials

	Renal Trials				Cardiac Trial	
	CellCept 2 g/day (n=501)	CellCept 3 g/day (n=490)	Placebo (n=166)	Azathioprine 1 to 2 mg/kg/day or 100 to 150 mg/day (n=326)	CellCept 3 g/day (n=289)	Azathioprine 5 to 3 mg/kg/day (n=289)
Lymphoma/ lymphoproliferative disease	0.6%	1.0%	0.0%	0.3%	0.7%	2.1%
Non-melanoma skin carcinoma	4.0	1.6	0.0	2.4	4.2	2.8
Other malignancy	0.8	1.4	1.8	1.8	2.1	2.1

Opportunistic Infections in Prevention of Renal Rejection Trials

USA Study Combined with Europe/Canada/Australia Study

	CellCept 2 g/day (n=336)	CellCept 3 g/day (n=330)	Azathioprine 1 to 2 mg/kg/day or 100 to 150 mg/day (n=326)
Herpes simplex	16.7%	20.0%	19.0%
CMV			
viremia/syndrome	13.4	12.4	13.8
tissue invasive disease	8.3	11.5	6.1
Herpes zoster	6.0	7.6	5.8
Candida			
fungemia/disseminated	0.6	0.6	0.3
tissue invasive disease	0.6	0.6	0.3
Aspergillus/Mucor invasive disease	0.3	0.9	0.3
Pneumocystis carinii	0.3	0.0	1.2

Europe Study

	CellCept 2 g/day (n=165)	CellCept 3 g/day (n=160)	Placebo (n=166)
Herpes simplex	15.2%	12.5%	6.0%
CMV			
viremia/syndrome	15.2	15.0	13.3
tissue invasive disease	3.6	7.5	2.4
Herpes zoster	6.7	6.9	2.4
Candida			
fungemia/disseminated	0.0	0.6	0.0
tissue invasive disease	0.0	0.6	0.0
Pneumocystis carinii	0.0	0.0	2.4

Opportunistic Infections in Prevention of Cardiac Rejection Trial

	CellCept 3 g/day (n=289)	Azathioprine 1.5 to 3 mg/kg/day (n=289)
Herpes simplex	20.8%	14.5%
CMV		
viremia/syndrome	12.1	10.0
tissue invasive disease	11.4	8.7
CMV infection	2.8	2.8
CMV urine	2.4	2.8
CMV nasal secretions	0.3	0.0
CMV saliva	0.3	0.0
Herpes zoster	10.7	5.9
Herpes zoster cutaneous disease	10.0	5.5
Herpes zoster visceral disease	0.7	0.3
Candida	18.7	17.6
mucocutaneous	18.0	17.3
urinary tract infection	0.7	1.0
fungemia/disseminated disease	0.7	0.3
invasive tissue disease	0.0	0.3
Cryptococcosis	0.7	0.3
Aspergillus/Mucor	2.1	2.1
Aspergillus pulmonary or sinus invasive	0.7	1.4
Aspergillus disseminated or metastatic	0.3	1.0
Aspergillus cutaneous	0.7	0.0
Aspergillus sputum	0.3	0.3
Pneumocystis carinii	0.0	1.7
Listeriosis	0.0	0.7

DOSAGE AND ADMINISTRATION

The initial dose of CellCept should be given orally as soon as possible following renal or cardiac transplantation. A dose of 1.0 g administered twice a day (daily dose of 2 g) is recommended for use in renal transplant patients. Although a dose of 1.5 g administered twice daily (daily dose of 3 g) was used in clinical trials and was shown to be safe and effective, no efficacy advantage could be established for renal transplant patients. Patients receiving 2 g/day of CellCept demonstrated an overall better safety profile than did patients receiving 3 g/day of CellCept.

Continued on next page

Cellcept—Cont.

A dose of 1.5 g administered twice a day (daily dose of 3 g) is recommended for use in cardiac transplant patients.

Food had no effect on MPA AUC, but has been shown to decrease MPA C_{max} by 40%. It is recommended that CellCept be administered on an empty stomach.

Dosage Adjustments: In renal transplant patients with severe chronic renal impairment (GFR <25 mL/min/1.73m²) outside of the immediate posttransplant period, doses of CellCept greater than 1 g administered twice a day should be avoided. These patients should also be carefully observed. No dose adjustments are needed in renal transplant patients experiencing delayed graft function postoperatively (see CLINICAL PHARMACOLOGY: *Pharmacokinetics* and PRECAUTIONS: *General*).

No data are available for cardiac transplant patients with severe chronic renal impairment. CellCept may be used for cardiac transplant patients with severe chronic renal impairment if the potential benefits outweigh the potential risks.

If neutropenia develops (ANC <1.3 × 10³/µL), dosing with CellCept should be interrupted or the dose reduced, appropriate diagnostic tests performed, and the patient managed appropriately (see WARNINGS, ADVERSE REACTIONS, and PRECAUTIONS: *Laboratory Tests*).

HANDLING AND DISPOSAL

Because mycophenolate mofetil has demonstrated teratogenic effects in rats and rabbits, CellCept tablets should not be crushed and CellCept capsules should not be opened or crushed. Avoid inhalation or direct contact with skin or mucous membranes of the powder contained in CellCept capsules. If such contact occurs, wash thoroughly with soap and water; rinse eyes with plain water.

HOW SUPPLIED

CellCept capsules are blue-brown, two-piece hard gelatin capsules, printed in black with "CellCept 250" on the blue cap and "Roche" on the brown body. Supplied in the following presentations:

NDC Number	Size
NDC 0004-0259-01	Bottle of 100
NDC 0004-0259-43	Bottle of 500

CellCept tablets are lavender-colored, caplet-shaped, film-coated tablets printed in black with "CellCept 500" on one side and "Roche" on the other. Supplied in the following presentations:

NDC Number	Size
NDC 0004-0260-01	Bottle of 100
NDC 0004-0260-43	Bottle of 500

Storage: Store at 15° to 30°C (59° to 86°F). Tablets should be dispensed in light-resistant containers, such as the manufacturer's original containers.

CAUTION: Federal (USA) law prohibits dispensing without a prescription.

Manufactured by Syntex Puerto Rico, Inc., Humacao, Puerto Rico 00791

Revised: February 1998

Shown in Product Identification Guide, page 334

CYTOVENE®-IV   ℞
(ganciclovir sodium for injection)
FOR INTRAVENOUS INFUSION ONLY

CYTOVENE®
(ganciclovir capsules)
FOR ORAL ADMINISTRATION

The following text is complete prescribing information based on official labeling in effect June 1998.

WARNING: THE CLINICAL TOXICITY OF CYTOVENE AND CYTOVENE-IV INCLUDES GRANULOCYTOPENIA, ANEMIA AND THROMBOCYTOPENIA. IN ANIMAL STUDIES GANCICLOVIR WAS CARCINOGENIC, TERATOGENIC AND CAUSED ASPERMATOGENESIS. CYTOVENE-IV IS INDICATED FOR USE *ONLY* IN THE TREATMENT OF CYTOMEGALOVIRUS (CMV) RETINITIS IN IMMUNOCOMPROMISED PATIENTS AND FOR THE PREVENTION OF CMV DISEASE IN TRANSPLANT PATIENTS AT RISK FOR CMV DISEASE.

CYTOVENE CAPSULES ARE INDICATED *ONLY* FOR PREVENTION OF CMV DISEASE IN PATIENTS WITH ADVANCED HIV INFECTION AT RISK FOR CMV DISEASE, FOR MAINTENANCE TREATMENT OF CMV RETINITIS IN IMMUNOCOMPROMISED PATIENTS, AND FOR PREVENTION OF CMV DISEASE IN SOLID ORGAN TRANSPLANT RECIPIENTS (see INDICATIONS AND USAGE).

BECAUSE CYTOVENE CAPSULES ARE ASSOCIATED WITH A RISK OF MORE RAPID RATE OF CMV RETINITIS PROGRESSION, THEY SHOULD BE USED AS MAINTENANCE TREATMENT ONLY IN THOSE PATIENTS FOR WHOM THIS RISK IS BALANCED BY THE BENEFIT ASSOCIATED WITH AVOIDING DAILY INTRAVENOUS INFUSIONS.

DESCRIPTION

Ganciclovir is a synthetic guanine derivative active against cytomegalovirus (CMV). CYTOVENE-IV and CYTOVENE are the brand names for ganciclovir sodium for injection and ganciclovir capsules, respectively.

CYTOVENE-IV is available as sterile lyophilized powder in strength of 500 mg per vial for intravenous administration only. Each vial of CYTOVENE-IV contains the equivalent of 500 mg ganciclovir as the sodium salt (46 mg sodium). Reconstitution with 10 mL of Sterile Water for Injection, USP, yields a solution with pH 11 and a ganciclovir concentration of approximately 50 mg/mL. Further dilution in an appropriate intravenous solution must be performed before infusion (see DOSAGE AND ADMINISTRATION).

CYTOVENE is available as 250 mg and 500 mg capsules. Each capsule contains 250 mg or 500 mg ganciclovir, respectively, and inactive ingredients croscarmellose sodium, magnesium stearate and povidone. Both hard gelatin shells consist of gelatin, titanium dioxide, yellow iron oxide and FD&C Blue No. 2.

Ganciclovir is a white to off-white crystalline powder with a molecular formula of $C_9H_{13}N_5O_4$ and a molecular weight of 255.23. The chemical name for ganciclovir is 9-[[2-hydroxy-1-(hydroxymethyl)ethoxy]methyl]guanine. Ganciclovir is a polar hydrophilic compound with a solubility of 2.6 mg/mL in water at 25°C and an n-octanol/water partition coefficient of 0.022. The pK_as for ganciclovir are 2.2 and 9.4.

Ganciclovir, when formulated as monosodium salt in the IV dosage form, is a white to off-white lyophilized powder with a molecular formula of $C_9H_{12}N_5NaO_4$, and a molecular weight of 277.22. The chemical name for ganciclovir sodium is 9-[[2-hydroxy-1-(hydroxymethyl) ethoxy]methyl]guanine, monosodium salt. The lyophilized powder has an aqueous solubility of greater than 50 mg/mL at 25°C. At physiological pH, ganciclovir sodium exists as the un-ionized form with a solubility of approximately 6 mg/mL at 37°C.

All doses in this insert are specified in terms of ganciclovir.

VIROLOGY

Mechanism of Action: Ganciclovir is an acyclic nucleoside analogue of 2′-deoxyguanosine that inhibits replication of herpes viruses. Ganciclovir has been shown to be active against cytomegalovirus (CMV) and herpes simplex virus (HSV) in human clinical studies.

To achieve anti-CMV activity, ganciclovir is phosphorylated first to the monophosphate form by a CMV-encoded (UL97 gene) protein kinase homologue, then to the di- and triphosphate forms by cellular kinases. Ganciclovir triphosphate concentrations may be 100-fold greater in CMV-infected than in uninfected cells, indicating preferential phosphorylation in infected cells. Ganciclovir triphosphate, once formed, persists for days in the CMV-infected cell. Ganciclovir triphosphate is believed to inhibit viral DNA synthesis by (1) competitive inhibition of viral DNA polymerases; and (2) incorporation into viral DNA, resulting in eventual termination of viral DNA elongation.

Antiviral Activity: The median concentration of ganciclovir that inhibits CMV replication (IC$_{50}$) in vitro (laboratory strains or clinical isolates) has ranged from 0.02 to 3.48 µg/mL. Ganciclovir inhibits mammalian cell proliferation (CIC$_{50}$) in vitro at higher concentrations ranging from 30 to 725 µg/mL. Bone marrow-derived colony-forming cells are more sensitive (CIC$_{50}$ 0.028 to 0.7 µg/mL). The relationship of in vitro sensitivity of CMV to ganciclovir and clinical response has not been established.

Clinical Antiviral Effect of CYTOVENE-IV and CYTOVENE Capsules: CYTOVENE-IV: In a study of CYTOVENE-IV treatment of life- or sight-threatening CMV disease in immunocompromised patients, 121 of 314 patients had CMV cultured within 7 days prior to treatment and sequential posttreatment viral cultures of urine, blood, throat and/or semen. As judged by conversion to culture negativity, or a greater than 100-fold decrease in in vitro CMV titer, at least 83% of patients had a virologic response with a median response time of 7 to 15 days.

Antiviral activity of CYTOVENE-IV was demonstrated in two randomized studies for the prevention of CMV disease in transplant recipients (see table below).

[See table below]

CYTOVENE Capsules: In trials comparing CYTOVENE-IV with CYTOVENE capsules for the maintenance treatment of CMV retinitis in patients with AIDS, serial urine cultures and other available cultures (semen, biopsy specimens, blood and others) showed that a small proportion of patients remained culture-positive during maintenance therapy with no statistically significant differences in CMV isolation rates between treatment groups.

A study of CYTOVENE capsules (1000 mg q8h) for prevention of CMV disease in individuals with advanced HIV infection (ICM 1654) evaluated antiviral activity as measured by CMV isolation in culture; most cultures were from urine. At baseline, 40% (176/436) and 44% (92/210) of ganciclovir and placebo recipients, respectively, had positive cultures (urine or blood). After 2 months on treatment, 10% vs 44% of ganciclovir vs placebo recipients had positive cultures.

Viral Resistance: The current working definition of CMV resistance to ganciclovir in in vitro assays is IC$_{50}$ >3.0 µg/mL (12.0 µM). CMV resistance to ganciclovir has been observed in individuals with AIDS and CMV retinitis who have never received ganciclovir therapy. Viral resistance has also been observed in patients receiving prolonged treatment for CMV retinitis with CYTOVENE-IV. In a controlled study of oral ganciclovir for prevention of AIDS-associated CMV disease, 364 individuals had one or more cultures performed after at least 90 days of ganciclovir treatment. Of these, 113 had at least one positive culture. The last available isolate from each subject was tested for reduced sensitivity, and 2 of 40 were found to be resistant to ganciclovir. These resistant isolates were associated with subsequent treatment failure for retinitis.

The possibility of viral resistance should be considered in patients who show poor clinical response or experience persistent viral excretion during therapy. The principal mechanism of resistance to ganciclovir in CMV is the decreased ability to form the active triphosphate moiety; resistant viruses have been described that contain mutations in the UL97 gene of CMV that controls phosphorylation of ganciclovir. Mutations in the viral DNA polymerase have also been reported to confer viral resistance to ganciclovir.

CLINICAL PHARMACOLOGY

Pharmacokinetics:
BECAUSE THE MAJOR ELIMINATION PATHWAY FOR GANCICLOVIR IS RENAL, DOSAGE REDUCTIONS ACCORDING TO CREATININE CLEARANCE ARE REQUIRED FOR CYTOVENE-IV AND SHOULD BE CONSIDERED FOR CYTOVENE CAPSULES. FOR DOSING INSTRUCTIONS IN PATIENTS WITH RENAL IMPAIRMENT, REFER TO DOSAGE AND ADMINISTRATION.

Absorption: The absolute bioavailability of oral ganciclovir under fasting conditions was approximately 5% (n=6) and following food was 6% to 9% (n=32). When ganciclovir was administered orally with food at a total daily dosage of 3 g/day (500 mg q3h, 6 times daily and 1000 mg tid), the steady-state absorption as measured by area under the serum concentration vs time curve (AUC) over 24 hours and maximum serum concentrations (C$_{max}$) were similar following both regimens with an AUC$_{0-24}$ of 15.9 ± 4.2 (mean ± SD) and 15.4 ± 4.3 µg·hr/mL and C$_{max}$ of 1.02 ± 0.24 and 1.18 ± 0.36 µg/mL, respectively (n=16).

At the end of a 1-hour intravenous infusion of 5 mg/kg ganciclovir, total AUC ranged between 22.1 ± 3.2 (n=16) and 26.8 ± 6.1 µg·hr/mL (n=16) and C$_{max}$ ranged between 8.27 ± 1.02 (n=16) and 9.0 ± 1.4 µg/mL (n=16).

Food Effects: When CYTOVENE capsules were given with a meal containing 602 calories and 46.5% fat at a dosage of 1000 mg every 8 hours to 20 HIV-positive subjects, the steady-state AUC increased by 22 ± 22% (range: -6% to 68%) and there was a significant prolongation of time to peak serum concentrations (T$_{max}$) from 1.8 ± 0.8 to 3.0 ± 0.6 hours and a higher C$_{max}$ (0.85 ± 0.25 vs 0.96 ± 0.27 µg/mL) (n=20).

Distribution: The steady-state volume of distribution of ganciclovir after intravenous administration was 0.74 ± 0.15 L/kg (n=98). For CYTOVENE capsules, no correlation was observed between AUC and reciprocal weight (range: 55 to 128 kg); oral dosing according to weight is not required. Cerebrospinal fluid concentrations obtained 0.25 to 5.67 hours postdose in 3 patients who received 2.5 mg/kg ganciclovir intravenously q8h or q12h ranged from 0.31 to 0.68 µg/mL representing 24% to 70% of the respective plasma concentrations. Binding to plasma proteins was 1% to 2% over ganciclovir concentrations of 0.5 and 51 µg/mL.

	Patients With Positive CMV Cultures			
	Heart Allograft* (n=147)		Bone Marrow Allograft (n=72)	
Time	CYTOVENE-IV†	Placebo	CYTOVENE-IV‡	Placebo
Pretreatment	1/67 (2%)	5/64 (8%)	37/37 (100%)	35/35 (100%)
Week 2	2/75 (3%)	11/67 (16%)	2/31 (6%)	19/28 (68%)
Week 4	3/66 (5%)	28/66 (43%)	0/24 (0%)	16/20 (80%)

* CMV seropositive or receiving graft from seropositive donor
† 5 mg/kg bid for 14 days followed by 6 mg/kg qd for 5 days/week for 14 days
‡ 5 mg/kg bid for 7 days followed by 5 mg/kg qd until day 100 posttransplant

Estimated Creatinine Clearance (mL/min)	n	Dose	Clearance (mL/min) Mean ± SD	Half-life (hours) Mean ± SD
50–79	4	3.2 – 5 mg/kg	128 ± 63	4.6 ± 1.4
25–49	3	3 – 5 mg/kg	57 ± 8	4.4 ± 0.4
<25	3	1.25 – 5 mg/kg	30 ± 13	10.7 ± 5.7

Metabolism: Following oral administration of a single 1000 mg dose of ^{14}C-labeled ganciclovir, 86 ± 3% of the administered dose was recovered in the feces and 5 ± 1% was recovered in the urine (n=4). No metabolite accounted for more than 1% to 2% of the radioactivity recovered in urine or feces.

Elimination: When administered intravenously, ganciclovir exhibits linear pharmacokinetics over the range of 1.6 to 5.0 mg/kg and when administered orally, it exhibits linear kinetics up to a total daily dose of 4 g/day. Renal excretion of unchanged drug by glomerular filtration and active tubular secretion is the major route of elimination of ganciclovir. In patients with normal renal function, 91.3 ± 5.0% (n=4) of intravenously administered ganciclovir was recovered unmetabolized in the urine. Systemic clearance of intravenously administered ganciclovir was 3.52 ± 0.80 mL/min/kg (n=98) while renal clearance was 3.20 ± 0.80 mL/min/kg (n=47), accounting for 91 ± 11% of the systemic clearance (n=47). After oral administration of ganciclovir, steady-state is achieved within 24 hours. Renal clearance following oral administration was 3.1 ± 1.2 mL/min/kg (n=22). Half-life was 3.5 ± 0.9 hours (n=98) following IV administration and 4.8 ± 0.9 hours (n=39) following oral administration.

Special Populations: *Renal Impairment:* The pharmacokinetics following intravenous administration of CYTOVENE-IV solution were evaluated in 10 immunocompromised patients with renal impairment who received doses ranging from 1.25 to 5.0 mg/kg.
[See table above]
The pharmacokinetics of ganciclovir following oral administration of CYTOVENE capsules were evaluated in 44 patients, who were either solid organ transplant recipients or HIV positive. Apparent oral clearance of ganciclovir decreased and AUC_{0-24h} increased with diminishing renal function (as expressed by creatinine clearance). Based on these observations, it is necessary to modify the dosage of ganciclovir in patients with renal impairment (see DOSAGE AND ADMINISTRATION).
Hemodialysis reduces plasma concentrations of ganciclovir by about 50% after both intravenous and oral administration.

Race/Ethnicity and Gender: The effects of race/ethnicity and gender were studied in subjects receiving a dose regimen of 1000 mg every 8 hours. Although the numbers of blacks (16%) and Hispanics (20%) were small, there appeared to be a trend towards a lower steady-state C_{max} and AUC_{0-8} in these subpopulations as compared to Caucasians. No definitive conclusions regarding gender differences could be made because of the small number of females (12%); however, no differences between males and females were observed.

Pediatrics: Ganciclovir pharmacokinetics were studied in 27 neonates, aged 2 to 49 days. At an intravenous dose of 4 mg/kg (n=14) or 6 mg/kg (n=13), the pharmacokinetic parameters were, respectively, C_{max} of 5.5 ± 1.6 and 7.0 ± 1.6 μg/mL, systemic clearance of 3.14 ± 1.75 and 3.56 ± 1.27 mL/min/kg, and $t_{1/2}$ of 2.4 hours (harmonic mean) for both. Ganciclovir phrmacokinetics were also studied in 10 pediatric patients, aged 9 months to 12 years. The pharmacokinetic characteristics of ganciclovir were the same after single and multiple (q12h) intravenous doses (5 mg/kg). The steady-state volume of distribution was 0.64 ± 0.22 L/kg, C_{max} was 7.9 ± 3.9 μg/mL, systemic clearance was 4.7 ± 2.2 mL/min/kg, and $t_{1/2}$ was 2.4 ± 0.7 hours. The pharmacokinetics of intravenous ganciclovir in pediatric patients are similar to those observed in adults.

Elderly: No studies have been conducted in adults older than 65 years of age.

INDICATIONS AND USAGE

CYTOVENE-IV is indicated for the treatment of CMV retinitis in immunocompromised patients, including patients with acquired immunodeficiency syndrome (AIDS). CYTOVENE-IV is also indicated for the prevention of CMV disease in transplant recipients at risk for CMV disease (see CLINICAL TRIALS).
CYTOVENE capsules are indicated for the prevention of CMV disease in solid organ transplant recipients and in individuals with advanced HIV infection at risk for developing CMV disease. CYTOVENE capsules are also indicated as an alternative to the intravenous formulation for maintenance treatment of CMV retinitis in immunocompromised patients, including patients with AIDS, in whom retinitis is stable following appropriate induction therapy and for whom the risk of more rapid progression is balanced by the benefit associated with avoiding daily IV infusions (see CLINICAL TRIALS).
SAFETY AND EFFICACY OF **CYTOVENE-IV** AND **CYTOVENE** HAVE NOT BEEN ESTABLISHED FOR CONGENITAL OR NEONATAL CMV DISEASE; NOR FOR THE TREATMENT OF ESTABLISHED CMV DISEASE OTHER THAN RETINITIS; NOR FOR USE IN NON-IMMUNOCOMPROMISED INDIVIDUALS. THE SAFETY AND EFFICACY OF **CYTOVENE** CAPSULES HAVE NOT BEEN ESTABLISHED FOR TREATING ANY MANIFESTATION OF CMV DISEASE OTHER THAN MAINTENANCE TREATMENT OF CMV RETINITIS.

CLINICAL TRIALS

1. Treatment of CMV Retinitis
The diagnosis of CMV retinitis should be made by indirect ophthalmoscopy. Other conditions in the differential diagnosis of CMV retinitis include candidiasis, toxoplasmosis, histoplasmosis, retinal scars and cotton wool spots, any of which may produce a retinal appearance similar to CMV. For this reason it is essential that the diagnosis of CMV be established by an ophthalmologist familiar with the retinal presentation of these conditions. The diagnosis of CMV retinitis may be supported by culture of CMV from urine, blood, throat or other sites, but a negative CMV culture does not rule out CMV retinitis.

Studies With CYTOVENE-IV: In a retrospective, non-randomized, single-center analysis of 41 patients with AIDS and CMV retinitis diagnosed by ophthalmologic examination between August 1983 and April 1988, treatment with CYTOVENE-IV solution resulted in a significant delay in mean (median) time to first retinitis progression compared to untreated controls [105 (71) days from diagnosis vs 35 (29) days from diagnosis]. Patients in this series received induction treatment of CYTOVENE-IV 5 mg/kg bid for 14 to 21 days followed by maintenance treatment with either 5 mg/kg once daily, 7 days per week or 6 mg/kg once daily, 5 days per week (see DOSAGE AND ADMINISTRATION).

In a controlled, randomized study conducted between February 1989 and December 1990,[1] immediate treatment with CYTOVENE-IV was compared to delayed treatment in 42 patients with AIDS and peripheral CMV retinitis; 35 of 42 patients (13 in the immediate-treatment group and 22 in the delayed-treatment group) were included in the analysis of time to retinitis progression. Based on masked assessment of fundus photographs, the mean [95% CI] and median [95% CI] times to progression of retinitis were 66 days [39, 94] and 50 days [40, 84], respectively, in the immediate-treatment group compared to 19 days [11, 27] and 13.5 days [8, 18], respectively, in the delayed-treatment group.

Studies Comparing CYTOVENE Capsules to CYTOVENE-IV: [See table below]

ICM 1653: In this randomized, open-label, parallel group trial, conducted between March 1991 and November 1992, patients with AIDS and newly diagnosed CMV retinitis received a 3-week induction course of CYTOVENE-IV solution, 5 mg/kg bid for 14 days followed by 5 mg/kg once daily for 1 additional week.[2] Following the 21-day intravenous induction course, patients with stable CMV retinitis were randomized to receive 20 weeks of maintenance treatment with either CYTOVENE-IV solution, 5 mg/kg once daily, or CYTOVENE capsules, 500 mg 6 times daily (3000 mg/day). The study showed that the mean [95% CI] and median [95% CI] times to progression of CMV retinitis, as assessed by masked reading of fundus photographs, were 57 days [44, 70] and 29 days [28, 43], respectively, for patients on oral therapy compared to 62 days [50, 73] and 49 days [29, 61], respectively, for patients on intravenous therapy. The difference [95% CI] in the mean time to progression between the oral and intravenous therapies (oral - IV) was -5 days [-22, 12]. See Figure 1 for comparison of the proportion of patients remaining free of progression over time.

ICM 1774: In this three-arm, randomized, open-label, parallel group trial, conducted between June 1991 and August 1993, patients with AIDS and stable CMV retinitis following from 4 weeks to 4 months of treatment with CYTOVENE-IV solution were randomized to receive maintenance treatment with CYTOVENE-IV solution, 5 mg/kg once daily, CYTOVENE capsules, 500 mg 6 times daily, or CYTOVENE capsules, 1000 mg tid for 20 weeks. The study showed that the mean [95% CI] and median [95% CI] times to progression of CMV retinitis, as assessed by masked reading of fundus photographs, were 54 days [48, 60] and 42 days [31, 54], respectively, for patients on oral therapy compared to 66 days [56, 76] and 54 days [41, 69], respectively, for patients on intravenous therapy. The difference [95% CI] in the mean time to progression between the oral and intravenous therapies (oral - IV) was -12 days [-24, 0]. See Figure 2 for comparison of the proportion of patients remaining free of progression over time.

AVI 034: In this randomized, open-label, parallel group trial, conducted between June 1991 and February 1993, patients with AIDS and newly diagnosed (81%) or previously treated (19%) CMV retinitis who had tolerated 10 to 21 days of induction treatment with CYTOVENE-IV, 5 mg/kg twice daily, were randomized to receive 20 weeks of maintenance treatment with either CYTOVENE capsules, 500 mg 6 times daily or CYTOVENE-IV solution, 5 mg/kg/day.[3] The mean [95% CI] and median [95% CI] times to progression of CMV retinitis, as assessed by masked reading of fundus photographs, were 51 days [44, 57] and 41 days [31, 45], respectively, for patients on oral therapy compared to 62 days [52, 72] and 60 days [42, 83], respectively, for patients on intravenous therapy. The difference [95% CI] in the mean time to progression between the oral and intravenous therapies (oral - IV) was -11 days [-24, 1]. See Figure 3 for comparison of the proportion of patients remaining free of progression over time.

Comparison of other CMV retinitis outcomes between oral and IV formulations (development of bilateral retinitis, progression into Zone 1, and deterioration of visual acuity), while not definitive, showed no marked differences between treatment groups in these studies. Because of low event rates among these endpoints, these studies are underpowered to rule out significant differences in these endpoints.

Population Characteristics in Studies ICM 1653, ICM 1774 and AVI 034		ICM 1653 (n=121)	ICM 1774 (n=225)	AVI 034 (n=159)
Median age (years) Range		38 24–62	37 22–56	39 23–62
Sex	Males	116 (96%)	222 (99%)	148 (93%)
	Females	5 (4%)	3 (1%)	10 (6%)
Ethnicity	Asian	3 (3%)	5 (2%)	7 (4%)
	Black	11 (9%)	9 (4%)	3 (2%)
	Caucasian	98 (81%)	186 (83%)	140 (88%)
	Other	9 (7%)	25 (11%)	8 (5%)
Median CD_4 Count Range		9.5 0 – 141	7.0 0 – 80	10.0 0 – 320
Mean (SD) Observation Time (days)		107.9 (43.0)	97.6 (42.5)	80.9 (47.0)

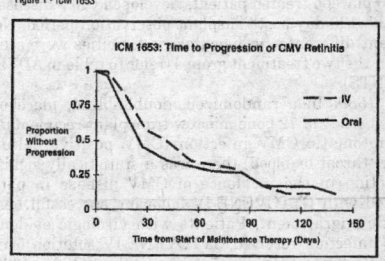

Figure 1 - ICM 1653

ICM 1653: Time to Progression of CMV Retinitis

Continued on next page

Cytovene—Cont.

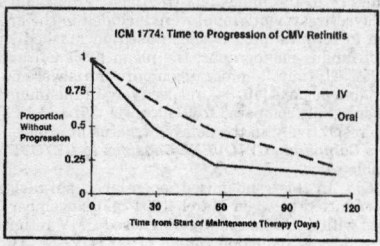

Figure 2 - ICM 1774

ICM 1774: Time to Progression of CMV Retinitis

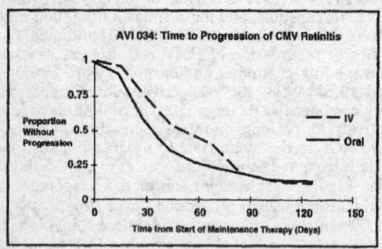

Figure 3 - AVI 034

AVI 034: Time to Progression of CMV Retinitis

2. Prevention of CMV Disease in Subjects With AIDS

ICM 1654: In a double-blind study conducted between November 1992 and July 1994, 725 subjects with AIDS, who were CMV seropositive and/or culture positive, were randomized to receive CYTOVENE capsules, 1000 mg, every 8 hours, or placebo.[4] The study population had a median age of 38 years (range: 21 to 69); were 99% male; were 82% Caucasian, 10% Hispanic, 7% African-American and 1% Asian; and had a median CD_4 count of 21 (range: 0 to 100). The mean observation time was 351 days (range: 5 to 621). As shown in the following table, significantly more placebo recipients developed CMV disease.

Incidence of CMV Disease at 6, 12 and 18 Months After Enrollment (Kaplan-Meier Estimates)

	Incidence (Number Still At Risk)	
	CMV Disease	
	Ganciclovir	Placebo
6 months	8% (397)	11% (190)
12 months	14% (225)	26% (92)
18 months	20% (27)	39% (9)

3. Prevention of CMV Disease In Transplant Recipients

CYTOVENE-IV: CYTOVENE-IV was evaluated in three randomized, controlled trials of prevention of CMV disease in organ transplant recipients.

ICM 1496: In a randomized, double-blind, placebo-controlled study of 149 heart transplant recipients[5] at risk for CMV infection (CMV seropositive or a seronegative recipient of an organ from a CMV seropositive donor), there was a statistically significant reduction in the overall incidence of CMV disease in patients treated with CYTOVENE-IV. Immediately posttransplant, patients received CYTOVENE-IV solution 5 mg/kg bid for 14 days followed by 6 mg/kg qd for 5 days/week for an additional 14 days. Twelve of the 76 (16%) patients treated with CYTOVENE-IV vs 31 of the 73 (43%) placebo-treated patients developed CMV disease during the 120-day posttransplant observation period. No significant differences in hematologic toxicities were seen between the two treatment groups (refer to table in ADVERSE EVENTS).

ICM 1689: In a randomized, double-blind, placebo-controlled study of 72 bone marrow transplant recipients[6] with asymptomatic CMV infection (CMV positive culture of urine, throat or blood) there was a statistically significant reduction in the incidence of CMV disease in patients treated with CYTOVENE-IV following successful hematopoietic engraftment. Patients with virologic evidence of CMV infection received CYTOVENE-IV solution 5 mg/kg bid for 7 days followed by 5 mg/kg qd through day 100 posttransplant. One of the 37 (3%) patients treated with CYTOVENE-IV vs 15 of the 35 (43%) placebo-treated patients developed CMV disease during the study. At 6 months posttransplant, there continued to be a statistically significant reduction in the incidence of CMV disease in patients treated with CYTOVENE-IV. Six of 37 (16%) patients treated with CYTOVENE-IV vs 15 of the 35 (43%) placebo-treated patients developed disease through 6 months posttransplant. The overall rate of survival was statistically significantly higher in the group treated with CYTOVENE-IV, both at day 100 and day 180 posttransplant. Although the differences in hematologic toxicities were not statistically significant, the incidence of neutropenia was higher in the group treated with CYTOVENE-IV (refer to table in ADVERSE EVENTS).

ICM 1570: A second, randomized, unblinded study evaluated 40 allogeneic bone marrow transplant recipients at risk for CMV disease.[7] Patients underwent bronchoscopy and bronchoalveolar lavage (BAL) on day 35 posttransplant. Patients with histologic, immunologic or virologic evidence of CMV infection in the lung were then randomized to observation or treatment with CYTOVENE-IV solution (5 mg/kg bid for 14 days followed by 5 mg/kg qd 5 days/week until day 120). Four of 20 (20%) patients treated with CYTOVENE-IV and 14 of 20 (70%) control patients developed interstitial pneumonia. The incidence of CMV disease was significantly lower in the group treated with CYTOVENE-IV, consistent with the results observed in ICM 1689.

CYTOVENE Capsules: GAN040: CYTOVENE capsules were evaluated in a randomized, double-blind, placebo-controlled study of 304 orthotopic liver transplant recipients who were CMV seropositive or recipients of an organ from a seropositive donor. Administration of CYTOVENE capsules (1000 mg three times daily) or matching placebo commenced as soon as patients were able to take medication by mouth, but no later than 10 days following transplantation, and continued through 14 weeks after transplantation. Dosing was adjusted for patients with an estimated creatinine clearance <50 mL/min. The incidence of CMV disease at 6 months is summarized in the table below.

[See table at top of page]

CYTOVENE capsules significantly reduced the 6-month incidence of CMV disease in patients at increased risk of CMV disease, including seronegative recipients of organs from seropositive donors (15% [3/21] with CYTOVENE capsules vs 44% [11/25] with placebo), and patients receiving antilymphocyte antibodies (5% [2/44] with CYTOVENE capsules vs 33% [12/37] with placebo). The incidence of HSV infection at 6 months was 4% (5/150) in ganciclovir vs 24% (36/154) in placebo recipients (relative risk: 0.13; 95% CI: 0.05, 0.32).

CONTRAINDICATIONS

CYTOVENE-IV and CYTOVENE are contraindicated in patients with hypersensitivity to ganciclovir or acyclovir.

WARNINGS

Hematologic: CYTOVENE-IV and CYTOVENE should not be administered if the absolute neutrophil count is less than 500 cells/µL or the platelet count is less than 25,000 cells/µL. Granulocytopenia (neutropenia), anemia and thrombocytopenia have been observed in patients treated with CYTOVENE-IV and CYTOVENE. The frequency and severity of these events vary widely in different patient populations (see ADVERSE EVENTS).

CYTOVENE-IV and CYTOVENE should, therefore, be used with caution in patients with pre-existing cytopenias or with a history of cytopenic reactions to other drugs, chemicals or irradiation. Granulocytopenia usually occurs during the first or second week of treatment but may occur at any time during treatment. Cell counts usually begin to recover within 3 to 7 days of discontinuing drug. Colony-stimulating factors have been shown to increase neutrophil and white blood cell counts in patients receiving CYTOVENE-IV solution for treatment of CMV retinitis.

Impairment of Fertility: Animal data indicate that administration of ganciclovir causes inhibition of spermatogenesis and subsequent infertility. These effects were reversible at lower doses and irreversible at higher doses (see PRECAUTIONS: *Carcinogenesis, Mutagenesis* and *Impairment of Fertility*). Although data in humans have not been obtained regarding this effect, it is considered probable that ganciclovir at the recommended doses causes temporary or permanent inhibition of spermatogenesis. Animal data also indicate that suppression of fertility in females may occur.

Teratogenesis: Because of the mutagenic and teratogenic potential of ganciclovir, women of childbearing potential should be advised to use effective contraception during treatment. Similarly, men should be advised to practice barrier contraception during and for at least 90 days following treatment with CYTOVENE-IV or CYTOVENE (see *Pregnancy:* Category C).

PRECAUTIONS

General: In clinical studies with CYTOVENE-IV, the maximum single dose administered was 6 mg/kg by intravenous infusion over 1 hour. Larger doses have resulted in increased toxicity. It is likely that more rapid infusions would also result in increased toxicity (see OVERDOSAGE). Administration of CYTOVENE-IV solution should be accompanied by adequate hydration.

Initially reconstituted solutions of CYTOVENE-IV have a high pH (pH 11). Despite further dilution in intravenous fluids, phlebitis and/or pain may occur at the site of intravenous infusion. Care must be taken to infuse solutions containing CYTOVENE-IV only into veins with adequate blood flow to permit rapid dilution and distribution (see DOSAGE AND ADMINISTRATION).

Since ganciclovir is excreted by the kidneys, normal clearance depends on adequate renal function. IF RENAL FUNCTION IS IMPAIRED, DOSAGE ADJUSTMENTS ARE REQUIRED FOR CYTOVENE-IV AND SHOULD BE CONSIDERED FOR CYTOVENE CAPSULES. Such adjustments should be based on measured or estimated creatinine clearance values (see DOSAGE AND ADMINISTRATION).

Information for Patients: All patients should be informed that the major toxicities of ganciclovir are granulocytopenia (neutropenia), anemia and thrombocytopenia and that dose modifications may be required, including discontinuation. The importance of close monitoring of blood counts while on therapy should be emphasized. Patients should be informed that ganciclovir has been associated with elevations in serum creatinine.

Patients should be instructed to take CYTOVENE capsules with food to maximize bioavailability.

Patients should be advised that ganciclovir has caused decreased sperm production in animals and may cause infertility in humans. Women of childbearing potential should be advised that ganciclovir causes birth defects in animals and should not be used during pregnancy. Women of childbearing potential should be advised to use effective contraception during treatment with CYTOVENE-IV or CYTOVENE. Similarly, men should be advised to practice barrier contraception during and for at least 90 days following treatment with CYTOVENE-IV or CYTOVENE.

Patients should be advised that ganciclovir causes tumors in animals. Although there is no information from human studies, ganciclovir should be considered a potential carcinogen.

All HIV+ Patients: These patients may be receiving zidovudine (Retrovir®*). Patients should be counseled that treatment with both ganciclovir and zidovudine simultaneously may not be tolerated by some patients and may result in severe granulocytopenia (neutropenia). Patients with AIDS may be receiving didanosine (Videx®†). Patients should be counseled that concomitant treatment with both ganciclovir and didanosine can cause didanosine serum concentrations to be significantly increased.

HIV+ Patients With CMV Retinitis: Ganciclovir is not a cure for CMV retinitis, and immunocompromised patients may continue to experience progression of retinitis during or following treatment. Patients should be advised to have ophthalmologic follow-up examinations at a minimum of every 4 to 6 weeks while being treated with CYTOVENE-IV or CYTOVENE. Some patients will require more frequent follow-up.

Transplant Recipients: Transplant recipients should be counseled regarding the high frequency of impaired renal function in transplant recipients who received

Incidence of CMV Disease at 6 Months (Kaplan-Meier Estimates)

CMV Disease at 6 months	Ganciclovir (n=150)	Placebo (n=154)	Relative Risk (95% CI)
CMV Disease,* N (%)	7 (4.8%)	29 (18.9%)	0.22 (0.10, 0.51)
CMV syndrome†	6 (4.1%)	19 (12.4%)	
CMV hepatitis	1 (0.7%)	9 (5.9%)	
CMV GI disease	0 (0.0%)	3 (2.0%)	
CMV lung disease	0 (0.0%)	4 (2.6%)	

* One or more CMV endpoints
† CMV syndrome: CMV viremia and unexplained fever, accompanied by malaise and/or neutropenia.

CYTOVENE-IV solution in controlled clinical trials, particularly in patients receiving concomitant administration of nephrotoxic agents such as cyclosporine and amphotericin B. Although the specific mechanism of this toxicity, which in most cases was reversible, has not been determined, the higher rate of renal impairment in patients receiving CYTOVENE-IV solution compared with those who received placebo in the same trials may indicate that CYTOVENE-IV played a significant role.

Laboratory Testing: Due to the frequency of neutropenia, anemia and thrombocytopenia in patients receiving CYTOVENE-IV and CYTOVENE (see ADVERSE EVENTS), it is recommended that complete blood counts and platelet counts be performed frequently, especially in patients in whom ganciclovir or other nucleoside analogues have previously resulted in leukopenia or in whom neutrophil counts are less than 1000 cells/μL at the beginning of treatment. Increased serum creatinine levels have been observed in trials evaluating both CYTOVENE-IV and CYTOVENE. Patients should have serum creatinine or creatinine clearance values monitored carefully to allow for dosage adjustments in renally impaired patients (see DOSAGE AND ADMINISTRATION).

Drug Interactions: *Didanosine:* At an oral dose of 1000 mg of CYTOVENE every 8 hours and didanosine, 200 mg every 12 hours, the steady-state didanosine AUC_{0-12} increased 111 ± 114% (range: 10% to 493%) when didanosine was administered either 2 hours prior to or concurrent with administration of CYTOVENE (n=12 patients, 23 observations). A decrease in steady-state ganciclovir AUC of 21 ± 17% (range: -44% to 5%) was observed when didanosine was administered 2 hours prior to administration of CYTOVENE, but ganciclovir AUC was not affected by the presence of didanosine when the two drugs were administered simultaneously (n=12). There were no significant changes in renal clearance for either drug.

When the standard intravenous ganciclovir induction dose (5 mg/kg infused over 1 hour every 12 hours) was coadministered with didanosine at a dose of 200 mg orally every 12 hours, the steady-state didanosine AUC_{0-12} increased 70 ± 40% (range: 3% to 121%, n=11) and C_{max} increased 49 ± 48% (range: -28% to 125%). In a separate study, when the standard intravenous ganciclovir maintenance dose (5 mg/kg infused over 1 hour every 24 hours) was coadministered with didanosine at a dose of 200 mg orally every 12 hours, didanosine AUC_{0-12} increased 50 ± 26% (range: 22% to 110%, n=11) and C_{max} increased 36 ± 36% (range: -27% to 94%) over the first didanosine dosing interval. Didanosine plasma concentrations (AUC_{12-24}) were unchanged during the dosing intervals when ganciclovir was not coadministered. Ganciclovir pharmacokinetics were not affected by didanosine. In neither study were there significant changes in the renal clearance of either drug.

Zidovudine: At an oral dose of 1000 mg of CYTOVENE every 8 hours, mean steady-state ganciclovir AUC_{0-8} decreased 17 ± 25% (range: -52% to 23%) in the presence of zidovudine, 100 mg every 4 hours (n=12). Steady-state zidovudine AUC_{0-4} increased 19 ± 27% (range: -11% to 74%) in the presence of ganciclovir.

Since both zidovudine and ganciclovir have the potential to cause neutropenia and anemia, some patients may not tolerate concomitant therapy with these drugs at full dosage.

Probenecid: At an oral dose of 1000 mg of CYTOVENE every 8 hours (n=10), ganciclovir AUC_{0-8} increased 53 ± 91% (range: -14% to 299%) in the presence of probenecid, 500 mg every 6 hours. Renal clearance of ganciclovir decreased 22 ± 20% (range: -54% to -4%), which is consistent with an interaction involving competition for renal tubular secretion.

Imipenem-cilastatin: Generalized seizures have been reported in patients who received ganciclovir and imipenem-cilastatin. These drugs should not be used concomitantly unless the potential benefits outweigh the risks.

Other Medications: It is possible that drugs that inhibit replication of rapidly dividing cell populations such as bone marrow, spermatogonia and germinal layers of skin and gastrointestinal mucosa may have additive toxicity when administered concomitantly with ganciclovir. Therefore, drugs such as dapsone, pentamidine, flucytosine, vincristine, vinblastine, adriamycin, amphotericin B, trimethoprim/sulfamethoxazole combinations or other nucleoside analogues, should be considered for concomitant use with ganciclovir only if the potential benefits are judged to outweigh the risks.

No formal drug interaction studies of CYTOVENE-IV or CYTOVENE and drugs commonly used in transplant recipients have been conducted. Increases in serum creatinine were observed in patients treated with CYTOVENE-IV plus either cyclosporine or amphotericin B, drugs with known potential for nephrotoxicity (see ADVERSE EVENTS). In a retrospective analysis of 93 liver allograft recipients receiving ganciclovir (5 mg/kg infused over 1 hour every 12 hours) and oral cyclosporine (at therapeutic doses), there was no evidence of an effect on cyclosporine whole blood concentrations.

Carcinogenesis, Mutagenesis‡: Ganciclovir was carcinogenic in the mouse at oral doses of 20 and 1000 mg/kg/day

Laboratory Data:

Selected Laboratory Abnormalities in Trials for Treatment of CMV Retinitis and Prevention of CMV Diseases

	CMV Retinitis Treatment*		CMV Disease Prevention§	
Treatment	CYTOVENE Capsules† 3000 mg/day	CYTOVENE-IV‡ 5 mg/kg/day	CYTOVENE Capsules‖ 3000 mg/day	Placebo¶
Subjects, number	320	175	478	234
Neutropenia:				
<500 ANC/μL	18%	25%	10%	6%
500 – <749	17%	14%	16%	7%
750 – <1000	19%	26%	22%	16%
Anemia:				
Hemoglobin:				
<6.5 g/dL	2%	5%	1%	<1%
6.5 – <8.0	10%	16%	5%	3%
8.0 – <9.5	25%	26%	15%	16%
Maximum Serum Creatinine:				
≥2.5 mg/dL	1%	2%	1%	2%
≥1.5 – <2.5	12%	14%	19%	11%

* Pooled data from Treatment Studies, ICM 1653. Study ICM 1774 and Study AVI 034
† Mean time on therapy = 91 days, including allowed reinduction treatment periods
‡ Mean time on therapy = 103 days, including allowed reinduction treatment periods
§ Data from Prevention Study, ICM 1654
‖ Mean time on ganciclovir = 269 days
¶ Mean time on placebo = 240 days
(See discussion of clinical trials under INDICATIONS AND USAGE.)

(approximately 0.1× and 1.4×, respectively, the mean drug exposure in humans following the recommended intravenous dose of 5 mg/kg, based on area under the plasma concentration curve [AUC] comparisons). At the dose of 1000 mg/kg/day there was a significant increase in the incidence of tumors of the preputial gland in males, forestomach (nonglandular mucosa) in males and females, and reproductive tissues (ovaries, uterus, mammary gland, clitoral gland and vagina) and liver in females. At the dose of 20 mg/kg/day, a slightly increased incidence of tumors was noted in the preputial and harderian glands in males, forestomach in males and females, and liver in females. No carcinogenic effect was observed in mice administered ganciclovir at 1 mg/kg/day (estimated as 0.01× the human dose based on AUC comparison). Except for histiocytic sarcoma of the liver, ganciclovir-induced tumors were generally of epithelial or vascular origin. Although the preputial and clitoral glands, forestomach and harderian glands of mice do not have human counterparts, ganciclovir should be considered a potential carcinogen in humans.

Ganciclovir increased mutations in mouse lymphoma cells and DNA damage in human lymphocytes in vitro at concentrations between 50 to 500 and 250 to 2000 μg/mL, respectively. In the mouse micronucleus assay, ganciclovir was clastogenic at doses of 150 and 500 mg/kg (IV) (2.8 to 10× human exposure based on AUC) but not 50 mg/kg (exposure approximately comparable to the human based on AUC). Ganciclovir was not mutagenic in the Ames Salmonella assay at concentrations of 500 to 5000 μg/mL.

Impairment of Fertility‡: Ganciclovir caused decreased mating behavior, decreased fertility, and an increased incidence of embryolethality in female mice following intravenous doses of 90 mg/kg/day (approximately 1.7× the mean drug exposure in humans following the dose of 5 mg/kg, based on AUC comparisons). Ganciclovir caused decreased fertility in male mice and hypospermatogenesis in mice and dogs following daily oral or intravenous administration of doses ranging from 0.2 to 10 mg/kg. Systemic drug exposure (AUC) at the lowest dose showing toxicity in each species ranged from 0.03 to 0.1× the AUC of the recommended human intravenous dose.

***Pregnancy:* Category C‡:** Ganciclovir has been shown to be embryotoxic in rabbits and mice following intravenous administration and teratogenic in rabbits. Fetal resorptions were present in at least 85% of rabbits and mice administered 60 mg/kg/day and 108 mg/kg/day (2× the human exposure based on AUC comparisons), respectively. Effects observed in rabbits included: fetal growth retardation, embryolethality, teratogenicity and/or maternal toxicity. Teratogenic changes included cleft palate, anophthalmia/microphthalmia, aplastic organs (kidney and pancreas), hydrocephaly and brachygnathia. In mice, effects observed were maternal/fetal toxicity and embryolethality.

Daily intravenous doses of 90 mg/kg administered to female mice prior to mating, during gestation, and during lactation caused hypoplasia of the testes and seminal vesicles in the month-old male offspring, as well as pathologic changes in the nonglandular region of the stomach (see *Carcinogenesis, Mutagenesis*). The drug exposure in mice as estimated by the AUC was approximately 1.7× the human AUC.

Ganciclovir may be teratogenic or embryotoxic at dose levels recommended for human use. There are no adequate and well-controlled studies in pregnant women. CYTOVENE-IV or CYTOVENE should be used during pregnancy only if the potential benefits justify the potential risk to the fetus.

‡Footnote: All dose comparisons presented in the *Carcinogenesis, Mutagenesis, Impairment of Fertility* and *Pregnancy* subsections are based on the human AUC following administration of a single 5 mg/kg intravenous infusion of CYTOVENE-IV as used during the maintenance phase of treatment. Compared with the single 5 mg/kg intravenous infusion, human exposure is doubled during the intravenous induction phase (5 mg/kg bid) and approximately halved during maintenance treatment with CYTOVENE capsules (1000 mg tid). The cross-species dose comparisons should be divided by 2 for intravenous induction treatment with CYTOVENE-IV and multiplied by 2 for CYTOVENE capsules.

Nursing Mothers: It is not known whether ganciclovir is excreted in human milk. However, many drugs are excreted in human milk and, because carcinogenic and teratogenic effects occurred in animals treated with ganciclovir, the possibility of serious adverse reactions from ganciclovir in nursing infants is considered likely (see *Pregnancy:* Category C). Mothers should be instructed to discontinue nursing if they are receiving CYTOVENE-IV or CYTOVENE. The minimum interval before nursing can safely be resumed after the last dose of CYTOVENE-IV or CYTOVENE is unknown.

Pediatric Use: **SAFETY AND EFFICACY OF CYTOVENE-IV AND CYTOVENE IN PEDIATRIC PATIENTS HAVE NOT BEEN ESTABLISHED. THE USE OF CYTOVENE-IV OR CYTOVENE IN THE PEDIATRIC POPULATION WARRANTS EXTREME CAUTION DUE TO THE PROBABILITY OF LONG-TERM CARCINOGENICITY AND REPRODUCTIVE TOXICITY. ADMINISTRATION TO PEDIATRIC PATIENTS SHOULD BE UNDERTAKEN ONLY AFTER CAREFUL EVALUATION AND ONLY IF THE POTENTIAL BENEFITS OF TREATMENT OUTWEIGH THE RISKS.**

The spectrum of adverse events reported in 120 immunocompromised pediatric clinical trial participants with serious CMV infections receiving CYTOVENE-IV solution were similar to those reported in adults. Granulocytopenia (17%) and thrombocytopenia (10%) were the most common adverse events reported.

Sixteen pediatric patients (8 months to 15 years of age) with life- or sight-threatening CMV infections were evaluated in an open-label, CYTOVENE-IV solution, pharmacokinetics study. Adverse events reported for more than one pediatric patient were as follows: hypokalemia (4/16, 25%), abnormal kidney function (3/16, 19%), sepsis (3/16, 19%), thrombocytopenia (3/16, 19%), leukopenia (2/16, 13%), coagulation disorder (2/16, 13%), hypertension (2/16, 13%), pneumonia (2/16, 13%) and immune system disorder (2/16, 13%).

There has been very limited clinical experience using CYTOVENE-IV for the treatment of CMV retinitis in patients under the age of 12 years. Two pediatric patients (ages 9 and 5 years) showed improvement or stabilization of retinitis for 23 and 9 months, respectively. These pediatric patients received induction treatment with 2.5 mg/kg tid followed by maintenance therapy with 6 to 6.5 mg/kg once per day, 5 to 7 days per week. When retinitis progressed

Continued on next page

Cytovene—Cont.

during once-daily maintenance therapy, both pediatric patients were treated with the 5 mg/kg bid regimen. Two other pediatric patients (ages 2.5 and 4 years) who received similar induction regimens showed only partial or no response to treatment. Another pediatric patient, a 6-year-old with T-cell dysfunction, showed stabilization of retinitis for 3 months while receiving continuous infusions of CYTOVENE-IV at doses of 2 to 5 mg/kg/24 hours. Continuous infusion treatment was discontinued due to granulocytopenia.

Eleven of the 72 patients in the placebo-controlled trial in bone marrow transplant recipients were pediatric patients, ranging in age from 3 to 10 years (5 treated with CYTOVENE-IV and 6 with placebo). Five of the pediatric patients treated with CYTOVENE-IV received 5 mg/kg intravenously bid for up to 7 days; 4 patients went on to receive 5 mg/kg qd up to day 100 posttransplant. Results were similar to those observed in adult transplant recipients treated with CYTOVENE-IV. Two of the 6 placebo-treated pediatric patients developed CMV pneumonia vs none of the 5 patients treated with CYTOVENE-IV. The spectrum of adverse events in the pediatric group was similar to that observed in the adult patients.

CYTOVENE capsules have not been studied in pediatric patients under age 13.

Use in Patients With Renal Impairment: CYTOVENE-IV and CYTOVENE should be used with caution in patients with impaired renal function because the half-life and plasma/serum concentrations of ganciclovir will be increased due to reduced renal clearance (see DOSAGE AND ADMINISTRATION and ADVERSE EVENTS: *Renal Toxicity*). Hemodialysis has been shown to reduce plasma levels of ganciclovir by approximately 50%.

Use in Elderly Patients: The pharmacokinetic profiles of CYTOVENE-IV and CYTOVENE in elderly patients have not been established. Since elderly individuals frequently have a reduced glomerular filtration rate, particular attention should be paid to assessing renal function before and during administration of CYTOVENE-IV or CYTOVENE (see DOSAGE AND ADMINISTRATION).

ADVERSE EVENTS

Adverse events that occurred during clinical trials of CYTOVENE-IV solution and CYTOVENE capsules are summarized below, according to the participating study subject population.

Subjects With AIDS: Three controlled, randomized, phase 3 trials comparing CYTOVENE-IV and CYTOVENE capsules for maintenance treatment of CMV retinitis have been completed. During these trials, CYTOVENE-IV or CYTOVENE capsules were prematurely discontinued in 9% of subjects because of adverse events. In a placebo-controlled, randomized, phase 3 trial of CYTOVENE capsules for prevention of CMV disease in AIDS, treatment was prematurely discontinued because of adverse events, new or worsening intercurrent illness, or laboratory abnormalities in 19.5% of subjects treated with CYTOVENE capsules and 16% of subjects receiving placebo. Laboratory data and adverse events reported during the conduct of these controlled trials are summarized below.

[See table at top of previous page]

Adverse Events: The following table shows selected adverse events reported in 5% or more of the subjects in three controlled clinical trials during treatment with either CYTOVENE-IV solution (5 mg/kg/day) or CYTOVENE capsules (3000 mg/day), and in one controlled clinical trial in which CYTOVENE capsules (3000 mg/day) were compared to placebo for the prevention of CMV disease.

[See first table above]

The following events were frequently observed in clinical trials but occurred with equal or greater frequency in placebo-treated subjects: abdominal pain, nausea, flatulence, pneumonia, paresthesia, rash.

Retinal Detachment: Retinal detachment has been observed in subjects with CMV retinitis both before and after initiation of therapy with ganciclovir. Its relationship to therapy with ganciclovir is unknown. Retinal detachment occurred in 11% of patients treated with CYTOVENE-IV solution and in 8% of patients treated with CYTOVENE capsules. Patients with CMV retinitis should have frequent ophthalmologic evaluations to monitor the status of their retinitis and to detect any other retinal pathology.

Transplant Recipients: There have been three controlled clinical trials of CYTOVENE-IV solution and one controlled clinical trial of CYTOVENE capsules for the prevention of CMV disease in transplant recipients. Laboratory data and adverse events reported during these trials are summarized below.

Laboratory Data: The following table shows the frequency of granulocytopenia (neutropenia) and thrombocytopenia observed:

[See second table above]

The following table shows the frequency of elevated serum creatinine values in these controlled clinical trials:

Selected Adverse Events Reported ≥5% of Subjects in Three Randomized Phase 3 Studies Comparing CYTOVENE Capsules to CYTOVENE-IV Solution for Maintenance Treatment of CMV Retinitis and in One Phase 3 Randomized Study Comparing Cytovene Capsules to Placebo for Prevention of CMV Disease

Body System	Adverse Event	Maintenance Treatment Studies		Prevention Study	
		Capsules (n=326)	IV (n=179)	Capsules (n=478)	Placebo (n=234)
Body as a Whole	Fever	38%	48%	35%	33%
	Infection	9%	13%	8%	4%
	Chills	7%	10%	7%	4%
	Sepsis	4%	15%	3%	2%
Digestive System	Diarrhea	41%	44%	48%	42%
	Anorexia	15%	14%	19%	16%
	Vomiting	13%	13%	14%	11%
Hemic and Lymphatic System	Leukopenia	29%	41%	17%	9%
	Anemia	19%	25%	9%	7%
	Thrombocytopenia	6%	6%	3%	1%
Nervous System	Neuropathy	8%	9%	21%	15%
Other	Sweating	11%	12%	14%	12%
	Pruritus	6%	5%	10%	9%
Catheter Related*	Total Catheter Events	6%	22%	–	–
	Catheter Infection	4%	9%	–	–
	Catheter Sepsis	1%	8%	–	–

* Some of these events also appear under other body systems.

Controlled Trials – Transplant Recipients

	CYTOVENE-IV				CYTOVENE Capsules	
	Heart Allograft*		Bone Marrow Allograft†		Liver Allograft‡	
	CYTOVENE-IV (n=76)	Placebo (n=73)	CYTOVENE-IV (n=57)	Control (n=55)	CYTOVENE Capsules (n=150)	Placebo (n=154)
Neutropenia						
Minimum ANC <500/μL	4%	3%	12%	6%	3%	1%
Minimum ANC 500–1000/μL	3%	8%	29%	17%	3%	2%
TOTAL ANC ≤1000/μL	7%	11%	41%	23%	6%	3%
Thrombocytopenia						
Platelet count <25,000/μL	3%	1%	32%	28%	0%	3%
Platelet count 25,000–50,000/μL	5%	3%	25%	37%	5%	3%
TOTAL Platelet ≤50,000/μL	8%	4%	57%	65%	5%	6%

* Study ICM 1496: Mean duration of treatment = 28 days
† Study ICM 1570 and ICM 1689. Mean duration of treatment = 45 days
‡ Study GAN040. Mean duration of ganciclovir treatment = 82 days
(See discussion of clinical trials under INDICATIONS AND USAGE.)

[See table at top of next page]
In 3 out of 4 trials, patients receiving either CYTOVENE-IV solution or CYTOVENE capsules had elevated serum creatinine levels when compared to those receiving placebo. Most patients in these studies also received cyclosporine. The mechanism of impairment of renal function is not known. However, careful monitoring of renal function during therapy with CYTOVENE-IV solution or CYTOVENE capsules is essential, especially for those patients receiving concomitant agents that may cause nephrotoxicity.

General: Other adverse events that were thought to be "probably" or "possibly" related to CYTOVENE-IV solution or CYTOVENE capsules in controlled clinical studies in either subjects with AIDS or transplant recipients are listed below. These events all occurred in at least 3 subjects.

Body as a Whole: abdomen enlarged, asthenia, chest pain, edema, headache, injection site inflammation, malaise, pain
Digestive System: abnormal liver function test, aphthous stomatitis, constipation, dyspepsia, eructation
Hemic and Lymphatic System: pancytopenia
Respiratory System: cough increased, dyspnea
Nervous System: abnormal dreams, anxiety, confusion, depression, dizziness, dry mouth, insomnia, seizures, somnolence, thinking abnormal, tremor
Skin and Appendages: alopecia, dry skin
Special Senses: abnormal vision, taste perversion, tinnitus, vitreous disorder

Metabolic and Nutritional Disorders: creatinine increased, SGOT increased, SGPT increased, weight loss
Cardiovascular System: hypertension, phlebitis, vasodilatation
Urogenital System: creatinine clearance decreased, kidney failure, kidney function abnormal, urinary frequency
Musculoskeletal System: arthralgia, leg cramps, myalgia, myasthenia
The following adverse events reported in patients receiving ganciclovir may be potentially fatal: gastrointestinal perforation, multiple organ failure, pancreatitis and sepsis.

Adverse Events Reported During Postmarketing Experience With CYTOVENE-IV and CYTOVENE Capsules: The following events have been identified during post-approval use of the drug. Because they are reported voluntarily from a population of unknown size, estimates of frequency cannot be made. These events have been chosen for inclusion due to either the seriousness, frequency of reporting, the apparent causal connection or a combination of these factors:

acidosis, allergic reaction, anaphylactic reaction, arthritis, bronchospasm, cardiac arrest, cardiac conduction abnormality, cataracts, cholelithiasis, cholestasis, congenital anomaly, dry eyes, dysesthesia, dysphasia, elevated triglyceride levels, encephalopathy, exfoliative dermatitis, extrapyramidal reaction, facial palsy, hallucinations, hemolytic anemia, hemolytic uremic syndrome, hepatic failure, hepatitis, hypercalcemia, hyponatremia, inappropriate serum ADH, in-

Controlled Trials – Transplant Recipients

	CYTOVENE-IV						CYTOVENE Capsules	
Maximum Serum Creatinine Levels	Heart Allograft ICM 1496		Bone Marrow Allograft ICM 1570		Bone Marrow Allograft ICM 1689		Liver Allograft Study 040	
	CYTOVENE-IV (n=76)	Placebo (n=73)	CYTOVENE-IV (n=20)	Control (n=20)	CYTOVENE-IV (n=37)	Placebo (n=35)	CYTOVENE Capsules (n=150)	Placebo (n=154)
Serum Creatinine ≥2.5 mg/dL	18%	4%	20%	0%	0%	0%	16%	10%
Serum Creatinine ≥1.5 –<2.5 mg/dL	58%	69%	50%	35%	43%	44%	39%	42%

fertility, intestinal ulceration, intracranial hypertension, irritability, loss of memory, loss of sense of smell, myelopathy, oculomotor nerve paralysis, peripheral ischemia, pulmonary fibrosis, renal tubular disorder, rhabdomyolysis, Stevens-Johnson syndrome, stroke, testicular hypotrophy, Torsades de Pointes, vasculitis, ventricular tachycardia

OVERDOSAGE
CYTOVENE-IV: Overdosage with CYTOVENE-IV has been reported in 17 patients (13 adults and 4 children under 2 years of age). Five patients experienced no adverse events following overdosage at the following doses: 7 doses of 11 mg/kg over a 3-day period (adult), single dose of 3500 mg (adult), single dose of 500 mg (72.5 mg/kg) followed by 48 hours of peritoneal dialysis (4-month-old), single dose of approximately 60 mg/kg followed by exchange transfusion (18-month-old), 2 doses of 500 mg instead of 31 mg (21-month-old).
Irreversible pancytopenia developed in 1 adult with AIDS and CMV colitis after receiving 3000 mg of CYTOVENE-IV solution on each of 2 consecutive days. He experienced worsening GI symptoms and acute renal failure that required short-term dialysis. Pancytopenia developed and persisted until his death from a malignancy several months later. Other adverse events reported following overdosage included: persistent bone marrow suppression (1 adult with neutropenia and thrombocytopenia after a single dose of 6000 mg), reversible neutropenia or granulocytopenia (4 adults, overdoses ranging from 8 mg/kg daily for 4 days to a single dose of 25 mg/kg), hepatitis (1 adult receiving 10 mg/kg daily, and one 2 kg infant after a single 40 mg dose), renal toxicity (1 adult with transient worsening of hematuria after a single 500 mg dose, and 1 adult with elevated creatinine (5.2 mg/dL) after a single 5000 to 7000 mg dose), and seizure (1 adult with known seizure disorder after 3 days of 9 mg/kg). In addition, 1 adult received 0.4 mL (instead of 0.1 mL) CYTOVENE-IV solution by intravitreal injection, and experienced temporary loss of vision and central retinal artery occlusion secondary to increased intraocular pressure related to the injected fluid volume.
CYTOVENE Capsules: There have been no reports of overdosage with CYTOVENE capsules. Doses as high as 6000 mg/day, given either as 1000 mg 6 times daily or as 2000 mg tid, did not result in overt toxicity other than transient neutropenia. Daily doses of more than 6000 mg have not been studied.

Since ganciclovir is dialyzable, dialysis may be useful in reducing serum concentrations. Adequate hydration should be maintained. The use of hematopoietic growth factors should be considered.

DOSAGE AND ADMINISTRATION
CAUTION—DO NOT ADMINISTER CYTOVENE-IV SOLUTION BY RAPID OR BOLUS INTRAVENOUS INJECTION. THE TOXICITY OF CYTOVENE-IV MAY BE INCREASED AS A RESULT OF EXCESSIVE PLASMA LEVELS.
CAUTION—INTRAMUSCULAR OR SUBCUTANEOUS INJECTION OF RECONSTITUTED CYTOVENE-IV SOLUTION MAY RESULT IN SEVERE TISSUE IRRITATION DUE TO HIGH pH (11).
Dosage: THE RECOMMENDED DOSE FOR CYTOVENE-IV SOLUTION AND CYTOVENE CAPSULES SHOULD NOT BE EXCEEDED. THE RECOMMENDED INFUSION RATE FOR CYTOVENE-IV SOLUTION SHOULD NOT BE EXCEEDED.
For Treatment of CMV Retinitis in Patients With Normal Renal Function:
1. Induction Treatment
The recommended initial dosage for patients with normal renal function is 5 mg/kg (given intravenously at a constant rate over 1 hour) every 12 hours for 14 to 21 days. CYTOVENE capsules should not be used for induction treatment.
2. Maintenance Treatment
CYTOVENE-IV: Following induction treatment, the recommended maintenance dosage of CYTOVENE-IV solution is 5 mg/kg given as a constant-rate intravenous infusion over 1 hour once daily, 7 days per week or 6 mg/kg once daily, 5 days per week.
CYTOVENE Capsules: Following induction treatment, the recommended maintenance dosage of CYTOVENE capsules is 1000 mg tid with food. Alternatively, the dosing regimen of 500 mg 6 times daily every 3 hours with food, during waking hours, may be used.
For patients who experience progression of CMV retinitis while receiving maintenance treatment with either formulation of ganciclovir, reinduction treatment is recommended.
For the Prevention of CMV Disease in Patients With Advanced HIV Infection and Normal Renal Function:
CYTOVENE Capsules: The recommended prophylactic dose of CYTOVENE capsules is 1000 mg tid with food.

For the Prevention of CMV Disease in Transplant Recipients With Normal Renal Function:
CYTOVENE-IV: The recommended initial dosage of CYTOVENE-IV solution for patients with normal renal function is 5 mg/kg (given intravenously at a constant rate over 1 hour) every 12 hours for 7 to 14 days, followed by 5 mg/kg once daily, 7 days per week or 6 mg/kg once daily, 5 days per week.
CYTOVENE Capsules: The recommended prophylactic dosage of CYTOVENE capsules is 1000 mg tid with food.
The duration of treatment with CYTOVENE-IV solution and CYTOVENE capsules in transplant recipients is dependent upon the duration and degree of immunosuppression. In controlled clinical trials in bone marrow allograft recipients, treatment with CYTOVENE-IV was continued until day 100 to 120 posttransplantation. CMV disease occurred in several patients who discontinued treatment with CYTOVENE-IV solution prematurely. In heart allograft recipients, the onset of newly diagnosed CMV disease occurred after treatment with CYTOVENE-IV was stopped at day 28 posttransplant, suggesting that continued dosing may be necessary to prevent late occurrence of CMV disease in this patient population. In a controlled clinical trial of liver allograft recipients, treatment with CYTOVENE capsules was continued through week 14 posttransplantation (see INDICATIONS AND USAGE section for a more detailed discussion).
Renal Impairment:
CYTOVENE-IV: For patients with impairment of renal function, refer to the table below for recommended doses of CYTOVENE-IV solution and adjust the dosing interval as indicated:
[See first table below]
Dosing for patients undergoing hemodialysis should not exceed 1.25 mg/kg 3 times per week, following each hemodialysis session. CYTOVENE-IV should be given shortly after completion of the hemodialysis session, since hemodialysis has been shown to reduce plasma levels by approximately 50%.
CYTOVENE Capsules: In patients with renal impairment, the dose of CYTOVENE capsules should be modified as shown below:
[See second table below]
Patient Monitoring: Due to the frequency of granulocytopenia, anemia and thrombocytopenia in patients receiving ganciclovir (see ADVERSE EVENTS), it is recommended that complete blood counts and platelet counts be performed frequently, especially in patients in whom ganciclovir or other nucleoside analogues have previously resulted in cytopenia, or in whom neutrophil counts are less than 1000 cells/µL at the beginning of treatment. Patients should have serum creatinine or creatinine clearance values followed carefully to allow for dosage adjustments in renally impaired patients (see DOSAGE AND ADMINISTRATION).
Reduction of Dose: Dosage reductions in renally impaired patients are required for CYTOVENE-IV and should be considered for CYTOVENE capsules (see *Renal Impairment*). Dosage reductions should also be considered for those with neutropenia, anemia and/or thrombocytopenia (see ADVERSE EVENTS). Ganciclovir should not be administered in patients with severe neutropenia (ANC less than 500/µL) or severe thrombocytopenia (platelets less than 25,000/µL).
Method of Preparation of CYTOVENE IV Solution: Each 10 mL clear glass vial contains ganciclovir sodium equivalent to 500 mg of ganciclovir and 46 mg of sodium. The contents of the vial should be prepared for administration in the following manner:
1. Reconstituted Solution:
   a. Reconstitute lyophilized CYTOVENE-IV by injecting 10 mL of Sterile Water for Injection, USP, into the vial. DO NOT USE BACTERIOSTATIC WATER FOR INJECTION CONTAINING PARABENS. IT IS INCOMPATIBLE WITH CYTOVENE-IV AND MAY CAUSE PRECIPITATION.

Creatinine Clearance* (mL/min)	CYTOVENE-IV Induction Dose (mg/kg)	Dosing Interval (hours)	CYTOVENE-IV Maintenance Dose (mg/kg)	Dosing Interval (hours)
≥70	5.0	12	5.0	24
50 – 69	2.5	12	2.5	24
25 – 49	2.5	24	1.25	24
10 – 24	1.25	24	0.625	24
<10	1.25	3 times per week, following hemodialysis	0.625	3 times per week, following hemodialysis

*Creatinine clearance can be related to serum creatinine by the formulas given below.

Creatinine Clearance* mL/min	CYTOVENE Capsule Dosages	
≥70	1000 mg tid or	500 mg q3h, 6x/day
50 – 69	1500 mg qd or	500 mg tid
25 – 49	1000 mg qd or	500 mg bid
10 – 24	500 mg qd	
<10	500 mg 3 times per week, following hemodialysis	

* Creatinine clearance can be related to serum creatinine by the following formulas:

Creatinine clearance for males = $\dfrac{(140 - \text{age [yrs]}) (\text{body wt [kg]})}{(72) (\text{serum creatinine [mg/dL]})}$

Creatinine clearance for females = $0.85 \times$ male value

Continued on next page

Cytovene—Cont.

b. Shake the vial to dissolve the drug.

c. Visually inspect the reconstituted solution for particulate matter and discoloration prior to proceeding with infusion solution. Discard the vial if particulate matter or discoloration is observed.

d. Reconstituted solution in the vial is stable at room temperature for 12 hours. It should not be refrigerated.

2. *Infusion Solution:*

Based on patient weight, the appropriate volume of the reconstituted solution (ganciclovir concentration 50 mg/mL) should be removed from the vial and added to an acceptable (see below) infusion fluid (typically 100 mL) for delivery over the course of 1 hour. Infusion concentrations greater than 10 mg/mL are not recommended. The following infusion fluids have been determined to be chemically and physically compatible with CYTOVENE-IV solution: 0.9% Sodium Chloride, 5% Dextrose, Ringer's Injection and Lactated Ringer's Injection, USP.

CYTOVENE-IV, when reconstituted with sterile water for injection, further diluted with 0.9% sodium chloride injection, and stored refrigerated at 5°C in polyvinyl chloride (PVC) bags, remains physically and chemically stable for 14 days.

However, because CYTOVENE-IV is reconstituted with nonbacteriostatic sterile water, it is recommended that the infusion solution be used within 24 hours of dilution to reduce the risk of bacterial contamination. The infusion should be refrigerated. Freezing is not recommended.

Handling and Disposal: Caution should be exercised in the handling and preparation of solutions of CYTOVENE-IV and in the handling of CYTOVENE capsules. Solutions of CYTOVENE-IV are alkaline (pH 11). Avoid direct contact with the skin or mucous membranes of the powder contained in CYTOVENE capsules or of CYTOVENE-IV solutions. If such contact occurs, wash thoroughly with soap and water; rinse eyes thoroughly with plain water. CYTOVENE capsules should not be opened or crushed.

Because ganciclovir shares some of the properties of antitumor agents (ie, carcinogenicity and mutagenicity), consideration should be given to handling and disposal according to guidelines issued for antineoplastic drugs. Several guidelines on this subject have been published.[8–10]

There is no general agreement that all of the procedures recommended in the guidelines are necessary or appropriate.

HOW SUPPLIED

CYTOVENE®-IV (ganciclovir sodium for injection) is supplied in 10 mL sterile vials, each containing ganciclovir sodium equivalent to 500 mg of ganciclovir, in cartons of 25 (NDC 0004-6940-03).

Store vials at temperatures below 40°C (104°F).

CYTOVENE® (ganciclovir capsules) 250 mg are two-pieced, size No. 1, opaque green hard gelatin capsules with ROCHE and CYTOVENE 250 mg imprinted on the capsules in dark blue ink and with two blue lines partially encircling the capsule body. Each capsule contains 250 mg of ganciclovir as a white to off-white powder. CYTOVENE capsules are supplied as follows: Bottles of 180 capsules (NDC 0004-0269-48).

CYTOVENE® (ganciclovir capsules) 500 mg are two-pieced, size No. 0 elongated, opaque yellow/opaque green hard gelatin capsules with ROCHE and CYTOVENE 500 mg imprinted on the capsules in dark blue ink and with two blue lines partially encircling the capsule body. Each capsule contains 500 mg of ganciclovir as a white to off-white powder. CYTOVENE capsules are supplied as follows:

Bottles of 180 capsules (NDC 0004-0278-48).

Store between 5° and 25°C (41° and 77°F).

*Retrovir is a registered trademark of Glaxo Wellcome.

†Videx is a registered trademark of Bristol-Meyers Squibb.

REFERENCES

1. Spector SA, Weingeis T, Pollard R, et al. A randomized, controlled study of intravenous ganciclovir therapy for cytomegalovirus peripheral retinitis in patients with AIDS. *J Inf Dis.* 1993; 168:557–563. **2.** Drew WL, Ives D, Lalezari JP, et al. Oral ganciclovir as maintenance treatment for cytomegalovirus retinitis in patients with AIDS. *New Engl J Med.* 1995; 333:615–620. **3.** The Oral Ganciclovir European and Australian Cooperative Study Group. Intravenous vs oral ganciclovir: European/Australian comparative study of efficacy and safety in the prevention of cytomegalovirus retinitis recurrence in patients with AIDS. *AIDS.* 1995; 9:471–477. **4.** Spector SA, McKinley GF, Lalezari JP, Samo T, et al. Oral ganciclovir for the prevention of cytomegalovirus disease in persons with AIDS. *New Engl J Med.* 1996; 334: 1491–1497. **5.** Merigan TC, Renlund DG, Keay S, et al. A controlled trial of ganciclovir to prevent cytomegalovirus disease after heart transplantation. *New Engl J Med.* 1992;

326:1182–1186. **6.** Goodrich JM, Mori M, Gleaves CA, et al. Early treatment with ganciclovir to prevent cytomegalovirus disease after allogeneic bone marrow transplantation. *New Engl J Med.* 1991; 325:1601–1607. **7.** Schmidt GM, Horak DA, Niland JC, et al. The City of Hope-Stanford-Syntex CMV Study Group. A randomized, controlled trial of prophylactic ganciclovir for cytomegalovirus pulmonary infection in recipients of allogeneic bone marrow transplants. *New Engl J Med.* 1991; 15:1005–1011. **8.** Recommendations for the Safe Handling of Cytotoxic Drugs. US Department of Health and Human Services, National Institutes of Health, Bethesda, MD, September, 1992. NIH Publication No. 92–2621. **9.** American Society of Hospital Pharmacists technical assistance bulletin on handling cytotoxic and hazardous drugs. *Am J Hosp Pharm.* 1990; 47:1033–1049. **10.** Controlling Occupational Exposures to Hazardous Drugs. US Department of Labor. Occupational Health and Safety Administration. OSHA Technical Manual. Section V - Chapter 3, September 22, 1995.

CYTOVENE-IV for intravenous infusion manufactured by Parkedale Pharmaceuticals, Inc., Rochester, MI 48307 and CYTOVENE Capsules for oral administration manufactured by Syntex Puerto Rico, Inc., Humacao, Puerto Rico 00791 for:

Roche Pharmaceuticals

Roche Laboratories Inc.
340 Kingsland Street
Nutley, New Jersey 07110-1199

Revised: May 1998

Shown in Product Identification Guide, page 334

DEMADEX®

℞

[dē'-mă-dex]
(torsemide)
TABLETS
INJECTION

The following text is complete prescribing information based on official labeling in effect June 1998.

DESCRIPTION

DEMADEX® (torsemide) is a diuretic of the pyridine-sulfonylurea class. Its chemical name is 1-isopropyl-3-[(4-*m*-toluidino-3-pyridyl) sulfonyl]urea.

Its empirical formula is $C_{16}H_{20}N_4O_3S$, its pKa is 7.1, and its molecular weight is 348.43.

Torsemide is a white to off-white crystalline powder. The tablets for oral administration also contain lactose NF, crospovidone NF, povidone USP, microcrystalline cellulose NF, and magnesium stearate NF. Torsemide ampuls for intravenous injection contain a sterile solution of torsemide (10 mg/mL), polyethylene glycol-400 NF, tromethamine USP, and sodium hydroxide NF (as needed to adjust pH) in water for injection USP.

CLINICAL PHARMACOLOGY

Mechanism of Action: Micropuncture studies in animals have shown that torsemide acts from within the lumen of the thick ascending portion of the loop of Henle, where it inhibits the Na$^+$/K$^+$/2Cl$^-$-carrier system. Clinical pharmacology studies have confirmed this site of action in humans, and effects in other segments of the nephron have not been demonstrated. Diuretic activity thus correlates better with the rate of drug excretion in the urine than with the concentration in the blood.

Torsemide increases the urinary excretion of sodium, chloride, and water, but it does not significantly alter glomerular filtration rate, renal plasma flow, or acid-base balance.

Pharmacokinetics and Metabolism: The bioavailability of DEMADEX tablets is approximately 80%, with little intersubject variation; the 90% confidence interval is 75% to 89%. The drug is absorbed with little first-pass metabolism, and the serum concentration reaches its peak (C_{max}) within 1 hour after oral administration. C_{max} and area under the serum concentration-time curve (AUC) after oral administration are proportional to dose over the range of 2.5 mg to 200 mg. Simultaneous food intake delays the time to C_{max} by about 30 minutes, but overall bioavailability (AUC) and diuretic activity are unchanged. Absorption is essentially unaffected by renal or hepatic dysfunction.

The volume of distribution of torsemide is 12 liters to 15 liters in normal adults or in patients with mild to moderate renal failure or congestive heart failure. In patients with hepatic cirrhosis, the volume of distribution is approximately doubled.

In normal subjects the elimination half-life of torsemide is approximately 3.5 hours. Torsemide is cleared from the circulation by both hepatic metabolism (approximately 80% of total clearance) and excretion into the urine (approximately 20% of total clearance in patients with normal renal function). The major metabolite in humans is the carboxylic acid derivative, which is biologically inactive. Two of the lesser metabolites possess some diuretic activity, but for practical purposes metabolism terminates the action of the drug.

Because torsemide is extensively bound to plasma protein (>99%), very little enters tubular urine via glomerular fil-

tration. Most renal clearance of torsemide occurs via active secretion of the drug by the proximal tubules into tubular urine.

In patients with decompensated congestive heart failure, hepatic and renal clearance are both reduced, probably because of hepatic congestion and decreased renal plasma flow, respectively. The total clearance of torsemide is approximately 50% of that seen in healthy volunteers, and the plasma half-life and AUC are correspondingly increased. Because of reduced renal clearance, a smaller fraction of any given dose is delivered to the intraluminal site of action, so at any given dose there is less natriuresis in patients with congestive heart failure than in normal subjects.

In patients with renal failure, renal clearance of torsemide is markedly decreased but total plasma clearance is not significantly altered. A smaller fraction of the administered dose is delivered to the intraluminal site of action, and the natriuretic action of any given dose of diuretic is reduced. A diuretic response in renal failure may still be achieved if patients are given higher doses. The total plasma clearance and elimination half-life of torsemide remain normal under the conditions of impaired renal function because metabolic elimination by the liver remains intact.

In patients with hepatic cirrhosis, the volume of distribution, plasma half-life, and renal clearance are all increased, but total clearance is unchanged.

The pharmacokinetic profile of torsemide in healthy elderly subjects is similar to that in young subjects except for a decrease in renal clearance related to the decline in renal function that commonly occurs with aging. However, total plasma clearance and elimination half-life remain unchanged.

Clinical Effects: The diuretic effects of DEMADEX begin within 10 minutes of intravenous dosing and peak within the first hour. With oral dosing, the onset of diuresis occurs within 1 hour and the peak effect occurs during the first or second hour. Independent of the route of administration, diuresis lasts about 6 to 8 hours. In healthy subjects given single doses, the dose-response relationship for sodium excretion is linear over the dose range of 2.5 mg to 20 mg. The increase in potassium excretion is negligible after a single dose of up to 10 mg and only slight (5 mEq to 15 mEq) after a single dose of 20 mg.

Congestive Heart Failure: DEMADEX has been studied in controlled trials in patients with New York Heart Association Class II to Class IV congestive heart failure. Patients who received 10 mg to 20 mg of daily DEMADEX in these studies achieved significantly greater reductions in weight and edema than did patients who received placebo.

Nonanuric Renal Failure: In single-dose studies in patients with nonanuric renal failure, high doses of DEMADEX (20 mg to 200 mg) caused marked increases in water and sodium excretion. In patients with nonanuric renal failure, severe enough to require hemodialysis, chronic treatment with up to 200 mg of daily DEMADEX has not been shown to change steady-state fluid retention. When patients in a study of acute renal failure received total daily doses of 520 mg to 1200 mg of DEMADEX, 19% experienced seizures. Ninety-six patients were treated in this study; 6/32 treated with torsemide experienced seizures, 6/32 treated with comparably high doses of furosemide experienced seizures, and 1/32 treated with placebo experienced a seizure.

Hepatic Cirrhosis: When given with aldosterone antagonists, DEMADEX also caused increases in sodium and fluid excretion in patients with edema or ascites due to hepatic cirrhosis. Urinary sodium excretion rate relative to the urinary excretion rate of DEMADEX is less in cirrhotic patients than in healthy subjects (possibly because of the hyperaldosteronism and resultant sodium retention that are characteristic of portal hypertension and ascites). However, because of the increased renal clearance of DEMADEX in patients with hepatic cirrhosis, these factors tend to balance each other, and the result is an overall natriuretic response that is similar to that seen in healthy subjects. Chronic use of any diuretic in hepatic disease has not been studied in adequate and well-controlled trials.

Essential Hypertension: In patients with essential hypertension, DEMADEX has been shown in controlled studies to lower blood pressure when administered once a day at doses of 5 mg to 10 mg. The antihypertensive effect is near maximal after 4 to 6 weeks of treatment, but it may continue to increase for up to 12 weeks. Systolic and diastolic supine and standing blood pressures are all reduced. There is no significant orthostatic effect, and there is only a minimal peak-trough difference in blood pressure reduction.

The antihypertensive effects of DEMADEX are, like those of other diuretics, on the average greater in black patients (a low-renin population) than in nonblack patients.

When DEMADEX is first administered, daily urinary sodium excretion increases for at least a week. With chronic administration, however, daily sodium loss comes into balance with dietary sodium intake. If the administration of

DEMADEX is suddenly stopped, blood pressure returns to pretreatment levels over several days, without overshoot. DEMADEX has been administered together with β-adrenergic blocking agents, ACE inhibitors, and calcium-channel blockers. Adverse drug interactions have not been observed, and special dosage adjustment has not been necessary.

INDICATIONS AND USAGE

DEMADEX is indicated for the treatment of edema associated with congestive heart failure, renal disease, or hepatic disease. Use of torsemide has been found to be effective for the treatment of edema associated with chronic renal failure. Chronic use of any diuretic in hepatic disease has not been studied in adequate and well-controlled trials.
DEMADEX intravenous injection is indicated when a rapid onset of diuresis is desired or when oral administration is impractical.
DEMADEX is indicated for the treatment of hypertension alone or in combination with other antihypertensive agents.

CONTRAINDICATIONS

DEMADEX is contraindicated in patients with known hypersensitivity to DEMADEX or to sulfonylureas. DEMADEX is contraindicated in patients who are anuric.

WARNINGS

Hepatic Disease With Cirrhosis and Ascites: DEMADEX should be used with caution in patients with hepatic disease with cirrhosis and ascites, since sudden alterations of fluid and electrolyte balance may precipitate hepatic coma. In these patients, diuresis with DEMADEX (or any other diuretic) is best initiated in the hospital. To prevent hypokalemia and metabolic alkalosis, an aldosterone antagonist or potassium-sparing drug should be used concomitantly with DEMADEX.
Ototoxicity: Tinnitus and hearing loss (usually reversible) have been observed after rapid intravenous injection of other loop diuretics and have also been observed after oral DEMADEX. It is not certain that these events were attributable to DEMADEX. Ototoxicity has also been seen in animal studies when very high plasma levels of torsemide were induced. Administered intravenously, DEMADEX should be injected slowly over 2 minutes, and single doses should not exceed 200 mg.
Volume and Electrolyte Depletion: Patients receiving diuretics should be observed for clinical evidence of electrolyte imbalance, hypovolemia, or prerenal azotemia. Symptoms of these disturbances may include one or more of the following: dryness of the mouth, thirst, weakness, lethargy, drowsiness, restlessness, muscle pains or cramps, muscular fatigue, hypotension, oliguria, tachycardia, nausea, and vomiting. Excessive diuresis may cause dehydration, blood-volume reduction, and possibly thrombosis and embolism, especially in elderly patients. In patients who develop fluid and electrolyte imbalances, hypovolemia, or prerenal azotemia, the observed laboratory changes may include hyper- or hyponatremia, hyper- or hypochloremia, hyper- or hypokalemia, acid-base abnormalities, and increased blood urea nitrogen (BUN). If any of these occur, DEMADEX should be discontinued until the situation is corrected; DEMADEX may be restarted at a lower dose.
In controlled studies in the United States, DEMADEX was administered to hypertensive patients at doses of 5 mg or 10 mg daily. After 6 weeks at these doses, the mean decrease in serum potassium was approximately 0.1 mEq/L. The percentage of patients who had a serum potassium level below 3.5 mEq/L at any time during the studies was essentially the same in patients who received DEMADEX (1.5%) as in those who received placebo (3%). In patients followed for 1 year, there was no further change in mean serum potassium levels. In patients with congestive heart failure, hepatic cirrhosis, or renal disease treated with DEMADEX at doses higher than those studied in United States antihypertensive trials, hypokalemia was observed with greater frequency, in a dose-related manner.
In patients with cardiovascular disease, especially those receiving digitalis glycosides, diuretic-induced hypokalemia may be a risk factor for the development of arrhythmias. The risk of hypokalemia is greatest in patients with cirrhosis of the liver, in patients experiencing a brisk diuresis, in patients who are receiving inadequate oral intake of electrolytes, and in patients receiving concomitant therapy with corticosteroids or ACTH.
Periodic monitoring of serum potassium and other electrolytes is advised in patients treated with DEMADEX.

PRECAUTIONS

Laboratory Values: *Potassium:* See WARNINGS.
Calcium: Single doses of DEMADEX increased the urinary excretion of calcium by normal subjects, but serum calcium levels were slightly increased in 4- to 6-week hypertension trials. In a long-term study of patients with congestive heart failure, the average 1-year change in serum calcium was a decrease of 0.10 mg/dL (0.02 mmol/L). Among 426 patients treated with DEMADEX for an average of 11 months, hypocalcemia was not reported as an adverse event.
Magnesium: Single doses of DEMADEX caused healthy volunteers to increase their urinary excretion of magnesium, but serum magnesium levels were slightly increased in 4- to 6-week hypertension trials. In long-term hypertension studies, the average 1-year change in serum magnesium was an increase of 0.03 mg/dL (0.01 mmol/L). Among 426 patients treated with DEMADEX for an average of 11 months, one case of hypomagnesemia (1.3 mg/dL (0.53 mmol/L)) was reported as an adverse event.
In a long-term clinical study of DEMADEX in patients with congestive heart failure, the estimated annual change in serum magnesium was an increase of 0.2 mg/dL (0.08 mmol/L), but these data are confounded by the fact that many of these patients received magnesium supplements. In a 4-week study in which magnesium supplementation was not given, the rate of occurrence of serum magnesium levels below 1.7 mg/dL (0.70 mmol/L) was 6% and 9% in the groups receiving 5 mg and 10 mg of DEMADEX, respectively.
Blood Urea Nitrogen (BUN), Creatinine and Uric Acid: DEMADEX produces small dose-related increases in each of these laboratory values. In hypertensive patients who received 10 mg of DEMADEX daily for 6 weeks, the mean increase in blood urea nitrogen was 1.8 mg/dL (0.6 mmol/L), the mean increase in serum creatinine was 0.05 mg/dL (4 mmol/L), and the mean increase in serum uric acid was 1.2 mg/dL (70 mmol/L). Little further change occurred with long-term treatment, and all changes reversed when treatment was discontinued.
Symptomatic gout has been reported in patients receiving DEMADEX, but its incidence has been similar to that seen in patients receiving placebo.
Glucose: Hypertensive patients who received 10 mg of daily DEMADEX experienced a mean increase in serum glucose concentration of 5.5 mg/dL (0.3 mmol/L) after 6 weeks of therapy, with a further increase of 1.8 mg/dL (0.1 mmol/L) during the subsequent year. In long-term studies in diabetics, mean fasting glucose values were not significantly changed from baseline. Cases of hyperglycemia have been reported but are uncommon.
Serum Lipids: In the controlled short-term hypertension studies in the United States, daily doses of 5 mg, 10 mg, and 20 mg of DEMADEX were associated with increases in total plasma cholesterol of 4, 4, and 8 mg/dL (0.10 to 0.20 mmol/L), respectively. The changes subsided during chronic therapy.
In the same short-term hypertension studies, daily doses of 5 mg, 10 mg and 20 mg of DEMADEX were associated with mean increases in plasma triglycerides of 16, 13 and 71 mg/dL (0.15 to 0.80 mmol/L), respectively.
In long-term studies of 5 mg to 20 mg of DEMADEX daily, no clinically significant differences from baseline lipid values were observed after 1 year of therapy.
Other: In long-term studies in hypertensive patients, DEMADEX has been associated with small mean decreases in hemoglobin, hematocrit, and erythrocyte count and small mean increases in white blood cell count, platelet count, and serum alkaline phosphatase. Although statistically significant, all of these changes were medically inconsequential. No significant trends have been observed in any liver enzyme tests other than alkaline phosphatase.
Drug Interactions: In patients with essential hypertension, DEMADEX has been administered together with beta-blockers, ACE inhibitors, and calcium-channel blockers. In patients with congestive heart failure, DEMADEX has been administered together with digitalis glycosides, ACE inhibitors, and organic nitrates. None of these combined uses was associated with new or unexpected adverse events.
Torsemide does not affect the protein binding of glyburide or of warfarin, the anticoagulant effect of phenprocoumon (a related coumarin derivative), or the pharmacokinetics of digoxin or carvedilol (a vasodilator/beta-blocker). In healthy subjects, coadministration of DEMADEX was associated with significant reduction in the renal clearance of spironolactone, with corresponding increases in the AUC. However, clinical experience indicates that dosage adjustment of either agent is not required.
Because DEMADEX and salicylates compete for secretion by renal tubules, patients receiving high doses of salicylates may experience salicylate toxicity when DEMADEX is concomitantly administered. Also, although possible interactions between torsemide and nonsteroidal anti-inflammatory agents (including aspirin) have not been studied, coadministration of these agents with another loop diuretic (furosemide) has occasionally been associated with renal dysfunction.
The natriuretic effect of DEMADEX (like that of many other diuretics) is partially inhibited by the concomitant administration of indomethacin. This effect has been demonstrated for DEMADEX under conditions of dietary sodium restriction (50 mEq/day) but not in the presence of normal sodium intake (150 mEq/day).
The pharmacokinetic profile and diuretic activity of torsemide are not altered by cimetidine or spironolactone. Coadministration of digoxin is reported to increase the area under the curve for torsemide by 50%, but dose adjustment of DEMADEX is not necessary.
Concomitant use of torsemide and cholestyramine has not been studied in humans but, in a study in animals, coadministration of cholestyramine decreased the absorption of orally administered torsemide. If DEMADEX and cholestyramine are used concomitantly, simultaneous administration is not recommended.
Coadministration of probenecid reduces secretion of DEMADEX into the proximal tubule and thereby decreases the diuretic activity of DEMADEX.
Other diuretics are known to reduce the renal clearance of lithium, inducing a high risk of lithium toxicity, so coadministration of lithium and diuretics should be undertaken with great caution, if at all. Coadministration of lithium and DEMADEX has not been studied.
Other diuretics have been reported to increase the ototoxic potential of aminoglycoside antibiotics and of ethacrynic acid, especially in the presence of impaired renal function. These potential interactions with DEMADEX have not been studied.
Carcinogenesis, Mutagenesis and Impairment of Fertility: No overall increase in tumor incidence was found when torsemide was given to rats and mice throughout their lives at doses up to 9 mg/kg/day (rats) and 32 mg/kg/day (mice). On a body-weight basis, these doses are 27 to 96 times a human dose of 20 mg; on a body-surface-area basis, they are 5 to 8 times this dose. In the rat study, the high-dose female group demonstrated renal tubular injury, interstitial inflammation, and a statistically significant increase in renal adenomas and carcinomas. The tumor incidence in this group was, however, not much higher than the incidence sometimes seen in historical controls. Similar signs of chronic non-neoplastic renal injury have been reported in high-dose animal studies of other diuretics such as furosemide and hydrochlorothiazide.
No mutagenic activity was detected in any of a variety of in vivo and in vitro tests of torsemide and its major human metabolite. The tests included the Ames test in bacteria (with and without metabolic activation), tests for chromosome aberrations and sister-chromatid exchanges in human lymphocytes, tests for various nuclear anomalies in cells found in hamster and murine bone marrow, tests for unscheduled DNA synthesis in mice and rats, and others.
In doses up to 25 mg/kg/day (75 times a human dose of 20 mg on a body-weight basis; 13 times this dose on a body-surface-area basis), torsemide had no adverse effect on the reproductive performance of male or female rats.
Pregnancy: Pregnancy Category B. There was no fetotoxicity or teratogenicity in rats treated with up to 5 mg/kg/day of torsemide (on a mg/kg basis, this is 15 times a human dose of 20 mg/day; on a mg/m^2 basis, the animal dose is 10 times the human dose), or in rabbits, treated with 1.6 mg/kg/day (on a mg/kg basis, 5 times the human dose of 20 mg/kg/day; on a mg/m^2 basis, 1.7 times this dose). Fetal and maternal toxicity (decrease in average body weight, increase in fetal resorption and delayed fetal ossification) occurred in rabbits and rats given doses 4 (rabbits) and 5 (rats) times larger. Adequate and well-controlled studies have not been carried out in pregnant women. Because animal reproduction studies are not always predictive of human response, this drug should be used during pregnancy only if clearly needed.
Labor and Delivery: The effect of DEMADEX on labor and delivery is unknown.
Nursing Mothers: It is not known whether DEMADEX is excreted in human milk. Because many drugs are excreted in human milk, caution should be exercised when DEMADEX is administered to a nursing woman.
Pediatric Use: Safety and effectiveness in pediatric patients have not been established.
Administration of another loop diuretic to severely premature infants with edema due to patent ductus arteriosus and hyaline membrane disease has occasionally been associated with renal calcifications, sometimes barely visible on X-ray but sometimes in staghorn form, filling the renal pelves. Some of these calculi have been dissolved, and hypercalciuria has been reported to have decreased, when chlorothiazide has been coadministered along with the loop diuretic. In other premature neonates with hyaline membrane disease, another loop diuretic has been reported to increase the risk of persistent patent ductus arteriosus, possibly through a prostaglandin-E-mediated process. The use of DEMADEX in such patients has not been studied.
Geriatric Use: Of the total number of patients who received DEMADEX in United States clinical studies, 24% were 65 or older while about 4% were 75 or older. No specific age-related differences in effectiveness or safety were observed between younger patients and elderly patients.

ADVERSE REACTIONS

At the time of approval, DEMADEX had been evaluated for safety in approximately 4000 subjects: over 800 of these subjects received DEMADEX for at least 6 months, and over 380 were treated for more than 1 year. Among these sub-

Continued on next page

Demadex—Cont.

jects were 564 who received DEMADEX during United States-based trials in which 274 other subjects received placebo.

The reported side effects of DEMADEX were generally transient, and there was no relationship between side effects and age, sex, race, or duration of therapy. Discontinuation of therapy due to side effects occurred in 3.5% of United States patients treated with DEMADEX and in 4.4% of patients treated with placebo. In studies conducted in the United States and Europe, discontinuation rates due to side effects were 3.0% (38/1250) with DEMADEX and 3.4% (13/380) with furosemide in patients with congestive heart failure, 2.0% (8/409) with DEMADEX and 4.8% (11/230) with furosemide in patients with renal insufficiency, and 7.6% (13/170) with DEMADEX and 0% (0/33) with furosemide in patients with cirrhosis.

The most common reasons for discontinuation of therapy with DEMADEX were (in descending order of frequency) dizziness, headache, nausea, weakness, vomiting, hyperglycemia, excessive urination, hyperuricemia, hypokalemia, excessive thirst, hypovolemia, impotence, esophageal hemorrhage, and dyspepsia. Dropout rates for these adverse events ranged from 0.1% to 0.5%.

The side effects considered possibly or probably related to study drug that occurred in United States placebo-controlled trials in more than 1% of patients treated with DEMADEX are shown in the table below.

Reactions Possibly or Probably Drug-Related United States Placebo-Controlled Studies Incidence (Percentages of Patients)

	DEMADEX (N=564)	Placebo (N=274)
Headache	7.3	9.1
Excessive Urination	6.7	2.2
Dizziness	3.2	4.0
Rhinitis	2.8	2.2
Asthenia	2.0	1.5
Diarrhea	2.0	1.1
ECG Abnormality	2.0	0.4
Cough Increase	2.0	1.5
Constipation	1.8	0.7
Nausea	1.8	0.4
Arthralgia	1.8	0.7
Dyspepsia	1.6	0.7
Sore Throat	1.6	0.7
Myalgia	1.6	1.5
Chest Pain	1.2	0.4
Insomnia	1.2	1.8
Edema	1.1	1.1
Nervousness	1.1	0.4

The daily doses of DEMADEX used in these trials ranged from 1.25 mg to 20 mg, with most patients receiving 5 mg to 10 mg; the duration of treatment ranged from 1 to 52 days, with a median of 41 days. Of the side effects listed in the table, only "excessive urination" occurred significantly more frequently in patients treated with DEMADEX than in patients treated with placebo. In the placebo-controlled hypertension studies whose design allowed side-effect rates to be attributed to dose, excessive urination was reported by 1% of patients receiving placebo, 4% of those treated with 5 mg of daily DEMADEX, and 15% of those treated with 10 mg. The complaint of excessive urination was generally not reported as an adverse event among patients who received DEMADEX for cardiac, renal, or hepatic failure.

Serious adverse events reported in the clinical studies for which a drug relationship could not be excluded were atrial fibrillation, chest pain, diarrhea, digitalis intoxication, gastrointestinal hemorrhage, hyperglycemia, hyperuricemia, hypokalemia, hypotension, hypovolemia, shunt thrombosis, rash, rectal bleeding, syncope, and ventricular tachycardia.

Angioedema has been reported in a patient exposed to DEMADEX who was later found to be allergic to sulfa drugs.

Of the adverse reactions during placebo-controlled trials listed without taking into account assessment of relatedness to drug therapy, arthritis and various other nonspecific musculoskeletal problems were more frequently reported in association with DEMADEX than with placebo, even though gout was somewhat more frequently associated with placebo. These reactions did not increase in frequency or severity with the dose of DEMADEX. One patient in the group treated with DEMADEX withdrew due to myalgia, and one in the placebo group withdrew due to gout.

Hypokalemia: See WARNINGS.

OVERDOSAGE

There is no human experience with overdoses of DEMADEX, but the signs and symptoms of overdosage can be anticipated to be those of excessive pharmacologic effect: dehydration, hypovolemia, hypotension, hyponatremia, hypokalemia, hypochloremic alkalosis, and hemoconcentration. Treatment of overdosage should consist of fluid and electrolyte replacement.

Laboratory determinations of serum levels of torsemide and its metabolites are not widely available.

No data are available to suggest physiological maneuvers (eg, maneuvers to change the pH of the urine) that might accelerate elimination of torsemide and its metabolites. Torsemide is not dialyzable, so hemodialysis will not accelerate elimination.

DOSAGE AND ADMINISTRATION

General: DEMADEX tablets may be given at any time in relation to a meal, as convenient. Special dosage adjustment in the elderly is not necessary.

Because of the high bioavailability of DEMADEX, oral and intravenous doses are therapeutically equivalent, so patients may be switched to and from the intravenous form with no change in dose. DEMADEX intravenous injection should be administered either slowly as a bolus over a period of 2 minutes or administered as a continuous infusion.

If DEMADEX is administered through an IV line, it is recommended that, as with other IV injections, the IV line be flushed with Normal Saline (Sodium Chloride Injection, USP) before and after administration. DEMADEX injection is formulated above pH 8.3. Flushing the line is recommended to avoid the potential for incompatibilities caused by differences in pH which could be indicated by color change, haziness or the formation of a precipitate in the solution.

If DEMADEX is administered as a continuous infusion, stability has been demonstrated through 24 hours at room temperature in plastic containers for the following fluids and concentrations:

200 mg DEMADEX (10 mg/mL) added to:
- 250 mL Dextrose 5% in water
- 250 mL 0.9% Sodium Chloride
- 500 mL 0.45% Sodium Chloride

50 mg DEMADEX (10 mg/mL) added to:
- 500 mL Dextrose 5% in water
- 500 mL 0.9% Sodium Chloride
- 500 mL 0.45% Sodium Chloride

Before administration, the solution of DEMADEX should be visually inspected for discoloration and particulate matter. If either is found, the ampul should not be used.

Congestive Heart Failure: The usual initial dose is 10 mg or 20 mg of once-daily oral or intravenous DEMADEX. If the diuretic response is inadequate, the dose should be titrated upward by approximately doubling until the desired diuretic response is obtained. Single doses higher than 200 mg have not been adequately studied.

Chronic Renal Failure: The usual initial dose of DEMADEX is 20 mg of once-daily oral or intravenous DEMADEX. If the diuretic response is inadequate, the dose should be titrated upward by approximately doubling until the desired diuretic response is obtained. Single doses higher than 200 mg have not been adequately studied.

Hepatic Cirrhosis: The usual initial dose is 5 mg or 10 mg of once-daily oral or intravenous DEMADEX, administered together with an aldosterone antagonist or a potassium-sparing diuretic. If the diuretic response is inadequate, the dose should be titrated upward by approximately doubling until the desired diuretic response is obtained. Single doses higher than 40 mg have not been adequately studied.

Chronic use of any diuretic in hepatic disease has not been studied in adequate and well-controlled trials.

Hypertension: The usual initial dose is 5 mg once daily. If the 5 mg dose does not provide adequate reduction in blood pressure within 4 to 6 weeks, the dose may be increased to 10 mg once daily. If the response to 10 mg is insufficient, an additional antihypertensive agent should be added to the treatment regimen.

HOW SUPPLIED

DEMADEX for oral administration is available as white, scored tablets containing 5 mg, 10 mg, 20 mg, or 100 mg of torsemide. The tablets are supplied in bottles and Tel-E-Dose®* packages of 100 as follows:

[See table below]

Each tablet is debossed on the scored side with the Boehringer Mannheim logo and 102, 103, 104, or 105 (for 5 mg, 10 mg, 20 mg, or 100 mg, respectively). On the opposite side, the tablet is debossed with 5, 10, 20, or 100 to indicate the dose.

Dose	*Shape*	*Bottle*	*Tel-E-Dose*
5 mg	oval	NDC 0004-0262-01	NDC 0004-0262-49
10 mg	oval	NDC 0004-0263-01	NDC 0004-0263-49
20 mg	oval	NDC 0004-0264-01	NDC 0004-0264-49
100 mg	capsule-shaped	NDC 0004-0265-01	NDC 0004-0265-49

DEMADEX for intravenous injection is supplied in clear ampuls containing 2 mL (20 mg, NDC 0004-0267-06) or 5 mL (50 mg, NDC 0004-0268-06) of a 10 mg/mL sterile solution.

Storage: Store all dosage forms at 15° to 30°C (59° to 86°F). Do not freeze.

*Tel-E-Dose is a registered trademark of Hoffmann-La Roche Inc.

Tablets manufactured by:
Boehringer Mannheim, GmbH, Mannheim, Germany
Ampuls manufactured by:
Abbott Laboratories, North Chicago, IL 60064

Revised: April 1998

Shown in Product Identification Guide, page 334

EC-NAPROSYN® ℞
(naproxen)
Delayed-Release Tablets

NAPROSYN® ℞
(naproxen)
Tablets

ANAPROX®/ANAPROX® DS ℞
[an' ă-prox]
(naproxen sodium)
Tablets

NAPROSYN® ℞
(naproxen)
Suspension

The following text is complete prescribing information based on official labeling in effect June 1998.

DESCRIPTION

Naproxen is a member of the arylacetic acid group of nonsteroidal anti-inflammatory drugs.

The chemical names for naproxen and naproxen sodium are (S)-6-methoxy-α-methyl-2-naphthaleneacetic acid and (S)-6-methoxy-α-methyl-2-naphthaleneacetic acid, sodium salt, respectively.

Naproxen is an odorless, white to off-white crystalline substance. It is lipid-soluble, practically insoluble in water at low pH and freely soluble in water at high pH. The octanol/water partition coefficient of naproxen at pH 7.4 is 1.6 to 1.8. Naproxen sodium is a white to creamy white, crystalline solid, freely soluble in water at neutral pH.

NAPROSYN (naproxen) Tablets contain 250 mg, 375 mg or 500 mg of naproxen and croscarmellose sodium, iron oxides, povidone and magnesium stearate.

EC-NAPROSYN (naproxen) Delayed-Release Tablets are enteric-coated tablets containing 375 mg or 500 mg of naproxen and croscarmellose sodium, povidone and magnesium stearate. The enteric coating dispersion contains methacrylic acid copolymer, talc, triethyl citrate, sodium hydroxide and purified water. The dispersion may also contain simethicone emulsion. The dissolution of this enteric-coated naproxen tablet is pH dependent with rapid dissolution above pH 6. There is no dissolution below pH 4.

Each ANAPROX 275 mg and ANAPROX DS 550 mg tablet contains naproxen sodium, the active ingredient, with magnesium stearate, microcrystalline cellulose, povidone and talc. The coating suspension for the ANAPROX 275 mg tablet may contain hydroxypropyl methylcellulose 2910, Opaspray K-1-4210A, polyethylene glycol 8000 or Opadry YS-1-4215. The coating suspension for the ANAPROX DS 550 mg tablet may contain hydroxypropyl methylcellulose 2910, Opaspray K-1-4227, polyethylene glycol 8000 or Opadry YS-1-4216.

NAPROSYN (naproxen) Suspension for oral administration contains 125 mg/5 mL of naproxen in a vehicle containing sucrose, magnesium aluminum silicate, sorbitol solution and sodium chloride (30 mg/5 mL, 1.5 mEq), methylparaben, fumaric acid, FD&C Yellow No. 6, imitation pineapple flavor, imitation orange flavor and purified water. The pH of the suspension ranges from 2.2 to 3.7.

CLINICAL PHARMACOLOGY

Naproxen is a nonsteroidal anti-inflammatory drug (NSAID) with analgesic and antipyretic properties. The sodium salt of naproxen has been developed as a more rapidly absorbed formulation of naproxen for use as an analgesic. The naproxen anion inhibits prostaglandin synthesis but beyond this its mode of action is unknown.

Pharmacokinetics: Naproxen itself is rapidly and completely absorbed from the gastrointestinal tract with an in vivo bioavailability of 95%. The different dosage forms of NAPROSYN are bioequivalent in terms of extent of absorption (AUC) and peak concentration (C_{max}); however, the products do differ in their pattern of absorption. These differences between naproxen products are related to both the chemical form of naproxen used and its formulation. Even with the observed differences in pattern of absorption, the

elimination half-life of naproxen is unchanged across products ranging from 12 to 17 hours. Steady-state levels of naproxen are reached in 4 to 5 days, and the degree of naproxen accumulation is consistent with this half-life. This suggests that the differences in pattern of release play only a negligible role in the attainment of steady-state plasma levels.

Absorption:

Immediate Release: After administration of NAPROSYN tablets, peak plasma levels are attained in 2 to 4 hours. After oral administration of ANAPROX, peak plasma levels are attained in 1 to 2 hours. The difference in rates between the two products is due to the increased aqueous solubility of the sodium salt of naproxen used in ANAPROX. Peak plasma levels of naproxen given as NAPROSYN Suspension are attained in 1 to 4 hours.

Delayed Release: EC-NAPROSYN is designed with a pH-sensitive coating to provide a barrier to disintegration in the acidic environment of the stomach and to lose integrity in the more neutral environment of the small intestine. The enteric polymer coating selected for EC-NAPROSYN dissolves above pH 6. When EC-NAPROSYN was given to fasted subjects, peak plasma levels were attained about 4 to 6 hours following the first dose (range: 2 to 12 hours). An in vivo study in man using radiolabeled EC-NAPROSYN tablets demonstrated that EC-NAPROSYN dissolves primarily in the small intestine rather than the stomach, so the absorption of the drug is delayed until the stomach is emptied.

When EC-NAPROSYN and NAPROSYN were given to fasted subjects (n=24) in a crossover study following 1 week of dosing, differences in time to peak plasma levels (T_{max}) were observed, but there were no differences in total absorption as measured by C_{max} and AUC:

[See table below]

Antacid Effects: When EC-NAPROSYN was given as a single dose with antacid (54 mEq buffering capacity), the peak plasma levels of naproxen were unchanged, but the time to peak was reduced (mean T_{max} fasted 5.6 hours, mean T_{max} with antacid 5 hours), although not significantly.

Food Effects: When EC-NAPROSYN was given as a single dose with food, peak plasma levels in most subjects were achieved in about 12 hours (range: 4 to 24 hours). Residence time in the small intestine until disintegration was independent of food intake. The presence of food prolonged the time the tablets remained in the stomach, time to first detectable serum naproxen levels, and time to maximal naproxen levels (T_{max}), but did not affect peak naproxen levels (C_{max}).

Distribution:

Naproxen has a volume of distribution of 0.16 L/kg. At therapeutic levels naproxen is greater than 99% albumin-bound. At doses of naproxen greater than 500 mg/day there is less than proportional increase in plasma levels due to an increase in clearance caused by saturation of plasma protein binding at higher doses (average trough C_{ss} 36.5, 49.2 and 56.4 mg/L with 500, 1000 and 1500 mg daily doses of naproxen). However, the concentration of unbound naproxen continues to increase proportionally to dose.

Metabolism:

Naproxen is extensively metabolized to 6-0-desmethyl naproxen, and both parent and metabolites do not induce metabolizing enzymes.

Elimination:

The clearance of naproxen is 0.13 mL/min/kg. Approximately 95% of the naproxen from any dose is excreted in the urine, primarily as naproxen (less than 1%), 6-0-desmethyl naproxen (less than 1%) or their conjugates (66% to 92%). The plasma half-life of the naproxen anion in humans ranges from 12 to 17 hours. The corresponding half-lives of both naproxen's metabolites and conjugates are shorter than 12 hours, and their rates of excretion have been found to coincide closely with the rate of naproxen disappearance from the plasma. In patients with renal failure metabolites may accumulate.

Special Populations:

Pediatric Patients: In pediatric patients aged 5 to 16 years with arthritis, plasma naproxen levels following a 5 mg/kg single dose of naproxen suspension (see DOSAGE AND ADMINISTRATION) were found to be similar to those found in normal adults following a 500 mg dose. The terminal half-life appears to be similar in pediatric and adult patients. Pharmacokinetic studies of naproxen were not performed in pediatric patients younger than 5 years of age. Pharmacokinetic parameters appear to be similar following administration of naproxen suspension or tablets in pediatric patients. EC-NAPROSYN has not been studied in subjects under the age of 18.

Renal Insufficiency: Naproxen pharmacokinetics has not been determined in subjects with renal insufficiency. Given that naproxen, its metabolites and conjugates are primarily excreted by the kidney, the potential exists for naproxen metabolites to accumulate in the presence of renal insufficiency.

CLINICAL STUDIES

General Information: Naproxen has been studied in patients with rheumatoid arthritis, osteoarthritis, juvenile arthritis, ankylosing spondylitis, tendonitis and bursitis, and acute gout. Improvement in patients treated for rheumatoid arthritis was demonstrated by a reduction in joint swelling, a reduction in duration of morning stiffness, a reduction in disease activity as assessed by both the investigator and patient, and by increased mobility as demonstrated by a reduction in walking time. Generally, response to naproxen has not been found to be dependent on age, sex, severity or duration of rheumatoid arthritis.

In patients with osteoarthritis, the therapeutic action of naproxen has been shown by a reduction in joint pain or tenderness, an increase in range of motion in knee joints, increased mobility as demonstrated by a reduction in walking time, and improvement in capacity to perform activities of daily living impaired by the disease.

In a clinical trial comparing standard formulations of naproxen 375 mg bid (750 mg a day) vs 750 mg bid (1500 mg/day), 9 patients in the 750 mg group terminated prematurely because of adverse events. Nineteen patients in the 1500 mg group terminated prematurely because of adverse events. Most of these adverse events were gastrointestinal events.

In clinical studies in patients with rheumatoid arthritis, osteoarthritis and juvenile arthritis, naproxen has been shown to be comparable to aspirin and indomethacin in controlling the aforementioned measures of disease activity, but the frequency and severity of the milder gastrointestinal adverse effects (nausea, dyspepsia, heartburn) and nervous system adverse effects (tinnitus, dizziness, lightheadedness) were less in naproxen-treated patients than in those treated with aspirin or indomethacin.

In patients with ankylosing spondylitis, naproxen has been shown to decrease night pain, morning stiffness and pain at rest. In double-blind studies the drug was shown to be as effective as aspirin, but with fewer side effects.

In patients with acute gout, a favorable response to naproxen was shown by significant clearing of inflammatory changes (eg, decrease in swelling, heat) within 24 to 48 hours, as well as by relief of pain and tenderness.

Naproxen has been studied in patients with mild to moderate pain secondary to postoperative, orthopedic, postpartum episiotomy and uterine contraction pain and dysmenorrhea. Onset of pain relief can begin within 1 hour in patients taking naproxen and within 30 minutes in patients taking naproxen sodium. Analgesic effect was shown by such measures as reduction of pain intensity scores, increase in pain relief scores, decrease in numbers of patients requiring additional analgesic medication, and delay in time to remedication. The analgesic effect has been found to last for up to 12 hours.

Naproxen may be used safely in combination with gold salts and/or corticosteroids; however, in controlled clinical trials, when added to the regimen of patients receiving corticosteroids, it did not appear to cause greater improvement over that seen with corticosteroids alone. Whether naproxen has a "steroid-sparing" effect has not been adequately studied. When added to the regimen of patients receiving gold salts, naproxen did result in greater improvement. Its use in combination with salicylates is not recommended because there is evidence that aspirin increases the rate of excretion of naproxen and data are inadequate to demonstrate that naproxen and aspirin produce greater improvement over that achieved with aspirin alone. In addition, as with other NSAIDs, the combination may result in higher frequency of adverse events than demonstrated for either product alone.

In ^{51}Cr blood loss and gastroscopy studies with normal volunteers, daily administration of 1000 mg of naproxen as 1000 mg of NAPROSYN (naproxen) or 1100 mg of ANAPROX (naproxen sodium) has been demonstrated to cause statistically significantly less gastric bleeding and erosion than 3250 mg of aspirin.

Three 6-week, double-blind, multicenter studies with EC-NAPROSYN (naproxen) (375 or 500 mg bid, n=385) and NAPROSYN (375 or 500 mg bid, n=279) were conducted comparing EC-NAPROSYN with NAPROSYN, including 355 rheumatoid arthritis and osteoarthritis patients who had a recent history of NSAID-related GI symptoms. These studies indicated that EC-NAPROSYN and NAPROSYN showed no significant differences in efficacy or safety and had similar prevalence of minor GI complaints. Individual patients, however, may find one formulation preferable to the other.

Five hundred and fifty-three patients received EC-NAPROSYN during long-term open label trials (mean length of treatment was 159 days). The rates for clinically-diagnosed peptic ulcers and GI bleeds were similar to what has been historically reported for long-term NSAID use.

INDIVIDUALIZATION OF DOSAGE

Although NAPROSYN, NAPROSYN Suspension, EC-NAPROSYN, ANAPROX and ANAPROX DS all circulate in the plasma as naproxen, they have pharmacokinetic differences that may affect onset of action. Onset of pain relief can begin within 30 minutes in patients taking naproxen sodium and within 1 hour in patients taking naproxen. Because EC-NAPROSYN dissolves in the small intestine rather than in the stomach, the absorption of the drug is delayed compared to the other naproxen formulations (see CLINICAL PHARMACOLOGY).

The recommended strategy for initiating therapy is to choose a formulation and a starting dose likely to be effective for the patient and then adjust the dosage based on observation of benefit and/or adverse events. A lower dose should be considered in patients with renal or hepatic impairment or in elderly patients (see PRECAUTIONS).

Analgesia/Dysmenorrhea/Bursitis and Tendonitis: Because the sodium salt of naproxen is more rapidly absorbed, ANAPROX/ANAPROX DS is recommended for the management of acute painful conditions when prompt onset of pain relief is desired. The recommended starting dose is 550 mg followed by 550 mg every 12 hours or 275 mg every 6 to 8 hours, as required. The initial total daily dose should not exceed 1375 mg of naproxen sodium. Thereafter, the total daily dose should not exceed 1100 mg of naproxen sodium. NAPROSYN may also be used for treatment of acute pain and dysmenorrhea. EC-NAPROSYN is not recommended for initial treatment of acute pain because absorption of naproxen is delayed compared to other naproxen-containing products (see CLINICAL PHARMACOLOGY and INDICATIONS AND USAGE).

Acute Gout: The recommended starting dose is 750 mg of NAPROSYN followed by 250 mg every 8 hours until the attack has subsided. ANAPROX may also be used at a starting dose of 825 mg followed by 275 mg every 8 hours as needed. EC-NAPROSYN is not recommended because of the delay in absorption (see CLINICAL PHARMACOLOGY).

Osteoarthritis/Rheumatoid Arthritis/Ankylosing Spondylitis: The recommended dose of naproxen is NAPROSYN or NAPROSYN Suspension 250 mg, 375 mg or 500 mg taken twice daily (morning and evening) or EC-NAPROSYN 375 mg or 500 mg taken twice daily. Naproxen sodium may also be used (see DOSAGE AND ADMINISTRATION).

During long-term administration the dose of naproxen may be adjusted up or down depending on the clinical response of the patient. A lower daily dose may suffice for long-term administration. In patients who tolerate lower doses well, the dose may be increased to 1500 mg per day when a higher level of anti-inflammatory/analgesic activity is required. When treating patients with naproxen 1500 mg/day (as NAPROSYN or 1650 mg of ANAPROX), the physician should observe sufficient increased clinical benefit to offset the potential increased risk. The morning and evening doses do not have to be equal in size and administration of the drug more frequently than twice daily does not generally make a difference in response (see CLINICAL PHARMACOLOGY).

Juvenile Arthritis: The use of NAPROSYN Suspension allows for more flexible dose titration. In pediatric patients, doses of 5 mg/kg/day produced plasma levels of naproxen similar to those seen in adults taking 500 mg of naproxen (see CLINICAL PHARMACOLOGY).

The recommended total daily dose is approximately 10 mg/kg given in two divided doses (ie, 5 mg/kg given twice a day) (see DOSAGE AND ADMINISTRATION).

INDICATIONS AND USAGE

Naproxen as NAPROSYN, EC-NAPROSYN, ANAPROX, ANAPROX DS or NAPROSYN Suspension are indicated for the treatment of rheumatoid arthritis, osteoarthritis, ankylosing spondylitis and juvenile arthritis.

Naproxen as NAPROSYN Suspension is recommended for juvenile rheumatoid arthritis in order to obtain the maximum dosage flexibility based on the patient's weight.

Naproxen as NAPROSYN, ANAPROX, ANAPROX DS and NAPROSYN Suspension are also indicated for the treatment of tendinitis, bursitis, acute gout, and for the management of pain and primary dysmenorrhea. EC-NAPROSYN is not recommended for initial treatment of acute pain because the absorption of naproxen is delayed compared to absorption from other naproxen-containing products (see CLINICAL PHARMACOLOGY and DOSAGE AND ADMINISTRATION).

	EC-NAPROSYN* 500 mg bid	NAPROSYN* 500 mg bid
C_{max} (μg/mL)	94.9 (18%)	97.4 (13%)
T_{max} (hours)	4 (39%)	1.9 (61%)
AUC_{0-12hr} (μg-hr/mL)	845 (20%)	767 (15%)

* Mean value (coefficient of variation)

Continued on next page

EC-Naprosyn/Anaprox—Cont.

CONTRAINDICATIONS

All naproxen products are contraindicated in patients who have had allergic reactions to prescription as well as to over-the-counter products containing naproxen. It is also contraindicated in patients in whom aspirin or other nonsteroidal anti-inflammatory/analgesic drugs induce the syndrome of asthma, rhinitis and nasal polyps. Both types of reactions have the potential of being fatal. Anaphylactoid reactions to naproxen, whether of the true allergic type or the pharmacologic idiosyncratic (eg, aspirin hypersensitivity syndrome) type, usually but not always occur in patients with a known history of such reactions. Therefore, careful questioning of patients for such things as asthma, nasal polyps, urticaria and hypotension associated with nonsteroidal anti-inflammatory drugs before starting therapy is important. In addition, if such symptoms occur during therapy, treatment should be discontinued.

WARNINGS

Risk of GI Ulceration, Bleeding and Perforation with NSAID Therapy: Serious gastrointestinal toxicity such as bleeding, ulceration and perforation can occur at any time, with or without warning symptoms, in patients treated chronically with NSAID therapy. Although minor upper gastrointestinal problems, such as dyspepsia, are common, usually developing early in therapy, physicians should remain alert for ulceration and bleeding in patients treated chronically with NSAIDs even in the absence of previous GI tract symptoms. In patients observed in clinical trials of several months to 2 years' duration, symptomatic upper GI ulcers, gross bleeding or perforation appear to occur in approximately 1% of patients treated for 3 to 6 months and in about 2% to 4% of patients treated for 1 year.

Physicians should inform patients about the signs and/or symptoms of serious GI toxicity and what steps to take if they occur.

Studies to date with all naproxen products have not identified any subset of patients not at risk of developing peptic ulceration and bleeding or any differences between different naproxen products in their propensity to cause peptic ulceration and bleeding. Except for a prior history of serious GI events and other risk factors known to be associated with peptic ulcer disease, such as alcoholism, smoking, etc., no risk factors (eg, age, sex) have been associated with increased risk. Elderly or debilitated patients seem to tolerate ulceration or bleeding less well than other individuals and most spontaneous reports of fatal GI events are in this population. Studies to date are inconclusive concerning the relative risk of various NSAIDs in causing such reactions. High doses of any NSAID probably carry a greater risk of these reactions, although controlled clinical trials showing this do not exist in most cases. In considering the use of relatively large doses (within the recommended dosage range), sufficient benefit should be anticipated to offset the potential increased risk of GI toxicity.

PRECAUTIONS

General: NAPROXEN-CONTAINING PRODUCTS SUCH AS NAPROSYN, EC-NAPROSYN, ANAPROX, ANAPROX DS, NAPROSYN SUSPENSION, ALEVE®, AND OTHER NAPROXEN PRODUCTS SHOULD NOT BE USED CONCOMITANTLY SINCE THEY ALL CIRCULATE IN THE PLASMA AS THE NAPROXEN ANION.

If the steroid dose is reduced or eliminated during therapy, the steroid dosage should be reduced slowly and the patients should be observed closely for any evidence of adverse effects, including adrenal insufficiency and exacerbation of symptoms of arthritis.

Patients with initial hemoglobin values of 10 grams or less who are to receive long-term therapy should have hemoglobin values determined periodically.

The antipyretic and anti-inflammatory activities of the drug may reduce fever and inflammation, thus diminishing their utility as diagnostic signs in detecting complications of presumed noninfectious, noninflammatory painful conditions.

Because of adverse eye findings in animal studies with drugs of this class, it is recommended that ophthalmic studies be carried out if any change or disturbance in vision occurs.

Renal Effects: As with other nonsteroidal anti-inflammatory drugs, long-term administration of naproxen to animals has resulted in renal papillary necrosis and other abnormal renal pathology. In humans, there have been reports of acute interstitial nephritis, hematuria, proteinuria and occasionally nephrotic syndrome associated with naproxen-containing products and other NSAIDs since they have been marketed.

A second form of renal toxicity has been seen in patients taking naproxen as well as other nonsteroidal anti-inflammatory drugs. In patients with prerenal conditions leading to a reduction in renal blood flow or blood volume, where the renal prostaglandins have a supportive role in the maintenance of renal perfusion, administration of a nonsteroidal anti-inflammatory drug may cause a dose-dependent reduc-tion in prostaglandin formation and precipitate overt renal decompensation. Patients at greatest risk of this reaction are those with impaired renal function, heart failure, liver dysfunction, those taking diuretics and the elderly. Discontinuation of nonsteroidal anti-inflammatory therapy is typically followed by recovery to the pretreatment state.

Naproxen and its metabolites are eliminated primarily by the kidneys; therefore, the drug should be used with caution in patients with significantly impaired renal function, and the monitoring of serum creatinine and/or creatinine clearance is advised in these patients. Caution should be used if the drug is given to patients with creatinine clearance of less than 20 mL/minute because accumulation of naproxen metabolites has been seen in such patients.

Chronic alcoholic liver disease and probably other diseases with decreased or abnormal plasma proteins (albumin) reduce the total plasma concentration of naproxen, but the plasma concentration of unbound naproxen is increased. Caution is advised when high doses are required and some adjustment of dosage may be required in these patients. It is prudent to use the lowest effective dose.

Studies indicate that although total plasma concentration of naproxen is unchanged, the unbound plasma fraction of naproxen is increased in the elderly. Caution is advised when high doses are required and some adjustment of dosage may be required in elderly patients. As with other drugs used in the elderly, it is prudent to use the lowest effective dose.

Hepatic Function: As with other nonsteroidal anti-inflammatory drugs, borderline elevations of one or more liver tests may occur in up to 15% of patients. These abnormalities may progress, may remain essentially unchanged, or may be transient with continued therapy. The SGPT (ALT) test is probably the most sensitive indicator of liver dysfunction. Meaningful (3 times the upper limit of normal) elevations of SGPT or SGOT (AST) occurred in controlled clinical trials in less than 1% of patients. A patient with symptoms and/or signs suggesting liver dysfunction or in whom an abnormal liver test has occurred, should be evaluated for evidence of the development of more severe hepatic reaction while on therapy with naproxen. Severe hepatic reactions, including jaundice and cases of fatal hepatitis, have been reported with naproxen as with other nonsteroidal anti-inflammatory drugs. Although such reactions are rare, if abnormal liver tests persist or worsen, if clinical signs and symptoms consistent with liver disease develop, or if systemic manifestations occur (eg, eosinophilia, rash, etc.), naproxen should be discontinued.

Fluid Retention and Edema: Peripheral edema has been observed in some patients receiving naproxen. Since each ANAPROX or ANAPROX DS tablet contains 25 mg or 50 mg of sodium (about 1 mEq per each 250 mg of naproxen), and each teaspoonful of NAPROSYN Suspension contains 39 mg (about 1.5 mEq per each 125 mg of naproxen) of sodium, this should be considered in patients whose overall intake of sodium must be severely restricted. For these reasons, ANAPROX, ANAPROX DS and NAPROSYN Suspension should be used with caution in patients with fluid retention, hypertension or heart failure.

Information for Patients: Naproxen, in NAPROSYN, EC-NAPROSYN, ANAPROX, ANAPROX DS and NAPROSYN Suspension, like other drugs of this class, is not free of side effects. The side effects of these formulations of naproxen can cause discomfort and, rarely, there are more serious side effects, such as gastrointestinal bleeding, which may result in hospitalization and even fatal outcomes.

NSAIDs (Nonsteroidal Anti-Inflammatory Drugs) are often essential agents in the management of arthritis and have a major role in the treatment of pain, but they also may be commonly employed for conditions that are less serious.

Physicians may wish to discuss with their patients the potential risks (see WARNINGS, PRECAUTIONS and ADVERSE REACTIONS) and likely benefits of naproxen treatment, particularly when it is used for less serious conditions where treatment without NSAIDs may represent an acceptable alternative to both the patient and physician.

Caution should be exercised by patients whose activities require alertness if they experience drowsiness, dizziness, vertigo or depression during therapy with naproxen.

Laboratory Tests: Because serious GI tract ulceration and bleeding can occur without warning symptoms, physicians should follow patients chronically treated with naproxen for signs and symptoms of ulceration and bleeding and should inform them of the importance of this follow-up and what they should do if certain signs and symptoms do appear (see WARNINGS: *Risk of GI Ulcerations, Bleeding and Perforation with NSAID Therapy*).

Drug Interactions: The use of NSAIDs in patients who are receiving ACE inhibitors may potentiate renal disease states (see PRECAUTIONS: *Renal Effects*).

In vitro studies have shown that naproxen anion, because of its affinity for protein, may displace from their binding sites other drugs that are also albumin-bound (see CLINICAL PHARMACOLOGY: *Pharmacokinetics*).

Theoretically, the naproxen anion itself could likewise be displaced. Short-term controlled studies failed to show that taking the drug significantly affects prothrombin times when administered to individuals on coumarin-type anticoagulants. Caution is advised nonetheless, since interactions have been seen with other nonsteroidal agents of this class. Similarly, patients receiving the drug and a hydantoin, sulfonamide or sulfonylurea should be observed for signs of toxicity to these drugs (see CLINICAL STUDIES: *General Information*).

Concomitant administration of naproxen and aspirin is not recommended because naproxen is displaced from its binding sites during the concomitant administration of aspirin, resulting in lower plasma concentrations and peak plasma levels.

The natriuretic effect of furosemide has been reported to be inhibited by some drugs of this class. Inhibition of renal lithium clearance leading to increases in plasma lithium concentrations has also been reported. Naproxen and other nonsteroidal anti-inflammatory drugs can reduce the antihypertensive effect of propranolol and other beta-blockers. Probenecid given concurrently increases naproxen anion plasma levels and extends its plasma half-life significantly. Caution should be used if naproxen is administered concomitantly with methotrexate. Naproxen, naproxen sodium and other nonsteroidal anti-inflammatory drugs have been reported to reduce the tubular secretion of methotrexate in an animal model, possibly increasing the toxicity of methotrexate.

Due to the gastric pH elevating effects of H2-blockers, sucralfate and intensive antacid therapy, concomitant administration of EC-NAPROSYN is not recommended.

Drug/Laboratory Test Interactions: Naproxen may decrease platelet aggregation and prolong bleeding time. This effect should be kept in mind when bleeding times are determined.

The administration of naproxen may result in increased urinary values for 17-ketogenic steroids because of an interaction between the drug and/or its metabolites with m-dinitrobenzene used in this assay. Although 17-hydroxy-corticosteroid measurements (Porter-Silber test) do not appear to be artifactually altered, it is suggested that therapy with naproxen be temporarily discontinued 72 hours before adrenal function tests are performed if the Porter-Silber test is to be used.

Naproxen may interfere with some urinary assays of 5-hydroxy indoleacetic acid (5HIAA).

Carcinogenesis: A 2-year study was performed in rats to evaluate the carcinogenic potential of naproxen at rat doses of 8, 16 and 24 mg/kg/day (50, 100 and 150 mg/m²). The maximum dose used was 0.28 times the systemic exposure to humans at the recommended dose. No evidence of tumorigenicity was found.

Pregnancy: *Teratogenic Effects:* **Pregnancy Category B.** Reproduction studies have been performed in rats at 20 mg/kg/day (125 mg/m²/day, 0.23 times the human systemic exposure), rabbits at 20 mg/kg/day (220 mg/m²/day, 0.27 times the human systemic exposure), and mice at 170 mg/kg/day (510 mg/m²/day, 0.28 times the human systemic exposure) with no evidence of impaired fertility or harm to the fetus due to the drug. There are no adequate and well-controlled studies in pregnant women. Because animal reproduction studies are not always predictive of human response, naproxen should not be used during pregnancy unless clearly needed.

Nonteratogenic Effects: There is some evidence to suggest that when inhibitors of prostaglandin synthesis are used to delay preterm labor there is an increased risk of neonatal complications such as necrotizing enterocolitis, patent ductus arteriosus and intracranial hemorrhage. Naproxen treatment given in late pregnancy to delay parturition has been associated with persistent pulmonary hypertension, renal dysfunction and abnormal prostaglandin E levels in preterm infants. Because of the known effect of drugs of this class on the human fetal cardiovascular system (closure of ductus arteriosus), use during third trimester should be avoided.

Nursing Mothers: The naproxen anion has been found in the milk of lactating women at a concentration of approximately 1% of that found in plasma. Because of the possible adverse effects of prostaglandin-inhibiting drugs on neonates, use in nursing mothers should be avoided.

Pediatric Use: Safety and effectiveness in pediatric patients below the age of 2 years have not been established. Pediatric dosing recommendations for juvenile arthritis are based on well-controlled studies (see DOSAGE AND ADMINISTRATION). There are no adequate effectiveness or dose-response data for other pediatric conditions, but the experience in juvenile arthritis and other use experience have established that single doses of 2.5 to 5 mg/kg (as naproxen suspension, see DOSAGE AND ADMINISTRATION), with total daily dose not exceeding 15 mg/kg/day, are well tolerated in pediatric patients over 2 years of age.

ADVERSE REACTIONS

The following adverse reactions are divided into three parts based on frequency and whether or not the possibility exists

NAPROSYN	250 mg or 375 mg or 500 mg	twice daily twice daily twice daily
ANAPROX	275 mg (naproxen 250 mg with 25 mg sodium)	twice daily
ANAPROX DS	550 mg (naproxen 500 mg with 50 mg sodium)	twice daily
NAPROSYN Suspension	250 mg (10 mL/2 tsp) or 375 mg (15 mL/3 tsp) or 500 mg (20 mL/4 tsp)	twice daily twice daily twice daily
EC-NAPROSYN	375 mg or 500 mg	twice daily twice daily

of a causal relationship between naproxen and these adverse events. In those reactions listed as "Probable Causal Relationship" there is at least 1 case for each adverse reaction where there is evidence to suggest that there is a causal relationship between drug usage and the reported event.
Adverse reactions reported in controlled clinical trials in 960 patients treated for rheumatoid arthritis or osteoarthritis are treated below. In general, reactions in patients treated chronically were reported 2 to 10 times more frequently than they were in short-term studies in the 962 patients treated for mild to moderate pain or for dysmenorrhea. The most frequent complaints reported related to the gastrointestinal tract.
A clinical study found gastrointestinal reactions to be more frequent and more severe in rheumatoid arthritis patients taking daily doses of 1500 mg naproxen compared to those taking 750 mg naproxen (see CLINICAL PHARMACOLOGY).
In controlled clinical trials with about 80 pediatric patients and in well-monitored, open-label studies with about 400 pediatric patients with juvenile arthritis treated with naproxen, the incidence of rash and prolonged bleeding times were increased, the incidence of gastrointestinal and central nervous system reactions were about the same, and the incidence of other reactions were lower in pediatric patients than in adults.
The following adverse reactions are divided into three parts based on frequency and causal relationship. Incidence greater than 1% (Probable Causal Relationship):
Gastrointestinal: constipation*, heartburn*, abdominal pain*, nausea*, dyspepsia, diarrhea, stomatitis
Central Nervous System: headache*, dizziness*, drowsiness*, lightheadedness, vertigo
Dermatologic: itching (pruritus)*, skin eruptions*, ecchymoses*, sweating, purpura
Special Senses: tinnitus*, hearing disturbances, visual disturbances
Cardiovascular: edema*, dyspnea*, palpitations
General: thirst
*Incidence of reported reaction between 3% and 9%. Those reactions occurring in less than 3% of the patients are unmarked.
Incidence less than 1% (Probable Causal Relationship):
The following adverse reactions were reported less frequently than 1% during controlled clinical trials and through voluntary reports since marketing. Those reactions observed through voluntary reporting since marketing are italicized.
Gastrointestinal: *abnormal liver function tests, colitis*, gastrointestinal bleeding and/or *perforation, hematemesis*, jaundice, pancreatitis, melena, vomiting
Renal: *glomerular nephritis, hematuria, hyperkalemia, interstitial nephritis, nephrotic syndrome, renal disease, renal failure, renal papillary necrosis*
Hematologic: agranulocytosis, *eosinophilia, granulocytopenia, leukopenia*, thrombocytopenia
Central Nervous System: *depression, dream abnormalities*, inability to concentrate, *insomnia, malaise, myalgia, muscle weakness*
Dermatologic: *alopecia, photosensitive dermatitis, urticaria*, skin rashes, *photosensitivity reactions resembling porphyria cutanea tarda, epidermolysis bullosa*
Special Senses: *hearing impairment*
Cardiovascular: *congestive heart failure*
Respiratory: *eosinophilic pneumonitis*
General: *anaphylactoid reactions, angioneurotic edema, menstrual disorders, pyrexia (chills and fever)*
Incidence less than 1% (Causal Relationship Unknown):
These observations are being listed to serve as alerting information to the physician.
Hematologic: *aplastic anemia, hemolytic anemia*
Central Nervous System: *aseptic meningitis, cognitive dysfunction*
Dermatologic: *epidermal necrolysis, erythema multiforme, Stevens-Johnson syndrome*
Gastrointestinal: *nonpeptic gastrointestinal ulceration, ulcerative stomatitis*
Cardiovascular: *vasculitis*
General: *hyperglycemia, hypoglycemia*

OVERDOSAGE

Significant naproxen overdosage may be characterized by drowsiness, heartburn, indigestion, nausea or vomiting. Because naproxen sodium may be rapidly absorbed, high and early blood levels should be anticipated. A few patients have experienced seizures, but it is not clear whether or not these were drug-related. It is not known what dose of the drug would be life-threatening. The oral LD_{50} of the drug is 543 mg/kg in rats, 1234 mg/kg in mice, 4110 mg/kg in hamsters, and greater than 1000 mg/kg in dogs.
Should a patient ingest a large number of tablets or a large volume of suspension, accidentally or purposefully, the stomach may be emptied and usual supportive measures employed. In animals 0.5 g/kg of activated charcoal was effective in reducing plasma levels of naproxen. Hemodialysis does not decrease the plasma concentration of naproxen because of the high degree of its protein binding.

DOSAGE AND ADMINISTRATION

Rheumatoid Arthritis, Osteoarthritis, and Ankylosing Spondylitis
[See table above]
To maintain the integrity of the enteric coating, the EC-NAPROSYN tablet should not be broken, crushed or chewed during ingestion.
During long-term administration, the dose of naproxen may be adjusted up or down depending on the clinical response of the patient. A lower daily dose may suffice for long-term administration. The morning and evening doses do not have to be equal in size and the administration of the drug more frequently than twice daily is not necessary.
In patients who tolerate lower doses well, the dose may be increased to naproxen 1500 mg per day for limited periods when a higher level of anti-inflammatory/analgesic activity is required. When treating such patients with naproxen 1500 mg/day, the physician should observe sufficient increased clinical benefits to offset the potential increased risk (see CLINICAL PHARMACOLOGY and INDIVIDUALIZATION OF DOSAGE).
Juvenile Arthritis: The recommended total daily dose of naproxen is approximately 10 mg/kg given in 2 divided doses (ie, 5 mg/kg given twice a day). A measuring cup marked in $^1/_2$ teaspoon and 2.5 milliliter increments is provided with the NAPROSYN Suspension. The following table may be used as a guide for dosing of NAPROSYN Suspension:

Patient's Weight	Dose	Administered as
13 kg (29 lb)	62.5 mg bid	2.5 mL (1/2 tsp) twice daily
25 kg (55 lb)	125 mg bid	5.0 mL (1 tsp) twice daily
38 kg (84 lb)	187.5 mg bid	7.5 mL (1 1/2 tsp) twice daily

Management of Pain, Primary Dysmenorrhea and Acute Tendonitis and Bursitis: The recommended starting dose is 550 mg of naproxen sodium as ANAPROX/ANAPROX DS followed by 550 mg every 12 hours or 275 mg every 6 to 8 hours as required. The initial total daily dose should not exceed 1375 mg of naproxen sodium. Thereafter, the total daily dose should not exceed 1100 mg of naproxen sodium. NAPROSYN may also be used but EC-NAPROSYN is not recommended for initial treatment of acute pain because absorption of naproxen is delayed compared to other naproxen containing products (see CLINICAL PHARMACOLOGY, INDICATIONS AND USAGE and INDIVIDUALIZATION OF DOSAGE).
Acute Gout: The recommended starting dose is 750 mg of NAPROSYN followed by 250 mg every 8 hours until the attack has subsided. ANAPROX may also be used at a starting dose of 825 mg followed by 275 mg every 8 hours. EC-NAPROSYN is not recommended because of the delay in absorption (see CLINICAL PHARMACOLOGY).

HOW SUPPLIED

NAPROSYN Tablets: 250 mg: round, yellow, biconvex, debossed with ROCHE on one side and NAPROSYN 250 on the other. Packaged in light-resistant bottles of 100 and 500.
100's (bottle): NDC 0004-6312-01; 500's (bottle): NDC 0004-6312-14.
375 mg: peach, capsule-shaped, debossed with NAPROSYN on one side and 375 on the other. Packaged in light-resistant bottles of 100 and 500.
100's (bottle): NDC 0004-6311-01; 500's (bottle): NDC 0004-6311-14.
500 mg: yellow, capsule-shaped, debossed with NAPROSYN on one side and 500 on the other. Packaged in light-resistant bottles of 100 and 500.
100's (bottle): NDC 0004-6310-01; 500's (bottle): NDC 0004-6310-14.
Store at 15° to 30°C (59° to 86°F) in well-closed containers; dispense in light-resistant containers.
NAPROSYN Suspension: 125 mg/5mL (contains 39 mg sodium, about 1.5 mEq/teaspoon): Available in 1 pint (473 mL) light-resistant bottles (NDC 0004-0028-28).
Store at 15° to 30°C (59° to 86°F); avoid excessive heat, above 40°C (104°F). Dispense in light-resistant containers.
EC-NAPROSYN Delayed-Release Tablets: 375 mg: white, capsule-shaped, imprinted with EC-NAPROSYN on one side and 375 on the other. Packaged in light-resistant bottles of 100.
100's (bottle): NDC 0004-6415-01.
500 mg: white, capsule-shaped, imprinted with EC-NAPROSYN on one side and 500 on the other. Packaged in light-resistant bottles of 100.
100's (bottle): NDC 0004-6416-01.
Store at 15° to 30°C (59° to 86°F) in well-closed containers; dispense in light-resistant containers.
ANAPROX Tablets: Naproxen sodium 275 mg: blue, biconvex oval-shaped, debossed with ROCHE on one side and 274 on the other. Packaged in bottles of 100 and 500.
100's (bottle): NDC 0004-6201-01; 500's (bottle): NDC 0004-6201-14.
Store at 15° to 30°C (59° to 86°F) in well-closed containers.
ANAPROX DS Tablets: Naproxen sodium 550 mg: dark blue, capsule-shaped, film-coated, debossed with ROCHE on one side and ANAPROX DS on the other. Packaged in bottles of 100 and 500.
100's (bottle): NDC 0004-6200-01; 500's (bottle): NDC 0004-6200-14.
Store at 15° to 30°C (59° to 86°F) in well-closed containers.
Naprosyn Suspension manufactured by Patheon Inc., Mississauga, Ontario, Canada L5N 7K9
Naprosyn Tablets, EC-Naprosyn Delayed-Release Tablets, Anaprox Tablets and Anaprox DS Tablets manufactured by Syntex Puerto Rico, Inc., Humacao, PR 00791
for:
Roche Pharmaceuticals
Roche Laboratories Inc.
340 Kingsland Street
Nutley, New Jersey 07110-1199

Revised: July 1998
Shown in Product Identification Guide, page 334 and 335

FORTOVASE™ ℞
(saquinavir)
SOFT GELATIN CAPSULES

The following text is complete prescribing information based on official labeling in effect June 1998.

DESCRIPTION

FORTOVASE brand of saquinavir is an inhibitor of the human immunodeficiency virus (HIV) protease. FORTOVASE is available as beige, opaque, soft gelatin capsules for oral administration in a 200-mg strength (as saquinavir free base). Each capsule also contains the inactive ingredients medium chain mono- and diglycerides, povidone and dl-alpha tocopherol. Each capsule shell contains gelatin and glycerol 85% with the following colorants: red iron oxide, yellow iron oxide and titanium dioxide. The chemical name for saquinavir is N-tert-butyl-decahydro-2-[2(R)-hydroxy-4-phenyl-3(S)-[[N-(2-quinolylcarbonyl)-L-asparaginyl]amino]butyl]-(4aS,8aS)-isoquinoline-3(S)-carboxamide which has a molecular formula $C_{38}H_{50}N_6O_5$ and a molecular weight of 670.86.
Saquinavir is a white to off-white powder and is insoluble in aqueous medium at 25°C.

MICROBIOLOGY

Mechanism of Action: Saquinavir is an inhibitor of HIV protease. HIV protease is an enzyme required for the proteolytic cleavage of viral polyprotein precursors into individual functional proteins found in infectious HIV. Saquinavir is a peptide-like substrate analogue that binds to the protease active site and inhibits the activity of the enzyme. Saquinavir inhibition prevents cleavage of the viral polyproteins resulting in the formation of immature noninfectious virus particles.
Antiviral Activity In Vitro: In vitro antiviral activity of saquinavir was assessed in lymphoblastoid and monocytic cell lines and in peripheral blood lymphocytes. Saquinavir inhibited HIV activity in both acutely and chronically in-

Continued on next page

Fortovase—Cont.

fected cells. IC_{50} and IC_{90} values (50% and 90% inhibitory concentrations) were in the range of 1 to 30 nM and 5 to 80 nM, respectively; however, these concentrations may be altered in the presence of human plasma due to protein binding of saquinavir. In cell culture saquinavir demonstrated additive to synergistic effects against HIV in double- and triple-combination regimens with reverse transcriptase inhibitors zidovudine, zalcitabine, didanosine, lamivudine, stavudine and nevirapine, without enhanced cytotoxicity. The relationship between in vitro susceptibility of HIV to saquinavir and inhibition of HIV replication in humans has not been established.

Drug Resistance: HIV isolates with reduced susceptibility to saquinavir (4-fold or greater increase in IC_{50} from baseline; ie, phenotypic resistance) have been selected in vitro. Genotypic analyses of these HIV isolates showed several mutations in the HIV-protease gene but only those at codons 48 (Gly→Val) and/or 90 (Leu→Met) were consistently associated with saquinavir resistance.

Isolates from selected patients with loss of antiviral activity and prolonged (range: 24 to 147 weeks) therapy with INVIRASE® (saquinavir mesylate) (alone or in combination with nucleoside analogues) showed reduced susceptibility to saquinavir. Genotypic analysis of these isolates showed that mutations at amino acid positions 48 and/or 90 of the HIV-protease gene were most consistently associated with saquinavir resistance. Other mutations in the protease gene were also observed. Mutations at codons 48 and 90 have not been detected in isolates from protease inhibitor naive patients.

In a study (NV15107) of treatment-experienced patients receiving FORTOVASE monotherapy (1200 mg tid) for 8 weeks followed by antiretroviral combination therapy for a period of 4 to 48 weeks (median 32 weeks), 10 of 32 patients showed genotypic changes associated with reduced susceptibility to saquinavir. However, for resistance evaluation virus could not be recovered from 11 of 32 patients.

In a study (NV15355) of treatment-naive patients receiving FORTOVASE in combination with two nucleoside analogues for a period of 16 weeks, 1 of 28 patient isolates showed genotypic changes at codon 71 and 90 in the HIV-protease gene.

Cross-resistance: Among protease inhibitors variable cross-resistance has been recognized. Analysis of saquinavir-resistant isolates from patients following prolonged (24 to 147 weeks) therapy with INVIRASE showed that a majority of patients had resistance to at least one of four other protease inhibitors (indinavir, nelfinavir, ritonavir, 141W94).

CLINICAL PHARMACOLOGY

Pharmacokinetics: The pharmacokinetic properties of saquinavir when administered as FORTOVASE have been evaluated in healthy volunteers (n=207) and HIV-infected patients (n=91) after single-oral doses (range: 300 mg to 1200 mg) and multiple-oral doses (range: 400 mg to 1200 mg tid). The disposition properties of saquinavir have been studied in healthy volunteers after intravenous doses of 6, 12, 36 or 72 mg (n=21).

ABSORPTION AND BIOAVAILABILITY IN ADULTS: Following multiple dosing of FORTOVASE (1200 mg tid) in HIV-infected patients in study NV15107, the mean steady-state area under the plasma concentration versus time curve (AUC) at week 3 was 7249 ng·h/mL (n=31) compared to 866 ng·h/mL (n=10) following multiple dosing with 600 mg tid of INVIRASE (Table 1). Preliminary results from a pharmacokinetic substudy of NV15182 showed a mean saquinavir AUC of 3485 (CV 66%) ng·h/mL (n=11) in patients sampled between weeks 61 to 69 of therapy (see PRECAUTIONS: *General*). While this mean AUC value was lower than that of the week 3 steady-state value for FORTOVASE (1200 mg tid) from study NV15107, it remained higher than the mean AUC value for INVIRASE in study NV15107.

Table 2. Effect of FORTOVASE on the Pharmacokinetics of Coadministered Drugs

Coadministered Drug	FORTOVASE Dose	N	% Change for Coadministered Drug	
			AUC (95%CI)	C_{max} (95%CI)
Clarithromycin 500 mg bid × 7 days	1200 mg tid × 7 days	12V		
Clarithromycin			↑ 45% (17-81%)	↑ 39% (10-76%)
14-OH clarithromycin metabolite			↓ 24% (5-40%)	↓ 34% (14-50%)
Nelfinavir 750-mg single dose	1200 mg tid × 4 days	14P	↑ 18% (5-33%)	↔
Ritonavir 400 mg bid × 14 days	400 mg bid × 14 days	8V	↔	↔
Terfenadine 60 mg bid × 11 days*	1200 mg tid × 4 days	12V		
Terfenadine			↑ 368% (257-514%)	↑ 253% (164-373%)
Terfenadine acid metabolite			↑ 120% (89-156%)	↑ 93% (59-133%)

↑ Denotes an average increase in exposure by the percentage indicated.
↓ Denotes an average decrease in exposure by the percentage indicated.
↔Denotes no statistically significant change in exposure was observed.
* FORTOVASE should not be coadministered with terfenadine (see PRECAUTIONS: *Drug Interactions*).
P Patient
V Healthy Volunteers.

Table 3. Effect of Coadministered Drugs on FORTOVASE and INVIRASE Pharmacokinetics

Coadministered Drug	FORTOVASE Dose	N	% Change for Saquinavir	
			AUC (95%CI)	C_{max} (95%CI)
Clarithromycin 500 mg bid × 7 days	1200 mg tid × 7 days	12V	↑ 177% (108-269%)	↑ 187% (105-300%)
Indinavir 800 mg q8h × 2 days	800-mg single dose	6V	↑ 620% (273-1288%)	↑ 551% (320-908%)
	1200-mg single dose	6V	↑ 364% (190-644%)	↑ 299% (138-568%)
Nelfinavir 750 mg × 4 days	1200-mg single dose	14P	↑ 392% (271-553%)	↑ 179% (105-280%)
Ritonavir 400 mg bid × 14 days*	400 mg bid × 14 days†	8V	↑ 121% (7-359%)	↑ 64%§

Coadministered Drug	INVIRASE Dose	N	% Change for Saquinavir	
			AUC (95%CI)	C_{max} (95%CI)
Delavirdine 400 mg tid × 14 days	600 mg tid × 21 days	13V	↑ 5-fold	Not available
Ketoconazole 200 mg qd × 6 days	600 mg tid × 6 days	12V	↑ 130% (58-235%)	↑ 147% (53-298%)
Nevirapine 200 mg bid × 21 days	600 mg tid × 7 days	23P	↓ 24% (1-42%)	↓ 28% (1-47%)
Ranitidine 150 mg × 2 doses	600-mg single dose	12V	↑ 67%§	↑ 74% (16-161%)
Rifabutin 300 mg qd × 14 days	600 mg tid × 14 days	12P	↓ 43% (29-53%)	↓ 30%§
Rifampin 600 mg qd × 7 days	600 mg tid × 14 days	12V	↓ 84% (79-88%)	↓ 79% (68-86%)
Ritonavir 400 mg bid steady state*	400 mg bid steady state‡	7P	↑ 1587% (808-3034%)	↑ 1277% (577-2702%)
Zalcitabine (ddC) 0.75 mg tid × 7 days	600 mg tid × 7 days	27P	↔	↔
Zidovudine (ZDV) 200 mg tid × > 7 days	600 mg tid × > 7 days	20P	↔	↔

↑ Denotes an average increase in exposure by the percentage indicated.
↓ Denotes an average decrease in exposure by the percentage indicated.
↔Denotes no statistically significant change in exposure was observed.
* When ritonavir was combined with the same dose of either INVIRASE or FORTOVASE, actual mean plasma exposures (AUC$_{12}$, 18.2 µg·h/mL, 20.0 µg·h/mL, respectively) were not significantly different.
† Compared to standard FORTOVASE 1200 mg tid regimen (n=33).
‡ Compared to standard INVIRASE 600 mg tid regimen (n=114).
§ Did not reach statistical significance.
P Patient
V Healthy Volunteers.

Table 1. Mean AUC$_8$ in Patients Treated With FORTOVASE and INVIRASE (Week 3)

Treatment	n	AUC$_8$ ng·h/mL	± SD
FORTOVASE			
1200 mg tid	31	7249	± 6174
INVIRASE			
600 mg tid	10	866	± 533

The absolute bioavailability of saquinavir administered as FORTOVASE has not been assessed. However, following single 600-mg doses, the relative bioavailability of saquinavir as FORTOVASE compared to saquinavir administered as INVIRASE was estimated as 331% (95% CI 207% to 530%). The absolute bioavailability of saquinavir administered as INVIRASE average 4% (CV 73%, range: 1% to 9%) in 8 healthy volunteers who received a single 600-mg dose of INVIRASE following a high-fat breakfast (48 g protein, 60 g carbohydrate, 57 g fat; 1006 kcal). In healthy volunteers receiving single doses of FORTOVASE (300 mg to 1200 mg) and in HIV-infected patients receiving multiple doses of FORTOVASE (400 mg to 1200 mg tid), a greater than dose-proportional increase in saquinavir plasma concentrations has been observed.

Comparison of pharmacokinetic parameters between single- and multiple-dose studies shows that following multiple dosing of FORTOVASE (1200 mg tid) in healthy male volunteers (n=18), the steady-state AUC was 80% (95% CI 22% to 176%) higher than that observed after a single 1200-mg dose (n=30).

HIV-infected patients administered FORTOVASE (1200 mg tid) had AUC and maximum plasma concentration (C$_{max}$) values approximately twice those observed in healthy volunteers receiving the same treatment regimen. The mean AUC values at week 1 were 4159 (CV 88%) and 8839 (CV 82%) ng·h/mL, and C$_{max}$ values were 1420 (CV 81%) and 2477 (CV 76%) ng/mL for healthy volunteers and HIV-infected patients, respectively.

FOOD EFFECT: The mean 12-hour AUC after a single 800-mg oral dose of saquinavir in healthy volunteers (n=12) was increased from 167 ng·h/mL (CV 45%), under fasting conditions, to 1120 ng·h/mL (CV 54%) when FORTOVASE was given with breakfast (48 g protein, 60 g carbohydrate, 57 g fat; 1006 kcal).

DISTRIBUTION IN ADULTS: The mean steady-state volume of distribution following intravenous administration of a 12-mg dose of saquinavir (n=8) was 700 L (CV 39%), suggesting saquinavir partitions into tissues. It has been shown that saquinavir, up to 30 μg/mL is approximately 97% bound to plasma proteins.

METABOLISM AND ELIMINATION IN ADULTS: In vitro studies using human liver microsomes have shown that the metabolism of saquinavir is cytochrome P450 mediated with the specific isoenzyme, CYP3A4, responsible for more than 90% of the hepatic metabolism. Based on in vitro studies, saquinavir is rapidly metabolized to a range of mono- and di-hydroxylated inactive compounds. In a mass balance study using 600 mg ^{14}C-saquinavir mesylate (n=8), 88% and 1% of the orally administered radioactivity was recovered in feces and urine, respectively, within 5 days of dosing. In an additional 4 subjects administered 10.5 mg ^{14}C-saquinavir intravenously, 81% and 3% of the intravenously administered radioactivity was recovered in feces and urine, respectively, within 5 days of dosing. In mass balance studies, 13% of circulating radioactivity in plasma was attributed to unchanged drug after oral administration and the remainder attributed to saquinavir metabolites. Following intravenous administration, 66% of circulating radioactivity was attributed to unchanged drug and the remainder attributed to saquinavir metabolites, suggesting that saquinavir undergoes extensive first-pass metabolism.

Systemic clearance of saquinavir was rapid, 1.14 L/h/kg (CV 12%) after intravenous doses of 6, 36 and 72 mg. The mean residence time of saquinavir was 7 hours (n=8).

SPECIAL POPULATIONS: Hepatic or Renal Impairment: Saquinavir pharmacokinetics in patients with hepatic or renal insufficiency has not been investigated (see PRECAUTIONS). Only 1% of saquinavir is excreted in the urine, so the impact of renal impairment on saquinavir elimination should be minimal.

Gender, Race and Age: The effect of gender was investigated in healthy volunteers receiving single 1200-mg doses of FORTOVASE (n=12 females, 18 males). No effect of gender was apparent on the pharmacokinetics of saquinavir in this study.

The effect of race on the pharmacokinetics of saquinavir when administered as FORTOVASE is unknown.

The pharmacokinetics of saquinavir when administered as FORTOVASE has not been investigated in patients >65 years of age or in pediatric patients (<16 years of age).

DRUG INTERACTIONS (see PRECAUTIONS: *Drug Interactions*): Several drug interaction studies have been completed with both INVIRASE and FORTOVASE. Results

from studies conducted with INVIRASE may not be applicable to FORTOVASE. Table 2 summarizes the effect of FORTOVASE on the geometric mean AUC and C$_{max}$ of coadministered drugs. Table 3 summarizes the effect of coadministered drugs on the geometric mean AUC and C$_{max}$ of saquinavir.

For information regarding clinical recommendations, see PRECAUTIONS: *Drug Interactions*.

[See tables 2 & 3 on previous page]

INDICATIONS AND USAGE

FORTOVASE is indicated for use in combination with other antiretroviral agents for the treatment of HIV infection. This indication is based on a study that showed a reduction in both mortality and AIDS-defining clinical events for patients who received INVIRASE in combination with HIVID® (zalcitabine) compared to patients who received either HIVID or INVIRASE alone. This indication is also based on studies that showed increased saquinavir concentrations and improved antiviral activity for FORTOVASE 1200 mg tid compared to INVIRASE 600 mg tid.

Description of Clinical Studies: *STUDIES WITH FORTOVASE (saquinavir)*:

Study NV15355: Efficacy Study

Study NV15355 is an ongoing, open-label, randomized, parallel study comparing FORTOVASE (n=90) and INVIRASE (n=81) in combination with two nucleoside reverse transcriptase inhibitors of choice in treatment-naive patients. The median age was 35 (range: 18 to 63), 92% of patients were male, and 68% were Caucasian. Mean baseline CD$_4$ cell count was 429 cells/mm^3, and mean baseline plasma HIV-RNA was 4.8 log$_{10}$ copies/mL.

At week 16, 60 patients on the FORTOVASE arm compared to 30 patients on the INVIRASE arm had plasma HIV RNA levels below the limit of assay quantification (<400 copies/mL, Amplicor HIV-1 Monitor™ Test).

At week 16, mean changes from baseline in CD$_4$ cell counts and plasma HIV-RNA levels between the two treatment arms were statistically indistinguishable. The mean change in CD$_4$ cell count was 97 cells/mm^3 for the FORTOVASE arm and 115 cells/mm^3 for the INVIRASE arm. The mean changes in plasma HIV-RNA levels are summarized in Figure 1.

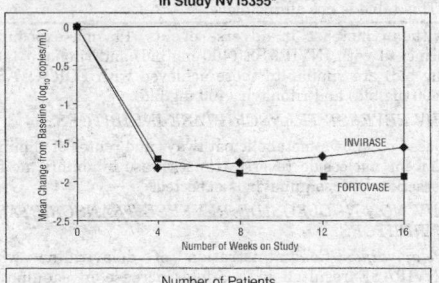

Figure 1. Mean Change from Baseline in Plasma HIV-RNA Levels in Study NV15355*

	Number of Patients				
Week	0	4	8	12	16
INVIRASE	81	74	71	75	69†
FORTOVASE	90	83	79	78	75†

* Amplicor HIV-1 Monitor™ Test. Limit of quantification = 400 copies/mL.
† By 16 weeks of therapy, 15 patients receiving FORTOVASE and 7 receiving INVIRASE had discontinued study treatment; 5 patients on INVIRASE had missing data at week 16.

Study NV15182: Safety Study

Study NV15182 was an open-label safety study of FORTOVASE in combination with other antiretroviral agents in 442 patients (median age 39 [range: 15 to 71], 90% male and 73% Caucasian). The mean baseline CD$_4$ cell count was 227 cells/mm^3 and mean baseline HIV-RNA was 4.14 log$_{10}$ copies/mL. The safety results from this study are displayed in the ADVERSE REACTIONS section.

STUDIES WITH INVIRASE (saquinavir mesylate):

Study NV14256: INVIRASE + HIVID Versus Either Monotherapy

Study NV14256 (North America) was a randomized, double-blind study comparing the combination of INVIRASE 600 mg tid + HIVID to HIVID monotherapy and INVIRASE monotherapy. The study accrued 970 patients, with median baseline CD$_4$ cell count at study entry of 170 cells/mm^3. Median duration of prior ZDV treatment was 17 months. Median duration of follow-up was 17 months. There were 88 first AIDS-defining events or deaths in the HIVID monotherapy group, 84 in the INVIRASE monotherapy group and 51 in the combination group. For survival there were 30 deaths in the HIVID group, 40 in the INVIRASE group and 11 deaths in the combination group.

The analysis of clinical endpoints from this study showed that the 18-month cumulative incidence of clinical disease progression to AIDS-defining event or death was 17.7% for patients randomized to INVIRASE + HIVID compared to

30.7% for patients randomized to HIVID monotherapy and 28.3% for patients randomized to INVIRASE monotherapy. The reduction in the number of clinical events for the combination regimen relative to both monotherapy regimens was statistically significant (see Figure 2 for Kaplan-Meier estimates of time to disease progression).

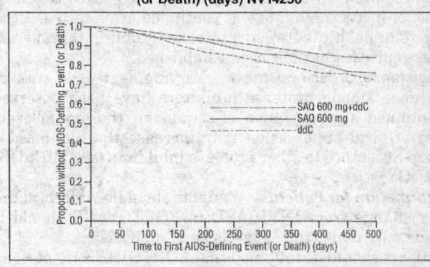

Figure 2. Time to First AIDS-Defining Event (or Death) (days) NV14256

The 18-month cumulative mortality was 4% for patients randomized to INVIRASE + HIVID, 8.9% for patients randomized to HIVID monotherapy and 12.6% for patients randomized to INVIRASE monotherapy. The reduction in the number of deaths for the combination regimen relative to both monotherapy regimens was statistically significant (see Figure 3 for Kaplan-Meier estimates of time to death).

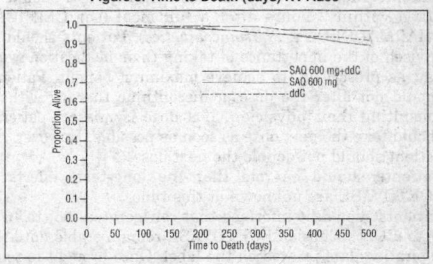

Figure 3. Time to Death (days) NV14256

CONTRAINDICATIONS

FORTOVASE is contraindicated in patients with clinically significant hypersensitivity to saquinavir or to any of the components contained in the capsule.

FORTOVASE should not be administered concurrently with terfenadine, cisapride, astemizole, triazolam, midazolam or ergot derivatives, because competition for CYP3A by saquinavir could result in inhibition of the metabolism of these drugs and create the potential for serious and/or life-threatening reactions such as cardiac arrhythmias or prolonged sedation (see PRECAUTIONS: *Drug Interactions*).

WARNINGS

New onset diabetes mellitus, exacerbation of pre-existing diabetes mellitus and hyperglycemia have been reported during post-marketing surveillance in HIV-infected patients receiving protease-inhibitor therapy. Some patients required either initiation or dose adjustments of insulin or oral hypoglycemic agents for the treatment of these events. In some cases diabetic ketoacidosis has occurred. In those patients who discontinued protease-inhibitor therapy, hyperglycemia persisted in some cases. Because these events have been reported voluntarily during clinical practice, estimates of frequency cannot be made and a causal relationship between protease-inhibitor therapy and these events has not been established.

PRECAUTIONS

General: If a serious or severe toxicity occurs during treatment with FORTOVASE, FORTOVASE should be interrupted until the etiology of the event is identified or the toxicity resolves. At that time, resumption of treatment with full-dose FORTOVASE may be considered.

Preliminary results from a pharmacokinetic substudy of NV15182 from patients sampled between weeks 61 to 69 of treatment showed that the mean saquinavir AUC was lower than the week 3 mean AUC from study NV15107. However, the mean AUC of saquinavir at week 61 to 69 remained higher than the mean AUC of INVIRASE in study NV15107 (see CLINICAL PHARMACOLOGY: *Pharmacokinetics*). The clinical significance of this finding is unknown.

Hepatic Insufficiency: Saquinavir is principally metabolized by the liver. Therefore, caution should be exercised when administering FORTOVASE to patients with hepatic insufficiency since patients with baseline liver function tests >5 times the upper limit of normal were not included in clinical studies. Although a causal relationship has not been established, there have been reports of exacerbation of chronic liver dysfunction, including portal hypertension, in patients

Continued on next page

Fortovase—Cont.

with underlying hepatitis B or C, cirrhosis or other underlying liver abnormalities.

Hemophilia: There have been reports of spontaneous bleeding in patients with hemophilia A and B treated with protease inhibitors. In some patients additional factor VIII was required. In the majority of reported cases treatment with protease inhibitors was continued or restarted. A causal relationship between protease-inhibitor therapy and these episodes has not been established.

Resistance/Cross-resistance: Varying degrees of cross-resistance among protease inhibitors have been observed. Continued administration of saquinavir therapy following loss of viral suppression may increase the likelihood of cross-resistance to other protease inhibitors (see MICROBIOLOGY).

Information for Patients: Patients should be informed that any change from INVIRASE to FORTOVASE should be made only under the supervision of a physician.

Patients should be informed that FORTOVASE is not a cure for HIV infection and that they may continue to contract illnesses associated with advanced HIV infection, including opportunistic infections. They should be informed that FORTOVASE therapy has not been shown to reduce the risk of transmitting HIV to others through sexual contact or blood contamination.

FORTOVASE may interact with some drugs; therefore, patients should be advised to report to their physician the use of any other prescription or nonprescription medication.

Patients should be advised that FORTOVASE should be taken within 2 hours after a full meal (see CLINICAL PHARMACOLOGY: *Pharmacokinetics*). Patients should be advised of the importance of taking their medication every day, as prescribed, to achieve maximum benefit. Patients should not alter the dose or discontinue therapy without consulting their physician. If a dose is missed, patients should take the next dose as soon as possible. However, the patient should not double the next dose.

Patients should be told that the long-term effects of FORTOVASE are unknown at this time.

Patients should be informed that refrigerated (36° to 46°F, 2° to 8°C) capsules of FORTOVASE remain stable until the expiration date printed on the label. Once brought to room temperature [at or below 77°F (25°C)], capsules should be used within 3 months.

Laboratory Tests: Clinical chemistry tests should be performed prior to initiating FORTOVASE therapy and at appropriate intervals thereafter. Elevated nonfasting triglyceride levels have been observed in patients in saquinavir trials. Triglyceride levels should be periodically monitored during therapy. For comprehensive information concerning laboratory test alterations associated with use of other antiretroviral therapies, physicians should refer to the complete product information for these drugs.

Drug Interactions: **Several drug interaction studies have been completed with both INVIRASE and FORTOVASE. Observations from drug interaction studies with INVIRASE may not be predictive for FORTOVASE.**

[See table above]

ANTIBIOTICS:

Clarithromycin: Coadministration of clarithromycin with FORTOVASE resulted in a 177% increase in saquinavir plasma AUC, a 45% increase in clarithromycin AUC and a 24% decrease in clarithromycin 14-OH metabolite AUC.

ANTIHISTAMINES:

Terfenadine: Coadministration of terfenadine with FORTOVASE resulted in increased terfenadine plasma levels; therefore, FORTOVASE should not be administered concurrently with terfenadine because of the potential for serious and/or life-threatening cardiac arrhythmias.

Astemizole: Because a similar interaction to that seen with terfenadine is likely from the coadministration of FORTOVASE and astemizole, FORTOVASE should not be administered concurrently with astemizole.

HIV PROTEASE INHIBITORS:

Indinavir: Coadministration of indinavir with FORTOVASE (1200-mg single dose) resulted in a 364% increase in saquinavir plasma AUC. Currently, there are no safety and efficacy data available from the use of this combination.

Nelfinavir: Coadministration of nelfinavir with FORTOVASE resulted in an 18% increase in nelfinavir plasma AUC and a 392% increase in saquinavir plasma AUC. Currently, there are no safety and efficacy data available from the use of this combination.

Ritonavir: Following approximately 4 weeks of a combination regimen of saquinavir (400 mg or 600 mg bid) and ritonavir (400 mg or 600 mg bid) in HIV-infected patients, saquinavir AUC values were at least 17-fold greater than historical AUC values from patients who received saquinavir 600 mg tid without ritonavir. When used in combination therapy for up to 24 weeks, doses greater than 400 mg bid of either ritonavir or saquinavir were associated

Drugs That Should Not Be Coadministered With FORTOVASE

Antihistamines	Astemizole, Terfenadine
Antimigraine	Ergot Derivatives
GI Motility Agents	Cisapride
Sedatives/Hypnotics	Midazolam, Triazolam

Clinically Significant Drug Interactions Which Decrease Saquinavir Plasma Concentrations

HIV Non-nucleoside Reverse Transcriptase Inhibitors	Nevirapine*
Antimycobacterial Agents	Rifabutin*, Rifampin*

Clinically Significant Drug Interactions Which Increase Saquinavir Plasma Concentrations

Antibiotics	Clarithromycin†
HIV Protease Inhibitors	Indinavir†, Ritonavir*† Nelfinavir†
HIV Non-nucleoside Reverse Transcriptase Inhibitors	Delavirdine*
Antifungal Agents	Ketoconazole*

Other Potential Drug Interactions‡

Anticonvulsants: Carbamazepine, Phenobarbital, Phenytoin	May decrease saquinavir plasma concentrations
Corticosteroids: Dexamethasone	May decrease saquinavir plasma concentrations

*Studied with INVIRASE.
†Studied with FORTOVASE.
‡This table is not all inclusive.

with an increase in adverse events. Plasma exposures achieved with INVIRASE (400 mg bid) and ritonavir (400 mg bid) are similar to those achieved with FORTOVASE (400 mg bid) and ritonavir (400 mg bid).

HIV REVERSE TRANSCRIPTASE INHIBITORS:

Based on known metabolic pathways and routes of elimination for nucleoside reverse transcriptase inhibitors, no interaction with saquinavir is expected.

HIV NON-NUCLEOSIDE REVERSE TRANSCRIPTASE INHIBITORS:

Delavirdine: Coadministration of delavirdine with INVIRASE resulted in a 5-fold increase in saquinavir plasma AUC. Currently there are limited safety and no efficacy data available from the use of this combination. In a small, preliminary study, hepatocellular enzyme elevations occurred in 13% of subjects during the first several weeks of the delavirdine and saquinavir combination (6% Grade 3 or 4). Hepatocellular changes should be monitored frequently if this combination is prescribed.

Nevirapine: Coadministration of nevirapine with INVIRASE resulted in a 24% decrease in saquinavir plasma AUC. Currently, there are no safety and efficacy data available from the use of this combination.

ANTIFUNGAL AGENTS:

Ketoconazole: Coadministration of ketoconazole with INVIRASE resulted in a 130% increase in saquinavir plasma AUC.

ANTIMYCOBACTERIAL AGENTS:

Rifabutin: Coadministration of rifabutin with INVIRASE resulted in a 43% decrease in saquinavir plasma AUC. Physicians should consider using an alternative to rifabutin when a patient is taking FORTOVASE.

Rifampin: Coadministration of rifampin with INVIRASE resulted in an 84% decrease in saquinavir plasma AUC. Physicians should consider using an alternative to rifampin when a patient is taking FORTOVASE.

H$_2$ ANTAGONISTS:

Ranitidine: Little or no change in the pharmacokinetics of INVIRASE was observed when coadministered with ranitidine. No significant interaction would be expected between FORTOVASE and ranitidine.

GI MOTILITY AGENTS:

Cisapride: Although no interaction study has been conducted, cisapride should not be administered concurrently with FORTOVASE because of the potential for serious and/or life-threatening cardiac arrhythmias.

Carcinogenesis, Mutagenesis and Impairment of Fertility: *Carcinogenesis:* Carcinogenicity studies in rats and mice have not yet been completed.

Mutagenesis: Mutagenicity and genotoxicity studies, with and without metabolic activation where appropriate, have shown that saquinavir has no mutagenic activity in vitro in either bacterial (Ames test) or mammalian cells (Chinese hamster lung V79/HPRT test). Saquinavir does not induce chromosomal damage in vivo in the mouse micronucleus assay or in vitro in human peripheral blood lymphocytes and does not induce primary DNA damage in vitro in the unscheduled DNA synthesis test.

Impairment of Fertility: Fertility and reproductive performance were not affected in rats at plasma exposures (AUC values) approximately 50% of those achieved in humans at the recommended dose.

Pregnancy: *Teratogenic Effects:* Category B. Reproduction studies conducted with saquinavir in rats have shown no embryotoxicity or teratogenicity at plasma exposures (AUC values) approximately 50% of those achieved in humans at the recommended dose or in rabbits at plasma exposures approximately 40% of those achieved at the recommended clinical dose of FORTOVASE. Distribution studies in these species showed that placental transfer of saquinavir is low (less than 5% of maternal plasma concentrations).

Studies in rats indicated that exposure to saquinavir from late pregnancy through lactation at plasma concentrations (AUC values) approximately 50% of those achieved in humans at the recommended dose of FORTOVASE had no effect on the survival, growth and development of offspring to weaning. Because animal reproduction studies are not always predictive of human response, FORTOVASE should only be used during pregnancy after taking into account the importance of the drug to the mother. Presently, there are no reports of women receiving FORTOVASE in clinical trials who became pregnant.

Nursing Mothers: The US Public Health Service Centers for Disease Control and Prevention advises HIV-infected women not to breastfeed to avoid postnatal transmission of HIV to a child who may not be infected. It is not known whether saquinavir is excreted in human milk.

Pediatric Use: Safety and effectiveness of FORTOVASE in HIV-infected pediatric patients younger than 16 years of age have not been established.

Geriatric Use: Safety and effectiveness of FORTOVASE in HIV-infected geriatric patients older than 65 years of age have not been established.

ADVERSE REACTIONS (see PRECAUTIONS)

The safety of FORTOVASE was studied in more than 500 patients who received the drug either alone or in combina-

Table 4. Percentage of Patients With Treatment-Emergent Adverse Events* of at Least Moderate Intensity, Occurring in ≥2% of Patients

ADVERSE EVENT	NV15182 (48 weeks) FORTOVASE + TOC† N=442	NV15355 (16 weeks) Naive Patients INVIRASE + 2 RTIs‡ N=81	NV15355 (16 weeks) Naive Patients FORTOVASE + 2 RTIs‡ N=90
GASTROINTESTINAL			
Diarrhea	19.9	12.3	15.6
Nausea	10.6	13.6	17.8
Abdominal Discomfort	8.6	4.9	13.3
Dyspepsia	8.4	—	8.9
Flatulence	5.7	7.4	12.2
Vomiting	2.9	1.2	4.4
Abdominal Pain	2.3	1.2	7.8
Constipation	—	—	3.3
BODY AS A WHOLE			
Fatigue	4.8	6.2	6.7
CENTRAL AND PERIPHERAL NERVOUS SYSTEM			
Headaches	5.0	4.9	8.9
PSYCHIATRIC DISORDERS			
Depression	2.7	—	—
Insomnia	—	1.2	5.6
Anxiety	—	2.5	2.2
Libido Disorder	—	—	2.2
SPECIAL SENSES DISORDERS			
Taste Alteration	—	1.2	4.4
MUSCULOSKELETAL DISORDERS			
Pain	—	3.7	3.3
DERMATOLOGICAL DISORDERS			
Eczema	—	2.5	—
Rash	—	2.5	—
Verruca	—	—	2.2

* Includes adverse events at least possibly related to study drug or of unknown intensity and/or relationship to treatment (corresponding to ACTG Grade 3 and 4).
† Antiretroviral Treatment of Choice.
‡ Reverse Transcriptase Inhibitor.

Table 5. Percentage of Patients With Marked Laboratory Abnormalities*

BIOCHEMISTRY	Limit	NV15182 (48 weeks) FORTOVASE + TOC† N=442	NV15355 (16 weeks) Naive Patients INVIRASE + 2 RTIs‡ N=81	NV15355 (16 weeks) Naive Patients FORTOVASE + 2 RTIs‡ N=90
Alkaline Phosphatase	>5 × ULN§	0.5	0.0	0.0
Calcium (high)	>12.5 mg/dL	0.2	0.0	0.0
Creatine Kinase	>4 × ULN§	7.8	0.0	4.8
Gamma GT	>5 × ULN§	5.7	2.6	7.1
Glucose (low)	<40 mg/dL	6.4	2.5	3.5
Glucose (high)	>250 mg/dL	1.4	1.3	1.2
Phosphate	<1.5 mg/dL	0.5	0.0	0.0
Potassium (high)	>6.5 mEq/L	2.7	0.0	1.2
Serum Amylase	>2 × ULN§	1.9	ND	ND
SGOT (AST)	>5 × ULN§	4.1	0.0	1.2
SGPT (ALT)	>5 × ULN§	5.7	1.3	2.3
Sodium (high)	>157 mEq/L	0.7	0.0	0.0
Total Bilirubin	>2.5 × ULN§	1.6	0.0	0.0
HEMATOLOGY				
Hemoglobin	<7.0 gm/dL	0.7	0.0	1.2
Absolute Neutrophil Count	<750 mm³	2.9	2.9	1.2
Platelets	<50,000 mm³	0.9	2.5	0.0

* ACTG Grade 3 or above.
† Antiretroviral Treatment of Choice.
‡ Reverse Transcriptase Inhibitor.
§ ULN = Upper limit of normal range.
ND Not done.

tion with other antiretroviral agents. The majority of treatment-related adverse events were of mild intensity. The most frequently reported treatment-emergent adverse events among patients receiving FORTOVASE in combination with other antiretroviral agents were diarrhea, nausea, abdominal discomfort and dyspepsia.

Clinical adverse events of at least moderate intensity which occurred in ≥2% of patients in studies NV15182 and NV15355 are summarized in Table 4. The median duration of treatment in studies NV15182 and NV15355 were 52 and 18 weeks, respectively. In NV15182, more than 300 patients were on treatment for approximately 1 year.

[See table 4 at left]

FORTOVASE did not appear to alter the pattern, frequency or severity of known major toxicities associated with the use of nucleoside analogues. Physicians should refer to the complete product information for other antiretroviral agents as appropriate for drug-associated adverse reactions to these other agents.

Rare occurrences of the following serious adverse experiences have been reported during clinical trials of FORTOVASE and/or INVIRASE and were considered at least possibly related to use of study drugs: confusion, ataxia and weakness; seizures; headache; acute myeloblastic leukemia; hemolytic anemia; thrombocytopenia; thrombocytopenia and intracranial hemorrhage leading to death; attempted suicide; Stevens-Johnson syndrome; bullous skin eruption and polyarthritis; severe cutaneous reaction associated with increased liver function tests; isolated elevation of transaminases, exacerbation of chronic liver disease with Grade 4 elevated liver function tests, jaundice, ascites, and right and left upper quadrant abdominal pain; pancreatitis leading to death; intestinal obstruction; portal hypertension; thrombophlebitis; peripheral vasoconstriction; drug fever; nephrolithiasis; and acute renal insufficiency.

Table 5 summarizes the percentage of patients with marked laboratory abnormalities in study NV15182 and NV15355 (median duration of treatment was 52 and 18 weeks, respectively). In study NV15182, by 48 weeks <1% of patients discontinued treatment due to laboratory abnormalities.

[See table 5 at left]

Additional marked lab abnormalities have been observed with INVIRASE. These include: calcium (low), phosphate (low), potassium (low), sodium (low).

Monotherapy and Combination Studies: Other clinical adverse experiences of any intensity, at least remotely related to FORTOVASE and INVIRASE, including those in <2% of patients, are listed below by body system.

Autonomic Nervous System: Mouth dry, night sweats, sweating increased

Body as a Whole: Allergic reaction, anorexia, appetite decreased, appetite disturbances, asthenia, chest pain, edema, fever, intoxication, malaise, olfactory disorder, pain body, pain pelvic, retrosternal pain, shivering, trauma, wasting syndrome, weakness generalized, weight decrease

Cardiovascular/Cerebrovascular: Cyanosis, heart murmur, heart rate disorder, heart valve disorder, hypertension, hypotension, stroke, syncope, vein distended

Central and Peripheral Nervous System: Ataxia, cerebral hemorrhage, confusion, convulsions, dizziness, dysarthria, dysesthesia, hyperesthesia, hyperreflexia, hyporeflexia, light-headed feeling, myelopolyradiculoneuritis, neuropathy, numbness extremities, numbness face, paresis, paresthesia, peripheral neuropathy, poliomyelitis, prickly sensation, progressive multifocal leukoencephalopathy, spasms, tremor, unconsciousness

Dermatological: Acne, alopecia, chalazion, dermatitis, dermatitis seborrheic, erythema, folliculitis, furunculosis, hair changes, hot flushes, nail disorder, papillomatosis, papular rash, photosensitivity reaction, pigment changes skin, parasites external, pruritus, psoriasis, rash maculopapular, rash pruritic, red face, skin disorder, skin nodule, skin syndrome, skin ulceration, urticaria, verruca, xeroderma

Endocrine/Metabolic: Dehydration, diabetes mellitus, hyperglycemia, hypoglycemia, hypothyroidism, thirst, triglyceride increase, weight increase

Gastrointestinal: Abdominal distention, bowel movements frequent, buccal mucosa ulceration, canker sores oral, cheilitis, colic abdominal, dysphagia, esophageal ulceration, esophagitis, eructation, fecal incontinence, feces blood-stained, feces discolored, gastralgia, gastritis, gastroesophageal reflux, gastrointestinal inflammation, gingivitis, glossitis, hemorrhage rectum, hemorrhoids, infectious diarrhea, melena, painful defecation, parotid disorder, pruritus ani, pyrosis, salivary glands disorder, stomach upset, stomatitis, taste unpleasant, toothache, tooth disorder, ulcer gastrointestinal

Hematologic: Anemia, neutropenia, pancytopenia, splenomegaly

Liver and Biliary: Cholangitis sclerosing, cholelithiasis, hepatitis, hepatomegaly, hepatosplenomegaly, jaundice, liver enzyme disorder, pancreatitis

Continued on next page

Fortovase—Cont.

Musculoskeletal: Arthralgia, arthritis, back pain, cramps leg, cramps muscle, lumbago, musculoskeletal disorders, myalgia, myopathy, pain facial, pain jaw, pain leg, pain musculoskeletal, stiffness, tissue changes

Neoplasm: Kaposi's sarcoma, tumor

Platelet, Bleeding, Clotting: Bleeding dermal, hemorrhage, microhemorrhages, thrombocytopenia

Psychiatric: Agitation, amnesia, anxiety attack, behavior disturbances, dreaming excessive, euphoria, hallucination, intellectual ability reduced, irritability, lethargy, overdose effect, psychic disorder, psychosis, somnolence, speech disorder

Reproductive System: Epididymitis, erectile impotence, impotence, menstrual disorder, menstrual irregularity, penis disorder, prostate enlarged, vaginal discharge

Resistance Mechanism: Abscess, angina tonsillaris, candidiasis, cellulitis, herpes simplex, herpes zoster, infection bacterial, infection mycotic, infection staphylococcal, infestation parasitic, influenza, lymphadenopathy, molluscum contagiosum, moniliasis

Respiratory: Asthma bronchial, bronchitis, cough, dyspnea, epistaxis, hemoptysis, laryngitis, pharyngitis, pneumonia, pulmonary disease, respiratory disorder, rhinitis, rhinitis allergic atopic, sinusitis, upper respiratory tract infection

Special Senses: Blepharitis, conjunctivitis, cytomegalovirus retinitis, dry eye syndrome, earache, ear pressure, eye irritation, hearing decreased, otitis, taste unpleasant, tinnitus, visual disturbance, xerophthalmia

Urinary System: Micturition disorder, nocturia, renal calculus, renal colic, urinary tract bleeding, urinary tract infection

OVERDOSAGE

Overdosage with FORTOVASE has not been reported. There were 2 patients who had overdoses with INVIRASE. No sequelae were noted in the first patient after ingesting 8 grams of INVIRASE as a single dose. The patient was treated with induction of emesis within 2 to 4 hours after ingestion. The second patient ingested 2.4 grams of INVIRASE in combination with 600 mg of ritonavir and experienced pain in the throat that lasted for 6 hours and then resolved.

DOSAGE AND ADMINISTRATION

The recommended dose of FORTOVASE is six 200-mg capsules orally, three times a day (1200 mg tid). FORTOVASE should be taken with a meal or up to 2 hours after a meal. When used in combination with nucleoside analogues, the dosage of FORTOVASE should not be reduced as this will lead to greater than dose proportional decreases in saquinavir plasma levels.

Patients should be advised that FORTOVASE, like other protease inhibitors, is recommended for use in combination with active antiretroviral therapy. Greater activity has been observed when new antiretroviral therapies are begun at the same time as FORTOVASE. As with all protease inhibitors, adherence to the prescribed regimen is strongly recommended. Concomitant therapy should be based on a patient's prior drug exposure.

Monitoring of Patients: Clinical chemistry tests should be performed prior to initiating FORTOVASE therapy and at appropriate intervals thereafter. For comprehensive patient monitoring recommendations for other antiretroviral therapies, physicians should refer to the complete product information for these drugs.

Dose Adjustment for Combination Therapy With FORTOVASE: For toxicities that may be associated with FORTOVASE, the drug should be interrupted. For recipients of combination therapy with FORTOVASE and other antiretroviral agents, dose adjustment of the other antiretroviral agents should be based on the known toxicity profile of the individual drug. Physicians should refer to the complete product information for these drugs for comprehensive dose adjustment recommendations and drug-associated adverse reactions.

HOW SUPPLIED

FORTOVASE 200-mg capsules are beige, opaque, soft gelatin capsules with ROCHE and 0246 imprinted on the capsule shell — bottles of 180 (NDC 0004-0246-48).

The capsules should be refrigerated at 36° to 46°F (2° to 8°C) in tightly closed bottles until dispensed.

For patient use, refrigerated (36° to 46°F, 2° to 8°C) capsules of FORTOVASE remain stable until the expiration date printed on the label. Once brought to room temperature [at or below 77°F (25°C)], capsules should be used within 3 months.

Active ingredient manufactured by:
F. Hoffmann-La Roche Ltd., Basel, Switzerland

Issued: November 1997

Shown in Product Identification Guide, page 334

STERILE
FUDR
[ef-u-dee-are]
brand of floxuridine

℞

The following text is complete prescribing information based on official labeling in effect June 1998.

> **WARNING**
>
> It is recommended that FUDR be given only by or under the supervision of a qualified physician who is experienced in cancer chemotherapy and intra-arterial drug therapy and is well versed in the use of potent antimetabolites.
>
> Because of the possibility of severe toxic reactions, all patients should be hospitalized for initiation of the first course of therapy.

DESCRIPTION

Sterile FUDR (floxuridine), an antineoplastic antimetabolite, is available as a sterile, nonpyrogenic, lyophilized powder for reconstitution. Each vial contains 500 mg of floxuridine which is to be reconstituted with 5 mL of sterile water for injection. An appropriate amount of reconstituted solution is then diluted with a parenteral solution for intra-arterial infusion (see DOSAGE AND ADMINISTRATION). Floxuridine is a fluorinated pyrimidine. Chemically, floxuridine is 2′-deoxy-5-fluorouridine with an empirical formula of $C_9H_{11}FN_2O_5$. It is a white to off-white odorless solid which is freely soluble in water.

The 2% aqueous solution has a pH of between 4.0 to 5.5. The molecular weight of floxuridine is 246.19.

CLINICAL PHARMACOLOGY

When FUDR is given by rapid intra-arterial injection it is apparently rapidly catabolized to 5-fluorouracil. Thus, rapid injection of FUDR produces the same toxic and antimetabolic effects as does 5-fluorouracil. The primary effect is to interfere with the synthesis of deoxyribonucleic acid (DNA) and to a lesser extent inhibit the formation of ribonucleic acid (RNA). However, when FUDR is given by continuous intra-arterial infusion its direct anabolism to FUDR-monophosphate is enhanced, thus increasing the inhibition of DNA.

Floxuridine is metabolized in the liver. The drug is excreted intact and as urea, fluorouracil, α-fluoro-β-ureidopropionic acid, dihydrofluorouracil, α-fluoro-β-guanidopropionic acid and α-fluoro-β-alanine in the urine; it is also expired as respiratory carbon dioxide. Pharmacokinetic data on intra-arterial infusion of FUDR are not available.

INDICATIONS AND USAGE

FUDR is effective in the palliative management of gastrointestinal adenocarcinoma metastatic to the liver, when given by continuous regional intra-arterial infusion in carefully selected patients who are considered incurable by surgery or other means. Patients with known disease extending beyond an area capable of infusion via a single artery should, except in unusual circumstances, be considered for systemic therapy with other chemotherapeutic agents.

CONTRAINDICATIONS

FUDR therapy is contraindicated for patients in a poor nutritional state, those with depressed bone marrow function or those with potentially serious infections.

WARNINGS

BECAUSE OF THE POSSIBILITY OF SEVERE TOXIC REACTIONS, ALL PATIENTS SHOULD BE HOSPITALIZED FOR THE FIRST COURSE OF THERAPY.

FUDR should be used with extreme caution in poor risk patients with impaired hepatic or renal function or a history of high-dose pelvic irradiation or previous use of alkylating agents. The drug is not intended as an adjuvant to surgery.

FUDR may cause fetal harm when administered to a pregnant woman. It has been shown to be teratogenic in the chick embryo, mouse (at doses of 2.5 to 100 mg/kg) and rat (at doses of 75 to 150 mg/kg). Malformations included cleft palates; skeletal defects; and deformed appendages, paws and tails. The dosages which were teratogenic in animals are 4.2 to 125 times the recommended human therapeutic dose.

There are no adequate and well-controlled studies with FUDR in pregnant women. If this drug is used during pregnancy or if the patient becomes pregnant while taking (receiving) this drug, the patient should be apprised of the potential hazard to the fetus. Women of childbearing potential should be advised to avoid becoming pregnant.

Combination Therapy: Any form of therapy which adds to the stress of the patient, interferes with nutrition or depresses bone marrow function will increase the toxicity of FUDR.

PRECAUTIONS

General: Sterile FUDR is a highly toxic drug with a narrow margin of safety. Therefore, patients should be carefully supervised since therapeutic response is unlikely to occur

---

without some evidence of toxicity. Severe hematological toxicity, gastrointestinal hemorrhage and even death may result from the use of FUDR despite meticulous selection of patients and careful adjustment of dosage. Although severe toxicity is more likely in poor risk patients, fatalities may be encountered occasionally even in patients in relatively good condition.

Therapy is to be discontinued promptly whenever one of the following signs of toxicity appears:
Myocardial ischemia
Stomatitis or esophagopharyngitis, at the first visible sign
Leukopenia (WBC under 3500) or a rapidly falling white blood count
Vomiting, intractable
Diarrhea, frequent bowel movements or watery stools
Gastrointestinal ulceration and bleeding
Thrombocytopenia (platelets under 100,000)
Hemorrhage from any site

Information For Patients: Patients should be informed of expected toxic effects, particularly oral manifestations. Patients should be alerted to the possibility of alopecia as a result of therapy and should be informed that it is usually a transient effect.

Laboratory Tests: Careful monitoring of the white blood count and platelet count is recommended.

Drug Interactions: See WARNINGS section.

Carcinogenesis, Mutagenesis, Impairment Of Fertility:

Carcinogenesis: Long-term studies in animals to evaluate the carcinogenic potential of floxuridine have not been conducted. On the basis of the available data, no evaluation can be made of the carcinogenic risk of FUDR to humans.

Mutagenesis: Oncogenic transformation of fibroblasts from mouse embryo has been induced in vitro by FUDR, but the relationship between oncogenicity and mutagenicity is not clear. Floxuridine has also been shown to be mutagenic in human leukocytes in vitro and in the *Drosophila* test system. In addition, 5-fluorouracil, to which floxuridine is catabolized when given by intra-arterial injection, has been shown to be mutagenic in in vitro tests.

Impairment Of Fertility: The effects of floxuridine on fertility and general reproductive performance have not been studied in animals. However, because floxuridine is catabolized to 5-fluorouracil, it should be noted that 5-fluorouracil has been shown to induce chromosomal aberrations and changes in chromosome organization of spermatogonia in rats at doses of 125 or 250 mg/kg, administered intraperitoneally.

Spermatogonial differentiation was also inhibited by fluorouracil, resulting in transient infertility. In female rats, fluorouracil, administered intraperitoneally at doses of 25 or 50 mg/kg during the preovulatory phase of oogenesis, significantly reduced the incidence of fertile matings, delayed the development of pre- and post-implantation embryos, increased the incidence of preimplantation lethality and induced chromosomal anomalies in these embryos. Compounds such as FUDR, which interfere with DNA, RNA and protein synthesis, might be expected to have adverse effects on gametogenesis.

Pregnancy: *Teratogenic Effects:* Pregnancy Category D (see WARNINGS). Floxuridine has been shown to be teratogenic in the chick embryo, mouse (at doses of 2.5 to 100 mg/kg) and rat (at doses of 75 to 150 mg/kg). Malformations included cleft palates, skeletal defects and deformed appendages, paws and tails. The dosages which were teratogenic in animals are 4.2 to 125 times the recommended human therapeutic dose.

There are no adequate and well-controlled studies with FUDR in pregnant women. While there is no evidence of teratogenicity in humans due to FUDR, it should be kept in mind that other drugs which inhibit DNA synthesis (eg, methotrexate and aminopterin) have been reported to be teratogenic in humans. FUDR should be used during pregnancy only if the potential benefit justifies the potential risk to the fetus.

Nonteratogenic Effects: Floxuridine has not been studied in animals for its effects on peri- and postnatal development. However, compounds which inhibit DNA, RNA and protein synthesis might be expected to have adverse effects on peri- and postnatal development.

Nursing Mothers: It is not known whether FUDR is excreted in human milk. Because FUDR inhibits DNA and RNA synthesis, mothers should not nurse while receiving this drug.

Pediatric Use: Safety and effectiveness in pediatric patients have not been established.

ADVERSE REACTIONS

Adverse reactions to the arterial infusion of FUDR are generally related to the procedural complications of regional arterial infusion.

The more common adverse reactions to the drug are nausea, vomiting, diarrhea, enteritis, stomatitis and localized erythema. The more common laboratory abnormalities are anemia, leukopenia, thrombocytopenia and elevations of alkaline phosphatase, serum transaminase, serum bilirubin and lactic dehydrogenase.

Other adverse reactions are:

Gastrointestinal: duodenal ulcer, duodenitis, gastritis, bleeding, gastroenteritis, glossitis, pharyngitis, anorexia, cramps, abdominal pain; possible intra- and extrahepatic biliary sclerosis, as well as acalculous cholecystitis.

Dermatologic: alopecia, dermatitis, nonspecific skin toxicity, rash.

Cardiovascular: myocardial ischemia.

Miscellaneous Clinical Reactions: fever, lethargy, malaise, weakness.

Laboratory Abnormalities: BSP, prothrombin, total proteins, sedimentation rate and thrombopenia.

Procedural Complications of Regional Arterial Infusion: arterial aneurysm; arterial ischemia; arterial thrombosis; embolism; fibromyositis; thrombophlebitis; hepatic necrosis; abscesses; infection at catheter site; bleeding at catheter site; catheter blocked, displaced or leaking.

The following adverse reactions have not been reported with FUDR but have been noted following the administration of 5-fluorouracil. While the possibility of these occurring following FUDR therapy is remote because of its regional administration, one should be alert for these reactions following the administration of FUDR because of the pharmacological similarity of these two drugs: pancytopenia, agranulocytosis, myocardial ischemia, angina, anaphylaxis, generalized allergic reactions, acute cerebellar syndrome, nystagmus, headache, dry skin, fissuring, photosensitivity, pruritic maculopapular rash, increased pigmentation of the skin, vein pigmentation, lacrimal duct stenosis, visual changes, lacrimation, photophobia, disorientation, confusion, euphoria, epistaxis and nail changes, including loss of nails.

OVERDOSAGE

The possibility of overdosage with FUDR is unlikely in view of the mode of administration. Nevertheless, the anticipated manifestations would be nausea, vomiting, diarrhea, gastrointestinal ulceration and bleeding, bone marrow depression (including thrombocytopenia, leukopenia and agranulocytosis). No specific antidotal therapy exists. Patients who have been exposed to an overdosage of FUDR should be monitored hematologically for at least 4 weeks. Should abnormalities appear, appropriate therapy should be utilized. The acute intravenous toxicity of floxuridine is as follows:

Species	LD_{50} (mg/kg $\pm$ S.E.)
Mouse	880 $\pm$ 51
Rat	670 $\pm$ 73
Rabbit	94 $\pm$ 19.6
Dog	157 $\pm$ 46

DOSAGE AND ADMINISTRATION

Each vial must be reconstituted with 5 mL of sterile water for injection to yield a solution containing approximately 100 mg of floxuridine/mL. The calculated daily dose(s) of the drug is then diluted with 5% dextrose or 0.9% sodium chloride injection to a volume appropriate for the infusion apparatus to be used. The administration of FUDR is best achieved with the use of an appropriate pump to overcome pressure in large arteries and to ensure a uniform rate of infusion.

Parenteral drug products should be inspected visually for particulate matter and discoloration prior to administration whenever solution and container permit.

The recommended therapeutic dosage schedule of FUDR by continuous arterial infusion is 0.1 to 0.6 mg/kg/day. The higher dosage ranges (0.4 mg to 0.6 mg) are usually employed for hepatic artery infusion because the liver metabolizes the drug, thus reducing the potential for systemic toxicity. Therapy can be given until adverse reactions appear. (See PRECAUTIONS section.) When these side effects have subsided, therapy may be resumed. The patient should be maintained on therapy as long as response to FUDR continues.

Procedures for proper handling and disposal of anticancer drugs should be considered. Several guidelines on this subject have been published.[1-6] There is no general agreement that all of the procedures recommended in the guidelines are necessary or appropriate.

HOW SUPPLIED

500 mg Sterile FUDR (floxuridine) powder in a 5-mL vial (NDC 0004-1935-08). This is to be reconstituted with 5 mL sterile water for injection.

The sterile powder should be stored at 59° to 86°F (15° to 30°C). Reconstituted vials should be stored under refrigeration (36° to 46°F, 2° to 8°C) for not more than 2 weeks.

REFERENCES

1. Recommendations for the safe handling of parenteral antineoplastic drugs. Washington, DC, US Government Printing Office NIH publication 83-2621.
2. AMA Council Report. Guidelines for handling parenteral antineoplastics. *JAMA.* Mar 15, 1985, 253:1590–1592.
3. National Study Commission on Cytotoxic Exposure: Recommendations for handling cytotoxic agents. Available from Louis P. Jeffrey, ScD, Director of Pharmacy Services, Rhode Island Hospital, 593 Eddy Street, Providence, Rhode Island 02902.
4. Clinical Oncological Society of Australia: Guidelines and recommendations for safe handling of antineoplastic agents. *Med J Aust.* Apr 30, 1983, 1:426–428.
5. Jones RB, Frank R, Mass T: Safe handling of chemotherapeutic agents: a report from the Mount Sinai Medical Center. *CA* Sept–Oct, 1983, 33:258–263.
6. ASHP technical assistance bulletin on handling cytotoxic drugs in hospitals. *Am J Hosp Pharm.* Jan, 1985, 42:131–137.

Revised: September 1997

HIVID® ℞
[*hiv' 'id*]
(zalcitabine)
TABLETS

The following text is complete prescribing information based on official labeling in effect June 1998.

> **WARNING:**
> THE USE OF HIVID HAS BEEN ASSOCIATED WITH SIGNIFICANT CLINICAL ADVERSE REACTIONS, SOME OF WHICH ARE POTENTIALLY FATAL. HIVID CAN CAUSE SEVERE PERIPHERAL NEUROPATHY AND BECAUSE OF THIS SHOULD BE USED WITH EXTREME CAUTION IN PATIENTS WITH PREEXISTING NEUROPATHY. HIVID MAY ALSO RARELY CAUSE PANCREATITIS AND PATIENTS WHO DEVELOP ANY SYMPTOMS SUGGESTIVE OF PANCREATITIS WHILE USING HIVID SHOULD HAVE THERAPY SUSPENDED IMMEDIATELY UNTIL THIS DIAGNOSIS IS EXCLUDED.
> RARE OCCURRENCES OF POTENTIALLY FATAL LACTIC ACIDOSIS IN THE ABSENCE OF HYPOXEMIA AND SEVERE HEPATOMEGALY WITH STEATOSIS HAVE BEEN REPORTED WITH THE USE OF NUCLEOSIDE ANALOGUES, INCLUDING ZIDOVUDINE AND HIVID. IN ADDITION, RARE CASES OF HEPATIC FAILURE AND DEATH CONSIDERED POSSIBLY RELATED TO UNDERLYING HEPATITIS B AND HIVID HAVE BEEN REPORTED (SEE WARNINGS AND PRECAUTIONS).

DESCRIPTION

HIVID is the Hoffmann-La Roche brand of zalcitabine [formerly called 2′,3′-dideoxycytidine (ddC)], a synthetic pyrimidine nucleoside analogue active against the human immunodeficiency virus (HIV). HIVID is available as film-coated tablets for oral administration in strengths of 0.375 mg and 0.750 mg. Each tablet also contains the inactive ingredients lactose, microcrystalline cellulose, croscarmellose sodium, magnesium stearate, hydroxypropyl methylcellulose, polyethylene glycol and polysorbate 80 along with the following colorant system: 0.375 mg tablet — synthetic brown, black, red and yellow iron oxides, and titanium dioxide; 0.750 mg tablet — synthetic black iron oxide and titanium dioxide. The chemical name for zalcitabine is 4-amino-1-beta-D-2′, 3′-dideoxyribofuranosyl-2-(1H)-pyrimidone or 2′,3′-dideoxycytidine with the molecular formula $C_9H_{13}N_3O_3$ and a molecular weight of 211.22.

Zalcitabine is a white to off-white crystalline powder with an aqueous solubility of 76.4 mg/mL at 25°C.

MICROBIOLOGY

Mechanism of Action: Zalcitabine is a synthetic nucleoside analogue of the naturally occurring nucleoside deoxycytidine, in which the 3′-hydroxyl group is replaced by hydrogen. Within cells, zalcitabine is converted to the active metabolite, dideoxycytidine 5′-triphosphate (ddCTP), by the sequential action of cellular enzymes. Dideoxycytidine 5′-triphosphate inhibits the activity of the HIV-reverse transcriptase both by competing for utilization of the natural substrate, deoxycytidine 5′-triphosphate (dCTP), and by its incorporation into viral DNA. The lack of a 3′-OH group in the incorporated nucleoside analogue prevents the formation of the 5′ to 3′ phosphodiester linkage essential for DNA chain elongation and, therefore, the viral DNA growth is terminated. The active metabolite, ddCTP, is also an inhibitor of cellular DNA polymerase-beta and mitochondrial DNA polymerase-gamma and has been reported to be incorporated into the DNA of cells in culture.

In Vitro HIV Susceptibility: The in vitro anti-HIV activity of zalcitabine was assessed by infecting cell lines of lymphoblastic and monocytic origin and peripheral blood lymphocytes with laboratory and clinical isolates of HIV. The IC50 and IC95 values (50% and 95% inhibitory concentration) were in the range of 30 to 500 nM and 100 to 1000 nM, respectively (1 nM = 0.21 ng/mL). Zalcitabine showed antiviral activity in all acute infections; however, activity was substantially less in chronically infected cells. In drug combination studies with zidovudine (ZDV) or saquinavir, zalcitabine showed additive to synergistic activity in cell culture. The relationship between the in vitro susceptibility of HIV to reverse-transcriptase inhibitors and the inhibition of HIV replication in humans has not been established.

Drug Resistance: HIV isolates with a reduction in sensitivity to zalcitabine (ddC) have been isolated from a small number of patients treated with HIVID by 1 year of therapy. Genetic analysis of these isolates showed point mutations (Lys 65 Arg or Asn, Thr 69 Asp, Leu 74 Val, Val 75 Thr or Ala, Met 184 Val or Tyr 215 Cys) in the pol gene that encodes for the reverse transcriptase. Combination therapy with HIVID and ZDV does not appear to prevent the emergence of zidovudine-resistant isolates.

Cross-resistance: The potential for cross-resistance between HIV-reverse transcriptase inhibitors and HIV-protease inhibitors is low because of the different enzyme targets involved. The point mutation at position 69 appears to be specific to ddC in its selection and effect. Additionally, the point mutations at positions 65, 74, 75 and 184 are associated with resistance to didanosine (ddI), that at position 75 with resistance to stavudine (d4T), and those at positions 65 (Lys to Arg) and 184 (Met to Val) with resistance to lamivudine (3TC). HIV isolates with multidrug resistance to ZDV, ddI, ddC, d4T and 3TC were recovered from a small number of patients treated for 1 year with the combination of ZDV, ddI or ddC. The pattern of resistance mutations in the combination therapy was different (Ala 62 Val, Val 75 Ile, Phe 77 Leu, Phe 116 Tyr and Gln 151 Met) from monotherapy with mutation 151 being most significant for multidrug resistance.

CLINICAL PHARMACOLOGY

Pharmacokinetics: The pharmacokinetics of zalcitabine has been evaluated in studies in HIV-infected patients following 0.01 mg/kg, 0.03 mg/kg and 1.5 mg oral doses, and a 1.5 mg intravenous dose administered as a 1-hour infusion. *Absorption and Bioavailability in Adults:* Following oral administration to HIV-infected patients, the mean absolute bioavailability of zalcitabine was >80% (30% CV, range 23% to 124%, n=19). The absorption rate of a 1.5 mg oral dose of zalcitabine (n=20) was reduced when administered with food. This resulted in a 39% decrease in mean maximum plasma concentrations (C_{max}) from 25.2 ng/mL (35% CV, range 11.6 to 37.5 ng/mL) to 15.5 ng/mL (24% CV, range 9.1 to 23.7 ng/mL), and a 2-fold increase in time to achieve maximum plasma concentrations from a mean of 0.8 hours under fasting conditions to 1.6 hours when the drug was given with food. The extent of absorption (as reflected by AUC) was decreased by 14%, from 72 ng•hr/mL (28% CV, range 43 to 119 ng•hr/mL) to 62 ng•hr/mL (23% CV, range 42 to 91 ng•hr/mL). The clinical relevance of these decreases is unknown. Absorption of zalcitabine does not appear to be reduced in patients with diarrhea not caused by an identified pathogen.

Distribution in Adults: The steady-state volume of distribution following intravenous administration of a 1.5 mg dose of zalcitabine averaged 0.534 ($\pm$ 0.127) L/kg (24% CV, range 0.304 to 0.734 L/kg, n=20). Cerebrospinal fluid obtained from 9 patients at 2 to 3.5 hours following 0.06 mg/kg or 0.09 mg/kg intravenous infusion showed measurable concentrations of zalcitabine. The CSF:plasma concentration ratio ranged from 9% to 37% (mean 20%), demonstrating penetration of the drug through the blood-brain barrier. The clinical relevance of these ratios has not been evaluated.

Metabolism and Elimination in Adults: Zalcitabine is phosphorylated intracellularly to zalcitabine triphosphate, the active substrate for HIV-reverse transcriptase. Concentrations of zalcitabine triphosphate are too low for quantitation following administration of therapeutic doses to humans.

Zalcitabine does not undergo a significant degree of metabolism by the liver. The primary metabolite of zalcitabine that has been identified is dideoxyuridine (ddU), which accounts for less than 15% of an oral dose in both urine and feces (n=4). Approximately 10% of an orally administered radiolabeled dose of zalcitabine appears in the feces (n=10), comprised primarily of unchanged drug and ddU. Renal excretion of unchanged drug appears to be the primary route of elimination, accounting for approximately 80% of an intravenous dose and 60% of an orally administered dose within 24 hours after dosing (n=19). The mean elimination half-life is 2 hours and generally ranges from 1 to 3 hours in individual patients. Total clearance following an intravenous dose averaged 285 mL/min (29% CV, range 165 to 447 mL/min, n=20). Renal clearance averaged approximately 235 mL/min or about 80% of total clearance (30% CV, range 129 to 348 mL/min, n=20). Renal clearance exceeds glomerular filtration rate suggesting renal tubular secretion contributes to the elimination of zalcitabine by the kidneys.

In patients with impaired kidney function, prolonged elimination of zalcitabine may be expected. Preliminary results from 7 patients with renal impairment (estimated creatinine clearance <55 mL/min) indicate that the half-life was prolonged (up to 8.5 hours) in these patients compared to those with normal renal function. Maximum plasma concentrations were higher in some patients after a single dose (see PRECAUTIONS).

Continued on next page

Hivid—Cont.

In patients with normal renal function, the pharmacokinetics of zalcitabine was not altered during 3 times daily multiple dosing (n=9). Accumulation of drug in plasma during this regimen was negligible. The drug was <4% bound to plasma proteins, indicating that drug interactions involving binding-site displacement are unlikely (see *Drug Interactions*).

Drug Interactions: *Zidovudine:* There was no significant pharmacokinetic interaction between zidovudine and zalcitabine when single doses of zalcitabine (1.5 mg) and zidovudine (200 mg) were coadministered to 12 HIV-positive patients.

Probenecid: Following administration of a single oral 1.5 mg dose of zalcitabine alone during probenecid treatment (500 mg at 8 and 2 hours before and 4 hours after zalcitabine dosing) to 12 HIV-positive patients, mean renal clearance decreased from 310 mL/min (28% CV) to 180 mL/min (22% CV) and AUC increased from 59 ng•hr/mL (27% CV) to 91 ng•hr/mL (22% CV), indicating an increase in exposure of approximately 50% to zalcitabine. Mean half-life of zalcitabine increased from 1.7 to 2.5 hours (see PRECAUTIONS).

Cimetidine: Administration of a single dose of 1.5 mg zalcitabine with a single dose of 800 mg cimetidine to 12 HIV-positive patients resulted in a decrease in renal clearance from 224 mL/min (27% CV) to 171 mL/min (39% CV) and an increase in AUC from 75 ng•hr/mL (29% CV) to 102 ng•hr/mL (35% CV) (see PRECAUTIONS) indicating an increase in exposure of approximately 36% to zalcitabine.

Maalox: Concomitant administration of Maalox TC (30 mL) with single dose of 1.5 mg zalcitabine to 12 HIV-positive patients resulted in a decrease in mean C_{max} from 25.2 ng/mL (28% CV) to 18.4 ng/mL (34% CV) and AUC from 75 ng•hr/mL (29% CV, n=10) to 58 ng•hr/mL (36% CV, n=10) indicating a decrease in bioavailability of approximately 25% to zalcitabine (see PRECAUTIONS).

Metoclopramide: Administration of a single dose of 1.5 mg zalcitabine with 20 mg metoclopramide (10 mg 1 hour before and 10 mg 4 hours after zalcitabine dose) to 12 HIV-positive patients resulted in a decrease in AUC from 69 ng•hr/mL (16% CV) to 62 ng•hr/mL (21% CV) indicating a decrease in bioavailability of approximately 10% (see PRECAUTIONS).

Loperamide: Administration of a single dose of 1.5 mg zalcitabine during loperamide treatment (4 mg 16 hours before zalcitabine, 2 mg at 10 and 4 hours before zalcitabine and 2 mg 2 hours after the zalcitabine dose) to 12 HIV-positive patients with diarrhea resulted in no significant pharmacokinetic interaction between zalcitabine and loperamide.

Pharmacokinetics in Pediatric Patients: For pharmacokinetic properties in pediatric patients, see PRECAUTIONS: *Pediatric Use.* Limited pharmacokinetic data have been reported for 5 HIV-positive pediatric patients using doses of 0.03 and 0.04 mg/kg HIVID administered orally every 6 hours.[1] The mean bioavailability of zalcitabine in these pediatric patients was 54% and mean apparent systemic clearance was 150 mL/min/m². Due to the small number of subjects and different analytical techniques, it is difficult to make comparisons between pediatric and adult data.

INDICATIONS AND USAGE

HIVID is indicated in combination with antiretroviral agents for the treatment of HIV infection. This indication is based on study results showing a reduction in the rate of disease progression (AIDS-defining events or death) in patients with limited prior antiretroviral therapy who were treated with the combination of HIVID and zidovudine (see *Description of Clinical Studies*). This indication is also based on a study showing a reduction in both mortality and AIDS-defining clinical events for patients who received INVIRASE® (saquinavir mesylate) in combination with HIVID compared to patients who received either HIVID or INVIRASE alone.

Description of Clinical Studies: The use of HIVID in combination with zidovudine is based on the clinical results from study ACTG 175. ACTG 175 was a randomized, double-blind, controlled trial that compared zidovudine 200 mg three times daily; didanosine 200 mg twice daily; zidovudine + didanosine; and zidovudine + HIVID 0.750 mg three times daily. A total of 2467 HIV-infected adults (mean baseline CD_4 count = 352 cells/mm³) with no prior AIDS-defining event enrolled with the following demographics: male (82%), Caucasian (70%), mean age of 35 years, asymptomatic HIV infection (81%) and prior antiretroviral use (57%, mean duration = 89.5 weeks). The overall mean duration of study treatment was 99 weeks. The incidence of AIDS-defining events or death is shown in the table below:
[See table 1 below]

Although no antiretroviral agent should be used as monotherapy, a description of CPCRA 002 is included here as it provides a comparison of the safety and efficacy of HIVID compared to ddI.

CPCRA 002 was a randomized, multicenter, open-label study in which HIVID was compared to ddI as treatment for patients with advanced HIV infection (median CD4 cell count = 37 cells/mm³) who were clinically intolerant to ZDV, or who had met criteria for having disease progression while receiving ZDV.[2] Patients in this study had a mean of 17.5 months of prior ZDV use. The median duration of treatment for both HIVID and ddI was 34 weeks. The results demonstrate that HIVID was at least as efficacious as ddI in terms of time to an AIDS-defining event or death, while for survival alone the results favored HIVID. However, most of the patients (66%) in either group had disease progression over the median 16 months of follow-up. Overall rates of study drug intolerance, discontinuation and adverse events were similar for the two groups, although the types of events were different.

A clinical study (N3300/ACTG 114) has demonstrated ZDV to be superior to HIVID as monotherapy for advanced HIV disease (CD4 cell count ≤200 cells/mm³) in previously untreated patients.[3,4] The final analysis of this study indicated that 134 patients (42%) in the HIVID group with a median follow-up of 85 weeks and 120 patients (38%) in the ZDV group with a median follow-up of 96 weeks died with a relative risk for mortality of ZDV to HIVID of 0.54.

CONTRAINDICATIONS

HIVID is contraindicated in patients with clinically significant hypersensitivity to zalcitabine or to any of the excipients contained in the tablets.

WARNINGS

SIGNIFICANT CLINICAL ADVERSE REACTIONS, SOME OF WHICH ARE POTENTIALLY FATAL, HAVE BEEN REPORTED WITH HIVID. PATIENTS WITH DECREASED CD4 CELL COUNTS APPEAR TO HAVE AN INCREASED INCIDENCE OF ADVERSE EVENTS.

1. Peripheral Neuropathy:

THE MAJOR CLINICAL TOXICITY OF HIVID IS PERIPHERAL NEUROPATHY, WHICH MAY OCCUR IN UP TO 1/3 OF PATIENTS WITH ADVANCED DISEASE TREATED WITH HIVID. The incidence in patients with less-advanced disease is lower.

HIVID-related peripheral neuropathy is a sensorimotor neuropathy characterized initially by numbness and burning dysesthesia involving the distal extremities. These symptoms may be followed by sharp shooting pains or severe continuous burning pain if the drug is not withdrawn. The neuropathy may progress to severe pain requiring narcotic analgesics and is potentially irreversible. In some patients, symptoms of neuropathy may initially progress despite discontinuation of HIVID. With prompt discontinuation of HIVID, the neuropathy is usually slowly reversible. There are no data regarding the use of HIVID in patients with preexisting peripheral neuropathy since these patients were excluded from clinical trials; therefore, HIVID should be used with extreme caution in these patients. Individuals

with moderate or severe peripheral neuropathy, as evidenced by symptoms accompanied by objective findings, are advised to avoid HIVID.

HIVID should be stopped promptly when moderate discomfort from numbness, tingling, burning or pain of the extremities progresses, or any related symptoms occur that are accompanied by an objective finding.

2. Pancreatitis:

PANCREATITIS, WHICH HAS BEEN FATAL IN SOME CASES, HAS BEEN OBSERVED WITH THE ADMINISTRATION OF HIVID. Pancreatitis is an uncommon complication of HIVID occurring in up to 1.1% of patients. Patients with a history of pancreatitis or known risk factors for the development of pancreatitis should be followed more closely while on HIVID therapy. Of 528 HIVID-treated patients enrolled in an expanded-access safety study (N3544), who had a history of prior pancreatitis or increased amylase, 28 (5.3%) developed pancreatitis and an additional 23 (4.4%) developed asymptomatic elevated serum amylase. Treatment with HIVID should be stopped immediately if clinical signs or symptoms (nausea, vomiting, abdominal pain) or if abnormalities in laboratory values (hyperamylasemia associated with dysglycemia, rising triglyceride level, decreasing serum calcium) suggestive of pancreatitis should occur. If clinical pancreatitis develops during HIVID administration, it is recommended that HIVID be permanently discontinued. Treatment with HIVID should also be interrupted if treatment with another drug known to cause pancreatitis (eg, intravenous pentamidine) is required (see *Drug Interactions*).

3. Hepatic Toxicity:

RARE OCCURRENCES OF POTENTIALLY FATAL LACTIC ACIDOSIS IN THE ABSENCE OF HYPOXEMIA AND SEVERE HEPATOMEGALY WITH STEATOSIS HAVE BEEN REPORTED WITH THE USE OF NUCLEOSIDE ANALOGUES, INCLUDING ZIDOVUDINE AND HIVID.[5,6] IN ADDITION, RARE CASES OF HEPATIC FAILURE AND DEATH CONSIDERED POSSIBLY RELATED TO UNDERLYING HEPATITIS B AND HIVID HAVE BEEN REPORTED. Treatment with HIVID in patients with preexisting liver disease, liver enzyme abnormalities, a history of ethanol abuse or hepatitis should be approached with caution. HIVID should be interrupted or discontinued in the setting of deterioration of liver function tests, hepatic steatosis, progressive hepatomegaly or unexplained lactic acidosis. In clinical trials, drug interruption was recommended if liver function tests exceeded >5 times the upper limit of normal.

4. Other Serious Toxicities:

a) *Oral Ulcers:* Severe oral ulcers occurred in up to 3% of patients receiving HIVID in CPCRA 002 and ACTG 175; less severe oral ulcerations have occurred at higher frequencies in other clinical trials.

b) *Esophageal Ulcers:* Infrequent cases of esophageal ulcers have also been attributed to HIVID therapy. Interruption of HIVID should be considered in patients who develop esophageal ulcers that do not respond to specific treatment for opportunistic pathogens in order to assess a possible relationship to HIVID.

c) *Cardiomyopathy/Congestive Heart Failure:* Cardiomyopathy and congestive heart failure in patients with AIDS have been associated with the use of nucleoside analogues. Infrequent cases have been reported in patients receiving HIVID. Treatment with HIVID in patients with baseline cardiomyopathy or history of congestive heart failure should be approached with caution.

d) *Anaphylactoid Reaction:* An anaphylactoid reaction was reported in a patient receiving both HIVID and zidovudine. In addition, there have been several reports of urticaria without other signs of anaphylaxis.

PRECAUTIONS

General:

1. *Renal Impairment:* Patients with renal impairment (estimated creatinine clearance <55 mL/min) may be at a greater risk of toxicity from HIVID due to decreased drug clearance. Dosage adjustment is recommended in these patients (see DOSAGE AND ADMINISTRATION).

2. *Lymphoma:* High doses of zalcitabine, administered for 3 months to $B_6C_3F_1$ mice (resulting in plasma concentrations over 1000 times those seen in patients taking the recommended doses of HIVID) induced an increased incidence of thymic lymphoma.[7] Although the pathogenesis of the effect is uncertain, a predisposition to chemically induced thymic lymphoma and high rates of spontaneous lymphoreticular neoplasms have previously been noted in this strain of mice.[8]

The incidence of lymphomas was reviewed in 13 comparative studies conducted by Roche, the NIAID and the NCI, as well as 7 Roche expanded-access studies that included HIVID. In 1 study, ACTG 155, a statistically significant increased rate of lymphomas was seen in patients receiving HIVID or combination HIVID and zidovudine compared to zidovudine alone (rates of 0, 1.3 and 2.3 per 100 person years for zidovudine, HIVID, and combination HIVID and zidovudine, respectively; log rank p-value=0.01, pooling

Table 1. First AIDS-defining Event or Death and Death Only by Study Arm and Antiretroviral Experience in ACTG 175

Antiretroviral Experience	Event	Treatment			
		zidovudine	zidovudine+ didanosine	zidovudine+ HIVID	didanosine
Overall	n	619	613	615	620
	AIDS/Death	96 (16%)	65 (11%)	76 (12%)	71 (11%)
	Death Only	54 (9%)	31 (5%)	40 (7%)	29 (5%)
Naive	n	269	263	267	268
	AIDS/Death	32 (12%)	20 (8%)	16 (6%)	23 (9%)
	Death Only	18 (7%)	11 (4%)	9 (3%)	11 (4%)
Experienced	n	350	350	348	352
	AIDS/Death	64 (18%)	45 (13%)	60 (17%)	48 (14%)
	Death Only	36 (10%)	20 (6%)	31 (9%)	18 (5%)

HIVID, and combination HIVID and zidovudine vs zidovudine, p-value=0.003). Based on review of the literature, the incidence of lymphomas in HIV-infected patients with advanced disease on zidovudine monotherapy would be expected to be approximately 1 to 2 per 100 person years of follow-up.

None of the other comparative studies evaluated showed a statistically significant difference in rates of lymphomas in patients receiving HIVID. In a large, controlled clinical trial (ACTG 175) HIVID in combination with zidovudine was not associated with an increase in the incidence of lymphoma over that seen with zidovudine monotherapy (6 of 615 and 9 of 619, respectively).

Patients receiving HIVID or any other antiretroviral therapy may continue to develop opportunistic infections and other complications of HIV infections, and therefore should remain under close clinical observation by physicians experienced in the treatment of patients with associated HIV diseases.

The duration of clinical benefit from antiretroviral therapy may be limited. Alterations in antiretroviral therapy should be considered in cases of disease progression, either clinical or as demonstrated by viral rebound (increase in HIV RNA after initial decline).

Information for Patients: Patients should be informed that HIVID is not a cure for HIV infection and that they may continue to acquire illnesses associated with advanced HIV infection, including opportunistic infections.

Patients should be told that there is currently no data demonstrating that HIVID therapy can reduce the risk of transmitting HIV to others through sexual contact or blood contamination.

Patients should be advised to take HIVID every day as prescribed. Patients should not alter the dose or discontinue therapy without consulting with their doctor. If a dose is missed, patients should take the dose as soon as possible and then return to their normal schedule. However, if a dose is skipped, the patient should not double the next dose.

Patients should be instructed that the major toxicity of HIVID is peripheral neuropathy. Pancreatitis and hepatic toxicity are other serious potentially life-threatening toxicities that have been reported in patients treated with HIVID. Patients should be advised of the early symptoms of these conditions and instructed to promptly report them to their physician. Since the development of peripheral neuropathy appears to be dose-related to HIVID, patients should be advised to follow their physicians' instructions regarding the prescribed dose.

Laboratory Tests: Complete blood counts and clinical chemistry tests should be performed prior to initiating HIVID therapy and at appropriate intervals thereafter. Baseline testing of serum amylase and triglyceride levels should be performed in individuals with a prior history of pancreatitis, increased amylase, those on parenteral nutrition or with a history of ethanol abuse.

Drug Interactions: The concomitant use of HIVID with drugs that have the potential to cause peripheral neuropathy should be avoided where possible. Drugs that have been associated with peripheral neuropathy include chloramphenicol, cisplatin, dapsone, disulfiram, ethionamide, glutethimide, gold, hydralazine, iodoquinol, isoniazid, metronidazole, nitrofurantoin, phenytoin, ribavirin and vincristine. Concomitant use of HIVID with didanosine is not recommended.

Treatment with HIVID should be interrupted when the use of a drug that has the potential to cause pancreatitis is required. Death due to fulminant pancreatitis possibly related to intravenous pentamidine has been reported. If intravenous pentamidine is required to treat *Pneumocystis carinii* pneumonia, treatment with HIVID should be interrupted (see WARNINGS).

Drugs such as amphotericin, foscarnet and aminoglycosides may increase the risk of developing peripheral neuropathy or other HIVID-associated toxicities by interfering with the renal clearance of zalcitabine (thereby raising systemic exposure). Patients who require the use of one of these drugs with HIVID should have frequent clinical and laboratory monitoring with dosage adjustment for any significant change in renal function. Concomitant administration of probenecid or cimetidine decreases the elimination of zalcitabine, most likely by inhibition of renal tubular secretion of zalcitabine. Patients receiving these drugs in combination with zalcitabine should be monitored for signs of toxicity and the dose of zalcitabine reduced if warranted.

Absorption of zalcitabine is moderately reduced (approximately 25%) when coadministered with magnesium/aluminum containing antacid products. The clinical significance of this reduction is not known, hence zalcitabine is not recommended to be ingested simultaneously with magnesium/aluminum containing antacids. Bioavailability is mildly reduced (approximately 10%) when zalcitabine and metoclopramide are coadministered (see CLINICAL PHARMACOLOGY: *Drug Interactions*).

Carcinogenesis, Mutagenesis and Impairment of Fertility: *Carcinogenesis:* Carcinogenicity studies in animals have not yet been completed.

Mutagenesis: There was no evidence of mutagenicity in Ames tests, Chinese Hamster lung cell tests and mouse lymphoma cell tests. An unscheduled DNA synthesis assay was performed in rat hepatocytes with no increases in DNA repair. An in vitro mammalian cell transformation assay was positive at doses of 500 mcg/mL and higher. Human peripheral blood lymphocytes were exposed to zalcitabine, with and without metabolic activation; at 1.5 mcg/mL and higher, dose-related increases in chromosomal aberration were seen. Oral doses of zalcitabine at 2500 and 4500 mg/kg were clastogenic in the mouse micronucleus assay.

Impairment of Fertility: Fertility and reproductive performance were assessed in rats at plasma concentrations up to 2142 times those achieved with the maximum recommended human dose (MRHD) based on AUC measurements. No adverse effects on rate of conception or general reproductive performance were observed. The highest dose was associated with embryolethality and evidence of teratogenicity. The next lower dose studied (plasma concentrations equivalent to 485 times the MRHD) was associated with a lower frequency of embryotoxicity but no teratogenicity. The fertility of F1 males was significantly reduced at a calculated dose of 2142 (but not 485) times the MRHD (based on AUC measurements) in a teratology study in which rat mothers were dosed on gestation days 7 to 15. No adverse effects were observed on the fertility of parents or F1 generation in the study of fertility and general reproductive performance or in the perinatal and postnatal reproduction study.

Pregnancy: *Teratogenic Effects:* Pregnancy Category C. Zalcitabine has been shown to be teratogenic in mice at calculated exposure levels of 1365 and 2730 times that of the MRHD (based on AUC measurements). In rats, zalcitabine was teratogenic at a calculated exposure level of 2142 times the MRHD but not at an exposure level of 485 times the MRHD. In a perinatal and postnatal study in the rat, a high incidence of hydrocephalus was observed in the F1 offspring derived from litters of dams treated with 1071 (but not 485) times the MRHD (based on AUC measurements). There are no adequate and well-controlled studies of zalcitabine in pregnant women. HIVID should be used during pregnancy only if the potential benefit justifies the potential risk to the fetus. Fertile women should not receive HIVID unless they are using effective contraception during therapy. If pregnancy occurs, physicians are encouraged to report such cases by calling (800) 526-6367.

Nonteratogenic Effects: Increased embryolethality was observed in pregnant mice at doses 2730 times the MRHD and in pregnant rats above 485 (but not 98) times the MRHD (based on AUC measurements). Average fetal body weight was significantly decreased in mice at doses of 1365 times the MRHD and in rats at 2142 times the MRHD (based on AUC measurements). In a perinatal and postnatal study, the learning and memory of a significant number of F1 offspring were impaired, and they tended to stay hyperactive for a longer period of time. These effects, observed at a calculated exposure level of 1071 (but not 485) times the MRHD (based on AUC measurements), were considered to result from extensive damage to or gross underdevelopment of the brain of these F1 offspring consistent with the finding of hydrocephalus.

Nursing Mothers: The US Public Health Service Centers for Disease Control and Prevention advises HIV-infected women not to breastfeed to avoid postnatal transmission of HIV to a child who may not yet be infected. It is not known whether zalcitabine is excreted in human milk.

Pediatric Use: *Pharmacokinetics in Pediatric Patients:* Limited pharmacokinetic data have been reported for 5 HIV-positive pediatric patients using doses of 0.03 and 0.04 mg/kg HIVID administered orally every 6 hours.[1] The mean bioavailability of zalcitabine in these pediatric patients was 54% and mean apparent systemic clearance was 150 mL/

Table 2. Percentage of Patients With Clinical Adverse Experience ≥ Grade 3[*,†] in ≥1% of Patients Receiving HIVID

| | CPCRA 002[*] ZDV Intolerant or Failure | | ACTG 175[‡] ZDV Naive/Experienced | |
| | HIVID 0.750 mg q8h | ddI 250 mg q12h | ZDV 200 mg q8h | HIVID+ZDV 0.750 mg q8h+200 mg q8h |
Body System/Adverse Event	n=237	n=230	n=619	n=615
Systemic				
Fatigue	3.8	2.6	2.7	2.3
Headache	2.1	1.3	2.4	2.6
Fever	1.7	0.4	2.7	2.9
Gastrointestinal				
Abdominal Pain	3.0	7.0	2.3	1.8
Oral Lesions/ Stomatitis§	3.0	0.0	0.6	1.5
Vomiting/ Nausea§	3.4	7.0	4.9	2.1
Diarrhea/ Constipation§	2.5	17.4	2.9	1.0
Hepatic				
Abnormal Hepatic Function	8.9	7.0	‖	‖
Neurological				
Convulsions	1.3	2.2		
Peripheral Neuropathy¶	28.3	13.0	3.1	3.3
Skin				
Rash/Pruritus/ Urticaria	3.4	3.9	1.8	1.6
Metabolic and Nutrition				
Pancreatitis	0.0	1.7	0.2	0.5
Psychological				
Depression	0.4	0.0	1.1	1.8
Musculoskeletal				
Painful/Swollen Joints	0.4	0.0	0.3	1.0

* Grade 2 Adverse Events possibly or probably related to treatment or unassessable were included if study drug dosage was changed or interrupted.

† Grade 3 severity: event causing marked limitation in activity, requiring medical care and possible hospitalization. Grade 4 severity: completely disabling, unable to care for self, requiring active medical intervention, probable hospitalization or hospice care.

‡All relationships.

§ Adverse experiences were combined to form this category.

‖See Table 3.

¶CPCRA 002 included patients who were dose-adjusted for Grade 2 events; ACTG 175 required dose adjustment for Grade 2 peripheral neuropathy but recorded only Grade 3 events.

Continued on next page

Hivid—Cont.

min/m^2. Due to the small number of subjects and different analytical techniques, it is difficult to make comparisons between pediatric and adult data.

Safety and effectiveness of HIVID in HIV-infected pediatric patients younger than 13 years of age has not been established.

Geriatric Use: Safety and effectiveness of HIVID in HIV-infected geriatric patients older than 65 years of age have not been established.

ADVERSE REACTIONS

(See WARNINGS.) Tables 2 and 3 summarize the clinical adverse events and laboratory abnormalities, respectively, that occurred in ≥1% of patients in the comparative monotherapy trial (CPCRA 002) of HIVID vs didanosine (ddI), and the comparative combination trial (ACTG 175) of zidovudine (ZDV) monotherapy vs HIVID and zidovudine combination therapy, respectively. Other studies have found a higher or lower incidence of adverse experiences depending upon disease status, generally being lower in patients with less advanced disease.

[See table 2 at top of previous page]

[See table 3 below]

Additional clinical adverse experiences associated with HIVID that occurred in <1% of patients in CPCRA 002 (at least possibly related, Grade 3 or higher), ACTG 175 (any relationship, Grade 3/4) or in other clinical studies are listed below by body system. Several of these events occurred in slightly higher rates in other studies. The incidence of adverse experiences varied in different studies, generally being lower in patients with less-advanced disease.

Body as a Whole: abnormal weight loss, asthenia, cachexia, chest tightness or pain, chills, cutaneous/allergic reaction, debilitation, difficulty moving, dry eyes/mouth, edema, facial pain or swelling, flank pain, flushing, increased sweating, lymphadenopathy, malaise, night sweats, pain, pelvic/groin pain, rigors.

Cardiovascular: abnormal cardiac movement, arrhythmia, atrial fibrillation, cardiac failure, cardiac dysrhythmias, cardiomyopathy, heart racing, hypertension, palpitation, subarachnoid hemorrhage, syncope, tachycardia, ventricular ectopy.

Endocrine/Metabolic: abnormal triglycerides, abnormal lipase, altered serum glucose, decreased bicarbonate, diabetes mellitus, glycosuria, gout, hot flushes, hypercalcemia, hyperkalemia, hyperlipemia, hypernatremia, hyperuricemia, hypocalcemia, hypoglycemia, hypokalemia, hypomagnesemia, hyponatremia, hypophosphatemia, increased nonprotein nitrogen.

Gastrointestinal: abdominal bloating or cramps, acute pancreatitis, anal/rectal pain, anorexia, bleeding gums, bloody or black stools, colitis, dental abscess, dry mouth, dyspepsia, dysphagia, enlarged abdomen, epigastric pain, eructation, esophageal pain, esophageal ulcers, esophagitis, flatulence, gagging with pills, gastritis, gastrointestinal hemorrhage, gingivitis, glossitis, gum disorder, heartburn, hemorrhagic pancreatitis, hemorrhoids, increased saliva, left quadrant pain, melena, mouth lesion, odynophagia, painful sore gums, painful swallowing, pancreatitis, rectal hemorrhage, rectal mass, rectal ulcers, salivary gland enlargement, sore tongue, sore throat, tongue disorder, tongue ulcer, toothache, unformed/loose stools, vomiting.

Hematologic: absolute neutrophil count alteration, anemia, epistaxis, decreased hematocrit, granulocytosis, hemoglobinemia, leukopenia, neutrophilia, platelet alteration, purpura, thrombus, unspecified hematologic toxicity, white blood cell alteration.

Hepatic: abnormal lactate dehydrogenase, bilirubinemia, cholecystitis, decreased alkaline phosphatase, hepatitis, hepatocellular damage, hepatomegaly, increased alkaline phosphatase.

Musculoskeletal: arthralgia, arthritis, arthropathy, arthrosis, back pain, backache, bone pains/aches, bursitis, cold extremities, extremity pain, joint inflammation, leg cramps, muscle aches, muscle weakness, muscle disorder, muscle stiffness, muscle cramps, myalgia, myopathy, myositis, neck pain, rib pain, stiff neck.

Neurological: abnormal coordination, aphasia, ataxia, Bell's palsy, confusion, decreased concentration, decreased neurological function, disequilibrium, dizziness, dysphonia, facial nerve palsy, focal motor seizures, grand mal seizure, hyperkinesia, hypertonia, hypokinesia, memory loss, migraine, neuralgia, neuritis, paralysis, seizures, speech disorder, status epilepticus, stupor, tremor, twitch, vertigo.

Psychological: acute psychotic disorder, acute stress reaction, agitation, amnesia, anxiety, confusion, decreased motivation, decreased sexual desire, depersonalization, emotional lability, euphoria, hallucination, impaired concentration, insomnia, manic reaction, mood swings, nervousness, paranoid state, somnolence, suicide attempt.

Respiratory: acute nasopharyngitis, chest congestion, coughing, cyanosis, difficulty breathing, dry nasal mucosa, dyspnea, flu-like symptoms, hemoptysis, nasal discharge, pharyngitis, rales/rhonchi, respiratory distress, sinus congestion, sinus pain, sinusitis, wheezing.

Skin: acne, alopecia, bullous eruptions, carbuncle/furuncle, cellulitis, cold sore, dermatitis, dry skin, dry rash desquamation, erythematous rash, exfoliative dermatitis, finger inflammation, follicular rash, impetigo, infection, itchy rash, lip blisters/lesions, macular/papular rash, maculopapular rash, moniliasis, mucocutaneous/skin disorder, nail disorder, photosensitivity reaction, pruritic disorder, pruritus, skin disorder, skin lesions, skin fissure, skin ulcer, urticaria.

Special Senses: abnormal vision, blurred vision, burning eyes, decreased taste, decreased vision, ear pain/problem, ear blockage, eye abnormality, eye inflammation, eye itching, eye pain, eye irritation, eye redness, eye hemorrhage, fluid in ears, hearing loss, increased tears, loss of taste, mucopurulent conjunctivitis, parosmia, photophobia, smell dysfunction, taste perversion, tinnitus, unequal-sized pupils, xerophthalmia, yellow sclera.

Urogenital: abnormal renal function, acute renal failure, albuminuria, bladder pain, dysuria, frequent urination, genital lesion/ulcer, increased blood urea nitrogen, increased creatinine, micturition frequency, nocturia, painful penis sore, pain on urination, penile edema, polyuria, renal cyst, renal calculus, testicular swelling, toxic nephropathy, urinary retention, vaginal itch, vaginal ulcer, vaginal pain, vaginal/cervix disorder, vaginal discharge.

OVERDOSAGE

Acute Overdosage: Inadvertent pediatric overdoses have occurred with doses up to 1.5 mg/kg HIVID. Pediatric patients had prompt gastric lavage and treatment with activated charcoal and had no sequelae. Mixed overdoses including HIVID and other drugs have led to drowsiness and vomiting (with HIVID or placebo, zidovudine and trimethoprim/sulfamethoxazole [TMP/SMX]), or increased GGT (with 18.75 mg HIVID with zidovudine and lormetazepam) or increased creatine phosphokinase (with HIVID or placebo, zidovudine, fluconazole, dapsone and wine). There is no experience with acute HIVID overdosage at higher doses and sequelae are unknown. There is no known antidote for HIVID overdosage. It is not known whether zalcitabine is dialyzable by peritoneal dialysis or hemodialysis.

Chronic Overdosage: In the early Phase 1 studies, all patients receiving zalcitabine at approximately 6 times the current total daily recommended dose experienced peripheral neuropathy by week 10. Eighty percent of patients who received approximately 2 times the current total daily recommended dose experienced peripheral neuropathy by week 12.

DOSAGE AND ADMINISTRATION

Patients should be advised that HIVID is recommended for use in combination with active antiretroviral therapy. Greater activity has been observed when new antiretroviral therapies are begun at the same time as HIVID. Concomitant therapy should be based on a patient's prior drug exposure. The recommended regimen is one 0.750 mg tablet of HIVID orally every 8 hours (2.25 mg HIVID total daily dose) in combination with other antiretroviral agents. Please refer to the complete product information for each of the other antiretroviral agents for the recommended doses of these agents. Based on preliminary data, the recommended HIVID dosage reduction for patients with impaired renal function is: creatinine clearance 10 to 40 mL/min: 0.750 mg of HIVID every 12 hours; creatinine clearance <10 mL/min: 0.750 mg of HIVID every 24 hours.

Monitoring of Patients: Complete blood counts and clinical chemistry tests should be performed prior to initiating HIVID therapy and at appropriate intervals thereafter. For comprehensive patient monitoring recommendations for other antiretroviral therapies, physicians should refer to the complete product information for these drugs. Serum amylase levels should be monitored in those individuals who have a history of elevated amylase, pancreatitis, ethanol abuse, who are on parenteral nutrition or who are otherwise at high risk of pancreatitis. Careful monitoring for signs or symptoms suggestive of peripheral neuropathy is recommended, particularly in individuals with a low CD4 cell count or who are at a greater risk of developing peripheral neuropathy while on therapy (see WARNINGS).

Dose Adjustment for HIVID: For toxicities that are likely to be associated with HIVID (eg, peripheral neuropathy, severe oral ulcers, pancreatitis, elevated liver function tests especially in patients with chronic Hepatitis B) HIVID should be interrupted or dose reduced. FOR SEVERE TOXICITIES OR THOSE PERSISTING AFTER DOSE REDUCTION, HIVID SHOULD BE INTERRUPTED. For recipients of combination therapy with HIVID and other antiretroviral agents, dose adjustments or interruption for each drug should be based on the known toxicity profile of the individual drugs. SEE INFORMATION FOR EACH DRUG USED IN COMBINATION FOR A DESCRIPTION OF KNOWN DRUG-ASSOCIATED ADVERSE REACTIONS.

Patients developing moderate discomfort with signs or symptoms of peripheral neuropathy should stop HIVID. HIVID-associated peripheral neuropathy may continue to worsen despite interruption of HIVID. HIVID should be reintroduced at 50% dose - 0.375 mg every 8 hours only if all findings related to peripheral neuropathy have improved to mild symptoms. HIVID should be permanently discontinued if patients experience severe discomfort related to peripheral neuropathy or moderate discomfort that progresses. If other moderate to severe clinical adverse reactions or laboratory abnormalities (such as increased liver function tests) occur, then HIVID and/or the other potential causative agent(s) should be interrupted until the adverse reaction abates. HIVID and/or the other potential causative agent(s) should then be carefully reintroduced at lower doses if appropriate. If adverse reactions recur at the reduced dose, therapy should be discontinued. The minimum effective dose of HIVID in combination with zidovudine for the treatment of adult patients with advanced HIV infection has not been established.

In patients with poor bone marrow reserve, particularly those patients with advanced symptomatic HIV disease, frequent monitoring of hematologic indices is recommended to detect serious anemia or granulocytopenia. Significant toxicities, such as anemia (hemoglobin of <7.5 gm/dL or reduction of >25% of baseline) and/or granulocytopenia (granulocyte count of <750 cells/mm^3 or reduction of >50% from baseline), may require a treatment interruption of HIVID and zidovudine until evidence of marrow recovery is observed. For less severe anemia or granulocytopenia, a reduction in daily dose of zidovudine in those patients receiving combination therapy may be adequate. In patients who experience hematologic toxicity, reduction in hemoglobin

Table 3. Percentage of Patients With Laboratory Abnormalities Protocol Grade 3/4

	CPCRA 002* ZDV Intolerant or Failure		ACTG 175 ZDV Naive/Experienced	
	HIVID 0.750 mg q8h n=237	ddI 250 mg q12h n=230	ZDV 200 mg q8h n=619	HIVID+ZDV 0.750 mg q8h+200 mg q8h n=615
Laboratory Abnormality				
Anemia (<7.5 gm/dL)	8.4	7.4	1.8	3.1
Leukopenia (<1500 cells/mm^3)	13.1	9.6	N/A	N/A
Eosinophilia (>1000 cells/mm^3 or 25%)	2.5	1.7	N/A	N/A
Neutropenia (<750 cells/mm^3)	16.9	11.7	1.9	4.2
Thrombocytopenia <50,000 cells/mm^3)	1.3	4.8	1.1	1.8
CPK Elevation* (>4 × ULN)	0.8	0.0	5.8	5.7
ALT (SGPT) (>5 × ULN)	N/A	N/A	3.6	5.0
AST (SGOT) (>5 × ULN)	7.6	5.7	2.9	4.1
Bilirubin (>2.5 × ULN)	0.8	0.9	0.5	1.0
GGT (>5 × ULN)	N/A	N/A	0.5	1.0
Amylase (>2 × ULN)	5.1	3.9	1.0	1.5
Hyperglycemia* (>250 mg/dL)	0.0	1.7	0.8	2.0

*Grade 3 or higher reported for CPCRA 002
N/A Not available

may occur as early as 2 to 4 weeks after initiation of therapy, and granulocytopenia usually occurs after 6 to 8 weeks of therapy. In patients who develop significant anemia, dose modification does not necessarily eliminate the need for transfusion. If marrow recovery occurs following dose modification, gradual increases in dose may be appropriate depending on hematologic indices and patient tolerance. For more details, refer to the complete product information for zidovudine.

HOW SUPPLIED

HIVID 0.375 mg tablets are oval, beige, film-coated tablets with "HIVID 0.375" imprinted on one side and "ROCHE" on the other side - bottles of 100 (NDC 0004-0220-01). HIVID 0.750 mg tablets are oval, gray, film-coated tablets with "HIVID 0.750" imprinted on one side and "ROCHE" on the other side - bottles of 100 (NDC 0004-0221-01).

The tablets should be stored in tightly closed bottles at 59° to 86°F (15° to 30°C).

REFERENCES

1. Pizzo PA, Butler K, Balis F, et al. Dideoxycytidine alone and in an alternating schedule with zidovudine in children with symptomatic human immunodeficiency virus infection. *J Pediatr.* 1990;117(5): 799–808.
2. Abrams DI, Goldman AI, Launer C, et al. A comparative trial of didanosine or zalcitabine after treatment with zidovudine in patients with human immunodeficiency virus infection. *N Engl J Med.* 1994;330(10): 657–662.
3. Follansbee S, Drew L, Olson R, et al. The efficacy of zalcitabine (ddC, HIVID) versus zidovudine (ZDV) as monotherapy in ZDV-naive patients with advanced HIV disease; a randomized, double-blind, comparative trial (ACTG 114; N3300). IXth International Conference on AIDS/IV STD World Congress, Berlin, Germany, June 7-11, 1993. Poster PO-B26-2113.
4. Remick S, Follansbee S, Olson R, et al. Safety and tolerance of zalcitabine (ddC, HIVID) in a double-blind comparative trial (ACTG 114; N3300). IXth International Conference on AIDS/IV STD World Congress, Berlin, Germany, June 7–11, 1993. Poster PO-B26-2115.
5. "Dear Doctor" letter, Burroughs Wellcome Co., June 1, 1993.
6. Food and Drug Administration Antiviral Drugs Advisory Committee Meeting, "Mitochondrial Damage Associated with Nucleoside Analogues," Rockville, MD, September 21, 1993.
7. Sanders VM, Elwell MR, Heath JE, et al. Induction of Thymic Lymphoma in Mice Administered the Dideoxynucleoside ddC. *Fundamental and Applied Toxicology.* 1995;27: 263–269.
8. Irons RD, Le AT, Som DB, et al. 2'3'-Dideoxycytidine-induced Thymic Lymphoma Correlates with Species-specific Suppression of a Subpopulation of Primitive Hematopoietic Progenitor Cells in Mouse but Not Rat or Human Bone Marrow. *J Clin Invest.* 1995;95: 2777–2782.

Revised: March 1998

Shown in Product Identification Guide, page 334

INVIRASE® ℞
(saquinavir mesylate)
CAPSULES

The following text is complete prescribing information based on official labeling in effect June 1998.

DESCRIPTION

INVIRASE brand of saquinavir mesylate is an inhibitor of the human immunodeficiency virus (HIV) protease. INVIRASE is available as light brown and green, opaque hard gelatin capsules for oral administration in a 200-mg strength (as saquinavir free base). Each capsule also contains the inactive ingredients lactose, microcrystalline cellulose, povidone K30, sodium starch glycolate, talc and magnesium stearate. Each capsule shell contains gelatin and water with the following dye systems: red iron oxide, yellow iron oxide, black iron oxide, FD&C Blue #2 and titanium dioxide. The chemical name for saquinavir mesylate is N-tert-butyl-decahydro-2- [2(R)-hydroxy-4-phenyl-3(S)-[[N-(2-quinolylcarbonyl)-L-asparaginyl]amino]butyl]-(4aS,8aS) -isoquinoline-3(S)-carboxamide methanesulfonate with a molecular formula $C_{38}H_{50}N_6O_5 \cdot CH_4O_3S$ and a molecular weight of 766.96. The molecular weight of the free base is 670.86.

Saquinavir mesylate is a white to off-white, very fine powder with an aqueous solubility of 2.22 mg/mL at 25°C.

CLINICAL PHARMACOLOGY

Mechanism of Action: HIV protease cleaves viral polyprotein precursors to generate functional proteins in HIV-infected cells. The cleavage of viral polyprotein precursors is essential for maturation of infectious virus. Saquinavir mesylate, henceforth referred to as saquinavir, is a synthetic peptide-like substrate analogue that inhibits the activity of HIV protease and prevents the cleavage of viral polyproteins.

Table 1. Frequency of Genotypic and Phenotypic Changes in Selected Patients Treated With Saquinavir

	Genotypic*		Phenotypic†	
	24 Week	1 Year	24 Week	1 Year
Monotherapy	3/8 (38%)	15/33 (45%)	2/22 (9%)	5/11 (45%)
Combination Therapy	5/30 (17%)	16/52 (31%)	0/23 (0%)	11/29 (38%)

*Double mutation (G48V and L90M) has occurred in 2 of 33 patients receiving monotherapy. The double mutation has not occurred with combination therapy.

†Phenotypic changes have been defined as at least a 10-fold change in sensitivity relative to baseline. In a few patients genotypic and phenotypic changes were unrelated.

Microbiology: *Antiviral Activity In Vitro:* The in vitro antiviral activity of saquinavir was assessed in lymphoblastoid and monocytic cell lines and in peripheral blood lymphocytes. Saquinavir inhibited HIV activity in both acutely and chronically infected cells. IC50 values (50% inhibitory concentration) were in the range of 1 to 30 nM. In cell culture saquinavir demonstrated additive to synergistic effects against HIV in double- and triple-combination regimens with reverse transcriptase inhibitors zidovudine (ZDV), zalcitabine (ddC) and didanosine (ddI), without enhanced cytotoxicity.

Resistance: HIV isolates with reduced susceptibility to saquinavir have been selected in vitro. Genotypic analyses of these isolates showed substitution mutations in the HIV protease at amino acid positions 48 (Glycine to Valine) and 90 (Leucine to Methionine).

Phenotypic and genotypic changes in HIV isolates from patients treated with saquinavir were also monitored in Phase 1/2 clinical trials. Phenotypic changes were defined as a 10-fold decrease in sensitivity from baseline. Two viral protease mutations (L90M and/or G48V, the former predominating) were found in virus from treated, but not untreated, patients. The incidence across studies of phenotypic and genotypic changes in the subsets of patients studied for a period of 16 to 74 weeks (median observation time approximately 1 year) is shown in Table 1. However, the clinical relevance of phenotypic and genotypic changes associated with saquinavir therapy has not been established.

[See table 1 above]

Cross-resistance to Other Antiretrovirals: The potential for HIV cross-resistance between protease inhibitors has not been fully explored. Therefore, it is unknown what effect saquinavir therapy will have on the activity of subsequent protease inhibitors. Cross-resistance between saquinavir and reverse transcriptase inhibitors is unlikely because of the different enzyme targets involved. ZDV-resistant HIV isolates have been shown to be sensitive to saquinavir in vitro.

Pharmacokinetics: The pharmacokinetic properties of saquinavir have been evaluated in healthy volunteers (n=351) and HIV-infected patients (n=270) after single- and multiple-oral doses of 25, 75, 200 and 600 mg tid and in healthy volunteers after intravenous doses of 6, 12, 36 or 72 mg (n=21).

ABSORPTION AND BIOAVAILABILITY IN ADULTS: Following multiple dosing (600 mg tid) in HIV-infected patients (n=30), the steady-state area under the plasma concentration versus time curve (AUC) was 2.5 times (95% CI 1.6 to 3.8) higher than that observed after a single dose. HIV-infected patients administered saquinavir 600 mg tid, with the instructions to take saquinavir after a meal or substantial snack, had AUC and maximum plasma concentration (C_{max}) values which were about twice those observed in healthy volunteers receiving the same treatment regimen (Table 2).

Table 2. Mean (%CV) AUC and C_{max} in Patients and Healthy Volunteers

	AUC_8 (dose interval) (ng·h/mL)	C_{max} (ng/mL)
Healthy Volunteers (n=6)	359.0 (46)	90.39 (49)
Patients (n=113)	757.2 (84)	253.3 (99)

Absolute bioavailability averaged 4% (CV 73%, range: 1% to 9%) in 8 healthy volunteers who received a single 600-mg dose (3 × 200 mg) of saquinavir following a high fat breakfast (48 g protein, 60 g carbohydrate, 57 g fat; 1006 kcal). The low bioavailability is thought to be due to a combination of incomplete absorption and extensive first-pass metabolism.

FOOD EFFECT: The mean 24-hour AUC after a single 600-mg oral dose (6 × 100 mg) in healthy volunteers (n=6) was increased from 24 ng·h/mL (CV 33%), under fasting conditions, to 161 ng·h/mL (CV 35%) when saquinavir was given following a high fat breakfast (48 g protein, 60 g carbohydrate, 57 g fat; 1006 kcal). Saquinavir 24-hour AUC and C_{max} (n=6) following the administration of a higher calorie meal (943 kcal, 54 g fat) were on average two times higher than after a lower calorie, lower fat meal (355 kcal, 8 g fat). The effect of food has been shown to persist for up to 2 hours.

DISTRIBUTION IN ADULTS: The mean steady-state volume of distribution following intravenous administration of a 12-mg dose of saquinavir (n=8) was 700 L (CV 39%), suggesting saquinavir partitions into tissues. Saquinavir was approximately 98% bound to plasma proteins over a concentration range of 15 to 700 ng/mL. In 2 patients receiving saquinavir 600 mg tid, cerebrospinal fluid concentrations were negligible when compared to concentrations from matching plasma samples.

METABOLISM AND ELIMINATION IN ADULTS: In vitro studies using human liver microsomes have shown that the metabolism of saquinavir is cytochrome P450 mediated with the specific isoenzyme, CYP3A4, responsible for more than 90% of the hepatic metabolism. Based on in vitro studies, saquinavir is rapidly metabolized to a range of mono- and di-hydroxylated inactive compounds. In a mass balance study using 600 mg ^{14}C-saquinavir (n=8), 88% and 1% of the orally administered radioactivity, was recovered in feces and urine, respectively, within 5 days of dosing. In an additional 4 subjects administered 10.5 mg ^{14}C-saquinavir intravenously, 81% and 3% of the intravenously administered radioactivity was recovered in feces and urine, respectively, within 5 days of dosing. In mass balance studies, 13% of circulating radioactivity in plasma was attributed to unchanged drug after oral administration and the remainder attributed to saquinavir metabolites. Following intravenous administration, 66% of circulating radioactivity was attributed to unchanged drug and the remainder attributed to saquinavir metabolites, suggesting that saquinavir undergoes extensive first-pass metabolism.

Systemic clearance of saquinavir was rapid, 1.14 L/h/kg (CV 12%) after intravenous doses of 6, 36 and 72 mg. The mean residence time of saquinavir was 7 hours (n=8).

SPECIAL POPULATIONS: Hepatic or Renal Impairment: Saquinavir pharmacokinetics in patients with hepatic or renal insufficiency has not been investigated (see PRECAUTIONS).

Gender, Race and Age: Pharmacokinetic data were available for 17 women in the Phase 1/2 studies. Pooled data did not reveal an apparent effect of gender on the pharmacokinetics of saquinavir.

The effect of race on the pharmacokinetics of saquinavir has not been evaluated, due to the small numbers of minorities for whom pharmacokinetic data were available.

Saquinavir pharmacokinetics has not been investigated in patients >65 years of age or in pediatric patients (<16 years).

DRUG INTERACTIONS: HIVID and ZDV: Concomitant use of INVIRASE with HIVID® (zalcitabine, ddC) and ZDV has been studied (as triple combination) in adults. Pharmacokinetic data suggest that the absorption, metabolism and elimination of each of these drugs are unchanged when they are used together.

Nelfinavir: In 14 HIV-positive patients, coadministration of nelfinavir (750 mg) with saquinavir (given as FORTOVASE, 1200 mg) resulted in an 18% (95% CI 5–33%) increase in nelfinavir plasma AUC and a 392% (95% CI 271–553%) increase in saquinavir plasma AUC (see PRECAUTIONS: *Drug Interactions*).

Ritonavir: Following approximately 4 weeks of a combination regimen of saquinavir (400 or 600 mg bid) and ritonavir (400 or 600 mg bid) in HIV-positive patients, saquinavir AUC and C_{max} values increased at least 17-fold (95% CI 9–31-fold) and 14-fold, respectively (see PRECAUTIONS: *Drug Interactions*).

Delavirdine: In 13 healthy volunteers, coadministration of saquinavir (600 mg tid) with delavirdine (400 mg tid) resulted in a 5-fold increase in saquinavir AUC. In 7 healthy volunteers, coadministration of saquinavir (600 mg tid) with delavirdine (400 mg tid) resulted in a 15 ± 16% decrease in delavirdine AUC (see PRECAUTIONS: *Drug Interactions*).

Nevirapine: In 23 HIV-positive patients, coadministration of saquinavir (600 mg tid) with nevirapine (200 mg bid) resulted in a 24% (95% CI 1–42%) and 28% (95% CI 1–47%) decrease in saquinavir plasma AUC and C_{max}, respectively (see PRECAUTIONS: *Drug Interactions*).

Ketoconazole: Concomitant administration of ketoconazole (200 mg qd) and saquinavir (600 mg tid) to 12 healthy volunteers resulted in steady-state saquinavir AUC and C_{max} values which were three times those seen with saquinavir alone. No dose adjustment is required when the two drugs are coadministered at the doses studied. Ketoconazole pharmacokinetics was unaffected by coadministration with saquinavir.

Continued on next page

Invirase—Cont.

Rifampin: Coadministration of rifampin (600 mg qd) and saquinavir (600 mg tid) to 12 healthy volunteers decreased the steady-state AUC and C_{max} of saquinavir by approximately 80%.

Rifabutin: Preliminary data from 12 HIV-infected patients indicate that the steady-state AUC of saquinavir (600 mg tid) was decreased by 40% when saquinavir was coadministered with rifabutin (300 mg qd).

INDICATIONS AND USAGE

INVIRASE in combination with other antiretroviral agents is indicated for the treatment of HIV infection. This indication is based on results from studies of surrogate marker responses and from a clinical study that showed a reduction in both mortality and AIDS-defining clinical events for patients who received INVIRASE in combination with HIVID compared to patients who received either HIVID or INVIRASE alone.

Description of Clinical Studies: *Patients With Advanced HIV Infection and Prior ZDV Therapy:* Study NV14256 (North America) was a randomized, double-blind study comparing the combination of INVIRASE 600 mg tid + HIVID to HIVID monotherapy and INVIRASE monotherapy. The study accrued 970 patients, with median baseline CD_4 cell count at study entry of 170 cells/mm³. Median duration of prior ZDV treatment was 17 months. Median duration of follow-up was 17 months. There were 88 first AIDS-defining events or deaths in the HIVID monotherapy group, 84 in the INVIRASE monotherapy group and 51 in the combination group. For survival there were 30 deaths in the HIVID group, 40 in the INVIRASE group and 11 deaths in the combination group.

The analysis of clinical endpoints from this study showed that the 18-month cumulative incidence of clinical disease progression to AIDS-defining event or death was 17.7% for patients randomized to INVIRASE + HIVID compared to 30.7% for patients randomized to HIVID monotherapy and 28.3% for patients randomized to INVIRASE monotherapy. The reduction in the number of clinical events for the combination regimen relative to both monotherapy regimens was statistically significant (see Figure 1 for Kaplan-Meier estimates of time to disease progression).

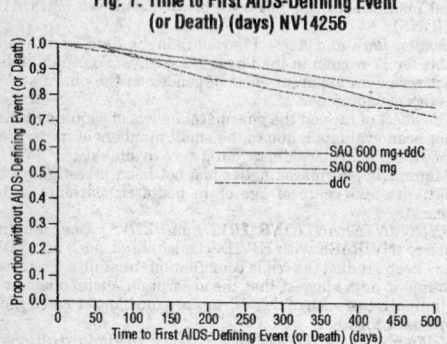

Fig. 1. Time to First AIDS-Defining Event (or Death) (days) NV14256

The 18-month cumulative mortality was 4% for patients randomized to INVIRASE + HIVID, 8.9% for patients randomized to HIVID monotherapy and 12.6% for patients randomized to INVIRASE monotherapy. The reduction in the number of deaths for the combination regimen relative to both monotherapy regimens was statistically significant (see Figure 2 for Kaplan-Meier estimates of time to death).
[See figure 2 at top of next column]

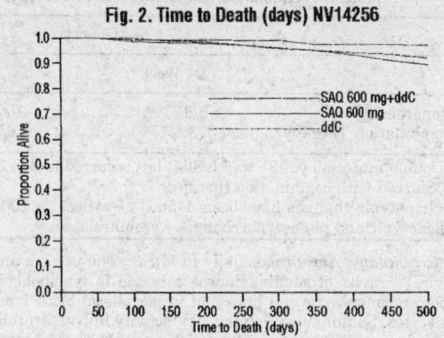

Fig. 2. Time to Death (days) NV14256

Figure 5 shows mean CD_4 changes over 48 weeks for the three treatment arms in study NV14256. Table 3 displays log RNA reductions at 16, 24 and 48 weeks among INVIRASE combination treatment arms in three clinical trials, including NV14256. Monotherapy arms are included for reference.

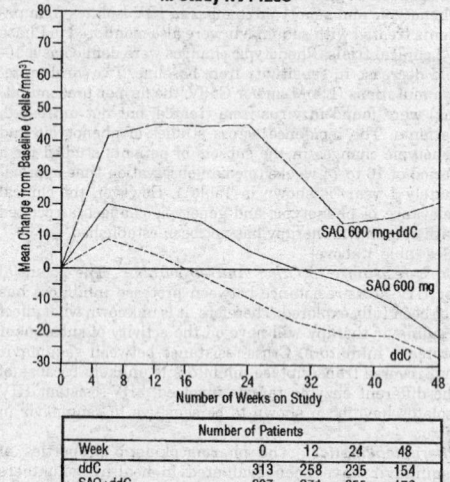

Fig. 5. Mean CD4 Changes (cells/mm³) from Baseline in Study NV14256

Number of Patients				
Week	0	12	24	48
ddC	313	258	235	154
SAQ+ddC	307	271	255	179
SAQ	317	263	242	175

[See table 3 below]
In ACTG229/NV14255, 295 patients (mean baseline CD_4=165) with prolonged ZDV treatment (median 713 days) were randomized to receive either INVIRASE 600 mg tid + HIVID + ZDV (triple combination), INVIRASE 600 mg tid + ZDV or HIVID + ZDV. In analyses of average CD_4 changes over 24 weeks, the triple combination produced greater increases in CD_4 cell counts (see Figure 4) compared to that of HIVID + ZDV. There were no significant differences in CD_4 changes among patients receiving INVIRASE + ZDV and HIVID + ZDV.
[See figure 4 at top of next column]
Comparisons of data across studies (NV14256 compared to ACTG229/NV14255) suggest that when INVIRASE was added to a regimen of prolonged prior zidovudine, there was little activity contributed by continuing ZDV.

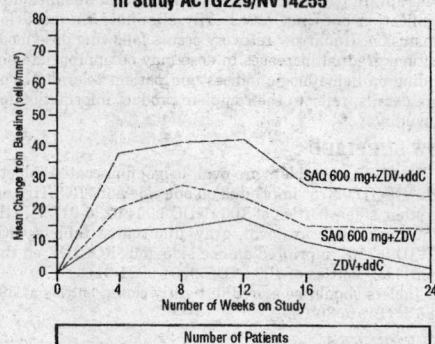

Fig. 4. Mean CD4 Changes (cells/mm³) from Baseline in Study ACTG229/NV14255

Number of Patients			
Week	0	12	24
ZDV+ddC	100	88	87
SAQ+ZDV	98	88	87
SAQ+ZDV+ddC	97	87	89

Advanced Patients Without Prior ZDV Therapy: A dose-ranging study (Italy, V13330) conducted in 92 ZDV-naive patients (mean baseline CD_4=179) studied INVIRASE at doses of 75 mg, 200 mg and 600 mg tid in combination with ZDV 200 mg tid compared to INVIRASE 600 mg tid alone and ZDV alone.

In analyses of average CD_4 changes over 16 weeks, treatment with the combination of INVIRASE 600 mg tid + ZDV produced greater CD_4 cell increases than ZDV monotherapy (see Figure 3). The CD_4 changes of ZDV in combination with doses of INVIRASE lower than 600 mg tid were no greater than that of ZDV alone.

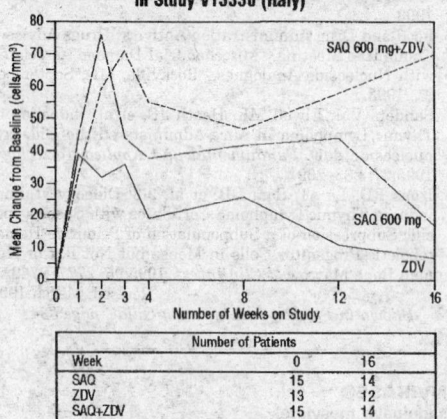

Fig. 3. Mean CD4 Changes (cells/mm³) from Baseline in Study V13330 (Italy)

Number of Patients		
Week	0	16
SAQ	15	14
ZDV	13	12
SAQ+ZDV	15	14

CONTRAINDICATIONS

INVIRASE is contraindicated in patients with clinically significant hypersensitivity to saquinavir or to any of the components contained in the capsule.

INVIRASE should not be administered concurrently with terfenadine, cisapride, astemizole, triazolam, midazolam or ergot derivatives. Inhibition of CYP3A4 by saquinavir could result in elevated plasma concentrations of these drugs, potentially causing serious or life-threatening reactions.

Table 3. Summary of Mean Log 10 Plasma RNA Results From Major INVIRASE Clinical Studies

	V13330 (Italy) Naive patients		NV14255/ACTG229 (USA) ZDV-experienced				NV14256 (North America) ZDV-experienced		
	ZDV	SAQ*	ZDV+SAQ	ZDV+ddC	ZDV+SAQ	ZDV+ddC+SAQ	ddC	SAQ	SAQ+ddC
n Enrolled	17	19	20	100	99	98	314	318	308
Prior ZDV									
n	—	—	—	99	98	97	305	315	304
Median Duration (days)	—	—	—	659	713	647	521	523	477
Log₁₀ Plasma RNA by PCR (copies/mL)									
n	17	19	20	100	97	96	300	307	294
Mean Baseline (n)	5.2 (17)	5.2 (19)	5.3 (20)	4.7 (100)	4.8 (97)	4.8 (96)	5.0 (300)	5.1 (307)	5.0 (294)
Mean Change from Baseline Week 16 (n)	−0.5 (15)	−0.2 (17)	−1.0 (17)	−0.3 (93)	0.0 (81)	−0.5 (86)	−0.4 (253)	−0.1 (262)	−0.6 (258)
Mean Change from Baseline Week 24 (n)	—	—	—	−0.2 (86)	0.0 (83)	−0.6 (84)	−0.3 (228)	−0.1 (244)	−0.6 (232)
Mean Change from Baseline Week 48 (n)	—	—	—	—	—	—	−0.3 (147)	−0.1 (167)	−0.6 (169)

*Saquinavir (SAQ) at 600 mg tid   —Indicates not applicable

WARNING: New onset diabetes mellitus, exacerbation of pre-existing diabetes mellitus and hyperglycemia have been reported during postmarketing surveillance in HIV-infected patients receiving protease inhibitor therapy. Some patients required either initiation or dose adjustments of insulin or oral hypoglycemic agents for treatment of these events. In some cases diabetic ketoacidosis has occurred. In those patients who discontinued protease inhibitor therapy, hyperglycemia persisted in some cases. Because these events have been reported voluntarily during clinical practice, estimates of frequency cannot be made and a causal relationship between protease inhibitor therapy and these events has not been established.

PRECAUTIONS

General: The safety profile of INVIRASE in pediatric patients younger than 16 years has not been established.

If a serious or severe toxicity occurs during treatment with INVIRASE, INVIRASE should be interrupted until the etiology of the event is identified or the toxicity resolves. At that time, resumption of treatment with full-dose INVIRASE may be considered. For nucleoside analogues used in combination with INVIRASE, physicians should refer to the complete product information for these drugs for dose adjustment recommendations and for information regarding drug-associated adverse reactions.

Caution should be exercised when administering INVIRASE to patients with hepatic insufficiency since patients with baseline liver function tests >5 times the upper limit of normal were not included in clinical studies. Although a causal relationship has not been established, exacerbation of chronic liver dysfunction, including portal hypertension, has been reported in patients with underlying hepatitis B or C, cirrhosis or other underlying liver abnormalities.

There have been reports of spontaneous bleeding in patients with hemophilia A and B treated with protease inhibitors. In some patients additional factor VIII was required. In the majority of reported cases treatment with protease inhibitors was continued or restarted. A causal relationship between protease inhibitor therapy and these episodes has not been established.

Resistance/Cross-resistance: The potential for HIV cross-resistance between protease inhibitors has not been fully explored. Therefore, it is unknown what effect saquinavir therapy will have on the activity of subsequent protease inhibitors (see *Microbiology*).

Information for Patients: Patients should be informed that INVIRASE is not a cure for HIV infection and that they may continue to acquire illnesses associated with advanced HIV infection, including opportunistic infections. Patients should be advised that INVIRASE should be used only in combination with an active nucleoside analogue regimen.

Patients should be told that the long-term effects of INVIRASE are unknown at this time. They should be informed that INVIRASE therapy has not been shown to reduce the risk of transmitting HIV to others through sexual contact or blood contamination.

Patients should be advised that INVIRASE should be taken within 2 hours after a full meal (see *Pharmacokinetics*). When INVIRASE is taken without food, concentrations of saquinavir in the blood are substantially reduced and may result in no antiviral activity.

Laboratory Tests: Clinical chemistry tests should be performed prior to initiating INVIRASE therapy and at appropriate intervals thereafter. For comprehensive information concerning laboratory test alterations associated with use of individual nucleoside analogues, physicians should refer to the complete product information for these drugs.

Drug Interactions: *METABOLIC ENZYME INDUCERS:* INVIRASE should not be administered concomitantly with rifampin, since rifampin decreases saquinavir concentrations by 80% (see *Pharmacokinetics*). Rifabutin also substantially reduces saquinavir plasma concentrations by 40%. Other drugs that induce CYP3A4 (eg, phenobarbital, phenytoin, dexamethasone, carbamazepine) may also reduce saquinavir plasma concentrations. If therapy with such drugs is warranted, physicians should consider using alternatives when a patient is taking INVIRASE.

OTHER POTENTIAL INTERACTIONS: Coadministration of terfenadine, astemizole or cisapride with drugs that are known to be potent inhibitors of the cytochrome P4503A pathway (ie, ketoconazole, itraconazole, etc.) may lead to elevated plasma concentrations of terfenadine, astemizole or cisapride, which may in turn prolong QT intervals leading to rare cases of serious cardiovascular adverse events. Although INVIRASE is not a strong inhibitor of cytochrome P4503A, pharmacokinetic interaction studies with INVIRASE and terfenadine, astemizole or cisapride have not been conducted. Physicians should use alternatives to terfenadine, astemizole or cisapride when a patient is taking INVIRASE. Other compounds that are substrates of CYP3A4 (eg, calcium channel blockers, clindamycin, dapsone, quinidine, triazolam) may have elevated plasma concentrations when coadministered with INVIRASE; therefore, patients should be monitored for toxicities associated with such drugs.

ANTI-HIV COMPOUNDS: Nelfinavir: Coadministration of nelfinavir with saquinavir (given as FORTOVASE, 1200 mg) resulted in an 18% increase in nelfinavir plasma AUC and a 4-fold increase in saquinavir plasma AUC. If used in combination with saquinavir hard-gelatin capsules at the recommended dose of 600 mg tid, no dose adjustments are needed. Currently, there are no safety and efficacy data available from the use of this combination.

Ritonavir: Following approximately 4 weeks of a combination regimen of saquinavir (400 or 600 mg bid) and ritonavir (400 or 600 mg bid) in HIV-positive patients, saquinavir AUC values were at least 17-fold greater than historical AUC values from patients who received saquinavir 600 mg tid without ritonavir. When used in combination therapy for up to 24 weeks, doses greater than 400 mg bid of either ritonavir or saquinavir were associated with an increase in adverse events.

Delavirdine: Saquinavir AUC increased 5-fold when delavirdine (400 mg tid) and saquinavir (600 mg tid) were administered in combination. Currently, there are limited safety and no efficacy data available from the use of this combination. In a small, preliminary study, hepatocellular enzyme elevations occurred in 15% of subjects during the first several weeks of the delavirdine and saquinavir combination (6% Grade 3 or 4). Hepatocellular enzymes (ALT/AST) should be monitored frequently if this combination is prescribed.

Nevirapine: Coadministration of nevirapine with INVIRASE resulted in a 24% decrease in saquinavir plasma AUC. Currently, there are no safety and efficacy data available from the use of this combination.

Carcinogenesis, Mutagenesis and Impairment of Fertility:
Carcinogenesis: Carcinogenicity studies in rats and mice have not yet been completed.

Mutagenesis: Mutagenicity and genotoxicity studies, with and without metabolic activation where appropriate, have shown that saquinavir has no mutagenic activity in vitro in either bacterial (Ames test) or mammalian cells (Chinese hamster lung V79/HPRT test). Saquinavir does not induce chromosomal damage in vivo in the mouse micronucleus assay or in vitro in human peripheral blood lymphocytes, and does not induce primary DNA damage in vitro in the unscheduled DNA synthesis test.

Impairment of Fertility: Fertility and reproductive performance were not affected in rats at plasma exposures (AUC values) up to five times those achieved in humans at the recommended dose.

Pregnancy: *Teratogenic Effects:* Category B. Reproduction studies conducted with saquinavir in rats have shown no embryotoxicity or teratogenicity at plasma exposures (AUC values) up to five times those achieved in humans at the recommended dose or in rabbits at plasma exposures four times those achieved at the recommended clinical dose. Studies in rats indicated that exposure to saquinavir from late pregnancy through lactation at plasma concentrations (AUC values) up to five times those achieved in humans at the recommended dose had no effect on the survival, growth and development of offspring to weaning. Because animal reproduction studies are not always predictive of human response, INVIRASE should be used during pregnancy after taking into account the importance of the drug to the mother. Presently, there are no reports of infants being born after women receiving INVIRASE in clinical trials became pregnant.

Nursing Mothers: The US Public Health Service Centers for Disease Control and Prevention advises HIV-infected women not to breastfeed to avoid postnatal transmission of HIV to a child who may not yet be infected. It is not known whether INVIRASE is excreted in human milk.

Pediatric Use: Safety and effectiveness of INVIRASE in HIV-infected pediatric patients younger than 16 years of age have not been established.

ADVERSE REACTIONS (see PRECAUTIONS)

The safety of INVIRASE was studied in patients who received the drug either alone or in combination with ZDV and/or HIVID (zalcitabine, ddC). The majority of adverse events were of mild intensity. The most frequently reported adverse events among patients receiving INVIRASE (excluding those toxicities known to be associated with ZDV and HIVID when used in combinations) were diarrhea, abdominal discomfort and nausea.

INVIRASE did not alter the pattern, frequency or severity of known major toxicities associated with the use of HIVID and/or ZDV. Physicians should refer to the complete product information for these drugs (or other antiretroviral agents as appropriate) for drug-associated adverse reactions to other nucleoside analogues.

In an open-label protocol, NV15114, in which 33 patients received treatment with INVIRASE, ZDV and lamivudine for 4 to 16 weeks, no unexpected toxicities were reported.

Table 4 lists clinical adverse events that occurred in ≥2% of patients receiving INVIRASE 600 mg tid alone or in combination with ZDV and/or HIVID in two trials. Median duration of treatment in NV14255/ACTG229 (triple-combination

study) was 48 weeks; median duration of treatment in NV14256 (double-combination study) was approximately 1 year.

[See table 4 on next page]

Rare occurrences of the following serious adverse experiences have been reported during clinical trials of INVIRASE and were considered at least possibly related to use of study drugs: confusion, ataxia and weakness; acute myeloblastic leukemia; hemolytic anemia; attempted suicide; Stevens-Johnson syndrome; seizures; severe cutaneous reaction associated with increased liver function tests; isolated elevation of transaminases; thrombophlebitis; headache; thrombocytopenia; exacerbation of chronic liver disease with Grade 4 elevated liver function tests, jaundice, ascites, and right and left upper quadrant abdominal pain; drug fever; bullous skin eruption and polyarthritis; pancreatitis leading to death; nephrolithiasis; thrombocytopenia and intracranial hemorrhage leading to death; peripheral vasoconstriction; portal hypertension; intestinal obstruction. These events were reported from a database of >6000 patients. Over 100 patients on saquinavir therapy have been followed for >2 years.

Table 5 shows the percentage of patients with marked laboratory abnormalities in studies NV14255/ACTG229 and NV14256. Marked laboratory abnormalities are defined as a Grade 3 or 4 abnormality in a patient with a normal baseline value or a Grade 4 abnormality in a patient with a Grade 1 abnormality at baseline (ACTG Grading System).

[See table 5 on next page]

Monotherapy and Combination Studies: Other clinical adverse experiences of any intensity, at least remotely related to INVIRASE, including those in <2% of patients on arms containing INVIRASE in studies NV14255/ACTG229 and NV14256, and those in smaller clinical trials, are listed below by body system.

Body as a Whole: Allergic reaction, anorexia, chest pain, edema, fatigue, fever, intoxication, parasites external, retrosternal pain, shivering, wasting syndrome, weakness generalized, weight decrease

Cardiovascular: Cyanosis, heart murmur, heart valve disorder, hypertension, hypotension, syncope, vein distended

Endocrine/Metabolic: Dehydration, diabetes mellitus, dry eye syndrome, hyperglycemia, weight increase, xerophthalmia

Gastrointestinal: Cheilitis, colic abdominal, constipation, dyspepsia, dysphagia, esophagitis, eructation, feces blood-stained, feces discolored, flatulence, gastralgia, gastritis, gastrointestinal inflammation, gingivitis, glossitis, hemorrhage rectum, hemorrhoids, hepatitis, hepatomegaly, hepatosplenomegaly, infectious diarrhea, jaundice, liver enzyme disorder, melena, pain pelvic, painful defecation, pancreatitis, parotid disorder, salivary glands disorder, stomach upset, stomatitis, toothache, tooth disorder, vomiting

Hematologic: Anemia, bleeding dermal, microhemorrhages, neutropenia, pancytopenia, splenomegaly, thrombocytopenia

Musculoskeletal: Arthralgia, arthritis, back pain, cramps leg, cramps muscle, creatine phosphokinase increased, musculoskeletal disorders, stiffness, tissue changes, trauma

Neurological: Ataxia, bowel movements frequent, confusion, convulsions, dysarthria, dysesthesia, heart rate disorder, hyperesthesia, hyperreflexia, hyporeflexia, light-headed feeling, mouth dry, myelopolyradiculoneuritis, numbness face, pain facial, paresis, poliomyelitis, prickly sensation, progressive multifocal leukoencephalopathy, spasms, tremor, unconsciousness

Psychological: Agitation, amnesia, anxiety, anxiety attack, depression, dreaming excessive, euphoria, hallucination, insomnia, intellectual ability reduced, irritability, lethargy, libido disorder, overdose effect, psychic disorder, psychosis, somnolence, speech disorder, suicide attempt

Reproductive System: Impotence, prostate enlarged, vaginal discharge

Resistance Mechanism: Abscess, angina tonsillaris, candidiasis, cellulitis, herpes simplex, herpes zoster, infection bacterial, infection mycotic, infection staphylococcal, influenza, lymphadenopathy, moniliasis, tumor

Respiratory: Bronchitis, cough, dyspnea, epistaxis, hemoptysis, laryngitis, pharyngitis, pneumonia, pulmonary disease, respiratory disorder, rhinitis, sinusitis, upper respiratory tract infection

Skin and Appendages: Acne, alopecia, chalazion, dermatitis, dermatitis seborrheic, eczema, erythema, folliculitis, furunculosis, hair changes, hot flushes, nail disorder, night sweats, papillomatosis, photosensitivity reaction, pigment changes skin, rash maculopapular, skin disorder, skin nodule, skin ulceration, sweating increased, urticaria, verruca, xeroderma

Special Senses: Blepharitis, earache, ear pressure, eye irritation, hearing decreased, otitis, taste alteration, tinnitus, visual disturbance

Urinary System: Micturition disorder, renal calculus, urinary tract bleeding, urinary tract infection

Continued on next page

Invirase—Cont.

OVERDOSAGE

No acute toxicities or sequelae were noted in 1 patient who ingested 8 grams of INVIRASE as a single dose. The patient was treated with induction of emesis within 2 to 4 hours after ingestion. In an exploratory Phase 2 study of oral dosing with INVIRASE at 7200 mg/day (1200 mg q4h), there were no serious toxicities reported through the first 25 weeks of treatment.

DOSAGE AND ADMINISTRATION

The recommended dose for INVIRASE in combination with a nucleoside analogue is three 200-mg capsules three times daily taken within 2 hours after a full meal. Please refer to the complete product information for each of the nucleoside analogues for the recommended doses of these agents. INVIRASE should be used only in combination with an active antiretroviral nucleoside analogue regimen. Concomitant therapy should be based on a patient's prior drug exposure.

Monitoring of Patients: Clinical chemistry tests should be performed prior to initiating INVIRASE therapy and at appropriate intervals thereafter. For comprehensive patient monitoring recommendations for other nucleoside analogues, physicians should refer to the complete product information for these drugs.

Dose Adjustment for Combination Therapy With INVIRASE: For toxicities that may be associated with INVIRASE, the drug should be interrupted. INVIRASE at doses less than 600 mg tid are not recommended since lower doses have not shown antiviral activity. For recipients of combination therapy with INVIRASE and nucleoside analogues, dose adjustment of the nucleoside analogue should be based on the known toxicity profile of the individual drug. Physicians should refer to the complete product information for these drugs for comprehensive dose adjustment recommendations and drug-associated adverse reactions of nucleoside analogues.

HOW SUPPLIED

INVIRASE 200-mg capsules are light brown and green opaque capsules with ROCHE and 0245 imprinted on the capsule shell – bottles of 270 (NDC 0004-0245-15).

The capsules should be stored at 59° to 86°F (15° to 30°C) in tightly closed bottles.

Table 4. Percentage of Patients, by Study Arm, With Clinical Adverse Experiences Considered at Least Possibly Related to Study Drug or of Unknown Relationship and of Moderate, Severe or Life-threatening Intensity, Occurring in ≥2% of Patients in NV14255/ACTG229 and NV14256

| ADVERSE EVENT | NV14255/ACTG229 | | | | NV14256 | |
	SAQ+ZDV n=99	SAQ+ddC+ZDV n=98	ddC+ZDV n=100	ddC n=325	SAQ n=327	SAQ+ddC n=318
GASTROINTESTINAL						
Diarrhea	3.0	1.0	—	0.9	4.9	4.4
Abdominal Discomfort	2.0	3.1	4.0	0.9	0.9	0.9
Nausea	—	3.1	3.0	1.5	2.4	0.9
Dyspepsia	1.0	1.0	2.0	0.6	0.9	0.9
Abdominal Pain	2.0	1.0	2.0	0.6	1.2	0.3
Mucosa Damage	—	—	4.0	—	—	0.3
Buccal Mucosa Ulceration	—	2.0	2.0	6.2	2.1	3.8
CENTRAL AND PERIPHERAL NERVOUS SYSTEM						
Headache	2.0	2.0	2.0	3.4	2.4	0.9
Paresthesia	2.0	3.1	4.0	1.2	0.3	0.3
Extremity Numbness	2.0	1.0	4.0	1.5	0.6	0.9
Dizziness	—	2.0	1.0	—	0.3	—
Peripheral Neuropathy	—	1.0	2.0	11.4	3.1	11.3
BODY AS A WHOLE						
Asthenia	6.1	9.2	10.0	—	0.3	—
Appetite Disturbances	—	1.0	2.0	—	—	—
SKIN AND APPENDAGES						
Rash	—	—	3.0	1.5	2.1	1.3
Pruritus	—	—	2.0	—	0.6	—
MUSCULOSKELETAL DISORDERS						
Musculoskeletal Pain	2.0	2.0	4.0	0.6	0.6	0.6
Myalgia	1.0	—	3.0	0.6	0.3	0.3

—Indicates no events reported

Table 5. Percentage of Patients, by Treatment Group, With Marked Laboratory Abnormalities* in NV14255/ACTG229 and NV14256

| | NV14255/ACTG229 | | | | NV14256 | |
	SAQ+ZDV n=99	SAQ+ddC+ZDV n=98	ddC+ZDV n=100	ddC n=325	SAQ n=327	SAQ+ddC n=318
BIOCHEMISTRY						
Calcium (high)	1	0	0	<1	0	0
Calcium (low)	—	—	—	<1	<1	0
Creatine Phosphokinase (high)	10	12	7	6	3	7
Glucose (high)	0	0	0	<1	1	1
Glucose (low)	0	0	0	5	5	5
Phosphate (low)	2	1	0	0	<1	<1
Potassium (high)	0	0	0	2	2	3
Potassium (low)	0	0	0	0	1	0
Serum Amylase (high)	2	1	1	2	1	1
SGOT (AST) (high)	2	2	0	2	2	3
SGPT (ALT) (high)	0	3	1	2	2	2
Sodium (high)	—	—	—	0	0	<1
Sodium (low)	—	—	—	0	<1	0
Total Bilirubin (high)	1	0	0	0	<1	1
Uric Acid	0	0	1	Not assessed	Not assessed	Not assessed
HEMATOLOGY						
Neutrophils (low)	2	2	8	1	1	1
Hemoglobin (low)	0	0	1	<1	<1	0
Platelets (low)	0	0	2	1	1	<1

* Marked Laboratory Abnormality defined as a shift from Grade 0 to at least Grade 3 or from Grade 1 to Grade 4 (ACTG Grading System)

Manufactured by F. Hoffmann-La Roche Ltd., Basel, Switzerland or Hoffmann-La Roche Laboratories Inc., Nutley, New Jersey

Revised: January 1998

Shown in Product Identification Guide, page 334

KLONOPIN®

℞

[klon 'o-pin]

(clonazepam)

TABLETS

The following text is complete prescribing information based on official labeling in effect June 1998.

DESCRIPTION

Klonopin, a benzodiazepine, is available as scored tablets with a K-shaped perforation containing 0.5 mg of clonazepam, and unscored tablets with a K-shaped perforation containing 1 mg or 2 mg of clonazepam. Klonopin is also available as round, scored tablets containing 0.5 mg, 1 mg or 2 mg clonazepam. Each tablet also contains lactose, magnesium stearate, microcrystalline cellulose and corn starch, with the following colorants: 0.5 mg—FD&C Yellow No. 6 Lake; 1 mg—FD&C Blue No. 1 Lake and FD&C Blue No. 2 Lake.

Chemically, clonazepam is 5-(2-chlorophenyl)-1,3-dihydro-7-nitro-2H-1,4-benzodiazepin-2-one. It is a light yellow crystalline powder. It has a molecular weight of 315.72.

CLINICAL PHARMACOLOGY

Pharmacodynamics: The precise mechanism by which clonazepam exerts its antiseizure and antipanic effects is unknown, although it is believed to be related to its ability to enhance the activity of gamma aminobutyric acid (GABA), the major inhibitory neurotransmitter in the central nervous system. Convulsions produced in rodents by pentylenetetrazol or, to a lesser extent, electrical stimulation are antagonized, as are convulsions produced by photic stimulation in susceptible baboons. A taming effect in aggressive primates, muscle weakness and hypnosis are also produced. In humans, clonazepam is capable of suppressing the spike and wave discharge in absence seizures (petit mal) and decreasing the frequency, amplitude, duration and spread of discharge in minor motor seizures.

Pharmacokinetics: Clonazepam is rapidly and completely absorbed after oral administration. The absolute bioavailability of clonazepam is about 90%. Maximum plasma concentrations of clonazepam are reached within 1 to 4 hours after oral administration. Clonazepam is approximately 85% bound to plasma proteins. Clonazepam is highly metabolized, with less than 2% unchanged clonazepam being excreted in the urine. Biotransformation occurs mainly by reduction of the 7-nitro group to the 4-amino derivative. This derivative can be acetylated, hydroxylated and glucuronidated. Cytochrome P-450 including CYP3A, may play an important role in clonazepam reduction and oxidation. The elimination half-life of clonazepam is typically 30 to 40 hours. Clonazepam pharmacokinetics are dose-independent throughout the dosing range. There is no evidence that clonazepam induces its own metabolism or that of other drugs in humans.

Pharmacokinetics in Demographic Subpopulations and in Disease States: Controlled studies examining the influence of gender and age on clonazepam pharmacokinetics have not been conducted, nor have the effects of renal or liver disease on clonazepam pharmacokinetics been studied. Because clonazepam undergoes hepatic metabolism, it is possible that liver disease will impair clonazepam elimination. Thus, caution should be exercised when administering clonazepam to these patients.

Clinical Trials: Panic Disorder: The effectiveness of Klonopin in the treatment of panic disorder was demonstrated in two double-blind, placebo-controlled studies of adult outpatients who had a primary diagnosis of panic disorder (DSM-IIIR) with or without agoraphobia. In these studies, Klonopin was shown to be significantly more effective than placebo in treating panic disorder on change from baseline in panic attack frequency, the Clinician's Global Impression Severity of Illness Score and the Clinician's Global Impression Improvement Score.

Study 1 was a 9-week, fixed-dose study involving Klonopin doses of 0.5, 1.0, 2.0, 3.0 or 4.0 mg/day or placebo. This study was conducted in four phases: a 1-week placebo lead-in, a 3-week upward titration, a 6-week fixed dose and a 7-week discontinuance phase. A significant difference from placebo was observed consistently only for the 1.0 mg/day group. The difference between the 1.0 mg dose group and placebo in reduction from baseline in the number of full panic attacks was approximately 1 panic attack per week. At endpoint, 74% of patients receiving clonazepam 1.0 mg/day were free of full panic attacks, compared to 56% of placebo-treated patients.

Study 2 was a 6-week, flexible-dose study involving Klonopin in a dose range of 0.5 to 4 mg/day or placebo. This study was conducted in three phases: a 1-week placebo lead-

in, a 6-week optimal-dose and a 6-week discontinuance phase. The mean clonazepam dose during the optimal dosing period was 2.3 mg/day. The difference between Klonopin and placebo in reduction from baseline in the number of full panic attacks was approximately 1 panic attack per week. At endpoint, 62% of patients receiving clonazepam were free of full panic attacks, compared to 37% of placebo-treated patients.

Subgroup analyses did not indicate that there were any differences in treatment outcomes as a function of race or gender.

INDICATIONS AND USAGE

Seizure Disorders: Klonopin is useful alone or as an adjunct in the treatment of the Lennox-Gastaut syndrome (petit mal variant), akinetic and myoclonic seizures. In patients with absence seizures (petit mal) who have failed to respond to succinimides, Klonopin may be useful.

In some studies, up to 30% of patients have shown a loss of anticonvulsant activity, often within 3 months of administration. In some cases, dosage adjustment may reestablish efficacy.

Panic Disorder: Klonopin is indicated for the treatment of panic disorder, with or without agoraphobia, as defined in DSM-IV. Panic disorder is characterized by the occurrence of unexpected panic attacks and associated concern about having additional attacks, worry about the implications or consequences of the attacks, and/or a significant change in behavior related to the attacks.

The efficacy of Klonopin was established in two 6- to 9-week trials in panic disorder patients whose diagnoses corresponded to the DSM-IIIR category of panic disorder (see CLINICAL PHARMACOLOGY: *Clinical Trials*).

Panic disorder (DSM-IV) is characterized by recurrent unexpected panic attacks, ie, a discrete period of intense fear or discomfort in which four (or more) of the following symptoms develop abruptly and reach a peak within 10 minutes: (1) palpitations, pounding heart or accelerated heart rate; (2) sweating; (3) trembling or shaking; (4) sensations of shortness of breath or smothering; (5) feeling of choking; (6) chest pain or discomfort; (7) nausea or abdominal distress; (8) feeling dizzy, unsteady, lightheaded or faint; (9) derealization (feelings of unreality) or depersonalization (being detached from oneself); (10) fear of losing control; (11) fear of dying; (12) paresthesias (numbness or tingling sensations); (13) chills or hot flushes.

The effectiveness of Klonopin in long-term use, that is, for more than 9 weeks, has not been systematically studied in controlled clinical trials. The physician who elects to use Klonopin for extended periods should periodically reevaluate the long-term usefulness of the drug for the individual patient (see DOSAGE AND ADMINISTRATION).

CONTRAINDICATIONS

Klonopin should not be used in patients with a history of sensitivity to benzodiazepines, nor in patients with clinical or biochemical evidence of significant liver disease. It may be used in patients with open angle glaucoma who are receiving appropriate therapy but is contraindicated in acute narrow angle glaucoma.

WARNINGS

Interference with Cognitive and Motor Performance: Since Klonopin produces CNS depression, patients receiving this drug should be cautioned against engaging in hazardous occupations requiring mental alertness, such as operating machinery or driving a motor vehicle. They should also be warned about the concomitant use of alcohol or other CNS-depressant drugs during Klonopin therapy (see *Drug Interactions* and *Information for Patients* under PRECAUTIONS).

Pregnancy Risks: Data from several sources raise concerns about the use of Klonopin during pregnancy.

Animal Findings: In three studies in which Klonopin was administered orally to pregnant rabbits at doses of 0.2, 1.0, 5.0 or 10.0 mg/kg/day (low dose approximately 0.2 times the maximum recommended human dose of 20 mg/day for seizure disorders and equivalent to the maximum dose of 4 mg/day for panic disorder, on a mg/m² basis) during the period of organogenesis, a similar pattern of malformations (cleft palate, open eyelid, fused sternebrae and limb defects) was observed in a low, non-dose-related incidence in exposed litters from all dosage groups. Reductions in maternal weight gain occurred at dosages of 5 mg/kg/day or greater and reduction in embryo-fetal growth occurred in one study at a dosage of 10 mg/kg/day. No adverse maternal or embryo-fetal effects were observed in mice and rats following administration during organogenesis of oral doses up to 15 mg/kg/day or 40 mg/kg/day, respectively (4 and 20 times the maximum recommended human dose of 20 mg/day for seizure disorders and 20 and 100 times the maximum dose of 4 mg/day for panic disorder, respectively, on a mg/m² basis).

General Concerns and Considerations About Anticonvulsants: Recent reports suggest an association between the use of anticonvulsant drugs by women with epilepsy and an elevated incidence of birth defects in children born to these women. Data are more extensive with respect to diphenylhydantoin and phenobarbital, but these are also the most

commonly prescribed anticonvulsants; less systematic or anecdotal reports suggest a possible similar association with the use of all known anticonvulsant drugs.

In children of women treated with drugs for epilepsy, reports suggesting an elevated incidence of birth defects cannot be regarded as adequate to prove a definite cause and effect relationship. There are intrinsic methodologic problems in obtaining adequate data on drug teratogenicity in humans; the possibility also exists that other factors (eg, genetic factors or the epileptic condition itself) may be more important than drug therapy in leading to birth defects. The great majority of mothers on anticonvulsant medication deliver normal infants. It is important to note that anticonvulsant drugs should not be discontinued in patients in whom the drug is administered to prevent seizures because of the strong possibility of precipitating status epilepticus with attendant hypoxia and threat to life. In individual cases where the severity and frequency of the seizure disorder are such that the removal of medication does not pose a serious threat to the patient, discontinuation of the drug may be considered prior to and during pregnancy; however, it cannot be said with any confidence that even mild seizures do not pose some hazards to the developing embryo or fetus.

General Concerns About Benzodiazepines: An increased risk of congenital malformations associated with the use of benzodiazepine drugs has been suggested in several studies. There may also be non-teratogenic risks associated with the use of benzodiazepines during pregnancy. There have been reports of neonatal flaccidity, respiratory and feeding difficulties, and hypothermia in children born to mothers who have been receiving benzodiazepines late in pregnancy. In addition, children born to mothers receiving benzodiazepines late in pregnancy may be at some risk of experiencing withdrawal symptoms during the postnatal period.

Advice Regarding the Use of Klonopin in Women of Childbearing Potential: In general, the use of Klonopin in women of childbearing potential, and more specifically during known pregnancy, should be considered only when the clinical situation warrants the risk to the fetus.

The specific considerations addressed above regarding the use of anticonvulsants for epilepsy in women of childbearing potential should be weighed in treating or counseling these women.

Because of experience with other members of the benzodiazepine class, Klonopin is assumed to be capable of causing an increased risk of congenital abnormalities when administered to a pregnant woman during the first trimester. Because use of these drugs is rarely a matter of urgency in the treatment of panic disorder, their use during the first trimester should almost always be avoided. The possibility that a woman of childbearing potential may be pregnant at the time of institution of therapy should be considered. If this drug is used during pregnancy, or if the patient becomes pregnant while taking this drug, the patient should be apprised of the potential hazard to the fetus. Patients should also be advised that if they become pregnant during therapy or intend to become pregnant, they should communicate with their physician about the desirability of discontinuing the drug.

Withdrawal Symptoms: Withdrawal symptoms of the barbiturate type have occurred after the discontinuation of benzodiazepines (see DRUG ABUSE AND DEPENDENCE section).

PRECAUTIONS

General: Worsening of Seizures: When used in patients in whom several different types of seizure disorders coexist, Klonopin may increase the incidence or precipitate the onset of generalized tonic-clonic seizures (grand mal). This may require the addition of appropriate anticonvulsants or an increase in their dosages. The concomitant use of valproic acid and Klonopin may produce absence status.

Laboratory Testing During Long-Term Therapy: Periodic blood counts and liver function tests are advisable during long-term therapy with Klonopin.

Risks of Abrupt Withdrawal: The abrupt withdrawal of Klonopin, particularly in those patients on long-term, high-dose therapy, may precipitate status epilepticus. Therefore, when discontinuing Klonopin, gradual withdrawal is essential. While Klonopin is being gradually withdrawn, the simultaneous substitution of another anticonvulsant may be indicated.

Caution in Renally Impaired Patients: Metabolites of Klonopin are excreted by the kidneys; to avoid their excess accumulation, caution should be exercised in the administration of the drug to patients with impaired renal function.

Hypersalivation: Klonopin may produce an increase in salivation. This should be considered before giving the drug to patients who have difficulty handling secretions. Because of this and the possibility of respiratory depression, Klonopin should be used with caution in patients with chronic respiratory diseases.

Information for Patients: Physicians are advised to discuss the following issues with patients for whom they prescribe Klonopin:

Dose Changes: To assure the safe and effective use of benzodiazepines, patients should be informed that, since benzodiazepines may produce psychological and physical dependence, it is advisable that they consult with their physician before either increasing the dose or abruptly discontinuing this drug.

Interference with Cognitive and Motor Performance: Because benzodiazepines have the potential to impair judgment, thinking or motor skills, patients should be cautioned about operating hazardous machinery, including automobiles, until they are reasonably certain that Klonopin therapy does not affect them adversely.

Pregnancy: Patients should be advised to notify their physician if they become pregnant or intend to become pregnant during therapy with Klonopin (see WARNINGS).

Nursing: Patients should be advised not to breastfeed an infant if they are taking Klonopin.

Concomitant Medication: Patients should be advised to inform their physicians if they are taking, or plan to take, any prescription or over-the-counter drugs, since there is a potential for interactions.

Alcohol: Patients should be advised to avoid alcohol while taking Klonopin.

Drug Interactions: *Effect of Clonazepam on the Pharmacokinetics of Other Drugs:* Clonazepam does not appear to alter the pharmacokinetics of phenytoin, carbamazepine or phenobarbital. The effect of clonazepam on the metabolism of other drugs has not been investigated.

Effect of Other Drugs on the Pharmacokinetics of Clonazepam: Ranitidine and propantheline, agents that decrease stomach acidity, do not greatly alter clonazepam pharmacokinetics. Fluoxetine does not affect the pharmacokinetics of clonazepam. Cytochrome P-450 inducers, such as phenytoin, carbamazepine and phenobarbital, induce clonazepam metabolism, causing an approximately 30% decrease in plasma clonazepam levels. Although clinical studies have not been performed, based on the involvement of the cytochrome P-450 3A family in clonazepam metabolism, inhibitors of this enzyme system, notably oral antifungal agents, should be used cautiously in patients receiving clonazepam.

Pharmacodynamic Interactions: The CNS-depressant action of the benzodiazepine class of drugs may be potentiated by alcohol, narcotics, barbiturates, nonbarbiturate hypnotics, antianxiety agents, the phenothiazines, thioxanthene and butyrophenone classes of antipsychotic agents, monoamine oxidase inhibitors and the tricyclic antidepressants, and by other anticonvulsant drugs.

Carcinogenesis, Mutagenesis, Impairment of Fertility: Carcinogenicity studies have not been conducted with clonazepam.

The data currently available are not sufficient to determine the genotoxic potential of clonazepam.

In a two-generation fertility study in which clonazepam was given orally to rats at 10 and 100 mg/kg/day (low dose approximately 5 times and 24 times the maximum recommended human dose of 20 mg/day for seizure disorder and 4 mg/day for panic disorder, respectively, on a mg/m² basis), there was a decrease in the number of pregnancies and in the number of offspring surviving until weaning.

Pregnancy: Teratogenic Effects: Pregnancy Category D (see WARNINGS).

Labor and Delivery: The effect of Klonopin on labor and delivery in humans has not been specifically studied; however, perinatal complications have been reported in children born to mothers who have been receiving benzodiazepines late in pregnancy, including findings suggestive of either excess benzodiazepine exposure or of withdrawal phenomena (see *Pregnancy Risks* under WARNINGS).

Nursing Mothers: Mothers receiving Klonopin should not breastfeed their infants.

Pediatric Use: Because of the possibility that adverse effects on physical or mental development could become apparent only after many years, a benefit-risk consideration of the long-term use of Klonopin is important in pediatric patients being treated for seizure disorder (see INDICATIONS and DOSAGE AND ADMINISTRATION sections).

Safety and effectiveness in pediatric patients with panic disorder below the age of 18 have not been established.

ADVERSE REACTIONS

The adverse experiences for Klonopin are provided separately for patients with seizure disorders and with panic disorder.

Seizure Disorders: The most frequently occurring side effects of Klonopin are referable to CNS depression. Experience in treatment of seizures has shown that drowsiness has occurred in approximately 50% of patients and ataxia in approximately 30%. In some cases, these may diminish with time; behavior problems have been noted in approximately 25% of patients. Others, listed by system, are:

Neurologic: Abnormal eye movements, aphonia, choreiform movements, coma, diplopia, dysarthria, dysdiadochokinesis, "glassy-eyed" appearance, headache, hemiparesis,

Continued on next page

Klonopin—Cont.

hypotonia, nystagmus, respiratory depression, slurred speech, tremor, vertigo.

Psychiatric: Confusion, depression, amnesia, hallucinations, hysteria, increased libido, insomnia, psychosis, suicidal attempt (the behavior effects are more likely to occur in patients with a history of psychiatric disturbances). The following paradoxical reactions have been observed: excitability, irritability, aggressive behavior, agitation, nervousness, hostility, anxiety, sleep disturbances, nightmares and vivid dreams.

Respiratory: Chest congestion, rhinorrhea, shortness of breath, hypersecretion in upper respiratory passages.

Cardiovascular: Palpitations.

Dermatologic: Hair loss, hirsutism, skin rash, ankle and facial edema.

Gastrointestinal: Anorexia, coated tongue, constipation, diarrhea, dry mouth, encopresis, gastritis, increased appetite, nausea, sore gums.

Genitourinary: Dysuria, enuresis, nocturia, urinary retention.

Musculoskeletal: Muscle weakness, pains.

Miscellaneous: Dehydration, general deterioration, fever, lymphadenopathy, weight loss or gain.

Hematopoietic: Anemia, leukopenia, thrombocytopenia, eosinophilia.

Hepatic: Hepatomegaly, transient elevations of serum transaminases and alkaline phosphatase.

Panic Disorder: Adverse events during exposure to Klonopin were obtained by spontaneous report and recorded by clinical investigators using terminology of their own choosing. Consequently, it is not possible to provide a meaningful estimate of the proportion of individuals experiencing adverse events without first grouping similar types of events into a smaller number of standardized event categories. In the tables and tabulations that follow, CIGY dictionary terminology has been used to classify reported adverse events, except in certain cases in which redundant terms were collapsed into more meaningful terms, as noted below. The stated frequencies of adverse events represent the proportion of individuals who experienced, at least once, a treatment-emergent adverse event of the type listed. An event was considered treatment-emergent if it occurred for the first time or worsened while receiving therapy following baseline evaluation.

Adverse Findings Observed in Short-Term, Placebo-Controlled Trials: Adverse Events Associated with Discontinuation of Treatment:

Overall, the incidence of discontinuation due to adverse events was 17% in Klonopin compared to 9% for placebo in the combined data of two 6- to 9-week trials. The most common events (≥1%) associated with discontinuation and a dropout rate twice or greater for Klonopin than that of placebo included the following:

Adverse Event	Klonopin (N=574)	Placebo (N=294)
Somnolence	7%	1%
Depression	4%	1%
Dizziness	1%	<1%
Nervousness	1%	0%
Ataxia	1%	0%
Intellectual Ability Reduced	1%	0%

Adverse Events Occurring at an Incidence of 1% or More Among Klonopin-Treated Patients:

Table 1 enumerates the incidence, rounded to the nearest percent, of treatment-emergent adverse events that occurred during acute therapy of panic disorder from a pool of two 6- to 9-week trials. Events reported in 1% or more of patients treated with Klonopin (doses ranging from 0.5 to 4 mg/day) and for which the incidence was greater than that in placebo-treated patients are included.

The prescriber should be aware that the figures in Table 1 cannot be used to predict the incidence of side effects in the course of usual medical practice where patient characteristics and other factors differ from those that prevailed in the clinical trials. Similarly, the cited frequencies cannot be compared with figures obtained from other clinical investigations involving different treatments, uses and investigators. The cited figures, however, do provide the prescribing physician with some basis for estimating the relative contribution of drug and nondrug factors to the side effect incidence in the population studied.

[See table 1 at left]

Commonly Observed Adverse Events:

Table 2. Incidence of Most Commonly Observed Adverse Events* in Acute Therapy in Pool of 6- to 9-Week Trials

Adverse Event (Roche Preferred Term)	Clonazepam (N=574)	Placebo (N=294)
Somnolence	37%	10%
Depression	7%	1%
Coordination Abnormal	6%	0%
Ataxia	5%	0%

*Treatment-emergent events for which the incidence in the clonazepam patients was ≥5% and at least twice that in the placebo patients.

Treatment-Emergent Depressive Symptoms: In the pool of two short-term placebo-controlled trials, adverse events classified under the preferred term "depression" were reported in 7% of Klonopin-treated patients compared to 1% of placebo-treated patients, without any clear pattern of dose relatedness. In these same trials, adverse events classified under the preferred term "depression" were reported as leading to discontinuation in 4% of Klonopin-treated patients compared to 1% of placebo-treated patients. While these findings are noteworthy, Hamilton Depression Rating Scale (HAM-D) data collected in these trials revealed a larger decline in HAM-D scores in the clonazepam group than the placebo group suggesting that clonazepam-treated patients were not experiencing a worsening or emergence of clinical depression.

Other Adverse Events Observed During the Premarketing Evaluation of Klonopin in Panic Disorder:

Following is a list of modified CIGY terms that reflect treatment-emergent adverse events reported by patients treated with Klonopin at multiple doses during clinical trials. All reported events are included except those already listed in Table 1 or elsewhere in labeling, those events for which a drug cause was remote, those event terms which were so general as to be uninformative, and events reported only once and which did not have a substantial probability of being acutely life-threatening. It is important to emphasize that, although the events occurred during treatment with Klonopin, they were not necessarily caused by it.

Events are further categorized by body system and listed in order of decreasing frequency. These adverse events were reported infrequently, which is defined as occurring in 1/100 to 1/1000 patients.

Table 1. Treatment-Emergent Adverse Event Incidence in 6- to 9-Week Placebo-Controlled Clinical Trials*

Clonazepam Maximum Daily Dose

Adverse Event by Body System	<1 mg n=96 %	1-<2 mg n=129 %	2-<3 mg n=113 %	≥3 mg n=235 %	All Klonopin Groups N=574 %	Placebo N=294 %
Central & Peripheral Nervous System						
Somnolence†	26	35	50	36	37	10
Dizziness	5	5	12	8	8	4
Coordination Abnormal†	1	2	7	9	6	0
Ataxia†	2	1	8	8	5	0
Dysarthria†	0	0	4	3	2	0
Psychiatric						
Depression	7	6	8	8	7	1
Memory Disturbance	2	5	2	5	4	2
Nervousness	1	4	3	4	3	2
Intellectual Ability Reduced	0	2	4	3	2	0
Emotional Lability	0	1	2	2	1	1
Libido Decreased	0	1	3	1	1	0
Confusion	0	2	2	1	1	0
Respiratory System						
Upper Respiratory Tract Infection†	10	10	7	6	8	4
Sinusitis	4	2	8	4	4	3
Rhinitis	3	2	4	2	2	1
Coughing	2	2	4	0	2	0
Pharyngitis	1	1	3	2	2	1
Bronchitis	1	0	2	2	1	1
Gastrointestinal System						
Constipation†	0	1	5	3	2	2
Appetite Decreased	1	1	0	3	1	1
Abdominal Pain†	2	2	2	0	1	1
Body as a Whole						
Fatigue	9	6	7	7	7	4
Allergic Reaction	3	1	4	2	2	1
Musculoskeletal						
Myalgia	2	1	4	0	1	1
Resistance Mechanism Disorders						
Influenza	3	2	5	5	4	3
Urinary System						
Micturition Frequency	1	2	2	1	1	0
Urinary Tract Infection†	0	0	2	2	1	0
Vision Disorders						
Blurred Vision	1	2	3	0	1	1
Reproductive Disorders‡						
Female						
Dysmenorrhea	0	6	5	2	3	2
Colpitis	4	0	2	1	1	1
Male						
Ejaculation Delayed	0	0	2	2	1	0
Impotence	3	0	2	1	1	0

* Events reported by at least 1% of patients treated with Klonopin and for which the incidence was greater than that for placebo.

† Indicates that the p-value for the dose-trend test (Cochran-Mantel-Haenszel) for adverse event incidence was ≤0.10.

‡ Denominators for events in gender-specific systems are n=240 (clonazepam), 102 (placebo) for male, and 334 (clonazepam), 192 (placebo) for female.

Body as a Whole: weight increase, accident, weight decrease, wound, edema, fever, shivering, abrasions, ankle edema, edema foot, edema periorbital, injury, malaise, pain, cellulitis, inflammation localized
Cardiovascular Disorders: chest pain, hypotension postural
Central and Peripheral Nervous System Disorders: migraine, paresthesia, drunkenness, feeling of enuresis, paresis, tremor, burning skin, falling, head fullness, hoarseness, hyperactivity, hypoesthesia, tongue thick, twitching
Gastrointestinal System Disorders: abdominal discomfort, gastrointestinal inflammation, stomach upset, toothache, flatulence, pyrosis, saliva increased, tooth disorder, bowel movements frequent, pain pelvic, dyspepsia, hemorrhoids
Hearing and Vestibular Disorders: vertigo, otitis, earache, motion sickness
Heart Rate and Rhythm Disorders: palpitation
Metabolic and Nutritional Disorders: thirst, gout
Musculoskeletal System Disorders: back pain, fracture traumatic, sprains and strains, pain leg, pain nape, cramps muscle, cramps leg, pain ankle, pain shoulder, tendinitis, arthralgia, hypertonia, lumbago, pain feet, pain jaw, pain knee, swelling knee
Platelet, Bleeding and Clotting Disorders: bleeding dermal
Psychiatric Disorders: insomnia, organic disinhibition, anxiety, depersonalization, dreaming excessive, libido loss, appetite increased, libido increased, reactions decreased, aggressive reaction, apathy, attention lack, excitement, feeling mad, hunger abnormal, illusion, nightmares, sleep disorder, suicide ideation, yawning
Reproductive Disorders, Female: breast pain, menstrual irregularity
Reproductive Disorders, Male: ejaculation decreased
Resistance Mechanism Disorders: infection mycotic, infection viral, infection streptococcal, herpes simplex infection, infectious mononucleosis, moniliasis
Respiratory System Disorders: sneezing excessive, asthmatic attack, dyspnea, nosebleed, pneumonia, pleurisy
Skin and Appendages Disorders: acne flare, alopecia, xeroderma, dermatitis contact, flushing, pruritus, pustular reaction, skin burns, skin disorder
Special Senses Other, Disorders: taste loss
Urinary System Disorders: dysuria, cystitis, polyuria, urinary incontinence, bladder dysfunction, urinary retention, urinary tract bleeding, urine discoloration
Vascular (Extracardiac) Disorders: thrombophlebitis leg
Vision Disorders: eye irritation, visual disturbance, diplopia, eye twitching, styes, visual field defect, xerophthalmia

DRUG ABUSE AND DEPENDENCE

Controlled Substance Class: Clonazepam is a Schedule IV controlled substance.

Physical and Psychological Dependence: Withdrawal symptoms, similar in character to those noted with barbiturates and alcohol (eg, convulsions, psychosis, hallucinations, behavioral disorder, tremor, abdominal and muscle cramps) have occurred following abrupt discontinuance of clonazepam. The more severe withdrawal symptoms have usually been limited to those patients who received excessive doses over an extended period of time. Generally milder withdrawal symptoms (eg, dysphoria and insomnia) have been reported following abrupt discontinuance of benzodiazepines taken continuously at therapeutic levels for several months. Consequently, after extended therapy, abrupt discontinuation should generally be avoided and a gradual dosage tapering schedule followed (see DOSAGE AND ADMINISTRATION section). Addiction-prone individuals (such as drug addicts or alcoholics) should be under careful surveillance when receiving clonazepam or other psychotropic agents because of the predisposition of such patients to habituation and dependence.

Following the short-term treatment of patients with panic disorder in Studies 1 and 2 (see CLINICAL PHARMACOLOGY: *Clinical Trials*), patients were gradually withdrawn during a 7-week downward-titration (discontinuance) period. Overall, the discontinuance period was associated with good tolerability and a very modest clinical deterioration, without evidence of a significant rebound phenomenon. However, there are not sufficient data from adequate and well-controlled long-term clonazepam studies in patients with panic disorder to accurately estimate the risks of withdrawal symptoms and dependence that may be associated with such use.

OVERDOSAGE

Human Experience: Symptoms of clonazepam overdosage, like those produced by other CNS depressants, include somnolence, confusion, coma and diminished reflexes.

Overdose Management: Treatment includes monitoring of respiration, pulse and blood pressure, general supportive measures and immediate gastric lavage. Intravenous fluids should be administered and an adequate airway maintained. Hypotension may be combated by the use of levarterenol or metaraminol. Dialysis is of no known value.

Flumazenil, a specific benzodiazepine-receptor antagonist, is indicated for the complete or partial reversal of the sedative effects of benzodiazepines and may be used in situations when an overdose with a benzodiazepine is known or suspected. Prior to the administration of flumazenil, necessary measures should be instituted to secure airway, ventilation and intravenous access. Flumazenil is intended as an adjunct to, not as a substitute for, proper management of benzodiazepine overdose. Patients treated with flumazenil should be monitored for resedation, respiratory depression and other residual benzodiazepine effects for an appropriate period after treatment. **The prescriber should be aware of a risk of seizure in association with flumazenil treatment, particularly in long-term benzodiazepine users and in cyclic antidepressant overdose.** The complete flumazenil package insert, including CONTRAINDICATIONS, WARNINGS and PRECAUTIONS, should be consulted prior to use.

Flumazenil is not indicated in patients with epilepsy who have been treated with benzodiazepines. Antagonism of the benzodiazepine effect in such patients may provoke seizures.

Serious sequelae are rare unless other drugs or alcohol have been taken concomitantly.

DOSAGE AND ADMINISTRATION

Seizure Disorders: *Adults*: The initial dose for adults with seizure disorders should not exceed 1.5 mg/day divided into three doses. Dosage may be increased in increments of 0.5 to 1 mg every 3 days until seizures are adequately controlled or until side effects preclude any further increase. Maintenance dosage must be individualized for each patient depending upon response. Maximum recommended daily dose is 20 mg.

The use of multiple anticonvulsants may result in an increase of depressant adverse effects. This should be considered before adding Klonopin to an existing anticonvulsant regimen.

Pediatric Patients: Klonopin is administered orally. In order to minimize drowsiness, the initial dose for infants and children (up to 10 years of age or 30 kg of body weight) should be between 0.01 and 0.03 mg/kg/day but not to exceed 0.05 mg/kg/day given in two or three divided doses. Dosage should be increased by no more than 0.25 to 0.5 mg every third day until a daily maintenance dose of 0.1 to 0.2 mg/kg of body weight has been reached, unless seizures are controlled or side effects preclude further increase. Whenever possible, the daily dose should be divided into three equal doses. If doses are not equally divided, the largest dose should be given before retiring.

Panic Disorder: *Adults*: The initial dose for adults with panic disorder is 0.25 mg bid. An increase to the target dose for most patients of 1 mg/day may be made after 3 days. The recommended dose of 1 mg/day is based on the results from a fixed dose study in which the optimal effect was seen at 1 mg/day. Higher doses of 2, 3 and 4 mg/day in that study were less effective than the 1 mg/day dose and were associated with more adverse effects. Nevertheless, it is possible that some individual patients may benefit from doses of up to a maximum dose of 4 mg/day, and in those instances, the dose may be increased in increments of 0.125 to 0.25 mg bid every 3 days until panic disorder is controlled or until side effects make further increases undesired. To reduce the inconvenience of somnolence, administration of one dose at bedtime may be desirable.

Treatment should be discontinued gradually, with a decrease of 0.125 mg bid every 3 days, until the drug is completely withdrawn.

There is no body of evidence available to answer the question of how long the patient treated with clonazepam should remain on it. Therefore, the physician who elects to use Klonopin for extended periods should periodically reevaluate the long-term usefulness of the drug for the individual patient.

Pediatric Patients: There is no clinical trial experience with Klonopin in panic disorder patients under 18 years of age.

HOW SUPPLIED

Scored tablets with a K-shaped perforation—0.5 mg, orange (NDC 0004-0068-01); and unscored tablets with a K-shaped perforation—1 mg, blue (NDC 0004-0058-01); 2 mg, white (NDC 0004-0098-01)—bottles of 100. Imprint on tablets:

0.5 mg—1/2 KLONOPIN (front)
ROCHE (scored side)

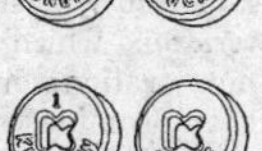

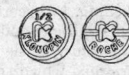

1 mg—1 KLONOPIN (front)
ROCHE (reverse side)

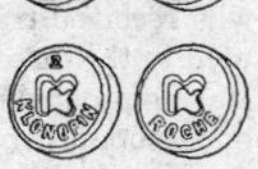

2 mg—2 KLONOPIN (front)
ROCHE (reverse side)

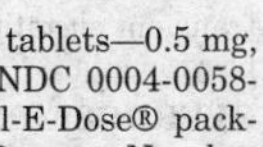

Klonopin is also available as round, scored tablets—0.5 mg, orange (NDC 0004-0068-50); 1 mg, blue (NDC 0004-0058-50); 2 mg, white (NDC 0004-0098-50)–Tel-E-Dose® packages of 100, available in boxes of four Reverse Number Packs of 25.

Store at 50° to 86°F (15° to 37°C).

Manufactured by Roche Pharma, Inc.

Manati, Puerto Rico 00674 or Roche Laboratories Inc. Nutley, New Jersey 07110-1199

Revised: October 1997

Shown in Product Identification Guide, page 334

LARIAM® ℞

[lar-é-um]

brand of mefloquine hydrochloride
TABLETS

The following text is complete prescribing information based on official labeling in effect June 1998.

DESCRIPTION

Lariam (mefloquine hydrochloride) is an antimalarial agent available as 250-mg tablets of mefloquine hydrochloride (equivalent to 228.0 mg of the free base) for oral administration.

Mefloquine hydrochloride is a 4-quinolinemethanol derivative with the specific chemical name of (R*, S*)-(±)-α-2-piperidinyl-2,8-bis (trifluoromethyl)-4-quinolinemethanol hydrochloride. It is a 2-aryl substituted chemical structural analog of quinine. The drug is a white to almost white crystalline compound, slightly soluble in water.

Mefloquine hydrochloride has a calculated molecular weight of 414.78.

The inactive ingredients are ammonium-calcium alginate, corn starch, crospovidone, lactose, magnesium stearate, microcrystalline cellulose, poloxamer #331 and talc.

CLINICAL PHARMACOLOGY

Mefloquine is an antimalarial agent which acts as a blood schizonticide. Its exact mechanism of action is not known.

Pharmacokinetic studies of mefloquine in healthy male subjects showed that a significant lagtime occurred after drug administration, and the terminal elimination half-life varied widely (13 to 24 days) with a mean of about 3 weeks. Mefloquine is a mixture of enantiomeric molecules whose rates of release, absorption, transport, action, degradation and elimination may differ. A valid pharmacokinetic model may not exist in such a case.

Additional studies in European subjects showed slightly greater concentrations of drug for longer periods of time. The absorption half-life was 0.36 to 2 hours, and the terminal elimination half-life was 15 to 33 days. The primary metabolite was identified and its concentrations were found to surpass the concentrations of mefloquine.

Multiple-dose kinetic studies confirmed the long elimination half-lives previously observed. The mean metabolite to mefloquine ratio measured at steady-state was found to range between 2.3 and 8.6.

The total clearance of the drug, which is essentially all hepatic, is approximately 30 mL/min. The volume of distribution, approximately 20 L/kg, indicates extensive distribution. The drug is highly bound (98%) to plasma proteins and concentrated in blood erythrocytes, the target cells in malaria, at a relatively constant erythrocyte-to-plasma concentration ratio of about 2.

The pharmacokinetics of mefloquine in patients with compromised renal function and compromised hepatic function have not been studied.

In vitro and *in vivo* studies showed no hemolysis associated with glucose-6-phosphate dehydrogenase deficiency. (See ANIMAL TOXICOLOGY for additional information.)

Microbiology: Strains of *Plasmodium falciparum* resistant to mefloquine have been reported.

INDICATIONS AND USAGE

Treatment of Acute Malaria Infections: Lariam is indicated for the treatment of mild to moderate acute malaria caused by mefloquine-susceptible strains of *P. falciparum* (both chloroquine-susceptible and resistant strains) or by *Plasmodium vivax*. There are insufficient clinical data to document the effect of mefloquine in malaria caused by *P. ovale* or *P. malariae*.

Note: Patients with acute *P. vivax* malaria, treated with Lariam, are at high risk of relapse because Lariam does not eliminate exoerythrocytic (hepatic phase) parasites. To avoid relapse, after initial treatment of the acute infection with Lariam, patients should subsequently be treated with an 8-aminoquinoline (eg, primaquine).

Prevention of Malaria: Lariam is indicated for the prophylaxis of *P. falciparum* and *P. vivax* malaria infections, including prophylaxis of chloroquine-resistant strains of *P. falciparum*.

CONTRAINDICATIONS

Use of this drug is contraindicated in patients with a known hypersensitivity to mefloquine or related compounds (eg, quinine).

Continued on next page

Lariam—Cont.

WARNINGS

In case of life-threatening, serious or overwhelming malaria infections due to *P. falciparum*, patients should be treated with an intravenous antimalarial drug. Following completion of intravenous treatment, Lariam may be given orally to complete the course of therapy.

Concomitant administration of Lariam and quinine, quinidine or drugs producing beta-adrenergic blockade may produce electrocardiographic abnormalities or cardiac arrest. Concomitant administration of Lariam and quinine or chloroquine may increase the risk of convulsions. Data on the use of halofantrine subsequent to administration of Lariam suggests a significant, potentially fatal, prolongation of the QTc interval of the ECG. Therefore, halofantrine should not be given simultaneously with or subsequent to Lariam. (see PRECAUTIONS: *Drug Interactions*.)

PRECAUTIONS

General: Caution should be exercised with regard to driving, piloting airplanes and operating machines, as dizziness, a disturbed sense of balance, neurological or psychiatric reactions have been reported during and following the use of Lariam. These effects may occur after therapy is discontinued due to the long half-life of the drug. During prophylactic use, if signs of unexplained anxiety, depression, restlessness or confusion are noticed, these may be considered prodromal to a more serious event. In these cases, the drug must be discontinued. Larium should be used with caution in patients with psychiatric disturbances because mefloquine use has been associated with emotional disturbances (see ADVERSE REACTIONS section).

This drug has not been administered for longer than 1 year. If the drug is to be administered for a prolonged period, periodic evaluations including liver function tests should be performed. Although retinal abnormalities seen in humans with long-term chloroquine use have not been observed with mefloquine use, long-term feeding of mefloquine to rats resulted in dose-related ocular lesions (retinal degeneration, retinal edema and lenticular opacity at 12.5 mg/kg/day and higher). (See ANIMAL TOXICOLOGY.) Therefore, periodic ophthalmic examinations are recommended.

Parenteral studies in animals show that mefloquine, a myocardial depressant, possesses 20% of the antifibrillatory action of quinidine and produces 50% of the increase in the PR interval reported with quinine. The effect of mefloquine on the compromised cardiovascular system has not been evaluated. However, transitory and clinically silent ECG alterations have been reported during the use of mefloquine. Alterations included sinus bradycardia, sinus arrhythmia, first degree AV-block, prolongation of the QTc interval and abnormal T waves (see also cardiovascular effects under PRECAUTIONS: *Drug Interactions* and ADVERSE REACTIONS). The benefits of Lariam therapy should be weighed against the possibility of adverse effects in patients with cardiac disease.

Laboratory Tests: Periodic evaluation of hepatic function should be performed during prolonged prophylaxis.

Drug Interactions: Drug-drug interactions with Lariam have not been explored in detail. There is one report of cardiopulmonary arrest, with full recovery, in a patient who was taking a beta blocker (propranolol), (see also WARNINGS and PRECAUTIONS: *General*). The effects of mefloquine on the compromised cardiovascular system have not been evaluated. The benefits of Lariam therapy should be weighed against the possibility of adverse effects in patients with cardiac disease.

Because of the danger of a potentially fatal prolongation of the QTc interval, halofantrine should not be given simultaneously with or subsequent to Lariam (see also WARNINGS).

Lariam should not be used concurrently with quinine or quinidine. If these drugs are to be used in the initial treatment of severe malaria, Lariam administration should be delayed at least 12 hours after the last dose.

Patients taking Lariam while taking valproic acid had loss of seizure control and lower than expected valproic acid blood levels. Therefore, patients concurrently taking antiseizure medication and Lariam should have the blood level of their antiseizure medication monitored and the dosage adjusted appropriately.

In clinical trials the concomitant administration of sulfadoxine and pyrimethamine did not alter the adverse reaction profile.

Carcinogenesis, Mutagenesis, Impairment of Fertility:

Carcinogenesis: The carcinogenic potential of mefloquine was studied in rats and mice in 2-year feeding studies at doses up to 30 mg/kg/day. No treatment-related increases in tumor of any type were noted.

Mutagenesis: The mutagenic potential of mefloquine was studied in a variety of assay systems including: Ames test, a host-mediated assay in mice, fluctuation tests and a mouse micronucleus assay. Several of these assays were performed

with and without prior metabolic activation. In no instance was evidence obtained for the mutagenicity of mefloquine.

Impairment of Fertility: Fertility studies in rats at doses of 5, 20 and 50 mg/kg/day of mefloquine have demonstrated adverse effects on fertility in the male at the high dose of 50 mg/kg/day, and in the female at doses of 20 and 50 mg/kg/day. Histopathological lesions were noted in the epididymides from male rats at doses of 20 and 50 mg/kg/day. Administration of 250 mg/week of mefloquine (base) in adult males for 22 weeks failed to reveal any deleterious effects on human spermatozoa.

Pregnancy: Teratogenic Effects. Pregnancy Category C. Mefloquine has been demonstrated to be teratogenic in rats and mice at a dose of 100 mg/kg/day. In rabbits, a high dose of 160 mg/kg/day was embryotoxic and teratogenic, and a dose of 80 mg/kg/day was teratogenic but not embryotoxic. There are no adequate and well-controlled studies in pregnant women. Mefloquine should be used during pregnancy only if the potential benefit justifies the potential risk to the fetus. Women of childbearing potential who are traveling to areas where malaria is endemic should be warned against becoming pregnant.

Nursing Mothers: Mefloquine is excreted in human milk. Based on a study in a few subjects, low concentrations (3% to 4%) of mefloquine were excreted in human milk following a dose equivalent to 250 mg of the free base. Because of the potential for serious adverse reactions in nursing infants from mefloquine, a decision should be made whether to discontinue the drug, taking into account the importance of the drug to the mother.

Pediatric Use: Safety and effectiveness in children have not been established. Two studies of mefloquine in children living in endemic areas for *P. falciparum* were conducted. All children in these studies had at least a low level of parasitemia and 18% to 40% had significant parasitemia with or without mild malaria symptoms. When given 20 to 30 mg/kg of mefloquine as a single dose, all children with fever became afebrile, and 92% of those with significant parasitemia had a satisfactory response to treatment. While incomplete follow-up was obtained in these studies, nausea and vomiting occurred in approximately 10% and 20%, respectively, and dizziness was seen in approximately 40% of children.

ADVERSE REACTIONS

Clinical: At the doses used for treatment of acute malaria infections, the symptoms possibly attributable to drug administration cannot be distinguished from those symptoms usually attributable to the disease itself.

Among subjects who received mefloquine for prophylaxis of malaria, the most frequently observed adverse experience was vomiting (3%). Dizziness, syncope, extrasystoles and other complaints affecting less than 1% were also reported. Among subjects who received mefloquine for treatment, the most frequently observed adverse experiences included: dizziness, myalgia, nausea, fever, headache, vomiting, chills, diarrhea, skin rash, abdominal pain, fatigue, loss of appetite and tinnitus. Those side effects occurring in less than 1% included bradycardia, hair loss, emotional problems, pruritus, asthenia, transient emotional disturbances and telogen effluvium (loss of resting hair). Seizures have also been reported.

Two serious adverse reactions were cardiopulmonary arrest in one patient shortly after ingesting a single prophylactic dose of mefloquine while concomitantly using propranolol (see WARNINGS and PRECAUTIONS), and encephalopathy of unknown etiology during prophylactic mefloquine administration. The relationship of encephalopathy to drug administration could not be clearly established.

Post Marketing: Post-marketing surveillance indicates that the same adverse experiences are reported during prophylaxis, as well as acute treatment.

The following additional adverse reactions have been reported during post-marketing surveillance: vertigo, visual disturbances, central nervous system disturbances (eg, psychotic manifestations, hallucinations, confusion, anxiety and depression), insomnia, abnormal dreams, forgetfulness, motor and sensory neuropathy, hypertension, hypotension, flushing, tachycardia, palpitations, uticaria, Stevens-Johnson syndrome and erythema multiforma.

Laboratory: The most frequently observed laboratory alterations which could be possibly attributable to drug administration were decreased hematocrit, transient elevation of transaminases, leukopenia and thrombocytopenia. These alterations were observed in patients with acute malaria who received treatment doses of the drug and were attributed to the disease itself.

During prophylactic administration of mefloquine to indigenous populations in malaria-endemic areas, the following occasional alterations in laboratory values were observed: transient elevation of transaminases, leukocytosis or thrombocytopenia.

OVERDOSAGE

The following procedure is recommended in case of overdosage: Induce vomiting or perform gastric lavage, as appropriate. Monitor cardiac function and neurologic and psychiatric

status for at least 24 hours. Provide symptomatic and intensive supportive treatment as required, particularly for cardiovascular disturbances. Treat vomiting or diarrhea with standard fluid therapy.

DOSAGE AND ADMINISTRATION (see INDICATIONS AND USAGE section):

(a) Treatment of mild to moderate malaria in adults caused by *P. vivax* or mefloquine-susceptible strains of *P. falciparum*—5 tablets (1250 mg) mefloquine hydrochloride to be given as a single oral dose. The drug should not be taken on an empty stomach and should be administered with at least 8 oz (240 mL) of water.

If a full treatment course has been administered without clinical cure, alternative treatment should be given. Similarly, if previous prophylaxis with mefloquine has failed, Larium should not be used for curative treatment.

Note: Patients with acute *P. vivax* malaria, treated with Lariam, are at high risk of relapse because Lariam does not eliminate exoerythrocytic (hepatic phase) parasites. To avoid relapse after initial treatment of the acute infection with Lariam, patients should subsequently be treated with an 8-aminoquinoline (eg, primaquine).

(b) Malaria prophylaxis—one 250 mg Lariam tablet once weekly.

Prophylactic drug administration should begin 1 week before departure to an endemic area. Subsequent weekly doses should always be taken on the same day of the week. To reduce the risk of malaria after leaving an endemic area, prophylaxis should be continued for 4 additional weeks. Tablets should not be taken on an empty stomach and should be administered with at least 8 oz (240 mL) of water.

HOW SUPPLIED

Lariam is available as scored, white, round tablets, containing 250 mg of mefloquine hydrochloride in Tel-E-Dose packages of 25 (NDC 0004-0172-02). Imprint on tablets: LARIAM 250 ROCHE.

Tablets should be stored at 15°–30°C (59°–86°F).

ANIMAL TOXICOLOGY

Ocular lesions were observed in rats fed mefloquine daily for 2 years. All surviving rats given 30 mg/kg/day had ocular lesions in both eyes characterized by retinal degeneration, opacity of the lens and retinal edema. Similar but less severe lesions were observed in 80% of female and 22% of male rats fed 12.5 mg/kg/day for 2 years. At doses of 5 mg/kg/day, only corneal lesions were observed. They occurred in 9% of rats studied.

Manufactured by
F. Hoffmann-La Roche & Co., Ltd.,
Basle, Switzerland   Revised: August 1994
Shown in Product Identification Guide, page 334

ROCALTROL®   ℞

[*ro-cal 'trol*]
brand of calcitriol
CAPSULES

The following text is complete prescribing information based on official labeling in effect June 1998.

DESCRIPTION

Rocaltrol (calcitriol) is a synthetic vitamin D analog which is active in the regulation of the absorption of calcium from the gastrointestinal tract and its utilization in the body. It is available in capsules containing 0.25 mcg or 0.5 mcg calcitriol. Each capsule also contains butylated hydroxyanisole (BHA), butylated hydroxytoluene (BHT) and fractionated triglyceride of coconut oil. Gelatin capsule shells contain glycerin, parabens (methyl and propyl) and sorbitol, with the following dye systems: 0.25 mcg—FD&C Yellow No. 6 and titanium dioxide; 0.5 mcg—FD&C Red No. 3, FD&C Yellow No. 6 and titanium dioxide.

Calcitriol is a colorless, crystalline compound which occurs naturally in humans. It has a calculated molecular weight of 416.65 and is soluble in organic solvents but relatively insoluble in water. Chemically, calcitriol is 9,10-seco(5Z,7E)-5,7,10(19)-cholestatriene-1α, 3β, 25-triol.

The other names frequently used for calcitriol are 1α,25-dihydroxycholecalciferol, 1,25-dihydroxyvitamin D_3, 1,25-DHCC, 1,25$(OH)_2D_3$ and 1,25-diOHC.

CLINICAL PHARMACOLOGY

Man's natural supply of vitamin D depends mainly on exposure to the ultraviolet rays of the sun for conversion of 7-dehydrocholesterol in the skin to vitamin D_3 (cholecalciferol). Vitamin D_3 must be metabolically activated in the liver and the kidney before it is fully active as a regulator of calcium and phosphorus metabolism at target tissues. The initial transformation of vitamin D_3 is catalyzed by a vitamin D_3-25-hydroxylase enzyme (25-OHase) present in the liver, and the product of this reaction is 25-hydroxyvitamin D_3 [25-$(OH)D_3$]. Hydroxylation of 25-$(OH)D_3$ occurs in the mitochondria of kidney tissue, activated by the renal 25-hydroxyvitamin D_3-1 alpha-hydroxylase (alpha-OHase), to produce

$1,25\text{-}(OH)_2D_3$ (calcitriol), the active form of vitamin D_3. Several metabolites of calcitriol have been identified which include:

1α, 25, $(OH)_2$-24-oxo-D_3
1α, 23,25$(OH)_3$-24-oxo-D_3
1α, 24R,25$(OH)_3D_3$
1α, 25R$(OH)_2$-26-23S-lactone D_3
1α, 25S,26$(OH)_3D_3$
1α, 25$(OH)_2$-23-oxo-D_3
1α, 25R,26$(OH)_3$-23-oxo-D_3
1α, (OH)24,25,26,27-tetranor-COOH-D_3

The two known sites of action of calcitriol are intestine and bone. A calcitriol receptor-binding protein appears to exist in the mucosa of human intestine. Additional evidence suggests that calcitriol may also act on the kidney and the parathyroid glands. Calcitriol is the most active known form of vitamin D_3 in stimulating intestinal calcium transport. In acutely uremic rats calcitriol has been shown to stimulate intestinal calcium absorption. The kidneys of uremic patients cannot adequately synthesize calcitriol, the active hormone formed from precursor vitamin D. Resultant hypocalcemia and secondary hyperparathyroidism are a major cause of the metabolic bone disease of renal failure. However, other bone-toxic substances which accumulate in uremia (eg, aluminum) may also contribute.

The beneficial effect of Rocaltrol in renal osteodystrophy appears to result from correction of hypocalcemia and secondary hyperparathyroidism. It is uncertain whether Rocaltrol produces other independent beneficial effects.

Calcitriol is rapidly absorbed from the intestine. Peak serum concentrations (above basal values) were reached within 3 to 6 hours following oral administration of single doses of 0.25 to 1.0 mcg of Rocaltrol. The half-life of calcitriol elimination from serum was found to range from 3 to 6 hours. Following a single oral dose of 0.5 mcg, mean serum concentrations of calcitriol rose from a baseline value of 40.0 ± 4.4 (S.D.) pg/ ml to 60.0 ± 4.4 pg/mL at 2 hours, and declined to 53.0 ± 6.9 at 4 hours, 50 ± 7.0 at 8 hours, 44 ± 4.6 at 12 hours and 41.5 ± 5.1 at 24 hours. The duration of pharmacologic activity of a single dose of calcitriol is about 3 to 5 days.

Calcitriol and other vitamin D metabolites are transported in blood, bound to specific plasma proteins. Enterohepatic recycling and biliary excretion of calcitriol occurs. Following intravenous administration of radiolabeled calcitriol in normal subjects, approximately 27% and 7% of the radioactivity appeared in the feces and urine, respectively, within 24 hours. When a 1-mcg oral dose of radiolabeled calcitriol was administered to normals, approximately 10% of the total radioactivity appeared in urine within 24 hours. Cumulative excretion of radioactivity on the sixth day following intravenous administration of radiolabeled calcitriol averaged 16% in urine and 49% in feces.

There is evidence that maternal calcitriol may enter the fetal circulation. Calcitriol may be excreted in human milk.

Pediatric Pharmacokinetics: The steady state pharmacokinetics of oral Rocaltrol were determined in a small group of pediatric patients (age range: 1.8 to 16 years) undergoing peritoneal dialysis. Rocaltrol was administered for two months at an average dose of 10.2 ng/kg (S.D. 5.5 ng/kg). In this pediatric population, mean C_{max} was 116 pmol/L, mean serum half-life was 27.4 hours, and mean clearance was 15.3 mL/hr/kg.[1]

INDICATIONS AND USAGE

Rocaltrol is indicated in the management of hypocalcemia and the resultant metabolic bone disease in patients undergoing chronic renal dialysis. In these patients, Rocaltrol administration enhances calcium absorption, reduces serum alkaline phosphatase levels and may reduce elevated parathyroid hormone levels and the histological manifestations of osteitis fibrosa cystica and defective mineralization.

Rocaltrol is also indicated in the management of hypocalcemia and its clinical manifestations in patients with postsurgical hypoparathyroidism, idiopathic hypoparathyroidism, and pseudohypoparathyroidism.

CONTRAINDICATIONS

Rocaltrol should not be given to patients with hypercalcemia or evidence of vitamin D toxicity.

WARNINGS

Since Rocaltrol is the most potent metabolite of vitamin D available, pharmacologic doses of vitamin D and its derivatives should be withheld during Rocaltrol treatment to avoid possible additive effects and hypercalcemia.

Both appropriate oral phosphate-binders and a low phosphate diet should be used to control serum phosphate levels in patients undergoing dialysis.

Magnesium-containing antacids and Rocaltrol should not be used concomitantly in patients on chronic renal dialysis because such use may lead to the development of hypermagnesemia.

Overdosage of any form of vitamin D is dangerous (see also OVERDOSAGE). Progressive hypercalcemia due to overdosage of vitamin D and its metabolites may be so severe as to require emergency attention. Chronic hypercalcemia can lead to generalized vascular calcification, nephrocalcinosis and other soft-tissue calcification. **The serum calcium times phospate (Ca × P) product should not be allowed to exceed 70.** Radiographic evaluation of suspect anatomical regions may be useful in the early detection of this condition.

Studies in dogs and rats given calcitriol for up to 26 weeks have shown that small increases of calcitriol above endogenous levels can lead to abnormalities of calcium metabolism with the potential for calcification of many tissues in the body.

PRECAUTIONS

General: Excessive dosage of Rocaltrol induces hypercalcemia and in some instances hypercalciuria; therefore, early in treatment during dosage adjustment, serum calcium should be determined twice weekly. In dialysis patients, a fall in serum alkaline phosphatase levels usually antedates the appearance of hypercalcemia and may be an indication of impending hypercalcemia. Should hypercalcemia develop, the drug should be discontinued immediately. Rocaltrol should be given cautiously to patients on digitalis, because hypercalcemia in such patients may precipitate cardiac arrhythmias.

In patients with normal renal function, chronic hypercalcemia may be associated with an increase in serum creatinine. While this is usually reversible, it is important in such patients to pay careful attention to those factors which may lead to hypercalcemia. Rocaltrol therapy should always be started at the lowest possible dose and should not be increased without careful monitoring of the serum calcium. An estimate of daily dietary calcium intake should be made and the intake adjusted when indicated.

Patients with normal renal function taking Rocaltrol should avoid dehydration. Adequate fluid intake should be maintained.

Information for the Patient: The patient and his or her parents or spouse should be informed about compliance with dosage instructions, adherence to instructions about diet and calcium supplementation and avoidance of the use of unapproved nonprescription drugs. Patients should also be carefully informed about the symptoms of hypercalcemia (see ADVERSE REACTIONS section).

Laboratory Tests: For dialysis patients, serum calcium, phosphorus, magnesium and alkaline phosphatase should be determined periodically. For hypoparathyroid patients, serum calcium, phosphorus and 24-hour urinary calcium should be determined periodically.

Drug Interactions: Cholestyramine has been reported to reduce intestinal absorption of fat-soluble vitamins; as such it may impair intestinal absorption of Rocaltrol. (Also see WARNINGS and PRECAUTIONS[General] sections.)

Carcinogenesis, Mutagenesis, Impairment of Fertility: Long-term studies in animals have not been conducted to evaluate the carcinogenic potential of Rocaltrol. There was no evidence of mutagenicity as studied by the Ames method. No significant effects of Rocaltrol on fertility and/or general reproductive performances were reported.

Pregnancy: Teratogenic Effects: Pregnancy Category C. Rocaltrol has been found to be teratogenic in rabbits when given in doses 4 and 15 times the dose recommended for human use. All 15 fetuses in 3 litters at these doses showed external and skeletal abnormalities. However, none of the other 23 litters (156 fetuses) showed significant abnormalities compared with controls. Teratogenicity studies in rats showed no evidence of teratogenic potential. There are no adequate and well-controlled studies in pregnant women. Rocaltrol should be used during pregnancy only if the potential benefit justifies the potential risk to the fetus.

Nonteratogenic Effects: In the rabbit, dosages of 0.3 mcg/kg/day administered on days 7 to 18 of gestation resulted in 19% maternal mortality, a decrease in mean fetal body weight and a reduced number of newborn surviving to 24 hours. A study of peri- and postnatal development in rats resulted in hypercalcemia in the offspring of dams given Rocaltrol at doses of 0.08 or 0.3 mcg/ kg/day, hypercalcemia and hypophosphatemia in dams at doses of 0.08 or 0.3 mcg/kg/day, and increased serum urea nitrogen in dams given Rocaltrol at a dose of 0.3 mcg/kg/day. In another study in rats, maternal weight gain was slightly reduced at a dose of 0.3 mcg/kg/day administered on days 7 to 15 of gestation.

The offspring of a woman administered 17 to 36 mcg/day of Rocaltrol (17 to 144 times the recommended dose) during pregnancy manifested mild hypercalcemia in the first 2 days of life which returned to normal at day 3.

Nursing Mothers: Calcitriol may be excreted in human milk. Because many drugs are excreted in human milk and because of the potential for serious adverse reactions from Rocaltrol in nursing infants, a mother should not nurse while taking this drug.

Pediatric Use: Safety and effectiveness of Rocaltrol in pediatric patients undergoing dialysis have not been established. Dosing guidelines have not been established for pediatric patients under 1 year of age with hypoparathyroidism or for pediatric patients less than 6 years of age with pseudohypoparathyroidism (see DOSAGE AND ADMINISTRATION: *Hypoparathyroidism*).

ADVERSE REACTIONS

Since Rocaltrol is believed to be the active hormone which exerts vitamin D activity in the body, adverse effects are, in general, similar to those encountered with excessive vitamin D intake. The early and late signs and symptoms of vitamin D intoxication associated with hypercalcemia include:

Early: Weakness, headache, somnolence, nausea, vomiting, dry mouth, constipation, muscle pain, bone pain and metallic taste.

Late: Polyuria, polydipsia, anorexia, weight loss, nocturia, conjunctivitis (calcific), pancreatitis, photophobia, rhinorrhea, pruritus, hyperthermia, decreased libido, elevated BUN, albuminuria, hypercholesterolemia, elevated SGOT and SGPT, ectopic calcification, nephrocalcinosis, hypertension, cardiac arrhythmias and, rarely, overt psychosis.

In clinical studies on hypoparathyroidism and pseudohypoparathyroidism, hypercalcemia was noted on at least one occasion in about 1 in 3 patients and hypercalciuria in about 1 in 7. Elevated serum creatinine levels were observed in about 1 in 6 patients (approximately one half of whom had normal levels at baseline).

One case of erythema multiforme and one case of allergic reaction (swelling of lips and hives all over the body) were confirmed by rechallenge.

OVERDOSAGE

Administration of Rocaltrol to patients in excess of their daily requirements can cause hypercalcemia, hypercalciuria and hyperphosphatemia. High intake of calcium and phosphate concomitant with Rocaltrol may lead to similar abnormalities. High levels of calcium in the dialysate bath may contribute to the hypercalcemia.

Treatment of Hypercalcemia and Overdosage: General treatment of hypercalcemia (greater than 1 mg/dL above the upper limit of the normal range) consists of immediate discontinuation of Rocaltrol therapy, institution of a low calcium diet and withdrawal of calcium supplements. Serum calcium levels should be determined daily until normocalcemia ensues. Hypercalcemia frequently resolves in 2 to 7 days. When serum calcium levels have returned to within normal limits, Rocaltrol therapy may be reinstituted at a dose of 0.25 mcg/day less than prior therapy. Serum calcium levels should be obtained at least twice weekly after all dosage changes and subsequent dosage titration. In dialysis patients, persistent or markedly elevated serum calcium levels may be corrected by dialysis against a calcium-free dialysate.

Treatment of Accidental Overdosage of Rocaltrol: The treatment of acute accidental overdosage of Rocaltrol should consist of general supportive measures. If drug ingestion is discovered within a relatively short time, induction of emesis or gastric lavage may be of benefit in preventing further absorption. If the drug has passed through the stomach, the administration of mineral oil may promote its fecal elimination. Serial serum electrolyte determinations (especially calcium), rate of urinary calcium excretion and assessment of electrocardiographic abnormalities due to hypercalcemia should be obtained. Such monitoring is critical in patients receiving digitalis. Discontinuation of supplemental calcium and a low calcium diet are also indicated in accidental overdosage. Due to the relatively short duration of the pharmacological action of calcitriol, further measures are probably unnecessary. Should, however, persistent and markedly elevated serum calcium levels occur, there are a variety of therapeutic alternatives which may be considered, depending on the patient's underlying condition. These include the use of drugs such as phosphates and corticosteroids as well as measures to induce an appropriate forced diuresis. The use of peritoneal dialysis against a calcium-free dialysate has also been reported.

DOSAGE AND ADMINISTRATION

The optimal daily dose of Rocaltrol must be carefully determined for each patient.

The effectiveness of Rocaltrol therapy is predicated on the assumption that each patient is receiving an adequate daily intake of calcium. The U.S. RDA for calcium in adults is 800 to 1200 mg. To ensure that each patient receives an adequate daily intake of calcium, the physician should either prescribe a calcium supplement or instruct the patient in proper dietary measures.

Dialysis Patients: The recommended initial dose of Rocaltrol is 0.25 mcg/day. If a satisfactory response in the biochemical parameters and clinical manifestations of the disease state is not observed, dosage may be increased by 0.25 mcg/day at 4- to 8-week intervals. During this titration period, serum calcium levels should be obtained at least twice weekly, and if hypercalcemia is noted, the drug should be immediately discontinued until normocalcemia ensues.

Patients with normal or only slightly reduced serum calcium levels may respond to Rocaltrol doses of 0.25 mcg every other day. Most patients undergoing hemodialysis respond to doses between 0.5 and 1 mcg/day.

Continued on next page

Rocaltrol—Cont.

Oral Rocaltrol may normalize plasma ionized calcium in some uremic patients, yet fail to suppress parathyroid hyperfunction. In these individuals with autonomous parathyroid hyperfunction, oral Rocaltrol may be useful to maintain normocalcemia, but has not been shown to be adequate treatment for hyperparathyroidism.

Hypoparathyroidism: The recommended initial dose of Rocaltrol is 0.25 mcg/day given in the morning. If a satisfactory response in the biochemical parameters and clinical manifestations of the disease is not observed, the dose may be increased at 2- to 4-week intervals. During the dosage titration period, serum calcium levels should be obtained at least twice weekly and, if hypercalcemia is noted, Rocaltrol should be immediately discontinued until normocalcemia ensues. Careful consideration should also be given to lowering the dietary calcium intake.

Most adult patients and pediatric patients age 6 years and older have responded to dosages in the range of 0.5 to 2 mcg daily. Pediatric patients in the 1–5 year age group with hypoparathyroidism have usually been given 0.25 to 0.75 mcg daily. The number of treated patients with pseudohypoparathyroidism less than 6 years of age is too small to make dosage recommendations.

HOW SUPPLIED

0.25 mcg calcitriol in soft gelatin, light orange, oval capsules, imprinted ROCALTROL 0.25 ROCHE; bottles of 30 (NDC 0004-0143-23), and bottles of 100, (NDC 0004-0143-01).

0.5 mcg calcitriol in soft gelatin, dark orange, oblong capsules, imprinted ROCALTROL 0.5 ROCHE; bottles of 100, (NDC 0004-0144-01).

Rocaltrol should be protected from heat and light.

REFERENCE

1. Jones CL, et al. Comparisons between oral and intraperitoneal 1.25–dihydroxyvitamin D, therapy in children treated with peritoneal dialysis. *Clin Nephrol.* 1994; 42:44–49.

Revised: March 1997

Shown in Product Identification Guide, page 335

ROCEPHIN®

[ro-sef ' in]

(ceftriaxone sodium)
FOR INJECTION

℞

The following text is complete prescribing information based on official labeling in effect June 1998.

DESCRIPTION

Rocephin is a sterile, semisynthetic, broad-spectrum cephalosporin antibiotic for intravenous or intramuscular administration. Ceftriaxone sodium is $(6R,7R)$-7-[2-(2-Amino-4-thiazolyl)glyoxylamido]-8-oxo-3-[[(1,2,5,6-tetrahydro-2-methyl-5,6-dioxo-as-triazin-3-yl)thio]methyl]-5-thia-1-azabicyclo[4.2.0]oct-2-ene-2-carboxylic acid, 7^2-(Z)-(O-methyloxime), disodium salt, sesquaterhydrate.

The chemical formula of ceftriaxone sodium is $C_{18} H_{16} N_8 Na_2 O_7 S_3$ 3.5 H_2O. It has a calculated molecular weight of 661.59.

Rocephin is a white to yellowish-orange crystalline powder which is readily soluble in water, sparingly soluble in methanol and very slightly soluble in ethanol. The pH of a 1% aqueous solution is approximately 6.7. The color of Rocephin solutions ranges from light yellow to amber, depending on the length of storage, concentration and diluent used.

Rocephin contains approximately 83 mg (3.6 mEq) of sodium per gram of ceftriaxone activity.

CLINICAL PHARMACOLOGY

Average plasma concentrations of ceftriaxone following a single 30-minute intravenous (IV) infusion of a 0.5, 1 or 2 gm dose and intramuscular (IM) administration of a single 0.5 (250 mg/mL or 350 mg/mL concentrations) or 1 gm dose in healthy subjects are presented in Table 1.

[See table 1 above]

Ceftriaxone was completely absorbed following IM administration with mean maximum plasma concentrations occurring between 2 and 3 hours postdosing. Multiple IV or IM doses ranging from 0.5 to 2 gm at 12- to 24-hour intervals resulted in 15% to 36% accumulation of ceftriaxone above single dose values.

Ceftriaxone concentrations in urine are high, as shown in Table 2.

[See table 2 at right]

Thirty-three to 67% of a ceftriaxone dose was excreted in the urine as unchanged drug and the remainder was secreted in the bile and ultimately found in the feces as microbiologically inactive compounds. After a 1 gm IV dose, average concentrations of ceftriaxone, determined from 1 to

---

TABLE 1 Ceftriaxone Plasma Concentrations After Single Dose Administration

Dose/Route	Average Plasma Concentrations (mcg/mL)								
	0.5 hr	1 hr	2 hr	4 hr	6 hr	8 hr	12 hr	16 hr	24 hr
0.5 gm IV*	82	59	48	37	29	23	15	10	5
0.5 gm IM 250 mg/mL	22	33	38	35	30	26	16	ND	5
0.5 gm IM 350 mg/mL	20	32	38	34	31	24	16	ND	5
1 gm IV*	151	111	88	67	53	43	28	18	9
1 gm IM	40	68	76	68	56	44	29	ND	ND
2 gm IV*	257	192	154	117	89	74	46	31	15

*IV doses were infused at a constant rate over 30 minutes.
ND = Not determined.

---

3 hours after dosing, were 581 mcg/mL in the gallbladder bile, 788 mcg/mL in the common duct bile, 898 mcg/mL in the cystic duct bile, 78.2 mcg/gm in the gallbladder wall and 62.1 mcg/mL in the concurrent plasma.

Over a 0.15 to 3 gm dose range in healthy adult subjects, the values of elimination half-life ranged from 5.8 to 8.7 hours; apparent volume of distribution from 5.78 to 13.5 L; plasma clearance from 0.58 to 1.45 L/hour; and renal clearance from 0.32 to 0.73 L/hour. Ceftriaxone is reversibly bound to human plasma proteins, and the binding decreased from a value of 95% bound at plasma concentrations of <25 mcg/mL to a value of 85% bound at 300 mcg/mL.

The average values of maximum plasma concentration, elimination half-life, plasma clearance and volume of distribution after a 50 mg/kg IV dose and after a 75 mg/kg IV dose in pediatric patients suffering from bacterial meningitis are shown in Table 3. Ceftriaxone penetrated the inflamed meninges of infants and children; CSF concentrations after a 50 mg/kg IV dose and after a 75 mg/kg IV dose are also shown in Table 3.

[See table 3 on next page]

Compared to that in healthy adult subjects, the pharmacokinetics of ceftriaxone were only minimally altered in elderly subjects and in patients with renal impairment or hepatic dysfunction (Table 4); therefore, dosage adjustments are not necessary for these patients with ceftriaxone dosages up to 2 gm per day. Ceftriaxone was not removed to any significant extent from the plasma by hemodialysis. In 6 of 26 dialysis patients, the elimination rate of ceftriaxone was markedly reduced, suggesting that plasma concentrations of ceftriaxone should be monitored in these patients to determine if dosage adjustments are necessary.

[See table 4 on next page]

Pharmacokinetics in the Middle Ear Fluid: In one study, total ceftriaxone concentrations (bound and unbound) were measured in middle ear fluid obtained during the insertion of tympanostomy tubes in 42 pediatric patients with otitis media. Sampling times were from 1 to 50 hours after a single intramuscular injection of 50 mg/kg of ceftriaxone. Mean (± SD) ceftriaxone levels in the middle ear reached a peak of 35 (± 12) µg/mL at 24 hours, and remained at 19 (± 7) µg/mL at 48 hours. Based on middle ear fluid ceftriaxone concentrations in the 23 to 25 hour and the 46 to 50 hour sampling time intervals, a half-life of 25 hours was calculated. Ceftriaxone is highly bound to plasma proteins. The extent of binding to proteins in the middle ear fluid is unknown.

Microbiology: The bactericidal activity of ceftriaxone results from inhibition of cell wall synthesis. Ceftriaxone has a high degree of stability in the presence of beta-lactamases, both penicillinases and cephalosporinases, of gram-negative and gram-positive bacteria. Ceftriaxone is usually active against the following microorganisms in vitro and in clinical infections (see INDICATIONS AND USAGE):

GRAM-NEGATIVE AEROBES:
Acinetobacter calcoaceticus
Enterobacter aerogenes
Enterobacter cloacae
Escherichia coli
Haemophilus influenzae (including ampicillin-resistant and beta-lactamase producing strains)
Haemophilus parainfluenzae
Klebsiella oxytoca

Klebsiella pneumoniae
Moraxella catarrhalis (including beta-lactamase producing strains)
Morganella morganii
Neisseria gonorrhoeae (including penicillinase- and nonpenicillinase-producing strains)
Neisseria meningitidis
Proteus mirabilis
Proteus vulgaris
Serratia marcescens
Ceftriaxone is also active against many strains of *Pseudomonas aeruginosa*.
Note: Many strains of the above organisms that are multiply resistant to other antibiotics, eg, penicillins, cephalosporins and aminoglycosides, are susceptible to ceftriaxone.
GRAM-POSITIVE AEROBES:
Staphylococcus aureus (including penicillinase-producing strains)
Staphylococcus epidermidis
Streptococcus pneumoniae
Streptococcus pyogenes
Viridans group streptococci
Note: Methicillin-resistant staphylococci are resistant to cephalosporins, including ceftriaxone. Most strains of Group D streptococci and enterococci, eg, *Enterococcus (Streptococcus) faecalis*, are resistant.
ANAEROBES:
Bacteroides fragilis
Clostridium species
Peptostreptococcus species
Note: Most strains of *C. difficile* are resistant.
Ceftriaxone also demonstrates in vitro activity against most strains of the following microorganisms, although the clinical significance is unknown:
GRAM-NEGATIVE AEROBES:
Citrobacter diversus
Citrobacter freundii
Providencia species (including *Providencia rettgeri*)
Salmonella species (including *S. typhi*)
Shigella species
GRAM-POSITIVE AEROBES:
Streptococcus agalactiae
ANAEROBES:
Bacteroides bivius
Bacteroides melaninogenicus

Susceptibility Tests: *Diffusion Techniques:* Quantitative methods that require the measurement of zone diameters give the most precise estimate of the susceptibility of bacteria to antimicrobial agents. One such standard procedure[1] which has been recommended for use with disks to test susceptibility of organisms to ceftriaxone uses a 30-mcg ceftriaxone disk. Interpretation involves the correlation of the diameters obtained in the disk test with the minimum inhibitory concentration (MIC) for ceftriaxone.

Reports from the laboratory giving results of the standardized single disk susceptibility test using a 30-mcg ceftriaxone disk should be interpreted for ceftriaxone according to the following criteria:

Zone Diameter (mm)		Interpretation
≥18	(S)	Susceptible
14–17	(MS)	Moderately Susceptible
≤13	(R)	Resistant

TABLE 2 Urinary Concentrations of Ceftriaxone After Single Dose Administration

Dose/Route	Average Urinary Concentrations (mcg/mL)					
	0–2 hr	2–4 hr	4–8 hr	8–12 hr	12–24 hr	24–48 hr
0.5 gm IV	526	366	142	87	70	15
0.5 gm IM	115	425	308	127	96	28
1 gm IV	995	855	293	147	132	32
1 gm IM	504	628	418	237	ND*	ND
2 gm IV	2692	1976	757	274	198	40

*ND = Not determined.

A report of "Susceptible" indicates that the pathogen is likely to be inhibited by generally achievable levels. A report of "Moderately Susceptible" suggests that the organism would be susceptible if high dosage (not to exceed 4 gm per day) is used or if the infection is confined to tissues or fluids in which high antimicrobial levels are attained. A report of "Resistant" indicates that achievable concentrations are unlikely to be inhibitory, and other therapy should be selected.

Standardized procedures require the use of laboratory control organisms. The 30-mcg ceftriaxone disk should give the following zone diameters:

Organism	Zone Diameter (mm)
Staphylococcus aureus ATCC® 25923	22–28
Escherichia coli ATCC® 25922	29–35
Pseudomonas aeruginosa ATCC® 27853	17–23

Dilution Techniques:

Use a standardized dilution method[2] (broth, agar, microdilution) or equivalent with ceftriaxone powder. The MIC values obtained should be interpreted according to the following criteria:

MIC (mcg/mL)	Interpretation
≤16	Susceptible
>16–<64	Moderately Susceptible
≥64	Resistant

As with standard diffusion techniques, dilution methods require the use of laboratory control organisms. Standard ceftriaxone powder should provide the following MIC values:

Organism	MIC (mcg/mL)
Staphylococcus aureus ATCC® 29213	1–8
Escherichia coli ATCC® 25922	0.03–0.12
Pseudomonas aeruginosa ATCC® 27853	8–32

INDICATIONS AND USAGE

Rocephin is indicated for the treatment of the following infections when caused by susceptible organisms:

LOWER RESPIRATORY TRACT INFECTIONS caused by *Streptococcus pneumoniae, Staphylococcus aureus, Haemophilus influenzae, Haemophilus parainfluenzae, Klebsiella pneumoniae, Escherichia coli, Enterobacter aerogenes, Proteus mirabilis* or *Serratia marcescens.*

ACUTE BACTERIAL OTITIS MEDIA caused by *Streptococcus pneumoniae, Haemophilus influenzae* (including beta-lactamase producing strains) or *Moraxella catarrhalis* (including beta-lactamase producing strains).

NOTE: In one study lower clinical cure rates were observed with a single dose of Rocephin compared to 10 days of oral therapy. In a second study comparable cure rates were observed between single dose Rocephin and the comparator. The potentially lower clinical cure rate of Rocephin should be balanced against the potential advantages of parenteral therapy (see CLINICAL STUDIES).

SKIN AND SKIN STRUCTURE INFECTIONS caused by *Staphylococcus aureus, Staphylococcus epidermidis, Streptococcus pyogenes, Viridans* group streptococci, *Escherichia coli, Enterobacter cloacae, Klebsiella oxytoca, Klebsiella pneumoniae, Proteus mirabilis, Morganella morganii*,*

*Pseudomonas aeruginosa, Serratia marcescens, Acinetobacter calcoaceticus, Bacteroides fragilis** or *Peptostreptococcus* species.

URINARY TRACT INFECTIONS (complicated and uncomplicated) caused by *Escherichia coli, Proteus mirabilis, Proteus vulgaris, Morganella morganii* or *Klebsiella pneumoniae.*

UNCOMPLICATED GONORRHEA (cervical/urethral and rectal) caused by *Neisseria gonorrhoeae,* including both penicillinase- and nonpenicillinase-producing strains, and pharyngeal gonorrhea caused by nonpenicillinase-producing strains of *Neisseria gonorrhoeae.*

PELVIC INFLAMMATORY DISEASE caused by *Neisseria gonorrhoeae.* Rocephin, like other cephalosporins, has no activity against *Chlamydia trachomatis.* Therefore, when cephalosporins are used in the treatment of patients with pelvic inflammatory disease and *C. trachomatis* is one of the suspected pathogens, appropriate antichlamydial coverage should be added.

BACTERIAL SEPTICEMIA caused by *Staphylococcus aureus, Streptococcus pneumoniae, Escherichia coli, Haemophilus influenzae* or *Klebsiella pneumoniae.*

BONE AND JOINT INFECTIONS caused by *Staphylococcus aureus, Streptococcus pneumoniae, Escherichia coli, Proteus mirabilis, Klebsiella pneumoniae* or *Enterobacter* species.

INTRA-ABDOMINAL INFECTIONS caused by *Escherichia coli, Klebsiella pneumoniae, Bacteroides fragilis, Clostridium* species (Note: most strains of *C. difficile* are resistant) or *Peptostreptococcus* species.

MENINGITIS caused by *Haemophilus influenzae, Neisseria meningitidis* or *Streptococcus pneumoniae.* Rocephin has also been used successfully in a limited number of cases of meningitis and shunt infection caused by *Staphylococcus epidermidis** and *Escherichia coli.**

*Efficacy for this organism in this organ system was studied in fewer than ten infections.

SURGICAL PROPHYLAXIS: The preoperative administration of a single 1 gm dose of Rocephin may reduce the incidence of postoperative infections in patients undergoing surgical procedures classified as contaminated or potentially contaminated (eg, vaginal or abdominal hysterectomy or cholecystectomy for chronic calculous cholecystitis in high-risk patients, such as those over 70 years of age, with acute cholecystitis not requiring therapeutic antimicrobials, obstructive jaundice or common duct bile stones) and in surgical patients for whom infection at the operative site would present serious risk (eg, during coronary artery bypass surgery). Although Rocephin has been shown to have been as effective as cefazolin in the prevention of infection following coronary artery bypass surgery, no placebo-controlled trials have been conducted to evaluate any cephalosporin antibiotic in the prevention of infection following coronary artery bypass surgery.

When administered prior to surgical procedures for which it is indicated, a single 1 gm dose of Rocephin provides protection from most infections due to susceptible organisms throughout the course of the procedure.

Before instituting treatment with Rocephin, appropriate specimens should be obtained for isolation of the causative organism and for determination of its susceptibility to the drug. Therapy may be instituted prior to obtaining results of susceptibility testing.

CONTRAINDICATIONS

Rocephin is contraindicated in patients with known allergy to the cephalosporin class of antibiotics.

WARNINGS

BEFORE THERAPY WITH ROCEPHIN IS INSTITUTED, CAREFUL INQUIRY SHOULD BE MADE TO DETERMINE WHETHER THE PATIENT HAS HAD PREVIOUS HYPERSENSITIVITY REACTIONS TO CEPHALOSPORINS, PENICILLINS OR OTHER DRUGS. THIS PRODUCT SHOULD BE GIVEN CAUTIOUSLY TO PENICILLIN-SENSITIVE PATIENTS. ANTIBIOTICS SHOULD BE ADMINISTERED WITH CAUTION TO ANY PATIENT WHO HAS DEMONSTRATED SOME FORM OF ALLERGY, PARTICULARLY TO DRUGS. SERIOUS ACUTE HYPERSENSITIVITY REACTIONS MAY REQUIRE THE USE OF SUBCUTANEOUS EPINEPHRINE AND OTHER EMERGENCY MEASURES.

Pseudomembranous colitis has been reported with nearly all antibacterial agents, including ceftriaxone, and may range in severity from mild to life-threatening. Therefore, it is important to consider this diagnosis in patients who present with diarrhea subsequent to the administration of antibacterial agents.

Treatment with antibacterial agents alters the normal flora of the colon and may permit overgrowth of clostridia. Studies indicate that a toxin produced by *Clostridium difficile* is one primary cause of "antibiotic-associated colitis."

After the diagnosis of pseudomembranous colitis has been established, appropriate therapeutic measures should be initiated. Mild cases of pseudomembranous colitis usually respond to drug discontinuation alone. In moderate to severe cases, consideration should be given to management with fluids and electrolytes, protein supplementation and treatment with an antibacterial drug clinically effective against *C. difficile* colitis.

PRECAUTIONS

General: Although transient elevations of BUN and serum creatinine have been observed, at the recommended dosages, the nephrotoxic potential of Rocephin is similar to that of other cephalosporins.

Ceftriaxone is excreted via both biliary and renal excretion (see CLINICAL PHARMACOLOGY). Therefore, patients with renal failure normally require no adjustment in dosage when usual doses of Rocephin are administered, but concentrations of drug in the serum should be monitored periodically. If evidence of accumulation exists, dosage should be decreased accordingly.

Dosage adjustments should not be necessary in patients with hepatic dysfunction; however, in patients with both hepatic dysfunction and significant renal disease, Rocephin dosage should not exceed 2 gm daily without close monitoring of serum concentrations.

Alterations in prothrombin times have occurred rarely in patients treated with Rocephin. Patients with impaired vitamin K synthesis or low vitamin K stores (eg, chronic hepatic disease and malnutrition) may require monitoring of prothrombin time during Rocephin treatment. Vitamin K administration (10 mg weekly) may be necessary if the prothrombin time is prolonged before or during therapy.

Prolonged use of Rocephin may result in overgrowth of non-susceptible organisms. Careful observation of the patient is essential. If superinfection occurs during therapy, appropriate measures should be taken.

Rocephin should be prescribed with caution in individuals with a history of gastrointestinal disease, especially colitis.

There have been reports of sonographic abnormalities in the gallbladder of patients treated with Rocephin; some of these patients also had symptoms of gallbladder disease. These abnormalities appear on sonography as an echo without acoustical shadowing suggesting sludge or as an echo with acoustical shadowing which may be misinterpreted as gallstones. The chemical nature of the sonographically detected material has been determined to be predominantly a ceftriaxone-calcium salt. **The condition appears to be transient and reversible upon discontinuation of Rocephin and institution of conservative management.** Therefore, Rocephin should be discontinued in patients who develop signs and symptoms suggestive of gallbladder disease and/or the sonographic findings described above.

Carcinogenesis, Mutagenesis, Impairment of Fertility: Carcinogenesis: Considering the maximum duration of treatment and the class of the compound, carcinogenicity studies with ceftriaxone in animals have not been performed. The maximum duration of animal toxicity studies was 6 months. *Mutagenesis:* Genetic toxicology tests included the Ames test, a micronucleus test and a test for chromosomal aberrations in human lymphocytes cultured in vitro with ceftriaxone. Ceftriaxone showed no potential for mutagenic activity in these studies.

Impairment of Fertility: Ceftriaxone produced no impairment of fertility when given intravenously to rats at daily doses up to 586 mg/kg/day, approximately 20 times the recommended clinical dose of 2 gm/day.

TABLE 3 Average Pharmacokinetic Parameters of Ceftriaxone in Pediatric Patients With Meningitis

	50 mg/kg IV	75 mg/kg IV
Maximum Plasma Concentrations (mcg/mL)	216	275
Elimination Half-life (hr)	4.6	4.3
Plasma Clearance (mL/hr/kg)	49	60
Volume of Distribution (mL/kg)	338	373
CSF Concentration—inflamed meninges (mcg/mL)	5.6	6.4
Range (mcg/mL)	1.3–18.5	1.3–44
Time after dose (hr)	3.7 (± 1.6)	3.3 (± 1.4)

TABLE 4 Average Pharmacokinetic Parameters of Ceftriaxone in Humans

Subject Group	Elimination Half-Life (hr)	Plasma Clearance (L/hr)	Volume of Distribution (L)
Healthy Subjects	5.8–8.7	0.58–1.45	5.8–13.5
Elderly Subjects (mean age, 70.5 yr)	8.9	0.83	10.7
Patients with renal impairment			
Hemodialysis patients (0–5 mL/min)*	14.7	0.65	13.7
Severe (5–15 mL/min)	15.7	0.56	12.5
Moderate (16–30 mL/min)	11.4	0.72	11.8
Mild (31–60 mL/min)	12.4	0.70	13.3
Patients with liver disease	8.8	1.1	13.6

*Creatinine clearance.

Continued on next page

Rocephin—Cont.

Pregnancy: Teratogenic Effects: Pregnancy Category B. Reproductive studies have been performed in mice and rats at doses up to 20 times the usual human dose and have no evidence of embryotoxicity, fetotoxicity or teratogenicity. In primates, no embryotoxicity or teratogenicity was demonstrated at a dose approximately 3 times the human dose. There are, however, no adequate and well-controlled studies in pregnant women. Because animal reproductive studies are not always predictive of human response, this drug should be used during pregnancy only if clearly needed.

Nonteratogenic Effects: In rats, in the Segment I (fertility and general reproduction) and Segment III (perinatal and postnatal) studies with intravenously administered ceftriaxone, no adverse effects were noted on various reproductive parameters during gestation and lactation, including postnatal growth, functional behavior and reproductive ability of the offspring, at doses of 586 mg/kg/day or less.

Nursing Mothers: Low concentrations of ceftriaxone are excreted in human milk. Caution should be exercised when Rocephin is administered to a nursing woman.

Pediatric Use: Safety and effectiveness of Rocephin in neonates, infants and children have been established for the dosages described in the DOSAGE AND ADMINISTRATION section. In vitro studies have shown that ceftriaxone, like some other cephalosporins, can displace bilirubin from serum albumin. Rocephin should not be administered to hyperbilirubinemic neonates, especially prematures.

ADVERSE REACTIONS

Rocephin is generally well tolerated. In clinical trials, the following adverse reactions, which were considered to be related to Rocephin therapy or of uncertain etiology, were observed:

LOCAL REACTIONS—pain, induration and tenderness was 1% overall. Phlebitis was reported in <1% after IV administration. The incidence of injection site reaction was 17% (3/17) after IM administration of 350 mg/mL and 5% (1/20) after IM administration of 250 mg/mL.

HYPERSENSITIVITY—rash (1.7%). Less frequently reported (<1%) were pruritus, fever or chills.

HEMATOLOGIC—eosinophilia (6%), thrombocytosis (5.1%) and leukopenia (2.1%). Less frequently reported (<1%) were anemia, hemolytic anemia, neutropenia, lymphopenia, thrombocytopenia and prolongation of the prothrombin time.

GASTROINTESTINAL—diarrhea (2.7%). Less frequently reported (<1%) were nausea or vomiting, and dysgeusia. The onset of pseudomembranous colitis symptoms may occur during or after antibacterial treatment (see WARNINGS).

HEPATIC—elevations of SGOT (3.1%) or SGPT (3.3%). Less frequently reported (<1%) were elevations of alkaline phosphatase and bilirubin.

RENAL—elevations of the BUN (1.2%). Less frequently reported (<1%) were elevations of creatinine and the presence of casts in the urine.

CENTRAL NERVOUS SYSTEM—headache or dizziness were reported occasionally (<1%).

GENITOURINARY—moniliasis or vaginitis were reported occasionally (<1%).

MISCELLANEOUS—diaphoresis and flushing were reported occasionally (<1%).

Other rarely observed adverse reactions (<0.1%) include leukocytosis, lymphocytosis, monocytosis, basophilia, a decrease in the prothrombin time, jaundice, gallbladder sludge, glycosuria, hematuria, anaphylaxis, bronchospasm, serum sickness, abdominal pain, colitis, flatulence, dyspepsia, palpitations and epistaxis.

DOSAGE AND ADMINISTRATION

Rocephin may be administered intravenously or intramuscularly.

ADULTS: The usual adult daily dose is 1 to 2 grams given once a day (or in equally divided doses twice a day) depending on the type and severity of infection. The total daily dose should not exceed 4 grams.

If *C. trachomatis* is a suspected pathogen, appropriate antichlamydial coverage should be added, because ceftriaxone sodium has no activity against this organism.

For the treatment of uncomplicated gonococcal infections, a single intramuscular dose of 250 mg is recommended.

For preoperative use (surgical prophylaxis), a single dose of 1 gram administered intravenously ½ to 2 hours before surgery is recommended.

PEDIATRIC PATIENTS: For the treatment of skin and skin structure infections, the recommended total daily dose is 50 to 75 mg/kg given once a day (or in equally divided doses twice a day). The total daily dose should not exceed 2 grams.

For the treatment of acute bacterial otitis media, a single intramuscular dose of 50 mg/kg (not to exceed 1 gram) is recommended (see INDICATIONS AND USAGE).

Diluent	Concentration mg/mL	Storage Room Temp. (25°C)	Storage Refrigerated (4°C)
Sterile Water for	100	3 days	10 days
Injection	250, 350	24 hours	3 days
0.9% Sodium	100	3 days	10 days
Chloride Solution	250, 350	24 hours	3 days
5% Dextrose	100	3 days	10 days
Solution	250, 350	24 hours	3 days
Bacteriostatic Water + 0.9%	100	24 hours	10 days
Benzyl Alcohol	250, 350	24 hours	3 days
1% Lidocaine Solution	100	24 hours	10 days
(without epinephrine)	250, 350	24 hours	3 days

Diluent	Storage Room Temp. (25°C)	Storage Refrigerated (4°C)
Sterile Water	3 days	10 days
0.9% Sodium Chloride Solution	3 days	10 days
5% Dextrose Solution	3 days	10 days
10% Dextrose Solution	3 days	10 days
5% Dextrose + 0.9% Sodium Chloride Solution*	3 days	Incompatible
5% Dextrose + 0.45% Sodium Chloride Solution	3 days	Incompatible

*Data available for 10 to 40 mg/mL concentrations in this diluent in PVC containers only.

For the treatment of serious miscellaneous infections other than meningitis, the recommended total daily dose is 50 to 75 mg/kg, given in divided doses every 12 hours. The total daily dose should not exceed 2 grams.

In the treatment of meningitis, it is recommended that the initial therapeutic dose be 100 mg/kg (not to exceed 4 grams). Thereafter, a total daily dose of 100 mg/kg/day (not to exceed 4 grams daily) is recommended. The daily dose may be administered once a day (or in equally divided doses every 12 hours). The usual duration of therapy is 7 to 14 days.

Generally, Rocephin therapy should be continued for at least 2 days after the signs and symptoms of infection have disappeared. The usual duration of therapy is 4 to 14 days; in complicated infections, longer therapy may be required. When treating infections caused by *Streptococcus pyogenes*, therapy should be continued for at least 10 days.

No dosage adjustment is necessary for patients with impairment of renal or hepatic function; however, blood levels should be monitored in patients with severe renal impairment (eg, dialysis patients) and in patients with both renal and hepatic dysfunctions.

DIRECTIONS FOR USE: Intramuscular Administration: Reconstitute Rocephin powder with the appropriate diluent (see COMPATIBILITY AND STABILITY section).

After reconstitution, each 1 mL of solution contains approximately 250 mg or 350 mg equivalent of ceftriaxone according to the amount of diluent indicated below. If required, more dilute solutions could be utilized. **A 350 mg/mL concentration is not recommended for the 250 mg vial since it may not be possible to withdraw the entire contents.** As with all intramuscular preparations, Rocephin should be injected well within the body of a relatively large muscle; aspiration helps to avoid unintentional injection into a blood vessel.

Vial Dosage Size	Amount of Diluent to be Added 250 mg/mL	350 mg/mL
250 mg	0.9 mL	—
500 mg	1.8 mL	1.0 mL
1 gm	3.6 mL	2.1 mL
2 gm	7.2 mL	4.2 mL

Intramuscular Convenience Kit: For the 500 mg vial, withdraw 1 mL of diluent, discard the remainder. Inject diluent into vial, shake vial thoroughly to form solution. Withdraw entire contents of vial into syringe to equal approximately 1.4 mL.

For 1 gm vial, withdraw entire contents of diluent (2.1 mL). Inject diluent into vial, shake vial thoroughly to form solution. Withdraw entire contents of vial into syringe to equal approximately 2.8 mL.

Intravenous Administration: Rocephin should be administered intravenously by infusion over a period of 30 minutes. Concentrations between 10 mg/mL and 40 mg/mL are recommended; however, lower concentrations may be used if desired. Reconstitute vials or "piggyback" bottles with an appropriate IV diluent (see COMPATIBILITY AND STABILITY section).

Vial Dosage Size	Amount of Diluent to be Added
250 mg	2.4 mL
500 mg	4.8 mL
1 gm	9.6 mL
2 gm	19.2 mL

After reconstitution, each 1 mL of solution contains approximately 100 mg equivalent of ceftriaxone. Withdraw entire contents and dilute to the desired concentration with the appropriate IV diluent.

Piggyback Bottle Dosage Size	Amount of Diluent to be Added
1 gm	10 mL
2 gm	20 mL

After reconstitution, further dilute to 50 mL or 100 mL volumes with the appropriate IV diluent.

COMPATIBILITY AND STABILITY: Rocephin sterile powder should be stored at room temperature—77°F (25°C)—or below and protected from light. After reconstitution, protection from normal light is not necessary. The color of solutions ranges from light yellow to amber, depending on the length of storage, concentration and diluent used.

Rocephin *intramuscular* solutions remain stable (loss of potency less than 10%) for the following time periods:
[See first table above]

Rocephin *intravenous* solutions, at concentrations of 10, 20 and 40 mg/mL, remain stable (loss of potency less than 10%) for the following time periods stored in glass or PVC containers:
[See second table above]

Similarly, Rocephin *intravenous* solutions, at concentrations of 100 mg/mL, remain stable in the IV piggyback glass containers for the above specified time periods.

The following *intravenous* Rocephin solutions are stable at room temperature (25°C) for 24 hours, at concentrations between 10 mg/mL and 40 mg/mL: Sodium Lactate (PVC container), 10% Invert Sugar (glass container), 5% Sodium Bicarbonate (glass container), Freamine III (glass container), Normosol-M in 5% Dextrose (glass and PVC containers), Ionosol-B in 5% Dextrose (glass container), 5% Mannitol (glass container), 10% Mannitol (glass container).

After the indicated stability time periods, unused portions of solutions should be discarded.

Rocephin reconstituted with 5% Dextrose or 0.9% Sodium Chloride solution at concentrations between 10 mg/mL and 40 mg/mL, and then stored in frozen state (−20°C) in PVC or polyolefin containers, remains stable for 26 weeks.

Frozen solutions should be thawed at room temperature before use. After thawing, unused portions should be discarded. **DO NOT REFREEZE.**

Rocephin solutions should *not* be physically mixed with or piggybacked into solutions containing other antimicrobial drugs or into diluent solutions other than those listed above, due to possible incompatibility.

ANIMAL PHARMACOLOGY

Concretions consisting of the precipitated calcium salt of ceftriaxone have been found in the gallbladder bile of dogs and baboons treated with ceftriaxone.

These appeared as a gritty sediment in dogs that received 100 mg/kg/day for 4 weeks. A similar phenomenon has been observed in baboons but only after a protracted dosing period (6 months) at higher dose levels (335 mg/kg/day or more). The likelihood of this occurrence in humans is considered to be low, since ceftriaxone has a greater plasma half-life in humans, the calcium salt of ceftriaxone is more soluble in human gallbladder bile and the calcium content of human gallbladder bile is relatively low.

HOW SUPPLIED

Rocephin is supplied as a sterile crystalline powder in glass vials and piggyback bottles. The following packages are available:

Vials containing 250 mg equivalent of ceftriaxone. Box of 1 (NDC 0004-1962-02) and box of 10 (NDC 0004-1962-01).
Vials containing 500 mg equivalent of ceftriaxone. Box of 1 (NDC 0004-1963-02) and box of 10 (NDC 0004-1963-01).

Clinical Efficacy in Evaluable Population

Study Day	Ceftriaxone Single Dose	Comparator – 10 days of Oral Therapy	95% Confidence Interval	Statistical Outcome
Study 1—US		amoxicillin/clavulanate		
14	74% (220/296)	82% (247/302)	(-14.4%, -0.5%)	Ceftriaxone is lower than control at study day 14 and 28.
28	58% (167/288)	67% (200/297)	(-17.5%, -1.2%)	
Study 2—US[3]		TMP-SMZ		
14	54% (113/210)	60% (124/206)	(-16.4%, 3.6%)	Ceftriaxone is equivalent to control at study day 14 and 28.
28	35% (73/206)	45% (93/205)	(-19.9%, 0.0%)	

	Study Day 13–15		Study Day 30+2	
Organism	No. Analyzed	No. Erad. (%)	No. Analyzed	No. Erad. (%)
S. pneumoniae	38	32 (84)	35	25 (71)
H. influenzae	33	28 (85)	31	22 (71)
M. catarrhalis	15	12 (80)	15	9 (60)

Vials containing 1 gm equivalent of ceftriaxone. Box of 1 (NDC 0004-1964-04) and box of 10 (NDC 0004-1964-01). Piggyback bottles containing 1 gm equivalent of ceftriaxone. Box of 1 (NDC 0004-1964-02).
Vials containing 2 gm equivalent of ceftriaxone. Box of 10 (NDC 0004-1965-01).
Piggyback bottles containing 2 gm equivalent of ceftriaxone. Box of 1 (NDC 0004-1965-02).
Bulk pharmacy containers, containing 10 gm equivalent of ceftriaxone. Box of 1 (NDC 0004-1971-01). NOT FOR DIRECT ADMINISTRATION.
Rocephin is also supplied in an Intramuscular Convenience Kit, available in two strengths, consisting of a vial of ceftriaxone sodium as a sterile crystalline powder and a vial of Xylocaine®-MPF 1% (lidocaine HCl Injection, USP).
The following strengths are available:
Kit containing 1 vial of 500 mg equivalent of ceftriaxone, plus 1 vial of 2.1 mL Xylocaine (NDC 0004-2014-92).
Kit containing 1 vial of 1 gm equivalent of ceftriaxone, plus 1 vial of 2.1 mL Xylocaine (NDC 0004-2013-92).
Xylocaine®-MPF 1% (lidocaine HCl Injection, USP) is manufactured for Roche Laboratories Inc. by Astra USA, Inc., Westborough, MA 01581.
Rocephin is also supplied as a sterile crystalline powder in ADD-Vantage®* Vials as follows:
ADD-Vantage Vials containing 1 gm equivalent of ceftriaxone. Box of 10 (NDC 0004-1964-05).
ADD-Vantage Vials containing 2 gm equivalent of ceftriaxone. Box of 10 (NDC 0004-1965-05).
Rocephin (ceftriaxone sodium injection), also supplied premixed as a frozen, iso-osmotic, sterile, nonpyrogenic solution of ceftriaxone sodium in 50 mL single dose Galaxy®† containers (PL 2040 plastic), is manufactured for Roche Laboratories Inc., by Baxter Healthcare Corporation, Deerfield, Illinois 60015. The following strengths are available:
1 gm equivalent of ceftriaxone, iso-osmotic with approximately 1.9 gm Dextrose Hydrous, USP, added (NDC 0004-2002-78).
2 gm equivalent of ceftriaxone, iso-osmotic with approximately 1.2 gm Dextrose Hydrous, USP, added (NDC 0004-2003-78).
NOTE: Store Rocephin in the frozen state at or below -20°C/-4°F.

*Registered trademark of Abbott Laboratories, Inc.
†Registered trademark of Baxter International Inc.

CLINICAL STUDIES

Clinical Trials in Pediatric Patients With Acute Bacterial Otitis Media: In two adequate and well controlled US clinical trials a single IM dose of ceftriaxone was compared with a 10 day course of oral antibiotic in pediatric patients between the ages of 3 months and 6 years. The clinical cure rates and statistical outcome appear in the table below:
[See first table above]
An open-label bacteriologic study of ceftriaxone without a comparator enrolled 108 pediatric patients, 79 of whom had positive baseline cultures for one or more of the common pathogens. The results of this study are tabulated as follows:
Week 2 and 4 Bacteriologic Eradication Rates in the Per Protocol Analysis in the Roche Bacteriologic Study by pathogen:
[See second table above]

REFERENCES

1. National Committee for Clinical Laboratory Standards, *Performance Standards for Antimicrobial Disk Susceptibility Tests.* 5th ed. Villanova, PA: 1993. Approved Standard NCCLS Document M2-A5, Vol. 13, No. 24. NCCLS.
2. National Committee for Clinical Laboratory Standards, *Methods for Dilution Antimicrobial Susceptibility Tests for Bacteria That Grow Aerobically.* 3rd ed. Villanova, PA: 1993. Approved Standard NCCLS Document M7-A3, Vol. 13, No. 25. NCCLS.
3. Barnett ED, Teele DW, Klein JO, et al. *Comparison of Ceftriaxone and Trimethoprim-Sulfamethoxazole for Acute Otitis Media.* Pediatrics. Vol. 99, No. 1, January 1997.

Revised: January 1998

ROFERON®-A
[ro-fear 'on]
(Interferon alfa-2a, recombinant) ℞

The following text is complete prescribing information based on official labeling in effect June 1998.

DESCRIPTION

Roferon-A (Interferon alfa-2a, recombinant) is a sterile protein product for use by injection. Roferon-A is manufactured by recombinant DNA technology that employs a genetically engineered *Escherichia coli* bacterium containing DNA that codes for the human protein. Interferon alfa-2a, recombinant is a highly purified protein containing 165 amino acids, and it has an approximate molecular weight of 19,000 daltons. The purification procedure includes affinity chromatography using a murine monoclonal antibody. Fermentation is carried out in a defined nutrient medium containing the antibiotic tetracycline hydrochloride, 5 mg/L. However, the presence of the antibiotic is not detectable in the final product. Roferon-A is supplied as an injectable solution or as a sterile powder for injection with its accompanying diluent.

Injectable Solution:
3 million IU (11.1 mcg/mL) Roferon-A per vial—The solution is colorless and each mL contains 3 MIU of Interferon alfa-2a, recombinant, 7.21 mg sodium chloride, 0.2 mg polysorbate 80, 10 mg benzyl alcohol as a preservative and 0.77 mg ammonium acetate.
6 million IU (22.2 mcg/mL) Roferon-A per vial—The solution is colorless and each mL contains 6 MIU of Interferon alfa-2a, recombinant, 7.21 mg sodium chloride, 0.2 mg polysorbate 80, 10 mg benzyl alcohol as a preservative and 0.77 mg ammonium acetate. This dosage form should not be used for the treatment of hairy cell leukemia.
9 million IU (33.3 mcg/0.9 mL) Roferon-A per vial—The solution is colorless and each 0.9 mL contains 9 MIU of Interferon alfa-2a, recombinant, 6.49 mg sodium chloride, 0.18 mg polysorbate 80, 9 mg benzyl alcohol as a preservative and 0.69 mg ammonium acetate.
18 million IU (66.7 mcg/3 mL) Roferon-A per vial—The solution is colorless and each mL contains 6 MIU of Interferon alfa-2a, recombinant, 7.21 mg sodium chloride, 0.2 mg polysorbate 80, 10 mg benzyl alcohol as a preservative and 0.77 mg ammonium acetate. Each 0.5 mL contains 3 MIU of Interferon alfa-2a, recombinant.
36 million IU (133.3 mcg/mL) Roferon-A per vial—The solution is colorless and each mL contains 36 MIU of Interferon alfa-2a, recombinant, 7.21 mg sodium chloride, 0.2 mg polysorbate 80, 10 mg benzyl alcohol as a preservative and 0.77 mg ammonium acetate. This dosage form should not be used for the treatment of hairy cell leukemia.
Based on the specific activity of 2.7×10^8 IU/mg protein, the corresponding quantities of Interferon alfa-2a, recombinant in the vials described above are approximately 3 MIU (11.1 mcg/mL), 6 MIU (22.2 mcg/mL), 9 MIU (33.3 mcg/0.9 mL), 18 MIU (66.7 mcg/3 mL) and 36 MIU (133.3 mcg/mL).
Sterile Powder for Injection:

18 million IU Roferon-A per vial—The powder is white to beige and when reconstituted with 3 mL of Diluent for Sterile Powder for Injection each 1 mL of reconstituted solution contains 6 MIU of Interferon alfa-2a, recombinant, 9 mg sodium chloride, 1.67 mg Albumin (Human) and 3.3 mg phenol as a preservative. Each 0.5 mL contains 3 MIU of Interferon alfa-2a, recombinant.
Diluent for Sterile Powder for Injection:
3 mL per vial—Each mL contains 6 mg sodium chloride and 3.3 mg phenol as a preservative.
The route of administration is subcutaneous or intramuscular.

CLINICAL PHARMACOLOGY

The mechanism by which Interferon alfa-2a, recombinant, or any other interferon, exerts antitumor or antiviral activity is not clearly understood. However, it is believed that direct antiproliferative action against tumor cells, inhibition of virus replication and modulation of the host immune response play important roles in antitumor and antiviral activity.
The biological activities of Interferon alfa-2a, recombinant are species-restricted, ie, they are expressed in a very limited number of species other than humans. As a consequence, preclinical evaluation of Interferon alfa-2a, recombinant has involved in vitro experiments with human cells and some in vivo experiments.[1] Using human cells in culture, Interferon alfa-2a, recombinant has been shown to have antiproliferative and immunomodulatory activities that are very similar to those of the mixture of interferon alfa subtypes produced by human leukocytes. In vivo, Interferon alfa-2a, recombinant has been shown to inhibit the growth of several human tumors growing in immunocompromised (nude) mice. Because of its species-restricted activity, it has not been possible to demonstrate antitumor activity in immunologically intact syngeneic tumor model systems, where effects on the host immune system would be observable. However, such antitumor activity has been repeatedly demonstrated with, for example, mouse interferon-alfa in transplantable mouse tumor systems. The clinical significance of these findings is unknown.
The metabolism of Interferon alfa-2a, recombinant is consistent with that of alfa interferons in general. Alfa interferons are totally filtered through the glomeruli and undergo rapid proteolytic degradation during tubular reabsorption, rendering a negligible reappearance of intact alfa interferon in the systemic circulation. Small amounts of radiolabeled Interferon alfa-2a, recombinant appear in the urine of isolated rat kidneys, suggesting near complete reabsorption of Interferon alfa-2a, recombinant catabolites. Liver metabolism and subsequent biliary excretion are considered minor pathways of elimination for alfa interferons.
The serum concentrations of Interferon alfa-2a, recombinant reflected a large intersubject variation in both healthy volunteers and patients with disseminated cancer.
In healthy people, Interferon alfa-2a, recombinant exhibited an elimination half-life of 3.7 to 8.5 hours (mean 5.1 hours), volume of distribution at steady-state of 0.223 to 0.748 L/kg (mean 0.400 L/kg) and a total body clearance of 2.14 to 3.62 mL/min/kg (mean 2.79 mL/min/kg) after a 36 MIU (2.2×10^8 pg) intravenous infusion. After intramuscular and subcutaneous administrations of 36 MIU, peak serum concentrations ranged from 1500 to 2580 pg/mL (mean 2020 pg/mL) at a mean time to peak of 3.8 hours and from 1250 to 2320 pg/mL (mean 1730 pg/mL) at a mean time to peak of 7.3 hours, respectively. The apparent fraction of the dose absorbed after intramuscular injection was greater than 80%. The pharmacokinetics of Interferon alfa-2a, recombinant after single intramuscular doses to patients with disseminated cancer were similar to those found in healthy volunteers. Dose proportional increases in serum concentrations were observed after single doses up to 198 MIU. There were no changes in the distribution or elimination of Interferon alfa-2a, recombinant during twice daily (0.5 to 36 MIU), once daily (1 to 54 MIU), or three times weekly (1 to 136 MIU) dosing regimens up to 28 days of dosing. Multiple intramuscular doses of Interferon alfa-2a, recombinant resulted in an accumulation of two to four times the single dose serum concentrations. There is no pharmacokinetic information in patients with chronic hepatitis C, hairy cell leukemia, AIDS-related Kaposi's sarcoma and chronic myelogenous leukemia.
Serum neutralizing activity, determined by a highly sensitive enzyme immunoassay, and a neutralization bioassay, was detected in approximately 25% of all patients who received Roferon-A.[2] Antibodies to human leukocyte interferon may occur spontaneously in certain clinical conditions (cancer, systemic lupus erythematosus, herpes zoster) in patients who have never received exogenous interferon.[3] The significance of the appearance of serum neutralizing activity is not known.
CLINICAL STUDIES: Studies have shown that Roferon-A can normalize serum ALT, improve liver histology and reduce viral load in patients with chronic hepatitis C. Other studies have shown that Roferon-A can produce clinically meaningful tumor regression or disease stabilization in patients with hairy cell leukemia or in patients with AIDS-

Continued on next page

Roferon-A—Cont.

related Kaposi's sarcoma.[4-6] In Ph-positive Chronic Myelogenous Leukemia, Roferon-A supplemented with intermittent chemotherapy has been shown to prolong overall survival and to delay disease progression compared to patients treated with chemotherapy alone.[7] In addition, Roferon-A has been shown to produce sustained complete cytogenetic responses in a small subset of patients with CML in chronic phase. The activity of Roferon-A in Ph-*negative* CML has not been determined.

EFFECTS ON CHRONIC HEPATITIS C: The safety and efficacy of Roferon-A was evaluated worldwide in multiple clinical trials involving a total of 1831 patients. Roferon-A was given three times a week (tiw) by subcutaneous (SC) or intramuscular injection (IM) in a variety of dosing regimens. Doses studied ranged from 1 MIU to 9 MIU and duration of treatment from 6 to 12 months. Observation periods following therapy ranged from 3 months to 4 years. The patients were 18 years of age or older, had a history of elevated levels of serum alanine aminotransferase (ALT) at least 1.5 times above normal, were positive for antibody to HCV, were tested negative for antibody to both HIV and HBV, and had hepatitis with or without cirrhosis in the absence of decompensated liver disease.

Therapy with Roferon-A resulted in normalization of serum ALT at the end of treatment and at the end of treatment-free follow-up. In two randomized, controlled trials those treated for 12 months were more likely to maintain normal serum ALT levels following discontinuation of therapy than those treated for 6 months. In addition, patients treated with higher doses more often experienced a complete response at the end of follow-up than did those treated with lower doses. Younger patients (eg, less than 35 years of age) and patients without cirrhosis on liver biopsy were more likely to respond completely to Roferon-A than those patients greater than 35 years of age or patients with cirrhosis on liver biopsy.

In all studies a complete response was defined as two consecutive normal serum ALT values at least 21 days apart at the end of treatment or at the end of follow-up. Forty-three percent (75 of 173) of patients receiving Roferon-A 3 MIU tiw for 12 months had reduction in serum ALT to normal levels at some point during therapy. However, only 23% had a complete response at the end of treatment. Approximately half of the patients receiving Roferon-A 3 MIU tiw for 12 months who had a complete response at the end of treatment subsequently relapsed (ie, recurrence of abnormal ALT) following cessation of therapy (see Table 1). In studies with long-term follow-up, 91% (39 of 43) of patients with normal ALTs at the end of 6 months of follow-up had persistently normal ALTs during continuous follow-up of up to 4 years. Of patients who relapsed during the follow-up period and were retreated at this dose, 90% (18/20) responded to treatment. Patients who fail to sustain a complete response following an initial course of therapy may benefit from retreatment with higher doses of Roferon-A.

A subset of patients had liver biopsies performed both before and after treatment with Roferon-A. An improvement in liver histology as assessed by Knodell Histology Activity Index was generally observed (see Table 2).

[See table 1 below]

[See table 2 at bottom of next page]

A retrospective subgroup analysis of 317 patients from two studies suggests a correlation between improvement in liver histology, durable serum ALT response rates, and decreased viral load as measured by the polymerase chain reaction (PCR).

EFFECTS ON HAIRY CELL LEUKEMIA: A multicenter US phase II study (N2752) enrolled 218 patients; 75 were evaluable for efficacy in a preliminary analysis; 218 patients were evaluable for safety. Patients were to receive a starting dose of Roferon-A up to 6 MIU/m^2/day, for an induction period of 4 to 6 months. Responding patients were to receive 12 months maintenance therapy.

During the first 1 to 2 months of treatment of patients with hairy cell leukemia, significant depression of hematopoiesis was likely to occur. Subsequently, there was improvement in circulating blood cell counts. Of the 75 patients who were evaluable for efficacy following at least 16 weeks of therapy, 46 (61%) achieved complete or partial response. Twenty-one patients (28%) had a minor remission, 8 (11%) remained stable, and none had worsening of disease. All patients who achieved either a complete or partial response had complete or partial normalization of all peripheral blood elements including hemoglobin level, white blood cell, neutrophil, monocyte and platelet counts with a concomitant decrease in peripheral blood and bone marrow hairy cells. Responding patients also exhibited a marked reduction in red blood cell and platelet transfusion requirements, a decrease in infectious episodes and improvement in performance status. The probability of survival for 2 years in patients receiving Roferon-A (94%) was statistically increased compared to a historical control group (75%).

EFFECTS ON AIDS-RELATED KAPOSI'S SARCOMA: In six studies with Roferon-A, doses of 3 to 54 MIU daily were evaluated for the treatment of AIDS-related Kaposi's sarcoma in more than 350 patients. Four dosage regimens of Roferon-A were evaluated for initial induction. Thirty-nine patients received 3 MIU daily; 99 patients received an escalating regimen of 3 MIU, 9 MIU and 18 MIU each daily for 3 days, followed by 36 MIU daily; 119 patients received 36 MIU daily; and 16 patients received doses greater than 36 MIU to a maximum of 54 MIU daily. An additional 91 patients received Roferon-A in combination with vinblastine. The best response rate associated with acceptable toxicity was observed when Roferon-A was administered as a single agent at a dose of 36 MIU daily. The escalating regimen of 3 to 36 MIU daily provided equivalent therapeutic benefit with some amelioration of acute toxicity in some patients. In AIDS-related Kaposi's sarcoma, lower doses were less effective in inducing tumor regression and doses higher than 36 MIU daily were associated with unacceptable toxicity.

As summarized in Table 3, the likelihood of response to Roferon-A varied with the clinical manifestations of human immunodeficiency virus (HIV) infection. Patients with prior opportunistic infection or B symptoms are unlikely to respond to treatment with Roferon-A.

Table 3.—Likelihood of Response to Roferon-A in Patients with AIDS-Related Kaposi's Sarcoma

	$CD_4(T_4)$ Lymphocyte Count	Objective Response Rate (%)		
No. Pts.*	(cells/mm^3)	CR	PR	Total
83	0–200	3.6	3.6	7.2
51	201–400	15.7	11.8	27.5
33	>400	24.2	21.2	45.4

In the 28 patients evaluated who had prior opportunistic infection or B symptoms, the response rate was 3.6%.

*Patients had no prior opportunistic infection or B symptoms. B symptoms include night sweats, weight loss of greater than 10% of body weight or 15 lbs, or fever greater than 100°F without an identifiable source of infection.

Patients who were otherwise asymptomatic, with no prior opportunistic infection and near-normal levels of CD_4 lymphocytes, experienced higher response rates. Responding patients with a baseline CD_4 lymphocyte count greater than 200 cells/mm^3 had a distinct survival advantage over both responding patients with a baseline CD_4 lymphocyte count of 200 cells/mm^3 or less and nonresponding patients regardless of their baseline CD_4 lymphocyte count. Median survival for responding patients with CD_4 lymphocyte counts of greater than 200 to 400 cells/mm^3 had not been reached but was greater than 32.7 months from the initiation of therapy. For responding patients with CD_4 lymphocyte counts of greater than 400 cells/mm^3, the median survival had not been reached but was greater than 29.5 months.

A classification system for staging AIDS-related Kaposi's sarcoma has been described based on location and extent of disease. In studies of Roferon-A, no difference was noted in response rates for patients with different stages of Kaposi's sarcoma. Likelihood of response was related to manifestations of HIV infection (baseline CD_4 lymphocyte count, prior opportunistic infection or B symptoms) and not to extent of tumor involvement. The median time to response was 2.7 months. The median duration of response for patients achieving a partial or complete response was 6.3 and 20.7 months, respectively. Complete and partial responses lasting in excess of 3 years have been observed. Therapy was discontinued because of progression of Kaposi's sarcoma, development of severe opportunistic infection or severe adverse effects. The median time to discontinuation of treatment was 12.5 months for responding patients and 2.3 months for patients who did not respond.

EFFECTS ON Ph-POSITIVE CHRONIC MYELOGENOUS LEUKEMIA (CML): Roferon-A was evaluated in two trials of patients with chronic phase CML. Study DM84-38 was a single center phase II study conducted at the MD Anderson Cancer Center, which enrolled 91 patients, 81% were previously treated, 82% were Ph positive, and 63% received Roferon-A within 1 year of diagnosis. Study MI400 was a multicenter randomized phase III study conducted in Italy by the Italian Cooperative Study Group on CML in 335 patients; 226 Roferon-A and 109 chemotherapy. Patients with Ph-positive, newly diagnosed or minimally treated CML were randomized (ratio 2:1) to either Roferon-A or conventional chemotherapy with either hydroxyurea or busulfan. In study DM84-38, patients started Roferon-A at 9 MIU/day, whereas in study MI400, it was progressively escalated from 3 to 9 MIU/day over the first month. In both trials, dose escalation for insufficient hematologic response, and dose attenuation or interruption for toxicity was permitted. No formal guidelines for dose attenuation were given in the chemotherapy arm of study MI400. In addition, in the Roferon-A arm, the MI400 protocol allowed the addition of intermittent single agent chemotherapy for insufficient hematologic response to Roferon-A alone. In this trial, 44% of the Roferon-A treated patients also received intermittent single agent chemotherapy at some time during the study. The two studies were analyzed according to uniform response criteria. For hematologic response: complete response (WBC $<9x10^9$/L, normalization of the differential with no immature forms in the peripheral blood, disappearance of splenomegaly), partial response (>50% decrease from baseline of WBC to $<20x10^9$/L). For cytogenetic response: complete response (0% Ph-positive metaphases), partial response (1% to 34% Ph-positive metaphases).

In study DM84-38, the median survival from initiation of Roferon-A was 47 months. In study MI400, the median survival for the patients on the interferon arm was 69 months, which was significantly better than the 55 months seen in the chemotherapy control group (48 patients in study MI400 proceeded to BMT and in study DM84-38, 15 patients proceeded to BMT). Roferon-A treatment significantly delayed disease progression to blastic phase as evidenced by a median time to disease progression of 69 months compared to 46 months with chemotherapy.

By multivariate analysis of prognostic factors associated with all 335 patients entered into the randomized study, treatment with Roferon-A (with or without intermittent additional chemotherapy; p=0.006), Sokal index[8] (p=0.006) and WBC (p=0.023) were the three variables associated with an improved survival, independent of other baseline characteristics (Karnofsky performance status and hemoglobin being the other factors entered into the model).

In study MI400, overall hematologic responses, [complete responses (CR) and partial responses (PR)], were observed in approximately 60% of patients treated with Roferon-A (40% CR, 20% PR), compared to 70% with chemotherapy (30% CR, 40% PR). The median time to reach a complete hematologic response was 5 months in the Roferon-A arm and 4 months in the chemotherapy arm. The overall cytogenetic response rate (CR+PR), in patients receiving Roferon-A, was 10% and 12% in studies MI400 and DM84-38, respectively, according to the intent-to-treat principle. In contrast, only 2% of the patients in the chemotherapy arm of study MI400 achieved a cytogenetic response (with no complete responses). Cytogenetic responses were observed only in patients who had complete hematologic responses. In study DM84-38, hematologic and cytogenetic response rates were higher in the subset of patients treated with Roferon-A within 1 year of diagnosis (76% and 17%, respectively) compared to the subset initiating Roferon-A therapy more than 1 year from diagnosis (29% and 4%, respectively). In an exploratory analysis, patients who achieved a cytogenetic response lived longer than those who did not.

Severe adverse events were observed in 66% and 31% of patients on study DM84-38 and MI400, respectively. Dose reduction and temporary cessation of therapy was required frequently. Permanent cessation of Roferon-A, due to intolerable side effects, was required in 15% and 23% of patients on studies DM84-38 and MI400, respectively (see ADVERSE REACTIONS).

Limited data are available on the use of Roferon-A in children with Ph-positive, adult-type CML. A published report on 15 children with CML suggests a safety profile similar to that seen in adult CML; clinical responses were also observed[9] (see DOSAGE AND ADMINISTRATION).

INDICATIONS AND USAGE

Roferon-A is indicated for the treatment of chronic hepatitis C, hairy cell leukemia and AIDS-related Kaposi's sarcoma in patients 18 years of age or older. In addition, it is indicated for chronic phase, Philadelphia chromosome (Ph) positive chronic myelogenous leukemia (CML) patients who are minimally pretreated (within 1 year of diagnosis).

FOR PATIENTS WITH CHRONIC HEPATITIS C: Roferon-A is indicated for use in patients with chronic hep-

Table 1.—Complete Biochemical Response (CR) at the End of Treatment and at the End of Follow-up*

Study No.	Treatment Duration (months)	Dose (MIU)	N	End of Treatment CR [% (95% CI)]	End of Follow-up CR [% (95% CI)]
1	12	Placebo	56	0	0
1	12	3	56	23	11
2	12	3	117	23	12
All	12	3	173	23 (17–30)	12 (7–17)

*All patients were followed for 6 months after the end of treatment.

atitis C diagnosed by HCV antibody and/or a history of exposure to hepatitis C who have compensated liver disease and are 18 years of age or older. A liver biopsy and a serum test for the presence of antibody to HCV should be performed to establish the diagnosis of chronic hepatitis C. Other causes of hepatitis, including hepatitis B, should be excluded prior to therapy with Roferon-A.

FOR PATIENTS WITH AIDS-RELATED KAPOSI'S SARCOMA: Roferon-A is indicated for the treatment of AIDS-related Kaposi's sarcoma in a select group of patients. In determining whether a patient should be treated, the physician should assess the likelihood of response based on the clinical manifestations of HIV infection, including prior opportunistic infections, presence of B symptoms, and CD_4 count, and the manifestations of Kaposi's sarcoma requiring treatment (see CLINICAL PHARMACOLOGY).

CONTRAINDICATIONS

Roferon-A is contraindicated in patients with known hypersensitivity to alfa interferon, mouse immunoglobulin or any component of the product. The injectable solutions contain benzyl alcohol and are contraindicated in any individual with a known allergy to that preservative.

WARNINGS

Roferon-A should be administered under the guidance of a qualified physician (see DOSAGE AND ADMINISTRATION). Appropriate management of the therapy and its complications is possible only when adequate facilities are readily available.

DEPRESSION AND SUICIDAL BEHAVIOR INCLUDING SUICIDAL IDEATION, SUICIDAL ATTEMPTS AND SUICIDES HAVE BEEN REPORTED IN ASSOCIATION WITH TREATMENT WITH ALFA INTERFERONS, INCLUDING ROFERON-A. Patients to be treated with Roferon-A should be informed that depression and suicidal ideation may be side effects of treatment and should be advised to report these side effects immediately to the prescribing physician. Patients receiving Roferon-A therapy should receive close monitoring for the occurrence of depressive symptomatology. Cessation of treatment should be considered for patients experiencing depression. Although dose reduction or treatment cessation may lead to resolution of the depressive symptomatology, depression may persist and suicides have occurred after withdrawing therapy (see PRECAUTIONS and ADVERSE REACTIONS).

Central nervous system adverse reactions have been reported in a number of patients. These reactions included decreased mental status, dizziness, impaired memory, agitation, manic behavior and psychotic reactions. More severe obtundation and coma have been rarely observed. Most of these abnormalities were mild and reversible within a few days to 3 weeks upon dose reduction or discontinuation of Roferon-A therapy. Careful periodic neuropsychiatric monitoring of all patients is recommended.

Roferon-A should be used with caution in patients with severe preexisting cardiac disease, severe renal or hepatic disease, seizure disorders and/or compromised central nervous system function.

Roferon-A should be administered with caution to patients with cardiac disease or with any history of cardiac illness. Acute, self-limited toxicities (ie, fever, chills) frequently associated with Roferon-A administration may exacerbate preexisting cardiac conditions. Rarely, myocardial infarction has occurred in patients receiving Roferon-A. Cases of cardiomyopathy have been observed on rare occasions in patients treated with alfa interferons.

Patients with a history of autoimmune hepatitis or a history of autoimmune disease and patients who are immunosuppressed transplant recipients should not be treated with Roferon-A. Controlled studies of Roferon-A therapy in patients with advanced cirrhosis and/or decompensated liver disease have not been performed. In chronic hepatitis C, initiation of alfa-interferon therapy, including Roferon-A, has been reported to cause transient liver abnormalities, which in patients with poorly compensated liver disease can result in increased ascites, hepatic failure or death.

Leukopenia and elevation of hepatic enzymes occurred frequently but were rarely dose-limiting. Thrombocytopenia occurred less frequently. Proteinuria and increased cells in urinary sediment were also seen infrequently. Dose-limiting hepatic or renal toxicities were unusual. Infrequently, severe renal toxicities, sometimes requiring renal dialysis, have been reported with alfa-interferon therapy alone or in combination with IL-2 (see PRECAUTIONS).

Infrequently, severe or fatal gastrointestinal hemorrhage has been reported in association with alfa-interferon therapy.

Caution should be exercised when administering Roferon-A to patients with myelosuppression or when Roferon-A is used in combination with other agents that are known to cause myelosuppression. Synergistic toxicity has been observed when Roferon-A is administered in combination with zidovudine (AZT).[10] The effects of Roferon-A when combined with other drugs used in the treatment of AIDS-related disease are not known.

Hyperglycemia has been observed rarely in patients treated with Roferon-A. Symptomatic patients should have their blood glucose measured and followed-up accordingly. Patients with diabetes mellitus may require adjustment of their anti-diabetic regimen.

Roferon-A should not be used for the treatment of visceral AIDS-related Kaposi's sarcoma associated with rapidly progressive or life-threatening disease.

The injectable solutions contain benzyl alcohol and should not be used by patients with a known allergy to benzyl alcohol. This product is not indicated for use in neonates or infants and should not be used by patients in that age group. There have been rare reports of death in neonates and infants associated with excessive exposure to benzyl alcohol. The amount of benzyl alcohol at which toxicity or adverse effects may occur in neonates or infants is not known (see CONTRAINDICATIONS).

PRECAUTIONS

General: In all instances where the use of Roferon-A is considered for chemotherapy, the physician must evaluate the need and usefulness of the drug against the risk of adverse reactions. Most adverse reactions are reversible if detected early. If severe reactions occur, the drug should be reduced in dosage or discontinued and appropriate corrective measures should be taken according to the clinical judgment of the physician. Reinstitution of Roferon-A therapy should be carried out with caution and with adequate consideration of the further need for the drug and, alertness to possible recurrence of toxicity. The minimum effective doses of Roferon-A for treatment of hairy cell leukemia, AIDS-related Kaposi's sarcoma and chronic myelogenous leukemia have not been established.

Variations in dosage and adverse reactions exist among different brands of Interferon. Therefore, do not use different brands of Interferon in a single treatment regimen.

Information for Patient: Patients should be cautioned not to change brands of Interferon without medical consultation, as a change in dosage may result. Patients should be informed regarding the potential benefits and risks attendant to the use of Roferon-A. If home use is determined to be desirable by the physician, instructions on appropriate use should be given, including review of the contents of the enclosed Patient Information Sheet. Patients should be well hydrated, especially during the initial stages of treatment. Patients should be thoroughly instructed in the importance of proper disposal procedures and cautioned against reusing syringes and needles. If home use is prescribed, a puncture-resistant container for the disposal of used syringes and needles should be supplied to the patient. The full container should be disposed of according to directions provided by the physician.

Patients receiving high-dose alfa interferon should be cautioned against performing tasks that require complete mental alertness such as operating machinery or driving a motor vehicle. Patients to be treated with Roferon-A should be informed that depression and suicidal ideation may be side effects of treatment and should be advised to report these side effects immediately to the prescribing physician.

Laboratory Tests: Complete blood with differential platelet counts and clinical chemistry tests should be performed before initiation of Roferon-A therapy and at appropriate periods during therapy. Since responses of hairy cell leukemia, AIDS-related Kaposi's sarcoma, chronic hepatitis C and chronic myelogenous leukemia are not generally observed for 1 to 3 months after initiation of treatment, very careful monitoring for severe depression of blood cell counts is warranted during the initial phase of treatment.

Those patients who have preexisting cardiac abnormalities and/or are in advanced stages of cancer should have electrocardiograms taken before and during the course of treatment.

For patients being treated for chronic hepatitis C, serum ALT should be evaluated before therapy to establish baselines and repeated at week 2 and monthly thereafter following initiation of therapy for monitoring clinical response. Patients with neutrophil count $<1500/mm^3$, platelet count $<75,000/mm^3$, hemoglobin <10 g/dL and creatinine >1.5 mg/dL were excluded from several major chronic hepatitis C studies; patients with these laboratory abnormalities should be carefully monitored if treated with Roferon-A.

Patients with preexisting thyroid abnormalities may be treated if normal thyroid stimulating hormone (TSH) levels can be maintained by medication. Testing of TSH levels in these patients is recommended at baseline and every 3 months following initiation of therapy.

Drug Interactions: Roferon-A has been reported to reduce the clearance of theophylline.[11,12] The clinical relevance of this interaction is presently unknown. Interactions between Roferon-A and other drugs have not been fully evaluated. Caution should be exercised when administering Roferon-A in combination with other potentially myelosuppressive agents (see WARNINGS).

Other Drug Interactions: Alfa Interferons may affect the oxidative metabolic process by reducing the activity of hepatic microsomal cytochrome enzymes in the P450 group. Although the clinical relevance is still unclear, this should be taken into account when prescribing concomitant therapy with drugs metabolized by this route.

The neurotoxic, hematotoxic or cardiotoxic effects of previously or concurrently administered drugs may be increased by interferons. Interactions could occur following concurrent administration of centrally acting drugs. Use of Roferon-A in conjunction with interleukin-2 may potentiate risks of renal failure.

Carcinogenesis, Mutagenesis, Impairment of Fertility:

Carcinogenesis: Roferon-A has not been tested for its carcinogenic potential.

Mutagenesis: A. Internal Studies — Ames tests using six different tester strains, with and without metabolic activation, were performed with Roferon-A up to a concentration of 1920 µg/plate. There was no evidence of mutagenicity.

Human lymphocyte cultures were treated in vitro with Roferon-A at noncytotoxic concentrations. No increase in the incidence of chromosomal damage was noted.

B. Published Studies — There are no published studies on the mutagenic potential of Roferon-A. However, a number of studies on the genotoxicity of human leukocyte interferon have been reported.

A chromosomal defect following the addition of human leukocyte interferon to lymphocyte cultures from a patient suffering from a lymphoproliferative disorder has been reported.

In contrast, other studies have failed to detect chromosomal abnormalities following treatment of lymphocyte cultures from healthy volunteers with human leukocyte interferon.

It has also been shown that human leukocyte interferon protects primary chick embryo fibroblasts from chromosomal aberrations produced by gamma rays.

Impairment of Fertility: Roferon-A has been studied for its effect on fertility in Macaca mulatta (rhesus monkeys). Nonpregnant rhesus females treated with Roferon-A at doses of 5 and 25 MIU/kg/day have shown menstrual cycle irregularities, including prolonged or shortened menstrual periods and erratic bleeding; these cycles were considered to be anovulatory on the basis that reduced progesterone levels were noted and that expected increases in preovulatory estrogen and luteinizing hormones were not observed. These monkeys returned to a normal menstrual rhythm following discontinuation of treatment.

Pregnancy: Teratogenic Effects: Pregnancy Category C. Roferon-A has been shown to demonstrate a statistically significant increase in abortifacient activity in rhesus monkeys when given at approximately 20 to 500 times the human dose. A study in pregnant rhesus monkeys treated with 1, 5 or 25 MIU/kg/day of Roferon-A in their early to midfetal period (days 22 to 70 of gestation) has failed to demonstrate teratogenic activity for Roferon-A.

There are no adequate and well-controlled studies in pregnant women.

Nonteratogenic Effects: Dose-related abortifacient activity was observed in pregnant rhesus monkeys treated with 1, 5 or 25 MIU/kg/day of Roferon-A in their early to midfetal period (days 22 to 70 of gestation). A late fetal period study (days 79 to 100 of gestation) is in progress and as yet there have been no reports of any increased rate of abortion.

Continued on next page

Table 2.—Histological Improvement* at the End of Treatment

Study No.	Treatment Duration (months)	Dose (MIU)	N†	Percent of Patients with Histologic Improvement at End of Treatment (95% CI)
1	12	Placebo	41	41 (26–58)
1	12	3	42	71
2	12	3	96	64
All	12	3	138	66 (57–74)

*As assessed by Knodell Histology Activity Index—HAI.
†Biopsy samples were not available for all of the enrolled patients.

Roferon-A—Cont.

Usage in Pregnancy: Safe use in human pregnancy has not been established. Therefore, Roferon-A should be used during pregnancy only if the potential benefit justifies the potential risk to the fetus. Information from primate studies showed dose-related menstrual irregularities and an increased incidence of spontaneous abortions. Decreases in serum estradiol and progesterone concentrations have been reported in women treated with human leukocyte interferon.[13] Therefore, fertile women should not receive Roferon-A unless they are using effective contraception during the therapy period.

Male fertility and teratologic evaluations have yielded no significant adverse effects to date.

Nursing Mothers: It is not known whether this drug is excreted in human milk. Because many drugs are excreted in human milk and because of the potential for serious adverse reactions in nursing infants from Roferon-A, a decision should be made whether to discontinue nursing or to discontinue the drug, taking into account the importance of the drug to the mother.

Pediatric Use: Use of Roferon-A in children with Ph-positive adult-type CML is supported by evidence from adequate and well-controlled studies of Roferon-A in adults with additional data from the literature on the use of alfa interferon in children with CML. A published report on 15 children with Ph-positive adult-type CML suggests a safety profile similar to that seen in adult CML; clinical responses were also observed[9] (see DOSAGE AND ADMINISTRATION).

For all other indications, safety and effectiveness have not been established in patients below the age of 18 years.

The injectable solutions are not indicated for use in neonates or infants and should not be used by patients in that age group (see WARNINGS).

ADVERSE REACTIONS

Depressive illness and suicidal behavior, including suicidal ideation and suicides, have been reported in association with the use of alfa interferon products. The incidence of reported depression has varied substantially among trials, possibly related to the underlying disease, dose, duration of therapy and degree of monitoring, but has been reported to be 15% or higher (see WARNINGS).

FOR PATIENTS WITH CHRONIC HEPATITIS C: The most frequent adverse experiences were reported to be possibly or probably related to therapy with 3 MIU tiw Roferon-A, were mostly mild to moderate in severity and manageable without the need for discontinuation of therapy. A relative increase in the incidence, severity and seriousness of adverse events was observed in patients receiving doses above 3 MIU tiw.

Adverse reactions associated with the 3 MIU dose include:

Flu-like Symptoms: Fatigue (58%), myalgia/arthralgia (51%), flu-like symptoms (33%), fever (28%), chills (23%), asthenia (6%), sweating (5%), leg cramps (3%) and malaise (1%).

Central and Peripheral Nervous System: Headache (52%), dizziness (13%), paresthesia (7%), confusion (7%), concentration impaired (4%) and change in taste or smell (3%).

Gastrointestinal: Nausea/vomiting (33%), diarrhea (20%), anorexia (14%), abdominal pain (12%), flatulence (3%), liver pain (3%), digestion impaired (2%) and gingival bleeding (2%).

Psychiatric: Depression (16%), irritability (15%), insomnia (14%), anxiety (5%) and behavior disturbances (3%).

Pulmonary and Cardiovascular: Dryness or inflammation of oropharynx (6%), epistaxis (4%), rhinitis (3%), arrhythmia (1%) and sinusitis (<1%).

Skin: Injection site reaction (29%), partial alopecia (19%), rash (8%), dry skin or pruritus (7%) and hematoma (1%).

Other: Conjunctivitis (4%), menstrual irregularity (2%) and visual acuity decreased (<1%).

Patients receiving 6 MIU tiw experienced a higher incidence of severe psychiatric events (9%) than those receiving 3 MIU tiw (6%) in two large US studies. In addition, more patients withdrew from these studies when receiving 6 MIU tiw (11%) than when receiving 3 MIU tiw (7%). Up to half of patients receiving 3 MIU or 6 MIU tiw withdrawing from the study experienced depression or other psychiatric adverse events. At higher doses anxiety, sleep disorders and irritability were observed more frequently. An increased incidence of fatigue, myalgia/arthralgia, headache, fever, chills, alopecia, sleep disturbances and dry skin or pruritus was also generally observed during treatment with higher doses of Roferon-A.

Generally there were fewer adverse events reported in the second 6 months of treatment than in the first 6 months for patients treated with 3 MIU tiw. Patients tolerant of initial therapy with Roferon-A generally tolerate re-treatment at the same dose, but tend to experience more adverse reactions at higher doses.

Infrequent adverse events (>1% but <3% incidence) included: cold feeling, cough, muscle cramps, diaphoresis, dyspnea, eye pain, reactivation of herpes simplex, lethargy, edema, sexual dysfunction, shaking, skin lesions, stomatitis, tooth disorder, urinary tract infection, weakness in extremities.

FOR PATIENTS WITH HAIRY CELL LEUKEMIA:

Constitutional (100%): Fever (92%), fatigue (86%), headache (64%), chills (64%), weight loss (33%), dizziness (21%) and flu-like symptoms (16%).

Integumentary (79%): Skin rash (44%), diaphoresis (22%), partial alopecia (17%), dry skin (17%) and pruritus (13%).

Musculoskeletal (73%): Myalgia (71%), joint or bone pain (25%) and arthritis or polyarthritis (5%).

Gastrointestinal (69%): Anorexia (43%), nausea/vomiting (39%) and diarrhea (34%).

Head and Neck (45%): Throat irritation (21%), rhinorrhea (12%) and sinusitis (11%).

Pulmonary (40%): Coughing (16%), dyspnea (12%) and pneumonia (11%).

Central Nervous System (39%): Dizziness (21%), depression (16%), sleep disturbance (10%), decreased mental status (10%), anxiety (6%), lethargy (6%), visual disturbance (6%) and confusion (5%).

Cardiovascular (39%): Chest pain (11%), edema (11%) and hypertension (11%).

Pain (34%): Pain (24%) and pain in back (16%).

Peripheral Nervous System (23%): Paresthesia (12%) and numbness (12%).

Rarely (<5%), central nervous system effects including gait disturbance, nervousness, syncope and vertigo, as well as cardiac adverse events including murmur, thrombophlebitis and hypotension were reported. Adverse experiences that occurred rarely, and may have been related to underlying disease, included ecchymosis, epistaxis, bleeding gums and petechiae. Urticaria and inflammation at the site of injection were also rarely observed.

FOR PATIENTS WITH AIDS-RELATED KAPOSI'S SARCOMA:

Flu-like Symptoms: Fatigue (95%), fever (74%), myalgia (69%), headache (66%), chills (41%) and arthralgia (24%).

Gastrointestinal: Anorexia (65%), nausea (51%), diarrhea (42%), emesis (17%) and abdominal pain (15%).

Central and Peripheral Nervous System: Dizziness (40%), decreased mental status (17%), depression (16%), paresthesia (8%), confusion (8%), diaphoresis (7%), visual disturbances (5%), sleep disturbances (5%) and numbness (3%).

Pulmonary and Cardiovascular: Coughing (27%), dyspnea (11%), edema (9%), chest pain (4%) and hypotension (4%).

Skin: Partial alopecia (22%), rash (11%) and dry skin or pruritus (5%).

Other: Weight loss (25%), change in taste (25%), dryness or inflammation of the oropharynx (14%), night sweats (8%) and rhinorrhea (4%).

Occasionally (<3%) nervous system effects including anxiety, nervousness, emotional lability, vertigo and forgetfulness, as well as cardiac adverse events, including palpitations and arrhythmia, were reported. Other adverse experiences that occurred occasionally (<3%) and may have been related to underlying disease, included sinusitis, constipation, chest congestion, pneumonia, urticaria and flatulence. Adverse experiences which occurred rarely (<1%) included ataxia, seizures, cyanosis, gastric distress, bronchospasm, pain at injection site, earache, eye irritation and rhinitis. Miscellaneous adverse experiences such as poor coordination, lethargy, muscle contractions, neuropathy, tremor, involuntary movement, syncope, aphasia, aphonia, dysarthria, amnesia, weakness and flushing of skin were observed in less than 0.5% of patients. Cases of cardiomyopathy have been observed on rare occasions in patients treated with alfa interferons.

FOR PATIENTS WITH CHRONIC MYELOGENOUS LEUKEMIA:

For patients with chronic myelogenous leukemia, the percentage of adverse events, whether related to drug therapy or not, experienced by patients treated with rIFNα-2a is given below. Severe adverse events were observed in 66% and 31% of patients on study DM84-38 and MI400, respectively. Dose reduction and temporary cessation of therapy were required frequently. Permanent cessation of Roferon-A, due to intolerable side effects, was required in 15% and 23% of patients on studies DM84-38 and MI400, respectively.

Flu-like Symptoms: Fever (92%), asthenia or fatigue (88%), myalgia (68%), chills (63%), arthralgia/bone pain (47%) and headache (44%).

Gastrointestinal: Anorexia (48%), nausea/vomiting (37%) and diarrhea (37%).

Central and Peripheral Nervous System: Headache (44%), depression (28%), decreased mental status (16%), dizziness (11%), sleep disturbances (11%), paresthesia (8%), involuntary movements (7%) and visual disturbance (6%).

Pulmonary and Cardiovascular: Coughing (19%), dyspnea (8%) and dysrhythmia (7%).

Skin: Hair changes (including alopecia) (18%), skin rash (18%), sweating (15%), dry skin (7%) and pruritus (7%).

Uncommon adverse events (< 4%) reported in clinical studies included chest pain, syncope, hypotension, impotence, alterations in taste or hearing, confusion, seizures, memory loss, disturbances of libido, bruising and coagulopathy. Miscellaneous adverse events that were rarely observed included Coombs' positive hemolytic anemia, aplastic anemia, hypothyroidism, cardiomyopathy, hypertriglyceridemia and bronchospasm.

IN OTHER INVESTIGATIONAL STUDIES OF ROFERON-A:

The following infrequent adverse events have been reported in one or more of the approved clinical indications as well as with the investigational use of Roferon-A (<5%): pancreatitis, colitis, gastrointestinal hemorrhage, stomatitis, thyroid dysfunction (including hypothyroidism and hyperthyroidism), diabetes (in some patients requiring insulin therapy), and pneumonitis (some cases responding to interferon cessation and corticosteroid therapy). In addition to the adverse experiences noted above, other adverse experiences that occurred included: abdominal fullness, hypermotility, hepatitis, gait disturbance, hallucinations, encephalopathy, psychomotor retardation, coma, stroke, transient ischemic attacks, dysphasia, sedation, apathy, irritability, hyperactivity, claustrophobia, loss of libido, congestive heart failure, myocardial infarction, Raynaud's phenomenon, hot flashes, tachypnea, ischemic retinopathy, excessive salivation and anaphylactic reactions. These adverse experiences occurred rarely (<1%).

The following events have been rarely observed (<3%) in some patients receiving Roferon-A: vasculitis, arthritis, hemolytic anemia and lupus erythematosus syndrome. The mechanism by which these events develop and their relationship to Roferon-A therapy are unclear. Similar events have been reported for other types of interferon.

ABNORMAL LABORATORY TEST VALUES: The percentage of patients with chronic hepatitis C, hairy cell leukemia, with AIDS-related Kaposi's sarcoma, and with chronic myelogenous leukemia who experienced a significant abnormal laboratory test value (*NCI or WHO grades III or IV*) at least once during their treatment with Roferon-A is shown in the following table:

[See table 4 at left]

CHRONIC HEPATITIS C: The incidence of neutropenia (*WHO grades III or IV*) was over twice as high in those treated with 6 MIU tiw (21%) as those treated with 3 MIU tiw (10%).

HAIRY CELL LEUKEMIA: Increases in serum phosphorus (≥1.6 mmol/L) and serum uric acid (≥9.1 mg/dL) were observed in 9% and 10% of patients, respectively. The in-

Table 4.—Significant Abnormal Laboratory Test Values

	Chronic Hepatitis C (n=203) 3 MIU tiw	Hairy Cell Leukemia (n=218)	AIDS-related Kaposi's Sarcoma (n=241)	Chronic Myelogenous Leukemia‡ US Study (n=91)	Chronic Myelogenous Leukemia‡ Non-US Study (n=219)
Leukopenia	1.5%	45%*	49%	20%	3%
Neutropenia	10%	68%*	52%	22%	0%
Thrombocytopenia	4.5%	62%*	35%	27%	5%
Anemia (Hb)	0%	31%*	27%	15%	4%
SGOT	NAP	9%	46%	5%	1%
Alk. Phosphatase	0%	3%	11%	3%	1%
LDH	NAP	<1%	10%	NA	NA
Proteinuria	0%	10%†	<1%	NA	NA

*In the majority of patients, initial hematologic laboratory test values were abnormal due to their underlying disease.
†Ten percent of the patients experienced a proteinuria >1+ at least once.
‡Patients enrolled in the two clinical studies receiving at least one dose of Roferon-A.
NAP=Not applicable.
NA=Not assessed.

crease in serum uric acid is likely to be related to the underlying disease. Decreases in serum calcium (≤1.9 mmol/L) and serum phosphorus (≤0.9 mmol/L) were seen in 28% and 22% of patients, respectively.

CHRONIC MYELOGENOUS LEUKEMIA: In the two clinical studies, a severe or life-threatening anemia was seen in up to 15% of patients. A severe or life-threatening leukopenia and thrombocytopenia were observed in up to 20% and 27% of patients, respectively. Changes were usually reversible when therapy was discontinued. One case of aplastic anemia and one case of Coombs' positive hemolytic anemia were seen in 310 patients treated with rIFNα-2a in clinical studies. Severe cytopenias led to discontinuation of therapy in 4% of all Roferon-A treated patients.

Transient increases in liver transaminases or alkaline phosphatase of any intensity were seen in up to 50% of patients during treatment with Roferon-A. Only 5% of patients had a severe or life-threatening increase in SGOT. In the clinical studies, such abnormalities required termination of therapy in less than 1% of patients.

DOSAGE AND ADMINISTRATION

The recommended dosages of Roferon-A differ for chronic hepatitis C, hairy cell leukemia, AIDS-related Kaposi's sarcoma and chronic myelogenous leukemia. See indication-specific dosages below.

Note: Parenteral drug products should be inspected visually for particulate matter and discoloration before administration, whenever solution and container permit.

CHRONIC HEPATITIS C: The recommended dosage of Roferon-A for the treatment of chronic hepatitis C is 3 MIU three times a week (tiw) administered subcutaneously or intramuscularly for 12 months (48 to 52 weeks). Normalization of serum ALT generally occurs within a few weeks after initiation of treatment in responders. Approximately 90% of patients who respond to Roferon-A do so within the first 3 months of treatment; however, patients responding to Roferon-A with a reduction in ALT should complete 12 months of treatment. Patients who have no response to Roferon-A within the first 3 months of therapy are not likely to respond with continued treatment; treatment discontinuation should be considered in these patients.

Patients who tolerate and partially or completely respond to therapy with Roferon-A but relapse following its discontinuation may be re-treated. Re-treatment with either 3 MIU tiw or with 6 MIU tiw for 6 to 12 months may be considered. Please see ADVERSE REACTIONS regarding the increased frequency of adverse reactions associated with treatment with higher doses.

Temporary dose reduction by 50% is recommended in patients who do not tolerate the prescribed dose. If adverse events resolve, treatment with the original prescribed dose can be re-initiated. In patients who cannot tolerate the reduced dose, cessation of therapy, at least temporarily, is recommended.

HAIRY CELL LEUKEMIA: Prior to initiation of therapy, tests should be performed to quantitate peripheral blood hemoglobin, platelets, granulocytes and hairy cells and bone marrow hairy cells. These parameters should be monitored periodically (eg, monthly) during treatment to determine whether response to treatment has occurred. If a patient does not respond within 6 months, treatment should be discontinued. If a response to treatment does occur, treatment should be continued until no further improvement is observed and these laboratory parameters have been stable for about 3 months. Patients with hairy cell leukemia have been treated for up to 24 consecutive months. The optimal duration of treatment for this disease has not been determined.

The induction dose of Roferon-A is 3 MIU daily for 16 to 24 weeks, administered as a subcutaneous or intramuscular injection. Subcutaneous administration is particularly suggested for, but not limited to, thrombocytopenic patients (platelet count <50,000) or for patients at risk for bleeding. The recommended maintenance dose is 3 MIU, three times a week (tiw). Dose reduction by one-half or withholding of individual doses may be needed when severe adverse reactions occur. The use of doses higher than 3 MIU is not recommended in hairy cell leukemia. The 36 MIU dosage form should not be used for the treatment of hairy cell leukemia.

AIDS-RELATED KAPOSI'S SARCOMA: Roferon-A is useful for the treatment of AIDS-related Kaposi's sarcoma in a select group of patients. In determining whether a patient should be treated, the physician should assess the likelihood of response based on the clinical manifestations of HIV infection and the manifestations of Kaposi's sarcoma requiring treatment (see CLINICAL PHARMACOLOGY).

Indicator lesion measurements and total lesion count should be performed before initiation of therapy. These parameters should be monitored periodically (eg, monthly) during treatment to determine whether response to treatment or disease stabilization has occurred. When disease stabilization or a response to treatment occurs, treatment should continue until there is no further evidence of tumor or until discontinuation is required because of a severe opportunistic infection or adverse effects. The optimal duration of treatment for this disease has not been determined.

The recommended induction dose of Roferon-A is 36 MIU daily for 10 to 12 weeks, administered as an intramuscular or subcutaneous injection. Subcutaneous administration is particularly suggested for, but not limited to, patients who are thrombocytopenic (platelet count <50,000) or who are at risk for bleeding. The recommended maintenance dose is 36 MIU, three times a week (tiw). If severe reactions occur, the dose should be modified (50% reduction) or therapy should be temporarily discontinued until the adverse reactions abate. An escalating schedule of 3 MIU, 9 MIU and 18 MIU each daily for 3 days followed by 36 MIU daily for the remainder of the 10- to 12-week induction period has also produced equivalent therapeutic benefit with some amelioration of the acute toxicity in some patients.

CHRONIC MYELOGENOUS LEUKEMIA: For patients with Ph-positive CML in chronic phase: Prior to initiation of therapy, a diagnosis of Philadelphia chromosome positive CML in chronic phase by the appropriate peripheral blood, bone marrow and other diagnostic testing should be made. Monitoring of hematologic parameters should be done regularly (eg, monthly). Since significant cytogenetic changes are not readily apparent until after hematologic response has occurred, and usually not until several months of therapy have elapsed, cytogenetic monitoring may be performed at less frequent intervals. Achievement of complete cytogenetic response has been observed up to 2 years following the start of Roferon-A treatment.

The recommended initial dose of Roferon-A is 9 MIU daily administered as a subcutaneous or intramuscular injection. Based on clinical experience,[3] short-term tolerance may be improved by gradually increasing the dose of Roferon-A over the first week of administration from 3 MIU daily for 3 days to 6 MIU daily for 3 days to the target dose of 9 MIU daily for the duration of the treatment period.

The optimal dose and duration of therapy have not yet been determined. Even though the median time to achieve a complete hematologic response was 5 months in study MI400, hematologic responses have been observed up to 18 months after treatment start. Treatment should be continued until disease progression. If severe side effects occur, a treatment interruption or a reduction in either the dose or the frequency of injections may be necessary to achieve the individual maximally tolerated dose (see PRECAUTIONS).

Limited data are available on the use of Roferon-A in children with CML. In one report of 15 children with Ph-positive, adult-type CML doses between 2.5 to 5 MIU/m^2/day given intramuscularly were tolerated.[9] In another study, severe adverse effects including deaths were noted in children with previously untreated, Ph-negative, juvenile CML, who received interferon doses of 30 MIU/m^2/day.[14]

HOW SUPPLIED

Single Use Injectable Solution:

3 million IU Roferon-A per vial—Each 1 mL contains 3 MIU of Interferon alfa-2a, recombinant, 7.21 mg sodium chloride, 0.2 mg polysorbate 80, 10 mg benzyl alcohol as a preservative and 0.77 mg ammonium acetate. Boxes of 1 (NDC 0004-2009-09).

6 million IU Roferon-A per vial—Each 1 mL contains 6 MIU of Interferon alfa-2a, recombinant, 7.21 mg sodium chloride, 0.2 mg polysorbate 80, 10 mg benzyl alcohol as a preservative and 0.77 mg ammonium acetate. This dosage form should not be used for the treatment of hairy cell leukemia. Boxes of 1 (NDC 0004-2007-09).

9 million IU Roferon-A per vial—Each 0.9 mL contains 9 MIU of Interferon alfa-2a, recombinant, 6.49 mg sodium chloride, 0.18 mg polysorbate 80, 9 mg benzyl alcohol as a preservative and 0.69 mg ammonium acetate. For single dose administration, withdraw 0.9 mL using a 1 mL syringe. Also can be used as a multidose vial. Boxes of 1 (NDC 0004-2010-09).

36 million IU Roferon-A per vial—Each 1 mL contains 36 MIU of Interferon alfa-2a, recombinant, 7.21 mg sodium chloride, 0.2 mg polysorbate 80, 10 mg benzyl alcohol as a preservative and 0.77 mg ammonium acetate. This dosage form should not be used for the treatment of hairy cell leukemia. Boxes of 1 (NDC 0004-2012-09).

Multidose Injectable Solution:

9 million IU Roferon-A per vial—Each 0.3 mL contains 3 MIU of Interferon alfa-2a, recombinant, 2.16 mg sodium chloride, 0.06 mg polysorbate 80, 3 mg benzyl alcohol as a preservative and 0.23 mg ammonium acetate. Also can be used as a single use vial. Once the vial is entered, it must be used within 30 days. The 9 MIU multidose vial contains an average of 13 MIU of Interferon alfa-2a, recombinant in order to provide the delivery of three 0.3 mL doses, each containing 3 MIU of Roferon-A Interferon alfa-2a, recombinant for injection. Boxes of 1 (NDC 0004-2010-09).

18 million IU Roferon-A per vial— Each 1 mL contains 6 MIU of Interferon alfa-2a, recombinant, 7.21 mg sodium chloride, 0.2 mg polysorbate 80, 10 mg benzyl alcohol as a preservative and 0.77 mg ammonium acetate. Each 0.5 mL contains 3 MIU of Interferon alfa-2a, recombinant. Once the vial is entered, it must be used within 30 days. The 18 MIU multidose vial contains an average of 22.8 MIU of Interferon alfa-2a, recombinant in order to provide the delivery of six 0.5 mL doses, each containing 3 MIU of Roferon-A Interferon alfa-2a, recombinant for injection. Boxes of 1 (NDC 0004-2011-09).

Sterile Powder for Injection:

18 million IU Roferon-A per vial—Reconstitute with 3 mL diluent and swirl gently to dissolve. When reconstituted with accompanying Diluent for Roferon-A, each 1 mL of reconstituted solution contains 6 MIU Interferon alfa-2a, recombinant, 9 mg sodium chloride, 1.67 mg Albumin (Human) and 3.3 mg phenol as a preservative. Each 0.5 mL contains 3 MIU of Interferon alfa-2a, recombinant. Once the powder is reconstituted, it must be used within 30 days. Boxes of 1 (NDC 0004-1993-09).

Storage: The sterile powder and its accompanying diluent, the reconstituted solution and the injectable solution should be stored in the refrigerator at 36° to 46°F (2° to 8°C). Do *not* freeze or shake.

REFERENCES

1. Trown PW, et al. *Cancer.* 1986; 57(suppl):1648-1656. 2. Itri LM, et al. *Cancer.* 1987; 59:668-674.3. Jones GJ, Itri LM. *Cancer.* 1986; 57(suppl):1709-1715. 4. Foon KA, et al. *Blood.* 1984; 64(suppl 1):164a. 5. Quesada Jr, et al. *Cancer.* 1986; 57(suppl):1678-1680. 6. Krown SE, et al. *N Eng J Med.* 1984; 308:1071-1076. 7. The Italian Cooperative Study Group on CML. *N Engl J Med.* 1994; 330:820-825. 8. Sokal JE, et al. *Blood.* 1984; 63(4):789-799. 9. Dow LW, et al. *Cancer.* 1991; 68:1678-1684. 10. Krown SE, et al. *Proc Am Soc Clin Oncol.* 1988; 7:1. 11. Williams SJ, et al. *Lancet.* 1987; 2:939-941. 12. Jonkman JHG, et al. *Br J Clin Pharmacol.* 1989; 2(27):795-802. 13. Kauppila A, et al. *Int J Cancer.* 1982; 29:291-294. 14. Maybee D, et al. *Proc Annu Meet Am Soc Clin Oncol.* 1992; 11:A950.

Revised: May 1997

ROMAZICON® ℞

[ro-mäs 'ĕ-kōn]

(flumazenil)

INJECTION

The following text is complete prescribing information based on official labeling in effect June 1998.

DESCRIPTION

ROMAZICON® (flumazenil) is a benzodiazepine receptor antagonist. Chemically, flumazenil is ethyl 8-fluoro-5,6-dihydro-5-methyl-6-oxo-4H-imidazo [1,5-a](1,4) benzodiazepine-3-carboxylate. Flumazenil has an imidazobenzodiazepine structure and a calculated molecular weight of 303.3.

Flumazenil is a white to off-white crystalline compound with an octanol:buffer partition coefficient of 14 to 1 at pH 7.4. It is insoluble in water but slightly soluble in acidic aqueous solutions. ROMAZICON is available as a sterile parenteral dosage form for intravenous administration. Each mL contains 0.1 mg of flumazenil compounded with 1.8 mg of methylparaben, 0.2 mg of propylparaben, 0.9% sodium chloride, 0.01% edetate disodium, and 0.01% acetic acid; the pH is adjusted to approximately 4 with hydrochloric acid and/or, if necessary, sodium hydroxide.

CLINICAL PHARMACOLOGY

Flumazenil, an imidazobenzodiazepine derivative, antagonizes the actions of benzodiazepines on the central nervous system. Flumazenil competitively inhibits the activity at the benzodiazepine recognition site on the GABA/benzodiazepine receptor complex. Flumazenil is a weak partial agonist in some animal models of activity, but has little or no agonist activity in man. Flumazenil does not antagonize the central nervous system effects of drugs affecting GABA-ergic neurons by means other than the benzodiazepine receptor (including ethanol, barbiturates, or general anesthetics) and does not reverse the effects of opioids.

PHARMACODYNAMICS: Intravenous ROMAZICON has been shown to antagonize sedation, impairment of recall, psychomotor impairment and ventilatory depression produced by benzodiazepines in healthy human volunteers.

The duration and degree of reversal of benzodiazepine effects are related to the dose and plasma concentrations of flumazenil as shown in the following data from a study in normal volunteers.

Continued on next page

Romazicon—Cont.

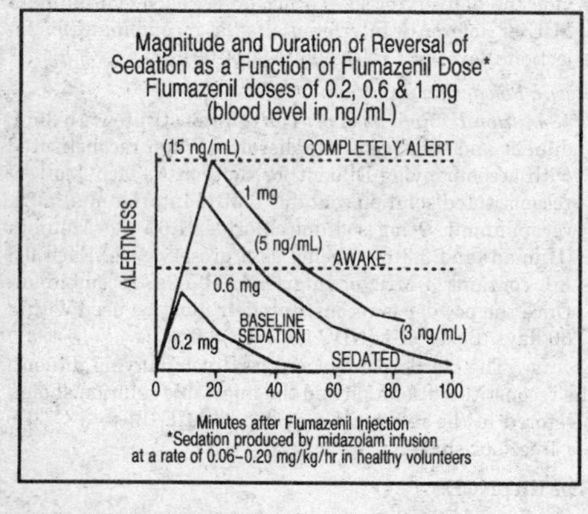
Magnitude and Duration of Reversal of
Sedation as a Function of Flumazenil Dose*
Flumazenil doses of 0.2, 0.6 & 1 mg
(blood level in ng/mL)
(15 ng/mL)
COMPLETELY ALERT
1 mg
(5 ng/mL)
AWAKE
0.6 mg
ALERTNESS
BASELINE SEDATION
(3 ng/mL)
0.2 mg
SEDATED
0
20
40
60
80
100
Minutes after Flumazenil Injection
*Sedation produced by midazolam infusion
at a rate of 0.06–0.20 mg/kg/hr in healthy volunteers

Generally, doses of approximately 0.1 to 0.2 mg (corresponding to peak plasma levels of 3 to 6 ng/mL) produce partial antagonism, whereas higher doses of 0.4 to 1 mg (peak plasma levels of 12 to 28 ng/mL) usually produce complete antagonism in patients who have received the usual sedating doses of benzodiazepines. The onset of reversal is usually evident within 1 to 2 minutes after the injection is completed. Eighty percent response will be reached within 3 minutes, with the peak effect occurring at 6 to 10 minutes. The duration and degree of reversal are related to the plasma concentration of the sedating benzodiazepine as well as the dose of ROMAZICON given.

In healthy volunteers, ROMAZICON did not alter intraocular pressure when given alone and reversed the decrease in intraocular pressure seen after administration of midazolam.

PHARMACOKINETICS: After IV administration, plasma concentrations of flumazenil follow a two compartment open pharmacokinetic model with an initial distribution half-life of 7 to 15 minutes and a terminal half-life of 41 to 79 minutes. Peak concentrations of flumazenil are proportional to dose, with an apparent initial volume of distribution of 0.5 L/kg. After redistribution the apparent volume of distribution (V_{ss}) ranges from 0.77 to 1.60L/kg. Protein binding is approximately 50% and the drug shows no preferential partitioning into red blood cells.

Flumazenil is a highly extracted drug. Clearance of flumazenil occurs primarily by hepatic metabolism and is dependent on hepatic blood flow. In pharmacokinetic studies of normal volunteers, total clearance ranges from 0.7 to 1.3 L/hr/kg, with less than 1% of the administered dose eliminated unchanged in the urine. The major metabolites of flumazenil identified in urine are the de-ethylated free acid and its glucuronide conjugate. In preclinical studies there was no evidence of pharmacologic activity exhibited by the de-ethylated free acid. Elimination of radiolabelled drug is essentially complete within 72 hours, with 90% to 95% of the radioactivity appearing in urine and 5% to 10% in the feces.

Pharmacokinetic Parameters Following a 5-minute infusion of a total of 1 mg of ROMAZICON Mean (Coefficient of variation, Range)

C_{max}(ng/mL)	24 (38%, 11–43)
AUC (ng·hr/mL)	15 (22%, 10–22)
V_{ss}(L/kg)	1 (24%, 0.8–1.6)
Cl (L/hr/kg)	1 (20%, 0.7–1.4)
Half-life (min)	54 (21%, 41–79)

The pharmacokinetics of flumazenil are not significantly affected by gender, age, renal failure (creatinine clearance <10mL/min), or hemodialysis beginning 1 hour after drug administration. Mean total clearance is decreased to 40% to 60% of normal in patients with moderate liver dysfunction and to 25% of normal in patients with severe liver dysfunction compared with age-matched healthy subjects. This results in a prolongation of the half-life from 0.8 hours in healthy subjects to 1.3 hours in patients with moderate hepatic impairment and 2.4 hours in severely impaired patients. Ingestion of food during an intravenous infusion of the drug results in a 50% increase in clearance, most likely due to the increased hepatic blood flow that accompanies a meal. The pharmacokinetic profile of flumazenil is unaltered in the presence of benzodiazepine agonists and the kinetic profiles of those benzodiazepines are unaltered by flumazenil.

CLINICAL TRIALS

ROMAZICON has been administered to reverse the effects of benzodiazepines in conscious sedation, general anesthesia, and the management of suspected benzodiazepine overdose.

CONSCIOUS SEDATION: ROMAZICON was studied in four trials in 970 patients who received an average of 30 mg diazepam or 10 mg midazolam for sedation (with or without a narcotic) in conjunction with both inpatient and outpatient diagnostic or surgical procedures. ROMAZICON was effective in reversing the sedating and psychomotor effects of the benzodiazepine, however, amnesia was less completely and less consistently reversed. In these studies, ROMAZICON was administered as an initial dose of 0.4 mg I.V. (two doses of 0.2 mg) with additional 0.2 mg doses as needed to achieve complete awakening, up to a maximum total dose of 1 mg.

Seventy-eight percent of patients receiving flumazenil responded by becoming completely alert. Of those patients, approximately half responded to doses of 0.4 to 0.6 mg, while the other half responded to doses of 0.8 to 1 mg. Adverse effects were infrequent in patients who received 1 mg of ROMAZICON or less, although injection site pain, agitation and anxiety did occur. Reversal of sedation was not associated with any increase in the frequency of inadequate analgesia or increase in narcotic demand in these studies. While most patients remained alert throughout the 3 hour post-procedure observation period, resedation was observed to occur in 3% to 9% of the patients, and was most common in patients who had received high doses of benzodiazepine. (See PRECAUTIONS.)

GENERAL ANESTHESIA: ROMAZICON was studied in four trials in 644 patients who received midazolam as an induction and/or maintenance agent in both balanced and inhalational anesthesia. Midazolam was generally administered in doses ranging from 5 to 80 mg, alone and/or in conjunction with muscle relaxants, nitrous oxide, regional or local anaesthetics, narcotics and/or inhalational anesthetics. Flumazenil was given as an initial dose of 0.2 mg IV, with additional 0.2 mg doses as needed to reach a complete response, up to a maximum total dose of 1 mg. These doses were effective in reversing sedation and restoring psychomotor function, but did not completely restore memory as tested by picture recall. ROMAZICON was not as effective in the reversal of sedation in patients who had received multiple anesthetic agents in addition to benzodiazepines.

Eighty-one percent of patients sedated with midazolam responded to flumazenil by becoming completely alert or just slightly drowsy. Of those patients, 36% responded to doses of 0.4 to 0.6 mg, while 64% responded to doses of 0.8 to 1 mg.

Resedation in patients who responded to ROMAZICON occurred in 10% to 15% of patients studied and was more common with larger doses of midazolam (>20 mg), long procedures (>60 minutes) and use of neuromuscular blocking agents. (See PRECAUTIONS.)

MANAGEMENT OF SUSPECTED BENZODIAZEPINE OVERDOSE: ROMAZICON was studied in two trials in 497 patients who were presumed to have taken an overdose of a benzodiazepine, either alone or in combination with a variety of other agents. In these trials, 299 patients were proven to have taken a benzodiazepine as part of the overdose, and 80% of the 148 who received ROMAZICON responded by an improvement in level of consciousness. Of the patients who responded to flumazenil, 75% responded to a total dose of 1 to 3 mg.

Reversal of sedation was associated with an increased frequency of symptoms of CNS excitation. Of the patients treated with flumazenil, 1% to 3% were treated for agitation or anxiety. Serious side effects were uncommon, but six seizures were observed in 446 patients treated with flumazenil in these studies. Four of these 6 patients had ingested a large dose of cyclic antidepressants, which increased the risk of seizures. (See WARNINGS.)

INDIVIDUALIZATION OF DOSAGE

GENERAL PRINCIPLES: The serious adverse effects of ROMAZICON are related to the reversal of benzodiazepine effects. Using more than the minimally effective dose of ROMAZICON is tolerated by most patients but may complicate the management of patients who are physically dependent on benzodiazepines or patients who are depending on benzodiazepines for therapeutic effect (such as suppression of seizures in cyclic antidepressant overdose).

In high-risk patients, it is important to administer the smallest amount of ROMAZICON that is effective. The 1-minute wait between individual doses in the dose-titration recommended for general clinical populations may be too short for high-risk patients. This is because it takes 6 to 10 minutes for any single dose of flumazenil to reach full effects. Practitioners should slow the rate of administration of ROMAZICON administered to high-risk patients as recommended below.

ANESTHESIA AND CONSCIOUS SEDATION: ROMAZICON is well tolerated at the recommended doses in individuals who have no tolerance to (or dependence on) benzodiazepines. The recommended dosages and titration rates in anesthesia and conscious sedation (0.2 to 1 mg given at 0.2 mg/min) are well tolerated in patients receiving the drug for reversal of a single benzodiazepine exposure in most clinical settings (see Adverse Events). The major risk will be resedation because the duration of effect of a long-acting (or large dose of a short-acting) benzodiazepine may exceed that of ROMAZICON. Resedation may be treated by giving a repeat dose at no less than 20-minute intervals. For repeat treatment, no more than 1 mg (at 0.2 mg/min doses) should be given at any one time and no more than 3 mg should be given in any one hour.

OVERDOSE PATIENTS: The risk of confusion, agitation, emotional lability and perceptual distortion with the doses recommended in patients with benzodiazepine overdose (3 to 5 mg administered as 0.5 mg/min) may be greater than that expected with lower doses and slower administration. The recommended doses represent a compromise between a desirable slow awakening and the need for prompt response and a persistent effect in the overdose situation. If circumstances permit, the physician may elect to use the 0.2 mg/minute titration rate to slowly awaken the patient over 5 to 10 minutes, which may help to reduce signs and symptoms on emergence.

ROMAZICON has no effect in cases where benzodiazepines are not responsible for sedation. Once doses of 3 to 5 mg have been reached without clinical response, additional ROMAZICON is likely to have no effect.

PATIENTS TOLERANT TO BENZODIAZEPINES: ROMAZICON may cause benzodiazepine withdrawal symptoms in individuals who have been taking benzodiazepines long enough to have some degree of tolerance. Patients who had been taking benzodiazepines prior to entry into the ROMAZICON trials who were given flumazenil in doses over 1 mg experienced withdrawal-like events 2 to 5 times more frequently than patients who received less than 1 mg.

In patients who may have tolerance to benzodiazepines, as indicated by clinical history or by the need for larger than usual doses of benzodiazepine, slower titration rates of 0.1 mg/min and lower total doses may help reduce the frequency of emergent confusion and agitation. In such cases special care must be taken to monitor the patients for resedation because of the lower doses of ROMAZICON used.

PATIENTS PHYSICALLY DEPENDENT ON BENZODIAZEPINES: ROMAZICON is known to precipitate withdrawal seizures in patients who are physically dependent on benzodiazepines, even if such dependence was established in a relatively few days of high dose sedation in Intensive Care Unit environments. The risk of either seizures or resedation in such cases is high and patients have experienced seizures before regaining consciousness. ROMAZICON should be used in such settings with extreme caution, since the use of flumazenil in this situation has not been studied and no information as to dose and rate of titration is available. ROMAZICON should be used in such patients only if the potential benefits of using the drug outweigh the risks of precipitated seizures. Physicians are directed to the scientific literature for the most current information in this area.

INDICATIONS AND USAGE

ROMAZICON is indicated for the complete or partial reversal of the sedative effects of benzodiazepines in cases where general anesthesia has been induced and/or maintained with benzodiazepines, where sedation has been produced with benzodiazepines for diagnostic and therapeutic procedures, and for the management of benzodiazepine overdose.

CONTRAINDICATIONS

ROMAZICON is contraindicated:

- in patients with a known hypersensitivity to flumazenil or to benzodiazepines.
- in patients who have been given a benzodiazepine for control of a potentially life-threatening condition (*e.g.* control of intracranial pressure or status epilepticus).
- in patients who are showing signs of serious cyclic antidepressant overdose. (See WARNINGS.)

WARNINGS

THE USE OF ROMAZICON HAS BEEN ASSOCIATED WITH THE OCCURRENCE OF SEIZURES.
THESE ARE MOST FREQUENT IN PATIENTS WHO HAVE BEEN ON BENZODIAZEPINES FOR LONG-TERM SEDATION OR IN OVERDOSE CASES WHERE PATIENTS ARE SHOWING SIGNS OF SERIOUS CYCLIC ANTIDEPRESSANT OVERDOSE.
PRACTITIONERS SHOULD INDIVIDUALIZE THE DOSAGE OF ROMAZICON AND BE PREPARED TO MANAGE SEIZURES.

Risk of Seizures: The reversal of benzodiazepine effects may be associated with the onset of seizures in certain high-risk populations. Possible risk factors for seizures include: concurrent major sedative-hypnotic drug withdrawal, recent therapy with repeated doses of parenteral benzodiazepines, myoclonic jerking or seizure activity prior to flumazenil administration in overdose cases, or concurrent cyclic anti-depressant poisoning.

ROMAZICON is not recommended in cases of serious cyclic antidepressant poisoning, as manifested by motor abnormalities (twitching, rigidity, focal seizure), dysrhythmia (wide QRS, ventricular dysrhythmia, heart block), anticholinergic signs (mydriasis, dry mucosa, hypo-peristalsis), and cardiovascular collapse at presentation. In such cases ROMAZICON should be withheld and the patient should be allowed to remain sedated (with ventilatory and circulatory support as needed) until the signs of antidepressant toxicity have subsided. Treatment with ROMAZICON has no known benefit to the seriously ill mixed-overdose pa-

tient other than reversing sedation and should not be used in cases where seizures (from any cause) are likely.

Most convulsions associated with flumazenil administration require treatment and have been successfully managed with benzodiazepines, phenytoin or barbiturates. Because of the presence of flumazenil, higher than usual doses of benzodiazepines may be required.

HYPOVENTILATION: Patients who have received ROMAZICON for the reversal of benzodiazepine effects (after conscious sedation or general anesthesia) should be monitored for resedation, respiratory depression, or other residual benzodiazepine effects for an appropriate period (up to 120 minutes) based on the dose and duration of effect of the benzodiazepine employed.

This is because ROMAZICON has not been established in patients as an effective treatment for hypoventilation due to benzodiazepine administration. In healthy male volunteers, ROMAZICON is capable of reversing benzodiazepine-induced depression of the ventilatory responses to hypercapnia and hypoxia after a benzodiazepine alone. However, such depression may recur because the ventilatory effects of typical doses of ROMAZICON (1 mg or less) may wear off before the effects of many benzodiazepines. The effects of ROMAZICON on ventilatory response following sedation with a benzodiazepine in combination with an opioid are inconsistent and have not been adequately studied. The availability of flumazenil does not diminish the need for prompt detection of hypoventilation and the ability to effectively intervene by establishing an airway and assisting ventilation.

Overdose cases should always be monitored for resedation until the patients are stable and resedation in unlikely.

PRECAUTIONS

RETURN OF SEDATION: ROMAZICON may be expected to improve the alertness of patients recovering from a procedure involving sedation or anesthesia with benzodiazepines, but should not be substituted for an adequate period of post-procedure monitoring. The availability of ROMAZICON does not reduce the risks associated with the use of large doses of benzodiazepines for sedation.

Patients should be monitored for resedation, respiratory depression (See WARNINGS), or other persistent or recurrent agonist effects for an adequate period of time after administration of ROMAZICON.

Resedation is least likely in cases where ROMAZICON is administered to reverse a low dose of a short-acting benzodiazepine (<10 mg midazolam). It is most likely in cases where a large single or cumulative dose of a benzodiazepine has been given in the course of a long procedure along with neuromuscular blocking agents and multiple anesthetic agents.

Profound resedation was observed in 1% to 3% of patients in the clinical studies. In clinical situations where resedation must be prevented, physicians may wish to repeat the initial dose (up to 1 mg of ROMAZICON given at 0.2 mg/min) at 30 minutes and possibly again at 60 minutes. This dosage schedule, although not studied in clinical trials, was effective in preventing resedation in a pharmacologic study in normal volunteers.

USE IN THE ICU: ROMAZICON should be used with caution in the Intensive Care Unit because of the increased risk of unrecognized benzodiazepine dependence in such settings. ROMAZICON may produce convulsions in patients physically dependent on benzodiazepines. (See INDIVIDUALIZATION OF DOSAGE AND WARNINGS.)

Administration of ROMAZICON to diagnose benzodiazepine-induced sedation in the Intensive Care Unit is not recommended due to the risk of adverse events as described above. In addition, the prognostic significance of a patient's failure to respond to flumazenil in cases confounded by metabolic disorder, traumatic injury, drugs other than benzodiazepines, or any other reasons not associated with benzodiazepine receptor occupancy is not known.

USE IN OVERDOSE: ROMAZICON is intended as an adjunct to, not as a substitute for, proper management of airway, assisted breathing, circulatory access and support, internal decontamination by lavage and charcoal, and adequate clinical evaluation.

Necessary measures should be instituted to secure airway, ventilation and intravenous access prior to administering flumazenil. Upon arousal patients may attempt to withdraw endotracheal tubes and/or intravenous lines as the result of confusion and agitation following awakening.

HEAD INJURY: ROMAZICON should be used with caution in patients with head injury as it may be capable of precipitating convulsions or altering cerebral blood flow in patients receiving benzodiazepines. It should be used only by practitioners prepared to manage such complications should they occur.

USE WITH NEUROMUSCULAR BLOCKING AGENTS: ROMAZICON should not be used until the effects of neuromuscular blockade have been fully reversed.

USE IN PSYCHIATRIC PATIENTS: ROMAZICON has been reported to provoke panic attacks in patients with a history of panic disorder.

PAIN ON INJECTION: To minimize the likelihood of pain or inflammation at the injection site, ROMAZICON should be administered through a freely flowing intravenous infusion into a large vein. Local irritation may occur following extravasation into perivascular tissues.

USE IN RESPIRATORY DISEASE: The primary treatment of patients with serious lung disease who experience serious respiratory depression due to benzodiazepines should be appropriate ventilatory support (See PRECAUTIONS) rather than the administration of ROMAZICON. Flumazenil is capable of partially reversing benzodiazepine-induced alterations in ventilatory drive in healthy volunteers, but has not been shown to be clinically effective.

USE IN CARDIOVASCULAR DISEASE: ROMAZICON did not increase the work of the heart when used to reverse benzodiazepines in cardiac patients when given at a rate of 0.1 mg/min in total doses of less than 0.5 mg in studies reported in the clinical literature. Flumazenil alone had no significant effects on cardiovascular parameters when administered to patients with stable ischemic heart disease.

USE IN LIVER DISEASE: The clearance of ROMAZICON is reduced to 40% to 60% of normal in patients with mild to moderate hepatic disease and to 25% of normal in patients with severe hepatic dysfunction. (See PHARMACOKINETICS.) While the dose of flumazenil used for initial reversal of benzodiazepine effects is not affected, repeat doses of the drug in liver disease should be reduced in size or frequency.

USE IN DRUG AND ALCOHOL DEPENDENT PATIENTS: ROMAZICON should be used with caution in patients with alcoholism and other drug dependencies due to the increased frequency of benzodiazepine tolerance and dependence observed in these patient populations. ROMAZICON is not recommended either as a treatment for benzodiazepine dependence or for the management of protracted benzodiazepine abstinence syndromes, as such use has not been studied.

The administration of flumazenil can precipitate benzodiazepine withdrawal in animals and man. This has been seen in healthy volunteers treated with therapeutic doses of oral lorazepam for up to 2 weeks who exhibited effects such as hot flushes, agitation and tremor when treated with cumulative doses of up to 3 mg doses of flumazenil.

Similar adverse experiences suggestive of flumazenil precipitation of benzodiazepine withdrawal have occurred in some patients in clinical trials. Such patients had a short-lived syndrome characterized by dizziness, mild confusion, emotional lability, agitation (with signs and symptoms of anxiety), and mild sensory distortions. This response was dose-related, most common at doses above 1 mg, rarely required treatment other than reassurance and was usually short lived. When required (5 to 10 cases), these patients were successfully treated with usual doses of a barbiturate, a benzodiazepine, or other sedative drug.

Practitioners should assume that flumazenil administration may trigger dose-dependent withdrawal syndromes in patients with established physical dependence on benzodiazepines and may complicate the management of withdrawal syndromes for alcohol, barbiturates and cross-tolerant sedatives.

DRUG INTERACTIONS

Interaction with central nervous system depressants other than benzodiazepines has not been specifically studied; however, no deleterious interactions were seen when ROMAZICON was administered after narcotics, inhalational anesthetics, muscle relaxants and muscle relaxant antagonists administered in conjunction with sedation or anesthesia.

Particular caution is necessary when using ROMAZICON in cases of mixed drug overdosage since the toxic effects (such as convulsions and cardiac dysrhythmias) of other drugs taken in overdose (especially cyclic antidepressants) may emerge with the reversal of the benzodiazepine effect by flumazenil. (See WARNINGS.)

The pharmacokinetics of benzodiazepines are unaltered in the presence of flumazenil.

USE IN AMBULATORY PATIENTS: The effects of ROMAZICON may wear off before a long-acting benzodiazepine is completely cleared from the body. In general, if a patient shows no signs of sedation within 2 hours after a 1 mg dose of flumazenil, serious resedation at a later time is unlikely. An adequate period of observation must be provided for any patient in whom either long-acting benzodiazepines (such as diazepam) or large doses of short-acting benzodiazepines (such as >10 mg of midazolam) have been used. (See INDIVIDUALIZATION OF DOSAGE.)

Because of the increased risk of adverse reactions in patients who have been taking benzodiazepines on a regular basis, it is particularly important that physicians query carefully about benzodiazepine, alcohol and sedative use as part of the history prior to any procedure in which the use of ROMAZICON is planned. (See DRUG AND ALCOHOL DEPENDENT PATIENTS.)

INFORMATION FOR PATIENTS: ROMAZICON does not consistently reverse amnesia. Patients cannot be expected to remember information told to them in the post-procedure

period and instructions given to patients should be reinforced in writing or given to a responsible family member. Physicians are advised to discuss with their patients, both before surgery and at discharge, that although the patient may feel alert at the time of discharge, the effects of the benzodiazepine may recur. As a result, the patient should be instructed, preferably in writing, that their memory and judgment may be impaired and specifically advised:

1. Not to engage in any activities requiring complete alertness, and not to operate hazardous machinery or a motor vehicle until at least 18 to 24 hours after discharge, and it is certain no residual sedative effects of the benzodiazepine remain.
2. Not to take any alcohol or non-prescription drugs for 18 to 24 hours after flumazenil administration or if the effects of the benzodiazepine persist.

LABORATORY TESTS: No specific laboratory tests are recommended to follow the patient's response or to identify possible adverse reactions.

DRUG/LABORATORY TEST INTERACTIONS: The possible interaction of flumazenil with commonly used laboratory tests has not been evaluated.

CARCINOGENESIS, MUTAGENESIS, IMPAIRMENT OF FERTILITY: Carcinogenesis: No studies in animals to evaluate the carcinogenic potential of flumazenil have been conducted.

Mutagenesis: No evidence for mutagenicity was noted in the Ames test using five different tester strains. Assays for mutagenic potential in *S. cerevisiae* D7 and in Chinese hamster cells were considered to be negative as were blastogenesis assays *in vitro* in peripheral human lymphocytes and *in vivo* in a mouse micronucleus assay. Flumazenil caused a slight increase in unscheduled DNA synthesis in rat hepatocyte culture at concentrations which were also cytotoxic; no increase in DNA repair was observed in male mouse germ cells in an *in vivo* DNA repair assay.

Impairment of fertility: A reproduction study in male and female rats did not show any impairment of fertility at oral dosages of 125 mg/kg/day. From the available data on the area under the curve (AUC) in animals and man the dose represented 120 × the human exposure from a maximum recommended intravenous dose of 5 mg.

PREGNANCY: CATEGORY C. There are no adequate and well-controlled studies of the use of flumazenil in pregnant women. Flumazenil should be used during pregnancy only if the potential benefit justifies the potential risk to the fetus. Teratogenic Effects: Flumazenil has been studied for teratogenicity in rats and rabbits following oral treatments of up to 150 mg/kg/day. The treatments during the major organogenesis were on days 6 to 15 of gestation in the rat and days 6 to 18 of gestation in the rabbit. No teratogenic effects were observed in rats or rabbits at 150 mg/kg; the dose, based on the available data on the area under the plasma concentration-time curve (AUC) represented 120 × to 600 × the human exposure from a maximum recommended intravenous dose of 5 mg in humans. In rabbits, embryocidal effects (as evidenced by increased pre-implantation and post-implantation losses) were observed at 50 mg/kg or 200 × the human exposure from a maximum recommended intravenous dose of 5 mg. The no-effect dose of 15 mg/kg in rabbits represents 60 × the human exposure.

Nonteratogenic Effects: An animal reproduction study was conducted in rats at oral dosages of 5, 25 and 125 mg/kg/day of flumazenil. Pup survival was decreased during the lactating period, pup liver weight at weaning was increased for the high-dose group (125 mg/kg/day) and incisor eruption and ear opening in the offspring were delayed; the delay in ear opening was associated with a delay in the appearance of the auditory startle response. No treatment-related adverse effects were noted for the other dose groups. Based on the available data from AUC, the effect level (125 mg/kg), represents 120 × the human exposure from 5 mg, the maximum recommended intravenous dose in humans. The no-effect level represents 24 × the human exposure from an intravenous dose of 5 mg.

LABOR AND DELIVERY: The use of ROMAZICON to reverse the effects of benzodiazepines used during labor and delivery is not recommended because the effects of the drug in the newborn are unknown.

NURSING MOTHERS: Caution should be exercised when deciding to administer ROMAZICON to a nursing woman because it is not known whether flumazenil is excreted in human milk.

PEDIATRIC USE: ROMAZICON is not recommended for use in children (either for the reversal of sedation, the management of overdose or the resuscitation of the newborn), as no clinical studies have been performed to determine the risks, benefits and dosages to be used.

Continued on next page

Romazicon—Cont.

GERIATRIC USE: The pharmacokinetics of flumazenil have been studied in the elderly and are not significantly different from younger patients. Several studies of ROMAZICON in patients over the age of 65 and one study in patients over the age of 80 suggest that while the doses of benzodiazepine used to induce sedation should be reduced, ordinary doses of ROMAZICON may be used for reversal.

ADVERSE REACTIONS

SERIOUS ADVERSE REACTIONS: Deaths have occurred in patients who received ROMAZICON in a variety of clinical settings. The majority of deaths occurred in patients with serious underlying disease or in patients who had ingested large amounts of non-benzodiazepine drugs, (usually cyclic antidepressants) as part of an overdose.

Serious adverse events have occurred in all clinical settings, and convulsions are the most common serious adverse event reported. ROMAZICON administration has been associated with the onset of convulsions in patients who are relying on benzodiazepine effects to control seizures, are physically dependent on benzodiazepines, or who have ingested large doses of other drugs. (See WARNINGS.)

Two of the 446 patients who received ROMAZICON in controlled clinical trials for the management of a benzodiazepine overdosage had cardiac dysrhythmias (1 ventricular tachycardia, 1 junctional tachycardia).

ADVERSE EVENTS IN CLINICAL STUDIES: The following adverse reactions were considered to be related to ROMAZICON administration (both alone and for the reversal of benzodiazepine effects) and were reported in studies involving 1875 individuals who received flumazenil in controlled trials. Adverse events most frequently associated with flumazenil alone were limited to dizziness, injection site pain, increased sweating, headache and abnormal or blurred vision (3% to 9%).

BODY AS A WHOLE: Fatigue (asthenia, malaise), Headache, Injection Site Pain*, Injection Site Reaction (thrombophlebitis, skin abnormality, rash)

CARDIOVASCULAR SYSTEM: Cutaneous vasodilation (sweating, flushing, hot flushes)

DIGESTIVE SYSTEM: Nausea and Vomiting (11%)

NERVOUS SYSTEM: Agitation (anxiety, nervousness, dry mouth, tremor, palpitations, insomnia, dyspnea, hyperventilation)*, Dizziness (vertigo, ataxia) (10%), Emotional lability (crying abnormal, depersonalization, euphoria, increased tears, depression, dysphoria, paranoia).

SPECIAL SENSES: Abnormal Vision (visual field defect, diplopia), Paresthesia (sensation abnormal, hypoesthesia)

All adverse reactions occurred in 1% to 3% of cases unless otherwise marked.
*indicates reaction in 3% to 9% of cases.
Observed percentage reported if greater than 9%.

The following adverse events were observed infrequently (less than 1%) in the clinical studies, but were judged as probably related to ROMAZICON administration and/or reversal of benzodiazepine effects:

NERVOUS SYSTEM: Confusion (difficulty concentrating, delirium), Convulsions (See WARNINGS), Somnolence (stupor)

SPECIAL SENSES: Abnormal Hearing (transient hearing impairment, hyperacusis, tinnitus).

The following adverse events occurred with frequencies less than 1% in the clinical trials. Their relationship to ROMAZICON administration is unknown, but they are included as alerting information for the physician.

BODY AS A WHOLE: Rigors, shivering.

CARDIOVASCULAR: Arrythmia (atrial, nodal, ventricular extrasystoles), bradycardia, tachycardia, hypertension, chest pain.

DIGESTIVE SYSTEM: Hiccup.

NERVOUS SYSTEM: Speech disorder (dysphonia, thick tongue).

Not included in this list is operative site pain that occurred with the same frequency in patients receiving placebo as in patients receiving flumazenil for reversal of sedation following a surgical procedure.

DRUG ABUSE AND DEPENDENCE

ROMAZICON acts as a benzodiazepine antagonist, blocks the effects of benzodiazepines in animals and man, antagonizes benzodiazepine reinforcement in animal models, produces dysphoria in normal subjects, and has had no reported abuse in foreign marketing. Although ROMAZICON has a benzodiazepine-like structure it does not act as a benzodiazepine agonist in man and is not a controlled substance.

OVERDOSAGE

Large intravenous doses of ROMAZICON, when administered to healthy normal volunteers in the absence of a benzodiazepine agonist, produced no serious adverse reactions, severe signs or symptoms, or clinically significant laboratory test abnormalities. In clinical studies, most adverse reactions to flumazenil were an extension of the pharmacologic effects of the drug in reversing benzodiazepine effects. Reversal with an excessively high dose of ROMAZICON may produce anxiety, agitation, increased muscle tone, hyperesthesia and possibly convulsions. Convulsions have been treated with barbiturates, benzodiazepines and phenytoin, generally with prompt resolution of the seizures. (See WARNINGS.)

DOSE AND ADMINISTRATION

ROMAZICON is recommended for intravenous use only. It is compatible with 5% dextrose in water, lactated Ringer's and normal saline solutions. If ROMAZICON is drawn into a syringe or mixed with any of these solutions, it should be discarded after 24 hours. For optimum sterility, ROMAZICON should remain in the vial until just before use. As with all parenteral drug products, ROMAZICON should be inspected visually for particulate matter and discoloration prior to administration, whenever solution and container permit.

To minimize the likelihood of pain at the injection site, ROMAZICON should be administered through a freely running intravenous infusion into a large vein.

REVERSAL OF CONSCIOUS SEDATION OR IN GENERAL ANESTHESIA: For the reversal of the sedative effects of benzodiazepines administered for conscious sedation or general anesthesia, the recommended initial dose of ROMAZICON is 0.2 mg (2 mL) administered intravenously over 15 seconds. If the desired level of consciousness is not obtained after waiting an additional 45 seconds, a further dose of 0.2 mg (2 mL) can be injected and repeated at 60-second intervals where necessary (up to a maximum of 4 additional times) to a maximum total dose of 1 mg (10 mL). The dose should be individualized based on the patient's response, with most patients responding to doses of 0.6 to 1 mg. (See INDIVIDUALIZATION OF DOSAGE.)

In the event of resedation, repeated doses may be administered at 20 minute intervals as needed. For repeat treatment, no more than 1 mg (given as 0.2 mg/min) should be administered at any one time, and no more than 3 mg should be given in any one hour.

It is recommended that ROMAZICON be administered as the series of small injections described (not as a single bolus injection) to allow the practitioner to control the reversal of sedation to the approximate endpoint desired and to minimize the possibility of adverse effects. (See INDIVIDUALIZATION OF DOSAGE.)

MANAGEMENT OF SUSPECTED BENZODIAZEPINE OVERDOSE: For initial management of a known or suspected benzodiazepine overdose, the recommended initial dose of ROMAZICON is 0.2 mg (2 mL) administered intravenously over 30 seconds. If the desired level of consciousness is not obtained after waiting 30 seconds, a further dose of 0.3 mg (3 mL) can be administered over another 30 seconds. Further doses of 0.5 mg (5 mL) can be administered over 30 seconds at 1-minute intervals up to a cumulative dose of 3 mg.

Do not rush the administration of ROMAZICON. Patients should have a secure airway and intravenous access before administration of the drug and be awakened gradually. (See PRECAUTIONS.)

Most patients with benzodiazepine overdose will respond to a cumulative dose of 1–3 mg of ROMAZICON, and doses beyond 3 mg do not reliably produce additional effects. On rare occasions, patients with a partial response at 3 mg may require additional titration up to a total dose of 5 mg (administered slowly in the same manner).

If a patient has not responded 5 minutes after receiving a cumulative dose of 5 mg ROMAZICON, the major cause of sedation is likely not to be due to benzodiazepines, and additional ROMAZICON is likely to have no effect.

In the event of resedation, repeated doses may be given at 20-minute intervals if needed. For repeat treatment, no more than 1 mg (given as 0.5 mg/min) should be given at any one time and no more than 3 mg should be given in any one hour.

SAFETY AND HANDLING: ROMAZICON is supplied in sealed dosage forms and poses no known risk to the health care provider. Routine care should be taken to avoid aerosol generation when preparing syringes for injection, and spilled medication should be rinsed from the skin with cool water.

HOW SUPPLIED

5 mL multiple-use vials containing 0.1 mg/mL flumazenil: Boxes of 10 (NDC 0004-6911-06).

10 mL multiple-use vials containing 0.1 mg/mL flumazenil: Boxes of 10 (NDC 0004-6912-06).

Store at 59° to 86°F (15° to 30°C).

Revised: October 1994

SORIATANE® ℞

[sŏr 'ĭa tane]
(acitretin)
CAPSULES

The following text is complete prescribing information based on official labeling in effect June 1998.

CONTRAINDICATIONS AND WARNINGS: Soriatane must not be used by females who are pregnant, or who intend to become pregnant during therapy or at any time for at least 3 years following discontinuation of therapy. Soriatane also must not be used by females who may not use reliable contraception while undergoing treatment or for at least 3 years following discontinuation of treatment. Acitretin is a metabolite of etretinate (Tegison®), and major human fetal abnormalities have been reported with the administration of etretinate and acitretin. Potentially, any fetus exposed can be affected.

Clinical evidence has shown that concurrent ingestion of acitretin and ethanol has been associated with the formation of etretinate, which has a longer elimination half-life than acitretin. Because the longer elimination half-life of etretinate would increase the duration of teratogenic potential for female patients, ethanol must not be ingested by female patients either during treatment with Soriatane or for 2 months after cessation of therapy. This allows for elimination of acitretin, thus removing the substrate for transesterification to etretinate. The mechanism of the metabolic process for conversion of acitretin to etretinate has not been fully defined. It is not known whether substances other than ethanol are associated with transesterification.

Acitretin has been shown to be embryotoxic and/or teratogenic in rabbits, mice, and rats at doses approximately 0.6, 3 and 15 times the maximum recommended therapeutic dose, respectively.

Major human fetal abnormalities associated with etretinate and/or acitretin administration have been reported including meningomyelocele, meningoencephalocele, multiple synostoses, facial dysmorphia, syndactylies, absence of terminal phalanges, malformations of hip, ankle and forearm, low set ears, high palate, decreased cranial volume, cardiovascular malformation and alterations of the skull and cervical vertebrae on x-ray.

Females of reproductive potential must not be given Soriatane until pregnancy is excluded. It is contraindicated in females of reproductive potential unless the patient meets ALL of the following conditions:

- **has severe psoriasis and is unresponsive to other therapies or whose clinical condition contraindicates the use of other treatments;**
- **has received both oral and written warnings of the hazards of taking Soriatane during pregnancy;**
- **has received both oral and written warnings of the risk of possible contraception failure and of the need to use two reliable forms of contraception simultaneously both during therapy and for at least 3 years *after* discontinuation of therapy and has acknowledged in writing her understanding of these warnings and of the need for using dual contraceptive methods (unless the patient has undergone a hysterectomy or practices abstinence);**
- **has had a negative serum or urine pregnancy test with a sensitivity of at least 50 mIU/mL within 1 week prior to beginning therapy;**
- **will begin therapy only on the second or third day of the next normal menstrual period;**
- **is capable of complying with the mandatory contraceptive measures; and**
- **is reliable in understanding and carrying out instructions.**

A prescription for Soriatane should not be issued by the physician until a report of a negative pregnancy test has been obtained and the patient has begun her menstrual period. Pregnancy testing and contraception counseling should be repeated on a regular basis. To encourage compliance with this recommendation, the physician should prescribe a limited supply of the drug. Effective contraception must be used for at least 1 month before beginning Soriatane therapy, during therapy and for at least 3 years following discontinuation of therapy even where there has been a history of infertility, unless due to hysterectomy. It is recommended that two reliable forms of contraception be used simultaneously unless abstinence is the chosen method. Patients who have undergone tubal ligation should use a second form of contraception.

It is not known whether residual acitretin in seminal fluid poses risk to a fetus while a male patient is taking the drug or after it is discontinued. There have been five pregnancies reported in which the male partner was undergoing Soriatane treatment. One pregnancy resulted in a normal infant. Two pregnancies ended in

spontaneous abortions. In another case, the fetus had bilateral cystic hygromas and multiple cardiopulmonary malformations. The relationship of these malformations to the drug is unknown. The outcome of the fifth case is unknown.

Samples of seminal fluid from 3 male patients treated with acitretin and 6 male patients treated with etretinate have been assayed for the presence of acitretin. The maximum concentration of acitretin observed in the seminal fluid of these men was 12.5 ng/mL. Assuming an ejaculate volume of 10 mL, the amount of drug transferred in semen would be 125 ng, which is 1/200,000 of a single 25 mg capsule.

Females who have taken Tegison (etretinate) must continue to follow the contraceptive recommendations for Tegison.

Acitretin, the active metabolite of etretinate, is teratogenic and is contraindicated during pregnancy. The risk of severe fetal malformations is well established when systemic retinoids are taken during pregnancy. Pregnancy must also be prevented after stopping acitretin therapy, while the drug is being eliminated to below a threshold blood concentration that would be associated with an increased incidence of birth defects. Because this threshold has not been established for acitretin in humans and because elimination rates vary among patients, the duration of posttherapy contraception to achieve adequate elimination cannot be calculated precisely. It is strongly recommended that contraception be continued for at least 3 years after stopping treatment with acitretin, based on the following considerations:

- **◇ In the absence of transesterification to form etretinate, greater than 98% of the acitretin would be eliminated within 2 months, assuming a mean elimination half-life of 49 hours.**
- **◇ In cases where etretinate is formed, as has been demonstrated with concomitant administration of acitretin and ethanol,**
  - **greater than 98% of the etretinate formed would be eliminated in 2 years, assuming a mean elimination half-life of 120 days.**
  - **greater than 98% of the etretinate formed would be eliminated in 3 years, based on the longest demonstrated elimination half-life of 168 days. However, etretinate was found in plasma and subcutaneous fat in one patient reported to have had sporadic alcohol intake, 52 months after she stopped acitretin therapy.[1]**
- **◇ An increased incidence of birth defects was estimated based on a limited number of cases which have been reported to Roche, which were identified before the outcome was known, and where pregnancy occurred during the time interval when the patient was being treated with acitretin or etretinate. For cases identified after the outcome was known, severe birth defects have been reported where pregnancy occurred during the time interval when the patient was being treated with acitretin or etretinate.**
- **◇ There have been 202 cases reported before the outcome was known where pregnancy occurred after the last dose of etretinate or acitretin. Fetal outcome remained unknown in approximately one-half of these cases, of which 62 were terminated and 11 were spontaneous abortions. Fetal outcome is known for 103 of these prospectively reported cases. Fifteen of the outcomes were abnormal: hernia, hypocalcemia, hypotonia, undescended testicle, laparoschisis, absent hand/wrist, clubfoot, ichthyosis, apnea/anemia, placental disorder/death and premature birth (5). Birth defects have also been reported retrospectively (ie, after the outcome was known). Among the retrospectively reported cases where pregnancy occurred more than 2 years after the last dose of etretinate or acitretin, there are 2 normal outcomes, 3 unknown outcomes and 7 abnormal outcomes. The 7 abnormal outcomes reported are: malformation unspecified, aplasia of the forearm, stillbirth, right ventricular/aortic duct defect, heart malformation unspecified, and chromosomal disorder (2). For these listed reports, the relationship of the birth defects to the drug is unknown.**

If pregnancy does occur during Soriatane therapy or at any time for at least 3 years following discontinuation of Soriatane therapy, the physician and patient should discuss the possible effects on the pregnancy.

Soriatane should be prescribed only by physicians who have special competence in the diagnosis and treatment of severe psoriasis, are experienced in the use of systemic retinoids, and understand the risk of teratogenicity.

DESCRIPTION

Soriatane (acitretin), a retinoid, is available in 10 mg and 25 mg gelatin capsules for oral administration. Chemically, acitretin is all-*trans*-9-(4-methoxy-2,3,6-trimethylphenyl)-3,7-dimethyl-2,4,6,8-nonatetraenoic acid. It is a metabolite of etretinate and is related to both retinoic acid and retinol (vitamin A). It is a yellow to greenish-yellow powder with a molecular weight of 326.44.

Table 1. Adverse Events Frequently Reported During Clinical Trials
Percent of Patients Reporting (N=525)

BODY SYSTEM	>75%	50% to 75%	25% to 50%	10% to 25%
Mucous Membranes	Cheilitis		Rhinitis	Dry mouth Epistaxis
Skin and Appendages		Alopecia Skin peeling	Dry skin Nail disorder Pruritus	Erythematous rash Hyperesthesia Paresthesia Paronychia Skin atrophy Sticky skin
Eye Disorders				Xerophthalmia
Musculoskeletal				Arthralgia Spinal hyperostosis (progression of existing lesions)
CNS				Rigors

Each capsule contains acitretin, microcrystalline cellulose, sodium ascorbate, gelatin, black monogramming ink and maltodextrin (a mixture of polysaccharides).

Gelatin capsule shells contain gelatin, parabens (methyl and propyl), iron oxide (yellow, black, and red), and titanium dioxide. They may also contain benzyl alcohol, butyl paraben, carboxymethylcellulose sodium, edetate calcium disodium, potassium sorbate and/or sodium propionate.

CLINICAL PHARMACOLOGY

The mechanism of action of Soriatane is unknown.

Pharmacokinetics: *Absorption:* Oral absorption of acitretin is optimal when given with food. For this reason, acitretin was given with food in all of the following studies. After administration of a single 50 mg oral dose of acitretin to 18 healthy subjects, maximum plasma concentrations ranged from 196 to 728 ng/mL (mean 416 ng/mL) and were achieved in 2 to 5 hours (mean 2.7 hours). The oral absorption of acitretin is linear and proportional with increasing doses from 25 to 100 mg. Approximately 72% (range 47% to 109%) of the administered dose was absorbed after a single 50 mg dose of acitretin was given to 12 healthy subjects.

Distribution: Acitretin is more than 99.9% bound to plasma proteins, primarily albumin.

Metabolism (see Pharmacokinetic Drug Interactions: Ethanol): Following oral absorption, acitretin undergoes extensive metabolism and interconversion by simple isomerization to its 13-*cis* form (*cis*-acitretin). The formation of *cis*-acitretin relative to parent compound is not altered by dose or fed/fast conditions of oral administration of acitretin. Both parent compound and isomer are further metabolized into chain-shortened breakdown products and conjugates which are excreted.

Following multiple-dose administration of acitretin, steady-state concentrations of acitretin and *cis*-acitretin in plasma are achieved within approximately 3 weeks.

Elimination: The chain-shortened metabolites and conjugates of acitretin and *cis*-acitretin are ultimately excreted in the feces (34% to 54%) and urine (16% to 53%). The terminal elimination half-life of acitretin following multiple-dose administration is 49 hours (range 33 to 96 hours), and that of *cis*-acitretin under the same conditions is 63 hours (range 28 to 157 hours). The accumulation ratio of the parent compound is 1.2; that of *cis*-acitretin is 6.6.

Special Populations: *Psoriasis:* In an 8-week study of acitretin pharmacokinetics in patients with psoriasis, mean steady-state trough concentrations of acitretin increased in a dose proportional manner with dosages ranging from 10 to 50 mg daily. Acitretin plasma concentrations were nonmeasurable (<4 ng/mL) in all patients 3 weeks after cessation of therapy.

Elderly: In a multiple-dose study in healthy young (n=6) and elderly (n=8) subjects, a two-fold increase in acitretin plasma concentrations were seen in elderly subjects, although the elimination half-life did not change.

Renal Failure: Plasma concentrations of acitretin were significantly (59.3%) lower in end-stage renal failure subjects (n=6) when compared to age-matched controls, following single 50 mg oral doses. Acitretin was not removed by hemodialysis in these subjects.

Pharmacokinetic Drug Interactions (see also boxed CONTRAINDICATIONS AND WARNINGS and PRECAUTIONS: *Drug Interactions*): In studies of in vivo pharmacokinetic drug interactions, no interaction was seen between acitretin and cimetidine, digoxin, phenprocoumon or glyburide.

Ethanol: Clinical evidence has shown that etretinate (a retinoid with a much longer half-life, see below) can be formed with concurrent ingestion of acitretin and ethanol. In a two-way crossover study, all 10 subjects formed etretinate with concurrent ingestion of a single 100 mg oral dose of acitretin during a 3-hour period of ethanol ingestion (total ethanol, approximately 1.4 g/kg body weight). A mean peak etretinate concentration of 59 ng/mL (range 22 to 105 ng/mL) was observed, and extrapolation of AUC values indicated that the formation of etretinate in this study was comparable to a single 5 mg oral dose of etretinate. There was no detectable formation of etretinate when a single 100 mg oral dose of acitretin was administered without concurrent ethanol ingestion, although the formation of etretinate without concurrent ethanol ingestion cannot be excluded (see boxed CONTRAINDICATIONS AND WARNINGS). Of 93 evaluable psoriatic patients on acitretin therapy in several foreign studies (10 to 80 mg/day), 16% had measurable etretinate levels (>5 ng/mL).

Etretinate has a much longer elimination half-life compared to that of acitretin. In one study the apparent mean terminal half-life after 6 months of therapy was approximately 120 days (range 84 to 168 days). In another study of 47 patients treated chronically with etretinate, 5 had detectable serum drug levels (in the range of 0.5 to 12 ng/mL) 2.1 to 2.9 years after therapy was discontinued. The long half-life appears to be due to storage of etretinate in adipose tissue.

Progestin-only Contraceptives: It has not been established if there is a pharmacokinetic interaction between acitretin and combined oral contraceptives. However, it *has been* established that acitretin interferes with the contraceptive effect of microdosed progestin preparations.[2] *It is not known whether other progestational contraceptives, such as implants and injectables, are inadequate methods of contraception during acitretin therapy.*

INDICATIONS AND USAGE

Soriatane is indicated for the treatment of severe psoriasis, including the erythrodermic and generalized pustular types, in adults. Because of significant adverse effects associated with its use, Soriatane should be prescribed only by physicians knowledgeable in the systemic use of retinoids. In females of reproductive potential, Soriatane should be reserved for patients who are unresponsive to other therapies or whose clinical condition contraindicates the use of other treatments.

Most patients experience relapse of psoriasis after discontinuing therapy. Subsequent courses, when clinically indicated, have produced results similar to the initial course of therapy.

CONTRAINDICATIONS

Pregnancy Category X (see boxed CONTRAINDICATIONS AND WARNINGS)

WARNINGS

(See also boxed CONTRAINDICATIONS AND WARNINGS)

Hepatotoxicity: **Of the 525 patients treated in US clinical trials, 2 had clinical jaundice with elevated serum bilirubin and transaminases considered related to Soriatane treatment. Liver function test results in these patients returned to normal after Soriatane was discontinued. Two of the 1289 patients treated in European clinical trials developed biopsy-confirmed toxic hepatitis. A second biopsy in one of these patients revealed nodule formation suggestive of cirrhosis. One patient in a Canadian clinical trial of 63 patients developed a three-fold increase of transaminases. A liver biopsy of this patient showed mild lobular disarray, multifocal hepatocyte loss and mild triaditis of the portal**

Continued on next page

Soriatane—Cont.

tracts compatible with acute reversible hepatic injury. The patient's transaminase levels returned to normal 2 months after Soriatane was discontinued.

The potential of acitretin therapy to induce hepatotoxicity was prospectively evaluated using liver biopsies in an open-label study of 128 patients. Pretreatment and posttreatment biopsies were available for 87 patients. A comparison of liver biopsy findings before and after therapy revealed 49 (58%) patients showed no change, 21 (25%) improved and 14 (17%) patients had a worsening of their liver biopsy status. For 6 patients, the classification changed from class 0 (no pathology) to class I (normal fatty infiltration; nuclear variability and portal inflammation; both mild); for 7 patients, the change was from class I to class II (fatty infiltration, nuclear variability, portal inflammation and focal necrosis; all moderate to severe); and for 1 patient, the change was from class II to class IIIb (fibrosis, moderate to severe). No correlation could be found between liver function test result abnormalities and the change in liver biopsy status, and no cumulative dose relationship was found.

Elevations of AST (SGOT), ALT (SGPT), GGT (GGTP) or LDH have occurred in approximately 1 in 3 patients treated with Soriatane. Of the 525 patients treated in clinical trials in the US, treatment was discontinued in 20 (3.8%) due to elevated liver function test results. If hepatotoxicity is suspected during treatment with Soriatane, the drug should be discontinued and the etiology further investigated.

Ten of 652 patients treated in US clinical trials of etretinate, of which acitretin is the active metabolite, had clinical or histologic hepatitis considered to be possibly or probably related to etretinate treatment. There have been reports of hepatitis-related deaths worldwide; a few of these patients had received etretinate for a month or less before presenting with hepatic symptoms or signs.

Pancreatitis: Lipid elevations occur in 25% to 50% of patients treated with acitretin. Triglyceride increases sufficient to be associated with pancreatitis are much less common, although fatal fulminant pancreatitis has been reported for one patient.

Pseudotumor cerebri: Soriatane and other retinoids administered orally have been associated with cases of pseudotumor cerebri (benign intracranial hypertension). Some of these events involved concomitant use of isotretinoin and tetracyclines. However, the event seen in a single Soriatane patient was not associated with tetracycline use. Early signs and symptoms include papilledema, headache, nausea and vomiting and visual disturbances. Patients with these signs and symptoms should be examined for papilledema and, if present, should discontinue Soriatane immediately and be referred for neurological evaluation and care.

Ophthalmologic Effects: The eyes and vision of 329 patients treated with Soriatane were examined by ophthalmologists. The findings included dry eyes (23%), irritation of eyes (9%) and brow and lash loss (5%). The following were reported in less than 5% of patients: Bell's Palsy, blepharitis and/or crusting of lids, blurred vision, conjunctivitis, corneal epithelial abnormality, cortical cataract, decreased night vision, diplopia, itchy eyes or eyelids, nuclear cataract, pannus, papilledema, photophobia, posterior subcapsular cataract, recurrent sties and subepithelial corneal lesions.

Any patient treated with Soriatane who is experiencing visual difficulties should discontinue the drug and undergo ophthalmologic evaluation.

Hyperostosis: In clinical trials with Soriatane, patients were prospectively evaluated for evidence of development or change in bony abnormalities of the vertebral column, knees and ankles.

Vertebral Results: Of 380 patients treated with Soriatane, 15% had preexisting abnormalities of the spine which showed new changes or progression of preexisting findings. Changes included degenerative spurs, anterior bridging of spinal vertebrae, diffuse idiopathic skeletal hyperostosis, ligament calcification and narrowing and destruction of a cervical disc space.

De novo changes (formation of small spurs) were seen in 3 patients after 1 1/2 to 2 1/2 years.

Skeletal Appendicular Results: Six of 128 patients treated with Soriatane showed abnormalities in the knees and ankles before treatment that progressed during treatment. In 5, these changes involved the formation of additional spurs or enlargement of existing spurs. The sixth patient had degenerative joint disease which worsened. No patients developed spurs de novo. Clinical complaints did not predict radiographic changes.

Lipids: Blood lipid determinations should be performed before Soriatane is administered and again at intervals of 1 to

Table 2. Adverse Events Less Frequently Reported During Clinical Trials
(Some of Which May Bear No Relationship to Therapy)
Percent of Patients Reporting (N=525)

BODY SYSTEM	1% to 10%	<1%
Mucous Membranes	Gingival bleeding Gingivitis Increased saliva Stomatitis Thirst Ulcerative stomatitis	Altered saliva Anal disorder Gum hyperplasia Hemorrhage Pharyngitis
Skin and Appendages	Abnormal skin odor Abnormal hair texture Bullous eruption Cold/clammy skin Dermatitis Increased sweating Infection Psoriasiform rash Purpura Pyogenic granuloma Rash Seborrhea Skin fissures Skin ulceration Sunburn	Acne Breast pain Cyst Eczema Fungal infection Furunculosis Hair discoloration Herpes simplex Hyperkeratosis Hypertrichosis Hypoesthesia Impaired healing Otitis media Otitis externa Photosensitivity reaction Psoriasis aggravated Scleroderma Skin nodule Skin hypertrophy Skin disorder Skin irritation Sweat gland disorder Urticaria Verrucae
Eye Disorders	Abnormal/blurred vision Blepharitis Conjunctivitis/irritation Corneal epithelial abnormality Decreased night vision/ night blindness Eye abnormality Eye pain Photophobia	Abnormal lacrimation Chalazion Conjunctival hemorrhage Corneal ulceration Diplopia Ectropion Itchy eyes and lids Papilledema Recurrent sties Subepithelial corneal lesions

Musculoskeletal	Arthritis
	Arthrosis
	Back pain
	
	Hypertonia
	Myalgia
	Osteodynia
	Peripheral joint hyperostosis
	   (progression of existing lesions)
		Bone disorder
		Olecranon bursitis
		Spinal hyperostosis
		   (new lesions)
		Tendinitis

CNS	Headache Pain	Abnormal gait Migraine Neuritis Pseudotumor cerebri (intracranial hypertension)
Gastrointestinal	Abdominal pain Diarrhea Nausea Tongue disorder	Constipation Dyspepsia Esophagitis Gastritis Gastroenteritis Glossitis Hemorrhoids Melena Tenesmus Tongue ulceration
Special Senses/Other	Earache Taste perversion Tinnitus	Ceruminosis Deafness Taste loss
Psychiatric	Depression Insomnia Somnolence	Anxiety Dysphonia Libido decreased Nervousness
Respiratory	Sinusitis	Coughing Increased sputum Laryngitis
Urinary		Abnormal urine Dysuria Penis disorder
Reproductive		Atrophic vaginitis Leukorrhea

Continued on next page

Table 2 (continued)

BODY SYSTEM	1% to 10%	<1%
Cardiovascular	Flushing	Chest pain Cyanosis Increased bleeding time Intermittent claudication Peripheral ischemia
Body as a Whole	Anorexia Edema Fatigue Hot flashes Increased appetite	Alcohol tolerance Dizziness Fever Influenza-like symptoms Malaise Moniliasis Muscle weakness Weight increase
Liver and Biliary		Hepatic function abnormal Hepatitis Jaundice

2 weeks until the lipid response to the drug is established, usually within 4 to 8 weeks. In patients receiving Soriatane during clinical trials, 66% and 33% experienced elevation in triglycerides and cholesterol, respectively. Decreased high density lipoproteins (HDL) occurred in 40%. These effects of Soriatane were generally reversible upon cessation of therapy.

Patients with an increased tendency to develop hypertriglyceridemia included those with diabetes mellitus, obesity, increased alcohol intake or a familial history of these conditions.

Hypertriglyceridemia and lowered HDL may increase a patient's cardiovascular risk status. In addition, elevation of serum triglycerides to greater than 800 mg/dL has been associated with fatal fulminant pancreatitis. Therefore, dietary modifications, reduction in Soriatane dose, or drug therapy should be employed to control significant elevations of triglycerides.

Animal Studies: Subchronic and chronic toxicity studies in rats and dogs revealed dose-related, reversible signs of intolerance typical of retinoids. In rats, decreased body weight gain and increases in serum cholesterol, triglycerides, lipoproteins and alkaline phosphatase were observed; fractures and evidence of healed fractures were also noted. In dogs, signs of intolerance included erythema, skin hypertrophy/hyperplasia and testicular changes. In dogs, the dosages studied were as much as ten times the recommended human dosage; in rats, one to two times. Most of the side effects were readily reversible after cessation of treatment, except for epiphyseal ossification.

Acitretin shares with vitamin A and other retinoids the potential to cause malformations in the offspring of various species, including mouse, rat and rabbit, even at dosage levels recommended for humans. Since acitretin is teratogenic in animals at human dosage levels, females of reproductive potential must not be treated if pregnancy cannot be excluded.

PRECAUTIONS

General: Caution is advised in patients with severely impaired liver or kidney function (see CLINICAL PHARMACOLOGY). Soriatane should not be given to patients who are sensitive to parabens, which are used as preservatives in the gelatin capsule.

Information for Patients: Females of reproductive potential should be advised that they must not be pregnant when Soriatane therapy is initiated and that they should use effective contraception for at least 1 month prior to Soriatane therapy, and while taking Soriatane. Acitretin, the active metabolite of etretinate, is teratogenic and is contraindicated during pregnancy. The risk of severe fetal malformation is well established when systemic retinoids are taken during pregnancy. Pregnancy must also be prevented after stopping acitretin therapy, while the drug is being eliminated to below a threshold blood concentration that would be associated with an increased incidence of birth defects. Because this threshold has not been established for acitretin in humans and because elimination rates vary among patients, the duration of posttherapy contraception to achieve adequate elimination cannot be calculated precisely. It is strongly recommended that contraception be continued for at least 3 years after stopping treatment with acitretin, based on the following considerations:

◊ In the absence of transesterification to form etretinate, greater than 98% of the acitretin would be eliminated within 2 months, assuming a mean elimination half-life of 49 hours.

◊ In cases where etretinate is formed, as has been demonstrated with concomitant administration of acitretin and ethanol,

  • greater than 98% of the etretinate formed would be eliminated in 2 years, assuming a mean elimination half-life of 120 days.

  • greater than 98% of the etretinate formed would be eliminated in 3 years, based on the longest demonstrated elimination half-life of 168 days. However, etretinate was found in plasma and subcutaneous fat in one patient reported to have had sporadic alcohol intake, 52 months after she stopped acitretin therapy.[1]

◊ An increased incidence of birth defects was estimated based on a limited number of cases which have been reported to Roche, which were identified before the outcome was known, and where pregnancy occurred during the time interval when the patient was being treated with acitretin or etretinate. For cases identified after the outcome was known, severe birth defects have been reported where pregnancy occurred during the time interval when the patient was being treated with acitretin or etretinate.

◊ There have been 202 cases reported before the outcome was known where pregnancy occurred *after* the last dose of etretinate or acitretin. Fetal outcome remained unknown in approximately one-half of these cases, of which 62 were terminated and 11 were spontaneous abortions. Fetal outcome is known for 103 of these prospectively reported cases. Fifteen of the outcomes were abnormal: hernia, hypocalcemia, hypotonia, undescended testicle, laparoschisis, absent hand/wrist, clubfoot, ichthyosis, apnea/anemia, placental disorder/death and premature birth (5). Birth defects have also been reported retrospectively (ie, after the outcome was known). Among the retrospectively reported cases where pregnancy occurred more than 2 years after the last dose of etretinate or acitretin, there are 2 normal outcomes, 3 unknown outcomes and 7 abnormal outcomes. The 7 abnormal outcomes reported are: malformation unspecified, aplasia of the forearm, stillbirth, right ventricular/aortic duct defect, heart malformation unspecified, and chromosomal disorder (2). For these listed reports, the relationship of the birth defects to the drug is unknown.

Females of reproductive potential should also be advised that they must not ingest beverages or products containing ethanol while taking Soriatane and for 2 months after Soriatane treatment has been discontinued. This allows for elimination of the acitretin which can be converted to etretinate in the presence of alcohol. They should be advised that certain methods of birth control can fail, including tubal ligation and microdosed progestin "minipill" preparations. Data from one patient who received a very low-dosed progestin contraceptive (levonorgestrel 0.03 mg) had a significant increase of the progesterone level after three menstrual cycles during acitretin treatment.[2] Female patients should sign a consent form prior to beginning Soriatane therapy (see boxed CONTRAINDICATIONS AND WARNINGS).

Because of the relationship of Soriatane to vitamin A, patients should be advised against taking vitamin A supplements in excess of minimum recommended daily allowances to avoid possible additive toxic effects.

Patients should be advised that a transient worsening of psoriasis is sometimes seen during the initial treatment period.

Patients should be advised that they may have to wait 2 or 3 months before they get the full benefit of Soriatane.

Patients should be advised that they may experience decreased tolerance to contact lenses during the treatment period.

It is recommended that patients not donate blood during and for 3 years following therapy.

Patients should avoid the use of sun lamps and excessive exposure to sunlight because the effects of UV light are enhanced by retinoid therapy.

Patients should be advised that they must not give their Soriatane capsules to any other person.

Laboratory Tests: In clinical studies, the incidence of hypertriglyceridemia was 66%, hypercholesterolemia was 33%

and that of decreased HDL was 40%. Pretreatment and follow-up measurements should be obtained under fasting conditions. It is recommended that these tests be performed weekly or every other week until the lipid response to Soriatane has stabilized (see WARNINGS).

Elevations of AST (SGOT), ALT (SGPT) or LDH were experienced by approximately 1 in 3 patients treated with Soriatane. It is recommended that these tests be performed prior to initiation of Soriatane therapy, at 1- to 2-week intervals until stable and thereafter at intervals as clinically indicated.

Certain patients receiving retinoids have experienced problems in the control of their blood sugar. In addition, new cases of diabetes have been diagnosed during retinoid therapy, although no causal relationship has been established.

Drug Interactions: Clinical evidence has shown that etretinate can be formed with concurrent ingestion of acitretin and ethanol (see boxed CONTRAINDICATIONS AND WARNINGS and CLINICAL PHARMACOLOGY: *Pharmacokinetics*).

In a study of 7 healthy male volunteers, acitretin treatment enhanced clearance of blood glucose in the presence of glibenclamide (a sulfonylurea similar to chlorpropamide) in 3 of the 7 subjects. Repeating the study with 6 healthy male volunteers in the absence of glibenclamide did not detect an effect of acitretin on glucose tolerance. Careful supervision of diabetic patients under treatment with Soriatane is recommended (see CLINICAL PHARMACOLOGY: *Pharmacokinetics* and DOSAGE AND ADMINISTRATION).

There may be the possibility of an increased risk of hepatotoxicity in patients treated with etretinate and methotrexate concomitantly. Consequently, the concomitant use of Soriatane and methotrexate should be avoided.

There appears to be no pharmacokinetic interaction between acitretin and cimetidine, digoxin, phenprocoumon or glyburide.

It has not been established if there is a pharmacokinetic interaction between acitretin and combined oral contraceptives. However, it *has* been established that acitretin interferes with the contraceptive effect of microdosed progestin "minipill" preparations. *It is not known whether other progestational contraceptives, such as implants and injectables, may be inadequate methods of contraception during acitretin therapy.*

Carcinogenesis, Mutagenesis and Impairment of Fertility: Carcinogenesis: A carcinogenesis study of acitretin in Wistar rats, at doses up to 2 mg/kg/day administered 7 days/week for 104 weeks, has been completed. There were no neoplastic lesions observed that were considered to have been related to treatment with acitretin. A carcinogenesis study in mice has been completed with etretinate, the ethyl ester of acitretin. Blood level data obtained during this study demonstrated that etretinate was metabolized to acitretin and that blood levels of acitretin exceeded those of etretinate at all times studied. In the etretinate study, an increased incidence of blood vessel tumors (hemangiomas and hemangiosarcomas at several different sites) was noted in male, but not female, mice at doses approximately 5.7 to 7.1 times the maximum recommended human therapeutic dose. *Mutagenesis:* Acitretin was evaluated for mutagenic potential in the Ames test, in the Chinese hamster (V79/HGPRT) assay, in unscheduled DNA synthesis assays using rat hepatocytes and human fibroblasts and in an in vivo mouse micronucleus assay. No evidence of mutagenicity of acitretin was demonstrated in any of these assays.

Impairment of Fertility: In a fertility study in rats, the fertility of treated animals was not impaired at the highest dosage of acitretin tested, 3 mg/kg/day (approximately three times the maximum recommended therapeutic dose). Chronic toxicity studies in dogs revealed testicular changes (reversible mild to moderate spermatogenic arrest and appearance of multinucleated giant cells) in the highest dosage group (50 then 30 mg/kg/day).

No decreases in sperm count or concentration and no changes in sperm motility or morphology were noted in 31 men (17 psoriatic patients, 8 patients with disorders of keratinization and 6 healthy volunteers) given 30 to 50 mg/day of acitretin for at least 12 weeks. In these studies, no deleterious effects were seen on either testosterone production, LH or FSH in any of the 31 men.[3-5] No deleterious effects were seen on the hypothalamic-pituitary axis in any of the 18 men where it was measured.[3,4]

Pregnancy: Teratogenic Effects: **Pregnancy Category X (see boxed CONTRAINDICATIONS AND WARNINGS).**

Effective contraception must be used by female patients of reproductive potential for at least 1 month before beginning Soriatane therapy, during therapy and for at least 3 years following discontinuation of therapy. This warning applies even where there has been a history of infertility, unless due to hysterectomy.

In a study in which acitretin was administered to male rats only at a dosage of 5 mg/kg/day for 10 weeks (approximate duration of one spermatogenic cycle) prior to and during mating with untreated female rats, no teratogenic effects were observed in the progeny.

Samples of seminal fluid from 3 male patients treated with acitretin and 6 male patients treated with etretinate have been assayed for the presence of acitretin. The maximum concentration of acitretin observed in the seminal fluid of

Continued on next page

Soriatane—Cont.

these men was 12.5 ng/mL. Assuming an ejaculate volume of 10 mL, the amount of drug transferred in semen would be 125 ng, which is 1/200,000 of a single 25 mg capsule.

It is not known whether residual acitretin in seminal fluid poses risk to a fetus while a male patient is taking the drug or after it is discontinued. There have been five pregnancies reported in which the male partner was undergoing Soriatane treatment. One pregnancy resulted in a normal infant. Two pregnancies ended in spontaneous abortions. In one case the fetus had bilateral cystic hygromas and multiple cardiopulmonary malformations: the relationship of these malformations to the drug is unknown. The outcome of the fifth case is unknown.

Nonteratogenic Effects: In rats dosed at 3 mg/kg/day (approximately three times the maximum recommended therapeutic dose), slightly decreased pup survival and delayed incisor eruption were noted. At the next lowest dose tested, 1 mg/kg/day, no treatment-related adverse effects were observed.

Nursing Mothers: Studies on lactating rats have shown that etretinate is excreted in the milk. However, it is not known whether either etretinate or acitretin is excreted in human milk. However, nursing mothers should not receive Soriatane because of the potential for excretion in milk and serious adverse reactions in nursing infants.

Pediatric Use: No clinical studies have been conducted in pediatric patients. Therefore, safety and effectiveness in pediatric patients have not been established. Ossification of interosseous ligaments and tendons of the extremities, skeletal hyperostoses and premature epiphyseal closure have been reported with other systemic retinoids. While it is not known that these occurrences are more severe or more frequent in children, there is concern in pediatric patients because of the implications for growth potential.

ADVERSE EVENTS

During clinical trials with acitretin, 513/525 (98%) of patients reported a total of 3545 adverse events. One-hundred sixteen patients left studies prematurely, primarily because of adverse experiences involving the mucous membranes and skin. Three patients died. Two of the deaths were not drug related (pancreatic adenocarcinoma and lung cancer); the other patient died of an acute myocardial infarction, considered remotely related to drug therapy.

In clinical trials, Soriatane has been associated with elevations in liver function test results or triglyceride levels and hepatitis. A case of fatal fulminant pancreatitis has been reported during Soriatane therapy.

Soriatane has also been associated with a case of pseudotumor cerebri (see WARNINGS). One case of myopathy with peripheral neuropathy has been reported during Soriatane therapy. Both conditions improved with discontinuation of the drug.

Hypervitaminosis A produces a wide spectrum of signs and symptoms primarily of the mucocutaneous, musculoskeletal, hepatic, and central nervous systems. Many of the clinical adverse reactions reported to date with Soriatane administration resemble those of the hypervitaminosis A syndrome. The tables below list by body system and frequency the adverse events reported during clinical trials of 525 patients with psoriasis.

[See table 1 at top of page 2705]

[See table 2 at top of page 2706 and on previous page]

Laboratory: Soriatane therapy induces changes in liver function tests in a significant number of patients. Elevations of AST (SGOT), ALT (SGPT) or LDH were experienced by approximately 1 in 3 patients treated with Soriatane. In most patients, elevations were slight to moderate and returned to normal either during continuation of therapy or after cessation of treatment. In patients receiving Soriatane during clinical trials, 66% and 33% experienced elevation in triglycerides and cholesterol, respectively. Decreased high density lipoproteins (HDL) occurred in 40% (see WARNINGS).

Table 3 lists the laboratory abnormalities reported during clinical trials.

[See table 3 above]

OVERDOSAGE

One overdose case has been reported. A 32-year-old mentally handicapped male with Darier's disease took 21 × 25 mg capsules (525 mg single dose). He vomited several hours later but experienced no other ill effects. His therapeutic treatment was continued. The acute oral toxicity (LD$_{50}$) of acitretin in both mice and rats was greater than 4000 mg/kg.

DOSAGE AND ADMINISTRATION

There is intersubject variation in the pharmacokinetics, clinical efficacy and incidence of side effects with Soriatane. A number of the more common side effects are dose related. Individualization of dosage is required to achieve maximum therapeutic response while minimizing side effects. Soriatane therapy should be initiated at 25 or 50 mg per day, given as a single dose with the main meal. Maintenance doses of 25 to 50 mg per day may be given after initial response to treatment; although, in general, therapy should be terminated when lesions have resolved sufficiently. Relapses may be treated as outlined for initial therapy.

Females who have taken Tegison (etretinate) must continue to follow the contraceptive recommendations for Tegison.

HOW SUPPLIED

Brown and white capsules, 10 mg, imprinted SORIATANE 10 ROCHE; Prescription Paks of 30 (NDC 0004-0213-57).

Brown and yellow capsules, 25 mg, imprinted SORIATANE 25 ROCHE; Prescription Paks of 30 (NDC 0004-0214-57).

Store between 15° and 25°C (59° and 77°F). Protect from light. Avoid exposure to high temperatures and humidity after the bottle is opened.

REFERENCES:

1. Maier H, Honigsmann H: Concentration of etretinate in plasma and subcutaneous fat after long-term acitretin. *Lancet* 348:1107, 1996.
2. Berbis Ph, et al.: *Arch Dermatol Res* (1988) 280:388-389.
3. Sigg C, et al.: Andrological investigations in patients treated with etretin. *Dermatologica* 175:48-49, 1987.
4. Parsch EM, et al.: Andrological investigation in men treated with acitretin (Ro 10-1670). *Andrologia* 22:479-482, 1990.
5. Kadar L, et al.: Spermatological investigations in psoriatic patients treated with acitretin. In: Pharmacology of Retinoids in the Skin; Reichert U. et al., ed, KARGER, Basel, vol. 3, pp 253-254, 1988.

PATIENT INFORMATION/CONSENT:

IMPORTANT INFORMATION AND WARNINGS FOR *ALL* PATIENTS:

Small amounts of Soriatane have been detected in the ejaculate of males taking Soriatane. The amount of Soriatane detected corresponds to less than 1/200,000 of a 25 mg dose. You should discuss any questions you have about this information with your physician.

Alcohol intake can cause Soriatane to be changed into a related drug, etretinate, which may not leave the body for many years.

In addition, you must not donate blood during your treatment with Soriatane and for 3 years after you stop taking Soriatane.

It is recommended that you and your doctor schedule appointments regularly to check your body's response to Soriatane. For your health and well-being, be sure to keep your appointments as scheduled.

Do not give your Soriatane capsules to any other person.

IMPORTANT INFORMATION AND WARNINGS FOR *FEMALE* PATIENTS:

Soriatane must not be used by females who are pregnant or who may become pregnant while undergoing treatment or at any time for at least 3 years after treatment is discontinued.

If you do become pregnant during Soriatane therapy, or at any time for at least 3 years after you stop taking Soriatane, you should discuss with your physician the possible effects on the pregnancy.

Soriatane can cause severe birth defects if it is taken when a female is pregnant. In addition, birth defects have occurred in babies of females who became pregnant after stopping Soriatane treatment. Therefore:

• you must not be pregnant when you start taking Soriatane,

• you must not become pregnant while you are taking Soriatane,

• you must wait at least 3 years after you stop taking Soriatane before becoming pregnant.

Alcohol must be avoided during the entire Soriatane treatment course and for 2 months after you stop taking Soriatane. This is because alcohol intake can cause Soriatane to be changed into a related drug, etretinate.

Table 3. Abnormal Laboratory Test Results Reported During Clinical Trials
Percent of Patients Reporting

BODY SYSTEM	50% to 75%	25% to 50%	10% to 25%	1% to 10%
Hematologic		Increased reticulocytes	Decreased: – Hematocrit – Hemoglobin – WBC Increased: – Haptoglobin – Neutrophils – WBC	Increased: – Bands – Basophils – Eosinophils – Hematocrit – Hemoglobin – Lymphocytes – Monocytes Decreased: – Haptoglobin – Lymphocytes – Neutrophils – Reticulocytes Increased or decreased: – Platelets – RBC
Electrolytes			Increased: – Phosphorus – Potassium – Sodium Increased and decreased magnesium	Decreased: – Phosphorus – Potassium – Sodium Increased and decreased: – Calcium – Chloride
Renal			Increased uric acid	Increased: – BUN – Creatinine
Hepatic		Increased: – Cholesterol – LDH – SGOT – SGPT Decreased HDL cholesterol	Increased: – Alkaline phosphatase – Direct bilirubin – GGTP	Increased: – Globulin – Total bilirubin – Total protein Increased and decreased Serum albumin
Urinary		WBC in urine	Acetonuria Hematuria RBC in urine	Glycosuria Proteinuria
Miscellaneous	Increased triglycerides	Increased: – CPK – Fasting blood sugar	Decreased: fasting blood sugar High occult blood	Increased and decreased iron

Etretinate may not leave the body for many years and, like Soriatane, can cause severe birth defects. It is recommended that you and your doctor schedule appointments regularly to repeat the pregnancy test and check your body's response to Soriatane. For your health and well-being, be sure to keep your appointments as scheduled.

In addition, you must not donate blood during your treatment with Soriatane and for 3 years after you stop taking Soriatane.

Do not give your Soriatane capsules to any other person.

THE CONSENT FOR *FEMALE* PATIENTS:

My treatment with Soriatane has been personally explained to me by Dr. _____. The following points of information, among others, have been specifically discussed and made clear:

1. I,_____,
(Patient's Name)
understand that Soriatane is used to treat severe psoriasis that is unresponsive to other therapies.
INITIALS: _____

2. I understand that severe birth defects related to treatment with Soriatane have occurred in babies of women who have taken Soriatane during pregnancy. In addition, birth defects have occurred in babies of women who became pregnant after stopping Soriatane treatment.
INITIALS: _____

3. I understand that I must not be pregnant when I start taking Soriatane.
INITIALS: _____

4. I understand that I must not become pregnant while I am taking Soriatane.
INITIALS: _____

5. I understand that I must wait at least 3 years after I stop taking Soriatane before becoming pregnant.
INITIALS: _____

6. I have been told by my doctor that effective birth control (contraception) must be used for at least 1 month before starting Soriatane, for the entire duration of Soriatane therapy and for at least 3 years after Soriatane treatment has stopped. My doctor has told me that I must either abstain from sexual intercourse or use two reliable kinds of birth control at the same time. I have also been told that any method of birth control can fail, including tubal ligation or microdosed progestin "minipill" preparations. I must use two forms of reliable birth control simultaneously, even if I think I cannot become pregnant, unless I abstain from sexual intercourse or have had a hysterectomy.
INITIALS: _____

7. I understand that if I have taken Tegison (etretinate), I must continue to follow the birth control (contraception) recommendations for Tegison.
INITIALS: _____

8. I know that I must have a blood or urine test done by my doctor that shows I am not pregnant within 1 week before starting Soriatane. I understand that I must wait until the second or third day of my next normal menstrual period before starting Soriatane.
INITIALS: _____

9. My doctor has told me that I can participate in the "Patient Referral" program for an initial free pregnancy test and birth control counseling session by a consulting physician.
INITIALS: _____

10. I know that I must immediately stop taking Soriatane if I become pregnant and immediately contact my doctor to discuss possible effects on the pregnancy. I also know that I must immediately contact my doctor if I become pregnant at any time for at least 3 years after stopping Soriatane.
INITIALS: _____

11. I have carefully read the Soriatane patient brochure, "Important information concerning your treatment with Soriatane," given to me by my doctor. I understand all of its contents and have talked over any questions I have with my doctor.
INITIALS: _____

12. I am not now pregnant, nor do I plan to become pregnant while taking Soriatane and for at least 3 years after I have completely finished taking Soriatane.
INITIALS: _____

13. I know that I must avoid ingesting any beverage or product that contains alcohol during the entire Soriatane treatment course and for 2 months after I have completely finished taking Soriatane.
INITIALS: _____

14. I understand that if I consume any beverage or product that contains alcohol during my treatment with Soriatane or during the 2 months after I stop taking Soriatane, the risk of birth defects will persist for a longer period of time.
INITIALS: _____

15. I have been told not to donate blood during my treatment with Soriatane and for 3 years after I have completely finished taking Soriatane.
INITIALS: _____

I now authorize Dr. _____
to begin my treatment with Soriatane.

Patient signature, Parent or Guardian signature if patient is a minor   Date

Address _____

Telephone Number _____
I have fully explained to the patient, _____, the nature and purpose of the treatment described above and the teratogenic risk. I have asked the patient if there are any questions regarding treatment with Soriatane and have answered those questions to the best of my ability.

Physician signature   Date
Issued: August 1997
Shown in Product Identification Guide, page 335

TASMAR®
(tolcapone)
TABLETS   ℞

The following text is complete prescribing information based on official labeling in effect June 1998.

DESCRIPTION

TASMAR® is available as tablets containing 100 mg or 200 mg tolcapone.

Tolcapone, an inhibitor of catechol-*O*-methyltransferase (COMT), is used in the treatment of Parkinson's disease as an adjunct to levodopa/carbidopa therapy. It is a yellow, odorless, non-hygroscopic, crystalline compound with a relative molecular mass of 273.25. The chemical name of tolcapone is 3,4-dihydroxy-4′-methyl-5-nitrobenzophenone. Its empirical formula is $C_{14}H_{11}NO_5$.

Inactive ingredients: Core: lactose monohydrate, microcrystalline cellulose, dibasic calcium phosphate anhydrous, povidone K-30, sodium starch glycolate, talc and magnesium stearate. Film coating: hydroxypropyl methyl cellulose, titanium dioxide, talc, ethylcellulose, triacetin and sodium lauryl sulfate, with the following dye systems: 100 mg—yellow and red iron oxide; 200 mg—red iron oxide.

CLINICAL PHARMACOLOGY

Mechanism of Action: Tolcapone is a selective and reversible inhibitor of catechol-*O*-methyltransferase (COMT).

In mammals, COMT is distributed throughout various organs. The highest activities are in the liver and kidney. COMT also occurs in the heart, lung, smooth and skeletal muscles, intestinal tract, reproductive organs, various glands, adipose tissue, skin, blood cells and neuronal tissues, especially in glial cells. COMT catalyzes the transfer of the methyl group of S-adenosyl-L-methionine to the phenolic group of substrates that contain a catechol structure. Physiological substrates of COMT include dopa, catecholamines (dopamine, norepinephrine, epinephrine) and their hydroxylated metabolites. The function of COMT is the elimination of biologically active catechols and some other hydroxylated metabolites. In the presence of a decarboxylase inhibitor, COMT becomes the major metabolizing enzyme for levodopa catalyzing the metabolism to 3-methoxy-4-hydroxy-L-phenylalanine (3-OMD) in the brain and periphery.

The precise mechanism of action of tolcapone is unknown, but it is believed to be related to its ability to inhibit COMT and alter the plasma pharmacokinetics of levodopa. When tolcapone is given in conjunction with levodopa and an aromatic amino acid decarboxylase inhibitor, such as carbidopa, plasma levels of levodopa are more sustained than after administration of levodopa and an aromatic amino acid decarboxylase inhibitor alone. It is believed that these sustained plasma levels of levodopa result in more constant dopaminergic stimulation in the brain, leading to greater effects on the signs and symptoms of Parkinson's disease in patients as well as increased levodopa adverse effects, sometimes requiring a decrease in the dose of levodopa. Tolcapone enters the CNS to a minimal extent, but has been shown to inhibit central COMT activity in animals.

Pharmacodynamics: *COMT Activity in Erythrocytes:* Studies in healthy volunteers have shown that tolcapone reversibly inhibits human erythrocyte catechol-*O*-methyltransferase (COMT) activity after oral administration. The inhibition is closely related to plasma tolcapone concentrations. With a 200 mg single dose of tolcapone, maximum inhibition of erythrocyte COMT activity is on average greater than 80%. During multiple dosing with tolcapone (200 mg tid), erythrocyte COMT inhibition at trough tolcapone blood concentrations is 30% to 45%.

Effect on the Pharmacokinetics of Levodopa and its Metabolites: When tolcapone is administered together with levodopa/carbidopa, it increases the relative bioavailability (AUC) of levodopa by approximately twofold. This is due to a decrease in levodopa clearance resulting in a prolongation

of the terminal elimination half-life of levodopa (from approximately 2 hours to 3.5 hours). In general, the average peak levodopa plasma concentration (C_{max}) and the time of its occurrence (T_{max}) are unaffected. The onset of effect occurs after the first administration and is maintained during long-term treatment. Studies in healthy volunteers and Parkinson's disease patients have confirmed that the maximal effect occurs with 100 mg to 200 mg tolcapone. Plasma levels of 3-OMD are markedly and dose-dependently decreased by tolcapone when given with levodopa/carbidopa. Population pharmacokinetic analyses in patients with Parkinson's disease have shown the same effects of tolcapone on levodopa plasma concentrations that occur in healthy volunteers.

Pharmacokinetics of Tolcapone: Tolcapone pharmacokinetics are linear over the dose range of 50 mg to 400 mg, independent of levodopa/carbidopa coadministration. The elimination half-life of tolcapone is 2 to 3 hours and there is no significant accumulation. With tid dosing of 100 mg or 200 mg, C_{max} is approximately 3 µg/mL and 6 µg/mL, respectively.

Absorption: Tolcapone is rapidly absorbed, with a T_{max} of approximately 2 hours. The absolute bioavailability following oral administration is about 65%. Food given within 1 hour before and 2 hours after dosing of tolcapone decreases the relative bioavailability by 10% to 20% (see DOSAGE AND ADMINISTRATION).

Distribution: The steady-state volume of distribution of tolcapone is small (9 L). Tolcapone does not distribute widely into tissues due to its high plasma protein binding. The plasma protein binding of tolcapone is >99.9% over the concentration range of 0.32 to 210 µg/mL. In vitro experiments have shown that tolcapone binds mainly to serum albumin.

Metabolism and Elimination: Tolcapone is almost completely metabolized prior to excretion, with only a very small amount (0.5% of dose) found unchanged in urine. The main metabolic pathway of tolcapone is glucuronidation; the glucuronide conjugate is inactive. In addition, the compound is methylated by COMT to 3-*O*-methyl-tolcapone. Tolcapone is metabolized to a primary alcohol (hydroxylation of the methyl group), which is subsequently oxidized to the carboxylic acid. In vitro experiments suggest that the oxidation may be catalyzed by cytochrome P450 3A4 and P450 2A6. The reduction to an amine and subsequent *N*-acetylation occur to a minor extent. After oral administration of a ^{14}C-labeled dose of tolcapone, 60% of labeled material is excreted in urine and 40% in feces.

Tolcapone is a low-extraction ratio drug (extraction ratio = 0.15) with a moderate systemic clearance of about 7L/h.

Special Populations: Tolcapone pharmacokinetics are independent of sex, age, body weight, and race (Japanese, Black and Caucasian). Polymorphic metabolism is unlikely based on the metabolic pathways involved.

Hepatic Impairment: A study in patients with hepatic impairment has shown that moderate non-cirrhotic liver disease had no impact on the pharmacokinetics of tolcapone. In patients with moderate cirrhotic liver disease (Child-Pugh Class B), however, clearance and volume of distribution of unbound tolcapone was reduced by almost 50%. This reduction may increase the average concentration of unbound drug by twofold (see DOSAGE AND ADMINISTRATION).

Renal Impairment: The pharmacokinetics of tolcapone have not been investigated in a specific renal impairment study. However, the relationship of renal function and tolcapone pharmacokinetics has been investigated using population pharmacokinetics during clinical trials. The data of more than 400 patients have confirmed that over a wide range of creatinine clearance values (30 mL/min to 130 mL/min) the pharmacokinetics of tolcapone are unaffected by renal function. This could be explained by the fact that only a negligible amount of unchanged tolcapone (0.5%) is excreted in the urine. The glucuronide conjugate of tolcapone is mainly excreted in the urine but is also excreted in the bile. Accumulation of this stable and inactive metabolite should not present a risk in renally impaired patients with creatinine clearance above 25 mL/min (see DOSAGE AND ADMINISTRATION). Given the very high protein binding of tolcapone, no significant removal of the drug by hemodialysis would be expected.

Drug Interactions: See PRECAUTIONS: *Drug Interactions*.

Clinical Studies: The effectiveness of TASMAR as an adjunct to levodopa in the treatment of Parkinson's disease was established in three multicenter randomized controlled trials of 13 to 26 weeks duration, supported by four 6-week trials whose results were consistent with those of the longer trials. In two of the longer trials, tolcapone was evaluated in patients whose Parkinson's disease was characterized by deterioration in their response to levodopa at the end of a dosing interval (so-called fluctuating patients with wearing-off phenomena). In the remaining trial, tolcapone was evaluated in patients whose response to levodopa was relatively stable (so-called non-fluctuators).

Continued on next page

Tasmar—Cont.

Fluctuating Patients: In two 3-month trials, patients with documented episodes of wearing-off phenomena, despite optimum levodopa therapy, were randomized to receive placebo, tolcapone 100 mg tid or 200 mg tid. The formal double-blind portion of the trial was 3 months long, and the primary outcome was a comparison between treatments in the change from baseline in the amount of time spent "On" (a period of relatively good functioning) and "Off" (a period of relatively poor functioning). Patients recorded periodically, throughout the duration of the trial, the time spent in each of these states.

In addition to the primary outcome, patients were also assessed using sub-parts of the Unified Parkinson's Disease Rating Scale (UPDRS), a frequently used multi-item rating scale intended to evaluate mentation (Part I), activities of daily living (Part II), motor function (Part III), complications of therapy (Part IV), and disease staging (Part V & VI); an Investigator's Global Assessment of Change (IGA), a subjective scale designed to assess global functioning in 5 areas of Parkinson's disease; the Sickness Impact Profile (SIP), a multi-item scale in 12 domains designed to assess the patient's functioning in multiple areas; and the change in daily levodopa/carbidopa dose.

In one of the studies, 202 patients were randomized in 11 centers in the United States and Canada. In this trial, all patients were receiving concomitant levodopa and carbidopa. In the second trial, 177 patients were randomized in 24 centers in Europe. In this trial, all patients were receiving concomitant levodopa and benserazide.

The following tables display the results of these 2 trials:

[See table 1 at right]

[See table 2 at right]

Effects on "Off" time and levodopa dose did not differ by age or sex.

Non-fluctuating Patients: In this study, 298 patients with idiopathic Parkinson's disease on stable doses of levodopa/carbidopa who were not experiencing wearing-off phenomena were randomized to placebo, tolcapone 100 mg tid, or tolcapone 200 mg tid for 6 months at 20 centers in the United States and Canada. The primary measure of effectiveness was the Activities of Daily Living portion (Subscale II) of the UPDRS. In addition, the change in daily levodopa dose, other subscales of the UPDRS, and the SIP were assessed as secondary measures. The results are displayed in the following table:

[See table 3 at top of next page]

Effects on Activities of Daily Living did not differ by age or sex.

INDICATIONS

TASMAR is indicated as an adjunct to levodopa and carbidopa for the treatment of the signs and symptoms of idiopathic Parkinson's disease.

The effectiveness of TASMAR was demonstrated in randomized controlled trials in patients receiving concomitant levodopa therapy with carbidopa or another aromatic amino acid decarboxylase inhibitor who experienced end of dose wearing-off phenomena as well as in patients who did not experience such phenomena (see CLINICAL PHARMACOLOGY: *Clinical Trials*).

CONTRAINDICATIONS

TASMAR tablets are contraindicated in patients who have demonstrated hypersensitivity to the drug or its ingredients.

WARNINGS

Monoamine oxidase (MAO) and COMT are the two major enzyme systems involved in the metabolism of catecholamines. It is theoretically possible, therefore, that the combination of TASMAR and a non-selective MAO inhibitor (eg, phenelzine and tranylcypromine) would result in inhibition of the majority of the pathways responsible for normal catecholamine metabolism. For this reason, patients should ordinarily not be treated concomitantly with TASMAR and a non-selective MAO inhibitor.

Tolcapone can be taken concomitantly with a selective MAO-B inhibitor (eg, selegiline).

PRECAUTIONS

Hypotension/Syncope: Dopaminergic therapy in Parkinson's disease patients has been associated with orthostatic hypotension. Tolcapone enhances levodopa bioavailability and, therefore, may increase the occurrence of orthostatic hypotension. In TASMAR clinical trials, orthostatic hypotension was documented at least once in 8%, 14% and 13% of the patients treated with placebo, 100 mg and 200 mg TASMAR tid, respectively. A total of 2%, 5% and 4% of the patients treated with placebo, 100 mg and 200 mg TASMAR tid, respectively, reported orthostatic symptoms at some time during their treatment and also had at least one episode of orthostatic hypotension documented (however, the episode of orthostatic symptoms itself was invariably not accompanied by vital sign measurements). Patients with orthostasis at baseline were more likely than patients with-

Table 1.
US/Canadian Fluctuator Study

Primary Measure

	Baseline (hrs)	Change from Baseline at Month 3 (hrs)	p-value*
*Hours of Wake Time "Off"****			
placebo	6.2	−1.2	—
100 mg tid	6.4	−2.0	0.169
200 mg tid	5.9	−3.0	<0.001
*Hours of Wake Time "On"****			
placebo	8.7	1.4	—
100 mg tid	8.1	2.0	0.267
200 mg tid	9.1	2.9	0.008

Secondary Measures

	Baseline	Change from Baseline at Month 3	p-value*
Levodopa Total Daily Dose (mg)			
placebo	948	16	—
100 mg tid	788	−166	<0.001
200 mg tid	865	−207	<0.001
Global (overall) % Improved			
placebo	—	42	—
100 mg tid	—	71	<0.001
200 mg tid	—	91	<0.001
UPDRS Motor			
placebo	19.5	−0.4	—
100 mg tid	17.6	−1.9	0.217
200 mg tid	20.6	−2.0	0.210
UPDRS ADL			
placebo	7.5	−0.3	—
100 mg tid	7.7	−0.8	0.487
200 mg tid	8.3	0.2	0.412
SIP (total)			
placebo	14.7	−2.2	—
100 mg tid	14.9	−0.4	0.210
200 mg tid	17.6	−0.3	0.216

*Compared to placebo.
**Hours "Off" or "On" are based on the percent of waking day "Off" or "On", assuming a 16-hour waking day.

Table 2.
European Fluctuator Study

Primary Measure

	Baseline (hrs)	Change from Baseline at Month 3 (hrs)	p-value*
*Hours of Wake Time "Off"****			
placebo	6.1	−0.7	—
100 mg tid	6.5	−2.0	0.008
200 mg tid	6.0	−1.6	0.081
*Hours of Wake Time "On"****			
placebo	8.5	−0.1	—
100 mg tid	8.1	1.7	0.003
200 mg tid	8.4	1.7	0.003

Secondary Measures

	Baseline	Change from Baseline at Month 3	p-value*
Levodopa Total Daily Dose (mg)			
placebo	660	−29	—
100 mg tid	667	−109	0.025
200 mg tid	675	−122	0.010
Global (overall) % Improved			
placebo	—	37	—
100 mg tid	—	70	0.003
200 mg tid	—	78	<0.001
UPDRS Motor			
placebo	24.0	−2.1	—
100 mg tid	22.4	−4.2	0.163
200 mg tid	22.4	−6.5	0.004
UPDRS ADL			
placebo	7.9	−0.5	—
100 mg tid	7.5	−0.9	0.408
200 mg tid	7.7	−1.3	0.097
SIP (total)			
placebo	21.6	−0.9	—
100 mg tid	16.6	−1.9	0.419
200 mg tid	18.4	−4.2	0.011

*Compared to placebo.
**Hours "Off" or "On" are based on the percent of waking day "Off" or "On", assuming a 16-hour waking day.

Table 3.
US/Canadian Non-fluctuator Study

Primary Measure

	Baseline	Change from Baseline at Month 6	p-value*
UPDRS ADL			
placebo	8.5	0.1	—
100 mg tid	7.5	-1.4	<0.001
200 mg tid	7.9	-1.6	<0.001

Secondary Measures

	Baseline	Change from Baseline at Month 6	p-value*
Levodopa Total Daily Dose (mg)			
placebo	364	47	—
100 mg tid	370	-21	<0.001
200 mg tid	381	-32	<0.001
UPDRS Motor			
placebo	19.7	0.1	—
100 mg tid	17.3	-2.0	0.018
200 mg tid	16.0	-2.3	0.008
Sip (total)			
placebo	6.9	0.4	—
100 mg tid	7.3	-0.9	0.044
200 mg tid	7.3	-0.7	0.078
Percent of Patients who Developed Fluctuations			
placebo	—	26	—
100 mg tid	—	19	0.297
200 mg tid	—	14	0.047

* Compared to placebo.

out symptoms to have orthostatic hypotension during the study, irrespective of treatment group. In addition, the effect was greater in tolcapone-treated patients than in placebo-treated patients. Baseline treatment with dopamine agonists or selegiline did not appear to increase the likelihood of experiencing orthostatic hypotension when treated with TASMAR. Approximately 0.7% of the patients treated with TASMAR (5% of patients who were documented to have had at least one episode of orthostatic hypotension) eventually withdrew from treatment due to adverse events presumably related to hypotension.

In controlled Phase 3 trials, approximately 5%, 4% and 3% of tolcapone 200 mg tid, 100 mg tid and placebo patients, respectively, reported at least one episode of syncope. Reports of syncope were generally more frequent in patients in all three treatment groups who had an episode of documented hypotension (although the episodes of syncope, obtained by history, were themselves not documented with vital sign measurement) compared to patients who did not have any episodes of documented hypotension.

Diarrhea: In clinical trials, diarrhea developed in approximately 8%, 16% and 18% of patients treated with placebo, 100 mg and 200 mg TASMAR tid, respectively. While diarrhea was generally regarded as mild to moderate in severity, approximately 3% to 4% of patients on tolcapone had diarrhea which was regarded as severe. Diarrhea was the adverse event which most commonly led to discontinuation, with approximately 1%, 5% and 6% of patients treated with placebo, 100 mg and 200 mg TASMAR tid, respectively, withdrawing from the trials prematurely. Discontinuing TASMAR for diarrhea was related to the severity of the symptom. Diarrhea resulted in withdrawal in approximately 8%, 40% and 70% of patients with mild, moderate and severe diarrhea, respectively. Although diarrhea generally resolved after discontinuation of TASMAR, it led to hospitalization in 0.3%, 0.7% and 1.7% of patients in the placebo, 100 mg and 200 mg TASMAR tid groups.

Typically, diarrhea presents 6 to 12 weeks after tolcapone is started, but it may appear as early as 2 weeks and as late as many months after the initiation of treatment. Clinical trial data suggested that diarrhea associated with tolcapone use may sometimes be associated with anorexia (decreased appetite).

No consistent description of tolcapone-induced diarrhea has been derived from clinical trial data, and the mechanism of action is currently unknown.

It is recommended that all cases of persistent diarrhea should be followed up with an appropriate work-up (including occult blood samples).

Hallucinations: In clinical trials, hallucinations developed in approximately 5%, 8% and 10% of patients treated with placebo, 100 mg and 200 mg TASMAR tid, respectively. Hallucinations led to drug discontinuation and premature withdrawal from clinical trials in 0.3%, 1.4% and 1.0% of patients treated with placebo, 100 mg and 200 mg TASMAR tid, respectively. Hallucinations led to hospitalization in

0.0%, 1.7% and 0.0% of patients in the placebo, 100 mg and 200 mg TASMAR tid groups, respectively.

In general, hallucinations present shortly after the initiation of therapy with tolcapone (typically within the first 2 weeks). Clinical trial data suggest that hallucinations associated with tolcapone use may be responsive to levodopa dose reduction. Patients whose hallucinations resolved had a mean levodopa dose reduction of 175 mg to 200 mg (20% to 25%) after the onset of the hallucinations. Hallucinations were commonly accompanied by confusion and to a lesser extent sleep disorder (insomnia) and excessive dreaming.

Dyskinesia: TASMAR may potentiate the dopaminergic side effects of levodopa and may cause and/or exacerbate preexisting dyskinesia. Although decreasing the dose of levodopa may ameliorate this side effect, many patients in controlled trials continued to experience frequent dyskinesias despite a reduction in their dose of levodopa. The rates of withdrawal for dyskinesia were 0.0%, 0.3% and 1.0% for placebo, 100 mg and 200 mg TASMAR tid, respectively.

Renal and Hepatic: Renal Impairment: No dosage adjustment is needed in patients with mild to moderate renal impairment, however, patients with severe renal impairment should be treated with caution (see CLINICAL PHARMACOLOGY: *Pharmacokinetics of Tolcapone* and DOSAGE AND ADMINISTRATION).

Renal Toxicity: When rats were dosed daily for 1 or 2 years (exposures 6 times the human exposure or greater) there was a high incidence of proximal tubule cell damage consisting of degeneration, single cell necrosis, hyperplasia, karyocytomegaly and atypical nuclei. These effects were not associated with changes in clinical chemistry parameters, and there is no established method for monitoring for the possible occurrence of these lesions in humans. Although it has been speculated that these toxicities may occur as the result of a species-specific mechanism, experiments which would confirm that theory have not been conducted.

Hepatic Impairment: Patients with moderate non-cirrhotic liver disease need no adjustment of dose. Patients with moderate cirrhotic liver disease have reduced clearance of unbound tolcapone by almost 50%, increasing the average concentration of unbound drug by about twofold. Dosage should be reduced in such patients (see CLINICAL PHARMACOLOGY: *Pharmacokinetics of Tolcapone* and DOSAGE AND ADMINISTRATION). Patients with severe liver impairment should be treated with caution.

Hepatic Enzyme Abnormalities: In Phase 3 controlled trials, increases to more than 3 times the upper limit of normal in ALT or AST occurred in approximately 1% of patients at 100 mg tid and 3% of patients at 200 mg tid. Females were more likely than males to have an increase in hepatic enzymes (approximately 5% vs 2%). Approximately one third of patients with elevated enzymes had diarrhea. Increases to more than 8 times the upper limit of normal in hepatic enzymes occurred in 0.3% at 100 mg tid and 0.7% at 200 mg tid. Elevated enzymes led to discontinuation in 0.3% and 1.7% of patients treated with 100 mg tid and 200 mg

tid, respectively. Elevations usually occurred within 6 weeks to 6 months of starting treatment. In about half the cases with elevated hepatic enzymes, enzyme levels returned to baseline values within 1 to 3 months while patients continued TASMAR treatment. When treatment was discontinued, enzymes generally declined within 2 to 3 weeks but in some cases took as long as 1 to 2 months to return to normal.

One patient, a 55-year-old woman who had received treatment with tolcapone 200 mg tid for 53 days, had the onset of diarrhea followed 4 days later by yellowing of the skin and eyes. She died 7 days after the onset of the diarrhea. No liver function tests were performed after the onset of symptoms.

It is recommended that liver enzymes be monitored monthly during the first 3 months of TASMAR treatment, and every 6 weeks for the next 3 months of treatment. Tolcapone should be discontinued for enzyme elevations greater than or equal to 5 times the upper limit of normal or at the appearance of jaundice (see PRECAUTIONS: *Laboratory Tests*).

Hematuria: The rates of hematuria in placebo-controlled trials were approximately 2%, 4% and 5% in placebo, 100 mg and 200 mg TASMAR tid, respectively. The etiology of the increase with TASMAR has not always been explained (for example, by urinary tract infection or coumadin therapy). In placebo-controlled trials in the United States (N=593) rates of microscopically confirmed hematuria were approximately 3%, 2% and 2% in placebo, 100 mg and 200 mg TASMAR tid, respectively.

Events Reported With Dopaminergic Therapy: The events listed below are known to be associated with the use of drugs that increase dopaminergic activity, although they are most often associated with the use of direct dopamine agonists. While cases of Withdrawal Emergent Hyperpyrexia and Confusion have been reported in association with tolcapone withdrawal (see below), the expected incidence of fibrotic complications is so low that even if tolcapone caused these complications at rates similar to those attributable to other dopaminergic therapies, it is unlikely that even a single example would have been detected in a cohort of the size exposed to tolcapone.

Withdrawal Emergent Hyperpyrexia and Confusion: Four cases of a symptom complex resembling the neuroleptic malignant syndrome (characterized by elevated temperature, muscular rigidity, and altered consciousness), similar to that reported in association with the rapid dose reduction or withdrawal of other dopaminergic drugs, have been reported in association with the abrupt withdrawal or lowering of the dose of tolcapone. In 3 of these cases, CPK was elevated as well. One patient died, and the other 3 patients recovered over periods of approximately 2, 4 and 6 weeks.

Fibrotic Complications: Cases of retroperitoneal fibrosis, pulmonary infiltrates, pleural effusion, and pleural thickening have been reported in some patients treated with ergot derived dopaminergic agents. While these complications may resolve when the drug is discontinued, complete resolution does not always occur. Although these adverse events are believed to be related to the ergoline structure of these compounds, whether other, nonergot derived drugs (eg, tolcapone) that increase dopaminergic activity can cause them is unknown.

Three cases of pleural effusion, one with pulmonary fibrosis, occurred during clinical trials. These patients were also on concomitant dopamine agonists (pergolide or bromocriptine) and had a prior history of cardiac disease or pulmonary pathology (nonmalignant lung lesion).

Information for Patients: Patients should be instructed to take TASMAR only as prescribed.

Patients should be informed that hallucinations can occur. Patients should be advised that they may develop postural (orthostatic) hypotension with or without symptoms such as dizziness, nausea, syncope, and sometimes sweating. Hypotension may occur more frequently during initial therapy. Accordingly, patients should be cautioned against rising rapidly after sitting or lying down, especially if they have been doing so for prolonged periods, and especially at the initiation of treatment with TASMAR.

Patients should be advised that they should neither drive a car nor operate other complex machinery until they have gained sufficient experience on TASMAR to gauge whether or not it affects their mental and/or motor performance adversely. Because of the possible additive sedative effects, caution should be used when patients are taking other CNS depressants in combination with TASMAR.

Patients should be informed that nausea may occur, especially at the initiation of treatment with TASMAR.

Patients should be advised of the possibility of an increase in dyskinesia and/or dystonia.

Although TASMAR has not been shown to be teratogenic in animals, it is always given in conjunction with levodopa/carbidopa, which is known to cause visceral and skeletal malformations in the rabbit. Accordingly, patients should be

Continued on next page

Tasmar—Cont.

advised to notify their physicians if they become pregnant or intend to become pregnant during therapy (see PRECAUTIONS: *Pregnancy*).

Tolcapone is excreted into maternal milk in rats. Because of the possibility that tolcapone may be excreted into human maternal milk, patients should be advised to notify their physicians if they intend to breastfeed or are breastfeeding an infant.

Laboratory Tests: It is recommended that transaminases be monitored monthly for the first 3 months of treatment with TASMAR, after which LFTs should be monitored every 6 weeks for the next 3 months. If elevations occur, and a decision is made to continue to treat the patient, more frequent monitoring of complete liver function is recommended. Treatment should be discontinued if ALT exceeds 5 × ULN or if jaundice develops.

Special Populations: Parkinson's disease patients with moderate to severe liver impairment or severe renal impairment should be treated with caution (see DOSAGE AND ADMINISTRATION).

Drug Interactions: *Protein Binding:* Although tolcapone is highly protein bound, in vitro studies have shown that tolcapone at a concentration of 50 μg/mL did not displace other highly protein-bound drugs from their binding sites at therapeutic concentrations. The experiments included warfarin (0.5 to 7.2 μg/mL), phenytoin (4.0 to 38.7 μg/mL), tolbutamide (24.5 to 96.1 μg/mL) and digitoxin (9.0 to 27.0 μg/mL).

Drugs Metabolized by Catechol-O-methyltransferase (COMT): Tolcapone may influence the pharmacokinetics of drugs metabolized by COMT. However, no effects were seen on the pharmacokinetics of the COMT substrate carbidopa. The effect of tolcapone on the pharmacokinetics of other drugs of this class such as α-methyldopa, dobutamine, apomorphine, and isoproterenol has not been evaluated. A dose reduction of such compounds should be considered when they are coadministered with tolcapone.

Effect of Tolcapone on the Metabolism of Other Drugs: In vitro experiments have been performed to assess the potential of tolcapone to interact with isoenzymes of cytochrome P450 (CYP). No relevant interactions with substrates for CYP 2A6 (coumadin), CYP 1A2 (caffeine), CYP 3A4 (midazolam, terfenadine, cyclosporine), CYP 2C19 (S-mephenytoin) and CYP 2D6 (desipramine) were observed in vitro. The absence of an interaction with desipramine, a drug metabolized by cytochrome P450 2D6, was also confirmed in an in vivo study where tolcapone did not change the pharmacokinetics of desipramine.

Due to its affinity to cytochrome P450 2C9 in vitro, tolcapone may interfere with drugs, whose clearance is dependent on this metabolic pathway, such as tolbutamide and warfarin. However, in an in vivo interaction study, tolcapone did not change the pharmacokinetics of tolbutamide. Therefore, clinically relevant interactions involving cytochrome P450 2C9 appear unlikely. Similarly, tolcapone did not affect the pharmacokinetics of desipramine, a drug metabolized by cytochrome P450 2D6, indicating that interactions with drugs metabolized by that enzyme are unlikely. Since clinical information is limited regarding the combination of warfarin and tolcapone, coagulation parameters should be monitored when these two drugs are coadministered.

Drugs That Increase Catecholamines: Tolcapone did not influence the effect of ephedrine, an indirect sympathomimetic, on hemodynamic parameters or plasma catecholamine levels, either at rest or during exercise. Since tolcapone did not alter the tolerability of ephedrine, these drugs can be coadministered.

When TASMAR was given together with levodopa/carbidopa and desipramine, there was no significant change in blood pressure, pulse rate and plasma concentrations of desipramine. Overall, the frequency of adverse events increased slightly. These adverse events were predictable based on the known adverse reactions to each of the three drugs individually. Therefore, caution should be exercised when desipramine is administered to Parkinson's disease patients being treated with TASMAR and levodopa/carbidopa.

In clinical trials, patients receiving TASMAR/levodopa preparations reported a similar adverse event profile independent of whether or not they were also concomitantly administered selegiline (a selective MAO-B inhibitor).

Carcinogenesis, Mutagenesis and Impairment of Fertility:

Carcinogenesis: Carcinogenicity studies in which tolcapone was administered in the diet were conducted in mice and rats. Mice were treated for 80 (female) or 95 (male) weeks with doses of 100, 300 and 800 mg/kg/day, equivalent to 0.8, 1.6 and 4 times human exposure (AUC = 80 μg·hr/mL) at the recommended daily clinical dose of 600 mg.

Rats were treated for 104 weeks with doses of 50, 250 and 450 mg/kg/day. Tolcapone exposures were 1, 6.3 and 13 times the human exposure in male rats and 1.7, 11.8 and 26.4 times the human exposure in female rats. There was an increased incidence of uterine adenocarcinomas in female rats at exposure equivalent to 26.4 times the human exposure. There was evidence of renal tubular injury and renal tubular tumor formation in rats. A low incidence of renal tubular cell adenomas occurred in middle- and high-dose female rats; tubular cell carcinomas occurred in middle- and high-dose male and high-dose female rats, with a statistically significant increase in high-dose males. Exposures were equivalent to 6.3 (males) or 11.8 (females) times the human exposure or greater; no renal tumors were observed at exposures of 1 (males) or 1.7 (females) times the human exposure. Minimal-to-marked damage to the renal tubules, consisting of proximal tubule cell degeneration, single cell necrosis, hyperplasia and karyocytomegaly, occurred at the doses associated with renal tumors. Renal tubule damage, characterized by proximal tubule cell degeneration and the presence of atypical nuclei, as well as one adenocarcinoma in a high-dose male, were observed in a 1-year study in rats receiving doses of tolcapone of 150 and 450 mg/kg/day. These histopathological changes suggest the possibility that renal tumor formation might be secondary to chronic cell damage and sustained repair, but this relationship has not been established, and the relevance of these findings to humans is not known. There was no evidence of carcinogenic effects in the long-term mouse study. The carcinogenic potential of tolcapone in combination with levodopa/carbidopa has not been examined.

Mutagenesis: Tolcapone was clastogenic in the in vitro mouse lymphoma/thymidine kinase assay in the presence of metabolic activation. Tolcapone was not mutagenic in the Ames test, the in vitro V79/HPRT gene mutation assay, or the unscheduled DNA synthesis assay. It was not clastogenic in an in vitro chromosomal aberration assay in cultured human lymphocytes, or an in vivo micronucleus assay in mice.

Impairment of Fertility: Tolcapone did not affect fertility and general reproductive performance in rats at doses up to 300 mg/kg/day (5.7 times the human dose on a mg/m^2 basis).

Pregnancy: Pregnancy Category C. Tolcapone, when administered alone during organogenesis, was not teratogenic at doses of up to 300 mg/kg/day in rats or up to 400 mg/kg/day in rabbits (5.7 times and 15 times the recommended daily clinical dose of 600 mg, on a mg/m^2 basis, respectively). In rabbits, however, an increased rate of abortion occurred at a dose of 100 mg/kg/day (3.7 times the daily clinical dose on a mg/m^2 basis) or greater. Evidence of maternal toxicity (decreased weight gain, death) was observed at 300 mg/kg in rats and 400 mg/kg in rabbits. When tolcapone was administered to female rats during the last part of gestation and throughout lactation, decreased litter size and impaired growth and learning performance in female pups were observed at a dose of 250/150 mg/kg/day (dose reduced from 250 to 150 mg/kg/day during late gestation due to high rate of maternal mortality; equivalent to 4.8/2.9 times the clinical dose on a mg/m^2 basis).

Tolcapone is always given concomitantly with levodopa/carbidopa, which is known to cause visceral and skeletal malformations in rabbits. The combination of tolcapone (100 mg/kg/day) with levodopa/carbidopa (80/20 mg/kg/day) produced an increased incidence of fetal malformations (primarily external and skeletal digit defects) compared to levodopa/carbidopa alone when pregnant rabbits were treated throughout organogenesis. Plasma exposures to tolcapone (based on AUC) were 0.5 times the expected human exposure, and plasma exposures to levodopa were 6 times higher than those in humans under therapeutic conditions. In a combination embryo-fetal development study in rats, fetal body weights were reduced by the combination of tolcapone (10, 30 and 50 mg/kg/day) and levodopa/carbidopa (120/30 mg/kg/day) and by levodopa/carbidopa alone. Tolcapone exposures were 0.5 times expected human exposure or greater; levodopa exposures were 21 times expected human exposure or greater. The high dose of 50 mg/kg/day of tolcapone given alone was not associated with reduced fetal body weight (plasma exposures of 1.4 times the expected human exposure).

There is no experience from clinical studies regarding the use of TASMAR in pregnant women. Therefore, TASMAR should be used during pregnancy only if the potential benefit justifies the potential risk to the fetus.

Nursing Women: In animal studies, tolcapone was excreted into maternal rat milk.

It is not known whether tolcapone is excreted in human milk. Because many drugs are excreted in human milk, caution should be exercised when tolcapone is administered to a nursing woman.

Pediatric Use: There is no identified potential use of tolcapone in pediatric patients.

ADVERSE REACTIONS

During the pre-marketing development of tolcapone, two distinct patient populations were studied, patients with end-of-dose wearing-off phenomena and patients with stable responses to levodopa therapy. All patients received concomitant treatment with levodopa preparations, however, and were similar in other clinical aspects. Adverse events are, therefore, shown for these two populations combined.

The most commonly observed adverse events (>5%) in the double-blind, placebo-controlled trials (N=892) associated with the use of TASMAR not seen at an equivalent frequency among the placebo-treated patients were dyskinesia, nausea, sleep disorder, dystonia, dreaming excessive, anorexia, cramps muscle, orthostatic complaints, somnolence, diarrhea, confusion, dizziness, headache, hallucination, vomiting, constipation, fatigue, upper respiratory tract infection, falling, sweating increased, urinary tract infection, xerostomia, abdominal pain, urine discoloration.

Approximately 16% of the 592 patients who participated in the double-blind, placebo-controlled trials discontinued treatment due to adverse events compared to 10% of the 298 patients who received placebo. Diarrhea was by far the most frequent cause of discontinuation (approximately 6% in tolcapone patients vs 1% on placebo).

Adverse Event Incidence in Controlled Clinical Studies: Table 4 lists treatment emergent adverse events that occurred in at least 1% of patients treated with tolcapone participating in the double-blind, placebo-controlled studies and were numerically more common in at least one of the tolcapone groups. In these studies, either tolcapone or placebo were added to levodopa/carbidopa (or benserazide).

The prescriber should be aware that these figures cannot be used to predict the incidence of adverse events in the course of usual medical practice where patient characteristics and other factors differ from those that prevailed in the clinical studies. Similarly, the cited frequencies cannot be compared with figures obtained from other clinical investigations involving different treatments, uses, and investigators. However, the cited figures do provide the prescriber with some basis for estimating the relative contribution of drug and nondrug factors to the adverse events incidence rate in the population studied.

Table 4.
Summary of Patients With Adverse Events After Start of Trial Drug Administration

(At Least 1% in TASMAR Group and at Least One TASMAR Dose Group > Placebo)

	Placebo	Tolcapone tid	
		100 mg	200 mg
	N = 298	N = 296	N = 298
Adverse Events	(%)	(%)	(%)
Dyskinesia	20	42	51
Nausea	18	30	35
Sleep Disorder	18	24	25
Dystonia	17	19	22
Dreaming Excessive	17	21	16
Anorexia	13	19	23
Cramps Muscle	17	17	18
Orthostatic Complaints	14	17	17
Somnolence	13	18	14
Diarrhea	8	16	18
Confusion	9	11	10
Dizziness	10	13	6
Headache	7	10	11
Hallucination	5	8	10
Vomiting	4	8	10
Constipation	5	6	8
Fatigue	6	7	3
Upper Respiratory Tract Infection	3	5	7
Falling	4	4	6
Sweating Increased	2	4	7
Urinary Tract Infection	4	5	5
Xerostomia	2	5	6
Abdominal Pain	3	5	6
Syncope	3	4	5
Urine Discoloration	1	2	7
Dyspepsia	2	4	3
Influenza	2	3	4
Dyspnea	2	3	3
Balance Loss	2	3	2
Flatulence	2	2	4
Hyperkinesia	1	3	2
Chest Pain	1	3	1
Hypotension	1	2	2
Paresthesia	2	3	1
Stiffness	1	2	2
Arthritis	1	2	1
Chest Discomfort	1	1	2
Hypokinesia	1	1	3
Micturition Disorder	1	2	1
Pain Neck	1	2	2
Burning	0	2	1
Sinus Congestion	0	2	1
Agitation	0	1	1
Bleeding Dermal	0	1	1
Irritability	0	1	1
Mental Deficiency	0	1	1
Hyperactivity	0	1	1
Malaise	0	1	0

Panic Reaction	0	1	0
Tumor Skin	0	1	0
Cataract	0	1	0
Euphoria	0	1	0
Fever	0	0	1
Alopecia	0	1	0
Eye Inflamed	0	1	0
Hypertonia	0	0	1
Tumor Uterus	0	1	0

Other events reported by 1% or more of patients treated with TASMAR but that were equally or more frequent in the placebo group were arthralgia, pain limbs, anxiety, micturition frequency, fractures, vision blurred, pneumonia, paresis, lethargy, asthenia, edema peripheral, gait abnormal, taste alteration, weight decrease and sinusitis.

Effects of Gender and Age on Adverse Reactions: Experience in clinical trials have suggested that patients greater than 75 years of age may be more likely to develop hallucinations than patients less than 75 years of age, while patients over 75 may be less likely to develop dystonia. Females may be more likely to develop somnolence than males.

Other Adverse Events Observed During All Trials in Patients With Parkinson's Disease: TASMAR has been administered in 1536 patients with Parkinson's disease in clinical trials. During these trials, all adverse events were recorded by the clinical investigators using terminology of their own choosing. To provide a meaningful estimate of the proportion of individuals having adverse events, similar types of adverse events were grouped into a smaller number of standardized categories using COSTART dictionary terminology. These categories are used in the listing below.

All reported events that occurred at least twice (or once for serious or potentially serious events), except those already listed above, trivial events and terms too vague to be meaningful are included, without regard to determination of a causal relationship to TASMAR.

Events are further classified within body system categories and enumerated in order of decreasing frequency using the following definitions: frequent adverse events are defined as those occurring in at least 1/100 patients; infrequent adverse events are defined as those occurring in between 1/100 and 1/1000 patients; and rare adverse events are defined as those occurring in fewer than 1/1000 patients.

Nervous System—frequent: depression, hypesthesia, tremor, speech disorder, vertigo, emotional lability; *infrequent:* neuralgia, amnesia, extrapyramidal syndrome, hostility, libido increased, manic reaction, nervousness, paranoid reaction, cerebral ischemia, cerebrovascular accident, delusions, libido decreased, neuropathy, apathy, choreoathetosis, myoclonus, psychosis, thinking abnormal, twitching; *rare:* antisocial reaction, delirium, encephalopathy, hemiplegia, meningitis.

Digestive System—frequent: tooth disorder; *infrequent:* dysphagia, gastrointestinal hemorrhage, gastroenteritis, mouth ulceration, increased salivation, abnormal stools, esophagitis, cholelithiasis, colitis, tongue disorder, rectal disorder; *rare:* cholecystitis, duodenal ulcer, gastrointestinal carcinoma, stomach atony.

Body as a Whole—frequent: flank pain, accidental injury, abdominal pain, infection; *infrequent:* hernia, pain, allergic reaction, cellulitis, infection fungal, viral infection, carcinoma, chills, infection bacterial, neoplasm, abscess, face edema; *rare:* death.

Cardiovascular System—frequent: palpitation; *infrequent:* hypertension, vasodilation, angina pectoris, heart failure, atrial fibrillation, tachycardia, migraine, aortic stenosis, arrhythmia, arteriospasm, bradycardia, cerebral hemorrhage, coronary artery disorder, heart arrest, myocardial infarct, myocardial ischemia, pulmonary embolus; *rare:* arteriosclerosis, cardiovascular disorder, pericardial effusion, thrombosis.

Musculoskeletal System—frequent: myalgia; *infrequent:* tenosynovitis, arthrosis, joint disorder.

Urogenital System—frequent: urinary incontinence, impotence; *infrequent:* prostatic disorder, dysuria, nocturia, polyuria, urinary retention, urinary tract disorder, hematuria, kidney calculus, prostatic carcinoma, breast neoplasm, oliguria, uterine atony, uterine disorder, vaginitis; *rare:* bladder calculus, ovarian carcinoma, uterine hemorrhage.

Respiratory System—frequent: bronchitis, pharyngitis; *infrequent:* cough increased, rhinitis, asthma, epistaxis, hyperventilation, laryngitis, hiccup; *rare:* apnea, hypoxia, lung edema.

Skin and Appendages—frequent: rash; *infrequent:* herpes zoster, pruritus, seborrhea, skin discoloration, eczema, erythema multiforme, skin disorder, furunculosis, herpes simplex, urticaria.

Special Senses—frequent: tinnitus; *infrequent:* diplopia, ear pain, eye hemorrhage, eye pain, lacrimation disorder, otitis media, parosmia; *rare:* glaucoma.

Metabolic and Nutritional—infrequent: edema, hypercholesteremia, thirst, dehydration.

Hemic and Lymphatic System—infrequent: anemia; *rare:* leukemia, thrombocytopenia.

Endocrine System—infrequent: diabetes mellitus.

Unclassified—infrequent: surgical procedure.

DRUG ABUSE AND DEPENDENCE

Tolcapone is not a controlled substance.

Studies conducted in rats and monkeys did not reveal any potential for physical or psychological dependence. Although clinical trials have not revealed any evidence of the potential for abuse, tolerance or physical dependence, systematic studies in humans designed to evaluate these effects have not been performed.

OVERDOSAGE

The highest dose of tolcapone administered to humans was 800 mg tid, with and without levodopa/carbidopa coadministration. This was in a 1-week study in elderly, healthy volunteers. The peak plasma concentrations of tolcapone at this dose were on average 30 μg/mL (compared to 3 μg/mL and 6 μg/mL with 100 mg and 200 mg tolcapone, respectively). Nausea, vomiting and dizziness were observed, particularly in combination with levodopa/carbidopa.

The threshold for the lethal plasma concentration for tolcapone based on animal data is >100 μg/mL. Respiratory difficulties were observed in rats at high oral (gavage) and intravenous doses and in dogs with rapidly injected intravenous doses.

Management of Overdose: Hospitalization is advised. General supportive care is indicated. Based on the physicochemical properties of the compound, hemodialysis is unlikely to be of benefit.

DOSAGE AND ADMINISTRATION

Therapy with TASMAR may be initiated with 100 mg or 200 mg tid, always as an adjunct to levodopa/carbidopa therapy. Although clinical trial data suggest that initial treatment with 200 mg tid (a daily dose of 600 mg) is reasonably well tolerated, the prescriber may wish to begin treatment with 100 mg tid because of the potential for increased dopaminergic side effects (eg, dyskinesias) and the possible necessary adjustment of the concomitant levodopa/carbidopa dose. In clinical trials, the first dose of the day of TASMAR was always taken together with the first dose of the day of levodopa/carbidopa, and the subsequent doses of TASMAR were given approximately 6 and 12 hours later.

In clinical trials, the majority of patients required a decrease in their daily levodopa dose if their daily dose of levodopa was >600 mg or if patients had moderate or severe dyskinesias before beginning treatment.

The maximum recommended dose of TASMAR is 600 mg a day, given as tid dosing. To optimize an individual patient's response, reductions in daily levodopa dose may be necessary. In clinical trials, the average reduction in daily levodopa dose was about 30% in those patients requiring a levodopa dose reduction. (Greater than 70% of patients with levodopa doses above 600 mg daily required such a reduction.)

The safety and effectiveness of daily doses greater than 600 mg, or of single doses greater than 200 mg, have not been systematically evaluated.

TASMAR can be combined with both the immediate and sustained release formulations of levodopa/carbidopa.

TASMAR may be taken with or without food (see CLINICAL PHARMACOLOGY).

Patients With Impaired Renal or Hepatic Function: Patients with moderate to severe cirrhosis of the liver should not be escalated to 200 mg TASMAR tid (see CLINICAL PHARMACOLOGY).

No dose adjustment of TASMAR is recommended for patients with mild to moderate renal impairment. The safety of tolcapone has not been examined in subjects who had creatinine clearance less than 25 mL/min (see CLINICAL PHARMACOLOGY).

HOW SUPPLIED

TASMAR is supplied as film-coated tablets containing 100 mg or 200 mg tolcapone. The 100 mg beige tablet and the 200 mg reddish-brown tablet are hexagonal and biconvex. Imprinted with black ink on one side of the tablet is TASMAR and the tablet strength (100 or 200), on the other side is ROCHE.

TASMAR 100 mg Tablets: bottles of 90 (NDC 0004-5920-01).
TASMAR 200 mg Tablets: bottles of 90 (NDC 0004-5921-01).

Storage: Store at controlled room temperature 20° to 25°C (68° to 77°F) in tight containers as defined in USP/NF.

Issued: January 1998

Shown in Product Identification Guide, page 335

TICLID® ℞

[tye'klid]

(ticlopidine hydrochloride)

Tablets

The following text is complete prescribing information based on official labeling in effect June 1998.

WARNING: TICLID can cause life-threatening hematological adverse reactions, including neutropenia/agranulocytosis and thrombotic thrombocytopenic purpura (TTP).

Neutropenia/Agranulocytosis: **Among 2048 patients in clinical trials, there were 50 cases (2.4%) of neutropenia (less than 1200 neutrophils/mm^3), and the neutrophil count was below 450/mm^3 in 17 of these patients (0.8% of the total population).**

TTP: **Thrombotic thrombocytopenic purpura was not seen during clinical trials, but US physicians reported about 100 cases between 1992 and 1997. Based on an estimated patient exposure of 2 million to 4 million, and assuming an event reporting rate of 10% (the true rate is not known), the incidence of ticlopidine-associated TTP may be as high as one case in every 2000 to 4000 patients exposed.**

Monitoring of Clinical and Hematologic Status: **Severe hematological adverse reactions may occur within a few days of the start of therapy. The incidence of TTP peaks after about 3 to 4 weeks of therapy and neutropenia peaks at approximately 4 to 6 weeks with both declining thereafter. Only a few cases have arisen after more than 3 months of treatment.**

Hematological adverse reactions cannot be reliably predicted by any identified demographic or clinical characteristics. During the first 3 months of treatment, patients receiving TICLID must, therefore, be hematologically and clinically monitored for evidence of neutropenia or TTP. If any such evidence is seen, TICLID should be immediately discontinued.

The detection and treatment of ticlopidine-associated hematological adverse reactions are further described under WARNINGS.

DESCRIPTION

TICLID (ticlopidine hydrochloride) is a platelet aggregation inhibitor. Chemically it is 5-[(2-chlorophenyl)methyl]-4,5,6,7-tetrahydrothieno [3,2-c] pyridine hydrochloride.

Ticlopidine hydrochloride is a white crystalline solid. It is freely soluble in water and self-buffers to a pH of 3.6. It also dissolves freely in methanol, is sparingly soluble in methylene chloride and ethanol, slightly soluble in acetone and insoluble in a buffer solution of pH 6.3. It has a molecular weight of 300.25.

TICLID tablets for oral administration are provided as white, oval, film-coated, blue-imprinted tablets containing 250 mg of ticlopidine hydrochloride. Each tablet also contains citric acid, magnesium stearate, microcrystalline cellulose, povidone, starch and stearic acid as inactive ingredients. The white film-coating contains hydroxypropylmethyl cellulose, polyethylene glycol and titanium dioxide. Each tablet is printed with blue ink, which includes FD&C Blue #1 aluminum lake as the colorant. The tablets are identified with Ticlid on one side and 250 on the reverse side.

CLINICAL PHARMACOLOGY

Mechanism of Action: When taken orally, ticlopidine hydrochloride causes a time- and dose-dependent inhibition of both platelet aggregation and release of platelet granule constituents, as well as a prolongation of bleeding time. The intact drug has no significant in vitro activity at the concentrations attained in vivo; and, although analysis of urine and plasma indicates at least 20 metabolites, no metabolite which accounts for the activity of ticlopidine has been isolated.

Ticlopidine hydrochloride, after oral ingestion, interferes with platelet membrane function by inhibiting ADP-induced platelet-fibrinogen binding and subsequent platelet-platelet interactions. The effect on platelet function is irreversible for the life of the platelet, as shown both by persistent inhibition of fibrinogen binding after washing platelets ex vivo and by inhibition of platelet aggregation after resuspension of platelets in buffered medium.

Pharmacokinetics and Metabolism: After oral administration of a single 250-mg dose, ticlopidine hydrochloride is rapidly absorbed with peak plasma levels occurring at approximately 2 hours after dosing and is extensively metabolized. Absorption is greater than 80%. Administration after meals results in a 20% increase in the AUC of ticlopidine.

Ticlopidine hydrochloride displays nonlinear pharmacokinetics and clearance decreases markedly on repeated dosing. In older volunteers the apparent half-life of ticlopidine after a single 250-mg dose is about 12.6 hours; with repeat dosing at 250 mg bid, the terminal elimination half-life rises to 4 to 5 days and steady-state levels of ticlopidine hydrochloride in plasma are obtained after approximately 14 to 21 days.

Ticlopidine hydrochloride binds reversibly (98%) to plasma proteins, mainly to serum albumin and lipoproteins. The binding to albumin and lipoproteins is nonsaturable over a wide concentration range. Ticlopidine also binds to alpha-1 acid glycoprotein. At concentrations attained with the recommended dose, only 15% or less ticlopidine in plasma is bound to this protein.

Ticlopidine hydrochloride is metabolized extensively by the liver; only trace amounts of intact drug are detected in the

Continued on next page

Ticlid—Cont.

urine. Following an oral dose of radioactive ticlopidine hydrochloride administered in solution, 60% of the radioactivity is recovered in the urine and 23% in the feces. Approximately 1/3 of the dose excreted in the feces is intact ticlopidine hydrochloride, possibly excreted in the bile. Ticlopidine hydrochloride is a minor component in plasma (5%) after a single dose, but at steady-state is the major component (15%). Approximately 40% to 50% of the radioactive metabolites circulating in plasma are covalently bound to plasma proteins, probably by acylation.

Clearance of ticlopidine decreases with age. Steady-state trough values in elderly patients (mean age 70 years) are about twice those in younger volunteer populations.

Hepatically Impaired Patients: The effect of decreased hepatic function on the pharmacokinetics of TICLID was studied in 17 patients with advanced cirrhosis. The average plasma concentration of ticlopidine in these subjects was slightly higher than that seen in older subjects in a separate trial (see CONTRAINDICATIONS).

Renally Impaired Patients: Patients with mildly (Ccr 50 to 80 mL/min) or moderately (Ccr 20 to 50 mL/min) impaired renal function were compared to normal subjects (Ccr 80 to 150 mL/min) in a study of the pharmacokinetic and platelet pharmacodynamic effects of TICLID (250 mg bid) for 11 days. Concentrations of unchanged TICLID were measured after a single 250-mg dose and after the final 250-mg dose on Day 11.

AUC values of ticlopidine increased by 28% and 60% in mild and moderately impaired patients, respectively, and plasma clearance decreased by 37% and 52%, respectively, but there were no statistically significant differences in ADP-induced platelet aggregation. In this small study (26 patients), bleeding times showed significant prolongation only in the moderately impaired patients.

Pharmacodynamics: In healthy volunteers over the age of 50, substantial inhibition (over 50%) of ADP-induced platelet aggregation is detected within 4 days after administration of ticlopidine hydrochloride 250 mg bid, and maximum platelet aggregation inhibition (60% to 70%) is achieved after 8 to 11 days. Lower doses cause less, and more delayed, platelet aggregation inhibition, while doses above 250 mg bid give little additional effect on platelet aggregation but an increased rate of adverse effects. The dose of 250 mg bid is the only dose that has been evaluated in controlled clinical trials.

After discontinuation of ticlopidine hydrochloride, bleeding time and other platelet function tests return to normal within 2 weeks, in the majority of patients.

At the recommended therapeutic dose (250 mg bid), ticlopidine hydrochloride has no known significant pharmacological actions in man other than inhibition of platelet function and prolongation of the bleeding time.

CLINICAL TRIALS

The effect of ticlopidine on the risk of stroke and cardiovascular events was studied in two multicenter, randomized, double-blind trials.

1. Study in Patients Experiencing Stroke Precursors: In a trial comparing ticlopidine and aspirin (The Ticlopidine Aspirin Stroke Study or TASS), 3069 patients (1987 men, 1082 women) who had experienced such stroke precursors as transient ischemic attack (TIA), transient monocular blindness (amaurosis fugax), reversible ischemic neurological deficit or minor stroke, were randomized to ticlopidine 250 mg bid or aspirin 650 mg bid. The study was designed to follow patients for at least 2 years and up to 5 years.

Over the duration of the study, TICLID significantly reduced the risk of fatal and nonfatal stroke by 24% (p = .011) from 18.1 to 13.8 per 100 patients followed for 5 years, compared to aspirin. During the first year, when the risk of stroke is greatest, the reduction in risk of stroke (fatal and nonfatal) compared to aspirin was 48%; the reduction was similar in men and women.

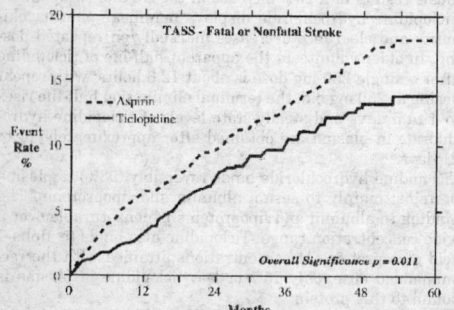

2. Study in Patients Who Had a Completed Atherothrombotic Stroke: In a trial comparing ticlopidine with placebo

(The Canadian American Ticlopidine Study or CATS) 1073 patients who had experienced a previous atherothrombotic stroke were treated with TICLID 250 mg bid or placebo for up to 3 years.

TICLID significantly reduced the overall risk of stroke by 24% (p = .017) from 24.6 to 18.6 per 100 patients followed for 3 years, compared to placebo. During the first year the reduction in risk of fatal and nonfatal stroke over placebo was 33%.

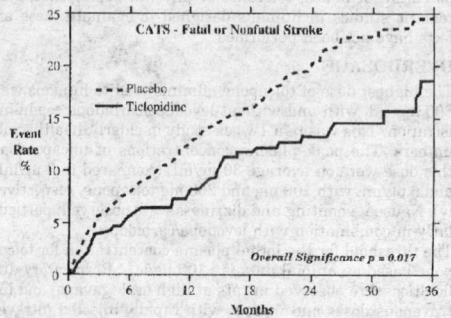

INDICATIONS AND USAGE

TICLID is indicated to reduce the risk of thrombotic stroke (fatal or nonfatal) in patients who have experienced stroke precursors, and in patients who have had a completed thrombotic stroke.

Because TICLID is associated with a risk of life-threatening blood dyscrasias including thrombotic thrombocytopenic purpura (TTP) and neutropenia/agranulocytosis (see BOXED WARNING and WARNINGS), TICLID should be reserved for patients who are intolerant or allergic to aspirin therapy or who have failed aspirin therapy.

CONTRAINDICATIONS

The use of TICLID is contraindicated in the following conditions:
- Hypersensitivity to the drug
- Presence of hematopoietic disorders such as neutropenia and thrombocytopenia or a past history of TTP
- Presence of a hemostatic disorder or active pathological bleeding (such as bleeding peptic ulcer or intracranial bleeding)
- Patients with severe liver impairment

WARNINGS

Hematological Adverse Reactions: *Neutropenia:* Neutropenia may occur suddenly. Bone-marrow examination typically shows a reduction in myeloid precursors. After withdrawal of ticlopidine, the neutrophil count usually rises to >1200/mm³ within 1 to 3 weeks.

Thrombocytopenia: Rarely, thrombocytopenia may occur in isolation or together with neutropenia.

Thrombotic Thrombocytopenic Purpura (TTP): TTP is characterized by thrombocytopenia, microangiopathic hemolytic anemia (schistocytes [fragmented RBCs] seen on peripheral smear), neurological findings, renal dysfunction, and fever. The signs and symptoms can occur in any order, in particular, clinical symptoms may precede laboratory findings by hours or days. With **prompt** treatment (often including plasmapheresis), 70% to 80% of patients will survive with minimal or no sequelae. Because platelet transfusions may accelerate thrombosis in patients with TTP on ticlopidine, they should, if possible, be avoided.

Monitoring for Hematologic Adverse Reactions: Starting just before initiating treatment and continuing through the third month of therapy, patients receiving TICLID must be monitored every 2 weeks. Because of ticlopidine's long plasma half-life, patients who discontinue ticlopidine during this 3-month period should continue to be monitored for 2 weeks after discontinuation. More frequent monitoring, and monitoring after the first 3 months of therapy, is necessary only in patients with clinical signs (eg, signs or symptoms suggestive of infection) or laboratory signs (eg, neutrophil count less than 70% of the baseline count, decrease in hematocrit or platelet count) that suggest incipient hematological adverse reactions.

Clinically, fever might suggest either neutropenia or TTP; TTP might also be suggested by weakness, pallor, petechiae or purpura, dark urine (due to blood, bile pigments, or hemoglobin) or jaundice, or neurological changes. Patients should be told to discontinue TICLID and to contact the physician immediately upon the occurrence of any of these findings.

Laboratory monitoring should include a complete blood count, with special attention to the absolute neutrophil count (WBC × % neutrophils), platelet count, and the appearance of the peripheral smear. Ticlopidine is occasionally associated with thrombocytopenia unrelated to TTP. Any acute, unexplained reduction in **hemoglobin** or platelet count should prompt further investigation for a diagnosis of

TTP, and the appearance of **schistocytes** (fragmented RBCs) on the smear should be treated as presumptive evidence of TTP. If there are laboratory signs of TTP, or if the neutrophil count is confirmed to be <1200/mm³, then the drug should be discontinued.

Other Hematological Effects: Rare cases of agranulocytosis, pancytopenia or aplastic anemia have been reported in postmarketing experience, some of which have been fatal. All forms of hematological adverse reactions are potentially fatal.

Cholesterol Elevation: TICLID therapy causes increased serum cholesterol and triglycerides. Serum total cholesterol levels are increased 8% to 10% within 1 month of therapy and persist at that level. The ratios of the lipoprotein subfractions are unchanged.

Anticoagulant Drugs: The tolerance and safety of coadministration of TICLID with heparin, oral anticoagulants or fibrinolytic agents have not been established. If a patient is switched from an anticoagulant or fibrinolytic drug to TICLID, the former drug should be discontinued prior to TICLID administration.

PRECAUTIONS

General: TICLID should be used with caution in patients who may be at risk of increased bleeding from trauma, surgery or pathological conditions. If it is desired to eliminate the antiplatelet effects of TICLID prior to elective surgery, the drug should be discontinued 10 to 14 days prior to surgery. Several controlled clinical studies have found increased surgical blood loss in patients undergoing surgery during treatment with ticlopidine. In TASS and CATS it was recommended that patients have ticlopidine discontinued prior to elective surgery. Several hundred patients underwent surgery during the trials, and no excessive surgical bleeding was reported.

Prolonged bleeding time is normalized within 2 hours after administration of 20 mg methylprednisolone IV. Platelet transfusions may also be used to reverse the effect of TICLID on bleeding. Because platelet transfusions may accelerate thrombosis in patients with TTP on ticlopidine, they should, if possible, be avoided.

GI Bleeding: TICLID prolongs template bleeding time. The drug should be used with caution in patients who have lesions with a propensity to bleed (such as ulcers). Drugs that might induce such lesions should be used with caution in patients on TICLID (see CONTRAINDICATIONS).

Use in Hepatically Impaired Patients: Since ticlopidine is metabolized by the liver, dosing of TICLID or other drugs metabolized in the liver may require adjustment upon starting or stopping concomitant therapy. Because of limited experience in patients with severe hepatic disease, who may have bleeding diatheses, the use of TICLID is not recommended in this population (see CLINICAL PHARMACOLOGY and CONTRAINDICATIONS).

Use in Renally Impaired Patients: There is limited experience in patients with renal impairment. Decreased plasma clearance, increased AUC values and prolonged bleeding times can occur in renally impaired patients. In controlled clinical trials no unexpected problems have been encountered in patients having mild renal impairment, and there is no experience with dosage adjustment in patients with greater degrees of renal impairment. Nevertheless, for renally impaired patients, it may be necessary to reduce the dosage of ticlopidine or discontinue it altogether if hemorrhagic or hematopoietic problems are encountered (see CLINICAL PHARMACOLOGY).

Information for the Patient (see PPI): Patients should be told that a decrease in the number of white blood cells (neutropenia) or platelets (thrombocytopenia) can occur with TICLID, especially during the first 3 months of treatment and that neutropenia, if it is severe, can result in an increased risk of infection. They should be told it is critically important to obtain the scheduled blood tests to detect neutropenia or thrombocytopenia. Patients should also be reminded to contact their physicians if they experience any indication of infection such as fever, chills, or sore throat, any of which might be a consequence of neutropenia. Thrombocytopenia may be part of a syndrome called TTP. Symptoms and signs of TTP, such as fever, weakness, difficulty speaking, seizures, yellowing of skin or eyes, dark or bloody urine, pallor or petechiae (pinpoint hemorrhagic spots on the skin), should be reported immediately.

All patients should be told that it may take them longer than usual to stop bleeding when they take TICLID and that they should report any unusual bleeding to their physician. Patients should tell physicians and dentists that they are taking TICLID before any surgery is scheduled and before any new drug is prescribed.

Patients should be told to promptly report side effects of TICLID such as severe or persistent diarrhea, skin rashes or subcutaneous bleeding or any signs of cholestasis, such as yellow skin or sclera, dark urine, or light-colored stools. Patients should be told to take TICLID with food or just after eating in order to minimize gastrointestinal discomfort.

Laboratory Tests: *Liver Function:* TICLID therapy has been associated with elevations of alkaline phosphatase and

transaminases, which generally occurred within 1 to 4 months of therapy initiation. In controlled clinical trials the incidence of elevated alkaline phosphatase (greater than two times upper limit of normal) was 7.6% in ticlopidine patients, 6% in placebo patients and 2.5% in aspirin patients. The incidence of elevated AST (SGOT) (greater than two times upper limit of normal) was 3.1% in ticlopidine patients, 4% in placebo patients and 2.1% in aspirin patients. No progressive increases were observed in closely monitored clinical trials (eg, no transaminase greater than 10 times the upper limit of normal was seen), but most patients with these abnormalities had therapy discontinued. Occasionally patients had developed minor elevations in bilirubin.

Based on postmarketing and clinical trial experience, liver function testing, including SGPT and GGTP, should be considered whenever liver dysfunction is suspected, particularly during the first 4 months of treatment.

Drug Interactions: Therapeutic doses of TICLID caused a 30% increase in the plasma half-life of antipyrine and may cause analogous effects on similarly metabolized drugs. Therefore, the dose of drugs metabolized by hepatic microsomal enzymes with low therapeutic ratios or being given to patients with hepatic impairment may require adjustment to maintain optimal therapeutic blood levels when starting or stopping concomitant therapy with ticlopidine. Studies of specific drug interactions yielded the following results:

Aspirin and Other NSAIDs: Ticlopidine potentiates the effect of aspirin or other NSAIDs on platelet aggregation. The safety of concomitant use of ticlopidine with aspirin or other NSAIDs has not been established. Aspirin did not modify the ticlopidine-mediated inhibition of ADP-induced platelet aggregation, but ticlopidine potentiated the effect of aspirin on collagen-induced platelet aggregation. Concomitant use of aspirin and ticlopidine is not recommended (see PRECAUTIONS: *GI Bleeding*).

Antacids: Administration of TICLID after antacids resulted in an 18% decrease in plasma levels of ticlopidine.

Cimetidine: Chronic administration of cimetidine reduced the clearance of a single dose of TICLID by 50%.

Digoxin: Coadministration of TICLID with digoxin resulted in a slight decrease (approximately 15%) in digoxin plasma levels. Little or no change in therapeutic efficacy of digoxin would be expected.

Theophylline: In normal volunteers, concomitant administration of TICLID resulted in a significant increase in the theophylline elimination half-life from 8.6 to 12.2 hours and a comparable reduction in total plasma clearance of theophylline.

Phenobarbital: In 6 normal volunteers, the inhibitory effects of TICLID on platelet aggregation were not altered by chronic administration of phenobarbital.

Phenytoin: In vitro studies demonstrated that ticlopidine does not alter the plasma protein binding of phenytoin. However, the protein binding interactions of ticlopidine and its metabolites have not been studied in vivo. Several cases of elevated phenytoin plasma levels with associated somnolence and lethargy have been reported following coadministration with TICLID. Caution should be exercised in coadministering this drug with TICLID, and it may be useful to remeasure phenytoin blood concentrations.

Propranolol: In vitro studies demonstrated that ticlopidine does not alter the plasma protein binding of propranolol. However, the protein binding interactions of ticlopidine and its metabolites have not been studied in vivo. Caution should be exercised in coadministering this drug with TICLID.

Other Concomitant Therapy: Although specific interaction studies were not performed, in clinical studies TICLID was used concomitantly with beta blockers, calcium channel blockers and diuretics without evidence of clinically significant adverse interactions (see PRECAUTIONS).

Food Interaction: The oral bioavailability of ticlopidine is increased by 20% when taken after a meal. Administration of TICLID with food is recommended to maximize gastrointestinal tolerance. In controlled trials TICLID was taken with meals.

Carcinogenesis, Mutagenesis, Impairment of Fertility: In a 2-year oral carcinogenicity study in rats, ticlopidine at daily doses of up to 100 mg/kg (610 mg/m^2) was not tumorigenic. For a 70-kg person (1.73m^2 body surface area) the dose represents 14 times the recommended clinical dose on a mg/kg basis and two times the clinical dose on body surface area basis. In a 78-week oral carcinogenicity study in mice, ticlopidine at daily doses up to 275 mg/kg (1180 mg/m^2) was not tumorigenic. The dose represents 40 times the recommended clinical dose on a mg/kg basis and four times the clinical dose on body surface area basis.

Ticlopidine was not mutagenic in vitro in the Ames test, the rat hepatocyte DNA-repair assay, or the Chinese-hamster fibroblast chromosomal aberration test; or in vivo in the mouse spermatozoid morphology test, the Chinese-hamster micronucleus test, or the Chinese-hamster bone-marrow-cell sister-chromatid exchange test. Ticlopidine was found to have no effect on fertility of male and female rats at oral doses up to 400 mg/kg/day.

Pregnancy: *Teratogenic Effects:* Pregnancy: Category B. Teratology studies have been conducted in mice (doses up to 200 mg/kg/day), rats (doses up to 400 mg/kg/day) and rabbits (doses up to 200 mg/kg/day). Doses of 400 mg/kg in rats, 200 mg/kg/day in mice and 100 mg/kg in rabbits produced maternal toxicity, as well as fetal toxicity, but there was no evidence of a teratogenic potential of ticlopidine. There are, however, no adequate and well-controlled studies in pregnant women. Because animal reproduction studies are not always predictive of a human response, this drug should be used during pregnancy only if clearly needed.

Nursing Mothers: Studies in rats have shown ticlopidine is excreted in the milk. It is not known whether this drug is excreted in human milk. Because many drugs are excreted in human milk and because of the potential for serious adverse reactions in nursing infants from ticlopidine, a decision should be made whether to discontinue nursing or to discontinue the drug, taking into account the importance of the drug to the mother.

Pediatric Use: Safety and effectiveness in pediatric patients have not been established.

Geriatric Use: Clearance of ticlopidine is somewhat lower in elderly patients and trough levels are increased. The major clinical trials with TICLID were conducted in an elderly population with an average age of 64 years. Of the total number of patients in the therapeutic trials, 45% of patients were over 65 years old and 12% were over 75 years old. No overall differences in effectiveness or safety were observed between these patients and younger patients, and other reported clinical experience has not identified differences in responses between the elderly and younger patients, but greater sensitivity of some older individuals cannot be ruled out.

ADVERSE REACTIONS

Adverse reactions were relatively frequent with over 50% of patients reporting at least one. Most (30% to 40%) involved the gastrointestinal tract. Most adverse effects are mild, but 21% of patients discontinued therapy because of an adverse event, principally diarrhea, rash, nausea, vomiting, GI pain and neutropenia. Most adverse effects occur early in the course of treatment, but a new onset of adverse effects can occur after several months.

The incidence rates of adverse events listed in the following table were derived from multicenter, controlled clinical trials described above comparing TICLID, placebo and aspirin over study periods of up to 5.8 years. Adverse events considered by the investigator to be probably drug-related that occurred in at least 1% of patients treated with TICLID are shown in the following table:

Percent of Patients With Adverse Events in Controlled Studies

Event	TICLID (n = 2048) Incidence		Aspirin (n = 1527) Incidence		Placebo (n = 536) Incidence	
Any Events	*60.0*	*(20.9)*	*53.2*	*(14.5)*	*34.3*	*(6.1)*
Diarrhea	12.5	(6.3)	5.2	(1.8)	4.5	(1.7)
Nausea	7.0	(2.6)	6.2	(1.9)	1.7	(0.9)
Dyspepsia	7.0	(1.1)	9.0	(2.0)	0.9	(0.2)
Rash	5.1	(3.4)	1.5	(0.8)	0.6	(0.9)
GI Pain	3.7	(1.9)	5.6	(2.7)	1.3	(0.4)
Neutropenia	2.4	(1.3)	0.8	(0.1)	1.1	(0.4)
Purpura	2.2	(0.2)	1.6	(0.1)	0.0	(0.0)
Vomiting	1.9	(1.4)	1.4	(0.9)	0.9	(0.4)
Flatulence	1.5	(0.1)	1.4	(0.3)	0.0	(0.0)
Pruritus	1.3	(0.8)	0.3	(0.1)	0.0	(0.0)
Dizziness	1.1	(0.4)	0.5	(0.4)	0.0	(0.0)
Anorexia	1.0	(0.4)	0.5	(0.3)	0.0	(0.0)
Abnormal Liver Function Test	1.0	(0.7)	0.3	(0.3)	0.0	(0.0)

Incidence of discontinuation, regardless of relationship to therapy, is shown in parentheses.

Hematological: Neutropenia/thrombocytopenia, TTP (see BOXED WARNING and WARNINGS), agranulocytosis, eosinophilia, pancytopenia, thrombocytosis and bone-marrow depression have been reported.

Gastrointestinal: TICLID therapy has been associated with a variety of gastrointestinal complaints including diarrhea and nausea. The majority of cases are mild, but about 13% of patients discontinued therapy because of these. They usually occur within 3 months of initiation of therapy and typically are resolved within 1 to 2 weeks without discontinuation of therapy. If the effect is severe or persistent, therapy should be discontinued. In some cases of severe or bloody diarrhea, colitis was later diagnosed.

Hemorrhagic: TICLID has been associated with increased bleeding, spontaneous posttraumatic bleeding and perioperative bleeding including, but not limited to, gastrointestinal bleeding. It has also been associated with a number of bleeding complications such as ecchymosis, epistaxis, hematuria and conjunctival hemorrhage.

Intracerebral bleeding was rare in clinical trials with TICLID, with an incidence no greater than that seen with comparator agents (ticlopidine 0.5%, aspirin 0.6%, placebo 0.75%). It has also been reported postmarketing.

Rash: Ticlopidine has been associated with a maculopapular or urticarial rash (often with pruritus). Rash usually occurs within 3 months of initiation of therapy with a mean onset time of 11 days. If drug is discontinued, recovery occurs within several days. Many rashes do not recur on drug rechallenge. There have been rare reports of severe rashes, including Stevens-Johnson syndrome, erythema multiforme and exfoliative dermatitis.

Less Frequent Adverse Reactions (Probably Related): Clinical adverse experiences occurring in 0.5% to 1% of patients in the controlled trials include:

Digestive System: GI fullness
Skin and Appendages: urticaria
Nervous System: headache
Body as a Whole: asthenia, pain
Hemostatic System: epistaxis
Special Senses: tinnitus

In addition, rarer, relatively serious events have also been reported from postmarketing experience: Hemolytic anemia with reticulocytosis, aplastic anemia, immune thrombocytopenia, hepatitis, hepatocellular jaundice, cholestatic jaundice, hepatic necrosis, peptic ulcer, renal failure, nephrotic syndrome, hyponatremia, vasculitis, sepsis, angioedema, allergic pneumonitis, systemic lupus (positive ANA), peripheral neuropathy, serum sickness, arthropathy and myositis.

OVERDOSAGE

One case of deliberate overdosage with TICLID has been reported by a foreign postmarketing surveillance program. A 38-year-old male took a single 6000-mg dose of TICLID (equivalent to 24 standard 250-mg tablets). The only abnormalities reported were increased bleeding time and increased SGPT. No special therapy was instituted and the patient recovered without sequelae.

Single oral doses of ticlopidine at 1600 mg/kg and 500 mg/kg were lethal to rats and mice, respectively. Symptoms of acute toxicity were GI hemorrhage, convulsions, hypothermia, dyspnea, loss of equilibrium and abnormal gait.

DOSAGE AND ADMINISTRATION

The recommended dose of TICLID is 250 mg bid taken with food. Other doses have not been studied in controlled trials for these indications.

HOW SUPPLIED

TICLID is available in white, oval, film-coated 250-mg tablets, printed in blue with Ticlid on one side and 250 on the other. They are provided in unit of use bottles of 30 tablets (NDC 0004-0018-23) and 60 tablets (NDC 0004-0018-22) and 500 tablets (NDC 0004-0018-14).

Store at 15° to 30°C (59° to 86°F).

IMPORTANT INFORMATION ABOUT TICLID (ticlopidine HCl) TABLETS

The information in this leaflet is intended to help you use TICLID safely. Please read the leaflet carefully. Although it does not contain all the detailed medical information that is provided to your doctor, it provides facts about TICLID that are important for you to know. If you still have questions after reading this leaflet or if you have questions at any time during your treatment with TICLID, check with your doctor.

Special Warning for Users of TICLID/Necessary Blood Tests: TICLID is recommended to help reduce your risk of having a stroke, but only for patients who have had a stroke or early stroke warning symptoms while on aspirin, or for those who have these symptoms but are intolerant or allergic to aspirin.

TICLID is not prescribed for those who can take aspirin to prevent a stroke because TICLID can cause life-threatening blood problems. **Getting your blood tests done and reporting symptoms to your doctor as soon as possible can avoid serious complications.**

The white cells of the blood that fight infection may drop to dangerous levels (a condition called neutropenia). This occurs in about 2.4% (1 in 40) of people on ticlopidine. You should be on the lookout for signs of infection such as fever, chills or sore throat. If this problem is caught early, it can almost always be reversed, but if undetected it can be fatal.

Another problem that has occurred in some patients taking ticlopidine is a decrease in cells called platelets (a condition called thrombocytopenia). This may occur as part of a syndrome that includes injury to red blood cells, causing anemia, kidney abnormalities, neurologic changes and fever. This condition is called TTP and can be fatal.

Things you should watch for as possible early signs of TTP are yellow skin or eye color, pinpoint dots (rash) on the skin, pale color, fever, weakness on a side of the body, or dark urine. **If any of these occur, contact your doctor immediately.**

Continued on next page

Ticlid—Cont.

Both complications occur most frequently in the first 90 days after TICLID is started. To make sure you don't develop either of these problems, your doctor will arrange for you to have your blood tested before you start taking TICLID and then every 2 weeks for the first 3 months you are on TICLID. If detected, neutropenia and thrombocytopenia can almost always be reversed. It is essential that you keep your appointments for the blood tests and that you call your doctor immediately if you have any indication that you may have TTP or neutropenia. If you stop taking TICLID for any reason within the first 3 months, you will still need to have your blood tested for an additional 2 weeks after you have stopped taking TICLID.

Other Warnings and Precautions: A few people may develop jaundice while being treated with TICLID. The signs of jaundice are yellowing of the skin or the whites of the eyes or consistent darkening of the urine or lightening in the color of the stools. These symptoms should be reported to your physician promptly.

If any of the symptoms described above for neutropenia, TTP or jaundice occur, contact your doctor immediately.

TICLID should be used only as directed by your doctor. Do not give TICLID to anyone else. **Keep TICLID out of reach of children!**

Some people may have such side effects as diarrhea, skin rash, stomach or intestinal discomfort. If any of these problems are persistent, or if you are concerned about them, bring them to your doctor's attention.

It may take longer than usual to stop bleeding when taking TICLID. Tell your doctor if you have any more bleeding or bruising than usual, and, if you have emergency surgery, be sure to let your doctor or dentist know that you are taking TICLID. Also, tell your doctor well in advance of any planned surgery (including tooth extraction), because he or she may recommend that you stop taking TICLID temporarily.

How TICLID Works: A stroke occurs when a clot (or thrombus) forms in a blood vessel in the brain or forms in another part of the body and breaks off, then travels to the brain (an embolus). In both cases the blood supply to part of the brain is blocked and that part of the brain is damaged. TICLID works by making the blood less likely to clot, although not so much less that it causes you to become likely to bleed, unless you have a bleeding disorder or some injury (such as a bleeding ulcer of the stomach or intestine) that is especially likely to bleed.

Who Should Not Take TICLID? Contact your doctor immediately and do not take TICLID if:

- you have an allergic reaction to TICLID
- you have a blood disorder or a serious bleeding problem, such as a bleeding stomach ulcer
- you have previously been told you had TTP
- you have severe liver disease or other liver problems
- you are pregnant or you are planning to become pregnant
- you are breastfeeding

Copyright © 1998 by Roche Laboratories Inc. All rights reserved.

Manufactured by Syntex Puerto Rico, Inc.
Humacao, Puerto Rico 00791
or Oread Inc.
Palo Alto, California 94304

Revised: June 1998

Shown in Product Information Guide, page 335

TORADOL® IV/IM ℞

[tō rah-dol]

(ketorolac tromethamine injection)

TORADOL® ORAL

(ketorolac tromethamine tablets)

The following text is complete prescribing information based on official labeling in effect June 1998.

WARNING

TORADOL, a nonsteroidal anti-inflammatory drug (NSAID), is indicated for the short-term (up to 5 days) management of moderately severe acute pain that requires analgesia at the opioid level. It is NOT indicated for minor or chronic painful conditions. TORADOL is a potent NSAID analgesic, and its administration carries many risks. The resulting NSAID-related adverse events can be serious in certain patients for whom TORADOL is indicated, especially when the drug is used inappropriately. Increasing the dose of TORADOL beyond the label recommendations will not provide better efficacy but will result in increasing the risk of developing serious adverse events.

GASTROINTESTINAL EFFECTS

- TORADOL can cause peptic ulcers, gastrointestinal bleeding and/or perforation. Therefore, TORADOL is CONTRAINDICATED in patients with active peptic ulcer disease, in patients with recent gastrointestinal bleeding or perforation, and in patients with a history of peptic ulcer disease or gastrointestinal bleeding.

RENAL EFFECTS

- TORADOL is CONTRAINDICATED in patients with advanced renal impairment and in patients at risk for renal failure due to volume depletion (see WARNINGS).

RISK OF BLEEDING

- TORADOL inhibits platelet function and is, therefore, CONTRAINDICATED in patients with suspected or confirmed cerebrovascular bleeding, patients with hemorrhagic diathesis, incomplete hemostasis and those at high risk of bleeding (see WARNINGS and PRECAUTIONS).
- TORADOL is CONTRAINDICATED as prophylactic analgesic before any major surgery and is CONTRAINDICATED intraoperatively when hemostasis is critical because of the increased risk of bleeding.

HYPERSENSITIVITY

- Hypersensitivity reactions, ranging from bronchospasm to anaphylactic shock, have occurred and appropriate counteractive measures must be available when administering the first dose of TORADOL IV/IM (see CONTRAINDICATIONS and WARNINGS). TORADOL is CONTRAINDICATED in patients with previously demonstrated hypersensitivity to ketorolac tromethamine or allergic manifestations to aspirin or other nonsteroidal anti-inflammatory drugs (NSAIDs).

INTRATHECAL OR EPIDURAL ADMINISTRATION

- TORADOL is CONTRAINDICATED for intrathecal or epidural administration due to its alcohol content.

LABOR, DELIVERY AND NURSING

- The use of TORADOL in labor and delivery is CONTRAINDICATED because it may adversely affect fetal circulation and inhibit uterine contractions.
- The use of TORADOL is CONTRAINDICATED in nursing mothers because of the potential adverse effects of prostaglandin-inhibiting drugs on neonates.

CONCOMITANT USE WITH NSAIDs

- TORADOL is CONTRAINDICATED in patients currently receiving ASA or NSAIDs because of the cumulative risk of inducing serious NSAID-related side effects.

DOSAGE AND ADMINISTRATION

TORADOL ORAL

- TORADOL ORAL is indicated only as continuation therapy to TORADOL IV/IM, and the combined duration of use of TORADOL IV/IM and TORADOL ORAL is not to exceed 5 days because of the increased risk of serious adverse events.
- The recommended total daily dose of TORADOL ORAL (maximum 40 mg) is significantly lower than for TORADOL IV/IM (maximum 120 mg) (see DOSAGE AND ADMINISTRATION and *Transition from TORADOL IV/IM to TORADOL ORAL*).

SPECIAL POPULATIONS

- Dosage should be adjusted for patients 65 years or older, for patients under 50 kg (110 lbs) of body weight (see DOSAGE AND ADMINISTRATION) and for patients with moderately elevated serum creatinine (see WARNINGS). Doses of TORADOL IV/IM are not to exceed 60 mg (total dose per day) in these patients.

DESCRIPTION

TORADOL (ketorolac tromethamine) is a member of the pyrrolo-pyrrole group of nonsteroidal anti-inflammatory drugs (NSAIDs). The chemical name for ketorolac tromethamine is (±)-5-benzoyl-2,3-dihydro-1H-pyrrolizine-1-carboxylic acid, compound with 2-amino-2-(hydroxymethyl)-1,3-propanediol.

TORADOL is a racemic mixture of [−]S and [+]R ketorolac tromethamine. Ketorolac tromethamine may exist in three crystal forms. All forms are equally soluble in water. Ketorolac tromethamine has a pKa of 3.5 and an n-octanol/water partition coefficient of 0.26. The molecular weight of ketorolac tromethamine is 376.41.

TORADOL is available for intravenous (IV) or intramuscular (IM) administration as: 15 mg in 1 mL (1.5%) and 30 mg in 1 mL (3%) in sterile solution; 60 mg in 2 mL (3%) of ketorolac tromethamine in sterile solution is available for IM administration only. For the TUBEX syringe units, the solutions contain 10% (w/v) alcohol, USP, and 6.68 mg, 4.35 mg and 8.70 mg, respectively, of sodium chloride in sterile water. For the vials, the solutions contain 0.1% citric acid, 10% (w/v) alcohol, USP, and 6.68 mg, 4.35 mg and 8.70 mg, respectively, of sodium chloride in sterile water. The pH is adjusted with sodium hydroxide or hydrochloric acid, and the solutions are packaged with nitrogen. The sterile solutions are clear and slightly yellow in color.

TORADOL ORAL is available as round, white, film-coated, red-printed tablets. Each tablet contains 10 mg ketorolac tromethamine, the active ingredient, with added lactose, magnesium stearate and microcrystalline cellulose. The white film-coating contains hydroxypropyl methylcellulose, polyethylene glycol and titanium dioxide. The tablets are printed with red ink that includes FD&C Red #40 Aluminum lake as the colorant. There is a large T printed on both sides of the tablet, as well as the word TORADOL on one side, and the word ROCHE on the other.

CLINICAL PHARMACOLOGY

Pharmacodynamics: Ketorolac tromethamine is a nonsteroidal anti-inflammatory drug (NSAID). Ketorolac tromethamine inhibits synthesis of prostaglandins and may be considered a peripherally acting analgesic. The biological activity of ketorolac tromethamine is associated with the S-form. Ketorolac tromethamine possesses no sedative or anxiolytic properties.

Pain relief was statistically different after TORADOL dosing from that of placebo at 1/2 hour (the first time point at which it was measured) following the largest recommended doses of TORADOL and by 1 hour following the smallest recommended doses. The peak analgesic effect occurred within 2 to 3 hours and was not statistically significantly different over the recommended dosage range of TORADOL. The greatest difference between large and small doses of TORADOL by either route was in the duration of analgesia.

Pharmacokinetics: Ketorolac tromethamine is a racemic mixture of [−]S- and [+]R-enantiomeric forms, with the S-form having analgesic activity.

Comparison of IV, IM and Oral Pharmacokinetics: The pharmacokinetics of ketorolac tromethamine, following IV, IM and oral doses of TORADOL, are compared in Table 1. The extent of bioavailability following administration of the oral and IM forms of TORADOL was equal to that following an IV bolus.

Linear Kinetics: Following administration of single ORAL, IM or IV doses of TORADOL in the recommended dosage ranges, the clearance of the racemate does not change. This implies that the pharmacokinetics of ketorolac tromethamine in humans, following single or multiple IM, IV or recommended oral doses of TORADOL, are linear. At the higher recommended doses, there is a proportional increase in the concentrations of free and bound racemate.

Binding and Distribution: The ketorolac tromethamine racemate has been shown to be highly protein bound (99%). Nevertheless, even plasma concentrations as high as 10 µg/mL will only occupy approximately 5% of the albumin binding sites. Thus, the unbound fraction for each enantiomer will be constant over the therapeutic range. A decrease in serum albumin, however, will result in increased free drug concentrations.

The mean apparent volume (Vβ) of ketorolac tromethamine following complete distribution was approximately 13 liters. This parameter was determined from single-dose data.

Metabolism: Ketorolac tromethamine is largely metabolized in the liver. The metabolic products are hydroxylated and conjugated forms of the parent drug. The products of metabolism, and some unchanged drug, are excreted in the urine.

Clearance and Excretion: A single-dose study with 10 mg TORADOL (n=9) demonstrated that the S-enantiomer is cleared approximately two times faster than the R-enantiomer and that the clearance was independent of the route of administration. This means that the ratio of S/R plasma concentrations decreases with time after each dose. There is little or no inversion of the R- to S- form in humans. The clearance of the racemate in normal subjects, elderly individuals and in hepatically and renally impaired patients is outlined in Table 2.

The half-life of the ketorolac tromethamine S-enantiomer was approximately 2.5 hours (SD ± 0.4) compared with 5 hours (SD ± 1.7) for the R-enantiomer. In other studies, the half-life for the racemate has been reported to lie within the range of 5 to 6 hours.

Accumulation: TORADOL administered as an IV bolus every 6 hours for 5 days to healthy subjects (n=13), showed no significant difference in C_{max} on Day 1 and Day 5. Trough levels averaged 0.29 µg/mL (SD ± 0.13) on Day 1 and 0.55 µg/mL (SD ± 0.23) on Day 6. Steady state was approached after the fourth dose.

Accumulation of ketorolac tromethamine has not been studied in special populations (elderly patients, renal failure patients or hepatic disease patients).

Effect of Food: Oral administration of TORADOL after a high-fat meal resulted in decreased peak and delayed time-to-peak concentrations of ketorolac tromethamine by about 1 hour. Antacids did not affect the extent of absorption.

Kinetics in Special Populations: Elderly Patients: Based on single-dose data only, the half-life of the ketorolac tromethamine racemate increased from 5 to 7 hours in the elderly (65 to 78 years) compared with young healthy volunteers (24 to 35 years) (see Table 2). There was little difference in the C_{max} for the two groups (elderly, 2.52 µg/mL ± 0.77; young, 2.99 µg/mL ± 1.03) (see PRECAUTIONS—*Use in the Elderly*).

Renally Impaired Patients: Based on single-dose data only, the mean half-life of ketorolac tromethamine in renally impaired patients is between 6 and 19 hours and is dependent on the extent of the impairment. There is poor correlation between creatinine clearance and total ketorolac tromethamine clearance in the elderly and populations with renal impairment (r=0.5).

Table 1
Table of Approximate Average Pharmacokinetic Parameters (Mean ± SD) Following Oral, Intramuscular and Intravenous Doses of TORADOL

Pharmacokinetic Parameters (units)	Oral* 10 mg	Oral* 15 mg	Intramuscular† 30 mg	Intramuscular† 60 mg	Intravenous Bolus‡ 15 mg	Intravenous Bolus‡ 30 mg
Bioavailability (extent)			100%			
T_{max}[1] (min)	44 ± 34	33 ± 21§	44 ± 29	33 ± 21§	1.1 ± 0.7§	2.9 ± 1.8
C_{max}[2] (µg/mL) [single-dose]	0.87 ± 0.22	1.14 ± 0.32§	2.42 ± 0.68	4.55 ± 1.27§	2.47 ± 0.51§	4.65 ± 0.96
C_{max} (µg/mL) [steady state qid]	1.05 ± 0.26§	1.56 ± 0.44§	3.11 ± 0.87§	N/A"	3.09 ± 1.17§	6.85 ± 2.61
C_{min}[3] (µg/mL) [steady state qid]	0.29 ± 0.07§	0.47 ± 0.13§	0.93 ± 0.26§	N/A	0.61 ± 0.21§	1.04 ± 0.35
C_{avg}[4] (µg/mL) [steady state qid]	0.59 ± 0.20§	0.94 ± 0.29§	1.88 ± 0.59§	N/A	1.09 ± 0.30§	2.17 ± 0.59
Vβ[5](L/kg)	——0.175 ± 0.039——					0.210 ± 0.044

% Dose metabolized = <50 % Dose excreted in feces = 6 [1]Time-to-peak plasma concentration

% Dose excreted in urine = 91 % Plasma protein binding = 99 [2]Peak plasma concentration

[3]Trough plasma concentration

* Derived from PO pharmacokinetic studies in 77 normal fasted volunteers

† Derived from IM pharmacokinetic studies in 54 normal volunteers [4]Average plasma concentration

‡ Derived from IV pharmacokinetic studies in 24 normal volunteers [5]Volume of distribution

§ Mean value was simulated from observed plasma concentration data and standard deviation was simulated from percent coefficient of variation for observed C_{max} and T_{max} data

" Not applicable because 60 mg is only recommended as a single dose

In patients with renal disease, the AUC_∞ of each enantiomer increased by approximately 100% compared with healthy volunteers. The volume of distribution doubles for the S-enantiomer and increases by 1/5th for the R-enantiomer. The increase in volume of distribution of ketorolac tromethamine implies an increase in unbound fraction. The AUC_∞-ratio of the ketorolac tromethamine enantiomers in healthy subjects and patients remained similar, indicating there was no selective excretion of either enantiomer in patients compared to healthy subjects (see WARNINGS—*Renal Effects*).

Hepatic Effects: There was no significant difference in estimates of half-life, AUC_∞ and C_{max} in 7 patients with liver disease compared to healthy volunteers (see PRECAUTIONS—*Hepatic Effects*).

Clinical Studies: The analgesic efficacy of intramuscularly, intravenously and orally administered TORADOL was investigated in two postoperative pain models: general surgery (orthopedic, gynecologic and abdominal) and oral surgery (removal of impacted third molars). The studies were double-blind, single- and multiple-dose, parallel trial designs in patients with moderate to severe pain at baseline. TORADOL[IV/IM] was compared as follows: IM to meperidine or morphine administered intramuscularly and IV to morphine administered either directly IV or through a PCA (Patient-Controlled Analgesia) pump.

Short-Term Use (up to 5 days) Studies: In the comparisons of intramuscular administration during the first hour, the onset of analgesic action was similar for TORADOL and the narcotics, but the duration of analgesia was longer with TORADOL than with the opioid comparators meperidine or morphine.

[See table 1 at left]

[See table 2 at left]

In a multidose, postoperative (general surgery) double-blind trial of TORADOL[IM] 30 mg versus morphine 6 and 12 mg IM, each drug given on an as needed basis for up to 5 days, the overall analgesic effect of TORADOL[IM] 30 mg was between that of morphine 6 and 12 mg. The majority of patients treated with either TORADOL or morphine were dosed for up to 3 days; a small percentage of patients received 5 days of dosing.

In clinical settings where perioperative morphine was allowed, TORADOL[IV] 30 mg, given once or twice as needed, provided analgesia comparable to morphine 4 mg IV once or twice as needed.

There was relatively limited experience with 5 consecutive days of TORADOL[IV] use in controlled clinical trials, as most patients were given the drug for 3 days or less. The adverse events seen with IV-administered TORADOL were similar to those observed with IM-administered TORADOL, as would be expected based on the similar pharmacokinetics and bioequivalence (AUC, clearance, plasma half-life) of IV and IM routes of TORADOL administration.

Clinical Studies with Concomitant Use of Opioids: Clinical studies in postoperative pain management have demonstrated that TORADOL[IV/IM], when used in combination with opioids, significantly reduced opioid consumption. This combination may be useful in the subpopulation of patients especially prone to opioid-related complications. TORADOL and narcotics should not be administered in the same syringe.

In a postoperative study, where all patients received morphine by a PCA device, patients treated with TORADOL[IV] as fixed intermittent boluses (eg, 30 mg initial dose followed by 15 mg q3h), required significantly less morphine (26%) than the placebo group. Analgesia was significantly superior, at various postdosing pain assessment times, in the patients receiving TORADOL[IV] plus PCA morphine as compared to patients receiving PCA-administered morphine alone.

Postmarketing Surveillance Study: A large postmarketing observational, nonrandomized study, involving approximately 10,000 patients receiving TORADOL, demonstrated that the risk of clinically serious gastrointestinal (GI) bleeding was dose-dependent (see Tables 3A and 3B). This was particularly true in elderly patients who received an average daily dose greater than 60 mg/day of TORADOL (Table 3A).

Table 2
The Influence of Age, Liver and Kidney Function, on the Clearance and Terminal Half-life of TORADOL (IM[1] and ORAL[2])

Type of Subjects	Total Clearance [In L/h/kg][3] IM Mean (range)	Total Clearance [In L/h/kg][3] ORAL Mean (range)	Terminal Half-life [In hours] IM Mean (range)	Terminal Half-life [In hours] ORAL Mean (range)
Normal Subjects IM (n=54) mean age=32, range=18–60 Oral (n=77) mean age=32, range=20–60	0.023 (0.010–0.046)	0.025 (0.013–0.050)	5.3 (3.5–9.2)	5.3 (2.4–9.0)
Healthy Elderly Subjects IM (n=13), Oral (n=12) mean age=72, range=65–78	0.019 (0.013–0.034)	0.024 (0.018–0.034)	7.0 (4.7–8.6)	6.1 (4.3–7.6)
Patients with Hepatic Dysfunction IM and Oral (n=7) mean age=51, range 43–64	0.029 (0.013–0.066)	0.033 (0.019–0.051)	5.4 (2.2–6.9)	4.5 (1.6–7.6)
Patients with Renal Impairment IM (n=25), Oral (n=9) serum creatinine:1.9–5.0 mg/dL, mean age (IM)=54, range=35–71 mean age (Oral)=57, range=39–70	0.015 (0.005–0.043)	0.016 (0.007–0.052)	10.3 (5.9–19.2)	10.8 (3.4–18.9)
Renal Dialysis Patients IM and Oral (n=9) mean age=40, range 27–63	0.016 (0.003–0.036)	—	13.6 (8.0–39.1)	—

[1]Estimated from 30 mg single IM doses of ketorolac tromethamine
[2]Estimated from 10 mg single oral doses of ketorolac tromethamine
[3]Liters/hour/kilogram
IV Administration: In normal subjects (n=37), the total clearance of 30 mg IV-administered TORADOL was 0.030 (0.017–0.051) L/h/kg. The terminal half-life was 5.6 (4.0–7.9) hours.

Table 3
Incidence of Clinically Serious GI Bleeding as Related to Age, Total Daily Dose, and History of GI Perforation, Ulcer, Bleeding (PUB) after up to 5 Days of Treatment with TORADOL[IV/IM]

A. Patients without History of PUB

Age of Patients	Total Daily Dose of TORADOL[IV/IM] ≤60 mg	>60 to 90 mg	>90 to 120 mg	>120 mg
<65 years of age	0.4%	0.4%	0.9%	4.6%
≥65 years of age	1.2%	2.8%	2.2%	7.7%

B. Patients with History of PUB

Age of Patients	Total Daily Dose of TORADOL[IV/IM] ≤60 mg	>60 to 90 mg	>90 to 120 mg	>120 mg
<65 years of age	2.1%	4.6%	7.8%	15.4%
≥65 years of age	4.7%	3.7%	2.8%	25.0%

INDICATIONS AND USAGE

TORADOL is indicated for the short-term (≤5 days) management of moderately severe acute pain that requires analgesia at the opioid level, usually in a postoperative setting. Therapy should always be initiated with TORADOL[IV/IM], and TORADOL[ORAL] is to be used only as continuation treatment, if necessary. Combined use of TORADOL[IV/IM] and TORADOL[ORAL] is not to exceed 5 days of use because of the potential of increasing the frequency and severity of adverse reactions associated with the recommended doses (see WARNINGS, PRECAUTIONS, DOSAGE AND ADMINIS-

Continued on next page

Toradol—Cont.

TRATION and ADVERSE REACTIONS). Patients should be switched to alternative analgesics as soon as possible, but TORADOL therapy is not to exceed 5 days.

TORADOL$^{IV/IM}$ has been used concomitantly with morphine and meperidine and has shown an opioid-sparing effect. For breakthrough pain, it is recommended to supplement the lower end of the TORADOL$^{IV/IM}$ dosage range with low doses of narcotics prn, unless otherwise contraindicated. TORADOL$^{IV/IM}$ and narcotics should not be administered in the same syringe (see DOSAGE AND ADMINISTRATION: *Pharmaceutical Information for TORADOL$^{IV/IM}$*).

CONTRAINDICATIONS

(see also Boxed WARNING):

- TORADOL is CONTRAINDICATED in patients with active peptic ulcer disease, in patients with recent gastrointestinal bleeding or perforation and in patients with a history of peptic ulcer disease or gastrointestinal bleeding.
- TORADOL is CONTRAINDICATED in patients with advanced renal impairment or in patients at risk for renal failure due to volume depletion (see WARNINGS for correction of volume depletion).
- TORADOL is CONTRAINDICATED in labor and delivery because, through its prostaglandin synthesis inhibitory effect, it may adversely affect fetal circulation and inhibit uterine contractions, thus increasing the risk of uterine hemorrhage.
- The use of TORADOL is CONTRAINDICATED in nursing mothers because of the potential adverse effects of prostaglandin-inhibiting drugs on neonates.
- TORADOL is CONTRAINDICATED in patients with previously demonstrated hypersensitivity to ketorolac tromethamine, allergic manifestations to aspirin or other nonsteroidal anti-inflammatory drugs (NSAIDs).
- TORADOL is CONTRAINDICATED as prophylactic analgesic before any major surgery and is CONTRAINDICATED intraoperatively when hemostasis is critical because of the increased risk of bleeding.
- TORADOL inhibits platelet function and is, therefore, CONTRAINDICATED in patients with suspected or confirmed cerebrovascular bleeding, hemorrhagic diathesis, incomplete hemostasis and those at high risk of bleeding (see WARNINGS and PRECAUTIONS).
- TORADOL is CONTRAINDICATED in patients currently receiving ASA or NSAIDs because of the cumulative risks of inducing serious NSAID-related adverse events.
- TORADOL$^{IV/IM}$ is CONTRAINDICATED for neuraxial (epidural or intrathecal) administration due to its alcohol content.
- The concomitant use of TORADOL and probenecid is CONTRAINDICATED .

WARNINGS

(see also Boxed WARNING):

The combined use of TORADOL$^{IV/IM}$ and TORADOL^{ORAL} is not to exceed 5 days.

The most serious risks associated with TORADOL are:

- *Gastrointestinal Ulcerations, Bleeding and Perforation:* TORADOL is CONTRAINDICATED in patients with previously documented peptic ulcers and/or GI bleeding. Serious gastrointestinal toxicity, such as bleeding, ulceration and perforation, can occur at any time, with or without warning symptoms, in patients treated with TORADOL. Studies to date with NSAIDs have not identified any subset of patients not at risk of developing peptic ulceration and bleeding. Elderly or debilitated patients seem to tolerate ulceration or bleeding less well than other individuals, and most spontaneous reports of fatal GI events are in this population. Postmarketing experience with parenterally administered TORADOL suggests that there may be a greater risk of gastrointestinal ulcerations, bleeding and perforation in the elderly.

The incidence and severity of gastrointestinal complications increases with increasing dose of, and duration of treatment with, TORADOL. In a nonrandomized, in-hospital postmarketing surveillance study comparing parenteral TORADOL to parenteral opioids, higher rates of clinically serious GI bleeding were seen in patients <65 years of age who received an average total daily dose of more than 90 mg of TORADOL$^{IV/IM}$ per day (see CLINICAL PHARMACOLOGY: *Postmarketing Surveillance Study*).

The same study showed that elderly (≥65 years of age) and debilitated patients are more susceptible to gastrointestinal complications. A history of peptic ulcer disease was revealed as another risk factor that increases the possibility of developing serious gastrointestinal complications during TORADOL therapy (see Tables 3A and 3B).

- *Impaired Renal Function: TORADOL should be used with caution in patients with impaired renal function or a history of kidney disease because it is a potent inhibitor of prostaglandin synthesis.* Renal toxicity with TORADOL has been seen in patients with conditions leading to a reduction in blood volume and/or renal blood flow where renal prostaglandins have a supportive role in the main-

tenance of renal perfusion. In these patients administration of TORADOL may cause a dose-dependent reduction in renal prostaglandin formation and may precipitate acute renal failure. Patients at greatest risk of this reaction are those with impaired renal function, dehydration, heart failure, liver dysfunction, those taking diuretics and the elderly. Discontinuation of TORADOL therapy is usually followed by recovery to the pretreatment state.

Renal Effects: TORADOL and its metabolites are eliminated primarily by the kidneys, which, in patients with reduced creatinine clearance, will result in diminished clearance of the drug (see CLINICAL PHARMACOLOGY). Therefore, TORADOL should be used with caution in patients with impaired renal function (see DOSAGE AND ADMINISTRATION) and such patients should be followed closely. With the use of TORADOL, there have been reports of acute renal failure, nephritis and nephrotic syndrome.

Because patients with underlying renal insufficiency are at increased risk of developing acute renal failure, the risks and benefits should be assessed prior to giving TORADOL to these patients. Hence, in patients with moderately elevated serum creatinine, it is recommended that the daily dose of TORADOL$^{IV/IM}$ be reduced by half, not to exceed 60 mg/day. TORADOL IS CONTRAINDICATED IN PATIENTS WITH SERUM CREATININE CONCENTRATIONS INDICATING ADVANCED RENAL IMPAIRMENT (see CONTRAINDICATIONS).

Hypovolemia should be corrected before treatment with TORADOL is initiated.

- *Fluid Retention and Edema:* Fluid retention, edema, retention of NaCl, oliguria, elevations of serum urea nitrogen and creatinine have been reported in clinical trials with TORADOL. Therefore, TORADOL should be used only very cautiously in patients with cardiac decompensation, hypertension or similar conditions.

- *Hemorrhage:* Because prostaglandins play an important role in hemostasis and NSAIDs affect platelet aggregation as well, use of TORADOL in patients who have coagulation disorders should be undertaken very cautiously, and those patients should be carefully monitored. Patients on therapeutic doses of anticoagulants (eg, heparin or dicumarol derivatives) have an increased risk of bleeding complications if given TORADOL concurrently; therefore, physicians should administer such concomitant therapy only extremely cautiously. The concurrent use of TORADOL and prophylactic low-dose heparin (2500 to 5000 units q12h), warfarin and dextrans have not been studied extensively, but may also be associated with an increased risk of bleeding. Until data from such studies are available, physicians should carefully weigh the benefits against the risks and use such concomitant therapy in these patients only extremely cautiously. In patients who receive anticoagulants for any reason, there is an increased risk of intramuscular hematoma formation from administered TORADOL^{IM} (see PRECAUTIONS: *Drug Interactions*). Patients receiving therapy that affects hemostasis should be monitored closely.

In postmarketing experience, postoperative hematomas and other signs of wound bleeding have been reported in association with the perioperative use of TORADOL$^{IV/IM}$. Therefore, perioperative use of TORADOL should be avoided and postoperative use be undertaken with caution when hemostasis is critical (see WARNINGS and PRECAUTIONS).

- *Anaphylactoid Reactions:* Anaphylactoid reactions may occur in patients without a known previous exposure or hypersensitivity to aspirin, TORADOL or other NSAIDs, or in individuals with a history of angioedema, bronchospastic reactivity (eg, asthma) and nasal polyps. Anaphylactoid reactions, like anaphylaxis, may have a fatal outcome.

PRECAUTIONS

General:

- *Hepatic Effects: TORADOL should be used with caution in patients with impaired hepatic function or a history of liver disease.* Treatment with TORADOL may cause elevations of liver enzymes, and, in patients with preexisting liver dysfunction, it may lead to the development of a more severe hepatic reaction. The administration of TORADOL should be discontinued in patients in whom an abnormal liver test has occurred as a result of TORADOL therapy.

- *Hematologic Effects:* TORADOL inhibits platelet aggregation and may prolong bleeding time; therefore, it is contraindicated as a preoperative medication, and caution should be used when hemostasis is critical. Unlike aspirin, the inhibition of platelet function by TORADOL disappears within 24 to 48 hours after the drug is discontinued. TORADOL does not appear to affect platelet count, prothrombin time (PT) or partial thromboplastin time (PTT). In controlled clinical studies, where TORADOL was administered intramuscularly or intravenously postoperatively, the incidence of clinically significant postoperative bleeding was 0.4% for TORADOL compared to 0.2% in the control groups receiving narcotic analgesics.

Information for Patients: TORADOL is a potent NSAID and may cause serious side effects such as gastrointestinal bleeding or kidney failure, which may result in hospitalization and even fatal outcome.

Physicians, when prescribing TORADOL, should inform their patients of the potential risks of TORADOL treatment (see Boxed WARNING, WARNINGS, PRECAUTIONS and ADVERSE REACTIONS sections). *Advise patients not to give TORADOL^{ORAL} to other family members and to discard any unused drug.*

Remember that the total duration of TORADOL therapy is not to exceed 5 days.

Drug Interactions: Ketorolac is highly bound to human plasma protein (mean 99.2%).

The in vitro binding of *warfarin* to plasma proteins is only slightly reduced by ketorolac tromethamine (99.5% control vs 99.3%) when ketorolac plasma concentrations reach 5 to 10 µg/mL. Ketorolac does not alter *digoxin* protein binding. In vitro studies indicate that, at therapeutic concentrations of *salicylate* (300 µg/mL), the binding of ketorolac was reduced from approximately 99.2% to 97.5%, representing a potential twofold increase in unbound ketorolac plasma levels. Therapeutic concentrations of *digoxin, warfarin, ibuprofen, naproxen, piroxicam, acetaminophen, phenytoin* and *tolbutamide* did not alter ketorolac tromethamine protein binding.

In a study involving 12 volunteers, TORADOL^{ORAL} was coadministered with a single dose of 25 mg *warfarin*, causing no significant changes in pharmacokinetics or pharmacodynamics of warfarin. In another study, TORADOL$^{IV/IM}$ was given with two doses of 5000 U of *heparin* to 11 healthy volunteers, resulting in a mean template bleeding time of 6.4 minutes (3.2 to 11.4 min) compared to a mean of 6.0 minutes (3.4 to 7.5 min) for heparin alone and 5.1 minutes (3.5 to 8.5 min) for placebo. Although these results do not indicate a significant interaction between TORADOL and warfarin or heparin, the administration of TORADOL to patients taking anticoagulants should be done extremely cautiously, and patients should be closely monitored (see WARNINGS and PRECAUTIONS).

TORADOL$^{IV/IM}$ reduced the diuretic response to *furosemide* in normovolemic healthy subjects by approximately 20% (mean sodium and urinary output decreased 17%).

Concomitant administration of TORADOL^{ORAL} and *probenecid* resulted in decreased clearance of ketorolac and significant increases in ketorolac plasma levels (total AUC increased approximately threefold from 5.4 to 17.8 µg/h/mL) and terminal half-life increased approximately twofold from 6.6 to 15.1 hours. Therefore, concomitant use of TORADOL and probenecid is contraindicated.

Inhibition of renal *lithium* clearance, leading to an increase in plasma lithium concentration, has been reported with some prostaglandin synthesis-inhibiting drugs. The effect of TORADOL on plasma lithium has not been studied, but cases of increased lithium plasma levels during TORADOL therapy have been reported.

Concomitant administration of *methotrexate* and some NSAIDs has been reported to reduce the clearance of methotrexate, enhancing the toxicity of methotrexate. The effect of TORADOL on methotrexate clearance has not been studied.

In postmarketing experience there have been reports of a possible interaction between TORADOL$^{IV/IM}$ and *nondepolarizing muscle relaxants* that resulted in apnea. The concurrent use of TORADOL with muscle relaxants has not been formally studied.

Concomitant use of *ACE inhibitors* may increase the risk of renal impairment, particularly in volume-depleted patients. Sporadic cases of seizures have been reported during concomitant use of TORADOL and *antiepileptic drugs* (phenytoin, carbamazepine).

Hallucinations have been reported when TORADOL was used in patients taking *psychoactive drugs* (fluoxetine, thiothixene, alprazolam).

TORADOL$^{IV/IM}$ has been administered concurrently with *morphine* in several clinical trials of postoperative pain without evidence of adverse interactions. Do not mix TORADOL and morphine in the same syringe.

There is no evidence in animal or human studies that TORADOL induces or inhibits hepatic enzymes capable of metabolizing itself or other drugs.

Carcinogenesis, Mutagenesis and Impairment of Fertility: An 18-month study in mice with oral doses of ketorolac tromethamine at 2 mg/kg/day (0.9 times the human systemic exposure at the recommended IM or IV dose of 30 mg qid, based on area-under-the-plasma-concentration curve [AUC]), and a 24-month study in rats at 5 mg/kg/day (0.5 times the human AUC) showed no evidence of tumorigenicity.

Ketorolac tromethamine was not mutagenic in the Ames test, unscheduled DNA synthesis and repair, and in forward mutation assays. Ketorolac tromethamine did not cause chromosome breakage in the in vivo mouse micronucleus assay. At 1590 µg/mL and at higher concentrations, ketorolac tromethamine increased the incidence of chromosomal aberrations in Chinese hamster ovarian cells.

Impairment of fertility did not occur in male or female rats at oral doses of 9 mg/kg (0.9 times the human AUC) and 16 mg/kg (1.6 times the human AUC) of ketorolac tromethamine, respectively.

Pregnancy: Pregnancy Category C. Reproduction studies have been performed during organogenesis using daily oral doses of ketorolac tromethamine at 3.6 mg/kg (0.37 times the human AUC) in rabbits and at 10 mg/kg (1.0 times the human AUC) in rats. Results of these studies did not reveal evidence of teratogenicity to the fetus. Oral doses of ketorolac tromethamine at 1.5 mg/kg (0.14 times the human AUC), administered after gestation Day 17, caused dystocia and higher pup mortality in rats. There are no adequate and well-controlled studies of TORADOL in pregnant women. TORADOL should be used during pregnancy only if the potential benefit justifies the potential risk to the fetus.

Labor and Delivery: The use of TORADOL is contraindicated in labor and delivery because, through its prostaglandin synthesis inhibitory effect, it may adversely affect fetal circulation and inhibit uterine contractions, thus increasing the risk of uterine hemorrhage (see CONTRAINDICATIONS).

Lactation and Nursing: After a single administration of 10 mg of TORADOL^{ORAL} to humans, the maximum milk concentration observed was 7.3 ng/mL, and the maximum milk-to-plasma ratio was 0.037. After 1 day of dosing (qid), the maximum milk concentration was 7.9 ng/mL, and the maximum milk-to-plasma ratio was 0.025. Because of the possible adverse effects of prostaglandin-inhibiting drugs on neonates, use in nursing mothers is contraindicated.

Pediatric Use: Safety and efficacy in children (less than 16 years of age) have not been established. Therefore, use of TORADOL in children is not recommended.

Use in the Elderly (≥65 years of age): Because ketorolac tromethamine may be cleared more slowly by the elderly (see CLINICAL PHARMACOLOGY) who are also more sensitive to the adverse effects of NSAIDs (see WARNINGS: *Renal Effects*), extra caution and reduced dosages (see DOSAGE AND ADMINISTRATION) must be used when treating the elderly with TORADOL$^{IV/IM}$. The lower end of the TORADOL$^{IV/IM}$ dosage range is recommended for patients over 65 years of age, and total daily dose is not to exceed 60 mg. The incidence and severity of gastrointestinal complications increases with increasing dose of, and duration of treatment with, TORADOL.

ADVERSE REACTIONS

Adverse reaction rates increase with higher doses of TORADOL. Practitioners should be alert for the severe complications of treatment with TORADOL, such as GI ulceration, bleeding and perforation, postoperative bleeding, acute renal failure, anaphylactic and anaphylactoid reactions and liver failure (see Boxed WARNING, WARNINGS, PRECAUTIONS and DOSAGE AND ADMINISTRATION). These NSAID-related complications can be serious in certain patients for whom TORADOL is indicated, especially when the drug is used inappropriately.

The Adverse Reactions Listed Below Were Reported In Clinical Trials As Probably Related To TORADOL:

• ***Incidence Greater Than 1%***

Percentage of incidence in parentheses for those events reported in 3% or more patients.

Body as a Whole: edema (4%)
Cardiovascular: hypertension
Dermatologic: pruritus, rash
Gastrointestinal: nausea (12%), dyspepsia (12%), gastrointestinal pain (13%), diarrhea (7%), constipation, flatulence, gastrointestinal fullness, vomiting, stomatitis
Hemic and Lymphatic: purpura
Nervous System: headache (17%), drowsiness (6%), dizziness (7%), sweating
Injection-site pain was reported by 2% of patients in multidose studies.

• ***Incidence 1% or Less***

Body as a Whole: weight gain, fever, infections, asthenia
Cardiovascular: palpitation, pallor, syncope
Dermatologic: urticaria
Gastrointestinal: gastritis, rectal bleeding, eructation, anorexia, increased appetite
Hemic and Lymphatic: epistaxis, anemia, eosinophilia
Nervous System: tremors, abnormal dreams, hallucinations, euphoria, extrapyramidal symptoms, vertigo, paresthesia, depression, insomnia, nervousness, excessive thirst, dry mouth, abnormal thinking, inability to concentrate, hyperkinesis, stupor
Respiratory: dyspnea, pulmonary edema, rhinitis, cough
Special Senses: abnormal taste, abnormal vision, blurred vision, tinnitus, hearing loss
Urogenital: hematuria, proteinuria, oliguria, urinary retention, polyuria, increased urinary frequency

The Following Adverse Events Were Reported From Postmarketing Experience:

Body as a Whole: hypersensitivity reactions such as anaphylaxis, anaphylactoid reaction, laryngeal edema, tongue edema (see Boxed WARNING, WARNINGS), myalgia
Cardiovascular: hypotension, flushing
Dermatologic: Lyell's syndrome, Stevens-Johnson syndrome, exfoliative dermatitis, maculopapular rash, urticaria
Gastrointestinal: peptic ulceration, GI hemorrhage, GI perforation (see Boxed WARNING, WARNINGS), melena, acute pancreatitis
Hemic and Lymphatic: postoperative wound hemorrhage (rarely requiring blood transfusion—see Boxed WARNING, WARNINGS and PRECAUTIONS), thrombocytopenia, leukopenia
Hepatic: hepatitis, liver failure, cholestatic jaundice
Nervous System: convulsions, psychosis, aseptic meningitis
Respiratory: asthma, bronchospasm
Urogenital: acute renal failure (see Boxed WARNING, WARNINGS), flank pain with or without hematuria and/or azotemia, nephritis, hyponatremia, hyperkalemia, hemolytic uremic syndrome

OVERDOSAGE

In controlled overdosage, daily doses of 360 mg of TORADOL$^{IV/IM}$ given for 5 days (three times the highest recommended dose), caused abdominal pain and peptic ulcers which healed after discontinuation of dosing. Metabolic acidosis has been reported following intentional overdosage. Dialysis does not significantly clear ketorolac tromethamine from the blood stream.

DOSAGE AND ADMINISTRATION

THE COMBINED DURATION OF USE OF TORADOL$^{IV/IM}$ AND TORADOL^{ORAL} IS NOT TO EXCEED 5 DAYS.
THE USE OF TORADOL^{ORAL} IS ONLY INDICATED AS CONTINUATION THERAPY TO TORADOL$^{IV/IM}$.

TORADOL$^{IV/IM}$

TORADOL$^{IV/IM}$ may be used as a single or multiple dose on a regular or prn schedule for the management of moderately severe acute pain that requires analgesia at the opioid level, usually in a postoperative setting. Hypovolemia should be corrected prior to the administration of TORADOL (see WARNINGS: *Renal Effects*). Patients should be switched to alternative analgesics as soon as possible, but TORADOL therapy is not to exceed 5 days.

When administering TORADOL$^{IV/IM}$, the IV bolus must be given over no less than 15 seconds. The IM administration should be given slowly and deeply into the muscle. The analgesic effect begins in 30 minutes with maximum effect in 1 to 2 hours after dosing IV or IM. Duration of analgesic effect is usually 4 to 6 hours.

Single-Dose Treatment: The Following Regimen Should Be Limited To Single Administration Use Only

IM Dosing:

- *Patients <65 years of age: One dose of 60 mg.*
- *Patients ≥65 years of age, renally impaired and/or less than 50 kg (110 lbs) of body weight: One dose of 30 mg.*

IV Dosing:

- *Patients <65 years of age: One dose of 30 mg.*
- *Patients ≥65 years of age, renally impaired and/or less than 50 kg (110 lbs) of body weight: One dose of 15 mg.*

Multiple-Dose Treatment (IV or IM)

- *Patients <65 years of age:* The recommended dose is 30 mg TORADOL$^{IV/IM}$ every 6 hours. The maximum daily dose should not exceed 120 mg.
- *For Patients ≥65 years of age, renally impaired patients (see WARNINGS) and patients less than 50 kg (110 lbs):* The recommended dose is 15 mg TORADOL$^{IV/IM}$ every 6 hours. The maximum daily dose for these populations should not exceed 60 mg.

For breakthrough pain do not increase the dose or the frequency of TORADOL. Consideration should be given to supplementing these regimens with low doses of opioids prn unless otherwise contraindicated.

Pharmaceutical Information for TORADOL$^{IV/IM}$: Parenteral drug products should be inspected visually for particulate matter and discoloration prior to administration whenever solution and container permit.

TORADOL$^{IV/IM}$ should not be mixed in a small volume (eg, in a syringe) with morphine sulfate, meperidine hydrochloride, promethazine hydrochloride or hydroxyzine hydrochloride; this will result in precipitation of ketorolac from solution.

TORADOL^{ORAL} is indicated ONLY as continuation therapy to TORADOL$^{IV/IM}$ for the management of moderately severe acute pain that requires analgesia at the opioid level (see also PRECAUTIONS: *Information for Patients*).

Transition from TORADOL$^{IV/IM}$ to TORADOL^{ORAL}: The recommended TORADOL^{ORAL} dose is as follows:

- *Patients <65 years of age:* 2 tablets as a first oral dose for patients who received **60 mg IM single dose, 30 mg IV single dose or 30 mg multiple dose.** TORADOL$^{IV/IM}$ followed by 1 tablet TORADOL^{ORAL} every 4 to 6 hours, not to exceed 40 mg/24 h of TORADOL^{ORAL}
- *Patients ≥65 years of age, renally impaired and/or less than 50 kg (110 lbs) of body weight:* 1 tablet as a first oral dose for patients who received **30 mg IM single dose, 15 mg IV single dose or 15 mg multiple dose.** TORADOL$^{IV/IM}$ followed by 1 tablet TORADOL^{ORAL} every 4 to 6 hours, not to exceed 40 mg/24 h of TORADOL^{ORAL}.

Shortening the recommended dosing intervals may result in increased frequency and severity of adverse reactions.

The maximum combined duration of use (parenteral and oral TORADOL) is limited to 5 days.

The TUBEX® BLUNT POINTE™ Sterile Cartridge Unit is suitable for substances to be administered intravenously only. It is intended for use with injection sets specifically manufactured as "needle-less" injection systems. TUBEX® BLUNT POINTE™ is compatible with Abbott's LifeShield® prepierced reseal injection site, Baxter's InterLink® Injection Site, and B. Braun Medical's SafSite® Reflux Valve. Consult manufacturer's recommendations regarding "Directions for Use" of the "needle-less" system. It is also intended for admixture with, and convenient administration of, various medicaments when using Drug Vial Adapters for "needle-less" injection systems.

The TUBEX® Sterile Cartridge-Needle Unit and sterile vial are suitable for substances to be administered intravenously and intramuscularly.

HOW SUPPLIED

TORADOL$^{IV/IM}$ for intramuscular or intravenous use is available in a TUBEX® Cartridge-Needle Unit or a sterial vial:

15 mg: 15 mg/mL, 1 mL TUBEX® Sterile Cartridge-Needle Unit (22 gauge × 1-1/4 inch needle) box of 10 (NDC 0004-6921-06) or 1 mL fill per 2 mL single use vial, box of 10 (NDC 0004-6925-06).

30 mg: 30 mg/mL, 1 mL TUBEX® Sterile Cartridge-Needle Unit (22 gauge × 1-1/4 inch needle) box of 10 (NDC 0004-6923-06) or 1 mL fill per 2 mL single use vial, box of 10 (NDC 0004-6926-06).

For IM Single-Dose Use Only Not Intended for IV Use—60 mg: 30 mg/mL, 2 mL TUBEX® Sterile Cartridge-Needle Unit (22 gauge × 1-1/4 inch needle) box of 1 (NDC 0004-6924-09 or 2 mL fill per 2 mL single use vial, box of 1 (NDC 0004-6927-09).

TORADOL^{IV} for intravenous use is available in a TUBEX® BLUNT POINTE™ Sterile Cartridge Unit:

15 mg: 15 mg/mL, 1 mL TUBEX® BLUNT POINTE™ Sterile Cartridge Unit, box of 10 (NDC 0004-6920-06).

30 mg: 30 mg/mL, 1 mL TUBEX® BLUNT POINTE™ Sterile Cartridge Unit, box of 10 (NDC 0004-6922-06).

Syringes manufactured by Wyeth Laboratories, Inc., Philadelphia, PA 19101 for Roche Laboratories Inc., Nutley, NJ 07110.

Vials manufactured by Hoffmann-La Roche Inc., Nutley, NJ 07110.

Store at 15° to 30°C (59° to 86°F) with protection from light.

TORADOL^{ORAL} 10 mg tablets are available in bottles of 100 tablets (NDC 0004-0273-01).

Store bottles at 15° to 30°C (59° to 86°F).

Manufactured by Syntex Puerto Rico, Inc., Humacao, PR 00791

TUBEX® Injector

NOTE: The TUBEX® Injector is reusable: do not discard.

TUBEX® Sterile Cartridge-Needle Unit
DIRECTIONS FOR USE

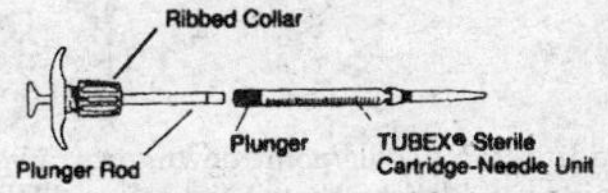

TUBEX® BLUNT POINTE™ Sterile Cartridge Unit
DIRECTIONS FOR USE:

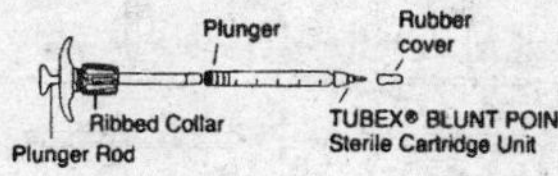

TUBEX® BLUNT POINTE™ Sterile Cartridge Unit is intended for use with injection sets specifically manufactured as "needle-less" injection systems.

TUBEX® BLUNT POINTE™ Sterile Cartridge Unit is compatible with Abbott's LifeShield® prepierced reseal injection site, Baxter's InterLink® Injection Site and B. Braun Medical's SafSite® Reflux Valve. Consult manufacturer's recommendations regarding "Directions for Use" of the "needle-less" injection system.

To load a TUBEX® Sterile Cartridge Unit into the TUBEX® Injector

1. Turn the ribbed collar to the "OPEN" position until it stops.

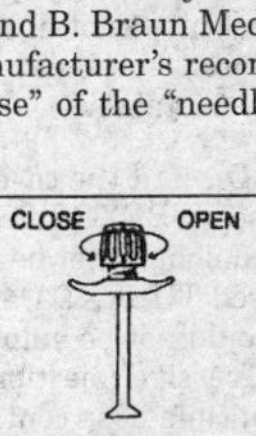

Continued on next page

Toradol—Cont.

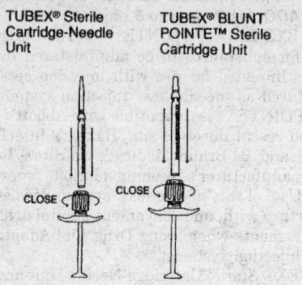

TUBEX® Sterile Cartridge-Needle Unit

TUBEX® BLUNT POINTE™ Sterile Cartridge Unit

CLOSE   CLOSE

2. Hold the Injector with the open end up and fully insert the TUBEX® Sterile Cartridge Unit. Firmly tighten the ribbed collar in the direction of the "CLOSE" arrow.

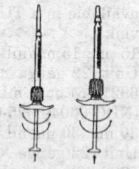

3. Thread the plunger rod into the plunger of the TUBEX® Sterile Cartridge Unit until slight resistance is felt. The Injector is now ready for use in the usual manner.

To administer TUBEX® Sterile Cartridge-Needle Units
Method of administration is the same as with conventional syringe. Remove needle cover by grasping it securely; twist and pull. Introduce needle into patient, aspirate by pulling back slightly on the plunger, and inject.

To administer TUBEX® BLUNT POINTE™ Sterile Cartridge Units
"Needle-less" IV set administration is similar to administration with conventional syringes. Remove rubber cover by grasping it securely; twist and pull. For B. Braun Medical's SafSite® Reflux Valves, aseptically swab the luer slip fitting of the BLUNT POINTE™ sterile cartridge tip assembly with a sterile, individually wrapped, saturated 70% Isopropyl Alcohol swab. This action will remove the lubricant coating from the tip to facilitate a tight seal. Introduce TUBEX® BLUNT POINTE™ Sterile Cartridge Unit into the "needle-less" IV set as per manufacturer's "Directions for Use."

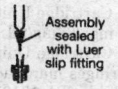

Assembly sealed with Luer slip fitting

To remove the empty TUBEX® Cartridge Unit and dispose into a vertical disposal container
1. Do not recap the needle/point. Disengage the plunger rod.

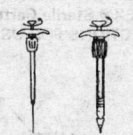

2. Hold the Injector, needle/point down, over a vertical disposal container and loosen the ribbed collar. TUBEX® Cartridge Unit will drop into the container.

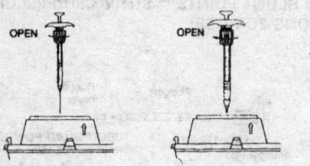

OPEN   OPEN

3. Discard the cover.

To remove the empty TUBEX® Cartridge Unit and dispose into a horizontal (mailbox) disposal container
1. Do not recap the needle/point. Disengage the plunger rod.
2. Open the horizontal (mailbox) disposal container. Insert TUBEX® Cartridge Unit, needle/point pointing down, halfway into container. Close the container lid on cartridge. Loosen ribbed collar; TUBEX® Cartridge Unit will drop into the container.

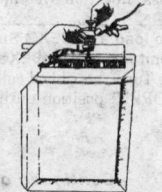

3. Discard the cover.
The TUBEX® Injector is reusable and should not be discarded.
Used TUBEX® Cartridge Units should not be employed for successive injections or as multiple-dose containers. They are intended to be used only once and discarded.

NOTE: Any graduated markings on TUBEX® Sterile Cartridge Units are to be used only as a guide in mixing, withdrawing, or administering measured doses.
Wyeth-Ayerst does not recommend and will not accept responsibility for the use of any cartridge-needle units or needle-less units other than TUBEX® Cartridge Units in the TUBEX® Injector.

Revised August 1997
Shown in Product Identification Guide, page 335

VERSED®
[ver-sed ']
midazolam HCl
INJECTION

^(IV)

The following text is complete prescribing information based on official labeling in effect June 1998.

WARNING
Adults and Pediatrics: Intravenous VERSED has been associated with respiratory depression and respiratory arrest, especially when used for sedation in noncritical care settings. In some cases, where this was not recognized promptly and treated effectively, death or hypoxic encephalopathy has resulted. Intravenous VERSED should be used only in hospital or ambulatory care settings, including physicians' and dental offices, that provide for continuous monitoring of respiratory and cardiac function, ie, pulse oximetry. Immediate availability of resuscitative drugs and age- and size-appropriate equipment for bag/valve/mask ventilation and intubation, and personnel trained in their use and skilled in airway management should be assured (see WARNINGS). For deeply sedated pediatric patients, a dedicated individual, other than the practitioner performing the procedure, should monitor the patient throughout the procedure.
The initial intravenous dose for sedation in adult patients may be as little as 1 mg, but should not exceed 2.5 mg in a normal healthy adult. Lower doses are necessary for older (over 60 years) or debilitated patients and in patients receiving concomitant narcotics or other central nervous system (CNS) depressants. The initial dose and all subsequent doses should always be titrated slowly; administer over at least 2 minutes and allow an additional 2 or more minutes to fully evaluate the sedative effect. The use of the 1 mg/mL formulation or dilution of the 1 mg/mL or 5 mg/mL formulation is recommended to facilitate slower injection. Doses of sedative medications in pediatric patients must be calculated on a mg/kg basis, and initial doses and all subsequent doses should always be titrated slowly. The initial pediatric dose of VERSED for sedation/anxiolysis/amnesia is age, procedure, and route dependent (see DOSAGE AND ADMINISTRATION for complete dosing information).
Neonates: VERSED should not be administered by rapid injection in the neonatal population. Severe hypotension and seizures have been reported following rapid IV administration, particularly with concomitant use of fentanyl (see DOSAGE AND ADMINISTRATION for complete information).

DESCRIPTION
VERSED is a water-soluble benzodiazepine available as a sterile, nonpyrogenic parenteral dosage form for intravenous or intramuscular injection. Each mL contains midazolam hydrochloride equivalent to 1 mg or 5 mg midazolam compounded with 0.8% sodium chloride and 0.01% edetate disodium, with 1% benzyl alcohol as preservative; the pH is adjusted to approximately 3 with hydrochloric acid and, if necessary, sodium hydroxide.
Midazolam is a white to light yellow crystalline compound, insoluble in water. The hydrochloride salt of midazolam, which is formed *in situ*, is soluble in aqueous solutions. Chemically, midazolam HCl is 8-chloro-6-(2-fluorophenyl)-1-methyl-4H-imidazo[1,5-a][1,4]benzodiazepine hydrochloride. Midazolam hydrochloride has the empirical formula $C_{18}H_{13}ClFN_3 \cdot HCl$, a calculated molecular weight of 362.25 and the following structural formula:
[See chemical structure at top of next column]

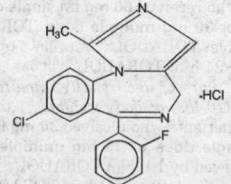

CLINICAL PHARMACOLOGY
VERSED is a short-acting benzodiazepine central nervous system (CNS) depressant.
The effects of VERSED on the CNS are dependent on the dose administered, the route of administration, and the presence or absence of other medications. Onset time of sedative effects after IM administration in adults is 15 minutes, with peak sedation occurring 30 to 60 minutes following injection. In one adult study, when tested the following day, 73% of the patients who received VERSED intramuscularly had no recall of memory cards shown 30 minutes following drug administration; 40% had no recall of the memory cards shown 60 minutes following drug administration. Onset time of sedative effects in the pediatric population begins within 5 minutes and peaks at 15 to 30 minutes depending upon the dose administered. In pediatric patients, up to 85% had no recall of pictures shown after receiving intramuscular VERSED compared with 5% of the placebo controls.
Sedation in adult and pediatric patients is achieved within 3 to 5 minutes after intravenous (IV) injection; the time of onset is affected by total dose administered and the concurrent administration of narcotic premedication. Seventy-one percent of the adult patients in endoscopy studies had no recall of introduction of the endoscope; 82% of the patients had no recall of withdrawal of the endoscope. In one study of pediatric patients undergoing lumbar puncture or bone marrow aspiration, 88% of patients had impaired recall vs 9% of the placebo controls. In another pediatric oncology study, 91% of VERSED treated patients were amnestic compared with 35% of patients who had received fentanyl alone. When VERSED is given IV as an anesthetic induction agent, induction of anesthesia occurs in approximately 1.5 minutes when narcotic premedication has been administered and in 2 to 2.5 minutes without narcotic premedication or other sedative premedication. Some impairment in a test of memory was noted in 90% of the patients studied. A dose response study of pediatric patients premedicated with 1.0 mg/kg intramuscular (IM) meperidine found that only 4 out of 6 pediatric patients who received 600 µg/kg IV VERSED lost consciousness, with eye closing at 108 ± 140 seconds. This group was compared with pediatric patients who were given thiopental 5 mg/kg IV; 6 out of 6 closed their eyes at 20 ± 3.2 seconds. VERSED did not dependably induce anesthesia at this dose despite concomitant opioid administration in pediatric patients.
VERSED, used as directed, does not delay awakening from general anesthesia in adults. Gross tests of recovery after awakening (orientation, ability to stand and walk, suitability for discharge from the recovery room, return to baseline Trieger competency) usually indicate recovery within 2 hours but recovery may take up to 6 hours in some cases. When compared with patients who received thiopental, patients who received midazolam generally recovered at a slightly slower rate. Recovery from anesthesia or sedation for procedures in pediatric patients depends on the dose of VERSED administered, coadministration of other medications causing CNS depression and duration of the procedure.
In patients without intracranial lesions, induction of general anesthesia with IV VERSED is associated with a moderate decrease in cerebrospinal fluid pressure (lumbar puncture measurements), similar to that observed following IV thiopental. Preliminary data in neurosurgical patients with normal intracranial pressure but decreased compliance (subarachnoid screw measurements) show comparable elevations of intracranial pressure with VERSED and with thiopental during intubation. No similar studies have been reported in pediatric patients.
The usual recommended intramuscular premedicating doses of VERSED do not depress the ventilatory response to carbon dioxide stimulation to a clinically significant extent in adults. Intravenous induction doses of VERSED depress the ventilatory response to carbon dioxide stimulation for 15 minutes or more beyond the duration of ventilatory depression following administration of thiopental in adults. Impairment of ventilatory response to carbon dioxide is more marked in adult patients with chronic obstructive pulmonary disease (COPD). Sedation with IV VERSED does not adversely affect the mechanics of respiration (resistance, static recoil, most lung volume measurements); total lung capacity and peak expiratory flow decrease significantly but static compliance and maximum expiratory flow at 50% of awake total lung capacity (V_{max}) increase. In one study of pediatric patients under general anesthesia, intramuscular VERSED (100 or 200 µg/kg) was shown to depress the response to carbon dioxide in a dose-related manner.
In cardiac hemodynamic studies in adults, IV induction of general anesthesia with VERSED was associated with a slight to moderate decrease in mean arterial pressure, cardiac output, stroke volume and systemic vascular resis-

tance. Slow heart rates (less than 65/minute), particularly in patients taking propranolol for angina, tended to rise slightly; faster heart rates (eg, 85/minute) tended to slow slightly. In pediatric patients, a comparison of IV VERSED (500 µg/kg) with propofol (2.5 mg/kg) revealed a mean 15% decrease in systolic blood pressure in patients who had received IV VERSED vs a mean 25% decrease in systolic blood pressure following propofol.

Pharmacokinetics: Midazolam's activity is primarily due to the parent drug. Elimination of the parent drug takes place via hepatic metabolism of midazolam to hydroxylated metabolites that are conjugated and excreted in the urine. Six single-dose pharmacokinetic studies involving healthy adults yield pharmacokinetic parameters for midazolam in the following ranges: volume of distribution (Vd), 1.0 to 3.1 L/kg; elimination half-life, 1.8 to 6.4 hours (mean approximately 3 hours); total clearance (Cl), 0.25 to 0.54 L/hr/kg. In a parallel group study, there was no difference in the clearance, in subjects administered 0.15 mg/kg (n=4) and 0.30 mg/kg (n=4) IV doses indicating linear kinetics. The clearance was successively reduced by approximately 30% at doses of 0.45 mg/kg (n=4) and 0.6 mg/kg (n=5) indicating non-linear kinetics in this dose range.

Absorption: The absolute bioavailability of the intramuscular route was greater than 90% in a crossover study in which healthy subjects (n=17) were administered a 7.5 mg IV or IM dose. The mean peak concentration (C_{max}) and time to peak (T_{max}) following the IM dose was 90 ng/mL (20% CV) and 0.5 hour (50% CV). C_{max} for the 1-hydroxy metabolite following the IM dose was 8 ng/mL (T_{max}=1.0 hour).

Following IM administration, C_{max} for midazolam and its 1-hydroxy metabolite were approximately one-half of those achieved after intravenous injection.

Distribution: The volume of distribution (Vd) determined from six single-dose pharmacokinetic studies involving healthy adults ranged from 1.0 to 3.1 L/kg. Female gender, old age, and obesity are associated with increased values of midazolam Vd. In humans, midazolam has been shown to cross the placenta and enter into fetal circulation and has been detected in human milk and CSF (see *Special Populations*).

In adults and pediatric patients older than 1 year, midazolam is approximately 97% bound to plasma protein, principally albumin.

Metabolism: In vitro studies with human liver microsomes indicate that the biotransformation of midazolam is mediated by cytochrome P450 3A4. This cytochrome also appears to be present in gastrointestinal tract mucosa as well as liver. Sixty to seventy percent of the biotransformation products is 1-hydroxy-midazolam (also termed alpha-hydroxy-midazolam) while 4-hydroxy-midazolam constitutes 5% or less. Small amounts of a dihydroxy derivative have also been detected but not quantified. The principal urinary excretion products are glucuronide conjugates of the hydroxylated derivatives.

Drugs that inhibit the activity of cytochrome P450 3A4 may inhibit midazolam clearance and elevate steady-state midazolam concentrations.

Studies of the intravenous administration of 1-hydroxy-midazolam in humans suggest that 1-hydroxy-midazolam is at least as potent as the parent compound and may contribute to the net pharmacologic activity of midazolam. In vitro studies have demonstrated that the affinities of 1- and 4-hydroxy-midazolam for the benzodiazepine receptor are approximately 20% and 7%, respectively, relative to midazolam.

Excretion: Clearance of midazolam is reduced in association with old age, congestive heart failure, liver disease (cirrhosis) or conditions which diminish cardiac output and hepatic blood flow.

The principal urinary excretion product is 1-hydroxy-midazolam in the form of a glucuronide conjugate; smaller amounts of the glucuronide conjugates of 4-hydroxy- and dihydroxy-midazolam are detected as well. The amount of midazolam excreted unchanged in the urine after a single IV dose is less than 0.5% (n=5). Following a single IV infusion in 5 healthy volunteers, 45% to 57% of the dose was excreted in the urine as 1-hydroxymethyl midazolam conjugate.

Pharmacokinetics-Continuous Infusion: The pharmacokinetic profile of midazolam following continuous infusion, based on 282 adult subjects, has been shown to be similar to that following single-dose administration for subjects of comparable age, gender, body habitus and health status. However, midazolam can accumulate in peripheral tissues with continuous infusion. The effects of accumulation are greater after long-term infusions than after short-term infusions. The effects of accumulation can be reduced by maintaining the lowest midazolam infusion rate that produces satisfactory sedation.

Infrequent hypotensive episodes have occurred during continuous infusion; however, neither the time to onset nor the duration of the episode appeared to be related to plasma concentrations of midazolam or alpha-hydroxy-midazolam.

Further, there does not appear to be an increased chance of occurrence of a hypotensive episode with increased loading doses.

Patients with renal impairment may have longer elimination half-lives for midazolam (see *Special Populations: Renal Failure*).

Special Populations: Changes in the pharmacokinetic profile of midazolam due to drug interactions, physiological variables, etc., may result in changes in the plasma concentration-time profile and pharmacological response to midazolam in these patients. For example, patients with acute renal failure appear to have a longer elimination half-life for midazolam and may experience delayed recovery (see *Special Populations: Renal Failure*). In other groups, the relationship between prolonged half-life and duration of effect has not been established.

Pediatrics and Neonates: In pediatric patients aged 1 year and older, the pharmacokinetic properties following a single dose of VERSED reported in 10 separate studies of midazolam are similar to those in adults. Weight-normalized clearance is similar or higher (0.19 to 0.80 L/hr/kg) than in adults and the terminal elimination half-life (0.78 to 3.3 hours) is similar to or shorter than in adults. The pharmacokinetic properties during and following continuous intravenous infusion in pediatric patients in the operating room as an adjunct to general anesthesia and in the intensive care environment are similar to those in adults.

In seriously ill neonates, however, the terminal elimination half-life of midazolam is substantially prolonged (6.5 to 12.0 hours) and the clearance reduced (0.07 to 0.12 L/hr/kg) compared to healthy adults or other groups of pediatric patients. It cannot be determined if these differences are due to age, immature organ function or metabolic pathways, underlying illness or debility.

Obese: In a study comparing normals (n=20) and obese patients (n=20) the mean half-life was greater in the obese group (5.9 vs 2.3 hours). This was due to an increase of approximately 50% in the Vd corrected for total body weight. The clearance was not significantly different between groups.

Geriatric: In three parallel group studies, the pharmacokinetics of midazolam administered IV or IM were compared in young (mean age 29, n=52) and healthy elderly subjects (mean age 73, n=53). Plasma half-life was approximately two-fold higher in the elderly. The mean Vd based on total body weight increased consistently between 15% to 100% in the elderly. The mean Cl decreased approximately 25% in the elderly in two studies and was similar to that of the younger patients in the other.

Congestive Heart Failure: In patients suffering from congestive heart failure, there appeared to be a two-fold increase in the elimination half-life, a 25% decrease in the plasma clearance and a 40% increase in the volume of distribution of midazolam.

Hepatic Insufficiency: Midazolam pharmacokinetics were studied after an IV single dose (0.075 mg/kg) was administered to 7 patients with biopsy proven alcoholic cirrhosis and 8 control patients. The mean half-life of midazolam increased 2.5-fold in the alcoholic patients. Clearance was reduced by 50% and the Vd increased by 20%. In another study in 21 male patients with cirrhosis, without ascites and with normal kidney function as determined by creatinine clearance, no changes in the pharmacokinetics of midazolam or 1-hydroxy-midazolam were observed when compared to healthy individuals.

Renal Failure: Patients with renal impairment may have longer elimination half-lives for midazolam and its metabolites which may result in slower recovery. Midazolam and 1-hydroxy-midazolam pharmacokinetics in 6 ICU patients who developed acute renal failure (ARF) were compared with a normal renal function control group. Midazolam was administered as an infusion (5 to 15 mg/hr). Midazolam clearance was reduced (1.9 vs 2.8 mL/min/kg) and the half-life was prolonged (7.6 vs 13 hours) in the ARF patients. The renal clearance of the 1-hydroxy-midazolam glucuronide was prolonged in the ARF group (4 vs 136 mL/min) and the half-life was prolonged (12 vs >25 hours). Plasma levels accumulated in all ARF patients to about ten times that of the parent drug. The relationship between accumulating metabolite levels and prolonged sedation is unclear.

In a study of chronic renal failure patients (n=15) receiving a single IV dose, there was a two-fold increase in the clearance and volume of distribution but the half-life remained unchanged. Metabolite levels were not studied.

Plasma Concentration-Effect Relationship: Concentration-effect relationships (after an IV dose) have been demonstrated for a variety of pharmacodynamic measures (eg, reaction time, eye movement, sedation) and are associated with extensive intersubject variability. Logistic regression analysis of sedation scores and steady-state plasma concentration indicated that at plasma concentrations greater than 100 ng/mL there was at least a 50% probability that patients would be sedated, but respond to verbal commands (sedation score = 3). At 200 ng/mL there was at least a 50% probability that patients would be asleep, but respond to glabellar tap (sedation score = 4).

Drug Interactions: For information concerning pharmacokinetic drug interactions with VERSED, (see PRECAUTIONS).

INDICATIONS

Injectable VERSED is indicated:
- intramuscularly or intravenously for preoperative sedation/anxiolysis/amnesia;
- intravenously as an agent for sedation/anxiolysis/amnesia prior to or during diagnostic, therapeutic or endoscopic procedures, such as bronchoscopy, gastroscopy, cystoscopy, coronary angiography, cardiac catheterization, oncology procedures, radiologic procedures, suture of lacerations and other procedures either alone or in combination with other CNS depressants;
- intravenously for induction of general anesthesia, before administration of other anesthetic agents. With the use of narcotic premedication, induction of anesthesia can be attained within a relatively narrow dose range and in a short period of time. Intravenous VERSED can also be used as a component of intravenous supplementation of nitrous oxide and oxygen (balanced anesthesia);
- continuous intravenous infusion for sedation of intubated and mechanically ventilated patients as a component of anesthesia or during treatment in a critical care setting.

VERSED is associated with a high incidence of partial or complete impairment of recall for the next several hours (see CLINICAL PHARMACOLOGY).

CONTRAINDICATIONS

Injectable VERSED is contraindicated in patients with a known hypersensitivity to the drug. Benzodiazepines are contraindicated in patients with acute narrow-angle glaucoma. Benzodiazepines may be used in patients with open-angle glaucoma only if they are receiving appropriate therapy. Measurements of intraocular pressure in patients without eye disease show a moderate lowering following induction with VERSED; patients with glaucoma have not been studied.

VERSED is not intended for intrathecal or epidural administration due to the presence of the preservative benzyl alcohol in the dosage form.

WARNINGS

VERSED must never be used without individualization of dosage particularly when used with other medications capable of producing central nervous system depression. Prior to the intravenous administration of VERSED in any dose, the immediate availability of oxygen, resuscitative drugs, age- and size-appropriate equipment for bag/valve/mask ventilation and intubation, and skilled personnel for the maintenance of a patent airway and support of ventilation should be ensured. Patients should be continuously monitored with some means of detection for early signs of hypoventilation, airway obstruction, or apnea, ie, pulse oximetry. Hypoventilation, airway obstruction, and apnea can lead to hypoxia and/or cardiac arrest unless effective countermeasures are taken immediately. The immediate availability of specific reversal agents (flumazenil) is highly recommended. Vital signs should continue to be monitored during the recovery period. Because intravenous VERSED depresses respiration (see CLINICAL PHARMACOLOGY) and because opioid agonists and other sedatives can add to this depression, VERSED should be administered as an induction agent only by a person trained in general anesthesia and should be used for sedation/anxiolysis/amnesia only in the presence of personnel skilled in early detection of hypoventilation, maintaining a patent airway and supporting ventilation. **When used for sedation/anxiolysis/amnesia, VERSED should always be titrated slowly in adult or pediatric patients.** Adverse hemodynamic events have been reported in pediatric patients with cardiovascular instability; rapid intravenous administration should also be avoided in this population (see DOSAGE AND ADMINISTRATION for complete information).

Serious cardiorespiratory adverse events have occurred after administration of VERSED. These have included respiratory depression, airway obstruction, oxygen desaturation, apnea, respiratory arrest and/or cardiac arrest, sometimes resulting in death or permanent neurologic injury. There have also been rare reports of hypotensive episodes requiring treatment during or after diagnostic or surgical manipulations particularly in adult or pediatric patients with hemodynamic instability. Hypotension occurred more frequently in the sedation studies in patients premedicated with a narcotic.

Reactions such as agitation, involuntary movements (including tonic/clonic movements and muscle tremor), hyperactivity and combativeness have been reported in both adult and pediatric patients. These reactions may be due to inadequate or excessive dosing or improper administration of VERSED; however, consideration should be given to the possibility of cerebral hypoxia or true paradoxical reactions. Should such reactions occur, the response to each dose of VERSED and all other drugs, including local anesthetics,

Continued on next page

Versed—Cont.

should be evaluated before proceeding. Reversal of such responses with flumazenil has been reported in pediatric patients.

Concomitant use of barbiturates, alcohol or other central nervous system depressants may increase the risk of hypoventilation, airway obstruction, desaturation, or apnea and may contribute to profound and/or prolonged drug effect. Narcotic premedication also depresses the ventilatory response to carbon dioxide stimulation.

Higher risk adult and pediatric surgical patients, elderly patients and debilitated adult and pediatric patients require lower dosages, whether or not concomitant sedating medications have been administered. Adult or pediatric patients with COPD are unusually sensitive to the respiratory depressant effect of VERSED. Pediatric and adult patients undergoing procedures involving the upper airway such as upper endoscopy or dental care, are particularly vulnerable to episodes of desaturation and hypoventilation due to partial airway obstruction. Adult and pediatric patients with chronic renal failure and patients with congestive heart failure eliminate midazolam more slowly (see CLINICAL PHARMACOLOGY). Because elderly patients frequently have inefficient function of one or more organ systems and because dosage requirements have been shown to decrease with age, reduced initial dosage of VERSED is recommended, and the possibility of profound and/or prolonged effect should be considered.

Injectable VERSED should not be administered to adult or pediatric patients in shock or coma, or in acute alcohol intoxication with depression of vital signs. Particular care should be exercised in the use of intravenous VERSED in adult or pediatric patients with uncompensated acute illnesses, such as severe fluid or electrolyte disturbances.

There have been limited reports of intra-arterial injection of VERSED. Adverse events have included local reactions, as well as isolated reports of seizure activity in which no clear causal relationship was established. Precautions against unintended intra-arterial injection should be taken. Extravasation should also be avoided.

The safety and efficacy of VERSED following nonintravenous and nonintramuscular routes of administration have not been established. VERSED should only be administered intramuscularly or intravenously.

The decision as to when patients who have received injectable VERSED, particularly on an outpatient basis, may again engage in activities requiring complete mental alertness, operate hazardous machinery or drive a motor vehicle must be individualized. Gross tests of recovery from the effects of VERSED (see CLINICAL PHARMACOLOGY) cannot be relied upon to predict reaction time under stress. It is recommended that no patient operate hazardous machinery or a motor vehicle until the effects of the drug, such as drowsiness, have subsided or until one full day after anesthesia and surgery, whichever is longer. For pediatric patients, particular care should be taken to assure safe ambulation.

Usage in Pregnancy: **An increased risk of congenital malformations associated with the use of benzodiazepine drugs (diazepam and chlordiazepoxide) has been suggested in several studies. If this drug is used during pregnancy, the patient should be apprised of the potential hazard to the fetus.**

Withdrawal symptoms of the barbiturate type have occurred after the discontinuation of benzodiazepines (see DRUG ABUSE AND DEPENDENCE section).

Usage in Preterm Infants and Neonates: Rapid injection should be avoided in the neonatal population. VERSED administered rapidly as an intravenous injection (less than 2 minutes) has been associated with severe hypotension in neonates, particularly when the patient has also received fentanyl. Likewise, severe hypotension has been observed in neonates receiving a continuous infusion of midazolam who then receive a rapid intravenous injection of fentanyl. Seizures have been reported in several neonates following rapid intravenous administration.

The neonate also has reduced and/or immature organ function and is also vulnerable to profound and/or prolonged respiratory effects of VERSED.

Exposure to excessive amounts of benzyl alcohol has been associated with toxicity (hypotension, metabolic acidosis), particularly in neonates, and an increased incidence of kernicterus, particularly in small preterm infants. There have been rare reports of deaths, primarily in preterm infants, associated with exposure to excessive amounts of benzyl alcohol. The amount of benzyl alcohol from medications is usually considered negligible compared to that received in flush solutions containing benzyl alcohol. Administration of high dosages of medications (including VERSED) containing this preservative must take into account the total amount of benzyl alcohol administered. The recommended dosage range of VERSED for preterm and term infants includes amounts of benzyl alcohol well below that associated with toxicity; however, the amount of benzyl alcohol at which toxicity may occur is not known. If the patient requires more than the recommended dosages or other medications containing this preservative, the practitioner must consider the daily metabolic load of benzyl alcohol from these combined sources.

PRECAUTIONS

General: Intravenous doses of VERSED should be decreased for elderly and for debilitated patients (see WARNINGS and DOSAGE AND ADMINISTRATION). These patients will also probably take longer to recover completely after VERSED administration for the induction of anesthesia.

VERSED does not protect against the increase in intracranial pressure or against the heart rate rise and/or blood pressure rise associated with endotracheal intubation under light general anesthesia.

Use With Other CNS Depressants: The efficacy and safety of VERSED in clinical use are functions of the dose administered, the clinical status of the individual patient, and the use of concomitant medications capable of depressing the CNS. Anticipated effects range from mild sedation to deep levels of sedation virtually equivalent to a state of general anesthesia where the patient may require external support of vital functions. Care must be taken to individualize and carefully titrate the dose of VERSED to the patient's underlying medical/surgical conditions, administer to the desired effect being certain to wait an adequate time for peak CNS effects of both VERSED and concomitant medications, and have the personnel and size-appropriate equipment and facilities available for monitoring and intervention (see Boxed WARNING, WARNINGS and DOSAGE AND ADMINISTRATION). Practitioners administering VERSED must have the skills necessary to manage reasonably foreseeable adverse effects, particularly skills in airway management. For information regarding withdrawal (see DRUG ABUSE AND DEPENDENCE).

Information for Patients: To assure safe and effective use of benzodiazepines, the following information and instructions should be communicated to the patient when appropriate:

1. Inform your physician about any alcohol consumption and medicine you are now taking, especially blood pressure medication and antibiotics, including drugs you buy without a prescription. Alcohol has an increased effect when consumed with benzodiazepines; therefore, caution should be exercised regarding simultaneous ingestion of alcohol during benzodiazepine treatment.
2. Inform your physician if you are pregnant or are planning to become pregnant.
3. Inform your physician if you are nursing.
4. Patients should be informed of the pharmacological effects of VERSED, such as sedation and amnesia, which in some patients may be profound. The decision as to when patients who have received injectable VERSED, particularly on an outpatient basis, may again engage in activities requiring complete mental alertness, operate hazardous machinery or drive a motor vehicle must be individualized.
5. Patients receiving continuous infusion of midazolam in critical care settings over an extended period of time, may experience symptoms of withdrawal following abrupt discontinuation.

Drug Interactions: The sedative effect of intravenous VERSED is accentuated by any concomitantly administered medication, which depresses the central nervous system, particularly narcotics (eg, morphine, meperidine and fentanyl) and also secobarbital and droperidol. Consequently, the dosage of VERSED should be adjusted according to the type and amount of concomitant medications administered and the desired clinical response (see DOSAGE AND ADMINISTRATION).

Caution is advised when midazolam is administered concomitantly with drugs that are known to inhibit the P450 3A4 enzyme system such as cimetidine (not ranitidine), erythromycin, diltiazem, verapamil, ketoconazole and itraconazole. These drug interactions may result in prolonged sedation due to a decrease in plasma clearance of midazolam.

The effect of single oral doses of 800 mg cimetidine and 300 mg ranitidine on steady-state concentrations of midazolam was examined in a randomized crossover study (n=8). Cimetidine increased the mean midazolam steady-state concentration from 57 to 71 ng/mL. Ranitidine increased the mean steady-state concentration to 62 ng/mL. No change in choice reaction time or sedation index was detected after dosing with the H2 receptor antagonists.

In a placebo-controlled study, erythromycin administered as a 500 mg dose, tid, for 1 week (n=6), reduced the clearance of midazolam following a single 0.5 mg/kg IV dose. The half-life was approximately doubled.

The effects of diltiazem (60 mg tid) and verapamil (80 mg tid) on the pharmacokinetics and pharmacodynamics of midazolam were investigated in a three-way crossover study (n=9). The half-life of midazolam increased from 5 to 7 hours when midazolam was taken in conjunction with verapamil or diltiazem. No interaction was observed in healthy subjects between midazolam and nifedipine.

A moderate reduction in induction dosage requirements of thiopental (about 15%) has been noted following use of intramuscular VERSED for premedication in adults.

The intravenous administration of VERSED decreases the minimum alveolar concentration (MAC) of halothane required for general anesthesia. This decrease correlates with the dose of VERSED administered; no similar studies have been carried out in pediatric patients but there is no scientific reason to expect that pediatric patients would respond differently than adults.

Although the possibility of minor interactive effects has not been fully studied, VERSED and pancuronium have been used together in patients without noting clinically significant changes in dosage, onset or duration in adults. VERSED does not protect against the characteristic circulatory changes noted after administration of succinylcholine or pancuronium and does not protect against the increased intracranial pressure noted following administration of succinylcholine. VERSED does not cause a clinically significant change in dosage, onset or duration of a single intubating dose of succinylcholine; no similar studies have been carried out in pediatric patients but there is no scientific reason to expect that pediatric patients would respond differently than adults.

No significant adverse interactions with commonly used premedications or drugs used during anesthesia and surgery (including atropine, scopolamine, glycopyrrolate, diazepam, hydroxyzine, d-tubocurarine, succinylcholine and other nondepolarizing muscle relaxants) or topical local anesthetics (including lidocaine, dyclonine HCl and Cetacaine) have been observed in adults or pediatric patients. In neonates, however, severe hypotension has been reported with concomitant administration of fentanyl. This effect has been observed in neonates on an infusion of midazolam who received a rapid injection of fentanyl and in patients on an infusion of fentanyl who have received a rapid injection of midazolam.

Drug/Laboratory Test Interactions: Midazolam has not been shown to interfere with results obtained in clinical laboratory tests.

Carcinogenesis, Mutagenesis and Impairment of Fertility:
Carcinogenesis: Midazolam maleate was administered with diet in mice and rats for 2 years at dosages of 1, 9 and 80 mg/kg/day. In female mice in the highest dose group there was a marked increase in the incidence of hepatic tumors. In high-dose male rats there was a small but statistically significant increase in benign thyroid follicular cell tumors. Dosages of 9 mg/kg/day of midazolam maleate (25 times a human dose of 0.35 mg/kg) do not increase the incidence of tumors. The pathogenesis of induction of these tumors is not known. These tumors were found after chronic administration, whereas human use will ordinarily be of single or several doses.

Mutagenesis: Midazolam did not have mutagenic activity in *Salmonella typhimurium* (5 bacterial strains), Chinese hamster lung cells (V79), human lymphocytes or in the micronucleus test in mice.

Impairment of Fertility: A reproduction study in male and female rats did not show any impairment of fertility at dosages up to 10 times the human IV dose of 0.35 mg/kg.

Pregnancy: *Teratogenic Effects:* Pregnancy Category D (see WARNINGS).

Segment II teratology studies, performed with midazolam maleate injectable in rabbits and rats at 5 and 10 times the human dose of 0.35 mg/kg, did not show evidence of teratogenicity.

Nonteratogenic Effects: Studies in rats showed no adverse effects on reproductive parameters during gestation and lactation. Dosages tested were approximately 10 times the human dose of 0.35 mg/kg.

Labor and Delivery: In humans, measurable levels of midazolam were found in maternal venous serum, umbilical venous and arterial serum and amniotic fluid, indicating placental transfer of the drug. Following intramuscular administration of 0.05 mg/kg of midazolam, both the venous and the umbilical arterial serum concentrations were lower than maternal concentrations.

The use of injectable VERSED in obstetrics has not been evaluated in clinical studies. Because midazolam is transferred transplacentally and because other benzodiazepines given in the last weeks of pregnancy have resulted in neonatal CNS depression, VERSED is not recommended for obstetrical use.

Nursing Mothers: Midazolam is excreted in human milk. Caution should be exercised when VERSED is administered to a nursing woman.

Pediatric Use: The safety and efficacy of VERSED for sedation/anxiolysis/amnesia following single dose intramuscular administration, intravenously by intermittent injections and continuous infusion have been established in pediatric and neonatal patients. For specific safety monitoring and dosage guidelines (see Boxed WARNING, CLINICAL PHARMACOLOGY, INDICATIONS, WARNINGS, PRECAUTIONS, ADVERSE REACTIONS, OVERDOSAGE and DOSAGE AND ADMINISTRATION). UNLIKE ADULT PATIENTS, PEDIATRIC PATIENTS GENERALLY RECEIVE

INCREMENTS OF VERSED ON A MG/KG BASIS. As a group, pediatric patients generally require higher dosages of VERSED (mg/kg) than do adults. Younger (less than six years) pediatric patients may require higher dosages (mg/kg) than older pediatric patients, and may require closer monitoring. In obese PEDIATRIC PATIENTS, the dose should be calculated based on ideal body weight. When VERSED is given in conjunction with opioids or other sedatives, the potential for respiratory depression, airway obstruction, or hypoventilation is increased. The health care practitioner who uses this medication in pediatric patients should be aware of and follow accepted professional guidelines for pediatric sedation appropriate to their situation. VERSED should not be administered by rapid injection in the neonatal population. Severe hypotension and seizures have been reported following rapid IV administration, particularly with concomitant use of fentanyl.

ADVERSE REACTIONS

See WARNINGS concerning serious cardiorespiratory events and possible paradoxical reactions. Fluctuations in vital signs were the most frequently seen findings following parenteral administration of VERSED in adults and included decreased tidal volume and/or respiratory rate decrease (23.3% of patients following IV and 10.8% of patients following IM administration) and apnea (15.4% of patients following IV administration), as well as variations in blood pressure and pulse rate. The majority of serious adverse effects, particularly those associated with oxygenation and ventilation, have been reported when VERSED is administered with other medications capable of depressing the central nervous system. **The incidence of such events is higher in patients undergoing procedures involving the airway without the protective effect of an endotracheal tube (eg, upper endoscopy and dental procedures).**

Adults: The following additional adverse reactions were reported after intramuscular administration:

headache (1.3%)	*Local effects at IM Injection site*
	pain (3.7%)
	induration (0.5%)
	redness (0.5%)
	muscle stiffness (0.3%)

Administration of IM VERSED to elderly and/or higher risk surgical patients has been associated with rare reports of death under circumstances compatible with cardiorespiratory depression. In most of these cases, the patients also received other central nervous system depressants capable of depressing respiration, especially narcotics (see DOSAGE AND ADMINISTRATION).

The following additional adverse reactions were reported subsequent to intravenous administration as a single sedative/anxiolytic/amnestic agent in adult patients:

hiccoughs (3.9%)	*Local effects at the IV site*
nausea (2.8%)	tenderness (5.6%)
vomiting (2.6%)	pain during injection (5.0%)
coughing (1.3%)	redness (2.6%)
"oversedation" (1.6%)	induration (1.7%)
headache (1.5%)	phlebitis (0.4%)
drowsiness (1.2%)	

Pediatric Patients: The following adverse events related to the use of IV VERSED in pediatric patients were reported in the medical literature: desaturation 4.6%, apnea 2.8%, hypotension 2.7%, paradoxical reactions 2.0%, hiccough 1.2%, seizure-like activity 1.1% and nystagmus 1.1%. The majority of airway-related events occurred in patients receiving other CNS depressing medications and in patients where VERSED was not used as a single sedating agent.

Neonates: For information concerning hypotensive episodes and seizures following the administration of VERSED to neonates (see Boxed WARNING, CONTRAINDICATIONS, WARNINGS and PRECAUTIONS).

Other adverse experiences, observed mainly following IV injection as a single sedative/anxiolytic/amnesia agent and occurring at an incidence of <1.0% in adult and pediatric patients, are as follows:

Respiratory: Laryngospasm, bronchospasm, dyspnea, hyperventilation, wheezing, shallow respirations, airway obstruction, tachypnea

Cardiovascular: Bigeminy, premature ventricular contractions, vasovagal episode, bradycardia, tachycardia, nodal rhythm

Gastrointestinal: Acid taste, excessive salivation, retching

CNS/Neuromuscular: Retrograde amnesia, euphoria, hallucination, confusion, argumentativeness, nervousness, anxiety, grogginess, restlessness, emergence delirium or agitation, prolonged emergence from anesthesia, dreaming during emergence, sleep disturbance, insomnia, nightmares, athetoid movements, seizure-like activity, ataxia, dizziness, dysphoria, slurred speech, dysphonia, paresthesia

Special Senses: Blurred vision, diplopia, nystagmus, pinpoint pupils, cyclic movements of eyelids, visual disturbance, difficulty focusing eyes, ears blocked, loss of balance, light-headedness

Integumentary: Hive-like elevation at injection site, swelling or feeling of burning, warmth or coldness at injection site

Hypersensitivity: Allergic reactions including anaphylactoid reactions, hives, rash, pruritus

Miscellaneous: Yawning, lethargy, chills, weakness, toothache, faint feeling, hematoma

DRUG ABUSE AND DEPENDENCE

Midazolam is subject to Schedule IV control under the Controlled Substances Act of 1970.

Midazolam was actively self-administered in primate models used to assess the positive reinforcing effects of psychoactive drugs.

Midazolam produced physical dependence of a mild to moderate intensity in cynomolgus monkeys after 5 to 10 weeks of administration. Available data concerning the drug abuse and dependence potential of midazolam suggest that its abuse potential is at least equivalent to that of diazepam. Withdrawal symptoms, similar in character to those noted with barbiturates and alcohol (convulsions, hallucinations, tremor, abdominal and muscle cramps, vomiting and sweating), have occurred following abrupt discontinuation of benzodiazepines, including midazolam. Abdominal distention, nausea, vomiting, and tachycardia are prominent symptoms of withdrawal in infants. The more severe withdrawal symptoms have usually been limited to those patients who had received excessive doses over an extended period of time. Generally milder withdrawal symptoms (eg, dysphoria and insomnia) have been reported following abrupt discontinuance of benzodiazepines taken continuously at therapeutic levels for several months. Consequently, after extended therapy, abrupt discontinuation should generally be avoided and a gradual dosage tapering schedule followed. There is no consensus in the medical literature regarding tapering schedules; therefore, practitioners are advised to individualize therapy to meet patient's needs. In some case reports, patients who have had severe withdrawal reactions due to abrupt discontinuation of high-dose long-term midazolam, have been successfully weaned off of midazolam over a period of several days.

OVERDOSAGE

The manifestations of VERSED overdosage reported are similar to those observed with other benzodiazepines, including sedation, somnolence, confusion, impaired coordination, diminished reflexes, coma and untoward effects on vital signs. No evidence of specific organ toxicity from VERSED overdosage has been reported.

Treatment of Overdosage: Treatment of injectable VERSED overdosage is the same as that followed for overdosage with other benzodiazepines. Respiration, pulse rate and blood pressure should be monitored and general supportive measures should be employed. Attention should be given to the maintenance of a patent airway and support of ventilation, including administration of oxygen. An intravenous infusion should be started. Should hypotension develop, treatment may include intravenous fluid therapy, repositioning, judicious use of vasopressors appropriate to the clinical situation, if indicated, and other appropriate countermeasures. There is no information as to whether peritoneal dialysis, forced diuresis or hemodialysis are of any value in the treatment of midazolam overdosage.

Flumazenil, a specific benzodiazepine-receptor antagonist, is indicated for the complete or partial reversal of the sedative effects of benzodiazepines and may be used in situations when an overdose with a benzodiazepine is known or suspected. There are anecdotal reports of reversal of adverse hemodynamic responses associated with VERSED following administration of flumazenil to pediatric patients. Prior to the administration of flumazenil, necessary measures should be instituted to secure the airway, assure adequate ventilation, and establish adequate intravenous access. Flumazenil is intended as an adjunct to, not as a substitute for, proper management of benzodiazepine overdose. Patients treated with flumazenil should be monitored for resedation, respiratory depression and other residual benzodiazepine effects for an appropriate period after treatment. **Flumazenil will only reverse benzodiazepine-induced effects but will not reverse the effects of other concomitant medications.** The reversal of benzodiazepine effects may be associated with the onset of seizures in certain high-risk patients. **The prescriber should be aware of a risk of seizure in association with flumazenil treatment, particularly in long-term benzodiazepine users and in cyclic antidepressant overdose.** The complete flumazenil package insert, including CONTRAINDICATIONS, WARNINGS and PRECAUTIONS, should be consulted prior to use.

DOSAGE AND ADMINISTRATION

VERSED is a potent sedative agent that requires slow administration and individualization of dosage. Clinical experience has shown VERSED to be 3 to 4 times as potent per mg as diazepam. BECAUSE SERIOUS AND LIFE-THREATENING CARDIORESPIRATORY ADVERSE EVENTS HAVE BEEN REPORTED, PROVISION FOR MONITORING, DETECTION AND CORRECTION OF THESE REACTIONS MUST BE MADE FOR EVERY PATIENT TO WHOM VERSED INJECTION IS ADMINISTERED, REGARDLESS OF AGE OR HEALTH STATUS. Excessive single doses or rapid intrave-

nous administration may result in respiratory depression, airway obstruction and/or arrest. The potential for these latter effects is increased in debilitated patients, those receiving concomitant medications capable of depressing the CNS, and patients without an endotracheal tube but undergoing a procedure involving the upper airway such as endoscopy or dental (see Boxed WARNING and WARNINGS).

Reactions such as agitation, involuntary movements, hyperactivity and combativeness have been reported in adult and pediatric patients. Should such reactions occur, caution should be exercised before continuing administration of VERSED (see WARNINGS).

VERSED should only be administered IM or IV (see WARNINGS).

Care should be taken to avoid intra-arterial injection or extravasation (see WARNINGS).

VERSED Injection may be mixed in the same syringe with the following frequently used premedications: morphine sulfate, meperidine, atropine sulfate or scopolamine. VERSED, at a concentration of 0.5 mg/mL, is compatible with 5% dextrose in water and 0.9% sodium chloride for up to 24 hours and with lactated Ringer's solution for up to 4 hours. Both the 1 mg/mL and 5 mg/mL formulations of VERSED may be diluted with 0.9% sodium chloride or 5% dextrose in water.

MONITORING: Patient response to sedative agents, and resultant respiratory status, is variable. Regardless of the intended level of sedation or route of administration, sedation is a continuum; a patient may move easily from light to deep sedation, with potential loss of protective reflexes. This is especially true in pediatric patients. Sedative doses should be individually titrated, taking into account patient age, clinical status and concomitant use of other CNS depressants. Continuous monitoring of respiratory and cardiac function is required (ie, pulse oximetry).

Adults and Pediatrics: Sedation guidelines recommend a careful presedation history to determine how a patient's underlying medical conditions or concomitant medications might affect their response to sedation/analgesia as well as a physical examination including a focused examination of the airway for abnormalities. Further recommendations include appropriate presedation fasting.

Titration to effect with multiple small doses is essential for safe administration. It should be noted that adequate time to achieve peak central nervous system effect (3 to 5 minutes) for midazolam should be allowed between doses to minimize the potential for oversedation. Sufficient time must elapse between doses of concomitant sedative medications to allow the effect of each dose to be assessed before subsequent drug administration. This is an important consideration for all patients who receive intravenous VERSED.

Immediate availability of resuscitative drugs and *age- and size-appropriate* equipment and personnel trained in their use and skilled in airway management should be assured (see WARNINGS).

Pediatrics: For deeply sedated pediatric patients a dedicated individual, other than the practitioner performing the procedure, should monitor the patient throughout the procedure.

Intravenous access is not thought to be necessary for all pediatric patients sedated for a diagnostic or therapeutic procedure because in some cases the difficulty of gaining IV access would defeat the purpose of sedating the child; rather, emphasis should be placed upon having the intravenous equipment available and a practitioner skilled in establishing vascular access in pediatric patients immediately available.

USUAL ADULT DOSE

INTRAMUSCULARLY

For preoperative sedation/anxiolysis/amnesia (induction of sleepiness or drowsiness and relief of apprehension and to impair memory of perioperative events).	The recommended premedication dose of VERSED for good risk (ASA Physical Status I & II) adult patients below the age of 60 years is 0.07 to 0.08 mg/kg IM (approximately 5 mg IM) administered up to 1 hour before surgery.
For intramuscular use, VERSED should be injected deep in a large muscle mass.	The dose must be individualized and reduced when IM VERSED is administered to patients with chronic obstructive pulmonary disease, other higher risk surgical patients, patients 60 or more years of age, and patients who have received concomitant narcotics or other CNS depressants (see ADVERSE REACTIONS). In a study of patients 60 years or older, who did not receive

Versed—Cont.

concomitant administration of narcotics, 2 to 3 mg (0.02 to 0.05 mg/kg) of VERSED produced adequate sedation during the preoperative period. The dose of 1 mg IM VERSED may suffice for some older patients if the anticipated intensity and duration of sedation is less critical. As with any potential respiratory depressant, these patients require observation for signs of cardiorespiratory depression after receiving IM VERSED. Onset is within 15 minutes, peaking at 30 to 60 minutes. It can be administered concomitantly with atropine sulfate or scopolamine hydrochloride and reduced doses of narcotics.

INTRAVENOUSLY

Sedation/anxiolysis/amnesia for procedures (see INDICATIONS): Narcotic premedication results in less variability in patient response and a reduction in dosage of VERSED. For peroral procedures, the use of an appropriate topical anesthetic is recommended. For bronchoscopic procedures, the use of narcotic premedication is recommended.

VERSED 1 mg/mL formulation is recommended for sedation/anxiolysis/ amnesia for procedures to facilitate slower injection. Both the 1 mg/mL and the 5 mg/mL formulations may be diluted with 0.9% sodium chloride or 5% dextrose in water.

When used for sedation/ anxiolysis/amnesia for a procedure, dosage must be individualized and titrated. VERSED should always be titrated slowly; administer over at least 2 minutes and allow an additional 2 or more minutes to fully evaluate the sedative effect. Individual response will vary with age, physical status and concomitant medications, but may also vary independent of these factors. (see WARNINGS concerning cardiac/respiratory arrest/ airway obstruction/ hypoventilation.)

1. *Healthy Adults Below the Age of 60:* Titrate slowly to the desired effect (eg, the initiation of slurred speech). Some patients may respond to as little as 1 mg. No more than 2.5 mg should be given over a period of at least 2 minutes. Wait an additional 2 or more minutes to fully evaluate the sedative effect. If further titration is necessary, continue to titrate, using small increments, to the appropriate level of sedation. Wait an additional 2 or more minutes after each increment to fully evaluate the sedative effect. A total dose greater than 5 mg is not usually necessary to reach the desired endpoint. If narcotic premedication or other CNS depressants are used, patients will require approximately 30% less VERSED than unpremedicated patients.

2. *Patients Age 60 or Older, and Debilitated or Chronically Ill Patients:* Because the danger of hypoventilation, airway obstruction, or apnea is greater in elderly patients and those with chronic disease states or decreased pulmonary reserve, and because the peak effect may take longer in these patients, increments should be smaller and the rate of injection slower. Titrate slowly to the desired effect (eg, the initiation of slurred speech). Some patients may respond to as little as 1 mg. No more than 1.5 mg should be given over a period of no less than 2 minutes. Wait an additional 2 or more minutes to fully evaluate the sedative effect. If additional titration is necessary, it should be given at a rate of no more than 1 mg over a period of 2 minutes, waiting an additional 2 or more minutes each time to fully evaluate the sedative effect. Total doses greater than 3.5 mg are not usually necessary. If concomitant CNS depressant premedications are used in these patients, they will require at least 50% less VERSED than healthy young unpremedicated patients.

3. *Maintenance Dose:* Additional doses to maintain the desired level of sedation may be given in increments of 25% of the dose used to first reach the sedative endpoint, but again only by slow titration, especially in the elderly and chronically ill or debilitated patient. These additional doses should be given only after a thorough clinical evaluation clearly indicates the need for additional sedation.

Induction of Anesthesia: For induction of general anesthesia, before administration of other anesthetic agents.

Individual response to the drug is variable, particularly when a narcotic premedication is not used. The dosage should be titrated to the desired effect according to the patient's age and clinical status. When VERSED is used before other intravenous agents for induction of anesthesia, the initial dose of each agent may be significantly reduced, at times to as low as 25% of the usual initial dose of the individual agents.
Unpremedicated Patients: In the absence of premedication, an average adult under the age of 55 years will usually require an initial dose of 0.3 to 0.35 mg/kg for induction, administered over 20 to 30 seconds and allowing 2 minutes for effect. If needed to complete induction, increments of approximately 25% of the patient's initial dose may be used; induction may instead be completed with inhalational anesthetics. In resistant cases, up to 0.6 mg/kg total dose may be used for induction, but such larger doses may prolong recovery.

Unpremedicated patients over the age of 55 years usually require less VERSED for induction; an initial dose of 0.3 mg/kg is recommended. Unpremedicated patients with severe systemic disease or other debilitation usually require less VERSED for induction. An initial dose of 0.2 to 0.25 mg/kg will usually suffice; in some cases, as little as 0.15 mg/kg may suffice.
Premedicated Patients: When the patient has received sedative or narcotic premedication, particularly narcotic premedication, the range of recommended doses is 0.15 to 0.35 mg/kg. In average adults below the age of 55 years, a dose of 0.25 mg/kg, administered over 20 to 30 seconds and allowing 2 minutes for effect, will usually suffice. The initial dose of 0.2 mg/kg is recommended for good risk (ASA I & II) surgical patients over the age of 55 years. In some patients with severe systemic disease or debilitation, as little as 0.15 mg/kg may suffice. Narcotic premedication frequently used during clinical trials included fentanyl (1.5 to 2 µg/kg IV, administered 5 minutes before induction), morphine (dosage individualized, up to 0.15 mg/kg IM), and meperidine (dosage individualized, up to 1 mg/kg IM). Sedative premedications were hydroxyzine pamoate (100 mg orally) and sodium secobarbital (200 mg orally). Except for intravenous fentanyl, administered 5 minutes before induction, all other premedications should be administered approximately 1 hour prior to the time anticipated for VERSED induction.

Injectable VERSED can also be used during maintenance of anesthesia, for surgical procedures, as a component of balanced anesthesia. Effective narcotic premedication is especially recommended in such cases.

Incremental injections of approximately 25% of the induction dose should be given in response to signs of lightening of anesthesia and repeated as necessary.

CONTINUOUS INFUSION

For continuous infusion, VERSED 5 mg/mL formulation is recommended diluted to a concentration of 0.5 mg/mL with 0.9% sodium chloride or 5% dextrose in water.

Usual Adult Dose: If a loading dose is necessary to rapidly initiate sedation, 0.01 to 0.05 mg/kg (approximately 0.5 to 4.0 mg for a typical adult) may be given slowly or infused over several minutes. This dose may be repeated at 10 to 15 minute intervals until adequate sedation is achieved. For maintenance of sedation, the usual initial infusion rate is 0.02 to 0.10 mg/kg/hr (1 to 7 mg/hr). Higher loading or maintenance infusion rates may occasionally be required in some patients. The lowest recommended doses should be used in patients with residual effects from anesthetic drugs, or in those

concurrently receiving other sedatives or opioids. Individual response to VERSED is variable. The infusion rate should be titrated to the desired level of sedation, taking into account the patient's age, clinical status and current medications. In general, VERSED should be infused at the lowest rate that produces the desired level of sedation. Assessment of sedation should be performed at regular intervals and the VERSED infusion rate adjusted up or down by 25% to 50% of the initial infusion rate so as to assure adequate titration of sedation level. Larger adjustments or even a small incremental dose may be necessary if rapid changes in the level of sedation are indicated. In addition, the infusion rate should be decreased by 10% to 25% every few hours to find the minimum effective infusion rate. Finding the minimum effective infusion rate decreases the potential accumulation of midazolam and provides for the most rapid recovery once the infusion is terminated. Patients who exhibit agitation, hypertension, or tachycardia in response to noxious stimulation, but who are otherwise adequately sedated, may benefit from concurrent administration of an opioid analgesic. Addition of an opioid will generally reduce the minimum effective VERSED infusion rate.

OBSERVER'S ASSESSMENT OF ALERTNESS/SEDATION (OAA/S)

Assessment Categories

Responsiveness	Speech	Facial Expression	Eyes	Composite Score
Responds readily to name spoken in normal tone	normal	normal	clear, no ptosis	5 (alert)
Lethargic response to name spoken in normal tone	mild slowing or thickening	mild relaxation	glazed or mild ptosis (less than half the eye)	4
Responds only after name is called loudly and/or repeatedly	slurring or prominent slowing	marked relaxation (slack jaw)	glazed and marked ptosis (half the eye or more)	3
Responds only after mild prodding or shaking	few recognizable words	—	—	2
Does not respond to mild prodding or shaking	—	—	—	1 (deep sleep)

FREQUENCY OF OBSERVER'S ASSESSMENT OF ALERTNESS/SEDATION COMPOSITE SCORES IN ONE STUDY OF PEDIATRIC PATIENTS UNDERGOING PROCEDURES WITH INTRAVENOUS MIDAZOLAM FOR SEDATION

Age Range (years)	n	OAA/S Score				
		1 (deep sleep)	2	3	4	5 (alert)
1–2	16	6 (38%)	4 (25%)	3 (19%)	3 (19%)	0
>2–5	22	9 (41%)	5 (23%)	8 (36%)	0	0
>5–12	34	1 (3%)	6 (18%)	22 (65%)	5 (15%)	0
>12–17	18	0	4 (22%)	14 (78%)	0	0
Total (1–17)	90	16 (18%)	19 (21%)	47 (52%)	8 (9%)	0

PEDIATRIC PATIENTS

UNLIKE ADULT PATIENTS, PEDIATRIC PATIENTS GENERALLY RECEIVE INCREMENTS OF VERSED ON A MG/KG BASIS. As a group, pediatric patients generally require higher dosages of VERSED (mg/kg) than do adults. Younger (less than six years) pediatric patients may require higher dosages (mg/kg) than older pediatric patients, and may require close monitoring (see tables below). In obese PEDIATRIC PATIENTS, the dose should be calculated based on ideal body weight. When VERSED is given in conjunction with opioids or other sedatives, the potential for respiratory depression, airway obstruction, or hypoventilation is increased. For appropriate patient monitoring (see Boxed WARNING, WARNINGS, *MONITORING* subsection of DOSAGE AND ADMINISTRATION). The health care practitioner who uses this medication in pediatric patients should be aware of and follow accepted professional guidelines for pediatric sedation appropriate to their situation.

[See table above]

INTRAMUSCULARLY

For sedation/anxiolysis/amnesia prior to anesthesia or for procedures, intramuscular VERSED can be used to sedate pediatric patients to faciliate less traumatic insertion of an intravenous catheter for titration of additional medication.

INTRAVENOUSLY BY INTERMITTENT INJECTION

For sedation/anxiolysis/amnesia prior to and during procedures or prior to anesthesia.

USUAL PEDIATRIC DOSE (NON-NEONATAL)

Sedation after intramuscular VERSED is age and dose dependent: higher doses may result in deeper and more prolonged sedation. Doses of 0.1 to 0.15 mg/kg are usually effective and do not prolong emergence from general anesthesia. For more anxious patients, doses up to 0.5 mg/kg have been used. Although not systematically studied, the total dose usually does not exceed 10 mg. If VERSED is given with an opioid, the initial dose of each must be reduced.

USUAL PEDIATRIC DOSE (NON-NEONATAL)

It should be recognized that the depth of sedation/anxiolysis needed for pediatric patients depends on the type of procedure to be performed. For example, simple light sedation/anxiolysis in the preoperative period is quite different from the deep sedation and analgesia required for an endoscopic procedure in a child. For this reason, there is a broad range of dosage. For all pediatric patients, regardless of the indications for sedation/anxiolysis, it is vital to titrate VERSED and other concomitant medications slowly to the desired clinical effect. The initial dose of VERSED should be administered over 2 to 3 minutes. Since VERSED is water soluble, it takes approximately three times longer than diazepam to achieve peak EEG effects, therefore one must wait an additional 2 to 3 minutes to fully evaluate the sedative effect before initiating a

procedure or repeating a dose. If further sedation is necessary, continue to titrate with small increments until the appropriate level of sedation is achieved. If other medications capable of depressing the CNS are coadministered, the peak effect of those concomitant medications must be considered and the dose of VERSED adjusted. The importance of drug titration to effect is vital to the safe sedation/anxlysis of the pediatric patient. The total dose of VERSED will depend on patient response, the type and duration of the procedure, as well as the type and dose of concomitant medications.

1. *Pediatric Patients Less Than 6 Months of Age:* Limited information is available in non-intubated pediatric patients less than 6 months of age. It is uncertain when the patient transfers from neonatal physiology to pediatric physiology, therefore the dosing recommendations are unclear. Pediatric patients less than 6 months of age are particularly vulnerable to airway obstruction and hypoventilation, therefore titration with small increments to clinical effect and careful monitoring are essential.

2. *Pediatric Patients 6 Months to 5 Years of Age:* Initial dose 0.05 to 0.1 mg/kg; total dose up to 0.6 mg/kg may be necessary to reach the desired endpoint but usually does not exceed 6 mg. Prolonged sedation and risk of

Versed—Cont.

hypoventilation may be associated with the higher doses.

3. *Pediatric Patients 6 to 12 Years of Age:* Initial dose 0.025 to 0.05 mg/kg; total dose up to 0.4 mg/kg may be needed to reach the desired endpoint but usually does not exceed 10 mg. Prolonged sedation and risk of hypoventilation may be associated with the higher doses.

4. *Pediatric Patients 12 to 16 Years of Age:* Should be dosed as adults. Prolonged sedation may be associated with higher doses; some patients in this age range will require higher than recommended adult doses but the total dose usually does not exceed 10 mg. The dose of VERSED must be reduced in patients premedicated with opioid or other sedative agents including VERSED. Higher risk or debilitated patients may require lower dosages whether or not concomitant sedating medications have been administered (see WARNINGS).

CONTINUOUS INTRAVENOUS INFUSION
For sedation/anxiolysis/amnesia in critical care settings.

USUAL PEDIATRIC DOSE (NON-NEONATAL)
To initiate sedation, an intravenous loading dose of 0.05 to 0.2 mg/kg administered over at least 2 to 3 minutes can be used to establish the desired clinical effect IN PATIENTS WHOSE TRACHEA IS INTUBATED. (VERSED should not be administered as a rapid intravenous dose.) This loading dose may be followed by a continuous intravenous infusion to maintain the effect. An infusion of VERSED has been used in patients whose trachea was intubated but who were allowed to breathe spontaneously. Assisted ventilation is recommended for pediatric patients who are receiving other central nervous system depressant medications such as opioids. Based on pharmacokinetic parameters and reported clinical experience, continuous intravenous infusions of VERSED should be initiated at a rate of 0.06 to 0.12 mg/kg/hr (1 to 2 µg/kg/min). The rate of infusion can be increased or decreased (generally by 25% of the initial or subsequent infusion rate) as required, or supplemental intravenous doses of VERSED can be administered to increase or maintain the desired effect. Frequent assessment at regular intervals using standard pain/sedation scales is recommended. Drug elimination may be delayed in patients receiving erythromycin and/or other P450 3A4 enzyme inhibitors (see PRECAUTIONS: *Drug*

CONTINUOUS INTRAVENOUS INFUSION
For sedation in critical care settings.

Interactions) and in patients with liver dysfunction, low cardiac output (especially those requiring inotropic support), and in neonates. Hypotension may be observed in patients who are critically ill, particularly those receiving opioids and/or when VERSED is rapidly administered. When initiating an infusion with VERSED in hemodynamically compromised patients, the usual loading dose of VERSED should be titrated in small increments and the patient monitored for hemodynamic instability (eg, hypotension). These patients are also vulnerable to the respiratory depressant effects of VERSED and require careful monitoring of respiratory rate and oxygen saturation.

USUAL NEONATAL DOSE
Based on pharmacokinetic parameters and reported clinical experience in preterm and term neonates WHOSE TRACHEA WAS INTUBATED, continuous intravenous infusions of VERSED should be initiated at a rate of 0.03 mg/kg/hr (0.5 µg/kg/min) in neonates <32 weeks and 0.06 mg/kg/hr (1 µg/kg/min) in neonates >32 weeks. Intravenous loading doses should not be used in neonates, rather the infusion may be run more rapidly for the first several hours to establish therapeutic plasma levels. The rate of infusion should be carefully and frequently reassessed, particularly after the first 24 hours so as to administer the lowest possible effective dose and reduce the potential for drug accumulation. This is particularly important because of the potential for adverse effects related to metabolism of the benzyl alcohol (see WARNINGS: *Usage in Preterm Infants and Neonates*). Hypotension may be observed in patients who are critically ill and in preterm and term infants, particularly those receiving fentanyl and/or when VERSED is administered rapidly. Due to an increased risk of apnea, extreme caution is advised when sedating preterm and former preterm patients whose trachea is not intubated.

Note: Parenteral drug products should be inspected visually for particulate matter and discoloration prior to administration, whenever solution and container permit.

HOW SUPPLIED
Package configurations containing midazolam hydrochloride equivalent to **5 mg midazolam/mL**:
1-mL vials (5 mg) — boxes of 10 (NDC 0004-1974-01);* 2-mL vials (10 mg) — boxes of 10 (NDC 0004-1973-01);† 5-mL vials (25 mg) — boxes of 10 (NDC 0004-1975-01);† 10-mL vials (50 mg) — boxes of 10 (NDC 0004-1946-01);† 2-mL Tel-E-Ject® disposable syringes (10 mg) box of 1 (NDC 0004-1947-09); — package of 10 boxes (NDC 0004-1947-01).*
Package configurations containing midazolam hydrochloride equivalent to **1 mg midazolam/mL**:
2-mL vials (2 mg) — boxes of 10 (NDC 0004-1998-06);† 5-mL vials (5 mg) — boxes of 10 (NDC 0004-1999-01);† 10-mL vials (10 mg) — boxes of 10 (NDC 0004-2000-06).†
Store at 59° to 86°F (15° to 30° C).

*Manufactured by Hoffmann-LaRoche Inc., Nutley, New Jersey 07110. Distributed by Roche Laboratories Inc., Nutley, New Jersey 07110.
†Manufactured by Roche Pharma, Inc., Humacao, Puerto Rico 00791 or Hoffmann-LaRoche Inc., Nutley, New Jersey 07110. Distributed by Roche Laboratories Inc., Nutley, New Jersey 07110.

Revised: June 1998

VESANOID®
[ves 'ă noid]
(tretinoin)
CAPSULES

R

The following text is complete prescribing information based on official labeling in effect June 1998.

> ### WARNINGS:
>
> 1. *Experienced Physician and Institution:* Patients with acute promyelocytic leukemia (APL) are at high risk in general and can have severe adverse reactions to VESANOID (tretinoin). VESANOID should therefore be administered under the supervision of a physician who is experienced in the management of patients with acute leukemia and in a facility with laboratory and supportive services sufficient to monitor drug tolerance and protect and maintain a patient compromised by drug toxicity, including respiratory compromise. Use of VESANOID requires that the physician concludes that the possible benefit to the patient outweighs the following known adverse effects of the therapy.
>
> 2. *Retinoic Acid-APL Syndrome:* About 25% of patients with APL treated with VESANOID have experienced a syndrome called the retinoic-acid-APL (RA-APL) syndrome characterized by fever, dyspnea, weight gain, radiographic pulmonary infiltrates and pleural or pericardial effusions. This syndrome has occasionally been accompanied by impaired myocardial contractility and episodic hypotension. It has been observed with or without concomitant leukocytosis. Endotracheal intubation and mechanical ventilation have been required in some cases due to progressive hypoxemia, and several patients have expired with multiorgan failure. The syndrome generally occurs during the first month of treatment, with some cases reported following the first dose of VESANOID.
>
> The management of the syndrome has not been defined rigorously, but high-dose steroids given at the first suspicion of the RA-APL syndrome appear to reduce morbidity and mortality. At the first signs suggestive of the syndrome (unexplained fever, dyspnea and/or weight gain, abnormal chest auscultatory findings or radiographic abnormalities), high-dose steroids (dexamethasone 10 mg intravenously administered every 12 hours for 3 days or until the resolution of symptoms) should be immediately initiated, irrespective of the leukocyte count. The majority of patients do not require termination of VESANOID therapy during treatment of the RA-APL syndrome.
>
> 3. *Leukocytosis at Presentation and Rapidly Evolving Leukocytosis During VESANOID Treatment:* During VESANOID treatment about 40% of patients will develop rapidly evolving leukocytosis. Patients who present with high WBC at diagnosis (>5×10⁹/L) have an increased risk of a further rapid increase in WBC counts. Rapidly evolving leukocytosis is associated with a higher risk of life-threatening complications. If signs and symptoms of the RA-APL syndrome are present together with leukocytosis, treatment with high-dose steroids should be initiated immediately. Some investigators routinely add chemotherapy to VESANOID treatment in the case of patients presenting with a WBC count of >5×10⁹/L or in the case of a rapid increase in WBC count for patients leukopenic at start of treatment, and have reported a lower incidence of the RA-APL syndrome. Consideration could be given to adding full-dose chemotherapy (including an anthracycline if not contraindicated) to the VESANOID therapy on day 1 or 2 for patients presenting with a WBC count of >5×10⁹/L, or immediately, for patients presenting with a WBC count of <5×10⁹/L, if the WBC count reaches >6×10⁹/L by day 5, or ≥10×10⁹/L by day 10, or ≥15×10⁹/L by day 28.
>
> 4. *Teratogenic Effects. Pregnancy Category D—see WARNINGS.* There is a high risk that a severely deformed infant will result if VESANOID is administered during pregnancy. If, nonetheless, it is determined that VESANOID represents the best available treatment for a pregnant woman or a woman of childbearing potential, it must be assured that the patient has received full information and warnings of the

risk to the fetus if she were to be pregnant and of the risk of possible contraception failure and has been instructed in the need to use two reliable forms of contraception simultaneously during therapy and for 1 month following discontinuation of therapy, and has acknowledged her understanding of the need for using dual contraception, unless abstinence is the chosen method.

Within 1 week prior to the institution of VESANOID therapy, the patient should have blood or urine collected for a serum or urine pregnancy test with a sensitivity of at least 50 mIU/L. When possible VESANOID therapy should be delayed until a negative result from this test is obtained. When a delay is not possible the patient should be placed on two reliable forms of contraception. Pregnancy testing and contraception counseling should be repeated monthly throughout the period of VESANOID treatment.

DESCRIPTION

VESANOID (tretinoin) is a retinoid that induces maturation of acute promyelocytic leukemia (APL) cells in culture. It is available in a 10 mg soft gelatin capsule for oral administration. Each capsule also contains beeswax, butylated hydroxyanisole, edetate disodium, hydrogenated soybean oil flakes, hydrogenated vegetable oils and soybean oil. The gelatin capsule shell contains glycerin, yellow iron oxide, red iron oxide, titanium dioxide, methylparaben and propylparaben.

Chemically, tretinoin is all-*trans* retinoic acid and is related to retinol (Vitamin A). It is a yellow to light orange crystalline powder with a molecular weight of 300.44.

CLINICAL PHARMACOLOGY

Mechanism of Action: Tretinoin is not a cytolytic agent but instead induces cytodifferentiation and decreased proliferation of APL cells in culture and in vivo. In APL patients, tretinoin treatment produces an initial maturation of the primitive promyelocytes derived from the leukemic clone, followed by a repopulation of the bone marrow and peripheral blood by normal, polyclonal hematopoietic cells in patients achieving complete remission (CR). The exact mechanism of action of tretinoin in APL is unknown.

PHARMACOKINETICS

Tretinoin activity is primarily due to the parent drug. In human pharmacokinetics studies, orally administered drug was well absorbed into the systemic circulation, with approximately two-thirds of the administered radiolabel recovered in the urine. The terminal elimination half-life of tretinoin following initial dosing is 0.5 to 2 hours in patients with APL. There is evidence that tretinoin induces its own metabolism. Plasma tretinoin concentrations decrease on average to one-third of their day 1 values during 1 week of continuous therapy. Mean ± SD peak tretinoin concentrations decreased from 394 ± 89 to 138 ± 139 ng/mL, while area under the curve (AUC) values decreased from 537 ± 191 ng·h/mL to 249 ± 185 ng·h/mL during 45 mg/m^2 daily dosing in 7 APL patients. Increasing the dose to "correct" for this change has not increased response.

Absorption: A single 45 mg/m^2 (80 mg) oral dose to APL patients resulted in a mean ± SD peak tretinoin concentration of 347 ± 266 ng/mL. Time to reach peak concentration was between 1 and 2 hours.

Distribution: The apparent volume of distribution of tretinoin has not been determined. Tretinoin is greater than 95% bound in plasma, predominately to albumin. Plasma protein binding remains constant over the concentration range of 10 to 500 ng/mL.

Metabolism: Tretinoin metabolites have been identified in plasma and urine. Cytochrome P450 (CYP) enzymes have been implicated in the oxidative metabolism of tretinoin. Metabolites include 13-*cis* retinoic acid, 4-oxo *trans* retinoic acid, 4-oxo *cis* retinoic acid, and 4-oxo *trans* retinoic acid glucuronide. In APL patients, daily administration of a 45 mg/m^2 dose of tretinoin resulted in an approximately tenfold increase in the urinary excretion of 4-oxo *trans* retinoic acid glucuronide after 2 to 6 weeks of continuous dosing, when compared to baseline values.

Excretion: Studies with radiolabeled drug have demonstrated that after the oral administration of 2.75 and 50 mg doses of tretinoin, greater than 90% of the radioactivity was recovered in the urine and feces. Based upon data from 3 subjects, approximately 63% of radioactivity was recovered in the urine within 72 hours and 31% appeared in the feces within 6 days.

Special Populations: The pharmacokinetics of tretinoin have not been separately evaluated in women, in members of different ethnic groups, or in individuals with renal or hepatic insufficiency.

Drug-Drug Interactions: In 13 patients who had received daily doses of tretinoin for 4 consecutive weeks, administration of ketoconazole (400 to 1200 mg oral dose) 1 hour prior to the administration of the tretinoin dose on day 29 led to a 72% increase (218 ± 224 versus 375 ± 285 ng·h/mL) in tretinoin mean plasma AUC. The precise CYP system involved in these interactions has not been specified; CYP, 3A4, 2C8 and 2E have been implicated in various preliminary reports.

Clinical Studies: VESANOID has been investigated in 114 previously treated APL patients and in 67 previously untreated ("de novo") patients in one open-label, uncontrolled single investigator clinical study (Memorial Sloan-Kettering Cancer Center [MSKCC]) and in two cohorts of compassionate cases treated by multiple investigators under the auspices of the National Cancer Institute (NCI). All patients received 45 mg/m^2/day as a divided oral dose for up to 90 days or 30 days beyond the day that CR was reached. Results are shown in the following table:

[See table above]

	MSKCC		NCI Cohort 1		NCI Cohort 2	
	Relapsed	De Novo	Relapsed*	De Novo	Relapsed	De Novo†
	n=20	n=15	n=48	n=14	n=46	n=38
Complete Remission	16 (80%)	11 (73%)	24 (50%)	5 (36%)	24 (52%)	26 (68%)
Median Survival (Mo)	10.8	NR	5.8	0.5	8.8	NR
Median Follow-up (Mo)	9.9	42.9	5.6	1.2	8.0	13.1
RA-APL Syndrome	4 (20%)	5 (33%)	10 (21%)	6 (43%)	NA	NA

NR = Not Reached
NA = Not Available
* Including 9 chemorefractory patients
† Including 8 patients who received chemotherapy but failed to enter remission

The median time to CR was between 40 and 50 days (range: 2 to 120 days). Most patients in these studies received cytotoxic chemotherapy during the remission phase. These results compare to the 30% to 50% CR rate and ≤6 month median survival reported for cytotoxic chemotherapy of APL in the treatment of relapse.

Ten of 15 pediatric cases achieved CR (8 of 10 males and 2 of 5 females). There were insufficient patients of black, Hispanic or Asian derivation to estimate relative response rates in these groups, but responses were seen in each category. Responses were seen in 3 of 4 patients for whom cytogenetic analysis failed to detect the t(15;17) translocation typically seen in APL. The t(15;17) translocation results in the PML/RARα gene, which appears necessary for this disease. Molecular genetic studies were not conducted in these cases, but it is likely they represent cases with a masked translocation giving rise to PML/RARα. Responses to tretinoin have not been observed in cases in which PML/RARα fusion has been shown to be absent.

INDICATIONS AND USAGE

VESANOID (tretinoin) capsules are indicated for the induction of remission in patients with acute promyelocytic leukemia (APL), French-American-British (FAB) classification M3 (including the M3 variant), characterized by the presence of the t(15;17) translocation and/or the presence of the PML/RARα gene who are refractory to, or who have relapsed from, anthracycline chemotherapy, or for whom anthracycline-based chemotherapy is contraindicated. VESANOID is for the induction of remission only. The optimal consolidation or maintenance regimens have not been defined, but all patients should receive an accepted form of remission consolidation and/or maintenance therapy for APL after completion of induction therapy with VESANOID.

CONTRAINDICATIONS

VESANOID is contraindicated in patients with a known hypersensitivity to retinoids. VESANOID should not be given to patients who are sensitive to parabens, which are used as preservatives in the gelatin capsule.

WARNINGS

Pregnancy Category D—see boxed WARNINGS: Tretinoin has teratogenic and embryotoxic effects in mice, rats, hamsters, rabbits and pigtail monkeys, and may be expected to cause fetal harm when administered to a pregnant woman. Tretinoin causes fetal resorptions and a decrease in live fetuses in all animals studied. Gross external, soft tissue and skeletal alterations occurred at doses higher than 0.7 mg/kg/day in mice, 2 mg/kg/day in rats, 7 mg/kg/day in hamsters, and at a dose of 10 mg/kg/day, the only dose tested, in pigtail monkeys (about $^1/_{20}$, $^1/_4$, and $^1/_2$ and 4 times the human dose, respectively, on a mg/m^2 basis).

There are no adequate and well controlled studies in pregnant women. Although experience with humans administered VESANOID is extremely limited, increased spontaneous abortions and major human fetal abnormalities related to the use of other retinoids have been documented in humans.

Reported defects include abnormalities of the CNS, musculoskeletal system, external ear, eye, thymus and great vessels; and facial dysmorphia, cleft palate, and parathyroid hormone deficiency. Some of these abnormalities were fatal. Cases of IQ scores less than 85, with or without obvious CNS abnormalities, have also been reported. All fetuses exposed during pregnancy can be affected and at the present time there is no antepartum means of determining which fetuses are and are not affected.

Effective contraception must be used by all females during VESANOID therapy and for 1 month following discontinuation of therapy. Contraception must be used even when there is a history of infertility or menopause, unless a hysterectomy has been performed. Whenever contraception is required, it is recommended that two reliable forms of contraception be used simultaneously, unless abstinence is the chosen method. If pregnancy does occur during treatment, the physician and patient should discuss the desirability of continuing or terminating the pregnancy.

Patients without the t(15;17) Translocation: Initiation of therapy with VESANOID may be based on the morphological diagnosis of acute promyelocytic leukemia. Confirmation of the diagnosis of APL should be sought by detection of the t(15;17) genetic marker by cytogenetic studies. If these are negative, PML/RARα fusion should be sought using molecular diagnostic techniques. The response rate of other AML subtypes to VESANOID has not been demonstrated; therefore, patients who lack the genetic marker should be considered for alternative treatment.

Retinoic Acid-APL (RA-APL) Syndrome: In up to 25% of patients with APL treated with VESANOID, a syndrome occurs which can be fatal (see boxed WARNINGS and ADVERSE REACTIONS).

Leukocytosis at Presentation and Rapidly Evolving Leukocytosis During VESANOID Treatment: (see boxed WARNINGS).

Pseudotumor Cerebri: Retinoids, including VESANOID, have been associated with pseudotumor cerebri (benign intracranial hypertension), especially in pediatric patients. Early signs and symptoms of pseudotumor cerebri include papilledema, headache, nausea and vomiting and visual disturbances. Patients with these symptoms should be evaluated for pseudotumor cerebri, and, if present, appropriate care should be instituted in concert with neurological assessment.

Lipids: Up to 60% of patients experienced hypercholesterolemia and/or hypertriglyceridemia, which were reversible upon completion of treatment. The clinical consequences of temporary elevation of triglycerides and cholesterol are unknown, but venous thrombosis and myocardial infarction have been reported in patients who ordinarily are at low risk for such complications.

Elevated Liver Function Test Results: Elevated liver function test results occur in 50% to 60% of patients during treatment. Liver function test results should be carefully monitored during treatment and consideration be given to a temporary withdrawal of VESANOID if test results reach greater than five times the upper limit of normal values. However, the majority of these abnormalities resolve without interruption of VESANOID or after completion of treatment.

PRECAUTIONS

General: VESANOID has potentially significant toxic side effects in APL patients. Patients undergoing therapy should be closely observed for signs of respiratory compromise and/or leukocytosis (see boxed WARNINGS). Supportive care appropriate for APL patients; eg, prophylaxis for bleeding, prompt therapy for infection, should be maintained during therapy with VESANOID.

Laboratory Tests: The patient's hematologic profile, coagulation profile, liver function test results, and triglyceride and cholesterol levels should be monitored frequently.

Drug Interactions: Limited clinical data on potential drug interactions are available. As VESANOID is metabolized by the hepatic CYP system, there is a potential for alteration of pharmacokinetics parameters in patients administered concomitant medications that are also inducers or inhibitors of this system. Medications that generally induce hepatic CYP enzymes include rifampicin, glucocorticoids, phenobarbital and pentobarbital. Medications that generally inhibit hepatic CYP enzymes include ketoconazole, cimetidine, erythromycin, verapamil, diltiazem and cyclosporin. To date there are no data to suggest that co-use with these medications increases or decreases either efficacy or toxicity of VESANOID.

Effect of Food: No data on the effect of food on the absorption of VESANOID are available. The absorption of retinoids as a class has been shown to be enhanced when taken together with food.

Continued on next page

Vesanoid—Cont.

Carcinogenesis, Mutagenesis and Impairment of Fertility: No long-term carcinogenicity studies with tretinoin have been conducted. In short-term carcinogenicity studies, tretinoin at a dose of 30 mg/kg/day (about 2 times the human dose on a mg/m^2 basis) was shown to increase the rate of diethylnitrosamine (DEN)-induced mouse liver adenomas and carcinomas. Tretinoin was negative when tested in the Ames and Chinese hamster V79 cell HGPRT assays for mutagenicity. A twofold increase in the sister chromatid exchange (SCE) has been demonstrated in human diploid fibroblasts, but other chromosome aberration assays, including an in vitro assay in human peripheral lymphocytes and an in vivo mouse micronucleus assay, did not show a clastogenic or aneuploidogenic effect. Adverse effects on fertility and reproductive performance were not observed in studies conducted in rats at doses up to 5 mg/kg/day (about $^2/_3$ the human dose on a mg/m^2 basis). In a 6-week toxicology study in dogs, minimal to marked testicular degeneration, with increased numbers of immature spermatozoa, were observed at 10 mg/kg/day (about 4 times the equivalent human dose in mg/m^2).
Nursing Mothers: It is not known whether this drug is excreted in human milk. Because many drugs are excreted in human milk, and because of the potential for serious adverse reactions from VESANOID in nursing infants, mothers should discontinue nursing prior to taking this drug.
Pediatric Use: There are limited clinical data on the pediatric use of VESANOID. Of 15 pediatric patients (age range: 1 to 16 years) treated with VESANOID, the incidence of complete remission was 67%. Safety and effectiveness in pediatric patients below the age of 1 year have not been established. Some pediatric patients experience severe headache and pseudotumor cerebri, requiring analgesic treatment and lumbar puncture for relief. Increased caution is recommended in the treatment of pediatric patients. Dose reduction may be considered for pediatric patients experiencing serious and/or intolerable toxicity; however, the efficacy and safety of VESANOID at doses lower than 45 mg/m^2/day have not been evaluated in the pediatric population.

ADVERSE REACTIONS

Virtually all patients experience some drug related toxicity, especially headache, fever, weakness, and fatigue. These adverse effects are seldom permanent or irreversible nor do they usually require interruption of therapy. Some of the adverse events are common in patients with APL, including hemorrhage, infections, gastrointestinal hemorrhage, disseminated intravascular coagulation, pneumonia, septicemia, and cerebral hemorrhage. The following describes the adverse events, regardless of drug relationship, that were observed in patients treated with VESANOID.
Typical Retinoid Toxicity: The most frequently reported adverse events were similar to those described in patients taking high doses of vitamin A and included headache (86% of patients), fever (83%), skin/mucous membrane dryness (77%), bone pain (77%), nausea/vomiting (57%), rash (54%), mucositis (26%), pruritus (20%), increased sweating (20%), visual disturbances (17%), ocular disorders (17%), alopecia (14%), skin changes (14%), changed visual acuity (6%), bone inflammation (3%), visual field defects (3%).
RA-APL Syndrome: APL patients treated with VESANOID have experienced a syndrome characterized by fever, dyspnea, weight gain, radiographic pulmonary infiltrates and pleural or pericardial effusions. This syndrome has occasionally been accompanied by impaired myocardial contractility and episodic hypotension and has been observed with or without concomitant leukocytosis. Some patients have expired due to progressive hypoxemia and multiorgan failure. The syndrome generally occurs during the first month of treatment, with some cases reported following the first dose of VESANOID. The management of the syndrome has not been defined rigorously, but high-dose steroids given at the first signs of the syndrome appear to reduce morbidity and mortality. Treatment with dexamethasone, 10 mg intravenously administered every 12 hours for 3 days or until resolution of symptoms, should be initiated without delay at the first suspicion of symptoms (one or more of the following: fever, dyspnea, weight gain, abnormal chest auscultatory findings or radiographic abnormalities). Sixty percent or more of patients treated with VESANOID may require high-dose steroids because of these symptoms. The majority of patients do not require termination of VESANOID therapy during treatment of the syndrome.
Body as a Whole: General disorders related to VESANOID administration and/or associated with APL included malaise (66%), shivering (63%), hemorrhage (60%), infections (58%), peripheral edema (52%), pain (37%), chest discomfort (32%), edema (29%), disseminated intravascular coagulation (26%), weight increase (23%), injection site reactions (17%), anorexia (17%), weight decrease (17%), myalgia (14%), flank pain (9%), cellulitis (8%), face edema (6%), fluid imbalance (6%), pallor (6%), lymph disorders (6%), acidosis (3%), hypothermia (3%), ascites (3%).
Respiratory System Disorders: Respiratory system disorders were commonly reported in APL patients administered VESANOID. The majority of these events are symptoms of the RA-APL syndrome (see boxed WARNING). Respiratory system adverse events included upper respiratory tract disorders (63%), dyspnea (60%), respiratory insufficiency (26%), pleural effusion (20%), pneumonia (14%), rales (14%), expiratory wheezing (14%), lower respiratory tract disorders (9%), pulmonary infiltration (6%), bronchial asthma (3%), pulmonary edema (3%), larynx edema (3%), unspecified pulmonary disease (3%).
Ear Disorders: Ear disorders were consistently reported, with earache or feeling of fullness in the ears reported by 23% of the patients. Hearing loss and other unspecified auricular disorders were observed in 6% of patients, with infrequent (<1%) reports of irreversible hearing loss.
Gastrointestinal Disorders: GI disorders included GI hemorrhage (34%), abdominal pain (31%), other gastrointestinal disorders (26%), diarrhea (23%), constipation (17%), dyspepsia (14%), abdominal distention (11%), hepatosplenomegaly (9%), hepatitis (3%), ulcer (3%), unspecified liver disorder (3%).
Cardiovascular and Heart Rate and Rhythm Disorders: Arrhythmias (23%), flushing (23%), hypotension (14%), hypertension (11%), phlebitis (11%), cardiac failure (6%) and for 3% of patients: cardiac arrest, myocardial infarction, enlarged heart, heart murmur, ischemia, stroke, myocarditis, pericarditis, pulmonary hypertension, secondary cardiomyopathy.
Central and Peripheral Nervous System Disorders and Psychiatric: Dizziness (20%), paresthesias (17%), anxiety (17%), insomnia (14%), depression (14%), confusion (11%), cerebral hemorrhage (9%), intracranial hypertension (9%), agitation (9%), hallucination (6%) and for 3% of patients: abnormal gait, agnosia, aphasia, asterixis, cerebellar edema, cerebellar disorders, convulsions, coma, CNS depression, dysarthria, encephalopathy, facial paralysis, hemiplegia, hyporeflexia, hypotaxia, no light reflex, neurologic reaction, spinal cord disorder, tremor, leg weakness, unconsciousness, dementia, forgetfulness, somnolence, slow speech.
Urinary System Disorders: Renal insufficiency (11%), dysuria (9%), acute renal failure (3%), micturition frequency (3%), renal tubular necrosis (3%), enlarged prostate (3%).
Miscellaneous Adverse Events: Isolated cases of erythema nodosum, basophilia and hyperhistaminemia, Sweet's syndrome, organomegaly, hypercalcemia, pancreatitis and myositis have been reported.

OVERDOSAGE

There has been no experience with acute overdosage in humans. The maximal tolerated dose in patients with myelodysplastic syndrome or solid tumors was 195 mg/m^2/day. The maximal tolerated dose in pediatric patients was lower at 60 mg/m^2/day. Overdosage with other retinoids has been associated with transient headache, facial flushing, cheilosis, abdominal pain, dizziness and ataxia. These symptoms have quickly resolved without apparent residual effects.

DOSAGE AND ADMINISTRATION

The recommended dose is 45 mg/m^2/day administered as two evenly divided doses until complete remission is documented. Therapy should be discontinued 30 days after achievement of complete remission or after 90 days of treatment, whichever occurs first.
If after initiation of treatment of VESANOID the presence of the t(15;17) translocation is not confirmed by cytogenetics and/or by polymerase chain reaction studies and the patient has not responded to VESANOID, alternative therapy appropriate for acute myelogenous leukemia should be considered.
VESANOID is for the induction of remission only. Optimal consolidation or maintenance regimens have not been determined. All patients should therefore receive a standard consolidation and/or maintenance chemotherapy regimen for APL after induction therapy with VESANOID, unless otherwise contraindicated.

HOW SUPPLIED

VESANOID is supplied as 10 mg capsules, two-tone (lengthwise), orange-yellow and reddish-brown and imprinted VESANOID 10 ROCHE. Supplied in high density polyethylene, opaque Prescription Pak Bottles of 100 capsules with child-resistant closure (NDC 0004-0250-01).
Store at 15°C to 30°C (59°F to 86°F). Protect from light.
Issued: November 1995
Shown in Product Identification Guide, page 335

XELODA™
(capecitabine)
TABLETS
℞

DESCRIPTION

XELODA (capecitabine) is a fluoropyrimidine carbamate with antineoplastic activity. It is an orally administered systemic prodrug of 5′-deoxy-5-fluorouridine (5′-DFUR) which is converted to 5-fluorouracil.
The chemical name for capecitabine is 5′-deoxy-5-fluoro-N-[(pentyloxy)carbonyl]-cytidine and a molecular weight of 359.35. Capecitabine has the following structural formula:

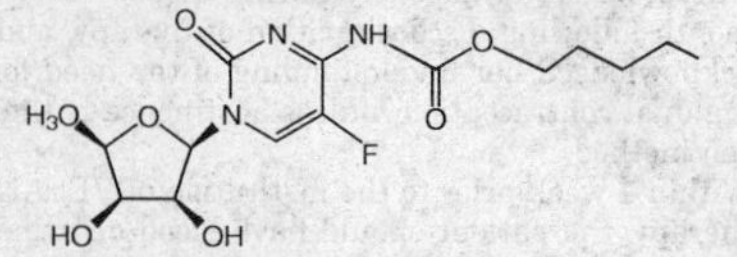

Capecitabine is a white to off-white crystalline powder with an aqueous solubility of 26 mg/mL at 20°C.
XELODA is supplied as biconvex, oblong film-coated tablets for oral administration. Each light peach-colored tablet contains 150 mg capecitabine and each peach-colored tablet contains 500 mg capecitabine. The inactive ingredients in XELODA include: anhydrous lactose, croscarmellose sodium, hydroxypropyl methylcellulose, microcrystalline cellulose, magnesium stearate and purified water. The peach or light peach film coating contains hydroxypropyl methylcellulose, talc, titanium dioxide, and synthetic yellow and red iron oxides.

CLINICAL PHARMACOLOGY

Capecitabine is relatively non-cytotoxic in vitro. This drug is enzymatically converted to 5-fluorouracil (5-FU) in vivo.
Bioactivation: Capecitabine is readily absorbed from the gastrointestinal tract. In the liver, a 60 kDa carboxyesterase hydrolyzes much of the compound to 5′-deoxy-5-fluorocytidine (5′-DFCR). Cytidine deaminase, an enzyme found in most tissues, including tumors, subsequently converts 5′-DFCR to 5′-deoxy-5-fluorouridine (5′-DFUR). The enzyme, thymidine phosphorylase (dThdPase), then hydrolyzes 5′-DFUR to the active drug 5-FU. Many tissues throughout the body express thymidine phosphorylase. Some human carcinomas express this enzyme in higher concentrations than surrounding normal tissues.

Metabolic Pathway of capecitabine to 5-FU

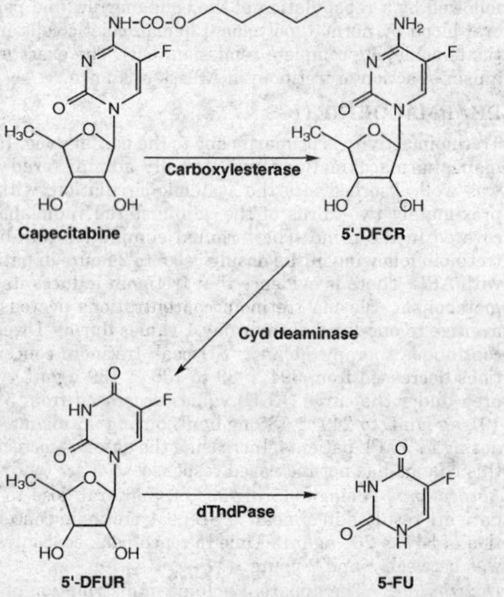

Mechanism of Action: Both normal and tumor cells metabolize 5-FU to 5-fluoro-2-deoxyuridine monophosphate (FdUMP) and 5-fluorouridine triphosphate (FUTP). These metabolites cause cell injury by two different mechanisms. First, FdUMP and the folate cofactor, N^{5-10}-methylenetetrahydrofolate, bind to thymidylate synthase (TS) to form a covalently bound ternary complex. This binding inhibits the formation of thymidylate from uracil. Thymidylate is the necessary precursor of thymidine triphosphate, which is essential for the synthesis of DNA, so that a deficiency of this compound can inhibit cell division. Second, nuclear transcriptional enzymes can mistakenly incorporate FUTP in place of uridine triphosphate (UTP) during the synthesis of RNA. This metabolic error can interfere with RNA processing and protein synthesis.
Pharmacokinetics in Colorectal Tumors and Adjacent Healthy Tissue: Following oral administration of capecitabine 7 days before surgery in patients with colorectal cancer, the median ratio of 5-FU concentration in colorectal tumors to adjacent tissues was 2.9 (range from 0.9 to 8.0). These ratios have not been evaluated in breast cancer patients or compared to 5-FU infusion.
Human Pharmacokinetics: The pharmacokinetics of XELODA and its metabolites have been evaluated in about 200 cancer patients over a dosage range of 500 to 3500 mg/m^2/day. Over this range, the pharmacokinetics of capecitabine and its metabolite, 5′-DFCR were dose proportional and did not change over time. The increases in the AUCs of 5′-DFUR and 5-FU, however, were greater than proportional to the increase in dose and the AUC of 5-FU was 34% higher on day 14 than on day 1. The elimination half-life of both

parent capecitabine and 5-FU was about 3/4 of an hour. The inter-patient variability in the C_{max} and AUC of 5-FU was greater than 85%.

Absorption, Distribution, Metabolism and Excretion: Capecitabine reached peak blood levels in about 1.5 hours (T_{max}) with peak 5-FU levels occurring slightly later, at 2 hours. Food reduced both the rate and extent of absorption of capecitabine with mean C_{max} and $AUC_{0-\infty}$ decreased by 60% and 35%, respectively. The C_{max} and $AUC_{0-\infty}$ of 5-FU were also reduced by food by 43% and 21%, respectively. Food delayed T_{max} of both parent and 5-FU by 1.5 hours (see PRECAUTIONS and DOSAGE AND ADMINISTRATION). Plasma protein binding of capecitabine and its metabolites is less than 60% and is not concentration-dependent. Capecitabine was primarily bound to human albumin (approximately 35%).

Capecitabine is extensively metabolized enzymatically to 5-FU. The enzyme dihydropyrimidine dehydrogenase hydrogenates 5-FU, the product of capecitabine metabolism, to the much less toxic 5-fluoro-5,6-dihydro-fluorouracil (FUH_2). Dihydropyrimidinase cleaves the pyrimidine ring to yield 5-fluoro-ureido-propionic acid (FUPA). Finally, β-ureido-propionase cleaves FUPA to α-fluoro-β-alanine (FBAL) which is cleared in the urine.

Over 70% of the administered capecitabine dose is recovered in urine as drug-related species, about 50% of it as FBAL.

Special Populations:

Age, Gender and Ethnicity: No formal studies were conducted to examine the effect of age or gender or ethnicity on the pharmacokinetics of capecitabine and its metabolites.

Hepatic Insufficiency: XELODA has been evaluated in 13 patients with mild to moderate hepatic dysfunction due to liver metastases defined by a composite score including bilirubin, AST/ALT and alkaline phosphatase following a single 1255 mg/m^2 dose of capecitabine. Both $AUC_{0-\infty}$ and C_{max} of capecitabine increased by 60% in patients with hepatic dysfunction compared to patients with normal hepatic function (n = 14). The $AUC_{0-\infty}$ and C_{max} of 5-FU was not affected. In patients with mild to moderate hepatic dysfunction due to liver metastases, caution should be exercised when XELODA is administered. The effect of severe hepatic dysfunction on XELODA is not known (see PRECAUTIONS and DOSAGE AND ADMINISTRATION).

Renal Insufficiency: No formal pharmacokinetic study was conducted in patients with renal impairment (see PRECAUTIONS).

Drug-Drug Interactions:

Drugs Metabolized by Cytochrome P450 Enzymes: In vitro enzymatic studies with human liver microsomes indicated that capecitabine and 5'-DFUR had no inhibitory effects on substrates of cytochrome P450 for the major isoenzymes such as 1A2, 2A6, 3A4, 2C9, 2C19, 2D6, and 2E1, suggesting a low likelihood of interactions with drugs metabolized by cytochrome P450 enzymes.

Antacid: When Maalox®* (20 mL), an aluminum hydroxide- and magnesium hydroxide-containing antacid, was administered immediately after capecitabine (1250 mg/m^2, n=12 cancer patients), AUC and C_{max} increased by 16% and 35%, respectively, for capecitabine and by 18% and 22%, respectively, for 5'-DFCR. No effect was observed on the other three major metabolites (5'-DFUR, 5-FU, FBAL) of capecitabine.

XELODA has a low potential for pharmacokinetic interactions related to plasma protein binding.

CLINICAL STUDIES

In a phase 1 study with XELODA in patients with solid tumors, the maximum tolerated dose as a single agent was 3000 mg/m^2 when administered daily for 2 weeks, followed by a 1-week rest period. The dose-limiting toxicities were diarrhea and leukopenia.

Breast Carcinoma: The antitumor activity of XELODA was evaluated in an open-label single-arm trial conducted in 24 centers in the US and Canada. A total of 162 patients with stage IV breast cancer were enrolled. The primary endpoint was tumor response rate in patients with measurable disease, with response defined as a ≥50% decrease in sum of the products of the perpendicular diameters of bidimensionally measurable disease for at least 1 month. XELODA was administered at a daily dose of 2510 mg/m^2 for 2 weeks followed by a 1-week rest period and given as 3-week cycles. The baseline demographics and clinical characteristics for all patients (n=162) and those with measurable disease (N=135) are shown in the table below. Resistance was defined as progressive disease while on treatment, with or without an initial response, or relapse within 6 months of completing treatment with an anthracycline-containing adjuvant chemotherapy regimen.

[See table 1 above]

Antitumor responses for patients with disease resistant to both paclitaxel and an anthracycline are shown in the table below.

[See table 2 above]

For the subgroup of 43 patients who were doubly resistant, the median time to progression was 102 days and the me-

Table 1. Baseline Demographics and Clinical Characteristics

	Patients With Measurable Disease (n=135)	All Patients (n=162)
Age (median, years)	55	56
Karnofsky PS	90	90
No. Disease Sites		
1–2	43 (32%)	60 (37%)
3–4	63 (46%)	69 (43%)
>5	29 (22%)	34 (21%)
Dominant Site of Disease		
Visceral[1]	101 (75%)	110 (68%)
Soft Tissue	30 (22%)	35 (22%)
Bone	4 (3%)	17 (10%)
Prior Chemotherapy		
Paclitaxel	135 (100%)	162 (100%)
Anthracycline[2]	122 (90%)	147 (91%)
5-FU	110 (81%)	133 (82%)
Resistance to Paclitaxel	103 (76%)	124 (77%)
Resistance to an Anthracycline[2]	55 (41%)	67 (41%)
Resistance to both Paclitaxel and an Anthracycline[2]	43 (32%)	51 (31%)

[1] Lung, pleura, liver, peritoneum
[2] Includes 2 patients treated with an anthracenedione

Table 2. Response Rates in Doubly-Resistant Patients

	Resistance to Both Paclitaxel and an Anthracycline (n=43)
CR	0
PR[1]	11
CR + PR[1]	11
Response Rate[1] (95% C.I.)	25.6% (13.5, 41.2)
Duration of Response,[1] Median in days[2] (Range)	154 (63 to 233)

[1] Includes 2 patients treated with an anthracenedione
[2] From date of first response

dian survival was 255 days. The objective response rate in this population was supported by a response rate of 18.5% (1 CR, 24 PRs) in the overall population of 135 patients with measurable disease, who were less resistant to chemotherapy (see Table 1). The median time to progression was 90 days and the median survival was 306 days.

INDICATIONS AND USAGE

XELODA is indicated for the treatment of patients with metastatic breast cancer resistant to both paclitaxel and an anthracycline-containing chemotherapy regimen or resistant to paclitaxel and for whom further anthracycline therapy is not indicated, eg, patients who have received cumulative doses of 400 mg/m^2 of doxorubicin or doxorubicin equivalents. Resistance is defined as progressive disease while on treatment, with or without an initial response, or relapse within 6 months of completing treatment with an anthracycline-containing adjuvant regimen.

This indication is based on demonstration of a response rate. No results are available from controlled trials that demonstrate a clinical benefit resulting from treatment, such as improvement in disease-related symptoms, disease progression, or survival.

CONTRAINDICATIONS

XELODA is contraindicated in patients who have a known hypersensitivity to 5-fluorouracil.

WARNINGS

Diarrhea: XELODA can induce diarrhea, sometimes severe. Patients with severe diarrhea should be carefully monitored and given fluid and electrolyte replacement if they become dehydrated. The median time to first occurrence of grade 2–4 diarrhea was 31 days (range from 1 to 322 days). National Cancer Institute of Canada (NCIC) grade 2 diarrhea is defined as an increase of 4 to 6 stools/day or nocturnal stools, grade 3 diarrhea as an increase of 7 to 9 stools/day or incontinence and malabsorption, and grade 4 diarrhea as an increase of ≥10 stools/day or grossly bloody diarrhea or the need for parenteral support. If grade

2, 3 or 4 diarrhea occurs, administration of XELODA should be immediately interrupted until the diarrhea resolves or decreases in intensity to grade 1. Following grade 3 or 4 diarrhea, subsequent doses of XELODA should be decreased (see DOSAGE AND ADMINISTRATION). Standard antidiarrheal treatments (eg, loperamide) are recommended. Necrotizing enterocolitis (typhlitis) has been reported.

Geriatric Patients (gastrointestinal toxicity): Patients ≥80 years old may experience a greater incidence of gastrointestinal grade 3 or 4 adverse events (see PRECAUTIONS: *Geriatric Use*). Among the 14 patients 80 years of age and greater treated with capecitabine, three (21.4%), three (21.4%) and one (7.1%) patients experienced reversible grade 3 or 4 diarrhea, nausea and vomiting, respectively. Among the 313 patients age 60 to 79 years old, the incidence of gastrointestinal toxicity was similar to that in the overall population.

Pregnancy: XELODA may cause fetal harm when given to a pregnant woman. Capecitabine at doses of 198 mg/kg/day during organogenesis caused teratogenic malformations and embryo death in mice. In separate pharmacokinetic studies, this dose in mice produced 5'-DFUR AUC values about 0.2 times the corresponding values in patients administered the recommended daily dose. Teratogenic malformations in mice included cleft palate, anophthalmia, microphthalmia, oligodactyly, polydactyly, syndactyly, kinky tail and dilation of cerebral ventricles. At doses of 90 mg/kg/day, capecitabine given to pregnant monkeys during organogenesis caused fetal death. This dose produced 5'-DFUR AUC values about 0.6 times the corresponding values in patients administered the recommended daily dose. There are no adequate and well-controlled studies in pregnant women using XELODA. If the drug is used during pregnancy, or if the patient becomes pregnant while receiving this drug, the patient should be apprised of the potential hazard to the fetus. Women of childbearing potential should be advised to avoid becoming pregnant while receiving treatment with XELODA.

Continued on next page

Xeloda—Cont.

PRECAUTIONS

General: Patients receiving therapy with XELODA should be monitored by a physician experienced in the use of cancer chemotherapeutic agents. Most adverse events are reversible and do not need to result in discontinuation, although doses may need to be withheld or reduced (see DOSAGE AND ADMINISTRATION).

Hand-and-Foot Syndrome: Hand-and-foot syndrome (palmar-plantar erythrodysesthesia or chemotherapy induced acral erythema) is characterized by the following: numbness, dysesthesia/paresthesia, tingling, painless or painful swelling, erythema, desquamation, blistering and severe pain. Grade 2 hand-and-foot syndrome is defined as painful erythema and swelling of the hands and/or feet that results in discomfort affecting the patient's activities of daily living. Grade 3 hand-and-foot syndrome is defined as moist desquamation, ulceration, blistering and severe pain of the hands and/or feet that results in severe discomfort that causes the patient to be unable to work or perform activities of daily living. If grade 2 or 3 hand-and-foot syndrome occurs, administration of XELODA should be interrupted until the event resolves or decreases in intensity to grade 1. Following grade 3 hand-and-foot syndrome, subsequent doses of XELODA should be decreased (see DOSAGE AND ADMINISTRATION).

Cardiac: There has been cardiotoxicity associated with fluorinated pyrimidine therapy, including myocardial infarction, angina, dysrhythmias, cardiogenic shock, sudden death and electrocardiograph changes. These adverse events may be more common in patients with a prior history of coronary artery disease.

Hepatic Insufficiency: Patients with mild to moderate hepatic dysfunction due to liver metastases should be carefully monitored when XELODA is administered. The effect of severe hepatic dysfunction on the disposition of XELODA is not known (see CLINICAL PHARMACOLOGY and DOSAGE AND ADMINISTRATION).

Hyperbilirubinemia: Grade 3 or 4 hyperbilirubinemia occurred in 17% (n=97) of 570 patients with either metastatic breast or colorectal cancer who received a dose of 2510 mg/m² daily for 2 weeks followed by a 1-week rest period. Of 339 patients who had hepatic metastases at baseline and 231 patients without hepatic metastases at baseline, grade 3 or 4 hyperbilirubinemia occurred in 21.2% and 10.4%, respectively. Seventy-four (76%) of the 97 patients with grade 3 or 4 hyperbilirubinemia also had concurrent elevations in alkaline phosphatase and/or hepatic transaminases; 6% of these were grade 3 or 4. Only 4 patients (4%) had elevated hepatic transaminases without a concurrent elevation in alkaline phosphatase. If drug related grade 2–4 elevations in bilirubin occur, administration of XELODA should be immediately interrupted until the hyperbilirubinemia resolves or decreases in intensity to grade 1. NCIC grade 2 hyperbilirubinemia is defined as 1.5 × normal, grade 3 hyperbilirubinemia as 1.5–3 × normal and grade 4 hyperbilirubinemia as >3 × normal. (See recommended dose modifications under DOSAGE AND ADMINISTRATION.)

Renal Insufficiency: There is little experience in patients with renal impairment. Physicians should exercise caution when XELODA is administered (see DOSAGE AND ADMINISTRATION).

Hematologic: In 570 patients with either metastatic breast or colorectal cancer who received a dose of 2510 mg/m² administered daily for 2 weeks followed by a 1-week rest period, 4%, 2%, and 3% of patients had grade 3 or 4 neutropenia, thrombocytopenia and decreases in hemoglobin, respectively.

Carcinogenesis, Mutagenesis and Impairment of Fertility: Long-term studies in animals to evaluate the carcinogenic potential of capecitabine have not been conducted. Capecitabine was not mutagenic in vitro to bacteria (Ames test) or mammalian cells (Chinese hamster V79/HPRT gene mutation assay). Capecitabine was clastogenic in vitro to human peripheral blood lymphocytes but not clastogenic in vivo to mouse bone marrow (micronucleus test). Fluorouracil causes mutations in bacteria and yeast. Fluorouracil also causes chromosomal abnormalities in the mouse micronucleus test in vivo.

Impairment of Fertility: In studies of fertility and general reproductive performance in mice, oral capecitabine doses of 760 mg/kg/day disturbed estrus and consequently caused a decrease in fertility. In mice that became pregnant, no fetuses survived this dose. The disturbance in estrus was reversible. In males, this dose caused degenerative changes in the testes, including decreases in the number of spermatocytes and spermatids. In separate pharmacokinetic studies, this dose in mice produced 5'-DFUR AUC values about 0.7 times the corresponding values in patients administered the recommended daily dose.

Information for Patients (see Patient Package Insert): Patients and patients' caregivers should be informed of the expected adverse effects of XELODA, particularly nausea, vomiting, diarrhea, and hand-and-foot syndrome, and

should be made aware that patient-specific dose adaptations during therapy are expected and necessary (see DOSAGE AND ADMINISTRATION). Patients should be encouraged to recognize the common grade 2 toxicities associated with XELODA treatment.

Diarrhea: Patients experiencing grade 2 diarrhea (an increase of 4 to 6 stools/day or nocturnal stools) or greater should be instructed to stop taking XELODA immediately. Standard antidiarrheal treatments (eg, loperamide) are recommended.

Nausea: Patients experiencing grade 2 nausea (food intake significantly decreased but able to eat intermittently) or greater should be instructed to stop taking XELODA immediately. Initiation of symptomatic treatment is recommended.

Vomiting: Patients experiencing grade 2 vomiting (2 to 5 episodes in a 24-hour period) or greater should be instructed to stop taking XELODA immediately. Initiation of symptomatic treatment is recommended.

Hand-and-Foot Syndrome: Patients experiencing grade 2 hand-and-foot syndrome (painful erythema and swelling of the hands and/or feet that results in discomfort affecting the patients' activities of daily living) or greater should be instructed to stop taking XELODA immediately.

Stomatitis: Patients experiencing grade 2 stomatitis (painful erythema, edema or ulcers of the mouth or tongue, but able to eat) or greater should be instructed to stop taking XELODA immediately. Initiation of symptomatic treatment is recommended (see DOSAGE AND ADMINISTRATION).

Fever and Neutropenia: Patients who develop a fever of 100.5°F or greater or other evidence of potential infection should be instructed to call their physician.

Drug-Food Interaction: In all clinical trials, patients were instructed to administer XELODA within 30 minutes after a meal. Since current safety and efficacy data are based upon administration with food, it is recommended that XELODA

be administered with food (see DOSAGE AND ADMINISTRATION).

Drug-Drug Interactions: Antacid: The effect of an aluminum hydroxide- and magnesium hydroxide-containing antacid (Maalox)* on the pharmacokinetics of capecitabine was investigated in 12 cancer patients. There was a small increase in plasma concentrations of capecitabine and one metabolite (5'DFCR); there was no effect on the 3 major metabolites (5'DFUR, 5-FU and FBAL).

Leucovorin: The concentration of 5-fluorouracil is increased and its toxicity may be enhanced by leucovorin. Deaths from severe enterocolitis, diarrhea, and dehydration have been reported in elderly patients receiving weekly leucovorin and fluorouracil.

Pregnancy: Teratogenic Effects: Category D (see WARNINGS). Women of childbearing potential should be advised to avoid becoming pregnant while receiving treatment with XELODA.

Nursing Women: It is not known whether the drug is excreted in human milk. Because many drugs are excreted in human milk and because of the potential for serious adverse reactions in nursing infants, it is recommended that nursing be discontinued when receiving XELODA therapy.

Pediatric Use: The safety and effectiveness of XELODA in persons <18 years of age have not been established.

Geriatric Use: No separate studies have been conducted to examine the effect of age on the pharmacokinetics of capecitabine and its metabolites. Patients ≥80 years old may experience a greater incidence of gastrointestinal grade 3 or 4 adverse events (see WARNINGS). Among the 14 patients 80 years of age and greater treated with capecitabine, 21.4%, 21.4% and 7.1% experienced grade 3 or 4 diarrhea, nausea and vomiting, respectively. Among the 313 patients 60 to 79 years old, the incidence was similar to the overall population.

Table 3. Percent Incidence of Adverse Events Considered Remotely, Possibly or Probably Related to Treatment in ≥5% of Patients

Adverse Event	Phase 2 Trial in Stage IV Breast Cancer (n=162)			Overall Safety Database (n=570)		
Body System/ Adverse Event	Total	Grade 3	Grade 4	Total	Grade 3	Grade 4
GI						
Diarrhea	57	12	3	50	11	2
Nausea	53	4	–	44	4	–
Vomiting	37	4	–	26	3	–
Stomatitis	24	7	–	23	4	–
Abdominal pain	20	4	–	17	4	–
Constipation	15	1	–	9	1	–
Dyspepsia	8	–	–	6	–	–
Skin and Subcutaneous						
Hand-and-Foot Syndrome	57	11	–	45	13	–
Dermatitis	37	1	–	31	1	–
Nail disorder	7	–	–	4	–	–
General						
Fatigue	41	8	–	34	5	–
Pyrexia	12	1	–	10	–	–
Pain in limb	6	1	–	4	–	–
Neurological						
Paraesthesia	21	1	–	12	–	–
Headache	9	1	–	7	1	–
Dizziness	8	–	–	5	–	–
Insomnia	8	–	–	3	–	–
Metabolism						
Anorexia	23	3	–	20	2	–
Dehydration	7	4	1	5	2	1
Eye						
Eye irritation	15	–	–	10	–	–
Musculoskeletal						
Myalgia	9	–	–	4	–	–
Cardiac						
Edema	9	1	–	6	–	–
Blood						
Neutropenia	26	2	2	22	3	2
Thrombocytopenia	24	3	1	21	1	1
Anemia	72	3	1	74	2	1
Lymphopenia	94	44	15	94	36	10
Hepatobiliary						
Hyperbilirubinemia	22	9	2	34	14	3

–Not observed or applicable.

Table 4. XELODA Dose Calculation According to Body Surface Area

Dose level 2500 mg/m^2/day		Number of tablets to be taken at each dose (morning and evening)	
Surface Area (m^2)	Total Daily* Dose (mg)	150 mg	500 mg
≤ 1.24	3000	0	3
1.25 – 1.36	3300	1	3
1.37 – 1.51	3600	2	3
1.52 – 1.64	4000	0	4
1.65 – 1.76	4300	1	4
1.77 – 1.91	4600	2	4
1.92 – 2.04	5000	0	5
2.05 – 2.17	5300	1	5
≥ 2.18	5600	2	5

*Total Daily Dose divided by 2 to allow equal morning and evening doses.

Table 5. Recommended Dose Modifications

Toxicity NCIC Grades*	During a Course of Therapy	Dose Adjustment for Next Cycle (% of starting dose)
• Grade 1	Maintain dose level	Maintain dose level
• Grade 2		
-1st appearance	Interrupt until resolved to grade 0–1	100%
-2nd appearance	Interrupt until resolved to grade 0–1	75%
-3rd appearance	Interrupt until resolved to grade 0–1	50%
-4th appearance	Discontinue treatment permanently	
• Grade 3		
-1st appearance	Interrupt until resolved to grade 0–1	75%
-2nd appearance	Interrupt until resolved to grade 0–1	50%
-3rd appearance	Discontinue treatment permanently	
• Grade 4		
-1st appearance	Discontinue permanently or If physician deems it to be in the patient's best interest to continue, interrupt until resolved to grade 0–1	50%

* National Cancer Institute of Canada Common Toxicity Criteria were used except for the Hand-and-Foot Syndrome (see PRECAUTIONS).

The elderly may be pharmacodynamically more sensitive to the toxic effects of 5-FU. Physicians should pay particular attention to monitoring the adverse effects of XELODA in the elderly.

ADVERSE REACTIONS

The following table shows the adverse events occurring in ≥5% of patients reported as at least remotely related to the administration of XELODA. Rates are rounded to the nearest whole number. The data are shown both for the study in stage IV breast cancer and for a group of 570 patients with breast and colorectal cancer who received a dose of 2510 mg/m^2 administered daily for 2 weeks followed by a 1-week rest period. The 570 patients were enrolled in 6 clinical trials (162 from the breast cancer trial described under Clinical Studies, 73 other patients with breast cancer and 325 patients with colorectal cancer). The mean duration of treatment was 121 days. A total of 71 patients (13%) discontinued treatment because of adverse events/intercurrent illness.
[See table 3 at top of previous page]
Shown below by body system are the adverse events in <5% of patients reported as related to the administration of XELODA and that were clinically at least remotely relevant. In parentheses is the incidence of grade 3 or 4 occurrences of each adverse event.
Gastrointestinal: intestinal obstruction (1.1), rectal bleeding (0.4), GI hemorrhage (0.2), esophagitis (0.4), gastritis, colitis, duodenitis, haematemesis, necrotizing enterocolitis

Skin: increased sweating (0.2), photosensitivity (0.2), radiation recall syndrome (0.2)
General: chest pain (0.2)
Neurological: ataxia (0.4), encephalopathy (0.2), depressed level of consciousness (0.2), loss of consciousness (0.2)
Metabolism: cachexia (0.4), hypertriglyceridemia (0.2)
Respiratory: dyspnea (0.5), epistaxis (0.2), bronchospasm (0.2), respiratory distress (0.2)
Infections: oral candidiasis (0.2), upper respiratory tract infection (0.2), urinary tract infection (0.2), bronchitis (0.2), pneumonia (0.2), sepsis (0.4), bronchopneumonia (0.2), gastroenteritis (0.2), gastrointestinal candidiasis (0.2), laryngitis (0.2), esophageal candidiasis (0.2)
Musculoskeletal: bone pain (0.2), joint stiffness (0.2)
Cardiac: angina pectoris (0.2), cardiomyopathy
Vascular: hypotension (0.2), hypertension (0.2), venous phlebitis and thrombophlebitis (0.2), deep venous thrombosis (0.7), lymphoedema (0.2), pulmonary embolism (0.4), cerebrovascular accident (0.2)
Blood: coagulation disorder (0.2), idiopathic thrombocytopenic purpura (0.2), pancytopenia (0.2)
Psychiatric: confusion (0.2)
Renal and Urinary: nocturia (0.2)
Hepato-Biliary: hepatic fibrosis (0.2), cholestatic hepatitis (0.2), hepatitis (0.2)
Immune System: drug hypersensitivity (0.2)

OVERDOSAGE

Acute: Based on experience in animals and in humans treated up to doses of 3514 mg/m^2/day, the anticipated manifestations of acute overdose would be nausea, vomiting, diarrhea, gastrointestinal irritation and bleeding, and bone marrow depression. Medical management of overdose should include customary supportive medical interventions aimed at correcting the presenting clinical manifestations. Although no clinical experience has been reported, dialysis may be of benefit in reducing circulating concentrations of 5'-DFUR, a low-molecular weight metabolite of the parent compound.

Single doses of XELODA were not lethal to mice, rats, and monkeys at doses up to 2000 mg/kg (2.4, 4.8, and 9.6 times the recommended human daily dose on a mg/m^2 basis).

DOSAGE AND ADMINISTRATION

The recommended dose of XELODA is 2500 mg/m^2 administered orally daily with food for 2 weeks followed by a 1-week rest period given as 3 week cycles. The XELODA daily dose is given orally in two divided doses (approximately 12 hours apart) at the end of a meal. XELODA tablets should be swallowed with water. The following table displays the total daily dose by body surface area and the number of tablets to be taken at each dose.
[See table 4 above]
Dose Modification Guidelines: Patients should be carefully monitored for toxicity. Toxicity due to XELODA administration may be managed by symptomatic treatment, dose interruptions and adjustment of XELODA dose. Once the dose has been reduced it should not be increased at a later time.
[See table 5 above]
Dosage modifications are not recommended for grade 1 events. Therapy with XELODA should be interrupted upon the occurrence of a grade 2 or 3 adverse experience. Once the adverse event has resolved or decreased in intensity to grade 1, then XELODA therapy may be restarted at full dose or as adjusted according to the above table. If a grade 4 experience occurs, therapy should be discontinued or interrupted until resolved or decreased to grade 1, and therapy should be restarted at 50% of the original dose. Doses of capecitabine omitted for toxicity are not replaced or restored; instead the patient should resume the planned treatment cycles.

Adjustment of Starting Dose in Special Populations:
Hepatic Impairment: In patients with mild to moderate hepatic dysfunction due to liver metastases, no starting dose adjustment is necessary; however, patients should be carefully monitored. Patients with severe hepatic dysfunction have not been studied.
Renal Impairment: Insufficient data are available in patients with renal impairment to provide a dosage recommendation.
Geriatrics: The elderly may be pharmacodynamically more sensitive to the toxic effects of 5-FU and therefore, physicians should exercise caution in monitoring the effects of XELODA in the elderly. Insufficient data are available to provide a dosage recommendation.

HOW SUPPLIED

XELODA is supplied as biconvex, oblong film-coated tablets, available in bottles as follows:

Continued on next page

Xeloda—Cont.

150 mg
color: light peach
engraving: XELODA on one side, 150 on the other
150 mg tablets packaged in bottles of 120 (NDC 0004-1100-51)
500 mg
color: peach
engraving: XELODA on one side, 500 on the other
500 mg tablets packaged in bottles of 240 (NDC 0004-1101-16)
Storage Conditions: **Store at 25°C (77°F); excursions permitted to 15° to 30°C (59° to 86°F), keep tightly closed.** [See USP Controlled Room Temperature]
Caution: Federal law prohibits dispensing without a prescription.
*Maalox is a registered trademark of Novartis.

PATIENT PACKAGE INSERT (text only):

Patient Information About XELODA™ (capecitabine) Tablets

This information will help you learn more about XELODA™ (capecitabine) Tablets. It cannot, however, cover all possible precautions or side effects associated with XELODA nor does it list all the benefits and risks of XELODA. Your doctor should always be your first choice for detailed information about your medical condition and your treatment. Be sure to ask your doctor about any questions you may have.

What is XELODA?

- XELODA [zeh-LOE-duh] is an oral medication for the treatment of advanced breast cancer resistant to treatment with paclitaxel [pak-lih-TAK-sil] and an anthracycline [ann-thruh-SYE-kleen]-containing chemotherapy regimen. Paclitaxel is also known as Taxol®*. Anthracyclines include Adriamycin®† or doxorubicin.
- XELODA tablets come in two strengths: 150 mg (light peach) and 500 mg (peach).

How does XELODA work?

XELODA is converted in the body to the substance 5-fluorouracil. In some patients, this substance kills cancer cells and decreases the size of the tumor.

Who should not take XELODA?

- Patients allergic to 5-fluorouracil.
- Studies in animals suggest that XELODA may cause serious harm to an unborn child. No studies have been done with pregnant women. If you are pregnant, be sure to discuss with your doctor whether XELODA is right for you. Also, tell your doctor if you are nursing.

How should I take XELODA?

Your doctor will prescribe a dose and treatment regimen that is right for *you*. Your doctor may want you to take a combination of *150 mg* and *500 mg* tablets for each dose. If a combination of tablets is prescribed, it is very important that you correctly identify the tablets. Taking the wrong tablets could result in an overdose (too much medication) or underdose (too little medication). The 150 mg tablets are light peach in color and have 150 engraved on one side. The 500 mg tablets are peach in color and have 500 engraved on one side.

- Take the tablets in the combination prescribed by your doctor for your **morning and evening** doses.
- Take the tablets within **30 minutes after the end of a meal** (breakfast and dinner).
- XELODA tablets should be **swallowed with water.**
- It is important that you take all your medication as prescribed by your doctor.
- If you are taking the vitamin folic acid, please inform your doctor.

How long will I have to take XELODA?

It is recommended that XELODA be taken for 14 days followed by a 7-day rest period (no drug) given as a 21-day cycle. Your doctor will determine how many cycles of treatment you will need.

What if I miss a dose?

If you miss a dose of XELODA, do not take the missed dose at all and do not double the next one. Instead, continue your regular dosing schedule and check with your doctor.

What are the most common side effects of XELODA?

The most common side effects of XELODA are:

- diarrhea, nausea, vomiting, stomatitis (sores in mouth and throat), abdominal pain, constipation, loss of appetite or decreased appetite, and dehydration (excessive water loss from the body).
- hand-and-foot syndrome (palms of the hands or soles of the feet tingle, become numb, painful, swollen or red), rash, dry or itchy skin.
- tiredness, weakness, dizziness, headache, and fever.

When should I call my doctor?

It is important that you **CONTACT YOUR DOCTOR IMMEDIATELY** if you experience the following side effects. This will help reduce the likelihood that the side effect will continue or become serious.

Your doctor may instruct you to decrease the dose and/or temporarily discontinue treatment with XELODA.

STOP taking XELODA immediately and contact your doctor if any of these symptoms occur:

- ***Diarrhea:*** if you have more than 4 bowel movements each day or any diarrhea at night.
- ***Vomiting:*** if you vomit more than once in a 24-hour time period.
- ***Nausea:*** if you lose your appetite, and the amount of food you eat each day is much less than usual.
- ***Stomatitis:*** if you have pain, redness, swelling or sores in your mouth.
- ***Hand-and-foot syndrome:*** if you have pain, swelling, or redness of hands and/or feet.
- ***Fever or Infection:*** if you have a temperature of 100.5°F or greater, or other evidence of infection.

If caught early, most of these side effects usually improve within 2 to 3 days after you stop taking XELODA. If they don't improve within 2 to 3 days, call your doctor again. After side effects have improved, your doctor will tell you whether to start taking XELODA again or what dose to use.

How should I store and use XELODA?

- Never share XELODA with anyone.
- XELODA should be stored at normal room temperature (about 65° to 85°F).
- Keep this and all other medications out of the reach of children.
- In case of accidental ingestion or if you suspect that more than the prescribed dose of this medication has been taken, contact your doctor or local poison control center or emergency room IMMEDIATELY.
- Medicines are sometimes prescribed for uses other than those listed in this leaflet. If you have any questions or concerns, or want more information about XELODA, contact your doctor or pharmacist.

*Taxol is a registered trademark of Bristol-Myers Squibb Company.
†Adriamycin is a registered trademark of Pharmacia & Upjohn Company.

Issued: April 1998

Shown in Product Identification Guide, page 335

ZENAPAX® ℞
(Daclizumab)
STERILE CONCENTRATE FOR INJECTION

The following text is complete prescribing information based on official labeling in effect June 1998.

WARNING:
Only physicians experienced in immunosuppressive therapy and management of organ transplant patients should prescribe ZENAPAX® (Daclizumab). The physician responsible for ZENAPAX administration should have complete information requisite for the follow-up of the patient. Patients receiving the drug should be managed in facilities equipped and staffed with adequate laboratory and supportive medical resources.

DESCRIPTION

ZENAPAX® (Daclizumab) is an immunosuppressive, humanized IgG1 monoclonal antibody produced by recombinant DNA technology that binds specifically to the alpha subunit (p55 alpha, CD25, or Tac subunit) of the human high-affinity interleukin-2 (IL-2) receptor that is expressed on the surface of activated lymphocytes.

Daclizumab is a composite of human (90%) and murine (10%) antibody sequences. The human sequences were derived from the constant domains of human IgG1 and the variable framework regions of the Eu myeloma antibody. The murine sequences were derived from the complementarity-determining regions of a murine anti-Tac antibody. The molecular weight predicted from DNA sequencing is 144 kilodaltons.

ZENAPAX 25 mg/5mL is supplied as a clear, sterile, colorless concentrate for further dilution and intravenous administration. Each milliliter of ZENAPAX contains 5 mg of Daclizumab and 3.6 mg sodium phosphate monobasic monohydrate, 11 mg sodium phosphate dibasic heptahydrate, 4.6 mg sodium chloride, 0.2 mg polysorbate 80 and may contain hydrochloric acid or sodium hydroxide to adjust the pH to 6.9. No preservatives are added.

CLINICAL PHARMACOLOGY

Mechanism of Action: Daclizumab functions as an IL-2 receptor antagonist that binds with high affinity to the Tac subunit of the high affinity IL-2 receptor complex and inhibits IL-2 binding. Daclizumab binding is highly specific for Tac, which is expressed on activated but not resting lymphocytes. Administration of ZENAPAX inhibits IL-2–mediated activation of lymphocytes, a critical pathway in the cellular immune response involved in allograft rejection.

While in the circulation, ZENAPAX impairs the response of the immune system to antigenic challenges. Whether the ability to respond to repeated or ongoing challenges with those antigens returns to normal after ZENAPAX is cleared is unknown (see PRECAUTIONS).

Pharmacokinetics: In clinical trials involving renal allograft patients treated with a 1 mg/kg IV dose of ZENAPAX every 14 days for a total of five doses, peak serum concentration (mean ± SD) rose between the first dose (21 ± 14 μg/mL) and fifth dose (32 ± 22 μg/mL). The mean trough serum concentration before the fifth dose was 7.6 ± 4.0 μg/mL. In vitro and in vivo data suggest that serum levels of 5 to 10 μg/mL are necessary for saturation of the Tac subunit of the IL-2 receptors to block the responses of activated T lymphocytes.

Population pharmacokinetic analysis of the data using a two-compartment open model gave the following values for a reference patient (45-year-old male Caucasian patient with a body weight of 80 kg and no proteinuria): systemic clearance = 15 mL/hour, volume of central compartment = 2.5 liter, volume of peripheral compartment = 3.4 liter. The estimated terminal elimination half-life for the reference patient was 20 days (480 hours), which is similar to the terminal elimination half-life for human IgG (18 to 23 days). Bayesian estimates of terminal elimination half-life ranged from 11 to 38 days for the 123 patients included in the population analysis.

The influence of body weight on systemic clearance supports the dosing of ZENAPAX on a milligram per kilogram (mg/kg) basis. For patients studied, this dosing maintained drug exposure within 30% of the reference exposure. Covariate analyses showed that no dosage adjustments based on age, race, gender or degree of proteinuria, are required for renal allograft patients. The estimated interpatient variability (percent coefficient of variation) in systemic clearance and central volume of distribution were 15% and 27%, respectively.

Pharmacodynamics: At the recommended dosage regimen, Daclizumab saturates the Tac subunit of the IL-2 receptor for approximately 120 days post-transplant. The duration of clinically significant IL-2 receptor blockade after the recommended course of ZENAPAX is not known. No significant changes to circulating lymphocyte numbers or cell phenotypes were observed by flow cytometry. Cytokine release syndrome has not been observed after ZENAPAX administration.

CLINICAL STUDIES

The safety and efficacy of ZENAPAX for the prophylaxis of acute organ rejection in adult patients receiving their first cadaveric kidney transplant were assessed in two randomized, double-blind, placebo-controlled, multicenter trials. These trials compared a dose of 1.0 mg/kg of ZENAPAX with placebo when each was administered as part of standard immunosuppressive regimens containing either cyclosporine and corticosteroids (double-therapy trial, no US sites) or cyclosporine, corticosteroids, and azathioprine (triple-

Table 1. Efficacy Parameters

	Triple-therapy Regimen (cyclosporine, corticosteroids, and azathioprine)			**Double-therapy Regimen** (cyclosporine and corticosteroids)		
	Placebo (N=134)	**ZENAPAX (N=126)**	**p-value**	**Placebo (N=134)**	**ZENAPAX (N=141)**	**p-value**
Primary Endpoint						
Incidence of biopsy-proven acute rejection at 6 months						
No. of patients	47 (35%)	28 (22%)	0.03	63 (47%)	39 (28%)	0.001
Secondary Endpoints						
Incidence of biopsy-proven acute rejection at 1 year						
No. of patients	51 (38%)	35 (28%)	0.09	65 (49%)	39 (28%)	<0.001
Patient survival at 1 year post-transplant						
No. of patients	129 (96%)	123 (98%)	0.51	126 (94%)	140 (99%)	0.01
Graft survival at 1 year post-transplant						
No. of patients with functioning graft	121 (90%)	120 (95%)	0.08	111 (83%)	124 (88%)	0.30

therapy trial, predominantly US sites) to prevent acute renal allograft rejection. ZENAPAX dosing was initiated within 24 hours pretransplant, with subsequent doses given every 14 days for a total of five doses.

The primary efficacy endpoint of both trials was the proportion of patients who developed a biopsy-proven acute rejection episode within the first 6 months following transplantation. As shown in Table 1, this incidence was significantly lower in the ZENAPAX-treated group in both the double-therapy and triple-therapy trials.

[See table 1 at bottom of previous page]

No difference in patient survival was observed in the triple-therapy study between ZENAPAX- and placebo-treated patients. Treatment with ZENAPAX was associated with better patient survival at 1 year post-transplant in the double-therapy study.

The incidence of delayed graft function was no different between placebo-treated and ZENAPAX-treated patients in either study. No difference in graft function was observed 1 year post-transplant in either study between placebo-treated and ZENAPAX-treated patients.

In a randomized, double-blind study, ZENAPAX (50 patients) or placebo (25 patients) was added to an immunosuppressive regimen of cyclosporine, mycophenolate mofetil, and steroids to assess tolerability, pharmacokinetics, and drug interactions. The addition of ZENAPAX to an immunosuppressive regimen of cyclosporine, mycophenolate mofetil, and steroids did not result in an increased incidence of adverse events or a change in the types of adverse events reported. The incidence of the combined endpoint of biopsy-proven or clinically presumptive acute rejection was 20% (5 of 25 patients) in the placebo group and 12% (6 of 50 patients) in the ZENAPAX group. Although numerically lower, the difference in acute rejection was not significant.

INDICATION AND USAGE

ZENAPAX is indicated for the prophylaxis of acute organ rejection in patients receiving renal transplants. It is used as part of an immunosuppressive regimen that includes cyclosporine and corticosteroids.

CONTRAINDICATION

ZENAPAX is contraindicated in patients with known hypersensitivity to Daclizumab or to any components of this product.

WARNINGS

See Boxed WARNING.

ZENAPAX should be administered under qualified medical supervision. Patients should be informed of the potential benefits of therapy and the risks associated with administration of immunosuppressive therapy.

While the incidence of lymphoproliferative disorders and opportunistic infections, in the limited clinical trial experience, was no higher in ZENAPAX-treated patients compared with placebo-treated patients, patients on immunosuppressive therapy are at increased risk for developing lymphoproliferative disorders and opportunistic infections and should be monitored accordingly.

Anaphylactoid reactions following the administration of ZENAPAX have not been observed but can occur following the administration of proteins. Medications for the treatment of severe hypersensitivity reactions should, therefore, be available for immediate use.

PRECAUTIONS

General: It is not known whether ZENAPAX use will have a long-term effect on the ability of the immune system to respond to antigens first encountered during ZENAPAX-induced immunosuppression.

Re-administration of ZENAPAX after an initial course of therapy has not been studied in humans. The potential risks of such re-administration, specifically those associated with immunosuppression and/or the occurrence of anaphylaxis/anaphylactoid reactions, are not known.

Immunogenicity: Low titers of anti-idiotype antibodies to Daclizumab were detected in the ZENAPAX-treated patients with an overall incidence of 8.4%. No antibodies that affected efficacy, safety, serum Daclizumab levels or any other clinically relevant parameter examined were detected.

Drug Interactions: The following medications have been administered in clinical trials with ZENAPAX with no incremental increase in adverse reactions: cyclosporine, mycophenolate mofetil, ganciclovir, acyclovir, azathioprine, and corticosteroids. Very limited experience exists with the use of ZENAPAX concomitantly with tacrolimus, muromonab-CD3, antithymocyte globulin, and antilymphocyte globulin. In renal allograft recipients treated with ZENAPAX and mycophenolate mofetil, no pharmacokinetic interaction between Daclizumab and mycophenolic acid, the active metabolite of mycophenolate mofetil, was observed.

Carcinogenesis, Mutagenesis and Impairment of Fertility: Long-term studies to evaluate the carcinogenic potential of ZENAPAX have not been performed. ZENAPAX was not genotoxic in the Ames or the V79 chromosomal aberration assays, with or without metabolic activation. The effect of ZENAPAX on fertility is not known, because animal repro-

duction studies have not been conducted with ZENAPAX (see WARNINGS and ADVERSE REACTIONS).

Pregnancy: Pregnancy Category C: Animal reproduction studies have not been conducted with ZENAPAX. Therefore, it is not known whether ZENAPAX can cause fetal harm when administered to pregnant women or can affect reproductive capacity. In general, IgG molecules are known to cross the placental barrier. ZENAPAX should not be used in pregnant women unless the potential benefit justifies the potential risk to the fetus. Women of childbearing potential should use effective contraception before beginning ZENAPAX therapy, during therapy, and for 4 months after completion of ZENAPAX therapy.

Nursing Mothers: It is not known whether ZENAPAX is excreted in human milk. Because many drugs are excreted in human milk, including human antibodies, and because of the potential for adverse reactions, a decision should be made to discontinue nursing or to discontinue the drug, taking into account the importance of the drug to the mother.

Pediatric Use: No adequate and well-controlled studies have been completed in pediatric patients. The preliminary results of an ongoing safety and pharmacokinetic study (N=25) in pediatric patients (median age: 12 years of age, range: 11 months to 17 years of age; 11 months to 5 years = 7 patients; 6 years to 12 years = 6 patients; 13 years to 17 years = 12 patients) treated with ZENAPAX in addition to standard immunosuppressive agents including mycophenolate mofetil, cyclosporine, tacrolimus, azathioprine, and corticosteroids indicate that the most frequently reported adverse events were hypertension (48%), post-operative (post-traumatic) pain (44%), diarrhea (36%), and vomiting (32%). The reported rates of hypertension and dehydration were higher for pediatric patients than for adult patients. It is not known whether the immune response to vaccines, infection, and other antigenic stimuli administered or encountered during ZENAPAX therapy is impaired or whether such response will remain impaired after ZENAPAX therapy.

The preliminary pharmacokinetic results from this ongoing study in pediatric patients indicate Daclizumab serum levels (N=6) appear to be somewhat lower in pediatric renal transplant patients than in adult transplant patients administered the same dosing regimen. However, Daclizumab levels in these pediatric patients were sufficient to saturate the Tac subunit of the IL-2 receptor on lymphocytes as measured by flow cytometry (N=24). The Tac subunit of the IL-2 receptor was saturated immediately after the first dose of 1.0 mg/kg of Daclizumab and remained saturated for at least the first 3 months post-transplant. Saturation of the Tac subunit of the IL-2 receptor was similar to that observed in adult patients receiving the same dose regimen.

Geriatric Use: Clinical studies of ZENAPAX did not include sufficient numbers of subjects age 65 and older to determine whether they respond differently from younger subjects. Caution must be used in giving immunosuppressive drugs to elderly patients.

ADVERSE REACTIONS

The safety of ZENAPAX was determined in four clinical studies, three of which were randomized controlled clinical trials, in 629 patients receiving renal allografts of whom 336 received ZENAPAX and 293 received placebo. All patients received concomitant cyclosporine and corticosteroids.

ZENAPAX did not appear to alter the pattern, frequency or severity of known major toxicities associated with the use of immunosuppressive drugs.

Adverse events were reported by 95% of the patients in the placebo-treated group and 96% of the patients in the ZENAPAX-treated group. The proportion of patients prematurely withdrawn from the combined studies because of adverse events was 8.5% in the placebo-treated group and 8.6% in the ZENAPAX-treated group.

ZENAPAX did not increase the number of serious adverse events observed compared with placebo. The most frequently reported adverse events were gastrointestinal disorders, which were reported with equal frequency in ZENAPAX- (67%) and placebo-treated (68%) patient groups. The incidence and types of adverse events were similar in both placebo-treated and ZENAPAX-treated patients. The following adverse events occurred in ≥5% of ZENAPAX-treated patients. These events included: *Gastrointestinal System:* constipation, nausea, diarrhea, vomiting, abdominal pain, pyrosis, dyspepsia, abdominal distention, epigastric pain not food-related; *Metabolic and Nutritional:* edema extremities, edema; *Central and Peripheral Nervous System:* tremor, headache, dizziness; *Urinary System:* oliguria, dysuria, renal tubular necrosis; *Body as a Whole—General:* post-traumatic pain, chest pain, fever, pain, fatigue; *Autonomic Nervous System:* hypertension, hypotension, aggravated hypertension; *Respiratory System:* dyspnea, pulmonary edema, coughing; *Skin and Appendages:* impaired wound healing without infection, acne; *Psychiatric:* insomnia; *Musculoskeletal System:* musculoskeletal pain, back pain; *Heart Rate and Rhythm:* tachycardia; *Vascular Extracardiac:* thrombosis; *Platelet, Bleeding and Clotting Disorders:* bleeding; *Hemic and Lymphatic:* lymphocele.

The following adverse events occurred in <5% and ≥2% of ZENAPAX-treated patients. These included: *Gastrointestinal System:* flatulence, gastritis, hemorrhoids; *Metabolic and Nutritional:* fluid overload, diabetes mellitus, dehydration; *Urinary System:* renal damage, hydronephrosis, urinary tract bleeding, urinary tract disorder, renal insufficiency; *Body as a Whole—General:* shivering, generalized weakness; *Central and Peripheral Nervous System:* urinary retention, leg cramps, prickly sensation; *Respiratory System:* atelectasis, congestion, pharyngitis, rhinitis, hypoxia, rales, abnormal breath sounds, pleural effusion; *Skin and Appendages:* pruritus, hirsutism, rash, night sweats, increased sweating; *Psychiatric:* depression, anxiety; *Musculoskeletal System:* arthralgia, myalgia; *Vision:* vision blurred; *Application Site:* application site reaction.

Incidence of Malignancies: One year after treatment, the incidence of malignancies was 2.7% in the placebo group compared with 1.5% in the ZENAPAX group. Addition of ZENAPAX did not increase the number of post-transplant lymphomas, which occurred with a frequency of <1% in both placebo-treated and ZENAPAX-treated groups.

Hyperglycemia: No differences in abnormal hematologic or chemical laboratory test results were seen between placebo-treated and ZENAPAX-treated groups with the exception of fasting blood glucose. Fasting blood glucose was measured in a small number of placebo- and ZENAPAX-treated patients. A total of 16% (10 of 64 patients) of placebo-treated and 32% (28 of 88 patients) of ZENAPAX-treated patients had high fasting blood glucose values. Most of these high values occurred either on the first day post-transplant when patients received high doses of corticosteroids or in patients with diabetes.

Incidence of Infectious Episodes: The overall incidence of infectious episodes, including viral infections, fungal infections, bacteremia and septicemia, and pneumonia, was not higher in ZENAPAX-treated patients than in placebo-treated patients. The types of infections reported were similar in both the ZENAPAX-treated and the placebo-treated groups. Cytomegalovirus infection was reported in 16% of the patients in the placebo group and 13% of the patients in the ZENAPAX group. One exception was cellulitis and wound infections, which occurred in 4.1% of placebo-treated and 8.4% of ZENAPAX-treated patients. At 1 year post-transplant, 7 placebo patients and only 1 ZENAPAX-treated patient had died of an infection.

OVERDOSAGE

There have not been any reports of overdoses with ZENAPAX. A maximum tolerated dose has not been determined in patients. A dose of 1.5 mg/kg has been administered to bone marrow transplant recipients without any associated adverse events.

DOSAGE AND ADMINISTRATION

ZENAPAX is used as part of an immunosuppressive regimen that includes cyclosporine and corticosteroids. The recommended dose for ZENAPAX is 1.0 mg/kg. The calculated volume of ZENAPAX should be mixed with 50 mL of sterile 0.9% sodium chloride solution and administered via a peripheral or central vein over a 15-minute period.

Based on the clinical trials, the standard course of ZENAPAX therapy is five doses. The first dose should be given no more than 24 hours before transplantation. The four remaining doses should be given at intervals of 14 days.

No dosage adjustment is necessary for patients with severe renal impairment. No dosage adjustments based on other identified covariates (age, gender, proteinuria, race) are required for renal allograft patients. No data are available for administration in patients with severe hepatic impairment.

Instructions for Administration:

- ZENAPAX IS NOT FOR DIRECT INJECTION. The calculated volume should be diluted in 50 mL of sterile 0.9% sodium chloride solution before intravenous administration to patients. When mixing the solution, gently invert the bag in order to avoid foaming; DO NOT SHAKE.
- Parenteral drug products should be inspected visually for particulate matter and discoloration before administration. If particulate matter is present or the solution colored, do not use.
- Care must be taken to assure sterility of the prepared solution, since the drug product does not contain any antimicrobial preservative or bacteriostatic agents.
- ZENAPAX is a colorless solution provided as a single-use vial; any unused portion of the drug should be discarded.
- Once the infusion is prepared, it should be administered intravenously within 4 hours. If it must be held longer, it should be refrigerated between 2° to 8°C (36° to 46°F) for up to 24 hours. After 24 hours, the prepared solution should be discarded.
- No incompatibility between ZENAPAX and polyvinyl chloride or polyethylene bags or infusion sets has been observed. No data are available concerning the incompatibility of ZENAPAX with other drug substances. However, other drug substances should not be added or infused simultaneously through the same intravenous line.

Continued on next page

Zenapax—Cont.

HOW SUPPLIED

ZENAPAX is supplied in single-use glass vials. Each vial contains 25 mg of Daclizumab in 5 mL of solution (NDC 0004-0501-09). Vials should be stored between the temperatures of 2° to 8°C (36° to 46°F); do not shake or freeze. Protect undiluted solution against direct light. Diluted medication is stable for 24 hours at 4°C or for 4 hours at room temperature.

Issued: December 1997

EDUCATIONAL MATERIAL

Please contact your Roche representative concerning availability of educational programs and material.

Roche Pharmaceuticals

Roche Products Inc.
Manati, Puerto Rico 00674

Direct Medical Inquiries to:
Roche Laboratories Inc
(800) 526-6367
Direct Customer Service (Distribution) Inquiries to:
Roche Laboratories Inc
(800) 526-0625

VALIUM® Ⓒ
[val 'ee-um]
brand of diazepam
INJECTION

The following text is complete prescribing information based on official labeling in effect June 1998.

DESCRIPTION

Each mL contains 5 mg diazepam compounded with 40% propylene glycol, 10% ethyl alcohol, 5% sodium benzoate and benzoic acid as buffers, and 1.5% benzyl alcohol as preservative.

Diazepam is a benzodiazepine derivative developed through original Roche research. Chemically, diazepam is 7-chloro-1, 3-dihydro-1-methyl-5-phenyl-2H-1,4-benzodiazepin-2-one. It is a colorless crystalline compound, insoluble in water and has a molecular weight of 284.74.

ACTIONS

In animals, diazepam appears to act on parts of the limbic system, the thalamus and hypothalamus, and induces calming effects. Diazepam, unlike chlorpromazine and reserpine, has no demonstrable peripheral autonomic blocking action, nor does it produce extrapyramidal side effects; however, animals treated with diazepam do have a transient ataxia at higher doses. Diazepam was found to have transient cardiovascular depressor effects in dogs. Long-term experiments in rats revealed no disturbances of endocrine function. Injections into animals have produced localized irritation of tissue surrounding injection sites and some thickening of veins after intravenous use.

INDICATIONS

Valium is indicated for the management of anxiety disorders or for the short-term relief of the symptoms of anxiety. Anxiety or tension associated with the stress of everyday life usually does not require treatment with an anxiolytic.

In acute alcohol withdrawal, Valium may be useful in the symptomatic relief of acute agitation, tremor, impending or acute delirium tremens and hallucinosis.

As an adjunct prior to endoscopic procedures if apprehension, anxiety or acute stress reactions are present, and to diminish the patient's recall of the procedures. (See WARNINGS.)

Valium is a useful adjunct for the relief of skeletal muscle spasm due to reflex spasm to local pathology (such as inflammation of the muscles or joints, or secondary to trauma); spasticity caused by upper motor neuron disorders (such as cerebral palsy and paraplegia); athetosis; stiff-man syndrome; and tetanus.

Valium Injection is a useful adjunct in status epilepticus and severe recurrent convulsive seizures.

Valium is a useful premedication (the IM route is preferred) for relief of anxiety and tension in patients who are to undergo surgical procedures. Intravenously, prior to cardioversion for the relief of anxiety and tension and to diminish the patient's recall of the procedure.

CONTRAINDICATIONS

Valium Injection is contraindicated in patients with a known hypersensitivity to this drug; acute narrow angle glaucoma; and open angle glaucoma unless patients are receiving appropriate therapy.

WARNINGS

When used intravenously, the following procedures should be undertaken to reduce the possibility of venous thrombosis, phlebitis, local irritation, swelling, and, rarely, vascular impairment: the solution should be injected slowly, taking at least 1 minute for each 5 mg (1 mL) given; do not use small veins, such as those on the dorsum of the hand or wrist; extreme care should be taken to avoid intra-arterial administration or extravasation.

Do not mix or dilute Valium with other solutions or drugs in syringe or infusion flask. If it is not feasible to administer Valium directly IV, it may be injected slowly through the infusion tubing as close as possible to the vein insertion.

Extreme care must be used in administering Valium Injection, particularly by the IV route, to the elderly, to very ill patients and to those with limited pulmonary reserve because of the possibility that apnea and/or cardiac arrest may occur. Concomitant use of barbiturates, alcohol or other central nervous system depressants increases depression with increased risk of apnea. Resuscitative equipment including that necessary to support respiration should be readily available.

When Valium is used with a narcotic analgesic, the dosage of the narcotic should be reduced by at least one-third and administered in small increments. In some cases the use of a narcotic may not be necessary.

Valium Injection should not be administered to patients in shock, coma or in acute alcoholic intoxication with depression of vital signs. As is true of most CNS-acting drugs, patients receiving Valium should be cautioned against engaging in hazardous occupations requiring complete mental alertness, such as operating machinery or driving a motor vehicle.

Tonic status epilepticus has been precipitated in patients treated with IV Valium for petit mal status or petit mal variant status.

Usage in Pregnancy: **An increased risk of congenital malformations associated with the use of minor tranquilizers (diazepam, meprobamate and chlordiazepoxide) during the first trimester of pregnancy has been suggested in several studies. Because use of these drugs is rarely a matter of urgency, their use during this period should almost always be avoided. The possibility that a woman of childbearing potential may be pregnant at the time of institution of therapy should be considered. Patients should be advised that if they become pregnant during therapy or intend to become pregnant they should communicate with their physicians about the desirability of discontinuing the drug.**

In humans, measurable amounts of diazepam were found in maternal and cord blood, indicating placental transfer of the drug. Until additional information is available, Valium Injection is not recommended for obstetrical use.

Withdrawal symptoms of the barbiturate type have occurred after the discontinuation of benzodiazepines (see DRUG ABUSE AND DEPENDENCE section).

PRECAUTIONS

Although seizures may be brought under control promptly, a significant proportion of patients experience a return to seizure activity, presumably due to the short-lived effect of Valium after IV administration. The physician should be prepared to readminister the drug. However, Valium is not recommended for maintenance, and once seizures are brought under control, consideration should be given to the administration of agents useful in longer term control of seizures.

If Valium is to be combined with other psychotropic agents or anticonvulsant drugs, careful consideration should be given to the pharmacology of the agents to be employed—particularly with known compounds which may potentiate the action of Valium, such as phenothiazines, narcotics, barbiturates, MAO inhibitors and other antidepressants. In highly anxious patients with evidence of accompanying depression, particularly those who may have suicidal tendencies, protective measures may be necessary. The usual precautions in treating patients with impaired hepatic function should be observed. Metabolites of Valium are excreted by the kidney; to avoid their excess accumulation, caution should be exercised in the administration to patients with compromised kidney function.

Since an increase in cough reflex and laryngospasm may occur with peroral endoscopic procedures, the use of a topical anesthetic agent and the availability of necessary countermeasures are recommended.

Until additional information is available, diazepam injection is not recommended for obstetrical use.

Valium Injection has produced hypotension or muscular weakness in some patients particularly when used with narcotics, barbiturates or alcohol.

Lower doses (usually 2 mg to 5 mg) should be used for elderly and debilitated patients.

The clearance of Valium and certain other benzodiazepines can be delayed in association with Tagamet (cimetidine) administration. The clinical significance of this is unclear.

Pediatric Use: Safety and effectiveness in pediatric patients below the age of 30 days have not been established. Prolonged central nervous system depression has been observed in neonates, apparently due to inability to biotransform Valium into inactive metabolites.

In pediatric use, in order to obtain maximal clinical effect with the minimum amount of drug and thus to reduce the risk of hazardous side effects, such as apnea or prolonged periods of somnolence, it is recommended that the drug be given slowly over a 3-minute period in a dosage not to exceed 0.25 mg/kg. After an interval of 15 to 30 minutes the initial dosage can be safely repeated. If, however, relief of symptoms is not obtained after a third administration, adjunctive therapy appropriate to the condition being treated is recommended.

ADVERSE REACTIONS

Side effects most commonly reported were drowsiness, fatigue and ataxia; venous thrombosis and phlebitis at the site of injection. Other adverse reactions less frequently reported include: *CNS:* confusion, depression, dysarthria, headache, hypoactivity, slurred speech, syncope, tremor, vertigo. *GI:* constipation, nausea. *GU:* incontinence, changes in libido, urinary retention. *Cardiovascular:* bradycardia, cardiovascular collapse, hypotension. *EENT:* blurred vision, diplopia, nystagmus. *Skin:* urticaria, skin rash. *Other:* hiccups, changes in salivation, neutropenia, jaundice.

Paradoxical reactions such as acute hyperexcited states, anxiety, hallucinations, increased muscle spasticity, insomnia, rage, sleep disturbances and stimulation have been reported; should these occur, use of the drug should be discontinued. Minor changes in EEG patterns, usually low-voltage fast activity, have been observed in patients during and after Valium therapy and are of no known significance.

In peroral endoscopic procedures, coughing, depressed respiration, dyspnea, hyperventilation, laryngospasm and pain in throat or chest have been reported.

Because of isolated reports of neutropenia and jaundice, periodic blood counts and liver function tests are advisable during long-term therapy.

DRUG ABUSE AND DEPENDENCE

Withdrawal symptoms, similar in character to those noted with barbiturates and alcohol (convulsions, tremor, abdominal and muscle cramps, vomiting and sweating), have occurred following abrupt discontinuance of diazepam. The more severe withdrawal symptoms have usually been limited to those patients who had received excessive doses over an extended period of time. Generally milder withdrawal symptoms (eg, dysphoria and insomnia) have been reported following abrupt discontinuance of benzodiazepines taken continuously at therapeutic levels for several months. Consequently, after extended therapy, abrupt discontinuation should generally be avoided and a gradual dosage tapering schedule followed. Addiction-prone individuals (such as drug addicts or alcoholics) should be under careful surveillance when receiving diazepam or other psychotropic agents because of the predisposition of such patients to habituation and dependence.

DOSAGE AND ADMINISTRATION

Dosage should be individualized for maximum beneficial effect. The usual recommended dose in adults ranges from 2 mg to 20 mg IM or IV, depending on the indication and its severity. In some conditions, eg, tetanus, larger doses may be required. (See dosage for specific indications.) In acute conditions the injection may be repeated within 1 hour although an interval of 3 to 4 hours is usually satisfactory. Lower doses (usually 2 mg to 5 mg) and slow increase in dosage should be used for elderly or debilitated patients and when other sedative drugs are administered (see WARNINGS and ADVERSE REACTIONS).

For dosage in pediatric patients above the age of 30 days, see the specific indications below. When intravenous use is indicated, facilities for respiratory assistance should be readily available.

Intramuscular: Valium Injection should be injected deeply into the muscle.

Intravenous Use: (See WARNINGS and PRECAUTIONS: *Pediatric Use.*) The solution should be injected slowly, taking at least 1 minute for each 5 mg (1 mL) given. Do not use small veins, such as those on the dorsum of the hand or wrist. Extreme care should be taken to avoid intra-arterial administration or extravasation.

Do not mix or dilute Valium with other solutions or drugs in syringe or infusion flask. If it is not feasible to administer Valium directly IV, it may be injected slowly through the infusion tubing as close as possible to the vein insertion.

[See table at top of next page]

USUAL ADULT DOSAGE		DOSAGE RANGE IN PEDIATRIC PATIENTS (IV administration should be made slowly)
Moderate Anxiety Disorders and Symptoms of Anxiety.	2 mg to 5 mg, IM or IV. Repeat in 3 to 4 hours, if necessary.	
Severe Anxiety Disorders and Symptoms of Anxiety.	5 mg to 10 mg, IM or IV. Repeat in 3 to 4 hours, if necessary.	
Acute Alcohol Withdrawal: As an aid in symptomatic relief of acute agitation, tremor, impending or acute delirium tremens and hallucinosis.	10 mg, IM or IV initially, then 5 mg to 10 mg in 3 to 4 hours, if necessary.	
Endoscopic Procedures: Adjunctively, if apprehension, anxiety or acute stress reactions are present prior to endoscopic procedures. Dosage of narcotics should be reduced by at least a third and in some cases may be omitted. See *Precautions* for peroral procedures.	Titrate IV dosage to desired sedative response, such as slurring of speech, with slow administration immediately prior to the procedure. Generally 10 mg or less is adequate, but up to 20 mg IV may be given, particularly when concomitant narcotics are omitted. If IV cannot be used, 5 mg to 10 mg IM approximately 30 minutes prior to the procedure.	
Muscle Spasm: Associated with local pathology, cerebral palsy, athetosis, stiff-man syndrome or tetanus.	5 mg to 10 mg, IM or IV initially, then 5 mg to 10 mg in 3 to 4 hours, if necessary. For tetanus, larger doses may be required.	For tetanus in pediatric patients between 30 days and 5 years of age, 1 mg to 2 mg IM or IV, slowly, repeated every 3 to 4 hours as necessary. In pediatric patients 5 years or older, 5 mg to 10 mg repeated every 3 to 4 hours may be required to control tetanus spasms. Respiratory assistance should be available.
Status Epilepticus and Severe Recurrent Convulsive Seizures: In the convulsing patient, the IV route is by far preferred. This injection should be administered slowly. However, if IV administration is impossible, the IM route may be used.	5 mg to 10 mg initially (IV preferred). This injection may be repeated if necessary at 10 to 15 minute intervals up to a maximum dose of 30 mg. If necessary, therapy with Valium may be repeated in 2 to 4 hours; however, residual active metabolites may persist, and readministration should be made with this consideration. Extreme caution must be exercised with individuals with chronic lung disease or unstable cardiovascular status.	Pediatric patients between the ages of 30 days and 5 years, 0.2 mg to 0.5 mg slowly every 2 to 5 minutes up to a maximum of 5 mg (IV preferred). Pediatric patients 5 years or older, 1 mg every 2 to 5 minutes up to a maximum of 10 mg (slow IV administration preferred). Repeat in 2 to 4 hours if necessary. EEG monitoring of the seizure may be helpful.
Preoperative Medication: To relieve anxiety and tension. (If atropine, scopolamine or other premedications are desired, they must be administered in separate syringes.)	10 mg, IM (preferred route), before surgery.	
Cardioversion: To relieve anxiety and tension and to reduce recall of procedure.	5 mg to 15 mg, IV, within 5 to 10 minutes prior to the procedure.	

Once the acute symptomatology has been properly controlled with Valium Injection, the patient may be placed on oral therapy with Valium if further treatment is required.

Management of Overdosage:
Manifestations of Valium overdosage include somnolence, confusion, coma and diminished reflexes. Respiration, pulse and blood pressure should be monitored, as in all cases of drug overdosage, although, in general, these effects have been minimal. General supportive measures should be employed, along with intravenous fluids, and an adequate airway maintained. Hypotension may be combated by the use of Levophed® (levarterenol) or Aramine (metaraminol). Dialysis is of limited value.
Flumazenil, a specific benzodiazepine-receptor antagonist, is indicated for the complete or partial reversal of the sedative effects of benzodiazepines and may be used in situations when an overdose with a benzodiazepine is known or suspected. Prior to the administration of flumazenil, necessary measures should be instituted to secure airway, ventilation and intravenous access. Flumazenil is intended as an adjunct to, not as a substitute for, proper management of benzodiazepine overdose. Patients treated with flumazenil should be monitored for resedation, respiratory depression and other residual benzodiazepine effects for an appropriate period after treatment. **The prescriber should be aware of a risk of seizure in association with flumazenil treatment, particularly in long-term benzodiazepine users and cyclic antidepressant overdose.** The complete flumazenil package insert, including CONTRAINDICATIONS, WARNINGS and PRECAUTIONS, should be consulted prior to use.

HOW SUPPLIED

Ampuls, 2 mL, boxes of 10 (NDC 0140-1931-06); *Vials,* 10 mL, boxes of 1 (NDC 0140-1932-06). *Tel-E-Ject ®* (disposable syringes), 2 mL, boxes of 10 (NDC 0140-1933-06).

ANIMAL PHARMACOLOGY

Oral LD$_{50}$ of diazepam is 720 mg/kg in mice and 1240 mg/kg in rats. Intraperitoneal administration of 400 mg/kg to a monkey resulted in death on the sixth day.

Reproduction Studies: A series of rat reproduction studies was performed with diazepam in oral doses of 1, 10, 80 and 100 mg/kg given for periods ranging from 60 to 228 days prior to mating. At 100 mg/kg there was a decrease in the number of pregnancies and surviving offspring in these rats. These effects may be attributable to prolonged sedative activity, resulting in lack of interest in mating and lessened maternal nursing and care of the young. Neonatal survival of rats at doses lower than 100 mg/kg was within normal limits. Several neonates, both controls and experimentals, in these rat reproduction studies showed skeletal or other defects. Further studies in rats at doses up to and including 80 mg/kg/day did not reveal significant teratological effects on the offspring. Rabbits were maintained on doses of 1, 2, 5 and 8 mg/kg from day 6 through day 18 of gestation. No adverse effects on reproduction and no teratological changes were noted.

Manufactured by Hoffmann-La Roche Inc., Nutley N.J. 07110

Revised: April 1997

VALIUM®   Ⓒ
[val 'ee-um]
brand of diazepam
TABLETS

The following text is complete prescribing information based on official labeling in effect June 1998.

DESCRIPTION

Valium (diazepam) is a benzodiazepine derivative developed through original Roche research. Chemically, diazepam is 7-chloro-1,3-dihydro-1-methyl -5- phenyl-2H-1,4-benzodiazepin-2-one. It is a colorless crystalline compound, insoluble in water and has a molecular weight of 284.74.

Valium 5-mg tablets contain FD&C Yellow No. 6 and D&C Yellow No. 10 dyes. Valium 10-mg tablets contain FD&C Blue No. 1 dye. Valium 2-mg tablets contain no dye.

PHARMACOLOGY

In animals, Valium appears to act on parts of the limbic system, the thalamus and hypothalamus, and induces calming effects. Valium, unlike chlorpromazine and reserpine, has no demonstrable peripheral autonomic blocking action, nor does it produce extrapyramidal side effects; however, animals treated with Valium do have a transient ataxia at higher doses. Valium was found to have transient cardiovascular depressor effects in dogs. Long-term experiments in rats revealed no disturbances of endocrine function.

Oral LD$_{50}$ of diazepam is 720 mg/kg in mice and 1240 mg/kg in rats. Intraperitoneal administration of 400 mg/kg to a monkey resulted in death on the sixth day.

Reproduction Studies: A series of rat reproduction studies was performed with diazepam in oral doses of 1, 10, 80 and 100 mg/kg. At 100 mg/kg there was a decrease in the number of pregnancies and surviving offspring in these rats. Neonatal survival of rats at doses lower than 100 mg/kg was within normal limits. Several neonates in these rat reproduction studies showed skeletal or other defects. Further studies in rats at doses up to and including 80 mg/kg/day did not reveal teratological effects on the offspring.

In humans, measurable blood levels of Valium were obtained in maternal and cord blood, indicating placental transfer of the drug.

INDICATIONS

Valium is indicated for the management of anxiety disorders or for the short-term relief of the symptoms of anxiety. Anxiety or tension associated with the stress of everyday life usually does not require treatment with an anxiolytic. In acute alcohol withdrawal, Valium may be useful in the symptomatic relief of acute agitation, tremor, impending or acute delirium tremens and hallucinosis.

Valium is a useful adjunct for the relief of skeletal muscle spasm due to reflex spasm to local pathology (such as inflammation of the muscles or joints, or secondary to trauma); spasticity caused by upper motor neuron disorders (such as cerebral palsy and paraplegia); athetosis; and stiff-man syndrome.

Oral Valium may be used adjunctively in convulsive disorders, although it has not proved useful as the sole therapy. The effectiveness of Valium in long-term use, that is, more than 4 months, has not been assessed by systematic clinical studies. The physician should periodically reassess the usefulness of the drug for the individual patient.

CONTRAINDICATIONS

Valium is contraindicated in patients with a known hypersensitivity to this drug and, because of lack of sufficient clinical experience, in pediatric patients under 6 months of age. It may be used in patients with open angle glaucoma who are receiving appropriate therapy, but is contraindicated in acute narrow angle glaucoma.

WARNINGS

Valium is not of value in the treatment of psychotic patients and should not be employed in lieu of appropriate treatment. As is true of most preparations containing CNS-acting drugs, patients receiving Valium should be cautioned against engaging in hazardous occupations requiring complete mental alertness such as operating machinery or driving a motor vehicle.

As with other agents which have anticonvulsant activity, when Valium is used as an adjunct in treating convulsive disorders, the possibility of an increase in the frequency and/or severity of grand mal seizures may require an increase in the dosage of standard anticonvulsant medication.

Continued on next page

Valium Tablets—Cont.

Abrupt withdrawal of Valium in such cases may also be associated with a temporary increase in the frequency and/or severity of seizures.

Since Valium has a central nervous system depressant effect, patients should be advised against the simultaneous ingestion of alcohol and other CNS-depressant drugs during Valium therapy.

> *Usage in Pregnancy:* **An increased risk of congenital malformations associated with the use of minor tranquilizers (diazepam, meprobamate and chlordiazepoxide) during the first trimester of pregnancy has been suggested in several studies. Because use of these drugs is rarely a matter of urgency, their use during this period should almost always be avoided. The possibility that a woman of childbearing potential may be pregnant at the time of institution of therapy should be considered. Patients should be advised that if they become pregnant during therapy or intend to become pregnant they should communicate with their physicians about the desirability of discontinuing the drug.**

Management of Overdosage: Manifestations of Valium overdosage include somnolence, confusion, coma and diminished reflexes. Respiration, pulse and blood pressure should be monitored, as in all cases of drug overdosage, although, in general, these effects have been minimal following overdosage. General supportive measures should be employed, along with immediate gastric lavage. Intravenous fluids should be administered and an adequate airway maintained. Hypotension may be combated by the use of Levophed® (levarterenol) or Aramine (metaraminol). Dialysis is of limited value. As with the management of intentional overdosage with any drug, it should be borne in mind that multiple agents may have been ingested.

Flumazenil, a specific benzodiazepine-receptor antagonist, is indicated for the complete or partial reversal of the sedative effects of benzodiazepines and may be used in situations when an overdose with a benzodiazepine is known or suspected. Prior to the administration of flumazenil, necessary measures should be instituted to secure airway, ventilation, and intravenous access. Flumazenil is intended as an adjunct to, not as a substitute for, proper management of benzodiazepine overdose. Patients treated with flumazenil should be monitored for resedation, respiratory depression and other residual benzodiazepine effects for an appropriate period after treatment. **The prescriber should be aware of a risk of seizure in association with flumazenil treatment, particularly in long-term benzodiazepine users and in cyclic antidepressant overdose.** The complete flumazenil package insert, including CONTRAINDICATIONS, WARNINGS and PRECAUTIONS, should be consulted prior to use.

Withdrawal symptoms of the barbiturate type have occurred after the discontinuation of benzodiazepines. (See DRUG ABUSE AND DEPENDENCE section.)

PRECAUTIONS

If Valium is to be combined with other psychotropic agents or anticonvulsant drugs, careful consideration should be given to the pharmacology of the agents to be employed—particularly with known compounds which may potentiate the action of Valium, such as phenothiazines, narcotics, barbiturates, MAO inhibitors and other antidepressants. The usual precautions are indicated for severely depressed patients or those in whom there is any evidence of latent depression; particularly the recognition that suicidal tendencies may be present and protective measures may be necessary. The usual precautions in treating patients with impaired renal or hepatic function should be observed.

In elderly and debilitated patients, it is recommended that the dosage be limited to the smallest effective amount to preclude the development of ataxia or oversedation (2 mg to $2\frac{1}{2}$ mg once or twice daily, initially, to be increased gradually as needed and tolerated).

The clearance of Valium and certain other benzodiazepines can be delayed in association with Tagamet (cimetidine) administration. The clinical significance of this is unclear.

Information for Patients: To assure the safe and effective use of benzodiazepines, patients should be informed that, since benzodiazepines may produce psychological and physical dependence, it is advisable that they consult with their physician before either increasing the dose or abruptly discontinuing this drug.

Pediatric Use: Safety and effectiveness in pediatric patients below the age of 6 months have not been established.

ADVERSE REACTIONS

Side effects most commonly reported were drowsiness, fatigue and ataxia. Infrequently encountered were confusion, constipation, depression, diplopia, dysarthria, headache, hypotension, incontinence, jaundice, changes in libido, nausea, changes in salivation, skin rash, slurred speech, tremor, urinary retention, vertigo and blurred vision. Paradoxical reactions such as acute hyperexcited states, anxiety, hallucinations, increased muscle spasticity, insomnia, rage,

sleep disturbances and stimulation have been reported; should these occur, use of the drug should be discontinued. Because of isolated reports of neutropenia and jaundice, periodic blood counts and liver function tests are advisable during long-term therapy. Minor changes in EEG patterns, usually low-voltage fast activity, have been observed in patients during and after Valium therapy and are of no known significance.

DRUG ABUSE AND DEPENDENCE

Withdrawal symptoms, similar in character to those noted with barbiturates and alcohol (convulsions, tremor, abdominal and muscle cramps, vomiting and sweating), have occurred following abrupt discontinuance of diazepam. The more severe withdrawal symptoms have usually been limited to those patients who had received excessive doses over an extended period of time. Generally milder withdrawal symptoms (eg, dysphoria and insomnia) have been reported following abrupt discontinuation of benzodiazepines taken continuously at therapeutic levels for several months. Consequently, after extended therapy, abrupt discontinuation should generally be avoided and a gradual dosage tapering schedule followed. Addiction-prone individuals (such as drug addicts or alcoholics) should be under careful surveillance when receiving diazepam or other psychotropic agents because of the predisposition of such patients to habituation and dependence.

DOSAGE AND ADMINISTRATION

Dosage should be individualized for maximum beneficial effect. While the usual daily dosages given below will meet the needs of most patients, there will be some who may require higher doses. In such cases dosage should be increased cautiously to avoid adverse effects.

	USUAL DAILY DOSE
ADULTS:	
Management of Anxiety Disorders and Relief of Symptoms of Anxiety.	Depending upon severity of symptoms—2 mg to 10 mg, 2 to 4 times daily
Symptomatic Relief in Acute Alcohol Withdrawal.	10 mg, 3 or 4 times during the first 24 hours, reducing to 5 mg, 3 or 4 times daily as needed
Adjunctively for Relief of Skeletal Muscle Spasm.	2 mg to 10 mg, 3 or 4 times daily
Adjunctively in Convulsive Disorders.	2 mg to 10 mg, 2 to 4 times daily
Geriatric Patients, or in the presence of debilitating disease.	2 mg to $2\frac{1}{2}$ mg, 1 or 2 times daily initially; increase gradually as needed and tolerated
PEDIATRIC PATIENTS:	
Because of varied responses to CNS-acting drugs, initiate therapy with lowest dose and increase as required. Not for use in pediatric patients under 6 months.	1 mg to $2\frac{1}{2}$ mg, 3 or 4 times daily initially; increase gradually as needed and tolerated

HOW SUPPLIED

For oral administration, round, scored tablets with a cut out "V" design—2 mg, white—bottles of 100 (NDC 0140-0004-01) and 500 (NDC 0140-0004-14); 5 mg, yellow—bottles of 100 (NDC 0140-0005-01) and 500 (NDC 0140-0005-14); 10 mg, blue—bottles of 100 (NDC 0140-0006-01) and 500 (NDC 0140-0006-14).

Imprint on tablets:

2 mg:
2 VALIUM® (front)
ROCHE (scored side)

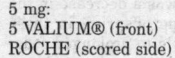

5 mg:
5 VALIUM® (front)
ROCHE (scored side)

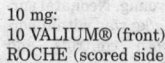

10 mg:
10 VALIUM® (front)
ROCHE (scored side)

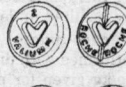
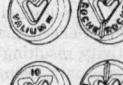

Revised: April 1997
Shown in Product Identification Guide, page 335

Roerig Division
see Pfizer Inc

Ross Products Division
**ABBOTT LABORATORIES INC.
COLUMBUS, OH 43215-1724**

Direct Inquiries to:
1-800-227-5767

CLEAR EYES®   OTC
[*klēr īz*]
Lubricant Eye Redness Reliever Drops

(See PDR For Ophthalmology.)

CLEAR EYES® ACR   OTC
[*klēr īz*]
Astringent/Lubricant Eye Redness Reliever Drops

(See PDR For Ophthalmology.)

CLEAR EYES® CLR   OTC
[*klēr īz*]
**Soothing drops
Contact Lens Relief**

(See PDR For Ophthalmology.)

EAR DROPS BY MURINE®   OTC
See Murine Ear Wax Removal System/Murine Ear Drops

MURINE TEARS®   OTC
[*mur 'ēn*]
Lubricant Eye Drops

(See PDR For Ophthalmology.)

MURINE TEARS® PLUS   OTC
[*mur 'ēn*]
Lubricant Redness Reliever Eye Drops

(See PDR For Ophthalmology.)

MURINE® EAR WAX REMOVAL SYSTEM/MURINE® EAR DROPS   OTC
[*mur 'ēn*]
Carbamide Peroxide Ear Wax Removal Aid

PEDIALYTE®   OTC
[*pē 'dē-ah-līt''*]
Oral Electrolyte Maintenance Solution

USAGE

To quickly restore fluid and minerals lost in diarrhea and vomiting; for maintenance of water and electrolytes following corrective parenteral therapy for severe diarrhea. Pedialyte is designed to promote fluid absorption more effectively than common household beverages.

Features:
- Ready To Use—no mixing or dilution necessary.
- Balanced electrolytes to replace diarrheal stool losses and provide maintenance requirements.
- Provides glucose to promote sodium and water absorption.
- Unflavored form available for young infants; fruit-flavored, bubble gum-flavored and grape-flavored forms available to enhance compliance in older infants and children.
- Freezer Pops (2.1-fl-oz Pedialyte per sleeve) available in Cherry, Orange, Grape and Blue Raspberry Flavors to encourage compliance with fluid intake recommendations for children 1 year of age and older.
- Plastic liter bottles are resealable, easy to pour and easy to measure.
- Widely available in grocery, drug and discount stores.

Pedialyte, Rehydralyte Administration Guide*

For Infants and Young Children

Age	2 Weeks	3	6	9	1	1½	2	2½	3	3½	4	5	6
		Months							Years				
Approximate Weight†													
(lb)	7	13	17	20	23	25	28	30	32	35	38	41	46
(kg)	3.2	6.0	7.8	9.2	10.2	11.4	12.6	13.6	14.6	16.0	17.0	18.7	20.7
PEDIALYTE fl oz/day for maintenance**	13 to 16	28 to 32	34 to 40	38 to 44	41 to 46	45 to 50	48 to 53	51 to 56	54 to 58	56 to 60	57 to 62	59 to 66	62 to 69
REHYDRALYTE fl oz/day for Replacement for 5% Dehydration (including maintenance)**	18 to 21	38 to 42	47 to 53	53 to 59	58 to 63	64 to 69	69 to 74	74 to 79	78 to 82	83 to 87	85 to 90	90 to 97	96 to 104
REHYDRALYTE fl oz/day for Replacement for 10% Dehydration (including maintenance)**	23 to 26	48 to 52	60 to 66	68 to 74	75 to 80	83 to 88	90 to 95	97 to 102	102 to 106	110 to 114	113 to 118	121 to 128	131 to 138

* Administration Guide does not apply to infants less than 1 week of age. For children over 6 years, maintenance intakes may exceed 2 liters daily.

** Fluid intake in guide is total fluid requirement from oral electrolyte solution, formula or other fluids, but does not take into account ongoing stool losses. Fluid loss in the stool should be replaced by consumption of an amount of Pedialyte or Rehydralyte equal to stool losses in addition to fluid maintenance requirement in this Administration Guide. Pedialyte Freezer Pops are to be used with Pedialyte Oral Electrolyte Maintenance Solution or other appropriate fluids to help prevent dehydration.

† Weight based on the 50th percentile of weight for age of the National Center for Health Statistics (NCHS) reference growth data. Hamill PVV, Drizd TA, Johnson CL, et al: Physical growth: National Center for Health Statistics percentiles. *Am J Clin Nutr* 1979;32:607-629.

1. Extrapolated from Barness L: Nutrition and nutritional disorders, in Behrman RE, Kliegman RM, Nelson WE, Vaughan VC III: *Nelson Textbook of Pediatrics,* ed 14. Philadelphia: WB Saunders Co, 1992, pp 105-107.

AVAILABILITY

Ready To Use:

1 Qt 1.8-fl-oz (1 L) plastic bottles; 8 per case; Unflavored, No. 00336; Fruit Flavor, No. 00365; Bubble Gum Flavor, No. 51752; Grape Flavor, No. 00240.

8-fl-oz (237 mL) bottles; 4 six-packs per case; Unflavored, No. 00160 (retail); 4-fl-oz (118 mL) glass bottles; 48 per case; Unflavored No. 51856 (hospital). 2.1-fl-oz sleeve Freezer Pops; 8 sixteen-sleeve boxes per case; Grape, Cherry, Orange and Blue Raspberry, No. 00245.

DOSAGE

Refer to Administration Guide to restore fluid and minerals lost in diarrhea and vomiting (Pedialyte Oral Electrolyte Maintenance Solution) and for management of mild to moderate dehydration secondary to moderate to severe diarrhea (Rehydralyte® Oral Electrolyte Rehydration Solution). Pedialyte or Rehydralyte should be offered frequently in amounts tolerated. Total daily intake should be adjusted to meet individual needs, based on thirst and response to therapy. The following suggested intakes for maintenance are based on water requirements for ordinary energy expenditure.[1] For dehydrated children, the suggested intakes are for replacement and for maintenance, based on a fluid deficit of 5% or 10% of body weight (including maintenance requirement). The fluid deficit should be replaced as quickly as possible, usually in the first 4 to 6 hours.

[See table above]

INGREDIENTS:

Unflavored: (Pareve,Ⓤ) Water, dextrose, potassium citrate, sodium chloride and sodium citrate.

Fruit Flavor: (Pareve,Ⓤ) Water, dextrose; less than 2% of: fructose, citric acid, natural and artificial fruit flavors, potassium citrate, sodium chloride, sodium citrate, aspartame and Yellow 6.

Grape Flavor: (Pareve,Ⓤ) Water, dextrose; less than 2% of: fructose, citric acid, potassium citrate, sodium chloride, artificial grape flavor, sodium citrate, aspartame, Red 40 and Blue 1.

Bubble Gum Flavor: (Pareve,Ⓤ) Water, dextrose; less than 2% of: fructose, citric acid, potassium citrate, sodium chloride, sodium citrate, artificial bubble gum flavor, aspartame and Red 40.

Freezer Pops: (Pareve,Ⓤ) Water, dextrose; less than 2% of: citric acid, sodium chloride, sodium carboxymethylcellulose, potassium citrate, aspartame, potassium sorbate and sodium benzoate; **Grape** also contains: Natural and artificial grape flavor, Red 40 and Blue 1; **Cherry** also contains: Natural and artificial cherry flavor and Red 40; **Orange** also contains: Natural and artificial orange flavor, Yellow 6 and Red 40; **Blue Raspberry** also contains: Natural and artificial blue raspberry flavor and Blue 1.

PHENYLKETONURICS: Pedialyte products that include aspartame contain Phenylalanine.

	Per 8 Fl Oz	Per Liter
Provides:		
Sodium (mEq)	10.6	45
Potassium (mEq)	4.7	20
Chloride (mEq)	8.3	35
Citrate (mEq)	7.1	30
Carbohydrate (g)	5.9	25
Calories	24	100

(FAN 3434)

PEDIAZOLE®   ℞
(8030)
erythromycin ethylsuccinate
and sulfisoxazole acetyl
for oral suspension

DESCRIPTION

Pediazole is a combination of erythromycin ethylsuccinate, USP, and sulfisoxazole acetyl, USP. When reconstituted with water as directed on the label, the granules form a white, strawberry-banana flavor suspension that provides the equivalent of 200 mg erythromycin activity and the equivalent of 600 mg of sulfisoxazole activity per teaspoonful (5 mL).

Erythromycin is produced by a strain of *Saccaropolyspora erythraea* and belongs to the macrolide group of antibiotics. It is basic and readily forms salts and esters. Erythromycin ethylsuccinate is the 2′-ethylsuccinyl ester of erythromycin. It is essentially a tasteless form of the antibiotic suitable for oral administration, particularly in suspension dosage forms. The chemical name is erythromycin 2′-(ethyl succinate). Erythromycin ethylsuccinate has the following structural formula:

Sulfisoxazole acetyl or N¹-acetyl sulfisoxazole is an ester of sulfisoxazole. Chemically, sulfisoxazole is N-(3,4-Dimethyl-5-isoxazolyl)-N-sulfanilylacetamide. Sulfisoxazole acetyl has the following structural formula:

[See chemical structure at top of next column]

Inactive Ingredients: Citric acid, magnesium aluminum silicate, poloxamer, sodium carboxymethylcellulose, sodium citrate, sucrose and artificial flavoring.

CLINICAL PHARMACOLOGY

Orally administered erythromycin ethylsuccinate suspensions are readily and reliably absorbed. Erythromycin ethylsuccinate products have demonstrated rapid and consistent absorption in both fasting and nonfasting conditions. However, higher serum concentrations are obtained when these products are given with food. Bioavailability data are available from Ross Products Division. Erythromycin is largely bound to plasma proteins. After absorption, erythromycin diffuses readily into most body fluids. In the absence of meningeal inflammation, low concentrations are normally achieved in the spinal fluid, but the passage of the drug across the blood-brain barrier increases in meningitis. Erythromycin crosses the placental barrier and is excreted in human milk. Erythromycin is not removed by peritoneal dialysis or hemodialysis.

In the presence of normal hepatic function, erythromycin is concentrated in the liver and is excreted in the bile; the effect of hepatic dysfunction on biliary excretion of erythromycin is not known. After oral administration, less than 5% of the administered dose can be recovered in the active form in the urine.

Wide variation in blood levels may result following identical doses of a sulfonamide. Blood levels should be measured in patients receiving these drugs for serious infections. Free sulfonamide blood levels of 50 to 150 mcg/mL may be considered therapeutically effective for most infections, with blood levels of 120 to 150 mcg/mL being optimal for serious infections. The maximum sulfonamide level should be 200 mcg/mL, because adverse reactions occur more frequently above this concentration.

Following oral administration, sulfisoxazole is rapidly and completely absorbed; the small intestine is the major site of absorption, but some of the drug is absorbed from the stomach. Sulfonamides are present in the blood as free, conjugated (acetylated and possibly other forms), and protein-bound forms. The amount present as "free" drug is considered to be the therapeutically active form. Approximately 85% of a dose of sulfisoxazole is bound to plasma proteins, primarily to albumin; 65% to 72% of the unbound portion is in the nonacetylated form.

Maximum plasma concentrations of intact sulfisoxazole following a single 2-g oral dose of sulfisoxazole to healthy adult volunteers ranged from 127 to 211 mcg/mL (mean, 169 mcg/mL), and the time of peak plasma concentration ranged from 1 to 4 hours (mean, 2.5 hours). The elimination half-life of sulfisoxazole ranged from 4.6 to 7.8 hours after oral administration. The elimination of sulfisoxazole has been shown to be slower in elderly subjects (63 to 75 years) with diminished renal function (creatine clearance 37 to 68 mL/min).[1] After multiple-dose oral administration of 500 mg q.i.d. to healthy volunteers, the average steady-state plasma concentrations of intact sulfisoxazole ranged from 49.9 to 88.8 mcg/mL (mean, 63.4 mcg/mL).[2]

Sulfisoxazole and its acetylated metabolites are excreted primarily by the kidneys through glomerular filtration. Concentrations of sulfisoxazole are considerably higher in the urine than in the blood. The mean urinary recovery following oral administration of sulfisoxazole is 97% within 48 hours; 52% of this is intact drug, and the remainder is the N⁴-acetylated metabolite.

Sulfisoxazole is distributed only in extracellular body fluids. It is excreted in human milk. It readily crosses the placental barrier. In healthy subjects, cerebrospinal fluid concentrations of sulfisoxazole vary; in patients with meningitis, however, concentrations of free drug in cerebrospinal fluid as high as 94 mcg/mL have been reported.

Microbiology:

Pediazole has been formulated to contain sulfisoxazole for concomitant use with erythromycin.

Erythromycin acts by inhibition of protein synthesis by binding 50 S ribosomal subunits of susceptible organisms. It does not affect nucleic acid synthesis. Antagonism has been demonstrated *in vitro* between erythromycin and clindamycin, lincomycin, and chloramphenicol.

The sulfonamides are bacteriostatic agents, and the spectrum of activity is similar for all. Sulfonamides inhibit bacterial synthesis of dihydrofolic acid by preventing the condensation of the pteridine with *para*-aminobenzoic acid

Continued on next page

Pediazole—Cont.

through competitive inhibition of the enzyme dihydropteroate synthetase. Resistant strains have altered dihydropteroate synthetase with reduced affinity for sulfonamides or produce increased quantities of *para*-aminobenzoic acid.

Susceptibility Testing:

Quantitative methods that require measurement of zone diameter give the most precise estimates of the susceptibility of bacteria to antimicrobial agents. One such standardized single-disc procedure[3] has been recommended for use with discs to test susceptibility to erythromycin and sulfisoxazole. Interpretation involves correlation of the zone diameters obtained in the disc test with minimal inhibitory concentration (MIC) values for erythromycin.

If the standardized procedure of disc susceptibility is used, a 15-mcg erythromycin disc should give a zone diameter of at least 18 mm when tested against an erythromycin-susceptible bacterial strain, and a 250-300 mcg sulfisoxazole disc should give a zone diameter of at least 17 mm when tested against a sulfisoxazole-susceptible bacterial strain.

In vitro sulfonamide susceptibility tests are not always reliable because media containing excessive amounts of thymidine are capable of reversing the inhibitory effect of sulfonamides, which may result in false resistant reports. The tests must be carefully coordinated with bacteriological and clinical responses. When the patient is already taking sulfonamides, follow-up cultures should have aminobenzoic acid added to the isolation media but not to subsequent susceptibility test media.

INDICATIONS AND USAGE

For treatment of ACUTE OTITIS MEDIA in children that is caused by susceptible strains of *Haemophilus influenzae*.

CONTRAINDICATIONS

Pediazole is contraindicated in the following patient populations:

Patients with a known hypersensitivity to either of its components, children younger than 2 months, pregnant women *at term*, and mothers nursing infants less than 2 months of age.

Use in pregnant women at term, in children less than 2 months of age, and in mothers nursing infants less than 2 months of age is contraindicated because sulfonamides may promote kernicterus in the newborn by displacing bilirubin from plasma proteins.

Erythromycin is contraindicated in patients taking terfenadine. (**See PRECAUTIONS—Drug Interactions.**)

WARNINGS

FATALITIES ASSOCIATED WITH THE ADMINISTRATION OF SULFONAMIDES, ALTHOUGH RARE, HAVE OCCURRED DUE TO SEVERE REACTIONS INCLUDING STEVENS-JOHNSON SYNDROME, TOXIC EPIDERMAL NECROLYSIS, FULMINANT HEPATIC NECROSIS, AGRANULOCYTOSIS, APLASTIC ANEMIA, AND OTHER BLOOD DYSCRASIAS.

SULFONAMIDES, INCLUDING SULFONAMIDE-CONTAINING PRODUCTS SUCH AS PEDIAZOLE, SHOULD BE DISCONTINUED AT THE FIRST APPEARANCE OF SKIN RASH OR ANY SIGN OF ADVERSE REACTION. In rare instances, a skin rash may be followed by a more severe reaction, such as Stevens-Johnson syndrome, toxic epidermal necrolysis, hepatic necrosis, and serious blood disorders. (**See PRECAUTIONS.**)

Clinical signs such as sore throat, fever, pallor, rash, purpura, or jaundice may be early indications of serious reactions.

There have been reports of hepatic dysfunction with or without jaundice, occurring in patients receiving oral erythromycin products.

Cough, shortness of breath, and pulmonary infiltrates are hypersensitivity reactions of the respiratory tract that have been reported in association with sulfonamide treatment.

The sulfonamides should not be used for the treatment of group A beta-hemolytic streptococcal infections. In an established infection, they will not eradicate the streptococcus and, therefore, will not prevent sequelae such as rheumatic fever.

Pseudomembranous colitis has been reported with nearly all antibacterial agents, including Pediazole, and may range in severity from mild to life-threatening. Therefore, it is important to consider this diagnosis in patients who present with diarrhea subsequent to the administration of antibacterial agents.

Treatment with antibacterial agents alters the normal flora of the colon and may permit overgrowth of clostridia. Studies indicate that a toxin produced by *Clostridium difficile* is one primary cause of "antibiotic-associated colitis."

After diagnosis of pseudomembranous colitis has been established, therapeutic measures should be initiated. Mild cases of pseudomembranous colitis usually respond to drug discontinuation alone. In moderate to severe cases, consideration should be given to management with fluids and electrolytes, protein supplementation, and treatment with an antibacterial drug clinically effective against *Clostridium difficile* colitis.

There have been reports suggesting that erythromycin does not reach the fetus in adequate concentration to prevent congenital syphilis. Infants born to women treated during pregnancy with erythromycin for early syphilis should be treated with an appropriate penicillin regimen.

Rhabdomyolysis with or without renal impairment has been reported in seriously ill patients receiving erythromycin concomitantly with lovastatin. Therefore, patients receiving concomitant lovastatin and erythromycin should be carefully monitored for creatine kinase (CK) and serum transaminase levels. (See package insert for lovastatin.)

PRECAUTIONS

General: Erythromycin is principally excreted by the liver. Caution should be exercised when erythromycin is administered to patients with impaired hepatic function. (**See CLINICAL PHARMACOLOGY and WARNING sections.**)

Prolonged or repeated use of erythromycin may result in an overgrowth of nonsusceptible bacteria or fungi. If superinfection occurs, erythromycin should be discontinued and appropriate therapy instituted.

There have been reports that erythromycin may aggravate the weakness of patients with myasthenia gravis.

When indicated, incision and drainage or other surgical procedures should be performed in conjunction with antibiotic therapy.

Sulfonamides should be given with caution to patients with impaired renal or hepatic function and to those with severe allergy or bronchial asthma. In glucose-6-phosphate dehydrogenase-deficient individuals, hemolysis may occur; this reaction is frequently dose-related.

Information for Patients: Patients should maintain an adequate fluid intake to prevent crystalluria and stone formation.

Laboratory Tests: Complete blood counts should be done frequently in patients receiving sulfonamides. If a significant reduction in the count of any formed blood element is noted, Pediazole should be discontinued. Urinalysis with careful microscopic examination and renal function tests should be performed during therapy, particularly for those patients with impaired renal function. Blood levels should be measured in patients receiving a sulfonamide for serious infections. (**See INDICATIONS AND USAGE.**)

Drug/laboratory Test Interactions: Erythromycin interferes with the fluorometric determination of urinary catecholamines.

Drug Interactions: Erythromycin use in patients who are receiving high doses of theophylline may be associated with an increase in serum theophylline levels and potential theophylline toxicity. In case of theophylline toxicity and/or elevated serum theophylline levels, the dose of theophylline should be reduced while the patient is receiving concomitant erythromycin therapy.

Concomitant administration of erythromycin and digoxin has been reported to result in elevated digoxin serum levels. There have been reports of increased anticoagulant effects when erythromycin and oral anticoagulants were used concomitantly. Increased anticoagulation effects due to this drug may be more pronounced in the elderly.

Concurrent use of erythromycin and ergotamine or dihydroergotamine has been associated in some patients with acute ergot toxicity characterized by severe peripheral vasospasm and dysesthesia.

Erythromycin has been reported to decrease the clearance of triazolam and midazolam and thus may increase the pharmacologic effect of these benzodiazepines.

The use of erythromycin in patients concurrently taking drugs metabolized by the cytochrome P450 system may be associated with elevations in serum levels of these other drugs. There have been reports of interactions of erythromycin with carbamazepine, cyclosporine, hexobarbital, phenytoin, alfentanil, diisopyramide, lovastatin, and bromocriptine. Serum concentrations of drugs metabolized by the cytochrome P450 system should be monitored closely in patients concurrently receiving erythromycin.

Erythromycin significantly alters the metabolism of terfenadine when taken concomitantly. Rare cases of serious cardiovascular adverse events, including death, cardiac arrest, torsades de pointes, and other ventricular arrhythmias, have been observed. (**See CONTRAINDICATIONS.**)

It has been reported that sulfisoxazole may prolong the prothrombin time in patients who are receiving the anticoagulant warfarin. This interaction should be kept in mind when Pediazole is given to patients already on anticoagulant therapy, and the coagulation time should be reassessed.

It has been proposed that sulfisoxazole competes with thiopental for plasma protein binding. In one study involving 48 patients, intravenous sulfisoxazole resulted in a decrease in the amount of thiopental required for anesthesia and in a shortening of the awakening time. It is not known whether chronic oral doses of sulfisoxazole have a similar effect. Until more is known about this interaction, physicians should be aware that patients receiving sulfisoxazole might require less thiopental for anesthesia.

Sulfonamides can displace methotrexate from plasma protein binding sites, thus increasing free methotrexate concentrations. Studies in man have shown sulfisoxazole infusions to decrease plasma protein-bound methotrexate by one fourth.

Sulfisoxazole can also potentiate the blood-sugar-lowering activity of sulfonylureas.

Carcinogenesis, Mutagenesis, Impairment of Fertility:

Carcinogenesis: Pediazole has not undergone adequate trials relating to carcinogenicity; each component, however, has been evaluated separately. Long-term (21 month) oral studies conducted in rats with erythromycin ethylsuccinate did not provide evidence of tumorigenicity. Sulfisoxazole was not carcinogenic in either sex when administered to mice by gavage for 103 weeks at dosages up to approximately 18 times the recommended human dose or to rats at 4 times the human dose. Rats appear to be especially susceptible to the goitrogenic effects of sulfonamides, and long-term administration of sulfonamides has resulted in thyroid malignancies in this species.

Mutagenesis: There are no studies available that adequately evaluate the mutagenic potential of Pediazole or either of its components. However, sulfisoxazole was not observed to be mutagenic in *E. coli* Sd-4-73 when tested in the absence of a metabolic activating system. There was no apparent effect on male or female fertility in rats fed erythromycin (base) at levels up to 0.25% of diet.

Impairment of Fertility: Pediazole has not undergone adequate trials relating to impairment of fertility. In a reproduction study in rats given 7 times the human dose per day of sulfisoxazole, no effects were observed regarding mating behavior, conception rate or fertility index (percent pregnant).

Pregnancy: Teratogenic Effects. Pregnancy Category C. At dosages 7 times the human daily dose, sulfisoxazole was not teratogenic in either rats or rabbits. However, in two other teratogenicity studies, cleft palates developed in both rats and mice after administration of 5 to 9 times the human therapeutic dose of sulfisoxazole.

There is no evidence of teratogenicity or any other adverse effect on reproduction in female rats fed erythromycin base (up to 0.25% of diet) prior to and during mating, during gestation, and through weaning of two successive litters. There are, however, no adequate and well-controlled studies in pregnant women. Because animal reproduction studies are not always predictive of human response, this drug should be used during pregnancy only if clearly needed. Erythromycin has been reported to cross the placental barrier in humans, but fetal plasma levels are generally low.

There are no adequate or well-controlled studies of Pediazole in either laboratory animals or in pregnant women. It is not known whether Pediazole can cause fetal harm when administered to a pregnant woman prior to term or can affect reproduction capacity. Pediazole should be used during pregnancy only if the potential benefit justifies the potential risk to the fetus.

Nonteratogenic Effects: Kernicterus may occur in the newborn as a result of treatment of a pregnant woman *at term* with sulfonamides. (**See CONTRAINDICATIONS.**)

Labor and Delivery: The effects of erythromycin and sulfisoxazole on labor and delivery are unknown.

Nursing Mothers: Both erythromycin and sulfisoxazole are excreted in human milk. **Because of the potential for the development of kernicterus in neonates due to the displacement of bilirubin from plasma proteins by sulfisoxazole, a decision should be made whether to discontinue nursing or discontinue the drug, taking into account the importance of the drug to the mother. (See CONTRAINDICATIONS.)**

Pediatric Use: **See INDICATIONS AND USAGE and DOSAGE AND ADMINISTRATION** sections. Not for use in children under 2 months of age. (**See CONTRAINDICATIONS.**)

ADVERSE REACTIONS

Erythromycin ethylsuccinate: The most frequent side effects of oral erythromycin preparations are gastrointestinal and are dose-related. They include nausea, vomiting, abdominal pain, diarrhea and anorexia. Symptoms of hepatic dysfunction and/or abnormal liver-function test results may occur (**see WARNINGS section**). Pseudomembranous colitis has been rarely reported in association with erythromycin therapy.

Allergic reactions ranging from urticaria and mild skin eruptions to anaphylaxis have occurred.

There have been isolated reports of reversible hearing loss occurring chiefly in patients with renal insufficiency and in patients receiving high doses of erythromycin.

Onset of pseudomembranous colitis symptoms may occur during or after antibiotic treatment. (**See WARNINGS.**)

Sulfisoxazole acetyl: Included in the listing that follows are adverse reactions that have been reported with other

sulfonamide products: pharmacologic similarities require that each of the reactions be considered with Pediazole administration.

Allergic/Dermatologic: Anaphylaxis, erythema multiforme (Stevens-Johnson syndrome), toxic epidermal necrolysis (Lyell's syndrome), exfoliative dermatitis, angioedema, arteritis, vasculitis, allergic myocarditis, serum sickness, rash, urticaria, pruritus, photosensitivity, and conjunctival and scleral injection. In addition, periarteritis nodosa and systemic lupus erythematosus have been reported. **(See WARNINGS.)**

Cardiovascular: Tachycardia, palpitations, syncope, and cyanosis.

Rarely, erythromycin has been associated with the production of ventricular arrhythmias, including ventricular tachycardia and torsade de pointes, in individuals with prolonged QT intervals.

Endocrine: The sulfonamides bear certain chemical similarities to some goitrogens, diuretics (acetazolamide and the thiazides) and oral hypoglycemic agents. Cross-sensitivity may exist with these agents. Developments of goiter, diuresis, and hypoglycemia have occurred rarely in patients receiving sulfonamides.

Gastrointestinal: Hepatitis, hepatocellular necrosis, jaundice, pseudomembranous colitis, nausea, emesis, anorexia, abdominal pain, diarrhea, gastrointestinal hemorrhage, melena, flatulence, glossitis, stomatitis, salivary gland enlargement, and pancreatitis. Onset of pseudomembranous colitis symptoms may occur during or after treatment with sulfisoxazole, a component of Pediazole. **(See WARNINGS.)**

The sulfisoxazole acetyl component of Pediazole has been reported to cause increased elevation of liver-associated enzymes in patients with hepatitis.

Genitourinary: Crystalluria, hematuria, BUN and creatinine elevations, nephritis, and toxic nephrosis with oliguria and anuria. Acute renal failure and urinary retention have also been reported.

The frequency of renal complications, commonly associated with some sulfonamides, is lower in patients receiving the more soluble sulfonamides such as sulfisoxazole.

Hematologic: Leukopenia, agranulocytosis, aplastic anemia, thrombocytopenia, purpura, hemolytic anemia, eosinophilia, clotting disorders including hypoprothrombinemia and hypofibrinogenemia, sulfhemoglobinemia, and methemoglobinemia.

Neurologic: Headache, dizziness, peripheral neuritis, paresthesia, convulsions, tinnitus, vertigo, ataxia, and intracranial hypertension.

Psychiatric: Psychosis, hallucinations, disorientation, depression, and anxiety.

Respiratory: Cough, shortness of breath, and pulmonary infiltrates. **(See WARNINGS.)**

Vascular: Angioedema, arteritis, and vasculitis.

Miscellaneous: Edema (including periorbital), pyrexia, drowsiness, weakness, fatigue, lassitude, rigors, flushing, hearing loss, insomnia, and pneumonitis.

OVERDOSAGE

No information is available on a specific result of overdose with Pediazole. Overdosage of erythromycin should be handled with the prompt elimination of unabsorbed drug and all other appropriate measures. Erythromycin is not removed by peritoneal dialysis or hemodialysis.

The amount of a single dose of sulfisoxazole that is either associated with symptoms of overdosage or is likely to be life-threatening has not been reported. Signs and symptoms of overdosage reported with sulfonamides include anorexia, colic, nausea, vomiting, dizziness, headache, drowsiness and unconsciousness. Pyrexia, hematuria and crystalluria may be noted. Blood dyscrasias and jaundice are potential late manifestations of overdosage.

General principles of treatment include the immediate discontinuation of the drug, instituting gastric lavage or emesis, forcing oral fluids, and administering intravenous fluids if urine output is low and renal function is normal. The patient should be monitored with blood counts and appropriate blood chemistries, including electrolytes. If the patient becomes cyanotic, the possibility of methemoglobinemia should be considered and, if present, the condition should be treated appropriately with intravenous 1% methylene blue. If a significant blood dyscrasia or jaundice occurs, specific therapy should be instituted for these complications. Peritoneal dialysis is not effective, and hemodialysis is only moderately effective in removing sulfonamides.

The acute toxicity of sulfisoxazole in animals is as follows:

Species	$LD_{50} \pm$ S.E. · (mg/kg)
mouse	5700 ± 235
rats	>10,000
rabbits	>2000

DOSAGE AND ADMINISTRATION

PEDIAZOLE SHOULD NOT BE ADMINISTERED TO INFANTS UNDER 2 MONTHS OF AGE BECAUSE OF CONTRAINDICATIONS OF SYSTEMIC SULFONAMIDES IN THIS AGE GROUP.

For Acute Otitis Media in Children: The dose of Pediazole can be calculated based on the erythromycin component (50 mg/kg/day) or the sulfisoxazole component (150 mg/kg/day to a maximum of 6 g/day). The total daily dose of Pediazole should be administered in equally divided doses three or four times a day for 10 days. Pediazole may be administered without regard to meals.

The following approximate dosage schedules are recommended for using Pediazole:

Children: Two months of age or older

FOUR-TIMES-A-DAY SCHEDULE

Weight	Dose—every 6 hours
Less than 8 kg (<18 lbs)	Adjust dosage by body weight
8 kg (18 lbs)	$^1/_2$ teaspoonful (2.5 mL)
16 kg (35 lbs)	1 teaspoonful (5 mL)
24 kg (53 lbs)	$1^1/_2$ teaspoonfuls (7.5 mL)
Over 32 kg (over 70 lbs)	2 teaspoonfuls (10 mL)

THREE-TIMES-A-DAY SCHEDULE

Weight	Dose—every 8 hours
Less than 6 kg (<13 lbs)	Adjust dosage by body weight
6 kg (13 lbs)	$^1/_2$ teaspoonful (2.5 mL)
12 kg (26 lbs)	1 teaspoonful (5 mL)
18 kg (40 lbs)	$1^1/_2$ teaspoonfuls (7.5 mL)
24 kg (53 lbs)	2 teaspoonfuls (10 mL)
Over 30 kg (over 66 lbs)	$2^1/_2$ teaspoonfuls (12.5 mL)

TO PATIENT: Shake before using. Oversize bottle provides shake space. Keep tightly closed. Store in the refrigerator. Use within 14 days. Unused portion should be discarded after 14 days.

HOW SUPPLIED

Pediazole Suspension is available for teaspoon dosage in 100-mL (**NDC** 0074-8030-13), 150-mL (**NDC** 0074-8030-43), 200-mL (**NDC** 0074-8030-53) and 250-mL (**NDC** 0074-8030-73) bottles, in the form of granules to be reconstituted with water. The suspension provides erythromycin ethylsuccinate equivalent to 200 mg erythromycin activity and sulfisoxazole acetyl equivalent to 600 mg sulfisoxazole per teaspoonful (5 mL).

Before mixing, store below 86°F (30°C).

REFERENCES

1. Biovert A, Barbeau G, Belanger PM: Pharmacokinetics of sulfisoxazole in young and elderly subjects. *Gerontology* 1984; 30:125-131.
2. Oie S, Gambertoglio JG, Fleckenstein L: Comparison of the disposition of total and unbound sulfisoxazole after single and multiple dosing. *J Pharmacokinet Biopharm* 1982; 10:157-172.
3. National Committee for Clinical Laboratory Standards: *Performance Standards for Antimicrobial Disk Susceptibility Tests,* ed. 4. Approved Standard NCCLS Document M2-A4, Vol 10, No. 7. Villanova, Pa: NCCLS, 1990.

July 1994

PEDIASURE®   OTC
[pē 'dē-ah-shur″]
Complete Liquid Nutrition

USAGE

As a nutritionally complete, balanced, enteral formula especially designed for tube or oral feeding of children 1 to 10 years of age. Also available with fiber. The fiber level in PediaSure With Fiber helps maintain bowel function. May be used as the sole source of nutrition or as a supplement. PediaSure meets or exceeds 100% of the NAS-NRC RDAs for protein, vitamins and minerals for children 1 to 6 years of age in 1000 mL (approx. 34 fl oz), and for children 7 to 10 years of age in 1300 mL (approx. 44 fl oz). Calcium:phosphate ratio of 1.2:1 meets recommendations by the American Academy of Pediatrics Committee on Nutrition (AAP-CON) for growing children. Fortified with biotin, choline, inositol, taurine and carnitine.

Not for parenteral use.

Not intended for infants under 1 year of age unless specified by a doctor.

AVAILABILITY
Ready To Use:
8-fl-oz (237 mL) cans: 24 per case; Vanilla, No. 00373 (retail), Vanilla, No. 51804 (institution); Chocolate No. 51812 (retail), Chocolate, No. 51882 (institution); Strawberry, No. 51810 (retail), Strawberry, No. 51880 (institution); Banana Cream, No. 51808 (retail), Banana Cream, No. 51884 (institution); PediaSure With Fiber, Vanilla, No. 50652 (retail), Vanilla No. 51806 (institution).

COMPOSITION

Ready To Use PediaSure Vanilla. (Other flavors have similar composition and nutrient values. For specific information, see product labels.)

INGREDIENTS

Ⓦ-D Water, Maltodextrin (Corn), Sugar (Sucrose), Sodium Caseinate, High-Oleic Safflower Oil, Soy Oil, Fractionated Coconut Oil (Medium-Chain Triglycerides), Whey Protein Concentrate; less than 0.5% of: Calcium Phosphate Tribasic, Natural and Artificial Flavor, Potassium Citrate, Magnesium Chloride, Cellulose Gel, Potassium Phosphate Dibasic, Potassium Chloride, Soy Lecithin, Mono- and Diglycerides, Choline Chloride, Carrageenan, Ascorbic Acid, Cellulose Gum, m-Inositol, Taurine, Ferrous Sulfate, Zinc Sulfate, Niacinamide, Alpha-Tocopheryl Acetate, L-Carnitine, Calcium Pantothenate, Thiamine Chloride Hydrochloride, Pyridoxine Hydrochloride, Riboflavin, Manganese Sulfate, Cupric Sulfate, Vitamin A Palmitate, Folic Acid, Biotin, Potassium Iodide, Sodium Selenate, Sodium Molybdate, Phylloquinone, Vitamin D_3 and Cyanocobalamin. PediaSure With Fiber also contains soy fiber.

NUTRIENTS (PER 8 FL OZ):

Energy	237	Cal
Protein	7.1	g
Fat	11.8	g
Carbohydrate	26 (26.9)*	g
L-Carnitine	4	mg
Taurine	17	mg
Water	200	g

VITAMINS/MINERALS PER 8 FL OZ:

Vitamin A	610	IU
Vitamin D	120	IU
Vitamin E	5.4	IU
Vitamin K	9.0	mcg
Vitamin C	24	mg
Folic Acid	88	mcg
Thiamin (Vit B_1)	0.64	mg
Riboflavin (Vit B_2)	0.50	mg
Vitamin B_6	0.62	mg
Vitamin B_{12}	1.4	mcg
Niacin	4.0	mg
Choline	71	mg
Biotin	76	mcg
Pantothenic Acid	2.4	mg
Inositol	19	mg
Sodium	90	mg
Potassium	310	mg
Chloride	240	mg
Calcium	230	mg
Phosphorus	190	mg
Magnesium	47	mg
Iodine	23	mcg
Manganese	0.24	mg
Copper	0.24	mg
Zinc	2.8	mg
Iron	3.3	mg
Chromium	7.1	mcg
Molybdenum	8.5	mcg
Selenium	5.4	mcg

*PediaSure With Fiber includes soy fiber (a source of dietary fiber that provides 1.2 calories and 1.2 g of total dietary fiber).

(FAN 3480-01)

ROSS METABOLIC FORMULA SYSTEM

CALCILO XD®
Low-Calcium/Vitamin D-Free
Infant Formula With Iron
USAGE:

For use in the nutrition support of infants with hypercalcemia, as may occur in infants with Williams syndrome, or in management of infants with osteopetrosis and when a low-calcium/vitamin D-free formula is needed.

Powder: 14.1-oz (400-g) cans; measuring scoop enclosed; 6 per case; No. 00378.

Continued on next page

Ross Metabolic Formula Sys.—Cont.

CYCLINEX®-1
Amino Acid-Modified Medical Food With Iron
USAGE:
When a nonessential amino acid-free medical food is needed for nutrition support of infants and toddlers with a defect in a urea cycle enzyme or with gyrate atrophy of the choroid and retina.
Powder: 12.3-oz (350-g) cans; 6 per case; No. 51144.

CYCLINEX®-2
Amino Acid-Modified Medical Food
USAGE:
When a nonessential amino acid-free medical food is needed for nutrition support of children and adults with a defect in a urea cycle enzyme or with gyrate atrophy of the choroid and retina.
Powder: 11.4-oz (325-g) cans; 6 per case; No. 51146.

FLAVONEX® Flavored Energy Supplement
USAGE:
With amino acid-modified medical foods for children and adults.
Powder: Red Punch, 21.1-oz (600-g) cans; 6 per case; No. 51530. Grapefruit, 21.1-oz (600-g) cans; 6 per case; No. 51280.

GLUTAREX®-1
Amino Acid-Modified Medical Food With Iron
USAGE:
When a lysine- and tryptophan-free medical food is needed for nutrition support of infants and toddlers with glutaric aciduria type I.
Powder: 12.3-oz (350-g) cans; 6 per case; No. 51140.

GLUTAREX®-2
Amino Acid-Modified Medical Food
USAGE:
When a lysine- and tryptophan-free medical food is needed for nutrition support of children and adults with glutaric aciduria type I.
Powder: 11.4-oz (325-g) cans; 6 per case; No. 51142.

HOMINEX®-1
Amino Acid-Modified Medical Food With Iron
USAGE:
When a methionine-free medical food is needed for nutrition support of infants and toddlers with vitamin B_6-nonresponsive homocystinuria or hypermethioninemia.
Powder: 12.3-oz (350-g) cans; 6 per case; No. 51116.

HOMINEX®-2
Amino Acid-Modified Medical Food
USAGE:
When a methionine-free medical food is needed for nutrition support of children and adults with vitamin B_6-nonresponsive homocystinuria or hypermethioninemia.
Powder: 11.4-oz (325-g) cans; 6 per case; No. 51118.

I-VALEX®-1
Amino Acid-Modified Medical Food With Iron
USAGE:
When a leucine-free medical food is needed for nutrition support of infants and toddlers with isovaleric acidemia or other disorders of leucine catabolism.
Powder: 12.3-oz (350-g) cans; 6 per case; No. 51136.

I-VALEX®-2
Amino Acid-Modified Medical Food
USAGE:
When a leucine-free medical food is needed for nutrition support of children and adults with isovaleric acidemia or other disorders of leucine catabolism.
Powder: 11.4-oz (325-g) cans; 6 per case; No. 51138.

KETONEX®-1
Amino Acid-Modified Medical Food With Iron
USAGE:
When a branched-chain amino acid-free medical food is needed for nutrition support of infants and toddlers with branched-chain ketoaciduria (maple syrup urine disease—MSUD).
Powder: 12.3-oz (350-g) cans; 6 per case; No. 51112.

KETONEX®-2
Amino Acid-Modified Medical Food
USAGE:
When a branched-chain amino acid-free medical food is needed for nutrition support of children and adults with branched-chain ketoaciduria (maple syrup urine disease—MSUD).

Powder: 11.4-oz (325-g) cans; 6 per case; No. 51114.

PHENEX™-1
Amino Acid-Modified Medical Food With Iron
USAGE:
When a phenylalanine-free medical food is needed for nutrition support of infants and toddlers with phenylketonuria (PKU) or hyperphenylalaninemia.
Powder: 12.3-oz (350-g) cans; 6 per case; No. 51120.

PHENEX™-2
Amino Acid-Modified Medical Food
USAGE:
When a phenylalanine-free medical food is needed for nutrition support of children and adults with phenylketonuria (PKU) or hyperphenylalaninemia.
Powder: 11.4-oz (325-g) cans; 6 per case; No. 51122.

PRO-PHREE®
Protein-Free Energy Module With Iron, Vitamins & Minerals
USAGE:
When a protein-free medical food is indicated for nutrition support of infants and toddlers requiring reduced protein intake, specific mixture of L-amino acids or increased energy, minerals and vitamins.
Powder: 12.3-oz (350-g) cans; 6 per case; No. 51148.

PROPIMEX®-1
Amino Acid-Modified Medical Food With Iron
USAGE:
When a methionine- and valine-free, low-isoleucine and low-threonine medical food is needed for nutrition support of infants and toddlers with propionic or methylmalonic acidemia.
Powder: 12.3-oz (350-g) cans; 6 per case; No. 51132.

PROPIMEX®-2
Amino Acid-Modified Medical Food
USAGE:
When a methionine- and valine-free, low-isoleucine and low-threonine medical food is needed for nutrition support of children and adults with propionic or methylmalonic acidemia.
Powder: 11.4-oz (325-g) cans; 6 per case; No. 51134.

PROVIMIN®
Protein-Vitamin-Mineral
Formula Component With Iron
USAGE:
For use in the management of patients who require a formula modified in carbohydrate and fat.
Powder: 5.3-oz (150-g) cans; 6 per case; No. 50260.

RCF®
Ross Carbohydrate Free
Soy Formula Base With Iron
USAGE:
For use in the dietary management of persons unable to tolerate the type or amount of carbohydrate in milk or conventional infant formulas; or with seizure disorders requiring a ketogenic diet. This product has been formulated to contain no carbohydrate, which must be added before feeding.
Concentrated Liquid: 13-fl-oz (384-mL) cans; 12 per case; No. 00108.

SIMILAC® PM 60/40
[sim 'e-lak]
Low-Iron Infant Formula
USAGE:
For infants in the lower range of homeostatic capacity; those who are predisposed to hypocalcemia; and those whose renal, digestive or cardiovascular functions would benefit from lowered mineral levels.
Powder: 1-lb (454-g) cans, measuring scoop enclosed; 6 per case; No. 00850.
For hospital use, Similac PM 60/40 Powder is available in the Ross Hospital Formula System.

TYROMEX®-1
Amino Acid-Modified Medical Food With Iron
USAGE:
When a phenylalanine-, tyrosine- and methionine-free medical food is needed for nutrition support of infants and toddlers with tyrosinemia type I.
Powder: 12.3-oz (350-g) cans; 6 per case; No. 51128.

TYREX®-2
Amino Acid-Modified Medical Food
USAGE:
When a phenylalanine- and tyrosine-free medical food is needed for nutrition support of children and adults with tyrosinemia type II.
Powder: 11.4-oz (325-g) cans; 6 per case; No. 51126.

SELSUN® Rx
[sel 'sun]
(2.5% selenium sulfide lotion, USP)

℞

DESCRIPTION
A liquid antiseborrheic, antifungal preparation for topical application. Contains: Selenium sulfide 2 $^1/_2$% w/v in aqueous suspension; also contains: bentonite, lauric diethanolamide, ethylene glycol monostearate, titanium dioxide, amphoteric-2, sodium lauryl sulfate, sodium phosphate (monobasic), glyceryl monoricinoleate, citric acid, captan and perfume.

CLINICAL PHARMACOLOGY
Selenium sulfide appears to have a cytostatic effect on cells of the epidermis and follicular epithelium, reducing corneocyte production.

INDICATIONS AND USAGE
Treatment of tinea versicolor, seborrheic dermatitis of scalp and treatment of dandruff.

CONTRAINDICATIONS
Not to be used by patients allergic to ingredients.

PRECAUTIONS
General: Not to be used when inflammation or exudation is present as increased absorption may occur.
Information for Patients: See Warnings and Precautions section under Application Instructions.
Carcinogenesis: Dermal application of 25% and 50% solutions of 2.5% selenium sulfide lotion on mice over an 88 week period, indicated no carcinogenic effects.
Pregnancy: WHEN USED FOR THE TREATMENT OF TINEA VERSICOLOR, SELSUN IS CLASSIFIED AS PREGNANCY CATEGORY C. Animal reproduction studies have not been conducted with SELSUN. It is also not known whether SELSUN can cause fetal harm when applied to body surfaces of a pregnant woman or can affect reproduction capacity. Under ordinary circumstances SELSUN should not be used for the treatment of tinea versicolor in pregnant women.
Pediatric Use: Safety and effectiveness in infants have not been established.

ADVERSE REACTIONS
In decreasing order of severity: skin irritation; occasional reports of increase in normal hair loss; discoloration of hair (can be avoided or minimized by thorough rinsing of hair after treatment). As with other shampoos, oiliness or dryness of hair and scalp may occur.

OVERDOSAGE
Accidental Oral Ingestion:
No documented reports of serious toxicity in humans resulting from acute ingestion of SELSUN, however, acute toxicity studies in animals suggest that ingestion of large amounts could result in potential human toxicity. Evacuation of the stomach contents should be considered in cases of acute oral ingestion.

DOSAGE AND ADMINISTRATION
See application instructions.
Treatment of tinea versicolor: Apply to affected areas and lather with a small amount of water. Allow product to remain on skin for 10 minutes, then rinse thoroughly. Repeat procedure once a day for 7 days.
Treatment of seborrheic dermatitis and dandruff: Usually two applications each week for two weeks will afford control. After this, may be used at less frequent intervals—weekly, every two weeks, or every 3 or 4 weeks in some cases. Should not be applied more frequently than required to maintain control.
APPLICATION INSTRUCTIONS: Keep tightly capped.
Shake well before using. Product may damage jewelry; remove jewelry before use.
For treatment of tinea versicolor:
1. Apply to affected areas and lather with a small amount of water.
2. Allow to remain on skin for 10 minutes.
3. Rinse body thoroughly.
4. Repeat this procedure once a day for 7 days.
For treatment of dandruff and seborrheic dermatitis of the scalp:
1. Massage about 1 or 2 teaspoonfuls of shampoo into wet scalp.
2. Allow to remain on scalp for 2 to 3 minutes.
3. Rinse scalp thoroughly.
4. Repeat application and rinse thoroughly.
5. After treatment, wash hands well.
6. Repeat treatments as directed by physician.
WARNINGS AND PRECAUTIONS
For External Use Only. Do not use on broken skin or inflamed areas. If allergic reactions occur, discontinue use. Avoid getting shampoo in eyes or in contact with genital area and skin folds as it may cause irritation and burning. These areas should be thoroughly rinsed after application. Keep this and all medicines out of reach of children.

Store below 86°F (30°C).

HOW SUPPLIED
4-fl-oz bottles (NDC 0074-2660-04).
(.2960)

SELSUN BLUE® OTC
[sel 'sun]
**Dandruff Shampoo
(selenium sulfide lotion, 1%)**

SURVANTA® ℞
**beractant
intratracheal suspension**

**Sterile Suspension
For Intratracheal Use Only**

DESCRIPTION
SURVANTA® (beractant) Intratracheal Suspension is a sterile, non-pyrogenic pulmonary surfactant intended for intratracheal use only. It is a natural bovine lung extract containing phospholipids, neutral lipids, fatty acids, and surfactant-associated proteins to which colfosceril palmitate (dipalmitoylphosphatidylcholine), palmitic acid, and tripalmitin are added to standardize the composition and to mimic surface-tension lowering properties of natural lung surfactant. The resulting composition provides 25 mg/mL phospholipids (including 11.0-15.5 mg/mL disaturated phosphatidylcholine), 0.5-1.75 mg/mL triglycerides, 1.4-3.5 mg/mL free fatty acids, and less than 1.0 mg/mL protein. It is suspended in 0.9% sodium chloride solution, and heat-sterilized. SURVANTA contains no preservatives. Its protein content consists of two hydrophobic, low molecular weight, surfactant-associated proteins commonly known as SP-B and SP-C. It does not contain the hydrophilic, large molecular weight surfactant-associated protein known as SP-A.
Each mL of SURVANTA contains 25 mg of phospholipids. It is an off-white to light brown liquid supplied in single-use glass vials containing 8 mL (200 mg phospholipids).

CLINICAL PHARMACOLOGY
Endogenous pulmonary surfactant lowers surface tension on alveolar surfaces during respiration and stabilizes the alveoli against collapse at resting transpulmonary pressures. Deficiency of pulmonary surfactant causes Respiratory Distress Syndrome (RDS) in premature infants. SURVANTA replenishes surfactant and restores surface activity to the lungs of these infants.

Activity
In vitro, SURVANTA reproducibly lowers minimum surface tension to less than 8 dynes/cm as measured by the pulsating bubble surfactometer and Wilhelmy Surface Balance. *In situ*, SURVANTA restores pulmonary compliance to excised rat lungs artificially made surfactant-deficient. *In vivo*, single SURVANTA doses improve lung pressure-volume measurements, lung compliance, and oxygenation in premature rabbits and sheep.

Animal Metabolism
SURVANTA is administered directly to the target organ, the lungs, where biophysical effects occur at the alveolar surface. In surfactant-deficient premature rabbits and lambs, alveolar clearance of radio-labelled lipid components of SURVANTA is rapid. Most of the dose becomes lung-associated within hours of administration, and the lipids enter endogenous surfactant pathways of reutilization and recycling. In surfactant-sufficient adult animals, SURVANTA clearance is more rapid than in premature and young animals. There is less reutilization and recycling of surfactant in adult animals.
Limited animal experiments have not found effects of SURVANTA on endogenous surfactant metabolism. Precursor incorporation and subsequent secretion of saturated phosphatidylcholine in premature sheep are not changed by SURVANTA treatments.
No information is available about the metabolic fate of the surfactant-associated proteins in SURVANTA. The metabolic disposition in humans has not been studied.

Clinical Studies
Clinical effects of SURVANTA were demonstrated in six single-dose and four multiple-dose randomized, multicenter, controlled clinical trials involving approximately 1700 infants. Three open trials, including a Treatment IND, involved more than 8500 infants. Each dose of SURVANTA in all studies was 100 mg phospholipids/kg birth weight and was based on published experience with Surfactant TA, a lyophilized powder dosage form of SURVANTA having the same composition.

Prevention Studies
Infants of 600-1250 g birth weight and 23 to 29 weeks estimated gestational age were enrolled in two *multiple-dose* studies. A dose of SURVANTA was given within 15 minutes of birth to prevent the development of RDS. Up to three ad-

ditional doses in the first 48 hours, as often as every 6 hours, were given if RDS subsequently developed and infants required mechanical ventilation with an $FiO_2 \geq 0.30$. Results of the studies at 28 days of age are shown in Table 1.

TABLE 1

Study 1

	SURVANTA	Control	P-Value
Number infants studied	119	124	
Incidence of RDS (%)	27.6	63.5	<0.001
Death due to RDS (%)	2.5	19.5	<0.001
Death or BPD due to RDS (%)	48.7	52.8	0.536
Death due to any cause (%)	7.6	22.8	0.001
Air Leaks[a](%)	5.9	21.7	0.001
Pulmonary interstitial emphysema (%)	20.8	40.0	0.001

Study 2[b]

	SURVANTA	Control	P-Value
Number infants studied	91	96	
Incidence of RDS (%)	28.6	48.3	0.007
Death due to RDS (%)	1.1	10.5	0.006
Death or BPD due to RDS (%)	27.5	44.2	0.018
Death due to any cause[c](%)	16.5	13.7	0.633
Air Leaks[a](%)	14.5	19.6	0.374
Pulmonary interstitial emphysema (%)	26.5	33.2	0.298

[a] Pneumothorax or pneumopericardium
[b] Study discontinued when Treatment IND initiated
[c] No cause of death in the SURVANTA group was significantly increased; the higher number of deaths in this group was due to the sum of all causes.

Rescue Studies
Infants of 600-1750 g birth weight with RDS requiring mechanical ventilation and an $FiO_2 \geq 0.40$ were enrolled in two *multiple-dose* rescue studies. The initial dose of SURVANTA was given after RDS developed and before 8 hours of age. Infants could receive up to three additional doses in the first 48 hours, as often as every 6 hours, if they required mechanical ventilation and an $FiO_2 \geq 0.30$. Results of the studies at 28 days of age are shown in Table 2.

TABLE 2

Study 3[a]

	SURVANTA	Control	P-Value
Number infants studied	198	193	
Death due to RDS (%)	11.6	18.1	0.071
Death or BPD due to RDS (%)	59.1	66.8	0.102
Death due to any cause (%)	21.7	26.4	0.285
Air Leaks[b](%)	11.8	29.5	<0.001
Pulmonary interstitial emphysema (%)	16.3	34.0	<0.001

Study 4

	SURVANTA	Control	P-Value
Number infants studied	204	203	
Death due to RDS (%)	6.4	22.3	<0.001
Death or BPD due to RDS (%)	43.6	63.4	<0.001
Death due to any cause (%)	15.2	28.2	0.001
Air Leaks[b] (%)	11.2	22.2	0.005
Pulmonary interstitial emphysema (%)	20.8	44.4	<0.001

[a] Study discontinued when Treatment IND initiated
[b] Pneumothorax or pneumopericardium

Acute Clinical Effects
Marked improvements in oxygenation may occur within minutes of administration of SURVANTA.
All controlled clinical studies with SURVANTA provided information regarding the acute effects of SURVANTA on the arterial-alveolar oxygen ratio (a/APO$_2$), FiO$_2$, and mean airway pressure (MAP) during the first 48 to 72 hours of life. Significant improvements in these variables were sustained for 48-72 hours in SURVANTA-treated infants in four sin-

gle-dose and two multiple-dose rescue studies and in two multiple-dose prevention studies. In the single-dose prevention studies, FiO$_2$ improved significantly.

INDICATIONS AND USAGE
SURVANTA is indicated for prevention and treatment ("rescue") of Respiratory Distress Syndrome (RDS) (hyaline membrane disease) in premature infants. SURVANTA significantly reduces the incidence of RDS, mortality due to RDS and air leak complications.

Prevention
In premature infants less than 1250 g birth weight or with evidence of surfactant deficiency, give SURVANTA as soon as possible, preferably within 15 minutes of birth.

Rescue
To treat infants with RDS confirmed by x-ray and requiring mechanical ventilation, give SURVANTA as soon as possible, preferably by 8 hours of age.

CONTRAINDICATIONS
None known.

WARNINGS
SURVANTA is intended for intratracheal use only.
SURVANTA CAN RAPIDLY AFFECT OXYGENATION AND LUNG COMPLIANCE. Therefore, its use should be restricted to a highly supervised clinical setting with immediate availability of clinicians experienced with intubation, ventilator management, and general care of premature infants. Infants receiving SURVANTA should be frequently monitored with arterial or transcutaneous measurement of systemic oxygen and carbon dioxide.
DURING THE DOSING PROCEDURE, TRANSIENT EPISODES OF BRADYCARDIA AND DECREASED OXYGEN SATURATION HAVE BEEN REPORTED. If these occur, stop the dosing procedure and initiate appropriate measures to alleviate the condition. After stabilization, resume the dosing procedure.

PRECAUTIONS
General
Rales and moist breath sounds can occur transiently after administration. Endotracheal suctioning or other remedial action is not necessary unless clear-cut signs of airway obstruction are present.
Increased probability of post-treatment nosocomial sepsis in SURVANTA-treated infants was observed in the controlled clinical trials (Table 3). The increased risk for sepsis among SURVANTA-treated infants was not associated with increased mortality among these infants. The causative organisms were similar in treated and control infants. There was no significant difference between groups in the rate of post-treatment infections other than sepsis.
Use of SURVANTA in infants less than 600 g birth weight or greater than 1750 g birth weight has not been evaluated in controlled trials. There is no controlled experience with use of SURVANTA in conjunction with experimental therapies for RDS (eg, high-frequency ventilation or extracorporeal membrane oxygenation).
No information is available on the effects of doses other than 100 mg phospholipids/kg, more than four doses, dosing more frequently than every 6 hours, or administration after 48 hours of age.

Carcinogenesis, Mutagenesis, Impairment of Fertility
Carcinogenicity studies have not been performed with SURVANTA. SURVANTA was negative when tested in the Ames test for mutagenicity. Using the maximum feasible dose volume, SURVANTA up to 500 mg phospholipids/kg/day (approximately one-third the premature infant dose based on mg/m^2/day) was administered subcutaneously to newborn rats for 5 days. The rats reproduced normally and there were no observable adverse effects in their offspring.

ADVERSE REACTIONS
The most commonly reported adverse experiences were associated with the dosing procedure. In the multiple-dose controlled clinical trials, each dose of SURVANTA was divided into four quarter-doses which were instilled through a catheter inserted into the endotracheal tube by briefly disconnecting the endotracheal tube from the ventilator. Transient bradycardia occurred with 11.9% of doses. Oxygen desaturation occurred with 9.8% of doses.
Other reactions during the dosing procedure occurred with fewer than 1% of doses and included endotracheal tube reflux, pallor, vasoconstriction, hypotension, endotracheal tube blockage, hypertension, hypocarbia, hypercarbia, and apnea. No deaths occurred during the dosing procedure, and all reactions resolved with symptomatic treatment.
The occurrence of concurrent illnesses common in premature infants was evaluated in the controlled trials. The rates in all controlled studies are in Table 3.

Continued on next page

Survanta—Cont.

TABLE 3

	All Controlled Studies		
Concurrent Event	SURVANTA (%)	Control (%)	P-Value[a]
Patent ductus arteriosus	46.9	47.1	0.814
Intracranial hemorrhage	48.1	45.2	0.241
Severe intracranial hemorrhage	24.1	23.3	0.693
Pulmonary air leaks	10.9	24.7	<0.001
Pulmonary interstitial emphysema	20.2	38.4	<0.001
Necrotizing enterocolitis	6.1	5.3	0.427
Apnea	65.4	59.6	0.283
Severe apnea	46.1	42.5	0.114
Post-treatment sepsis	20.7	16.1	0.019
Post-treatment infection	10.2	9.1	0.345
Pulmonary hemorrhage	7.2	5.3	0.166

[a]*P*-value comparing groups in controlled studies

When all controlled studies were pooled, there was no difference in intracranial hemorrhage. However, in one of the single-dose rescue studies and one of the multiple-dose prevention studies, the rate of intracranial hemorrhage was significantly higher in SURVANTA patients than control patients (63.3% *v* 30.8%, $P=0.001$; and 48.8% *v* 34.2%, $P=0.047$, respectively). The rate in a Treatment IND involving approximately 8100 infants was lower than in the controlled trials.

In the controlled clinical trials, there was no effect of SURVANTA on results of common laboratory tests: white blood cell count and serum sodium, potassium, bilirubin, creatinine.

More than 4300 pretreatment and posttreatment serum samples from approximately 1500 patients were tested by Western Blot Immunoassay for antibodies to surfactant-associated proteins SP-B and SP-C. No IgG or or IgM antibodies were detected.

Several other complications are known to occur in premature infants. The following conditions were reported in the controlled clinical studies. The rates of the complications were not different in treated and control infants, and none of the complications were attributed to SURVANTA.

Respiratory: lung consolidation, blood from the endotracheal tube, deterioration after weaning, respiratory decompensation, subglottic stenosis, paralyzed diaphragm, respiratory failure.

Cardiovascular: hypotension, hypertension, tachycardia, ventricular tachycardia, aortic thrombosis, cardiac failure, cardio-respiratory arrest, increased apical pulse, persistent fetal circulation, air embolism, total anomalous pulmonary venous return.

Gastrointestinal: abdominal distention, hemorrhage, intestinal perforations, volvulus, bowel infarct, feeding intolerance, hepatic failure, stress ulcer.

Renal: renal failure, hematuria.

Hematologic: coagulopathy, thrombocytopenia, disseminated intravascular coagulation.

Central Nervous System: seizures.

Endocrine/Metabolic: adrenal hemorrhage, inappropriate ADH secretion, hyperphosphatemia.

Musculoskeletal: inguinal hernia.

Systemic: fever, deterioration.

Follow-Up Evaluations

To date, no long-term complications or sequelae of SURVANTA therapy have been found.

Single-Dose Studies

Six-month adjusted-age follow-up evaluations of 232 infants (115 treated) demonstrated no clinically important differences between treatment groups in pulmonary and neurologic sequelae, incidence or severity of retinopathy of prematurity, rehospitalizations, growth, or allergic manifestations.

Multiple-Dose Studies

Six-month adjusted age follow-up evaluations have been completed in 631 (345 treated) of 916 surviving infants. There were significantly less cerebral palsy and need for supplemental oxygen in SURVANTA infants than controls. Wheezing at the time of examination was significantly more frequent among SURVANTA infants, although there was no difference in bronchodilator therapy.

Final twelve-month follow-up data from the multiple-dose studies are available from 521 (272 treated) of 909 surviving infants. There was significantly less wheezing in SURVANTA infants than controls, in contrast to the six-month results. There was no difference in the incidence of cerebral palsy at twelve months.

Twenty-four month adjusted age evaluations were completed in 429 (226 treated) of 906 surviving infants. There were significantly fewer SURVANTA infants with rhonchi, wheezing, and tachypnea at the time of examination. No other differences were found.

OVERDOSAGE

Overdosage with SURVANTA has not been reported. Based on animal data, overdosage might result in acute airway obstruction. Treatment should be symptomatic and supportive.

Rales and moist breath sounds can transiently occur after SURVANTA is given, and do not indicate overdosage. Endotracheal suctioning or other remedial action is not required unless clear-cut signs of airway obstruction are present.

DOSAGE AND ADMINISTRATION

FOR INTRATRACHEAL ADMINISTRATION ONLY.

SURVANTA should be administered by or under the supervision of clinicians experienced in intubation, ventilator management, and general care of premature infants.

Marked improvements in oxygenation may occur within minutes of administration of SURVANTA. Therefore, frequent and careful clinical observation and monitoring of systemic oxygenation are essential to avoid hyperoxia.

Review of audiovisual instructional materials describing dosage and administration procedures is recommended before using SURVANTA. Materials are available upon request from Ross Products Division.

Dosage

Each dose of SURVANTA is 100 mg of phospholipids/kg birth weight (4 mL/kg). The SURVANTA DOSING CHART shows the total dosage for a range of birth weights.

SURVANTA DOSING CHART

WEIGHT (grams)	TOTAL DOSE (mL)	WEIGHT (grams)	TOTAL DOSE (mL)
600- 650	2.6	1301-1350	5.4
651- 700	2.8	1351-1400	5.6
701- 750	3.0	1401-1450	5.8
751- 800	3.2	1451-1500	6.0
801- 850	3.4	1501-1550	6.2
851- 900	3.6	1551-1600	6.4
901- 950	3.8	1601-1650	6.6
951-1000	4.0	1651-1700	6.8
1001-1050	4.2	1701-1750	7.0
1051-1100	4.4	1751-1800	7.2
1101-1150	4.6	1801-1850	7.4
1151-1200	4.8	1851-1900	7.6
1201-1250	5.0	1901-1950	7.8
1251-1300	5.2	1951-2000	8.0

Four doses of SURVANTA can be administered in the first 48 hours of life. Doses should be given no more frequently than every 6 hours.

Directions for Use

SURVANTA should be inspected visually for discoloration prior to administration. The color of SURVANTA is off-white to light brown. If settling occurs during storage, swirl the vial gently (DO NOT SHAKE) to redisperse. Some foaming at the surface may occur during handling and is inherent in the nature of the product.

SURVANTA is stored refrigerated (2-8°C). Before administration, SURVANTA should be warmed by standing at room temperature for at least 20 minutes or warmed in the hand for at least 8 minutes. ARTIFICIAL WARMING METHODS SHOULD NOT BE USED. If a prevention dose is to be given, preparation of SURVANTA should begin before the infant's birth.

Unopened, unused vials of SURVANTA that have been warmed to room temperature may be returned to the refrigerator within 8 hours of warming, and stored for future use. Drug should not be warmed and returned to the refrigerator more than once. Each single-use vial of SURVANTA should be entered only once. Used vials with residual drug should be discarded.

SURVANTA DOES NOT REQUIRE RECONSTITUTION OR SONICATION BEFORE USE.

Dosing Procedures

General

SURVANTA is administered intratracheally by instillation through a 5 French end-hole catheter. The catheter can be inserted into the infant's endotracheal tube without interrupting ventilation by passing the catheter through a neonatal suction valve attached to the endotracheal tube. Alternatively, SURVANTA can be instilled through the catheter by briefly disconnecting the endotracheal tube from the ventilator.

The neonatal suction valve used for administering SURVANTA should be a type that allows entry of the catheter into the endotracheal tube without interrupting ventilation and also maintains a closed airway circuit system by sealing the valve around the catheter.

If the neonatal suction valve is used, the catheter should be rigid enough to pass easily into the endotracheal tube. A very soft and pliable catheter may twist or curl within the neonatal suction valve. The length of the catheter should be shortened so that the tip of the catheter protrudes just beyond the end of the endotracheal tube above the infant's carina. SURVANTA should not be instilled into a mainstem bronchus.

To ensure homogenous distribution of SURVANTA throughout the lungs, each dose is divided into *four quarter-doses.* Each quarter-dose is administered with the infant in a different position. The recommended positions are:

- Head and body inclined 5–10° down, head turned to the right
- Head and body inclined 5–10° down, head turned to the left
- Head and body inclined 5–10° up, head turned to the right
- Head and body inclined 5–10° up, head turned to the left

The dosing procedure is facilitated if one person administers the dose while another person positions and monitors the infant.

First Dose

Determine the total dose of SURVANTA from the SURVANTA DOSING CHART based on the infant's birth weight. Slowly withdraw the entire contents of the vial into a plastic syringe through a large-gauge needle (eg, at least 20 gauge). DO NOT FILTER SURVANTA AND AVOID SHAKING.

Attach the premeasured 5 French end-hole catheter to the syringe. Fill the catheter with SURVANTA. Discard excess SURVANTA through the catheter so that only the total dose to be given remains in the syringe.

BEFORE ADMINISTERING SURVANTA, assure proper placement and patency of the endotracheal tube. At the discretion of the clinician, the endotracheal tube may be suctioned before administering SURVANTA. The infant should be allowed to stabilize before proceeding with dosing.

In the prevention strategy, weigh, intubate and stabilize the infant. Administer the dose as soon as possible after birth, preferably within 15 minutes. Position the infant appropriately and gently inject the first quarter-dose through the catheter over 2-3 seconds.

After administration of the first quarter-dose, remove the catheter from the endotracheal tube. Manually ventilate with a hand-bag with sufficient oxygen to prevent cyanosis, at a rate of 60 breaths/minute, and sufficient positive pressure to provide adequate air exchange and chest wall excursion.

In the rescue strategy, the first dose should be given as soon as possible after the infant is placed on a ventilator for management of RDS. In the clinical trials, immediately before instilling the first quarter-dose, the infant's ventilator settings were changed to rate 60/minute, inspiratory time 0.5 second, and FiO_2 1.0.

Position the infant appropriately and gently inject the first quarter-dose through the catheter over 2–3 seconds. After administration of the first quarter-dose, remove the catheter from the endotracheal tube and continue mechanical ventilation.

In both strategies, ventilate the infant for at least 30 seconds or until stable. Reposition the infant for instillation of the next quarter-dose.

Instill the remaining quarter-doses using the same procedures. After instillation of each quarter-dose, remove the catheter and ventilate for at least 30 seconds or until the infant is stabilized. After instillation of the final quarter-dose, remove the catheter without flushing it. Do not suction the infant for 1 hour after dosing unless signs of significant airway obstruction occur.

AFTER COMPLETION OF THE DOSING PROCEDURE, RESUME USUAL VENTILATOR MANAGEMENT AND CLINICAL CARE.

Repeat Doses

The dosage of SURVANTA for repeat doses is also 100 mg phospholipids/kg and is based on the infant's birth weight. The infant should not be reweighed for determination of the SURVANTA dosage. Use the SURVANTA DOSING CHART to determine the total dosage.

The need for additional doses of SURVANTA is determined by evidence of continuing respiratory distress. Using the following criteria for redosing, significant reductions in mortality due to RDS were observed in the multiple-dose clinical trials with SURVANTA.

Dose no sooner than 6 hours after the preceding dose if the infant remains intubated and requires at least 30% inspired oxygen to maintain a PaO_2 less than or equal to 80 torr.

Radiographic confirmation of RDS should be obtained before administering additional doses to those who received a prevention dose.

Prepare SURVANTA and position the infant for administration of each quarter-dose as previously described. After instillation of each quarter-dose, remove the dosing catheter from the endotracheal tube and ventilate the infant for at least 30 seconds or until stable.

In the clinical studies, ventilator settings used to administer repeat doses were different than those used for the first dose. For repeat doses, the FiO_2 was increased by 0.20 or an amount sufficient to prevent cyanosis. The ventilator delivered a rate of 30/minute with an inspiratory time less than

1.0 second. If the infant's pretreatment rate was 30 or greater, it was left unchanged during SURVANTA instillation.
Manual hand-bag ventilation should not be used to administer repeat doses. DURING THE DOSING PROCEDURE, VENTILATOR SETTINGS MAY BE ADJUSTED AT THE DISCRETION OF THE CLINICIAN TO MAINTAIN APPROPRIATE OXYGENATION AND VENTILATION. AFTER COMPLETION OF THE DOSING PROCEDURE, RESUME USUAL VENTILATOR MANAGEMENT AND CLINICAL CARE.

Dosing Precautions
If an infant experiences bradycardia or oxygen desaturation during the dosing procedure, stop the dosing procedure and initiate appropriate measures to alleviate the condition. After the infant has stabilized, resume the dosing procedure. Rales and moist breath sounds can occur transiently after administration of SURVANTA. Endotracheal suctioning or other remedial action is unnecessary unless clear-cut signs of airway obstruction are present.

HOW SUPPLIED
SURVANTA (beractant) Intratracheal Suspension is supplied in single-use glass vials containing 8 mL of SURVANTA (NDC 0074-1040-08). Each milliliter contains 25 mg of phospholipids (200 mg phospholipids/8 mL) suspended in 0.9% sodium chloride solution. The color is off-white to light brown.
Store unopened vials at refrigeration temperature (2-8°C). Protect from light. Store vials in carton until ready for use. Vials are for single use only. Upon opening, discard unused drug.
April, 1995

TRONOLANE® OTC
[tron 'e-lān]
Anesthetic Cream for Hemorrhoids
Hemorrhoidal Suppositories

PEDIAFLOR® Drops ℞
Sodium Fluoride Oral Solution, USP
1.7 fl oz (50 mL) bottles, calibrated dropper

VI-DAYLIN® ADC VITAMINS Drops OTC
Dietary Supplement of
Vitamins A,D, and C
50 mL Spil-gard bottles, calibrated dropper

VI-DAYLIN® ADC VITAMINS + IRON OTC
Drops
Dietary Supplement of Vitamins A,D, and C
with Iron
50 mL Spil-gard bottles, calibrated dropper

VI-DAYLIN® MULTIVITAMIN DROPS OTC
Multivitamin Supplement
50 mL Spil-gard Bottles, calibrated dropper

VI-DAYLIN® MULTIVITAMIN + IRON OTC
Drops
Multivitamin/Iron Supplement
50 mL Spil-gard bottles, calibrated dropper

VI-DAYLIN®/F ADC VITAMINS ℞
Drops With Fluoride
ADC Vitamins/Fluoride
50 mL Spil-gard bottles, calibrated dropper

VI-DAYLIN®/F ADC VITAMINS + IRON ℞
Drops With Fluoride
ADC Vitamins/Fluoride/Iron Supplement
50 mL Spil-gard bottles, calibrated dropper

VI-DAYLIN®/F MULTIVITAMIN ℞
Drops With Fluoride
Multivitamins/Fluoride
50 mL Spil-gard bottles, calibrated dropper

VI-DAYLIN®/F MULTIVITAMIN + IRON ℞
Drops With Fluoride
Multivitamins/Fluoride/Iron Supplement
50 mL Spil-gard bottles, calibrated dropper

VI-DAYLIN® MULTIVITAMIN OTC
Chewable Tablets
Multivitamin Supplement
100 tablet bottles

VI-DAYLIN® MULTIVITAMIN + IRON OTC
Chewable Tablets
Multivitamin/Iron Supplement
100 tablet bottles

VI-DAYLIN®/F MULTIVITAMIN ℞
Chewable Tablets With Fluoride
Multivitamins/Fluoride
100 tablet bottles

VI-DAYLIN®/F MULTIVITAMIN + IRON ℞
Chewable Tablets With Fluoride
Multivitamins/Fluoride/Iron
100 tablet bottles

VI-DAYLIN® MULTIVITAMIN Liquid OTC
Multivitamin Supplement
16-fl-oz (473 mL) bottles
8-fl-oz (237 mL) bottles

VI-DAYLIN® MULTIVITAMIN + IRON OTC
Liquid
Multivitamin/Iron Supplement
16-fl-oz (473 mL) bottles
8-fl-oz (237 mL) bottles

Roxane Laboratories, Inc.
P.O. 16532
COLUMBUS, OH 43216-6532

Direct Inquiries to:
Professional Services Department
P.O. 16532
Columbus, OH 43216-6532
(800) 848-0120
(614) 276-4000

ROXANE LABORATORIES, INC
PRODUCT LIST

Acetaminophen Oral Solution USP (Cherry) 160mg/5mL, 325mg/10.15mL, 650mg/20.3mL
Acetaminophen Tablets USP 325mg, 500mg
Acetaminophen 120mg and Codeine Phosphate 12mg Oral per 5 mL Solution USP
Acetaminophen 300mg and Codeine Phosphate 30mg Tablets USP
Acetylcysteine Solution USP 10%, 20%
Acyclovir Capsules 200 mg
Aluminum Hydroxide Gel USP (Flavored) 2700mg/30mL, 450mg/5mL
Aluminum Hydroxide, Concentrate 2700mg/20mL, 4050mg/30mL, 675mg/5mL
Alumina and Magnesia Oral Suspension USP 30 mL
Alumina, Magnesia, and Simethicone Oral Suspension USP I 15mL, 30mL
Aminophylline Oral Solution USP 105mg/5mL, 210mg/10mL, 315mg/15mL
Aromatic Cascara Fluidextract USP 5mL
Aromatic Castor Oil USP 30mL, 60mL
Azathioprine Tablets USP 50mg
Calcium Carbonate Tablets USP 1250mg
Calcium Carbonate Oral Suspension 1250mg/5mL
Calcium Gluconate Tablets USP 500mg
Castor Oil USP 30mL, 60mL
Chlorpromazine HCl Intensol™ 30 mg/mL, 100 mg/mL
Cimetidine HCl Oral Solution 300 mg/5mL, 400 mg/6.7 mL
Cocaine Hydrochloride Topical Solution 4%,10%
Cocaine HCl Viscous Topical Solution 4%, 10%
Codeine Phosphate Oral Solution 15mg/5mL
Codeine Sulfate Tablets USP 15mg, 30mg, 60mg
Dexamethasone Intensol™ 1 mg/mL
Dexamethasone Oral Solution 0.5mg/5mL, 2mg/20mL
Dexamethasone Tablets USP 0.5 mg, 0.75mg, 1mg, 1.5mg, 2mg, 4mg, 6mg
Diazepam Intensol™ Oral Solution (Concentrate)
Diazepam Oral Solution 5 mg/5 mL, 10 mg/10 mL
Diclofenac Sodium Tablets 25mg, 50mg, 75mg
Diflunisal Tablets USP 250mg, 500mg
Digoxin Elixir USP 0.05mg/mL, 0.125mg/2.5mL, 0.25mg/5mL
DHT™ Tablets (Dihydrotachysterol Tablets USP) 0.125mg, 0.2mg, 0.4mg
DHT™ Intensol™ 0.2 mg/mL
Diluent (Flavored) for Oral Use
Diphenhydramine Hydrochloride Elixir USP 25mg/10mL
Diphenoxylate Hydrochloride and Atropine Sulfate Oral Solution USP 2mg/4mL, 2.5mg/5mL, 5mg/10mL
Docusate Sodium Syrup USP 50mg/15mL, 100mg/30mL
Duraclon™ Injection (Clonidine Hydrochloride)
Ferrous Sulfate Oral Solution USP 300mg/5mL
Ferrous Sulfate Tablets USP 300mg
Furosemide Oral Solution 10mg/mL, 40mg/5mL
Furosemide Tablets USP 20mg, 40mg, 80mg
Guaifenesin Syrup USP 100mg/5mL, 200mg/10mL, 300mg/15mL
Haloperidol Intensol™ Oral Solution (Concentrate) 2mg/mL
Haloperidol Tablets USP 0.5 mg, 1 mg, 2 mg, 5 mg, 10 mg and 20 mg
Hydrochlorothiazide Oral Solution 50mg/5mL
Hydromorphone Hydrochloride Tablets USP 2mg, 4mg

Hydroxyurea Capsules USP 500mg
Indomethacin Oral Suspension USP 25mg/5mL
Ipecac Syrup USP 15mL, 30mL
Ipratropium Bromide Inhalation Solution UDV 0.02%
Isoetharine Inhalation Solution 1%
Kaolin-Pectin Suspension
Lactulose Solution USP 10gm/15mL
Leucovorin Calcium Tablets 5mg., 10mg, 15mg, 25mg
Levorphanol Tartrate Tablets USP 2 mg
Lidocaine Viscous 2%
Lidocaine Hydrochloride Topical Solution USP 4%
Lithium Carbonate Capsules USP 150mg, 300mg, 600mg
Lithium Carbonate Tablets USP 300mg
Lithium Citrate Syrup USP 8mEq per 5 mL, 16mEq per 10mL
Loperamide Hydrochloride Capsules USP 2mg
Loperamide Hydrochloride Oral Solution 1mg/5mL, 2mg/10mL
Lorazepam Intensol™ Oral Concentrate 2mg/mL
Marinol® (Dronabinol) Capsules 2.5 mg, 5 mg, 10 mg
Megestrol Acetate Tablets USP 20mg, 40mg
Meperidine Hydrochloride Tablets USP 50mg, 100mg
Meperidine Hydrochloride Syrup USP 50mg/5mL
Metaproterenol Sulfate Inhalation Solution 0.4%, 0.6%
Methadone Hydrochloride Intensol™ Oral Solution (Concentrate) USP 10mg/mL
Methadone Hydrochloride Tablets USP 5mg, 10mg
Methadone Hydrochloride Oral Solution USP 5mg/5mL, 10mg/5mL
Methadone HCl USP Powder 50 g/100 g
Methotrexate Tablets USP 2.5mg
Metoclopramide Intensol™ Metoclopramide Hydrochloride Oral Solution (Concentrate) 10mg/mL
Metoclopramide Oral Solution USP 5mg/5mL, 10mg/10mL
Mexiletine Hydrochloride Capsules USP 150mg, 200mg, 250mg
Milk of Magnesia USP 30mL
Milk of Magnesia Concentrated Flavored 10mL
Milk of Magnesia—Cascara Suspension Concentrated 15mL
Milk of Magnesia—Mineral Oil Emulsion 30mL
Milk of Magnesia—Mineral Oil Emulsion (Flavored) 30mL
Mineral Oil, Topical Light USP 10mL, 30mL
Mineral Oil USP 30mL
Morphine Sulfate Tablets 15mg, 30mg
Morphine Sulfate Oral Solution 10mg/5mL, 20mg/10mL, 20mg/5mL
Naproxen Oral Suspension USP 125mg/5mL
Naproxen Sodium Tablets USP 275mg, 550mg
Naproxen Tablets USP 250mg, 375mg, 500mg
Neomycin Sulfate Tablets USP 500mg
Oramorph® SR Tablets (Morphine Sulfate Sustained Release Tablets) 15mg, 30mg, 60mg, 100mg
Phenobarbital Elixir USP 20mg/5mL, 30mg/7.5mL
Phenobarbital Tablets USP 15mg, 30mg, 60mg, 100mg
Potassium Chloride Oral Solution USP 10%, 20%
Potassium Iodide Oral Solution USP (Saturated) 1g/mL
Prednisone Intensol™ Oral Solution (Concentrate) 5mg/mL
Prednisone Oral Solution 5mg/5mL
Prednisone Tablets USP 1mg, 2.5mg, 5mg, 10mg, 20mg, 50mg
Prelu-2® (Phendimetrazine Tartrate) 105mg
Propantheline Bromide Tablets USP 15mg
Propranolol HCl Intensol™ Oral Solution (Concentrate) 80mg/mL
Propranolol Hydrochloride Oral Solution 20mg/5mL and 40mg/5 mL
Pseudoephedrine Hydrochloride Tablets USP 30mg, 60mg
Quinidine Sulfate Tablets USP 200 mg/300 mg
Ranitidine Tablets USP 150mg, 300mg
Roxanol™ Morphine Sulfate Concentrated Oral Solution 20mg/mL
Roxanol 100™ Morphine Sulfate Concentrated Oral Solution 100mg/5mL
Roxanol-T™ Morphine Sulfate Concentrated Oral Solution (tinted-fruit mint flavored) 20mg/mL
Roxicet™ Oral Solution (Oxycodone Hydrochloride 5mg and Acetaminophen 325mg/5mL)
Roxicet™ Tablets (Oxycodone and Acetaminophen Tablets USP 5mg/325mg)
Roxicet™ 5/500 Caplets (Oxycodone and Acetaminophen Tablets USP 5mg/500mg)
Roxicodone™ Oral Solution (Oxycodone Hydrochloride Oral Solution USP 5mg/5mL)
Roxicodone™ Tablets (Oxycodone Tablets USP 5mg)
Roxicodone Intensol™ (Oxycodone HCl Concentrated Oral Solution) 20mg/mL
Roxilox™ Capsules (Oxycodone and Acetaminophen Capsules USP) 5mg/500mg
Roxiprin™ Tablets (Oxycodone Hydrochloride 4.5mg, Oxycodone Terephthalate 0.38mg, and Aspirin 325mg Tablets USP)

Continued on next page

Product List—Cont.

Saliva Substitute
Sodium Chloride Inhalation Solution USP (Normal Saline) Sterile 0.9% 3mL, 5mL
Sodium Polystyrene Sulfonate Suspension USP 60mL, and 120mL Enema Package, 200 mL Enema Package
Theophylline Oral Solution 80mg/15mL, 100mg/18.75mL, 160mg/30mL
Torecan® Injection (Thiethylperazine Malate Injection USP) 10mg
Torecan® Tablets (Thiethylperazine Maleate Tablets USP) 10mg
Triazolam Tablets USP 0.125mg, 0.25mg
Viramune Tablets 200mg

AZATHIOPRINE ℞
TABLETS USP 50 MG
COMPLETE PRESCRIBING INFORMATION

WARNING: Chronic immunosuppression with this purine antimetabolite increases *risk of neoplasia* in humans. Physicians using this drug should be very familiar with this risk as well as with the mutagenic potential to both men and women and with possible hematologic toxicities. See **WARNINGS**.

DESCRIPTION

Azathioprine, an immunosuppressive antimetabolite, is available in tablet form for oral administration. Each scored tablet contains 50 mg azathioprine and the inactive ingredients anhydrous lactose, starch (corn), povidone, magnesium stearate and stearic acid.

Azathioprine is chemically 6-[(1-methyl-4-nitroimidazol-5-yl)thio]purine. The structural formula of azathioprine is:

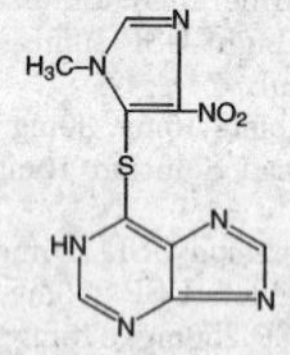

$C_9H_7N_7O_2S$
M. W. 277.26

It is an imidazolyl derivative of 6-mercaptopurine and many of its biological effects are similar to those of the parent compound.

Azathioprine is insoluble in water, but may be dissolved with addition of one molar equivalent of alkali. The sodium salt of azathioprine is sufficiently soluble to make a 10 mg/mL water solution which is stable for 24 hours of 59° to 77°F (15° to 25°C). Azathioprine is stable in solution at neutral or acid pH but hydrolysis to mercaptopurine occurs in excess sodium hydroxide (0.1N), especially on warming. Conversion to mercaptopurine also occurs in the presence of sulfhydryl compounds such as cysteine, glutathione and hydrogen sulfide.

CLINICAL PHARMACOLOGY AND ACTIONS

Metabolism[1]: Azathioprine is well absorbed following oral administration. Maximum serum radioactivity occurs at one to two hours after oral ^{35}S-azathioprine and decays with a half-life of five hours. This is not an estimate of the half-life of azathioprine itself but is the decay rate of all ^{35}S-containing metabolites of the drug. Because of extensive metabolism, only a fraction of the radioactivity is present as azathioprine. Usual doses produce blood levels of azathioprine, and of mercaptopurine derived from it, which are low (<1 μg/mL). Blood levels are of little predictive value for therapy since the magnitude and duration of clinical effects correlate with thiopurine nucleotide levels in tissues rather than with plasma drug levels. Azathioprine and mercaptopurine are moderately bound to serum proteins (30%) and are partially dialyzable.

Azathioprine is cleaved *in vito* to mercaptopurine. Both compounds are rapidly eliminated from blood and are oxidized or methylated in erythrocytes and liver; no azathioprine or mercaptopurine is detectable in urine after eight hours. Conversion to inactive 6-thiouric acid by xanthine oxidase is an important degradative pathway, and the inhibition of this pathway in patients receiving allopurinol is the basis for the azathioprine dosage reduction required in these patients (see **Drug Interactions** under **PRECAUTIONS**). Proportions of metabolites are different in individual patients, and this presumably accounts for variable magnitude and duration of drug effects. Renal clearance is probably not important in predicting biological effectiveness or toxicities, although dose reduction is practiced in patients with poor renal function.

Homograft Survival[1,2]: Summary information from transplant centers and registries indicates relatively universal use of azathioprine with or without other immunosuppressive agents.[3,4,5] Although the use of azathioprine for inhibition of renal homograft rejection is well established, the mechanism(s) for this action are somewhat obscure. The drug suppresses hypersensitivities of the cell-mediated type and causes variable alterations in antibody production. Suppression of T-cell effects, including ablation of T-cell suppression is dependent on the temporal relationship to antigenic stimulus or engraftment. This agent has little effect on established graft rejections or secondary responses.

Alterations in specific immune responses or immunologic functions in transplant recipients are difficult to relate specifically to immunosuppression by azathioprine. These patients have subnormal responses to vaccines, low numbers of T-cells, and abnormal phagocytosis by peripheral blood cells, but their mitogenic responses, serum immunoglobulins and secondary antibody responses are usually normal.

Immunoinflammatory Response: Azathioprine suppresses disease manifestations as well as underlying pathology in animal models of auto-immune disease. For example, the severity of adjuvant arthritis is reduced by azathioprine.

The mechanisms whereby azathioprine affects auto-immune diseases are not known. Azathioprine is immunosuppressive, delayed hypersensitivity and cellular cytotoxicity tests being suppressed to a greater degree than are antibody responses. In the rat model of adjuvant arthritis, azathioprine has been shown to inhibit the lymph node hyperplasia which preceded the onset of the signs of the disease. Both the immunosuppressive and therapeutic effects in animal models are dose-related. Azathioprine is considered a slow-acting drug and effects may persist after the drug has been discontinued.

INDICATIONS AND USAGE

Azathioprine is indicated as an adjunct for the prevention of rejection in renal homotransplantation. It is also indicated for the management of severe, active rheumatoid arthritis unresponsive to rest, aspirin or other nonsteroidal anti-inflammatory drugs, or to agents in the class of which gold is an example.

Renal Homotransplantation: Azathioprine is indicated as an adjunct for the prevention of rejection in renal homotransplantation. Experience with over 16,000 transplants shows a five-year patient survival of 35% to 55%, but this is dependent on donor, match of HLA antigens, antidonor or anti B-cell alloantigen antibody and other variables. The effect of azathioprine on these variables has not been tested in controlled trials.

Rheumatoid Arthritis[6,7]: Azathioprine is indicated only in adult patients meeting criteria for classic or definite rheumatoid arthritis as specified by the American Rheumatism Association.[8] Azathioprine should be restricted to patients with severe, active and erosive disease not responsive to conventional management including rest, aspirin or other non-steroidal drugs or to agents in the class of which gold is an example. Rest, physiotherapy and salicylates should be continued while azathioprine is given, but it may be possible to reduce the dose of corticosteroids in patients on azathioprine. The combined use of azathioprine with gold, antimalarials or penicillamine has not been studied for either added benefit or unexpected adverse effects. The use azathioprine with these agents cannot be recommended.

CONTRAINDICATIONS

Azathioprine should not be given to patients who have shown hypersensitivity to the drug.

Azathioprine should not be used to treating rheumatoid arthritis in pregnant women.

Patients with rheumatoid arthritis previously treated with alkylating agents (cyclophosphamide, chlorambucil, melphalan or others) may have a prohibitive risk of neoplasia if treated with azathioprine.[9]

WARNINGS

Severe *leukopenia and/or thrombocytopenia* may occur in patients on azathioprine. Macrocytic anemia and severe bone marrow depression may also occur. Hematologic toxicities are dose related and may be more severe in renal transplant patients whose homograft is undergoing rejection. It is suggested that patients on azathioprine have complete blood counts, including platelet counts, weekly during the first month, twice monthly for the second and third months of treatment, then monthly or more frequently if dosage alterations or other therapy changes are necessary. Delayed hematologic suppression may occur. Prompt reduction in dosage or temporary withdrawal of the drug may be necessary if there is a rapid fall in, or persistently low leukocyte count or other evidence of bone marrow depression. Leukopenia does not correlate with therapeutic effect; therefore the dose should not be increased intentionally to lower the white blood cell count.

Serious infections are a constant hazard for patients on chronic immunosuppression, especially for homograft recipients. Fungal, viral, bacterial and protozoal infections may be fatal and should be treated vigorously. Reduction of azathioprine dosage and/or use of other drugs should be considered.

Azathioprine is mutagenic in animals and humans, carcinogenic in animals, and may increase the patient's *risk of neoplasia*. Renal transplant patients are known to have an increased risk of malignancy, predominantly skin cancer and reticulum cell or lymphomatous tumors.[10] The risk of post-transplant lymphomas may be increased in patients who receive aggressive treatment with immunosuppressive drugs.[11] The degree of immunosuppression is determined not only by the immunosuppressive regimen but also by a number of other patient factors. The number of immunosuppressive agents may not necessarily increase the risk of post-transplant lymphomas. However, transplant patients who receive multiple immunosuppressive agents may be at risk for over-immunosuppression; therefore, immunosuppressive drug therapy should be maintained at the lowest effective levels. Information is available on the spontaneous neoplasia risk in rheumatoid arthritis,[12,13] and on neoplasia following immunosuppressive therapy of other autoimmune diseases.[14,15] It has not been possible to define the precise risk of neoplasia due to azathioprine.[16] The data suggest the risk may be elevated in patients with rheumatoid arthritis, though lower than for renal transplant patients.[11,13] However, acute myelogenous leukemia as well as solid tumors have been reported in patients with rheumatoid arthritis who have received azathioprine. Data on neoplasia in patients receiving azathioprine can be found under **ADVERSE REACTIONS**.

Azathioprine has been reported to cause temporary depression in spermatogenesis and reduction in sperm viability and sperm count in mice at doses 10 times the human therapeutic dose[17]; a reduced percentage of fertile matings occurred when animals received 5 mg/kg.[18]

Pregnancy: "Pregnancy Category D": Azathioprine can cause fetal harm when administered to a pregnant woman. Azathioprine should not be given during pregnancy without careful weighing of risk versus benefit. Whenever possible, use of azathioprine in pregnant patients should be avoided. This drug should not be used for treating rheumatoid arthritis in pregnant women.[19]

Azathioprine is teratogenic in rabbits and mice when given in doses equivalent to the human dose (5 mg/kg daily). Abnormalities included skeletal malformations and visceral anomalies.[18]

Limited immunologic and other abnormalities have occurred in a few infants born of renal allograft recipients on azathioprine. In a detailed case report,[20] documented lymphopenia, diminished IgG and IgM levels, CMV infection, and a decreased thymic shadow were noted in an infant born to a mother receiving 150 mg azathioprine and 30 mg prednisone daily throughout pregnancy. At ten weeks most features were normalized. DeWitte et al[21] reported pancytopenia and severe immune deficiency in a pre-term infant whose mother received 125 mg azathioprine and 12.5 mg prednisone daily. There have been two published reports of abnormal physical findings. Williamson and Karp[22] described an infant born with preaxial polydactyly whose mother received azathioprine 200 mg daily and prednisone 20 mg every other day during pregnancy. Tallent et al[23] described an infant with a large myelomeringocele in the upper lumbar region, bilateral dislocated hips, and bilateral talipes equinovarus. The father was on long-term azathioprine therapy.

Benefit versus risk must be weighed carefully before use of azathioprine in patients of reproductive potential. There are no adequate and well-controlled studies in pregnant women. If this drug is used during pregnancy or if the patient becomes pregnant while taking this drug, the patient should be apprised of the potential hazard to the fetus. Women of childbearing age should be advised to avoid becoming pregnant.

PRECAUTIONS

General: A gastrointestinal hypersensitivity reaction characterized by severe nausea and vomiting has been reported.[24,25,26] These symptoms may also be accompanied by diarrhea, rash, fever, malaise, myalgias, elevations in liver enzymes, and occasionally, hypotension. Symptoms of gastrointestinal toxicity most often develop within the first several weeks of azathioprine therapy and are reversible upon discontinuation of the drug. The reaction can recur within hours after rechallenge with a single dose of azathioprine.

Information for Patients:
Patients being started on azathioprine should be informed of the necessity of periodic blood counts while they are receiving the drug and should be encouraged to report any unusual bleeding or bruising to their physician. They should be informed of the danger of infection while receiving azathioprine and encouraged to report signs and symptoms of infection to their physician. Careful dosage instructions should be given to the patient, especially when azathioprine

is being administered in the presence of impaired renal function or concomitantly with allopurinol (see **DOSAGE AND ADMINISTRATION** and **Drug Interactions** under **PRECAUTIONS**). Patients should be advised of the potential risks of the use of azathioprine during pregnancy and during the nursing period. The increased risk of neoplasia following azathioprine therapy should be explained to the patient.

Laboratory Tests: See **WARNINGS** and **ADVERSE REACTIONS**.

Drug Interactions:

Use with Allopurinol: The principal pathway for detoxification of azathioprine is inhibited by allopurinol. Patients receiving azathioprine and allopurinol concomitantly should have a dose reduction of azathioprine, to approximately $^1/_3$ to $^1/_4$ the usual dose.

Use with Other Agents Affecting Myelopoesis: Drugs which may effect leukocyte production, including co-trimoxazole, may lead to exaggerated leukopenia, especially in renal transplant recipients.[27]

Use with Angiotensin Converting Enzyme Inhibitors: The use of angiotensin converting enzyme inhibitors to control hypertension in patients on azathioprine has been reported to induce severe leukopenia.[28]

Carcinogenesis, Mutagenesis, Impairment of Fertility: See **WARNINGS** section.

Pregnancy: Teratogenic Effect. Pregnancy Category D. See **WARNINGS** section.

Nursing Mothers: The use of azathioprine in nursing mothers is not recommended. Azathioprine or its metabolites are transferred at low levels, both transplacentally and in breast milk.[29,30,31] Because of the potential for tumorigenicity shown for azathioprine, a decision should be made whether to discontinue nursing or discontinue the drug, taking into account the importance of the drug to the mother.

Pediatric Use: Safety and efficacy of azathioprine in children have not been established.

ADVERSE REACTIONS

The principal and potentially serious toxic effects of azathioprine are hematologic and gastrointestinal. The risks of secondary infection and neoplasia are also significant (see **WARNINGS**). The frequency and severity of adverse reactions depend on the dose and duration of azathioprine as well as on the patient's underlying disease or concomitant therapies. The incidence of hematologic toxicities and neoplasia encountered in groups of renal hemograft recipients is significantly higher than that in studies employing azathioprine for rheumatoid arthritis. The relative incidences in clinical studies are summarized below:

Toxicity	Renal Homograft	Rheumatoid Arthritis
Leukopenia		
Any Degree	>50%	28%
<2500/mm^3	16%	5.3%
Infections	20%	<1%
Neoplasia		*
Lymphoma	0.5%	
Others	2.8%	

*Data on the rate and risk of neoplasia among persons with rheumatoid arthritis treated with azathioprine are limited. The incidence of lymphoproliferative disease in patients with RA appears to be significantly higher than that in the general population.[12] In one completed study, the rate of lymphoproliferative disease in RA patients receiving higher than recommended doses of azathioprine (5 mg/kg/day) was 1.8 cases per 1000 patient years of follow-up compared with 0.8 cases per 1000 patient years of follow-up, in those not receiving azathioprine.[13] However, the proportion of the increased risk attributable to the azathioprine dosage or to other therapies (i.e., alkylating agents) received by azathioprine-treated patients cannot be determined.

Hematologic: Leukopenia and/or thrombocytopenia are dose dependent and may occur late in the course of azathioprine therapy. Dose reduction or temporary withdrawal allows reversal of these toxicities. Infection may occur as a secondary manifestation of bone marrow suppression or leukopenia, but the incidence of infection in renal homotransplantation is 30 to 60 times that in rheumatoid arthritis. Macrocytic anemia and/or bleeding have been reported in two patients on azathioprine.

Gastrointestinal: Nausea and vomiting may occur within the first few months of azathioprine therapy, and occurred in approximately 12% of 676 rheumatoid arthritis patients. The frequency of gastric disturbance can be reduced by administration of the drug in divided doses and/or after meals. However, in some patients, nausea and vomiting may be severe and may be accompanied by symptoms such as diarrhea, fever, malaise, and myalgias (see **PRECAUTIONS**). Vomiting with abdominal pain may occur rarely with a hypersensitivity pancreatitis. Hepatotoxicity manifest by elevation of serum alkaline phosphatase, bilrubin and/or serum transaminases is known to occur following azathioprine use, primarily in allograft recipients. Hepatotoxicity has been uncommon (less than 1%) in rheumatoid arthritis patients. Hepatotoxicity following transplantation most often occurs within 6 months of transplantation and is generally reversible after interruption of azathioprine. A rare, but life-threatening hepatic veno-occlusive disease associated with chronic administration of azathioprine has been described in transplant patients and in one patient receiving azathioprine for panuveitis.[32,33,34] Periodic measurement of serum transaminases, alkaline phosphatase and bilirubin is indicated for early detection of hepatotoxicity. If hepatic veno-occlusive disease is clinically suspected, azathioprine should be permanently withdrawn.

Others: Additional side effects of low frequency have been recorded. These include skin rashes (approximately 2%), alopecia, fever, arthralgias, diarrhea, steatorrhea and negative nitrogen balance (all less than 1%).

OVERDOSAGE

The oral LD_{50}s for single doses of azathioprine in mice and rats are 2500 mg/kg and 400 mg/kg, respectively. Very large doses of this antimetabolite may lead to marrow hypoplasia, bleeding, infection, and death. About 30% of azathioprine is bound to serum proteins, but approximately 45% is removed during an 8 hour hemodialysis.[35] A single case has been reported of a renal transplant patient who ingested a single dose of 7500 mg azathioprine. The immediate toxic reactions were nausea, vomiting, and diarrhea, followed by mild leukopenia, and mild abnormalities in liver function. The white blood cell count, SGOT, and bilirubin returned to normal six days after the overdose.

DOSAGE AND ADMINISTRATION

Renal Homotransplantation: The dose of azathioprine required to prevent rejection and minimize toxicity will vary with individual patients; this necessitates careful management. Initial dose is usually 3 to 5 mg/kg daily, beginning at the time of transplant. Azathioprine is usually given as a single daily dose on the day of, and in a minority of cases one to three days before, transplantation. Azathioprine is often initiated with the intravenous administration of the sodium salt, with subsequent use of tablets (at the same dose level) after the post-operative period. Intravenous administration of the sodium salt is indicated only in patients unable to tolerate oral medications. Dose reduction to maintenance levels of 1 to 3 mg/kg daily is usually possible. The dose of azathioprine should not be increased to toxic levels because of threatened rejection. Discontinuation may be necessary for severe hematologic or other toxicity, even if rejection of the homograft may be a consequence of drug withdrawal.

Rheumatoid Arthritis: Azathioprine is usually given on a daily basis. The initial dose should be approximately 1.0 mg/kg (50 to 100 mg) given as a single dose or on a twice daily schedule. The dose may be increased, beginning at six to eight weeks and thereafter by steps at four-week intervals, if there are no serious toxicities and if initial response is unsatisfactory. Dose increments should be 0.5 mg/kg daily, up to a maximum dose of 2.5 mg/kg/day. Therapeutic response occurs after several weeks of treatment, usually six to eight; an adequate trial should be a minimum of 12 weeks. Patients not improved after twelve weeks can be considered refractory. Azathioprine may be continued long-term in patients with clinical response, but patients should be monitored carefully, and gradual dosage reduction should be attempted to reduce risk of toxicities.

Maintenance therapy should be at the lowest effective dose, and the dose given can be lowered decrementally with changes of 0.5 mg/kg or approximately 25 mg daily every four weeks while other therapy is kept constant. The optimum duration of maintenance azathioprine has not been determined. Azathioprine can be discontinued abruptly, but delayed effects are possible.

Use in Renal Dysfunction: Relatively oliguric patients, especially those with tubular necrosis in the immediate post-cadaveric transplant period, may have delayed clearance of azathioprine or its metabolites, may be particularly sensitive to this drug and may require lower doses.

Procedures for proper handling and disposal of this immunosuppressive antimetabolite drug should be considered. Several guidelines on this subject have been published.[36–42] There is no general agreement that all of the procedures recommended in the guidelines are necessary or appropriate.

HOW SUPPLIED

Azathioprine Tablets USP, 50 mg
Yellow, round, scored tablets (identified 54 043)
NDC 0054-8084-25: Unit dose, 10 tablets per strip, 10 strips per shelf pack, 10 shelf packs per shipper.
NDC 0054-4084-25: Bottles of 100 tablets.

Caution: Federal law prohibits dispensing without prescription.

Store between 15°C–25°C (59°–77°F)
Protect From Light
Protect From Moisture
Dispense in tight, light resistant container as defined in the USP/NF.

REFERENCES

1. Elion GB, Hitchings GH. Azathioprine In: Sartorelli AC, Johns DG, eds. *Antineoplastic and Immunosuppressive Agents Pt II.* New York, NY:Springer Verlag; 1975:chap 48.
2. McIntosh J, Hansen P, Ziegler J, Penny R. Defective immune and phagocytic functions in uraemia and renal transplantation. *Int Arch Allergy Appl Immunol.* 1976;15:544-549.
3. Renal Transplant Registry Advisory Committee. The 12th report of the Human Renal Transplant Registry. JAMA. 1975;233:787-796.
4. McGeown M. Immunosuppression for kidney transplantation. *Lancet.* 1973;1:310-312.
5. Simmons RL, Thompson EJ, Yunis EJ, et al. 115 Patients with first cadaver kidney transplants followed two to seven and a half years: a multifactorial analysis. *Am J Med.* 1977;62:234-242.
6. Fye K, Talal N. Cytotoxic drugs in the treatment of rheumatoid arthritis. *Ration Drug Ther.* 1975;9(4):1-5.
7. Davis JD, Muss HB, Turner RA. Cytotoxic agents in the treatment of rheumatoid arthritis. *South Med J.* 1978;71:58-64.
8. McEwen C. the diagnosis and differential diagnosis of rheumatoid arthritis. In: Hollander JL, ed. *Arthritis and Allied Conditions: A Textbook of Rheumatology.* 8th ed. Philadelphia, PA: Lea and Febiger; 1972:403-418.
9. Hoover R, Fraumeni, JF. Drug-induced cancer. *Cancer.* 1981;47(5):1071-1080.
10. Hoover R, Fraumeni JF Jr. Risk of cancer in renal transplant recipients. *Lancet.* 1973;2:55-57.
11. Wilkenson AH, Smith JL, Hunsicker LG, et al. Increased frequency of post-transplant lymphomas in patients treated with cyclosporine, azathioprine, and prednisone. *Transplantation.* 1989;47:293-296.
12. Prior P, Symmons DP, Hawkins CF, et al. Cancer morbidity in rheumatoid arthritis. *Ann Rheum Dis* 1984;43:128-131.
13. Silman AJ, Petrie J, Hazelman B, et al. Lymphoproliferative cancer and other malignancy in patients with rheumatoid arthritis treated with azathioprine: a 20 year follow up study. *Ann Rheum Dis.* 1988;47:988-992.
14. Louie S, Schwartz RS. Immunodeficiency and pathogenesis of lymphoma and leukemia. *Semin Hematol.* 1978;15:117-138.
15. Wang KK, Czaja AJ, Beaver SJ, et al. Extra hepatic malignancy following long-term immunosuppressive therapy of severe hepatitis B surface antigen-negative chronic active hepatitis. *Hepatology.* 1989;10:39-43.
16. Sieber SM, Adamson RH. Toxicity of antineoplastic agents in man: chromosomal aberrations, antifertility effects, congenital malformations and carcinogenic potential. In: Klein G, Weinhouse S, eds. *Advances in Cancer Research,* v.22. New York, NY: Academic Press; 1975: 57-155.
17. Clark JM. The mutagenicity of azathioprine in mice, *Drosophila Melanogaster* and *Neurospora Crassa. Mut Res.* 1975;28(1):87-99.
18. Data on file at Burroughs Wellcome Co.
19. Tagatz GE, Simmons RL. Pregnancy after renal transplantation. *Ann Intern Med.* 1975;82:113-114, Editorial Notes.
20. Coté CJ, Meuwissen HJ, Pickering RJ. Effects on the neonate of prednisone and azathioprine administered to the mother during pregnancy. *J Pediatr.* 1974;85(3):324-328.
21. DeWitte DB, Buick MK, Stephen EC, et al. Neonatal pancytopenia and severe combined immunodeficiency associated with antenatal administration of azathioprine and prednisone. *J Pediatr.* 1984;105(4):625-628.
22. Williamson RA, Karp LE. Azathioprine teratogenicity: review of the literature and case report. *Obstet Gynecol.* 1981;58:247-250.
23. Tallent MB, Simmons RL, Najarian JS. Birth defects in child of male recipient of kidney transplant. *JAMA.* 1970;211(11):1854-1855.
24. Assini JF, Hamilton R, Strosberg JM. Adverse reactions to azathioprine mimicking gastroenteritis. *J Rheumatol.* 1986;13:1117-1118.
25. Cochrane D, Adamson AR, Halsey JP. Adverse reactions to azathioprine mimicking gastroenteritis. *J Rheumatol.* 1987;14:1075.
26. Cox J, Daneshmend JK, Hawkey CJ, et al. Devastating diarrhea caused by azathioprine: management difficulty in inflammatory bowel disease. *Gut.* 1988;29(5):686-688.

Continued on next page

Azathioprine—Cont.

27. Bradley PP, Warden GD, Maxwell JG, et al. Neutropenia and thrombocytopenia in renal allograft recipients treated with trimethoprim-sulfamethoxazole. *Ann Int Med.* 1980;93:560-562.

28. Kirchertz EJ, Grone HJ, Rieger J, et al. Successful low dose captopril rechallenge following drug-induced leucopenia. *Lancet.* 1981;8234:1362-1363.

29. Nelson D, Bugge C. Data on file, Burroughs Wellcome Co.

30. Saarikoski S, Seppälä M. Immunosuppression during pregnancy: transmission of azathioprine and its metabolites from the mother to the fetus. *Am J Obstet Gynecol.* 1973;115:1100-1106.

31. Coulam CB, Moyer TP, Jiang NS, et al. Breast-feeding after renal transplantation. *Transplant Proc.* 1982;14: 605-609.

32. Read AE, Wiesner RH, LaBrecque DR, et al. Hepatic veno-occlusive disease associated with renal transplantation and azathioprine therapy. *Ann Intern Med.* 1986;104:651-655.

33. Katzka DA, Saul SH, Jorkasky D, Sigal H, Reynolds JC, Soloway RD. Azathioprine and hepatic venocclusive disease in renal transplant patients. *Gastroenterology.* 1986;90:446-454.

34. Weitz H, Gokel JM, Loeschke K, et al. Veno-occlusive disease of the liver in patients receiving immunosuppressive therapy. *Virchows Arch A.* 1982;395:245-256.

35. Schusziarra V, Ziekursch V, Schlamp R, et al. Pharmacokinetics of azathioprine under haemodialysis. *Int J Clin Pharmacol Biopharm.* 1976;14(4):298-302.

36. Recommendations for the safe handling of parenteral antineoplastic drugs. Washington, DC: Division of Safety, National Institutes of Health; 1983. US Dept of Health and Human Service publication NIH 83-2621.

37. AMA Council on Scientific Affairs. Guidelines for handling parenteral antineoplastics. *JAMA* 1985;253:1590-1591.

38. National Study Commission on Cytotoxic Exposure. Recommendations for handling cytotoxic agents. 1984. Available from Louis P. Jeffrey, ScD, Director of Pharmacy Services, Rhode Island Hospital, 593 Eddy Street, Providence, Rhode Island 02902.

39. Clinical Oncological Society of Australia. Guidelines and recommendations for safe handling of antineoplastic agents. *Med J Australia.* 1983;1:426-428.

40. Jones RB, Frank R, Mass T. Safe handling of chemotherapeutic agents: a report from the Mount Sinai Medical Center. *CA-A Cancer J for Clin.* 1983;33(Sept/Oct):258-263.

41. American Society of Hospital Pharmacists. ASHP technical assistance bulletin on handling cytotoxic and hazardous drugs. *Am J Hosp Pharm.* 1990;47:1033-1049.

42. Yodaiken RE, Bennett D. OSHA work-practice guidelines for personnel dealing with cytotoxic (antineoplastic) drugs. *Am J Hosp Pharm.* 1986;43:1193-1204.

4042500   Revised October 1995
105
© RLI, 1995.
Roxane Laboratories, Inc.
Columbus, Ohio 43216

DHT™
Dihydrotachysterol
Tablets USP and Intensol™   ℞

DESCRIPTION
Each tablet contains:
Dihydrotachysterol .... 0.125 mg, 0.2 mg, or 0.4 mg
Each mL of Intensol contains:
Dihydrotachysterol .... 0.2 mg
Dihydrotachysterol is a synthetic reduction product of tachysterol, a close isomer of vitamin D. Chemically Dihydrotachysterol is *9,10- Secoergosta-5,7,22-tri-en-3β- ol.*
Dihydrotachysterol acts as a blood calcium regulator.

CLINICAL PHARMACOLOGY
Dihydrotachysterol is hydroxylated in the liver to 25-hydroxydihydrotachysterol, which is the major circulating active form of the drug. It does not undergo further hydroxylation by the kidney and therefore is the analogue of 1,25-dihydroxyvitamin D. Dihydrotachysterol is effective in the elevation of serum calcium by stimulating intestinal calcium absorption and mobilizing bone calcium in the absence of parathyroid hormone and of functioning renal tissue. Dihydrotachysterol also increases renal phosphate excretion. In contrast to parathyroid extract, Dihydrotachysterol is active when taken orally, exerts a slow but persistent effect, and may be used for long periods without increasing the dosage or causing tolerance. Dihydrotachysterol is faster-acting than pharmacologic doses of vitamin D and is less persistent after cessation of treatment, thus decreasing the risk of accumulation and of hypercalcemia.

INDICATIONS AND USAGE
Dihydrotachysterol is indicated for the treatment of acute, chronic, and latent forms of postoperative tetany, idiopathic tetany, and hypoparathyroidism.

CONTRAINDICATIONS
Contraindicated in patients with hypercalcemia, abnormal sensitivity to the effects of vitamin D, and hypervitaminosis D.

PRECAUTIONS
General: The difference between therapeutic dose and intoxicating dose may be small in any patient and therefore dosage must be individualized and periodically reevaluated. In patients with renal osteodystrophy accompanied by hyperphosphatemia, maintenance of a normal serum phosphorus level by dietary phosphate restriction and/or administration of aluminum gels as intestinal phosphate binders is essential to prevent metastatic calcification.
Because of its effect on serum calcium, Dihydrotachysterol should be administered to pregnant patients or to patients with renal stones only when, in the judgment of the physician, the potential benefits outweigh the possible hazards.
Laboratory tests: **To prevent hypercalcemia, treatment should always be controlled by regular determinations of blood calcium level, which should be maintained within the normal range.**
Drug interactions: Administration of thiazide diuretics to hypoparathyroid patients who are concurrently being treated with Dihydrotachysterol may cause hypercalcemia.
Pregnancy: Teratogenic effects—Pregnancy Category C: Animal reproduction studies have shown fetal abnormalities in several species associated with hypervitaminosis D. These are similar to the supravalvular aortic stenosis syndrome described in infants by Black in England (1963). This syndrome was characterized by supravalvular aortic stenosis, elfin facies, and mental retardation.
There are no adequate and well-controlled studies in pregnant women. Dihydrotachysterol should be used during pregnancy only if the potential benefit justifies the potential risk to the fetus.
Nursing mothers: It is not known whether this drug is excreted in human milk. Because many drugs are excreted in human milk, caution should be exercised when Dihydrotachysterol is administered to a nursing woman.

OVERDOSAGE
The effects of Dihydrotachysterol can persist for up to one month after cessation of treatment.
Manifestations: Toxicity associated with Dihydrotachysterol is similar to that seen with large doses of vitamin D. Overdosage is manifested by symptoms of hypercalcemia, i.e., weakness, headache, anorexia, nausea, vomiting, abdominal cramps, diarrhea, constipation, vertigo, tinnitus, ataxia, hypotonia, lethargy, depression, amnesia, disorientation, hallucinations, syncope, and coma. Impairment of renal function may result in polyuria, polydipsia, and albuminuria. Widespread calcification of soft tissues, including heart, blood vessels, kidneys, and lungs, can occur. Death can result from cardiovascular or renal failure.
Treatment: Treatment of overdosage consists of withdrawal of Dihydrotachysterol, bed rest, liberal intake of fluids, a low-calcium diet, and administration of a laxative. Hypercalcemic crisis with dehydration, stupor, coma, and azotemia requires more vigorous treatment. The first step should be hydration of the patient. Intravenous saline may quickly and significantly increase urinary calcium excretion. A loop diuretic (furosemide or ethacrynic acid) may be given with the saline infusion to further increase renal calcium excretion. Other reported therapeutic measures include dialysis or the administration of citrates, sulfates, phosphates, corticosteroids, EDTA (ethylenediaminetetraacetic acids), and mithramycin via appropriate regimens.

DOSAGE AND ADMINISTRATION
The dosage depends on the nature and seriousness of the disorder and should be adapted to each individual patient. Serum calcium levels should be maintained between 9 to 10 mg per 100 mL.
The following dosage schedule will serve as a guide:
Initial dose: 0.8 mg to 2.4 mg daily for several days.
Maintenance dose: 0.2 mg to 1.0 mg daily as required for normal serum calcium levels. The average maintenance dose is 0.6 mg daily. This dose may be supplemented with 10 to 15 grams of calcium lactate or gluconate by mouth daily.

HOW SUPPLIED
0.125 mg white tablets. (identified 54 280)
NDC 0054-8172-25: Unit dose, 10 tablets per strip, 10 strips per shelf pack, 10 shelf packs per shipper.
NDC 0054-4190-19: Bottles of 50 tablets.
0.2 mg pink tablets. (identified 54 903)
NDC 0054-8182-25: Unit dose, 10 tablets per strip, 10 strips per shelf pack, 10 shelf packs per shipper.
NDC 0054-4189-25: Bottles of 100 tablets.

0.4 mg white tablets. (identified 54 772)
NDC 0054-4191-19: Bottles of 50 tablets.
Intensol 0.2 mg/mL
NDC 0054-3170-44: Bottles of 30 mL with calibrated dropper (graduated 0.25 mL to 1.0 mL)
4049201   Revised October 1994
104

DOLOPHINE® HYDROCHLORIDE   Ⓒ ℞
Methodone Hydrochloride
Tablets USP 5 mg, 10 mg
Methadone Hydrochloride
Injection USP 10 mg per mL

(WARNING: May be habit forming)

> CONDITIONS FOR DISTRIBUTION AND
> USE OF METHADONE PRODUCTS:
> Code of Federal Regulations,
>   Title 21, Sec. 291.505
>
> METHADONE PRODUCTS, WHEN USED FOR TREATMENT OF NARCOTIC ADDICTION IN DETOXIFICATION OR MAINTENANCE PROGRAMS, SHALL BE DISPENSED ONLY BY APPROVED HOSPITAL PHARMACIES, APPROVED COMMUNITY PHARMACIES, AND MAINTENANCE PROGRAMS APPROVED BY THE FOOD AND DRUG ADMINISTRATION AND THE DESIGNATED STATE AUTHORITY.
>   APPROVED MAINTENANCE PROGRAMS SHALL DISPENSE AND USE METHADONE IN ORAL FORM ONLY AND ACCORDING TO THE TREATMENT REQUIREMENTS STIPULATED IN THE FEDERAL METHADONE REGULATIONS (21 CFR 291.505).
>   FAILURE TO ABIDE BY THE REQUIREMENTS IN THESE REGULATIONS MAY RESULT IN CRIMINAL PROSECUTION, SEIZURE OF THE DRUG SUPPLY, REVOCATION OF THE PROGRAM APPROVAL, AND INJUNCTION PRECLUDING OPERATION OF THE PROGRAM.
>   A METHADONE PRODUCT, WHEN USED AS AN ANALGESIC, MAY BE DISPENSED IN ANY LICENSED PHARMACY.

DESCRIPTION
Chemically, Methadone Hydrochloride is 3-Heptanone, 6-(dimethylamino)-4,4-diphenyl-, hydrochloride, which can be represented by the following structural formula:

$C_{21}H_{27}NO \cdot HCl$ M.W. 345.91

Each tablet for oral administration contains:
Methadone Hydrochloride .... 5 mg, 10 mg
(Warning: May be habit forming)
Each mL contains methadone hydrochloride 10 mg (0.029 mmol) and sodium chloride 0.9%. Sodium hydroxide and/or hydrochloric acid may have been added during manufacture to adjust the pH. The 20 mL vials also contain chlorobutanol (chloroform derivative), 0.5%, as a preservative.
Inactive Ingredients:
The tablets contain magnesium stearate, cellulose, starch (corn), lactose, sucrose and talc. The 10 mg tablet also contains acacia.

HOW SUPPLIED
DOLOPHINE HYDROCHLORIDE®
(Methadone Hydrochloride Tablets USP)
5 mg tablets (Identified 54 162).
NDC 0054-4216-25: Bottles of 100 tablets.
10 mg tablets (Identified 54 549).
NDC 0054-4217-25: Bottles of 100 tablets.
DOLOPHINE HYDROCHLORIDE®
(Methadone Hydrochloride Injection USP)
10 mg per mL, Multiple-Dose Vials.
NDC 0054-1218-42: Single 20 mL multiple-dose vials.
Store at Controlled Room Temperature 15°–30°C (59°–86°F)
Protect from light.
Dispense in a tight, light-resistant container as defined in the USP/NF.
Caution: Federal law prohibits dispensing without prescription.
March 1995

DURACLON™ ℞

[*dŭră clŏn*]

clonidine hydrochloride injection

> **NOTE: Duraclon™ (epidural clonidine) is not recommended for obstetrical, post-partum, or peri-operative pain management. The risk of hemodynamic instability, especially hypotension and bradycardia, from epidural clonidine may be unacceptable in these patients. However, in a rare obstetrical, post-partum or peri-operative patient, potential benefits may outweigh the possible risks.**

DESCRIPTION

Duraclon (clonidine hydrochloride injection) is a centrally-acting analgesic for use in continuous epidural infusion devices.

Clonidine Hydrochloride, USP, is an imidazoline derivative and exists as a mesomeric compound. The chemical names are Benzenamine, 2,6-dichloro-N-2-imidazolindinylidene-monohydrochloride and 2-[(2, 6-dichlorophenyl)imino]imidazolidine monohydrochloride. The following is the structural formula:

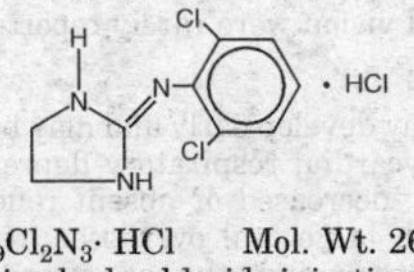

$C_9H_9Cl_2N_3$· HCl Mol. Wt. 266.56

Duraclon (clonidine hydrochloride injection) is supplied as a clear, colorless, preservative-free, pyrogen-free, aqueous sterile solution (pH 5 to 7) in a single-dose, 10 mL vial. Each mL of solution contains 100 mcg of Clonidine Hydrochloride, USP and 9 mg Sodium Chloride, USP in Water for Injection, USP. Hydrochloric Acid and/or Sodium Hydroxide may have been added for pH adjustment. Each 10 mL vial contains 1 mg (1000 mcg) of clonidine hydrochloride.

CLINICAL PHARMACOLOGY

Mechanism of Action

Epidurally administered clonidine produces dose-dependent analgesia not antagonized by opiate antagonists. The analgesia is limited to the body regions innervated by the spinal segments where analgesic concentrations of clonidine are present. Clonidine is thought to produce analgesia at presynaptic and postjunctional alpha-2-adrenoceptors in the spinal cord by preventing pain signal transmission to the brain.

Pharmacokinetics

Following a 10 minute intravenous infusion of 300 mcg clonidine HCl to five male volunteers, plasma clonidine levels showed an initial rapid distribution phase (mean±SD $t_{1/2}$=11±9 minutes) followed by a slower elimination phase ($t_{1/2}$=9±2 hours) over 24 hours. Clonidine's total body clearance (CL) was 219±92 mL/min.

Following a 700 mcg clonidine HCl epidural dose given over five minutes to four male and five female volunteers, peak clonidine plasma levels (4.4±1.4 ng/mL) were obtained in 19±27 minutes. The plasma elimination half-life was determined to be 22±15 hours following sample collection for 24 hours. CL was 190±70 mL/min. In cerebral spinal fluid (CSF), peak clonidine levels (418±255 ng/mL) were achieved in 26±11 minutes. The clonidine CSF elimination half-life was 1.3±0.5 hours when samples were collected for 6 hours. Compared to men, women had a lower mean plasma clearance, longer mean plasma half-life, and higher mean peak level of clonidine in both plasma and CSF.

In cancer patients who received 14 days of clonidine HCl epidural infusion (rate=30 mcg/hr) plus morphine by patient-controlled analgesia (PCA), steady state clonidine plasma concentrations of 2.2±1.1 and 2.4±1.4 ng/mL were obtained on dosing days 7 and 14, respectively. CL was 279±184 and 272±163 mL/min on these days. CSF concentrations were not determined in these patients.

Distribution

Clonidine is highly lipid soluble and readily distributes into extravascular sites including the central nervous system. Clonidine's volume of distribution is 2.1±0.4 L/kg. The binding of clonidine to plasma protein is primarily to albumin and varies between 20 and 40% *in vitro*. Epidurally administered clonidine readily partitions into plasma via the epidural veins and attains systemic concentrations (0.5–2.0 ng/mL) that are associated with a hypotensive effect mediated by the central nervous system.

Excretion

Following an intravenous dose of ^{14}C-clonidine, 72% of the administered dose was excreted in urine in 96 hours of which 40–50% was unchanged clonidine. Renal clearance for clonidine was determined to be 133±66 mL/min. In a study where ^{14}C-clonidine was given to subjects with varying degrees of kidney function, elimination half-lives varied (17.5 to 41 hours) as a function of creatinine clearance. In subjects undergoing hemodialysis only 5% of body clonidine stores was removed.

Metabolism

In humans, clonidine metabolism follows minor pathways with the major metabolite, p-hydroxyclonidine, being present at less than 10% of the concentration of unchanged drug in urine.

Special Populations

The pharmacokinetics of epidurally administered clonidine has not been studied in the pediatric population or in patients with renal or hepatic disease.

Clinical Trials

In a double-blind, randomized study of cancer patients with severe intractable pain below the C4 dermatome not controlled by morphine, 38 patients were randomized to an epidural infusion of Duraclon plus epidural morphine, whereas 47 subjects received epidural placebo plus epidural morphine. Both groups were allowed rescue doses of epidural morphine. Successful analgesia, defined as a decrease in either morphine use or Visual Analog Score (VAS) pain, was significantly more common with epidural clonidine than placebo (45% vs 21%, p=0.016). Only the subgroup of 36 patients with "neuropathic" pain, characterized by the investigator as well-localized, burning, shooting, or electric-like pain in a dermatomal or peripheral nerve distribution had significant analgesic effects relative to placebo in this study. The most frequent adverse events with clonidine were hypotension (45% vs 11% for placebo, p< 0.001), postural hypotension (32% vs 0%, p< 0.001), dizziness (13% vs 4%, p=0.234), anxiety (11% vs 2%, p=0.168) and dry mouth (13% vs 9%, p=0.505). Both mean blood pressure and heart rate were reduced in the clonidine group. At the conclusion of the two week study period in the clinical trial, all patients were abrubtly withdrawn from study drug or placebo. Four patients of the clonidine group suffered rebound hypertension upon withdrawal of clonidine; one of these patients suffered a cerebrovascular accident. Asymptomatic bradycardia was noted in one clonidine patient.

INDICATIONS AND USAGE

Duraclon is indicated in combination with opiates for the treatment of severe pain in cancer patients that is not adequately relieved by opioid analgesics alone. Epidural clonidine is more likely to be effective in patients with neuropathic pain than somatic or visceral pain (see ***Clinical Trials***).

The safety of this drug product has only been established in a highly selected group of cancer patients, and only after an adequate trial of opioid analgesia. Other use is of unproven safety and is not recommended. In a rare patient, the potential benefits may outweigh the known risks (see **WARNINGS**).

CONTRAINDICATIONS

Duraclon is contraindicated in patients with a history of sensitization or allergic reactions to clonidine. Epidural administration is contraindicated in the presence of an injection site infection, in patients on anticoagulant therapy, and in those with a bleeding diathesis. Administration of Duraclon above the C4 dermatome is contraindicated since there are no adequate safety data to support such use. (See **WARNINGS**).

WARNINGS

Use in Postoperative or Obstetrical Analgesia

Duraclon (epidural clonidine) is not recommended for obstetrical, post-partum, or perioperative pain management. The risk of hemodynamic instability, especially hypotension and bradycardia, from epidural clonidine may be unacceptable in these patients.

Hypotension

Because severe hypotension may follow the administration of clonidine, it should be used with caution in all patients. It is not recommended in most patients with severe cardiovascular disease or in those who are otherwise hemodynamically unstable. The benefit of its administration in these patients should be carefully balanced against the potential risks resulting from hypotension.

Vital signs should be monitored frequently, especially during the first few days of epidural clonidine therapy. When clonidine is infused into the upper thoracic spinal segments, more pronounced decreases in the blood pressure may be seen.

Clonidine decreases sympathetic outflow from the central nervous system resulting in decreases in peripheral resistance, renal vascular resistance, heart rate, and blood pressure. However, in the absence of profound hypotension, renal blood flow and glomerular filtration rate remain essentially unchanged.

In the pivotal double-blind, randomized study of cancer patients, where 38 subjects were administered epidural Duraclon at 30 mcg/hr in addition to epidural morphine, hypotension occurred in 45% of subjects. Most episodes of hypotension occurred within the first four days after beginning epidural clonidine. However, hypotensive episodes occurred throughout the duration of the trial. There was a tendency for these episodes to occur more commonly in women, and in those with higher serum clonidine levels. Patients experiencing hypotension also tended to weigh less than those who did not experience hypotension. The hypotension usually responded to intravenous fluids and, if necessary, parenteral ephedrine.

Published reports on the use of epidural clonidine for intraoperative or postoperative analgesia also show a consistent and marked hypotensive response to clonidine. Severe hypotension may occur even if intravenous fluid pretreatment is given.

Withdrawal

Sudden cessation of clonidine treatment, regardless of the route of administration, has, in some cases, resulted in symptoms such as nervousness, agitation, headache, and tremor, accompanied or followed by a rapid rise in blood pressure. The likelihood of such reactions appears to be greater after administration of higher doses or with concomitant beta-blocker treatment. Special caution is therefore advised in these situations. Rare instances of hypertensive encephalopathy, cerebrovascular accidents and death have been reported with abrupt clonidine withdrawal. Patients with a history of hypertension and/or other underlying cardiovascular conditions may be at particular risk of the consequences of abrupt discontinuation of clonidine. In the pivotal double-blind, randomized cancer pain study, four of 38 subjects receiving 720 mcg of clonidine per day experienced rebound hypertension following abrupt withdrawal. One of these patients with rebound hypertension subsequently experienced a cerebrovascular accident.

Careful monitoring of infusion pump function and inspection of catheter tubing for obstruction or dislodgment can help reduce the risk of inadvertent abrupt withdrawal of epidural clonidine. Patients should notify their physician immediately if clonidine administration is inadvertently interrupted for any reason. Patients should also be instructed not to discontinue therapy without consulting their physician.

When discontinuing therapy with epidural clonidine, the physician should reduce the dose gradually over 2 to 4 days to avoid withdrawal symptoms.

An excessive rise in blood pressure following discontinuation of epidural clonidine can be treated by administration of clonidine or by intravenous phentolamine. If therapy is to be discontinued in patients receiving a beta-blocker and clonidine concurrently, the beta-blocker should be withdrawn several days before the gradual discontinuation of epidural clonidine.

Infections

Infections related to implantable epidural catheters pose a serious risk. Evaluation of fever in a patient receiving epidural clonidine should include the possibility of a catheter-related infection such as meningitis or epidural abscess.

PRECAUTIONS

General

Cardiac Effects: Epidural clonidine frequently causes decreases in heart rate. Symptomatic bradycardia can be treated with atropine. Rarely, atrioventricular block greater than first degree has been reported. Clonidine does not alter the hemodynamic response to exercise, but may mask the increase in heart rate associated with hypovolemia.

Respiratory Depression and Sedation: Clonidine administration may result in sedation through the activation of alpha-adrenoceptors in the brainstem. High doses of clonidine cause sedation and ventilatory abnormalities that are usually mild. Tolerance to these effects can develop with chronic administration. These effects have been reported with bolus doses that are significantly larger than the infusion rate recommended for treating cancer patients.

Depression: Depression has been seen in a small percentage of patients treated with oral or transdermal clonidine. Depression commonly occurs in cancer patients and may be exacerbated by treatment with clonidine. Patients, especially those with a known history of affective disorders, should be monitored for the signs and symptoms of depression.

Pain of Visceral or Somatic Origin: In the clinical investigations, at doses tested, Duraclon was most effective in well-localized, "neuropathic" pain that was characterized as electrical, burning, or shooting in nature, and which was localized to a dermatomal or peripheral nerve distribution. Duraclon may be less effective, or possibly ineffective in the treatment of pain that is diffuse, poorly localized, or visceral in origin.

Information for Patients

Patients should be instructed about the risks of rebound hypotension and warned not to discontinue clonidine except under the supervision of a physician. Patients should notify their physician immediately if clonidine administration is inadvertently interrupted for any reason. Patients who engage in potentially hazardous activities, such as operating machinery or driving, should be advised of the potential sedative and hypotensive effects of epidural clonidine. They should also be informed that sedative effects may be increased by CNS-depressing drugs such as alcohol and barbiturates, and that hypotensive effects may be increased by opiates.

Continued on next page

Duraclon—Cont.

Drug Interactions

Clonidine may potentiate the CNS-depressive effect of alcohol, barbiturates or other sedating drugs. Narcotic analgesics may potentiate the hypotensive effects of clonidine. Tricyclic antidepressants may antagonize the hypotensive effects of clonidine. The effects of tricyclic antidepressants on clonidine's analgesic actions are not known.

Beta blockers may exacerbate the hypertensive response seen with clonidine withdrawal. Also, due to the potential for additive effects such as bradycardia and AV block, caution is warranted in patients receiving clonidine with agents known to affect sinus node function or AV nodal conduction, e.g., digitalis, calcium channel blockers, and beta-blockers.

There is one reported case of a patient with acute delirium associated with the simultaneous use of fluphenazine and oral clonidine. Symptoms resolved when clonidine was withdrawn and recurred when the patient was rechallenged with clonidine.

Epidural clonidine may prolong the duration of pharmacologic effects of epidural local anesthetics, including both sensory and motor blockade.

Carcinogenesis, Mutagenesism, Impairment of Fertility

In a 132-week study in rats, clonidine hydrochloride administered as a dietary admixture at 5–8 times (based on body surface area) the 50 mcg/kg maximum recommended daily human dose (MRDHD) for hypertension did not show any carcinogenic potential. Clonidine was inactive in the Ames test of mutagenicity.

Fertility of male or female rats was unaffected by oral clonidine hydrochloride doses as high as 150 mcg/kg, or about 0.5 times the MRDHD. Fertility of female rats did, however, appear to be affected in another experiment at oral dose levels of 500–2000 mcg/kg, or 2–7 times the MRDHD.

Usage in Pregnancy/Teratogenic Effects

PREGNANCY CATEGORY C: Reproduction studies in rabbits at clonidine hydrochloride doses up to approximately the MRDHD revealed no evidence of teratogenic or embryotoxic potential. In rats, however, doses as low as one-third the MRDHD were associated with increased resorptions in a study in which dams were treated continuously from 2 months prior to mating. Increased resorptions were not associated with treatment with the same or higher doses up to 0.5 times the MRDHD when dams were treated on days 6–15 of gestation. Increased resorptions were observed at higher levels (7-times the MRDHD) in rats and mice treated on days 1–14 of gestation.

Clonidine readily crosses the placenta and its concentrations are equal in maternal and umbilical cord plasma; amniotic fluid concentrations can be 4-times those found in serum. There are no adequate and well-controlled studies in pregnant women during early gestation when organ formation takes place. Studies using epidural clonidine during labor have demonstrated no apparent adverse effects on the infant at the time of delivery. However, these studies did not monitor the infants for hemodynamic effects in the days following delivery. Clonidine hydrochloride injection should be used during pregnancy only if the potential benefits justify the potential risk to the fetus.

Labor and Delivery

There are no adequate controlled clinical trials evaluating the safety, efficacy, and dosing of Duraclon in obstetrical settings. Because maternal perfusion of the placenta is critically dependent on blood pressure, use of Duraclon as an analgesic during labor and delivery is not indicated (see **WARNINGS**).

Nursing Mothers

Concentrations of clonidine in human breast milk are approximately twice those found in maternal plasma. Caution should be exercised when clonidine is administered to a nursing women. Because of the potential for severe adverse reactions in nursing infants, a decision should be made to either discontinue nursing or to discontinue clonidine.

Pediatric Use

The safety and effectiveness of Duraclon in this limited indication and clinical population have been established in patients old enough to tolerate placement and management of an epidural catheter, based on evidence from adequate and well controlled studies in adults and experience with the use of clonidine in the pediatric age group for other indications. The use of Duraclon should be restricted to pediatric patients with severe intractable pain from malignancy that is unresponsive to epidural or spinal opiates or other more conventional analgesic techniques. The starting dose of Duraclon should be selected on per kilogram basis (0.5 mcg per kg per hour) and cautiously adjusted based on the clinical response.

ADVERSE REACTIONS

Adverse reactions seen during continuous epidural clonidine infusion are dose-dependent and typical for a compound of this pharmacological class. The adverse events most frequently reported in the pivotal controlled clinical trial of continuous epidural clonidine administration consisted of hypotension, postural hypotension, decreased heart rate, rebound hypertension, dry mouth, nausea, confusion, dizziness, somnolence, and fever. Hypotension is the adverse event that most frequently requires treatment. The hypotension is usually responsive to intravenous fluids and, if necessary, parenterally-administered ephedrine. Hypotension was observed more frequently in women and in lower weight patients, but no dose-related response was established.

Implantable epidural catheters are associated with a risk of catheter-related infections, including meningitis and/or epidural abscess. The risk depends on the clinical situation and the type of catheter used, but catheter related infections occur in 5%–20% of patients, depending on the kind of catheter used, catheter placement techniques, quality of catheter care, and length of catheter placement.

The inadvertent intrathecal administration of clonidine has not been associated with a significantly increased risk of adverse events, but there are inadequate safety and efficacy data to support the use of intrathecal clonidine.

Epidural clonidine was compared to placebo in a two week double-blind study of 85 terminal cancer patients with intractable pain receiving epidural morphine. The following adverse events were reported in two or more patients and may be related to administration of either Duraclon or morphine.

Incidence of Adverse Events in the Two-Week Trial

Adverse Events	Clonidine N = 38 n (%)	Placebo N = 47 n (%)
Total Number of Patients Who Experienced At Least One Adverse Event	37 (97.4)	38 (80.5)
Hypotension	17 (44.8)	5 (10.6)
Postural Hypotension	12 (31.6)	0 (0)
Dry Mouth	5 (13.2)	4 (8.5)
Nausea	5 (13.2)	10 (21.3)
Somnolence	5 (13.2)	10 (21.3)
Dizziness	5 (13.2)	2 (4.3)
Confusion	5 (13.2)	5 (10.6)
Vomiting	4 (10.5)	7 (14.9)
Nausea/Vomiting	3 (7.9)	1 (2.1)
Sweating	2 (5.3)	0 (0)
Chest Pain	2 (5.3)	0 (0)
Hallucination	2 (5.3)	1 (2.1)
Tinnitus	2 (5.3)	0 (0)
Constipation	1 (2.6)	2 (4.3)
Tachycardia	1 (2.6)	2 (4.3)
Hypoventilation	1 (2.6)	2 (4.3)

An open label long-term extension of the above trial was performed. Thirty-two subjects received epidural clonidine and morphine for up to 94 weeks with a median dosing period of 10 weeks. The following adverse events (and percent incidence) were reported: hypotension/postural hypotension (47%); nausea (13%); anxiety/confusion (38%); somnolence (25%); urinary tract infection (22%); constipation, dyspnea, fever, infection (6% each); asthenia, hyperaesthesia, pain, skin ulcer, and vomiting (5% each). Eighteen percent of subjects discontinued this study as a result of catheter-related problems (infections, accidental dislodging, etc.), and one subject developed meningitis, possibly as a result of a catheter-related infection. In this study, rebound hypertension was not assessed, and ECG and laboratory data were not systematically sought.

The following adverse reactions have also been reported with the use of any dosage form of clonidine. In many cases patients were receiving concomitant medication and a causal relationship has not been established:

Body as a Whole: Weakness, 10%; fatigue, 4%; headache and withdrawal syndrome, each 1%. Also reported were pallor, a weakly positive Coomb's test, and increased sensitivity to alcohol.

Cardiovascular: Palpitations and tachycardia, and bradycardia, each 0.5%. Syncope, Raynaud's phenomenon, congestive heart failure, and electrocardiographic abnormalities (i.e., sinus node arrest, functional bradycardia, high degree AV block) have been reported rarely. Rare cases of sinus bradycardia and atrioventricular block have been reported, both with and without the use of concomitant digitalis.

Central Nervous System: Nervousness and agitation, 3%; mental depression, 1%; insomnia, 0.5%. Cerebrovascular accidents, other behavioral changes, vivid dreams or nightmares, restlessness, and delirium have been reported rarely.

Dermatological: Rash, 1%; pruritus, 0.7%; hives, angioneurotic edema and urticaria, 0.5%; alopecia, 0.2%.

Gastrointestinal: Anorexia and malaise, each 1%; mild transient abnormalities in liver function tests, 1%; hepatitis, parotitis, ileus and pseudoobstruction, and abdominal pain, rarely.

Genitourinary: Decreased sexual activity, impotence, and libido, 3%; nocturia, about 1%; difficulty in micturition, about 0.2%; urinary retention, about 0.1%.

Hematologic: Thrombocytopenia, rarely.

Metabolic: Weight gain, 0.1%; gynecomastia, 1%; transient elevation of glucose or serum phosphatase, rarely.

Musculoskeletal: Muscle or joint pain, about 0.6%; leg cramps, 0.3%.

Oro-otolaryngeal: Dryness of the nasal mucosa was rarely reported.

Ophthalmological: Dryness of the eyes, burning of the eyes and blurred vision were rarely reported.

OVERDOSAGE

Hypertension may develop early and may be followed by hypotension, bradycardia, respiratory depression, hypothermia, drowsiness, decreased or absent reflexes, irritability, and miosis. With large oral overdoses, reversible cardiac conduction defects or arrhythmias, apnea, coma, and seizures have been reported. As little as 100 mcg of oral clonidine has produced signs of toxicity in pediatric patients.

There is no specific antidote for clonidine overdosage. Supportive care may include atropine sulfate for bradycardia, intravenous fluids and/or vasopressor agents for hypotension. Hypertension associated with overdosage has been treated with intravenous furosemide, diazoxide, or alpha-blocking agents such as phentolamine.

Naloxone may be a useful adjunct in the treatment of clonidine-induced respiratory depression, hypotension, and/or coma; blood pressure should be monitored since the administration of naloxone has occasionally resulted in paradoxical hypertension. Tolazoline administration has yielded inconsistent results and is not recommended as first-line therapy. Dialysis is not likely to significantly enhance the elimination of clonidine.

The largest overdose reported to date involved a 28-year old white male who ingested 100 mg of clonidine hydrochloride powder. This patient developed hypertension followed by hypotension, bradycardia, apnea, hallucinations, semicoma, and premature ventricular contractions. The patient fully recovered after intensive treatment. Plasma clonidine levels were 60 ng/mL after 1 hour, 190 ng/mL after 1.5 hours, 370 ng/mL after 2 hours, and 120 ng/mL after 5.5 and 6.5 hours. In mice and rats, the oral LD50 of clonidine is 206 and 465 mg/kg, respectively.

DOSAGE AND ADMINISTRATION

The recommended starting dose of Duraclon for continuous epidural infusion is 30 mcg/hr. Although dosage may be titrated up or down depending on pain relief and occurrence of adverse events, experience with dosage rates above 40 mcg/hr is limited.

Familiarization with the continuous epidural infusion device is essential. Patients receiving epidural clonidine from a continuous infusion device should be closely monitored for the first few days to assess their response.

Renal Impairment: Dosage should be adjusted according to the degree of renal impairment, and patients should be carefully monitored. Since only a minimal amount of clonidine is removed during routine hemodialysis, there is no need to give supplemental clonidine following dialysis.

Duraclon must *not* be used with a preservative.

HOW SUPPLIED

Product No.	NDC No.
400110	0054-8233-01 Duraclon™ (clonidine hydrochloride injection) is supplied as 100 mcg/mL solution in 10 mL vials, packaged individually.

Store at controlled room temperature 15°–30°C (59°–86°F).

Preservative Free. Discard unused portion.

CAUTION: Federal law prohibits dispensing without prescription.

Manufactured for:
Roxane Laboratories, Inc.
By: Fujisawa USA, Inc.
Deerfield, IL 60015-2548
45632/Issued: September 1996
Roxane Laboratories, Inc.
Columbus, Ohio 43216

HYDROXYUREA CAPSULES USP ℞
500 mg

DESCRIPTION
Hydroxyurea Capsules USP is an antineoplastic agent, available for oral use as capsules containing 500 mg of hydroxyurea. Inactive ingredients: lactose monohydrate, dibasic sodium phosphate, magnesium stearate, citric acid, and gelatin capsules containing D&C Yellow No. 10, FD&C Blue No. 1, D&C Red No. 33, FD&C Red No. 40, gelatin, and titanium dioxide.
Hydroxyurea occurs as an essentially tasteless, white crystalline powder. Its chemical formula is $CH_4N_2O_2$ and it has a molecular weight of 76.05.

CLINICAL PHARMACOLOGY
Mechanism of Action:
The precise mechanism by which hydroxyurea produces its cytotoxic effects cannot, at present, be described. However, the reports of various studies in tissue culture in rats and man lend support to the hypothesis that hydroxyurea causes an immediate inhibition of DNA synthesis without interfering with the synthesis of ribonucleic acid or of protein. This hypothesis explains why, under certain conditions, hydroxyurea may induce teratogenic effects.
Three mechanisms of action have been postulated for the increased effectiveness of concomitant use of hydroxyurea therapy with irradiation on squamous cell (epidermoid) carcinomas of the head and neck. *In vitro* studies utilizing Chinese hamster cells suggest that hydroxyurea (1) is lethal to normally radioresistant S-stage cells, and (2) holds other cells of the cell cycle in the G1 or pre-DNA synthesis stage where they are most susceptible to the effects of irradiation. The third mechanism of action has been theorized on the basis of in vitro studies of HeLa cells: it appears that hydroxyurea, by inhibition of DNA synthesis, hinders the normal repair process of cells damaged but not killed by irradiation, thereby decreasing their survival rate; RNA and protein syntheses have shown no alteration.
Absorption, Metabolism, Fate and Excretion:
After oral administration in man, hydroxyurea is readily absorbed from the gastrointestinal tract. The drug reaches peak serum concentrations within 2 hours; by 24 hours the concentration in the serum is essentially zero. Approximately 80 percent of an oral or intravenous dose of 7 to 30 mg/kg may be recovered in the urine within 12 hours.
Animal Pharmacology and Toxicology:
The oral LD_{50} of hydroxyurea is 7330 mg/kg in mice and 5780 mg/kg in rats, given as a single dose.
In subacute and chronic toxicity studies in the rat, the most consistent pathological findings were an apparent dose-related mild to moderate bone marrow hypoplasia as well as pulmonary congestion and mottling of the lungs. At the highest dosage levels (1260 mg/kg/day for 37 days then 2520 mg/kg/day for 40 days), testicular atrophy with absence of spermatogenesis occurred; in several animals, hepatic cell damage with fatty metamorphosis was noted. In the dog, mild to marked bone marrow depression was a consistent finding except at the lower dosage levels. Additionally, at the higher dose levels (140 to 420 mg or 140 to 1260 mg/kg/week given 3 or 7 days weekly for 12 weeks), growth retardation, slightly increased blood glucose values, and hemosiderosis of the liver or spleen were found; reversible spermatogenic arrest was noted. In the monkey, bone marrow depression, lymphoid atrophy of the spleen, and degenerative changes in the epithelium of the small and large intestines were found. At the higher, often lethal, doses (400 to 800 mg/kg/day for 7 to 15 days), hemorrhage and congestion were found in the lungs, brain, and urinary tract. Cardiovascular effects (changes in heart rate, blood pressure, orthostatic hypotension, EKG changes) and hematological changes (slight hemolysis, slight methemoglobinemia) were observed in some species of laboratory animals at doses exceeding clinical levels.

INDICATIONS AND USAGE
Significant tumor response to hydroxyurea has been demonstrated in melanoma, resistant chronic myelocytic leukemia, and recurrent, metastatic, or inoperable carcinoma of the ovary.
Hydroxyurea used concomitantly with irradiation therapy is intended for use in the local control of primary squamous cell (epidermoid) carcinomas of the head and neck, excluding the lip.

CONTRAINDICATIONS
Hydroxyurea is contraindicated in patients with marked bone marrow depression, i.e., leukopenia (<2500 WBC) or thrombocytopenia (<100,000), or severe anemia.

WARNINGS
Treatment with hydroxyurea should not be initiated if bone marrow function is markedly depressed (see **CONTRAINDICATIONS**). Bone marrow suppression may occur, and leukopenia is generally its first and most common manifestation. Thrombocytopenia and anemia occur less often, and are seldom seen without a preceding leukopenia. However, the recovery from myelosuppression is rapid when therapy is interrupted. It should be borne in mind that bone marrow depression is more likely in patients who have previously received radiotherapy or cytotoxic cancer chemotherapeutic agents; hydroxyurea should be used cautiously in such patients.
Patients who have received irradiation therapy in the past may have an exacerbation of postirradiation erythema.
Severe anemia must be corrected with whole blood replacement before initiating therapy with hydroxyurea.
Erythrocytic abnormalities: megaloblastic erythropoiesis, which is self-limiting, is often seen early in the course of hydroxyurea therapy. The morphologic change resembles pernicious anemia, but is not related to vitamin B12 or folic acid deficiency. Hydroxyurea may also delay plasma iron clearance and reduce the rate of iron utilization by erythrocytes, but it does not appear to alter the red blood cell survival time.
Hydroxyurea should be used with caution in patients with marked renal dysfunction.
Elderly patients may be more sensitive to the effects of hydroxyurea, and may require a lower dose regimen.
Usage In Pregnancy:
Drugs which affect DNA synthesis, such as hydroxyurea, may be potential mutagenic agents. The physician should carefully consider this possibility before administering this drug to male or female patients who may contemplate conception.
Hydroxyurea is a known teratogenic agent in animals. Therefore, hydroxyurea should not be used in women who are or may become pregnant unless in the judgment of the physician the potential benefits outweigh the possible hazards.

PRECAUTIONS
Therapy with hydroxyurea requires close supervision. The complete status of the blood, including bone marrow examination, if indicated, as well as kidney function and liver function should be determined prior to, and repeatedly during, treatment. The determination of the hemoglobin level, total leukocyte counts, and platelet counts should be performed at least once a week throughout the course of hydroxyurea therapy. If the white blood cell count decreases to less than 2500/mm^3, or the platelet count to less than 100,000/mm^3, therapy should be interrupted until the values rise significantly toward normal levels. Anemia, if it occurs, should be managed with whole blood replacement, without interrupting hydroxyurea therapy.
Information for Patients:
Patients who take the drug by emptying the contents of the capsule into water (see **DOSAGE AND ADMINISTRATION**) should be reminded that this is a potent medication that must be handled with care. Patients must be cautioned not to allow the powder to come in contact with the skin or mucous membranes, and must be told not to inhale the powder when opening the capsules. If the powder is spilled, it should be immediately wiped up with a damp towel and disposed of, as should the empty capsules. The medication particularly open capsules, should be kept away from children and pets.

ADVERSE REACTIONS
Adverse reactions have been primarily bone marrow depression (leukopenia, anemia, and occasionally thrombocytopenia) and less frequently gastrointestinal symptoms (stomatitis, anorexia, nausea, vomiting, diarrhea, and constipation), and dermatological reactions such as maculopapular rash and facial erythema. Dysuria and alopecia occur very rarely. Large doses may produce moderate drowsiness. Neurological disturbances have occurred extremely rarely and were limited to headache, dizziness, disorientation, hallucinations, and convulsions. Hydroxyurea occasionally may cause temporary impairment of renal tubular function accompanied by elevations in serum uric acid, BUN, and creatinine levels. Abnormal BSP retention has been reported. Fever, chills, malaise, and elevation of hepatic enzymes have also been reported.
Adverse reactions observed with combined hydroxyurea and irradiation therapy are similar to those reported with the use of hydroxyurea alone. These effects primarily include bone marrow depression (anemia and leukopenia), and gastric irritation. Almost all patients receiving an adequate course of combined hydroxyurea and irradiation therapy will demonstrate concurrent leukopenia. Platelet depression (<100,000 cells/mm^3) has occurred rarely and only in the presence of marked leukopenia. Gastric distress has also been reported with irradiation alone and in combination with hydroxyurea therapy.
It should be borne in mind that therapeutic doses of irradiation alone produce the same adverse reactions as hydroxyurea; combined therapy may cause an increase in the incidence and severity of these side effects.
Although inflammation of the mucous membranes at the irradiated site (mucositis) is attributed to irradiation alone, some investigators believe that the more sever cases are due to combination therapy.
The association of hydroxyurea with the with the development of acute pulmonary reactions consisting of diffuse pulmonary infiltrates, fever and dyspnea has been rarely reported.

DOSAGE AND ADMINISTRATION
Because of the rarity of melanoma, resistant chronic myelocytic leukemia, carcinoma of the ovary, and carcinomas of the head and neck in children, dosage regimens have not been established.
All dosage should be based on the patient's actual or ideal weight, whichever is less.
NOTE: If the patient prefers, or is unable to swallow capsules, the contents of the capsules may be emptied into a glass of water and taken immediately. Some inert material used as a vehicle in the capsules may not dissolve, and may float on the surface.

SOLID TUMORS
Intermittent Therapy
80 mg/kg administered orally as a *single* dose every *third* day
Continuous Therapy
20 to 30 mg/kg administered orally as a *single* dose *daily*
The intermittent dosage schedule offers the advantage of reduced toxicity since patients on this dosage regimen have rarely required complete discontinuance of therapy because of toxicity.
Concomitant Therapy with Irradiation
(Carcinoma of the head and neck)
80 mg/kg administered orally as a *single* dose every *third* day
Administration of hydroxyurea should be begun at least seven days before initiation of irradiation and continued during radiotherapy as well as indefinitely afterwards provided that the patient may be kept under adequate observation and evidences no unusual or severe reactions.
Irradiation should be given at the maximum dose considered appropriate for the particular therapeutic situation; adjustment of irradiation dosage is not usually necessary when hydroxyurea is used concomitantly.

RESISTANT CHRONIC MYELOCYTIC LEUKEMIA
Until the intermittent therapy regimen has been evaluated: CONTINUOUS therapy (20 to 30 mg/kg administered orally as a *single* dose *daily*) is recommended.
An adequate trial period for determining the antineoplastic effectiveness of hydroxyurea is six weeks of therapy. When there is regression in tumor size or arrest in tumor growth, therapy should be continued indefinitely. Therapy should be interrupted if the white blood cell count drops below 2500/mm^3, or the platelet count below 100,000/mm^3. In these cases, the counts should be rechecked after three days and therapy resumed when the counts rise significantly toward normal values. Since the hematopoietic rebound is prompt, it is usually necessary to omit only a few doses. If prompt rebound has not occurred during combined hydroxyurea and irradiation therapy, irradiation may also be interrupted. However, the need for postponement of irradiation has been rare; radiotherapy has usually been continued using the recommended dosage and technique. Anemia, if it occurs, should be corrected with whole blood replacement, without interrupting hydroxyurea therapy. Because hematopoiesis may be compromised by extensive irradiation or by other antineoplastic agents, it is recommended that hydroxyurea be administered cautiously to patients who have recently received extensive radiation therapy or chemotherapy with other cytotoxic drugs.
Pain or discomfort from inflammation of the mucous membranes at the irradiated site (mucositis) is usually controlled by measures such as topical anesthetics and orally administered analgesics. If the reaction is severe, hydroxyurea therapy may be temporarily interrupted; if it is extremely severe, irradiation dosage may, in addition, be temporarily postponed. However, it has rarely been necessary to terminate these therapies.
Severe gastric distress, such as nausea, vomiting, and anorexia, resulting from combined therapy may usually be controlled by temporary interruption of hydroxyurea administration; rarely has the additional interruption of irradiation been necessary.
Procedures for proper handling and disposal of antineoplastic drugs should be considered. Several guidelines on this subject have been published.[1–7] there is no general agreement that all of the procedures recommended in the guidelines are necessary or appropriate.

HOW SUPPLIED
500 mg dark green/flesh opaque capsules
(Capsules Identified: 54 072)
NDC 0054-8247-25: Unit dose, 10 capsules per strip, 10 strips per shelf pack, 10 shelf packs per shipper.
NDC 0054-2247-25: Bottles of 100 capsules.

Continued on next page

Hydroxyurea—Cont.

Store at controlled Room Temperature 15°-30°C (59°-86°F). Avoid excessive heat.
Keep tightly closed.
Caution: Federal law prohibits dispensing without prescription.
4054290 Revised August 1997
087
© RLI, 1997

REFERENCES

1. Recommendations for the safe handling of parenteral antineoplastic drugs. NIH Publication No. 83-2621. Available from Superintendent of Documents, US Government Printing Office, Washington, DC, 20402.
2. AMA Council Report: Guidelines for handling parenteral antineoplastics. JAMA 253:1590-1592, 1985.
3. National Study Commission on Cytotoxic Exposure-Recommendations for Handling Cytotoxic Agents. Available from Louis P Jeffrey, ScD, Chairman, National Study Commission on Cytotoxic Exposure, Massachusetts College of Pharmacy and Allied Health Science, 179 Longwood Ave., Boston, Massachusetts, 02115.
4. Clinical Oncological Society of Australia: Guidelines and recommendations for safe handling of antineoplastic agents. Med J Australia 1:426–428, 1983.
5. Jones RB, et al: Safe handling of chemotherapeutic agents: a report from the Mount Sinai Medical Center. Ca: A Cancer J for Clinicians 133:258-263, 1983.
6. American Society of Hospital Pharmacists Technical Assistance Bulletin on Handling Cytotoxic and Hazardous Drugs. Am J Hosp Pharm 1990; 47:1033-1049.
7. OSHA Work-Practice Guidelines for Personnel Dealing with Cytotoxic (Antineoplastic) Drugs, Am J Hosp Pharm 1986; 43:1193-1204.

IPRATROPIUM BROMIDE INHALATION SOLUTION, 0.02% ℞

Prescribing Information

DESCRIPTION

The active ingredient, ipratropium bromide monohydrate, is an anticholinergic bronchodilator chemically described as 8-azoniabicyclo [3.2.1]-octane, 3-(3-hydroxy-1-oxo-2-phenylpropoxy)-8-methyl-8-(1-methylethyl)-, bromide, monohydrate (*endo, syn*)-, (±)-; a synthetic quarternary ammonium compound, chemically related to atropine.

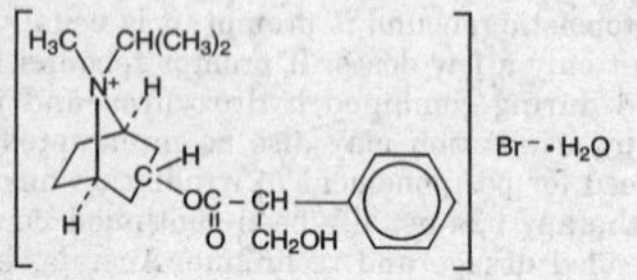

Ipratropium Bromide $C_{20}H_{30}BrNO_3{\cdot}H_2O$ Mol. Wt. 430.4

Ipratropium bromide is a white crystalline substance, freely soluble in water and lower alcohols. It is a quarternary ammonium compound and thus exists in an ionized state in aqueous solutions. It is relatively insoluble in non-polar media.

Ipratropium Bromide Inhalation Solution is administered by oral inhalation with the aid of a nebulizer. It contains ipratropium bromide 0.02% (anhydrous basis) in a sterile, preservative-free, isotonic saline solution, pH-adjusted to 3.4 (3 to 4) with hydrochloric acid.

HOW SUPPLIED

Ipratropium Bromide Inhalation Solution Unit-Dose Vial is supplied as a 0.02% clear, colorless solution containing 2.5 mL.
NDC 0054-8402-11 25 vials in a single foil pouch
NDC 0054-8402-13 30 vials in a single foil pouch
NDC 0054-8402-21 60 vials (two foil pouches 30 vials per pouch)
Each vial is made from a low-density polyethylene (LDPE) resin.
Store between 59°F (15°C) and 86°F (30°C).
Protect from light.
Store unused vials in the foli pouch.
ATTENTION PHARMACIST: Detach "Patient's Instructions for Use" from Package Insert and dispense with solution.
Caution: Federal law prohibits dispensing without prescription.

Licensed from Boehringer Ingelheim International GmbH
Manufactured by
Roxane Laboratories, Inc., Columbus OH 43228
Distributed by
Roxane Laoratories, Inc.
Columbus, Ohio 43216
4054320 Revised October 1997
107
©RLI, 1997

LITHIUM CARBONATE ℞

CAPSULES USP 150 mg, 300 mg, and 600 mg
TABLETS USP 300 mg

> **WARNING**
> **Lithium toxicity is closely related to serum lithium levels, and can occur at doses close to therapeutic levels. Facilities for prompt and accurate serum lithium determinations should be available before initiating therapy.**

DESCRIPTION

Each tablet for oral administration contains:
Lithium Carbonate .... 300 mg
Each capsule for oral administration contains:
Lithium Carbonate .... 150 mg, 300 mg, or 600 mg
Inactive Ingredients:
The capsules contain talc, gelatin, FD&C Red No. 40, titanium dioxide, and the imprinting ink contains FD&C Blue No. 2, FD&C Yellow No. 6, FD&C Red No. 40, synthetic black iron oxide, and pharmaceutical glaze. The tablets contain calcium stearate, microcrystalline cellulose, povidone, sodium lauryl sulfate, and sodium starch glycolate.
Lithium Carbonate is a white, light alkaline powder with molecular formula Li_2CO_3 and molecular weight 73.89. Lithium is an element of the alkali-metal group with atomic number 3, atomic weight 6.94 and an emission line at 671 nm on the flame photometer. Lithium acts as an antimanic.

CLINICAL PHARMACOLOGY

Preclinical studies have shown that lithium alters sodium transport in nerve and muscle cells and effects a shift toward intraneuronal metabolism of catecholamines, but the specific biochemical mechanism of lithium action in mania is unknown.

INDICATIONS AND USAGE

Lithium carbonate is indicated in the treatment of manic episodes of Bipolar Disorder. Bipolar Disorder, Manic (DSM-III) is equivalent to Manic Depressive illness, Manic, in the older DSM-II terminology.
Lithium is also indicated as a maintenance treatment for individuals with a diagnosis of Bipolar Disorder. Maintenance therapy reduces the frequency of manic episodes and diminishes the intensity of those episodes which may occur. Typical symptoms of mania include pressure of speech, motor hyperactivity, reduced need for sleep, flight of ideas, grandiosity, or poor judgment, aggressiveness, and possibly hostility. When given to a patient experiencing a manic episode, lithium may produce a normalization of symptomatology within 1 to 3 weeks.

CONTRAINDICATIONS

Lithium should generally not be given to patients with significant renal or cardiovascular disease, severe debilitation or dehydration, or sodium depletion, and to patients receiving diuretics, since the risk of lithium toxicity is very high in such patients. If the psychiatric indication is life-threatening, and if such a patient fails to respond to other measures, lithium treatment may be undertaken with extreme caution, including daily serum lithium determinations and adjustment to the usually low doses ordinarily tolerated by these individuals. In such instances, hospitalization is a necessity.

WARNINGS

Lithium may cause fetal harm when administered to a pregnant woman. There have been reports of lithium having adverse effects on nidation in rats, embryo viability in mice, and metabolism in-vitro of rat testis and human spermatozoa have been attributed to lithium, as have teratogenicity in submammalian species and cleft palates in mice. Studies in rats, rabbits and monkeys have shown no evidence of lithium-induced teratology. Data from lithium birth registries suggest an increase in cardiac and other anomalies, especially Ebstein's anomaly. If the patient becomes pregnant while taking lithium, she should be apprised of the potential risk to the fetus. If possible, lithium should be withdrawn for at least the first trimester unless it is determined that this would seriously endanger the mother.
Chronic lithium therapy may be associated with diminution of renal concentrating ability, occasionally presenting as nephrogenic diabetes insipidus, with polyuria and polydipsia. Such patients should be carefully managed to avoid dehydration with resulting lithium retention and toxicity. This condition is usually reversible when lithium is discontinued. Morphologic changes with glomerular and interstitial fibrosis and nephron-atrophy have been reported in patients on chronic lithium therapy. Morphologic changes have been seen in bipolar patients never exposed to lithium. The relationship between renal functional and morphologic changes and their association with lithium therapy has not been established. To date, lithium in therapeutic doses has not been reported to cause end-stage renal disease.
When kidney function is assessed, for baseline data prior to starting lithium therapy or thereafter, routine urinalysis and other tests may be used to evaluate tubular function (e.g., urine specific gravity or osmolality following a period of water deprivation, or 24-hour urine volume) and glomerular function (e.g., serum creatinine or creatinine clearance). During lithium therapy, progressive or sudden changes in renal function, even within the normal range, indicate the need for reevaluation of treatment.
Lithium toxicity is closely related to serum lithium levels, and can occur at doses close to therapeutic levels (see DOSAGE AND ADMINISTRATION).

PRECAUTIONS

General: The ability to tolerate lithium is greater during the acute manic phase and decreases when manic symptoms subside (See DOSAGE AND ADMINISTRATION).
The distribution space of lithium approximates that of total body water. Lithium is primarily excreted in urine with insignificant excretion in feces. Renal excretion of lithium is proportional to its plasma concentration. The half-life of elimination of lithium is approximately 24 hours. Lithium decreases sodium reabsorption by the renal tubules which could lead to sodium depletion. Therefore, it is essential for the patient to maintain a normal diet, including salt, and an adequate fluid intake (2500-3000 mL) at least during the initial stabilization period. Decreased tolerance to lithium has been reported to ensue from protracted sweating or diarrhea and, if such occur, supplemental fluid and salt should be administered.
In addition to sweating and diarrhea, concomitant infection with elevated temperatures may also necessitate a temporary reduction or cessation of medication.
Previously existing underlying thyroid disorders do not necessarily constitute a contraindication to lithium treatment; where hypothyroidism exists, careful monitoring of thyroid function during lithium stabilization and maintenance allows for correction of changing thyroid parameters, if any. Where hypothyroidism occurs during lithium stabilization and maintenance, supplemental thyroid treatment may be used.
Information for the patients: Outpatients and their families should be warned that the patient must discontinue lithium therapy and contact his physician if such clinical signs of lithium toxicity as diarrhea, vomiting, tremor, mild ataxia, drowsiness, or muscular weakness occur.
Lithium may impair mental and/or physical abilities. Caution patients about activities requiring alertness (e.g., operating vehicles or machinery).
Drug interactions: Combined use of haloperidol and lithium: An encephalopathic syndrome (characterized by weakness, lethargy, fever, tremulousness and confusion, extrapyramidal symptoms, leucocytosis, elevated serum enzymes, BUN and FBS) followed by irreversible brain damage has occurred in a few patients treated with lithium plus haloperidol. A causal relationship between these events and the concomitant administration of lithium and haloperidol has not been established; however, patients receiving such combined therapy should be monitored closely for early evidence of neurological toxicity and treatment discontinued promptly if such signs appear.
The possibility of similar adverse interactions with other antipsychotic medication exists.
Lithium may prolong the effects of neuromuscular blocking agents. Therefore, neuromuscular blocking agents should be given with caution to patients receiving lithium.
Indomethacin and piroxicam have been reported to increase significantly steady state plasma lithium levels. In some cases lithium toxicity has resulted from such interactions. There is also evidence that other non-steroidal, anti-inflammatory agents may have a similar effect. When such combinations are used, increased plasma lithium level monitoring is recommended.
Caution should be used when lithium and diuretics or angiotensin converting enzyme (ACE) inhibitors are used concomitantly because sodium loss may reduce the renal clearance of lithium and increase serum lithium levels with risk of lithium toxicity. When such combinations are used, the lithium dosage may need to be decreased, and more frequent monitoring of lithium plasma levels is recommended.
Pregnancy: Teratogenic effects—Pregnancy Category D, See "Warnings" section.
Nursing mothers: Lithium is excreted in human milk. Nursing should not be undertaken during lithium therapy except in rare and unusual circumstances where, in the view of the physician, the potential benefits to the mother outweigh possible hazards to the child.

Usage in Children: Since information regarding the safety and effectiveness of lithium in children under 12 years of age is not available, its use in such patients is not recommended at this time. There has been a report of a transient syndrome of acute dystonia and hyperreflexia occurring in a 15 kg child who ingested 300 mg lithium carbonate.

ADVERSE REACTIONS

Lithium toxicity: The likelihood of toxicity increases with increasing serum lithium levels. Serum lithium levels greater than 1.5 mEq/l carry a greater risk than lower levels. However, patients sensitive to lithium may exhibit toxic signs at serum levels below 1.5 mEq/l.

Diarrhea, vomiting, drowsiness, muscular weakness and lack of coordination may be early signs of lithium toxicity, and can occur at lithium levels below 2.0 mEq/l. At higher levels, giddiness, ataxia, blurred vision, tinnitus and a large output of dilute urine may be seen. Serum lithium levels above 3.0 mEq/l may produce a complex clinical picture involving multiple organs and organ systems. Serum lithium levels should not be permitted to exceed 2.0 mEq/l during the acute treatment phase.

Fine hand tremor, polyuria and mild thirst may occur during initial therapy for the acute manic phase, and may persist throughout treatment. Transient and mild nausea and general discomfort may also appear during the first few days of lithium administration.

These side effects are an inconvenience rather than a disabling condition, and usually subside with continued treatment or a temporary reduction or cessation of dosage. If persistent, a cessation of dosage is indicated.

The following adverse reactions have been reported and do not appear to be directly related to serum lithium levels.

Neuromuscular: tremor, muscle hyperirritability (fasciculations, twitching, clonic movements of whole limbs), ataxia, choreo-athetotic movements, hyperactive deep tendon reflexes.

Central Nervous System: Blackout spells, epileptiform seizures, slurred speech, dizziness, vertigo, incontinence of urine or feces, somnolence, psychomotor retardation, restlessness, confusion, stupor, coma, acute dystonia, downbeat nystagmus.

Cardiovascular: cardiac arrhythmia, hypotension, peripheral circulatory collapse, sinus node dysfunction with severe bradycardia (which may result in syncope).

Neurological: Cases of pseudotumor cerebri (increased intracranial pressure and papilledema) have been reported with lithium use. If undetected, this condition may result in enlargement of the blind spot, constriction of visual fields and eventual blindness due to optic atrophy. Lithium should be discontinued, if clinically possible, if this syndrome occurs.

Gastrointestinal: anorexia, nausea, vomiting, diarrhea.

Genitourinary: albuminuria, oliguria, polyuria, glycosuria.

Dermatologic: drying and thinning of hair, anesthesia of skin, chronic folliculitis, xerosis cutis, alopecia and exacerbation of psoriasis.

Autonomic Nervous System: blurred vision, dry mouth.

Thyroid Abnormalities: euthyroid goiter and/or hypothyroidism (including myxedema) accompanied by lower T_3 and T_4. Iodine 131 uptake may be elevated. (See PRECAUTIONS). Paradoxically, rare cases of hyperthyroidism have been reported.

EEG Changes: diffuse slowing, widening of frequency spectrum, potentiation and disorganization of background rhythm.

EKG Changes: reversible flattening, isoelectricity or inversion of T-waves.

Miscellaneous: fatigue, lethargy, transient scotomata, dehydration, weight loss, tendency to sleep.

Miscellaneous reactions unrelated to dosage are: transient electroencephalographic and electrocardiographic changes, leucocytosis, headache, diffuse nontoxic goiter with or without hypothyroidism, transient hyperglycemia, generalized pruritis with or without rash, cutaneous ulcers, albuminuria, worsening of organic brain syndromes, excessive weight gain, edematous swelling of ankles or wrists, and thirst or polyuria, sometimes resembling diabetes insipidus, and metallic taste.

A single report has been received of the development of painful discoloration of fingers and toes and coldness of the extremities within one day of the starting of treatment of lithium. The mechanism through which these symptoms (resembling Raynaud's Syndrome) developed is not known. Recovery followed discontinuance.

OVERDOSAGE

The toxic levels for lithium are close to the therapeutic levels. It is therefore important that patients and their families be cautioned to watch for early symptoms and to discontinue the drug and inform the physician should they occur. Toxic symptoms are listed in detail under ADVERSE REACTIONS.

Treatment: No specific antidote for lithium poisoning is known. Early symptoms of lithium toxicity can usually be treated by reduction or cessation of dosage of the drug and resumption of the treatment at a lower dose after 24 to 48 hours. In severe cases of lithium poisoning, the first and foremost goal of treatment consists of elimination of this ion from the patient.

Treatment is essentially the same as that used in barbiturate poisoning: 1) gastric lavage, 2) correction of fluid and electrolyte imbalance and 3) regulation of kidney functioning. Urea, mannitol, and aminophylline all produce significant increases in lithium excretion. Hemodialysis is an effective and rapid means of removing the ion from the severely toxic patient. Infection prophylaxis, regular chest X-rays, and preservation of adequate respiration are essential.

DOSAGE AND ADMINISTRATION

Acute Mania: Optimal patient response to Lithium Carbonate usually can be established and maintained with 600 mg t.i.d. Such doses will normally produce an effective serum lithium level ranging between 1.0 and 1.5 mEq/l. Dosage must be individualized according to serum levels and clinical response. Regular monitoring of the patient's clinical state and of serum lithium levels is necessary. Serum levels should be determined twice per week during the acute phase, and until the serum level and clinical condition of the patient have been stabilized.

Long-term Control: The desirable serum lithium levels are 0.6 to 1.2 mEq/l. Dosage will vary from one individual to another, but usually 300 mg t.i.d. or q.i.d. will maintain this level. Serum lithium levels in uncomplicated cases receiving maintenance therapy during remission should be monitored at least every two months.

Patients abnormally sensitive to lithium may exhibit toxic signs at serum levels of 1.0 to 1.5 mEq/l. Elderly patients often respond to reduced dosage, and may exhibit signs of toxicity at serum levels ordinarily tolerated by other patients.

N.B.: Blood samples for serum lithium determination should be drawn immediately prior to the next dose when lithium concentrations are relatively stable (i.e., 8–12 hours after the previous dose.) Total reliance must not be placed on serum levels alone. Accurate patient evaluation requires both clinical and laboratory analysis.

HOW SUPPLIED

Lithium Carbonate Tablets USP

300 mg white, scored tablets (Identified 54 452)

NDC 0054-8528-25: Unit dose, 10 tablets per strip, 10 strips per shelf pack, 10 shelf packs per shipper.
(For Institutional Use Only).
NDC 0054-4527-25: Bottles of 100 tablets.
NDC 0054-4527-31: Bottles of 1000 tablets.

Lithium Carbonate Capsules USP

150 mg white opaque colored capsules (size 4) (Identified 54 213).

NDC 0054-8526-25: Unit dose, 10 capsules per strip, 10 strips per shelf pack, 10 shelf packs per shipper.
(For Institutional Use Only).
NDC 0054-2526-25: Bottles of 100 capsules.

300 mg flesh-colored capsules (size 2) (Identified 54 463).

NDC 0054-8527-25: Unit dose, 10 capsules per strip, 10 strips per shelf pack, 10 shelf packs per shipper.
(For Institutional Use Only).
NDC 0054-2527-25: Bottles of 100 capsules.
NDC 0054-2527-31: Bottles of 1000 capsules.

600 mg white opaque/flesh colored capsules (size 0) (Identified 54 702).

NDC 0054-8531-25: Unit dose, 10 capsules per strip, 10 strips per shelf pack, 10 shelf packs per shipper.
(For Institutional Use Only.)
NDC 0054-2531-25: Bottles of 100 capsules.
NDC 0054-2531-31: Bottles of 1000 capsules.

Caution: Federal law prohibits dispensing without prescription.

4055500
084 Revised August 1994

LITHIUM CITRATE SYRUP USP ℞

8 mEq of Lithium per 5 mL, 16mEq of Lithium per 10 mL
SUGAR FREE
FOR ORAL ADMINISTRATION ONLY

DESCRIPTION

Lithium Citrate Syrup is a palatable oral dosage form of lithium ion. Lithium citrate is prepared in solution from lithium hydroxide and citric acid in a ratio approximating di-lithium citrate:

Each 5 mL of Lithium Citrate Syrup contains 8 mEq of lithium ion (Li+), equivalent to the amount of lithium in 300 mg of lithium carbonate and alcohol 0.3% v/v.

Inactive ingredients:

The syrup contains alcohol, sorbitol, flavoring, water, and other ingredients.

Lithium is an element of the alkali-metal group with atomic number 3, atomic weight 6.94, and an emission line at 671 nm on the flame photometer.

HOW SUPPLIED

Lithium Citrate Syrup, 8 mEq per 5 mL

NDC 0054-8529-04: Unit dose Patient Cup™ filled to deliver 5 mL, ten 5 mL Patient Cups™ per shelf pack, ten shelf packs per shipper. (For Institutional Use Only).
NDC 0054-3527-63: Bottles of 500 mL.

Lithium Citrate Syrup, 16 mEq per 10 mL

NDC 0054-8530-04: Unit dose Patient Cup™ filled to deliver 10 mL, ten 10 mL Patient Cups™ per shelf pack, ten shelf packs per shipper. (For Institutional Use Only).

Refer to Lithium Carbonate Capsules and Tablets heading for complete text.

MARINOL® Ⓒ ℞

(dronabinol)
Capsules

Dronabinol is a cannabinoid designated chemically as (6a*R*-*trans*)-6a,7,8,10a-tetrahydro-6,6,9-trimethyl-3-pentyl-6*H*-dibenzo[*b,d*]pyran-1-ol. Dronabinol has the following empirical and structural formula:

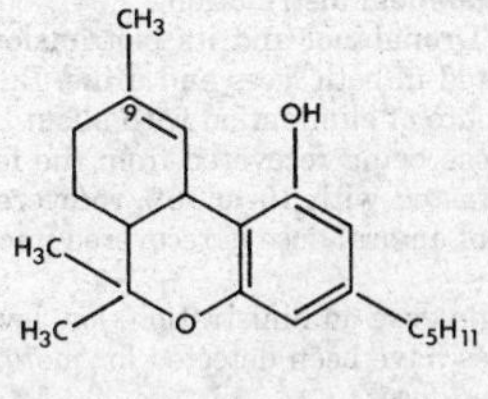

$C_{21}H_{30}O_2$ (molecular weight = 314.47)

Dronabinol, delta-9-tetrahydrocannabinol (delta-9-THC), is naturally-occurring and has been extracted from *Cannabis sativa* L. (marijuana).

Dronabinol is also chemically synthesized and is a light-yellow resinous oil that is sticky at room temperature and hardens upon refrigeration. Dronabinol is insoluble in water and is formulated in sesame oil. It has a pK_a of 10.6 and an octanol-water partition coefficient: 6,000:1 at pH 7.

Capsules for oral administration: Marinol is supplied as round, soft gelatin capsules containing either 2.5 mg, 5 mg, or 10 mg dronabinol. Each Marinol capsule is formulated with the following inactive ingredients: sesame oil, gelatin, glycerin, methylparaben, propylparaben, FD&C Yellow No. 6 (5 mg and 10 mg), and titanium dioxide.

CLINICAL PHARMACOLOGY

Dronabinol is an orally active cannabinoid which, like other cannabinoids, has complex effects on the central nervous system (CNS), including central sympathomimetic activity. Cannabinoid receptors have been discovered in neural tissues. These receptors may play a role in mediating the effects of dronabinol and other cannabinoids.

Pharmacodynamics: Dronabinol-induced sympathomimetic activity may result in tachycardia and/or conjunctival injection. Its effects on blood pressure are inconsistent, but occasional subjects have experienced orthostatic hypotension and/or syncope upon abrupt standing.

Dronabinol also demonstrates reversible effects on appetite, mood, cognition, memory, and perception. These phenomena appear to be dose-related, increasing in frequency with higher dosages, and subject to great interpatient variability.

After oral administration, dronabinol has an onset of action of approximately 0.5 to 1 hours and peak effect at 2 to 4 hours. Duration of action of psychoactive effects is 4 to 6 hours, but the appetite stimulant effect of dronabinol may continue for 24 hours or longer after administration.

Tachyphylaxis and tolerance develop to some of the pharmacologic effects of dronabinol and other cannabinoids with chronic use, suggesting an indirect effect on sympathetic neurons. In a study of the pharacodynamics of chronic dronabinol exposure, healthy male volunteers (N = 12) received 210 mg/day dronabinol, administered orally in divided doses, for 16 days. An initial tachycardia induced by dronabinol was replaced successively by normal sinus rhythm and then bradycardia. A decrease in supine blood pressure, made worse by standing, was also observed initially. These volunteers developed tolerance to the cardiovascular and subjective adverse CNS effects of dronabinol within 12 days of treatment initiation.

Tachyphylaxis and tolerance do not, however, appear to develop to the appetite stimulant effect of Marinol. In studies involving patients with Aquired Immune Deficiency Syndrome (AIDS), the appetite stimulant effect of Marinol has been sustained for up to five months in clinical trials, at dosages ranging from 2.5 mg/day to 20 mg/day.

Pharmacokinetics:

Absorption and Distribution: Marinol (dronabinol) is almost completely absorbed (90 to 95%) after single oral doses. Due to the combined effects of first pass hepatic me-

Continued on next page

Marinol—Cont.

tabolism and high lipid solubility, only 10 to 20% of the administered dose reaches the systemic circulation. Dronabinol has a large apparent volume of distribution, approximately 10 L/kg, because of its lipid solubility. The plasma protein binding of dronabinol and its metabolites is approximately 97%.

The elimination phase of dronabinol can be described using a two compartment model with an initial (alpha) half-life of about 4 hours and a terminal (beta) half-life of 25 to 36 hours. Because of its large volume of distribution, dronabinol and its metabolites may be excreted at low levels for prolonged periods of time.

Metabolism: Dronabinol undergoes extensive first-pass hepatic metabolism, primarily by microsomal hydroxylation, yielding both active and inactive metabolites. Dronabinol and its principal active metabolite, 11-OH-delta-9-THC, are present in approximately equal concentrations in plasma. Concentrations of both parent drug and metabolite peak at approximately 2 to 4 hours after oral dosing and decline over several days. Values for clearance average about 0.2 L/kg-hr, but are highly variable due to the complexity of cannabinoid distribution.

Elimination: Dronabinol and its biotransformation products are excreted in both feces and urine. Biliary excretion is the major route of elimination with about half of a radiolabeled oral dose being recovered from the feces within 72 hours as contrasted with 10 to 15% recovered from urine. Less than 5% of an oral dose is recovered unchanged in the feces.

Following single dose administration, low levels of dronabinol metabolites have been detected for more than 5 weeks in the urine and feces.

In a study of Marinol involving AIDS patients, urinary cannabinoid/creatinine concentration ratios were studied biweekly over a six week period. The urinary cannabinoid/creatinine ratio was closely correlated with dose. No increase in the cannabinoid/creatinine ratio was observed after the first two weeks of treatment, indicating that steady-state cannabinoid levels had been reached. This conclusion is consistent with predictions based on the observed terminal half-life of dronabinol.

Special Populations: The pharmacokinetic profile of Marinol has not been investigated in either pediatric or geriatric patients.

CLINICAL TRIALS

Appetite Stimulation: The appetite stimulant effect of Marinol (dronabinol) in the treatment of AIDS-related anorexia associated with weight loss was studied in a randomized, double-blind, placebo-controlled study involving 139 patients. The initial dosage of Marinol in all patients was 5 mg/day, administered in doses of 2.5 mg one hour before lunch and one hour before supper. In pilot studies, early morning administration of Marinol appeared to have been associated with an increased frequency of adverse experiences, as compared to dosing later in the day. The effect of Marinol on appetite, weight, mood, and nausea was measured at scheduled intervals during the six-week treatment period. Side effects (feeling high, dizziness, confusion, somnolence) occurred in 13 ot 72 patients (18%) at this dosage level and the dosage was reduced to 2.5 mg/day, administered as a single dose at supper or bedtime.

As compared to placebo, Marinol treatment resulted in a statistically significant improvement in appetite as measured by visual analog scale (see figure). Trends toward improved body weight and mood, and decreases in nausea were also seen.

After completing the 6-week study, patients were allowed to continue treatment with Marinol in an open-label study, in which there was a sustained improvement in appetite. [See figure at top of next column]

Antiemetic: Marinol (dronabinol) treatment of chemotherapy-induced emesis was evaluated in 454 patients with cancer, who received a total of 750 courses of treatment of various malignancies. The antiemetic efficacy of Marinol was greatest in patients receiving cytotoxic therapy with MOPP for Hodgkin's and non-Hodgkin's lymphomas. Marinol dosages ranged from 2.5 mg/day to 40 mg/day, administered in equally divided doses every four to six hours (four times daily). As indicated in the following table, escalating the Marinol dose about 7 mg/m² increased the frequency of adverse experiences, with no additional antiemetic benefit. [See table below]

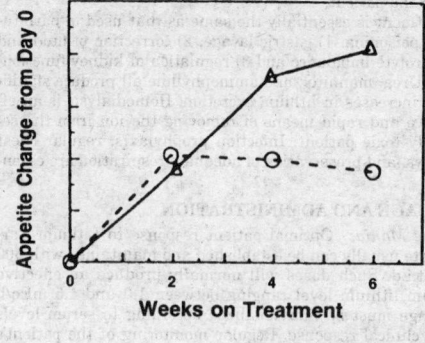

Appetite Change from Baseline

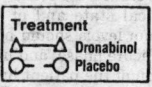

Treatment
△ — △ Dronabinol
○ — ○ Placebo

Combination antiemetic therapy with Marinol and a phenothiazine (prochlorperazine) may result in synergistic or additive antiemetic effects and attenuate the toxicities associated with each of the agents.

INDIVIDUALIZATION OF DOSAGES

The pharmacologic effects of Marinol (dronabinol) are dose-related and subject to considerable interpatient variability. Therefore, dosage individualization is critical in achieving the maximum benefit of Marinol treatment.

Appetite Stimulation: In the clinical trials, the majority of patients were treated with 5 mg/day Marinol, although the dosages ranged from 2.5 to 20 mg/day. For an adult:

1. Begin with 2.5 mg before lunch and 2.5 mg before supper. If CNS symptoms (feeling high, dizziness, confusion, somnolence) do occur, they usually resolve in 1 to 3 days with continued dosage.

2. If CNS symptoms are severe or persistent, reduce the dose to 2.5 mg before supper. If symptoms continue to be a problem, taking the single dose in the evening or at bedtime may reduce their severity.

3. When adverse effects are absent or minimal and further therapeutic effect is desired, increase the dose to 2.5 mg before lunch and 5 mg before supper or 5 and 5 mg. Although most patients respond to 2.5 mg twice daily, 10 mg twice daily has been tolerated in about half of the patients in appetite stimulation studies.

The pharmacologic effects of Marinol are reversible upon treatment cessation.

Antiemetic: Most patients respond to 5 mg three or four times daily. Dosage may be escalated during a chemotherapy cycle or at subsequent cycles, based upon initial results. Therapy should be initiated at the lowest recommended dosage and titrated to clinical response. Administration of Marinol with phenothiazines, such as prochlorperazine, has resulted in improved efficacy as compared to either drug alone, without additional toxicity.

Pediatrics: Marinol is not recommended for AIDS-related anorexia in pediatric patients because it has not been studied in this population. The pediatric dosage for the treatment of chemotherapy-induced emesis is the same as in adults. Caution is recommended in prescribing Marinol for children because of the psychoactive effects.

Geriatrics: Caution is advised in prescribing Marinol in elderly patients because they are generally more sensitive to the psychoactive effects of drugs. In antiemetic studies, no difference in tolerance or efficacy was apparent in patients >55 years old.

INDICATIONS AND USAGE

Marinol (dronabinol) is indicated for the treatment of:

1. anorexia associated with weight loss in patients with AIDS; and

2. nausea and vomiting associated with cancer chemotherapy in patients who have failed to respond adequately to conventional antiemetic treatments.

CONTRAINDICATIONS

Marinol (dronabinol) is contraindicated in any patient who has a history of hypersensitivity to any cannabinoid or sesame oil.

WARNINGS

Marinol (dronabinol) is a medication with a potential for abuse. Physcians and pharmacies should use the same care in prescribing and accounting for Marinol as they would with morphine or other drugs controlled under Schedule II (CII) of the Controlled Substances Act. Because of the risk of diversion, it is recommended that prescriptions be limited to the amount necessary for the period between clinic visits. Patients receiving treatment with Marinol should be specifically warned not to drive, operate machinery, or engage in any hazardous activity until it is established that they are able to tolerate the drug and to perform such tasks safely.

PRECAUTIONS

General: The risk/benefit ratio of Marinol (dronabinol) use should be carefully evaluated in patients with the following medical conditions because of individual variation in response and tolerance to the effects of Marinol.

Marinol should be used with caution in patients with cardiac disorders because of occasional hypotension, possible hypertension, syncope, or tachycardia (see CLINICAL PHARMACOLOGY).

Marinol should be used with caution in patients with a history of substance abuse, including alcohol abuse or dependence, because they may be more prone to abuse Marinol as well. Multiple substance abuse is common and marijuana, which contains the same active compound, is a frequently abused substance.

Marinol should be used with caution and careful psychiatric monitoring in patients with mania, depression, or schizophrenia because Marinol may exacerbate these illnesses.

Marinol should be used with caution in patients receiving concomitant therapy with sedatives, hypnotics or other psychoactive drugs because of the potential for additive or synergistic CNS effects.

Marinol should be used with caution in pregnant patients, nursing mothers, or pediatric patients because it has not been studied in these patient populations.

Marinol should be used with caution for treatment of anorexia and weight loss in elderly patients with AIDS because they may be more sensitive to the psychoactive effects and because its use in these patients has not been studied.

Information for Patients: Patients receiving treatment with Marinol (dronabinol) should be alerted to the potential for additive central nervous system depression if Marinol is used concomitantly with alcohol or other CNS depressants such as benzodiazepines and barbiturates.

Patients receiving treatment with Marinol should be specifically warned not to drive, operate machinery, or engage in any hazardous activity until it is established that they are able to tolerate the drug and to perform such tasks safely. Patients using Marinol should be advised of possible changes in mood and other adverse behavioral effects of the drug so as to avoid panic in the event of such manifestations. Patients should remain under the supervision of a responsible adult during initial use of marinol and following dosage adjustments.

Drug Interactions: In studies involving patients with AIDS and/or cancer, Marinol (dronabinol) has been coadministered with a variety of medications (e.g., cytotoxic agents, anti-infective agents, sedatives, or opioid analgesics) without resulting in any clinically significant drug/drug interactions. Although no drug/drug interactions were discovered during the clinical trials of Marinol, cannabinoids may interact with other medications through both metabolic and pharmacodynamic mechanisms. Dronabinol is highly protein bound to plasma proteins, and therefore, might displace other protein-bound drugs. Although this displacement has not been confirmed in vivo, practitioners should monitor patients for a change in dosage requirements when administering dronabinol to patients receiving other highly protein-bound drugs. Published reports of drug/drug interactions involving cannabinoids are summarized in the following table.

CONCOMITANT DRUG	CLINICAL EFFECT(S)
Amphetamines, cocaine, other sympathomimetic agents	Additive hypertension, tachycardia, possibly cardiotoxicity
Atropine, scopolamine, antihistamines, other anticholergic agents	Additive or super-additive tachycardia, drowsiness
Amitriptyline, amoxapine, desipramine, other tricyclic antidepressants	Additive tachycardia, hypertension, drowsiness
Barbiturates, benzodiazepines, ethanol, lithium, opiods, buspirone, antihistamines, muscle relaxants, other CNS depressants	Additive drowsiness and CNS depression

Marinol Dose: Response Frequency and Adverse Experience*
(N = 750 treatment courses)

Marinol Dose	Response Frequency (%)			Adverse Events Frequency (%)		
	Complete	Partial	Poor	None	Nondysphoric	Dysphoric
<7 mg/m²	36	32	32	23	65	12
>7 mg/m²	33	31	36	13	58	28

Disulfiram	A reversible hypomanic reaction was reported in a 28 y/o man who smoked marijuana; confirmed by dechallenge and rechallenge
Fluoxetine	A 21 y/o female with depression and bullimia receiving 20 mg/day fluoxetine × 4 wks became hypomanic after smoking marijuana; symptoms resolved after 4 days
Antipurine, barbiturates	Decreased clearance of these agents, presumably via competitive inhibition of metabolism
Theophylline	Increased theophylline metabolism reported with smoking of marijuana; effect similar to that following smoking tobacco

Carcinogenesis, Mutagenesis, Impairment of Fertility: Carcinogenicity studies have not been performed with dronabinol. Mutagenicity testing of dronabinol was negative in an Ames test. In a long-term study (77 days) in rats, oral administration of dronabinol at doses of 30 to 150 mg/m^2, equivalent to 0.3 to 1.5 times maximum recommended human dose (MRHD) of 90 mg/m^2/day in cancer patients or 2 to 10 times MRHD of 15 mg/m^2/day in AIDS patients, reduced ventral prostate, seminal vesicle and epididymal weights and caused a decrease in seminal fluid volume. Decreases in spermatogenesis, number of developing germ cells, and number of Leydig cells in the testis were also observed. However, sperm count, mating success and testosterone levels were not affected. The significance of these animal findings in humans is not known.

Pregnancy: Pregnancy Category C. Reproduction studies with dronabinol have been performed in mice at 15 to 450 mg/m^2, equivalent to 0.2 to 5 times maximum recommended human dose (MRHD) of 90 mg/m^2/day in cancer patients or 1 to 30 times MRHD of 15 mg/m^2/day in AIDS patients, and in rats at 74 to 295 mg/m^2 (equivalent to 0.8 to 3 times MRHD of 90 mg/m^2 in cancer patients or 5 to 20 times MRHD of 15 mg/m^2/day in AIDS patients). These studies have revealed no evidence of teratogenicity due to dronabinol. At these dosages in mice and rats, dronabinol decreased maternal weight gain and number of viable pups and increased fetal mortality and early resorptions. Such effects were dose dependent and less apparent at lower doses which produced less maternal toxicity. There are no adequate and well-controlled studies in pregnant women. Dronabinol should be used only if the potential benefit justifies the potential risk to the fetus.

Nursing Mothers: Use of Marinol is not recommended in nursing mothers since, in addition to the secretion of HIV virus in breast milk, dronabinol is concentrated in and secreted in human breast milk and is absorbed by the nursing baby.

ADVERSE REACTIONS

Adverse experiences information summarized in the tables below was derived from well-controlled clinical trials conducted in the US and US territories involving 474 patients exposed to Marinol (dronabinol). Studies of AIDS-related weight loss included 157 patients receiving dronabinol at a dose of 2.5 mg twice daily and 67 receiving placebo. Studies of different durations were combined by considering the first occurrence of events during the first 28 days. Studies of nausea and vomiting related to cancer chemotherapy included 317 patients receiving dronabinol and 68 receiving placebo.

A cannabinoid dose-related "high" (easy laughing, elation and heightened awareness) has been reported by patients receiving marinol in both the antiemetic (24%) and the lower dose appetite stimulant clinical trials (8%) (see CLINICAL TRIALS).

The most frequently reported adverse experiences in patients with AIDS during placebo-controlled clinical trials involved the CNS and were reported by 33% of patients receiving Marinol. About 25% of patients reported a minor CNS adverse event during the first 2 weeks and about 4% reported such an event each week for the next 6 weeks thereafter.

PROBABLY CAUSALLY RELATED: Incidence greater than 1%.

Rates derived from clinical trials in AIDS-related anorexia (N=157) and chemotherapy-related nausea (N=317). Rates were generally higher in the anti-emetic use (given in parentheses).

Body as a whole: Asthenia.
Cardiovascular: Palpitations, tachycardia, vasodilation/facial flush.
Digestive: Abdominal pain*, nausea*, vomiting*.
Nervous system: (Amnesia), anxiety/nervousness, (ataxia), confusion, depersonalization, dizziness*, euphoria*, (hallucination), paranoid reaction*, somnolence*, thinking abnormal*.

*Incidence of events 3% to 10%

PROBABLY CAUSALLY RELATED: Incidence less than 1%.

Event rates derived from clinical trials in AIDS-related anorexia (N=157) and chemotherapy-related nausea (N=317).

Cardiovascular: Conjunctivitis*, hypotension*.
Digestive: Diarrhea*, fecal incontinence.
Musculoskeletal: Myalgias.
Nervous system: Depression, nightmares, speech difficulties, tinnitus.
Skin and Appendages: Flushing*.
Special senses: Vision difficulties.

*Incidence of events 0.3% to 1%.

CAUSAL RELATIONSHIP UNKNOWN: Incidence less than 1%

The clinical significance of the association of these events with Marinol treatment is unknown, but they are reported as alerting information for the clinician.

Body as a whole: Chills, headache, malaise.
Digestive: Anorexia, hepatic enzyme elevation.
Respiratory: Cough, rhinitis, sinusitis.
Skin and Appendages: Sweating.

DRUG ABUSE AND DEPENDENCE

Marinol (dronabinol) is one of the psychoactive compounds present in cannabis, and is abusable and controlled Schedule II (CII) under the Controlled Substances Act. Both psychological and physiological dependence have been noted in healthy individuals receiving dronabinol, but addiction is uncommon and has only been seen after prolonged high dose administration.

Chronic abuse of cannabis has been associated with decrements in motivation, cognition, judgement, and perception. The etiology of these impairments is unknown, but may be associated with the complex process of addiction rather than an isolated effect of the drug. No such decrements in physchological, social or neurological status have been associated with the administration of Marinol for therapeutic purposes.

In an open-label study in patients with AIDS who received Marinol for up to five months, no abuse, diversion or systematic change in personality or social functioning were observed despite the inclusion of a substantial number of patients with a past history of drug abuse.

An abstinence syndrome has been reported after the abrupt discontinuation of dronabinol in volunteers receiving dosages of 210 mg/day for 12 to 16 consecutive days. Within 12 hours after discontinuation, these volunteers manifested symptoms such as irritability, insomnia, and restlessness. By approximately 24 hours post-dronabinol discontinuation, withdrawal symptoms intensified to include "hot flashes", sweating, rhinorrhea, loose stools, hiccoughs and anorexia. These withdrawal symptoms gradually dissipated over the next 48 hours. Electroencephalographic changes consistent with the effects of drug withdrawal (hyperexcitation) were recorded in patients after abrupt dechallenge. Patients also complained of disturbed sleep for several weeks after discontinuing therapy with high dosages of dronabinol.

OVERDOSAGE

Signs and symptoms following MILD Marinol (dronabinol) intoxication include drowsiness, euphoria, heightened sensory awareness, altered time perception, reddened conjunctiva, dry mouth and tachycardia; following MODERATE intoxication include memory impairment, depersonalization, mood alteration, urinary retention, and reduced bowel motility; and following SEVERE intoxication include decreased motor coordination, lethargy, slurred speech, and postural hypotension. Apprehensive patients may experience panic reactions and seizures may occur in patients with existing seizure disorders.

The estimated lethal human dose of intravenous dronabinol is 30 mg/kg (2100 mg/70kg). Significant CNS symptoms in antiemetic studies followed oral doses of 0.4 mg/kg (28 mg/70kg) of Marinol.

Management: A potentially serious oral ingestion, if recent, should be managed with gut decontamination. In unconscious patients with a secure airway, instill activated charcoal (30 to 100 g in adults, 1 to 2 g/kg in infants) via a nasogastric tube. A saline cathartic or sorbitol may be added to the first dose of activated charcoal. Patients experiencing depressive, hallucinatory or psychotic reactions should be placed in a quiet area and offered reassurance. Benzodiazepines (5 to 10 mg diazepam *po*) may be used for treatment of extreme agitation. Hypotension usually responds to Trendelenburg position and IV fluids. Pressors are rarely required.

DOSAGE AND ADMINISTRATION

Appetite stimulation: Initially, 2.5 mg Marinol (dronabinol) should be administered orally twice daily (b.i.d.), before lunch and supper. For patients unable to tolerate this 5 mg/day dosage of Marinol, the dosage can be reduced to 2.5 mg/day, administered as a single dose in the evening or at bedtime. If clinically indicated and in the absence of significant adverse effects, the dosage may be gradually increased to a maximum of 20 mg/day Marinol, administered in divided oral doses. Caution should be exercised in escalating the dosage of Marinol because of the increased frequency of dose-related adverse experiences at higher dosage (see PRECAUTIONS).

Antiemetic: Marinol is best administered at an initial dose of 5 mg/m^2, given 1 to 3 hours prior to the administration of chemotherapy, then every 2 to 4 hours after chemotherapy is given, for a total of 4 to 6 doses/day. Should the 5 mg/m^2 dose prove to be ineffective, and in the absence of significant side effects, the dose may be escalated by 2.5 mg/m^2 increments to a maximum of 15 mg/m^2 per dose. Caution should be exercised in dose escalation, however, as the incidence of disturbing psychiatric symptoms increases significantly at maximum dose (see PRECAUTIONS).

SAFETY AND HANDLING

Marinol (dronabinol) should be packaged in a well-closed container and stored in a cool environment between 8° and 15°C (46° and 59°F). Protect from freezing. No particular hazard to health care workers handling the capsules has been identified.

Access to abusable drugs such as Marinol presents an occupational hazard for addiction in the health care industry. Routine procedures for handling controlled substances developed to protect the public may not be adequate to protect health care workers. Implementation of more effective accounting procedures and measures to appropriately restrict access to drugs of this class may minimize the risk of self-administration by health care providers.

HOW SUPPLIED

MARINOL® CAPSULES (dronabinol solution in sesame oil in soft gelatin capsules)

2.5 mg white capsules (identified RL).
NDC 0054-2601-11: Bottles of 25 capsules.
NDC 0054-2601-21: Bottles of 60 capsules.
NDC 0054-2601-25: Bottles of 100 capsules.

5 mg dark brown capsules (identified RL).
NDC 0054-2602-11: Bottles of 25 capsules.
NDC 0054-2602-25: Bottles of 100 capsules.

10 mg orange capsules (identified RL).
NDC 0054-2603-11: Bottles of 25 capsules.
NDC 0054-2603-21: Bottles of 60 capsules.

MARINOL® is a registered trademark of Unimed Pharmaceuticals, Inc. and is marketed by Roxane Laboratories, Inc. under license from Unimed Pharmaceuticals, Inc.
Manufactured by Banner Pharmacaps, Inc.
Chatsworth CA 91311

DEA ORDER FORM REQUIRED
Rx only

4056050 **Revised June 1998**
068 © RLI, 1998
Roxane
Laboratories, Inc.
Columbus, Ohio 43216

Shown in Product Identification Guide, page 335

METHADONE HYDROCHLORIDE CII ℞

[*mĕth 'ă-dōn hī-drō- klō-rīd*]
DISKETS® (dispersible tablets)
Tablets, USP
(See also **Dolophine® Hydrochloride**)

(WARNING: May be habit forming)

CONDITIONS FOR DISTRIBUTION AND USE OF METHADONE PRODUCTS:
Code of Federal Regulations,
Title 21, Sec. 291.505

METHADONE PRODUCTS, WHEN USED FOR TREATMENT OF NARCOTIC ADDICTION IN DETOXIFICATION OR MAINTENANCE PROGRAMS, SHALL BE DISPENSED ONLY BY APPROVED HOSPITAL PHARMACIES, APPROVED COMMUNITY PHARMACIES, AND MAINTENANCE PROGRAMS APPROVED BY THE FOOD AND DRUG ADMINISTRATION AND THE DESIGNATED STATE AUTHORITY.

Continued on next page

Methadone HCl Diskets—Cont.

APPROVED MAINTENANCE PROGRAMS SHALL DISPENSE AND USE METHADONE IN ORAL FORM ONLY AND ACCORDING TO THE TREATMENT REQUIREMENTS STIPULATED IN THE FEDERAL METHADONE REGULATIONS (21 CFR 291.505).

FAILURE TO ABIDE BY THE REQUIREMENTS IN THESE REGULATIONS MAY RESULT IN CRIMINAL PROSECUTION, SEIZURE OF THE DRUG SUPPLY, REVOCATION OF THE PROGRAM APPROVAL, AND INJUNCTION PRECLUDING OPERATION OF THE PROGRAM.

DESCRIPTION

Each tablet for oral administration contains:
Methadone Hydrochloride .... 40 mg
(Warning: May be habit forming)
Inactive Ingredients:
The dispersible tablets contain magnesium stearate, microcrystalline cellulose, and starch (corn). The Diskets® contain cellulose, FD&C Yellow No. 6, flavors, magnesium stearate, potassium phosphate, silicon dioxide, cornstarch, and stearic acid.

Methadone hydrochloride is a white crystalline material which is water soluble. However, the methadone hydrochloride dispersible tablets have been specially formulated with insoluble excipients to deter the use of this drug by injection.

Chemically, Methadone Hydrochloride is 6-(Dimethylamino)-4,4-diphenyl-3-heptanone hydrochloride, which can be represented by the following structural formula:

$C_{21}H_{27}NO \cdot HCl$ M.W. 345.91

HOW SUPPLIED

Methadone Hydrochloride
Tablets USP (Dispersible), 40 mg
40 mg white cross-scored tablets (Identified 54 843).
NDC 0054-8547-25: Unit dose, 20 tablets per card (reverse numbered), 5 cards per shipper.
NDC 0054-4547-25: Bottles of 100 tablets.
Methadone Hydrochloride
Tablets USP, 40 mg Diskets®
40 mg peach-colored, cross-scored tablets (Identified 54 883).
NDC 0054-4538-25: Bottles of 100 tablets.
Store at Controlled Room Temperature 15°–30°C (59°–86°F)
Dispense in a well-closed container as defined in the USP/NF, with a child-resistant closure.
Caution: Federal law prohibits dispensing without prescription.
The Diskets® are manufactured for Roxane Laboratories by Eli Lilly and Company (Indianapolis, IN 46285).
4056070

025   Revised
                                                    February 1995
© RLl. 1995.

METHADONE HYDROCHLORIDE Ⓒ ℞
Oral Concentrate USP
10 mg per mL
For Methadone Treatment Programs Only

(Warning: May be habit forming)

CONDITIONS FOR DISTRIBUTION
AND USE OF METHADONE PRODUCTS:
Code of Federal Regulations,
Title 21, Sec. 291.505

METHADONE PRODUCTS, WHEN USED FOR TREATMENT OF NARCOTIC ADDICTION IN DETOXIFICATION OR MAINTENANCE PROGRAMS, SHALL BE DISPENSED ONLY BY APPROVED HOSPITAL PHARMACIES, APPROVED COMMUNITY PHARMACIES, AND MAINTENANCE PROGRAMS APPROVED BY THE FOOD AND DRUG ADMINISTRATION AND THE DESIGNATED STATE AUTHORITY.
APPROVED MAINTENANCE PROGRAMS SHALL DISPENSE AND USE METHADONE IN ORAL FORM ONLY AND ACCORDING TO THE TREATMENT REQUIREMENTS STIPULATED IN THE FEDERAL METHADONE REGULATIONS (21 CFR 291.505).
FAILURE TO ABIDE BY THE REQUIREMENTS IN THESE REGULATIONS MAY RESULT IN CRIMINAL PROSECUTION, SEIZURE OF THE DRUG SUPPLY, REVOCATION OF THE PROGRAM APPROVAL, AND INJUNCTION PRECLUDING OPERATION OF THE PROGRAM.

DESCRIPTION

Each mL for oral administration contains:
Methadone Hydrochloride .... 10 mg
(Warning: May be habit forming)
Inactive ingredients: sodium benzoate, citric acid, and water.

CLINICAL PHARMACOLOGY

Methadone Hydrochloride is a synthetic narcotic analgesic with multiple actions quantitatively similar to those of morphine, the most prominent of which involve the central nervous system and organs composed of smooth muscle. The principal actions of therapeutic value are analgesia and sedation, detoxification or maintenance in narcotic addiction. The methadone abstinence syndrome, although qualitatively similar to that of morphine, differs in that the onset is slower, the course is more prolonged, and the symptoms are less severe.
When administered orally, methadone is approximately one-half as potent as when given parenterally. Oral administration results in a delay of the onset, a lowering of the peak, and an increase in the duration of analgesic effect.

INDICATIONS AND USAGE

1. Detoxification treatment of narcotic addiction (heroin or other morphine-like drugs).
2. Maintenance treatment of narcotic addiction (heroin or other morphine-like drugs), in conjunction with appropriate social and medical services.

NOTE
If methadone is administered for treatment of heroin dependence for more than three weeks, the procedure passes from treatment of the acute withdrawal syndrome (detoxification) to maintenance therapy. Maintenance treatment is permitted to be undertaken only by approved methadone programs. This does not preclude the maintenance treatment of an addict who is hospitalized for medical conditions other than addiction and who requires temporary maintenance during the critical period of his stay or whose enrollment has been verified in a program which has approval for maintenance treatment with methadone.

CONTRAINDICATIONS

Hypersensitivity to methadone.

WARNINGS

Methadone Hydrochloride Oral Concentrate is for oral administration only. This preparation must not be injected. It is recommended that Methadone Hydrochloride Oral Concentrate, if dispensed, be packaged in child-resistant containers and kept out of the reach of children to prevent accidental ingestion.

Methadone Hydrochloride, a narcotic, is a Schedule II controlled substance under the Federal Controlled Substances Act. Appropriate security measures should be taken to safeguard stocks of methadone against diversion.

DRUG DEPENDENCE-METHADONE CAN PRODUCT DRUG DEPENDENCE OF THE MORPHINE TYPE AND, THEREFORE, HAS THE POTENTIAL FOR BEING ABUSED. PSYCHIC DEPENDENCE, PHYSICAL DEPENDENCE, AND TOLERANCE MAY DEVELOP UPON REPEATED ADMINISTRATION OF METHADONE, AND IT SHOULD BE PRESCRIBED AND ADMINISTERED WITH THE SAME DEGREE OF CAUTION APPROPRIATE TO THE USE OF MORPHINE.
Interaction with Other Central-Nervous-System Depressants—Methadone should be used with caution and in reduced dosage in patients who are concurrently receiving other narcotic analgesics, general anesthetics, phenothiazines, other tranquilizers, sedative-hyponotics, tricyclic an-

tidepressants, and other C.N.S. depressants (including alcohol). Respiratory depression, hypotension, and profound sedation or coma may result.
Anxiety—Since methadone, as used by tolerant subjects at a constant maintenance dosage, is not a tranquilizer, patients who are maintained on this drug will react to life problems and stresses with the same symptoms of anxiety as do other individuals. The physician should not confuse such symptoms with those of narcotic abstinence and should not attempt to treat anxiety by increasing the dosage of methadone. The action of methadone in maintenance treatment is limited to the control of narcotic symptoms and is ineffective for relief of general anxiety.
Head Injury and Increased Intracranial Pressure—The respiratory depressant effects of methadone and its capacity to elevate cerebrospinal-fluid pressure may be markedly exaggerated in the presence of increased intracranial pressure. Furthermore, narcotics produce side effects that may obscure the clinical course of patients with head injuries. In such patients, methadone must be used with caution and only if it is deemed essential.
Asthma and Other Respiratory Conditions—Methadone should be used with caution in patients having an acute asthmatic attack, in those with chronic obstructive pulmonary disease or cor pulmonale, and in individuals with a substantially decreased respiratory reserve, preexisting respiratory depression, hypoxia, or hypercapnia. In such patients, even usual therapeutic doses of narcotics may decrease respiratory drive while simultaneously increasing airway resistance to the point of apnea.
Hypotensive Effect—The administration of methadone may result in severe hypotension in an individual whose ability to maintain his blood pressure has already been compromised by a depleted blood volume or concurrent administration of such drugs as the phenothiazines or certain anesthetics.
Use in Ambulatory Patients—Methadone may impair the mental and/or physical abilities required for the performance of potentially hazardous tasks, such as driving a car or operating machinery. The patient should be cautioned accordingly.
Methadone, like other narcotics, may produce orthostatic hypotension in ambulatory patients.
Use in Pregnancy—Safe use in pregnancy has not been established in relation to possible adverse effects on fetal development. Therefore, methadone should not be used in pregnant women unless, in the judgment of the physician, the potential benefits outweigh the possible hazards.

PRECAUTIONS

Interaction with Pentazocine—Patients who are addicted to heroin or who are on the methadone maintenance program may experience withdrawal symptoms when given pentazocine.
Interaction with Rifampin—The concurrent administration of rifampin may possibly reduce the blood concentration of methadone to a degree sufficient to produce withdrawal symptoms. The mechanism by which rifampin may decrease blood concentrations of methadone is not fully understood although enhanced microsomal drug-metabolized enzymes may influence drug disposition.
Interaction with Monoamine Oxidase (MAO) Inhibitors—Therapeutic doses of meperidine have precipitated severe reactions in patients concurrently receiving monoamine oxidase inhibitors or those who have received such agents within 14 days. Similar reactions thus far have not been reported with methadone; but if the use of methadone is necessary in such patients, a sensitivity test should be performed in which repeated small incremental doses are administered over the course of several hours while the patient's condition and vital signs are under careful observation.
Acute Abdominal Conditions—The administration of methadone or other narcotics may obscure the diagnosis or clinical course of patients with acute abdominal conditions.
Special-Risk Patients—Methadone should be given with caution and the initial dose should be reduced in certain patients, such as the elderly or debilitated and those with severe impairment of hepatic or renal function, hypothyroidism, Addison's disease, prostatic hypertrophy, or urethral stricture.

ADVERSE REACTIONS

Heroin Withdrawal—During the induction phase of methadone maintenance treatment, patients are being withdrawn from heroin and may therefore show typical withdrawal symptoms, which should be differentiated from methadone-induced side effects. They may exhibit some or all of the following symptoms associated with acute withdrawal from heroin or other opiates: lacrimation, rhinorrhea, sneezing, yawning, excessive perspiration, goose-flesh, fever, chilliness alternating with flushing, restlessness, irritability, "sleepy yen", weakness, anxiety, depression, dilated pupils, tremors, tachycardia, abdominal cramps, body aches, involuntary twitching and kicking movements, anorexia, nausea, vomiting, diarrhea, intestinal spasms, and weight loss.

Initial Administration—Initially, the dosage of methadone should be carefully titrated to the individual. Induction too rapid for the patient's sensitivity is more likely to produce the following effects.

THE MAJOR HAZARDS OF METHADONE, AS OF OTHER NARCOTIC ANALGESICS, ARE RESPIRATORY DEPRESSION AND, TO A LESSER DEGREE, CIRCULATORY DEPRESSION. RESPIRATORY ARREST, SHOCK, AND CARDIAC ARREST HAVE OCCURRED.

The most frequently observed adverse reactions include lightheadedness, dizziness, sedation, nausea, vomiting, and sweating. These effects seem to be more prominent in ambulatory patients and in those who are not suffering severe chronic pain. In such individuals, lower doses are advisable. Some adverse reactions may be alleviated in the ambulatory patient if he lies down.

Other adverse reactions include the following:

Central Nervous System—Euphoria, dysphoria, weakness, headache, insomnia, agitation, disorientation, and visual disturbances.

Gastrointestinal—Dry mouth, anorexia, constipation and biliary tract spasm.

Cardiovascular—Flushing of the face, bradycardia, palpitation, faintness, and syncope.

Genito-Urinary—Urinary retention or hesitancy, antidiuretic effect, and reduced libido and/or potency.

Allergic—Pruritus, urticaria, other skin rashes, edema, and, rarely hemorrhagic urticaria.

Maintenance on a Stabilized Dose—During prolonged administration of methadone, as in a methadone maintenance treatment program, there is a gradual, yet progressive disappearance of side effects over a period of several weeks. However, constipation and sweating often persist.

OVERDOSAGE

Symptoms—Serious overdosage of methadone is characterized by respiratory depression (a decrease in respiratory rate and/or tidal volume, Cheyne-Stokes respiration, cyanosis), extreme somnolence progressing to stupor or coma, maximally constricted pupils, skeletal-muscle flaccidity, cold and clammy skin, and, sometimes, bradycardia and hypotension. In severe overdosage, particularly by the intravenous route, apnea, circulatory collapse, cardiac arrest, and death may occur.

Treatment—Primary attention should be given to the reestablishment of adequate respiratory exchange through provision of a patent airway and institution of assisted or controlled ventilation. If a non-tolerant person, especially a child, takes a large dose of methadone, effective narcotic antagonists are available to counter-act the potentially lethal respiratory depression. THE PHYSICIAN MUST REMEMBER, HOWEVER, THAT METHADONE IS A LONG-ACTING DEPRESSANT (THIRTY-SIX TO FORTY-EIGHT HOURS), WHEREAS THE ANTAGONISTS ACT FOR MUCH SHORTER PERIODS (ONE TO THREE HOURS). The patient must, therefore, be monitored continuously for recurrence of respiratory depression and treated repeatedly with the narcotic antagonist as needed. If the diagnosis is correct and respiratory depression is due only to overdosage of methadone, the use of respiratory stimulants is not indicated.

An antagonist should not be administered in the absence of clinically significant respiratory or cardiovascular depression. Intravenously administered narcotic antagonists, naloxone hydrochloride, nalorphine hydrochloride, or levallorphan tartrate are the drugs of choice to reverse signs of intoxication. These agents should be given repeatedly until the patient's status remains satisfactory. The hazard that the narcotic antagonist will further depress respiration is less likely with the use of naloxone.

Oxygen, intravenous fluids, vasopressors, and other supportive measures should be employed as indicated.

NOTE: IN AN INDIVIDUAL PHYSICALLY DEPENDENT ON NARCOTICS, THE ADMINISTRATION OF THE USUAL DOSE OF A NARCOTIC ANTAGONIST WILL PRECIPITATE AN ACUTE WITHDRAWAL SYNDROME. THE SEVERITY OF THIS SYNDROME WILL DEPEND ON THE DEGREE OF PHYSICAL DEPENDENCE AND THE DOSE OF THE ANTAGONIST ADMINISTERED. THE USE OF A NARCOTIC ANTAGONIST IN SUCH A PERSON SHOULD BE AVOIDED IF POSSIBLE. IF IT MUST BE USED TO TREAT SERIOUS RESPIRATORY DEPRESSION IN THE PHYSICALLY DEPENDENT PATIENT, THE ANTAGONIST SHOULD BE ADMINISTERED WITH EXTREME CARE AND BY TITRATION WITH SMALLER THAN USUAL DOSES OF THE ANTAGONIST.

DOSAGE AND ADMINISTRATION

For Detoxification Treatment—THE DRUG SHALL BE ADMINISTERED DAILY UNDER CLOSE SUPERVISION AS FOLLOWS:

A detoxification treatment course shall not exceed 21 days and may not be repeated earlier than four weeks after completion of the preceding course.

In detoxification, the patient may receive methadone when there are significant symptoms of withdrawal. The dosage schedules indicated below are recommended but could be varied in accordance with clinical judgment. Initially, a single oral dose of 15 to 20 mg of methadone will often be sufficient to suppress withdrawal symptoms. Additional methadone may be provided if withdrawal symptoms are not suppressed or if symptoms reappear. When patients are physically dependent on high doses, it may be necessary to exceed these levels. Forty mg per day in single or divided doses will usually constitute an adequate stabilizing dosage level. Stabilization can be continued for two to three days, and then the amount of methadone normally will be gradually decreased. The rate at which methadone is decreased will be determined separately with each patient. The dose of methadone can be decreased on a daily basis or at two-day intervals, but the amount of intake shall always be sufficient to keep withdrawal symptoms at a tolerable level. In hospitalized patients, a daily reduction of 20 percent of the total daily dose may be tolerated and may cause little discomfort. In ambulatory patients, a somewhat slower schedule may be needed. If methadone is administered for more than three weeks, the procedure is considered to have progressed from detoxification or treatment of the acute withdrawal syndrome to maintenance treatment, even though the goal and intent may be eventual total withdrawal.

For Maintenance Treatment—In maintenance treatment of respiratory depression, or other effects of acute intoxication. It is important that the initial dosage be adjusted on an individual basis to the narcotic tolerance of the new patient. If such a patient has been a heavy user of heroin up to the day of admission, he/she may be given 20 mg 4 to 8 hours later or 40 mg in a single oral dose. If the patient enters treatment with little or no narcotic tolerance (e.g., if he/she has recently been released from jail or other confinement), the initial dosage may be one-half these quantities. When there is any doubt, the smaller dose should be used initially. The patient should then be kept under observation, and, if symptoms of abstinence are distressing, additional 10 mg doses may be administered as needed. Subsequently, the dosage should be adjusted individually, as tolerated and required, up to a level of 120 mg daily. The patient will initially ingest the drug under observation daily, or at least 6 days a week, for the first 3 months. After demonstrating satisfactory adherence to the program regulations for at least 3 months, the patient may be permitted to reduce to 3 times weekly the occasions when he/she must ingest the drug under observation. The patient shall receive no more than a 2-day take-home supply. With continuing adherence to the program's requirements for at least 2 years, he/she may then be permitted twice-weekly visits to the program for drug ingestion under observation, with a 3-day take-home supply. A daily dose of 120 mg or more shall be justified in the medical record. Prior approval from state authority and the Food and Drug Administration is required for any dose above 120 mg administered at the clinic and for any dose above 100 mg to be taken at home. A regular review of dosage level should be made by the responsible physician, with careful consideration given to reduction of dosage as indicated on an individual basis. A new dosage level is only a test level until stability is achieved.

Special Considerations for a Pregnant Patient–Caution shall be taken in the maintenance treatment of pregnant patients. Dosage levels should be kept as low as possible if continued methadone treatment is deemed necessary. It is the responsibility of the program sponsor to assure that each female patient be fully informed concerning the possible risks to a pregnant woman or her unborn child from the use of methadone.

Special Limitations-
Treatment of Patients Under Age 18

1. The safety and effectiveness of methadone for use in the treatment of adolescents have not been proved by adequate clinical study. Special procedures are therefore necessary to assure that patients under age 16 will not be admitted to a program and that patients between 16 and 18 years of age will be admitted to maintenance treatment only under limited conditions.

2. Patients between 16 and 18 years of age who were enrolled and under treatment in approved programs on December 15, 1972, may continue in maintenance treatment. No new patients between 16 and 18 years of age may be admitted to a maintenance treatment program after March 15, 1973, unless a parent, legal guardian, or responsible adult designated by the state authority completes and signs Form FD 2635, "Consent for Methadone Treatment".

Methadone treatment of new patients between the ages of 16 and 18 years will be permitted after December 15, 1972, only with a documented history of 2 or more unsuccessful attempts at detoxification and a documented history of dependence on heroin or other morphine-like

drugs beginning 2 years or more prior to application for treatment. No patient under age 16 may be continued or started on methadone treatment after December 15, 1972, but these patients may be detoxified and retained in the program in a drug-free state for follow-up and aftercare.

3. Patients under age 18 who are not placed on maintenance treatment may be detoxified. Detoxification may not exceed 3 weeks. A repeat episode of detoxification may not be initiated until 4 weeks after the completion of the previous detoxification.

HOW SUPPLIED

Methadone Hydrochloride Oral Concentrate USP
10 mg per mL
Clear, flavorless solution.
NDC 0054-3553-67: Bottles of 1 quart (946 mL).
Store at Controlled Room Temperature
15°–30°C (59°–86°F)
Protect from light.
Dispense in a tight, light-resistant container as defined in the USP/NF.
Caution: Federal law prohibits dispensing without prescription.
4056322   Revised January 1996
016
© RLI, 1996.
Roxane
Laboratories, Inc.
Columbus, Ohio 43216

METHADONE HYDROCHLORIDE   Ⓒ ℞
ORAL SOLUTION USP
TABLETS USP

(WARNING: May be habit forming)

CONDITIONS FOR DISTRIBUTION AND
USE OF METHADONE PRODUCTS:
Code of Federal Regulations,
Title 21, Sec. 291.505

METHADONE PRODUCTS, WHEN USED FOR TREATMENT OF NARCOTIC ADDICTION IN DETOXIFICATION OR MAINTENANCE PROGRAMS, SHALL BE DISPENSED ONLY BY APPROVED HOSPITAL PHARMACIES, APPROVED COMMUNITY PHARMACIES, AND MAINTENANCE PROGRAMS APPROVED BY THE FOOD AND DRUG ADMINISTRATION AND THE DESIGNATED STATE AUTHORITY.

APPROVED MAINTENANCE PROGRAMS SHALL DISPENSE AND USE METHADONE IN ORAL FORM ONLY AND ACCORDING TO THE TREATMENT REQUIREMENTS STIPULATED IN THE FEDERAL METHADONE REGULATIONS (21 CFR 291.505).

FAILURE TO ABIDE BY THE REQUIREMENTS IN THESE REGULATIONS MAY RESULT IN CRIMINAL PROSECUTION, SEIZURE OF THE DRUG SUPPLY, REVOCATION OF THE PROGRAM APPROVAL, AND INJUNCTION PRECLUDING OPERATION OF THE PROGRAM.

A METHADONE PRODUCT, WHEN USED AS AN ANALGESIC, MAY BE DISPENSED IN ANY LICENSED PHARMACY.

DESCRIPTION

Each 5 mL of Methadone Hydrochloride Oral Solution contains:
Methadone Hydrochloride .... 5 mg or 10 mg
(**Warning:** May be habit forming)
Alcohol 8%
Each tablet for oral administration contains:
Methadone Hydrochloride .... 5 mg or 10 mg
(**Warning:** May be habit forming)

Inactive Ingredients:
The oral solution contains alcohol, FD&C Red No. 40, FD&C Yellow No. 6, flavoring, glycol, sorbitol, water, and other ingredients.
The tablets contain magnesium stearate, microcrystalline cellulose, and starch (corn).
Chemically, Methadone Hydrochloride is 3-Heptanone, 6-(dimethylamino)-4,4-diphenyl-, hydrochloride.
Methadone Hydrochloride acts as a narcotic analgesic.

CLINICAL PHARMACOLOGY

Methadone Hydrochloride is a synthetic narcotic analgesic with multiple actions quantitatively similar to those of morphine, the most prominent of which involve the central nervous system and organs composed of smooth muscle. The principal actions of therapeutic value are analgesia and se-

Continued on next page

Methadone HCl Sol./Tab.—Cont.

dation and detoxification or temporary maintenance in narcotic addiction. The methadone abstinence syndrome, although qualitatively similar to that of morphine, differs in that the onset is slower, the course is more prolonged, and the symptoms are less severe.

When administered orally, methadone is approximately one-half as potent as when given parenterally. Oral administration results in a delay of the onset, a lowering of the peak, and an increase in the duration of analgesic effect.

INDICATIONS AND USAGE

Methadone Hydrochloride is indicated for relief of severe pain, for detoxification treatment of narcotic addiction, and for temporary maintenance treatment of narcotic addiction.

Note

If methadone is administered for treatment of heroin dependence for more than three weeks, the procedure passes from treatment of the acute withdrawal syndrome (detoxification) to maintenance therapy. Maintenance treatment is permitted to be undertaken only by approved methadone programs. This does not preclude the maintenance treatment of an addict who is hospitalized for medical conditions other than addiction and who requires temporary maintenance during the critical period of his stay or whose enrollment has been verified in a program which has approval for maintenance treatment with methadone.

CONTRAINDICATIONS

Hypersensitivity to methadone.

WARNINGS

Methadone Hydrochloride Tablets are for oral administration only and *must not* be used for injection. It is recommended that Methadone Hydrochloride Tablets, if dispensed, be packaged in child-resistant containers and kept out of the reach of children to prevent accidental ingestion.

Methadone Hydrochloride, a narcotic, is a Schedule II controlled substance under the Federal Controlled Substances Act. Appropriate security measures should be taken to safeguard stocks of methadone against diversion.

DRUG DEPENDENCE — METHADONE CAN PRODUCE DRUG DEPENDENCE OF THE MORPHINE TYPE AND, THEREFORE, HAS THE POTENTIAL FOR BEING ABUSED. PSYCHIC DEPENDENCE, PHYSICAL DEPENDENCE, AND TOLERANCE MAY DEVELOP UPON REPEATED ADMINISTRATION OF METHADONE, AND IT SHOULD BE PRESCRIBED AND ADMINISTERED WITH THE SAME DEGREE OF CAUTION APPROPRIATE TO THE USE OF MORPHINE.

Interaction with Other Central-Nervous-System Depressants—Methadone should be used with caution and in reduced dosage in patients who are concurrently receiving other narcotic analgesics, general anesthetics, phenothiazines, other tranquilizers, sedative-hypnotics, tricyclic antidepressants, and other C.N.S. depressants (including alcohol). Respiratory depression, hypotension, and profound sedation or coma may result.

Anxiety—Since methadone, as used by tolerant subjects at a constant maintenance dosage, is not a tranquilizer, patients who are maintained on this drug will react to life problems and stresses with the same symptoms of anxiety as do other individuals. The physician should not confuse such symptoms with those of narcotic abstinence and should not attempt to treat anxiety by increasing the dosage of methadone. The action of methadone in maintenance treatment is limited to the control of narcotic symptoms and is ineffective for relief of general anxiety.

Head Injury and Increased Intracranial Pressure—The respiratory depressant effects of methadone and its capacity to elevate cerebrospinal-fluid pressure may be markedly exaggerated in the presence of increased intracranial pressure. Furthermore, narcotics produce side effects that may obscure the clinical course of patients with head injuries. In such patients, methadone must be used with caution and only if it is deemed essential.

Asthma and Other Respiratory Conditions—Methadone should be used with caution in patients having an acute asthmatic attack, in those with chronic obstructive pulmonary disease or cor pulmonale, and in individuals with a substantially decreased respiratory reserve, preexisting respiratory depression, hypoxia, or hypercapnia. In such patients, even usual therapeutic doses of narcotics may decrease respiratory drive while simultaneously increasing airway resistance to the point of apnea.

Hypotensive Effect—The administration of methadone may result in severe hypotension in an individual whose ability to maintain his blood pressure has already been compromised by a depleted blood volume or concurrent administration of such drugs as the phenothiazines or certain anesthetics.

Use in Ambulatory Patients—Methadone may impair the mental and/or physical abilities required for the performance of potentially hazardous tasks, such as driving a car or operating machinery. The patient should be cautioned accordingly.

Methadone, like other narcotics, may produce orthostatic hypotension in ambulatory patients.

Use in Pregnancy—Safe use in pregnancy has not been established in relation to possible adverse effects on fetal development. Therefore, methadone should not be used in pregnant women unless, in the judgment of the physician, the potential benefits outweigh the possible hazards.

Methadone is not recommended for obstetric analgesia because its long duration of action increases the probability of respiratory depression in the newborn.

Use in Children—Methadone is not recommended for use as an analgesic in children, since documented clinical experience has been insufficient to establish a suitable dosage regimen for the pediatric age group.

PRECAUTIONS

Interaction with Pentazocine—**Patients who are addicted to heroin or who are on the methadone maintenance program may experience withdrawal symptoms when given pentazocine.**

Interaction with Rifampin—The concurrent administration of rifampin may possibly reduce the blood concentration of methadone. The mechanism by which rifampin may decrease blood concentrations of methadone is not fully understood, although enhanced microsomal drug-metabolized enzymes may influence drug disposition.

Acute Abdominal Conditions—The administration of methadone or other narcotics may obscure the diagnosis or clinical course in patients with acute abdominal conditions.

Interaction with Monoamine Oxidase (MAO) Inhibitors—Therapeutic doses of meperidine have precipitated severe reactions in patients concurrently receiving monoamine oxidase inhibitors or those who have received such agents within 14 days. Similar reactions thus far have not been reported with methadone; but if the use of methadone is necessary in such patients, a sensitivity test should be performed in which repeated small incremental doses are administered over the course of several hours while the patient's condition and vital signs are under careful observation.

Special-Risk Patients—Methadone should be given with caution and the initial dose should be reduced in certain patients, such as the elderly or debilitated and those with severe impairment of hepatic or renal function, hypothyroidism, Addison's disease, prostatic hypertrophy, or urethral stricture.

ADVERSE REACTIONS

THE MAJOR HAZARDS OF METHADONE, AS OF OTHER NARCOTIC ANALGESICS, ARE RESPIRATORY DEPRESSION AND, TO A LESSER DEGREE, CIRCULATORY DEPRESSION. RESPIRATORY ARREST, SHOCK, AND CARDIAC ARREST HAVE OCCURRED.

The most frequently observed adverse reactions include lightheadedness, dizziness, sedation, nausea, vomiting, and sweating. These effects seem to be more prominent in ambulatory patients and in those who are not suffering severe chronic pain. In such individuals, lower doses are advisable. Some adverse reactions may be alleviated in the ambulatory patient if he lies down.

Other adverse reactions include the following:

Central Nervous System—Euphoria, dysphoria, weakness, headache, insomnia, agitation, disorientation, and visual disturbances.

Gastrointestinal—Dry mouth, anorexia, constipation, and biliary tract spasm.

Cardiovascular—Flushing of the face, bradycardia, palpitation, faintness, and syncope.

Genitourinary—Urinary retention or hesitancy, antidiuretic effect, and reduced libido and/or potency.

Allergic—Pruritus, urticaria, other skin rashes, edema, and, rarely, hemorrhagic urticaria.

ADMINISTRATION AND DOSAGE

For relief of Severe Pain—Dosage should be adjusted according to the severity of the pain and the response of the patient. Occasionally it may be necessary to exceed the usual dosage recommended in cases of exceptionally severe chronic pain or in those patients who have become tolerant to the analgesic effect of narcotics.

The usual adult dose is 2.5 mg to 10 mg every three to four hours as necessary.

For Detoxification Treatment—THE DRUG SHALL BE ADMINISTERED DAILY UNDER CLOSE SUPERVISION AS FOLLOWS:

A detoxification treatment course shall not exceed 21 days and may not be repeated earlier than four weeks after completion of the preceding course.

The oral form of administration is preferred. However, if the patient is unable to ingest oral medication, he may be started on the parenteral form initially.

In detoxification, the patient may receive methadone when there are significant symptoms of withdrawal. The dosage schedules indicated below are recommended but could be varied in accordance with clinical judgment. Initially, a single dose of 15 to 20 mg of methadone will often be sufficient to suppress withdrawal symptoms. Additional methadone may be provided if withdrawal symptoms are not suppressed or if symptoms reappear. When patients are physically dependent on high doses, it may be necessary to exceed these levels. Forty mg per day in single or divided doses will usually constitute an adequate stabilizing dosage level. Stabilization can be continued for two to three days, and then the amount of methadone normally will be gradually decreased. The rate at which methadone is decreased will be determined separately for each patient. The dose of methadone can be decreased on a daily basis or at two-day intervals, but the amount of intake shall always be sufficient to keep withdrawal symptoms at a tolerable level. In hospitalized patients, a daily reduction of 20 percent of the total dose may be tolerated and may cause little discomfort. In ambulatory patients, a somewhat slower schedule may be needed. If methadone is administered for more than three weeks, the procedure is considered to have progressed from detoxification or treatment of the acute withdrawal syndrome to maintenance treatment, even though the goal and intent may be eventual total withdrawal.

OVERDOSAGE

Symptoms—Serious overdosage of methadone is characterized by respiratory depression (a decrease in respiratory rate and/or tidal volume, Cheyne-Stokes respiration, cyanosis), extreme somnolence progressing to stupor or coma, maximally constricted pupils, skeletal-muscle flaccidity, cold and clammy skin, and sometimes, bradycardia and hypotension. In severe overdosage, particularly by the intravenous route, apnea, circulatory collapse, cardiac arrest, and death may occur.

Treatment—Primary attention should be given to the reestablishment of adequate respiratory exchange through provision of a patent airway and institution of assisted or controlled ventilation. If a nontolerant person, especially a child, takes a large dose of methadone, effective narcotic antagonists are available to counteract the potentially lethal respiratory depression. **The physician must remember, however, that methadone is a long-acting depressant (36 to 48 hours), whereas the antagonists act for much shorter periods (one to three hours).** The patient must, therefore, be monitored continuously for recurrence of respiratory depression and treated repeatedly with the narcotic antagonist as needed. If the diagnosis is correct and respiratory depression is due only to overdosage of methadone, the use of other respiratory stimulants is not indicated.

An antagonist should not be administered in the absence of clinically significant respiratory or cardiovascular depression. Intravenously administered narcotic antagonists (naloxone and nalorphine) are the drugs of choice to reverse signs of intoxication. These agents should be given repeatedly until the patient's status remains satisfactory. The hazard that the narcotic agent will further depress respiration is less likely with the use of naloxone.

Oxygen, intravenous fluids, vasopressors, and other supportive measures should be employed as indicated.

Note

IN AN INDIVIDUAL PHYSICALLY DEPENDENT ON NARCOTICS, THE ADMINISTRATION OF THE USUAL DOSE OF A NARCOTIC ANTAGONIST WILL PRECIPITATE AN ACUTE WITHDRAWAL SYNDROME. THE SEVERITY OF THIS SYNDROME WILL DEPEND ON THE DEGREE OF PHYSICAL DEPENDENCE AND THE DOSE OF THE ANTAGONIST ADMINISTERED. THE USE OF A NARCOTIC ANTAGONIST IN SUCH A PERSON SHOULD BE AVOIDED IF POSSIBLE. IF IT MUST BE USED TO TREAT SERIOUS RESPIRATORY DEPRESSION IN THE PHYSICALLY DEPENDENT PATIENT, THE ANTAGONIST SHOULD BE ADMINISTERED WITH EXTREME CARE AND BY TITRATION WITH SMALLER THAN USUAL DOSES OF THE ANTAGONIST.

HOW SUPPLIED

Methadone Hydrochloride Oral Solution USP
Clear, orange-colored, citrus-flavored solution
5 mg per 5 mL
NDC 0054-3555-63: Bottles of 500 mL
10 mg per 5 mL
NDC 0054-3556-63: Bottles of 500 mL
Methadone Hydrochloride Tablets USP
5 mg white, scored identified (54 210) tablets.
NDC 0054-4570-25: Bottle of 100 tablets.
NDC 0054-8553-24: Unit dose, 25 tablets per card (reverse numbered), 4 cards per shipper.
10 mg white, scored identified (54 142) tablets.
NDC 0054-4571-25: Bottle of 100 tablets.
NDC 0054-8554-24: Unit dose, 25 tablets per card (reverse numbered), 4 cards per shipper.

ORAMORPH SR® Ⓒ ℞
(MORPHINE SULFATE)
SUSTAINED RELEASE TABLETS
15 mg, 30 mg, 60 mg, 100 mg
(WARNING: May be habit forming.)

NOTE

THIS IS A SUSTAINED RELEASE DOSAGE FORM. PATIENT SHOULD BE INSTRUCTED TO SWALLOW THE TABLET AS A WHOLE; THE TABLE SHOULD NOT BE BROKEN IN HALF, NOR SHOULD IT BE CRUSHED OR CHEWED.
THE SUSTAINED RELEASE OF MORPHINE FROM ORAMORPH SR SHOULD BE TAKEN INTO CONSIDERATION IN EVENT OF ADVERSE REACTIONS OR OVERDOSAGE.

DESCRIPTION

Each tablet for oral administration contains:
Morphine sulfate .... 15 mg, 30 mg, 60 mg, or 100 mg
(**WARNING:** May be habit forming)
in a tablet that provides for sustained release of the medication.

Morphine sulfate occurs as white, feathery, silky crystals, cubical masses of crystals, or white crystalline powder; it is soluble in water and slightly soluble in alcohol. Morphine has a pKa of 7.9, with an octanol/water partition coefficient of 1.42 at pH 7.4. At this pH, the tertiary amino group is mostly ionized, making the molecule water-soluble. Morphine is significantly more water-soluble than any other opioid in clinical use.

Chemically, morphine sulfate is 7,8-didehydro-4,5α-epoxy-17-methyl-morphinian-3,6α-diol sulfate (2:1)(salt) pentahydrate, and has the following structural formula:

Each ORAMORPH SR Tablet contains 15 mg, 30 mg, 60 mg, or 100 mg Morphine Sulfate USP. Inactive ingredients: Lactose, Hydroxypropyl Methylcellulose, Colloidal Silicon Dioxide, and Stearic Acid.

CLINICAL PHARMACOLOGY

Morphine is the prototype of many narcotic drugs that interact predeominantly with the opioid μ-receptor. These μ-binding sites are discretely distributed in the human brain, with high densities in the posterior amygdala, hypothalamus, thalamus, nucleus caudatus, putamen, and certain cortical areas. They are also found on the terminal axons of primary afferents with laminae I and II (substantia gelatinosa) of the spinal cord and in the spinal nucleus of the trigeminal nerve.

In clinical settings, morphine exerts its principal pharmacological effect on the central nervous system and gastrointestinal tract. Its primary actions of therapeutic value are analgesia and sedation. Morphine appears to increase the patient's tolerance for pain and to decrease discomfort, although the presence of the pain itself may still be recognized. In addition to analgesia, alterations in mood, euphoria and dysphoria, and drowsiness commonly occur.

Morphine depresses various respiratory centers, depresses the cough reflex, and constricts the pupils. Analgesically effective blood levels of morphine may cause nausea and vomiting directly by stimulating the chemoreceptor trigger zone, but nausea and vomiting are significantly more common in ambulatory than in recumbent patients, as is postural syncope.

Morphine increases the tone and decreases the propulsive contractions of the smooth muscle of the gastrointestinal tract. The resultant prolongation in gastrointestinal transit time is responsible for the constipating effect of morphine. Because morphine may increase biliary-tract pressure, some patients with biliary colic may experience worsening rather than relief of pain.

While morphine generally increases the tone of urinary-tract smooth muscle, the net effect tends to be variable, in some cases producing urinary urgency, in others, difficulty in urination.

In therapeutic doses, morphine does not usually exert major effects on the cardiovascular system. Some patients, however, exhibit a propensity to develop orthostatic hypotension and fainting. Rapid intravenous injection is more likely to precipitate a fall in blood pressure than oral dosing.

Morphine can cause histamine release, which appears to be responsible for dilation of cutaneous blood vessels, with resulting flushing of the face and neck, pruritus, and sweating.

PHARMACOKINETICS

ORAMORPH SR Tablets are a sustained release oral dosage form of morphine sulfate. Only about 40% of the administered dose reaches the central compartment because of first-pass effect (i.e., metabolism in the gut wall and liver). Once absorbed, morphine is distributed to skeletal muscle, kidneys, liver, intestinal tract, lungs, spleen and brain. Morphine also crosses the placental membrane and has been found in breast milk.

For all practical purposes, virtually all morphine is converted to glucuronide metabolites; only a small fraction (less than 5%) of absorbed morphine is demethylated. Among these glucuronide metabolites, morphine-3-glucuronide is present in the highest plasma concentration following oral administration; a smaller fraction is converted to morphine-6-glucuronide, which has the greater analgesic activity of these two metabolites.

The glucuronide system has a high capacity and is not easily saturated, even in disease. Therefore, the rate of delivery of morphine to the gut and liver does not influence the total and/or the relative quantities of the various metabolites formed.

The pharmacokinetic parameters following oral administration of ORAMORPH SR, presented in the table below, show considerable inter-subject variation, but are representative of average values reported in the literature. The volume of distribution (Vd) for morphine is 4 liters per kilogram (L/kg), and the terminal elimination half-life is approximately 2 to 4 hours.
[See table above]

Following the administration of conventional, immediate-release, oral morphine products, approximately 50% of the morphine that will ever reach the central compartment, reaches it within 30 minutes. Following the administration of an equal amount of ORAMORPH SR to normal volunteers, however, 50% of absorption occurs, on average, after 1.5 hours.

The possible effect of food upon the systemic bioavailability of ORAMORPH SR has not been evaluated.

Although variation in the physico-mechanical properties of a formulation of an oral morphine drug product can affect both its absolute bioavailability and its absorption rate constant (k_a), morphine distribution and clearance are unchanged, as they are fundamental properties of morphine in the organism. However, in chronic use, the possibility of shifts in metabolite-to-parent drug ratios cannot be excluded.

When immediate-release oral morphine or ORAMORPH SR is given on a fixed dosing regimen, steady-state is achieved in about one or two days.

For a given dose and dosing interval, the Area-Under-the-Curve (AUC) and average blood concentration of morphine at steady-state (C_{SS}) will be independent of the type of oral formulation administered, as long as the formulations have the same absolute bioavailability. The absorption rate of a formulation will, however, affect the maximum (C_{max}) and minimum (C_{min}) plasma concentrations and the time between administration and their occurrence. For any fixed dose and dosing interval, ORAMORPH SR will have, at steady-state, a lower C_{max} and a higher C_{min} than conventional immediate-release morphine, which might be a therapeutic advantage in chronic pain control (see also PHARMACODYNAMICS).

The clearance of morphine occurs primarily as renal excretion of morphine-3-glucuronide. A small amount of the glucuronide conjugate is excreted in the bile, and there is some minor enterohepatic recycling; about 10% of the glucuronide conjugate is excreted in the feces. Because morphine is essentially metabolized in the liver, the effects of renal disease on morphine's clearance are not likely to be pronounced. As with any drug, however, caution should be taken to guard against unanticipated accumulation if renal and/or hepatic function is seriously impaired.

PHARMACODYNAMICS

In clinical settings, morphine's primary actions of therapeutic value are analgesia and sedation. Opiate analgesia involves at least three anatomical areas of the central nervous system: the periaqueductal-periventricular gray matter, the ventromedial medulla, and the spinal cord. Morphine appears to increase the patient's tolerance for pain, and to decrease the discomfort, although the presence of pain itself may still be recognized.

While there is considerable variability in the relationship between morphine blood concentration and analgesic response, effective analgesia probably will not occur below some minimum blood level in a given patient. The minimum effective blood level for analgesia will vary among patients, especially among patients who have been previously treated with potent μ-agonist opioids. Similarly, there is considerable variability in the relationship between morphine plasma concentration and untoward clinical responses, but higher concentrations are more likely to be toxic.

In contrast to immediate-release morphine, after dosing with ORAMORPH SR, the morphine blood levels show reduced fluctuation between peak and trough plasma levels; that means that they are more centered within the theoretical 'therapeutic window'. On the other hand, the reduced fluctuation in morphine plasma concentration might conceivably affect other phenomena, as for example, the rate of tolerance induction.

ORAMORPH SR is an analgesic intended for patients who require chronic morphine analgesia and who will have, in consequence, markedly different degrees of pharmacodynamic tolerance for opioid drugs. Morphine and similar opioids induce tolerance to their effects, so that a shortening of the duration of satisfactory analgesia may be the first sign of an increase in tolerance.

Once patients are started on morphine, the dose required for satisfactory analgesia will rise, with the rate of development of tolerance varying, depending on the patient's prior narcotic use, level of pain, degree of anxiety, use of other CNS-active drugs, circulatory status, total daily dose, and the dosing interval.

INDICATIONS AND USAGE

ORAMORPH SR is indicated for the relief of pain in patients who require opioid analgesics for more than a few days.

Continued on next page

TABLE OF APPROXIMATE[1] AVERAGE PHARMACOKINETIC PARAMETERS FOLLOWING ORAL DOSING OF ORAMORPH SR ®

Pharmacokinetic Parameter [scientific notation] (unit)	Dose of 2 × 15 mg	30 mg	60 mg	100 mg
Bioavailability (oral compared to injectable)	approximately 40%			
Time-to-peak plasma concentration {T_{max}}(h) — mean (range)	3.7 (1–6)	3.8 (1–7)	3.8 (2–7)	3.6 (1.5–12)
Peak plasma concentration {C_{max}} (ng/mL) [single dose] — mean (range)	11.1 (6.5–16.2)	9.9 (5.0–18.6)	16.1 (10.0–25.3)	27.4 14.1–46.1)
Volume of distribution (calculated from mean clearance and terminal half-life) {$Vd(\beta)$} (L/kg) — mean	4 L/kg			

Dose metabolized = approximately 90%
Morphine metabolites (%) = morphine-3-glucuronide (55–75%), morphine-6-glucuronide (1–5%)

[1]Derived from pharmacokinetic studies in 24 normal volunteers

Oramorph SR—Cont.

CONTRAINDICATIONS

ORAMORPH SR is contraindicated in patients with respiratory depression in the absence of resuscitative equipment, in patients with acute or severe bronchial asthma and in patients with known hypersensitivity to morphine.

ORAMORPH SR is contraindicated in any patient who has or is suspected of having a paralytic ileus.

WARNINGS

IMPAIRED RESPIRATION:

Respiratory depression is the chief hazard of all morphine preparations. Respiratory depression occurs more frequently in the elderly and debilitated patients, as well as in those suffering from conditions accompanied by hypoxia or hypercapnia when even moderate therapeutic doses may dangerously decrease pulmonary ventiliation.

Morphine should be used with extreme caution in patients who have a decreased respiratory reserve (e.g., emphysema, severe obesity, kyphoscoliosis, or paralysis of the phrenic nerve). ORAMORPH SR should not be given in cases of chronic asthma, upper airway obstruction, or in any other chronic pulmonary disorder without due consideration of the known risk of acute respiratory failure following morphine administration in such patients.

DRUG ABUSE AND DEPENDENCE

CONTROLLED SUBSTANCE:

Morphine sulfate is a Schedule II narcotic under the United States Controlled Substance Act (21 U.S.C. 801–886).

Morphine is the most commonly cited prototype for narcotic substances that possess an addiction-forming or addition-sustaining liability. A patient may be at risk for developing a dependence to morphine if used improperly or for overly long periods of time. As with all potent opioids which are μ-agonists, tolerance as well as psychological and physical dependence to morphine may develop irrespective of the route of administration (oral, intravenous, intramuscular, intrathecal, epidural). Individuals with a prior history of opioid or other substance abuse or dependence, being more apt to respond to eurphorogenic and reinforcing properties of morphine, would be considered to be at greater risk.

Care must be taken to avert withdrawal symptoms when morphine is discontinued abruptly or upon administration of a narcotic antagonist.

PRECAUTIONS

General Precautions:

Selection of patients for treatment with ORAMORPH SR should be governed by the same principles that apply to the use of morphine or other potent opioid analgesics. Narcotic analgesics are drugs that have a narrow therapeutic index in the old, the sick, and the infirm, i.e., the very population in which their use is indicated. Physicians should individualize treatment with ORAMORPH SR in every case, weighing the need for analgesia against the risk of serious or fatal reactions to the drug.

Use in Patients with Increased Intracranial Pressure or with Head Injury:

ORAMORPH SR should be used with extreme caution in patients with increased intracranial pressure or with head injury. The respiratory depressant effects of morphine (increased pCO_2) may result in elevation of cerebrospinal fluid pressure and may thus be markedly exaggerated in the presence of head injury, other intracranial lesions, or a pre-existing increased intracranial pressure. Morphine produces effects which may obscure neurologic signs of further increases in pressure in patients with head injuries. Pupillary changes (miosis), associated with morphine, may conceal the existence, extent, and course of intracranial pathology.

Use in Hepatic or Renal Disease:

The clearance of morphine may be reduced in patients with hepatic dysfunction, while the clearance of its metabolites may be decreased in renal dysfunction. This will be manifested by both, a prolonged elimination half-life and the accumulation of levels of either morphine or its metabolites in excess of those produced in normals, with the potential for an increase of adverse effects (see WARNINGS and ADVERSE REACTIONS). These changes in morphine pharmacodynamics, in patients with hepatic or renal dysfunctions, should be considered when adjusting the dose and dosage intervals, taking also into account the slow-release character of ORAMORPH SR.

Drug Interactions:

Use with Other Central Nervous System Depressants:

The depressant effects of morphine are potentiated by the presence of other CNS depressants such as alcohol, sedatives, antihistaminics, or psychotropic drugs. Use of neuroleptics in conjunction with oral morphine may increase the risk of respiratory depression, hypotension and profound sedation or coma.

Interaction with Mixed Agonist/Antagonist Opioid Analgesics:

Agonist/antagonist analgesics (i.e., pentazocine, nalbuphine, butorphanol, or buprenorphine) should NOT be administered to patients who have received or are receiving a course of therapy with a pure opioid agonist analgesic. In these patients, the mixed agonist/antagonist may alter the analgesic effect or may precipitate withdrawal symptoms.

Carcinogenesis, Mutagenesis, Impairment of Fertility:

Studies of morphine sulfate in animals to evaluate the drug's carcinogenic and mutagenic potential or the effect on fertility have not been conducted.

Pregnancy:

Teratogenic Effects—Category C: There are no well-controlled studies in women, but marketing experience does not include any evidence of adverse effects on the fetus following routine (short-term) clinical use of morphine sulfate products. Although there is no clearly defined risk, such experience cannot exclude the possibility of infrequent or subtle damage to the human fetus.

ORAMORPH SR should be used in pregnant women only when clearly needed. (See also: PRECAUTIONS: Labor and Delivery, and DRUG ABUSE AND DEPENDENCE CONTROLLED SUBSTANCE.)

Nonteratogenic Effects:

Infants born from mothers who have been taking morphine chronically may exhibit withdrawal symptoms.

Labor and Delivery:

ORAMORPH SR is not recommended for use in women during and immediately prior to labor. Occasionally, opioid analgesics may prolong labor through actions which temporarily reduce the strength, duration and frequency of uterine contractions.

Neonates, whose mothers received opioid analgesics during labor, should be observed closely for signs of respiratory depression. A specific narcotic antagonist, naloxone, should be available for reversal of narcotic-induced respiratory depression in the neonate.

Nursing Mothers:

ORAMORPH SR should not be given to nursing mothers because morphine is excreted in maternal milk. Effects on the nursing infant are not known, but withdrawal symptoms can occur in breast-fed infants when maternal administration of morphine sulfate is stopped.

Pediatric Use:

ORAMORPH SR has not been evaluated in children. Its use in the pediatric population is, therefore, not recommended.

Use in the Aged:

The pharmacodynamic effects of morphine in the aged are more variable than in the younger population. Patients will vary widely in the effective initial dose, rate of development of tolerance, and the frequency and magnitude of associated adverse effects as the dose is increased. Individualization of doses must receive careful attention in elderly patients.

Information for Patients:

If clinically advisable, patients receiving ORAMORPH SR brand or morphine sulfate sustained release tablets, should be given the following instructions by the physician:

1. Morphine may produce psychological and/or physical dependence. For this reason, the dose of the drug should not be increased without consulting a physician.
2. Morphine may impair mental and/or physical ability required for the performance of potentially hazardous tasks (e.g., driving, operating machinery).
3. Morphine should not be taken with alcohol or other CNS depressants (sleep aids, tranquilizers) because additive effects, including CNS depression, may occur. A physician should be consulted if other prescription and/or over-the-counter medications are currently being used or are prescribed for future use.
4. For women of childbearing potential, who become or are planning to become pregnant, a physician should be consulted regarding analgesics and other drug use.

ADVERSE REACTIONS

> **NOTE:** THE SUSTAINED RELEASE OF MORPHINE FROM ORAMORPH SR SHOULD BE TAKEN INTO CONSIDERATION IN THE EVENT OF OCCURRING ADVERSE REACTIONS.

Adverse reactions caused by morphine are essentially those observed with other opioid analgesics. They include the following *major hazards:* **respiratory depression,** and less frequently, **circulatory depression, apnea, shock** and **cardiac arrest** secondary to respiratory and/or circulatory depression.

Most Frequently Observed Reactions:

Constipation, nausea, vomiting, lightheadedness, dizziness sedation, dysphoria, euphoria, and sweating. Some of these effects seem to be more prominent in ambulatory patients and in those not experiencing severe pain. Some adverse reactions in ambulatory patients may be alleviated if the patient is in a supine position.

Less Frequently Observed Reactions:

Body as a Whole: Edema, antidiuretic effect, chills, muscle tremor, muscle rigidity.

Cardiovascular: Flushing of the face, tachycardia, bradycardia, palpitation, faintness, syncope, hypotension, hypertension.

Gastrointestinal: Dry mouth, biliary tract spasm, laryngospasm, anorexia, diarrhea, cramps, taste alterations.

Genitourinary: Urine retention or hesitance, reduced libido and/or potency.

Nervous System: Weakness, headache, agitation, tremor, uncoordinated muscle movements, seizure, paresthesia, alterations of mood (nervousness, apprehension, depression, floating feelings), dreams, transient hallucination and disorientation, visual disturbances, insomnia, increased intracranial pressure.

Skin: Pruritus, urticaria and other skin rashes.

Special Senses: Blurred vision, nystagmus, diplopia, miosis.

DRUG ABUSE AND DEPENDENCE

Opioid analgesics may cause psychological and physical dependence (see WARNINGS). Physical dependence results in withdrawal symptoms in patients who abruptly discontinue the drug, or these symptoms may be precipitated through the administration of drugs with antagonistic activity, e.g., naloxone or mixed agonist/antagonist analgesics (pentazocine, etc.; see also OVERDOSAGE). Physical dependence usually does not occur, to a clinically significant degree, until several weeks of continued opioid usage. Tolerance, in which increasingly larger doses are required to produce the same degree of analgesia, is initially manifested by a shortened duration of a analgesic effect and, subsequently, by decreases in the intensity of analgesia. In patients with chronic pain, as well as in opioid-tolerant cancer patients, the administration of ORAMORPH SR (morphine sulfate) should be guided by the degree of tolerance manifested. Physical dependence, *per se,* is not ordinarily a concern when one is dealing with opioid-tolerant patients whose pain and suffering is associated with an irreversible illness.

If ORAMORPH SR is abruptly discontinued, an abstinence syndrome may occur. Withdrawal symptoms, in patients dependent on morphine, begin shortly before the time of the next scheduled dose, reaching a peak at 36 to 72 hours after the last dose, and then slowly subside over a period of 7 to 10 days. Symptoms include yawning, sweating, lacrimation, rhinorrhea, restless sleep, dilated pupils, gooseflesh, irritability, tremor, nausea, vomiting, and diarrhea.

Treatment of the abstinence syndrome is primarily symptomatic and supportive, including maintenance of proper fluid and electrolyte balance. If withdrawal has inadvertently been precipitated in a patient who requires narcotics for pain management, the withdrawal syndrome can be terminated rapidly by the administration of an appropriate dose of a pure agonist opioid, such as morphine. The degree of physical dependence of a patient on ORAMORPH SR can be intentionally reduced by a gradual reduction of dosage and symptomatic treatment of withdrawal symptomatology.

OVERDOSAGE

> **NOTE:** THE SUSTAINED RELEASE OF MORPHINE FROM **ORAMORPH SR** SHOULD BE TAKEN INTO CONSIDERATION IN THE EVENT OF AN OVERDOSAGE.

Overdosage of morphine is characterized by respiratory depression, with or without concomitant CNS depression. Since respiratory arrest may result either through direct depression of the respiratory center, or as the result of hypoxia, primary attention should be given to the establishment of adequate respiratory exchange through provision of a patent airway and institution of assisted, or controlled, ventilation. The narcotic antagonist, naloxone, is a specific antidote. An initial dose of 0.4 to 2 mg of naloxone should be administered intravenously, simultaneously with respiratory resuscitation. If the desired degree of counteraction and improvement in respiratory function is not obtained, naloxone may be repeated at 2 to 3 minute intervals. If no response is observed after 10 mg of naloxone has been administered, the diagnosis of narcotic-induced, or partial narcotic-induced, toxicity should be questioned. Intramuscular or subcutaneous administration may be used if the intravenous route is not available.

As the duration of effect of naloxone is considerably shorter than that of ORAMORPH SR, repeated administration may be necessary. Patients should be closely observed for evidence of renarcotization.

> NOTE: In a individual physically dependent on opioids, administration of the usual dose of the antagonist will precipitate an acute withdrawal syndrome. The severity of the withdrawal syndrome produced will depend on the degree of physical dependence and the dose of the antagonist administered. Use of a narcotic antagonist in such a person should be avoided. If necessary to treat serious respiratory depression in a physically dependent patient, the antagonist should be administered with extreme care and by titration with smaller than usual dose of the antagonist.

When indicated, gut decontamination should be performed via emesis and/or activated charcoal (60 to 100 g in adults, 1

to 2 g/kg in children) with cathartic. Since ORAMORPH SR is a sustained release product, absorption may be expected to continue for many hours, particularly following an overdose, combined with decreased peristaltic activity of the gastrointestinal tract.

Supportive measures (including oxygen, vasopressors) should be employed in the management of circulatory shock and pulmonary edema accompanying overdose as indicated. Cardiac arrest or arrhythmias may require cardiac massage or defibrillation.

DOSAGE AND ADMINISTRATION

(See also: CLINICAL PHARMACOLOGY, WARNINGS and PRECAUTIONS sections.)

NOTE: ORAMORPH SR TABLET MUST BE SWALLOWED WHOLE. DO NOT BREAK THE TABLET IN HALF. DO NOT CRUSH OR CHEW. TAKING BROKEN, CHEWED OR CRUSHED TABLETS COULD LEAD TO THE RAPID RELEASE AND ABSORPTION OF A POTENTIALLY TOXIC DOSE OF MORPHINE.

ORAMORPH SR is intended for use in patients who require more than several days of continuous treatment with a potent opioid analgesic. The sustained release nature of the formulation allows it to be administered on a more convenient schedule than conventional immediate-release oral morphine products (see CLINICAL PHARMACOLOGY—PHARMACOKINETICS). However, ORAMORPH SR does not release morphine continuously over the course of a dosing interval. The administration of single doses of ORAMORPH SR on a q12h dosing schedule will result in peak and trough plasma levels similar to those following an identical daily dose of morphine administered using conventional oral formulations on a q4h regimen. If pain is not controlled for a full 12 hours, then the dosing interval should be shortened, but to no less than 8 hours.

As with any potent opioid, it is critical to adjust the dosing regimen for each patient individually, taking into account the patient's prior analgesic treatment experience. Although it is not possible to enumerate every condition that is important to the selection of the initial dose and dosing interval of ORAMORPH SR, attention should be given to (1) the daily dose, potency and characteristics of a pure agonist, or mixed agonist-antagonist, the patient has been taking previously, (2) the reliability of the relative potentcy estimate to calculate the dose of morphine needed [N.B.: potency estimates may vary with the route of administration], (3) the fact that roughly only 40% of the morphine sulfate in ORAMORPH SR becomes available after pre-systemic metabolization in the intestinal wall and liver, (4) the degree of opioid tolerance, and (5) the general condition and medical status of the patient.

The following dosing recommendation for ORAMORPH SR therefore, can only be considered suggested approaches to the series of clinical decisions in the management of pain of an individual patient.

Conversion from Conventional Immediate-Release Oral Morphine to ORAMORPH SR:

A patient's daily morphine requirement is established by using the Daily Oral Morphine Requirement of the immediate-release formulation which gives the Daily Oral Morphine Requirement for ORAMORPH SR. Since ORAMORPH SR is given on an 'every 12 hour' schedule, the single dose of ORAMORPH SR is half of the Daily Oral Morphine Requirement. Dose and dosing interval is adjusted as needed (see discussion below). For initial conversion, the 30 mg tablet strength is recommended for patients with a daily morphine requirement of 120 mg or less.

Conversion from Parental Morphine or Other Opioid Analgesics (parental or oral) to ORAMORPH SR:

Because of uncertainty about relative estimates of opioid potency and cross tolerance, as well as intersubject variation, initial dosing regimens should be conservative, i.e., an underestimation of the 24-hour oral morphine requirement is preferred to an overestimate. To this end, initial individual doses of ORAMORPH SR should be estimated conservatively. In patients whose daily morphine requirements are expected to be less than or equal to 120 mg per day, the 30 mg tablet strength is recommended for the initial titration period. Once a stable dose regimen is reached, the patient can be converted to the 60 mg or 100 mg tablet strength, as appropriate.

Estimates of the relative potency of opioids are only approximate, and are influenced by route of administration, individual patient differences, and possibly, by the patient's medical condition. Consequently, it is difficult to recommend any precise rule for converting a patient to ORAMORPH SR directly. However, the following general points should be considered:

1. *Parenteral to oral morphine ratio:* Estimates of the oral-to-parenteral potency of morphine vary. Some authorities suggest that a dose of morphine only 3 times the daily parenteral morphine requirement may be sufficient in chronic use settings. (3 times the Daily Parenteral Morphine Requirement = the Daily Oral Morphine Requirement)
2. *Oral parenteral or oral opioids to oral morphine:* Because of a lack of reliable relative potency assays, specific recommendations are not possible. In general, it is safer to underestimate the Total Daily Dose of ORAMORPH SR required and rely upon *ad hoc* supplementation to deal with inadequate analgesia (see discussion which follows).

Use of ORAMORPH SR as the First Opioid Analgesic:

There has been no systematic evaluation of ORAMORPH SR as an initial opioid analgesic in the management of pain. Because it may be more difficult to titrate a patient using a sustained release morphine, it is ordinarily advisable to begin treatment using an immediate release formulation.

Considerations in the Adjustment of Dosing Regimens.

Whatever the approach, if signs of excessive opioid effects are observed early in a dosing interval, the next dose should be reduced. If this adjustment leads to inadequate analgesia, i.e., 'breakthrough' pain occurs late in the dosing interval, the dosing interval may be shortened. Alternatively, a supplemental dose of a short-acting analgesic may be given. As experience is gained, adjustments can be made to obtain an appropriate balance between pain relief, opioid side effects and the convenience of the dosing schedule.

In adjusting dose requirements, it is recommended that the dosing interval never be extended beyond 12 hours, because the administration of very large single doses of ORAMORPH SR may lead to acute overdosage.

For patients with low daily morphine requirements, the 15 mg tablet should be used. In this regard, adjustment in dose should NOT be attempted by breaking or crushing the tablets. ORAMORPH SR tablets are intended to be swallowed whole.

Conversion from ORAMORPH SR to Parenteral Opioids:

When converting a patient from ORAMORPH SR to parenteral opioids, it is best to assume that the parenteral to oral potency relationship is high. NOTE THAT THIS IS THE CONVERSE OF THE STRATEGY USED WHEN THE DIRECTION OF CONVERSION IS FROM THE PARENTERAL TO ORAL FORMULATIONS. IN BOTH CASES, HOWEVER, THE AIM IS TO ESTIMATE THE NEW DOSE CONSERVATIVELY. For example, to estimate the required 24-hour dose of morphine for IM use, one could employ a conversion of 1 mg of morphine IM for every 6 mg of morphine as ORAMORPH SR. Of course, the IM 24-hour dose would have to be divided by six and administered on a q4h regimen. This approach is recommended because it is least likely to cause overdosage.

HOW SUPPLIED

ORAMORPH SR® (Morphine Sulfate)

Sustained Release Tablets

15 mg white tablets (Identified 54 782)

[Embossed with 15]

NDC 0054-8790-24: Unit dose, 25 tablets per card (reverse numbered), 4 cards per shipper.

NDC 0054-4790-25: Bottles of 100 tablets.

NDC 0054-4790-29: Bottles of 500 tablets.

30 mg white tablets (Identified 54 409)

[Embossed with 30]

NDC 0054-8805-24: Unit dose, 25 tablets per card (reverse numbered), 4 cards per shipper.

NDC 0054-4805-19: Bottles of 50 tablets.

NDC 0054-4805-25: Bottles of 100 tablets.

NDC 0054-4805-27: Bottles of 250 tablets.

60 mg white tablets (Identified 54 933)

[Embossed with 60]

NDC 0054-8792-11: Unit dose, 25 tablets per card (reverse numbered), 1 card per shipper.

NDC 0054-4792-25: Bottles of 100 tablets.

100 mg white tablets (Identified 54 862)

[Embossed with 100]

NDC 0054-8793-11: Unit dose, 25 tablets per card (reverse numbered), 1 card per shipper.

NDC 0054-4793-25: Bottles of 100 tablets.

DEA Order Form Required.

Dispense in a tight, light-resistant container.

Storage: ORAMORPH SR Tablets should be stored in unopened containers at or below room temperature.

Caution: Federal law prohibits dispensing without prescription. Federal law prohibits the transfer of this drug to any person other than the patient for whom it was prescribed.

Safety and Handling Instructions:

ORAMORPH SR is supplied as tablets that pose little risk of direct exposure to health care personnel and should be handled and disposed of in accordance with hospital policy. Patients and their families should be instructed to dispose of ORAMORPH SR tablets, that are no longer needed, down the toilet.

4073305 Revised February 1995

025

Roxane

Laboratories, Inc.

Columbus, Ohio 43216

Shown in Product Identification Guide, page 335

ORLAAM® CII ℞

Levomethadyl Acetate Hydrochloride Oral Solution

(Warning: May be habit forming.)

CONDITIONS FOR DISTRIBUTION AND USE OF ORLAAM (21 CFR 291.505)

ORLAAM, used for the treatment of narcotic addiction, shall be dispensed only by treatment programs approved by FDA, DEA and the designated state authority. Approved treatment programs shall dispense and use ORLAAM in oral form only and according to the treatment requirements stipulated in Federal regulations. Failure to abide by these requirements may result in injunction precluding operation of the program, seizure of the drug supply, revocation of the program approval, and possible criminal prosecution.

ORLAAM has no recommended uses outside of the treatment of opiate addiction.

DESCRIPTION

ORLAAM (brand of levomethadyl acetate hydrochloride) is a synthetic opiate agonist. Chemically, it is levo-alpha-6-dimethylamino-4, 4-diphenyl-3-heptyl acetate hydrochloride, $C_{23}H_{31}NO_2$ • HCl. It is also known as levo-alpha-acetymethadol hydrochloride (LAAM). The structural formula is:

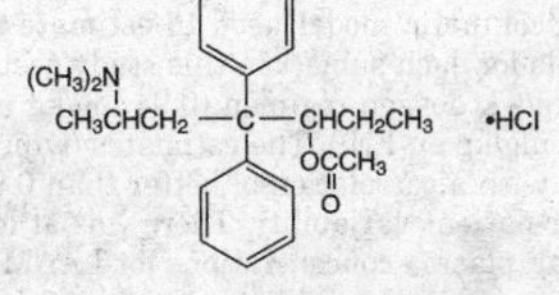

The compound is a white crystalline powder, soluble in water (>15 mg/mL), ethanol, and methyl ethyl ketone. The octanol:water partition coefficient of LAAM is 405:1 at physiologic pH. Doses of ORLAAM (LAAM) are always expressed as the weight of the hydrochloride salt (molecular weight 389.95).

ORLAAM is an aqueous solution which is diluted for oral administration. Each one mL of ORLAAM contains: Levomethadyl acetate hydrochloride (LAAM) 10 mg.

Inactive ingredients: methylparaben, propylparaben, hydrochloric acid, and water.

CLINICAL PHARMACOLOGY

LAAM is a synthetic opioid agonist with actions qualitatively similar to morphine (a prototypic mu agonist) and affecting the central nervous system (CNS) and smooth muscle. Principal actions include analgesia and sedation. Tolerance to these effects develops with repeated use. An abstinence syndrome generally occurs upon cessation of chronic administration similar to that observed with other opiates, but with slower onset, more prolonged course, and less severe symptoms.

LAAM exerts its clinical effects in the treatment of opiate abuse through two mechanisms. First, LAAM cross-substitutes for opiates of the morphine-type, suppressing symptoms of withdrawal in opiate-dependent individuals. Second, chronic oral administration of LAAM can produce sufficient tolerance to block the subjective "high" of usual doses of parenterally administered opiates.

LAAM is metabolized by N-demethylation to nor-LAAM and dinor-LAAM, which are also opioid agonists. These metabolities are more potent than the parent drug. The opiod effect which occurs when LAAM is administered is slower in onset and longer in duration (72 hours) than that of methadone (24 hours). This extended duration of action allows three-times-weekly administration (see CLINICAL TRIALS).

PHARMACODYNAMICS

The duration of action of a single dose of LAAM is due to the sum of the opioid activity of the parent drug and its metabolites. A single dose of orally administered LAAM has an onset of opioid effects averaging 2 to 4 hours of ingestion and a duration of action of 48 to 72 hours (as measured by pupillary constriction and suppression of abstinence signs). LAAM cross-substitutes for opiates like morphine in opiate-dependent individuals, suppressing symptom of withdrawal from these compounds. Single oral doses of 30 to 60 mg of LAAM eliminate signs of abstinence for 24 to 48 hours in individuals maintained on high doses of morphine who are abruptly withdrawn. At higher doses (80 mg and above), suppression of withdrawal can increase to 48 to 72 hours in most individuals.

Repeated oral administration of LAAM can produce sufficient tolerance to block the effects of parenterally administered opiates. Chronic oral administration of 70 to 100 mg of

Continued on next page

Orlaam—Cont.

LAAM three times weekly produces tolerance which blocks the "high" of a 25 mg dose of intravenously administered heroin for up to 72 hours; maintenance on lower does (50 mg) of LAAM produces only partial blockage for the same period.

PHARMACOKINETICS

Absorption

LAAM is rapidly absorbed from an oral solution. Plasma levels are detectable within 15 to 30 minutes after ingestion and reach their peak within 1.5 to 2 hours at steady-state. LAAM undergoes first-pass metabolism to its demethylated metabolite nor-LAAM, which is sequentially N-demethylated to dinor-LAAM. Both metabolites are active and contribute to the extent and duration of ORLAAM's clinical activity (see PHARMACODYNAMICS).

Pharmacokinetic Model

The steady-state pharmacokinetics of LAAM were modeled from a study in 25 health adult addicts using three-times-a-week dosing over a 15-day observation period. LAAM and its metabolites were found to follow a multu-compartment model with extensive tissue distribution (Vd - 20 L/kg). LAAM had a clearance of about 0.22 L/kg/hr, mostly by conversion to nor-LAAM. Kinetic studies of the pure metabolites in man have not yet provided accurate estimates of their clearance in the absence of the precursor, but the half-lives observed in this study were 2.6 days for LAAM, approximately 2 days for non-LAAM, and approximately 4 days for dinor-LAAM.

The pharmacokinetic model used to estimate steady-state plasma levels for each subject in this study assumed a common 3 mg/kg/wk dosage regimen (0.94 mg/kg on Mon. and Wed., 1.125 mg/kg on Fri.). The estimates (which fit the observed data with a correlation of better than 0.95) revealed a large inter-patient variability. There was at least a 5-fold range in peak plasma concentrations for LAAM and its metabolites across the 25 subjects over the 72-hour interval from Friday to Monday on a 3-times-a-week dosage regimen. Table 1 contains these estimates of peak and trough plasma concentrations of LAAM, nor-LAAM, and dinor-LAAM.

Table 1: Peak and Trough Estimated Steady-State Plasma Concentrations During the 72 Hour Interval (Friday to Monday) for 65-kg Patient Given 3 mg/kg/Week on Mon./Wed./Fri.

	LAAM Mean (CV)	Nor-LAAM Mean (CV)	Dinor-LAAM Mean (CV)
Cmax(ng/mL)*	204 (34%)	173 (34%)	114 (28%)
Cmin(ng/mL)**	36 (62%)	85 (58%)	96 (34%)

* Following Friday Morning Does
** Prior to Monday Morning Dose

Figure 1: Simulated Steady-State Plasma Concentrations of LAAM, Nor-LAAM and Dinor-LAAM following Thrice Weekly Dosing with ORLAAM

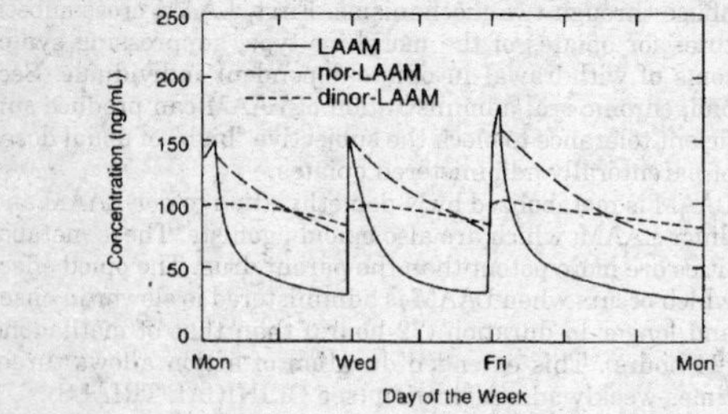

Metabolism and Elimination

As noted above, the information of nor-LAAM and dinor-LAAM is by sequential demethylation, such that dinor-LAAM is formed from nor-LAAM, not directly from LAAM. While N-demethylation is the primary route of metabolism, minor pathways of elimination include direct excretion and deacetylation to methadol, nor-methadol, and dinor-methadol.

Special Populations

Gender

An analysis of the data from the above study showed some differences in the plasma clearance of LAAM in 8 females versus 17 males. Males showed a trend toward a slower conversion of LAAM to nor-LAAM, which may alter the plasma concentration profile of LAAM and its active opioid metabolites. Although this effect was much smaller than the observed inter-individual differences, physicians should be alert to a possible gender difference (see INDIVIDUALIZATION OF DOSAGE).

Hepatic and Renal Disease

At the present time no pharmacokinetics studies have been carried out in subjects with clinically significant hepatic insufficiency or serious renal impairment. Since both the pharmacokinetics and pharmacodynamics of opiate agonists may be altered in these subjects, and any additional risks of ORLAAM therapy are not well understood in such patients, physicians may choose to manage such patients with methadone due to its simpler metabolic profile.

CLINICAL TRIALS

ORLAAM has been studied in 2666 street addicts and 3319 methadone maintenance patients, including 5697 males and 288 females. During the course of 27 studies, 4610 patients received orally administered ORLAAM for up to three years in thrice-weekly doses ranging from 10 to 140 mg. Twenty-one studies provide the primary evidence upon which the dosing recommendations for ORLAAM are based. The vast majority of patients who received ORLAAM were treated on a thrice-weekly basis, typically on Mondays, Wednesdays and Fridays (Mon./Wed./Fri.), although every-other-day dosing schedules were used in some settings. Most of the sites dosing patients with LAAM on a 3-times-a-week (Mon./Wed./Fri. or Tues./Thurs./Sat.) schedule increased the dose prior to the 72-hour inter-dose interval by 20 to 40% to obtain coverage for the full 72 hours.

In controlled clinical trials, treatment with ORLAAM was found to be comparable to treatment with methadone with respect to reduction in use of illicit opioids. ORLAAM doses in the range of 60 to 100 mg 3-times-a-week reduced the average frequency of urine samples positive for opiates to 15–20%, as did therapy with 50 to 100 mg a day of methadone. There was a trend for more patients to drop out of ORLAAM therapy than methadone therapy in the first 4 weeks of treatment (16% dropouts for ORLAAM v. 12% for methadone), but the dropout rates for both treatments rapidly declined and both were in the range of 1 to 2% per week for the remaining patients by the third month of the studies. Global ratings of patient acceptability and response to treatment were similar for both LAAM and methadone.

In the Phase III studies, ORLAAM tended to be more effective in patients perceived by staff to benefit from a reduced frequency of clinic visits and less effective in patients perceived as needing the added support of daily clinic visits.

Four independent studies were concerned with other research objectives, including induction regimens, methadone-to-ORLAAM (and ORLAAM-to-methadone) crossover ratios, and detoxification. This research involved 800 adults (including 11 females), approximately 440 of whom were methadone maintenance patients. The results of these studies, as well as the results of a nationwide Phase III usage study of 623 patients (including 204 females) in 25 representative clinics across the country, are reflected in the dosing recommendations.

INDIVIDUALIZATION OF DOSAGE

ORLAAM is intended for use as part of a comprehensive treatment plan for narcotic dependence of the opioid type. Supplying narcotic drugs to narcotic addicts for the treatment of addiction without appropriate medical evaluation, treatment planning, and counseling has not been shown to be effective, and is a violation of the law except in special circumstances.

The therapeutic goal early in treatment with ORLAAM is to reduce illicit opioid use. The dose of ORLAAM should be chosen and adjusted as needed to provide a dose that is high enough to suppress drug withdrawal, illicit drug seeking and usage, and related high-risk behavior. If opioid side effects persist once illicit dry use is controlled, the dose of ORLAAM may require further adjustment later in treatment to minimize adverse effects.

Physicians should be alert to patient differences in levels of opioid tolerance and inter-patient variability in the absorption, distribution and metabolism of both ORLAAM and its metabolites. As with methadone, an important contribution to continued abuse of illicit drugs is an inadequate dose of the treatment medication.

Initial dosage adjustment with ORLAAM is complex due to its delayed onset of action. If the starting dose is too high or if the dose is escalated too rapidly for the patient's level of tolerance, symptoms characteristic of excessive opioid effect may occur, i.e., poor concentration, sedation, and orthostatic hypotension. Patients should be watched for such symptoms, and the dose should be lowered if they appear. In rare instances, serious symptoms of narcotic overdosage may occur, leading to profound CNS and respiratory depression.

ORLAAM and its metabolites quickly accumulate to toxic levels if the doses intended for 3-times-a-week dosing are given too frequently. The recommended doses are intended for every-other-day or 3-times-a-week dosing and **should not be given daily.**

The recommended initial dose for patients with low or unknown tolerance to opioids is 20 to 40 mg **three-times-a-week** or **every-other-day**. Successive doses may be increased by 5 to 10 mg. At least two weeks are needed to achieve a clinical plateau after a dosage adjustment. Adjustment to a dosing schedule is dependent upon the rate at which an individual develops tolerance to the increaseing level of ORLAAM (and its metabolites) as well as the time required for ORLAAM and its metabolites to accumulate to steady-state levels.

The goal of dosage titration is to suppress narcotic withdrawal while avoiding excessive opioid effects due to the build-up of long-acting metabolites. It may be safer to provide extra counseling and support rather than to attempt to completely suppress a patient's withdrawal or narcotic hunger during the first week or two of therapy. On the other hand, there is the ever-present danger that patients who receive sub-therapeutic starting doses will supplement with street drugs, resulting in overdose. Patients should be strongly warned against this practice. Later in the titration process, dosage adjustments are better made on a weekly basis whenever possible.

For patients on methadone maintenance whose level of tolerance is known, the recommended initial dose of ORLAAM is 1.2 to 1.3 times the patient's daily dose of methadone, not to exceed 120 mg. Care should be taken not to adjust the dose too frequently thereafter (usually 5 to 10 mg changes every second or third dose) since increasing the dose too rapidly may result in oversedation.

One major advantage of ORLAAM therapy is reduction in need for daily clinic visits and for take-home medication. In some patients, ORLAAM may not provide adequate suppression of withdrawal for a full 72 hours. For such individuals, several therapeutic options are available: (1) extra support and an explanation of reasons for the effect, (2) increasing the dose given prior to the 72-hour interval, (3) switching to an every-other-day dosing schedule, (4) dispensing a supplemental methadone dose.

Most patients do not experience withdrawal during 72-hour inter-dose interval after reaching pharmacological steady-state **with** or **without** adjustment of the Friday dose. If additional opioids are required, small doses of supplemental methadone should be given rather than giving ORLAAM on two consecutive days. Take-home doses of methadone always pose a risk in this setting and physicians should carefully weigh the potential therapeutic benefit against the risk of diversion (see DOSAGE AND ADMINISTRATION).

Patients should receive extra support and counseling and be warned against supplementing street drugs as they make the switch from methadone to ORLAAM. The variability in the clearance of LAAM, nor-LAAM, and dinor-LAAM and clinical experience suggest that there will be a small number of patients who require either lower or higher doses than those recommended.

DURATION OF ORLAAM THERAPY

There is no information from controlled clinical trials as to the appropriate duration of ORLAAM therapy. There are reports from investigators that some patients on ORLAAM may experience less variation in opioid effects and have less drug craving than with methadone, so ORLAAM should be considered for patients who need long-term maintenance during social and vocational rehabilitation.

When a patient has eliminated illicit drug use, achieved social and occupational stability, and made lifestyle changes to reduce the risk of relapse, consideration may be given to discontinuation of ORLAAM therapy. Such a decision should be carefully considered as part of an individualized treatment plan. Stable long-term ORLAAM therapy is preferable to repeated cycles of premature discontinuation of medication followed by relapse to uncontrolled addiction.

A patient is most likely to remain abstinent if discontinuation of medication is attempted after the achievement of behavioral objectives and is accompanied by appropriate non-pharmacological support. The rate of dose reduction should vary according to patient's response. Discontinuation of ORLAAM therapy for administrative reasons or because of adverse reactions to the drug should be managed as described below under DOSAGE AND ADMINISTRATION.

INDICATIONS

ORLAAM is indicated for the management of opiate dependence.

CONTRAINDICATIONS

The only known contraindication in the treatment of opiate dependence is hypersensitivity to LAAM.

ORLAAM is not recommended for any use other than for the treatment of opioid dependence (see WARNINGS).

WARNINGS

Administration of ORLAAM on a daily basis has led to excessive drug accumulation and risk of fatal overdose. ORLAAM has only been studied on a thrice-weekly or every-other-day dosing regimen. Routine daily dosing after a patient has been inducted onto ORLAAM treatment is not allowed by current treatment regulations. Any decision to administer ORLAAM more frequently than every other day for any reason should be approached with extreme caution. Even then only very small doses (5 to 10 mg) should be considered.

Risk of Overdose: Analysis of some of the deaths from overdose observed in the development of ORLAAM has shown that when ORLAAM is diverted into channels of abuse, the uninformed addict can become impatient with the slow onset of ORLAAM (2 to 4 hours) and take illicit drugs, resulting in a potentially lethal combined overdose when the peak ORLAAM effect develops. Due to these risks of diversion and accidental death, ORLAAM has been approved for use only when **dispensed** by a licensed facility and is not given in take-home doses.

Use of Narcotic Antagonist: In an individual receiving ORLAAM, the administration of the usual dose of a narcotic antagonist may precipitate an acute withdrawal syndrome. The severity of this syndrome depends on the dose of the antagonist administered and the patient's level of physical dependence. Narcotic antagonist should be used in patients receiving ORLAAM only if needed. If a narcotic antagonist is used to treat respiratory depression in the physically dependent patient, it should be administered with care and titration should begin with much smaller-than-usual doses (0.1 to 0.2 mg recommended). If the desired effect is not achieved, escalating doses may be administered every 2 to 3 minutes. If a cumulative dose of 10 mg of naloxone has been given without effect, further administration is unlikely to be of benefit (see OVERDOSAGE).

If the patient does respond to narcotic antagonist, physicians should remember that naloxone has a much shorter duration of action than ORLAAM. Such patients should remain under prolonged observation rather than being allowed to leave emergency treatment, since ORLAAM's action will outlast naloxone-induced reversal, putting the unsupervised patient at risk of relapse, a return of respiratory depression and possible death if continuing medical attention is not avaiable. Use of other parenteral opioid antagonists may be appropriate in some cases, but only if the dosage of such drugs can be readily titrated. Oral naltrexone would not be appropriate for the treatment of ORLAAM overdose, as it has been associated with the precipitation of prolonged opioid withdrawal symptoms when used in overdose settings.

Warnings to Patients:

> Patients must be warned that the peak activity of ORLAAM is not immediate, and that use or abuse of other psychoactive drugs, including alcohol, may result in **fatal** overdose, especially with the first few doses of ORLAAM, either during initation of treatment of after a lapse in treatment.

Use in High Risk Patients: Suicide attempts with opiates, especially in combination with tricyclic antidepressants, alcohol, and other CNS active agents, are part of the clinical pattern of addiction. Although outpatient therapy with ORLAAM and other drugs of this class is usually associated with a reduction in the risk of suicide, such risk is not eliminated. Individualized evaluation and treatment planning, including hospitalization, should be considered for patients who continue to exhibit uncontrolled drug use and persistent high-risk behavior despite adequate pharmacotherapy.

PRECAUTIONS

Initial Administration and Dosage Adjustment: Due to the long half-lives of ORLAAM and its metabolites, patients will not feel the full effects of the medication for at least several days. Consequently, extra care is needed when starting patients on ORLAAM and when making initial dosage adjustments (see INDIVIDUALIZATION OF DOSAGE and DOSAGE AND ADMINISTRATION)

Use In Ambulatory Patients: Initiation of therapy or excessive doses of ORLAAM may impair the mental and/or physical abilities required for performance of potentially hazardous tasks, such as driving a car or operating machinery. Patients should be warned not to engage in such activities if their alertness and behavior are affected. Most patients show no detectable impairment of ordinary tasks on ORLAAM therapy.

Head Injury and Increased Intracranial Pressure: The respiratory depressant effects of narcotics and their capacity to elevate cerebrospinal fluid pressure may be markedly exaggerated in the presence of increased intracranial pressure. Furthermore, narcotics produce side effects that may make it difficult to evaluate the clinical course of patients with head injuries. In view of LAAM's profile as a mu agonist, it should be used with extreme caution and only if deemed essential in such patients.

Asthma and Other Respiratory Conditions: ORLAAM, as with other opioids, should be used with caution in patients with asthma, in those with chronic obstructive pulmonary disease or cor pulmonale, and in individuals with a substantially decreased respiratory reserve, preexisting respiratory depression, hypoxia, or hypercapnea. In such patients, even usual therapeutic doses of narcotics may decrease respiratory drive while simultaneously increasing airway resistance to the point of apnea.

Special Risk Patients: Opioids should be given with caution and at reduced initial dose in certain patients, such as the elderly or debilitated and those with significant hepatic or renal dysfunction, hypothyroidism, Addison's Disease, prostatic hypertrophy, or urethral stricture.

Effects on Cardiac Conduction: ORLAAM has been shown to prolong the ST segment of the electrocardiogram in beagle dogs dosed five days a week. Serial EKGs performed in a pharmacokinetics study showed a prolongation of the QTc interval in some patients which was not associated with dose.

Such a prolongation of the QTc interval has been seen with other opioids, and it is not known if this is an effect specific to a LAAM or if it is also seen with methadone. In either case, careful monitoring is recommended when using ORLAAM in patients with a history of known cardiac conduction defects, those taking medications affecting cardiac conduction and in other cases where an unusual risk of dysrhythmia is suggested by history or physical examination. This information is provided to alert the prescribing physician, and is not intended to deter the appropriate use of opioid agonists in patients with a history of cardiac disease. No adverse cardiac events have been associated with ORLAAM therapy in clinical study of the drug, and the risk of morbidity from treatment with either methadone or LAAM is less than the risk of morbidity from untreated addiction.

Acute Abdominal Conditions: As with other mu agonists, treatment with ORLAAM may obscure the diagnosis or clinical course in patients with acute abdominal conditions.

DRUG INTERACTIONS

Polydrug and Alcohol Abusers—Patients who are known to abuse sedatives, tranquilizers, propoxyphene, antidepressants, benzodiazepines, and alcohol should be warned of the risk of serious overdose if these substances are taken while on ORAAM maintenance.

Interaction with Narcotic Antagonists, Mixed Agonists/Antagonists, Partial Agonists, and Pure Agonists—As with other mu agonists, patients maintained on ORLAAM may experience withdrawal symptoms when administered pure narcotic antagonists, mixed agonist/antagonists or partial agonists such as naloxone, naltrexone, pentazocine, nalbuphine, butorphanol, and buprenorphine.

In addition, agonists such as meperidine and propoxyphene, which are N-demethylated to long-acting, excitatory metabolites, should not be used by patients taking ORLAAM because they would be ineffective unless given in such high doses that the risk of toxic effects of the metabolites becomes unacceptable.

Anesthesia and Analgesia—Patients receiving ORLAAM will develop a similar level of tolerance for opioids as patients receiving methadone. Anesthetists and other practitioners should be prepared to adjust their management of these patients accordingly.

Other Drug Interactions—The anti-tuberculosis drug rifampin has been found to produce a marked (50%) reduction in serum methadone levels, leading to the appearance of symptoms of withdrawal in well-stabilized methadone maintenance patients. Similar effects on serum methadone levels have been observed for carbamazepine, phenobarbital, and phenytoin, The presumed mechanism for this effect is the induction of methadone metabolizing enzymes. Since ORLAAM is metabolized into a **more** active metabolite, nor-LAAM, administration of these drugs may **increase** ORLAAM's peak activity and/or **shorten** its duration of action. Conversely, drugs like erythromycin, cimetidine, and antifungal drugs like ketoconazole that inhibit hepatic metabolism, may **slow** the onset, **lower** the activity, and/or **increase** the duration of action of ORLAAM. Caution and close observation of patients receiving these drugs are advised to allow early detection of any need to adjust the dose or dosing interval.

Information for Patients:

Patients should be provided the patient package insert for ORLAAM if they are new to the drug, and in addition should be advised that:

ORLAAM, unlike methadone, is not to be taken daily, and daily use of the usual doses will lead to serious overdose. ORLAAM is slow acting and patients should be alerted to the risk of abusing any psychoactive drug, including alcohol, while on ORLAAM therapy. This is particularly important during the first 7 to 10 days of treatment, before ORLAAM has had time to exert its full pharmacologic effect.

In addition to being warned of the delay in onset of ORLAAM, patients who are transferring from ORLAAM to methadone should be informed that they should wait 48 hours after the last dose of ORLAAM before ingesting their first dose of methadone or other narcotic (see DOSAGE AND ADMINISTRATION)

Patients should inform their adult family members that, in the event of overdose, the treating physician or emergency room staff should be told that the patient is being treated with ORLAAM, a long-acting opioid which is likely to outlast naloxone-induced reversal and which requires prolonged observation and careful monitoring. In addition, the treating physician or emergency room staff should be informed that the patient is physically dependent on narcotics and that naloxone should be administered with care so as to minimize any precipitated abstinence syndrome.

As with most mu agonists, ORLAAM may interact with other CNS depressants and should be used with caution, and in reduced dosage, in patients concurrently receiving other narcotic analgesics, antihistamines, benzodiazepines, phenothiazines or other major tranquilizers, anxiolytics, sedative-hypnotics, tricyclic antidepressants, and other CNS depressants, including alcohol. Patients should be warned of the importance of reporting the use of any of these compounds to their physicians, as serious side effects could result, including respiratory depression, hypotension, profound sedation or coma.

Carcinogenesis, Mutagenesis and Impairment of Fertility: Two-year carcinogenicity studies with LAAM in rats at 13 mg/kg (77 mg/m^2) and in mice at 30 mg/kg (90 mg/m^2) given orally in the diet did not show carcinogenic changes. LAAM is not mutagenic in the Ames test, the unscheduled DNA synthesis and repair test mouse lymphoma cells in vitro, or chromosal aberration tests in rats in vivo. LAAM tested positive in the forward mutation assay in N. crassa at 150 μg/mL in vitro and in the heritable translocation assay in mice at 21 mg/kg (63 mg/m^2). The clinical significance of these findings is not known.

Chronic treatment with LAAM at 80 mg three times a week did not produce chromosomal aberrations in peripheral human lymphocytes. Effects of LAAM on fertility in animals has not been fully evaluated.

Use in Pregnancy: Pregnancy Category C

Animal reproduction studies are not complete and there are no clinical data on the safety of ORLAAM in pregnancy. For these reasons, ORLAAM is not recommended for use in pregnancy. Women who may become pregnant should be advised of the risks of ORLAAM therapy and of the desirability of discontinuing ORLAAM prior to a planned pregnancy. Current regulations mandate monthly pregnancy tests in female patients of childbearing potential who are using ORLAAM.

If a female patient becomes pregnant on ORLAAM despite these precautions, it is recommended she be transferred to methadone for the remainder of the pregnancy (see TRANSFER FROM ORLAAM TO METHADONE, in DOSAGE AND ADMINISTRATION). If it appears wiser to continue a specific patient on ORLAAM, the physician should be alert to possible respiratory depression of the newborn and other perinatal complications (see Labor and Delivery).

Labor and Delivery: The effects of ORLAAM on labor and delivery are not known. Like other mu agonist opioids, however, ORLAAM is expected to produce respiratory depression and a possible neonatal dependence syndrome with a delayed emergence of withdrawal symptoms. Use of ORLAAM in labor and delivery is not recommended unless, in the opinion of the treating physician, the potential benefits outweigh the possible hazards.

Nursing Mothers: The effects of LAAM on infants of nursing mothers have not been studied. It is not known if LAAM is excreted in human milk in sufficient concentration to affect an infant. Use of ORLAAM in nursing mothers is not recommended unless, in the opinion of the treating physician, the potential benefits outweigh the possible hazards.

Pediatric Use: The use of ORLAAM in addicts under 18 years of age has not been studied. Its use is not recommended and is contrary to current regulations.

ADVERSE REACTIONS

Physicians should be alert to palpitations, syncope, or other symptoms suggestive of episodes of irregular cardiac rhythm in patients taking ORLAAM and promptly evaluate such cases (see Effects on Cardiac Conduction in PRECAUTIONS).

Heroin or Methadone Withdrawal Reactions—Patients presenting for ORLAAM treatment are frequently in withdrawal from heroin or other opiates. They may display typical withdrawal symptoms which should be differentiated from ORLAAM's side effects. Patients may exhibit some or all of the following signs and symptoms associated with withdrawal from opiates: lacrimation, rhinorrhea, sneezing, yawning, perspiration, gooseflesh, fever, chilliness alternating with flushing, restlessness, irritability, insomnia, weakness, anxiety, depression, dilated pupils, tremors, tachycardia, abdominal cramps, body aches, anorexia, nausea, vomiting, diarrhea, and weight loss. Control of such symptoms is a primary goal of therapy. However, because of the slow onset and long half-lives of ORLAAM, nor-LAAM and dinor-LAAM, overly aggresive increases in dosage to control these withdrawal symptoms with ORLAAM may result in overdose (see INDIVIDUALIZATION OF DOSAGE).

Signs and Symptoms of ORLAAM Excess—The interaction between the development and maintenance of opioid tolerance and ORLAAM dose can be complex. Dose reduction is recommended in cases where patients develop signs and symptoms of excessive ORLAAM effect, characterized by complaints of "feeling wired", poor concentration, drowsiness, and possibly dizziness on standing.

Continued on next page

Orlaam—Cont.

ORLAAM Withdrawal—Patients may experience withdrawal symptoms (nasal congestion, abdominal symptoms, diarrhea, muscle aches, anxiety) over the 72-hour dosing interval if the dose of ORLAAM is too low. This may be managed as described under INDIVIDUALIZATION OF DOSAGE, but physicians should be alert to the possible need for dose or dose schedule adjustments if patients complain of weekend withdrawal symptoms in the last day of the 72-hour dosing interval.

Adverse Reactions on Stable Therapy:

The following adverse events were observed in the 25-site, 623-patient usage study in male and female opiate addicts (see CLINICAL TRIALS). These signs and symptoms were reported during the second and third months of treatment with ORLAAM, and were considered severe enough to require medical evaluation. In this study, both questionnaires and spontaneous reports were used to gather information. Questionnaire-elicited symptom frequencies were about five times as frequent as the spontaneous reporting frequencies given below.

Incidence greater than 1%, Probably Causally Related

Body of a Whole—	Asthenia*, back pain chills, edema, hot flashes (males 2:1), flu syndrome and malaise (11%).
Gastrointestinal—	Abdominal pain*, constipation*, diarrhea, dry mouth, nausea and vomiting.
Musculoskeletal—	Arthralgia*
Nervous System—	Abnormal dreams, anxiety, decreased sex drive, depression, euphoria, headache, hypesthesia, insomnia (9.1%), nervousness*, somnolence.
Respiratory—	Cough, rhinitis, and yawning.
Skin/appendages—	Rash, sweating*.
Special Senses—	Blurred vision.
Urogenital—	Difficult ejaculation*, impotence*.

*Reactions in 3–9% of patients; reactions in 1–3% are unmarked.

Incidence less than 1%, Probably Causally Related

Cardiovascular—	Postural hypotension.
Musculoskeletal—	Myalgia.
Special Senses—	Tearing.

Causal Relationship Unknown

These reactions were reported with low frequency in controlled and uncontrolled studies of LAAM, are not known to be causally related to the administration of the drug, and are provided as alerting information for physicians.

Cardiovascular—	Hypertension, prolongation of the QT interval, non-specific ST-T wave changes.
Hepatic—	Hepatitis and abnormal liver function tests.
Urogenital—	Amenorrhea, pyuria.

DRUG DEPENDENCE

ORLAAM is a Schedule II controlled substance under the Federal Controlled Substances Act. ORLAAM produces dependence of the morphine-type and has potential for abuse. Tolerance and physical dependence will develop upon repeated administration. As with methadone and any other narcotic administered to narcotic addicts. ORLAAM is at risk for diversion and illicit use, and should be handled accordingly (see WARNINGS).

OVERDOSE

Signs and Symptoms: All but a few cases of ORLAAM overdose have involved multiple drugs. Overdose on ORLAAM alone is rare and has always been the result of too frequent (daily) dosing. Overdose is primarily of concern in persons not tolerant to opiates, since in such individuals a dose of 20 to 40 mg of ORLAAM may cause somnolence, and a larger initial dose may cause serious overdose. Tolerant individuals will generally not show symptoms unless higher doses are administered.

In ORLAAM overdose, as with other mu agonist opioids, the following signs and symptoms should be anticipated: respiratory depression (decrease in respiratory rate and/or tidal volume. Cheyne-Stokes respiration, cyanosis), extreme somnolence progressing to stupor or coma, maximally constricted pupils, skeletal muscle flaccidity, cold and clammy skin, bradycardia, and hypotension. In severe overdose, apnea, circulatory collapse, pulmonary edema, cardiac arrest and death may occur.

Treatment: In the case of ORLAAM overdose, protect the patient's airway and support ventilation and circulation. Absorption of ORLAAM from the gastrointestinal tract may be decreased by gastric emptying and/or administration of activated charcoal. (Safeguard the patient's airway when employing gastric emptying or administering charcoal in any patient with diminished consciousness). Forced diuresis, peritoneal dialysis, hemodialysis, or charcoal hemoperfusion are unlikely to be beneficial for ORLAAM overdose due to its high lipid solubility and large volume of distribution.

In managing ORLAAM overdose, the physician should consider the possibility of multiple drugs, the interaction between drugs, and any unusual drug kinetics in the patient. Naloxone may be given to antagonize opiate effects, but the airway must be secured as vomiting may ensue. If possible, naloxone should be titrated to clinical effect rather than given as a large single bolus, since rapid reversal of opioid effects by large naloxone doses can cause severe precipitated withdrawal effects that may include cardiac instability. If a patient has received a total of 10 mg of naloxone withoutclinical response, the diagnosis of opioid overdose is unlikely.

If the patient does respond to naloxone, the physician should remember that the duration of ORLAAM activity is much longer (days) than that of naloxone (minutes) and repeated dosing with or continuous intravenous infusion of naloxone is likely to be required. Use of oral naltrexone in this setting is not recommended because it may precipitate prolonged opioid withdrawal symptoms (see Use of Narcotic Antagonists).

DOSAGE AND ADMINISTRATION

ORLAAM produces opioid effects and a high degree of opioid tolerance that inhibits drug-seeking behavior and blocks the euphoria produced by the usual doses of heroin. The dose of ORLAAM in each patient should be adjusted to achieve the optimal therapeutic benefit with acceptable adverse opioid effects (see INDIVIDUALIZATION OF DOSAGE).

ORLAAM must always be diluted before administration, and should be mixed with diluent prior to dispensing. To avoid confusion between prepared doses of ORLAAM and methadone, the liquid used to dilute ORLAAM should be a different color from that used to dilute methadone in any specific clinic setting.

ORLAAM DOSING

Dosing Schedules:

ORLAAM is usually administered three times a week, either on Monday, Wednesday and Friday, or on Tuesday, Thursday and Saturday. If withdrawal is a problem during the 72-hour inter-dose interval, the preceding dose may be increased. In some cases, an every-other-day schedule may be appropriate (see INDIVIDUALIZATION OF DOSAGE). The usual doses of ORLAAM must not be given on consecutive days because of the risk of fatal overdose. No dose mentioned in this label is **ever** meant to be given as a daily dose (see WARNINGS).

INDUCTION

The initial dose of ORLAAM for street addicts should be 20 to 40 mg. Each subsequent dose, administered at 48- or 72-hour intervals, may be adjusted in increments of 5 to 10 mg until a pharmacokinetic and pharmacodynamic steady-state is reached, usually within 1 or 2 weeks (see INDIVIDUALIZATION OF DOSAGE).

Patients dependent on methadone may require higher initial doses of ORLAAM. The suggested initial 3-times-a-week dose of ORLAAM for such patients is 1.2 to 1.3 times the daily methadone maintenance dose being replaced. This initial dose should not exceed 120 mg and subsequent doses, administered at 48- or 72-hour intervals, should be adjusted according to clinical response.

Most patients can tolerate the 72-hour inter-dose interval during the induction period. Some patients may require additional intervention (see INDIVIDUALIZATION OF DOSAGE). If additional opioids are required, supplemental methadone in small doses should be given rather than giving ORLAAM on two consecutive days. Take-home doses of methadone always pose a risk in this setting and physicians should carefully weigh the potential therapeutic benefit against the risk of diversion.

In some cases, where the degree of tolerance is unknown, patients can be started on methadone to facilitate more rapid titration to an effective dose, then converted to ORLAAM after a few weeks of methadone therapy.

The crossover from methadone to ORLAAM should be accomplished in a single dose; complete transfer to ORLAAM is simpler and preferable to more complex regimens involving escalating doses of ORLAAM and decreasing doses of methadone.

Dosage should be carefully titrated to the individual; induction too rapid for the patient's level of tolerance may result in overdose. Serious hazards, as seen in association with all narcotic analgesics, are respiratory depression and, to a lesser extent, circulatory depression.

MAINTENANCE

Most patients will be stabilized on doses in the range of 60 to 90 mg, 3-times-a-week. Doses as low as 10 mg and as high as 140 mg three times a week have been given in clinical studies.

Supplemental dosing over the 72-hour inter-dose interval (weekend) is rarely needed. For example, if a patient on a Mon./Wed./Fri. schedule complains of withdrawal on Sundays, the recommended dosage adjustment is to increase the Friday dose in 5 to 10 mg increments up to 40% over the Mon./Wed. dose or to a maximum of 140 mg.

If withdrawal symptoms persist after adjustment of dose, consideration may be given to every-other-day dosing if clinic hours permit. If the clinic is not opern seven days a week and every-other day dosing is not practical, the patient's schedule may be adjusted so the 72-hour interval occurrs during the week and the patient can come to the clinic to receive a supplemental dose of methadone (see INDIVIDUALIZATION OF DOSAGE).

The maximum **total** amount of ORLAAM recommended for any patient is 140-140-140 mg or 130-130-180 mg on a thrice-weekly schedule or 140 mg every other day.

PLANNED TEMPORARY INTERRUPTION OF ORLAAM MAINTENANCE

ORLAAM take-home doses are not permitted by regulation. Thus, several circumstances may cause the planned temporary discontinuation of treatment with ORLAAM. Patients eligible for one or more take-home doses of methadone, who are unable to attend the clinic for their next regularly scheduled ORLAAM dose because of illness, personal or family crisis, other hardships, travel and/or state/federal holidays, may be temporarily transferred directly to methadone.

Patients meeting these criteria may receive one or more methadone doses. Methadone doses should be 80% of the patient's Monday/Wednesday ORLAAM dose (e.g., patients receiving 80-80-100 mg of ORLAAM on a Monday/Wednesday/Friday regimen would be transferred to a daily methadone dose of 64 mg). The first dose of methadone should be ingested no sooner than 48 hours after the last ORLAAM dose. The number of takehome methadone doses should be **two less** than the number of days of expected absence and should not exceed, in any case, the number of take-homes allowed in the methadone regulations.

Upon return to clinic, patients should resume ORLAAM maintenance following the same dosage regimen used prior to the temporary interruption (see above). If more than 48 hours has elapsed since their last methadone dose, patients should be reinducted on ORLAAM at a dose determined by clinical and/or toxicological evaluation of the patient by the physician.

REINDUCTION AFTER AN UNPLANNED LAPSE IN DOSING;

Following a lapse of one ORLAAM dose:

1) If a patient comes to the clinic to be dosed **on the day following a missed scheduled dose** (misses Monday, arrives Tuesday), the regular Monday dose should be administered on Tuesday, with the scheduled Wednesday dose administered on Thursday and the Friday dose given on Saturday. The patient's regular schedule may be resumed the following Monday (misses Wednesday, receives the regular dose on Thursday and Saturday, and returns to the regular Monday/Wednesday/Friday dosing schedule the next week).
2) If a patient misses one dose and comes to the clinic **on the day of the next scheduled dose** (misses Monday, arrives Wednesday), the usual dose will be well tolerated in most instances, although a reduced dose may be appropriate in selected cases.

Following a lapse of more than one ORLAAM dose:

Patients should be reinducted at an initial dose of $^1/_2$ or $^3/_4$ their previous ORLAAM dose, followed by increases of 5 to 10 mg every dosing day (48- or 72-hours intervals) until their previous maintenance dose is achieved. Patients who have been off of ORLAAM treatment for more than a week should be reinducted.

TRANSFER FROM ORLAAM TO METHADONE

Patients maintained on ORLAAM may be transferred directly to methadone. Because of the difference between the two compounds' metabolites and their pharmacological half-lives, it is recommended that methadone be started on a daily dose at 80% of the ORLAAM dose being replaced; the initial methadone dose must be given no sooner than 48 hours after the last ORLAAM dose. Subsequent increases or decreases of 5 to 10 mg in the daily methadone dose may be given to control symptoms or withdrawal or, less likely, symptoms of excessive sedation, in accordance with clinical observations.

DETOXIFICATION FROM ORLAAM

There is a limited experience with detoxifying patients from ORLAAM in a systematic manner, and both gradual reduction (5 to 10% a week) and abrupt withdrawal schedules have been used successfully. The decision to discontinue ORLAAM therapy should be made as part of a comprehensive treatment plan (see INDIVIDUALIZATION OF DOSAGE).

SAFETY AND HANDLING

ORLAAM is a solution of a potent narcotic (LAAM). There are no known specific hazards associated with dermal and aerosol exposure to ORLAAM. In case of accidental dermal exposure, promptly remove contaminated clothing and rinse the affected skin with cool water.

For the first six to twelve months, sales of ORLAAM will be restricted to clinics that have received training in its use, until there is general knowledge about how to use the drug

safely. Since ORLAAM can be potentially dangerous if diverted, appropriate security measures should be taken to safeguard stock of ORLAAM as required by 21 CFR 1301.74 & 1304.28.

HOW SUPPLIED

ORLAAM Oral Solution (10 mg/mL) is a clear, colorless liquid supplied in plastic bottles as follows:
NDC 0054-3649-63: 500 mL per bottle
Store at controlled room temperature, 15°-30°C (59°-86°F). Protect from direct sunlight. Retain in original carton until needed for use.
ORLAAM is compatible with the materials used in most dispensing systems. Information about obtaining appropriate dispensing systems suitable for use with ORLAAM is available from the manufacturer upon request.
Roxane Laboratories, Inc.
Columbus Ohio 43216
Revised June 1996
066
© RLI, 1996

ROXANOL™ Ⓒ ℞
[*rox ′-ĕ-nŭl*]
ROXANOL™–T
ROXANOL 100™
ROXANOL™ UD 30 mg
MORPHINE SULFATE
(IMMEDIATE RELEASE)
ORAL SOLUTION (CONCENTRATE)
ROXANOL™ UD 10 mg, 20 mg
MORPHINE SULFATE
(IMMEDIATE RELEASE)
ORAL SOLUTION

DESCRIPTION

Each mL of Roxanol™ contains:
Morphine Sulfate .... 20 mg
Each mL of Roxanol™–T contains:
Morphine Sulfate .... 20 mg
Solution is also tinted/flavored
Each 5 mL of Roxanol 100™ contains:
Morphine Sulfate .... 100 mg
Each 2.5 mL of Rescudose™ contains:
Morphine Sulfate .... 10 mg
Each vial of Roxanol™ UD contains:
Morphine Sulfate .... 10 mg, 20 mg or 30 mg

CLINICAL PHARMACOLOGY

The major effects of morphine are on the central nervous system and the bowel. Opioids act as agonists, interacting with stereospecific and saturable binding sites or receptors in the brain and other tissues.
Morphine is about two-thirds absorbed from the gastrointestinal tract with the maximum analgesic effect occurring 60 minutes post administration.

INDICATIONS AND USAGE

Morphine is indicated for the relief of severe acute and severe chronic pain.

CONTRAINDICATIONS

Hypersensitivity to morphine; respiratory insufficiency or depression; severe CNS depression; attack of bronchial asthma; heart failure secondary to chronic lung disease; cardiac arrhythmias; increased intracranial or cerebrospinal pressure; head injuries; brain tumor; acute alcoholism; delirium tremens; convulsive disorders; after biliary tract surgery; suspected surgical abdomen; surgical anastomosis; concomitantly with MAO inhibitors or within 14 days of such treatment.

WARNINGS

Morphine can cause tolerance, psychological and physical dependence. Withdrawal will occur on abrupt discontinuation or administration of a narcotic antagonist.
Interaction with Other Central-Nervous-System Depressants—Morphine should be used with caution and in reduced dosage in patients who are concurrently receiving other narcotic analgesics, general anesthetics, phenothiazines, other tranquilizers, sedative-hypnotics, tricyclic antidepressants, and other CNS depressants (including alcohol). Respiratory depression, hypotension, and profound sedation or coma may result.

PRECAUTIONS

General:
Head Injury and Increased Intracranial Pressure—The respiratory depressant effects of morphine and its capacity to elevate cerebrospinal-fluid pressure may be markedly exaggerated in the presence of increased intracranial pressure. Furthermore, narcotics produce side effects that may obscure the clinical course of patients with head injuries. In such patients, morphine must be used with caution and only if it is deemed essential.
Asthma and Other Respiratory Conditions—Morphine should be used with caution in patients having an acute asthmatic attack, in those with chronic obstructive pulmonary disease or cor pulmonale, and in individuals with a substantially decreased respiratory reserve, preexisting respiratory depression, hypoxia, or hypercapnia. In such patients, even usual therapeutic doses of narcotics may decrease respiratory drive while simultaneously increasing airway resistance to the point of apnea.
Hypotensive Effect—The administration of morphine may result in severe hypotension in an individual whose ability to maintain his blood pressure has already been compromised by a depleted blood volume or concurrent administration of such drugs as the phenothiazines or certain anesthetics.
Special-Risk Patients—Morphine should be given with caution and the initial dose should be reduced in certain patients, such as the elderly or debilitated and those with severe impairment of hepatic or renal function, hypothyroidism, Addison's disease, prostatic hypertrophy, or urethral stricture.
Acute Abdominal Conditions—The administration of morphine or other narcotics may obscure the diagnosis or clinical course in patients with acute abdominal conditions.
Information for patients:
Use in Ambulatory Patients—Morphine may impair the mental and/or physical abilities required for the performance of potentially hazardous tasks, such as driving a car or operating machinery. The patient should be cautioned accordingly.
Morphine, like other narcotics, may produce orthostatic hypotension in ambulatory patients.
Patients should be cautioned about the combined effects of alcohol or other central nervous system depressants with morphine.
Drug interactions:
Generally, effects of morphine may be potentiated by alkalizing agents and antagonized by acidifying agents. Analgesic effect of morphine is potentiated by chlorpromazine and methocarbamol. CNS depressants such as anaesthetics, hypnotics, barbiturates, phenothiazines, chloral hydrate, glutethimide, sedatives, MAO inhibitors (including procarbazine hydrochloride), antihistamines, β-blockers (propranolol), alcohol, furazolidone and other narcotics may enhance the depressant effects of morphine.
Morphine may increase anticoagulant activity of coumarin and other anticoagulants.
Carcinogenicity/Mutagenicity:
Long-term studies to determine the carcinogenic and mutagenic potential of morphine are not available.
Pregnancy:
Teratogenic Effects—Pregnancy Category C: Animal production studies have not been conducted with morphine. It is also not known whether morphine can cause fetal harm when administered to a pregnant woman or can affect reproduction capacity. Morphine should be given to a pregnant woman only if clearly needed.
Labor and Delivery:
Morphine readily crosses the placental barrier and, if administered during labor, may lead to respiratory depression in the neonate.
Nursing Mothers:
Morphine has been detected in human milk. For this reason, caution should be exercised when morphine is administered to a nursing woman.
Pediatric Usage:
Safety and effectiveness in children have not been established.

ADVERSE REACTIONS

THE MAJOR HAZARDS OF MORPHINE, AS OF OTHER NARCOTIC ANALGESICS, ARE RESPIRATORY DEPRESSION AND, TO A LESSER DEGREE, CIRCULATORY DEPRESSION, RESPIRATORY ARREST, SHOCK, AND CARDIAC ARREST HAVE OCCURRED.
The most frequently observed adverse reactions include lightheadedness, dizziness, sedation, nausea, vomiting, and sweating. These effects seem to be more prominent in ambulatory patients and in those who are not suffering severe pain. In such individuals, lower doses are advisable. Some adverse reactions may be alleviated in the ambulatory patient if he lies down.
Other adverse reactions include the following:
Central Nervous System—Euphoria, dysphoria, weakness, headache, insomnia, agitation, disorientation, and visual disturbances.
Gastrointestinal—Dry mouth, anorexia, constipation, and biliary tract spasm.
Cardiovascular—Flushing of the face, bradycardia, palpitation, faintness, and syncope.
Allergic—Pruritus, urticaria, other skin rashes, edema, and, rarely hemorrhagic urticaria.
Treatment of the most frequent adverse reactions:
Constipation—Ample intake of water or other liquids should be encouraged. Concomitant administration of a stool softener and a peristaltic stimulant with the narcotic analgesic can be an effective preventive measure for those patients in need of therapeutics. If elimination does not occur for two days, an enema should be administered to prevent impaction.
In the event diarrhea occurs, seepage around a fecal impaction is a possible cause to consider before antidiarrheal measures are employed.
Nausea and Vomiting—Phenothiazines and antihistamines can be effective treatments for nausea of the medullary and vestibular sources respectively. However, these drugs may potentiate the side effects of the narcotics or the antinauseant.
Drowsiness (sedation)—Once pain control is achieved, undesirable sedation can be minimized by titrating the dosage to a level that just maintains a tolerable pain or pain free state.

DRUG ABUSE AND DEPENDENCE

Morphine Sulfate, narcotic, is a Schedule II controlled substance under the Federal Controlled Substance Act. As with other narcotics, some patients may develop a physical and psychological dependence on morphine. They may increase dosage without consulting a physician and subsequently may develop a physical dependence on the drug. In such cases, abrupt discontinuance may precipitate typical withdrawal symptoms, including convulsions. Therefore the drug should be withdrawn gradually from any patient known to be taking excessive dosages over a long period of time.
In treating the terminally ill patient the benefit of pain relief may outweigh the possibility of drug dependence. The chance of drug dependence is substantially reduced when the patient is placed on scheduled narcotic programs instead of a "pain to relief-of-pain" cycle typical of a PRN regimen.

OVERDOSAGE

Signs and Symptoms: Serious overdose with morphine is characterized by respiratory depression (a decrease in respiratory rate and/or tidal volume, Cheyne-Stokes respiration, cyanosis), extreme somnolence progressing to stupor or coma, skeletal muscle flaccidity, cold or clammy skin, and sometimes bradycardia and hypotension. In severe overdosage, apnea, circulatory collapse, cardiac arrest and death may occur.
Treatment: Primary attention should be given to the reestablishment of adequate respiratory exchange through provision of a patent airway and the institution of assisted or controlled ventilation. The narcotic antagonist naloxone is a specific antidote against respiratory depression which may result from overdosage or unusual sensitivity to narcotics, including morphine. Therefore, an appropriate dose of naloxone (usual initial adult dose: 0.4 mg) should be administered, preferably by the intravenous route and simultaneously with efforts at respiratory resuscitation. Since the duration of action of morphine may exceed that of the antagonist, the patient should be kept under continued surveillance and repeated doses of the antagonist should be administered as needed to maintain adequate respiration.
An antagonist should not be administered in the absence of clinically significant respiratory or cardiovascular depression.
Oxygen, intravenous fluids, vasopressors and other supportive measures should be employed as indicated.
Gastric emptying may be useful in removing unabsorbed drug.

DOSAGE AND ADMINISTRATION

Usual Adult Oral Dose: 10 to 30 mg every 4 hours or as directed by physician. Dosage is a patient dependent variable, therefore increased dosage may be required to achieve adequate analgesia.
For control of severe, chronic pain in patients with certain terminal disease, this drug should be administered on a regularly scheduled basis, every 4 hours, at the lowest dosage level that will achieve adequate analgesia.
Note: Medication may suppress respiration in the elderly, the very ill, and those patients with respiratory problems, therefore lower doses may be required.
Morphine Dosage Reduction: During the first two to three days of effective pain relief, the patient may sleep for many hours. This can be misinterpreted as the effect of excessive analgesic dosing rather than the first sign of relief in a pain exhausted patient. The dose, therefore, should be maintained for at least three days before reduction, if respiratory activity and other vital signs are adequate.
Following successful relief of severe pain, periodic attempts to reduce the narcotic dose should be made. Smaller doses or complete discontinuation of the narcotic analgesic may become feasible due to a physiologic change or the improved mental state of the patient.

Continued on next page

Roxanol—Cont.

HOW SUPPLIED
Roxanol™
Morphine Sulfate (Immediate Release)
Oral Solution (Concentrate)
20 mg per mL
NDC 0054-3751-44: Bottles of 30 mL with calibrated dropper.
NDC 0054-3751-50: Bottles of 120 mL with calibrated dropper.
Roxanol™–T
Morphine Sulfate (Immediate Release)
Oral Solution (Concentrate)
20 mg per mL (tinted/flavored)
NDC 0054-3774-44: Bottles of 30 mL with calibrated dropper.
NDC 0054-3774-50: Bottles of 120 mL with calibrated dropper.
Roxanol 100™
Morphine Sulfate (Immediate Release)
Oral Solution (Concentrate)
100 mg per 5 mL
NDC 0054-3751-58: Bottles of 240 mL with calibrated patient spoon.
Roxanol™ UD
Morphine Sulfate (Immediate Release)
Oral Solution
10 mg per 2.5 mL
NDC 0054-8781-11: Unit dose vial of 2.5 mL (10 mg Morphine Sulfate).
25 reverse number vials per carton.
20 mg per 5 mL
NDC 0054-8785-11: Unit dose vial of 5 mL (20 mg Morphine Sulfate).
25 reverse number vials per carton.
Morphine Sulfate (Immediate Release)
Oral Solution (Concentrate)
30 mg per 1.5 mL
NDC 0054-8788-11: Unit dose vial of 1.5 mL (30 mg Morphine Sulfate).
25 reverse number vials per carton.

DEA Order Form Required
Rx only.
4073001
048
©RLI, 1998.
Revised April 1998

Shown in Product Identification Guide, page 335

ROXICET™ Tablets Ⓒ ℞
[rox-ē-cĕt]
Oxycodone and Acetaminophen Tablets USP
(Oxycodone Hydrochloride 5 mg and Acetaminophen 325 mg)
  (WARNING: May be habit forming)
ROXICET™ Oral Solution Ⓒ ℞
Oxycodone and Acetaminophen Oral Solution
(Oxycodone Hydrochloride 5 mg and Acetaminophen 325 mg Oral Solution per 5 mL)
  (WARNING: May be habit forming)
ROXICET 5/500™ Caplet Ⓒ ℞
Oxycodone and Acetaminophen Tablets USP
(Oxycodone Hydrochloride 5 mg and Acetaminophen 500 mg)
  (WARNING: May be habit forming)

DESCRIPTION
Each tablet contains:
Oxycodone Hydrochloride+ .... 5 mg
Acetaminophen .... 325 mg
Each 5 mL contains:
Oxycodone Hydrochloride+ .... 5 mg
Acetaminophen .... 325 mg
Alcohol 0.4%
Each caplet contains:
Oxycodone Hydrochloride+ .... 5 mg
Acetaminophen .... 500 mg
(+5 mg Oxycodone HCl is equivalent to 4.4815 mg Oxycodone.)

HOW SUPPLIED
ROXICET™ Tablets, Oxycodone and Acetaminophen Tablets USP (Oxycodone Hydrochloride 5 mg and Acetaminophen 325 mg) white scored tablets (Identified 54 543).
NDC 0054-8650-24: Unit dose, 25 tablets per card (reverse numbered), 4 cards per shipper.
NDC 0054-4650-25: Bottles of 100 tablets.
NDC 0054-4650-29: Bottles of 500 tablets.
ROXICET™ Oral Solution,
Oxycodone and Acetaminophen Oral Solution
(Oxycodone Hydrochloride 5 mg and Acetaminophen 325 mg Oral Solution per 5 mL)

NDC 0054-8648-16: Unit dose Patient Cups™ filled to deliver 5 mL (Oxycodone Hydrochloride 5 mg, Acetaminophen 325 mg), ten 5 mL Patient Cups™ per shelf pack, 4 shelf packs per shipper.
NDC 0054-3686-63: Bottles of 500 mL.
ROXICET 5/500™ Caplets,
Oxycodone and Acetaminophen Tablets USP
(Oxycodone Hydrochloride 5 mg and Acetaminophen 500 mg), white scored capsule-shaped tablets (Identified 54 730).
NDC 0054-8784-24: Unit dose, 25 caplets per card (reverse numbered), 4 cards per shipper.
NDC 0054-4784-25: Bottles of 100 caplets.
Store at Controlled Room Temperature (15°–30°C (59°–86°F).
DEA Order Form Required.
Caution: Federal law prohibits dispensing without prescription.

ROXICODONE™ Ⓒ ℞
[rox-ē-cō-dōne]
(oxycodone hydrochloride)
Tablets USP, Oral Solution USP, and Intensol™

DESCRIPTION
Each tablet contains:
Oxycodone Hydrochloride   5 mg
Each 5 mL Oral Solution contains:
Oxycodone Hydrochloride   5 mg
Each mL Intensol™ contains:
Oxycodone Hydrochloride   20 mg
Inactive Ingredients:
The tablets contain microcrystalline cellulose and stearic acid.
The oral solution contains alcohol, FD&C Red No. 40, flavoring, glycol, sorbitol, water, and other ingredients.
The Intensol™ contains citric acid, sodium benzoate, and water.
Oxycodone is 14-hydroxydihydrocodeinone, a white odorless crystalline powder which is derived from the opium alkaloid, thebaine.

ACTIONS
The analgesic ingredient, oxycodone, is a semisynthetic narcotic with multiple actions qualitatively similar to those of morphine; the most prominent of these involve the central nervous system and organs composed of smooth muscle. The principal actions of therapeutic value of oxycodone are analgesia and sedation.
Oxycodone is similar to codeine and methadone in that it retains at least one half of its analgesic activity when administered orally.

INDICATIONS
For the relief of moderate to moderately severe pain.

CONTRAINDICATIONS
Hypersensitivity to oxycodone.

WARNINGS
Drug Dependence: Oxycodone can produce drug dependence of the morphine type, and therefore, has the potential for being abused. Psychic dependence, physical dependence and tolerance may develop upon repeated administration of this drug, and it should be prescribed and administered with the same degree of caution appropriate to the use of other oral narcotic-containing medications. Like other narcotic-containing medications, this drug is subject to the Federal Controlled Substances Act.
Usage in Ambulatory Patients: Oxycodone may impair the mental and/or physical abilities required for the performance of potentially hazardous tasks such as driving a car or operating machinery. The patient using this drug should be cautioned accordingly.
Interaction with Other Central Nervous System Depressants: Patients receiving other narcotic analgesics, general anesthetics, phenothiazines, other tranquilizers, sedative-hypnotics or other CNS depressants (including alcohol) concomitantly with oxycodone hydrochloride may exhibit an additive CNS depression. When such combined therapy is contemplated, the dose of one or both agents should be reduced.
Usage In Pregnancy: Safe use in pregnancy has not been established relative to possible adverse effects on fetal development. Therefore, this drug should not be used in pregnant women unless, in the judgment of the physician, the potential benefits outweigh the possible hazards.
Usage In Children: This drug should not be administered to children.

PRECAUTIONS
Head Injury and Increased Intracranial Pressure: The respiratory depressant effects of narcotics and their capacity to elevate cerebrospinal fluid pressure may be markedly exaggerated in the presence of head injury, other intracranial lesions or a pre-existing increase in intracranial pressure. Furthermore, narcotics produce adverse reactions which may obscure the clinical course of patients with head injuries.
Acute Abdominal Conditions: The administration of this drug or other narcotics may obscure the diagnosis or clinical course in patients with acute abdominal conditions.
Special Risk Patients: This drug should be given with caution to certain patients such as the elderly, or debilitated, and those with severe impairment of hepatic or renal function, hypothyroidism, Addison's disease and prostatic hypertrophy or urethral stricture.

ADVERSE REACTIONS
The most frequently observed adverse reactions include light headedness, dizziness, sedation, nausea and vomiting. These effects seem to be more prominent in ambulatory than in nonambulatory patients, and some of these adverse reactions may be alleviated if the patient lies down.
Other adverse reactions include euphoria, dysphoria, constipation, skin rash and pruritus.

DOSAGE AND ADMINISTRATION
The usual adult oral dose is 10 to 30 mg every 4 hours as needed for pain or as directed by physician. The dose must be individually adjusted according to severity of pain, patient response and patient size. More severe pain may require 30 mg or more every 4 hours. If the pain increases in severity, analgesia is not adequate or tolerance occurs, a gradual increase in dosage may be required.
For control of severe, chronic pain in patients with certain terminal diseases, this drug should be administered on a regularly scheduled basis, every 4 hours, at the lowest dosage level that will achieve adequate analgesia.

DRUG INTERACTIONS
The CNS depressant effects of oxycodone hydrochloride may be additive with that of other CNS depressants. SeeWARNINGS.

MANAGEMENT OF OVERDOSAGE
Signs and Symptoms: Serious overdose of oxycodone hydrochloride is characterized by respiratory depression (a decrease in respiratory rate and/or tidal volume, Cheyne-Stokes respiration, cyanosis), extreme somnolence progressing to stupor or coma, skeletal muscle flaccidity, cold and clammy skin, and sometimes bradycardia and hypotension. In severe overdosage, apnea, circulatory collapse, cardiac arrest and death may occur.
Treatment: Primary attention should be given to the reestablishment of adequate respiratory exchange through provision of a patent airway and the institution of assisted or controlled ventilation. The narcotic antagonist naloxone is a specific antidote against respiratory depression which may result from overdosage or unusual sensitivity to narcotics, including oxycodone. Therefore, an appropriate dose of naloxone (usual initial adult dose: 0.4 mg) should be administered, preferably by the intravenous route, simultaneously with efforts at respiratory resuscitation. Since the duration of action of oxycodone may exceed that of the antagonist, the patient should be kept under continued surveillance and repeated doses of the antagonist should be administered as needed to maintain adequate respiration.
An antagonist should not be administered in the absence of clinically significant respiratory or cardiovascular depression.
Oxygen, intravenous fluids, vasopressors and other supportive measures should be employed as indicated.
Gastric emptying may be useful in removing unabsorbed drug.

HOW SUPPLIED
5 mg white scored tablets. (Identified 54 582).
NDC 0054-8657-24: Unit dose, 25 tablets per card (reverse numbered), 4 cards per shipper.
NDC 0054-4657-25: Bottles of 100 tablets.
5 mg per 5 mL Oral Solution.
NDC 0054-8545-16: Unit dose Patient Cups™ filled to deliver 5 mL (oxycodone hydrochloride 5 mg), ten 5 mL Patient Cups™ per shelf pack, 4 shelf packs per shipper.
NDC 0054-3682-63: Bottles of 500 mL.
20 mg per mL Intensol™
(Concentrated Oral Solution)
NDC 0054-3683-44: Bottles of 30 mL with calibrated dropper [graduations of 0.25 mL (5 mg), 0.5 mL (10 mg), 0.75 mL (15 mg), and 1 mL (20 mg) on the dropper].
DEA Order Form Required
Rx only.
Revised June 1998
4064401
068
© RLI, 1998.

SODIUM POLYSTYRENE SULFONATE SUSPENSION USP ℞

CATION-EXCHANGE RESIN

DESCRIPTION

Sodium Polystyrene Sulfonate Suspension USP can be administered orally or in an enema and contains the following per 60 mL:

sodium polystyrene sulfonate USP	15 g
sorbitol	14.1 g
alcohol	0.1%

The suspension is cherry/carmel-flavored and also contains citric acid, flavors, magnesium aluminum silicate, methylparaben, propylene glycol, propylparaben, saccharin sodium, and purified water. Hydrochloric acid and/or sodium hydroxide may have been added during manufacture to adjust the pH.

Sodium Polystyrene Sulfonate is a benzene, diethenyl-, polymer with ethenylbenzene, sulfonated, sodium salt.

The sodium content of the suspension is 1500 mg (65 mEq) per 60 mL. It is a brown, slightly viscous suspension with an *in-vitro* exchange capacity of approximately 3.1 mEq (*in-vivo* approximately 1 mEq) of potassium per 4 mL (1 gram) of suspension.

CLINICAL PHARMACOLOGY

As the resin passes along the intestine or is retained in the colon after administration by enema, the sodium ions are partially released and are replaced by potassium ions. For the most part, this action occurs in the large intestine, which excretes potassium ions to a greater degree than does the small intestine. The efficiency of this process is limited and unpredictably variable. It commonly approximates the order of 33%, but the range is so large that definite indices of electrolyte balance must be clearly monitored. Metabolic data are unavailable.

INDICATIONS AND USAGE

Sodium Polystyrene Sulfonate suspension is indicated to treatment of hyperkalemia.

CONTRAINDICATIONS

Sodium Polystyrene Sulfonate suspension is contraindicated in patients with hypokalema or those patients who are hypersensitive to it.

WARNINGS

Alternative Therapy in Severe Hyperkalemia:

Since the effective lowering of serum potassium with Sodium Polystyrene Sulfonate may take hours to days, treatment with this drug alone may be insufficient to rapidly correct severe hyperkalemia associated with states of rapid tissue breakdown (e.g., burns and renal failure) or hyperkalemia so marked as to constitute a medical emergency. Therefore, other definite measures, including dialysis, should always be considered and may be imperative.

Hypokalemia:

Serious potassium deficiency can occur from Sodium Polystyrene Sulfonate therapy. The effect must be carefully controlled by frequent serum potassium determination within each 24 hour period. Since intracellular potassium deficiency is not always reflected by serum potassium levels, the level at which treatment with Sodium Polystyrene Sulfonate should be discontinued must be determined individually for each patient. Important aids in making this determination are the patient's clinical condition and electrocardiogram. Early clinical signs of severe hypokalemia include a pattern of irritable confusion and delayed thought processes. Electocardiographically, severe hypokalemia is often associated with a lengthened Q-T interval, widening, flattening, or inversion of the T wave, and prominent U waves. Also, cardiac arrhythmias may occur, such as premature atrial, nodal, and ventricular contractions, and supraventricular and ventricular tachycardias. The toxic effects of digitalis are likely to be exaggerated. Marked hypokalemia can also be manifested by severe muscle weakness, at times extending into frank paralysis.

Electrolyte Disturbances:

Like all cation-exchange resins, Sodium Polystyrene Sulfonate is not totally selective (for potassium) in its actions, and small amounts of other cations such as magnesium and calcium can also be lost during treatment. Accordingly, patients receiving Sodium Polystyrene Sulfonate should be monitored for all applicable electrolyte disturbances.

Systemic Alkalosis:

Systemic alkalosis has been reported after cation-exchange resins were administered orally in combination with nonabsorbable cation-donating antacids and laxatives such as magnesium hydroxide and aluminum carbonate. Magnesium hydroxide should not be administered with Sodium Polystyrene Sulfonate. One case of grand mal seizure has been reported in a patient with chronic hypocalcemia of renal failure who was given Sodium Polystyrene Sulfonate with magnesium hydroxide as a laxative. (See PRECAUTIONS, Drug Interactions).

PRECAUTIONS

Caution is advised when Sodium Polystyrene Sulfonate is administered to patients who cannot tolerate even a small increase in sodium loads (i.e., severe congestive heart failure, severe hypertension, or marked edema). In such instances compensatory restriction of sodium intake from other sources may be indicated.

If constipation occurs, patients should be treated with sorbitol (from 10 to 20 mL of 70% syrup every 2 hours or as needed to produce 1 to 2 watery stools daily) a measure which also reduces any tendency to fecal impaction.

Drug Interactions:

Antacids: The simultaneous oral administration of Sodium Polystyrene Sulfonate suspension with nonabsorbable cation-donating antacids and laxatives may reduce the resin's potassium exchange capability.

Systemic alkalosis has been reported after cation-exchange resins were administered orally in combination with nonabsorbable cation-donating antacids and laxatives such as magnesium hydroxide and aluminum carbonate. Magnesium hydroxide should not be administered with Sodium Polystyrene Sulfonate suspension. One case of grand mal seizure has been reported in a patient with chronic hypocalcemia of renal failure who was given Sodium Polystyrene Sulfonate with magnesium hydroxide as a laxative. Intestinal obstruction due to concretions of aluminum hydroxide when used in combination with Sodium Polystyrene Sulfonate has been reported.

Digitalis: The toxic effects of digitalis on the heart, especially various ventricular arrhythmias and A-V nodal dissociation, are likely to be exaggerated by hypokalemia, even in the face of serum digoxin concentrations in the "normal range". (See WARNINGS.)

Carcinogenesis, Mutagenesis, Impairment of Fertility:

Studies have not been performed.

Pregnancy Category C: Animal reproduction studies have not been conducted with Sodium Polystyrene Sulfonate. It is also not known whether Sodium Polystyrene Sulfonate can cause fetal harm when administered to a pregnant woman or can affect reproduction capacity. Sodium Polystyrene Sulfonate should be given to a pregnant woman only if clearly needed.

Nursing Mothers: It is not known whether this drug is excreted in human milk. Because many drugs are excreted in human milk, caution should be exercised when Sodium Polystyrene Sulfonate is administered to a nursing woman.

ADVERSE REACTIONS

Sodium Polystyrene Sulfonate may cause some degree of gastric irritation. Anorexia, nausea, vomiting, and constipation may occur especially if high doses are given. Also, hypokalemia, hypocalcemia, and significant sodium retention may occur. Occasionally diarrhea develops. Large doses in elderly individuals may cause fecal impaction (see PRECAUTIONS). This effect may be obviated through usage of the resin in enemas as described under DOSAGE AND ADMINISTRATION. Rare instances of colonic necrosis have been reported. Intestinal obstruction due to concretions of aluminum hydroxide, when used in combination with Sodium Polystyrene Sulfonate, has been reported.

DOSAGE AND ADMINISTRATION

Oral Administration

The average daily adult dose is 15 g (60 mL) to 60 g (240 mL) of suspension. This is best provided by administering 15 g (60 mL) of Sodium Polystyrene Sulfonate suspension one to four times daily. Each 60 mL of Sodium Polystyrene Sulfonate suspension contains 1500 mg (65 mEq) of sodium. Since the *in-vivo* efficiency of sodium-potassium exchange resins is approximately 33%, about one-third of the resin's actual sodium content is being delivered to the body.

In smaller children and infants, lower doses should be employed by using as a guide a rate of 1 mEq of potassium per gram of resin as the basis of calculation.

The suspension may be introduced into the stomach through a plastic tube and, if desired, mixed with a diet appropriate for a patient in renal failure.

Rectal Administration:

The suspension may also be given, although with less effective results, as a retention enema for adults of 30 g (120 mL) to 50 g (200 mL) every six hours. The enema should be retained as long as possible and followed by a cleansing enema.

After an initial cleansing enema, a soft, large size (French 28) rubber tube is inserted into the rectum for a distance of 20 cm, with the tip well into the sigmoid colon and taped in place. The suspension is introduced at body temperature by gravity. The suspension is flushed with 50 or 100 mL of fluid, following which the tube is clamped and left in place. If back leakage occurs, the hips are elevated on pillows or a knee-chest position is taken temporarily. The suspension is kept in the sigmoid colon for several hours, if possible. Then the colon is irrigated with a nonsodium-containing solution at body temperature in order to remove the resin. Two quarts of flushing solution may be necessary. The returns are drained constantly through a Y tube connection. Particular attention should be paid to this cleansing enema when sorbitol has been used.

The intensity and duration of therapy depend upon the severity and resistance of hyperkalemia.

HOW SUPPLIED

Sodium Polystyrene Sulfonate Suspension USP, 15 g per 60 mL (an amber-colored, cherry/caramel-flavored suspension)

NDC 0054-8816-11: Unit dose bottle filled to deliver 60 mL, 10 bottles per shipper.

NDC 0054-8815-01: Unit dose enema bottle filled to contain 120 mL (for use in delivering the suspension rectally through appropriate tubing).

NDC 0054-8817-55: Unit dose enema bottle filled to contain 200 mL (for use in delivering the suspension rectally through appropriate tubing).

NDC 0054-3805-63: Bottle of 500 mL.

Note: Sodium Polystyrene Sulfonate suspension should not be heated for to do so may alter the exchange properties of the resin.

SHAKE WELL BEFORE USING

Dispense in a tight container as defined in the USP/NF.

Store at Controlled Room Temperature 15°–30°C (59°–86°F).

Caution: Federal law prohibits dispensing without prescription.

4073705 **Revised September 1997**

097

Roxane Laboratories, Inc.
Columbus, Ohio 43216

TORECAN® ℞

(thiethylperazine maleate tablets USP)
(thiethylperazine malate injection USP)
(for intramuscular use only)

Caution: Federal law prohibits dispensing without prescription.

DESCRIPTION

Torecan® (thiethylperazine) is a phenothiazine. Thiethylperazine is characterized by a substituted thioethyl group at position 2 in the phenothiazine nucleus, and a piperazine moiety in the side chain. The chemical designation is: 2-ethyl-mercapto-10-[3'(1"-methyl-piperazinyl-4")-propyl-1']phenothiazine. Thiethylperazine has the following structural formula:

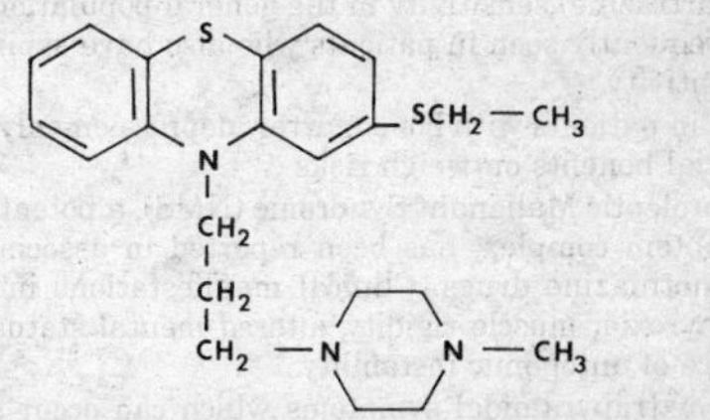

Tablet, 10 mg, for oral administration

ACTIVE INGREDIENT: thiethylperazine maleate USP, 10 mg. *INACTIVE INGREDIENTS:* acacia, carnauba wax, FD&C Yellow No. 5 aluminum lake (tartrazine), FD&C Yellow No. 6 aluminum lake, gelatin, lactose, magnesium stearate, povidone, sodium benzoate, sorbitol, starch, stearic acid, sucrose, talc, titanium dioxide.

Ampul, 2 ml, for intramuscular administration

ACTIVE INGREDIENT: thiethylperazine malate USP, 10 mg per 2 ml. *INACTIVE INGREDIENTS:* sodium metabisulfite NF, 0.5 mg; ascorbic acid USP, 2.0 mg; sorbitol NF, 40 mg; carbon dioxide gas q.s.; water for injection USP, q.s. to 2 ml.

ACTIONS

The pharmacodynamic action of Torecan® (thiethylperazine) in humans is unknown. However, a direct action of Torecan on both the CTZ and the vomiting center may be concluded from induced vomiting experiments in animals.

INDICATIONS

Torecan® (thiethylperazine) is indicated for the relief of nausea and vomiting.

CONTRAINDICATIONS

Severe central nervous system (CNS) depression and comatose states.

In patients who have demonstrated a hypersensitivity reaction (e.g., blood dyscrasias, jaundice) to phenothiazines.

Because severe hypotension has been reported after the intravenous administration of phenothiazines, this route of administration is contraindicated.

Usage in Pregnancy: Torecan® (thiethylperazine) is contraindicated in pregnancy.

Continued on next page

Torecan—Cont.

WARNINGS

Torecan® (thiethylperazine) injection contains sodium metabisulfite, a sulfite that may cause allergic-type reactions including anaphylactic symptoms and life-threatening or less severe asthmatic episodes in certain susceptible people. The overall prevalence of sulfite sensitivity in the general population is unknown and probably low. Sulfite sensitivity is seen more frequently in asthmatic than in nonasthmatic people.

Phenothiazines are capable of potentiating CNS depressants (e.g., anesthetics, opiates, alcohol, etc.) as well as atropine and phosphorus insecticides.

Since Torecan® (thiethylperazine) may impair mental and/or physical ability required in the performance of potentially hazardous tasks such as driving a car or operating machinery, it is recommended that patients be warned accordingly.

Postoperative Nausea and Vomiting: With the use of this drug to control postoperative nausea and vomiting occurring in patients undergoing elective surgical procedures, restlessness and postoperative CNS depression during anesthesia recovery may occur. Possible postoperative complications of a severe degree of any of the known reactions of this class of drug must be considered. Postural hypotension may occur after an initial injection, rarely with the tablet or suppository.

The administration of epinephrine should be avoided in the treatment of drug-induced hypotension in view of the fact that phenothiazines may induce a reversed epinephrine effect on occasion.

Should a vasoconstrictive agent be required, the most suitable are norepinephrine bitartrate and phenylephrine.

The use of this drug has not been studied following intracardiac and intracranial surgery.

PRECAUTIONS

Abnormal movements such as extrapyramidal symptoms (E.P.S.) (e.g., dystonia, torticollis, dysphasia, oculogyric crises, akathisia) have occurred. Convulsions have also been reported. The varied symptom complex is more likely to occur in young adults and children. Extrapyramidal effects must be treated by reduction of dosage or cessation of medication.

Torecan® (thiethylperazine) tablets contain FD&C Yellow No. 5 (tartrazine) which may cause allergic-type reactions (including bronchial asthma) in certain susceptible individuals. Although the overall incidence of FD&C Yellow No. 5 (tartrazine) sensitivity in the general population is low, it is frequently seen in patients who also have aspirin hypersensitivity.

Use in patients with bone marrow depression only when potential benefits outweigh risks.

Neuroleptic Malignant Syndrome (NMS), a potentially fatal symptom complex, has been reported in association with phenothiazine drugs. Clinical manifestations include: hyperpyrexia, muscle rigidity, altered mental status and evidence of autonomic instability.

The extrapyramidal symptoms which can occur secondary to TORECAN® (thiethylperazine) may be confused with the central nervous system signs of an undiagnosed primary disease responsible for the vomiting, e.g., Reye's Syndrome or other encephalopathy. The use of TORECAN® (thiethylperazine) and other potential hepatotoxins should be avoided in children and adolescents whose signs and symptoms suggest Reye's Syndrome.

Phenothiazine drugs may cause elevated prolactin levels that persist during chronic administration. Since approximately one-third of human breast cancers are prolactin-dependent *in vitro,* this elevation is of potential importance if phenothiazine drug administration is contemplated in a patient with a previously-detected breast cancer. Neither clinical nor epidemiologic studies to date, however, have shown an association between the chronic administration of phenothiazine drugs and mammary tumorigenesis.

Postoperative Nausea and Vomiting: When used in the treatment of the nausea and/or vomiting associated with anesthesia and surgery, it is recommended that Torecan® (thiethylperazine) should be administered by deep intramuscular injection at or shortly before the termination of anesthesia.

Information for Patients: Patients receiving TORECAN® (thiethylperazine) should be cautioned about possible combined effects with alcohol and other CNS depressants. Patients should be cautioned not to operate machinery or drive a motor vehicle after ingesting the drug.

Drug Interactions: Phenothiazines are capable of potentiating CNS depressants (e.g., barbiturates, anesthetics, opiates, alcohol, etc.) as well as atropine and phosphorus insecticides.

Laboratory Test Interactions: The usual precautions should be observed in patients with impaired renal or hepatic function.

Nursing Mothers: Information is not available concerning the excretion of TORECAN® (thiethylperazine) in the milk of nursing mothers. As a general rule, nursing should not be undertaken while the patient is on a drug, since many drugs are excreted in human milk.

Pediatric Use: Safety and effectiveness in pediatric patients have not been established.

ADVERSE REACTIONS

Central Nervous System: Serious: Convulsions have been reported. Extrapyramidal symptoms (E.P.S.) may occur, such as dystonia, torticollis, oculogyric crises, akathisia and gait disturbances. Others: Occasional cases of dizziness, headache, fever and restlessness have been reported.

Drowsiness may occur on occasion, following an initial injection. Generally this effect tends to subside with continued therapy or is usually alleviated by a reduction in dosage.

Autonomic Nervous System: Dryness of the mouth and nose, blurred vision, tinnitus. An occasional case of sialorrhea together with altered gustatory sensation has been observed.

Endocrine System: Peripheral edema of the arms, hands and face.

Hepatotoxicity: An occasional case of cholestatic jaundice has been observed.

Other: An occasional case of cerebral vascular spasm and trigeminal neuralgia has been reported.

Phenothiazine Derivatives: The physician should be aware that the following have occurred with one or more phenothiazines and should be considered whenever one of these drugs is used:

Blood Dyscrasias Serious—Agranulocytosis, leukopenia, thrombocytopenia, aplastic anemia, pancytopenia. Other—Eosinophilia, leukocytosis.

Autonomic Reactions Miosis, obstipation, anorexia, paralytic ileus.

Cutaneous Reactions Serious—Erythema, exfoliative dermatitis, contact dermatitis.

Hepatotoxicity Serious—Jaundice, biliary stasis.

Cardiovascular Effects Serious—Hypotension, rarely leading to cardiac arrest; electrocardiographic (ECG) changes.

Extrapyramidal Symptoms Serious—Akathisia, agitation, motor restlessness, dystonic reactions, trismus, torticollis, opisthotonos, oculogyric crises, tremor, muscular rigidity, akinesia—some of which have persisted for several months or years especially in patients of advanced age with brain damage.

Endocrine Disturbances Menstrual irregularities, altered libido, gynecomastia, weight gain. False positive pregnancy tests have been reported.

Urinary Disturbances Retention, incontinence.

Allergic Reactions Serious—Fever, laryngeal edema, angioneurotic edema, asthma.

Others: Hyperpyrexia, Behavioral effects suggestive of a paradoxical reaction have been reported. These include excitement, bizarre dreams, aggravation of psychoses and toxic confusional states. While there is no evidence at present that ECG changes observed in patients receiving phenothiazines are in any way precursors of any significant disturbance of cardiac rhythm, it should be noted that sudden and unexpected deaths apparently due to cardiac arrest have been reported in a few instances in hospitalized psychotic patients previously showing characteristic ECG changes. A peculiar skin-eye syndrome has also been recognized as a side effect following long-term treatment with certain phenothiazines. This reaction is marked by progressive pigmentation of areas of the skin or conjunctiva and/or accompanied by discoloration of the exposed sclera and cornea. Opacities of the anterior lens and cornea described as irregular or stellate in shape have also been reported.

DRUG ABUSE AND DEPENDENCE

TORECAN® (thiethylperazine) is not a controlled substance.

OVERDOSAGE

Manifestations of acute overdosage of TORECAN® (thiethylperazine) can be expected to reflect the CNS effects of the drug and include extrapyramidal symptoms (E.P.S.), confusion and convulsions with reduced or absent reflexes, respiratory depression and hypotension. If the patient is conscious, vomiting should be induced mechanically or with emetics. Gastric lavage should be employed utilizing concurrently a cuffed endotracheal tube if the patient is unconscious to prevent aspiration and pulmonary complications. Maintenance of adequate pulmonary ventilation is essential. The use of pressor agents intravenously may be necessary to combat hypotension. The administration of epinephrine should be avoided since phenothiazines may induce a reversed epinephrine effect. The most suitable vasoconstrictive agents are norepinephrine and phenylephrine. Fluids should be administered intravenously to encourage diuresis. The value of dialysis has not been determined. If excitation occurs, barbiturates should not be used. It should be borne in mind that multiple agents may have been ingested.

DOSAGE AND ADMINISTRATION

Adult: Usual daily dose range is 10 mg to 30 mg. *ORAL:* One tablet one to three times daily. *INTRAMUSCULAR:* 2 ml IM, one to three times daily. (See PRECAUTIONS.)

Pediatric Patients: Appropriate dosage of Torecan® (thiethylperazine) has not been determined in pediatric patients.

HOW SUPPLIED

Tablets Each tablet contains 10 mg thiethylperazine maleate, USP.

NDC 0054-8748-25: Unit dose tablets, 10 tablets per strip, 10 strips per shelf pack.

NDC 0054-4748-25: Bottles of 100 tablets.

Storage: Below 86°F (30°C). Dispense in a tight, light-resistant container as defined in the USP/NF.

Ampuls: Each 2 ml ampul contains in aqueous solution 10 mg thiethylperazine malate, USP.

NDC 0054-1701-07: Boxes of 20 ampules

NDC 0054-1701-25: Boxes of 100 ampules

Storage: Below 86 °F (30°C); protect from light.

Administer only if clear and colorless.

Manufactured by
Sandoz Pharmaceuticals Corporation
East Hanover, NJ 07936
Distributed by
Roxane Laboratories Inc.
Columbus OH 43216
Revised 01/97
30293902

VIRAMUNE® ℞

(nevirapine) Tablets
200 mg

> **WARNING**
> SEVERE AND LIFE-THREATENING SKIN REACTIONS (STEVENS-JOHNSON SYNDROME, TOXIC EPIDERMAL NECROLYSIS), INCLUDING FATAL CASES HAVE OCCURRED IN PATIENTS WITH VIRAMUNE®. (See WARNINGS)
> SEVERE AND LIFE-THREATENING HEPATOTOXICITY, INCLUDING FATAL HEPATIC NECROSIS, HAS OCCURED IN PATIENTS TREATED WITH VIRAMUNE®. (See WARNINGS)
> RESISTANT VIRUS EMERGES RAPIDLY AND UNIFORMLY WHEN VIRAMUNE® IS ADMINISTERED AS MONOTHERAPY. THEREFORE, VIRAMUNE® SHOULD ALWAYS BE ADMINISTERED IN COMBINATION WITH ANTIRETROVIRAL AGENTS.

DESCRIPTION

VIRAMUNE® is the brand name for nevirapine (NVP), a non-nucleoside reverse transcriptase inhibitor with activity against Human Immunodeficiency Virus Type 1 (HIV-1). Nevirapine is structurally a member of the dipyridodiazepinone chemical class of compounds.

VIRAMUNE® is available as tablets for oral administration. Each tablet contains 200 mg of nevirapine and the inactive ingredients microcrystalline cellulose, lactose monohydrate, povidone, sodium starch glycolate, colloidal silicon dioxide and magnesium stearate.

The chemical name of nevirapine is 11-cyclopropyl-5,11-dihydro-4-methyl-6H-dipyrido [3,2b:2′,3′-][1,4] diazepin-6-one. Nevirapine is a white to off-white crystalline powder with the molecular weight of 266.3 and the molecular formula $C_{15}H_{14}N_4O$. Nevirapine has the following structural formula:

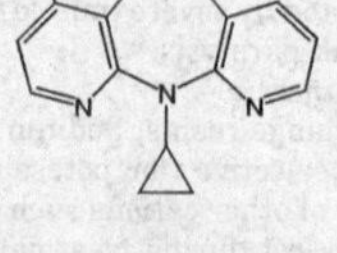

MICROBIOLOGY

Mechanism of Action: Nevirapine is a non-nucleoside reverse transcriptase inhibitor (NNRTI) of HIV-1. Nevirapine binds directly to reverse transcriptase (RT) and blocks the RNA-dependent and DNA-dependent DNA polymerase activities by causing a disruption of the enzyme's catalytic site. The activity of nevirapine does not compete with template or nucleoside triphosphates. HIV-2 RT and eukaryotic DNA polymerases (such as human DNA polymerases α, β, γ or δ) are not inhibited by nevirapine.

In Vitro HIV Susceptibility: The relationship between *in vitro* susceptibility of HIV-1 to nevirapine and the inhibition

of HIV-1 replication in humans has not been established. The *in vitro* antiviral activity of nevirapine was measured in peripheral blood mononuclear cells, monocyte derived macrophages, and lymphoblastoid cell lines. IC_{50} values (50% inhibitory concentration) ranged from 10–100 nM against laboratory and clinical isolates of HIV-1. In cell culture, nevirapine demonstrated additive to synergistic activity against HIV in drug combination regimens with zidovudine (ZDV), didanosine (ddI), stavudine (d4T), lamivudine (3TC), saquinavir, and indinavir.

Resistance: HIV isolates with reduced susceptibility (100-250-fold) to nevirapine emerge *in vitro*. Genotypic analysis showed mutations in the HIV RT gene at amino acid positions 181 and/or 106 depending upon the virus strain and cell line employed. Time to emergence of nevirapine resistance *in vitro* was not altered when selection included nevirapine in combination with several other NNRTIs.

Phenotypic and genotypic changes in HIV-1 isolates from patients treated with either nevirapine (n=24) or nevirapine and ZDV (n=14) were monitored in Phase I/II trials over 1 to ≥12 weeks. After 1 week of nevirapine monotherapy, isolates from 3/3 patients had decreased susceptibility to nevirapine *in vitro* ; one or more of the RT mutations at amino acid positions 103, 106, 108, 181, 188 and 190 were detected in some patients as early as 2 weeks after therapy initiation. By week eight of nevirapine monotherapy, 100% of the patients tested (n=24) had HIV isolates with a >100-fold decrease in susceptibility to nevirapine *in vitro* compared to baseline, and had one or more of the nevirapine-associated RT resistance mutations; 19 of 24 patients (80%) had isolates with a position 181 mutation regardless of dose. Nevirapine+ZDV combination therapy did not alter the emergence rate of nevirapine-resistant virus or the magnitude of nevirapine resistance *in vitro* ; however, a different RT mutation pattern, predominantly distributed amongst amino acid positions 103, 106, 188, and 190, was observed. In patients (6 of 14) whose baseline isolates possessed a wild type RT gene, nevirapine+ZDV combination therapy did not appear to delay emergence of ZDV-resistant RT mutations. The clinical relevance of phenotypic and genotypic changes associated with nevirapine therapy has not been established.

Cross-resistance: Rapid emergence of HIV strains which are cross-resistant to NNRTIs has been observed *in vitro*. Data on cross-resistance between the NNRTI nevirapine and nucleoside analogue RT inhibitors are very limited. In four patients, ZDV-resistant isolates tested *in vitro* retained susceptibility to nevirapine and in six patients, nevirapine-resistant isolates were susceptible to ZDV and ddI. Cross-resistance between nevirapine and HIV protease inhibitors is unlikely because the enzyme targets involved are different.

ANIMAL PHARMACOLOGY

Animal studies have shown that nevirapine is widely distributed to nearly all tissues and readily crosses the blood-brain barrier.

CLINICAL PHARMACOLOGY

Absorption and Bioavailability in Adults: Nevirapine is readily absorbed (>90%) after oral administration in healthy volunteers and in adults with HIV-1 infection. Absolute bioavailablility in 12 healthy adults following single-dose administration was 93 ± 9% (mean ± SD) for a 50 mg tablet and 91 ± 8% for an oral solution. Peak plasma nevirapine concentrations of 2 ± 0.4 µg/mL (7.5 µM) were attained by 4 hours following a single 200 mg dose. Following multiple doses, nevirapine peak concentrations appear to increase linearly in the dose range of 200 to 400 mg/day. Steady state through nevirapine concentrations of 4.5 ± 1.9 µg/mL (17 ± 7 µM), (n = 242) were attained at 400 mg/day. When VIRAMUNE® (200 mg) was administered to 24 healthy adults (12 female, 12 male), with either a high fat breakfast (857 kcal, 50 g fat, 53% of calories from fat) or antacid (Maalox® 30 mL), the extent of nevirapine absorption (AUC) was comparable to that observed under fasting conditions. In a separate study in HIV-1 infected patients (n=6), nevirapine steady-state systemic exposure (AUC_T) was not significantly altered by ddI, which is formulated with an alkaline buffering agent. VIRAMUNE® may be administered with or without food, antacid or ddI.

Distribution: Nevirapine is highly lipophilic and essentially nonionized at physiologic pH. Following intravenous administration to healthy adults, the apparent volume of distribution (Vdss) of nevirapine was 1.21 ± 0.09 L/kg, suggesting that nevirapine is widely distributed in humans. Nevirapine readily crosses the placenta and is found in breast milk. (See PRECAUTIONS, *Nursing Mothers*) Nevirapine is about 60% bound to plasma proteins in the plasma concentration range of 1–10 µg/mL. Nevirapine concentrations in human cerebrospinal fluid (n=6) were 45% (±5%) of the concentrations in plasma; this ratio is approximately equal to the fraction not bound to plasma protein.

Metabolism/Elimination: *In vivo* studies in humans and *in vitro* studies with human liver microsomes have shown that nevirapine is extensively biotransformed via cytochrome P450 (oxidative) metabolism to several hydroxylated metabolites. *In vitro* studies with human liver microsomes suggest that oxidative metabolism of nevirapine is mediated primarily by cytochrome P450 isozymes from the CYP3A family, although other isozymes may have a secondary role. In a mass balance/excretion study in eight healthy male volunteers dosed to steady state with nevirapine 200 mg given twice daily followed by a single 50 mg dose of ^{14}C-nevirapine, approximately 91.4 ± 10.5% of the radiolabeled dose was recovered, with urine (81.3 ± 11.1%) representing the primary route of excretion compared to feces (10.1 ± 1.5%). Greater than 80% of the radioactivity in urine was made up of glucuronide conjugates of hydroxylated metabolites. Thus cytochrome P450 metabolism, glucuronide conjugation, and urinary excretion of glucuronidated metabolites represent the primary route of nevirapine biotransformation and elimination in humans. Only a small fraction (<5%) of the radioactivity in urine (representing <3% of the total dose) was made up of parent compound; therefore, renal excretion plays a minor role in elimination of the parent compound.

Nevirapine has been shown to be an inducer of hepatic cytochrome P450 metabolic enzymes. The pharmacokinetics of autoinduction are characterized by an approximately 1.5 to 2 fold increase in the apparent oral clearance of nevirapine as treatment continues from a single dose to two-to-four weeks of dosing with 200–400 mg/day. Autoinduction also results in a corresponding decrease in the terminal phase half-life of nevirapine in plasma from approximately 45 hours (single dose) to approximately 25–30 hours following multiple dosing with 200–400 mg/day.

Special Populations: **Renal/Hepatic Dysfunction:** The pharmacokinetics of nevirapine have not been evaluated in patients with either renal or hepatic dysfunction.

Gender: In one Phase I study in healthy volunteers (15 females, 15 males), the weight-adjusted apparent volume of distribution (Vdss/F) of nevirapine was higher in the female subjects (1.54 L/kg) compared to the males (1.38 L/kg), suggesting that nevirapine was distributed more extensively in the female subjects. However, this difference was offset by a slightly shorter terminal-phase half-life in the females resulting in no significant gender difference in nevirapine oral clearance or plasma concentrations following either single- or multiple-dose adminstration(s).

Race: An evaluation of nevirapine plasma concentrations (pooled data from several clinical trials) from HIV-1 infected patients (27 Black, 24 Hispanic, 189 Caucasian) revealed no marked difference in nevirapine steady-state trough concentrations (median Cminss = 4.7 µg/mL Black, 3.8 µg/mL Hispanic, 4.3 µg/mL Caucasian) with long-term nevirapine treatment at 400 mg/day. However, the pharmacokinetics of nevirapine have not been evaluated specifically for the effects of ethnicity.

Age: Nevirapine pharmacokinetics in HIV-1 infected adults do not appear to change with age (range 18–68 years); however, nevirapine has not been extensively evaluated in patients beyond the age of 55 years. Nevirapine is metabolized more rapidly in pediatric patients than in adults. (See PRECAUTIONS, *Pediatric Use*)

Drug Interactions: *Nucleoside Analogues:* No dosage adjustments are required when VIRAMUNE® is taken in combination with ZDV, ddI, or zalcitabine (ddC). Results from studies in HIV-1 infected patients who were administered VIRAMUNE® with different combinations of ddI or ddC, on a background of ZDV therapy, indicated that no clinically significant pharmacokinetic interactions occurred when the nucleoside analogues were administered in combination with VIRAMUNE®.

Protease Inhibitors: In the following three studies, VIRAMUNE® was given 200 mg once daily for two weeks followed by 200 mg twice daily for 28 days:

Ritonavir: No dosage adjustments are required when VIRAMUNE® is taken in combination with ritonavir. Results from a 49-day study in HIV-infected patients (n=14) administered VIRAMUNE® and ritonavir (600 mg b.i.d. [using a gradual dose escalation regimen]) indicated that their coadministration did not affect ritonavir ACU or Cmax. Comparison of nevirapine pharmacokinetics from this study to historical data suggested that coadministration did not affect the pharmacokinetics of nevirapine.

Indinavir: Results from a 36-day study in HIV-infected patients (n=19) administered VIRAMUNE® and Indinavir (800 mg q8h) indicated that their coadministration led to a 28% mean decrease (95% Cl -39, -16) in indinavir AUC and an 11% mean decrease (95% Cl -49, +59) in indinavir Cmax. The clinical significance of this interaction is not known. Comparison of nevirapine pharmacokinetics from this study to historical data suggested that coadministration did not affect the pharmacokinetics of nevirapine.

Saquinavir: Results from a 42-day study in HIV-infected patients (n=23) administered VIRAMUNE® and saquinavir (hard gelatin capsules, 600 mg t.i.d.) indicated that their coadministration led to a 24% mean decrease (95% Cl -42, -1) in saquinavir AUC and a 28% mean decrease (95% Cl -47, -1) in saquinavir Cmax. The clinical significance of this interaction is not known. Coadministration did not affect the pharmacokinetics of nevirapine.

In vitro: Studies using human liver microsomes indicated that the formation of nevirapine hydroxylated metabolites was not affected by the presence of dapsone, rifabutin, rifampin, and trimethoprim/sulfamethoxazole. Ketoconazole significantly inhibited the formation of nevirapine hydroxylated metabolites.

In vivo: ketoconazole: VIRAMUNE® and ketoconazole should not be administered concomitantly. Ketoconazole and Cmax decreased by a median 63% (95% Cl -95, +33) and 40% (95% Cl -52, +11), respectively, in HIV-infected patients (n=22) who were given VIRAMUNE® 200 mg once daily for two weeks followed by 200 mg twice daily for two weeks along with ketoconazole 400 mg daily. (See PRECAUTIONS, *Drug Interactions*) Comparison of the pharmacokinetics from this study to historical data suggested that coadministration with ketoconazole may result in a 15–30% increase in nevirapine plasma concentrations. The clinical significance of this observation is not known.

Monitoring of nevirapine plasma concentrations in patients who received long-term VIRAMUNE® treatment indicate that steady-state nevirapine through plasma concentrations were elevated in patients who received cimetidine (+21%, n=11) and macrolides (+12%, n=24), known inhibitors of CYP3A.

Steady-state nevirapine trough concentrations were reduced in patients who received rifabutin (-16%, n=19) and rifampin (-37%, n=3), known inducers of CYP3A. Nevirapine is an inducer of CYP3A, with maximal induction occurring within 2–4 weeks of initiating multiple-dose therapy. Other compounds that are substrates of CYP3A may have decreased plasma concentrations when co-administered with VIRAMUNE®. Therefore, careful monitoring of the therapeutic effectiveness of CYP3A-metabolized drugs is recommended when taken in combination with VIRAMUNE®. (See PRECAUTIONS, *Drug Interactions*, for recommendations regarding rifampin, rifabutin and oral contraceptives)

INDICATIONS AND USAGE

VIRAMUNE® (nevirapine) is indicated for use in combination with other antiretroviral agents for the treatment of HIV-1 infection. This indication is based on analysis of changes in surrogate endpoints. At present, there are no results from controlled clinical trials evaluating the effect of VIRAMUNE® in combination with other antiretroviral agents on the clinical progression of HIV-1 infection, such as the incidence of opportunistic infections or survival.

Resistant virus emerges rapidly and uniformly when VIRAMUNE® is administered as monotherapy. Therefore, VIRAMUNE® should always be administered in combination with at least one additional antiretroviral agent.

Description of Clinical Studies: Patients with a prior history of nucleoside therapy: ACTG 241 compared treatment with VIRAMUNE®+ZDV+ddI versus ZDV+ddI in 398 HIV-1-infected patients (median age 38 years, 74% Caucasian, 80% male) with CD4+ cell counts ≤350 cells/mm^3 (mean 153 cells/mm^3) and a mean baseline plasma HIV-1 RNA concentration of 4.59 $\log_{10}$ copies/mL (38,905 copies/mL), who had received at least 6 months of nucleoside therapy prior to enrollment (median 115 weeks). Treatment doses were VIRAMUNE®, 200 mg daily for two weeks, followed by 200 mg twice daily, or placebo; ZDV, 200 mg three times daily; ddI, 200 mg twice daily. Mean changes in CD4+ cell counts are shown in Figure 1. For 198 patients in the virology substudy, mean HIV-1 RNA concentration changes from baseline are shown in Figure 2.

Figure 1: Mean Change From Baseline for CD4+ Cell Count (absolute number of CD4+ cells/mm^3), Trial ACTG 241

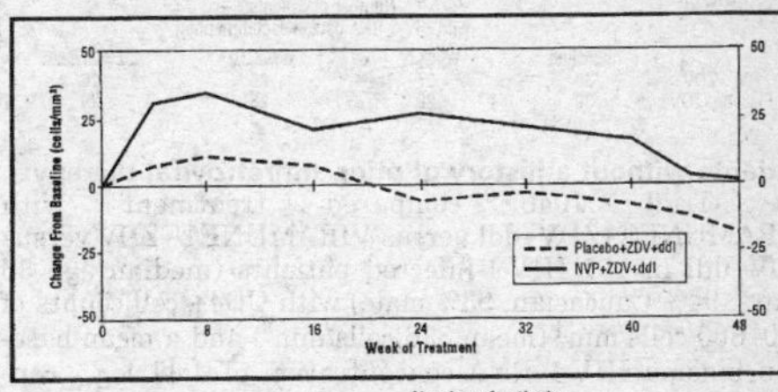

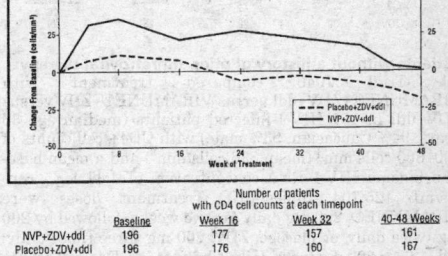

Number of patients with CD4 cell counts at each timepoint

	Baseline	Week 16	Week 32	40-48 Weeks
NVP+ZDV+ddI	196	177	157	161
Placebo+ZDV+ddI	196	176	160	167

[See figure 2 at top of next column]

Trial B1 1037 compared treatment with VIRAMUNE®+ZDV versus ZDV in 60 HIV-1- infected patients (median age 33 years, 70% Caucasian, 93% male) with CD4+ cell counts between 200 and 500 cells/mm^3 (mean 373 cells/mm^3) and a mean baseline plasma HIV-1

Continued on next page

Viramune—Cont.

Figure 2: Mean Change From Baseline in HIV-1 RNA* Concentrations (log_{10} copies/mL), Virology Sub-study of Trial ACTG 241

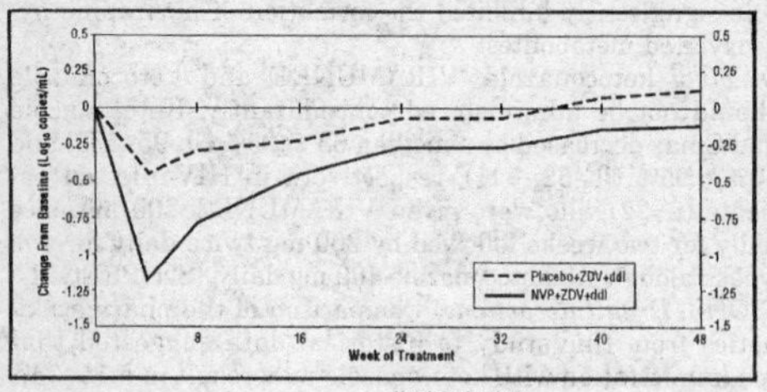

Number of patients with HIV-1 RNA data at each timepoint

	Baseline	Week 16	Week 32	40-48 Weeks
NVP+ZDV+ddI	95	84	75	74
Placebo+ZDV+ddI	93	82	75	75

* the clinical significance of changes in serum viral RNA measurements during treatment with VIRAMUNE® has not been established

RNA concentration of 4.24 log_{10} copies/mL (17,378 copies/mL), who had received between 3 and 24 months of prior ZDV therapy (median 35 weeks). Treatment doses were VIRAMUNE® 200 mg daily for 2 weeks, followed by 200 mg twice daily, or placebo; ZDV, 500–600 mg/day. Mean changes in CD4+ cell counts are shown in Figure 3. Mean HIV-1 RNA concentration changes from baseline are shown in Figure 4.

Figure 3: Mean Change From Baseline for CD4+ Cell Count (absolute number of CD4+ cells/mm^3), Trial B1 1037

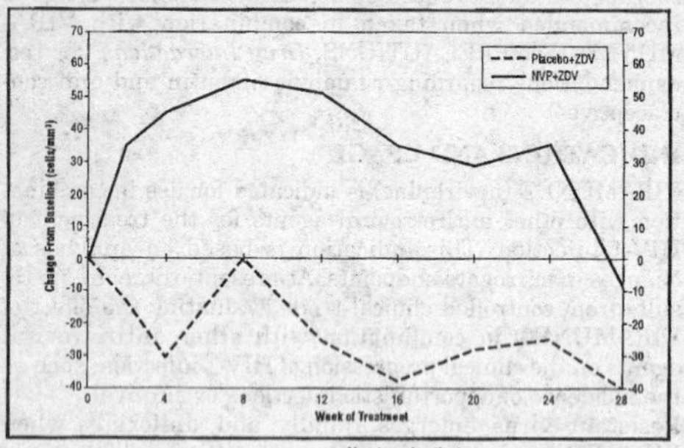

Number of patients with CD4 cell counts at each timepoint

	Baseline	Week 8	Week 16	20-28 Weeks
NVP+ZDV	30	28	26	26
Placebo+ZDV	30	30	28	29

Figure 4: Mean Change From Baseline for HIV-1 RNA Concentrations (log_{10} copies/mL), Trial B1 1037

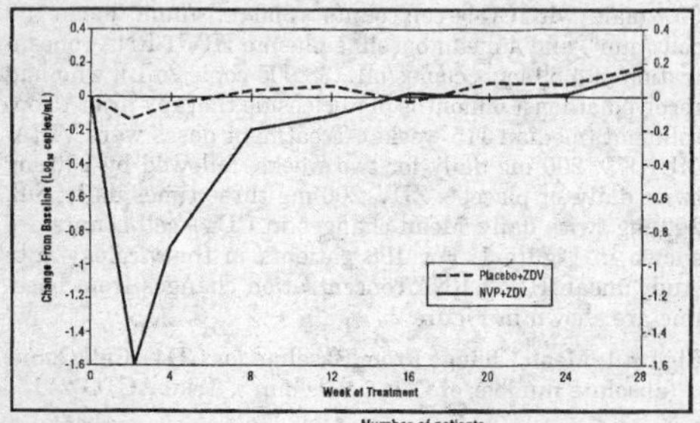

Number of patients with HIV-1 RNA data at each timepoint

	Baseline	Week 8	Week 16	20-28 Weeks
NVP+ZDV	30	27	26	26
Placebo+ZDV	30	29	28	29

Patients without a history of prior antiretroviral therapy: B1 Trial 1046 compared treatment with VIRAMUNE®+ZDV+ddI versus VIRAMUNE®+ZDV versus ZDV+ddI in 151 HIV-1-infected patients (median age 36 years, 94% Caucasian, 93% male) with CD4+ cell counts of 200–600 cells/mm^3 (mean 376 cells/mm^3) and a mean baseline plasma HIV-1 RNA concentration of 4.41 log_{10} copies/mL (25,704 copies/mL). Treatment doses were VIRAMUNE®, 200 mg daily for two weeks, followed by 200 mg twice daily, or placebo; ZDV, 200 mg three times daily; ddI, 125 or 200 mg twice daily. Changes in CD4+ cell counts at 24 weeks: mean levels of CD4+ cell counts in those randomized to VIRAMUNE®+ZDV+ddI and ZDV+ddI remained significantly above baseline; however there was no significant difference between these arms. Changes in HIV-1 viral RNA at 24 weeks: there was no significant difference as measured by mean changes in plasma viral RNA between those randomized to VIRAMUNE®+ZDV+ddI and ZDV+ddI. However, the proportion of patients whose HIV-1 RNA decreased below the limit of detection (400 copies/mL) was significantly greater for the VIRAMUNE®+ZDV+ddI group (27/36 or 75%), when compared to the ZDV+ddI group (18/39 or 46%) or the VIRAMUNE®+ZDV group (0/28 or 0%); the clinical significance of this finding is unknown.

CONTRAINDICATIONS

VIRAMUNE® is contraindicated in patients with clinically significant hypersensitivity to any of the components contained in the tablet.

WARNINGS

Severe and life-threatening skin reactions have occurred in patients treated with VIRAMUNE®, including Stevens-Johnson syndrome and toxic epidermal necrolysis. Fatal cases of toxic epidermal necrolysis have been reported. VIRAMUNE® must be discontinued in patients developing a severe rash or a rash accompanied by constitutional symptoms such as fever, blistering, oral lesions, conjunctivitis, swelling, muscle or joint aches, or general malaise. (See PRECAUTIONS, *Information for Patients*; ADVERSE REACTIONS) VIRAMUNE® therapy must be initiated with a 14-day lead-in period of 200 mg/day, which has been shown to reduce the frequency of rash. If rash is observed during this lead-in period, dose escalation should not occur until the rash has resolved. (See DOSAGE AND ADMINISTRATION)

Severe or life-threatening hepatoxicity, including fatal fulminant hepatitis (transaminase elevations, with or without hyperbilirubinemia, prolonged partial thromboplastin time, or eosinophilia), has occurred in patients treated with VIRAMUNE®. Some of these cases began in the first few weeks of therapy, and some were accompanied by rash. VIRAMUNE® administration should be interrupted in patients experiencing moderate or severe ALT or AST abnormalities until these return to baseline values. VIRAMUNE® should be permanently discontinued if liver function abnormalities recur upon readministration. Monitoring of ALT and AST is strongly recommended, especially during the first six months of VIRAMUNE® treatment. (See PRECAUTIONS, *Information for Patients*; ADVERSE REACTIONS; DOSAGE AND ADMINISTRATION)

PRECAUTIONS

General: Nevirapine is extensively metabolized by the liver and nevirapine metabolites are extensively eliminated by the kidney. However, the pharmacokinetics of nevirapine have not been evaluated in patients with either hepatic or renal dysfunction. Therefore, VIRAMUNE® should be used with caution in these patient populations.

The duration of clinical benefit from antiretroviral therapy may be limited. Patients receiving VIRAMUNE® or any other antiretroviral therapy may continue to develop opportunistic infections and other complications of HIV infection, and therefore should remain under close clinical observation by physicians experienced in the treatment of patients with associatied HIV diseases.

When administering VIRAMUNE® as part of an antiretroviral regimen, the complete product information for each therapeutic component should be consulted before initiation of treatment.

Drug Interactions: The induction of CYP3A by nevirapine may result in lower plasma concentrations of other concomitantly administered drugs that are extensively metabolized by CYP3A. (See CLINICAL PHARMACOLOGY) Thus, if a patient has been stabilized on a dosage regimen for a drug metabolized by CYP3A, and begins treatment with VIRAMUNE®, dose adjustments may be necessary.

Rifampin/Rifabutin: There are insufficient data to assess whether dose adjustments are necessary when nevirapine and rifampin or rifabutin are coadministered. Therefore, these drugs should only be used in combination if clearly indicated and with careful monitoring.

Ketoconazole: VIRAMUNE® and ketoconazole should not be administered concomitantly. Coadministration of nevirapine and ketoconazole resulted in a significant reduction in ketoconazole plasma concentrations. (See CLINICAL PHARMACOLOGY, Drug Interactions)

Oral Contraceptives: There are no clinical data on the effects of nevirapine on the pharmacokinetics of oral contraceptives. Nevirapine may decrease plasma concentrations of oral contraceptives (also other hormonal contraceptives); therefore, these drugs should not be administered concomitantly with VIRAMUNE®.

Information for Patients: **Patients should be instructed that the major toxicity of VIRAMUNE® is rash and should be advised to promptly notify their physician of any rash.** The majority of rashes associated with VIRAMUNE® occur within the first 6 weeks of initiation of therapy. Patients should be instructed that if any rash occurs during the two-week lead-in period, the VIRAMUNE® dose should not be escalated until the rash resolves. Any patient experiencing severe rash or a rash accompanied by constitutional symptoms such as fever, blistering, oral lesions, conjunctivitis, swelling, muscle or joint aches, or general malaise should immediately discontinue medication and consult a physician.

Patients should be instructed that abnormal liver function tests and cases of clinical hepatitis, including fatal fulminant hepatitis, have been reported with VIRAMUNE®. Liver function tests should be monitored, especially during the first six months of therapy. VIRAMUNE® administration should be interrupted in patients experiencing moderate or severe liver function test abnormalities, until liver function tests return to baseline values; VIRAMUNE® should be permanently discontinued if liver function abnormalities recur upon readministration. Patients should be instructed to consult their physicians immediately should symptoms of hepatitis occur.

Oral contraceptives and other hormonal methods of birth control should not be used as a method of contraception in women taking VIRAMUNE®. (See PRECAUTIONS, Drug Interactions)

Patients should be informed that VIRAMUNE® therapy has not been shown to reduce the risk of transmission of HIV-1 to others through sexual contact or blood contamination. The long term effects of VIRAMUNE® are unknown at this time.

VIRAMUNE® is not a cure for HIV-1 infection; patients may continue to experience illnesses associated with advanced HIV-1 infection, including opportunistic infections. Treatment with VIRAMUNE® has not been shown to reduce the incidence or frequency of such illnesses; patients should be advised to remain under the care of a physician when using VIRAMUNE®.

Patients should be informed to take VIRAMUNE® every day as prescribed. Patients should not alter the dose without consulting their doctor. If a dose is missed, patients should take the next dose as soon as possible. However, if a dose is skipped, the patient should not double the next dose. Patients should be advised to report to their doctor the use of any other medications.

Carcinogenesis, Mutagenesis, Impairment of Fertility: Long-term carcinogenicity studies of nevirapine in animals are currently in progress. In genetic toxicology assays, nevirapine showed no evidence of mutagenic or clastogenic activity in a battery of *in vitro* and *in vivo* assays including microbial assays for gene mutation (Ames: Salmonella strains and *E. coli*), mammalian cell gene mutation assays (CHO/HGPRT), cytogenic assays using a Chinese hamster ovary cell line and a mouse bone marrow micronucleus assay following oral administration. In reproductive toxicology studies, evidence of impaired fertility was seen in female rats at doses providing systemic exposure, based on AUC, approximately equivalent to that provided with the recommended clinical dose of VIRAMUNE®.

Pregnancy: Pregnancy Category C: No observable teratogenicity was detected in reproductive studies performed in pregnant rats and rabbits. In rats, a significant decrease in fetal body weight occurred at doses providing systemic exposure approximately 50% higher, based on AUC, than that seen at the recommended human clinical dose. The maternal and developmental no-observable-effect level dosages in rats and rabbits produced systemic exposures approximately equivalent to or approximately 50% higher, respectively, than those seen at the recommended daily human dose, based on AUC. There are no adequate and well-controlled studies in pregnant women. VIRAMUNE® should be used during pregnancy only if the potential benefit justifies the potential risk to the fetus.

Nursing Mothers: Preliminary results from an ongoing pharmacokinetic study (ACTG 250) of 10 HIV-1-infected pregnant women who were administered a single oral dose of 100 or 200 mg VIRAMUNE® at a median of 5.8 hours before delivery, indicate that nevirapine readily crosses the placenta and is found in breast milk. Consistent with the recommendation by the U.S. Public Health Service Centers for Disease Control and Prevention that HIV-infected mothers not breast-feed their infants to avoid risking postnatal transmission of HIV, mothers should discontinue nursing if they are receiving VIRAMUNE®.

Pediatric Use: Safety and effectiveness of VIRAMUNE® in pediatric patients have not been established.

VIRAMUNE® has been studied in two open-label, uncontrolled trials (B1 882, B1 892) in 37 HIV-1-infected pediatric patients with a median age of 0.9 years (range: 0.1 to 15 years) who were treated for a median duration of 20.7 months. Seven patients developed rashes while receiving VIRAMUNE®. In an ongoing, controlled trial of VIRAMUNE® combination therapy in HIV-1-infected pediatric patients (ACTG 245), one of approximately 288 patients treated with VIRAMUNE® experienced Stevens-Johnson syndrome.

Because there are no data on multi-dose pharmacokinetics in children, no recommendation on dosing can be made. Based on single-dose pharmacokinetics in 9 HIV-1-infected pediatric patients (age 9 mos. to 14 years) who were administered nevirapine in a suspension formulation, it appears that oral clearance is approximately 2-fold greater in children when compared to adults.

ADVERSE REACTIONS

The most frequently reported adverse events related to VIRAMUNE® therapy were rash, fever, nausea, headache, and abnormal liver function tests.

Table 1: Percentage of Patients with Rashes in Controlled Trials[a]

	ACTG 241[b]		BI 1037		BI 1011		COMBINED DATA	
	NVP+ZDV+ddl	ZDV+ddl	NVP+ZDV	ZDV	NVP+ZDV	ZDV	NVP	CONTROL
n	197	201	30	30	25	24	252	255
Rash events of all Grades and all causality	39.6%	23.9%	26.7%	6.7%	32.0%	4.2%	37.3%	20.0%
Grade 3 or 4 rash events; all causality	8.1%	1.5%	3.3%	0%	8.0%	0%	7.6%	1.2%

[a] At recommended dose of one 200 mg tablet daily for the first 14 days followed by one 200 mg tablet twice daily
[b] Trial ACTG 241 was designed to report Grade 3/4 (severe or life-threatening) events; except for several pre-specified events including rash for which all grades are reported

Table 2: Comparative Incidence of Selected Drug-Related Events in Controlled Trials

	ACTG 241		Trial BI 1037 and BI 1011	
	Grade 3/4 Events		All severities	
	NVP+ZDV+ddl	ZDV+ddl	NVP+ZDV	ZDV alone
Number of Patients	197	201	55	30
Overall incidence of related adverse events	31%	23%	42%	33%
Rash	8	2	20	3
Fever	3	3	11	3
Nausea	5	4	9	3
Headache	3	3	11	0
Diarrhea	2	2	0	0
Abdominal pain	1	2	2	0
Ulcerative stomatitis	0	0	4	0
Peripheral neuropathy	0	2	0	0
Paraesthesia	1	0	2	0
Myalgia	1	0	2	7
Hepatitis	1	0	4	0

Table 3: Percentaage of Patients with Marked Laboratory Abnormalities

	Data combined for controlled trials ACTG 241, BI 1037 & BI 1011	
	VIRAMUNE® n=252	Control n=255
Hematology		
Decreased Hg (<8.0 g/dL)	1.2%	2.0%
Decreased plateletes (<50,000/mm^3)	0.8	0.8
Decreased neutrophils (<750/mm^3)	11.1	10.2
Blood chemistry		
Increased ALT (>250 U/L)	3.4	3.5
Increased AST (>250 U/L)	2.0	2.4
Increased GGT (>450 U/L)	2.4	1.2
Increased total bilirubin (>2.5 mg/dL)	0.4	1.2

The major clinical toxicity of VIRAMUNE® is rash, with VIRAMUNE®-attributable rash occuring in 17% of patients in combination regimens in Phase II/III controlled studies. Thirty-seven percent of patients treated with VIRAMUNE® experienced rash compared with 20% of patients treated in control groups of either ZDV+ddl or ZDV alone (Table 1). Severe or life-threatening rash occurred in 7.6% of VIRAMUNE®-treated patients compared with 1.2% of patients treated in the control groups.

Rashes are usually mild to moderate, maculopapular erythematous cutaneous eruptions, with or without pruritus, located on the trunk, face and extremities. The majority of severe rashes occurred within the first 28 days of treatment; 25% of the patients with severe rashes required hospitalization; and one patient required surgical intervention. All patients recovered. Overall, 7% of patients discontinued VIRAMUNE® due to rash.
[See table 1 above]

Table 2 lists treatment-related clinical adverse events that occurred in patients receiving VIRAMUNE® in ACTG 241 and in Trials BI 1037 and BI 1011.
[See table 2 above]

Laboratory Abnormalities: Table 3 summarizes marked laboratory abnormalities occurring in three controlled studies.
[See table 3 above]
Asymptomatic elevations in GGT levels are more frequent in VIRAMUNE® recipientss than in controls. Because clinical hepatitis has been reported in VIRAMUNE®-treated patients, monitoring of ALT (SGPT) and AST (SGOT) is strongly recommended, especially during the first six months of VIRAMUNE® treatment. (See WARNINGS)

OVERDOSAGE

There is no known antidote for VIRAMUNE® overdosage. Cases of VIRAMUNE® overdose at doses ranging from 800 to 1800 mg per day for up to 15 days have been reported. Patients have experienced events including edema, erythema nodosum, fatigue, fever, headache, insomnia, nausea, pulmonary infiltrates, rash, vertigo, vomiting and weight decrease. All events subsided following discontinuation of VIRAMUNE®.

DOSAGE AND ADMINISTRATION

The recommended dose for VIRAMUNE® is one 200 mg tablet daily for the first 14 days (**this lead-in period should be used because it has been found to lessen the frequency of rash**), followed by one 200 mg tablet twice daily, in combination with antiretroviral agents. For concomitantly administered antiretroviral therapy, the manufacturer's recommended dosage and monitoring should be followed.
Monitoring of Patients: Clinical chemistry tests, which include liver function tests, should be performed prior to initiating VIRAMUNE® therapy and at appropriate intervals during therapy. (See WARNINGS)
Dosage Adjustment: **VIRAMUNE® should be discontinued if patients experience severe rash or a rash accompanied by constitutional findings. (See WARNINGS) Patients experiencing rash during the 14-day lead-in period of 200 mg/ day should not have their VIRAMUNE® dose increased until the rash has resolved. (See PRECAUTIONS, *Information for Patients*)**
VIRAMUNE® administration should be interrupted in patients experiencing moderate or severe liver function test abnormalities (excluding GGT), until the liver function test elevations have returned to baseline. VIRAMUNE® may then be restarted at 200 mg per day. Increasing the daily dose to 200 mg twice daily should be done with caution, after extended observation. VIRAMUNE® should be permanently discontinued if moderate or severe liver function test abnormalities recur. (See WARNINGS)
Patients who interrupt VIRAMUNE® dosing for more than 7 days should restart the recommended dosing, using one 200 mg tablet daily for the first 14 days (lead-in) followed by one 200 mg tablet twice daily.
No data are available to recommend a dosage of VIRAMUNE® in patients with hepatic dysfunction, renal insufficiency, or undergoing dialysis.

HOW SUPPLIED

VIRAMUNE® (nevirapine) Tablets, 200 mg, are white, oval, biconvex tablets, 9.3 mm × 19.1 mm. One side is embossed with "54 193", with a single bisect separating the "54" and "193". The opposite side has a single bisect.
VIRAMUNE® Tablets are supplied in bottles of 100 (NDC 0054-4647-25), bottles of 60 (NDC 0054-4647-21), and individually blister-sealed unit-dose cartons of 100 tablets as 10 × 10 cards (NDC 0054-8647-25).
Store at 15°C–30°C (59°F–86°F). The bottles should be kept tightly closed.
Manufactured by:
Boehringer Ingelheim Pharmaceuticals, Inc.
Ridgefield, CT 06877
Distributed by:
Roxane Laboratories, Inc.
Columbus, OH 43216
Rx only
FPL 6/98
Shown in Product Identification Guide, page 335

EDUCATIONAL MATERIAL

Booklets
"Oral Morphine in Advanced Cancer," Robert G. Twycross and Sylvia A. Lack. Practical guidelines on the considerations which must be taken into account when initiating oral morphine therapy, free to physicians and pharmacists. "Oral Morphine—Information for Patients, Families, and Friends," Robert G. Twycross and Sylvia A. Lack, free to physicians, pharmacists, and patients.

For information on over-the-counter drugs, consult **PDR For Nonprescription Drugs**.

Rystan Company, Inc.
47 CENTER AVENUE
P.O. BOX 214
LITTLE FALLS, NJ 07424-0214

Direct Inquiries to:
Professional Services Department
(973) 256-3737

CHLORESIUM®   OTC
[klor-eez 'ium]
Ointment and Solution
Healing and Deodorizing Agent

COMPOSITION

Ointment: 0.5% Chlorophyllin Copper Complex Sodium,
USP in a hydrophilic base. Solution: 0.2% Chlorophyllin
Copper Complex Sodium, USP in isotonic saline solution.

ACTIONS AND USES

To promote healing and to relieve itching and discomfort of
minor wounds, burns, surface ulcers, cuts, abrasions and
skin irritations. To reduce malodors in wounds and surface
ulcers.

ADMINISTRATION AND DOSAGE

Ointment: Apply generously and cover with an appropriate
dressing, or as directed by physician. Dressings preferably
changed no more often than every 48 to 72 hours. Solution:
Apply full strength as continuous wet dressing, or as directed by physician.

SIDE EFFECTS

CHLORESIUM Ointment and Solution are soothing and
nontoxic. Sensitivity reactions are extremely rare, and only
a few instances of slight itching or irritation have been reported.

HOW SUPPLIED

Ointment: 1 oz and 4 oz tubes, 1 lb. jars (NDC 0263-5155-01
and -04, -16). Solution: 8 fl oz and 32 fl oz bottles (NDC
0263-5158-08 and -32).

DERIFIL® Tablets   OTC
[der 'ah-fil]
Internal Deodorant

COMPOSITION

Active ingredient: 100 mg Chlorophyllin Copper Complex
Sodium, USP per tablet.
Inactive ingredients: Dextrose USP, Hydrogenated Vegetable Oil NF, Hydroxypropyl Methylcellulose USP, Microcrystalline Cellulose NF, Peppermint Powder, Polyethylene Glycol NF, Sodium Chloride USP.

INDICATIONS

Oral deodorant for internal use: 1. An aid to reduce fecal
odor due to incontinence, 2. An aid to reduce odor from a
colostomy or ileostomy.

DIRECTIONS

Adults and children 12 years of age and over: Oral dosage is
one to two tablets daily in divided doses as required. If odor
is not controlled, take up to one additional tablet daily in
divided doses as required. The smallest effective dose
should be used. Do not exceed 3 tablets daily. Children under 12 years of age: consult a doctor. In ostomies, tablets
may be either taken by mouth or placed in the appliance.

SIDE EFFECTS

When used as directed, no toxic effects have been reported.
As with any drug, do not exceed the recommended dosage. A
temporary mild laxative effect may be noted, and the fecal
discharge is commonly stained dark green.

WARNING

If cramps or diarrhea occurs, reduce the dosage. If symptoms persist, consult your doctor.

HOW SUPPLIED

Dark green, round, film-coated tablet with "D" on one side
and score on other. Each tablet contains 100 mg Chlorophyllin Copper Complex Sodium, USP. Bottles of 30 (NDC
87900-500-13), 100 (NDC 87900-500-10), 1000 tablets (NDC
87900-500-11) and blister pack of 40 tablets (NDC 87900-
500-14).

3/97

PANAFIL® Ointment   ℞
[pan 'ah-fil]
Papain-Urea-Chlorophyllin Copper Complex Sodium
Debriding-Healing Ointment

CAUTION
Federal law prohibits dispensing without prescription.

DESCRIPTION

PANAFIL® Ointment is an enzymatic debriding-healing
ointment which contains standardized Papain, USP (NOT
LESS THAN 521,700 USP units per gram of ointment);
Urea USP 10% and Chlorophyllin Copper Complex Sodium,
USP 0.5% in a hydrophilic base. Inactive ingredients are
Purified Water, USP; Propylene Glycol, USP; White Petro-
latum, USP; Stearyl Alcohol, NF; Polyoxyl 40 Stearate, NF;
Sorbitan Monostearate, NF; Boric Acid, NF; Chlorobutanol
(Anhydrous), NF as a preservative; Sodium Borate, NF.

CLINICAL PHARMACOLOGY

Papain, the proteolytic enzyme derived from the fruit of
carica papaya, is a potent digestant of nonviable protein
matter, but is harmless to viable tissue. It has the unique
advantage of being active over a wide pH range, 3 to 12.
Despite its recognized value as a digestive agent, papain is
relatively ineffective when used alone as a debriding agent,
primarily because it requires the presence of activators to
exert its digestive function.
In PANAFIL® Ointment, Urea is combined with papain to
provide two supplementary chemical actions: 1) to expose by
solvent action the activators of papain (sulfhydryl groups)
which are always present, but not necessarily accessible, in
the nonviable tissue or debris of lesions, and 2) to denature
the nonviable protein matter in lesions and thereby render
it more susceptible to enzymatic digestion. In pharmacologic studies involving digestion of beef powder, Miller[1]
showed that the combination of papain and urea produced
twice as much digestion as papain alone.
Chlorophyllin Copper Complex Sodium adds healing action
to the cleansing action of the proteolytic papain-urea combination. The basic wound-healing properties of Chlorophyllin Copper Complex Sodium are promotion of healthy
granulations, control of local inflammation and reduction of
wound odors.[2] Specifically, Chlorophyllin Copper Complex
Sodium inhibits the hemagglutinating and inflammatory
properties of protein degradation products in the wound, including the products of enzymatic digestion, thus providing
an additional protective factor.[1,3] The incorporation of Chlorophyllin Copper Complex Sodium in PANAFIL® Ointment
permits its continuous use for as long as desired to help produce and then maintain a clean wound base and to promote
healing.

INDICATIONS AND USES

PANAFIL® Ointment is suggested for treatment of acute
and chronic lesions such as varicose, diabetic and decubitus
ulcers, burns, postoperative wounds, pilonidal cyst wounds,
carbuncles and miscellaneous traumatic or infected
wounds.
PANAFIL® Ointment is applied continuously throughout
treatment of these conditions (1) for enzymatic debridement
of necrotic tissue and liquefaction of fibrinous, purulent debris, (2) to **keep** the wound clean, and simultaneously (3) to
promote normal healing.

CONTRAINDICATIONS
None known.

PRECAUTIONS
See Dosage and Administration.
Not to be used in eyes.

ADVERSE REACTIONS

PANAFIL® Ointment is generally well tolerated and nonirritating. A small percentage of patients may experience a
transient "burning" sensation on application of the ointment. Occasionally, the profuse exudate resulting from enzymatic digestion may cause irritation. In such cases, more
frequent changes of dressings until exudate diminishes will
alleviate discomfort.

DOSAGE AND ADMINISTRATION

Apply PANAFIL® Ointment directly to lesion and cover
with appropriate dressing. When practicable, daily or twice
daily changes of dressings are preferred. Longer intervals
between redressings (two or three days) have proved satisfactory, and PANAFIL® Ointment may be applied under
pressure dressings. At each redressing, the lesion should be
irrigated with isotonic saline solution or other mild cleansing solution (except hydrogen peroxide solution, which may
inactivate the papain) to remove any accumulation of liquefied necrotic material.

NOTE

Papain may also be inactivated by the salts of heavy metals
(lead, silver, mercury, etc.). Contact with medications containing these metals should be avoided.

HOW SUPPLIED

Available on prescription only in 1 oz tube (NDC 0263-5145-
01) and 1 lb jar (NDC 0263-5145-16).

REFERENCES
1–3. Data on file.   5/97

Shown in Product Identification Guide, page 335

PANAFIL®-WHITE   ℞
[pan' ah-fil]
Papain-Urea Debriding Ointment

CAUTION
Federal law prohibits dispensing without prescription.

DESCRIPTION

PANAFIL-WHITE Ointment is an enzymatic debriding
ointment containing standardized Papain, USP (NOT LESS
THAN 521,700 USP units per gram of ointment) and Urea
USP 10% in a hydrophilic base.
Inactive ingredients are Purified Water, USP; Propylene
Glycol, USP; White Petrolatum, USP; Stearyl Alcohol, NF;
Sorbitan Monostearate, NF; Polyoxyl 40 Stearate, NF; Boric
Acid, NF; Sodium Borate, NF; Chlorobutanol (Anhydrous),
NF as a preservative.

CLINICAL PHARMACOLOGY

Papain, the proteolytic enzyme from the fruit of carica papaya, is a potent digestant of nonviable protein matter, but
is harmless to viable tissue. It has the unique advantage of
being active over a wide pH range, 3 to 12. Despite its recognized value as a digestive agent, papain is relatively ineffective when used alone as a debriding agent, primarily
because it requires the presence of activators to exert its digestive function.
In PANAFIL-WHITE, urea is combined with papain to provide two supplementary chemical actions: 1) to expose by
solvent action the activators of papain (sulfhydryl groups)
which are always present, but not necessarily accessible, in
the nonviable tissue or debris of lesions, and 2) to denature
the nonviable protein matter in lesions and thereby render
it more susceptible to enzymatic digestion. In pharmacologic studies involving digestion of beef powder, Miller[1]
showed that the combination of papain and urea produced
twice as much digestion as papain alone.

INDICATIONS AND USES

PANAFIL-WHITE is indicated for debridement of necrotic
tissue and liquefaction of pus in acute and chronic lesions
such as decubitus, varicose and diabetic ulcers, burns, postoperative wounds, pilonidal cyst wounds, carbuncles and
miscellaneous traumatic or infected wounds.

CONTRAINDICATIONS
None known

PRECAUTIONS
See Dosage and Administration.
Not to be used in eyes.

ADVERSE REACTIONS

PANAFIL-WHITE is generally well tolerated and nonirritating. A small percentage of patients may experience a
transient "burning" sensation on application of the ointment. Occasionally, the profuse exudate resulting from
enzymatic digestion may cause irritation. In such cases, more
frequent changes of dressings until exudate diminishes will
alleviate discomfort.

DOSAGE AND ADMINISTRATION

Apply PANAFIL-WHITE directly to lesion and cover with
appropriate dressing. Daily or twice daily changes of dressings are preferred. At each redressing, the lesion should be
irrigated with isotonic saline solution, or other mild cleansing solution (except hydrogen peroxide solution, which may
inactivate the papain) to remove any accumulation of liquefied necrotic material.

NOTE

Papain may also be inactivated by the salts of heavy metals
(lead, silver, mercury, etc.). Contact with medications containing these metals should be avoided.

HOW SUPPLIED

Available on prescription only in 1 oz tubes. (NDC 0263-
5148-01)

REFERENCE
1. Data on file.

5/97

Shown in Product Identification Guide, page 335

PROPHYLLIN® CCC   OTC
[pro-fil 'in]
Topical, Emollient Ointment

ACTIVE INGREDIENT white petrolatum, USP. **Other ingredients**: purified water, USP; stearyl alcohol, NF; propylene

glycol, USP; sodium propionate, NF; polyoxyl 40 stearate, NF; methylparaben, NF: fragrance and chlorophyllin copper complex sodium, USP.

INDICATIONS

Helps prevent and temporarily protects chafed, chapped, cracked, or windburned skin and lips. Soothes irritated skin.

DIRECTIONS

Spread generously over area several times daily and upon retiring.

WARNING

For external use only. Avoid contact with the eyes. If condition worsens, or does not improve within seven days, consult a physician. Not to be applied over deep or puncture wounds, infections or lacerations; consult a physician. Keep this and all drugs out of reach of children. In case of accidental ingestion, contact a poison control center or a physician immediately.

HOW SUPPLIED

1 oz tube, (NDC 0263-5085-01)

11/93   Made in U.S.A.

SCS Pharmaceuticals

BOX 5110
CHICAGO, IL 60680

Direct Inquiries to:
(800) 323-1603

For Medical Information Contact:
Generally:
G.D. Searle & Co.
Healthcare Information Services
5200 Old Orchard Road
Skokie, IL 60077
In Emergencies:
Outside IL:
(800) 323-4204 (business hours)
(847) 982-7000 (at other times)
Within IL:
(847) 982-7000

Sales and Ordering:
(800) 323-1603

Alphabetic Product Listing
Product, ID #, (NDC*), Form, Strength
Flagyl, I.V., 1804, Vial (partial fill, lyoph. pwd.), 500 mg
Flagyl I.V. RTU, 1847, Plastic Container, 500 mg/100 ml
Levora® (levonorgestrel and ethinyl estradiol tablets 0.15 mg/30 mg)
Piroxicam USP, 5752, Tablet, 10 mg
Piroxicam USP, 5762, Tablet, 20 mg

*When the product ID # is not the same as the NDC #, the NDC # appears in parentheses.

Product Information Available on Request
Levora® (levonorgestrel and ethinyl estradiol tablets USP)
Piroxicam Tablets USP   ℞

*When the product ID # is not the same as the NDC #, the NDC # appears in parentheses.

FLAGYL® I.V.   ℞
[*flaj 'yl*]
(metronidazole hydrochloride)

FLAGYL® I.V. RTU®   ℞
(metronidazole injection USP) Ready-to-Use
STERILE
For Intravenous Infusion Only

> **WARNING**
> Metronidazole has been shown to be carcinogenic in mice and rats (see *Precautions*). Its use, therefore, should be reserved for the conditions described in the *Indications and Usage* section below.

DESCRIPTION

Flagyl I.V., sterile (metronidazole hydrochloride), and Flagyl I.V. RTU, sterile (metronidazole), are parenteral dosage forms of the synthetic antibacterial agents 1-(β-hydroxyethyl)-2-methyl-5-nitroimidazole hydrochloride and 1-(β-hydroxyethyl)-2-methyl-5-nitroimidazole, respectively.
[See chemical structure at top of next column]

metronidazole   metronidazole
hydrochloride

Each single-dose vial of lyophilized Flagyl I.V. contains sterile, nonpyrogenic metronidazole hydrochloride, equivalent to 500 mg metronidazole, and 415 mg mannitol.

Each Flagyl I.V. RTU 100-ml single-dose plastic container contains a sterile, nonpyrogenic, isotonic, buffered solution of 500 mg metronidazole, 47.6 mg sodium phosphate, 22.9 mg citric acid, and 790 mg sodium chloride in Water for Injection USP. Flagyl I.V. RTU has a tonicity of 310 mOsm/L and a pH of 5 to 7. Each container contains 14 mEq of sodium.

The plastic container is fabricated from a specially formulated polyvinyl chloride plastic. Water can permeate from inside the container into the overwrap in amounts insufficiento affect the solution significantly. Solutions in contact with the plastic container can leach out certain of its chemical components in very small amounts within the expiration period, eg, di 2-ethylhexyl phthalate (DEHP), up to 5 parts per million. However, the safety of the plastic has been confirmed in tests in animals according to USP biological tests for plastic containers as well as by tissue culture toxicity studies.

CLINICAL PHARMACOLOGY

Metronidazole is a synthetic antibacterial compound. Disposition of metronidazole in the body is similar for both oral and intravenous dosage forms, with an average elimination half-life in healthy humans of 8 hours.

The major route of elimination of metronidazole and its metabolites is via the urine (60–80% of the dose), with fecal excretion accounting for 6–15% of the dose. The metabolites that appear in the urine result primarily from side-chain oxidation [1-(β-hydroxyethyl) -2- hydroxymethyl-5- nitroimidazole and 2-methyl-5-nitroimidazole-1-yl-acetic acid] and glucuronide conjugation, with unchanged metronidazole accounting for approximately 20% of the total. Renal clearance of metronidazole is approximately 10 mL/min/$1.73~m^2$.

Metronidazole is the major component appearing in the plasma, with lesser quantities of the 2-hydroxymethyl metabolite also being present. Less than 20% of the circulating metronidazole is bound to plasma proteins. Both the parent compound and the metabolite possess *in vitro* bactericidal activity against most strains of anaerobic bacteria.

Metronidazole appears in cerebrospinal fluid, saliva, and breast milk in concentrations similar to those found in plasma. Bactericidal concentrations of metronidazole have also been detected in pus from hepatic abscesses.

Plasma concentrations of metronidazole are proportional to the administered dose. An 8-hour intravenous infusion of 100–4,000 mg of metronidazole in normal subjects showed a linear relationship between dose and peak plasma concentration.

In patients treated with Flagyl I.V., using a dosage regimen of 15 mg/kg loading dose followed 6 hours later by 7.5 mg/kg every six hours, peak steady-state plasma concentrations of metronidazole averaged 25 mcg/mL with trough (minimum) concentrations averaging 18 mcg/mL.

Decreased renal function does not alter the single-dose pharmacokinetics of metronidazole. However, plasma clearance of metronidazole is decreased in patients with decreased liver function.

In one study newborn infants appeared to demonstrate diminished capacity to eliminate metronidazole. The elimination half-life, measured during the first 3 days of life, was inversely related to gestational age. In infants whose gestational ages were between 28 and 40 weeks, the corresponding elimination half-lives ranged from 109 to 22.5 hours.

Microbiology: Metronidazole is active *in vitro* against most obligate anaerobes, but does not appear to possess any clinically relevant activity against facultative anaerobes or obligate aerobes. Against susceptible organisms, metronidazole is generally bactericidal at concentrations equal to or slightly higher than the minimal inhibitory concentrations. Metronidazole has been shown to have *in vitro* and clinical activity against the following organisms:

Anaerobic gram-negative bacilli, including:
  Bacteroides species, including the *Bacteroides fragilis* group (B. fragilis, B. distasonis, B. ovatus, B. thetaiotaomicron, B. vulgatus)
  Fusobacterium species
Anaerobic gram-positive bacilli, including:
  Clostridium species and susceptible strains of *Eubacterium*
Anaerobic gram-positive cocci, including:
  Peptococcus species
  Peptostreptococcus species

Susceptibility Tests: Bacteriologic studies should be performed to determine the causative organisms and their susceptibility to metronidazole; however, the rapid, routine susceptibility testing of individual isolates of anaerobic bacteria is not always practical, and therapy may be started while awaiting these results.

Quantitative methods give the most accurate estimates of susceptibility to antibacterial drugs. A standardized agar dilution method and a broth microdilution method are recommended.[1]

Control strains are recommended for standardized susceptibility testing. Each time the test is performed, one or more of the following strains should be included: *Clostridium perfringens* ATCC 13124, *Bacteroides fragilis* ATCC 25285, and *Bacteroides thetaiotaomicron* ATCC 29741. The mode metronidazole MICs for those three strains are reported to be 0.25, 0.25, and 0.5 mcg/mL, respectively.

A clinical laboratory test is considered under acceptable control if the results of the control strains are within one doubling dilution of the mode MICs reported for metronidazole.

A bacterial isolate may be considered susceptible if the MIC value for metronidazole is not more than 16 mcg/mL. An organism is considered resistant if the MIC is greater than 16 mcg/mL. A report of "resistant" from the laboratory indicates that the infecting organism is not likely to respond to therapy.

INDICATIONS AND USAGE
Treatment of Anaerobic Infections

Flagyl I.V. (metronidazole hydrochloride) and Flagyl I.V. RTU (metronidazole) are indicated in the treatment of serious infections caused by susceptible anaerobic bacteria. Indicated surgical procedures should be performed in conjunction with Flagyl I.V. or Flagyl I.V. RTU therapy. In a mixed aerobic and anaerobic infection, antibiotics appropriate for the treatment of the aerobic infection should be used in addition to Flagyl I.V. or Flagyl I.V. RTU.

Flagyl I.V. and Flagyl I.V. RTU are effective in *Bacteroides fragilis* infections resistant to clindamycin, chloramphenicol, and penicillin.

INTRA-ABDOMINAL INFECTIONS, including peritonitis, intra-abdominal abscess, and liver abscess, caused by *Bacteroides* species including the *B. fragilis* group (*B. fragilis, B. distasonis, B. ovatus, B. thetaiotaomicron, B. vulgatus*), *Clostridium* species, *Eubacterium* species, *Peptococcus* species, and *Peptostreptococcus* species.

SKIN AND SKIN STRUCTURE INFECTIONS caused by *Bacteroides* species including the *B. fragilis* group, *Clostridium* species, *Peptococcus* species, *Peptostreptococcus* species, and *Fusobacterium* species.

GYNECOLOGIC INFECTIONS, including endometritis, endomyometritis, tubo-ovarian abscess, and postsurgical vaginal cuff infection, caused by *Bacteroides* species including the *B. fragilis* group, *Clostridium* species, *Peptococcus* species, and *Peptostreptococcus* species.

BACTERIAL SEPTICEMIA caused by *Bacteroides* species including the *B. fragilis* group, and *Clostridium* species.

BONE AND JOINT INFECTIONS, as adjunctive therapy, caused by *Bacteroides* species including the *B. fragilis* group.

CENTRAL NERVOUS SYSTEM (CNS) INFECTIONS, including meningitis and brain abscess, caused by *Bacteroides* species including the *B. fragilis* group.

LOWER RESPIRATORY TRACT INFECTIONS, including pneumonia, empyema, and lung abscess, caused by *Bacteroides* species including the *B. fragilis* group.

ENDOCARDITIS caused by *Bacteroides* species including the *B. fragilis* group.

Prophylaxis

The prophylactic administration of Flagyl I.V. or Flagyl I.V. RTU preoperatively, intraoperatively, and postoperatively may reduce the incidence of postoperative infection in patients undergoing elective colorectal surgery which is classified as contaminated or potentially contaminated.

Prophylactic use of Flagyl I.V. or Flagyl I.V. RTU should be discontinued within 12 hours after surgery. If there are signs of infection, specimens for cultures should be obtained for the identification of the causative organism(s) so that appropriate therapy may be given (see *Dosage and Administration*).

CONTRAINDICATIONS

Flagyl I.V. and Flagyl I.V. RTU are contraindicated in patients with a prior history of hypersensitivity to metronidazole or other nitroimidazole derivatives.

WARNINGS

Convulsive Seizures and Peripheral Neuropathy: Convulsive seizures and peripheral neuropathy, the latter characterized mainly by numbness or paresthesia of an extremity, have been reported in patients treated with metronidazole. The appearance of abnormal neurologic signs demands the prompt evaluation of the benefit/risk ratio of the continuation of therapy.

Continued on next page

Flagyl I.V.—Cont.

PRECAUTIONS

General: Patients with severe hepatic disease metabolize metronidazole slowly, with resultant accumulation of metronidazole and its metabolites in the plasma. Accordingly, for such patients, doses below those usually recommended should be administered cautiously.

Administration of solutions containing sodium ions may result in sodium retention. Care should be taken when administering Flagyl I.V. RTU to patients receiving corticosteroids or to patients predisposed to edema.

Known or previously unrecognized candidiasis may present more prominent symptoms during therapy with Flagyl I.V. or Flagyl I.V. RTU and requires treatment with a candidicidal agent.

Laboratory Tests: Metronidazole is a nitroimidazole, and Flagyl I.V. or Flagyl I.V. RTU should be used with care in patients with evidence of or history of blood dyscrasia. A mild leukopenia has been observed during its administration; however, no persistent hematologic abnormalities attributable to metronidazole have been observed in clinical studies. Total and differential leukocyte counts are recommended before and after therapy.

Drug Interactions: Metronidazole has been reported to potentiate the anticoagulant effect of warfarin and other oral coumarin anticoagulants, resulting in a prolongation of prothrombin time. This possible drug interaction should be considered when Flagyl I.V. or Flagyl I.V. RTU is prescribed for patients on this type of anticoagulant therapy.

The simultaneous administration of drugs that induce microsomal liver enzymes, such as phenytoin or phenobarbital, may accelerate the elimination of metronidazole, resulting in reduced plasma levels; impaired clearance of phenytoin has also been reported.

The simultaneous administration of drugs that decrease microsomal liver enzyme activity, such as cimetidine, may prolong the half-life and decrease plasma clearance of metronidazole.

Alcoholic beverages should not be consumed during metronidazole therapy because abdominal cramps, nausea, vomiting, headaches, and flushing may occur.

Psychotic reactions have been reported in alcoholic patients who are using metronidazole and disulfiram concurrently. Metronidazole should not be given to patients who have taken disulfiram within the last two weeks.

Drug/Laboratory Test Interactions: Metronidazole may interfere with certain types of determinations of serum chemistry values, such as aspartate aminotransferase (AST, SGOT), alanine aminotransferase (ALT, SGPT), lactate dehydrogenase (LDH), triglycerides, and hexokinase glucose. Values of zero may be observed. All of the assays in which interference has been reported involve enzymatic coupling of the assay to oxidation-reduction of nicotine adenine dinucleotide (NAD$^+$ ⇌ NADH). Interference is due to the similarity in absorbance peaks of NADH (340 nm) and metronidazole (322 nm) at pH 7.

Carcinogenesis, Mutagenesis, Impairment of Fertility: Tumorigenicity in Rodents—Metronidazole has shown evidence of carcinogenic activity in studies involving chronic, oral administration in mice and rats, but similar studies in the hamster gave negative results. Also, metronidazole has shown mutagenic activity in a number of *in vitro* assay systems, but studies in mammals (*in vivo*) failed to demonstrate a potential for genetic damage.

Pregnancy: Teratogenic Effects—Pregnancy Category B. Metronidazole crosses the placental barrier and enters the fetal circulation rapidly. Reproduction studies have been performed in rats at doses up to five times the human dose and have revealed no evidence of impaired fertility or harm to the fetus due to metronidazole. Metronidazole administered intraperitoneally to pregnant mice at approximately the human dose caused fetotoxicity; administered orally to pregnant mice, no fetotoxicity was observed. There are, however, no adequate and well-controlled studies in pregnant women. Because animal reproduction studies are not always predictive of human response, and because metronidazole is a carcinogen in rodents, these drugs should be used during pregnancy only if clearly needed.

Nursing Mothers: Because of the potential for tumorigenicity shown for metronidazole in mouse and rat studies, a decision should be made whether to discontinue nursing or to discontinue the drug, taking into account the importance of the drug to the mother. Metronidazole is secreted in breast milk in concentrations similar to those found in plasma.

Pediatric Use: Safety and effectiveness in pediatric patients have not been established.

ADVERSE REACTIONS

Two serious adverse reactions reported in patients treated with Flagyl I.V. or Flagyl I.V. RTU have been convulsive seizures and peripheral neuropathy, the latter characterized mainly by numbness or paresthesia of an extremity. Since persistent peripheral neuropathy has been reported in some patients receiving prolonged oral administration of Flagyl® (metronidazole), patients should be observed carefully if neurologic symptoms occur and a prompt evaluation made of the benefit/risk ratio of the continuation of therapy.

The following reactions have also been reported during treatment with Flagyl I.V. (metronidazole hydrochloride) or Flagyl I.V. RTU (metronidazole):

Gastrointestinal: Nausea, vomiting, abdominal discomfort, diarrhea, and an unpleasant metallic taste.

Hematopoietic: Reversible neutropenia (leukopenia).

Dermatologic: Erythematous rash and pruritus.

Central Nervous System: Headache, dizziness, syncope, ataxia, and confusion.

Local Reactions: Thrombophlebitis after intravenous infusion. This reaction can be minimized or avoided by avoiding prolonged use of indwelling intravenous catheters.

Other: Fever. Instances of a darkened urine have also been reported, and this manifestation has been the subject of a special investigation. Although the pigment which is probably responsible for this phenomenon has not been positively identified, it is almost certainly a metabolite of metronidazole and seems to have no clinical significance.

The following adverse reactions have been reported during treatment with oral Flagyl (metronidazole):

Gastrointestinal: Nausea, sometimes accompanied by headache, anorexia, and occasionally vomiting; diarrhea, epigastric distress, abdominal cramping, and constipation.

Mouth: A sharp, unpleasant metallic taste is not unusual. Furry tongue, glossitis, and stomatitis have occurred; these may be associated with a sudden overgrowth of *Candida* which may occur during effective therapy.

Hematopoietic: Reversible neutropenia (leukopenia); rarely, reversible thrombocytopenia.

Cardiovascular: Flattening of the T-wave may be seen in electrocardiographic tracings.

Central Nervous System: Convulsive seizures, peripheral neuropathy, dizziness, vertigo, incoordination, ataxia, confusion, irritability, depression, weakness, and insomnia.

Hypersensitivity: Urticaria, erythematous rash, flushing, nasal congestion, dryness of the mouth (or vagina or vulva), and fever.

Renal: Dysuria, cystitis, polyuria, incontinence, a sense of pelvic pressure, and darkened urine.

Other: Proliferation of *Candida* in the vagina, dyspareunia, decrease of libido, proctitis, and fleeting joint pains sometimes resembling "serum sickness." If patients receiving metronidazole drink alcoholic beverages, they may experience abdominal distress, nausea, vomiting, flushing, or headache. A modification of the taste of alcoholic beverages has also been reported. Rare cases of pancreatitis, which abated on withdrawal of the drug, have been reported.

Crohn's disease patients are known to have an increased incidence of gastrointestinal and certain extraintestinal cancers. There have been some reports in the medical literature of breast and colon cancer in Crohn's disease patients who have been treated with metronidazole at high doses for extended periods of time. A cause and effect relationship has not been established. Crohn's disease is not an approved indication for Flagyl I.V. or Flagyl I.V. RTU.

OVERDOSAGE

Use of dosages of Flagyl I.V. (metronidazole hydrochloride) higher than those recommended has been reported. These include the use of 27 mg/kg three times a day for 20 days, and the use of 75 mg/kg as a single loading dose followed by 7.5 mg/kg maintenance doses. No adverse reactions were reported in either of the two cases.

Single oral doses of metronidazole, up to 15 g, have been reported in suicide attempts and accidental overdoses. Symptoms reported include nausea, vomiting, and ataxia.

Oral metronidazole has been studied as a radiation sensitizer in the treatment of malignant tumors. Neurotoxic effects, including seizures and peripheral neuropathy, have been reported after 5 to 7 days of doses of 6 to 10.4 g every other day.

Treatment: There is no specific antidote for overdose; therefore, management of the patient should consist of symptomatic and supportive therapy.

DOSAGE AND ADMINISTRATION

In elderly patients the pharmacokinetics of metronidazole may be altered and therefore monitoring of serum levels may be necessary to adjust the metronidazole dosage accordingly.

Treatment of Anaerobic Infections

The recommended dosage schedule for *adults* is:

Loading dose:

15 mg/kg infused over 1 hour (approximately 1 g for a 70-kg adult).

Maintenance Dose:

7.5 mg/kg infused over one hour every 6 hours (approximately 500 mg for a 70-kg adult). The first maintenance dose should be instituted 6 hours following the initiation of the loading dose.

Parenteral therapy may be changed to oral Flagyl (metronidazole) when conditions warrant, based upon the severity of the disease and the response of the patient to Flagyl I.V. or Flagyl I.V. RTU (metronidazole) treatment. The usual adult oral dosage is 7.5 mg/kg every 6 hours.

A maximum of 4 g should not be exceeded during a 24-hour period.

Patients with severe hepatic disease metabolize metronidazole slowly, with resultant accumulation of metronidazole and its metabolites in the plasma. Accordingly, for such patients, doses below those usually recommended should be administered cautiously. Close monitoring of plasma metronidazole levels[2] and toxicity is recommended.

In patients receiving Flagyl I.V. or Flagyl I.V. RTU in whom gastric secretions are continuously removed by nasogastric aspiration, sufficient metronidazole may be removed in the aspirate to cause a reduction in serum levels.

The dose of Flagyl I.V. or Flagyl I.V. RTU should not be specifically reduced in anuric patients since accumulated metabolites may be rapidly removed by dialysis.

The usual duration of therapy is 7 to 10 days; however, infections of the bone and joint, lower respiratory tract, and endocardium may require longer treatment.

Prophylaxis

For surgical prophylactic use, to prevent postoperative infection in contaminated or potentially contaminated colorectal surgery, the recommended dosage schedule for adults is:

a. 15 mg/kg infused over 30 to 60 minutes and completed approximately 1 hour before surgery; followed by

b. 7.5 mg/kg infused over 30 to 60 minutes at 6 and 12 hours after the initial dose.

It is important that (1) administration of the initial preoperative dose be completed approximately one hour before surgery so that adequate drug levels are present in the serum and tissues at the time of initial incision, and (2) Flagyl I.V. or Flagyl I.V. RTU be administered, if necessary, at 6-hour intervals to maintain effective drug levels. Prophylactic use of Flagyl I.V. or Flagyl I.V. RTU should be limited to the day of surgery only, following the above guidelines.

CAUTION: Flagyl I.V. (metronidazole hydrochloride) or Flagyl I.V. RTU (metronidazole) is to be administered by slow intravenous drip infusion only, either as a continuous or intermittent infusion. I.V. admixtures containing metronidazole and other drugs should be avoided. Additives should not be introduced into the Flagyl I.V. RTU solution. If used with a primary intravenous fluid system, the primary solution should be discontinued during metronidazole infusion. DO NOT USE EQUIPMENT CONTAINING ALUMINUM (EG, NEEDLES, CANNULAE) THAT WOULD COME IN CONTACT WITH THE DRUG SOLUTION.

FLAGYL I.V.

Flagyl I.V. cannot be given by direct intravenous injection (I.V. bolus) because of the low pH (0.5 to 2.0) of the reconstituted product. FLAGYL I.V. MUST BE FURTHER DILUTED AND NEUTRALIZED FOR I.V. INFUSION.

Flagyl I.V. is prepared for use in two steps:
NOTE: ORDER OF MIXING IS IMPORTANT
A. Reconstitution
B. Dilution in intravenous solution followed by pH neutralization with sodium bicarbonate injection into the dilution.

Reconstitution: To prepare the solution, add 4.4 mL of one of the following diluents and mix thoroughly: Sterile Water for Injection, USP; Bacteriostatic Water for Injection, USP; 0.9% Sodium Chloride Injection, USP; or Bacteriostatic 0.9% Sodium Chloride Injection, USP. The resultant approximate withdrawal volume is 5.0 mL with an approximate concentration of 100 mg/mL.

The pH of the reconstituted product will be in the range of 0.5 to 2.0. Reconstituted Flagyl I.V. is clear, and pale yellow to yellow-green in color.

Dilution in Intravenous Solutions: Properly reconstituted Flagyl I.V. (metronidazole hydrochloride) may be added to a glass or plastic I.V. container not to exceed a concentration of 8 mg/mL. Any of the following intravenous solutions may be used: 0.9% Sodium Chloride Injection, USP; 5% Dextrose Injection, USP; or Lactated Ringer's Injection, USP.

NEUTRALIZATION IS REQUIRED PRIOR TO ADMINISTRATION.

The final product should be mixed thoroughly and used within 24 hours.

Neutralization For Intravenous Infusion: Neutralize the intravenous solution containing Flagyl I.V. with approximately 5 mEq of sodium bicarbonate injection for each 500 mg of Flagyl I.V. used. Mix thoroughly. The pH of the neutralized intravenous solution will be approximately 6.0 to 7.0. Carbon dioxide gas will be generated with neutralization. It may be necessary to relieve gas pressure within the container.

Note: When the contents of one vial (500 mg) are diluted and neutralized to 100 mL, the resultant concentration is 5 mg/mL. Do not exceed an 8 mg/mL concentration of Flagyl I.V. in the neutralized intravenous solution, since neutralization will decrease the aqueous solubility and precipitation may occur. DO NOT REFRIGERATE NEUTRALIZED SOLUTIONS; otherwise, precipitation may occur.

Storage and Stability: Reconstituted vials of Flagyl I.V. are chemically stable for 96 hours when stored below 86°F (30°C) in room light.

Use diluted and neutralized intravenous solutions containing Flagyl I.V. within 24 hours of mixing.

FLAGYL I.V. RTU

Flagyl I.V. RTU is a ready-to-use isotonic solution. **NO DILUTION OR BUFFERING IS REQUIRED.** Do not refrigerate. Each container of Flagyl I.V. RTU contains 14 mEq of sodium.

Directions for use of plastic container:

CAUTION: Do not use plastic containers in series connections. Such use could result in air embolism due to residual air (approximately 15 mL) being drawn from the primary container before administration of the fluid from the secondary container is complete.

To open. Tear overwrap down side at slit and remove solution container. Some opacity of the plastic due to moisture absorption during the sterilization process may be observed. This is normal and does not affect the solution quality or safety. The opacity will diminish gradually. Check for minute leaks by squeezing inner bag firmLy. If leaks are found discard solution as sterility may be impaired.

Preparation for administration:

1. Suspend container from eyelet support.
2. Remove plastic protector from outlet port at bottom of container.
3. Attach administration set. Refer to complete directions accompanying set.

Parenteral drug products should be inspected visually for particulate matter and discoloration prior to administration, whenever solution and container permit. Do not use if cloudy or precipitated or if the seal is not intact.

Use sterile equipment. It is recommended that the intravenous administration apparatus be replaced at least once every 24 hours.

HOW SUPPLIED

FLAGYL I.V.

Flagyl I.V., sterile (metronidazole hydrochloride), is supplied in single-dose lyophilized vials each containing 500 mg metronidazole equivalent, individually packaged in cartons of 10 vials.

Flagyl I.V., prior to reconstitution, should be stored below 86°F (30°C) and protected from light.

FLAGYL I.V. RTU

Flagyl I.V. RTU, sterile (metronidazole), is supplied in 100-mL single-dose plastic containers, each containing an isotonic, buffered solution of 500 mg metronidazole, individually packaged in boxes of 24.

Flagyl I.V. RTU should be stored at controlled room temperature, 59° to 77° F (15° to 25°C), and protected from light during storage.

1. Proposed standard: PSM-11—Proposed Reference Dilution Procedure for Antimicrobic Susceptibility Testing of Anaerobic Bacteria, National Committee for Clinical Laboratory Standards; and Sutter, et al.: Collaborative Evaluation of a Proposed Reference Dilution Method of Susceptibility Testing of Anaerobic Bacteria, Antimicrob. Agents Chemother. *16:* 495–502 (Oct.) 1979; and Tally, et al.: *In Vitro* Activity of Thienamycin, Antimicrob. Agents Chemother. *14:* 436–438 (Sept.) 1978.

2. Ralph, E.D., and Kirby, W.M.M.: Bioassay of Metronidazole With Either Anaerobic or Aerobic Incubation, J. Infect. Dis. *132:* 587–591 (Nov.) 1975; or Gulaid, et al.: Determination of Metronidazole and Its Major Metabolites in Biological Fluids by High Pressure Liquid Chromatography, Br. J. Clin. Pharmacol. *6:* 430–432, 1978.

4/16/97•A05034-9

For EMERGENCY telephone numbers, consult the **Manufacturers' Index**.

Sandoz Pharmaceuticals Corporation

PLEASE NOTE:

Due to the merger of CibaGeneva Pharmaceuticals and Sandoz Pharmaceuticals Corporation, please refer to **Novartis Pharmaceuticals Corporation** for branded product information and Geneva Pharmaceuticals, Inc. for branded generic product information.

Sanofi Pharmaceuticals, Inc.
90 PARK AVENUE
NEW YORK, NY 10016

Direct Inquiries to:
(212) 551-4000

For Medical Information Contact:
Product Information Services
(800) 446-6267

Sales and Ordering:
East Coast: (800) 223-1062
West Coast: (800) 223-5511

ARALEN® Hydrochloride
brand of chloroquine hydrochloride
injection, USP   ℞

> **For Malaria and**
> **Extraintestinal Amebiasis**

> **WARNING: PHYSICIANS SHOULD COMPLETELY FAMILIARIZE THEMSELVES WITH THE COMPLETE CONTENTS OF THIS LEAFLET BEFORE PRESCRIBING ARALEN.**

DESCRIPTION

Parenteral solution, each mL containing 50 mg of the dihydrochloride salt equivalent to 40 mg of chloroquine base. ARALEN hydrochloride, a 4-aminoquinoline compound, is chemically 7- (Chloro - 4 - [[4 - diethylamino) - 1 - methylbutyl] amino]-quinoline dihydrochloride, a white, crystalline substance, freely soluble in water.

ACTIONS

The compound is a highly active antimalarial and amebicidal agent.

ARALEN hydrochloride has been found to be highly active against the erythrocytic forms of *Plasmodium vivax* and *malariae* and most strains of *Plasmodium falciparum* (but not the gametocytes of *P. falciparum).* The precise mechanism of action of the drug is not known.

ARALEN hydrochloride does not prevent relapses in patients with vivax or malariae malaria because it is not effective against exoerythrocytic forms of the parasite, nor will it prevent vivax or malariae infection when administered as a prophylactic. It is highly effective as a suppressive agent in patients with vivax or malariae malaria, in terminating acute attacks, and significantly lengthening the interval between treatment and relapse. In patients with falciparum malaria it abolishes the acute attack and effects complete cure of the infection, unless due to a resistant strain of *P. falciparum.*

INDICATIONS

ARALEN hydrochloride is indicated for the treatment of extraintestinal amebiasis and for treatment of acute attacks of malaria due to *P. vivax, P. malariae, P. ovale,* and susceptible strains of *P. falciparum* when oral therapy is not feasible.

CONTRAINDICATIONS

Use of this drug is contraindicated in the presence of retinal or visual field changes either attributable to 4- aminoquinoline compounds or to any other etiology, and in patients with known hypersensitivity to 4-aminoquinoline compounds. However, in the treatment of acute attacks of malaria caused by susceptible strains of plasmodia, the physician may elect to use this drug after carefully weighing the possible benefits and risks to the patient.

WARNINGS

Children and infants are extremely susceptible to adverse effects from an overdose of parenteral ARALEN and sudden deaths have been recorded after such administration. In no instance should the single dose of parenteral ARALEN administered to infants or children exceed 5 mg base per kg. In recent years it has been found that certain strains of P. falciparum have become resistant to 4-aminoquinoline com-

pounds (including chloroquine and hydroxychloroquine) as shown by the fact that normally adequate doses have failed to prevent or cure clinical malaria or parasitemia. Treatment with quinine or other specific forms of therapy is therefore advised for patients infected with a resistant strain of parasites.

Use of ARALEN should be avoided in patients with psoriasis, for it may precipitate a severe attack of psoriasis. Some authors consider the use of 4-aminoquinoline compounds contraindicated in patients with porphyria since the condition may be exacerbated.

Irreversible retinal damage has been observed in some patients who had received long-term or high-dosage 4-aminoquinoline therapy. Retinopathy has been reported to be dose related.

If there is any indication (past or present) of abnormality in the visual acuity, visual field, or retinal macular areas (such as pigmentary changes, loss of foveal reflex), or any visual symptoms (such as light flashes and streaks) which are not fully explainable by difficulties of accommodation or corneal opacities, the drug should be discontinued immediately and the patient closely observed for possible progression. Retinal changes (and visual disturbances) may progress even after cessation of therapy.

Usage in Pregnancy. Usage of this drug during pregnancy should be avoided except in the suppression or treatment of malaria when in the judgment of the physician the benefit outweighs the possible hazard. It should be noted that radioactively tagged chloroquine administered intravenously to pregnant pigmented CBA mice passed rapidly across the placenta, accumulated selectively in the melanin structures of the fetal eyes and was retained in the ocular tissues for five months after the drug had been eliminated from the rest of the body.[1]

PRECAUTIONS

Since the drug is known to concentrate in the liver, it should be used with caution in patients with hepatic disease or alcoholism or in conjunction with known hepatotoxic drugs. The drug should be administered with caution to patients having G-6-PD (glucose-6-phosphate dehydrogenase) deficiency.

ADVERSE REACTIONS

Respiratory depression, cardiovascular collapse, shock, convulsions, and death have been reported with overdoses of ARALEN hydrochloride, brand of chloroquine hydrochloride injection, especially in infants and children.

Any of the adverse reactions associated with short-term oral administration of chloroquine phosphate must be considered a possibility with chloroquine hydrochloride. Cardiovascular effects, such as hypotension and electrocardiographic changes (particularly inversion or depression of the T-wave, widening of the QRS complex), have rarely been noted in patients receiving usual antimalarial doses of the drug. Mild and transient headache, pruritus, psychic stimulation, visual disturbances (blurring of vision and difficulty of focusing or accommodation), pleomorphic skin eruptions, and gastrointestinal complaints (anorexia, nausea, vomiting, diarrhea, abdominal cramps) have been observed.

Instances of convulsive seizures associated with oral chloroquine therapy in patients with extraintestinal amebiasis have been reported.

A few cases of a nerve type of deafness have been reported after prolonged therapy, usually in high doses. Tinnitus and reduced hearing have been reported, in a patient with preexistent auditory damage, after administration of only 500 mg once a week for a few months. Since neuromyopathy, blood dyscrasias, lichen planus-like eruptions, and skin and mucosal pigmentary changes have been noted during prolonged oral therapy, their occurrence with this dosage form is possible.

Patients with retinal changes may be asymptomatic, especially in early cases, or may complain of nyctalopia and scotomatous vision with field defects of paracentral, pericentral ring types, and typically temporal scotomas, eg, difficulty in reading with words tending to disappear, seeing only half an object, misty vision, and fog before the eyes. Rarely scotomatous vision may occur without observable retinal changes.

DOSAGE AND ADMINISTRATION

Malaria — **Adult Dose.** An initial dose of 4 mL or 5 mL (160 mg to 200 mg chloroquine base) may be injected intramuscularly and repeated in 6 hours if necessary. The total parenteral dosage in the first 24 hours should not exceed

Continued on next page

This product information was prepared in September 1998. On these and other products of Sanofi Pharmaceuticals, Inc., detailed information may be obtained on a current basis by direct inquiry to Product Information Services, 90 Park Avenue, New York, NY 10016 (toll free 1-800-446-6267).

Aralen Hydrochloride—Cont.

800 mg chloroquine base. Treatment by mouth should be started as soon as practicable and continued until a course of approximately 1.5 g of base in 3 days is completed.

Pediatric Dose. Infants and children are extremely susceptible to overdosage of parenteral ARALEN. Severe reactions and deaths have occurred. In the pediatric age range, parenteral ARALEN dosage should be calculated in proportion to the adult dose based upon body weight. The recommended single dose in infants and children is 5 mg base per kg. This dose may be repeated in 6 hours; however, the total dose in any 24 hour period should not exceed 10 mg base per kg of body weight. Parenteral administration should be terminated and oral therapy instituted as soon as possible.

Extraintestinal Amebiasis —In adult patients not able to tolerate oral therapy, from 4 mL to 5 mL (160 mg to 200 mg chloroquine base) may be injected daily for 10 to 12 days. Oral administration should be substituted or resumed as soon as possible.

OVERDOSAGE

Inadvertent toxic doses may produce respiratory depression or shock with hypotension. Respiratory depression is treated by artificial respiration and administration of oxygen. In shock with hypotension, a potent vasopressor, such as NEO-SYNEPHRINE® hydrochloride, brand of phenylephrine hydrochloride, USP, should be given intramuscularly in doses of 2 mg to 5 mg.

HOW SUPPLIED

Ampuls of 5 mL, box of 5 (NDC 0024-0074-01)

REFERENCE

Ullberg S, Lindquist N G, Sjostrand S E: Accumulation of chorio-retinotoxic drugs in the foetal eye. *Nature* 1970; 227: 1257.

ASW-3

ARALEN® Phosphate ℞
brand of chloroquine phosphate tablets, USP

> **For Malaria and**
> **Extraintestinal Amebiasis**

> **WARNING**
> PHYSICIANS SHOULD COMPLETELY FAMILIARIZE THEMSELVES WITH THE COMPLETE CONTENTS OF THIS LEAFLET BEFORE PRESCRIBING ARALEN.

DESCRIPTION

ARALEN phosphate, brand of chloroquine phosphate, USP, is a 4-aminoquinoline compound for oral administration. It is a white, odorless, bitter tasting, crystalline substance, freely soluble in water.

ARALEN phosphate is an antimalarial and amebicidal drug.

Chemically, it is 7-chloro- 4-[[4- (diethylamino) -1-methylbutyl]amino] quinoline phosphate (1:2).

Inactive Ingredients: Carnauba Wax, Colloidal Silicon Dioxide, D&C Red No 27, Dibasic Calcium Phosphate, Hydroxypropyl Methylcellulose, Magnesium Stearate, Microcrystalline Cellulose, Polyethylene Glycol, Polysorbate 80, Pregelatinized Starch, Sodium Starch Glycolate, Stearic Acid, Titanium Dioxide.

CLINICAL PHARMACOLOGY

ARALEN phosphate has been found to be highly active against the erythrocytic forms of *Plasmodium vivax* and *Plasmodium malariae* and most strains of *Plasmodium falciparum* (but not the gametocytes of *P. falciparum*).

The mechanism of plasmodicidal action of chloroquine is not completely certain. While the drug can inhibit certain enzymes, its effect is believed to result, at least in part, from its interaction with DNA.

Chloroquine is rapidly and almost completely absorbed from the gastrointestinal tract, and only a small proportion of the administered dose is found in the stools. Approximately 55% of the drug in the plasma is bound to nondiffusible plasma constituents. Excretion of chloroquine is quite slow, but is increased by acidification of the urine. Chloroquine is deposited in the tissues in considerable amounts. In animals, from 200 to 700 times the plasma concentration may be found in the liver, spleen, kidney, and lung; leukocytes also concentrate the drug. The brain and spinal cord, in contrast, contain only 10 to 30 times the amount present in plasma. Chloroquine undergoes appreciable degradation in the body. The main metabolite is desethylchloroquine, which accounts for one fourth of the total material appearing in the urine; bisdesethylchloroquine, a carboxylic acid derivative, and other metabolic products as yet uncharacterized are

found in small amounts. Slightly more than half of the urinary drug products can be accounted for as unchanged chloroquine.

Microbiology

ARALEN phosphate has been found to be highly active against the erythrocytic forms of *Plasmodium vivax* and *malariae* and most strains of *Plasmodium falciparum* (but not the gametocytes of *P. falciparum*). The precise mechanism of action of the drug is not known.

In vitro studies with trophozoites of *Entamoeba histolytica* have demonstrated that ARALEN phosphate also possesses amebicidal activity comparable to that of emetine.

INDICATIONS AND USAGE

ARALEN phosphate, brand of chloroquine phosphate, is indicated for the suppressive treatment and for acute attacks of malaria due to *P. vivax, P. malariae, P. ovale,* and susceptible strains of *P. falciparum.* The drug is also indicated for the treatment of extraintestinal amebiasis.

ARALEN phosphate does not prevent relapses in patients with vivax or malariae malaria because it is not effective against exoerythrocytic forms of the parasite, nor will it prevent vivax or malariae infection when administered as a prophylactic. It is highly effective as a suppressive agent in patients with vivax or malariae malaria, in terminating acute attacks, and significantly lengthening the interval between treatment and relapse. In patients with falciparum malaria it abolishes the acute attack and effects complete cure of the infection, unless due to a resistant strain of *P. falciparum.*

CONTRAINDICATIONS

Use of this drug is contraindicated in the presence of retinal or visual field changes either attributable to 4-aminoquinoline compounds or to any other etiology, and, in patients with known hypersensitivity to 4-aminoquinoline compounds. However, in the treatment of acute attacks of malaria caused by susceptible strains of plasmodia, the physician may elect to use this drug after carefully weighing the possible benefits and risks to the patient.

WARNINGS

In recent years it has been found that certain strains of *P. falciparum* have become resistant to 4-aminoquinoline compounds (including chloroquine and hydroxychloroquine) as shown by the fact that normally adequate doses have failed to prevent or cure clinical malaria or parasitemia. Treatment with quinine or other specific forms of therapy is therefore advised for patients infected with a resistant strain of parasites.

Irreversible retinal damage has been observed in some patients who had received long-term or high-dosage 4-aminoquinoline therapy. Retinopathy has been reported to be dose related.

When prolonged therapy with any antimalarial compound is contemplated, initial (base line) and periodic ophthalmologic examinations (including visual acuity, expert slit-lamp, funduscopic, and visual field tests) should be performed.

If there is any indication (past or present) of abnormality in the visual acuity, visual field, or retinal macular areas (such as pigmentary changes, loss of foveal reflex), or any visual symptoms (such as light flashes and streaks) which are not fully explainable by difficulties of accommodation or corneal opacities, the drug should be discontinued immediately and the patient closely observed for possible progression. Retinal changes (and visual disturbances) may progress even after cessation of therapy.

All patients on long-term therapy with this preparation should be questioned and examined periodically, including testing knee and ankle reflexes, to detect any evidence of muscular weakness. If weakness occurs, discontinue the drug.

A number of fatalities have been reported following the accidental ingestion of chloroquine, sometimes in relatively small doses (0.75 g or 1 g chloroquine phosphate in one 3-year-old child). Patients should be strongly warned to keep this drug out of the reach of children because they are especially sensitive to the 4-aminoquinoline compounds.

Use of ARALEN phosphate, brand of chloroquine phosphate tablets, in patients with psoriasis may precipitate a severe attack of psoriasis. When used in patients with porphyria the condition may be exacerbated. The drug should not be used in these conditions unless in the judgment of the physician the benefit to the patient outweighs the possible hazard.

PRECAUTIONS

General

If any severe blood disorder appears which is not attributable to the disease under treatment, discontinuance of the drug should be considered.

Since this drug is known to concentrate in the liver, it should be used with caution in patients with hepatic disease or alcoholism or in conjunction with known hepatotoxic drugs.

The drug should be administered with caution to patients having G-6-PD (glucose-6-phosphate dehydrogenase) deficiency.

Laboratory Tests

Complete blood cell counts should be made periodically if patients are given prolonged therapy.

Nursing Mothers

Because of the potential for serious adverse reactions in nursing infants from chloroquine, a decision should be made whether to discontinue nursing or to discontinue the drug, taking into account the importance of the drug to the mother.

Pediatric Use

See WARNINGS and DOSAGE AND ADMINISTRATION.

ADVERSE REACTIONS

Ocular reactions: Irreversible retinal damage in patients receiving long-term or high-dosage 4-aminoquinoline therapy; visual disturbances (blurring of vision and difficulty of focusing or accommodation); nyctalopia; scotomatous vision with field defects of paracentral, pericentral ring types, and typically temporal scotomas, eg, difficulty in reading with words tending to disappear, seeing half an object, misty vision, and fog before the eyes.

Neuromuscular reactions: Convulsive seizures.

Auditory reactions: Nerve type deafness; tinnitus, reduced hearing in patients with preexisting auditory damage.

Gastrointestinal reactions: Anorexia, nausea, vomiting, diarrhea, abdominal cramps.

Dermatologic reactions: Pleomorphic skin eruptions, skin and mucosal pigmentary changes; lichen planus-like eruptions, pruritus, and hair loss.

CNS reactions: Mild and transient headache, psychic stimulation.

Cardiovascular reactions: Rarely, hypotension, electrocardiographic change.

OVERDOSAGE

Symptoms: Chloroquine is very rapidly and completely absorbed after ingestion. Toxic doses of chloroquine can be fatal. As little as 1 g may be fatal in children. Toxic symptoms can occur within minutes. These consist of headache, drowsiness, visual disturbances, nausea and vomiting, cardiovascular collapse, and convulsions followed by sudden and early respiratory and cardiac arrest. The electrocardiogram may reveal atrial standstill, nodal rhythm, prolonged intraventricular conduction time, and progressive bradycardia leading to ventricular fibrillation and/or arrest.

Treatment: Treatment is symptomatic and must be prompt with immediate evacuation of the stomach by emesis (at home, before transportation to the hospital) or gastric lavage until the stomach is completely emptied. If finely powdered, activated charcoal is introduced by stomach tube, after lavage, and within 30 minutes after ingestion of the antimalarial, it may inhibit further intestinal absorption of the drug. To be effective, the dose of activated charcoal should be at least five times the estimated dose of chloroquine ingested.

Convulsions, if present, should be controlled before attempting gastric lavage. If due to cerebral stimulation, cautious administration of an ultra short-acting barbiturate may be tried but, if due to anoxia, it should be corrected by oxygen administration and artificial respiration. In shock with hypotension, a potent vasopressor should be administered. Because of the importance of supporting respiration, tracheal intubation or tracheostomy, followed by gastric lavage, may also be necessary. Peritoneal dialysis and exchange transfusions have also been suggested to reduce the level of the drug in the blood.

A patient who survives the acute phase and is asymptomatic should be closely observed for at least six hours. Fluids may be forced, and sufficient ammonium chloride (8 g daily in divided doses for adults) may be administered for a few days to acidify the urine to help promote urinary excretion in cases of both overdosage or sensitivity.

DOSAGE AND ADMINISTRATION

The dosage of chloroquine phosphate is often expressed or calculated as the base. Each 500 mg tablet of ARALEN phosphate, brand of chloroquine phosphate, is equivalent to 300 mg base. In infants and children the dosage is preferably calculated on the body weight.

Malaria: Suppression—**Adult Dose:** 500 mg (= 300 mg base) on exactly the same day of each week.

Pediatric Dose: The weekly suppressive dosage is 5 mg calculated as base, per kg of body weight, but should not exceed the adult dose regardless of weight.

If circumstances permit, suppressive therapy should begin two weeks prior to exposure. However, failing this in adults, an initial double (loading) dose of 1 g (= 600 mg base), or in children 10 mg base/kg may be taken in two divided doses, six hours apart. The suppressive therapy should be continued for eight weeks after leaving the endemic area.

For Treatment of Acute Attack

Adults: An initial dose of 1 g (= 600 mg base) followed by an additional 500 mg (= 300 mg base) after six to eight

hours and a single dose of 500 mg (= 300 mg base) on each of two consecutive days. This represents a total dose of 2.5 g chloroquine phosphate or 1.5 g base in three days.

The dosage for adults may also be calculated on the basis of body weight; this method is preferred for infants and children. A total dose representing 25 mg of base per kg of body weight is administered in three days, as follows:

First dose: 10 mg base per kg (but not exceeding a single dose of 600 mg base).

Second dose: 5 mg base per kg (but not exceeding a single dose of 300 mg base) 6 hours after first dose.

Third dose: 5 mg base per kg 18 hours after second dose.

Fourth dose: 5 mg base per kg 24 hours after third dose.

For radical cure of *vivax* and *malariae* malaria concomitant therapy with an 8-aminoquinoline compound is necessary.

Extraintestinal Amebiasis: Adults, 1 g (600 mg base) daily for two days, followed by 500 mg (300 mg base) daily for at least two to three weeks. Treatment is usually combined with an effective intestinal amebicide.

HOW SUPPLIED

Tablets of 500 mg (= 300 mg base), bottles of 25 (NDC 0024-0084-01).

Pink, film-coated convex tablets, $^1/_2$ inch in diameter with an uncoated core, containing 500 mg chloroquine phosphate, equivalent to 300 mg of chloroquine base.

ASW-2

Shown in Product Identification Guide, page 335

AVAPRO®
(irbesartan) Tablets

R

CAUTION: FEDERAL LAW PROHIBITS DISPENSING WITHOUT PRESCRIPTION

USE IN PREGNANCY
When used in pregnancy during the second and third trimesters, drugs that act directly on the renin-angiotensin system can cause injury and even death to the developing fetus. When pregnancy is detected, AVAPRO should be discontinued as soon as possible. See **WARNINGS: Fetal/Neonatal Morbidity and Mortality.**

DESCRIPTION

AVAPRO* (irbesartan) is an angiotensin II receptor (AT₁ subtype) antagonist.

Irbesartan is a non-peptide compound, chemically described as a 2-butyl-3-[[2′- (1*H*-tetrazol-5-yl) [1, 1′-biphenyl]-4-yl]methyl]-1,3-diazaspiro [4,4] non-1-en-4-one.

Its empirical formula is $C_{25}H_{28}N_6O$, and the structural formula:

Irbesartan is a white to off-white crystalline powder with a molecular weight of 428.5. It is a nonpolar compound with a partition coefficient (octanol/water) of 10.1 at pH of 7.4. Irbesartan is slightly soluble in alcohol and methylene chloride and practically insoluble in water.

AVAPRO is available for oral administration in unscored tablets containing 75 mg, 150 mg, or 300 mg of irbesartan. Inactive ingredients include: lactose, microcrystalline cellulose, pregelatinized starch, croscarmellose sodium, poloxamer 188, silicon dioxide and magnesium stearate.

CLINICAL PHARMACOLOGY
Mechanism of Action

Angiotensin II is a potent vasoconstrictor formed from angiotensin I in a reaction catalyzed by angiotensin-converting enzyme (ACE, kininase II). Angiotensin II is the principal pressor agent of the renin-angiotensin system (RAS) and also stimulates aldosterone synthesis and secretion by adrenal cortex, cardiac contraction, renal resorption of sodium, activity of sympathetic nervous system, and smooth muscle cell growth. Irbesartan blocks the vasoconstrictor and aldosterone-secreting effects of angiotensin II by selectively binding to the AT₁ angiotensin II receptor. There is also an AT₂ receptor in many tissues, but it is not involved in cardiovascular homeostasis.

Irbesartan is a specific competitive antagonist of AT₁ receptors with a much greater affinity (more than 8500-fold) for

the AT₁ receptor than for the AT₂ receptor and no agonist activity.

Blockade of the AT₁ receptor removes the negative feedback of angiotensin II on renin secretion, but the resulting increased plasma renin activity and circulating angiotensin II do not overcome the effects of irbesartan on blood pressure. Irbesartan does not inhibit ACE or renin or affect other hormone receptors or ion channels known to be involved in the cardiovascular regulation of blood pressure and sodium homeostasis. Because irbesartan does not inhibit ACE, it does not affect the response to bradykinin; whether this has clinical relevance is not known.

Pharmacokinetics

Irbesartan is an orally active agent that does not require biotransformation into an active form. The oral absorption of irbesartan is rapid and complete with an average absolute bioavailability of 60–80%. Following oral administration of AVAPRO, peak plasma concentrations of irbesartan are attained at 1.5–2 hours after dosing. Food does not affect the bioavailability of AVAPRO.

Irbesartan exhibits linear pharmacokinetics over the therapeutic dose range.

The terminal elimination half-life of irbesartan averaged 11–15 hours. Steady-state concentrations are achieved within 3 days. Limited accumulation of irbesartan (<20%) is observed in plasma upon repeated once-daily dosing.

Metabolism and Elimination

Irbesartan is metabolized via glucuronide conjugation and oxidation. Following oral or intravenous administration of ¹⁴C-labeled irbesartan, more than 80% of the circulating plasma radioactivity is attributable to unchanged irbesartan. The primary circulating metabolite is the inactive irbesartan glucuronide conjugate (approximately 6%). The remaining oxidative metabolites do not add appreciably to irbesartan's pharmacologic activity.

Irbesartan and its metabolites are excreted by both biliary and renal routes. Following either oral or intravenous administration of ¹⁴C-labeled irbesartan, about 20% of radioactivity is recovered in the urine and the remainder in the feces, as irbesartan or irbesartan glucuronide.

In vitro studies of irbesartan oxidation by cytochrome P450 isoenzymes indicated irbesartan was oxidized primarily by 2C9; metabolism by 3A4 was negligible. Irbesartan was neither metabolized by, nor did it substantially induce or inhibit, isoenzymes commonly associated with drug metabolism (1A1, 1A2, 2A6, 2B6, 2D6, 2E1). There was no induction or inhibition of 3A4.

Distribution

Irbesartan is 90% bound to serum proteins (primarily albumin and α_1-acid glycoprotein) with negligible binding to cellular components of blood. The average volume of distribution is 53–93 liters. Total plasma and renal clearances are in the range of 157–176 and 3.0-3.5 mL/min, respectively. With repetitive dosing, irbesartan accumulates to no clinically relevant extent.

Studies in animals indicate that radiolabeled irbesartan weakly crosses the blood brain barrier and placenta. Irbesartan is excreted in the milk of lactating rats.

* Registered trademark of Sanofi

Special Populations

Pediatric: Irbesartan pharmacokinetics have not been investigated in patients <18 years of age.

Gender: No gender related differences in pharmacokinetics were observed in healthy elderly (age 65–80 years) or in healthy young (age 18–40 years) subjects. In studies of hypertensive patients, there was no gender difference in half-life or accumulation, but somewhat higher plasma concentrations of irbesartan were observed in females (11–44%). No gender-related dosage adjustment is necessary.

Geriatric: In elderly subjects (age 65–80 years), irbesartan elimination half-life was not significantly altered, but AUC and C_{max} values were about 20–50% greater than those of young subjects (age 18–40 years). No dosage adjustment is necessary in the elderly.

Race: In healthy black subjects, irbesartan AUC values were approximately 25% greater than whites; there was no difference in C_{max} values.

Renal Insufficiency: The pharmacokinetics of irbesartan were not altered in patients with renal impairment or in patients on hemodialysis. Irbesartan is not removed by hemodialysis. No dosage adjustment is necessary in patients with mild to severe renal impairment unless a patient with renal impairment is also volume depleted. (See **WARNINGS: Hypotension in Volume- or Salt-depleted Patients** and **DOSAGE AND ADMINISTRATION.**)

Hepatic Insufficiency: The pharmacokinetics of irbesartan following repeated oral administration were not significantly affected in patients with mild to moderate cirrhosis of the liver. No dosage adjustment is necessary in patients with hepatic insufficiency.

Drug Interactions: (See **PRECAUTIONS: Drug Interactions.**)

Pharmacodynamics

In healthy subjects, single oral irbesartan doses of up to 300 mg produced dose-dependent inhibition of the pressor effect

of angiotensin II infusions. Inhibition was complete (100%) 4 hours following oral doses of 150 mg or 300 mg and partial inhibition was sustained for 24 hours (60% and 40% at 300 mg and 150 mg, respectively).

In hypertensive patients, angiotensin II receptor inhibition following chronic administration of irbesartan causes a 1.5–2 fold rise in angiotensin II plasma concentration and a 2–3 fold increase in plasma renin levels. Aldosterone plasma concentrations generally decline following irbesartan administration, but serum potassium levels are not significantly affected at recommended doses.

In hypertensive patients, chronic oral doses of irbesartan (up to 300 mg) had no effect on glomerular filtration rate, renal plasma flow or filtration rate, renal plasma flow or filtration fraction. In multiple dose studies in hypertensive patients, there were no clinically important effects on fasting triglycerides, total cholesterol, HDL-cholesterol, or fasting glucose concentrations. There was no effect on serum uric acid during chronic oral administration, and no uricosuric effect.

Clinical Studies

The antihypertensive effects of AVAPRO (irbesatan) were examined in seven (7) major placebo-controlled 8–12 week trials in patients with baseline diastolic blood pressures of 95–110 mmHg. Doses of 1–900 mg were included in these trials in order to fully explore the dose-range of irbesartan. These studies allowed comparison of once- or twice-daily regimens at 150 mg/day, comparisons of peak and trough effects, and comparisons of response by gender, age, and race. Two of the seven placebo-controlled trials identified above examined the antihypertensive effects of irbesartan and hydrochlorothiazide in combination.

The seven (7) studies of irbesartan monotherapy included a total of 1915 patients randomized to irbesartan (1–900 mg) and 611 patients randomized to placebo. Once-daily doses of 150 and 300 mg provided statistically and clinically significant decreases in systolic and diastolic blood pressure with trough (24 hours post-dose) effects after 6–12 weeks of treatment compared to placebo, of about 8–10/5–6 and 8–12/5–8 mmHg, respectively. No further increase in effect was seen at dosages greater than 300 mg. The dose-response relationships for effects on systolic and diastolic pressure are shown in Figures 1 and 2.

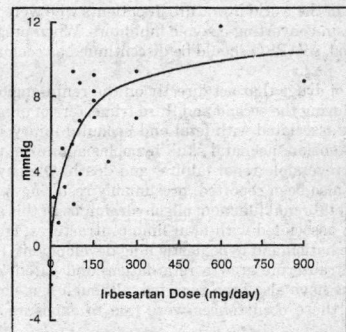

Figure 1. Placebo-subtracted reduction in trough SeSBP; integrated analysis

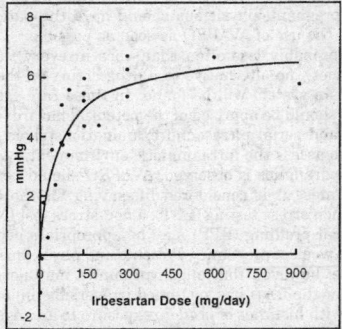

Figure 2. Placebo-subtracted reduction in trough SeDBP; integrated analysis

Continued on next page

This product information was prepared in September 1998. On these and other products of Sanofi Pharmaceuticals, Inc., detailed information may be obtained on a current basis by direct inquiry to Product Information Services, 90 Park Avenue, New York, NY 10016 (toll free 1-800-446-6267).

Avapro—Cont.

Once-daily administration of therapeutic doses of irbesartan gave peak effects at around 3–6 hours and, in one ambulatory blood pressure monitoring study, again around 14 hours. This was seen with both once-daily and twice-daily dosing. Trough-to-peak ratios by systolic and diastolic response were generally between 60–70%. In a continuous blood pressure monitoring study, once-daily dosing with 150 mg gave trough and mean 24-hour responses similar to those observed in patients receiving twice-daily dosing at the same total daily dose.

In controlled trials, the addition of irbesartan to hydrochlorothiazide doses of 6.25, 12.5, or 25 mg produced further dose-related reductions in blood pressure similar to those achieved with the same monotherapy dose of irbesartan. HCTZ aldo had an approximately additive effect.

Analysis of age, gender, and race subgroups of patients showed that men and women, and patients over and under 65 years of age, had generally similar responses. Irbesartan was effective in reducing blood pressure regardless of race, although the effect was somewhat less in blacks (usually a low-renin population).

The effect of irbesartan is apparent after the first dose and it is close to its full observed effect at 2 weeks. At the end of an 8-week exposure, about 2/3 of the antihypertensive effect was still present one week after the last dose. Rebound hypertension was not observed. There was essentially no change in average heart rate in irbesartan-treated patients in controlled trials.

INDICATIONS AND USAGE

AVAPRO (irbesartan) is indicated for the treatment of hypertension. It may be used alone or in combination with other antihypertensive agents.

CONTRAINDICATIONS

AVAPRO is contraindicated in patients who are hypersensitive to any component of this product.

WARNINGS

Fetal/Neonatal Morbidity and Mortality

Drugs that act directly on the renin-angiotensin system can cause fetal and neonatal morbidity and death when administered to pregnant women. Several dozen cases have been reported in the world literature in patients who were taking angiotensin-converting-enzyme inhibitors. When pregnancy is detected, AVAPRO should be discontinued as soon as possible.

The use of drugs that act directly on the renin-angiotensin system during the second and third trimesters of pregnancy has been associated with fetal and neonatal injury, including hypotension, neonatal skull hypoplasia, anuria, reversible or irreversible renal failure, and death. Oligohydramnios has also been reported, presumably resulting from decreased fetal renal function; oligohydramnios in this setting has been associated with fetal limb contractures, craniofacial deformation and hypoplastic lung development. Prematurity, intrauterine growth retardation, and patent ductus arteriosus have also been reported, although it is not clear whether these occurrences were due to exposure to the drug.

These adverse effects do not appear to have resulted from intrauterine drug exposure that has been limited to the first trimester.

Mothers whose embryos and fetuses are exposed to an angiotensin II receptor antagonist only during the first remester should be so informed. Nonetheless, when patients become pregnant, physicians should have the patient discontinue the use of AVAPRO as soon as possible.

Rarely (probably less often than once in every thousand pregnancies), no alternative to a drug acting on the renin-angiotensin system will be found. In these rare cases, the mothers should be apprised of the potential hazards to their fetuses, and serial ultrasound examinations shold be performed to assess the intraamniotic environment.

If oligohydramnios is observed, AVAPRO should be discontinued unless it is considered life-saving for the mother. Contraction stress testing (CST), a non-stress test (NST), or biophysical profiling (BPP) may be appropriate depending upon the week of pregnancy. Patients and physicians should be aware, however, that oligohydramnios may not appear until after the fetus has sustained irreversible injury.

Infants with histories of *in utero* exposure to an angiotensin II receptor antagonist should be closely observed for hypotension, oliguria, and hyperkalemia. If oliguria occurs, attention should be directed toward support of blood pressure and renal perfusion. Exchange transfusion or dialysis may be required as means of reversing hypotension and/or substituting for disordered renal function.

When pregnant rats were treated with irbesartan from day 0 to day 20 of gestation (oral doses of 50, 180, and 650 mg/kg/day), increased incidences of renal pelvic cavitation, hydroureter and/or absence of renal papilla were observed in fetuses at doses ≥50 mg/kg/day [approximately equivalent to the maximum recommended human dose (MRHD), 300 mg/day, on a body surface area basis]. Subcutaneous edema was observed in fetuses at doses ≥180 mg/kg/day (about 4 times the MRHD on a body surface area basis). As these anomalies were not observed in rats in which irbesartan exposure (oral doses of 50, 150 and 450 mg/kg/day) was limited to gestation days 6–15, they appear to reflect late gestational effects of the drug. In pregnant rabbits, oral doses of 30 mg irbesartan/kg/day were associated with maternal mortality and abortion. Surviving females receiving this dose (about 1.5 times the MRHD of a body surface area basis) had a slight increase in early resorptions and a corresponding decrease in live fetuses. Irbesartan was found to cross the placental barrier in rats and rabbits.

Radioactivity was present in the rat and rabbit fetus during late gestation and in rat milk following oral doses of radiolabeled irbesartan.

Hypotension in Volume- or Salt-depleted Patients

Excessive reduction of blood pressure was rarely seen (<0.1%) in patients with uncomplicated hypertension. Initiation of antihypertensive therapy may cause symptomatic hypotension in patients with intravascular volume- or sodium-depletion, e.g., in patients treated virgorously with diuretics or in patients on dialysis. Such volume depletion should be corrected prior to administration of AVAPRO (irbesartan), or a low starting dose should be used (see **DOSAGE AND ADMINISTRATION**).

If hypotension occurs, the patient should be placed in the supine position and, if necessary, given an intravenous infusion of normal saline. A transient hypotensive response is not a contraindication to further treatment, which usually can be continued without difficulty once the blood pressure has stabilized.

PRECAUTIONS

Impaired Renal Function

As a consequence of inhibiting the renin-angiotensin-aldosterone system, changes in renal function may be anticipated in susceptible individuals. In patients whose renal function may depend on the activity of the renin-angiotensin-aldosterone system (e.g., patients with severe congestive heart failure), treatment with angiotensin-converting-enzyme inhibitors has been associated with oliguria and/or progressive azotemia and (rarely) with acute renal failure and/or death. AVAPRO would be expected to behave similarly. In studies of ACE inhibitors in patients with unilateral or bilateral renal artery stenosis, increases in serum creatinine or BUN have been reported. There has been no known use of AVAPRO in patients with unilateral or bilateral renal artery stenosis, but a similar effect should be anticipated.

Information for Patients

Pregnancy: Female patients of childbearing age should be told about the consequences of second- and third-trimester exposure to drugs that act on the renin-angiotensin system, and they should also be told that these consequences do not appear to have resulted from intrauterine drug exposure that has been limited to the first trimester. These patients should be asked to report pregnancies to their physicians as soon as possible.

Drug Interactions

No significant drug-drug pharmacokinetic (or pharmacodynamic) interactions have been found in interaction studies with hydrochlorothiazide, digoxin, warfarin, and nifedipine. *In vitro* studies show significant inhibition of the formation of oxidized irbesartan metabolites with the known cytochrome CYP 2C9 substrates/inhibitors sulphenazole, tolbutamide and nifedipine. However, in clinical studies the consequences of concomitant irbesartan on the pharmacodynamics of warfarin were negligible. Based on *in vitro* data, no interaction would be expected with drugs whose metabolism is dependent upon cytochrome P450 isozymes 1A1, 1A2, 2A6, 2B6, 2D6, 2E1, or 3A4.

In separate studies of patients receiving maintenance doses of warfarin, hydrochlorothiazide, or digoxin, irbesartan administration for 7 days had no effect on the pharmacodynamics of warfarin (prothrombin time) or pharmacokinetics of digoxin. The pharmacokinetics of irbesartan were not affected by coadministration of nifedipine or hydrochlorothiazide.

Carcinogenesis, Mutagenesis, Impairment of Fertility

No evidence of carcinogenicity was observed when irbesartan was administered at doses of up to 500/1000 mg/kg/day (males/females, respectively) in rats and 1000 mg/kg/day in mice for up to two years. For male and female rats, 500 mg/kg/day provided an average systemic exposure to irbesartan (AUC_{0-24h}, bound plus unbound) about 3 and 11 times, respectively, the average systemic exposure in humans receiving the maximum recommended dose (MRD) of 300 mg irbesartan/day, whereas 1000 mg/kg/day (administered to females only) provided an average systemic exposure about 21 times that reported for humans at the MRD. For male and female mice, 1000 mg/kg/day provided an exposure to irbesartan about 3 and 5 times, respectively, the human exposure at 300 mg/day.

Irbesartan was not mutagenic in a battery of *in vitro* tests (Ames microbial test, rat hepatocyte DNA repair test, V79 mammalian-cell forward gene-mutation assay). Irbesartan was negative in several tests for induction of chromosomal aberrations (*in vitro*—human lymphocyte assay; *in vivo*—mouse micronucleus study).

Irbesartan had no adverse effects on fertility or mating of male or female rats at oral doses ≤650 mg/kg/day, the highest dose providing a systemic exposure to irbesartan (AUC_{0-24h}, bound plus unbound) about 5 times that found in humans receiving the maximum recommended dose of 300 mg/day.

Pregnancy

Pregnancy Categories C (first trimester) and D (second and third trimester).

See **WARNINGS: Fetal/Neonatal Morbidity and Mortality.**

Nursing Mothers

It is not known whether irbesartan is excreted in human milk, but irbesartan or some metabolite of irbesartan is secreted at low concentration in the milk of lactating rats. Because of the potential for adverse effects on the nursing infant, a decision should be made whether to discontinue nursing or discontinue the drug, taking into account the importance of the drug to the mother.

Pediatric Use

Safety and effectiveness in pediatric patients have not been established.

Geriatric Use

Of the total number of patients receiving AVAPRO (irbesartan) in controlled clinical studies, 911 patients (18.5%) were 65 years and over, while 150 patients (3.0%) were 75 years and over. No overall differences in effectiveness or safety were observed between these patients and younger patients, but greater sensitivity of some older individuals cannot be ruled out.

ADVERSE REACTIONS

AVAPRO has been evaluated for safety in more than 4300 patients with hypertension and about 5000 subjects overall. This experience includes 1303 patients treated for over 6 months and 407 patients for 1 year or more. Treatment with AVAPRO was well-tolerated, with an incidence of adverse events similar to placebo. These events generally were mild and transient with no relationship to the doses of AVAPRO.

In placebo-controlled clinical trials, discontinuation of therapy due to a clinical adverse event was required in 3.3 percent of patients treated with AVAPRO, versus 4.5 percent of patients given placebo.

In placebo-controlled clinical trials, the adverse event experiences that occurred in at least 1% of patients treated with AVAPRO (n=1965) and at a higher incidence versus placebo (n=641) included diarrhea (3% vs. 2%), dyspepsia/heartburn (2% vs. 1%), musculoskeletal trauma (2% vs. 1%), fatigue (4% vs. 3%), and upper respiratory infection (9% vs. 6%). None of these differences were significant.

The following adverse events occurred at an incidence of 1% or greater in patients treated with irbesartan, but were at least as frequent or more frequent in patients recieving placebo: abdominal pain, anxiety/nervousness, chest pain, dizziness, edema, headache, influenza, musculoskeletal pain, pharyngitis, nausea/vomiting, rash, rhinitis, sinus abnormailty, tachycardia and urinary tract infection.

Irbesartan use was not associated with an increased incidence of dry cough, as is typically associated with ACE inhibitor use. In placebo controlled studies, the incidence of cough in irbesartan treated patients was 2.8% versus 2.7% in patients receiving placebo.

The incidence of hypotension or orthostatic hypotension was low in irbesartan treated patients (0.4%), unrelated to dosage, and similar to the incidence among placebo treated patients (0.2%). Dizziness, syncope, and vertigo were reported with equal or less frequency in patients receiving irbesartan compared with placebo.

In addition, the following potentially important events occurred in less than 1% of the 1965 patients and at least 5 patients (0.3%) receiving irbesartan in clinical studies, and those less frequent, clinically significant events (listed by body system). It cannot be determined whether these events were causally related to irbesartan:

Body as a Whole: fever, chills, facial edema, upper extremity edema;

Cardiovascular: flushing, hypertension, cardiac murmur, myocardial infarction, angina pectoris, arrhythmic/conduction disorder, cardio-respiratory arrest, heart failure, hypertensive crisis;

Dermatologic: pruritus, dermatitis, ecchymosis, erythema face, urticaria;

Endocrine/Metabolic/Electrolyte Imbalances: sexual dysfunction, libido change, gout;

Gastrointestinal: constipation, oral lesion, gastroenteritis, flatulence, abdominal distention;

Musculoskeletal/Connective Tissue: extremity swelling, muscle cramp, arthritis, muscle ache, musculoskeletal chest pain, joint stiffness, bursitis, muscle weakness;

	75 mg	150 mg	300 mg
Debossing	2771	2772	2773
Bottle of 30	0087-2771-31	0087-2772-31	0089-2773-31
Bottle of 90	0087-2771-32	0087-2772-32	0087-2773-32
Bottle of 500	0087-2771-15	0087-2772-15	0087-2773-15
Blister of 100	0087-2771-35	0087-2772-35	0087-2773-35

Nervous System: sleep disturbance, numbness, somnolence, emotional disturbance, depression, paresthesia, tremor, transient ischemic attack, cerebrovascular accident;
Renal/Genitourinary: abnormal urination, prostate disorder;
Respiratory: epistaxis, tracheobronchitis, congestion, pulmonary congestion, dyspnea, wheezing;
Special Senses: vision disturbance, hearing abnormality, ear infection, ear pain, conjunctivitis, other eye disturbance, eyelid abnormality, ear abnormality.

Laboratory Test Findings

In controlled clinical trials, clincally important differences in laboratory tests were rarely associated with administration of AVAPRO.

Creatinine, Blood Urea Nitrogen: Minor increases in blood urea nitrogen (BUN) or serum creatinine were observed in less than 0.7% of patients with essential hypertension treated with AVAPRO alone versus 0.9% on placebo. (See **PRECAUTIONS: Impaired Renal Function.**)

Hematologic: Mean decreases in hemoglobin of 0.2 g/dL were observed in 0.2% of patients receiving AVAPRO compared to 0.3% of placebo treated patients. Neutropenia (<1000 cells/mm^3) occurred at similar frequencies among patients receiving AVAPRO (0.3%) and placebo treated patients (0.5%).

OVERDOSAGE

No data are available in regard to overdosage in humans. However, daily doses of 900 mg for 8 weeks were well-tolerated. The most likely manifestations of overdosage are expected to be hypotension and tachycardia; bradycardia might also occur from overdose. Irbesartan is not removed by hemodialysis.

To obtain up-to-date information about the treatment of overdosage, a good resource is a certified Regional Poison-Control Center. Telephone numbers of certified poison-control centers are listed in the *Physicians' Desk Reference* (PDR). In managing overdose, consider the possibilities of multiple-drug interactions, drug-drug interactions, and unusual drug kinetics in the patient.

Laboratory determinations of serum levels of irbesartan are not widely available, and such determinations have, in any event, no known established role in the management of irbesartan overdose.

Acute oral toxicity studies with irbesartan in mice and rats indicated acute lethal doses were in excess of 2000 mg/kg, about 25- and 50-fold the maximum recommended human dose (300 mg) on a mg/m^2 basis, respectively.

DOSAGE AND ADMINISTRATION

The recommended initial dose of AVAPRO is 150 mg once daily. Patients requiring further reduction in blood pressure should be titrated to 300 mg once daily.

A low dose of a diuretic may be added, if blood pressure is not controlled by AVAPRO alone. Hydrochlorothiazide has been shown to have an additive effect (see **CLINICAL PHARMACOLOGY: Clinical Studies**). Patients not adequately treated by the maximum dose of 300 mg once daily are unlikely to derive additional benefit from a higher dose or twice-daily dosing.

No dosage adjustment is necessary in elderly patients, or in patients with hepatic impairment or mild to severe renal impairment.

AVAPRO may be administered with other antihypertensive agents.

AVAPRO may be administered with or without food.

Volume- and Salt-depleted Patients

A lower initial dose or AVAPRO (75 mg) is recommended in patients with depletion of intravascular volume or salt (e.g., patients treated vigorously with diuretics or on hemodialysis) (see **WARNINGS: Hypotension in Volume- of Salt-depleted Patients**).

HOW SUPPLIED

AVAPRO® (irbesartan) is available as white to off-white biconvex oval tablets, debossed with a heart shape on one side and a portion of the NDC code on the other. Unit-of-use bottles contain 30, 90, or 500 tablets and blister packs contain 100 tablets, as follows:

[See table above]

Storage

Store at a temperature between 15° C and 30° C (59° F and 85° F) [USP].

Manufactured and Distributed by:
Bristol-Myers Squibb Company
Princeton, NJ 08543-4500

Comarketed by:
Sanofi Pharmaceuticals, Inc.
New York, NY 10016
Issued October 1997 P0617-00

Shown in Product Identification Guide, page 335

BRONCHOLATE® SYRUP ℞

Each teaspoonful (5 ml) orange flavored syrup contains:
Ephedrine HCl .... 6.25 mg
Guaifenesin .... 100.00 mg

HOW SUPPLIED

Bottles of 16 oz.

CHEMET® ℞
SUCCIMER

DESCRIPTION

CHEMET (succimer) is an orally active, heavy metal chelating agent. The chemical name for succimer is *meso* 2, 3-dimercaptosuccinic acid (DMSA). Its empirical formula is $C_4H_6O_4S_2$ and molecular weight is 182.2. The *meso*-structural formula is:

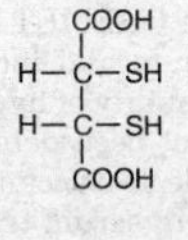

Succimer is a white crystalline powder with an unpleasant, characteristic mercaptan odor and taste.

Each CHEMET opaque white capsule for oral administration, contains beads coated with 100 mg of succimer and is imprinted black with CHEMET 100. Inactive ingredients in medicated beads are: povidone, sodium starch glycolate, starch and sucrose. Inactive ingredients in capsule are: gelatin, iron oxide, titanium dioxide and other ingredients.

CLINICAL PHARMACOLOGY

Succimer is a lead chelator; it forms water soluble chelates and, consequently, increases the urinary excretion of lead.

Preclinical Toxicology: In an ongoing six month chronic oral toxicity study in dogs, thrombocytopenia was observed in animals receiving succimer at 80 or 140 mg/kg/day after three months of dosing. Preliminary gross pathology findings in the affected dogs included ecchymoses in a number of organs. No depressed platelet counts were observed in dogs receiving succimer at 10 mg/kg/day for three months. Platelets were not enumerated in previous oral toxicity studies up to 28 days. In those studies, daily doses of succimer up to 200 mg/kg/day did not produce any significant overt toxicity in rats and dogs. However, six and twenty-eight day oral toxicity studies in dogs have shown that doses of 300 mg/kg/ day or higher were toxic and lethal to some dogs. Kidney and gastrointestinal tract were the major target organs for succimer toxicity. Toxicity was manifested by anorexia, emesis, mucoid and/or bloody diarrhea, increased blood urea nitrogen concentration, increased SGPT, SGOT and alkaline phosphatase levels, renal tubular necrosis, purulent nephritis and severe gastrointestinal bleeding and ulceration. Deaths were due to renal failure.

Pharmacokinetics: In a study performed in healthy adult volunteers, after a single dose of ^{14}C-succimer at 16, 32, or 48 mg/kg, absorption was rapid but variable with peak blood radioactivity levels between one and two hours. On average, 49% of the radiolabeled dose was excreted: 39% in the feces, 9% in the urine and 1% as carbon dioxide from the lungs. Since fecal excretion probably represented non-absorbed drug, most of the absorbed drug was excreted by the kidneys. The apparent elimination half-life of the radiolabeled material in the blood was about two days.

In other studies of healthy adult volunteers receiving a single oral dose of 10 mg/kg, the chemical analysis of succimer and its metabolites in the urine showed that succimer was rapidly and extensively metabolized. Approximately 25% of the administered dose was excreted in the urine with the peak blood level and urinary excretion occurring between two and four hours. Of the total amount of drug eliminated in the urine, approximately 90% was eliminated in altered form as mixed succimer-cysteine disulfides; the remaining 10% was eliminated unchanged. The majority of mixed disulfides consisted of succimer in disulfide linkages with two molecules of L-cysteine, the remaining disulfides contained one L-cysteine per succimer molecule.

Pharmacodynamics: Dose ranging studies were performed in 18 men with blood lead levels of 44–96 µg/dL. Three groups of 6 patients received either 10.0, 6.7 or 3.3 mg/kg succimer orally every 8 hours for 5 days. After five days the mean blood levels of the three groups decreased 72.5%, 58.3% and 35.5% respectively. The mean urinary lead excretions in the initial 24 hours were 28.6, 18.6 and 12.3 times the pretreatment 24 hour urinary lead excretion. As the chelatable pool was reduced during therapy, urinary lead output decreased. A mean of 19 mg of lead was excreted during a five-day course of 30 mg/kg/day succimer. Clinical symptoms, such as headache and colic and biochemical indices of lead toxicity also improved. Decrease in urinary excretion of d-aminolevulinic acid (ALA) and coproporphyrin paralleled the improvement in erythrocyte d-aminolevulinic acid dehydratase (ALA-D). Three control patients with lead poisoning of similar severity received $CaNa_2$ EDTA intravenously at a dose of 50 mg/kg/day for five days. The mean blood lead level decreased 47.4% and the mean urinary lead excretion was 21 mg in the control patients.

Effect on Essential Minerals: In the above studies succimer had no significant effect on the urinary elimination of iron, calcium or magnesium. Zinc excretion doubled during treatment. The effect of succimer on the excretion of essential minerals was small compared to that of $CaNa_2$ EDTA, which can induce more than a ten-fold increase in urinary excretion of zinc and doubling of copper and iron excretion.

Efficacy: A dose ranging study was performed in 15 pediatric patients aged 2 to 7 years with blood lead levels of 30–49 µg/dL and positive $CaNa_2$ EDTA lead mobilization tests. Each group of five patients received 350, 233 or 116 mg/m^2 succimer every 8 hours for 5 days. These doses corresponded to 10, 6.7 and 3.3 mg/kg. Six control patients received 1000 mg/m^2/day $CaNa_2$ EDTA intravenously for 5 days. Following therapy, the mean blood lead levels decreased 78, 63 and 42% respectively in the three groups treated with succimer. The response of the 350 mg/m^2 every 8 hours (10 mg/kg q 8 hr) group was significantly better than that of the other succimer treated groups as well as that of the control group, whose mean blood lead level fell 48%. No adverse reactions or changes in essential mineral excretion were reported in the succimer treated groups. In the $CaNa_2$ EDTA treated group, the cumulative amount of urinary lead excreted was slightly but significantly greater than in the succimer group. After $CaNa_2$ EDTA, the urinary excretion of copper, zinc, iron and calcium were significantly increased.

As with other chelators, both adults and pediatric patients experienced a rebound in blood lead levels after discontinuation of CHEMET. In these studies, after treatment with a dose of 350 mg/m^2 (10 mg/kg) every 8 hours for five days, the mean lead level rebounded and plateaued at 60–85% of pretreatment levels two weeks after therapy. The rebound plateau was somewhat higher with lower doses of succimer and with intravenous $CaNa_2$ EDTA.

In an attempt to control rebound of blood lead levels, 19 pediatric patients, ages 1–7 years, with blood lead levels of 42–67 µg/dL, were treated with 350 mg/m^2 succimer every 8 hours for five days and then divided into three groups. One group was followed for two weeks with no further therapy, the second group was treated for two weeks with 350 mg/m^2 daily, and the third with 350 mg/m^2 every 12 hours. After the initial 5 days of therapy, the mean blood lead level in all subjects declined 61%. While the untreated group and the group treated with 350 mg/m^2 daily experienced rebound during the ensuing two weeks, the group who received the 350 mg/ m^2 every 12 hours experienced no such rebound during the treatment period and less rebound following cessation of therapy.

In another study, ten pediatric patients, ages 21 to 72 months, with blood lead levels of 30–57 µg/dL were treated with succimer 350 mg/m^2 every eight hours for five days followed by an additional 19–22 days of therapy at a dose of 350 mg/m^2 every 12 hours. The mean blood lead levels decreased and remained stable at under 15 µg/dL during the extended dosing period.

In addition to the controlled studies, approximately 250 patients with lead poisoning have been treated with succimer either orally or parenterally in open U.S. and foreign studies with similar results reported. Succimer has been used for the treatment of lead poisoning in one patient with sickle cell anemia and in five patients with glucose-6-phosphodehydrogenase (G6PD) deficiency without adverse reactions.

Continued on next page

This product information was prepared in September 1998. On these and other products of Sanofi Pharmaceuticals, Inc., detailed information may be obtained on a current basis by direct inquiry to Product Information Services, 90 Park Avenue, New York, NY 10016 (toll free 1-800-446-6267).

Chemet—Cont.

Lead Encephalopathy: Three adults with lead encephalopathy have been reported in the literature to have improved with succimer therapy. However, data are not available regarding the use of succimer for the treatment of this rare and sometimes fatal complication of lead poisoning in pediatric patients.

Other Heavy Metal Poisoning: No controlled clinical studies have been conducted with succimer in poisoning with other heavy metals. A limited number of patients have received succimer for mercury or arsenic poisoning. These patients showed increased urinary excretion of the heavy metal and varying degrees of symptomatic improvement.

INDICATIONS AND USAGE

CHEMET is indicated for the treatment of lead poisoning in pediatric patients with blood lead levels above 45 µg/dL. CHEMET is not indicated for prophylaxis of lead poisoning in a lead-containing environment; the use of CHEMET should always be accompanied by identification and removal of the source of the lead exposure.

CONTRAINDICATIONS

CHEMET should not be administered to patients with a history of allergy to the drug.

WARNINGS

Keep out of reach of pediatric patients. CHEMET is not a substitute for effective abatement of lead exposure.

Mild to moderate neutropenia has been observed in some patients receiving succimer. While a causal relationship to succimer has not been definitely established, neutropenia has been reported with other drugs in the same chemical class. A complete blood count with white blood cell differential and direct platelet counts should be obtained prior to and weekly during treatment with succimer. Therapy should either be withheld or discontinued if the absolute neutrophil count (ANC) is below 1200/µL and the patient followed closely to document recovery of the ANC to above 1500/µL or to the patient's baseline neutrophil count. There is limited experience with reexposure in patients who have developed neutropenia. Therefore, such patients should be rechallenged only if the benefit of succimer therapy clearly outweighs the potential risk of another episode of neutropenia and then only with careful patient monitoring.

Patients treated with succimer should be instructed to promptly report any signs of infection. If infection is suspected, the above laboratory tests should be conducted immediately.

PRECAUTIONS

The extent of clinical experience with CHEMET is limited. Therefore, patients should be carefully observed during treatment.

General: Elevated blood lead levels and associated symptoms may return rapidly after discontinuation of CHEMET because of redistribution of lead from bone stores to soft tissues and blood. After therapy, patients should be monitored for rebound of blood lead levels, by measuring blood lead levels at least once weekly until stable. However, the severity of lead intoxication (as measured by the initial blood lead level and the rate and degree of rebound of blood lead) should be used as a guide for more frequent blood lead monitoring.

All patients undergoing treatment should be adequately hydrated. Caution should be exercised in using CHEMET therapy in patients with compromised renal function. Limited data suggests that CHEMET is dialyzable, but that the lead chelates are not.

Transient mild elevations of serum transaminases have been observed in 6–10% of patients during the course of succimer therapy. Serum transaminases should be monitored before the start of therapy and at least weekly during therapy. Patients with a history of liver disease should be monitored closely. No data are available regarding the metabolism of succimer in patients with liver disease.

Clinical experience with repeated courses is limited. The safety of uninterrupted dosing longer than three weeks has not been established and it is not recommended.

The possibility of allergic or other mucocutaneous reactions to the drug must be borne in mind on readministration (as well as during initial courses). Patients requiring repeated courses of CHEMET should be monitored during each treatment course. One patient experienced recurrent mucocutaneous vesicular eruptions of increasing severity affecting the oral mucosa, the external urethral meatus and the perianal area on the third, fourth and fifth courses of the drug. The reaction resolved between courses and upon discontinuation of therapy.

Information for Patients: Patients should be instructed to maintain adequate fluid intake. If rash occurs, patients should consult their physician. Patients should be instructed to promptly report any indication of infection, which may be a sign of neutropenia (see WARNINGS and ADVERSE REACTIONS).

In young pediatric patients unable to swallow capsules, the contents of the capsule can be administered in a small amount of food (see DOSAGE AND ADMINISTRATION).

Drug Interaction: CHEMET is not known to interact with other drugs including iron supplements; interactions have not been systematically studied. Concomitant administration of CHEMET with other chelation therapy, such as $CaNa_2$ EDTA is not recommended.

Drug/Laboratory Tests Interaction: Succimer may interfere with serum and urinary laboratory tests. *In vitro* studies have shown succimer to cause false positive results for ketones in urine using nitroprusside reagents such as Ketostix® and falsely decreased measurements of serum uric acid and CPK.

Carcinogenesis, Mutagenesis and Impairment of Fertility: CHEMET has not been tested for carcinogenic potential in long-term animal studies. CHEMET has not been tested in animals for its effect on fertility and reproductive performance in males and females. It was not mutagenic in the Ames bacterial assay and in the mammalian cell forward gene mutation assay.

Pregnancy: *Teratogenic Effects —Pregnancy Category C.* CHEMET has been shown to be teratogenic and fetotoxic in pregnant mice when given subcutaneously in a dose range of 410 to 1640 mg/kg/day during the period of organogenesis. There are no adequate and well controlled studies in pregnant women. CHEMET should be used during pregnancy only if the potential benefit justifies the potential risk to the fetus.

Nursing Mothers: It is not known whether this drug is excreted in human milk. Because many drugs and heavy metals are excreted in human milk, nursing mothers requiring CHEMET therapy should be discouraged from nursing their infants.

Pediatric Use: Refer to the INDICATIONS and DOSAGE AND ADMINISTRATION sections. Safety and efficacy in pediatric patients less than 12 months of age have not been established.

ADVERSE REACTIONS

Clinical experience with CHEMET has been limited. Consequently, the full spectrum and incidence of adverse reactions including the possibility of hypersensitivity or idiosyncratic reactions have not been determined. The most common events attributable to succimer, i.e., gastrointestinal symptoms or increases in serum transaminases, have been observed in about 10% of patients (see PRECAUTIONS). Rashes, some necessitating discontinuation of therapy, have been reported in about 4% of patients. If rash occurs, other causes (e.g. measles) should be considered before ascribing the reaction to succimer. Rechallenge with succimer may be considered if lead levels are high enough to warrant retreatment. One allergic mucocutaneous reaction has been reported on repeated administration of the drug (See PRECAUTIONS). Mild to moderate neutropenia has been observed in some patients receiving succimer (see WARNINGS). Table I presents adverse events reported with the administration of succimer for the treatment of lead and other heavy metal intoxication.

TABLE I
INCIDENCE OF ADVERSE EVENTS IN DOMESTIC STUDIES REGARDLESS OF ATTRIBUTION OR SUCCIMER DOSAGE

	Pediatric Patients (191)		Adults (134)	
	%	(n)	%	(n)
Digestive:	12.0	23	20.9	28
Nausea, vomiting, diarrhea, appetite loss, hemorrhoidal symptoms, loose stools, metallic taste in mouth.				
Body as a Whole:	5.2	10	15.7	21
Back pain, abdominal cramps, stomach pains, head pain, rib pain, chills, flank pain, fever, flu-like symptoms, heavy head/tired, head cold, headache, moniliasis.				
Metabolic:	4.2	8	10.4	14
Elevated SGPT, SGOT, alkaline phosphatase, elevated serum cholesterol.				
Nervous:	1.0	2	12.7	17
Drowsiness, dizziness, sensorimotor neuropathy, sleepiness, paresthesia.				
Skin and Appendages:	2.6	5	11.2	15
Papular rash, herpetic rash, rash, mucocutaneous eruptions, pruritus.				
Special Senses:	1.0	2	3.7	5
Cloudy film in eye, ears plugged, otitis media, eyes watery.				
Respiratory:	3.7	7	0.7	1
Throat sore, rhinorrhea, nasal congestion, cough.				
Urogenital:	0.0	—	3.7	5
Decreased urination, voiding difficulty, proteinuria increased.				
Cardiovascular:	0.0	—	1.8	2
Arrhythmia				
Heme/Lymphatic:	0.5*	1	1.5*	2
Mild to moderate neutropenia Increased platelet count, intermittent eosinophilia.				
Musculoskeletal:	0.0	—	3.0	4
Kneecap pain, leg pains.				

* Does not include neutropenia - see WARNINGS

OVERDOSAGE

Doses of 2300 mg/kg in the rat and 2400 mg/kg in the mouse produced ataxia, convulsions, labored respiration and frequently death. No case of overdosage has been reported in humans. Limited data indicate that succimer is dialyzable. In case of acute overdosage, induction of vomiting or gastric lavage followed by administration of an activated charcoal slurry and appropriate supportive therapy are recommended.

DOSAGE AND ADMINISTRATION

Start dosage at 10 mg/kg or 350 mg/m^2 every eight hours for five days. Initiation of therapy at higher doses is not recommended. (See Table II for Dosing chart and number of capsules.) Reduce frequency of administration to 10 mg/kg or 350 mg/m^2 every 12 hours (two-thirds of initial daily dosage) for an additional two weeks of therapy. A course of treatment lasts 19 days. Repeated courses may be necessary if indicated by weekly monitoring of blood lead concentration. A minimum of two weeks between courses is recommended unless blood lead levels indicate the need for more prompt treatment.

TABLE II
CHEMET (SUCCIMER) PEDIATRIC DOSING CHART

LBS	KG	DOSE (MG)*	Number of CAPSULES*
18–35	8–15	100	1
36–55	16–23	200	2
56–75	24–34	300	3
76–100	35–44	400	4
>100	>45	500	5

* To be administered every 8 hours for 5 days, followed by dosing every 12 hours for 14 days.

In young pediatric patients who cannot swallow capsules, CHEMET can be administered by separating the capsule and sprinkling the medicated beads on a small amount of soft food or putting them in a spoon and following with fruit drink.

Identification of the source of lead in the pediatric patient's environment and its abatement are critical to a successful therapy outcome. Chelation therapy is not a substitute for preventing further exposure to lead and should not be used to permit continued exposure to lead.

Patients who have received $CaNa_2$ EDTA with or without BAL may use CHEMET for subsequent treatment after an interval of four weeks. Data on the concomitant use of CHEMET with $CaNa_2$ EDTA with or without BAL are not available, and such use is not recommended.

HOW SUPPLIED

100 mg capsules in bottle of 100 (NDC 0024-0333-01)

Storage: Store between 15°C and 25°C and avoid excessive heat.

CAUTION: Federal law prohibits dispensing without prescription. Revised September, 1997.

HPG11506-01-1295BP

Shown in Product Identification Guide, page 335

DANOCRINE® ℞
DANAZOL, USP

DESCRIPTION

DANOCRINE, brand of danazol, is a synthetic steroid derived from ethisterone. It is a white to pale yellow crystalline powder, practically insoluble or insoluble in water, and sparingly soluble in alcohol. Chemically, danazol is 17α-Pregna-2,4-dien-20-yno [2,3-*d*]-isoxazol-17-ol. The molecular formula is $C_{22}H_{27}NO_2$. It has a molecular weight of 337.46 and the following structural formula:

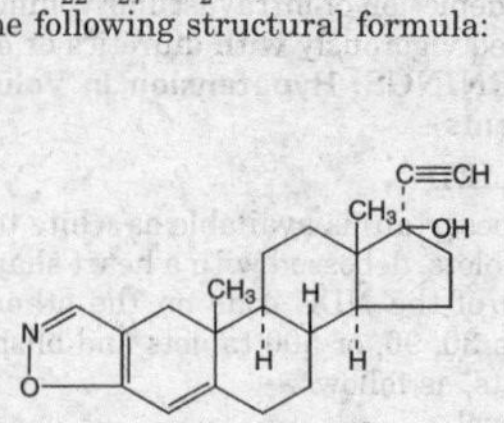

Danocrine capsules for oral administration contain 50 mg, 100 mg or 200 mg danazol.

Inactive Ingredients: Corn Starch, Lactose, Magnesium Stearate, Talc. Capsules 50 mg, 100 mg and 200 mg contain

D&C Yellow #10, FD&C Red #40, Gelatin, Silicon Dioxide, Sodium Lauryl Sulfate, Titanium Dioxide. The 50 mg and 200 mg capsules also contain D&C Red #28.

CLINICAL PHARMACOLOGY

DANOCRINE suppresses the pituitary-ovarian axis. This suppression is probably a combination of depressed hypothalamic-pituitary response to lowered estrogen production, the alteration of sex steroid metabolism, and interaction of danazol with sex hormone receptors. The only other demonstrable hormonal effect is weak androgenic activity. DANOCRINE depresses the output of both follicle-stimulating hormone (FSH) and luteinizing hormone (LH).

Recent evidence suggests a direct inhibitory effect at gonadal sites and a binding of DANOCRINE to receptors of gonadal steroids at target organs. In addition, DANOCRINE has been shown to significantly decrease IgG, IgM and IgA levels, as well as phospholipid and IgG isotope autoantibodies in patients with endometriosis and associated elevations of autoantibodies, suggesting this could be another mechanism by which it facilitates regression of the disease.

Bioavailability studies indicate that blood levels do not increase proportionally with increases in the administered dose. When the dose of DANOCRINE is doubled the increase in plasma levels is only about 35% to 40%.

Separate single dosing of 100 mg and 200 mg capsules of DANOCRINE to female volunteers showed that both the extent of availability and the maximum plasma concentration increased by three-to-four fold, respectively, following a meal (> 30 grams of fat), when compared to the fasted state. Further, food also delayed mean time to peak concentration of DANOCRINE by about 30 minutes.

In the treatment of endometriosis, DANOCRINE alters the normal and ectopic endometrial tissue so that it becomes inactive and atrophic. Complete resolution of endometrial lesions occurs in the majority of cases.

Changes in vaginal cytology and cervical mucus reflect the suppressive effect of DANOCRINE on the pituitary-ovarian axis.

In the treatment of fibrocystic breast disease, DANOCRINE usually produces partial to complete disappearance of nodularity and complete relief of pain and tenderness. Changes in the menstrual pattern may occur.

Generally, the pituitary-suppressive action of DANOCRINE is reversible. Ovulation and cyclic bleeding usually return within 60 to 90 days when therapy with DANOCRINE is discontinued.

In the treatment of hereditary angioedema, DANOCRINE at effective doses prevents attacks of the disease characterized by episodic edema of the abdominal viscera, extremities, face, and airway which may be disabling and, if the airway is involved, fatal. In addition, DANOCRINE corrects partially or completely the primary biochemical abnormality of hereditary angioedema by increasing the levels of the deficient C1 esterase inhibitor (C1EI). As a result of this action the serum levels of the C4 component of the complement system are also increased.

INDICATIONS AND USAGE

Endometriosis. DANOCRINE is indicated for the treatment of endometriosis amenable to hormonal management.

Fibrocystic Breast Disease. Most cases of symptomatic fibrocystic breast disease may be treated by simple measures (e.g., padded brassieres and analgesics).

In infrequent patients, symptoms of pain and tenderness may be severe enough to warrant treatment by suppression of ovarian function. DANOCRINE is usually effective in decreasing nodularity, pain, and tenderness. It should be stressed to the patient that this treatment is not innocuous in that it involves considerable alterations of hormone levels and that recurrence of symptoms is very common after cessation of therapy.

Hereditary Angioedema. DANOCRINE is indicated for the prevention of attacks of angioedema of all types (cutaneous, abdominal, laryngeal) in males and females.

CONTRAINDICATIONS

DANOCRINE should not be administered to patients with:
1. Undiagnosed abnormal genital bleeding.
2. Markedly impaired hepatic, renal, or cardiac function.
3. Pregnancy. (See WARNINGS.)
4. Breast feeding.
5. Porphyria—DANOCRINE can induce ALA synthetase activity and hence porphyrin metabolism.

WARNINGS

Use of danazol in pregnancy is contraindicated. A sensitive test (e.g., beta subunit test if available) capable of determining early pregnancy is recommended immediately prior to start of therapy. Additionally a non-hormonal method of contraception should be used during therapy. If a patient becomes pregnant while taking danazol, administration of the drug should be discontinued and the patient should be apprised of the potential risk to the fetus. Exposure to danazol in utero may

result in androgenic effects on the female fetus; reports of clitoral hypertrophy, labial fusion, urogenital sinus defect, vaginal atresia, and ambiguous genitalia have been received. (See PRECAUTIONS: Pregnancy, Teratogenic Effects.)

Thromboembolism, thrombotic and thrombophlebitic events including sagittal sinus thrombosis and life-threatening or fatal strokes have been reported.

Experience with long-term therapy with danazol is limited. Peliosis hepatis and benign hepatic adenoma have been observed with long-term use. Peliosis hepatis and hepatic adenoma may be silent until complicated by acute, potentially life-threatening intra-abdominal hemorrhage. The physician therefore should be alert to this possibility. Attempts should be made to determine the lowest dose that will provide adequate protection. If the drug was begun at a time of exacerbation of hereditary angioneurotic edema due to trauma, stress or other cause, periodic attempts to decrease or withdraw therapy should be considered.

Danazol has been associated with several cases of benign intracranial hypertension also known as pseudotumor cerebri. Early signs and symptoms of benign intracranial hypertension include papilledema, headache, nausea and vomiting, and visual disturbances. Patients with these symptoms should be screened for papilledema and, if present, the patients should be advised to discontinue danazol immediately and be referred to a neurologist for further diagnosis and care.

A temporary alteration of lipoproteins in the form of decreased high density lipoproteins and possibly increased low density lipoproteins has been reported during danazol therapy. These alterations may be marked, and prescribers should consider the potential impact on the risk of atherosclerosis and coronary artery disease in accordance with the potential benefit of the therapy to the patient.

Before initiating therapy of fibrocystic breast disease with DANOCRINE, carcinoma of the breast should be excluded. However, nodularity, pain, tenderness due to fibrocystic breast disease may prevent recognition of underlying carcinoma before treatment is begun. Therefore, if any nodule persists or enlarges during treatment, carcinoma should be considered and ruled out.

Patients should be watched closely for signs of androgenic effects some of which may not be reversible even when drug administration is stopped.

PRECAUTIONS

Because DANOCRINE may cause some degree of fluid retention, conditions that might be influenced by this factor, such as epilepsy, migraine, or cardiac or renal dysfunction, require careful observation.

Since hepatic dysfunction manifested by modest increases in serum transaminase levels has been reported in patients treated with DANOCRINE, periodic liver function tests should be performed (see WARNINGS and ADVERSE REACTIONS).

Administration of danazol has been reported to cause exacerbation of the manifestations of acute intermittent porphyria. (See CONTRAINDICATIONS.)

Drug Interactions: Prolongation of prothrombin time occurs in patients stabilized on warfarin. Therapy with danazol may cause an increase in carbamazepine levels in patients taking both drugs.

Laboratory Tests: Danazol treatment may interfere with laboratory determinations of testosterone, androstenedione and dehydroepiandrosterone.

Carcinogenesis, Mutagenesis, Impairment of Fertility: No valid studies have been performed to assess the carcinogenicity of DANOCRINE.

Pregnancy, Teratogenic Effects: (See CONTRAINDICATIONS.) Pregnancy Category X. DANOCRINE administered orally to pregnant rats from the 6th through the 15th day of gestation at doses up to 250 mg/kg/day (7–15 times the human dose) did not result in drug-induced embryotoxicity or teratogenicity, nor difference in litter size, viability or weight of offspring compared to controls. In rabbits, the administration of DANOCRINE on days 6–18 of gestation at doses of 60 mg/kg/day and above (2–4 times the human dose) resulted in inhibition of fetal development.

Nursing Mothers: (See CONTRAINDICATIONS.)

Pediatric Use: Safety and effectiveness in children have not been established.

ADVERSE REACTIONS

The following events have been reported in association with the use of DANOCRINE:

Androgen like effects include weight gain, acne and seborrhea. Mild hirsutism, edema, hair loss, voice change, which may take the form of hoarseness, sore throat or of instability or deepening of pitch, may occur and may persist after cessation of therapy. Hypertrophy of the clitoris is rare.

Other possible endocrine effects include menstrual disturbances in the form of spotting, alteration of the timing of the cycle and amenorrhea. Although cyclical bleeding and ovu-

lation usually return within 60–90 days after discontinuation of therapy with DANOCRINE, persistent amenorrhea has occasionally been reported.

Flushing, sweating, vaginal dryness and irritation and reduction in breast size, may reflect lowering of estrogen. Nervousness and emotional lability have been reported. In the male a modest reduction in spermatogenesis may be evident during treatment. Abnormalities in semen volume, viscosity, sperm count, and motility may occur in patients receiving long-term therapy.

Hepatic dysfunction, as evidenced by reversible elevated serum enzymes and/or jaundice, has been reported in patients receiving a daily dosage of DANOCRINE of 400 mg or more. It is recommended that patients receiving DANOCRINE be monitored for hepatic dysfunction by laboratory tests and clinical observation. Serious hepatic toxicity including cholestatic jaundice, peliosis hepatis, and hepatic adenoma have been reported. (See WARNINGS and PRECAUTIONS.)

Abnormalities in laboratory tests may occur during therapy with DANOCRINE including CPK, glucose tolerance, glucagon, thyroid binding globulin, sex hormone binding globulin, other plasma proteins, lipids and lipoproteins.

The following reactions have been reported, a causal relationship to the administration of DANOCRINE has neither been confirmed nor refuted; *allergic:* urticaria, pruritus and rarely, nasal congestion; *CNS effects:* headache, nervousness and emotional lability, dizziness and fainting, depression, fatigue, sleep disorders, tremor, paresthesias, weakness, visual disturbances, and rarely, benign intracranial hypertension, anxiety, changes in appetite, chills, and rarely convulsions, Guillain-Barre syndrome; *gastrointestinal:* gastroenteritis, nausea, vomiting, constipation, and rarely, pancreatitis; *musculoskeletal:* muscle cramps or spasms, or pains, joint pain, joint lockup, joint swelling, pain in back, neck, or extremities, and rarely, carpal tunnel syndrome which may be secondary to fluid retention; *genitourinary:* hematuria, prolonged posttherapy amenorrhea; *hematologic:* an increase in red cell and platelet count. Reversible erythrocytosis, leukocytosis or polycythemia may be provoked. Eosinophilia, leukopenia and thrombocytopenia have also been noted. *Skin:* rashes (maculopapular, vesicular, papular, purpuric, petechial), and rarely, sun sensitivity, Stevens-Johnson syndrome; *other:* increased insulin requirements in diabetic patients, change in libido, elevation in blood pressure, and rarely, cataracts, bleeding gums, fever, pelvic pain, nipple discharge. Malignant liver tumors have been reported in rare instances, after long-term use.

DOSAGE AND ADMINISTRATION

Endometriosis. In moderate to severe disease, or in patients infertile due to endometriosis, a starting dose of 800 mg given in two divided doses is recommended. Amenorrhea and rapid response to painful symptoms is best achieved at this dosage level. Gradual downward titration to a dose sufficient to maintain amenorrhea may be considered depending upon patient response. For mild cases, an initial daily dose of 200 mg to 400 mg given in two divided doses is recommended and may be adjusted depending on patient response. **Therapy should begin during menstruation. Otherwise, appropriate tests should be performed to ensure that the patient is not pregnant while on therapy with DANOCRINE. (See CONTRAINDICATIONS and WARNINGS.) It is essential that therapy continue uninterrupted for 3 to 6 months but may be extended to 9 months if necessary.** After termination of therapy, if symptoms recur, treatment can be reinstituted.

Fibrocystic Breast Disease. The total daily dosage of DANOCRINE for fibrocystic breast disease ranges from 100 mg to 400 mg given in two divided doses depending upon patient response. **Therapy should begin during menstruation. Otherwise, appropriate tests should be performed to ensure that the patient is not pregnant while on therapy with DANOCRINE.** A nonhormonal method of contraception is recommended when DANOCRINE is administered at this dose, since ovulation may not be suppressed.

In most instances, breast pain and tenderness are significantly relieved by the first month and eliminated in 2 to 3 months. Usually elimination of nodularity requires 4 to 6 months of uninterrupted therapy. Regular menstrual patterns, irregular menstrual patterns, and amenorrhea each occur in approximately one-third of patients treated with 100 mg of DANOCRINE. Irregular menstrual patterns and amenorrhea are observed more frequently with higher doses. Clinical studies have demonstrated that 50% of patients may show evidence of recurrence of symptoms within one year. In this event, treatment may be reinstated.

Continued on next page

This product information was prepared in September 1998. On these and other products of Sanofi Pharmaceuticals, Inc., detailed information may be obtained on a current basis by direct inquiry to Product Information Services, 90 Park Avenue, New York, NY 10016 (toll free 1-800-446-6267).

Danocrine—Cont.

Hereditary Angioedema. The dosage requirements for continuous treatment of hereditary angioedema with DANOCRINE should be individualized on the basis of the clinical response of the patient. It is recommended that the patient be started on 200 mg, two or three times a day. After a favorable initial response is obtained in terms of prevention of episodes of edematous attacks, the proper continuing dosage should be determined by decreasing the dosage by 50% or less at intervals of one to three months or longer if frequency of attacks prior to treatment dictates. If an attack occurs, the daily dosage may be increased by up to 200 mg. During the dose adjusting phase, close monitoring of the patient's response is indicated, particularly if the patient has a history of airway involvement.

HOW SUPPLIED

Capsules of 200 mg (orange), bottles of 60 (NDC 0024-0305-60).
Capsules of 200 mg (orange), bottles of 100 (NDC 0024-0305-06).
Capsules of 100 mg (yellow), bottles of 100 (NDC 0024-0304-06).
Capsules of 50 mg (orange and white), bottles of 100 (NDC 0024-0303-06).
Store at controlled room temperature, 15° C to 30° C (59° F to 86° F).
Caution: Federal law prohibits dispensing without prescription.

DSW-5 E (O)

Shown in Product Identification Guide, page 335

DEMEROL® Ⓒ℞
MEPERIDINE HYDROCHLORIDE, USP
WARNING: May be habit forming

DESCRIPTION

Meperidine hydrochloride is ethyl 1-methyl-4-phenylisonipecotate hydrochloride, a white crystalline substance with a melting point of 186° C to 189° C. It is readily soluble in water and has a neutral reaction and a slightly bitter taste. The solution is not decomposed by a short period of boiling.
The syrup is a pleasant-tasting, nonalcoholic, banana-flavored solution containing 50 mg of DEMEROL, brand of meperidine hydrochloride, per 5 mL teaspoon (25 drops contain 13 mg of DEMEROL). The tablets contain 50 mg or 100 mg of the analgesic.
Inactive Ingredients—TABLETS: Calcium Sulfate, Dibasic Calcium Phosphate, Starch, Stearic Acid, Talc. SYRUP: Benzoic Acid, Flavor, Liquid Glucose, Purified Water, Saccharin Sodium.

CLINICAL PHARMACOLOGY

Meperidine hydrochloride is a narcotic analgesic with multiple actions qualitatively similar to those of morphine; the most prominent of these involve the central nervous system and organs composed of smooth muscle. The principal actions of therapeutic value are analgesia and sedation.
There is some evidence which suggests that meperidine may produce less smooth muscle spasm, constipation, and depression of the cough reflex than equianalgesic doses of morphine. Meperidine, in 60 mg to 80 mg parenteral doses, is approximately equivalent in analgesic effect to 10 mg of morphine. The onset of action is slightly more rapid than with morphine, and the duration of action is slightly shorter. Meperidine is significantly less effective by the oral than by the parenteral route, but the exact ratio of oral to parenteral effectiveness is unknown.

INDICATIONS AND USAGE

For the relief of moderate to severe pain

CONTRAINDICATIONS

Hypersensitivity to meperidine.
Meperidine is contraindicated in patients who are receiving monoamine oxidase (MAO) inhibitors or those who have recently received such agents. Therapeutic doses of meperdine have occasionally precipitated unpredictable, severe, and occasionally fatal reactions in patients who have received such agents within 14 days. The mechanism of these reactions is unclear, but may be related to a preexisting hyperphenylalaninemia. Some have been characterized by coma, severe respiratory depression, cyanosis, and hypotension, and have resembled the syndrome of acute narcotic overdose. In other reactions the predominant manifestations have been hyperexcitability, convulsions, tachycardia, hyperpyrexia, and hypertension. Although it is not known that other narcotics are free of the risk of such reactions, virtually all of the reported reactions have occurred with meperidine. If a narcotic is needed in such patients, a sensitivity test should be performed in which repeated, small, incremental doses of morphine are administered over the course of several hours while the patient's condition and vital signs are under careful observation. (Intravenous hydrocortisone or prednisolone have been used to treat severe reactions, with the addition of intravenous chlorpromazine in those cases exhibiting hypertension and hyperpyrexia. The usefulness and safety of narcotic antagonists in the treatment of these reactions is unknown.)

WARNINGS

Drug Dependence. Meperidine can produce drug dependence of the morphine type and therefore has the potential for being abused. Psychic dependence, physical dependence, and tolerance may develop upon repeated administration of meperidine, and it should be prescribed and administered with the same degree of caution appropriate to the use of morphine. Like other narcotics, meperidine is subject to the provisions of the Federal narcotic laws.
Interaction with Other Central Nervous System Depressants. MEPERIDINE SHOULD BE USED WITH GREAT CAUTION AND IN REDUCED DOSAGE IN PATIENTS WHO ARE CONCURRENTLY RECEIVING OTHER NARCOTIC ANALGESICS, GENERAL ANESTHETICS, PHENOTHIAZINES, OTHER TRANQUILIZERS (SEE DOSAGE AND ADMINISTRATION), SEDATIVE-HYPNOTICS (INCLUDING BARBITUATES), TRICYCLIC ANTIDEPRESSANTS AND OTHER CNS DEPRESSANTS (INCLUDING ALCOHOL). RESPIRATORY DEPRESSION, HYPOTENSION, AND PROFOUND SEDATION OR COMA MAY RESULT.
Head Injury and Increased Intracranial Pressure. The respiratory depressant effects of meperidine and its capacity to elevate cerebrospinal fluid pressure may be markedly exaggerated in the presence of head injury, other intracranial lesions, or a preexisting increase in intracranial pressure. Furthermore, narcotics produce adverse reactions which may obscure the clinical course of patients with head injuries. In such patients, meperidine must be used with extreme caution and only if its use is deemed essential.
Asthma and Other Respiratory Conditions. Meperidine should be used with extreme caution in patients having an acute asthmatic attack, patients with chronic obstructive pulmonary disease or cor pulmonale, patients having a substantially decreased respiratory reserve, and patients with preexisting respiratory depression, hypoxia, or hypercapnia. In such patients, even usual therapeutic doses of narcotics may decrease respiratory drive while simultaneously increasing airway resistance to the point of apnea.
Hypotensive Effect. The administration of meperidine may result in severe hypotension in the postoperative patient or any individual whose ability to maintain blood pressure has been compromised by a depleted blood volume or the administration of drugs such as the phenothiazines or certain anesthetics.
Usage in Ambulatory Patients. Meperidine may impair the mental and/or physical abilities required for the performance of potentially hazardous tasks such as driving a car or operating machinery. The patient should be cautioned accordingly.
Meperidine, like other narcotics, may produce orthostatic hypotension in ambulatory patients.
Usage in Pregnancy and Lactation. Meperidine should not be used in pregnant women prior to the labor period, unless in the judgment of the physician the potential benefits outweigh the possible hazards, because safe use in pregnancy prior to labor has not been established relative to possible adverse effects on fetal development.
Meperidine crosses the placental barrier and can produce depression of respiration and psychophysiologic functions in the newborn. Resuscitation may be required (see section on OVERDOSAGE).
Meperidine appears in the milk of nursing mothers receiving the drug.

PRECAUTIONS

Supraventricular Tachycardias. Meperidine should be used with caution in patients with atrial flutter and other supraventricular tachycardias because of a possible vagolytic action which may produce a significant increase in the ventricular response rate.
Convulsions. Meperidine may aggravate preexisting convulsions in patients with convulsive disorders. If dosage is escalated substantially above recommended levels because of tolerance development, convulsions may occur in indivduals without a history of convulsive disorders.
Acute Abdominal Conditions. The administration of meperidine or other narcotics may obscure the diagnosis or clinical course in patients with acute abdominal conditions.
Special Risk Patients. Meperidine should be given with caution and the initial dose should be reduced in certain patients such as the elderly or debilitated, and those with severe impairment of hepatic or renal function, hypothyroidism, Addison's disease, and prostatic hypertrophy or urethral stricture.
Pregnancy. For usage during pregnancy see WARNINGS.
Nursing Mothers. See WARNINGS

ADVERSE REACTIONS

The major hazards of meperidine, as with other narcotic analgesics, are respiratory depression and, to a lesser degree, circulatory depression; respiratory arrest, shock, and cardiac arrest have occurred.
The most frequently observed adverse reactions include lightheadedness, dizziness, sedation, nausea, vomiting, and sweating. These effects seem to be more prominent in ambulatory patients and in those who are not experiencing severe pain. In such individuals, lower doses are advisable. Some adverse reactions in ambulatory patients may be alleviated if the patient lies down.
Other adverse reactions include:
Nervous System. Euphoria, dysphoria, weakness, headache, agitation, tremor, uncoordinated muscle movements, severe convulsions, transient hallucinations and disorientation, visual disturbances.
Gastrointestinal. Dry mouth, constipation, biliary tract spasm.
Cardiovascular. Flushing of the face, tachycardia, bradycardia, palpitation, hypotension (see WARNINGS), syncope, phlebitis following intravenous injection.
Genitourinary. Urinary retention.
Allergic. Pruritus, urticaria, other skin rashes, wheal and flare over the vein with intravenous injection.
Other. Pain at injection site; local tissue irritation and induration following subcutaneous injection, particularly when repeated; antidiuretic effect.

DOSAGE AND ADMINISTRATION

For Relief of Pain

Dosage should be adjusted according to the severity of the pain and the response of the patient. Meperidine is less effective orally than on parenteral administration. The dose of DEMEROL should be proportionately reduced (usually by 25 to 50 percent) when administered concomitantly with phenothiazines and many other tranquilizers since they potentiate the action of DEMEROL.
Adults. The usual dosage is 50 mg to 150 mg, or orally, every 3 or 4 hours as necessary.
Pediatric Patients. The usual dosage is 0.5 mg/lb to 0.8 mg/lb, or orally, up to the adult dose, every 3 or 4 hours as necessary.
Each dose of the syrup should be taken in one-half glass of water, since if taken undiluted, it may exert a slight topical anesthetic effect on mucous membranes.

OVERDOSAGE

Symptoms. Serious overdosage with meperidine is characterized by respiratory depression (a decrease in respiratory rate and/or tidal volume, Cheyne-Stokes respiration, cyanosis), extreme somnolence progressing to stupor or coma, skeletal muscle flaccidity, cold and clammy skin, and sometimes bradycardia and hypotension. In severe overdosage, particularly by the intravenous route, apnea, circulatory collapse, cardiac arrest, and death may occur.
Treatment. Primary attention should be given to the reestablishment of adequate respiratory exchange through provision of a patent airway and institution of assisted or controlled ventilation. The narcotic antagonist, naloxone hydrochloride, is a specific antidote against respiratory depression which may result from overdosage or unusual sensitivity to narcotics, including meperidine. Therefore, an appropriate dose of this antagonist should be administered, preferably by the intravenous route, simultaneously with efforts at respiratory resuscitation.
An antagonist should not be administered in the absence of clinically significant respiratory or cardiovascular depression.
Oxygen, intravenous fluids, vasopressors, and other supportive measures should be employed as indicated.
In cases of overdosage with DEMEROL tablets, the stomach should be evacuated by emesis or gastric lavage.
NOTE: In an individual physically dependent on narcotics, the administration of the usual dose of a narcotic antagonist will precipitate an acute withdrawal syndrome. The severity of this syndrome will depend on the degree of physical dependence and the dose of antagonist administered. The use of narcotic antagonists in such individuals should be avoided if possible. If a narcotic antagonist must be used to treat serious respiratory depression in the physically dependent patient, the antagonist should be administered with extreme care and only one-fifth to one-tenth the usual initial dose administered.

HOW SUPPLIED

For Oral Use

Tablets are white, round and convex: the 50 mg tablet is scored.

Tablets of 50 mg.
bottles of 100 (NDC 0024-0335-04),
bottles of 500 (NDC 0024-0335-06),
Hospital Blister Pak of 25 (NDC 0024-0335-02).
100 mg: bottles of 100 (NDC 0024-0337-04),
bottles of 500 (NDC 0024-0337-06),

Syrup

Nonalcoholic, banana-flavored 50 mg per 5 mL teaspoon, bottles of 16 fl oz (NDC 0024-0332-06).
Store at room temperature up to 25° C (77° F), excursions permitted to 15°–30°C (59°–86°F) [See USP controlled Room Temperature].

CAUTION: Federal law prohibits dispensing without prescription.

DSW-3 G(0)

Shown in Product Identification Guide, page 335

DYNABAC®
(dirithromycin tablets)

℞

DESCRIPTION

Dynabac® (dirithromycin tablets) contains the semi-synthetic macrolide antibiotic dirithromycin for oral administration. It is a pro-drug which is converted non-enzymatically during intestinal absorption into the microbiologically active moiety erythromycylamine.

Chemically, dirithromycin is designated (9S)-9-Deox-11-deoxy-9,11-[imino[(1R)-2-(2-methoxyethoxy)-ethylidene]oxy]erythromycin and has the molecular formula $C_{42}H_{78}N_2O_{14}$. Its molecular weight is 835.09. The structural formula is:

Chemically, erythromycylamine is designated 9-(S)-9-amino-9-deoxo-erythromycin and has a molecular formula of $C_{37}H_{70}N_2O_{12}$. Its molecular weight is 743.97. The structural formula is:

CLINICAL PHARMACOLOGY

Pharmacokinetics

Absorption—Dirithromycin is rapidly absorbed and converted by nonenzymatic hydrolysis to the microbiologically active compound erythromycylamine. The absolute bioavailability of the oral formulation is approximately 10%. The pharmacokinetic parameters of erythromycylamine in plasma after single- and multiple-dose oral administration of two 250-mg of Dynabac tablets once daily for 10 days in 10 fasting healthy subjects (19 to 50 years of age) were as follows:

[See first table above]

Distribution—The protein binding of erythromycylamine ranges from 15% to 30%. Erythromycylamine is widely distributed throughout the body with a mean apparent volume of distribution (V_{Dss}) of 800 L (504 to 1,041 L).

Rapid distribution of erythromycylamine into tissues and high concentrations within cells result in significantly higher concentrations in tissues than in plasma or serum. There are no data available on cerebrospinal fluid penetration.

[See table 1 above]

Metabolism and Excretion—Erythromycylamine is primarily eliminated in the bile and undergoes little or no hepatic metabolism. Thus, the primary route of elimination is fecal/hepatic with 81% to 97% of the dose eliminated in this manner. Approximately 2% of the administered dose is eliminated through the kidney, mainly within the first 36 hours following drug administration.

The mean plasma half-life of erythromycylamine was estimated to be about 8 h (2 to 36 h), while a mean urinary terminal elimination half-life of about 44 h (16 to 65 h) and a mean apparent total body clearance of approximately 23 L/h (20 to 32 L/h) were observed in patients with normal renal function.

Food Effect on Absorption—**Dynabac tablets should be administered with food or within an hour of having eaten.**

Pharmacokinetic Parameter (n=10 subjects)	Mean (1 S.D.)			
	Day 1		Day 10	
C_{max} (µg/mL)	0.3	(0.2)	0.4	(0.2)
T_{max} (h)	3.9	(3.9)	4.1	(1.3)
AUC_{0-24h} (ug•h/mL)	0.9	(0.7)	1.8	(1.1)

Table 1
Steady-State Tissue Concentrations of Erythromycylamine Following
Two 250-mg Tablets (500 mg) of Dynabac Given Orally Once Daily

Tissue	Time After Last Dose (h)	Mean Tissue Concentration (µg/g or µg/10⁷ cells)	Corresponding Mean Plasma or Serum Concentration (µg/mL)	Tissue Plasma (Serum) Ratio
Tonsil	14	3.47	0.17	20.4
Healthy lung	12	3.79	0.13	29.2
Pathologic/infected lung	12	3.85	0.13	29.6
Infected bronchial secretions	48	2.15	0.31	6.9
Infected bronchial mucosa	12	1.70	0.13	13.1
	48	2.59	0.31	8.4
	72	1.74	0.33	5.3
Alveolar Macrophages	5	0.37	0.35	1.1

High tissue concentrations should not be interpreted to be quantitatively related to clinical efficacy. Erythromycytamine is concentrated in all lysosomes, which have a low organelle pH at which drug activity is reduced.

The effect of food on the bioavailability of dirithromycin was evaluated following oral administration of two 250-mg Dynabac tablets 1 or 4 hours before food and immediately after a standard breakfast. Results obtained indicated a slight increase in the absorption of erythromycylamine when dirithromycin tablets were administered after food, while a significant decrease in C_{max} (33%) and AUC (31%) occurred when administer 1 hour before food. The effects of high and low fat meals on the bioavailability of dirithromycin were also investigated. The results showed that the amount of dietary fat had little or no effect on the bioavailability of dirithromycin.

Special Populations:

Hepatic Insufficiency—In patients with mild (Child's Grade A) hepatic impairment, mean peak serum concentration, AUC, and volume of distribution increased somewhat with multiple-dose administration; however, based on the magnitude of these changes, no dosage adjustment should be necessary in patients with mildly impaired hepatic function. The pharmacokinetics of dirithromycin in patients with moderate or severe impairment in hepatic function (Child's Grade B or greater) have not been studied.

Renal Insufficiency—The mean peak plasma concentration (C_{max}) and AUC tended to increase as creatinine clearance decreased; however, based on data available to date, no dosage adjustment should be necessary in patients with impaired renal function, including dialysis patients.

Geriatric Patients—In a multiple-dose study in which 19 healthy elderly subjects (65 to 83 years of age) were given two 250-mg Dynabac tablets every day for 10 days, C_{max} and AUC tended to increase with age; however, neither C_{max} nor AUC was statistically or clinically significantly altered with age. Therefore, based on these pharmacokinetic results, no dosage adjustment should be necessary in the elderly patients.

Microbiology:

Erythromycylamine, the microbiologically active product of dirithromycin hydrolysis, exerts its activity by binding to the 50S ribosomal subunits of susceptible mircoorganisms resulting in inhibition of protein synthesis.

Dirithromycin/erythromycylamine has been shown to be active against most strains of the following microorganisms both *in vitro* and in clinical infections as described in the **INDICATIONS AND USAGE** section:

Aerobic gram-positive microorganisms
Staphylococcus aureus (methicillin-susceptible strains only)
Streptococcus pneumoniae
Streptococcus pyogenes

Aerobic gram-negative microorganisms
Haemophilus influenzae
Legionella pneumophila
Moraxella catarrhalis

Other microorganisms
Mycoplasma pneumoniae

The following *in vitro* data are available, **but their clinical significance is unknown.**

Dirithromycin exhibits *in vitro* minimum inhibitory concentrations (MIC's) of 0.5 µg/mL or less against most (≥90%) strains of streptococci and MIC's of 2 µg/mL or less against most (≥90%) strains of the other microorganisms in the following list; however, the safety and effectiveness of dirithromycin in treating clinical infections due to these microorganisms have not been established in adequate and well-controlled trials.

Aerobic gram-positive microorganisms
Listeria monocytogenes
Streptococci, groups C, F, and G
Streptococcus agalactiae
Viridans group streptococci

Aerobic gram-negative microorganisms
Bordatella pertussis

Anaerobic microorganisms
Propionibacterium acnes

NOTE: Microorganisms that are resistant to other macrolides are cross-resistant to dirithromycin/erythromycylamine. Enterococci and most strains of methicillin-resistant staphylococci are resistant to macrolides.

Susceptibility Tests:

Dilution Techniques:

Quantitative methods are used to determine antimicrobial minimum inhibitory concentrations (MIC's). These MIC's provide estimates of the susceptibility of bacteria to antimicrobial compounds. The MIC's should be determined using a standardized procedure. Standardized procedures are based on a dilution method[1] (broth or agar) or equivalent with standardized inoculum concentrations and standardized concentrations of dirithromycin powder. The MIC values should be interpreted according to the following criteria:

For testing aerobic microorganisms other than *Haemophilus influenzae* and streptococci:

MIC (µ/mL)	Interpretation
≤2	Susceptible (S)
4	Intermediate (I)
≥8	Resistant (R)

For testing *Haemophilus influenzae*[a]:

MIC (µg/mL)	Interpretation
≤8	Susceptible (S)
16	Intermediate (I)
≥32	Resistant (R)

[a]These interpretive standards are applicable only to broth microdilution susceptibility tests with *Haemophilus influenzae* using *Haemophilus* Test Medium[1] and incubated aerobically.

For testing streptococci including *Streptococcus pneumonia*[b]:

MIC (µg/mL)	Interpretation
≤0.5	Susceptible (S)
1	Intermediate (I)
≥2	Resistant (R)

[b]These interpretive standards are applicable only to broth microdilution susceptibility tests using cation-adjusted Mueller-Hinton broth with 2–5% lysed horse blood.

Continued on next page

This product information was prepared in September 1998. On these and other products of Sanofi Pharmaceuticals, Inc., detailed information may be obtained on a current basis by direct inquiry to Product Information Services, 90 Park Avenue, New York, NY 10016 (toll free 1-800-446-6267).

Dynabac—Cont.

Microorganism	MIC Range (µg/mL)
Haemophilus influenzae ATOCC 49247[c]	8.0–32
Staphylococcus aureus ATCC 29213	1.0–4.0
*Streptococcus pneumoniae*ATCC 49619[d]	0.06–0.25

[c]This quality control range is applicable only to *H. influenzae* ATCC 49247 tested by a broth microdilution procedure using *Haemophilus* Test Medium (HTM)[1] and aerobically incubated.
[d]This quality control range is applicable only to *S. pneumoniae* ATCC 49619 tested by a broth microdilution procedure using cation-adjusted Mueller-Hinton broth with 2–5% lysed horse blood.

Microorganism	Zone Diameter (mm)
Staphylococcus aureus ATCC 25923	18–26
*Streptococcus pneumoniae*ATCC 49619[f]	18–25

[f]This quality control range is applicable only to *S. pneumoniae* ATCC 49619 tested by a disk diffusion procedure using Mueller-Hinton agar supplemented with 5% sheep blood and incubated in 5% CO_2.

A report of "Susceptible" indicates that the pathogen is likely to be inhibited if the antimicrobial compound in blood reaches the concentration usually achievable. A report of "Intermediate" indicates that the result should be considered equivocal, and, if the microorganism is not fully susceptible to alternative, clinically feasible drugs, the test should be repeated. This category implies possible clinical applicability in body sites where the drug is physiologically concentrated or in situations where high dosage of drug can be used. This category also provides a buffer zone which prevents small uncontrolled technical factors from causing major discrepancies in interpretation. A report of "Resistant" indicates that the pathogen is not likely to be inhibited if the antimicrobial compound in the blood reaches the concentration usually achievable; other therapy should be selected.

Standardized susceptibility test procedures require the use of laboratory control microorganisms to control the technical aspects of the laboratory procedures. Standardized dirithromycin powder should provide the following MIC values:
[See first table above]

Diffusion Techniques:
Quantitative methods that require measurement of zone diameters also provide reproducible estimates of the susceptibility of bacteria to antimicrobial compounds. One such standardized procedure[2] requires the use of standardized inoculum concentrations. This procedure uses paper disks impregnated with 15-µg dirithromycin to test the susceptibility of microorganisms to dirithromycin.
Reports from the laboratory providing results of the standard single-disk susceptibility test with a 15-µg dirithromycin disk should be interpreted according to the following criteria:
For testing aerobic microorganisms other than *Haemophilus influenzae* and streptococci:

Zone Diameter (mm)	Interpretation
≥19	Susceptible (S)
16–18	Intermediate (I)
≤15	Resistant (R)

For testing streptococci including *Streptococcus pneumoniae*[e]:

Zone Diameter (mm)	Interpretation
≥18	Susceptible (S)
14–17	Intermediate (I)
≤13	Resistant (R)

[d]These zone diameter standards for streptococci are applicable only to tests performed using Mueller-Hinton agar supplemented with 5% sheep blood incubated in 5% CO_2.

Due to the lack of standardized methodology and interpretive criteria, it is impossible at present to determine if strains of *Haemophilus* are susceptible or are resistant to dirithromycin/erythromycylamine using the disk diffusion assay.
Interpretation should be as stated above for results using dilution techniques. Interpretation involves correlation of the diameter obtained in the disk test with MIC for dirithromycin.
As with standardized dilution techniques, diffusion methods require the use of laboratory control microorganisms that are used to control the technical aspects of the laboratory procedures. For the diffusion technique, the 15-µg dirithromycin disk should provide the following zone diameters in these laboratory quality control strains:
[See second table above]

INDICATIONS AND USAGE

Dynabac (dirithromycin tablets) is indicated for the treatment of individuals age 12 years and older with mild-to-moderate infections caused by susceptible strains of the designated microorganisms in the specific conditions listed below. **Dirithromycin should not be used in patients with known, suspected, or potential bacteremias as serum levels are inadequate to provide antibacterial coverage of the blood stream.**

Acute Bacterial Exacerbation of Chronic Bronchitis due to *Haemophilus influenzae, Moraxella catarrhalis,* or *Streptococcus pneumoniae.*

Secondary Bacterial Infection of Acute Bronchitis due to *Moraxella catarrhalis* or *Streptococcus pneumoniae.*

Community-Acquired Pneumonia due to *Legionella pneumophila, Mycoplasma pneumoniae,* or *Streptococcus pneumoniae.*

Pharyngitis/Tonsilitis due to *Streptococcus pyogenes.*

NOTE: The usual drug of choice in the treatment and prevention of streptococcal infections and the prophylaxis of rheumatic fever is penicillin. Dynabac generally is effective in the eradication of *S. pyogenes* from the nasopharynx; however, data establishing the efficacy of Dynabac in the subsequent prevention of rheumatic fever are not available at present.

Uncomplicated Skin and Skin Structure Infections due to *Staphylococcus aureus* (methicillin-susceptible strains) or *Streptococcus pyogenes.* (Abscesses usually require surgical drainage.)

CONTRAINDICATIONS

Dynabac is contraindicated in patients with known hypersensitivity to dirithromycin, erythromycin, or any other macrolide antibiotic.

WARNINGS

In a prospective study involving 6 healthy male volunteers, dirithromycin did not affect the metabolism of terfenadine. These six volunteers received terfenadine alone (60 mg twice daily) for 8 days, followed by terfenadine in combination with dirithromycin (500 mg once daily) for 10 days. (Both drugs were thus dosed to steady state.) The pharmacokinetics of terfenadine and its acid metabolite and the electrocardiographic QT_c interval were measured during both periods: with terfenadine alone, and with terfenadine plus dirithromycin. In five men, terfenadine levels were undetectable (<5 ng/mL) throughout the study; in one man, the C_{max} of terfenadine was 8.1 ng/mL with terfenadine alone and 7.2 ng/mL with terfenadine plus dirithromycin. The mean C_{max}, T_{max} and AUC of the acid metabolite of terfenadine were not significantly changed. The mean QT_c interval (msec) was 369 with terfenadine alone and 367 with terfenadine plus dirithromycin.

Serious cardiac dysrhythmias, some resulting in death, have occurred in patients receiving terfenadine concomitantly with other macrolide antibiotics. In addition, most macrolides are contraindicated in patients receiving terfenadine therapy who have pre-existing cardiac abnormalities (arrhythmia, bradycardia, QT_c interval prolongation, ischemic heart disease, congestive heart failure, etc.) or electrolyte disturbances. Until further use data are available, it is prudent to monitor the terfenadine levels when dirithromycin and terfenadine are coadministered. (See terfenadine package insert.)

Dirithromycin should not be used in patients with known, suspected, or potential bacteremias as serum levels are inadequate to provide antibacterial coverage of the blood stream.

Pseudomembranous colitis has been reported with nearly all antibacterial agents, including dirithromycin, and may range in severity from mild to life-threatening. Therefore, it is important to consider this diagnosis in patients who present with diarrhea subsequent to the administration of antibacterial agents.

Treatment with antibacterial agents alters the normal flora of the colon and may permit overgrowth of clostridia. Studies indicate that a toxin produced by *Clostridium difficile* is a primary cause of "antibiotic-associated colitis."

After the diagnosis of pseudomembranous colitis has been established, therapeutic measures should be initiated. Mild cases of pseudomembranous colitis usually respond to discontinuation of the drug alone. In moderate-to-severe cases, consideration should be given to management with fluids and electrolytes, protein supplementation, and treatment with an antibacterial drug clinically effective against *C. difficile* colitis.

PRECAUTIONS

Hepatic Insufficiency—Because dirithromycin/erythromycylamine is principally eliminated via the liver and because no data exist regarding the safety of administering dirithromycin to patients with Child's Grade B or greater hepatic impairment, Dynabac should be administered to such patients only when absolutely necessary. No dosage adjustment should be necessary in patients with mildly impaired hepatic function. (See **CLINICAL PHARMACOLOGY** section.)

Information to Patients—Dynabac tablets should be taken with food or within one hour of having eaten. They should not be cut, chewed, or crushed.

Drug Interactions:

Terfenadine—See **WARNINGS.**

Theophylline—Following co-administration of two 250-mg dirithromycin tablets administered once daily with 200-mg theophylline tablets administered twice daily for 10 days to 14 healthy subjects, the steady-state plasma concentration of theophylline was not significantly altered. In general, most patients treated with dirithromycin who are receiving concomitant theophylline therapy *may* not require empiric adjustment of theophylline dosage or monitoring of theophylline plasma concentrations. However, theophylline plasma concentrations should be monitored, with dosage adjustment as appropriate, in patients whose pulmonary disease requires maintaining a given theophylline plasma concentration for optimal pulmonary function or in patients with theophylline concentrations at the higher end of the therapeutic range.

Antacids or H_2 receptor antagonists—When dirithromycin is administered immediately following antacids or H_2-receptor antagonists, the absorption of dirithromycin is slightly enhanced.

The following drug interactions have been reported with erythromycin products. It is presently not known whether these same drug interactions occur with dirithromycin. **Until further data are available regarding the potential interaction of dirithromycin with these compounds, caution should be used during coadministration.**

Triazolam—Erythromycin has been reported to decrease the clearance of triazolam and, thus, may increase the pharmacologic effect of triazolam.

Digoxin—Concomitant administration of erythromycin and digoxin has been reported to result in elevated digoxin serum levels.

Anticoagulants—There have been reports of increased anticoagulant effects when erythromycin and oral anticoagulants were used concomitantly. Increased anticoagulation effects due to a drug interactions with erythromycin may be more pronounced in the elderly.

Ergotamine—Concurrent use of erythromycin and ergotamine or dihydroergotamine has been associated in some patients with acute ergot toxicity characterized by severe peripheral vasospasm and dysesthesia.

Other drugs—Drug interactions have been reported with concomitant administration of erythromycin and other medications, including cyclosporine, hexobarbital, carbamazepine, alfentanil, disopyramide, phenytoin, bromocriptine, valproate, astemizole, and lovastatin.

Carcinogenesis, Mutagenesis, Impairment of Fertility—Lifetime studies in animals to evaluate carcinogenic potential have not been performed with dirithromycin.

No mutagenic potential was demonstrated when dirithromycin was used in standard tests of genotoxicity, which included the following bacterial mutation tests *in vitro* and *in vivo* mammalian systems:

Bacterial Reverse-Mutation Test (Ames test)
DNA repair (UDS) in rat hepatocytes
Chinese hamster lung fibroblasts (V79) test
Micronucleus test in mice
Sister-chromatid exchange—human lymphocytes
Sister-chromatid exchange—Chinese hamsters
Mouse Lymphoma Assay

Table 2
Adverse Clinical Reactions
(Incidence equal to or greater than 1%)
Clinical Trials - North America

ADVERSE REACTION	DIRITHROMYCIN		ERYTHROMYCIN	
	7–14 Day (n=1894)	5-Day (n=932)	7–14 Day (n=1894)	7-Day (n=932)
Abdominal pain	9.7%	7.1%	7.5%	6.2%
Headache	8.6%	7.7%	8.2%	7.6%
Nausea	8.3%	5.9%	7.5%	8.7%
Diarrhea	7.7%	6.7%	7.3%	9.4%
Vomiting	3.0%	1.1%	2.8%	1.3%
Dyspepsia	2.6%	4.1%	2.1%	2.7%
Dizziness/vertigo	2.3%	2.1%	2.3%	2.0%
Pain (non-specific)	2.2%	2.9%	1.6%	3.0%
Asthenia	2.0%	1.4%	1.9%	1.4%
Gastrointestinal disorder	1.6%	0	1.4%	0.2%
Increased Cough	1.5%	0.2%	2.6%	0.5%
Flatulence	1.5%	1.0%	1.5%	1.6%
Rash	1.4%	1.6%	2.6%	1.4%
Dyspnea	1.2%	1.8%	1.2%	1.6%
Pruritus/Urticaria	1.2%	0.5%	1.0%	0.6%
Insomnia	1.0%	0.9%	0.7%	1.1%
Vaginitis	0.4%	1.2%	0.6%	0.6%

Table 3
Adverse Laboratory Reactions
(Incidence equal to or greater than 1%)
Clinical Trials - North America

ADVERSE REACTIONS	DIRITHROMYCIN		ERYTHROMYCIN	
	7–14 Day (n=1894)	5-Day (n=932)	7–14 Day (n=1894)	7-Day (n=932)
Platelet count *increased*	3.8%	0.7%	4.8%	1.4%
Potassium *increased*	2.6%	0	0.0%	0
Bicarbonate *decreased*	1.4%	0	2.0%	0
CPK *increased*	1.2%	0.8%	0.9%	0.7%
Eosinophils *increased*	1.2%	0.9%	0.6%	0.9%
Seg Neutrophils *increased*	1.2%	1.7%	1.3%	2.3%
Leucocytes *increased*	0.8%	1.5%	0.9%	1.2%

Table 4
Recommended Dosage Schedule for Dynabac
(12 years of age and older)

Infection (Mild to Moderate Severity)	Dose	Frequency	Duration (days)
Acute Bacterial Exacerbations of Chronic Bronchitis due to *Haemophilus influenzae, Moraxella catarrhalis,* or *Streptococcus pneumonia*	500 mg	q day	5-7
Secondary Bacterial Infection of Acute Bronchitis due to *M. Catarrhalis* or *S. pneumoniae*	500 mg	q day	7
Community-Acquired Pneumonia due to *Legionella pneumophila, Mycoplasma pneumoniae,* or *S. pneumoniae*	500 mg	q day	14
Pharyngitis/Tonsillitis due to *Streptococcus pyogenes*	500 mg	q day	10
Uncomplicated Skin and Skin Structure Infections due to *Staphylococcus aureus* (methicillin-susceptible) or *S pyogenes*	500 mg	q day	5–7

In rats, fertility and reproductive performance were not affected when dirithromycin was administered at doses up to 21 times the maximum recommended human dose on a mg/m² basis.

Pregnancy: Teratogenic Effects. Pregnancy Category C—Teratology studies conducted in rats at doses up to 21 times the maximum recommended human dose on a mg/m² basis and in rabbits at doses up to 4 times the maximum recommended human dose on a mg/m² basis have revealed no evidence of impaired fertility or harm to the fetus due to dirithromycin administration. An additional teratology study in CD-1 mice demonstrated that fetal weight was significantly depressed at the 1000 mg/kg dose (8 times the maximum recommended human dose on a mg/m² basis), and there was an increased occurrence of incomplete ossification among these fetuses—a manifestation of retarded development. This decrease in ossification was also seen in rats given 1000 mg/kg/day for 2 weeks prior to mating, throughout the mating period, and throughout gestation.

There are no adequate and well-controlled studies in pregnant women. Dirithromycin should be used during pregnancy only if the potential benefit justifies the potential risk to the fetus.

Labor and Delivery—Dirithromycin has not been studied for use during labor and delivery. Treatment with dirithromycin should be given during labor and delivery only if clearly needed.

Nursing Mothers—It is not known whether either dirithromycin or erythromycylamine is excreted in human milk. It is known that dirithromycin is excreted in the milk of lactating rodents and that other drugs of this class are excreted in human milk. Because many drugs are excreted in human milk, caution should be exercised when dirithromycin is administered to a nursing woman.

Pediatric Use—Safety and effectiveness in pediatric patients below the age of 12 years have not been established.

Geriatric Use—In a clinical pharmacology study, 19 healthy geriatric volunteers (65 to 83 years of age) with normal renal and hepatic function had no statistically significant differences in AUC or C_{max} when compared with 10 healthy volunteers (19 to 50 years of age). In clinical trials in geriatric patients who received the usual recommended adult dose (500 mg q.d. P.O.), clinical efficacy and safety were comparable with results in non-geriatric adult patients.

ADVERSE REACTIONS

Clinical Trials: In clinical trials, 3299 patients were treated with dirithromycin 500 mg q.d. P.O. for approximately 7 to 14 days. There were no deaths or permanent disabilities thought related directly to drug toxicity. Eighty-seven (2.6%) patients discontinued medication due to adverse reactions. Thirty-five (40%) of the 87 patients who discontinued therapy did so because of nausea or abdominal pain.

In additional clinical trials conducted in North America, 932 patients were treated with dirithromycin 500 mg q.d. for 5 days. There were no deaths or permanent disabilities thought to be related directly to drug toxicity. Thirty-five (3.8%) patients discontinued medication due to adverse reactions. Fifteen (43%) of the 35 patients who discontinued therapy did so because of nausea or abdominal pain.

The following adverse clinical and laboratory reactions were reported during the dirithromycin clinical trials conducted in North America (n=1894 patients treated for 7–14 days and 932 patients treated for 5 days). (See Tables 2 and 3.)
[See table 2 at left]

Adverse reactions occurring during all clinical trials with dirithromycin with an incidence of less than 1% but greater than 0.1% included the following (listed alphabetically): Abnormal stools, allergic reaction, amblyopia, anorexia, constipation, dehydration, dry mouth, dysmenorrhea, dysphagia, edema, epistaxis, eye disorder (not further defined), fever, flu syndrome, gastritis, gastroenteritis, hemoptysis, hyperventilation, insomnia, malaise, mouth ulceration, myalgia, myasthenia, neck pain, nervousness, palpitation, paresthesia, peripheral edema, somnolence, sweating, syncope, taste perversion, thirst, tinnitus, tremor, urinary frequency, vaginal moniliasis, vaginitis, vasodilatation.
[See table 3 at left]

Adverse laboratory reactions occurring during all clinical trials with dirithromycin with an incidence of less than 1% but greater than 0.1% included the following (listed alphabetically):

Decreased:
Albumin, chloride, hematocrit, hemoglobin, lymphocytes, segmented neutrophils, phosphorus, platelet count, serum alkaline phosphatase, serum uric acid, and total protein.

Increased:
Alkaline phosphatase, ALT, AST, basophils, calcium, creatinine, GGT, leukocyte count, lymphocytes, hematocrit, hemoglobin, monocytes, phosphorous, total bilirubin, and uric acid.

Macrolide-class adverse reactions—Although not observed in patients treated with dirithromycin in clinical trials, the following adverse reactions and altered laboratory test results have been reported in patients treated with macrolide antibiotics:

Bullous fixed eruptions or serious allergic reactions, including anaphylaxis, have been reported. A few cases of transient deafness have been reported with high doses of oral erythromycin. Rarely, cholestatic hepatitis has been reported. In individuals with prolonged QT intervals, erythromycin has been associated, rarely, with the production of ventricular arrhythmias, including ventricular tachycardia and torsade de pointes.

OVERDOSAGE

The toxic symptoms following an overdose of a macrolide antibiotic may include nausea, vomiting, epigastric distress, and diarrhea. Forced diuresis, peritoneal dialysis, hemodialysis, or hemoperfusion have not been established as beneficial for an overdose of dirithromycin. Hemodialysis has been shown to be ineffective in hastening the elimination of erythromycylamine from plasma in patients with chronic renal failure.

DOSAGE AND ADMINISTRATION

Dynabac (dirithromycin tablets) should be administered with food or within 1 hour of having eaten. (See CLINICAL PHARMACOLOGY, *Food Effect on Absorption.***) Dynabac tablets should not be cut, crushed, or chewed.**
[See table 4 at left]

HOW SUPPLIED

Dynabac® (dirithromycin tablets) are available in:
The 250 mg tablets are white, enteric-coated, elliptical-shaped, imprinted with "DYNABAC" and "UC5364."
They are available as follows:
Bottles of 60   NDC 0024-0490-60 (UC5394)
Store at controlled room temperature, 15° to 30°C (59°to 86°F).

ANIMAL PHARMACOLOGY AND TOXICOLOGY

Cardiac and skeletal muscle lesions occurred in rats in studies up to three months by the intravenous route and in six-month studies in the rat and the dog by the oral route. While no target organ toxicity was identified in three-month oral studies, both cardiac and skeletal muscles were identified as target tissues after one-month intravenous studies in rats. Histologic changes from oral dosing occurred only after more than four months of treatment in rats and after six months in dogs. These findings were associated with high tissue-to-plasma concentration ratios of antimicrobial activity. The extensive drug uptake by tissues was reversible upon termination of treatment. Lesions in cardiac and skel-

Continued on next page

This product information was prepared in September 1998. On these and other products of Sanofi Pharmaceuticals, Inc., detailed information may be obtained on a current basis by direct inquiry to Product Information Services, 90 Park Avenue, New York, NY 10016 (toll free 1-800-446-6267).

Dynabac—Cont.

etal muscle also were reversed upon termination of treatment. Dirithromycin and/or its microbiologically active metabolite appeared to accumulate in tissues with time. Despite the drug uptake in rat tissues at high multiples (approximately 14 times the anticipated clinical dose in mg/m^2), there were no lesions in this species until oral treatment was extended beyond four months.

REFERENCES
1. National Committee for Clinical Laboratory Standards. Methods for Dilution Antimicrobial Susceptibility Tests for Bacteria that Grow Aerobically—Fourth Edition. Approved Standard NCCLS Document M7-A4, Vol. 17, No. 2, NCCLS, Wayne, PA, January, 1997.
2. National Committee for Clinical Laboratory Standards. Performance Standards for Antimicrobial Disk Susceptibility Tests—Sixth Edition. Approved Standard NCCLS Document M3-A6, Vol. 17, No. 1, NCCLS, Wayne, PA, January, 1997.

CAUTION:
Federal (USA) law prohibits dispensing without prescription.
Literature revised December 22, 1997

sanofi
Distributed by Sanofi Pharmaceuticals, Inc.
New York, NY 10016
Manufactured by Eli Lily and Company
Indianapolis, IN 46285, USA
PV 2594 UCP

Shown in Product Identification Guide, page 335

HISTUSSIN® D   Ⅲ℞

DESCRIPTION
Each 5ml teaspoonful of HISTUSSIN® D for oral use contains:
Hydrocodone Bitartrate .... 5 mg
  (Warning: May be habit forming)
Pseudoephedrine
Hydrochloride .... 60 mg

Antitussive-Decongestant Liquid.

Hydrocodone bitartrate is an opiod analgesic and antitussive. It occurs as fine white crystals or as crystalline powder, and is light sensitive. The chemical name is 4,5,epoxy-3-methoxy-17-methylmorphinan-6-one tartrate (1:1) hydrate (2:5). Its structural formula is shown below:

$C_{18}H_{21}NO_3 \cdot C_4H_6 \cdot 2.5H_2O$ MW 494.5

Pseudoephedrine hydrochloride is a nasal decongestant (vasoconstrictor) which occurs as fine white to off-white crystals or powder having a characteristic odor. The chemical name is α [1- (methylamino) ethyl] - benzenemethanol hydrochloride. Its chemical structure is shown below:

$C_{10}H_{15}NO \cdot HCl$ MW 201.7

CLINICAL PHARMACOLOGY
Hydrocodone is a semi-synthetic narcotic antitussive with multiple actions qualitatively similar to those of codeine. Most of these involve the central nervous system and smooth muscle. The precise mechanism of action of hydrocodone is not known; however, hydrocodone is believed to act directly on the cough center. In excessive doses, hydrocodone, like other opiates, will depress respiration. The effects of hydrocodone in therapeutic doses on the cardiovascular system are negligible. Hydrocodone can produce miosis, euphoria, physical and psychic dependence.
Following a 10 mg oral dose of hydrocodone administered to five adult male subjects, the mean peak serum concentration was 23.6 ± 5.2 ng/mL. Maximum serum levels were achieved at 1.3 ± 0.3 hours.[1] Hydrocodone exhibits a complex pattern of metabolism including O-demethylation, N-demethylation, and 6-keto reduction to the corresponding 6-α and 6-β-hydroxy metabolites.[2]

Pseudoephedrine acts as an indirect sympathomimetic agent by stimulating sympathetic (adrenergic) nerve endings to release norepinephrine. Norepinephrine in turn stimulates alpha and beta receptors throughout the body. The action of pseudoephedrine hydrochloride is apparently more specific for the blood vessels of the upper respiratory tract and less specific for the blood vessels of the systemic circulation. The vasoconstriction produced in the respiratory tract results in the shrinking of swollen tissues in the sinuses and nasal passages. Little, if any, rebound congestion has been reported upon withdrawal of orally administered pseudoephedrine.

Pseudoephedrine is rapidly and almost completely absorbed from the gastrointestinal tract. Considerable variation in elimination half-life has been observed (4.3 to 8 hours), which is attributed to individual differences in absorption, as well as excretion. Excretion rates are altered by urine pH, increasing with acidification, and decreasing with alkalization. As a result, mean half-life is approximately 3 hours at a urinary pH of 5, and increases to 16 hours at a urinary pH of 8. Approximately 43% to 96% of an administered dose is excreted unchanged in the urine; the remainder is apparently metabolized in the liver to inactive compounds by N-demethylation, parahydroxylation, and oxidative deamination.[3] The drug is distributed widely throughout body tissues and fluids including fetal tissue, breast milk, and the central nervous system.

INDICATIONS AND USAGE
For the symptomatic relief of cough accompanying upper respiratory tract congestion associated with the common cold, influenza, bronchitis and sinusitis.

CONTRAINDICATIONS
HISTUSSIN D is contraindicated in patients with severe hypertension, severe coronary artery disease, and in patients receiving MAO inhibitors.
Hypersensitivity: HISTUSSIN D is contraindicated in patients with hypersensitivity or a history of an iodiosyncratic reaction to sympathomimetic amines, phenanthrene derivatives, or to any other formula ingredients.

WARNINGS
Hydrocodone should be prescribed and administered with the same degree of caution as all oral medications containing a narcotic-analgesic. Extreme caution should be exercised in the use of hydrocodone in patients with severe respiratory impairment or patients with impaired respiratory drive.
If sympathomimetic amines are used in patients with hypertension, diabetes mellitus, ischemic heart disease, hyperthyroidism, increased intraocular pressure or prostatic hypertrophy, caution should be exercised (see CONTRAINDICATIONS). Sympathomimetic amines may produce central nervous system stimulation with convulsions or cardiovascular collapse with accompanying hypotension. DO NOT EXCEED RECOMMENDED DOSAGE.
Use in elderly: Elderly patients (60 years and older) are more likely to have adverse reactions to sympathomimetic amines. Overdosage in this age group may cause hallucinations, convulsions, CNS depression and death.

PRECAUTIONS
General: Caution should be exercised if used in patients with diabetes, hypertension, cardiovascular disease, sensitivity to ephedrine, or decreased respiratory drive (see CONTRAINDICATIONS).
Information for Patients: Hydrocodone may produce drowsiness. Persons who perform hazardous tasks requiring mental alertness or physical coordination should be cautioned accordingly. Concomitant use of hydrocodone with tranquilizers, alcohol or other depressants may produce additive depressant effects.
Do not exceed the prescribed dosage.
Drug Interactions: Hydrocodone may potentiate the effects of other narcotics, general anesthetics, tranquilizers, sedatives and hypnotics, tricyclic antidepressants, MAO inhibitors, alcohol, and other CNS depressants. Beta adrenergic blockers and MAO inhibitors potentiate the sympathomimetic effects of pseudoephedrine. Sympathomimetic amines may reduce the antihypertensive effects of methyldopa, mecamylamine, and reserpine alkaloids.
Hydrocodone-FDA Pregnancy Category C. Hydrocodone has been shown to be teratogenic in hamsters when given in doses 700 times the human dose. There are no adequate and well-controlled studies in pregnant women. HISTUSSIN D should be used during pregnancy only if the potential benefit justifies the potential risk to the fetus.
Pseudoephedrine-FDA Pregnancy Category B. Pseudoephedrine studies were conducted in rats at doses up to 150 times the human dose. No evidence of teratogenic harm to the fetus was observed. However, pseudoephedrine reduced average weight, length and rate of skeletal ossification in the animal fetus. There are, however, no adequate and well-controlled studies in pregnant women. Because animal re-

production studies are not always predictive of human response, this drug should be used during pregnancy only if clearly needed.
Nursing Mothers: Because of the potential for a series adverse reaction from sympathomimetic amines in nursing infants, pseudoephedrine is contraindicated in nursing mothers.

ADVERSE REACTIONS
The most frequent side effects are gastrointestinal upset, nausea, drowsiness and constipation.
Individuals sensitive to pseudoephedrine may display ephedrine-like reactions such as tachycardia, palpitations, headache, dizziness or nausea. Sympathomimetic drugs have been associated with certain untoward reactions including fear, anxiety, tenseness, restlessness, tremor, weakness, pallor, respiratory difficulty, dysuria, insomnia, hallucinations, convulsions, CNS depression, arrhythmias, and cardiovascular collapse with hypotension. Patient idiosyncrasy to adrenergic agents may be manifested by insomnia, dizziness, weakness, tremor or arrhythmias.

DRUG ABUSE AND DEPENDENCE
Controlled Substance: Hydrocodone in HISTUSSIN D mixture is controlled by the Drug Enforcement Administration. HISTUSSIN D is a Schedule III controlled substance.
Abuse: Hydrocodone is a narcotic drug related to codeine with roughly three times the abuse potential of codeine on a weight basis.
Dependence: Hydrocodone can produce drug dependence of the morphine type. Psychic dependence, physical dependence and tolerance may develop if dosage recommendations are greatly exceeded over a prolonged period of time.
Overdosage: Acute overdosage with HISTUSSIN D may produce variable clinical signs as hydrocodone produces CNS depression and cardiovascular depression while pseudoephedrine produces CNS stimulation and variable cardiovascular effects. Hydrocodone is likely to be responsible for most of the severe reactions from overdosage. Pressor amines should be used with great caution when taking pseudoephedrine. Patients with signs of stimulation should be treated conservatively and depressant medications should be avoided if possible because of potential drug interaction with hydrocodone.

DOSAGE AND ADMINISTRATION
Adults and children over 90 lb.–1 teaspoonful (5 ml); children 50 to 90 lb.–½ teaspoonful; children 25 to 50 lb.–¼ teaspoonful. May be given four times a day as needed. May be taken with meals.

HOW SUPPLIED
HISTUSSIN D liquid is supplied as a deep red syrup with a wild cherry/black raspberry flavor.
Pints NDC 0024-0864-16.
KEEP THIS AND ALL DRUGS OUT OF THE REACH OF CHILDREN. IN CASE OF ACCIDENTAL OVERDOSE, SEEK PROFESSIONAL ASSISTANCE OR CONTACT A POISON CONTROL CENTER IMMEDIATELY.

CAUTION: Federal law prohibits dispensing without prescription.

Store at controlled room temperature.
DISPENSE IN CHILD RESISTANT CONTAINERS.

REFERENCES
1. Barnhart, J.W. & Caldwell, W.J. (1977) Gas chromatographic determination of hydrocodone in serum. *J Chromatogr*, 130:243–249.
2. Cone, E.J. & Darwin, W.D. (1978) Simultaneous determination of hydromorphone, hydrocodone and their 6alpha- and 6beta-hydroxy metabolites in urine using selected ion recording with methane chemical ionization. *Biomed Mass Spectrom*, 5, 291.
3. Kanfer, I., Dowse, R. & Vuma, V. (1993) Pharmacokinetics of oral decongestants. *Pharmacotherapy*, 13, 116S–128S, discussion 143.

HPG12267-01-0697SP
086416-7671
Manufactured for
Sanofi Pharmaceuticals, Inc.
New York, NY 10016
by Forest Pharmaceuticals, Inc.
St. Louis, MO 63045
Copyright © 1997 Sanofi Pharmaceuticals, Inc.
All rights reserved.

HSW-20

HISTUSSIN® HC   Ⅲ℞

Each 5 ml orange/pineapple flavored alcohol-free, sugar-free orange syrup contains:
Hydrocodone Bitartrate .... 2.5 mg
  (Warning: May be habit forming.)
Phenylephrine Hydrochloride .... 5.0 mg
Chlorpheniramine Maleate .... 2.0 mg

HOW SUPPLIED

Bottles of 16 oz.
NDC 0024-0860-16

HYALGAN® ℞
(Sodium Hyaluronate)
LABELING

CAUTION

Federal law restricts this device to sale by or on the order of a physician.

DESCRIPTION

Hyalgan® is a viscous solution consisting of a high molecular weight (500,000–730,000 daltons) fraction of purified natural sodium hyaluronate in buffered physiological sodium chloride, having a pH of 6.8–7.5. The sodium hyaluronate is extracted from rooster combs. Hyaluronic acid is a natural complex sugar of the glycosaminoglycan family and is a long-chain polymer containing repeating disaccharide units of Na-glucuronate-N-acetyglucosamine.

INDICATIONS

Hyalgan® is indicated for the treatment of pain in osteoarthritis (OA) of the knee in patients who have failed to respond adequately to conservative nonpharmacologic therapy, and to simple analgesics, e.g., acetaminophen.

CONTRAINDICATIONS

• Do not administer to patients with known hypersensitivity to hyaluronate preparations.
• Intra-articular injections are contraindicated in cases of infections or skin diseases in the area of the injection site.

WARNINGS

• Do not concomitantly use disinfectants containing quaternary ammonium salts for skin preparation because hyaluronic acid can precipitate in their presence.
• Anaphylactoid and allergic reactions have been reported with this product. See Adverse Events Section for more detail.
• Transient increases in inflammation in the injected knee following Hyalgan® injection in some patients with inflammatory arthritis such as rheumatoid arthritis or gouty arthritis have been reported.

PRECAUTIONS

General

• The effectiveness of a single treatment cycle of less than 5 injections has not been established. Pain relief may not be seen until after the fifth injection.
• The safety and effectiveness of the use of Hyalgan® in joints other than the knee have not been established.
• The safety and effectiveness of the use of Hyalgan® concomitantly with other intra-articular injectables have not been established.
• Use caution when injecting Hyalgan® into patients who are allergic to avian proteins, feathers, and egg products.
• Strict aseptic administration technique must be followed.
• **STERILE CONTENTS.** The vial/syringe is intended for single use. The contents of the vial must be used immediately once the container has been opened. Discard any unused Hyalgan®.
• Do not use Hyalgan® if the package is opened or damaged. Store in the original packaging (protected from light) below 77° F (25° C). DO NOT FREEZE.
• Remove joint effusion, if present, before injecting Hyalgan®.

Information for Patients

• Provide patients with a copy of the Patient Information prior to use.
• Transient pain and/or swelling of the injected joint may occur after intra-articular injection of Hyalgan®.
• As with invasive joint procedure, it is recommended that the patient avoid any strenuous activities or prolonged (i.e., more than 1 hour) weight-bearing activities such as jogging or tennis within 48 hours following the intra-articular injection.
• The safety and effectiveness of repeat treatment cycles of Hyalgan® have not been established.

Use in Specific Populations

• **Pregnancy:** *Teratogenic Effects*- Reproductive toxicity studies, including multigeneration studies, have been performed in rats, and rabbits at doses up to 11 times the anticipated human dose (1.43 mg/kg per treatment cycle) and have revealed no evidence of impaired fertility or harm to the experimental animal fetus due to intra-articular injections of Hyalgan®. Animal reproduction studies are not always predictive of human response. The safety and effectiveness of Hyalgan® have not been established in pregnant women.
• **Nursing Mothers:** It is not known if Hyalgan® is excreted in human milk. The safety and effectiveness of Hyalgan® have not been established in lactating women.
• **Pediatrics:** The safety and effectiveness of Hyalgan® have not been demonstrated in children.

TABLE 3
Demographic Characteristics of all randomized subjects

DEMOGRAPHIC VARIABLE	TREATMENT			
	Hyalgan® N = 164	Placebo N = 168	Naproxen N = 163	TOTAL N = 495
AGE (years):				
Mean	63.5	64.3	63.2	63.7
SD	10.1	10.0	9.2	9.8
Range	41–90	44–85	40–80	40–90
Gender [N (%)]:				
Female	99 (60.3)	91 (54.1)	99 (60.7)	289 (58.4)
Male	65 (39.6)	77 (45.8)	64 (39.3)	206 (41.6)
Race [N (%)]:				
Caucasion	137 (83.6)	135 (80.4)	133 (81.6)	405 (81.8)
Black	23 (14.0)	32 (19.0)	25 (15.3)	80 (16.2)
Other	4 (4.2)	1 (1.0)	5 (3.1)	10 (2.0)
Height (cm):				
Mean	167.8	168.6	167.6	168.0
SD	8.8	10.7	11.9	10.5
Range	145–190	142–193	102–198	102–198
Weight (kg):				
Mean	88.4	88.1	89.7	88.7
SD	18.0	18.2	18.4	18.2
Range	46–139	49–170	45–150	45–170
NSAIDs Use (N, %)	107 (65.2)	117 (69.6)	113 (69.3)	337 (68.1)
Use of Assistive Devices (N, %)	35 (21.3)	34 (20.2)	32 (19.6)	101 (20.4)
Physical Therapy (N, %)	20 (12.2)	17 (10.1)	25 (15.3)	62 (12.5)

Legend: cm = centimeters; kg = kilograms; SD = standard deviation

ADVERSE EVENTS

Hyalgan® was investigated in a pivotal clinical investigation conducted in the United States in which there were three arms (164 subjects treated with Hyalgan®; 168 with placebo; and 163 with naproxen) (refer to Table 1). Common adverse events reported for the Hyalgan®-treated subjects were gastrointestinal complaints, injection site pain, knee swelling/effusion, local skin reactions (rash, ecchymosis), pruritus, and headache. Swelling and effusion, local skin reactions (ecchymosis and rash), and headache occurred at equal frequency in the Hyalgan®- and placebo-treated groups. Hyalgan®-treated subjects had 48/164 (29%) incidents of gastrointestinal complaints that were not statistically different from the placebo-treated group. A statistically significant difference in the occurrence of pain at the injection site was noted in the Hyalgan®-treated subjects: 38/164 (23%) in comparison to 22/168 (13%) in the placebo-treated subjects (p = 0.022). There were 6/164 (4%) premature discontinuations in Hyalgan®-treated subjects due to injection site pain in comparison to 1/168 (<1%) in the placebo-treated subjects. These differences were not statistically significant.
Two (2/164, 1.2%) Hyalgan®-treated subjects and 3/168 (1.8%) placebo-treated subjects were reported to have positive bacterial cultures of effusion aspirated from the treated knee. The two Hyalgan®-treated subjects and two of the placebo-treated subjects did not exhibit evidence of infection clinically or subsequently and were not treated with antibiotics. One of the placebo-treated subjects was hospitalized and received presumptive treatment for septic arthritis.
Hyalgan® has been in clinical use in Europe since 1987. Analysis of the adverse events that have been reported with the use of Hyalgan® in Europe reveals that most of the events are related to local symptoms such as pain, swelling/effusion, and warmth or redness at the injection site. In the two events reported as anaphylactoid reactions, Hyalgan® treatment was discontinued and both had favorable outcomes. Three cases of allergic reactions were reported in which the patients were discontinued from Hyalgan® treatment and the incidents resolved. Seven cases of fever were reported in which three of the cases were reported to be associated with local reactions; pyogenic arthritis was reported to be ruled out in these three cases. All the fever patients were discontinued from Hyalgan® treatment and all incidents resolved. One incident of shock (which was described as a "hypotensive crisis") was reported. The incident resolved and Hyalgan® treatment was continued.

TABLE 1
Incidence[1] of Adverse Events Occurring in More than 5% of All Subjects

Adverse Event	Hyalgan® N = 164	Placebo N = 168
Gastrointestinal Complaints[2]	48 (29%)	59 (36%)
Injection site pain[3]	38 (23%)[4]	22 (13%)
Headache	30 (18%)	29 (17%)
Local skin[5]	23 (14%)	17 (10%)
Local joint pain and swelling[6]	21 (13%)	22 (13%)
Pruritus (local)	12 (7%)	7 (4%)

Notes: [1]Number and % of subjects
[2]Severe in 4 Hyalgan®-treated subjects and 4 placebo-treated subjects
[3]Severe in 5 Hyalgan®-treated subjects and 2 placebo-treated subjects
[4]Statistically significant (p=0.02)
[5]Includes ecchymosis and rash
[6]Severe in 2 Hyalgan®-treated subjects (1.2%) and 1 placebo-treated subject

CLINICAL STUDY

The use of Hyalgan® as a treatment for pain in OA of the knee was investigated in a multicenter clinical trial conducted in the United States.

Study Design

This study was a double-masked, placebo and naproxen-controlled, multicenter prospective clinical trial with three treatment arms, as summarized in Table 2. A total of 495

Continued on next page

This product information was prepared in September 1998. On these and other products of Sanofi Pharmaceuticals, Inc., detailed information may be obtained on a current basis by direct inquiry to Product Information Services, 90 Park Avenue, New York, NY 10016 (toll free 1-800-446-6267).

Hyalgan—Cont.

subjects with moderate to severe pain was randomized (at baseline evaluation) into three treatment groups in a ratio of 1:1:1 Hyalgan®, placebo, or naproxen.
[See table 2 below]

Patient Population and Demographics

The demographics of trial participants were comparable across treatment groups with regard to age, sex, race, height, weight, history, of osteoarthritis, prior use of NSAIDs, prior physical therapy, and use of assistive devices (refer to Table 3).
[See table 3 at top of previous page]

Evaluation Schedule

After meeting initial screening requirements NSAID therapy was discontinued. After 2 weeks, all subjects returned for baseline evaluations. The baseline evaluation included assessment of three primary effectiveness criteria; measurement of pain during a 50-foot walk test using a 100 mm Visual Analog Scale (VAS), a categorical assessment (0 = none to 5 = disabled) of pain, as assessed by a masked evaluator, during the 48 hours preceding the visit, and a categorical assessment (0 = none to 5 = disabled) of pain, as assessed by the subject, during the 48 hours preceding the visit.

All subjects who completed the NSAID washout period and met all entry requirements received their first injection after randomization. All subjects received subcutaneous lidocaine injections. Intra-articular injections (Hyalgan®, placebo) were administered weekly for a total of 5 injections (Weeks 0–4). The naproxen group received 500 mg of naproxen to be taken b.i.d. for 26 weeks.

Subsequent visits and evaluations took place at Weeks 5, 9, 12, 16, 21, and 26. Safety and effectiveness criteria were assessed and recorded at these time periods.

Clinical Results

For this trial, overall success for effectiveness was defined as meeting all four of the success criteria listed in Table 4 using scores from week 26. The criteria were met (refer to Tables 4 through 8).
[See table 4 below]
[See tables 5 & 6 above]
[See tables 7 & 8 at top of next page]

Additional Analyses

a. An analysis of study completers was performed as follows: Success was defined as 1) achieving a 20 mm decrease in the VAS for the 50-foot walk test by Week 5, and 2) maintaining this improvement through Week 26. In this analysis greater proportions of Hyalgan®-treated subjects (59/105, 56%) than either placebo- (47/115, 41%) or naproxen-treated subjects (51/113, 45%) were successful under this definition. The Hyalgan®-placebo comparison was statistically significant (p = 0.031, Fisher's Exact Test).

b. *Categorical Assessment of Pain – Subjects:* A longitudinal analysis of categorical assessment of pain by the subject, which analyzed the percentage of subjects who attained success revealed that a significantly higher percentage of Hyalgan®-treated subjects as compared to the placebo-treated

TABLE 5
ANCOVA of 50-Foot Walk Test (mm) VAS by Week for all Completed Subjects

	Week							
	3	4	5	9	12	16	21	26
Adjusted Means Hyalgan®	27.23	21.54	19.29	20.04	20.26	20.83	18.44	17.88
Placebo	32.35	28.57	25.67	24.28	26.66	25.44	24.77	26.73
Hyalgan® versus Placebo	5.13	7.03	6.39	4.24	6.40	4.61	6.33	8.846
p-value	0.06	0.01	0.01	0.1	0.03	0.1	0.02	0.004

TABLE 6
Masked Evaluators' Categorical Assessments of Pain for Completed Subjects in Prior 48 Hours: Level of Pain by Treatment Group at Baseline and Week 26

	NUMBER (%) OF SUBJECTS IN CATEGORY					
	Hyalgan®		Placebo		Naproxen	
	Baseline	Week 26	Baseline	Week 26	Baseline	Week 26
None (0)	0 (0.0)	27 (25.7)	0 (0.0)	15 (13.0)	0 (0.0)	17 (15.0)
Slight (1)	1 (1.0)	23 (21.9)	0 (0.0)	27 (23.5)	0 (0.0)	32 (28.3)
Mild (2)	2 (1.9)	24 (22.9)	2 (1.7)	29 (25.2)	2 (1.8)	27 (23.9)
Moderate (3)	69 (65.7)	26 (24.8)	85 (73.9)	34 (29.6)	79 (70.5)	28 (24.8)
Marked (4)	33 (31.4)	5 (4.8)	28 (24.3)	10 (8.7)	31 (27.7)	9 (8.0)
TOTAL	105 (100)	105 (100)	115 (100)	115 (100)	112* (100)	113 (100)

*One Naproxen treated subject was missing a Baseline assessment.

TABLE 2 STUDY DESIGN

Routes of Administration	Hyalgan®	Placebo	Naproxen
s.c.	Lidocaine (1%)	Lidocaine (1%)	Lidocaine (1%)
i.a.*	Hyalgan® (20 mg/2 mL)	Phosphate-Buffered Saline (2 mL)	none
p.o./b.i.d.	Placebo for naproxen capsules	Placebo for naproxen capsules	Naproxen capsules (500 mg)
p.o./p.r.n.(not to exceed 4 grams/day)	Acetaminophen	Acetaminophen	Acetaminophen

Legend: s.c. = subcutaneous; i.a. = intra-articular; p.o.= by mouth; b.i.d. = twice a day; p.r.n. = as needed
*Synovial fluid was aspirated (when present) in the Hyalgan® and placebo groups.

TABLE 4
Clinical Results

Evaluation	Success Criteria	Results
100 mm VAS or pain during 50 foot walk.	A statistically significant (alpha = 0.05) reduction on mean VAS for Hyalgan® when compared to placebo at Week 26. This difference was also to exceed one fourth of the Standard Deviation of the mean change from baseline	At Week 26, this difference between the Hyalgan®-treated group and the placebo-treated group adjusted means was 8.85 mm (p = 0.0043), which is a difference of approximately one-third of a standard deviation (Table 5).
Masked Evaluator Categorical Assessment of subject pain (O=none to 5=disabled) during the 48 hours preceding visits.	The number of Hyalgan®-treated subjects showing improvement at Week 26 was to be concordant with the VAS results, however, not required to be independently statistically significant.	At Week 26 the masked evaluator's categorical assessment of pain indicated that the Hyalgan®-treated subjects experienced less pain than the placebo-treated subjects (Table 6).
Subjects' Categorical Assessment of pain (O=none to 5=disabled) during the 48 hours preceding visits.	The number of Hyalgan®-treated subjects showing improvement at Week 26 was to be concordant with the VAS results; however, not required to be independently statistically significant.	At Week 26 the subjects' categorical assessment of pain indicated that the Hyalgan®-treated subjects experienced less pain than the placebo-treated subjects (Table 7).
Magnitude of the observed effect for Hyalgan® versus placebo on both the VAS and the categorical pain assessments	At Week 26 the magnitude of the observed effect for Hyalgan®-versus placebo on both the VAS and the categorical pain assessments were to be at least 50% of those observed for the naproxen group.	The improvement in pain on the VAS exhibited by the Hyalgan®-treated group relative to the placebo-treated group were at least 50% of the benefits exhibited by the naproxen-treated group relative to the placebo treated group. The results of the categorical assessments by the masked evaluator and the subject indicated that improvement of the Hyalgan®-treated group relative to the placebo-treated group was at least 50% of the benefits exhibited by the naproxen-treated group relative to the placebo-treated group (Table 8).

TABLE 7
Subjects' Categorical Assessments of Pain For Completed Subjects in Prior 48 Hours: Level of Pain by Treatment Group at Baseline and Week 26

| | NUMBER (%) OF SUBJECTS IN CATEGORY | | | | | |
| | Hyalgan® | | Placebo | | Naproxen | |
	Baseline	Week 26	Baseline	Week 26	Baseline	Week 26
None (0)	1 (1.0)	23 (21.9)	0 (0.0)	14 (12.2)	0 (0.0)	13 (11.5)
Slight (1)	2 (1.9)	27 (25.7)	0 (0.0)	24 (20.9)	1 (0.9)	31 (27.4)
Mild (2)	6 (5.7)	19 (18.1)	8 (7.0)	24 (20.9)	7 (6.2)	26 (23.0)
Moderate (3)	62 (59.0)	26 (24.8)	78 (67.8)	40 (34.8)	72 (63.7)	31 (27.4)
Marked (4)	34 (32.4)	10 (9.5)	29 (25.2)	13 (11.3)	33 (29.2)	12 (10.6)
TOTAL	105 (100)	105 (100)	115 (100)	115 (100)	113 (100)	113 (100)

TABLE 8
Halgan® Effect as a Percentage of the Naproxen-Placebo Difference

Assessment	Hyalgan® (HYL)	Placebo (PLA)	Naproxen (NAP)	HYL-PLA	NAP-HYL	NAP-PLA	(HYL-PLA) % of (NAP-PLA)
VAS for 50 foot Walk Baseline Adjusted Mean Effect Sizes From ANCOVA				-8.85 mm on a 100 mm VAS	4.12 mm on a 100 mm VAS	-4.73* mm on a 100 mm VAS	187%
% of Subjects Improved by Masked Evaluators	78.1	69.6	73.2	8.5	-4.9	3.6	236%
% of Subjects Improved by Subjects	73.3	62.6	67.3	10.7	-6.0	4.7	228%

*Imputed as (NAP-HYL)+(HYL-PLA).
Note that Effectiveness Success Criterion D is satisfied since ((HYL-PLA) % of (NAP-PLA))>50% for all three of the above pain assessments.

subjects (55/105, 52% vs 43/115, 37%, p = 0.030, Fisher's Exact Test) achieved success (an improvement of greater than or equal to one point on the five-point scale) and maintained this success from Week 5 until Week 26.

Safety
In order for the product to be considered safe, the incidence of severe swelling and pain consequent to intra-articular injection should be less than 5%. This criterion was met as indicated in Table 1. See the Adverse Events Section.

DETAILED DEVICE DESCRIPTION
Each vial or syringe contains:

Sodium Hyaluronate	20.0 mg
Sodium chloride	17.0 mg
Monobasic sodium phosphate	
• 2H$_2$O	0.1 mg
Dibasic sodium phosphate • 12H$_2$O	1.2 mg
Water for injection	q.s.* to 2.0 mL

*q.s. = up to

HOW SUPPLIED
Hyalgan® is supplied as a sterile, non-pyrogenic solution in 2 mL vials or 2 mL pre-filled syringes.

DIRECTIONS FOR USE
Hyalgan® is administered by intra-articular injection once a week (1 week apart), for a total of five injections.

Precaution: Do not use Hyalgan® if the package is opened or damaged. Store in the original packaging (protected from light) below 77° F (25° C). DO NOT FREEZE.

Precaution: Strict aseptic administration technique must be followed.

Warning: Do not concomitantly use disinfectants containing quaternary ammonium salts for skin preparation because hyaluronic acid can precipitate in their presence.

Inject subcutaneous lidocaine or similar local anesthetic prior to injection of Hyalgan®.

Precaution: Remove joint effusion, if present, before injection of Hyalgan®.

Do not use the same syringe for removing joint effusion and for injecting Hyalgan®.

Take care to remove the tip cap of the syringe and needle aseptically.

Inject Hyalgan® into the joint through a 20-gauge needle.

Precaution: The vial/syringe is intended for single use. The contents of the vial must be used immediately once the container has been opened. Discard any unused Hyalgan®. Inject the full 2 mL in one knee only. If treatment is bilateral, a separate vial should be used for each knee.

MANUFACTURED BY
FIDIA S.p.A.
Via Ponte della Fabbrica 3/A
35031 Abano Terme, Padua (PD), Italy

DISTRIBUTED BY
Sanofi Pharmaceuticals, Inc.
90 Park Avenue
New York, NY 10016

Shown in Product Identification Guide, page 335

ISUPREL®
ISOPROTERENOL HYDROCHLORIDE INHALATION AEROSOL, USP
In MISTOMETER® oral inhaler

℞

DESCRIPTION
ISUPREL, isoproterenol hydrochloride, MISTOMETER is a beta agonist sympathomimetic bronchodilator. Mistometer® is a complete nebulizing unit consisting of a plastic-coated glass vial of aerosol solution, detachable plastic mouthpiece with built-in nebulizer, and protective cap. The vial contains isoproterenol hydrochloride 0.25% (w/w) with inert ingredients of alcohol 33% (w/w) and ascorbic acid 0.1% (w/w) and, as propellants, dichlorodifluoromethane and dichlorotetrafluoroethane.

Isoproternol hydrochloride is a racemic compound with a molecular weight of 247.72 and a molecular formula $C_{11}H_{17}NO_3 \cdot HCl$. Chemically, isoproterenol hydrochloride is 3,4-Dihydroxy-α-[(isopropylamino)methyl]benzyl alcohol hydrochloride and has the following structural formula:
[See chemical structure at top of next column]

$$HO-\text{(benzene ring)}-CH-CH_2-NHCH(CH_3)_2 \cdot HCl$$
$$\underset{OH}{|}$$

The contents permit the delivery of not less than 200 actuations from the 11.2 g (10 mL) vial and not less than 300 actuations from the 16.8 g (15 mL) vial. The MISTOMETER delivers a measured dose of 103 mcg of the bronchodilator in a fine, even mist for inhalation.

CLINICAL PHARMACOLOGY
ISUPREL relaxes bronchial spasm and facilitates expectoration of pulmonary secretions by acting almost exclusively on beta receptors. It is frequently effective when epinephrine and other drugs fail, and it has a wide margin of safety. ISUPREL is readily absorbed when given as an aerosol. It is metabolized primarily in the liver and other tissues by catechol-O-methyltransferase (COMT).

Recent studies in laboratory animals (minipigs, rodents, and dogs) recorded the occurrence of cardiac arrhythmias and sudden death (with histologic evidence of myocardial necrosis) when beta agonists and methylxanthines were concomitantly administered. The significance of these findings when applied to human usage is currently unknown.

INDICATIONS AND USAGE
ISUPREL is indicated for the relief of bronchospasm associated with acute and chronic asthma and reversible bronchospasm which may be associated with chronic bronchitis or emphysema.

CONTRAINDICATIONS
Use of isoproterenol in patients with preexisting cardiac arrhythmias associated with tachycardia is generally considered contraindicated because the cardiac stimulant effect of the drug may aggravate such disorders. The use of this medication is contraindicated in those patients who have a known hypersensitivity to isoproterenol or to any of the other components of this drug.

WARNINGS
Excessive use of an adrenergic aerosol should be discouraged as it may lose its effectiveness.

In patients with status asthmaticus and abnormal blood gas tensions, improvement in vital capacity and in blood gas tensions may not accompany apparent relief of bronchospasm. Facilities for administering oxygen mixtures and ventilatory assistance are necessary for such patients.

Occasional patients have been reported to develop severe paradoxical airway resistance with repeated, excessive use of isoproterenol inhalation preparations. The cause of this refractory state is unknown. It is advisable that in such instances the use of this preparation be discontinued immediately and alternative therapy instituted, since in the reported cases the patients did not respond to other forms of therapy until the drug was withdrawn.

Deaths have been reported following excessive use of isoproterenol inhalation preparations and the exact cause is unknown. Cardiac arrest was noted in several instances.

PRECAUTIONS
General
Isoproterenol should be used with caution in patients with cardiovascular disorders including coronary insufficiency, diabetes, or hyperthyroidism, and in persons sensitive to sympathomimetic amines.

A single treatment with the ISUPREL MISTOMETER is usually sufficient for controlling isolated attacks of asthma. Any patient who requires more than three aerosol treatments within a 24-hour period should be under the close supervision of a physician. Further therapy with the bronchodilator aerosol alone is inadvisable when three to five treatments within six to twelve hours produce minimal or no relief.

Information for Patients
Do not inhale more often than directed by your physician. Read enclosed instructions before using (see attachment to insert). Do not exceed the dose prescribed by your physician. If difficulty in breathing persists, contact your physician immediately. Avoid spraying in eyes. Contents under pressure. Do not break or incinerate. Do not store at temperatures above 120° F. Keep out of reach of children.

Drug Interactions
Epinephrine should not be administered concomitantly with ISUPREL, as both drugs are direct cardiac stimulants and their combined effects may induce serious arrhythmia. If desired they may, however, be alternated, provided an interval of at least four hours has elapsed.

Carcinogenesis, Mutagenesis, Impairment of Fertility
Long-term chronic toxicity studies in animals have not been done to evaluate isoproterenol in these areas.

Continued on next page

This product information was prepared in September 1998. On these and other products of Sanofi Pharmaceuticals, Inc., detailed information may be obtained on a current basis by direct inquiry to Product Information Services, 90 Park Avenue, New York, NY 10016 (toll free 1-800-446-6267).

Isuprel Mistometer—Cont.

Pregnancy Category C
Animal reproduction studies have not been conducted with isoproterenol hydrochloride. It is also not known whether isoproterenol hydrochloride can cause fetal harm when administered to a pregnant woman or can affect reproduction capacity. Isoproterenol hydrochloride should be given to a pregnant woman only if clearly needed.

Nursing Mothers
It is not known whether this drug is excreted in human milk. Because many drugs are excreted in human milk, caution should be exercised when isoproterenol hydrochloride is administered to a nursing woman.

Pediatric Use
In general, the technique of ISUPREL MISTOMETER in administration to children is similar to that of adults, since children's smaller ventilatory exchange capacity automatically provides proportionally smaller aerosol intake.

ADVERSE REACTIONS

The mist from the ISUPREL MISTOMETER contains alcohol but is generally very well tolerated. An occasional patient may experience some transient throat irritation which has been attributed to the alcohol content.

Serious reactions to ISUPREL, brand of isoproterenol hydrochloride inhalation aerosol, are infrequent. The following reactions, however, have been reported:

CNS: Nervousness, headache, dizziness, weakness.

Gastrointestinal: Nausea, vomiting.

Cardiovascular: Tachycardia, palpitations, precordial distress, anginal-type pain.

Other: Flushing of the skin, tremor, and sweating.

The inhalation route is usually accompanied by a minimum of side effects. These untoward reactions disappear quickly and do not, as a rule, inconvenience the patient to the extent that the drug must be discontinued. No cumulative effects have been reported.

OVERDOSAGE

Overdosage of ISUPREL may produce signs and symptoms typical of excessive sympathomimetic effects, including tachycardia, palpitations, nervousness, nausea, and vomiting. Excessive use of adrenergic aerosols may result in loss of effectiveness or severe paradoxical airway resistance. Cardiac arrest has been noted in several instances. In all cases of overdose or excessive use of ISUPREL, the drug should be discontinued immediately and vital functions supported until the patient is stabilized. It is not known whether isoproterenol hydrochloride is dialyzable.

The acute oral LD_{50} in mice is 3,850 mg/kg ± 1,190 mg/kg of pure drug in solution (isoproterenol hydrochloride). In dogs, the toxic dose is 1,000 times the therapeutic dose. Converted to the amount used clinically in man, this would be about 2,500 times the therapeutic dose.

DOSAGE AND ADMINISTRATION

Acute Bronchial Asthma: Hold the MISTOMETER in an inverted position. Close lips and teeth around open end of mouthpiece. Breathe out, expelling as much air from the lungs as possible; then inhale deeply while pressing down on the bottle to activate spray mechanism. Try to hold breath for a few seconds before exhaling. Wait one full minute in order to determine the effect before considering a second inhalation. A treatment may be repeated up to 5 times daily if necessary. (See PRECAUTIONS.) If carefully instructed, children quickly learn to keep the stream of mist clear of the teeth and tongue, thereby assuring inhalation into the lungs. Occlusion of the nares of very young children may be advisable to make inhalation certain.

Warm water should be run through the mouthpiece once daily to wash it and prevent clogging.

The mouthpiece may also be sanitized by immersion in alcohol.

Bronchospasm in Chronic Obstructive Lung Disease: The MISTOMETER provides a convenient aerosol method for delivering ISUPREL, brand of isoproterenol hydrochloride inhalation aerosol. The treatment described above for Acute Bronchial Asthma may be repeated at not less than 3 to 4 hour intervals as part of a programmed regimen of treatment of obstructive lung disease complicated by a reversible bronchospastic component. One application from the MISTOMETER may be regarded as equivalent in effectiveness to 5 to 7 operations of a hand-bulb nebulizer using a 1:100 solution.

Pediatric Dosage
In general, the technique of ISUPREL MISTOMETER in administration to children is similar to that of adults, since children's smaller ventilatory exchange capacity automatically provides proportionally smaller aerosol intake.

HOW SUPPLIED

ISUPREL MISTOMETER is supplied in a plastic coated glass vial as a metered dose aerosol providing 103 mcg of isoproterenol hydrochloride per actuation. There are 200 actuations per 10 mL.

Vial of 16.8 g (15 mL) with oral nebulizer
(NDC 0024-0878-01)

Refill only, 16.8 g (15 mL)
(NDC 0024-0879-01)

Store at room temperature up to 30° C (86° F).

Caution: Federal law prohibits dispensing without prescription.

Note: The indented statement below is required by the Federal government's Clean Air Act for all products containing or manufactured with chlorofluorocarbons (CFC's).

> **WARNING: Contains dichlorodifluoromethane and dichlorotetrafluoroethane, substances which harm public health and environment by destroying ozone in the upper atmosphere.**

A notice similar to the above WARNING has been placed in the information for the patient of this product pursuant to EPA regulations.

ISW-4C

ISUPREL® Hydrochloride ℞
ISOPROTERENOL
INHALATION SOLUTION, USP
SOLUTION 1:200
SOLUTION 1:100

Potent Bronchodilator

DESCRIPTION

ISUPREL, brand of isoproterenol inhalation solution, is a beta agonist sympathomimetic bronchodilator.

Solution 1:200 contains isoproterenol hydrochloride 5 mg/mL.

Inactive Ingredients: Chlorobutanol 0.5 percent and Sodium Metabisulfite 0.3 percent as preservatives, Citric Acid, Glycerin, Purified Water, and Sodium Chloride.

Solution 1:100 contains isoproterenol hydrochloride 10 mg/mL.

Inactive Ingredients: Chlorobutanol 0.5 percent and Sodium Metabisulfite 0.3 percent as preservatives, Citric Acid, Purified Water, Saccharin Sodium, Sodium Chloride, and Sodium Citrate.

Isoproterenol hydrochloride is soluble in water (1 g isoproterenol hydrochloride dissolves in 3 mL H_2O). The solutions have a pH range of 3 to 4.5.

Isoproterenol hydrochloride is a racemic compound with a molecular weight of 247.72 and the molecular formula $C_{11}H_{17}NO_3 \cdot HCl$.

Chemically, isoproterenol hydrochloride is 3,4-Dihydroxy-α-[(isopropylamino)methyl]benzyl alcohol hydrochloride and has the following structural formula:

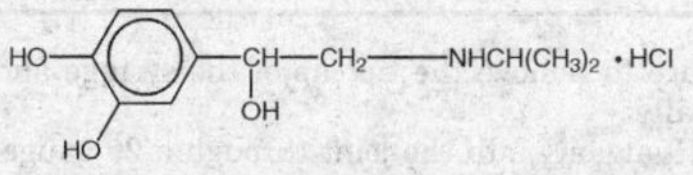

The air in the bottles has been displaced by nitrogen gas.

CLINICAL PHARMACOLOGY

ISUPREL relaxes bronchial spasm and facilitates expectoration of pulmonary secretions by acting almost exclusively on beta receptors.

ISUPREL is readily absorbed when given as an aerosol. It is metabolized primarily in the liver and other tissues by catechol-0-methyltransferase (CONT).

Recent studies in laboratory animals (minipigs, rodents, and dogs) recorded the occurrence of cardiac arrhythmias and sudden death (with histologic evidence of myocardial necrosis) when beta agonists and methylxanthines were concomitantly administered. The significance of these findings when applied to human usage is currently unknown.

INDICATIONS AND USAGE

ISUPREL is indicated for the relief of bronchospasm associated with acute and chronic asthma and reversible bronchospasm which may be associated with chronic bronchitis or emphysema.

CONTRAINDICATION

Use of isoproterenol in patients with preexisting cardiac arrhythmias associated with tachycardia is generally considered contraindicated because the cardiac stimulant effect of the drug may aggravate such disorders.

WARNINGS

Excessive use of an adrenergic aerosol should be discouraged as it may lose its effectiveness.

Isoproterenol administration as a solution for nebulization has been associated with a decrease in arterial pO_2 in asthmatic patients as a result of ventilation-perfusion abnormalities despite improvement in airway obstruction. The clinical significance of this relative hypoxemia is unclear.

As with other inhaled beta adrenergic agonists, ISUPREL can produce paradoxical bronchospasm, that can be life threatening. If this occurs, the product should be discontinued immediately and alternative therapy instituted.

Deaths have been reported following excessive use of isoproterenol inhalation preparations and the exact cause is unknown. Cardiac arrest was noted in several instances. It is therefore essential that the physician instruct the patient in the need for further evaluation if his/her asthma worsens.

Contains sodium metabisulfite, a sulfite that may cause allergic-type reactions including anaphylactic symptoms and life-threatening or less severe asthmatic episodes in certain susceptible people. The overall prevalence of sulfite sensitivity in the general population is unknown and probably low. Sulfite sensitivity is seen more frequently in asthmatic than in nonasthmatic people.

PRECAUTIONS

ISUPREL, as with all sympathomimetic amines, should be used with caution in patients with cardiovascular disorders, especially coronary insufficiency, cardiac arrhythmias, and hypertension; in patients with convulsive disorders, hyperthyroidism, or diabetes mellitus; and in patients who are unusually responsive to sympathomimetic amines. Clinically significant changes in systolic and diastolic blood pressure have been seen in some patients after use of any beta adrenergic bronchodilator.

Any patient who requires more than three aerosol treatments within a 24-hour period should be under the close supervision of his physician. Further therapy with the bronchodilator aerosol alone is inadvisable when three to five treatments within six to twelve hours produce minimal or no relief.

When compressed oxygen is employed as the aerosol propellant, the percentage of oxygen used should be determined by the patient's individual requirements to avoid depression of respiratory drive.

Drug Interactions:
Other sympathomimetic aerosol bronchodilators or epinephrine should not be used concomitantly with ISUPREL. If additional adrenergic drugs are to be administered by any route to the patient using ISUPREL, they should be used with caution to avoid deleterious cardiovascular effects.

Beta adrenergic agonists should be administered with caution to patients being treated with MAO inhibitors or tricyclic antidepressants since the action of the beta adrenergic agonists on the vascular system may be potentiated.

Beta receptor blocking agents and ISUPREL inhibit the effects of each other.

Carcinogenesis, Mutagenesis, Impairment of Fertility: Long-term chronic toxicity studies in animals have not been done to evaluate isoproterenol in these areas.

Pregnancy Category C: Animal reproduction studies have not been conducted with isoproterenol hydrochloride. It is also not known whether isoproterenol hydrochloride can cause fetal harm when administered to a pregnant woman or can affect reproduction capacity. Isoproterenol hydrochloride should be given to a pregnant woman only if clearly needed.

Nursing Mothers: It is not known whether this drug is excreted in human milk. Because many drugs are excreted in human milk, caution should be exercised when isoproterenol hydrochloride is administered to a nursing woman.

Pediatric Use: In general, the technique of isoproterenol hydrochloride solution in administration to children is similar to that of adults, since children's smaller ventilatory exchange capacity automatically provides proportionally smaller aerosol intake. However, it is generally recommended that the 1:200 solution (rather than the 1:100) be used for an acute attack of bronchospasm, and no more than 0.25 mL of the 1:200 solution should be used for each 10 to 15 minute programmed treatment in chronic bronchospastic disease.

ADVERSE REACTIONS

Serious reactions to ISUPREL are infrequent. The following reactions, however, have been reported:

CNS: Nervousness, headache, dizziness, weakness.

Gastrointestinal: Nausea, vomiting.

Cardiovascular: Tachycardia, palpitations, precordial distress, anginal-type pain.

Other: Flushing of the skin, tremor, and sweating.

The inhalation route is usually accompanied by a minimum of side effects. These untoward reactions disappear quickly and do not as a rule, inconvenience the patient to the extent that the drug must be discontinued. No cumulative effects have been reported.

OVERDOSAGE

Overdosage of ISUPREL may produce signs and symptoms typical of excessive sympathomimetic effects, including tachycardia, palpitations, nervousness, nausea, and vomiting. Excessive use of adrenergic aerosols may result in loss of effectiveness or severe paradoxical airway resistance. Cardiac arrest has been noted in several instances. In all cases of overdose or excessive use of ISUPREL, the drug should be discontinued immediately and vital functions supported until the patient is stabilized. It is not known whether isoproterenol hydrochloride is dialyzable.

The acute oral LD_{50} in mice is 3,850 mg/kg ± 1,190 mg/kg of pure drug in solution (isoproterenol hydrochloride). In dogs,

the toxic dose is 1,000 times the therapeutic dose. Converted to the amount used clinically in man, this would be about 2,500 times the therapeutic dose.

DOSAGE AND ADMINISTRATION

ISUPREL can be administered as an aerosol mist by hand-bulb nebulizer, compressed air or oxygen operated nebulizer, or by intermittent positive pressure breathing (IPPB) devices. The method of delivery, and the treatment regimen employed in the management of the reversible bronchospastic element accompanying bronchial asthma, chronic bronchitis, and chronic obstructive lung diseases, will depend on such factors as the severity of the bronchospasm, patient age, tolerance to the medication, complicating cardiopulmonary conditions, and whether therapy is for an intermittent acute attack of bronchospasm or is part of a programmed treatment regimen for constant bronchospasm.

Acute Bronchial Asthma. *Hand-Bulb Nebulizer*—Depending on the frequency of treatment and the type of nebulizer used, a volume of solution of ISUPREL, sufficient for not more than one day's treatment, should be placed in the nebulizer using the dropper provided. In time, the patient can learn to adjust the volume required. For adults and children, the 1:200 solution is administered by hand-bulb nebulization in a dosage of 5 to 15 deep inhalations (using an all glass or plastic nebulizer). In adults, the 1:100 solution may be used if a stronger solution seems to be indicated. The dose is 3 to 7 deep inhalations. If after about 5 to 10 minutes inadequate relief is observed, these doses may be repeated one more time. If the acute attack recurs, treatments may be repeated up to 5 times daily if necessary. (See PRECAUTIONS.)

Bronchospasm in Chronic Obstructive Lung Disease. *Hand-Bulb Nebulizer*—A solution of 1:200 or 1:100 of ISUPREL may be administered daily at not less than 3 to 4 hour intervals for subacute bronchospastic attacks or as part of a programmed treatment regimen in patients with chronic obstructive lung disease with a reversible bronchospastic component. An adequate dose is usually 5 to 15 deep inhalations, using the 1:200 solution. Some patients with severe attacks of bronchospasm may require 3 to 7 deep inhalations using the 1:100 solution of ISUPREL.

Nebulization by Compressed Air or Oxygen—A method often used in patients with severe chronic obstructive lung disease is to deliver the isoproterenol mist in more dilute form over a longer period of time. The purpose is, not so much to increase the dose supplied, as to achieve progressively deeper bronchodilatation and thus insure that the mist achieves maximum penetration of the finer bronchioles. In this method, 0.5 mL of a 1:200 solution of ISUPREL is diluted to 2 mL to 2.5 mL with water or isotonic saline to achieve a use concentration of 1:800 to 1:1000. If desired, 0.25 mL of the 1:100 solution may be similarly diluted to achieve the same use concentration. The diluted solution is placed in a nebulizer (e.g. DeVilbiss #640 unit) connected to either a source of compressed air or oxygen. The flow rate is regulated to suit the particular nebulizer so that the diluted solution of ISUPREL will be delivered over approximately 10 to 20 minutes. A treatment may be repeated up to 5 times daily if necessary. Although the total delivered dose of ISUPREL is somewhat higher than with the treatment regimen employing the hand-bulb nebulizer, patients usually tolerate it well because of the greater dilution and longer application-time factors.

Intermittent Positive Pressure Breathing (IPPB)—Diluted solutions of 1:200 or 1:100 of ISUPREL are used in a programmed regimen for the treatment of reversible bronchospasm in patients with chronic obstructive lung disease who require intermittent positive pressure breathing therapy. These devices generally have a small nebulizer, usually of 3 mL to 5 mL capacity, on a patient-operated side arm. The effectiveness of IPPB therapy is greatly enhanced by the simultaneous use of aerosolized bronchodilators. As with compressed air or oxygen operated nebulizers, the usual regimen is to place 0.5 mL of 1:200 solution of ISUPREL diluted to 2 mL to 2.5 mL with water or isotonic saline in the nebulizer cup and follow the IPPB manufacturer's operating instructions. IPPB-bronchodilator treatments are usually administered over 15 to 20 minutes, up to 5 times daily if necessary.

Pediatric Dosage: In general, the technique of isoproterenol hydrochloride solution in administration to children is similar to that of adults, since children's smaller ventilatory exchange capacity automatically provides proportionally smaller aerosol intake. However, it is generally recommended that the 1:200 solution (rather than the 1:100) be used for an acute attack of bronchospasm, and no more than 0.25 mL of the 1:200 solution should be used for each 10 to 15 minute programmed treatment in chronic bronchospastic disease.

HOW SUPPLIED

Solution 1:100 contains isoproterenol hydrochloride 1% (10 mg/mL).

Solution 1:200 contains isoproterenol hydrochloride 0.5% (5 mg/mL).

Solution 1:100
bottle of 10 mL **NDC** 0024-0873-01
Solution 1:200
bottle of 10 mL **NDC** 0024-0871-01

Do not use the inhalation solutions if their color is pinkish to brownish or if they contain a precipitate.

Protect from light.

Store at controlled room temperature 15° C to 30° C (59° F to 86° F).

ISW-3B

KAYEXALATE® ℞

brand of sodium polystyrene sulfonate, USP

Cation-Exchange Resin

DESCRIPTION

KAYEXALATE, brand of sodium polystyrene sulfonate, is a benzene, diethenyl- polymer, with ethenylbenzene, sulfonated, sodium salt and has the following structural formula:

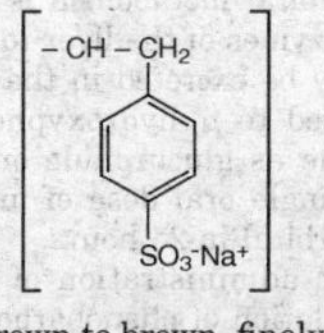

The drug is a light brown to brown, finely ground, powdered form of sodium polystyrene sulfonate, a cation-exchange resin prepared in the sodium phase with an *in vitro* exchange capacity of approximately 3.1 mEq (*in vivo* approximately 1 mEq) of potassium per gram. The sodium content is approximately 100 mg (4.1 mEq) per gram of the drug. It can be administered orally or in an enema.

CLINICAL PHARMACOLOGY

As the resin passes along the intestine or is retained in the colon after administration by enema, the sodium ions are partially released and are replaced by potassium ions. For the most part, this action occurs in the large intestine, which excretes potassium ions to a greater degree than does the small intestine. The efficiency of this process is limited and unpredictably variable. It commonly approximates the order of 33 percent but the range is so large that definitive indices of electrolyte balance must be clearly monitored. Metabolic data are unavailable.

INDICATION AND USAGE

KAYEXALATE is indicated for the treatment of hyperkalemia.

CONTRAINDICATIONS

KAYEXALATE is contraindicated in patients with hypokalemia or those patients who are hypersensitive to it.

WARNINGS

Alternative Therapy in Severe Hyperkalemia:
Since effective lowering of serum potassium with KAYEXALATE may take hours to days, treatment with this drug alone may be insufficient to rapidly correct severe hyperkalemia associated with states of rapid tissue breakdown (e.g., burns and renal failure) or hyperkalemia so marked as to constitute a medical emergency. Therefore, other definitive measures, including dialysis, should always be considered and may be imperative.

Hypokalemia: Serious potassium deficiency can occur from therapy with KAYEXALATE. The effect must be carefully controlled by frequent serum potassium determinations within each 24-hour period. Since intracellular potassium deficiency is not always reflected by serum potassium levels, the level at which treatment with KAYEXALATE should be discontinued must be determined individually for each patient. Important aids in making this determination are the patient's clinical condition and electrocardiogram. Early clinical signs of severe hypokalemia include a pattern of irritable confusion and delayed thought processes. Electrocardiographically, severe hypokalemia is often associated with a lengthened Q-T interval, widening, flattening, or inversion of the T wave, and prominent U waves. Also, cardiac arrhythmias may occur, such as premature atrial, nodal, and ventricular contractions, and supraventricular and ventricular tachycardias. The toxic effects of digitalis are likely to be exaggerated. Marked hypokalemia can also be manifested by severe muscle weakness, at times extending into frank paralysis.

Electrolyte Disturbances: Like all cation-exchange resins, KAYEXALATE is not totally selective (for potassium) in its actions, and small amounts of other cations such as magnesium and calcium can also be lost during treatment. Accordingly, patients receiving KAYEXALATE should be monitored for all applicable electrolyte disturbances.

Systemic Alkalosis: Systemic alkalosis has been reported after cation-exchange resins were administered orally in combination with nonabsorbable cation-donating antacids and laxatives such as magnesium hydroxide and aluminum carbonate. Magnesium hydroxide should not be administered with KAYEXALATE. One case of grand mal seizure has been reported in a patient with chronic hypocalcemia of renal failure who was given KAYEXALATE with magnesium hydroxide as laxative. (See PRECAUTIONS, Drug Interactions.)

PRECAUTIONS

Caution is advised when KAYEXALATE is administered to patients who cannot tolerate even a small increase in sodium loads (ie, severe congestive heart failure, severe hypertension, or marked edema). In such instances compensatory restriction of sodium intake from other sources may be indicated.

If constipation occurs, patients should be treated with sorbitol (from 10 mL to 20 mL of 70 percent syrup every two hours or as needed to produce one or two watery stools daily), a measure which also reduces any tendency to fecal impaction.

Drug Interactions

Antacids: The simultaneous oral administration of KAYEXALATE with nonabsorbable cation-donating antacids and laxatives may reduce the resin's potassium exchange capability.

Systemic alkalosis has been reported after cation-exchange resins were administered orally in combination with nonabsorbable cation-donating antacids and laxatives such as magnesium hydroxide and aluminum carbonate. Magnesium hydroxide should not be administered with KAYEXALATE. One case of grand mal seizure has been reported in a patient with chronic hypocalcemia of renal failure who was given KAYEXALATE with magnesium hydroxide as a laxative.

Intestinal obstruction due to concretions of aluminum hydroxide when used in combination with KAYEXALATE has been reported.

Digitalis: The toxic effects of digitalis on the heart, especially various ventricular arrhythmias and A-V nodal dissociation, are likely to be exaggerated by hypokalemia, even in the face of serum digoxin concentrations in the "normal range". (See WARNINGS.)

Carcinogenesis, Mutagenesis, Impairment of Fertility

Studies have not been performed.

Pregnancy Category C

Animal reproduction studies have not been conducted with KAYEXALATE. It is also not known whether KAYEXALATE can cause fetal harm when administered to a pregnant woman or can affect reproduction capacity. KAYEXALATE should be given to a pregnant woman only if clearly needed.

Nursing Mothers

It is not known whether this drug is excreted in human milk. Because many drugs are excreted in human milk, caution should be exercised when KAYEXALATE is administered to a nursing woman.

ADVERSE REACTIONS

KAYEXALATE may cause some degree of gastric irritation. Anorexia, nausea, vomiting, and constipation may occur especially if high doses are given. Also, hypokalemia, hypocalcemia, and significant sodium retention may occur. Occasionally diarrhea develops. Large doses in elderly individuals may cause fecal impaction (see PRECAUTIONS). This effect may be obviated through usage of the resin in enemas as described under DOSAGE AND ADMINISTRATION. Rare instances of colonic necrosis have been reported. Intestinal obstruction due to concretions of aluminum hydroxide, when used in combination with KAYEXALATE, has been reported.

DOSAGE AND ADMINISTRATION

Suspension of this drug should be freshly prepared and not stored beyond 24 hours.

The average daily adult dose of the resin is 15 g to 60 g. This is best provided by administering 15 g (approximately 4 *level* teaspoons) of KAYEXALATE one to four times daily. One gram of KAYEXALATE contains 4.1 mEq of sodium; one level teaspoon contains approximately 3.5 g of KAYEXALATE and 15 mEq of sodium. (A heaping teaspoon may contain as much as 10 g to 12 g of KAYEXALATE.) Since the *in vivo* efficiency of sodium-potassium exchange resins is approximately 33 percent, about one third of the resin's actual sodium content is being delivered to the body.

Continued on next page

This product information was prepared in September 1998. On these and other products of Sanofi Pharmaceuticals, Inc., detailed information may be obtained on a current basis by direct inquiry to Product Information Services, 90 Park Avenue, New York, NY 10016 (toll free 1-800-446-6267).

Kayexalate—Cont.

In smaller children and infants, lower doses should be employed by using as a guide a rate of 1 mEq of potassium per gram of resin as the basis for calculation.
Each dose should be given as a suspension in a small quantity of water or, for greater palatability, in syrup. The amount of fluid usually ranges from 20 mL to 100 mL, depending on the dose, or may be simply determined by allowing 3 mL to 4 mL per gram of resin. Sorbitol may be administered in order to combat constipation.
The resin may be introduced into the stomach through a plastic tube and, if desired, mixed with a diet appropriate for a patient in renal failure.
The resin may also be given, although with less effective results, in an enema consisting (for adults) of 30 g to 50 g every six hours. Each dose is administered as a warm emulsion (at body temperature) in 100 mL of aqueous vehicle, such as sorbitol. The emulsion should be agitated gently during administration. The enema should be retained as long as possible and followed by a cleansing enema.
After an initial cleansing enema, a soft, large size (French 28) rubber tube is inserted into the rectum for a distance of about 20 cm, with the tip well into the sigmoid colon, and taped in place. The resin is then suspended in the appropriate amount of aqueous vehicle at body temperature and introduced by gravity, while the particles are kept in suspension by stirring. The suspension is flushed with 50 mL or 100 mL of fluid, following which the tube is clamped and left in place. If back leakage occurs, the hips are elevated on pillows or a knee-chest position is taken temporarily. A somewhat thicker suspension may be used, but care should be taken that no paste is formed, because the latter has a greatly reduced exchange surface and will be particularly ineffective if deposited in the rectal ampulla. The suspension is kept in the sigmoid colon for several hours, if possible. Then, the colon is irrigated with nonsodium containing solution at body temperature in order to remove the resin. Two quarts of flushing solution may be necessary. The returns are drained constantly through a Y tube connection. Particular attention should be paid to this cleansing enema when sorbitol has been used.
The intensity and duration of therapy depend upon the severity and resistance of hyperkalemia.
KAYEXALATE should not be heated for to do so may alter the exchange properties of the resin.

HOW SUPPLIED

Store at room temperature.
KAYEXALATE is available as a cream to light brown, finely ground powder in jars of 1 pound (453.6g), NDC 0024-1075-01.
Caution: Federal law prohibits dispensing without prescription.

KSW-1A

MEBARAL® CIV ℞
Brand of MEPHOBARBITAL TABLETS, USP

DESCRIPTION

Mephobarbital, 5-Ethyl-1-methyl-5-phenylbarbituric acid, is a barbiturate with sedative, hypnotic, and anticonvulsant properties. It occurs as a white, nearly odorless, tasteless powder and is slightly soluble in water and in alcohol.
MEBARAL is available as tablets for oral administration.
The structural formula is:

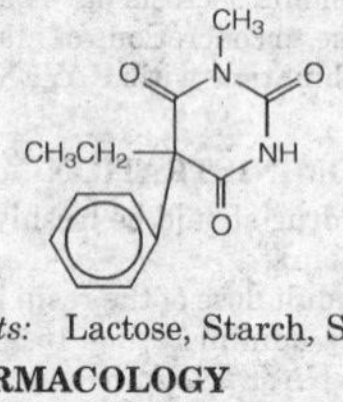

Inactive Ingredients: Lactose, Starch, Stearic Acid, Talc.

CLINICAL PHARMACOLOGY

Barbiturates are capable of producing all levels of CNS mood alteration from excitation to mild sedation, to hypnosis, and deep coma. Overdosage can produce death. In high enough therapeutic doses, barbiturates induce anesthesia.
Barbiturates depress the sensory cortex, decrease motor activity, alter cerebellar function, and produce drowsiness, sedation, and hypnosis.
Barbiturates are respiratory depressants. The degree of respiratory depression is dependent upon dose. With hypnotic doses, respiratory depression produced by barbiturates is similar to that which occurs during physiologic sleep with slight decrease in blood pressure and heart rate.
Studies in laboratory animals have shown that barbiturates cause reduction in the tone and contractility of the uterus, ureters, and urinary bladder. However, concentrations of the drugs required to produce this effect in humans are not reached with sedative-hypnotic doses.
Barbiturates do not impair normal hepatic function, but have been shown to induce liver microsomal enzymes, thus increasing and/or altering the metabolism of barbiturates and other drugs. (See PRECAUTIONS—Drug Interactions.)
MEBARAL exerts a strong sedative and anticonvulsant action but has a relatively mild hypnotic effect. It reduces the incidence of epileptic seizures in grand mal and petit mal. MEBARAL usually causes little or no drowsiness or lassitude. Hence, when it is used as a sedative or anticonvulsant, patients usually become more calm, more cheerful, and better adjusted to their surroundings without clouding of mental faculties. MEBARAL is reported to produce less sedation than does phenobarbital.
Barbiturates are weak acids that are absorbed and rapidly distributed to all tissues and fluids with high concentrations in the brain, liver, and kidneys. Lipid solubility of the barbiturates is the dominant factor in their distribution within the body. Barbiturates are bound to plasma and tissue proteins to a varying degree with the degree of binding increasing directly as a function of lipid solubility.
Approximately 50% of an oral dose of mephobarbital is absorbed from the gastrointestinal tract. Therapeutic plasma concentrations for mephobarbital have not been established nor has the half-life been determined. Following oral administration, the onset of action of the drug is 30 to 60 minutes and the duration of action is 10 to 16 hours. The primary route of mephobarbital metabolism is N-demethylation by the microsomal enzymes of the liver to form phenobarbital. Phenobarbital may be excreted in the urine unchanged or further metabolized to *p*-hydroxyphenobarbital and excreted in the urine as glucuronide or sulfate conjugates. About 75% of a single oral dose of mephobarbital is converted to phenobarbital in 24 hours.
Therefore, chronic administration of mephobarbital may lead to an accumulation of phenobarbital (not mephobarbital) in plasma. It has not been determined whether mephobarbital or phenobarbital is the active agent during long-time mephobarbital therapy.

INDICATIONS AND USAGE

MEBARAL is indicated for use as a sedative for the relief of anxiety, tension, and apprehension, and as an anticonvulsant for the treatment of grand mal and petit mal epilepsy.

CONTRAINDICATIONS

Hypersensitivity to any barbiturate. Manifest or latent porphyria.

WARNINGS

Habit Forming
Barbiturates may be habit forming. Tolerance, psychological, and physical dependence may occur with continued use. (See DRUG ABUSE AND DEPENDENCE and CLINICAL PHARMACOLOGY.) Patients who have psychological dependence on barbiturates may increase the dosage or decrease the dosage interval without consulting a physician and may subsequently develop a physical dependence on barbiturates. To minimize the possibility of overdosage or the development of dependence, the prescribing and dispensing of sedative-hypnotic barbiturates should be limited to the amount required for the interval until the next appointment. Abrupt cessation after prolonged use in the dependent person may result in withdrawal symptoms, including delirium, convulsions, and possibly death. Barbiturates should be withdrawn gradually from any patient known to be taking excessive dosage over long periods of time. (See DRUG ABUSE AND DEPENDENCE.)

Acute or Chronic Pain
Caution should be exercised when barbiturates are administered to patients with acute or chronic pain, because paradoxical excitement could be induced or important symptoms could be masked. However, the use of barbiturates as sedatives in the postoperative surgical period and as adjuncts to cancer chemotherapy is well established.

Use in Pregnancy
Barbiturates can cause fetal damage when administered to a pregnant woman. Retrospective, case-controlled studies have suggested a connection between the maternal consumption of barbiturates and a higher than expected incidence of fetal abnormalities. Following oral or parenteral administration, barbiturates readily cross the placental barrier and are distributed throughout fetal tissues with highest concentrations found in the placenta, fetal liver, and brain. Fetal blood levels approach maternal blood levels following parenteral administration.
Withdrawal symptoms occur in infants born to mothers who receive barbiturates throughout the last trimester of pregnancy. (See DRUG ABUSE AND DEPENDENCE.) If this drug is used during pregnancy, or if the patient becomes pregnant while taking this drug, the patient should be apprised of the potential hazard to the fetus.

Synergistic Effects
The concomitant use of alcohol or other CNS depressants may produce additive CNS depressant effects.

PRECAUTIONS

General
Barbiturates may be habit forming. Tolerance and psychological and physical dependence may occur with continuing use. (See DRUG ABUSE AND DEPENDENCE.) Barbiturates should be administered with caution, if at all, to patients who are mentally depressed, have suicidal tendencies, or a history of drug abuse.
Elderly or debilitated patients may react to barbiturates with marked excitement, depression, and confusion. In some persons, barbiturates repeatedly produce excitement rather than depression.
In patients with hepatic damage, barbiturates should be administered with caution and initially in reduced doses. Barbiturates should not be administered to patients showing the premonitory signs of hepatic coma.
Status epilepticus may result from the abrupt discontinuation of MEBARAL, even when administered in small daily doses in the treatment of epilepsy.
Caution and careful adjustment of dosage are required when MEBARAL is used in patients with impaired renal, cardiac, or respiratory function and in patients with myasthenia gravis and myxedema. The least quantity feasible should be prescribed or dispensed at any one time in order to minimize the possibility of acute or chronic overdosage.
Vitamin D Deficiency: MEBARAL may increase vitamin D requirements, possibly by increasing vitamin D metabolism via enzyme induction. Rarely, rickets and osteomalacia have been reported following prolonged use of barbiturates.
Vitamin K: Bleeding in the early neonatal period due to coagulation defects may follow exposure to anticonvulsant drugs *in utero;* therefore, vitamin K should be given to the mother before delivery or to the child at birth.

Information for the Patient
Practitioners should give the following information and instructions to patients receiving barbiturates.

1. The use of barbiturates carries with it an associated risk of psychological and/or physical dependence. The patient should be warned against increasing the dose of the drug without consulting a physician.
2. Barbiturates may impair mental and/or physical abilities required for the performance of potentially hazardous tasks. (e.g., driving, operating machinery, etc.)
3. Alcohol should not be consumed while taking barbiturates. Concurrent use of the barbiturates with other CNS depressants (e.g., alcohol, narcotics, tranquilizers, and antihistamines) may result in additional CNS depressant effects.

Laboratory Tests
Prolonged therapy with barbiturates should be accompanied by periodic laboratory evaluation of organ systems, including hematopoietic, renal, and hepatic systems. (See PRECAUTIONS [General] and ADVERSE REACTIONS.)

Drug Interactions
Most reports of clinically significant drug interactions occurring with the barbiturates have involved phenobarbital. However, the application of these data to other barbiturates appears valid and warrants serial blood level determinations of the relevant drugs when there are multiple therapies.
1. *Anticoagulants.* Phenobarbital lowers the plasma levels of dicumarol (name previously used: bishydroxycoumarin) and causes a decrease in anticoagulant activity as measured by the prothrombin time. Barbiturates can induce hepatic microsomal enzymes resulting in increased metabolism and decreased anticoagulant response of oral anticoagulants (eg, warfarin, acenocoumarol, dicumarol, and phenprocoumon). Patients stabilized on anticoagulant therapy may require dosage adjustments if barbiturates are added to or withdrawn from their dosage regimen.
2. *Corticosteroids.* Barbiturates appear to enhance the metabolism of exogenous corticosteroids probably through the induction of hepatic microsomal enzymes. Patients stabilized on corticosteroid therapy may require dosage adjustments if barbiturates are added to or withdrawn from their dosage regimen.
3. *Griseofulvin.* Phenobarbital appears to interfere with the absorption of orally administered griseofulvin, thus decreasing its blood level. The effect of the resultant decreased blood levels of griseofulvin on therapeutic response has not been established. However, it would be preferable to avoid concomitant administration of these drugs.
4. *Doxycycline.* Phenobarbital has been shown to shorten the half-life of doxycycline for as long as 2 weeks after barbiturate therapy is discontinued.
This mechanism is probably through the induction of hepatic microsomal enzymes that metabolize the antibiotic. If phenobarbital and doxycycline are administered concurrently, the clinical response to doxycycline should be monitored closely.
5. *Phenytoin, Sodium Valproate, Valproic Acid.* The effect of barbiturates on the metabolism of phenytoin appears to be variable. Some investigators report an accelerating effect, while others report no effect. Because the effect of barbiturates on the metabolism of phenytoin is not predictable, phenytoin and barbiturate blood levels should be monitored more frequently if these drugs are given concurrently. Sodium valproate and valproic acid appear to decrease barbi-

turate metabolism; therefore, barbiturate blood levels should be monitored and appropriate dosage adjustments made as indicated.

6. *Central Nervous System Depressants.* The concomitant use of other central nervous system depressants, including other sedatives or hypnotics, antihistamines, tranquilizers, or alcohol, may produce additive depressant effects.

7. *Monoamine Oxidase Inhibitors (MAOI).* MAOI prolong the effects of barbiturates probably because metabolism of the barbiturate is inhibited.

8. *Estradiol, Estrone, Progesterone, and other Steroidal Hormones.* Pretreatment with or concurrent administration of phenobarbital may decrease the effect of estradiol by increasing its metabolism. There have been reports of patients treated with antiepileptic drugs (e.g. phenobarbital) who become pregnant while taking oral contraceptives. An alternant contraceptive method might be suggested to women taking phenobarbital.

Carcinogenesis

Animal Data. Phenobarbital sodium is carcinogenic in mice and rats after lifetime administration. In mice, it produced benign and malignant liver cell tumors. In rats, benign liver cell tumors were observed very late in life. Phenobarbital is the major metabolite of MEBARAL.

Human Data. In a 29-year epidemiological study of 9,136 patients who were treated on an anticonvulsant protocol which included phenobarbital, results indicated a higher than normal incidence of hepatic carcinoma. Previously, some of these patients were treated with thorotrast, a drug which is known to produce hepatic carcinomas. Thus, this study did not provide sufficient evidence that phenobarbital sodium is carcinogenic in humans. Phenobarbital is the major metabolite of MEBARAL.

A retrospective study of 84 children with brain tumors matched to 73 normal controls and 78 cancer controls (malignant disease other than brain tumors) suggested an association between exposure to barbiturates prenatally and an increased incidence of brain tumors.

Pregnancy

Teratogenic Effects. Pregnancy Category D—See WARNINGS—Use in Pregnancy.

Nonteratogenic Effects. Reports of infants suffering from long-term barbiturate exposure *in utero* included the acute withdrawal syndrome of seizures and hyperirritability from birth to a delayed onset of up to 14 days. (See DRUG ABUSE AND DEPENDENCE.)

Labor and Delivery.

Hypnotic doses of these barbiturates do not appear to significantly impair uterine activity during labor. Full anesthetic doses of barbiturates decrease the force and frequency of uterine contractions. Administration of sedative-hypnotic barbiturates to the mother during labor may result in respiratory depression in the newborn. Premature infants are particularly susceptible to the depressant effects of barbiturates. If barbiturates are used during labor and delivery, resuscitation equipment should be available.

Data are currently not available to evaluate the effect of these barbiturates when forceps delivery or other intervention is necessary. Also, data are not available to determine the effect of these barbiturates on the later growth, development, and functional maturation of the child.

Nursing Mothers.

Caution should be exercised when a barbiturate is administered to a nursing woman since small amounts of barbiturates are excreted in the milk.

ADVERSE REACTIONS

The following adverse reactions and their incidence were compiled from surveillance of thousands of hospitalized patients. Because such patients may be less aware of certain of the milder adverse effects of barbiturates, the incidence of these reactions may be somewhat higher in fully ambulatory patients.

More than 1 in 100 Patients. The most common adverse reaction estimated to occur at a rate of 1 to 3 patients per 100 is:

Nervous System: Somnolence.

Less than 1 in 100 Patients. Adverse reactions estimated to occur at a rate of less than 1 in 100 patients listed below, grouped by organ system, and by decreasing order of occurrence are:

Nervous System: Agitation, confusion, hyperkinesia, ataxia, CNS depression, nightmares, nervousness, psychiatric disturbance, hallucinations, insomnia, anxiety, dizziness, thinking abnormality.

Respiratory System: Hypoventilation, apnea.

Cardiovascular System: Bradycardia, hypotension, syncope.

Digestive System: Nausea, vomiting, constipation.

Other Reported Reactions: Headache, hypersensitivity reactions (angioedema, skin rashes, exfoliative dermatitis), fever, liver damage, megaloblastic anemia following chronic phenobarbital use.

DRUG ABUSE AND DEPENDENCE

Mephobarbital is a controlled substance in Narcotic Schedule IV. Barbiturates may be habit forming. Tolerance, psy-

chological dependence, and physical dependence may occur especially following prolonged use of high doses of barbiturates. As tolerance to barbiturates develops, the amount needed to maintain the same level of intoxication increases; tolerance to a fatal dosage, however, does not increase more than two-fold. As this occurs, the margin between an intoxicating dosage and fatal dosage becomes smaller.

Symptoms of acute intoxication with barbiturates include unsteady gait, slurred speech, and sustained nystagmus. Mental signs of chronic intoxication include confusion, poor judgment, irritability, insomnia, and somatic complaints. Symptoms of barbiturate dependence are similar to those of chronic alcoholism. If an individual appears to be intoxicated with alcohol to a degree that is radically disproportionate to the amount of alcohol in his or her blood the use of barbiturates should be suspected. The lethal dose of a barbiturate is far less if alcohol is also ingested.

The symptoms of barbiturate withdrawal can be severe and may cause death. Minor withdrawal symptoms may appear 8 to 12 hours after the last dose of a barbiturate. These symptoms usually appear in the following order: anxiety, muscle twitching, tremor of hands and fingers, progressive weakness, dizziness, distortion in visual perception, nausea, vomiting, insomnia, and orthostatic hypotension. Major withdrawal symptoms (convulsions and delirium) may occur within 16 hours and last up to 5 days after abrupt cessation of these drugs. Intensity of withdrawal symptoms gradually declines over a period of approximately 15 days. Individuals susceptible to a barbiturate abuse and dependence include alcoholics and opiate abusers, as well as other sedative-hypnotic and amphetamine abusers.

Drug dependence to barbiturates arises from repeated administration of a barbiturate or agent with barbiturate-like effect on a continuous basis, generally in amounts exceeding therapeutic dose levels. The characteristics of drug dependence to barbiturates include: (a) a strong desire or need to continue taking the drug; (b) a tendency to increase the dose; (c) a psychic dependence on the effects of the drug related to subjective and individual appreciation of those effects; and (d) a physical dependence on the effects of the drug requiring its presence for maintenance of homeostasis and resulting in a definite, characteristic, and self-limited abstinence syndrome when the drug is withdrawn.

Treatment of barbiturate dependence consists of cautious and gradual withdrawal of the drug. Barbiturate-dependent patients can be withdrawn by using a number of different withdrawal regimens. In all cases withdrawal takes an extended period of time. One method involves substituting a 30 mg dose of phenobarbital for each 100 mg to 200 mg dose of barbiturate that the patient has been taking. The total daily amount of phenobarbital is then administered in 3 to 4 divided doses, not to exceed 600 mg daily. Should signs of withdrawal occur on the first day of treatment, a loading dose of 100 mg to 200 mg of phenobarbital may be administered IM in addition to the oral dose. After stabilization on phenobarbital, the total daily dose is decreased by 30 mg a day as long as withdrawal is proceeding smoothly. A modification of this regimen involves initiating treatment at the patient's regular dosage level and decreasing the daily dosage by 10% if tolerated by the patient.

Infants physically dependent on barbiturates may be given phenobarbital 3 mg/kg/day to 10 mg/kg/day. After withdrawal symptoms (hyperactivity, disturbed sleep, tremors, hyperreflexia) are relieved, the dosage of phenobarbital should be gradually decreased and completely withdrawn over a 2-week period.

OVERDOSAGE

The toxic dose of barbiturates varies considerably. In general, an oral dose of 1 g of most barbiturates produces serious poisoning in an adult. Death commonly occurs after 2 g to 10 g of ingested barbiturate. Barbiturate intoxication may be confused with alcoholism, bromide intoxication, and with various neurological disorders.

Acute overdosage with barbiturates is manifested by CNS and respiratory depression which may progress to Cheyne-Stokes respiration, areflexia, constriction of the pupils to a slight degree (though in severe poisoning they may show paralytic dilation), oliguria, tachycardia, hypotension, lowered body temperature, and coma. Typical shock syndrome (apnea, circulatory collapse, respiratory arrest, and death) may occur.

In extreme overdose, all electrical activity in the brain may cease, in which case a "flat" EEG normally equated with clinical death cannot be accepted. This effect is fully reversible unless hypoxic damage occurs. Consideration should be given to the possibility of barbiturate intoxication even in situations that appear to involve trauma.

Complications such as pneumonia, pulmonary edema, cardiac arrhythmias, congestive heart failure, and renal failure may occur. Uremia may increase CNS sensitivity to barbiturates if renal function is impaired. Differential diagnosis should include hypoglycemia, head trauma, cerebrovascular accidents, convulsive states, and diabetic coma.

Treatment of overdosage is mainly supportive and consists of the following:

1. Maintenance of an adequate airway, with assisted respiration and oxygen administration as necessary.
2. Monitoring of vital signs and fluid balance.
3. If the patient is conscious and has not lost the gag reflex, emesis may be induced with ipecac. Care should be taken to prevent pulmonary aspiration of vomitus. After completion of vomiting, 30 g activated charcoal in a glass of water may be administered.
4. If emesis is contraindicated, gastric lavage may be performed with a cuffed endotracheal tube in place with the patient in the face down position. Activated charcoal may be left in the emptied stomach and a saline cathartic administered.
5. Fluid therapy and other standard treatment for shock, if needed.
6. If renal function is normal, forced diuresis may aid in the elimination of the barbiturate. Alkalinization of the urine increases renal excretion of some barbiturates, including mephobarbital (which is metabolized to phenobarbital).
7. Although not recommended as a routine procedure, hemodialysis may be used in severe barbiturate intoxications or if the patient is anuric or in shock.
8. Patient should be rolled from side to side every 30 minutes.
9. Antibiotics should be given if pneumonia is suspected.
10. Appropriate nursing care to prevent hypostatic pneumonia, decubiti aspiration, and other complications of patients with altered states of consciousness.

DOSAGE AND ADMINISTRATION

Epilepsy: Average dose for adults: 400 mg to 600 mg (6 grains to 9 grains) daily; children under 5 years: 16 mg to 32 mg ($^1/_4$ grain to $^1/_2$ grain) three or four times daily; children over 5 years: 32 mg to 64 mg ($^1/_2$ grain to 1 grain) three or four times daily. MEBARAL is best taken at bedtime if seizures generally occur at night, and during the day if attacks are diurnal.

Treatment should be started with a small dose which is gradually increased over four or five days until the optimum dosage is determined. If the patient has been taking some other antiepileptic drug, it should be tapered off as the doses of MEBARAL are increased, to guard against the temporary marked attacks that may occur when any treatment for epilepsy is changed abruptly. Similarly, when the dose is to be lowered to a maintenance level or to be discontinued, the amount should be reduced gradually over four or five days.

Special Patient Population. Dosage should be reduced in the elderly or debilitated because these patients may be more sensitive to barbiturates. Dosage should be reduced for patients with impaired renal function or hepatic disease.

Combination with Other Drugs: MEBARAL may be used in combination with phenobarbital, either in the form of alternating courses or concurrently. When the two drugs are used at the same time, the dose should be about one-half the amount of each used alone. The average daily dose for an adult is from 50 mg to 100 mg ($^3/_4$ grain to $1^1/_2$ grains) of phenobarbital and from 200 mg to 300 mg (3 grains to $4^1/_2$ grains) of MEBARAL.

MEBARAL may also be used with phenytoin sodium; in some cases, combined therapy appears to give better results than either agent used alone, since phenytoin sodium is particularly effective for the psychomotor types of seizure but relatively ineffective for petit mal. When the drugs are employed concurrently, a reduced dose of phenytoin sodium is advisable, but the full dose of MEBARAL may be given. Satisfactory results have been obtained with an average daily dose of 230 mg ($3^1/_2$ grains) of phenytoin sodium plus about 600 mg (9 grains) of MEBARAL.

Sedation: Adults: 32 mg to 100 mg ($^1/_2$ grain to $1^1/_2$ grains)—optimum dose, 50 mg ($^3/_4$ grain)—three to four times daily. Children: 16 mg to 32 mg ($^1/_4$ grain to $^1/_2$ grain) three to four times daily.

HOW SUPPLIED

Tablets—white, round, convex and the 32 mg and 50 mg tablets are scored.

32 mg ($^1/_2$ grain), bottles of 250
(NDC 0024-1231-05)
50 mg ($^3/_4$ grain), bottles of 250
(NDC 0024-1232-05)
100 mg ($1^1/_2$ grains), bottles of 250
(NDC 0024-1233-05)

Store at room temperature up to 25° C (77° F).

Caution: Federal law prohibits dispensing without prescription.

MSW-9B

Continued on next page

This product information was prepared in September 1998. On these and other products of Sanofi Pharmaceuticals, Inc., detailed information may be obtained on a current basis by direct inquiry to Product Information Services, 90 Park Avenue, New York, NY 10016 (toll free 1-800-446-6267).

NegGram® ℞

NALIDIXIC ACID, USP

DESCRIPTION

NegGram®, brand of nalidixic acid, is a quinolone antibacterial agent for oral administration. Nalidixic acid is 1-ethyl-1, 4-dihydro-7-methyl-4-oxo-1, 8-naphthyridine-3-carboxylic acid. It a pale yellow, crystalline substance and a very weak organic acid.

Nalidixic acid has the following structural formula:

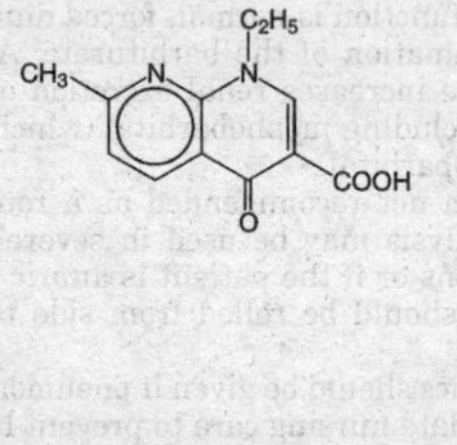

Inactive Ingredients—SUSPENSION: Carbomer 934P, FD&C Red #40, Flavor, Parabens, Purified Water, Saccharin Sodium, Sodium Chloride, Sorbitol Solution. CAPLETS: Hydrogenated Vegetable Oil, Methylcellulose, Microcrystalline Cellulose, Sodium Lauryl Sulfate, Yellow Ferric Oxide.

CLINICAL PHARMACOLOGY

Following oral administration, NegGram is rapidly absorbed from the gastrointestinal tract, partially metabolized in the liver, and rapidly excreted through the kidneys. Unchanged nalidixic acid appears in the urine along with an active metabolite, hydroxynalidixic acid, which has antibacterial activity similar to that of nalidixic acid. Other metabolites include glucuronic acid conjugates of nalidixic acid and hydroxy nalidixic acid, and the dicarboxylic acid derivative. The hydroxy metabolite represents 30 percent of the biologically active drug in the blood and 85 percent in the urine. Peak serum levels of active drug average approximately 20 mcg to 40 mcg per mL (90 percent protein bound), one to two hours after administration of a 1 g dose to a fasting normal individual, with a half-life of about 90 minutes. Peak urine levels of active drug average approximately 150 mcg to 200 mcg per mL, three to four hours after administration, with a half-life of about six hours. Approximately four percent of NegGram is excreted in the feces. Traces of nalidixic acid were found in blood and urine of an infant whose mother had received the drug during the last trimester of pregnancy. (See PRECAUTIONS—Drug Interactions.)

Microbiology

NegGram has marked antibacterial activity against gram-negative bacteria including *Enterobacter* species, *Escherichia coli, Morganella Morganii; Proteus Mirabilis, Proteus vulgaris,* and *Providencia rettgeri. Pseudomonas* species are generally resistant to the drug. NegGram is bactericidal and is effective over the entire urinary pH range. Conventional chromosomal resistance to NegGram taken in full dosage has been reported to emerge in approximately 2 to 14 percent of patients during treatment; however, bacterial resistance to NegGram has not been shown to be transferable via R factor.

Susceptibility Test

Diffusion Techniques: Quantitative methods that require measurement of zone diameters give the most precise estimates of antibacterial susceptibility. One such procedure recommended for use with a disc containing 30 mcg of nalidixic acid is the National Committee for Clinical Laboratory Standards (NCCLS) approved procedure. Only organisms from urinary tract infections should be tested. Results of laboratory tests using 30 mcg nalidixic acid discs should be interpreted using the following criteria:

Zone Diameter (mm)	Interpretation
≥ 19	(S) Susceptible
14–18	(I) Intermediate
≤ 13	(R) Resistant

Dilution Techniques: Broth and agar dilution methods, such as those recommended by the NCCLS, may be used to determine the minimum inhibitory concentration (MIC) of nalidixic acid. MIC test results should be interpreted according to the following criteria:

MIC (mcg/mL)	Interpretation
≤16	(S) Susceptible
≥32	(R) Resistant

For any susceptibility test, a report of "susceptible" indicates that the pathogen is likely to respond to nalidixic acid therapy. A report of "resistant" indicates that the pathogen is not likely to respond. A report of "intermediate" generally indicates that the test result is equivocal.

The Quality Control strains should have the following assigned daily ranges for nalidixic acid:

QC Strains
E. Coli
(ATCC 25922)

Disc Zone Diameter
22–28

MIC (mcg/mL)
1.0–4.0

INDICATIONS AND USAGE

NegGram is indicated for the treatment of urinary tract infections caused by susceptible gram-negative microorganisms, including the majority of *E. Coli, Enterobacter* species, *Klebsiella* species, and *Proteus* species. Disc susceptibility testing with the 30 mcg disc should be performed prior to administration of the drug, and during treatment if clinical response warrants.

CONTRAINDICATIONS

NegGram is contraindicated in patients with known hypersensitivity to nalidixic acid and in patients with a history of convulsive disorders.

WARNINGS

Central Nervous System (CNS) effects including convulsions, increased intracranial pressure, and toxic psychosis have been reported with nalidixic acid therapy. Convulsive seizures have been reported with other drugs in this class. Quinolones may also cause CNS stimulation which may lead to tremor, restlessness, lightheadedness, confusion, and hallucinations. Therefore, nalidixic acid should be used with caution in patients with known or suspected CNS disorders, such as, cerebral arteriosclerosis or epilepsy, or other factors which predispose seizures. (See ADVERSE REACTIONS.) If these reactions occur in patients receiving nalidixic acid, the drug should be discontinued and appropriate measures instituted.

Serious and occasionally fatal hypersensitivity (anaphylactoid) reactions, some following the first dose, have been reported in patients receiving quinolone therapy. Some reactions were accompanied by cardiovascular collapse, loss of consciousness, tingling, pharyngeal or facial edema, dyspnea, urticaria, and itching. Only a few patients had a history of hypersensitivity reactions. Serious anaphylactoid reactions required immediate emergency treatment with epinephrine. Oxygen, intravenous steroids, and airway management, including intubation, should be administered as indicated.

Nalidixic acid and other members of the quinolone drug class have been shown to cause arthropathy in juvenile animals. (See PRECAUTIONS and ANIMAL PHARMACOLOGY.)

Pseudomembranous colitis has been reported with nearly all antibacterial agents, including quinolones, and may range in severity from mild to life-threatening. Therefore, it is important to consider this diagnosis in patients who present with diarrhea subsequent to the administration of antibacterial agents.

Treatment with antibacterial agents alters the normal flora of the colon and may permit overgrowth of clostridia. Studies indicate that a toxin produced by *Clostridium difficile* is one primary cause of "antibiotic-associated colitis".

After the diagnosis of pseudomembranous colitis has been established, therapeutic measures should be initiated. Mild cases of pseudomembranous colitis usually respond to drug discontinuation alone. In moderate to severe cases, consideration should be given to management with fluids and electrolytes, protein supplementation, and treatment with an antibacterial drug clinically effective against *C. difficile* colitis.

PRECAUTIONS

General

Blood counts and renal and liver function tests should be performed periodically if treatment is continued for more than two weeks. NegGram should be used with caution in patients with liver disease, epilepsy, or severe cerebral arteriosclerosis. (See WARNINGS.) While caution should be used in patients with severe renal failure, therapeutic concentrations of NegGram in the urine, without increased toxicity due to drug accumulation in the blood, have been observed in patients on full dosage with creatinine clearances as low as 2 mL/minute to 8 mL/minute.

Moderate to severe phototoxicity reactions have been observed in patients who are exposed to direct sunlight while receiving NegGram or other members of this drug class. Excessive sunlight should be avoided. Therapy should be discontinued if phototoxicity occurs.

If bacterial resistance to NegGram emerges during treatment, it usually does so within 48 hours, permitting rapid change to another antimicrobial. Therefore, if the clinical response is unsatisfactory or if relapse occurs, cultures and sensitivity tests should be repeated. Underdosage with NegGram during initial treatment (with less than 4 g per day for adults) may predispose to emergence of bacterial resistance. (See DOSAGE AND ADMINISTRATION.)

Information for Patients

Patients should be advised NegGram may be taken with or without meals. Patients should be advised to drink fluids liberally and not take antacids.

Patients should be advised that quinolones may be associated with hypersensitivity reactions, even following a single dose, and to discontinue the drug at the first sign of a skin rash or other allergic reactions.

Quinolones may cause dizziness and lightheadedness, therefore, patients should know how they react to NegGram before they operate an automobile or machinery or engage in activities requiring mental alertness or coordination.

Patients should be advised that quinolones may increase the effects of theophylline and caffeine. There is a possibility of caffeine accumulation when products containing caffeine are consumed while taking quinolones. Patients should be advised to avoid excessive sunlight or artificial ultraviolet light while receiving nalidixic acid and to discontinue therapy if phototoxicity occurs.

Drug Interactions

Elevated plasma levels of theophylline have been reported with concomitant quinolone use. There have been reports of theophylline-related side effects in patients on concomitant therapy with quinolones and theophylline. Therefore, monitoring of theophylline plasma levels should be considered and dosage of theophylline adjusted, as required.

Quinolones have been shown to interfere with the metabolism of caffeine. This may lead to reduced clearance of caffeine and the prolongation of its plasma half-life.

Quinolones, including nalidixic acid, may enhance the effects of the oral anticoagulant warfarin or its derivatives. When these products are administered concomitantly, prothrombin time or other suitable coagulation test should be closely monitored.

Nitrofurantoin interferes with the therapeutic action of nalidixic acid.

Antacids containing magnesium, aluminum, or calcium; sucralfate or divalent or trivalent cations such as iron; and multivitamins containing zinc may substantially interfere with the absorption of quinolones, resulting in urine levels considerably lower than desired. They should not be given concomitantly or within two hours of the administration of quinolones.

Elevated serum levels of cyclosporine have been reported with the concomitant use of some quinolones and cyclosporine. Therefore, cyclosporine serum levels should be monitored and appropriate cyclosporine dosage adjustments made when these drugs are used concomitantly.

Drug Laboratory Test Interactions

When Benedict's or Fehling's solution or Clinitest® Reagent Tablets are used to test the urine of patients taking NegGram, a false-positive reaction for glucose may be obtained, due to the liberation of glucuronic acid from the metabolites excreted. However, a colorimetric test for glucose based on an enzyme reaction (e.g., with Clinistix® Reagent Strips or Tes-Tape®) does not give a false-positive reaction to the liberated glucuronic acid.

Incorrect values may be obtained for urinary 17-keto and ketogenic steroids in patients receiving NegGram, because of an interaction between the drug and the *m*-dinitrobenzene used in the usual assay method. In such cases, the Porter-Silber test for 17-hydroxycorticoids may be used.

Carcinogenesis, Mutagenesis, Impairment of Fertility

In lifetime studies in the rat given nalidixic acid in the diet, there was an increased incidence of preputial gland neoplasms in the treated males and clitoral gland neoplasms in the treated females. Studies in mice in which nalidixic acid was administered in the feed for two years, or was given in the feed for 76 weeks followed by no treatment for 9 weeks, gave equivocal evidence of carcinogenic activity.

Nalidixic acid was tested in the Ames bacterial mutagenicity test (maximum dose 33 mcg/plate) and the mouse lymphoma assay (L5178Y/TK; maximum dose 100 mcg/mL) with and without metabolic activation, and results were negative.

Pregnancy: Teratogenic Effects.

Pregnancy Category C.

NegGram has been shown to be teratogenic and embryocidal in rats when given in oral doses six times the human dose. NegGram also prolonged the duration of pregnancy especially at four times the clinical dose. There are no adequate and well-controlled studies in pregnant women. Since nalidixic acid, like other drugs in this class, causes arthropathy in immature animals, NegGram should be used during pregnancy only if the potential benefit justifies the potential risk to the fetus. (See WARNINGS and ANIMAL PHARMACOLOGY.)

Nursing Mothers

It is not known whether NegGram is excreted in human milk. Because other drugs are excreted in human milk and because of the potential for serious adverse reactions in nursing infants from NegGram, a decision should be made

whether to discontinue nursing or to discontinue the drug taking into account the importance of the drug to the mother.

Pediatric Use

Safety and effectiveness in infants below the age of three months have not been established.

Usage in Patients Under 18 Years of Age

Toxicological studies have shown that nalidixic acid and related drugs can produce erosions of the cartilage in weight-bearing joints and other signs of arthropathy in immature animals of most species tested. No such joint lesions have been reported in humans to date. Nevertheless, until the significance of this finding is clarified, this drug should only be used in patients under 18 years of age when the potential benefit justifies the potential risk. (See WARNINGS and ANIMAL PHARMACOLOGY.)

ADVERSE REACTIONS

Reactions reported after oral administration of NegGram include the following.

CNS effects: drowsiness, weakness, headache, and dizziness and vertigo. Reversible subjective visual disturbances without objective findings have occurred infrequently (generally with each dose during the first few days of treatment). These reactions include overbrightness of lights, change in color perception, difficulty in focusing, decrease in visual acuity, and double vision. They usually disappeared promptly when dosage was reduced or therapy was discontinued. Toxic psychosis or brief convulsions have been reported rarely, usually following excessive doses. In general, the convulsions have occurred in patients with predisposing factors such as epilepsy or cerebral arteriosclerosis. In infants and children receiving therapeutic doses of NegGram, increased intracranial pressure with bulging anterior fontanel, papilledema, and headache has occasionally been observed. A few cases of 6th cranial nerve palsy have been reported. Although the mechanisms of these reactions are unknown, the signs and symptoms usually disappeared rapidly with no sequelae when treatment was discontinued.

Gastrointestinal: abdominal pain, nausea, vomiting, and diarrhea.

Allergic: rash, pruritus, urticaria, angioedema, eosinophilia, arthralgia with joint stiffness and swelling, and anaphylactoid reaction. Erythema Multiforme and Stevens-Johnson syndrome have been reported with nalidixic acid and other drugs in this class. Rash was the most frequently reported adverse reaction. Photosensitivity reactions consisting of erythema and bullae on exposed skin surfaces usually resolve completely in 2 weeks to 2 months after NegGram is discontinued; however, bullae may continue to appear with successive exposures to sunlight or with mild skin trauma for up to 3 months after discontinuation of drug. (See PRECAUTIONS.)

Other: rarely, cholestasis, paresthesia, metabolic acidosis, thrombocytopenia, leukopenia, or hemolytic anemia, sometimes associated with glucose 6-phosphate dehydrogenase deficiency.

OVERDOSAGE

Manifestations: Toxic psychosis, convulsions, increased intracranial pressure, or metabolic acidosis may occur in patients taking more than the recommended dosage. Vomiting, nausea, and lethargy may also occur following overdosage.

Treatment: Reactions are short-lived (two or three hours) because the drug is rapidly excreted. If overdosage is noted early, gastric lavage is indicated. If absorption has occurred, increased fluid administration is advisable and supportive measures such as oxygen and means of artificial respiration should be available. Although anticonvulsant therapy has not been used in the few instances of overdosage reported, it may be indicated in a severe case.

DOSAGE AND ADMINISTRATION

Adults. The recommended dosage for initial therapy in adults is 1 g administered four times daily for one or two weeks (total daily dose, 4 g). For prolonged therapy, the total daily dose may be reduced to 2 g after the initial treatment period. Underdosage during initial treatment may predispose to emergence of bacterial resistance.

Children. Until further experience is gained, NegGram should not be administered to infants younger than three months. Dosage in children 12 years of age and under should be calculated on the basis of body weight. The recommended total daily dosage for initial therapy is 25 mg/lb/day (55 mg/kg/day), administered in four equally divided doses. For prolonged therapy, the total daily dose may be reduced to 15 mg/lb/day (33 mg/kg/day). NegGram Suspension or NegGram Caplets of 250 mg may be used. One 250 mg tablet is equivalent to one teaspoon (5 mL) of the Suspension.

HOW SUPPLIED

Suspension (250 mg/5 mL tsp), raspberry flavored, bottles of 1 pint (NDC 0024-1318-06)

Caplets of 1 g, light buff-colored capsule-shaped tablets, bottles of 100 (NDC 0024-1323-04)

Caplets of 500 mg, light buff-colored capsule-shaped tablets, bottles of 56 (NDC 0024-1322-03) 500 (NDC 0024-1322-06)

Caplets of 250 mg, light buff-colored capsule-shaped tablets, bottles of 56 (NDC 0024-1321-03)

Store suspension at room temperature up to 25° C (77° F).

Store caplets at room temperature, up to 30° C (86° F).

ANIMAL PHARMACOLOGY

NegGram (nalidixic acid) and related drugs have been shown to cause arthropathy in juvenile animals of most species tested. (See WARNINGS.)

Long-term administration of nalidixic acid to rats resulted in retinal degeneration and cataracts.

Hydroxynalidixic acid, the principal metabolite of NegGram, did not produce any oculotoxic effects at any dosage level in seven species of animals including three primate species. However, oral administration of this metabolite in high doses has been shown to have oculotoxic potential, namely in dogs and cats where it produced retinal degeneration upon prolonged administration leading, in some cases, to blindness.

In experiments with NegGram itself, little if any such activity could be elicited in either dogs or cats. Sensitivity to CNS side effects in these species limited the doses of NegGram that could be used; this factor, together with a low conversion rate to the hydroxy metabolite in these species, may explain the absence of these effects.

NSW-6 C (0)

Shown in Product Identification Guide, page 335

NEO–SYNEPHRINE® Hydrochloride ℞
brand of phenylephrine hydrochloride
ophthalmic solution, USP
Vasoconstrictor and Mydriatic
SOLUTIONS 2.5% AND 10%
VISCOUS SOLUTION 10%

For Use in Ophthalmology

WARNING: PHYSICIANS SHOULD COMPLETELY FAMILIARIZE THEMSELVES WITH THE COMPLETE CONTENTS OF THIS LEAFLET BEFORE PRESCRIBING NEO-SYNEPHRINE.

DESCRIPTION

NEO-SYNEPHRINE hydrochloride, brand of phenylephrine hydrochloride ophthalmic solution, is a sterile solution used as a vasoconstrictor and mydriatic for use in ophthalmology. NEO-SYNEPHRINE hydrochloride is a synthetic sympathomimetic compound structurally similar to epinephrine and ephedrine.

Phenylephrine hydrochloride is (–)-*m* -Hydroxy-α-[(methylamino)methyl] benzyl alcohol hydrochloride, and has the following structural formula:

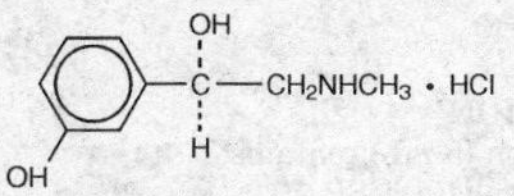

CLINICAL PHARMACOLOGY

NEO-SYNEPHRINE possesses predominantly α-adrenergic effects. In the eye, phenylephrine acts locally as a potent vasoconstrictor and mydriatic, by constricting ophthalmic blood vessels and the radial muscle of the iris.

The ophthalmologic usefulness of NEO-SYNEPHRINE hydrochloride is due to its rapid effect and moderately prolonged action, as well as to the fact that it produces no compensatory vasodilatation.

The action of different concentrations of ophthalmic solutions of NEO-SYNEPHRINE hydrochloride is shown in the following table:

Strength of solution (%)	Mydriasis		Paralysis of accommodation
	Maximal (minutes)	Recovery time (hours)	
2.5	15–60	3	trace
10	10–60	6	slight

Although rare, systemic absorption of sufficient quantities of phenylephrine may lead to systemic α-adrenergic effects, such as rise in blood pressure which may be accompanied by a reflex atropine-sensitive bradycardia.

INDICATIONS AND USAGE

NEO-SYNEPHRINE hydrochloride is recommended for use as a decongestant and vasoconstrictor and for pupil dilatation in uveitis (posterior synechiae), wide angle glaucoma, prior to surgery, refraction, ophthalmoscopic examination, and diagnostic procedures.

CONTRAINDICATIONS

Ophthalmic solutions of NEO-SYNEPHRINE hydrochloride are contraindicated in persons with narrow angle glaucoma (and in those individuals who are hypersensitive to NEO-SYNEPHRINE). NEO-SYNEPHRINE hydrochloride 10 percent ophthalmic solutions are contraindicated in infants and in patients with aneurysms.

WARNINGS

There have been rare reports associating the use of NEO-SYNEPHRINE 10 percent ophthalmic solutions with the development of serious cardiovascular reactions, including ventricular arrhythmias and myocardial infarctions. These episodes, some ending fatally, have usually occurred in elderly patients with preexisting cardiovascular diseases.

PRECAUTIONS

Exceeding recommended dosages or applying NEO-SYNEPHRINE hydrochloride ophthalmic solutions to the instrumented, traumatized, diseased or postsurgical eye or adnexa, or to patients with suppressed lacrimation, as during anesthesia, may result in the absorption of sufficient quantities of phenylephrine to produce a systemic vasopressor response.

A significant elevation in blood pressure is rare but has been reported following conjunctival instillation of recommended doses of NEO-SYNEPHRINE 10 percent ophthalmic solutions. Caution, therefore, should be exercised in administering the 10 percent solutions to children of low body weight, the elderly, and patients with insulin-dependent diabetes, hypertension, hyperthyroidism, generalized arteriosclerosis, or cardiovascular disease. The posttreatment blood pressure of these patients, and any patients who develop symptoms, should be carefully monitored.

Ordinarily, any mydriatic, including NEO-SYNEPHRINE hydrochloride, solution, is contraindicated in patients with glaucoma, since it may occasionally raise intraocular pressure. However, when temporary dilatation of the pupil may free adhesions or when vasoconstriction of intrinsic vessels may lower intraocular tension, these advantages may temporarily outweigh the danger from coincident dilatation of the pupil.

Rebound miosis has been reported in older persons one day after receiving NEO-SYNEPHRINE hydrochloride ophthalmic solutions, and reinstillation of the drug produced a reduction in mydriasis. This may be of clinical importance in dilating the pupils of older subjects prior to retinal detachment or cataract surgery.

Due to a strong action of the drug on the dilator muscle, older individuals may also develop transient pigment floaters in the aqueous humor 30 to 45 minutes following the administration of NEO-SYNEPHRINE hydrochloride ophthalmic solutions. The appearance may be similar to anterior uveitis or to a microscopic hyphema.

To prevent pain, a drop of suitable topical anesthetic may be applied before using the 10 percent ophthalmic solution.

Drug Interaction: As with all other adrenergic drugs, when NEO-SYNEPHRINE 10 percent ophthalmic solutions or 2.5 percent ophthalmic solution is administered simultaneously with, or up to 21 days after, administration of monoamine oxidase (MAO) inhibitors, careful supervision and adjustment of dosages are required since exaggerated adrenergic effects may occur. The pressor response of adrenergic agents may also be potentiated by tricyclic antidepressants, propranolol, reserpine, guanethidine, methyldopa, and atropine-like drugs.

It has been reported that the concomitant use of NEO-SYNEPHRINE 10 percent ophthalmic solutions and systemic beta blockers has caused acute hypertension and, in one case, the rupture of a congenital cerebral aneurysm. NEO-SYNEPHRINE may potentiate the cardiovascular depressant effects of potent inhalation anesthetic agents.

Carcinogenesis, Mutagenesis, Impairment of Fertility: No long-term animal studies have been done to evaluate the potential of NEO-SYNEPHRINE in these areas.

Pregnancy Category C: Animal reproduction studies have not been conducted with NEO-SYNEPHRINE. It is also not known whether NEO-SYNEPHRINE can cause fetal harm when administered to a pregnant woman or can affect reproduction capacity. NEO-SYNEPHRINE should be given to a pregnant woman only if clearly needed.

Nursing Mothers: It is not known whether this drug is excreted in milk; many are. Caution should be exercised when NEO-SYNEPHRINE hydrochloride ophthalmic solution is administered to a nursing woman.

Continued on next page

This product information was prepared in September 1998. On these and other products of Sanofi Pharmaceuticals, Inc., detailed information may be obtained on a current basis by direct inquiry to Product Information Services, 90 Park Avenue, New York, NY 10016 (toll free 1-800-446-6267).

Neo-Synephrine Solutions—Cont.

Pediatric Use: NEO-SYNEPHRINE hydrochloride 10 percent ophthalmic solutions are contraindicated in infants. (See CONTRAINDICATIONS.) For use in older children see DOSAGE AND ADMINISTRATION.

Exceeding recommended dosages or applying NEO-SYNEPHRINE hydrochloride ophthalmic solutions to the instrumented, traumatized, diseased or postsurgical eye or adnexa, or to patients with suppressed lacrimation, as during anesthesia, may result in the absorption of sufficient quantities of phenylephrine to produce a systemic vasopressor response.

The hypertensive effects of phenylephrine may be treated with an alpha-adrenergic blocking agent such as phentolamine mesylate, 5 mg to 10 mg intravenously, repeated as necessary.

The oral LD_{50} of phenylephrine in the rat: 350 mg/kg, in the mouse: 120 mg/kg.

DOSAGE AND ADMINISTRATION

Prolonged exposure to air or strong light may cause oxidation and discoloration. Do not use if solution is brown or contains a precipitate.

Vasoconstriction and Pupil Dilatation

NEO-SYNEPHRINE hydrochloride 10 percent ophthalmic solutions are especially useful when rapid and powerful dilatation of the pupil and reduction of congestion in the capillary bed are desired. A drop of a suitable topical anesthetic may be applied, followed in a few minutes by 1 drop of the NEO-SYNEPHRINE hydrochloride 10 percent ophthalmic solutions on the upper limbus. The anesthetic prevents stinging and consequent dilution of the solution by lacrimation. It may occasionally be necessary to repeat the instillation after one hour, again preceded by the use of the topical anesthetic.

Uveitis: Posterior Synechiae

NEO-SYNEPHRINE hydrochloride 10 percent ophthalmic solutions may be used in patients with uveitis when synechiae are present or may develop. The formation of synechiae may be prevented by the use of the 10 percent ophthalmic solutions and atropine to produce wide dilatation of the pupil. It should be emphasized, however, that the vasoconstrictor effect of NEO-SYNEPHRINE hydrochloride may be antagonistic to the increase of local blood flow in uveal infection.

To free recently formed posterior synechiae, 1 drop of the 10 percent ophthalmic solutions may be applied to the upper surface of the cornea. On the following day, treatment may be continued if necessary. In the interim, hot compresses should be applied for five or ten minutes three times a day, with 1 drop of a 1 or 2 percent solution of atropine sulfate before and after each series of compresses.

Glaucoma

In certain patients with glaucoma, temporary reduction of intraocular tension may be attained by producing vasoconstriction of the intraocular vessels; this may be accomplished by placing 1 drop of the 10 percent ophthalmic solutions on the upper surface of the cornea. This treatment may be repeated as often as necessary.

NEO-SYNEPHRINE hydrochloride, may be used with miotics in patients with wide angle glaucoma. It reduces the difficulties experienced by the patient because of the small field produced by miosis, and still it permits and often supports the effect of the miotic in lowering the intraocular pressure. Hence, there may be marked improvement in visual acuity after using NEO-SYNEPHRINE hydrochloride in conjunction with miotic drugs.

Surgery

When a short-acting mydriatic is needed for wide dilatation of the pupil before intraocular surgery, the 10 percent ophthalmic solutions or 2.5 percent ophthalmic solution may be applied topically from 30 to 60 minutes before the operation.

Refraction

Prior to determination of refractive errors, NEO-SYNEPHRINE hydrochloride 2.5 percent ophthalmic solution may be used effectively with homatropine hydrobromide, atropine sulfate, or a combination of homatropine and cocaine hydrochloride.

For *adults,* a drop of the preferred cycloplegic is placed in each eye, followed in five minutes by 1 drop of NEO-SYNEPHRINE hydrochloride 2.5 percent ophthalmic solution and in ten minutes by another drop of the cycloplegic. In 50 to 60 minutes, the eyes are ready for refraction.

For *children,* a drop of atropine sulfate 1 percent is placed in each eye, followed in 10 to 15 minutes by 1 drop of NEO-SYNEPHRINE hydrochloride 2.5 percent ophthalmic solution and in five to ten minutes by a second drop of atropine sulfate 1 percent. In one to two hours, the eyes are ready for refraction.

For a "one application method," NEO-SYNEPHRINE hydrochloride 2.5 percent ophthalmic solution may be combined with a cycloplegic to elicit synergistic action. The additive effect varies depending on the patient. Therefore, when using a "one application method," it may be desirable to increase the concentration of the cycloplegic.

Ophthalmoscopic Examination

One drop of NEO-SYNEPHRINE hydrochloride 2.5 percent ophthalmic solution is placed in each eye. Sufficient mydriasis to permit examination is produced in 15 to 30 minutes. Dilatation lasts from one to three hours.

Diagnostic Procedures

Provocative Test for Angle Block in Patients with Glaucoma: The 2.5 percent ophthalmic solution may be used as a provocative test when latent increased intraocular pressure is suspected. Tension is measured before application of NEO-SYNEPHRINE hydrochloride and again after dilatation. A 3 to 5 mm of mercury rise in pressure suggests the presence of angle block in patients with glaucoma; however, failure to obtain such a rise does not preclude the presence of glaucoma from other causes.

Shadow Test (Retinoscopy): When dilatation of the pupil without cycloplegic action is desired for the shadow test, the 2.5 percent ophthalmic solution may be used alone.

Blanching Test: One or 2 drops of the 2.5 percent ophthalmic solution should be applied to the injected eye. After five minutes, examine for perilimbal blanching. If blanching occurs, the congestion is superficial and probably does not indicate iritis.

HOW SUPPLIED

In Mono-Drop ® (plastic dropper) bottle:

Low surface tension solutions

2.5 percent ophthalmic solution —
NEO-SYNEPHRINE hydrochloride, 2.5 percent in a sterile, isotonic, buffered, low surface tension vehicle with sodium phosphate, sodium biphosphate, boric acid, and, as antiseptic preservative, benzalkonium chloride, NF, 1:7500. The pH is adjusted with phosphoric acid or sodium hydroxide.
Bottles of 15 mL (NDC 0024-1358-01)

10 percent ophthalmic solution —
NEO-SYNEPHRINE hydrochloride 10 percent in a sterile, buffered, low surface tension vehicle with sodium phosphate, sodium biphosphate, and, as antiseptic preservative, benzalkonium chloride 1:10,000. The pH is adjusted with phosphoric acid or sodium hydroxide.
Bottles of 5 mL (NDC 0024-1359-01)

Viscous solution

10 percent ophthalmic solution —
NEO-SYNEPHRINE hydrochloride 10 percent in a sterile, buffered, viscous vehicle with sodium phosphate, sodium biphosphate, methylcellulose, and, as antiseptic preservative, benzalkonium chloride 1:10,000. The pH is adjusted with phosphoric acid or sodium hydroxide.
Bottles of 5 mL (NDC 0024-1362-01)

Store at 25°C (77°F); excursions permitted to 15°C–30°C (59°F–86°F) [see USP Controlled Room Temperature]

Revised January 1998

NSW-5-C

PEDIACOF® Ⓒ℞

DESCRIPTION

Each teaspoon (5 mL) contains:

Codeine phosphate, USP	5.0 mg
(Warning: May be habit forming.)	
Phenylephrine hydrochloride, USP	2.5 mg
Chlorpheniramine maleate, USP	0.75 mg
Potassium iodide, USP	75.0 mg

with sodium benzoate 0.2% as preservative and alcohol 5%.

Inactive Ingredients: Alcohol, Citric Acid, FD&C Red #40, Flavor, Glycerin, Liquid Glucose, Purified Water, Saccharin Sodium, Sodium Benzoate.

HOW SUPPLIED

Raspberry flavored syrup

Bottle of 16 fl oz (**NDC** 0024-1509-06)

Store at room temperature up to 25° C (77° F)

Available on prescription only.

For complete prescribing information see package insert or contact Product Information Services. Revised May 1997

PSW-10B

pHisoHex® ℞

brand of hexachlorophene detergent cleanser

sudsing antibacterial soapless skin cleanser

DESCRIPTION

pHisoHex, brand of hexachlorophene detergent cleanser, is an antibacterial sudsing emulsion for topical administration. pHisoHex contains a colloidal dispersion of hexachlorophene 3% (w/w) in a stable emulsion consisting of entsufon sodium, petrolatum, lanolin cholesterols, methylcellulose, polyethylene glycol, polyethylene glycol monostearate, lauryl myristyl diethanolamide, sodium benzoate, and water. pH is adjusted with hydrochloric acid. Entsufon sodium is a synthetic detergent.

Chemically, hexachlorophene is Phenol, 2,2′-methylenebis[3,4,6-trichloro-].

CLINICAL PHARMACOLOGY

pHisoHex is a bacteriostatic cleansing agent. It cleanses the skin thoroughly and has bacteriostatic action against staphylococci and other gram-positive bacteria. Cumulative antibacterial action develops with repeated use. Cleansing with alcohol or soaps containing alcohol removes the antibacterial residue.

Detectable blood levels of hexachlorophene following absorption through intact skin have been found in subjects who regularly scrubbed with hexachlorophene emulsion 3%. (See **WARNINGS** for additional information.)

pHisoHex has the same slight acidity as normal skin (pH value 5.0 to 6.0).

INDICATIONS AND USAGE

pHisoHex is indicated for use as a surgical scrub and a bacteriostatic skin cleanser. It may also be used to control an outbreak of gram-positive infection where other infection control procedures have been unsuccessful. Use only as long as necessary for infection control.

CONTRAINDICATIONS

pHisoHex should not be used on burned or denuded skin.

It should not be used as an occlusive dressing, wet pack, or lotion.

It should not be used routinely for prophylactic total body bathing.

It should not be used as a vaginal pack or tampon, or on any mucous membranes.

pHisoHex should not be used on persons with sensitivity to any of its components. It should not be used on persons who have demonstrated primary light sensitivity to halogenated phenol derivatives because of the possibility of cross-sensitivity to hexachlorophene.

WARNINGS

RINSE THOROUGHLY AFTER EACH USE. Patients should be closely monitored and use should be immediately discontinued at the first sign of any of the symptoms described below. Rapid absorption of hexachlorophene may occur with resultant toxic blood levels when preparations containing hexachlorophene are applied to skin lesions such as ichthyosis congenita, the dermatitis of Letterer-Siwe's syndrome, or other generalized dermatological conditions. Application to burns has also produced neurotoxicity and death.

pHisoHex SHOULD BE DISCONTINUED PROMPTLY IF SIGNS OR SYMPTOMS OF CEREBRAL IRRITABILITY OCCUR.

Infants, especially premature infants or those with dermatoses, are particularly susceptible to hexachlorophene absorption. Systemic toxicity may be manifested by signs of stimulation (irritation) of the central nervous system, sometimes with convulsions.

Infants have developed dermatitis, irritability, generalized clonic muscular contractions and decerebrate rigidity following application of a 6 percent hexachlorophene powder. Examination of brainstems of those infants revealed vacuolization like that which can be produced in newborn experimental animals following repeated topical application of 3 percent hexachlorophene. Moreover, a study of histologic sections of premature infants who died of unrelated causes has shown a positive correlation between hexachlorophene baths and lesions in white matter of brains.

PRECAUTIONS

General

Avoid accidental contact of pHisoHex with the eyes.

If contact occurs, promptly rinse thoroughly with water. To assist in the detection of ocular irritation, applications to the head and periorbital skin areas should be performed only in responsive patients with unanesthetized eyes.

RINSE THOROUGHLY AFTER USE, especially from sensitive areas such as the scrotum and perineum.

pHisoHex is intended for external use only. If swallowed, pHisoHex is harmful, especially to infants and children. **pHisoHex should not be poured into measuring cups, medicine bottles, or similar containers since it may be mistaken for baby formula or other medications.**

Carcinogenesis, Mutagenesis, Impairment of Fertility

Carcinogenicity studies in animals: Hexachlorophene was tested in one experiment in rats by oral administration; it had no carcinogenic effect.

Hexachlorophene was not mutagenic in *Salmonella typhimurium* and was negative in a dominant lethal assay in male mice. Cytogenetic tests with cultured human lymphocytes were also negative.

Human data: No case reports or epidemiological studies were available.

Impairment of fertility: Topical exposure of neonatal rats to 3% hexachlorophene solution caused reduced fertility in 7-month-old males, due to inability to ejaculate.

Embryotoxicity and Teratogenicity

Placental transfer of hexachlorophene has been demonstrated in rats.

Hexachlorophene is embryotoxic and produces some terato-genic effects.

Pregnancy Category C

There are no adequate and well-controlled studies in pregnant women. Hexachlorophene should be used during pregnancy only if the potential benefit justifies potential risk to the fetus.

Hexachlorophene has been shown to be teratogenic and embryotoxic in rats when given by mouth or instilled into the vagina in large doses.

Administration of 500 mg/kg diet or 20 to 30 mg/kg bw/day by gavage to rats caused some malformations (angulated ribs, cleft palate, micro- and anophthalmia) and reduction in litter size.

Placental transfer and excretion in milk of hexachlorophene has been demonstrated in rats.

In another study, doses of up to 50 mg/kg diet failed to produce any effects in 3 generations of rats. Hexachlorophene did not interfere with reproduction in hamsters.

Nursing Mothers

It is not known whether this drug is excreted in human milk. Because many drugs are excreted in human milk and because of the potential for serious adverse reactions in nursing infants from hexachlorophene, a decision should be made whether to discontinue nursing or to discontinue the drug taking into account the importance of the drug to the mother.

Pediatric Use

pHisoHex, brand of hexachlorophene detergent cleanser, should not be used routinely for bathing infants. See **WARNINGS.** For premature infants: see **WARNINGS.**

ADVERSE REACTIONS

Adverse reactions to pHisoHex may include dermatitis and photosensitivity. Sensitivity to hexachlorophene is rare; however, persons who have developed photoallergy to similar compounds also may become sensitive to hexachlorophene.

In persons with highly sensitive skin the use of pHisoHex may at times produce a reaction characterized by redness and/or mild scaling or dryness, especially when it is combined with such mechanical factors as excessive rubbing or exposure to heat or cold.

OVERDOSAGE

The accidental ingestion of pHisoHex in amounts from 1 oz to 4 oz has caused anorexia, vomiting, abdominal cramps, diarrhea, dehydration, convulsions, hypotension, and shock, and in several reported instances, fatalities.

If patients are seen early, the stomach should be evacuated by emesis or gastric lavage. Olive oil or vegetable oil (60 mL or 2 fl oz) may then be given to delay absorption of hexachlorophene, followed by a saline cathartic to hasten removal. Treatment is symptomatic and supportive; intravenous fluids (5 percent dextrose in physiologic saline solution) may be given for dehydration. Any other electrolyte derangement should be corrected. If marked hypotension occurs, vasopressor therapy is indicated. Use of opiates may be considered if gastrointestinal symptoms (cramping, diarrhea) are severe. Scheduled medical or surgical procedures should be postponed until the patient's condition has been evaluated and stabilized.

DOSAGE AND ADMINISTRATION

Surgical Hand Scrub

1. Wet hands and forearms with water. Apply approximately 5 mL of pHisoHex over the hands and rub into a copious lather by adding small amounts of water. Spread suds over hands and forearms and scrub well with a wet brush for 3 minutes. Pay particular attention to the nails and interdigital spaces. A separate nail cleaner may be used. *Rinse thoroughly* under running water.
2. Apply 5 mL of pHisoHex to hands again and scrub as above for another 3 minutes. *Rinse thoroughly* with running water and dry.
3. For repeat surgical scrubs during the day, scrub thoroughly with the same amount of pHisoHex for 3 minutes only. *Rinse thoroughly* with water and dry.

Bacteriostatic Cleansing

Wet hands with water. Dispense approximately 5 mL of pHisoHex into the palm, work up a lather with water and apply to area to be cleansed.

Rinse thoroughly after each washing.

INFANT CARE: pHisoHex should not be used routinely for bathing infants. See **WARNINGS.**

PREMATURE INFANTS: See **WARNINGS.**

Use of baby skin products containing alcohol may decrease the antibacterial action of pHisoHex, brand of hexachlorophene detergent cleanser.

HOW SUPPLIED

pHisoHex is available in plastic squeeze bottle of 5 ounces (NDC 0024-1535-02) and 1 pint (NDC 0024-1535-06); in plastic bottle of 1 gallon (NDC 0024-1535-08) and $\frac{1}{4}$ oz (8 mL) unit packets, box of 50 (NDC 0024-1535-05).

The following, specially constructed, refillable dispensers made with metals and plastics compatible with pHisoHex can also be supplied: 16 oz hand operated wall dispensers;

30 oz pedal operated wall dispensers; 30 oz pedal operated wall dispenser with stand; portable stand with two 30 oz pedal operated dispensers.

Prolonged direct exposure of pHisoHex to strong light may cause brownish surface discoloration but does not affect its antibacterial or detergent properties. Shaking will disperse the color. If pHisoHex is spilled or splashed on porous surfaces, rinse off to avoid discoloration.

---

pHisoHex should not be dispensed from, or stored in, containers with ordinary metal parts. A special type of stainless steel must be used or undesirable discoloration of the product or oxidation of metal may occur. Specially designed dispensers for hospital or office use may be obtained through your local dealer.

Directions for Cleaning Dispensers: Before initial installation and use, run an antiseptic, such as an aqueous solution of benzalkonium chloride, NF, 1:500 to 1:750, or alcohol, through the working parts; rinse with sterile water. At weekly intervals thereafter, remove dispenser and pour off remainder of pHisoHex emulsion. Rinse empty dispenser with water. Run water through the working parts by operating the dispenser. Sanitize as described above. Rinse thoroughly with sterile water.

ANIMAL TOXICITY

The oral LD$_{50}$ of hexachlorophene in male rats is 66 mg/kg bw, in females 56 mg/kg bw, and in weanling rats 120 mg/kg bw.

In suckling rats (10-days old), it is 9 mg/kg bw.

PSW-9B

PHOTOFRIN® ℞
(porfimer sodium) for Injection

DESCRIPTION

PHOTOFRIN® (porfimer sodium) for Injection is a photosensitizing agent used in the photodynamic therapy (PDT) of tumors. Following reconstitution of the freeze-dried product with 5% Dextrose Injection (USP) or 0.9% Sodium Chloride Injection (USP), it is injected intravenously. This is followed 40–50 hours later by illumination of the tumor with laser light (630 nm wavelength). PHOTOFRIN® is not a single chemical entity; it is a mixture of oligomers formed by ether and ester linkages of up to eight porphyrin units. It is a dark red to reddish brown cake or powder. Each vial of PHOTOFRIN® contains 75 mg of porfimer sodium as a sterile freeze-dried cake or powder. Hydrochloric Acid and/or Sodium Hydroxide may be added during manufacture to adjust pH. There are no preservatives or other additives. The structural formula below is representative of the components present in PHOTOFRIN®.

[See chemical structure at bottom of next page]

CLINICAL PHARMACOLOGY

Pharmacology

The cytotoxic and antitumor actions of PHOTOFRIN® are light and oxygen dependent. Photodynamic therapy (PDT) with PHOTOFRIN® is a two-stage process. The first stage is the intravenous injection of PHOTOFRIN®. Clearance from a variety of tissues occurs over 40–72 hours, but tumors, skin, and organs of the reticuloendothelial system (including liver and spleen) retain PHOTOFRIN® for a longer period. Illumination with 630 nm wavelength laser light constitutes the second stage of therapy. Tumor selectivity in treatment occurs through a combination of selective retention of PHOTOFRIN® and selective delivery of light. Cellular damage caused by PHOTOFRIN® PDT is a consequence of the propagation of radical reactions. Radical initiation may occur after PHOTOFRIN® absorbs light to form a porphyrin excited state. Spin transfer from PHOTOFRIN® to molecular oxygen may then generate singlet oxygen. Subsequent radical reactions can form superoxide and hydroxyl radicals. Tumor death also occurs through ischemic necrosis secondary to vascular occlusion that appears to be partly mediated by thromboxane A$_2$ release. The laser treatment induces a photochemical, not a thermal, effect. The necrotic reaction and associated inflammatory responses may evolve over several days.

Pharmacokinetics

Following a 2 mg/kg dose of porfimer sodium to 4 male cancer patients, the average peak plasma concentration was 15 ± 3 mcg/mL, the elimination half-life was 250 ± 285 hours, the steady-state volume of distribution was 0.49 ± 0.28 L/kg, and the total plasma clearance was 0.051 ± 0.035 mL/min/kg. The mean plasma concentration at 48 hours was 2.6 ± 0.4 mcg/mL. The influence of impaired hepatic function on PHOTOFRIN® disposition has not been evaluated. PHOTOFRIN® was approximately 90% protein bound in human serum, studied in vitro. The binding was independent of concentration over the concentration range of 20–100 mcg/mL.

Clinical Studies

Clinical studies of PDT with PHOTOFRIN® were conducted in patients with obstructing esophageal and endobronchial nonsmall cell lung cancers and in patients with early-stage radiologically occult endobronchial cancer. In all clinical studies, the method of PDT administration was essentially identical. A course of therapy consisted of one injection of PHOTOFRIN® (2 mg/kg administered as a slow intravenous injection over 3–5 minutes) followed by up to two non-thermal applications of 630 nm laser light. Doses of 300 J/cm of tumor length were used in esophageal cancer. Doses of 200 J/cm were used in endobronchial cancer for both palliation of obstructing cancer and treatment of superficial lesions. The first application of light occurred 40–50 hours after injection. Debridement of residua was performed via endoscopy/bronchoscopy 96–120 hours after injection, after which any residual tumor could be retreated with a second laser light application at the same dose used for the initial treatment. Additional courses of PDT with PHOTOFRIN® were allowed after 1 month, up to a maximum of three courses.

Esophageal Cancer

PDT with PHOTOFRIN® was utilized in a multicenter, single-arm study in 17 patients with completely obstructing esophageal carcinoma. Assessments were made at 1 week and 1 month after the last treatment procedure. As shown in Table 1, after a single course of therapy, 94% of patients obtained an objective tumor response and 76% of patients experienced some palliation of their dysphagia. On average, before treatment these patients had difficulty swallowing liquids, even saliva. After one course of therapy, there was a statistically significant improvement in mean dysphagia grade (1.5 units, p<0.05) and 13 of 17 patients could swallow liquids without difficulty 1 week and/or 1 month after treatment. Based on all courses, three patients achieved a complete tumor response (CR). In two of these patients, the CR was documented only at Week 1 as they had no further assessments. The third patient achieved a CR after a second course of therapy, which was supported by negative histopathology and maintained for the entire follow-up of 6 months.

Of the 17 treated patients, 11 (65%) received clinically important benefit from PDT. Clinically important benefit was defined hierarchically as a complete tumor response (3 patients), achievement of normal swallowing (2 patients went from Grade 5 dysphagia to Grade 1), or achievement of a marked improvement of two or more grades of dysphagia with minimal adverse reactions (6 patients). The median duration of benefit in these patients was 69+ days. Duration of benefit was calculated only for the period with documented evidence of improvement. All of these patients were still in response at their last assessment and, therefore, the estimate of 69 days is conservative. The median survival for these 11 patients was 115 days.

TABLE 1.

Course 1 Efficacy Results in Patients with Completely Obstructing Esophageal Cancer

	PDT n=17
IMPROVEMENT[a] IN DYSPHAGIA (% of Patients)	
Week 1	71%
Month 1	47%
Any assessment[b]	76%
MEAN DYSPHAGIA GRADE[c] AT BASELINE	4.6
MEAN IMPROVEMENT[c] IN DYSPHAGIA GRADE (units)	
Week 1	1.4
Month 1	1.5
OBJECTIVE TUMOR RESPONSE[d] (% of Patients)	
Week 1	82%
Month 1	35%[e]
Any Assessment[b]	94%
MEAN NUMBER OF LASER APPLICATIONS PER PATIENT	1.4

[a] Patients with at least a one-grade improvement in dysphagia grade
[b] Week 1 or Month 1

Continued on next page

This product information was prepared in September 1998. On these and other products of Sanofi Pharmaceuticals, Inc., detailed information may be obtained on a current basis by direct inquiry to Product Information Services, 90 Park Avenue, New York, NY 10016 (toll free 1-800-446-6267).

Photofrin—Cont.

[c] Dysphagia Scale:
Grade 1 = normal swallowing, Grade 2 = difficulty swallowing some hard solids; can swallow semisolides, Grade 3 = unable to swallow any solids; can swallow liquids, Grade 4 = difficulty swallowing liquids, Grade 5 = unable to swallow saliva

[d] CR+PR, CR = complete response (absence of endoscopically visible tumor), PR = partial response (appearance of a visible lumen)

[e] Eight of the 17 treated patients did not have assessments at Month 1.

Endobronchial Cancer

The efficacy of PHOTOFRIN® PDT was evaluated in the treatment of microinvasive endobronchial tumors in 62 inoperable patients in three noncomparative studies. Microinvasive lung cancer is defined histologically as disease which invades beyond the basement membrane but not through or into the cartilage. For 11 of the 62 patients, it was clearly documented that surgery and radiotherapy were not indicated. These 11 patients were all inoperable for medical or technical reasons. Radiotherapy was not indicated due to prior high-dose radiotherapy (7 patients), poor pulmonary function (2 patients), multifocal multilobar disease (1 patient), and poor medical condition (1 patient). As shown in Table 2, the complete tumor response rate, biopsy-proven at least 3 months after treatment, was 50%, median time to tumor recurrence was more than 2.7 years, median survival was 2.9 years and disease-specific survival was 4.1 years.

TABLE 2

Overall Efficacy Results in Patients with Superficial Endobronchial Tumors

EFFICACY PARAMETER	PDT n=11	n=62
COMPLETE TUMOR RESPONSE, BIOPSY-PROVEN AT 3 MONTHS		
Number of Patients (%)	3 (27%)	31 (50%)[a]
TIME TO TUMOR RECURRENCE IN PATIENTS WITH COMPLETE RESPONSE		
Number of Patients (%) with Recurrences	1 (33%)	11 (35%)
Median Time to Tumor Recurrence		>2.7 years
[95% Confidence Interval]		[1.6,–[b]]
SURVIVAL		
Number of Patients (%) who Died of Any Cause	4 (36%)	32 (52%)
Median Survival		2.9 years
[95% Confidence Interval]		[2.1, 5.7]
DISEASE-SPECIFIC SURVIVAL		
Number of Patients (%) who Died of Lung Cancer	3 (27%)	22 (35%)
Median Disease-Specific Survival		4.1 years
[95% Confidence Interval]		[2.5,–[b]]

[a] Not included are an additional 18 patients (6 patients not eligible for surgery or radiotherapy) who had complete tumor responses which were documented earlier than 3 months after treatment.

[b] The upper limit of the confidence interval could not be estimated due to an insufficient number of patients whose tumors recurred (Time to Tumor Recurrence) or who died (Survival).

INDICATIONS AND USAGE

Photodynamic therapy with PHOTOFRIN® is indicated for:
— palliation of patients with completely obstructing esophageal cancer, or of patients with partially obstructing esophageal cancer who, in the opinion of their physician, cannot be satisfactorily treated with Nd:YAG laser therapy.
— treatment of microinvasive endobronchial nonsmall cell lung cancer in patients for whom surgery and radiotherapy are not indicated.

CONTRAINDICATIONS

PHOTOFRIN® is contraindicated in patients with porphyria or in patients with known allergies to porphyrins.
PDT is contraindicated in patients with an existing tracheoesophageal or bronchoesophageal fistula.
PDT is contraindicated in patients with tumors eroding into a major blood vessel.

WARNINGS

If the esophageal tumor is eroding into the trachea or bronchial tree, the likelihood of tracheoesophageal or bronchoesophageal fistula resulting from treatment is sufficiently high that PDT is not recommended.

Patients with esophageal varices should be treated with extreme caution. Light should not be given directly to the variceal area because of the high risk of bleeding.

If the endobronchial tumor invades deeply into the bronchial wall, the possibility exists for fistula formation upon resolution of tumor.

PDT should be used with extreme caution for endobronchial tumors in locations where treatment-induced inflammation could obstruct the main airway, e.g., long or circumferential tumors of the trachea, tumors of the carina that involve both mainstem bronchi circumferentially, or circumferential tumors in the mainstem bronchus in patients with prior pneumonectomy.

Following injection with PHOTOFRIN® precautions must be taken to avoid exposure of skin and eyes to direct sunlight or bright indoor light (see PRECAUTIONS, General Precautions and Information for Patients).

PRECAUTIONS

General Precautions and Information for Patients
Photosensitivity

All patients who receive PHOTOFRIN® will be photosensitive and must observe precautions to avoid exposure of skin and eyes to direct sunlight or bright indoor light (from examination lamps, including dental lamps, operating room lamps, unshaded light bulbs at close proximity, etc.) for 30 days. The photosensitivity is due to residual drug which will be present in all parts of the skin. Exposure of the skin to ambient indoor light is, however, beneficial because the remaining drug will be inactivated gradually and safely through a photobleaching reaction. Therefore, patients should not stay in a darkened room during this period and should be encouraged to expose their skin to ambient indoor light. The level of photosensitivity will vary for different areas of the body, depending on the extent of previous exposure to light. Before exposing any area of skin to direct sunlight or bright indoor light, the patient should test it for residual photosensitivity. A small area of skin should be exposed to sunlight for 10 minutes. If no photosensitivity reaction (erythema, edema, blistering) occurs within 24 hours, the patient can gradually resume normal outdoor activities, initially continuing to exercise caution and gradually allowing increased exposure. If some photosensitivity reaction occurs with the limited skin test, the patient should continue precautions for another 2 weeks before retesting. The tissue around the eyes may be more sensitive, and therefore, it is not recommended that the face be used for testing. If patients travel to a different geographical area with greater sunshine, they should retest their level of photosensitivity. UV (ultraviolet) sunscreens are of no value in protecting against photosensitivity reactions because photoactivation is caused by visible light.

Ocular Sensitivity

Ocular discomfort, commonly described as sensitivity to sun, bright lights, or car headlights, has been reported in patients who received PHOTOFRIN®. For 30 days, when outdoors, patients should wear dark sunglasses which have an average white light transmittance of <4%.

Use Before or After Radiotherapy

If PDT is to be used before or after radiotherapy, sufficient time should be allotted between the two therapies to ensure that the inflammatory response produced by the first treatment has subsided before commencing the second treatment. The inflammatory response from PDT will depend on tumor size and extent of surrounding normal tissue that receives light. It is recommended that 2 to 4 weeks be allowed after PDT before commencing radiotherapy. Similarly, if PDT is to be given after radiotherapy, the acute inflammatory reaction from radiotherapy usually subsides within 4 weeks after completing radiotherapy, after which PDT may be given.

Patients with obstructing lung cancer who have received prior radiation therapy have a higher incidence of fatal hemoptysis after PDT (see ADVERSE REACTIONS).

Chest Pain

As a result of PDT treatment, patients may complain of substernal chest pain because of inflammatory responses within the area of treatment. Such pain may be of sufficient intensity to warrant the short-term prescription of opiate analgesics.

Respiratory Distress

Patients with endobronchial lesions must be closely monitored between the laser light therapy and the mandatory debridement bronchoscopy for any evidence of respiratory distress. Inflammation, mucositis, and necrotic debris may cause obstruction of the airway. If respiratory distress occurs, the physician should be prepared to carry out immediate bronchoscopy to remove secretions and debris to open the airway.

Avoidance of Pregnancy

Women of childbearing potential should practice an effective method of contraception during therapy (see Pregnancy).

Drug Interactions

There have been no formal interaction studies of PHOTOFRIN® and any other drugs. However, it is possible that concomitant use of other photosensitizing agents (e.g., tetracyclines, sulfonamides, phenothiazines, sulfonylurea hypoglycemic agents, thiazide diuretics, and griseofulvin) could increase the photosensitivity reaction.

PHOTOFRIN® PDT causes direct intracellular damage by initiating radical chain reactions that damage intracellular membranes and mitochondria. Tissue damage also results from ischemia secondary to vasoconstriction, platelet activation and aggregation and clotting. Research in animals and in cell culture has suggested that many drugs could influence the effects of PDT, possible examples of which are described below. There are no human data that support or rebut these possibilities.

Compounds that quench active oxygen species or scavenge radicals, such as dimethyl sulfoxide, b-carotene, ethanol, formate and mannitol would be expected to decrease PDT activity. Preclinical data also suggest that tissue ischemia, allopurinol, calcium channel blockers and some prostaglandin synthesis inhibitors could interfere with PHOTOFRIN® PDT. Drugs that decrease clotting, vasoconstriction or platelet aggregation, e.g., thromboxane A_2 inhibitors, could decrease the efficacy of PDT. Glucocorticoid hormones given before or concomitant with PDT may decrease the efficacy of the treatment.

Carcinogenesis, Mutagenesis, Impairment of Fertility

No long-term studies have been conducted to evaluate the carcinogenic potential of PHOTOFRIN®. In vitro, PHOTOFRIN® PDT did not cause mutations in the Ames test, nor did it cause chromosome aberrations or mutations (HGPRT locus) in Chinese hamster ovary (CHO) cells. PHOTOFRIN® caused <2-fold, but significant, increases in sister chromatid exchange in CHO cells irradiated with visible light and a 3-fold increase in Chinese hamster lung fibroblasts irradiated with near UV light. PHOTOFRIN® PDT caused an increase in thymidine kinase mutants and DNA-protein crosslinks in mouse L5178Y cells, but not mouse LYR83 cells. PHOTOFRIN® PDT caused a light-dose dependant increase in DNA-strand breaks in malignant human cervical carcinoma cells, but not in normal cells. The mutagenicity of PHOTOFRIN® without light has not been adequately determined. In vivo, PHOTOFRIN® did not cause chromosomal aberrations in the mouse micronucleus test.

PHOTOFRIN® given to male and female rats intravenously, at 4 mg/kg/d (0.32 times the clinical dose on a mg/m^2 basis) before conception and through Day 7 of pregnancy caused no impairment of fertility. In this study, long-term dosing with PHOTOFRIN® caused discoloration of testes and ovaries and hypertrophy of the testes. PHOTOFRIN® also caused decreased body weight in the parent rats.

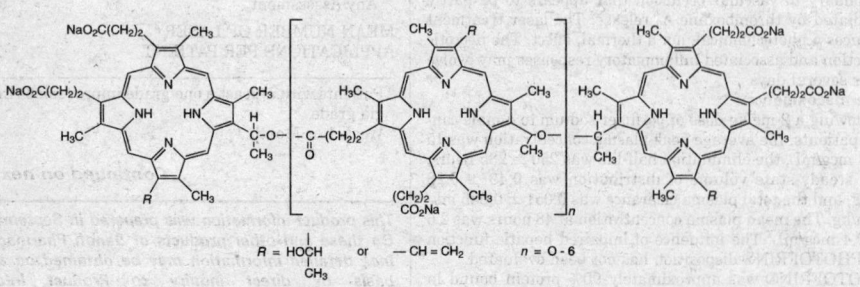

$R = HOCH$ or $-CH = CH_2$ $n = 0-6$
CH_3

Pregnancy: Pregnancy Category C

There are no adequate and well-controlled studies in pregnant women. PHOTOFRIN® should be used during pregnancy only if the potential benefit justifies the potential risk to the fetus.

PHOTOFRIN® given to rat dams during fetal organogenesis intravenously at 8 mg/kg/d (0.64 times the clinical dose on a mg/m² basis) for 10 days caused no major malformations or developmental changes. This dose caused maternal and fetal toxicity resulting in increased resorptions, decreased litter size, delayed ossification, and reduced fetal weight. PHOTOFRIN® caused no major malformations when given to rabbits intravenously during organogenesis at 4 mg/kg/d (0.65 times the clinical dose on a mg/m² basis) for 13 days. This dose caused maternal toxicity resulting in increased resorptions, decreased litter size, and reduced fetal body weight.

PHOTOFRIN® given to rats during late pregnancy through lactation intravenously at 4 mg/kg/d (0.32 times the clinical dose on a mg/m² basis) for at least 42 days caused a reversible decrease in growth of offspring. Parturition was unaffected.

Nursing Mothers

It is not known whether this drug is excreted in human milk. Because many drugs are excreted in human milk and because of the potential for serious adverse reactions in nursing infants from PHOTOFRIN®, women receiving PHOTOFRIN® must not breast feed.

Pediatric Use

Safety and effectiveness in children have not been established.

Use in Elderly Patients

Approximately 70% of the patients treated with PDT using PHOTOFRIN® in clinical trials were over 60 years of age. There was no apparent difference in effectiveness or safety in these patients compared to younger people. Dose modification based upon age is not required.

ADVERSE REACTIONS

Systemically induced effects associated with PDT with PHOTOFRIN® consist of photosensitivity and mild constipation. All patients who receive PHOTOFRIN® will be photosensitive and must observe precautions to avoid sunlight and bright indoor light (see PRECAUTIONS). Photosensitivity reactions (mostly mild erythema on the face and hands) occurred in approximately 20% of patients treated with PHOTOFRIN®.

Most toxicities associated with this therapy are local effects seen in the region of illumination and occasionally in surrounding tissues. The local adverse reactions are characteristic of an inflammatory response induced by the photodynamic effect.

Esophageal Carcinoma

The following adverse events were reported in at least 5% of patients treated with PHOTOFRIN® PDT, who had completely or partially obstructing esophageal cancer. Table 3 presents data from 88 patients who received the currently marketed formulation. The relationship of many of these adverse events to PDT with PHOTOFRIN® is uncertain.

TABLE 3.

Adverse Events Reported in 5% or More of Patients with Obstructing Esophageal Cancer

BODY SYSTEM/ Adverse Event	Number (%) of Patients n=88	
Patients with at Least One Adverse Event	84	(95)
AUTONOMIC NERVOUS SYSTEM		
Hypertension	5	(6)
Hypotension	6	(7)
BODY AS A WHOLE		
Asthenia	5	(6)
Back pain	10	(11)
Chest pain	19	(22)
Chest pain (substernal)	4	(5)
Edema generalized	4	(5)
Edema peripheral	6	(7)
Fever	27	(31)
Pain	19	(22)
Surgical complication	4	(5)
CARDIOVASCULAR		
Cardiac failure	6	(7)
GASTROINTESTINAL		
Abdominal pain	18	(20)
Constipation	21	(24)
Diarrhea	4	(5)
Dyspepsia	5	(6)
Dysphagia	9	(10)
Eructation	4	(5)
Esophageal edema	7	(8)
Esophageal tumor bleeding	7	(8)
Esophageal stricture	5	(6)
Esophagitis	4	(5)
Hematemesis	7	(8)
Melena	4	(5)
Nausea	21	(24)
Vomiting	15	(17)
HEART RATE/RHYTHM		
Atrial fibrillation	9	(10)
Tachycardia	5	(6)
METABOLIC & NUTRITIONAL		
Dehydration	6	(7)
Weight decrease	8	(9)
PSYCHIATRIC		
Anorexia	7	(8)
Anxiety	6	(7)
Confusion	7	(8)
Insomnia	12	(14)
RED BLOOD CELL		
Anemia	28	(32)
RESISTANCE MECHANISM		
Moniliasis	8	(9)
RESPIRATORY		
Coughing	6	(7)
Dyspnea	18	(20)
Pharyngitis	10	(11)
Pleural effusion	28	(32)
Pneumonia	16	(18)
Respiratory insufficiency	9	(10)
Tracheoesophageal fistula	5	(6)
SKIN & APPENDAGES		
Photosensitivity reaction	17	(19)
URINARY		
Urinary tract infection	6	(7)

Location of the tumor was a prognostic factor for three adverse events: upper-third of the esophagus (esophageal edema), middle-third (atrial fibrillation), and lower-third, the most vascular region (anemia). Also, patients with large tumors (>10 cm) were more likely to experience anemia. Two of 17 patients with complete esophageal obstruction from tumor experienced esophageal perforations which were considered to be possibly treatment associated; these perforations occurred during subsequent endoscopies.

Serious and other notable adverse events observed in less than 5% of PDT-treated patients with obstructing esophageal cancer in the clinical studies include the following; their relationship to therapy is uncertain. In the gastrointestinal system, esophageal perforation, gastric ulcer, ileus, jaundice, and peritonitis have occurred. Sepsis has been reported occasionally. Cardiovascular events have included angina pectoris, bradycardia, myocardial infarction, sick sinus syndrome, and supraventricular tachycardia. Respiratory events of bronchitis, bronchospasm, laryngotracheal edema, pneumonitis, pulmonary hemorrhage, pulmonary edema, respiratory failure, and stridor have occurred. The temporal relationship of some gastrointestinal, cardiovascular and respiratory events to the administration of light was suggestive of mediastinal inflammation in some patients. Vision-related events of abnormal vision, diplopia, eye pain and photophobia have been reported.

Endobronchial Cancer

The following adverse events were reported in at least 5% of patients with superficial tumors (microinvasive or carcinoma in situ) who received the currently marketed formulation.

TABLE 4

Adverse Events Reported in 5% or More of Patients with Superficial Endobronchial Tumors

BODY SYSTEM/ Adverse Event	Number (%) of Patients n=90	
Patients with at Least One Adverse Event	44	(49)
Photosensitivity reaction	20	(22)
Coughing	8	(9)
Dyspnea	6	(7)
Edema	16	(18)
Exudate	20	(22)
Obstruction	19	(21)
Stricture	10	(11)
Ulceration	8	(9)

In patients with superficial endobronchial tumors, 44 of 90 patients (49%) experienced an adverse event, two-thirds of which were related to the respiratory system. The most common reaction to therapy was a mucositis reaction in one-fifth of the patients which manifested as edema, exudate, and obstruction. The obstruction (mucus plug) is easily removed with suction or forceps. Mucositis can be minimized by avoiding exposure of normal tissue to excessive light (see PRECAUTIONS). Three patients experienced life-threatening dyspnea: one was given a double dose of light, one was treated concurrently in both mainstem bronchi and the other had had prior pneumonectomy and was treated in the sole remaining main airway (see WARNINGS). Stent placement was required in 3% of the patients due to endobronchial stricture.

Fatal hemoptysis occurred within 30 days of treatment in one patient with superficial tumors (1%) and in 4% of patients who participated in studies of obstructing tumors. While massive hemoptysis is a sign of progressive disease, it can also result from resolution of a tumor which has eroded into a pulmonary artery. Treatment of tumors eroding a blood vessel is contraindicated (see CONTRAINDICATIONS).

Patients who have received radiation therapy have a higher incidence of fatal hemoptysis after treatment with PDT and after other forms of local treatment. In controlled studies comparing PDT to Nd:YAG laser for palliation of obstructing lung cancer, the incidence of fatal hemoptysis in patients previously treated with radiotherapy was 21% (6/29) in patients treated with PDT and 10% (3/29) in patients treated with Nd:YAG. In patients with no prior radiotherapy, the overall incidence of fatal hemoptysis was less than 1%.

Laboratory Abnormalities

In patients with esophageal cancer, PDT with PHOTOFRIN® may result in anemia due to tumor bleeding. No consistent effects were observed for other parameters or in patients with endobronchial carcinoma.

OVERDOSAGE

PHOTOFRIN® Overdose

There is no information on overdosage situations involving PHOTOFRIN®. Higher than recommended drug doses of two 2 mg/kg doses given two days apart (10 patients) and three 2 mg/kg doses given within two weeks (1 patient), were tolerated without notable adverse reactions. Effects of overdosage on the duration of photosensitivity are unknown. Laser treatment should not be given if an overdose of PHOTOFRIN® is administered. In the event of an overdose, patients should protect their eyes and skin from direct sunlight or bright indoor lights for 30 days. At this time, patients should test for residual photosensitivity (see PRECAUTIONS). PHOTOFRIN® is not dialyzable.

Overdose of Laser Light Following PHOTOFRIN® Injection

Light doses of two to three times the recommended dose have been administered to a few patients with superficial endobronchial tumors. One patient experienced life-threatening dyspnea and the others had no notable complications. Increased symptoms and damage to normal tissue might be expected following an overdose of light.

DOSAGE AND ADMINISTRATION

Photodynamic therapy with PHOTOFRIN® is a two-stage process requiring administration of both drug and light. The first stage of PDT is the intravenous injection of PHOTOFRIN® at 2 mg/kg. Illumination with laser light 40–50 hours following injection with PHOTOFRIN® constitutes the second stage of therapy. A second laser light application may be given 96–120 hours after injection, preceded by gentle debridement of residual tumor (see Administration of Laser Light). In clinical studies, debridement via endoscopy was required 2 days after the initial light application. Standard endoscopic techniques are used for light administration and debridement. Practitioners should be fully familiar with the patient's condition and trained in the safe and efficacious treatment of esophageal or endobronchial cancer using photodynamic therapy with PHOTOFRIN® and associated light delivery devices.

Patients may receive a second course of PDT a minimum of 30 days after the initial therapy; up to three courses of PDT (each separated by a minimum of 30 days) can be given. Before each course of treatment, patients with esophageal cancer should be evaluated for the presence of a tracheoesophageal or bronchoesophageal fistula (see CONTRAINDICATIONS). In patients with endobronchial lesions who have recently undergone radiotherapy, sufficient time (approximately 4 weeks) should be allowed between the therapies to ensure that the acute inflammation produced by radiotherapy has subsided prior to PDT (see PRECAUTIONS, Use

Continued on next page

This product information was prepared in September 1998. On these and other products of Sanofi Pharmaceuticals, Inc., detailed information may be obtained on a current basis by direct inquiry to Product Information Services, 90 Park Avenue, New York, NY 10016 (toll free 1-800-446-6267).

Photofrin—Cont.

Before or After Radiotherapy). All patients should be evaluated for the possibility that the tumor may be eroding into a major blood vessel (see CONTRAINDICATIONS).

PHOTOFRIN® Administration

PHOTOFRIN® should be administered as a single slow intravenous injection over 3 to 5 minutes at 2 mg/kg body weight. Reconstitute each vial of PHOTOFRIN® with 31.8 mL of either 5% Dextrose Injection (USP) or 0.9% Sodium Chloride Injection (USP), resulting in a final concentration of 2.5 mg/mL. Shake well until dissolved. Do not mix PHOTOFRIN® with other drugs in the same solution. PHOTOFRIN®, reconstituted with 5% Dextrose Injection (USP) or with 0.9% Sodium Chloride Injection (USP), has a pH in the range of 7 to 8. PHOTOFRIN® has been formulated with an overage to deliver the 75 mg labeled quantity. **The reconstituted product should be protected from bright light and used immediately.** Reconstituted PHOTOFRIN® is an opaque solution, in which detection of particulate matter by visual inspection is extremely difficult. Reconstituted PHOTOFRIN®, however, like all parenteral drug products, should be inspected visually for particulate matter and discoloration prior to administration whenever solution and container permit.

Precautions should be taken to prevent extravasation at the injection site. If extravasation occurs, care must be taken to protect the area from light. There is no known benefit from injecting the extravasation site with another substance.

Administration of Laser Light

Initiate 630 nm wavelength laser light delivery to the patient 40–50 hours following injection with PHOTOFRIN®. A second laser light treatment may be given as early as 96 hours or as late as 120 hours after the initial injection with PHOTOFRIN®. No further injection of PHOTOFRIN® should be given for such retreatment with laser light. Before providing a second laser light treatment, the residual tumor should be debrided. Vigorous debridement may cause esophageal tumor bleeding.

The laser system must be approved for delivery of a stable power output at a wavelength of 630 ± 3 nm. Light is delivered to the tumor by cylindrical OPTIGUIDE™ fiber optic diffusers passed through the operating channel of an endoscope/bronchoscope. Instructions for use of the fiber optic and the selected laser system should be read carefully before use. OPTIGUIDE™ cylindrical diffusers are available in several lengths. The choice of diffuser tip length depends on the length of the tumor. Diffuser length should be sized to avoid exposure of nonmalignant tissue to light and to prevent overlapping of previously treated malignant tissue. Photoactivation of PHOTOFRIN® is controlled by the total light dose delivered:

In the treatment of esophageal cancer, a light dose of 300 joules/cm of tumor length should be delivered. The total power output at the fiber tip is set to deliver the appropriate light dose using exposure times of 12 minutes and 30 seconds.

In the treatment of endobronchial cancer, the light dose should be 200 joules/cm of tumor length. The total power output at the fiber tip is set to deliver the appropriate light dose using exposure times of 8 minutes and 20 seconds. For noncircumferential endobronchial tumors that are soft enough to penetrate, interstitial fiber placement is preferred to intraluminal activation, since this method results in less exposure of the normal bronchial mucosa to light. It is important to perform a debridement 2 to 3 days after each light injection to minimize the potential for obstruction caused by necrotic debris (see PRECAUTIONS).

Refer to the OPTIGUIDE™ instructions for use for complete instructions concerning the fiber optic diffuser.

HOW SUPPLIED

PHOTOFRIN® (porfimer sodium) for Injection is supplied as a freeze-dried cake or powder as follows:

NDC 0024-1550-01 — 75 mg vial

PHOTOFRIN® freeze-dried cake or powder should be stored at Controlled Room Temperature 20–25° C (68–77° F) [see USP].

Spills and Disposal

Spills of PHOTOFRIN® should be wiped up with a damp cloth. Skin and eye contact should be avoided due to the potential for photosensitivity reactions upon exposure to light; use of rubber gloves and eye protection is recommended. All contaminated materials should be disposed of in a polyethylene bag in a manner consistent with local regulations.

Accidental Exposure

PHOTOFRIN® is neither a primary ocular irritant nor a primary dermal irritant. However, because of its potential to induce photosensitivity, PHOTOFRIN® might be an eye and/or skin irritant in the presence of bright light. It is important to avoid contact with the eyes and skin during prep‑ ar‑ and/or administration. As with therapeutic overdos‑ overexposed person must be protected from bright

...Therapeutics Inc.
...d by

LEDERLE PARENTERALS, INC.
Carolina, Puerto Rico 00987
for
QLT PHOTOTHERAPEUTICS INC.
Seattle, WA 98101
Distributed by Sanofi Pharmaceuticals, Inc.
New York, NY 10016
For inquiries call 1-800-446-6267
Revised July 1998

PLAQUENIL® ℞
HYDROXYCHLOROQUINE SULFATE, USP

> **WARNING**
> PHYSICIANS SHOULD COMPLETELY FAMILIARIZE THEMSELVES WITH THE COMPLETE CONTENTS OF THIS LEAFLET BEFORE PRESCRIBING HYDROXYCHLO-ROQUINE.

DESCRIPTION

Hydroxychloroquine sulfate is a colorless crystalline solid, soluble in water to at least 20 percent; chemically the drug is 2-[[4-[(7-Chloro-4- quinolyl) amino] pentyl] ethylamino] ethanol sulfate (1:1).

Plaquenil (hydroxychloroquine sulfate) tablets contain 200 mg hydroxychloroquine sulfate, equivalent to 155 mg base, and are for oral administration.

Inactive Ingredients: Dibasic Calcium Phosphate, Hydroxypropyl Methylcellulose, Magnesium Stearate, Polyethylene glycol 400, Polysorbate 80, Starch, Titanium Dioxide.

ACTIONS

The drug possesses antimalarial actions and also exerts a beneficial effect in lupus erythematosus (chronic discoid or systemic) and acute or chronic rheumatoid arthritis. The precise mechanism of action is not known.

INDICATIONS

PLAQUENIL is indicated for the suppressive treatment and treatment of acute attacks of malaria due to *Plasmodium vivax, P. malariae, P. ovale*, and susceptible strains of *P. falciparum*. It is also indicated for the treatment of discoid and systemic lupus erythematosus, and rheumatoid arthritis.

CONTRAINDICATIONS

Use of this drug is contraindicated (1) in the presence of retinal or visual field changes attributable to any 4-aminoquinoline compound, (2) in patients with known hypersensitivity to 4-aminoquinoline compounds, and (3) for long-term therapy in children.

WARNINGS, General

PLAQUENIL is not effective against chloroquine-resistant strains of *P. falciparum*.

Children are especially sensitive to the 4-aminoquinoline compounds. A number of fatalities have been reported following the accidental ingestion of chloroquine, sometimes in relatively small doses (0.75 g or 1 g in one 3- year-old child). Patients should be strongly warned to keep these drugs out of the reach of children.

Use of PLAQUENIL in patients with psoriasis may precipitate a severe attack of psoriasis. When used in patients with porphyria the condition may be exacerbated. The preparation should not be used in these conditions unless in the judgment of the physician the benefit to the patient outweighs the possible hazard.

Usage in Pregnancy—Usage of this drug during pregnancy should be avoided except in the suppression or treatment of malaria when in the judgment of the physician the benefit outweighs the possible hazard. It should be noted that radioactively-tagged chloroquine administered intravenously to pregnant, pigmented CBA mice passed rapidly across the placenta. It accumulated selectively in the melanin structures of the fetal eyes and was retained in the ocular tissues for five months after the drug had been eliminated from the rest of the body.

PRECAUTIONS, General

Antimalarial compounds should be used with caution in patients with hepatic disease or alcoholism or in conjunction with known hepatotoxic drugs.

Periodic blood cell counts should be made if patients are given prolonged therapy. If any severe blood disorder appears which is not attributable to the disease under treatment, discontinuation of the drug should be considered. The drug should be administered with caution in patients having G-6-PD (glucose-6-phosphate dehydrogenase) deficiency.

OVERDOSAGE

The 4-aminoquinoline compounds are very rapidly and completely absorbed after ingestion, and in accidental overdosage, or rarely with lower doses in hypersensitive patients, toxic symptoms may occur within 30 minutes. These consist of headache, drowsiness, visual disturbances, cardiovascular collapse, and convulsions, followed by sudden and early respiratory and cardiac arrest. The electrocardiogram may reveal atrial standstill, nodal rhythm, prolonged intraventricular conduction time, and progressive bradycardia leading to ventricular fibrillation and/or arrest. Treatment is symptomatic and must be prompt with immediate evacuation of the stomach by emesis (at home, before transportation to the hospital) or gastric lavage until the stomach is completely emptied. If finely powdered, activated charcoal is introduced by the stomach tube, after lavage, and within 30 minutes after ingestion of the tablets, it may inhibit further intestinal absorption of the drug. To be effective, the dose of activated charcoal should be at least five times the estimated dose of hydroxychloroquine ingested. Convulsions, if present, should be controlled before attempting gastric lavage. If due to cerebral stimulation, cautious administration of an ultrashort-acting barbiturate may be tried but, if due to anoxia, it should be corrected by oxygen administration, artificial respiration or, in shock with hypotension, by vasopressor therapy. Because of the importance of supporting respiration, tracheal intubation or tracheostomy, followed by gastric lavage, may also be necessary. Exchange transfusions have been used to reduce the level of 4-aminoquinoline drug in the blood.

A patient who survives the acute phase and is asymptomatic should be closely observed for at least six hours. Fluids may be forced, and sufficient ammonium chloride (8 g daily in divided doses for adults) may be administered for a few days to acidify the urine to help promote urinary excretion in cases of both overdosage and sensitivity.

> **MALARIA**

ACTIONS

Like chloroquine phosphate, USP, PLAQUENIL is highly active against the erythrocytic forms of *P. vivax* and *malariae* and most strains of *P. falciparum* (but not the gametocytes of *P. falciparum*).

PLAQUENIL does not prevent relapses in patients with *vivax* or *malariae* malaria because it is not effective against exo-erythrocytic forms of the parasite, nor will it prevent *vivax* or *malariae* infection when administered as a prophylactic. It is highly effective as a suppressive agent in patients with *vivax* or *malariae* malaria, in terminating acute attacks, and significantly lengthening the interval between treatment and relapse. In patients with *falciparum* malaria, it abolishes the acute attack and effects complete cure of the infection, unless due to a resistant strain of *P. falciparum*.

INDICATIONS

PLAQUENIL is indicated for the treatment of acute attacks and suppression of malaria.

WARNING

In recent years, it has been found that certain strains of *P. falciparum* have become resistant to 4-aminoquinoline compounds (including hydroxychloroquine) as shown by the fact that normally adequate doses have failed to prevent or cure clinical malaria or parasitemia. Treatment with quinine or other specific forms of therapy is therefore advised for patients infected with a resistant strain of parasites.

ADVERSE REACTIONS

Following the administration in doses adequate for the treatment of an acute malarial attack, mild and transient headache, dizziness, and gastrointestinal complaints (diarrhea, anorexia, nausea, abdominal cramps and, on rare occasions, vomiting) may occur.

DOSAGE AND ADMINISTRATION

One tablet of 200 mg of hydroxychloroquine sulfate is equivalent to 155 mg base.

Malaria: Suppression—*In adults*, 400 mg (=310 mg base) on exactly the same day of each week. *In infants and children*, the weekly suppressive dosage is 5 mg, calculated as base, per kg of body weight, but should not exceed the adult dose regardless of weight.

If circumstances permit, suppressive therapy should begin two weeks prior to exposure. However, failing this, in adults an initial double (loading) dose of 800 mg (= 620 mg base), or in children 10 mg base/kg may be taken in two divided doses, six hours apart. The suppressive therapy should be continued for eight weeks after leaving the endemic area.

Treatment of the acute attack—*In adults*, an initial dose of 800 mg (= 620 mg base) followed by 400 mg (= 310 mg base) in six to eight hours and 400 mg (= 310 mg base) on each of two consecutive days (total 2 g hydroxychloroquine sulfate or 1.55 g base). An alternative method, employing a single dose of 800 mg (= 620 mg base), has also proved effective.

The dosage for adults may also be calculated on the basis of body weight; this method is preferred for infants and children. A total dose representing 25 mg of base per kg of body weight is administered in three days, as follows:

First dose: 10 mg base per kg (but not exceeding a single dose of 620 mg base).
Second dose: 5 mg base per kg (but not exceeding a single dose of 310 mg base) 6 hours after first dose.
Third dose: 5 mg base per kg 18 hours after second dose.
Fourth dose: 5 mg base per kg 24 hours after third dose.
For radical cure of *vivax* and *malariae* malaria concomitant therapy with an 8-aminoquinoline compound is necessary.

LUPUS ERYTHEMATOSUS AND RHEUMATOID ARTHRITIS

INDICATIONS

PLAQUENIL is useful in patients with the following disorders who have not responded satisfactorily to drugs with less potential for serious side effects: lupus erythematosus (chronic discoid and systemic) and acute or chronic rheumatoid arthritis.

WARNINGS

PHYSICIANS SHOULD COMPLETELY FAMILIARIZE THEMSELVES WITH THE COMPLETE CONTENTS OF THIS LEAFLET BEFORE PRESCRIBING PLAQUENIL.
Irreversible retinal damage has been observed in some patients who had received long-term or high-dosage 4-aminoquinoline therapy for discoid and systemic lupus erythematosus, or rheumatoid arthritis. Retinopathy has been reported to be dose related.
When prolonged therapy with any antimalarial compound is contemplated, initial (base line) and periodic (every three months) ophthalmologic examinations (including visual acuity, expert slit-lamp, funduscopic, and visual field tests) should be performed.
If there is any indication of abnormality in the visual acuity, visual field, or retinal macular areas (such as pigmentary changes, loss of foveal reflex), or any visual symptoms (such as light flashes and streaks) which are not fully explainable by difficulties of accommodation or corneal opacities, the drug should be discontinued immediately and the patient closely observed for possible progression. Retinal changes (and visual disturbances) may progress even after cessation of therapy.
All patients on long-term therapy with this preparation should be questioned and examined periodically, including the testing of knee and ankle reflexes, to detect any evidence of muscular weakness. If weakness occurs, discontinue the drug.
In the treatment of rheumatoid arthritis, if objective improvement (such as reduced joint swelling, increased mobility) does not occur within six months, the drug should be discontinued. Safe use of the drug in the treatment of juvenile arthritis has not been established.

PRECAUTIONS

Dermatologic reactions to PLAQUENIL may occur and, therefore, proper care should be exercised when it is administered to any patient receiving a drug with a significant tendency to produce dermatitis.
The methods recommended for early diagnosis of "chloroquine retinopathy" consist of (1) funduscopic examination of the macula for fine pigmentary disturbances or loss of the foveal reflex and (2) examination of the central visual field with a small red test object for pericentral or paracentral scotoma or determination of retinal thresholds to red. Any unexplained visual symptoms, such as light flashes or streaks should also be regarded with suspicion as possible manifestations of retinopathy.
If serious toxic symptoms occur from overdosage or sensitivity, it has been suggested that ammonium chloride (8 g daily in divided doses for adults) be administered orally three or four days a week for several months after therapy has been stopped, as acidification of the urine increases renal excretion of the 4-aminoquinoline compounds by 20 to 90 percent. However, caution must be exercised in patients with impaired renal function and/or metabolic acidosis.

ADVERSE REACTIONS

Not all of the following reactions have been observed with every 4-aminoquinoline compound during long-term therapy, but they have been reported with one or more and should be borne in mind when drugs of this class are administered. Adverse effects with different compounds vary in type and frequency.
CNS Reactions: Irritability, nervousness, emotional changes, nightmares, psychosis, headache, dizziness, vertigo, tinnitus, nystagmus, nerve deafness, convulsions, ataxia.
Neuromuscular Reactions: Extraocular muscle palsies, skeletal muscle weakness, absent or hypoactive deep tendon reflexes.
Ocular Reactions:
A. *Ciliary body:* Disturbance of accommodation with symptoms of blurred vision. This reaction is dose related and reversible with cessation of therapy.
B. *Cornea:* Transient edema, punctate to lineal opacities, decreased corneal sensitivity. The corneal changes, with or without accompanying symptoms (blurred vision, halos around lights, photophobia), are fairly common, but reversible. Corneal deposits may appear as early as three weeks following initiation of therapy.
The incidence of corneal changes and visual side effects appears to be considerably lower with hydroxychloroquine than with chloroquine.
C. *Retina:*
Macula: Edema, atrophy, abnormal pigmentation (mild pigment stippling to a "bull's-eye" appearance), loss of foveal reflex, increased macular recovery time following exposure to a bright light (photo-stress test), elevated retinal threshold to red light in macular, paramacular, and peripheral retinal areas.
Other fundus changes include optic disc pallor and atrophy, attenuation of retinal arterioles, fine granular pigmentary disturbances in the peripheral retina and prominent choroidal patterns in advanced stage.
D. *Visual field defects:* pericentral or paracentral scotoma, central scotoma with decreased visual acuity, rarely field constriction.
The most common visual symptoms attributed to the retinopathy are: reading and seeing difficulties (words, letters, or parts of objects missing), photophobia, blurred distance vision, missing or blacked out areas in the central or peripheral visual field, light flashes and streaks.
Retinopathy appears to be dose related and has occurred within several months (rarely) to several years of daily therapy; a small number of cases have been reported several years after antimalarial drug therapy was discontinued. It has not been noted during prolonged use of weekly doses of the 4-aminoquinoline compounds for suppression of malaria.
Patients with retinal changes may have visual symptoms or may be asymptomatic (with or without visual field changes). Rarely scotomatous vision or field defects may occur without obvious retinal change.
Retinopathy may progress even after the drug is discontinued. In a number of patients, early retinopathy (macular pigmentation sometimes with central field defects) diminished or regressed completely after therapy was discontinued. Paracentral scotoma to red targets (sometimes called "premaculopathy") is indicative of early retinal dysfunction which is usually reversible with cessation of therapy.
A small number of cases of retinal changes have been reported as occurring in patients who received only hydroxychloroquine. These usually consisted of alteration in retinal pigmentation which was detected on periodic ophthalmologic examination; visual field defects were also present in some instances. A case of delayed retinopathy has been reported with loss of vision starting one year after administration of hydroxychloroquine had been discontinued.
Dermatologic Reactions: Bleaching of hair, alopecia, pruritus, skin and mucosal pigmentation, skin eruptions (urticarial, morbilliform, lichenoid, maculopapular, purpuric, erythema annulare centrifugum and exfoliative dermatitis).
Hematologic Reactions: Various blood dyscrasias such as aplastic anemia, agranulocytosis, leukopenia, thrombocytopenia (hemolysis in individuals with glucose-6-phosphate dehydrogenase (G-6-PD) deficiency).
Gastrointestinal Reactions: Anorexia, nausea, vomiting, diarrhea, and abdominal cramps.
Miscellaneous Reactions: Weight loss, lassitude, exacerbation or precipitation of porphyria and nonlight-sensitive psoriasis.
Cardiomyopathy has been rarely reported and the relationship to hydroxychloroquine is unclear.

DOSAGE AND ADMINISTRATION

One tablet of hydroxychloroquine sulfate, 200 mg, is equivalent to 155 mg base.
Lupus erythematosus —Initially, the average *adult* dose is 400 mg (=310 mg base) once or twice daily. This may be continued for several weeks or months, depending on the response of the patient. For prolonged maintenance therapy, a smaller dose, from 200 mg to 400 mg (= 155 mg to 310 mg base) daily will frequently suffice.
The incidence of retinopathy has been reported to be higher when this maintenance dose is exceeded.
Rheumatoid arthritis —The compound is cumulative in action and will require several weeks to exert its beneficial therapeutic effects, whereas minor side effects may occur relatively early. Several months of therapy may be required before maximum effects can be obtained. If objective improvement (such as reduced joint swelling, increased mobility) does not occur within six months, the drug should be discontinued. Safe use of the drug in the treatment of juvenile rheumatoid arthritis has not been established.
Initial dosage —In ***adults,*** from 400 mg to 600 mg (=310 mg to 465 mg base) daily, each dose to be taken with a meal or a glass of milk. In a small percentage of patients, troublesome side effects may require temporary reduction of the initial dosage. Later (usually from five to ten days), the dose may gradually be increased to the optimum response level, often without return of side effects.
Maintenance dosage —When a good response is obtained (usually in four to twelve weeks), the dosage is reduced by 50 percent and continued at a usual maintenance level of 200 mg to 400 mg (=155 mg to 310 mg base) daily, each dose to be taken with a meal or a glass of milk. The incidence of retinopathy has been reported to be higher when this maintenance dose is exceeded.
Should a relapse occur after medication is withdrawn, therapy may be resumed or continued on an intermittent schedule if there are no ocular contraindications.
Corticosteroids and salicylates may be used in conjunction with this compound, and they can generally be decreased gradually in dosage or eliminated after the drug has been used for several weeks. When gradual reduction of steroid dosage is indicated, it may be done by reducing every four to five days the dose of cortisone by no more than from 5 mg to 15 mg; of hydrocortisone from 5 mg to 10 mg; of prednisolone and prednisone from 1 mg to 2.5 mg; of methylprednisolone and triamcinolone from 1 mg to 2 mg; and of dexamethasone from 0.25 mg to 0.5 mg.

HOW SUPPLIED

Plaquenil tablets are white, to off-white film coated tablets, each containing 200 mg hydroxychloroquine sulfate (equivalent to 155 mg base). Bottles of 100 tablets (NDC 0024-1562-10).
Dispense in a tight, light-resistant container as defined in the official compendia.
Store at room temperature up to 30°C (86°F).
Caution: Federal law prohibits dispensing without prescription.

PSW-5B

Shown in Product Identification Guide, page 335

PLAVIX® ℞
clopidogrel bisulfate tablets

DESCRIPTION

PLAVIX (clopidogrel bisulfate) is an inhibitor of ADP-induced platelet aggregation acting by direct inhibition of adenosine diphosphate (ADP) binding to its receptor and of the subsequent ADP-mediated activation of the glycoprotein GPIIb/IIIa complex. Chemically it is methyl (+)-(*S*)-α-(2-chlorophenyl)-6,7-dihydrothieno[3,2-c]pyridine-5(4*H*)-acetate sulfate (1:1). The empirical formula of clopidogrel bisulfate is $C_{16}H_{16}Cl\ NO_2S \bullet H_2SO_4$ and its molecular weight is 419.9.
The structural formula is as follows:

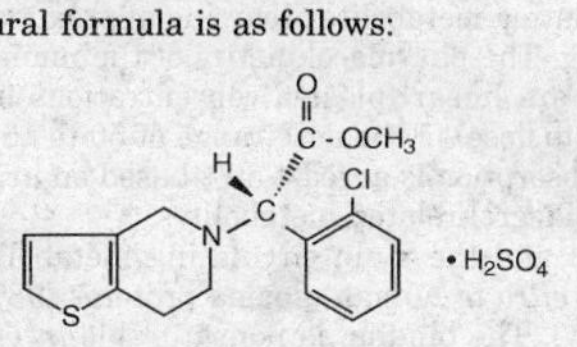

Clopidogrel bisulfate is a white to off-white powder. It is practically insoluble in water at neutral pH but freely soluble at pH 1. It also dissolves freely in methanol, dissolves sparingly in methylene chloride, and is practically insoluble in ethyl ether. It has a specific optical rotation of about +56°.
PLAVIX for oral administration is provided as pink, round, biconvex, engraved film-coated tablets containing 97.875 mg of clopidogrel bisulfate which is the molar equivalent of 75 mg of clopidogrel base.
Each tablet contains anhydrous lactose, hydrogenated castor oil, microcrystalline cellulose, polyethylene glycol 6000 and pregelatinized starch as inactive ingredients. The pink film coating contains ferric oxide (red), hydroxypropyl methylcellulose 2910, polyethylene glycol 6000 and titanium dioxide. The tablets are polished with Carnauba wax.

CLINICAL PHARMACOLOGY

Mechanism of Action
Clopidogrel is an inhibitor of platelet aggregation. A variety of drugs that inhibit platelet function have been shown to decrease morbid events in people with established atherosclerotic cardiovascular disease as evidenced by stroke or transient ischemic attacks, myocardial infarction, or need for bypass or angioplasty. This indicates that platelets participate in the initiation and/or evolution of these events and that inhibiting them can reduce the event rate.
Pharmacodynamic Properties
Clopidogrel selectively inhibits the binding of adenosine diphosphate (ADP) to its platelet receptor and the subsequent

Continued on next page

This product information was prepared in September 1998. On these and other products of Sanofi Pharmaceuticals, Inc., detailed information may be obtained on a current basis by direct inquiry to Product Information Services, 90 Park Avenue, New York, NY 10016 (toll free 1-800-446-6267).

Plavix—Cont.

ADP-mediated activation of the glycoprotein GPIIb/IIIa complex, thereby inhibiting platelet aggregation. Biotransformation of clopidogrel is necessary to produce inhibition of platelet aggregation, but an active metabolite responsible for the activity of the drug has not been isolated. Clopidogrel also inhibits platelet aggregation induced by agonists other than ADP by blocking the amplification of platelet activation by released ADP. Clopidogrel does not inhibit phosphodiesterase activity.

Clopidogrel acts by irreversibly modifying the platelet ADP receptor. Consequently, platelets exposed to clopidogrel are affected for the remainder of their lifespan.

Dose dependent inhibition of platelet aggregation can be seen 2 hours after single oral doses of PLAVIX. Repeated doses of 75 mg PLAVIX per day inhibit ADP-induced platelet aggregation on the first day, and inhibition reaches steady state between Day 3 and Day 7. At steady state, the average inhibition level observed with a dose of 75 mg PLAVIX per day was between 40% and 60%. Platelet aggregation and bleeding time gradually return to baseline values after treatment is discontinued, generally in about 5 days.

Pharmacokinetics and Metabolism

After repeated 75–mg oral doses of clopidogrel (base), plasma concentrations of the parent compound, which has no platelet inhibiting effect, are very low and are generally below the quantification limit (0.00025 mg/L) beyond 2 hours after dosing. Clopidogrel is extensively metabolized by the liver. The main circulating metabolite is the carboxylic acid derivative, and it too has no effect on platelet aggregation. It represents about 85% of the circulating drug-related compounds in plasma.

Following an oral dose of ^{14}C-labeled clopidogrel in humans, approximately 50% was excreted in the urine and approximately 46% in the feces in the 5 days after dosing. The elimination half-life of the main circulating metabolite was 8 hours after single and repeated administration. Covalent binding to platelets accounted for 2% of radiolabel with a half-life of 11 days.

Effect of Food: Administration of PLAVIX (clopidogrel bisulfate) with meals did not significantly modify the bioavailability of clopidogrel as assessed by the pharmacokinetics of the main circulating metabolite.

Absorption and Distribution: Clopidogrel is rapidly absorbed after oral administration of repeated doses of 75 mg clopidogrel (base), with peak plasma levels ($\cong 3$ mg/L) of the main circulating metabolite occurring approximately 1 hour after dosing. The pharmacokinetics of the main circulating metabolite are linear (plasma concentrations increased in proportion to dose) in the dose range of 50 to 150 mg of clopidogrel. Absorption is at least 50% based on urinary excretion of clopidogrel-related metabolites.

Clopidogrel and the main circulating metabolite bind reversibly *in vitro* to human plasma proteins (98% and 94%, respectively). The binding is nonsaturable *in vitro* up to a concentration of 100 µg/mL.

Metabolism and Elimination: In vitro and in vivo, clopidogrel undergoes rapid hydrolysis into its carboxylic acid derivative. In plasma and urine, the glucuronide of the carboxylic acid derivative is also observed.

Special Populations

Geriatric Patients: Plasma concentrations of the main circulating metabolite are significantly higher in elderly (≥ 75 years) compared to young healthy volunteers but these higher plasma levels were not associated with differences in platelet aggregation and bleeding time. No dosage adjustment is needed for the elderly.

Renally Impaired Patients: After repeated doses of 75 mg PLAVIX per day, plasma levels of the main circulating metabolite were lower in patients with severe renal impairment (creatinine clearance from 5 to 15 mL/min) compared to subjects with moderate renal impairment (creatinine clearance 30 to 60 mL/min) or healthy subjects. Although inhibition of ADP-induced platelet aggregation was lower (25%) than that observed in healthy volunteers, the prolongation of bleeding time was similar to healthy volunteers receiving 75 mg of PLAVIX per day. No dosage adjustment is needed in renally impaired patients.

Gender: No significant difference was observed in the plasma levels of the main circulating metabolite between males and females. In a small study comparing men and women, less inhibition of ADP-induced platelet aggregation was observed in women, but there was no difference in prolongation of bleeding time. In the large, controlled clinical study (Clopidogrel vs. Aspirin in Patients at Risk of Ischemic Events; CAPRIE), the incidence of clinical outcome events, other adverse clinical events, and abnormal clinical laboratory parameters was similar in men and women.

Race: Pharmacokinetic differences due to race have not been studied.

CLINICAL STUDIES

The evidence for the efficacy of PLAVIX is derived from CAPRIE (Clopidogrel vs. Aspirin in Patients at

Risk of Ischemic Events) trial. This was a 19,185-patient, 304-center, international, randomized, double-blind, parallel-group study comparing PLAVIX (75 mg daily) to aspirin (325 mg daily). The patients randomized had: 1) recent histories of myocardial infarction (within 35 days); 2) recent histories of ischemic stroke (within 6 months) with at least a week of residual neurological signs; or 3) objectively established peripheral arterial disease. Patients received randomized treatment for an average of 1.6 years (maximum of 3 years).

The trial's primary outcome was the time to first occurrence of new ischemic stroke (fatal or not), new myocardial infarction (fatal or not), or other vascular death. Deaths not easily attributable to nonvascular causes were all classified as vascular.

Outcome Events of the Primary Analysis

Patients	PLAVIX 9599	apririn 9586
IS (fatal or not)	438 (4.56%)	461 (4.81%)
MI (fatal or not)	275 (2.86%)	333 (3.47%)
Other vascular death	226 (2.35%)	226 (2.36%)
Total	939 (9.78%)	1020 (10.64%)

As shown in the table, PLAVIX (clopidogrel bisulfate) was associated with a lower incidence of outcome events of every kind. The overall risk reduction (9.78% vs. 10.64%) was 8.7%, P=0.045. Similar results were obtained when all-cause mortality and all-cause strokes were counted instead of vascular mortality and ischemic strokes (risk reduction 6.9%). In patients who survived an on-study stroke or myocardial infarction, the incidence of subsequent events was again lower in the PLAVIX group.

The curves showing the overall event rate are shown in the figure. The event curves separated early and continued to diverge over the 3-year follow-up period.

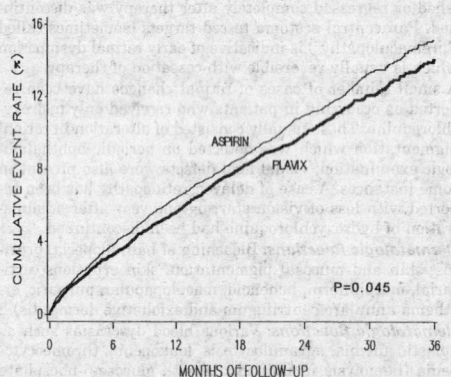

FATAL OR NON–FATAL VASCULAR EVENTS

P=0.045

MONTHS OF FOLLOW-UP

Although the statistical significance favoring PLAVIX over aspirin was marginal (P=0.045), and represents the result of a single trial that has not been replicated, the comparator drug, aspirin, is itself effective (vs. placebo) in reducing cardiovascular events in patients with recent myocardial infarction or stroke. Thus, the difference between PLAVIX and placebo, although not measured directly, is substantial. The CAPRIE trial included a population that was randomized on the basis of 3 entry criteria. The efficacy of PLAVIX relative to aspirin was heterogeneous across these randomized subgroups (P=0.043). It is not clear whether this difference is real or a chance occurrence. Although the CAPRIE trial was not designed to evaluate the relative benefit of PLAVIX over aspirin in the individual patient subgroups, the benefit appeared to be strongest in patients who were enrolled because of peripheral vascular disease (especially those who also had a history of myocardial infarction) and weaker in stroke patients. In patients who were enrolled in the trial on the sole basis of a recent myocardial infarction, PLAVIX was not numerically superior to aspirin.

In the meta-analyses of studies of aspirin vs. placebo in patients similar to those in CAPRIE, aspirin was associated with a reduced incidence of atherothrombotic events. There was a suggestion of heterogeneity in these studies too, with the effect strongest in patients with a history of myocardial infarction, weaker in patients with a history of stroke, and not discernible in patients with a history of peripheral vascular disease. With respect to the inferred comparison of PLAVIX to placebo, there is no indication of heterogeneity.

INDICATIONS AND USAGE

PLAVIX (clopidogrel bisulfate) is indicated for the reduction of atherosclerotic events (myocardial infarction, stroke, and vascular death) in patients with atherosclerosis documented by recent stroke, recent myocardial infarction, or established peripheral arterial disease.

CONTRAINDICATIONS

The use of PLAVIX is contraindicated in the following conditions:
- Hypersensitivity to the drug substance or any component of the product.
- Active pathological bleeding such as peptic ulcer or intracranial hemorrhage.

WARNINGS

None.

PRECAUTIONS

General

As with other anti-platelet agents, PLAVIX should be used with caution in patients who may be at risk of increased bleeding from trauma, surgery, or other pathological conditions. If a patient is to undergo elective surgery and an antiplatelet effect is not desired, PLAVIX should be discontinued 7 days prior to surgery.

GI Bleeding: PLAVIX prolongs the bleeding time. In CAPRIE, PLAVIX was associated with a rate of gastrointestinal bleeding of 2.0%, vs. 2.7% on aspirin. PLAVIX should be used with caution in patients who have lesions with a propensity to bleed (such as ulcers). Drugs that might induce such lesions (such as aspirin and other nonsteroidal anti-inflammatory drugs [NSAIDs]) should be used with caution in patients taking PLAVIX.

Use in Hepatically Impaired Patients: Experience is limited in patients with severe hepatic disease, who may have bleeding diatheses. PLAVIX should be used with caution in this population.

Information for Patients

Patients should be told that it may take them longer than usual to stop bleeding when they take PLAVIX, and that they should report any unusual bleeding to their physician. Patients should inform physicians and dentists that they are taking PLAVIX before any surgery is scheduled or before any new drug is taken.

Drug Interactions

Study of specific drug interactions yielded the following results:

Aspirin: Aspirin did not modify the clopidogrel-mediated inhibition of ADP-induced platelet aggregation. Concomitant administration of 500 mg of aspirin twice a day for 1 day did not significantly increase the prolongation of bleeding time induced by PLAVIX. PLAVIX potentiated the effect of aspirin on collagen-induced platelet aggregation. The safety of chronic concomitant administration of aspirin and PLAVIX has not been established.

Heparin: In a study in healthy volunteers, PLAVIX did not necessitate modification of the heparin dose or alter the effect of heparin on coagulation. Coadministration of heparin had no effect on inhibition of platelet aggregation induced by PLAVIX. The safety of this combination has not been established, however, and concomitant use should be undertaken with caution.

Nonsteroidal Anti-Inflammatory Drugs (NSAIDs): In healthy volunteers receiving naproxen, concomitant administration of PLAVIX was associated with increased occult gastrointestinal blood loss. NSAIDs and PLAVIX should be coadministered with caution.

Warfarin: The safety of the coadministration of PLAVIX with warfarin has not been established. Consequently, concomitant administration of these two agents should be undertaken with caution. (See **Precautions - General**).

Other Concomitant Therapy: No clinically significant pharmacodynamic interactions were observed when PLAVIX was coadministered with **atenolol, nifedipine**, or both atenolol and nifedipine. The pharmacodynamic activity of PLAVIX was also not significantly influenced by the coadministration of **phenobarbital, cimetidine** or **estrogen**.

The pharmacokinetics of **digoxin** or **theophylline** were not modified by the coadministration of PLAVIX (clopidogrel bisulfate).

At high concentrations *in vitro*, clopidogrel inhibits P_{450} (2C9). Accordingly, PLAVIX may interfere with the metabolism of **phenytoin, tamoxifen, tolbutamide, warfarin, torsemide, fluvastatin**, and many **nonsteroidal anti-inflammatory agents**, but there are no data with which to predict the magnitude of these interactions. Caution should be used when any of these drugs is coadministered with PLAVIX.

In addition to the above specific interaction studies, patients entered into CAPRIE received a variety of concomitant medications **including diuretics, beta-blocking agents, angiotensin converting enzyme inhibitors, calcium antagonists, cholesterol lowering agents, coronary vasodilators, antidiabetic agents, antiepileptic agents** and **hormone replacement therapy** without evidence of clinically significant adverse interactions.

Drug/Laboratory Test Interactions

None known.

Carcinogenesis, Mutagenesis, Impairment of Fertility

There was no evidence of tumorigenicity when clopidogrel was administered for 78 weeks to mice and 104 weeks to rats at dosages up to 77 mg/kg per day, which afforded plasma exposures >25 times that in humans at the recommended daily dose of 75 mg.

Clopidogrel was not genotoxic in four *in vitro* tests (Ames test, DNA-repair test in rat hepatocytes, gene mutation assay in Chinese hamster fibroblasts, and metaphase chromo-

some analysis of human lymphocytes) and in one *in vivo* test (micronucleus test by oral route in mice).

Clopidogrel was found to have no effect on fertility of male and female rats at oral doses up to 400 mg/kg per day (52 times the recommended human dose on a mg/m² basis).

Pregnancy

Pregnancy Category B. Reproduction studies performed in rats and rabbits at doses up to 500 and 300 mg/kg/day (respectively, 65 and 78 times the recommended daily human dose on a mg/m² basis), revealed no evidence of impaired fertility or fetotoxicity due to clopidogrel. There are, however, no adequate and well-controlled studies in pregnant women. Because animal reproduction studies are not always predictive of a human response, PLAVIX should be used during pregnancy only if clearly needed.

Nursing Mothers

Studies in rats have shown that clopidogrel and/or its metabolites are excreted in the milk. It is not known whether this drug is excreted in human milk. Because many drugs are excreted in human milk and because of the potential for serious adverse reactions in nursing infants, a decision should be made whether to discontinue nursing or to discontinue the drug, taking into account the importance of the drug to the nursing woman.

Pediatric Use

Safety and effectiveness in the pediatric population have not been established.

ADVERSE REACTIONS

PLAVIX has been evaluated for safety in more than 11,300 patients, including over 7,000 patients treated for 1 year or more. The overall tolerability of PLAVIX was similar to that of aspirin regardless of age, gender and race, with an approximately equal incidence (13%) of patients withdrawing from treatment because of adverse reactions. The clinically important adverse events observed in CAPRIE are discussed below.

Hemorrhagic: In patients receiving PLAVIX in CAPRIE, gastrointestinal hemorrhage occurred at a rate of 2.0%, and required hospitalization in 0.7%. In patients receiving aspirin, the corresponding rates were 2.7% and 1.1%, respectively. The incidence of intracranial hemorrhage was 0.4% for PLAVIX compared to 0.5% for aspirin.

Neutropenia/agranulocytosis: Ticlopidine, a drug chemically similar to PLAVIX, is associated with a 0.8% rate of severe neutropenia (less than 450 neutrophils/µL). Patients in CAPRIE (see Clinical Trials) were intensively monitored for neutropenia. Severe neutropenia was observed in six patients, four on PLAVIX and two on aspirin. Two of the 9599 patients who received PLAVIX and none of the 9586 patients who received aspirin had neutrophil counts of zero. One of the four PLAVIX patients was receiving cytotoxic chemotherapy, and another recovered and returned to the trial after only temporarily interrupting treatment with PLAVIX.

Although the risk of myelotoxicity with PLAVIX thus appears to be quite low, this possibility should be considerd when a patient receiving PLAVIX demonstrates fever or other sign of infection.

Gastrointestinal: Overall, the incidence of gastrointestinal events (e.g. abdominal pain, dyspepsia, gastritis and constipation) in patients receiving PLAVIX (clopidogrel bisulfate) was 27.1%, compared to 29.8% in those receiving aspirin.

The incidence of peptic, gastric or duodenal ulcers was 0.7% for PLAVIX and 1.2% for aspirin.

Cases of diarrhea were reported in 4.5% of patients in the PLAVIX group compared to 3.4% in the aspirin group. However, these were rarely severe (PLAVIX=0.2% and aspirin=0.1%).

The incidence of patients withdrawing from treatment because of gastrointestinal adverse reactions was 3.2% for PLAVIX and 4.0% for aspirin.

Rash and Other Skin Disorders: The incidence of skin and appendage disorders in patients receiving PLAVIX was 15.8% (0.7% serious); the corresponding rate in aspirin patients was 13.1% (0.5% serious).

The overall incidence of patients withdrawing from treatment because of skin and appendage disorders adverse reactions was 1.5% for PLAVIX and 0.8% for aspirin.

Adverse events occurring in ≥2.5% of patients on PLAVIX in the CAPRIE controlled clinical trial are shown below regardless of relationship to PLAVIX. The median duration of therapy was 20 months, with a maximum of 3 years.

Adverse Events Occurring in ≥2.5% of PLAVIX Patients

Body System Event	PLAVIX [n=9599] % Incidence (% Discontinuation)	Aspirin [n=9586] % Incidence (% Discontinuation)
Body as a Whole - general disorders		
Chest Pain	8.3 (0.2)	8.3 (0.3)
Accidental Injury	7.9 (0.1)	7.3 (0.1)
Influenza-like symptoms	7.5 (<0.1)	7.0 (<0.1)
Pain	6.4 (0.1)	6.3 (0.1)
Fatigue	3.3 (0.1)	3.4 (0.1)
Cardiovascular disorders, general		
Edema	4.1 (<0.1)	4.5 (<0.1)
Hypertension	4.3 (<0.1)	5.1 (<0.1)
Central & peripheral nervous system disorders		
Headache	7.6 (0.3)	7.2 (0.3)
Dizziness	6.2 (0.2)	6.7 (0.3)
Gastrointestinal system disorders		
Abdominal pain	5.6 (0.7)	7.1 (1.0)
Dyspepsia	5.2 (0.6)	6.1 (0.7)
Diarrhea	4.5 (0.4)	3.4 (0.3)
Nausea	3.4 (0.5)	3.8 (0.4)
Metabolic & nutritional disorders		
Hypercholesterolemia	4.0 (0)	4.4 (<0.1)
Musculo-skeletal system disorders		
Arthralgia	6.3 (0.1)	6.2 (0.1)
Back Pain	5.8 (0.1)	5.3 (<0.1)
Platelet, bleeding, & clotting disorders		
Purpura	5.3 (0.3)	3.7 (0.1)
Epistaxis	2.9 (0.2)	2.5 (0.1)
Psychiatric disorders		
Depression	3.6 (0.1)	3.9 (0.2)
Respiratory system disorders		
Upper resp tract infection	8.7 (<0.1)	8.3 (<0.1)
Dyspnea	4.5 (<0.1)	4.7 (0.1)
Rhinitis	4.2 (0.1)	4.2 (<0.1)
Bronchitis	3.7 (0.1)	3.7 (0)
Coughing	3.1 (<0.1)	2.7 (<0.1)
Skin & appendage disorders		
Rash	4.2 (0.5)	3.5 (0.2)
Pruritus	3.3 (0.3)	1.6 (0.1)
Urinary system disorders		
Urinary tract infection	3.1 (0)	3.5 (0.1)

Incidence of discontinuation, regardless of relationship to therapy, is shown in parentheses.

Other adverse experiences of potential importance occurring in 1% to 2.5% of patients receiving PLAVIX (clopidogrel bisulfate) in the CAPRIE controlled clinical trial are listed below regardless of relationship to PLAVIX. In general, the incidence of these events was similar in the aspirin-treated group.

Autonomic Nervous System Disorders: Syncope, Palpitation. *Body as a Whole - general disorders:* Asthenia, Hernia. *Cardiovascular disorders:* Cardiac failure. *Central and peripheral nervous system disorders:* Cramps legs, Hypoaesthesia, Neuralgia, Paraesthesia, Vertigo. *Gastrointestinal system disorders:* Constipation, Vomiting. *Heart rate and rhythm disorders:* Fibrillation atrial. *Liver and biliary system disorders:* Hepatic enzymes increased. *Metabolic and nutritional disorders:* Gout, hyperuricemia, non-protein nitrogen (NPN) increased. *Musculo-skeletal system disorders:* Arthritis, Arthrosis. *Platelet, bleeding & clotting disorders:* GI hemorrhage, hematoma, platelets decreased. *Psychiatric disorders:* Anxiety, Insomnia. *Red blood cell disorders:* Anemia. *Respiratory system disorders:* Pneumonia, Sinusitis. *Skin and appendage disorders:* Eczema, Skin ulceration. *Urinary system disorders:* Cystitis. *Vision disorders:* Cataract, Conjunctivitis.

Other potentially serious adverse events which may be of clinical interest but were rarely reported (<1%) in patients who received PLAVIX are listed below regardless of relationship to PLAVIX. In general, the incidence of these events was similar in the aspirin group.

Body as a whole: Allergic reaction, necrosis ischemic. *Cardiovascular disorders:* Edema generalized. *Gastrointestinal system disorders:* Gastric ulcer perforated, gastritis hemorrhagic, upper GI ulcer hemorrhagic. *Liver and Biliary system disorders:* Bilirubinemia, hepatitis infectious, liver fatty. *Platelet, bleeding and clotting disorders:* hemarthrosis, hematuria, hemoptysis, hemorrhage intracranial, hemorrhage retroperitoneal, hemorrhage of operative wound, ocular hemorrhage, pulmonary hemorrhage, purpura allergic, thrombocytopenia. *Red blood cell disorders:* Anemia aplastic, anemia hypochromic. *Reproductive disorders, female:* Menorrhagia. *Respiratory system disorders:* Hemothorax. *Skin and appendage disorders:* Bullous eruption, rash erythematous, rash maculopapular, urticaria. *White cell and reticuloendothelial system disorders:* Agranulocytosis, granulocytopenia, leukemia, leukopenia, neutrophils decreased.

OVERDOSAGE

One case of deliberate overdosage with PLAVIX was reported in the large, controlled clinical study. A 34-year-old woman took a single 1,050-mg dose of PLAVIX (equivalent to 14 standard 75-mg tablets). There were no associated adverse events. No special therapy was instituted, and she recovered without sequelae.

No adverse events were reported after single oral administration of 600 mg (equivalent to 8 standard 75-mg tablets) of PLAVIX in healthy volunteers. The bleeding time was prolonged by a factor of 1.7, which is similar to that typically observed with the therapeutic dose of 75 mg of PLAVIX per day.

A single oral dose or clopidogrel at 1500 or 2000 mg/kg was lethal to mice and to rats and at 3000 mg/kg to baboons. Symptoms of acute toxicity were vomiting (in baboons), prostration, difficult breathing, and gastrointestinal hemorrhage in all species.

Recommendations About Specific Treatment:

Based on biological plausibility, platelet transfusion may be appropriate to reverse the pharmacological effects of PLAVIX if quick reversal is required.

DOSAGE AND ADMINISTRATION

The recommended dose of PLAVIX is 75 mg once daily with or without food.

No dosage adjustment is necessary for elderly patients or patients with renal disease. (See **Clinical Pharmacology: Special Populations**.)

HOW SUPPLIED

PLAVIX (clopidogrel bisulfate) is available as a pink, round, biconvex, film-coated tablet engraved with "75" on one side. Tablets are provided as follows:

NDC 63653-1171-6 bottles of 30
NDC 63653-1171-1 bottles of 90
NDC 63653-1171-5 bottles of 500
NDC 63653-1171-3 blisters of 100

Storage

Store at 25°C (77°F); excursions permitted to 15°-30°C (59°-86°F) [See USP Controlled Room Temperature]

Manufactured by:
Sanofi Pharmaceuticals, Inc.
New York, NY 10016
Distributed by:
Bristol-Myers Squibb/Sanofi Pharmaceuticals Partnership
New York, NY 10016
PLAVIX® is a registered trademark of Sanofi

Revised May, 1998

J4-643B 51-006857-02

Shown in Product Identification Guide, page 335

POLY–HISTINE CS® ℂ ℞

Each 5 ml raspberry/strawberry flavored alcohol-free, red syrup contains:

Codeine Phosphate	10.0 mg
(Warning: May be habit forming.)	
Phenylpropanolamine HCl	12.5 mg
Brompheniramine Maleate	2.0 mg

HOW SUPPLIED

Bottles of 16 oz.
NDC 0024-1633-16

POLY–HISTINE ELIXIR® ℞

Each teaspoonful (5 ml) lemon-lime flavored green elixir contains:

Phenyltoloxamine Citrate	4.0 mg
Pyrilamine Maleate	4.0 mg
Pheniramine Maleate	4.0 mg
Alcohol	4%

HOW SUPPLIED

Bottles of 16 oz.
NDC 0024-1647-16

POLY–HISTINE-D® CAPSULES ℞

Each timed release* half red, half clear capsule with SANOFI printed on both halves contains:

Phenylpropanolamine HCl	50.0 mg

Continued on next page

This product information was prepared in September 1998. On these and other products of Sanofi Pharmaceuticals, Inc., detailed information may be obtained on a current basis by direct inquiry to Product Information Services, 90 Park Avenue, New York, NY 10016 (toll free 1-800-446-6267).

Poly-Histine-D Capsules—Cont.

Phenyltoloxamine Citrate	16.0 mg
Pyrilamine Maleate	16.0 mg
Pheniramine Maleate	16.0 mg

* In a special base to provide prolonged therapeutic action.

HOW SUPPLIED

Bottles of 100.
NDC 0024-1656-01
Shown in Product Identification Guide, page 335

POLY–HISTINE–D® ELIXIR ℞

Each teaspoonful (5 ml) wild cherry flavored red elixir contains:

Phenylpropanolamine HCl	12.5 mg
Phenyltoloxamine Citrate	4.0 mg
Pyrilamine Maleate	4.0 mg
Pheniramine Maleate	4.0 mg
Alcohol	4%

HOW SUPPLIED

Bottles of 16 oz.
NDC 0024-1662-16

POLY–HISTINE–D® PED CAPS ℞

Each timed release* clear capsule with SANOFI printed on both halves contains:

Phenylpropanolamine HCl	25 mg
Phenyltoloxamine Citrate	8 mg
Pyrilamine Maleate	8 mg
Pheniramine Maleate	8 mg

* In a special base to provide prolonged therapeutic action.

HOW SUPPLIED

Bottles of 100.
NDC 0024-1658-01
Shown in Product Identification Guide, page 335

POLY–HISTINE DM® SYRUP ℞

Each 5 ml black-raspberry flavored alcohol-free, sugar free purple syrup contains:

Dextromethorphan HBr	10.0 mg
Phenylpropanolamine HCl	12.5 mg
Brompheniramine Maleate	2.0 mg

HOW SUPPLIED

Bottles of 16 oz.
NDC 0024-1686-16

PRENATE® ULTRA™ TABLETS ℞
PRENATAL VITAMINS

DESCRIPTION

PRENATE® ULTRA™ is a white dye-free oval oil-and-water-soluble multivitamin/multimineral tablet which contains UltraDense™ calcium citrate and MicroIron II™ carbonyl iron. The tablet is embossed "sanofi" on one side and "P" bisect "N" on the other side.

Each tablet contains:

Elemental Iron (carbonyl iron)	90 mg
Iodine (potassium iodide)	150 mcg
Calcium (calcium citrate)	200 mg
Copper (cupric oxide)	2 mg
Zinc (zinc oxide)	25 mg
Folic Acid	1 mg
Vitamin A‡	2700 IU
Vitamin D3 (cholecalciferol)	400 IU
Vitamin E (dl-alpha tocopheryl acetate)	30 IU
Vitamin C (ascorbic acid)	120 mg
Vitamin B1 (thiamine mononitrate)	3 mg
Vitamin B2 (riboflavin)	3.4 mg
Vitamin B6 (pyridoxine HCl)	20 mg
Vitamin B12 (cyanocobalamin)	12 mcg
Niacinamide	20 mg
Docusate Sodium	50 mg

‡Input as Vitamin A palmitate and beta carotene.

INDICATIONS

PRENATE ULTRA is a multivitamin/multimineral nutritional supplement indicated for use in improving the nutritional status of women throughout pregnancy and in the postnatal period for both lactating and nonlactating mothers. PRENATE ULTRA can also be beneficial in improving the nutritional status of women prior to conception.

CONTRAINDICATIONS

This product is contraindicated in patients with a known hypersensitivity to any of the ingredients.

> **WARNING**
> Accidental overdose of iron-containing products is a leading cause of fatal poisoning in children under 6. Keep this product out of reach of children. In case of accidental overdose, call a doctor or poison control center immediately.

Folic acid alone is improper therapy in the treatment of pernicious anemia and other megaloblastic anemias where vitamin B12 is deficient.

NOTICE

Contact with moisture may produce surface discoloration or erosion of the tablet.

PRECAUTIONS

Folic acid in doses above 0.1 mg daily may obscure pernicious anemia in that hematologic remission can occur while neurological manifestations progress.

ADVERSE REACTIONS

Allergic sensitization has been reported following both oral and parenteral administration of folic acid.

DOSAGE AND ADMINISTRATION

One tablet daily or as directed by a physician.

HOW SUPPLIED

100's — NDC 0024-1730-01
DISPENSE IN A TIGHT, LIGHT RESISTANT CONTAINER AS DEFINED BY THE USP/NF WITH A CHILD RESISTANT CLOSURE.
KEEP THIS AND ALL DRUGS OUT OF THE REACH OF CHILDREN.
Store at controlled room temperature.
PRENATE ULTRA STARTER KIT CONTAINS A SEVEN-DAY BLISTER PACK OF PRENATAL VITAMINS PLUS A PRENATAL CARE BOOKLET.
Mfg. for Sanofi Pharmaceuticals, Inc.
New York, NY 10016
by Mission Pharmacal Co.
San Antonio, TX 78296

Shown in Product Identification Guide, page 335

PRIMACOR® ℞
MILRINONE LACTATE INJECTION

DESCRIPTION

PRIMACOR, brand of milrinone lactate injection, is a member of a new class of bipyridine inotropic/vasodilator agents with phosphodiesterase inhibitor activity, distinct from digitalis glycosides or catecholamines. PRIMACOR (milrinone lactate) is designated chemically as 1,6-dihydro-2-methyl-6-oxo-[3,4'-bipyridine]-5-carbonitrile lactate and has the following structure:

Milrinone is an off-white to tan crystalline compound with a molecular weight of 211.2 and an empirical formula of $C_{12}H_9N_3O$. It is slightly soluble in methanol, and very slightly soluble in chloroform and in water. As the lactate salt, it is stable and colorless to pale yellow in solution. PRIMACOR is available as sterile aqueous solutions of the lactate salt of milrinone for injection or infusion intravenously.

Sterile, single-dose vials: Single-dose vials of 10 and 20 mL contain in each mL milrinone lactate equivalent to 1 mg milrinone and 47 mg Dextrose, Anhydrous, USP, in Water for Injection, USP. The pH is adjusted to between 3.2 and 4.0 with lactic acid or sodium hydroxide. The total concentration of lactic acid can vary between 0.95 mg/mL and 1.29 mg/mL. These vials require preparation of dilutions prior to administration to patients intravenously.

Pre-Mix Flexible Container: The Flexible Container provides a ready-to-use dilution of milrinone in a volume of 100 and 200 mL of 5% Dextrose Injection. Each mL contains milrinone lactate equivalent to 200 mcg milrinone. The nominal concentration of lactic acid is 0.282 mg/mL. Each mL also contains 49.4 mg Dextrose, Anhydrous, USP. The pH is adjusted to between 3.2 and 4.0 with lactic acid or sodium hydroxide. The flexible plastic container is comprised of polyvinyl chloride with a foil overwrap. Water can permeate the plastic into the overwrap, but the amount is insufficient to significantly affect the pre-mix solution.

CLINICAL PHARMACOLOGY

PRIMACOR is a positive inotrope and vasodilator, with little chronotropic activity different in structure and mode of action from either the digitalis glycosides or catecholamines.

PRIMACOR, at relevant inotropic and vasorelaxant concentrations, is a selective inhibitor of peak III cAMP phosphodiesterase isozyme in cardiac and vascular muscle. This inhibitory action is consistent with cAMP mediated increases in intracellular ionized calcium and contractile force in cardiac muscle, as well as with cAMP dependent contractile protein phosphorylation and relaxation in vascular muscle. Additional experimental evidence also indicates that PRIMACOR is not a beta-adrenergic agonist nor does it inhibit sodium-potassium adenosine triphosphatase activity as do the digitalis glycosides.

Clinical studies in patients with congestive heart failure have shown that PRIMACOR produces dose-related and plasma drug concentration-related increases in the maximum rate of increase of left ventricular pressure. Studies in normal subjects have shown that PRIMACOR produces increases in the slope of the left ventricular pressure-dimension relationship, indicating a direct inotropic effect of the drug. PRIMACOR also produces dose-related and plasma concentration-related increases in forearm blood flow in patients with congestive heart failure, indicating a direct arterial vasodilator activity of the drug.

Both the inotropic and vasodilatory effects have been observed over the therapeutic range of plasma milrinone concentrations of 100 ng/mL to 300 ng/mL.

In addition to increasing myocardial contractility, PRIMACOR improves diastolic function as evidenced by improvements in left ventricular diastolic relaxation.

A further clinical perspective was obtained in a single, multi-center, double-blind trial of the chronic administration of oral milrinone. Patients with New York Heart Association Class III and IV heart failure and left ventricular ejection fraction of less than 35% were randomized to placebo (N=527) or oral milrinone (40 mg daily, N=561) and followed for a median of six months. The oral milrinone treatment group had statistically significantly increased all-cause mortality and cardiovascular mortality. This finding in patients on oral milrinone was not apparent during the initial period of chronic treatment (15 days) in either the overall patient population or in the NYHA Class IV subgroup.

The acute administration of intravenous milrinone has also been evaluated in clinical trials in excess of 1600 patients, with chronic heart failure, associated with cardiac surgery, and heart failure associated with myocardial infarction. The total number of deaths, either on therapy or shortly thereafter (24 hours) was 15, less than 0.9%, few of which were thought to be drug-related.

Pharmacokinetics

Following intravenous injections of 12.5 mcg/kg to 125 mcg/kg to congestive heart failure patients, PRIMACOR had a volume of distribution of 0.38 liters/kg, a mean terminal elimination half-life of 2.3 hours, and a clearance of 0.13 liters/kg/hr. Following intravenous infusions of 0.20 mcg/kg/min to 0.70 mcg/kg/min to congestive heart failure patients, the drug had a volume of distribution of about 0.45 liters/kg, a mean terminal elimination half-life of 2.4 hours, and a clearance of 0.14 liters/kg/hr. These pharmacokinetic parameters were not dose-dependent, and the area under the plasma concentration versus time curve following injections was significantly dose-dependent.

PRIMACOR has been shown (by equilibrium dialysis) to be approximately 70% bound to human plasma protein.

The primary route of excretion of PRIMACOR in man is via the urine. The major urinary excretions of orally administered PRIMACOR in man are milrinone (83%) and its 0-glucuronide metabolite (12%). Elimination in normal subjects via the urine is rapid, with approximately 60% recovered within the first two hours following dosing and approximately 90% recovered within the first eight hours following dosing. The mean renal clearance of PRIMACOR is approximately 0.3 liters/min, indicative of active secretion.

Pharmacodynamics

In patients with depressed myocardial function, PRIMACOR produced a prompt increase in cardiac output and decreases in pulmonary capillary wedge pressure and vascular resistance, without a significant increase in heart rate or myocardial oxygen consumption. These hemodynamic improvements were dose and plasma milrinone concentration related. Hemodynamic improvement during intravenous therapy with PRIMACOR was accompanied by clinical symptomatic improvement, as measured by changes in New York Heart Association classification. The great majority of patients experience improvements in hemodynamic function within 5 to 15 minutes of the initiation of therapy. In studies in congestive heart failure patients, PRIMACOR when administered as a loading injection followed by a

maintenance infusion produced significant mean initial increases in cardiac index of 25 percent, 38 percent, and 42 percent at dose regimens of 37.5 mcg/kg/0.375 mcg/kg/min, 50 mcg/kg/0.50 mcg/kg/min, and 75 mcg/kg/0.75 mcg/kg/min, respectively. Over the same range of loading injections and maintenance infusions, pulmonary capillary wedge pressure significantly decreased by 20 percent, 23 percent, and 36 percent, respectively, while systemic vascular resistance significantly decreased by 17 percent, 21 percent, and 37 percent. The heart rate was generally unchanged (increases of 3, 3 and 10 percent, respectively). Mean arterial pressure fell by up to 5 percent at the two lower dose regimens, but by 17 percent at the highest dose. Patients evaluated for 48 hours maintained improvements in hemodynamic function, with no evidence of diminished response (tachyphylaxis). A smaller number of patients have received infusions of PRIMACOR for periods up to 72 hours without evidence of tachyphylaxis.

The duration of therapy should depend upon patient responsiveness. Patients have been maintained on infusions of PRIMACOR for up to 5 days.

PRIMACOR has a favorable inotropic effect in fully digitalized patients without causing signs of glycoside toxicity. Theoretically, in cases of atrial flutter/fibrillation, it is possible that PRIMACOR may increase ventricular response rate because of its slight enhancement of AV node conduction. In these cases, digitalis should be considered prior to the institution of therapy with PRIMACOR.

Improvement in left ventricular function in patients with ischemic heart disease has been observed. The improvement has occurred without inducing symptoms or electrocardiographic signs of myocardial ischemia.

The steady-state plasma milrinone concentrations after approximately 6 to 12 hours of unchanging maintenance infusion of 0.50 mcg/kg/min are approximately 200 ng/mL. Near maximum favorable effects of PRIMACOR on cardiac output and pulmonary capillary wedge pressure are seen at plasma milrinone concentrations in the 150 ng/mL to 250 ng/mL range.

INDICATIONS AND USAGE

PRIMACOR is indicated for the short-term intravenous therapy of congestive heart failure. The majority of experience with intravenous PRIMACOR has been in patients receiving digoxin and diuretics.

In some patients injections of PRIMACOR and oral PRIMACOR have been shown to increase ventricular ectopy, including nonsustained ventricular tachycardia. Patients receiving PRIMACOR should be closely monitored during infusion.

CONTRAINDICATIONS

PRIMACOR is contraindicated in patients who are hypersensitive to it.

PRECAUTIONS

General

PRIMACOR should not be used in patients with severe obstructive aortic or pulmonic valvular disease in lieu of surgical relief of the obstruction. Like other inotropic agents, it may aggravate outflow tract obstruction in hypertrophic subaortic stenosis.

Supraventricular and ventricular arrhythmias have been observed in the high-risk population treated. In some patients, injections of PRIMACOR and oral PRIMACOR have been shown to increase ventricular ectopy, including nonsustained ventricular tachycardia. The potential for arrhythmia, present in congestive heart failure itself, may be increased by many drugs or combinations of drugs. Patients receiving PRIMACOR should be closely monitored during infusion.

PRIMACOR produces a slight shortening of AV node conduction time, indicating a potential for an increased ventricular response rate in patients with atrial flutter/fibrillation which is not controlled with digitalis therapy.

During therapy with PRIMACOR, blood pressure and heart rate should be monitored and the rate of infusion slowed or stopped in patients showing excessive decreases in blood pressure.

If prior vigorous diuretic therapy is suspected to have caused significant decreases in cardiac filling pressure, PRIMACOR should be cautiously administered with monitoring of blood pressure, heart rate, and clinical symptomatology.

USE IN ACUTE MYOCARDIAL INFARCTION

No clinical studies have been conducted in patients in the acute phase of post myocardial infarction. Until further clinical experience with this class of drugs is gained, PRIMACOR is not recommended in these patients.

Laboratory Tests

Fluid and Electrolytes: Fluid and electrolyte changes and renal function should be carefully monitored during therapy with PRIMACOR. Improvement in cardiac output with resultant diuresis may necessitate a reduction in the dose of diuretic. Potassium loss due to excessive diuresis may predispose digitalized patients to arrhythmias. Therefore, hypokalemia should be corrected by potassium supplementation in advance of or during use of PRIMACOR.

MAINTENANCE DOSE

	Infusion Rate	Total Daily Dose (24 Hours)	
Minimum	0. 375 mcg/kg/min	0.59 mg/kg	Administer as a
Standard	0. 50 mcg/kg/min	0.77 mg/kg	continuous
Maximum	0. 75 mcg/kg/min	1.13 mg/kg	intravenous infusion.

PRIMACOR Infusion Rate (mL/hr) Using 200 mcg/mL Concentration

Maintenance Dose (mcg/kg/min)	Patient Body Weight (kg) 30	40	50	60	70	80	90	100	110	120
0.375	3.4	4.5	5.6	6.8	7.9	9.0	10.1	11.3	12.4	13.5
0.400	3.6	4.8	6.0	7.2	8.4	9.6	10.8	12.0	13.2	14.4
0.500	4.5	6.0	7.5	9.0	10.5	12.0	13.5	15.0	16.5	18.0
0.600	5.4	7.2	9.0	10.8	12.6	14.4	16.2	18.0	19.8	21.6
0.700	6.3	8.4	10.5	12.6	14.7	16.8	18.9	21.0	23.1	25.2
0.750	6.8	9.0	11.3	13.5	15.8	18.0	20.3	22.5	24.8	27.0

Drug Interactions

No untoward clinical manifestations have been observed in limited experience with patients in whom PRIMACOR was used concurrently with the following drugs: digitalis glycosides; lidocaine, quinidine; hydralazine, prazosin; isosorbide dinitrate, nitroglycerin; chlorthalidone, furosemide, hydrochlorothiazide, spironolactone; captopril; heparin, warfarin, diazepam, insulin; and potassium supplements.

Chemical Interactions

There is an immediate chemical interaction which is evidenced by the formation of a precipitate when furosemide is injected into an intravenous line of an infusion of PRIMACOR. Therefore, furosemide should not be administered in intravenous lines containing PRIMACOR.

Carcinogenesis, Mutagenesis, Impairment of Fertility

Twenty-four months of oral administration of PRIMACOR to mice at doses up to 40 mg/kg/day (about 50 times the human oral therapeutic dose in a 50 kg patient) was unassociated with evidence of carcinogenic potential. Neither was there evidence of carcinogenic potential when PRIMACOR was orally administered to rats at doses up to 5 mg/kg/day (about 6 times the human oral therapeutic dose) for twenty-four months or at 25 mg/kg/day (about 30 times the human oral therapeutic dose) for up to 18 months in males and 20 months in females. Whereas the Chinese Hamster Ovary Chromosome Aberration Assay was positive in the presence of a metabolic activation system, results from the Ames Test, the Mouse Lymphoma Assay, the Micronucleus Test, and the in vivo Rat Bone Marrow Metaphase Analysis indicated an absence of mutagenic potential. In reproductive performance studies in rats, PRIMACOR had no effect on male or female fertility at oral doses up to 32 mg/kg/day.

Animal Toxicity

Oral and intravenous administration of toxic dosages of PRIMACOR to rats and dogs resulted in myocardial degeneration/fibrosis and endocardial hemorrhage, principally affecting the left ventricular papillary muscles. Coronary vascular lesions characterized by periarterial edema and inflammation have been observed in dogs only. The myocardial/endocardial changes are similar to those produced by beta-adrenergic receptor agonists such as isoproterenol, while the vascular changes are similar to those produced by minoxidil and hydralazine. Doses within the recommended clinical dose range (up to 1.13 mg/kg/day) for congestive heart failure patients have not produced significant adverse effects in animals.

Pregnancy Category C

Oral administration of PRIMACOR to pregnant rats and rabbits during organogenesis produced no evidence of teratogenicity at dose levels up to 40 mg/kg/day and 12 mg/kg/day, respectively. PRIMACOR did not appear to be teratogenic when administered intravenously to pregnant rats at doses up to 3 mg/kg/day (about 2.5 times the maximum recommended clinical intravenous dose) or pregnant rabbits at doses up to 12 mg/kg/day, although an increased resorption rate was apparent at both 8 mg/kg/day, 12 mg/kg/day (intravenous) in the latter species. There are no adequate and well-controlled studies in pregnant women. PRIMACOR should be used during pregnancy only if the potential benefit justifies the potential risk to the fetus.

Nursing Mothers

Caution should be exercised when PRIMACOR is administered to nursing women, since it is not known whether it is excreted in human milk.

Pediatric Use

Safety and effectiveness in pediatric patients have not been established.

Use in Elderly Patients

There are no special dosage recommendations for the elderly patient. Ninety percent of all patients administered PRIMACOR in clinical studies were within the age range of 45 to 70 years, with a mean age of 61 years. Patients in all age groups demonstrated clinically and statistically significant responses. No age-related effects on the incidence of adverse reactions have been observed. Controlled pharmacokinetic studies have not disclosed any age-related effects on the distribution and elimination of PRIMACOR.

ADVERSE REACTIONS

Cardiovascular Effects: In patients receiving PRIMACOR in Phase II and III clinical trials, ventricular arrhythmias were reported in 12.1%: Ventricular ectopic activity, 8.5%; nonsustained ventricular tachycardia, 2.8%; sustained ventricular tachycardia, 1% and ventricular fibrillation, 0.2%(2 patients experienced more than one type of arrhythmia). Holter recordings demonstrated that in some patients injection of PRIMACOR increased ventricular ectopy, including nonsustained ventricular tachycardia. Life-threatening arrhythmias were infrequent and when present have been associated with certain underlying factors such as preexisting arrhythmias, metabolic abnormalities (e.g. hypokalemia), abnormal digoxin levels and catheter insertion. PRIMACOR was not shown to be arrhythmogenic in an electrophysiology study. Supraventricular arrhythmias were reported in 3.8% of the patients receiving PRIMACOR. The incidence of both supraventricular and ventricular arrhythmias has not been related to the dose or plasma milrinone concentration.

Other cardiovascular adverse reactions include hypotension, 2.9% and angina/chest pain, 1.2%.

CNS Effects

Headaches, usually mild to moderate in severity, have been reported in 2.9% of patients receiving PRIMACOR.

Other Effects

Other adverse reactions reported, but not definitely related to the administration of PRIMACOR include hypokalemia, 0.6%; tremor, 0.4%; and thrombocytopenia, 0.4%.

Isolated spontaneous reports of bronchospasm have been received.

OVERDOSAGE

Doses of PRIMACOR may produce hypotension because of its vasodilator effect. If this occurs, administration of PRIMACOR should be reduced or temporarily discontinued until the patient's condition stabilizes. No specific antidote is known, but general measures for circulatory support should be taken.

DOSAGE AND ADMINISTRATION

PRIMACOR should be administered with a loading dose followed by a continuous infusion (maintenance dose) according to the following guidelines:

LOADING DOSE

50 mcg/kg: Administer slowly over 10 minutes

The table below shows the loading dose in milliliters (mL) of PRIMACOR (1 mg/mL) by patient body weight (kg).

Loading Dose (mL) Using 1 mg/mL Concentration

Patient Body Weight (kg)

kg	30	40	50	60	70	80	90	100	110	120
mL	1.5	2.0	2.5	3.0	3.5	4.0	4.5	5.0	5.5	6.0

Continued on next page

This product information was prepared in September 1998. On these and other products of Sanofi Pharmaceuticals, Inc., detailed information may be obtained on a current basis by direct inquiry to Product Information Services, 90 Park Avenue, New York, NY 10016 (toll free 1-800-446-6267).

Consult 1999 PDR® supplements and future editions for revisions

Primacor—Cont.

The loading dose may be given undiluted, but diluting to a rounded total volume of 10 or 20 mL (see Maintenance Dose for diluents) may simplify the visualization of the injection rate.
[See first table at top of previous page]
PRIMACOR drawn from vials should be diluted prior to maintenance dose administration. The diluents that may be used are 0.45% Sodium Chloride Injection USP, 0.9% Sodium Chloride Injection USP, or 5% Dextrose Injection USP. The table below shows the volume of diluent in milliliters (mL) that must be used to achieve 200 mcg/mL concentration for infusion, and the resultant total volumes.

Desired Infusion Concentration mcg/mL	PRIMACOR 1 mg/mL (mL)	Diluent (mL)	Total Volume (mL)
200	10	40	50
200	20	80	100

The infusion rate should be adjusted according to hemodynamic and clinical response. Patients should be closely monitored. In controlled clinical studies, most patients showed an improvement in hemodynamic status as evidenced by increases in cardiac output and reductions in pulmonary capillary wedge pressure.
Note: See **"Dosage Adjustment in Renally Impaired Patients."** Dosage may be titrated to the maximum hemodynamic effect and should not exceed 1.13 mg/kg/day. Duration of therapy should depend upon patient responsiveness.
The maintenance dose in mL/hr by patient body weight (kg) may be determined by reference to the following table.
Note: **PRIMACOR supplied in 100 mL and 200 mL Flexible Containers (200 mcg/mL in 5% Dextrose Injection) need not be diluted prior to use.**
[See second table at top of previous page]
When administering PRIMACOR (milrinone lactate) by continuous infusion, it is advisable to use a calibrated electronic infusion device.
The Flexible Container has a concentration of milrinone equivalent to 200 mcg/mL in 5% Dextrose Injection and is more convenient to use than dilutions prepared from the vials. To use the Flexible Container, tear the overwrap at the notch and remove the Pre-Mix solution container. Squeeze the container firmly to check for leaks. Discard the container if leaks are found since the sterility of the product could be affected. Do not add supplementary medication. To prepare the container for administration of PRIMACOR intravenously, use aseptic techniques.

1) The flow control clamp of the administration set is closed.
2) The cover of the outlet port at the bottom of the container is removed.
3) Noting the full directions on the administration set carton, the piercing pin of the set is inserted into the port with a twisting motion until it is firmly seated.
4) The container is suspended on the hanger.
5) The drip chamber is squeezed and released to establish the fill level.
6) The flow control clamp is opened to expel air from the set, and then closed.
7) The set is attached to the venipuncture device, primed, and if not indwelling, the venipuncture is performed.
8) The rate of administration is controlled with the flow control clamp. WARNING- DO NOT USE IN SERIES CONNECTIONS. Caution: Do not use plastic containers in series connections. Such use could result in air embolism due to residual air being drawn from the primary container before administration of the fluid from the secondary container is complete.

Intravenous drug products should be inspected visually and should not be used if particulate matter or discoloration is present.

Dosage Adjustment in Renally Impaired Patients

Data obtained from patients with severe renal impairment (creatinine clearance = 0 to 30 mL/min) but without congestive heart failure have demonstrated that the presence of renal impairment significantly increases the terminal elimination half-life of PRIMACOR. Reductions in infusion rate may be necessary in patients with renal impairment. For patients with clinical evidence of renal impairment, the recommended infusion rate can be obtained from the following table:

Creatinine Clearance (mL/min/1.73 m^2)	Infusion Rate (mcg/kg/min)
5	0.20
10	0.23
20	0.28
30	0.33
40	0.38
50	0.43

HOW SUPPLIED

PRIMACOR is supplied as 10 mL (1 mg/mL) NDC 0024-1200-10, box of 10 and 20 mL (1 mg/mL) NDC 0024-1200-20, and 50 mL (1 mg/mL) NDC 0024-1200-50, box of 10 single-dose vials containing a sterile, clear, colorless to pale yellow solution. Each mL contains milrinone lactate equivalent to 1 mg milrinone.
PRIMACOR is also supplied as Carpuject® sterile cartridge Unit with InterLink® System Cannula, 5 mL (1 mg/mL) NDC 0024-1200-06 in 5 mL cartridges, box of 10. Each mL contains milrinone lactate equivalent to 1 mg milrinone.
PRIMACOR is also supplied as **CARPUJECT** sterile cartridge Unit (22-gauge, 1 $^1/_4$ Inch Needle) 5 mL (1 mg/mL) NDC 0024-1200-05 in 5 mL cartridges, box of 10. Each mL contains milrinone lactate equivalent to 1 mg milrinone.
Store at controlled room temperature 15° C to 30° C (59° F to 86° F). Avoid freezing.
The following **PRIMACOR Flexible Containers** are also supplied:
100 mL (200 mcg/mL) NDC 0024-1203-01 in 5% Dextrose injection
200 mL (200 mcg/mL) NDC 0024-1203-02 in 5% Dextrose injection
Exposure of pharmaceutical products to heat should be minimized. Avoid excessive heat. Protect from freezing. It is recommended that the Flexible Containers be stored at room temperature, 25° C (77° F), however, brief exposure up to 40° C (104° F) does not adversely affect the product.
Caution: Federal law prohibitis dispensing without prescription.
PRIMACOR 10 and 20 mL vials are manufactured by Nycomed Puerto Rico Inc., Barceloneta Puerto Rico 00617.
InterLink® is a Trademark of Baxter International, Inc.
U.S. Pat. Nos. 5,158,554; 5,171,234; 5,188,620; Pat. Pending
PRIMACOR is manufactured for Sanofi Pharmaceuticals, Inc. by Abbott Laboratories, North Chicago, IL 60064

PSW-10(A)

Shown in Product Identification Guide, page 335

SKELID® ℞
[skel 'id]
(tiludronate disodium)

DESCRIPTION

SKELID is a bisphosphonate characterized by a (4-chlorophenylthio) group on the carbon atom of the basic P-C-P structure common to all bisphosphonates. Its generic name is tiludronate disodium. Tiludronate disodium is the hydrated hemihydrate form of the disodium salt of tiludronic acid. Its chemical name is [[(4-Chlorophenyl) thio]methylene]bis [phosphonic acid], disodium salt, and its structural formula is as follows:

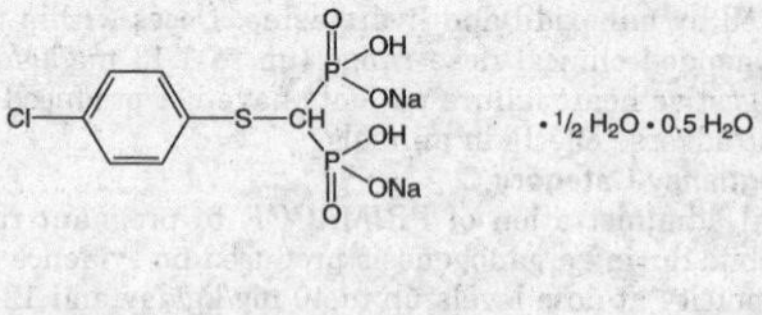

tiludronate disodium
(molecular weight 380.6)

SKELID tablets for oral administration contain 240 mg tiludronate disodium, which is the molar equivalent of 200 mg tiludronic acid. SKELID tablets also contain sodium lauryl sulfate, hydroxypropyl methylcellulose 2910, crospovidone, magnesium stearate, and lactose monohydrate.

CLINICAL PHARMACOLOGY

Mechanism of Action

In vitro studies indicate that tiludronate disodium acts primarily on bone through a mechanism that involves inhibition of osteoclastic activity with a probable reduction in the enzymatic and transport processes that lead to resorption of the mineralized matrix.
Bone resorption occurs following recruitment, activation, and polarization of osteoclasts. Tiludronate disodium appears to inhibit osteoclasts through at least two mechanisms: disruption of the cytoskeletal ring structure, possibly by inhibition of protein-tyrosine-phosphatase, thus leading to detachment of osteoclasts from the bone surface and the inhibition of the osteoclastic proton pump.

Pharmacokinetics

Absorption

Relative to an intravenous (IV) reference dose, the mean oral bioavailability of tiludronate disodium in healthy male subjects was 6% after an oral dose equivalent to 400 mg tiludronic acid administered after an overnight fast and 4 hours before a standard breakfast. In single-dose studies, bioavailability was reduced by 90% when an oral dose equivalent to 400 mg tiludronic acid was administered with, or 2 hours after, a standard breakfast compared to the same dose administered after an overnight fast and 4 hours before a standard breakfast. However, in clinical studies, efficacy was seen when SKELID was dosed at least 2 hours before or after meals.
After administration of a single dose equivalent to 400 mg tiludronic acid to healthy male subjects, tiludronic acid was rapidly absorbed with peak plasma concentrations of approximately 3 mg/L occurring within 2 hours. In pagetic patients, after repeated administration of doses equivalent to 400 mg/day tiludronic acid (2 hours before or 2 hours after a meal) for durations of 12 days to 12 weeks, average plasma concentrations of tiludronic acid occurring between 1 and 2 hours after dosing ranged between 1 and 4.6 mg/L.

Distribution

Animal pharmacology studies in rats demonstrate that tiludronic acid is widely distributed to bone and soft tissues. Over a period of days, loss of drug occurs from most tissues with the exception of bone and cartilage. Tiludronate is then slowly released from bone with a half-life in rats of 30 days or longer depending on the status of bone turnover.
After oral administration of doses equivalent to 400 mg/day tiludronic acid to nonpagetic patients with osteoarthrosis, the steady state in bone was not reached after 30 days of dosing.
At plasma concentrations between 1 and 10 mg/L, tiludronic acid was approximately 90% bound to human serum protein (mainly albumin).

Metabolism

In laboratory animals, tiludronic acid undergoes little if any metabolism. *In vitro*, tiludronic acid is not metabolized in human liver microsomes and hepatocytes.

Elimination

The principal route of elimination of tiludronic acid is in the urine. After IV administration to healthy volunteers, approximately 60% of the dose was excreted in the urine as tiludronic acid within 13 days. Renal clearance is dose independent and is approximately 10 mL/min in healthy subjects. In pagetic patients treated with doses equivalent to 400 mg/day tiludronic acid for 12 days, the mean apparent plasma elimination half-life was approximately 150 hours. The elimination rate from human bone is unknown.

Special Populations

Geriatric: No dosage adjustment in elderly patients is necessary. Plasma concentrations of tiludronic acid were higher in elderly pagetic patients (≥65 years of age); however, this difference was not clinically significant.
Pediatric: SKELID pharmacokinetics have not been investigated in subjects under the age of 18 years.
Gender: There were no clinically significant differences in plasma concentrations after repeated administration of tiludronate disodium to male and female pagetic patients.
Race: Pharmacokinetic differences due to race have not been studied.
Renal Insufficiency: SKELID is not recommended for patients with severe renal failure (creatinine clearance <30 mL/min) due to lack of clinical experience. After a single oral dose equivalent to 400 mg tiludronic acid, subjects with creatinine clearance between 11 and 18 mL/min had C_{max} values (approximately 3 mg/L) in the range of healthy volunteers. However, the plasma elimination half-life was approximately 205 hours, which is longer than that observed in pagetic patients after repeated doses (150 hours) and healthy subjects after single doses (50 hours). These values were obtained in a cross-study comparison between healthy volunteers and pagetic patients.
Hepatic Insufficiency: No dosage adjustment is needed. Since tiludronate undergoes little or no metabolism, no studies were conducted in subjects with hepatic insufficiency.
Drug-Drug Interactions: (See also PRECAUTIONS, Drug Interactions.) The bioavailability of SKELID is decreased 80% by calcium, when calcium and SKELID are administered at the same time, and 60% by some aluminum- or magnesium-containing antacids, when administered 1 hour before SKELID. Aspirin may decrease bioavailability of SKELID by up to 50% when taken 2 hours after SKELID. The bioavailability of SKELID is increased 2–4 fold by indomethacin and is not significantly altered by coadministration of diclofenac. The pharmacokinetic parameters of digoxin are not significantly modified by SKELID coadministration. *In vitro* studies show that tiludronate disodium does not displace warfarin from its binding site on protein.

Summary of Pharmacokinetic Parameters in the Normal Population

Parameter	Mean (SD)
Absolute bioavailability of two 200-mg tablets taken 4 hrs before standard breakfast	6% (2%)*
Time to peak plasma concentration (taken 4 hrs before first meal of day, n=151)	1.5 (0.9) hr
Maximum plasma concentration after a single 400-mg dose (taken 4 hrs before first meal of day, n=151)	2.66 (1.22) mg/L
Renal Clearance after IV administration of 20-mg dose	0.54 (0.14) L/hr

*Bioavailability was reduced by 90% when this oral dose was administered with, or 2 hours after, a standard breakfast.

Pharmacodynamics

Paget's disease of bone is a chronic, focal skeletal disorder characterized by greatly increased and disorderly bone remodeling. Excessive osteoclastic bone resorption is followed by osteoblastic new bone formation, leading to the replacement of the normal bone architecture by disorganized, enlarged, and weakened bone structure.

Clinical manifestations of Paget's disease range from no symptoms to severe bone pain, bone deformity, pathological fractures, and neurological and other complications. Serum alkaline phosphatase, the most frequently used biochemical index of disease activity, provides an objective measure of disease severity and response to therapy.

In pagetic patients treated with SKELID 400 mg/day for 3 months, changes in urinary hydroxyproline, a biochemical marker of bone resorption, and in serum alkaline phosphatase, a marker of bone formation, indicate a reduction toward normal in the rate of bone turnover. In addition, reduced numbers of osteoclasts by histomorphometric analysis and radiological improvement of lytic lesions indicate that SKELID can suppress the pagetic disease process.

Clinical Studies

The efficacy of SKELID 400 mg/day treatment was demonstrated in two randomized, double-blind, placebo-controlled multicenter studies and one positive-controlled study. All three studies included male and female patients with Paget's disease of the bone (radiograph examination and level of serum alkaline phosphatase [SAP] at least twice the upper normal limit). In one placebo-controlled study, conducted in North America, patients were randomly assigned to receive a daily dose of placebo or 200 or 400 mg/day SKELID for 3 months followed by an additional 12 weeks without treatment. A second placebo-controlled study of similar design was conducted in the UK.

A positive-controlled study was conducted in Europe with treatment groups of 400 mg/day SKELID for 3 months with a 3-month treatment-free follow-up, 400 mg/day SKELID for 6 months, and 400 mg/day etidronate for 6 months. In all of these studies, the efficacy of SKELID was primarily assessed by SAP activity after 3 and 6 months.

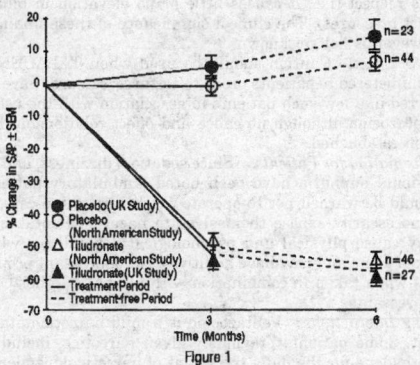

Figure 1

In the placebo-controlled trials, suppression of SAP levels was statistically significantly greater with 400 mg/day SKELID both at the end of treatment (3 months) and on follow-up (6 months) than with placebo (See Figure 1). The proportion of patients demonstrating at least a 50% reduction in SAP at 3 months with 400 mg/day SKELID was 61% in the North American study and 52% in the UK study. [See figure 2 at top of next column]

In the positive-controlled trial, six months after the start of dosing, the decrease in SAP levels in patients who ceased dosing after a 3-month course of SKELID was significantly

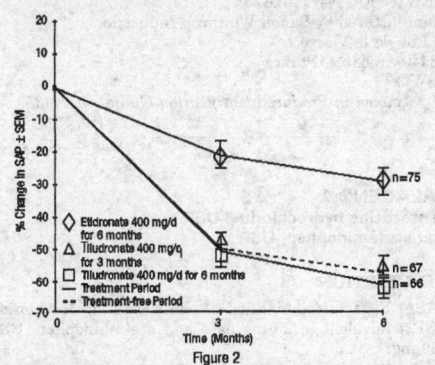

Figure 2

greater than with 6 months of etidronate 400 mg/day, and was equivalent to levels in patients who completed a 6-month course of SKELID (See Figure 2).

Treatment effects of SKELID were similar, regardless of pagetic patients' baseline SAP level, gender or age in the population studied.

Histomorphometry of the bone was studied in pagetic and nonpagetic patients (34 biopsies in pagetic patients and 41 biopsies in nonpagetic patients). Bone biopsy results in nonpagetic bone confirmed that SKELID did not impair bone remodeling or induce a significant decline in bone turnover. Results obtained in pagetic and nonpagetic bone indicated no evidence of osteomalacia or accumulation of unmineralized osteoid, and there was no reduction in the mineralization rate.

INDICATIONS AND USAGE

SKELID is indicated for treatment of Paget's disease of bone (osteitis deformans).

Treatment is indicated in patients with Paget's disease of bone (1) who have a level of serum alkaline phosphatase (SAP) at least twice the upper limit of normal, or (2) who are symptomatic, or (3) who are at risk for future complications of their disease.

CONTRAINDICATION

SKELID is contraindicated in individuals with known hypersensitivity to any component of this product.

WARNINGS

Bisphosphonates may cause upper gastrointestinal disorders, such as dysphagia, esophagitis, esophageal ulcer, and gastric ulcer (See ADVERSE REACTIONS).

PRECAUTIONS

General

SKELID is not recommended for patients with severe renal failure, for example, those with creatinine clearance <30 mL/min (see CLINICAL PHARMACOLOGY, Renal Insufficiency).

Information for Patients

Patients receiving SKELID should be instructed to:
1. Take SKELID with 6 to 8 ounces of plain water.
2. SKELID should not be taken within 2 hours of food.
3. Maintain adequate vitamin D and calcium intake.
4. Calcium supplements, aspirin, and indomethacin should not be taken within 2 hours before or 2 hours after SKELID.
5. Aluminum- or magnesium-containing antacids, if needed, should be taken at least 2 hours after taking SKELID.

Drug Interactions

The bioavailability of SKELID is decreased 80% by calcium, when calcium and SKELID are administered at the same time, and 60% by some aluminum- or magnesium-containing antacids, when administered 1 hour before SKELID. Aspirin may decrease bioavailability of SKELID by up to 50% when taken 2 hours after SKELID. The bioavailability of SKELID is increased 2–4 fold by indomethacin but is not significantly altered by coadministration of diclofenac. The pharmacokinetic parameters of digoxin are not significantly modified by SKELID coadministration. In vitro studies show that tiludronate does not displace warfarin from its binding site on protein.

Carcinogenesis, Mutagenesis, Impairment of Fertility

Carcinogenicity studies have not yet been completed.

Tiludronate was not genotoxic in the following assays: an in vitro microbial mutagenesis assay with and without metabolic activation, a human lymphocyte assay, a yeast cell assay for forward mutation and mitotic crossing over, or the in vivo mouse micronucleus test.

Tiludronate had no effect on rat fertility (male or female) at exposures up to two times the 400 mg/day human dose, based on surface area, mg/m^2 (75 mg/kg/day tiludronic acid dose).

Pregnancy

Pregnancy Category C

In a teratology study in rabbits dosed during days 6-18 of gestation at 42 mg/kg/day and 130 mg/kg/day (2 and 5 times

the 400 mg/day human dose based on body surface area), there was dose-related scoliosis likely attributable to the pharmacologic properties of the drug.

Mice receiving 375 mg/kg/day tiludronic acid (7 times the 400 mg/day human dose based on body surface area, mg/m^2) for days 6–15 of gestation showed slight maternal toxicity (decreased body weight gain), increased postimplantation loss, decreased number of fetuses/dam, and decreased fetus body weight. Uncommon malformations of the paw (shortened or missing digits, blood blisters between or in place of digits) were present in six fetuses at 375 mg/kg/day, all from the same litter.

Maternal toxicity (decreased body weight) was also observed in a teratology study in rats dosed during days 6–18 of gestation at 375 mg/kg/day tiludronic acid (10 times the 400 mg/day human dose based on body surface area, mg/m^2). There were reduced percent implantations, increased postimplantation loss, and increased intra-uterine deaths in the rats. There were no teratogenic effects on fetuses.

Protracted parturition and maternal death, presumably due to hypocalcemia, occurred at 75 mg/kg/day tiludronic acid (two times the 400 mg/day human dose based on body surface area, mg/m^2) when rats were treated from day 15 of gestation to day 25 postpartum.

There are no adequate and well-controlled studies in pregnant women. SKELID should be used during pregnancy only if the potential benefit justifies the potential risk to the fetus.

Nursing Mothers

It is not known whether tiludronate is excreted in human milk. Because many drugs are excreted in human milk, caution should be exercised when SKELID is administered to a nursing woman.

Pediatric Use

Safety and effectiveness of SKELID in pediatric patients have not been established.

ADVERSE REACTIONS

The safety of SKELID has been studied in more than 1100 patients, and the adverse experience profile is similar between controlled and uncontrolled clinical trials. Adverse events occurring in placebo-controlled trials of pagetic patients treated with SKELID 400 mg/day are presented in the table below.

The most frequently occurring adverse events in patients who received SKELID 400 mg/day were in the gastrointestinal body system: nausea (9.3%), diarrhea (9.3%), and dyspepsia (5.3%).

Adverse events associated with SKELID usually have been mild, and generally have not required discontinuation of therapy. In two placebo-controlled trials, 1.3% of patients receiving 400 mg SKELID and 5.4% of patients receiving placebo discontinued therapy due to any clinical adverse event.

Adverse Events[a] (%) Reported[b] in > 2% of Pagetic Patients from Placebo-Controlled Studies

	SKELID 400 mg/day (n=75)	Placebo (n=74)
Body as a Whole		
Pain	21.3	23.0
Back Pain	8.0	8.1
Accidental Injury	4.0	2.7
Influenza-like Symptoms	4.0	5.4
Chest Pain	2.7	0
Peripheral Edema	2.7	1.4
Cardiovascular, General		
Dependent Edema	2.7	0
Central and Peripheral		
Nervous System		
Headache	6.7	12.2
Dizziness	4.0	6.8
Paresthesia	4.0	0
Endocrine		
Hyperparathyroidism	2.7	0
Gastrointestinal		
Diarrhea	9.3	4.1
Nausea	9.3	5.4
Dyspepsia	5.3	8.1
Vomiting	4.0	0
Flatulence	2.7	0
Tooth Disorder	2.7	1.4
Metabolic and Nutritional		
Vitamin D Deficiency	2.7	2.7

Continued on next page

This product information was prepared in September 1998. On these and other products of Sanofi Pharmaceuticals, Inc., detailed information may be obtained on a current basis by direct inquiry to Product Information Services, 90 Park Avenue, New York, NY 10016 (toll free 1-800-446-6267).

Skelid—Cont.

Musculoskeletal System		
Arthralgia	2.7	5.4
Arthrosis	2.7	0
Resistance Mechanism		
Infection	2.7	0
Respiratory System		
Rhinitis	5.3	0
Sinusitis	5.3	1.4
Upper Respiratory Tract		
Infection	5.3	14.9
Coughing	2.7	2.7
Pharyngitis	2.7	1.4
Skin and Appendage		
Rash	2.7	1.4
Skin Disorder	2.7	1.4
Vision		
Cataract	2.7	0
Conjunctivitis	2.7	0
Glaucoma	2.7	0

[a] Reported using WHO terminology
[b] All events reported, irrespective of causality

Other adverse events not listed in the table above but reported in ≥ 1% of pagetic patients treated with SKELID in all clinical trials of at least one month duration, regardless of dose and causality assessment, are listed below. The adverse event terms within each body system are listed in the order of decreasing frequency occurring in the population.
Body as a Whole: Asthenia, syncope, fatigue
Cardiovascular: Hypertension
Central and Peripheral Nervous Systems: Vertigo, involuntary muscle contractions
Gastrointestinal: Abdominal pain, constipation, dry mouth, gastritis
Musculoskeletal: Fracture pathological
Psychiatric: Anorexia, somnolence, anxiety, nervousness, insomnia
Respiratory System: Bronchitis
Skin and Appendages: Pruritus, increased sweating
Urinary System: Urinary tract infection
Vascular (extracardiac): Flushing
Stevens-Johnson type syndrome has been observed rarely; the causality relationship of this to SKELID has not been established.

OVERDOSAGE

Based on the known action of tiludronate, hypocalcemia is a potential consequence of SKELID overdose. In one patient with hypercalcemia of malignancy, intravenous administration of high doses of SKELID (800 mg/day total dose, 6 mg/kg/day for 2 days) was associated with acute renal failure and death.
No specific information is available on the treatment of overdose with SKELID. Dialysis would not be beneficial. Standard medical practices may be used to manage renal insufficiency or hypocalcemia, if signs of these develop.

DOSAGE AND ADMINISTRATION

A single 400-mg daily oral dose of SKELID, taken with 6 to 8 ounces of plain water only, should be administered for a period of 3 months. Beverages other than plain water (including mineral water), food (see below), and some medications (see PRECAUTIONS, Drug Interactions) are likely to reduce the absorption of SKELID (see CLINICAL PHARMACOLOGY, Pharmacokinetics).
SKELID should not be taken within 2 hours of food.
Calcium or mineral supplements should be taken at least 2 hours before or two hours after SKELID. Aluminum- or magnesium-containing antacids, if needed, should be taken at least two hours after taking SKELID.
SKELID should not be taken within 2 hours of indomethacin.
Following therapy, allow an interval of 3 months to assess response. Specific data regarding retreatment are limited, although results from uncontrolled studies indicate favorable biochemical improvement similar to initial SKELID treatment.

HOW SUPPLIED

SKELID (NDC 0024-1800-02) is supplied as white to practically white, biconvex round tablets containing 240 mg tiludronate disodium, which is the molar equivalent of 200 mg tiludronic acid. SKELID tablets are engraved with "S.W" on one side and "200" on the other side and packaged, in foil strips in cartons of 56 tablets per carton.
Storage
SKELID should be stored at 25° C (77° F); excursions permitted to 15° C to 30° C (59° F to 86° F) [see USP Controlled Room Temperature]. Tablets should not be removed from the foil strips until they are to be used.
Caution: Federal law prohibits dispensing without prescription.

Distributed by *Sanofi Pharmaceuticals, Inc.*
NEW YORK, NY 10016
Manufactured by Sanofi Winthrop Industrie
1, Rue de la Vierge
33440 Ambarès, France
SSW-3
Shown in Product Identification Guide, page 335

TALACEN® Ⓒⅳ ℞

Pentazocine hydrochloride, USP and acetaminophen, USP

DESCRIPTION

TALACEN is a combination of pentazocine hydrochloride, USP, equivalent to 25 mg base and acetaminophen, USP, 650 mg.
Pentazocine is a member of the benzazocine series (also known as the benzomorphan series). Chemically, pentazocine is 1,2,3,4,5,6-hexahydro-6,11-dimethyl-3-(3-methyl-2-butenyl)-2,6-methano-3-benzazocin-8-ol, a white, crystalline substance soluble in acidic aqueous solutions.
Chemically, acetaminophen is Acetamide, *N*- (4-hydroxyphenyl)-.
Pentazocine is an analgesic and acetaminophen is an analgesic and antipyretic.
TALACEN is a pale blue, scored caplet for oral administration.
Inactive Ingredients: Colloidal Silicon Dioxide, FD&C Blue #1, Gelatin, Microcrystalline Cellulose, Potassium Sorbate, Pregelatinized Starch, Sodium Lauryl Sulfate, Sodium Metabisulfite, Sodium Starch Glycolate, Stearic Acid.

CLINICAL PHARMACOLOGY

TALACEN is an analgesic possessing antipyretic actions.
Pentazocine is an analgesic with agonist/antagonist action which when administered orally is approximately equivalent on a mg for mg basis in analgesic effect to codeine.
Acetaminophen is an analgesic and antipyretic.
Onset of significant analgesia with pentazocine usually occurs between 15 and 30 minutes after oral administration, and duration of action is usually three hours or longer. Onset and duration of action and the degree of pain relief are related both to dose and the severity of pretreatment pain. Pentazocine weakly antagonizes the analgesic effects of morphine, meperidine, and phenazocine; in addition, it produces incomplete reversal of cardiovascular, respiratory, and behavioral depression induced by morphine and meperidine. Pentazocine has about 1/50 the antagonistic activity of nalorphine. It also has sedative activity.
Pentazocine is well absorbed from the gastrointestinal tract. Plasma levels closely correspond to the onset, duration, and intensity of analgesia. The time to mean peak concentration in 24 normal volunteers was 1.7 hours (range 0.5 to 4 hours) after oral administration and the mean plasma elimination half-life was 3.6 hours (range 1.5 to 10 hours).
The action of pentazocine is terminated for the most part by biotransformation in the liver with some free pentazocine excreted in the urine. The products of the oxidation of the terminal methyl groups and glucuronide conjugates are excreted by the kidney. Elimination of approximately 60% of the total dose occurs within 24 hours. Pentazocine passes the placental barrier.
Onset of significant analgesic and antipyretic activity of acetaminophen when administered orally occurs within 30 minutes and is maximal at approximately $2^1/_2$ hours. The pharmacological mode of action of acetaminophen is unknown at this time.
Acetaminophen is rapidly and almost completely absorbed from the gastrointestinal tract. In 24 normal volunteers the time to mean peak plasma concentration was 1 hour (range 0.25 to 3 hours) after oral administration and the mean plasma elimination half-life was 2.8 hours (range 2 to 4 hours).
The effect of pentazocine on acetaminophen plasma protein binding or vice versa has not been established. For acetaminophen there is little or no plasma protein binding at normal therapeutic doses. When toxic doses of acetaminophen are ingested and drug plasma levels exceed 90 mcg/mL, plasma binding may vary from 8% to 43%.
Acetaminophen is conjugated in the liver with glucuronic acid and to a lesser extent with sulfuric acid. Approximately 80% of acetaminophen is excreted in the urine after conjugation and about 3% is excreted unchanged. The drug is also conjugated to a lesser extent with cysteine and additionally metabolized by hydroxylation.
If TALACEN is taken every 4 hours over an extended period of time, accumulation of pentazocine and to a lesser extent, acetaminophen, may occur.

INDICATIONS AND USAGE

TALACEN is indicated for the relief of mild to moderate pain.

CONTRAINDICATIONS

TALACEN should not be administered to patients who are hypersensitive to either pentazocine or acetaminophen.

WARNINGS

Contains sodium metabisulfite, a sulfite that may cause allergic-type reactions including anaphylactic symptoms and life-threatening or less severe asthmatic episodes in certain susceptible people. The overall prevalence of sulfite sensitivity in the general population is unknown and probably low. Sulfite sensitivity is seen more frequently in asthmatic than in nonasthmatic people.
Head Injury and Increased Intracranial Pressure. As in the case of other potent analgesics, the potential of pentazocine for elevating cerebrospinal fluid pressure may be attributed to CO_2 retention due to the respiratory depressant effects of the drug. These effects may be markedly exaggerated in the presence of head injury, other intracranial lesions, or a preexisting increase in intracranial pressure. Furthermore, pentazocine can produce effects which may obscure the clinical course of patients with head injuries. In such patients, TALACEN must be used with extreme caution and only if its use is deemed essential.
Acute CNS Manifestations. Patients receiving therapeutic doses of pentazocine have experienced hallucinations (usually visual), disorientation, and confusion which have cleared spontaneously within a period of hours. The mechanism of this reaction is not known. Such patients should be closely observed and vital signs checked. If the drug is reinstituted, it should be done with caution since these acute CNS manifestations may recur.
There have been instances of psychological and physical dependence on parenteral pentazocine in patients with a history of drug abuse, and rarely, in patients without such a history. (See DRUG ABUSE AND DEPENDENCE.)
Due to the potential for increased CNS depressant effects, alcohol should be used with caution in patients who are currently receiving pentazocine.
Pentazocine may precipitate opioid abstinence symptoms in patients receiving courses of opiates for pain relief.

PRECAUTIONS

In prescribing TALACEN for chronic use, the physician should take precautions to avoid increases in dose by the patient.
Myocardial Infarction. As with all drugs, TALACEN should be used with caution in patients with myocardial infarction who have nausea or vomiting.
Certain Respiratory Conditions. Although respiratory depression has rarely been reported after oral administration of pentazocine, the drug should be administered with caution to patients with respiratory depression from any cause, severely limited respiratory reserve, severe bronchial asthma and other obstructive respiratory conditions, or cyanosis.
Impaired Renal or Hepatic Function. Decreased metabolism of the drug by the liver in extensive liver disease may predispose to accentuation of side effects. Although laboratory tests have not indicated that pentazocine causes or increases renal or hepatic impairment, the drug should be administered with caution to patients with such impairment. Since acetaminophen is metabolized by the liver, the question of the safety of its use in the presence of liver disease should be considered.
Biliary Surgery. Narcotic drug products are generally considered to elevate biliary tract pressure for varying periods following their administration. Some evidence suggests that pentazocine may differ from other marketed narcotics in this respect (i.e., it causes little or no elevation in biliary tract pressures). The clinical significance of these findings, however, is not yet known.
CNS Effect. Caution should be used when TALACEN is administered to patients prone to seizures; seizures have occurred in a few such patients in association with the use of pentazocine although no cause and effect relationship has been established.
Information for Patients. Since sedation, dizziness, and occasional euphoria have been noted, ambulatory patients should be warned not to operate machinery, drive cars, or unnecessarily expose themselves to hazards. Pentazocine may cause physical and psychological dependence when taken alone and may have additive CNS depressant properties when taken in combination with alcohol or other CNS depressants.
Drug Interactions. Pentazocine is a mild narcotic antagonist. Some patients previously given narcotics, including methadone for the daily treatment of narcotic dependence, have experienced withdrawal symptoms after receiving pentazocine.
Carcinogenesis, Mutagenesis, Impairment of Fertility. Carcinogenesis, mutagenesis, and impairment of fertility studies have not been done with this combination product.
Pentazocine, when administered orally or parenterally, had no adverse effect on either the reproductive capabilities or the course of pregnancy in rabbits and rats. Embryotoxic effects on the fetuses were not shown.
The daily administration of 4 mg/kg to 20 mg/kg pentazocine subcutaneously to female rats during a 14 day premating period and until the 13th day of pregnancy did not have any adverse effects on the fertility rate.

There is no evidence in long-term animal studies to demonstrate that pentazocine is carcinogenic.

Pregnancy Category C. Animal reproduction studies have not been conducted with TALACEN. It is also not known whether TALACEN can cause fetal harm when administered to pregnant women or can affect reproduction capacity. TALACEN should be given to pregnant women only if clearly needed. However, animal reproduction studies with pentazocine have not demonstrated teratogenic or embryotoxic effects.

Nonteratogenic Effects. There has been no experience in this regard with the combination pentazocine and acetaminophen. However, there have been rare reports of possible abstinence syndromes in newborns after prolonged use of pentazocine during pregnancy.

Labor and Delivery. Patients receiving pentazocine during labor have experienced no adverse effects other than those that occur with commonly used analgesics. TALACEN should be used with caution in women delivering premature infants. The effect of TALACEN on the mother and fetus, the duration of labor or delivery, the possibility that forceps delivery or other intervention or resuscitation of the newborn may be necessary, or the effect of TALACEN, on the later growth, development, and functional maturation of the child are unknown at the present time.

Nursing Mothers. It is not known whether this drug is excreted in human milk. Because many drugs are excreted in human milk, caution should be exercised when TALACEN is administered to a nursing woman.

Pediatric Use. Safety and effectiveness in pediatric patients below the age of 12 have not been established.

ADVERSE REACTIONS

Clinical experience with TALACEN has been insufficient to define all possible adverse reactions with this combination. However, reactions reported after oral administration of pentazocine hydrochloride in 50 mg dosage include *gastrointestinal:* nausea, vomiting, infrequently constipation; and rarely abdominal distress, anorexia, diarrhea. *CNS effects:* dizziness, lightheadedness, hallucinations, sedation, euphoria, headache, confusion, disorientation; infrequently weakness, disturbed dreams, insomnia, syncope, visual blurring and focusing difficulty, depression; and rarely tremor, irritability, excitement, tinnitus. *Autonomic:* sweating; infrequently flushing; and rarely chills. *Allergic:* infrequently rash; and rarely urticaria, edema of the face. *Cardiovascular:* infrequently decrease in blood pressure, tachycardia. *Hematologic:* rarely depression of white blood cells (especially granulocytes), which is usually reversible, moderate transient eosinophilia. *Other:* rarely respiratory depression, urinary retention, paresthesia, toxic epidermal necrolysis, and in one instance, an apparent anaphylactic reaction has been reported.

Numerous clinical studies have shown that acetaminophen, when taken in recommended doses, is relatively free of adverse effects in most age groups, even in the presence of a variety of disease states.

A few cases of hypersensitivity to acetaminophen have been reported, as manifested by skin rashes, thrombocytopenic purpura, rarely hemolytic anemia and agranulocytosis. Occasional individuals respond to ordinary doses with nausea and vomiting and diarrhea.

DRUG ABUSE AND DEPENDENCE

Controlled Substance. TALACEN is a Schedule IV controlled substance.

Abuse and Dependence. There have been some reports of dependence and of withdrawal symptoms with orally administered pentazocine. There have been recorded instances of psychological and physical dependence in patients using parenteral pentazocine. Abrupt discontinuance following the extended use of parenteral pentazocine has resulted in withdrawal symptoms. Patients with a history of drug dependence should be under close supervision while receiving TALACEN. There have been rare reports of possible abstinence syndromes in newborns after prolonged use of pentazocine during pregnancy.

Some tolerance to the analgesic and subjective effects of pentazocine develops with frequent and repeated use.

Drug addicts who are given closely spaced doses of pentazocine (e.g., 60 mg to 90 mg every 4 hours) develop physical dependence which is demonstrated by abrupt withdrawal or by administration of naloxone. The withdrawal symptoms exhibited after chronic doses of more than 500 mg of pentazocine per day have similar characteristics, but to a lesser degree, of opioid withdrawal and may be associated with drug seeking behavior.

OVERDOSAGE

Manifestations. Clinical experience with TALACEN has been insufficient to define the signs of overdosage with this product. It may be assumed that signs and symptoms of TALACEN overdose would be a combination of those observed with pentazocine overdose and acetaminophen overdose.

For pentazocine alone in single doses above 60 mg there have been reports of the occurrence of nalorphine-like psy-

chotomimetic effects such as anxiety, nightmares, strange thoughts, and hallucinations. Marked respiratory depression associated with increased blood pressure and tachycardia have also resulted from excessive doses as have dizziness, nausea, vomiting, lethargy, and paresthesias. The respiratory depression is antagonized by naloxone (see *Treatment*).

In acute acetaminophen overdosage, dose-dependent, potentially fatal hepatic necrosis is the most serious adverse effect. Renal tubular necrosis, hypoglycemic coma, and thrombocytopenia may also occur.

In adults, a single dose of 10 g to 15 g (200 mg/kg to 250 mg/kg) of acetaminophen may cause hepatotoxicity. A dose of 25 g or more is potentially fatal. The potential seriousness of the intoxication may not be evident during the first two days of acute acetaminophen poisoning. During the first 24 hours, nausea, vomiting, anorexia, and abdominal pain occur. These may persist for a week or more. Liver injury may become evident the second day, initial signs being elevation of serum transaminase and lactic dehydrogenase activity, increased serum bilirubin concentration, and prolongation of prothrombin time. Serum albumin concentration and alkaline phosphatase activity may remain normal. The hepatotoxicity may lead to encephalopathy, coma, and death. Transient azotemia is evident in a majority of patients and acute renal failure occurs in some.

There have been reports of glycosuria and impaired glucose tolerance, but hypoglycemia may also occur. Metabolic acidosis and metabolic alkalosis have been reported. Cerebral edema and nonspecific myocardial depression have also been noted. Biopsy reveals centrolobular necrosis with sparing of the periportal area. The hepatic lesions are reversible over a period of weeks or months in nonfatal cases.

The severity of the liver injury can be determined by measurement of the plasma half-time of acetaminophen during the first day of acute poisoning. If the half-time exceeds 4 hours, hepatic necrosis is likely and if the half-time is greater than 12 hours, hepatic coma will probably occur. Only minimal liver damage has developed when the serum concentration was below 120 mcg/mL at 12 hours after ingestion of the drug. If serum bilirubin concentration is greater than 4 mg/100 mL during the first 5 days, encephalopathy may occur.

The seven day oral LD_{50} value for TALACEN in mice is 3570 mg/kg.

Treatment. Oxygen, intravenous fluids, vasopressors, and other supportive measures should be employed as indicated. Assisted or controlled ventilation should also be considered. For respiratory depression due to overdosage or unusual sensitivity to TALACEN, parenteral naloxone is a specific and effective antagonist.

The toxic effects of acetaminophen may be prevented or minimized by antidotal therapy with N-acetylcysteine. In order to obtain the best possible results, N-acetylcysteine should be administered within approximately 16 hours of ingestion of the overdose.

For complete prescribing information for the approved use of acetylcysteine in the treatment of acetaminophen overdose, see package insert for MUCOMYST® (acetylcysteine) Bristol-Myers Squibb.

Vigorous supportive therapy is required in severe intoxication. Procedures to limit the continuing absorption of the drug must be readily performed since the hepatic injury is dose dependent and occurs early in the course of intoxication. Induction of vomiting or gastric lavage, followed by oral administration of activated charcoal should be done in all cases.

If hemodialysis can be initiated within the first 12 hours, it is advocated for patients with a plasma acetaminophen concentration exceeding 120 mcg/mL at 4 hours after ingestion of the drug.

DOSAGE AND ADMINISTRATION

Adult. The usual adult dose is 1 caplet every 4 hours as needed for pain relief, up to a maximum of 6 caplets per day. The usual duration of therapy is dependent upon the condition being treated but in any case should be reviewed regularly by the physician. The effect of meals on the rate and extent of bioavailability of both pentazocine and acetaminophen has not been documented.

HOW SUPPLIED

Caplets, pale blue, scored, each containing pentazocine hydrochloride equivalent to 25 mg base and acetaminophen 650 mg.

Bottles of 100 (NDC 0024-1937-04).

Unit Dose Dispenser Package of 250 (NDC 0024-1937-14), 10 sleeves of 25 caplets each.

Store at controlled room temperature 15° C to 30° C (59° F to 86° F).

Caution: Federal law prohibits dispensing without prescription.

TSW-6 B

Shown in Product Identification Guide, page 336

TALWIN® Compound
pentazocine hydrochloride and aspirin, USP

C_{IV} R

DESCRIPTION

TALWIN Compound is a combination of pentazocine hydrochloride, USP, equivalent to 12.5 mg base and aspirin, USP, 325 mg.

Pentazocine is a member of the benzazocine series (also known as the benzomorphan series). Chemically, pentazocine is 1, 2, 3, 4, 5, 6 -hexahydro - 6, 11-dimethyl-3-(3-methyl-2-butenyl)-2, 6-methano-3-benzazocin-8-ol, a white, crystalline substance soluble in acidic aqueous solutions and has the following structural formula:

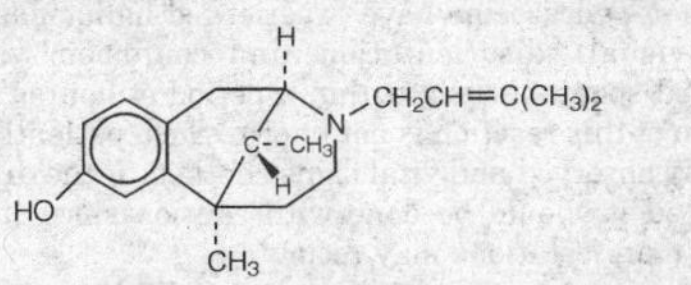

Chemically, aspirin is Benzoic acid, 2-(acetyloxy)- and has the following structural formula:

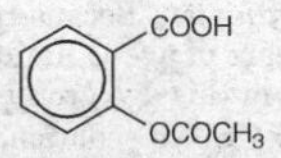

Inactive Ingredients: Magnesium Stearate, Microcrystalline Cellulose, Sodium Lauryl Sulfate, Starch.

CLINICAL PHARMACOLOGY

Pentazocine is a potent analgesic which when administered orally is approximately equivalent, on a mg for mg basis, in analgesic effect to codeine. Two caplets of TALWIN Compound when administered orally have the additive analgesic effect equivalent to 25 mg of TALWIN plus 650 mg of aspirin. TALWIN Compound provides the analgesic effects of pentazocine and the analgesic, anti-inflammatory, and antipyretic actions of aspirin.

Onset of significant analgesia usually occurs between 15 and 30 minutes after oral administration, and duration of action is usually three hours or longer. Onset and duration of action and the degree of pain relief are related both to dose and the severity of pretreatment pain. Pentazocine weakly antagonizes the analgesic effects of morphine, meperidine, and phenazocine; in addition, it produces incomplete reversal of cardiovascular, respiratory, and behavioral depression induced by morphine and meperidine. Pentazocine has about $^1/_{50}$ the antagonistic activity of nalorphine. It also has sedative activity.

INDICATION AND USAGE

For the relief of moderate pain

CONTRAINDICATIONS

TALWIN Compound should not be administered to patients who are hypersensitive to either pentazocine or salicylates, or in any situation where aspirin is contraindicated.

WARNINGS

Drug Dependence. There have been instances of psychological and physical dependence on parenteral pentazocine in patients with a history of drug abuse, and rarely, in patients without such a history. Abrupt discontinuance following the extended use of parenteral pentazocine has resulted in withdrawal symptoms. There have been a few reports of dependence and of withdrawal symptoms with orally administered pentazocine. Patients with a history of drug dependence should be under close supervision while receiving TALWIN Compound orally. There have been rare reports of possible abstinence syndromes in newborns after prolonged use of pentazocine during pregnancy.

In prescribing TALWIN Compound for chronic use, the physician should take precautions to avoid increases in dose by the patient and to prevent the use of the drug in anticipation of pain rather than for the relief of pain.

Head Injury and Increased Intracranial Pressure. The respiratory depressant effects of pentazocine and its potential for elevating cerebrospinal fluid pressure may be markedly exaggerated in the presence of head injury, other intracranial lesions, or a preexisting increase in intracranial pressure. Furthermore, pentazocine can produce effects which may obscure the clinical course of patients with head injuries. In such patients, TALWIN Compound must be used with extreme caution and only if its use is deemed essential.

Continued on next page

This product information was prepared in September 1998. On these and other products of Sanofi Pharmaceuticals, Inc., detailed information may be obtained on a current basis by direct inquiry to Product Information Services, 90 Park Avenue, New York, NY 10016 (toll free 1-800-446-6267).

Consult 1999 PDR® supplements and future editions for revisions

Talwin Compound—Cont.

Usage in Pregnancy. Safe use of pentazocine during pregnancy (other than labor) has not been established. Animal reproduction studies have not demonstrated teratogenic or embryotoxic effects. However, TALWIN Compound should be administered to pregnant patients (other than labor) only when, in the judgment of the physician, the potential benefits outweigh the possible hazards. Patients receiving pentazocine during labor have experienced no adverse effects other than those that occur with commonly used analgesics. TALWIN Compound, should be used with caution in women delivering premature infants.

Acute CNS Manifestations. Patients receiving therapeutic doses of pentazocine have experienced hallucinations (usually visual), disorientation, and confusion which have cleared spontaneously within a period of hours. The mechanism of this reaction is not known. Such patients should be closely observed and vital signs checked. If the drug is reinstituted it should be done with caution since these acute CNS manifestations may recur.

Due to the potential for increased CNS depressant effects, alcohol should be used with caution in patients who are currently receiving pentazocine.

Usage in pediatric patients. Because clinical experience in children under 12 years of age is limited, administration of TALWIN Compound in this age group is not recommended.

Ambulatory Patients. Since sedation, dizziness, and occasional euphoria have been noted, ambulatory patients should be warned not to operate machinery, drive cars, or unnecessarily expose themselves to hazards.

Other. Because of its aspirin content, TALWIN Compound should be used with caution in the presence of peptic ulcer, in conjunction with anticoagulant therapy, or in any situation where the effects of aspirin may be deleterious.

PRECAUTIONS

Certain Respiratory Conditions. Although respiratory depression has rarely been reported after oral administration of pentazocine, TALWIN Compound, should be administered with caution to patients with respiratory depression from any cause, severely limited respiratory reserve, severe bronchial asthma and other obstructive respiratory conditions, or cyanosis.

Impaired Renal or Hepatic Function. Decreased metabolism of the drug by the liver in extensive liver disease may predispose to accentuation of side effects. Although laboratory tests have not indicated that pentazocine causes or increases renal or hepatic impairment, TALWIN Compound should be administered with caution to patients with such impairment.

Myocardial Infarction. As with all drugs, TALWIN Compound should be used with caution in patients with myocardial infarction who have nausea or vomiting.

Biliary Surgery. Narcotic drug products are generally considered to elevate biliary tract pressure for varying periods following administration. Some evidence suggests that pentazocine may differ in this respect (i.e., it causes little or no elevation in biliary tract pressures). The clinical significance of these findings, however, is not yet known.

Patients Receiving Narcotics. Pentazocine is a mild narcotic antagonist. Some patients previously given narcotics, including methadone for the daily treatment of narcotic dependence, have experienced withdrawal symptoms after receiving pentazocine.

CNS Effect. Caution should be used when pentazocine is administered to patients prone to seizures. Seizures have occurred in a few such patients in association with the use of pentazocine although no cause and effect relationship has been established.

Pediatric Use. For usage in pediatric patients see WARNINGS.

ADVERSE REACTIONS

Reactions reported after oral administration of pentazocine or TALWIN Compound include *Gastrointestinal:* nausea, vomiting; infrequently constipation; and rarely abdominal distress, anorexia, diarrhea. *CNS Effects:* dizziness, lightheadedness, hallucinations, sedation, euphoria, headache, confusion, disorientation; infrequently weakness, disturbed dreams, insomnia, syncope, visual blurring and focusing difficulty, depression; and rarely tremor, irritability, excitement, tinnitus. *Autonomic:* sweating; infrequently flushing; and rarely chills. *Allergic:* infrequently rash; and rarely urticaria, edema of the face, and angioneurotic edema. *Cardiovascular:* infrequently decrease in blood pressure, tachycardia. *Hematologic:* rarely depression of white blood cells (especially granulocytes), which is usually reversible, moderate transient eosinophilia. *Other:* rarely respiratory depression, urinary retention, paresthesia, toxic epidermal necrolysis, and angioneurotic edema.

DOSAGE AND ADMINISTRATION

Adults. The usual adult dose is 2 caplets three or four times a day.

Pediatric Patients. Since clinical experience in pediatric patients under 12 years of age is limited, administration of TALWIN Compound in this age group is not recommended.

Duration of Therapy. Patients with chronic pain who receive pentazocine orally for prolonged periods have only rarely been reported to experience withdrawal symptoms when administration was abruptly discontinued (see WARNINGS). Tolerance to the analgesic effect of pentazocine has also been reported only rarely. Significant abnormalities of liver and kidney function tests have not been reported, even after prolonged administration of pentazocine.

OVERDOSAGE

Manifestations: Clinical experience with pentazocine overdosage has been insufficient to define the signs of this condition. Signs of salicylate overdosage include headache, dizziness, confusion, tinnitus, diaphoresis, thirst, nausea, vomiting, diarrhea, tachycardia, tachypnea, Kussmaul breathing, convulsions, and coma. Death is usually from respiratory failure.

Treatment: Treatment for overdosage of TALWIN Compound, should include treatment for salicylate poisoning as outlined in standard references.

Oxygen, intravenous fluids, vasopressors, and other supportive measures should be employed as indicated. Assisted or controlled ventilation should also be considered. For respiratory depression due to overdosage or unusual sensitivity to pentazocine, parenteral naloxone is a specific and effective antagonist.

HOW SUPPLIED

Caplets, white, each containing pentazocine hydrochloride equivalent to 12.5 mg base and aspirin 325 mg. Bottles of 100 (NDC 0024-1927-04).

Store at room temperature up to 30° C (86° F).

Caution: Federal law prohibits dispensing without prescription.

TSW-5 B

TALWIN® Nx ©IV ℞
pentazocine and naloxone hydrochlorides USP

Analgesic for Oral Use Only

> TALWIN® Nx is intended for oral use only. Severe, potentially lethal, reactions may result from misuse of TALWIN® Nx by injection either alone or in combination with other substances. (See DRUG ABUSE AND DEPENDENCE section.)

DESCRIPTION

TALWIN Nx contains pentazocine hydrochloride, USP, equivalent to 50 mg base and is a member of the benzazocine series (also known as the benzomorphan series), and naloxone hydrochloride, USP, equivalent to 0.5 mg base.

TALWIN Nx is an analgesic for oral administration.

Chemically, pentazocine hydrochloride is 1,2,3,4,5,6-Hexahydro -6,11 -dimethyl -3-(3-methyl-2-butenyl)-2, 6-methano-3-benzazocin-8-ol hydrochloride, a white, crystalline substance soluble in acidic aqueous solutions.

Chemically, naloxone hydrochloride is Morphinan-6-one, 4, 5-epoxy-3, 14-dihydroxy-17-(2-propenyl)-, hydrochloride, (5α)-. It is a slightly off-white powder, and is soluble in water and dilute acids.

Inactive Ingredients: Colloidal Silicon Dioxide, Dibasic Calcium Phosphate, D&C Yellow #10, FD&C Yellow #6, Magnesium Stearate, Microcrystalline Cellulose, Sodium Lauryl Sulfate, Starch.

CLINICAL PHARMACOLOGY

Pentazocine is a potent analgesic which when administered orally in a 50 mg dose appears equivalent in analgesic effect to 60 mg (1 grain) of codeine. Onset of significant analgesia usually occurs between 15 and 30 minutes after oral administration, and duration of action is usually three hours or longer. Onset and duration of action and the degree of pain relief are related both to dose and the severity of pretreatment pain. Pentazocine weakly antagonizes the analgesic effects of morphine and meperidine; in addition, it produces incomplete reversal of cardiovascular, respiratory, and behavioral depression induced by morphine and meperidine. Pentazocine has about 1/50 the antagonistic activity of nalorphine. It also has sedative activity.

Pentazocine is well absorbed from the gastrointestinal tract. Concentrations in plasma coincide closely with the onset, duration, and intensity of analgesia; peak values occur 1 to 3 hours after oral administration. The half-life in plasma is 2 to 3 hours.

Pentazocine is metabolized in the liver and excreted primarily in the urine. Pentazocine passes into the fetal circulation.

Naloxone when administered orally at 0.5 mg has no pharmacologic activity. Naloxone hydrochloride administered parenterally at the same dose is an effective antagonist to pentazocine and a pure antagonist to narcotic analgesics.

TALWIN Nx is a potent analgesic when administered orally. However, the presence of naloxone in TALWIN Nx will prevent the effect of pentazocine if the product is misused by injection.

Studies in animals indicate that the presence of naloxone does not affect pentazocine analgesia when the combination is given orally. If the combination is given by injection the action of pentazocine is neutralized.

INDICATIONS AND USAGE

> TALWIN® Nx is intended for oral use only. Severe, potentially lethal, reactions may result from misuse of TALWIN® Nx by injection either alone or in combination with other substances. (See DRUG ABUSE AND DEPENDENCE section.)

TALWIN Nx is indicated for the relief of moderate to severe pain.

TALWIN Nx is indicated for oral use only.

CONTRAINDICATIONS

TALWIN Nx should not be administered to patients who are hypersensitive to either pentazocine or naloxone.

WARNINGS

> TALWIN® Nx is intended for oral use only. Severe, potentially lethal, reactions may result from misuse of TALWIN® Nx by injection either alone or in combination with other substances. (See DRUG ABUSE AND DEPENDENCE section.)

Drug Dependence. Pentazocine can cause a physical and psychological dependence. (See DRUG ABUSE AND DEPENDENCE.)

Head Injury and Increased Intracranial Pressure. As in the case of other potent analgesics, the potential of pentazocine for elevating cerebrospinal fluid pressure may be attributed to CO_2 retention due to the respiratory depressant effects of the drug. These effects may be markedly exaggerated in the presence of head injury, other intracranial lesions, or a preexisting increase in intracranial pressure. Furthermore, pentazocine can produce effects which may obscure the clinical course of patients with head injuries. In such patients, pentazocine must be used wth extreme caution and only if its use is deemed essential.

Usage with Alcohol. Due to the potential for increased CNS depressant effects, alcohol should be used with caution in patients who are currently receiving pentazocine.

Patients Receiving Narcotics. Pentazocine is a mild narcotic antagonist. Some patients previously given narcotics, including methadone for the daily treatment of narcotic dependence, have experienced withdrawal symptoms after receiving pentazocine.

Certain Respiratory Conditions. Although respiratory depression has rarely been reported after oral administration of pentazocine, the drug should be administered with caution to patients with respiratory depression from any cause, severely limited respiratory reserve, severe bronchial asthma, and other obstructive respiratory conditions, or cyanosis.

Acute CNS Manifestations. Patients receiving therapeutic doses of pentazocine have experienced hallucinations (usually visual), disorientation, and confusion which have cleared spontaneously within a period of hours. The mechanism of this reaction is not known. Such patients should be very closely observed and vital signs checked. If the drug is reinstituted, it should be done with caution since these acute CNS manifestations may recur.

PRECAUTIONS

CNS Effect. Caution should be used when pentazocine is administered to patients prone to seizures; seizures have occurred in a few such patients in association with the use of pentazocine though no cause and effect relationship has been established.

Impaired Renal or Hepatic Function. Decreased metabolism of pentazocine by the liver in extensive liver disease may predispose to accentuation of side effects. Although laboratory tests have not indicated that pentazocine causes or increases renal or hepatic impairment, the drug should be administered with caution to patients with such impairment.

In prescribing pentazocine for long-term use, the physician should take precautions to avoid increases in dose by the patient.

Biliary Surgery. Narcotic drug products are generally considered to elevate biliary tract pressure for varying periods following their administration. Some evidence suggests that pentazocine may differ from other marketed narcotics in this respect (i.e., it causes little or no elevation in biliary tract pressures). The clinical significance of these findings, however, is not yet known.

Information for Patients. Since sedation, dizziness, and occasional euphoria have been noted, ambulatory patients

should be warned not to operate machinery, drive cars, or unnecessarily expose themselves to hazards. Pentazocine may cause physical and psychological dependence when taken alone and may have additive CNS depressant properties when taken in combination with alcohol or other CNS depressants.

Myocardial Infarction. As with all drugs, pentazocine should be used with caution in patients with myocardial infarction who have nausea or vomiting.

Drug Interactions. Usage with Alcohol: See WARNINGS.

Carcinogenesis, Mutagenesis, Impairment of Fertility. No long-term studies in animals to test for carcinogenesis have been performed with the components of TALWIN Nx.

Pregnancy Category C. Animal reproduction studies have not been conducted with TALWIN Nx. It is also not known whether TALWIN Nx can cause fetal harm when administered to pregnant women or can affect reproduction capacity. TALWIN Nx should be given to pregnant women only if clearly needed. However, animal reproduction studies with pentazocine have not demonstrated teratogenic or embryotoxic effects.

Labor and Delivery. Patients receiving pentazocine during labor have experienced no adverse effects other than those that occur with commonly used analgesics. TALWIN Nx should be used with caution in women delivering premature infants. The effect of TALWIN Nx on the mother and fetus, the duration of labor or delivery, the possibility that forceps delivery or other intervention or resuscitation of the newborn may be necessary, or the effect of TALWIN Nx on the later growth, development, and functional maturation of the child are unknown at the present time.

Nursing Mothers. It is not known whether this drug is excreted in human milk. Because many drugs are excreted in human milk, caution should be exercised when TALWIN Nx is administered to a nursing woman.

Pediatric Use. Safety and effectiveness in pediatric patients below the age of 12 years have not been established.

ADVERSE REACTIONS

Cardiovascular. Hypotension, tachycardia, syncope.

Respiratory. Rarely, respiratory depression.

Acute CNS Manifestations. Patients receiving therapeutic doses of pentazocine have experienced hallucinations (usually visual), disorientation, and confusion which have cleared spontaneously within a period of hours. The mechanism of this reaction is not known. Such patients should be closely observed and vital signs checked. If the drug is reinstituted it should be done with caution since these acute CNS manifestations may recur.

Other CNS Effects. Dizziness, lightheadedness, hallucinations, sedation, euphoria, headache, confusion, disorientation; infrequently weakness, disturbed dreams, insomnia, syncope, visual blurring and focusing difficulty, depression; and rarely tremor, irritability, excitement, tinnitus.

Autonomic. Sweating; infrequently flushing; and rarely chills.

Gastrointestinal. Nausea, vomiting, constipation, diarrhea, anorexia, rarely abdominal distress.

Allergic. Edema of the face; dermatitis, including pruritus; flushed skin, including plethora; infrequently rash, and rarely urticaria.

Ophthalmic. Visual blurring and focusing difficulty.

Hematologic. Depression of white blood cells (especially granulocytes), which is usually reversible, moderate transient eosinophilia.

Other. Headache, chills, insomnia, weakness, urinary retention, paresthesia.

DRUG ABUSE AND DEPENDENCE

Controlled Substance. TALWIN Nx is a Schedule IV controlled substance.

There have been some reports of dependence and of withdrawal symptoms with orally administered pentazocine. Patients with a history of drug dependence should be under close supervision while receiving pentazocine orally. There have been rare reports of possible abstinence syndromes in newborns after prolonged use of pentazocine during pregnancy.

There have been instances of psychological and physical dependence on parenteral pentazocine in patients with a history of drug abuse and rarely, in patients without such a history. Abrupt discontinuance following the extended use of parenteral pentazocine has resulted in withdrawal symptoms.

In prescribing pentazocine for chronic use, the physician should take precautions to avoid increases in dose by the patient.

The amount of naloxone present in TALWIN Nx (0.5 mg per tablet) has no action when taken orally and will not interfere with the pharmacologic action of pentazocine. However, this amount of naloxone given by injection has profound antagonistic action to narcotic analgesics.

Severe, even lethal, consequences may result from misuse of tablets by injection either alone or in combination with other substances, such as pulmonary emboli, vascular occlusion, ulceration and abscesses, and withdrawal symptoms in narcotic dependent individuals.

TALWIN Nx contains an opioid antagonist, naloxone (0.5 mg). Naloxone is inactive when administered orally at this dose, and its inclusion in TALWIN Nx is intended to curb a form of misuse of oral pentazocine. Parenterally, naloxone is an active narcotic antagonist. Thus, TALWIN Nx has a lower potential for parenteral misuse than the previous oral pentazocine formulation TALWIN® 50, (pentazocine hydrochloride tablets, USP). However, it is still subject to patient misuse and abuse by the oral route.

OVERDOSAGE

Manifestations. Clinical experience of overdosage with this oral medication has been insufficient to define the signs of this condition.

Treatment. Oxygen, intravenous fluids, vasopressors, and other supportive measures should be employed as indicated. Assisted or controlled ventilation should also be considered. For respiratory depression due to overdosage or unusual sensitivity to pentazocine, parenteral naloxone is a specific and effective antagonist.

DOSAGE AND ADMINISTRATION

> TALWIN® Nx is intended for oral use only. Severe, potentially lethal, reactions may result from misuse of TALWIN® Nx by injection either alone or in combination with other substances. (See DRUG ABUSE AND DEPENDENCE section.)

Adults. The usual initial adult dose is 1 tablet every three or four hours. This may be increased to 2 tablets when needed. Total daily dosage should not exceed 12 tablets.

When anti-inflammatory or antipyretic effects are desired in addition to analgesia, aspirin can be administered concomitantly with this product.

Pediatric Patients. Since clinical experience in pediatric patients under 12 years of age is limited, administration of this product in this age group is not recommended.

Duration of Therapy. Patients with chronic pain who receive TALWIN Nx orally for prolonged periods have only rarely been reported to experience withdrawal symptoms when administration was abruptly discontinued (see WARNINGS). Tolerance to the analgesic effect of pentazocine has also been reported only rarely. However, there is no long-term experience with the oral administration of TALWIN Nx.

HOW SUPPLIED

Tablets (oblong), yellow, scored, each containing pentazocine hydrochloride equivalent to 50 mg base and naloxone hydrochloride equivalent to 0.5 mg base.

Bottles of 100 (NDC 0024-1951-04).

Unit Dose Dispenser Package of 250 (NDC 0024-1951-24), 10 sleeves of 25 tablets each.

Store at controlled room temperature 15° C to 30° C (59° F to 80° F).

Caution: Federal law prohibits dispensing without prescription.

TSW-4 B

Shown in Product Identification Guide, page 336

WINSTROL® CIII ℞
stanozolol, USP

DESCRIPTION

WINSTROL, brand of stanozolol tablets, is an anabolic steroid, a synthetic derivative of testosterone. Each tablet for oral administration contains 2 mg of stanozolol. It is designated chemically as 17-methyl-2'*H*-5α-androst-2-eno[3,2-*c*]pyrazol-17β-ol, and has the following structural formula:

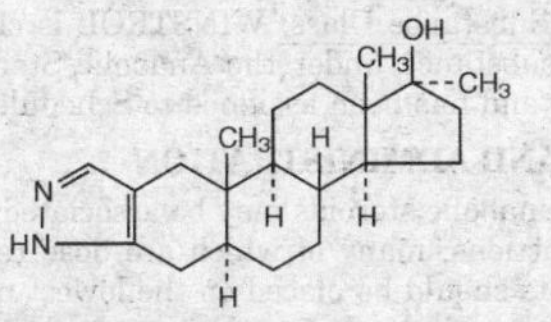

Inactive Ingredients: Dibasic Calcium Phosphate, D&C Red #28, FD&C Red #40, Lactose, Magnesium Stearate, Starch.

CLINICAL PHARMACOLOGY

Anabolic steroids are synthetic derivatives of testosterone. Certain clinical effects and adverse reactions demonstrate the androgenic properties of this class of drugs. Complete dissociation of anabolic and androgenic effects has not been achieved. The actions of anabolic steroids are therefore similar to those of male sex hormones with the possibility of causing serious disturbances of growth and sexual development if given to young children. They suppress the gonadotropic functions of the pituitary and may exert a direct effect upon the testes.

WINSTROL has been found to increase low-density lipoproteins and decrease high-density lipoproteins. These changes are not associated with any increase in total cholesterol or triglyceride levels and revert to normal on discontinuation of treatment.

Hereditary angioedema (HAE) is an autosomal dominant disorder caused by a deficient or nonfunctional C1 esterase inhibitor (C1 INH) and clinically characterized by episodes of swelling of the face, extremities, genitalia, bowel wall, and upper respiratory tract.

In small scale clinical studies, stanozolol was effective in controlling the frequency and severity of attacks of angioedema and in increasing serum levels of C1 INH and C4. WINSTROL is not effective in stopping HAE attacks while they are under way. The effect of WINSTROL on increasing serum levels of C1 INH and C4 may be related to an increase in protein anabolism.

INDICATIONS AND USAGE

Hereditary Angioedema. WINSTROL is indicated prophylactically to decrease the frequency and severity of attacks of angioedema.

CONTRAINDICATIONS

The use of WINSTROL is contraindicated in the following:

1. Male patients with carcinoma of the breast, or with known or suspected carcinoma of the prostate.
2. Carcinoma of the breast in females with hypercalcemia; androgenic anabolic steroids may stimulate osteolytic resorption of bone.
3. Nephrosis or the nephrotic phase of nephritis.
4. WINSTROL can cause fetal harm when administered to a pregnant woman.

WINSTROL is contraindicated in women who are or may become pregnant. If this drug is used during pregnancy, or if the patient becomes pregnant while taking this drug, the patient should be apprised of the potential hazard to the fetus.

WARNINGS

PELIOSIS HEPATIS, A CONDITION IN WHICH LIVER AND SOMETIMES SPLENIC TISSUE IS REPLACED WITH BLOOD-FILLED CYSTS, HAS BEEN REPORTED IN PATIENTS RECEIVING ANDROGENIC ANABOLIC STEROID THERAPY. THESE CYSTS ARE SOMETIMES PRESENT WITH MINIMAL HEPATIC DYSFUNCTION, BUT AT OTHER TIMES THEY HAVE BEEN ASSOCIATED WITH LIVER FAILURE. THEY ARE OFTEN NOT RECOGNIZED UNTIL LIFE-THREATENING LIVER FAILURE OR INTRA-ABDOMINAL HEMORRHAGE DEVELOPS. WITHDRAWAL OF DRUG USUALLY RESULTS IN COMPLETE DISAPPEARANCE OF LESIONS.

LIVER CELL TUMORS ARE ALSO REPORTED. MOST OFTEN THESE TUMORS ARE BENIGN AND ANDROGEN-DEPENDENT, BUT FATAL MALIGNANT TUMORS HAVE BEEN REPORTED. WITHDRAWAL OF DRUG OFTEN RESULTS IN REGRESSION OR CESSATION OF PROGRESSION OF THE TUMOR. HOWEVER, HEPATIC TUMORS ASSOCIATED WITH ANDROGENS OR ANABOLIC STEROIDS ARE MUCH MORE VASCULAR THAN OTHER HEPATIC TUMORS AND MAY BE SILENT UNTIL LIFE-THREATENING INTRA-ABDOMINAL HEMORRHAGE DEVELOPS.

BLOOD LIPID CHANGES THAT ARE KNOWN TO BE ASSOCIATED WITH INCREASED RISK OF ATHEROSCLEROSIS ARE SEEN IN PATIENTS TREATED WITH ANDROGENS AND ANABOLIC STEROIDS. THESE CHANGES INCLUDE DECREASED HIGH-DENSITY LIPOPROTEIN AND SOMETIMES INCREASED LOW-DENSITY LIPOPROTEIN. THE CHANGES MAY BE VERY MARKED AND COULD HAVE A SERIOUS IMPACT ON THE RISK OF ATHEROSCLEROSIS AND CORONARY ARTERY DISEASE.

Cholestatic hepatitis and jaundice occur with 17-alpha-alkylated androgens at relatively low doses. If cholestatic hepatitis with jaundice appears, the anabolic steroid should be discontinued. If liver function tests become abnormal, the patient should be monitored closely and the etiology determined. Generally, the anabolic steroid should be discontinued although in cases of mild abnormalities, the physician may elect to follow the patient carefully at a reduced drug dosage.

In patients with breast cancer, anabolic steroid therapy may cause hypercalcemia by stimulating osteolysis. In this case, the drug should be discontinued.

Continued on next page

This product information was prepared in September 1998. On these and other products of Sanofi Pharmaceuticals, Inc., detailed information may be obtained on a current basis by direct inquiry to Product Information Services, 90 Park Avenue, New York, NY 10016 (toll free 1-800-446-6267).

Winstrol—Cont.

Edema with or without congestive heart failure may be a serious complication in patients with preexisting cardiac, renal, or hepatic disease. Concomitant administration of adrenal cortical steroids or ACTH may add to the edema.

Geriatric male patients treated with androgenic anabolic steroids may be at an increased risk for the development of prostatic hypertrophy and prostatic carcinoma.

In children, anabolic steroid treatment may accelerate bone maturation without producing compensatory gain in linear growth. This adverse effect may result in compromised adult stature. The younger the child, the greater the risk of compromising final mature height. The effect on bone maturation should be monitored by assessing bone age of the wrist and hand every six months.

Anabolic steroids have not been shown to enhance athletic ability.

PRECAUTIONS

General
Anabolic steroids may cause suppression of clotting factors II, V, VII, and X, and an increase in prothrombin time. Women should be observed for signs of virilization (deepening of the voice, hirsutism, acne, and clitoromegaly). To prevent irreversible change, drug therapy must be discontinued, or the dosage significantly reduced when mild virilism is first detected. Such virilization is usual following androgenic anabolic steroid use at high doses. Some virilizing changes in women are irreversible even after prompt discontinuance of therapy and are not prevented by concomitant use of estrogens. Menstrual irregularities may also occur.

The insulin or oral hypoglycemic dosage may need adjustment in diabetic patients who receive anabolic steroids.

Information for the Patient. The physician should instruct patients to report any of the following side effects of androgens:

Adult or Adolescent Males. Too frequent or persistent erections of the penis, appearance or aggravation of acne.

Women. Hoarseness, acne, changes in menstrual periods, or more hair on the face.

All Patients. Any nausea, vomiting, changes in skin color, or ankle swelling.

Laboratory Tests. Women with disseminated breast carcinoma should have frequent determination of urine and serum calcium levels during the course of androgenic anabolic steroid therapy (see WARNINGS).

Because of the hepatotoxicity associated with the use of 17-alpha-alkylated androgens, liver function tests should be obtained periodically.

Periodic (every 6 months) x-ray examinations of bone age should be made during treatment of prepubertal patients to determine the rate of bone maturation and the effects of androgenic anabolic steroid therapy on the epiphyseal centers.

In common with other anabolic steroids, WINSTROL has been reported to lower the level of high-density lipoproteins and raise the level of low-density lipoproteins. These changes usually revert to normal on discontinuation of treatment. Increased low-density lipoproteins and decreased high-density lipoproteins are considered cardiovascular risk factors. Serum lipids and high-density lipoprotein cholesterol should be determined periodically.

Hemoglobin and hematocrit should be checked periodically for polycythemia in patients who are receiving high doses of anabolic steroids.

Drug Interaction. Anabolic steroids may increase sensitivity to anticoagulants; therefore, dosage of an anticoagulant may have to be decreased in order to maintain the prothrombin time at the desired therapeutic level.

Drug/Laboratory Test Interferences. Therapy with androgenic anabolic steroids may decrease levels of thyroxine-binding globulin resulting in decreased total T_4 serum levels and increase resin uptake of T_3 and T_4. Free thyroid hormone levels remain unchanged and there is no clinical evidence of thyroid dysfunction.

Carcinogenesis, Mutagenesis, Impairment of Fertility.
Animal data: Testosterone has been tested by subcutaneous injection and implantation in mice and rats. The implant induced cervical-uterine tumors in mice, which metastasized in some cases. There is suggestive evidence that injection of testosterone into some strains of female mice increases their susceptibility to hepatoma. Testosterone is also known to increase the number of tumors and decrease the degree of differentiation of chemically-induced carcinomas of the liver in rats.

Human data: There are rare reports of hepatocellular carcinoma in patients receiving long-term therapy with androgens in high doses. Withdrawal of the drugs did not lead to regression of the tumors in all cases.

Geriatric patients treated with androgens may be at an increased risk of developing prostatic hypertrophy and prostatic carcinoma although conclusive evidence to support this concept is lacking.

This compound has not been tested for mutagenic potential. However, as noted above, carcinogenic effects have been attributed to treatment with androgenic hormones. The potential carcinogenic effects likely occur through a hormonal mechanism rather than by a direct chemical interaction mechanism.

Impairment of fertility was not tested directly in animal species. However, as noted below under ADVERSE REACTIONS, oligospermia in males and amenorrhea in females are potential adverse effects of treatment with WINSTROL Tablets. Therefore, impairment of fertility is a possible outcome of treatment with WINSTROL.

Pregnancy Category X. See CONTRAINDICATIONS section.

Nursing Mothers. It is not known whether anabolic steroids are excreted in human milk. Many drugs are excreted in human milk and because of the potential for adverse reactions in nursing infants from WINSTROL, a decision should be made whether to discontinue nursing or discontinue the drug, taking into account the importance of the drug to the mother.

Pediatric Use. Anabolic agents may accelerate epiphyseal maturation more rapidly than linear growth in children, and the effect may continue for 6 months after the drug has been stopped. Therefore, therapy should be monitored by x-ray studies at 6 month intervals in order to avoid the risk of compromising the adult height. The safety and efficacy of WINSTROL in children with hereditary angioedema have not been established.

ADVERSE REACTIONS

Hepatic: Cholestatic jaundice with, rarely, hepatic necrosis and death. Hepatocellular neoplasms and peliosis hepatis have been reported in association with long-term androgenic-anabolic steroid therapy (see WARNINGS). Reversible changes in liver function tests also occur including increased bromsulphalein (BSP) retention and increases in serum bilirubin, glutamic oxaloacetic transaminase (SGOT), and alkaline phosphatase.

Genitourinary System: *In men. Prepubertal:* Phallic enlargement and increased frequency of erections.
Postpubertal: Inhibition of testicular function, testicular atrophy and oligospermia, impotence, chronic priapism, epididymitis and bladder irritability.
In women: Clitoral enlargement, menstrual irregularities.
In both sexes: Increased or decreased libido.

CNS: Habituation, excitation, insomnia, depression.

Gastrointestinal: Nausea, vomiting, diarrhea.

Hematologic: Bleeding in patients on concomitant anticoagulant therapy.

Breast: Gynecomastia.

Larynx: Deepening of the voice in women.

Hair: Hirsutism and male pattern baldness in women.

Skin: Acne (especially in women and prepubertal boys).

Skeletal: Premature closure of epiphyses in children (see PRECAUTIONS, **Pediatric Use**).

Fluid and Electrolytes: Edema, retention of serum electrolytes (sodium, chloride, potassium, phosphate, calcium).

Metabolic/Endocrine: Decreased glucose tolerance (see PRECAUTIONS), increased serum levels of low-density lipoproteins and decreased levels of high-density lipoproteins (see PRECAUTIONS, **Laboratory Tests**), increased creatine and creatinine excretion, increased serum levels of creatinine phosphokinase (CPK).

Some virilizing changes in women are irreversible even after prompt discontinuation of therapy and are not prevented by concomitant use of estrogens (see PRECAUTIONS).

DRUG ABUSE AND DEPENDENCE

Controlled Substance Class: WINSTROL is classified as a controlled substance under the Anabolic Steroids Control Act of 1990 and has been assigned to Schedule III.

DOSAGE AND ADMINISTRATION

The use of anabolic steroids may be associated with serious adverse reactions, many of which are dose related; therefore, patients should be placed on the lowest possible effective dose.

Hereditary Angioedema. The dosage requirements for continuous treatment of hereditary angioedema with WINSTROL should be individualized on the basis of the clinical response of the patient. It is recommended that the patient be started on 2 mg, three times a day. After a favorable initial response is obtained in terms of prevention of episodes of edematous attacks, the proper continuing dosage should be determined by decreasing the dosage at intervals of one to three months to a maintenance dosage of 2 mg a day. Some patients may be successfully managed on a 2 mg alternate day schedule. During the dose adjusting phase, close monitoring of the patient's response is indicated, particularly if the patient has a history of airway involvement.

The prophylactic dose of WINSTROL, to be used prior to dental extraction, or other traumatic or stressful situations has not been established and may be substantially larger. Attacks of hereditary angioedema are generally infrequent in childhood and the risks from stanozolol administration are substantially increased. Therefore, long-term prophylactic therapy with this drug is generally not recommended in children, and should only be undertaken with due consideration of the benefits and risks involved (see PRECAUTIONS, **Pediatric Use**).

HOW SUPPLIED

WINSTROL tablets for oral administration are pink, round tablets scored on one side.
Bottles of 100—NDC 0024-2253-04
Store at controlled room temperature 15° to 30° C (59° to 86° F)
Caution: Federal law prohibits dispensing without prescription.

WSW-1-D(O)

Shown in Product Identification Guide, page 336

ZEPHREX® TABLETS ℞

DESCRIPTION
ZEPHREX® is a white film coated, oval-shaped tablet with a bisect on one side and SANOFI with 460 below the name on the other side.
Each tablet contains:
Pseudoephedrine HCl .... 60 mg
Guaifenesin .... 400 mg

HOW SUPPLIED
100's NDC 0024-2624-01

ZEPHREX LA® TABLETS ℞

Each timed release* orange, oval-shaped tablet embossed with bock on one side and a Z bisect LA on the other side contains:
Pseudoephedrine HCl .... 120.0 mg
Guaifenesin .... 600.0 mg
* In a special base to provide prolonged therapeutic action.

HOW SUPPLIED
Bottles of 100.
NDC 0024-2627-02

Savage Laboratories®
a division of Altana Inc.
60 BAYLIS ROAD
MELVILLE, NY 11747

Direct Inquiries to:
Customer Service
(800) 231-0206
FAX: (516) 454-0732

For Medical Information Contact:
Dr. Arnold Yeadon
(516) 454-9071
FAX: (516) 454-6389

AXOCET® ℞
(Butalbital and Acetaminophen capsules)

DESCRIPTION
AXOCET® are opaque grey capsules imprinted with Savage logo and 0198. Each capsule contains Butalbital USP, 50 mg and Acetaminophen USP, 650 mg.
(WARNING—May be habit forming)

HOW SUPPLIED
AXOCET® Capsules are supplied as follows:
Bottle of 100, NDC 0281-0198-17

CHROMAGEN® ℞
[kro "mah-jen]
Soft Gelatin Capsules

DESCRIPTION
Each maroon soft gelatin capsule contains ferrous fumarate USP, 200 mg (66 mg elemental iron), ascorbic acid USP, 250 mg, cyanocobalamin USP, 10 mcg, desiccated stomach substance 100 mg (Contains: Intrinsic factor).

HOW SUPPLIED
Chromagen Capsules are supplied as follows:
NDC 0281-4285-18, Unit Dose Box 100

CHROMAGEN® FA ℞
SOFT GELATIN CAPSULES

DESCRIPTION

CONTENTS: Each maroon and brown soft gelatin capsule contains: ferrous fumarate USP, 200 mg (66 mg elemental iron), ascorbic acid USP, 250 mg, folic acid USP, 1 mg, cyanocobalamin USP, 10 mcg.

DISCUSSION: The amount of elemental iron and the absorption of the iron components of commercial iron preparations vary widely. It is further established that certain "accessory components" may be included to enhance absorption and utilization of iron. Chromagen® FA Capsules are formulated to provide the essential factors for a complete, versatile hematinic.

ACTIONS

HIGH ELEMENTAL IRON CONTENT: Ferrous fumarate, used in Chromagen® FA Capsules, is an organic iron complex which has the highest elemental iron content of any hematinic salt - 33%. This compares with 20% for ferrous sulfate (heptahydrate) and 13% for ferrous gluconate.[1,2]

MORE COMPLETE ABSORPTION: It has been repeatedly shown that ascorbic acid, when given in sufficient amounts, can increase the absorption of ferrous iron from the gastrointestinal tract.[3,4,5,6,7,8,9] The absorption-promoting effect is mainly due to the reducing action of ascorbic acid within the gastrointestinal lumen, which helps to prevent or delay the formation of insoluble or less dissociated ferric compounds.[3] Iron absorption has been shown to increase sharply with increasing amounts of ascorbic acid, showing a gain in absorption of approximately 40% at 250 mg. Above 250 mg, the gain becomes insignificant, with an additional gain of only approximately 8% at 500 mg.[3] Each Chromagen® FA Capsule contains 250 mg of ascorbic acid, believed to be the optimal amount.

PROMOTES MOVEMENT OF PLASMA IRON: Ascorbic acid also plays an important role in the movement of plasma iron to storage depots in the tissues.[10] The action, which leads to the transport of plasma iron to ferritin, presumably involves its reducing effect, converting transferrin iron from the ferric to the ferrous state.[5] There is also evidence that ascorbic acid improves iron utilization, presumably as a further result of its reducing action,[6, 9] and some evidence that it may have a direct effect upon erythropoiesis. Ascorbic acid is further alleged to enhance the conversion of folic acid to a more physiologically active form, folinic acid, which would make it even more important in the treatment of anemia since it would aid in the utilization of dietary folic acid.[11]

EXCELLENT ORAL TOLERATION: Ferrous fumarate is used in Chromagen® FA Capsules because it is less likely to cause the gastric disturbances so often associated with oral iron therapy. Ferrous fumarate has a low ionization constant and high solubility in the entire pH range of the gastrointestinal tract. It does not precipitate proteins or have the astringency of more ionizable forms of iron, and does not interfere with proteolytic or diastatic activities of the digestive system. Because of excellent oral toleration, Chromagen® FA Capsules can usually be administered between meals when iron absorption is maximal.

FOLIC ACID SUPPLEMENTATION: The use of supplemental folic acid may be indicated in patients with increased requirements for this vitamin, such as iron deficiency anemia. Folic acid administration may reduce the risk of neural tube defects in the developing fetus.[12] Folic acid has also been shown to reduce circulating homocysteine levels in the blood.[15,16] Folate as 5-methyltetrahydrofolate and B_{12} as methylcobalamin are involved in the remethylation reaction of homocysteine to methionine.[17,18] Elevated homocysteine plasma levels are associated with increased risk of preeclampsia, neural tube defects, myocardial infarction and artherosclerosis.[19–23]

TOXICITY: Ferrous fumarate was found to be the least toxic of three popular oral iron salts, with an oral LD_{50} of 630 mg/kg. In the same report, the LD_{50} of ferrous gluconate was reported to be 320 mg/kg and ferrous sulfate 230 mg/kg.[1,13]

INDICATIONS

For the treatment of all anemias responsive to oral iron therapy, such as hypochromic anemia associated with pregnancy, chronic or acute blood loss, dietary restriction, metabolic disease and post-surgical convalescence.

CONTRAINDICATIONS

Hemochromatosis and hemosiderosis are contraindications to iron therapy. Folic acid is contraindicated in patients with pernicious anemia (see **PRECAUTIONS**).

> **WARNING**
> Accidental overdose of iron-containing products is a leading cause of fatal poisoning in children under 6. Keep this product out of reach of children. In case of accidental overdose, call a doctor or poison control center immediately.

PRECAUTIONS

Folic acid should not be prescribed until the diagnosis of pernicious anemia has been eliminated, since it can alleviate the hematologic manifestations, while allowing neurological damage to continue undetected.[14]

ADVERSE REACTIONS

Average capsule doses in sensitive individuals or excessive dosage may cause nausea, skin rash, vomiting, diarrhea, precordial pain, or flushing of the face and extremities.

DOSAGE AND ADMINISTRATION

Usual adult dose is 1 soft gelatin capsule daily

HOW SUPPLIED

Capsules: NDC 0281-0259-18, Unit Dose Box 100

CAUTION: Federal law prohibits dispensing without prescription.

BIBLIOGRAPHY

[1]Berk, M.S. and Novich, M.A.: "Treatment of Iron Deficiency Anemia With Ferrous Fumarate," Am. J. Obst. & Gynec., 203–206, 1962. [2]Shapleigh, J.B., and Montgomery, A.:Am. Pract. & Dig. Treat. 10–461, 1959. [3]Brise, H. and Hallberg, L.: "Effect of Ascorbic Acid on Iron Absorption," Acta. Med. Scand. 171:376, 51–58, 1962. [4]New Drugs, p. 309, AMA, Chicago, 1966. [5]Mazur, A., Green, S. and Carleton, A,: "Mechanism of Plasma Iron Incorporation into Hepatic Ferritin," J. Bio. Chem. 3:595–603, 1960. [6]Greenberg, S.M., Tucker, A. E., Mathues, H and J.D.: "Iron Absorption and Metabolism, I. Interrelationship of Ascorbic Acid and Vitamin E," J. Nutrition 63:19–31, 1957. [7]Moore, C.V. and Dubach, R. "Observations on the Absorption of Iron from Foods Tagged with Radioiron" Trans. Assoc. Amer. Physic. 64:245, 1951. [8]Steinkamp, R. Dubach, R. and Moore, C.V.: "Studies in Iron Transportation and Metabolism,"Arch. Int. Med. 95:181, 1955. [9]Gorten, M. K. and Bradley, J. E.: "The Treatment of Nutritional Anemia in Infancy and Childhood with Oral Iron and Ascorbic Acid," J. Pediatrics, 45:1, 1954. [10]Mazur, A.: "Role of Ascorbic Acid in the Incorporation of Plasma Iron into Ferritin," Ann. N.Y. Acad. Sci, 92:223–229, 1961. [11]Cox, E.V. et al.: "The Anemia of Scurvy," Amer. J. Med. 42:220–227, 1967. [12]McEvoy, G.K., Ed.: AHFS Drug Information, p. 2667–2669, Am. Soc. Hosp. Pharm., Bethesda, 1996. [13]Berenbaum, M.C. et al.: Blood, 15:540, 1960. [14]Drug Information for the Health Care Professional, p.1365–1368, U. S. Pharmacopeial Conven., Rockville, 1995. [15]Franken DG, Boers GH, Blom HJ, Trijbels JM. "Effect of various regimens of vitamin B_6 and folic acid on mild hyperhomocysteinemia in vascular patients." J. Inherit. Metab. Dis. 1994; 17:159–62. [16]Brattstrom L, Israelsson B, Norrving B, et al. "Impaired homocysteine metabolism in early-onset cerebral and peripheral occlusive disease - effects of pyridoxine and folic acid treatment." Atherosclerosis 1990; 81: 2004–6. [17]Kang S. Wong PWK, Norusis M. "Homocysteinemia due to folate deficiency." Metabolism 1987; 36: 458–62. [18]Allen RH, Stabler SP, Savage DG, Lindernbaum J. "Diagnosis of cobalamin deficiency." IL usefulness of serum methylmalonic acid and total homocysteine concentrations. Am. J. Hematol. 1990; 34: 90–98. [19]Dekker GA, de Vries JI, Doelitzsch PM, Huijgens PC, von Blomberg BM, Jakobs, C, van Geijn HP. 1985. "Underlying disorder associated with severe early-onset preeclampsia." Am. J. Obstet. Gynecol. 173: 1042–1048. [20]Mills JL, McPartlin JM, Kirke PN, Lee YJ, Conley MR, Weir DG, Scott JM. 1995. "Homocysteine metabolism in pregnancies complicated by neural-tube defects." Lancet. 345: 149–151. [21]Steegers-Theunissen RP, Boers GH, Blom HJ, Nijhuis JG, Thomas CM, Borm GF, Eskes TK. 1995. "Neural tube defects and elevated homocysteine levels in amniotic fluid." Am. J. Obstet. Gynecol. 172: 1436–1441. [22]Landgren F, Israelsson B, Lindgren A, Hultberg B, Andersson A, Brattstrom L. 1995. "Plasma homocysteine in acute myocardial infarction: Homocysteine-lowering effect of folic acid." J. Intern. Med. 237: 381–388. [23]Mayer EL, Jacobsen DW, Robinson K. 1996. "Homocysteine and Coronary Atherosclerosis." J. Am. Coll. Cardiol. 27: 517–27.

Manufactured for:
SAVAGE LABORATORIES®
a division of Altana Inc.
MELVILLE, NEW YORK 11747

IF70259B
by: R.P. Scherer Corporation, St. Petersburg, Florida 33702
R3/97

Shown in Product Identification Guide, page 336

CHROMAGEN® FORTE ℞
SOFT GELATIN CAPSULES

DESCRIPTION

CONTENTS: Each brown soft gelatin capsule contains: ferrous fumarate USP, 460 mg (151 mg elemental iron), ascorbic acid USP, 60 mg, folic acid USP, 1 mg, cyanocobalamin USP, 10 mcg.

DISCUSSION: The amount of elemental iron and the absorption of the iron components of commercial iron preparations vary widely. It is further established that certain "accessory components" may be included to enhance absorption and utilization of iron. Chromagen® Forte Capsules are formulated to provide the essential factors for a complete, versatile hematinic.

ACTIONS

HIGH ELEMENTAL IRON CONTENT: Ferrous fumarate, used in Chromagen® Forte Capsules, is an organic iron complex which has the highest elemental iron content of any hematinic salt - 33%. This compares with 20% for ferrous sulfate (heptahydrate) and 13% for ferrous gluconate.[1,2] Chromagen® Forte contains 151 mg of elemental iron.

MORE COMPLETE ABSORPTION: It has been repeatedly shown that ascorbic acid, when given in sufficient amounts, can increase the absorption of ferrous iron from the gastrointestinal tract.[3–9] The absorption-promoting effect is mainly due to the reducing action of ascorbic acid within the gastrointestinal lumen, which helps to prevent or delay the formation of insoluble or less dissociated ferric compounds.[3]

PROMOTES MOVEMENT OF PLASMA IRON: Ascorbic acid also plays an important role in the movement of plasma iron to storage depots in the tissues.[10] The action, which leads to the transport of plasma iron to ferritin, presumably involves its reducing effect, converting transferrin iron from the ferric to the ferrous state.[5] There is also evidence that ascorbic acid improves iron utilization, presumably as a further result of its reducing action,[6,9] and some evidence that it may have a direct effect upon erythropoiesis. Ascorbic acid is further alleged to enhance the conversion of folic acid to a more physiologically active form, folinic acid, which would make it even more important in the treatment of anemia since it would aid in the utilization of dietary folic acid.[11]

EXCELLENT ORAL TOLERATION: Ferrous fumarate is used in Chromagen® Forte Capsules because it is less likely to cause the gastric disturbances so often associated with oral iron therapy. Ferrous fumarate has a low ionization constant and high solubility in the entire pH range of the gastrointestinal tract. It does not precipitate proteins or have the astringency of more ionizable forms of iron, and does not interfere with proteolytic or diastatic activities of the digestive system. Because of excellent oral toleration, Chromagen® Forte Capsules can usually be administered between meals when iron absorption is maximal.

FOLIC ACID SUPPLEMENTATION: The use of supplemental folic acid may be indicated in patients with increased requirements for this vitamin, such as iron deficiency anemia. Folic acid administration may reduce the risk of neural tube defects in the developing fetus.[12] Folic acid has also been shown to reduce circulating homocysteine levels in the blood.[13,14] Folate as 5-methyltetrahydrofolate and B_{12} as methylcobalamin are involved in the remethylation reaction of homocysteine to methionine.[15,16] Elevated homocysteine plasma levels are associated with increased risk of preeclampsia, neural tube defects, myocardial infarction and artherosclerosis.[17–21]

TOXICITY: Ferrous fumarate was found to be the least toxic of three popular oral iron salts, with an oral LD_{50} of 630 mg/kg. In the same report, the LD_{50} of ferrous gluconate was reported to be 320 mg/kg and ferrous sulfate 230 mg/kg.[1,22]

INDICATIONS

For the treatment of all anemias responsive to oral iron therapy, such as hypochromic anemia associated with pregnancy, chronic or acute blood loss, dietary restriction, metabolic disease and post-surgical convalescence.

CONTRAINDICATIONS

Hemochromatosis and hemosiderosis are contraindications to iron therapy. Folic acid is contraindicated in patients with pernicious anemia (see **PRECAUTIONS**).

> **WARNING**
> Accidental overdose of iron-containing products is a leading cause of fatal poisoning in children under 6. Keep this product out of reach of children. In case of accidental overdose, call a doctor or poison control center immediately.

PRECAUTIONS

Folic acid should not be prescribed until the diagnosis of pernicious anemia has been eliminated, since it can alleviate the hematologic manifestations, while allowing neurological damage to continue undetected.[23]

ADVERSE REACTIONS

Average capsule doses in sensitive individuals or excessive dosage may cause nausea, skin rash, vomiting, diarrhea, precordial pain, or flushing of the face and extremities.

DOSAGE AND ADMINISTRATION

Usual adult dose is 1–2 soft gelatin capsules daily, or as directed by a physician.

Continued on next page

Chromagen Forte—Cont.

HOW SUPPLIED

Capsules: NDC 0281-0262-18, Unit Dose Box 100

CAUTION: Federal law prohibits dispensing without prescription.

BIBLIOGRAPHY

[1]Berk, M.S. and Novich, M.A.: "Treatment of Iron Deficiency Anemia With Ferrous Fumarate," Am. J. Obst. & Gynec., 203–206, 1962. [2]Shapleigh, J.B., and Montgomery, A.:Am. Pract. & Dig. Treat. 10–461, 1959. [3]Brise, H. and Hallberg, L.: "Effect of Ascorbic Acid on Iron Absorption," Acta. Med. Scand.171:376, 51–58, 1962. [4]New Drugs, p. 309, AMA, Chicago, 1966. [5]Mazur, A., Green, S. and Carleton, A.: "Mechanism of Plasma Iron Incorporation into Hepatic Ferritin," J. Bio. Chem. 3:595–603, 1960. [6]Greenberg, S.M., Tucker, A. E., Mathues, H and J.D.: "Iron Absorption and Metabolism, I. Interrelationship of Ascorbic Acid and Vitamin E," J. Nutrition 63:19–31, 1957. [7]Moore, C.V. and Dubach, R. "Observations on the Absorption of Iron from Foods Tagged with Radioiron" Trans. Assoc. Amer. Physic. 64:245, 1951. [8]Steinkamp, R. Dubach, R. and Moore, C.V.: "Studies in Iron Transportation and Metabolism,"Arch. Int. Med. 95:181, 1955. [9]Gorten, M. K. and Bradley, J. E.: "The Treatment of Nutritional Anemia in Infancy and Childhood with Oral Iron and Ascorbic Acid," J. Pediatrics, 45:1, 1954. [10]Mazur, A.: "Role of Ascorbic Acid in the Incorporation of Plasma Iron into Ferritin," Ann. N.Y. Acad. Sci, 92:223–229, 1961. [11]Cox, E.V. et al.: "The Anemia of Scurvy," Amer. J. Med. 42:220–227, 1967. [12]McEvoy, G.K., Ed.: AHFS Drug Information, p. 2667-2669, Am. Soc. Hosp. Pharm., Bethesda, 1996. [13]Franken DG, Boers GH, Blom HJ, Trijbels JM. "Effect of various regimens of vitamin B_6 and folic acid on mild hyperhomocysteinemia in vascular patients." J. Inherit. Metab. Dis. 1994; 17:159–62. [14]Brattstrom L, Israelsson B, Norrving B, et al. "Impaired homocysteine metabolism in early-onset cerebral and peripheral occlusive disease—effects of pyridoxine and folic acid treatment." Atherosclerosis 1990; 81: 2004–6. [15]Kang S. Wong PWK, Norusis M. "Homocysteinemia due to folate deficiency." Metabolism 1987; 36: 458–62. [16]Allen RH, Stabler SP, Savage DG, Lindernbaum J. "Diagnosis of cobalamin deficiency." IL usefulness of serum methylmalonic acid and total homocysteine concentrations. Am. J. Hematol. 1990; 34: 90–98. [17]Dekker GA, de Vries JI, Doelitzsch PM, Huijgens PC, von Blomberg BM, Jakobs, C, van Geijn HP. 1985. "Underlying disorder associated with severe early-onset preeclampsia." Am. J. Obstet. Gynecol. 173: 1042–1048. [18]Mills JL, McPartlin JM, Kirke PN, Lee YJ, Conley MR, Weir DG, Scott JM. 1995. "Homocysteine metabolism in pregnancies complicated by neural-tube defects." Lancet. 345: 149–151. [19]Steegers-Theunissen RP, Boers GH, Blom HJ, Nijhuis JG, Thomas CM, Borm GF, Eskes TK. 1995. "Neural tube defects and elevated homocysteine levels in amniotic fluid." Am. J. Obstet. Gynecol. 172: 1436–1441. [20]Landgren F, Israelsson B, Lindgren A, Hultberg B, Andersson A, Brattstrom L. 1995. "Plasma homocysteine in acute myocardial infarction: Homocysteine-lowering effect of folic acid." J. Intern. Med. 237: 381–388. [21]Mayer EL, Jacobsen DW, Robinson K. 1996. "Homocysteine and Coronary Atherosclerosis." J. Am. Coll. Cardiol. 27: 517–27. [22]Berenbaum, M.C. et al.: Blood, 15:540, 1960. [23]Drug Information for the Health Care Professional, p.1365-1368, U. S. Pharmacopeial Conven., Rockville, 1995.

Manufactured for:
SAVAGE LABORATORIES®
a division of Altana Inc.
MELVILLE, NEW YORK 11747

IF70262C

by: R.P. Scherer Corporation, St. Petersburg, Florida 33702

R9/97

Shown in Product Identification Guide, page 336

DILOR® ℞
(Dyphylline tablets USP)

DESCRIPTION

Dilor® Tablets 200 mg
Each round, light blue, scored tablet contains dyphylline USP, 200 mg. Dyphylline is a white, extremely bitter, amorphous solid, freely soluble in water and soluble to the extent of 2 g/100 mL alcohol.
Dilor® Tablets 400 mg
Each round, white, scored tablet contains dyphylline 400 mg and the following inactive ingredients: colloidal silicon dioxide, corn starch, food starch, povidone, sodium lauryl sulfate, and stearic acid.
Dilor® Elixir
Each tablespoon (15 mL) contains dyphylline USP 160 mg in a mint flavored base containing the following: alcohol (18%), citric acid, glycerin, saccharin sodium, sorbitol, sucrose, purified water, artificial coloring and flavorings. Methylparaben and propylparaben added as preservatives.
Dilor® Injection
Each 2 mL ampule contains dyphylline USP, 500 mg (250 mg/mL), in water for injection USP, Sodium hydroxide NF used to adjust pH.

HOW SUPPLIED

Dilor® Tablets are supplied as follows:
NDC 0281-1115-53 Bottle of 100
NDC 0281-1115-57 Bottle of 1000
NDC 0281-1115-63 Unit dose, Box of 100
Dilor®-400 Tablets are supplied as follows:
NDC 0281-1116-53 Bottle of 100
NDC 0281-1116-57 Bottle of 1000
NDC 0281-1116-63 Unit dose box of 100
Dilor® Elixir (dyphylline elixir USP) 160 mg/15 mL, is available as follows: NDC 0281-1118-74 Pint
Dilor® Injection (dyphylline injection USP) 250 mg/mL is supplied as follows:
NDC 0281-1112-31 Box of 6 × 2 mL ampules

DILOR-G® ℞
(Dyphylline and Guaifenesin tablets USP)

DESCRIPTION

Each round, pink scored tablet contains dyphylline USP 200 mg and guaifenesin USP 200 mg and the following inactive ingredients: colloidal silicon dioxide, corn starch, food starch, povidone, stearic acid and artificial coloring.

Dilor-G® Liquid
Each teaspoon (5 mL) contains dyphylline USP 100 mg and guaifenesin USP 100 mg in a pale-pink, mint flavored base containing: citric acid, glycerin, saccharin sodium, sorbitol, sucrose, artificial coloring and flavoring, purified water, and sodium hydroxide to adjust pH. Methylparaben and propylparaben added as preservatives.

HOW SUPPLIED

Dilor-G® Tablets are supplied as follows:
NDC 0281-1124-53, Bottle of 100.
NDC 0281-1124-57, Bottle of 1000.
NDC 0281-1124-63, Unit dose, Box of 100.
Dilor-G® Liquid
NDC 0281-1127-74, Pint.

ETHIODOL® ℞
BRAND OF ETHIODIZED OIL INJECTION
A Low Viscosity Radio-Opaque Diagnostic Agent

NOT FOR INTRAVASCULAR, INTRATHECAL OR INTRABRONCHIAL USE

DESCRIPTION

Ethiodol, brand of ethiodized oil, is a sterile injectable radio-opaque diagnostic agent for use in hysterosalpingography and lymphography. It contains 37% iodine (475 mg/mL) organically combined with ethyl esters of the fatty acids (primarily as ethyl monoiodostearate and ethyl diiodostearate) of poppyseed oil. Stabilized with poppyseed oil, 1%. The precise structure of Ethiodol is unknown at this time. Ethiodol is a straw to amber colored, oily fluid, which because of simplified molecular structure, possesses a greatly reduced viscosity (1.280 specific gravity at 15°C yields viscosity of 0.5–1.0 poise). This high fluidity provides a new flexibility for radiographic exploration.

CLINICAL PHARMACOLOGY

There has been little detailed investigation of the metabolic fate of Ethiodol in either man or animals. However, the fate of Ethiodol following lymphangiography in dogs has been reported.[1] Koehler et al. employed I^{131}-tagged Ethiodol for lymphangiography in dogs and analyses of individual organs at various time intervals were done. The investigators reported an average of only 25% of the injected medium was retained in the lymphatics at the end of three days. An average of 50% was recovered from the lungs. They found the remainder of injected activity was fairly uniformly distributed throughout the body. Urinary excretion in the form of inorganic iodine was revealed as the chief mode of iodine loss from the system.

INDICATIONS

Ethiodol is indicated for use as a radio-opaque medium for hysterosalpingography and lymphography.

IN HYSTEROSALPINGOGRAPHY

CONTRAINDICATIONS

Ethiodol is contraindicated in patients hypersensitive to it. Ethiodol should not be injected intrathecally or intravascularly, or used in bronchography. A history of sensitivity to iodine contraindicates the use of Ethiodol; iodine is split off from fatty compounds and becomes free iodine in the body. Hysterosalpingography is contraindicated in intrauterine pregnancy, acute pelvic inflammatory disease, marked cervical erosion, endocervicitis in the presence of intrauterine bleeding, in the immediate pre-or postmenstrual phase, or within 30 days of curettage or conization.

WARNINGS

Ethiodol is not intended for use in bronchography and, therefore, is not to be introduced into the bronchial tree. A history of sensitivity to iodine or to other contrast materials is not an absolute contraindication to Ethiodol, but calls for extreme caution. All procedures utilizing contrast media carry a definite risk of adverse reactions. While most reactions are minor, life threatening and fatal reactions may occur without warning. The risk/benefit factor should always be carefully evaluated. At all times a fully equipped emergency cart and resuscitation equipment should be readily available, and personnel competent in recognizing and treating reactions of all severity should be on hand.

PRECAUTIONS

General: Since iodine-containing contrast materials may alter the results of certain thyroid function tests, such tests, if indicated, should be performed prior to the administration of this drug. Pulmonary embolization of the contrast material may occur if hysterosalpingography is performed under conditions which may lead to intravasation of the contrast materials. These conditions include uterine bleeding, recent curettage or conization and injection of the contrast material under excessive pressure.
Carcinogenesis, Mutagenesis, and Impairment of Fertility: Long-term studies in animals have not been performed to evaluate carcinogenic potential, mutagenesis, or whether Ethiodol can affect fertility in males or females.
Pregnancy Category C: Animal reproduction studies have not been conducted with Ethiodol. It is also not known whether Ethiodol can cause fetal harm when administered to a pregnant woman or can affect reproduction capacity. Ethiodol should be administered to a pregnant woman only if clearly needed.
Nursing Mothers: It is not known whether this drug is excreted in human milk. Because many drugs are excreted in human milk and because of the potential for serious adverse reactions in nursing infants from Ethiodol, a decision should be made whether to discontinue nursing or to discontinue the drug, taking into account the importance of the drug to the mother.

ADVERSE REACTIONS

Hypersensitivity reactions, foreign body reactions and exacerbation of pelvic inflammatory disease, although infrequent, have been reported. In an occasional patient, abdominal pains may occur. Such pains may be the result of tubal torsion, or possibly due to too rapid a rate of instillation or excessive pressure, or both. The condition is usually only transitory, lasting one or two hours at most, and may be relieved by the administration of any of the commonly used analgesics.

DOSAGE AND ADMINISTRATION

The hysterosalpingogram is preferably taken during the patient's preovulatory phase (as determined from her basal body temperature record) and not less than two days after cessation of her menstrual flow. It has been frequently observed that some bleeding will occur during or after the onset of pregnancy which cannot be distinguished by the patient from a normal menstrual period. In such cases a basal body temperature record will reveal a sustained high temperature phase, and thus enable an operator to avoid hysterosalpingography when a pregnancy may exist. Salpingography should not be performed if the blood is exuding from the cervical os (which occasionally occurs without the patient being aware of it) or if any gross evidence of endocervicitis exists.
Careful aseptic technique should be employed as for any operative procedure in which the uterus is entered. A self-retaining cannula should be used thereby permitting removal of the vaginal speculum so that the outline of the cervical canal may be seen in the film. The use of a radio-opaque aluminum speculum may be employed in patients where a lacerated or patulous cervix does not permit the use of a retaining cannula.
The radio-opaque agent is introduced under pressure and preferably with fluoroscopic control. A preliminary film is exposed and a skiagram is made after the injection of 5 mL of the agent. The pressure is raised to 80–90 mm Hg. In cases of normal bilateral tubal patency, the pressure falls immediately to below 60 mm Hg. The wet film may be viewed immediately and if both tubes are seen to "fill", the apparatus is removed and the procedure is finished, except for the 24 hour follow-up to establish whether or not "spill" into the peritoneal cavity has occurred.
Increments of 2 mL of the agent are injected and successive films exposed until tubal patency is established or until the patient's limit of tolerance to discomfort is reached. Few patients will complain of discomfort at pressures under 200 mm Hg.

IN LYMPHOGRAPHY

CONTRAINDICATIONS

Ethiodol is contraindicated in patients hypersensitive to it. Ethiodol should not be injected intrathecally or intravascu-

larly or introduced into the bronchial tree. Patients with known sensitivity to iodine should not have lymphography performed. Iodine is split off from fatty compounds and becomes free iodine in the body. Lymphography is contraindicated in patients with a right to left cardiac shunt, in patients with advanced pulmonary disease, especially those with alveolar-capillary block, and in patients who have had radiotherapy to the lungs.

WARNINGS

The use of intralymphatic Ethiodol presents a significant hazard in patients with pre-existing pulmonary disease characterized by a decrease in pulmonary diffusing capacity and/or pulmonary blood flow. A few fatalities have been noted in such patients. With reference to this potential complication, recent studies indicate a significant decrease in both pulmonary diffusing capacity and pulmonary capillary blood flow following Ethiodol lymphography without appreciable concomitant clinical manifestations. Also, care should be exercised in patients with other types of pulmonary disease in view of the more frequent incidence of overt pulmonary complications such as pulmonary infarction, in these groups. However, it is to be noted that pulmonary infarction, although rare, has occurred in patients without evidence of pre-existing pulmonary disease.

The safety of intralymphatic Ethiodol has not been established in pregnant women, and accordingly, its use should be restricted to such situations where it is deemed necessary.

PRECAUTIONS

General: Although subclinical pulmonary embolization occurs in a majority of patients following Ethiodol lymphography, clinical evidence of such embolization is infrequent and is usually of a transient nature. Such clinical manifestations are usually immediate, but may be delayed from a few hours to days. It would appear that it is advantageous to use the smallest volume of Ethiodol necessary for radiographic visualization. For this reason, and to prevent inadvertent venous administration, radiographic monitoring of patients is recommended during the injection of Ethiodol.

The timing and choice of anesthesia following Ethiodol injection may be influenced by consideration of the above noted decrease in pulmonary and capillary blood flow and diffusing capacity. It should be noted that although an average of 2 to 3 days was required for complete reversibility for such tests, an occasional patient required up to 12 days to return to baseline values.

PBI determination of thyroid uptake studies should be carried out prior to the lymphographic procedure because interference with these tests may be anticipated for as long as one year. In the presence of known iodine sensitivity, Ethiodol lymphography should be carried out with greatest precaution.

Carcinogenesis, Mutagenesis, and Impairment of Fertility: Long-term studies in animals have not been performed to evaluate carcinogenic potential, mutagenesis, or whether Ethiodol can affect fertility in males or females.

Pregnancy Category C: Animal reproduction studies have not been conducted with Ethiodol. It is also not known whether Ethiodol can cause fetal harm when administered to a pregnant woman or can affect reproduction capacity. Ethiodol should be administered to a pregnant woman only if clearly needed.

Nursing Mothers: It is not known whether this drug is excreted in human milk. Because many drugs are excreted in human milk and because of the potential for serious adverse reactions in nursing infants from Ethiodol, a decision should be made whether to discontinue nursing or to discontinue the drug, taking into account the importance of the drug to the mother.

ADVERSE REACTIONS

The occasional observation of pulmonary Ethiodol embolization (infarction) several hours after injection has been reported. This was noticed more frequently when excessive amounts of Ethiodol have been injected, in the presence of marked lymphatic obstruction or through accidental intravenous injection. Radiologic manifestations are fine, granular stippling throughout both lung fields. The clinical symptoms usually noted have been mild, consisting of moderate temperature elevation, dyspnea, and cough. However, severe acute symptoms developed in two patients both of whom were severely ill and required extensive care.[2] Fuchs[3] experienced 1 severe and 3 minor complications in a series of 20 bilateral procedures. Two are described by the author as cardiovascular collapse occurring at two hours respectively following the completion of the procedure. It was postulated that minute emboli may have been causative. Recovery was rapid and complete in both instances.

The occurrence of pulmonary invasion may be minimized if radiographic confirmation of intralymphatic (rather than venous) injection is secured, and the procedure discontinued when the medium becomes visible in the thoracic duct or the presence of lymphatic obstruction is noticed.

While rare, other side effects reported include transient fever, lymphangitis, iodism (headache, soreness of mouth and pharynx, coryza and skin rash), allergic dermatitis, and lipogranuloma formation. Delayed wound healing at the site of incision and secondary infection are occasionally seen, and can be prevented or minimized by adhering to a strict sterile technique.

Transient edema or temporary exacerbation of preexisting lymphedema, as well as thrombophlebitis have also been reported. In the extremely rare presence of concomitant lymphatic and inferior vena cava obstruction the contrast medium may be shunted partially to the liver, resulting in hepatic embolization. Also, when accidental intravenous administration of Ethiodol results in a considerable amount of this medium entering the circulation, embolization other than pulmonary may occur as reported in 2 cases.[4] Both cases developed a transient, psychotic-like manifestation, which in all probability stemmed from the entrance of fine oil droplets into the cerebral circulation. Recovery was uneventful and complete without evidence of neurological sequelae.

DOSAGE AND ADMINISTRATION

This method applies for both the upper and lower extremities. A lymphatic vessel is selected for cannulization.

The patient should be comfortably arranged in a supine position on a portable stretcher or an x-ray table. When available, a radiolucent pad will add to the patient's comfort during the one to two hours required for completion of the examination. It is important that the patient be in a cooperative state. Premedication might be advisable in the unusually apprehensive patient.

In the unusually restless patient, the extremities should be immobilized during the entire procedure to prevent displacement of the needle. Thomas splints have been satisfactorily employed for the legs and simple arm boards for the upper extremities. The cut-down and injection instruments and materials include the following:

Sterile pediatric cut-down set
Sterile towels for draping, sponges, etc.
Local anesthetic, such as procaine hydrochloride, and a syringe
Bactericidal painting solution
20 mL syringe containing 15 mL of Ethiodol with an 18 inch catheter to which is affixed a 27 or 30 gauge needle. (If bilateral lymphography is scheduled, two syringes should be prepared.)
A manually driven or motorized unit (a pressure regulated pump) to provide for slow injection.

Under local infiltration anesthesia, a transverse, curvilinear or longitudinal small skin incision should be made near the ankle or wrist (just lateral and distal to the first metatarsal head on the dorsum of the foot, or just over the "snuffbox" in the dorsum of the hand).

Upon superficial dissection (but not penetrating the subcutaneous layer of tissue) lymph vessels will be noted in the immediate subcutaneous tissue, while larger lymph vessel trunks are found in the extrafascial plane. The deeper lymph trunks will be easier to cannulate.

One lymph vessel is then exposed, avoiding circumferential dissection. The less manipulation performed, the better the results that will be obtained. The lymphatic, thus isolated, is then cannulated with a 27 or 30 gauge 5/8 inch needle, depending upon the size of the lymphatic selected for injection. It is rarely possible to cannulate with a needle greater than 27 gauge. Insertion of the needle through the skin flap before cannulating the lymphatic serves to reduce the movement of the needle within the vessel. Additional security of the needle in the lymphatic is obtained by strapping, with sterile tape, the polyethylene tubing to the patient's foot.

The injection should be started at a slow rate, i.e., 0.1 mL to 0.2 mL per minute. Radiographic monitoring either by fluoroscopy or serial radiographs after 1 mL to 2 mL has been injected, will confirm the proper intralymphatic placement of the needle, rule out accidental intravenous injection or extravasation of the medium by perforation or rupture of the lymphatic. Monitoring will also permit prompt termination of the procedure in the event that lymphatic blockage is present. In such situations, continuation of the injection will result in unnecessary introduction of contrast material in the venous system via the lymphovenous communication channels. If the injection is satisfactory, approximately 6 to 8 mL, are then injected. However, as soon as it becomes radiographically evident that Ethiodol has entered the thoracic duct, the procedure should be terminated to minimize entry of the contrast material into the subclavian vein. Two to four mL of Ethiodol injected into the upper extremity will suffice to demonstrate the axillary and supraclavicular nodes. In penile lymphography approximately 2 to 3 mL of Ethiodol is required. In infants and children, a minimum of 1 mL to a maximum of 6 mL should be employed.

The rate of speed at which the contrast material may be introduced varies and is dependent upon receptivity of the lymphatics in the individual patient. If the injection is proceeding at too rapid a rate, extravasation will be noted and the patient may refer to pain in the foot, leg or arm.

At the completion of the injection, anteroposterior roentgenograms are obtained of the legs or arms, thighs, pelvis, abdomen and chest (dorsal spine technique). Lateral or oblique views as well as laminograms are obtained when indicated. Follow-up films at 24 or 48 hours provide better demonstration of lymph nodes and permit more concise evaluation of nodal architecture.

As a general rule, the smallest possible amount of Ethiodol should be employed according to the anatomical area to be visualized. Therefore, and to prevent inadvertent venous administration, fluoroscopic monitoring or serial radiographic guidance of patients is recommended during the injection of Ethiodol.

Average dose in the adult patient for unilateral lymphography of the upper extremities is 2 to 4 mL; of lower extremities, 6 to 8 mL; of penile lymphography, 2 to 3 mL; of cervical lymphography, 1 to 2 mL.

In the pediatric patient, a minimum of 1 mL to a maximum of 6 mL may be employed according to the anatomical area to be visualized.

SUMMARY OF STEPS TO AVOID COMPLICATIONS IN LYMPHOGRAPHY[5]

1. Contraindicate patients:
   A. With a known hypersensitivity to Ethiodol
   B. With a right to left cardiac shunt
   C. With advanced pulmonary disease, especially those with alveolar-capillary block. Pulmonary gas diffusion studies should be done if in doubt.
   D. Who have had radiation therapy to the lungs
2. Proceed with caution:
   A. Patients having markedly advanced neoplastic disease with expected lymphatic obstruction.
   B. Patients having undergone previous surgery interrupting the lymphatic system.
   C. Patients having had deep radiation therapy to the examined area.
   If in those cases in which extreme caution should be exercised, lymphography is still necessary, a smaller dose of oily contrast medium with protracted injection time with less pressure and careful monitoring is required.
3. Skin testing should be done on all patients before submitting them to lymphography. Be aware of possible hypersensitivity to local anesthetics and skin disinfectants. Careful history taking is important.
4. Technique of cannulation: extravasation is to be avoided and/or detected early. The injection site should be included on the "scout film" or observed under image amplification fluoroscopy. The needle tip must remain visible in the incision wound.
5. Oily contrast materials: once opened, ampules should be discarded. Ampules of Ethiodol should not be used if the color has darkened or if particulate matter is present. The average dose for each foot in an adult is 5 to 6 mL; one-half as much for the upper extremity. The amount for children should be determined by careful monitoring. It should stay below 0.25 mL/kg.
6. Injection pressure should be regulated to deliver the average dose in no less than 11/4 hours. Continuous monitoring helps to determine the speed most appropriate for each individual. Sensation of pain is a warning of too high pressure.
7. Scout roentgenograms: if scout roentgenograms are used for monitoring, they should be developed and viewed immediately in order to apply corrective measures when needed; e.g., discontinuation of the study when one sees intravenous injection or lymphatico-venous anastomosis. Reduction of injection speed is needed if evidence of collateral circulation occurs or if the higher abdomino-aortic nodes do not opacify in spite of the usual injection pressure. This is highly suggestive of lymphatic obstruction. Scout roentgenograms should be taken more frequently in such cases.
8. Surgical technique: strict aseptic surgical technique is followed including the wearing of a face mask. Before suturing the incision wound, the remnants of the lymphatic vessels and loose tissue are removed and the wound well washed with saline to remove any possible oil. In case of reflux type lymphedema, the cannulated large lymphatic vessel may have to be closed by catgut to avoid development of a lymphocyst.

The patient is instructed to elevate the legs as often as possible to promote healing. The sutures are removed from the feet on the 10th day, and on the 5th or 6th from the hands.

HOW SUPPLIED

Ethiodol (ethiodized oil for injection) is supplied in a box of two 10 ml ampules, NDC 0281-7062-37.

Store at controlled room temperature 15°–30°C (59°–86°F). Protect from light. Remove from carton only upon use.

Parenteral drug products should be inspected visually for particulate matter and discoloration prior to administration, whenever solution and container permit. Ethiodol brand of ethiodized oil for injection is straw to amber color under normal conditions. (See **DESCRIPTION**).

Continued on next page

Ethiodol—Cont.

Caution: Federal law prohibits dispensing without prescription.

A development of Guerbet Laboratories.

BIBLIOGRAPHY
1. P. Ruben Koehler, M.D. et al.: "Body Distribution of Ethiodol Following Lymphangiography", Radiology, 1964, 82, 5 866-871.
2. Bronk, et. al.: "Oil Embolism in Lymphography", Radiation, 80:194, February 1963.
3. Fuchs, S.A., "Complications in Lymphography With Oily Contrast Media", Acta Radiol., 57:247, November 1962.
4. Viamonte, M. Jr., University of Miami, Jackson Memorial Hospital, Miami, Florida, Private Communication.
5. Kuisk, H., "Techniques of Lymphography and Principles of Interpretation", 1971, Warren H. Green, Inc., St. Louis, Missouri, 63105.

SAVAGE LABORATORIES®
a division of Altana Inc.
MELVILLE, NEW YORK 11747

IF77062D
#45
R4/98

EVAC-Q-KWIK®
OTC

DESCRIPTION
A bowel evacuant system comprised of three separate products that are intended to be administered sequentially at intervals intended to minimize the overlap of pharmacological activity.

Evac-Q-Mag® - (saline cathartic)
Electrolyte content of 250 mEq of magnesium, 21 mEq of potassium, and .95 mEq of sodium.

Evac-Q-Tabs® - (oral stimulant laxative)
Active Ingredient: each tablet contains Bisacodyl 5 mg.
Inactive Ingredients: Lactose anhydrous, magnesium stearate, stearic acid, sodium starch glycolate, microcrystalline cellulose, silicone dioxide colloidal, acacia, gelatin, pharmaceutical glaze, polyvinyl acetate phthalate, D&C yellow #10, FD&C yellow #6, corn starch, calcium sulfate, sugar, talc, titanium dioxide, beewax, carnauba wax, and other coating ingredients.

Evac-Q-Kwik® suppository -
Each suppository containing 10 mg of bisacodyl.

To promote the flushing of the G.I. tract. Together the products and the liquid comprise the bowel evacuant system.

HOW SUPPLIED
(NDC 0281-0297-76) Evac-Q-Kwik Kit

ILOPAN® INJECTION
Rx
(Dexpanthenol Preparation USP)

DESCRIPTION
ILOPAN® INJECTION contains dexpanthenol preparation USP (a mixture of dexpanthenol and pantolactone). Dexpanthenol is a derivative of pantothenic acid, a B complex vitamin. ILOPAN® INJECTION is a sterile aqueous solution indicated for use as a gastrointestinal stimulant.

HOW SUPPLIED
ILOPAN® INJECTION is available as follows:
NDC 0281-0306-95 2 mL Ampuls, Box of 25

MYTREX®
Rx
(Nystatin and Triamcinolone Acetonide Cream USP and Ointment USP)

DESCRIPTION
Each gram of MYTREX® Cream USP contains 100,000 USP Nystatin Units and 1 mg of triamcinolone acetonide in a cream base containing polyoxyethylene fatty alcohol ether, white petrolatum, glyceryl monostearate, polyethylene glycol 400 monostearate, sorbitol solution, simethicone emulsion, propylene glycol, aluminum hydroxide gel, polysorbate 60, titanium dioxide, and purified water. Hydrochloric acid or sodium hydroxide to adjust pH.
Each gram of MYTREX® Ointment contains 100,000 USP Nystatin Units and 1 mg of triamcinolone acetonide in a base of polyethylene and mineral oil.

HOW SUPPLIED
MYTREX® Cream
NDC 0281-0081-08 12 × 1.5 gram foilpac
NDC 0281-0081-15 15 gram tube
NDC 0281-0081-30 30 gram tube
NDC 0281-0081-60 60 gram tube

MYTREX® Ointment
NDC 0281-0089-15 15 gram tube
NDC 0281-0089-30 30 gram tube

NITROL® OINTMENT
Rx
(Nitroglycerin 2% Ointment)

DESCRIPTION
Nitroglycerin is 1,2,3 propanetriol trinitrate, an organic nitrate, whose structural nitrate formula is:

$$CH_2-ONO_2$$
$$CH-ONO_2$$
$$CH_2-ONO_2$$

and whose molecular weight is 227.09. The organic nitrates are vasodilators, active on both arteries and veins.
Nitrol® Ointment contains lactose and 2% nitroglycerin in a base of lanolin, white petrolatum and purified water. Each inch (2.5 cm), as squeezed from the tube, contains approximately 15 mg of nitroglycerin.

HOW SUPPLIED
NITROL® Ointment is supplied as follows. Package includes a supply of ruled applicators for convenient application.

60 gram tube - NDC 0281-0038-56

PANDEL®
Rx
(hydrocortisone probutate cream)
Cream, 0.1%

For Dermatologic Use Only
Not for Ophthalmic Use
DESCRIPTION
Pandel Cream contains hydrocortisone probutate, a synthetic adrenocorticosteroid, for dermatologic use. The topical corticosteroids constitute a class of primarily synthetic steroids used as anti-inflammatory and anti-pruritic agents. Hydrocortisone probutate is a tasteless and odorless white crystalline powder practically insoluble in hexane or water, slightly soluble in ether, and very soluble in dichloromethane, methanol and acetone. Chemically, it is 11β,17,21-trihydroxypregn-4-ene-3,20-dione 17-butyrate 21-propionate. The structural formula is:

Molecular Formula: $C_{28}H_{40}O_7$
M.W. = 488.62

Each gram of Pandel (hydrocortisone probutate cream) Cream, 0.1% contains: 1 mg of hydrocortisone probutate in a cream base of propylene glycol, white petrolatum, light mineral oil, stearyl alcohol, polysorbate 60, sorbitan monostearate, glyceryl monostearate, PEG-20 stearate, glyceryl stearate SE, methylparaben, butylparaben, citric acid, sodium citrate anhydrous, and purified water.

CLINICAL PHARMACOLOGY
Topical corticosteroids share anti-inflammatory, anti-pruritic and vasoconstrictive actions. The mechanism of anti-inflammatory activity of the topical corticosteroids is unclear. However, corticosteroids are thought to act by the induction of phospholipase A_2 inhibitory proteins, collectively called lipocortins. It is postulated that these proteins control the biosynthesis of potent mediators of inflammation such as prostaglandins and leukotrienes by inhibiting the release of their common precursor arachidonic acid. Arachidonic acid is released from membrane phospholipids by phospholipase A_2.

Pharmacokinetics: The extent of percutaneous absorption of topical corticosteroids is determined by many factors, including the vehicle and the integrity of the epidermal barrier. Use of occlusive dressings with hydrocortisone for up to 24 hours has not been shown to increase penetration; however, occlusion of hydrocortisone for 96 hours does markedly enhance penetration. Topical corticosteroids can be absorbed from normal intact skin. Inflammation and/or other disease processes in the skin increase percutaneous absorption.
Studies performed with Pandel (hydrocortisone probutate cream) Cream, 0.1% indicate that it is in the medium range of potency compared with other topical corticosteroids.

INDICATIONS AND USAGE
Pandel (hydrocortisone probutate cream) Cream, 0.1% is a medium potency corticosteroid indicated for the relief of the inflammatory and pruritic manifestations of corticosteroid-responsive dermatoses in patients 18 years of age or older.

CONTRAINDICATIONS
Pandel (hydrocortisone probutate cream) Cream, 0.1% is contraindicated in those patients who are hypersensitive to hydrocortisone probutate or to any of the components of the preparation.

PRECAUTIONS
General: Systemic absorption of topical corticosteroids can produce reversible hypothalamic-pituitary-adrenal (HPA) axis suppression with the potential for glucocorticosteroid insufficiency after withdrawal of treatment. Manifestations of Cushing's syndrome, hyperglycemia, and glucosuria can also be produced in some patients by systemic absorption of topical corticosteroids while on treatment.
Patients applying a topical steroid to a large surface area or to areas under occlusion should be evaluated periodically for evidence of HPA-axis suppression. This may be done by using the ACTH stimulation, A.M. plasma cortisol or urinary free cortisol tests.
If HPA axis suppression is noted, an attempt should be made to withdraw the drug, to reduce the frequency of application, or to substitute a less potent steroid. Recovery of HPA axis function is generally prompt and complete upon discontinuation of the drug. Infrequently, signs and symptoms of steroid withdrawal may occur, requiring supplemental systemic corticosteroids. For information on systemic supplementation, see prescribing information for those products.
Pediatric patients may be more susceptible to systemic toxicity from equivalent doses due to their larger skin surface to body mass ratios. (See **PRECAUTIONS-Pediatric Use**).
If irritation develops, Pandel (hydrocortisone probutate cream) Cream, 0.1% should be discontinued and appropriate therapy instituted. Allergic contact dermatitis with corticosteroids is usually diagnosed by observing a failure to heal rather than noting a clinical exacerbation, as observed with most topical products not containing corticosteroids.
If concomitant skin infections are present or develop, an appropriate antifungal or antibacterial agent should be used. If a favorable response does not occur promptly, use of Pandel (hydrocortisone probutate cream) Cream, 0.1% should be discontinued until the infection has been adequately controlled.

Information for Patients: Patients using Pandel (hydrocortisone probutate cream) Cream, 0.1% should receive the following information and instructions:
1. This medication is to be used as directed by the physician. It is for external use only. Avoid contact with the eyes.
2. This medication should not be used for any disorder other than that for which it was prescribed.
3. The treated skin area should not be bandaged or otherwise covered or wrapped so as to be occlusive, unless directed by the physician.
4. Patients should report to their physician any signs of local adverse reactions.
5. Parents of pediatric patients should be advised not to use Pandel (hydrocortisone probutate cream) Cream, 0.1% in the treatment of diaper dermatitis. Pandel (hydrocortisone probutate cream) Cream, 0.1% should not be applied in the diaper area as diapers or plastic pants may constitute occlusive dressings (See **DOSAGE AND ADMINISTRATION**).
6. This medication should not be used on the face, underarms, or groin areas unless directed by the physician.
7. As with other corticosteroids, therapy should be discontinued when control is achieved. If no improvement is seen within two weeks, contact the physician.

Laboratory Tests: The following tests may be helpful in evaluating if HPA axis suppression does occur:
ACTH stimulation test
A.M. plasma cortisol test
Urinary free cortisol test
Carcinogenesis, Mutagenesis and Impairment of Fertility: Long-term animal studies have not been performed to evaluate the carcinogenic potential or the effect on fertility of topical corticosteroids.
In two mutagenicity experiments using hydrocortisone probutate, negative responses were observed in the occurrence of micronuclei in the bone marrow of mice and in the Ames reverse mutation test bacterial assay-with and without metabolic activation.
Pregnancy: **Teratogenic Effects** —**Pregnancy Category C.** Corticosteroids have been shown to be teratogenic in laboratory animals when administered systemically at relatively low dosage levels. Some corticosteroids have been shown to be teratogenic after dermal application to laboratory animals.
Hydrocortisone probutate has not been tested for teratogenicity when applied topically; however, it is absorbed percutaneously, and studies in Wistar rats using the subcutaneous route resulted in teratogenicity at dose levels equal to or greater than 1 mg/kg. This dose is approximately 12 times the human average topical dose of Pandel Cream, 0.1% assuming 3% absorption and an application of 30 g/day on a 70 kg individual. Abnormalities seen included delayed ossi-

fication of the caudal vertebrae and other skeletal variations, cleft palate, umbilical hernia, edema, and exencephalia.

In rabbits, hydrocortisone probutate given by the subcutaneous route was teratogenic at doses equal to or greater than 0.1 mg/kg. This dose is approximately 2 times the human average topical dose of Pandel Cream, 0.1% assuming 3% absorption and an application of 30 g/day on a 70 kg individual. Abnormalities seen included delayed ossification of the caudal vertebrae and other skeletal abnormalities, cleft palate and increased fetal mortality.

The differences between the doses used in animal studies and the proposed human dose may not fully predict the human outcome. The animals received a bolus subcutaneous dose, whereas humans receive a dermal application, where absorption is lower and highly dependent on various factors (e.g., vehicle, integrity of epidermal barrier, occlusion).

There are no adequate and well-controlled studies of the teratogenic potential of hydrocortisone probutate in pregnant women. Although human epidemiological studies do not indicate an increased incidence of teratogenicity with the use of topical corticosteroids, Pandel Cream should be used during pregnancy only if the potential benefit justifies the potential risk to the fetus.

Nursing Mothers: Systemically administered corticosteroids appear in human milk and could suppress growth, interfere with endogenous corticosteroid production, or cause other untoward effects. It is not known whether topical administration of corticosteroids could result in sufficient systemic absorption to produce detectable quantities in human milk. Because many drugs are excreted in human milk, caution should be exercised when Pandel (hydrocortisone probutate cream) Cream, 0.1% is administered to a nursing woman.

Pediatric Use: Safety and effectiveness in pediatric patients have not been established. Because of a higher ratio of skin surface area to body mass, pediatric patients are at a greater risk than adults of HPA axis suppression and Cushing's syndrome when they are treated with topical corticosteroids. They are therefore also at a greater risk of adrenal insufficiency during and/or after withdrawal of treatment. Adverse effects including striae have been reported with inappropriate use of topical corticosteroids in infants and children.

Hypothalamic-pituitary-adrenal (HPA) axis suppression, Cushing's syndrome, linear growth retardation, delayed weight gain, and intracranial hypertension have been reported in children receiving topical corticosteroids. Manifestations of adrenal suppression in children include low plasma cortisol levels and an absence of response to ACTH stimulation. Manifestations of intracranial hypertension include bulging fontanelles, headaches, and bilateral papilledema.

ADVERSE REACTIONS

The most frequent adverse reactions reported for Pandel (hydrocortisone probutate cream) Cream, 0.1% have included burning in 4, stinging in 2, and moderate paresthesia in 1 out of 226 patients.

The following local adverse reactions are reported with topical corticosteroids, and they may occur more frequently with the use of occlusive dressings. These reactions are listed in an approximate decreasing order of occurrence: burning, itching, irritation, dryness, folliculitis, hypertrichosis, acneiform eruptions, hypopigmentation, perioral dermatitis, allergic contact dermatitis, secondary infections, skin atrophy, striae, miliaria.

OVERDOSAGE

Topically applied corticosteroids can be absorbed in sufficient amounts to produce systemic effects. (See **PRECAUTIONS**).

DOSAGE AND ADMINISTRATION

Apply a thin film of Pandel (hydrocortisone probutate cream) Cream, 0.1% to the affected area once or twice a day depending on the severity of the condition. Massage gently until the medication disappears.

Occlusive dressings may be used for the management of refractory lesions of psoriasis and other deep-seated dermatoses, such as localized neurodermatitis (lichen simplex chronicus).

As with other corticosteroids, therapy should be discontinued when control is achieved. If no improvement is seen within 2 weeks, reassessment of the diagnosis may be necessary. Pandel (hydrocortisone probutate cream) Cream, 0.1% should not be used with occlusive dressings unless directed by the physician. Pandel (hydrocortisone probutate cream) Cream, 0.1% should not be applied in the diaper area, as diapers or plastic pants may constitute occlusive dressings.

HOW SUPPLIED

Pandel (hydrocortisone probutate cream) Cream, 0.1%, a white to off-white opaque cream is supplied as follows:
15 g tubes (NDC 0281-0153-15)
45 g tubes (NDC 0281-0153-46)
80 g tubes (NDC 0281-0153-80)

Store at controlled room temperature 15°-30°C (59°-86°F).

CAUTION: Federal law prohibits dispensing without prescription.

SAVAGE LABORATORIES® I7153B / IF7153B
a division of Altana Inc. #104
MELVILLE, NEW YORK 11747 R1/98

Shown in Product Identification Guide, page 336

TYMPAGESIC® ℞
(Analgesic-Decongestant Ear Drops)

DESCRIPTION

TYMPAGESIC® Otic Solution, analgesic-decongestant ear drops, contains phenylephrine hydrochloride USP 0.25%, antipyrine USP 5%, benzocaine USP 5%, sodium metabisulfite and edetate disodium USP in propylene glycol USP.

HOW SUPPLIED

TYMPAGESIC® Otic Solution is supplied as follows:
13 mL amber glass bottle with dropper
NDC 0281-7363-39

Scandipharm, Inc.
22 INVERNESS CENTER PARKWAY
BIRMINGHAM, AL 35242

Direct Inquiries to:
Customer Services
(800) 950-8085
Fax: (205) 991-8426

For Medical Information Contact:
John R. Booth, R.Ph.
(205) 991-8085
Fax: (205) 991-9547

ULTRASE® ℞
[*ul 'trāce*]
(pancrelipase) Capsules
Enteric-Coated Microspheres

Prescribing Information

DESCRIPTION

ULTRASE® (pancrelipase) Capsules are orally administered capsules containing enteric-coated microspheres of porcine pancreatic enzyme concentrate, predominantly pancreatic lipase, amylase, and protease.

Each ULTRASE ® capsule contains:

Lipase	4,500 U.S.P. Units
Amylase	20,000 U.S.P. Units
Protease	25,000 U.S.P. Units

Inactive ingredients: povidone, talc, sugar, methacrylic acid copolymer (Type C), triethyl citrate, simethicone emulsion.

CLINICAL PHARMACOLOGY

ULTRASE® (pancrelipase) Capsules are designed to prevent inactivation by gastric acid thereby resulting in the delivery of high levels of biologically active enzymes into the duodenum. The enzymes catalyze the hydrolysis of fats into glycerol and fatty acids, starch into dextrins and sugars, and protein into proteoses and derived substances.

INDICATIONS AND USAGE

ULTRASE® (pancrelipase) Capsules are indicated for patients with partial or complete exocrine pancreatic insufficiency caused by:

- Cystic fibrosis
- Chronic pancreatitis due to alcohol use or other causes
- Surgery (pancreatico-duodenectomy or Whipple's procedure, with or without Wirsung duct injection, total pancreatectomy)
- Obstruction (pancreatic and biliary duct lithiasis, pancreatic and duodenal neoplasms, ductal stenosis)
- Other pancreatic disease (hereditary, post traumatic and allograft pancreatitis, hemochromatosis, Schwachman's Syndrome, lipomatosis, hyperparathyroidism)
- Poor mixing (Billroth II gastrectomy, other types of gastric bypass surgery, gastrinoma)

Pancrelipase capsules are effective in controlling steatorrhea.[1–9]

CONTRAINDICATIONS

Pancrelipase capsules are contraindicated in patients known to be hypersensitive to pork protein. Pancrelipase capsules are contraindicated in patients with acute pancreatitis or with acute exacerbations of chronic pancreatic diseases.

WARNINGS

Should hypersensitivity occur, discontinue medication and treat symptomatically.

PRECAUTIONS

General

TO PROTECT ENTERIC COATING, MICROSPHERES MUST NOT BE CRUSHED OR CHEWED. Where swallowing of capsules is difficult, they may be opened and the microspheres added to a small quantity of a soft food (e.g. applesauce, gelatin, etc.) that does not require chewing, and swallowed immediately. Contact of the microsphere with foods having a pH greater than 5.5 can dissolve the protective enteric shell.

Carcinogenesis, Mutagenesis, Impairment of Fertility

Long-term studies in animals have not been performed to evaluate carcinogenic potential. Methacrylic acid, a minor component of the methacrylic acid copolymer enteric-coating contained in ULTRASE® (pancrelipase) Capsules, has been reported to act as a teratogen in rat embryo cultures. However, the copolymer enteric-coating of ULTRASE® (pancrelipase) Capsules was not mutagenic by the Ames test, and it did not produce chromosome damage in a test for unscheduled DNA synthesis in rat hepatocytes.

Pregnancy : Category C.

Animal reproduction studies have not been conducted with ULTRASE® (pancrelipase) Capsules. It is not known whether ULTRASE® (pancrelipase) Capsules can cause fetal harm when administered to a pregnant woman or can affect reproduction capacity. ULTRASE® (pancrelipase) Capsules should be given to a pregnant woman only if the potential benefit outweighs the potential risk to the fetus.

Nursing Mothers

It is not known whether ULTRASE® (pancrelipase) is excreted in human milk. Because many drugs are excreted in human milk, caution should be exercised when ULTRASE® (pancrelipase) Capsules are administered to a nursing mother.

ADVERSE REACTIONS

The most frequently reported adverse reactions to products containing pancrelipase are gastrointestinal in nature. Less frequently, allergic-type reactions have also been observed. Extremely high doses of exogenous pancreatic enzymes have been associated with hyperuricosuria and hyperuricemia when the preparations given were pancrelipase in powdered or capsule form, or pancreatin in tablet form.

Colonic strictures have been reported in cystic fibrosis patients treated with both high- and lower-strength enzyme supplements.[10] A causal relationship has not been established. The possibility of bowel stricture should be considered if symptoms suggestive of gastrointestinal obstruction occur. Since impaired fluid secretion may be a factor in the development of intestinal obstruction, care should be taken to maintain adequate hydration, particularly in warm weather.[11]

"Fibrosing colonopathy" is a term used to describe a condition seen in patients with CF who have taken high amounts of pancreatic enzyme supplements (>6,000 lipase U/kg/meal). At its most advanced, this condition leads to colonic strictures.

1. In whom should one consider the diagnosis of fibrosing colonopathy?

a. Patients with cystic fibrosis who have evidence of partial or complete obstruction, bloody diarrhea or chylous ascites.

b. Patients who have two of the following three symptoms:
 abdominal pain
 ongoing diarrhea
 poor weight gain
 ESPECIALLY if they have:
 taken >6,000 lipase U/kg/meal
 age less than twelve years
 history of meconium ileus
 prior intestinal surgery
 history of recurrent DIOS
 "inflammatory bowel disease"[12]

DOSAGE AND ADMINISTRATION

The enzymatic activity of ULTRASE® (pancrelipase) Capsules is expressed in U.S.P. units. The smallest effective dose should be used. Dosage should be adjusted according to the severity of the exocrine pancreatic insufficiency. Begin therapy with one or two capsules with meals or snacks and adjust dosage according to symptoms.

The number of capsules or capsule strength given with meals and/or snacks should be estimated by assessing which dose minimizes steatorrhea and maintains good nutritional status. Dosages should be adjusted according to the response of the patient. Where swallowing of capsules is difficult, they may be opened and the microspheres added to a small quantity of a soft food (e.g. applesauce, gelatin, etc.) that does not require chewing, and swallowed immediately.

Continued on next page

Ultrase—Cont.

It is recommended that the total dose of pancrelipase being ingested for a meal or snack be dispersed equally (with fluids) before, during, and after the meal or snack.

SUGGESTION FOR THE USE OF PANCREATIC ENZYMES IN CYSTIC FIBROSIS [12]

1. Patients should be receiving optimal diet for age and clinical status, recognizing that those with failure to thrive or malnutrition require additional calories and other nutrients for catch-up growth.
2. Nutrition assessment should be a part of routine clinical evaluations.
3. Initial dosing of pancreatic enzyme supplements should begin with 500 lipase U/kg/meal using enteric-coated microcapsule products.
4. Patients should be reassessed 2–4 weeks after initiation of therapy. The following items should be assessed:
   Clinical status, e.g. abdominal symptoms and exam
   Nutritional intake and growth (height, weight, head circumference)
   Character of stools—greasy, oily (for information, not for decision making)
   Quantitative 72-hr fecal fat when indicated (perform on a normal diet for age)
   Fat soluble vitamin measures.
5. Corollaries to dosing suggestions:
   a. Dose may be increased in a stepwise fashion.
   b. Dose approaching 2,000 lipase U/kg/meal would indicate the need for further investigation (see below). Patients presently on higher doses should be reevaluated; either immediately decrease the dose or titrate down to a lower dose range at, or below, 2,000 lipase U/kg/meal. Doses >6,000 lipase U/kg/meal have been associated with colonic strictures.
   c. Pancreatic supplements mixed with applesauce or other acidic food substances should be administered immediately, not stored.
   d. Enteric-coated microcapsules should not be crushed.
   e. Enzyme doses (as lipase U/kg/meal) tend to decrease with advancing age.
   f. Patients should accept only product brands prescribed by CF Center staff.
   g. Adjustment of dosage is the responsibility of the CF Center staff. Patients should be advised not to adjust doses without consulting the CF Center staff. Changes in product may require an adjustment period.
   h. Complaints transmitted by phone should be investigated before dose is adjusted.
   i. Pancreatic supplements should be stored in a cool dry place and checked regularly for expiration date.

HOW SUPPLIED

ULTRASE ® (pancrelipase) Capsules

Gelatin capsules (opaque white and opaque white), imprinted "ULTRASE". Bottles of 100 (NDC 58914-045-10).

Store at controlled room temperature, between 15°C and 25°C (59°F and 77°F), in a dry place. Do not refrigerate.

REFERENCES

1. Delchier JC, Vidon N. *et al.* Fate of orally ingested enzymes in pancreatic insufficiency: comparison of two pancreatic enzyme preparations. *Aliment Pharmacol Therap.* 1991;5:365-378.
2. Duhamel JP, Vidailhet M, *et al.* Étude multicentrique comparative d'une nouvelle présentation de pancréatine en microgranules gastrorésistants dans l'insuffisance pancréatique exocrine de la mucoviscidose chez l'enfant. *Ann Pediatr.* 1988;35:69-74.
3. Dutta SK, Tilley DK. The pH-sensitive enteric-coated pancreatic enzyme preparations: an evaluation of therapeutic efficacy in adult patients with pancreatic insufficiency. *J Clin Gastroenterol.* 1983;5:51-54.
4. Dutta SK, Rubin J. Harvey J. Comparative evaluation of the therapeutic efficacy of a pH-sensitive enteric-coated pancreatic enzyme preparation with conventional pancreatic enzyme therapy in the treatment of exocrine pancreatic insufficiency. *Gastroenterol.* 1983;84: 476-482.
5. Gouerou H, Dain MP, *et al.* Alipase versus nonenteric-coated enzymes in pancreatic insufficiency. *Int J Pancreatol.* 1989;5:45-50.
6. Mischler EH, Parrell S, *et al.* Comparison of effectiveness of pancreatic enzyme preparations in cystic fibrosis. *Am J Dis Child.* 1982;136:1060-1063.
7. Salen G, Prakash A. Evaluation of enteric-coated microspheres for enzyme replacement therapy in adults with pancreatic insufficiency. *Cur Ther Res.* 1979;25:650-656.
8. Schneider MU, Knoll-Ruzicka ML, *et al.* Pancreatic enzyme replacement therapy: comparative effects of conventional and enteric-coated microspheric pancreatin and acid-stable fungal enzyme preparations on steatorrhea in chronic pancreatitis. *Hepato-gastroenterol.* 1985;32:97-102.
9. Halgreen H, Thorsgaard Pedersen N, Worning H. Symptomatic effect of pancreatic enzyme therapy in patients with chronic pancreatitis. *Scand J Gastroenterol.* 1986;21:104-108.
10. Smyth RL, van Velzen D, *et al.* Strictures of ascending colon in cystic fibrosis and high-strength pancreatic enzymes. *The Lancet.* 1994;343:85-86.
11. Lands L, Zinman R, *et al.* Pancreatic function testing in meconium disease in CF: two case reports. *J Ped Gastroenterol and Nut.* 1988;7:276-279.
12. Cystic Fibrosis Foundation Conference on Pancreatic Enzyme Supplementation in the Context of Fibrosing Colonopathy; Washington, D.C., March 23-24, 1995.

Marketed as ULTRASE® by:
Scandipharm, Inc.
22 Inverness Center Parkway
Birmingham, AL 35242
U.S.A.
Rx only
Rev. 3/98. Printed in U.S.A.

ULTRASE® is a registered trademark of Scandipharm, Inc. Manufactured by Eurand International, Milan, Italy, using its DIFFUCAPS® technology for Scandipharm, Inc.

Shown in Product Identification Guide, page 336

ULTRASE® MT ℞

[*ul 'trāce*]
(pancrelipase) Capsules
Enteric-Coated Minitablets

Prescribing Information

DESCRIPTION

ULTRASE® MT (pancrelipase) Capsules are orally administered capsules containing enteric-coated minitablets of porcine pancreatic enzyme concentrate, predominantly pancreatic lipase, amylase, and protease.

Each ULTRASE ® MT12 Capsule contains:	
Lipase	12,000 U.S.P. Units
Amylase	39,000 U.S.P. Units
Protease	39,000 U.S.P. Units
Each ULTRASE ® MT18 Capsule contains:	
Lipase	18,000 U.S.P. Units
Amylase	58,500 U.S.P. Units
Protease	58,500 U.S.P. Units
Each ULTRASE ® MT20 Capsule contains:	
Lipase	20,000 U.S.P. Units
Amylase	65,000 U.S.P. Units
Protease	65,000 U.S.P. Units

ULTRASE® MT (pancrelipase) Capsules contain an amount of pancrelipase equivalent to but not more than 125% of the labeled lipase activity expressed in U.S.P. Units.

Inactive ingredients: hydrogenated castor oil, silicon dioxide, sodium carboxymethylcellulose, magnesium stearate, microcrystalline cellulose, methacrylic acid copolymer (Type C), talc, simethicone, triethylcitrate, iron oxides and titanium oxide.

CLINICAL PHARMACOLOGY

ULTRASE® MT (pancrelipase) Capsules are designed to prevent inactivation by gastric acid thereby resulting in the delivery of high levels of biologically active enzymes into the duodenum. The enzymes catalyze the hydrolysis of fats into glycerol and fatty acids, starch into dextrins and sugars, and protein into proteoses and derived substances.

INDICATIONS AND USAGE

ULTRASE® MT (pancrelipase) Capsules are indicated for patients with partial or complete exocrine pancreatic insufficiency caused by:

- Cystic fibrosis
- Chronic pancreatitis due to alcohol use or other causes
- Surgery (pancreatico-duodenectomy or Whipple's procedure, with or without Wirsung duct injection, total pancreatectomy)
- Obstruction (pancreatic and biliary duct lithiasis, pancreatic and duodenal neoplasms, ductal stenosis)
- Other pancreatic disease (hereditary, post traumatic and allograft pancreatitis, hemochromatosis, Schwachman's Syndrome, lipomatosis, hyperparathyroidism)
- Poor mixing (Billroth II gastrectomy, other types of gastric bypass surgery, gastrinoma)

Pancrelipase capsules are effective in controlling steatorrhea.[1–9]

CONTRAINDICATIONS

Pancrelipase capsules are contraindicated in patients known to be hypersensitive to pork protein. Pancrelipase capsules are contraindicated in patients with acute pancreatitis or with acute exacerbations of chronic pancreatic diseases.

WARNINGS

Should hypersensitivity occur, discontinue medication and treat symptomatically.

PRECAUTIONS

General

TO PROTECT ENTERIC COATING, MINITABLETS MUST NOT BE CRUSHED OR CHEWED. Where swallowing of capsules is difficult, they may be opened and the minitablets added to a small quantity of a soft food (e.g. applesauce, gelatin, etc.) that does not require chewing, and swallowed immediately. Contact of the minitablet with foods having a pH greater than 5.5 can dissolve the protective enteric shell.

Carcinogenesis, Mutagenesis, Impairment of Fertility

Long-term studies in animals have not been performed to evaluate carcinogenic potential. Methacrylic acid, a minor component of the methacrylic acid copolymer enteric-coating contained in ULTRASE® MT (pancrelipase) Capsules, has been reported to act as a teratogen in rat embryo cultures. However, ULTRASE® MT (pancrelipase) Capsules have been shown to contain <0.001% of methacrylic acid, and the mammalian teratology studies in the rat and rabbit were negative.

The copolymer enteric-coating of ULTRASE® MT (pancrelipase) Capsules was not mutagenic by the Ames test, and it did not produce chromosome damage in a test for unscheduled DNA synthesis in rat hepatocytes.

Pregnancy: Category C.

Animal reproduction studies have not been conducted with ULTRASE® MT (pancrelipase) Capsules. It is not known whether ULTRASE® MT (pancrelipase) Capsules can cause fetal harm when administered to a pregnant woman or can affect reproduction capacity. ULTRASE® MT (pancrelipase) Capsules should be given to a pregnant woman only if the potential benefit outweighs the potential risk to the fetus.

Nursing Mothers

It is not known whether ULTRASE® MT (pancrelipase) is excreted in human milk. Because many drugs are excreted in human milk, caution should be exercised when ULTRASE® MT (pancrelipase) Capsules are administered to a nursing mother.

ADVERSE REACTIONS

The most frequently reported adverse reactions to pancrelipase-containing products are gastrointestinal in nature. Less frequently, allergic-type reactions have also been observed.

Extremely high doses of exogenous pancreatic enzymes have been associated with hyperuricosuria and hyperuricemia when the preparations given were pancrelipase in powdered or capsule form, or pancreatin in tablet form.

In two clinical studies with ULTRASE® MT in 193 patients with cystic fibrosis, the adverse events described were all gastrointestinal in nature and may actually represent symptoms of the underlying disease, such as abdominal pain/cramps (5.7%), diarrhea (3.6%), and greasy stools and flatulence (1.5% each). In a postmarketing trial with another enteric-coated formulation, 160 adverse events occurred in the 15,711 patients (0.97%) evaluated.[10] The most frequent events reported were diarrhea, skin reaction, and abdominal discomfort (0.2% each).

Colonic strictures have been reported in cystic fibrosis patients treated with both high- and lower-strength enzyme supplements.[11] A causal relationship has not been established. The possibility of bowel stricture should be considered if symptoms suggestive of gastrointestinal obstruction occur. Since impaired fluid secretion may be a factor in the development of intestinal obstruction, care should be taken to maintain adequate hydration, particularly in warm weather.[12]

"Fibrosing colonopathy" is a term used to describe a condition seen in patients with CF who have taken high amounts of pancreatic enzyme supplements (>6,000 lipase U/kg/meal). At its most advanced, this condition leads to colonic strictures.

1. In whom should one consider the diagnosis of fibrosing colonopathy?

a. Patients with cystic fibrosis who have evidence of partial or complete obstruction, bloody diarrhea or chylous ascites.

b. Patients who have two of the following three symptoms:
   abdominal pain
   ongoing diarrhea
   poor weight gain
   ESPECIALLY if they have:
   taken >6,000 lipase U/kg/meal
   age less than twelve years
   history of meconium ileus
   prior intestinal surgery
   history of recurrent DIOS
   "inflammatory bowel disease"[13]

DOSAGE AND ADMINISTRATION

The enzymatic activity of ULTRASE® MT (pancrelipase) Capsules is expressed in U.S.P. units. Each capsule contains the labeled amount of lipase activity and an overage of not more than 25%.

The smallest effective dose should be used. Dosage should be adjusted according to the severity of the exocrine pancreatic insufficiency. Begin therapy with one or two capsules

with meals or snacks and adjust dosage according to symptoms. The number of capsules or capsule strength given with meals and/or snacks should be estimated by assessing which dose minimizes steatorrhea and maintains good nutritional status. Dosages should be adjusted according to the response of the patient. Where swallowing of capsules is difficult, they may be opened and the minitablets added to a small quantity of a soft food (e.g. applesauce, gelatin, etc.) that does not require chewing, and swallowed immediately. It is recommended that the total dose of pancrelipase being ingested for a meal or snack be dispersed equally (with fluids) before, during, and after the meal or snack.

SUGGESTIONS FOR THE USE OF PANCREATIC ENZYMES IN CYSTIC FIBROSIS[13]

1. Patients should be receiving optimal diet for age and clinical status, recognizing that those with failure to thrive or malnutrition require additional calories and other nutrients for catch-up growth.

2. Nutrition assessment should be a part of routine clinical evaluations.

3. Initial dosing of pancreatic enzyme supplements should begin with 500 lipase U/kg/meal using enteric-coated microcapsule products.

4. Patients should be reassessed 2–4 weeks after initiation of therapy.
The following items should be assessed:
Clinical status, e.g. abdominal symptoms and exam
Nutritional intake and growth (height, weight, head circumference)
Character of stools—greasy, oily (for information, not for decision making)
Quantitative 72-hr fecal fat when indicated (perform on a normal diet for age)
Fat soluble vitamin measures.

5. Corollaries to dosing suggestions:
a. Dose may be increased in a stepwise fashion.
b. Dose approaching 2,000 lipase U/kg/meal would indicate the need for further investigation (see below). Patients presently on higher doses should be reevaluated; either immediately decrease the dose or titrate down to a lower dose range at, or below, 2,000 lipase U/kg/meal. Doses >6,000 lipase U/kg/meal have been associated with colonic strictures.
c. Pancreatic supplements mixed with applesauce or other acidic food substances should be administered immediately, not stored.
d. Enteric-coated microcapsules should not be crushed.
e. Enzyme doses (as lipase U/kg/meal) tend to decrease with advancing age.
f. Patient should accept only product brands prescribed by CF Center staff.
g. Adjustment of dosage is the responsibility of the CF Center staff. Patients should be advised not to adjust doses without consulting the CF Center staff. Changes in product may require an adjustment period.
h. Complaints transmitted by phone should be investigated before dose is adjusted.
i. Pancreatic supplements should be stored in a cool dry place and checked regularly for expiration date.

HOW SUPPLIED

ULTRASE ® MT12 (pancrelipase) Capsules
Gelatin capsules (white and yellow), imprinted "ULTRASE MT12". Bottles of 100 (NDC 58914-002-10).

ULTRASE ® MT18 (pancrelipase) Capsules
Gelatin capsules (gray and white), imprinted "ULTRASE MT18". Bottles of 100 (NDC 58914-018-10).

ULTRASE ® MT20 (pancrelipase) Capsules
Gelatin capsules (light gray and yellow), imprinted "ULTRASE MT20". Bottles of 100 (NDC 58914-004-10), and bottles of 500 (NDC 58914-004-50).

Store at controlled room temperature, between 15°C and 25°C (59°F and 77°F), in a dry place. Do not refrigerate.

REFERENCES

1. Delchier JC, Vidon N, *et al.* Fate of orally ingested enzymes in pancreatic insufficiency: comparison of two pancreatic enzyme preparations. *Aliment Pharmacol Therap.* 1991;5:365–378.

2. Duhamel JP, Vidailhet M, *et al.* Étude multicentrique comparative d'une nouvelle présentation de pancréatine en microgranules gastrorésistants dans l'insuffisance pancréatique exocrine de la mucoviscidose chez l'enfant. *Ann Pediatr.* 1988;35:69–74.

3. Dutta SK, Tilley DK. The pH-sensitive enteric-coated pancreatic enzyme preparations: an evaluation of therapeutic efficacy in adult patients with pancreatic insufficiency. *J Clin Gastroenterol.* 1983;5:51–54.

4. Dutta SK, Rubin J, Harvey J. Comparative evaluation of the therapeutic efficacy of a pH-sensitive enteric-coated pancreatic enzyme preparation with conventional pancreatic enzyme therapy in the treatment of exocrine pancreatic insufficiency. *Gastroenterol.* 1983;84:476–482.

5. Gouerou H, Dain MP, *et al.* Alipase versus nonenteric-coated enzymes in pancreatic insufficiency. *Int J Pancreatol.* 1989;5:45–50.

6. Mischler EH, Parrell S, *et al.* Comparison of effectiveness of pancreatic enzyme preparations in cystic fibrosis. *Am J Dis Child.* 1982;136:1060–1063.

7. Salen G, Prakash A. Evaluation of enteric-coated microspheres for enzyme replacement therapy in adults with pancreatic insufficiency. *Cur Ther Res.* 1979;25:650–656.

8. Schneider MU, Knoll-Ruzicka ML, *et al.* Pancreatic enzyme replacement therapy: comparative effects of conventional and enteric-coated microspheric pancreatin and acid-stable fungal enzyme preparations on steatorrhea in chronic pancreatitis. *Hepato-gastroenterol.* 1985;32:97–102.

9. Halgreen H, Thorsgaard Pedersen N, Worning H. Symptomatic effect of pancreatic enzyme therapy in patients with chronic pancreatitis. *Scand J Gastroenterol.* 1986;21:104–108.

10. Gretzmacher I, Rüther HG. Maldigestion. *Therapiewoche.* 1983;33:6776–6782.

11. Smyth RL, van Velzen D, *et al.* Strictures of ascending colon in cystic fibrosis and high-strength pancreatic enzymes. *The Lancet.* 1994;343:85–86.

12. Lands L, Zinman R, *et al.* Pancreatic function testing in meconium disease in CF: two case reports. *J Ped Gastroenterol and Nut.* 1988;7:276–279.

13. Cystic Fibrosis Foundation Conference on Pancreatic Enzyme Supplementation in the Context of Fibrosing Colonopathy; Washington, D.C., March 23–24, 1995.

Marketed as ULTRASE® by:
Scandipharm, Inc.
22 Inverness Center Parkway
Birmingham, AL 35242
U.S.A.

Rx only
Rev. 3/98.
ULTRASE® is a registered trademark of Scandipharm, Inc. Manufactured by Eurand International, Milan, Italy, using its Eurand MINITABS® technology for Scandipharm, Inc.
Shown in Product Identification Guide, page 336

Schein Pharmaceutical, Inc.
100 CAMPUS DRIVE
FLORHAM PARK, NJ 07932

Direct Inquiries to:
Customer Service
(800) 356-5790
FAX: 800-760-9224

For Medical Information Contact:
(800) 548-6236 (24 Hours)

INFeD®
(IRON DEXTRAN INJECTION, USP)

℞

WARNING
THE PARENTERAL USE OF COMPLEXES OF IRON AND CARBOHYDRATES HAS RESULTED IN ANAPHYLACTIC-TYPE REACTIONS. DEATHS ASSOCIATED WITH SUCH ADMINISTRATION HAVE BEEN REPORTED. THEREFORE, INFeD SHOULD BE USED ONLY IN THOSE PATIENTS IN WHOM THE INDICATIONS HAVE BEEN CLEARLY ESTABLISHED AND LABORATORY INVESTIGATIONS CONFIRM AN IRON DEFICIENT STATE NOT AMENABLE TO ORAL IRON THERAPY.

DESCRIPTION

INFeD (iron dextran injection, USP) is a dark brown, slightly viscous sterile liquid complex of ferric hydroxide and dextran for intravenous or intramuscular use.

Each mL contains the equivalent of 50 mg of elemental iron (as an iron dextran complex), approximately 0.9% sodium chloride, in water for injection. Sodium hydroxide and/or hydrochloric acid may have been used to adjust pH. The pH of the solution is between 5.2 and 6.5.

The iron dextran complex has an average apparent molecular weight of 165,000 g/mole with a range of approximately +/− 10%.

Therapeutic Class: Hematinic

CLINICAL PHARMACOLOGY

General: After intramuscular injection, iron dextran is absorbed from the injection site into the capillaries and the lymphatic system. Circulating iron dextran is removed from the plasma by cells of the reticuloendothelial system, which split the complex into its components of iron and dextran. The iron is immediately bound to the available protein moieties to form hemosiderin or ferritin, the physiological forms of iron, or to a lesser extent to transferrin. This iron which is subject to physiological control replenishes hemoglobin and depleted iron stores.

Dextran, a polyglucose, is either metabolized or excreted. Negligible amounts of iron are lost via the urinary or alimentary pathways after administration of iron dextran.

The major portion of intramuscular injections of iron dextran is absorbed within 72 hours; most of the remaining iron is absorbed over the ensuing 3 to 4 weeks.

Various studies involving intravenously administered ^{59}Fe iron dextran to iron deficient subjects, some of whom had coexisting diseases, have yielded half-life values ranging from 5 hours to more than 20 hours. The 5-hour value was determined for ^{59}Fe iron dextran from a study that used laboratory methods to separate the circulating ^{59}Fe iron dextran from the transferrin-bound [59]Fe. The 20-hour value reflects a half-life determined by measuring total ^{59}Fe, both circulating and bound. It should be understood that these half-life values do not represent clearance of iron from the body. Iron is not easily eliminated from the body and accumulation of iron can be toxic.

In vitro studies have shown that removal of iron dextran by dialysis is negligible.[1,2] Six different dialyzer membranes were investigated (polysulfone, cuprophane, cellulose acetate, cellulose triacetate, polymethylmethacrylate and polyacrylonitrile), including those considered high efficiency and high flux.

INDICATIONS AND USAGE

Intravenous or intramuscular injections of iron dextran are indicated for treatment of patients with documented iron deficiency in whom oral administration is unsatisfactory or impossible.

CONTRAINDICATIONS

Hypersensitivity to the product. All anemias not associated with iron deficiency.

WARNINGS

See BOXED WARNING.
A risk of carcinogenesis may attend the intramuscular injection of iron-carbohydrate complexes. Such complexes have been found under experimental conditions to produce sarcoma when large doses or small doses injected repeatedly at the same site were given to rats, mice, and rabbits, and possibly in hamsters.

The long latent period between the injection of a potential carcinogen and the appearance of a tumor makes it impossible to measure accurately the risk in man. There have, however, been several reports in the literature describing tumors at the injection site in humans who had previously received intramuscular injections of iron-carbohydrate complexes.

Large intravenous doses, such as used with total dose infusions (TDI), have been associated with an increased incidence of adverse effects. The adverse effects frequently are delayed (1–2 days) reactions typified by one or more of the following symptoms; arthralgia, backache, chills, dizziness, moderate to high fever, headache, malaise, myalgia, nausea, and vomiting. The onset is usually 24–48 hours after administration and symptoms generally subside within 3–4 days. These symptoms have also been reported following intramuscular injection and generally subside within 3–7 days. The etiology of these reactions is not known. The potential for a delayed reaction must be considered when estimating the risk/benefit of treatment.

The maximum daily dose should not exceed 2 mL undiluted iron dextran.

This preparation should be used with extreme care in patients with serious impairment of liver function.

It should not be used during the acute phase of infectious kidney disease.

Adverse reactions experienced following administration of INFeD may exacerbate cardiovascular complications in patients with pre-existing cardiovascular disease.

PRECAUTIONS

General: Unwarranted therapy with parenteral iron will cause excess storage of iron with the consequent possibility of exogenous hemosiderosis. Such iron overload is particularly apt to occur in patients with hemoglobinopathies and other refractory anemias that might be erroneously diagnosed as iron deficiency anemias.

INFeD should be used with caution in individuals with histories of significant allergies and/or asthma.

Anaphylaxis and other hypersensitivity reactions have been reported after uneventful test doses as well as therapeutic doses of iron dextran injection. Therefore, administration of subsequent test doses during therapy should be considered. (See DOSAGE AND ADMINISTRATION: Administration.)

Epinephrine should be immediately available in the event of acute hypersensitivity reactions. (Usual adult dose: 0.5 mL of a 1:1000 solution, by subcutaneous or intramuscular injection.)

Continued on next page

INFeD—Cont.

Note: Patients using beta-blocking agents may not respond adequately to epinephrine. Isoproterenol or similar beta-agonist agents may be required in these patients.

Patients with rheumatoid arthritis may have an acute exacerbation of joint pain and swelling following the administration of INFeD.

Reports in the literature from countries outside the United States (in particular, New Zealand) have suggested that the use of intramuscular iron dextran in neonates has been associated with an increased incidence of gram-negative sepsis, primarily due to *E. Coli.*

Information For Patients: Patients should be advised of the potential adverse reactions associated with the use of INFeD.

Drug/Laboratory Test Interactions: Large doses of iron dextran (5 mL or more) have been reported to give a brown color to serum from a blood sample drawn 4 hours after administration.

The drug may cause falsely elevated values of serum bilirubin and falsely decreased values of serum calcium.

Serum iron determinations (especially by colorimetric assays) may not be meaningful for 3 weeks following the administration of iron dextran.

Serum ferritin peaks approximately 7 to 9 days after an intravenous dose of INFeD and slowly returns to baseline after about 3 weeks.

Examination of the bone marrow for iron stores may not be meaningful for prolonged periods following iron dextran therapy because residual iron dextran may remain in the reticuloendothelial cells.

Bone scans involving 99m Tc-diphosphonate have been reported to show a dense, crescentic area of activity in the buttocks, following the contour of the iliac crest, 1 to 6 days after intramuscular injections of iron dextran.

Bone scans with 99m Tc-labeled bone seeking agents, in the presence of high serum ferritin levels or following iron dextran infusions, have been reported to show reduction of bony uptake, marked renal activity, and excessive blood pool and soft tissue accumulation.

Carcinogenesis, Mutagenesis, Impairment Of Fertility: See WARNINGS.

Pregnancy: *Pregnancy Category C:* Iron dextran has been shown to be teratogenic and embryocidal in mice, rats, rabbits, dogs, and monkeys when given in doses of about 3 times the maximum human dose.

No consistent adverse fetal effects were observed in mice, rats, rabbits, dogs and monkeys at doses of 50 mg iron/kg or less. Fetal and maternal toxicity has been reported in monkeys at a total intravenous dose of 90 mg iron/kg over a 14 day period. Similar effects were observed in mice and rats on administration of a single dose of 125 mg iron/kg. Fetal abnormalities in rats and dogs were observed at doses of 250 mg iron/kg and higher. The animals used in these tests were not iron deficient. There are no adequate and well-controlled studies in pregnant women. INFeD should be used during pregnancy only if the potential benefit justifies the potential risk to the fetus.

Placental Transfer: Various animal studies and studies in pregnant humans have demonstrated inconclusive results with respect to the placental transfer of iron dextran as iron dextran. It appears that some iron does reach the fetus, but the form in which it crosses the placenta is not clear.

Nursing Mothers: Caution should be exercised when INFeD is administered to a nursing woman. Traces of unmetabolized iron dextran are excreted in human milk.

Pediatric Use: Not recommended for use in infants under 4 months of age (See DOSAGE AND ADMINISTRATION.)

ADVERSE REACTIONS

Severe/Fatal: Anaphylactic reactions have been reported with the use of iron dextran injection; on occasions these reactions have been fatal. Such reactions, which occur most often within the first several minutes of administration, have been generally characterized by sudden onset of respiratory difficulty and/or cardiovascular collapse. (See boxed WARNING and PRECAUTIONS: General, pertaining to immediate availability of epinephrine.)

Cardiovascular: Chest pain, chest tightness, shock, cardiac arrest, hypotension, hypertension, tachycardia, bradycardia, flushing, arrhythmias. (Flushing and hypotension may occur from too rapid injections by the intravenous route.)

Dermatologic: Urticaria, pruritus, purpura, rash, cyanosis.

Gastrointestinal: Abdominal pain, nausea, vomiting, diarrhea.

Hematologic/lymphatic: Leucocytosis, lymphadenopathy.

Musculoskeletal/soft tissue: Arthralgia, arthritis (may represent reactivation in patients with quiescent rheumatoid arthritis—See PRECAUTIONS: General), myalgia; backache; sterile abscess, atrophy/fibrosis (intramuscular injection site); brown skin and/or underlying tissue discoloration (staining), soreness or pain at or near intramuscular injection sites; cellulitis; swelling; inflammation; local phlebitis at or near intravenous injection site.

Neurologic: Convulsions, seizures, syncope, headache, weakness, unresponsiveness, paresthesia, febrile episodes, chills, dizziness, disorientation, numbness, unconsciousness.

Respiratory: Respiratory arrest, dyspnea, bronchospasm, wheezing.

Urologic: Hematuria.

Delayed reactions: Arthralgia, backache, chills, dizziness, fever, headache, malaise, myalgia, nausea, vomiting (See WARNINGS.).

Miscellaneous: Febrile episodes, sweating, shivering, chills, malaise, altered taste.

OVERDOSAGE

Overdosage with iron dextran is unlikely to be associated with any acute manifestations. Dosages of iron dextran in excess of the requirements for restoration of hemoglobin and replenishment of iron stores may lead to hemosiderosis. Periodic monitoring of serum ferritin levels may be helpful in recognizing a deleterious progressive accumulation of iron resulting from impaired uptake of iron from the reticuloendothelial system in concurrent medical conditions such as chronic renal failure, Hodgkin's disease, and rheumatoid arthritis. The LD_{50} of iron dextran is not less than 500 mg/kg in the mouse.

DOSAGE AND ADMINISTRATION

Oral iron should be discontinued prior to administration of INFeD.

Dosage:

I. *Iron Deficiency Anemia:* Periodic hematologic determination (hemoglobin and hematocrit) is a simple and accurate technique for monitoring hematological response, and should be used as a guide in therapy. It should be recognized that iron storage may lag behind the appearance of normal blood morphology. Serum iron, total iron binding capacity (TIBC) and percent saturation of transferrin are other important tests for detecting and monitoring the iron deficient state.

After administration of iron dextran complex, evidence of a therapeutic response can be seen in a few days as an increase in the reticulocyte count.

Although serum ferritin is usually a good guide to body iron stores, the correlation of body iron stores and serum ferritin may not be valid in patients on chronic renal dialysis who are also receiving iron dextran complex.

Although there are significant variations in body build and weight distribution among males and females, the accompanying table and formula represent a convenient means for estimating the total iron required. This total iron requirement reflects the amount of iron needed to restore hemoglobin concentration to normal or near normal levels plus an additional allowance to provide adequate replenishment of iron stores in most individuals with moderately or severely reduced levels of hemoglobin. It should be remembered that iron deficiency anemia will not appear until essentially all iron stores have been depleted. Therapy, thus, should aim at not only replenishment of hemoglobin iron but iron stores as well.

Factors contributing to the formula are shown below. [See tables at left]

The total amount of INFeD in mL required to treat the anemia and replenish iron stores may be approximated as follows:

Adults and Children over 15 kg (33 lbs): See Dosage Table.

Alternatively the total dose may be calculated:

Dose (mL) = 0.0442 (Desired Hb − Observed Hb) × LBW + (0.26 × LBW)

Based on: Desired Hb = the target Hb in g/dl.

Observed Hb = the patient's current hemoglobin in g/dl.

LBW = Lean body weight in kg. A patient's lean body weight (or actual body weight if less than lean body weight) should be utilized when determining dosage.

For males: LBW = 50 kg + 2.3 kg for each inch of patient's height over 5 feet

mg blood iron	=	mL blood		×	g hemoglobin	×	mg iron
lb body weight		lb body weight			mL blood		g hemoglobin

a) Blood volume .... 65 mL/kg body weight

b) Normal hemoglobin (males and females)
   over 15 kg (33 lbs) .... 14.8 g/dl
   15 kg (33 lbs) or less .... 12.0 g/dl

c) Iron content of hemoglobin ... 0.34%

d) Hemoglobin deficit

e) Weight

Based on the above factors, individuals with normal hemoglobin levels will have approximately 33 mg of blood iron per kilogram of body weight (15 mg/lb).

Note: The table and accompanying formula are applicable for dosage determinations only in patients with iron deficiency anemia; they are not to be used for dosage determinations in patients requiring iron replacement for blood loss.

TOTAL INFeD® REQUIREMENT FOR HEMOGLOBIN RESTORATION AND IRON STORES REPLACEMENT*

PATIENT LEAN BODY WEIGHT		Milliliter Requirement of INFeD Based On Observed Hemoglobin of							
kg	lb	3 (g/dl)	4 (g/dl)	5 (g/dl)	6 (g/dl)	7 (g/dl)	8 (g/dl)	9 (g/dl)	10 (g/dl)
5	11	3	3	3	3	2	2	2	2
10	22	7	6	6	5	5	4	4	3
15	33	10	9	9	8	7	7	6	5
20	44	16	15	14	13	12	11	10	9
25	55	20	18	17	16	15	14	13	12
30	66	23	22	21	19	18	17	15	14
35	77	27	26	24	23	21	20	18	17
40	88	31	29	28	26	24	22	21	19
45	99	35	33	31	29	27	25	23	21
50	110	39	37	35	32	30	28	26	24
55	121	43	41	38	36	33	31	28	26
60	132	47	44	42	39	36	34	31	28
65	143	51	48	45	42	39	36	34	31
70	154	55	52	49	45	42	39	36	33
75	165	59	55	52	49	45	42	39	35
80	176	63	59	55	52	48	45	41	38
85	187	66	63	59	55	51	48	44	40
90	198	70	66	62	58	54	50	46	42
95	209	74	70	66	62	57	53	49	45
100	220	78	74	69	65	60	56	52	47
105	231	82	77	73	68	63	59	54	50
110	242	86	81	76	71	67	62	57	52
115	253	90	85	80	75	70	64	59	54
120	264	94	88	83	78	73	67	62	57

* Table values were calculated based on a normal adult hemoglobin of 14.8 g/dl for weights greater than 15 kg (33 lbs) and a hemoglobin of 12.0 g/dl for weights less than or equal to 15 kg (33 lbs).

For females: LBW = 45.5 kg + 2.3 kg for each inch of patient's height over 5 feet

To calculate a patient's weight in kg when lbs are known:

$$\frac{\text{patient's weight in pounds}}{2.2} = \text{weight in kilograms}$$

Children 5–15 kg (11–33 lbs): See Dosage Table.

INFeD should not normally be given in the first four months of life. (See PRECAUTIONS: Pediatric Use.)

Alternatively the total dose may be calculated:

Dose (mL) = 0.0442 (Desired Hb−Observed Hb) × W + (0.26 × W)

Based on: Desired Hb = the target Hb in g/dl. (Normal Hb for Children 15 kg or less is 12 g/dl.)

W = Weight in kg.

To calculate a patient's weight in kg when lbs are known:

$$\frac{\text{patient's weight in pounds}}{2.2} = \text{weight in kilograms}$$

II. Iron Replacement for Blood Loss: Some individuals sustain blood losses on an intermittent or repetitive basis. Such blood losses may occur periodically in patients with hemorrhagic diatheses (familial telangiectasia; hemophilia; gastrointestinal bleeding) and on a repetitive basis from procedures such as renal hemodialysis.

Iron therapy in these patients should be directed toward replacement of the equivalent amount of iron represented in the blood loss. The table and formula described under **I. Iron Deficiency Anemia** are **not** applicable for simple iron replacement values.

Quantitative estimates of the individual's periodic blood loss and hematocrit during the bleeding episode provide a convenient method for the calculation of the required iron dose.

The formula shown below is based on the approximation that 1 mL of normocytic, normochromic red cells contains 1 mg of elemental iron:

Replacement iron (in mg) = Blood loss (in mL) × hematocrit

Example:　　Blood loss of 500 mL with 20% hematocrit
　　　　　　Replacement Iron = 500 × 0.20 = 100 mg

$$\text{INFeD dose} = \frac{100 \text{ mg}}{50} = 2 \text{ mL}$$

Administration: The total amount of INFeD required for the treatment of iron deficiency anemia or iron replacement for blood loss is determined from the table or appropriate formula. (See Dosage.)

1. *Intravenous Injection*—PRIOR TO RECEIVING THEIR FIRST INFeD THERAPEUTIC DOSE, ALL PATIENTS SHOULD BE GIVEN AN INTRAVENOUS TEST DOSE OF 0.5 mL. (See PRECAUTIONS: General.) THE TEST DOSE SHOULD BE ADMINISTERED AT A GRADUAL RATE OVER AT LEAST 30 SECONDS. Although anaphylactic reactions known to occur following INFeD administration are usually evident within a few minutes, or sooner, it is recommended that a period of an hour or longer elapse before the remainder of the initial therapeutic dose is given.

Individual doses of 2 mL or less may be given on a daily basis until the calculated total amount required has been reached. INFeD is given undiluted at a **slow gradual rate** not to exceed 50 mg (1 mL) per minute.

2. *Intramuscular Injection*—PRIOR TO RECEIVING THEIR FIRST INFeD THERAPEUTIC DOSE, ALL PATIENTS SHOULD BE GIVEN AN INTRAMUSCULAR TEST DOSE OF 0.5 mL. (See PRECAUTIONS: General.) The test dose should be administered in the same recommended test site and by the same technique as described in the last paragraph of this section. Although anaphylactic reactions known to occur following INFeD administration are usually evident within a few minutes or sooner, it is recommended that at least an hour or longer elapse before the remainder of the initial therapeutic dose is given.

If no adverse reactions are observed, INFeD can be given according to the following schedule until the calculated total amount required has been reached. Each day's dose should ordinarily not exceed 0.5 mL (25 mg of iron) for infants under 5 kg (11 lbs); 1.0 mL (50 mg of iron) for children under 10 kg (22 lbs); and 2.0 mL (100 mg of iron) for other patients.

INFeD should be injected only into the muscle mass of the upper outer quadrant of the buttock—never into the arm or other exposed areas—and should be injected deeply, with a 2-inch or 3-inch 19 or 20 gauge needle. If the patient is standing, he/she should be bearing his/her weight on the leg opposite the injection site, or if in bed, he/she should be in the lateral position with injection site uppermost. To avoid injection or leakage into the subcutaneous tissue, a Z-track technique (displacement of the skin laterally prior to injection) is recommended.

NOTE: Do not mix INFeD with other medications or add to parenteral nutrition solutions for intravenous infusion.

Parenteral drug products should be inspected visually for particulate matter and discoloration prior to administration, whenever the solution and container permit.

HOW SUPPLIED

INFeD® (Iron Dextran Injection, USP) containing 50 mg of elemental iron per mL, is available in 2 mL single dose amber vials (for intramuscular or intravenous use) in cartons of 10 (NDC 0364-3012-47).

Store at controlled room temperature 15°–30°C (59°–86°F).

CAUTION: Federal law prohibits dispensing without prescription.

REFERENCES

1. Hatton RC, Portales IT, Finlay A, Ross EA. Removal of Iron Dextran by Hemodialysis: An In Vitro Study. Am J Kid Dis. 1995; 26(2):327–330.
2. Manuel MA, Stewart WK, St. Clair Neill GD, Hutchinson F. Loss of Iron - Dextran through Cuprophane Membrane of a Disposable Coil Dialyser. Nephron. 1972; 9:94–98.

Literature revised: September 1996
Product No.: 1001-02

SCHEIN PHARMACEUTICAL, INC.
Florham Park, NJ 07932 USA

Shown in Product Identification Guide, page 336

Schering Corporation
a wholly-owned subsidiary of Schering-Plough Corporation
GALLOPING HILL ROAD
KENILWORTH, NJ 07033

Direct Inquiries to:
(908) 298-4000
CUSTOMER SERVICE:
(800) 222-7579
FAX: (908) 820-6400

For Medical Information Contact:
Schering Laboratories
Drug Information Services
2000 Galloping Hill Road
Kenilworth, NJ 07033
(800) 526-4099
FAX: (908) 298-2188

Product Identification Codes

To provide quick and positive identification of Schering Products, we have imprinted the product identification number of the National Drug Code on most tablets and capsules. In some cases, identification letters also appear. Additionally, the following telephone numbers are provided for inquiries:

Drug Information Services
9:00 AM to 5:00 PM EST
1-800-526-4099
After regular hours and on weekends: (908) 298-4000

CEDAX®　　　　　　　　　　　　　　　　R
(ceftibuten capsules)
and
(ceftibuten for oral suspension)
FOR ORAL USE ONLY

PRODUCT INFORMATION

DESCRIPTION

CEDAX (ceftibuten capsules) and (ceftibuten for oral suspension) contain the active ingredient ceftibuten as ceftibuten dihydrate. Ceftibuten dihydrate is a semisynthetic cephalosporin antibiotic for oral administration. Chemically, it is (+)-(6R,7R)-7-[(Z)-2-(2-Amino-4-thiazoly)-4-carboxycrotonamido]-8-oxo-5-thia-1-azabicyclo[4.2.0]oct-2-ene-2-carboxylic acid, dihydrate. Its molecular formula is $C_{15}H_{14}N_4O_6S_2 \cdot 2H_2O$. Its molecular weight is 446.43 as the dihydrate.

Ceftibuten dihydrate has the following structural formula:

・ 2H₂O

CEDAX Capsules contain ceftibuten dihydrate equivalent to 400 mg of ceftibuten. Inactive ingredients contained in

the capsule formulation include: magnesium stearate, microcrystalline cellulose, and sodium starch glycolate. The capsule shell and/or band contains gelatin, sodium lauryl sulfate, titanium dioxide, and polysorbate 80. The capsule shell may also contain benzyl alcohol, sodium propionate, edetate calcium disodium, butylparaben, propylparaben, and methylparaben.

CEDAX Oral Suspension after reconstitution contains ceftibuten dihydrate equivalent to either 90 mg of ceftibuten per 5 mL or 180 mg of ceftibuten per 5 mL. CEDAX Oral Suspension is cherry flavored and contains the inactive ingredients: cherry flavoring, polysorbate 80, silcon dioxide, simethicone, sodium benzoate, sucrose (approximately 1 g/5 mL), titanium dioxide, and xanthan gum.

CLINICAL PHARMACOLOGY

PHARMACOKINETICS

Absorption:

　　　　　　　CEDAX CAPSULES

Ceftibuten is rapidly absorbed after oral administration of CEDAX Capsules. The plasma concentrations and pharmacokinetic parameters of ceftibuten after a single 400-mg dose of CEDAX Capsules to 12 healthy adult male volunteers (20 to 39 years of age) are displayed in the table below. When CEDAX Capsules were administered once daily for 7 days, the average C_{max} was 17.9 μg/mL on day 7. Therefore, ceftibuten accumulation in plasma is about 20% at steady state.

　　　　　CEDAX ORAL SUSPENSION

Ceftibuten is rapidly absorbed after oral administration of CEDAX Oral Suspension. The plasma concentrations and pharmacokinetic parameters of ceftibuten after a single 9-mg/kg dose of CEDAX Oral Suspension to 32 fasting pediatric patients (6 months to 12 years of age) are displayed in the following table:

[See table at bottom of next page]

The absolute bioavailability of CEDAX Oral Suspension has not been determined. The plasma concentrations of ceftibuten in pediatric patients are dose proportional following single doses of CEDAX Capsules of 200 mg and 400 mg and of CEDAX Oral Suspension between 4.5 mg/kg and 9 mg/kg.

Distribution:

　　　　　　　CEDAX CAPSULES

The average apparent volume of distribution (V/F) of ceftibuten in 6 adult subjects is 0.21 L/kg (± 1 SD = 0.03 L/kg).

　　　　　CEDAX ORAL SUSPENSION

The average apparent volume of distribution (V/F) of ceftibuten in 32 fasting pediatric patients is 0.5 L/kg (± 1 SD = 0.2 L/kg).

Protein Binding:

Ceftibuten is 65% bound to plasma proteins. The protein binding is independent of plasma ceftibuten concentration.

Tissue Penetration:

Bronchial secretions: In a study of 15 adults administered a single 400-mg dose of ceftibuten and scheduled to undergo bronchoscopy, the mean concentrations in epithelial lining fluid and bronchial mucosa were 15% and 37%, respectively, of the plasma concentrations.

Sputum: Ceftibuten sputum levels average approximately 7% of the concomitant plasma ceftibuten level. In a study of 24 adults administered ceftibuten 200 mg bid or 400 mg qd, the average C_{max} in sputum (1.5 μg/mL) occurred at 2 hours postdose and the average C_{max} in plasma (17 μg/mL) occurred at 2 hours postdose.

Middle-ear fluid (MEF): In a study of 12 pediatric patients administered 9 mg/kg, ceftibuten MEF area under the curve (AUC) averaged approximately 70% of the plasma AUC. In the same study, C_{max} values were 14.3 ± 2.7 μg/mL in MEF at 4 hours postdose and 14.5 ± 3.7 μg/mL in plasma at 2 hours postdose.

Tonsillar tissue: Data on ceftibuten penetration into tonsillar tissue are not available.

Cerebrospinal fluid: Data on ceftibuten penetration into cerebrospinal fluid are not available.

Metabolism and Excretion:

A study with radiolabeled ceftibuten administered to 6 healthy adult male volunteers demonstrated that *cis*-ceftibuten is the predominant component in both plasma and urine. About 10% of ceftibuten is converted to the *trans*-isomer. The *trans*-isomer is approximately $\frac{1}{8}$ as antimicrobially potent as the *cis*-isomer.

Ceftibuten is excreted in the urine; 95% of the administered radioactivity was recovered either in urine or feces. In 6 healthy adult male volunteers, approximately 56% of the administered dose of ceftibuten was recovered from urine and 39% from the feces within 24 hours. Because renal excretion is a significant pathway of elimination, patients

Continued on next page

Information on Schering products appearing on these pages is effective as of August 15, 1998.

Cedax—Cont.

with renal dysfunction and patients undergoing hemodialysis require dosage adjustment (see **DOSAGE AND ADMINISTRATION**).

Food Effect on Absorption:

Food affects the bioavailability of ceftibuten from CEDAX Capsules and CEDAX Oral Suspension.

The effect of food on the bioavailability of CEDAX Capsules was evaluated in 26 healthy adult male volunteers who ingested 400 mg of CEDAX Capsules after an overnight fast or immediately after a standardized breakfast. Results showed that food delays the time of C_{max} by 1.75 hours, decreases the C_{max} by 18%, and decreases the extent of absorption (AUC) by 8%.

The effect of food on the bioavailability of CEDAX Oral Suspension was evaluated in 18 healthy adult male volunteers who ingested 400 mg of CEDAX Oral Suspension after an overnight fast or immediately after a standardized breakfast. Results obtained demonstrated a decrease in C_{max} of 26% and an AUC of 17% when CEDAX Oral Suspension was administered with a high-fat breakfast, and a decrease in C_{max} of 17% and in AUC of 12% when CEDAX Oral Suspension was administered with a low-calorie nonfat breakfast (see **PRECAUTIONS**).

Bioequivalence of Dosage Formulations:

A study in 18 healthy adult male volunteers demonstrated that a 400-mg dose of CEDAX Capsules produced equivalent concentrations to a 400-mg dose of CEDAX Oral Suspension. Average C_{max} values were 15.6 (3.1) μg/mL for the capsule and 17.0 (3.2) μg/mL for the suspension. Average AUC values were 80.1 (14.4) μg•hr/mL for the capsule and 87.0 (12.2) μg•hr/mL for the suspension.

Special Populations:

Geriatric patients: Ceftibuten pharmacokinetics have been investigated in elderly (65 years of age and older) men (n = 8) and women (n = 4). Each volunteer received ceftibuten 200-mg capsules twice daily for 3½ days. The average C_{max} was 17.5 (3.7) μg/mL after 3½ days of dosing compared to 12.9 (2.1) μg/mL after the first dose; ceftibuten accumulation in plasma was 40% at steady state. Information regarding the renal function of these volunteers was not available; therefore, the significance of this finding for clinical use of CEDAX Capsules in elderly patients is not clear. Ceftibuten dosage adjustment in elderly patients may be necessary (see **DOSAGE AND ADMINISTRATION**).

Patients with renal insufficiency: Ceftibuten pharmacokinetics have been investigated in adult patients with renal dysfunction. The ceftibuten plasma half-life increased and apparent total clearance (Cl/F) decreased proportionally with increasing degree of renal dysfunction. In 6 patients with moderate renal dysfunction (creatinine clearance 30 to 49 mL/min), the plasma half-life of ceftibuten increased to 7.1 hours and Cl/F decreased to 30 mL/min. In 6 patients with severe renal dysfunction (creatinine clearance 5 to 29 mL/min), the half-life increased to 13.4 hours and Cl/F decreased to 16 mL/min. In 6 functionally anephric patients (creatinine clearance <5 mL/min), the half-life increased to 22.3 hours and Cl/F decreased to 11 mL/min (a 7- to 8-fold change compared to healthy volunteers). Hemodialysis removed 65% of the drug from the blood in 2 to 4 hours. These changes serve as the basis for dosage adjustment recommendations in adult patients with mild to severe renal dysfunction (see **DOSAGE AND ADMINISTRATION**).

Microbiology:

Ceftibuten exerts its bactericidal action by binding to essential target proteins of the bacterial cell wall. This binding leads to inhibition of cell-wall synthesis.

Ceftibuten is stable in the presence of most plasmid-mediated beta-lactamases, but it is not stable in the presence of chromosomally-mediated cephalosporinases produced in organisms such as *Bacteroides, Citrobacter, Enterobacter, Morganella,* and *Serratia.* Like other beta-lactam agents, ceftibuten should not be used against strains resistant to beta-lactams due to general mechanisms such as permeability or penicillin-binding protein changes like penicillin-resistant, *S. pneumoniae.*

Ceftibuten has been shown to be active against most strains of the following organisms both *in vitro* and in clinical infections (see **INDICATIONS AND USAGE**):

Gram-positive aerobes:

Streptococcus pneumoniae (penicillin-susceptible strains only)

Streptococcus pyogenes

Gram-negative aerobes:

Haemophilus influenzae (including β-lactamase-producing strains)

Moraxella catarrhalis (including β-lactamase-producing strains)

There are no known organisms which are potential pathogens in the indications approved for ceftibuten for which ceftibuten exhibits *in vitro* activity but for which the safety and efficacy of ceftibuten in treating clinical infections due to these organisms, have not been established in adequate and well-controlled trials.

NOTE: Ceftibuten is INACTIVE *in vitro* against *Acinetobacter, Bordetella, Campylobacter, Enterobacter, Enterococcus, Flavobacterium, Hafnia, Listeria, Pseudomonas, Staphylococcus,* and *Streptococcus* (except *pneumoniae* and *pyogenes*) species. In addition, it shows little *in vitro* activity against most anaerobes, including most species of *Bacteroides.*

Susceptibility testing:

Dilution Techniques: Quantitative methods are used to determine antimicrobial minimal inhibitory concentrations (MICs). These MICs provide estimates of the susceptibility of bacteria to antimicrobial compounds. The MICs should be determined using a standardized procedure. Standardized procedures are based on a dilution method (broth, agar, or microdilution) or equivalent with standardized inoculum concentrations and standardized concentrations of ceftibuten powder. The MIC values should be interpreted according to the following criteria when testing *Haemophilus* species using Haemophilus Test Media (HTM):

MIC (μg/mL)	Interpretation
≤2	(S) Susceptible

The current absence of resistant strains precludes defining any categories other than "Susceptible". Strains yielding results suggestive of a "Nonsusceptible" category should be submitted to a reference laboratory for further testing.

A report of "Susceptible" implies that an infection due to the strain may be appropriately treated with the dosage of antimicrobial agent recommended for that type of infection and infecting species, unless otherwise contraindicated. Ceftibuten is indicated for penicillin-susceptible only strains of *Streptococcus pneumoniae.* A pneumococcal isolate that is susceptible to penicillin (MIC ≤0.06 μg/mL) can be considered susceptible to ceftibuten for approved indications. Testing of ceftibuten against penicillin-intermediate or penicillin-resistant isolates is not recommended. Reliable interpretive criteria for ceftibuten are not currently available. Physicians should be informed that clinical response rates with ceftibuten may be lower in strains that are not penicillin-susceptible.

Standardized susceptibility test procedures require the use of laboratory control microorganisms to control the technical aspect of laboratory procedures. Standard ceftibuten powder should provide the following MIC values:

Organism	MIC range (μg/mL)
Haemophilus influenzae ATCC 49247	0.25–1.0

Diffusion Techniques: Quantitative methods that require measurement of zone diameters also provide estimates of the susceptibility of bacteria to antimicrobial compounds. One such standardized procedure requires the use of standardized inoculum concentrations. This procedure uses paper disks impregnated with 30 μg of ceftibuten to test the susceptibility of microorganisms to ceftibuten.

Reports from the laboratory providing results of the standard single-disk susceptibility test with a 30-μg ceftibuten disk should be interpreted according to the following criteria when testing *Haemophilus* species using Haemophilus Test Media (HTM):

Zone diameter (mm)	Interpretation
≥28	(S) Susceptible

The current absence of resistant strains precludes defining any categories other than "Susceptible". Strains yielding results suggestive of a "Nonsusceptible" category should be submitted to a reference laboratory for further testing. Interpretation should be as stated above for results using dilution techniques.

Ceftibuten is indicated for penicillin-susceptible only strains of *Streptococcus pneumoniae.* Pneumococcal isolates with oxacillin zone sizes of ≥20 mm are susceptible to penicillin and can be considered susceptible for approved indications. Reliable disk diffusion tests for ceftibuten do not yet exist.

As with standardized dilution techniques, diffusion methods require the use of laboratory control microorganisms that are used to control the technical aspects of the laboratory procedures. For the diffusion technique, the 30-μg ceftibuten disk should provide the following zone diameters in these laboratory test quality control strains:

Organism	Zone diameter (mm)
Haemophilus influenzae ATCC 49247	29–35

Cephalosporin-class disks should not be used to test for susceptibility to ceftibuten.

INDICATIONS AND USAGE

CEDAX (ceftibuten) is indicated for the treatment of individuals with mild-to-moderate infections caused by susceptible strains of the designated microorganisms in the specific conditions listed below (see **DOSAGE AND ADMINISTRATION** and **CLINICAL STUDIES** section).

Acute Bacterial Exacerbations of Chronic Bronchitis due to *Haemophilus influenzae* (including β-lactamase-producing strains), *Moraxella catarrhalis* (including β-lactamase-producing strains), or *Streptococcus pneumoniae* (penicillin-susceptible strains only).

NOTE: In acute bacterial exacerbations of chronic bronchitis clinical trials where *Moraxella catarrhalis* was isolated from infected sputum at baseline, ceftibuten clinical efficacy was 22% less than control.

Acute Bacterial Otitis Media due to *Haemophilus influenzae* (including β-lactamase-producing strains), *Moraxella catarrhalis* (including β-lactamase-producing strains), or *Streptococcus pyogenes.*

NOTE: Although ceftibuten used empirically was equivalent to comparators in the treatment of clinically and/or microbiologically documented acute otitis media, the efficacy against *Streptococcus pneumoniae* was 23% less than control. Therefore, ceftibuten should be given empirically **only** when adequate antimicrobial coverage against *Streptococcus pneumoniae* has been previously administered.

Pharyngitis and Tonsillitis due to *Streptococcus pyogenes.*

NOTE: Only penicillin by the intramuscular route of administration has been shown to be effective in the prophylaxis of rheumatic fever. Ceftibuten is generally effective in the eradication of *Streptococcus pyogenes* from the oropharynx; however, data establishing the efficacy of the CEDAX product for the prophylaxis of subsequent rheumatic fever are not available.

Parameter	Average Plasma Concentration (in μg/mL of ceftibuten after a single 400-mg dose) and Derived Pharmacokinetic Parameters (± 1 SD) (n = 12 healthy adult males)	Average Plasma Concentration (in μg/mL of ceftibuten after a single 9-mg/kg dose) and Derived Pharmacokinetic Parameters (± 1 SD) (n = 32 pediatric patients)
1.0 h	6.1 (5.1)	9.3 (6.3)
1.5 h	9.9 (5.9)	8.6 (4.4)
2.0 h	11.3 (5.2)	11.2 (4.6)
3.0 h	13.3 (3.0)	9.0 (3.4)
4.0 h	11.2 (2.9)	6.6 (3.1)
6.0 h	5.8 (1.6)	3.8 (2.5)
8.0 h	3.2 (1.0)	1.6 (1.3)
12.0 h	1.1 (0.4)	0.5 (0.4)
C_{max}, μg/mL	15.0 (3.3)	13.4 (4.9)
T_{max}, h	2.6 (0.9)	2.0 (1.0)
AUC, μg•h/mL	73.7 (16.0)	56.0 (16.9)
$T^{1/2}$ h	2.4 (0.2)	2.0 (0.6)
Total body clearance (Cl/F) mL/min/kg	1.3 (0.3)	2.9 (0.7)

CONTRAINDICATIONS

CEDAX (ceftibuten) is contraindicated in patients with known allergy to the cephalosporin group of antibiotics.

WARNINGS

BEFORE THERAPY WITH THE CEDAX PRODUCT IS INSTITUTED, CAREFUL INQUIRY SHOULD BE MADE TO DETERMINE WHETHER THE PATIENT HAS HAD PREVIOUS HYPERSENSITIVITY REACTIONS TO CEFTIBUTEN, OTHER CEPHALOSPORINS, PENICILLINS, OR OTHER DRUGS. IF THIS PRODUCT IS TO BE GIVEN TO PENICILLIN-SENSITIVE PATIENTS, CAUTION SHOULD BE EXERCISED BECAUSE CROSS HYPERSENSITIVITY AMONG BETA-LACTAM ANTIBIOTICS HAS BEEN CLEARLY DOCUMENTED AND MAY OCCUR IN UP TO 10% OF PATIENTS WITH A HISTORY OF PENICILLIN ALLERGY. IF AN ALLERGIC REACTION TO THE CEDAX PRODUCT OCCURS, DISCONTINUE THE DRUG. SERIOUS ACUTE HYPERSENSITIVITY REACTIONS MAY REQUIRE TREATMENT WITH EPINEPHRINE AND OTHER EMERGENCY MEASURES, INCLUDING OXYGEN, INTRAVENOUS FLUIDS, INTRAVENOUS ANTIHISTAMINES, CORTICOSTEROIDS, PRESSOR AMINES, AND AIRWAY MANAGEMENT, AS CLINICALLY INDICATED.

Pseudomembranous colitis has been reported with nearly all antibacterial agents, including ceftibuten, and may range in severity from mild to life threatening. Therefore, it is important to consider this diagnosis in patients who present with diarrhea subsequent to the administration of antibacterial agents.

Treatment with antibacterial agents alters normal flora of the colon and may permit overgrowth of clostridia. Studies indicate that a toxin produced by *Clostridium difficile* is one primary cause of "antibiotic-associated colitis".

After the diagnosis of pseudomembranous colitis has been established, appropriate therapeutic measures should be initiated. Mild cases of pseudomembranous colitis usually respond to drug discontinuation alone. In moderate to severe cases, consideration should be given to management with fluids and electrolytes, protein supplementation, and treatment with an antibacterial drug clinically effective against *Clostridium difficile*.

PRECAUTIONS

General:

As with other broad-spectrum antibiotics, prolonged treatment may result in the possible emergence and overgrowth of resistant organisms. Careful observation of the patient is essential. If superinfection occurs during therapy, appropriate measures should be taken.

The dose of ceftibuten may require adjustment in patients with varying degrees of renal insufficiency, particularly in patients with creatinine clearance less than 50 mL/min or undergoing hemodialysis (see **DOSAGE AND ADMINISTRATION**). Ceftibuten is readily dialyzable. Dialysis patients should be monitored carefully, and administration of ceftibuten should occur immediately following dialysis. Ceftibuten should be prescribed with caution to individuals with a history of gastrointestinal disease, particularly colitis.

Information to Patients:

Patients should be informed that:

- If the patient is diabetic, he/she should be informed that CEDAX Oral Suspension contains 1 gram sucrose per teaspoon of suspension.
- CEDAX Oral Suspension should be taken at least 2 hours before a meal or at least 1 hour after a meal (see **CLINICAL PHARMACOLOGY, Food Effect on Absorption**).

Drug Interactions:

Theophylline: Twelve healthy male volunteers were administered one 200-mg ceftibuten capsule twice daily for 6 days. With the morning dose of ceftibuten on day 6, each volunteer received a single intravenous infusion of theophylline (4 mg/kg). The pharmacokinetics of theophylline were not altered. The effect of ceftibuten on the pharmacokinetics of theophylline administered orally has not been investigated.

Antacids or H₂-receptor antagonists: The effect of increased gastric pH on the bioavailability of ceftibuten was evaluated in 18 healthy adult volunteers. Each volunteer was administered one 400-mg ceftibuten capsule. A single dose of liquid antacid did not affect the C_{max} or AUC of ceftibuten; however, 150 mg of ranitidine q12h for 3 days increased the ceftibuten C_{max} by 23% and ceftibuten AUC by 16%. The clinical relevance of these increases is not known.

Drug/Laboratory Test Interactions:

There have been no chemical or laboratory test interactions with ceftibuten noted to date. False-positive direct Coombs' tests have been reported during treatment with other cephalosporins. Therefore, it should be recognized that a positive Coombs' test could be due to the drug. The results of assays using red cells from healthy subjects to determine whether ceftibuten would cause direct Coombs' reactions *in vitro* showed no positive reaction at ceftibuten concentrations as high as 40 μg/mL.

Carcinogenesis, Mutagenesis, Impairment of Fertility:

Long-term animal studies have not been performed to evaluate the carcinogenic potential of ceftibuten. No mutagenic effects were seen in the following studies: *in vitro* chromosome assay in human lymphocytes, *in vivo* chromosome assay in mouse bone marrow cells, Chinese Hamster Ovary (CHO) cell point mutation assay at the hypoxanthine-guanine phosphoribosyl transferase (HGPRT) locus, and in a bacterial reversion point mutation test (Ames). No impairment of fertility occurred when rats were administered ceftibuten orally up to 2000 mg/kg/day (approximately 43 times the human dose based on mg/m²/day).

Pregnancy Teratogenic effects: Pregnancy Category B:

Ceftibuten was not teratogenic in the pregnant rat at oral doses up to 400 mg/kg/day (approximately 8.6 times the human dose based on mg/m²/day). Ceftibuten was not teratogenic in the pregnant rabbit at oral doses up to 40 mg/kg/day (approximately 1.5 times the human dose based on mg/m²/day) and has revealed no evidence of harm to the fetus. There are no adequate and well-controlled studies in pregnant women. Because animal reproduction studies are not always predictive of human response, this drug should be used during pregnancy only if clearly needed.

Labor and Delivery:

Ceftibuten has not been studied for use during labor and delivery. Its use during such clinical situations should be weighed in terms of potential risk and benefit to both mother and fetus.

Nursing Mothers:

It is not known whether ceftibuten (at recommended dosages) is excreted in human milk. Because many drugs are excreted in human milk, caution should be exercised when ceftibuten is administered to a nursing woman.

Pediatric Use:

The safety and efficacy of ceftibuten in infants less than 6 months of age has not been established.

Geriatric Patients:

The usual adult dosage recommendation may be followed for patients in this age group. However, these patients should be monitored closely, particularly their renal function, as dosage adjustment may be required.

ADVERSE EVENTS

Clinical Trials:

CEDAX CAPSULES (adult patients)

In clinical trials, 1728 adult patients (1092 US and 636 International) were treated with the recommended dose of ceftibuten capsules (400 mg per day). There were no deaths or permanent disabilities thought due to drug toxicity in any of the patients in these studies. Thirty-six of 1728 (2%) patients discontinued medication due to adverse events thought by the investigators to be possibly, probably, or almost certainly related to drug toxicity. The discontinuations were primarily for gastrointestinal disturbances, usually diarrhea, vomiting, or nausea. Six of 1728 (0.3%) patients were discontinued due to rash or pruritus thought related to ceftibuten administration.

In the US trials, the following adverse events were thought by the investigators to be possibly, probably, or almost certainly related to ceftibuten capsules in multiple-dose clinical trials (n = 1092 ceftibuten-treated patients).

[See first and second tables above]

ADVERSE REACTIONS CEFTIBUTEN CAPSULES US CLINICAL TRIALS IN ADULT PATIENTS (n = 1092)

Incidence equal to or greater than 1%	Nausea	4%
	Headache	3%
	Diarrhea	3%
	Dyspepsia	2%
	Dizziness	1%
	Abdominal pain	1%
	Vomiting	1%
Incidence less than 1% but greater than 0.1%	Anorexia, Constipation, Dry mouth, Dyspnea, Dysuria, Eructation, Fatigue, Flatulence, Loose stools, Moniliasis, Nasal congestion, Paresthesia, Pruritus, Rash, Somnolence, Taste perversion, Urticaria, Vaginitis	

LABORATORY VALUE CHANGES* CEFTIBUTEN CAPSULES US CLINICAL TRIALS IN ADULT PATIENTS

Incidence equal to or greater than 1%	↑ BUN	4%
	↑ Eosinophils	3%
	↓ Hemoglobin	2%
	↑ ALT (SGPT)	1%
	↑ Bilirubin	1%
Incidence less than 1% but greater than 0.1%	↑ Alk phosphatase ↑ Creatinine ↑ Platelets ↓ Platelets ↓ Leukocytes ↑ AST (SGOT)	

*Changes in laboratory values with possible clinical significance regardless of whether or not the investigator thought that the change was due to drug toxicity.

ADVERSE REACTIONS CEFTIBUTEN ORAL SUSPENSION US CLINICAL TRIALS IN PEDIATRIC PATIENTS (n = 772)

Incidence equal to or greater than 1%	Diarrhea*	4%
	Vomiting	2%
	Abdominal pain	2%
	Loose stools	2%
Incidence less than 1% but greater than 0.1%	Agitation, Anorexia, Dehydration, Diaper dermatitis, Dizziness, Dyspepsia, Fever, Headache, Hematuria, Hyperkinesia, Insomnia, Irritability, Nausea, Pruritus, Rash, Rigors, Urticaria	

*NOTE: The incidence of diarrhea in pediatric patients ≤2 years old was 8% (23/301) compared with 2% (9/471) in pediatric patients >2 years old.

Continued on next page

Information on Schering products appearing on these pages is effective as of August 15, 1998.

Cedax—Cont.

CEDAX ORAL SUSPENSION (pediatric patients)
In clinical trials, 1152 pediatric patients (772 US and 380 international), 97% of whom were younger than 12 years of age, were treated with the recommended dose of ceftibuten (9 mg/kg once daily up to a maximum dose of 400 mg per day) for 10 days. There were no deaths, life-threatening adverse events, or permanent disabilities in any of the patients in these studies. Eight of 1152 (<1%) patients discontinued medication due to adverse events thought by the investigators to be possibly, probably, or almost certainly related to drug toxicity. The discontinuations were primarily (7 out of 8) for gastrointestinal disturbances, usually diarrhea or vomiting. One patient was discontinued due to a cutaneous rash thought possibly related to ceftibuten administration.
In the US trials, the following adverse events were thought by the investigators to be possibly, probably, or almost certainly related to ceftibuten oral suspension in multiple-dose clinical trials (n = 772 ceftibuten-treated patients).
[See third table on previous page]
[See first table above]

In Post-marketing Experience:
The following adverse experiences have been reported during worldwide post-marketing surveillance: aphasia, jaundice, melena, psychosis, serum sickness-like reactions, stridor, and toxic epidermal necrolysis.

Cephalosporin-class Adverse Reactions:
In addition to the adverse reactions listed above that have been observed in patients treated with ceftibuten capsules, the following adverse events and altered laboratory tests have been reported for cephalosporin-class antibiotics:
allergic reactions, anaphylaxis, drug fever, Stevens-Johnson syndrome, renal dysfunction, toxic nephropathy, hepatic cholestasis, aplastic anemia, hemolytic anemia, hemorrhage, false-positive test for urinary glucose, neutropenia, pancytopenia, and agranulocytosis. Pseudomembranous colitis; onset of symptoms may occur during or after antibiotic treatment (see **WARNINGS**).
Several cephalosporins have been implicated in triggering seizures, particularly in patients with renal impairment when the dosage was not reduced (see **DOSAGE AND ADMINISTRATION** and **OVERDOSAGE**). If seizures associated with drug therapy occur, the drug should be discontinued. Anticonvulsant therapy can be given if clinically indicated.

OVERDOSAGE

Overdosage of cephalosporins can cause cerebral irritation leading to convulsions. Ceftibuten is readily dialyzable and significant quantities (65% of plasma concentrations) can be removed from the circulation by a single hemodialysis session. Information does not exist with regard to removal of ceftibuten by peritoneal dialysis.

DOSAGE AND ADMINISTRATION

The recommended doses of CEDAX Oral Suspension are presented in the table below. **CEDAX Oral Suspension must be administered at least 2 hours before or 1 hour after a meal.**
[See second table above]

CEFTIBUTEN ORAL SUSPENSION PEDIATRIC DOSAGE CHART

CHILD'S WEIGHT	90 mg/5 mL	180 mg/5 mL
10 kg 22 lbs	1 tsp QD	1/2 tsp QD
20 kg 44 lbs	2 tsp QD	1 tsp QD
40 kg 88 lbs	4 tsp QD	2 tsp QD

Pediatric patients weighing more than 45 kg should receive the maximum daily dose of 400 mg.
Renal Impairment:
CEDAX Capsules and CEDAX Oral Suspension may be administered at normal doses in the presence of impaired renal function with creatinine clearance of 50 mL/min or greater. The recommendations for dosing in patients with varying degrees of renal insufficiency are presented in the following table.

Creatinine Clearance (mL/min)	Recommended Dosing Schedules
>50	9 mg/kg or 400 mg Q24h (normal dosing schedule)
30–49	4.5 mg/kg or 200 mg Q24h
5–29	2.25 mg/kg or 100 mg Q24h

LABORATORY VALUE CHANGES* CEFTIBUTEN ORAL SUSPENSION US CLINICAL TRIALS IN PEDIATRIC PATIENTS

Incidence equal to or greater than 1%	↑ Eosinophils	3%
	↑ BUN	2%
	↓ Hemoglobin	1%
	↑ Platelets	1%
Incidence less than 1% but greater than 0.1%	↑ ALT (SGPT)	
	↑ AST (SGOT)	
	↑ Alk phosphatase	
	↑ Bilirubin	
	↑ Creatinine	

*Changes in laboratory values with possible clinical significance regardless of whether or not the investigator thought that the change was due to drug toxicity.

Type of infection (as qualified in the **INDICATIONS AND USAGE** section of this labeling)	Daily Maximum Dose	Dose and Frequency	Duration
ADULTS (12 years of age and older): Acute Bacterial Exacerbations of Chronic Bronchitis due to *H. influenzae* (including β-lactamase-producing strains), *M. catarrhalis* (including β-lactamase-producing strains), or *Streptococcus pneumoniae* (penicillin-susceptible strains only). (See **INDICATIONS AND USAGE - NOTE.**) Pharyngitis and tonsillitis due to *S. pyogenes.* Acute Bacterial Otitis Media due to *H. influenzae* (including β-lactamase-producing strains), *M. catarrhalis* (including β-lactamase-producing strains). or *S. pyogenes.* (See **INDICATIONS AND USAGE - NOTE.**)	400 mg	400 mg QD	10 days
PEDIATRIC PATIENTS: Pharyngitis and tonsilitis due to *S. pyogenes.* Acute Bacterial Otitis Media due to *H. influenzae* (including β-lactamase-producing strains), and *M. Catarrhalis* (including β-lactamase-producing strains), or *S. pyogenes.* (See **INDICATIONS AND USAGE - NOTE.**)	400 mg	9 mg/kg QD	10 days

DIRECTIONS FOR MIXING CEDAX ORAL SUSPENSION

Final Concentration	Bottle Size	Amount of Water	Directions
90 mg per 5 mL	30 mL	Suspend in 28 mL of water	First tap the bottle to loosen powder. Then add water in two portions, shaking well after each aliquot.
	60 mL	Suspend in 53 mL of water	
	90 mL	Suspend in 78 mL of water	
	120 mL	Suspend in 103 mL of water	
180 mg per 5 mL	30 mL	Suspend in 28 mL of water	
	60 mL	Suspend in 53 mL of water	
	120 mL	Suspend in 103 mL of water	

BACTERIOLOGICAL OUTCOME ACUTE BACTERIAL EXACERBATIONS OF CHRONIC BRONCHITIS

Bacteriological Eradication Rates	Ceftibuten 400 mg QD	Control
Haemophilus influenzae	45/62 (73%)	26/36 (72%)
H. parainfluenzae	10/10	4/6
Moraxella catarrhalis	33/46 (72%)	32/34 (94%)
Streptococcus pneumoniae	23/35 (66%)	14/20 (70%)

BACTERIOLOGICAL OUTCOME ACUTE BACTERIAL OTITIS MEDIA

Bacteriological Eradication Rates	Ceftibuten 9 mg/kg QD	Control
Haemophilus influenzae	56/67 (81%)	29/38 (76%)
Moraxella catarrhalis	20/26 (77%)	13/17 (77%)
Streptococcus pneumoniae	68/105 (65%)	35/40 (88%)
Streptococcus pyogenes	13/15 (87%)	5/5

Hemodialysis Patients:
In patients undergoing hemodialysis two or three times weekly, a single 400-mg dose of ceftibuten capsules or a single dose of 9 mg/kg (maximum of 400 mg of ceftibuten) oral suspension may be administered at the end of each hemodialysis session.

Directions for Mixing CEDAX Oral Suspension:
[See third table at top of previous page]
After mixing, the suspension may be kept for 14 days and must be stored in the refrigerator. Keep tightly closed. Shake well before each use. Discard any unused portion after 14 days.

HOW SUPPLIED

CEDAX Capsules, containing 400 mg of ceftibuten (as ceftibuten dihydrate) are white, opaque capsules imprinted with the product name and strength, are available as follows:
20 Capsules/Bottle (NDC 0085-0691-01)
100 Capsules/Bottle (NDC 0085-0691-02)
Unit-dose dispensing (10 strips of 4 capsules each) (NDC 0085-0691-03)
Store the capsules between 2° and 25°C (36° and 77°F). Replace cap securely after each opening.
CEDAX Oral Suspension is an off-white to cream-colored powder that, when reconstituted as directed, contains either ceftibuten equivalent to 90 mg/5 mL or 180 mg/5 mL, supplied as follows:

90 mg/5 mL
18 mg/mL 30-mL Bottle (NDC 0085-0777-03)
18 mg/mL 60-mL Bottle (NDC 0085-0777-01)
18 mg/mL 90-mL Bottle (NDC 0085-0777-04)
18 mg/mL 120-mL Bottle (NDC 0085-0777-02)

180 mg/5 mL
36 mg/mL 30-mL Bottle (NDC 0085-0834-03)
36 mg/mL 60-mL Bottle (NDC 0085-0834-01)
36 mg/mL 120-mL Bottle (NDC 0085-0834-02)

Prior to reconstitution, the powder must be stored between 2° and 25°C (36° and 77°F). Once it is reconstituted, the oral suspension is stable for 14 days when stored in the refrigerator between 2° and 8°C (36° and 46°F).

CLINICAL STUDIES

Acute Bacterial Exacerbations of Chronic Bronchitis:
Three clinical trials (two domestic, the third abroad) have been conducted testing ceftibuten in the treatment of acute exacerbations of chronic bronchitis (AECB). Overall, the clinical outcome among patients who had signs and symptoms of AECB, who had a gram stain showing a predominance of PMNs and few epithelial cells, and who were evaluated at approximately 1 to 2 weeks after completing therapy were equivalent to comparators. The bacterial eradication rates of specific pathogens are presented below.
[See fourth table at top of previous page]

Acute Bacterial Otitis Media:
Four clinical trials (three domestic, the fourth abroad) have been conducted testing ceftibuten in the treatment of acute bacterial otitis media. Overall, the clinical outcome among patients who had signs and symptoms of acute bacterial otitis media and who were evaluated at approximately 1 to 2 weeks after completing therapy were equivalent to comparators. Tympanocentesis was performed on patients in three of the above-mentioned studies; the bacterial eradication rates of specific pathogens are presented below.
[See fifth table at top of previous page]

REFERENCES

1. National Committee for Clinical Laboratory Standards. Methods for Dilution Antimicrobial Susceptibility Tests for Bacteria that Grow Aerobically – Third Edition. Approved Standard NCCLS Document M7-A3, Vol. 13, No. 25, NCCLS, Villanova, PA. December, 1993.
2. National Committee for Clinical Laboratory Standards. Performance Standards for Antimicrobial Disk Susceptibility Tests-Fifth Edition. Approved Standard NCCLS Document M2-A5, Vol. 13, No. 24, NCCLS, Villanova, PA. December, 1993.

Schering Corporation
Kenilworth, NJ 07033 USA
Licensed by Shionogi and Co., Ltd., Japan
Copyright © 1995, 1997, 1998, Schering Corporation. All rights reserved.
Rev. 8/97 B-18890658
18890950T

Shown in Product Identification Guide, page 336

CELESTONE® SOLUSPAN®* ℞
brand of betamethasone sodium phosphate and betamethasone acetate Injectable Suspension, USP**
6 mg per mL
*brand of rapid and repository injectable.
FORMERLY **CELESTONE® SOLUSPAN®*
Suspension, USP

DESCRIPTION

Each mL of CELESTONE SOLUSPAN* Injectable Suspension contains: 3.0 mg betamethasone as betamethasone sodium phosphate; 3.0 mg betamethasone acetate; 7.1 mg dibasic sodium phosphate; 3.4 mg monobasic sodium phosphate; 0.1 mg edetate disodium; and 0.2 mg benzalkonium chloride. It is a sterile, aqueous suspension with a pH between 6.8 and 7.2.
The formula for betamethasone sodium phosphate is $C_{22}H_{28}FNa_2O_8P$ with a molecular weight of 516.41. Chemically it is 9-Fluoro-11β,17,21-trihydroxy-16β-methylpregna-1,4-diene-3,20-dione 21-(disodium phosphate).
The formula for betamethasone acetate is $C_{24}H_{31}FO_6$ with a molecular weight of 434.50. Chemically it is 9-Fluoro-11β,17,21-trihydroxy-16β-methylpregna-1,4-diene-3,20-dione 21-acetate.
The chemical structures for betamethasone sodium phosphate and betamethasone acetate are as follows:

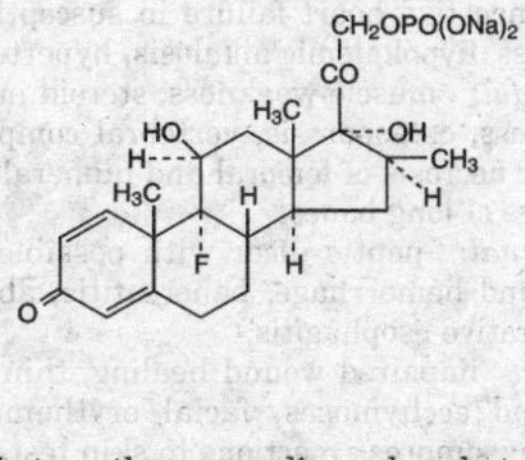
betamethasone sodium phosphate

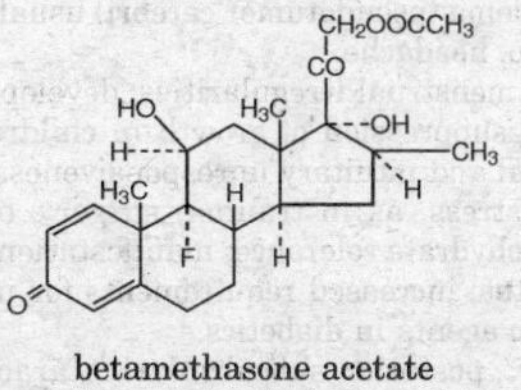
betamethasone acetate

Betamethasone sodium phosphate is a white to practically white, odorless powder, and is hygroscopic. It is freely soluble in water and in methanol, but is practically insoluble in acetone and in chloroform.
Betamethasone acetate is a white to creamy white, odorless powder that sinters and resolidifies at about 165°C, and remelts at about 200°C–220°C with decomposition. It is practically insoluble in water, but freely soluble in acetone, and is soluble in alcohol and in chloroform.

ACTIONS

Naturally occurring glucocorticoids (hydrocortisone), which also have salt-retaining properties, are used as replacement therapy in adrenocortical deficiency states. Their synthetic analogs are primarily used for their potent anti-inflammatory effects in disorders of many organ systems.
Betamethasone sodium phosphate, a soluble ester, provides prompt activity, while betamethasone acetate is only slightly soluble and affords sustained activity.
Glucocorticoids cause profound and varied metabolic effects. In addition, they modify the body's immune responses to diverse stimuli.

INDICATIONS

When oral therapy is not feasible and the strength, dosage form, and route of administration of the drug reasonably lend the preparation to the treatment of the condition, CELESTONE SOLUSPAN Injectable Suspension for intramuscular use is indicated as follows:
Endocrine disorders: Primary or secondary adrenocortical insufficiency (hydrocortisone or cortisone is the drug of choice; synthetic analogs may be used in conjunction with mineralocorticoids where applicable; in infancy mineralocorticoid supplementation is of particular importance).
Acute adrenocortical insufficiency (hydrocortisone or cortisone is the drug of choice; mineralocorticoid supplementation may be necessary, particularly when synthetic analogs are used); preoperatively and in the event of serious trauma or illness, in patients with known adrenal insufficiency or when adrenocortical reserve is doubtful; shock unresponsive to conventional therapy if adrenocortical insufficiency exists or is suspected; congenital adrenal hyperplasia; nonsuppurative thyroiditis; hypercalcemia associated with cancer.
Rheumatic disorders: As adjunctive therapy for short-term administration (to tide the patient over an acute episode or exacerbation) in: post-traumatic osteoarthritis; synovitis of osteoarthritis; rheumatoid arthritis, including juvenile rheumatoid arthritis (selected cases may require low-dose maintenance therapy); acute and subacute bursitis; epicondylitis; acute nonspecific tenosynovitis; acute gouty arthritis; psoriatic arthritis; ankylosing spondylitis.
Collagen diseases: During an exacerbation or as maintenance therapy in selected cases of systemic lupus erythematosus, acute rheumatic carditis.
Dermatologic diseases: Pemphigus, severe erythema multiforme (Stevens-Johnson syndrome), exfoliative dermatitis, bullous dermatitis herpetiformis, severe seborrheic dermatitis, severe psoriasis, mycosis fungoides.
Allergic states: Control of severe or incapacitating allergic conditions intractable to adequate trials of conventional treatment in: bronchial asthma, contact dermatitis, atopic dermatitis, serum sickness, seasonal or perennial allergic rhinitis, drug hypersensitivity reactions, urticarial transfusion reactions, acute noninfectious laryngeal edema (epinephrine is the drug of first choice).
Ophthalmic diseases: Severe acute and chronic allergic and inflammatory processes involving the eye, such as: herpes zoster ophthalmicus, iritis and iridocyclitis, chorioretinitis, diffuse posterior uveitis and choroiditis, optic neuritis, sympathetic ophthalmia, anterior segment inflammation, allergic conjunctivitis, allergic corneal marginal ulcers, keratitis.
Gastrointestinal diseases: To tide the patient over a critical period of disease in: ulcerative colitis—(systemic therapy), regional enteritis—(systemic therapy).
Respiratory diseases: Symptomatic sarcoidosis, berylliosis, fulminating or disseminated pulmonary tuberculosis when used concurrently with appropriate antituberculous chemotherapy, Loeffler's syndrome not manageable by other means, aspiration pneumonitis.
Hematologic disorders: Acquired (autoimmune) hemolytic anemia, secondary thrombocytopenia in adults, erythroblastopenia (RBC anemia), congenital (erythroid) hypoplastic anemia.
Neoplastic diseases: For palliative management of: leukemias and lymphomas in adults, acute leukemia of childhood.
Edematous states: To induce diuresis or remission of proteinuria in the nephrotic syndrome, without uremia, of the idiopathic type or that due to lupus erythematosus.
Miscellaneous: Tuberculous meningitis with subarachnoid block or impending block when used concurrently with appropriate antituberculous chemotherapy, trichinosis with neurologic or myocardial involvement.
When the strength and dosage form of the drug lend the preparation to the treatment of the condition, the **intra-articular or soft tissue administration** of CELESTONE SOLUSPAN Injectable Suspension is indicated as adjunctive therapy for short-term administration (to tide the patient over an acute episode or exacerbation) in: synovitis of osteoarthritis, rheumatoid arthritis, acute and subacute bursitis, acute gouty arthritis, epicondylitis, acute nonspecific tenosynovitis, post-traumatic osteoarthritis.
When the strength and dosage form of the drug lend the preparation to the treatment of the condition, the **intralesional administration** of CELESTONE SOLUSPAN Injectable Suspension is indicated for: keloids; localized hypertrophic, infiltrated, inflammatory lesions of: lichen planus, psoriatic plaques, granuloma annulare, and lichen simplex chronicus (neurodermatitis); discoid lupus erythematosus; necrobiosis lipoidica diabeticorum; alopecia areata.
CELESTONE SOLUSPAN Injectable Suspension may also be useful in cystic tumors of an aponeurosis or tendon (ganglia).

CONTRAINDICATIONS

CELESTONE SOLUSPAN Injectable Suspension is contraindicated in systemic fungal infections.

WARNINGS

CELESTONE SOLUSPAN Injectable Suspension should not be administered intravenously.
In patients on corticosteroid therapy subjected to any unusual stress, increased dosage of rapidly acting corticosteroids before, during, and after the stressful situation is indicated.
Corticosteroids may mask some signs of infection, and new infections may appear during their use. There may be decreased resistance and inability to localize infection when corticosteroids are used.
Prolonged use of corticosteroids may produce posterior subcapsular cataracts, glaucoma with possible damage to the optic nerves, and may enhance the establishment of secondary ocular infections due to fungi or viruses.
CELESTONE SOLUSPAN Injectable Suspension contains two betamethasone esters one of which, betamethasone sodium phosphate, disappears rapidly from the injection site. The potential for systemic effect produced by the soluble portion of CELESTONE SOLUSPAN Injectable Suspension should therefore be taken into account by the physician when using the drug.
Average and large doses of cortisone or hydrocortisone can cause elevation of blood pressure, salt and water retention, and increased excretion of potassium. These effects are less likely to occur with the synthetic derivatives except when

Continued on next page

Information on Schering products appearing on these pages is effective as of August 15, 1998.

Celestone Soluspan—Cont.

used in large doses. Dietary salt restriction and potassium supplementation may be necessary. All corticosteroids increase calcium excretion.

While on corticosteroid therapy patients should not be vaccinated against smallpox. Other immunization procedures should not be undertaken in patients who are on corticosteroids, especially in high doses, because of possible hazards of neurological complications and lack of antibody response.

Persons who are on drugs which suppress the immune system are more susceptible to infections than healthy individuals. Chickenpox and measles, for example, can have a more serious or even fatal course in non-immune children or adults on corticosteroids. In such children, or adults who have not had these diseases, particular care should be taken to avoid exposure. How the dose, route, and duration of corticosteroid administration affects the risk of developing a disseminated infection is not known. The contribution of the underlying disease and/or prior corticosteroid treatment to the risk is also not known. If exposed to chickenpox, prophylaxis with varicella-zoster immune globulin (VZIG) may be indicated. If exposed to measles, prophylaxis with pooled intramuscular immunoglobulin (IG) may be indicated. (See the respective package inserts for complete VZIG and IG prescribing information.) If chickenpox develops, treatment with antiviral agents may be considered.

Similarly, corticosteroids should be used with great care in patients with known or suspected *Strongyloides* (threadworm) infestation. In such patients, corticosteroid-induced immunosuppression may lead to *Strongyloides* hyperinfection and dissemination with widespread larval migration, often accompanied by severe enterocolitis and potentially fatal gram-negative septicemia.

The use of CELESTONE SOLUSPAN Injectable Suspension in active tuberculosis should be restricted to those cases of fulminating or disseminated tuberculosis in which the corticosteroid is used for the management of the disease in conjunction with appropriate antituberculous regimen.

If corticosteroids are indicated in patients with latent tuberculosis or tuberculin reactivity, close observation is necessary as reactivation of the disease may occur. During prolonged corticosteroid therapy, these patients should receive chemoprophylaxis.

Because rare instances of anaphylactoid reactions have occurred in patients receiving parenteral corticosteroid therapy, appropriate precautionary measures should be taken prior to administration, especially when the patient has a history of allergy to any drug.

Usage in pregnancy: Since adequate human reproduction studies have not been done with corticosteroids, the use of these drugs in pregnancy, nursing mothers, or women of childbearing potential requires that the possible benefits of the drug be weighed against the potential hazards to the mother and embryo or fetus. Infants born of mothers who have received substantial doses of corticosteroids during pregnancy should be carefully observed for signs of hypoadrenalism.

PRECAUTIONS

Information for Patients

Persons who are on immunosuppressant doses of corticosteroids should be warned to avoid exposure to chickenpox or measles. Patients should also be advised that if they are exposed, medical advice should be sought without delay.

General: Drug-induced secondary adrenocortical insufficiency may be minimized by gradual reduction of dosage. This type of relative insufficiency may persist for months after discontinuation of therapy; therefore, in any situation of stress occurring during that period, hormone therapy should be reinstituted. Since mineralocorticoid secretion may be impaired, salt and/or a mineralocorticoid should be administered concurrently.

There is an enhanced effect of corticosteroids in patients with hypothyroidism and in those with cirrhosis.

Corticosteroids should be used cautiously in patients with ocular herpes simplex for fear of corneal perforation.

The lowest possible dose of corticosteroid should be used to control the condition under treatment, and when reduction in dosage is possible, the reduction must be gradual.

Psychic derangements may appear when corticosteroids are used, ranging from euphoria, insomnia, mood swings, personality changes, and severe depression to frank psychotic manifestations. Also, existing emotional instability or psychotic tendencies may be aggravated by corticosteroids.

Aspirin should be used cautiously in conjunction with corticosteroids in hypoprothrombinemia.

Steroids should be used with caution in nonspecific ulcerative colitis, if there is a probability of impending perforation, abscess, or other pyogenic infection; also in diverticulitis, fresh intestinal anastomoses, active or latent peptic ulcer, renal insufficiency, hypertension, osteoporosis, and myasthenia gravis.

Growth and development of infants and children on prolonged corticosteroid therapy should be carefully followed.

The following additional precautions also apply for parenteral corticosteroids. **Intra-articular injection of a corticosteroid may produce systemic as well as local effects.**

Appropriate examination of any joint fluid present is necessary to exclude a septic process.

A marked increase in pain accompanied by local swelling, further restriction of joint motion, fever, and malaise are suggestive of septic arthritis. If this complication occurs and the diagnosis of sepsis is confirmed, appropriate antimicrobial therapy should be instituted.

Local injection of a steroid into a previously infected joint is to be avoided.

Corticosteroids should not be injected into unstable joints.

The slower rate of absorption by intramuscular administration should be recognized.

ADVERSE REACTIONS

Fluid and electrolyte disturbances: sodium retention, fluid retention, congestive heart failure in susceptible patients, potassium loss, hypokalemic alkalosis, hypertension.

Musculoskeletal: muscle weakness, steroid myopathy, loss of muscle mass, osteoporosis, vertebral compression fractures, aseptic necrosis of femoral and humeral heads, pathologic fracture of long bones.

Gastrointestinal: peptic ulcer with possible subsequent perforation and hemorrhage, pancreatitis, abdominal distention, ulcerative esophagitis.

Dermatologic: impaired wound healing, thin fragile skin, petechiae and ecchymoses, facial erythema, increased sweating, may suppress reactions to skin tests.

Neurological: convulsions, increased intracranial pressure with papilledema (pseudotumor cerebri) usually after treatment, vertigo, headache.

Endocrine: menstrual irregularities; development of cushingoid state; suppression of growth in children; secondary adrenocortical and pituitary unresponsiveness, particularly in times of stress, as in trauma, surgery, or illness: decreased carbohydrate tolerance; manifestations of latent diabetes mellitus; increased requirements for insulin or oral hypoglycemic agents in diabetics.

Ophthalmic: posterior subcabsular cataracts, increased intraocular pressure, glaucoma, exophthalmos.

Metabolic: negative nitrogen balance due to protein catabolism.

The following *additional* adverse reactions are related to parenteral corticosteroid therapy: rare instances of blindness associated with intralesional therapy around the face and head, hyperpigmentation or hypopigmentation, subcutaneous and cutaneous atrophy, sterile abscess, post-injection flare (following intra-articular use), charcot-like arthropathy.

DOSAGE AND ADMINISTRATION

The initial dosage of CELESTONE SOLUSPAN Injectable Suspension may vary from 0.5 to 9.0 mg per day depending on the specific disease entity being treated. In situations of less severity, lower doses will generally suffice while in selected patients higher initial doses may be required. Usually the parenteral dosage ranges are one-third to one-half the oral dose given every 12 hours. However, in certain overwhelming, acute, life-threatening situations, administration in dosages exceeding the usual dosages may be justified and may be in multiples of the oral dosages.

The initial dosage should be maintained or adjusted until a satisfactory response is noted. If after a reasonable period of time there is a lack of satisfactory clinical response, CELESTONE SOLUSPAN Injectable Suspension should be discontinued and the patient transferred to other appropriate therapy. *It Should Be Emphasized That Dosage Requirements Are Variable and Must Be Individualized on the Basis of the Disease Under Treatment and the Response of the Patient.* After a favorable response is noted, the proper maintenance dosage should be determined by decreasing the initial drug dosage in small decrements at appropriate time intervals until the lowest dosage which will maintain an adequate clinical response is reached. It should be kept in mind that constant monitoring is needed in regard to drug dosage. Included in the situations which may make dosage adjustments necessary are changes in clinical status secondary to remissions or exacerbations in the disease process, the patient's individual drug responsiveness, and the effect of patient exposure to stressful situations not directly related to the disease entity under treatment; in this latter situation it may be necessary to increase the dosage of CELESTONE SOLUSPAN Injectable Suspension for a period of time consistent with the patient's condition. If after long-term therapy the drug is to be stopped, it is recommended that it be withdrawn gradually rather than abruptly.

If coadministration of a local anesthetic is desired, CELESTONE SOLUSPAN Injectable Suspension may be mixed with 1% or 2% lidocaine hydrochloride, using the formulations which do not contain parabens. Similar local anesthetics may also be used. Diluents containing methylparaben, propylparaben, phenol, etc., should be avoided since these compounds may cause flocculation of the steroid. The required dose of CELESTONE SOLUSPAN Injectable Suspension is first withdrawn from the vial into the syringe. The local anesthetic is then drawn in, and the syringe shaken briefly. **Do not inject local anesthetics into the vial of CELESTONE SOLUSPAN Injectable Suspension.**

Bursitis, tenosynovitis, peritendinitis. In acute subdeltoid, subacromial, olecranon, and prepatellar bursitis, one intrabursal injection of 1.0 mL CELESTONE SOLUSPAN Injectable Suspension can relieve pain and restore full range of movement. Several intrabursal injections of corticosteroids are usually required in recurrent acute bursitis and in acute exacerbations of chronic bursitis. Partial relief of pain and some increase in mobility can be expected in both conditions after one or two injections. Chronic bursitis may be treated with reduced dosage once the acute condition is controlled. In tenosynovitis and tendinitis, three or four local injections at intervals of 1 to 2 weeks between injections are given in most cases. Injections should be made into the affected tendon sheaths rather than into the tendons themselves. In ganglions of joint capsules and tendon sheaths, injection of 0.5 mL directly into the ganglion cysts has produced marked reduction in the size of the lesions.

Rheumatoid arthritis and osteoarthritis. Following intra-articular administration of 0.5 to 2.0 mL of CELESTONE SOLUSPAN Injectable Suspension, relief of pain, soreness, and stiffness may be experienced. Duration of relief varies widely in both diseases. Intra-articular Injection—CELESTONE SOLUSPAN Injectable Suspension is well tolerated in joints and periarticular tissues. There is virtually no pain on injection, and the "secondary flare" that sometimes occurs a few hours after intra-articular injection of corticosteroids has not been reported with CELESTONE SOLUSPAN Injectable Suspension. Using sterile technique, a 20- to 24-gauge needle on an empty syringe is inserted into the synovial cavity, and a few drops of synovial fluid are withdrawn to confirm that the needle is in the joint. The aspirating syringe is replaced by a syringe containing CELESTONE SOLUSPAN Injectable Suspension and injection is then made into the joint.

Recommended Doses for Intra-articular Injection

Size of joint	Location	Dose (mL)
Very Large	Hip	1.0–2.0
Large	Knee, Ankle, Shoulder	1.0
Medium	Elbow, Wrist	0.5–1.0
Small (Metacarpophalangeal, interphalangeal) (Sternoclavicular)	Hand Chest	0.25–0.5

A portion of the administered dose of CELESTONE SOLUSPAN Injectable Suspension is absorbed systemically following intra-articular injection. In patients being treated concomitantly with oral or parenteral corticosteroids, especially those receiving large doses, the systemic absorption of the drug should be considered in determining intra-articular dosage.

Dermatologic conditions. In intralesional treatment, 0.2 mL/sq cm of CELESTONE SOLUSPAN Injectable Suspension is injected intradermally (not subcutaneously) using a tuberculin syringe with a 25-gauge, $^1/_2$-inch needle. Care should be taken to deposit a uniform depot of medication intradermally. A total of no more than 1.0 mL at weekly intervals is recommended.

Disorders of the foot. A tuberculin syringe with a 25-gauge, $^3/_4$-inch needle is suitable for most injections into the foot. The following doses are recommended at intervals of 3 days to a week.

Diagnosis	CELESTONE SOLUSPAN Injectable Suspension Dose (mL)
Bursitis	
under heloma durum or heloma molle	0.25–0.5
under calcaneal spur	0.5
over hallux rigidus or digiti quinti varus	0.5
Tenosynovitis, periostitis of cuboid	0.5
Acute gouty arthritis	0.5–1.0

HOW SUPPLIED

CELESTONE SOLUSPAN Injectable Suspension, 5 mL multiple-dose vial; box of one (NDC 0085-0566-05).

Shake well before using.
Store between 2° and 25°C (36° and 77°F).
Protect from light.
Schering Corporation
Kenilworth, NJ 07033 USA
Copyright © 1969, 1996, Schering Corporation.
All rights reserved.
Rev. 3/96 10229790

CLARITIN® ℞
brand of loratadine
TABLETS, SYRUP, and
RAPIDLY-DISINTEGRATING TABLETS

DESCRIPTION

Loratadine is a white to off-white powder not soluble in water, but very soluble in acetone, alcohol, and chloroform. It has a molecular weight of 382.89, and empirical formula of $C_{22}H_{23}ClN_2O_2$; its chemical name is ethyl 4-(8-chloro-5,6-dihydro-11*H*-benzo[5,6]cyclohepta[1,2-*b*]pyridin-11-ylidene)-1-piperidinecarboxylate and has the following structural formula:

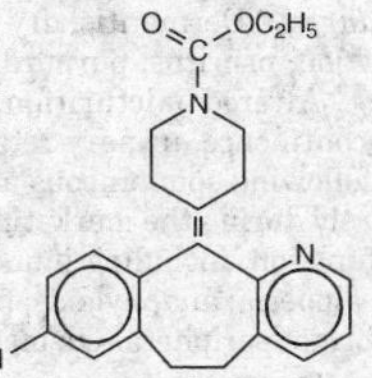

CLARITIN Tablets contain 10 mg micronized loratadine, an antihistamine, to be administered orally. They also contain the following inactive ingredients: corn starch, lactose, and magnesium stearate.

CLARITIN Syrup contains 1 mg/mL micronized loratadine, an antihistamine, to be administered orally. It also contains the following inactive ingredients: citric acid, artificial flavor, glycerin, propylene glycol, sodium benzoate, sugar, and water. The pH is between 2.5 and 3.1.

CLARITIN REDITABS (loratadine rapidly-disintegrating tablets) contain 10 mg micronized loratadine, an antihistamine, to be administered orally. It disintegrates in the mouth within seconds after placement on the tongue, allowing its contents to be subsequently swallowed with or without water. CLARITIN REDITABS (loratadine rapidly-disintegrating tablets) also contain the following inactive ingredients: citric acid, gelatin, mannitol, and mint flavor.

CLINICAL PHARMACOLOGY

Loratadine is a long-acting tricyclic antihistamine with selective peripheral histamine H_1-receptor antagonistic activity.

Human histamine skin wheal studies following single and repeated 10 mg oral doses of CLARITIN have shown that the drug exhibits an antihistaminic effect beginning within 1 to 3 hours, reaching a maximum at 8 to 12 hours, and lasting in excess of 24 hours. There was no evidence of tolerance to this effect after 28 days of dosing with CLARITIN.

Whole body autoradiographic studies in rats and monkeys, radiolabeled tissue distribution studies in mice and rats, and *in vivo* radioligand studies in mice have shown that neither loratadine nor its metabolites readily cross the blood-brain barrier. Radioligand binding studies with guinea pig pulmonary and brain H_1-receptors indicate that there was preferential binding to peripheral versus central nervous system H_1-receptors.

Repeated application of CLARITIN REDITABS (loratadine rapidly-disintegrating tablets) to the hamster cheek pouch did not cause local irritation.

Pharmacokinetics: Loratadine was rapidly absorbed following oral administration of 10 mg tablets, once daily for 10 days to healthy adult volunteers with times to maximum concentration (T_{max}) of 1.3 hours for loratadine and 2.5 hours for its major active metabolite, descarboethoxylortadine. Based on a cross-study comparison of single doses of loratadine syrup and tablets given to healthy adult volunteers, the plasma concentration profile of descarboethoxyloratadine for the two formulations is comparable. The pharmacokinetics of loratadine and descarboethoxyloratadine are independent of dose over the dose range of 10 to 40 mg and are not altered by the duration of treatment. In a single-dose study, food increased the systemic bioavailability (AUC) of loratadine and descarboethoxyloratadine by approximately 40% and 15%, respectively. The time to peak plasma concentration (T_{max}) of loratadine and descarboethoxyloratadine was delayed by 1 hour. Peak plasma concentrations (C_{max}) were not affected by food.

Pharmacokinetic studies showed that CLARITIN REDITABS (loratadine rapidly-disintegrating tablets) provide plasma concentrations of loratadine and descarboethoxyloratadine similar to those achieved with CLARITIN Tablets. Following administration of 10 mg loratadine once daily for 10 days with each dosage form in a randomized crossover comparison in 24 normal adult subjects, similar mean exposures (AUC) and peak plasma concentrations (C_{max}) of loratadine were observed. CLARITIN REDITABS (loratadine rapidly-disintegrating tablets) mean AUC and C_{max} were 11% and 6% greater than that of the CLARITIN Tablet values, respectively. Descarboethoxyloratadine bioequivalence was demonstrated between the two formulations. After 10 days of dosing, mean peak plasma concentrations were attained at 1.3 hours and 2.3 hours (T_{max}) for parent and metabolite, respectively.

In a single-dose study with CLARITIN REDITABS (loratadine rapidly-disintegrating tablets), food increased the AUC of loratadine by approximately 48% and did not appreciably affect the AUC of descarboethoxyloratadine. The times to peak plasma concentration (T_{max}) of loratadine and descarboethoxyloratadine were delayed by approximately 2.4 and 3.7 hours, respectively, when food was consumed prior to CLARITIN REDITABS (loratadine rapidly-disintegrating tablets) administration. Parent and metabolite peak concentrations (C_{max}) were not affected by food.

In a single-dose study with CLARITIN REDITABS (loratadine rapidly-disintegrating tablets) in 24 subjects, the AUC of loratadine was increased by 26% when administered without water compared to administration with water, while C_{max} was not substantially affected. The bioavailability of descarboethoxyloratadine was not different when administered without water.

Approximately 80% of the total loratadine dose administered can be found equally distributed between urine and feces in the form of metabolic products within 10 days. In nearly all patients, exposure (AUC) to the metabolite is greater than to the parent loratadine. The mean elimination half-lives in normal adult subjects (n = 54) were 8.4 hours (range = 3 to 20 hours) for loratadine and 28 hours (range = 8.8 to 92 hours) for descarboethoxyloratadine. Loratadine and descarboethoxyloratadine reached steady-state in most patients by approximately the fifth dosing day. There was considerable variability in the pharmacokinetic data in all studies of CLARITIN Tablets and Syrup, probably due to the extensive first-pass metabolism.

In vitro studies with human liver microsomes indicate that loratadine is metabolized to descarboethoxyloratadine predominantly by cytochrome P450 3A4 (CYP3A4) and, to a lesser extent, by cytochrome P450 2D6 (CYP2D6). In the presence of a CYP3A4 inhibitor ketoconazole, loratadine is metabolized to descarboethoxyloratadine predominantly by CYP2D6. Concurrent administration of loratadine with either ketoconazole, erythromycin (both CYP3A4 inhibitors), or cimetidine (CYP2D6 and CYP3A4 inhibitor) to healthy volunteers was associated with substantially increased plasma concentrations of loratadine (see **Drug Interactions** section).

The pharmacokinetic profile of loratadine in children in the 6- to 12-year age group is similar to that of adults. In a single-dose pharmacokinetic study of 13 pediatric volunteers (aged 8–12 years) given 10 mL of CLARITIN Syrup containing 10 mg loratadine, the ranges of individual subject values of pharmacokinetic parameters (AUC and C_{max}) were comparable to those following administration of a 10 mg tablet or syrup to adult volunteers.

Special Populations: In a study involving twelve healthy geriatric subjects (66 to 78 years old), the AUC and peak plasma levels (C_{max}) of both loratadine and descarboethoxyloratadine were approximately 50% greater than those observed in studies of younger subjects. The mean elimination half-lives for the geriatric subjects were 18.2 hours (range = 6.7 to 37 hours) for loratadine and 17.5 hours (range = 11 to 38 hours) for descarboethoxyloratadine.

In a study involving 12 subjects with chronic renal impairment (creatinine clearance ≤ 30 mL/min) both AUC and C_{max} increased by approximately 73% for loratadine and by 120% for descarboethoxyloratadine, as compared to 6 subjects with normal renal function (creatinine clearance ≥ 80 mL/min). The mean elimination half-lives of loratadine (7.6 hours) and descarboethoxyloratadine (23.9 hours) were not substantially different from that observed in normal subjects. Hemodialysis does not have an effect on the pharmacokinetics of loratadine or descarboethoxyloratadine in subjects with chronic renal impairment.

In seven patients with chronic alcoholic liver disease, the AUC and C_{max} of loratadine were double while the pharmacokinetic profile of descarboethoxyloratadine was not substantially different from that observed in other trials enrolling normal subjects. The elimination half-lives for loratadine and descarboethoxyloratadine were 24 hours and 37 hours, respectively, and increased with increasing severity of liver disease.

Clinical Trials: Clinical trials of CLARITIN Tablets involved over 10,700 patients, 12 years of age and older, who received either CLARITIN Tablets or another antihistamine and/or placebo in double-blind randomized controlled studies. In placebo-controlled trials, 10 mg once daily of CLARITIN Tablets was superior to placebo and similar to clemastine (1 mg BID) or terfenadine (60 mg BID) in effects on nasal and non-nasal symptoms of allergic rhinitis. In these studies somnolence occurred less frequently with CLARITIN Tablets than with clemastine and at about the same frequency as terfenadine or placebo. In studies with CLARITIN Tablets at doses 2 to 4 times higher than the recommended dose of 10 mg, a dose-related increase in the incidence of somnolence was observed. Therefore, some patients, particularly those with hepatic or renal impairment and the elderly, or those on medications that impair clearance of loratadine and its metabolites may experience somnolence. In addition, three placebo-controlled, double-blind, 2-week trials in 188 pediatric patients with seasonal allergic rhinitis aged 6 to 12 years, were conducted at doses of CLARITIN Syrup up to 10 mg once daily.

Clinical trials of CLARITIN REDITABS (loratadine rapidly-disintegrating tablets) involved over 1300 patients who received either CLARITIN REDITABS (loratadine rapidly-disintegrating tablets), CLARITIN Tablets, or placebo. In placebo-controlled trials, one CLARITIN REDITABS (loratadine rapidly-disintegrating tablets) once daily was superior to placebo and similar to CLARITIN Tablets in effects on nasal and non-nasal symptoms of seasonal allergic rhinitis.

Among those patients involved in double-blind, randomized, controlled studies of CLARITIN Tablets, approximately 1000 patients (age 12 and older), were enrolled in studies of chronic idiopathic urticaria. In placebo-controlled clinical trials, CLARITIN Tablets 10 mg once daily were superior to placebo in the management of chronic idiopathic urticaria, as demonstrated by reduction of associated itching, erythema, and hives. In these studies, the incidence of somnolence seen with CLARITIN Tablets was similar to that seen with placebo.

In a study in which CLARITIN Tablets were administered to adults at 4 times the clinical dose for 90 days, no clinically significant increase in the QT_c was seen on ECGs.

In a single-rising dose study in which doses up to 160 mg (16 times the clinical dose) were studied, loratadine did not cause any clinically significant changes on the QT_c interval in ECGs.

INDICATIONS AND USAGE

CLARITIN is indicated for the relief of nasal and non-nasal symptoms of seasonal allergic rhinitis and for the treatment of chronic idiopathic urticaria in patients 6 years of age or older.

CONTRAINDICATIONS

CLARITIN is contraindicated in patients who are hypersensitive to this medication or to any of its ingredients.

PRECAUTIONS

General: Patients with liver impairment or renal insufficiency (GFR < 30 mL/min) should be given a lower initial dose (10 mg every other day). (See **CLINICAL PHARMACOLOGY: Special Populations**).

Drug Interactions: Loratadine (10 mg once daily) has been coadministered with therapeutic doses of erythromycin, cimetidine, and ketoconazole in controlled clinical pharmacology studies in adult volunteers. Although increased plasma concentrations (AUC 0–24 hrs) of loratadine and/or descarboethoxyloratadine were observed following coadministration of loratadine with each of these drugs in normal volunteers (n = 24 in each study), there were no clinically relevant changes in the safety profile of loratadine, as assessed by electrocardiographic parameters, clinical laboratory tests, vital signs, and adverse events. There were no significant effects on QT_c intervals, and no reports of sedation or syncope. No effects on plasma concentrations of cimetidine or ketoconazole were observed. Plasma concentrations (AUC 0–24 hrs) of erythromycin decreased 15% with coadministration of loratadine relative to that observed with erythromycin alone. The clinical relevance of this difference is unknown. These above findings are summarized in the following table:

Effects on Plasma Concentrations (AUC 0-24 hrs) of Loratadine and Descarboethoxyloratadine After 10 Days of Coadministration (Loratadine 10 mg) in Normal Volunteers

	Loratadine	Descarbo-ethoxyloratadine
Erythromycin (500 mg Q8h)	+ 40%	+46%
Cimetidine (300 mg QID)	+103%	+ 6%
Ketoconazole (200 mg Q12h)	+307%	+73%

There does not appear to be an increase in adverse events in subjects who received oral contraceptives and loratadine.

Continued on next page

Information on Schering products appearing on these pages is effective as of August 15, 1998.

Claritin—Cont.

Carcinogenesis, Mutagenesis, and Impairment of Fertility: In an 18-month carcinogenicity study in mice and a 2-year study in rats, loratadine was administered in the diet at doses up to 40 mg/kg (mice) and 25 mg/kg (rats). In the carcinogenicity studies, pharmacokinetic assessments were carried out to determine animal exposure to the drug. AUC data demonstrated that the exposure of mice given 40 mg/kg of loratadine was 3.6 (loratadine) and 18 (descarboethoxyloratadine) times higher than in humans given the maximum recommended daily oral dose. Exposure of rats given 25 mg/kg of loratadine was 28 (loratadine) and 67 (descarboethoxyloratadine) times higher than in humans given the maximum recommended daily oral dose. Male mice given 40 mg/kg had a significantly higher incidence of hepatocellular tumors (combined adenomas and carcinomas) than concurrent controls. In rats, a significantly higher incidence of hepatocellular tumors (combined adenomas and carcinomas) was observed in males given 10 mg/kg and males and females given 25 mg/kg. The clinical significance of these findings during long-term use of CLARITIN is not known.

In mutagenicity studies, there was no evidence of mutagenic potential in reverse (Ames) or forward point mutation (CHO-HGPRT) assays, or in the assay for DNA damage (rat primary hepatocyte unscheduled DNA assay) or in two assays for chromosomal aberrations (human peripheral blood lymphocyte clastogenesis assay and the mouse bone marrow erythrocyte micronucleus assay). In the mouse lymphoma assay, a positive finding occurred in the nonactivated but not the activated phase of the study.

Decreased fertility in male rats, shown by lower female conception rates, occurred at an oral dose of 64 mg/kg (approximately 50 times the maximum recommended human daily oral dose on a mg/m^2 basis) and was reversible with cessation of dosing. Loratadine had no effect on male or female fertility or reproduction in the rat at an oral dose of approximately 24 mg/kg (approximately 20 times the maximum recommended human daily oral dose on a mg/m^2 basis).

Pregnancy Category B: There was no evidence of animal teratogenicity in studies performed in rats and rabbits at oral doses up to 96 mg/kg (approximately 75 times and 150 times, respectively, the maximum recommended human daily oral dose on a mg/m^2 basis). There are, however, no adequate and well-controlled studies in pregnant women. Because animal reproduction studies are not always predictive of human response, CLARITIN should be used during pregnancy only if clearly needed.

Nursing Mothers: Loratadine and its metabolite, descarboethoxyloratadine, pass easily into breast milk and achieve concentrations that are equivalent to plasma levels with an AUC$_{milk}$/AUC$_{plasma}$ ratio of 1.17 and 0.85 for loratadine and descarboethoxyloratadine, respectively. Following a single oral dose of a 40 mg, a small amount of loratadine and descarboethoxyloratadine was excreted into the breast milk (approximately 0.03% of 40 mg over 48 hours). A decision should be made whether to discontinue nursing or to discontinue the drug, taking into account the importance of the drug to the mother. Caution should be exercised when CLARITIN is administered to a nursing woman.

Pediatric Use: The safety of CLARITIN Syrup at a daily dose of 10 mg has been demonstrated in 188 pediatric patients 6–12 years of age in placebo-controlled 2-week trials. The effectiveness of CLARITIN for the treatment of seasonal allergic rhinitis and chronic idiopathic urticaria in this pediatric age group is based on an extrapolation of the demonstrated efficacy of CLARITIN in adults in these conditions and the likelihood that the disease course, pathophysiology, and the drug's effect are substantially similar to that of the adults. The recommended dose for the pediatric population is based on cross-study comparison of the pharmacokinetics of CLARITIN in adults and pediatric subjects and on the safety profile of loratadine in both adults and pediatric patients at doses equal to or higher than the recommended doses. The safety and effectiveness of CLARITIN in pediatric patients under 6 years of age have not been established.

ADVERSE REACTIONS

CLARITIN Tablets: Approximately 90,000 patients, aged 12 and older, received CLARITIN Tablets 10 mg once daily in controlled and uncontrolled studies. Placebo-controlled clinical trials at the recommended dose of 10 mg once a day varied from 2 weeks' to 6 months' duration. The rate of premature withdrawal from these trials was approximately 2% in both the treated and placebo groups.

[See first table below]

Adverse events reported in placebo-controlled chronic idiopathic urticaria trials were similar to those reported in allergic rhinitis studies.

Adverse event rates did not appear to differ significantly based on age, sex, or race, although the number of nonwhite subjects was relatively small.

CLARITIN REDITABS (loratadine rapidly-disintegrating tablets): Approximately 500 patients received CLARITIN REDITABS (loratadine rapidly-disintegrating tablets) in controlled clinical trials of 2 weeks' duration. In these studies, adverse events were similar in type and frequency to those seen with CLARITIN Tablets and placebo.

Administration of CLARITIN REDITABS (loratadine rapidly-disintegrating tablets) did not result in an increased reporting frequency of mouth or tongue irritation.

CLARITIN Syrup: Approximately 300 pediatric patients 6 to 12 years of age received 10 mg loratadine once daily in controlled clinical trials for a period of 8–15 days. Among these, 188 children were treated with 10 mg loratadine syrup once daily in placebo-controlled trials. Adverse events in these pediatric patients were observed to occur with type and frequency similar to those seen in the adult population. The rate of premature discontinuance due to adverse events among pediatric patients receiving loratadine 10 mg daily was less than 1%.

[See second table below]

In addition to those adverse events reported above (≥2%), the following adverse events have been reported in at least one patient in CLARITIN clinical trials in adult and pediatric patients:

Autonomic Nervous System: Altered lacrimation, altered salivation, flushing, hypoesthesia, impotence, increased sweating, thirst.
Body As A Whole: Angioneurotic edema, asthenia, back pain, blurred vision, chest pain, earache, eye pain, fever, leg cramps, malaise, rigors, tinnitus, viral infection, weight gain.
Cardiovascular System: Hypertension, hypotension, palpitations, supraventricular tachyarrhythmias, syncope, tachycardia.
Central and Peripheral Nervous System: Blepharospasm, dizziness, dysphonia, hypertonia, migraine, paresthesia, tremor, vertigo.
Gastrointestinal System: Altered taste, anorexia, constipation, diarrhea, dyspepsia, flatulence, gastritis, hiccup, increased appetite, nausea, stomatitis, toothache, vomiting.
Musculoskeletal System: Arthralgia, myalgia.
Psychiatric: Agitation, amnesia, anxiety, confusion, decreased libido, depression, impaired concentration, insomnia, irritability, paroniria.
Reproductive System: Breast pain, dysmenorrhea, menorrhagia, vaginitis.
Respiratory System: Bronchitis, bronchospasm, coughing, dyspnea, epistaxis, hemoptysis, laryngitis, nasal dryness, pharyngitis, sinusitis, sneezing.
Skin and Appendages: Dermatitis, dry hair, dry skin, photosensitivity reaction, pruritus, purpura, rash, urticaria.
Urinary System: Altered micturition, urinary discoloration, urinary incontinence, urinary retention.
In addition, the following spontaneous adverse events have been reported rarely during the marketing of loratadine: abnormal hepatic function, including jaundice, hepatitis, and hepatic necrosis; alopecia; anaphylaxis; breast enlargement; erythema multiforme; peripheral edema; and seizures.

DRUG ABUSE AND DEPENDENCE

There is no information to indicate that abuse or dependency occurs with CLARITIN.

OVERDOSAGE

In adults, somnolence, tachycardia, and headache have been reported with overdoses greater than 10 mg with the Tablet formulation (40 to 180 mg). Extrapyramidal signs and palpitations have been reported in children with overdoses of greater than 10 mg of CLARITIN Syrup. In the event of overdosage, general symptomatic and supportive measures should be instituted promptly and maintained for as long as necessary.

Treatment of overdosage would reasonably consist of emesis (ipecac syrup), except in patients with impaired consciousness, followed by the administration of activated charcoal to absorb any remaining drug. If vomiting is unsuccessful, or contraindicated, gastric lavage should be performed with normal saline. Saline cathartics may also be of value for rapid dilution of bowel contents. Loratadine is not eliminated by hemodialysis. It is not known if loratadine is eliminated by peritoneal dialysis.

No deaths occurred at oral doses up to 5000 mg/kg in rats and mice (greater than 2400 and 1200 times, respectively, the maximum recommended human daily oral dose on a mg/m^2 basis). Single oral doses of loratadine showed no effects in rats, mice, and monkeys at doses as high as 10 times the maximum recommended human daily oral dose on a mg/m^2 basis.

DOSAGE AND ADMINISTRATION

Adults and children 12 years of age and over: The recommended dose of CLARITIN is 10 mg once daily.

Children 6–11 years of age: The recommended dose of CLARITIN is 10 mg (2 teaspoonfuls) once daily.

In patients with liver failure or renal insufficiency (GFR <30 mL/min), one tablet or two teaspoonfuls every other day should be the starting dose.

Administration of CLARITIN REDITABS (loratadine rapidly-disintegrating tablets): Place CLARITIN REDITABS (loratadine rapidly-disintegrating tablets) on the tongue. Tablet disintegration occurs rapidly. Administer with or without water.

HOW SUPPLIED

CLARITIN Tablets: 10 mg, white to off-white compressed tablets; impressed with the product identification number "458" on one side and "CLARITIN 10" on the other; high-density polyethylene plastic bottles of 100 (NDC 0085-0458-03) and 500 (NDC 0085-0458-06). Also available, CLARITIN Unit-of-Use packages of 14 tablets (7 tablets per blister card) (NDC 0085-0458-01) and 30 tablets (10 tablets per blister card) (NDC 0085-0458-05); and 10 x 10 tablet Unit Dose-Hospital Pack (NDC 0085-0458-04).

Protect Unit-of-Use packaging and Unit Dose-Hospital Pack from excessive moisture.

Store between 2° and 30°C (36° and 86°F).

CLARITIN Syrup: Clear, colorless to light-yellow liquid, containing 1 mg loratadine per mL; amber glass bottles of 16 fluid ounces (NDC 0085-0612-02).

Store between 2° and 25°C (36° and 77°F).

CLARITIN REDITABS (loratadine rapidly-disintegrating tablets): CLARITIN REDITABS (loratadine rapidly-disinte-

REPORTED ADVERSE EVENTS WITH AN INCIDENCE OF MORE THAN 2% IN PLACEBO-CONTROLLED ALLERGIC RHINITIS CLINICAL TRIALS IN PATIENTS 12 YEARS OF AGE AND OLDER
PERCENT OF PATIENTS REPORTING

	LORATADINE 10 mg QD n = 1926	PLACEBO n = 2545	CLEMASTINE 1 mg BID n = 536	TERFENADINE 60 mg BID n = 684
Headache	12	11	8	8
Somnolence	8	6	22	9
Fatigue	4	3	10	2
Dry Mouth	3	2	4	3

ADVERSE EVENTS OCCURRING WITH A FREQUENCY OF ≥2% IN LORATADINE SYRUP-TREATED PATIENTS (6-12 YEARS OLD) IN PLACEBO-CONTROLLED TRIALS, AND MORE FREQUENTLY THAN IN THE PLACEBO GROUP
PERCENT OF PATIENTS REPORTING

	LORATADINE 10 mg QD n = 188	PLACEBO n = 262	CHLORPHENIRAMINE 2-4 mg BID/TID n = 170
Nervousness	4	2	2
Wheezing	4	2	5
Fatigue	3	2	5
Hyperkinesia	3	1	4
Abdominal Pain	2	0	0
Conjunctivitis	2	<1	1
Dysphonia	2	<1	0
Malaise	2	0	1
Upper Respiratory Tract Infection	2	<1	0

grating tablets), 10 mg, white to off-white blister-formed tablet: Unit-of-Use polyvinyl chloride blister packages of 30 tablets (3 laminated foil pouches, each containing one blister card of 10 tablets) supplied with Patient's Instructions for Use (NDC 0085-1128-02).

Keep CLARITIN REDITABS (loratadine rapidly-disintegrating tablets) in a dry place.

Store between 2° and 25°C (36° and 77°F). Use within 6 months of opening laminated foil pouch, and immediately upon opening individual tablet blister.

Schering Corporation
Kenilworth, NJ 07033 USA
Rev. 3/98

19628426T

CLARITIN REDITABS (loratadine rapidly-disintegrating tablets) are manufactured for Schering Corporation by Scherer DDS, England.

U.S. Patent Nos. 4,282,233 and 4,371,516.

Copyright © 1997, 1998, Schering Corporation. All rights reserved.

Shown in Product Identification Guide, page 336

CLARITIN-D® 12 HOUR ℞

brand of loratadine and pseudoephedrine sulfate, USP Extended Release Tablets

CAUTION: Federal Law Prohibits Dispensing Without Prescription

DESCRIPTION

CLARITIN-D 12 HOUR Extended Release Tablets contain 5 mg loratadine in the tablet coating for immediate release and 120 mg pseudoephedrine sulfate, USP equally distributed between the tablet coating for immediate release and the barrier-coated extended release core.

Loratadine is a white to off-white powder, not soluble in water, but very soluble in acetone, alcohol, and chloroform. Loratadine has a molecular weight of 382.89 and empirical formula of $C_{22}H_{23}ClN_2O_2$; the chemical name, ethyl 4-(8-chloro-5,6-dihydro-11*H*-benzo[5,6]cyclohepta[1,2-*b*]pyridin-11-ylidene)-1-piperidinecarboxylate; and has the following chemical structure:

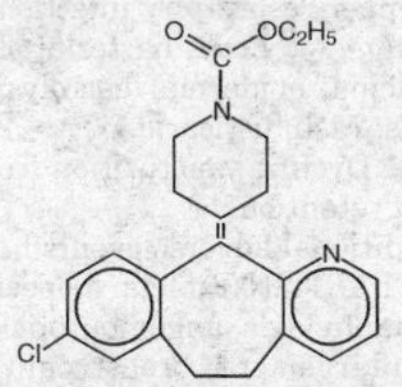

Pseudoephedrine sulfate is the synthetic salt of one of the naturally occurring dextrorotatory diastereomers of ephedrine and is classified as an indirect sympathomimetic amine. The empirical formula for pseudoephedrine sulfate is $(C_{10}H_{15}NO)_2 \cdot H_2SO_4$; the chemical name is [S-(R*,R*)]-α-[1(methylamino)ethyl] benzenemethanol sulfate (2:1) (salt), and the following chemical structure:

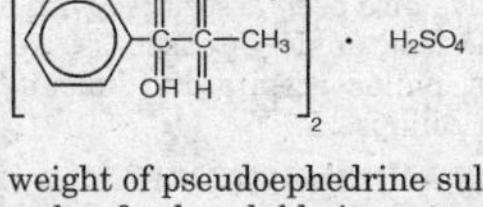

The molecular weight of pseudoephedrine sulfate is 428.54. It is a white powder, freely soluble in water and methanol and sparingly soluble in chloroform.

The inactive ingredients for CLARITIN-D 12 HOUR Extended Release Tablets are acacia, butylparaben, calcium sulfate, carnauba wax, corn starch, lactose, magnesium stearate, microcrystalline cellulose, neutral soap, oleic acid, povidone, rosin, sugar, talc, titanium dioxide, white wax, and zein.

CLINICAL PHARMACOLOGY

The following information is based upon studies of loratadine alone or pseudoephedrine alone, except as indicated.

Loratadine is a long-acting tricyclic antihistamine with selective peripheral histamine H_1-receptor antagonistic activity.

Human histamine skin wheal studies following single and repeated oral doses of loratadine have shown that the drug exhibits an antihistaminic effect beginning within 1 to 3 hours, reaching a maximum at 8 to 12 hours and lasting in excess of 24 hours. There was no evidence of tolerance to this effect developing after 28 days of dosing with loratadine.

Pharmacokinetic studies following single and multiple oral doses of loratadine in 115 volunteers showed that loratadine is rapidly absorbed and extensively metabolized to an active metabolite (descarboethoxyloratadine). Approximately 80% of the total dose administered can be found equally distributed between urine and feces in the form of metabolic products after 10 days. The mean elimination half-lives found in studies in normal adult subjects (n = 54) were 8.4 hours (range = 3 to 20 hours) for loratadine and 28 hours (range = 8.8 to 92 hours) for the major active metabolite (descarboethoxyloratadine). In nearly all patients, exposure (AUC) to the metabolite is greater than exposure to parent loratadine. Loratadine and descarboethoxyloratadine reached steady-state in most patients by approximately the fifth dosing day. The pharmacokinetics of loratadine and descarboethoxyloratadine are dose independent over the dose range of 10 to 40 mg and are not significantly altered by the duration of treatment.

In vitro studies with human liver microsomes indicate that loratadine is metabolized to descarboethoxyloratadine predominantly by P450 CYP3A4 and, to a lesser extent, by P450 CYP2D6. In the presence of a CYP3A4 inhibitor ketoconazole, loratadine is metabolized to descarboethoxyloratadine predominantly by CYP2D6. Concurrent administration of loratadine with either ketoconazole, erythromycin (both CYP3A4 inhibitors), or cimetidine (CYP2D6 and CYP3A4 inhibitor) to healthy volunteers was associated with significantly increased plasma concentrations of loratadine (see **Drug Interactions** section).

In a study involving twelve healthy geriatric subjects (66 to 78 years old), the AUC and peak plasma levels (C_{max}) of both loratadine and descarboethoxyloratadine were significantly higher (approximately 50% increased) than in studies of younger subjects. The mean elimination half-lives for the elderly subjects were 18.2 hours (range = 6.7 to 37 hours) for loratadine and 17.5 hours (range = 11 to 38 hours) for the active metabolite.

In the clinical efficacy studies, loratadine was administered before meals. In a single-dose study, food increased the AUC of loratadine by approximately 40% and of descarboethoxyloratadine by approximately 15%. The time of peak plasma concentration (T_{max}) of loratadine and descarboethoxyloratadine was delayed by 1 hour with a meal.

In patients with chronic renal impairment (creatinine clearance $\leq$ 30 mL/min) both the AUC and peak plasma levels (C_{max}) increased on average by approximately 73% for loratadine; and approximately by 120% for descarboethoxyloratadine, compared to individuals with normal renal function. The mean elimination half-lives of loratadine (7.6 hours) and descarboethoxyloratadine (23.9 hours) were not significantly different from that observed in normal subjects. Hemodialysis does not have an effect on the pharmacokinetics of loratadine or its active metabolite (descarboethoxyloratadine) in subjects with chronic renal impairment.

In patients with chronic alcoholic liver disease the AUC and peak plasma levels (C_{max}) of loratadine were double while the pharmacokinetic profile of the active metabolite (descarboethoxyloratadine) was not significantly changed from that in normals. The elimination half-lives for loratadine and descarboethoxyloratadine were 24 hours and 37 hours, respectively, and increased with increasing severity of liver disease.

There was considerable variability in the pharmacokinetic data in all studies of loratadine, probably due to the extensive first-pass metabolism. Individual histograms of area under the curve, clearance, and volume of distribution showed a log normal distribution with a 25-fold range in distribution in healthy subjects.

Loratadine is about 97% bound to plasma proteins at the expected concentrations (2.5 to 100 ng/mL) after a therapeutic dose. Loratadine does not affect the plasma protein binding of warfarin and digoxin. The metabolite descarboethoxyloratadine is 73% to 77% bound to plasma proteins (at 0.5 to 100 ng/mL).

Whole body autoradiographic studies in rats and monkeys, radiolabeled tissue distribution studies in mice and rats, and *in vivo* radioligand studies in mice have shown that neither loratadine nor its metabolites readily cross the blood-brain barrier. Radioligand binding studies with guinea pig pulmonary and brain H_1-receptors indicate that there was preferential binding to peripheral versus central nervous system H_1-receptors.

In a study in which loratadine alone was administered at four times the clinical dose for 90 days, no clinically significant increase in the QT_c was seen on ECGs.

Pseudoephedrine sulfate (d-isoephedrine sulfate) is an orally active sympathomimetic amine which exerts a decongestant action on the nasal mucosa. It is recognized as an effective agent for the relief of nasal congestion due to allergic rhinitis. Pseudoephedrine produces peripheral effects similar to those of ephedrine and central effects similar to, but less intense than, amphetamines. It has the potential for excitatory side effects.

The pseudoephedrine component of CLARITIN-D 12 HOUR Extended Release Tablets was absorbed at a similar rate and was equally available from the combination tablet as from a pseudoephedrine sulfate repetabs 120 mg tablet. Mean (%CV) steady-state peak plasma concentration of 464 ng/mL (22) was attained at 3.9 hours (50). The terminal half-life of pseudoephedrine from the combination tablet administered twice daily was 6.3 hours (23). The ingestion of food was found not to affect the absorption of pseudoephedrine from CLARITIN-D 12 HOUR Extended Release Tablets. Loratadine and pseudoephedrine sulfate do not influence the pharmacokinetics of each other when administered concomitantly.

Clinical Studies: Clinical trials of CLARITIN-D 12 HOUR Extended Release Tablets in seasonal allergic rhinitis involved approximately 3700 patients who received either the combination product, a comparative treatment, or placebo, in double-blind, randomized controlled studies. Four of the largest studies involved approximately 1600 patients in comparisons of the combination product, loratadine (5 mg bid), pseudoephedrine sulfate (120 mg bid), and placebo. Improvement in symptoms of seasonal allergic rhinitis for patients receiving CLARITIN-D 12 HOUR Extended Release Tablets was significantly greater than the improvement in those patients who received the individual components or placebo. The combination reduced the intensity of sneezing, rhinorrhea, nasal pruritus, and eye tearing more than pseudoephedrine and reduced the intensity of nasal congestion more than loratadine, demonstrating a contribution of each of the components. The onset of antihistamine and nasal decongestant actions occurred after the first dose of CLARITIN-D 12 HOUR Extended Release Tablets. CLARITIN-D 12 HOUR Extended Release Tablets were well tolerated, with a frequency of sedation similar to that seen with placebo, and an adverse event profile clinically similar to that of pseudoephedrine.

In a 6-week, placebo-controlled study of 193 patients with seasonal allergic rhinitis and concomitant mild to moderate asthma, CLARITIN-D 12 HOUR Extended Release Tablets twice daily improved seasonal allergic rhinitis signs and symptoms with no decrease in pulmonary function or adverse effect on asthma symptoms. This supports the safety of administering CLARITIN-D 12 HOUR Extended Release Tablets to seasonal allergic rhinitis patients with asthma.

INDICATIONS AND USAGE

CLARITIN-D 12 HOUR Extended Release Tablets are indicated for the relief of symptoms of seasonal allergic rhinitis. CLARITIN-D 12 HOUR Extended Release Tablets should be administered when both the antihistaminic properties of CLARITIN (loratadine) and the nasal decongestant activity of pseudoephedrine are desired (see **CLINICAL PHARMACOLOGY**).

CONTRAINDICATIONS

CLARITIN-D 12 HOUR Extended Release Tablets are contraindicated in patients who are hypersensitive to this medication or to any of its ingredients.

This product, due to its pseudoephedrine component, is contraindicated in patients with narrow-angle glaucoma or urinary retention, and in patients receiving monoamine oxidase (MAO) inhibitor therapy or within fourteen (14) days of stopping such treatment (see **Drug Interactions** section). It is also contraindicated in patients with severe hypertension, severe coronary artery disease, and in those who have shown hypersensitivity or idiosyncrasy to its components, to adrenergic agents, or to other drugs of similar chemical structures. Manifestations of patient idiosyncrasy to adrenergic agents include: insomnia, dizziness, weakness, tremor, or arrhythmias.

WARNINGS

CLARITIN-D 12 HOUR Extended Release Tablets should be used with caution in patients with hypertension, diabetes mellitus, ischemic heart disease, increased intraocular pressure, hyperthyroidism, renal impairment, or prostatic hypertrophy. Central nervous system stimulation with convulsions or cardiovascular collapse with accompanying hypotension may be produced by sympathomimetic amines.

Use in Patients Approximately 60 years and Older: The safety and efficacy of CLARITIN-D 12 HOUR Extended Release Tablets in patients greater than 60 years old have not been investigated in placebo-controlled clinical trials. The elderly are more likely to have adverse reactions to sympathomimetic amines.

PRECAUTIONS

General: Because the doses of this fixed combination product cannot be individually titrated and hepatic insufficiency results in a reduced clearance of loratadine to a much greater extent than pseudoephedrine, CLARITIN-D 12 HOUR Extended Release Tablets should generally be avoided in patients with hepatic insufficiency. Patients with renal insufficiency (GFR < 30 mL/min) should be given a lower initial dose (one tablet per day) because they have reduced clearance of loratadine and pseudoephedrine.

Information for Patients: Patients taking CLARITIN-D 12 HOUR Extended Release Tablets should receive the fol-

Continued on next page

Information on Schering products appearing on these pages is effective as of August 15, 1998.

Claritin-D 12 Hour—Cont.

lowing information: CLARITIN-D 12 HOUR Extended Release Tablets are prescribed for the relief of symptoms of seasonal allergic rhinitis. Patients should be instructed to take CLARITIN-D 12 HOUR Extended Release Tablets only as prescribed and not to exceed the prescribed dose. Patients should also be advised against the concurrent use of CLARITIN-D 12 HOUR Extended Release Tablets with over-the-counter antihistamines and decongestants.
This product should not be used by patients who are hypersensitive to it or to any of its ingredients. Due to its pseudoephedrine component, this product should not be used by patients with narrow-angle glaucoma, urinary retention, or by patients receiving a monoamine oxidase (MAO) inhibitor or within 14 days of stopping use of an MAO inhibitor. It also should not be used by patients with severe hypertension or severe coronary artery disease.
Patients who are or may become pregnant should be told that this product should be used in pregnancy or during lactation only if the potential benefit justifies the potential risk to the fetus or nursing infant.
Patients should be instructed not to break or chew the tablet.

Drug Interactions: No specific interaction studies have been conducted with CLARITIN-D 12 HOUR Extended Release Tablets. However, loratadine (10 mg once daily) has been safely coadministered with therapeutic doses of erythromycin, cimetidine, and ketoconazole in controlled clinical pharmacology studies. Although increased plasma concentrations (AUC 0–24 hrs) of loratadine and/or descarboethoxyloratadine were observed following coadministration of loratadine with each of these drugs in normal volunteers (n = 24 in each study), there were no clinically relevant changes in the safety profile of loratadine, as assessed by electrocardiographic parameters, clinical laboratory tests, vital signs, and adverse events. There were no significant effects on QT_c intervals, and no reports of sedation or syncope. No effects on plasma concentrations of cimetidine or ketoconazole were observed. Plasma concentrations (AUC 0–24 hrs) of erythromycin decreased 15% with coadministration of loratadine relative to that observed with erythromycin alone. The clinical relevance of this difference is unknown. These above findings are summarized in the following table:

Effects on Plasma Concentrations (AUC 0—24 hrs) of Loratadine and Descarboethoxyloratadine After 10 Days of Coadministration (Loratadine 10 mg) in Normal Volunteers

	Loratadine	Descarboethoxyloratadine
Erythromycin (500 mg Q8h)	+ 40%	+46%
Cimetidine (300 mg QID)	+103%	+ 6%
Ketoconazole (200 mg Q12h)	+307%	+73%

There does not appear to be an increase in adverse events in subjects who received oral contraceptives and loratadine.
CLARITIN-D 12 HOUR Extended Release Tablets (pseudoephedrine component) are contraindicated in patients taking monoamine oxidase inhibitors and for 2 weeks after stopping use of an MAO inhibitor. The antihypertensive effects of beta-adrenergic blocking agents, methyldopa, mecamylamine, reserpine, and veratrum alkaloids may be reduced by sympathomimetics. Increased ectopic pacemaker activity can occur when pseudoephedrine is used concomitantly with digitalis.

Drug/Laboratory Test Interactions: The *in vitro* addition of pseudoephedrine to sera containing the cardiac isoenzyme MB of serum creatinine phosphokinase progressively inhibits the activity of the enzyme. The inhibition becomes complete over 6 hours.

Carcinogenesis, Mutagenesis, Impairment of Fertility: There are no animal or laboratory studies on the combination product loratadine and pseudoephedrine sulfate to evaluate carcinogenesis, mutagenesis, or impairment of fertility.
In an 18-month oncogenicity study in mice and a 2-year study in rats loratadine was administered in the diet at doses up to 40 mg/kg (mice) and 25 mg/kg (rats). In the carcinogenicity studies pharmacokinetic assessments were carried out to determine animal exposure to the drug. AUC data demonstrated that the exposure of mice given 40 mg/kg of loratadine was 3.6 (loratadine) and 18 (active metabolite) times higher than a human given 10 mg/day. Exposure of rats given 25 mg/kg of loratadine was 28 (loratadine) and 67 (active metabolite) times higher than a human given 10 mg/day. Male mice given 40 mg/kg had a significantly higher incidence of hepatocellular tumors (combined adenomas and carcinomas) than concurrent controls. In rats, a significantly higher incidence of hepatocellular tumors (combined adenomas and carcinomas) was observed in males given 10 mg/kg and males and females given 25 mg/kg. The clinical significance of these findings during long-term use of loratadine is not known.
In mutagenicity studies with loratadine alone, there was no evidence of mutagenic potential in reverse (Ames) or forward point mutation (CHO-HGPRT) assays, or in the assay for DNA damage (Rat Primary Hepatocyte Unscheduled DNA Assay) or in two assays for chromosomal aberrations (Human Peripheral Blood Lymphocyte Clastogenesis Assay and the Mouse Bone Marrow Erythrocyte Micronucleus Assay). In the Mouse Lymphoma Assay, a positive finding occurred in the nonactivated but not the activated phase of the study.
Loratadine administration produced hepatic microsomal enzyme induction in the mouse at 40 mg/kg and rat at 25 mg/kg, but not at lower doses.
Decreased fertility in male rats, shown by lower female conception rates, occurred at approximately 64 mg/kg of loratadine and was reversible with cessation of dosing. Loratadine had no effect on male or female fertility or reproduction in the rat at doses approximately 24 mg/kg.

Pregnancy Category B: There was no evidence of animal teratogenicity in reproduction studies performed on rats and rabbits with this combination at oral doses up to 150 mg/kg (885 mg/m^2 or 5 times the recommended daily human dosage of 250 mg or 185 mg/m^2), and 120 mg/kg (1416 mg/m^2 or 8 times the recommended daily human dosage), respectively. There are, however, no adequate and well-controlled studies in pregnant women. Because animal reproduction studies are not always predictive of human response, CLARITIN-D 12 HOUR Extended Release Tablets should be used during pregnancy only if clearly needed.

Nursing Mothers: It is not known if this combination product is excreted in human milk. However, loratadine when administered alone and its metabolite descarboethoxyloratadine pass easily into breast milk and achieve concentrations that are equivalent to plasma levels, with an AUC_{milk}/AUC_{plasma} ratio of 1.17 and 0.85 for the parent and active metabolite, respectively. Following a single oral dose of 40 mg, a small amount of loratadine and metabolite was excreted into the breast milk (approximately 0.03% of 40 mg after 48 hours). Pseudoephedrine administered alone also distributes into breast milk of the lactating human female. Pseudoephedrine concentrations in milk are consistently higher than those in plasma. The total amount of drug in milk as judged by the area under the curve (AUC) is 2 to 3 times greater than in plasma. The fraction of a pseudoephedrine dose excreted in milk is estimated to be 0.4% to 0.7%. A decision should be made whether to discontinue nursing or to discontinue the drug, taking into account the importance of the drug to the mother. Caution should be exercised when CLARITIN-D 12 HOUR Extended Release Tablets are administered to a nursing woman.

Pediatric Use: Safety and effectiveness in children below the age of 12 years have not been established.

ADVERSE REACTIONS

Experience from controlled and uncontrolled clinical studies involving approximately 10,000 patients who received the combination of loratadine and pseudoephedrine sulfate for a period of up to 1 month provides information on adverse reactions. The usual dose was one tablet every 12 hours for up to 28 days.
In controlled clinical trials using the recommended dose of one tablet every 12 hours, the incidence of reported adverse events was similar to those reported with placebo, with the exception of insomnia (16%) and dry mouth (14%).
[See table below]

REPORTED ADVERSE EVENTS WITH AN INCIDENCE OF ≥2% ON CLARITIN-D 12 HOUR EXTENDED RELEASE TABLETS IN PLACEBO-CONTROLLED CLINICAL TRIALS PERCENT OF PATIENTS REPORTING

	CLARITIN-D® 12 HOUR n=1023	Loratadine n=543	Pseudo-ephedrine n=548	Placebo n=922
Headache	19	18	17	19
Insomnia	16	4	19	3
Dry Mouth	14	4	9	3
Somnolence	7	8	5	4
Nervousness	5	3	7	2
Dizziness	4	1	5	2
Fatigue	4	6	3	3
Dyspepsia	3	2	3	1
Nausea	3	2	3	2
Pharyngitis	3	3	2	3
Anorexia	2	1	2	1
Thirst	2	1	2	1

Adverse event rates did not appear to differ significantly based on age, sex, or race, although the number of nonwhite subjects was relatively small.
In addition to those adverse events reported above (≥2%), the following less frequent adverse events have been reported in at least one patient treated with CLARITIN-D 12 HOUR Extended Release Tablets:
Autonomic Nervous System: Abnormal lacrimation, dehydration, flushing, hypoesthesia, increased sweating, mydriasis.
Body As A Whole: Asthenia, back pain, blurred vision, chest pain, conjunctivitis, earache, ear infection, eye pain, fever, flu-like symptoms, leg cramps, lymphadenopathy, malaise, photophobia, rigors, tinnitus, viral infection, weight gain.
Cardiovascular System: Hypertension, hypotension, palpitations, peripheral edema, syncope, tachycardia, ventricular extrasystoles.
Central and Peripheral Nervous System: Dysphonia, hyperkinesia, hypertonia, migraine, paresthesia, tremors, vertigo.
Gastrointestinal System: Abdominal distension, abdominal distress, abdominal pain, altered taste, constipation, diarrhea, eructation, flatulence, gastritis, gingival bleeding, hemorrhoids, increased appetite, stomatitis, taste loss, tongue discoloration, toothache, vomiting.
Liver and Biliary System: Hepatic function abnormal.
Musculoskeletal System: Arthralgia, myalgia, torticollis.
Psychiatric: Aggressive reaction, agitation, anxiety, apathy, confusion, decreased libido, depression, emotional lability, euphoria, impaired concentration, irritability, paroniria.
Reproductive System: Dysmenorrhea, impotence, intermenstrual bleeding, vaginitis.
Respiratory System: Bronchitis, bronchospasm, chest congestion, coughing, dry throat, dyspnea, epistaxis, halitosis, nasal congestion, nasal irritation, sinusitis, sneezing, sputum increased, upper respiratory infection, wheezing.
Skin and Appendages: Acne, bacterial skin infection, dry skin, eczema, edema, epidermal necrolysis, erythema, hematoma, pruritus, rash, urticaria.
Urinary System: Dysuria, micturition frequency, nocturia, polyuria, urinary retention.
The following additional adverse events have been reported with the use of CLARITIN Tablets: alopecia, altered salivation, amnesia, anaphylaxis, angioneurotic edema, blepharospasm, breast enlargement, breast pain, dermatitis, dry hair, erythema multiforme, hemoptysis, hepatic necrosis, hepatitis, jaundice, laryngitis, menorrhagia, nasal dryness, photosensitivity reaction, purpura, seizures, supraventricular tachyarrhythmias, and urinary discoloration.
Pseudoephedrine may cause mild CNS stimulation in hypersensitive patients. Nervousness, excitability, restlessness, dizziness, weakness, or insomnia may occur. Headache, drowsiness, tachycardia, palpitation, pressor activity, and cardiac arrhythmias have been reported. Sympathomimetic drugs have also been associated with other untoward effects, such as fear, anxiety, tenseness, tremor, hallucinations, seizures, pallor, respiratory difficulty, dysuria, and cardiovascular collapse.

DRUG ABUSE AND DEPENDENCE

There is no information to indicate that abuse or dependency occurs with loratadine or the combination of loratadine and pseudoephedrine. Pseudoephedrine, like other central nervous system stimulants, has been abused. At high doses, subjects commonly experience an elevation of mood, a sense of increased energy and alertness, and decreased appetite. Some individuals become anxious, irritable, and loquacious. In addition to the marked euphoria, the user experiences a sense of markedly enhanced physical strength and mental capacity. With continued use, tolerance develops, the user increases the dose, and toxic signs and symptoms appear. Depression may follow rapid withdrawal.

OVERDOSAGE

In the event of overdosage, general symptomatic and supportive measures should be instituted promptly and maintained for as long as necessary. Treatment of overdosage would reasonably consist of emesis (ipecac syrup), except in patients with impaired consciousness, followed by the administration of activated charcoal to absorb any remaining drug. If vomiting is unsuccessful, or contraindicated, gastric lavage should be performed with normal saline. Saline cathartics may also be of value for rapid dilution of bowel contents. Loratadine is not eliminated by hemodialysis. It is not known if loratadine is eliminated by peritoneal dialysis. Somnolence, tachycardia, and headache have been reported with doses of 40 to 180 mg of CLARITIN Tablets. In large

doses, sympathomimetics may give rise to giddiness, headache, nausea, vomiting, sweating, thirst, tachycardia, precordial pain, palpitations, difficulty in micturition, muscular weakness and tenseness, anxiety, restlessness, and insomnia. Many patients can present a toxic psychosis with delusions and hallucinations. Some may develop cardiac arrhythmias, circulatory collapse, convulsions, coma, and respiratory failure.

The oral LD_{50} values for the mixture of the two drugs were greater than 525 and 1839 mg/kg in mice and rats, respectively. Oral LD_{50} values for loratadine were greater than 5000 mg/kg in rats and mice. Doses of loratadine as high as 10 times the recommended daily clinical dose showed no effect in rats, mice, and monkeys.

DOSAGE AND ADMINISTRATION

Adults and children 12 years of age and over: one tablet twice a day (every 12 hours). Because the doses of this fixed combination product cannot be individually titrated and hepatic insufficiency results in a reduced clearance of loratadine to a much greater extent than pseudoephedrine, CLARITIN-D 12 HOUR Extended Release Tablets should generally be avoided in patients with hepatic insufficiency. Patients with renal insufficiency (GFR < 30 mL/min) should be given a lower initial dose (one tablet per day) because they have reduced clearance of loratadine and pseudoephedrine.

HOW SUPPLIED

CLARITIN-D 12 HOUR Extended Release Tablets contain 5 mg loratadine and 120 mg pseudoephedrine sulfate. CLARITIN-D 12 HOUR Extended Release Tablets are white tablets branded in green with "CLARITIN-D", which are supplied in high density polyethylene bottles of 100 (NDC 0085-0635-01). Also available are CLARITIN-D 12 HOUR Extended Release Tablets Unit-of-Use packages of 30 tablets (3 packs of 10 tablets each) (NDC 0085-0635-05); and 10 × 10 tablets Unit Dose-Hospital Pack (NDC 0085-0635-04).

Keep Unit-of-Use packaging and Unit Dose-Hospital Pack in a dry place.

Store between 2° and 25°C (36° and 77°F).

Schering Corporation
Kenilworth, NJ 07033 USA
Rev. 2/97 17762656T

Copyright © 1994, 1995, 1996, 1997,
Schering Corporation. All rights reserved.

Shown in Product Identification Guide, page 336

CLARITIN-D® 24 HOUR ℞

brand of loratadine and pseudoephedrine sulfate, USP Extended Release Tablets

DESCRIPTION

CLARITIN-D® 24 HOUR (loratadine and pseudoephedrine sulfate, USP) Extended Release Tablets contain 10 mg loratadine in the tablet film coating for immediate release and 240 mg pseudoephedrine sulfate, USP in the tablet core which is released slowly allowing for once-daily administration.

Loratadine is a long-acting antihistamine having the empirical formula $C_{22}H_{23}ClN_2O_2$; the chemical name ethyl 4-(8-chloro-5,6-dihydro-11*H*-benzo[5,6']cyclohepta[1,2-*b*]pyridin-11-ylidene)-1-piperidinecarboxylate; and the following chemical structure:

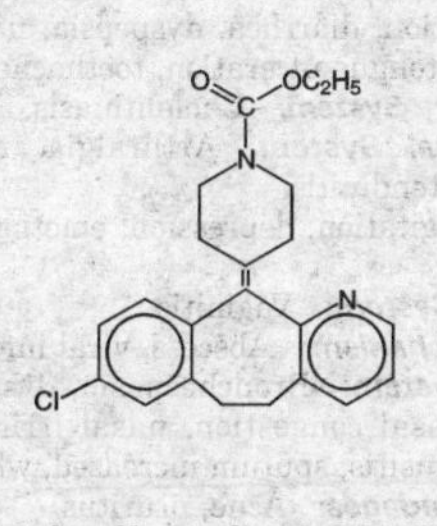

The molecular weight of loratadine is 382.89. It is a white to off-white powder, not soluble in water, but very soluble in acetone, alcohol, and chloroform.

Pseudoephedrine sulfate is the synthetic salt of one of the naturally occurring dextrorotatory diastereomers of ephedrine and is classified as an indirect sympathomimetic amine. The empirical formula for pseudoephedrine sulfate is $(C_{10}H_{15}NO)_2 \cdot H_2SO_4$; the chemical name is α-[1-(methylamino) ethyl]-[*S*-(*R**,*R**)]-benzenemethanol sulfate (2:1) (salt); and the chemical structure is:

[See chemical structure at top of next column]

The molecular weight of pseudoephedrine sulfate is 428.54. It is a white powder, freely soluble in water and methanol and sparingly soluble in chloroform.

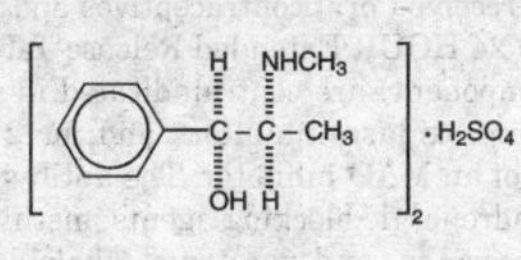

The inactive ingredients for CLARITIN-D 24 HOUR Extended Release Tablets are calcium phosphate, ethylcellulose, hydroxypropyl methylcellulose, magnesium stearate, polyethylene glycol, povidone, silicon dioxide, and titanium dioxide.

CLINICAL PHARMACOLOGY

The following information is based upon studies of loratadine alone or pseudoephedrine alone, except as indicated.

Loratadine is a long-acting tricyclic antihistamine with selective peripheral histamine H_1-receptor antagonistic activity.

Human histamine skin wheal studies following single and repeated oral doses of loratadine have shown that the drug exhibits an antihistaminic effect beginning within 1 to 3 hours, reaching a maximum at 8 to 12 hours, and lasting in excess of 24 hours. There was no evidence of tolerance to this effect developing after 28 days of dosing with loratadine.

Pharmacokinetic studies following single and multiple oral doses of loratadine in 115 volunteers showed that loratadine is rapidly absorbed and extensively metabolized to an active metabolite (descarboethoxyloratadine). Approximately 80% of the total dose administered can be found equally distributed between urine and feces in the form of metabolic products after 10 days. The mean elimination of half-lives found in studies in normal adult subjects (n = 54) were 8.4 hours (range = 3 to 20 hours) for loratadine and 28 hours (range = 8.8 to 92 hours) for the major active metabolite (descarboethoxyloratadine). In nearly all patients, exposure (AUC) to the metabolite is greater than exposure to parent loratadine. Loratadine and descarboethoxyloratadine reached steady state in most patients by approximately the fifth dosing day. The pharmacokinetics of loratadine and descarboethoxyloratadine are dose independent over the dose range of 10 to 40 mg and are not significantly altered by the duration of treatment.

In vitro studies with human liver microsomes indicate that loratadine is metabolized to descarboethoxyloratadine predominantly by P450 CYP3A4 and, to a lesser extent, by P450 CYP2D6. In the presence of a CYP3A4 inhibitor ketoconazole, loratadine is metabolized to descarboethoxyloratadine predominantly by CYP2D6. Concurrent administration of loratadine with either ketoconazole, erythromycin (both CYP3A4 inhibitors), or cimetidine (CYP2D6 and CYP3A4 inhibitor) to healthy volunteers was associated with significantly increased plasma concentrations of loratadine (see **Drug Interactions** section).

In a study involving 12 healthy geriatric subjects (66 to 78 years old), the AUC and peak plasma levels (C_{max}) of both loratadine and descarboethoxyloratadine were significantly higher (approximately 50% increased) than in the studies of younger subjects. The mean elimination half-lives for the elderly subjects were 18.2 hours (range = 6.7 to 37 hours) for loratadine and 17.5 hours (range = 11 to 38 hours) for the active metabolite.

In patients with chronic renal impairment (creatinine clearance ≤30 mL/min) both the AUC and peak plasma levels (C_{max}) increased on average by approximately 73% for loratadine; and approximately by 120% for descarboethoxyloratadine, compared to individuals with normal renal function. The mean elimination half-lives of loratadine (7.6 hours) and descarboethoxyloratadine (23.9 hours) were not significantly different from that observed in normal subjects. Hemodialysis does not have an effect on the pharmacokinetics of loratadine or its active metabolite (descarboethoxyloratadine) in subjects with chronic renal impairment.

In patients with chronic alcoholic liver disease the AUC and peak plasma levels (C_{max}) of loratadine were double while the pharmacokinetic profile of the active metabolite (descarboethoxyloratadine) was not significantly changed from that in normals. The elimination half-lives for loratadine and descarboethoxyloratadine were 24 hours and 37 hours, respectively, and increased with increasing severity of liver disease.

There was considerable variability in the pharmacokinetic data in all studies of loratadine, probably due to the extensive first-pass metabolism. Individual histograms of area under the curve, clearance, and volume of distribution showed a log normal distribution with a 25-fold range in distribution in healthy subjects.

Loratadine is about 97% bound to plasma proteins at the expected plasma concentrations (2.5 to 100 ng/mL) after a therapeutic dose. Loratadine does not affect the plasma protein binding of warfarin and digoxin. The metabolite descarboethoxyloratadine is 73% to 77% bound to plasma proteins (at 0.5 to 100 ng/mL).

Whole body autoradiographic studies in rats and monkeys, radiolabeled tissue distribution studies in mice and rats, and *in vivo* radioligand studies in mice have shown that neither loratadine nor its metabolites readily cross the blood-brain barrier. Radioligand binding studies with guinea pig pulmonary and brain H_1-receptors indicate that there was preferential binding to peripheral versus central nervous system H_1-receptors.

In a study in which loratadine alone was administered at four times the clinical dose for 90 days, no clinically significant increase in the QT_c was seen on ECGs.

Pseudophedrine sulfate (d-isoephedrine sulfate) is an orally active sympathomimetic amine which exerts a decongestant action on the nasal mucosa. It is recognized as an effective agent for the relief of nasal congestion due to allergic rhinitis. Pseudoephedrine produces peripheral effects similar to those of ephedrine and central effects similar to, but less intense than, amphetamines. It has the potential for excitatory side effects.

The bioavailability of loratadine and pseudoephedrine sulfate from CLARITIN-D 24 HOUR Extended Release Tablets is similar to that achieved with separate administration of the components. Coadministration of loratadine and pseudoephedrine does not significantly affect the bioavailability of either component.

In a single-dose study, food increased the AUC of loratadine by approximately 125% and C_{max} by approximately 80%. However, food did not significantly affect the pharmacokinetics of pseudoephedrine sulfate or descarboethoxyloratadine.

Clinical Studies: Clinical trials of CLARITIN-D 24 HOUR Extended Release Tablets involved a total of approximately 2000 patients with seasonal allergic rhinitis. One study involved 879 patients, who received either the combination product (loratadine 10 mg and pseudoephedrine sulfate 240 mg), loratadine (10 mg once daily) or pseudoephedrine sulfate (120 mg twice daily) alone, or placebo, in a double-blind randomized design. Improvement in nasal and non-nasal symptoms of seasonal allergic rhinitis including nasal congestion in patients receiving CLARITIN-D 24 HOUR Extended Release Tablets was significantly greater than in placebo recipients, and generally greater than that achieved with loratadine or pseudoephedrine sulfate alone. In this study, CLARITIN-D 24 HOUR Extended Release Tablets were well tolerated, with a frequency of sedation similar to that seen with placebo, and a frequency of nervousness and insomnia similar to that seen with pseudoephedrine sulfate given alone.

In another study of 469 patients, once-daily administration of CLARITIN-D 24 HOUR Extended Release Tablets provided effects similar to those achieved with twice-daily administration of CLARITIN-D 12 HOUR Extended Release Tablets, a combination product containing 5 mg loratadine plus 120 mg pseudoephedrine sulfate, USP, extended release.

The end of dosing interval efficacy of the pseudoephedrine component of CLARITIN-D 24 HOUR Extended Release Tablets on the symptom of nasal stuffiness was evaluated in a study of 695 patients who were randomized to receive CLARITIN-D 24 HOUR Extended Release Tablets, CLARITIN Tablets, or placebo. Patients who received CLARITIN-D 24 HOUR Extended Release Tablets had significantly more improvement in nasal stuffiness scores at the end of the dosing interval than those patients receiving CLARITIN Tablets or placebo throughout the course of the trial.

In a 6-week, placebo-controlled study of 193 patients with seasonal allergic rhinitis and concomitant mild to moderate asthma, CLARITIN-D 12 HOUR Extended Release Tablets twice daily improved seasonal allergic rhinitis signs and symptoms with no decrease in pulmonary function or adverse effect on asthma symptoms. This supports the safety of administering CLARITIN-D 24 HOUR Extended Release Tablets to seasonal rhinitis patients with asthma.

INDICATIONS AND USAGE

CLARITIN-D 24 HOUR Extended Release Tablets are indicated for the relief of symptoms of seasonal allergic rhinitis. CLARITIN-D 24 HOUR Extended Release Tablets should be administered when both the antihistaminic properties of CLARITIN® (loratadine) and the nasal decongestant activity of pseudoephedrine sulfate are desired (see **CLINICAL PHARMACOLOGY** section).

CONTRAINDICATIONS

CLARITIN-D 24 HOUR Extended Release Tablets are contraindicated in patients who are hypersensitive to this medication or to any of its ingredients.

Continued on next page

Information on Schering products appearing on these pages is effective as of August 15, 1998.

Claritin-D 24 Hour—Cont.

This product, due to its pseudoephedrine component, is contraindicated in patients with narrow-angle glaucoma or urinary retention, and in patients receiving monoamine oxidase (MAO) inhibitor therapy or within fourteen (14) days of stopping such treatment. (See **PRECAUTIONS: Drug Interactions** section.) It is also contraindicated in patients with severe hypertension, severe coronary artery disease, and in those who have shown hypersensitivity or idiosyncrasy to its components, to adrenergic agents, or to other drugs of similar chemical structures. Manifestations of patient idiosyncrasy to adrenergic agents include: insomnia dizziness, weakness, tremor, or arrhythmias.

WARNINGS

CLARITIN-D 24 HOUR Extended Release Tablets should be used with caution in patients with hypertension, diabetes mellitus, ischemic heart disease, increased intraocular pressure, hyperthyroidism, renal impairment, or prostatic hypertrophy. Central nervous system stimulation with convulsions or cardiovascular collapse with accompanying hypotension may be produced by sympathomimetic amines.
Use in Patients Approximately 60 Years of Age and Older: The safety and efficacy of CLARITIN-D 24 HOUR Extended Release Tablets in patients greater than 60 years old have not been investigated in placebo-controlled clinical trials. The elderly are more likely to have adverse reactions to sympathomimetic amines.

PRECAUTIONS

General: Because the doses of this fixed combination product cannot be individually titrated and hepatic insufficiency results in a reduced clearance of loratadine to a much greater extent than pseudoephedrine, CLARITIN-D 24 HOUR Extended Release Tablets should generally be avoided in patients with hepatic insufficiency. Patients with renal insufficiency (GFR <30 mL/min) should be given a lower initial dose (one tablet every other day) because they have reduced clearance of loratadine and pseudoephedrine.
Information for Patients: Patients taking CLARITIN-D 24 HOUR Extended Release Tablets should receive the following information: CLARITIN-D 24 HOUR Extended Release Tablets are prescribed for the relief of symptoms of seasonal allergic rhinitis. Patients should be instructed to take CLARITIN-D 24 HOUR Extended Release Tablets only as prescribed and not to exceed the prescribed dose. Patients should also be advised against the concurrent use of CLARITIN-D 24 HOUR Extended Release Tablets with over-the-counter antihistamines and decongestants. Patients who have a history of difficulty in swallowing tablets or who have known upper gastrointestinal narrowing or abnormal esophageal peristalsis should not use this product. This product should not be used by patients who are hypersensitive to it or to any of its ingredients. Due to its pseudoephedrine component, this product should not be used by patients with narrow-angle glaucoma, urinary retention, or by patients receiving a monoamine oxidase (MAO) inhibitor or within 14 days of stopping use of an MAO inhibitor. It also should not be used by patients with severe hypertension or severe coronary artery disease.
Patients who are or may become pregnant should be told that this product should be used in pregnancy or during lactation only if the potential benefit justifies the potential risk to the fetus or nursing infant.
Patients should be instructed not to break or chew the tablet and to take it with a glass of water.
Drug Interactions: No specific interaction studies have been conducted with CLARITIN-D 24 HOUR Extended Release Tablets. However, loratadine (10 mg once daily) has been safely coadministered with therapeutic doses of erythromycin, cimetidine, and ketoconazole in controlled clinical pharmacology studies. Although increased plasma concentrations (AUC 0–24 hrs) of loratadine and/or descarboethoxyloratadine were observed following coadministration of loratadine with each of these drugs in normal volunteers (n = 24 in each study), there were no clinically relevant changes in the safety profile of loratadine, as assessed by electrocardiographic parameters, clinical laboratory tests, vital signs, and adverse events. There were no significant effects on QT$_c$ intervals, and no reports of sedation or syncope. No effects on plasma concentrations of cimetidine or ketoconazole were observed. Plasma concentrations (AUC 0–24 hrs) of erythromycin decreased 15% with coadministration of loratadine relative to that observed with erythromycin alone. The clinical relevance of this difference is unknown. These above findings are summarized in the following table:

Effects on Plasma Concentrations (AUC 0-24 hrs) of Loratadine and Descarboethoxyloratadine After 10 Days of Coadministration (Loratadine 10 mg) in Normal Volunteers

	Loratadine	Descarboethoxy-loratadine
Erythromycin (500 mg Q8h)	+ 40%	+46%
Cimetidine (300 mg QID)	+103%	+ 6%
Ketoconazole (200 mg Q12h)	+307%	+73%

There does not appear to be an increase in adverse events in subjects who received oral contraceptives and loratadine. CLARITIN-D 24 HOUR Extended Release Tablets (pseudoephedrine component) are contraindicated in patients taking monoamine oxidase inhibitors and for 2 weeks after stopping use of an MAO inhibitor. The antihypertensive effects of beta-adrenergic blocking agents, methyldopa, mecamylamine, reserpine, and veratrum alkaloids may be reduced by sympathomimetics. Increased ectopic pacemaker activity can occur when pseudoephedrine is used concomitantly with digitalis.
Drug/Laboratory Test Interactions: The *in vitro* addition of pseudoephedrine to sera containing the cardiac isoenzyme MB of serum creatinine phosphokinase progressively inhibits the activity of the enzyme. The inhibition becomes complete over 6 hours.
Carcinogenesis, Mutagenesis, Impairment of Fertility: There are no animal or laboratory studies on the combination product loratadine and pseudoephedrine sulfate to evaluate carcinogenesis, mutagenesis, or impairment of fertility.
In an 18-month carcinogenicity study in mice and a 2-year study in rats loratadine was administered in the diet at doses up to 40 mg/kg (mice) and 25 mg/kg (rats). In the carcinogenicity studies pharmacokinetic assessments were carried out to determine animal exposure to the drug. AUC data demonstrated that the exposure of mice given 40 mg/kg of loratadine was 3.6 (loratadine) and 18 (active metabolite) times higher than in humans given the maximum recommended daily oral dose. Exposure of rats given 25 mg/kg of loratadine was 28 (loratadine) and 67 (active metabolite) times higher than in humans given the maximum recommended daily oral dose. Male mice given 40 mg/kg had a significantly higher incidence of hepatocellular tumors (combined adenomas and carcinomas) than concurrent controls. In rats, a significantly higher incidence of hepatocellular tumors (combined adenomas and carcinomas) was observed in males given 10 mg/kg and in males and females given 25 mg/kg. The clinical significance of these findings during long-term use of loratadine is not known.
Two-year feeding studies in mice and rats conducted under the auspices of the National Toxicology Programs (NTP) uncovered no evidence of carcinogenic potential of ephedrine sulfate at doses up to 10 and 27 mg/kg, respectively (approximately 16% and 100% of the maximum recommended human daily oral dose of pseudoephedrine sulfate on a mg/m^2 basis).
In mutagenicity studies with loratadine alone, there was no evidence of mutagenic potential in reverse (Ames) or forward point mutation (CHO-HGPRT) assays, or in the assay for DNA damage (Rat Primary Hepatocyte Unscheduled DNA Assay) or in two assays for chromosomal aberrations (Human Peripheral Blood Lymphocyte Clastogenesis Assay and the Mouse Bone Marrow Erythrocyte Micronucleus Assay). In the Mouse Lymphoma Assay, a positive finding occurred in the nonactivated but not the activated phase of the study.
Decreased fertility in male rats, shown by lower female conception rates, occurred at 64 mg/kg of loratadine (approximately 50 times the maximum recommended human daily oral dose based on mg/m^2) and was reversible with cessation of dosing. Loratadine had no effect on male or female fertility or reproduction in the rat at 24 mg/kg (approximately 20 times the maximum recommended human daily oral dose on a mg/m^2 basis).
Pregnancy Category B: The combination product loratadine and pseudoephedrine sulfate was evaluated for teratogenicity in rats and rabbits. There was no evidence of teratogenicity in reproduction studies with this combination of the same clinical ratio (1:24) at oral doses up to 150 mg/kg (approximately 5 times the maximum recommended human daily oral dose on a mg/m^2 basis) in rats, and 120 mg/kg (8 times the maximum recommended human daily oral dose on a mg/m^2 basis) in rabbits. Similarly, no evidence of animal teratogenicity in rats and rabbits was reported at oral doses up to 96 mg/kg of loratadine alone (approximately 75 and 150 times, respectively, the maximum human daily oral dose on a mg/m^2 basis). There are, however, no adequate and well-controlled studies in pregnant women. Because animal reproduction studies are not always predictive of human response, CLARITIN-D 24 HOUR Extended Release Tablets should be used during pregnancy only if clearly needed.
Nursing Mothers: It is not known if this combination product is excreted in human milk. However, loratadine when administered alone and its metabolite descarboethoxyloratadine pass easily into breast milk and achieve concentrations that are equivalent to plasma levels, with an AUC$_{milk}$/AUC$_{plasma}$ ratio of 1.17 and 0.85 for the parent and active metabolite, respectively. Following a single oral dose of 40 mg, a small amount of loratadine and metabolite was excreted into the breast milk (approximately 0.03% of 40 mg over 48 hours). Pseudoephedrine administered alone also distributes into breast milk of the lactating human female. Pseudoephedrine concentrations in milk are consistently higher than those in plasma. The total amount of drug in milk as judged by the area under the curve (AUC) is 2 to 3 times greater than in plasma. The fraction of a pseudoephedrine dose excreted in milk is estimated to be 0.4% to 0.7%. A decision should be made whether to discontinue nursing or to discontinue the drug, taking into account the importance of the drug to the mother. Caution should be exercised when CLARITIN-D 24 HOUR Extended Release Tablets are administered to a nursing woman.
Pediatric Use: Safety and effectiveness in children below the age of 12 years have not been established.

ADVERSE REACTIONS

Information on adverse reactions is provided from placebo-controlled studies involving over 2000 patients, 605 of whom received CLARITIN-D 24 HOUR Extended Release Tablets once daily for up to 2 weeks. In these studies, the incidence of adverse events reported with CLARITIN-D 24 HOUR Extended Release Tablets was similar to those reported with twice-daily (q12h) 120 mg sustained-release pseudoephedrine alone.

REPORTED ADVERSE EVENTS WITH AN INCIDENCE OF ≥2% IN CLARITIN-D 24 HOUR EXTENDED RELEASE TABLETS TREATMENT GROUP IN DOUBLE-BLIND, RANDOMIZED, PLACEBO-CONTROLLED CLINICAL TRIALS

PERCENT OF PATIENTS REPORTING

	CLARITIN-D® 24 HOUR (n=605)	Loratadine 10 mg (n=449)	Pseudo-ephedrine 120 mg q12h (n=220)	Placebo (n=605)
Dry Mouth	8	2	7	2
Somnolence	6	4	5	4
Insomnia	5	1	9	1
Pharyngitis	5	5	5	5
Dizziness	4	2	3	2
Coughing	3	2	3	1
Fatigue	3	4	1	2
Nausea	3	2	4	2
Nervousness	3	1	4	1
Anorexia	2	<1	2	0
Dysmenorrhea	2	2	2	1

Adverse events occurring in greater than or equal to 2% of CLARITIN-D 24 HOUR Extended Release Tablets-treated patients, but that were more common in the placebo-treated group, include headache.
Adverse events did not appear to significantly differ based on age, sex, or race, although the number of non-whites was relatively small.
In addition to those adverse events reported above, the following adverse events have been reported in fewer than 2% of patients who received CLARITIN-D 24 HOUR Extended Release Tablets:
Autonomic Nervous System: Altered lacrimation, flushing, increased sweating, mydriasis, thirst.
Body As A Whole: Abnormal vision, asthenia, back pain, chest pain, conjunctivitis, earache, eye pain, facial edema, fever, flu-like symptoms, leg cramps, lymphadenopathy, malaise, rigors, tinnitus.
Cardiovascular System: Hypertension, palpitation, tachycardia.
Central and Peripheral Nervous System: Convulsions, dysphonia, hyperkinesis, hypertonia, migraine, paresthesia, tremor.
Gastrointestinal System: Abdominal distension, altered taste, constipation, diarrhea, dyspepsia, flatulence, gastritis, stomatitis, tongue ulceration, toothache, vomiting.
Liver and Biliary System: Cholelithiasis.
Musculoskeletal System: Arthralgia, musculoskeletal pain, myalgia, tendinitis.
Psychiatric: Agitation, depression, emotional lability, irritability.
Reproductive System: Vaginitis.
Resistance Mechanism: Abscess, viral infection.
Respiratory System: Bronchospasm, dyspnea, epistaxis, hemoptysis, nasal congestion, nasal irritation, pleurisy, pneumonia, sinusitis, sputum increased, wheezing.
Skin and Appendages: Acne, pruritus.
Urinary System: Oliguria, micturition frequency, urinary retention, urinary tract infection.
Additional adverse events reported with the combination of loratadine and pseudoephedrine include abnormal hepatic function, aggressive reaction, anxiety, apathy, confusion, euphoria, paroniria, postural hypotension, syncope, urticaria, vertigo, weight gain.
The following additional adverse events have been reported with CLARITIN Tablets: abdominal distress, alopecia, altered micturition, altered salivation, amnesia, anaphylaxis, angioneurotic edema, blepharospasm, breast enlargement, breast pain, bronchitis, decreased libido, dermatitis, dry hair, dry skin, erythema multiforme, hypoesthesia, impaired concentration, impotence, increased appetite, laryn-

gitis, menorrhagia, nasal dryness, peripheral edema, photosensitivity reaction, purpura, rash, seizures, sneezing, supraventricular tachyarrhythmias, upper respiratory infection, urinary discoloration.

Pseudoephedrine may cause mild CNS stimulation in hypersensitive patients. Nervousness, excitability, restlessness, dizziness, weakness, or insomnia may occur. Headache, drowsiness, tachycardia, palpitation, pressor activity, and cardiac arrhythmias have been reported. Sympathomimetic drugs have also been associated with other untoward effects, such as fear, anxiety, tenseness, tremor, hallucinations, seizures, pallor, respiratory difficulty, dysuria, and cardiovascular collapse.

There have been rare postmarketing reports of mechanical upper gastrointestinal tract obstruction in patients taking CLARITIN-D 24 HOUR Extended Release Tablets. In many of these cases, patients have had a history of difficulty in swallowing tablets or have had known upper gastrointestinal narrowing or abnormal esophageal peristalsis.

DRUG ABUSE AND DEPENDENCE

There is no information to indicate that abuse or dependency occurs with loratadine. Pseudoephedrine, like other central nervous system stimulants, has been abused. At high doses, subjects commonly experience an elevation of mood, a sense of increased energy and alertness, and decreased appetite. Some individuals become anxious, irritable, and loquacious. In addition to the marked euphoria, the user experiences a sense of markedly enhanced physical strength and mental capacity. With continued use, tolerance develops, the user increases the dose, and toxic signs and symptoms appear. Depression may follow rapid withdrawal.

OVERDOSAGE

In the event of overdosage, general symptomatic and supportive measures should be instituted promptly and maintained for as long as necessary. Treatment of overdosage would reasonably consist of emesis (ipecac syrup), except in patients with impaired consciousness, followed by the administration of activated charcoal to absorb any remaining drug. If vomiting is unsuccessful, or contraindicated, gastric lavage should be performed with normal saline. Saline cathartics may also be of value for rapid dilution of bowel contents. Loratadine is not eliminated by hemodialysis. It is not known if loratadine is eliminated by peritoneal dialysis.

Somnolence, tachycardia, and headache have been reported with doses of 40 to 180 mg of loratadine. In large doses, sympathomimetics may give rise to giddiness, headache, nausea, vomiting, sweating, thirst, tachycardia, precordial pain, palpitations, difficulty in micturition, muscular weakness and tenseness, anxiety, restlessness, and insomnia. Many patients can present a toxic psychosis with delusions and hallucinations. Some may develop cardiac arrhythmias, circulatory collapse, convulsions, coma, and respiratory failure.

The oral median lethal dose for the mixture of the two drugs was greater than 525 of 1839 mg/kg in mice and rats, respectively (approximately 10 and 58 times the maximum recommended human daily oral dose on a mg/m^2 basis). The oral median lethal dose for loratadine was greater than 5000 mg/kg in rats and mice (greater than 2000 times the maximum recommended human daily oral dose on a mg/m^2 basis). Single oral doses of loratadine showed no effects in rats, mice, and monkeys at doses as high as 10 times the maximum recommended human daily oral dose on a mg/m^2 basis.

DOSAGE AND ADMINISTRATION

Adults and children 12 years of age and over: one tablet daily taken with a glass of water. Because the doses of this fixed combination product cannot be individually titrated and hepatic insufficiency results in a reduced clearance of loratadine to a much greater extent than pseudoephedrine, CLARITIN-D 24 HOUR Extended Release Tablets should generally be avoided in patients with hepatic insufficiency. Patients with renal insufficiency (GFR <30 mL/min) should be given a lower initial dose (one tablet every other day) because they have reduced clearance of loratadine and pseudoephedrine. Patients who have a history of difficulty in swallowing tablets or who have known upper gastrointestinal narrowing or abnormal esophageal peristalsis should not use this product (see **PRECAUTIONS**, **Information for Patients**, and **ADVERSE REACTIONS**).

HOW SUPPLIED

CLARITIN-D 24 HOUR Extended Release Tablets contain 10 mg loratadine in the tablet coating for immediate release and 240 mg pseudoephedrine sulfate, USP in an extended-release core. CLARITIN-D 24 HOUR Extended Release Tablets are white to off-white film-coated tablets branded in black with "CLARITIN-D 24 HOUR"; high-density polyethylene bottles of 100 (NDC 0085-0640-01) and polyvinyl chloride packages of 10 × 10 tablet Unit Dose-Hospital Pack (NDC 0085-0640-02).

Protect Unit Dose-Hospital Pack from light and store in a dry place. Store between 15° and 25°C (59° and 77°F).

U.S. Patent Nos. 5,314,697; 4,731,447; and 4,282,233.

Rev. 10/97 B-19428443
19410943T

Shown in Product Identification Guide, page 336

DIPROLENE® AF ℞

brand of augmented
betamethasone dipropionate*
CREAM 0.05%
(potency expressed as betamethasone)
*Vehicle augments the penetration of the steroid.
For Dermatologic Use Only–Not for Ophthalmic Use

DESCRIPTION

DIPROLENE® AF Cream contains betamethasone dipropionate, USP, a synthetic adrenocorticosteroid, for dermatologic use in an emollient base. Betamethasone, an analog of prednisolone, has a high degree of corticosteroid activity and a slight degree of mineralocorticoid activity. Betamethasone dipropionate is the 17,21-dipropionate ester of betamethasone.

Chemically, betamethasone dipropionate is 9-fluoro-11β, 17,21-trihydroxy-16β-methylpregna-1,4-diene-3,20-dione 17,21-dipropionate, with the empirical formula $C_{28}H_{37}FO_7$, a molecular weight of 504.6, and the following structural formula:

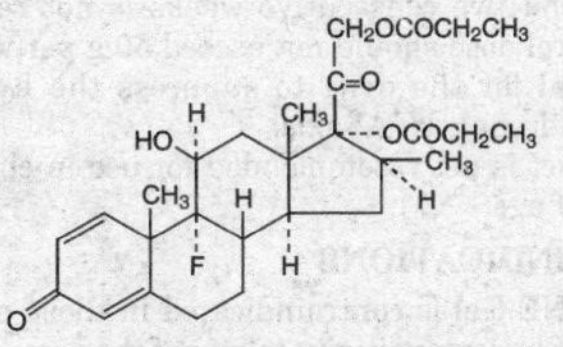

Betamethasone dipropionate is a white to creamy white, odorless crystalline powder, insoluble in water.

Each gram of DIPROLENE AF Cream 0.05% contains: 0.64 mg betamethasone dipropionate, USP (equivalent to 0.5 mg betamethasone) in an emollient cream base of purified water, chlorocresol, propylene glycol, white petrolatum, white wax, cyclomethicone, sorbitol solution, glyceryl monooleate, ceteareth-30, carbomer 940 and sodium hydroxide.

CLINICAL PHARMACOLOGY

The corticosteroids are a class of compounds comprising steroid hormones secreted by the adrenal cortex and their synthetic analogs. In pharmacologic doses, corticosteroids are used primarily for their anti-inflammatory and/or immunosuppressive effects.

Topical corticosteroids, such as betamethasone dipropionate, are effective in the treatment of corticosteroid-responsive dermatoses primarily because of their anti-inflammatory, anti-pruritic, and vasoconstrictive actions. However, while the physiologic, pharmacologic, and clinical effects of the corticosteroids are well-known, the exact mechanisms of their actions in each disease are uncertain. Betamethasone dipropionate, a corticosteroid, has been shown to have topical (dermatologic) and systemic pharmacologic and metabolic effects characteristic of this class of drugs.

Pharmacokinetics: The extent of percutaneous absorption of topical corticosteroids is determined by many factors including the vehicle, the integrity of the epidermal barrier, and the use of occlusive dressings. (See **DOSAGE AND ADMINISTRATION** section.)

Topical corticosteroids can be absorbed through normal intact skin. Inflammation and/or other disease processes in the skin may increase percutaneous absorption. Occlusive dressings substantially increase the percutaneous absorption of topical corticosteroids. (See **DOSAGE AND ADMINISTRATION** section.)

Once absorbed through the skin, topical corticosteroids enter pharmacokinetic pathways similar to systemically administered corticosteroids. Corticosteroids are bound to plasma proteins in varying degrees, are metabolized primarily in the liver and excreted by the kidneys. Some of the topical corticosteroids and their metabolites are also excreted into the bile.

DIPROLENE AF Cream was applied once daily at 7 grams per day for one week to diseased skin, in patients with psoriasis or atopic dermatitis, to study its effects on the hypothalamic-pituitary-adrenal (HPA) axis. The results suggested that the drug caused a slight lowering of adrenal corticosteroid secretion, although in no case did plasma cortisol levels go below the lower limit of the normal range.

INDICATIONS AND USAGE

DIPROLENE AF Cream is indicated for relief of the inflammatory and pruritic manifestations of corticosteroid-responsive dermatoses.

CONTRAINDICATIONS

DIPROLENE AF Cream is contraindicated in patients who are hypersensitive to betamethasone dipropionate, to other corticosteroids, or to any ingredient in this preparation.

PRECAUTIONS

General: Systemic absorption of topical corticosteroids has produced reversible HPA axis suppression, manifestations of Cushing's syndrome, hyperglycemia, and glucosuria in some patients.

Conditions which augment systemic absorption include the application of the more potent corticosteroids, use over large surface areas, prolonged use, and the addition of occlusive dressings. (See **DOSAGE AND ADMINISTRATION** section.)

Therefore, patients receiving a large dose of a potent topical steroid applied to a large surface area should be evaluated periodically for evidence of HPA axis suppression by using the urinary free cortisol and ACTH stimulation tests. If HPA axis suppression is noted, an attempt should be made to withdraw the drug, to reduce the frequency of application, or to substitute a less potent steroid.

Recovery of HPA axis function is generally prompt and complete upon discontinuation of the drug. Infrequently, signs and symptoms of steroid withdrawal may occur, requiring supplemental systemic corticosteroids.

Children may absorb proportionally larger amounts of topical corticosteroids and thus be more susceptible to systemic toxicity. (See **PRECAUTIONS—Pediatric Use.**)

If irritation develops, topical corticosteroids should be discontinued and appropriate therapy instituted.

In the presence of dermatological infections, the use of an appropriate antifungal or antibacterial agent should be instituted. If a favorable response does not occur promptly, the corticosteroid should be discontinued until the infection has been adequately controlled.

Information for Patients: Patients using topical corticosteroids should receive the following information and instructions. This information is intended to aid in the safe and effective use of this medication. It is not a disclosure of all possible adverse or intended effects.

1. This medication is to be used as directed by the physician and should not be used longer than the prescribed time period. It is for external use only. Avoid contact with the eyes.
2. Patients should be advised not to use this medication for any disorder other than that for which it was prescribed.
3. The treated skin area should not be bandaged or otherwise covered or wrapped as to be occlusive. (See **DOSAGE AND ADMINISTRATION** section.)
4. Patients should report any signs of local adverse reactions.

Laboratory Tests: The following tests may be helpful in evaluating HPA axis suppression:

Urinary free cortisol test
ACTH stimulation test

Carcinogenesis, Mutagenesis, and Impairment of Fertility: Long-term animal studies have not been performed to evaluate the carcinogenic potential or the effect on fertility of topically applied corticosteroids.

Studies to determine mutagenicity with prednisolone and hydrocortisone have revealed negative results.

Pregnancy Category C: Corticosteroids are generally teratogenic in laboratory animals when administered systemically at relatively low dosage levels. The more potent corticosteroids have been shown to be teratogenic after dermal application in laboratory animals. There are no adequate and well-controlled studies of the teratogenic effects of topically applied corticosteroids in pregnant women. Therefore, topical corticosteroids should be used during pregnancy only if the potential benefit justifies the potential risk to the fetus. Drugs of this class should not be used extensively on pregnant patients, in large amounts, or for prolonged periods of time.

Nursing Mothers: It is not known whether topical administration of corticosteroids can result in sufficient systemic absorption to produce detectable quantities in breast milk. Systemically administered corticosteroids are secreted into breast milk in quantities not likely to have a deleterious effect on the infant. Nevertheless, a decision should be made whether to discontinue nursing or to discontinue the drug, taking into account the importance of the drug to the mother.

Pediatric Use: Use of DIPROLENE AF Cream in children under 12 years is not recommended.

Pediatric patients may demonstrate greater susceptibility to topical corticosteroid-induced HPA axis suppression and Cushing's syndrome than mature patients because of a larger skin surface area to body weight ratio.

Continued on next page

Information on Schering products appearing on these pages is effective as of August 15, 1998.

Diprolene AF—Cont.

Hypothalamic-pituitary-adrenal (HPA) axis suppression, Cushing's syndrome, and intracranial hypertension have been reported in children receiving topical corticosteroids. Manifestations of adrenal suppression in children include linear growth retardation, delayed weight gain, low plasma cortisol levels, and absence of response to ACTH stimulation. Manifestations of intracranial hypertension include bulging fontanelles, headaches, and bilateral papilledema. Chronic corticosteroid therapy may interfere with the growth and development of children.

ADVERSE REACTIONS

The only local adverse reaction reported to be possibly or probably related to treatment with DIPROLENE AF Cream during controlled clinical studies was stinging. It occurred in 0.4% of the 242 patients or subjects involved in the studies.

The following local adverse reactions are reported infrequently when topical corticosteroids are used as recommended. These reactions are listed in an approximate decreasing order of occurrence: burning, itching, irritation, dryness, folliculitis, hypertrichosis, acneiform eruptions, hypopigmentation, perioral dermatitis, allergic contact dermatitis, maceration of the skin, secondary infection, skin atrophy, striae, miliaria.

OVERDOSAGE

Topically applied corticosteroids can be absorbed in sufficient amounts to produce systemic effects. (See **PRECAUTIONS**.)

DOSAGE AND ADMINISTRATION

Apply a thin film of DIPROLENE AF Cream to the affected skin areas once or twice daily. Treatment with DIPROLENE AF Cream should be limited to 45 g per week.

DIPROLENE AF Cream is not to be used with occlusive dressings.

HOW SUPPLIED

DIPROLENE AF Cream 0.05% is supplied in 15 g (NDC 0085-0517-01), and 50 g (NDC 0085-0517-04) tubes; boxes of one.

Store between 2° and 30°C (36° and 86°F).

Schering Corporation
Kenilworth, NJ 07033 USA
Rev. 7/95

18670305T

Copyright © 1987, 1991, 1994, 1995, Schering Corporation. All rights reserved.

Shown in Product Identification Guide, page 336

DIPROLENE® ℞

brand of augmented betamethasone dipropionate*
Gel 0.05%
(potency expressed as betamethasone)

*Vehicle augments the penetration of the steroid.

For Dermatologic Use Only—
Not for Ophthalmic Use

DESCRIPTION

DIPROLENE® Gel contains betamethasone dipropionate, USP, a synthetic fluorinated corticosteroid for topical dermatologic use. Betamethasone dipropionate is included in a class of compounds consisting primarily of synthetic corticosteroids for use topically as anti-inflammatory and antipruritic agents.

Chemically, betamethasone dipropionate is 9-fluoro-11β, 17,21-trihydroxy-16β-methylpregna-1,4-diene-3,20-dione 17, 21-dipropionate, with the empirical formula $C_{28}H_{37}FO_7$, a molecular weight of 504.6, and the following structural formula:

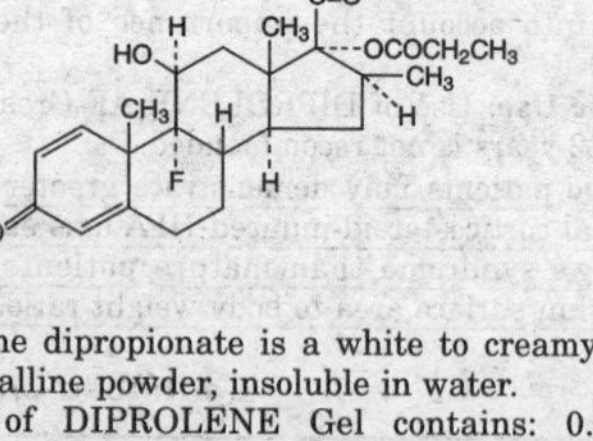

Betamethasone dipropionate is a white to creamy white, odorless crystalline powder, insoluble in water.

Each gram of DIPROLENE Gel contains: 0.64 mg betamethasone dipropionate, USP (equivalent to 0.5 mg betamethasone), in an augmented gel base of purified water, propylene glycol, carbomer 940, and sodium hydroxide.

CLINICAL PHARMACOLOGY

Like other topical corticosteroids, betamethasone dipropionate has anti-inflammatory, anti-pruritic, and vasoconstrictive properties. The mechanism of the anti-inflammatory activity of the topical steroids, in general, is unclear. However, corticosteroids are thought to act by the induction of phospholipase A_2 inhibitory proteins, collectively called lipocortins. It is postulated that these proteins control the biosynthesis of potent mediators of inflammation, such as prostaglandins and leukotrienes, by inhibiting the release of their common precursor, arachidonic acid. Arachidonic acid is released from membrane phospholipids by phospholipase A_2.

Pharmacokinetics: The extent of percutaneous absorption of topical corticosteroids is determined by many factors including the vehicle and the integrity of the epidermal barrier. Occlusive dressings with hydrocortisone for up to 24 hours have not been demonstrated to increase penetration; however, occlusion of hydrocortisone for 96 hours markedly enhances penetration. Topical corticosteroids can be absorbed from normal intact skin. In addition, inflammation and/or other disease processes in the skin may increase percutaneous absorption. Studies performed with DIPROLENE (augmented betamethasone dipropionate) Gel indicate that it is in the super-high range of potency as compared with other topical corticosteroids.

INDICATIONS AND USAGE

DIPROLENE Gel is a super-high potency corticosteroid indicated for the relief of the inflammatory and pruritic manifestations of corticosteroid-responsive dermatoses. Treatment beyond two consecutive weeks is not recommended, and the total dose should not exceed 50 g per week because of potential for the drug to suppress the hypothalamic-pituitary-adrenal (HPA) axis.

This product is not recommended for use in children under 12 years of age.

CONTRAINDICATIONS

DIPROLENE Gel is contraindicated in those patients with a history of hypersensitivity to any of the components of the preparation.

PRECAUTIONS

General: DIPROLENE Gel should not be used in the treatment of rosacea or perioral dermatitis, and it should not be used on the face, groin, or in the axillae.

Systemic absorption of topical corticosteroids can produce reversible hypothalamic-pituitary-adrenal (HPA) axis suppression with the potential for glucocorticosteroid insufficiency after withdrawal of treatment. Manifestations of Cushing's syndrome, hyperglycemia, and glucosuria can also be produced in some patients by systemic absorption of topical corticosteroids while on treatment.

At 7 g per day (applied once daily or as 3.5 g twice daily), DIPROLENE Gel was shown to cause inhibition of the HPA axis following application for one, two or three weeks to diseased skin in some patients with psoriasis or atopic dermatitis. These effects were reversible upon discontinuation of treatment.

Patients receiving DIPROLENE Gel applied to large areas should be evaluated periodically for evidence of HPA axis suppression. This may be done by using the ACTH-stimulation, morning plasma cortisol and urinary free-cortisol tests. Patients should not be treated with DIPROLENE Gel for more than 2 weeks at a time, and amounts greater than 50 g per week should not be used because of the potential for the drug to suppress the HPA axis.

If HPA axis suppression is noted, an attempt should be made to withdraw the drug, to reduce the frequency of application, or to substitute a less potent corticosteroid. Recovery of HPA axis function is generally prompt and complete upon discontinuation of topical corticosteroids. Infrequently, signs and symptoms of glucocorticosteroid insufficiency may occur, requiring supplemental systemic corticosteroids. For information on systemic supplementation, see prescribing information for systemic corticosteroids.

Children may be more susceptible to systemic toxicity from equivalent doses due to their larger skin surface to body mass ratios (see **PRECAUTIONS**—Pediatric Use).

If irritation develops, DIPROLENE Gel should be discontinued and appropriate therapy instituted. Allergic contact dermatitis with corticosteroids is usually diagnosed by observing failure to heal rather than noting clinical exacerbation as with most topical products not containing corticosteroids. Such an observation should be corroborated with appropriate diagnostic patch testing.

If concomitant fungal and/or bacterial skin infections are present or develop, an appropriate antifungal or antibacterial agent should be used. If a favorable response does not occur promptly, use of DIPROLENE Gel should be discontinued until the infection has been adequately controlled.

Information for Patients: Patients using topical corticosteroids should receive the following information and instructions:

1. The medication is to be used as directed by the physician. It is for external use only. Avoid contact with the eyes.
2. The medication should not be used for any disorder other than that for which it was prescribed.
3. The treated skin area should not be bandaged or otherwise covered or wrapped so as to be occlusive.
4. Patients should report to their physician any signs of local adverse reactions.

Laboratory Tests: The following tests may be helpful in evaluating patients for HPA axis suppression:

ACTH-stimulation test
Morning plasma-cortisol test
Urinary free-cortisol test

Carcinogenesis, Mutagenesis, and Impairment of Fertility: Long-term animal studies have not been performed to evaluate the carcinogenic potential of betamethasone dipropionate.

Studies in rabbits, mice and rats using intramuscular doses up to 1.0, 33 and 2.0 mg/kg, respectively, resulted in dose related increases in fetal resorptions in the rabbits and mice.

Pregnancy: Teratogenic Effects: Pregnancy Category C: Corticosteroids have been shown to be teratogenic in laboratory animals when administered systemically at relatively low dosage levels. Some corticosteroids have been shown to be teratogenic after dermal application to laboratory animals.

Betamethasone dipropionate has been shown to be teratogenic in rabbits when given by the intramuscular route at doses of 0.05 mg/kg. This dose is approximately 26 times the human topical dose of DIPROLENE Gel assuming human percutaneous absorption of approximately 3% and the use in a 70 kg person of 7 g per day. The abnormalities observed included umbilical hernias, cephalocele and cleft palate.

There are no adequate and well-controlled studies of the teratogenic potential of betamethasone dipropionate in pregnant women. Therefore, DIPROLENE Gel should be used during pregnancy only if the potential benefit justifies the potential risk to the fetus.

Nursing Mothers: Systemically administered corticosteroids appear in human milk and could suppress growth, interfere with endogenous corticosteroid production, or cause other untoward effects. It is not known whether topical administration of corticosteroids could result in sufficient systemic absorption to produce detectable quantities in human milk. Because many drugs are excreted in human milk, caution should be exercised when DIPROLENE Gel is administered to a nursing woman.

Pediatric Use: Safety and effectiveness of DIPROLENE Gel in children have not been established, therefore its use in children under 12 is not recommended. *Because of a higher ratio of skin surface area to body mass, children are at a greater risk than adults of HPA axis suppression when they are treated with topical corticosteroids. They are, therefore, also at greater risk of glucocorticosteroid insufficiency after withdrawal of treatment and of Cushing's syndrome while on treatment.* Adverse effects, including striae, have been reported with inappropriate use of topical corticosteroids in infants and children.

HPA axis suppression, Cushing's syndrome, and intracranial hypertension have been reported in children receiving topical corticosteroids. Manifestations of adrenal suppression in children include linear growth retardation, delayed weight gain, low plasma cortisol levels, and absence of response to ACTH stimulation. Manifestations of intracranial hypertension include bulging fontanelles, headaches, and bilateral papilledema.

ADVERSE REACTIONS

In controlled clinical trials, the total incidence of adverse events associated with the use of DIPROLENE (augmented betamethasone dipropionate) Gel was 10%. These included stinging or burning in 6% of patients, dry skin in 4% of patients, and pruritus in 2% of patients. Less frequently reported adverse reactions were irritation, skin atrophy, telangiectasia, erythema, cracking/tightening of the skin, follicular rash, and allergic contact dermatitis.

The following additional local adverse reactions are reported infrequently with topical corticosteroids, but may occur more frequently with super-high potency corticosteroids, such as DIPROLENE Gel. These reactions are listed in approximate decreasing order of occurrence: acneiform eruptions, hypopigmentation, perioral dermatitis, secondary infection, striae and miliaria.

OVERDOSAGE

Topically applied DIPROLENE Gel can be absorbed in sufficient amounts to produce systemic effects (see **PRECAUTIONS**).

DOSAGE AND ADMINISTRATION

Apply a thin layer of DIPROLENE Gel to the affected skin once or twice daily and rub in gently and completely.

DIPROLENE Gel is a super-high potency topical corticosteroid; therefore, treatment should be limited to two weeks, and amounts greater than 50 g per week should not be used.

DIPROLENE Gel should not be used with occlusive dressings.

HOW SUPPLIED

DIPROLENE Gel 0.05% is supplied in 15 g (NDC 0085-0634-01), and 50 g (NDC 0085-0634-03) tubes; boxes of one.
Store between 2° and 25°C (36° and 77°F).
Schering Corporation
Kenilworth, NJ 07033 USA
Rev. 6/95 **18671409T**
Copyright © 1991, 1994, 1995, Schering Corporation.
All rights reserved.
Shown in Product Identification Guide, page 336

DIPROLENE® ℞

brand of augmented betamethasone dipropionate*
Lotion 0.05%
(potency expressed as betamethasone)

*Vehicle augments the penetration of the steroid.
For Dermatologic Use Only—Not for Ophthalmic Use

DESCRIPTION

DIPROLENE® Lotion contains betamethasone dipropionate, USP, a synthetic adrenocorticosteroid, for dermatologic use. Betamethasone, an analog of prednisolone, has a high degree of corticosteroid activity and a slight degree of mineralocorticoid activity. Betamethasone dipropionate is the 17, 21-dipropionate ester of betamethasone.
Chemically, betamethasone dipropionate is 9-fluoro-11β, 17,21-trihydroxy -16β- methylpregna-1,4-diene-3,20-dione 17,21-dipropionate, with the empirical formula $C_{28}H_{37}FO_7$, a molecular weight of 504.6, and the following structural formula:

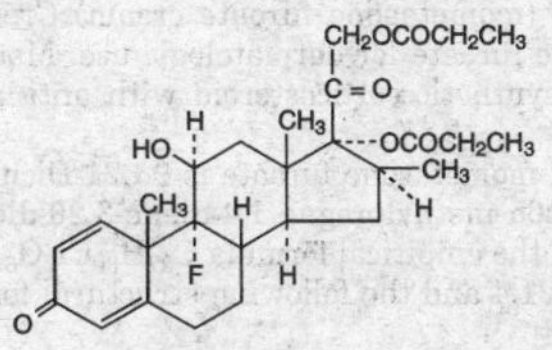

Betamethasone dipropionate is a white to creamy white, odorless crystalline powder, insoluble in water.
Each gram of DIPROLENE Lotion 0.05% contains: 0.64 mg betamethasone dipropionate, USP (equivalent to 0.5 mg betamethasone), in a lotion base of purified water, isopropyl alcohol (30%), hydroxypropylcellulose, propylene glycol, sodium phosphate; phosphoric acid and sodium hydroxide used to adjust the pH to 4.5.

CLINICAL PHARMACOLOGY

The corticosteroids are a class of compounds comprising steroid hormones secreted by the adrenal cortex and their synthetic analogs. In pharmacologic doses, corticosteroids are used primarily for their anti-inflammatory and/or immunosuppressive effects.
Topical corticosteroids, such as betamethasone dipropionate, are effective in the treatment of corticosteroid-responsive dermatoses primarily because of their anti-inflammatory, anti-pruritic, and vasoconstrictive actions. However, while the physiologic, pharmacologic, and clinical effects of the corticosteroids are well-known, the exact mechanisms of their actions in each disease are uncertain. Betamethasone dipropionate, a corticosteroid, has been shown to have topical (dermatologic) and systemic pharmacologic and metabolic effects characteristic of this class of drugs.
Pharmacokinetics The extent of percutaneous absorption of topical corticosteroids is determined by many factors including the vehicle, the integrity of the epidermal barrier, and the use of occlusive dressings. (See **DOSAGE AND ADMINISTRATION** section.)
Topical corticosteroids can be absorbed through normal intact skin. Inflammation and/or other disease processes in the skin may increase percutaneous absorption. Occlusive dressings substantially increase the percutaneous absorption of topical corticosteroids. (See **DOSAGE AND ADMINISTRATION** section.)
Once absorbed through the skin, topical corticosteroids enter pharmacokinetic pathways similar to systemically administered corticosteroids. Corticosteroids are bound to plasma proteins in varying degrees, are metabolized primarily in the liver and excreted by the kidneys. Some of the topical corticosteroids and their metabolites are also excreted into the bile.
DIPROLENE Lotion was applied once daily at 7 mL per day for 21 days to diseased skin (in patients with scalp psoriasis), to study its effects on the hypothalamic-pituitary-adrenal (HPA) axis. In 2 out of 11 patients, the drug lowered plasma cortisol levels below normal limits. Adrenal depression in these patients was transient, and returned to normal within a week. In one of these patients, plasma cortisol levels returned to normal while treatment continued.

INDICATIONS AND USAGE

DIPROLENE Lotion is indicated for treatment of the inflammatory and pruritic manifestations of moderate to severe corticosteroid-responsive dermatoses.
Treatment beyond two weeks is not recommended, and the total dosage should not exceed 50 mL per week because of potential for the drug to suppress the hypothalamic-pituitary-adrenal axis.

CONTRAINDICATIONS

DIPROLENE Lotion is contraindicated in patients who are hypersensitive to betamethasone dipropionate, to other corticosteroids, or to any ingredient in this preparation.

PRECAUTIONS

General DIPROLENE Lotion is a highly potent topical corticosteroid that has been shown to suppress the HPA axis at 7 mL per day.
Systemic absorption of topical corticosteroids has produced reversible HPA axis suppression, manifestations of Cushing's syndrome, hyperglycemia, and glucosuria in some patients.
Conditions which augment systemic absorption include the application of the more potent corticosteroids such as DIPROLENE, use over large surface areas, prolonged use, and the addition of occlusive dressings. (See **DOSAGE AND ADMINISTRATION** section.)
Therefore, patients receiving large doses of a potent topical steroid applied to a large surface area should be evaluated periodically for evidence of HPA axis suppression by using the urinary free cortisol and ACTH stimulation tests. If HPA axis suppression is noted, an attempt should be made to withdraw the drug, to reduce the frequency of application, or to substitute a less potent steroid.
Recovery of HPA axis function is generally prompt and complete upon discontinuation of the drug. Infrequently, signs and symptoms of steroid withdrawal may occur, requiring supplemental systemic corticosteroids.
Children may absorb proportionally larger amounts of topical corticosteroids and thus be more susceptible to systemic toxicity. (See **PRECAUTIONS—Pediatric Use.**)
If irritation develops, topical corticosteroids should be discontinued and appropriate therapy instituted.
In the presence of dermatological infections, the use of an appropriate antifungal or antibacterial agent should be instituted. If a favorable response does not occur promptly, the corticosteroid should be discontinued until the infection has been adequately controlled.
Information for Patients Patients using topical corticosteroids should receive the following information and instructions. This information is intended to aid in the safe and effective use of this medication. It is not a disclosure of all possible adverse or intended effects.

1. This medication is to be used as directed by the physician and should not be used longer than the prescribed time period. It is for external use only. Avoid contact with the eyes.
2. Patients should be advised not to use this medication for any disorder other than that for which it was prescribed.
3. The treated skin areas should not be bandaged or otherwise covered or wrapped so as to be occlusive. (See **DOSAGE AND ADMINISTRATION** section.)
4. Patients should report any sign of local adverse reactions.

Laboratory Tests The following tests may be helpful in evaluating HPA axis suppression:
Urinary free cortisol test
ACTH stimulation test
Carcinogenesis, Mutagenesis, and Impairment of Fertility Long-term animal studies have not been performed to evaluate the carcinogenic potential or the effect on fertility of topically applied corticosteroids.
Studies to determine mutagenicity with prednisolone and hydrocortisone have revealed negative results.
Pregnancy Category C Corticosteroids are generally teratogenic in laboratory animals when administered systemically at relatively low dosage levels. The more potent corticosteroids have been shown to be teratogenic after dermal application in laboratory animals. Betamethasone dipropionate has not been tested for teratogenicity by this route; however, it appears to be fairly well-absorbed percutaneously. There are no adequate and well-controlled studies of the teratogenic effects of topically applied corticosteroids in pregnant women. Therefore, topical corticosteroids should be used during pregnancy only if the potential benefit justifies the potential risk to the fetus. Drugs of this class should not be used extensively on pregnant patients, in large amounts, or for prolonged periods of time.
Nursing Mothers It is not known whether topical administration of corticosteroids can result in sufficient systemic absorption to produce detectable quantities in breast milk. Systemically administered corticosteroids are secreted into breast milk in quantities not likely to have a deleterious effect on the infant. Nevertheless, a decision should be made whether to discontinue nursing or to discontinue the drug, taking into account the importance of the drug to the mother.
Pediatric Use The safety and efficacy of DIPROLENE Lotion when used in children under 12 years of age have not been established.
Pediatric patients may demonstrate greater susceptibility to topical corticosteroid-induced HPA axis suppression, and Cushing's syndrome than mature patients because of a larger skin surface area to body weight ratio.
Hypothalamic-pituitary-adrenal (HPA) axis suppression, Cushing's syndrome, and intracranial hypertension have been reported in children receiving topical corticosteroids. Manifestations of adrenal suppression in children include linear growth retardation, delayed weight gain, low plasma cortisol levels, and absence of response to ACTH stimulation. Manifestations of intracranial hypertension include bulging fontanelles, headaches, and bilateral papilledema. Chronic corticosteroid therapy may interfere with the growth and development of children.

ADVERSE REACTIONS

The overall incidence of drug-related adverse reactions in the DIPROLENE Lotion clinical studies was 5%. The adverse reactions that were reported to be possibly or probably related to treatment with DIPROLENE Lotion during controlled clinical studies involving 327 patients or normal volunteers, were as follows: folliculitis occurred in 2%, burning and acneiform papules each occurred in 1%, and hyperesthesia and irritation each occurred in less than 1% of patients.
The following adverse reactions are also reported infrequently when topical corticosteroids are used as recommended. These reactions are listed in approximate decreasing order of occurrence: itching, dryness, hypertrichosis, hypopigmentation, perioral dermatitis, allergic contact dermatitis, maceration of the skin, secondary infection, skin atrophy, striae, miliaria.

OVERDOSAGE

Topically applied corticosteroids can be absorbed in sufficient amounts to produce systemic effects. (See **PRECAUTIONS.**)

DOSAGE AND ADMINISTRATION

Apply a few drops of DIPROLENE Lotion to the affected area once or twice daily and massage lightly until the lotion disappears. Treatment must be limited to 14 days, and amounts greater than 50 mL per week should not be used.
DIPROLENE Lotion is not to be used with occlusive dressings.

HOW SUPPLIED

DIPROLENE Lotion 0.05% is supplied in 30 mL (29 g) (NDC 0085-0962-01), and 60 mL (58 g) (NDC 0085-0962-02), plastic squeeze bottles; boxes of one.
Store between 2° and 25°C (36° and 77°F).
Schering Corporation
Kenilworth, NJ 07033 USA
Rev. 11/91 16566012
Copyright © 1988, 1992, Schering Corporation.
All rights reserved.

DIPROLENE® ℞

brand of augmented betamethasone dipropionate*
Ointment 0.05%
(potency expressed as betamethasone)
*Vehicle augments the penetration of the steroid.
For Dermatologic Use Only–
Not for Ophthalmic Use

DESCRIPTION

DIPROLENE Ointment contains betamethasone dipropionate, USP, a synthetic drenocorticosteroid, for dermatologic use. Betamethasone, an analog of prednisolone, has a high degree of corticosteroid activity and a slight degree of mineralocorticoid activity. Betamethasone dipropionate is the 17,21 - dipropionate ester of betamethasone.
Chemically, betamethasone dipropionate is 9-fluoro-11β, 17,21-trihydroxy-16β-methylpregna-1,4-diene -3,20- dione 17,21-dipropionate, with the empirical formula $C_{28}H_{37}FO_7$, a molecular weight of 504.6, and the following structural formula:
[See chemical structure at top of next column]
Betamethasone dipropionate is a white to creamy white, odorless crystalline powder, insoluble in water.

Continued on next page

Information on Schering products appearing on these pages is effective as of August 15, 1998.

Diprolene Ointment—Cont.

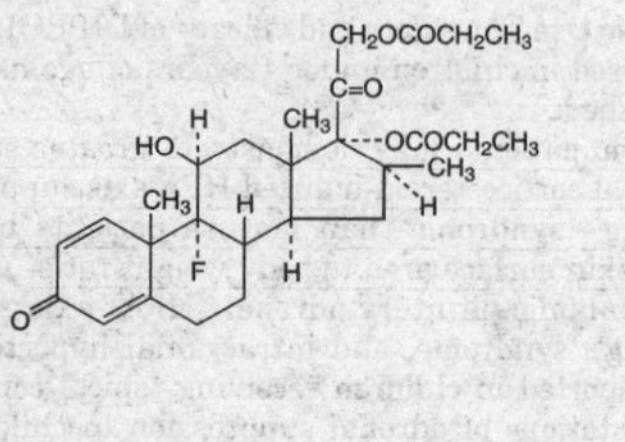

Each gram of DIPROLENE Ointment 0.05% contains: 0.64 mg betamethasone dipropionate, USP (equivalent to 0.5 mg betamethasone), in ACTIBASE®, an optimized vehicle of propylene glycol, propylene glycol stearate, white wax, and white petrolatum.

CLINICAL PHARMACOLOGY

The corticosteroids are a class of compounds comprising steroid hormones secreted by the adrenal cortex and their synthetic analogs. In pharmacologic doses, corticosteroids are used primarily for their anti-inflammatory and/or immunosuppressive effects.

Topical corticosteroids, such as betamethasone dipropionate, are effective in the treatment of corticosteroid-responsive dermatoses primarily because of their anti-inflammatory, anti-pruritic, and vasoconstrictive actions. However, while the physiologic, pharmacologic, and clinical effects of the corticosteroids are well known, the exact mechanisms of their actions in each disease are uncertain. Betamethasone dipropionate, a corticosteroid, has been shown to have topical (dermatologic) and systemic pharmacologic and metabolic effects characteristic of this class of drugs.

Pharmacokinetics The extent of percutaneous absorption of topical corticosteroids is determined by many factors including the vehicle, the integrity of the epidermal barrier, and the use of occlusive dressings. (See **DOSAGE AND ADMINISTRATION** section.)

Topical corticosteroids can be absorbed from normal intact skin. Inflammation and/or other disease processes in the skin may increase percutaneous absorption. Occlusive dressings substantially increase the percutaneous absorption of topical corticosteroids. (See **DOSAGE AND ADMINISTRATION** section.)

Once absorbed through the skin, topical corticosteroids enter pharmacokinetic pathways similar to systemically administered corticosteroids. Corticosteroids are bound to plasma proteins in varying degrees. Corticosteroids are metabolized primarily in the liver and are then excreted by the kidneys. Some of the topical corticosteroids and their metabolites are also excreted into the bile.

At 14 g per day, DIPROLENE Ointment was shown to depress the plasma levels of adrenal cortical hormones following repeated application to diseased skin in patients with psoriasis. Adrenal depression in these patients was transient, and rapidly returned to normal upon cessation of treatment. At 7 g per day (3.5 g bid), DIPROLENE Ointment was shown to cause minimal inhibition of the hypothalamic-pituitary-adrenal (HPA) axis when applied two times daily for 2 to 3 weeks, in normal patients and in patients with psoriasis and eczematous disorders.

With 6 to 7 g of DIPROLENE Ointment applied once daily for 3 weeks, no significant inhibition of the HPA axis was observed in patients with psoriasis and atopic dermatitis, as measured by plasma cortisol and 24-hour urinary 17-hydroxycorticosteroid levels.

INDICATIONS AND USAGE

DIPROLENE Ointment is indicated for relief of the inflammatory and pruritic manifestations of corticosteroid-responsive dermatoses.

CONTRAINDICATIONS

DIPROLENE Ointment is contraindicated in patients who are hypersensitive to betamethasone dipropionate, to other corticosteroids, or to any ingredient in this preparation.

PRECAUTIONS

General Systemic absorption of topical corticosteroids has produced reversible HPA axis suppression, manifestations of Cushing's syndrome, hyperglycemia, and glucosuria in some patients.

Conditions which augment systemic absorption include the application of the more potent corticosteroids, use over large surface areas, prolonged use, and the addition of occlusive dressings. (See **DOSAGE AND ADMINISTRATION** section.)

Therefore, patients receiving a large dose of a potent topical steroid applied to a large surface area should be evaluated periodically for evidence of HPA axis suppression by using the urinary free cortisol and ACTH stimulation tests. If HPA axis suppression is noted, an attempt should be made to withdraw the drug, to reduce the frequency of application, or to substitute a less potent steroid.

Recovery of HPA axis function is generally prompt and complete upon discontinuation of the drug. Infrequently, signs and symptoms of steroid withdrawal may occur, requiring supplemental systemic corticosteroids.

Children may absorb proportionally larger amounts of topical corticosteroids and thus be more susceptible to systemic toxicity. (See **PRECAUTIONS–Pediatric Use**.)

If irritation develops, topical corticosteroids should be discontinued and appropriate therapy instituted.

In the presence of dermatological infections, the use of an appropriate antifungal or antibacterial agent should be instituted. If a favorable response does not occur promptly, the corticosteroid should be discontinued until the infection has been adequately controlled.

Information for Patients Patients using topical corticosteroids should receive the following information and instructions:

1. This medication is to be used as directed by the physician and should not be used longer than the prescribed time period. It is for external use only. Avoid contact with the eyes.
2. Patients should be advised not to use this medication for any disorder other than that for which it was prescribed.
3. The treated skin area should not be bandaged or otherwise covered or wrapped as to be occlusive. (See **DOSAGE AND ADMINISTRATION** section.)
4. Patients should report any signs of local adverse reactions.

Laboratory Tests The following tests may be helpful in evaluating HPA axis suppression:

Urinary free cortisol test
ACTH stimulation test

Carcinogenesis, Mutagenesis, and Impairment of Fertility Long-term animal studies have not been performed to evaluate the carcinogenic potential or the effect on fertility of topically applied corticosteroids.

Studies to determine mutagenicity with prednisolone have revealed negative results.

Pregnancy Category C Corticosteroids are generally teratogenic in laboratory animals when administered systemically at relatively low dosage levels. The more potent corticosteroids have been shown to be teratogenic after dermal application in laboratory animals. There are no adequate and well-controlled studies of the teratogenic effects of topically applied corticosteroids in pregnant women. Therefore, topical corticosteroids should be used during pregnancy only if the potential benefit justifies the potential risk to the fetus. Drugs of this class should not be used extensively on pregnant patients, in large amounts, or for prolonged periods of time.

Nursing Mothers It is not known whether topical administration of corticosteroids could result in sufficient systemic absorption to produce detectable quantities in breast milk. Systemically administered corticosteroids are secreted into breast milk in quantities not likely to have a deleterious effect on the infant. Nevertheless, caution should be exercised when topical corticosteroids are prescribed for a nursing woman.

Pediatric Use Use of DIPROLENE Ointment in children under 12 years is not recommended.

Pediatric patients may demonstrate greater susceptibility to topical corticosteroid-induced HPA axis suppression and Cushing's syndrome than mature patients because of a larger skin surface area to body weight ratio.

Hypothalamic-pituitary-adrenal (HPA) axis suppression, Cushing's syndrome, and intracranial hypertension have been reported in children receiving topical corticosteroids. Manifestations of adrenal suppression in children include linear growth retardation, delayed weight gain, low plasma cortisol levels, and absence of response to ACTH stimulation. Manifestations of intracranial hypertension include bulging fontanelles, headaches, and bilateral papilledema.

Administration of topical corticosteroids to children should be limited to the least amount compatible with an effective therapeutic regimen. Chronic corticosteroid therapy may interfere with the growth and development of children.

ADVERSE REACTIONS

The local adverse reactions were reported with DIPROLENE Ointment applied either once or twice a day during clinical studies are as follows: erythema, 3 per 767 patients; folliculitis, 2 per 767 patients; pruritus, 2 per 767 patients; vesiculation, 1 per 767 patients.

The following local adverse reactions are reported infrequently when topical corticosteroids are used as recommended. These reactions are listed in an approximate decreasing order of occurrence: burning, itching, irritation, dryness, folliculitis, hypertrichosis, acneiform eruptions, hypopigmentation, perioral dermatitis, allergic contact dermatitis, maceration of the skin, secondary infection, skin atrophy, striae, miliaria.

Systemic absorption of topical corticosteroids has produced reversible HPA axis suppression, manifestations of Cushing's syndrome, hyperglycemia, and glucosuria in some patients.

OVERDOSAGE

Topically applied corticosteroids can be absorbed in sufficient amounts to produce systemic effects. (See **PRECAUTIONS**.)

DOSAGE AND ADMINISTRATION

Apply a thin film of DIPROLENE Ointment to the affected skin areas once or twice daily. Treatment with DIPROLENE Ointment should be limited to 45 g per week.

DIPROLENE Ointment is not to be used with occlusive dressings.

HOW SUPPLIED

DIPROLENE Ointment 0.05% is supplied in 15 g (NDC 0085-0575-02), and 50 g (NDC 0085-0575-05) tubes; boxes of one.

Store between 2° and 25°C (36° and 77°F).

Schering Corporation
Kenilworth, NJ 07033 USA
Rev. 7/95

18670500T

Copyright © 1983, 1991, 1994, 1995, Schering Corporation. All rights reserved.

Shown in Product Identification Guide, page 336

ELOCON® ℞

brand of mometasone furoate cream
Cream 0.1%
For Dermatologic Use Only
Not for Ophthalmic Use

DESCRIPTION

ELOCON® (mometasone furoate cream) Cream contains mometasone furoate for dermatologic use. Mometasone furoate is a synthetic corticosteroid with anti-inflammatory activity.

Chemically, mometasone furoate is 9α,21-Dichloro-11β, 17-dihydroxy-16α-methylpregna-1,4-diene-3,20-dione 17-(2-furoate), with the empirical formula $C_{27}H_{30}Cl_2O_6$, a molecular weight of 521.4 and the following structural formula:

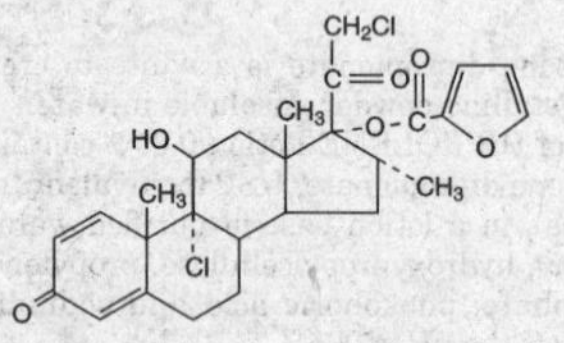

Mometasone furoate is a white to off-white powder practically insoluble in water, slightly soluble in octanol, and moderately soluble in ethyl alcohol.

Each gram of ELOCON Cream 0.1% contains: 1 mg mometasone furoate in a cream base of hexylene glycol, phosphoric acid, propylene glycol stearate, stearyl alcohol and ceteareth-20, titanium dioxide, aluminum starch octenylsuccinate, white wax, white petrolatum, and purified water.

CLINICAL PHARMACOLOGY

Like other topical corticosteroids, mometasone furoate has anti-inflammatory, anti-pruritic, and vasoconstrictive properties. The mechanism of the anti-inflammatory activity of the topical steroids, in general, is unclear. However, corticosteroids are thought to act by the induction of phospholipase A_2 inhibitory proteins, collectively called lipocortins. It is postulated that these proteins control the biosynthesis of potent mediators of inflammation such as prostaglandins and leukotrienes by inhibiting the release of their common precursor arachidonic acid. Arachidonic acid is released from membrane phospholipids by phospholipase A_2.

Pharmacokinetics The extent of percutaneous absorption of topical corticosteroids is determined by many factors including the vehicle and the integrity of the epidermal barrier. Occlusive dressings with hydrocortisone for up to 24 hours have not been demonstrated to increase penetration; however, occlusion of hydrocortisone for 96 hours markedly enhances penetration. Studies in humans indicate that approximately 0.4% of the applied dose of ELOCON Cream 0.1% enters the circulation after 8 hours of contact on normal skin without occlusion. Inflammation and/or other disease processes in the skin may increase percutaneous absorption.

Studies performed with ELOCON Cream indicate that it is in the medium range of potency as compared with other topical corticosteroids.

In a pediatric trial, 24 atopic dermatitis patients, of which 19 patients were age 2 to 12 years, were treated with ELOCON Cream 0.1% once daily. The majority of patients cleared within 3 weeks.

INDICATIONS AND USAGE

ELOCON Cream 0.1% is a medium potency corticosteroid indicated for the relief of the inflammatory and pruritic manifestations of corticosteroid-responsive dermatoses.

ELOCON (mometasone furoate cream) Cream may be used in pediatric patients 2 years of age or older, although the safety and efficacy of drug use for longer than 3 weeks have not been established (see **PRECAUTIONS–Pediatric Use**). Since safety and efficacy of ELOCON Cream have not been established in pediatric patients below 2 years of age, its use in this age group is not recommended.

CONTRAINDICATIONS

ELOCON Cream is contraindicated in those patients with a history of hypersensitivity to any of the components in the preparation.

PRECAUTIONS

General Systemic absorption of topical corticosteroids can produce reversible hypothalamic-pituitary-adrenal (HPA) axis suppression with the potential for glucocorticosteroid insufficiency after withdrawal of treatment. Manifestations of Cushing's syndrome, hyperglycemia, and glucosuria can also be produced in some patients by systemic absorption of topical corticosteroids while on treatment.

Patients applying a topical steroid to a large surface area or to areas under occlusion should be evaluated periodically for evidence of HPA axis suppression. This may be done by using the ACTH stimulation, A.M. plasma cortisol, and urinary free cortisol tests.

In a study evaluating the effects of mometasone furoate cream on the hypothalamic-pituitary-adrenal (HPA) axis, 15 grams were applied twice daily for 7 days to six adult patients with psoriasis or atopic dermatitis. The cream was applied without occlusion to at least 30% of the body surface. The results show that the drug caused a slight lowering of adrenal corticosteroid secretion.

If HPA axis suppression is noted, an attempt should be made to withdraw the drug, to reduce the frequency of application, or to substitute a less potent corticosteroid. Recovery of HPA axis function is generally prompt upon discontinuation of topical corticosteroids. Infrequently, signs and symptoms of glucocorticosteroid insufficiency may occur requiring supplemental systemic corticosteroids. For information on systemic supplementation, see Prescribing Information for those products.

Pediatric patients may be more susceptible to systemic toxicity from equivalent doses due to their larger skin surface to body mass ratios (see **PRECAUTIONS–Pediatric Use**).

If irritation develops, ELOCON Cream should be discontinued and appropriate therapy instituted. Allergic contact dermatitis with corticosteroids is usually diagnosed by observing a failure to heal rather than noting a clinical exacerbation as with most topical products not containing corticosteroids. Such an observation should be corroborated with appropriate diagnostic patch testing.

If concomitant skin infections are present or develop, an appropriate antifungal or antibacterial agent should be used. If a favorable response does not occur promptly, use of ELOCON Cream should be discontinued until the infection has been adequately controlled.

Information for Patients Patients using topical corticosteroids should receive the following information and instructions:

1. This medication is to be used as directed by the physician. It is for external use only. Avoid contact with the eyes.
2. This medication should not be used for any disorder other than that for which it was prescribed.
3. The treated skin area should not be bandaged or otherwise covered or wrapped so as to be occlusive unless directed by the physician.
4. Patients should report to their physician any signs of local adverse reactions.
5. Parents of pediatric patients should be advised not to use ELOCON Cream in the treatment of diaper dermatitis. ELOCON Cream should not be applied in the diaper area as diapers or plastic pants may constitute occlusive dressing (see **DOSAGE AND ADMINISTRATION**).
6. This medication should not be used on the face, underarms, or groin areas unless directed by the physician.
7. As with other corticosteroids, therapy should be discontinued when control is achieved. If no improvement is seen within 2 weeks, contact the physician.

Laboratory Tests The following tests may be helpful in evaluating patients for HPA axis suppression:

ACTH stimulation test
A.M. plasma cortisol test
Urinary free cortisol test

Carcinogenesis, Mutagenesis, and Impairment of Fertility In studies of the effect of mometasone furoate on fertility, pregnancy, and postnatal development in rats and rabbits, 25 rats were treated with doses up to 1.2 mg/kg of drug topically, and 15 rabbits with doses up to 0.3 mg/kg of drug topically. The drugs were left on the skin for 6 hours daily during gestation. At the highest dosage, the rat dams lost weight. One of the rabbit dams at the highest dosage had wrinkled skin, muscle wasting and aborted 5 fetuses.

Genetic toxicity studies with mometasone furoate, which included the Ames test, mouse lymphoma assay, and a micronucleus test did not reveal any mutagenic potential.

Long term animal studies have not been performed to evaluate the carcinogenic potential of ELOCON (mometasone furoate cream) Cream.

Pregnancy Teratogenic effects: Pregnancy Category C Corticosteroids have been shown to be teratogenic in laboratory animals when administered systemically at relatively low dosage levels. Some corticosteroids have been shown to be teratogenic after dermal application in laboratory animals.

Rat offspring of dams treated with 1.2 mg/kg of mometasone furoate topically (4 times the maximum dose in a 50 kg individual) displayed umbilical hernias, unossified sternebrae and vertebrae, and wavy ribs, as well as markedly depressed fetal growth. Rabbit offspring of dams treated with up to 0.3 mg/kg of mometasone furoate topically (the same dose as the maximum dose in a 50 kg individual) displayed flexed paws, umbilical hernias, and cleft palate. A 50 kg female using 1 gram of ELOCON Cream would apply approximately 0.023 mg/kg.

There are no adequate and well-controlled studies of the teratogenic potential of mometasone furoate in pregnant women. ELOCON Cream should be used during pregnancy only if the potential benefit justifies the potential risk to the fetus.

Nursing Mothers Systemtically administered corticosteroids appear in human milk and could suppress growth, interfere with endogenous corticosteroid production, or cause other untoward effects. It is not known whether topical administration of corticosteroids could result in sufficient systemic absorption to produce detectable quantities in human milk. Because many drugs are excreted in human milk, caution should be exercised when ELOCON Cream is administered to a nursing woman.

Pediatric Use ELOCON Cream may be used with caution in pediatric patients 2 years of age or older, although the safety and efficacy of drug use for longer than 3 weeks have not been established. Use of ELOCON Cream is supported by results from adequate and well-controlled studies in pediatric patients with corticosteroid-responsive dermatoses. Since safety and efficacy of ELOCON Cream have not been established in pediatric patients below 2 years of age, its use in this age group is not recommended. Because of a higher ratio of skin surface area to body mass, pediatric patients are at a greater risk than adults of HPA axis suppression and Cushing's syndrome when they are treated with topical corticosteroids. They are, therefore, also at greater risk of adrenal insufficiency during and/or after withdrawal of treatment. Pediatric patients may be more susceptible than adults to skin atrophy, including striae, when they are treated with topical corticosteroids. Pediatric patients applying topical corticosteroids to greater than 20% of body surface are at higher risk of HPA axis suppression.

HPA axis suppression, Cushing's syndrome, linear growth retardation, delayed weight gain, and intracranial hypertension have been reported in pediatric patients receiving topical corticosteroids. Manifestations of adrenal suppression in children include low plasma cortisol levels, and an absence of response to ACTH stimulation. Manifestations of intracranial hypertension include bulging fontanelles, headaches, and bilateral papilledema.

ELOCON (mometasone furoate cream) Cream should not be used in the treatment of diaper dermatitis.

ADVERSE REACTIONS

In controlled clinical studies involving 319 patients, the incidence of adverse reactions associated with the use of ELOCON Cream was 1.6%. Reported reactions included burning, pruritus, and skin atrophy. Reports of rosacea associated with the use of ELOCON Cream have also been received. In controlled clinical studies (n=74) involving pediatric patients 2 to 12 years of age, the incidence of adverse experiences associated with the use of ELOCON Cream was approximately 7%. Reported reactions included stinging, pruritus, and furunculosis.

The following additional local adverse reactions have been reported infrequently with topical corticosteroids, but may occur more frequently with the use of occlusive dressings. These reactions are listed in an approximate decreasing order of occurrence: irritation, dryness, folliculitis, hypertrichosis, acneiform eruptions, hypopigmentation, perioral dermatitis, allergic contact dermatitis, secondary infection, striae, and miliaria.

OVERDOSAGE

Topically applied ELOCON Cream can be absorbed in sufficient amounts to produce systemic effects (see **PRECAUTIONS**).

DOSAGE AND ADMINISTRATION

Apply a thin film of ELOCON Cream to the affected skin areas once daily.

ELOCON Cream may be used in pediatric patients 2 years of age or older. Safety and efficacy of ELOCON Cream in pediatric patients for more than 3 weeks of use have not been established. Use in pediatric patients under 2 years of age is not recommended.

As with other corticosteroids, therapy should be discontinued when control is achieved. If no improvement is seen within 2 weeks, reassessment of diagnosis may be necessary.

ELOCON Cream should not be used with occlusive dressings unless directed by a physician. ELOCON Cream should not be applied in the diaper area if the child still requires diapers or plastic pants as these garments may constitute occlusive dressing.

HOW SUPPLIED

ELOCON Cream 0.1% is supplied in 15 g (NDC 0085-0567-01) and 45 g (NDC 0085-0567-02) tubes; boxes of one.

Store ELOCON Cream between 2° and 25°C (36° and 77°F).

Schering Corporation
Kenilworth, NJ 07033 USA
Revised 8/95

18724308T

Copyright © 1987, 1991, 1994, 1995, Schering Corporation. All rights reserved.

ELOCON® ℞

brand of mometasone furoate
Lotion 0.1%
For Dermatologic Use Only
Not for Ophthalmic Use

DESCRIPTION

ELOCON Lotion 0.1% contains mometasone furoate for dermatologic use. Mometasone furoate is a synthetic corticosteroid with anti-inflammatory activity.

Chemically, mometasone furoate is 9α, 21-Dichloro-11β, 17-dihydroxy-16α-methylpregna-1, 4-diene-3, 20 dione 17-(2-furoate), with the empirical formula $C_{27}H_{30}Cl_2O_6$, a molecular weight of 521.4 and the following structural formula:

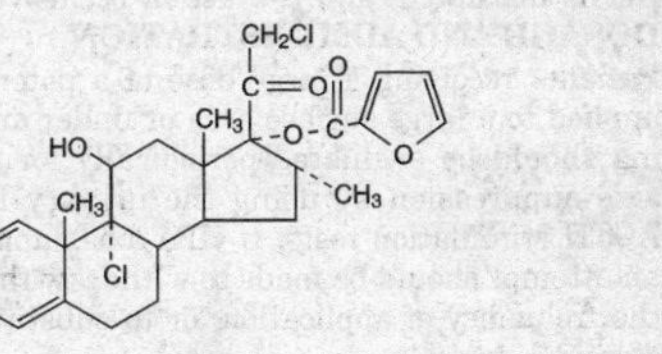

Mometasone furoate is a white to off-white powder practically insoluble in water, slightly soluble in octanol, and moderately soluble in ethyl alcohol.

Each gram of ELOCON Lotion 0.1% contains: 1 mg of mometasone furoate in a lotion base of isopropyl alcohol (40%), propylene glycol, hydroxypropylcellulose, sodium phosphate and water. May also contain phosphoric acid and sodium hydroxide used to adjust the pH to approximately 4.5.

CLINICAL PHARMACOLOGY

The corticosteroids are a class of compounds comprising steroid hormones secreted by the adrenal cortex and their synthetic analogs. In pharmacologic doses corticosteroids are used primarily for their anti-inflammatory and/or immunosuppressive effects.

Topical corticosteroids, such as mometasone furoate, are effective in the treatment of corticosteroid-responsive dermatoses primarily because of their anti-inflammatory, antipruritic, and vasoconstrictive actions. However, while the physiologic, pharmacologic, and clinical effects of the corticosteroids are well known, the exact mechanisms of their actions in each disease are uncertain. Mometasone furoate has been shown to have topical (dermatologic) and systemic pharmacologic and metabolic effects characteristic of this class of drugs.

Pharmacokinetics The extent of percutaneous absorption of topical corticosteroids is determined by many factors including the vehicle, the integrity of the epidermal barrier, and the use of occlusive dressings. (See **DOSAGE AND ADMINISTRATION.**) Topical corticosteroids can be absorbed from normal intact skin.

Continued on next page

Information on Schering products appearing on these pages is effective as of August 15, 1998.

Elocon Lotion—Cont.

A study using a radio-labelled ^3H mometasone furoate ointment (0.1%) formulation was performed in man to measure systemic absorption and excretion. Results showed that approximately 0.7% of the steroid was absorbed during 8 hours of contact, without occlusion, with intact skin of normal volunteers. A similar minimal degree of absorption of the corticosteroid from the lotion formulation would be anticipated.
Inflammation and/or disease processes in the skin increase percutaneous absorption. Occlusive dressings substantially increase the percutaneous absorption of topical corticosteroids. (See **DOSAGE AND ADMINISTRATION**.)
Mometasone furoate lotion was applied at 15 mL twice daily (30 mL per day) to diseased skin (patients with scalp and body psoriasis) of four patients for seven days, to study its effects on the hypothalamic-pituitary-adrenal (HPA) axis. Plasma cortisol levels for each of the four patients remained well within the normal range and changed little from baseline.
Once absorbed through the skin, topical corticosteroids are handled through pharmacokinetic pathways similar to systemically administered corticosteroids. Corticosteroids are bound to plasma proteins in varying degrees. Corticosteroids are metabolized primarily in the liver and are then excreted by the kidneys. Some of the topical corticosteroids and their metabolites are also excreted into the bile.

INDICATIONS AND USAGE

ELOCON Lotion is indicated for the relief of the inflammatory and pruritic manifestations of corticosteroid-responsive dermatoses.

CONTRAINDICATIONS

ELOCON Lotion is contraindicated in patients who are hypersensitive to mometasone furoate, to other corticosteroids, or to any ingredient in this preparation.

PRECAUTIONS

General Systemic absorption of potent topical corticosteroids has produced reversible hypothalamic-pituitary-adrenal (HPA) axis suppression, manifestations of Cushing's syndrome, hyperglycemia, and glucosuria in some patients. Conditions which augment systemic absorption include application of more potent steroids, use over large surface areas, prolonged use, use in areas where the epidermal barrier is disrupted, and the use of occlusive dressings. (See **DOSAGE AND ADMINISTRATION**.)
Patients receiving a large dose of a potent topical steroid applied to a large surface area or under an occlusive dressing should be evaluated periodically for evidence of HPA axis suppression by using the urinary free cortisol and ACTH stimulation tests. If HPA axis suppression is noted, an attempt should be made to withdraw the drug, to reduce the frequency of application, or to substitute a less potent steroid.
Recovery of HPA axis function is generally prompt and complete upon discontinuation of the drug. Infrequently, signs and symptoms of steroid withdrawal may occur, requiring supplemental systemic corticosteroids.
Children may absorb proportionally larger amounts of topical corticosteroids and thus be more susceptible to systemic toxicity. (See **PRECAUTIONS—Pediatric Use.**)
If irritation develops, topical corticosteroids should be discontinued and appropriate therapy instituted.
In the presence of dermatological infections, use of an appropriate antifungal or antibacterial agent should be instituted. If a favorable response does not occur promptly, the corticosteroid should be discontinued until the infection has been adequately controlled.
Information for Patients Patients using topical corticosteroids should receive the following information and instructions. This information is intended to aid in the safe and effective use of this medication. It is not a disclosure of all possible adverse or intended effects.
1. This medication is to be used as directed by the physician. It is for external use only. Avoid contact with the eyes.
2. Patients should be advised not to use this medication for any disorder other than that for which it was prescribed.
3. The treated skin area should not be bandaged or otherwise covered or wrapped as to be occlusive unless directed by the physician. (See **DOSAGE AND ADMINISTRATION**.)
4. Patients should report any signs of local adverse reactions.
5. Parents of pediatric patients should be advised not to use tight-fitting diapers or plastic pants on a child being treated in the diaper area, as these garments may constitute occlusive dressing. (See **DOSAGE AND ADMINISTRATION**.)
Laboratory Tests The following tests may be helpful in evaluating HPA axis suppression:
Urinary free cortisol test
ACTH stimulation test

Carcinogenesis, Mutagenesis, and Impairment of Fertility Long-term animal studies have not been performed to evaluate the carcinogenic potential or the effect on fertility of topical corticosteroids.
Genetic toxicity studies with mometasone furoate, which included the Ames test, mouse lymphoma assay, and a micronucleus test, did not reveal any mutagenic potential.
Pregnancy Category C Corticosteroids are generally teratogenic in laboratory animals when administered systemically at relatively low dosage levels. Corticosteroids have been shown to be teratogenic after dermal application in laboratory animals. There are no adequate and well-controlled studies of teratogenic effects from topically applied corticosteroids in pregnant women. Therefore, topical corticosteroids should be used during pregnancy only if the potential benefit justifies the potential risk to the fetus. Drugs of this class should not be used extensively on pregnant patients, in large amounts, or for prolonged periods.
Nursing Mothers It is not known whether topical administration of corticosteroids could result in sufficient systemic absorption to produce detectable quantities in breast milk. Systemically administered corticosteroids are secreted into breast milk in quantities not likely to have a deleterious effect on the infant. Nevertheless, a decision should be made whether to discontinue nursing or to discontinue the drug, taking into account the importance of the drug to the mother.
Pediatric Use Pediatric patients may demonstrate greater susceptibility to topical corticosteroid-induced HPA axis suppression and Cushing's syndrome than mature patients because of a larger skin surface area to body weight ratio.
Hypothalamic-pituitary-adrenal (HPA) axis suppression, Cushing's syndrome, and intracranial hypertension have been reported in children receiving topical corticosteroids. Manifestations of adrenal suppression in children include linear growth retardation, delayed weight gain, low plasma cortisol levels, and absence of response to ACTH stimulation. Manifestations of intracranial hypertension include bulging fontanelles, headaches, and bilateral papilledema. Administration of topical corticosteroids to children should be limited to the least amount compatible with an effective therapeutic regimen. Chronic corticosteroid therapy may interfere with the growth and development of children.

ADVERSE REACTIONS

The following local adverse reactions were reported with ELOCON Lotion during clinical studies with 209 patients: acneiform reaction, 2; burning, 4; and itching, 1. In an irritation/sensitization study with 156 normal subjects, folliculitis was reported in 4.
The following local adverse reactions have been reported infrequently when other topical dermatologic corticosteroids have been used as recommended. These reactions are listed in an approximate decreasing order of occurrence: burning, itching, irritation, dryness, folliculitis, hypertrichosis, acneiform eruptions, hypopigmentation, perioral dermatitis, allergic contact dermatitis, maceration of the skin, secondary infection, skin atrophy, striae, miliaria.

OVERDOSAGE

Topically applied corticosteroids can be absorbed in sufficient amounts to produce systemic effects. (See **PRECAUTIONS**.)

DOSAGE AND ADMINISTRATION

Apply a few drops of ELOCON Lotion to the affected areas once daily and massage lightly until it disappears. For the most effective and economical use, hold the nozzle of the bottle very close to the affected areas and gently squeeze.

HOW SUPPLIED

ELOCON Lotion 0.1% is supplied in 30 mL (27.5 g) (NDC-0085-0854-01) and 60 mL (55 g) (NDC-0085-0854-02) bottles; boxes of one.
Store ELOCON Lotion between 2° and 30°C (36° and 86°F).
Schering Corporation
Kenilworth, NJ 07033 USA
Rev. 11/93

17980904

ELOCON® ℞
brand of mometasone furoate ointment
Ointment 0.1%
For Dermatologic Use Only
Not for Ophthalmic Use

DESCRIPTION

ELOCON® (mometasone furoate ointment) Ointment contains mometasone furoate for dermatologic use. Mometasone furoate is a synthetic corticosteroid with anti-inflammatory activity.
Chemically, mometasone furoate is 9α,21-Dichloro-11β,17-dihydroxy-16α-methylpregna-1,4-diene-3,20-dione 17-(2-furoate), with the empirical formula $C_{27}H_{30}Cl_2O_6$, a molecular weight of 521.4 and the following structural formula:

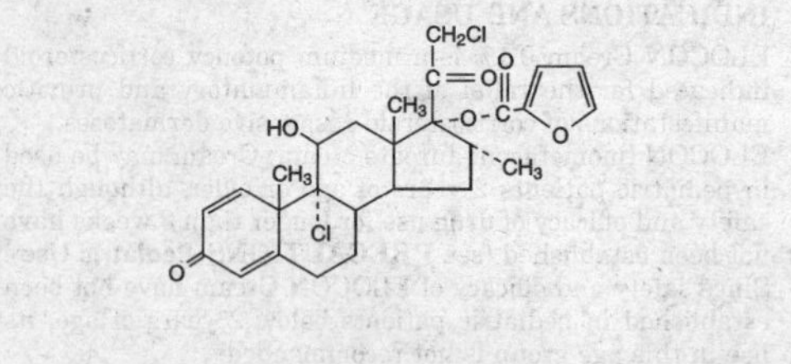

Mometasone furoate is a white to off-white powder practically insoluble in water, slightly soluble in octanol, and moderately soluble in ethyl alcohol.
Each gram of ELOCON Ointment 0.1% contains: 1 mg mometasone furoate in an ointment base of hexylene glycol, phosphoric acid, propylene glycol stearate, white wax, white petrolatum, and purified water.

CLINICAL PHARMACOLOGY

Like other topical corticosteroids, mometasone furoate has anti-inflammatory, antipruritic, and vasoconstrictive properties. The mechanism of the anti-inflammatory activity of the topical steroids, in general, is unclear. However, corticosteroids are thought to act by the induction of phospholipase A_2 inhibitory proteins, collectively called lipocortins. It is postulated that these proteins control the biosynthesis of potent mediators of inflammation such as prostaglandins and leukotrienes by inhibiting the release of their common precursor arachidonic acid. Arachidonic acid is released from membrane phospholipids by phospholipase A_2.
Pharmacokinetics The extent of percutaneous absorption of topical corticosteroids is determined by many factors including the vehicle and the integrity of the epidermal barrier. Occlusive dressings with hydrocortisone for up to 24 hours have not been demonstrated to increase penetration; however, occlusion of hydrocortisone for 96 hours markedly enhances penetration. Studies in humans indicate that approximately 0.7% of the applied dose of ELOCON Ointment 0.1% enters the circulation after 8 hours of contact on normal skin without occlusion. Inflammation and/or other disease processes in the skin may increase percutaneous absorption.
Studies performed with ELOCON Ointment indicate that it is in the medium range of potency as compared with other topical corticosteroids.
In a pediatric trial, 24 atopic dermatitis patients, of which 19 patients were age 2 to 12 years, were treated with ELOCON Cream 0.1% once daily. The majority of patients cleared within 3 weeks.

INDICATIONS AND USAGE

ELOCON Ointment 0.1% is a medium potency corticosteroid indicated for the relief of the inflammatory and pruritic manifestations of corticosteroid-responsive dermatoses.
ELOCON (mometasone furoate ointment) Ointment may be used in pediatric patients 2 years of age or older, although the safety and efficacy of drug use for longer than 3 weeks have not been established (see **PRECAUTIONS—Pediatric Use**). Since safety and efficacy of ELOCON Ointment have not been established in pediatric patients below 2 years of age, its use in this age group is not recommended.

CONTRAINDICATIONS

ELOCON Ointment is contraindicated in those patients with a history of hypersensitivity to any of the components in the preparation.

PRECAUTIONS

General Systemic absorption of topical corticosteroids can produce reversible hypothalamic-pituitary-adrenal (HPA) axis suppression with the potential for glucocorticosteroid insufficiency after withdrawal of treatment. Manifestations of Cushing's syndrome, hyperglycemia, and glucosuria can also be produced in some patients by systemic absorption of topical corticosteroids while on treatment.
Patients applying a topical steroid to a large surface area or areas under occlusion should be evaluated periodically for evidence of HPA axis suppression. This may be done by using the ACTH stimulation, A.M. plasma cortisol, and urinary free cortisol tests.
In a study evaluating the effects of mometasone furoate ointment on the hypothalamic-pituitary-adrenal (HPA) axis, 15 grams were applied twice daily for 7 days to six adult patients with psoriasis or atopic dermatitis. The ointment was applied without occlusion to at least 30% of the body surface. The results show that the drug caused a slight lowering of adrenal corticosteroid secretion.
If HPA axis suppression is noted, an attempt should be made to withdraw the drug, to reduce the frequency of application, or to substitute a less potent corticosteroid. Recovery of HPA axis function is generally prompt upon discon-

tinuation of topical corticosteroids. Infrequently, signs and symptoms of glucocorticosteroid insufficiency may occur requiring supplemental systemic corticosteroids. For information on systemic supplementation, see Prescribing Information for those products.

Pediatric patients may be more susceptible to systemic toxicity from equivalent doses due to their larger skin surface to body mass ratios (see **PRECAUTIONS–Pediatric Use**).

If irritation develops, ELOCON Ointment should be discontinued and appropriate therapy instituted. Allergic contact dermatitis with corticosteroids is usually diagnosed by observing failure to heal rather than noting a clinical exacerbation as with most topical products not containing corticosteroids. Such an observation should be corroborated with appropriate diagnostic patch testing.

If concomitant skin infections are present or develop, an appropriate antifugal or antibacterial agent should be used. If a favorable response does not occur promptly, use of ELOCON Ointment should be discontinued until the infection has been adequately controlled.

Information for Patients Patients using topical corticosteroids should receive the following information and instructions:

1. This medication is to be used as directed by the physician. It is for external use only. Avoid contact with the eyes.
2. This medication should not be used for any disorder other than that for which it was prescribed.
3. The treated skin area should not be bandaged or otherwise covered or wrapped so as to be occlusive unless directed by the physician.
4. Patients should report to their physician any signs of local adverse reactions.
5. Parents of pediatric patients should be advised not to use ELOCON Ointment in the treatment of diaper dermatitis. ELOCON Ointment should not be applied in the diaper area as diapers or plastic pants may constitute occlusive dressing (see **DOSAGE AND ADMINISTRATION**).
6. This medication should not be used on the face, underarms, or groin areas unless directed by the physician.
7. As with other corticosteroids, therapy should be discontinued when control is achieved. If no improvement is seen within 2 weeks, contact the physician.

Laboratory Tests The following tests may be helpful in evaluating patients for HPA axis suppression:

ACTH stimulation test
A.M. plasma cortisol test
Urinary free cortisol test

Carcinogenesis, Mutagenesis, and Impairment of Fertility In studies of the effect of mometasone furoate on fertility, pregnancy, and postnatal development in rats and rabbits, 25 rats were treated with doses up to 1.2 mg/kg of drug topically, and 15 rabbits with doses up to 0.3 mg/kg of drug topically. The drugs were left on the skin for 6 hours daily during gestation. At the highest dosage, the rat dams lost weight. One of the rabbit dams at the highest dosage had wrinkled skin, muscle wasting and aborted 5 fetuses.

Genetic toxicity studies with mometasone furoate, which included the Ames test, mouse lymphoma assay, and a micronucleus test did not reveal any mutagenic potential.

Long term animal studies have not been performed to evaluate the carcinogenic potential of ELOCON (mometasone furoate ointment) Ointment.

Pregnancy Teratogenic effects: Pregnancy Category C Corticosteroids have been shown to be teratogenic in laboratory animals when administered systemically at relatively low dosage levels. Some corticosteroids have been shown to be teratogenic after dermal application in laboratory animals. Rat offspring of dams treated with 1.2 mg/kg of mometasone furoate topically (4 times the maximum dose in a 50 kg individual) displayed umbilical hernias, unossified sternebrae and vertebrae, and wavy ribs, as well as markedly depressed fetal growth. Rabbit offspring of dams treated with up to 0.3 mg/kg of mometasone furoate topically (the same dose as the maximum dose in a 50 kg individual) displayed flexed paws, umbilical hernias, and cleft palate. A 50 kg female using 1 gram of ELOCON Ointment would apply approximately 0.023 mg/kg.

There are no adequate and well-controlled studies of the teratogenic potential of mometasone furoate in pregnant women. Therefore, ELOCON Ointment should be used during pregnancy only if the potential benefit justifies the potential risk to the fetus.

Nursing Mothers Systemically administered corticosteroids appear in human milk and could suppress growth, interfere with endogenous corticosteroid production, or cause other untoward effects. It is not known whether topical administration of corticosteroids could result in sufficient systemic absorption to produce detectable quantities in human milk. Because many drugs are excreted in human milk, caution should be exercised when ELOCON Ointment is administered to a nursing woman.

Pediatric Use ELOCON Ointment may be used with caution in pediatric patients 2 years of age or older, although the safety and efficacy of drug use for longer than 3 weeks have not been established. Use of ELOCON Ointment is supported by results from adequate and well-controlled studies in pediatric patients with corticosteroid-responsive dermatoses. Since safety and efficacy of ELOCON Ointment have not been established in pediatric patients below 2 years of age, its use in this age group is not recommended. Because of a higher ratio of skin surface area to body mass, pediatric patients are at a greater risk than adults of HPA axis suppression and Cushing's syndrome when they are treated with topical corticosteroids. They are, therefore, also at greater risk of glucocorticosteroid insufficiency during and/or after withdrawal of treatment. Pediatric patients may be more susceptible than adults to skin atrophy, including striae, when they are treated with topical corticosteroids. Pediatric patients applying topical corticosteroids to greater than 20% of body surface are at a higher risk of HPA axis suppression.

HPA axis suppression, Cushing's syndrome, linear growth retardation, delayed weight gain, and intracranial hypertension have been reported in children receiving topical corticosteroids. Manifestations of adrenal suppression in children include low plasma cortisol levels, and absence of response to ACTH stimulation. Manifestations of intracranial hypertension include bulging fontanelles, headaches, and bilateral papilledema.

ELOCON (mometasone furoate ointment) Ointment should not be used in the treatment of diaper dermatitis.

ADVERSE REACTIONS

In controlled clinical studies involving 812 patients, the incidence of adverse reactions associated with the use of ELOCON Ointment was 4.8%. Reported reactions included burning, pruritus, skin atrophy, tingling/stinging, and furunculosis. Reports of rosacea associated with the use of ELOCON Ointment have been received. In controlled clinical studies (n=74) involving pediatric patients 2 to 12 years of age, the incidence of adverse experiences associated with the use of ELOCON Cream is approximately 7%. Reported reactions included stinging, pruritus, and furunculosis.

The following additional local adverse reactions have been reported infrequently with topical corticosteroids, but may occur more frequently with the use of occlusive dressings. These reactions are listed in an approximate decreasing order of occurrence: irritation, dryness, folliculitis, hypertrichosis, acneiform eruptions, hypopigmentation, perioral dermatitis, allergic contact dermatitis, secondary infection, striae, and miliaria.

OVERDOSAGE

Topically applied ELOCON Ointment can be absorbed in sufficient amounts to produce systemic effects (see **PRECAUTIONS**).

DOSAGE AND ADMINISTRATION

Apply a thin film of ELOCON Ointment to the affected skin areas once daily. ELOCON Ointment may be used in pediatric patients 2 years of age or older. Safety and efficacy of ELOCON Ointment in pediatric patients for more than 3 weeks have not been established. Use in pediatric patients under 2 years of age is not recommended.

As with other corticosteroids, therapy should be discontinued when control is achieved. If no improvement is seen within 2 weeks, reassessment of diagnosis may be necessary.

ELOCON Ointment should not be used with occlusive dressings unless directed by a physician. ELOCON Ointment should not be applied in the diaper area if the child still requires diapers or plastic pants as these garments may constitute occlusive dressing.

HOW SUPPLIED

ELOCON Ointment 0.1% is supplied in 15 g (NDC 0085–0370–01) and 45 g (NDC 0085–0370–02) tubes; boxes of one.

Store ELOCON Ointment between 2° and 30°C (36° and 86°F).

Schering Corporation
Kenilworth, NJ 07033 USA
Revised 8/95

18724200T

Copyright © 1987, 1991, 1994, 1995, Schering Corporation. All rights reserved.

ETRAFON® ℞

brand of perphenazine and amitriptyline hydrochloride
ETRAFON 2-10 TABLETS (2-10), USP
ETRAFON TABLETS (2-25), USP
ETRAFON-FORTE TABLETS (4-25), USP

DESCRIPTION

ETRAFON Tablets contain perphenazine, USP and amitriptyline hydrochloride, USP. Perphenazine is a piperazinyl phenothiazine having the chemical formula, $C_{21}H_{26}ClN_3OS$. Amitriptyline hydrochloride is a dibenzocycloheptadiene derivative having the chemical formula, $C_{20}H_{23}N.HCl$.

ETRAFON Tablets are available in multiple strengths to afford dosage flexibility for optimum management. They are available as ETRAFON 2-10 Tablets, 2 mg perphenazine and 10 mg amitriptyline hydrochloride; ETRAFON Tablets, 2 mg perphenazine and 25 mg amitriptyline hydrochloride; ETRAFON-Forte Tablets, 4 mg perphenazine and 25 mg amitriptyline hydrochloride.

The inactive ingredients for ETRAFON 2-10 Tablets (2-10) include: acacia, butylparaben, calcium phosphate, calcium sulfate, carnauba wax, corn starch, D&C Yellow No. 10 Al Lake, FD&C Yellow No. 6 Al Lake, gelatin, lactose, magnesium stearate, potato starch, sugar, and white wax. May also contain talc.

The inactive ingredients for ETRAFON Tablets (2-25) include: acacia, butylparaben, calcium phosphate, calcium sulfate, carnauba wax, corn starch, D&C Red No. 30 Al Lake, FD&C Yellow No. 6 Al Lake, gelatin, lactose, magnesium stearate, potato starch, sugar, and white wax. May also contain talc.

The inactive ingredients for ETRAFON-Forte Tablets (4-25) include: acacia, butylparaben, calcium phosphate, calcium sulfate, carnauba wax, corn starch, FD&C Red No. 40 Al Lake, FD&C Yellow No. 6 Al Lake, gelatin, lactose, magnesium stearate, potato starch, sugar, and white wax. May also contain talc.

ACTIONS

ETRAFON Tablets combine the tranquilizing action of perphenazine with the antidepressant properties of amitriptyline hydrochloride. Perphenazine acts on the central nervous system, and has a greater behavioral potency than other phenothiazine derivatives whose side chains do not contain a piperazine moiety. Amitriptyline hydrochloride is a tricyclic antidepressant. While its mechanism of action in man is not known, it does not act primarily by stimulation of the central nervous system, and is not a monoamine oxidase (MAO) inhibitor.

INDICATIONS

ETRAFON Tablets are indicated for the treatment of patients with moderate to severe anxiety and/or agitation and depressed mood; patients with depression in whom anxiety and/or agitation are moderate or severe; patients with anxiety and depression associated with chronic physical disease; patients in whom depression and anxiety cannot be clearly differentiated.

Schizophrenic patients who have associated symptoms of depression should be considered for therapy with ETRAFON.

CONTRAINDICATIONS

ETRAFON Tablets are contraindicated in comatose or greatly obtunded patients and in patients receiving large doses of central nervous system depressants (barbiturates, alcohol, narcotics, analgesics, or antihistamines); in the presence of existing blood dyscrasias, bone marrow depression, or liver damage; and in patients who have shown hypersensitivity to ETRAFON Tablets, its components, or related compounds.

ETRAFON Tablets are also contraindicated in patients with suspected or established subcortical brain damage, with or without hypothalamic damage, since a hyperthermic reaction with temperatures in excess of 104°F may occur in such patients, sometimes not until 14 to 16 hours after drug administration. Total body ice-packing is recommended for such a reaction; antipyretics may also be useful.

ETRAFON Tablets should not be given concomitantly with a monoamine oxidase inhibiting compound. Hyperpyretic crises, severe convulsions, and deaths have occurred in patients receiving tricyclic antidepressant and monoamine oxidase inhibiting drugs simultaneously. In patients who have been receiving a monoamine oxidase inhibitor, it is recommended that 2 weeks or longer elapse before the start of treatment with ETRAFON Tablets to permit recovery from the effects of the MAO inhibitor and to avoid possible potentiation. Treatment with ETRAFON Tablets should be initiated cautiously in such patients, with gradual increase in dosage until a satisfactory response is obtained.

Amitriptyline hydrochloride is not recommended for use during the acute recovery phase following myocardial infarction.

WARNINGS

Tardive dyskinesia, a syndrome consisting of potentially irreversible, involuntary, dyskinetic movements, may develop in patients treated with neuroleptic (antipsychotic) drugs. Although the prevalence of the syndrome appears to be highest among the elderly, especially elderly women, it is impossible to rely upon prevalence estimates to predict, at the inception of neuroleptic treatment, which patients are

Continued on next page

Information on Schering products appearing on these pages is effective as of August 15, 1998.

Etrafon—Cont.

likely to develop the syndrome. Whether neuroleptic drug products differ in their potential to cause tardive dyskinesia is unknown.

Both the risk of developing the syndrome and the likelihood that it will become irreversible are believed to increase as the duration of treatment and the total cumulative dose of neuroleptic drugs administered to the patient increase. However, the syndrome can develop, although much less commonly, after relatively brief treatment periods at low doses.

There is no known treatment for established cases of tardive dyskinesia, although the syndrome may remit, partially or completely, if neuroleptic treatment is withdrawn. Neuroleptic treatment itself, however, may suppress (or partially suppress) the signs and symptoms of the syndrome, and thereby may possibly mask the underlying disease process. The effect that symptomatic suppression has upon the long-term course of the syndrome is unknown.

Given these considerations, neuroleptics should be prescribed in a manner that is most likely to minimize the occurrence of tardive dyskinesia. Chronic neuroleptic treatment should generally be reserved for patients who suffer from a chronic illness that, 1) is known to respond to neuroleptic drugs, and, 2) for whom alternative, equally effective, but potentially less harmful treatments are not available or appropriate. In patients who do require chronic treatment, the smallest dose and the shortest duration of treatment producing a satisfactory clinical response should be sought. The need for continued treatment should be reassessed periodically.

If signs and symptoms of tardive dyskinesia appear in a patient on neuroleptics, drug discontinuation should be considered. However, some patients may require treatment despite the presence of the syndrome.

(For further information about the description of tardive dyskinesia and its clinical detection, please refer to **Information for Patients** and **ADVERSE REACTIONS**.)

NEUROLEPTIC MALIGNANT SYNDROME (NMS) A potentially fatal symptom complex, sometimes referred to as Neuroleptic Malignant Syndrome (NMS), has been reported in association with antipsychotic drugs. Clinical manifestations of NMS are hyperpyrexia, muscle rigidity, altered mental status, and evidence of autonomic instability (irregular pulse or blood pressure, tachycardia, diaphoresis, and cardiac dysrhythmias).

The diagnostic evaluation of patients with this syndrome is complicated. In arriving at a diagnosis, it is important to identify cases where the clinical presentation includes both serious medical illness (eg, pneumonia, systemic infection, etc.) and untreated or inadequately treated extrapyramidal signs and symptoms (EPS). Other important considerations in the differential diagnosis include central anticholinergic toxicity, heat stroke, drug fever, and primarily central nervous system (CNS) pathology.

The management of NMS should include; 1) immediate discontinuation of antipsychotic drugs and other drugs not essential to concurrent therapy, 2) intensive symptomatic treatment and medical monitoring, and 3) treatment of any concomitant serious medical problems for which specific treatments are available. There is no general agreement about specific pharmacological treatment regimens for uncomplicated NMS.

If a patient requires antipsychotic drug treatment after recovery from NMS, the reintroduction of drug therapy should be carefully considered. The patient should be carefully monitored since recurrences of NMS have been reported.

Patients with cardiovascular disorders should be watched closely. Tricyclic antidepressant drugs, including amitriptyline hydrochloride, particularly when given in high doses, have been reported to produce arrhythmias, sinus tachycardia, and prolongation of the conduction time. Myocardial infarction and stroke have been reported with drugs of this class.

ETRAFON Tablets should not be given concomitantly with guanethidine or similarly acting compounds, since amitriptyline, like other tricyclic antidepressants, may block the antihypertensive effect of these compounds. If hypotension develops, epinephrine should not be administered since its action is blocked and partially reversed by perphenazine. If a vasopressor is needed, norepinephrine may be used. Severe, acute hypotension has occurred with the use of phenothiazines and is particularly likely to occur in patients with mitral insufficiency or pheochromocytoma. Rebound hypertension may occur in pheochromocytoma patients.

Perphenazine can lower the convulsive threshold in susceptible individuals; it should be used with caution in alcohol withdrawal and in patients with convulsive disorders. If the patient is being treated with an anticonvulsant agent, increased dosage of that agent may be required when ETRAFON Tablets are used concomitantly.

Because of the anticholinergic activity of amitriptyline hydrochloride, ETRAFON Tablets should be used with caution in patients with glaucoma, increased intraocular pressure,

and those in whom urinary retention is present or anticipated. In patients with angle-closure glaucoma, even average doses may precipitate an attack.

Close supervision is required when amitriptyline hydrochloride is given to hyperthyroid patients or those receiving thyroid medication.

ETRAFON Tablets may impair the mental and/or physical abilities required for the performance of potentially hazardous tasks, such as driving a car or operating machinery; the patient should be warned accordingly.

Usage in Children: Since a dosage for children has not been established, ETRAFON Tablets are not recommended for use in children.

Use in Pregnancy: Safe use of ETRAFON Tablets during pregnancy and lactation has not been established; therefore, in administering the drug to pregnant patients, nursing mothers, or women who may become pregnant, the possible benefits must be weighed against the possible hazards to mother and child.

PRECAUTIONS

The possibility of suicide in depressed patients remains during treatment and until significant remission occurs. This type of patient should not have access to large quantities of this drug.

Perphenazine

As with all phenothiazine compounds, perphenazine should not be used indiscriminately. Caution should be observed in giving it to patients who have previously exhibited severe adverse reactions to other phenothiazines. Some of the untoward actions of perphenazine tend to appear more frequently when high doses are used. However, as with other phenothiazine compounds, patients receiving perphenazine in any dosage should be kept under close supervision.

Neuroleptic drugs elevate prolactin levels; the elevation persists during chronic administration. Tissue culture experiments indicate that approximately one third of human breast cancers are prolactin dependent *in vitro*, a factor of potential importance if the prescription of these drugs is contemplated in a patient with a previously detected breast cancer. Although disturbances such as galactorrhea, amenorrhea, gynecomastia, and impotence have been reported, the clinical significance of elevated serum prolactin levels is unknown for most patients. An increase in mammary neoplasms has been found in rodents after chronic administration of neuroleptic drugs. Neither clinical studies nor epidemiologic studies conducted to date, however, have shown an association between chronic administration of these drugs and mammary tumorigenesis; the available evidence is considered too limited to be conclusive at this time.

The antiemetic effect of perphenazine may obscure signs of toxicity due to overdosage of other drugs, or render more difficult the diagnosis of disorders such as brain tumors or intestinal obstruction.

A significant, not otherwise explained, rise in body temperature may suggest individual intolerance to perphenazine, in which case ETRAFON Tablets should be discontinued.

Blood counts and hepatic and renal functions should be checked periodically. The appearance of signs of blood dyscrasias requires the discontinuance of the drug and institution of appropriate therapy. If abnormalities in hepatic tests occur, phenothiazine treatment should be discontinued. Renal function in patients on long-term therapy should be monitored; if blood urea nitrogen (BUN) becomes abnormal, treatment with the drug should be discontinued.

The use of phenothiazine derivatives in patients with diminished renal function should be undertaken with caution.

Use with caution in patients suffering from respiratory impairment due to acute pulmonary infections, or in chronic respiratory disorders such as severe asthma or emphysema.

In general, phenothiazines do not produce psychic dependence. Gastritis, nausea and vomiting, dizziness, and tremulousness have been reported following abrupt cessation of high-dose therapy. Reports suggest that these symptoms can be reduced by continuing concomitant antiparkinson agents for several weeks after the phenothiazine is withdrawn.

The possibility of liver damage, corneal and lenticular deposits, and irreversible dyskinesias should be kept in mind when patients are on long-term therapy.

Because photosensitivity has been reported, undue exposure to the sun should be avoided during phenothiazine treatment.

Information for Patients: This information is intended to aid in the safe and effective use of this medication. It is not a disclosure of all possible adverse or intended effects.

Given the likelihood that a substantial proportion of patients exposed chronically to neuroleptics will develop tardive dyskinesia, it is advised that all patients in whom chronic use is contemplated be given, if possible, full information about this risk. The decision to inform patients and/or their guardians must obviously take into account the clinical circumstances and the competency of the patient to understand the information provided.

Amitriptyline Hydrochloride

In manic-depressive psychosis, depressed patients may experience a shift toward the manic phase if they are treated with an antidepressant drug. Patients with paranoid symptomatology may have an exaggeration of such symptoms. The tranquilizing effect of ETRAFON Tablets has seemed to reduce the likelihood of this effect.

Both elevation and lowering of blood sugar levels have been reported.

The usefulness of amitriptyline in the treatment of depression has been amply demonstrated; however, it should be realized that abuse of amitriptyline among a narcotic-dependent population is not uncommon.

Drug Interactions: Drugs Metabolized by P450 2D6 — The biochemical activity of the drug metabolizing isozyme cytochrome P450 2D6 (debrisoquin hydroxylase) is reduced in a subset of the Caucasian population (about 7%–10% of Caucasians are so called "poor metabolizers"); reliable estimates of the prevalence of reduced P450 2D6 isozyme activity among Asian, African, and other populations are not yet available. Poor metabolizers have higher than expected plasma concentrations of tricyclic antidepressants (TCAs) when given usual doses. Depending on the fraction of drug metabolized by P450 2D6, the increase in plasma concentration may be small, or quite large (8-fold increase in plasma AUC of the TCA).

In addition, certain drugs inhibit the activity of this isozyme and make normal metabolizers resemble poor metabolizers. An individual who is stable on a given dose of TCA may become abruptly toxic when given one of these inhibiting drugs as concomitant therapy. The drugs that inhibit cytochrome P450 2D6 include some that are not metabolized by the enzyme (quinidine; cimetidine) and many that are substrates for P450 2D6 (many other antidepressants, phenothiazines, and the Type 1C antiarrhythmics propafenone and flecainide). While all the selective serotonin reuptake inhibitors (SSRIs), eg, fluoxetine, sertraline, and paroxetine, inhibit P450 2D6, they may vary in the extent of inhibition. The extent to which SSRI TCA interactions may pose clinical problems will depend on the degree of inhibition and the pharmacokinetics of the SSRI involved. Nevertheless, caution is indicated in the coadministration of TCAs with any of the SSRIs and also in switching from one class to the other. Of particular importance, sufficient time must elapse before initiating TCA treatment in a patient being withdrawn from fluoxetine, given the long half-life of the parent and active metabolite (at least 5 weeks may be necessary). Concomitant use of tricyclic antidepressants with drugs that can inhibit cytochrome P450 2D6 may require lower doses than usually prescribed for either the tricyclic antidepressant or the other drug. Furthermore, whenever one of these other drugs is withdrawn from co-therapy, an increased dose of tricyclic antidepressant may be required. It is desirable to monitor TCA plasma levels whenever a TCA is going to be coadministered with another drug known to be an inhibitor of P450 2D6.

Perphenazine

Patients on large doses of a phenothiazine drug who are undergoing surgery should be watched carefully for possible hypotensive phenomena. Morever, reduced amounts of anesthetics or central nervous system depressants may be necessary.

Since phenothiazines and central nervous system depressants (opiates, analgesics, antihistamines, barbiturates) can potentiate each other, less than the usual dosage of the added drug is recommended and caution is advised when they are administered concomitantly.

Use with caution in patients who are receiving atropine or related drugs because of additive anticholinergic effects and also in patients who will be exposed to extreme heat or organic phosphate insecticides.

The use of alcohol should be avoided, since additive effects and hypotension may occur. Patients should be cautioned that their response to alcohol may be increased while they are being treated with ETRAFON Tablets. The risk of suicide and the danger of overdose may be increased in patients who use alcohol excessively due to its potentiation of the drug's effect.

Amitriptyline Hydrochloride

When amitriptyline hydrochloride is given with anticholinergic agents or sympathomimetic drugs, including epinephrine combined with local anesthetics, close supervision and careful adjustment of dosages are required.

Paralytic ileus may occur in patients taking tricyclic antidepressants in combination with anticholinergic-type drugs.

Concurrent use of large doses of ethchlorvynol should be used with caution, since transient delirium has been reported in patients receiving this drug in combination with amitriptyline hydrochloride.

This drug may enhance the response to alcohol and the effects of barbiturates and other CNS depressants.

Concurrent administration of amitriptyline hydrochloride and electroshock therapy may increase the hazards of therapy. Such treatment should be limited to patients for whom it is essential.

Discontinue the drug several days before elective surgery, if possible.

Concurrent administration of cimetidine and tricyclic antidepressants can produce clinically significant increases in the plasma concentrations of the tricyclic antidepressant. Serious anticholinergic symptoms (severe dry mouth, urinary retention, blurred vision) have been associated with elevations in the serum levels of the tricyclic antidepressant when cimetidine is added to the drug regimen. Additionally, higher than expected steady-state serum concentrations of the tricyclic antidepressant have been observed when therapy is initiated in patients taking cimetidine.

Alternatively, decreases in the steady-state serum concentration of the tricyclic antidepressant have been reported in well-controlled patients on concurrent therapy upon discontinuance of cimetidine. The therapeutic efficacy of the tricyclic antidepressant may be compromised in these patients as the cimetidine is discontinued.

ADVERSE REACTIONS

Adverse reactions to ETRAFON Tablets are the same as those to its components, perphenazine and amitriptyline hydrochloride. There have been no reports of effects peculiar to the combination of these compenents in ETRAFON Tablets.

Perphenazine

Not all of the following adverse reactions have been reported with perphenazine; however, pharmacological similarities among various phenothiazine derivatives require that each be considered. With the piperazine group (of which perphenazine is an example), the extrapyramidal symptoms are more common, and others (eg, sedative effects, jaundice, and blood dyscrasias) are less frequently seen.

CNS Effects: *Extrapyramidal reactions:* opisthotonus, trismus, torticollis, retrocollis, aching and numbness of the limbs, motor restlessness, oculogyric crisis, hyperreflexia, dystonia, including protrusion, discoloration, aching and rounding of the tongue, tonic spasm of the masticatory muscles, tight feeling in the throat, slurred speech, dysphagia, akathisia, dyskinesia, parkinsonism, and ataxia. Their incidence and severity usually increase with an increase in dosage, but there is considerable individual variation in the tendency to develop such symptoms. Extrapyramidal symptoms can usually be controlled by the concomitant use of effective antiparkinsonian drugs, such as benztropine mesylate, and/or by reduction in dosage. In some instances, however, these extrapyramidal reactions may persist after discontinuation of treatment with perphenazine.

Persistant tardive dyskinesia: As with all antipsychotic agents, tardive dyskinesia may appear in some patients on long-term therapy or may appear after drug therapy has been discontinued. Although the risk appears to be greater in elderly patients on high-dose therapy, especially females, it may occur in either sex and in children. The symptoms are persistent and in some patients appear to be irreversible. The syndrome is characterized by rhythmical, involuntary movements of the tongue, face, mouth, or jaw (eg, protrusion of tongue, puffing of cheeks, puckering of mouth, chewing movements). Sometimes these may be accompanied by involuntary movements of the extremities. There is no known effective treatment for tardive dyskinesia; antiparkinsonism agents usually do not alleviate the symptoms of this syndrome. It is suggested that all antipsychotic agents be discontinued if these symptoms appear. Should it be necessary to reinstitute treatment, increase the dosage of the agent, or switch to a different antipsychotic agent, the syndrome may be masked. It has been reported that fine, vermicular movements of the tongue may be an early sign of the syndrome, and if the medication is stopped at that time the syndrome may not develop.

Other CNS effects include cerebral edema; abnormality of cerebrospinal fluid proteins; convulsive seizures, particularly in patients with EEG abnormalities or a history of such disorders; and headaches.

Neuroleptic malignant syndrome has been reported in patients treated with neuroleptic drugs (see **WARNINGS** section for further information).

Drowsiness may occur, particularly during the first or second week, after which it generally disappears. If troublesome, lower the dosage. Hypnotic effects appear to be minimal, especially in patients who are permitted to remain active.

Adverse behavioral effects include paradoxical exacerbation of psychotic symptoms, catatonic-like states, paranoid reactions, lethargy, paradoxical excitement, restlessness, hyperactivity, nocturnal confusion, bizarre dreams, and insomnia. Hyperreflexia has been reported in the newborn when a phenothiazine was used during pregnancy.

Autonomic Effects: dry mouth or salivation, nausea, vomiting, diarrhea, anorexia, constipation, obstipation, fecal impaction, urinary retention, frequency or incontinence, polyuria, bladder paralysis, nasal congestion, pallor, myosis, mydriasis, blurred vision, glaucoma, perspiration, hypertension, hypotension, and change in pulse rate occasionally may occur. Significant autonomic effects have been infrequent in patients receiving less than 24 mg perphenazine daily.

Adynamic ileus occasionally occurs with phenothiazine therapy and if severe, can result in complications and death. It is of particular concern in psychiatric patients, who may fail to seek treatment of the condition.

Allergic Effects: urticaria, erythema, eczema, exfoliative dermatitis, pruritus, photosensitivity, asthma, fever, anaphylactoid reactions, laryngeal edema, and angioneurotic edema; contact dermatitis in nursing personnel administering the drug; and in extremely rare instances, individual idiosyncrasy or hypersensitivity to phenothiazines has resulted in cerebral edema, circulatory collapse, and death.

Endocrine Effects: lactation, galactorrhea, moderate breast enlargement in females and gynecomastia in males on large doses; disturbances in the menstrual cycle, amenorrhea, changes in libido, inhibition of ejaculation, false-positive pregnancy tests, hyperglycemia, hypoglycemia, glycosuria, syndrome of inappropriate ADH (antidiuretic hormone) secretion.

Cardiovascular Effects: Postural hypotension, tachycardia (especially with sudden marked increase in dosage), bradycardia, cardiac arrest, faintness, and dizziness. Occasionally the hypotensive effect may produce a shock-like condition. ECG changes, nonspecific (quinidine-like effect), usually reversible, have been observed in some patients receiving phenothiazine tranquilizers.

Sudden death has occasionally been reported in patients who have received phenothiazines. In some cases, the death was apparently due to cardiac arrest; in others, the cause appeared to be asphyxia due to failure of the cough reflex. In some patients, the cause could not be determined nor could it be established that the death was due to the phenothiazine.

Hematological Effects: agranulocytosis, eosinophilia, leukopenia, hemolytic anemia, thrombocytopenic purpura, and pancytopenia. Most cases of agranulocytosis have occurred between the fourth and tenth weeks of therapy. Patients should be watched closely, especially during that period, for the sudden appearance of sore throat or signs of infection. If white blood cell and differential cell counts show significant cellular depression, discontinue the drug and start appropriate therapy. However, a slightly lowered white count is not in itself an indication to discontinue the drug.

Other Effects: Special considerations in long-term therapy include pigmentation of the skin, occurring chiefly in the exposed areas; ocular changes consisting of deposition of fine particulate matter in the cornea and lens, progressing in more severe cases to star-shaped lenticular opacities; epithelial keratopathies; and pigmentary retinopathy. Also noted: peripheral edema, reversed epinephrine effect, increase in PBI not attributable to an increase in thyroxine, parotid swelling (rare), hyperpyrexia, systemic lupus erythematosus-like syndrome, increases in appetite and weight, polyphagia, photophobia, and muscle weakness.

Liver damage (biliary stasis) may occur. Jaundice may occur, usually between the second and fourth weeks of treatment, and is regarded as a hypersensitivity reaction. Incidence is low. The clinical picture resembles infectious hepatitis but with laboratory features of obstructive jaundice. It is usually reversible; however, chronic jaundice has been reported.

Amitriptyline Hydrochloride

Although activation of latent schizophrenia has been reported with antidepressant drugs, including amitriptyline hydrochloride, it may be prevented with ETRAFON Tablets in some cases because of the antipsychotic effect of perphenazine. A few instances of epileptiform seizures have been reported in chronic schizophrenic patients during treatment with amitriptyline hydrochloride.

Note: Included in the listing which follows are a few adverse reactions which have not been reported with this specific drug. However, pharmacological similarities among the tricyclic antidepressant drugs require that each of the reactions be considered when amitriptyline hydrochloride is administered.

Allergic Effects: Rash, pruritus, urticaria, photosensitization, edema of face and tongue.

Anticholinergic Effects: Dry mouth, blurred vision, disturbance of accommodation, constipation, paralytic ileus, urinary retention, dilatation of urinary tract.

Cardiovascular Effects: Hypotension, hypertension, tachycardia, palpitations, myocardial infarction, arrhythmias, heart block, stroke.

CNS and Neuromuscular Effects: Confusional states, disturbed concentration, disorientation, delusions, hallucinations, excitement, jitteriness, anxiety, restlessness, insomnia, nighmares, numbness, tingling, and paresthesias of the extremities, peripheral neuropathy, incoordination, ataxia, tremors, seizures, alteration in EEG patterns, extrapyramidal symptoms, tinnitus.

Endocrine Effects: Testicular swelling and gynecomastia in the male, breast enlargement and galactorrhea in the female, increased or decreased libido, elevation and lowering of blood sugar levels, syndrome of inappropriate ADH (antidiuretic hormone) secretion.

Gastrointestinal Effects: Nausea, epigastric distress, heartburn, vomiting, anorexia, stomatitis, peculiar taste, diarrhea, jaundice, parotid swelling, black tongue. Rarely hepatitis has occurred (including altered liver function and jaundice).

Hematological Effects: Bone marrow depression, including agranulocytosis, leukopenia, eosinophilia, purpura, thrombocytopenia.

Other Effects: Dizziness, weakness, fatigue, headache, weight gain or loss, increased perspiration, urinary frequency, mydriasis, drowsiness, alopecia.

Withdrawal Symptoms: Abrupt cessation of treatment after prolonged administration may produce nausea, headache, and malaise. These are not indicative of addiction.

DOSAGE AND ADMINISTRATION

Initial Dosage

In psychoneurotic patients whose anxiety and depression warrant combined therapy, one ETRAFON Tablet (2-25) or one ETRAFON-Forte Tablet (4-25) three or four times a day is recommended.

In elderly patients and adolescents, a lower initial dosage may be needed. The dosage may then be adjusted cautiously to produce an adequate response.

In more severely ill patients with schizophrenia, two ETRAFON-Forte Tablets (4-25) three times a day are recommended as the initial dosage. If necessary, a fourth dose may be given at bedtime. The total daily dosage should not exceed eight tablets of any strength.

Maintenance Dosage

Depending on the condition being treated, the onset of therapeutic response may vary from a few days to a few weeks or even longer. After a satisfactory response is noted, dosage should be reduced to the smallest dose which is effective for relief of the symptoms for which ETRAFON Tablets are being administered. A useful maintenance dosage is one ETRAFON Tablet (2-25) or one ETRAFON-Forte Tablet (4-25) two to four times a day. In some patients, maintenance dosage is required for many months.

ETRAFON 2-10 Tablets (2-10) can be used to increase flexibility in adjusting maintenance dosage to the lowest amount consistent with relief of symptoms.

OVERDOSAGE*

Deaths may occur from overdosage with this class of drugs. Multiple drug ingestion (including alcohol) is common in deliberate overdose. As the management is complex and changing, it is recommended that the physician contact a poison control center for current information on treatment. Signs and symptoms of toxicity develop rapidly after overdose, therefore, hospital monitoring is required as soon as possible.

Manifestations: Overdosage of ETRAFON Tablets may cause any of the adverse reactions listed for perphenazine or amitriptyline hydrochloride.

Overdosage of perphenazine usually produces extrapyramidal symptoms such as dyskinesia and dystonia as described under **ADVERSE REACTIONS**, but this may be masked by the anticholinergic effects of amitriptyline. Other symptoms may include stupor or coma; children may have convulsive seizures.

Critical manifestations of tricyclic antidepressant overdose includes: cardiac dysrhythmias, severe hypotension, convulsions, and CNS depression, including coma. Changes in the electrocardiogram, particularly in QRS axis or width, are clinically significant indicators of tricyclic antidepressant toxicity. Other signs of overdose may include: confusion, disturbed concentration, transient visual hallucinations, dilated pupils, agitation, hyperactive reflexes, stupor, drowsiness, muscle rigidity, vomiting, hypothermia, hyperpyrexia, or any of the symptoms listed under **ADVERSE REACTIONS**.

Management: *General:* Obtain an ECG and immediately initiate cardiac monitoring. Protect the patient's airway, establish an intravenous line, and initiate gastric decontamination. A minimum of 6 hours of observation with cardiac monitoring and observation for signs of CNS or respiratory depression, hypotension, cardiac dysrhythmias and/or conduction blocks, and seizures is necessary. If signs of toxicity occur at any time during this period, extended monitoring is required. There are case reports of patients succumbing to fatal dysrhythmias late after overdose; these patients had clinical evidence of significant poisoning prior to death and most received inadequate gastrointestinal decontamination. Monitoring of plasma drug levels should not guide management of the patient.

Gastrointestinal Decontamination: All patients suspected of tricyclic antidepressant overdose should receive gastroin-

Continued on next page

Information on Schering products appearing on these pages is effective as of August 15, 1998.

Etrafon—Cont.

testinal decontamination. This should include large volume gastric lavage followed by activated charcoal. If consciousness is impaired, the airway should be secured prior to lavage. Emesis is contraindicated.
Cardiovascular: A maximal limb-lead QRS duration of ≥ 0.10 seconds may be the best indication of the severity of the overdose. Intravenous sodium bicarbonate should be used to maintain the serum pH in the range of 7.45 to 7.55. If the pH response is inadequate, hyperventilation may also be used. Concomitant use of hyperventilation and sodium bicarbonate should be done with extreme caution, with frequent pH monitoring. A pH >7.60 or a pCO_2 < 20 mm Hg is undesirable. Dysrhythmias unresponsive to sodium bicarbonate therapy/hyperventilation may respond to lidocaine, bretylium, or phenytoin. Type 1A and 1C antiarrhythmics are generally contraindicated (eg, quinidine, disopyramide, and procainamide).
In rare instances, hemoperfusion may be beneficial in acute refractory cardiovascular instability in patients with acute toxicity. However, hemodialysis, peritoneal dialysis, exchange transfusions, and forced diuresis generally have been reported as ineffective in tricyclic antidepressant poisoning.
CNS: In patients with CNS depression, early intubation is advised because of the potential for abrupt deterioration. Seizures should be controlled with benzodiazepines, or if these are ineffective, other anticonvulsants (eg, phenobarbital, phenytoin). Physostigmine is not recommended except to treat life-threatening symptoms that have been unresponsive to other therapies, and then only in consultation with a poison control center.
Psychiatric Follow-up: Since overdosage is often deliberate, patients may attempt suicide by other means during the recovery phase. Psychiatric referral may be appropriate.
Pediatric Management: The principles of management of child and adult overdosages are similar. It is strongly recommended that the physician contact the local poison control center for specific pediatric treatment.

HOW SUPPLIED

ETRAFON 2-10 Tablets (perphenazine 2 mg and amitriptyline hydrochloride 10 mg): deep yellow, sugar-coated tablets branded in blue-black with the Schering trademark and either product identification letters, ANA, or number, 287; bottles of 100 (NDC 0085-0287-04), and box of 100 for unit-dose dispensing (10 strips of 10 tablets each) (NDC 0085-0287-08).
ETRAFON Tablets (perphenazine 2 mg and amitriptyline hydrochloride 25 mg): pink, sugar-coated tablets branded in red with the Schering trademark and either product identification letters, ANC, or number, 598; bottles of 100 (NDC 0085-0598-04), and box of 100 for unit-dose dispensing (10 strips of 10 tablets each) (NDC 0085-0598-08).
ETRAFON-Forte Tablets (perphenazine 4 mg and amitriptyline hydrochloride 25 mg): red, sugar-coated tablets branded in blue with the Schering trademark and either product identification letters, ANE, or number, 720; bottles of 100 (NDC 0085-0720-04), and box of 100 for unit-dose dispensing (10 strips of 10 tablets each) (NDC 0085-0720-08).
Store ETRAFON 2-10, 2-25, 4-25 Tablets between 2° and 25°C (36° and 77°F). In addition, protect unit-dose packages from excessive moisture.
**Poisindex® Toxicologic Management.* Topic: Antidepressants, Tricyclic. Micromedex Inc. Vol 85.
ETRAFON®
brand of perphenazine and amitriptyline chloride
ETRAFON 2-10 TABLETS (2-10), USP
ETRAFON TABLETS (2-25), USP
ETRAFON-FORTE TABLETS (4-25), USP
Schering Corporation
Kenilworth, NJ 07033 USA
Rev. 5/96 16184586
Copyright © 1969, 1994, 1996, Schering Corporation.
All rights reserved.
Shown in Product Identification Guide, page 336

EULEXIN® ℞
brand of flutamide
Capsules

DESCRIPTION

EULEXIN Capsules contain flutamide, an acetanilid, nonsteroidal, orally active antiandrogen having the chemical name, 2-methyl-*N*-[4-nitro-3-(trifluoromethyl)phenyl] propanamide.
Each capsule contains 125 mg flutamide. The compound is a buff to yellow powder with a molecular weight of 276.2 and the following structural formula:
[See chemical structure at top of next column]
The inactive ingredients for EULEXIN Capsules include: corn starch, lactose, magnesium stearate, povidone, and so-

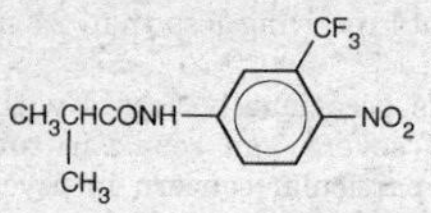

dium lauryl sulfate. Gelatin capsule shells may contain methylparaben, propylparaben, butylparaben, and the following dye systems: FD&C Blue 1, FD&C Yellow 6, and either FD&C Red 3 or FD&C Red 40 plus D&C Yellow 10, with titanium dioxide and other inactive ingredients.

CLINICAL PHARMACOLOGY

General: In animal studies, flutamide demonstrates potent antiandrogenic effects. It exerts its antiandrogenic action by inhibiting androgen uptake and/or by inhibiting nuclear binding of androgen in target tissues or both. Prostatic carcinoma is known to be androgen-sensitive and responds to treatment that counteracts the effect of androgen and/or removes the source of androgen, eg, castration. Elevations of plasma testosterone and estradiol levels have been noted following flutamide administration.
Pharmacokinetics:
Absorption: Analysis of plasma, urine, and feces following a single oral 200 mg dose of tritium-labeled flutamide to human volunteers showed that the drug is rapidly and completely absorbed. Following a single 250 mg oral dose to normal adult volunteers, the biologically active alpha-hydroxylated metabolite reaches maximum plasma concentrations in about 2 hours, indicating that it is rapidly formed from flutamide.
Distribution: In male rats neither flutamide nor any of its metabolites is preferentially accumulated in any tissue except the prostate after an oral 5 mg/kg dose of ^{14}C-flutamide. Total drug levels were highest 6 hours after drug administration in all tissues. Levels declined at roughly similar rates to low levels at 18 hours. The major metabolite was present at higher concentrations than flutamide in all tissues studied. Following a single 250 mg oral dose to normal adult volunteers, low plasma levels of flutamide were detected. The plasma half-life for the alpha-hydroxylated metabolite of flutamide is about 6 hours. Flutamide, *in vivo,* at steady-state plasma concentrations of 24 to 78 ng/mL, is 94% to 96% bound to plasma proteins. The active metabolite of flutamide, *in vivo,* at steady-state plasma concentrations of 1556 to 2284 ng/mL, is 92% to 94% bound to plasma proteins.
Metabolism: The composition of plasma radioactivity, following a single 200 mg oral dose of tritium-labeled flutamide to normal adult volunteers, showed that flutamide is rapidly and extensively metabolized, with flutamide comprising only 2.5% of plasma radioactivity 1 hour after administration. At least 6 metabolites have been identified in plasma. The major plasma metabolite is a biologically active alpha-hydroxylated derivative which accounts for 23% of the plasma tritium 1 hour after drug administration. The major urinary metabolite is 2-amino-5-nitro-4-(trifluoromethyl)phenol.
Excretion: Flutamide and its metabolites are excreted mainly in the urine with only 4.2% of the dose excreted in the feces over 72 hours.
[See table below]
Special Populations:
Geriatric: Following multiple oral dosing of 250 mg t.i.d. in normal geriatric volunteers, flutamide and its active metabolite approached steady-state plasma levels (based on pharmacokinetic simulations) after the fourth flutamide dose. The half-life of the active metabolite in geriatric volunteers after a single flutamide dose is about 8.1 hours and at steady state in 9.6 hours.
Race: There are no known alterations in flutamide absorption, distribution, metabolism, or excretion due to race.
Renal Impairment: Following a single 250 mg dose of flutamide administered to subjects with chronic renal insufficiency, there appeared to be no correlation between creatinine clearance and either C_{max} or AUC of flutamide. Renal impairment did not have an effect on the C_{max} or AUC of the biologically active alpha-hydroxylated metabolite of flutamide. In subjects with creatinine clearance of <29 mL/min, the half-life of the active metabolite was slightly prolonged. Flutamide and its active metabolite were not well dialyzed. Dose adjustment in patients with chronic renal insufficiency is not warranted.
Hepatic Impairment: No information on the pharmacokinetics of flutamide in hepatic impairment is available (see **WARNINGS, Hepatic Injury**).

Drug-Drug Interactions: Interactions between EULEXIN Capsules and LHRH-agonists have not occurred. Increases in prothrombin have been noted in patients receiving warfarin therapy (see **PRECAUTIONS**).
Clinical Studies: Flutamide has been demonstrated to interfere with testosterone at the cellular level. This can complement medical castration achieved with LHRH agonists which suppresses testicular androgen production by inhibiting luteinizing hormone secretion.
The effects of combination therapy have been evaluated in two studies. One study evaluated the effects of flutamide and an LHRH agonist as neoadjuvant therapy to radiation in stage B_2-C prostatic carcinoma and the other study evaluated flutamide and an LHRH agonist as the sole therapy in stage D_2 metastatic carcinoma.
Stage B_2-C Prostatic Carcinoma: The effects of hormonal treatment combined with radiation were studied in 466 patients (231 EULEXIN Capsules + LHRH-A + radiation, 235 radiation alone) with bulky primary tumors confined to the prostate (stage B_2) or extending beyond the capsule (stage C), with or without pelvic node involvement.
In this multicentered, controlled trial, administration of EULEXIN Capsules (250 mg t.i.d.) and goserelin acetate (3.6 mg depot) prior to and during radiation was associated with a significantly lower rate of local failure compared to radiation alone (16% vs 33% at 4 years, P<0.001). The combination therapy also resulted in a trend toward reduction in the incidence of distant metastases (27% vs 36% at 4 years, P =0.058). Median disease-free survival was significantly increased in patients who received complete hormonal therapy combined with radiation as compared to those patients who received radiation alone (4.4 vs 2.6 years, P<0.001). Inclusion of normal PSA level as a criterion for disease-free survival also resulted in significantly increased median disease-free survival in patients receiving the combination therapy (2.7 vs 1.5 years, P<0.001).
Stage D_2 Metastatic Carcinoma: To study the effects of combination therapy in metastatic disease, 617 patients (311 leuprolide + flutamide, 306 leuprolide + placebo) with previously untreated advanced prostatic carcinoma were enrolled in a large multicentered, controlled clinical trial. Three and one-half years after the study was initiated, median survival had been reached. The median actuarial survival time was 34.9 months for patients treated with leuprolide and flutamide versus 27.9 months for patients treated with leuprolide alone. This 7-month increment represents a 25% improvement in overall survival time with the flutamide therapy. Analysis of progression-free survival showed a 2.6 month improvement in patients who received leuprolide plus flutamide, a 19% increment over leuprolide and placebo.

INDICATIONS AND USAGE

EULEXIN Capsules are indicated for use in combination with LHRH agonists for the management of locally confined Stage B_2-C and Stage D_2 metastatic carcinoma of the prostate.
Stage B_2-C Prostatic Carcinoma: Treatment with EULEXIN Capsules and the LHRH agonist should start 8 weeks prior to initiating radiation therapy and continue during radiation therapy.
Stage D_2 Metastatic Carcinoma: To achieve benefit from treatment, EULEXIN Capsules should be initiated with the LHRH agonist and continued until progression.

CONTRAINDICATIONS

EULEXIN Capsules are contraindicated in patients who are hypersensitive to flutamide or any component of this preparation.

WARNINGS

Gynecomastia occurred in 9% of patients receiving flutamide together with medical castration.
Flutamide may cause fetal harm when administered to a pregnant woman. There was decreased 24-hour survival in the offspring of rats treated with flutamide at doses of 30, 100, or 200 mg/kg/day (approximately 3, 9, and 19 times the human dose) during pregnancy. A slight increase in minor variations in the development of the sternebrae and vertebrae was seen in fetuses of rats at the two higher doses. Feminization of the males also occurred at the two higher dose levels. There was a decreased survival rate in the offspring of rabbits receiving the highest dose (15 mg/kg/day; equal to 1.4 times the human dose).
Preclinical data from rats, cats, dogs and monkeys as well as clinical data in men, demonstrate that one metabolite of flutamide is 4-nitro-3-fluoro-methylaniline. Several toxicities consistent with aniline exposure including methemoglobinemia, hemolytic anemia, and cholestatic jaundice have been observed in animals and humans after flutamide administration. Methemoglobin levels should be monitored in

Plasma Pharmacokinetics of Flutamide and Hydroxyflutamide in Geriatric Volunteers (mean ± S)

	Single Dose		Steady State	
	Flutamide	Hydroxyflutamide	Flutamide	Hydroxyflutamide
C_{max} (ng/mL)	25.2 ± 34.2	894 ± 406	113 ± 213	1629 ± 586
Elimination half-life (hr)	—	8.1 ± 1.3	7.8	9.6 ± 2.5
T_{max} (hr)	1.9 ± 0.7	2.7 ± 1.0	1.3 ± 0.7	1.9 ± 0.6
C_{min} (ng/mL)	—	—	—	673 ± 316

patients susceptible to aniline toxicity (eg, persons with glucose-6-phosphate dehydrogenase deficiency or hemoglobin M disease as well as patients who smoke).

Serious cardiac lesions were observed in 2/10 beagle dogs receiving 25 mg/kg/day for 78 weeks and 3/16 receiving 40 mg/kg/day for 2–4 years. The lesions, indicative of chronic injury and repair processes, including chronic myxomatous degeneration, intra-atrial fibrosis, myocardial acidophilic degeneration, vasculitis, and perivasculitis. The doses at which these lesions occurred were associated with 2-hydroxyflutamide levels that were 1- to 12-fold greater than those observed in humans at therapeutic levels.

Hepatic Injury: Since transaminase abnormalities, cholestatic jaundice, hepatic necrosis, and hepatic encephalopathy have been reported with the use of flutamide, periodic liver function tests should be considered. (See **ADVERSE REACTIONS** section.) Appropriate laboratory testing should be done at the first symptom/sign of liver dysfunction (eg, pruritus, dark urine, persistent anorexia, jaundice, right upper quadrant tenderness, or unexplained "flu-like" symptoms). If the patient has clinically evident jaundice, in the absence of biopsy-confirmed liver metastases, EULEXIN therapy should be discontinued. In clinically asymptomatic patients, if transaminases increase over 2–3 times the upper limit of normal, treatment should be discontinued. The hepatic injury is usually reversible after discontinuation of therapy, and in some patients, after dosage reduction. However, there have been reports of death following severe hepatic injury associated with use of flutamide.

PRECAUTIONS

Information for Patients: Patients should be informed that EULEXIN Capsules and the drug used for medical castration should be administered concomitantly, and that they should not interrupt their dosing or stop taking these medications without consulting their physician.

Laboratory Tests: Regular assessment of serum Prostate Specific Antigen (PSA) may be helpful in monitoring the patient's response. If PSA levels rise significantly and consistently during EULEXIN therapy the patient should be evaluated for clinical progression. For patients who have objective progression of disease together with an elevated PSA, a treatment-free period of antiandrogen while continuing the LHRH analogue may be considered.

Since transaminase abnormalities, and rarely jaundice, have been reported with the use of EULEXIN Capsules, periodic liver function tests should be considered, eg, when the patient has jaundice or laboratory evidence of liver injury in the absence of liver metastases, EULEXIN therapy should be discontinued. Abnormalities are usually reversible upon discontinuation. See **WARNINGS, Hepatic Injury** above.

Drug Interactions: Increases in prothrombin time have been noted in patients receiving long-term warfarin therapy after flutamide was initiated. Therefore close monitoring of prothrombin time is recommended and adjustment of the anticoagulant dose may be necessary when EULEXIN Capsules are administered concomitantly with warfarin.

Carcinogenesis, Mutagenesis, Impairment of Fertility: In a 1-year dietary study in male rats, interstitial cell adenomas of the testes were present in 49% to 75% of all treated rats (daily oral doses of 10, 30, and 50 mg/kg/day were administered). These produce plasma C_{max} values that are 1, 2-3, and 4-fold, respectively, those associated with therapeutic doses in humans. In male rats similarly dosed for 1 year, tumors were still present after 1 year of a drug-free period, but the incidences were 43% to 47%. In a 2-year carcinogenicity study in male rats, daily administration of flutamide at these same doses produced testicular interstitial cell adenomas in 91% to 95% of all treated rats as opposed to 11% of untreated control rats. Mammary adenomas, adenocarcinomas, and fibroadenomas were increased in treated male rats at exposure levels that were 1- to 4-fold those observed during therapeutic dosing in humans. There are likewise reports of malignant breast neoplasms in men treated with EULEXIN Capsules (see **ADVERSE REACTIONS** section).

Flutamide did not demonstrate DNA modifying activity in the Ames *Salmonella*/microsome Mutagenesis Assay. Dominant lethal tests in rats were negative.

Reduced sperm counts were observed during a 6-week study of flutamide monotherapy in normal human volunteers.

Flutamide did not affect estrous cycles or interfere with the mating behavior of male and female rats when the drug was administered at 25 and 75 mg/kg/day prior to mating. Males treated with 150 mg/kg/day (30 times the minimum effective antiandrogenic dose) failed to mate; mating behavior returned to normal after dosing was stopped. Conception rates were decreased in all dosing groups. Suppression of spermatogenesis was observed in rats dosed for 52 weeks at approximately 3, 8, or 17 times the human dose and in dogs dosed for 78 weeks at 1.4, 2.3, and 3.7 times the human dose.

Pregnancy: *Pregnancy Category D.* See **WARNINGS** section.

Adverse Events During Acute Radiation Therapy
(within first 90 days of radiation therapy)

	(n=231) LHRH-A + EULEXIN Capsules + Radiation % All	(n=235) Radiation Only % All
Rectum/Large Bowel	80	76
Bladder	58	60
Skin	37	37

Adverse Events During Late Radiation Phase
(after 90 days of radiation therapy)

	(n=231) LHRH-A + EULEXIN Capsules + Radiation % All	(n=235) Radiation Only % All
Diarrhea	36	40
Cystitis	16	16
Rectal Bleeding	14	20
Proctitis	8	8
Hematuria	7	12

	(n=294) Flutamide + LHRH agonist % All	(n=285) Placebo + LHRH agonist % All
Hot Flashes	61	57
Loss of Libido	36	31
Impotence	33	29
Diarrhea	12	4
Nausea/Vomiting	11	10
Gynecomastia	9	11
Other	7	9
Other GI	6	4

ADVERSE REACTIONS

Stage B₂-C Prostatic Carcinoma: Treatment with EULEXIN Capsules and the LHRH agonist did not add substantially to the toxicity of radiation treatment alone. The following adverse experiences were reported during a multicenter clinical trial comparing EULEXIN Capsules + LHRH-A + radiation versus radiation alone. The most frequently reported (greater than 5%) adverse experiences are listed below.

[See first table above]

Additional adverse event data was collected for the combination therapy with radiation group over both the hormonal treatment and hormonal treatment plus radiation phases of the study. Adverse experiences occurring in more than 5% of patients in this group, over both parts of the study, were hot flashes (46%), diarrhea (40%), nausea (9%), and skin rash (8%).

Stage D₂ Metastatic Carcinoma: The following adverse experiences were reported during a multicenter clinical trial comparing EULEXIN Capsules + LHRH agonist versus placebo + LHRH agonist.

The most frequently reported (greater than 5%) adverse experiences during treatment with EULEXIN Capsules in combination with an LHRH agonist are listed in the table below. For comparison, adverse experiences seen with an LHRH agonist and placebo are also listed in the following table.

[See second table above]

As shown in the table, for both treatment groups, the most frequently occurring adverse experiences (hot flashes, impotence, loss of libido) were those known to be associated with low serum androgen levels and known to occur with LHRH agonists alone.

The only notable difference was the higher incidence of diarrhea in the flutamide + LHRH agonist group (12%), which was severe in 5% as opposed to the placebo + LHRH agonist (4%), which was severe in less than 1%.

In addition, the following adverse reactions were reported during treatment with flutamide + LHRH agonist. No causal relatedness of these reactions to drug treatment has been made, and some of the adverse experiences reported are those that commonly occur in elderly patients.

Cardiovascular System: hypertension in 1% of patients.
Central Nervous System: CNS (drowsiness/confusion/depression/anxiety/nervousness) reactions occurred in 1% of patients.
Gastrointestinal System: anorexia 4%, and other GI disorders occurred in 6% of patients.
Hematopoietic System: anemia occurred in 6%, leukopenia in 3%, and thrombocytopenia in 1% of patients.
Liver and Biliary System: hepatitis and jaundice in less than 1% of patients.
Skin: irritation at the injection site and rash occurred in 3% of patients.
Other: edema occurred in 4%, genitourinary and neuromuscular symptoms in 2%, and pulmonary symptoms in less than 1% of patients.

In addition, the following spontaneous adverse experiences have been reported during the marketing of flutamide: hemolytic anemia, macrocytic anemia, methemoglobinemia, photosensitivity reactions (including erythema, ulceration, bullous eruptions, and epidermal necrolysis), and urine discoloration. The urine was noted to change to an amber or yellow-green appearance which can be attributed to the flutamide and/or its metabolites. Also reported were cholestatic jaundice, hepatic encephalopathy, and hepatic necrosis. The hepatic conditions were usually reversible after discontinuing therapy; however, there have been reports of death following severe hepatic injury associated with use of flutamide.

Two reports of malignant breast neoplasms occurring in male patients being dosed with EULEXIN Capsules have been reported. One involved a pre-existing nodule which was first detected 3–4 months before initiation of EULEXIN monotherapy. After excision, this nodule was diagnosed as a poorly differentiated ductal carcinoma. The other report involved gynecomastia and a breast nodule noted 2 and 6 months, respectively, after initiation of EULEXIN monotherapy. The nodule was excised and diagnosed as a moderately differentiated invasive ductal tumor.

Abnormal Laboratory Test Values: Laboratory abnormalities including elevated SGOT, SGPT, bilirubin values, SGGT, BUN, and serum creatinine have been reported.

OVERDOSAGE

In animal studies with flutamide alone, signs of overdose included hypoactivity, piloerection, slow respiration, ataxia, and/or lacrimation, anorexia, tranquilization, emesis, and methemoglobinemia.

Clinical trials have been conducted with flutamide in doses up to 1500 mg per day for periods up to 36 weeks with no serious adverse effects reported. Those adverse reactions reported included gynecomastia, breast tenderness, and some increases in SGOT. The single dose of flutamide ordinarily associated with symptoms of overdose or considered to be life-threatening has not been established.

Since flutamide is highly protein bound, dialysis may not be of any use as treatment for overdose. As in the management of overdosage with any drug, it should be borne in mind that multiple agents may have been taken. If vomiting does not occur spontaneously, it should be induced if the patient is alert. General supportive care, including frequent monitoring of the vital signs and close observation of the patient, is indicated.

DOSAGE AND ADMINISTRATION

The recommended dosage is 2 capsules 3 times a day at 8-hour intervals for a total daily dose of 750 mg.

Continued on next page

Eulexin—Cont.

HOW SUPPLIED

EULEXIN Capsules, 125 mg, are available as opaque, two-toned brown capsules, imprinted with "Schering 525". They are supplied as follows:

NDC 0085-0525-05 - Bottles of 500
NDC 0085-0525-03 - Unit Dose packages of 100 (10 × 10's)
NDC 0085-0525-06 - Bottles of 180
Store between 2° and 30°C (36° and 86°F).
Protect the Unit Dose packages from excessive moisture.
Schering Corporation
Kenilworth, NJ 07033 USA
Rev. 6/96

18822415T

Copyright © 1989, 1996, Schering Corporation.
All rights reserved.
Shown in Product Identification Guide, page 336

FARESTON®
(toremifene citrate)
Tablets

℞

PRODUCT INFORMATION

DESCRIPTION

FARESTON (toremifene citrate) Tablets for oral administration each contain 88.5 mg of toremifene citrate, which is equivalent to 60 mg toremifene.
FARESTON is a nonsteroidal antiestrogen. The chemical name of toremifene is: 2-{p-[(Z)-4-chloro-1,2-diphenyl-1-butenyl]phenoxy]-N,N-dimethylethylamine citrate (1:1). The structural formula is:

and the molecular formula is $C_{26}H_{28}ClNO \cdot C_6H_8O_7$. The molecular weight of toremifene citrate is 598.10. The pK_a is 8.0. Water solubility at 37°C is 0.63 mg/mL and in 0.02N HCl at 37°C is 0.38 mg/mL.
FARESTON is available only as tablets for oral administration. Inactive ingredients: starch, lactose, povidone, sodium starch glycolate, magnesium stearate, microcrystalline cellulose, and colloidal silicon dioxide.

CLINICAL PHARMACOLOGY

Mechanism of Action: Toremifene is a nonsteroidal triphenylethylene derivative. Toremifene binds to estrogen receptors and may exert estrogenic, antiestrogenic, or both activities, depending upon the duration of treatment, animal species, gender, target organ, or endpoint selected. In general, however, nonsteroidal triphenylethylene derivatives are predominantly antiestrogenic in rats and humans and estrogenic in mice. In rats, toremifene causes regression of established dimethylbenzanthracene (DMBA)-induced mammary tumors. The antitumor effect of toremifene in breast cancer is believed to be mainly due to its antiestrogenic effects, ie, its ability to compete with estrogen for binding sites in the cancer, blocking the growth-stimulating effects of estrogen in the tumor.

Toremifene causes a decrease in the estradiol-induced vaginal cornification index in some postmenopausal women, indicative of its antiestrogenic activity. Toremifene also has estrogenic activity as shown by decreases in serum gonadotropin concentrations (FSH and LH).

Pharmacokinetics: The plasma concentration time profile of toremifene declines biexponentially after absorption with a mean distribution half-life of about 4 hours and an elimination half-life of about 5 days. Elimination half-lives of major metabolites, N-demethyltoremifene and (deaminohydroxy) toremifene were 6 and 4 days, respectively. Mean total clearance of toremifene was approximately 5 L/h.

Absorption and Distribution: Toremifene is well absorbed after oral administration and absorption is not influenced by food. Peak plasma concentrations are obtained within 3 hours. Toremifene displays linear pharmacokinetics after single oral doses of 10 to 680 mg. After multiple dosing, dose proportionality was observed for doses of 10 to 400 mg. Steady-state concentrations were reached in about 4–6 weeks. Toremifene has an apparent volume of distribution of 580 L and binds extensively (>99.5%) to serum proteins, mainly to albumin.

Metabolism and Excretion: Toremifene is extensively metabolized, principally by CYP3A4 to N-demethyltoremifene, which is also antiestrogenic but with weak *in vivo* antitumor potency. Serum concentrations of N-demethyltoremifene are 2 to 4 times higher than toremifene at steady state. Toremifene is eliminated as metabolites predominantly in the feces, with about 10% excreted in the urine during a 1-week period. Elimination of toremifene is slow, in part because of enterohepatic circulation.

Special Populations: *Renal Insufficiency:* The pharmacokinetics of toremifene and N-demethyltoremifene were similar in normals and in patients with impaired kidney function.
Hepatic insufficiency: The mean elimination half-life of toremifene was increased by less than twofold in 10 patients with hepatic impairment (cirrhosis or fibrosis) compared to subjects with normal hepatic function. The pharmacokinetics of N-demethyltoremifene were unchanged in these patients. Ten patients on anticonvulsants (phenobarbital, clonazepam, phenytoin, and carbamazepine) showed a twofold increase in clearance and a decrease in the elimination half-life of toremifene.
Geriatric patients: The pharmacokinetics of toremifene were studied in 10 healthy young males and 10 elderly females following a single 120 mg dose under fasting conditions. Increases in the elimination half-life (4.2 versus 7.2 days) and the volume of distribution (457 versus 627 L) of toremifene were seen in the elderly females without any change in clearance or AUC.
Race: The pharmacokinetics of toremifene in patients of different races has not been studied.
Drug-drug interactions: No formal drug-drug interaction studies with toremifene have been performed.

CLINICAL STUDIES

Three prospective, randomized, controlled clinical studies (North American, Eastern European, and Nordic) were conducted to evaluate the efficacy of FARESTON for the treatment of breast cancer in postmenopausal women. The patients were randomized to parallel groups receiving FARESTON 60 mg (FAR60) or tamoxifen 20 mg (TAM20) in the North American Study or tamoxifen 40 mg (TAM40) in the Eastern European and Nordic studies. The North American and Eastern European studies also included high-dose toremifene arms of 200 and 240 mg daily, respectively. The studies included postmenopausal patients with estrogen-receptor (ER) positive or estrogen-receptor (ER) unknown

metastatic breast cancer. The patients had at least one measurable or evaluable lesion. The primary efficacy variables were response rate (RR) and time to progression (TTP). Survival (S) was also determined. Ninety-five percent confidence intervals (95% CI) were calculated for the difference in RR between FAR60 and TAM groups and the hazard ratio (relative risk for an unfavorable event, such as disease progression or death) between TAM and FAR60 for TTP and S. Two of the 3 studies showed similar results for all effectiveness endpoints. However, the Nordic Study showed a longer time to progression for tamoxifen (see table).
[See table below]
The high-dose groups, toremifene 200 mg daily in the North American Study and 240 mg daily in the Eastern European Study, were not superior to the lower toremifene dose groups, with response rates of 22.6% and 28.7%, median times to progression of 5.6 and 6.1 months, and median survivals of 30.1 and 23.8 months, respectively. The median treatment duration in the three pivotal studies was 5 months (range 4.2–6.3 months).

INDICATIONS AND USAGE

FARESTON is indicated for the treatment of metastatic breast cancer in postmenopausal women with estrogen-receptor positive or unknown tumors.

CONTRAINDICATIONS

FARESTON is contraindicated in patients with known hypersensitivity to the drug.

WARNINGS

Hypercalcemia and Tumor Flare: As with other antiestrogens, hypercalcemia and tumor flare have been reported in some breast cancer patients with bone metastases during the first weeks of treatment with FARESTON. Tumor flare is a syndrome of diffuse musculoskeletal pain and erythema with increased size of tumor lesions that later regress. It is often accompanied by hypercalcemia. Tumor flare does not imply failure of treatment or represent tumor progression. If hypercalcemia occurs, appropriate measures should be instituted and if hypercalcemia is severe FARESTON treatment should be discontinued.
Tumorigenicity: Since most toremifene trials have been conducted in patients with metastatic disease, adequate data on the potential endometrial tumorigenicity of long-term treatment with FARESTON are not available. Endometrial hyperplasia has been reported. Some patients treated with FARESTON have developed endometrial cancer, but circumstances (short duration of treatment or prior antiestrogen treatment or premalignant conditions) make it difficult to establish the role of FARESTON.
Endometrial hyperplasia of the uterus was observed in monkeys following 52 weeks of treatment at ≥1 mg/kg and in dogs following 16 weeks of treatment at ≥3 mg/kg with toremifene (about 1/4 and 1.4 times, respectively, the daily maximum recommended human dose on a mg/m² basis).
Pregnancy: FARESTON may cause fetal harm when administered to pregnant women. Studies in rats at doses ≥1.0 mg/kg/day (about 1/4 the daily maximum recommended human dose on a mg/m²basis) administered during the period of organogenesis, have shown that toremifene is embryotoxic and fetotoxic, as indicated by intrauterine mortality, increased resorption, reduced fetal weight, and fetal anomalies; including malformation of limbs, incomplete ossification, misshapen bones, ribs/spine anomalies, hydroureter, hydronephrosis, testicular displacement, and subcutaneous edema. Fetal anomalies may have been a consequence of maternal toxicity. Toremifene has been shown to cross the placenta and accumulate in the rodent fetus.
In rodent models of fetal reproductive tract development, toremifene produced inhibition of uterine development in female pups similar to diethylstilbestrol (DES) and tamoxifen. The clinical relevance of these changes is not known. Embryotoxicity and fetotoxicity were observed in rabbits at doses ≥1.25 mg/kg/day and 2.5 mg/kg/day, respectively (about 1/3 and 2/3 the daily maximum recommended human dose on a mg/m² basis); fetal anomalies included incomplete ossification and anencephaly.
There are no studies in pregnant women. If FARESTON is used during pregnancy, or if the patient becomes pregnant while receiving this drug, the patient should be apprised of the potential hazard to the fetus or potential risk for loss of the pregnancy.

PRECAUTIONS

General: Patients with a history of thromboembolic diseases should generally not be treated with FARESTON. In general, patients with preexisting endometrial hyperplasia should not be given long-term FARESTON treatment. Patients with bone metastases should be monitored closely for hypercalcemia during the first weeks of treatment (see **WARNINGS**). Leukopenia and thrombocytopenia have been reported rarely; leukocyte and platelet counts should be monitored when using FARESTON in patients with leukopenia or thrombocytopenia.
Information for Patients: Vaginal bleeding has been reported in patients using FARESTON. Patients should be in-

CLINICAL STUDIES

Study	North American		Eastern European		Nordic	
Treatment Group	FAR60	TAM20	FAR60	TAM40	FAR60	TAM40
No. Patients	221	215	157	149	214	201
Responses						
CR[1] + PR[2]	14+33	11+30	7+25	3+28	19+48	19+56
RR[3] (CR + PR)%	21.3	19.1	20.4	20.8	31.3	37.3
Difference in RR	2.2		-0.4		-6.0	
95% CI[4]for						
Difference in RR	-5.8 to 10.2		-9.5 to 8.6		-15.1 to 3.1	
Time to Progression (TTP)						
Median TTP (mo.)	5.6	5.8	4.9	5.0	7.3	10.2
Hazard Ratio (TAM/FAR)	1.01		1.02		0.80	
95% CI[4]for						
Hazard Ratio (%)	0.81 to 1.26		0.79 to 1.31		0.64 to 1.00	
Survival (S)						
Median S (mo.)	33.6	34.0	25.4	23.4	33.0	38.7
Hazard Ratio (TAM/FAR)	0.94		0.96		0.94	
95% CI[4]for						
Hazard Ratio (%)	0.74 to 1.24		0.72 to 1.28		0.73 to 1.22	

[1]CR = complete response; [2]PR = partial response; [3]RR = response rate; [4]CI = confidence interval

formed about this and instructed to contact their physician if such bleeding occurs.

Patients with bone metastases should be informed about the typical signs and symptoms of hypercalcemia and instructed to contact their physician for further assessment if such signs or symptoms occur.

Laboratory Tests: Periodic complete blood counts, calcium levels, and liver function tests should be obtained.

Drug-drug Interactions: Drugs that decrease renal calcium excretion, eg, thiazide diuretics, may increase the risk of hypercalcemia in patients receiving FARESTON. There is a known interaction between antiestrogenic compounds of the triphenylethylene derivative class and coumarin-type anticoagulants (eg, warfarin), leading to an increased prothrombin time. When concomitant use of anticoagulants with FARESTON is necessary, careful monitoring of the prothrombin time is recommended.

Cytochrome P450 3A4 enzyme inducers, such as phenobarbital, phenytoin, and carbamazepine increase the rate of toremifene metabolism, lowering the steady-state concentration in serum. Metabolism of toremifene may be inhibited by drugs known to inhibit the CYP3A4-6 enzymes. Examples of such drugs are ketoconazole and similar antimycotics as well as erythromycin and similar macrolides. This interaction has not been studied and its clinical relevance is uncertain.

Carcinogenesis, Mutagenesis, and Impairment of Fertility: Conventional carcinogenesis studies in rats at doses of 0.12 to 12 mg/kg/day (about 1/100 to 1.5 times the daily maximum recommended human dose on a mg/m² basis) for up to 2 years did not show evidence of carcinogenicity. Studies in mice at doses of 1.0 to 30.0 mg/kg/day (about 1/15 to 2 times the daily maximum recommended human dose on a mg/m² basis) for up to 2 years revealed increased incidence of ovarian and testicular tumors, and increased incidence of osteoma and osteosarcoma. The significance of the mouse findings is uncertain because of the different role of estrogens in mice and the estrogenic effect of toremifene in mice. An increased incidence of ovarian and testicular tumors in mice has also been observed with other human antiestrogenic agents that have primarily estrogenic activity in mice.

Toremifene has not been shown to be mutagenic in *in vitro* tests (Ames and *E. coli* bacterial tests). Toremifene is clastogenic *in vitro* (chromosomal aberrations and micronuclei formation in human lymphoblastoid MCL-5 cells) and *in vivo* (chromosomal aberrations in rat hepatocytes). No significant adduct formation could be detected using ³²P postlabeling in liver DNA from rats administered toremifene when compared to tamoxifen at similar doses. A study in cultured human lymphocytes indicated that adducting activity of toremifene, detected by ³²P post-labeling, was about 1/6 that of tamoxifen at approximately equipotent concentrations. In addition, the DNA adducting activity of toremifene in salmon sperm, using ³²P post-labeling, was 1/6 and 1/4 that observed with tamoxifen at equivalent concentrations following activation by rat and human microsomal systems, respectively. However, toremifene exposure is fourfold the exposure of tamoxifen based on human AUC in serum at recommended clinical doses.

Toremifene produced impairment of fertility and conception in male and female rats at doses ≥25.0 and 0.14 mg/kg/day, respectively (about 3.5 times and 1/50 the daily maximum recommended human dose on a mg/m² basis). At these doses, sperm counts, fertility index, and conception rate were reduced in males with atrophy of seminal vesicles and prostate. In females, fertility and reproductive indices were markedly reduced with increased pre- and post-implantation loss. In addition, offspring of treated rats exhibited depressed reproductive indices. Toremifene produced ovarian atrophy in dogs administered doses ≥3 mg/kg/day (about 1.5 times the daily maximum recommended human dose on a mg/m² basis) for 16 weeks. Cystic ovaries and reduction in endometrial stromal cellularity were observed in monkeys at doses ≥1 mg/kg/day (about 1/4 the daily maximum recommended human dose on a mg/m² basis) for 52 weeks.

Pregnancy: *Pregnancy Category D:* (see **WARNINGS**).

Nursing mothers: Toremifene has been shown to be excreted in the milk of lactating rats. It is not known if this drug is excreted in human milk. (See **WARNINGS** and **PRECAUTIONS.**)

Pediatric use: There is no indication for use of FARESTON in pediatric patients.

Geriatric use: The median age in the three controlled studies ranged from 60 to 66 years. No significant age-related differences in FARESTON effectiveness or safety were noted.

Race: Fourteen percent of patients in the North American Study were non-caucasian. No significant race-related differences in FARESTON effectiveness or safety were noted.

ADVERSE REACTIONS

Adverse drug reactions are principally due to the antiestrogenic hormonal actions of FARESTON and typically occur at the beginning of treatment.

The incidences of the following eight clinical toxicities were prospectively assessed in the North American Study. The incidence reflects the toxicities that were considered by the investigator to be drug related or possibly drug related.

Adverse Events	North American		Eastern European		Nordic	
	FAR60 n=221(%)	TAM20 n=215(%)	FAR60 n=157(%)	TAM40 n=149(%)	FAR60 n=214(%)	TAM40 n=201(%)
Cardiac						
Cardiac Failure	2 (1)	1 (<1)	–	1 (<1)	2 (1)	3 (1.5)
Myocardial Infarction	2 (1)	3 (1.5)	1 (<1)	2 (1)	–	1 (<1)
Arrhythmia	–	–	–	–	3 (1.5)	1 (<1)
Angina Pectoris	–	–	1 (<1)	–	1 (<1)	2 (1)
Ocular*						
Cataracts	22 (10)	16 (7.5)	–	–	–	5 (3)
Dry Eyes	20 (9)	16 (7.5)	–	–	–	–
Abnormal Visual Fields	8 (4)	10 (5)	–	–	–	1 (<1)
Corneal Keratopathy	4 (2)	2 (1)	–	–	–	–
Glaucoma	3 (1.5)	2 (1)	1 (<1)	–	–	1 (<1)
Abnormal Vision/Diplopia	–	–	–	–	3 (1.5)	–
Thromboembolic						
Pulmonary Embolism	4 (2)	2 (1)	1 (<1)	–	–	1 (<1)
Thrombophlebitis	–	2 (1)	1 (<1)	1 (<1)	4 (2)	3 (1.5)
Thrombosis	–	1 (<1)	1 (<1)	–	3 (1.5)	4 (2)
CVA/TIA	1 (<1)	–	1 (<1)	–	4 (2)	4 (2)
Elevated Liver Tests**						
SGOT	11 (5)	4 (2)	30 (19)	22 (15)	32 (15)	35 (17)
Alkaline Phosphatase	41 (19)	24 (11)	16 (10)	13 (9)	18 (8)	31 (15)
Bilirubin	3 (1.5)	4 (2)	2 (1)	1 (<1)	2 (1)	3 (1.5)
Hypercalcemia	6 (3)	6 (3)	1 (<1)	–	–	–

* Most of the ocular abnormalities were observed in the North American Study in which on-study and biannual ophthalmic examinations were performed. No cases of retinopathy were observed in any arm.

** Elevated defined as follows: North American Study: SGOT >100 IU/L; alkaline phosphatase >200 IU/L; bilirubin >2 mg/dL. Eastern European and Nordic studies: SGOT, alkaline phosphatase, and bilirubin – WHO Grade 1 (1.25 times the upper limit of normal).

	North American Study	
	FAR60 n = 221	TAM20 n = 215
Hot Flashes	35%	30%
Sweating	20%	17%
Nausea	14%	15%
Vaginal Discharge	13%	16%
Dizziness	9%	7%
Edema	5%	5%
Vomiting	4%	2%
Vaginal Bleeding	2%	4%

Approximately 1% of patients receiving FARESTON (n = 592) in the three controlled studies discontinued treatment as a result of adverse events (nausea and vomiting, fatigue, thrombophlebitis, depression, lethargy, anorexia, ischemic attack, arthritis, pulmonary embolism, and myocardial infarction).

Serious adverse events occurring in patients receiving FARESTON in the three major trials are listed in the table below.

[See table at top of page]

Other adverse events of unclear causal relationship to FARESTON included leukopenia and thrombocytopenia, skin discoloration or dermatitis, constipation, dyspnea, paresis, tremor, vertigo, pruritus, anorexia, reversible corneal opacity (corneal verticulata), asthenia, alopecia, depression, jaundice, and rigors.

In the 200 and 240 mg FARESTON dose arms, the incidence of SGOT elevation and nausea was higher. Approximately 4% of patients were withdrawn for toxicity from the high-dose FARESTON treatment arms. Reasons for withdrawal included hypercalcemia, abnormal liver function tests, and one case each of toxic hepatitis, depression, dizziness, incoordination, ataxia, blurry vision, diffuse dermatitis, and a constellation of symptoms consisting of nausea, sweating, and tremor.

OVERDOSAGE

Lethality was observed in rats following single oral doses that were >1000 mg/kg (about 150 times the recommended human dose on a mg/m² basis) and was associated with gastric atony/dilatation leading to interference with digestion and adrenal enlargement.

Vertigo, headache, and dizziness were observed in healthy volunteer studies at a daily dose of 680 mg for 5 days. The symptoms occurred in two of the five subjects during the third day of the treatment and disappeared within 2 days of discontinuation of the drug. No immediate concomitant changes in any measured clinical chemistry parameters were found. In a study in postmenopausal breast cancer patients, toremifene 400 mg/m²/day caused dose-limiting nausea, vomiting, and dizziness, as well as reversible hallucinations and ataxia in one patient.

Theoretically, overdose may be manifested as an increase of antiestrogenic effects, such as hot flashes; estrogenic effects, such as vaginal bleeding; or nervous system disorders, such as vertigo, dizziness, ataxia, and nausea. There is no specific antidote and the treatment is symptomatic.

DOSAGE AND ADMINISTRATION

The dosage of FARESTON is 60 mg, once daily, orally. Treatment is generally continued until disease progression is observed.

HOW SUPPLIED

FARESTON Tablets, containing toremifene citrate in an amount equivalent to 60 mg of toremifene, are round, convex, unscored, uncoated, and white, or almost white. FARESTON Tablets are identified with TO 60 embossed on one side.

FARESTON Tablets are available as:
NDC 0085-1126-01 bottles of 30
NDC 0085-1126-02 bottles of 100
Store at 25°C (77°F). Protect from heat and light.

Schering Corporation
Kenilworth, NJ 07033 USA

1/97   19214907
Copyright © 1997, Schering Corporation. All rights reserved.

Shown in Product Identification Guide, page 336

FULVICIN® P/G   ℞
brand of ultramicrosize griseofulvin
Tablets, USP

DESCRIPTION

FULVICIN P/G Tablets contain ultra-microsize crystals of griseofulvin, an antibiotic derived from a species of *Penicillium*. Griseofulvin crystals are partly dissolved in polyethylene glycol 8000 and partly dispersed throughout the tablet matrix.

Each FULVICIN P/G Tablet contains 125 mg or 250 mg griseofulvin ultramicrosize.

Continued on next page

Information on Schering products appearing on these pages is effective as of August 15, 1998.

Fulvicin P/G—Cont.

The inactive ingredients for FULVICIN P/G Tablets, 125 or 250 mg, include: corn starch, lactose monohydrate, magnesium stearate, PEG, and sodium lauryl sulfate.

ACTIONS

Microbiology

Griseofulvin is fungistatic with *in vitro* activity against various species of *Microsporum, Epidermophyton,* and *Trichophyton.* It has no effect on bacteria or on other genera of fungi.

Human Pharmacology

Following oral administration, griseofulvin is deposited in the keratin precursor cells and has a greater affinity for diseased tissue. The drug is tightly bound to the new keratin which becomes highly resistant to fungal invasions.

The efficiency of gastrointestinal absorption of ultramicrocrystalline griseofulvin is approximately one and one-half times that of the conventional microsized griseofulvin. This factor permits the oral intake of two-thirds as much ultramicrocrystalline griseofulvin as the microsize form. However, there is currently no evidence that this lower dose confers any significant clinical differences with regard to safety and/or efficacy.

INDICATIONS

FULVICIN P/G Tablets are indicated for the treatment of ringworm infections of the skin, hair, and nails, namely: tinea corporis, tinea pedis, tinea cruris, tinea barbae, tinea capitis, tinea unguium (onychomycosis) when caused by one or more of the following genera of fungi: *Trichophyton rubrum, Trichophyton tonsurans, Trichophyton mentagrophytes, Trichophyton interdigitale, Trichophyton verrucosum, Trichophyton megninii, Trichophyton gallinae, Trichophyton crateriforme, Trichophyton sulphureum, Trichophyton schoenleinii, Microsporum audouini, Microsporum canis, Microsporum gypseum,* and *Epidermophyton floccosum.*

Note: Prior to therapy, the type of fungi responsible for the infection should be identified.

The use of this drug is not justified in minor or trivial infections which will respond to topical agents alone.

Griseofulvin is not effective in the following: bacterial infections, candidiasis (moniliasis), histoplasmosis, actinomycosis, sporotrichosis, chromoblastomycosis, coccidioidomycosis, North American blastomycosis, cryptococcosis (torulosis), tinea versicolor, and nocardiosis.

CONTRAINDICATIONS

This drug is contraindicated in patients with porphyria, hepatocellular failure, and in individuals with a history of hypersensitivity to griseofulvin.

Rare cases of conjoined twins have been reported in patients taking griseofulvin during the first trimester of pregnancy. Griseofulvin should not be prescribed to pregnant patients or to women contemplating pregnancy.

WARNINGS

Prophylactic Usage: Safety and efficacy of griseofulvin for phophylaxis of fungal infections have not been established. Since griseofulvin has demonstrated harmful effects *in vitro* on the genotype in bacteria, plants, and fungi, males should wait at least 6 months after completing griseofulvin therapy before fathering a child. Females should avoid risk of pregnancy while receiving griseofulvin therapy.

Animal Toxicology: Chronic feeding of griseofulvin, at levels ranging from 0.5–2.5% of the diet, resulted in the development of liver tumors in several strains of mice, particularly in males. Smaller particle sizes result in an enhanced effect. Lower oral dosage levels have not been tested. Subcutaneous administration of relatively small doses of griseofulvin once a week during the first 3 weeks of life has also been reported to induce hepatoma in mice. Thyroid tumors, mostly adenomas but some carcinomas, have been reported in male rats receiving griseofulvin at levels of 2.0%, 1.0%, and 0.2% of the diet, and in female rats, receiving the two higher dose levels. Although studies in other animal species have not yielded evidence of tumorigenicity, these studies were not of adequate design to form a basis for conclusions in this regard.

In subacute toxicity studies, orally administered griseofulvin produced hepatocellular necrosis in mice, but this has not been seen in other species. Disturbances in porphyrin metabolism have been reported in griseofulvin-treated laboratory animals. Griseofulvin has been reported to have a colchicine-like effect on mitosis and cocarcinogenicity with methylcholanthrene in cutaneous tumor induction in laboratory animals.

Griseofulvin interferes with chromosomal distribution during cell division, causing aneuploidy in plant and mammalian cells. These effects have been demonstrated *in vitro* at concentrations that may be achieved in the serum with the recommended therapeutic dosage.

Usage in Pregnancy: Griseofulvin should not be prescribed to pregnant patients or to women contemplating pregnancy (see **CONTRAINDICATIONS**).

Animal Reproduction Studies: It has been reported in the literature that griseofulvin was found to be embryotoxic and teratogenic on oral administration to pregnant rats. Pups with abnormalities have been reported in the litters of a few bitches treated with griseofulvin.

Suppression of spermatogenesis has been reported to occur in rats, but investigation in man failed to confirm this.

PRECAUTIONS

Patients on prolonged therapy with any potent medication should be under close observation. Periodic monitoring of organ system function, including renal, hepatic, and hematopoietic, should be done.

Since griseofulvin is derived from species of *Penicillium,* the possibility of cross-sensitivity with penicillin exists; however, known penicillin-sensitive patients have been treated without difficulty.

Since a photosensitivity reaction is occasionally associated with griseofulvin therapy, patients should be warned to avoid exposure to intense natural or artificial sunlight.

Lupus erythematosus or lupus-like syndromes, or exacerbation of existing lupus, have been reported in patients receiving griseofulvin.

Drug Interactions: Griseofulvin decreases the activity of warfarin-type anticoagulants so that patients receiving these drugs concomitantly may require dosage adjustment of the anticoagulant during and after griseofulvin therapy.

Barbiturates usually depress griseofulvin activity, and concomitant administration may require a dosage adjustment of the antifungal agent.

The effects of alcohol may be potentiated by griseofulvin, producing such effects as tachycardia and flush.

Griseofulvin may potentiate an increase in hepatic enzymes that metabolize estrogens at an increased rate, including the estrogen component of oral contraceptives, thereby causing possible decreased contraceptive effects and menstrual irregularities.

ADVERSE REACTIONS

When adverse reactions occur, they are most commonly of the hypersensitivity type, such as skin rashes and urticaria; and rarely, angioneurotic edema and epidermal necrolysis (Lyell's syndrome), and may necessitate withdrawal of therapy and appropriate countermeasures. Paresthesias of the hands and feet have been reported rarely after extended therapy. Other side effects reported occasionally are oral thrush, nausea, vomiting, epigastric distress, diarrhea, headache, fatigue, dizziness, insomnia, mental confusion, and impairment of performance of routine activities.

Proteinuria, nephrosis, leukopenia, hepatic toxicity, GI bleeding, and menstrual irregularities have been reported rarely. Administration of the drug should be discontinued if granulocytopenia occurs.

When rare, serious reactions occur with griseofulvin, they are usually associated with high dosages, long periods of therapy, or both.

DOSAGE AND ADMINISTRATION

Accurate diagnosis of the infecting organism is essential. Identification should be made either by direct microscopic examination of a mounting of infected tissue in a solution of potassium hydroxide or by culture on an appropriate medium.

Medication must be continued until the infecting organism is completely eradicated as indicated by appropriate clinical or laboratory examination. Representative treatment periods are tinea capitis, 4 to 6 weeks; tinea corporis, 2 to 4 weeks; tinea pedis, 4 to 8 weeks; tinea unguium—depending on rate of growth—fingernails, at least 4 months; toenails, at least 6 months.

General measures in regard to hygiene should be observed to control sources of infection or reinfection. Concomitant use of appropriate topical agents is usually required, particularly in treatment of tinea pedis. In some forms of athlete's foot, yeasts and bacteria may be involved as well as fungi. Griseofulvin will not eradicate the bacterial or monilial infection.

Adults: Daily administration of 375 mg (as a single dose or in divided amounts) will give a satisfactory response in most patients with tinea corporis, tinea cruris, and tinea capitis. For those fungus infections more difficult to eradicate, such as tinea pedis and tinea unguium, a divided dose of 750 mg is recommended.

Children: Approximately 3.3 mg per pound of body weight per day of ultramicrosize griseofulvin is an effective dose for most children. On this basis, the following dosage schedule is suggested: Children weighing 35 to 60 pounds—125 mg to 187.5 mg daily. Children weighing over 60 pounds—187.5 mg to 375 mg daily.

Children 2 years of age and younger—dosage has not been established.

Clinical experience with griseofulvin in children with tinea capitis indicates that a single daily dose is effective. Clinical relapse will occur if the medication is not continued until the infecting organism is eradicated.

HOW SUPPLIED

FULVICIN P/G Tablets, 125 mg, white, compressed, scored tablets impressed with the Schering trademark ® and product identification numbers, 228; bottle of 100 (NDC 0085-0228-03).

FULVICIN P/G Tablets, 250 mg, white, compressed, scored tablets impressed with the Schering trademark ® and product identification numbers, 507; bottle of 100 (NDC 0085-0507-03).

Store between 15° and 30°C (59° and 86°F).

FULVICIN® P/G
brand of ultramicrosize
griseofulvin
Tablets, USP

Schering Corporation
Kenilworth, NJ 07033 USA
Rev. 2/96 B-16184756

Copyright © 1976, 1992, 1993, 1996, Schering Corporation. All rights reserved.

Shown in Product Identification Guide, page 336

FULVICIN® P/G 165 and 330 ℞
brand of ultramicrosize griseofulvin
Tablets, USP

DESCRIPTION

FULVICIN P/G Tablets contain ultramicrosize crystals of griseofulvin, an antibiotic derived from a species of *Penicillium.* Griseofulvin crystals are partly dissovled in polyethylene glycol 8000 and partly dispersed throughout the tablet matrix.

Each FULVICIN P/G Tablet contains 165 mg or 330 mg ultramicrosize griseofulvin, USP.

The inactive ingredients for FULVICIN P/G 165 and 330 Tablets include: corn starch, lactose monohydrate, magnesium stearate, PEG, and sodium lauryl sulfate.

ACTIONS

Microbiology

Griseofulvin is fungistatic with *in vitro* against various species of *Microsporum, Epidermophyton,* and *Trichophyton.* It has no effect on bacteria or on other genera of fungi.

Human Pharmacology

Following oral administration, griseofulvin is deposited in the keratin precursor cells and has a greater affinity for diseased tissue. The drug is tightly bound to the new keratin which becomes highly resistant to fungal invasions.

The efficiency of gastrointestinal absorption of ultramicrocrystalline griseofulvin is approximately one and one-half times that of the conventional microsize griseofulvin. This factor permits the oral intake of two-thirds as much ultramicrocrystalline griseofulvin as the microsize form. However, there is currently no evidence that this lower dose confers any significant clinical differences with regard to safety and/or efficacy.

INDICATIONS

FULVICIN P/G Tablets are indicated for the treatment of ringworm infections of the skin, hair, and nails, namely: tinea corporis, tinea pedis, tinea cruris, tinea barbae, tinea capitis, tinea unguium (onychomycosis) when caused by one or more of the following genera of fungi: *Trichophyton rubrum, Trichophyton tonsurans, Trichophyton mentagrophytes, Trichophyton interdigitale, Trichophyton verrucosum, Trichophyton megninii, Trichophyton gallinae, Trichophyton crateriforme, Trichophyton sulphureum, Trichophyton schoenieinii, Microsporum audouini, Microsporum canis, Microsporum gypseum,* and *Epidermophyton floccosum.*

Note: Prior to therapy, the type of fungi responsible for the infection should be identified.

The use of this drug is not justified in minor or trivial infections which will respond to topical agents alone.

Griseofulvin is not effective in the following: bacterial infections, candidiasis (moniliasis), histoplasmosis, actinomycosis, sporotrichosis, chromoblastomycosis, coccidioidomycosis, North American blastomycosis, cryptococcosis (torulosis), tinea versicolor, and nocardiosis.

CONTRAINDICATIONS

This drug is contraindicated in patients with porphyria, hepatocellular failure, and in individuals with a history of hypersensitivity to griseofulvin.

Rare cases of conjoined twins have been reported in patients taking griseofulvin during the first trimester of pregnancy. Griseofulvin should not be prescribed to pregnant patients or to women contemplating pregnancy.

WARNINGS

Prophylactic Usage: Safety and efficacy of griseofulvin for prophylaxis of fungal infections have not been established. Since griseofulvin has demonstrated harmful effects *in vitro* on the genotype in bacteria, plants, and fungi, males should

wait at least 6 months after completing griseofulvin therapy before fathering a child. Females should avoid risk of pregnancy while receiving griseofulvin therapy.

Animal Toxicology: Chronic feeding of griseofulvin, at levels ranging from 0.5–2.5% of the diet, resulted in the development of liver tumors in several strains of mice, particularly in males. Smaller particle sizes results in an enhanced effect. Lower oral dosage levels have not been tested. Subcutaneous administration of relatively small doses of griseofulvin once a week during the first 3 weeks of life has also been reported to induce hepatomata in mice. Thyroid tumors, mostly adenomas but some carcinomas, have been reported in male rats receiving griseofulvin at levels of 2.0%, 1.0%, and 0.2% of the diet, and in female rats receiving the two higher dose levels. Although studies in other animal species have not yielded evidence of tumorigenicity, these studies were not of adequate design to form a basis for conclusions in this regard.

In subacute toxicity studies, orally administered griseofulvin produced hepatocellular necrosis in mice, but this has not been seen in other species. Disturbances in porphyrin metabolism have been reported in griseofulvin-treated laboratory animals. Griseofulvin has been reported to have a colchicine-like effect on mitosis an cocarcinogenicity with methylcholanthrene in cutaneous tumor induction in laboratory animals.

Griseofulvin interferes with chromosomal distribution during cell division, causing aneuploidy in plant and mammalian cells. These effects have been demonstrated *in vitro* at concentrations that may be achieved in the serum with the recommended therapeutic dosage.

Usage in Pregnancy: Griseofulvin should not be prescribed to pregnant patients or to women contemplating pregnancy (see **CONTRAINDICATIONS**).

Animal Reproduction Studies: It has been reported in the literature that griseofulvin was found to be embryotoxic and teratogenic on oral administration to pregnant rats. Pups with abnormalities have been reported in the litters of a few bitches treated with griseofulvin.

Suppression of spermatogenesis has been reported to occur in rats, but investigation in man failed to confirm this.

PRECAUTIONS

Patients on prolonged therapy with any potent medication should be under close observation. Periodic monitoring of organ system function, including renal, hepatic, and hematopoietic, should be done.

Since griseofulvin is derived from species of *Penicillium*, the possibility of cross-sensitivity with penicillin exists; however, known penicillin-sensitive patients have been treated without difficulty.

Since a photosensitivity reaction is occasionally associated with griseofulvin therapy, patients should be warned to avoid exposure to intense natural or artificial sunlight.

Lupus erythematosus or lupus-like syndromes, or exacerbation of existing lupus, have been reported in patients receiving griseofulvin.

Drug Interactions: Griseofulvin decreases the activity of warfarin-type anticoagulants so that patients receiving these drugs concomitantly may require dosage adjustment of the anticoagulant during and after griseofulvin therapy. Barbiturates usually depress griseofulvin activity, and concomitant administration may require a dosage adjustment of the antifungal agent.

The effects of alcohol may be potentiated by griseofulvin, producing such effect as tachycardia and flush.

Griseofulvin may potentiate an increase in hepatic enzymes that metabolize estrogens at an increased rate, including the estrogen component of oral contraceptives, thereby causing possible decreased contraceptive effects and menstrual irregularities.

ADVERSE REACTIONS

When adverse reactions occur, they are most commonly of the hypersensitivity type, such as skin rashes and urticaria; and rarely, angioneurotic edema and epidermal necrolysis (Lyell's syndrome), and may necessitate withdrawal of therapy and appropriate countermeasures. Paresthesias of the hands and feet have been reported rarely after extended therapy. Other side effects reported occasionally are oral thrush, nausea, vomiting, epigastric distress, diarrhea, headache, fatigue, dizziness, insomnia, mental confusion, and impairment of performance of routine activities.

Proteinuria, nephrosis, leukopenia, hepatic toxicity, GI bleeding, and menstrual irregularities have been reported rarely. Administration of the drug should be discontinued if granulocytopenia occurs.

When rare, serious reactions occur with griseofulvin, they are usually associated with high dosages, long periods of therapy, or both.

DOSAGE AND ADMINISTRATION

Accurate diagnosis of the infecting organism is essential. Identification should be made either by direct microscopic examination of a mounting of infected tissue in a solution of potassium hydroxide or by culture on an appropriate medium.

Medication must be continued until the infecting organism is completely eradicated as indicated by appropriate clinical or laboratory examination. Representative treatment periods are tinea capitis, 4 to 6 weeks; tinea corporis, 2 to 4 weeks; tinea pedis, 4 to 8 weeks; tinea unguium-depending on rate of growth-fingernails, at least 4 months; toenails, at least 6 months.

General measures in regard to hygiene should be observed to control sources of infection or reinfection. Concomitant use of appropriate topical agents is usually required, particularly in treatment of tinea pedis. In some forms of athlete's foot, yeasts and bacteria may be involved as well as fungi. Griseofulvin will not eradicate the bacterial or monilial infection.

Adults: Daily administration of 330 mg (as a single dose or in divided amounts) will give a satisfactory response in most patients with tinea corporis, tinea cruris, and tinea capitis. For those fungus infections more difficult to eradicate, such as tinea pedis and tinea unguium, a divided daily dosage of 660 mg is recommended.

Children: Approximately 3.3 mg per pound of body weight per day is an effective dose for most children. On this basis, the following dosage schedule is suggested: Children weighing 30 to 50 pounds-82.5 mg to 165 mg daily. Children weighing over 50 pounds-165 mg to 330 mg daily.

Children 2 years of age and younger-dosage has not been established.

Clinical experience with griseofulvin in children with tinea capitis indicates that a single daily dose is effective. Clinical relapse will occur if the medication is not continued until the infecting organism is eradicated.

HOW SUPPLIED

FULVICIN P/G 165 Tablets, 165 mg, off-white, oval, compressed, scored tablets impressed with the product name (FULVICIN P/G) and product identification numbers, 654; bottle of 100 (NDC 0085–0654–03).

FULVICIN P/G 330 Tablets, 330 mg, off-white, oval, compressed, scored tablets impressed with the product name (FULVICIN P/G) and product identification numbers, 352; bottle of 100 (NDC 0085–0352–03).

Store between 2° and 30° C (36° and 86°F).

FULVICIN® P/G 165 and 330

brand of ultramicrosize griseofulvin

Tablets, USP

Schering Corporation
Kenilworth, NJ 07033 USA
Rev. 6/96   16100145

Copyright © 1976, 1989, 1992, 1996, Schering Corporation. All rights reserved.

Shown in Product Identification Guide, page 336

GARAMYCIN®   ℞
brand of gentamicin sulfate
Cream, USP 0.1% and
Ointment, USP 0.1%
For Dermatologic Use Only–Not For Ophthalmic Use

DESCRIPTION

Each gram of GARAMYCIN **Cream** 0.1% contains 1.7 mg gentamicin sulfate, USP, equivalent to 1.0 mg gentamicin base, with 1.0 mg methylparaben and 4.0 mg butylparaben as preservatives, in a bland, emulsion-type vehicle composed of stearic acid, propylene glycol stearate, isopropyl myristate, propylene glycol, polysorbate 40, sorbitol solution and purified water.

Each gram of GARAMYCIN **Ointment** 0.1% contains 1.7 mg gentamicin sulfate, USP, equivalent to 1.0 mg gentamicin base, with 0.5 mg methylparaben and 0.1 mg propylparaben as preservatives in a bland, unctuous petrolatum base.

ACTIONS

GARAMYCIN, a wide-spectrum antibiotic, provides highly effective topical treatment in primary and secondary bacterial infections of the skin. GARAMYCIN may clear infections that have not responded to other topical antibiotic agents. In impetigo contagiosa and other primary skin infections, treatment three or four times daily with GARAMYCIN usually clears the lesions promptly. In secondary skin infections, GARAMYCIN facilitates the treatment of the underlying dermatosis by controlling the infection. Bacteria susceptible to the action of GARAMYCIN include sensitive strains of streptococci (group A beta-hemolytic, alpha-hemolytic), *Staphylococcus aureus* (coagulase-positive, coagulase-negative, and some penicillinase-producing strains), and the gram-negative bacteria, *Pseudomonas aeruginosa, Aerobacter aerogenes, Escherichia coli, Proteus vulgaris,* and *Klebsiella pneumoniae.*

INDICATIONS

Primary skin infections: Impetigo contagiosa, superficial folliculitis, ecthyma, furunculosis, sycosis barbae, and pyoderma gangrenosum. *Secondary skin infections:* Infectious eczematoid dermatitis, pustular acne, pustular psoriasis, infected seborrheic dermatitis, infected contact dermatitis

(including poison ivy), infected excoriations, and bacterial superinfections of fungal or viral infections. Note: GARAMYCIN is a bactericidal agent that is not effective against viruses or fungi in skin infections. GARAMYCIN is useful in the treatment of infected skin cysts and certain other skin abscesses when preceded by incision and drainage to permit adequate contact between the antibiotic and the infecting bacteria. Good results have been obtained in the treatment of infected stasis and other skin ulcers, infected superficial burns, paronychia, infected insect bites and stings, infected lacerations and abrasions, and wounds from minor surgery. Patients sensitive to neomycin can be treated with gentamicin, although regular observation of patients sensitive to topical antibiotics is advisable when such patients are treated with any topical antibiotic. GARAMYCIN **Ointment** helps retain moisture and has been useful in infection on dry eczematous or psoriatic skin. GARAMYCIN **Cream** is recommended for wet, oozing primary infections and greasy, secondary infections, such as pustular acne or infected seborrheic dermatitis. If a water-washable preparation is desired, GARAMYCIN **Cream** is preferable. GARAMYCIN **Ointment** and **Cream** have been used successfully in infants over one year of age, as well as in adults and children.

CONTRAINDICATIONS

This drug is contraindicated in individuals with a history of sensitivity reactions to any of its components.

PRECAUTIONS

Use of topical antibiotics occasionally allows overgrowth of nonsusceptible organisms, including fungi. If this occurs, or if irritation, sensitization, or superinfection develops, treatment with gentamicin should be discontinued and appropriate therapy instituted.

ADVERSE REACTIONS

In patients with dermatoses treated with gentamicin, irritation (erythema and pruritus) that did not usually require discontinuance of treatment has been reported in a small percentage of cases. There was no evidence of irritation or sensitization, however, in any of these patients patch-tested subsequently with gentamicin on normal skin. Possible photosensitization has been reported in several patients but could not be elicited in these patients by reapplication of gentamicin followed by exposure to ultraviolet radiation.

DOSAGE AND ADMINISTRATION

A small amount of GARAMYCIN **Cream** or **Ointment** should be applied gently to the lesions three or four times daily. The area treated may be covered with a gauze dressing if desired. In impetigo contagiosa, the crusts should be removed before application of GARAMYCIN to permit maximum contact between the antibiotic and the infection. Care should be exercised to avoid further contamination of the infected skin. Infected stasis ulcers have responded well to GARAMYCIN under gelatin packing.

HOW SUPPLIED

GARAMYCIN **Cream** 0.1% (NDC-0085-0008-05) and GARAMYCIN **Ointment** 0.1% (NDC-0085-0343-05), 15 g tubes.

Store between 2° and 30°C (36° and 86°F).

Schering Corporation
Kenilworth, NJ 07033 USA
Revised 7/91   11808654

Copyright © 1966, 1991, Schering Corporation. All rights reserved.

GARAMYCIN® Injectable   ℞
brand of gentamicin sulfate injection, USP
40 mg per mL
Each mL contains gentamicin sulfate, USP
equivalent to 40 mg gentamicin.
For Parenteral Administration

PRODUCT INFORMATION

WARNINGS
Patients treated with aminoglycosides should be under close clinical observation because of the potential toxicity associated with their use.   As with other aminoglycosides, GARAMYCIN Injectable is potentially nephrotoxic. The risk of nephrotoxicity is greater in patients with impaired renal function and in those who receive high dosage or prolonged therapy. Neurotoxicity manifested by ototoxicity, both vestibular and auditory, can occur in patients treated with GARAMYCIN Injectable, primarily in those with pre-

Continued on next page

Information on Schering products appearing on these pages is effective as of August 15, 1998.

Consult 1999 PDR® supplements and future editions for revisions

Garamycin Injectable—Cont.

existing renal damage and in patients with normal renal function treated with higher doses and/or for longer periods than recommended. Aminoglycoside-induced ototoxicity is usually irreversible. Other manifestations of neurotoxicity may include numbness, skin tingling, muscle twitching, and convulsions.

Renal and eighth cranial nerve function should be closely monitored, especially in patients with known or suspected reduced renal function at onset of therapy, and also in those whose renal function is initially normal but who develop signs of renal dysfunction during therapy. Urine should be examined for decreased specific gravity, increased excretion of protein, and the presence of cells or casts. Blood urea nitrogen, serum creatinine, or creatinine clearance should be determined periodically. When feasible, it is recommended that serial audiograms be obtained in patients old enough to be tested, particularly high-risk patients. Evidence of ototoxicity (dizziness, vertigo, ataxia, tinnitus, roaring in the ears, or hearing loss) or nephrotoxicity requires dosage adjustment or discontinuance of the drug. As with the other aminoglycosides, on rare occasions changes in renal and eighth cranial nerve function may not become manifest until soon after completion of therapy.

Serum concentrations of aminoglycosides should be monitored when feasible to assure adequate levels and to avoid potentially toxic levels. When monitoring gentamicin peak concentrations, dosage should be adjusted so that prolonged levels above 12 mcg/mL are avoided. When monitoring gentamicin trough concentrations, dosage should be adjusted so that levels above 2 mcg/mL are avoided. Excessive peak and/or trough serum concentrations of aminoglycosides may increase the risk of renal and eighth cranial nerve toxicity. In the event of overdose or toxic reactions, hemodialysis may aid in the removal of gentamicin from the blood, especially if renal function is, or becomes, compromised. The rate of removal of gentamicin is considerably less by peritoneal dialysis than by hemodialysis.

Concurrent and/or sequential systemic or topical use of other potentially neurotoxic and/or nephrotoxic drugs, such as cisplatin, cephaloridine, kanamycin, amikacin, neomycin, polymyxin B, colistin, paromomycin, streptomycin, tobramycin, vancomycin, and viomycin, should be avoided. Other factors which may increase patient risk of toxicity are advanced age and dehydration.

The concurrent use of gentamicin with potent diuretics, such as ethacrynic acid or furosemide, should be avoided, since certain diuretics by themselves may cause ototoxicity. In addition, when administered intravenously, diuretics may enhance aminoglycoside toxicity by altering the antibiotic concentration in serum and tissue.

DESCRIPTION

Gentamicin sulfate, USP, a water-soluble antibiotic of the aminoglycoside group, is derived from *Micromonospora purpurea*, an actinomycete. GARAMYCIN Injectable is a sterile, aqueous solution for parenteral administration. Each mL contains gentamicin sulfate, USP equivalent to 40 mg gentamicin base; 1.8 mg methylparaben and 0.2 mg propylparaben as preservatives; 3.2 mg sodium bisulfite; and 0.1 mg edetate disodium.

CLINICAL PHARMACOLOGY

After intramuscular administration of GARAMYCIN Injectable, peak serum concentrations usually occur between 30 and 60 minutes and serum levels are measurable for 6 to 8 hours. When gentamicin is administered by intravenous infusion over a 2-hour period, the serum concentrations are similar to those obtained by intramuscular administration. In patients with normal renal function, peak serum concentrations of gentamicin (mcg/mL) are usually up to four times the single intramuscular dose (mg/kg); for example, a 1.0 mg/kg injection in adults may be expected to result in a peak serum concentration up to 4 mcg/mL; a 1.5 mg/kg dose may produce levels up to 6 mcg/mL. While some variation is to be expected due to a number of variables such as age, body temperature, surface area, and physiologic differences, the individual patient given the same dose tends to have similar levels in repeated determinations. Gentamicin administered at 1.0 mg/kg every 8 hours for the usual 7- to 10-day treatment period to patients with normal renal function does not accumulate in the serum.

Gentamicin, like all aminoglycosides, may accumulate in the serum and tissues of patients treated with higher doses and/or for prolonged periods, particularly in the presence of impaired renal function. In adult patients, treatment with gentamicin dosages of 4 mg/kg/day or higher for 7 to 10 days may result in a slight, progressive rise in both peak and trough concentrations. In patients with impaired renal function, gentamicin is cleared from the body more slowly than in patients with normal renal function. The more severe the impairment, the slower the clearance. (Dosage must be adjusted.)

Since gentamicin is distributed in extracellular fluid, peak serum concentrations may be lower than usual in adult patients who have a large volume of this fluid. Serum concentrations of gentamicin in febrile patients may be lower than those in afebrile patients given the same dose. When body temperature returns to normal, serum concentrations of the drug may rise. Febrile and anemic states may be associated with a shorter than usual serum half-life. (Dosage adjustment is usually not necessary.) In severely burned patients, the half-life may be significantly decreased and resulting serum concentrations may be lower than anticipated from the mg/kg dose.

Protein-binding studies have indicated that the degree of gentamicin binding is low; depending upon the methods used for testing, this may be between 0% and 30%.

After initial administration to patients with normal renal function, generally 70% or more of the gentamicin dose is recoverable in the urine in 24 hours; concentrations in urine above 100 mcg/mL may be achieved. Little, if any, metabolic transformation occurs; the drug is excreted principally by glomerular filtration. After several days of treatment, the amount of gentamicin excreted in the urine approaches the daily dose administered. As with other aminoglycosides, a small amount of the gentamicin dose may be retained in the tissues, especially in the kidneys. Minute quantities of aminoglycosides have been detected in the urine weeks after drug administration was discontinued. Renal clearance of gentamicin is similar to that of endogenous creatinine.

In patients with marked impairment of renal function, there is a decrease in the concentration of aminoglycosides in urine and in their penetration into defective renal parenchyma. This decreased drug excretion, together with the potential nephrotoxicity of aminoglycosides, should be considered when treating such patients who have urinary tract infections.

Probenecid does not affect renal tubular transport of gentamicin.

The endogenous creatinine clearance rate and the serum creatinine level have a high correlation with the half-life of gentamicin in serum. Results of these tests may serve as guides for adjusting dosage in patients with renal impairment (see **DOSAGE AND ADMINISTRATION**).

Following parenteral administration, gentamicin can be detected in serum, lymph, tissues, sputum, and in pleural, synovial, and peritoneal fluids. Concentrations in renal cortex sometimes may be eight times higher than the usual serum levels. Concentrations in bile, in general, have been low and have suggested minimal biliary excretion. Gentamicin crosses the peritoneal as well as the placental membranes. Since aminoglycosides diffuse poorly into the subarachnoid space after parenteral administration, concentrations of gentamicin in cerebrospinal fluid are often low and dependent upon dose, rate of penetration, and degree of meningeal inflammation. There is minimal penetration of gentamicin into ocular tissues following intramuscular or intravenous administration.

Microbiology: *In vitro* tests have demonstrated that gentamicin is a bactericidal antibiotic which acts by inhibiting normal protein synthesis in susceptible microorganisms. It is active against a wide variety of pathogenic bacteria including *Escherichia coli*, *Proteus* species (indole-positive and indole-negative), *Pseudomonas aeruginosa*, species of the *Klebsiella-Enterobacter-Serratia* group. *Citrobacter* species, and *Staphylococcus* species (including penicillin- and methicillin-resistant strains). Gentamicin is also active *in vitro* against species of *Salmonella* and *Shigella*. The following bacteria are usually resistant to aminoglycosides: *Streptococcus pneumoniae*, most species of streptococci, particularly group D and anaerobic organisms, such as *Bacteroides* species or *Clostridium* species.

In vitro studies have shown that an aminoglycoside combined with an antibiotic that interferes with cell wall synthesis may act synergistically against some group D streptococcal strains. The combination of gentamicin and penicillin G has a synergistic bactericidal effect against virtually all strains of *Streptococcus faecalis* and its varieties (*S. faecalis* var. *liquifaciens*, *S. faecalis* var. *zymogenes*), *S. faecium* and *S. durans*. An enhanced killing effect against many of these strains has also been shown *in vitro* with combinations of gentamicin and ampicillin, carbenicillin, nafcillin, or oxacillin.

The combined effect of gentamicin and carbenicillin is synergistic for many strains of *Pseudomonas aeruginosa*. *In vitro* synergism against other gram-negative organisms has been shown with combinations of gentamicin and cephalosporins.

Gentamicin may be active against clinical isolates of bacteria resistant to other aminoglycosides. Bacteria resistant to one aminoglycoside may be resistant to one or more other aminoglycosides. Bacterial resistance to gentamicin is generally developed slowly.

Susceptibility Testing: If the disc method of susceptibility testing used is that described by Bauer *et al.* (*Am J Clin Path* 45:493, 1966; *Federal Register* 37:20525-20529, 1972), a disc containing 10 mcg of gentamicin should give a zone of inhibition of 15 mm or more to indicate susceptibility of the infecting organism. A zone of 12 mm or less indicates that the infecting organism is likely to be resistant. Zones greater than 12 mm and less than 15 mm indicate intermediate susceptibility. In certain conditions it may be desirable to do additional susceptibility testing by the tube or agar dilution method; gentamicin substance is available for this purpose.

INDICATIONS AND USAGE

GARAMYCIN Injectable is indicated in the treatment of serious infections caused by susceptible strains of the following microorganisms: *Pseudomonas aeruginosa*, *Proteus* species (indole-positive and indole-negative), *Escherichia coli*, *Klebsiella-Enterobacter-Serratia* species, *Citrobacter* species, and *Staphylococcus* species (coagulase-positive and coagulase-negative).

Clinical studies have shown GARAMYCIN Injectable to be effective in bacterial neonatal sepsis; bacterial septicemia; and serious bacterial infections of the central nervous system (meningitis), urinary tract, respiratory tract, gastrointestinal tract (including peritonitis), skin, bone and soft tissue (including burns). Aminoglycosides, including gentamicin, are not indicated in uncomplicated initial episodes of urinary tract infections unless the causative organisms are susceptible to these antibiotics and are not susceptible to antibiotics having less potential for toxicity.

Specimens for bacterial culture should be obtained to isolate and identify causative organisms and to determine their susceptibility to gentamicin.

GARAMYCIN Injectable may be considered as initial therapy in suspected or confirmed gram-negative infections, and therapy may be instituted before obtaining results of susceptibility testing. The decision to continue therapy with this drug should be based on the results of susceptibility tests, the severity of the infection, and the important additional concepts contained in the "**WARNINGS**" Box. If the causative organisms are resistant to gentamicin, other appropriate therapy should be instituted.

In serious infections when the causative organisms are unknown, GARAMYCIN Injectable may be administered as initial therapy in conjunction with a penicillin-type or cephalosporin-type drug before obtaining results of susceptibility testing. If anaerobic organisms are suspected as etiologic agents, consideration should be given to using other suitable antimicrobial therapy in conjunction with gentamicin. Following identification of the organism and its susceptibility, appropriate antibiotic therapy should then be continued. GARAMYCIN Injectable has been used effectively in combination with carbenicillin for the treatment of life-threatening infections caused by *Pseudomonas aeruginosa*. It has also been found effective when used in conjunction with a penicillin-type drug for the treatment of endocarditis caused by group D streptococci.

GARAMYCIN Injectable has also been shown to be effective in the treatment of serious staphylococcal infections. While not the antibiotic of first choice, GARAMYCIN Injectable may be considered when penicillins or other less potentially toxic drugs are contraindicated and bacterial susceptibility tests and clinical judgment indicate its use. It may also be considered in mixed infections caused by susceptible strains of staphylococci and gram-negative organisms.

In the neonate with suspected bacterial sepsis or staphylococcal pneumonia, a penicillin-type drug is also usually indicated as concomitant therapy with gentamicin.

CONTRAINDICATIONS

Hypersensitivity to gentamicin is a contraindication to its use. A history of hypersensitivity or serious toxic reactions to other aminoglycosides may contraindicate use of gentamicin because of the known cross-sensitivity of patients to drugs in this class.

WARNINGS

(See boxed **WARNINGS**.) Aminoglycosides can cause fetal harm when administered to a pregnant woman. Aminoglycoside antibiotics cross the placenta, and there have been several reports of total irreversible bilateral congenital deafness in children whose mothers received streptomycin during pregnancy. Serious side effects to mother, fetus, or newborn have not been reported in the treatment of pregnant women with other aminoglycosides. Animal reproduction studies conducted on rats and rabbits did not reveal evidence of impaired fertility or harm to the fetus due to gentamicin sulfate.

It is not known whether gentamicin sulfate can cause fetal harm when administered to a pregnant woman or can affect reproduction capacity. If gentamicin is used during pregnancy or if the patient becomes pregnant while taking gentamicin, she should be apprised of the potential hazard to the fetus.

GARAMYCIN Injectable contains sodium bisulfite, a sulfite that may cause allergic-type reactions including anaphylactic symptoms and life-threatening or less severe asthmatic episodes in certain susceptible people. The overall prevalence of sulfite sensitivity in the general population is unknown and probably low. Sulfite sensitivity is seen more frequently in asthmatic than in nonasthmatic people.

PRECAUTIONS

Neurotoxic and nephrotoxic antibiotics may be absorbed in significant quantities from body surfaces after local irrigation or application. The potential toxic effect of antibiotics administered in this fashion should be considered.

Increased nephrotoxicity has been reported following concomitant administration of aminoglycoside antibiotics and cephalosporins.

Neuromuscular blockade and respiratory paralysis have been reported in the cat receiving high doses (40 mg/kg) of gentamicin. The possibility of these phenomena occurring in man should be considered if aminoglycosides are administered by any route to patients receiving anesthetics, or to patients receiving neuromuscular blocking agents, such as succinylcholine, tubocurarine, or decamethonium, or in patients receiving massive transfusions of citrate-anticoagulated blood. If neuromuscular blockade occurs, calcium salts may reverse it.

Aminoglycosides should be used with caution in patients with neuromuscular disorders, such as myasthenia gravis, since these drugs may aggravate muscle weakness because of their potential curare-like effects on the neuromuscular junction. During or following gentamicin therapy, paresthesias, tetany, positive Chvostek and Trousseau signs, and mental confusion have been described in patients with hypomagnesemia, hypocalcemia, and hypokalemia. When this has occurred in infants, tetany and muscle weakness has been described. Both adults and infants required appropriate corrective electrolyte therapy.

Elderly patients may have reduced renal function which may not be evident in the results of routine screening tests, such as BUN or serum creatinine. A creatinine clearance determination may be more useful. Monitoring of renal function during treatment with gentamicin, as with other aminoglycosides, is particularly important in such patients. A Fanconi-like syndrome, with aminoaciduria and metabolic acidosis, has been reported in some adults and infants being given gentamicin injections.

Cross-allergenicity among aminoglycosides has been demonstrated.

Patients should be well hydrated during treatment.

Although the *in vitro* mixing of gentamicin and carbenicillin results in a rapid and significant inactivation of gentamicin, this interaction has not been demonstrated in patients with normal renal function who received both drugs by different routes of administration. A reduction in gentamicin serum half-life has been reported in patients with severe renal impairment receiving carbenicillin concomitantly with gentamicin.

Treatment with gentamicin may result in overgrowth of nonsusceptible organisms. If this occurs, appropriate therapy is indicated.

See "**WARNINGS**" Box regarding concurrent use of potent diuretics and regarding concurrent and/or sequential use of other neurotoxic and/or nephrotoxic antibiotics and for other essential information.

Usage in Pregnancy—Safety for use in pregnancy has not been established.

ADVERSE REACTIONS

Nephrotoxicity Adverse renal effects, as demonstrated by the presence of casts, cells, or protein in the urine or by rising BUN, NPN, serum creatinine or oliguria, have been reported. They occur more frequently in patients with a history of renal impairment and in patients treated for longer periods or with larger dosage than recommended.

Neurotoxicity Serious adverse effects on both vestibular and auditory branches of the eighth cranial nerve have been reported, primarily in patients with renal impairment (especially if dialysis is required) and in patients on high doses and/or prolonged therapy. Symptoms include dizziness, vertigo, ataxia, tinnitus, roaring in the ears and hearing loss, which, as with the other aminoglycosides, may be irreversible. Hearing loss is usually manifested initially by diminution of high-tone acuity. Other factors which may increase the risk of toxicity include excessive dosage, dehydration, and previous exposure to other ototoxic drugs.

Peripheral neuropathy or encephalopathy, including numbness, skin tingling, muscle twitching, convulsions, and a myasthenia gravis-like syndrome, have been reported.

Note: The risk of toxic reactions is low in patients with normal renal function who do not receive GARAMYCIN Injectable at higher doses or for longer periods of time than recommended.

Other reported adverse reactions possibly related to gentamicin include: respiratory depression, lethargy, confusion, depression, visual disturbances, decreased appetite, weight loss, and hypotension and hypertension; rash, itching, urticaria, generalized burning, laryngeal edema, anaphylactoid reactions, fever, and headache; nausea, vomiting, increased salivation, and stomatitis; purpura, pseudotumor cerebri, acute organic brain syndrome, pulmonary fibrosis, alopecia, joint pain, transient hepatomegaly, and splenomegaly.

Laboratory abnormalities possibly related to gentamicin include: increased levels of serum transaminase (SGOT, SGPT), serum LDH, and bilirubin; decreased serum calcium, magnesium, sodium, and potassium; anemia, leukopenia, granulocytopenia, transient agranulocytosis, eosinophilia, increased and decreased reticulocyte counts, and thrombocytopenia. While clinical laboratory test abnormalities may be isolated findings, they may also be associated with clinically related signs and symptoms. For example, tetany and muscle weakness may be associated with hypomagnesemia, hypocalcemia, and hypokalemia.

While local tolerance of GARAMYCIN Injectable is generally excellent, there has been an occasional report of pain at the injection site. Subcutaneous atrophy or fat necrosis suggesting local irritation has been reported rarely.

OVERDOSAGE

In the event of overdose or toxic reactions, hemodialysis may aid in the removal of gentamicin from the blood, and is especially important if renal function is, or becomes, compromised. The rate of removal of gentamicin is considerably less by peritoneal dialysis than it is by hemodialysis.

DOSAGE AND ADMINISTRATION

GARAMYCIN Injectable may be given intramuscularly or intravenously. The patient's pretreatment body weight should be obtained for calculation of correct dosage. The dosage of aminoglycosides in obese patients should be based on an estimate of the lean body mass. It is desirable to limit the duration of treatment with aminoglycosides to short term.

DOSAGE FOR PATIENTS WITH NORMAL RENAL FUNCTION

Adults: The recommended dosage of GARAMYCIN Injectable for patients with serious infections and normal renal function is 3 mg/kg/day, administered in three equal doses every 8 hours (Table I).

For patients with life-threatening infections, dosages up to 5 mg/kg/day may be administered in three or four equal doses. This dosage should be reduced to 3 mg/kg/day as soon as clinically indicated (Table I).

It is desirable to measure periodically both peak and trough serum concentrations of gentamicin when feasible during therapy to assure adequate but not excessive drug levels. For example, the peak concentration (at 30 to 60 minutes after intramuscular injection) is expected to be in the range of 4 to 6 mcg/mL. When monitoring peak concentrations after intramuscular or intravenous administration, dosage should be adjusted so that prolonged levels above 12 mcg/mL are avoided. When monitoring trough concentrations (just prior to the next dose), dosage should be adjusted so that levels above 2 mcg/mL are avoided. Determination of the adequacy of a serum level for a particular patient must take into consideration the susceptibility of the causative organism, the severity of the infection, and the status of the patient's host-defense mechanisms.

In patients with extensive burns, altered pharmacokinetics may result in reduced serum concentrations of aminoglycosides. In such patients treated with gentamicin, measurement of serum concentrations is recommended as a basis for dosage adjustment.

[See table above]

TABLE I
DOSAGE SCHEDULE GUIDE FOR ADULTS
WITH NORMAL RENAL FUNCTION
(Dosage at 8-Hour Intervals)
40 mg per mL

Patient's Weight* kg	(lb)	Usual Dose for Serious Infections 1 mg/kg q8h (3 mg/kg/day) mg/dose q8h	mL/dose	Dose For Life-Threatening Infections (Reduce As Soon As Clinically Indicated) 1.7 mg/kg q8h** (5 mg/kg/day) mg/dose q8h	mL/dose
40	(88)	40	1.0	66	1.6
45	(99)	45	1.1	75	1.9
50	(110)	50	1.25	83	2.1
55	(121)	55	1.4	91	2.25
60	(132)	60	1.5	100	2.5
65	(143)	65	1.6	108	2.7
70	(154)	70	1.75	116	2.9
75	(165)	75	1.9	125	3.1
80	(176)	80	2.0	133	3.3
85	(187)	85	2.1	141	3.5
90	(198)	90	2.25	150	3.75
95	(209)	95	2.4	158	4.0
100	(220)	100	2.5	166	4.2

* The dosage of aminoglycosides in obese patients should be based on an estimate of the lean body mass.

** For q6h schedules, dosage should be recalculated.

Children: 6 to 7.5 mg/kg/day. (2.0 to 2.5 mg/kg administered every 8 hours.)

Infants and Neonates: 7.5 mg/kg/day. (2.5 mg/kg administered every 8 hours.)

Premature or Full-Term Neonates One Week of Age or Less: 5 mg/kg/day. (2.5 mg/kg administered every 12 hours.)

The usual duration of treatment for all patients is 7 to 10 days. In difficult and complicated infections, a longer course of therapy may be necessary. In such cases, monitoring of renal, auditory, and vestibular functions is recommended, since toxicity is more apt to occur with treatment extended for more than 10 days. Dosage should be reduced if clinically indicated.

For Intravenous Administration

The intravenous administration of gentamicin may be particularly useful for treating patients with bacterial septicemia or those in shock. It may also be the preferred route of administration for some patients with congestive heart failure, hematologic disorders, severe burns, or those with reduced muscle mass. For intermittent intravenous administration in adults, a single dose of GARAMYCIN Injectable may be diluted in 50 to 200 mL of sterile isotonic saline solution or in a sterile solution of dextrose 5% in water; in infants and children, the volume of diluent should be less. The solution may be infused over a period of $^1/_2$ to 2 hours. The recommended dosage for intravenous and intramuscular administration is identical.

GARAMYCIN Injectable should not be physically premixed with other drugs, but should be administered separately in accordance with the recommended route of administration and dosage schedule.

DOSAGE FOR PATIENTS WITH IMPAIRED RENAL FUNCTION

Dosage must be adjusted in patients with impaired renal function to assure therapeutically adequate, but not excessive, blood levels. Whenever possible, serum concentrations of gentamicin should be monitored. One method of dosage adjustment is to increase the interval between administration of the usual doses. Since the serum creatinine concentration has a high correlation with the serum half-life of gentamicin, this laboratory test may provide guidance for adjustment of the interval between doses. The interval between doses (in hours) may be approximated by multiplying the serum creatinine level (mg/100 mL) by 8. For example, a patient weighing 60 kg with a serum creatinine level of 2.0 mg/100 mL could be given 60 mg (1 mg/kg) every 16 hours (2×8).

In patients with serious systemic infections and renal impairment, it may be desirable to administer the antibiotic more frequently but in reduced dosage. In such patients, serum concentrations of gentamicin should be measured so that adequate but not excessive levels result. A peak and trough concentration measured intermittently during therapy will provide optimal guidance for adjusting dosage. After the usual initial dose, a rough guide for determining reduced dosage at 8-hour intervals is to divide the normally recommended dose by the serum creatinine level (Table II). For example, after an initial dose of 60 mg (1.0 mg/kg), a patient weighing 60 kg with a serum creatinine level of 2.0 mg/100 mL could be given 30 mg every 8 hours (60÷2). It should be noted that the status of renal function may be changing over the course of the infectious process.

It is important to recognize that deteriorating renal function may require a greater reduction in dosage than that specified in the above guidelines for patients with stable renal impairment.

Continued on next page

Information on Schering products appearing on these pages is effective as of August 15, 1998.

Garamycin Injectable—Cont.

TABLE II
DOSAGE ADJUSTMENT GUIDE FOR PATIENTS WITH RENAL IMPAIRMENT
(Dosage at 8-Hour Intervals After the Usual Initial Dose)

Serum Creatinine (mg %)	Approximate Creatinine Clearance Rate (mL/min/1.73M^2)	Percent of Usual Doses Shown in Table I
≤ 1.0	>100	100
1.1–1.3	70–100	80
1.4–1.6	55–70	65
1.7–1.9	45–55	55
2.0–2.2	40–45	50
2.3–2.5	35–40	40
2.6–3.0	30–35	35
3.1–3.5	25–30	30
3.6–4.0	20–25	25
4.1–5.1	15–20	20
5.2–6.6	10–15	15
6.7–8.0	<10	10

In adults with renal failure undergoing hemodialysis, the amount of gentamicin removed from the blood may vary depending upon several factors including the dialysis method used. An 8-hour hemodialysis may reduce serum concentrations of gentamicin by approximately 50%. The recommended dosage at the end of each dialysis period is 1 to 1.7 mg/kg depending upon the severity of infection. In children, a dose of 2 mg/kg may be administered.

The above dosage schedules are not intended as rigid recommendations but are provided as guides to dosage when the measurement of gentamicin serum levels is not feasible.

A variety of methods is available to measure gentamicin concentrations in body fluids; these include microbiologic, enzymatic, and radioimmunoassay techniques.

HOW SUPPLIED

GARAMYCIN Injectable, 40 mg per mL, for parenteral administration, is supplied in 2 mL (80 mg) vials, boxes of 25 (NDC 0085-0069-04).

GARAMYCIN Injectable is a clear, stable solution that requires no refrigeration.

Store between 2° and 30°C (36° and 86°F).

Schering Corporation
Kenilworth, NJ 07033 USA
Rev. 5/96 17150839

Copyright © 1968, 1992, 1994, 1996, Schering Corporation. All rights reserved.

HYPERSTAT® I.V. ℞

brand of diazoxide, USP
Injection
For Intravenous Use In Hospitalized Patients Only

DESCRIPTION

HYPERSTAT I.V. Injection is a nondiuretic benzothiadiazine antihypertensive agent. Each ampule (20 ml) contains 300 mg diazoxide, USP, in a clear, sterile, colorless aqueous solution; the pH is adjusted to approximately 11.6 with sodium hydroxide.

Diazoxide has the following structural formula:

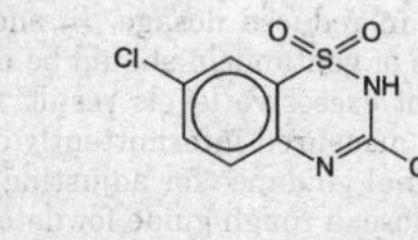

Diazoxide is 7-chloro-3-methyl-2*H*-1,2,4-benzothiadiazine 1,1-dioxide, with the empirical formula $C_8H_7ClN_2O_2S$, and the molecular weight 230.7. It is a white crystalline powder practically insoluble to sparingly soluble in water.

CLINICAL PHARMACOLOGY

HYPERSTAT I.V. Injection produces a prompt reduction of blood pressure in man by relaxing smooth muscle in the peripheral arterioles. Cardiac output is increased as blood pressure is reduced. Studies in animals demonstrate that coronary blood flow is maintained, while renal blood flow is increased after an initial decrease.

Transient hyperglycemia occurs in the majority of patients treated with HYPERSTAT, but usually requires treatment only in patients with diabetes mellitus. It will respond to the usual management measures, including insulin.

Blood glucose levels should be monitored, especially in patients with diabetes and in those requiring multiple injections of diazoxide. Cataracts have been observed in a few animals receiving repeated daily doses of intravenous diazoxide.

Since diazoxide causes sodium retention, repeated injections may precipitate edema and congestive heart failure. Increased volume of extracellular fluid may be a cause of treatment failure in nonresponsive patients. The increase in fluid volume characteristically responds to diuretic agents if adequate renal function exists. Concurrently administered thiazide diuretics may be expected to potentiate the antihypertensive and hyperuricemic actions of diazoxide. (See **Drug Interactions.**)

Diazoxide is extensively bound to serum protein (>90%). The plasma half-life is 28 ± 8.3 hours; however, the duration of its antihypertensive effect is variable, generally lasting less than 12 hours.

INDICATIONS AND USAGE

HYPERSTAT I.V. Injection is indicated for short-term use in the emergency reduction of blood pressure in severe, nonmalignant and malignant hypertension in hospitalized adults; and in acute severe hypertension in hospitalized children, when prompt and urgent decrease of diastolic pressure is required. Treatment with orally effective antihypertensive agents should not be instituted until blood pressure has stabilized. The use of HYPERSTAT I.V. Injection for longer than 10 days is not recommended.

HYPERSTAT I.V. Injection is ineffective against hypertension due to pheochromocytoma.

CONTRAINDICATIONS

HYPERSTAT I.V. Injection should not be used in the treatment of compensatory hypertension, such as that associated with aortic coarctation or arteriovenous shunt, and should not be used in patients hypersensitive to diazoxide, other thiazides, or other sulfonamide-derived drugs.

WARNINGS

Rapid Decrease of Blood Pressure Caution must be observed when reducing severely elevated blood pressure. Diazoxide should only be administered utilizing the new 150-mg minibolus dosage. The use of a 300-mg intravenous dose of diazoxide has been associated with angina and with myocardial and cerebral infarction. One instance of optic nerve infarction was reported when a 100-mmHg reduction in diastolic pressure occurred over ten minutes following a single 300-mg bolus. In one prospective trial conducted in patients with severe hypertension and coexistent coronary artery disease, a 50% incidence of ischemic changes in the electrocardiogram was observed following single 300-mg bolus injections of diazoxide. The desired blood pressure lowering should therefore be achieved over as long a period of time as is compatible with the patient's status. At least several hours and preferably one or two days is tentatively recommended.

Improved safety with equal efficacy can be achieved by administering HYPERSTAT I.V. Injection as a minibolus dose (1 to 3 mg/kg every 5 to 15 minutes up to a maximum of 150 mg in a single injection) until a diastolic blood pressure below 100 mmHg is achieved. HYPERSTAT I.V. Injection should not be administered in a bolus dose of 300 mg since this mode of administration is less predictable and less controllable than the minibolus dosage. If hypotension severe enough to require therapy results from the reduction in blood pressure, it will usually respond to the Trendelenberg maneuver. If necessary, sympathomimetic agents such as dopamine or norepinephrine may be administered.

Special attention is required for patients with diabetes mellitus and those in whom retention of salt and water may present serious problems.

Myocardial Lesions in Animals Intravenous administration of diazoxide in dogs has induced subendocardial necrosis and necrosis of papillary muscles. These lesions, which are also produced by other vasodilator drugs (i.e., hydralazine, minoxidil) and by catecholamines, are presumed to be related to anoxia resulting from a combination of reflex tachycardia and decreased perfusion.

PRECAUTIONS

General: HYPERSTAT (diazoxide) I.V. Injection is an effective antihypertensive agent requiring close monitoring of the patient's blood pressure at frequent intervals. Its administration may occasionally cause hypotension requiring treatment with sympathomimetic drugs. Therefore, HYPERSTAT I.V. Injection should be used primarily in the hospital or where adequate facilities exist to treat such untoward responses.

HYPERSTAT I.V. Injection should be administered only into a peripheral vein. Because the alkalinity of the solution is irritating to tissue, avoid extravascular injection or leakage. Subcutaneous administration has produced inflammation and pain without subsequent necrosis. If leakage into subcutaneous tissue occurs, the area should be treated with warm compresses and rest.

HYPERSTAT I.V. Injection should be used with care in patients who have impaired cerebral or cardiac circulation, that is, patients in whom abrupt reduction in blood pressure might be detrimental or those in whom mild tachycardia or decreased blood perfusion may be deleterious (see **WARNINGS**). Prolonged hypotension should be avoided so as not to aggravate preexisting renal failure.

Information for Patients: During and immediately following intravenous injection of HYPERSTAT I.V. Injection, the patient should remain supine.

Laboratory Tests: Diagnostic laboratory tests necessary to establish the patient's condition and status should be carried out prior to treatment with HYPERSTAT I.V. Injection. During and following treatment with HYPERSTAT I.V. Injection, laboratory tests to monitor the effects of treatment with this drug and the patient's condition should be done. Among the tests (not necessarily inclusive) are: hematologic (hematocrit, hemoglobin, white blood cell and platelet counts); metabolic (glucose, uric acid, total protein, albumin); electrolyte (sodium, potassium) and osmolality; renal function (creatinine, urine-protein); electrocardiogram.

Drug Interactions: Diazoxide is highly bound to serum protein. It can be expected to displace other substances which are also bound to protein, such as bilirubin or coumarin and its derivatives, resulting in higher blood levels of these substances.

An undesirable hypotension may result when diazoxide is administered to patients who have received other antihypertensive medication within six hours.

One patient in a clinical study exhibited excessive hypotension after concomitant administration of HYPERSTAT with hydralazine and methyldopa. An episode of maternal hypotension and fetal bradycardia occurred in a patient in labor who received both reserpine and hydralazine prior to administration of diazoxide. Neonatal hyperglycemia following intrapartum administration of HYPERSTAT I.V. Injection has also been reported.

HYPERSTAT I.V. Injection should not be administered within six hours of the administration of: hydralazine, reserpine, alphaprodine, methyldopa, beta-blockers, prazosin, minoxidil, the nitrites and other papaverine-like compounds.

Concomitant administration with thiazides or other commonly used diuretics may be expected to potentiate the hyperuricemic and antihypertensive effects of diazoxide.

Drug/Laboratory Test Interactions: The hyperglycemic and hyperuricemic effects of diazoxide preclude proper assessment of these metabolic states. Increased renin secretion, IgG concentrations and decreased cortisol secretion have also been noted. Diazoxide inhibits glucagon-stimulated insulin release and will cause a false-negative insulin response to glucagon. In the rat, dog, and monkey, diazoxide increased serum free fatty acids and decreased plasma insulin levels.

Carcinogenesis, Mutagenesis, Impairment of Fertility: No long-term animal dosing study has been done to evaluate the carcinogenic potential of diazoxide. No laboratory studies of mutagenic potential or animal studies of effects on fertility have been done.

Pregnancy Category C: Diazoxide has been shown to reduce fetal and/or pup survival; and to reduce fetal growth in rats, rabbits, and dogs at daily doses of 30, 21, or 10 mg/kg, respectively. In rats treated at term, diazoxide, at doses of 10 mg/kg and above, prolonged parturition.

The safety of HYPERSTAT I.V. Injection in pregnancy has not been established.

Nonteratogenic Effects: Diazoxide crosses the placental barrier and appears in cord blood. When given to the mother prior to delivery, the drug may produce fetal or neonatal hyperbilirubinemia, thrombocytopenia, altered carbohydrate metabolism, and possibly other side effects that have occurred in adults.

Labor and Delivery: HYPERSTAT I.V. Injection is not indicated for use in pregnancy. Intravenous administration of the drug during labor may cause cessation of uterine contractions, requiring administration of an oxytocic agent.

Nursing Mothers: Information is not available concerning the passage of HYPERSTAT in breast milk. Because many drugs are excreted in human milk and because of the potential for adverse reactions in nursing infants from diazoxide, a decision should be made whether to discontinue nursing or to discontinue the drug, taking into account the importance of the drug to the mother.

Pediatric Use: See **INDICATIONS AND USAGE.**

ADVERSE REACTIONS

It is reasonable to speculate that the currently recommended minibolus dosing regimen, which has replaced the 300-mg bolus dose in clinical practice, will result in adverse effects which are of similar character but of lesser frequency and severity.

In clinical experience with the rapid bolus administration of 300 mg, the most common adverse reactions reported were: hypotension (7%); nausea and vomiting (4%); dizziness and weakness (2%). Additional adverse reactions reported with bolus administration of 300 mg were as follows:

Cardiovascular: sodium and water retention after repeated injections, especially important in patients with impaired cardiac reserve; hypotension to shock levels; myocardial ischemia, usually transient and manifested by angina, atrial and ventricular arrhythmias, and marked electrocardiographic changes, but occasionally leading to myocardial infarction; optic nerve infarction following too rapid decrease in severely elevated blood pressure; supraventricular tachycardia and palpitation; bradycardia; chest discomfort or nonanginal "tightness in the chest."

Central Nervous System: cerebral ischemia, usually transient but occasionally leading to infarction and manifested by unconsciousness, convulsions, paralysis, confusion, or focal neurological deficit such as numbness of the hands; vasodilative phenomena, such as orthostatic hypotension, sweating, flushing, and generalized or localized sensations of warmth; various transient neurological findings secondary to alteration in regional blood flow to brain, such as headache (sometimes throbbing), dizziness, lightheadedness, sleepiness (also reported as lethargy, somnolence or drowsiness), euphoria or "funny feeling," ringing in the ears and momentary hearing loss, and weakness of short duration; apprehension or anxiety.

Gastrointestinal: rarely, acute pancreatitis; nausea, vomiting and/or abdominal discomfort; anorexia; alteration in taste; parotid swelling; salivation; dry mouth; lacrimation; ileus; constipation and diarrhea.

Other: hyperglycemia in diabetic patients, especially after repeated injections; hyperosmolar coma in an infant; transient hyperglycemia in nondiabetic patients; transient retention of nitrogenous wastes; various respiratory findings secondary to the relaxation of smooth muscle, such as dyspnea, cough and choking sensation; warmth or pain along the injected vein; cellulitis without sloughing and/or phlebitis at the injection site of extravasation; back pain and increased nocturia; hypersensitivity reactions, such as rash, leukopenia and fever; papilledema induced by plasma volume expansion secondary to the administration of diazoxide reported in a patient who had received eleven injections (300 mg/dose) over a 22-day period; malaise and blurred vision; transient cataract in an infant; hirsutism, and decreased libido.

OVERDOSAGE

Overdosage of HYPERSTAT I.V. Injection may cause an undesirable hypotension. Usually, this can be controlled with the Trendelenberg maneuver. If necessary, sympathomimetic agents, such as dopamine or norepinephrine, may be administered. Failure of blood pressure to rise in response to such agents suggests that the hypotension may have been caused by something other than diazoxide. Excessive hyperglycemia resulting from overdosage will respond to conventional therapy of hyperglycemia.

DOSAGE AND ADMINISTRATION

HYPERSTAT I.V. Injection was originally recommended for use by bolus administration of 300 mg. Recent studies have shown that minibolus administration of HYPERSTAT I.V. Injection, i.e., doses of 1 to 3 mg/kg repeated at intervals of 5 to 15 minutes is as effective in reducing blood pressure. Minibolus administration usually provides a more gradual reduction in blood pressure and thus may be expected to reduce the circulatory and neurological risks associated with acute hypotension.

HYPERSTAT I.V. Injection is administered undiluted and rapidly by intravenous injections of 1 to 3 mg/kg up to a maximum of 150 mg in a single injection. This dose may be repeated at intervals of 5 to 15 minutes until a satisfactory reduction in blood pressure (diastolic pressure below 100 mmHg) has been achieved.

With the patient recumbent, the calculated dose of HYPERSTAT I.V. Injection is administered intravenously in 30 seconds or less.

HYPERSTAT I.V. Injection should only be given into a peripheral vein. Do not administer it intramuscularly, subcutaneously, or into body cavities. Avoid extravasation of the drug into subcutaneous tissues.

Following the use of HYPERSTAT I.V. Injection, the blood pressure should be monitored closely until it has stabilized. Thereafter, measurements taken hourly during the balance of the effect should indicate any unusual response. A further decrease in blood pressure 30 minutes or more after injection should be investigated for causes other than the action of HYPERSTAT I.V. Injection. It is preferable that the patient remain supine for at least one hour after injection. In ambulatory patients, the blood pressure should also be measured with the patient standing before surveillance is ended.

Repeated administration of HYPERSTAT I.V. Injection at intervals of 4 to 24 hours usually will maintain the blood pressure below pretreatment levels until a regimen of oral antihypertensive medication can be instituted. The interval between injections may be adjusted by the duration of the response to each injection. It is usually unnecessary to continue treatment with HYPERSTAT I.V. Injection for more than four to five days.

Since repeated administration of HYPERSTAT I.V. Injection can lead to sodium and water retention, administration of a diuretic may be necessary both for maximal blood pressure reduction and to avoid congestive heart failure. (See **CLINICAL PHARMACOLOGY.**)

Parenteral drug products should be inspected visually for particulate matter and discoloration prior to administration, whenever solution and container permit.

HOW SUPPLIED

HYPERSTAT I.V. Injection is supplied in a 20-ml ampule, containing 300 mg diazoxide, in a clear, sterile, colorless, aqueous solution; box of one ampule (NDC 0085-0201-05). **Protect from light and freezing. Store between 2° and 30°C (36° and 86°F).**

Revised 2/85   11037496
Copyright ©1972, 1984, 1985. Schering Corporation. USA. All rights reserved.

INSPIREASE®   ℞
Drug Delivery System* for use with metered dose inhalers
* U.S. Patent 4,484,577

Instructions for use and care
Includes Instructions for Universal Mouthpiece and Actuation Aid

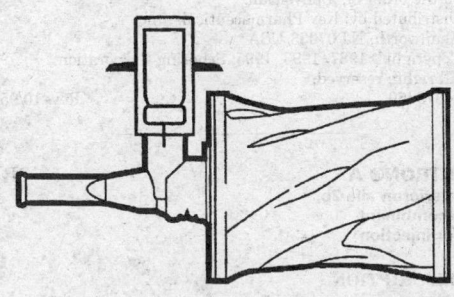

InspirEase® is a portable drug delivery system that helps "spray inhalers" (also known as metered–dose inhalers) deliver medication to the lungs. It is designed to improve the delivery of these medications by making it easier for you to use them.

If you are using a "spray inhaler" alone, you may not be getting all your medication. These "spray inhalers" provide a convenient and effective method for delivering drugs, but it is not easy to use them correctly. You must carefully time each breath while squeezing the "spray inhaler" downward. If your timing is incorrect, the full dose of medication may not be delivered deep within your lungs.

InspirEase makes it simpler to use your "spray inhaler" correctly. After you press down on your "spray inhaler," medication is released and stored in the compact bag, giving you the chance to breathe in the medication in two breaths. This does away with the need to carefully coordinate taking a breath and releasing the spray.

And InspirEase has a special feature to help teach you better breathing technique. When you are using it correctly (taking a slow, deep breath that helps get the medication deep within your lungs), the bag will collapse and you will *not* hear a whistling sound. However, if you breathe in too fast (a common mistake that can reduce the effectiveness of your treatment), you will hear a whistling sound.

This signals you to breathe slower.

Slow breathing and holding your breath after taking each dose of medication are necessary to obtain more complete relief. See diagram below:

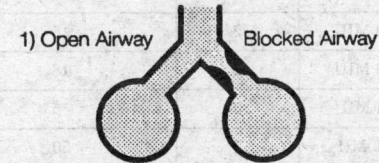

1) Open Airway   Blocked Airway

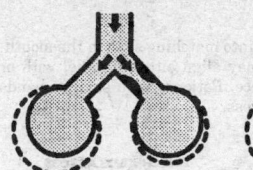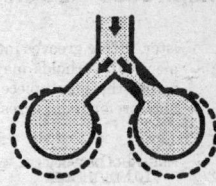

2) Fast breathing causes less lung expansion when you have a blocked airway.

Slow (optimal) breathing causes lung expansion to be more equal even if an airway is blocked.

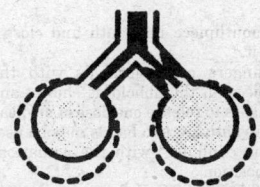

3) Aerosol drug delivered—Settling of drug on blocked airway with slow breathing, followed by breath holding, allows the airway to open.

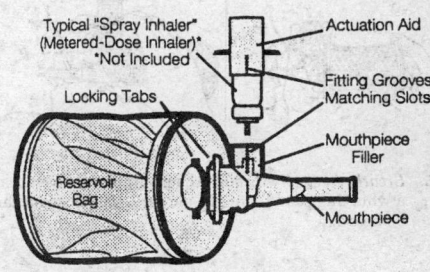

Typical "Spray Inhaler" (Metered-Dose Inhaler)*
*Not Included

Actuation Aid
Fitting Grooves Matching Slots
Locking Tabs
Reservoir Bag
Mouthpiece Filler
Mouthpiece

Contents
Your InspirEase® kit includes 3 replaceable reservoir bags, one actuation aid, and a *single universal mouthpiece* which can be used with both metal and white plastic stem inhalers.

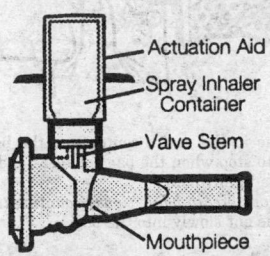

Actuation Aid
Spray Inhaler Container
Valve Stem
Mouthpiece

INSTRUCTIONS FOR USE

1. Connect the mouthpiece to the reservoir bag by lining up the *locking tabs* with the opening in the reservoir bag. Push in and twist to lock.

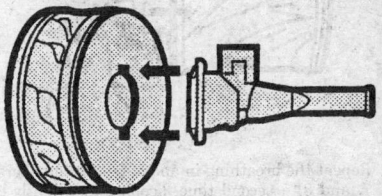

2. Untwist the reservoir bag gently to open it to its full size. Shake "spray inhaler" well before placing its stem in the *mouthpiece*. Make sure the stem sits in the center of the mouthpiece filler. Some inhalers may fit more loosely than others. This will not affect drug delivery. Place actuation aid over "spray inhaler" can-

Continued on next page

Inspirease—Cont.

ister, fitting grooves into matching slots in the mouthpiece. Fingerholds may align either parallel with or across the mouthpiece. Patients with smaller hands may prefer them across.

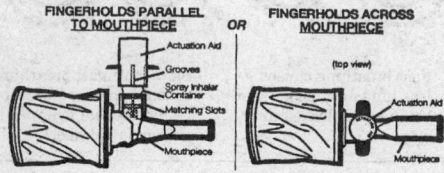

FINGERHOLDS PARALLEL TO MOUTHPIECE OR FINGERHOLDS ACROSS MOUTHPIECE

3. Place mouthpiece in mouth and close lips tightly around it.
4. Place fingers on fingerholds with thumb under mouthpiece on thumbhold as shown, and pull down with fingers to release one dose of medication into the bag. Alternatively, two hands may be used to actuate the "spray inhaler" with the actuation aid in the across position.
   IMPORTANT NOTE: Follow your physician's instructions regarding the number of doses you should take and when to take them.

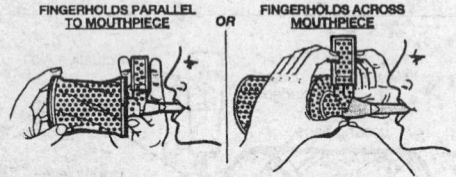

FINGERHOLDS PARALLEL TO MOUTHPIECE OR FINGERHOLDS ACROSS MOUTHPIECE

5. *Breathe in slowly* through the mouthpiece. If you hear a whistling sound, breathe slower until no sound can be heard.

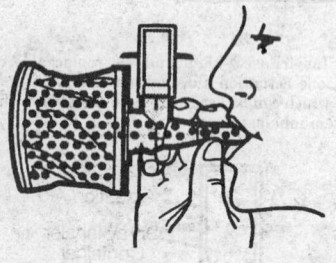

6. Breathe in the entire contents of the bag. You will know to stop when the bag collapses and you cannot breathe in anymore.
7. *Hold your breath while slowly counting to five.*
8. Breathe out slowly into the bag.

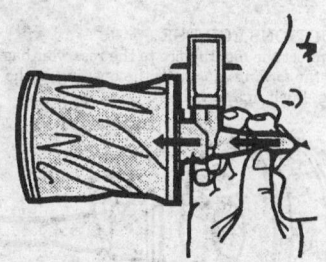

9. Repeat the breathing in and out steps (numbers 5, 6, 7, and 8) a second time, keeping lips tightly closed around the mouthpiece.
10. Remove the mouthpiece from your mouth. Unlock mouthpiece from the bag by untwisting and pulling out and store all components in carrying case.

How to tell if your "spray inhaler" is full or empty
Drop your "spray inhaler" into a pan of water. Its position in the water will tell you how much medication is left. See diagram below.
[See figure at top of next column]

Important Instructions
Clean mouthpiece thoroughly with warm (not hot) running water *at least* once a day. *The InspirEase® system is not dishwasher safe. Always clean by hand.*

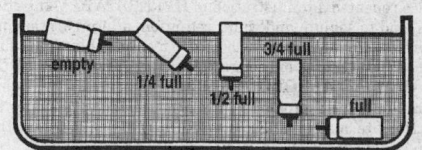

The clear plastic reed section of the mouthpiece should not be touched due to potential breakage. We recommend a visual inspection of the reed section for signs of breakage prior to each use. If reed breakage occurs, replace mouthpiece immediately; otherwise replace mouthpiece as needed every six months.

After cleaning, wait until mouthpiece is *completely dry* before storing in carrying case. Do not place near artificial heat such as dishwasher or oven.

We recommend that the reservoir bag be replaced every two to three weeks or as needed. *However, if there is a hole or tear in it, replace immediately.*

NOTE: You will need a physician's prescription for replacement bags or a new starter kit.

InspirEase is designed for use with most "spray inhaler" (metered-dose inhaler) containers currently available; for single-patient use and single-drug use.

The usual caution should be exercised in dosing medications and evaluating patient response. The prescribing information for the marketed MDIs varies with respect to dosing, administration, etc. We recommend that these be followed when using InspirEase.

CAUTION: Federal law restricts this device to sale by, or on the order of, a physician.

Distributed by: Key Pharmaceuticals, Inc.
Kenilworth, NJ 07033 USA
Copyright© 1987, 1993, 1995, Schering Corporation.
All rights reserved.
14379460   Rev. 10/95

INTRON® A
Interferon alfa-2b, recombinant For Injection

℞

DESCRIPTION
INTRON A Interferon alfa-2b, recombinant for intramuscular, subcutaneous, intralesional, or intravenous Injection is a purified sterile recombinant interferon product.

Interferon alfa-2b, recombinant for Injection has been classified as an alfa interferon and is a water-soluble protein with a molecular weight of 19,271 daltons produced by recombinant DNA techniques. It is obtained from the bacterial fermentation of a strain of *Escherichia coli* bearing a genetically engineered plasmid containing an interferon alfa-2b gene from human leukocytes. The fermentation is carried out in a defined nutrient medium containing the antibiotic tetracycline hydrochloride at a concentration of 5 to 10 mg/L; the presence of this antibiotic is not detectable in the final product. The specific activity of Interferon alfa-2b, recombinant is approximately 2.6×10^8 IU/mg protein as measured by the HPLC assay.
[See table below]

Prior to administration, the INTRON A Powder for Injection is to be reconstituted with the provided Diluent for INTRON A Interferon alfa-2b, recombinant for Injection (bacteriostatic water for injection) containing 0.9% benzyl alcohol as a preserative. (See **DOSAGE AND ADMINISTRATION.**) INTRON A Powder for Injection is a white to cream-colored powder.
[See tables at bottom of next page]

These packages do not require reconstitution prior to administration. (See **DOSAGE AND ADMINISTRATION.**) INTRON A Solution for Injection is a clear, colorless solution.

CLINICAL PHARMACOLOGY
General The interferons are a family of naturally occurring small proteins and glycoproteins with molecular weights of approximately 15,000 to 27,600 daltons produced and secreted by cells in response to viral infections and to synthetic or biological inducers.

Preclinical Pharmacology Interferons exert their cellular activities by binding to specific membrane receptors on the cell surface. Once bound to the cell membrane, interferons initiate a complex sequence of intracellular events. *In vitro* studies demonstrated that these include the induction of certain enzymes, suppression of cell proliferation, immunomodulating activities such as enhancement of the phagocytic activity of macrophages and augmentation of the specific cytotoxicity of lymphocytes for target cells, and inhibition of virus replication in virus-infected cells.

In a study using human hepatoblastoma cell line, HB 611, the *in vitro* antiviral activity of alfa interferon was demonstrated by its inhibition of hepatitis B virus (HBV) replication.

The correlation between these *in vitro* data and the clinical results is unknown. Any of these activities might contribute to interferon's therapeutic effects.

Pharmacokinetics The pharmacokinetics of INTRON A Interferon alfa-2b, recombinant for Injection were studied in 12 healthy male volunteers following single doses of 5 million IU/m^2 administered intramuscularly, subcutaneously, and as a 30-minute intravenous infusion in a crossover design. INTRON A concentrations were determined using a radioimmunoassay (RIA) with a detection limit equal to 10 IU/mL.

The mean serum INTRON A concentrations following intramuscular and subcutaneous injections were comparable. The maximum serum concentrations obtained via these routes were approximately 18 to 116 IU/mL and occurred 3 to 12 hours after administration. The elimination half-life of INTRON A Interferon alfa-2b, recombinant for Injection following both intramuscular and subcutaneous injections was approximately 2 to 3 hours. Serum concentrations were below the detection limit by 16 hours after the injections.

After intravenous administration, serum INTRON A concentrations peaked (135 to 273 IU/mL) by the end of the 30-minute infusion, then declined at a slightly more rapid rate than after intramuscular or subcutaneous drug administration, becoming undetectable 4 hours after the infusion. The elimination half-life was approximately 2 hours.

Urine INTRON A concentrations following a single dose (5 million IU/m^2) were not detectable after any of the parenteral routes of administration. This result was expected since preliminary studies with isolated and perfused rabbit kidneys have shown that the kidney may be the main site of interferon catabolism.

There are no pharmacokinetic data available for the intralesional route of administration.

Serum Neutralizing Antibodies In INTRON A treated patients tested for antibody activity in clinical trials, serum anti-interferon neutralizing antibodies were detected in 0% (0/90) of patients with hairy cell leukemia, 0.8% (2/260) of patients treated intralesionally for condylomata acuminata, and 4% (1/24) of patients with AIDS-Related Kaposi's Sarcoma. Serum neutralizing antibodies have been detected in <3% of patients treated with higher INTRON A doses in malignancies other than hairy cell leukemia or AIDS-Related Kaposi's Sarcoma. The clinical significance of the appearance of serum anti-interferon neutralizing activity in these indications is not known.

Powder for Injection				
Vial Strength	mL Diluent	Final Concentration after Reconstitution million IU/mL*	mg INTRON A[†] Interferon alfa-2b, recombinant	Route of Administration
3 MIU	1	3	0.012	IM, SC, IV
5 MU	1	5	0.019	IM, SC, IV
10 MIU	2	5	0.038	IM, SC, IV, IL[††]
18 MIU	1	18	0.069	IM, SC, IV
14 MIU	5	5	0.096	IM, SC, IV
50 MU	1	50	0.192	IM, SC, IV

* Each mL also contains 20 mg glycine, 2.3 mg sodium phosphate dibasic, 0.55 mg sodium phosphate monobasic, and 1.0 mg human albumin.
[†] Based on the specific activity of approximately 2.6×10^8 IU/mg protein, as mesured by HPLC assay.
[††]The 10 MIU vial for intralesional use should be reconstituted with 1 mL of the provided diluent.

Serum anti-interferon neutralizing antibodies were detected in 7% (12/168) of patients either during treatment or after completing 12 to 48 weeks of treatment with 3 million IU TIW of INTRON A therapy for chronic hepatitis C and in 13% (6/48) of patients who received INTRON A therapy for chronic hepatitis B at 5 million IU QD for 4 months, and in 3% (1/33) of patients treated at 10 million IU TIW. In patients with chronic hepatitis, the titers detected were low (18/19 with titers ≤1:40 and 1/19 with a titer of 1:160) and the appearance of serum anti-interferon neutralizing activity did not appear to affect safety or efficacy.

Hairy Cell Leukemia In clinical trials in patients with hairy cell leukemia, there was depression of hematopoiesis during the first 1 to 2 months of INTRON A treatment, resulting in reduced numbers of circulating red and white blood cells, and platelets. Subsequently, both splenectomized and nonsplenectomized patients achieved substantial and sustained improvements in granulocytes, platelets, and hemoglobin levels in 75% of treated patients and at least some improvement (minor responses) occurred in 90%. INTRON A treatment resulted in a decrease in bone marrow hypercellularity and hairy cell infiltrates. The hairy cell index (HCI), which represents the percent of bone marrow cellularity times the percent of hairy cell infiltrate, was ≥50% at the beginning of the study in 87% of patients. The percentage of patients with such an HCI decreased to 25% after 6 months and to 14% after 1 year. These results indicate that even though hematologic improvement had occurred earlier, prolonged INTRON A treatment may be required to obtain maximal reduction in tumor cell infiltrates in bone marrow.

The percentage of patients with hairy cell leukemia who required red blood cell or platelet transfusions decreased significantly during treatment and the percentage of patients with confirmed and serious infections declined as granulocyte counts improved. Reversal of splenomegaly and of clinically significant hypersplenism was demonstrated in some patients.

A study was conducted to assess the effects of extended INTRON A treatment on duration of response for patients who responded to initial therapy. In this study, 126 responding patients were randomized to receive additional INTRON A treatment for 6 months or observation for a comparable period, after 12 months of initial INTRON A therapy. During this 6-month period, 3% (2/66) of INTRON A treated patients relapsed compared with 18% (11/60) who were not treated. This represents a significant difference in time to relapse in favor of continued INTRON A treatment (p=0.006/0.01, Log Rank/Wilcoxon). Since a small proportion of the total population had relapsed, median time to relapse could not be estimated in either group. A similar pattern in relapses was seen when all randomized treatment, including that beyond 6 months, and available fol-

low-up data were assessed. The 15% (10/66) relapses among INTRON A patients occurred over a significantly longer period of time than the 40% (24/60) with observation (p=0.0002/0.0001, Log Rank/Wilcoxon). Median time to relapse was estimated, using the Kaplan-Meier method, to be 6.8 months in the observation group but could not be estimated in the INTRON A group.

Subsequent follow-up with a median time of approximately 40 months demonstrated an overall median survival of 87.8%. In a comparable historical control group followed for 24 months, overall median survival was approximately 40%.

Malignant Melanoma The safety and efficacy of INTRON A Interferon alfa-2b, recombinant for Injection was evaluated as adjuvant to surgical treatment in patients with melanoma who were free of disease (post-surgery) but at high risk for systemic recurrence. These included patients with lesions of Breslow thickness >4 mm, or patients with lesions of any Breslow thickness with primary or recurrent nodal involvement. In a randomized, controlled trial in 280 patients, 143 patients received INTRON A therapy at 20 million IU/m² intravenously five time per week for 4 weeks (induction phase) followed by 10 million IU/m² subcutaneously three times per week for 48 weeks (maintenance phase). INTRON A therapy was begun ≤56 days after surgical resection. The remaining 137 patients were observed.

INTRON A therapy produced a significant increase in relapse-free and overall survival. Median time to relapse for the INTRON A treated patients vs observation patients was 1.72 years vs 0.98 years (p<0.01, stratified Log Rank). The estimated 5-year relapse-free survival rate, using the Kaplan-Meier method, was 37% for INTRON A treated patients vs 26% for observation patients. Median overall survival time for INTRON A treated patients vs observation patients was 3.82 years vs 2.78 years (p=0.047, stratified Log Rank). The estimated 5-year overall survival rate, using the Kaplan-Meier method, was 46% for INTRON A treated patients vs 37% for observation patients.

Follicular Lymphoma The safety and efficacy of INTRON A in conjunction with CHVP, a combination chemotherapy regimen, was evaluated as initial treatment in patients with clinically aggressive, large tumor burden, Stage III/IV follicular Non-Hodgkin's Lymphoma. Large tumor burden was defined by the presence of any one of the following: a nodal or extranodal tumor mass with a diameter of >7 cm; involvement of at least three nodal sites (each with a diameter of >3 cm); systemic symptoms; splenomegaly; serous effusion, orbital or epidural involvement; ureteral compression; or leukemia.

In a randomized, controlled trial, 130 patients received CHVP therapy and 135 patients received CHVP therapy plus INTRON A therapy at 5 million IU subcutaneously three times weekly for the duration of 18 months. CHVP

chemotherapy consisted of cyclophosphamide 600 mg/m², doxorubicin 25 mg/m², and teniposide (VM-26) 60 mg/m², administered intravenously on Day 1 and prednisone at a daily dose of 40 mg/m² given orally on Days 1 to 5. Treatment consisted of six CHVP cycles administered monthly, followed by an additional 6 cycles administered every 2 months for 1 year. Patients in both treatment groups received a total of twelve CHVP cycles over 18 months.

The group receiving the combination of INTRON A therapy plus CHVP had a significantly longer progression-free survival (2.9 years vs 1.5 years, p=0.0001, Log Rank test). After a median follow-up of 6.1 years, the median survival for patients treated with CHVP alone was 5.5 years while median survival for patients treated with CHVP plus INTRON A therapy had not been reached (p=0.004, Log Rank test). In three additional published, randomized, controlled studies of the addition of interferon alfa to anthracycline-containing combination chemotherapy regimens,[1–3] the addition of interferon alfa was associated with significantly prolonged progression-free survival. Differences in overall survival were not consistently observed.

Condylomata Acuminata Condylomata acuminata (venereal or genital warts) are associated with infections of the human papilloma virus (HPV). The safety and efficacy of INTRON A Interferon alfa-2b, recombinant for Injection in the treatment of condylomata acuminata were evaluated in three controlled double-blind clinical trials. In these studies INTRON A doses of 1 million IU per lesion were administered intralesionally three times a week (TIW), in ≤5 lesions per patient for 3 weeks. The patients were observed for up to 16 weeks after completion of the full treatment course.

INTRON A treatment of condylomata was significantly more effective than placebo, as measured by disappearance of lesions, decreases in lesion size, and by an overall change in disease status. Of 192 INTRON A treated patients and 206 placebo treated patients who were evaluable for efficacy at the time of best response during the course of the study, 42% of INTRON A patients vs 17% of placebo patients experienced clearing of all treated lesions. Likewise 24% of INTRON A patients vs 8% of placebo patients experienced marked (≥75% to <100%) reduction in lesion size, 18% vs 9% experienced moderate (≥50% to ≤75%) reduction in lesion size, 10% vs 42% had a slight (<50%) reduction in lesion size, 5% vs 24% had no change in lesion size, and 0% vs 1% experienced exacerbation (p<0.001).

In one of these studies, 43% (54/125) of patients in whom multiple (≤3) lesions were treated, experienced complete clearing of all treated lesions during the course of the study. Of these patients, 81% remained cleared 16 weeks after treatment was initiated.

Patients who did not achieve total clearing of all their treated lesions had these same lesions treated with a second course of therapy. During this second course of treatment, 38% to 67% of patients had clearing of all treated lesions. The overall percentage of patients who had cleared all their treated lesions after two courses of treatment ranged from 57% to 85%.

INTRON A treated lesions showed improvement within 2 to 4 weeks after the start of treatment in the above study; maximal response to INTRON A therapy was noted 4 to 8 weeks after initiation of treatment.

The response to INTRON A therapy was better in patients who had condylomata for shorter durations than in patients with lesions for a longer duration.

Another study involved 97 patients in whom three lesions were treated with either an intralesional injection of 1.5 million IU of INTRON A Interferon alfa-2b, recombinant for Injection per lesion followed by a topical application of 25% podophyllin, or a topical application of 25% podophyllin alone. Treatment was given once a week for 3 weeks. The combined treatment of INTRON A Interferon alfa-2b, recombinant for Injection and podophyllin was shown to be significantly more effective than podophyllin alone, as determined by the number of patients whose lesions cleared. This significant difference in response was evident after the second treatment (Week 3) and continued through 8 weeks posttreatment. At the time of the patient's best response, 67% (33/49) of the INTRON A Interferon alfa-2b, recombinant for Injection and podophyllin treated patients had all three treated lesions clear while 42% (20/48) of the podophyllin treated patients had all three clear (p=0.003).

AIDS-Related Kaposi's Sarcoma The safety and efficacy of INTRON A Interferon alfa-2b, recombinant for Injection in the treatment of Kaposi's Sarcoma (KS), a common manifestation of the Acquired Immune Deficiency Syndrome (AIDS), were evaluated in clinical trials in 144 patients.

In one study, INTRON A doses of 30 million IU/m² were administered subcutaneously three times per week (TIW), to patients with AIDS-Related KS. Doses were adjusted for patient tolerance. The average weekly dose delivered in the

Solution Vials for Injection

Vial Strength	Final Concentration*	mg INTRON A[†] Interferon alfa-2b, recombinant	Route of Administration
3 MIU	3 million IU/0.5 mL	0.012	IM, SC
5 MIU	5 million IU/0.5 mL	0.019	IM, SC, IL
10 MIU	10 million IU/1.0 mL	0.038	IM, SC, IL
18[‡]MIU multidose	3 million IU/0.5 mL	0.088	IM, SC
25[¶]MIU multidose	5 million IU/0.5 mL	0.123	IM, SC, IL

* Each mL contains 7.5 mg sodium chloride, 1.8 mg sodium phosphate dibasic, 1.3 mg sodium phosphate monobasic, 0.1 mg edetate disodium, 0.1 mg polysorbate 80, and 1.5 mg m-cresol as a preservative.
† Based on the specific activity of approximately 2.6×10^8 IU/mg protein as measured by HLPC assay.
‡ This is a multidose vial which contains a total of 22.8 million IU of interferon alfa-2b, recombinant per 3.8 mL in order to provide the delivery of six 0.5-mL doses, each containing 3 million IU of INTRON A Interferon alfa-2b, recombinant for Injection (for a label strength of 18 million IU).
¶ This is a multidose vial which contains a total of 32.0 million IU of interferon alfa-2b, recombinant per 3.2 mL in order to provide the delivery of the 0.5-mL doses, each containing 5 million IU of INTRON A Interferon alfa-2b, recombinant for Injection (for a label strength of 25 million IU).

Solution in Multidose Pens for Injection

Pen Strength	Final Concentration*	INTRON A Dose Delivered (6 doses, 0.2 mL each)	mg INTRON A[†]	Route of Administration
18 MIU	22.5 MIU/1.5 mL	3 MIU/dose	0.087	SC
30 MIU	37.5 MIU/1.5 mL	5 MIU/dose	0.144	SC
60 MIU	75 MIU/1.5 mL	10 MIU/dose	0.288	SC

* Each mL also contains 7.5 mg sodium chloride, 1.8 mg sodium phosphate dibasic, 1.3 mg sodium phosphate monobasic, 0.1 mg edetate disodium, 0.1 mg polysorbate 80, and 1.5 mg m-cresol as a preservative.
† Based on the specific activity of approximately 2.6×10^8 IU/mg protein as measured by HPLC assay.

Continued on next page

Information on Schering products appearing on these pages is effective as of August 15, 1998.

Intron A—Cont.

first 4 weeks was 150 million IU; at the end of 12 weeks this averaged 110 million IU/week; and by 24 weeks averaged 75 million IU/week.

Forty-four percent of asymptomatic patients responded vs 7% of symptomatic patients. The median time to response was approximately 2 months and 1 month, respectively, for asymptomatic and symptomatic patients. The median duration of response was approximately 3 months and 1 month, respectively, for the asymptomatic and symptomatic patients. Baseline T4/T8 ratios were 0.46 for responders vs 0.33 for nonresponders.

In another study, INTRON A doses of 35 million IU were administered subcutaneously, daily (QD), for 12 weeks. Maintenance treatment, with every other day dosing (QOD), was continued for up to 1 year in patients achieving antitumor and antiviral responses. The median time to response was 2 months and the median duration of response was 5 months in the asymptomatic patients.

In all studies, the likelihood of response was greatest in patients with relatively intact immune systems as assessed by baseline CD4 counts (interchangeable with T4 counts). Results at doses of 30 million IU/m^2 TIW and 35 million IU/QD were subcutaneously similar and are provided together in TABLE 1. This table demonstrates the relationship of response to baseline CD4 count in both asymptomatic and symptomatic patients in the 30 million IU/m^2 TIW and the 35 million IU/QD treatment groups.

In the 30 million IU study group, 7% (5/72) of patients were complete responders and 22% (16/72) of the patients were partial responders. The 35 million IU study had 13% (3/23 patients) complete responders and 17% (4/23) partial responders.

For patients who received 30 million IU TIW, the median survival time was longer in patients with CD4 >200 (30.7 months) than in patients with CD4 ≤200 (8.9 months). Among responders, the median survival time was 22.6 months vs 9.7 months in nonresponders.

Chronic Hepatitis C The safety and efficacy of INTRON A Interferon alfa-2b, recombinant for Injection in the treatment of chronic hepatitis C was evaluated in 5 randomized clinical studies in which an INTRON A dose of 3 million IU three times a week (TIW) was assessed. The initial three studies were placebo-controlled trials that evaluated a 6-month (24 week) course of therapy. In each of the three studies, INTRON A therapy resulted in a reduction in serum alanine aminotransferase (ALT) in a greater proportion of patients vs control patients at the end of 6 months of dosing. During the 6 months of follow-up, approximately 50% of the patients who responded maintained their ALT response. A combined analysis comparing pretreatment and posttreatment liver biopsies revealed histological improvement in a statistically significantly greater proportion of INTRON A treated patients compared to controls.

Two additional studies have investigated longer treatment durations (up to 24 months).[5,6] Patients in the two studies to evaluate longer duration of treatment had hepatitis with or without cirrhosis in the absence of decompensated liver disease. Complete response to treatment was defined as normalization of the final two serum ALT levels during the treatment period. A sustained response was defined as a complete response at the end of the treatment period with sustained normal ALT values lasting at least 6 months following discontinuation of therapy.

In Study 1, all patients were initially treated with INTRON A 3 million IU TIW subcutaneously for 24 weeks (run-in-period). Patients who completed the initial 24-week treatment period were then randomly assigned to receive no further treatment or to receive 3 million IU TIW for an additional 48 weeks. In Study 2, patients who met the entry criteria were randomly assigned to receive INTRON A 3 million IU TIW subcutaneously for 24 weeks or to receive INTRON A 3 million IU TIW subcutaneously for 96 weeks. In both studies, patient follow-up was variable and some data collection was retrospective.

Results show that longer durations of INTRON A therapy improved the sustained response rate (see TABLE 2). In patients with complete responses (CR) to INTRON A therapy after 6 months of treatment (149/352 [42%]), responses were less often sustained if drug was discontinued (21/70 [30%]) than if it was continued for 18 to 24 months (44/79 [56%]). Of all patients randomized, the sustained response rate in the patients receiving 18 or 24 months of therapy was 22% and 26%, respectively, in the two trials. In patients who did not have a CR by 6 months, additional therapy did not result in significantly more responses, since almost all patients who responded to therapy did so within the first 16 weeks of treatment.

A subset (<50%) of patients from the combined extended dosing studies had liver biopsies performed both before and after INTRON A treatment. Improvement in necroinflammatory activity as assessed retrospectively by the Knodell (Study 1) and Scheuer (Study 2) Histology Activity Indices was observed in both studies. A higher number of patients (58%, 45/78) improved with extended therapy than with shorter (6 months) therapy (38%, 34/89) in this subset.

Chronic Hepatitis B The safety and efficacy of INTRON A Interferon alfa-2b, recombinant for Injection in the treatment of chronic hepatitis B were evaluated in three clinical trials in which INTRON A doses of 30 to 35 million IU per week were administered subcutaneously (SC), as either 5 million IU daily (QD), or 10 million IU three times a week (TIW) for 16 weeks vs no treatment. All patients were 18 years of age or older with compensated liver disease, and had chronic hepatitis B virus (HBV) infection (serum HBsAg positive for at least 6 months) and HBV replication (serum HBeAg positive). Patients were also serum HBV-DNA positive, an additional indicator of HBV replication, as measured by a research assay.[7,8] All patients had elevated serum alanine aminotransferase (ALT) and liver biopsy findings compatible with the diagnosis of chronic hepatitis. Patients with the presence of antibody to human immunodeficiency virus (anti-HIV) or antibody to hepatitis delta virus (anti-HDV) in the serum were excluded from the studies.

Virologic response to treatment was defined in these studies as a loss of serum markers of HBV replication (HBeAg and HBV DNA). Secondary parameters of response included loss of serum HBsAg, decreases in serum ALT, and improvement in liver histology.

In each of two randomized controlled studies, a significantly greater proportion of INTRON A treated patients exhibited a virologic response compared with untreated control patients (see TABLE 3). In a third study without a concurrent control group, a similar response rate to INTRON A therapy was observed. Pretreatment with prednisone, evaluated in two of the studies, did not improve the response rate and provided no additional benefit.

The response to INTRON A therapy was durable. No patient responding to INTRON A therapy at a dose of 5 million IU QD or 10 million IU TIW, relapsed during the follow-up period which ranged from 2 to 6 months after treatment ended. The loss of serum HBeAg and HBV DNA was maintained in 100% of 19 responding patients followed for 3.5 to 36 months after the end of therapy.

In a proportion of responding patients, loss of HBeAg was followed by the loss of HBsAg. HBsAg was lost in 27% (4/15) of patients who responded to INTRON A therapy at a dose of 5 million IU QD, and 35% (8/23) of patients who responded to 10 million IU TIW. No untreated control patient lost HBsAg in these studies.

In an ongoing study to assess the long-term durability of virologic response, 64 patients responding to INTRON A therapy have been followed for 1.1 to 6.6 years after treatment; 95% (61/64) remain serum HBeAg negative and 49% (30/61) have lost serum HBsAg.

INTRON A therapy resulted in normalization of serum ALT in a significantly greater proportion of treated patients compared to untreated patients in each of two controlled studies (see TABLE 4). In a third study without a concurrent control group, normalization of serum ALT was observed in 50% (12/24) of patients receiving INTRON A therapy.

Virologic response was associated with a reduction in serum ALT to normal or near normal (≤1.5 × the upper limit of normal) in 87% (13/15) of patients responding to INTRON A therapy at 5 million IU QD, and 100% (23/23) of patients responding to 10 million IU TIW.

Improvement in liver histology was evaluated in Studies 1 and 3 by comparison of pretreatment and 6-month post-treatment liver biopsies using the semiquantitative Knodell Histology Activity Index.[9] No statistically significant difference in liver histology was observed in treated patients compared to control patients in Study 1. Although statistically significant histological improvement from baseline was observed in treated patients in Study 3 (p≤0.01), there was no control group for comparison. Of those patients exhibiting a virologic response following treatment with 5 million IU QD or 10 million IU TIW, histological improvement was observed in 85% (17/20) compared to 36% (9/25) of patients who were not virologic responders. The histological improvement was due primarily to decreases in severity of necrosis, degeneration, and inflammation in the periportal, lobular, and portal regions of the liver (Knodell Categories I + II + III). Continued histological improvement was observed in four responding patients who lost serum HBsAg and were followed 2 to 4 years after the end of INTRON A therapy.[10]

TABLE 1

*RESPONSE BY BASELINE CD4 COUNT**
IN AIDS-RELATED KS PATIENTS
30 million IU/m^2
TIW, SC and 35 million IU QD, SC

	Asymptomatic		*Symptomatic*	
CD4<200	4/14	(29%)	0/19	(0%)
200≤CD4≤400	6/12	(50%) } 58%	0/5	(0%)
CD4>400	5/7	(71%)	0/0	(0%)

*Data for CD4, and asymptomatic and symptomatic classification were not available for all patients.

[See table 2 below]
[See table 3 at bottom of next page]
[See table 4 at bottom of next page]

INDICATIONS AND USAGE

Hairy Cell Leukemia INTRON A Interferon alfa-2b, recombinant for Injection is indicated for the treatment of patients 18 years of age or older with hairy cell leukemia.

Malignant Melanoma INTRON A Interferon alfa-2b, recombinant for Injection is indicated as adjuvant to surgical treatment in patients 18 years of age or older with malignant melanoma who are free of disease but at high risk for systemic recurrence, within 56 days of surgery.

Follicular Lymphoma INTRON A Interferon alfa-2b, recombinant for Injection is indicated for the initial treatment of clinically aggressive (see **Clinical Experience**) follicular Non-Hodgkin's Lymphoma in conjunction with anthracycline-containing combination chemotherapy in patients 18 years of age or older. Efficacy of INTRON A in patients with low-grade, low-tumor burden follicular Non-Hodgkin's Lymphoma has not been demonstrated.

Condylomata Acuminata INTRON A Interferon alfa-2b, recombinant for Injection is indicated for intralesional treatment of selected patients 18 years of age or older with condylomata acuminata involving external surfaces of the genital and perianal areas (see **DOSAGE AND ADMINISTRATION**).

The use of this product in adolescents has not been studied.

AIDS-Related Kaposi's Sarcoma INTRON A Interferon alfa-2b, recombinant for Injection is indicated for the treatment of selected patients 18 years of age or older with AIDS-Related Kaposi's Sarcoma. The likelihood of response to INTRON A therapy is greater in patients who are without systemic symptoms, who have limited lymphadenopathy and who have a relatively intact immune system as indicated by total CD4 count.

Chronic Hepatitis C INTRON A Interferon alfa-2b, recombinant for Injection is indicated for the treatment of chronic hepatitis C in patients 18 years of age or older with compensated liver disease who have a history of blood or blood-product exposure and/or are HCV antibody positive. Studies in these patients demonstrated that INTRON A therapy can produce clinically meaningful effects on this disease, manifested by normalization of serum alanine aminotransferase (ALT) and reduction in liver necrosis and degeneration.

A liver biopsy should be performed to establish the diagnosis of chronic hepatitis. Patients should be tested for the presence of antibody to HCV. Patients with other causes of chronic hepatitis, including autoimmune hepatitis, should be excluded. Prior to initiation of INTRON A therapy, the physician should establish that the patient has compensated liver disease. The following patient entrance criteria

TABLE 2

SUSTAINED ALT RESPONSE RATE VS DURATION OF THERAPY
IN CHRONIC HEPATITIS C PATIENTS
INTRON A 3 Million IU TIW
*Treatment Group *— Number of Patients (%)*

Study Number	*INTRON A 3 million IU 24 weeks of treatment*		*INTRON A 3 million IU 72 or 96 weeks of treatment†*		*Difference (Extended - 24 weeks) (95% CI)‡*	
	ALT response at the end of follow-up					
1	12/101	(12%)	23/104	(22%)	10%	(-3, 24)
2	9/67	(13%)	21/80	(26%)	13%	(-4, 30)
Combined Studies	**21/168**	**(12.5%)**	**44/184**	**(24%)**	**11.4%**	**(2, 21)**
	ALT response at the end of treatment					
1	40/101	(40%)	51/104	(49%)	—	
2	32/67	(48%)	35/80	(44%)	—	

* Intent to treat groups.
† Study 1: 72 weeks of treatment; Study 2: 96 weeks of treatment.
‡ Confidence intervals adjusted for multiple comparisons due to 3 treatment arms in the study.

for compensated liver disease were used in the clinical studies and should be considered before INTRON A treatment of patients with chronic hepatitis C:

- No history of hepatic encephalopathy, variceal bleeding, ascites, or other clinical signs of decompensation
- Bilirubin ≤2 mg/dL
- Albumin Stable and within normal limits
- Prothrombin Time <3 seconds prolonged
- WBC ≥3000/mm^3
- Platelets ≥70,000/mm^3

Serum creatinine should be normal or near normal.

Prior to initiation of INTRON A therapy, CBC and platelet counts should be evaluated in order to establish baselines for monitoring potential toxicity. These tests should be repeated at weeks 1 and 2 following initiation of INTRON A therapy, and monthly thereafter. Serum ALT should be evaluated at approximately 3-month intervals to assess response to treatment (see **DOSAGE AND ADMINISTRATION**).

Patients with preexisting thyroid abnormalities may be treated if thyroid-stimulating hormone (TSH) levels can be maintained in the normal range by medication. TSH levels must be within normal limits upon initiation of INTRON A treatment and TSH testing should be repeated at 3 and 6 months (see **PRECAUTIONS—Laboratory Tests**).

Chronic Hepatitis B INTRON A Interferon alfa-2b, recombinant for Injection is indicated for the treatment of chronic hepatitis B in patients 18 years of age or older with compensated liver disease and HBV replication. Patients must be serum HBsAg positive for at least 6 months and have HBV replication (serum HBeAg positive) with elevated serum ALT. Studies in these patients demonstrated that INTRON A therapy can produce virologic remission of this disease (loss of serum HBeAg), and normalization of serum aminotransferases. INTRON A therapy resulted in the loss of serum HBsAg in some responding patients.

Prior to initiation of INTRON A therapy, it is recommended that a liver biopsy be performed to establish the presence of chronic hepatitis and the extent of liver damage. The physician should establish that the patient has compensated liver disease. The following patient entrance criteria for compensated liver disease were used in the clinical studies and should be considered before INTRON A treatment of patients with chronic hepatitis B:

- No history of hepatic encephalopathy, variceal bleeding, ascites, or other signs of clinical decompensation
- Bilirubin Normal
- Albumin Stable and within normal limits
- Prothrombin Time <3 seconds prolonged
- WBC ≥4000/mm^3
- Platelets >100,000/mm^3

Patients with causes of chronic hepatitis other than chronic hepatitis B or chronic hepatitis C should not be treated with INTRON A Interferon alfa-2b, recombinant for Injection. CBC and platelet counts should be evaluated prior to initiation of INTRON A therapy in order to establish baselines for monitoring potential toxicity. These tests should be repeated at treatment weeks 1, 2, 4, 8, 12, and 16. Liver function tests, including serum ALT, albumin, and bilirubin, should be evaluated at treatment weeks 1, 2, 4, 8, 12, and 16. HBeAg, HBsAg, and ALT should be evaluated at the end of therapy, as well as 3- and 6-months posttherapy, since patients may become virologic responders during the 6-month period following the end of treatment. In clinical studies, 39% (15/38) of responding patients lost HBeAg 1 to 6 months following the end of INTRON A therapy. Of responding patients who lost HBsAg, 58% (7/12) did so 1- to 6-months posttreatment.

A transient increase in ALT ≥2 × baseline value (flare) can occur during INTRON A therapy for chronic hepatitis B. In clinical trials, this flare generally occurred 8 to 12 weeks after initiation of therapy and was more frequent in responders (63%, 24/38) than in nonresponders (27%, 13/48). However, elevations in bilirubin ≥3 mg/dL occurred infrequently (2%, 2/86) during therapy. When ALT flare occurs, in general, INTRON A therapy should be continued unless signs and symptoms of liver failure are observed. During ALT flare, clinical symptomatology and liver function tests including ALT, prothrombin time, alkaline phosphatase, albumin, and bilirubin, should be monitored at approximately 2-week intervals (see **WARNINGS**).

TABLE 3
*VIROLOGIC RESPONSE**
*IN **CHRONIC HEPATITIS B** PATIENTS*

Study Number	*Treatment Group†— Number of Patients (%)* INTRON A 5 million IU QD		*INTRON A 10 million IU TIW*		*Untreated Controls*		*P‡ Value*
1[7]	15/38	(39%)	—	—	3/42	(7%)	0.0009
2	—	—	10/24	(42%)	1/22	(5%)	0.005
3[8]	—	—	13/24§	(54%)	2/27	(7%)§	NA§
All Studies	**15/38**	**(39%)**	**23/48**	**(48%)**	**6/91**	**(7%)**	**—**

* Loss of HBeAg and HBV DNA by 6 months posttherapy.
† Patients pretreated with prednisone not shown.
‡ INTRON A treatment group vs untreated control.
§ Untreated control patients evaluated after 24-week observation period. A subgroup subsequently received INTRON A therapy. A direct comparison is not applicable (NA).

TABLE 4
*ALT RESPONSES**
*IN **CHRONIC HEPATITIS B** PATIENTS*

Study Number	*Treatment Group — Number of Patients (%)* INTRON A 5 million IU QD		*INTRON A 10 million IU TIW*		*Untreated Controls*		*P† Value*
1	16/38	(42%)	—	—	8/42	(19%)	0.03
2	—	—	10/24	(42%)	1/22	(5%)	0.0034
3	—	—	12/24‡	(50%)	2/27	(7%)‡	NA‡
All Studies	**16/38**	**(42%)**	**22/48**	**(46%)**	**11/91**	**(12%)**	**—**

* Reduction in serum ALT to normal by 6 months posttherapy.
† INTRON A treatment group *versus* untreated control.
‡ Untreated control patients evaluated after 24-week observation period. A subgroup subsequently received INTRON A therapy. A direct comparison is not applicable (NA).

DOSAGE AND ADMINISTRATION

IMPORTANT: INTRON A Interferon alfa-2b, recombinant for Injection dosing regimens are different for each of the following indications described in this section of the product information sheet. INTRON A Solution for Injection multidose pen contains a prefilled, multidose cartridge for subcutaneous administration. It is designed to deliver doses as required using a simple dial mechanism. The needles provided in the packaging should be used for the INTRON A Solution for Injection multidose pen only. A new needle is to be used each time a dose is delivered using the pen. Each INTRON A Solution for Injection multidose pen is for individual patient use only.

Hairy Cell Leukemia The recommended dosage of INTRON A Interferon alfa-2b, recombinant for Injection for the treatment of hairy cell leukemia is 2 million IU/m^2 administered intramuscularly (see **WARNINGS**) or subcutaneously 3 times a week for up to 6 months. The 50 million IU strength of the INTRON A Powder for Injection is not to be used for the treatment of hairy cell leukemia. Higher doses are not recommended. Responding patients may benefit from continued treatment.

If severe adverse reactions develop, the dosage should be modified (50% reduction) or therapy should be temporarily discontinued until the adverse reactions abate. If persistent or recurrent intolerance develops following adequate dosage adjustment, or disease progresses, INTRON A treatment should be discontinued. The minimum effective INTRON A dose has not been established.

Malignant Melanoma The recommended INTRON A treatment regimen includes induction treatment 5 consecutive days per week for 4 weeks as an intravenous (IV) infusion at a dose of 20 million IU/m^2, followed by maintenance treatment three times per week for 48 weeks as a subcutaneous (SC) injection, at a dose of 10 million IU/m^2.

In the clinical trial, the median daily INTRON A doses administered to patients were 19.1 million IU/m^2 during the induction phase and 9.1 million IU/m^2 during the maintenance phase.

Regular laboratory testing should be performed to monitor laboratory abnormalities for the purposes of dose modification (see **PRECAUTIONS—Laboratory Tests**). If adverse reactions develop during INTRON A treatment, particularly if granulocytes decrease to <500/mm^3 or SGPT/SGOT rises to >5 × upper limit of normal, treatment should be temporarily discontinued until the adverse reactions abate. INTRON A treatment should be restarted at 50% of the previous dose. If intolerance persists after dose adjustments or if granulocytes decrease to <250/mm^3 or SGPT/SGOT rises to >10 × upper limit of normal, INTRON A therapy should be discontinued.

Follicular Lymphoma The recommended dosage of INTRON A Interferon alfa-2b, recombinant for Injection is 5 million IU subcutaneously three times per week for up to 18 months in conjunction with an anthracycline-containing chemotherapy regimen.

In published reports, the doses of myelosuppressive drugs were reduced by 25% from those utilized in a full-dose CHOP regimen, and cycle length increased by 33% (eg, from 21 to 28 days) when an alfa interferon was added to the regimen.[1,4] The dosing regimen should be modified for evidence of serious toxicity. The following dose modification guidelines for hematologic toxicity were used in the clinical trial: the chemotherapy regimen was delayed if either the neutrophil count was <1,500/mm^3 or the platelet count was <75,000/mm^3. Administration of INTRON A was temporarily interrupted for a neutrophil count <1,000/mm^3, or a platelet count <50,000/mm^3, or reduced by 50% to 2.5 MIU TIW for a neutrophil count >1,000/mm^3 but <1,500/mm^3. Reinstitution of the initial INTRON A dose (5 million IU TIW) was tolerated after resolution of hematologic toxicity (≥1,500/mm^3).

INTRON A therapy should be discontinued if SGOT exceeds >5 × the upper limit of normal or serum creatinine >2.0 mg/dL. (See **WARNINGS**.)

Condylomata Acuminata The 10 million IU vial of INTRON A Powder for Injection must be reconstituted with 1 mL of Diluent for INTRON A Interferon alfa-2b, recombinant for Injection (bacteriostatic water for injection). Do not reconstitute the 10 million IU vial of INTRON A Powder for Injection with more than 1 mL of diluent since the injection would be subpotent. Do not use the 3 million, 5 million, 18 million, 25 million, or 50 million IU vials of INTRON A Powder for Injection for the treatment of condylomata acuminata since the resulting reconstituted solution would be either hypertonic or an inappropriate concentration. Do not use the 3 million IU vial or the 18 million IU multidose vial of INTRON A Solution for Injection for the intralesional treatment of condylomata acuminata since the concentrations are inappropriate for such use.

Inject 1.0 million IU of INTRON A Interferon alfa-2b, recombinant for Injection (either 0.1 mL of reconstituted 10 million IU INTRON A Powder for Injection or 0.1 mL of the 5 million IU, 10 million IU, or 25 million IU strengths of INTRON A Solution for Injection, each having a final concentration of 10 million IU/mL) into each lesion three times per week on alternate days, for 3 weeks. The injection should be administered intralesionally using a Tuberculin or similar syringe and a 25- to 30-gauge needle. The needle should be directed at the center of the base of the wart and at an angle almost parallel to the plane of the skin (approximating that in the commonly used PPD test). This will deliver the interferon to the dermal core of the lesion, infiltrating the lesion and causing a small wheal. Care should be taken not to go beneath the lesion too deeply; subcutaneous injection should be avoided, since this area is below the base of the lesion. Do not inject too superficially since this will result in possible leakage, infiltrating only the keratinized layer, and not the dermal core. As many as 5 lesions can be treated at one time. To reduce side effects, INTRON A injections may be administered in the evening, when possible. Additionally, acetaminophen may be administered at the time of injection to alleviate some of the potential side effects.

The maximum response usually occurs 4 to 8 weeks after initiation of the first treatment course. If results at 12 to 16 weeks after the initial treatment course has concluded are not satisfactory, a second course of treatment using the above dosage schedule may be instituted providing that clinical symptoms and signs, or changes in laboratory parameters (liver function tests, WBC, and platelets) do not preclude such a course of action.

Patients with six to ten condylomata may receive a second (sequential) course of treatment at the above dosage schedule, to treat up to five additional condylomata per course of treatment. Patients with greater than ten condylomata may receive additional sequences depending on how large a number of condylomata are present.

AIDS-Related Kaposi's Sarcoma The recommended INTRON A dosage is 30 million IU/m^2 three times a week

Continued on next page

Information on Schering products appearing on these pages is effective as of August 15, 1998.

Intron A—Cont.

administered subcutaneously or intramuscularly. The 18 million and 25 million IU multidose strengths of the INTRON A Solution for Injection should not be used for the treatment of AIDS-Related Kaposi's Sarcoma since the concentrations are inappropriate.

The selected dosage regimen should be maintained unless the disease progresses rapidly or severe intolerance is manifested. If severe adverse reactions develop, the dosage should be modified (50% reduction) or therapy should be temporarily discontinued until the adverse reactions abate. When patients initiate therapy at 30 million IU/m² TIW, the average dose tolerated at the end of 12 weeks of therapy is 110 million IU/week and 75 million IU/week at the end of 24 weeks of therapy.

When disease stabilization or a response to treatment occurs, treatment should continue until there is no further evidence of tumor or until discontinuation is required by evidence of a severe opportunistic infection or adverse effect.

Chronic Hepatitis C The recommended dosage of INTRON A Interferon alfa-2b, recombinant for Injection for the treatment of chronic hepatitis C is 3 million IU three times a week (TIW) administered subcutaneously or intramuscularly. In patients tolerating therapy with normalization of ALT at 16 weeks of treatment, INTRON A therapy should be extended to 18 to 24 months (72 to 96 weeks) at 3 million IU TIW to improve the sustained response rate (see **CLINICAL PHARMACOLOGY—Chronic Hepatitis C**). Patients who do not normalize their ALTs after 16 weeks of therapy rarely achieve a sustained response with extension of treatment. Consideration should be given to discontinuing these patients from therapy.

If severe adverse reactions develop during INTRON A treatment, the dose should be modified (50% reduction) or therapy should be temporarily discontinued until the adverse reactions abate. If intolerance persists after dose adjustment, INTRON A therapy should be discontinued.

Chronic Hepatitis B The recommended dosage of INTRON A Interferon alfa-2b, recombinant for Injection for the treatment of chronic hepatitis B is 30 to 35 million IU per week, administered subcutaneously or intramuscularly, either as 5 million IU daily (QD) or as 10 million IU three times a week (TIW) for 16 weeks.

If severe adverse reactions or laboratory abnormalities develop during INTRON A therapy the dose should be modified (50% reduction), or discontinued if appropriate, until the adverse reactions abate. If intolerance persists after dose adjustment, INTRON A therapy should be discontinued.

For patients with decreases in granulocyte or platelet counts, the following guidelines for dose modification were used in the clinical trials:

INTRON A Dose	Granulocyte Count	Platelet Count
Reduce 50%	<750/mm³	<50,000/mm³
Interrupt	<500/mm³	<30,000/mm³

INTRON A therapy was resumed at up to 100% of the initial dose when granulocyte and/or platelet counts returned to normal or baseline values.

At the discretion of the physician, the patient may self-administer the medication. (See illustrated **PATIENT INFORMATION SHEET** for instructions.)

Preparation and Administration of INTRON A Interferon alfa-2b, recombinant Powder to Injection for Intramuscular, Subcutaneous, or Intralesional Administration

Reconstitution of INTRON A Powder for Injection Inject the amount of Diluent for INTRON A Interferon alfa-2b, recombinant for Injection (bacteriostatic water for injection) stated in the chart below (diluent is supplied in either a vial or syringe, see **HOW SUPPLIED** below), into the INTRON A vial. Swirl gently to hasten complete dissolution of the powder. The appropriate INTRON A dose should then be withdrawn and injected subcutaneously, subcutaneously, or intralesionally. (See **PATIENT INFORMATION SHEET** for detailed instructions.) After preparation and administration of the INTRON A injection, it is essential to follow the procedure for proper disposal of syringes and needles. (See **PATIENT INFORMATION SHEET** for detailed instructions.)

Preparation and Administration of INTRON A Interferon alfa-2b, recombinant Powder for Injection for Intravenous Infusion

The infusion solution should be prepared immediately prior to use. Based on the desired dose, the appropriate vial strength(s) of INTRON A Interferon alfa-2b, recombinant Powder for Injection should be reconstituted with the diluent provided. The appropriate INTRON A dose should then be withdrawn and injected into a 100-mL bag of 0.9% Sodium Chloride Injection, USP. The final concentration of INTRON A Interferon alfa-2b, recombinant for Injection should be not less than 10 million IU/100 mL. The prepared solution should be infused over a 20-minute period.

[See first table above]

Stability INTRON A Interferon alfa-2b, recombinant Powder for Injection provided in vials ranging from 3 to 50 million IU per vial, is stable at 45°C (113°F) for up to 7 days. After reconstitution with Diluent for INTRON A Interferon alfa-2b, recombinant for Injection (bacteriostatic water for injection) the solution is stable for 1 month at 2° to 8°C (36° to 46°F). The reconstituted solution is clear and colorless to light yellow.

Preparation and Administration of INTRON A Interferon alfa-2b, recombinant Solution for Injection

The 3 million IU, 5 million IU, and 10 million IU vials, and the 18 million and 25 million IU multidose vials of INTRON A Solution for Injection do not require reconstitution prior to administration. The solution is clear and colorless. The appropriate INTRON A dose should be withdrawn from the vial and injected intramuscularly, subcutaneously, or intralesionally (5 million IU and 10 million IU vials, and 25 million IU multidose vials only). After administration of INTRON A Solution for Injection, it is essential to follow the procedure for proper disposal of syringes and needles. (See **PATIENT INFORMATION SHEET** for detailed instructions.)

[See second table above]

[See third table above]

IMPORTANT: The 3 million IU vial and the 18 million IU multidose vial of INTRON A Solution for Injection are **not** to be used for chronic hepatitis B or condylomata acuminata. **The multidose pen should not be used for condylomata acuminata.** The 10 million IU vial of INTRON A Solution for Injection should not be used for chronic hepatitis C.

INTRON A Interferon alfa-2b, recombinant Powder for Injection

	3 million IU	5 million IU	10 million IU	18 million IU	25 million IU	50 million IU‡
Chronic Hepatitis B		1 mL	1 mL			
Chronic Hepatitis C	1 mL					
Hairy Cell Leukemia	1 mL	1 mL	2 mL		5 mL	
AIDS-Related Kaposi's Sarcoma						1 mL
Condylomata Acuminata			1 mL**			
Malignant Melanoma induction phase† maintenance phase	1 mL* 1 mL*	1 mL 1 mL	1 mL 1 mL	1 mL 1 mL	5 mL	1 mL 1 mL
Follicular Lymphoma	1 mL	1 mL	1 mL		5 mL	

* Use only for dose reduction.
** IMPORTANT: For patients with condylomata acuminata, reconstitute the 10 million IU vial with only 1 mL of the diluent provided to reach a final concentration of 10 million IU/mL to be administered intralesionally.
† Based on the desired dose, the appropriate vial strengths should be reconstituted and administered intravenously.
‡ This vial strength should be used only for the treatment of patients with AIDS-Related Kaposi's Sarcoma or malignant melanoma since the concentration is inappropriate for all other indications.

INTRON A Interferon alfa-2b, recombinant Solution for Injection

	3 million IU	5 million IU	10 million IU	18 million IU multidose*	25 million IU multidose†
Chronic Hepatitis B		✔	✔		✔§
Chronic Hepatitis C	✔			✔	
Hairy Cell Leukemia	✔	✔	✔	✔	✔
Condylomata Acuminata		✔	✔		✔
Malignant Melanoma	✔‡	✔	✔	✔‡	✔¶
Follicular Lymphoma		✔			✔

* This is a multidose vial which contains a total of 22.8 million IU of interferon alfa-2b, recombinant per 3.8 mL in order to provide the delivery of six 0.5-mL doses, each containing 3 million IU of INTRON A Interferon alfa-2b, recombinant for Injection (for a label strength of 18 million IU).
† This is a multidose vial which contains a total of 32 million IU of interferon alfa-2b, recombinant per 3.2 mL in order to provide the delivery of five 0.5-mL doses, each containing 5 million IU of INTRON A Interferon alfa-2b, recombinant for Injection (for a label strength of 25 million IU).
‡ Use only for dose reduction.
§ Use only for the 5 MIU daily regimen.
¶ Use only for maintenance treatment.

INTRON A Interferon alfa-2b, recombinant Solution in Multidose Pens

	3 million IU/0.2 mL*	5 million IU/0.2 mL**	10 million IU/0.2 mL***
Chronic Hepatitis B		✔	✔
Chronic Hepatitis C	✔		
Hairy Cell Leukemia	✔	✔	
Malignant Melanoma			✔
Follicular Lymphoma		✔	

* The 3 million IU multidose pen contains a total of 22.5 million IU of interferon alfa-2b, recombinant per 1.5 mL in order to provide delivery of six 0.2-mL doses each containing 3 million IU of interferon alfa-2b, recombinant Solution for Injection (for a label strength of 18 million IU).
** The 5 million IU multidose pen contains a total of 37.5 million IU of interferon alfa-2b, recombinant per 1.5 mL in order to provide delivery of six 0.2-mL doses each containing 5 million IU of interferon alfa-2b, recombinant Solution for Injection (for a label strength of 30 million IU).
***The 10 million IU multidose pen contains a total of 75 million IU of interferon alfa-2b, recombinant per 1.5 mL in order to provide delivery of six 0.2-mL doses each containing 10 million IU of interferon alfa-2b, recombinant Solution for Injection (for a label strength of 60 million IU).

INTRON A Solution for Injection should not be used for AIDS-Related Kaposi's Sarcoma since the concentrations are inappropriate. INTRON A Solution for Injection is not recommended for intravenous administration and should not be used for the induction phase of malignant melanoma. (See **DOSAGE AND ADMINISTRATION—Condylomata Acuminata; DOSAGE AND ADMINISTRATION—AIDS-Related Kaposi's Sarcoma.**)

Parenteral drug products should be inspected visually for particulate matter and discoloration prior to administration, whenever solution and container permit. INTRON A Interferon alfa-2b, recombinant for Injection may be administered using either sterilized glass or plastic disposable syringes.

Stability INTRON A Interferon alfa-2b, recombinant Solution for Injection multidose pens provided in strengths ranging from 18 to 60 million IU per pen is stable at 30°C (86°F) for up to 2 days. INTRON A Interferon alfa-2b, recombinant Solution for Injection provided in vials ranging from 3 to 25 million IU per vial, is stable at 35°C (95°F) for up to 7 days and at 30°C (86°F) for up to 14 days. The solution is clear and colorless.

INTRON A SOLUTION FOR INJECTION IS NOT RECOMMENDED FOR INTRAVENOUS ADMINISTRATION.

CONTRAINDICATIONS

INTRON A Interferon alfa-2b, recombinant for Injection is contraindicated in patients with a history of hypersensitivity to interferon alfa or any component of the injection.

WARNINGS

General Moderate to severe adverse experiences may require modification of the patient's dosage regimen, or in some cases termination of INTRON A therapy. Because of the fever and other "flu-like" symptoms associated with INTRON A administration, it should be used cautiously in patients with debilitating medical conditions, such as those with a history of pulmonary disease (eg, chronic obstructive pulmonary disease), or diabetes mellitus prone to ketoacidosis. Caution should also be observed in patients with coagulation disorders (eg, thrombophlebitis, pulmonary embolism) or severe myelosuppression.

Patients with platelet counts of less than 50,000/mm^3 should not be administered INTRON A Interferon alfa-2b, recombinant for Injection intramuscularly, but instead by subcutaneous administration.

INTRON A therapy should be used cautiously in patients with a history of cardiovascular disease. Those patients with a history of myocardial infarction and/or previous or current arrhythmic disorder who require INTRON A therapy should be closely monitored (see **Laboratory Tests**). Cardiovascular adverse experiences, which include hypotension, arrhythmia, or tachycardia of 150 beats per minute or greater, and rarely, cardiomyopathy and myocardial infarction have been observed in some INTRON A treated patients. Some patients with these adverse events had no history of cardiovascular disease. Transient cardiomyopathy was reported in approximately 2% of the AIDS-Related Kaposi's Sarcoma patients treated with INTRON A Interferon alfa-2b, recombinant for Injection. Hypotension may occur during INTRON A administration, or up to 2 days post-therapy, and may require supportive therapy including fluid replacement to maintain intravascular volume.

Supraventricular arrhythmias occurred rarely and appeared to be correlated with preexisting conditions and prior therapy with cardiotoxic agents. These adverse experiences were controlled by modifying the dose or discontinuing treatment, but may require specific additional therapy. DEPRESSION AND SUICIDAL BEHAVIOR INCLUDING SUICIDAL IDEATION, SUICIDAL ATTEMPTS, AND COMPLETED SUICIDES HAVE BEEN REPORTED IN ASSOCIATION WITH TREATMENT WITH ALFA INTERFERONS, INCLUDING INTRON A THERAPY. Patients with a preexisting psychiatric condition, especially depression, or a history of severe psychiatric disorder should not be treated with INTRON A Interferon alfa-2b, recombinant for Injection.[11] INTRON A therapy should be discontinued for any patient developing severe depression or other psychiatric disorder during treatment. Obtundation and coma have also been observed in some patients, usually elderly, treated at higher doses. While these effects are usually rapidly reversible upon discontinuation of therapy, full resolution of symptoms has taken up to 3 weeks in a few severe episodes. Narcotics, hypnotics, or sedatives may be used concurrently with caution and patients should be closely monitored until the adverse effects have resolved.

Infrequently, patients receiving INTRON A therapy developed thyroid abnormalities, either hypothyroid or hyperthyroid. The mechanism by which INTRON A Interferon alfa-2b, recombinant for Injection may alter thyroid status is unknown. Patients with preexisting thyroid abnormalities whose thyroid function cannot be maintained in the normal range by medication should not be treated with INTRON A Interferon alfa-2b, recombinant for Injection. Prior to initiation of INTRON A therapy, serum TSH should be evaluated. Patients developing symptoms consistent with possible thyroid dysfunction during the course of INTRON A therapy should have their thyroid function evaluated and appropriate treatment instituted. Therapy should be discontinued for patients developing thyroid abnormalities during treatment whose thyroid function cannot be normalized by medication. Discontinuation of INTRON A therapy has not always reversed thyroid dysfunction occurring during treatment.

Hepatotoxicity, including fatality, has been observed in interferon alfa treated patients, including those treated with INTRON A Interferon alfa-2b, recombinant for Injection. Any patient developing liver function abnormalities during treatment should be monitored closely and if appropriate, treatment should be discontinued.

Pulmonary infiltrates, pneumonitis and pneumonia, including fatality, have been observed in interferon alfa treated patients, including those treated with INTRON A Interferon alfa-2b, recombinant for Injection. The etiologic explanation for these pulmonary findings has yet to be established. Any patient developing fever, cough, dyspnea, or other respiratory symptoms should have a chest X-ray taken. If the chest X-ray shows pulmonary infiltrates or there is evidence of pulmonary function impairment, the patient should be closely monitored, and, if appropriate, interferon alfa treatment should be discontinued. While this has been reported more often in patients with chronic hepatitis C treated with interferon alfa, it has also been reported in patients with oncologic diseases treated with interferon alfa.

Retinal hemorrhages, cotton-wool spots, and retinal artery or vein obstruction have been observed rarely in patients treated with interferon alfa, including those treated with INTRON A Interferon alfa-2b, recombinant for Injection. The etiologic explanation for these findings has not yet been established. These events appear to occur after use of the drug for several months, but also have been reported after shorter treatment periods. Diabetes mellitus or hypertension have been present in some patients. Any patient complaining of changes in visual acuity or visual fields, or reporting other ophthalmologic symptoms during treatment with INTRON A Interferon alfa-2b, recombinant for Injection, should have an eye examination. Because the retinal events may have to be differentiated from those seen with diabetic or hypertensive retinopathy, a baseline ocular examination is recommended prior to treatment with interferon in patients with diabetes mellitus or hypertension.

Rare cases of autoimmune diseases including thrombocytopenia, vasculitis, Raynaud's phenomenon, rheumatoid arthritis, lupus erythematosus, and rhabdomyolysis have been observed in patients treated with alfa interferons, including patients treated with INTRON A Interferon alfa-2b, recombinant for Injection. In very rare cases the event resulted in fatality. The mechanism by which these events develop and their relationship to interferon alfa therapy is not clear. Any patient developing an autoimmune disorder during treatment should be closely monitored and, if appropriate, treatment should be discontinued.

Diabetes mellitus and hyperglycemia have been observed rarely in patients treated with INTRON A Interferon alfa-2b, recombinant for Injection. Symptomatic patients should have their blood glucose measured and followed up accordingly. Patients with diabetes mellitus may require adjustment of their antidiabetic regimen.

The 50 million IU strength of the INTRON A Powder for Injection is not to be used for the treatment of hairy cell leukemia, condylomata acuminata, follicular lymphoma, chronic hepatitis C, or chronic hepatitis B. The 3 million, 5 million, 18 million, and 25 million IU strengths of the INTRON A Powder for Injection are not to be used for the intralesional treatment of condylomata acuminata since the dilution required for the intralesional use would result in a hypertonic solution.

The INTRON A multidose pens, the 3 million IU vial, and the 18 million IU multidose vial of INTRON A Solution for Injection are not to be used for the treatment of condylomata acuminata. The INTRON A multidose pens and the 18 million and 25 million IU multidose vials of INTRON A Solution for Injection are not to be used for the treatment of AIDS-Related Kaposi's Sarcoma. INTRON A Solution for Injection is not recommended for the intravenous treatment of malignant melanoma.

AIDS-Related Kaposi's Sarcoma INTRON A therapy should not be used for patients with rapidly progressive visceral disease (see **CLINICAL PHARMACOLOGY**). Also of note, there may be synergistic adverse effects between INTRON A Interferon alfa-2b, recombinant for Injection and zidovudine. Patients receiving concomitant zidovudine have had a higher incidence of neutropenia than that expected with zidovudine alone. Careful monitoring of the WBC count is indicated in all patients who are myelosuppressed and in all patients receiving other myelosuppressive medications. The effects of INTRON A Interferon alfa-2b, recombinant for Injection when combined with other drugs used in the treatment of AIDS-Related disease are unknown.

Chronic Hepatitis C and Chronic Hepatitis B Patients with decompensated liver disease, autoimmune hepatitis or a history of autoimmune disease, and patients who are immunosuppressed transplant recipients should not be treated with INTRON A Interferon alfa-2b, recombinant for Injection. There are reports of worsening liver disease, including jaundice, hepatic encephalopathy, hepatic failure, and death following INTRON A therapy in such patients. Therapy should be discontinued for any patient developing signs and symptoms of liver failure.

Chronic hepatitis B patients with evidence of decreasing hepatic synthetic functions, such as decreasing albumin levels or prolongation of prothrombin time, who nevertheless meet the entry criteria to start therapy, may be at increased risk of clinical decompensation if a flare of aminotransferases occurs during INTRON A treatment. In such patients, if increases in ALT occur during INTRON A therapy for chronic hepatitis B, they should be followed carefully including close monitoring of clinical symptomatology and liver function tests, including ALT, prothrombin time, alkaline phosphatase, albumin, and bilirubin. In considering these patients for INTRON A therapy, the potential risks must be evaluated against the potential benefits of treatment.

PRECAUTIONS

General Acute serious hypersensitivity reactions (eg, urticaria, angioedema, bronchoconstriction, anaphylaxis) have been observed rarely in INTRON A treated patients; if such an acute reaction develops, the drug should be discontinued immediately and appropriate medical therapy instituted. Transient rashes have occurred in some patients following injection, but have not necessitated treatment interruption. While fever may be related to the flu-like syndrome reported commonly in patients treated with interferon, other causes of persistent fever should be ruled out.

There have been reports of interferon, including INTRON A Interferon alfa-2b, recombinant for Injection, exacerbating preexisting psoriasis; therefore, INTRON A therapy should be used in these patients only if the potential benefit justifies the potential risk.

Variations in dosage, routes of administration, and adverse reactions exist among different brands of interferon. Therefore, do not use different brands of interferon in any single treatment regimen.

Drug Interactions Interactions between INTRON A Interferon alfa-2b, recombinant for Injection and other drugs have not been fully evaluated. Caution should be exercised when administering INTRON A therapy in combination with other potentially myelosuppressive agents such as zidovudine. Concomitant use of alfa interferon and theophylline decreases theophylline clearance resulting in a 100% increase in serum theophylline levels.

Information for Patients Patients receiving INTRON A treatment should be directed in its appropriate use, informed of benefits and risks associated with treatment, and referred to the PATIENT INFORMATION SHEET. This information is intended to aid in the safe and effective use of this medication. It is not a disclosure of all possible adverse or intended effects.

If home use is prescribed, a puncture-resistant container for the disposal of used syringes and needles should be supplied to the patient. Patients should be thoroughly instructed in the importance of proper disposal and cautioned against any reuse of needles and syringes. The full container should be disposed of according to the directions provided by the physician (see PATIENT INFORMATION SHEET).

Patients should be cautioned not to change brands of interferon without medical consultation as a change in dosage may result.

Patients receiving high INTRON A doses should be cautioned against performing tasks that would require complete mental alertness, such as operating machinery or driving a motor vehicle.

The most common adverse experiences occurring with INTRON A therapy are "flu-like" symptoms, such as fever, headache, fatigue, anorexia, nausea, or vomiting (see **ADVERSE REACTIONS**) and appear to decrease in severity as treatment continues. Some of these "flu-like" symptoms may be minimized by bedtime administration. Antipyretics may be used to prevent or partially alleviate the fever and headache. Another common adverse experience is thinning of the hair.

It is advised that patients be well hydrated, especially during the initial stages of treatment.

Laboratory Tests In addition to those tests normally required for monitoring patients, the following laboratory tests are recommended for all patients on INTRON A therapy, prior to beginning treatment and then periodically thereafter.

- Standard hematologic tests—including hemoglobin, complete and differential white blood cell counts, and platelet count.

- Blood chemistries—electrolytes, liver function tests, and TSH.

Continued on next page

Information on Schering products appearing on these pages is effective as of August 15, 1998.

Consult 1999 PDR® supplements and future editions for revisions

TREATMENT-RELATED ADVERSE EXPERIENCES BY INDICATION
Dosing Regimens
Percentage (%) of Patients*

ADVERSE EXPERIENCE	MALIGNANT MELANOMA 20 MIU/m² Induction (IV) 10 MIU/m² Maintenance (SC)	FOLLICULAR LYMPHOMA 5 MIU TIW/SC	HAIRY CELL LEUKEMIA 2 MIU/m² TIW/SC	CONDYLOMATA ACUMINATA 1 MIU/lesion	AIDS-RELATED KAPOSI'S SARCOMA 30 MIU/m² TIW/SC	AIDS-RELATED KAPOSI'S SARCOMA 35 MIU/QD/SC	CHRONIC HEPATITIS C‖ 3 MIU TIW	CHRONIC HEPATITIS B 5 MIU QD	CHRONIC HEPATITIS B 10 MIU TIW
	N=143	N=135	N=145	N=352	N=74	N=29	N=183	N=101	N=78

Application-Site Disorders

injection site inflammation	—	1	20	—	—	—	5	3	—
other (<5%)	burning, injection site bleeding, injection site pain, injection site reaction, itching								

Blood Disorders (<5%) anemia, granulocytopenia, hemolytic anemia, leukopenia, lymphocytosis, neutropenia (9% in chronic hepatitis C), thrombocytopenia (10% in chronic hepatitis C) (bleeding 8% in malignant melanoma), thrombocytopenic purpura

Body as a Whole

facial edema	—	1	—	<1	—	10	<1	3	1
weight decrease	3	13	<1	<1	5	3	10	2	5
other (≤5%)	allergic reaction, cachexia, dehydration, earache, hernia, edema, hypercalcemia, hyperglycemia, hypothermia, inflammation nonspecific, lymphadenitis, lymphadenopathy, mastitis, periorbital edema, poor peripheral circulation, peripheral edema (6% in follicular lymphoma), phlebitis superficial, scrotal/penile edema, thirst, weakness, weight increase								

Cardiovascular System Disorders (<5%) angina, arrhythmia, atrial fibrillation, bradycardia, cardiac failure, cardiomegaly, cardiomyopathy, coronary artery disorder, extrasystoles, heart valve disorder, hematoma, hypertension (9% in chronic hepatitis C), hypotension, palpitations, phlebitis, postural hypotension, pulmonary embolism, Raynaud's disease, tachycardia, thrombosis, varicose vein

Endocrine System Disorders (<5%) aggravation of diabetes mellitus, goiter, gynecomastia, hyperglycemia, hyperthyroidism, hypertriglyceridemia, hypothyroidism, virilism

Flu-like Symptoms

fever	81	56	68	56	47	55	34	66	86
headache	62	21	39	47	36	21	43	61	44
chills	54	—	46	45	—	—	—	—	—
myalgia	75	16	39	44	34	28	43	59	40
fatigue	96	8	61	18	84	48	23	75	69
increased sweating	6	13	8	2	4	21	4	1	1
asthenia	—	63	7	—	11	—	40	5	15
rigors	2	7	—	—	30	14	16	38	42
arthralgia	6	8	8	9	—	3	16	19	8
dizziness	23	—	12	9	7	24	9	13	10
influenza-like symptoms	10	—	37	—	45	79	26	5	—
back pain	—	15	19	6	1	3	—	—	—
dry mouth	1	2	19	—	22	28	5	6	5
chest pain	2	8	<1	<1	1	28	4	4	—
malaise	6	—	—	14	5	—	13	9	6
pain (unspecified)	15	9	18	3	3	3	—	—	—
other (<5%)	chest pain substernal, rhinitis, rhinorrhea								

Gastrointestinal System Disorders

diarrhea	35	19	18	2	18	45	13	19	8
anorexia	69	21	19	1	38	41	14	43	53
nausea	66	24	21	17	28	21	19	50	33
taste alteration	24	2	13	<1	5	7	2	10	—
abdominal pain	2	20	<5	1	5	21	16	5	4
loose stools	—	1	—	<1	—	10	2	2	—
vomiting	†	32	6	2	11	14	8	7	10
constipation	1	14	<1	—	1	10	4	5	—
gingivitis	2‡	7‡	—	—	—	14	—	1	—
dyspepsia	—	2	—	2	4	—	7	3	8
other (<5%)	abdominal ascites, abdominal distension, colitis, dysphagia, eructation, esophagitis, flatulence, gallstones, gastric ulcer, gastritis, gastroenteritis, gastrointestinal disorder (7% in follicular lymphoma), gastrointestinal hemorrhage, gastrointestinal mucosal discoloration, gingival bleeding, gum hyperplasia, halitosis, hemorrhoids, increased appetite, increased saliva, intestinal disorder, melena, mouth ulceration, mucositis, oral hemorrhage, oral leukoplakia, rectal bleeding after stool, rectal hemorrhage, stomatitis, stomatitis ulcerative, taste loss, tongue disorder, tooth disorder								

Liver and Biliary System Disorders (<5%) abnormal hepatic function tests, biliary pain, bilirubinemia, hepatitis, increased lactate dehydrogenase, increased transaminases (SGOT/SGPT) (elevated SGOT 63% in malignant melanoma and 24% in follicular lymphoma), jaundice, right upper quadrant pain (15% in chronic hepatitis C), and very rarely, hepatic encephalopathy, hepatic failure, and death

Musculoskeletal System Disorders

musculoskeletal pain	—	18	—	—	—	—	21	9	1
other (<5%)	arteritis, arthritis, arthritis aggravated, arthrosis, bone disorder, bone pain, carpal tunnel syndrome, hyporeflexia, leg cramps, muscle atrophy, muscle weakness, polyarteritis nodosa, tendinitis, rheumatoid arthritis, spondylitis								

Nervous System and Psychiatric Disorders

depression	40	9	6	3	9	28	19	17	6
paresthesia	13	13	6	1	3	21	5	6	3
impaired concentration	—	1	—	<1	3	14	3	8	5
amnesia	§	1	<5	—	—	14	—	—	—
confusion	8	2	<5	4	12	10	1	—	—
hypoesthesia	—	1	<5	1	—	10	—	—	—
irritability	1	1	—	—	—	—	13	16	12
somnolence	1	2	<5	3	3	—	33¶	14	9
anxiety	1	9	5	<1	1	3	5	2	—
insomnia	5	4	—	<1	3	3	12	11	6
nervousness	1	1	—	1	—	3	2	3	—
decreased libido	1	—	<5	—	—	—	1	5	1
other (<5%)	abnormal coordination, abnormal dreaming, abnormal gait, abnormal thinking, aggravated depression, aggressive reaction, agitation, alcohol intolerance, apathy, aphasia, ataxia, Bell's palsy, CNS dysfunction, coma, convulsions, dysphonia, emotional lability, extrapyramidal disorder, feeling of ebriety, flushing, hearing disorder, hearing impairment, hot flashes, hyperesthesia, hyperkinesia, hypertonia, hypokinesia, impaired consciousness, labyrinthine disorder, loss of consciousness, manic depression, manic reaction, migraine, neuralgia, neuritis, neuropathy, neurosis, paresis, paroniria, parosmia, personality disorder, polyneuropathy, psychosis, speech disorder, stroke, suicide attempt, syncope, tinnitus, tremor, vertigo (8% in follicular lymphoma)								

Reproduction System Disorders (<5%)	amenorrhea (12% in follicular lymphoma), dysmenorrhea, impotence, leukorrhea, menorrhagia, menstrual irregularity, pelvic pain, penis disorder, sexual dysfunction, uterine bleeding, vaginal dryness								
Resistance Mechanism Disorders									
moniliasis	—	1	—	<1	—	17	—	1	5
herpes simplex	1	2	—	—	—	3	1	—	—
other (<5%)	abscess, conjunctivitis, fungal infection, hemophilus, herpes zoster, infection, infection bacterial, infection nonspecific (7% in follicular lymphoma), infection parasitic, otitis media, sepsis, stye, trichomonas, upper respiratory tract infection, viral infection (7% in chronic hepatitis C)								
Respiratory System Disorders									
dyspnea	15	14	<1	—	1	34	3	5	—
coughing	6	13	<1	—	—	31	1	4	—
pharyngitis	2	8	<5	1	1	31	3	7	1
sinusitis	1	4	—	—	—	21	2	—	—
nonproductive coughing	2	7	—	—	—	14	0	1	—
nasal congestion	1	7	—	1	—	10	<1	4	—
other (<5%)	bronchitis, (10% in follicular lymphoma), bronchospasm, cyanosis, epistaxis, hemoptysis, hypoventilation, laryngitis, lung fibrosis, pleural effusion, orthopnea, pleural pain, pneumonia, pneumothorax, rales, respiratory disorder, respiratory insufficiency, sneezing, tonsillitis, tracheitis, wheezing								
Skin and Appendages Disorders									
dermatitis	1	—	8	—	—	—	2	1	—
alopecia	29	23	8	—	12	31	28	26	38
pruritus	—	10	11	1	7	—	9	6	4
rash	19	13	25	—	9	10	5	8	1
dry skin	1	3	9	—	9	10	4	3	—
other (<5%)	abnormal hair texture, acne, cellulitis, cyanosis of the hand, cold and clammy skin, dermatitis lichenoides, eczema, epidermal necrolysis, erythema, erythema nodosum, folliculitis, furunculosis, increased hair growth, lacrimal gland disorder, lacrimation, lipoma, maculopapular rash, melanosis, nail disorders, nonherpetic cold sores, pallor, peripheral ischemia, photosensitivity, psoriasis, psoriasis aggravated, purpura (5% in chronic hepatitis C), rash erythematous, sebaceous cyst, skin depigmentation, skin discoloration, skin nodule, urticaria, vitiligo								
Urinary System Disorders (<5%)	albumin/protein in urine, cystitis, dysuria, hematuria, incontinence, increased BUN, micturition disorder, micturition frequency, nocturia, polyuria (10% in follicular lymphoma), renal insufficiency, urinary tract infection (5% in chronic hepatitis C)								
Vision Disorders (<5%)	abnormal vision, blurred vision, diplopia, dry eyes, eye pain, nystagmus, photophobia								

* Dash (—) indicates not reported
† Vomiting was reported with nausea as a single term
‡ Includes stomatitis/mucositis
§ Amnesia was reported with confusion as a single term
‖ Percentages based upon a summary of all adverse events during 18 to 24 months of treatment
¶ Predominantly lethargy

Those patients who have preexisting cardiac abnormalities and/or are in advanced stages of cancer should have electrocardiograms taken prior to and during the course of treatment.

Mild-to-moderate leukopenia and elevated serum liver enzyme (SGOT) levels have been reported with intralesional administration of INTRON A Interferon alfa-2b, recombinant for Injection (see **ADVERSE REACTIONS**); therefore, the monitoring of these laboratory parameters should be considered.

Baseline chest X-rays are suggested and should be repeated if clinically indicated.

For malignant melanoma patients, differential WBC count and liver function tests should be monitored weekly during the induction phase of therapy and monthly during the maintenance phase of therapy.

For specific recommendations in chronic hepatitis C and chronic hepatitis B, see **INDICATIONS AND USAGE**.

Carcinogenesis, Mutagenesis, Impairment of Fertility: Studies with INTRON A Interferon alfa-2b, recombinant for Injection have not been performed to determine carcinogenicity.

Interferon may impair fertility. In studies of interferon administration in nonhuman primates, menstrual cycle abnormalities have been observed. Decreases in serum estradiol and progesterone concentrations have been reported in women treated with human leukocyte interferon.[12] Therefore, fertile women should not receive INTRON A therapy unless they are using effective contraception during the therapy period. INTRON A therapy should be used with caution in fertile men.

Mutagenicity studies have demonstrated that INTRON A Interferon alfa-2b, recombinant for Injection is not mutagenic.

Studies in mice (0.1, 1.0 million IU/day), rats (4, 20, 100 million IU/kg/day), and cynomolgus monkeys (1.1 million IU/kg/day; 0.25, 0.75, 2.5 million IU/kg/day) injected with INTRON A Interferon alfa-2b, recombinant for Injection for up to 9 days, 3 months, and 1 month, respectively, have revealed no evidence of toxicity. However, in cynomolgus monkeys (4, 20, 100 million IU/kg/day) injected daily for 3 months with INTRON A Interferon alfa-2b, recombinant for Injection toxicity was observed at the mid and high doses and mortality was observed at the high dose.

However, due to the known species-specificity of interferon, the effects in animals are unlikely to be predictive of those in man.

Pregnancy Category C INTRON A Interferon alfa-2b, recombinant for Injection has been shown to have abortifacient effects in Macaca mulatta (rhesus monkeys) at 7.5, 15, and 30 million IU/kg (90, 180, and 360 times the intramuscular or subcutaneous dose of 2 million IU/m². Although abortion was observed in all dose groups, it was only statistically significant at the mid- and high-dose groups. There are no adequate and well-controlled studies in pregnant

women. INTRON A therapy should be used during pregnancy only if the potential benefit justifies the potential risk to the fetus.

Nursing Mothers It is not known whether this drug is excreted in human milk. However, studies in mice have shown that mouse interferons are excreted into the milk. Because of the potential for serious adverse reactions from the drug in nursing infants, a decision should be made whether to discontinue nursing or to discontinue INTRON A therapy, taking into account the importance of the drug to the mother.

Pediatric Use Safety and effectiveness have not been established in patients below the age of 18 years.

ADVERSE REACTIONS

General The adverse experiences listed below were reported to be possibly or probably related to INTRON A therapy during clinical trials. Most of these adverse reactions were mild to moderate in severity and were manageable. Some were transient and most diminished with continued therapy.

The most frequently reported adverse reactions were "flu-like" symptoms, particularly fever, headache, chills, myalgia, and fatigue. More severe toxicities are observed generally at higher doses and may be difficult for patients to tolerate.

In addition, the following spontaneous adverse experiences have been reported during the marketing surveillance of INTRON A Interferon alfa-2b, recombinant for Injection: nephrotic syndrome, pancreatitis, renal failure, and renal insufficiency.

[See table at top of previous page and above]

Hairy Cell Leukemia The adverse reactions most frequently reported during clinical trials in 145 patients with hairy cell leukemia were the "flu-like" symptoms of fever (68%), fatigue (61%), and chills (46%).

Malignant Melanoma The INTRON A dose was modified because of adverse events in 65% (n=93) of the patients. INTRON A therapy was discontinued because of adverse events in 8% of the patients during induction and 18% of the patients during maintenance. The most frequently reported adverse reaction was fatigue which was observed in 96% of patients. Other adverse reactions that were recorded in >20% of INTRON A treated patients included neutropenia (92%), fever (81%), myalgia (75%), anorexia (69%), vomiting/nausea (66%), increased SGOT (63%), headache (62%), chills (54%), depression (40%), diarrhea (35%), alopecia (29%), altered taste sensation (24%), dizziness/vertigo (23%), and anemia (22%).

Adverse reactions classified as severe or life threatening (ECOG Toxicity Criteria grade 3 or 4) were recorded in 66% and 14% of INTRON A treated patients, respectively. Severe adverse reactions recorded in >10% of INTRON A treated patients included neutropenia/leukopenia (26%), fatigue

(23%), fever (18%), myalgia (17%), headache (17%), chills (16%), and increased SGOT (14%). Grade 4 fatigue was recorded in 4% and grade 4 depression was recorded in 2% of INTRON A treated patients. No other grade 4 AE was reported in more than 2 INTRON A treated patients. Lethal hepatotoxicity occurred in 2 INTRON A treated patients early in the clinical trial. No subsequent lethal hepatotoxicities were observed with adequate monitoring of liver function tests (see **PRECAUTIONS—Laboratory Tests**).

Follicular Lymphoma Ninety-six percent of patients treated with CHVP plus INTRON A therapy and 91% of patients treated with CHVP alone reported an adverse event of any severity. Asthenia, fever, neutropenia, increased hepatic enzymes, alopecia, headache, anorexia, "flu-like" symptoms, myalgia, dyspnea, thrombocytopenia, paresthesia, and polyuria occurred more frequently in the CHVP plus INTRON A treated patients than in patients treated with CHVP alone. Adverse reactions classified as severe or life threatening (World Health Organization grade 3 or 4) recorded in >5% of CHVP plus INTRON A treated patients included neutropenia (34%), asthenia (10%), and vomiting (10%). The incidence of neutropenic infection was 6% in CHVP plus INTRON A vs 2% in CHVP alone. One patient in each treatment group required hospitalization.

Twenty-eight percent of CHVP plus INTRON A treated patients has a temporary modification/interruption of their INTRON A therapy, but only 13 patients (10%) permanently stopped INTRON A therapy because of toxicity. There were 4 deaths on study; two patients committed suicide in the CHVP plus INTRON A arm and two patients in the CHVP arm had unwitnessed sudden death. Three patients with hepatitis B (one of whom also had alcoholic cirrhosis) developed hepatotoxicity leading to discontinuation of INTRON A. Other reasons for discontinuation included intolerable asthenia (5/135), severe flu symptoms (2/135), and one patient each with exacerbation of ankylosing spondylitis, psychosis, and decreased ejection fraction.

Condylomata Acuminata Eighty-eight percent (311/352) of patients treated with INTRON A Interferon alfa-2b, recombinant for Injection for condylomata acuminata who were evaluable for safety, reported an adverse reaction during treatment. The incidence of the adverse reactions reported increased when the number of treated lesions increased from one to five. All 40 patients who had five warts treated, reported some type of adverse reaction during treatment.

Adverse reactions and abnormal laboratory test values reported by patients who were retreated were qualitatively and quantitatively similar to those reported during the initial INTRON A treatment period.

Continued on next page

Information on Schering products appearing on these pages is effective as of August 15, 1998.

Intron A—Cont.

AIDS-Related Kaposi's Sarcoma In patients with AIDS-Related Kaposi's Sarcoma, some type of adverse reaction occurred in 100% of the 74 patients treated with 30 million IU/m² three times a week and in 97% of the 29 patients treated with 35 million IU per day.

Of these adverse reactions, those classified as severe (World Health Organization grade 3 or 4) were reported in 27% to 55% of patients. Severe adverse reactions in the 30 million IU/m² TIW study included: fatigue (20%), influenza-like symptoms (15%), anorexia (12%), dry mouth (4%), headache (4%), confusion (3%), fever (3%), myalgia (3%), and nausea and vomiting (1% each). Severe adverse reactions for patients who received the 35 million IU QD included: fever (24%), fatigue (17%), influenza-like symptoms (14%), dyspnea (14%), headache (10%), pharyngitis (7%), and ataxia, confusion, dysphagia, GI hemorrhage, abnormal hepatic function, increased SGOT, myalgia, cardiomyopathy, face edema, depression, emotional lability, suicide attempt, chest pain, and coughing (1 patient each). Overall, the incidence of severe toxicity was higher among patients who received the 35 million IU per day dose.

Chronic Hepatitis C Two studies of extended treatment (18 to 24 months) with INTRON A Interferon alfa-2b, recombinant for Injection show that approximately 95% of all patients treated experience some type of adverse event and that patients treated for extended duration continue to experience adverse events throughout treatment. Most adverse events reported are mild to moderate in severity. However, 29/152 (19%) of patients treated for 18 to 24 months experienced a serious adverse event compared to 11/163 (7%) of those treated for 6 months. Adverse events which occur or persist during extended treatment are similar in type and severity to those occurring during short-course therapy.

Of the patients achieving a complete response after 6 months of therapy, 12/79 (15%) subsequently discontinued INTRON A treatment during extended therapy because of adverse events, and 23/79 (29%) experienced severe adverse events (WHO grade 3 or 4) during extended therapy.

Chronic Hepatitis B In patients with chronic hepatitis B, some type of adverse reaction occurred in 98% of the 101 patients treated at 5 million IU QD and 90% of the 78 patients treated at 10 million IU TIW. Most of these adverse reactions were mild to moderate in severity, were manageable, and were reversible following the end of therapy.

Adverse reactions classified as severe (causing a significant interference with normal daily activities or clinical state) were reported in 21% to 44% of patients. The severe adverse reactions reported most frequently were the "flu-like" symptoms of fever (28%), fatigue (15%), headache (5%), myalgia (4%), rigors (4%), and other severe "flu-like" symptoms which occurred in 1% to 3% of patients. Other severe adverse reactions occurring in more than one patient were alopecia (8%), anorexia (6%), depression (3%), nausea (3%), and vomiting (2%).

To manage side effects, the dose was reduced, or INTRON A therapy was interrupted in 25% to 38% of patients. Five percent of patients discontinued treatment due to adverse experiences.

[See table below]

HOW SUPPLIED

INTRON A Interferon alfa-2b, recombinant Powder for Injection INTRON A Interferon alfa-2b, recombinant Powder for Injection, 3 million IU per vial and Diluent for INTRON A Interferon alfa-2b, recombinant for Injection (bacteriostatic water for injection) 1 mL per vial; boxes containing 1 INTRON A vial and 1 vial of INTRON A Diluent (NDC 0085-0647-03).

INTRON A Interferon alfa-2b, recombinant Powder for Injection INTRON® A, Pak-3, containing 6 INTRON A vials, 3 million IU per vial, and 6 syringes of Diluent for INTRON A Interferon alfa-2b, recombinant for Injection (bacteriostatic water for injection) 1 mL per syringe for chronic hepatitis C (NDC 0085-0647-05).

INTRON A Interferon alfa-2b, recombinant Powder for Injection, 5 million IU per vial and Diluent for INTRON A Interferon alfa-2b, recombinant for Injection (bacteriostatic water for injection) 1 mL per vial; boxes containing 1 INTRON A vial and 1 vial of INTRON A Diluent (NDC 0085-0120-02).

INTRON A Interferon alfa-2b, recombinant Powder for Injection, 10 million IU per vial and Diluent for INTRON A Interferon alfa-2b, recombinant for Injection (bacteriostatic water for injection) 2 mL per vial; boxes containing 1 INTRON A vial and 1 vial of INTRON A Diluent (NDC 0085-0571-02).

INTRON A Interferon alfa-2b, recombinant Powder for Injection, 18 million IU per vial and Diluent for INTRON A Interferon alfa-2b, recombinant for Injection (bacteriostatic water for injection) 1 mL per vial; boxes containing 1 vial of INTRON A and 1 vial of INTRON A Diluent (NDC 0085-1110-01).

INTRON A Interferon alfa-2b, recombinant Powder for Injection, 25 million IU per vial and Diluent for INTRON A Interferon alfa-2b, recombinant for Injection (bacteriostatic water for injection) 5 mL per vial; boxes containing 1 INTRON A vial and 1 vial of INTRON A Diluent (NDC 0085-0285-02).

INTRON A Interferon alfa-2b, recombinant Powder for Injection, 50 million IU per vial and Diluent for INTRON A Interferon alfa-2b, recombinant for Injection (bacteriostatic water for injection) 1 mL per vial; boxes containing 1 INTRON A vial and 1 vial of INTRON A Diluent (NDC 0085-0539-01).

Store INTRON A Interferon alfa-2b, recombinant Powder for Injection both before and after reconstitution between 2° and 8°C (36° and 46°F).

INTRON A Interferon alfa-2b, recombinant Solution for Injection INTRON A Interferon alfa-2b, recombinant Solution for Injection, 6 doses of 3 million IU (18 million IU) multidose pen (22.5 million IU per 1.5 mL per pen); boxes containing 1 INTRON A multidose pen, six disposable needles and alcohol swabs (NDC 0085-1242-01).

INTRON A Interferon alfa-2b, recombinant Solution for Injection, 6 doses of 5 million IU (30 million IU) multidose pen (37.5 million IU per 1.5 mL per pen); boxes containing 1 INTRON A multidose pen, six disposible needles and alcohol swabs (NDC 0085-1235-01).

INTRON A Interferon alfa-2b, recombinant Solution for Injection, 6 doses of 10 million IU (60 million IU) multidose pen (75 million IU per 1.5 mL per pen); boxes containing 1 INTRON A multidose pen, six disposable needles and alcohol swabs (NDC 0085-1254-01).

INTRON A Interferon alfa-2b, recombinant Solution for Injection, 3 million IU per 0.5 mL per vial; boxes containing 1 vial of INTRON A Solution for Injection (NDC 0085-1184-01).

INTRON A Interferon alfa-2b, recombinant Solution for Injection INTRON® A, Pak-3, containing 6 INTRON A vials, 3 million IU per vial, and 6 syringes (NDC 0085-1184-02).

INTRON A Interferon alfa-2b, recombinant Solution for Injection, 5 million IU per 0.5 mL per vial; boxes containing 1 vial of INTRON A Solution for Injection (NDC 0085-1191-01).

INTRON A Interferon alfa-2b, recombinant Solution for Injection INTRON® A, Pak-5, containing 6 INTRON A vials, 5 million IU per vial, and 6 syringes (NDC 0085-1191-02).

INTRON A Interferon alfa-2b, recombinant Solution for Injection, 10 million IU per 1.0 mL per vial; boxes containing 1 vial of INTRON A Solution for Injection (NDC 0085-1179-01).

INTRON A Interferon alfa-2b, recombinant Solution for Injection INTRON® A, Pak-10, containing 6 INTRON A vials, 10 million IU per vial, and 6 syringes (NDC 0085-1179-02).

INTRON A Interferon alfa-2b, recombinant Solution for Injection, 18 million IU multidose vial (22.8 million IU per 3.8 mL per vial); boxes containing 1 vial of INTRON A Solution for Injection (NDC 0085-1168-01).

INTRON A Interferon alfa-2b, recombinant Solution for Injection, 25 million IU multidose vial (32 million IU per 3.2 mL per vial); boxes containing 1 vial of INTRON A Solution for Injection (NDC 0085-1133-01).

Store INTRON A Interferon alfa-2b, recombinant Solution for Injection between 2° and 8°C (36° and 46°F).

References:
1. Smalley R, et al. *N Engl J Med.* 1922;327:1336–1341.
2. Aviles A, et al. *Leukemia and Lymphoma.* 1996;20:495–499.
3. Unterhalt M, et al. *Blood* 1996;88 (10Suppl 1):1744A.
4. Schiller J, et al. *J Biol Response Mod.* 1989;8:252–261.
5. Poynard T, et al. *N Engl J Med.* 1995;332:(22)1457–1462.
6. Lin R, et al *J Hepatol.*1995;23:487–496.
7. Perrillo R, et al. *N Engl J Med.* 1990;323:295–301.
8. Perez V, et al. *J Hepatol* 1990;11:S113–S117.
9. Knodell R, et al. *Hepatology.* 1981;1:431–435.
10. Perrillo R, et al. *Ann Intern Med.* 1991;115:113–115.
11. Renault P, et al. *Arch Intern Med* 1987;147:1577–1580.
12. Kauppila A, et al. *Int J Cancer.* 1982;29:291–294.

ABNORMAL LABORATORY TEST VALUES BY INDICATION
Dosing Regimens
Percentage (%) of Patients

Laboratory Tests	MALIGNANT MELANOMA 20 MIU/m² Induction (IV) 10 MIU/m² Maintenance (SC)	FOLLICULAR LYMPHOMA 5 MIU TIW/SC	HAIRY CELL LEUKEMIA 2 MIU/m² TIW/SC	CONDYLOMATA ACUMINATA 1 MIU/ lesion	AIDS-RELATED KAPOSI'S SARCOMA 30 MIU/m² TIW/SC	AIDS-RELATED KAPOSI'S SARCOMA 35 MIU/ QD/SC	CHRONIC HEPATITIS C 3 MIU TIW	CHRONIC HEPATITIS B 5 MIU QD	CHRONIC HEPATITIS B 10 MIU TIW
	N=143	N=135	N=145	N=352	N=69-73	N=26-28	N=140-171	N=101	N=78
Hemoglobin	22	8	NA	—	1	15	26¶	32*	23*
White Blood Cell Count	‖	—	NA	17	10	22	26†	68†	34†
Platelet Count	15	13	NA	—	0	8	15‡	12‡	5‡
Serum Creatinine	3	2	0	—	—	—	6	3	0
Alkaline Phosphatase	13	—	4	—	—	—	—	8	4
Lactate Dehydrogenase	1	—	0	—	—	—	—	—	—
Serum Urea Nitrogen	12	4	0	—	—	—	—	2	0
SGOT	63	24	4	12	11	41	—	—	—
SGPT	2	—	13	—	10	15	—	—	—
Granulocyte Count									
• Total	92	36	NA	—	31	39	45§	75¶	61¶
• 1000-<1500/mm³	66	—	—	—	—	—	32	30	32
• 750-<1000/mm³	—	21	—	—	—	—	10	24	18
• 500-<750/mm³	25	—	—	—	—	—	1	17	9
• <500/mm³	1	13	—	—	—	—	2	4	2

NA – Not Applicable–Patients' initial hematologic laboratory test values were abnormal due to their condition.
* Decrease of ≥2 g/dL
† Decrease to <3000/mm³
‡ Decrease to <70,000/mm³
§ Neutrophils plus bands
‖ White Blood Cell Count was reported as neutropenia
¶ Decrease of ≥2 g/dL; 20% 2-<3 g/dL; 6% ≥3g/dL

Schering Corporation
Kenilworth, NJ 07033 USA
Rev 3/98
U.S. Patents 4,530,901 & 4,496,537
Copyright © 1986, 1995, 1996, 1998, Schering Corporation.
All rights reserved.

18766167

LOTRIMIN®   ℞
brand of clotrimazole
   Cream, USP 1%*
   Lotion, USP 1%*
   Topical Solution, USP 1%*
For Dermatologic Use Only—
Not For Ophthalmic Use

*These preparations are also available without a prescription as LOTRIMIN AF.

DESCRIPTION
LOTRIMIN products contain clotrimazole, USP, a synthetic antifungal agent having the chemical name 1-(o-Chloro-α,α-diphenylbenzyl)imidazole; the empirical formula, $C_{22}H_{17}ClN_2$; a molecular weight of 344.84; and the chemical structure:

Clotrimazole is an odorless, white crystalline substance. It is practically insoluble in water, sparingly soluble in ether and very soluble in polyethylene glycol 400, ethanol, and chloroform.
Each gram of LOTRIMIN **Cream** contains 10 mg clotrimazole, USP in a vanishing cream base of benzyl alcohol, cetearyl alcohol, cetyl esters wax, octyldodecanol, polysorbate, sorbitan monostearate, and water.
Each gram of LOTRIMIN **Lotion** contains 10 mg clotrimazole, USP dispersed in an emulsion vehicle composed of benzyl alcohol, cetearyl alcohol, cetyl esters wax, octyldodecanol, polysorbate, sodium phosphate, sorbitan monostearate, and water.
Each mL of LOTRIMIN **Topical Solution** contains 10 mg clotrimazole, USP in a nonaqueous vehicle of PEG.

CLINICAL PHARMACOLOGY
Clotrimazole is a broad-spectrum antifungal agent that is used for the treatment of dermal infections caused by various species of pathogenic dermatophytes, yeasts, and *Malassezia furfur*. The primary action of clotrimazole is against dividing and growing organisms.
In vitro, clotrimazole exhibits fungistatic and fungicidal activity against isolates of *Trichophyton rubrum, Trichophyton mentagrophytes, Epidermophyton floccosum, Microsporum canis,* and *Candida* species, including *Candida albicans*. In general, the *in vitro* activity of clotrimazole corresponds to that of tolnaftate and griseofulvin against the mycelia of dermatophytes (*Trichophyton, Microsporum,* and *Epidermophyton*), and to that of the polyenes (amphotericin B and nystatin) against budding fungi (*Candida*). Using an *in vivo* (mouse) and an *in vitro* (mouse kidney homogenate) testing system, clotrimazole and miconazole were equally effective in preventing the growth of the pseudomycelia and mycelia of *Candida albicans*.
Strains of fungi having a natural resistance to clotrimazole are rare. Only a single isolate of *Candida guilliermondi* has been reported to have primary resistance to clotrimazole. No single-step or multiple-step resistance to clotrimazole has developed during successive passages of *Candida albicans* and *Trichophyton mentagrophytes*. No appreciable change in sensitivity was detected after successive passages of isolates of *C. albicans, C. krusei,* or *C. pseudotropicalis* in liquid or solid media containing clotrimazole. Also, resistance could not be developed in chemically induced mutant strains of polyene-resistant isolates of *C. albicans*. Slight, reversible resistance was noted in three isolates of *C. albicans* tested by one investigator. There is a single report that records the clinical emergence of a *C. albicans* strain with considerable resistance to flucytosine and miconazole, and with cross-resistance to clotrimazole; the strain remained sensitive to nystatin and amphotericin B.
In studies of the mechanism of action, the minimum fungicidal concentration of clotrimazole caused leakage of intracellular phosphorus compounds into the ambient medium with concomitant breakdown of cellular nucleic acids and accelerated potassium efflux. Both these events began rapidly and extensively after addition of the drug.

Clotrimazole appears to be well absorbed in humans following oral administration and is eliminated mainly as inactive metabolites. Following topical and vaginal administration, however, clotrimazole appears to be minimally absorbed.
Six hours after the application of radioactive clotrimazole 1% cream and 1% solution onto intact and acutely inflamed skin, the concentration of clotrimazole varied from 100 mcg/cm³ in the stratum corneum to 0.5 to 1 mcg/cm³ in the stratum reticulare, and 0.1 mcg/cm³ in the subcutis. No measurable amount of radioactivity (≤0.001 mcg/mL) was found in the serum within 48 hours after application under occlusive dressing of 0.5 mL of the solution or 0.8 g of the cream. Only 0.5% or less of the applied radioactivity was excreted in the urine.
Following intravaginal administration of 100 mg ¹⁴C-clotrimazole vaginal tablets to nine adult females, an average peak serum level, corresponding to only 0.03 µg equivalents/mL of clotrimazole, was reached 1 to 2 days after application. After intravaginal administration of 5 g of 1% ¹⁴C-clotrimazole vaginal cream containing 50 mg active drug, to five subjects (one with candidal colpitis), serum levels corresponding to approximately 0.01 µg equivalents/mL were reached between 8 and 24 hours after application.

INDICATIONS AND USAGE
Prescription LOTRIMIN (clotrimazole cream, lotion, and solution 1%) products are indicated for the topical treatment of candidiasis due to *Candida albicans* and tinea versicolor due to *Malassezia furfur*.
These formulations are also available as the LOTRIMIN AF (clotrimazole cream, lotion, and solution 1%) line of nonprescription products which are indicated for the topical treatment of the following dermal infections: tinea pedis, tinea cruris, and tinea corporis due to *Trichophyton rubrum, Trichophyton mentagrophytes, Epidermophyton floccosum,* and *Microsporum canis*.

CONTRAINDICATIONS
LOTRIMIN products are contraindicated in individuals who have shown hypersensitivity to any of their components.

WARNINGS
LOTRIMIN products are not for ophthalmic use.

PRECAUTIONS
General: If irritation or sensitivity develops with the use of clotrimazole, treatment should be discontinued and appropriate therapy instituted.
Information For Patients: This information is intended to aid in the safe and effective use of this medication. It is not a disclosure of all possible adverse or intended effects.
The patient should be advised to:
1. Use the medication for the full treatment time even though the symptoms may have improved. Notify the physician if there is no improvement after 4 weeks of treatment.
2. Inform the physician if the area of application shows signs of increased irritation (redness, itching, burning, blistering, swelling, oozing) indicative of possible sensitization.
3. Avoid sources of infection or reinfection.
Laboratory Tests: If there is lack of response to clotrimazole, appropriate microbiological studies should be repeated to confirm the diagnosis and rule out other pathogens before instituting another course of antimycotic therapy.
Drug Interactions: Synergism or antagonism between clotrimazole and nystatin, or amphotericin B, or flucytosine against strains of *C. albicans* has not been reported.
Carcinogenesis, Mutagenesis, Impairment of Fertility: An 18-month oral dosing study with clotrimazole in rats has not revealed any carcinogenic effect.
In tests for mutagenesis, chromosomes of the spermatophores of Chinese hamsters which had been exposed to clotrimazole were examined for structural changes during the metaphase. Prior to testing, the hamsters had received five oral clotrimazole doses of 100 mg/kg body weight. The results of this study showed that clotrimazole had no mutagenic effect.
Usage in Pregnancy: Pregnancy Category B: The disposition of ¹⁴C-clotrimazole has been studied in humans and animals. Clotrimazole is very poorly absorbed following dermal application or intravaginal administration to humans. (See **CLINICAL PHARMACOLOGY.**)
In clinical trials, use of vaginally applied clotrimazole in pregnant women in their second and third trimesters has not been associated with ill effects. There are, however, no adequate and well-controlled studies in pregnant women during the first trimester of pregnancy.
Studies in pregnant rats with intravaginal doses up to 100 mg/kg have revealed no evidence of harm to the fetus due to clotrimazole.
High oral doses of clotrimazole in rats and mice ranging from 50 to 120 mg/kg resulted in embryotoxicity (possibly secondary to maternal toxicity), impairment of mating, decreased litter size and number of viable young and decreased pup survival to weaning. However, clotrimazole was not teratogenic in mice, rabbits, and rats at oral doses up to

200, 180, and 100 mg/kg, respectively. Oral absorption in the rat amounts to approximately 90% of the administered dose.
Because animal reproduction studies are not always predictive of human response, this drug should be used only if clearly indicated during the first trimester of pregnancy.
Nursing Mothers: It is not known whether this drug is excreted in human milk. Because many drugs are excreted in human milk, caution should be exercised when clotrimazole is used by a nursing woman.
Pediatric Use: Safety and effectiveness in children have been established for clotrimazole when used as indicated and in the recommended dosage.

ADVERSE REACTIONS
The following adverse reactions have been reported in connection with the use of clotrimazole: erythema, stinging, blistering, peeling, edema, pruritus, urticaria, burning, and general irritation of the skin.

OVERDOSAGE
Acute overdosage with topical application of clotrimazole is unlikely and would not be expected to lead to a life-threatening situation.

DOSAGE AND ADMINISTRATION
Gently massage sufficient LOTRIMIN into the affected and surrounding skin areas twice a day, in the morning and evening.
Clinical improvement, with relief of pruritus, usually occurs within the first week of treatment with LOTRIMIN. If the patient shows no clinical improvement after 4 weeks of treatment with LOTRIMIN, the diagnosis should be reviewed.

HOW SUPPLIED
LOTRIMIN Cream 1% is supplied in 15, 30, 45, and 90-g tubes (NDC 0085-0613-02, 05, 04, 03, respectively); boxes of one.
Store between 2° and 30°C (36° and 86°F).
LOTRIMIN Lotion 1% is supplied in 30-mL bottles (NDC 0085-0707-02); boxes of one.
Store between 2° and 25°C (36° and 77°F).
Shake well before using.
LOTRIMIN Topical Solution 1% is supplied in 10-mL and 30-mL plastic bottles (NDC 0085-0182-02, 04, respectively); boxes of one.
Store between 2° and 30°C (36° and 86°F).
Rev. 11/93
Copyright © 1984, 1991, 1993, 1994,
Schering Corporation.
All rights reserved.
17981005

LOTRISONE®   ℞
brand of clotrimazole
and betamethasone
dipropionate
Cream, USP

For Dermatologic Use Only—
Not for Ophthalmic Use

DESCRIPTION
LOTRISONE Cream contains a combination of clotrimazole, USP, a synthetic antifungal agent, and betamethasone dipropionate, USP, a synthetic corticosteroid, for dermatologic use.
Chemically, clotrimazole is 1-(o-Chloro-α,α-diphenyl-benzyl) imidazole, with the empirical formula $C_{22}H_{17}ClN_2$, a molecular weight of 344.8, and the following structural formula:

Clotrimazole is an odorless, white crystalline powder, insoluble in water and soluble in ethanol.
Betamethasone dipropionate has the chemical name 9-Fluoro-11β, 17,21-trihydroxy-16β-methylpregna-1,4-diene-3,20-dione 17,21-dipropionate, with the empirical formula $C_{28}H_{37}FO_7$, a molecular weight of 504.6, and the following structural formula:
[See chemical structure at top of next column]

Continued on next page

Lotrisone—Cont.

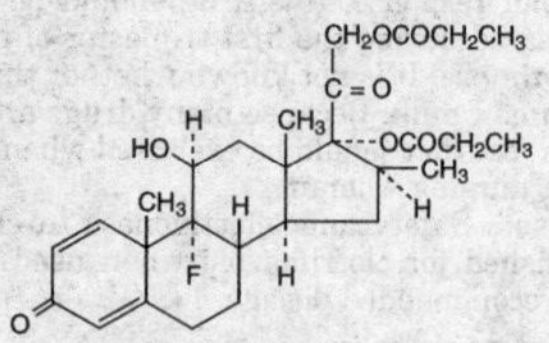

Betamethasone dipropionate is a white to creamy white, odorless crystalline powder, insoluble in water.

Each gram of LOTRISONE Cream contains 10.0 mg clotrimazole, USP, and 0.64 mg betamethasone dipropionate, USP (equivalent to 0.5 mg betamethasone), in a hydrophilic emollient cream consisting of purified water, mineral oil, white petrolatum, cetearyl alcohol, ceteareth-30, propylene glycol, sodium phosphate monobasic, and phosphoric acid; benzyl alcohol as preservative.

LOTRISONE is a smooth, uniform, white to off-white cream.

CLINICAL PHARMACOLOGY

Clotrimazole

Clotrimazole is a broad-spectrum, antifungal agent that is used for the treatment of dermal infections caused by various species of pathogenic dermatophytes, yeasts, and *Malassezia furfur.* The primary action of clotrimazole is against dividing and growing organisms.

In vitro, clotrimazole exhibits fungistatic and fungicidal activity against isolates of *Trichophyton rubrum, Trichophyton mentagrophytes, Epidermophyton floccosum,* and *Microsporum canis.* In general, the *in vitro* activity of clotrimazole corresponds to that of tolnaftate and griseofulvin against the mycelia of dermatophytes (*Trichophyton, Microsporum,* and *Epidermophyton*).

In vivo studies in guinea pigs infected with *Trichophyton mentagrophytes* have shown no measurable loss of clotrimazole activity due to combination with betamethasone dipropionate.

Strains of fungi having a natural resistance to clotrimazole have not been reported.

No single-step or multiple-step resistance to clotrimazole has developed during successive passages of *Trichophyton mentagrophytes.*

In studies of the mechanism of action in fungal cultures, the minimum fungicidal concentration of clotrimazole caused leakage of intracellular phosphorous compounds into the ambient medium with concomitant breakdown of cellular nucleic acids, and accelerated potassium efflux. Both of these events began rapidly and extensively after addition of the drug to the cultures.

Clotrimazole appears to be minimally absorbed following topical application to the skin. Six hours after the application of radioactive clotrimazole 1% cream and 1% solution onto intact and acutely inflamed skin, the concentration of clotrimazole varied from 100 mcg/cm^3 in the stratum corneum, to 0.5 to 1 mcg/cm^3 in the stratum reticulare, and 0.1 mcg/cm^3 in the subcutis. No measureable amount of radioactivity (<0.001 mcg/mL) was found in the serum within 48 hours after application under occlusive dressing of 0.5 mL of the solution or 0.8 g of the cream.

Betamethasone dipropionate

Betamethasone dipropionate, a corticosteroid, is effective in the treatment of corticosteroid-responsive dermatoses primarily because of its anti-inflammatory, anti-pruritic, and vasoconstrictive actions. However, while the physiologic, pharmacologic, and clinical effects of corticosteroids are well known, the exact mechanisms of their actions in each disease are uncertain. Betamethasone dipropionate, a corticosteroid, has been shown to have topical (dermatologic) and systemic pharmacologic and metabolic effects characteristic of this class of drugs.

Pharmacokinetics The extent of percutaneous absorption of topical corticosteroids is determined by many factors including the vehicle, the integrity of the epidermal barrier, and the use of occlusive dressings. (See **DOSAGE AND ADMINISTRATION** section.)

Topical corticosteroids can be absorbed from normal intact skin. Inflammation and/or other disease processes in the skin increase percutaneous absorption. Occlusive dressings substantially increase the percutaneous absorption of topical corticosteroids. (See **DOSAGE AND ADMINISTRATION** section.)

Once absorbed through the skin, topical corticosteroids are handled through pharmacokinetic pathways similar to systemically administered corticosteroids. Corticosteroids are bound to plasma proteins in varying degrees. Corticosteroids are metabolized primarily in the liver and are then excreted by the kidneys. Some of the topical corticosteroids and their metabolites are also excreted into the bile.

Clotrimazole and betamethasone dipropionate

In clinical studies of tinea corporis, tinea cruris, and tinea pedis, patients treated with LOTRISONE Cream showed a better clinical response at the first return visit than patients treated with clotrimazole cream. In tinea corporis and tinea cruris, the patient returned three days after starting treatment, and in tinea pedis, after one week. Mycological cure rates observed in patients treated with LOTRISONE Cream were as good as or better than in those patients treated with clotrimazole cream.

In these same clinical studies, patients treated with LOTRISONE Cream showed statistically significantly better clinical responses and mycological cure rates when compared with patients treated with betamethasone dipropionate cream.

INDICATIONS AND USAGE

LOTRISONE Cream is indicated for the topical treatment of the following dermal infections: tinea pedis, tinea cruris, and tinea corporis due to *Trichophyton rubrum, Trichophyton mentagrophytes, Epidermophyton floccosum,* and *Microsporum canis.*

CONTRAINDICATIONS

LOTRISONE Cream is contraindicated in patients who are sensitive to clotrimazole, betamethasone dipropionate, other corticosteroids or imidazoles, or to any ingredient in this preparation.

PRECAUTIONS

General Systemic absorption of topical corticosteroids has produced reversible hypothalamic-pituitary-adrenal (HPA) axis suppression, manifestations of Cushing's syndrome, hyperglycemia, and glucosuria in some patients.

Conditions which augment systemic absorption include the application of the more potent steroids, use over large surface areas, prolonged use, and the addition of occlusive dressings. (See **DOSAGE AND ADMINISTRATION** section.)

Therefore, patients receiving a large dose of a potent topical steroid applied to a large surface area should be evaluated periodically for evidence of HPA axis suppression by using the urinary free cortisol and ACTH stimulation tests. If HPA axis suppression is noted, an attempt should be made to withdraw the drug, to reduce the frequency of application, or to substitute a less potent steroid.

Recovery of HPA axis function is generally prompt and complete upon discontinuation of the drug. Infrequently, signs and symptoms of steroid withdrawal may occur, requiring supplemental systemic corticosteroids.

Children may absorb proportionally larger amounts of topical corticosteroids and thus be more susceptible to systemic toxicity. (See **PRECAUTIONS-Pediatric Use.**)

If irritation or hypersensitivity develops with the use of LOTRISONE Cream, treatment should be discontinued and appropriate therapy instituted.

Information for Patients Patients using LOTRISONE Cream should receive the following information and instructions:

1. This medication is to be used as directed by the physician. It is for external use only. Avoid contact with the eyes.
2. The medication is to be used for the full prescribed treatment time, even though the symptoms may have improved. Notify the physician if there is no improvement after 1 week of treatment for tinea cruris or tinea corporis, or after 2 weeks for tinea pedis.
3. Patients should be advised not to use this medication for any disorder other than for which it was prescribed.
4. The treated skin areas should not be bandaged or otherwise covered or wrapped as to be occluded. (See **DOSAGE AND ADMINISTRATION** section.)
5. When using this medication in the groin area, patients should be advised to use the medication for 2 weeks only, and to apply the cream sparingly. The physician should be notified if the condition persists after 2 weeks. Patients should also be advised to wear loose fitting clothing. (See **DOSAGE AND ADMINISTRATION** section.)
6. Patients should report any signs of local adverse reactions.
7. Patients should avoid sources of infection or reinfection.

Laboratory Tests If there is a lack of response to LOTRISONE Cream, appropriate microbiological studies should be repeated to confirm the diagnosis and rule out other pathogens before instituting another course of antimycotic therapy.

The following tests may be helpful in evaluating HPA axis suppression due to the corticosteroid component:

Urinary free cortisol test
ACTH stimulation test

Carcinogenesis, Mutagenesis, Impairment of Fertility There are no animal or laboratory studies with the combination clotrimazole and betamethasone dipropionate to evaluate carcinogenesis, mutagenesis, or impairment of fertility.

An 18-month oral dosing study with clotrimazole in rats has not revealed any carcinogenic effect.

In tests for mutagenesis, chromosomes of the spermatophores of Chinese hamsters which had been exposed to clotrimazole were examined for structural changes during the metaphase. Prior to testing, the hamsters had received five oral clotrimazole doses of 100 mg/kg body weight. The results of this study showed that clotrimazole had no mutagenic effect.

Pregnancy Category C There have been no teratogenic studies performed with the combination clotrimazole and betamethasone dipropionate.

Studies in pregnant rats with intravaginal doses up to 100 mg/kg have revealed no evidence of harm to the fetus due to clotrimazole.

High oral doses of clotrimazole in rats and mice ranging from 50 to 120 mg/kg resulted in embryotoxicity (possibly secondary to maternal toxicity), impairment of mating, decreased litter size and number of viable young and decreased pup survival to weaning. However, clotrimazole was not teratogenic in mice, rabbits, and rats at oral doses up to 200, 180, and 100 mg/kg, respectively. Oral absorption in the rat amounts to approximately 90% of the administered dose.

Corticosteroids are generally teratogenic in laboratory animals when administered systemically at relatively low dosage levels. The more potent corticosteroids have been shown to be teratogenic after dermal application in laboratory animals.

There are no adequate and well-controlled studies in pregnant women on teratogenic effects from a topically applied combination of clotrimazole and betamethasone dipropionate. Therefore, LOTRISONE Cream should be used during pregnancy only if the potential benefit justifies the potential risk to the fetus.

Drugs containing corticosteroids should not be used extensively on pregnant patients, in large amounts, or for prolonged periods of time.

Nursing Mothers It is not known whether this drug is excreted in human milk. Because many drugs are excreted in human milk, caution should be exercised when LOTRISONE Cream is used by a nursing woman.

Pediatric Use Safety and effectiveness in children below the age of 12 have not been established with LOTRISONE Cream.

Pediatric patients may demonstrate greater susceptibility to topical corticosteroid-induced HPA axis suppression and Cushing's syndrome than mature patients because of a larger skin surface area to body weight ratio.

Hypothalamic-pituitary-adrenal (HPA) axis suppression, Cushing's syndrome, and intracranial hypertension have been reported in children receiving topical corticosteroids. Manifestations of adrenal suppression in children include linear growth retardation, delayed weight gain, low plasma cortisol levels, and absence of response to ACTH stimulation. Manifestations of intracranial hypertension include bulging fontanelles, headaches, and bilateral papilledema.

Administration of topical dermatologics containing a corticosteroid to children should be limited to the least amount compatible with an effective therapeutic regimen. Chronic corticosteroid therapy may interfere with the growth and development of children.

The use of LOTRISONE Cream in diaper dermatitis is not recommended.

ADVERSE REACTIONS

The following adverse reactions have been reported in connection with the use of LOTRISONE Cream: paresthesia in 5 of 270 patients, maculopapular rash, edema, and secondary infection, each in 1 of 270 patients.

Adverse reactions reported with the use of clotrimazole are as follows: erythema, stinging, blistering, peeling, edema, pruritus, urticaria, and general irritation of the skin.

The following local adverse reactions are reported infrequently when topical corticosteroids are used as recommended. These reactions are listed in an approximate decreasing order of occurrence: burning, itching, irritation, dryness, folliculitis, hypertrichosis, acneiform eruptions, hypopigmentation, perioral dermatitis, allergic contact dermatitis, maceration of the skin, secondary infection, skin atrophy, striae, and miliaria.

OVERDOSAGE

Acute overdosage with topical application of LOTRISONE Cream is unlikely and would not be expected to lead to a life-threatening situation.

Topically applied corticosteroids can be absorbed in sufficient amounts to produce systemic effects. (See **PRECAUTIONS.**)

DOSAGE AND ADMINISTRATION

Gently massage sufficient LOTRISONE Cream into the affected and surrounding skin areas twice a day, in the morning and evening, for 2 weeks in tinea cruris and tinea corporis and for 4 weeks in tinea pedis. The use of LOTRISONE Cream for longer than 4 weeks is not recommended.

Clinical improvement, with relief of erythema and pruritus, usually occurs within 3 to 5 days of treatment. If a patient

with tinea cruris or tinea corporis shows no clinical improvement after 1 week of treatment with LOTRISONE Cream, the diagnosis should be reviewed. In tinea pedis, the treatment should be applied for 2 weeks prior to making that decision.
Treatment with LOTRISONE Cream should be discontinued if the condition persists after 2 weeks in tinea cruris and tinea corporis, and after 4 weeks in tinea pedis. Alternate therapy may then be instituted with LOTRIMIN Cream, a product containing an antifungal only.
LOTRISONE Cream should not be used with occlusive dressings.

HOW SUPPLIED

LOTRISONE Cream is supplied in 15-gram (NDC 0085-0924-01), and 45-gram tubes (NDC 0085-0924-02); boxes of one.
Store between 2° and 30°C (36° and 86°F).
Rev. 1/94 17969609
Copyright © 1984, 1991, 1994, Schering Corporation. All rights reserved.

NASONEX® ℞

(mometasone furoate monohydrate)
Nasal Spray, 50 mcg*
FOR INTRANASAL USE ONLY
*calculated on the anhydrous basis

DESCRIPTION

Mometasone furoate monohydrate, the active component of NASONEX Nasal Spray, 50 mcg, is an anti-inflammatory corticosteroid having the chemical name, 9,21-Dichloro-11β,17-dihydroxy-16α-methylpregna-1,4-diene-3,20-dione 17-(2-furoate) monohydrate, and the following chemical structure:

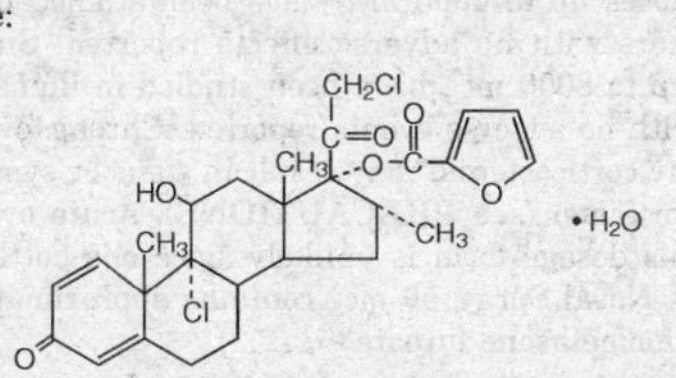

Mometasone furoate monohydrate is a white powder, with an empirical formula of $C_{27}H_{30}Cl_2O_6 \bullet H_2O$, and a molecular weight of 539.45. It is practically insoluble in water; slightly soluble in methanol, ethanol, and isopropanol; soluble in acetone and chloroform; and freely soluble in tetrahydrofuran. Its partition coefficient between octanol and water is greater than 5000.
NASONEX Nasal Spray, 50 mcg is a metered-dose, manual pump spray unit containing an aqueous suspension of mometasone furoate monohydrate equivalent to 0.05% w/w mometasone furoate calculated on the anhydrous basis; in an aqueous medium containing glycerin, microcrystalline cellulose and carboxymethylcellulose sodium, sodium citrate, 0.25% w/w phenylethyl alcohol, citric acid, benzalkonium chloride, and polysorbate 80. The pH is between 4.3 and 4.9.
After initial priming (10 actuations), each actuation of the pump delivers a metered spray containing 100 mg of suspension containing mometasone furoate monohydrate equivalent to 50 mcg of mometasone furoate calculated on the anhydrous basis. Each bottle of NASONEX Nasal Spray, 50 mcg provides 120 sprays.

CLINICAL PHARMACOLOGY

NASONEX Nasal Spray, 50 mcg is a corticosteroid demonstrating anti-inflammatory properties. The precise mechanism of corticosteroid action on allergic rhinitis is not known. Corticosteroids have been shown to have a wide range of effects on multiple cell types (eg, mast cells, eosinophils, neutrophils, macrophages, and lymphocytes) and mediators (eg, histamine, eicosanoids, leukotrienes, and cytokines) involved in inflammation.
Mometasone furoate demonstrated no mineralocorticoid, androgenic, antiandrogenic, or estrogenic activity in preclinical studies. After administration of a single intranasal dose of mometasone furoate to adult male rats, the highest drug levels were seen in the esophagus, trachea, nasal passage, and mouth.
In two clinical studies utilizing nasal antigen challenge, NASONEX Nasal Spray, 50 mcg decreased some markers of the early- and late-phase allergic response. These observations included decreases (vs placebo) in histamine and eosinophil cationic protein levels, and reductions (vs baseline) in eosinophils, neutrophils, and epithelial cell adhesion proteins. The clinical significance of these findings is not known.
The effect of NASONEX Nasal Spray, 50 mcg on nasal mucosa following 12 months of treatment was examined in 46 patients with allergic rhinitis. There was no evidence of atrophy and there was a marked reduction in intraepithelial eosinophilia and inflammatory cell infiltration (eg, eosinophils, lymphocytes, monocytes, neutrophils, and plasma cells).
Pharmacokinetics: ***Absorption:*** Mometasone furoate monohydrate administered as a nasal spray is virtually undetectable in plasma despite the use of a sensitive assay with a lower quantitation limit (LOQ) of 50 pcg/mL.
Metabolism: Studies have shown that any portion of a mometasone furoate dose which is swallowed and absorbed undergoes extensive metabolism to multiple metabolites.
Excretion: Following intravenous administration, the effective plasma elimination half-life of mometasone furoate is 5.8 hours. Any absorbed drug is excreted as metabolites mostly via the bile, and to a limited extent, into the urine.
Special Populations: The effects of renal impairment, hepatic impairment, age, or gender on mometasone furoate pharmacokinetics have not been adequately investigated.
Pharmacodynamics: Three clinical pharmacology studies have been conducted in humans to assess the effect of NASONEX Nasal Spray, 50 mcg at various doses on adrenal function. In one study, daily doses of 200 and 400 mcg of NASONEX Nasal Spray, 50 mcg and 10 mg of prednisone were compared to placebo in 64 patients with allergic rhinitis. Adrenal function before and after 36 consecutive days of treatment was assessed by measuring plasma cortisol levels following a 6-hour Cortrosyn (ACTH) infusion and by measuring 24-hour urinary-free cortisol levels. NASONEX Nasal Spray, 50 mcg, at both the 200 and 400 mcg dose, was not associated with a statistically significant decrease in mean plasma cortisol levels post-Cortrosyn infusion or a statistically significant decrease in the 24-hour urinary-free cortisol levels compared to placebo. A statistically significant decrease in the mean plasma cortisol levels post-Cortrosyn infusion and 24-hour urinary-free cortisol levels was detected in the prednisone treatment group compared to placebo.
A second study assessed adrenal response to NASONEX Nasal Spray, 50 mcg (400 and 1600 mcg/day), prednisone (10 mg/day), and placebo, administered for 29 days in 48 male volunteers. The 24-hour plasma cortisol area under the curve (AUC_{0-24}), during and after an 8-hour Cortrosyn infusion and 24-hour urinary-free cortisol levels were determined at baseline and after 29 days of treatment. No statistically significant differences of adrenal function were observed with NASONEX Nasal Spray, 50 mcg compared to placebo.
A third study evaluated single, rising doses of NASONEX Nasal Spray, 50 mcg (1000, 2000, and 4000 mcg/day), orally administered mometasone furoate (2000, 4000, and 8000 mcg/day), orally administered dexamethasone (200, 400, and 800 mcg/day), and placebo (administered at the end of each series of doses) in 24 male volunteers. Dose administrations were separated by at least 72 hours. Determination of serial plasma cortisol levels at 8 AM and for the 24-hour period following each treatment were used to calculate the plasma cortisol area under the curve (AUC_{0-24}). In addition, 24-hour urinary-free cortisol levels were collected prior to initial treatment administration and during the period immediately following each dose. No statistically significant decreases in the plasma cortisol AUC, 8 AM cortisol levels, or 24-hour urinary-free cortisol levels were observed in volunteers treated with either NASONEX Nasal Spray, 50 mcg or oral mometasone, as compared with placebo treatment. Conversely, nearly all volunteers treated with the 3 doses of dexamethasone demonstrated abnormal 8 AM cortisol levels (defined as a cortisol level <10 mcg/dL), reduced 24-hour plasma AUC values, and decreased 24-hour urinary-free cortisol levels, as compared to placebo treatment.
Clinical Studies: The efficacy and safety of NASONEX Nasal Spray, 50 mcg in the prophylaxis and treatment of seasonal allergic rhinitis and the treatment of perennial allergic rhinitis have been evaluated in 18 controlled trials, and one uncontrolled clinical trial, in approximately 3000 adults (age 17 to 85) and adolescents (age 12 to 16). This included 1757 males and 1453 females, including a total of 283 adolescents (182 boys and 101 girls) with seasonal allergic or perennial allergic rhinitis, treated with NASONEX Nasal Spray, 50 mcg at doses ranging from 50 to 800 mcg/day. The majority of patients were treated with 200 mcg/day. These trials evaluated the total nasal symptom scores that included stuffiness, rhinorrhea, itching, and sneezing. Patients treated with NASONEX Nasal Spray, 50 mcg 200 mcg/day had a significant decrease in total nasal symptom scores compared to placebo-treated patients. No additional benefit was observed for mometasone furoate doses greater than 200 mcg/day. A total of 350 patients have been treated with NASONEX Nasal Spray, 50 mcg for 1 year or longer.
In patients with seasonal allergic rhinitis, NASONEX Nasal Spray, 50 mcg demonstrated improvement in nasal symptoms (vs placebo) within 2 days after the first dose. Maximum benefit is usually achieved within 1 to 2 weeks after initiation of dosing.
Prophylaxis of seasonal allergic rhinitis for patients 12 years of age and older with NASONEX Nasal Spray, 50 mcg, given at a dose of 200 mcg/day, was evaluated in two clinical studies in 284 patients. These studies were designed such that patients received 4 weeks of prophylaxis with NASONEX Nasal Spray, 50 mcg prior to the anticipated onset of the pollen season, however, some patients received only 2 to 3 weeks of prophylaxis. Patients receiving 2 to 4 weeks of prophylaxis with NASONEX Nasal Spray, 50 mcg demonstrated a statistically significantly smaller mean increase in total nasal symptom scores with onset of the pollen season as compared to placebo patients.

INDICATIONS AND USAGE

NASONEX Nasal Spray, 50 mcg is indicated for the prophylaxis and treatment of the nasal symptoms of seasonal allergic rhinitis and the treatment of the nasal symptoms of perennial allergic rhinitis, in adults and children 12 years of age and older. In patients with a known seasonal allergen that precipitates nasal symptoms of seasonal allergic rhinitis, initiation of prophylaxis with NASONEX Nasal Spray, 50 mcg is recommended 2 to 4 weeks prior to the anticipated start of the pollen season.

CONTRAINDICATIONS

Hypersensitivity to any of the ingredients of this preparation contraindicates its use.

WARNINGS

The replacement of a systemic corticosteroid with a topical corticosteroid can be accompanied by signs of adrenal insufficiency and, in addition, some patients may experience symptoms of withdrawal; ie, joint and/or muscular pain, lassitude, and depression. Careful attention must be given when patients previously treated for prolonged periods with systemic corticosteroids are transferred to topical corticosteroids, with careful monitoring for acute adrenal insufficiency in response to stress. This is particularly important in those patients who have associated asthma or other clinical conditions where too rapid a decrease in systemic corticosteroid dosing may cause a severe exacerbation of their symptoms.
If recommended doses of intranasal corticosteroids are exceeded or if individuals are particularly sensitive or predisposed by virtue of recent systemic steroid therapy, symptoms of hypercorticism may occur, including very rare cases of menstrual irregularities, acneiform lesions, and cushingoid features. If such changes occur, topical corticosteroids should be discontinued slowly, consistent with accepted procedures for discontinuing oral steroid therapy.
Persons who are on drugs which suppress the immune system are more susceptible to infections than healthy individuals. Chickenpox and measles, for example, can have a more serious or even fatal course in nonimmune children or adults on corticosteroids. In such children or adults who have not had these diseases, particular care should be taken to avoid exposure. How the dose, route, and duration of corticosteroid administration affects the risk of developing a disseminated infection is not known. The contribution of the underlying disease and/or prior corticosteroid treatment to the risk is also not known. If exposed to chickenpox, prophylaxis with varicella zoster immune globin (VZIG) may be indicated. If exposed to measles, prophylaxis with pooled intramuscular immunoglobulin (IG) may be indicated. (See the respective package inserts for complete VZIG and IG prescribing information.) If chickenpox develops, treatment with antiviral agents may be considered.

PRECAUTIONS

General: In clinical studies with NASONEX Nasal Spray, 50 mcg, the development of localized infections of the nose and pharynx with *Candida albicans* has occurred only rarely. When such an infection develops, use of NASONEX Nasal Spray, 50 mcg should be discontinued and appropriate local or systemic therapy instituted, if needed.
Nasal corticosteroids should be used with caution, if at all, in patients with active or quiescent tuberculous infection of the respiratory tract, or in untreated fungal, bacterial, systemic viral infections, or ocular herpes simplex.
Rarely, immediate hypersensitivity reactions may occur after the intranasal administration of mometasone furoate monohydrate. Extreme rare instances of wheezing have been reported.
Rare instances of nasal septum perforation and increased intraocular pressure have also been reported following the intranasal application of aerosolized corticosteroids. As with any long-term topical treatment of the nasal cavity, patients using NASONEX Nasal Spray, 50 mcg over several months or longer should be examined periodically for possible changes in the nasal mucosa.
Because of the inhibitory effect of corticosteroids on wound healing, patients who have experienced recent nasal septum ulcers, nasal surgery, or nasal trauma should not use a nasal corticosteroid until healing has occurred.
Glaucoma and cataract formation was evaluated in one controlled study of 12 weeks' duration and one uncontrolled

Continued on next page

Information on Schering products appearing on these pages is effective as of August 15, 1998.

Nasonex—Cont.

study of 12 months' duration in patients treated with NASONEX Nasal Spray, 50 mcg at 200 mcg/day, using intraocular pressure measurements and slit lamp examination. No significant change from baseline was noted in the mean intraocular pressure measurements for the 141 NASONEX-treated patients in the 12-week study, as compared with 141 placebo-treated patients. No individual NASONEX-treated patient was noted to have developed a significant elevation in intraocular pressure or cataracts in this 12-week study. Likewise, no significant change from baseline was noted in the mean intraocular pressure measurements for the 139 NASONEX-treated patients in the 12-month study and again, no cataracts were detected in these patients. Nonetheless, nasal and inhaled corticosteroids have been associated with the development of glaucoma and/or cataracts. Therefore, close follow-up is warranted in patients with a change in vision and with a history of glaucoma and/or cataracts.

When nasal corticosteroids are used at excessive doses, systemic corticosteroid effects such as hypercorticism and adrenal suppression may appear. If such changes occur, NASONEX Nasal Spray, 50 mcg should be discontinued slowly, consistent with accepted procedures for discontinuing oral steroid therapy.

Information for Patients: Patients being treated with NASONEX Nasal Spray, 50 mcg should be given the following information and instructions. This information is intended to aid in the safe and effective use of this medication. It is not a disclosure of all intended or possible adverse effects. Patients should use NASONEX Nasal Spray, 50 mcg at regular intervals (once daily) since its effectiveness depends on regular use. Improvement in nasal symptoms of allergic rhinitis has been shown to occur within 2 days after the first dose. Maximum benefit is usually achieved within 1 to 2 weeks after initiation of dosing. Patients should take the medication as directed and should not increase the prescribed dosage by using it more than once a day in an attempt to increase its effectiveness. Patients should contact their physician if symptoms do not improve, or if the condition worsens. To assure proper use of this nasal spray, and to attain maximum benefit, patients should read and follow the accompanying Patient's Instructions for Use carefully. Patients should be cautioned not to spray NASONEX Nasal Spray, 50 mcg into the eyes.

Persons who are on immunosuppressant doses of corticosteroids should be warned to avoid exposure to chickenpox or measles, and patients should also be advised that if they are exposed, medical advice should be sought without delay.

Carcinogenesis, Mutagenesis, Impairment of Fertility: In Sprague Dawley rats, mometasone furoate demonstrated no statistically significant increase in the incidence of tumors at an inhalation dose of 67 mcg/kg (approximately 3 times the maximum recommended daily intranasal dose in adults on a mcg/m² basis). In Swiss CD-1 mice, mometasone furoate demonstrated no statistically significant increase in the incidence of tumors at an inhalation dose of 160 mcg/kg (approximately 4 times the maximum recommended daily intranasal dose in adults on a mcg/m² basis).

At cytotoxic doses, mometasone furoate produced an increase in chromosome aberrations in vitro in Chinese hamster ovary-cell cultures in the nonactivation phase, but not in the presence of rat liver S9 fraction. Mometasone furoate was not mutagenic in the mouse-lymphoma assay and the Salmonella/E. coli/mammalian microsome mutation assay, a Chinese hamster lung cell (CHL) chromosomal-aberrations assay, an in vivo mouse bone-marrow erythrocyte-micronucleus assay, a rat bone-marrow clastogenicity assay, and the mouse male germ-cell clastogenicity assay. Mometasone furoate also did not induce unscheduled DNA synthesis in vivo in rat hepatocytes.

In reproductive toxicity studies in rats, mometasone furoate administered subcutaneously caused prolonged gestation, prolonged and difficult labor, reduced offspring survival, and reduced maternal body weight gain following treatment at 15 mcg/kg (approximately ¾ the maximum recommended daily intranasal dose in adults on a mcg/m² basis). Impairment of fertility in rats was not produced by subcutaneous doses up to 15 mcg/kg.

Pregnancy: *Teratogenic Effects: Pregnancy Category C:* Mometasone furoate caused cleft palate in mice at subcutaneous doses of 60 and 180 mcg/kg, (approximately 2 and 4 times the maximum recommended daily intranasal dose in adults on a mcg/m² basis, respectively). Offspring survival was reduced in the 180 mcg/kg group. The nonteratogenic subcutaneous dose level in mice was 20 mcg/kg (approximately ½ the maximum recommended daily intranasal dose in adults on a mcg/m² basis).

In rabbits, mometasone furoate was teratogenic and caused flexed front paws at a topical dermal dose of 150 mcg/kg (approximately 14 times the maximum recommended daily intranasal dose in adults on a mcg/m² basis).

In rats, mometasone furoate produced umbilical hernia, cleft palate, and delayed ossification at a topical dermal

dose of 600 mcg/kg (approximately 30 times the maximum recommended daily intranasal dose in adults on a mcg/m² basis). At 1200 mcg/kg (approximately 60 times the maximum recommended daily intranasal dose in adults on a mcg/m² basis), microphthalmia, umbilical hernias, and delayed ossification were observed in rat pups.

In these teratogenicity studies, there were also reductions in maternal body weight gain and effects on fetal growth (lower fetal body weights and/or delayed ossification) in mice (60 and 180 mcg/kg), rabbits (150 mcg/kg), and rats (600 mcg/kg).

In an oral teratology study in rabbits, at 700 mcg/kg, (approximately 70 times the maximum recommended daily intranasal dose in adults on a mcg/m² basis), increased incidences of resorptions and malformations, including cleft palate and/or head malformations (hydrocephaly or domed head) were observed. Pregnancy failure was observed in most rabbits at 2800 mcg/kg (approximately 270 times the maximum recommended daily intranasal dose in adults on a mcg/m² basis).

There are no adequate, and well-controlled studies in pregnant women. NASONEX Nasal Spray, 50 mcg, like other corticosteroids, should be used during pregnancy only if the potential benefits justify the potential risk to the fetus. Experience with oral corticosteroids since their introduction in pharmacologic, as opposed to physiologic doses suggests that rodents are more prone to teratogenic effects from corticosteroids than humans. In addition, because there is a natural increase in corticosteroid production during pregnancy, most women will require a lower exogenous corticosteroid dose and many will not need corticosteroid treatment during pregnancy.

Nonteratogenic Effects: Hypoadrenalism may occur in infants born to women receiving corticosteroids during pregnancy. Such infants should be carefully monitored.

Nursing Mothers: It is not known if mometasone furoate is excreted in human milk. Because other corticosteroids are excreted in human milk, caution should be used when NASONEX Nasal Spray, 50 mcg is administered to nursing women.

Pediatric Use: Safety and effectiveness in children less than 12 years of age have not been established.

Geriatric Use: A total of 203 patients above 64 years of age (age range 64 to 85) have been treated with NASONEX Nasal Spray, 50 mcg for up to 3 months. The adverse reactions reported in this population were similar in type and incidence to those reported by younger patients.

ADVERSE REACTIONS

In controlled US and International clinical studies, a total of 3210 patients received treatment with NASONEX Nasal Spray, 50 mcg at doses of 50 to 800 mcg/day. The majority of patients (n = 2103) were treated with 200 mcg/day. A total of 350 patients have been treated for 1 year or longer. The overall incidence of adverse events for patients treated with NASONEX Nasal Spray, 50 mcg was comparable to patients treated with the vehicle placebo. Also, adverse events did not differ significantly based on age, sex, or race.

Three percent of patients in clinical trials discontinued treatment because of adverse events; this rate was similar for the vehicle and active comparators.

All adverse events reported by 5% or more of patients (regardless of relationship to treatment) who received NASONEX Nasal Spray, 50 mcg 200 mcg/day in clinical trials, and that were more common with NASONEX Nasal Spray, 50 mcg than placebo, are displayed in the table below.

[See table above]

Other adverse events which occurred in less than 5% but greater than or equal to 2% of mometasone-treated patients (regardless of relationship to treatment), and more frequently than in the placebo group included: arthralgia, asthma, bronchitis, chest pain, conjunctivitis, diarrhea, dyspepsia, earache, flu-like symptoms, myalgia, nausea, and rhinitis.

ADVERSE EVENTS FROM CONTROLLED CLINICAL TRIALS IN SEASONAL ALLERGIC AND PERENNIAL ALLERGIC RHINITIS (PERCENT OF PATIENTS REPORTING)

	NASONEX NASAL SPRAY, 50 mcg 200 mcg/day (N = 2103)	VEHICLE PLACEBO (N = 1671)
Headache	26	22
Viral Infection	14	11
Pharyngitis	12	10
Epistaxis/Blood-Tinged Mucus	11	6
Coughing	7	6
Upper Respiratory Tract Infection	6	2
Dysmenorrhea	5	3
Musculoskeletal Pain	5	3
Sinusitis	5	3

Rare cases of nasal ulcers and nasal and oral candidiasis were also reported in patients treated with NASONEX Nasal Spray, 50 mcg, primarily in patients treated for longer than 4 weeks.

OVERDOSAGE

There are no data available on the effects of acute or chronic overdosage with NASONEX Nasal Spray, 50 mcg. Because of low systemic bioavailability, and an absence of acute drug-related systemic findings in clinical studies, overdose is unlikely to require any therapy other than observation. Intranasal administration of 1600 mcg (8 times the recommended dose of NASONEX Nasal Spray, 50 mcg) daily for 29 days, to healthy human volunteers, was well tolerated with no increased incidence of adverse events. Single intranasal doses up to 4000 mcg have been studied in human volunteers with no adverse effects reported. Single oral doses up to 8000 mcg have been studied in human volunteers with no adverse events reported. Chronic overdosage with any corticosteroid may result in signs or symptoms of hypercorticism (see **PRECAUTIONS**). Acute overdosage with this dosage form is unlikely since one bottle of NASONEX Nasal Spray, 50 mcg contains approximately 8500 mcg of mometasone furoate.

DOSAGE AND ADMINISTRATION

Adults and Children 12 Years of Age and Older: The usual recommended dose for prophylaxis and treatment of the nasal symptoms of seasonal allergic rhinitis and treatment of the nasal symptoms of perennial allergic rhinitis is two sprays (50 mcg of mometasone furoate in each spray) in each nostril once daily (total daily dose of 200 mcg).

In patients with a known seasonal allergen that precipitates nasal symptoms of seasonal allergic rhinitis, prophylaxis with NASONEX Nasal Spray, 50 mcg (200 mcg/day) is recommended 2 to 4 weeks prior to the anticipated start of the pollen season.

Improvement in nasal symptoms generally occurs within 2 days after the first dose. Maximum benefit is usually achieved within 1 to 2 weeks. Patients should use NASONEX Nasal Spray, 50 mcg only once daily at a regular interval.

Prior to initial use of NASONEX Nasal Spray, 50 mcg, the pump must be primed by actuating ten times or until a fine spray appears. The pump may be stored unused for up to 1 week without repriming. If unused for more than 1 week, reprime by actuating two times, or until a fine spray appears.

Directions for Use: Illustrated Patient's Instructions for Use accompany each package of NASONEX Nasal Spray, 50 mcg.

HOW SUPPLIED

NASONEX (mometasone furoate monohydrate) Nasal Spray, 50 mcg is supplied in a white, high-density, polyethylene bottle fitted with a white metered-dose, manual spray pump, and teal-blue dust cap. It contains 17 g of product formulation, 120 sprays, each delivering 50 mcg of mometasone furoate per actuation. Supplied with Patient's Instructions for Use (NDC 0085-1197-01).

Store between 2° and 25°C (36° and 77°F). Protect from light.

When NASONEX Nasal Spray, 50 mcg is removed from its cardboard container, prolonged exposure of the product to direct light should be avoided. Brief exposure to light, as with normal use, is acceptable.

SHAKE WELL BEFORE EACH USE.

Schering Corporation
Kenilworth, NJ 07033 USA
Copyright © 1997, Schering Corporation. All rights reserved.

9/97
20109807T

NETROMYCIN® ℞
brand of netilmicin sulfate
Injection, USP 100 mg/ml

WARNINGS

Patients treated with aminoglycosides should be under close clinical observation because of the potential toxicity associated with the use of these drugs.

Netilmicin has potent neuromuscular blocking potential. Neuromuscular blockade and respiratory paralysis have been reported in animals receiving netilmicin. The possibility of these phenomena occurring in man should be considered if aminoglycosides are administered by any route to patients receiving neuromuscular blocking agents, such as succinylcholine, tubocurarine, or decamethonium, or to patients receiving massive transfusions of citrate-anticoagulated blood. If neuromuscular blockade occurs, calcium salts may lessen it, but mechanical respiratory assistance may also be necessary.

As with other aminoglycosides, netilmicin sulfate injection is potentially nephrotoxic. The risk is greater in patients with impaired renal function, in those who receive high dosage or prolonged therapy, and in the elderly.

Neurotoxicity manifested by ototoxicity, both vestibular and auditory, can occur in patients treated with netilmicin, primarily in those with preexisting renal damage and in patients treated with higher doses and/ or for longer periods than recommended. Aminoglycoside-induced ototoxicity is usually irreversible. Other manifestations of aminoglycoside-induced neurotoxicity include numbness, skin tingling, muscle twitching, and convulsions.

Renal and eighth cranial nerve functions should be closely monitored, especially in patients with known or suspected impairment of renal function either at onset of therapy or during therapy. Urine should be examined for increased excretion of protein, the presence of cells or casts, and decreased specific gravity. Serum creatinine concentration or blood urea nitrogen should be determined periodically. A more precise measure of glomerular filtration rate is a carefully conducted determination of creatinine clearance rate or, often more practically, an estimate of creatinine clearance based on published nomograms or equations. (See **DOSAGE AND ADMINISTRATION**.) When feasible it is recommended that serial audiograms be obtained in patients old enough to be tested, particularly in high-risk patients. The dosage of netilmicin should be reduced or administration discontinued if evidence of drug-induced auditory or vestibular toxicity (dizziness, vertigo, tinnitus, nystagmus, or hearing loss) develops during therapy. If evidence of nephrotoxicity occurs, dosage should be adjusted. (See **DOSAGE AND ADMINISTRATION, DOSAGE FOR IMPAIRED RENAL FUNCTION**.) As with the other aminoglycosides, on rare occasions changes in renal and eighth cranial nerve functions may not become manifest until soon after completion of therapy.

Serum concentrations of aminoglycosides should be monitored when feasible to assure adequate levels and to avoid potentially toxic levels. After administration of an appropriate dose of netilmicin, peak serum concentrations occur approximately 30 to 60 minutes after an intramuscular injection or at the end of a one hour intravenous infusion. Dosage should be adjusted so that prolonged peak serum concentrations above 16 mcg/ml are avoided.

When monitoring trough concentrations, dosage should be adjusted so that levels above 4 mcg/ml are avoided. Excessive peak and/or trough serum concentrations of aminoglycosides may increase the risk of renal and eighth cranial nerve toxicity. In the event of overdose or toxic reactions, hemodialysis may aid in removal of netilmicin from the blood, especially if renal function is, or becomes, compromised. Removal of netilmicin by peritoneal dialysis is at a rate considerably less than by hemodialysis.

Concurrent and/or sequential systemic or topical use of other potentially neurotoxic and/or nephrotoxic drugs, such as: cephaloridine, amphotericin B, streptomycin, kanamycin, acyclovir, gentamicin, tobramycin, amikacin, neomycin, vancomycin, bacitracin, polymixin B, colistin, paromomycin, viomycin, or cisplatin should be avoided. The concurrent use of aminoglycosides with potent diuretics, such as ethacrynic acid or furosemide, should be avoided since certain diuretics by themselves may cause ototoxicity. In addition, when administered intravenously, diuretics may enhance aminoglycoside toxicity by altering the antibiotic concentration in the serum and tissues. Other factors which may increase patient risk of toxicity are advanced age and dehydration.

DESCRIPTION

NETROMYCIN Injection contains netilmicin sulfate, USP in clear, sterile aqueous solution with a pH range of 3.5 to 6.0 for intramuscular or intravenous administration. Netilmicin is a semisynthetic, water-soluble antibiotic of the aminoglycoside group, derived from sisomicin. Its chemical name is: *O*-3-Deoxy-4-*C* -methyl-3-(methylamino)- β -L-arabinopyranosyl (1→4)-*O*-[2,6-diamino-2,3,4,6-tetradeoxy-α-D-*glycero*-hex-4-enopyranosyl-(1→6)]-2-deoxy-N^3-ethyl-L-streptamine sulfate (2:5) (salt), having the following structural formula:

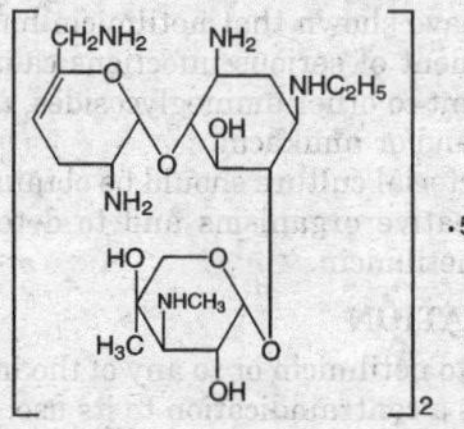

Each ml of NETROMYCIN Injection contains netilmicin sulfate, USP equivalent to 100 mg netilmicin; 10 mg benzyl alcohol as a preservative; 0.1 mg edetate disodium; 2.4 mg sodium metabisulfite; 0.8 mg sodium sulfite; and water for injection, q.s.

CLINICAL PHARMACOLOGY

Netilmicin is rapidly and completely absorbed after intramuscular injection. Peak serum levels, after intramuscular injection, usually occur within 30 to 60 minutes and levels are measurable for 12 hours. In adult volunteers with normal renal function, peak serum concentrations of netilmicin in mcg/ml are usually about 3 to 3.5 times the single intramuscular dose in mg/kg. For example, a dose of 2.0 mg/kg may be expected to result in a peak serum concentration of approximately 7 mcg/ml. At eight or more hours after administration of a dose in the recommended range, serum levels are usually less than 3 mcg/ml. When a single dose of netilmicin is administered by 60-minute intravenous infusion, the peak serum concentrations are similar to those obtained by intramuscular administration. Following a rapid intravenous injection of netilmicin, levels in serum may be transiently 2 to 3 times higher than those of the 60-minute infusion. Netilmicin rapidly distributes to tissues.

The half-life of netilmicin after single doses is usually 2 to 2.5 hours, a half-life which is very similar to that of gentamicin, and is independent of the route of administration. The half-life increases as the dose increases (e.g., 2.2 hours after a 1 mg/kg dose to 3 hours after a 3 mg/kg dose). Approximately 80% of the administered dose is excreted in the urine within 24 hours; the urine netilmicin concentration after a dose often exceeds 100 mcg/ml. There is no evidence of metabolic transformation of netilmicin. The drug is excreted principally by glomerular filtration. Probenecid does not affect renal tubular transport of aminoglycosides. The volume of distribution of netilmicin is approximately 20% of body weight; total body clearance is about 80 ml/min and renal clearance is about 60 ml/min. In multiple-dose studies in volunteers when the drug was administered every 12 hours at doses ranging from 1.0 to 4.0 mg/kg, steady-state levels were obtained by the second day.

The serum levels at steady-state were less than 20% higher than those of the first dose. As with other aminoglycosides, the half-life of netilmicin increases, and its renal clearance decreases with decreasing renal function.

The endogenous creatinine clearance rate and the serum creatinine level have a high correlation with the half-life of netilmicin. Results of these tests can serve as a guide for adjusting dosage in patients with renal impairment.

In patients with marked impairment of renal function, there is a decrease in the concentration of aminoglycosides in urine and in their penetration into defective renal parenchyma. This should be considered when treating patients with urinary tract infections. In one study of adults with renal failure undergoing hemodialysis, netilmicin serum levels were reduced by approximately 63% over an 8-hour dialysis session. Shorter dialysis sessions will remove less drug. No hemodialysis information is available for children. Aminoglycosides are also removed by peritoneal dialysis but at a rate considerably less than by hemodialysis.

Since netilmicin is distributed in extracellular fluid, peak serum concentrations may be lower than usual in patients whose extracellular fluid volume is expanded (e.g., patients with edema or ascites). Serum concentrations of aminoglycosides in febrile patients may be lower than those in afebrile patients given the same dose. When body temperature returns to normal, serum concentrations of the drug may rise. Both febrile and anemic states may be associated with a shorter than usual half-life. (Dosage adjustment is usually not necessary.)

In severely burned patients, the half-life of aminoglycosides may be significantly decreased, and serum concentrations resulting from a particular dose may be lower than anticipated.

The elimination half-life of netilmicin in neonates during the first week of life is inversely correlated with body weight, ranging from approximately 8 hours for neonates weighing 1.5 to 2.0 kg to approximately 4.5 hours for 3.0 to 4.0 kg neonates. The elimination half-life of infants and children 6 weeks of age and older is 1.5 to 2.0 hours.

Following parenteral administration, aminoglycosides can be detected in serum, tissues, and sputum and in pericardial, pleural, synovial, and peritoneal fluids. A variety of methods are available to measure netilmicin concentrations in body fluids; these include microbiologic, enzymatic, and radioimmunoassay techniques. Concentrations in renal cortex may be markedly higher than the usual serum levels.

Minute quantities of aminoglycosides have been detected in the urine for up to 30 days after discontinuing administration. Hepatic secretion is minimal. As with all aminoglycosides, netilmicin diffuses poorly into the subarachnoid space after parenteral administration. Concentrations of netilmicin in cerebrospinal fluid are often low and dependent upon dose and the degree of meningeal inflammation. Netilmicin crosses the placenta and has been detected in cord blood and in the fetus. Studies in nursing mothers indicate that small amounts of the drug are excreted in breast milk. Netilmicin is poorly absorbed from the intact gastrointestinal tract after oral administration. As with other aminoglycosides, the binding of netilmicin to serum proteins is low (0–30%).

Microbiology: Netilmicin is a rapidly acting, broad-spectrum bactericidal antibiotic which appears to act by inhibiting normal protein synthesis in susceptible microorganisms. Netilmicin is active *in vitro* against a wide variety of pathogenic bacteria, primarily gram-negative bacilli and also a few gram-positive organisms including *Citrobacter, Enterobacter, Escherichia coli, Klebsiella* species, *Proteus mirabilis, Pseudomonas aeruginosa, Salmonella* species, *Shigella* species, and *Staphylococcus* species (penicillin- and methicillin-resistant strains).

Netilmicin is also active *in vitro* against some isolates of *Acinetobacter* and *Neisseria* species, indole-positive *Proteus* species, *Pseudomonas* and *Serratia* species. In addition, netilmicin is active *in vitro* against many strains which have acquired resistance to other aminoglycosides. Such resistance is usually caused by aminoglycoside modifying (inactivating) enzymes. In general, netilmicin is active against organisms which inactivate aminoglycosides by either phosphorylation or adenylylation; it has variable activity against acetylating strains, depending on the specific type. For example, the susceptibility of *Serratia* species producing a combination of adenylylating and acetylating enzymes varies according to the level of acetylating enzyme present. Netilmicin is active *in vitro* against certain strains of gram-negative bacteria resistant to gentamicin and tobramycin: *Citrobacter, Enterobacter* species, *Escherichia coli, Klebsiella, Proteus* (indole-positive), *Pseudomonas, Salmonella,* and *Shigella* species. Netilmicin is active *in vitro* against certain staphylococci resistant to amikacin and tobramycin. Like other aminoglycosides, netilmicin is not active against bacteria with reduced permeability to this class of antibiotics.

Most species of streptococci and anaerobic organisms, such as *Bacteroides* and *Clostridium* species, are resistant to aminoglycosides.

The *in vitro* activity of netilmicin and of other aminoglycosides is affected by media pH, protein content, divalent cation concentration, and inoculum size.

Netilmicin acts synergistically *in vitro* with members of the penicillin class of antibiotics against *Streptococcus faecalis.* It also acts synergistically with those penicillins which are active alone against many strains of *Pseudomonas.* In addition, many, but not all isolates of *Serratia* which are resistant to multiple antibiotics, are inhibited by synergistic combinations of netilmicin with carbenicillin, azlocillin, mezlocillin, cefamandole, cefotaxime, or moxalactam. Tests for antibiotic synergy are necessary.

Susceptibility Testing: Quantitative methods that require measurements of zone diameters give the most precise estimates of antibiotic susceptibility. One such procedure has been recommended for use with discs to test susceptibility to netilmicin. Interpretation involves correlation of the diameters obtained in the disc test with minimal inhibitory concentration (MIC) values for netilmicin.

Reports from the laboratory giving results of the standardized single disc susceptibility test (Bauer, et al. Am J Clin Path 1966; 45:493 and Federal Register 37:20525–20529, 1972), using a 30 mcg netilmicin disc should be interpreted according to the following criteria:

Continued on next page

Information on Schering products appearing on these pages is effective as of August 15, 1998.

Netromycin—Cont.

Organisms producing zones of 15 mm or greater, or MIC's of 8.0 mcg or less are considered susceptible, indicating that the tested organism is likely to respond to therapy.

Resistant organisms produce zones of 12 mm or less or MIC's of 16 mcg or greater. A report of "resistant" from the laboratory indicates that the infecting organism is not likely to respond to therapy.

Zones greater than 12 mm and less than 15 mm, or MIC's of greater than 8.0 mcg and less than 16 mcg, indicate intermediate susceptibility. A report of "intermediate" susceptibility suggests that the organism would be susceptible if the infection is confined to tissues and fluids (e.g., urine), in which high antibiotic levels are attained.

Control organisms are recommended for susceptibility testing. Each time the test is performed one or more of the following organisms should be included: *Escherichia coli* ATCC 25922, *Staphylococcus aureus* ATCC 25923, and *Pseudomonas aeruginosa* ATCC 27853. The control organisms should produce zones of inhibition within the following ranges:

Escherichia coli (ATCC 25922) 22–30 mm

Staphylococcus aureus (ATCC 25923) 22–31 mm

Pseudomonas aeruginosa (ATCC 27853) 17–23 mm

In certain circumstances, particularly with strains of *Pseudomonas aeruginosa*, it may be desirable to do additional susceptibility testing by the tube or agar dilution method. Netilmicin sulfate powder, a diagnostic reagent, is available for this purpose.

The MIC values of netilmicin for the control strains are the following:

Escherichia coli (ATCC 25922) 0.25–0.5 mcg/ml

Staphylococcus aureus (ATCC 25923) 0.125–0.25 mcg/ml

Pseudomonas aeruginosa (ATCC 27853) 4–8 mcg/ml in media supplemented with calcium and magnesium.

INDICATIONS AND USAGE

Netilmicin sulfate injection is indicated for the short-term treatment of patients of all ages, including neonates, infants, and children with serious or life-threatening bacterial infections caused by susceptible strains of the designated microorganisms in the diseases listed below:

COMPLICATED URINARY TRACT infections caused by *Escherichia coli, Klebsiella pneumoniae, Pseudomonas aeruginosa, Enterobacter* species, *Proteus mirabilis, Proteus* species (indole-positive), *Serratia** and *Citrobacter* species, and *Staphylococcus aureus.***

SEPTICEMIA caused by *Escherichia coli, Klebsiella pneumoniae, Pseudomonas aeruginosa, Enterobacter* and *Serratia** species, and *Proteus mirabilis.*

SKIN AND SKIN STRUCTURE infections caused by *Escherichia coli, Klebsiella pneumoniae, Pseudomonas aeruginosa, Enterobacter* and *Serratia** species. *Proteus mirabilis, Proteus* species (indole-positive), and *Staphylococcus aureus*** (pencillinase- and non-penicillinase- producing strains).

INTRA-ABDOMINAL infections including peritonitis and intra-abdominal abscess caused by *Escherichia coli, Klebsiella pneumoniae, Pseudomonas aeruginosa, Enterobacter* species, *Proteus mirabilis, Proteus* species (indole-positive), and *Staphylococcus aureus*** (penicillinase- and non-penicillinase-producing strains).

LOWER RESPIRATORY TRACT infections caused by *Escherichia coli, Klebsiella pneumoniae, Pseudomonas aeruginosa, Enterobacter* and *Serratia** species, *Proteus mirabilis, Proteus* species (indole-positive), and *Staphylococcus aureus*** (penicillinase- and non-penicillinase-producing strains).

*(See **Microbiology** Section.)

**While not the antibiotic class of first choice, aminoglycosides, including netilmicin, may be considered for the treatment of serious staphylococcal infections when penicillins or other less potentially toxic drugs are contraindicated and bacterial susceptibility tests and clinical judgment indicate their use. They may also be considered in mixed infections caused by susceptible strains of staphylococci and gram-negative organisms.

Aminoglycosides are indicated for those infections for which less potentially toxic antimicrobial agents are ineffective or contraindicated. They are not indicated in the treatment of uncomplicated initial episodes of urinary tract infection unless the causative organisms are resistant to antimicrobial agents having less potential toxicity.

Netilmicin sulfate injection may be considered as initial therapy in suspected or confirmed gram-negative infections, and therapy may be instituted before obtaining results of susceptibility testing. The decision to continue therapy with netilmicin should be based on the results of susceptibility tests, the severity of the infection, and the important additional concepts contained in the "**WARNINGS** Box" above. If the causative organisms are resistant to netilmicin, other appropriate therapy should be instituted.

In serious infections when the causative organisms are unknown, netilmicin may be administered as initial therapy in conjunction with a penicillin-type or cephalosporin-type drug before obtaining results of susceptibility testing. In neonates with suspected sepsis, a penicillin-type drug is also usually indicated as concomitant therapy with netilmicin. If anaerobic organisms are suspected as etiologic agents, other suitable antimicrobial therapy should also be given. Following identification of the organism and its susceptibility, appropriate antibiotic therapy should then be continued.

Netilmicin sulfate injection has been used effectively in combination with carbenicillin or ticarcillin for the treatment of life-threatening infections caused by *Pseudomonas aeruginosa.*

Clinical studies have shown that netilmicin has been effective in the treatment of serious infections caused by some organisms resistant to other aminoglycosides, *i.e.,* gentamicin, tobramycin, and/or amikacin.

Specimens for bacterial culture should be obtained to isolate and identify causative organisms and to determine their susceptibility to netilmicin.

CONTRAINDICATION

Hypersensitivity to netilmicin or to any of the ingredients of the preparation is a contraindication to its use. See **WARNINGS** if patient is hypersensitive to another aminoglycoside.

WARNINGS

(See "**WARNINGS** Box" above.) If the patient has a history of hypersensitivity or serious toxic reaction to another aminoglycoside, netilmicin should be used very cautiously, if at all, because cross-sensitivity to drugs in this class has been reported.

Aminoglycosides can cause fetal harm when administered to a pregnant woman. Aminoglycoside antibiotics cross the placenta and there have been several reports of total irreversible bilateral congenital deafness in children whose mothers received streptomycin during pregnancy. Although serious side effects to fetus or newborn have not been reported in the treatment of pregnant women with other aminoglycosides, the potential for harm exists. Reproduction studies of netilmicin have been performed in rats and rabbits using intramuscular and subcutaneous doses approximately 13–15 times the highest adult human dose and have revealed no evidence of impairment of fertility or harm to the fetus. Moreover, there was no evidence of ototoxicity in the offspring of rats treated subcutaneously with netilmicin throughout pregnancy and during the subsequent lactation period. It is not known whether netilmicin sulfate can cause fetal harm when administered to a pregnant woman or can affect reproduction capacity. However, if this drug is used during pregnancy, or if the patient becomes pregnant while taking this drug, the patient should be apprised of the potential hazard to the fetus.

NETROMYCIN Injection contains sodium metabisulfite and sodium sulfite, which may cause allergic-type reactions including anaphylactic symptoms and life-threatening or less severe asthmatic episodes in certain susceptible people. The overall prevalence of sulfite sensitivity in the general population is unknown and probably low. Sulfite sensitivity is seen more frequently in asthmatic than in nonasthmatic people.

PRECAUTIONS

General: Neurotoxic and nephrotoxic antibiotics may be almost completely absorbed from body surfaces (except the urinary bladder) after local irrigation and after topical application during surgical procedures. The potential toxic effects of antibiotics administered in this fashion (neuromuscular blockade, respiratory paralysis, oto- and nephrotoxicity) should be considered. (See "**WARNINGS** Box.")

Increased nephrotoxicity has been reported following concomitant administration of aminoglycoside antibiotics with some cephalosporins.

Aminoglycosides should be used with caution in patients with neuromuscular disorders, such as myasthenia gravis, or infant botulism, since these drugs may aggravate muscle weakness because of their potential curare-like effect on the neuromuscular junction.

During or following netilmicin therapy, parasthesias, tetany, positive Chvostek and Trousseau signs, and mental confusion have been described in patients with hypomagnesemia, hypocalcemia, and hypokalemia. When this has occurred in infants, tetany and muscle weakness has been described. Both adults and infants required appropriate corrective electrolyte therapy.

Elderly patients may have reduced renal function which may not be evident in the results of routine screening tests, such as BUN or serum creatinine levels. Determination of creatinine clearance or an estimate based on published nomograms or equations may be more useful. Monitoring of renal function during treatment with netilmicin, as with other aminoglycosides, is particularly important in such patients. A Fanconi-like syndrome, with aminoaciduria and metabolic acidosis, has been reported in some adults and infants being given netilmicin injections.

Patients should be well hydrated during treatment.

Treatment with netilmicin may result in overgrowth of non-susceptible organisms. If this occurs, appropriate therapy is indicated.

Laboratory Tests: *Tests of renal function:* Urine should be examined periodically for increased excretion of protein and the presence of cells and casts, keeping in mind the effects of the primary illness on these tests. One or more of the following laboratory measurements should be obtained at the onset of therapy, periodically during therapy, and at, or shortly after, the end of therapy:

• creatinine clearance rate (either carefully measured or estimated from published nomograms or equations based on the patient's age, sex, body weight, and serum creatinine concentration) (preferred over BUN);

• serum creatinine concentration (preferred over BUN);

• blood urea nitrogen (BUN).

More frequent testing is desirable if renal function is changing.

See also "**PRECAUTIONS, General**" above regarding elderly patients.

Test of eighth cranial nerve functions: Serial audiometric tests are suggested, particularly when renal function is impaired and/or prolonged aminoglycoside therapy is required; such tests should also be repeated periodically after treatment if there is evidence of a hearing deficit or vestibular abnormality before or during therapy, or when consecutive or concomitant use of other potentially ototoxic drugs is unavoidable.

Drug Interactions: *In vitro* mixing of an aminoglycoside with beta-lactam-type antibiotics (penicillins or cephalosporins) may result in a significant mutual inactivation. Even when an aminoglycoside and a penicillin-type drug are administered separately by different routes, a reduction in aminoglycoside serum half-life or serum levels has been reported in patients with impaired renal function and in some patients with normal renal function. Usually, such inactivation of the aminoglycoside is clinically significant only in patients with severely impaired renal function. (See also "Drug/Laboratory Test Interactions.") See "**WARNINGS** Box" regarding concurrent use of potent diuretics, concurrent and/or sequential use of other neurotoxic and/or nephrotoxic antibiotics, and for other essential information.

See also "**PRECAUTIONS, General.**"

Drug/Laboratory Test Interactions: Concomitant cephalosporin therapy may spuriously elevate creatinine determinations.

The inactivation between aminoglycosides and beta-lactam antibiotics described in "Drug Interactions" may continue in specimens of body fluids collected for assay, resulting in inaccurate, false low aminoglycoside readings. Such specimens should be properly handled, *i.e.,* assayed promptly, frozen, or treated with beta-lactamase.

Carcinogenesis, Mutagenesis, Impairment of Fertility: Lifetime carcinogenicity tests have been undertaken in the mouse and rat and no drug-related tumors were observed. Similarly, mutagenesis tests with netilmicin have proven negative, and no impairment in fertility has been observed in the rat.

Pregnancy Category D: (See **WARNINGS** Section.)

Nursing Mothers: Clinical studies in nursing mothers indicate that small amounts of netilmicin are excreted in breast milk. Because of the potential for serious adverse reactions from aminoglycosides in nursing infants, a decision should be made whether to discontinue nursing or to discontinue the drug, taking into account the importance of the drug to the mother.

Pediatric Use: Aminoglycosides should be used with caution in prematures and neonates because of the renal immaturity of these patients and the resulting prolongation of serum half-life of these drugs (also see **DOSAGE AND ADMINISTRATION** for use in Neonates and Children).

ADVERSE REACTIONS

Nephrotoxicity—Adverse renal effects due to netilmicin were reported in 7 per 100 patients.

They were demonstrated by a rise in serum creatinine and may have been accompanied by oliguria; the presence of casts, cells or protein in the urine; by rising levels of BUN; or by decreasing creatinine clearance rates. These effects occurred more frequently in the elderly, in patients with a history of renal impairment, and in patients treated for longer periods or with larger doses than recommended. While permanent impairment of renal function may occur following aminoglycoside therapy, observed renal impairment associated with netilmicin was usually mild and reversible after treatment ended while the drug was being excreted.

Neurotoxicity—Adverse effects on both the auditory and vestibular branches of the eighth cranial nerves have been reported.

Audiometric changes associated with netilmicin occurred in approximately 4 per 100 patients. Subjective netilmicin-related hearing loss occurred in about 1 per 250 patients. Vestibular abnormalities related to netilmicin were seen in 1 per 150 patients. Factors which may increase the risk of aminoglycoside-induced ototoxicity include renal impairment (especially if dialysis is required), excessive dosage,

TABLE I

DOSAGE GUIDE FOR ADULTS WITH NORMAL RENAL FUNCTION

Patient's Weight*		For Complicated Urinary Tract Infections, Give 3.0–4.0 mg/kg/day as 1.5–2.0 mg/kg	For Serious Systemic Infections Give 4.0–6.5 mg/kg/day as	
			1.3–2.2 mg/kg or 2.0–3.25 mg/kg	
kg	(lb)	EVERY 12 HOURS mg/dose	EVERY 8 HOURS mg/dose	EVERY 12 HOURS mg/dose
40	(88)	60– 80	52– 88	80–130
45	(99)	68– 90	59– 99	90–146
50	(110)	75–100	65–110	100–163
55	(121)	83–110	72–121	110–179
60	(132)	90–120	78–132	120–195
65	(143)	98–130	85–143	130–211
70	(154)	105–140	91–154	140–228
75	(165)	113–150	98–165	150–244
80	(176)	120–160	104–176	160–260
85	(187)	128–170	111–187	170–276
90	(198)	135–180	117–198	180–293
95	(209)	143–190	124–209	190–309
100	(220)	150–200	130–220	200–325

* The dosage of aminoglycosides in obese patients should be based on an estimate of the lean body mass.

dehydration, concomitant administration of ethacrynic acid or furosemide, or previous exposure to other ototoxic drugs. Peripheral neuropathy or encephalopathy including numbness, skin tingling, muscle twitching, convulsions, and myasthenia gravis-like syndrome have been reported.

Symptoms include dizziness, vertigo, tinnitus, nystagmus, and hearing loss. Aminoglycoside-induced ototoxicity is usually irreversible. Cochlear damage is usually manifested initially by small changes in audiometric test results at the higher frequencies and may not be associated with subjective hearing loss. Vestibular dysfunction is usually manifested by nystagmus, vertigo, nausea, vomiting, or acute Meniere's syndrome.

The risk of toxic reactions is low in patients with normal renal function who do not receive netilmicin injection at higher doses or for longer periods of time than recommended. Some patients who have had previous neurotoxic reactions to other aminoglycosides have been treated with netilmicin without further neurotoxicity.

Neuromuscular blockade manifested as acute muscular paralysis and apnea can occur following treatment with aminoglycosides. (See "WARNINGS Box.")

The approximate incidence of other reported adverse reactions to netilmicin injection follows: increased levels of serum transaminase (SGOT or SGPT), alkaline phosphatase, or bilirubin in 15 patients per 1000; rash or itching in 4 or 5 patients per 1000; eosinophilia in 4 patients per 1000; thrombocytosis in 2 patients per 1000; prolonged prothrombin time in 1 patient per 1000; fever in 1 patient per 1000. Fewer than one patient per 1000 was reported to have netilmicin-related anemia, leukopenia, thrombocytopenia, leukemoid reaction, immature circulating white blood cells,

hyperkalemia, vomiting, diarrhea, palpitations, hypotension, headache, disorientation, blurred vision, or paresthesias. Local tolerance to intramuscular injection and intravenous infusion of netilmicin is generally excellent, but approximately four patients per 1000 have had severe pain, and similar numbers had induration or hematomas.

OVERDOSAGE

In the event of overdosage or toxic reaction, netilmicin can be removed from the blood by hemodialysis, and is especially important if renal function is, or becomes, compromised. Although there is no specific information concerning removal of netilmicin by peritoneal dialysis, other aminoglycosides are known to be removed by this method but at a rate considerably less than by hemodialysis.

DOSAGE AND ADMINISTRATION

Netilmicin injection may be given intramuscularly or intravenously. (See CLINICAL PHARMACOLOGY.) The recommended dosage for both methods of administration is identical.

The patient's pretreatment body weight should be obtained for calculation of correct dosage. The dosage of aminoglycosides in obese patients should be based on an estimate of the lean body mass.

The status of renal function should be estimated by measurement of the serum creatinine concentration or calculation of the endogenous creatinine clearance rate. The blood urea nitrogen (BUN) level is much less reliable for this purpose. Reassessment of renal function should be made periodically during therapy.

In patients with extensive body surface burns, altered pharmacokinetics may result in reduced serum concentrations of aminoglycosides. Measurement of netilmicin serum concentrations is particularly important as a basis for dosage adjustment in such patients.

Duration of Treatment: It is desirable to limit the duration of treatment with aminoglycosides to short-term whenever feasible. The usual duration of treatment for all patients is seven to fourteen days. In complicated infections, a longer course of therapy may be necessary. Although prolonged courses of netilmicin injection have been well tolerated, it is particularly important that patients treated for longer than the usual period be carefully monitored for changes in renal, auditory, and vestibular functions. Dosage should be adjusted if clinically indicated.

Measurement of Serum Concentrations: It is desirable to measure both peak and trough serum concentrations of netilmicin to determine the adequacy and safety of the administered dosage.

When such measurements are feasible, they should be carried out periodically during therapy. Peak serum concentrations are expected to range from 4 to 12 mcg/ml. Dosage should be adjusted to attain the desired peak and trough concentrations and to avoid prolonged peak serum concentrations above 16 mcg/ml. When monitoring trough concentrations (just prior to the next dose), dosage should be adjusted so that levels above 4 mcg/ml are avoided. Interpatient variation of aminoglycoside serum concentrations occurs in patients with normal or abnormal renal function. Generally, desirable peak and trough concentrations will be in the range of 6–10 and 0.5–2 mcg/ml, respectively.

Determination of the adequacy of a serum level for a particular patient must take into consideration the susceptibility of the causative organism, the severity of the infection, and the status of the patient's host-defense mechanisms.

The dosage recommendations which follow are not intended as rigid schedules, but are provided as guides for initial therapy, or for when the measurement of netilmicin serum levels during therapy is not feasible.

DOSAGE FOR PATIENTS WITH NORMAL RENAL FUNCTION

Table I shows the recommended dosage of netilmicin injection for patients of various ages with normal renal function. [See table I above]

Although a causal relationship has not been established, administration of injections preserved with benzyl alcohol has been associated with toxicity in neonates. Caution should be used when NETROMYCIN Injection (100 mg/ml) is administered to neonates and children.

  Neonates (less than 6 weeks): 4.0 to 6.5 mg/kg/day given as 2.0 to 3.25 mg/kg every 12 hours.

  Infants and Children (6 weeks through 12 years): 5.5 to 8.0 mg/kg/day given either as 1.8 to 2.7 mg/kg every 8 hours, or as 2.7 to 4.0 mg/kg every 12 hours.

DOSAGE FOR PATIENTS WITH IMPAIRED RENAL FUNCTION

Dosage must be individualized in patients with impaired renal function to ensure therapeutic levels are attained. There

Continued on next page

TABLE II
LARGE VOLUME PARENTERAL SOLUTIONS IN WHICH NETILMICIN SULFATE IS STABLE

Products/Compositions Tested	Other Trade Names and Manufacturers
	(Solutions of Same Composition)
Sterile Water for Injection 0.9% Sodium Chloride Injection alone or with 5% Dextrose	
5% or 10% Dextrose Injection in Water, or 5% Dextrose in Polysal Injection, or 5% Dextrose with Electrolyte #48 or #75	
Ringer's and Lactated Ringer's, and Lactated Ringer's with 5% Dextrose Injection	
10% Travert with Electrolyte #2 or #3 Injection (Travenol)	Electrolyte #3 (Cooke & Crowley's Solution) with 10% Inverted Sugar Injection (Cutter)
Isolyte E, M, or P with 5% Dextrose Injection	
10% Dextran 40 or 6% Dextran 75 in 5% Dextrose Injection	
Plasma-Lyte 56 or 148 Injection with 5% Dextrose (Travenol)	Normosol-M or R in D5-W (Abbott), Isolyte H or S with 5% Dextrose (McGaw), Polyonic R-148 or M-56 with 5% Dextrose (Cutter)
Plasma-Lyte M Injection 5% Dextrose (Travenol)	Polysal M with 5% Dextrose (Cutter)
Ionosol B in D5-W	
5% Amigen Injection alone or with 5% Dextrose	
Normosol-R	Polyonic R-148 (Cutter), Isolyte S (McGaw), Plasma-Lyte 148 Injection in Water (Travenol)
Polysal (Plain)	
Aminosol 5% Injection	
Fre-Amine II 8.5% Injection	
Plasma-Lyte 148 Injection (approx. pH 7.4) (Travenol)	Normosol-R pH 7.4 (Abbott)
10% Fructose Injection	

Information on Schering products appearing on these pages is effective as of August 15, 1998.

Netromycin—Cont.

are several methods of doing this; however, dosage adjustment based upon the measurement of serum drug concentrations during treatment is the most accurate.

If netilmicin serum concentrations are not available and renal function is stable, serum creatinine and creatinine clearance values are the most reliable, readily available indicators of the degree of renal impairment for use as a guide for dosage adjustment.

It is also important to recognize that deteriorating renal function may require a greater reduction in dosage than that specified in the guidelines given below for patients with stable renal impairment.

The initial or loading dose is the same as that for a patient with normal renal function. A number of methods are available to adjust the total daily dosage for the degree of renal impairment. Three suggested methods are:

1) Divide the suggested dosage value for patients with normal renal function from Table I above by the serum creatinine level to obtain the adjusted size of each dose.
2) If the creatinine clearance rate is known or can be estimated from the serum creatinine levels using the formula given below, the adjusted daily dose of netilmicin may be determined by multiplying the dose given in Table I by:

$$\frac{\text{Patient's Creatinine Clearance Rate}}{\text{Normal Creatinine Clearance Rate}}$$

3) Alternatively, the following graph may be used to obtain the percentage of the dose selected from Table I, which should be administered at 8-hour intervals:

REDUCED DOSAGE GRAPH

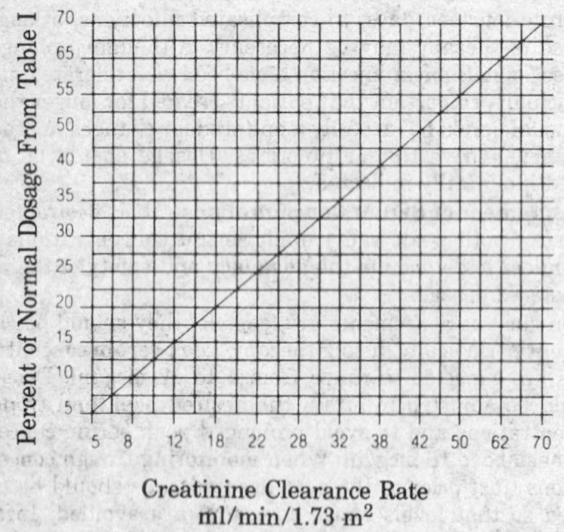

Creatinine clearance can be estimated from serum creatinine levels by the following formula for adult males; multiply by 0.85 for adult females (Nephron, 1976; 16:31–41):

$$C_{cr} = \frac{(140 - \text{Age})(\text{Wt. Kg})}{72 \times S_{cr}(\text{mg/100 ml})}$$

The adjusted total daily dose may be administered as one dose at 24-hour intervals, or as 2 or 3 equally divided doses at 12-hour or 8-hour intervals, respectively. Generally, each individual dose should not exceed 3.25 mg/kg. In adults with renal failure who are undergoing hemodialysis, the amount of netilmicin removed from the blood may vary depending upon the dialysis equipment and methods used. (See **CLINICAL PHARMACOLOGY**.) In adults, a dose of 2.0 mg/kg at the end of each dialysis period is recommended until the results of tests measuring netilmicin serum levels become available. Dosage should then be appropriately adjusted based on these tests.

ALTERNATE DOSING METHOD FOR PATIENTS WITH NORMAL OR IMPAIRED RENAL FUNCTION

An alternate method of determining a dosage regimen (dose and dosing interval) applicable to all ages and all states of renal function (both normal and abnormal) is to employ pharmacokinetic parameters derived from measurements of serum concentrations.

Following the administration of an initial dose of netilmicin and the determination of drug serum concentrations in post-infusion blood samples, the drug's half-life and the patient's elimination rate constant and volume of distribution can be calculated. Desired peak and trough serum levels for a particular patient are then selected by taking into consideration the susceptibility of the causative organism, the severity of infection, and the status of the patient's host-defense mechanisms. The dosage regimen (dose and dosing interval) is then determined using standardized formulae and the appropriate computer program, and the dosage regimen can be adjusted to the nearest practical interval and amount.

ADDITION OF NETILMICIN SULFATE TO VARIOUS INTRAVENOUS PREPARATIONS

In adults, a single dose of netilmicin injection may be diluted in 50 to 200 ml of one of the parenteral solutions listed below. In infants and children, the volume of diluent should be less according to the fluid requirements of the patient. The solution may be infused over a period of one-half to two hours.

Tested at concentrations of 2.1 to 3.0 mg/ml, netilmicin sulfate has been shown to be stable in the following large volume parenteral solutions for up to 72 hours when stored in glass containers, both when refrigerated and at room temperature. Use after this time period is not recommended.

[See table II at bottom of previous page]

Parenteral drug products should be inspected visually for particulate matter and discoloration prior to administration, whenever solution and container permit.

HOW SUPPLIED

NETROMYCIN Injection 100 mg/ml is supplied in 1.5 ml vials, box of 10 (NDC 0085-0264-02). **Store between 2° and 30°C (36° and 86°F).**

ANIMAL PHARMACOLOGY AND/OR ANIMAL TOXICOLOGY

Netilmicin sulfate, administered by the intravenous and intramuscular routes, has been compared to kanamycin, sisomicin, gentamicin, amikacin, and tobramycin in studies ranging in duration from two weeks to three months. Among the aminoglycosides, netilmicin is one of the more potent neuromuscular-blocking agents; however, in six different species, netilmicin sulfate has proven to be the least nephrotoxic and ototoxic of these aminoglycosides, using morphological as well as functional end points. In the clinical trials nephrotoxicity and ototoxicity occurred at about the same frequency in netilmicin-treated patients as in those treated with other aminoglycosides.

Schering Biochem Corporation,
Manati, Puerto Rico 00701
An Affiliate of Schering Corporation,
Kenilworth, NJ 07033

Revised 1/87 12759568

An Affiliate of Schering Corporation,
Kenilworth, NJ 07033

Revised 1/87 12759568

Copyright © 1980, 1983, 1984, 1987, Schering Corporation, USA. All rights reserved.

NORMODYNE® ℞

brand of labetalol hydrochloride, USP
Injection

DESCRIPTION

NORMODYNE (labetalol HCl) is an adrenergic receptor blocking agent that has both selective alpha$_1$- and nonselective beta-adrenergic receptor blocking actions in a single substance.

Labetalol HCl is a racemate, chemically designated as 5-[1-hydroxy-2-[(1-methyl-3-phenylpropyl) amino] ethyl]salicylamide monohydrochloride, and has the following structure:

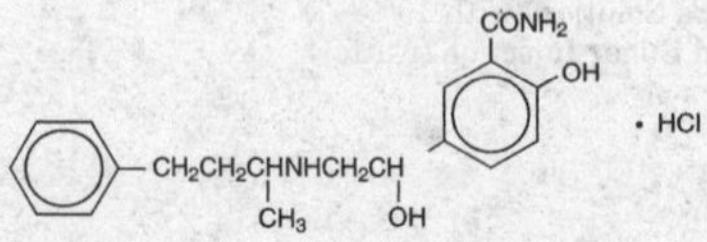

Labetalol HCl has the empirical formula $C_{19}H_{24}N_2O_3 \cdot HCl$ and a molecular weight of 364.9. It has two asymmetric centers and therefore exists as a molecular complex of two diastereoisomeric pairs. Dilevalol, the R,R′ stereoisomer, makes up 25% of racemic labetalol.

Labetalol HCl is a white or off-white crystalline powder, soluble in water.

NORMODYNE (labetalol HCl) Injection is a clear, colorless to light yellow aqueous sterile isotonic solution for intravenous injection. It has a pH range of 3.0 to 4.0. Each mL contains 5 mg labetalol HCl, USP, 45 mg anhydrous dextrose, 0.10 mg edetate disodium; 0.80 mg methylparaben and 0.10 mg propylparaben as preservatives; citric acid monohydrate and sodium hydroxide, as necessary, to bring the solution into the pH range.

CLINICAL PHARMACOLOGY

NORMODYNE (labetalol HCl) combines both selective, competitive alpha$_1$-adrenergic blocking and nonselective, competitive beta-adrenergic blocking activity in a single substance. In man, the ratios of alpha- to beta-blockade have been estimated to be approximately 1:3 and 1:7 following oral and intravenous administration, respectively. Beta$_2$-agonist activity has been demonstrated in animals with minimal beta$_1$-agonist (ISA) activity detected. In animals, at doses greater than those required for alpha- or beta-adrenergic blockade, a membrane-stabilizing effect has been demonstrated.

Pharmacodynamics The capacity of labetalol HCl to block alpha-receptors in man has been demonstrated by attenuation of the pressor effect of phenylephrine and by a significant reduction of the pressor response caused by immersing the hand in ice-cold water ("cold-pressor test"). Labetalol HCl's beta$_1$-receptor blockade in man was demonstrated by a small decrease in the resting heart rate, attenuation of tachycardia produced by isoproterenol or exercise, and by attenuation of the reflex tachycardia to the hypotension produced by amyl nitrite. Beta$_2$-receptor blockade was demonstrated by inhibition of the isoproterenol-induced fall in diastolic blood pressure. Both the alpha- and beta-blocking actions of orally administered labetalol HCl contribute to a decrease in blood pressure in hypertensive patients. Labetalol HCl consistently, in dose-related fashion, blunted increases in exercise-induced blood pressure and heart rate, and in their double product. The pulmonary circulation during exercise was not affected by labetalol HCl dosing.

Single oral doses of labetalol HCl administered in patients with coronary artery disease had no significant effect on sinus rate, intraventricular conduction, or QRS duration. The AV conduction time was modestly prolonged in 2 of 7 patients. In another study, intravenous labetalol HCl slightly prolonged AV nodal conduction time and atrial effective refractory period with only small changes in heart rate. The effects on AV nodal refractoriness were inconsistent.

Labetalol HCl produces dose-related falls in blood pressure without reflex tachycardia and without significant reduction in heart rate, presumably through a mixture of its alpha-blocking and beta-blocking effects. Hemodynamic effects are variable with small nonsignificant changes in cardiac output seen in some studies but not others, and small decreases in total peripheral resistance. Elevated plasma renins are reduced.

Doses of labetalol HCl that controlled hypertension did not affect renal function in mild to severe hypertensive patients with normal renal function.

Due to the alpha$_1$-receptor blocking activity of labetalol HCl, blood pressure is lowered more in the standing than in the supine position, and symptoms of postural hypotension can occur. During dosing with intravenous labetalol HCl, the contribution of the postural component should be considered when positioning patients for treatment, and patients should not be allowed to move to an erect position unmonitored until their ability to do so is established.

In a clinical pharmacologic study in severe hypertensives, an initial 0.25 mg/kg injection of labetalol HCl, administered to patients in the supine position, decreased blood pressure by an average of 11/7 mmHg. Additional injections of 0.5 mg/kg at 15-minute intervals up to a total cumulative dose of 1.75 mg/kg of labetalol HCl caused further dose-related decreases in blood pressure. Some patients required cumulative doses of up to 3.25 mg/kg. The maximal effect of each dose level occurred within 5 minutes. Following discontinuation of intravenous treatment with labetalol HCl, the blood pressure rose gradually and progressively, approaching pretreatment baseline values within an average of 16–18 hours in the majority of patients.

Similar results were obtained in the treatment of patients with severe hypertension requiring urgent blood pressure reduction with an initial dose of 20 mg (which corresponds to 0.25 mg/kg for an 80 kg patient) followed by additional doses of either 40 or 80 mg at 10-minute intervals to achieve the desired effect or up to a cumulative dose of 300 mg.

Labetalol HCl administered as a continuous intravenous infusion, with a mean dose of 136 mg (27 to 300 mg) over a period of 2 to 3 hours (mean of 2 hours and 39 minutes) lowered the blood pressure by an average of 60/35 mmHg.

Exacerbation of angina and, in some cases, myocardial infarction and ventricular dysrhythmias have been reported after abrupt discontinuation of therapy with beta-adrenergic blocking agents in patients with coronary artery disease. Abrupt withdrawal of these agents in patients without coronary artery disease has resulted in transient symptoms, including tremulousness, sweating, palpitation, headache, and malaise. Several mechanisms have been proposed to explain these phenomena, among them increased sensitivity to catecholamines because of increased numbers of beta-receptors.

Although beta-adrenergic receptor blockade is useful in the treatment of angina and hypertension, there are also situations in which sympathetic stimulation is vital. For example, in patients with severely damaged hearts, adequate ventricular function may depend on sympathetic drive. Beta-adrenergic blockade may worsen AV block by preventing the necessary facilitating effects of sympathetic activity on conduction. Beta$_2$-adrenergic blockade results in passive bronchial constriction by interfering with endogenous adrenergic bronchodilator activity in patients subject to bronchospasm and may also interfere with exogenous bronchodilators in such patients.

Pharmacokinetics and Metabolism Following intravenous infusion, the elimination half-life is about 5.5 hours and the total body clearance is approximately 33 mL/min/kg. The plasma half-life of labetalol following oral administration is about 6 to 8 hours. In patients with decreased hepatic or renal function, the elimination half-life of labetalol is not altered; however, the relative bioavailability in hepatically impaired patients is increased due to decreased "first-pass" metabolism.

The metabolism of labetalol is mainly through conjugation to glucuronide metabolites. These metabolites are present in plasma and are excreted in the urine and, via the bile, into the feces. Approximately 55% to 60% of a dose appears in the urine as conjugates or unchanged labetalol within the first 24 hours of dosing.

Labetalol has been shown to cross the placental barrier in humans. Only negligible amounts of the drug crossed the blood-brain barrier in animal studies. Labetalol is approximately 50% protein bound. Neither hemodialysis nor peritoneal dialysis removes a significant amount of labetalol HCl from the general circulation (<1%).

INDICATIONS AND USAGE

NORMODYNE (labetalol HCl) Injection is indicated for control of blood pressure in severe hypertension.

CONTRAINDICATIONS

NORMODYNE (labetalol HCl) Injection is contraindicated in bronchial asthma, overt cardiac failure, greater than first degree heart block, cardiogenic shock, severe bradycardia, other conditions associated with severe and prolonged hypotension, and in patients with a history of hypersensitivity to any component of the product (see **WARNINGS**).

WARNINGS

Hepatic Injury Severe hepatocellular injury, confirmed by rechallenge in at least one case, occurs rarely with labetalol therapy. The hepatic injury is usually reversible, but hepatic necrosis and death have been reported. Injury has occurred after both short- and long-term treatment and may be slowly progressive despite minimal symptomatology. Similar hepatic events have been reported with a related compound, dilevalol HCl, including two deaths. Dilevalol HCl is one of the four isomers of labetalol HCl. Thus, for patients taking labetalol, periodic determination of suitable hepatic laboratory tests would be appropriate. Laboratory testing should also be done at the very first symptom or sign of liver dysfunction (eg, pruritus, dark urine, persistent anorexia, jaundice, right upper quadrant tenderness, or unexplained "flu-like" symptoms). If the patient has jaundice or laboratory evidence of liver injury, labetalol HCl should be stopped and not restarted.

Cardiac Failure Sympathetic stimulation is a vital component supporting circulatory function in congestive heart failure. Beta-blockade carries a potential hazard of further depressing myocardial contractility and precipitating more severe failure. Although beta-blockers should be avoided in overt congestive heart failure, if necessary, labetalol HCl can be used with caution in patients with a history of heart failure who are well compensated. Congestive heart failure has been observed in patients receiving labetalol HCl. Labetalol HCl does not abolish the inotropic action of digitalis on heart muscle.

In Patients Without a History of Cardiac Failure In patients with latent cardiac insufficiency, continued depression of the myocardium with beta-blocking agents over a period of time can lead, in some cases, to cardiac failure. At the first sign or symptom of impending cardiac failure, patients should be fully digitalized and/or be given a diuretic, and the response observed closely. If cardiac failure continues, despite adequate digitalization and diuretic, NORMODYNE (labetalol HCl) therapy should be withdrawn (gradually if possible).

Ischemic Heart Disease Angina pectoris has not been reported upon labetalol HCl discontinuation. However, following abrupt cessation of therapy with some beta-blocking agents in patients with coronary artery disease, exacerbations of angina pectoris and, in some cases, myocardial infarction have been reported. Therefore, such patients should be cautioned againt interruption of therapy without the physician's advice. Even in the absence of overt angina pectoris, when discontinuation of NORMODYNE (labetalol HCl) is planned, the patient should be carefully observed and should be advised to limit physical activity. If angina markedly worsens or acute coronary insufficiency develops, NORMODYNE (labetalol HCl) administration should be reinstituted promptly, at least temporarily, and other measures appropriate for the management of unstable angina should be taken.

Nonallergic Bronchospasm (eg, chronic bronchitis and emphysema) Since NORMODYNE (labetalol HCl) Injection at the usual intravenous therapeutic doses has not been studied in patients with nonallergic bronchospastic disease, it should not be used in such patients.

Pheochromocytoma Intravenous labetalol HCl has been shown to be effective in lowering the blood pressure and relieving symptoms in patients with pheochromocytoma; higher than usual doses may be required. However, paradoxical hypertensive responses have been reported in a few patients with this tumor; therefore, use caution when administering labetalol HCl to patients with pheochromocytoma.

Diabetes Mellitus and Hypoglycemia Beta-adrenergic blockade may prevent the appearance of premonitory signs and symptoms (eg, tachycardia) of acute hypoglycemia. This is especially important with labile diabetics. Beta-blockade also reduces the release of insulin in response to hyperglycemia; it may therefore be necessary to adjust the dose of antidiabetic drugs.

Major Surgery The necessity or desirability of withdrawing beta-blocking therapy prior to major surgery is controversial. Protracted severe hypotension and difficulty in restarting or maintaining a heartbeat have been reported with beta-blockers. The effect of labetalol HCl's alpha-adrenergic activity has not been evaluated in this setting.

Several deaths have occurred when NORMODYNE (labetalol HCl) Injection was used during surgery (including when used in cases to control bleeding).

A synergism between labetalol HCl and halothane anesthesia has been shown (see **PRECAUTIONS-Drug Interactions**).

Rapid Decreases of Blood Pressure Caution must be observed when reducing severely elevated blood pressure. Although such findings have not been reported with intravenous labetalol HCl, a number of adverse reactions, including cerebral infarction, optic nerve infarction, angina, and ischemic changes in the electrocardiogram, have been reported with other agents when severely elevated blood pressure was reduced over time courses of several hours to as long as 1 or 2 days. The desired blood pressure lowering should therefore be achieved over as long a period of time as is compatible with the patient's status.

PRECAUTIONS

General: *Impaired Hepatic Function* may diminish metabolism of NORMODYNE (labetalol HCl) Injection.

Following Coronary Artery Bypass Surgery In one uncontrolled study, patients with low cardiac indices and elevated systemic vascular resistance following intravenous labetalol HCl experienced significant declines in cardiac output with little change in systemic vascular resistance. One of these patients developed hypotension following labetalol HCl treatment. Therefore, use of labetalol HCl should be avoided in such patients.

High-Dose Labetalol HCl Administration of up to 3 g/d as an infusion for up to 2 to 3 days has been anecdotally reported; several patients experienced hypotension or bradycardia (see **DOSAGE AND ADMINISTRATION**).

Hypotension Symptomatic postural hypotension (incidence 58%) is likely to occur if patients are tilted or allowed to assume the upright position within 3 hours of receiving NORMODYNE (labetalol HCl) Injection. Therefore, the patient's ability to tolerate an upright position should be established before permitting any ambulation.

Jaundice or Hepatic Dysfunction (see **WARNINGS**).

Information for Patients: The following information is intended to aid in the safe and effective use of this medication. It is not a disclosure of all possible adverse or intended effects. During and immediately following (for up to 3 hours) NORMODYNE (labetalol HCl) Injection, the patient should remain supine. Subsequently, the patient should be advised on how to proceed gradually to become ambulatory, and should be observed at the time of first ambulation.

When the patient is started on NORMODYNE (labetalol HCl) Tablets, following adequate control of blood pressure with NORMODYNE (labetalol HCl) Injection, appropriate directions for titration of dosage should be provided (see **DOSAGE AND ADMINISTRATION**).

As with all drugs with beta-blocking activity, certain advice to patients being treated with labetalol HCl is warranted: While no incident of the abrupt withdrawal phenomenon (exacerbation of angina pectoris) has been reported with labetalol HCl, dosing with NORMODYNE (labetalol HCl) Tablets should not be interrupted or discontinued without a physician's advice. Patients being treated with NORMODYNE (labetalol HCl) Tablets should consult a physican at any signs or symptoms of impending cardiac failure or hepatic dysfunction (see **WARNINGS**). Also, transient scalp tingling may occur, usually when treatment with NORMODYNE (labetalol HCl) Tablets is initiated (see **ADVERSE REACTIONS**).

Laboratory Tests: Routine laboratory tests are ordinarily not required before or after intravenous labetalol HCl. In patients with concomitant illnesses, such as impaired renal function, appropriate tests should be done to monitor these conditions.

Drug Interactions: Since NORMODYNE (labetalol HCl) Injection may be administered to patients already being treated with other medications, including other antihypertensive agents, careful monitoring of these patients is necessary to detect and treat promptly any undesired effect from concomitant administration.

In one survey, 2.3% of patients taking labetalol HCl orally in combination with tricyclic antidepressants experienced tremor as compared to 0.7% reported to occur with labetalol HCl alone. The contribution of each of the treatments to this adverse reaction is unknown but the possibility of a drug interaction cannot be excluded.

Drugs possessing beta-blocking properties can blunt the bronchodilator effect of beta-receptor agonist drugs in patients with bronchospasm; therefore, doses greater than the normal antiasthmatic dose of beta-agonist bronchodilator drugs may be required.

Cimetidine has been shown to increase the bioavailability of labetalol HCl administered orally. Since this could be explained either by enhanced absorption or by an alteration of hepatic metabolism of labetalol HCl, special care should be used in establishing the dose required for blood pressure control in such patients.

Synergism has been shown between halothane anesthesia and intravenously administered labetalol HCl. During controlled hypotensive anesthesia using labetalol HCl in association with halothane, high concentrations (3% or above) of halothane should not be used because the degree of hypotension will be increased and because of the possibility of a large reduction in cardiac output and an increase in central venous pressure. The anesthesiologist should be informed when a patient is receiving labetalol HCl.

Labetalol HCl blunts the reflex tachycardia produced by nitroglycerin without preventing its hypotensive effect. If labetalol HCl is used with nitroglycerin in patients with angina pectoris, additional antihypertensive effects may occur.

Care should be taken if labetalol HCl is used concomitantly with calcium antagonists of the verapamil type.

When drug products that are alkaline, such as furosemide, have been administered in combination with labetalol, a white precipitate has been noted. Therefore, these drugs should be administered in the same infusion line.

Risk of Anaphylactic Reaction While taking beta-blockers, patients with a history of severe anaphylactic reactions to a variety of allergens may be more reactive to repeated challenge, either accidental, diagnostic, or therapeutic. Such patients may be unresponsive to the usual doses of epinephrine used to treat allergic reactions.

Drug/Laboratory Test Interactions: The presence of labetalol metabolites in the urine may result in falsely elevated levels of urinary catecholamines, metanephrine, normetanephrine, and vanillylmandelic acid (VMA) when measured by fluorimetric or photometric methods. In screening patients suspected of having a pheochromocytoma and being treated with labetalol HCl, a specific method, such as a high-performance liquid chromatographic assay with solid phase extraction (eg, *J Chromatogr*. 385: 241, 1987) should be employed in determining levels of catecholamines.

Labetalol HCl has also been reported to produce a false-positive test for amphetamine when screening urine for the presence of drugs using the commercially available assay methods Toxi-Lab A® (thin-layer chromatographic assay) and Emit-d.a.u.® (radioenzymatic assay). When patients being treated with labetalol HCl have a positive urine test for amphetamine using these techniques, confirmation should be made by using more specific methods, such as a gas chromatographic-mass spectrometer technique.

Carcinogenesis, Mutagenesis, Impairment of Fertility: Long-term oral dosing studies with labetalol HCl for 18 months in mice and for 2 years in rats showed no evidence of carcinogenesis. Studies with labetalol HCl, using dominant lethal assays in rats and mice, and exposing microorganisms according to modified Ames tests, showed no evidence of mutagenesis.

Pregnancy Category C: Teratogenic studies have been performed with labetalol HCl in rats and rabbits at oral doses up to approximately 6 and 4 times the maximum recommended human dose (MRHD), respectively. No reproducible evidence of fetal malformations was observed. Increased fetal resorptions were seen in both species at doses approximating the MRHD. A teratology study performed with labetalol HCl in rabbits at intravenous doses up to 1.7 times the MRHD revealed no evidence of drug-related harm to the fetus. There are no adequate and well-controlled studies in pregnant women. Labetalol HCl should be used during pregnancy only if the potential benefit justifies the potential risk to the fetus.

Nonteratogenic Effects: Hypotension, bradycardia, hypoglycemia, and respiratory depression have been reported in infants of mothers who were treated with labetalol HCl for hypertension during pregnancy. Oral administration of labetalol to rats during late gestation through weaning at doses of 2 to 4 times the MRHD caused a decrease in neonatal survival.

Continued on next page

Information on Schering products appearing on these pages is effective as of August 15, 1998.

Normodyne—Cont.

Labor and Delivery: Labetalol HCl given to pregnant women with hypertension did not appear to affect the usual course of labor and delivery.

Nursing Mothers: Small amounts of labetalol (approximately 0.004% of the maternal dose) are excreted in human milk. Caution should be exercised when NORMODYNE (labetalol HCl) Injection is administered to a nursing woman.

Pediatric Use: Safety and effectiveness in children have not been established.

ADVERSE REACTIONS

NORMODYNE (labetalol HCl) Injection is usually well tolerated. Most adverse events have been mild and transient and in controlled trials involving 92 patients did not require labetalol HCl withdrawal. Symptomatic postural hypotension (incidence 58%) is likely to occur if patients are tilted or allowed to assume the upright position within 3 hours of receiving NORMODYNE (labetalol HCl) Injection. Moderate hypotension occurred in 1 of 100 patients while supine. Increased sweating was noted in 4 of 100 patients, and flushing occurred in 1 of 100 patients.

The following also were reported with NORMODYNE (labetalol, HCl) Injection with the incidence per 100 patients as noted:

Cardiovascular System Ventricular arrhythmias in 1.

Central and Peripheral Nervous System Dizziness in 9; tingling of the scalp/skin 7; hypoesthesia (numbness) and vertigo, 1 each.

Gastrointestinal System Nausea in 13; vomiting 4; dyspepsia and taste distortion, 1 each.

Metabolic Disorders Transient increases in blood urea nitrogen and serum creatinine levels occurred in 8 of 100 patients; these were associated with drops in blood pressure, generally in patients with prior renal insufficiency.

Psychiatric Disorders Somnolence/yawning in 3.

Respiratory System Wheezing in 1.

Skin Pruritus in 1.

The incidence of adverse reactions depends upon the dose of labetalol HCl. The largest experience is with oral labetalol HCl (see NORMODYNE (labetalol HCl) Tablet Product Information for details). Certain of the side effects increased with increasing oral dose as shown in the table below which depicts the entire U.S. therapeutic trials data base for adverse reactions that are clearly or possibly dose related.

[See table below]

In addition, a number of other less common adverse events have been reported:

Cardiovascular Hypotension, and rarely, syncope, bradycardia, heart block.

Liver and Biliary System Hepatic necrosis, hepatitis, cholestatic jaundice, elevated liver function tests.

Hypersensitivity Rare reports of hypersensitivity (eg, rash, urticaria, pruritus, angioedema, dyspnea) and anaphylactoid reactions.

The oculomucocutaneous syndrome associated with the beta-blocker practolol has not been reported with labetalol HCl during investigational use and extensive foreign marketing experience.

Clinical Laboratory Tests: Among patients dosed with NORMODYNE (labetalol HCl) Tablets, there have been reversible increases of serum transaminases in 4% of patients tested, and more rarely, reversible increases in blood urea.

OVERDOSAGE

Overdosage with NORMODYNE (labetalol HCl) Injection causes excessive hypotension that is posture sensitive, and sometimes, excessive bradycardia. Patients should be placed supine and their legs raised if necessary to improve the blood supply to the brain. If overdosage with labetalol HCl follows oral ingestion, gastric lavage or pharmacologically induced emesis (using syrup of ipecac) may be useful for removal of the drug shortly after ingestion. The following additional measures should be employed if necessary: *Excessive bradycardia*–administer atropine or epinephrine. *Cardiac failure*–administer a digitalis glycoside and a diuretic. Dopamine or dobutamine may also be useful. *Hypotension*–administer vasopressors, eg, norepinephrine. There is pharmacological evidence that norepinephrine may be the drug of choice. *Bronchospasm*–administer epinephrine and/or an aerosolized beta$_2$-agonist. *Seizures*–administer diazepam.

In severe beta-blocker overdose resulting in hypotension and/or bradycardia, glucagon has been shown to be effective when administered in large doses (5 to 10 mg rapidly over 30 seconds, followed by continuous infusion of 5 mg/hr that can be reduced as the patient improves).

Neither hemodialysis nor peritoneal dialysis removes a significant amount of labetalol HCl from the general circulation (<1%).

The oral LD_{50} value of labetalol HCl in the mouse is approximately 600 mg/kg and in the rat is greater than 2 g/kg. The intravenous LD_{50} in these species is 50 to 60 mg/kg.

DOSAGE AND ADMINISTRATION

NORMODYNE (labetalol HCl) Injection is intended for intravenous use in hospitalized patients. DOSAGE MUST BE INDIVIDUALIZED depending upon the severity of hypertension and the response of the patient during dosing.

Patients should always be kept in a supine position during the period of intravenous drug administration. A substantial fall in blood pressure on standing should be expected in these patients. The patient's ability to tolerate an upright position should be established before permitting any ambulation, such as using toilet facilities.

Either of two methods of administration of NORMODYNE (labetalol HCl) Injection may be used: a) repeated intravenous injections, b) slow continuous infusion.

Repeated Intravenous Injection: Initially, NORMODYNE (labetalol HCl) Injection should be given in a dose of 20 mg labetalol HCl (which corresponds to 0.25 mg/kg for an 80 kg patient) by slow intravenous injection over a 2-minute period.

Immediately before the injection and at 5 and 10 minutes after injection, supine blood pressure should be measured to evaluate response. Additional injections of 40 mg or 80 mg can be given at 10-minute intervals until a desired supine blood pressure is achieved or a total of 300 mg labetalol HCl has been injected. The maximum effect usually occurs within 5 minutes of each injection.

Slow Continuous Infusion: NORMODYNE (labetalol HCl) Injection is prepared for intravenous continuous infusion by diluting the contents with commonly used intravenous fluids (see below). Examples of methods of preparing the infusion solution are:

The contents of either two 20-mL vials (40 mL), or one 40-mL vial, are added to 160 mL of a commonly used intravenous fluid such that the resultant 200 mL of solution contains 200 mg of labetalol HCl, 1 mg/mL. The diluted solution should be administered at a rate of 2 mL/min to deliver 2 mg/min.

Alternatively, the contents of either two 20-mL vials (40 mL), or one 40-mL vial, of NORMODYNE (labetalol HCl) Injection are added to 250 mL of a commonly used intravenous fluid. The resultant solution will contain 200 mg of labetalol HCl, approximately 2 mg/3 mL. The diluted solution should be administered at a rate of 3 mL/min to deliver approximately 2 mg/min.

The rate of infusion of the diluted solution may be adjusted according to the blood pressure response, at the discretion of the physician. To facilitate a desired rate of infusion, the diluted solution can be infused using a controlled administered mechanism, eg, graduated burette or mechanically driven infusion pump.

Since the half-life of labetalol is 5 to 8 hours, steady-state blood levels (in the face of a constant rate of infusion) would not be reached during the usual infusion time period. The infusion should be continued until a satisfactory response is obtained and should then be stopped and oral labetalol HCl started (see below). The effective intravenous dose is usually in the range of 50 to 200 mg. A total dose of up to 300 mg may be required in some patients.

Blood Pressure Monitoring: The blood pressure should be monitored during and after completion of the infusion or intravenous injections. Rapid or excessive falls in either systolic or diastolic blood pressure during intravenous treatment should be avoided. In patients with excessive systolic hypertension, the decrease in systolic pressure should be used as indicator of effectiveness in addition to the response of the diastolic pressure.

Initiation of Dosing with NORMODYNE (labetalol HCl) Tablets: Subsequent oral dosing with NORMODYNE (labetalol HCl) Tablets should begin when it has been established that the supine diastolic blood pressure has begun to rise. The recommended initial dose is 200 mg, followed in 6–12 hours by an additional dose of 200 or 400 mg, depending on the blood pressure response. Thereafter, *inpatient titration with NORMODYNE (labetalol HCl) Tablets* may proceed as follows:

Inpatient Titration Instructions

Regimen	Daily Dose*
200 mg b.i.d.	400 mg
400 mg b.i.d.	800 mg
800 mg b.i.d.	1600 mg
1200 mg b.i.d.	2400 mg

*If needed, the total daily dose may be given in three divided doses.

While in the hospital, the dosage of NORMODYNE (labetalol HCl) Tablets may be increased at 1-day intervals to achieve the desired blood pressure reduction.

For subsequent outpatient titration or maintenance dosing see NORMODYNE (labetalol HCl) Tablets Product Information **DOSAGE AND ADMINISTRATION** for additional recommendations.

Compatibility with commonly used intravenous fluids:

Parental drug products should be inspected visually for particulate matter and discoloration prior to administration, whenever solution and container permit.

NORMODYNE (labetalol HCl) Injection was tested for compatibility with commonly used intravenous fluids at final concentrations of 1.25 mg to 3.75 mg labetalol HCl per mL of the mixture. NORMODYNE (labetalol HCl) Injection was found to be compatible with and stable (for 24 hours refrigerated or at room temperature) in mixtures with the following solutions:

Ringers Injection, USP
Lactated Ringers Injection, USP
5% Dextrose and Ringers Injection
5% Lactated Ringers and 5% Dextrose Injection
5% Dextrose Injection, USP
0.9% Sodium Chloride Injection, USP
5% Dextrose and 0.2% Sodium Chloride Injection, USP
2.5% Dextrose and 0.45% Sodium Chloride Injection, USP
5% Dextrose and 0.9% Sodium Chloride Injection, USP
5% Dextrose and 0.33% Sodium Chloride Injection, USP

NORMODYNE (labetalol HCl) Injection was NOT compatible with 5% Sodium Bicarbonate Injection, USP.

HOW SUPPLIED

NORMODYNE (labetalol HCl) Injection, 5 mg/mL, is supplied in:

20 mL (100 mg) (NDC 0085-0362-07) multi-dose vial, box of 1 and

40 mL (200 mg) (NDC 0085-0362-06) multi-dose vial, box of 1

4 mL (20 mg) (NDC 0085-0362-08) single-dose, prefilled, disposable syringe, box of 1 and

8 mL (40 mg) (NDC 0085-0362-09) single-dose, prefilled, disposable syringe, box of 1.

Store between 2° and 30°C (36° and 86°F). Protect from freezing. Protect syringe from light.

Note: To ensure patient safety, the needle and the prefilled syringes should be handled with care and should be destroyed and discarded if damaged in any manner. If the cannula is bent, not attempt should be made to straighten it. To prevent needle-stick injuries, needles should not be recapped, purposely bent, or broken by hand.

Only the prefilled syringes are manufactured for Schering Corporation by:

Meridian Medical
Technologies, Inc.,
Columbia, MD 21046

Key Pharmaceuticals, Inc.
Kenilworth, NJ 07033 USA

Rev. 2/97 B-19881504

Copyright © 1984, 1996, 1997, Schering Corporation. All rights reserved.

Shown in Product Identification Guide, page 336

Labetalol HCl Daily Dose (mg)	200	300	400	600	800	900	1200	1600	2400
Number of Patients	522	181	606	608	503	117	411	242	175
Dizziness (%)	2	3	3	3	5	1	9	13	16
Fatigue	2	1	4	4	5	3	7	6	10
Nausea	<1	0	1	2	4	0	7	11	19
Vomiting	0	0	<1	<1	<1	0	1	2	3
Dyspepsia	1	0	2	1	1	0	2	2	4
Paresthesias	2	0	2	2	1	1	2	5	5
Nasal Stuffiness	1	1	2	2	2	2	4	5	6
Ejaculation Failure	0	2	1	2	3	0	4	3	5
Impotence	1	1	1	1	2	4	3	4	3
Edema	1	0	1	1	1	0	1	2	2

NORMODYNE® ℞

brand of
labetalol hydrochloride
Tablets, USP

DESCRIPTION

NORMODYNE (labetalol HCl) is an adrenergic receptor blocking agent that has both selective alpha$_1$-and non-selective beta-adrenergic receptor blocking actions in a single substance.

Labetalol HCl is a racemate, chemically designated as 5-[1-hydroxy-2-[(1-methyl-3-phenylpropyl) amino] ethyl]salicylamide monohydrochloride, and has the following structure:

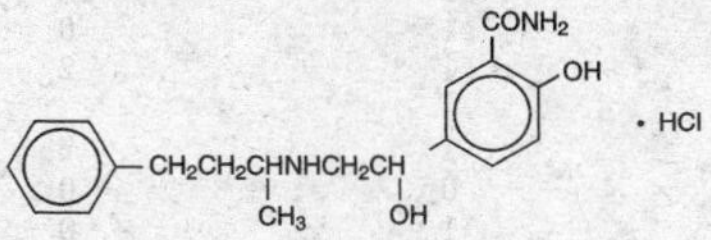

Labetalol HCl has the empirical formula $C_{19}H_{24}N_2O_3 \cdot HCl$ and a molecular weight of 364.9. It has two asymmetric centers and therefore exists as a molecular complex of two diastereoisomeric pairs. Dilevalol, the R,R' stereoisomer, makes up 25% of racemic labetalol.

Labetalol HCl is a white or off-white crystalline powder, soluble in water.

NORMODYNE Tablets contain 100 mg, 200 mg, or 300 mg labetalol HCl, USP and are taken orally.

The inactive ingredients for NORMODYNE Tablets, 100 mg, include: corn starch, FD&C Blue No. 2 Al Lake, FD&C Yellow No. 6 Al Lake, hydroxypropyl methylcellulose, lactose, magnesium stearate, methylparaben, PEG, and propylparaben. May also contain: potato starch and wheat starch.

The inactive ingredients for NORMODYNE Tablets, 200 mg, include: corn starch, hydroxypropyl methylcellulose, lactose, magnesium stearate, methylparaben, PEG, propylparaben, and titanium dioxide. May also contain: potato starch and wheat starch.

The inactive ingredients for NORMODYNE Tablets, 300 mg, include: corn starch, FD&C Blue No. 2 Al Lake, hydroxypropyl methylcellulose, lactose, magnesium stearate, methylparaben, PEG, and propylparaben. May also contain: potato starch and wheat starch.

CLINICAL PHARMACOLOGY

NORMODYNE (labetalol HCl) combines both selective, competitive alpha$_1$-adrenergic blocking and nonselective, competitive beta-adrenergic blocking activity in a single substance. In man, the ratios of alpha- to beta-blockade have been estimated to be approximately 1:3 and 1:7 following oral and intravenous administration, respectively. Beta$_2$-agonist activity has been demonstrated in animals with minimal beta$_1$-agonist (ISA) activity detected. In animals, at doses greater than those required for alpha- or beta-adrenergic blockade, a membrane-stabilizing effect has been demonstrated.

Pharmacodynamics The capacity of labetalol HCl to block alpha receptors in man has been demonstrated by attenuation of the pressor effect of phenylephrine and by a significant reduction of the pressor response caused by immersing the hand in ice-cold water ("cold-pressor test"). Labetalol HCl's beta$_1$-receptor blockade in man was demonstrated by a small decrease in the resting heart rate, attenuation of tachycardia produced by isoproterenol or exercise, and by attenuation of the reflex tachycardia to the hypotension produced by amyl nitrite. Beta$_2$-receptor blockade was demonstrated by inhibition of the isoproterenol-induced fall in diastolic blood pressure. Both the alpha- and beta-blocking actions of orally administered labetalol HCl contribute to a decrease in blood pressure in hypertensive patients. Labetalol HCl consistently, in dose-related fashion, blunted increases in exercise-induced blood pressure and heart rate, and in their double product. The pulmonary circulation during exercise was not affected by labetalol HCl dosing.

Single oral doses of labetalol HCl administered in patients with coronary artery disease had no significant effect on sinus rate, intraventricular conduction, or QRS duration. The AV conduction time was modestly prolonged in 2 of 7 patients. In another study, intravenous labetalol HCl slightly prolonged AV nodal conduction time and atrial effective refractory period with only small changes in heart rate. The effects on AV nodal refractoriness were inconsistent.

Labetalol HCl produces dose-related falls in blood pressure without reflex tachycardia and without significant reduction in heart rate, presumably through a mixture of its alpha-blocking and beta-blocking effects. Hemodynamic effects are variable with small nonsignificant changes in cardiac output seen in some studies but not others, and small decreases in total peripheral resistance. Elevated plasma renins are reduced.

Doses of labetalol HCl that controlled hypertension did not affect renal function in mild to severe hypertensive patients with normal renal function.

Due to the alpha$_1$-receptor blocking activity of labetalol HCl, blood pressure is lowered more in the standing than in the supine position, and symptoms of postural hypotension (2%), including rare instances of syncope, can occur. Following oral administration, when postural hypotension has occurred, it has been transient and is uncommon when the recommended starting dose and titration increments are closely followed (see **DOSAGE AND ADMINISTRATION**). Symptomatic postural hypotension is most likely to occur 2 to 4 hours after a dose, especially following the use of large initial doses or upon large changes in dose.

The peak effects of single oral doses of labetalol HCl occur within 2 to 4 hours. The duration of effect depends upon dose, lasting at least 8 hours following single oral doses of 100 mg and more than 12 hours following single oral doses of 300 mg. The maximum, steady-state blood pressure response upon oral, twice-a-day dosing occurs within 24 to 72 hours.

The antihypertensive effect of labetalol has a linear correlation with the logarithm of labetalol plasma concentration, and there is also a linear correlation between the reduction in exercise-induced tachycardia occurring at 2 hours after oral administration of labetalol HCl and the logarithm of the plasma concentration.

About 70% of the maximum beta-blocking effect is present for 5 hours after the administration of a single oral dose of 400 mg, with suggestion that about 40% remains at 8 hours.

The anti-anginal efficacy of labetalol HCl has not been studied. In 37 patients with hypertension and coronary artery disease, labetalol HCl did not increase the incidence or severity of angina attacks.

Exacerbation of angina and, in some cases, myocardial infarction and ventricular dysrhythmias have been reported after abrupt discontinuation of therapy with beta-adrenergic blocking agents in patients with coronary artery disease. Abrupt withdrawal of these agents in patients without coronary artery disease has resulted in transient symptoms, including tremulousness, sweating, palpitation, headache, and malaise. Several mechanisms have been proposed to explain these phenomena, among them increased sensitivity to catecholamines because of increased numbers of beta receptors.

Although beta-adrenergic receptor blockade is useful in the treatment of angina and hypertension, there are also situations in which sympathetic stimulation is vital. For example, in patients with severely damaged hearts, adequate ventricular function may depend on sympathetic drive. Beta-adrenergic blockade may worsen AV block by preventing the necessary facilitating effects of sympathetic activity on conduction. Beta$_2$-adrenergic blockade results in passive bronchial constriction by interfering with endogenous adrenergic bronchodilator activity in patients subject to bronchospasm and may also interfere with exogenous bronchodilators in such patients.

Pharmacokinetics and Metabolism Labetalol HCl is completely absorbed from the gastrointestinal tract with peak plasma levels occurring 1 to 2 hours after oral administration. The relative bioavailability of labetalol HCl tablets compared to an oral solution is 100%. The absolute bioavailability (fraction of drug reaching systemic circulation) of labetalol when compared to an intravenous infusion is 25%; this is due to extensive "first-pass" metabolism. Despite "first-pass" metabolism there is a linear relationship between oral doses of 100 to 3000 mg and peak plasma levels. The absolute bioavailability of labetalol is increased when administered with food.

The plasma half-life of labetalol following oral administration is about 6 to 8 hours. Steady-state plasma levels of labetalol during repetitive dosing are reached by about the third day of dosing. In patients with decreased hepatic or renal function, the elimination half-life of labetalol is not altered; however, the relative bioavailability in hepatically impaired patients is increased due to decreased "first-pass" metabolism.

The metabolism of labetalol is mainly through conjugation to glucuronide metabolites. These metabolites are present in plasma and are excreted in the urine and, via the bile, into the feces. Approximately 55% to 60% of a dose appears in the urine as conjugates or unchanged labetalol within the first 24 hours of dosing.

Labetalol has been shown to cross the placental barrier in humans. Only negligible amounts of the drug crossed the blood-brain barrier in animal studies. Labetalol is approximately 50% protein bound. Neither hemodialysis nor peritoneal dialysis removes a significant amount of labetalol HCl from the general circulation (<1%).

INDICATIONS AND USAGE

NORMODYNE (labetalol HCl) Tablets are indicated in the management of hypertension. NORMODYNE Tablets may be used alone or in combination with other antihypertensive agents, especially thiazide and loop diuretics.

CONTRAINDICATIONS

NORMODYNE (labetalol HCl) Tablets are contraindicated in bronchial asthma, overt cardiac failure, greater than first degree heart block, cardiogenic shock, severe bradycardia, other conditions associated with severe and prolonged hypotension, and in patients with a history of hypersensitivity to any component of the product (see **WARNINGS**).

WARNINGS

Hepatic Injury Severe hepatocellular injury, confirmed by rechallenge in at least one case, occurs rarely with labetalol therapy. The hepatic injury is usually reversible, but hepatic necrosis and death have been reported. Injury has occurred after both short- and long-term treatment and may be slowly progressive despite minimal symptomatology. Similar hepatic events have been reported with a related compound, dilevalol HCl, including two deaths. Dilevalol HCl is one of the four isomers of labetalol HCl. Thus, for patients taking labetalol, periodic determination of suitable hepatic laboratory tests would be appropriate. Laboratory testing should also be done at the very first symptom or sign of liver dysfunction (eg, pruritis, dark urine, persistent anorexia, jaundice, right upper quadrant tenderness, or unexplained "flu-like" symptoms). If the patient has jaundice or laboratory evidence of liver injury, labetalol HCl should be stopped and not restarted.

Cardiac Failure Sympathetic stimulation is a vital component supporting circulatory function in congestive heart failure. Beta blockade carries a potential hazard of further depressing myocardial contractility and precipitating more severe failure. Although beta-blockers should be avoided in overt congestive heart failure, if necessary, labetalol HCl can be used with caution in patients with a history of heart failure who are well-compensated. Congestive heart failure has been observed in patients receiving labetalol HCl. Labetalol HCl does not abolish the inotropic action of digitalis on heart muscle.

In Patients Without a History of Cardiac Failure In patients with latent cardiac insufficiency, continued depression of the myocardium with beta-blocking agents over a period of time can, in some cases, lead to cardiac failure. At the first sign or symptom of impending cardiac failure, patients should be fully digitalized and/or be given a diuretic, and the response observed closely. If cardiac failure continues, despite adequate digitalization and diuretic, NORMODYNE (labetalol HCl) therapy should be withdrawn (gradually if possible).

Exacerbation of Ischemic Heart Disease Following Abrupt Withdrawal Angina pectoris has not been reported upon labetalol HCl discontinuation. However, hypersensitivity to catecholamines has been observed in patients withdrawn from beta-blocker therapy; exacerbation of angina and, in some cases, myocardial infarction have occurred after *abrupt* discontinuation of such therapy. When discontinuing chronically administered NORMODYNE (labetalol HCl), particularly in patients with ischemic heart disease, the dosage should be gradually reduced over a period of 1 to 2 weeks and the patient should be carefully monitored. If angina markedly worsens or acute coronary insufficiency develops, NORMODYNE (labetalol HCl) administration should be reinstituted promptly, at least temporarily, and other measures appropriate for the management of unstable angina should be taken. Patients should be warned against interruption or discontinuation of therapy without the physician's advice. Because coronary artery disease is common and may be unrecognized, it may be prudent not to discontinue NORMODYNE (labetalol HCl) therapy abruptly even in patients treated only for hypertension.

Nonallergic bronchospasm (eg, chronic bronchitis and emphysema) patients with bronchospastic disease should, in general, not receive beta-blockers. NORMODYNE (labetalol HCl) may be used with caution, however, in patients who do not respond to, or cannot tolerate, other antihypertensive agents. It is prudent, if NORMODYNE (labetalol HCl) is used, to use the smallest effective dose, so that inhibition of endogenous or exogenous beta-agonists is minimized.

Pheochromocytoma Labetalol HCl has been shown to be effective in lowering the blood pressure and relieving symptoms in patients with pheochromocytoma. However, paradoxical hypertensive responses have been reported in a few patients with this tumor; therefore, use caution when administering labetalol HCl to patients with pheochromocytoma.

Diabetes Mellitus and Hypoglycemia Beta-adrenergic blockade may prevent the appearance of premonitory signs and symptoms (eg, tachycardia) of acute hypoglycemia. This is especially important with labile diabetics. Beta-blockade also reduces the release of insulin in response to hyperglycemia; it may therefore be necessary to adjust the dose of antidiabetic drugs.

Major Surgery The necessity or desirability of withdrawing beta-blocking therapy prior to major surgery is controversial. Protracted severe hypotension and difficulty in restarting or maintaining a heartbeat have been reported with beta-blockers. The effect of labetalol HCl's alpha-adrenergic activity has not been evaluated in this setting.

A synergism between labetalol HCl and halothane anesthesia has been shown (see **PRECAUTIONS–Drug Interactions**).

PRECAUTIONS

General *Impaired Hepatic Function* NORMODYNE (labetalol HCl) Tablets should be used with caution in patients with impaired hepatic function since metabolism of the drug may be diminished.

Jaundice or Hepatic Dysfunction (see **WARNINGS**).

Continued on next page

Information on Schering products appearing on these pages is effective as of August 15, 1998.

Normodyne Tablets—Cont.

Information for Patients
As with all drugs with beta-blocking activity, certain advice to patients being treated with labetalol HCl is warranted. This information is intended to aid in the safe and effective use of this medication. It is not a disclosure of all possible adverse or intended effects. While no incident of the abrupt withdrawal phenomenon (exacerbation of angina pectoris) has been reported with labetalol HCl, dosing with NORMODYNE (labetalol HCl) Tablets should not be interrupted or discontinued without a physician's advice. Patients being treated with NORMODYNE (labetalol HCl) Tablets should consult a physician at any signs or symptoms of impending cardiac failure or hepatic dysfunction (see **WARNINGS**). Also, transient scalp tingling may occur, usually when treatment with NORMODYNE (labetalol HCl) Tablets is initiated (see **ADVERSE REACTIONS**).

Laboratory Tests
As with any new drug given over prolonged periods, laboratory parameters should be observed over regular intervals. In patients with concomitant illnesses, such as impaired renal function, appropriate tests should be done to monitor these conditions.

Drug Interactions
In one survey, 2.3% of patients taking labetalol HCl in combination with tricyclic antidepressants experienced tremor as compared to 0.7% reported to occur with labetalol HCl alone. The contribution of each of the treatments to this adverse reaction is unknown but the possibility of a drug interaction cannot be excluded.

Drugs possessing beta-blocking properties can blunt the bronchodilator effect of beta-receptor agonist drugs in patients with bronchospasm; therefore, doses greater than the normal anti-asthmatic dose of beta-agonist bronchodilator drugs may be required.

Cimetidine has been shown to increase the bioavailability of labetalol HCl. Since this could be explained either by enhanced absorption or by an alteration of hepatic metabolism of labetalol HCl, special care should be used in establishing the dose required for blood pressure control in such patients.

Synergism has been shown between halothane anesthesia and intravenously administered labetalol HCl. During controlled hypotensive anesthesia using labetalol HCl in association with halothane, high concentrations (3% or above) of halothane should not be used because the degree of hypotension will be increased and because of the possibility of a large reduction in cardiac output and an increase in central venous pressure. The anesthesiologist should be informed when a patient is receiving labetalol HCl.

Labetalol HCl blunts the reflex tachycardia produced by nitroglycerin without preventing its hypotensive effect. If labetalol HCl is used with nitroglycerin in patients with angina pectoris, additional antihypertensive effects may occur. Care should be taken if labetalol HCl is used concomitantly with calcium antagonists of the verapamil type.

Risk of Anaphylactic Reaction While taking beta-blockers, patients with a history of severe anaphylactic reaction to a variety of allergens may be more reactive to repeated challenge, either accidental, diagnostic, or therapeutic. Such patients may be unresponsive to the usual doses of epinephrine used to treat allergic reaction.

Drug/Laboratory Test Interactions
The presence of labetalol metabolites in the urine may result in falsely elevated levels of urinary catecholamines, metanephrine, normetanephrine, and vanillylmandelic acid (VMA) when measured by fluorimetric or photometric methods. In screening patients suspected of having a pheochromocytoma and being treated with labetalol HCl, a specific method, such as a high performance liquid chromatographic assay with solid phase extraction (eg, *J Chromatogr* 385: 241,1987) should be employed in determining levels of catecholamines.

Labetalol HCl has also been reported to produce a false-positive test for amphetamine when screening urine for the presence of drugs using the commercially available assay methods Toxi-Lab A® (thin-layer chromatographic assay) and Emit-d.a.u.® (radioenzymatic assay). When patients being treated with labetalol HCl have a positive urine test for amphetamine using these techniques, confirmation should be made by using more specific methods, such as a gas chromatographic-mass spectrometer technique.

Carcinogenesis, Mutagenesis, Impairment of Fertility
Long-term oral dosing studies with labetalol HCl for 18 months in mice and for 2 years in rats showed no evidence of carcinogenesis. Studies with labetalol HCl, using dominant lethal assays in rats and mice, and exposing microorganisms according to modified Ames tests, showed no evidence of mutagenesis.

Pregnancy Category C
Teratogenic studies have been performed with labetalol HCl in rats and rabbits at oral doses up to approximately 6 and 4 times the maximum recommended human dose (MRHD), respectively. No reproducible evidence of fetal malforma-

tions was observed. Increased fetal resorptions were seen in both species at doses approximating the MRHD. A teratology study performed with labetalol HCl in rabbits at intravenous doses up to 1.7 times the MRHD revealed no evidence of drug-related harm to the fetus. There are no adequate and well-controlled studies in pregnant women. Labetalol HCl should be used during pregnancy only if the potential benefit justifies the potential risk to the fetus.

Nonteratogenic Effects
Hypotension, bradycardia, hypoglycemia, and respiratory depression have been reported in infants of mothers who were treated with labetalol HCl for hypertension during pregnancy. Oral administration of labetalol to rats during late gestation through weaning at doses of 2 to 4 times the MRHD caused a decrease in neonatal survival.

Labor and Delivery
Labetalol HCl given to pregnant women with hypertension did not appear to affect the usual course of labor and delivery.

Nursing Mothers
Small amounts of labetalol (approximately 0.004% of the maternal dose) are excreted in human milk. Caution should be exercised when NORMODYNE (labetalol HCl) Tablets are administered to a nursing woman.

Pediatric Use
Safety and effectiveness in children have not been established.

ADVERSE REACTIONS
Most adverse effects are mild, transient and occur early in the course of treatment. In controlled clinical trials of 3 to 4 months duration, discontinuation of NORMODYNE (labetalol HCl) Tablets due to one or more adverse effects was required in 7% of all patients. In these same trials, beta-blocker control agents led to discontinuation in 8% to 10% of patients, and a centrally acting alpha-agonist in 30% of patients.

The incidence rates of adverse reactions listed in the following table were derived from multicenter controlled clinical trials, comparing labetalol HCl, placebo, metoprolol, and propranolol, over treatment periods of 3 and 4 months. Where the frequency of adverse effects for labetalol HCl and placebo is similar, causal relationship is uncertain. The rates are based on adverse reactions considered probably

drug related by the investigator. If all reports are considered, the rates are somewhat higher (eg, dizziness 20%, nausea 14%, fatigue 11%), but the overall conclusions are unchanged.
[See table above]

The adverse effects were reported spontaneously and are representative of the incidence of adverse effects that may be observed in a properly selected hypertensive patient population, ie, a group excluding patients with bronchospastic disease, overt congestive heart failure, or other contraindications to beta-blocker therapy.

Clinical trials also included studies utilizing daily doses up to 2400 mg in more severely hypertensive patients. Certain of the side effects increased with increasing dose as shown in the table below which depicts the entire U.S. therapeutic trials data base for adverse reactions that are clearly or possibly drug related.
[See table below]

In addition, a number of other less common adverse events have been reported:
Body as a Whole Fever.
Cardiovascular Hypotension, and rarely, syncope, bradycardia, heart block.
Central and Peripheral Nervous Systems Paresthesias, most frequently described as scalp tingling. In most cases, it was mild, transient and usually occurred at the beginning of treatment.
Collagen Disorders Systemic lupus erythematosus; positive antinuclear factor (ANF).
Eyes Dry eyes.
Immunological System Antimitochondrial antibodies.
Liver and Biliary System Hepatic necrosis; hepatitis; cholestatic jaundice; elevated liver function tests.
Musculoskeletal System Muscle cramps; toxic myopathy.
Respiratory System Bronchospasm.
Skin and Appendages Rashes of various types, such as generalized maculopapular; lichenoid; urticarial; bullous lichen planus; psoriaform; facial erythema; Peyronie's disease; reversible alopecia.
Urinary System Difficulty in micturition, including acute urinary bladder retention.
Hypersensitivity Rare reports of hypersensitivity (eg, rash, urticaria, pruritus, angioedema, dyspnea) and anaphylactoid reactions.

	Labetalol HCl (N=227) %	Placebo (N=98) %	Propranolol (N=84) %	Metoprolol (N=49) %
Body as a whole				
fatigue	5	0	12	12
asthenia	1	1	1	0
headache	2	1	1	2
Gastrointestinal				
nausea	6	1	1	2
vomiting	<1	0	0	0
dyspepsia	3	1	1	0
abdominal pain	0	0	1	2
diarrhea	<1	0	2	0
taste distortion	1	0	0	0
Central and Peripheral Nervous Systems				
dizziness	11	3	4	4
paresthesias	<1	0	0	0
drowsiness	<1	2	2	2
Autonomic Nervous System				
nasal stuffiness	3	0	0	0
ejaculation failure	2	0	0	0
impotence	1	0	1	3
increased sweating	<1	0	0	0
Cardiovascular				
edema	1	0	0	0
postural hypotension	1	0	0	0
bradycardia	0	0	5	12
Respiratory				
dyspnea	2	0	1	2
Skin				
rash	1	0	0	0
Special Senses				
vision abnormality	1	0	0	0
vertigo	2	1	0	0

Labetalol HCl

Daily Dose (mg)	200	300	400	600	800	900	1200	1600	2400
Number of Patients	522	181	606	608	503	117	411	242	175
Dizziness (%)	2	3	3	3	5	1	9	13	16
Fatigue	2	1	4	4	5	3	7	6	10
Nausea	<1	0	1	2	4	0	7	11	19
Vomiting	0	0	<1	<1	<1	0	1	2	3
Dyspepsia	1	0	2	1	1	0	2	2	4
Paresthesias	0	0	2	2	1	0	2	5	5
Nasal Stuffiness	1	1	2	2	2	2	4	5	6
Ejaculation Failure	0	2	1	2	3	0	4	3	5
Impotence	1	1	1	1	2	4	3	4	3
Edema	1	1	1	1	1	0	1	2	2

Following approval for marketing in the United Kingdom, a monitored release survey involving approximately 6,800 patients was conducted for further safety and efficacy evaluation of this product. Results of this survey indicate that the type, severity, and incidence of adverse effects were comparable to those cited above.

Potential Adverse Effects

In addition, other adverse effects not listed above have been reported with other beta-adrenergic blocking agents.

Central Nervous System Reversible mental depression progressing to catatonia; an acute reversible syndrome characterized by disorientation for time and place, short-term memory loss, emotional lability, slightly clouded sensorium, and decreased performance on neuropsychometrics.

Cardiovascular Intensification of AV block (see **CONTRAINDICATIONS).**

Allergic Fever combined with aching and sore throat; laryngospasm; respiratory distress.

Hematologic Agranulocytosis; thrombocytopenic or nonthrombocytopenic purpura.

Gastrointestinal Mesenteric artery thrombosis; ischemic colitis.

The oculomucocutaneous syndrome associated with the beta-blocker practolol has not been reported with labetalol HCl.

Clinical Laboratory Tests

There have been reversible increases of serum transaminases in 4% of patients treated with labetalol HCl and tested, and more rarely, reversible increases in blood urea.

OVERDOSAGE

Overdosage with NORMODYNE (labetalol HCl) Tablets causes excessive hypotension that is posture sensitive, and sometimes, excessive bradycardia. Patients should be placed supine and their legs raised if necessary to improve the blood supply to the brain. If overdosage with labetalol HCl follows oral ingestion, gastric lavage or pharmacologically induced emesis (using syrup of ipecac) may be useful for removal of the drug shortly after ingestion. The following additional measures should be employed if necessary: *Excessive bradycardia* —administer atropine or epinephrine. *Cardiac failure*—administer a digitalis glycoside and a diuretic. Dopamine or dobutamine may also be useful. *Hypotension* —administer vasopressors, eg, norepinephrine. There is pharmacological evidence that norepinephrine may be the drug of choice. *Bronchospasm* —administer epinephrine and/or an aerosolized beta$_2$-agonist. *Seizures* —administer diazepam.

In severe beta-blocker overdose resulting in hypotension and/or bradycardia, glucagon has been shown to be effective when administered in large doses (5 to 10 mg rapidly over 30 seconds, followed by continuous infusion of 5 mg/hr that can be reduced as the patient improves).

Neither hemodialysis nor peritoneal dialysis removes a significant amount of labetalol HCl from the general circulation (<1%).

The oral LD_{50} value of labetalol HCl in the mouse is approximately 600 mg/kg and in the rat is greater than 2 g/kg. The intravenous LD_{50} in these species is 50 to 60 mg/kg.

DOSAGE AND ADMINISTRATION

DOSAGE MUST BE INDIVIDUALIZED. The recommended initial dose is 100 mg twice daily whether used alone or added to a diuretic regimen. After 2 or 3 days, using standing blood pressure as an indicator, dosage may be titrated in increments of 100 mg b.i.d. every 2 or 3 days. The usual maintenance dosage of labetalol HCl is between 200 and 400 mg twice daily.

Since the full antihypertensive effect of labetalol HCl is usually seen within the first 1 to 3 hours of the initial dose or dose increment, the assurance of a lack of an exaggerated hypotensive response can be clinically established in the office setting. The antihypertensive effects of continued dosing can be measured at subsequent visits, approximately 12 hours after a dose, to determine whether further titration is necessary.

Patients with severe hypertension may require from 1200 mg to 2400 mg per day, with or without thiazide diuretics. Should side effects (principally nausea or dizziness) occur with these doses administered b.i.d., the same total daily dose administered t.i.d. may improve tolerability and facilitate further titration. Titration increments should not exceed 200 mg b.i.d..

When a diuretic is added, an additive antihypertensive effect can be expected. In some cases this may necessitate a labetalol HCl dosage adjustment. As with most antihypertensive drugs, optimal dosages of NORMODYNE (labetalol HCl) Tablets are usually lower in patients also receiving a diuretic.

When transferring patients from other antihypertensive drugs, NORMODYNE (labetalol HCl) Tablets should be introduced as recommended and the dosage of the existing therapy progressively decreased.

HOW SUPPLIED

NORMODYNE (labetalol HCl) Tablets, 100 mg, light-brown, round, scored, film-coated tablets engraved on one side with Schering and product identification numbers 244, and on the other side the number 100 for the strength and "NORMODYNE"; bottles of 100 (NDC-0085-0244-04), bottles of 500 (NDC-0085-0244-05), bottles of 1000 (NDC-0085-0244-07), and box of 100 for unit-dose dispensing (NDC-0085-0244-08).

NORMODYNE (labetalol HCl) Tablets, 200 mg, white, round, scored, film-coated tablets engraved on one side with Schering and product identification numbers 752, and on the other side the number 200 for the strength and "NORMODYNE"; bottles of 100 (NDC-0085-0752-04), bottles of 500 (NDC-0085-0752-05), bottles of 1000 (NDC-0085-0752-07), box of 100 for unit-dose dispensing (NDC-0085-0752-08).

NORMODYNE (labetalol HCl) Tablets, 300 mg, blue, round, film-coated tablets engraved on one side with Schering and product identification numbers 438, and on the other side the number 300 for the strength and "NORMODYNE"; bottles of 100 (NDC-0085-0438-03), bottles of 500 (NDC-0085-0438-05), box of 100 for unit-dose dispensing (NDC-0085-0438-06).

NORMODYNE (labetalol HCl) Tablets should be stored between 2° and 30°C (36° and 86°F).

NORMODYNE (labetalol HCl) Tablets in the unit-dose boxes should be protected from excessive moisture.

Key Pharmaceuticals, Inc.
Kenilworth, NJ 07033 USA
Rev. 5/94 16833525

Shown in Product Identification Guide, page 336

PROVENTIL® ℞

brand of albuterol, USP
Inhalation Aerosol
Bronchodilator Aerosol
FOR ORAL INHALATION ONLY

DESCRIPTION

The active component of PROVENTIL Inhalation Aerosol is albuterol, USP racemic (α^1-[(*tert* -butylamino)methyl]-4-hydroxy-*m*-xylene-α,α'-diol), a relatively selective beta$_2$-adrenergic bronchodilator, having the chemical structure:

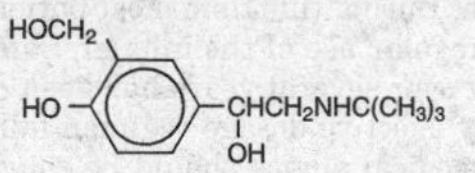

Albuterol is the official generic name in the United States. The World Health Organization recommended name for the drug is salbutamol. The molecular weight of albuterol is 239.3, and the empirical formula is $C_{13}H_{21}NO_3$. Albuterol is a white to off-white crystalline solid. It is soluble in ethanol, sparingly soluble in water, and very soluble in chloroform. PROVENTIL Inhalation Aerosol is a metered-dose aerosol unit for oral inhalation. It contains a microcrystalline suspension of albuterol in propellants (trichloromonofluoromethane and dichlorodifluoromethane) with oleic acid. Each actuation delivers from the mouthpiece 90 mcg of albuterol, USP. Each canister provides at least 200 inhalations.

CLINICAL PHARMACOLOGY

In vitro studies and *in vivo* pharmacologic studies have demonstrated that albuterol has a preferential effect on beta$_2$-adrenergic receptors compared with isoproterenol. While it is recognized that beta$_2$-adrenergic receptors are the predominant receptors in bronchial smooth muscle, recent data indicate that there is a population of beta$_2$-receptors in the human heart existing in a concentration between 10% and 50%. The precise function of these, however, is not yet established.

The pharmacologic effects of beta-adrenergic agonist drugs, including albuterol, are at least in part attributable to stimulation through beta-adrenergic receptors of intracellular adenyl cyclase, the enzyme which catalyzes the conversion of adenosine triphosphate (ATP) to cyclic-3′, 5′-adenosine monophosphate (c-AMP). Increased c-AMP levels are associated with relaxation of bronchial smooth muscle and inhibition of release of mediators of immediate hypersensitivity from cells, especially from mast cells.

Albuterol has been shown in most controlled clinical trials to have more effect on the respiratory tract, in the form of bronchial smooth muscle relaxation, than isoproterenol at comparable doses while producing fewer cardiovascular effects. Controlled clinical studies and other clinical experience have shown that inhaled albuterol, like other beta-adrenergic agonist drugs, can produce a significant cardiovascular effect in some patients, as measured by pulse rate, blood pressure, symptoms, and/or ECG changes.

Albuterol is longer acting than isoproterenol by any route of administration in most patients because it is not a substrate for the cellular uptake processes for catecholamines nor for catechol-*O* -methyl transferase.

Because of its gradual absorption from the bronchi, systemic levels of albuterol are low after inhalation of recommended doses. Studies undertaken with four subjects administered tritiated albuterol resulted in maximum plasma concentrations occurring within 2 to 4 hours. Due to the sensitivity of the assay method, the metabolic rate and half-life of elimination of albuterol in plasma could not be determined. However, urinary excretion provided data indicating that albuterol has an elimination half-life of 3.8 hours. Approximately 72% of the inhaled dose is excreted within 24 hours in the urine, and consists of 28% of unchanged drug and 44% as metabolite.

Results of animal studies show that albuterol does not pass the blood-brain barrier.

Recent studies in laboratory animals (minipigs, rodents, and dogs) recorded the occurrence of cardiac arrhythmias and sudden death (with histologic evidence of myocardial necrosis) when beta-agonists and methylxanthines were administered concurrently. The significance of these findings when applied to humans is currently unknown.

The effects of rising doses of albuterol and isoproterenol aerosols were studied in volunteers and asthmatic patients. Results in normal volunteers indicated that albuterol is $^1/_2$ to $^1/_4$ as active as isoproterenol in producing increases in heart rate. In asthmatic patients similar cardiovascular differentiation between the two drugs was also seen.

INDICATIONS AND USAGE

PROVENTIL Inhalation Aerosol is indicated for the prevention and relief of bronchospasm in patients with reversible obstructive airway disease, and for the prevention of exercise-induced bronchospasm.

In controlled clinical trials the onset of improvement in pulmonary function was within 15 minutes, as determined by both maximal midexpiratory flow rate (MMEF) and FEV_1. MMEF measurements also showed that near maximum improvement in pulmonary function generally occurs within 60 to 90 minutes, following 2 inhalations of albuterol and that clinically significant improvement generally continues for 3 to 4 hours in most patients. In clinical trials, some patients with asthma showed a therapeutic response (defined by maintaining FEV_1 values 15% or more above baseline) which was still apparent at 6 hours. Continued effectiveness of albuterol was demonstrated over a 13-week period in these same trials.

In clinical studies, 2 inhalations of albuterol taken approximately 15 minutes prior to exercise prevented exercise-induced bronchospasm, as demonstrated by the maintenance of FEV_1 within 80% of baseline values in the majority of patients. One of these studies also evaluated the duration of the prophylactic effect to repeated exercise challenges, which was evident at 4 hours in the majority of patients, and at 6 hours in approximately one-third of the patients.

CONTRAINDICATIONS

PROVENTIL Inhalation Aerosol is contraindicated in patients with a history of hypersensitivity to any of its components.

WARNINGS

As with other inhaled beta-adrenergic agonists, PROVENTIL Inhalation Aerosol can produce paradoxical bronchospasm that can be life-threatening. If it occurs, the preparation should be discontinued immediately and alternative therapy instituted.

Fatalities have been reported in association with excessive use of inhaled sympathomimetic drugs. The exact cause of death is unknown, but cardiac arrest following the unexpected development of a severe acute asthmatic crisis and subsequent hypoxia is suspected.

Immediate hypersensitivity reactions may occur after administration of albuterol inhalation aerosol, as demonstrated by rare cases of urticaria, angioedema, rash, bronchospasm, anaphylaxis, and oropharyngeal edema.

The contents of PROVENTIL Inhalation Aerosol are under pressure. Do not puncture. Do not use or store near heat or open flame. Exposure to temperatures above 120°F may cause bursting. Never throw container into fire or incinerator. Keep out of reach of children.

Continued on next page

Information on Schering products appearing on these pages is effective as of August 15, 1998.

Proventil Aerosol—Cont.

PRECAUTIONS

General: Albuterol, as with all sympathomimetic amines, should be used with caution in patients with cardiovascular disorders, especially coronary insufficiency, cardiac arrhythmias, and hypertension; in patients with convulsive disorders, hyperthyroidism, or diabetes mellitus; and in patients who are unusually responsive to sympathomimetic amines.

Large doses of intravenous albuterol have been reported to aggravate preexisting diabetes and ketoacidosis. Additionally, beta-agonists, including albuterol, when given intraveneously may cause a decrease in serum potassium, possibly through intracellular shunting. The relevance of this observation to the use of PROVENTIL Inhalation Aerosol is unknown, since the aerosol dose is much lower than the doses given intravenously.

Although there have been no reports concerning the use of PROVENTIL Inhalation Aerosol during labor and delivery, it has been reported that high doses of albuterol administered intravenously inhibit uterine contractions. Although this effect is extremely unlikely as a consequence of aerosol use, it should be kept in mind.

Information For Patients: The action of PROVENTIL Inhalation Aerosol may last up to 6 hours and therefore it should not be used more frequently than recommended. Increasing the number or frequency of doses without consulting your physician can be dangerous. If recommended dosage does not provide relief of symptoms or symptoms become worse, seek immediate medical attention. While taking PROVENTIL Inhalation Aerosol, other inhaled medicines should not be used unless prescribed.

See Illustrated Patient's Instructions For Use.

Drug Interactions: Other sympathomimetic aerosol bronchodilators should not be used concomitantly with albuterol. If additional adrenergic drugs are to be administered by any route, they should be used with caution to avoid deleterious cardiovascular effects.

Albuterol should be administered with caution to patients being treated with monoamine oxidase inhibitors or tricyclic antidepressants, since the action of albuterol on the vascular system may be potentiated.

Beta-receptor blocking agents and albuterol inhibit the effect of each other.

Since albuterol may lower serum potassium, care should be taken in patients also using other drugs which lower serum potassium as the effects may be additive.

Carcinogenesis, Mutagenesis, and Impairment of Fertility: In a 2-year study in the rat, albuterol sulfate caused a significant dose-related increase in the incidence of benign leiomyomas of the mesovarium at doses corresponding to 111, 555, and 2,800 times the maximum human inhalational dose. In another study this effect was blocked by the coadministration of propranolol. The relevance of these findings to humans is not known. An 18-month study in mice revealed no evidence of tumorigenicity. Studies with albuterol revealed no evidence of mutagenesis. Reproduction studies in rats revealed no evidence of impaired fertility.

Teratogenic Effects — Pregnancy Category C: Albuterol has been shown to be teratogenic in mice when given in doses corresponding to 14 times the human dose. There are no adequate and well-controlled studies in pregnant women. Albuterol should be used during pregnancy only if the potential benefit justifies the potential risk to the fetus. A reproduction study in CD-1 mice with albuterol (0.025, 0.25, and 2.5 mg/kg, corresponding to 1.4, 14, and 140 times the maximum human inhalational dose) showed cleft palate formation in 5 of 111 (4.5%) fetuses at 0.25 mg/kg and in 10 of 108 (9.3 %) fetuses at 2.5 mg/kg. None were observed at 0.025 mg/kg. Cleft palate also occurred in 22 of 72 (30.5%) fetuses treated with 2.5 mg/kg isoproterenol (positive control). A reproduction study in Stride Dutch rabbits revealed cranioschisis in 7 of 19 (37%) fetuses at 50 mg/kg, corresponding to 2,800 times the maximum human inhalational dose of albuterol. During marketing, various congenital anomalies, including cleft palate and limb defects, have been reported in the offspring of patients being treated with albuterol. Some of the mothers were taking multiple medications during their pregnancies. Because no consistent pattern of defects can be discerned, a relationship between albuterol use and congenital anomalies cannot be established.

Nursing Mothers: It is not known whether this drug is excreted in human milk. Because of the potential for tumorigenicity shown for albuterol in animal studies, a decision should be made whether to discontinue nursing or to discontinue the drug, taking into account the importance of the drug to the mother.

Pediatric Use: Safety and effectiveness in children below the age of 12 years have not been established.

ADVERSE REACTIONS

The adverse reactions of albuterol are similar in nature to those of other sympathomimetic agents, although the incidence of certain cardiovascular effects is less with albuterol. A 13-week double-blind study compared albuterol and isoproterenol aerosols in 147 asthmatic patients. The results of this study showed that the incidence of cardiovascular effects was: palpitations, less than 10 per 100 with albuterol and less than 15 per 100 with isoproterenol; tachycardia, 10 per 100 with both albuterol and isoproterenol; and increased blood pressure, less than 5 per 100 with both albuterol and isoproterenol. In the same study, both drugs caused tremor or nausea in less than 15 patients per 100; dizziness or heartburn in less than 5 per 100 patients. Nervousness occurred in less than 10 per 100 patients receiving albuterol and in less than 15 per 100 patients receiving isoproterenol.

Rare cases of urticaria, angioedema, rash, bronchospasm, and oropharyngeal edema have been reported after the use of inhaled albuterol.

In addition, albuterol, like other sympathomimetic agents, can cause adverse reactions such as hypertension, angina, vomiting, vertigo, central nervous system stimulation, insomnia, headache, unusual taste, and drying or irritation of the oropharynx.

OVERDOSAGE

Manifestations of overdosage may include anginal pain, hypertension, hypokalemia, and exaggeration of the pharmacological effects listed in **ADVERSE REACTIONS.**

As with all sympathomimetic aerosol medications, cardiac arrest and even death may be associated with abuse.

The oral LD_{50} in male and female rats and mice was greater than 2,000 mg/kg. The aerosol LD_{50} could not be determined.

Dialysis is not appropriate treatment for overdosage of PROVENTIL Inhalation Aerosol. The judicious use of a cardioselective beta-receptor blocker, such as metoprolol tartrate, is suggested, bearing in mind the danger of inducing an asthmatic attack.

DOSAGE AND ADMINISTRATION

For treatment of acute episodes of bronchospasm or prevention of asthmatic symptoms, the usual dosage for adults and children 12 years and older is 2 inhalations repeated every 4 to 6 hours; in some patients, 1 inhalation every 4 hours may be sufficient. More frequent administration or a larger number of inhalations is not recommended. For maintenance therapy or prevention of exacerbation of bronchospasm, 2 inhalations, 4 times a day should be sufficient.

The use of PROVENTIL Inhalation Aerosol can be continued as medically indicated to control recurring bouts of bronchospasm. During this time most patients gain optimal benefit from regular use of the inhaler. Safe usage for periods extending over several years has been documented.

If a previously effective dosage regimen fails to provide the usual relief, medical advice should be sought immediately, as this is often a sign of seriously worsening asthma which would require reassessment of therapy.

Exercise-Induced Bronchospasm Prevention: The usual dosage for adults and children 12 years and older is 2 inhalations, 15 minutes prior to exercise.

For treatment, see above.

HOW SUPPLIED

PROVENTIL Inhalation Aerosol, 17.0 g canister box of one (NDC-0085-0614-02); and 6.8 g canister for institutional use only, box of one (NDC-0085-0615-10). Each actuation delivers 90 mcg of albuterol from the mouthpiece. Each canister is supplied with an oral adapter and Patient's Instructions. PROVENTIL Inhalation Aerosol REFILL canister, 17.0 g, with Patient's Instructions; box of one (NDC-0085-0614-03).

Store between 15° and 30°C (59° and 86°F). Failure to use the product within this temperature range may result in improper dosing. Shake well before using.

NOTE: The indented statement below is required by the Federal government's Clean Air Act for all products containing or manufactured with chlorofluorocarbons (CFCs).

> **WARNING:** Contains dichlorodifluoromethane (CFC-11) and trichloromonofluoromethane (CFC-12), substances which harm public health and the environment by destroying ozone in the upper atmosphere.

A notice similar to the above WARNING has been placed in the "Patient's Instructions for Use" portion of this package insert pursuant to EPA regulations.

Rev. 10/94 18206811

Copyright © 1981, 1993, 1995, Schering Corporation. All rights reserved.

PROVENTIL® ℞

brand of albuterol sulfate, USP
Solution for Inhalation 0.5%*
(*Potency expressed as albuterol)

DESCRIPTION

PROVENTIL Solution for Inhalation contains albuterol sulfate, USP, the racemic form of albuterol and a relatively selective $beta_2$-adrenergic bronchodilator (see **CLINICAL PHARMACOLOGY** section below). Albuterol sulfate has the chemical name α^1-[(*tert* -Butylamino) methyl]-4-hydroxy-*m*-xylene-α,α′-diol sulfate (2:1) (salt), and the following chemical structure:

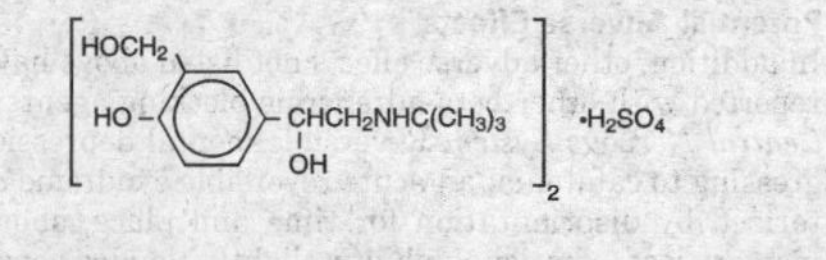
HOCH2
HO
CHCH2NHC(CH3)3
OH
•H2SO4
2

Albuterol sulfate has a molecular weight of 576.7 and the empirical formula $(C_{13}H_{21}NO_3)_2 \cdot H_2SO_4$. Albuterol sulfate is a white crystalline powder, soluble in water and slightly soluble in ethanol.

The World Health Organization's recommended name for albuterol base is salbutamol.

PROVENTIL Solution for Inhalation 0.5% is in concentrated form. Dilute 0.5 mL of the solution to 3 mL with sterile normal saline solution prior to administration.

Each mL of PROVENTIL Solution for Inhalation 0.5% contains 5 mg of albuterol (as 6.0 mg of albuterol sulfate) in an aqueous solution containing benzalkonium chloride; sulfuric acid is used to adjust the pH between 3 and 5. PROVENTIL Solution for Inhalation 0.5% contains no sulfiting agents. It is supplied in 20 mL bottles.

PROVENTIL Solution for Inhalation is a clear, colorless to light yellow solution.

CLINICAL PHARMACOLOGY

The prime action of beta-adrenergic drugs is to stimulate adenyl cyclase, the enzyme which catalyzes the formation of cyclic-3′,5′-adenosine monophosphate (cyclic AMP) from adenosine triphosphate (ATP). The cyclic AMP thus formed mediates the cellular responses. *In vitro* studies and *in vivo* pharmacologic studies have demonstrated that albuterol has a preferential effect on $beta_2$-adrenergic receptors compared with isoproterenol. While it is recognized that $beta_2$-adrenergic receptors are the predominant receptors in bronchial smooth muscle, recent data indicate that 10% to 50% of the beta receptors in the human heart may be $beta_2$ receptors. The precise function of these receptors, however, is not yet established. Albuterol has been shown in most controlled clinical trials to have more effect on the respiratory tract, in the form of bronchial smooth muscle relaxation, than isoproterenol at comparable doses while producing fewer cardiovascular effects. Controlled clinical studies and other clinical experience have shown that inhaled albuterol, like other beta-adrenergic agonist drugs, can produce a significant cardiovascular effect in some patients, as measured by pulse rate, blood pressure, symptoms, and/or ECG changes.

Albuterol is longer acting than isoproterenol in most patients by any route of administration because it is not a substrate for the cellular uptake processes for catecholamines nor for catechol-*O* -methyl transferase.

Studies in asthmatic patients have shown that less than 20% of a single albuterol dose was absorbed following either IPPB or nebulizer administration; the remaining amount was recovered from the nebulizer and apparatus and expired air. Most of the absorbed dose was recovered in the urine 24 hours after drug administration. Following a 3.0 mg dose of nebulized albuterol, the maximum albuterol plasma level at 0.5 hour was 2.1 ng/mL (range 1.4 to 3.2 ng/mL). There was a significant dose-related response in FEV_1 and peak flow rate (PFR). It has been demonstrated that following oral administration of 4 mg albuterol, the elimination half-life was 5 to 6 hours.

Animal studies show that albuterol does not pass the blood-brain barrier. Recent studies in laboratory animals (minipigs, rodents, and dogs) recorded the occurrence of cardiac arrhythmias and sudden death (with histologic evidence of myocardial necrosis) when beta-agonists and methylxanthines were administered concurrently. The significance of these findings when applied to humans is currently unknown.

In controlled clinical trials, most patients exhibited an onset of improvement in pulmonary function within 5 minutes as determined by FEV_1. FEV_1 measurements also showed that the maximum average improvement in pulmonary function usually occurred at approximately 1 hour following inhalation of 2.5 mg of albuterol by compressor-nebulizer, and remained close to peak for 2 hours. Clinically significant improvement in pulmonary function (defined as maintenance of a 15% or more increase in FEV_1 over baseline values) continued for 3 to 4 hours in most patients and in some patients continued up to 6 hours.

In repetitive dose studies, continued effectiveness was demonstrated throughout the 3-month period of treatment in some patients.

INDICATIONS AND USAGE

PROVENTIL Solution for Inhalation is indicated for the relief of bronchospasm in patients with reversible obstructive airway disease and acute attacks of bronchospasm.

CONTRAINDICATIONS

PROVENTIL Solution for Inhalation is contraindicated in patients with a history of hypersensitivity to any of its components.

WARNINGS

As with other inhaled beta-adrenergic agonists, PROVENTIL Solution for Inhalation can produce paradoxical bronchospasm, which can be life threatening. If it occurs, the preparation should be discontinued immediately and alternative therapy instituted.

Fatalities have been reported in association with excessive use of inhaled sympathomimetic drugs and with the home use of sympathomimetic nebulizers. It is, therefore, essential that the physician instruct the patient in the need for further evaluation if his/her asthma becomes worse. In individual patients, any $beta_2$-adrenergic agonist, including albuterol inhalation solution and solution for inhalation, may have a clinically significant cardiac effect.

Immediate hypersensitivity reactions may occur after administration of albuterol as demonstrated by rare cases of urticaria, angioedema, rash, bronchospasm, and oropharyngeal edema.

PRECAUTIONS

General: Albuterol, as with all sympathomimetic amines, should be used with caution in patients with cardiovascular disorders, especially coronary insufficiency, cardiac arrhythmias and hypertension, in patients with convulsive disorders, hyperthyroidism or diabetes mellitus, and in patients who are unusually responsive to sympathomimetic amines.

Large doses of intravenous albuterol have been reported to aggravate preexisting diabetes mellitus and ketoacidosis. Additionally, beta-agonists, including albuterol, when given intravenously may cause a decrease in serum potassium, possibly through intracellular shunting. The decrease is usually transient, not requiring supplementation. The relevance of these observations to the use of PROVENTIL Solution for Inhalation is unknown.

To avoid contaminating the multi-dose bottle of PROVENTIL Solution for Inhalation, proper aseptic technique should be used when withdrawing and delivering the dose into the nebulizer.

Information For Patients: The action of PROVENTIL Solution for Inhalation may last up to 6 hours and therefore it should not be used more frequently than recommended. Do not increase the dose or frequency of medication without medical consultation. If symptoms get worse, medical consultation should be sought promptly. While taking PROVENTIL Solution for Inhalation, other anti-asthma medicines should not be used unless prescribed.

Drug stability and safety of PROVENTIL Solution for Inhalation when mixed with other drugs in a nebulizer have not been established.

See illustrated **"Patient's Instructions for Use."**

Drug Interactions: Other sympathomimetic aerosol bronchodilators or epinephrine should not be used concomitantly with albuterol.

Albuterol should be administered with extreme caution to patients being treated with monoamine oxidase inhibitors or tricyclic antidepressants, since the action of albuterol on the vascular system may be potentiated.

Beta-receptor blocking agents and albuterol inhibit the effect of each other.

Since albuterol may lower serum potassium, care should be taken in patients also using other drugs which lower serum potassium as the effects may be additive.

Carcinogenesis, Mutagenesis, and Impairment of Fertility: Albuterol sulfate, like other agents in its class, caused a significant dose-related increase in the incidence of benign leiomyomas of the mesovarium in a 2-year study in the rat, at oral doses corresponding to 10, 50, and 250 times the maximum human nebulizer dose. In another study, this effect was blocked by the coadministration of propranolol. The relevance of these findings to humans is not known. An 18-month study in mice and a lifetime study in hamsters revealed no evidence of tumorigenicity. Studies with albuterol revealed no evidence of mutagenesis. Reproduction studies in rats revealed no evidence of impaired fertility.

Teratogenic Effects—Pregnancy Category C: Albuterol has been shown to be teratogenic in mice when given subcutaneously in doses corresponding to the human nebulization dose. There are no adequate and well-controlled studies in pregnant women. Albuterol should be used during pregnancy only if the potential benefit justifies the potential risk to the fetus. A reproduction study in CD-1 mice with albuterol (0.025, 0.25, and 2.5 mg/kg subcutaneously, corresponding to 0.1, 1, and 12.5 times the maximum human nebulization dose, respectively) showed cleft palate formation in 5 of 111 (4.5%) fetuses at 0.25 mg/kg and in 10 of 108 (9.3%) fetuses at 2.5 mg/kg. None were observed at 0.025 mg/kg. Cleft palate also occurred in 22 of 72 (30.5%) fetuses treated with 2.5 mg/kg isoproterenol (positive control). A reproduction study in Stride Dutch rabbits revealed cranioschisis in 7 of 19 (37%) fetuses at 50 mg/kg, corresponding to 250 times the maximum human nebulization dose. During marketing, various congenital anomalies, including cleft palate and limb defects, have been reported in the offspring of patients being treated with albuterol. Some of the mothers were taking multiple medications during their pregnancies. Because no consistent pattern of defects can be discerned, a relationship between albuterol use and congenital anomalies cannot be established.

Labor and Delivery: Oral albuterol has been shown to delay preterm labor in some reports. There are presently no well-controlled studies which demonstrate that it will stop preterm labor or prevent labor at term. Therefore, cautious use of PROVENTIL Solution for Inhalation is required in pregnant patients when given for relief of bronchospasm so as to avoid interference with uterine contractibility.

Nursing Mothers: It is not known whether this drug is excreted in human milk. Because of the potential for tumorigenicity shown for albuterol in some animal studies, a decision should be made whether to discontinue nursing or to discontinue the drug, taking into account the importance of the drug to the mother.

Pediatric Use: Safety and effectiveness of albuterol inhalation solution and solution for inhalation in children below the age of 12 years have not been established.

ADVERSE REACTIONS

The results of clinical trials with PROVENTIL Solution for Inhalation in 135 patients showed the following side effects which were considered probably or possibly drug related:

Central Nervous System: tremors (20%), dizziness (7%), nervousness (4%), headache (3%), insomnia (1%).

Gastrointestinal: nausea (4%), dyspepsia (1%).

Ear, Nose, Throat: pharyngitis (<1%), nasal congestion (1%).

Cardiovascular: tachycardia (1%), hypertension (1%).

Respiratory: bronchospasm (8%), cough (4%), bronchitis (4%), wheezing (1%).

No clinically relevant laboratory abnormalities related to PROVENTIL Solution for Inhalation administration were determined in these studies.

In comparing the adverse reactions reported for patients treated with PROVENTIL Solution for Inhalation with those of patients treated with isoproterenol during clinical trials of 3 months, the following moderate to severe reactions, as judged by the investigators, were reported. This table does not include mild reactions.

Percent Incidence of Moderate To Severe Adverse Reactions

Reaction	Albuterol N=65	Isoproterenol N=65
Central Nervous System		
Tremors	10.7%	13.8%
Headache	3.1%	1.5%
Insomnia	3.1%	1.5%
Cardiovascular		
Hypertension	3.1%	3.1%
Arrhythmias	0%	3.0%
* Palpitation	0%	22.0%
Respiratory		
† Bronchospasm	15.4%	18.0%
Cough	3.1%	5.0%
Bronchitis	1.5%	5.0%
Wheeze	1.5%	1.5%
Sputum Increase	1.5%	1.5%
Dyspnea	1.5%	1.5%
Gastrointestinal		
Nausea	3.1%	0%
Dyspepsia	1.5%	0%
Systemic		
Malaise	1.5%	0%

* The finding of no arrhythmias and no palpitations after albuterol administration in this clinical study should not be interpreted as indicating that these adverse effects cannot occur after the administration of inhaled albuterol.

† In most cases of bronchospasm, this item was generally used to describe exacerbations in the underlying pulmonary disease.

Rare cases of urticaria, angioedema, rash, bronchospasm, and oropharyngeal edema have been reported after the use of inhaled albuterol.

OVERDOSAGE

Manifestations of overdosage may include anginal pain, hypertension, hypokalemia, and exaggeration of the pharmacological effects listed in **ADVERSE REACTIONS.**

The oral LD_{50} in rats and mice was greater than 2,000 mg/kg. The inhalational LD_{50} could not be determined.

There is insufficient evidence to determine if dialysis is beneficial for overdosage of PROVENTIL Solution for Inhalation.

DOSAGE AND ADMINISTRATION

The usual dosage for adults and children 12 years and older is 2.5 mg of albuterol administered 3 to 4 times daily by nebulization. More frequent administration or higher doses are not recommended. To administer 2.5 mg of albuterol, dilute 0.5 mL of the 0.5% solution for inhalation to a total volume of 3 mL with sterile normal saline solution and administer by nebulization. The flow rate is regulated to suit the particular nebulizer so that the PROVENTIL Solution for Inhalation will be delivered over approximately 5 to 15 minutes.

Drug stability and safety of PROVENTIL Solution for Inhalation when mixed with other drugs in a nebulizer have not been established.

The use of PROVENTIL Solution for Inhalation can be continued as medically indicated to control recurring bouts of bronchospasm. During treatment, most patients gain optimum benefit from regular use of the nebulizer solution.

If a previously effective dosage regimen fails to provide the usual relief, medical advice should be sought immediately, as this is often a sign of seriously worsening asthma which would require reassessment of therapy.

HOW SUPPLIED

PROVENTIL Solution for Inhalation 0.5%, is a clear, colorless to light yellow solution, and is supplied in amber glass bottles of 20 mL fill (NDC-0085-0208-02) with accompanying calibrated dropper; boxes of one. **Store between 2° and 25°C (36 ° and 77°F).**

Rev 10/94 17979914

Copyright © 1986, 1993, 1995, Schering Corporation.
All rights reserved.

PROVENTIL® ℞

brand of albuterol sulfate, USP
Inhalation Solution 0.083%*
(*Potency expressed as albuterol)

DESCRIPTION

PROVENTIL Inhalation Solution contains albuterol sulfate, USP, the racemic form of albuterol, a relatively selective $beta_2$-adrenergic bronchodilator (see **CLINICAL PHARMACOLOGY** section below). Albuterol sulfate has the chemical name (α^1-[(*tert*-Butylamino) methyl]-4-hydroxy-*m*-xylene-α,α'-diol sulfate (2:1) (salt), and the following chemical structure:

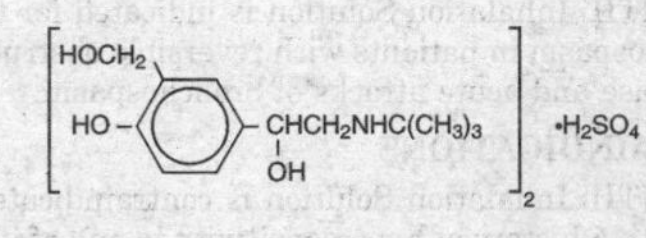

Albuterol sulfate has a molecular weight of 576.7 and the empirical formula $(C_{13}H_{21}NO_3)_2 \cdot H_2SO_4$. Albuterol sulfate is a white crystalline powder, soluble in water and slightly soluble in ethanol.

The World Health Organization recommended name for albuterol base is salbutamol.

Each mL of PROVENTIL Inhalation Solution 0.083% contains 0.83 mg of albuterol (as 1.0 mg of albuterol sulfate) in an isotonic aqueous solution containing sodium chloride and benzalkonium chloride; sulfuric acid is used to adjust the pH between 3 and 5. The 0.083% solution requires no dilution prior to administration. PROVENTIL Inhalation Solution 0.083% contains no sulfiting agents. It is supplied in 3 mL bottles for unit-dose dispensing.

PROVENTIL Inhalation Solution is a clear, colorless to light yellow solution.

CLINICAL PHAMACOLOGY

The prime action of beta-adrenergic drugs is to stimulate adenyl cyclase, the enzyme which catalyzes the formation of cyclic-3′,5′-adenosine monophosphate (cyclic AMP) from adenosine triphosphate (ATP). The cyclic AMP thus formed mediates the cellular responses. *In vitro* studies and *in vivo* pharmacologic studies have demonstrated that albuterol has a preferential effect on $beta_2$-adrenergic receptors compared with isoproterenol. While it is recognized that $beta_2$-adrenergic receptors are the predominant receptors in bronchial smooth muscle, recent data indicate that 10% to 50% of the beta receptors in the human heart may be $beta_2$ receptors. The precise function of these receptors, however, is not yet established. Albuterol has been shown in most controlled clinical trials to have more effect on the respiratory

Continued on next page

Information on Schering products appearing on these pages is effective as of August 15, 1998.

Proventil Solution—Cont.

tract, in the form of bronchial smooth muscle relaxation, than isoproterenol at comparable doses while producing fewer cardiovascular effects. Controlled clinical studies and other clinical experience have shown that inhaled albuterol, like other beta-adrenergic agonist drugs, can produce a significant cardiovascular effect in some patients, as measured by pulse rate, blood pressure, symptoms, and/or ECG changes.

Albuterol is longer acting than isoproterenol in most patients by any route of administration because it is not a substrate for the cellular uptake processes for catecholamines nor for catechol-O-methyl transferase.

Studies in asthmatic patients have shown that less than 20% of a single albuterol dose was absorbed following either IPPB or nebulizer administration; the remaining amount was recovered from the nebulizer and apparatus and expired air. Most of the absorbed dose was recovered in the urine 24 hours after drug administration. Following a 3.0 mg dose of nebulized albuterol, the maximum albuterol plasma level at 0.5 hour was 2.1 ng/mL (range 1.4 to 3.2 ng/mL). There was a significant dose-related response in FEV_1 and peak flow rate (PFR). It has been demonstrated that following oral administration of 4 mg albuterol, the elimination half-life was 5 to 6 hours.

Animal studies show that albuterol does not pass the blood-brain barrier. Recent studies in laboratory animals (minipigs, rodents, and dogs) recorded the occurrence of cardiac arrhythmias and sudden death (with histologic evidence of myocardial necrosis) when beta-agonists and methylxanthines were administered concurrently. The significance of these findings when applied to humans is currently unknown.

In controlled clinical trials, most patients exhibited an onset of improvement in pulmonary function within 5 minutes as determined by FEV_1. FEV_1 measurements also showed that the maximum average improvement in pulmonary function usually occurred at approximately 1 hour following inhalation of 2.5 mg of albuterol by compressor-nebulizer, and remained close to peak for 2 hours. Clinically significant improvement in pulmonary function (defined as maintenance of a 15% or more increase in FEV_1 over baseline values) continued for 3 to 4 hours in most patients and in some patients continued up to 6 hours.

In repetitive dose studies, continued effectiveness was demonstrated throughout the 3-month period of treatment in some patients.

INDICATIONS AND USAGE

PROVENTIL Inhalation Solution is indicated for the relief of bronchospasm in patients with reversible obstructive airway disease and acute attacks of bronchospasm.

CONTRAINDICATIONS

PROVENTIL Inhalation Solution is contraindicated in patients with a history of hypersensitivity to any of its components.

WARNINGS

As with other inhaled beta-adrenergic agonists, PROVENTIL Inhalation Solution can produce paradoxical bronchospasm, which can be life threatening. If it occurs, the preparation should be discontinued immediately and alternative therapy instituted.

Fatalities have been reported in association with excessive use of inhaled sympathomimetic drugs and with the home use of sympathomimetic nebulizers. It is, therefore, essential that the physician instruct the patient in the need for further evaluation if his/her asthma becomes worse. In individual patients, any beta₂-adrenergic agonist, including albuterol inhalation solution and solution for inhalation, may have a clinically significant cardiac effect.

Immediate hypersensitivity reactions may occur after administration of albuterol as demonstrated by rare cases of urticaria, angioedema, rash, bronchospasm, and oropharyngeal edema.

PRECAUTIONS

General: Albuterol, as with all sympathomimetic amines, should be used with caution in patients with cardiovascular disorders, especially coronary insufficiency, cardiac arrhythmias and hypertension, in patients with convulsive disorders, hyperthyroidism or diabetes mellitus, and in patients who are unusually responsive to sympathomimetic amines. Large doses of intravenous albuterol have been reported to aggravate preexisting diabetes mellitus and ketoacidosis. Additionally, beta-agonists, including albuterol, when given intravenously may cause a decrease in serum potassium, possibly through intracellular shunting. The decrease is usually transient, not requiring supplementation. The relevance of these observations to the use of PROVENTIL Inhalation Solution is unknown.

Information For Patients: The action of PROVENTIL Inhalation Solution may last up to 6 hours and therefore it should not be used more frequently than recommended. Do not increase the dose or frequency of medication without

medical consultation. If symptoms get worse, medical consultation should be sought promptly. While taking PROVENTIL Inhalation Solution, other anti-asthma medicines should not be used unless prescribed.

Drug stability and safety of PROVENTIL Inhalation Solution when mixed with other drugs in a nebulizer have not been established.

See illustrated **"Patient's Instructions for Use."**

Drug Interactions: Other sympathomimetic aerosol bronchodilators or epinephrine should not be used concomitantly with albuterol.

Albuterol should be administered with extreme caution to patients being treated with monoamine oxidase inhibitors or tricyclic antidepressants, since the action of albuterol on the vascular system may be potentiated.

Beta-receptor blocking agents and albuterol inhibit the effect of each other.

Since albuterol may lower serum potassium, care should be taken in patients also using other drugs which lower serum potassium as the effects may be additive.

Carcinogenesis, Mutagenesis, and Impairment of Fertility: Albuterol sulfate, like other agents in its class, caused a significant dose-related increase in the incidence of benign leiomyomas of the mesovarium in a 2-year study in the rat, at oral doses corresponding to 10, 50, and 250 times the maximum human nebulizer dose. In another study, this effect was blocked by the coadministration of propranolol. The relevance of these findings to humans is not known. An 18-month study in mice and a lifetime study in hamsters revealed no evidence of tumorigenicity. Studies with albuterol revealed no evidence of mutagenesis. Reproduction studies in rats revealed no evidence of impaired fertility.

Teratogenic Effects—Pregnancy Category C: Albuterol has been shown to be teratogenic in mice when given subcutaneously in doses corresponding to the human nebulization dose. There are no adequate and well-controlled studies in pregnant women. Albuterol should be used during pregnancy only if the potential benefit justifies the potential risk to the fetus. A reproduction study in CD-1 mice with albuterol (0.025, 0.25, and 2.5 mg/kg subcutaneously, corresponding to 0.1, 1, and 12.5 times the maximum human nebulization dose, respectively) showed cleft palate formation in 5 of 111 (4.5%) fetuses at 0.25 mg/kg and in 10 of 108 (9.3%) fetuses at 2.5 mg/kg. None were observed at 0.025 mg/kg. Cleft palate also occurred in 22 of 72 (30.5%) fetuses treated with 2.5 mg/kg isoproterenol (positive control). A reproduction study in Stride Dutch rabbits revealed cranioschisis in 7 of 19 (37%) fetuses at 50 mg/kg, corresponding to 250 times the maximum human nebulization dose. During marketing, various congenital anomalies, including cleft palate and limb defects, have been reported in the offspring of patients being treated with albuterol. Some of the mothers were taking multiple medications during their pregnancies. Because no consistent pattern of defects can be discerned, a relationship between albuterol use and congenital anomalies cannot be established.

Labor and Delivery: Oral albuterol has been shown to delay preterm labor in some reports. There are presently no well-controlled studies which demonstrate that it will stop preterm labor or prevent labor at term. Therefore, cautious use of PROVENTIL Inhalation Solution is required in pregnant patients when given for relief of bronchospasm so as to avoid interference with uterine contractility.

Nursing Mothers: It is not known whether this drug is excreted in human milk. Because of the potential for tumorigenicity shown for albuterol in some animal studies, a decision should be made whether to discontinue nursing or to discontinue the drug, taking into account the importance of the drug to the mother.

Pediatric Use: Safety and effectiveness of albuterol inhalation solution and solution for inhalation in children below the age of 12 years have not been established.

ADVERSE REACTIONS

The results of clinical trials with PROVENTIL Inhalation Solution in 135 patients showed the following side effects which were considered probably or possibly drug related:

Central Nervous System: tremors (20%), dizziness (7%), nervousness (4%), headache (3%), insomnia (1%).

Gastrointestinal: nausea (4%), dyspepsia (1%).

Ear, Nose and Throat: pharyngitis (<1%), nasal congestion (1%).

Cardiovascular: tachycardia (1%), hypertension (1%).

Respiratory: bronchospasm (8%), cough (4%), bronchitis (4%), wheezing (1%).

No clinically relevant laboratory abnormalities related to PROVENTIL Inhalation Solution administration were determined in these studies.

In comparing the adverse reactions reported for patients treated with PROVENTIL Inhalation Solution with those of patients treated with isoproterenol during clinical trials of 3 months, the following moderate to severe reactions, as judged by the investigators, were reported. This table does not include mild reactions.

Incidence of Moderate To Severe Reactions

Reaction	Albuterol N=65	Isoproterenol N=65
Central Nervous System		
Tremors	10.7%	13.8%
Headache	3.1%	1.5%
Insomnia	3.1%	1.5%
Cardiovascular		
Hypertension	3.1%	3.1%
Arrhythmias	0%	3.0%
* Palpitation	0%	22.0%
Respiratory		
** Bronchospasm	15.4%	18.0%
Cough	3.1%	5.0%
Bronchitis	1.5%	5.0%
Wheeze	1.5%	1.5%
Sputum Increase	1.5%	1.5%
Dyspnea	1.5%	1.5%
Gastrointestinal		
Nausea	3.1%	0%
Dyspepsia	1.5%	0%
Systemic		
Malaise	1.5%	0%

* The finding of no arrhythmias and no palpitations after albuterol administration in this clinical study should not be interpreted as indicating that these adverse effects cannot occur after the administration of inhaled albuterol.

** In most cases of bronchospasm, this term was generally used to describe exacerbations in the underlying pulmonary disease.

Rare cases of urticaria, angioedema, rash, bronchospasm, and oropharyngeal edema have been reported after the use of inhaled albuterol.

OVERDOSAGE

Manifestations of overdosage may include anginal pain, hypertension, hypokalemia, and exaggeration of the pharmacological effects listed in **ADVERSE REACTIONS.**

The oral LD_{50} in rats and mice was greater than 2,000 mg/kg. The inhalational LD_{50} could not be determined.

There is insufficient evidence to determine if dialysis is beneficial for overdosage of PROVENTIL Inhalation Solution.

DOSAGE AND ADMINISTRATION

The usual dosage for adults and children 12 years and older is 2.5 mg of albuterol administered 3 to 4 times daily by nebulization. More frequent administration or higher doses are not recommended. To administer 2.5 mg of albuterol, administer the contents of one unit-dose bottle (3 mL of 0.083% nebulizer solution) by nebulization. The flow rate is regulated to suit the particular nebulizer so that the PROVENTIL Inhalation Solution will be delivered over approximately 5 to 15 minutes.

Drug stability and safety of PROVENTIL Inhalation Solution when mixed with other drugs in a nebulizer have not been established.

The use of PROVENTIL Inhalation Solution can be continued as medically indicated to control recurring bouts of bronchospasm. During treatment, most patients gain optimum benefit from regular use of the nebulizer solution.

If a previously effective dosage regimen fails to provide the usual relief, medical advice should be sought immediately, as this is often a sign of seriously worsening asthma which would require reassessment of therapy.

HOW SUPPLIED

PROVENTIL Inhalation Solution 0.083% is a clear, colorless to light yellow solution, and is supplied in unit-dose HDPE (high density polyethylene) bottles of 3 mL fill each, boxes of 25 (NDC-0085-0209-01). **Store between 2° and 25°C (36° and 77°F).**

Rev. 10/94   17253832

Copyright © 1986, 1993, 1995, Schering Corporation. All rights reserved.

PROVENTIL®   ℞

brand of albuterol sulfate, USP
Syrup

DESCRIPTION

PROVENTIL Syrup contains albuterol sulfate, USP, the racemic form of albuterol and a relatively selective beta₂-adrenergic bronchodilator. Albuterol sulfate has the chemical name α^1-[(*tert*-Butylamino)methyl]-4-hydroxy-*m*-xylene-α,α′-diol sulfate (2:1) (salt), and the following chemical structure:

[See chemical structure at top of next column]

Albuterol sulfate has a molecular weight of 576.7 and the empirical formula $(C_{13}H_{21}NO_3)_2 \cdot H_2SO_4$. Albuterol sulfate is a white crystalline powder, soluble in water and slightly soluble in ethanol.

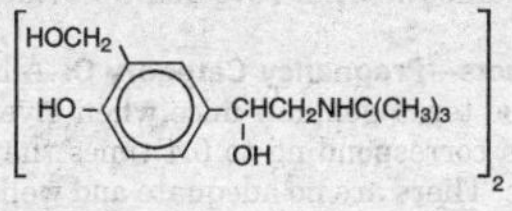

The World Health Organization recommended name for albuterol base is salbutamol.
PROVENTIL Syrup contains 2 mg of albuterol as 2.4 mg of albuterol sulfate in each teaspoonful (5 mL).
The inactive ingredients for PROVENTIL Syrup include: citric acid, FD&C Yellow No. 6, flavor, hydroxypropyl methylcellulose, saccharin, sodium benzoate, sodium citrate, and water.

CLINICAL PHARMACOLOGY

The prime action of beta-adrenergic drugs is to stimulate adenyl cyclase, the enzyme which catalyzes the formation of cyclic-3′,5′-adenosine monophosphate (cyclic AMP) from adenosine triphosphate (ATP). The cyclic AMP thus formed mediates the cellular responses. Based on pharmacologic studies in animals, albuterol appears to exert direct and preferential action on beta$_2$-adrenoceptors including those of the bronchial tree and uterus, and may have less cardiac stimulant effect than isoproterenol, when given in the usual recommended dose.
Albuterol is longer acting than isoproterenol in most patients by any route of administration because it is not a substrate for the cellular uptake processes for catecholamines nor for catechol-*O*-methyl transferase.
After oral administration of 10 mL PROVENTIL Syrup (4 mg albuterol) in normal volunteers, albuterol is rapidly absorbed. Maximum plasma albuterol concentrations of about 18 ng/mL are achieved within 2 hours and the drug is eliminated with a half-life of about 5 hours. In other studies, the analysis of urine samples of patients given 8 mg tritiated albuterol orally showed that 76% of the dose was excreted over 3 days, with the majority of the dose being excreted within the first 24 hours. Sixty percent of this radioactivity was shown to be the metabolite. Feces collected over this period contained 4% of the administered dose.
Animal studies show that albuterol does not pass the blood-brain barrier.

INDICATIONS AND USAGE

PROVENTIL Syrup is indicated for the relief of bronchospasm in adults and in children 2 years of age and older with reversible obstructive airway disease.
In controlled clinical trials in patients with asthma, the onset of improvement in pulmonary function, as measured by maximal midexpiratory flow rate (MMEF) and forced expiratory volume in one second (FEV$_1$), was within 30 minutes after a dose of PROVENTIL Syrup. Peak improvement of pulmonary function occurred between 2 and 3 hours. In a controlled clinical trial involving 55 children, clinically significant improvement (defined as maintenance of mean values over baseline of 15% or 20% or more in the FEV$_1$ and MMEF respectively) continued to be recorded up to 6 hours. No decrease in the effectiveness was reported in one uncontrolled study of 32 children who took PROVENTIL Syrup for a 3-month period.

CONTRAINDICATIONS

PROVENTIL Syrup is contraindicated in patients with a history of hypersensitivity to any of its components.

WARNINGS

Immediate hypersensitivity reactions may occur after administration of albuterol, as demonstrated by rare cases of anaphylaxis, angioedema, oropharyngeal edema, bronchospasm, urticaria, and rash.
Rarely, erythema multiforme and Stevens-Johnson syndrome have been associated with the administration of albuterol sulfate syrup in children.

PRECAUTIONS

General: Although albuterol usually has minimal effects on the beta$_1$-adrenoceptors of the cardiovascular system at the recommended dosage, occasionally the usual cardiovascular and CNS stimulatory effects common to all sympathomimetic agents have been seen with patients treated with albuterol necessitating discontinuation. Therefore, albuterol, as with all sympathomimetic amines, should be used with caution in patients with cardiovascular disorders, including coronary insufficiency, cardiac arrhythmias, and hypertension; in patients with convulsive disorders, hyperthyroidism, or diabetes mellitus, and in patients who are unusually responsive to sympathomimetic amines.
Large doses of intravenous albuterol have been reported to aggravate preexisting diabetes mellitus and ketoacidosis. Additionally, albuterol and other beta-agonists, when given intravenously, may cause a decrease in serum potassium, possibly through intracellular shunting. The decrease is usually transient, not requiring supplementation. The relevance of these observations to the use of PROVENTIL Syrup is unknown.

Information for Patients: The action of PROVENTIL Syrup may last up to 6 hours and therefore it should not be taken more frequently than recommended. Do not increase the dose or frequency of medication without medical consultation. If symptoms get worse, medical consultation should be sought promptly. If pregnant or nursing, consult with your physician.

Drug Interactions: The concomitant use of PROVENTIL Syrup and other oral sympathomimetic agents is not recommended since such combined use may lead to deleterious cardiovascular effects. This recommendation does not preclude the judicious use of an aerosol bronchodilator of the adrenergic stimulant type in patients receiving PROVENTIL Syrup. Such concomitant use, however, should be individualized and not given on a routine basis. If regular coadministration is required, then alternative therapy should be considered.
Albuterol should be administered with extreme caution to patients being treated with monoamine oxidase inhibitors or tricyclic antidepressants, since the action of albuterol on the vascular system may be potentiated.
Beta-receptor blocking agents and albuterol inhibit the effect of each other.
Since albuterol may lower serum potassium, care should be taken in patients also using other drugs which lower serum potassium as the effects may be additive.
After single-dose administration of albuterol to normal volunteers who had received digoxin for 10 days, a 16%–22% decrease in serum digoxin levels was demonstrated. The clinical significance of these findings for patients with obstructive airway disease who are receiving albuterol and digoxin on a chronic basis is unclear.
Nevertheless, it would be prudent to carefully evaluate the serum digoxin levels in patients who are concurrently receiving digoxin and albuterol.

Carcinogenesis, Mutagenesis, and Impairment of Fertility: Albuterol sulfate, like other agents in its class, caused a significant dose-related increase in the incidence of benign leiomyomas of the mesovarium in a 2-year study in the rat, at doses corresponding to 2, 9, and 46 times the maximum human (child weighing 21 kg) oral dose. In another study this effect was blocked by the coadministration of propranolol. The relevance of these findings to humans is not known. An 18-month study in mice and a lifetime study in hamsters revealed no evidence of tumorigenicity. Studies with albuterol revealed no evidence of mutagenesis. Reproduction studies in rats revealed no evidence of impaired fertility.

Teratogenic Effects—Pregnancy Category C: Albuterol has been shown to be teratogenic in mice when given subcutaneously in doses corresponding to 0.2 times the maximum human (child weighing 21 kg) oral dose. There are no adequate and well-controlled studies in pregnant women. Albuterol should be used during pregnancy only if the potential benefit justifies the potential risk to the fetus. A reproduction study in CD-1 mice with albuterol showed cleft palate formation in 5 of 111 (4.5%) fetuses at 0.25 mg/kg and in 10 of 108 (9.3%) fetuses at 2.5 mg/kg; none was observed at 0.025 mg/kg. Cleft palate also occurred in 22 of 72 (30.5%) fetuses treated with 2.5 mg/kg isoproterenol (positive control). A reproduction study in Stride Dutch rabbits revealed cranioschisis in 7 of 19 (37%) fetuses at 50 mg/kg, corresponding to 46 times the maximum human (child weighing 21 kg) oral dose of albuterol sulfate. During marketing, various congenital anomalies, including cleft palate and limb defects, have been reported in the offspring of patients being treated with albuterol. Some of the mothers were taking multiple medications during their pregnancies. Because no consistent pattern of defects can be discerned, a relationship between albuterol use and congenital anomalies cannot be established.

Labor and Delivery: Oral albuterol has been shown to delay preterm labor in some reports. There are presently no well-controlled studies which demonstrate that it will stop preterm labor or prevent labor at term. Therefore, cautious use of PROVENTIL Syrup is required in pregnant patients when given for relief of bronchospasm so as to avoid interference with uterine contractibility. Use in such patients should be restricted to those patients in whom the benefits clearly outweigh the risks.

Nursing Mothers: It is not known whether this drug is excreted in human milk. Because of the potential for tumorigenicity shown for albuterol in animal studies, a decision should be made whether to discontinue nursing or to discontinue the drug, taking into account the importance of the drug to the mother.

Pediatric Use: Safety and effectiveness in children below the age of 2 years have not yet been adequately demonstrated.

ADVERSE REACTIONS

The adverse reactions to albuterol are similar in nature to those of other sympathomimetic agents. The most frequent adverse reactions to PROVENTIL Syrup in adults and older children were tremor, 10 of 100 patients; nervousness and shakiness, each 9 of 100 patients. Other reported adverse reactions were headache, 4 of 100 patients; dizziness and increased appetite, each 3 of 100 patients; hyperactivity and excitement, each 2 of 100 patients; tachycardia, epistaxis, irritable behavior, and sleeplessness, each 1 of 100 patients. The following adverse effects occurred in less than 1 of 100 patients each: muscle spasm; disturbed sleep; epigastric pain; cough; palpitations; stomach ache; irritable behavior; dilated pupils; sweating; chest pain; weakness.
In young children 2 to 6 years of age, some adverse reactions were noted more frequently than in adults and older children. Excitement was noted in approximately 20% of patients and nervousness in 15%. Hyperkinesia occurred in 4% of patients; insomnia, tachycardia, and gastrointestinal symptoms in 2% each. Anorexia, emotional lability, pallor, fatigue, and conjunctivitis were seen in 1%.
In addition, albuterol, like other sympathomimetic agents, can cause adverse reactions such as hypertension, angina, vomiting, vertigo, central nervous system stimulation, unusual taste, and drying or irritation of the oropharynx.
The reactions are generally transient in nature, and it is usually not necessary to discontinue treatment with PROVENTIL Syrup. In selected cases, however, dosage may be reduced temporarily; after the reaction has subsided, dosage should be increased in small increments to the optimal dosage.

OVERDOSAGE

Manifestations of overdosage include anginal pain, hypertension, hypokalemia, and exaggeration of the effects listed in **ADVERSE REACTIONS.**
The oral LD_{50} in rats and mice was greater than 2,000 mg/kg. Dialysis is not appropriate treatment for overdosage of PROVENTIL Syrup. The judicious use of a cardioselective beta-receptor blocker, such as metoprolol tartrate, is suggested, bearing in mind the danger of inducing an asthmatic attack.

DOSAGE AND ADMINISTRATION

The following dosages of PROVENTIL Syrup are expressed in terms of albuterol base.
Usual Dose The usual starting dosage for adults and children over 14 years of age is 2 mg (1 teaspoonful) or 4 mg (2 teaspoonsful) three or four times a day.
The usual starting dosage for children 6 to 14 years of age is 2 mg (1 teaspoonful) three or four times a day.
For children 2 to 6 years of age, dosing should be initiated at 0.1 mg/kg of body weight three times a day. This starting dosage should not exceed 2 mg (1 teaspoonful) three times a day.
Dosage Adjustment For adults and children above age 14, a dosage above 4 mg four times a day should be used *only* when the patient fails to respond. If a favorable response does not occur, the dosage may be cautiously increased stepwise, but the dosage should not exceed 8 mg four times a day.
For children from 6 to 14 years of age who fail to respond to the initial starting dosage of 2 mg four times a day, the dosage may be cautiously increased stepwise, but not to exceed 24 mg per day (given in divided doses).
For children 2 to 6 years of age who do not respond satisfactorily to the initial dosage, the dose may be increased stepwise to 0.2 mg/kg of body weight three times a day, but not to exceed a maximum of 4 mg (2 teaspoonsful) given three times a day.
For elderly patients and those sensitive to beta-adrenergic stimulation, the initial dosage should be restricted to 2 mg three or four times a day and individually adjusted thereafter.

HOW SUPPLIED

PROVENTIL Syrup, a clear orange-yellow liquid with a strawberry flavor, contains 2 mg albuterol as the sulfate per 5 mL; bottles of 16 fluid ounces (NDC 0085-0315-02).
Store between 2° and 30°C (36° and 86°F).
Rev. 10/94 17979329
Copyright © 1982, 1992, 1993, 1995, Schering Corporation. All rights reserved.

PROVENTIL® ℞
brand of albuterol sulfate, USP
REPETABS® brand of
extended-release Tablets
PROVENTIL®
brand of albuterol sulfate, USP
Tablets

DESCRIPTION

PROVENTIL REPETABS Tablets and PROVENTIL Tablets contain albuterol sulfate, USP, the racemic form of albuterol and a relatively selective beta$_2$-adrenergic bronchodilator.

Continued on next page

Information on Schering products appearing on these pages is effective as of August 15, 1998.

Proventil Tabs/Repetabs—Cont.

Albuterol sulfate has the chemical name α^1-[(*tert*-Butylamino)methyl]-4-hydroxy-*m*-xylene-α, α′-diol sulfate (2:1) (salt), and the following chemical structure:

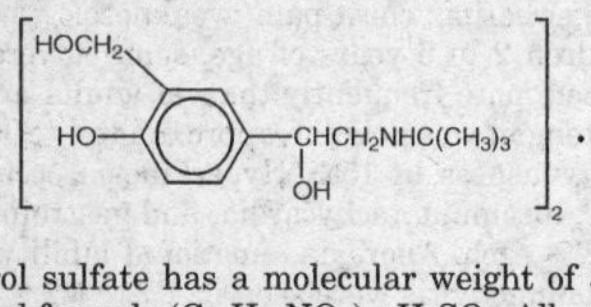

Albuterol sulfate has a molecular weight of 576.7 and the empirical formula $(C_{13}H_{21}NO_3)_2 \bullet H_2SO_4$. Albuterol sulfate is a white crystalline powder, soluble in water and slightly soluble in ethanol.

The World Health Organization recommended name for albuterol base is salbutamol.

Each PROVENTIL REPETABS Tablet contains a total of 4 mg (2 mg in the coating for immediate release and 2 mg in the core for release after several hours) of albuterol as 4.8 mg of albuterol sulfate.

Each PROVENTIL Tablet contains 2 or 4 mg of albuterol as 2.4 and 4.8 mg of albuterol sulfate, respectively.

The inactive ingredients for PROVENTIL REPETABS Tablets include: acacia, butylparaben, calcium phosphate, calcium sulfate, carnauba wax, corn starch, lactose, magnesium stearate, neutral soap, oleic acid, rosin, sugar, talc, titanium dioxide, white wax, and zein.

The inactive ingredients for PROVENTIL Tablets, 2 and 4 mg include: corn starch, lactose, and magnesium stearate.

CLINICAL PHARMACOLOGY

In vitro studies and *in vivo* pharmacologic studies have demonstrated that PROVENTIL has a preferential effect on $beta_2$-adrenergic receptors compared with isoproterenol. While it is recognized that $beta_2$-adrenergic receptors are the predominant receptors in bronchial smooth muscle, recent data indicate that there is a population of $beta_2$-receptors in the human heart, existing in a concentration between 10% and 50%. The precise function of these receptors, however, is not yet established.

Animal studies show that albuterol does not pass the blood-brain barrier. Studies in laboratory animals (minipigs, rodents, and dogs) recorded the occurrence of cardiac arrhythmias and sudden death (with histologic evidence of myocardial necrosis) when beta-agonists and methylxanthines were administered concurrently. The significance of these findings when applied to humans is currently unknown.

Albuterol is longer acting than isoproterenol in most patients by any route of administration because it is not a substrate for the cellular uptake processes for catecholamines nor for catechol-*O*-methyl transferase.

Pharmacokinetics and Disposition: Albuterol is rapidly and well absorbed following oral administration. In studies involving normal volunteers, the mean steady-state peak and trough plasma levels of albuterol were 6.7 and 3.8 ng/mL, respectively, following dosing with a 2 mg PROVENTIL Tablet every 6 hours and 14.8 and 8.6 ng/mL, respectively, following dosing with a 4 mg PROVENTIL Tablet every 6 hours. Maximum albuterol plasma levels are usually obtained between 2 and 3 hours after dosing and the elimination half-life is 5 to 6 hours. These data indicate that albuterol, administered orally, is dose proportional and exhibits dose independent pharmacokinetics.

PROVENTIL REPETABS Tablets have been formulated to provide a duration of action of up to 12 hours. In studies conducted in normal adult volunteers, the mean steady-state peak and trough plasma levels of albuterol were 6.5 and 3.0 ng/mL, respectively, following dosing with a 4 mg PROVENTIL REPETABS Tablet every 12 hours. In addition, it has been shown that administration of a 4 mg PROVENTIL REPETABS Tablet every 12 hours, and a 2 mg PROVENTIL Tablet every 6 hours for 5 days gave comparable peak albuterol levels and similar extent of absorption at steady state.

In other studies, the analysis of urine samples of subjects given tritiated albuterol (4 to 10 mg) orally showed that 65% to 90% of the dose was excreted over 3 days, with the majority of the dose being excreted within the first 24 hours. Sixty percent of this radioactivity was shown to be the metabolite of albuterol. Feces collected over this period contained 4% of the administered dose.

Clinical Studies: In controlled clinical trials in patients with asthma, the onset of improvement in pulmonary function, as measured by maximal mid-expiratory flow rate, MMEF, was noted within 30 minutes after a dose of PROVENTIL Tablets with peak improvement occurring between 2 and 3 hours. In controlled clinical trials, in which measurements were conducted for 6 hours, significant clinical improvement in pulmonary function (defined as maintaining a 15% or more increase in FEV_1 and a 20% or more increase in MMEF over baseline values) was observed in 60% of patients at 4 hours and in 40% at 6 hours. In other single-dose, controlled clinical trials, clinically significant improvement was observed in at least 40% of the patients at 8 hours with the 4 mg PROVENTIL Tablet. No decrease in the effectiveness of PROVENTIL Tablets has been reported in patients who received long-term treatment with the drug in uncontrolled studies for periods up to 6 months.

In another controlled clinical study in adult asthmatic patients, it has been demonstrated that the initiation of therapy with either the 4 mg PROVENTIL REPETABS Tablet dosed every 12 hours, or the 2 mg PROVENTIL Tablet dosed every 6 hours, achieve therapeutically equivalent effects.

INDICATIONS AND USAGE

PROVENTIL REPETABS Tablets and PROVENTIL Tablets are indicated for the relief of bronchospasm in patients 6 years of age or older with reversible obstructive airway disease.

CONTRAINDICATIONS

PROVENTIL REPETABS Tablets and PROVENTIL Tablets are contraindicated in patients with a history of hypersensitivity to any of their components.

PRECAUTIONS

General: Since albuterol is a sympathomimetic amine, it should be used with caution in patients with cardiovascular disorders, including ischemic heart disease, hypertension, or cardiac arrhythmias, in patients with hyperthyroidism or diabetes mellitus, and in patients who are unusually responsive to sympathomimetic amines or who have convulsive disorders. Significant changes in systolic and diastolic blood pressure could be expected to occur in some patients after use of any beta adrenergic bronchodilator.

Large doses of intravenous albuterol have been reported to aggravate preexisting diabetes mellitus and ketoacidosis. Additionally, albuterol and other beta agonists, when given intravenously, may cause a decrease in serum potassium, possibly through intracellular shunting. The decrease is usually transient not requiring supplementation. The relevance of these observations to the use of PROVENTIL REPETABS Tablets and PROVENTIL Tablets is unknown.

Information for Patients: Patients being treated with PROVENTIL REPETABS Tablets or PROVENTIL Tablets should receive the following information and instructions. This information is intended to aid in the safe and effective use of this medication. It is not a disclosure of all possible adverse or intended effects.

PROVENTIL REPETABS Tablets should not be chewed, crushed, or mixed in food.

PROVENTIL REPETABS Tablets and PROVENTIL Tablets should not be taken more frequently than recommended. Do not increase the dose or frequency of either medication, or add other medications to your therapy without medical consultation. If symptoms get worse, medical consultation should be sought promptly. If pregnant or nursing, consult with your physician.

Drug Interactions: The concomitant use of PROVENTIL REPETABS Tablets or PROVENTIL Tablets and other oral sympathomimetic agents is not recommended since such combined use may lead to deleterious cardiovascular effects. This recommendation does not preclude the judicious use of an aerosol bronchodilator of the adrenergic stimulant type in patients receiving PROVENTIL REPETABS Tablets or PROVENTIL Tablets. Such concomitant use, however, should be individualized and not given on a routine basis. If regular coadministration is required, then alternative therapy should be considered.

Albuterol should be administered with extreme caution to patients being treated with monoamine oxidase inhibitors or tricyclic antidepressants, since the action of albuterol on the vascular system may be potentiated.

Beta-receptor blocking agents and albuterol inhibit the effect of each other.

Since albuterol may lower serum potassium, care should be taken in patients also using other drugs which lower serum potassium as the effects may be additive.

After single-dose administration of albuterol to normal volunteers who had received digoxin for 10 days, a 16% to 22% decrease in serum digoxin levels was demonstrated. The clinical significance of these findings for patients with obstructive airway disease who are receiving albuterol and digoxin on a chronic basis is unclear. Nevertheless, it would be prudent to carefully evaluate the serum digoxin levels in patients who are concurrently receiving digoxin and albuterol.

Carcinogenesis, Mutagenesis, and Impairment of Fertility: Albuterol sulfate, like other agents in its class, caused a significant dose-related increase in the incidence of benign leiomyomas of the mesovarium in a 2-year study in the rat, at doses corresponding to 3, 16 and 78 times the maximum human oral dose. In another study this effect was blocked by the coadministration of propranolol. The relevance of these findings to humans is not known. An 18-month study in mice and a lifetime study in hamsters revealed no evidence of tumorigenicity. Studies with albuterol revealed no evidence of mutagenesis. Reproduction studies in rats revealed no evidence of impaired fertility.

Teratogenic Effects—Pregnancy Category C: Albuterol has been shown to be teratogenic in mice when given subcutaneously in doses corresponding to 0.4 times the maximum human oral dose. There are no adequate and well-controlled studies in pregnant women. Albuterol should be used during pregnancy only if the potential benefit justifies the potential risk to the fetus. A reproduction study in CD-1 mice with albuterol showed cleft palate formation in 5 of 111 (4.5%) fetuses at 0.25 mg/kg and in 10 of 108 (9.3%) fetuses at 2.5 mg/kg; none were observed at 0.025 mg/kg. Cleft palate also occurred in 22 of 72 (30.5%) fetuses treated with 2.5 mg/kg isoproterenol (positive control). A reproduction study in Stride Dutch rabbits revealed cranioschisis in 7 of 19 (37%) fetuses of 50 mg/kg, corresponding to 78 times the maximum human oral dose of albuterol.

During marketing, various congenital anomalies, including cleft palate and limb defects, have been reported in the offspring of patients being treated with albuterol. Some of the mothers were taking multiple medications during their pregnancies. Because no consistent pattern of defects can be discerned a relationship between albuterol use and congenital anomalies cannot be established.

Labor and Delivery: Oral albuterol has been shown to delay preterm labor in some reports. There are presently no well-controlled studies which demonstrate what it will stop preterm labor or prevent labor at term. Therefore, cautious use of PROVENTIL REPETABS Tablets or PROVENTIL Tablets is required in pregnant patients when given for relief of bronchospasm so as to avoid interference with uterine contractibility.

Nursing Mothers: It is not known whether this drug is excreted in human milk. Because of the potential for tumorigenicity shown for albuterol in some animal studies, a decision should be made whether to discontinue nursing or to discontinue the drug, taking into account the importance of the drug to the mother.

Pediatric Use: The safety and effectiveness of PROVENTIL Tablets and PROVENTIL REPETABS Tablets have been established in pediatric patients 6 years of age and older. Use of PROVENTIL REPETABS Tablets in these age groups is supported by evidence from adequate and well-controlled studies of PROVENTIL REPETABS Tablets in adults; the likelihood that the disease course, pathophysiology, and the drug's effect in pediatric and adult patients are substantially similar; the established safety and effectiveness of PROVENTIL Tablets in pediatric patients 6 years of age and older; and one clinical trial that provides evidence of the safety of PROVENTIL REPETABS Tablets in pediatric patients aged 6 to 12 years. The recommended dose of PROVENTIL REPETABS Tablets for the pediatric population is based upon the recommended pediatric dosing of PROVENTIL Tablets and pharmacokinetic studies in adults showing PROVENTIL REPETABS Tablets to have similar peak albuterol levels (ie, C_{max}) and exposures (ie, AUC) as PROVENTIL Tablets administered every 6 hours at one-half of the PROVENTIL REPETABS Tablets dose.

Safety and effectiveness in pediatric patients below the age of 6 years have not been established for PROVENTIL Tablets and PROVENTIL REPETABS Tablets.

ADVERSE REACTIONS

The adverse reactions to albuterol are similar in nature to those of other sympathomimetic agents. The most frequent adverse reactions to PROVENTIL Tablets were nervousness and tremor, with each occurring in approximately 20 of 100 patients (20%). Other reported reactions were headache, 7 of 100 patients (7%); tachycardia and palpitations, 5 of 100 patients (5%); muscle cramps, 3 of 100 patients (3%); insomnia, nausea, weakness, and dizziness, each occurred in 2 of 100 patients (2%). Drowsiness, flushing, restlessness, irritability, chest discomfort, and difficulty in micturition each occurred in less than 1 of 100 patients (less than 1%).

In a clinical study of 1 week duration in adults, comparing a 4 mg PROVENTIL REPETABS Tablet administered every 12 hours to a 2 mg PROVENTIL Tablet administered every 6 hours, the following adverse reactions considered to be possibly or probably treatment related were reported: nervousness in 1 of 50 (2%) and 3 of 50 patients (6%) for PROVENTIL REPETABS Tablets and PROVENTIL Tablets, respectively; nausea in 2 of 50 (4%) for both; vomiting in 1 of 50 (2%) and 2 of 50 (4%) for PROVENTIL REPETABS Tablets and PROVENTIL Tablets, respectively; somnolence in 1 of 50 (2%) for both. The following adverse reactions were reported for PROVENTIL Tablets only: tremor in 3 of 50 patients (6%); tinnitus, dyspepsia, and rash each occurred in 1 of 50 patients (2%).

Although not reported for PROVENTIL REPETABS Tablets in the above study in adults, there have been reports of tremor in other trials. When all clinical experience is considered, the incidence of tremor is approximately the same as that seen with PROVENTIL Tablets.

A placebo-controlled trial of 4 weeks duration in 157 mild-to-moderate asthmatic children aged 6 to 12 years, demon-

strated the safety of escalating doses of PROVENTIL REPETABS Tablets. In this study, the starting dose of PROVENTIL REPETABS Tablets was 4 mg twice daily. Patients were advanced to a maximum of 12 mg PROVENTIL REPETABS Tablets twice daily by the investigator, based on patient tolerance and response. Only one of the 79 children treated with PROVENTIL REPETABS Tablets was advanced to the maximum daily dose of 12 mg twice daily. The following treatment-related adverse events occurred in more than 5% of treated patients and were greater in PROVENTIL REPETABS Tablets patients when compared to placebo: headache (22% PROVENTIL REPETABS Tablets, 9% placebo); tremor (10% PROVENTIL REPETABS Tablets, 1% placebo); tachycardia and palpitations (8% PROVENTIL REPETABS Tablets, 1% placebo); insomnia (11% PROVENTIL REPETABS Tablets, 5% placebo); and nervousness (13% PROVENTIL REPETABS Tablets, 6% placebo). Other adverse events were noted in 5% or fewer patients, or had equal or greater rates of occurrence in placebo patients than in PROVENTIL REPETABS Tablets patients.

In addition to those adverse reactions reported above, albuterol, like other sympathomimetic agents, can cause adverse reactions such as hypertension, angina, vomiting, vertigo, central nervous system stimulation, unusual taste, and drying or irritation of the oropharynx.

The reactions are generally transient in nature, and it is usually not necessary to discontinue treatment with PROVENTIL REPETABS Tablets or PROVENTIL Tablets. In selected cases, however, dosage may be reduced temporarily; after the reaction has subsided, dosage should be increased in small increments to the optimal dosage.

OVERDOSAGE

Manifestations of overdosage include anginal pain, hypertension, hypokalemia, and exaggeration of the pharmacological effects listed in **ADVERSE REACTIONS.**

The oral LD_{50} in rats and mice was greater than 2,000 mg/kg.

There is insufficient evidence to determine if dialysis is beneficial for overdosage of PROVENTIL REPETABS Tablets or PROVENTIL Tablets.

DOSAGE AND ADMINISTRATION

The following dosages of PROVENTIL REPETABS Tablets and PROVENTIL Tablets are expressed in terms of albuterol base.

PROVENTIL REPETABS Tablets

Usual Dose: **Pediatric Patients 6 to 11 years of age:** The usual starting dosage of PROVENTIL REPETABS Tablets is 4 mg (one tablet) every 12 hours.

Adults and Pediatric Patients 12 years and over: The usual starting dosage of PROVENTIL REPETABS Tablets is 4 or 8 mg (one or two tablets) every 12 hours.

Dosage Adjustment in Pediatric Patients aged 6 to 11 years: Doses of PROVENTIL REPETABS Tablets above 4 mg twice a day should be used only when the patient fails to respond to this dose while on otherwise optimized asthma therapy. In such instances, the PROVENTIL REPETABS Tablets dose may be increased cautiously stepwise as tolerated if a favorable response does not occur with the 4 mg twice daily initial dose. The maximum recommended dose of PROVENTIL REPETABS Tablets in pediatric patients aged 6 to 11 years is 12 mg twice a day.

Dosage Adjustment in Adults and Pediatric Patients 12 years of age and over: Doses of PROVENTIL REPETABS Tablets above 8 mg twice a day should be used only when the patient fails to respond to this dose while on otherwise optimized asthma therapy. The PROVENTIL REPETABS Tablets dose may be increased cautiously stepwise as tolerated if a favorable response does not occur with the 8 mg twice daily dose. The maximum recommended dose of PROVENTIL REPETABS Tablets in adults and pediatric patients over 12 years of age is 16 mg twice a day.

Switching to PROVENTIL REPETABS Tablets: Patients currently maintained on PROVENTIL Tablets can be switched to PROVENTIL REPETABS Tablets. For example, the administration of a 4 mg PROVENTIL REPETABS Tablet every 12 hours is clinically comparable to one 2 mg PROVENTIL Tablet every 6 hours. Multiples of this regimen up to the maximum recommended daily dose also apply.

PROVENTIL Tablets

Usual Dose: **Pediatric Patients 6 to 12 years of age:** The usual starting dosage for pediatric patients 6 to 12 years of age is 2 mg three or four times a day.

Adults and Pediatric Patients 12 years and over: The usual starting dosage for adults and pediatric patients 12 years and over is 2 mg or 4 mg three or four times a day.

Dosage Adjustment: For pediatric patients from 6 to 12 years of age who fail to respond to the initial starting dosage of 2 mg four times a day, the dosage may be cautiously increased stepwise, but not to exceed 24 mg per day (given in divided doses).

For adults and pediatric patients 12 years and over, a dosage above 4 mg four times a day should be used only when the patient fails to respond to lower doses. The dose should be increased cautiously stepwise up to a maximum of 8 mg four times a day as tolerated if a favorable response does not occur with the 4 mg initial dose.

Elderly Patients and Those Sensitive to Beta-Adrenergic Stimulators: An initial dosage of 2 mg three or four times a day is recommended for elderly patients and for those with a history of unusual sensitivity to beta-adrenergic stimulators. If adequate bronchodilation is not obtained, dosage may be increased gradually to as much as 8 mg three or four times a day.

The total daily dose should not exceed 24 mg per day in pediatric patients from 6 to 12 years of age, and 32 mg per day in adults and pediatric patients 12 years and over.

HOW SUPPLIED

PROVENTIL REPETABS Tablets, 4 mg albuterol as the sulfate (2 mg in the coating for immediate release and 2 mg in the core for release after several hours), white, round, coated tablets, branded in red on one side with the Schering trademark and product identification numbers, 431, bottles of 100 (NDC 0085-0431-02) and 500 (NDC 0085-0431-03) and boxes of 100 for unit dose dispensing (NDC 0085-0431-04).

PROVENTIL Tablets, 2 mg albuterol as the sulfate, white, round, compressed tablets, impressed with the product name (PROVENTIL) and the number 2 on one side, and product identification numbers, 252, and scored on the other, bottles of 100 (NDC 0085-0252-02) and 500 (NDC 0085-0252-03).

PROVENTIL Tablets, 4 mg albuterol as the sulfate, white, round, compressed tablets, impressed with the product name (PROVENTIL) and the number 4 on one side, and product identification numbers, 573, and scored on the other, bottles of 100 (NDC 0085-0573-02) and 500 (NDC 0085-0573-03).

Store PROVENTIL REPETABS Tablets between 2° and 25°C (36° and 77°F), and PROVENTIL Tablets between 2° and 30°C (36° and 86°F). Protect PROVENTIL REPETABS Tablets in the unit dose box from excessive moisture.

Schering Corporation
Kenilworth, NJ 07033 USA

Rev. 10/97 B-17543334

Shown in Product Identification Guide, page 336

PROVENTIL® HFA ℞

(Albuterol Sulfate Inhalation Aerosol)
FOR ORAL INHALATION ONLY

Prescribing Information

DESCRIPTION

The active component of PROVENTIL HFA (Albuterol Sulfate Inhalation Aerosol) is albuterol sulfate, USP racemic a[1]-[(*tert*-Butylamino)methyl]-4-hydroxy-m-xylene-α, α′-diol sulfate (2:1)(salt), a relatively selective $beta_2$-adrenergic bronchodilator.

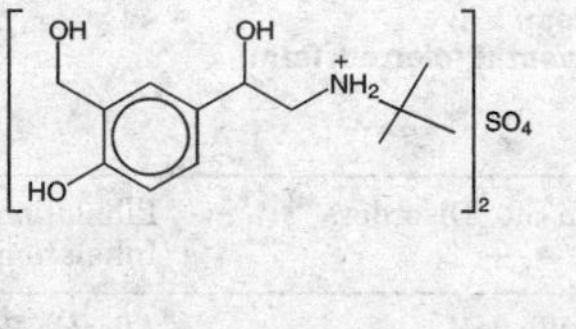

Albuterol sulfate is the official generic name in the United States. The World Health Organization recommended name for the drug is salbutamol sulfate. The molecular weight of albuterol sulfate is 576.7, and the empirical formula is $(C_{13}H_{21}NO_3)_2{\cdot}H_2SO_4$. Albuterol sulfate is a white to off-white crystalline solid. It is soluble in water and slightly soluble in ethanol. PROVENTIL HFA (Albuterol Sulfate Inhalation Aerosol) is a pressurized metered-dose aerosol unit for oral inhalation. It contains a microcrystalline suspension of albuterol sulfate in propellant HFA-134a (1,1,1,2-tetrafluoroethane), ethanol, and oleic acid.

Each actuation delivers 120 mcg albuterol sulfate, USP from the valve and 108 mcg albuterol sulfate, USP from the mouthpiece (equivalent to 90 mcg of albuterol base from the mouthpiece). Each canister provides 200 inhalations (pharmacy pack) or 100 inhalations (institutional pack).

This product does not contain chlorofluorocarbons (CFCs) as the propellant.

CLINICAL PHARMACOLOGY

Mechanism of Action *In vitro* studies and *in vivo* pharmacologic studies have demonstrated that albuterol has a preferential effect on $beta_2$-adrenergic receptors compared with isoproterenol. While it is recognized that $beta_2$-adrenergic receptors are the predominant receptors on bronchial smooth muscle, recent data indicate that there is a population of $beta_2$ receptors in the human heart which comprise between 10% and 50% of cardiac beta-adrenergic receptors. The precise function of these receptors, however, is not yet established. (See **WARNINGS** for **Cardiovascular Effects.**)

Activation of $beta_2$-adrenergic receptors on airway smooth muscle leads to the activation of adenylcyclase and to an increase in the intracellular concentration of cyclic-3′,5′-adenosine monophosphate (cyclic AMP). This increase of cyclic AMP leads to the activation of protein kinase A, which inhibits the phosphorylation of myosin and lowers intracellular ionic calcium concentrations, resulting in relaxation. Albuterol relaxes the smooth muscles of all airways, from the trachea to the terminal bronchioles. Albuterol acts as a functional antagonist to relax the airway irrespective of the spasmogen involved, thus protecting against all bronchoconstrictor challenges. Increased cyclic AMP concentrations are also associated with the inhibition of release of mediators from mast cells in the airway.

Albuterol has been shown in most clinical trials to have more bronchial smooth muscle relaxation effect than isoproterenol at comparable doses while producing fewer cardiovascular effects. However, all beta-adrenergic drugs, including albuterol sulfate, can produce a significant cardiovascular effect in some patients.

Preclinical Intravenous albuterol studies in rats have demonstrated that albuterol crosses the blood-brain barrier and reaches brain concentrations amounting to about 5% of the plasma concentrations. In structures outside the blood-brain barrier (pineal and pituitary glands), the drug achieves concentrations of more than 100 times those in whole brain.

Studies in pregnant rats with tritiated albuterol have demonstrated that approximately 10% of the circulating maternal drug is transferred to the fetus. Disposition in fetal lungs is comparable to maternal lungs, but fetal liver disposition is 1% of maternal liver levels.

Studies in laboratory animals (minipigs, rodents, and dogs) have demonstrated the occurrence of cardiac arrhythmias and sudden death (with histologic evidence of myocardial necrosis) when β-agonists and methylxanthines were administered concurrently. The significance of these findings when applied to humans is unknown.

Propellant HFA-134a is devoid of pharmacological activity except at very high doses in animals (380 – 1300 times the maximum human exposure based on comparisons of AUC values), primarily producing ataxia, tremors, dyspnea, or salivation. These are similar to effects produced by the structurally related chlorofluorocarbons (CFCs), which have been used extensively in metered dose inhalers.

In animals and humans, propellant HFA-134a was found to be rapidly absorbed and rapidly eliminated, with an elimination half-life of 3–27 minutes in animals and 5–7 minutes in humans. Time to maximum plasma concentration (T_{max}) and mean residence time are both extremely short leading to a transient appearance of HFA-134a in the blood with no evidence of accumulation.

Pharmacokinetics In a single-dose bioavailability study which enrolled 6 healthy, male volunteers, transient low albuterol levels (close to the lower limit of quantitation) were obtained after administration of two puffs from both PROVENTIL HFA (Albuterol Sulfate Inhalation Aerosol) and a CFC 11/12 propelled albuterol inhaler. No formal pharmacokinetic analyses were possible for either treatment, but systemic albuterol levels appeared similar.

Clinical Trials In a 12-week, randomized, double-blind, double-dummy, active- and placebo-controlled trial, 565 patients with asthma were evaluated for the bronchodilator efficacy of PROVENTIL HFA (Albuterol Sulfate Inhalation Aerosol) (193 patients) in comparison to a CFC 11/12 propelled albuterol inhaler (186 patients) and an HFA-134a placebo inhaler (186 patients).

Serial FEV_1 measurements (shown below as percent change from test-day baseline) demonstrated that two inhalations of PROVENTIL HFA (Albuterol Sulfate Inhalation Aerosol) produced significantly greater improvement in pulmonary function than placebo and produced outcomes which were clinically comparable to a CFC 11/12 propelled albuterol inhaler.

The mean time to onset of a 15 percent increase in FEV_1 was 6 minutes and the mean time to peak effect was 50 to 55 minutes. The mean duration of effect as measured by a 15 percent increase in FEV_1 was 3 hours. In some patients, duration of effect was as long as 6 hours.

[See figure at top of next column]

Continued on next page

Information on Schering products appearing on these pages is effective as of August 15, 1998.

Proventil/HFA—Cont.

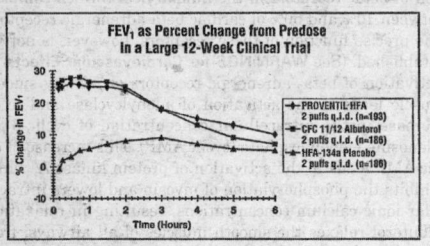

**FEV₁ as Percent Change from Predose
in a Large 12-Week Clinical Trial**

INDICATIONS AND USAGE

PROVENTIL HFA (Albuterol Sulfate Inhalation Aerosol) is indicated for the treatment or prevention of bronchospasm in patients 12 years of age and older with reversible obstructive airway disease.

CONTRAINDICATIONS

PROVENTIL HFA (Albuterol Sulfate Inhalation Aerosol) is contraindicated in patients with a history of hypersensitivity to any of its components.

WARNINGS

1. Paradoxical Bronchospasm: Inhaled albuterol sulfate can produce paradoxical bronchospasm that may be life threatening. If paradoxical bronchospasm occurs, PROVENTIL HFA (Albuterol Sulfate Inhalation Aerosol) should be discontinued immediately and alternative therapy instituted. It should be recognized that paradoxical bronchospasm, when associated with inhaled formulations, frequently occurs with the first use of a new canister.

2. Deterioration of Asthma: Asthma may deteriorate acutely over a period of hours or chronically over several days or longer. If the patient needs more doses of PROVENTIL HFA (Albuterol Sulfate Inhalation Aerosol) than usual, this may be a marker of destabilization of asthma and requires re-evaluation of the patient and treatment regimen, giving special consideration to the possible need for anti-inflammatory treatment, eg, corticosteroids.

3. Use of Anti-inflammatory Agents: The use of beta-adrenergic-agonist bronchodilators alone may not be adequate to control asthma in many patients. Early consideration should be given to adding anti-inflammatory agents, eg, corticosteroids, to the therapeutic regimen.

4. Cardiovascular Effects: PROVENTIL HFA (Albuterol Sulfate Inhalation Aerosol), like other beta-adrenergic agonists, can produce clinically significant cardiovascular effects in some patients as measured by pulse rate, blood pressure, and/or symptoms. Although such effects are uncommon after administration of PROVENTIL HFA (Albuterol Sulfate Inhalation Aerosol) at recommended doses, if they occur, the drug may need to be discontinued. In addition, beta agonists have been reported to produce ECG changes, such as flattening of the T wave, prolongation of the QTc interval, and ST segment depression. The clinical significance of these findings is unknown. Therefore, PROVENTIL HFA (Albuterol Sulfate Inhalation Aerosol), like all sympathomimetic amines, should be used with caution in patients with cardiovascular disorders, especially coronary insufficiency, cardiac arrhythmias, and hypertension.

5. Do Not Exceed Recommended Dose: Fatalities have been reported in association with excessive use of inhaled sympathomimetic drugs in patients with asthma. The exact cause of death is unknown, but cardiac arrest following an unexpected development of a severe acute asthmatic crisis and subsequent hypoxia is suspected.

6. Immediate Hypersensitivity Reactions: Immediate hypersensitivity reactions may occur after administration of albuterol sulfate, as demonstrated by rare cases of urticaria, angioedema, rash, bronchospasm, anaphylaxis, and oropharyngeal edema.

PRECAUTIONS

General Preparations containing sympathomimetic amines such as albuterol sulfate should be used with caution in patients who are unusually responsive to such agents and in patients with convulsive disorders, hyperthyroidism, or diabetes.

Beta-adrenergic-agonist medications may produce significant hypokalemia in some patients, possibly through intracellular shunting, which has the potential to produce adverse cardiovascular effects. The decrease is usually transient, not requiring supplementation.

Information for Patients See illustrated Patient's Instructions for Use. SHAKE WELL BEFORE USING. Patients should be given the following information:
KEEPING THE PLASTIC MOUTHPIECE CLEAN IS VERY IMPORTANT TO PREVENT MEDICATION BUILD-UP AND BLOCKAGE. THE MOUTHPIECE SHOULD BE WASHED, SHAKEN TO REMOVE EXCESS

WATER, AND AIR DRIED THOROUGHLY AT LEAST ONCE A WEEK. INHALER MAY CEASE TO DELIVER MEDICATION IF NOT PROPERLY CLEANED.
The mouthpiece should be cleaned (with the canister removed) by running warm water through the top and bottom for 30 seconds at least once a week. The mouthpiece must be shaken to remove excess water, then air dried thoroughly (such as overnight). Blockage from medication build-up or improper medication delivery may result from failure to thoroughly air dry the mouthpiece.
If the mouthpiece should become blocked (little or no medication coming out of the mouthpiece), the blockage may be removed by washing as described above.
If it is necessary to use the inhaler before it is completely dry, shake off excess water, replace canister, test spray twice away from face, and take the prescribed dose. After such use, the mouthpiece should be rewashed and allowed to air dry thoroughly.
The action of PROVENTIL HFA (Albuterol Sulfate Inhalation Aerosol) should last up to 4 to 6 hours. PROVENTIL HFA (Albuterol Sulfate Inhalation Aerosol) should not be used more frequently than recommended. Do not increase the number of puffs or frequency of doses of PROVENTIL HFA (Albuterol Sulfate Inhalation Aerosol) without consulting your physician. If you find that treatment with PROVENTIL HFA (Albuterol Sulfate Inhalation Aerosol) becomes less effective for symptomatic relief, your symptoms become worse, and/or you need to use the product more frequently than usual, medical attention should be sought immediately. While you are taking PROVENTIL HFA (Albuterol Sulfate Inhalation Aerosol), other inhaled drugs should be taken only as directed by your physician. If you are pregnant or nursing, contact your physician about use of PROVENTIL HFA (Albuterol Sulfate Inhalation Aerosol).
Common adverse effects of treatment with inhaled albuterol include palpitations, chest pain, rapid heart rate, tremor, or nervousness. Effective and safe use of PROVENTIL HFA (Albuterol Sulfate Inhalation Aerosol) includes an understanding of the way that it should be administered. Use PROVENTIL HFA (Albuterol Sulfate Inhalation Aerosol) only with the actuator supplied with the product. Discard the canister after 200 sprays have been used. (See Patient's Instructions for Use.)

Drug Interactions

1. Beta Blockers: Beta-adrenergic-receptor blocking agents not only block the pulmonary effect of beta agonists, such as PROVENTIL HFA (Albuterol Sulfate Inhalation Aerosol), but may produce severe bronchospasm in asthmatic patients. Therefore, patients with asthma should not normally be treated with beta blockers. However, under certain circumstances, eg, as prophylaxis after myocardial infarction, there may be no acceptable alternatives to the use of beta-adrenergic-blocking agents in patients with asthma. In this setting, cardioselective beta blockers could be considered, although they should be administered with caution.

2. Diuretics: The ECG changes and/or hypokalemia which may result from the administration of nonpotassium sparing diuretics (such as loop or thiazide diuretics) can be

acutely worsened by beta agonists, especially when the recommended dose of the beta agonist is exceeded. Although the clinical significance of these effects is not known, caution is advised in the coadministration of beta agonists with nonpotassium sparing diuretics.

3. Digoxin: Mean decreases of 16% and 22% in serum digoxin levels were demonstrated after single dose intravenous and oral administration of albuterol, respectively, to normal volunteers who had received digoxin for 10 days. The clinical significance of these findings for patients with obstructive airway disease who are receiving albuterol and digoxin on a chronic basis is unclear; however, careful evaluation of serum digoxin levels is recommended in patients who are currently receiving digoxin and albuterol.

4. Monoamine oxidase inhibitors or tricyclic antidepressants: PROVENTIL HFA (Albuterol Sulfate Inhalation Aerosol) should be administered with extreme caution to patients being treated with monoamine oxidase inhibitors or tricyclic antidepressants, or within 2 weeks of discontinuation of such agents, because the action of albuterol on the cardiovascular system may be potentiated.

Carcinogenesis, Mutagenesis, and Impairment of Fertility
In a 2-year study in rats, albuterol sulfate caused a significant dose-related increase in the incidence of benign leiomyomas of the mesovarium at oral dietary doses of 2, 10, and 50 mg/kg/day (approximately 12, 60, and 300 times the maximum recommended human daily inhalation dose on a mg/m² basis). In another study this effect was blocked by the coadministration of propranolol. The relevance of these findings to humans is not known. An 18-month study in mice at dietary doses up to 500 mg/kg/day (approximately 1560 times the maximum recommended human daily inhalation dose on a mg/m² basis) revealed no evidence of tumorigenicity. Studies with albuterol revealed no evidence of mutagenesis in rats at oral doses up to 50 mg/kg (approximately 300 times the maximum recommended human daily inhalation dose on a mg/m² basis).

Teratogenic Effects—Pregnancy Category C
Albuterol has been shown to be teratogenic in mice. A reproduction study in CD-1 mice given albuterol sulfate subcutaneously (0.025, 0.25, and 2.5 mg/kg) showed cleft palate formation in 5 of 111 (4.5%) fetuses at 0.25 mg/kg (approximately equal to the maximum recommended human daily inhalation dose on a mg/m² basis) and in 10 of 108 (9.3%) fetuses at 2.5 mg/kg (approximately 10 times the maximum recommended human daily inhalation dose on a mg/m² basis). None was observed at 0.025 mg/kg (approximately one tenth the maximum recommended human daily inhalation dose on a mg/m² basis). Cleft palate also occurred in 22 of 72 (30.5%) fetuses treated with 2.5 mg/kg isoproterenol (positive control). A reproduction study with oral albuterol in Stride Dutch rabbits revealed cranioschisis in 7 of 19 (37%) fetuses at 50 mg/kg (approximately 600 times the maximum recommended human daily inhalation dose on a mg/m² basis).
In a separate inhalation reproduction study in rats using albuterol sulfate/HFA-134a formulation, albuterol sulfate did not exhibit any teratogenic effects at 10.5 mg/kg/day (approximately 65 times the maximum recommended human daily inhalation dose on a mg/m² basis).

Adverse Experience Incidences (% of patients) in a Large 12-week Clinical Trial*				
Body System/ Adverse Event (Preferred Term)		**PROVENTIL HFA (Albuterol Sulfate Inhalation Aerosol) (N = 193)**	**CFC 11/12 Propelled Albuterol Inhaler (N = 186)**	**HFA-134a Placebo Inhaler (N = 186)**
Application Site Disorders	Inhalation Site Sensation	6	9	2
	Inhalation Taste Sensation	4	3	3
Body as a Whole	Allergic Reaction/Symptoms	6	4	<1
	Back Pain	4	2	3
	Fever	6	2	5
Central and Peripheral Nervous System	Tremor	7	8	2
Gastrointestinal System	Nausea	10	9	5
	Vomiting	7	2	3
Heart Rate and Rhythm Disorder	Tachycardia	7	2	<1
Psychiatric Disorders	Nervousness	7	9	3
Respiratory System Disorders	Respiratory Disorder (unspecified)	6	4	5
	Rhinitis	16	22	14
	Upper Resp Tract Infection	21	20	18
Urinary System Disorder	Urinary Tract Infection	3	4	2

* This table includes all adverse events (whether considered by the investigator drug related or unrelated to drug) which occurred at an incidence rate of at least 3.0% in the PROVENTIL HFA (Albuterol Sulfate Inhalation Aerosol) group and more frequently in the PROVENTIL HFA (Albuterol Sulfate Inhalation Aerosol) group than in the HFA-134a placebo inhaler group.

There are, however, no adequate and well-controlled studies of PROVENTIL HFA (Albuterol Sulfate Inhalation Aerosol) or albuterol sulfate in pregnant women. Because animal reproduction studies are not always predictive of human response, PROVENTIL HFA (Albuterol Sulfate Inhalation Aerosol) should be used during pregnancy only if the potential benefit justifies the potential risk to the fetus.

Various congenital anomalies, including cleft palate and limb defects, have been reported in the offspring of patients being treated with albuterol. Some of the mothers were taking multiple medications during their pregnancies. Because no consistent pattern of defects can be discerned, a relationship between albuterol use and congenital anomalies cannot be established.

Use in Labor and Delivery

Because of the potential for beta-agonist interference with uterine contractility, use of PROVENTIL HFA (Albuterol Sulfate Inhalation Aerosol) for relief of bronchospasm during labor should be restricted to those patients in whom the benefits clearly outweigh the risk.

Nursing Mothers

Plasma levels of albuterol sulfate and HFA-134a after inhaled therapeutic doses are very low in humans, but it is not known whether the components of PROVENTIL HFA (Albuterol Sulfate Inhalation Aerosol) are excreted in human milk.

Because of the potential for tumorigenicity shown for albuterol in animal studies and lack of experience with the use of PROVENTIL HFA (Albuterol Sulfate Inhalation Aerosol) by nursing mothers, a decision should be made whether to discontinue nursing or to discontinue the drug, taking into account the importance of the drug to the mother. Caution should be exercised when albuterol sulfate is administered to a nursing woman.

Pediatrics

The safety and effectiveness of PROVENTIL HFA (Albuterol Sulfate Inhalation Aerosol) in children below the age of 12 years have not been established.

Geriatrics

PROVENTIL HFA (Albuterol Sulfate Inhalation Aerosol) has not been studied in a geriatric population. As with other beta$_2$-agonists, special caution should be observed when using PROVENTIL HFA (Albuterol Sulfate Inhalation Aerosol) in elderly patients who have concomitant cardiovascular disease that could be adversely affected by this class of drug.

ADVERSE REACTIONS

Adverse reaction information concerning PROVENTIL HFA (Albuterol Sulfate Inhalation Aerosol) is derived from a 12-week, double-blind, double-dummy study which compared PROVENTIL HFA (Albuterol Sulfate Inhalation Aerosol), a CFC 11/12 propelled albuterol inhaler, and an HFA-134a placebo inhaler in 565 asthmatic patients. The following table lists the incidence of all adverse events (whether considered by the investigator drug related or unrelated to drug) from this study which occurred at a rate of 3% or greater in the PROVENTIL HFA (Albuterol Sulfate Inhalation Aerosol) treatment group and more frequently in the PROVENTIL HFA (Albuterol Sulfate Inhalation Aerosol) treatment group than in the placebo group. Overall, the incidence and nature of the adverse reactions reported for PROVENTIL HFA (Albuterol Sulfate Inhalation Aerosol) and a CFC 11/12 propelled albuterol inhaler were comparable.

[See table at bottom of previous page]

Adverse events reported by less than 3% of the patients receiving PROVENTIL HFA (Albuterol Sulfate Inhalation Aerosol), and by a greater proportion of PROVENTIL HFA (Albuterol Sulfate Inhalation Aerosol) patients than placebo patients, which have the potential to be related to PROVENTIL HFA (Albuterol Sulfate Inhalation Aerosol) include: dysphonia, increased sweating, dry mouth, chest pain, edema, rigors, ataxia, leg cramps, hyperkinesia, eructation, flatulence, tinnitus, diabetes mellitus, anxiety, depression, somnolence, rash. Palpitation and dizziness have also been observed with PROVENTIL HFA.

In small, cumulative dose studies, tremor, nervousness, and headache appeared to be dose related.

Rare cases of urticaria, angioedema, rash, bronchospasm, and oropharyngeal edema have been reported after the use of inhaled albuterol. In addition, albuterol, like other sympathomimetic agents, can cause adverse reactions such as hypertension, angina, vertigo, central nervous system stimulation, insomnia, headache, and drying or irritation of the oropharynx.

OVERDOSAGE

The expected symptoms with overdosage are those of excessive beta stimulation and/or occurrence or exaggeration of any of the symptoms listed under **ADVERSE REACTIONS,** eg, seizures, angina, hypertension or hypotension, tachycardia, arrhythmias, nervousness, headache, tremor, dry mouth, palpitation, nausea, dizziness, fatigue, malaise, and insomnia. Hypokalemia may also occur. As with all sympathomimetic medications, cardiac arrest and even death may be associated with abuse of PROVENTIL HFA (Albuterol Sulfate Inhalation Aerosol).

The oral median lethal dose of albuterol sulfate in mice and rats was greater than 2,000 mg/kg (approximately 6,000 and 12,000 times the maximum recommended human daily inhalation dose, respectively, on a mg/m^2 basis). The inhalation median lethal dose could not be determined.

Treatment consists of discontinuation of PROVENTIL HFA (Albuterol Sulfate Inhalation Aerosol) together with appropriate symptomatic therapy. The judicious use of a cardioselective beta-receptor blocker may be considered, bearing in mind that such medication can produce bronchospasm. There is insufficient evidence to determine if dialysis is beneficial for overdosage of PROVENTIL HFA (Albuterol Sulfate Inhalation Aerosol).

DOSAGE AND ADMINISTRATION

For treatment of acute episodes of bronchospasm or prevention of asthmatic symptoms, the usual dosage for adults and children 12 years and older is 2 inhalations repeated every 4 to 6 hours. More frequent administration or a larger number of inhalations is not recommended. In some patients, 1 inhalation every 4 hours may be sufficient. Each actuation of PROVENTIL HFA (Albuterol Sulfate Inhalation Aerosol) delivers 108 mcg of albuterol sulfate (equivalent to 90 mcg of albuterol base) from the mouthpiece.

To maintain proper use of this product it is important that the mouthpiece be washed and dried thoroughly at least once a week. The inhaler may cease to deliver medication if not properly cleaned and dried thoroughly. **See Information for Patients.** Keeping the plastic mouthpiece clean is very important to prevent medication build-up and blockage. The inhaler may cease to deliver medication if not properly cleaned and air dried thoroughly. If the mouthpiece becomes blocked, washing the mouthpiece will remove the blockage.

HOW SUPPLIED

PROVENTIL HFA (Albuterol Sulfate Inhalation Aerosol) is supplied as a pressurized aluminum canister with a yellow plastic actuator and orange dust cap. Each actuation delivers 120 mcg of albuterol sulfate from the valve and 108 mcg of albuterol sulfate from the mouthpiece (equivalent to 90 mcg of albuterol base). Canisters with a labeled net weight of 6.7 g contain 200 inhalations (Pharmacy Pack: NDC 0085-1132-01); 3.7 g labeled canisters contain 100 inhalations (Institutional Pack: NDC 0085-1132-02).

CAUTION

Federal law prohibits dispensing without prescription. Store between 15° and 25°C (59° and 77°F). For best results, canister should be at room temperature before use.

SHAKE WELL BEFORE USING.

PROVENTIL HFA (Albuterol Sulfate Inhalation Aerosol) should be used only with the actuator provided. The actuator should not be used with other aerosol medications. Avoid spraying in eyes. Contents under pressure. Do not puncture or incinerate. Exposure to temperatures above 120°F may cause bursting. Keep out of reach of children. PROVENTIL HFA (Albuterol Sulfate Inhalation Aerosol) does not contain chlorofluorocarbons (CFCs) as the propellant.

Developed and Manufactured by
3M Health Care Limited
Loughborough UK
or
3M Pharmaceuticals
Northridge, CA 91324
for
Key Pharmaceuticals, Inc.
Kenilworth, NJ 07033 USA
Copyright © 1996, 1997, Key Pharmaceuticals, Inc. All rights reserved.
Rev. 6/97   19863816-NPI

PROVENTIL® HFA   ℞
(Albuterol Sulfate Inhalation Aerosol)
Attention Pharmacist: Detach "Patient's Instructions for Use" from package insert and dispense with the product.
Patient's Instructions For Use

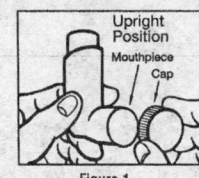

Upright Position
Mouthpiece
Cap

Figure 1

[See figure 2 at top of next column]

Before using your PROVENTIL HFA (Albuterol Sulfate Inhalation Aerosol), read complete instructions carefully.

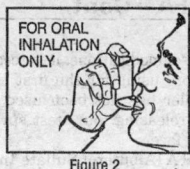

FOR ORAL INHALATION ONLY

Figure 2

Please note that **CFC** indicates that this inhalation aerosol does not contain chlorofluorocarbons (CFCs) as the propellant.

1. SHAKE THE INHALER WELL immediately before each use. **Then remove the cap from the mouthpiece** (see Figure 1). **Check mouthpiece for foreign objects prior to use.** Make sure the canister is fully inserted into the actuator.
2. BREATHE OUT FULLY THROUGH THE MOUTH, expelling as much air from your lungs as possible. Place the mouthpiece fully into the mouth holding the inhaler in its upright position (see Figure 2) and closing the lips around it.
3. WHILE BREATHING IN DEEPLY AND SLOWLY THROUGH THE MOUTH, FULLY DEPRESS THE TOP OF THE METAL CANISTER with your index finger (see Figure 2).
4. HOLD YOUR BREATH AS LONG AS POSSIBLE, up to 10 seconds. Before breathing out, remove the inhaler from your mouth and release your finger from the canister.
5. If your physician has prescribed additional puffs, wait 1 minute, shake the inhaler again and repeat steps 2 through 4. Replace the cap after use.
6. KEEPING THE PLASTIC MOUTHPIECE CLEAN IS EXTREMELY IMPORTANT TO PREVENT MEDICATION BUILD-UP AND BLOCKAGE. THE MOUTHPIECE SHOULD BE WASHED, SHAKEN TO REMOVE EXCESS WATER, AND AIR DRIED THOROUGHLY AT LEAST ONCE A WEEK. INHALER MAY STOP SPRAYING IF NOT PROPERLY CLEANED.

Routine cleaning instructions:

Step 1. To clean, remove the canister and mouthpiece cap. Wash the mouthpiece through the top and bottom with warm running water for 30 seconds at least once a week (see Figure A). **Never immerse the metal canister in water.**

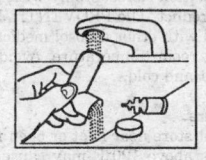

Figure A
Wash mouthpiece under warm running water

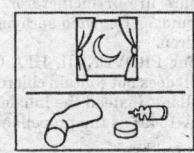

Figure B
Allow mouthpiece to air dry, such as overnight

not blocked

blocked

Figure C
When blocked little or no medicine comes out

Step 2. To dry, shake off excess water and let the mouthpiece air dry thoroughly, such as overnight (see Figure B). When the mouthpiece is dry, replace the canister and the mouthpiece cap. Blockage from medication build-up is more likely to occur if the mouthpiece is not allowed to air dry thoroughly.

IF YOUR INHALER HAS BECOME BLOCKED (little or no medication coming out of the mouthpiece, see Figure C), wash the mouthpiece as described in STEP 1 and air dry thoroughly as described in STEP 2.

IF YOU NEED TO USE YOUR INHALER BEFORE IT IS COMPLETELY DRY, SHAKE OFF EXCESS WATER, replace the canister, and test spray twice into the air, away from your face, to remove most of the water remaining in the mouthpiece. Then take your dose as prescribed. **After such use, rewash and air dry thoroughly as described in STEPS 1 and 2.**

Continued on next page

Information on Schering products appearing on these pages is effective as of August 15, 1998.

Proventil/HFA—Cont.

7. As with all aerosol medications, it is recommended to test the inhaler before using for the first time and in cases where the inhaler has not been used for more than 2 weeks. Test by releasing four "test sprays" into the air, away from your face.

8. PROVENTIL HFA (Albuterol Sulfate Inhalation Aerosol) will deliver at least 200 sprays. However, after 200 sprays, the amount of drug delivered per spray may not be consistent. You should keep track of the number of sprays used from each canister of PROVENTIL HFA (Albuterol Sulfate Inhalation Aerosol) and discard the canister after 200 sprays.

You may notice a slightly different taste or spray force than you are used to with PROVENTIL HFA (Albuterol Sulfate Inhalation Aerosol), compared to other albuterol inhalation aerosol products.

DOSAGE

Use only as directed by your physician.

WARNINGS

The action of PROVENTIL HFA (Albuterol Sulfate Inhalation Aerosol) should last up to 4 to 6 hours. PROVENTIL HFA (Albuterol Sulfate Inhalation Aerosol) should not be used more frequently than recommended. Do not increase the number of puffs or frequency of doses of PROVENTIL HFA (Albuterol Sulfate Inhalation Aerosol) without consulting your physician. If you find that treatment with PROVENTIL HFA (Albuterol Sulfate Inhalation Aerosol) becomes less effective for symptomatic relief, your symptoms become worse, and/or you need to use the product more frequently than usual, medical attention should be sought immediately. While you are taking PROVENTIL HFA (Albuterol Sulfate Inhalation Aerosol), other inhaled drugs should be taken only as directed by your physician. If you are pregnant or nursing, contact your physician about the use of PROVENTIL HFA (Albuterol Sulfate Inhalation Aerosol).

Common adverse effects of treatment with PROVENTIL HFA (Albuterol Sulfate Inhalation Aerosol) include palpitations, chest pain, rapid heart rate, tremor, or nervousness. Effective and safe use of PROVENTIL HFA (Albuterol Sulfate Inhalation Aerosol) includes an understanding of the way that it should be administered. Use PROVENTIL HFA (Albuterol Sulfate Inhalation Aerosol) only with the actuator supplied with the product. The PROVENTIL HFA actuator should not be used with other aerosol medications.

For best results use at room temperature. Avoid exposing product to extreme heat and cold.

Shake well before use.

Contents Under Pressure.

Do not puncture. Do not store near heat or open flame. Exposure to temperatures above 120°F may cause bursting. Never throw container into fire or incinerator. Store between 15° and 25°C (59° and 77°F). Avoid spraying in eyes. Keep out of reach of children.

Further Information: Your PROVENTIL HFA (Albuterol Sulfate Inhalation Aerosol) does not contain chlorofluorocarbons (CFCs) as the propellant. Instead the inhaler contains a hydrofluoroalkane (HFA-134a) as the propellant.

Developed and Manufactured by
3M Health Care Limited
Loughborough UK
or
3M Pharmaceuticals
Northridge, CA 91324
for
Key Pharmaceuticals, Inc.
Kenilworth, NJ 07033 USA
Copyright © 1996, 1997, Key Pharmaceuticals, Inc. All rights reserved.
Rev. 6/97   19863816
U.S. Patent 5,225,183

REBETRON™   ℞
Combination Therapy *containing*
REBETOL® (ribavirin, USP) Capsules *and*
INTRON® A (interferon alfa-2b, recombinant) Injection

PRODUCT INFORMATION

Combination REBETOL/INTRON A therapy is contraindicated in women who are pregnant. Women of childbearing potential and men must use effective contraception during treatment and during the 6-month posttreatment follow-up period. Significant teratogenic and/or embryocidal potential has been demonstrated for ribavirin in all animal species studied. See **CONTRAINDICATIONS**.

DESCRIPTION
INTRON® A

INTRON A is Schering Corporation's brand name for interferon alfa-2b, recombinant, a purified sterile recombinant interferon product.

Interferon alfa-2b, recombinant has been classified as an alpha interferon and is a water-soluble protein with a molecular weight of 19,271 daltons produced by recombinant DNA techniques. It is obtained from the bacterial fermentation of a strain of *Escherichia coli* bearing a genetically engineered plasmid containing an interferon alfa-2b gene from human leukocytes. The fermentation is carried out in a defined nutrient medium containing the antibiotic tetracycline hydrochloride at a concentration of 5 to 10 mg/L; the presence of this antibiotic is not detectable in the final product. INTRON A Injection is a clear, colorless solution. The 3 million IU vial of INTRON A Injection contains 3 million IU of interferon alfa-2b, recombinant per 0.5 mL. The 18 million IU multidose vial of INTRON A Injection contains a total of 22.8 million IU of interferon alfa-2b, recombinant per 3.8 mL (3 million IU/0.5 mL) in order to provide the delivery of six 0.5-mL doses, each containing 3 million IU of INTRON A (for a label strength of 18 million IU). The 18 million IU INTRON A Injection multidose pen contains a total of 22.5 million IU of interferon alfa-2b, recombinant per 1.5 mL (3 million IU/0.2 mL) in order to provide the delivery of six 0.2-mL doses, each containing 3 million IU of INTRON A (for a label strength of 18 million IU). Each mL also contains 7.5 mg sodium chloride, 1.8 mg sodium phosphate dibasic, 1.3 mg sodium phosphate monobasic, 0.1 mg edetate disodium, 0.1 mg polysorbate 80, and 1.5 mg m-cresol as a preservative.

Based on the specific activity of approximately 2.6×10^8 IU/mg protein as measured by HPLC assay, the corresponding quantities of interferon alfa-2b, recombinant in the vials and pen described above are approximately 0.012 mg, 0.088 mg, and 0.087 mg protein, respectively.

REBETOL®

REBETOL is Schering Corporation's brand name for ribavirin, a nucleoside analog with antiviral activity. The chemical name of ribavirin is 1-β-D-ribofuranosyl-1H-1,2,4-triazole-3-carboxamide and has the following structural formula:

Ribavirin is a white, crystalline powder. It is freely soluble in water and slightly soluble in anhydrous alcohol. The empirical formula is $C_8H_{12}N_4O_5$ and the molecular weight is 244.21.

REBETOL Capsules consist of a white powder in a white, opaque, gelatin capsule. Each capsule contains 200 mg ribavirin and the inactive ingredients microcrystalline cellulose, lactose monohydrate, croscarmellose sodium, and magnesium stearate. The capsule shell consists of gelatin, sodium lauryl sulfate, silicon dioxide, and titanium dioxide. The capsule is printed with edible blue pharmaceutical ink which is made of shellac, anhydrous ethyl alcohol, isopropyl alcohol, n-butyl alcohol, propyllene glycol, ammonium hydroxide, and FD&C Blue #2 aluminum lake.

Mechanism of Action

Interferon alfa-2b, recombinant / Ribavirin The mechanism of inhibition of hepatitis C virus (HCV) RNA by combination therapy with INTRON A and REBETOL has not been established.

CLINICAL PHARMACOLOGY
Pharmacokinetics

Interferon alfa-2b, recombinant Single- and multiple-dose pharmacokinetic properties of INTRON A are summarized in **TABLE 1**. Following a single 3 million IU (MIU) subcutaneous dose in 12 patients with chronic hepatitis C, mean (% CV*) serum concentrations peaked at 7 (44%) hours. Following 4 weeks of subcutaneous dosing with MIU three times a week (TIW), interferon serum concentrations were undetectable predose. However, a twofold increase in bioavailability was noted upon multiple dosing of interferon; the reason for this is unknown. Mean half-life values following single and multiple dose administrations were 6.8 (24%) hours and 6.5 (29%) hours, respectively.

Ribavirin Single- and multiple-dose pharmacokinetic properties in adults with chronic hepatitis C are summarized in Table 1. Ribavirin was rapidly and extensively absorbed following oral administration. However, due to first-pass metabolism, the absolute bioavailability averaged 64% (44%). There was a linear relationship between dose and AUC_{tf} (AUC from time zero to last measurable concentration) following single doses of 200–1200 mg ribavirin. The relationship between dose and C_{max} was curvilinear, tending to asymptote above single doses of 400–600 mg.

Upon multiple oral dosing, based on $AUC12_{hr}$, a sixfold accumulation of ribavirin was observed in plasma. Following oral dosing with 600 mg BID, steady-state was reached by approximately 4 weeks, with mean steady-state plasma concentrations of 2200 (37%) ng/mL. Upon discontinuation of dosing, the mean half-life was 298 (30%) hours, which probably reflects slow elimination from nonplasma compartments.

Effect of Food on Absorption of Ribavirin Both AUC_{tf} and C_{max} increased by 70% when REBETOL was administered with a high-fat meal (841 kcal, 53.8 g fat, 31.6 g protein, and 57.4 g carbohydrate) in a single-dose pharmacokinetic study. There are insufficient data to address the clinical relevance of these results. Clinical efficacy studies were conducted without instructions with respect to food consumption. (See **DOSAGE AND ADMINISTRATION**.)

Effect of Antacid on Absorption of Ribavirin Coadministration with an antacid containing magnesium, aluminum, and simethicone (Mylanta®) resulted in a 14% decrease in mean ribavirin AUC_{tf}. The clinical relevance of results, from this single-dose study is unknown.

[See table 1 below]

Ribavirin transport into nonplasma compartments has been most extensively studied in red blood cells, and has been identified to be primarily via an e_s-type equilibrative nucleoside transporter. This type of transporter is present on virtually all cell types and may account for the extensive volume of distribution. Ribavirin does not bind to plasma proteins.

Ribavirin has two pathways of metabolism: (i) a reversible phosphorylation pathway in nucleated cells; and (ii) a degradative pathway involving deribosylation and amide hydrolysis to yield a triazole carboxylic acid metabolite. Ribavirin and its triazole carboxamide and triazole carboxylic acid metabolites are excreted renally. After oral administration of 600 mg of ^{14}C-ribavirin, approximately 61% and 12% of the radioactivity was eliminated in the urine and feces, respectively, in 336 hours. Unchanged ribavirin accounted for 17% of the administered dose.

Results of *in vitro* studies using both human and rat liver microsome preparations indicated little or no cytochrome P450 enzyme-mediated metabolism of ribavirin with minimal potential for P450 enzyme-based drug interactions.

No pharmacokinetic interactions were noted between INTRON A and REBETOL Capsules in a multiple-dose pharmacokinetic study.

Special Populations

Renal Dysfunction The pharmacokinetics of ribavirin were assessed after administration of a single oral dose (400 mg)

TABLE 1. Mean (% CV) Pharmacokinetic Parameters for INTRON A and REBETOL When Administered Individually to Adults with Chronic Hepatitis C

Parameter	INTRON (N=12)		REBETOL (N=12)	
	Single Dose 3 MIU	Multiple Dose 3 MIU TIW	Single Dose 600 mg	Multiple Dose 600 mg BID
T_{max} (hr)	7 (44)	5 (37)	1.7 (46)***	3 (60)
C_{max} *	13.9 (32)	29.7 (33)	782 (37)	3680 (85)
AUC_{cf} **	142 (43)	333 (39)	13400 (48)	228000 (25)
$T_{1/2}$ (hr)	6.9 (24)	6.5 (29)	43.6 (47)	298 (30)
Apparent Volume of Distribution (L)			2825 (9)†	
Apparent Clearance (L/hr)	14.3 (17)		38.2 (40)	
Absolute Bioavailability			64% (44)‡	

* IU/mL for INTRON A and ng/mL for REBETOL
** IU.hr/mL for NITRON A and ng.hr/mL for REBETOL
† data obtained from a single-dose pharmacokinetic study using ^{14}C labeled ribavirin; N=5
‡ N=6
*** N=11

TABLE 2. Patients with Virologic and Histologic Responses*

	US Study		International Study	
	INTRON A plus REBETOL (N=77)	INTRON A plus Placebo (N=76)	INTRON A plus REBETOL (N=96)	INTRON A plus Placebo (N=96)
Virological Response				
-Responder[1]	33 (43)	3 (4)	46 (48)	5 (5)
-Nonresponder	36 (47)	66 (87)	45 (47)	91 (95)
-Missing	8 (10)	7 (9)	5 (5)	0 (0)
Histological Response				
-Improvement[2]	38 (49)	27 (36)	49 (51)	30 (31)
-No improvement	23 (30)	37 (49)	29 (30)	44 (46)
-Missing	16 (21)	12 (16)	18 (19)	22 (23)

* Number (%) of patients.
[1] Defined as HCV RNA below limit of detection using a research based RT-PCR assay at end of treatment and during follow-up period.
[2] Defined as posttreatment (end of follow-up) -pretreatment liver biopsy Knodell HAI score (I+II+III) improvement of ≥2 points.

TABLE 3. Selected Treatment-Emergent Adverse Events: Treated Relapse Patients

	Percentage of Patients			
	US Study		International Study	
Patients Reporting Adverse Events*	INTRON A plus REBETOL (N=77)	INTRON A plus Placebo (N=76)	INTRON A plus REBETOL (N=96)	INTRON A plus Placebo (N=96)
Application Site Disorders				
injection site inflammation	6	8	5	4
injection site reaction	5	3	0	3
Body as a Whole-General Disorders				
headache	66	68	47	43
fatigue	60	53	35	28
rigors	43	37	13	8
fever	32	36	31	30
influenza-like symptoms	13	13	29	32
asthenia	10	4	27	26
chest pain	6	7	1	5
Central & Peripheral Nervous System Disorders				
dizziness	26	21	9	5
Gastrointestinal System Disorders				
nausea	47	33	25	9
anorexia	21	14	19	11
dyspepsia	16	9	6	8
vomiting	12	8	6	1
Musculoskeletal System Disorders				
myalgia	61	58	30	24
arthralgia	29	29	15	18
musculoskeletal pain	22	28	18	18
Psychiatric Disorders				
insomnia	26	25	16	21
irritability	25	20	8	10
depression	23	14	10	8
emotional lability	12	8	7	3
concentration impaired	10	12	4	2
nervousness	5	4	7	1
Respiratory System Disorders				
dyspnea	17	12	11	1
sinusitus	12	7	3	1
Skin and Appendages Disorders				
alopecia	27	26	17	11
rash	21	5	6	4
pruritus	13	4	13	8
Special Senses, Other Disorders				
taste perversion	6	5	9	2

*Patients reporting one or more adverse events. A patient may have reported more than one adverse event within a body system/organ class category.

of ribavirin to subjects with varying degrees of renal dysfunction. The mean AUC_{tf} value was threefold greater in subjects with creatinine clearance values between 10 to 30 mL/min when compared to control subjects (creatinine clearance >90 mL/min). This appears to be due to reduction of apparent clearance in these patients. Ribavirin was not removed by hemodialysis. REBETOL is not recommended for patients with severe renal impairment (see **WARNINGS**).

Hepatic Dysfunction The effect of hepatic dysfunction was assessed after a single oral dose of ribavirin (600 mg). The mean AUC_{tf} values were not significantly different in subjects with mild, moderate, or severe hepatic dysfunction (Child-Pugh Classification A, B, or C) when compared to control subjects. However, the mean C_{max} values increased with severity of hepatic dysfunction and was twofold greater in subjects with severe hepatic dysfunction when compared to control subjects.

Pediatric Patients Pharmacokinetic evaluations for pediatric subjects have not been performed.

Elderly Patients Pharmacokinetic evaluations for elderly subjects have not been performed.

Gender There were no clinically significant pharmacokinetic differences noted in a single-dose study of eighteen male and eighteen female subjects.

*In this section of the label, numbers in parenthesis indicate % coefficient of variation.

INDICATIONS AND USAGE

The combination therapy of REBETOL (ribavirin, USP) Capsules with INTRON A (interferon alfa-2b, recombinant) Injection is indicated for the treatment of chronic hepatitis C in patients with compensated liver disease who have relapsed following alpha interferon therapy.

Description of Clinical Studies
Patients with compensated chronic hepatitis C and detectable HCV RNA (assessed by a central laboratory using a research based RT-PCR assay) who had relapsed following one or two courses of interferon therapy (defined as abnormal serum ALT levels) were enrolled into two multicenter, double-blind trials (US and International) and randomized to receive REBETOL 1200 mg/day (1000 mg/day for patients weighing ≤75 kg) plus INTRON A 3 MIU TIW or INTRON A plus placebo for 24 weeks followed by 24 weeks of off-therapy follow-up. The US study enrolled and treated 153 patients who, at baseline, were 67% male, 92% caucasian with a mean Knodell HAI score (I+II+III) of 6.8, and 58% genotype 1. The international study, conducted in Europe, Israel, Canada, and Australia, enrolled and treated 192 patients (64% male, 95% caucasian, mean Knodell score 6.6, and 56% genotype 1).

Study results are summarized in **TABLE 2.**

[See table 2 above]

Virologic and histologic response rates to therapy were similar in both male and female patients.

CONTRAINDICATIONS

Combination REBETOL/INTRON A therapy must not be used by women who are or may become pregnant. Combination REBETOL/INTRON A therapy should not be initiated until a report of a negative pregnancy test has been obtained. Women of childbearing potential and men must use effective contraception during treatment and during the 6-month posttreatment follow-up period. Significant teratogenic and/or embryocidal potential has been demonstrated for ribavirin in all animal species in which adequate studies have been conducted. These effects occurred at doses as low as one twentieth of the recommended human dose of REBETOL. If pregnancy occurs in a patient or partner of a patient during treatment or during the 6 months after treatment cessation, physicians are encouraged to report such cases by calling (800) 727-7064.

REBETOL Capsules in combination with INTRON A Injection is contraindicated in patients with a history of hypersensitivity to alpha interferons and/or ribavirin or any component of the injection and/or capsule.

Patients with autoimmune hepatitis must not be treated with combination REBETOL/INTRON A therapy.

WARNINGS
Anemia

ANEMIA (HEMOGLOBIN <10 G/DL) WAS OBSERVED IN 10% OF REBETOL/INTRON A-TREATED PATIENTS IN CLINICAL TRIALS (SEE ADVERSE REACTIONS LABORATORY VALUES - HEMOGLOBIN). ANEMIA OCCURRED WITHIN 1-2 WEEKS OF INITIATION OF RIBAVIRIN THERAPY. BECAUSE OF THIS INITIAL ACUTE DROP IN HEMOGLOBIN, IT IS ADVISED THAT COMPLETE BLOOD COUNTS (CBC) SHOULD BE OBTAINED PRETREATMENT AND AT WEEK 2 AND WEEK 4 OF THERAPY OR MORE FREQUENTLY IF CLINICALLY INDICATED. PATIENTS SHOULD THEN BE FOLLOWED AS CLINICALLY APPROPRIATE.

The anemia associated with REBETOL/INTRON A therapy may result in deterioration of cardiac function and/or exacerbation of the symptoms of coronary disease. Patients should be assessed before initiation of therapy and should be appropriately monitored during therapy. If there is any deterioration of cardiovascular status, therapy should be suspended or discontinued. (See **DOSAGE AND ADMINISTRATION**.) Because cardiac disease may be worsened by drug induced anemia, patients with a history of significant

Continued on next page

Information on Schering products appearing on these pages is effective as of August 15, 1998.

Rebetron—Cont.

or unstable cardiac disease should not use combination RE-BETOL/INTRON A therapy. (See **ADVERSE REACTIONS**.)

Similarly, patients with hemoglobinopathies (eg, thalassemia, sickle-cell anemia) should not be treated with combination REBETOL/INTRON A therapy.

Psychiatric

SEVERE PSYCHIATRIC ADVERSE EVENTS, INCLUDING DEPRESSION AND SUICIDAL BEHAVIOR (SUICIDAL IDEATION, SUICIDAL ATTEMPTS, AND SUICIDES) HAVE OCCURRED DURING REBETOL/INTRON A THERAPY AND WITH INTERFERON MONOTHERAPY, BOTH IN PATIENTS WITH AND WITHOUT A PREVIOUS PSYCHIATRIC ILLNESS. REBETOL/INTRON A therapy should be used with extreme caution in patients with a history of pre-existing psychiatric disorders who report a history of severe depression, and physicians should monitor all patients for evidence of depression. In severe cases, therapy should be stopped and psychiatric intervention sought. In general, the adverse events resolve on cessation of therapy; however, adjunctive psychiatric medications may be required. (See **ADVERSE REACTIONS**.)

Pulmonary

Pulmonary symptoms, including dyspnea, pulmonary infiltrates, pneumonitis and pneumonia, including fatality, have been reported during therapy with REBETOL/INTRON A. If there is evidence of pulmonary infiltrates or pulmonary function impairment, the patient should be closely monitored, and, if appropriate, combination REBETOL/INTRON A treatment should be discontinued.

Other

- Combination REBETOL/INTRON A therapy should be used with caution in patients with creatinine clearance <50 mL/min.
- Diabetes mellitus and hyperglycemia have been observed in patients treated with INTRON A.
- Ophthalmologic disorders have been reported with treatment with alpha interferons. Investigators using alpha interferons have reported the occurrence of retinal hemorrhages, cotton wool spots, and retinal artery or vein obstruction in rare instances. Any patient complaining of loss of visual acuity or visual field should have an eye examination. Because these ocular events may occur in conjunction with other disease states, a visual exam prior to initiation of combination REBETOL/INTRON A therapy is recommended in patients with diabetes mellitus or hypertension.
- Acute serious hypersensitivity reactions (eg, urticaria, angioedema, bronchoconstriction, anaphylaxis) have been observed in INTRON A-treated patients; if such an acute reaction develops, combination REBETOL/INTRON A therapy should be discontinued immediately and appropriate medical therapy instituted.
- Combination REBETOL/INTRON A therapy should be discontinued for patients developing thyroid abnormalities during treatment whose thyroid function cannot be controlled by medication.

PRECAUTIONS

Exacerbation of autoimmune disease has been reported in patients receiving alpha interferon therapy. REBETOL/INTRON A therapy should be used with caution in patients with other autoimmune disorders.

There have been reports of interferon, including INTRON A, exacerbating pre-existing psoriasis; therefore, combination REBETOL/INTRON A therapy should be used in these patients only if the potential benefit justifies the potential risk.

The safety and efficacy of REBETOL/INTRON A therapy has not been established in organ transplant patients, decompensated hepatitis C patients, patients who are nonresponders or naive to interferon therapy, or patients coinfected with HBV or HIV.

REBETOL monotherapy is not effective for the treatment of chronic hepatitis C and should not be used for this indication.

Information for Patients

Combination REBETOL/INTRON A therapy should not be initiated until a report of a negative pregnancy test has been obtained. It is also recommended that the patient be advised of the need to perform a pregnancy test monthly during therapy and for 6 months posttherapy. Women of childbearing potential must be counseled about use of adequate contraception prior to initiating therapy. Patients (male and female) should be advised to practice adequate contraception during combination REBETOL/INTRON A therapy and should be advised to notify the physician in the event of a pregnancy. (See **CONTRAINDICATIONS**.)

If pregnancy does occur during treatment or during 6 months posttherapy, the patient must be advised of the significant teratogenic risk of REBETOL therapy to the fetus. Patients, or partners of patients, should report any pregnancy that occurs during treatment or within 6 months af-

ter treatment cessation to their physician immediately. Physicians are encouraged to report such cases by calling (800) 727-7064.

Patients receiving combination REBETOL/INTRON A treatment should be directed in its appropriate use, informed of the benefits and risks associated with treatment, and referred to the **MEDICATION GUIDE**. There are no data evaluating whether REBETOL/INTRON A therapy will prevent transmission of infection to others.

If home use is prescribed, a puncture-resistant container for the disposal of used syringes and needles should be supplied to the patient. Patients should be thoroughly instructed in the importance of proper disposal and cautioned against any reuse of needles and syringes. The full container should be disposed of according to the directions provided by the physician (see **MEDICATION GUIDE**).

The most common adverse experiences occurring with combination REBETOL/INTRON A therapy are "flu-like" symptoms, such as headache, fatigue, myalgia, and fever (see **ADVERSE REACTIONS**) and appear to decrease in severity as treatment continues. Some of these "flu-like" symptoms may be minimized by bedtime administration of INTRON A therapy. Antipyretics should be considered to prevent or partially alleviate the fever and headache. Another common adverse experience associated with INTRON A therapy is thinning of the hair.

Patients should be advised that laboratory evaluations are required prior to starting therapy and periodically thereafter (see **Laboratory tests**). It is advised that patients be well hydrated, especially during the initial stages of treatment.

Laboratory Tests The following laboratory tests are recommended for all patients on combination REBETOL/INTRON A therapy, prior to beginning treatment and then periodically thereafter.

- Standard hematologic tests - including hemoglobin (pretreatment, week 2 and week 4 of therapy, and as clinically appropriate [see **WARNINGS**]), complete and differential white blood cell counts, and platelet count.
- Blood chemistries - liver function tests and TSH.
- Pregnancy - including monthly monitoring for women of childbearing potential.

Carcinogenesis and Mutagenesis Carcinogenicity studies with interferon alfa-2b, recombinant have not been performed because neutralizing activity appears in the serum after multiple dosing in all of the animal species tested. Adequate studies to assess the carcinogenic potential of ribavirin in animals have not been conducted. However, ribavirin is a nucleoside analog that has produced positive findings in multiple *in vitro* and animal *in vivo* genotoxicity assays, and should be considered a potential carcinogen. Further studies to assess the carcinogenic potential of ribavirin in animals are ongoing.

TABLE 4. Selected Hematologic Values During Treatment with REBETOL plus INTRON A

	Percentage of Patients			
	US Study		International Study	
	INTRON A plus REBETOL (N=77)	INTRON A plus Placebo (N=76)	INTRON A plus REBETOL (N=95)	INTRON A plus Placebo (N=96)
Hemoglobin (g/dL)				
9.5–10.9	21	3	24	1
8.0–9.4	4	0	1	0
6.5–7.9	0	0	0	0
<6.5	0	0	0	0
Leukocytes × 10⁹/L				
2.0–2.9	45	26	34	6
1.5–1.9	5	3	2	1
1.0–1.4	0	0	0	0
<1.0	0	0	0	0
Neutrophils × 10⁹/L				
1.0–1.49	42	34	32	31
0.75–0.99	16	18	12	6
0.5–0.74	8	4	6	0
<0.5	5	8	0	2
Platelets × 10⁹/L				
70–99	6	12	6	6
50–69	0	5	1	3
<49	0	0	0	0
Total Bilirubin (mg/dL)				
1.5–3.0	21	7	13	0
3.1–6.0	3	0	3	0
6.1–12.0	0	0	0	0
>12.0	0	0	0	0

In the above table the leukocytes, neutrophils, and platelets values are expressed as $\times 10^9$/L.

TABLE 5. Recommended Dosing

Body Weight	REBETOL Capsules	INTRON A Injection
≤75 kg	2 × 200 mg capsules AM, 3 × 200 mg capsules PM p.o.	3 million IU 3 times weekly s.c.
> 75 kg	3 × 200 mg capsules AM, 3 × 200 mg capsules PM p.o.	3 million IU 3 times weekly s.c.

TABLE 6. Guidelines for Dose Modifications

	Dose Reduction* REBETOL - 600 mg daily INTRON A - 1.5 million IU TIW	Permanent Discontinuation of Treatment REBETOL and INTRON A
Hemoglobin	<10 g/dL (REBETOL)	<8.5 g/dL
	Cardiac History Patients Only. **≥2 g/dL decrease during any 4-week period during treatment (REBETOL/INTRON A)**	**Cardiac History Patients Only.** **<12 g/dL after 4 weeks of dose reduction**
White blood count	<1.5 × 10⁹/L (INTRON A)	<1.0 ×10⁹/L
Neutrophil count	<0.75 ×10⁹/L (INTRON A)	<0.5 ×10⁹/L
Platelet count	<50 ×10⁹/L (INTRON A)	<25 ×10⁹/L

*Study medication to be dose reduced is shown in parenthesis.

Vial/Pen Label Strength	Fill Volume	Concentration
3 million IU vial	0.5 mL	3 million IU/0.5 mL
18 million IU multidose vial†	3.8 mL	3 million IU/0.5 mL
18 million IU multidose pen‡	1.5 mL	3 million IU/0.2 mL

† This is a multidose vial which contains a total of 22.8 million IU of interferon alfa-2b, recombinant per 3.8 mL in order to provide the delivery of six 0.5-mL doses, each containing 3 million IU of INTRON A (for a label strength of 18 milion IU).

‡ This is a multidose pen which contains a total of 22.5 million IU of interferon alfa-2b, recombinant per 1.5 mL in order to provide the delivery of six 0.2-mL doses, each containing 3 million IU of INTRON A (for a label strength of 18 million IU).

	Each REBETRON Combination Package Consists of:	
For Patients ≤75 kg	A box containing 6 vials of INTRON A Injection (3 million IU in 0.5 mL per vial) and 6 syringes and alcohol swabs. Two boxes containing 35 REBETOL Capsules each for a total of 70 capsules (5 capsules per blister card).	(NDC 0085-1241-02)
	One 18 million IU multidose vial of INTRON A Injection (22.8 million IU per 3.8 mL; 3 million IU/0.5 mL) and 6 syringes and alcohol swabs. Two boxes containing 35 REBETOL Capsules each for a total of 70 capsules (5 capsules per blister card).	(NDC 0085-1236-02)
	One 18 million IU INTRON A Injection multidose pen (22.5 million IU per 1.5 mL; 3 million IU/0.2 mL) and 6 disposable needles and alcohol swabs. Two boxes containing 35 REBETOL Capsules each for a total of 70 capsules (5 capsules per blister card).	(NDC 0085-1258-02)
For Patients <75 kg	A box containing 6 vials of INTRON A Injection (3 million IU in 0.5 mL per vial) and 6 syringes and alcohol swabs. Two boxes containing 42 REBETOL Capsules each for a total of 84 capsules (6 capsules per blister card).	(NDC 0085-1241-01)
	One 18 million IU multidose vial of INTRON A Injection (22.8 million IU per 3.8 mL; 3 million IU/0.5 mL) and 6 syringes and alcohol swabs. Two boxes containing 42 REBETOL Capsules each for a total of 84 capsules (6 capsules per blister card).	(NDC 0085-1236-01)
	One 18 million IU INTRON A Injection multidose pen (22.5 million IU per 3.8 mL; 3 million IU/0.2 mL) and 6 disposable needles and alcohol swabs. two boxes containing 42 REBETOL Capsules each for a total of 84 capsules (6 capsules per blister card).	(NDC 0085-1258-01)
For REBETOL Dose Reduction	A box containing 6 vials of INTRON A Injection (3 million IU in 0.5 mL per vial) and 6 syringes and alcohol swabs. One box containing 42 REBETOL Capsules (6 capsules per blister card).	(NDC 0085-1241-03)
	One 18 million IU multidose vial of INTRON A Injection (22.8 million IU per 3.8 mL; 3 million IU/0.5 mL) and 6 syringes and alcohol swabs. One box containing 42 REBETOL Capsules (6 capsules per blister card)	(NDC 0085-1236-03)
	One 18 million IU INTRON A Injection multidose pen (22.5 million IU per 1.5 mL; 3 million IU/.2 mL) and 6 disposable needles and alcohol swabs. One box containing 42 REBETOL Capsules (6 capsules per blister card)	(NDC 0085-1258-03)

Mutagenicity studies have demonstrated that interferon alfa-2b, recombinant is not mutagenic. Ribavirin demonstrated increased incidences of mutation and cell transformation in multiple genotoxicity assays. Ribavirin was active in the Balb/3T3 *In Vitro* Cell Transformation Assay. Mutagenic activity was obsered in the mouse lymphoma assay, and at doses of 20–200 mg/kg (estimated human equivalent of 1.67–16.7 mg/kg, based on body surface area adjustment for a 60 kg adult; 0.1–1 X the maximum recommended human 24-hour dose of ribavirin) in a mouse micronucleus assay. A dominant lethal assay in rats was negative, indicating that if mutations occurred in rats they were not transmitted through male gametes.

Impairment of Fertility No reproductive toxicology studies have been performed using interferon alfa-2b, recombinant in combination with ribavirin. However, evidence provided below for interferon alfa-2b, recombinant and ribavirin when administered alone indicate that both agents have adverse effects on reproduction. It should be assumed that the effects produced by either agent alone will also be caused by the combination of the two agents. Interferons may impair human fertility. In studies of interferon alfa-2b, recombinant administration in nonhuman primates, menstrual cycle abnormalities have been observed. Decreases in serum estradiol and progesterone concentrations have been reported in women treated with human leukocyte interferon. In addition, ribavirin demonstrated significant embryotoxic and/or teratogenic effects at doses well below the recom-

mended human dose in all animal species in which adequate studies have been conducted.

Fertile women should not receive combination REBETOL/INTRON A therapy unless they are using effective contraception during the therapy period. Based on a multiple dose t₁/₂ of 12 days, effective contraception should be utilized for 6 months posttherapy (eg, 15 half-lives of clearance for ribavirin).

Combination REBETOL/INTRON A therapy should be used with caution in fertile men. In a study in mice to evaluate the time course and reversibility of ribavirin-induced testicular degeneration at doses of 35 to 150 mg/kg/day (estimated human equivalent of 2.92–12.5 mg/kg/day, based on body surface area adjustment for a 60 kg adult; 0.2–0.8 X the maximum human 24–hour dose of ribavirin) administered for 3 or 6 months, abnormalities in sperm occurred. Upon cessation of treatment, essentially total recovery from ribavirin-induced testicular toxicity was apparent within 1 or 2 spermatogenesis cycles. A follow-up study to further assess these findings is ongoing.

Animal Toxicology Long-term studies in the mouse and rat (18–24 months; doses of 20–75 and 10–40 mg/kg/day, respectively [estimated human equivalent doses of 1.67–6.25 and 1.43–5.71 mg/kg/day, respectively, based on body surface area adjustment for a 60 kg adult; approximately 0.1–0.4 X the maximum human 24-hour dose of ribavirin] have demonstrated a relationship between chronic ribavirin exposure and increased incidences of vascular lesions (microscopic

hemorrhages) in mice. In rats, retinal degeneration occurred in controls, but the incidence was increased in ribavirin-treated rats.

Pregnancy Category X (see **CONTRAINDICATIONS**) Interferon alfa-2b, recombinant has been shown to have abortifacient effects in *Macaca mulatta* (rhesus monkeys) at 15 and 30 million IU/kg (estimated human equivalent of 5 and 10 million IU/kg, based on body surface area adjustment for a 60 kg adult). There are no adequate and well-controlled studies in pregnant women.

Ribavirin produced significant embryotoxic and/or teratogenic effects in all animal species in which adequate studies have been conducted. Malformations of the skull, palate, eye, jaw, limbs, skeleton, and gastrointestinal tract were noted. The incidence and severity of teratogenic effects increased with escalation of the drug dose. Survival of fetuses and offspring was reduced. In conventional embryotoxicity/teratogenicity studies in rats and rabbits, observed no effect dose levels were well below those for proposed clinical use (0.3 mg/kg/day for both the rat and rabbit; approximately 0.06 X the recommended human 24-hour dose of ribavirin). No maternal toxicity nor effects on offspring were observed in a peri/postnatal toxicity study in rats dosed orally at up to 1 mg/kg/day (estimated human equivalent dose of 0.17 mg/kg based on body surface area adjustment for a 60 kg adult; approximately 0.01 X the maximum recommended human 24-hour dose of ribavirin).

Treatment and Posttreatment: Potential Risk to the Fetus Ribavirin is known to accumulate in intracellular components from where it is cleared very slowly. It is not known whether ribavirin contained in sperm will exert a potential teratogenic effect upon fertilization of the ova. In a study in rats, it was concluded that dominant lethality was not induced by ribavirin at doses up to 200 mg/kg for 5 days (estimated human equivalent doses of 7.14–28.6 mg/kg, based on body surface area adjustment or a 60 kg adult; up to 1.7 X the maximum recommended human dose of ribavirin). However, because of the potential human teratogenic effects of ribavirin exposure to the fetus, male patients should be advised to take every precaution to avoid risk of pregnancy for their female partners.

It is advised that male patients be counseled to practice effective contraception during treatment with combination REBETOL/INTRON A therapy and for the 6-month posttherapy period (eg, 15 half-lives for ribavirin clearance from the body).

Women of childbearing potential should not receive combination REBETOL/INTRON A therapy unless they are using effective contraception during the therapy period. In addition, effective contraception should be utilized for 6 months posttherapy based on a multiple dose t₁/₂ of ribavirin of 12 days.

If pregnancy occurs in a patient or partner of a patient during treatment or during the 6 months after treatment cessation, physicians are encouraged to report such cases by calling (800) 727–7064.

Nursing Mothers It is not known whether REBETOL and INTRON A are excreted in human milk. However, studies in mice have shown that mouse interferons are excreted into the milk. Because of the potential for serious adverse reactions from the drugs in nursing infants, a decision should be made whether to discontinue nursing or to discontinue combination REBETOL/INTRON A therapy, taking into account the importance of the therapy to the mother.

Pediatric Use Safety and effectiveness in pediatric patients below the age of 18 years have not been established. (See **INDICATIONS AND USAGE.**)

ADVERSE REACTIONS

The safety of combination REBETOL/INTRON A therapy was evaluated in controlled trials of 173 HCV-infected patients who had relapsed after interferon therapy. (See *Description of Clinical Studies*.) Overall, 6% of patients discontinued therapy due to adverse events in the combination arm compared to 3% in the interferon arm.

The primary toxicity of ribavirin is anemia. Reductions in hemoglobin levels occurred within the first 1–2 weeks of therapy (see **WARNINGS**). Cardiac and pulmonary events associated with anemia occurred in approximately 10% of patients treated with REBETOL/INTRON A. (See **WARNINGS.**)

Psychiatric events, most commonly insomnia, depression, and irritability occurred in 53% (91/173) of patients. Suicidal behavior (ideation, attempts, and suicides) occurred in < 1% of patients. (See **WARNINGS.**)

Selected treatment-emergent adverse events that occurred with ≥5% incidence are provided in **Table 3** by treatment group.

[See table 3 at top of page 2881]

Laboratory Values Changes in selected hematologic values (hemoglobin, white blood cells, neutrophils, and platelets) during combination REBETOL/INTRON A treatment are described below (see **TABLE 4**).

Hemoglobin Hemoglobin decreases among patients on combination therapy began at Week 1, with stabilization by

Continued on next page

Information on Schering products appearing on these pages is effective as of August 15, 1998.

Rebetron—Cont.

Week 4. The mean maximum decrease from baseline was 2.8 g/dL in the US study and 2.6 g/dL in the International study. Hemoglobin values returned to pretreatment levels within 4–8 weeks of cessation of therapy in most patients.

Neutrophils There were decreases in neutrophil counts in both the combination REBETOL/INTRON A and INTRON A plus placebo dose groups. The mean maximum decrease in neutrophil count in the US study was 1.3×10^9 /L and in the International study was 1.6×10^9 /L. Neutrophil counts returned to pretreatment levels within 4 weeks of cessation of therapy in most patients.

Platelets Mean platelet values remained in the normal range of $150–450 \times 10^9$/L during combination REBETOL/INTRON A and INTRON A plus placebo therapy; however, mean platelet values were approximately 10% lower in the INTRON A plus placebo group than the REBETOL/INTRON A group. Mean platelet values returned to baseline levels within 4 weeks after treatment discontinuation.

Thyroid Function Of patients who entered the studies without thyroid abnormalities, approximately 1% to 2% developed thyroid abnormalities requiring clinical intervention.

Bilirubin and Uric Acid Increases in both bilirubin and uric acid, associated with hemolysis, were noted in clinical trials. Most were moderate biochemical changes and were reversed within 4 weeks after treatment discontinuation. This observation occurs most frequently in patients with a previous diagnosis of Gilbert's syndrome. This has not been associated with hepatic dysfunction or clinical morbidity.

[See table 4 at top of page 2882]

OVERDOSAGE

In combination REBETOL/INTRON A clinical trials, the maximum overdose reported was a dose of 39 million units of INTRON A (13 subcutaneous injections of 3 million IU each) taken with 10 g of REBETOL (fifty 200-mg capsules) in an investigator-initiated trial. The patient was observed for 2 days in the emergency room during which time no adverse event from the overdose was noted.

DOSAGE AND ADMINISTRATION

INTRON A Injection should be administered subcutaneously and REBETOL Capsules should be administered orally (see **TABLE 5**).

The recommended dose of REBETOL depends on the patient's body weight. The recommended doses of REBETOL and INTRON A are given in **TABLE 5** and should be administered for a period of 6 months (24 weeks). The safety and efficacy of the combination of REBETOL and INTRON A therapy have not been established beyond 6 months of treatment.

[See table 5 on page 2882]

REBETOL may be administered without regard to food. (See **CLINICAL PHARMACOLOGY**.)

Variations in dosage, routes of administration, and adverse reactions exist among different brands of interferon. There is no information regarding the use of REBETOL Capsules with other interferons.

Dose Modifications **(TABLE 6)**

If severe adverse reactions or laboratory abnormalities develop during combination REBETOL/INTRON A therapy the dose should be modified, or discontinued if appropriate, until the adverse reactions abate. If intolerance persists after dose adjustment, REBETOL/INTRON A therapy should be discontinued.

REBETOL/INTRON A therapy should be administered with caution to patients with pre-existing cardiac disease. Patients should be assessed before commencement of therapy and should be appropriately monitored during therapy. If there is any deterioration of cardiovascular status, therapy should be stopped. (See **WARNINGS**.)

For patients with a history of stable cardiovascular disease, a permanent dose reduction is required if the hemoglobin decreases by ≥2 g/dL during any 4-week period. In addition, for these cardiac history patients, if the hemoglobin remains <12 g/dL after 4 weeks on a reduced dose, the patient should discontinue combination REBETOL/INTRON A therapy.

It is recommended that a patient whose hemoglobin level falls below 10 g/dL have his/her REBETOL dose reduced to 600 mg daily (1 × 200 mg capsule AM, 2 × 200 mg capsules PM). A patient whose hemoglobin level falls below 8.5 g/dL should be permanently discontinued from REBETOL/INTRON A therapy. (See **WARNINGS**.)

It is recommended that a patient who experiences moderate depression (persistent low mood, loss of interest, poor self image, and/or hopelessness) have his/her INTRON A dose temporarily reduced and/or be considered for medical therapy. A patient experiencing severe depression or suicidal ideation/attempt should be discontinued from REBETOL/INTRON A therapy and followed closely with appropriate medical management. (See **WARNINGS**.)

[See table 6 on page 2882]

Administration of INTRON A Injection
At the discretion of the physician, the patient may self-administer the INTRON A.
(See illustrated **MEDICATION GUIDE** for instructions.)

The INTRON A Injection is supplied as a clear and colorless solution. The appropriate INTRON A dose should be withdrawn from the vial or set on the multidose pen and injected subcutaneously. After administration of INTRON A Injection, it is essential to follow the procedure for proper disposal of syringes and needles. (See **MEDICATION GUIDE** for detailed instructions.)

[See first table at top of previous page]

Parenteral drug products should be inspected visually for particulate matter and discoloration prior to administration, whenever solution and container permit. INTRON A Injection may be administered using either sterilized glass or plastic disposable syringes.

Stability INTRON A Injection provided in vials is stable at 35°C (95°F) for up to 7 days and at 30°C (86°F) for up to 14 days. INTRON A Injection provided in a multidose pen is stable at 30°C (86°F) for up to 2 days. The solution is clear and colorless.

HOW SUPPLIED

REBETOL 200-mg Capsules are white, opaque capsules with REBETOL, 200 mg, and the Schering Corporation logo imprinted on the capsule shell; the capsules are packaged in blisters.

INTRON A Injection is a clear, colorless solution packaged in single dose and multidose vials, and a multidose pen.

INTRON A Injection and REBETOL Capsules are available in the following combination package presentations:

[See second table at top of previous page]

STORAGE CONDITIONS

Store the REBETOL Capsules plus INTRON A Injection combination package refrigerated between 2° and 8°C (36° and 46°F).

When separated, the individual carton of REBETOL Capsules should be stored refrigerated between 2° and 8°C (36° and 46°F) or at 25°C (77°F); excursions are permitted between 15° and 30°C (59° and 86°F).

When separated, the individual carton or vial of INTRON A Injection and the INTRON A multidose pen should be stored refrigerated between 2° and 8°C (36° and 46°F).

Schering Corporation
Kenilworth, NJ 07033 USA
U.S. Patents 4,530,901 & 4,211,771
Copyright © 1998, Schering Corporation. All rights reserved.

21617601 5/98

SOLGANAL®   ℞
brand of aurothioglucose
Injectable Suspension*
FOR INTRAMUSCULAR
INJECTION ONLY—
NOT FOR INTRAVENOUS USE
* FORMERLY SOLGANAL® Suspension, USP

PRODUCT INFORMATION

WARNINGS

> Physicians planning to use SOLGANAL Injectable Suspension should thoroughly familiarize themselves with its toxicity and its benefits. The possibility of toxic reactions should always be explained to the patient before starting therapy. Patients should be warned to report promptly any symptom suggesting toxicity. Before **each** injection of SOLGANAL Injectable Suspension, the physician should review the results of laboratory work and see the patient to determine the presence or absence of adverse reactions, since some of these can be severe or even fatal.

DESCRIPTION

SOLGANAL (aurothioglucose) is a sterile suspension, for **intramuscular injection only**. SOLGANAL Injectable Suspension is an antiarthritic agent which is absorbed gradually following intramuscular injection, producing a therapeutically desired prolonged effect.

Each mL contains 50 mg of aurothiolglucose in sterile sesame oil with 2% aluminum monostearate; 1 mg propylparaben is added as preservative. Aurothioglucose contains approximately 50% gold by weight.

The empirical formula for aurothioglucose is $C_6H_{11}AuO_5S$; the molecular weight is 392.18. Chemically it is (1-Thio-D-glucopyranosato) gold, with the following structural formula:
[See chemical structure at top of next column]
Aurothioglucose is a nearly odorless, yellow powder which is stable in air. An aqueous solution is unstable on long stand-

---

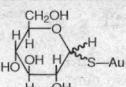

ing. Aurothiolglucose is freely soluble in water but practically insoluble in acetone, in alcohol, in chloroform, and in ether.

CLINICAL PHARMACOLOGY

Although the mechanism of action is not well understood, gold compounds have been reported to decrease synovial inflammation and retard cartilage and bone destruction.

Gold is absorbed from injection sites, reaching peak concentration in blood in 4 to 6 hours. Following a single intramuscular injection of 50 mg SOLGANAL Injectable Suspension in each of two subjects, peak serum levels were about 235 mcg/dL in one patient and 450 mcg/dL in the other. In plasma, 95% is bound to the albumin fraction. Approximately 70% of the gold is eliminated in the urine and approximately 30% in the feces. When a standard weekly treatment schedule is followed approximately 40% of the administered dose is excreted each week, and the remainder is excreted over a longer period. The biological half-life of gold salts following a single 50 mg dose has been reported to range from 3 to 27 days. Following successive weekly doses, the half-life increases and may be 14 to 40 days after the third dose and up to 168 days after the eleventh weekly dose.

After the initial injection, the serum level of gold rises sharply and declines over the next week. Peak levels with aqueous preparations are higher and decline faster than those with oily preparations. Weekly administration produces a continuous rise in the basal value for several months, after which the serum level becomes relatively stable. After a standard weekly dose, considerable individual variation in the levels of gold has been found. A steady decline in gold levels occurs when the interval between injections is lengthened, and small amounts may be found in the serum for months after discontinuation of therapy. The incidence of toxic reactions is apparently unrelated to the plasma level of gold, but it may be related to the cumulative body content of gold.

Storage of gold in human tissues is dependent upon organ mass as well as upon the concentration of gold. Therefore, tissues having the highest gold levels (weight/weight) do not necessarily contain the greatest total amounts of gold. The major depots, in decreasing order of total gold content, are the bone marrow, liver, skin, and bone, accounting for approximately 85% of body gold. The highest concentrations of gold are found in the lymph nodes, adrenal glands, liver, kidneys, bone marrow, and spleen. Relatively small concentrations are found in articular structures.

Gold passes the blood-brain barrier in hamsters.

Transfer of gold across the human placenta at the twentieth week of pregnancy has been documented. The placenta showed numerous gold deposits and smaller amounts were detected in the fetal liver and kidneys; other tissues provided no evidence of gold deposition.

Gold is excreted into human milk in significant amounts and trace amounts can be demonstrated in the blood of nursing infants. (See **PRECAUTIONS**, *Nursing Mothers*.)

INDICATIONS AND USAGE

SOLGANAL Injectable Suspension is indicated for the adjunctive treatment of early active rheumatoid arthritis (both of the adult and juvenile types) not adequately controlled by other anti-inflammatory agents and conservative measures. In chronic, advanced cases of rheumatoid arthritis, gold therapy is less valuable.

Antirheumatic measures such as salicylates and other anti-inflammatory drugs (both steroidal and nonsteroidal) may be continued after initiation of gold therapy. After improvement commences, these measures may be discontinued slowly as symptoms permit. (See **PRECAUTIONS**, *Laboratory Tests* and **DOSAGE AND ADMINISTRATION**.)

CONTRAINDICATIONS

A history of known hypersensitivity to any component of SOLGANAL Injectable Suspension contraindicates its use. Gold therapy is contraindicated in patients with uncontrolled diabetes mellitus, severe debilitation, systemic lupus erythematosus, renal disease, hepatic dysfunction, uncontrolled congestive heart failure, marked hypertension, agranulocytosis, other blood dyscrasias, or hemorrhagic diathesis; or if there is a history of infectious hepatitis. Patients who recently have had radiation, and those who have developed severe toxicity from previous exposure to gold or other heavy metals should not receive SOLGANAL Injectable Suspension.

Urticaria, eczema, and colitis are also contraindications.

Gold therapy is usually contraindicated in pregnancy. (See **PRECAUTIONS**, *Usage in Pregnancy*.)

Gold salts should not be used with penicillamine (see **MANAGEMENT OF ADVERSE REACTIONS**) or antimalarials. The safety of coadministration with immunosuppressive agents other than corticosteroids has not been established.

WARNINGS

The following signs should be considered danger signals of gold toxicity, and no additional injection should be given unless further studies reveal some other cause for their pres-

ence; rapid reduction of hemoglobin, leukopenia (WBC below 4000/cu mm), eosinophilia above 5%, platelet count below 100,000/cu mm, albuminuria, hematuria, pruritus, dermatitis, stomatitis, jaundice, and petechiae.

Effects that may occur immediately following an injection, or at any time during gold therapy, include: anaphylactic shock, syncope, bradycardia, thickening of the tongue, difficulty in swallowing and breathing, and angioneurotic edema. If such effects are observed, treatment with SOLGANAL Injectable Suspension should be discontinued.

Tolerance to gold usually decreases with advancing age. Diabetes mellitus or congestive heart failure should be under control before gold therapy is instituted.

SOLGANAL Injectable Suspension should be used with extreme caution in patients with: skin rash, hypersensitivity to other medications, or a history of renal or liver disease.

PRECAUTIONS

General: Before **each** injection, the physician should personally check the patient for adverse reactions and inquiry should be made regarding pruritus, rash, sore mouth, indigestion, and metallic taste. The patient should be observed for at least 15 minutes following each injection. (See also *Laboratory Tests.*)

Patients with HLA-D locus histocompatibility antigens DRw2 and DRw3 may have a genetic predisposition to develop certain toxic reactions, such as proteniuria, during treatment with gold or D-penicillamine.

SOLGANAL Injectable Suspension should be used with caution in patients with compromised cardiovascular or cerebral circulation.

Information for Patients:

1. Promptly report to the physician any unusual symptoms such as pruritus (itching), rash, sore mouth, indigestion, or metallic taste.
2. Increased joint pain may occur for 1 or 2 days after an injection and usually subsides after the first few injections.
3. Exposure to sunlight or artificial ultraviolet light should be minimized.
4. Careful oral hygiene is recommended in conjunction with therapy.
5. Patients should be aware of potential hazards if they become pregnant while receiving gold therapy. (See *Usage in Pregnancy.*)

Laboratory Tests: Before treatment is started, a complete blood count, platelet count, and urinalysis should be done to serve as reference points. Since gold therapy is usually contraindicated in pregnant patients, pregnancy should be ruled out before treatment is started. Throughout the treatment period, urinalysis should be repeated prior to each injection, and complete blood cell and platelet counts should be performed every 2 weeks. A platelet count is indicated any time that purpura or ecchymosis occurs.

Drug Interactions: Drug interactions have not been reported. (See **CONTRAINDICATIONS.**)

Carcinogenesis, Mutagenesis, and Impairment of Fertility: Renal adenomas developed in rats receiving an injectable gold product similar to SOLGANAL Injectable Suspension at doses of 2 mg/kg weekly for 46 weeks, followed by 6 mg/kg daily for 47 weeks. These doses were higher and administered more frequently than the recommended human doses. The adenomas were similar histologically to those produced by chronic administration of other gold compounds and heavy metals, such as lead or nickel.

Renal tubular cell neoplasia consisting of renal adenoma and adenocarcinoma was noted in a dose-response relationship in another study in rats using daily intramuscular doses of 3 mg/kg and 6 mg/kg for up to 2 years. These doses were higher and were administered more frequently than the recommended human doses. In this same study, sarcomas at the injection site occurred in some rats but their numbers were not sufficient to demonstrate a dose-response relationship.

No report of renal adenoma or sarcoma at the injection site in man in association with the use of SOLGANAL Injectable Suspension has been received.

Gold compounds have not been studied for evaluation of mutagenesis.

Gold sodium thiomalate given subcutaneously did not adversely affect fertility or reproductive performance.

Usage in Pregnancy: Gold therapy is usually contraindicated in pregnant patients. The patient should be warned about the hazards of becoming pregnant while on gold therapy. Rheumatoid arthritis frequently improves when the patient becomes pregnant, thereby eliminating the need for gold therapy. The potential nephrotoxicity of gold should not be superimposed on the inceased renal burden which normally occurs in pregnancy and hence, gold therapy should be discontinued upon recognition of pregnancy unless continued use is required in an individual case. The slow excretion of gold and its persistence in body tissues after discontinuation of treatment should be kept in mind when a woman of childbearing potential being treated with gold plans to become pregnant.

Pregnancy Category C: Gold sodium thiomalate administered subcutaneously, a route not used clinically, has been shown to be teratogenic during the organogenic period in rats and rabbits when given in doses 140 and 175 times, respectively, the usual human dose. Hydrocephalus and microphthalmia were the malformations observed in rats when gold sodium thiomalate was administerd at a dose of 25 mg/kg/day from day 6 through day 15 of gestation. In rabbits, limb defects and gastroschisis were the malformations observed when gold sodium thiomalate was administered at doses of 20 to 45 mg/kg/day from day 6 through day 18 of gestation.

Gold compounds administered orally to rabbits from days 6 through 18 of pregnancy resulted in the occurrence of abdominal defects, such as gastroschisis and umbilical hernia; anomalies of the brain, heart, lung, and skeleton; and microphthalmia.

The administration of excessive doses of gold-containing compounds during pregnancy in the above studies was toxic to the mothers and their embryos; the embryotoxic effects probably were secondary to maternal toxicity. Therefore, the significance of these findings in relation to human use is unknown.

There are no adequate and well-controlled studies with SOLGANAL Injectable Suspension in pregnant women. Extensive clinical experience with SOLGANAL Injectable Suspension has not demonstrated human teratogenicity.

Nursing Mothers: Gold has been demonstrated in the milk of lactating mothers. In one patient, a total dose of 135 mg of gold thioglucose was given during the postpartum period. Samples of the maternal milk and urine, and samples of red blood cells and serum of the mother and child were evaluated by atomic absorption spectrophotometry. Trace amounts of gold appeared in the serum and red blood cells of the nursing offspring. It has been postulated that this may be the cause of unexplained rashes, nephritis, hepatitis, and hematologic aberrations in the nursing infants of mothers treated with gold. Because of the potential for serious adverse reactions in nursing infants, a decision should be made whether to discontinue nursing or to discontinue the gold therapy, taking into account the importance of the drug to the mother. The slow excretion of gold and its persistence in the mother after discontinuation of treatment should be kept in mind.

Pediatric Use: Safety and effectiveness in children below the age of 6 years have not been established.

ADVERSE REACTIONS

Adverse reactions to gold therapy may occur at any time during treatment or many months after therapy has been discontinued. The incidence of toxic reactions is apparently unrelated to the plasma level of gold, but it may be related to the cumulative body content of gold. Higher than conventional dosage schedules may increase the occurrence and severity of toxicity. Severe effects are most common after 300 to 500 mg have been administered.

Cutaneous Reactions: Dermatitis is the most common reaction. Pruritus should be considered a warning signal of an impending cutaneous reaction. Erythema and occasionally the more severe reactions such as papular, vesicular, and exfoliative dermatitis leading to alopecia and shedding of the nails may occur. Chrysiasis (gray-to-blue pigmentation) has been reported, especially on photoexposed areas. Gold dermatitis may be aggravated by exposure to sunlight, or an actinic rash may develop.

Mucous Membrane Reactions: Stomatitis is the second most common adverse reaction. Shallow ulcers on the buccal membranes, on the borders of the tongue, and on the palate; diffuse glossitis; or gingivitis may be preceded by the sensation of metallic taste. Careful oral hygiene is recommended. Inflammation of the upper respiratory tract, pharyngitis, gastritis, colitis, tracheitis, and vaginitis have also been reported. Conjunctivitis is rare.

Renal Reactions: Nephrotic syndrome or glomerulitis with hematuria, which is usually relatively mild, subsides completely if recognized early and treatment is discontinued. These reactions become severe and chronic if gold therapy is continued after their onset. Therefore, it is important to perform a urinalysis before each injection and to discontinue treatment promptly if proteinuria or hematuria develops.

Hematologic Reactions: Although rare, blood dyscrasias, including granulocytopenia, agranulocytosis, thrombocytopenia with or without purpura, leukopenia, eosinophilia, panmyelopathy, hemorrhagic diathesis, and hypoplastic and aplastic anemia, have been reported. These actions may occur separately or in combination.

Nitritoid and Allergic Reactions: These reactions, which may rarely occur with SOLGANAL Injectable Suspension and which resemble anaphylactoid effects, include flushing, fainting, dizziness, sweating, malaise, weakness, nausea, and vomiting.

Miscellaneous Reactions: On rare occasions, gastrointestinal symptoms, ie, nausea, vomiting, colic, anorexia, abdominal cramps, diarrhea, ulcerative enterocolitis, and headache have been reported.

There have been rare reports of iritis and corneal ulcers. Transient, asymptomatic gold deposits in the cornea or conjunctiva may occur.

Other reported reactions include encephalitis, immunological destruction of the synovia, EEG abnormalities, intrahepatic cholestasis, hepatitis with jaundice, toxic hepatitis, acute yellow atrophy, peripheral neuritis, gold bronchitis, pulmonary injury manifested by interstitial pneumonitis or fibrosis, fever, and partial or complete hair loss.

Less common but more severe effects that may occur shortly after an injection or at any time during gold therapy include: anaphylactic shock, syncope, bradycardia, thickening of the tongue, difficulty in swallowing and breathing, and angioneurotic edema. If they are observed, treatment with SOLGANAL Injectable Suspension should be discontinued.

Arthralgia may occur for 1 or 2 days after an injection and usually subsides after the first few injections. The mechanism of the transient increase in rheumatic symptoms after injection of gold (the so-called nonvasomotor postinjection reaction) is unknown. These reactions are usually mild but occasionally may be so severe that treatment is stopped prematurely.

MANAGEMENT OF ADVERSE REACTIONS

In the event of toxic reactions, gold therapy should be discontinued immediately.

In the presence of mild reactions, it may be sufficient to discontinue the administration of SOLGANAL Injectable Suspension for a short period and then to resume treatment with smaller doses.

Dematitis and pruritus may respond to soothing lotions, other appropriate antipruritic treatment, or topical glucocorticoids.

If dermatitis or stomatitis becomes severe or spreads, systemic glucocorticoid treatment may be indicated. For renal, hematologic, and most other adverse reactions, glucocorticoids may be required in larger doses and for a longer time than for dermatologic reactions. Often this treatment may be required for many months because of the slow elimination of gold from the body.

If severe adverse reactions do not improve with steroid treatment in patients who receive large doses of gold, a chelating agent, such as dimercaprol (BAL), may be used. In one case, it was reported that penicillamine was beneficial in the treatment of gold-induced thrombocytopenia. Adjunctive use of an anabolic steroid with other drugs (ie, BAL, penicillamine, and corticosteroids) may contribute to recovery of bone marrow deficiency.

In the presence of severe or idiosyncratic reactions, treatment with SOLGANAL Injectable Suspension should not be reinstituted.

OVERDOSAGE

Overdosage resulting from too rapid increases in dosing with SOLGANAL Injectable Suspension will be manifested by rapid appearance of toxic reactions, particularly those relating to renal damage, such as hematuria, proteinuria, and to hematologic effects, such as thrombocytopenia and granulocytopenia. Other toxic effects, including fever, nausea, vomiting, diarrhea, and various skin disorders such as papulovesicular lesions, urticaria, and exfoliative dermatitis, all attended with severe pruritus, may develop. Treatment consists of prompt discontinuation of the medication, and early administration of dimercaprol. Specific supportive therapy should be given for the renal and hematologic complications. (See also **MANAGEMENT OF ADVERSE REACTIONS.**)

DOSAGE AND ADMINISTRATION

Adults—The usual dosage schedule for the intramuscular administration of SOLGANAL Injectable Suspension is as follows: first dose, 10 mg; second and third doses, 25 mg; fourth and subsequent doses, 50 mg. The interval between doses is 1 week. The 50 mg dose is continued at weekly intervals until 0.8 to 1.0 g SOLGANAL Injectable Suspension has been given. If the patient has improved and has exhibited no sign of toxicity. the 50 mg dose may be continued many months longer, at 3- to 4-week intervals. A weekly dose above 50 mg is usually unnecessary and contraindicated; the tendency in gold therapy is toward lower dosage. With this in mind, it may eventually be established that a 25 mg dose is the one of choice. If no improvement has been demonstrated after a total administration of 1.0 g of SOLGANAL Injectable Suspension, the necessity for gold therapy should be reevaluated.

Children 6 to 12 years—one fourth of the adult dose, governed chiefly by body weight, not to exceed 25 mg per dose.

SOLGANAL Injectable Suspension should be injected **intramuscularly** (preferably intragluteally), **never intravenously.** The patient should be lying down and should remain recumbent for approximately 10 minutes after the injection. The

Continued on next page

Information on Schering products appearing on these pages is effective as of August 15, 1998.

Solganal—Cont.

vial should be thoroughly shaken in order to suspend all of the active material. Heating the vial to body temperature (by immersion in warm water) will facilitate drawing the suspension into the syringe. An 18-guage, 1¹/₂-inch needle is recommended for depositing the preparation deep into the muscular tissue. For obese patients, an 18-gauge, 2-inch needle may be used. The site usually selected for injection is the upper outer quadrant of the gluteal region.

NOTE: Shake the vial in horizontal position before the dose is withdrawn. Needle and syringe must be dry. The patient should be observed for at least 15 minutes following each injection.

HOW SUPPLIED

SOLGANAL Injectable Suspension is available in 10 mL multiple-dose vials containing 5% (50 mg/mL) aurothioglucose; box of one (NDC 0085-0460-03).

Shake well before using. Store between 0° and 30°C (32° and 86°F). Protect from light. Store in carton until contents are used.

Schering Corporation
Kenilworth, NJ 07033 USA
Rev. 3/96   13288518
Copyright © 1963, 1984, 1996, Schering Corporation.
All rights reserved.

TRILAFON®
brand of perphenazine, USP
   Tablets
   Concentrate
   Injection

℞

DESCRIPTION

TRILAFON products contain perphenazine, USP (4-[3-(2-chlorophenothiazin-10-yl)propyl]-1-piperazineethanol), a piperazinyl phenothiazine having the chemical formula, $C_{21}H_{26}ClN_3OS$. They are available as **Tablets**, 2, 4, 8, and 16 mg; **Concentrate**, 16 mg perphenazine per 5 mL and alcohol less than 0.1%; and **Injection**, perphenazine 5 mg per 1 mL. The inactive ingredients for TRILAFON **Tablets**, 2, 4, 8, and 16 mg. include: acacia, black iron oxide, butylparaben, calcium phosphate, calcium sulfate, carnauba wax, corn starch, gelatin, lactose, magnesium stearate, potato starch, sugar, titanium dioxide, white wax and other ingredients. May also contain talc.

The inactive ingredients for TRILAFON **Concentrate** include: alcohol, citric acid, flavors, menthol, sodium phosphate, sorbitol, sugar, and water.

The inactive ingredients for TRILAFON **Injection** include: citric acid, sodium bisulfite, sodium hydroxide, and water.

ACTIONS

Perphenazine has actions at all levels of the central nervous system, particularly the hypothalamus. However, the site and mechanism of action of therapeutic effect are not known.

INDICATIONS

Perphenazine is indicated for use in the management of the manifestations of psychotic disorders; and for the control of severe nausea and vomiting in adults.

TRILAFON has not been shown effective for the management of behavioral complications in patients with mental retardation.

CONTRAINDICATIONS

TRILAFON products are contraindicated in comatose or greatly obtunded patients and in patients receiving large doses of central nervous system depressants (barbiturates, alcohol, narcotics, analgesics, or antihistamines); in the presence of existing blood dyscrasias, bone marrow depression, or liver damage; and in patients who have shown hypersensitivity to TRILAFON products, their components, or related compounds.

TRILAFON products are also contraindicated in patients with suspected or established subcortical brain damage, with or without hypothalamic damage, since a hyperthermic reaction with temperatures in excess of 104°F may occur in such patients, sometimes not until 14 to 16 hours after drug administration. Total body ice-packing is recommended for such a reaction; antipyretics may also be useful.

WARNINGS

Tardive dyskinesia, a syndrome consisting of potentially irreversible, involuntary, dyskinetic movements, may develop in patients treated with neuroleptic (antipsychotic) drugs. Although the prevalence of the syndrome appears to be highest among the elderly, especially elderly women, it is impossible to rely upon prevalence estimates to predict, at the inception of neuroleptic treatment, which patients are likely to develop the syndrome. Whether neuroleptic drug products differ in their potential to cause tardive dyskinesia is unknown.

Both the risk of developing the syndrome and the likelihood that it will become irreversible are believed to increase as the duration of treatment and the total cumulative dose of neuroleptic drugs administered to the patient increase. However, the syndrome can develop, although much less commonly, after relatively brief treatment periods at low doses.

There is no known treatment for established cases of tardive dyskinesia, although the syndrome may remit, partially or completely, if neuroleptic treatment is withdrawn. Neuroleptic treatment itself, however, may suppress (or partially suppress) the signs and symptoms of the syndrome, and thereby may possibly mask the underlying disease process. The effect that symptomatic suppression has upon the long-term course of the syndrome is unknown.

Given these considerations, neuroleptics should be prescribed in a manner that is most likely to minimize the occurrence of tardive dyskinesia. Chronic neuroleptic treatment should generally be reserved for patients who suffer from a chronic illness that, 1) is known to respond to neuroleptic drugs, and 2) for whom alternative, equally effective, but potentially less harmful treatments are not available or appropriate. In patients who do require chronic treatment, the smallest dose and the shortest duration of treatment producing a satisfactory clinical response should be sought. The need for continued treatment should be reassessed periodically.

If signs and symptoms of tardive dyskinesia appear in a patient on neuroleptics, drug discontinuation should be considered. However, some patients may require treatment despite the presence of the syndrome.

(For further information about the description of tardive dyskinesia and its clinical detection, please refer to **Information for Patients** and **ADVERSE REACTIONS**.)

TRILAFON **Injection** contains sodium bisulfite, a sulfite that may cause allergic-type reactions including anaphylactic symptoms and life-threatening or less severe asthmatic episodes in certain susceptible people. The overall prevalence of sulfite sensitivity is seen more frequently in asthmatic than in nonasthmatic people.

NEUROLEPTIC MALIGNANT SYNDROME (NMS)

A potentially fatal symptom complex sometimes referred to as Neuroleptic Malignant Syndrome (NMS), has been reported in association with antipsychotic drugs. Clinical manifestations of NMS are hyperpyrexia, muscle rigidity, altered mental status and evidence of autonomic instability (irregular pulse or blood pressure, tachycardia, diaphoresis, and cardiac dysrhythmias).

The diagnostic evaluation of patients with this syndrome is complicated. In arriving at a diagnosis, it is important to identify cases where the clinical presentation includes both serious medical illness (e.g., pneumonia, systemic infection, etc.) and untreated or inadequately treated extrapyramidal signs and symptoms (EPS). Other important considerations in the differential diagnosis include central anticholinergic toxicity, heat stroke, drug fever and primary central nervous system (CNS) pathology.

The management of NMS should include 1) immediate discontinuation of antipsychotic drugs and other drugs not essential to concurrent therapy, 2) intensive symptomatic treatment and medical monitoring, and 3) treatment of any concomitant serious medical problems for which specific treatments are available. There is no general agreement about specific pharmacological treatment regimens for uncomplicated NMS.

If a patient requires antipsychotic drug treatment after recovery from NMS, the reintroduction of drug therapy should be carefully considered. The patient should be carefully monitored, since recurrences of NMS have been reported.

If hypotension develops, epinephrine should not be administered since its action is blocked and partially reversed by perphenazine. If a vasopressor is needed, norepinephrine may be used. Severe, acute hypotension has occurred with the use of phenothiazines and is particularly likely to occur in patients with mitral insufficiency or pheochromocytoma. Rebound hypertension may occur in pheochromocytoma patients.

TRILAFON products can lower the convulsive threshold in susceptible individuals; they should be used with caution in alcohol withdrawal and in patients with convulsive disorders. If the patient is being treated with an anticonvulsant agent, increased dosage of that agent may be required when TRILAFON products are used concomitantly.

TRILAFON products should be used with caution in patients with psychic depression.

Perphenazine may impair the mental and/or physical abilities required for the performance of hazardous tasks such as driving a car or operating machinery; therefore, the patient should be warned accordingly.

TRILAFON products are not recommended for children under 12 years of age.

Usage in Pregnancy: Safe use of TRILAFON during pregnancy and lactation has not been established; therefore, in administering the drug to pregnant patients, nursing mothers, or women who may become pregnant, the possible benefits must be weighed against the possible hazards to mother and child.

PRECAUTIONS

The possibility of suicide in depressed patients remains during treatment and until significant remission occurs. This type of patient should not have access to large quantities of this drug.

As with all phenothiazine compounds, perphenazine should not be used indiscriminately. Caution should be observed in giving it to patients who have previously exhibited severe adverse reactions to other phenothiazines. Some of the untoward actions of perphenazine tend to appear more frequently when high doses are used. However, as with other phenothiazine compounds, patients receiving TRILAFON products in any dosage should be kept under close supervision.

Neuroleptic drugs elevate prolactin levels; the elevation persists during chronic administration. Tissue culture experiments indicate that approximately one-third of human breast cancers are prolactin dependent *in vitro*, a factor of potential importance if the prescription of these drugs is contemplated in a patient with a previously detected breast cancer. Although disturbances such as galactorrhea, amenorrhea, gynecomastia, and impotence have been reported, the clinical significance of elevated serum prolactin levels is unknown for most patients. An increase in mammary neoplasms has been found in rodents after chronic administration of neuroleptic drugs. Neither clinical studies nor epidemiologic studies conducted to date, however, have shown an association between chronic administration of these drugs and mammary tumorigenesis; the available evidence is considered too limited to be conclusive at this time.

The antiemetic effect of perphenazine may obscure signs of toxicity due to overdosage of other drugs, or render more difficult the diagnosis of disorders such as brain tumors or intestinal obstruction.

A significant, not otherwise explained, rise in body temperature may suggest individual intolerance to perphenazine, in which case it should be discontinued.

Patients on large doses of a phenothiazine drug who are undergoing surgery should be watched carefully for possible hypotensive phenomena. Moreover, reduced amounts of anesthetics or central nervous system depressants may be necessary.

Since phenothiazines and central nervous system depressants (opiates, analgesics, antihistamines, barbiturates) can potentiate each other, less than the usual dosage of the added drug is recommended and caution is advised when they are administered concomitantly.

Use with caution in patients who are receiving atropine or related drugs because of additive anticholinergic effects and also in patients who will be exposed to extreme heat or phosphorus insecticides.

The use of alcohol should be avoided, since additive effects and hypotension may occur. Patients should be cautioned that their response to alcohol may be increased while they are being treated with TRILAFON products. The risk of suicide and the danger of overdose may be increased in patients who use alcohol excessively due to its potentiation of the drug's effect.

Blood counts and hepatic and renal functions should be checked periodically. The appearance of signs of blood dyscrasias requires the discontinuance of the drug and institution of appropriate therapy. If abnormalities in hepatic tests occur, phenothiazine treatment should be discontinued. Renal function in patients on long-term therapy should be monitored; if blood urea nitrogen (BUN) becomes abnormal, treatment with the drug should be discontinued.

The use of phenothiazine derivatives in patients with diminished renal function should be undertaken with caution.

Use with caution in patients suffering from respiratory impairment due to acute pulmonary infections, or in chronic respiratory disorders such as severe asthma or emphysema.

In general, phenothiazines, including perphenazine, do not produce psychic dependence. Gastritis, nausea and vomiting, dizziness, and tremulousness have been reported following abrupt cessation of high-dose therapy. Reports suggest that these symptoms can be reduced by continuing concomitant antiparkinson agents for several weeks after the phenothiazine is withdrawn.

The possibility of liver damage, corneal and lenticular deposits, and irreversible dyskinesias should be kept in mind when patients are on long-term therapy.

Because photosensitivity has been reported, undue exposure to the sun should be avoided during phenothiazine treatment.

Information for Patients: This information is intended to aid in the safe and effective use of this medication. It is not a disclosure of all possible adverse or intended effects.

Given the likelihood that a substantial proportion of patients exposed chronically to neuroleptics will develop tardive dyskinesia, it is advised that all patients in whom chronic use is contemplated be given, if possible, full information about this risk. The decision to inform patients

and/or their guardians must obviously take into account the clinical circumstances and the competency of the patient to understand the information provided.

ADVERSE REACTIONS

Not all of the following adverse reactions have been reported with this specific drug; however, pharmacological similarities among various phenothiazine derivatives require that each be considered. With the piperazine group (of which perphenazine is an example), the extrapyramidal symptoms are more common, and others (e.g., sedative effects, jaundice, and blood dyscrasias) are less frequently seen.

CNS Effects: *Extrapyramidal reactions:* opisthotonus, trismus, torticollis, retrocollis, aching and numbness of the limbs, motor restlessness, oculogyric crisis, hyperreflexia, dystonia, including protrusion, discoloration, aching and rounding of the tongue, tonic spasm of the masticatory muscles, tight feeling in the throat, slurred speech, dysphagia, akathisia, dyskinesia, parkinsonism, and ataxia. Their incidence and severity usually increase with an increase in dosage, but there is considerable individual variation in the tendency to develop such symptoms. Extrapyramidal symptoms can usually be controlled by the concomitant use of effective antiparkinsonian drugs, such as benztropine mesylate, and/or by reduction in dosage. In some instances, however, these extrapyramidal reactions may persist after discontinuation of treatment with perphenazine.

Persistent tardive dyskinesia: As with all antipsychotic agents, tardive dyskinesia may appear in some patients on long-term therapy or may appear after drug therapy has been discontinued. Although the risk appears to be greater in elderly patients on high-dose therapy, especially females, it may occur in either sex and in children. The symptoms are persistent and in some patients appear to be irreversible. The syndrome is characterized by rhythmical, involuntary movements of the tongue, face, mouth or jaw (e.g., protrusion of tongue, puffing of cheeks, puckering of mouth, chewing movements). Sometimes these may be accompanied by involuntary movements of the extremities. There is no known effective treatment for tardive dyskinesia; antiparkinsonism agents usually do not alleviate the symptoms of this syndrome. It is suggested that all antipsychotic agents be discontinued if these symptoms appear. Should it be necessary to reinstitute treatment, or increase the dosage of the agent, or switch to a different antipsychotic agent, the syndrome may be masked. It has been reported that fine, vermicular movements of the tongue may be an early sign of the syndrome, and if the medication is stopped at that time the syndrome may not develop.

Other CNS effects include cerebral edema; abnormality of cerebrospinal fluid proteins; convulsive seizures, particularly in patients with EEG abnormalities or a history of such disorders, and headaches.

Neuroleptic malignant syndrome has been reported in patients treated with neuroleptic drugs (see **WARNINGS** for further information).

Drowsiness may occur, particularly during the first or second week, after which it generally disappears. If troublesome, lower the dosage. Hypnotic effects appear to be minimal, especially in patients who are permitted to remain active.

Adverse behavioral effects include paradoxical exacerbation of psychotic symptoms, catatonic-like states, paranoid reactions, lethargy, paradoxical excitement, restlessness, hyperactivity, nocturnal confusion, bizarre dreams, and insomnia.

Hyperreflexia has been reported in the newborn when a phenothiazine was used during pregnancy.

Autonomic Effects: dry mouth or salivation, nausea, vomiting, diarrhea, anorexia, constipation, obstipation, fecal impaction, urinary retention, frequency or incontinence, bladder paralysis, polyuria, nasal congestion, pallor, myosis, mydriasis, blurred vision, glaucoma, perspiration, hypertension, hypotension, and change in pulse rate occasionally may occur. Significant autonomic effects have been infrequent in patients receiving less than 24 mg perphenazine daily.

Adynamic ileus occasionally occurs with phenothiazine therapy and if severe can result in complications and death. It is of particular concern in psychiatric patients, who may fail to seek treatment of the condition.

Allergic Effects: urticaria, erythema, eczema, exfoliative dermatitis, pruritus, photosensitivity, asthma, fever, anaphylactoid reactions, laryngeal edema; and angioneurotic edema; contact dermatitis in nursing personnel administering the drug; and in extremely rare instances, individual idiosyncrasy or hypersensitivity to phenothiazines has resulted in cerebral edema, circulatory collapse, and death.

Endocrine Effects: lactation, galactorrhea, moderate breast enlargement in females and gynecomastia in males on large doses, disturbances in the menstrual cycle, amenorrhea, changes in libido, inhibition of ejaculation, syndrome of inappropriate ADH (antidiuretic hormone) secretion, false positive pregnancy tests, hyperglycemia, hypoglycemia, glycosuria.

Cardiovascular Effects: postural hypotension, tachycardia (especially with sudden marked increase in dosage), bradycardia, cardiac arrest, faintness, and dizziness. Occasionally the hypotensive effect may produce a shock-like condition. ECG changes, nonspecific (quinidine-like effect) usually reversible, have been observed in some patients receiving phenothiazine tranquilizers.

Sudden death has occasionally been reported in patients who have received phenothiazines. In some cases the death was apparently due to cardiac arrest; in others, the cause appeared to be asphyxia due to failure of the cough reflex. In some patients, the cause could not be determined nor could it be established that the death was due to the phenothiazine.

Hematological Effects: agranulocytosis, eosinophilia, leukopenia, hemolytic anemia, thrombocytopenic purpura, and pancytopenia. Most cases of agranulocytosis have occurred between the fourth and tenth weeks of therapy. Patients should be watched closely, especially during that period, for the sudden appearance of sore throat or signs of infection. If white blood cell and differential cell counts show significant cellular depression, discontinue the drug and start appropriate therapy. However, a slightly lowered white count is not in itself an indication to discontinue the drug.

Other Effects: Special considerations in long-term therapy include pigmentation of the skin, occurring chiefly in the exposed areas; ocular changes consisting of deposition of fine particulate matter in the cornea and lens, progressing in more severe cases to star-shaped lenticular opacities; epithelial keratopathies; and pigmentary retinopathy. Also noted: peripheral edema, reversed epinephrine effect, increase in PBI not attributable to an increase in thyroxine, parotid swelling (rare), hyperpyrexia, systemic lupus erythematosus-like syndrome, increases in appetite and weight, polyphagia, photophobia, and muscle weakness.

Liver damage (biliary stasis) may occur. Jaundice may occur, usually between the second and fourth weeks of treatment, and is regarded as a hypersensitivity reaction. Incidence is low. The clinical picture resembles infectious hepatitis but with laboratory features of obstructive jaundice. It is usually reversible; however, chronic jaundice has been reported.

Side effects with intramuscular TRILAFON **Injection** have been infrequent and transient. Dizziness or significant hypotension after treatment with TRILAFON **Injection** is a rare occurrence.

DOSAGE AND ADMINISTRATION

Dosage must be individualized and adjusted according to the severity of the condition and the response obtained. As with all potent drugs, the best dose is the lowest dose that will produce the desired clinical effect. Since extrapyramidal symptoms increase in frequency and severity with increased dosage, it is important to employ the lowest effective dose. These symptoms have disappeared upon reduction of dosage, withdrawal of the drug, or administration of an antiparkinsonian agent.

Prolonged administration of doses exceeding 24 mg daily should be reserved for hospitalized patients or patients under continued observation for early detection and management of adverse reactions. An antiparkinsonian agent, such as trihexyphenidyl hydrochloride or benztropine mesylate, is valuable in controlling drug-induced extrapyramidal symptoms.

TRILAFON **Tablets**

Suggested dosages for **Tablets** for various conditions follow:

Moderately disturbed nonhospitalized psychotic patients: **Tablets** 4 to 8 mg t.i.d. initially; reduce as soon as possible to minimum effective dosage.

Hospitalized psychotic patients: **Tablets** 8 to 16 mg b.i.d. to q.i.d.; avoid dosages in excess of 64 mg daily.

Severe nausea and vomiting in adults: **Tablets** 8 to 16 mg daily in divided doses; 24 mg occasionally may be necessary; early dosage reduction is desirable.

TRILAFON **Injection—**Intramuscular Administration

The injection is used when rapid effect and prompt control of acute or intractable conditions is required or when oral administration is not feasible. TRILAFON **Injection,** administered by deep intramuscular injection, is well tolerated. The injection should be given with the patient seated or recumbent, and the patient should be observed for a short period after administration.

Therapeutic effect is usually evidenced in 10 minutes and is maximal in 1 to 2 hours. The average duration of effective action is 6 hours, occasionally 12 to 24 hours.

Pediatric dosage has not yet been established. Children over 12 years may receive the lowest limit of adult dosage.

The usual initial dose is 5 mg (1 mL). This may be repeated every 6 hours. Ordinarily, the total daily dosage should not exceed 15 mg in ambulatory patients or 30 mg in hospitalized patients. When required for satisfactory control of symptoms in severe conditions, an initial 10-mg intramuscular dose may be given. Patients should be placed on oral therapy as soon as practicable. Generally, this may be achieved within 24 hours. In some instances, however, patients have been maintained on injectable therapy for several months. It has been established that TRILAFON **Injection** is more potent than TRILAFON **Tablets.** Therefore, equal or higher dosage should be used when the patient is transferred to oral therapy after receiving the injection.

Psychotic conditions: While 5 mg of the **Injection** has a definite tranquilizing effect, it may be necessary to use 10-mg doses to initiate therapy in severely agitated states. Most patients will be controlled and amendable to oral therapy within a maximum of 24 to 48 hours. Acute conditions (hysteria, panic reaction) often respond well to a single dose, whereas in chronic conditions, several injections may be required. When transferring patients to oral therapy, it is suggested that increased dosage be employed to maintain adequate clinical control. This should be followed by gradual reduction to the minimal maintenance dose which is effective.

Severe nausea and vomiting in adults: To obtain rapid control of vomiting, administer 5 mg (1 mL); in rare instances it may be necessary to increase the dose to 10 mg; in general, higher doses should be given only to hospitalized patients.

Intravenous Administration

The intravenous administration of TRILAFON **Injection** is seldom required. This route of administration should be used with particular caution and care, and only when absolutely necessary to control severe vomiting, intractable hiccoughs, or acute conditions, such as violent retching during surgery. Its use should be limited to recumbent hospitalized adults in doses not exceeding 5 mg. When employed in this manner, intravenous injection ordinarily should be given as a diluted solution by either fractional injection or a slow drip infusion. In the surgical patient, slow infusion of not more than 5 mg is preferred. When administered in divided doses, TRILAFON **Injection** should be diluted to 0.5 mg/mL (1 mL mixed with 9 mL of physiologic saline solution), and not more than 1 mg per injection given at not less than one-to two-minute intervals. Intravenous injection should be discontinued as soon as symptoms are controlled and should not exceed 5 mg. The possibility of hypotensive and extrapyramidal side effects should be considered and appropriate means for management kept available. Blood pressure and pulse should be monitored continuously during intravenous administration. Pharmacologic and clinical studies indicate that intravenous administration of norepinephrine should be useful in alleviating the hypotensive effect.

TRILAFON **Concentrate**

In hospitalized psychotic patients, the usual dosage range is 8 to 16 mg b.i.d. to q.i.d., depending on the severity of symptoms and individual response. Although a number of investigators have employed higher dosage, a total daily dose of more than 64 mg ordinarily is not required. The **Concentrate** should be diluted only with water, saline, Seven-Up, homogenized milk, carbonated orange drink, and pineapple, apricot, prune, orange. V-8, tomato, and grapefruit juices. Trilafon **Concentrate** should not be mixed with beverages containing caffeine (coffee, cola), tannics (tea), or pectinates (apple juice), since physical incompatibility may result. Suggested dilution is approximately two fluid ounces of diluent for each 5 mL (16 mg) teaspoonful of TRILAFON **Concentrate.** For convenience in measuring smaller doses, a graduated dropper marked to measure 8 mg or 4 mg is supplied with each bottle.

OVERDOSAGE

In the event of overdosage, emergency treatment should be started immediately. All patients suspected of having taken an overdose should be hospitalized as soon as possible.

Manifestations Overdosage of perphenazine primarily involves the extrapyramidal mechanism and produces the same side effects described under **ADVERSE REACTIONS**, but to a more marked degree. It is usually evidenced by stupor or coma; children may have convulsive seizures.

Treatment Treatment is symptomatic and supportive. There is no specific antidote. The patient should be induced to vomit even if emesis has occurred spontaneously. Pharmacologic vomiting by the administration of ipecac syrup is a preferred method. It should be noted that ipecac has a central mode of action in addition to its local gastric irritant properties, and the central mode of action may be blocked by the antiemetic effect of TRILAFON products. Vomiting should not be induced in patients with impaired consciousness. The action of ipecac is facilitated by physical activity and by the administration of 8 to 12 fluid ounces of water. If emesis does not occur within 15 minutes, the dose of ipecac should be repeated. Precautions against aspiration must be taken, especially in infants and children. Following emesis, any drug remaining in the stomach may be adsorbed by activated charcoal administered as a slurry with water. If vomiting is unsuccessful or contraindicated, gastric lavage should be performed. Isotonic and one-half isotonic saline

Continued on next page

Information on Schering products appearing on these pages is effective as of August 15, 1998.

Trilafon—Cont.

are the lavage solutions of choice. Saline cathartics, such as milk of magnesia, draw water into the bowel by osmosis and therefore, may be valuable for their action in rapid dilution of bowel content.
Standard measures (oxygen, intravenous fluids, corticosteroids) should be used to manage circulatory shock or metabolic acidosis. An open airway and adequate fluid intake should be maintained. Body temperature should be regulated. Hypothermia is expected, but severe hyperthermia may occur and must be treated vigorously. (See **CONTRAINDICATIONS**.)
An electrocardiogram should be taken and close monitoring of cardiac function instituted if there is any sign of abnormality. Cardiac arrhythmias may be treated with neostigmine, pyridostigmine, or propranolol. Digitalis should be considered for cardiac failure. Close monitoring of cardiac function is advisable for not less than five days. Vasopressors such as norepinephrine may be used to treat hypotension, but epinephrine should NOT be used.
Anticonvulsants (an inhalation anesthetic, diazepam, or paraldehyde) are recommended for control of convulsions, since perphenazine increases the central nervous system depressant action, but not the anticonvulsant action of barbiturates.
If acute parkinson-like symptoms result from perphenazine intoxication, benztropine mesylate or diphenydramine may be administered.
Central nervous system depression may be treated with nonconvulsant doses of CNS stimulants. Avoid stimulants that may cause convulsions (e.g., picrotoxin and pentylenetetrazol).
Signs of arousal may not occur for 48 hours.
Dialysis is of no value because of low plasma concentrations of the drug.
Since overdosage is often deliberate, patients may attempt suicide by other means during the recovery phase. Deaths by deliberate or accidental overdosage have occurred with this class of drugs.

HOW SUPPLIED

TRILAFON **Tablets** (2 mg): gray, sugar-coated tablets branded in black with the Schering trademark and either product identification letters, ADH, or numbers, 705, bottles of 100 (NDC 0085-0705-04). **Store between 2° and 25°C (36° and 77°F).**
TRILAFON **Tablets** (4 mg): gray, sugar-coated tablets branded in green with the Schering trademark and either product identification letters, ADK, or numbers, 940; bottles of 100 (NDC 0085-0940-05). **Store between 2° and 25°C (36° and 77°F).**
TRILAFON **Tablets** (8 mg): gray, sugar-coated tablets branded in blue with the Schering trademark and either product identification letters, ADJ, or numbers, 313; bottles of 100 (NDC 0085-0313-05). **Store between 2° and 25°C (36° and 77°F).**
TRILAFON **Tablets** (16 mg): gray, sugar-coated tablets branded in red with the Schering trademark and either product identification letters, ADM, or numbers, 077; bottles of 100 (NDC 0085-0077-05). **Store between 2° and 25°C (36° and 77°F).**
TRILAFON **Concentrate,** 16 mg per 5 mL, 4 fluid ounce (118 mL) bottle with graduated dropper (NDC 0085-0363-02). The **Concentrate** is light-sensitive and should be dispensed in amber bottles. **Protect from light. Store between 2° and 30°C (36° and 86°F). Shake well before using. Store in carton until completely used.**
TRILAFON **Injection,** 5 mg per mL, 1-mL ampul for intramuscular or intravenous use, box of 100 (NDC 0085-0012-04). Keep package closed to protect from light. Exposure may cause discoloration. Slight yellowish discoloration will not alter potency or therapeutic efficacy; if markedly discolored, ampul should be discarded. **Protect from light. Store in carton until completely used.**
TRILAFON®
brand of perphenazine, USP
Tablets, Concentrate,
Injection
Schering Corporation
Kenilworth, NJ 07033 USA
Revised 11/93 17978900
Copyright © 1969, 1991, 1994, Schering Corporation.
All rights reserved.
Shown in Product Identification Guide, page 336

VANCENASE® POCKETHALER® ℞
(beclomethasone dipropionate nasal aerosol)
For Nasal Inhalation Only

DESCRIPTION

Beclomethasone dipropionate, USP, the active component of VANCENASE POCKETHALER (beclomethasone dipropionate nasal aerosol) is an anti-inflammatory steroid having the chemical name, 9-Chloro-11β,17,21-trihydroxy-16β-methylpregna-1,4-diene-3,20-dione 17,21-dipropionate, and the following formula:

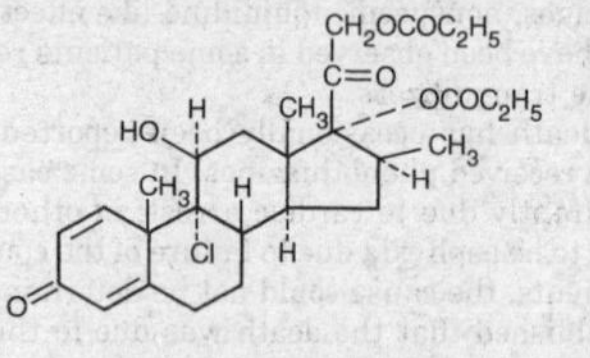

Beclomethasone dipropionate is a white to creamy-white, odorless powder with a molecular weight of 521.25. It is very slightly soluble in water, very soluble in chloroform, and freely soluble in acetone and in alcohol.
VANCENASE POCKETHALER (beclomethasone dipropionate nasal aersol) is a metered-dose aerosol unit containing a microcrystalline suspension of beclomethasone dipropionate-trichloromonofluoromethane clathrate in a mixture of propellants (trichloromonofluoromethane and dichlorodifluoromethane) with oleic acid. Each canister contains beclomethasone dipropionate-trichloromonofluoromethane clathrate having a molecular proportion of beclomethasone dipropionate to trichloromonofluoromethane between 3:1 and 3:2. Each actuation delivers from the nasal adapter a quantityofclathrateequivalentto42mcgofbeclomethasonedipropionate, USP. The contents of one canister provide at least 200 metered doses.

CLINICAL PHARMACOLOGY

Beclomethasone 17,21-dipropionate is a diester of beclomethasone, a synthetic halogenated corticosteroid. Animal studies showed that beclomethasone dipropionate has potent glucocorticoid and weak mineralocorticoid activity. The mechanisms for the anti-inflammatory action of beclomethasone dipropionate are unknown. The precise mechanism of the aerosolized drug's action in the nose is also unknown. Biopsies of nasal mucosa obtained during clinical studies showed no histopathologic changes when beclomethasone dipropionate was administered intranasally.
The effects of beclomethasone dipropionate on hypothalamic-pituitary-adrenal (HPA) function have been evaluated in adult volunteers by other routes of administration. Studies are currently being undertaken with beclomethasone dipropionate by the intransal route, which may demonstrate that there is more or that there is less absorption by this route of administration. There was no suppression of early morning plasma cortisol concentrations when beclomethasone dipropionate was administered in a dose of 1000 mcg/day for 1 month as an oral aerosol or for 3 days by intramuscular injection. However, partial suppression of plasma cortisol concentration was observed when beclomethasone dipropionate was administered in doses of 2000 mcg/day either by oral aerosol or intramuscularly. Immediate suppression of plasma cortisol concentrations was observed after single doses of 4000 mcg of beclomethasone dipropionate. Suppression of HPA function (reduction of early morning plasma cortisol levels) has been reported in adult patients who received 1600 mcg daily doses of oral beclomethasone dipropionate for 1 month. In clinical studies using beclomethasone dipropionate intranasally, there was no evidence of adrenal insufficiency.
Beclomethasone dipropionate is sparingly soluble. When given by nasal inhalation in the form of an aqueous or aerosolized suspension, the drug is deposited primarily in the nasal passages. A portion of the drug is swallowed. Absorption occurs rapidly from all respiratory and gastrointestinal tissues. There is no evidence of tissue storage of beclomethasone dipropionate or its metabolities. *In vitro* studies have shown that tissue other than the liver (lung slices) can rapidly metabolize beclomethasone dipropionate to beclomethasone 17-monopropionate and more slowly to free beclomethasone (which has very weak anti-inflammatory activity). However, irrespective of the route of entry, the principal route of excretion of the drug and its metabolites is the feces. In humans, 12% to 15% of an orally administered dose of beclomethasone dipropionate is excreted in the urine as both conjugated and free metabolites of the drug.
Studies have shown that the degree of binding to plasma proteins is 87%.

INDICATIONS AND USAGE

VANCENASE POCKETHALER (beclomethasone dipropionate nasal aerosol) is indicated for the relief of the symptoms of seasonal or perennial rhinitis in those cases poorly responsive to conventional treatment.
VANCENASE POCKETHALER (beclomethasone dipropionate nasal aeroasol) is also indicated for the prevention of recurrence of nasal polyps following surgical removal.
Clinical studies in seasonal and perennial rhinitis have shown that improvement is usually apparent within a few days. However symptomatic relief may not occur in some patients for as long as 2 weeks. Although systemic effects are minimal at recommended doses, VANCENASE treatment should not be continued beyond 3 weeks in the absence of significant symptomatic improvement. VANCENASE treatment should not be used in the presence of untreated, localized infection involving the nasal mucosa.
Clinical studies have shown that treatment of the symptoms associated with nasal polyps may have to be continued for several weeks or more before a therapeutic result can be fully assessed. Recurrence of symptoms due to polyps can occur after stopping treatment, depending on the severity of the disease.

CONTRAINDICATIONS

Hypersensitivity to any of the ingredients of this preparation contraindicates its use.

WARNINGS

The replacement of a systemic corticosteroid with VANCENASE POCKETHALER (beclomethasone dipropionate nasal aerosol) can be accompanied by signs of adrenal insufficiency.
Careful attention must be given when patients, previously treated for prolonged periods with systemic corticosteroids, are transferred to VANCENASE POCKETHALER (beclomethasone dipropionate nasal aerosol). This is particularly important in those patients who have associated asthma or other clinical conditions, where too rapid a decrease in systemic corticosteroids may cause a severe excerbation of their symptoms.
Studies have shown that the combined administration of alternate day prednisone systemic treatment and orally inhaled beclomethasone increased the likelihood of HPA suppression compared to a therapeutic dose of either one alone. Therefore, VANCENASE treatment should be used with caution in patients already on alternate day prednisone regimens for any disease.
If recommended doses of intranasal beclomethasone are exceeded or if individuals are particularly sensitive or predisposed by virtue of recent systemic steroid therapy, symptoms of hypercorticism may occur, including very rare cases of menstrual irregularities, acneiform lesions, and cushingoid features. If such changes occur, VANCENASE POCKETHALER (beclomethasone dipropionate nasal aerosol) should be discontinued slowly, consistent with accepted procedures for discontinuing oral steroid therapy.
Persons who are on drugs which suppress the immune system are more susceptible to infections than healthy individuals. Chickenpox and measles, for example, can have a more serious or even fatal course in nonimmune pediatric patients or adults on corticosteroids. In such pediatric patients or adults who have not had these diseases, particular care should be taken to avoid exposure. How the dose, route, and duration of corticosteroid administration affects the risk of developing a disseminated infection is not known. The contribution of the underlying disease and/or prior corticosteroid treatment to the risk is also not known. If exposed to chickenpox, prophylaxis with varicella-zoster immune globulin (VZIG) may be indicated. If exposed to measles, prophylaxis with pooled intramuscular immunoglobulin (IG) may be indicated. (See the respective package inserts for complete VZIG and IG prescribing information.) If chickenpox develops, treatment with antiviral agents may be considered.

PRECAUTIONS

General: During withdrawal from oral steroids, some patients may experience symptoms of withdrawal, eg, joint and/or muscular pain, lassitude, and depression.
Extremely rare instances of nasal septum perforation and increased intraocular pressure have been reported following the intranasal application of aerosolized corticosteroids.
In clinical studies with beclomethasone dipropionate administered intranasally, the development of localized infections of the nose and pharynx with *Candida albicans* has occurred only rarely. When such an infection develops, it may require treatment with appropriate local therapy or discontinuance of treatment with VANCENASE POCKETHALER (beclomethasone dipropionate nasal aerosol).
Beclomethasone dipropionate is absorbed into the circulation. Use of excessive doses of VANCENASE POCKETHALER (beclomethasone dipropionate nasal aerosol) may suppress HPA function.
VANCENASE treatment should be used with caution, if at all, in patients with active or quiescent tuberculous infections of the respiratory tract, or in untreated fungal, bacterial, systemic viral infections, or ocular herpes simplex.
For VANCENASE POCKETHALER (beclomethasone dipropionate nasal aerosol) to be effective in the treatment of nasal polyps, the aerosol must be able to enter the nose. Therefore, treatment of nasal polyps with VANCENASE POCKETHALER (beclomethasone dipropionate nasal aerosol) should be considered adjunctive therapy to surgical removal and/or the use of other medications which will permit effective penetration of the VANCENASE product into the nose. Nasal polyps may recur after any form of treatment. As with any long-term treatment, patients using VANCENASE treatment over several months or longer should be examined periodically for possible changes in the nasal mucosa.

Because of the inhibitory effect of corticosteroids on wound healing, patients who have experienced recent nasal septum ulcers, nasal surgery, or trauma should not use a nasal corticosteroid until healing has occurred.
Although systemic effects have been minimal with recommended doses, this potential increases with excessive doses. Therefore, larger than recommended doses should be avoided.
Information for Patients: Patients should use VANCENASE POCKETHALER (beclomethasone dipropionate nasal aerosol) at regular intervals since its effectiveness depends on its regular use. The patient should take the medication as directed. It is not acutely effective and the prescribed dosage should not be increased. Instead, nasal vasoconstrictors or oral antihistamines may be needed until the effects of VANCENASE POCKETHALER (beclomethasone dipropionate nasal aerosol) are fully manifested. One to 2 weeks may pass before full reflief is obtained. The patient should contact the doctor if symptoms do not improve, if the condition worsens, or if sneezing or nasal irritation occurs. For the proper use of this unit and to attain maximum improvement, the patient should read and follow the accompanying PATIENT'S INSTRUCTIONS carefully.
Persons who are on immunosuppressant doses of corticosteroids should be warned to avoid exposure to chickenpox or measles. Patients should also be advised that if they are exposed, medical advice should be sought without delay.
Carcinogenesis, Mutagenesis, Impairment of Fertility: Treatment of rats for a total of 95 weeks, 13 weeks by inhalation and 82 weeks by the oral route, resulted in no evidence of carcinogenic activity. Mutagenic studies have not been performed.
Impairment of fertility, as evidenced by inhibition of the estrous cycle in dogs, was observed following treatment by the oral route. No inhibition of the estrous cycle in dogs was seen following treatment with beclomethasone dipropionate by the inhalation route.
Pregnancy Category C: Like other corticoids, parenteral (subcutaneous) beclomethasone dipropionate has been shown to be teratogenic and embryocidal in the mouse and rabbit when given in doses approximately ten times the human dose. In these studies, beclomethasone was found to produce fetal resorption, cleft palate, agnathia, microstomia, absence of tongue, delayed ossification, and agenesis of the thymus. No teratogenic or embryocidal effects have been seen in the rat when beclomethasone dipropionate was administered by inhalation at ten times the human dose or orally at 1000 times the human dose. There are no adequate and well-controlled studies in pregnant women. Beclomethasone dipropionate should be used during pregnancy only if the potential benefit justifies the potential risk to the fetus.
Nonteratogenic Effects: Hypoadrenalism may occur in infants born of mothers receiving corticosteroids during pregnancy. Such infants should be carefully observed.
Nursing Mothers: It is not known whether beclomethasone dipropionate is excreted in human milk. Because other corticosteroids are excreted in human milk, caution should be exercised when VANCENASE POCKETHALER (beclomethasone dipropionate nasal aersol) is administered to nursing women.
Pediatric Use: Safety and effectiveness in pediatric patients below the age of 6 years have not been established.

ADVERSE REACTIONS

In general, side effects in clinical studies have been primarily associated with the nasal mucous membranes. Adverse reactions reported in controlled clinical trials and in long-term open studies in patients treated with VANCENASE Nasal Inhaler are described below.
Sensations of irritation and burning in the nose (11 per 100 patients) following the use of VANCENASE Nasal Inhaler have been reported. Also, occasional sneezing attacks (10 per 100 patients) have occurred immediately following the use of the intranasal inhaler. This symptom may be more common in children.
Rhinorrhea may occur occasionally (1 per 100 patients).
Localized infections of the nose and pharynx with *Candida albicans* have occurred rarely (See **PRECAUTIONS**).
Transient episodes of epistaxis or bloody discharge from the nose have been reported in 2 per 100 patients.
Ulceration of the nasal mucosa has been reported rarely.
Extremely rare instances of nasal septum perforation have been reported following the intranasal application of aerosolized corticosteroids. Rare cases of immediate and delayed hypersensitivity reactions, including urticaria, angioedema, rash, and bronchospasm have been reported following the oral and intransal inhalation of beclomethasone.
Increased intraocular pressure has been reported rarely. (See **PRECAUTIONS**.)
Systemic corticosteroid side effects were not reported during controlled clinical trials. If recommended doses are exceeded, however, or if individuals are particularly sensitive, symptoms of hypercorticism, ie, Cushing's syndrome could occur.

DOSAGE AND ADMINISTRATION

Adults and Pediatric Patients 12 Years of Age and Over: The usual dosage is one inhalation (42 mcg) in each nostril two to four times a day (total dose 168–336 mcg/day). Patients can often be maintained on a maximum dose of one inhalation in each nostril three times a day (252 mcg/day).
Pediatric Patients 6 to 12 Years of Age: The usual dosage is one inhalation in each nostril three times a day (252 mcg/day). VANCENASE POCKETHALER (beclomethasone dipropionate nasal aerosol) is not recommended for pediatric patients below 6 years of age since safety and efficacy studies have not been conducted in this age group.
In patients who respond to VANCENASE POCKETHALER (beclomethasone dipropionate nasal aerosol), an improvement of the symptoms of seasonal or perennial rhinitis usually becomes apparent within a few days after the start of VANCENASE POCKETHALER (beclomethasone dipropionate nasal aerosol) therapy. However, symptomatic relief may not occur in some patients for as long as 2 weeks. VANCENASE POCKETHALER (beclomethasone dipropionate nasal aerosol) should not be continued beyond 3 weeks in the absence of significant symptomatic improvment.
The therapeutic effects of corticosteroids, unlike those of decongestants, on seasonal or perennial rhinitis or on nasal polyps are not immediate. This should be explained to the patient in advance in order to ensure cooperation and continuation of treatment with the prescribed dosage regimen. VANCENASE POCKETHALER (beclomethasone dipropionate nasal aerosol) is not recommended for pediatric patients below 6 years of age.
In the presence of excessive nasal mucus secretion or edema of the nasal mucosa, the drug may fail to reach the site of intended action. In such cases it is advisable to use a nasal vasoconstrictor during the first 2 to 3 days of VANCENASE POCKETHALER (beclomethasone dipropionate nasal aerosol) therapy.
Directions for Use: Illustrated PATIENT'S INSTRUCTIONS for proper use accompany each package of VANCENASE POCKETHALER (beclomethasone dipropionate nasal aerosol).
CONTENTS UNDER PRESSURE. Do not puncture. Do not use or store near heat or open flame. Exposure to temperatures above 120°F may cause bursting. Never throw container into fire or incinerator. Keep out of reach of children.

OVERDOSAGE

When used at excessive doses, systemic corticosteroid effects such as hypercorticism and adrenal suppression may appear. If such changes occur, VANCENASE POCKETHALER (beclomethasone dipropionate nasal aerosol) should be discontinued slowly consistent with accepted procedures for discontinued oral steroid therapy.
The oral LD_{50} of beclomethasone dipropionate is greater than 1 g/kg in rodents. One canister of VANCENASE POCKETHALER (beclomethasone dipropionate nasal aerosol) contains 8.4 mg of beclomethasone dipropionate; therefore acute overdosage is unlikely.

HOW SUPPLIED

VANCENASE POCKETHALER (beclomethasone dipropionate nasal aerosol), 7 g canister; box of one. Supplied with nasal adapter and PATIENT'S INSTRUCTIONS (NDC 0085-0649-02).
Store between 15° and 30°C (59° and 86°F). Protect from moisture and unusual temperature fluctuations. Shake well before using. Failure to use the product within this temperature range may result in improper dosing.
Note: The intended statement below is required by the Federal government's Clean Air Act for all products containing or manufactured with chlorofluorocarbons (CFCs).
WARNING: Contains dichlorodifluoromethane (CFC-11) and trichloromonofluoromethane (CFC-12), substances which harm public health and the environment by destroying ozone in the upper atmosphere.
A notice similar to the above WARNING has been placed in the "Patient's Instructions for Use" portion of this package insert pursuant to EPA regulations.
Schering Corporation
Kenilworth, NJ 07033 USA
Rev. 4/97 B-19529614

Shown in Product Identification Guide, page 336

VANCENASE® AQ ℞

brand of beclomethasone dipropionate, monohydrate
Nasal Spray 0.042%*
FOR INTRANASAL USE ONLY
***calculated on the dried basis**

DESCRIPTION

Beclomethasone dipropionate, monohydrate, the active component of VANCENASE AQ Nasal Spray, is an anti-inflammatory steroid having the chemical name, 9-Chloro-11β, 17, 21-trihydroxy-16 β-methylpregna-1, 4-diene-3, 20-dione 17, 21-dipropionate, monohydrate and the following chemical structure:

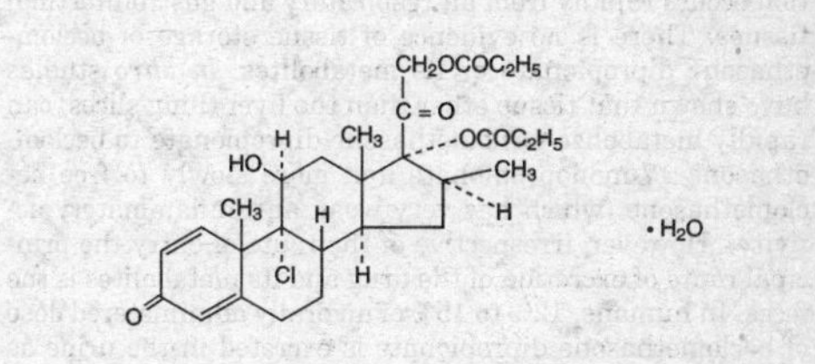

Beclomethasone dipropionate, monohydrate is a white to creamy-white, odorless powder with a molecular weight of 539.06. It is very slightly soluble in water; very soluble in chloroform; and freely soluble in acetone and in alcohol.
VANCENASE AQ Nasal Spray is a metered-dose, manual pump spray unit containing a microcrystalline suspension of beclomethasone dipropionate, monohydrate equivalent to 0.042% w/w beclomethasone dipropionate calculated on the dried basis in an aqueous medium containing microcrystalline cellulose and carboxymethylcellulose sodium, dextrose, benzalkonium chloride, polysorbate 80, and 0.25% v/w phenylethyl alcohol; hydrochloric acid may be added to adjust pH. The pH is between 4.5 and 7.0.
After initial priming (3 to 4 actuations), each actuation of the pump delivers from the nasal adapter 100 mg of suspension containing beclomethasone dipropionate, monohydrate equivalent to 42 mcg beclomethasone dipropionate. Each bottle of VANCENASE AQ Nasal Spray will provide at least 200 metered doses.

CLINICAL PHARMACOLOGY

Beclomethasone 17, 21-dipropionate is a diester of beclomethasone, a synthetic halogenated corticosteroid. Animal studies show that beclomethasone dipropionate has potent glucocorticosteroid and weak mineralocorticosteroid activity. The mechanisms for the anti-inflammatory action of beclomethasone dipropionate are unknown. The precise mechanism of the aerosolized drug's action in the nose is also unknown. Biopsies of nasal mucosa obtained during clinical studies showed no histopathologic changes when beclomethasone dipropionate was administered intranasally.
The effects of beclomethasone dipropionate on hypothalamic-pituitary-adrenal (HPA) function have been evaluated in adult volunteers by other routes of administration. Studies with beclomethasone dipropionate by the intranasal route may demonstrate that there is more or that there is less absorption by this route of administration. There was no suppression of early morning plasma cortisol concentrations when beclomethasone dipropionate was administered in a dose of 1000 mcg/day for 1 month as an oral aerosol or for 3 days by intramuscular injection. However, partial suppression of plasma cortisol concentration was observed when beclomethasone dipropionate was administered in doses of 2000 mcg/day either by oral aerosol or intramuscular injection. Immediate suppression of plasma cortisol concentrations was observed after single doses of 4000 mcg of beclomethasone dipropionate. Suppression of HPA function (reduction of early morning plasma cortisol levels) has been reported in adult patients who received 1600 mcg daily doses of oral beclomethasone dipropionate for 1 month. In clinical studies using beclomethasone dipropionate aerosol intranasally, there was no evidence of adrenal insufficiency. The effect of VANCENASE AQ Nasal Spray on HPA function was not evaluated but would not be expected to differ from intranasal beclomethasone dipropionate aerosol.
In one study in asthmatic children, the administration of inhaled beclomethasone at recommended daily doses for at least 1 year was associated with a reduction in nocturnal cortisol secretion. The clinical significance of this finding is not clear. It reinforces other evidence, however, that topical beclomethasone may be absorbed in amounts that can have systemic effects and that physicians should be alert for evidence of systemic effects, especially in chronically treated patients (see **PRECAUTIONS**).

Continued on next page

Information on Schering products appearing on these pages is effective as of August 15, 1998.

Vancenase AQ—Cont.

Beclomethasone dipropionate is sparingly soluble. When given by nasal inhalation in the form of an aqueous or aerosolized suspension, the drug is deposited primarily in the nasal passages. A portion of the drug is swallowed. Absorption occurs rapidly from all respiratory and gastrointestinal tissues. There is no evidence of tissue storage of beclomethasone dipropionate or its metabolites. In vitro studies have shown that tissue other than the liver (lung slices) can rapidly metabolize beclomethasone dipropionate to beclomethasone 17-monopropionate and more slowly to free beclomethasone (which has very weak anti-inflammatory activity). However, irrespective of the route of entry the principal route of excretion of the drug and its metabolites is the feces. In humans, 12% to 15% of an orally administered dose of beclomethasone dipropionate is excreted in the urine as both conjugated and free metabolites of the drug.

Studies have shown that the degree of binding to plasma proteins is 87%.

INDICATIONS AND USAGE

VANCENASE AQ Nasal Spray is indicated for the relief of the symptoms of seasonal or perennial allergic and non-allergic (vasomotor) rhinitis. Results from two clinical trials have shown that significant symptomatic relief was obtained within 3 days. However, symptomatic relief may not occur in some patients for as long as 2 weeks. VANCENASE AQ Nasal Spray should not be continued beyond 3 weeks in the absence of significant symptomatic improvement. VANCENASE AQ Nasal Spray should not be used in the presence of untreated localized infection involving the nasal mucosa.

VANCENASE AQ Nasal Spray is also indicated for the prevention of recurrence of nasal polyps following surgical removal.

Clinical studies have shown that treatment of the symptoms associated with nasal polyps may have to be continued for several weeks or more before a therapeutic result can be fully assessed. Recurrence of symptoms due to polyps can occur after stopping treatment, depending on the severity of the disease.

CONTRAINDICATIONS

Hypersensitivity to any of the ingredients of this preparation contraindicates its use.

WARNINGS

The replacement of a systemic corticosteroid with VANCENASE AQ Nasal Spray can be accompanied by signs of adrenal insufficiency.

When transferred to VANCENASE AQ Nasal Spray, careful attention must be given to patients previously treated for prolonged periods with systemic corticosteroids. This is particularly important in those patients who have associated asthma or other clinical conditions, where too rapid a decrease in systemic corticosteroids may cause a severe exacerbation of their symptoms.

Studies have shown that the combined administration of alternate day prednisone systemic treatment and orally inhaled beclomethasone increased the likelihood of HPA suppression compared to a therapeutic dose of either one alone. Therefore, VANCENASE AQ Nasal Spray treatment should be used with caution in patients already on alternate day prednisone regimens for any disease.

If recommended doses of intranasal beclomethasone are exceeded or if individuals are particularly sensitive or predisposed by virtue of recent systemic steroid therapy, symptoms of hypercorticism may occur, including very rare cases of menstrual irregularities, acneiform lesions, and cushingoid features. If such changes occur, VANCENASE AQ Nasal Spray should be discontinued slowly, consistent with accepted procedures for discontinuing oral steroid therapy. Persons who are on drugs which suppress the immune system are more susceptible to infections than healthy individuals. Chickenpox and measles, for example, can have a more serious or even fatal course in non-immune children or adults on corticosteroids. In such children or adults who have not had these diseases, particular care should be taken to avoid exposure. How the dose, route and duration of corticosteroid administration affects the risk of developing a disseminated infection is not known. The contribution of the underlying disease and/or prior corticosteroid treatment to the risk is also not known. If exposed to chickenpox, prophylaxis with varicella-zoster immune globulin (VZIG) may be indicated. If exposed to measles, prophylaxis with pooled intramuscular immunoglobulin (IG) may be indicated. (See the respective package inserts for complete VZIG and IG prescribing information.) If chickenpox develops, treatment with antiviral agents may be considered.

PRECAUTIONS

General: During withdrawal from oral steroids, some patients may experience symptoms of withdrawal, eg, joint and/or muscular pain, lassitude, and depression. Rarely, immediate hypersensitivity reactions may occur after the intranasal administration of beclomethasone.

Extremely rare instances of wheezing, nasal septum perforation, and increased intraocular pressure have been reported following the intranasal application of aerosolized corticosteroids. Although these have not been observed in clinical trials with VANCENASE AQ Nasal Spray, vigilance should be maintained.

In clinical studies with beclomethasone dipropionate administered intranasally, the development of localized infections of the nose and pharynx with *Candida albicans* has occurred only rarely. When such an infection develops, it may require treatment with appropriate local therapy or discontinuance of treatment with VANCENASE AQ Nasal Spray.

If persistent nasopharyngeal irritation occurs, it may be an indication for stopping VANCENASE AQ Nasal Spray.

Beclomethasone dipropionate is absorbed into the circulation. Use of excessive doses of VANCENASE AQ Nasal Spray may suppress HPA function.

VANCENASE AQ Nasal Spray should be used with caution, if at all, in patients with active or quiescent tuberculous infections of the respiratory tract, or in untreated fungal, bacterial, systemic viral infections, or ocular herpes simplex.

For VANCENASE AQ Nasal Spray to be effective in the treatment of nasal polyps, the spray must be able to enter the nose. Therefore, treatment of nasal polyps with VANCENASE AQ Nasal Spray should be considered adjunctive therapy to surgical removal and/or the use of other medications which will permit effective penetration of VANCENASE AQ Nasal Spray into the nose. Nasal polyps may recur after any form of treatment.

As with any long-term treatment, patients using VANCENASE AQ Nasal Spray over several months or longer should be examined periodically for possible changes in the nasal mucosa.

Because of the inhibitory effect of corticosteroids on wound healing, patients who have experienced recent nasal septal ulcers, nasal surgery, or trauma should not use a nasal corticosteroid until healing has occurred.

Although systemic effects have been minimal with recommended doses, this potential increases with excessive doses. Therefore, larger than recommended doses should be avoided.

Information for Patients: Patients being treated with VANCENASE AQ Nasal Spray should receive the following information and instructions. This information is intended to aid in the safe and effective use of medication. It is not a disclosure of all possible adverse or intended effects. Patients should use VANCENASE AQ Nasal Spray at regular intervals since its effectiveness depends on its regular use. The patient should take the medication as directed. It is not acutely effective and the prescribed dosage should not be increased. Instead, nasal vasoconstrictors or oral antihistamines may be needed until the effects of VANCENASE AQ Nasal Spray are fully manifested. One to 2 weeks may pass before full relief is obtained. The patient should contact the physician if symptoms do not improve, or if the condition worsens, or if sneezing or nasal irritation occurs. For the proper use of this unit and to attain maximum improvement, the patient should read and follow the accompanying Patient's Instructions carefully.

Patients who are on immunosuppressant doses of corticosteroids should be warned to avoid exposure to chickenpox or measles. Patients should also be advised that if they are exposed, medical advice should be sought without delay.

Carcinogenesis, Mutagenesis, Impairment of Fertility: Treatment of rats for a total of 95 weeks, 13 weeks by inhalation and 82 weeks by the oral route, resulted in no evidence of carcinogenic activity. Mutagenic studies have not been performed.

Impairment of fertility, as evidenced by inhibition of the estrous cycle in dogs, was observed following treatment by the oral route. No inhibition of the estrous cycle in dogs was seen following treatment with beclomethasone dipropionate by the inhalation route.

Pregnancy Category C: Like other corticosteroids, parenteral (subcutaneous) beclomethasone dipropionate has been shown to be teratogenic and embryocidal in the mouse and rabbit when given in doses approximately ten times the human dose. In these studies beclomethasone was found to produce fetal resorption, cleft palate, agnathia, microstomia, absence of tongue, delayed ossification, and agenesis of the thymus. No teratogenic or embryocidal effects have been seen in the rat when beclomethasone dipropionate was administered by inhalation at ten times the human dose or orally at 1000 times the human dose. There are no adequate and well-controlled studies in pregnant women. Beclomethasone dipropionate should be used during pregnancy only if the potential benefit justifies the potential risk to the fetus.

Nonteratogenic Effects: Hypoadrenalism may occur in infants born of mothers receiving corticosteroids during pregnancy. Such infants should be carefully observed.

Nursing Mothers: It is not known whether beclomethasone dipropionate is excreted in human milk. Because other corticosteroids are excreted in human milk, caution should be exercised when VANCENASE AQ Nasal Spray is administered to nursing women.

Pediatric Use: Safety and effectiveness in children below the age of 6 years have not been established.

ADVERSE REACTIONS

In general, side effects in clinical studies have been primarily associated with irritation of the nasal mucous membranes. Rarely, immediate hypersensitivity reactions may occur after the intranasal administration of beclomethasone dipropionate.

Adverse reactions reported in controlled clinical trials and open studies in patients treated with VANCENASE AQ Nasal Spray are described below.

Mild, transient nasopharyngeal irritation following the use of beclomethasone aqueous nasal spray has been reported in up to 24% of patients treated, including occasional sneezing attacks (about 4%) occurring immediately following use of the inhaler. In patients experiencing these symptoms, none had to discontinue treatment. The incidence of irritation and sneezing was approximately the same in the group of patients who received placebo in these studies, implying that these complaints may be related to vehicle components of the formulation.

Fewer than 5 per 100 patients reported headache, nausea, or lightheadedness following the use of VANCENASE AQ (beclomethasone dipropionate, monohydrate) Nasal Spray. Fewer than 3 per 100 patients reported nasal stuffiness, nosebleeds, rhinorrhea, and tearing eyes.

Extremely rare instances of wheezing, nasal septum perforation, and increased intraocular pressure have been reported following the intranasal administration of aerosolized corticosteroids (see **PRECAUTIONS**).

OVERDOSAGE

When used at excessive doses, systemic corticosteroid effects such as hypercorticism and adrenal suppression may appear. If such changes occur, VANCENASE AQ Nasal Spray should be discontinued slowly consistent with accepted procedures for discontinuing oral steroid therapy. The oral LD_{50} of beclomethasone dipropionate is greater than 1 g/kg in rodents. One bottle of VANCENASE AQ Nasal Spray contains beclomethasone dipropionate, monohydrate equivalent to 10.5 mg of beclomethasone dipropionate; therefore, acute overdosage is unlikely.

DOSAGE AND ADMINISTRATION

Adults and Children 6 Years of Age and Over: The usual dosage is 1 or 2 inhalations (42-84 mcg) in each nostril 2 times a day (total dose 168-336 mcg/day).

In patients who respond to VANCENASE AQ Nasal Spray, an improvement of the symptoms of seasonal or perennial rhinitis usually becomes apparent within a few days after the start of VANCENASE AQ Nasal Spray therapy. However, symptomatic relief may not occur in some patients for as long as 2 weeks. VANCENASE AQ Nasal Spray should not be continued beyond 3 weeks in the absence of significant symptomatic improvement.

The therapeutic effects of corticosteroids, unlike those of decongestants on seasonal or perennial rhinitis, or on nasal polyps, are not immediate. This should be explained to the patient in advance in order to ensure cooperation and continuation of treatment with the prescribed dosing regimen. VANCENASE AQ Nasal Spray is not recommended for children below 6 years of age.

In the presence of excessive nasal mucus secretion or edema of the nasal mucosa, the drug may fail to reach the site of intended action. In such cases it is advisable to use a nasal vasoconstrictor during the first 2 to 3 days of VANCENASE AQ Nasal Spray therapy.

Directions for Use: Illustrated Patient's Instructions for proper use accompany each package of VANCENASE AQ Nasal Spray.

HOW SUPPLIED

VANCENASE AQ (beclomethasone dipropionate, monohydrate) Nasal Spray 0.042%*, 25 g bottle; box of one. Supplied with nasal pump unit and dust cap; and Patient's Instructions (NDC 0085-0259-02).

* calculated on the dried basis

Store between 2° and 25°C (36° and 77°F).

SHAKE WELL BEFORE USING

Rev. 6/94   17905414

Copyright © 1993, 1994, Schering Corporation, Kenilworth, NJ 07033 USA. All rights reserved.

Shown in Product Identification Guide, page 336

VANCENASE® AQ 84 mcg   ℞
(beclomethasone
dipropionate, monohydrate)
Nasal Spray
FOR INTRANASAL USE ONLY

DESCRIPTION

Beclomethasone dipropionate, monohydrate, the active component of VANCENASE AQ 84 mcg Nasal Spray, is an anti-inflammatory steroid having the chemical name,

9-Chloro-11β, 17,21-trihydroxy-16β-methylpregna-1, 4-diene-3, 20-dione 17,21-dipropionate, monohydrate and the following chemical structure:

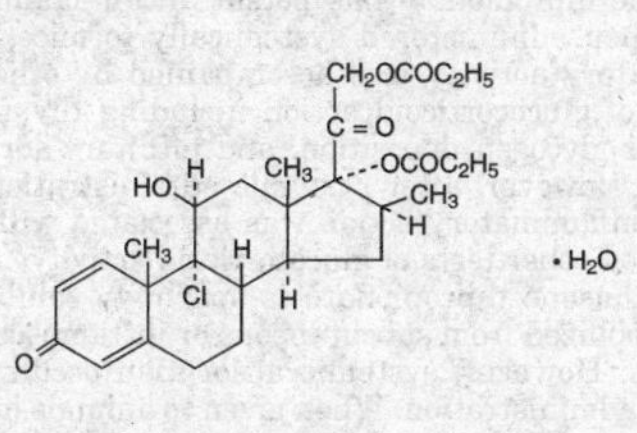

Beclomethasone dipropionate, monohydrate, is a white to creamy-white, odorless powder with a molecular formula of $C_{28}H_{37}ClO_7 \cdot H_2O$ and a molecular weight of 539.06. It is very slightly soluble in water; very soluble in chloroform; and freely soluble in acetone and in alcohol.

After initial priming (at least 6 actuations) of VANCENASE AQ 84 mcg Nasal Spray, each actuation of the pump delivers 100 mg of suspension containing beclomethasone dipropionate, monohydrate equivalent to 84 mcg beclomethasone dipropionate. Each bottle of VANCENASE AQ 84 mcg Nasal Spray will provide at least 120 actuations.

VANCENASE AQ 84 mcg Nasal Spray is a metered-dose, manual pump spray unit containing a suspension of beclomethasone dipropionate, monohydrate equivalent to 0.084% w/w beclomethasone dipropionate in an aqueous medium containing microcrystalline cellulose, carboxymethylcellulose sodium, dextrose, benzalkonium chloride, polysorbate 80, and phenylethyl alcohol. The suspension is formulated at a target pH of 6.4, with a range of 5.5 to 6.8 over its shelf life.

CLINICAL PHARMACOLOGY

Beclomethasone 17,21-dipropionate is a diester of beclomethasone, a synthetic halogenated corticosteroid. Animal studies show that beclomethasone dipropionate has potent glucocorticosteroid and weak mineralcorticosteroid activity. The mechanisms for the anti-inflammatory action of beclomethasone dipropionate are unknown. The precise mechanism of the aerosolized drug's action in the nose is also unknown. Biopsies of nasal mucosa obtained during clinical studies (duration of treatment from 1 to 6 years at doses up to 336 mcg/day) showed no histopathologic changes when beclomethasone dipropionate was administered intranasally.

In a study evaluating the hypothalamic-pituitary-adrenal (HPA) effects of 336 mcg/day beclomethasone dipropionate administered intranasally for 36 consecutive days via aqueous suspension, there was no statistically significant difference in cortisol suppression between beclomethasone dipropionate 336 mcg once daily, beclomethasone dipropionate 168 mcg twice daily, and placebo. Plasma cortisol response to 6-hour cosyntropin stimulation was attenuated in control patients who received oral prednisone 10 mg daily.

The effects of beclomethasone dipropionate on HPA function have also been evaluated in adult volunteers by other routes of administration. There was no suppression of early morning plasma cortisol concentrations when beclomethasone dipropionate was administered in a dose of 1000 mcg/day for 1 month as an oral aerosol or for 3 days by intramuscular injection. However, partial suppression of plasma cortisol concentration was observed when beclomethasone dipropionate was administered in doses of 2000 mcg/day either by oral aerosol or intramuscular injection. Immediate suppression of plasma cortisol concentrations was observed after single doses of 4000 mcg of beclomethasone dipropionate. Suppression of HPA function (reduction of early morning plasma cortisol levels) has been reported in adult patients who received 1600 mcg daily doses of oral beclomethasone dipropionate for 1 month.

In one study of pediatric patients with asthma, the administration of inhaled beclomethasone dipropionate at recommended daily doses for at least 1 year was associated with a reduction in nocturnal cortisol secretion. The clinical significance of this finding is not clear. It reinforces other evidence, however, that topical beclomethasone dipropionate may be absorbed in amounts that can have systemic effects and that physicians should be alert for evidence of systemic effects, especially in chronically treated patients (see **PRECAUTIONS**).

Beclomethasone dipropionate is sparingly soluble. When given by nasal inhalation in the form of an aqueous or aerosolized suspension, the drug is deposited primarily in the nasal passages. A portion of the drug is swallowed. Absorption occurs rapidly from all respiratory and gastrointestinal tissues. There is no evidence of tissue storage of beclomethasone dipropionate or its metabolites. *In vitro* studies have shown that tissue other than the liver (lung slices) can rapidly metabolize beclomethasone dipropionate to beclomethasone 17-monopropionate and more slowly to free beclomethasone (which has very weak anti-inflammatory activity). However, irrespective of the route of entry, the principal route of excretion is the feces. In humans, 12% to 15% of an orally administered dose of beclomethasone dipropionate is excreted in the urine. The drug is excreted in both urine and feces as free and conjugated polar metabolites.

Studies have shown that the degree of binding to plasma proteins is 87%.

In clinical trials with VANCENASE AQ 84 mcg Nasal Spray in patients with seasonal allergic rhinitis, 336 mcg of beclomethasone dipropionate once daily was superior to placebo with respect to effects on nasal symptoms. In a study comparing VANCENASE AQ 84 mcg Nasal Spray once daily with beclomethasone dipropionate 42 mcg nasal spray twice daily, each delivering a total daily dose of 336 mcg beclomethasone dipropionate, both regimens were comparable with respect to effects on physician-rated nasal symptoms. In this study, a significant advantage over placebo was observed for both regimens within 3 days of the start of treatment.

INDICATIONS AND USAGE

VANCENASE AQ 84 mcg Nasal Spray is indicated for the relief of symptoms of allergic and nonallergic (vasomotor) rhinitis. Results from clinical trials of intranasal beclomethasone dipropionate in patients with seasonal allergic rhinitis have shown that significant symptom relief was obtained in most patients within 3 days. However, symptom relief may not occur in some patients for as long as 2 weeks. VANCENASE AQ 84 mcg Nasal Spray should not be continued beyond 3 weeks in the absence of significant symptom improvement. VANCENASE AQ 84 mcg Nasal Spray should not be used in the presence of untreated localized infection involving the nasal mucosa.

VANCENASE AQ 84 mcg Nasal Spray is also indicated for the prevention of recurrence of nasal polyps following surgical removal.

Clinical studies with beclomethasone dipropionate 42 mcg nasal spray have shown that treatment of the symptoms associated with nasal polyps may have to be continued for several weeks or more before a therapeutic result can be fully assessed. Recurrence of symptoms due to polyps can occur after stopping treatment, depending on the severity of the disease.

CONTRAINDICATIONS

Hypersensitivity to any of the ingredients of this preparation contraindicates its use.

WARNINGS

The replacement of a systemic corticosteroid with VANCENASE AQ 84 mcg Nasal Spray can be accompanied by signs of adrenal insufficiency.

When transferred to VANCENASE AQ 84 mcg Nasal Spray, careful attention must be given to patients previously treated for prolonged periods with systemic corticosteroids. This is particularly important in those patients who have associated asthma or other clinical conditions, where too rapid a decrease in systemic corticosteroids may cause a severe exacerbation of their symptoms.

If recommended doses of intranasal beclomethasone dipropionate are exceeded or if individuals are particularly sensitive or predisposed by virtue of recent systemic steroid therapy, symptoms of hypercorticism may occur, including very rare cases of menstrual irregularities, acneiform lesions, and cushingoid features. If such changes occur, VANCENASE AQ 84 mcg Nasal Spray should be discontinued slowly, consistent with accepted procedures for discontinuing oral steroid therapy.

Persons who are on drugs which suppress the immune system are more susceptible to infections than healthy individuals. Chickenpox and measles, for example, can have a more serious or even fatal course in nonimmune pediatric or adult patients on corticosteroids. In such pediatric or adult patients who have not had these diseases, particular care should be taken to avoid exposure. How the dose, route, and duration of corticosteroid administration affects the risk of developing a disseminated infection is not known. The contribution of the underlying disease and/or prior corticosteroid treatment to the risk is also not known. If exposed to chickenpox, prophylaxis with varicella-zoster immune globulin (VZIG) may be indicated. If exposed to measles, prophylaxis with pooled intramuscular immunoglobulin (IG) may be indicated. (See the respective package inserts for complete VZIG and IG prescribing information.) If chickenpox develops, treatment with antiviral agents may be considered.

PRECAUTIONS

General: During withdrawal from oral steroids, some patients may experience symptoms of withdrawal, eg, joint and/or muscular pain, lassitude, and depression.

Rarely, immediate hypersensitivity reactions may occur after the intranasal administration of beclomethasone. Rare instances of nasal septum perforation have been reported. Rare instances of wheezing and increased intraocular pressure have been reported following the intranasal application of aerosolized corticosteroids. Although these have not been observed in clinical trials with VANCENASE AQ 84 mcg Nasal Spray, vigilance should be maintained.

In clinical studies with beclomethasone dipropionate administered intranasally, the development of localized infections of the nose and pharynx with *Candida albicans* has occurred only rarely. When such an infection develops, use of VANCENASE AQ 84 mcg Nasal Spray should be discontinued and appropriate local or systemic therapy instituted, if needed.

If persistent nasopharyngeal irritation occurs, VANCENASE AQ 84 mcg Nasal Spray should be discontinued.

Beclomethasone dipropionate is absorbed into the circulation. Use of excessive doses of VANCENASE AQ 84 mcg Nasal Spray may suppress HPA function.

VANCENASE AQ 84 mcg Nasal Spray should be used with caution, if at all, in patients with active or quiescent tuberculous infections of the respiratory tract, or in untreated fungal, bacterial, systemic viral infections, or ocular herpes simplex.

For VANCENASE AQ 84 mcg Nasal Spray to be effective in the treatment of nasal polyps, the spray must be able to enter the nose. Therefore, treatment of nasal polyps with VANCENASE AQ 84 mcg Nasal Spray should be considered adjunctive therapy to surgical removal and/or the use of other medications which will permit effective penetration of VANCENASE AQ 84 mcg Nasal Spray into the nose. Nasal polyps may recur after any form of treatment.

As with any long-term treatment, patients using VANCENASE AQ 84 mcg Nasal Spray over several months or longer should be examined periodically for possible changes in the nasal mucosa.

Because of the inhibitory effect of corticosteroids on wound healing, patients who have experienced recent nasal septum ulcers, nasal surgery, or trauma should not use a corticosteroid intranasally until healing has occurred.

Although systemic effects have been minimal with recommended doses, this potential increases with excessive doses. Therefore, larger than recommended doses should be avoided.

Information for Patients: Patients being treated with VANCENASE AQ 84 mcg Nasal Spray should receive the following information and instructions. This information is intended to aid in the safe and effective use of this medication. It is not a disclosure of all possible adverse or intended effects. Patients should use VANCENASE AQ 84 mcg Nasal Spray ONLY once daily at a regular interval. Improvement usually becomes apparent within 3 days after the start of therapy. However, 1 to 2 weeks may pass before full relief is obtained. Since VANCENASE AQ 84 mcg Nasal Spray is not immediately effective, the prescribed dosage of VANCENASE AQ 84 mcg Nasal Spray should not be increased by using it more often than once a day in an attempt to increase its efficacy. Instead, nasal vasoconstrictors or oral antihistamines may be needed until the effects of VANCENASE AQ 84 mcg Nasal Spray are fully manifested. The patient should contact the physician if symptoms do not improve, or if the condition worsens, or if sneezing or nasal irritation occurs. For the proper use of this unit and to attain maximum benefit, the patient should read and follow the accompanying Patient's Instructions carefully.

Patients should be warned not to spray VANCENASE AQ 84 mcg Nasal Spray into the eyes.

Persons who are on immunosuppressant doses of corticosteroids should be warned to avoid exposure to chickenpox or measles, and patients should also be advised that if they are exposed, medical advice should be sought without delay.

Carcinogenesis, Mutagenesis, Impairment of Fertility: The carcinogenicity of beclomethasone dipropionate was evaluated in rats which were treated for a total of 95 weeks, 13 weeks at inhalation doses up to 0.4 mg/kg/day and the remaining 82 weeks at combined oral and inhalation doses up to 2.4 mg/kg/day (approximately 40 times the maximum recommended human daily intranasal dose on a mg/m^2 basis). There was no evidence of carcinogenicity in this study. Studies to assess the mutagenic potential of beclomethasone dipropionate have not been conducted. Impairment of fertility, as evidenced by inhibition of the estrous cycle in dogs, was observed following treatment by the oral route at a dose of 0.5 mg/kg/day (approximately 40 times the maximum recommended human daily intranasal dose on a mg/m^2 basis). No inhibition of the estrous cycle in dogs was seen following 12 months of exposure to beclomethasone dipropionate by the inhalation route at an estimated weekly dose of 2.3 mg/kg (approximately 26 times the maximum recommended human weekly intranasal dose on a mg/m^2 basis).

Pregnancy Category C: Like other corticosteroids, parenteral (subcutaneous) beclomethasone dipropionate has been

Continued on next page

Information on Schering products appearing on these pages is effective as of August 15, 1998.

Consult 1999 PDR® supplements and future editions for revisions

Vancenase AQ 84 mcg—Cont.

shown to be teratogenic and embryocidal in the mouse and rabbit when given at a dose of 0.1 mg/kg/day in mice and at a dose of 0.25 mg/kg/day in rabbits (approximately 1.2 times the maximum recommended human daily intranasal dose on a mg/m^2 basis). No teratogenic or embryocidal effects have been seen in rats treated with beclomethasone by combined inhalation and oral administration at doses of 0.1 mg/kg/day and 10 mg/kg/day, respectively (approximately 250 times the maximum recommended human daily intranasal dose on a mg/m^2 basis). There are no adequate and well-controlled studies in pregnant women. Beclomethasone dipropionate should be used during pregnancy only if the potential benefit justifies the potential risk to the fetus.

Nonteratogenic Effects: Hypoadrenalism may occur in infants born of mothers receiving corticosteroids during pregnancy. Such infants should be carefully observed.

Nursing Mothers: It is not known whether beclomethasone dipropionate is excreted in human milk. Because other corticosteroids are excreted in human milk, caution should be exercised when VANCENASE AQ 84 mcg Nasal Spray is administered to nursing women.

Pediatric Use: Safety and effectiveness of VANCENASE AQ 84 mcg Nasal Spray in pediatric patients below the age of 6 years have not been established.

ADVERSE REACTIONS

In clinical studies with intranasally administered beclomethasone dipropionate, adverse effects have primarily been related to irritation of the nasal mucous membranes. Rarely, immediate hypersensitivity reactions may occur after intranasal administration of beclomethasone dipropionate.

Clinical trials of VANCENASE AQ 84 mcg Nasal Spray included 187 patients who received VANCENASE AQ 84 mcg Nasal Spray, 127 patients who received beclomethasone dipropionate 42 mcg nasal spray, and 192 patients who received vehicle placebo. The incidence and nature of adverse events with VANCENASE AQ 84 mcg Nasal Spray (336 mcg beclomethasone dipropionate once daily) was comparable to that seen with beclomethasone dipropionate 42 mcg nasal spray (168 mcg beclomethasone dipropionate twice daily) and with vehicle placebo. Adverse events reported by 2% or more of patients (regardless of relationship to treatment) who received VANCENASE AQ 84 mcg Nasal Spray in clinical trials and that were more common with VANCENASE AQ 84 mcg Nasal Spray than with placebo are displayed in the table below.

ADVERSE EVENTS FROM CONTROLLED CLINICAL TRIALS IN SEASONAL ALLERGIC RHINITIS

	VANCENASE AQ 84 mcg Once daily (N=187)	BECLOMETHASONE DIPROPIONATE 42 mcg Twice daily (N=127)	VEHICLE PLACEBO (N=192)
Headache	34%	33%	32%
Pharyngitis	12%	11%	6%
Coughing	6%	6%	5%
Epistaxis	5%	2%	4%
Nasal burning	5%	4%	3%
Pain	4%	2%	1%
Conjunctivitis	2%	2%	1%
Myalgia	2%	1%	1%
Tinnitus	2%	3%	0%

Rare cases of ulceration of the nasal mucosa and instances of nasal septum perforation have been reported following the intranasal administration of beclomethasone dipropionate (see **PRECAUTIONS**).

Rare instances of wheezing and increased intraocular pressure have been reported following the intranasal administration of aerosolized corticosteroids (see **PRECAUTIONS**).

Single cases each of aseptic necrosis of the femoral head and of nasal fungal infection with erosion through the cribriform plate have been reported after long-term administration of beclomethasone dipropionate nasal spray.

OVERDOSAGE

When used at excessive doses, systemic corticosteroid effects such as hypercorticism and adrenal suppression may appear. If such changes occur, VANCENASE AQ 84 mcg Nasal Spray should be discontinued slowly consistent with accepted procedures for discontinuing oral steroid therapy. The oral median lethal dose of beclomethasone dipropionate is greater than 1 g/kg in mice and rats (approximately 7000 times and 14,000 times, respectively, the maximum recommended human daily intranasal dose on a mg/m^2 basis). One bottle of VANCENASE AQ 84 mcg Nasal Spray contains beclomethasone dipropionate, monohydrate equivalent to 16.0 mg of beclomethasone dipropionate; therefore, acute overdosage is unlikely.

DOSAGE AND ADMINISTRATION

Adults and Pediatric Patients 6 Years of Age and Over: The usual dosage of VANCENASE AQ 84 mcg Nasal Spray is 1 or 2 inhalations in each nostril once daily (total dose 168–336 mcg/day).

In patients who respond to VANCENASE AQ 84 mcg Nasal Spray, an improvement of the symptoms of allergic rhinitis usually becomes apparent within a few days after the start of therapy. Patients should use VANCENASE AQ 84 mcg Nasal Spray ONLY once daily at a regular interval. VANCENASE AQ 84 mcg Nasal Spray is not acutely effective, therefore, the prescribed dosage of VANCENASE AQ 84 mcg Nasal Spray should not be increased by using it more often than once daily. Symptom relief may not occur in some patients for as long as 2 weeks. VANCENASE AQ 84 mcg Nasal Spray should not be continued beyond 3 weeks in the absence of significant symptom improvement.

Since the therapeutic effects of corticosteroids, unlike those of a decongestant on allergic rhinitis or on nasal polyps, are not immediate, this should be explained to the patient in advance in order to ensure cooperation and continuation of treatment with the prescribed dosage regimen.

VANCENASE AQ 84 mcg Nasal Spray is not recommended for pediatric patients below 6 years of age.

In the presence of excessive nasal mucus secretion or edema of the nasal mucosa, the drug may fail to reach the sites of intended action. In such cases it is advisable to use a topical or oral nasal vasoconstrictor/decongestant during the first 2 to 3 days of VANCENASE AQ 84 mcg Nasal Spray therapy.

Prior to initial use of VANCENASE AQ 84 mcg Nasal Spray, the pump must be primed by actuating six times or until a fine spray appears. If the pump is unused for more than 4 days, repriming may be necessary. To reprime the unit, spray once or until a fine spray appears.

Directions for Use: Illustrated Patient's Instructions for proper use accompany each package of VANCENASE AQ 84 mcg Nasal Spray.

HOW SUPPLIED

VANCENASE AQ 84 mcg (beclomethasone dipropionate, monohydrate) Nasal Spray, 19 g net weight, 120 actuations, white high-density polyethylene bottle fitted with a white metered-dose nasal spray pump, maroon safety clip, and white dust cap; box of one. Supplied with Patient's Instructions for Use (NDC 0085-1049-01).

Store between 2° and 25°C (36° and 77°F).
SHAKE WELL BEFORE EACH USE.

Schering Corporation
Kenilworth, NJ 07033 USA

Copyright © 1996, 1997, Schering Corporation. All rights reserved.

Rev. 4/97
B-18802333
18780941T

Shown in Product Identification Guide, page 336

VANCERIL® 42 mcg ℞
(beclomethasone dipropionate, 42 mcg)
Inhalation Aerosol

For Oral Inhalation Only

DESCRIPTION

Beclomethasone dipropionate, USP, the active component of VANCERIL 42 mcg Inhalation Aerosol, is an anti-inflammatory steroid having the chemical name 9-Chloro-11β,17,21-trihydroxy-16β-methylpregna-1,4-diene-3,20-dione 17,21-dipropionate.

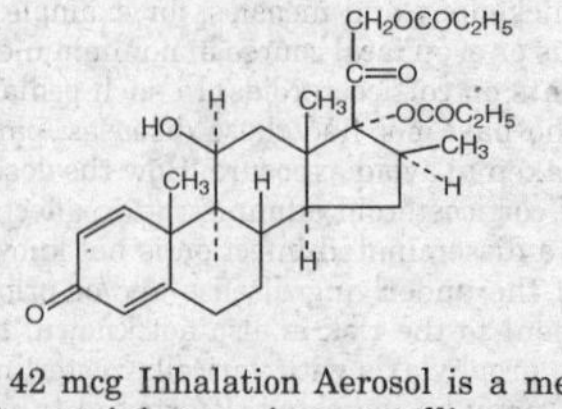

VANCERIL 42 mcg Inhalation Aerosol is a metered-dose aerosol unit containing a microcrystalline suspension of beclomethasone dipropionate-trichloromonofluoromethane clathrate in a mixture of propellants (trichloromonofluoromethane and dichlorodifluoromethane) with oleic acid. Each canister contains beclomethasone dipropionate-trichloromonofluoromethane clathrate having a molecular proportion of beclomethasone dipropionate, USP, to trichloromonofluoromethane between 3:1 and 3:2. Each actuation delivers from the mouthpiece a quantity of clathrate equivalent to 42 mcg of beclomethasone dipropionate, USP. The contents of one canister provide at least 200 oral inhalations.

CLINICAL PHARMACOLOGY

Beclomethasone 17, 21-dipropionate is a diester of beclomethasone, a synthetic corticosteroid which is chemically related to dexamethasone. Beclomethasone differs from dexamethasone only in having a chlorine at the 9-alpha in place of a fluorine and in having a 16β-methyl group instead of a 16 alpha-methyl group. Animal studies show that beclomethasone dipropionate has potent anti-inflammatory activity. When administered systemically to mice, the anti-inflammatory activity was accompanied by other typical features of glucocorticoid action including thymic involution, liver glycogen deposition, and pituitary-adrenal suppression. However, after systemic administration to rats, the anti-inflammatory action was associated with little or no effect on other tests of glucocorticoid activity.

Beclomethasone dipropionate is sparingly soluble and is poorly mobilized from subcutaneous or intramuscular injection sites. However, systemic absorption occurs after all routes of administration. When given to animals in the form of an aerosolized suspension of the trichloromonofluoromethane clathrate, the drug is deposited in the mouth and nasal passages, the trachea and principal bronchi, and in the lung; a considerable portion of the drug is also swallowed. Absorption occurs rapidly from all respiratory and gastrointestinal tissues, as indicated by the rapid clearance of radioactivity labeled drug from local tissues and appearance of tracer in the circulation. There is no evidence of tissue storage of beclomethasone dipropionate or its metabolites. Lung slices can metabolize beclomethasone dipropionate rapidly to beclomethasone 17-monopropionate and more slowly to free beclomethasone (which has very weak anti-inflammatory activity). However, irrespective of the route of administration (injection, oral, or aerosol), the principal route of excretion of the drug and its metabolites is the feces. Less than 10% of the drug and its metabolites is excreted in the urine. In humans, 12% to 15% of an orally administered dose of beclomethasone dipropionate is excreted in the urine as both conjugated and free metabolites of the drug.

The mechanisms responsible for the anti-inflammatory action of beclomethasone dipropionate are unknown. The precise mechanism of the aerosolized drug's action in the lung is also unknown.

INDICATIONS

VANCERIL 42 mcg Inhalation Aerosol is indicated only for patients who required chronic treatment with corticosteroids for control of the symptoms of bronchial asthma. Such patients would include those already receiving systemic corticosteroids, and selected patients who are inadequately controlled on a nonsteroid regimen and in whom steroid therapy has been withheld because of concern over potential adverse effects.

VANCERIL 42 mcg Inhalation Aerosol is NOT indicated:

1. For relief of asthma which can be controlled by bronchodilators and other nonsteroid medications.
2. In patients who require systemic corticosteroid treatment infrequently.
3. In the treatment of nonasthmatic bronchitis.

CONTRAINDICATIONS

VANCERIL 42 mcg Inhalation Aerosol is contraindicated in the primary treatment of status asthmaticus or other acute episodes of asthma where intensive measures are required. Hypersensitivity to any of the ingredients of this preparation contraindicates its use.

WARNINGS

Particular care is needed in patients who are transferred from systemically active corticosteroids to VANCERIL 42 mcg Inhalation Aerosol because deaths due to adrenal insufficiency have occurred in asthmatic patients during and after transfer from systemic corticosteroids to aerosol beclomethasone dipropionate. After withdrawal from systemic corticosteroids, a number of months are required for recovery of hypothalamic-pituitary-adrenal (HPA) function. During this period of HPA suppression, patients may exhibit signs and symptoms of adrenal insufficiency when exposed to trauma, surgery, or infections, particularly gastroenteritis. Although VANCERIL 42 mcg Inhalation Aerosol may provide control of asthmatic symptoms during these episodes, it does NOT provide the systemic steroid which is necessary for coping with these emergencies.

During periods of stress or a severe asthmatic attack, patients who have been withdrawn from systemic corticosteroids should be instructed to resume systemic steroids (in large doses) immediately and to contact their physician for further instruction. These patients should also be instructed to carry a warning card indicating that they may need supplementary systemic steroids during periods of stress or a severe asthma attack. To assess the risk of adrenal insufficiency in emergency situations, routine tests of adrenal cortical function, including measurement of early morning resting cortisol levels, should be performed periodically in all patients. An early morning resting cortisol level may be accepted as normal only if it falls at or near the normal mean level.

Localized infections with *Candida albicans* or *Aspergillus niger* have occurred frequently in the mouth and pharynx and occasionally in the larynx. Positive cultures for oral *Candida* may be present in up to 75% of patients. Although the frequency of clinically apparent infection is considerably lower, these infections may require treatment with appropriate antifungal therapy or discontinuance of treatment with VANCERIL 42 mcg Inhalation Aerosol.

VANCERIL 42 mcg Inhalation Aerosol is not to be regarded as a bronchodilator and is not indicated for rapid relief of bronchospasm.

Patients should be instructed to contact their physician immediately when episodes of asthma which are not responsive to bronchodilators occur during the course of treatment with VANCERIL 42 mcg Inhalation Aerosol. During such episodes, patients may require therapy with systemic corticosteroids.

There is no evidence that control of asthma can be achieved by the administration of VANCERIL 42 mcg Inhalation Aerosol in amounts greater than the recommended doses.

Transfer of patients from systemic steroid therapy to VANCERIL 42 mcg Inhalation Aerosol may unmask allergic conditions previously suppressed by the systemic steroid therapy, eg, rhinitis, conjunctivitis, and eczema.

Persons who are on drugs which suppress the immune system are more susceptible to infections than healthy individuals. Chickenpox and measles, for example, can have a more serious or even fatal course in nonimmune children or adults on corticosteroids. In such children or adults who have not had these diseases, particular care should be taken to avoid exposure. How the dose, route, and duration of corticosteroid administration affects the risk of developing a disseminated infection is not known. The contribution of the underlying disease and/or prior corticosteroid treatment to the risk is also not known. If exposed to chickenpox, prophylaxis with varicella-zoster immune globulin (VZIG) may be indicated. If exposed to measles, prophylaxis with pooled intramuscular immunoglobulin (IG) may be indicated. (See the respective package inserts for complete VZIG and IG prescribing information.) If chickenpox develops, treatment with antiviral agents may be considered.

PRECAUTIONS

During withdrawal from oral steroids, some patients may experience symptoms of systemically active steroid withdrawal, eg, joint and/or muscular pain, lassitude and depression, despite maintenance or even improvement of respiratory function. (See **DOSAGE AND ADMINISTRATION** for details.)

In responsive patients, beclomethasone dipropionate may permit control of asthmatic symptoms without suppression of HPA function, as discussed below. (See **CLINICAL STUDIES.**) Since beclomethasone dipropionate is absorbed into the circulation and can be systemically active, the beneficial effects of VANCERIL 42 mcg Inhalation Aerosol in minimizing or preventing HPA dysfunction may be expected only when recommended dosages are not exceeded.

The long-term effects of beclomethasone dipropionate in human subjects are still unknown. In particular, the local effects of the agent on developmental or immunologic processes in the mouth, pharynx, trachea, and lung are unknown. There is also no information about the possible long-term systemic effects of the agent.

The potential effects of VANCERIL 42 mcg Inhalation Aerosol on acute, recurrent, or chronic pulmonary infections, including active or quiescent tuberculosis, are not known. Similarly, the potential effects of long-term administration of the drug on lung or other tissues are unknown.

Pulmonary infiltrates with eosinophilia may occur in patients on VANCERIL 42 mcg Inhalation Aerosol therapy. Although it is possible that in some patients this state may become manifest because of systemic steroid withdrawal when inhalational steroids are administered, a causative role for beclomethasone dipropionate and/or its vehicle cannot be ruled out.

Use in Pregnancy: Glucocorticoids are known teratogens in rodent species and beclomethasone dipropionate is no exception.

Teratology studies were done in rats, mice, and rabbits treated with subcutaneous beclomethasone dipropionate. Beclomethasone dipropionate was found to produce fetal resorptions, cleft palate, agnathia, microstomia, absence of tongue, delayed ossification, and partial agenesis of the thymus. Well-controlled trials relating to fetal risk in humans are not available. Glucocorticoids are secreted in human milk. It is not known whether belcomethasone dipropionate would be secreted in human milk but it is safe to assume that it is likely. The use of beclomethasone dipropionate in pregnancy, nursing mothers, or women of childbearing potential requires that the possible benefits of the drug be weighed against the potential hazards to the mother, embryo, or fetus. Infants born of mothers who have received substantial doses of corticosteroids during pregnancy should be carefully observed for hypoadrenalism.

Information for Patients: Persons who are on immunosuppressant doses of corticosteroids should be warned to avoid exposure to chickenpox or measles. Patients should also be advised that if they are exposed, medical advice should be sought without delay.

ADVERSE REACTIONS

Deaths due to adrenal insufficiency have occurred in asthmatic patients during and after transfer from systemic corticosteroids to aerosol beclomethasone dipropionate. (See **WARNINGS.**)

Suppression of HPA function (reduction of early morning plasma cortisol levels) has been reported in adult patients who received 1600 mcg daily doses of VANCERIL 42 mcg Inhalation Aerosol for 1 month. A few patients on VANCERIL 42 mcg Inhalation Aerosol have complained of hoarseness or dry mouth.

Rare cases of immediate and delayed hypersensitivity reactions, including urticaria, angioedema, rash, and bronchospasm have been reported following the oral and intranasal inhalation of beclomethasone.

DOSAGE AND ADMINISTRATION

Adults: The usual recommended dosage is two inhalations (84 mcg) given three or four times a day. Alternatively, four inhalations (168 mcg) given twice daily has been shown to be effective in some patients. In patients with severe asthma, it is advisable to start with 12 to 16 inhalations a day and adjust the dosage downward according to the response of the patient. The maximal daily intake should not exceed 20 inhalations, 840 mcg (0.84 mg), in adults.

Children 6 to 12 Years of Age: The usual recommended dosage is one or two inhalations (42 to 84 mcg) given three or four times a day according to the response of the patient. Alternatively, four inhalations (168 mcg) given twice daily has been shown to be effective in some patients. The maximal daily intake should not exceed ten inhalations, 420 mcg (0.42 mcg), in children 6 to 12 years of age. Insufficient clinical data exist with respect to the administration of VANCERIL 42 mcg Inhalation Aerosol in children below the age of 6.

Rinsing the mouth after inhalation is advised.

Patients receiving bronchodilators by inhalation should be advised to use the bronchodilator before VANCERIL 42 mcg Inhalation Aerosol in order to enhance penetration of beclomethasone dipropionate into the bronchial tree. After use of an aerosol bronchodilator, several minutes should elapse before use of the VANCERIL 42 mcg Inhalation Aerosol to reduce the potential toxicity from the inhaled fluorocarbon propellants in the two aerosols.

Different considerations must be given to the following groups of patients in order to obtain the full therapeutic benefit of VANCERIL 42 mcg Inhalation Aerosol.

Patients Not Receiving Systemic Steroids: The use of VANCERIL 42 mcg Inhalation Aerosol is straightforward in patients who are inadequately controlled with nonsteroid medications but in whom systemic steroid therapy has been withheld because of concern over potential adverse reactions. In patients who respond to VANCERIL, an improvement in pulmonary function is usually apparent within 1 to 4 weeks after the start of VANCERIL 42 mcg Inhalation Aerosol.

Patients Receiving Systemic Steroids: In those patients dependent on systemic steroids, transfer to VANCERIL 42 mcg Inhalation Aerosol and subsequent management may be more difficult because of recovery from impaired adrenal function is usually slow. Such suppression has been known to last for up to 12 months. Clinical studies, however, have demonstrated that VANCERIL may be effective in the management of these asthmatic patients and may permit replacement or significant reduction in the dosage of systemic corticosteriods.

The patient's asthma should be reasonably stable before treatment with VANCERIL 42 mcg Inhalation Aerosol is started. Initially, the aerosol should be used concurrently with the patient's usual maintenance dose of systemic steroid. After approximately 1 week, gradual withdrawal of the systemic steroid is started by reducing the daily or alternate daily dose. The next reduction is made after an interval of 1 or 2 weeks, depending on the response of the patient. Generally, these decrements should not exceed 2.5 mg of prednisone or its equivalent. A slow rate of withdrawal cannot be overemphasized. During withdrawal, some patients may experience symptoms of systemically active steroid withdrawal, eg, joint and/or muscular pain, lassitude and depression, despite maintenance or even improvement of respiratory function. Such patients should be encouraged to continue with the inhaler but should be watched carefully for objective signs of adrenal insufficiency, such as hypotension and weight loss. If evidence of adrenal insufficiency occurs, the systemic steroid dose should be boosted temporarily thereafter further withdrawal should continue more slowly.

During periods of stress or a severe asthma attack, transfer patients will require supplementary treatment with systemic steroids. Exacerbations of asthma which occur during the course of treatment with VANCERIL 42 mcg Inhalation Aerosol should be treated with a short course of systemic steroid which is gradually tapered as these symptoms subside. There is no evidence that control of asthma can be achieved by administration of VANCERIL in amounts greater than the recommended doses.

Directions for Use: Illustrated Patient's Instructions for proper use accompany each package of VANCERIL 42 mcg Inhalation Aerosol.

CONTENTS UNDER PRESSURE. Do not puncture. Do not use or store near heat or open flame. Exposure to temperatures above 120°F may cause bursting. Never throw container into fire or incinerator. Keep out of reach of children.

HOW SUPPLIED

VANCERIL 42 mcg Inhalation Aerosol 16.8 g canister supplied with an oral adapter and Patient's Instructions; box of one (NDC 0085-0736-04). Institutional Pack for Inpatient Use Only: VANCERIL 42 mcg Inhalation Aerosol 6.7 g canister supplied with an oral adapter and Patient's Instructions; box of one (NDC 0085-0738-01).

Store between 15° and 30°C (59° and 86°F). Protect from moisture and unusual temperature fluctuations. Shake well before using. Failure to use the product within this temperature range may result in improper dosing.

Note: The indented statement below is required by the Federal government's Clean Air Act for all products containing or manufactured with chlorofluorocarbons (CFCs).

> **WARNING**: Contains dichlorodifluoromethane (CFC-11) and trichloromonofluoromethane (CFC-12), substances which harm public health and the environment by destroying ozone in the upper atmosphere.

A notice similar to the above WARNING has been placed in the "Patient's Instructions" portion of this package insert pursuant to EPA regulations.

ANIMAL PHARMACOLOGY AND TOXICOLOGY

Studies in a number of animal species including rats, rabbits, and dogs have shown no unusual toxicity during acute experiments. However, the effects of beclomethasone dipropionate in producing signs of glucocorticoid excess during chronic administration by various routes were dose related.

CLINICAL STUDIES

The effects of beclomethasone dipropionate on hypothalamic-pituitary-adrenal (HPA) function have been evaluated in adult volunteers. There was no suppression of early morning plasma cortisol concentrations when beclomethasone dipropionate was administered at a dose of 1000 mcg/day for 1 month as an aerosol or for 3 days by intramuscular injection. However, partial suppression of plasma cortisol concentration was observed when beclomethasone dipropionate was administered at doses of 2000 mcg/day either intramuscularly or by aerosol. Immediate suppression of plasma cortisol concentrations was observed after single doses of 4000 mcg of beclomethasone dipropionate.

In one study, the effects of beclomethasone dipropionate on HPA function were examined in patients with asthma. There was no change in basal early morning plasma cortisol concentrations or in the cortisol responses to tetracosactrin (ACTH 1:24) stimulation after daily administration of 400, 800, or 1200 mcg of beclomethasone dipropionate for 28 days. After daily administration of 1600 mcg each day for 28 days, there was a slight reduction in basal cortisol concentrations and a statistically significant ($p < .01$) reduction in plasma cortisol responses to tetracosactrin stimulation. The effects of a more prolonged period of beclomethasone dipropionate administration on HPA function have not been evaluated. However, a number of investigators have noted that when systemic corticosteroid therapy in asthmatic subjects can be replaced with recommended doses of beclomethasone dipropionate, there is gradual recovery of endogenous cortisol concentrations to the normal range. There is still no documented evidence of recovery from other adverse systemic corticosteroid-induced reactions during prolonged therapy of patients with beclomethasone dipropionate.

Clinical experience has shown that some patients with bronchial asthma who require corticosteroid therapy for control of symptoms can be partially or completely withdrawn from systemic corticosteroid if therapy with beclomethasone dipropionate aerosol is substituted. Beclomethasone dipropionate aerosol is not effective for all patients with bronchial asthma or at all stages of the disease in a given patient.

The early clinical experience has revealed several new problems which may be associated with the use of beclomethasone dipropionate by inhalation for treatment of patients with bronchial asthma:

1. There is a risk of adrenal insufficiency when patients are transferred from systemic corticosteroids to aerosol beclomethasone dipropionate. Although the aerosol may provide adequate control of asthma during the transfer period, it does not provide the systemic steroid which is needed dur-

Continued on next page

Information on Schering products appearing on these pages is effective as of August 15, 1998.

Vanceril 42 mcg—Cont.

ing acute stress situations. Deaths due to adrenal insufficiency have occurred in asthmatic patients during and after transfer from systemic corticosteroids to aerosol beclomethasone dipropionate. (See **WARNINGS.**)

2. Transfer of patients from systemic steroid therapy to beclomethasone dipropionate aerosol may unmask allergic conditions which were previously controlled by the systemic steroid therapy, eg, rhinitis, conjunctivitis, and eczema.

3. Localized infections with *Candida albicans* or *Aspergillus niger* have occurred frequently in the mouth and pharynx and occasionally in the larynx. It has been reported that up to 75% of the patients who receive prolonged treatment with beclomethasone dipropionate have positive oral cultures for *Candida albicans*. The incidence of clinically apparent infection is considerably lower but may require therapy with appropriate antifungal agents or discontinuation of treatment with beclomethasone dipropionate aerosol.

The long-term effects of beclomethasone dipropionate in human subjects are still unknown. In particular, the local effects of the agent on developmental or immunologic processes in the mouth, pharynx, trachea, and lung are unknown. There is also no information about the possible longterm systemic effects of the agent. The possible relevance of the data in animal studies to results in human subjects cannot be evaluated.

Schering Corporation
Kenilworth, NJ 07033 USA

Rev. 4/97 B-20108908

Copyright © 1973, 1995, 1996, 1997, Schering Corporation. All rights reserved.

VANCERIL® 42 mcg

(beclomethasone dipropionate, 42 mcg) Inhalation Aerosol

For Oral Inhalation Only

PATIENT'S INSTRUCTIONS

It is important that you read these instructions before using your VANCERIL 42 mcg Inhalation Aerosol. Correct and regular use of the inhaler will prevent or lessen the severity of asthma attacks.

1. SHAKE THE INHALER WELL and remove the plastic cap (see Figure 1).

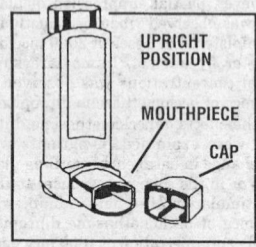

UPRIGHT POSITION

MOUTHPIECE

CAP

Figure 1

2. As with all aerosol medications, it is recommended to "test spray" into the air before using for the first time and in cases where the aerosol has not been used for a prolonged period of time.

3. BREATHE OUT AS FULLY AS YOU COMFORTABLY CAN. Hold the inhaler in the upright position and put the mouthpiece into your mouth (see Figure 2). Close your lips around the mouthpiece, *keeping your tongue below it.*

4. WHILE BREATHING IN DEEPLY, PRESS DOWN ON

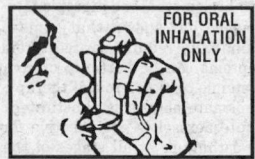

FOR ORAL INHALATION ONLY

Figure 2

THE CAN WITH YOUR FIRST FINGER. When you have finished breathing in, hold your breath as long as you comfortably can.

5. TAKE YOUR FINGER OFF THE CAN and remove the inhaler from your mouth. Breathe out gently.

6. If your physician has told you to take more than one inhalation per treatment, wait 1 minute between puffs. Shake the inhaler well and repeat steps 3 through 5.

7. It is recommended that you rinse your mouth thoroughly with water, gargle, or drink water after inhalation(s), whenever possible.

8. CLEAN YOUR INHALER AT LEAST ONCE A DAY. Remove the can and rinse the plastic case and cap in warm

running water. Dry the case and cap and gently replace the metal canister into the case with a twisting motion. Put the cap on the mouthpiece.

9. DISCARD THE CANISTER AFTER the date calculated by your physician or pharmacist. The correct amount of medication in each inhalation cannot be assured after a specified number of inhalations even though the canister is not completely empty. Before the discard date you should consult your physician to determine whether a refill is needed. Just as you should not take extra doses without consulting your physician, you also should not stop VANCERIL without consulting your physician.

IMPORTANT: VANCERIL 42 mcg Inhalation Aerosol is preventive therapy for asthma and must be used regularly and at the times your physician has prescribed. DO NOT CONFUSE VANCERIL 42 mcg Inhalation Aerosol WITH OTHER ASTHMA MEDICATION. VANCERIL 42 mcg Inhalation Aerosol WILL NOT PROVIDE IMMEDIATE RELIEF IF YOU ARE HAVING AN ATTACK. Your physician will decide whether other medication is needed should you require immediate relief. If you also use another medicine by inhalation, you should consult your physician for instructions on when to use it in relation to using VANCERIL. If this is the first time you will be using VANCERIL 42 mcg Inhalation Aerosol, it may take from 1 to 4 weeks before you feel the full benefits.

Dosage: Use only as directed by your physician.

Contents under pressure. Do not puncture. Do not use or store near heat or open flame. Exposure to temperatures above 120°F may cause bursting. Never throw container into fire or incinerator. Keep out of reach of children.

Store between 15° and 30°C (59° and 86°F). Protect from moisture and unusual temperature fluctuations. Shake well before using. Failure to use the product within this temperature range may result in improper dosing.

Note: The indented statement below is required by the Federal government's Clean Air Act for all products containing or manufactured with chlorofluorocarbons (CFCs).

This product contains dichlorodifluoromethane (CFC-11) and trichloromonofluoromethane (CFC-12), substances which harm the environment by destroying ozone in the upper atmosphere.

Your physician has determined that this product is likely to help your personal health. USE THIS PRODUCT AS DIRECTED, UNLESS INSTRUCTED TO DO OTHERWISE BY YOUR PHYSICIAN. If you have any questions about alternatives, consult with your physician.

Schering Corporation
Kenilworth, NJ 07033 USA

Copyright © 1973, 1995, 1996, 1997,
Schering Corporation.

All rights reserved. Rev. 4/97

Shown in Product Identification Guide, page 336

VANCERIL® 84 mcg ℞
DOUBLE STRENGTH
(beclomethasone dipropionate, 84 mcg)
Inhalation Aerosol

For Oral Inhalation Only

DESCRIPTION

Beclomethasone dipropionate, USP, the active component of VANCERIL 84 mcg DOUBLE STRENGTH Inhalation Aerosol, is an anti-inflammatory corticosteroid having the chemical name 9-Chloro-11β,17,21-trihydroxy-16β-methylpregna-1,4-diene-3,20-dione 17,21-dipropionate. Beclomethasone 17,21-dipropionate is a diester of beclomethasone, a synthetic corticosteroid which is chemically related to dexamethasone. Beclomethasone differs from dexamethasone only in having a chlorine at the 9α carbon in place of fluorine and in having a 16β-methyl group instead of a 16α-methyl group.

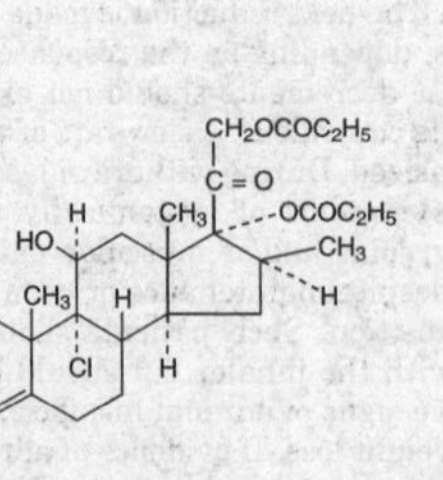

$CH_2OCOC_2H_5$
$C = O$
CH_3 ---OCOC$_2$H$_5$
HO
CH_3 CH_3
Cl H
O

Beclomethasone dipropionate is a white to creamy white, odorless powder with a molecular formula of $C_{28}H_{37}ClO_7$, and a molecular weight of 521.05. It is very slightly soluble in water, very soluble in chloroform, and freely soluble in acetone and in alcohol.

VANCERIL 84 mcg DOUBLE STRENGTH Inhalation Aerosol is a pressurized metered-dose aerosol unit containing a

microcrystalline suspension of beclomethasone dipropionate-trichloromonofluoromethane clathrate in a mixture of propellants (trichloromonofluoromethane and dichlorodifluoromethane) with oleic acid. Each canister contains beclomethasone dipropionate-trichloromonofluoromethane clathrate having a molecular proportion of beclomethasone dipropionate, USP, to trichloromonofluoromethane between 3:1 and 3:2. Each actuation delivers a quantity of clathrate equivalent to 84 mcg of beclomethasone dipropionate, USP from the mouthpiece and 100 mcg of beclomethasone dipropionate from the valve. The contents of the 5.4 g and 12.2 g canisters provide 40 and 120 oral inhalations, respectively (see HOW SUPPLIED)

CLINICAL PHARMACOLOGY

Animal studies showed that beclomethasone dipropionate has potent anti-inflammatory activity. When administered systemically to mice, the anti-inflammatory activity was accompanied by other typical features of glucocorticoid action including thymic involution, liver glycogen deposition, and pituitary-adrenal suppression. However, after systemic administration to rats, the anti-inflammatory action was associated with little or no effect on other tests of glucocorticoid activity.

Beclomethasone dipropionate is sparingly soluble and is poorly mobilized from subcutaneous or intramuscular injection sites. However, systemic absorption occurs after all routes of administration. When given to animals in the form of an aerosolized suspension of the trichloromonofluoromethane clathrate, the drug is deposited in the mouth and nasal passages, the trachea and principal bronchi, and in the lung; a considerable portion of the drug is also swallowed. Absorption occurs rapidly from all respiratory and gastrointestinal tissues, as indicated by the rapid clearance of radioactively labeled drug from local tissues and appearance of tracer in the circulation. There is no evidence of tissue storage of beclomethasone dipropionate or its metabolites. Lung slices can metabolize beclomethasone dipropionate rapidly to beclomethasone 17-monopropionate and more slowly to free beclomethasone (which has very weak anti-inflammatory activity). However, irrespective of the route of administration (injection, oral, or aerosol), the principal route of excretion of the drug and its metabolites is the feces. Less than 10% of the drug and its metabolites is excreted in the urine. In humans, 12% to 15% of an orally administered dose of beclomethasone dipropionate was excreted in the urine as both conjugated and free metabolites of the drug.

The mechanisms responsible for the anti-inflammatory action of beclomethasone dipropionate are unknown. The precise mechanism of the aerosolized drug's action in the lung is also unknown.

Clinical Trials: The efficacy of VANCERIL 84 mcg DOUBLE STRENGTH Inhalation Aerosol was compared with VANCERIL Inhaler (42 mcg/actuation) in a 28-day, randomized, parallel-group, double-blind, placebo-controlled study in patients with moderate to severe asthma. A total of 336 mcg/day of each VANCERIL formulation or placebo was administered based on BID dosing. FEV_1 at endpoint (last valid visit for each patient) was regarded as the primary measure of efficacy. VANCERIL 84 mcg DOUBLE STRENGTH Inhalation Aerosol and VANCERIL Inhaler were both significantly more effective ($p≤0.01$) than placebo in improving FEV_1 at all time points, but were not significantly different from each other at any time point ($p>0.05$). Thus VANCERIL 84 mcg DOUBLE STRENGTH Inhalation Aerosol administered twice daily to give a total daily dose of 336 mcg was comparable in efficacy to VANCERIL Inhaler when administered at the same total daily dose.

The effects of beclomethasone dipropionate on hypothalamic-pituitary-adrenal (HPA) function have been evaluated in adult volunteers. There was no suppression of early morning plasma cortisol concentrations when beclomethasone dipropionate was administered at a dose of 840 mcg/day for 1 month as an aerosol or 1000 mcg/day for 3 days by intramuscular injection. However, partial suppression of plasma cortisol concentration was observed when beclomethasone dipropionate was administered at doses of 2000 mcg/day intramuscularly or 1680 mcg/day by aerosol. Immediate suppression of plasma cortisol concentrations was observed after single doses of 4000 mcg of beclomethasone dipropionate intramuscularly.

The potential for VANCERIL 84 mcg DOUBLE STRENGTH Inhalation Aerosol (84 mcg/actuation) to cause HPA axis suppression was compared with VANCERIL Inhaler (42 mcg/actuation) in a randomized, parallel, placebo- and positive-controlled study. Sixty-four adult patients with moderate asthma received doses of either: 1) 420 mcg twice daily of VANCERIL 84 mcg DOUBLE STRENGTH; 2) 420 mcg twice daily of VANCERIL Inhaler; 3) 10 mg of prednisone orally; or 4) placebo, for 35.5 days. The potential for HPA axis suppression was evaluated via a cosyntropin stimulation test administered on the 36th day. In response to a 6-hour cosyntropin 250 mcg infusion, there was no evidence of HPA axis suppression associated with either VANCERIL 84 mcg DOUBLE STRENGTH Inhalation Aerosol or

VANCERIL Inhaler preparations as compared with placebo. However, there were significant (p≤0.01) attenuations of the plasma cortisol concentration responses to cosyntropin stimulation in the prednisone-treated group compared with the placebo-treated group.

In another study with VANCERIL Inhaler, the effects of beclomethasone dipropionate on HPA function were examined in patients with asthma. There was no change in basal early morning plasma cortisol concentrations or in the cortisol responses to tetracosactrin (ACTH 1:24) stimulation after daily aerosol administration of 336, 672, or 1008 mcg of beclomethasone dipropionate for 28 days. After daily aerosol administration of 1344 mcg for 28 days, there was a slight reduction in basal cortisol concentrations and a statistically significant (p<0.01) reduction in plasma cortisol responses to tetracosactrin stimulation. The effects of a more prolonged period of beclomethasone dipropionate administration on HPA function have not been evaluated.

Clinical experience has shown that some patients with asthma who require corticosteroid therapy for control of symptoms can be partially or completely withdrawn from systemic corticosteroid if therapy with beclomethasone dipropionate aerosol is substituted. Beclomethasone dipropionate aerosol is not effective for all patients with asthma or at all stages of the disease in a given patient.

INDICATIONS

VANCERIL 84 mcg DOUBLE STRENGTH Inhalation Aerosol is indicated in the maintenance treatment of asthma as prophylactic therapy. VANCERIL 84 mcg DOUBLE STRENGTH Inhalation Aerosol is also indicated for asthma patients who require systemic corticosteroid administration, where adding VANCERIL 84 mcg DOUBLE STRENGTH Inhalation Aerosol may reduce or eliminate the need for systemic corticosteroids.

VANCERIL 84 mcg DOUBLE STRENGTH Inhalation Aerosol is NOT indicated for the relief of acute bronchospasm.

CONTRAINDICATIONS

VANCERIL 84 mcg DOUBLE STRENGTH Inhalation Aerosol is contraindicated in the primary treatment of status asthmaticus or other acute episodes of asthma where intensive measures are required.

Hypersensitivity to any of the ingredients of this preparation contraindicates its use.

WARNINGS

Particular care is needed in patients who are transferred from systemically active corticosteroids to VANCERIL 84 mcg DOUBLE STRENGTH Inhalation Aerosol because deaths due to adrenal insufficiency have occurred in asthmatic patients during and after transfer from systemic corticosteroids to aerosol beclomethasone dipropionate. After withdrawal from systemic corticosteroids, a number of months are required for recovery of hypothalamic-pituitary-adrenal (HPA) function. During this period of HPA suppression, patients may exhibit signs and symptoms of adrenal insufficiency when exposed to trauma, surgery, or infections, particularly gastroenteritis. Although VANCERIL 84 mcg DOUBLE STRENGTH Inhalation Aerosol may provide control of asthmatic symptoms during these episodes, it does NOT provide the systemic steroid which is necessary for coping with these emergencies.

During periods of stress or a severe asthmatic attack, patients who have been withdrawn from systemic corticosteroids should be instructed to resume systemic corticosteroids (in large doses) immediately and to contact their physician for further instruction. These patients should also be instructed to carry a warning card indicating that they may need supplementary systemic steroids during periods of stress or a severe asthma attack. To assess the risk of adrenal insufficiency in emergency situations, routine tests of adrenal cortical function, including measurement of early morning resting cortisol levels, should be performed periodically in all patients. An early morning resting cortisol level may be accepted as normal only if it falls at or near the normal mean level.

Localized infections with *Candida albicans* or *Aspergillus niger* have occurred in the mouth and pharynx and occasionally in the larynx. Positive cultures for oral *Candida* may be present in up to 75% of patients. Although the frequency of clinically apparent infection is considerably lower, these infections can develop with any inhaled corticosteroid and may require treatment with appropriate antifungal therapy or discontinuance of treatment with VANCERIL 84 mcg DOUBLE STRENGTH Inhalation Aerosol.

VANCERIL 84 mcg DOUBLE STRENGTH Inhalation Aerosol is not a bronchodilator and is, therefore, not indicated for rapid relief of bronchospasm.

Patients should be instructed to contact their physician immediately when episodes of asthma which are not responsive to bronchodilators occur during the course of treatment with VANCERIL 84 mcg DOUBLE STRENGTH Inhalation Aerosol. During such episodes, patients may require therapy with systemic corticosteroids.

Transfer of patients from systemic corticosteroid therapy to VANCERIL 84 mcg DOUBLE STRENGTH Inhalation Aerosol may unmask allergic conditions previously suppressed by the systemic corticosteroid therapy, eg, rhinitis, conjunctivitis, and eczema.

Patients who are on drugs which suppress the immune system are more susceptible to infections than healthy individuals. Chickenpox and measles, for example, can have a more serious or even fatal course in non-immune children or adults on corticosteroids. In children or adults who have not had these diseases, particular care should be taken to avoid exposure to these infectious agents. How the dose, route, and duration of corticosteroid administration affects the risk of developing disseminated infection is not known. The contribution of underlying disease and/or prior corticosteroid treatment to the risk of developing more severe infection is also not known. If exposed to chickenpox, prophylaxis with varicella-zoster immune globulin (VZIG) may be indicated. If exposed to measles, prophylaxis with pooled intramuscular immunoglobulin (IG) may be indicated. (See the respective package inserts for complete VZIG and IG prescribing information.) If chickenpox develops, treatment with antiviral agents may be considered.

Avoid spraying in eyes.

PRECAUTIONS

During withdrawal from oral corticosteroids, some patients may experience symptoms of systemically active corticosteroid withdrawal, eg, joint and/or muscular pain, lassitude and depression, despite maintenance or even improvement of respiratory function. (See **DOSAGE AND ADMINISTRATION** for details.)

In responsive patients, beclomethasone dipropionate may permit control of asthmatic symptoms without suppression of HPA function, as discussed above. (See **CLINICAL PHARMACOLOGY**.) Since inhaled beclomethasone dipropionate is absorbed into the circulation and can be systemically active, lack of HPA suppression by VANCERIL 84 mcg DOUBLE STRENGTH Inhalation Aerosol may be expected only when recommended dosages are not exceeded.

The long-term local and systemic effects of VANCERIL 84 mcg DOUBLE STRENGTH Inhalation Aerosol in human subjects are still not fully known. In particular, the effects resulting from chronic use of the agent on developmental or immunologic processes in the mouth, pharynx, trachea, and lung are unknown.

Inhaled corticosteroids should be used with caution, if at all, in patients with active or quiescent tuberculous infection of the respiratory tract; untreated systemic fungal, bacterial, parasitic, or viral infections; or ocular herpes simplex.

Pulmonary infiltrates with eosinophilia may occur in patients receiving orally inhaled beclomethasone dipropionate. Although it is possible that in some patients this state may become manifest because of systemic corticosteroid withdrawal when inhalational corticosteroids are administered, a causative role for beclomethasone dipropionate and/or its vehicle cannot be ruled out.

Carcinogenesis, Mutagenesis, Impairment of Fertility: The carcinogenicity of beclomethasone dipropionate was evaluated in rats which were exposed for a total of 95 weeks, 13 weeks at inhalation doses up to 0.4 mg/kg/day and the remaining 82 weeks at combined oral and inhalation doses up to 2.4 mg/kg/day. There was no evidence of carcinogenicity in this study at the highest dose which is approximately 23 times the maximum recommended human daily inhalation dose on a mg/m^2 basis. Impairment of fertility, as evidenced by inhibition of the estrous cycle in dogs, was observed following treatment by the oral route at a dose of 0.5 mg/kg/day which is approximately 16 times the maximum recommended human daily inhalation dose on a mg/m^2 basis. No inhibition of the estrous cycle in dogs was seen following 12 months of exposure to beclomethasone dipropionate by the inhalation route at an estimated daily dose of 0.33 mg/kg (approximately 11 times the maximum recommended human daily inhalation dose on a mg/m^2 basis).

Pregnancy Category C: Like other corticosteroids, parenteral (subcutaneous) beclomethasone dipropionate was teratogenic and embryocidal in the mouse and rabbit when given at a dose of 0.1 mg/kg/day in mice or at a dose of 0.025 mg/kg/day in rabbits. These doses in mice and rabbits were approximately one-half the maximum recommended human daily inhalation dose on a mg/m^2 basis. No teratogenicity or embryocidal effects were seen in rats when exposed to an inhalation dose of 0.1 mg/kg plus oral doses of up to 10 mg/kg/day for a combined daily dose of 10.1 mg/kg (approximately 97 times the maximum recommended human daily inhalation dose on a mg/m^2 basis). There are no adequate and well-controlled studies in pregnant women. Beclomethasone dipropionate should be used during pregnancy only if the potential benefit justifies the potential risk to the fetus.

Nursing Mothers: Corticosteroids are secreted in human milk. Because of the potential for serious adverse reactions in nursing infants from VANCERIL 84 mcg DOUBLE STRENGTH Inhalation Aerosol, a decision should be made whether to discontinue nursing or to discontinue the drug, taking into account the importance of the drug to the mother.

Pediatric Use: Safety and effectiveness in pediatric patients below the age of 6 years have not been established.

Information for Patients: Patients being treated with VANCERIL 84 mcg DOUBLE STRENGTH Inhalation Aerosol should receive the following information and instructions. This information is intended to aid them in the safe and effective use of this medication. It is not a disclosure of all possible adverse or intended effects.

Patients should use VANCERIL 84 mcg DOUBLE STRENGTH Inhalation Aerosol at regular intervals as directed. Results of clinical trials indicated significant improvement may occur within the first day or two of treatment; however, the full benefit may not be achieved until treatment has been administered for 1 to 2 weeks or longer. The patient should not increase the prescribed dosage but should contact the physician if symptoms do not improve or if the condition worsens.

Patients should be warned to avoid exposure to chickenpox or measles. Patients should be advised that if they are exposed, medical advice should be sought without delay.

Patients should also be advised that VANCERIL 84 mcg DOUBLE STRENGTH Inhalation Aerosol is not intended for use in the treatment of acute asthma. Patients should be instructed to contact their physician immediately if there is any deterioration of their asthma.

Patients should be advised to rinse his/her mouth each time after using VANCERIL 84 mcg DOUBLE STRENGTH Inhalation Aerosol.

VANCERIL 84 mcg DOUBLE STRENGTH Inhalation Aerosol should not be stopped abruptly. If discontinuing use of VANCERIL 84 mcg DOUBLE STRENGTH Inhalation Aerosol is necessary, the patient's physician should be contacted immediately.

ADVERSE REACTIONS

In a 4-week, randomized, double-blind, placebo-controlled clinical trial, the incidence of adverse events reported for VANCERIL 84 mcg DOUBLE STRENGTH Inhalation Aerosol was similar to that reported for placebo. Adverse event rates did not appear to differ significantly based on age, sex, or race. Adverse events that were reported by 2% or more of patients receiving VANCERIL 84 mcg DOUBLE STRENGTH Inhalation Aerosol (regardless of relationship to treatment) and that occurred more frequently than placebo are displayed in the following table.

In a 4-week, randomized, double-blind clinical study, there were no reports of oral candidiasis in patients receiving VANCERIL 84 mcg DOUBLE STRENGTH Inhalation Aerosol (0/103) (see **WARNINGS**).

ADVERSE EVENTS FROM A 4-WEEK PLACEBO-CONTROLLED CLINICAL TRIAL IN PATIENTS WITH ASTHMA

PERCENT OF PATIENTS REPORTING

	VANCERIL 84 mcg DOUBLE STRENGTH Inhalation Aerosol (336 mcg/day) n=103	VANCERIL Inhaler (336 mcg/day) n=104	Vehicle Placebo n=109
Headache	22	27	18
Pharyngitis	14	11	8
Coughing	9	7	4
Infection (Viral)	8	5	6
Nasal Congestion	6	5	2
Dysmenorrhea	4	0	3
Sinusitis	4	3	3
Dyspepsia	3	6	2
Fatigue	3	2	2
Influenza-like Symptoms	3	<1	0
Sneezing	3	2	0
Eczema	2	0	0
Pruritus	2	0	<1
Respiratory Disorder	2	0	0

Continued on next page

Information on Schering products appearing on these pages is effective as of August 15, 1998.

Vanceril 84 mcg—Cont.

In addition to those adverse events reported in the table above, the following adverse events have been reported in fewer than 2% of patients (regardless of relationship to treatment).

Autonomic Nervous System: Lacrimation.
Body as a Whole: Increased allergy symptoms, chest pain, fever, rigors.
Gastrointestinal System: Diarrhea, nausea, rectal hemorrhage.
Hearing and Vestibular: Earache.
Heart Rate and Rhythm: Tachycardia.
Musculoskeletal: Arthralgia, pain.
Psychiatric: Depression, insomnia.
Respiratory System: Bronchitis, bronchospasm, chest congestion, dysphonia, upper respiratory infection.
Skin and Appendages: Rash, skin discoloration, urticaria.
Special Senses: Taste perversion.
Urinary System: Urinary tract infection.
Vascular (Extracardiac): Migraine.
White Cell and Reticuloendothelial System: Lymphadenopathy.

Deaths due to adrenal insufficiency have occurred in asthmatic patients during and after transfer from systemic corticosteroids to aerosol beclomethasone dipropionate. (See **WARNINGS.**)

Suppression of HPA function (reduction of early morning plasma cortisol levels) has been reported in adult patients who received 1344 mcg daily doses (approximately twice the maximum recommended daily dose) of beclomethasone dipropionate by oral inhalation for 1 month. Some patients receiving orally inhaled beclomethasone dipropionate have complained of hoarseness or dry mouth.

Rare cases of immediate and delayed hypersensitivity reactions, including urticaria, angioedema, rash, and bronchospasm have been reported following the oral and intranasal inhalation of beclomethasone.

Rare cases of hypercorticism, adrenal insufficiency, growth inhibitory effects, cataracts, glaucoma, and hyperglycemia have been reported with inhaled corticosteroids.

OVERDOSAGE

There were no deaths over 15 days following the oral administration of a single dose of 3000 mg/kg in mice, 2000 mg/kg in rats, and 1000 mg/kg in rabbits. The doses in mice, rats, and rabbits were 14,500, 19,300, and 19,300 times, respectively, the maximum recommended human daily inhalation dose on a mg/m^2 basis.

DOSAGE AND ADMINISTRATION

VANCERIL 84 mcg DOUBLE STRENGTH Inhalation Aerosol should be test sprayed 2 times into the air before using for the first time and in cases where the product has not been used for more than 7 days.

Adults: The usual recommended dosage is two inhalations (168 mcg) given twice daily. In patients with severe asthma, it is advisable to start with 6 to 8 inhalations a day and adjust the dosage downward according to the response of the patient. The maximal daily intake should not exceed 10 inhalations, 840 mcg (0.84 mg), in adults.

Children 6 to 12 Years of Age: The usual recommended dosage is two inhalations (168 mcg) given twice daily. The maximal daily intake should not exceed 5 inhalations, 420 mcg (0.42 mg), in children 6 to 12 years of age. Insufficient clinical data exist with respect to the administration of VANCERIL 84 mcg DOUBLE STRENGTH Inhalation Aerosol in children below the age of 6.

Rinsing the mouth after inhalation is advised.

Different considerations must be given to the following groups of patients in order to obtain the full therapeutic benefit of VANCERIL 84 mcg DOUBLE STRENGTH Inhalation Aerosol.

Patients Not Receiving Systemic Corticosteroids Patients who require maintenance therapy of their asthma may benefit from treatment with VANCERIL 84 mcg DOUBLE STRENGTH Inhalation Aerosol at the doses recommended above. In patients who respond to VANCERIL 84 mcg DOUBLE STRENGTH Inhalation Aerosol, improvement in pulmonary function is usually apparent within 1 to 4 weeks after the start of therapy. Once the desired effect is achieved, consideration should be given to tapering to the lowest effective dose.

Patients Maintained on Systemic Corticosteroids Clinical studies have shown that beclomethasone dipropionate may be effective in the management of asthmatics dependent or maintained on systemic corticosteroids and may permit replacement or significant reduction in the dosage of systemic corticosteroids.

The patient's asthma should be reasonably stable before treatment with VANCERIL 84 mcg DOUBLE STRENGTH Inhalation Aerosol is started. Initially, VANCERIL 84 mcg DOUBLE STRENGTH Inhalation Aerosol should be used concurrently with the patient's usual maintenance dose of systemic corticosteroid. After approximately 1 week, gradual withdrawal of the systemic corticosteroid is started by

reducing the daily or alternate daily dose. Reductions may be made after an interval of 1 or 2 weeks, depending on the response of the patient. A slow rate of withdrawal is strongly recommended. Generally, these decrements should not exceed 2.5 mg of prednisone or its equivalent. During withdrawal, some patients may experience symptoms of systemic corticosteroid withdrawal, eg, joint and/or muscular pain, lassitude and depression, despite maintenance or even improvement in pulmonary function. Such patients should be encouraged to continue with the inhaler but should be monitored for objective signs of adrenal insufficiency. If evidence of adrenal insufficiency occurs, the systemic corticosteroid doses should be increased temporarily and thereafter withdrawal should continue more slowly.

During periods of stress or a severe asthma attack, transfer patients may require supplementary treatment with systemic corticosteroids.

Directions for Use: Illustrated Patient's Instructions for Use accompany each package of VANCERIL 84 mcg DOUBLE STRENGTH Inhalation Aerosol.

CONTENTS UNDER PRESSURE. Do not puncture. Do not use or store near heat or open flame. Exposure to temperatures above 120°F may cause bursting. Never throw container into fire or incinerator. Keep out of reach of children.

HOW SUPPLIED

VANCERIL 84 mcg DOUBLE STRENGTH Inhalation Aerosol 12.2 g canisters containing 120 metered inhalations, in boxes of one (NDC 0085-1112-01), and 5.4 g canisters containing 40 metered inhalations for Institutional Use only, in boxes of one (NDC 0085-1112-02). Each canister is supplied with a dark-pink plastic actuator with a maroon cap and Patient's Instructions for Use. Each actuation delivers an amount of beclomethasone dipropionate-trichloromonofluoromethane clathrate equivalent to 84 mcg of beclomethasone dipropionate from the mouthpiece and 100 mcg of beclomethasone dipropionate from the valve.

The VANCERIL 84 mcg DOUBLE STRENGTH Inhalation Aerosol canister should only be used with the VANCERIL 84 mcg DOUBLE STRENGTH Inhalation Aerosol mouthpiece and this mouthpiece should not be used with any other inhalation drug product.

The correct amount of medication in each inhalation cannot be assured after 120 actuations from the 12.2 g canister or 40 actuations from the 5.4 g canister even though the canister is not completely empty. The canister should be discarded when the labeled number of actuations have been used.

Store at 15°–30°C (59°–86°F). Protect from moisture and unusual temperature fluctuations. Failure to use the product within this temperature range may result in improper dosing. For optimal results, the canister should be at room temperature before use. Shake well before using. Once canister is removed from the moisture protective package the product must be used within 6 months.

Note: The indented statement below is required by the Federal government's Clean Air Act for all products containing or manufactured with chlorofluorocarbons (CFCs).

> **WARNING:** Contains dichlorodifluoromethane (CFC-12) and trichloromonofluoromethane (CFC-11), substances which harm public health and the environment by destroying ozone in the upper atmosphere.

A notice similar to the above **WARNING** has been placed in the "Patient's Instructions for Use" portion of this package insert pursuant to Environmental Protection Agency (EPA) regulations. The patient's warning states that the patient should consult his or her physician if there are questions about alternatives.

Schering/Key
Kenilworth, NJ 07033 USA
Copyright © 1996, Schering Corporation. All rights reserved.
12/96   18691426T

IDENTIFICATION PROBLEM?
Turn to the **Product Identification Guide,**
where you'll find more than
1600 products pictured in actual
size and full color.

Schwarz Pharma, Inc.
5600 W. COUNTY LINE ROAD
P.O. BOX 2038
MILWAUKEE, WI 53201

For Medical Information Contact:
Schwarz Pharma, Inc.
Drug Safety and Information
(414) 238-9994
(800) 558-5114

CALCIFEROL™ Products
[kal-si 'fur-ol]

CALCIFEROL™ Drops   OTC
(ergocalciferol oral solution USP)
8,000 USP Units/mL

CALCIFEROL™ Tablets   ℞
(ergocalciferol tablets USP)
50,000 USP Units

CALCIFEROL™ in Oil Injection   ℞
(ergocalciferol)
500,000 Units/mL

CODICLEAR® DH SYRUP   Ⓒ ℞
[kō 'dī-klēr "]

DESCRIPTION

A clear, colorless, sweet-tasting syrup for oral administration, which is alcohol-free, dye-free and sugar-free. Contains no parabens.

Each teaspoonful (5 mL) contains:
Hydrocodone* Bitartrate .... 5 mg
(*Warning—May be habit forming)
Guaifenesin .... 100 mg
This product contains ingredients of the following therapeutic classes: antitussive and expectorant.

CAUTION

Federal law prohibits dispensing without prescription.

INACTIVE INGREDIENTS

Benzoic Acid, Citric Acid, Flavors, Glycerin, Polyethylene Glycol, Povidone, Propylene Glycol, Purified Water, Saccharin Sodium, Sodium Citrate and Sorbitol.

CLINICAL PHARMACOLOGY

Hydrocodone bitartrate is a potent antitussive which causes suppression of the cough reflex by a direct action on the cough center. Hydrocodone is approximately three times as potent as codeine on a weight basis, and has a higher addiction potential. Guaifenesin is used as an expectorant. It is thought to increase mucous flow in the lung by stimulation of gastric mucosal reflexes.

INDICATIONS

For the temporary relief of dry, non-productive cough associated with upper and lower respiratory tract congestion.

CONTRAINDICATIONS

Hypersensitivity to hydrocodone or guaifenesin. Hydrocodone is contraindicated in the presence of increased intracranial pressure and whenever ventilatory function is depressed.

WARNINGS

Hydrocodone can produce drug dependence and therefore has the potential for being abused. CODICLEAR® DH should be prescribed and administered with the degree of caution appropriate for this type product.

PRECAUTIONS

General: The hydrocodone in this product may exhibit additive effects with other CNS depressants, including alcohol. Respiratory depression can be a real hazard so caution should be used, especially in patients with chronic obstructive pulmonary disease.

Information for Patients: The hydrocodone may cause drowsiness and ambulatory patients who operate machinery or motor vehicles should be cautioned accordingly.

Drug Interactions: Patients receiving other narcotic analgesics, general anesthetics, phenothiazines, other tranquilizers, sedative hypnotics or other CNS depressants (including alcohol) concomitantly with hydrocodone may exhibit an additive CNS depression. When such combined therapy is contemplated the dose of one or both agents should be reduced. (See WARNINGS.)

Laboratory Interactions: The metabolite of guaifenesin has been found to produce an apparent increase in urinary 5-hydroxyindoleacetic acid, and guaifenesin therefore may interfere with the interpretation of this test for the diagno-

sis of carcinoid syndrome. Guaifenesin administration should be discontinued 24 hours prior to the collection of urine specimens for the determination of 5-hydroxyindoleacetic acid.

Usage in Pregnancy: Pregnancy Category C. Hydrocodone has been shown to be teratogenic in hamsters when given in doses 700 times the human dose. There are no adequate and well-controlled studies in pregnant women. CODICLEAR® DH Syrup should be used during pregnancy only if the potential benefit justifies the potential risk to the fetus.

Pediatric Use: Safety and effectiveness in pediatric patients under 6 years of age have not been established.

ADVERSE REACTIONS

Adverse reactions include drowsiness, lassitude, nausea, giddiness, constipation, respiratory depression and addiction.

DRUG ABUSE AND DEPENDENCE

This product is a Schedule III Controlled Sustance. Because of the hydrocodone content, some abuse might be expected. Psychic dependence, physical dependence and tolerance may develop upon repeated administration. It should be prescribed and administered with the degree of caution appropriate for this type product.

OVERDOSAGE

Symptoms of overdosage include respiratory depression, extreme somnolence progressing to stupor or coma, skeletal muscle flaccidity, cold and clammy skin and other symptoms common with narcotic overdosage.

Primary treatment consists of insuring adequate respiration through provision of a patent airway and the institution of assisted or controlled ventilation. Naloxone hydrochloride should be administered in small intravenous doses (consult specific product labeling before use). In addition, oxygen, intravenous fluids, vasopressors and other supportive measures should be employed as indicated. Gastric emptying may be useful in removing unabsorbed drug. Activated charcoal may also be of benefit.

DOSAGE AND ADMINISTRATION

Usual Adult Dose—One teaspoonful (5 mL) after meals and at bedtime, not less than 4 hours apart (not to exceed 6 teaspoonsful in a 24 hour period.) Treatment should be initiated with one teaspoonful and subsequent doses, up to a maximum single dose of 3 teaspoonsful, adjusted if required.

Usual Pediatric Dose—Over 12 years: Initial dose 1 teaspoonful; maximum single dose, 2 teaspoonsful. 6 to 12 years: Initial dose $1/2$ teaspoonful: maximum single dose, 1 teaspoonful.

HOW SUPPLIED

Bottles of 4 fl oz	NDC 0131-5134-64
Bottles of one pint	NDC 0131-5134-70

DISPENSE IN A TIGHT CONTAINER AS DEFINED IN THE USP/NF, WITH A CHILD-RESISTANT CLOSURE. STORE AT CONTROLLED ROOM TEMPERATURE AS DEFINED IN THE USP/NF.

PC3180A   Rev. 10/97

CODIMAL® DH SYRUP   Ⓒ Ⅲ ℞
[kō 'di-mahl "]

DESCRIPTION

A red colored, sweet-tasting syrup for oral administration. Each teaspoonful (5 mL) contains:

Hydrocodone Bitartrate .... 1.66 mg
  (Warning—May be habit forming)
Phenylephrine Hydrochloride .... 5 mg
Pyrilamine Maleate .... 8.33 mg
This product contains ingredients of the following therapeutic classes: antitussive, nasal decongestant and antihistamine.

Inactive Ingredients: Benzoic Acid, Citric Acid Anhydrous, F.D.&C. Red #40, Flavors, Menthol, Propylene Glycol, Sodium Citrate, Sucrose and Thymol.

CLINICAL PHARMACOLOGY

Hydrocodone bitartrate is a potent antitussive which causes suppression of the cough reflex by a direct action on the cough center. Hydrocodone is approximately three times as potent as codeine on a weight basis, and has a higher addiction potential also. Phenylephrine hydrochloride is a sympathomimetic which acts predominantly on alpha receptors and has little action on beta receptors. It therefore functions as an oral nasal decongestant with minimal CNS stimulation. Pyrilamine maleate is an antihistamine used in suppressing symptoms of allergic rhinitis. However, it is more prone to cause drowsiness than some other antihistamines.

INDICATIONS

Temporary relief of cough, nasal congestion, and other symptoms associated with colds, or seasonal or perennial allergic vasomotor rhinitis (hay fever).

CONTRAINDICATIONS

Patients with severe hypertension, severe coronary artery disease, in patients on MAO inhibitor therapy and in nursing mothers. Also contraindicated in patients, with narrow-angle glaucoma, urinary retention, peptic ulcer or in patients with a hypersensitivity to any of its ingredients.

WARNINGS

Considerable caution should be exercised in patients with hypertension, diabetes mellitus, ischemic heart disease, hyperthyroidism, increased intraocular pressure and prostatic hypertrophy. The elderly (60 years or older) are more likely to exhibit adverse reactions. Antihistamines may cause excitability, especially in children. At dosages higher than the recommended dose, nervousness, dizziness or sleeplessness, may occur. Hydrocodone can produce drug dependence and therefore has the potential for being abused.

PRECAUTIONS

General: Caution should be exercised in patients with high blood pressure, heart disease, diabetes or thyroid disease. The antihistamines and hydrocodone in this product may exhibit additive effects with other CNS depressants, including alcohol.

Information for Patients: The hydrocodone and antihistamines may cause drowsiness and ambulatory patients who operate machinery or motor vehicles should be cautioned accordingly.

Drug Interactions: MAO inhibitors and beta adrenergic blockers may increase the effects of sympathomimetics. Sympathomimetics may reduce the antihypertensive effects of methyldopa, mecamylamine, reserpine and veratrum alkaloids. Concomitant use of hydrocodone and antihistamines with alcohol and other CNS depressants may have an additive effect.

Pregnancy: Pregnancy Category C: Hydrocodone has been shown to be teratogenic in hamsters when given doses 700 times the human dose. There are no adequate and well-controlled studies in pregnant women. Codimal® DH should be used during pregnancy only if the potential benefit justifies the potential risk to the fetus.

ADVERSE REACTIONS

Adverse reactions include drowsiness, lassitude, nausea, giddiness, dryness of mouth, blurred vision, cardiac palpitations, flushing, increased irritability or excitement (especially in pediatric patients).

DRUG ABUSE AND DEPENDENCE

This product is a Schedule III controlled substance. Because of the hydrocodone content, some abuse may be expected. Psychic dependence, physical dependence, and tolerance may develop upon repeated administration. It should be prescribed and administered with the degree of caution appropriate for this type product.

DOSAGE AND ADMINISTRATION

Adults and pediatric patients 12 years of age and older — 1 to 2 teaspoonfuls every 4 hours. Pediatric patients, 6 to 12 years of age — 1 teaspoonful every 4 hours. Pediatric patients, 2 to 6 years of age — $1/2$ teaspoonful every 4 hours. Under 2 years: Narcotic antitussives are not recommended for use in pediatric patients under 2 years of age. Pediatric patients under 2 years may be more susceptible to the respiratory depressant effects of narcotics, including respiratory arrest, coma, and death. However, dosages based on hydrocodone, 0.3 mg/kg/24 hours divided into four equal doses have been suggested.

CAUTION: Federal law prohibits dispensing without prescription.

HOW SUPPLIED

A red, pleasantly flavored, sweet-tasting syrup available in bottles of:

4 fl oz	NDC 0131-5129-64
1 pint	NDC 0131-5129-70
1 gallon	NDC 0131-5129-72

DISPENSE IN A TIGHT CONTAINER AS DEFINED IN USP/NF WITH A CHILD-RESISTANT CLOSURE. STORE AT CONTROLLED ROOM TEMPERATURE 15°–30°C (59°–86°F).

PC3285   Rev. 10/97

CODIMAL® DM SYRUP   OTC
[kō ' di-mahl "]

DESCRIPTION

Each teaspoonful (5 mL) of CODIMAL® DM contains: Dextromethorphan hydrobromide 10 mg.; Phenylephrine hydrochloride 5 mg; Pyrilamine maleate 8.33 mg.

INACTIVE INGREDIENTS: Benzoic Acid, Citric Acid, Flavors, Menthol, Propylene Glycol, Saccharin Sodium, Sodium Citrate, Sorbitol and Water. Alcohol-Free, Dye-Free, Sugar-Free.

HOW SUPPLIED

Codimal® DM (Clear Syrup)
4 oz-NDC # 0131-5131-64
Pint-NDC# 0131-5131-70
Gallon-NDC# 0131-5131-72
For full information see product labeling.

CODIMAL® PH SYRUP   Ⓒ ℞
[kō ' di-mahl "]

DESCRIPTION

Each teaspoonful (5 mL) of CODIMAL® PH contains: Codeine Phosphate 10 mg (Warning-May be habit forming); Phenylephrine Hydrochloride 5 mg.; Pyrilamine Maleate 8.33 mg.

INACTIVE INGREDIENTS: Benzoic Acid, Citric Acid, FD&C Red #40, Flavors, Propylene Glycol, Sodium Citrate and Sucrose. Alcohol-Free.

HOW SUPPLIED

Codimal® PH (Red Syrup)
4 oz-NDC# 0131-5038-64
Pint-NDC# 0131-5038-70
Gallon-NDC# 0131-5038-72

COLYTE® and COLYTE®-FLAVORED   ℞
(PEG-3350 & ELECTROLYTES) For Oral Solution
For Gastrointestinal Lavage

DESCRIPTION

COLYTE® and COLYTE®-FLAVORED are colon lavage preparations provided as water-soluble components for solution. In solution each COLYTE® and COLYTE®-FLAVORED preparation delivers the following, in grams per liter.

Polyethylene glycol 3350	60.00
Sodium chloride	1.46
Potassium chloride	0.745
Sodium bicarbonate	1.68
Sodium sulfate	5.68
Flavor ingredients (COLYTE®-FLAVORED)	0.463

When dissolved in sufficient water to make 4 liters, the final solution contains 125 mEq/L sodium, 10 mEq/L potassium, 20 mEq/L bicarbonate, 80 mEq/L sulfate, 35 mEq/L chloride and 18 mEq/L polyethylene glycol 3350. The reconstituted solution is isosmotic and has a mildly salty taste. COLYTE® and COLYTE®-FLAVORED are administered orally or via nasogastric tube.

CLINICAL PHARMACOLOGY

COLYTE® and COLYTE®-FLAVORED cleanse the bowel by induction of diarrhea. The osmotic activity of Polyethylene Glycol 3350, in combination with the electrolyte concentration, results in virtually no net absorption or excretion of ions or water. Accordingly, large volumes may be administered without significant changes in fluid and electrolyte balance.

INDICATIONS AND USAGE

COLYTE® and COLYTE®-FLAVORED are indicated for bowel cleansing prior to colonoscopy or barium enema X-ray examination.

CONTRAINDICATIONS

COLYTE® and COLYTE®-FLAVORED are contraindicated in patients with ileus, gastric retention, gastrointestinal obstruction, bowel perforation, toxic colitis and toxic megacolon.

WARNINGS

No additional ingredients (e.g., flavorings) should be added to the solution. COLYTE® and COLYTE®-FLAVORED should be used with caution in patients with severe ulcerative colitis.

PRECAUTIONS

General: Patients with impaired gag reflex, unconscious or semiconscious patients and patients prone to regurgitation or aspiration should be observed during the administration of COLYTE® or COLYTE®-FLAVORED, especially if it is administered via nasogastric tube.

If gastrointestinal obstruction or perforation is suspected appropriate studies should be performed to rule out these conditions before administration of COLYTE® or COLYTE®-FLAVORED.

INFORMATION FOR PATIENTS

COLYTE® and COLYTE®-FLAVORED produce a watery stool which cleanses the bowel prior to examination.

For best results, no solid food should be ingested during the 3 to 4 hour period prior to the initiation of COLYTE® or

Continued on next page

Colyte/Colyte-Flavored—Cont.

COLYTE®-FLAVORED administration. In no case should solid foods be eaten within 2 hours of drinking COLYTE® or COLYTE®-FLAVORED.
The rate of administration is 240 ml (8 fl. oz.) every 10 minutes. Rapid drinking of each portion is preferred rather than drinking small amounts continuously. The first bowel movement should occur approximately one hour after the start of COLYTE® or COLYTE®-FLAVORED administration.
Administration of COLYTE® or COLYTE®-FLAVORED should be continued until the watery stool is clear and free of solid matter. This normally requires the consumption of approximately 3–4 liters (3–4 quarts), although more or less may be required in some patients. The unused portion should be discarded.

DRUG INTERACTIONS

Oral medication administered within one hour of the start of administration of COLYTE® or COLYTE®-FLAVORED may be flushed from the gastrointestinal tract and not absorbed.

CARCINOGENESIS, MUTAGENESIS, IMPAIRMENT OF FERTILITY

Studies to evaluate carcinogenic or mutagenic potential or potential to adversely affect male or female fertility have not been performed.

PREGNANCY

Category C. Animal reproduction studies have not been conducted with COLYTE® (PEG-3350 & ELECTROLYTES For Oral Solution) or COLYTE®-FLAVORED, and it is not known whether COLYTE® or COLYTE®-FLAVORED can affect reproductive capacity or harm the fetus when administered to a pregnant patient. COLYTE® or COLYTE®-FLAVORED should be given to a pregnant patient only if clearly needed.

PEDIATRIC USE

Safety and effectiveness in pediatric patients have not been established.

ADVERSE REACTIONS

Nausea, abdominal fullness and bloating are the most frequent adverse reactions, occurring in up to 50% of patients. Abdominal cramps, vomiting and anal irritation occur less frequently. These adverse reactions are transient. Isolated cases of urticaria, rhinorrhea and dermatitis have been reported which may represent allergic reactions.

DOSAGE AND ADMINISTRATION

COLYTE® or COLYTE®-FLAVORED can be administered orally or by nasogastric tube. Patients should fast at least 3 hours prior to administration. A one hour waiting period after the appearance of clear liquid stool should be allowed prior to examination to complete bowel evacuation. No foods except clear liquids should be permitted prior to examination after COLYTE® or COLYTE®-FLAVORED administration.

ORAL

The recommended adult oral dose is 240 ml (8 fl. oz.) every 10 minutes (see INFORMATION FOR PATIENTS). Lavage is complete when fecal discharge is clear. Lavage is usually complete after the ingestion of 3–4 liters.

NASOGASTRIC TUBE

COLYTE® or COLYTE®-FLAVORED is administered at a rate of 20–30 ml per minute (1.2–1.8 L/hour).

PREPARATION OF COLYTE® or COLYTE®-FLAVORED SOLUTION:

4 Liter: Add tap water to FILL line. Replace cap tightly and mix or shake well until all ingredients have dissolved. (No additional ingredients, e.g., flavorings, should be added to the solution.)
One Gallon: The preparation is made by dissolving the contents of the bottle in a food-grade container, in a sufficient quantity of water to produce the final volume according to package directions. (No additional ingredients, e.g., flavorings, should be added to the solution.) Mix well.

HOW SUPPLIED

COLYTE® and COLYTE®-FLAVORED are supplied in 4 liter (NDC 0091-4401-23 and NDC 0091-4403-05, respectively) and 18 oz. (NDC 0091-4401-49 and NDC 0091-4403-13, respectively) bottles in powdered form, for oral administration as a solution. Each contains the following:

4 liter, (NDC 0091-4401-23 and NDC 0091-4403-05): polyethylene glycol 3350 240 g, sodium chloride 5.84 g, potassium chloride 2.98 g, sodium bicarbonate 6.72 g, sodium sulfate (anhydrous) 22.72 g, flavor ingredients (COLYTE®-FLAVORED only) 1.85 g, in a bottle.

18 oz., (NDC 0091-4401-49 and NDC 0091-4403-13): polyethylene glycol 3350 227.10 g, sodium chloride 5.53 g, potassium chloride 2.82 g, sodium bicarbonate 6.36 g, sodium sulfate (anhydrous) 21.50 g, flavor ingredients (COLYTE®-FLAVORED only) 1.75 g, in a bottle.

Store powder at controlled room temperature 15°–30°C (59°–86°F).
CAUTION: Federal law prohibits dispensing without prescription.
KEEP RECONSTITUTED SOLUTION REFRIGERATED. USE WITHIN 48 HOURS. DISCARD UNUSED PORTION.
PD2198A Rev. 8/96
Shown in Product Identification Guide, pages 336 and 337

CORTIFOAM® ℞
(hydrocortisone acetate) 10%
Rectal Foam

DESCRIPTION

CORTIFOAM® (hydrocortisone acetate) 10% Rectal Foam contains hydrocortisone acetate 10% in a base containing propylene glycol, emulsifying wax, polyoxyethylene-10-stearyl ether, cetyl alcohol, methylparaben, propylparaben, trolamine, purified water and inert propellants: isobutane and propane.
Each application delivers approximately 900 mg of foam containing 80 mg of hydrocortisone (90 mg of hydrocortisone acetate).
Molecular weight: Hydrocortisone acetate 404.51
Solubility of hydrocortisone acetate in water: 1 mg/100 mL
Chemical name: Pregn-4-ene-3,20-dione, 21-(acetyloxy)-11, 17-dihydroxy-, (11β)-.

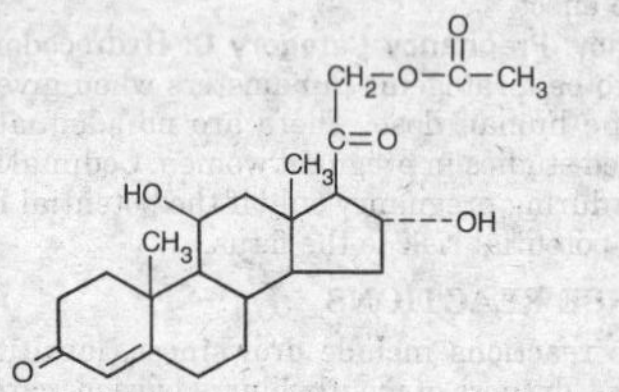

CLINICAL PHARMACOLOGY

CORTIFOAM provides effective topical administration of an anti-inflammatory corticosteroid as adjunctive therapy of ulcerative proctitis.

INDICATIONS AND USAGE

CORTIFOAM is indicated as adjunctive therapy in the topical treatment of ulcerative proctitis of the distal portion of the rectum in patients who cannot retain hydrocortisone or other corticosteroid enemas. Direct observations of methylene blue-containing foam have shown staining about 10 centimeters into the rectum.

CONTRAINDICATIONS

Local contraindications to the use of intrarectal steroids include obstruction, abscess, perforation, peritonitis, fresh intestinal anastomoses, extensive fistulas and sinus tracts. Tuberculosis (active, latent or questionably healed), ocular herpes simplex and acute psychosis are usually considered absolute contraindications to the use of corticosteroids. Relative contraindications include active peptic ulcer, acute glomerulonephritis, myasthenia gravis, osteoporosis, diverticulitis, thrombophlebitis, psychic disturbances, pregnancy, diabetes, hyperthyroidism, acute coronary disease, hypertension, limited cardiac reserve, and local or systemic infections, including fungal or exanthematous diseases. Where these conditions exist, the expected benefits from steroid therapy must be weighed against the risks involved in its use. Pregnancy is a relative contraindication to corticosteroids, particularly during third trimester. If corticosteroids must be administered in pregnancy, watch newborn infant closely for signs of hypoadrenalism, and administer appropriate therapy if needed.

WARNINGS

Do not insert any part of the aerosol container directly into the anus. Contents of the container are under pressure. Do not burn or puncture the aerosol container. Store at room temperature and not over 120° F. Because CORTIFOAM is not expelled, systemic hydrocortisone absorption may be greater from CORTIFOAM than from corticosteroid enema formulations. If there is not evidence of clinical or proctologic improvement within two or three weeks after starting CORTIFOAM therapy, or if the patient's condition worsens, discontinue the drug.
Persons who are on drugs which suppress the immune system are more susceptible to infections than healthy individuals. Chickenpox and measles, for example, can have a more serious or even fatal course in non-immune pediatric patients or adults on corticosteroids. In such pediatric patients or adults who have not had these diseases, particular care should be taken to avoid exposure. How the dose, route and duration of corticosteroid administration affects the risk of developing a disseminated infection is not known. The contribution of the underlying disease and/or prior corticosteroid treatment to the risk is also not known. If exposed to chickenpox, prophylaxis with varicella zoster immune globulin (VZIG) may be indicated. If exposed to measles, prophylaxis with pooled intramuscular immunoglobulin (IG) may be indicated. (See the respective package inserts for complete VZIG and IG prescribing information). If chickenpox develops, treatment with antiviral agents may be considered.

PRECAUTIONS

General
Steroid therapy should be administered with caution in patients with severe ulcerative disease because these patients are predisposed to perforation of the bowel wall. Where surgery is imminent, it is hazardous to wait more than a few days for a satisfactory response to medical treatment. General precautions common to all corticosteroid therapy should be observed during treatment with CORTIFOAM. These include gradual withdrawal of therapy to allow for possible adrenal insufficiency and awareness to possible growth suppression in pediatric patients. Patients should be kept under close observation, for, as with all drugs, rare individuals may react unfavorably under certain conditions. If severe reactions or idiosyncrasies occur, steroids should be discontinued immediately and appropriate measures instituted. Do not employ in immediate or early postoperative period following ileorectostomy.
Information for patients
Persons who are on immunosuppressant doses of corticosteroids should be warned to avoid exposure to chickenpox or measles. Patients should also be advised that if they are exposed, medical advice should be sought without delay.
Pediatric Use
Safety and effectiveness in pediatric patients have not been established. (Please see **WARNINGS** and **ADVERSE REACTIONS** for additional information.)

ADVERSE REACTIONS

Corticosteroid therapy may produce side effects which include moon face, fluid retention, excessive appetite and weight gain, abnormal fat deposits, mental symptoms, hypertrichosis, acne, ecchymosis, increased sweating, pigmentation, dry scaly skin, thinning scalp hair, thrombophlebitis, decreased resistance to infection, negative nitrogen balance with delayed bone and wound healing, menstrual disorders, neuropathy, peptic ulcer, decreased glucose tolerance, hypopotassemia, adrenal insufficiency, necrotizing angiitis, hypertension, pancreatitis and increased intraocular pressure. In pediatric patients, suppression of growth may occur. Increased intracranial pressure may occur and possibly account for headache, insomnia and fatigue. Subcapsular cataracts may result from prolonged usage. Long-term use of all corticosteroids results in catabolic effects characterized by negative protein and calcium balance. Osteoporosis, spontaneous fractures and aseptic necrosis of the hip and humerus may occur as part of this catabolic phenomenon. Where hypopotassemia and other symptoms associated with fluid and electrolyte imbalance call for potassium supplementation and salt poor or salt-free diets, these may be instituted and are compatible with diet requirements for ulcerative proctitis.

DOSAGE AND ADMINISTRATION

Usual dose is one applicatorful once or twice daily for two or three weeks, and every second day thereafter, administered rectally. Directions for use, below and on the carton, describe how to use the aerosol container and applicator. Satisfactory response usually occurs within five to seven days marked by a decrease in symptoms. Symptomatic improvement in ulcerative proctitis should not be used as the sole criterion for evaluating efficacy. Sigmoidoscopy is also recommended to judge dosage adjustment, duration of therapy and rate of improvement.

Directions For Use
1) Shake foam container vigorously for 5–10 seconds before each use. **Do not remove container cap during use of the product. 2)** Hold container upright on a level surface and gently place the tip of the applicator onto the nose of the container cap. CONTAINER MUST BE HELD UPRIGHT TO OBTAIN PROPER FLOW OF MEDICATION. **3)** Gently withdraw applicator plunger past the fill line on the applicator barrel. **4)** To fill applicator barrel, press down slowly on cap flanges and release, pause, and allow foam to enter and expand in applicator barrel. Repeat until foam in the applicator reaches fill line. Remove applicator from container cap. Allow some foam to remain on the applicator tip. **5)** Hold applicator firmly by barrel, making sure thumb and middle finger are positioned securely underneath and resting against barrel wings. Place index finger over the plunger. Gently insert tip into anus. Once in place, push plunger to expel foam, then withdraw applicator. **CAUTION:** Do not insert any part of the aerosol container directly into the anus. Apply to anus only with enclosed applicator. **6)** After each use, applicator parts should be pulled apart for

thorough cleaning with warm water. The container cap and underlying tip should also be pulled apart and rinsed to help prevent build-up of foam and possible blockage.

HOW SUPPLIED

CORTIFOAM is supplied in an aerosol container with a special rectal applicator. Each applicator delivers approximately 900 mg of foam containing approximately 80 mg of hydrocortisone as 90 mg of hydrocortisone acetate. When used correctly, the aerosol container will deliver a minimum of 14 applications.

NDC 0091-0695-20   15 g

Store upright at controlled room temperature 15°–30°C (59°–86°F).

DO NOT REFRIGERATE.

CAUTION: Federal law prohibits dispensing without prescription.

PC2080   Rev. 3/96

Shown in Product Identification Guide, page 337

DEPONIT®   ℞

[dĕp 'ō-nĭt]

(nitroglycerin transdermal delivery system)

DESCRIPTION

Nitroglycerin is 1,2,3-propanetriol trinitrate, an organic nitrate whose structural formula is:

$$
\begin{array}{c}
H_2CONO_2 \\
| \\
HCONO_2 \\
| \\
H_2CONO_2
\end{array}
$$

and whose molecular weight is 227.09. The organic nitrates are vasodilators, active on both arteries and veins.

The Deponit transdermal system is a flat unit designed to provide continuous controlled release of nitroglycerin through intact skin. The rate of release of nitroglycerin is linearly dependent upon the area of the applied system; each cm^2 of applied system delivers approximately 0.013 mg of nitroglycerin per hour. Thus, the 16 cm^2 and 32 cm^2 systems deliver approximately 0.2 and 0.4 mg of nitroglycerin per hour, respectively.

The remainder of the nitroglycerin in each system serves as a reservoir and is not delivered in normal use. After 12 hours, for example, each system has delivered 15% of its original content of nitroglycerin.

Deponit contains nitroglycerin in a matrix composed of lactose, plasticizer, medical adhesive, polyisobutylene and aluminized plastic for controlled release of the active agent through the skin into the systemic circulation. The 16 cm^2 and 32 cm^2 systems contain 16 mg and 32 mg of nitroglycerin, respectively.

The Deponit system is approximately 0.3 mm thick, insoluble in water, and, as illustrated below, consists of two main elements:

1. A flexible, flesh-colored waterproof covering foil.
2. A multilayered adhesive film that constitutes simultaneously the drug reservoir and the release-control system.

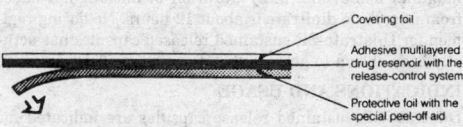

The system is protected by an aluminum foil which has a patented S-shaped opening to facilitate its removal prior to use of the system. Prior to use, the protective foil is removed from the adhesive surface.

CLINICAL PHARMACOLOGY

The principal pharmacological action of nitroglycerin is relaxation of vascular smooth muscle and consequent dilatation of peripheral arteries and veins, especially the latter. Dilatation of the veins promotes peripheral pooling of blood and decreases venous return to the heart, thereby reducing left ventricular end-diastolic pressure and pulmonary capillary wedge pressure (preload). Arteriolar relaxation reduces systemic vascular resistance, systolic arterial pressure, and mean arterial pressure (afterload). Dilatation of the coronary arteries also occurs. The relative importance of preload reduction, afterload reduction and coronary dilatation remains undefined.

Dosing regimens for most chronically used drugs are designed to provide plasma concentrations that are continuously greater than a minimally effective concentration. This strategy is inappropriate for organic nitrates. Several well-controlled clinical trials have used exercise testing to assess the anti-anginal efficacy of continuously-delivered nitrates. In the large majority of these trials, active agents were in-

Nitroglycerin Transdermal Rated Release in vivo	Total Nitroglycerin in System	System Size	Carton Size	NDC
0.2 mg/hr	16 mg	16 cm^2	30	0091-4195-01
			30*	0091-4195-31
			100*	0091-4195-11
0.4 mg/hr	32 mg	32 cm^2	30	0091-4196-01
			30*	0091-4196-31
			100*	0091-4196-11

---

*Institutional Package

distinguishable from placebo after 24 hours (or less) of continuous therapy. Attempts to overcome nitrate tolerance by dose escalation, even in doses far in excess of those used acutely, have consistently failed. Only after nitrates have been absent from the body for several hours has their antianginal efficacy been restored.

Pharmacokinetics:

The volume of distribution of nitroglycerin is about 3 L/kg, and nitroglycerin is cleared from this volume at extremely rapid rates, with a resulting serum half-life of about 3 minutes. The observed clearance rates (close to 1 L/kg/min) greatly exceed hepatic blood flow; known sites of extrahepatic metabolism include red blood cells and vascular walls. The first products in the metabolism of nitroglycerin are inorganic nitrate and the 1,2- and 1,3-dinitroglycerols. The dinitrates are less effective vasodilators than nitroglycerin, but they are longer-lived in the serum, and their net contribution to the overall effect of chronic nitroglycerin regimens is not known. The dinitrates are further metabolized to (non-vasoactive) mononitrates and, ultimately, to glycerol and carbon dioxide.

To avoid development of tolerance to nitroglycerin, drug-free intervals of 10–12 hours are known to be sufficient; shorter intervals have not been well studied. In one well-controlled clinical trial, subjects receiving nitroglycerin appeared to exhibit a rebound or withdrawal effect, so that their exercise tolerance at the end of the daily drug-free interval was *less* than that exhibited by the parallel group receiving placebo.

In healthy volunteers, steady-state plasma concentrations of nitroglycerin are reached by about two hours after application of a patch and are maintained for the duration of wearing the system (observations have been limited to 24 hours). Upon removal of the patch, the plasma concentration declines with a half-life of about an hour.

Clinical trials:

Regimens in which nitroglycerin patches were worn for 12 hours daily have been studied in well-controlled trials up to 4 weeks in duration. Starting about 2 hours after application and continuing until 10–12 hours after application, patches that deliver at least 0.4 mg of nitroglycerin per hour have consistently demonstrated greater anti-anginal activity than placebo. Lower-dose patches have not been as well studied, but in one large, well-controlled trial in which higher-dose patches were also studied, patches delivering 0.2 mg/hr had significantly *less* anti-anginal activity than placebo.

It is reasonable to believe that the rate of nitroglycerin absorption from patches may vary with the site of application, but this relationship has not been adequately studied. The onset of action of transdermal nitroglycerin is not sufficiently rapid for this product to be useful in aborting an acute anginal episode.

INDICATIONS AND USAGE

Transdermal nitroglycerin is indicated for the prevention of angina pectoris due to coronary artery disease. The onset of action of transdermal nitroglycerin is not sufficiently rapid for this product to be useful in aborting an acute attack.

CONTRAINDICATIONS

Allergic reactions to organic nitrates are extremely rare, but they do occur. Nitroglycerin is contraindicated in patients who are allergic to it. Allergy to the adhesives used in nitroglycerin patches has also been reported, and it similarly constitutes a contraindication to the use of this product.

WARNINGS

The benefits of transdermal nitroglycerin in patients with acute myocardial infarction or congestive heart failure have not been established. If one elects to use nitroglycerin in these conditions, careful clinical or hemodynamic monitoring must be used to avoid the hazards of hypotension and tachycardia.

A cardioverter/defibrillator should not be discharged through a paddle electrode that overlies a Deponit patch. The arcing that may be seen in this situation is harmless in itself, but it may be associated with local current concentration that can cause damage to the paddles and burns to the patient.

PRECAUTIONS

General:

Severe hypotension, particularly with upright posture, may occur with even small doses of nitroglycerin. This drug

should therefore be used with caution in patients who may be volume depleted or who, for whatever reason, are already hypotensive. Hypotension induced by nitroglycerin may be accompanied by paradoxical bradycardia and increased angina pectoris.

Nitrate therapy may aggravate the angina caused by hypertrophic cardiomyopathy.

As tolerance to other forms of nitroglycerin develops, the effect of sublingual nitroglycerin on exercise tolerance, although still observable, is somewhat blunted.

In industrial workers who have had long-term exposure to unknown (presumably high) doses of organic nitrates, tolerance clearly occurs. Chest pain, acute myocardial infarction, and even sudden death have occurred during temporary withdrawal of nitrates from these workers, demonstrating the existence of true physical dependence.

Several clinical trials in patients with angina pectoris have evaluated nitroglycerin regimens which incorporated a 10–12 hour nitrate-free interval. In some of these trials, an increase in the frequency of anginal attacks during the nitrate-free interval was observed in a small number of patients. In one trial, patients demonstrated decreased exercise tolerance at the end of the nitrate-free interval. Hemodynamic rebound has been observed only rarely; on the other hand, few studies were so designed that rebound, if it had occurred, would have been detected. The importance of these observations to the routine, clinical use of transdermal nitroglycerin is unknown.

Information for Patients:

Daily headaches sometimes accompany treatment with nitroglycerin. In patients who get these headaches, the headaches may be a marker of the activity of the drug. Patients should resist the temptation to avoid headaches by altering the schedule of their treatment with nitroglycerin, since loss of headache may be associated with simultaneous loss of antianginal efficacy.

Treatment with nitroglycerin may be associated with lightheadedness on standing, especially just after rising from a recumbent or seated position. This effect may be more frequent in patients who have also consumed alcohol.

After normal use, there is enough residual nitroglycerin in discarded patches that they are a potential hazard to children and pets.

A patient leaflet is supplied with the systems.

Drug Interactions:

The vasodilating effects of nitroglycerin may be additive with those of other vasodilators. Alcohol, in particular, has been found to exhibit additive effects of this variety.

Carcinogenesis, Mutagenesis, Impairment of Fertility:

Studies to evaluate the carcinogenic or mutagenic potential of nitroglycerin have not been performed. Nitroglycerin's effect upon reproductive capacity is similarly unknown.

Pregnancy —Pregnancy Category C:

Animal reproduction studies have not been conducted with nitroglycerin. It is also not known whether nitroglycerin can cause fetal harm when administered to a pregnant woman or whether it can affect reproductive capacity. Nitroglycerin should be given to a pregnant woman only if clearly needed.

Nursing Mothers:

It is not known whether nitroglycerin is excreted in human milk. Because many drugs are excreted in human milk, caution should be exercised when nitroglycerin is administered to a nursing woman.

Pediatric use:

Safety and effectiveness in pediatric patients have not been established.

ADVERSE REACTIONS

Adverse reactions to nitroglycerin are generally dose-related, and almost all of these reactions are the result of nitroglycerin's activity as a vasodilator. Headache, which may be severe, is the most commonly reported side effect. Headache may be recurrent with each daily dose, especially at higher doses. Transient episodes of lightheadedness, occasionally related to blood pressure changes, may also occur. Hypotension occurs infrequently, but in some patients it may be severe enough to warrant discontinuation of therapy. Syncope, crescendo angina, and rebound hypertension have been reported but are uncommon.

Allergic reactions to nitroglycerin are also uncommon, and the great majority of those reported have been cases of con-

Continued on next page

Deponit—Cont.

tact dermatitis or fixed drug eruptions in patients receiving nitroglycerin in ointments or patches. There have been a few reports of genuine anaphylactoid reactions, and these reactions can probably occur in patients receiving nitroglycerin by any route.
Extremely rarely, ordinary doses of organic nitrates have caused methemoglobinemia in normal-seeming patients; for further discussion of its diagnosis and treatment see OVERDOSAGE.
Application-site irritation may occur but is rarely severe.
In two placebo-controlled trials of intermittent therapy with nitroglycerin patches at 0.2 to 0.8 mg/hr, the most frequent adverse reactions among 307 subjects were as follows:

	placebo	patch
headache	18%	63%
lightheadedness	4%	6%
hypotension and/or syncope	0%	4%
increased angina	2%	2%

OVERDOSAGE:

Hemodynamic Effects:
The ill effects of nitroglycerin overdose are generally the results of nitroglycerin's capacity to induce vasodilatation, venous pooling, reduced cardiac output, and hypotension. These hemodynamic changes may have protean manifestations, including increased intracranial pressure, with any or all of persistent throbbing headache, confusion, and moderate fever, vertigo; palpitations; visual disturbances; nausea and vomiting (possibly with colic and even bloody diarrhea); syncope (especially in the upright posture); air hunger and dyspnea, later followed by reduced ventilatory effort; diaphoresis, with the skin either flushed or cold and clammy; heart block and bradycardia; paralysis; coma; seizures; and death.
Laboratory determinations of serum levels of nitroglycerin and its metabolites are not widely available, and such determinations have, in any event, no established role in the management of nitroglycerin overdose.
No data are available to suggest physiological maneuvers (e.g. maneuvers to change the pH of the urine) that might accelerate elimination of nitroglycerin and its active metabolites. Similarly, it is not known which—if any—of these substances can usefully be removed from the body by hemodialysis.
No specific antagonist to the vasodilator effects of nitroglycerin is known, and no intervention has been subject to controlled study as a therapy of nitroglycerin overdose. Because the hypotension associated with nitroglycerin overdose is the result of venodilatation and arterial hypovolemia, prudent therapy in this situation should be directed toward increase in central fluid volume. Passive elevation of the patient's legs may be sufficient, but intravenous infusion of normal saline or similar fluid may also be necessary.
The use of epinephrine or other arterial vasoconstrictors in this setting is likely to do more harm than good.
In patients with renal disease or congestive heart failure, therapy resulting in central volume expansion is not without hazard. Treatment of nitroglycerin overdose in these patients may be subtle and difficult, and invasive monitoring may be required.
Methemoglobinemia:
Nitrate ions liberated during metabolism of nitroglycerin can oxidize hemoglobin into methemoglobin. Even in patients totally without cytochrome b_5 reductase activity, however, and even assuming that the nitrate moieties of nitroglycerin are quantitatively applied to oxidation of hemoglobin, about 1 mg/kg of nitroglycerin should be required before any of these patients manifests clinically significant (≥10%) methemoglobinemia. In patients with normal reductase function, significant production of methemoglobin should require even larger doses of nitroglycerin. In one study in which 36 patients received 2–4 weeks of continuous nitroglycerin therapy at 3.1 to 4.4 mg/hr, the average methemoglobin level measured was 0.2%; this was comparable to that observed in parallel patients who received placebo. Notwithstanding these observations, there are case reports of significant methemoglobinemia in association with moderate overdoses of organic nitrates. None of the affected patients had been thought to be unusually susceptible. Methemoglobin levels are available from most clinical laboratories. The diagnosis should be suspected in patients who exhibit signs of impaired oxygen delivery despite adequate cardiac output and adequate arterial pO_2. Classically, methemoglobinemic blood is described as chocolate brown, without color change on exposure to air. When methemoglobinemia is diagnosed, the treatment of choice is methylene blue, 1–2 mg/kg intravenously.

DOSAGE AND ADMINISTRATION

The suggested starting dose is between 0.2 mg/hr and 0.4 mg/hr. Doses between 0.4 mg/hr and 0.8 mg/hr have shown continued effectiveness for 10–12 hours daily for at least one month (the longest period studied) of intermittent administration. Although the minimum nitrate-free interval has not been defined, data show that a nitrate-free interval of 10–12 hours is sufficient (see CLINICAL PHARMACOLOGY). Thus, an appropriate dosing schedule for nitroglycerin patches would include a daily patch-on period of 12–14 hours and a daily patch-off period of 10–12 hours.
Although some well controlled clinical trials using exercise tolerance testing have shown maintenance of effectiveness when patches are worn continuously, the large majority of such controlled trials have shown the development of tolerance (i.e., complete loss of effect) within the first 24 hours after therapy was initiated. Dose adjustment, even to levels much higher than generally used, did not restore efficacy.

HOW SUPPLIED

Deponit (nitroglycerin transdermal delivery system) is packaged in cartons containing unit doses of flesh-colored systems on aluminum backings. See table below.
[See table at top of previous page]
Store at room temperature not above 25° C (77° F). Do not refrigerate.
CAUTION: Federal law prohibits dispensing without prescription.
PC1954A Rev. 7/96
Shown in Product Identification Guide, page 337.

DILATRATE®-SR ℞

[dī 'lă-trāt]
(isosorbide dinitrate)
Sustained Release Capsules
40 mg

DESCRIPTION

Isosorbide dinitrate (ISDN) is 1,4:3,6-dianhydro-D-glucitol 2,5 dinitrate, an organic nitrate whose structural formula is

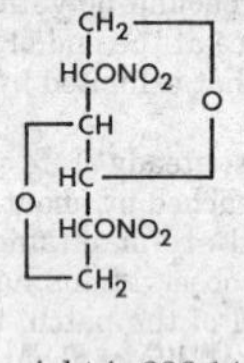

and whose molecular weight is 236.14. The organic nitrates are vasodilators, active on both arteries and veins. Each Dilatrate-SR sustained release capsule contains 40 mg of isosorbide dinitrate, in a microdialysis delivery system that causes the active drug to be released over an extended period. Each capsule also contains ethylcellulose, lactose, pharmaceutical glaze, starch, sucrose and talc. The capsule shells contain D&C Red 33, D&C Yellow 10, gelatin and titanium dioxide.

CLINICAL PHARMACOLOGY

The principal pharmacological action of isosorbide dinitrate is relaxation of vascular smooth muscle and consequent dilatation of peripheral arteries and veins, especially the latter. Dilatation of the veins promotes peripheral pooling of blood and decreases venous return to the heart, thereby reducing left ventricular end-diastolic pressure and pulmonary capillary wedge pressure (preload). Arteriolar relaxation reduces systemic vascular resistance, systolic arterial pressure, and mean arterial pressure (afterload). Dilatation of the coronary arteries also occurs. The relative importance of preload reduction, afterload reduction, and coronary dilatation remains undefined.
Dosing regimens for most chronically used drugs are designed to provide plasma concentrations that are continuously greater than a minimally effective concentration. This strategy is inappropriate for organic nitrates. Several well-controlled clinical trials have used exercise testing to assess the antianginal efficacy of continuously-delivered nitrates. In the large majority of these trials, active agents were no more effective than placebo after 24 hours (or less) of continuous therapy. Attempts to overcome nitrate tolerance by dose escalation, even to doses far in excess of those used acutely, have consistently failed. Only after nitrates have been absent from the body for several hours has their antianginal efficacy been restored.
Pharmacokinetics:
The kinetics of absorption of isosorbide dinitrate from Dilatrate-SR sustained release capsules have not been well studied. Studies of immediate-release formulations of ISDN have found highly variable bioavailability (10 to 90%), with extensive first-pass metabolism in the liver. Most such studies have observed progressive increases in bioavailability during chronic therapy; it is not known whether similar increases in bioavailability appear during the course of chronic therapy with Dilatrate-SR sustained release capsules.
Once absorbed, the distribution volume of isosorbide dinitrate is 2–4 L/kg and this volume is cleared at the rate of 2–4 L/min, so ISDN's half-life in serum is about an hour. Since the clearance exceeds hepatic blood flow, considerable extrahepatic metabolism must also occur. Clearance is affected primarily by denitration to the 2-mononitrate (15 to 25%) and the 5- mononitrate (75 to 85%).
Both metabolites have biological activity, especially the 5-mononitrate. With an overall half-life of about 5 hours, the 5-mononitrate is cleared from the serum by denitration to isosorbide; glucuronidation to the 5-mononitrate glucuronide; and denitration/hydration to sorbitol. The 2-mononitrate has been less well studied, but it appears to participate in the same metabolic pathways, with a half-life of about 2 hours.
The interdosing interval sufficient to avoid tolerance to ISDN has not been well defined. Studies of nitroglycerin (an organic nitrate with a very short half-life) have shown that dosing intervals of 10–12 hours are usually sufficient to prevent or attenuate tolerance. Dosing intervals that have succeeded in avoiding tolerance during trials of moderate doses (e.g. 30 mg) of immediate release ISDN have generally been somewhat longer (at least 14 hours), but this is consistent with the longer half-lives of ISDN and its active metabolites.
An interdosing interval sufficient to avoid tolerance with Dilatrate-SR has not been demonstrated. In an eccentric dosing study, 40 mg capsules of Dilatrate-SR were administered daily at 0800 and 1400 hours. After two weeks of this regimen, Dilatrate-SR was statistically indistinguishable from placebo. Thus, the necessary interdosing interval sufficient to avoid tolerance remains unknown, but it must be greater than 18 hours.
Few well-controlled clinical trials of organic nitrates have been designed to detect rebound or withdrawal effects. In one such trial, however, subjects receiving nitroglycerin had less exercise tolerance at the end of the daily interdosing interval than the parallel group receiving placebo. The incidence, magnitude, and clinical significance of similar phenomena in patients receiving ISDN have not been studied.
Clinical trials:
In clinical trials, extended-release oral isosorbide dinitrate has been administered in a variety of regimens, with total daily doses ranging from 40 to 160 mg. A controlled trial using a single 40 mg sustained-release oral dose of isosorbide dinitrate (Dilatrate-SR) has demonstrated effective reductions in exercise-related angina for up to 8 hours. Antianginal activity is present about 1 hour after dosing.
Adequate multiple-dose trials of Dilatrate-SR sustained release capsules have not been reported.
Most controlled trials of multiple-dose immediate-release oral ISDN taken every 12 hours (or more frequently) for several weeks have shown statistically significant antianginal efficacy for only 2 hours after dosing. Once-daily regimens, and regimens with one daily interdosing interval of at least 14 hours (e.g., a regimen providing doses at 0800, 1400 and 1800 hours), have shown efficacy after the first dose of each day that was similar to that shown in the single dose studies cited above. The efficacy of subsequent doses has not been demonstrated. From large, well-controlled studies of other nitrates, it is reasonable to believe that the maximal achievable daily duration of antianginal effect from isosorbide dinitrate is about 12 hours. No dosing regimen for Dilatrate-SR sustained released capsules has actually been shown to achieve this duration of effect.

INDICATIONS AND USAGE

Dilatrate-SR sustained release capsules are indicated for the prevention of angina pectoris due to coronary artery disease. The onset of action of controlled-release oral isosorbide dinitrate is not sufficiently rapid for this product to be useful in aborting an acute anginal episode.

CONTRAINDICATIONS

Allergic reactions to organic nitrates are extremely rare, but they do occur. Isosorbide dinitrate is contraindicated in patients who are allergic to it.

WARNINGS

The benefits of extended-release oral isosorbide dinitrate in patients with acute myocardial infarction or congestive heart failure have not been established. If one elects to use isosorbide dinitrate in these conditions, careful clinical or hemodynamic monitoring must be used to avoid the hazards of hypotension and tachycardia. Because the effects of extended-release oral isosorbide dinitrate are so difficult to terminate rapidly, this formulation is not recommended in these settings.

PRECAUTIONS

General:
Severe hypotension, particularly with upright posture, may occur with even small doses of isosorbide dinitrate. This drug should therefore be used with caution in patients who

may be volume depleted or who, for whatever reason, are already hypotensive. Hypotension induced by isosorbide dinitrate may be accompanied by paradoxical bradycardia and increased angina pectoris.

Nitrate therapy may aggravate the angina caused by hypertrophic cardiomyopathy.

As tolerance to isosorbide dinitrate develops, the effect of sublingual nitroglycerin on exercise tolerance, although still observable, is somewhat blunted.

Some clinical trials in angina patients have provided nitroglycerin for about 12 continuous hours of every 24-hour day. During the interdosing intervals in some of these trials, anginal attacks have been more easily provoked than before treatment and patients have demonstrated hemodynamic rebound and decreased exercise tolerance. The importance of these observations to the routine, clinical use of controlled-release oral isosorbide dinitrate is not known.

In industrial workers who have had long-term exposure to unknown (presumably high) doses of organic nitrates, tolerance clearly occurs. Chest pain, acute myocardial infarction, and even sudden death have occurred during temporary withdrawal of nitrates from these workers demonstrating the existence of true physical dependence.

Information for Patients:

Patients should be told that the antianginal efficacy of isosorbide dinitrate is strongly related to its dosing regimen, so the prescribed schedule of dosing should be followed carefully. In particular, daily headaches sometimes accompany treatment with isosorbide dinitrate. In patients who get these headaches, the headaches are a marker of the activity of the drug. Patients should resist the temptation to avoid headaches by altering the schedule of their treatment with isosorbide dinitrate, since loss of headache may be associated with simultaneous loss of antianginal efficacy. Aspirin and/or acetaminophen, on the other hand, often successfully relieve isosorbide dinitrate-induced headaches with no deleterious effect on isosorbide dinitrate's antianginal efficacy.

Treatment with isosorbide dinitrate may be associated with lightheadedness on standing, especially just after rising from a recumbent or seated position. This effect may be more frequent in patients who have also consumed alcohol.

Drug Interactions:

The vasodilating effects of isosorbide dinitrate may be additive with those of other vasodilators. Alcohol, in particular, has been found to exhibit additive effects of this variety.

Carcinogenesis, Mutagenesis and Impairment of Fertility:

No long-term studies in animals have been performed to evaluate the carcinogenic potential of isosorbide dinitrate. In a modified two-litter reproduction study, there was no remarkable gross pathology and no altered fertility or gestation among rats fed isosorbide dinitrate at 25 or 100 mg/kg/day.

Pregnancy Category C:

At oral doses 35 and 150 times the daily Maximum Recommended Human Dose (MRHD), isosorbide dinitrate has been shown to cause a dose related increase in embryotoxicity (increase in mummified pups) in rabbits. There are no adequate, well-controlled studies in pregnant women. Isosorbide dinitrate should be used during pregnancy only if the potential benefit justifies the potential risk to the fetus.

Nursing Mothers:

It is not known whether isosorbide dinitrate is excreted in human milk. Because many drugs are excreted in human milk, caution should be exercised when isosorbide dinitrate is administered to a nursing woman.

Pediatric Use:

Safety and effectiveness in pediatric patients have not been established.

ADVERSE REACTIONS

Adverse reactions to isosorbide dinitrate are generally dose related, and almost all of these reactions are the result of isosorbide dinitrate's activity as a vasodilator. Headache, which may be severe, is the most commonly reported side effect. Headache may be recurrent with each daily dose, especially at higher doses. Transient episodes of lightheadedness, occasionally related to blood pressure changes, may also occur. Hypotension occurs infrequently, but in some patients it may be severe enough to warrant discontinuation of therapy. Syncope, crescendo angina, and rebound hypertension have been reported but are uncommon.

Extremely rarely, ordinary doses of organic nitrates have caused methemoglobinemia in normal-seeming patients. Methemoglobinemia is so infrequent at these doses that further discussion of its diagnosis and treatment is deferred (see OVERDOSAGE).

Data are not available to allow estimation of the frequency of adverse reactions during treatment with Dilatrate-SR sustained release capsules.

OVERDOSAGE

Hemodynamic Effects:

The ill effects of isosorbide dinitrate overdose are generally the results of isosorbide dinitrate's capacity to induce vasodilatation, venous pooling, reduced cardiac output, and hypotension. These hemodynamic changes may have protean manifestations, including increased intracranial pressure, with any or all of persistent throbbing headache, confusion, and moderate fever; vertigo; palpitations; visual disturbances; nausea and vomiting (possibly with colic and even bloody diarrhea); syncope (especially in the upright posture); air hunger and dyspnea, later followed by reduced ventilatory effort; diaphoresis, with the skin either flushed or cold and clammy; heart block and bradycardia; paralysis; coma; seizures and death.

Laboratory determinations of serum levels of isosorbide dinitrate and its metabolites are not widely available, and such determinations have, in any event, no established role in the management of isosorbide dinitrate overdose.

There are no data suggesting what dose of isosorbide dinitrate is likely to be life-threatening in humans. In rats, the median acute lethal dose (LD50) was found to be 1100 mg/kg.

No data are available to suggest physiological maneuvers (e.g., maneuvers to change the pH of the urine) might accelerate elimination of isosorbide dinitrate and its active metabolites. Similarly, it is not known which, if any, of these substances can usefully be removed from the body by hemodialysis.

No specific antagonist to the vasodilator effects of isosorbide dinitrate is known, and no intervention has been subject to controlled study as a therapy of isosorbide dinitrate overdose. Because the hypotension associated with isosorbide dinitrate overdose is the result of venodilatation and arterial hypovolemia, prudent therapy in this situation should be directed toward increase in central fluid volume. Passive elevation of the patient's legs may be sufficient, but intravenous infusion of normal saline or similar fluid may also be necessary. The use of epinephrine or other arterial vasoconstrictors in this setting is likely to do more harm than good. In patients with renal disease or congestive heart failure, therapy resulting in central volume expansion is not without hazard. Treatment of isosorbide dinitrate overdose in these patients may be subtle and difficult, and invasive monitoring may be required.

Methemoglobinemia:

Nitrate ions liberated during metabolism of isosorbide dinitrate can oxidize hemoglobin into methemoglobin. Even in patients totally without cytochrome b5 reductase activity, however, and even assuming that the nitrate moieties of isosorbide dinitrate are quantitatively applied to oxidation of hemoglobin, about 1 mg/kg of isosorbide dinitrate should be required before any of these patients manifests clinically significant (> 10%) methemoglobinemia. In patients with normal reductase function, significant production of methemoglobin should require even larger doses of isosorbide dinitrate. In one study in which 36 patients received 2–4 weeks of continuous nitroglycerin therapy at 3.1 to 4.4 mg/hr (equivalent, in total administered dose of nitrate ions, to 4.8–6.9 mg of bioavailable isosorbide dinitrate per hour), the average methemoglobin level measured was 0.2%; this was comparable to that observed in parallel patients who received placebo.

Notwithstanding these observations, there are case reports of significant methemoglobinemia in association with moderate overdoses of organic nitrates. None of the affected patients had been thought to be unusually susceptible.

Methemoglobin levels are available from most clinical laboratories. The diagnosis should be suspected in patients who exhibit signs of impaired oxygen delivery despite adequate cardiac output and adequate arterial p02. Classically, methemoglobinemic blood is described as chocolate brown, without color change on exposure to air.

When methemoglobinemia is diagnosed, the treatment of choice is methylene blue, 1–2 mg/kg intravenously.

DOSAGE AND ADMINISTRATION

As noted above (CLINICAL PHARMACOLOGY), multiple studies with ISDN and other nitrates have shown that maintenance of continuous 24-hour plasma levels results in refractory tolerance. Every dosing regimen for organic nitrates including Dilatrate-SR must provide a daily nitrate-free interval to avoid the development of tolerance. To achieve the necessary nitrate-free interval with immediate-release oral ISDN, it appears that at least one of the daily interdose intervals must be at least 14 hours long. The necessary interdose interval for Dilatrate-SR has not been clearly identified, but it must be greater than 18 hours.

As noted under Clinical Pharmacology, only one trial has ever studied the use of extended-release isosorbide dinitrate for more than one dose. In that trial, 40 mg of Dilatrate-SR was administered twice daily in doses given 6 hours apart. After 4 weeks, Dilatrate-SR could not be distinguished from placebo.

Large controlled studies with other nitrates suggest that no dosing regimen with Dilatrate-SR should be expected to provide more than about 12 hours of continuous antianginal efficacy per day.

In clinical trials, immediate-release oral isosorbide dinitrate has been administered in a variety of regimens, with total daily doses ranging from 30 to 480 mg.

Do not exceed 160 mg (4 capsules) per day.

HOW SUPPLIED

Dilatrate®-SR (isosorbide dinitrate) 40 mg Sustained Release Capsules are opaque pink and colorless capsules with white beadlets and are imprinted "Schwarz" and "0920". They are supplied as follows:

Bottles of 60	NDC 0091-0920-02
Bottles of 100	NDC 0091-0920-01

Store at controlled room temperature 15°–30°C (59°–86°F) in a dry place.

CAUTION: Federal law prohibits dispensing without prescription.

PC2088B Rev. 4/97

EDEX™ ℞

[ē-'*deks*]

(alprostadil for injection)
For Intracavernous Use Only
Sterile Powder in Vials
Sterile Powder and Diluent in Cartridges

Rx Only

DESCRIPTION

EDEX (alprostadil for injection) is a sterile, pyrogen-free powder for intracavernous administration after reconstitution with sterile 0.9% sodium chloride. EDEX is lyophilized in single-dose vials containing either 6.225, 12.45, 24.90 or 49.80 mcg (micrograms) of alprostadil, also known as prostaglandin E_1 (PGE_1), an endogenous substance, in an alfadex (α-cyclodextrin) inclusion complex. Lactose comprises the remainder of the dry powder in each vial. The EDEX vials are supplied in four strengths: 5 mcg vial (6.225 mcg alprostadil, 201.275 mcg α-cyclodextrin, 56.3 mg lactose anhydrous); 10 mcg vial (12.45 mcg alprostadil, 402.55 mcg α-cyclodextrin, 56.3 mg lactose anhydrous); 20 mcg vial (24.90 mcg alprostadil, 805.10 mcg α-cyclodextrin, 56.3 mg lactose anhydrous); 40 mcg vial (49.80 mcg alprostadil, 1610.2 mcg α-cyclodextrin, 56.3 mg lactose anhydrous).

EDEX is also lyophilized in single-dose, dual-chamber cartridges intended for use with the reusable EDEX injection device. One chamber of the cartridge contains alprostadil, alfadex and lactose as a sterile, pyrogen-free powder. The other chamber contains 1.075 mL of sterile 0.9% sodium chloride. The EDEX cartridges are supplied in three strengths: 10 mcg cartridge (10.75 mcg alprostadil, 347.55 mcg α-cyclodextrin, 51.06 mg lactose); 20 mcg cartridge (21.5 mcg alprostadil, 695.2 mcg α-cyclodextrin, 51.06 mg lactose); 40 mcg cartridge (43.0 mcg alprostadil, 1,390.3 mcg α-cyclodextrin, 51.06 mg lactose). The EDEX injection device is used to reconstitute the sterile powder in one chamber with the sterile 0.9% sodium chloride in the other chamber. After reconstitution, the EDEX injection device is used to administer the intracavernous injection of alprostadil.

The chemical name for alprostadil is (1R,2R,3R)-3-Hydroxy-2-[(E)-(3S)-3-hydroxy-1-octenyl]-5-oxocyclopentane heptanoic acid. The empirical formula is $C_{20}H_{34}O_5$ and the molecular weight is 354.49. The chemical structure is:

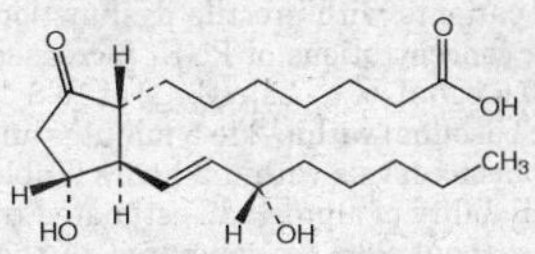

The α-cyclodextrin inclusion complex improves the water solubility of alprostadil. The empirical formula of α-cyclodextrin is $C_{36}H_{60}O_{30}$ and the molecular weight is 972.85. The chemical structure is:

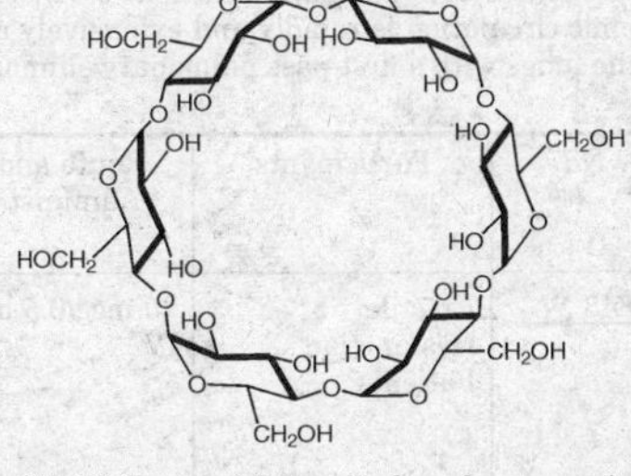

Alprostadil alfadex is a white, odorless, hygroscopic powder. It is freely soluble in water and practically insoluble in ethanol, ethyl acetate and ether. After reconstitution, the active ingredient, alprostadil, immediately dissociates from the α-cyclodextrin inclusion complex. The reconstituted solution is clear and colorless and has a pH between 4.0 and 8.0. When the single-dose vial containing either 6.225, 12.45, 24.90, or 49.80 mcg of alprostadil is reconstituted with 1.2 mL of sterile 0.9% sodium chloride, the deliverable amount

Continued on next page

Edex—Cont.

of alprostadil in each milliliter is 5, 10, 20, or 40 micrograms, respectively. When the single-dose, dual-chamber cartridge containing either 10.75, 21.5 or 43.0 mcg of alprostadil is placed into the EDEX injection device and reconstituted, the deliverable amount of alprostadil in each milliliter is 10, 20, or 40 micrograms, respectively.

CLINICAL PHARMACOLOGY

Alprostadil (PGE_1) is one of the prostaglandins, a family of naturally occurring acidic lipids with various pharmacological effects. Endogenous PGE_1 is derived from dihomo-gamma-linolenic acid, a fatty acid found within the phospholipids of cellular membranes. As an endogenous substance, PGE_1 exerts its biological effects either directly or indirectly by regulating and modifying the synthesis and effects of other hormones and mediators.

Mode of Action

Alprostadil is a smooth muscle relaxant. Precontracted isolated preparations of the human corpus cavernosum, corpus spongiosum and cavernous artery are relaxed by alprostadil. Alprostadil has been shown to bind to specific receptors in human penile tissue. Two types of receptors that differ in their PGE_1 binding affinity have been identified. The binding of alprostadil to its receptors is accompanied by an increase in intracellular cAMP levels. Human cavernous smooth muscle cells respond to alprostadil by releasing intracellular calcium into the surrounding medium. Smooth muscle relaxation is associated with a reduction of the cytoplasmic free calcium concentration. Alprostadil also attenuates presynaptic noradrenaline release in the corpus cavernosum which is essential for the maintenance of a flaccid and non-erect penis.

Alprostadil induces erection by relaxation of trabecular smooth muscle and by dilation of cavernous arteries. This leads to expansion of lacunar spaces and entrapment of blood by compressing the venules against the tunica albuginea, a process referred to as the corporal veno-occlusive mechanism.

Pharmacokinetics

Alpha-Cyclodextrin

After reconstitution, PGE_1 immediately dissociates from the α-cyclodextrin inclusion complex; the *in vivo* disposition of both components occurs independently after administration. After intravenous infusion of radiolabeled α-cyclodextrin to healthy volunteers, the radiolabeled components were rapidly eliminated within 24-hours, urine accounting for 81–83% of radioactivity and feces for 0.1%. There was no evidence of significant accumulation of radiolabeled α-cyclodextrin in the body even after 7 days of repeated intravenous injection. After intracavernous administration in monkeys, radiolabeled α-cyclodextrin was rapidly distributed from the injection site with less than 0.1% of the dose remaining in the penis 1 hour after administration. There was no evidence of tissue retention of radiolabeled α-cyclodextrin in monkeys.

Alprostadil

Absorption: After intracavernous injection of 20 mcg of EDEX in 24 patients with erectile dysfunction, mean systemic plasma concentrations of PGE_1 increased from baseline of 0.8 ± 0.6 pg/mL to a peak (C_{max}) of 16.8 ± 18.9 pg/mL (corrected for baseline) within 2 to 5 minutes and dropped to endogenous plasma levels within 2 hours (Table 1). The absolute bioavailability of alprostadil estimated from systemic exposure was about 98% as compared to the same dose given by a short-term intravenous infusion.

Distribution: The volume of distribution for PGE_1 was not estimated. Approximately 93% of PGE_1 found in plasma is protein-bound.

Metabolism: PGE_1 is metabolized in the corpus cavernosum after intracavernous administration. PGE_1 entering the systemic circulation is rapidly and extensively metabolized in the lungs with a first-pass pulmonary elimination of 60 to 90% of PGE_1. Enzymatic oxidation of the C15-hydroxy group followed by reduction of the C13, 14-double bond produces the primary metabolites, 15-keto-PGE_1, 15-keto-PGE_0, and PGE_0. 15-keto-PGE_1 has only been detected *in vitro* in homogenized lung preparations, whereas 15-keto-PGE_0 and PGE_0 have been measured in plasma. Unlike the 15-keto metabolites which are less pharmacologically active than the parent compound, PGE_0 is similar in potency to PGE_1 *in vitro* using isolated animal organs.

After intracavernous injection of 20 mcg of EDEX to 24 patients with erectile dysfunction, mean systemic plasma 15-keto-PGE_0 levels increased within 7 minutes from endogenous levels of 12.9 ± 11.8 pg/mL to a C_{max} of 421 ± 337 pg/mL (corrected for baseline) followed by a decrease to baseline levels in several hours. Mean systemic plasma PGE_0 levels increased within 20 minutes from endogenous levels of 0.6 ± 0.5 pg/mL to a C_{max} of 3.9 ± 2.3 pg/mL (corrected for baseline) followed by a decrease to baseline levels in several hours.

Excretion: After further degradation of PGE_1 by beta and omega oxidation, the main metabolites are excreted primarily in urine (88%) and feces (12%) over 72 hours, and total excretion is essentially complete (92%) within 24 hours after administration. No unchanged PGE_1 has been found in the urine and there is no evidence of tissue retention of PGE_1 and its metabolites. After intracavernous injection of 20 mcg of EDEX in patients with erectile dysfunction, the terminal half-lives ($T_{1/2}$) of 15-keto-PGE_0 and PGE_0 were calculated to be 40.9 ± 16.5 minutes and 63.2 ± 31.1 minutes, respectively. The terminal half-life of PGE_1 in healthy volunteers was calculated to be around 9–11 minutes which is consistent with that reported in the literature (8 minutes).

Mean total body clearance of PGE_1 in patients with erectile dysfunction was calculated to be around 115 L/min after an intravenous infusion of 20 mcg alprostadil. The above value exceeded cardiac output indicating extensive and rapid elimination of PGE_1 in the lungs and/or blood.

Special Populations

Geriatric: The potential effect of age on the pharmacokinetics of alprostadil has not been formally evaluated.

Race: The potential influence of race on the pharmacokinetics of alprostadil has not been formally evaluated.

Hepatic Insufficiency: In a study in symptomatic subjects with impaired hepatic function and age/weight/sex-matched healthy volunteers, 120 mcg of alprostadil was administered by intravenous infusion over 2 hours. The mean C_{max} value of PGE_1 in hepatically impaired patients was 96% higher than in healthy volunteers. Mean C_{max} values of both 15-keto-PGE_0 and PGE_0 increased 65% as compared to those in healthy volunteers. The terminal half-lives of PGE_1, PGE_0, and 15-keto PGE_0 and plasma albumin levels were similar in patients compared to healthy volunteers. Due to the fact that PGE_1 is primarily metabolized in the lung, the observed differences between hepatically impaired subjects and healthy volunteers were not anticipated; the mechanism responsible for the observed discrepancies is not known.

Renal Impairment: In a study in symptomatic subjects with end-stage renal disease undergoing hemodialysis and age/weight/sex-matched healthy volunteers, 120 mcg of alprostadil was administered by intravenous infusion over 2 hours. The mean C_{max} value of PGE_1 in renally impaired patients was 37% lower as compared to that in healthy volunteers whereas mean C_{max} values of 15-keto-PGE_0 and PGE_0 in these patients increased 104% and 145%, respectively as compared to those in healthy volunteers. The terminal half-lives of PGE_1, PGE_0 and 15-keto-PGE_0 and plasma albumin levels were similar in these patients vs healthy volunteers. The mechanism responsible for the observed discrepancies between renally impaired subjects and healthy volunteers is not known.

Pulmonary Disease: The pulmonary extraction of alprostadil following intravascular administration was reduced by 15% (66 ± 3.6% vs 78 ± 2.3%) in patients with acute respiratory distress syndrome (ARDS) compared with a group of patients with normal respiratory function who were undergoing cardiopulmonary bypass surgery. Pulmonary clearance was found to vary as a function of cardiac output and pulmonary intrinsic clearance in a group of 14 patients with ARDS or at risk of developing ARDS following trauma or sepsis. In this study, the pulmonary extraction efficiency of alprostadil ranged from subnormal (11%) to normal (90%), with an overall mean of 67%.

Drug-Drug Interactions: In clinical trials, concomitant use of agents such as antihypertensive drugs, diuretics, antidiabetic agents (including insulin), or nonsteroidal anti-inflammatory drugs had no apparent effect on the efficacy or safety of EDEX.

Aspirin, Warfarin, Digoxin, Glyburide: Several drug-drug interaction studies have been conducted with alprostadil alone or in combination with aspirin, digoxin or warfarin in healthy volunteers and with glyburide in subjects with stable, non-insulin dependent diabetes mellitus. The pharmacokinetic profiles of aspirin, warfarin, digoxin, and glyburide were not affected by concomitant administration of alprostadil. There were no clinically important changes or trends in pharmacodynamic parameters for these drugs.

Heparin: The pharmacokinetic and pharmacodynamic interaction between alprostadil intravenous infusion, 90 mcg over 3 hours, and heparin (5,000 IU) was evaluated in 12 healthy volunteers. Alprostadil had a significant effect on the pharmacodynamics of heparin resulting in a 140% increase in partial thromboplastin time and a 120% increase in thrombin time. Therefore, caution should be exercised with concomitant administration of heparin and EDEX.

[See table below]

Clinical Studies

In two studies [Protocol numbers KU-620-001 (Study 1) and KU-620-002 (Study 2)], the safety and efficacy of EDEX were evaluated in 347 men with a diagnosis of erectile dysfunction due to vasculogenic, neurogenic and/or mixed etiology. Each study consisted of three phases: an in-office dose-titration phase, a two-week double-blind cross-over phase at home, and an open-label at home treatment phase that lasted for 12 months (Study 1) or six months (Study 2). During the dose-titration phase, individualized optimum doses of EDEX were established. Erectile response was measured by the Buckling Test to assess axial penile rigidity. A positive Buckling Test was achieved if the erect penis was able to support an axial load of 1.0 kg without buckling of the penile shaft. During the subsequent two-week double-blind, cross-over phase, patients self-injected EDEX or placebo at home. Thereafter, patients continued to perform self-injections of open-label EDEX for six or 12 months, and the occurrence of an erection sufficient for sexual intercourse was documented following each injection.

Results

Study 1: One hundred fourteen men with a mean age of 53 years (range 22 to 65 years) were enrolled in the first phase. The mean optimum dose was 13.8 mcg (range 1 to 20 mcg). Seventy-six percent (87/114) of patients had an erection with a positive penile Buckling Test. Among the 71% (81/114) of patients who entered the placebo-controlled phase, an erection sufficient for sexual intercourse was achieved in 74% (60/81) of patients following EDEX injection compared to 7% (6/81) of patients following placebo injection. The mean duration of erection following EDEX was 56.9 minutes compared to 4.0 minutes following placebo. Among the 65% (74/114) of patients who entered the open-label treatment phase, the mean rate of response with an erection sufficient for sexual intercourse was 88.9% through 12 months. The average dose of EDEX remained essentially unchanged throughout the study duration.

Study 2: Two hundred thirty-three men with a mean age of 59.8 years (range 23 to 74 years) were enrolled in the first phase. The mean optimum dose was 25.9 mcg (range 1 to 40 mcg). Seventy-three percent (171/233) of patients had an

Study No.	Participants	Route and Dose Administration	Drug/ Metabolites	C_{max} [1] [pg/mL]	T_{max} [min]	AUC [2] [pg·min/mL]	Total Clearance [3] [L/min]	$T_{1/2}$ [4] [min]
PHAKI 848	Erectile Dysfunction Patients	20 mcg/0.5 hr IV	PGE_1	7.09 ± 3.12	25.5 ± 4.8	174 ± 101	115	—
			15-keto-PGE_0	471 ± 88	30.0 ± 1.2	13705 ± 2559	—	15.6 ± 5.6
			PGE_0	7.10 ± 2.19	32.2 ± 2.4	380 ± 115	—	39.8 ± 26.3
		20 mcg/IC	PGE_1	16.8 ± 18.9	4.8 ± 3.3	173 ± 115	—	—
			15-keto-PGE_0	421 ± 337	9.7 ± 7.7	10500 ± 4101	—	40.9 ± 16.5
			PGE_0	3.9 ± 2.3	20.3 ± 12.6	252 ± 134	—	63.2 ± 31.1

[1] Baseline-corrected data.
[2] $AUC_{0\text{-}150}$ for IV infusion and $AUC_{0\text{-}120}$ for IC injection.
[3] Calculated as IV dose/$AUC_{0\text{-}150}$ (IV).
[4] Apparent terminal half-life.

erection with a positive penile Buckling Test. Among the 60% (141/233) of patients who entered the placebo-controlled phase, an erection sufficient for sexual intercourse was achieved in 73% (103/141) of patients following EDEX injection compared to 13% (18/141) of patients following placebo injection. The mean duration of erection following EDEX was 59.0 minutes compared to 7.6 minutes following placebo. Among the 60% (139/233) of patients who entered the open-label treatment phase, the mean rate of response with an erection sufficient for intercourse was 85.3% through six months. The average dose of EDEX remained essentially unchanged throughout the study duration.

INDICATIONS AND USAGE
EDEX is indicated for the treatment of erectile dysfunction due to neurogenic, vasculogenic, psychogenic, or mixed etiology.

CONTRAINDICATIONS
EDEX should not be used in patients who have a known hypersensitivity to alprostadil or other prostaglandins, in patients who have conditions that might predispose them to priapism, such as sickle cell anemia or trait, multiple myeloma, or leukemia, or in patients with anatomical deformation of the penis, such as angulation, cavernosal fibrosis, or Peyronie's disease. **Patients with penile implants should not be treated with EDEX.**

EDEX should not be used in men for whom sexual activity is inadvisable or contraindicated.

EDEX should not be used in women and children and is not for use in newborns.

WARNINGS
Prolonged erections greater than four hours in duration occurred in 4% of all patients treated up to 24 months. The incidence of priapism (erections greater than 6 hours in duration) was <1% with long-term use for up to 24 months. In the majority of cases, spontaneous detumescence occurred. Pharmacologic intervention and/or aspiration of blood from the corpora was necessary in 1.6% of 311 patients with prolonged erections/priapism. To minimize the chances of prolonged erection or priapism, EDEX should be titrated slowly to the lowest effective dose (see DOSAGE AND ADMINISTRATION). The patient must be instructed to immediately report to his prescribing physician or, if unavailable, to seek immediate medical assistance for any erection that persists longer than six hours. If priapism is not treated immediately, penile tissue damage and permanent loss of potency may result.

PRECAUTIONS
General
1) Intracavernous injections of EDEX can lead to increased peripheral blood levels of PGE_1 and its metabolites, especially in those patients with significant corpora cavernosa venous leakage. Increased peripheral blood levels of PGE_1 and its metabolites may lead to hypotension and/or dizziness.

2) Regular follow-up of patients, with careful examination of the penis at the start of therapy and at regular intervals (e.g. 3 months), is strongly recommended to identify any penile changes. The overall incidence of penile fibrosis, including Peyronie's disease, reported in clinical studies up to 24 months with EDEX was 7.8%. Treatment with EDEX should be discontinued in patients who develop penile angulation, cavernosal fibrosis, or Peyronie's disease. Treatment can be resumed if the penile abnormality subsides.

3) The safety and efficacy of combinations of EDEX and other vasoactive agents have not been systematically studied. Therefore, the use of such combinations is not recommended.

4) After injection of the EDEX solution, compression of the injection site for five minutes, or until bleeding stops, is necessary. Patients on anticoagulants, such as warfarin or heparin, may have increased propensity for bleeding after intracavernous injection.

5) Underlying treatable medical causes of erectile dysfunction should be diagnosed and treated prior to initiation of therapy with EDEX.

6) **The patient should be instructed not to reuse or to share needles, syringes, vials or cartridges. As with all prescription medicines, the patient should not allow anyone else to use his medicine.**

7) *Drug Interactions*
The pharmacodynamic interaction between heparin (5,000 IU) and alprostadil intravenous infusion (90 mcg over 3 hours) was investigated. The results indicate significant changes in partial thromboplastin time (140% increase) and thrombin time (120% increase). Therefore, caution should be exercised with concomitant administration of heparin and EDEX.

(Also, see drug-drug interaction studies in CLINICAL PHARMACOLOGY, Pharmacokinetics subsection.)

Information for Patients
To ensure safe and effective use of EDEX, the patient should be thoroughly instructed and trained in the self-injection technique before he begins intracavernous treatment with EDEX at home. The desirable dose should be established in

the physician's office. The instructions for preparation of the EDEX solution should be carefully followed. The reconstituted solution may initially appear cloudy due to small air bubbles. Do not use the solution if it remains cloudy, contains precipitates, or is discolored. The reconstituted solution should be gently mixed, not shaken. A patient information pamphlet is included in each package of EDEX vials, kits and cartridges.

EDEX should be used immediately after reconstitution. The patient should follow the instructions in the patient information pamphlet to limit the possibility of bacterial contamination. The reconstituted vial or cartridge is designed for one use only and should be discarded after use.

The EDEX vial and cartridge contain a solid layer or lyophilized cake of dry white powder approximately 3/16" in thickness for the vial and 3/8" in thickness for the cartridge. A normal cake may appear cracked or crumbled. If the vial or cartridge is damaged, the cake may shrink in size. Do not use the vial or cartridge if they appear damaged or the cake is substantially reduced in size.

EDEX vials: If the dosage prescribed is less than 1 mL of EDEX solution, the patient will not need to withdraw the entire amount of drug solution from the vial to reach the prescribed dose. **The needles must be properly discarded after use; they must not be reused or shared with other persons.**

EDEX cartridges: If the dosage prescribed is less than 1 mL of EDEX solution, excess solution will be expelled through the needle as the plunger is pushed and the upper rim of the top stopper reaches the correct volume mark for the prescribed dose. **The needle must be properly discarded after use; it must not be reused or shared with other persons.**

The dose of EDEX that is established in the physician's office should not be changed by the patient without consulting the physician. The patient may expect an erection to occur within 5 to 20 minutes. A standard treatment goal is to produce an erection lasting no longer than 1 hour. EDEX should be used no more than 3 times per week, with at least 24 hours between each use.

Patients should be aware of possible side effects of therapy with EDEX; the most frequently occurring is penile pain during and/or after injection, usually mild to moderate in severity. A potentially serious adverse reaction with intracavernous therapy is priapism. Accordingly, the patient should be instructed to contact the physician's office immediately or, if unavailable, to seek immediate medical assistance if an erection persists for longer than 6 hours.

The patient should report any penile pain that was not present before or that increased in intensity, as well as the occurrence of nodules or hard tissue in the penis to his physician as soon as possible. As with any injection, infection is possible. Patients should be instructed to report to the physician any penile redness, swelling, tenderness or curvature of the erect penis. The patient must visit the physician's office for regular checkups for assessment of the therapeutic benefit and safety of treatment with EDEX.

Note: Individuals who are sexually active should be counseled about the protective measures that are necessary to guard against the spread of sexually transmitted diseases, including the human immunodeficiency virus (HIV). Use of intracavernous EDEX offers no protection from the transmission of sexually transmitted or blood-borne diseases. The injection of EDEX can induce a small amount of bleeding at the site of injection. In patients infected with blood-borne diseases, this could increase the risk of transmission of blood-borne diseases between partners.

Carcinogenesis, Mutagenesis, Impairment of Fertility
Long-term carcinogenicity studies have not been conducted. Alprostadil showed no evidence of mutagenicity in three *in vitro* assays including the AMES bacterial reverse mutation assay, a forward gene mutation assay in Chinese hamster lung (V79) cells, and a chromosome aberration assay in human peripheral lymphocytes. Alprostadil did not produce damage to chromosomes or the mitotic apparatus in the *in vivo* rat micronucleus test.

Alprostadil did not cause any adverse effects on fertility or general reproductive performance when administered intraperitoneally to male or female rats at dose levels from 2 to 200 mcg/kg/day. The high dose of 200 mcg/kg/day is about 300 times the maximum recommended human dose (MRHD) on a body weight basis. The human dose of EDEX is <1 mcg/kg (MRHD is 40 mcg and the calculation assumes a 60 kg subject).

Pregnancy, Nursing Mothers and Pediatric Use
EDEX is not indicated for use in women or pediatric patients.

Geriatric Use
Of the approximately 1,065 patients who entered the in-office dose-titration period in clinical studies, 25% were 65 years or older. In clinical studies, geriatric patients required, on average, higher minimally effective doses and had a higher rate of lack of effect (optimum dose not determined). Overall differences in safety were not observed between these geriatric patients and younger patients. Geriatric patients should be dosed and titrated according to the same DOSAGE AND ADMINISTRATION recommendations as younger patients, and the lowest possible effective dose should always be used.

ADVERSE REACTIONS
EDEX, administered by intracavernous injection in doses ranging from 1 to 40 mcg per injection for periods up to 24 months, has been evaluated in clinical trials for safety in over 1,065 patients with erectile dysfunction. Discontinuation of therapy due to a side effect in clinical trials was required in approximately 9% of patients treated with EDEX and in <1% of patients treated with placebo.

Local Adverse Reactions
The following local adverse reactions were reported in studies including 1,065 patients treated with EDEX for up to two years.

Penile Pain: With use of up to 24 months, penile pain was reported at least once by 29% of patients during injection, 35% of patients during erection, and by 30% of patients after erection. On a per injection basis, 15% of injections were associated with penile pain. Penile pain was judged by patients to be mild in intensity for 80% of painful injections, moderate in intensity for 16% of painful injections, and severe in intensity for 4% of painful injections. The frequency of penile pain reports decreased over time; forty-one percent of the patients experienced pain during the first 2 months and 3% of the patients experienced pain during months 21–24. In placebo-controlled studies, penile pain was reported by 31% of patients after EDEX and by 9% of patients after placebo injection.

Prolonged Erection/Priapism: Prolonged erections greater than four hours in duration occurred in 4% of all patients treated up to 24 months. In placebo-controlled studies, 3% of patients treated with EDEX and <1% of patients treated with placebo reported prolonged erections greater than four hours. The incidence of priapism (erections greater than 6 hours in duration) was <1% with long-term use for up to 24 months. In the majority of cases, spontaneous detumescence occurred. A higher incidence of prolonged erections was found in younger patients (<40 years), nondiabetic patients, and patients with psychogenic etiology of erectile dysfunction. (See WARNINGS.)

Hematoma/Ecchymosis: In patients treated with EDEX for up to 24 months, local bleeding, hematoma and ecchymosis were observed in 15%, 5% and 4% of patients, respectively. In placebo-controlled studies, the frequency of local bleeding was 6% with injection of EDEX and 3% with injection of placebo. In most cases, these reactions were attributed to faulty injection technique.

**Local Adverse Reactions
Reported by ≥1% of Patients
All Study Periods***

Local Reaction	EDEX (N = 1065) n (%)
Penile pain during injection	305 (29)
Penile pain during erection	368 (35)
Penile pain after erection	317 (30)
Penile pain (other)**	116 (11)
Prolonged erection	
> 4 ≤ 6 Hours	44 (4)
> 6 Hours	6 (<1)
Bleeding	158 (15)
Hematoma	56 (5)
Ecchymosis	44 (4)
Penile angulation	72 (7)
Penile fibrosis	52 (5)
Cavernous body fibrosis	20 (2)
Peyronie's disease	11 (1)
Faulty injection technique***	59 (6)
Penis disorder	28 (3)
Erythema	17 (2)

* Protocol Numbers KU-620-001, KU-620-002, KU-620-003, F-8653.
** Penile pain reported without an association to injection site or erection, such as pain in penis and scrotum, pain in glans penis, and burning penile pain.
*** Examples include injection into glans penis, urethra or subcutaneously.

Systemic Adverse Experiences
The following systemic adverse experiences were reported in controlled and uncontrolled studies in ≥1% of patients treated for up to 24 months with EDEX.

**Systemic Adverse Experiences Reported
by ≥1% of Patients***

BODY SYSTEM Adverse Experience	EDEX N = 1065 n (%)
RESPIRATORY	
Upper respiratory tract infection	58 (5)
Sinusitis	14 (1)

Continued on next page

Edex—Cont.

BODY AS A WHOLE	
Influenza-like symptoms	35 (3)
Headache	20 (2)
Infection	18 (2)
Pain	16 (2)

MUSCULOSKELETAL	
Back pain	23 (2)
Leg pain	13 (1)

CARDIOVASCULAR	
Hypertension	17 (2)
Myocardial infarction	13 (1)
Abnormal ECG	12 (1)

METABOLIC/NUTRITIONAL	
Hypertriglyceridemia	17 (2)
Hypercholesterolemia	12 (1)
Hyperglycemia	12 (1)

UROGENITAL	
Prostate disorder	15 (1)
Testicular pain	13 (1)
Inguinal hernia	11 (1)

DERMATOLOGIC	
Skin disorder	14 (1)

SPECIAL SENSES	
Abnormal vision	11 (1)

*Protocol Numbers KU-620-001, KU-620-002, KU-620-003, F-8653.

Hemodynamic changes, manifested as increases or decreases in blood pressure and pulse rate, were observed during clinical studies but did not appear to be dose-dependent. Four patients (<1%) reported clinical symptoms of hypotension such as dizziness or syncope.

EDEX had no clinically important effect on serum or urine laboratory tests.

OVERDOSAGE

Limited data are available in regard to EDEX overdose in humans. Systemic reactions are uncommon with intracavernous injection of EDEX. Hypotension occurred in less than 1% of patients treated with EDEX. A single dose rising tolerance study in healthy volunteers indicated that single **intravenous** doses of alprostadil from 1 to 120 mcg were well tolerated. Beginning with a 40 mcg bolus **intravenous** dose, the frequency of drug-related systemic adverse events increased in a dose-dependent manner, characterized mainly by facial flushing.

The primary symptom of an EDEX overdose is a prolonged erection or priapism. Because of the potential for tissue hypoxia and possible necrosis, it is strongly recommended to treat an erection lasting more than 6 hours. **The patient is strongly encouraged to go to the nearest emergency room if his personal physician is not available.**

In the event of an overdose, supportive therapy according to the presence of other symptoms is recommended.

DOSAGE AND ADMINISTRATION

EDEX in the Treatment of Erectile Dysfunction
The dosage range of EDEX for the treatment of erectile dysfunction is 1 to 40 mcg. The intracavernous injection should be given over a 5 to 10 second interval. In a study with a dose range of 1 to 20 mcg of EDEX, the mean dose was 10.7 mcg at the end of the dose titration period. In two studies with a dose range of 1 to 40 mcg of EDEX, the mean dose was 21.9 mcg at the end of the dose titration period. Doses greater than 40 mcg have not been studied. A 1/2 inch, 27 or 30 gauge needle is generally recommended for the intracavernous injection. The patient is advised not to exceed the optimum EDEX dose which was determined in the doctor's office. The lowest possible effective dose should always be used.

Initial Titration in Physician's Office
Erectile Dysfunction of Vasculogenic, Psychogenic, or Mixed Etiology: Dosage titration should be initiated at 2.5 micrograms of alprostadil. If there is a partial response, the dose may be increased by 2.5 micrograms to a dose of 5 micrograms and then in increments of 5 to 10 micrograms, depending upon erectile response, until the dose that produces an erection suitable for intercourse and not exceeding a duration of 1 hour is reached. If there is no response to the initial 2.5-microgram dose, the second dose may be increased to 7.5 micrograms, followed by increments of 5 to 10 micrograms. The patient must stay in the physician's office until complete detumescence occurs. If there is no response, then the next higher dose may be given within 1 hour. If there is a response, then there should be at least a 1-day interval before the next dose is given.

Erectile Dysfunction of Pure Neurogenic Etiology (Spinal Cord Injury): Dosage titration should be initiated at 1.25

micrograms of alprostadil using the EDEX vial. The dose may be increased by 1.25 micrograms to a dose of 2.5 micrograms, followed by an increment of 2.5 micrograms to a dose of 5 micrograms, and then in 5-microgram increments until the dose that produces an erection suitable for intercourse and not exceeding a duration of 1 hour is reached. The patient must stay in the physician's office until complete detumescence occurs. If there is no response, then the next higher dose may be given within 1 hour. If there is a response, then there should be at least a 1-day interval before the next dose is given.

At-Home (Maintenance Therapy) Dosing Instructions
The first injections of EDEX must be done at the physician's office by medically trained personnel. Self-injection therapy by the patient can be started only after the patient is properly instructed and well trained in the self-injection technique. When using the single-dose vials, the physician should instruct the patient on the appropriate needles to use for reconstitution and injection. The physician should instruct the patient to discard any needles which become bent during the reconstitution or self-injection procedure as these needles may break. The physician should make a careful assessment of the patient's skills and competence with the self-injection procedure. The intracavernous injection must be done under sterile conditions. The site of injection is usually along the lateral aspect of the proximal third of the penis. Visible veins should be avoided. The side of the penis that is injected and the site of injection must be alternated. The injection site must be cleansed with an alcohol swab before injection.

The dose of EDEX that is selected for self-injection treatment should provide the patient with an erection that is satisfactory for sexual intercourse and that is maintained for no longer than 1 hour. If the duration of erection is longer than 1 hour, the dose of EDEX should be reduced. The lowest effective dose should be used at home. Self-injection therapy for use at home should be initiated at the dose that was determined in the physician's office. Dose adjustment may be required and should be made only after consultation with the physician.

Careful and continuous follow-up of the patient while in the self-injection program must be exercised. This is especially true for the initial self-injections, since adjustments in the dose of EDEX may be needed. The recommended frequency of injection is no more than 3 times weekly, with at least 24 hours between each dose. **The reconstituted EDEX vial or cartridge and the needles are intended for single use only and should be discarded after use.** The user should be instructed in the proper disposal of the syringes, needles, vials or cartridges.

While on self-injection treatment, it is recommended that the patient visit the prescribing physician's office every 3 months. At that time, the efficacy and safety of the therapy should be assessed, and the dose of EDEX should be adjusted, if needed.

The patient is instructed to follow the enclosed patient information pamphlet.

Preparation of Solution
The EDEX vial is intended for intracavernous injection only after reconstitution of the powder with 1.2 mL of sterile 0.9% sodium chloride. The EDEX diluent (sterile 0.9% sodium chloride) in the pre-filled syringe supplied in the kit is only for reconstitution of the dry powder in the EDEX vial. The EDEX injection device is used to reconstitute the single-dose, dual-chamber cartridge. The threaded portion of the plunger is used to force the sterile 0.9% sodium chloride (1.075 mL) in one chamber into the chamber containing alprostadil. After reconstitution, the EDEX injection device is used to administer the intracavernous injection of alprostadil. The reusable EDEX injection device is for use only with the cartridges and needles included in the EDEX Cartridge Starter Pack or Refill Pack.

Prepare the EDEX solution immediately before use. Do not administer unless solution is clear. Do not add any drugs or solutions to the EDEX solution. Discard any unused solution remaining in the vial. The reconstituted solution should not be stored.

The EDEX vial and cartridge contain a solid layer or lyophilized cake of dry white powder approximately 3/16" in thickness for the vial and 3/8" in thickness for the cartridge. A normal cake may appear cracked or crumbled. If the vial or cartridge is damaged, the cake may shrink in size. Do not use the vial or cartridge if they appear damaged or the cake is substantially reduced in size.

Parenteral drug products should be inspected visually for particulate matter and discoloration prior to administration. The reconstituted solution may initially appear cloudy due to small air bubbles. Do not use the solution if it remains cloudy, contains precipitates, or is discolored.

CAUTION: Do not reuse any solution remaining in the vial due to the possibility of bacterial contamination.

Administration
EDEX is given as an intracavernous injection over a 5 to 10 second interval. See patient information for EDEX.

Stability
The single-dose vials and the single-dose, ignore-chamber cartridges should be reconstituted only when it is certain

that the patient is ready to administer the drug. The reconstituted drug solution should be used immediately after reconstitution. Any solution remaining in the vial should be discarded.

HOW SUPPLIED

EDEX (alprostadil for injection) is supplied as a white, sterile, lyophilized powder in single-dose vials containing either 6.225, 12.45, 24.90 or 49.80 mcg of alprostadil. When reconstituted with 1.2 mL of sterile 0.9% sodium chloride, the deliverable amount of alprostadil in each milliliter is 5, 10, 20 or 40 micrograms, respectively. The single-dose vials are supplied individually in a package of six or in a kit which also contains a syringe pre-filled with 1.2 mL of sterile 0.9% sodium chloride, one plunger rod, a 1/2 inch 27 gauge needle, a 1/2 inch 30 gauge needle, one alcohol swab for the top of the vial, one alcohol swab for the injection site and tape to secure the kit after use.

EDEX is supplied in the following packages:
Individual Vials

5 mcg	6 Individual Vials	NDC 0091-1005-06
10 mcg	6 Individual Vials	NDC 0091-1010-06
20 mcg	6 Individual Vials	NDC 0091-1020-06
40 mcg	6 Individual Vials	NDC 0091-1040-06

Kits (include one EDEX vial, one pre-filled diluent syringe, two needles and two alcohol swabs)

5 mcg	4 Kits	NDC 0091-1005-44
10 mcg	4 Kits	NDC 0091-1010-44
20 mcg	4 Kits	NDC 0091-1020-44
40 mcg	4 Kits	NDC 0091-1040-44

EDEX is also available in single-dose, dual-chamber cartridges intended for use with the reusable EDEX injection device. One chamber of the cartridge contains 10.75, 21.5 or 43.0 mcg of alprostadil as a white, sterile, lyophilized powder. The other chamber contains 1.075 mL of sterile 0.9% sodium chloride. When the cartridge is placed into the EDEX injection device and reconstituted, the deliverable amount of alprostadil in each milliliter is 10, 20, or 40 micrograms, respectively. EDEX Cartridge Starter Pack contains one reusable EDEX injection device, two single-dose, dual-chamber cartridges, two ½ inch, 29 gauge (0.33 mm x 12.7 mm) needles, and four alcohol swabs. EDEX Cartridge Refill Pack contains two single-dose, dual-chamber cartridges, two ½ inch, 29 gauge (0.33 mm x 12.7 mm) needles, and four alcohol swabs.

The EDEX cartridges are supplied in the following packages:
EDEX Cartridge Starter Pack (includes one injection device, two cartridges, two needles and four alcohol swabs)

10 mcg	1 Starter Pack	NDC 0091-1110-11
20 mcg	1 Starter Pack	NDC 0091-1120-11
40 mcg	1 Starter Pack	NDC 0091-1140-11

EDEX Cartridge Refill Pack (includes two cartridges, two needles and four alcohol swabs)

10 mcg	1 Refill Pack	NDC 0091-1027-22
20 mcg	1 Refill Pack	NDC 0091-1029-22
40 mcg	1 Refill Pack	NDC 0091-1032-22

Store at 25°C (77°F); excursions permitted between 15°–30°C (59°–86°F).
PC3556   6/98

PATIENT INFORMATION FOR EDEX KIT

Please read carefully before using.

EDEX can only be obtained with a prescription from your doctor. You or your partner should be fully trained on the proper injection technique before using EDEX at home. Be sure to use only the dose prescribed by your doctor.

This leaflet provides a summary of information about your medicine. Please read this information carefully before you prepare the EDEX solution.

Carefully follow the instructions for administration which are described below. For further information or advice, ask your doctor or pharmacist.

Please keep this information in case you need to refer to it again.

Erectile Dysfunction: Causes and Treatments

There are several causes of erectile dysfunction, commonly known as impotence. These include impaired blood circulation in the penis, nerve damage, hormonal imbalances, excessive alcohol use, emotional problems, and certain medications that you may be taking for other conditions.

Smoking has an adverse effect on erectile function by accentuating the effects of other risk factors such as blood vessel disease or high blood pressure. Erectile dysfunction is often due to more than one of these causes.

Treatment for erectile dysfunction includes penile injections, medical devices that produce an erection, surgical procedures (eg, penile bypass or implants), hormone treatment, psychological counseling, lifestyle changes, or a change in medication. You should not stop taking any prescription medications, unless told to do so by your doctor. Your doctor has prescribed EDEX, a penile injection, to treat your erectile dysfunction.

Use of EDEX
EDEX is injected into a specific area of the penis (see injection directions below) and should produce an erection in 5 to 20 minutes. The erection can be expected to last up to one hour. You should not use EDEX more than three times a week. Injections should be administered at least 24 hours apart.

Ideally, the injection should be administered just prior to foreplay. If your partner experiences insufficient vaginal lubrication or painful vaginal sensations during intercourse, the use of a lubricant may be helpful.

Who should NOT use EDEX?
Men who have conditions that might result in long-lasting erections should not use EDEX. Some of these conditions include sickle cell anemia or trait, leukemia, and tumor of the bone marrow (multiple myeloma). If you have any of these conditions, consult your doctor.

Men with penile implants, severe penile curvature, or those who have been advised not to engage in sexual activity should not use EDEX. EDEX should not be used by women or children.

What are the risks of using EDEX?
Erections that last more than 6 hours can cause serious damage to the penile tissue and may result in permanent impotence.

Call the prescribing physician or, if unavailable, seek professional help immediately if you still have an erection 6 hours after injection. Various treatment options for reversing a prolonged erection are available.

A common side effect of EDEX is mild to moderate pain during injection. The erection may also be associated with a painful sensation. If you experience severe pain, contact the prescribing physician.

Call your doctor if you notice any redness, lumps, swelling, tenderness, or curvature of the erect penis.

A small amount of bleeding at the injection site may occur. To prevent bruising, apply firm pressure to the injection site for 5 minutes. Tell your doctor if you have a condition or are taking a medicine that interferes with blood clotting.

NOTE: EDEX offers no protection from the transmission of sexually transmitted diseases such as HIV (the virus that causes AIDS). Small amounts of bleeding at the injection site can increase the risk of transmission of blood-borne diseases between partners.

There is no approved injectable treatment using multiple medications. In addition, there are no data on the efficacy and safety of these combinations.

PATIENT INSTRUCTIONS FOR SELF-INJECTION
EDEX Kit Supplies
(See Figure A)

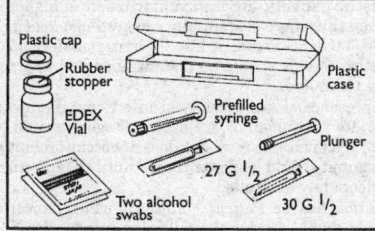

Figure A

Your kit should contain the following items:
Patient Information for EDEX
One EDEX vial
One syringe prefilled with 1.2 mL of diluent (sterile 0.9% sodium chloride)
One plunger rod
A 27 gauge $\frac{1}{2}$ inch sterile needle (27 G $\frac{1}{2}$)
A 30 gauge $\frac{1}{2}$ inch sterile needle (30 G $\frac{1}{2}$)
Two alcohol swabs
Tape

Storage and Handling
1. Store at room temperature between 15°-30°C (59°-86°F). As with any drug product, extremes in temperature should be avoided. When traveling, do not store in checked luggage during air travel or leave in a closed automobile.
2. EDEX solution should be used immediately after reconstitution.
3. Discard unused EDEX solution.

IMPORTANT: To maintain sterility and avoid contamination, follow these directions carefully.

Self-injection Procedure
Before using EDEX, you should be properly trained by your doctor. Your doctor should instruct you on the appropriate needles to use for reconstitution and injection. Mix EDEX just prior to injection. Your dose has been customized for your individual needs. Use only the dose prescribed by your doctor. Have a clean area available to assemble the items necessary for your EDEX injection.

READ THE INSTRUCTIONS COMPLETELY BEFORE STARTING YOUR SELF-INJECTION PROCEDURE.

Prepare EDEX Solution
1. Wash your hands thoroughly with soap and water and dry them with a clean towel.
2. Pick up the prefilled syringe by grasping the syringe barrel. Insert the plunger rod into the open end of the syringe. Attach the threaded end of the plunger rod to the rubber stopper by turning clockwise (Figure B).

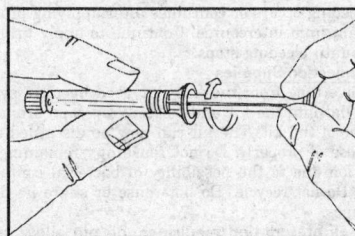

Figure B

Remove the cap from the syringe tip (Figure C).

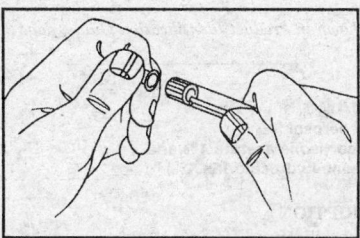

Figure C

Be careful not to accidentally push the plunger or touch the sterile syringe tip.
3. While holding the uncapped syringe, pick up the gray wrapper containing the capped 27 G $\frac{1}{2}$ needle and open it carefully by pulling the wrapper tabs back to expose the base of the needle (Figure D).

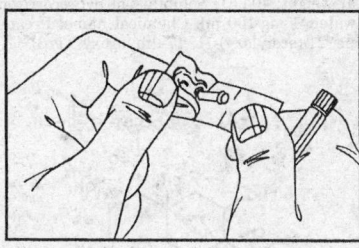

Figure D

Do not touch the sterile base of the needle.
4. Attach the needle to the syringe tip (turn clockwise) (Figure E).

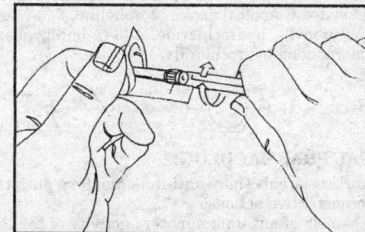

Figure E

Do not remove the needle cap. Set the syringe and needle down on a clean, level surface.
5. Remove the plastic cap from the EDEX vial.
6. Cleanse the rubber stopper on the EDEX vial by wiping it with an alcohol swab. Discard this alcohol swab.

7. Pick up the syringe barrel (not the plunger), hold horizontally, and carefully remove the needle cap (Figure F).

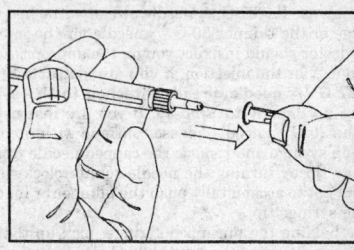

Figure F

Do not discard the needle cap; you will need to use it later. Do not touch the exposed needle or allow the needle to touch anything.
8. Insert the needle through the center of the vial's rubber stopper. Push down on the syringe plunger to expel all the diluent into the vial (Figure G).

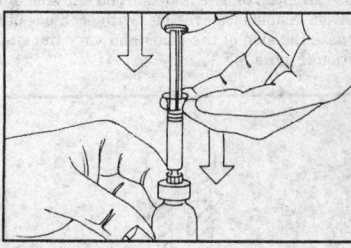

Figure G

Do not remove the needle from the vial. Holding the syringe and vial as a unit, gently swirl vial to mix and dissolve the drug. Do not shake the solution. Swirl until solution is clear. Do not use the solution if it is cloudy, colored, or contains particles.
9. With needle still inserted in the vial, turn the vial and needle/syringe upside down and hold firmly in one hand. Keeping the needle tip below the level of fluid, slowly withdraw the plunger until the amount of the solution is level with the dosage volume your doctor prescribed (Figure H).

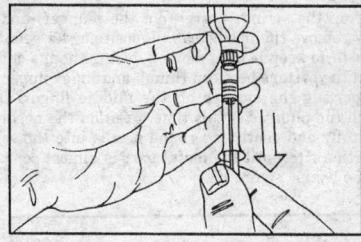

Figure H

If air bubbles appear in the syringe, withdraw more than your prescribed dose. Gently tap the side of the syringe barrel with your finger until trapped air bubbles float to the top of the solution (Figure I).

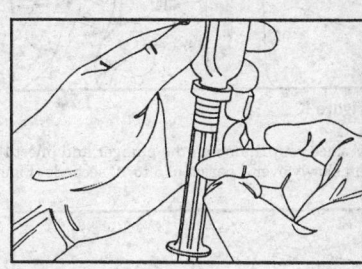

Figure I

Push the plunger to expel air and to reach the correct volume mark for your prescribed dose. If you do not have the correct dose, completely expel the solution back into the vial and slowly withdraw your dose again. **Note: If the dosage prescribed by your doctor is less than 1 mL of EDEX solution, you will not need to withdraw the entire amount of drug solution to reach your prescribed dose.**
10. Remove the needle/syringe from the EDEX vial by grasping the syringe barrel (not the plunger). Recap the needle and set the syringe down on a clean, level surface.

Continued on next page

Edex—Cont.

11. You may use the 27 G $^1/_2$ needle already attached to the syringe or the thinner 30 G $^1/_2$ needle for the injection. Your doctor should instruct you on the appropriate needle to use for the injection. **If you are instructed to use the 27 G $^1/_2$ needle already attached to the syringe, please go directly to *Step 15*.** If you are instructed to use the 30 G $^1/_2$ needle, please continue with *Step 12*.

12. Pick up syringe and remove the capped needle from the syringe tip by turning the needle counterclockwise. Be careful not to accidentally push the plunger or touch the sterile syringe tip.

13. While holding the uncapped syringe, pick up the beige wrapper containing the capped 30 G $^1/_2$ needle and open it carefully by pulling the wrapper tabs back to expose the base of the needle. Do not touch the sterile base of the needle.

14. Attach the needle to the syringe tip (turn clockwise). Do not remove the needle cap. Set the syringe and needle down on a clean, level surface.

Select Injection Site

15. Choose an injection site mid-shaft on one side of the penis. Avoid visible blood vessels. With each use of EDEX, alternate the side of the penis and vary the site of the injection (Figure J).

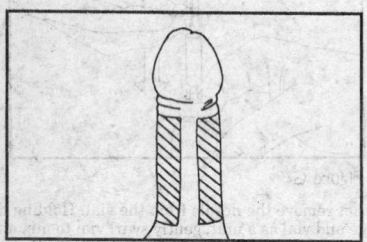

Figure J

If your penis is not circumcised, pull the foreskin back. Grasping the head of the penis with your thumb and forefinger, stretch it lengthwise along your thigh so that you can clearly see the selected injection site. Wipe the injection site with a new alcohol swab. Do not discard this swab; you will need to use it later.

Inject EDEX

16. Pick up the syringe barrel (not the plunger) and carefully remove the needle cap. Reposition the penis as in *Step 15* to keep it from moving during the injection.

17. Hold the syringe between thumb and index finger while supporting the syringe on the middle finger. Do not touch the plunger at this time. Position the needle horizontally and gently insert the needle into the selected injection site until the metal part is almost completely in the penis (Figure K).

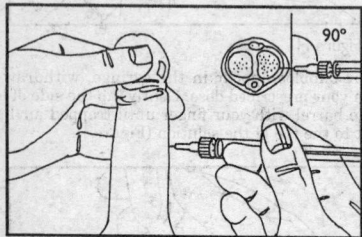

Figure K

Now place your thumb on the plunger and inject the solution slowly over a period of 5 to 10 seconds (Figure L).

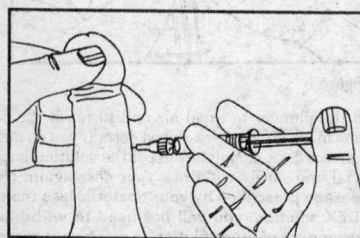

Figure L

18. If the solution does not inject easily, or if you immediately experience a burning pain at the injection site, reposition the needle by advancing it slightly or by withdrawing it until the solution can be injected easily and painlessly.

19. Withdraw needle from penis. Immediately apply firm but gentle pressure with the alcohol swab to injection site for five minutes to prevent bruising (Figure M).

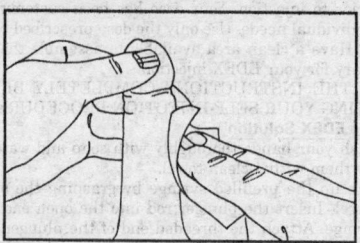

Figure M

If bleeding occurs or continues after applying pressure, abstain from intercourse. Continue to apply firm pressure until bleeding stops.

Discard Injection Supplies

20. Remove tape from the kit. Put used needles, syringe, and vial into the kit and close. Wrap tape around the center of the kit. The kit can now be discarded safely. Dispose of properly. Do not reuse any remaining drug solution due to the possibility of bacterial contamination. Do not recycle. Do not reuse or share needles or syringes.

As with all prescription medicines, do not allow anyone else to use your medication. Proper injection technique and individual dose titration are essential for the safe use of this product.

CAUTION: Federal law prohibits dispensing without prescription.

PC2505   6/96

Shown in Product Identification Guide, page 337

EPIFOAM®   ℞
topical aerosol
(hydrocortisone acetate 1% and
pramoxine hydrochloride 1%)

DESCRIPTION

A topical corticosteroid in an aerosol foam containing hydrocortisone acetate 1% and pramoxine hydrochloride 1% in a base containing: propylene glycol, cetyl alcohol, glyceryl monostearate and PEG 100 stearate blend, laureth-23, polyoxyl-40 stearate, methylparaben, propylparaben, trolamine, hydrochloric acid to adjust pH, purified water, propellants (inert): isobutane and propane.

EPIFOAM® contains a synthetic steroid used as an anti-inflammatory and antipruritic agent, and a local anesthetic.

Hydrocortisone acetate

Molecular weight: 404.51. Solubility of hydrocortisone acetate in water: 1 mg/100 ml. Chemical name: Pregn-4-ene-3,20-dione, 21-(acetyloxy)-11, 17-dihydroxy- (11β).

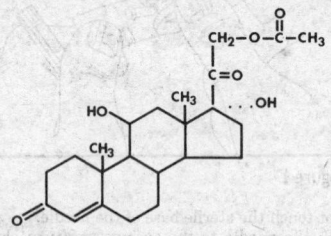

Pramoxine hydrochloride

Molecular weight: 329.87. Pramoxine hydrochloride is freely soluble in water. Chemical name: Morpholine, 4-[3-(4-butoxyphenoxy) propyl]-, hydrochloride, 4-[3-(*p*-butoxyphenoxy) propyl] morpholine hydrochloride.

$$CH_3CH_2CH_2CH_2O \!-\!\bigcirc\!-\!OCH_2CH_2CH_2N\bigcirc C^+HCl$$

CLINICAL PHARMACOLOGY

Topical corticosteroids share anti-inflammatory, antipruritic and vasoconstrictive actions.

The mechanism of anti-inflammatory activity of the topical corticosteroids is unclear. Various laboratory methods, including vasoconstrictor assays, are used to compare and predict potencies and/or clinical efficacies of the topical corticosteroids. There is some evidence to suggest that a recognizable correlation exists between vasoconstrictor potency and therapeutic efficacy in man.

PRAMOXINE HYDROCHLORIDE: A surface or local anesthetic which is not chemically related to the "caine" types of local anesthetics. Its unique chemical structure is likely to minimize the danger of cross-sensitivity reactions in patients allergic to other local anesthetics.

Pharmacokinetics: The extent of percutaneous absorption of topical corticosteroids is determined by many factors including the vehicle, the integrity of the epidermal barrier, and the use of occlusive dressings.

Topical corticosteroids can be absorbed from normal intact skin. Inflammation and/or disease processes in the skin increase the percutaneous absorption of topical corticosteroids. Occlusive dressings substantially increase the percutaneous absorption of topical corticosteroids. Thus, occlusive dressings may be a valuable therapeutic adjunct for treatment of resistant dermatoses. (See DOSAGE AND ADMINISTRATION.)

Once absorbed through the skin, topical corticosteroids are handled through pharmacokinetic pathways similar to systemically administered corticosteroids. Corticosteroids are bound to plasma proteins in varying degrees. Corticosteroids are metabolized primarily in the liver and are then excreted by the kidneys. Some of the topical corticosteroids and their metabolites are also excreted into the bile.

INDICATIONS AND USAGE

Topical corticosteroids are indicated for the relief of the inflammatory and pruritic manifestations of corticosteroid-responsive dermatoses.

CONTRAINDICATIONS

Topical corticosteroid products are contraindicated in those patients with a history of hypersensitivity to any of the components of the preparation.

WARNINGS

Not for prolonged use. If redness, pain, irritation or swelling persists, discontinue use and consult a physician. Contents of the container are under pressure. Do not puncture or incinerate. Do not store at temperatures above 120°F. Keep this and all medicines out of the reach of children.

PRECAUTIONS

General: Systemic absorption of topical corticosteroids has produced reversible hypothalamic-pituitary-adrenal (HPA) axis suppression, manifestations of Cushing's syndrome, hyperglycemia and glucosuria in some patients.

Conditions which augment systemic absorption include the application of the more potent steroids, use over large surface areas, prolonged use and the addition of occlusive dressings.

Therefore, patients receiving a large dose of a potent topical steroid applied to a large surface area or under an occlusive dressing should be evaluated periodically for evidence of HPA axis suppression by using the urinary free cortisol and ACTH stimulation tests. If HPA axis suppression is noted, an attempt should be made to withdraw the drug, to reduce the frequency of application, or to substitute a less potent steroid.

Recovery of HPA axis function is generally prompt and complete upon discontinuation of the drug. Infrequently, signs and symptoms of steroid withdrawal may occur, requiring supplemental systemic corticosteroids.

In pediatric patients, absorption may result in higher blood levels and thus more susceptibility to systemic toxicity. (See PRECAUTIONS—Pediatric Use.) If irritation develops, topical corticosteroids should be discontinued and appropriate therapy instituted.

In the presence of dermatological infections, the use of an appropriate antifungal or antibacterial agent should be instituted. If a favorable response does not occur promptly, the corticosteroid should be discontinued until the infection has been adequately controlled.

Information for the Patient: Patients using topical corticosteroids should receive the following information and instructions:

1. This medication is to be used as directed by the physician. It is for external use only. Avoid contact with the eyes.

2. Do not use this medication for any disorder other than for which it has been prescribed.

3. The treated skin area should not be bandaged or otherwise covered or wrapped as to be occlusive unless directed by the physician.

4. Report any signs of local adverse reactions especially under occlusive dressings.

5. Do not use any tight fitting diapers or plastic pants on a pediatric patient being treated in the diaper area, as these garments may constitute occlusive dressings.

Laboratory Tests: The following tests may be helpful in evaluating the HPA axis suppression:

Urinary free cortisol test

ACTH stimulation test

Carcinogenesis, Mutagenesis, and Impairment of Fertility: Long-term animal studies have not been performed to evaluate carcinogenic potential or the effect on fertility of topical corticosteroids.

Studies to determine mutagenicity with prednisolone and hydrocortisone have revealed negative results.

Pregnancy Category C: Corticosteroids are generally teratogenic in laboratory animals when administered systemically at relatively low dosage levels. The more potent corticosteroids have been shown to be teratogenic after dermal application in laboratory animals. There are no adequate and well-controlled studies in pregnant women of teratogenic effects from topically applied corticosteroids. Therefore, topical corticosteroids should be used during pregnancy only if the potential benefit justifies the potential risk to the fetus. Drugs of this class should not be used extensively on pregnant patients, in large amounts, or for prolonged periods of time.

Nursing Mothers: It is not known whether topical administration of corticosteroids could result in sufficient systemic absorption to produce detectable quantities in breast milk. Systemically administered corticosteroids are secreted into breast milk in quantities not likely to have a deleterious effect on the infant. Caution should be exercised when any topical corticosteroids are administered to a nursing woman.

Pediatric Use: PEDIATRIC PATIENTS MAY DEMONSTRATE GREATER SUSCEPTIBILITY TO TOPICAL CORTICOSTEROID-INDUCED HPA AXIS SUPPRESSION AND CUSHING'S SYNDROME THAN MATURE PATIENTS BECAUSE OF A LARGER SKIN SURFACE AREA TO BODY WEIGHT RATIO.

Hypothalamic-pituitary-adrenal (HPA) axis suppression, Cushing's syndrome and intracranial hypertension have been reported in pediatric patients receiving topical corticosteroids. Manifestations of adrenal suppression in pediatric patients include linear growth retardation, delayed weight gain, low plasma cortisone levels and absence of response to ACTH stimulation. Manifestations of intracranial hypertension include bulging fontanelles, headaches and bilateral papilledema.

Administration of topical corticosteroids to pediatric patients should be limited to the least amount compatible with an effective therapeutic regimen. Chronic corticosteroid therapy may interfere with the growth and development of pediatric patients.

ADVERSE REACTIONS

The following local adverse reactions are reported infrequently with topical corticosteroids, but may occur more frequently with the use of occlusive dressings. These reactions are listed in an approximately decreasing order of occurrence: Burning, Itching, Irritation, Dryness, Folliculitis, Hypertrichosis, Acneiform eruptions, Hypopigmentation, Perioral dermatitis, Allergic contact dermatitis, Maceration of the skin, Secondary infection, Skin atrophy, Striae, Miliaria.

OVERDOSAGE

Topically applied corticosteroids can be absorbed in sufficient amounts to produce systemic effects. (See PRECAUTIONS.)

DOSAGE AND ADMINISTRATION

Apply to affected area 3 to 4 times daily.
Occlusive dressings may be used for the management of psoriasis or recalcitrant conditions. If an infection develops, the use of occlusive dressings should be discontinued and appropriate antimicrobial therapy instituted.
DIRECTIONS FOR USE:
1. Shake the container vigorously for 5–10 seconds before each use.
2. While holding container upright, prime the container by pressing down several times on container cap until foam appears. Apply a small amount directly to affected area 3–4 times daily depending on severity of the condition. Alternatively, dispense a small amount to a pad and apply to affected areas.
   NOTE: The aerosol container should never be inserted into vagina or anus.
3. The container and cap should be disassembled and rinsed with warm water after use.

HOW SUPPLIED

EPIFOAM® is supplied in 10 g pressurized cans.
10 g   (NDC 0091-0740-10)
Store upright at controlled room temperature 15°–30°C (59°–86°F). Do not refrigerate.
CAUTION: Federal law prohibits dispensing without prescription.
PC2202A   Rev. 10/96
Shown in Product Identification Guide, page 337

KUTRASE® Capsules   ℞
[*qū 'trās*]

DESCRIPTION

KUTRASE® Capsules contain four standardized digestive enzymes: lipase, amylase, protease, cellulase, and hyoscyamine sulfate USP and phenyltoloxamine citrate. Lipase, amylase, protease and cellulase are derived from fungal, plant and animal sources and are oral digestive enzyme supplements. Hyoscyamine sulfate USP is one of the principal anticholinergic/antispasmodic components of belladonna alkaloids. Phenyltoloxamine citrate is a non-barbiturate sedative. Each capsule contains:

lipase	1,200 USP Units
amylase	30 mg
protease	6 mg
cellulase	2 mg
hyoscyamine sulfate USP	0.0625 mg
phenyltoloxamine citrate	15 mg

Each capsule also contains as inactive ingredients: D&C yellow #10, ethylcellulose, FD&C green #3, FD&C yellow #6, gelatin, lactose, magnesium stearate, titanium dioxide, vanillin and other ingredients.

CLINICAL PHARMACOLOGY

Diminution of secretions from exocrine glands is often a result of the normal aging process. KUTRASE provides a balanced combination of natural proteolytic, amylolytic, cellulolytic and lipolytic enzymes to enhance digestion of proteins, starch and fat in the gastrointestinal tract. These enzymes do not exert any systemic pharmacologic effects. KUTRASE should be considered an enzyme supplement and not an enzyme replacement therapy. Enzymes in KUTRASE are basically derived from fungal and plant sources and possess a broad spectrum of pH activity. Enzymes are promptly released from the capsule and are bioavailable for digestion of food in the stomach and intestines. Hyoscyamine sulfate provides a potent spasmolytic effect in reducing gastrointestinal hypermotility and intestinal spasm. A mild sedative effect is provided by phenyltoloxamine citrate.

INDICATIONS AND USAGE

KUTRASE is indicated for the relief of the symptoms of functional indigestion devoid of organic pathology commonly referred to as nervous indigestion and colloquially as "butterflies". The symptoms are bloating, gas, and fullness.

CONTRAINDICATIONS

KUTRASE is contraindicated in patients with glaucoma, obstructive uropathy, obstructive disease of the gastrointestinal tract (as in achalasia, pyloroduodenal stenosis), paralytic ileus, intestinal atony of elderly or debilitated patients, unstable cardiovascular status in acute hemorrhage, severe ulcerative colitis, toxic megacolon complicating ulcerative colitis, or myasthenia gravis. KUTRASE is contraindicated in patients known to be hypersensitive to pork protein and in patients with acute pancreatitis or with acute exacerbations of chronic pancreatic diseases.

WARNINGS

Do not administer to patients who are allergic to pork products. Should hypersensitivity occur, discontinue medication and treat symptomatically. In the presence of high environmental temperature, heat prostration can occur with drug use (fever and heat stroke due to decreased sweating). Diarrhea may be an early symptom of incomplete intestinal obstruction, especially in patients with ileostomy or colostomy. In this instance, treatment with this drug would be inappropriate. KUTRASE may produce drowsiness, dizziness or blurred vision. In this event, the patient should be warned not to engage in activities requiring mental alertness such as operating a motor vehicle or other machinery or to perform hazardous work while taking this drug.

PRECAUTIONS

General:
Use with caution in patients with autonomic neuropathy, hyperthyroidism, coronary heart disease, congestive heart failure, cardiac arrhythmias, hypertension and renal disease. Investigate any tachycardia before giving any anticholinergic drug since they may increase the heart rate. Use with caution in patients with hiatal hernia associated with reflux esophagitis.
Information for Patients:
If capsules are opened, avoid inhalation of the powder. Sensitive individuals may experience allergic reactions.
Carcinogenesis, Mutagenesis, Impairment of Fertility:
Long-term studies in animals have not been performed to evaluate the carcinogenic, mutagenic or impairment of fertility potential of KUTRASE.
Pregnancy-Pregnancy Category C:
Animal reproduction studies have not been conducted with KUTRASE. It is also not known whether KUTRASE can cause fetal harm when administered to a pregnant woman or can affect reproduction capacity. KUTRASE should be given to a pregnant woman only if clearly needed.
Nursing Mothers:
Hyoscyamine sulfate is excreted in human milk. It is not known whether the enzymes or phenyltoloxamine citrate are excreted in human milk. Caution should be exercised when KUTRASE is administered to a nursing woman.

ADVERSE REACTIONS

Occasionally a slight looseness of the stools may be noticed. If so, dosage should be reduced. Finely powdered pancreatic enzyme may be irritating to the mucous membranes and respiratory tract. Inhalation of the airborne powder may precipitate an asthma attack in sensitive individuals. Other adverse reactions may include dryness of the mouth; urinary hesitancy and retention; blurred vision; tachycardia; palpitations; mydriasis; cycloplegia; increased ocular tension; loss of taste; headache; nervousness; drowsiness; weakness; dizziness; insomnia; nausea; vomiting; impotence; suppression of lactation; constipation; bloated feeling; allergic reactions or drug idiosyncrasies; urticaria and other dermal manifestations; ataxia; speech disturbance; some degree of mental confusion and/or excitement (especially in elderly persons); and decreased sweating.

OVERDOSAGE

The signs and symptoms of overdose are headache, nausea, vomiting, blurred vision, dilated pupils, hot dry skin, dizziness, dryness of the mouth, difficulty in swallowing and CNS stimulation.
Measures to be taken are immediate lavage of the stomach and injection of physostigmine 0.5 to 2 mg intravenously and repeated as necessary up to a total of 5 mg. Fever may be treated symptomatically. Excitement to a degree which demands attention may be managed with sodium thiopental 2% solution given slowly intravenously. In the event of paralysis of the respiratory muscles, artificial respiration should be instituted.

DOSAGE AND ADMINISTRATION

1 or 2 capsules taken with each meal or snack. Dosage may be adjusted according to the conditions and severity of symptoms to assure symptomatic control with a minimum of adverse effects.

HOW SUPPLIED

KUTRASE Capsules are green and white capsules and are imprinted "SCHWARZ" and "475."
Bottles of 100 capsules   NDC 0091-3475-01
Store at controlled room temperature 15°–30°C (59°–86°F).
Protect from high humidity.
CAUTION: Federal law prohibits dispensing without prescription.
PC0203H   Rev. 11/96

KU-ZYME® Capsules   ℞
[*qū ' zīm*]

DESCRIPTION

KU-ZYME® Capsules contain four standardized enzymes: lipase, amylase, protease and cellulase. They are derived from fungal, plant and animal sources and are designed for oral digestive enzyme supplement therapy.
Each capsule contains

lipase	1,200 USP Units
amylase	30 mg
protease	6 mg
cellulase	2 mg

Each capsule also contains as inactive ingredients: D&C Yellow #10, FD&C Yellow #6, gelatin, lactose, magnesium stearate, synthetic red iron oxide, titanium dioxide, and vanillin.

CLINICAL PHARMACOLOGY

Diminution of secretions from exocrine glands is often a result of the normal aging process. KU-ZYME provides a balanced combination of natural proteolytic, amylolytic, cellulolytic and lipolytic enzymes to enhance digestion of proteins, starch and fat in the gastrointestinal tract. These enzymes do not exert any systemic pharmacologic effects. KU-ZYME should be considered an enzyme supplement and not an enzyme replacement therapy. Enzymes in KU-ZYME are basically derived from fungal and plant sources and possess a broad spectrum of pH activity. Enzymes are promptly released from the capsule and are bioavailable for digestion of food in the stomach and intestines.

INDICATIONS AND USAGE

For the relief of functional indigestion when due to enzyme deficiency or imbalance. KU-ZYME relieves symptoms due to faulty digestion including the sensation of fullness after meals, dyspepsia, flatulence, abdominal distention and intolerance to certain foods.

CONTRAINDICATIONS

KU-ZYME is contraindicated in patients known to be hypersensitive to pork protein and in patients with acute pancreatitis or with acute exacerbations of chronic pancreatic diseases.

Continued on next page

Ku-Zyme—Cont.

WARNINGS

Do not administer to patients who are allergic to pork products. Should hypersensitivity occur, discontinue medication and treat symptomatically.

PRECAUTIONS

Information for Patients:
If capsules are opened, avoid inhalation of the powder. Sensitive individuals may experience allergic reactions.
Carcinogenesis, Mutagenesis, Impairment of Fertility:
Long-term studies in animals have not been performed to evaluate carcinogenic, mutagenic or impairment of fertility potential of KU-ZYME.
Pregnancy-Pregnancy Category C:
Animal reproduction studies have not been conducted with KU-ZYME. It is also not known whether KU-ZYME can cause fetal harm when administered to a pregnant woman or can affect reproduction capacity. KU-ZYME should be given to a pregnant woman only if clearly needed.
Nursing Mothers:
It is not known whether KU-ZYME is excreted in human milk. Because many drugs are excreted in human milk, caution should be exercised when KU-ZYME is administered to a nursing woman.

ADVERSE REACTIONS

Virtually unknown. Occasionally, a slight looseness of stools may be noticed. If so, dosage should be reduced. Finely powdered pancreatic enzyme may be irritating to the mucous membranes and respiratory tract. Inhalation of the airborne powder may precipitate an asthma attack in sensitive individuals.

OVERDOSAGE

No systemic toxicity occurs. Excessive dosage may, however, produce a laxative effect.

DOSAGE AND ADMINISTRATION

1 or 2 capsules taken with each meal or snack. Dosage may be adjusted depending on individual requirements for relief of symptoms due to digestive enzyme deficiency. In patients who experience difficulty in swallowing the capsule, it may be opened and the contents sprinkled on the food. When opening the capsules, avoid inhalation of the powder (see PRECAUTIONS and ADVERSE REACTIONS).

HOW SUPPLIED

KU-ZYME Capsules are yellow and white capsules and are imprinted "SCHWARZ" and "522".
Bottles of 100 capsules NDC 0091-3522-01
Store at controlled room temperature 15°–30°C (59°–86°F).
Protect from high humidity.
CAUTION: Federal law prohibits dispensing without prescription.
PC0208H Rev. 11/96

KU-ZYME® HP Capsules ℞

[qū ' zīm]
(pancrelipase capsules USP)

DESCRIPTION

KU-ZYME® HP Capsules (pancrelipase capsules USP) contain standardized lipase, amylase and protease obtained from hog pancreas and are designed for oral digestive enzyme replacement therapy. Each capsule contains:

lipase	8,000 USP Units
protease	30,000 USP Units
amylase	30,000 USP Units

Each capsule also contains as inactive ingredients: gelatin, lactose, magnesium stearate, titanium dioxide and other ingredients.

CLINICAL PHARMACOLOGY

Pancrelipase USP is a pancreatic enzyme concentrate, which hydrolyzes fats to glycerol and fatty acids, changes protein into proteoses and derived substances, and converts starch into dextrins and sugars. The administration of pancrelipase reduces the fat and nitrogen content in the stool. Pancreatic enzymes are normally secreted in great excess. Generally, steatorrhea and malabsorption occur only after a 90% or greater reduction in secretion of lipase and proteolytic enzymes. It has been estimated that approximately 8,000 units of lipase per hour should be delivered into the duodenum postprandially. Even if all the enzymes taken orally reached the proximal intestine in active form, ingestion of 24,000 units of lipase (8,000 units per hour) for 3 postprandial hours would be required. If one could deliver sufficient pancreatic enzymes to the small intestine, malabsorption could be corrected. It is rarely possible to achieve complete relief of steatorrhea although major improvement in fat absorption can be achieved in most patients.

INDICATIONS AND USAGE

KU-ZYME HP is effective in patients with deficient exocrine pancreatic secretions. Thus, KU-ZYME HP may be used as enzyme replacement therapy in cystic fibrosis, chronic pancreatitis, post pancreatectomy, in ductal obstructions caused by cancer of the pancreas, pancreatic insufficiency and for steatorrhea of malabsorption syndrome and post gastrectomy (Billroth II and Total). May also be used as a presumptive test for pancreatic function, especially in pancreatic insufficiency due to chronic pancreatitis.

CONTRAINDICATIONS

KU-ZYME HP is contraindicated in patients known to be hypersensitive to pork protein and in patients with acute pancreatitis or with acute exacerbations of chronic pancreatic diseases.

WARNINGS

Pancreatic exocrine replacement therapy should not delay or supplant treatment of the primary disorder. Should hypersensitivity occur, discontinue medication and treat symptomatically.

PRECAUTIONS

Information for Patients:
If capsules are opened, avoid inhalation of the powder. Sensitive individuals may experience allergic reactions.
Drug Interactions:
The serum iron response to oral iron may be decreased by concomitant administration of pancreatic extracts.
Carcinogenesis, Mutagenesis, Impairment of Fertility:
Long-term studies in animals have not been performed to evaluate the carcinogenic, mutagenic or impairment of fertility potential of KU-ZYME HP.
Pregnancy-Pregnancy Category C:
Animal reproduction studies have not been conducted with KU-ZYME HP. It is also not known whether KU-ZYME HP can cause fetal harm when administered to a pregnant woman or can affect reproduction capacity. KU-ZYME HP should be given to a pregnant woman only if clearly needed.
Nursing Mothers:
It is not known whether KU-ZYME HP is excreted in human milk. Because many drugs are excreted in human milk, caution should be exercised when KU-ZYME HP is administered to a nursing woman.

ADVERSE REACTIONS

High doses may cause nausea, abdominal cramps and/or diarrhea in certain patients. Finely powdered pancreatic enzyme concentrate may be irritating to the mucous membranes and respiratory tract. Inhalation of the airborne powder may precipitate an asthma attack in sensitive individuals. Extremely high doses of exogenous pancreatic enzymes have been associated with hyperuricemia and hyperuricosuria.

DOSAGE AND ADMINISTRATION

1 to 3 capsules taken with each meal or snack. Dosage may be adjusted depending on individual requirements for control of steatorrhea. In severe deficiencies the dose may be increased to 8 capsules with meals or the frequency of administration may increase to hourly intervals if nausea, cramps and/or diarrhea do not occur.

HOW SUPPLIED

KU-ZYME® HP Capsules (pancrelipase capsules USP) are white opaque capsules and are imprinted "SCHWARZ" and "525."
Bottles of 100 capsules NDC 0091-3525-01
Store at a temperature not exceeding 25°C (77°F).
Protect from high humidity.
CAUTION: Federal law prohibits dispensing without prescription.
PC0190F Rev. 11/96

LEVATOL® ℞

[lev 'a-tol]
(penbutolol sulfate) 20 mg
TABLETS

DESCRIPTION

Levatol® (penbutolol sulfate) is a synthetic β-receptor antagonist for oral administration. The chemical name of penbutolol sulfate is (S)-1-tert-butylamino-3-(o-cyclopentylphenoxy)-2-propanol sulfate. It is provided as the levorotatory isomer. The empirical formula for penbutolol sulfate is $C_{36}H_{60}N_2O_8S$. Its molecular weight is 680.94. A dose of 20 mg is equivalent to 29.4 μmol. The structural formula is as follows:
[See chemical structure at top of next column]
Penbutolol is a white, odorless, crystalline powder. Levatol is available as tablets for oral administration. Each tablet contains 20 mg of penbutolol sulfate. It also contains corn starch, D&C Yellow No. 10, lactose, magnesium stearate, povidone, silicon dioxide, talc, titanium dioxide, and other inactive ingredients.

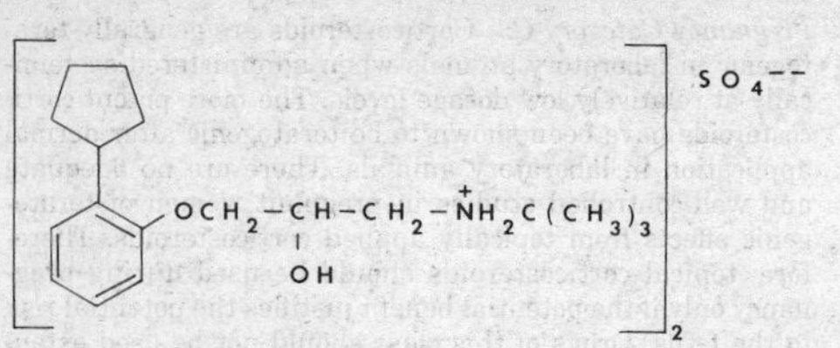

CLINICAL PHARMACOLOGY

Penbutolol is a β-1, β-2 (nonselective) adrenergic receptor antagonist. Experimental studies showed a dose-dependent increase in heart rate in reserpinized (norepinephrine-depleted) rats given penbutolol intravenously at doses of 0.25 to 1.0 mg/kg, suggesting that penbutolol has some intrinsic sympathomimetic activity. In human studies, however, heart rate decreases have been similar to those seen with propranolol.
Penbutolol antagonizes the heart rate effects of exercise and infused isoproterenol. The β-blocking potency of penbutolol is approximately 4 times that of propranolol. An oral dose of less than 10 mg will reduce exercise-induced tachycardia to one-half its usual level; maximum antagonism follows doses of 10 to 20 mg. The peak effect is between 1.5 and 3 hours after oral administration. The duration of effect exceeds 20 hours during a once-daily dosing regimen. During chronic administration of penbutolol, the duration of antihypertensive effects permits a once-daily dosage schedule.
Acute hemodynamic effects of penbutolol have been studied following single intravenous doses between 0.1 and 4 mg. The cardiovascular responses included significant reductions in heart rate, left ventricular maximum dP/dt, cardiac output, stroke volume index, stroke work, and stroke work index. Systolic pressure and mean arterial pressure were reduced, and total peripheral resistance was increased.
Chronic administration of penbutolol to hypertensive patients results in the hemodynamic pattern typical of β-adrenergic blocking drugs: a reduction in cardiac index, heart rate, systolic and diastolic blood pressures, and the product of heart rate and mean arterial pressure both at rest and with all levels of exercise, without significant change in total peripheral resistance. Penbutolol causes a reduction in left ventricular contractility. Penbutolol decreases glomerular filtration rate, but not significantly.
Clinical trial doses of 10 to 80 mg per day in single daily doses have reduced supine and standing systolic and diastolic blood pressures. In most studies, effects were small, generally a change in blood pressure 5 to 8/3 to 5 mm Hg greater than seen with a placebo measured 24 hours after dosing. It is not clear whether this relatively small effect reflects a characteristic of penbutolol or the particular population studied (the population had relatively mild hypertension but did not appear unusual in others respects). In a direct comparison of penbutolol with adequate doses of twice daily propranolol, no difference in blood pressure effect was seen. In a comparison of placebo and 10-, 20- and 40-mg single daily doses of penbutolol, no significant dose-related difference was seen in response to active drug at 6 weeks, but compared to the 10-mg dose, the two larger doses showed greater effects at 2 and 4 weeks and reached their maximum effect at 2 weeks. In several studies, dose increases from 40 to 80 mg were without additional effect on blood pressure. Response rates to penbutolol are unaffected by sex or age but are greater in caucasians than blacks.
Penbutolol decreases plasma renin activity in normal subjects and in patients with essential and renovascular hypertension. The mechanisms of the antihypertensive actions of β-receptor antagonists have not been established. However, factors that may be involved are: (1) competitive antagonism of catecholamines at peripheral adrenergic receptor sites (especially cardiac) that leads to decreased cardiac output; (2) a central nervous system (CNS) action that results in a decrease in tonic sympathetic neural outflow to the periphery; and (3) a reduction of renin secretion through blockade of β-receptors involved in release of renin from the kidneys.
Penbutolol dose dependently increases the RR and QT intervals. There is no influence on the PR, QRS or QT c (corrected) intervals.
Pharmacokinetics: Following oral administration, penbutolol is rapidly and completely absorbed. Peak plasma concentrations of penbutolol occur between 2 and 3 hours after oral administration and are proportional to single and multiple doses between 10 and 40 mg once a day. The average plasma elimination half-life of penbutolol is approximately 5 hours in normal subjects. There is no significant difference in the plasma half-life of penbutolol in healthy elderly persons or patients on renal dialysis. Twelve to 24 hours after oral administration of doses up to 120 mg, plasma concentrations of parent drug are 0% to 10% of the peak level. No accumulation of penbutolol is observed in hypertensive patients after 8 days of therapy at doses of 40 mg daily or 20 mg twice a day. Penbutolol is approximately 80% to 98% bound to plasma proteins.

The metabolism of penbutolol in humans involves conjugation and oxidation. The metabolites are excreted principally in the urine. When radiolabeled penbutolol was administered to humans, approximately 90% of the radioactivity was excreted in the urine. Approximately $1/6$ of the dose of penbutolol was recovered as penbutolol conjugate, while the remaining fraction was not identified. Conjugated penbutolol has a plasma elimination half-life of approximately 20 hours in healthy persons, 25 hours in healthy elderly persons and 100 hours in patients on renal dialysis. Thus, accumulation of penbutolol conjugate may be expected upon multiple-dosing in renal insufficiency. An oxidative metabolite of penbutolol, 4-hydroxy penbutolol, has been identified in small quantities in plasma and urine. It is $1/8$ to $1/15$ times as active as the parent compound in blocking isoproterenol-induced β-adrenergic receptor responses in isolated guinea-pig trachea and is $1/8$ to 1 times as potent in anesthetized dogs.

INDICATIONS AND USAGE

Levatol is indicated in the treatment of mild to moderate arterial hypertension. It may be used alone or in combination with other antihypertensive agents, especially thiazide-type diuretics.

CONTRAINDICATIONS

Levatol is contraindicated in patients with cardiogenic shock, sinus bradycardia, second and third degree atrioventricular conduction block, bronchial asthma, and those with known hypersensitivity to this product (*see* WARNINGS).

WARNINGS

Cardiac Failure: Sympathetic stimulation may be essential for supporting circulatory function in patients with heart failure, and its inhibition by β-adrenergic receptor blockade may precipitate more severe failure. Although β-blockers should be avoided in overt congestive heart failure, Levatol can, if necessary, be used with caution in patients with a history of cardiac failure who are well compensated, on treatment with vasodilators, digitalis and/or diuretics. Both digitalis and penbutolol slow AV conduction. Beta-adrenergic receptor antagonists do not inhibit the inotropic action of digitalis on heart muscle. If cardiac failure persists, treatment with Levatol should be discontinued.

Patients Without History of Cardiac Failure: Continued depression of the myocardium with β-blocking agents over a period of time can, in some cases, lead to cardiac failure. At the first evidence of heart failure, patients receiving Levatol should be given appropriate treatment, and the response should be closely observed. If cardiac failure continues despite adequate intervention with appropriate drugs, Levatol should be withdrawn (gradually, if possible).

Exacerbation of Ischemic Heart Disease Following Abrupt Withdrawal: Hypersensitivity to catecholamines has been observed in patients who were withdrawn from therapy with β-blocking agents; exacerbation of angina and, in some cases, myocardial infarction have occurred after abrupt discontinuation of such therapy. When discontinuing Levatol, particularly in patients with ischemic heart disease, the dosage should be reduced gradually over a period of 1 to 2 weeks and the patient should be monitored carefully. If angina becomes more pronounced or acute coronary insufficiency develops, administration of Levatol should be reinstated promptly, at least on a temporary basis, and appropriate measures should be taken for the management of unstable angina. Patients should be warned against interruption or discontinuation of therapy without the physician's advice. Because coronary artery disease is common and may not be recognized, it may not be prudent to discontinue Levatol abruptly, even in patients who are being treated only for hypertension.

Nonallergic Bronchospasm (e.g., chronic bronchitis, emphysema): Levatol is contraindicated in bronchial asthma. In general, patients with bronchospastic diseases should not receive β-blockers. Levatol should be administered with caution because it may block bronchodilation produced by endogenous catecholamine stimulation of β-2 receptors.

Anesthesia and Major Surgery: The necessity, or desirability, of withdrawal of a β-blocking therapy prior to major surgery is controversial. Beta-adrenergic receptor blockade impairs the ability of the heart to respond to β-adrenergically mediated reflex stimuli. Although this might be of benefit in preventing arrhythmic response, the risk of excessive myocardial depression during general anesthesia may be enhanced and difficulty in restarting and maintaining the heart beat has been reported with β-blockers. If treatment is continued, particular care should be taken when using anesthetic agents that depress the myocardium, such as ether, cyclopropane, and trichloroethylene, and it is prudent to use the lowest possible dose of Levatol. Levatol like other β-blockers, is a competitive inhibitor of β-receptor agonists, and its effect on the heart can be reversed by cautious administration of such agents (e.g., dobutamine or isoproterenol—see Overdose). Manifestations of excessive vagal tone (e.g., profound bradycardia, hypotension) may be corrected with atropine 1 to 3 mg IV in divided doses.

Diabetes Mellitus and Hypoglycemia: Beta-adrenergic receptor blockade may prevent the appearance of signs and symptoms of acute hypoglycemia, such as tachycardia and blood pressure changes. This is especially important in patients with labile diabetes. Beta-blockade also reduces the release of insulin in response to hyperglycemia; therefore, it may be necessary to adjust the dose of hypoglycemic drugs. Beta-adrenergic blockade may also impair the homeostatic response to hypoglycemia; in that event, the spontaneous recovery from hypoglycemia may be delayed during treatment with β-adrenergic receptor antagonists.

Thyrotoxicosis: Beta-adrenergic blockade may mask certain clinical signs (e.g., tachycardia) of hyperthyrodism. Patients suspected of developing thyrotoxicosis should be managed carefully to avoid abrupt withdrawal of β-adrenergic receptor blockers that might precipitate a thyroid storm.

PRECAUTIONS

Information for Patients: Patients, especially those with evidence of coronary artery insufficiency, should be warned against interruption or discontinuation of Levatol without the physician's advice. Although cardiac failure rarely occurs in properly selected patients, those being treated with β-adrenergic receptor antagonists should be advised of the symptoms of heart failure and to report such symptoms immediately, should they develop.

Drug Interactions: Levatol has been used in combination with hydrochlorothiazide in at least 100 patients without unexpected adverse reactions.

In one study, the combination of penbutolol and alcohol increased the number of errors in the eye-hand psychomotor function test.

Penbutolol increases the volume of distribution of lidocaine in normal subjects. This could result in a requirement for higher loading doses of lidocaine.

Cimetidine has no effect on the clearance of penbutolol. The major metabolite of penbutolol is a glucuronide, and it has been shown that cimetidine does not inhibit glucuronidation.

Synergistic hypotensive effects, bradycardia, and arrhythmias have been reported in some patients receiving β-adrenergic blocking agents when an oral calcium antagonist was added to the treatment regimen.

Generally, Levatol should not be used in patients receiving catecholamine-depleting drugs.

Risk of Anaphylactic Reaction: While taking β-blockers, patients with a history of severe anaphylactic reaction to a variety of allergens may be more reactive to repeated challenge, either accidental, diagnostic, or therapeutic. Such patients may be unresponsive to the usual doses of epinephrine used to treat allergic reaction.

Carcinogenesis, Mutagenesis, and Impairment of Fertility: There was no evidence of carcinogenicity observed in a 21-month study in mice or a 2-year study in rats. Mice were given penbutolol in the diet for 18 months at doses up to 395 mg/kg/day (about 500 times the Maximum Recommended Human Dose (MRHD) of 40 mg in a 50 kg person). Rats were given 141 mg/kg/day for the same length of time. Mice were observed for 3 months and rats for 5.5 to 7 months after termination of treatment before necropsy was performed.

No evidence of mutagenic activity of penbutolol was seen in the *Salmonella* mutagenicity test (Ames test), the point mutation induction test (*Saccharomyces*) and the micronucleus test.

Penbutolol had no adverse effects on fertility or general reproductive performance in mice and rats at oral doses up to 172 mg/kg/day.

Pregnancy—Teratogenic Effects: Pregnancy Category C: Teratology studies in rats and rabbits revealed no teratogenic effects related to treatment with penbutolol at oral doses up to 200 mg/kg/day (250 times the MRHD). In rabbits, a slight increase in the intrauterine fetal mortality and a reduced 24-hour offspring survival rate were observed in the groups treated with 125 mg/kg/day (156 times the MRHD) but not in the groups treated with 0.2 and 5 mg (0.25 to 6 times the MRHD).

There are no adequate and well-controlled studies in pregnant women. Levatol should be used during pregnancy only if the potential benefit justifies the potential risk to the fetus.

Nonteratogenic Effects: In a perinatal and postnatal study in rats, the pup body weight and pup survival rate were reduced at the highest dose level of 160 mg/kg/day (200 times the MRHD).

Nursing Mothers: It is not known whether Levatol is excreted in human milk. Because many drugs are excreted in human milk, caution should be exercised when Levatol is administered to a nursing woman.

Pediatric Use: Safety and effectiveness of Levatol in pediatric patients have not been established.

ADVERSE REACTIONS

Levatol is usually well tolerated in properly selected patients. Most adverse effects observed during clinical trials have been mild and reversible.

Table 1 lists the adverse reactions reported from 4 controlled studies conducted in the United States involving once-a-day administration of Levatol (at doses ranging from 10 to 120 mg) as monotherapy or in combination with hydrochlorothiazide. Levatol doses above 40 mg/day are not, however, recommended. The table includes only those events where the prevalence rate in the Levatol group was at least 1.5%, or where the reaction is of particular interest.

Table 1.
ADVERSE REACTIONS DURING CONTROLLED U.S. STUDIES

Body System Experience	Penbutolol (N = 628) %	Placebo (N = 212) %	Propranolol (N = 266) %
Body as a Whole			
Asthenia	1.6	0.9	4.9
Pain, chest	2.4	2.8	2.3
Pain, limb	2.4	1.4	1.5
Digestive System			
Diarrhea	3.3	1.9	2.6
Nausea	4.3	0.9	2.3
Dyspepsia	2.7	1.4	5.3
Nervous System			
Dizziness	4.9	2.4	4.2
Fatigue	4.4	1.9	2.6
Headache	7.8	6.1	7.5
Insomnia	1.9	0.9	2.6
Respiratory System			
Cough	2.1	0.5	1.1
Dyspnea	2.1	1.4	3.4
Upper respiratory infection	2.5	3.3	4.9
Skin and Appendages			
Sweating, excessive	1.6	0.5	2.3
Urogenital System			
Impotence, sexual	0.5	0.0	0.8

Table 2.
DISCONTINUATIONS DURING CONTROLLED U.S. STUDIES

Body System Experience	Penbutolol (N = 628) %	Placebo (N = 212) %	Propranolol (N = 266) %
Body as a Whole			
Asthenia	0.6	0.0	0.4
Pain, chest	0.6	1.4	0.4
Digestive System			
Nausea	0.8	0.0	0.8
Nervous System			
Depression	0.6	0.5	0.8
Dizziness	0.6	0.0	0.4
Fatigue	0.5	0.5	0.0
Headache	0.6	0.5	0.4

Continued on next page

Levatol—Cont.

Over a dose range from 10 to 40 mg, once a day, fatigue, nausea, and sexual impotence occurred at a greater frequency as the dose was increased.

[See table 1 at top of previous page]

In a double-blind clinical trial comparing Levatol (40 mg and greater once a day) and propranolol (40 mg or more twice a day), heart rates of less than 60 beats/min. were recorded at least once in 25% of the patients in the group receiving Levatol and in 37% of the patients in the propranolol group. Corresponding figures for heart rates of less than 50 beats/min. were 1.2% and 6%, respectively. No symptoms associated with bradycardia were reported.

Discontinuations of Levatol because of adverse reactions have ranged between 2.4% and 6.9% of patients in double-blind, parallel, controlled clinical trials, as compared to 1.8% to 4.1% in the corresponding control groups that were given placebo. The frequency and severity of adverse reactions have not increased during long-term administration of Levatol. The prevalence of adverse reactions reported from 4 controlled clinical trials (referred to in Table 1) as reasons for discontinuation of therapy by ≥0.5% of the Levatol group is listed in Table 2.

[See table 2 on previous page]

Potential Adverse Effects: In addition, certain adverse effects not listed above have been reported with other β-blocking agents and should also be considered as potential adverse effects of Levatol.

Central Nervous System: Reversible mental depression progressing to catatonia (an acute syndrome characterized by disorientation for time and place), short-term memory loss, emotional lability, slightly clouded sensorium, and decreased performance (neuropsychometrics).

Cardiovascular: Intensification of AV block (*see* CONTRAINDICATIONS).

Allergic: Erythematous rash, fever combined with aching and sore throat, laryngospasm, and respiratory distress.

Hematologic: Agranulocytosis, nonthrombocytopenic, and thrombocytopenic purpura.

Gastrointestinal: Mesenteric arterial thrombosis and ischemic colitis.

Miscellaneous: Reversible alopecia and Peyronie's disease. The oculomucocutaneous syndrome associated with the β-blocker practolol has not been reported with Levatol during investigational use and extensive foreign clinical experience.

OVERDOSAGE

There is no actual experience with Levatol overdose. The signs and symptoms that would be expected with overdosage of β-adrenergic receptor antagonists are symptomatic bradycardia, hypotension, bronchospasm, and acute cardiac failure. In addition to discontinuation of Levatol, gastric emptying, and close observation of the patient, the following measures might be considered as appropriate:

Excessive Bradycardia: Administer atropine sulfate to induce vagal blockade. If bradycardia persists, intravenous isoproterenol hydrochloride may be administered cautiously; larger than usual doses may be needed. In refractory cases, the use of a transvenous cardiac pacemaker may be necessary.

Hypotension: Sympathomimetic drug therapy, such as dopamine, dobutamine, or levarterenol, may be considered if hypotension persists despite correction of bradycardia. In refractory cases, administration of glucagon hydrochloride has been reported to be useful.

Bronchospasm: A β-2-agonist or isoproterenol hydrochloride may be administered. Additional therapy with aminophylline may be considered.

Acute Cardiac Failure: Institute conventional therapy immediately. Intravenous administration of dobutamine and glucagon hydrochloride has been reported to be useful.

Heart Block (Second or Third Degree): Isoproterenol hydrochloride or a transvenous cardiac pacemaker may be used.

DOSAGE AND ADMINISTRATION

The usual starting and maintenance dose of Levatol used alone or in combination with other antihypertensive agents, such as thiazide-type diuretics, is 20 mg given once daily. Doses of 40 mg and 80 mg have been well-tolerated but have not been shown to give a greater antihypertensive effect. The full effect of a 20- or 40-mg dose is seen by the end of 2 weeks. A dose of 10 mg also lowers blood pressure, but the full effect is not seen for 4 to 6 weeks.

HOW SUPPLIED

Levatol® (penbutolol sulfate) 20 mg tablets are yellow, scored, capsule-shaped and engraved "RC22". They are supplied as follows:

Bottles of 100   NDC 0091-4500-15

Store at controlled room temperature 15°–30°C (59°–86°F). Keep tightly closed and protect from light.

CAUTION: Federal law prohibits dispensing without prescription.

ANIMAL TOXICOLOGY

Studies in rats indicated that the combination of penbutolol, triamterene, and hydrochlorothiazide (up to 40, 50 and 25 mg/kg, respectively) increased the incidence and severity of renal tubular dilation and regeneration when compared to that in rats treated only with triamterene and hydrochlorothiazide. Dogs administered the same doses of triamterene and hydrochlorothiazide alone and in combination with penbutolol had an increase in serum alkaline phosphatase and serum alanine transferase, but there were no gross or microscopic abnormalities observed. No significant toxicologic findings were observed in rats and dogs treated with a combination of penbutolol and hydrochlorothiazide.

PC2077   Rev. 7/95

LEVSIN® PRODUCTS   ℞
[lev 'sin]
(hyoscyamine sulfate USP)
LEVBID® Extended-Release Tablets
LEVSIN®/SL Tablets
LEVSIN® Tablets
LEVSIN® Elixir
LEVSIN® Drops
(Oral Solution)
LEVSIN® Injection
LEVSINEX® TIMECAPS™

DESCRIPTION

LEVSIN® (hyoscyamine sulfate USP) is one of the principal anticholinergic/antispasmodic components of belladonna alkaloids. The empirical formula is $(C_{17}H_{23}NO_3)_2 \cdot H_2SO_4 \cdot 2H_2O$ and the molecular weight is 712.85. Chemically, it is benzeneacetic acid, α-(hydroxymethyl)-,8-methyl-8-azabicyclo [3.2.1.] oct-3-yl ester, [3(S)-endo]-, sulfate (2:1), dihydrate.

LEVBID Extended-Release Tablets contain 0.375 mg of hyoscyamine sulfate in a formulation designed for oral b.i.d. dosage. Each LEVBID Extended-Release Tablet also contains as inactive ingredients: lactose, magnesium stearate, FD&C yellow #6 and other ingredients.

LEVSIN/SL Tablets contain 0.125 mg hyoscyamine sulfate formulated for sublingual administration. However, the tablets may be chewed or taken orally. Each tablet also contains as inactive ingredients: colloidal silicon dioxide, dextrates, FD&C Green #3, flavor, mannitol, and stearic acid.

LEVSIN Tablets contain 0.125 mg hyoscyamine sulfate formulated for oral administration. Each tablet also contains as inactive ingredients: acacia, confectioner's sugar, corn starch, lactose, powdered cellulose and stearic acid.

LEVSIN Elixir contains 0.125 mg hyoscyamine sulfate per 5 mL with 20% alcohol for oral administration. LEVSIN Elixir also contains as inactive ingredients: FD&C Red #40, FD&C Yellow #6, flavor, glycerin, purified water, sorbitol solution and sucrose.

LEVSIN Drops contain 0.125 mg hyoscyamine sulfate per mL with 5% alcohol for oral administration. LEVSIN Drops also contain as inactive ingredients: FD&C Red #40, FD&C Yellow #6, flavor, glycerin, purified water, sodium citrate, sorbitol solution, and sucrose.

LEVSIN Injection is a sterile solution containing 0.5 mg hyoscyamine sulfate per mL. The 1 mL ampuls contain as inactive ingredients: water for injection, pH is adjusted with hydrochloric acid when necessary.

LEVSINEX TIMECAPS contain 0.375 mg hyoscyamine sulfate in an extended-release formulation designed for oral b.i.d. dosage. Each capsule also contains as inactive ingredients: corn starch, D&C Red #28, FD&C Blue #1, FD&C Blue #2, FD&C Red #40, FD&C Yellow #6, gelatin, sucrose, titanium dioxide and other ingredients.

CLINICAL PHARMACOLOGY

LEVSIN inhibits specifically the actions of acetylcholine on structures innervated by postganglionic cholinergic nerves and on smooth muscles that respond to acetylcholine but lack cholinergic innervation. These peripheral cholinergic receptors are present in the autonomic effector cells of the smooth muscle, the cardiac muscle, the sinoatrial node, the atrioventricular node, and the exocrine glands. At therapeutic doses, it is completely devoid of any action on autonomic ganglia. LEVSIN inhibits gastrointestinal propulsive motility and decreases gastric acid secretion. LEVSIN also controls excessive pharyngeal, tracheal and bronchial secretions.

LEVSIN is absorbed totally and completely by sublingual administration as well as oral administration. Once absorbed, LEVSIN disappears rapidly from the blood and is distributed throughout the entire body. The half-life of LEVSIN is 2 to 3½ hours. LEVSIN is partly hydrolyzed to tropic acid and tropine but the majority of the drug is excreted in the urine unchanged within the first 12 hours. Only traces of this drug are found in breast milk. LEVSIN passes the blood brain barrier and the placental barrier.

LEVBID releases 0.375 mg hyoscyamine sulfate at a controlled and predictable rate for 12 hours. Peak blood levels occur in approximately 4 hours and the apparent plasma elimination half-life is approximately 9 hours. The relative bioavailability of the extended-release tablet is approximately 92% that of the immediate-release tablet. Tablets may not completely disintegrate and may be excreted by some patients.

LEVSINEX TIMECAPS release 0.375 mg hyoscyamine sulfate at a controlled and predictable rate for 12 hours. Peak blood levels occur in 3 to 4 hours and the apparent plasma elimination half-life is 5 to 6 hours.

INDICATIONS AND USAGE

LEVSIN is effective as adjunctive therapy in the treatment of peptic ulcer. It can also be used to control gastric secretion, visceral spasm, and hypermotility in spastic colitis, spastic bladder, cystitis, pylorospasm, and associated abdominal cramps. May be used in functional intestinal disorders to reduce symptoms such as those seen in mild dysenteries, diverticulitis, and acute enterocolitis. For use as adjunctive therapy in the treatment of irritable bowel syndrome (irritable colon, spastic colon, mucous colitis) and functional gastrointestinal disorders. Also used as adjunctive therapy in the treatment of neurogenic bladder and neurogenic bowel disturbances (including the splenic flexure syndrome and neurogenic colon). Also used in the treatment of infant colic (elixir and drops). LEVSIN is indicated along with morphine or other narcotics in symptomatic relief of biliary and renal colic; as a "drying agent" in the relief of symptoms of acute rhinitis; in the therapy of parkinsonism to reduce rigidity and tremors and to control associated sialorrhea and hyperhidrosis. May be used in the therapy of poisoning by anticholinesterase agents.

Parenterally administered LEVSIN is also effective in reducing gastrointestinal motility to facilitate diagnostic procedures such as endoscopy or hypotonic duodenography. LEVSIN may be used to reduce pain and hypersecretion in pancreatitis. LEVSIN may also be used in certain cases of partial heart block associated with vagal activity.

IN ANESTHESIA:

LEVSIN Injection is indicated as a pre-operative antimuscarinic to reduce salivary, tracheobronchial, and pharyngeal secretions; to reduce the volume and acidity of gastric secretions; and to block cardiac vagal inhibitory reflexes during induction of anesthesia and intubation. LEVSIN protects against the peripheral muscarinic effects such as bradycardia and excessive secretions produced by halogenated hydrocarbons and cholinergic agents such as physostigmine, neostigmine, and pyridostigmine given to reverse the actions of curariform agents.

IN UROLOGY:

LEVSIN Injection may also be used intravenously to improve radiologic visibility of the kidneys. It is also indicated along with morphine or other narcotics in symptomatic relief of biliary and renal colic.

CONTRAINDICATIONS

Glaucoma; obstructive uropathy (for example, bladder neck obstruction due to prostatic hypertrophy); obstructive disease of the gastrointestinal tract (as in achalasia, pyloroduodenal stenosis); paralytic ileus, intestinal atony of elderly or debilitated patients; unstable cardiovascular status in acute hemorrhage; severe ulcerative colitis; toxic megacolon complicating ulcerative colitis; myasthenia gravis.

WARNINGS

In the presence of high environmental temperature, heat prostration can occur with drug use (fever and heat stroke due to decreased sweating). Diarrhea may be an early symptom of incomplete intestinal obstruction, especially in patients with ileostomy or colostomy. In this instance, treatment with this drug would be inappropriate and possibly harmful. Like other anticholinergic agents, LEVSIN may produce drowsiness, dizziness or blurred vision. In this event, the patient should be warned not to engage in activities requiring mental alertness such as operating a motor vehicle or other machinery or to perform hazardous work while taking this drug.

Psychosis has been reported in sensitive individuals given anticholinergic drugs. CNS signs and symptoms inlude confusion, disorientation, short term memory loss, hallucinations, dysarthria, ataxia, coma, euphoria, decreased anxiety, fatigue, insomnia, agitation and mannerisms, and inappropriate affect. These CNS signs and symptoms usually resolve within 12 to 48 hours after discontinuation of the drug.

PRECAUTIONS

General:

Use with caution in patients with: autonomic neuropathy, hyperthyroidism, coronary heart disease, congestive heart failure, cardiac arrhythmias, hypertension and renal disease. Investigate any tachycardia before giving any anticholinergic drug since they may increase the heart rate. Use with caution in patients with hiatal hernia associated with reflux esophagitis.

Information for Patients:
Like other anticholinergic agents, LEVSIN may produce drowsiness, dizziness or blurred vision. In this event, the patient should be warned not to engage in activities requiring mental alertness such as operating a motor vehicle or other machinery or to perform hazardous work while taking this drug.
Use of LEVSIN may decrease sweating resulting in heat prostration, fever or heat stroke; febrile patients or those who may be exposed to elevated environmental temperatures should use caution.
LEVBID Tablets may not completely disintegrate and may be excreted by some patients.
Drug Interactions:
Additive adverse effects resulting from cholinergic blockade may occur when LEVSIN is administered concomitantly with other antimuscarinics, amantadine, haloperidol, phenothiazines, monoamine oxidase (MAO) inhibitors, tricyclic antidepressants or some antihistamines.
Antacids may interfere with the absorption of LEVSIN. Administer LEVSIN before meals; antacids after meals.
Carcinogenesis, Mutagenesis, Impairment of Fertility:
No long-term studies in animals have been performed to determine the carcinogenic, mutagenic or impairment of fertility potential of LEVSIN; however, 40 years of marketing experience with hyoscyamine sulfate shows no demonstrable evidence of a problem.
Pregnancy—Pregnancy Category C:
Animal reproduction studies have not been conducted with LEVSIN. It is also not known whether LEVSIN can cause fetal harm when administered to a pregnant woman or can affect reproduction capacity. LEVSIN should be given to a pregnant woman only if clearly needed.
Nursing Mothers:
LEVSIN is excreted in human milk. Caution should be exercised when LEVSIN is administered to a nursing woman.

ADVERSE REACTIONS

Not all of the following adverse reactions have been reported with hyoscyamine sulfate. The following adverse reactions have been reported for pharmacologically similar drugs with anticholinergic/antispasmodic action. Adverse reactions may include dryness of the mouth; urinary hesitancy and retention; blurred vision; tachycardia; palpitations; mydriasis; cycloplegia; increased ocular tension; loss of taste; headache; nervousness; drowsiness; weakness; dizziness; insomnia; nausea; vomiting; impotence; suppression of lactation; constipation; bloated feeling; allergic reactions or drug idiosyncrasies; urticaria and other dermal manifestations; ataxia; speech disturbance; some degree of mental confusion and/or excitement (especially in elderly persons); and decreased sweating.

OVERDOSAGE

The signs and symptoms of overdose are headache, nausea, vomiting, blurred vision, dilated pupils, hot dry skin, dizziness, dryness of the mouth, difficulty in swallowing and CNS stimulation.
Measures to be taken are immediate lavage of the stomach and injection of physostigmine 0.5 to 2 mg intravenously and repeated as necessary up to a total of 5 mg. Fever may be treated symptomatically (tepid water sponge baths, hypothermic blanket). Excitement to a degree which demands attention may be managed with sodium thiopental 2% solution given slowly intravenously or chloral hydrate (100–200 mL of a 2% solution) by rectal infusion. In the event of progression of the curare-like effect to paralysis of the respiratory muscles, artificial respiration should be instituted and maintained until effective respiratory action returns.
In rats, the LD_{50} for LEVSIN is 375 mg/kg. LEVSIN is dialyzable.

DOSAGE AND ADMINISTRATION

Dosage may be adjusted according to the conditions and severity of symptoms.
LEVBID Extended-Release Tablets: *Adults and pediatric patients 12 years of age and older:* 1 to 2 tablets every 12 hours. Tablets are scored and may be broken to allow for dose titration if needed. Do not crush or chew tablets. Do not exceed 4 tablets in 24 hours.
LEVSIN/SL Tablets: The tablets may be taken sublingually, orally or chewed. *Adults and pediatric patients 12 years of age and older:* 1 to 2 tablets every four hours or as needed. Do not exceed 12 tablets in 24 hours. *Pediatric patients 2 to under 12 years of age:* $^1/_2$ to 1 tablet every four hours or as needed. Do not exceed 6 tablets in 24 hours.
LEVSIN Tablets: *Adults and pediatric patients 12 years of age and older:* 1 to 2 tablets every four hours or as needed. Do not exceed 12 tablets in 24 hours.
Pediatric patients 2 to under 12 years of age: $^1/_2$ to 1 tablet every four hours or as needed. Do not exceed 6 tablets in 24 hours.
LEVSIN Elixir: *Adults and pediatric patients 12 years of age and older:* 1 to 2 teaspoonfuls every four hours or as needed. Do not exceed 12 teaspoonfuls in 24 hours.
Pediatric patients 2 to under 12 years of age:
Please see the following dosage guide based on body weight. The doses may be repeated every four hours or as needed. Do not exceed 6 teaspoonfuls in 24 hours.

Body Weight	Usual Dose
10 kg (22 lb)	$^1/_4$ tsp (1.25 mL)
20 kg (44 lb)	$^1/_2$ tsp (2.5 mL)
40 kg (88 lb)	$^3/_4$ tsp (3.75 mL)
50 kg (110 lb)	1 tsp (5 mL)

LEVSIN Drops: *Adults and pediatric patients 12 years of age and older:* 1 to 2 mL every four hours or as needed. Do not exceed 12 mL in 24 hours.
Pediatric patients 2 to under 12 years of age: $^1/_4$ to 1 mL every four hours or as needed. Do not exceed 6 mL in 24 hours.
Pediatric patients under 2 years of age: The following dosage guide is based upon body weight. The doses may be repeated every four hours or as needed.

Body Weight	Usual Dose	Do Not Exceed in 24 Hours
3.4 kg (7.5 lb)	4 drops	24 drops
5 kg (11 lb)	5 drops	30 drops
7 kg (15 lb)	6 drops	36 drops
10 kg (22 lb)	8 drops	48 drops

LEVSIN Injection: The dose may be administered subcutaneously, intramuscularly, or intravenously without dilution. As with all parenteral drug products, LEVSIN Injection should be inspected visually for particulate matter and discoloration prior to administration whenever solution and container permit.
Gastrointestinal Disorders: The usual adult recommended dose is 0.5 to 1 mL (0.25 to 0.5 mg). Some patients may need only a single dose; others may require administration two, three, or four times a day at four hour intervals.
Diagnostic Procedures: The usual adult recommended dose is 0.5 to 1 mL (0.25 to 0.5 mg) administered intravenously 5 to 10 minutes prior to the diagnostic procedure.
Anesthesia: Adults and pediatric patients over 2 years of age: As a pre-anesthetic medication, the recommended dose is 5 µg (0.005 mg) per kg of body weight. This dose is usually given 30 to 60 minutes prior to the anticipated time of induction of anesthesia or at the time the pre-anesthetic narcotic or sedatives are administered.
LEVSIN Injection may be used during surgery to reduce drug-induced bradycardia. It should be administered intravenously in increments of 0.25 mL and repeated as needed.
To achieve reversal of neuromuscular blockade, the recommended dose is 0.2 mg (0.4 mL) LEVSIN Injection for every 1 mg neostigmine or the equivalent dose of physostigmine or pyridostigmine.
LEVSINEX TIMECAPS: *Adults and pediatric patients 12 years of age and older:* 1 to 2 capsules every 12 hours. Dosage may be adjusted to 1 capsule every 8 hours if needed. Do not exceed 4 capsules in 24 hours.

HOW SUPPLIED

LEVBID Extended-Release Tablets (hyoscyamine sulfate, 0.375 mg) are light orange, capsule-shaped, scored tablets. They are coded SP538.

Bottles of 100 tablets	NDC 0091-3538-01
Bottles of 500 tablets	NDC 0091-3538-05

LEVSIN/SL Tablets (hyoscyamine sulfate tablets USP, 0.125 mg) are pale blue-green, peppermint-flavored, octagonal shaped, scored, and imprinted with "SCHWARZ" on one side and "532" on the other.

Bottles of 100 tablets	NDC 0091-3532-01
Bottles of 500 tablets	NDC 0091-3532-05

LEVSIN Tablets (hyoscyamine sulfate tablets USP, 0.125 mg) are white, scored and imprinted with "SCHWARZ" on one side and "531" on the other.

Bottles of 100 tablets	NDC 0091-3531-01
Bottles of 500 tablets	NDC 0091-3531-05

LEVSIN Elixir (hyoscyamine sulfate elixir USP, 0.125 mg/ 5 mL) is orange colored and flavored and contains 20% alcohol.

Pint (473 mL) bottles	NDC 0091-4532-16

LEVSIN Drops (hyoscyamine sulfate oral solution USP, 0.125 mg/mL) are orange colored and flavored.

15 mL Dropper bottles	NDC 0091-4538-15

LEVSIN Injection (hyoscyamine sulfate injection USP, 0.5 mg/mL) is a clear, colorless and sterile solution.

1 mL ampuls-Box of 5	NDC 0091-1536-05

LEVSINEX TIMECAPS (hyoscyamine sulfate USP, 0.375 mg, extended-release) are brown and clear capsules containing brown and white beadlets. They are imprinted "SCHWARZ" and "537."

Bottles of 100 capsules	NDC 0091-3537-01
Bottles of 500 capsules	NDC 0091-3537-05

Store at controlled room temperature 15°–30°C (59°–86°F).
CAUTION: Federal law prohibits dispensing without prescription.

Shown in Product Identification Guide, page 337

MONOKET® TABLETS ℞

[*män'-o-ket*]
(isosorbide mononitrate)

DESCRIPTION

MONOKET, an organic nitrate, is a vasodilator with effects on both arteries and veins. The empirical formula is $C_6H_9NO_6$ and the molecular weight is 191.14. The chemical name for MONOKET is 1,4:3,6-Dianhydro-D-glucitol 5-nitrate and the compound has the following structural formula:

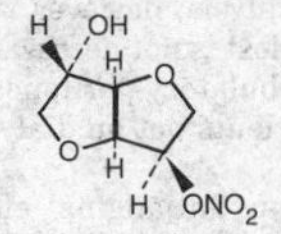

MONOKET is available in 10 mg and 20 mg tablets. Each tablet also contains as inactive ingredients: lactose, talc, colloidal silicon dioxide, starch, microcrystalline cellulose and aluminum stearate.

CLINICAL PHARMACOLOGY

Isosorbide mononitrate is the major active metabolite of isosorbide dinitrate (ISDN), and most of the clinical activity of the dinitrate is attributable to the mononitrate.
The principal pharmacological action of isosorbide mononitrate is relaxation of vascular smooth muscle and consequent dilatation of peripheral arteries and veins, especially the latter. Dilatation of the veins promotes peripheral pooling of blood and decreases venous return to the heart, thereby reducing left ventricular end-diastolic pressure and pulmonary capillary wedge pressure (preload). Arteriolar relaxation reduces systemic vascular resistance, systolic arterial pressure, and mean arterial pressure (afterload). Dilatation of the coronary arteries also occurs. The relative importance of preload reduction, afterload reduction and coronary dilatation remains undefined.
Pharmacodynamics:
Dosing regimens for most chronically used drugs are designed to provide plasma concentrations that are continuously greater than a minimally effective concentration. This strategy is inappropriate for organic nitrates. Several well-controlled clinical trials have used exercise testing to assess the antianginal efficacy of continuously-delivered nitrates. In the large majority of these trials, active agents were indistinguishable from placebo after 24 hours (or less) of continuous therapy. Attempts to overcome tolerance by dose escalation, even to doses far in excess of those used acutely, have consistently failed. Only after nitrates have been absent from the body for several hours has their antianginal efficacy been restored.
The drug-free interval sufficient to avoid tolerance to isosorbide mononitrate has not been completely defined. In the only regimen of twice-daily isosorbide mononitrate that has been shown to avoid development of tolerance, the two doses of MONOKET Tablets are given 7 hours apart, so there is a gap of 17 hours between the second dose of each day and the first dose of the next day. Taking account of the relatively long half-life of isosorbide mononitrate this result is consistent with those obtained for other organic nitrates.
The asymmetric twice daily regimen of MONOKET Tablets successfully avoided significant rebound/withdrawal effects. The incidence and magnitude of such phenomena have appeared, in studies of other nitrates, to be highly dependent upon the schedule of nitrate administration.
Pharmacokinetics:
MONOKET is rapidly and completely absorbed from the gastrointestinal tract. In humans, MONOKET is not subject to first pass metabolism in the liver. The absolute bioavailability of isosorbide mononitrate from MONOKET Tablets is nearly 100%. Peak plasma concentrations usually occur in about 30–60 minutes. MONOKET exhibits dose proportionality over the recommended dose range. Food does not significantly affect the absorption or bioavailability of MONOKET. Metoprolol coadministration did not change the pharmacokinetics of MONOKET. The volume of distribution is approximately 0.6 L/Kg. Plasma protein binding of MONOKET was found to be less than 5%.
When radiolabelled isosorbide mononitrate was administered to humans in order to elucidate the metabolic fate, about half of the dose was found denitrated and renally excreted as isosorbide and sorbitol. One quarter of the dose was accounted for as conjugates of the parent drug in the urine. None of these metabolites is vasoactive. Only 2% of the dose was excreted as unchanged drug.
The overall elimination half-life of MONOKET is about 5 hours. The rate of clearance is the same in healthy young adults, in patients with various degrees of renal, hepatic or cardiac dysfunction and in the elderly. When radiolabelled isosorbide mononitrate was administered to humans, 93%

Continued on next page

Monoket—Cont.

of the dose was excreted within 48 hours into the urine. Renal excretion was virtually complete after 5 days; fecal excretion amounted to only 1% of the dose.

MONOKET has no known effect on renal and hepatic function. In patients with varying degrees of renal failure, dosage adjustment does not appear necessary. In patients with liver cirrhosis, the pharmacokinetic parameters after a single dose of MONOKET were similar to the values found in healthy volunteers.

Isosorbide mononitrate is significantly removed from the blood during hemodialysis; however, an additional dose to compensate for drug lost is not necessary. In patients undergoing continuous ambulatory peritoneal dialysis, blood levels are similar to patients not on dialysis.

Clinical Trials:

The acute and chronic antianginal efficacy of MONOKET has been confirmed in clinical trials. The clinical efficacy of MONOKET was studied in 21 stable angina pectoris patients. After single dose administration of MONOKET, 20 mg, the exercise capacity was increased by 42.7% after one hour, 29.6% after 6 hours and by 25% after eight hours when compared to placebo. Controlled trials of single doses of MONOKET Tablets have demonstrated that antianginal activity is present about 1 hour after dosing, with peak effect seen from 1–4 hours after dosing.

In one multicenter placebo-controlled trial, MONOKET was found to be safe and effective during acute and chronic (3 weeks) treatment of angina pectoris. Two hundred fourteen (214) patients were enrolled in the trial; 54 patients were randomized to receive placebo and 106 patients were randomized to receive 10 or 20 mg of MONOKET twice daily seven hours apart. The largest effect of MONOKET, compared to placebo, was on day one—dose one. Although 14 hours after the first dose of day 14, the increase in exercise tolerance due to MONOKET was statistically significant, the increase was about half of that seen 2 hours after the first dose of day one. On day 21, two hours after the first dose the effect of MONOKET was 60 to 70% of that seen on day one.

INDICATIONS AND USAGE

MONOKET is indicated for the prevention and treatment of angina pectoris due to coronary artery disease. The onset of action of oral isosorbide mononitrate is not sufficiently rapid for this product to be useful in aborting an acute anginal episode.

CONTRAINDICATIONS

Allergic reactions to organic nitrates are extremely rare, but they do occur. Isosorbide mononitrate is contraindicated in patients who are allergic to it.

WARNINGS

The benefits of isosorbide mononitrate in patients with acute myocardial infarction or congestive heart failure have not been established. Because the effects of isosorbide mononitrate are difficult to terminate rapidly, this drug is not recommended in these settings.

If isosorbide mononitrate is used in these conditions, careful clinical or hemodynamic monitoring must be used to avoid the hazards of hypotension and tachycardia.

PRECAUTIONS

General:

Severe hypotension, particularly with upright posture, may occur with even small doses of isosorbide mononitrate. This drug should therefore be used with caution in patients who may be volume depleted or who, for whatever reason, are already hypotensive. Hypotension induced by isosorbide mononitrate may be accompanied by paradoxical bradycardia and increased angina pectoris.

Nitrate therapy may aggravate the angina caused by hypertrophic cardiomyopathy.

In industrial workers who have had long-term exposure to unknown (presumably high) doses of organic nitrates, tolerance clearly occurs. Chest pain, acute myocardial infarction, and even sudden death have occurred during temporary withdrawal of nitrates from these workers, demonstrating the existence of true physical dependence. The importance of these observations to the routine, clinical use of oral isosorbide mononitrate is not known.

Information for Patients:

Patients should be told that the antianginal efficacy of MONOKET Tablets can be maintained by carefully following the prescribed schedule of dosing (two doses taken seven hours apart). For most patients, this can be accomplished by taking the first dose on awakening and the second dose 7 hours later.

As with other nitrates, daily headaches sometimes accompany treatment with isosorbide mononitrate. In patients who get these headaches, the headaches are a marker of the activity of the drug. Patients should resist the temptation to avoid headaches by altering the schedule of their treatment with isosorbide mononitrate, since loss of headache may be associated with simultaneous loss of antianginal efficacy.

Aspirin and/or acetaminophen, on the other hand, often successfully relieve isosorbide mononitrate-induced headaches with no deleterious effect on isosorbide mononitrate's antianginal efficacy.

Treatment with isosorbide mononitrate may be associated with light-headedness on standing, especially just after rising from a recumbent or seated position. This effect may be more frequent in patients who have also consumed alcohol.

Drug Interactions:

The vasodilating effects of isosorbide mononitrate may be additive with those of other vasodilators. Alcohol, in particular, has been found to exhibit additive effects of this variety.

Marked symptomatic orthostatic hypotension has been reported when calcium channel blockers and organic nitrates were used in combination. Dose adjustments of either class of agents may be necessary.

Carcinogenesis, Mutagenesis, Impairment of Fertility:

No evidence of carcinogenicity was observed in rats exposed to isosorbide mononitrate in their diets at doses of up to 900 mg/kg/day for the first six months and 500 mg/kg/day for the remaining duration of a study in which males were dosed for up to 121 weeks and females were dosed for up to 137 weeks. No evidence of mutagenicity was seen *in vitro* in the Salmonella test (Ames test), in human peripheral lymphocytes, in Chinese hamster cells (V79) or, *in vivo* in the rat micronucleus test. In a study on the fertility and breeding capacity of two generations of rats, MONOKET had no adverse effects on fertility or general reproductive performance with oral doses up to 120 mg/kg/day. A dose of 360 mg/kg/day was associated with increased mortality in treated males and females and a reduced fertility index. (See table at end of *Pregnancy* section for animal-to-human dosage comparisons.)

Pregnancy:

Teratogenic Effects:

Pregnancy Category B: Reproduction studies performed in rats and rabbits at doses of up to 540 and 810 mg/kg/day, respectively, have revealed no evidence of harm to the fetus due to isosorbide mononitrate. There are, however, no adequate and well-controlled studies in pregnant women. Because animal reproduction studies are not always predictive of human response, MONOKET should be used during pregnancy only if clearly needed.

Nonteratogenic Effects:

Birth weights, neonatal survival and development, and incidence of stillbirths were adversely affected when pregnant rats were administered oral doses of 540 (but not 270) mg isosorbide mononitrate/kg/day during late gestation and lactation. This dose was associated with decreased maternal body weight gain and decreased maternal motor activity.

Species	Daily Dose (mg/kg)	Multiple of MRHD* Based on: Body Weight	Body Surface
Rabbit	810	1013	375
Rat	900	1125	195
	540	675	117
	500	625	108
	360	450	78
	270	338	59

Calculations assume a human weight of 50 kg and human body surface area of 1.46 m^2, a rabbit weight of 2 kg and rabbit body surface area of 0.163 m^2, and a rat weight of 150 g and rat body surface area of 0.025 m^2. *Maximum recommended human dose (MRHD) is 20 mg bid.

Nursing Mothers:

It is not known whether isosorbide mononitrate is excreted in human milk. Because many drugs are excreted in human milk, caution should be exercised when isosorbide mononitrate is administered to a nursing woman.

Pediatric Use:

Safety and effectiveness of isosorbide mononitrate in pediatric patients have not been established.

ADVERSE REACTIONS

Headache is the most frequent side effect and was the cause of 2% of all dropouts from controlled-clinical trials. Headache decreased in incidence after the first few days of therapy.

The following table shows the frequency of adverse reactions observed in 1% or more of subjects in 6 placebo-controlled trials, conducted in the United States and abroad. The same table shows the frequency of withdrawal for these adverse reactions. In many cases the adverse reactions were of uncertain relation to drug treatment.

[See table below]

Other adverse reactions, each reported by fewer than 1% of exposed patients, and in many cases of uncertain relation to drug treatment, were:

Cardiovascular: acute myocardial infarction, apoplexy, arrhythmias, bradycardia, edema, hypertension, hypotension, pallor, palpitations, tachycardia.

Dermatologic: sweating.

Gastrointestinal: anorexia, dry mouth, dyspepsia, thirst, vomiting, decreased weight.

Genitourinary: prostatic disorder.

Miscellaneous: amblyopia, back pain, bitter taste, muscle cramps, neck pain, paresthesia, susurrus aurium.

Neurologic: anxiety, impaired concentration, depression, insomnia, nervousness, nightmares, restlessness, tremor, vertigo.

Respiratory: asthma, dyspnea, sinusitis.

Extremely rarely, ordinary doses of organic nitrates have caused methemoglobinemia in normal-seeming patients; for further discussion of its diagnosis and treatment see under **Overdosage.**

OVERDOSAGE

Hemodynamic Effects:

The ill effects of isosorbide mononitrate overdose are generally the results of isosorbide mononitrate's capacity to induce vasodilatation, venous pooling, reduced cardiac output, and hypotension. These hemodynamic changes may have protean manifestations, including increased intracranial pressure, with any or all of persistent throbbing headache, confusion, and moderate fever; vertigo; palpitations; visual disturbances; nausea and vomiting (possibly with colic and even bloody diarrhea); syncope (especially in the upright posture); air hunger and dyspnea, later followed by reduced ventilatory effort; diaphoresis, with the skin either flushed or cold and clammy; heart block and bradycardia; paralysis; coma; seizures and death.

Laboratory determinations of serum levels of isosorbide mononitrate and its metabolites are not widely available, and such determinations have, in any event, no established role in the management of isosorbide mononitrate overdose.

There are no data suggesting what dose of isosorbide mononitrate is likely to be life-threatening in humans. In rats and mice, there is significant lethality at oral doses of 1965 mg/kg and 2581 mg/kg, respectively.

No data are available to suggest physiological maneuvers (e.g., maneuvers to change the pH of the urine) that might

Frequency of Adverse Reactions (Discontinuations)*

6 Placebo-Controlled Studies

Dose	Placebo	5 mg	10 mg	20 mg
Patients	160	54	52	159
Headache	6% (0%)	17% (0%)	13% (0%)	35% (5%)
Fatigue	2% (0%)	0% (0%)	4% (0%)	1% (0%)
Upper Respiratory				
Infection	<1% (0%)	0% (0%)	4% (0%)	1% (0%)
Pain	<1% (0%)	4% (0%)	0% (0%)	<1% (0%)
Dizziness	1% (0%)	0% (0%)	0% (0%)	4% (0%)
Nausea	<1% (0%)	0% (0%)	0% (0%)	3% (2%)
Inceased Cough	<1% (0%)	0% (0%)	2% (0%)	<1% (0%)
Rash	0% (0%)	2% (2%)	0% (0%)	<1% (0%)
Abdominal Pain	<1% (0%)	0% (0%)	2% (0%)	0% (0%)
Allergic Reaction	0% (0%)	0% (0%)	2% (0%)	0% (0%)
Cardiovascular				
Disorder	0% (0%)	2% (0%)	0% (0%)	0% (0%)
Chest Pain	<1% (0%)	0% (0%)	2% (0%)	<1% (0%)
Diarrhea	0% (0%)	0% (0%)	2% (0%)	0% (0%)
Flushing	0% (0%)	0% (0%)	2% (0%)	0% (0%)
Emotional Lability	0% (0%)	2% (0%)	0% (0%)	0% (0%)
Pruritus	1% (0%)	2% (2%)	0% (0%)	0% (0%)

*Some individuals discontinued for multiple reasons.

accelerate elimination of isosorbide mononitrate. Isosorbide mononitrate is significantly removed from the blood during hemodialysis.
No specific antagonist to the vasodilator effects of isosorbide mononitrate is known, and no intervention has been subject to controlled study as a therapy of isosorbide mononitrate overdose. Because the hypotension associated with isosorbide mononitrate overdose is the result of venodilatation and arterial hypovolemia, prudent therapy in this situation should be directed toward an increase in central fluid volume. Passive elevation of the patient's legs may be sufficient, but intravenous infusion of normal saline or similar fluid may also be necessary.
The use of epinephrine or other arterial vasoconstrictors in this setting is likely to do more harm than good.
In patients with renal disease or congestive heart failure, therapy resulting in central volume expansion is not without hazard. Treatment of isosorbide mononitrate overdose in these patients may be subtle and difficult, and invasive monitoring may be required.
Methemoglobinemia:
Methemoglobinemia has been reported in patients receiving other organic nitrates, and it probably could also occur as a side effect of isosorbide mononitrate. Certainly nitrate ions liberated during metabolism of isosorbide mononitrate can oxidize hemoglobin into methemoglobin. Even in patients totally without cytochrome b_5 reductase activity, however, and even assuming that the nitrate moiety of isosorbide mononitrate is quantitatively applied to oxidation of hemoglobin, about 2 mg/kg of isosorbide mononitrate should be required before any of these patients manifests clinically significant ($\geq$10%) methemoglobinemia. In patients with normal reductase function, significant production of methemoglobin should require even larger doses of isosorbide mononitrate. In one study in which 36 patients received 2–4 weeks of continuous nitroglycerin therapy at 3.1 to 4.4 mg/hr (equivalent, in total administered dose of nitrate ions, to 7.8–11.1 mg of isosorbide mononitrate per hour), the average methemoglobin level measured was 0.2%; this was comparable to that observed in parallel patients who received placebo.
Notwithstanding these observations, there are case reports of significant methemoglobinemia in association with moderate overdoses of organic nitrates. None of the affected patients had been thought to be unusually susceptible.
Methemoglobin levels are available from most clinical laboratories. The diagnosis should be suspected in patients who exhibit signs of impaired oxygen delivery despite adequate cardiac output and adequate arterial pO_2. Classically, methemoglobinemic blood is described as chocolate brown, without color change on exposure to air.
When methemoglobinemia is diagnosed, the treatment of choice is methylene blue, 1–2 mg/kg intravenously.

DOSAGE AND ADMINISTRATION

The recommended regimen of MONOKET Tablets is 20 mg twice daily, with the doses seven hours apart. A starting dose of 5 mg ($^1/_2$ tablet of the 10 mg dosing strength) might be appropriate for persons of particularly small stature but should be increased to at least 10 mg by the second or third day of therapy. Dosage adjustments are not necessary for elderly patients or patients with altered hepatic or renal function.
As noted above (**Clinical Pharmacology**), multiple studies of organic nitrates have shown that maintenance of continuous 24-hour plasma levels results in refractory tolerance. The asymmetric (2 doses, 7 hours apart) dosing regimen for MONOKET Tablets provides a daily nitrate-free interval to minimize the development of tolerance.
As also noted under **Clinical Pharmacology,** well-controlled studies have shown that tolerance to MONOKET Tablets occurs to some extent when using the twice-daily regimen in which the two doses are given seven hours apart. This regimen has been shown to have antianginal efficacy beginning one hour after the first dose and lasting at least seven hours after the second dose. The duration (if any) of antianginal activity beyond fourteen hours has not been studied.
In clinical trials, MONOKET has been administered in a variety of regimens and doses. Doses above 20 mg twice a day (with the doses seven hours apart) have not been adequately studied. Doses of 5 mg twice a day are clearly effective (effectiveness based on exercise tolerance) for only the first day of a twice-a-day (with doses 7 hours apart) regimen.

HOW SUPPLIED

MONOKET® (isosorbide mononitrate) 10mg Tablets are white, round, scored and engraved "10" on one side and engraved "SCHWARZ 610" on the other. They are supplied as follows:
Bottles of 100 NDC 0091-3610-01
MONOKET® (isosorbide mononitrate) 20 mg Tablets are white, round, scored and engraved "20" on one side and engraved "SCHWARZ 620" on the other. They are supplied as follows:
Bottles of 60 NDC 0091-3620-60
Bottles of 100 NDC 0091-3620-01
Bottles of 180 NDC 0091-3620-18
Unit Dose Packages of 100 NDC 0091-3620-11
Store at controlled room temperature 15°–30°C (59°–86°F). Keep tightly closed.
CAUTION: Federal law prohibits dispensing without prescription.
PC0786F Rev. 12/97
Shown in Product Identification Guide, page 337

NASCOBAL™ ℞

[*nās'cobal*]
(Cyanocobalamin, USP)
Gel for Intranasal Administration

DESCRIPTION

Cyanocobalamin is a synthetic form of vitamin B_{12} with equivalent vitamin B_{12} activity. The chemical name is 5,6-dimethyl-benzimidazolyl cyanocobamide. The cobalt content is 4.35%. The molecular formula is $C_{63}H_{88}CoN_{14}O_{14}P$, which corresponds to a molecular weight of 1355.38 and the following structural formula:

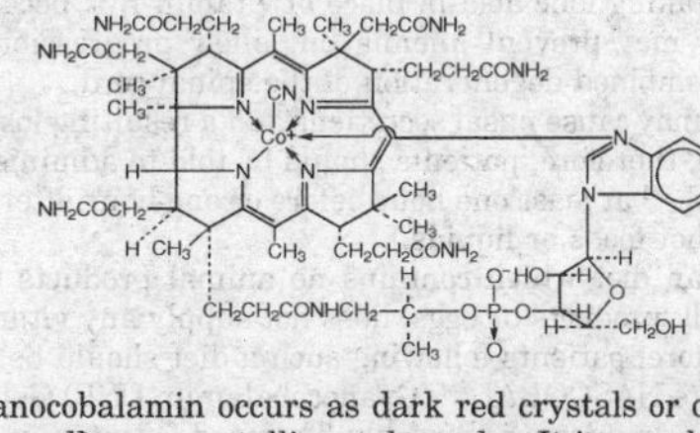

Cyanocobalamin occurs as dark red crystals or orthorhombic needles or crystalline red powder. It is very hygroscopic in the anhydrous form, and sparingly to moderately soluble in water (1:80). Its pharmacologic activity is destroyed by heavy metals (iron) and strong oxidizing or reducing agents (vitamin C), but not by autoclaving for short periods of time (15–20 minutes) at 121°C. The vitamin B_{12} coenzymes are very unstable in light.
NASCOBAL™ (Cyanocobalamin, USP) Gel for Intranasal Administration is a solution of Cyanocobalamin, USP (vitamin B_{12}) for administration as a metered gel to the nasal mucosa. Each bottle of NASCOBAL™ contains 5 mL of a 500 mcg/0.1 mL gel solution of cyanocobalamin with methylcellulose, sodium citrate, citric acid, glycerin, benzalkonium chloride in purified water. The gel solution has a pH between 4.5 and 5.5. The gel pump unit must be fully primed (see Patient Instructions) prior to initial use. After initial priming, each metered gel delivers an average of 500 mcg of cyanocobalamin and the 5 mL bottle will deliver 8 doses of NASCOBAL™. If not used for 48 hours or longer, the unit must be reprimed (see Patient Instructions).

CLINICAL PHARMACOLOGY

GENERAL PHARMACOLOGY AND MECHANISM OF ACTION

Vitamin B_{12} is essential to growth, cell reproduction, hematopoiesis, and nucleoprotein and myelin synthesis. Cells characterized by rapid division (e.g., epithelial cells, bone marrow, myeloid cells) appear to have the greatest requirement for vitamin B_{12}. Vitamin B_{12} can be converted to coenzyme B_{12} in tissues, and as such is essential for conversion of methylmalonate to succinate and synthesis of methionine from homocysteine, a reaction which also requires folate. In the absence of coenzyme B_{12}, tetrahydrofolate cannot be regenerated from its inactive storage form, 5-methyl tetrahydrofolate, and a functional folate deficiency occurs. Vitamin B_{12} also may be involved in maintaining sulfhydryl (SH) groups in the reduced form required by many SH-activated enzyme systems. Through these reactions, vitamin B_{12} is associated with fat and carbohydrate metabolism and protein synthesis. Vitamin B_{12} deficiency results in megaloblastic anemia, GI lesions, and neurologic damage that begins with an inability to produce myelin and is followed by gradual degeneration of the axon and nerve head.
Cyanocobalamin is the most stable and widely used form of vitamin B_{12}, and has hematopoietic activity apparently identical to that of the antianemia factor in purified liver extract. The information below, describing the clinical pharmacology of cyanocobalamin, has been derived from studies with injectable vitamin B_{12}.
Vitamin B_{12} is quantitatively and rapidly absorbed from intramuscular and subcutaneous sites of injection. It is bound to plasma proteins and stored in the liver. Vitamin B_{12} is excreted in the bile and undergoes some enterohepatic recycling. Absorbed vitamin B_{12} is transported via specific B_{12} binding proteins, transcobalamin I and II, to the various tissues. The liver is the main organ for vitamin B_{12} storage.
Parenteral (intramuscular) administration of vitamin B_{12} completely reverses the megaloblastic anemia and GI symptoms of vitamin B_{12} deficiency; the degree of improvement in neurologic symptoms depends on the duration and severity of the lesions, although progression of the lesions is immediately arrested.
Gastrointestinal absorption of vitamin B_{12} depends on the presence of sufficient intrinsic factor and calcium ions. Intrinsic factor deficiency causes pernicious anemia, which may be associated with subacute combined degeneration of the spinal cord. Prompt parenteral administration of vitamin B_{12} prevents progression of neurologic damage.
The average diet supplies about 4 to 15 mcg/day of vitamin B_{12} in a protein-bound form that is available for absorption after normal digestion. Vitamin B_{12} is not present in foods of plant origin, but is abundant in foods of animal origin. In people with normal absorption, deficiencies have been reported only in strict vegetarians who consume no products of animal origin (including no milk products or eggs).
Vitamin B_{12} is bound to intrinsic factor during transit through the stomach; separation occurs in the terminal ileum in the presence of calcium, and vitamin B_{12} enters the mucosal cell for absorption. It is then transported by the transcobalamin binding proteins. A small amount (approximately 1% of the total amount ingested) is absorbed by simple diffusion, but this mechanism is adequate only with very large doses. Oral absorption is considered too undependable to rely on in patients with pernicious anemia or other conditions resulting in malabsorption of vitamin B_{12}.
Colchicine, para-aminosalicylic acid, and heavy alcohol intake for longer than 2 weeks may produce malabsorption of vitamin B_{12}.

PHARMACOKINETICS

Absorption
In a bioavailability study in 24 pernicious anemia patients comparing B_{12} nasal gel to intramuscular B_{12}, peak concentrations of B_{12} after intranasal administration were reached in 1–2 hours. The average peak concentration of B_{12} after intranasal administration was 1,414 $\pm$ 1,003 pg/mL. The bioavailability of the nasal gel relative to an intramuscular injection was found to be 8.9% (90% confidence intervals 7.1–11.2%).
In pernicious anemia patients, once weekly intranasal dosing with 500 mcg B_{12} resulted in a consistent increase in pre-dose serum B_{12} levels during one month of treatment ($p < 0.003$) above that seen one month after 100 mcg intramuscular dose (Figure).
Distribution
In the blood, B_{12} is bound to transcobalamin II, a specific B-globulin carrier protein, and is distributed and stored primarily in the liver and bone marrow.
Elimination
About 3–8 mcg of B_{12} is secreted into the GI tract daily via the bile; in normal subjects with sufficient intrinsic factor, all but about 1 mcg is re-absorbed. When B_{12} is administered in doses which saturate the binding capacity of plasma proteins and the liver, the unbound B_{12} is rapidly eliminated in the urine. Retention of B_{12} in the body is dose-dependent. About 80–90% of an intramuscular dose up to 50 mcg is retained in the body; this percentage drops to 55% for a 100 mcg dose, and decreases to 15% when a 1000 mcg dose is given.

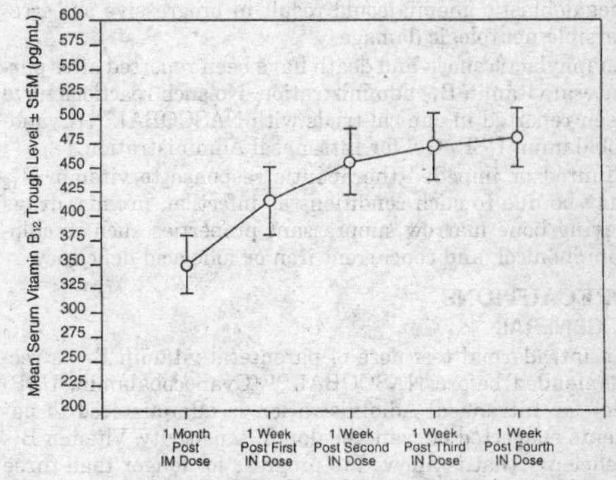

Figure. Vitamin B_{12} Serum Trough Levels After Intramuscular Solution (IM) of 100 mcg and Nasal Gel (IN) Administration of 500 mcg Cyanocobalamin After Weekly Doses.

INDICATIONS AND USAGE

NASCOBAL™ (Cyanocobalamin, USP) Gel for Intranasal Administration is indicated for the maintenance of the hematologic status of patients who are in remission following intramuscular vitamin B_{12} therapy for the following conditions:

I. Pernicious anemia. Indicated only in patients who are in hematologic remission with no nervous system involvement.
II. Dietary deficiency of vitamin B_{12} occurring in strict vegetarians. (Isolated vitamin B_{12} deficiency is very rare).
III. Malabsorption of vitamin B_{12} resulting from structural or functional damage to the stomach, where intrinsic factor is secreted or to the ileum, where intrinsic factor facilitates vitamin B_{12} absorption. These conditions include tropical sprue, and nontropical sprue (Idiopathic

Continued on next page

Nascobal—Cont.

steatorrhea, gluten-induced enteropathy). Folate deficiency in these patients is usually more severe than vitamin B_{12} deficiency.

IV. Inadequate secretion of intrinsic factor, resulting from lesions that destroy the gastric mucosa (ingestion of corrosives, extensive neoplasia), and a number of conditions associated with a variable degree of gastric atrophy (such as multiple sclerosis, certain endocrine disorders, iron deficiency, and subtotal gastrectomy). Total gastrectomy always produces vitamin B_{12} deficiency. Structural lesions leading to vitamin B_{12} deficiency include regional ileitis, ileal resections, malignancies, etc.

V. Competition for vitamin B_{12} by intestinal parasites or bacteria.

The fish tapeworm (Diphyllobothrium latum) absorbs huge quantities of vitamin B_{12} and infested patients often have associated gastric atrophy. The blind-loop syndrome may produce deficiency of vitamin B_{12} or folate.

VI. Inadequate utilization of vitamin B_{12}. This may occur if antimetabolites for the vitamin are employed in the treatment of neoplasia.

It may be possible to treat the underlying disease by surgical correction of anatomic lesions leading to small bowel bacterial overgrowth, expulsion of fish tapeworm, discontinuation of drugs leading to vitamin malabsorption (see "Drug/Laboratory Test Interactions"), use of a gluten-free diet in nontropical sprue, or administration of antibiotics in tropical sprue. Such measures remove the need for long-term administration of vitamin B_{12}.

Requirements of vitamin B_{12} in excess of normal (due to pregnancy, thyrotoxicosis, hemolytic anemia, hemorrhage, malignancy, hepatic and renal disease) can usually be met with intranasal or oral supplementation.

NASCOBAL™ (Cyanocobalamin, USP) Gel for Intranasal Administration has only been tested in patients with vitamin B_{12} malabsorption who have received prior intramuscular cyanocobalamin treatment and are in hematologic remission.

NASCOBAL™ (Cyanocobalamin, USP) Gel for Intranasal Administration is not suitable for the vitamin B_{12} absorption test (Schilling Test).

CONTRAINDICATION

Sensitivity to cobalt and/or vitamin B_{12} or any component of the medication is a contraindication.

WARNINGS

Patients with early Leber's disease (hereditary optic nerve atrophy) who were treated with vitamin B_{12} suffered severe and swift optic atrophy.

Hypokalemia and sudden death may occur in severe megaloblastic anemia which is treated intensely with vitamin B_{12}. Folic acid is not a substitute for vitamin B_{12} although it may improve vitamin B_{12}-deficient megaloblastic anemia. Exclusive use of folic acid in treating vitamin B_{12}-deficient megaloblastic anemia could result in progressive and irreversible neurologic damage.

Anaphylactic shock and death have been reported after parenteral vitamin B_{12} administration. No such reactions have been reported in clinical trials with NASCOBAL™ (Cyanocobalamin, USP) Gel for Intranasal Administration.

Blunted or impeded therapeutic response to vitamin B_{12} may be due to such conditions as infection, uremia, drugs having bone marrow suppressant properties such as chloramphenicol, and concurrent iron or folic acid deficiency.

PRECAUTIONS

1. GENERAL

An intradermal test dose of parenteral vitamin B_{12} is recommended before NASCOBAL™ (Cyanocobalamin, USP) Gel for Intranasal Administration is administered to patients suspected of cyanocobalamin sensitivity. Vitamin B_{12} deficiency that is allowed to progress for longer than three months may produce permanent degenerative lesions of the spinal cord. Doses of folic acid greater than 0.1 mg per day may result in hematologic remission in patients with vitamin B_{12} deficiency. Neurologic manifestations will not be prevented with folic acid, and if not treated with vitamin B_{12}, irreversible damage will result.

Doses of vitamin B_{12} exceeding 10 mcg daily may produce hematologic response in patients with folate deficiency. Indiscriminate administration may mask the true diagnosis. The validity of diagnostic vitamin B_{12} or folic acid blood assays could be compromised by medications, and this should be considered before relying on such tests for therapy.

Vitamin B_{12} is not a substitute for folic acid and since it might improve folic acid deficient megaloblastic anemia, indiscriminate use of vitamin B_{12} could mask the true diagnosis.

Hypokalemia and thrombocytosis could occur upon conversion of severe megaloblastic to normal erythropoiesis with vitamin B_{12} therapy. Therefore, serum potassium levels and the platelet count should be monitored carefully during therapy.

Vitamin B_{12} deficiency may suppress the signs of polycythemia vera. Treatment with vitamin B_{12} may unmask this condition.

If a patient is not properly maintained with NASCOBAL™ (Cyanocobalamin, USP) Gel for Intranasal Administration, intramuscular vitamin B_{12} is necessary for adequate treatment of the patient. No single regimen fits all cases, and the status of the patient observed in follow-up is the final criterion for adequacy of therapy.

The effectiveness of NASCOBAL™ (Cyanocobalamin, USP) Gel for Intranasal Administration in patients with nasal congestion, allergic rhinitis and upper respiratory infections has not been determined. Therefore, treatment with NASCOBAL™ should be deferred until symptoms have subsided.

2. INFORMATION FOR PATIENTS

Patients with pernicious anemia should be instructed that they will require weekly intranasal administration of NASCOBAL™ (Cyanocobalamin, USP) Gel for Intranasal Administration for the remainder of their lives. Failure to do so will result in return of the anemia and in development of incapacitating and irreversible damage to the nerves of the spinal cord. Also, patients should be warned about the danger of taking folic acid in place of vitamin B_{12}, because the former may prevent anemia but allow progression of subacute combined degeneration of the spinal cord.

(Hot foods may cause nasal secretions and a resulting loss of medication; therefore, patients should be told to administer NASCOBAL™ at least one hour before or one hour after ingestion of hot foods or liquids.)

A vegetarian diet which contains no animal products (including milk products or eggs) does not supply any vitamin B_{12}. Therefore, patients following such a diet should be advised to take NASCOBAL™ (Cyanocobalamin, USP) Gel for Intranasal Administration weekly. The need for vitamin B_{12} is increased by pregnancy and lactation. Deficiency has been recognized in infants of vegetarian mothers who were breast fed, even though the mothers had no symptoms of deficiency at the time.

The patient should also understand the importance of returning for follow-up blood tests every 3 to 6 months to confirm adequacy of the therapy. Careful instructions on the actuator assembly, priming of the actuator and nasal administration of NASCOBAL™ (Cyanocobalamin, USP) Gel for Intranasal Administration should be given to the patient. Although instructions for patients are supplied with individual bottles, procedures for use should be demonstrated to each patient.

3. LABORATORY TESTS

Hematocrit, reticulocyte count, vitamin B_{12}, folate and iron levels should be obtained prior to treatment. If folate levels are low, folic acid should also be administered. All hematologic parameters should be normal when beginning treatment with NASCOBAL™ (Cyanocobalamin, USP) Gel for Intranasal Administration.

Vitamin B_{12} blood levels and peripheral blood counts must be monitored initially at one month after the start of treatment with NASCOBAL™, and then at intervals of 3 to 6 months.

A decline in the serum levels of B_{12} after one month of treatment with B_{12} nasal gel may indicate that the dose may need to be adjusted upward. Patients should be seen one month after each dose adjustment; continued low levels of serum B_{12} may indicate that the patient is not a candidate for this mode of administration.

Patients with pernicious anemia have about 3 times the incidence of carcinoma of the stomach as in the general population, so appropriate tests for this condition should be carried out when indicated.

4. DRUG/LABORATORY TEST INTERACTIONS

Persons taking most antibiotics, methotrexate or pyrimethamine invalidate folic acid and vitamin B_{12} diagnostic blood assays.

Colchicine, para-aminosalicylic acid and heavy alcohol intake for longer than 2 weeks may produce malabsorption of vitamin B_{12}.

5. CARCINOGENESIS, MUTAGENESIS, IMPAIRMENT OF FERTILITY

Long-term studies in animals to evaluate carcinogenic potential have not been done. There is no evidence from long-

Table. Adverse Experiences by Body System, Number of Patients and Number of Occurrences by Treatment Following Intramuscular and Intranasal Administration of Cyanocobalamin.

Body System	Adverse Experience	Number of Patients (Occurrences)	
		Vitamin B_{12} Nasal Gel, 500 mcg N=24	Intramuscular Vitamin B_{12}, 100 mcg N=25
Body as a Whole	Asthenia	1 (1)	4 (4)
	Back Pain	0 (0)	1 (1)
	Generalized Pain	0 (0)	2 (3)
	Headache	1 (2)*	5 (11)
	Infection[a]	3 (4)	3 (3)
Cardiovascular System	Peripheral Vascular Disorder	0 (0)	1 (1)
Digestive System	Dyspepsia	0 (0)	1 (2)
	Glossitis	1 (1)	0 (0)
	Nausea	1 (1)*	1 (1)
	Nausea & Vomiting	0 (0)	1 (1)
	Vomiting	0 (0)	1 (1)
Musculoskeletal System	Arthritis	0 (0)	2 (2)
	Myalgia	0 (0)	1 (1)
Nervous System	Abnormal Gait	0 (0)	1 (1)
	Anxiety	0 (0)	1 (1)*
	Dizziness	0 (0)	3 (3)
	Hypoesthesia	0 (0)	1 (1)
	Incoordination	0 (0)	1 (2)*
	Nervousness	0 (0)	1 (3)*
	Paresthesia	1 (1)	1 (1)
Respiratory System	Dyspnea	0 (0)	1 (1)
	Rhinitis	1 (1)*	2 (2)

[a] Sore throat, common cold

* There may be a possible relationship between these adverse experiences and the study drugs. These adverse experiences could have also been produced by the patient's clinical state or other concomitant therapy.

term use in patients with pernicious anemia that vitamin B_{12} is carcinogenic. Pernicious anemia is associated with an increased incidence of carcinoma of the stomach, but this is believed to be related to the underlying pathology and not to treatment with vitamin B_{12}.

6. PREGNANCY

Pregnancy Category C: Animal reproduction studies have not been conducted with vitamin B_{12}. It is also not known whether vitamin B_{12} can cause fetal harm when administered to a pregnant woman or can affect reproduction capacity. Adequate and well-controlled studies have not been done in pregnant women. However, vitamin B_{12} is an essential vitamin and requirements are increased during pregnancy. Amounts of vitamin B_{12} that are recommended by the Food and Nutrition Board, National Academy of Science-National Research Council for pregnant women (4 mcg daily) should be consumed during pregnancy.

7. NURSING MOTHERS

Vitamin B_{12} appears in the milk of nursing mothers in concentrations which approximate the mother's vitamin B_{12} blood level. Amounts of vitamin B_{12} that are recommended by the Food and Nutrition Board, National Academy of Science-National Research Council for lactating women (4 mcg daily) should be consumed during lactation.

8. PEDIATRIC USE

Intake in children should be in the amount (0.5 to 3 mcg daily) recommended by the Food and Nutrition Board, National Academy of Science-National Research Council.

ADVERSE REACTIONS

The incidence of adverse experiences described in the Table below are based on data from a short-term clinical trial in vitamin B_{12} deficient patients in hematologic remission receiving NASCOBAL™ (Cyanocobalamin, USP) Gel for Intranasal Administration (N=24) and intramuscular vitamin B_{12} (N=25).

[See table at bottom of previous page]

The intensity of the reported adverse experiences following the administration of NASCOBAL™ (Cyanocobalamin, USP) Gel for Intranasal Administration and intramuscular vitamin B_{12} were generally mild. One patient reported severe headache following intramuscular dosing. Similarly, a few adverse experiences of moderate intensity were reported following intramuscular dosing (two headaches and rhinitis; one dyspepsia, arthritis, and dizziness), and dosing with NASCOBAL™ (Cyanocobalamin, USP) Gel for Intranasal Administration (one headache, infection, and paresthesia).

The majority of the reported adverse experiences following dosing with NASCOBAL™ (Cyanocobalamin, USP) Gel for Intranasal Administration and intramuscular vitamin B_{12} were judged to be intercurrent events. For the other reported adverse experiences, the relationship to study drug was judged as "possible" or "remote". Of the adverse experiences judged to be of "possible" relationship to the study drug, anxiety, incoordination, and nervousness were reported following intramuscular vitamin B_{12} and headache, nausea, and rhinitis were reported following dosing with NASCOBAL™ (Cyanocobalamin, USP) Gel for Intranasal Administration.

The following adverse reactions have been reported with parenteral vitamin B_{12}:

Generalized:	Anaphylactic shock and death (See warnings and precautions).
Cardiovascular:	Pulmonary edema and congestive heart failure early in treatment; peripheral vascular thrombosis.
Hematological:	Polycythemia vera.
Gastrointestinal:	Mild transient diarrhea.
Dermatological:	Itching; transitory exanthema.
Miscellaneous:	Feeling of swelling of the entire body.

OVERDOSAGE

No overdosage has been reported with NASCOBAL™ (Cyanocobalamin, USP) Gel for Intranasal Administration or parenteral vitamin B_{12}.

DOSAGE AND ADMINISTRATION

The recommended initial dose of NASCOBAL™ (Cyanocobalamin, USP) Gel for Intranasal Administration in patients with vitamin B_{12} malabsorption who are in remission following injectable vitamin B_{12} therapy is 500 mcg administered intranasally once weekly. Patients should be in hematologic remission before treatment with NASCOBAL™ (Cyanocobalamin, USP) Gel for Intranasal Administration. See LABORATORY TESTS for monitoring B_{12} levels and adjustment of dosage.

HOW SUPPLIED

NASCOBAL™ (Cyanocobalamin, USP) Gel for Intranasal Administration is available as a metered dose gel in 5 mL glass bottles. It is available in a dosage strength of 500 mcg per actuation (0.1 mL/actuation). A screw-on actuator is provided. This actuator, following priming, will deliver 0.1 mL of the gel. NASCOBAL™ (Cyanocobalamin, USP) Gel for Intranasal Administration is provided in a sealed prescription vial containing a metered dose nasal gel actuator with dust cover, a bottle of nasal gel solution, and a patient instruction leaflet. One bottle will deliver 8 doses (NDC 0091-7033-12).

PHARMACIST ASSEMBLY INSTRUCTIONS FOR NASCOBAL™ (CYANOCOBALAMIN, USP) GEL FOR INTRANASAL ADMINISTRATION

The pharmacist should assemble NASCOBAL™ (Cyanocobalamin, USP) Gel for Intranasal Administration prior to dispensing to the patient, according to the following instructions:

1. Break the protective seal, open the prescription vial, and remove the gel actuator and gel solution bottle.
2. Assemble NASCOBAL™ by first unscrewing the white cap from the gel solution bottle and screwing the actuator unit tightly onto the bottle. Make sure the clear dust cover is on the pump unit.
3. Return the NASCOBAL™ bottle to the prescription vial for dispensing to the patient.

STORAGE CONDITIONS

Protect from light. Keep covered in prescription vial until ready to use. Store at room temperature 15°C to 30°C (59°F to 86°F). Protect from freezing.

CAUTION

Federal law prohibits dispensing without prescription.
PC3137   Rev. 7/97

PATIENT INSTRUCTIONS

Take medication as directed by your physician. For proper use of the gel actuator, read the following instructions carefully.

NOTE: THE VIAL IS PREFILLED TO DELIVER EIGHT SINGLE 500 mcg DOSES. (THE DOSE IS 500 mcg — ONE DOSE IN ONE NOSTRIL.)

THE UNIT MUST BE PRIMED WITH THREE STROKES IF NOT USED FOR 48 HOURS OR LONGER.

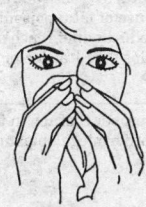

Fig 1
1. Blow nose gently to clear both nostrils. (Fig 1)

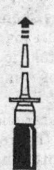

Fig 2
2. Pull Clear cover off pump unit. (Fig 2)

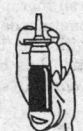

Fig 3
3. Prime NASCOBAL™ by placing nozzle between first and second finger with thumb on the bottom of bottle. Pump gel unit FIRMLY AND QUICKLY until the gel droplet appears (up to 7–8 strokes). Then prime actuator an additional 2 times. (Fig 3)

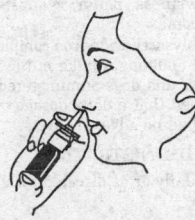

Fig 4
4. Insert tip approximately 1cm into one nostril, pointing the tip toward the back of the nose. (Fig 4)

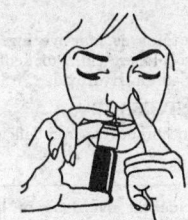

Fig 5
5. Close other nostril with your forefinger and tilt head slightly forward. (Fig 5)

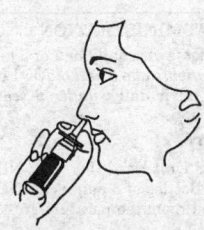

Fig 6
6. Pump gel unit firmly and quickly by pushing down on the "finger grips" of the pump unit and against the thumb at the bottom of the bottle. Sniff gently with your mouth closed. (Fig 6)

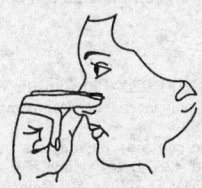

Fig 7
7. After dosing, remove pump unit from nose. Massage the dosed nostril gently a few seconds. (Fig 7)
8. Clean the nozzle of the gel pump by wiping with a clean tissue after use. Replace clear cover on pump unit (Fig 2) after each dose.
Follow this procedure for each dose.
9. Apply once into one nostril unless your doctor has directed you to apply NASCOBAL™ into both nostrils.
When not in use, store gel unit in container.
NASCOBAL™ should not be used by anyone other than the person for whom it was prescribed. To prevent this, and to reduce the chance of children taking the drug it is important to properly dispose of any excess NASCOBAL™ as soon as it is no longer needed.
The best way to safely dispose of the unit is to unscrew the cap, rinse the bottle and gel pump assembly under a water faucet, and dispose of the parts in a waste can or any container inaccessible to children.

> **USUAL DOSE: ONE Dose. Dose ONLY ONCE into ONLY ONE nostril. DO NOT dose into both nostrils unless directed by your doctor. DO NOT repeat sooner than directed by your doctor.**

> **KEEP OUT OF REACH OF CHILDREN**

PCL3139   7/97
Shown in Product Identification Guide, page 337

NIFEREX® TABLETS/ELIXIR   OTC
[*ni 'fer"ex*]
(polysaccharide-iron complex, as cell-contracted akaganéite)

DESCRIPTION

NIFEREX Film Coated Tablets contain 50 mg elemental iron. Each 5 mL (teaspoonful) NIFEREX Elixir contains 100 mg elemental iron.
Each tablet also contains as inactive ingredients: Castor Oil, Hydroxypropyl Cellulose, FD&C Blue #1 Aluminum Lake, FD&C Red #40 Aluminum Lake, FD&C Yellow #6 Aluminum Lake, Hydroxypropyl Methylcellulose, Lactose, Magnesium Stearate, Microcrystalline Cellulose, Pharmaceutical Glaze, Polyethylene Glycol, Povidone, Propylene Glycol, Sodium Starch Glycolate, Titanium Dioxide.

Continued on next page

Niferex—Cont.

The elixir also contains as inactive ingredients: Alcohol 10%, Flavor, Hydrochloric Acid, Purified Water, Sorbitol. May also contain: Sodium Hydroxide.

INDICATIONS AND USAGE

For treatment of uncomplicated iron deficiency anemias.

WARNINGS

> WARNING: Accidental overdose of iron-containing products is a leading cause of fatal poisoning in children under 6. Keep this product out of reach of children. In case of accidental overdose, call a doctor or poison control center immediately.

DOSAGE AND ADMINISTRATION

Adults: 1 or 2 tablets twice daily, *or* 1 or 2 teaspoonfuls elixir daily. *Pediatric patients age 6 and older:* 1 or 2 tablets daily, or 1 or 2 teaspoonfuls elixir daily; *under 6 years of age,* as directed by a physician.

HOW SUPPLIED

NIFEREX Tablets Unit Dose 100   NDC 0131-2200-86
NIFEREX Elixir Bottles of 8 ounces   NDC 0131-5066-68
Store at controlled room temperature 15°–30°C (59°–86°F).

NIFEREX®-150 CAPSULES   OTC
[ni ' fer " ex]
(polysaccharide-iron complex, as cell-contracted akaganéite)

DESCRIPTION

Each bead–filled NIFEREX-150 Capsule contains 150 mg elemental iron as polysaccharide-iron complex, as cell–contracted akaganéite.
Each capsule also contains as inactive ingredients: D&C Red #7, D&C Red #28, D&C Yellow #10, FD&C Blue #1, FD&C Red #40, FD&C Yellow #6, Gelatin, Hydrogenated Castor Oil, Pharmaceutical Glaze, Povidone, Sodium Lauryl Sulfate, Starch, Sucrose, Titanium Dioxide. May contain: Silicon Dioxide.

INDICATIONS AND USAGE

For treatment of uncomplicated iron deficiency anemias.

WARNINGS

> WARNING: Accidental overdose of iron-containing products is a leading cause of fatal poisoning in children under 6. Keep this product out of reach of children. In case of accidental overdose, call a doctor or poison control center immediately.

DOSAGE AND ADMINISTRATION

Adults: 1 or 2 capsules daily.

HOW SUPPLIED

NIFEREX-150 Capsules are orange and clear capsules containing brown beads. The capsules are imprinted "SP" and "4220". They are supplied as follows:
Unit Dose 100   NDC 0131-4220-09
Store at controlled room temperature 15°–30°C (59°–86°F).
CR2912A   7/97
Shown in Product Identification Guide, page 337

NIFEREX®-150 FORTE CAPSULES   ℞
[ni 'fer "ex for 'ta]

DESCRIPTION

Each bead-filled capsule for oral administration contains:
Iron (elemental) .... 150 mg
(polysaccharide-iron complex, as cell-contracted akaganéite)
Folic Acid .... 1 mg
Vitamin B$_{12}$ (cyanocobalamin) .... 25 mcg
Each capsule also contains the following inactive ingredients: corn starch, D&C Red #7, D&C Red #28, FD&C Blue #1, FD&C Red #40, FD&C Yellow #6, gelatin, hydrogenated castor oil, pharmaceutical glaze, povidone, sodium lauryl sulfate, sucrose, and titanium dioxide. It may contain: silicon dioxide.
NIFEREX® (polysaccharide-iron complex, as cell-contracted akaganéite) is the product of ferric iron complexed to a low molecular weight polysaccharide. This polysaccharide is produced by the extensive hydrolysis of starch. NIFEREX® is a dark brown powder which dissolves in water to form a very dark brown solution. It is virtually tasteless and odorless. Because it is an organic complex, it contains no free ions.

CLINICAL PHARMACOLOGY

Iron is an essential component in the formation of hemoglobin. Adequate amounts of iron are necessary for effective erythropoiesis. Iron also serves as a cofactor of several essential enzymes, including cytochromes that are involved in electron transport. A radioisotope tracer study in man demonstrated that absorption of NIFEREX® Elixir is comparable to ferrous sulfate elixir. Clinical studies demonstrate that NIFEREX® produces good hematopoietic response as shown by increases in hemoglobin and hematocrit in pediatric and elderly patients. NIFEREX® is effective in maintaining the hematopoietic status in end-stage renal disease patients receiving epoetin alfa therapy.
Folic acid is required for nucleoprotein synthesis and the maintenance of normal erythropoiesis. Folic acid is converted in the liver and plasma to its metabolically active form, tetrahydrofolic acid, by dihydrofolate reductase.
Vitamin B$_{12}$ is required for the maintenance of normal erythropoiesis, nucleoprotein and myelin synthesis, cell reproduction and normal growth. Intrinsic factor, a glycoprotein secreted by the gastric mucosa, is required for active absorption of Vitamin B$_{12}$ from the gastrointestinal tract.

INDICATIONS AND USAGE

NIFEREX®-150 FORTE is indicated for the prevention and treatment of iron deficiency anemia and/or nutritional megaloblastic anemias.

CONTRAINDICATIONS

NIFEREX®-150 FORTE is contraindicated in patients with a known hypersensitivity to any of the components of this product. Hemochromatosis and hemosiderosis are contraindications to iron therapy.

WARNINGS

> WARNING: Accidental overdose of iron-containing products is a leading cause of fatal poisoning in children under 6. Keep this product out of reach of children. In case of accidental overdose, call a doctor or poison control center immediately.

Folic acid alone is improper therapy in the treatment of pernicious anemia and other megaloblastic anemias where Vitamin B$_{12}$ is deficient.

PRECAUTIONS

General:
The type of anemia and the underlying cause or causes should be determined before starting therapy with NIFEREX®-150 FORTE. Since the anemia may be a result of a systemic disturbance, such as recurrent blood loss, the underlying cause or causes should be corrected, if possible. Folic acid in doses above 0.1 mg daily may obscure pernicious anemia in that hematologic remission can occur while neurological manifestations remain progressive.
Information for Patients:
As with all oral iron preparations, NIFEREX®-150 FORTE should be stored out of the reach of children to guard against accidental iron poisoning. Patients should not exceed the recommended dosage unless directed by the physician. Patients should be informed that iron therapy can cause black or dark stools.

ADVERSE REACTIONS

Adverse reactions with iron therapy may include constipation, diarrhea, nausea, vomiting, dark stools and abdominal pain. Adverse reactions with iron therapy are usually transient. Allergic sensitization has been reported following both oral and parenteral administration of folic acid.

OVERDOSAGE

ACCIDENTAL OVERDOSE OF IRON-CONTAINING PRODUCTS IS A LEADING CAUSE OF FATAL POISONING IN CHILDREN UNDER 6. KEEP THIS PRODUCT OUT OF REACH OF CHILDREN. IN CASE OF ACCIDENTAL OVERDOSE, CALL A DOCTOR OR POISON CONTROL CENTER IMMEDIATELY.
The clinical course of acute iron overdosage can be variable. Initial symptoms may include abdominal pain, nausea, vomiting, diarrhea, tarry stools, melena, hematemesis, hypotension, tachycardia, metabolic acidosis, hyperglycemia, dehydration, drowsiness, pallor, cyanosis, lassitude, seizures, shock and coma.
The oral LD$_{50}$ of polysaccharide-iron complex was estimated to be greater than 5000 mg iron/kg in the rat. Chronic toxicity studies in rats and dogs administered polysaccharide-iron complex showed that a daily dosage of 250 mg iron/kg for three months had no adverse effects.

DOSAGE AND ADMINISTRATION

Adults: 1 capsule daily or as directed by a physician.

HOW SUPPLIED

NIFEREX®-150 FORTE Capsules are red and clear capsules containing brown beads. The capsules are imprinted "SP" and "4330". They are supplied as follows:
Unit Dose 100   NDC 0131-4330-86

Store at controlled room temperature 15°–30°C (59°–86°F).
CAUTION: Federal law prohibits dispensing without prescription.
PC2995A   Rev. 9/97
Shown in Product Identification Guide, page 337

NIFEREX®—PN TABLETS   ℞
[ni 'fer "ex]

Rx Only

DESCRIPTION

NIFEREX-PN Tablets contain ingredients of the following classes: vitamins and minerals. Each blue, film-coated tablet for oral administration contains:
Iron (elemental) .... 60 mg
(polysaccharide-iron complex, as cell-contracted akaganéite)
Folic Acid .... 1 mg
Vitamin C (as sodium ascorbate) .... 50 mg
Vitamin B$_{12}$ (cyanocobalamin) .... 3 mcg
Vitamin A .... 4000 IU
Vitamin D .... 400 IU
Vitamin B$_1$ (as thiamine mononitrate) .... 2.43 mg
Vitamin B$_2$ (riboflavin) .... 3 mg
Vitamin B$_6$ (as pyridoxine hydrochloride) .... 1.64 mg
Niacinamide .... 10 mg
Calcium (as calcium carbonate) .... 125 mg
Zinc (as zinc sulfate) .... 18 mg
Each tablet also contains the following inactive ingredients: castor oil, corn starch, FD&C Blue #1 (Lake), gelatin, hydrogenated vegetable oil, hydroxypropyl cellulose, hydroxypropyl methylcellulose, magnesium stearate, microcrystalline cellulose, pharmaceutical glaze, polyethylene glycol, povidone, propylene glycol and titanium dioxide.
NIFEREX® (polysaccharide-iron complex, as cell-contracted akaganéite) is the product of ferric iron complexed to a low molecular weight polysaccharide. This polysaccharide is produced by the extensive hydrolysis of starch. NIFEREX® is a dark brown powder which dissolves in water to form a very dark brown solution. It is virtually tasteless and odorless. Because it is an organic complex, it contains no free ions.

CLINICAL PHARMACOLOGY

This product is formulated to meet the vitamin and mineral needs of the pregnant or lactating patient with special consideration given to adequate amounts of the hematopoietic factors: iron, folic acid and cyanocobalamin. Calcium is included in the formula to help supply the increased requirements of this mineral. Sixty (60) mg of elemental iron is available in the form of NIFEREX® (polysaccharide-iron complex, as cell–contracted akaganéite). A radioisotope tracer study in man demonstrated that absorption of NIFEREX® Elixir is comparable to that of ferrous sulfate elixir. In addition, folic acid and cyanocobalamin are included to prevent or treat pregnancy-related megaloblastic anemia.

INDICATIONS AND USAGE

NIFEREX®-PN is indicated for the prevention and/or treatment of dietary vitamin and mineral deficiencies associated with pregnancy and lactation.

CONTRAINDICATIONS

NIFEREX®-PN is contraindicated in patients with a known hypersensitivity to any of the components of this product. Hemochromatosis and hemosiderosis are contraindications to iron therapy.

WARNINGS

> WARNING: Accidental overdose of iron-containing products is a leading cause of fatal poisoning in children under 6. Keep this product out of reach of children. In case of accidental overdose, call a doctor or poison control center immediately.

Folic acid alone is improper therapy in the treatment of pernicious anemia and other megaloblastic anemias where Vitamin B$_{12}$ is deficient.

PRECAUTIONS

General:
Folic acid in doses above 0.1 mg daily may obscure pernicious anemia, in that hematologic remission can occur while neurological manifestations remain progressive. Vitamin A, in high doses, may be associated with birth defects.
Information for Patients:
As with all oral iron preparations, NIFEREX®-PN should be stored out of the reach of children to guard against accidental iron poisoning. Patients should not exceed the recommended dosage unless directed by the physician. Patients should be informed that iron therapy can cause black or dark stools.

ADVERSE REACTIONS

Adverse reactions with iron therapy may include constipation, diarrhea, nausea, vomiting, dark stools and abdominal pain. Adverse reactions with iron therapy are usually transient. Allergic sensitization has been reported following both oral and parenteral administration of folic acid.

OVERDOSAGE

ACCIDENTAL OVERDOSE OF IRON-CONTAINING PRODUCTS IS A LEADING CAUSE OF FATAL POISONING IN CHILDREN UNDER 6. KEEP THIS PRODUCT OUT OF REACH OF CHILDREN. IN CASE OF ACCIDENTAL OVERDOSE, CALL A DOCTOR OR POISON CONTROL CENTER IMMEDIATELY.

The clinical course of acute iron overdosage can be variable. Initial symptoms may include abdominal pain, nausea, vomiting, diarrhea, tarry stools, melena, hematemesis, hypotension, tachycardia, metabolic acidosis, hyperglycemia, dehydration, drowsiness, pallor, cyanosis, lassitude, seizures, shock and coma.

The oral LD_{50} of polysaccharide-iron complex was estimated to be greater than 5000 mg iron/kg in the rat. Chronic toxicity studies in rats and dogs administered polysaccharide-iron complex showed that a daily dosage of 250 mg iron/kg for three months had no adverse effects.

DOSAGE AND ADMINISTRATION

Adults: 1 tablet daily or as directed by a physician.

HOW SUPPLIED

NIFEREX®-PN Tablets are blue, oval, film-coated tablets debossed with "131/05" on one side and "SP2209" on the other. They are supplied as follows:

Unit Dose 100 NDC 0131-2209-09

Store at controlled room temperature 15°–30°C (59°–86°F).

PC2622C Rev. 5/98

Shown in Product Identification Guide, page 337

NIFEREX®-PN FORTE TABLETS ℞

[ni 'fer "ex]

Rx Only

DESCRIPTION

NIFEREX®-PN FORTE Tablets contain ingredients of the following classes: vitamins and minerals. Each white, film-coated tablet for oral administration contains:

Iron (elemental)	60 mg
(polysaccharide-iron complex, as cell-contracted akaganéite)	
Vitamin A	5000 IU
Vitamin D	400 IU
Vitamin E (as dl-alpha-tocopheryl acetate)	30 IU
Vitamin C (ascorbic acid)	80 mg
Folic acid	1 mg
Vitamin B_1 (as thiamine mononitrate)	3 mg
Vitamin B_2 (riboflavin)	3.4 mg
Vitamin B_6 (as pyridoxine hydrochloride)	4 mg
Niacinamide	20 mg
Vitamin B_{12} (cyanocobalamin)	12 mcg
Calcium (as calcium carbonate)	250 mg
Iodine (as potassium iodide)	200 mcg
Magnesium (as magnesium oxide)	10 mg
Copper (as cupric oxide)	2 mg
Zinc (as zinc sulfate)	25 mg

Each tablet also contains the following inactive ingredients: castor oil, corn starch, ethyl cellulose, flavor, gelatin, hydrogenated vegetable oil, hydroxypropyl cellulose, hydroxypropyl methylcellulose, magnesium stearate, microcrystalline cellulose, pharmaceutical glaze, polyethylene glycol, povidone, propylene glycol, silicon dioxide, sodium benzoate, sorbic acid and titanium dioxide.

NIFEREX® (polysaccharide-iron complex, as cell-contracted akaganéite) is the product of ferric iron complexed to a low molecular weight polysaccharide. This polysaccharide is produced by the extensive hydrolysis of starch. NIFEREX® is a dark brown powder which dissolves in water to form a very dark brown solution. It is virtually tasteless and odorless. Because it is an organic complex, it contains no free ions.

CLINICAL PHARMACOLOGY

This product is formulated to meet the vitamin and mineral needs of the pregnant or lactating patient with special consideration given to adequate amounts of the hematopoietic factors: iron, folic acid and cyanocobalamin. Calcium is included in the formula to help supply the increased requirements of this mineral. Sixty (60) mg of elemental iron is available in the form of NIFEREX® (polysaccharide-iron complex, as cell–contracted akaganéite). A radioisotope tracer study in man demonstrated that absorption of NIFEREX® Elixir is comparable to ferrous sulfate elixir. In addition, folic acid and cyanocobalamin are included to prevent or treat pregnancy-related megaloblastic anemia.

INDICATIONS AND USAGE

NIFEREX®-PN FORTE is indicated for the prevention and/or treatment of dietary vitamin and mineral deficiencies associated with pregnancy and lactation.

CONTRAINDICATIONS

NIFEREX®-PN FORTE is contraindicated in patients with a known hypersensitivity to any of the components of this product. Hemochromatosis and hemosiderosis are contraindications to iron therapy.

WARNINGS

> WARNING: Accidental overdose of iron-containing products is a leading cause of fatal poisoning in children under 6. Keep this product out of reach of children. In case of accidental overdose, call a doctor or poison control center immediately.

Folic acid alone is improper therapy in the treatment of pernicious anemia and other megaloblastic anemias where Vitamin B_{12} is deficient.

PRECAUTIONS

General:

Folic acid in doses above 0.1 mg daily may obscure pernicious anemia in that hematologic remission can occur while neurological manifestations remain progressive. Vitamin A, in high doses, may be associated with birth defects.

Information for Patients:

As with all oral iron preparations, NIFEREX®-PN FORTE should be stored out of the reach of children to guard against accidental poisoning. Patients should not exceed the recommended dosage unless directed by the physician. Patients should be informed that iron therapy can cause black or dark stools.

ADVERSE REACTIONS

Adverse reactions with iron therapy may include constipation, diarrhea, nausea, vomiting, dark stools and abdominal pain. Adverse reactions with iron therapy are usually transient. Allergic sensitization has been reported following both oral and parenteral administration of folic acid.

OVERDOSAGE

ACCIDENTAL OVERDOSE OF IRON-CONTAINING PRODUCTS IS A LEADING CAUSE OF FATAL POISONING IN CHILDREN UNDER 6. KEEP THIS PRODUCT OUT OF REACH OF CHILDREN. IN CASE OF ACCIDENTAL OVERDOSE, CALL A DOCTOR OR POISON CONTROL CENTER IMMEDIATELY.

The clinical course of acute iron overdosage can be variable. Initial symptoms may include abdominal pain, nausea, vomiting, diarrhea, tarry stools, melena, hematemesis, hypotension, tachycardia, metabolic acidosis, hyperglycemia, dehydration, drowsiness, pallor, cyanosis, lassitude, seizures, shock and coma.

The oral LD_{50} of polysaccharide-iron complex was estimated to be greater than 5000 mg iron/kg in the rat. Chronic toxicity studies in rats and dogs administered polysaccharide-iron complex showed that a daily dosage of 250 mg iron/kg for three months had no adverse effects.

DOSAGE AND ADMINISTRATION

Adults: 1 tablet daily or as directed by a physician.

HOW SUPPLIED

NIFEREX®-PN FORTE Tablets are white, capsule shaped, scored, film-coated tablets debossed with "SP2309" on the unscored side and 1/0 on the scored side. They are supplied as follows:

Unit Dose 100 NDC 0131-2309-09

Store at controlled room temperature 15°–30°C (59°–86°F).

PC2623C Rev. 5/98

Shown in Product Identification Guide, page 337

PROCTOCREAM®•HC 2.5% ℞

(hydrocortisone cream USP, 2.5%)
[topical]

DESCRIPTION

proctoCream®•HC 2.5% contains Hydrocortisone [Pregn-4-ene-3, 20-dione, 11, 17,21-trihydroxy-, (11β)-] with the molecular formula $C_{21}H_{30}O_5$ and a molecular weight of 362.47, CAS 50-23-7. Each gram for topical administration contains: 25 mg of hydrocortisone in a base of glyceryl monostearate, polyoxyl 40 stearate, glycerin, paraffin, stearyl alcohol, isopropyl palmitate, sorbitan monostearate, benzyl alcohol, potassium sorbate, lactic acid, and purified water. [See chemical structure at top of next column]

CLINICAL PHARMACOLOGY

Topical corticosteroids share anti-inflammatory, anti-pruritic and vasoconstrictive actions.

The mechanism of anti-inflammatory activity of the topical corticosteroids is unclear. Various laboratory methods, including vasoconstrictor assays, are used to compare and predict potencies and/or clinical efficacies of the topical corticosteroids. There is some evidence to suggest that a recognizable correlation exists between vasoconstrictor potency and therapeutic efficacy in man.

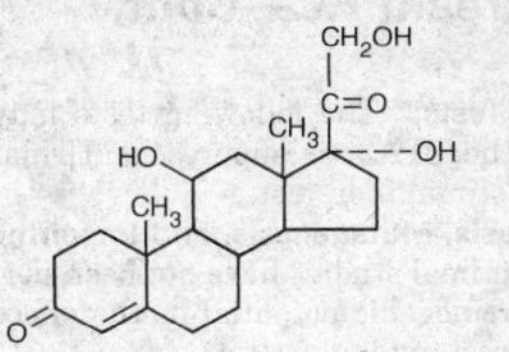

Pharmacokinetics: The extent of percutaneous absorption of topical corticosteroids is determined by many factors including the vehicle, the integrity of the epidermal barrier, and the use of occlusive dressings.

Topical corticosteroids can be absorbed from normal intact skin. Inflammation and/or other disease processes in the skin increase percutaneous absorption.

Occlusive dressings substantially increase the percutaneous absorption of topical corticosteroids. Thus, occlusive dressings may be a valuable therapeutic adjunct for treatment of resistant dermatoses. (See **DOSAGE AND ADMINISTRATION**).

Once absorbed through the skin, topical corticosteroids are handled through pharmacokinetic pathways similar to systemically administered corticosteroids. Corticosteroids are bound to plasma proteins in varying degrees. Corticosteroids are metobolized primarily in the liver and are then excreted by the kidneys. Some of the topical corticosteroids and their metabolites are also excreted into the bile.

INDICATIONS AND USAGE

Topical corticosteroids are indicated for the relief of the inflammatory and pruritic manifestations of corticosteroid-responsive dermatoses.

CONTRAINDICATIONS

Topical corticosteroids are contraindicated in those patients with a history of hypersensitivity to any of the components of the preparation.

PRECAUTIONS

General:

Systemic absorption of topical corticosteroids has produced reversible hypothalamic-pituitary-adrenal (HPA) axis suppression, manifestations of Cushing's syndrome, hyperglycemia, and glucosuria in some patients.

Conditions which augment systemic absorption include the application of the more potent steroids, use over large surface areas, prolonged use, and the addition of occlusive dressings.

Therefore, patients receiving a large dose of a potent topical steroid applied to a large surface area or under an occlusive dressing should be evaluated periodically for evidence of HPA axis suppression by using the urinary free cortisol and ACTH stimulation tests. If HPA axis suppression is noted, an attempt should be made to withdraw the drug, to reduce the frequency of application, or to substitute a less potent steroid.

Recovery of HPA axis function is generally prompt and complete upon discontinuation of the drug.

Infrequently, signs and symptoms of steroid withdrawal may occur, requiring supplemental systemic corticosteroids.

Children may absorb proportionally larger amounts of topical corticosteroids and thus be more susceptible to systemic toxicity (See **PRECAUTIONS—Pediatric Use**).

If irritation develops, topical corticosteroids should be discontinued and appropriate therapy instituted.

In the presence of dermatological infections, the use of an appropriate antifungal or antibacterial agent should be instituted. If a favorable response does not occur promptly, the corticosteroid should be discontinued until the infection has been adequately controlled.

Information for the Patient: Patients using topical corticosteroids should receive the following information and instructions:

1. This medication is to be used as directed by the physician. It is for external use only. Avoid contact with the eyes.
2. Patients should be advised not to use this medication for any disorder other than for which it was prescribed.
3. The treated skin area should not be bandaged or otherwise covered or wrapped so as to be occlusive unless directed by the physician.
4. Patients should report any signs of local adverses reactions especially under occlusive dressing.
5. Parents of pediatric patients should be advised not to use tight-fitting diapers or plastic pants on a child being treated in the diaper area, as these garments may constitute occlusive dressings.

Continued on next page

Proctocream HC—Cont.

Laboratory Tests: The following tests may be helpful in evaluating the HPA axis suppression:Urinary free cortisol test; ACTH stimulation test.

Carcinogenesis, Mutagenesis, and Impairment of Fertility: Long-term animal studies have not been performed to evaluate the carcinogenic potential or the effect on fertility of topical corticosteroids.

Studies to determine mutagenicity with prednisolone and hydrocortisone have revealed negative results.

Pregnancy: Teratogenic Effects — *Pregnancy Category C* Corticosteroids are generally teratogenic in laboratory animals when administered systemically at relatively low dosage levels. The more potent corticosteroids have been shown to be teratogenic after dermal application in laboratory animals. There are no adequate and well-controlled studies in pregnant women on teratogenic effects from topically applied corticosteroids. Therefore, topical corticosteroids should be used during pregnancy only if the potential benefit justifies the potential risk to the fetus. Drugs of this class should not be used extensively on pregnant patients, in large amounts, or for prolonged periods of time.

Nursing Mothers: It is not known whether topical administration of corticosteroids could result in sufficient systemic absorption to produce detectable quantities in breast milk. Systemically administered corticosteroids are secreted into breast milk in quantities *not* likely to have a deleterious effect on the infant. Nevertheless, caution should be exercised when topical corticosteroids are administered to a nursing woman.

Pediatric Use: *Pediatric patients may demonstrate greater susceptibility to topical corticosteroid-induced hypothalamic-pituitary-adrenal (HPA) axis suppression and Cushing's syndrome than mature patients because of a larger skin surface area to body weight ratio.*

Hypothalamic-pituitary-adrenal (HPA) axis suppression, Cushing's syndrome, and intracranial hypertension have been reported in pediatric patients receiving topical corticosteroids. Manisfestations of adrenal suppression in pediatric patients include linear growth retardation, delayed weight gain, low plasma cortisol levels, and absence of response to ACTH stimulation. Manifestations of intracranial hypertension include bulging fontanelles, headaches, and bilateral papilledema.

Administration of topical corticosteroids to pediatric patients should be limited to the least amount compatible with an effective therapeutic regimen. Chronic corticosteroid therapy may interfere with the growth and development of pediatric patients.

ADVERSE REACTIONS

The following local adverse reactions are reported infrequently with topical corticosteroids, but may occur more frequently with the use of occlusive dressings. These reactions are listed in an approximate decreasing order of occurrence: burning, itching, irritation, dryness, folliculitis, hypertrichosis, acneiform eruptions, hypopigmentation, perioral dermatitis, allergic contact dermatitis, maceration of the skin, secondary infection, skin atrophy, striae and miliaria.

OVERDOSAGE

Topically applied corticosteroids can be absorbed in sufficient amounts to produce systemic effects (See **PRECAUTIONS**).

DOSAGE AND ADMINISTRATION

Apply to the affected area as a thin film 2 to 4 times daily depending on the severity of the condition.

Occlusive dressings may be used for the management of psoriasis or recalcitrant conditions.

If an infection develops, the use of occlusive dressings should be discontinued and appropriate antimicrobial therapy instituted.

HOW SUPPLIED

proctoCream®•HC 2.5% (hydrocortisone cream USP, 2.5%) is supplied in 30 gram tubes.

30 g NDC 0091-4640-24

Store at controlled room temperature 15°-30°C (59°-86°F).

CAUTION: Federal law prohibits dispensing without prescription.

PC2178 Rev. 12/95

Shown in Product Identification Guide, page 337

PROCTOFOAM®–HC ℞

(hydrocortisone acetate 1%
and pramoxine hydrochloride 1%)
TOPICAL AEROSOL

DESCRIPTION

ProctoFoam HC (hydrocortisone acetate 1% and pramoxine hydrochloride 1%) is a topical aerosol foam for anal use containing hydrocortisone acetate 1% and pramoxine hydrochloride 1% in a hydrophilic base containing cetyl alcohol, emulsifying wax, methylparaben, polyoxyethylene-10 stearyl ether, propylene glycol, propylparaben, purified water, trolamine, and inert propellants: isobutane and propane. PROCTOFOAM®-HC contains a synthetic corticosteroid used as an anti-inflammatory/antipruritic agent, and a local anesthetic.

Hydrocortisone acetate

Molecular weight: 404.51. Solubility of hydrocortisone acetate in water: 1mg/100mL.

Chemical name: Pregn-4-ene-3,20-dione, 21-(acetyloxy)-11, 17-dihydroxy-,(11β)-.

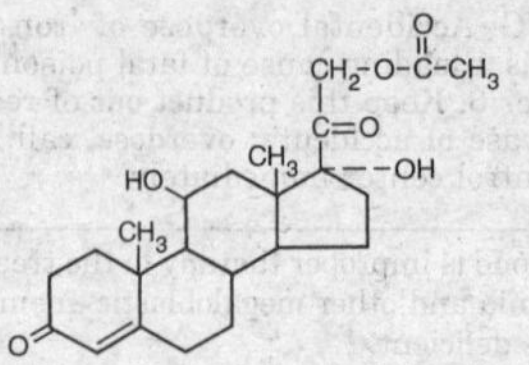

Pramoxine hydrochloride

Molecular weight: 329.87. Pramoxine hydrochloride is freely soluble in water.

Chemical name: Morpholine, 4-[3-(4-butoxyphenoxy) propyl]-, hydrochloride.

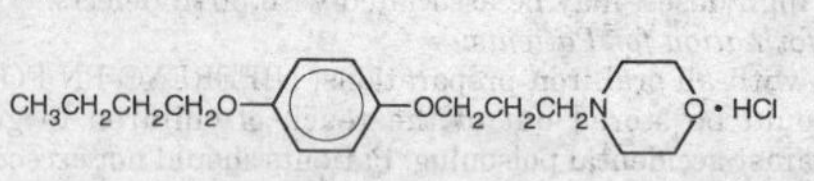

CLINICAL PHARMACOLOGY

Topical corticosteroids share anti-inflammatory, antipruritic and vasoconstrictive actions.

The mechanism of anti-inflammatory activity of the topical corticosteroids is unclear. Various laboratory methods, including vasoconstrictor assays, are used to compare and predict potencies and/or clinical efficacies of the topical corticosteroids. There is some evidence to suggest that a recognizable correlation exists between vasoconstrictor potency and therapeutic efficacy in man.

Pramoxine hydrochloride is a surface or local anesthetic which is not chemically related to the "caine" types of local anesthetics. Its unique chemical structure is likely to minimize the danger of cross-sensitivity reactions in patients allergic to other local anesthetics.

Pharmacokinetics: The extent of percutaneous absorption of topical corticosteroids is determined by many factors including the vehicle, the integrity of the epidermal barrier, and the use of occlusive dressings.

Topical corticosteroids can be absorbed through normal intact skin. Inflammation and/or other disease processes in the skin increase the percutaneous absorption of topical corticosteroids. Occlusive dressings substantially increase the percutaneous absorption of topical corticosteroids. Thus, occlusive dressings may be a valuable therapeutic adjunct for treatment of resistant dermatoses. (See DOSAGE AND ADMINISTRATION.)

Once absorbed through the skin, topical corticosteroids are handled through pharmacokinetic pathways similar to systemically administered corticosteroids. Corticosteroids are bound to plasma proteins in varying degrees. Corticosteroids are metabolized primarily in the liver and are then excreted by the kidneys. Some of the topical corticosteroids and their metabolites are also excreted into the bile.

INDICATIONS AND USAGE

ProctoFoam HC is indicated for the relief of the inflammatory and pruritic manifestations of corticosteroid-responsive dermatoses of the anal region.

CONTRAINDICATIONS

Topical corticosteroid products are contraindicated in those patients with a history of hypersensitivity to any of the components of the preparation.

WARNINGS

Do not insert any part of the aerosol container directly into the anus. Avoid contact with the eyes. Contents of the container are under pressure. Do not incinerate or puncture the aerosol container. Do not store at temperatures above 39°C (120°F). If there is no evidence of clinical improvement within two or three weeks after starting ProctoFoam HC therapy, or if the patient's condition worsens discontinue the drug. Keep this and all medicines out of the reach of children.

PRECAUTIONS

General: Systemic absorption of topical corticosteroids has produced reversible hypothalamic-pituitary-adrenal (HPA) axis suppression, manifestations of Cushing's syndrome, hyperglycemia, and glucosuria in some patients.

Conditions which augment systemic absorption include the application of the more potent steroids, use over large surface areas, prolonged use, and the addition of occlusive dressings. Therefore, patients receiving a large dose of a potent topical steroid applied to a large surface area or under an occlusive dressing should be evaluated periodically for evidence of HPA axis suppression by using the urinary free cortisol and ACTH stimulation tests. If HPA axis suppression is noted, an attempt should be made to withdraw the drug, to reduce the frequency of application, or to substitute a less potent steroid.

Recovery of HPA axis function is generally prompt and complete upon discontinuation of the drug. Infrequently, signs and symptoms of steroid withdrawal may occur, requiring supplemental systemic corticosteroids.

Pediatric patients may absorb proportionally larger amounts of topical corticosteroids and thus be more susceptible to systemic toxicity. (see PRECAUTIONS – *Pediatric Use.*)

If irritation develops, topical corticosteroids should be discontinued and appropriate therapy instituted.

In the presence of dermatological infections, the use of an appropriate antifungal or antibacterial agent should be instituted. If a favorable response does not occur promptly, the corticosteroid should be discontinued until the infection has been adequately controlled.

Information for the Patient: Patients using topical corticosteroids should receive the following information and instructions:

1. This medication is to be used as directed by the physician. It is for anal or perianal use only. Avoid contact with the eyes.
2. Be advised not to use this medication for any disorder other than for which it has been prescribed.
3. Report any signs of adverse reactions.

Laboratory Tests: The following tests may be helpful in evaluating the HPA axis suppression:

Urinary free cortisol test
ACTH stimulation test

Carcinogenesis, Mutagenesis, and Impairment of Fertility: Long-term animal studies have not been performed to evaluate the carcinogenic potential or the effect on fertility of topical corticosteroids.

Studies to determine mutagenicity with prednisolone and hydrocortisone have revealed negative results.

Pregnancy: Teratogenic Effects. Pregnancy Category C. Corticosteroids are generally teratogenic in laboratory animals when administered systemically at relatively low dosage levels. The more potent corticosteroids have been shown to be teratogenic after dermal application in laboratory animals. There are no adequate, well-controlled studies of teratogenic effects from topically applied corticosteroids in pregnant women. Therefore, topical corticosteroids should be used during pregnancy only if the potential benefit justifies the potential risk to the fetus. Drugs of this class should not be used extensively on pregnant patients, in large amounts, or for prolonged periods of time.

Nursing Mothers: It is not known whether topical administration of corticosteroids could result in sufficient systemic absorption to produce detectable quantities in breast milk. Systemically administered corticosteroids are secreted into breast milk in quantities *not* likely to have a deleterious effect on the infant. Nevertheless, caution should be exercised when topical corticosteroids are administered to a nursing woman.

Pediatric Use: Pediatric patients may demonstrate greater susceptibility to topical corticosteroid-induced HPA axis suppression and Cushing's syndrome than mature patients because of a larger skin surface area to body weight ratio.

Hypothalamic-pituitary-adrenal (HPA) axis suppression, Cushing's syndrome, and intracranial hypertension have been reported in pediatric patients receiving topical corticosteroids. Manifestations of adrenal suppression in pediatric patients include linear growth retardation, delayed weight gain, low plasma cortisol levels, and absense of response to ACTH stimulation. Manifestations of intracranial hypertension include bulging fontanelles, headaches, and bilateral papilledema.

Administration of topical corticosteroids to pediatric patients should be limited to the least amount compatible with an effective therapeutic regimen. Chronic corticosteroid therapy may interfere with the growth and development of pediatric patients.

ADVERSE REACTIONS

The following local adverse reactions are reported infrequently with topical corticosteroids, but may occur more frequently with the use of occlusive dressings. These reactions are listed in an approximate decreasing order of occurrence: burning, itching, irritation, dryness, folliculitis, hypertrichosis, acneiform eruptions, hypopigmentation, perioral dermatitis, allergic contact dermatitis, maceration of the skin, secondary infection, skin atrophy, striae and miliaria.

OVERDOSAGE

Topically applied corticosteroids can be absorbed in sufficient amounts to produce systemic effects. (See PRECAUTIONS.)

DOSAGE AND ADMINISTRATION

Apply to affected area 3 to 4 times daily. Use the applicator supplied for anal administration. For perianal use, transfer a small quantity to a tissue and rub in gently.

Directions for Use.

1. Shake the container vigorously for 5–10 seconds before each use. Do not remove container cap during use of the product.
2. Hold the container upright on a level surface and gently place the tip of the applicator onto the nose of the container cap. CONTAINER MUST BE HELD UPRIGHT TO OBTAIN PROPER FLOW OF MEDICATION.
3. Gently withdraw applicator plunger past the fill line on the applicator barrel.
4. Prime the container by placing the index and middle fingers on the container cap flanges, press down slowly on flanges and then release. Repeat until foam appears.
5. To fill applicator barrel, press down slowly on cap flanges and release, pause, and allow foam to enter and expand in applicator barrel. Repeat until foam in applicator reaches fill line. Remove applicator from container cap.
6. Hold applicator firmly by barrel, making sure thumb and middle finger are positioned securely underneath and resting against barrel wings. Place index finger over plunger. Gently insert tip into anus. Once in place, push plunger to expel foam, then withdraw applicator. CAUTION: Do not insert any part of the aerosol container directly into the anus. Apply to anus only with enclosed applicator. Do not insert any part of the applicator past the anus into the rectum.
7. After each use, applicator parts should be pulled apart for thorough cleaning with warm water. The container cap and underlying tip should also be pulled apart and rinsed to help prevent build-up of foam and possible blockage.

HOW SUPPLIED

PROCTOFOAM®-HC is supplied in an aerosol container with a special anal applicator. When used correctly, the aerosol container will deliver a minimum of 14 applications. **Store upright at controlled room temperature 15°–30°C (59°–86°F). Do not refrigerate.**

NDC 0091-0690-10 10g

CAUTION: Federal law prohibits dispensing without prescription.

PC2585A Rev. 10/97

Shown in Product Identification Guide, page 337

UNIRETIC™ ℞

[*yü-nə-retic*]

(moexipril hydrochloride/hydrochlorothiazide)
Tablets
7.5 mg/12.5 mg
15 mg/25 mg

USE IN PREGNANCY

When used in pregnancy during the second and third trimesters, ACE inhibitors can cause injury and even death to the developing fetus. When pregnancy is detected, UNIRETIC should be discontinued as soon as possible. **See WARNINGS, Fetal/Neonatal Morbidity and Mortality.**

DESCRIPTION

UNIRETIC (moexipril hydrochloride/hydrochlorothiazide) is a combination of an angiotensin-converting enzyme (ACE) inhibitor, moexipril hydrochloride, and a diuretic, hydrochlorothiazide. Moexipril hydrochloride is a fine white to off-white powder. It is soluble (about 10% weight-to-volume) in distilled water at room temperature. It has the empirical formula $C_{27}H_{34}N_2O_7 \cdot HCl$ and a molecular weight of 535.04. It is chemically described as [3S-[2[R*(R*)],3R*]]-2-[2-[[1-(Ethoxycarbonyl)-3-phenylpropyl]amino]-1-oxopropyl]-1,2,3,4-tetrahydro-6,7-dimethoxy-3-isoquinolinecarboxylic acid, monohydrochloride. Moexipril hydrochloride is a non-sulfhydryl containing precursor of the active ACE inhibitor moexiprilat and its structural formula is:

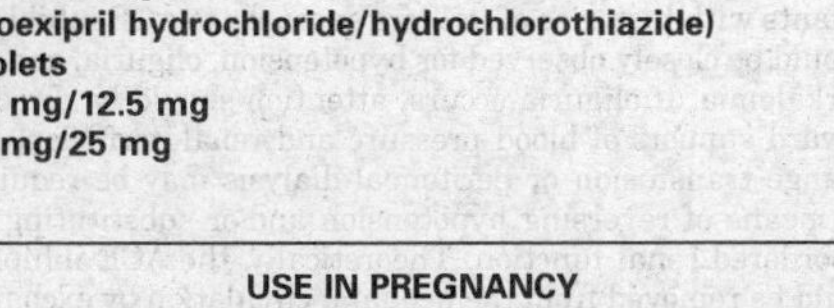

Hydrochlorothiazide is a white, or practically white, crystalline powder. It is slightly soluble in water, freely soluble in sodium hydroxide solution, in n-butylamine and in dimethylformamide. Hydrochlorothiazide has the empirical formula $C_7H_8ClN_3O_4S_2$ and a molecular weight of 297.75. It is chemically described as 2*H*-1,2,4-Benzothiadiazine-7-sulfonamide, 6-chloro-3,4-dihydro-, 1,1-dioxide. Hydrochlorothiazide is a thiazide diuretic and its structural formula is: [See chemical structure at top of next column]

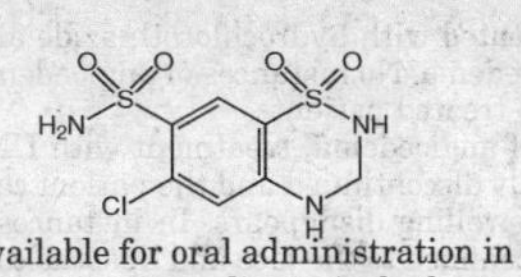

UNIRETIC is available for oral administration in two tablet strengths. The inactive ingredients in both strengths are lactose, magnesium oxide, crospovidone, magnesium stearate and gelatin. The film coating in both strengths contains hydroxypropyl methylcellulose, hydroxypropyl cellulose, polyethylene glycol 6000, magnesium stearate, titanium dioxide and ferric oxide.

CLINICAL PHARMACOLOGY

Mechanism of Action

Moexipril Hydrochloride

Moexipril hydrochloride is a prodrug for moexiprilat, which inhibits ACE in humans and animals. The mechanism through which moexiprilat lowers blood pressure is believed to be primarily inhibition of ACE activity. ACE is a peptidyl dipeptidase that catalyzes the conversion of the inactive decapeptide angiotensin I to the vasoconstrictor substance angiotensin II. Angiotensin II is a potent peripheral vasoconstrictor that also stimulates aldosterone secretion by the adrenal cortex and provides negative feedback on renin secretion. ACE is identical to kininase II, an enzyme that degrades bradykinin, an endothelium-dependent vasodilator. Moexiprilat is about 1000 times as potent as moexipril in inhibiting ACE and kininase II. Inhibition of ACE results in decreased angiotensin II formation, leading to decreased vasoconstriction, increased plasma renin activity, and decreased aldosterone secretion. The latter results in diuresis and natriuresis and a small increase in serum potassium concentration (mean increases of about 0.25 mEq/L were seen when moexipril was used alone).

Whether increased levels of bradykinin, a potent vasodepressor peptide, play a role in the therapeutic effects of moexipril remains to be elucidated. Although the principal mechanism of moexipril in blood pressure reduction is believed to be through the renin-angiotensin-aldosterone system, ACE inhibitors have some effect on blood pressure even in apparent low-renin hypertension. As is the case with other ACE inhibitors, however, the antihypertensive effect of moexipril is smaller in black patients, a predominantly low-renin population, than in nonblack hypertensive patients. Although moexipril monotherapy is less effective in blacks than in nonblacks, the efficacy of combination therapy appears to be independent of race.

Hydrochlorothiazide

Hydrochlorothiazide is a thiazide diuretic and antihypertensive. Thiazides affect the distal renal tubular mechanisms of electrolyte reabsorption, directly increasing excretion of sodium and chloride in approximately equivalent amounts. Indirectly, the diuretic action of hydrochlorothiazide reduces plasma volume, with consequent increases in plasma renin activity, increases in aldosterone secretion, increases in urinary potassium loss, and decreases in serum potassium. The renin-aldosterone link is mediated by angiotensin, so coadministration of an ACE inhibitor tends to reverse the potassium loss associated with these diuretics. The mechanism of the antihypertensive effect of thiazides is unknown.

Pharmacokinetics

Moexipril-Hydrochlorothiazide

Following oral administration of UNIRETIC, the moexipril peak plasma concentration was reached within 0.8 hour and the peak plasma concentration of moexiprilat occurred 1.6 hours after administration. After reaching the peak plasma level (C_{max}), moexiprilat plasma concentrations decreased biphasically. After administration of UNIRETIC, renal excretion of unchanged hydrochlorothiazide is about 60% in 24 hours. The pharmacokinetics of moexipril and hydrochlorothiazide after administration of UNIRETIC are not different, respectively, from the pharmacokinetics of moexipril and hydrochlorothiazide from immediate-release monotherapy formulations.

Moexipril Hydrochloride

Moexipril's antihypertensive activity is almost entirely due to its deesterified metabolite, moexiprilat. Bioavailability of oral moexipril is about 13% compared to intravenous (I.V.) moexipril (both measuring the metabolite moexiprilat), and is markedly affected by food, which reduces C_{max} and AUC (see Absorption). Moexipril should therefore be taken in a fasting state. The time of peak plasma concentration (T_{max}) of moexiprilat is about $1^1/_2$ hours and elimination half-life ($t_{1/2}$) is estimated at 2 to 9 hours in various studies, the variability reflecting a complex elimination pattern that is not simply exponential. Like all ACE inhibitors, moexiprilat has a prolonged terminal elimination phase, presumably reflecting slow release of drug bound to the ACE. Accumulation of moexiprilat with repeated dosing is minimal, about 30%, compatible with a functional elimination $t_{1/2}$ of about 12 hours. Over the dose range of 7.5 to 30 mg, pharmacokinetics are approximately dose proportional.

Absorption: Moexipril is incompletely absorbed, with bioavailability as moexiprilat of about 13%. Bioavailability varies with formulation and food intake which reduces C_{max} and AUC of moexiprilat by about 70% and 40% respectively after the ingestion of a low-fat breakfast or by 80% and 50% respectively after the ingestion of a high-fat breakfast.

Distribution: The clearance (CL) for moexipril is 441 mL/min and for moexiprilat 232 mL/min with a $t_{1/2}$ of 1.3 and 9.8 hours, respectively. Moexiprilat is about 50% protein bound. The volume of distribution of moexiprilat is about 2.8 L/kg.

Metabolism and Excretion: Moexipril is relatively rapidly converted to its active metabolite moexiprilat, but persists longer than some other ACE inhibitor prodrugs, such that its $t_{1/2}$ is over one hour and it has a significant AUC. Both moexipril and moexiprilat are converted to diketopiperazine derivatives and unidentified metabolites. After I.V. administration of moexipril, about 40% of the dose appears in urine as moexiprilat, about 26% as moexipril, with small amounts of the metabolites; about 20% of the I.V. dose appears in feces, principally as moexiprilat. After oral administration, only about 7% of the dose appears in urine as moexiprilat, about 1% as moexipril, with about 5% as other metabolites. Fifty-two percent of the dose is recovered in feces as moexiprilat and 1% as moexipril.

Special Populations:

Decreased Renal Function: The effective elimination $t_{1/2}$ and AUC of both moexipril and moexiprilat are increased with decreasing renal function. There is insufficient information available to characterize this relationship fully, but at creatinine clearances in the range of 10 to 40 mL/min, the $t_{1/2}$ of moexiprilat is increased by a factor of 3 to 4.

Decreased Hepatic Function: In patients with mild to moderate cirrhosis given single 15-mg doses of moexipril, the C_{max} of moexipril was increased by about 50% and the AUC increased by about 120%, while the C_{max} for moexiprilat was decreased by about 50% and the AUC increased by almost 300%.

Elderly Patients: In elderly male subjects (65–80 years old) with clinically normal renal and hepatic function, the AUC and C_{max} of moexiprilat are about 30% greater than in younger subjects (19–42 years old).

Pharmacokinetic Interactions With Other Drugs: No clinically important pharmacokinetic interactions occurred when moexipril was administered concomitantly with hydrochlorothiazide, digoxin, or cimetidine.

Hydrochlorothiazide

Absorption: After oral administration, 60–80% of a single dose of hydrochlorothiazide is absorbed. The reported studies of food effects on hydrochlorothiazide absorption have been inconclusive. The absorption of hydrochlorothiazide is reported to be reduced by 50% in patients with congestive heart failure. Hydrochlorothiazide exhibits dose proportionality over the dose range of 12.5 to 75 mg.

Distribution: The apparent volume of distribution has been observed to vary between 1.5–4.2 L/kg. Hydrochlorothiazide accumulates in red blood cells, so that whole blood levels are higher than those measured in plasma. Equilibrium between whole blood levels and plasma levels is reached 4 hours after oral administration. Hydrochlorothiazide crosses the placental barrier. Hydrochlorothiazide has a protein binding of 21–24%.

Metabolism and Excretion: Hydrochlorothiazide is not metabolized. Hydrochlorothiazide is eliminated rapidly by the kidney. More than 60 percent of the oral dose is eliminated unchanged within 24 hours. When plasma levels have been followed for at least 24 hours, the plasma half-life has been observed to vary between 5.6 and 14.8 hours. The renal clearance has been observed to vary between 3.1–5.5 mL/min/kg.

Special Populations:

Decreased Renal Function: In a study of patients with impaired renal function (mean creatinine clearance of 19 mL/min), the elimination half-life of hydrochlorothiazide was increased to 21 hours.

Pharmacokinetic Interactions With Other Drugs: Coadministration of propantheline or guanabenz increased the absorption of hydrochlorothiazide and coadministration of cholestyramine or colestipol decreased the absorption of hydrochlorothiazide.

Pharmacodynamics and Clinical Effect

Moexipril—Hydrochlorothiazide

In UNIRETIC clinical trials using moexipril doses of 3.75–30 mg and hydrochlorothiazide doses of 3.125–50 mg, the antihypertensive effects were sustained for at least 24 hours and they increased with increasing dose of either component. The extent of blood pressure reduction seen with UNIRETIC was approximately additive as compared to monotherapy of each component. The antihypertensive effects of UNIRETIC continue during therapy for up to 24 months. The effectiveness of UNIRETIC was not significantly influenced by patient age or gender. Although moexipril monotherapy is less effective in blacks than in nonblacks, the efficacy of UNIRETIC appears to be independent of race.

Continued on next page

Uniretic—Cont.

By blocking the renin-angiotensin-aldosterone axis, administration of moexipril tends to reduce the potassium loss associated with hydrochlorothiazide. In UNIRETIC controlled clinical trials, the average change in serum potassium was near zero in subjects who received 3.75/6.25 mg or 7.5/12.5 mg, but subjects who received 15/25 mg experienced a mild decrease in serum potassium, similar to that experienced by subjects who received hydrochlorothiazide 25 mg monotherapy.

Moexipril Hydrochloride

Single and multiple doses of 15 mg or more of moexipril give sustained inhibition of plasma ACE activity of 80–90%, beginning within 2 hours and lasting 24 hours (80%).

In controlled trials, the peak effects of orally administered moexipril increased with the dose administered over a dose range of 7.5 to 60 mg, given once a day. Antihypertensive effects were first detectable about 1 hour after dosing, with a peak effect between 3 and 6 hours after dosing. Just before dosing (i.e., at trough), the antihypertensive effects were less prominently related to dose and the antihypertensive effect tended to diminish during the 24-hour dosing interval when the drug was administered once a day.

In multiple-dose studies in the dose range of 7.5 to 30 mg once daily, moexipril lowered sitting blood pressure at trough by 4-11/3-6 mmHg more than placebo, a tendency toward increased response with higher doses. These effects are typical of ACE inhibitors; there are no trials of adequate size comparing moexipril with other antihypertensive agents.

Higher doses of moexipril generally leave a greater fraction of the peak blood pressure effect still present at trough. During dose titration, any decision as to the adequacy of a dosing regimen should be based on trough blood pressure measurements. If diastolic blood pressure control is not adequate at the end of the dosing interval, the dose can be increased or given as a divided (BID) regimen.

During chronic therapy, the antihypertensive effect of any dose of moexipril is generally evident within 2 weeks of treatment, with maximal reduction after 4 weeks. The antihypertensive effects of moexipril have been proven to continue during therapy for up to 24 months.

Moexipril, like other ACE inhibitors, is less effective in decreasing trough blood pressures in blacks than in nonblacks. Placebo-corrected trough group diastolic blood pressure effects in blacks in the proposed dose range were +1 to −3 mmHg compared with responses in nonblacks of −4 to −6 mmHg.

The effectiveness of moexipril was not significantly influenced by patient age, gender, or weight. Moexipril has been shown to have antihypertensive activity in both pre- and postmenopausal women who have participated in placebo-controlled clinical trials.

INDICATIONS AND USAGE

UNIRETIC is indicated for treatment of patients with hypertension. **This fixed combination is not indicated for the initial therapy of hypertension (see DOSAGE AND ADMINISTRATION).**

In using UNIRETIC, consideration should be given to the fact that another ACE inhibitor, captopril, has caused agranulocytosis, particularly in patients with renal impairment or collagen-vascular disease. Available data are insufficient to show that UNIRETIC does not have a similar risk (see WARNINGS, Neutropenia/Agranulocytosis). In addition, ACE inhibitors, for which adequate data are available, cause a higher rate of angioedema in black than in nonblack patients (see WARNINGS, Angioedema).

CONTRAINDICATIONS

UNIRETIC is contraindicated in patients who are hypersensitive to any component of this product and in patients with a history of angioedema related to previous treatment with an ACE inhibitor. Because of the hydrochlorothiazide component, this product is contraindicated in patients with anuria or hypersensitivity to other sulfonamide-derived drugs. Hypersensitivity reactions are more likely to occur in patients with a history of allergy or bronchial asthma.

WARNINGS

Anaphylactoid and Possibly Related Reactions

Presumably because angiotensin-converting enzyme inhibitors affect the metabolism of eicosanoids and polypeptides, including endogenous bradykinin, patients receiving ACE inhibitors, including UNIRETIC, may be subject to a variety of adverse reactions, some of them serious.

Angioedema: Angioedema involving the face, extremities, lips, tongue, glottis, and/or larynx has been reported in patients treated with ACE inhibitors, including moexipril. Symptoms suggestive of angioedema or facial edema occurred in <0.5% of moexipril-treated patients in placebo-controlled trials. None of the cases were considered life-threatening and all resolved either without treatment or with medication (antihistamines or glucocorticoids). One

patient treated with hydrochlorothiazide alone experienced laryngeal edema. No instances of angioedema were reported in placebo-treated patients.

In cases of angioedema, treatment with UNIRETIC should be promptly discontinued and the patient carefully observed until the swelling disappears. In instances where swelling has been confined to the face and lips, the condition has generally resolved without treatment, although antihistamines have been useful in relieving symptoms.

Angioedema associated with involvement of the tongue, glottis, or larynx may be fatal due to airway obstruction. Appropriate therapy, e.g., subcutaneous epinephrine solution 1:1000 (0.3 to 0.5 mL) and/or measures to ensure a patent airway, should be promptly provided (see ADVERSE REACTIONS).

Anaphylactoid Reactions During Desensitization: Two patients undergoing desensitizing treatment with hymenoptera venom while receiving ACE inhibitors sustained life-threatening anaphylactoid reactions. In the same patients, these reactions did not occur when ACE inhibitors were temporarily withheld, but they reappeared when the ACE inhibitors were inadvertently readministered.

Anaphylactoid Reactions During Membrane Exposure: Anaphylactoid reactions have been reported in patients dialyzed with high-flux membranes and treated concomitantly with an ACE inhibitor. Anaphylactoid reactions have also been reported in patients undergoing low-density lipoprotein apheresis with dextran sulfate absorption.

Hypotension

UNIRETIC can cause symptomatic hypotension, although, as with other ACE inhibitors, this is unusual in uncomplicated hypertensive patients treated with UNIRETIC alone. Symptomatic hypotension is most likely to occur in patients who have been salt- and/or volume-depleted as a result of prolonged diuretic therapy, dietary salt restriction, dialysis, diarrhea, or vomiting. Volume- and/or salt-depletion should be corrected before initiating therapy with UNIRETIC (see ADVERSE REACTIONS).

The thiazide component of UNIRETIC may potentiate the action of other antihypertensive drugs, especially ganglionic or peripheral adrenergic-blocking drugs. The antihypertensive effects of the thiazide component may also be enhanced in the postsympathectomy patient.

In patients with congestive heart failure, with or without associated renal insufficiency, ACE inhibitor therapy may cause excessive hypotension, which may be associated with oliguria or progressive azotemia, and rarely, with acute renal failure and death. In these patients, UNIRETIC therapy should be started under close medical supervision, and patients should be followed closely for the first two weeks of treatment and whenever the dose of UNIRETIC is increased. Care in avoiding hypotension should also be taken in patients with ischemic heart disease, aortic stenosis, or cerebrovascular disease, in whom an excessive decrease in blood pressure could result in a myocardial infarction or a cerebrovascular accident.

If hypotension occurs, the patient should be placed in a supine position and, if necessary, treated with an intravenous infusion of normal saline. UNIRETIC treatment usually can be continued following restoration of blood pressure and volume.

Impaired Renal Function

UNIRETIC should be used with caution in patients with severe renal disease. Thiazide diuretics may precipitate azotemia in such patients and the effects of repeated dosing may be cumulative.

As a consequence of inhibition of the renin-angiotensin-aldosterone system, changes in renal function may be anticipated in susceptible individuals. There is no clinical experience of UNIRETIC in the treatment of hypertension in patients with renal failure.

Some hypertensive patients with no apparent preexisting renal vascular disease have developed increases in blood urea nitrogen and serum creatinine, usually minor and transient, especially when moexipril has been given concomitantly with a thiazide diuretic. This is more likely to occur in patients with preexisting renal impairment. There may be a need for dose adjustment of UNIRETIC. **Evaluation of hypertensive patients should always include assessment of renal function** (see DOSAGE AND ADMINISTRATION).

In hypertensive patients with severe congestive heart failure, whose renal function may depend on the activity of the renin-angiotensin-aldosterone system, treatment with ACE inhibitors, including moexipril, may be associated with oliguria and/or progressive azotemia and, rarely, acute renal failure and/or death.

In hypertensive patients with unilateral or bilateral renal artery stenosis, increases in blood urea nitrogen and serum creatinine have been observed in some patients following ACE inhibitor therapy. These increases were almost always reversible upon discontinuation of the ACE inhibitor and/or diuretic therapy. In such patients, renal function should be monitored during the first few weeks of therapy.

Neutropenia/Agranulocytosis

Another ACE inhibitor, captopril, has been shown to cause agranulocytosis and bone marrow depression, rarely in pa-

tients with uncomplicated hypertension, but more frequently in hypertensive patients with renal impairment, especially if they also have a collagen-vascular disease such as systemic lupus erythematosus or scleroderma. Although there were no instances of severe neutropenia (absolute neutrophil count <500/mm³) among patients given moexipril, as with other ACE inhibitors, monitoring of white blood cell counts should be considered for patients who have collagen-vascular disease, especially if the disease is associated with impaired renal function. Available data from clinical trials of moexipril are insufficient to show that moexipril does not cause agranulocytosis at rates similar to captopril.

Fetal/Neonatal Morbidity and Mortality

ACE inhibitors can cause fetal and neonatal morbidity and death when administered to pregnant women. Several dozen cases have been reported in the world literature. When pregnancy is detected, ACE inhibitors should be discontinued as soon as possible.

The use of ACE inhibitors during the second and third trimesters of pregnancy has been associated with fetal and neonatal injury, including hypotension, neonatal skull hypoplasia, anuria, reversible or irreversible renal failure, and death. Oligohydramnios has also been reported, presumably resulting from decreased fetal renal function; oligohydramnios in this setting has been associated with fetal limb contractures, craniofacial deformation, and hypoplastic lung development. Prematurity, intrauterine growth retardation, and patent ductus arteriosus have also been reported, although it is not clear whether these were caused by the ACE inhibitor exposure.

Fetal and neonatal morbidity do not appear to have resulted from intrauterine ACE inhibitor exposure limited to the first trimester. Mothers who have used ACE inhibitors only during the first trimester should be informed of this. Nonetheless, when patients become pregnant, physicians should make every effort to discontinue the use of UNIRETIC as soon as possible.

Rarely (probably less often than once in every thousand pregnancies), no alternative to ACE inhibitors will be found. In these rare cases, the mothers should be apprised of the potential hazards to their fetuses, and serial ultrasound examinations should be performed to assess the intraamniotic environment.

If oligohydramnios is observed, UNIRETIC should be discontinued unless it is considered life-saving for the mother. Contraction stress testing (CST), a non-stress test (NST), or biophysical profiling (BPP) may be appropriate, depending upon the week of pregnancy. Patients and physicians should be aware, however, that oligohydramnios may not be detected until after the fetus has sustained irreversible injury. Infants with histories of *in utero* exposure to ACE inhibitors should be closely observed for hypotension, oliguria, and hyperkalemia. If oliguria occurs, attention should be directed toward support of blood pressure and renal perfusion. Exchange transfusion or peritoneal dialysis may be required as means of reversing hypotension and/or substituting for disordered renal function. Theoretically, the ACE inhibitor could be removed from the neonatal circulation by exchange transfusion, but no experience with this procedure has been reported.

Intrauterine exposure to thiazide diuretics is associated with fetal or neonatal jaundice, thrombocytopenia, and possibly other adverse reactions that have occurred in adults. Reproduction studies with the combination of moexipril hydrochloride and hydrochlorothiazide (ratio 7.5:12.5) indicated that the combination possessed no teratogenic properties up to the lethal dose of 800 mg/kg/day in rats and up to the maternotoxic dose of 160 mg/kg/day in rabbits.

Hepatic Failure

Rarely, ACE inhibitors have been associated with a syndrome that starts with cholestatic jaundice and progresses to fulminant hepatic necrosis and sometimes death. The mechanism of this syndrome is not understood. Patients receiving ACE inhibitors who develop jaundice or marked elevations of hepatic enzymes should discontinue the ACE inhibitor and receive appropriate medical follow-up.

Impaired Hepatic Function

UNIRETIC should be used with caution in patients with impaired hepatic function or progressive liver disease, since minor alterations of fluid and electrolyte balance may precipitate hepatic coma. In patients with mild to moderate cirrhosis given single 15 mg doses of moexipril, the C_{max} of moexipril was increased by about 50% and the AUC increased by about 120%, while the C_{max} for moexiprilat was decreased by about 50% and the AUC increased by almost 300%. No formal pharmacokinetic studies have been carried out with UNIRETIC in hypertensive patients with impaired liver function.

Systemic Lupus Erythematosus

Thiazide diuretics have been reported to cause exacerbation or activation of systemic lupus erythematosus.

PRECAUTIONS

General

Serum Electrolyte Imbalances: In clinical trials with moexipril monotherapy, persistent hyperkalemia (serum po-

tassium above 5.4 mEq/L) occurred in approximately 1.3% of hypertensive patients receiving moexipril. Risk factors for the development of hyperkalemia with ACE inhibitors include renal insufficiency, diabetes mellitus, and the concomitant use of potassium-sparing diuretics, potassium supplements, and/or potassium-containing salt substitutes. Treatment with thiazide diuretics has been associated with hypokalemia, hyponatremia, and hypochloremic alkalosis. These disturbances sometimes manifest as one or more of the following: dryness of mouth, thirst, weakness, lethargy, drowsiness, restlessness, muscle pains or cramps, muscular fatigue, hypotension, oliguria, tachycardia, nausea, and vomiting. Hypokalemia has also been reported to sensitize or exaggerate the response of the heart to the toxic effects of digitalis. The risk of hypokalemia is greatest in patients with cirrhosis of the liver, in patients experiencing a brisk diuresis, in patients who are receiving inadequate oral intake of electrolytes, and in patients receiving concomitant therapy with corticosteroids or ACTH.

The opposite effects of moexipril and hydrochlorothiazide on serum potassium will approximately counterbalance each other in many patients, so that little net effect upon serum potassium will be seen. Initial and periodic determinations of serum electrolytes to detect possible electrolyte imbalance should be performed at appropriate intervals.

Chloride deficits generally are mild and require specific treatment only under extraordinary circumstances (e.g., in liver disease or renal disease). Dilutional hyponatremia may occur in edematous patients; appropriate therapy is water restriction rather than administration of salt, except in rare instances when the hyponatremia is life-threatening. In actual salt depletion, appropriate replacement is the therapy of choice.

Calcium excretion is reduced by thiazides. In a few patients on prolonged thiazide therapy, pathological changes in the parathyroid gland have been seen, with hypercalcemia and hypophosphatemia. More serious complications of hyperparathyroidism (renal lithiasis, bone resorption, and peptic ulceration) have not been seen.

Thiazides enhance urinary excretion of magnesium and hypomagnesemia may result.

Other Metabolic Disturbances: Thiazide diuretics may reduce glucose tolerance and may raise serum levels of cholesterol, triglycerides, and uric acid. These effects are usually minor, but frank gout or overt diabetes may be precipitated in susceptible patients.

Surgery/Anesthesia: In patients undergoing major surgery or during anesthesia with agents that produce hypotension, moexipril may block the effects of compensatory renin release. If hypotension occurs in this setting and is considered to be due to this mechanism, it can be corrected by volume expansion.

Cough: Presumably due to the inhibition of the degradation of endogenous bradykinin, persistent nonproductive cough has been reported with all ACE inhibitors, always resolving after discontinuation of therapy. ACE inhibitor-induced cough should be considered in the differential diagnosis of cough. In placebo-controlled trials with UNIRETIC, cough was present in 3% of UNIRETIC patients and 1% of patients given placebo.

Information for Patients

Food: Patients should be advised to take UNIRETIC one hour before a meal (see CLINICAL PHARMACOLOGY and DOSAGE AND ADMINISTRATION).

Angioedema: Angioedema, including laryngeal edema, may occur with treatment with ACE inhibitors, usually occurring early in therapy (within the first month). Patients should be so advised and told to report immediately any signs or symptoms suggesting angioedema (swelling of the face, extremities, eyes, lips, tongue, difficulty in breathing) and to take no more drug until they have consulted with the prescribing physician.

Symptomatic Hypotension: Patients should be cautioned that lightheadedness can occur with UNIRETIC, especially during the first few days of therapy. If fainting occurs, the patient should stop taking UNIRETIC and consult the prescribing physician.

All patients should be cautioned that excessive perspiration and dehydration may lead to an excessive fall in blood pressure because of reduction in fluid volume. Other causes of volume depletion such as vomiting or diarrhea may also lead to a fall in blood pressure; patients should be advised to consult their physician if they develop these conditions.

Hyperkalemia: Patients should be told not to use potassium supplements or salt substitutes containing potassium without consulting their physician.

Neutropenia: Patients should be told to report promptly any indication of infection (e.g., sore throat, fever) that could be a sign of neutropenia.

Pregnancy: Female patients of childbearing age should be told about the consequences of second- and third-trimester exposure to ACE inhibitors and should also be told that these consequences do not appear to have resulted from intrauterine ACE inhibitor exposure that has been limited to the first trimester. Patients should be asked to report pregnancies to their physicians as soon as possible.

Drug Interactions

Potassium Supplements and Potassium-Sparing Diuretics: As noted above (*Serum Electrolyte Imbalances*), the net effect of UNIRETIC may be to elevate a patient's serum potassium (at low doses of hydrochlorothiazide), to reduce it (at high doses of hydrochlorothiazide), or to leave it unchanged. Potassium-sparing diuretics (spironolactone, amiloride, triamterene) or potassium supplements can increase the risk of hyperkalemia. If concomitant use of such agents is indicated, they should be given with caution, and the patient's serum potassium should be monitored.

Oral Anticoagulants: Interaction studies with warfarin failed to identify any clinically important effect of moexipril monotherapy on the serum concentrations of the anticoagulant or on its anticoagulant effect.

Lithium: Increased serum lithium levels and symptoms of lithium toxicity have been reported in patients receiving ACE inhibitors during therapy with lithium. Because renal clearance of lithium is reduced by thiazides, the risk of lithium toxicity is presumably raised further when, as in therapy with UNIRETIC, a thiazide diuretic is coadministered with the ACE inhibitor. These drugs should be coadministered with caution, and frequent monitoring of serum lithium levels is recommended.

Alcohol, Barbiturates, or Narcotics: Potentiation of orthostatic hypotension may occur in patients on thiazide diuretic therapy with concomitant use of alcohol, barbiturates, or narcotics.

Antidiabetic Agents: Use of thiazide diuretics concomitantly with antidiabetic agents (oral agents and insulin) may require dosage adjustment of the antidiabetic agent. Moexipril has been used in clinical trials concomitantly with oral hypoglycemic agents and there was no evidence of any clinically important adverse interactions.

Cholestyramine and Colestipol Resins: Absorption of hydrochlorothiazide is impaired in the presence of anionic exchange resins. Single doses of either cholestyramine or colestipol resins bind the hydrochlorothiazide and reduce its absorption from the gastrointestinal tract by up to 85% and 43%, respectively.

Corticosteroids, ACTH: Use of thiazide diuretics concomitantly with corticosteroids or ACTH may intensify electrolyte depletion, particularly hypokalemia.

Pressor Amines: Thiazide diuretics may decrease arterial responsiveness to pressor amines (eg. norepinephrine), but not enough to preclude effectiveness of the pressor agent for therapeutic use.

Skeletal Muscle Relaxants, Nondepolarizing: Thiazide diuretics may increase the responsiveness to tubocurarine.

Non-steroidal Anti-inflammatory Drugs: In some patients, the administration of a non-steroidal anti-inflammatory agent can reduce the diuretic, natriuretic, and antihypertensive effects of loop, potassium-sparing and thiazide diuretics. Thus, when UNIRETIC and non-steroidal antiinflammatory agents are used concomitantly, the patient should be observed closely to determine if the desired effect of the diuretic is obtained.

Other Agents: No clinically important pharmacokinetic interactions occurred when moexipril was administered concomitantly with digoxin or cimetidine.

Moexipril has been used in clinical trials concomitantly with calcium-channel-blocking agents, diuretics, H_2 blockers, digoxin, and cholesterol-lowering agents. There was no evidence of clinically important adverse interactions. In general, ACE inhibitors have less than additive effects with beta-adrenergic blockers, presumably because both work by inhibiting the renin-angiotensin system.

Coadministration of propantheline or guanabenz increased the absorption of hydrochlorothiazide.

Carcinogenesis, Mutagenesis, Impairment of Fertility
Moexipril Hydrochloride

No evidence of carcinogenicity was detected in long-term studies when moexipril was administered to mice and rats at doses up to 14 or 27.3 times the Maximum Recommended Human Dose (MRHD) on a mg/m² basis. No mutagenicity was detected in the Ames test and microbial reverse mutation assay, with and without metabolic activation, or in an *in vivo* nucleus anomaly test. However, increased chromosomal aberration frequency in Chinese hamster ovary (CHO) cells was detected under metabolic activation conditions at a 20-hour harvest time. Reproduction studies have been performed in rabbits at oral doses up to 0.7 times the MRHD on a mg/m² basis, and in rats up to 90.9 times the MRHD on a mg/m² basis. No indication of impaired fertility, reproductive toxicity, or teratogenicity was observed.

Hydrochlorothiazide

Under the auspices of the National Toxicology Program, rats and mice received hydrochlorothiazide in their feed for two years, at doses up to 600 mg/kg/day in mice and up to 100 mg/kg/day in rats. These studies uncovered no evidence of a carcinogenic potential of hydrochlorothiazide in rats or female mice, but there was equivocal evidence of hepatocarcinogenicity in male mice. Hydrochlorothiazide was not genotoxic in *in vitro* assays using strains TA 98, TA 100, TA 1535, TA 1537, and TA 1538 of *Salmonella typhimurium* (the Ames test); in the CHO test for chromosomal aberra-

tions; or in *in vivo* assays using mouse germinal cell chromosomes, Chinese hamster bone marrow chromosomes; and the *Drosophila* sex-linked recessive lethal trait gene. Positive test results were obtained in the *in vitro* CHO Sister Chromatid Exchange (clastogenicity) test and in the Mouse Lymphoma Cell (mutagenicity) assays, using concentrations of hydrochlorothiazide of 43-1300 mcg/mL. Positive test results were also obtained in the *Aspergillus nidulans* nondisjunction assay, using an unspecified concentration of hydrochlorothiazide.

Hydrochlorothiazide had no adverse effects on the fertility of mice and rats of either sex in studies wherein these species were exposed, via their diets, to doses up to 100 and 4 mg/kg/day, respectively, prior to mating and throughout gestation.

Pregnancy
Pregnancy Categories C (first trimester) and D (second and third trimesters).

See WARNINGS, Fetal/Neonatal Morbidity and Mortality.

Nursing Mothers

It is not known whether moexipril or moexiprilat is excreted in human milk. Thiazides are excreted in human milk. Because of the potential for serious adverse reactions in nursing infants from hydrochlorothiazide and the unknown effects of moexipril or moexiprilat in infants, a decision should be made whether to discontinue nursing or to discontinue UNIRETIC, taking into account the importance of the drug to the mother.

Geriatric Use

Of the patients who received UNIRETIC in controlled clinical studies, 24% were 65 years of age or older. No overall differences in effectiveness or safety were observed between these patients and younger patients. In elderly patients receiving moexipril, plasma levels of drug are slightly higher and renal clearance is reduced when compared to younger patients, but these effects did not have detectable consequences.

Pediatric Use

Safety and effectiveness of UNIRETIC in pediatric patients have not been established.

ADVERSE REACTIONS

UNIRETIC has been evaluated for safety in more than 1140 patients with hypertension with more than 120 treated for more than one year. UNIRETIC has not demonstrated a potential for causing adverse experiences different from those previously associated with other ACE inhibitor/diuretic combinations. The overall incidence of reported adverse events was slightly less in patients treated with UNIRETIC than patients treated with placebo.

Adverse experiences were usually mild and transient, and there was no relationship between adverse experiences and gender, race, age, or total daily dosage (except for serum potassium decreases at 50 mg hydrochlorothiazide) within the moexipril/hydrochlorothiazide dosage range of 3.75 mg/3.125 mg to 30 mg/50 mg. Discontinuation of therapy due to adverse experiences was required in 5.3% of patients treated with UNIRETIC and in 8.4% of patients treated with placebo. The most common reasons for discontinuation of therapy with UNIRETIC were cough (0.5%) and dizziness (0.5%).

All adverse experiences considered at least possibly related to treatment that occurred at any dose in placebo-controlled trials of once-daily dosing in more than 1% of patients treated with UNIRETIC and that were at least as frequent in the UNIRETIC group as in the placebo group are shown in the following table.

Adverse Events in Placebo-Controlled Trials

ADVERSE EVENT	UNIRETIC (N = 506) N (%)	PLACEBO (N = 202) N (%)
Cough	15 (3)	2 (1)
Dizziness	7 (1.4)	2 (1)
Fatigue	5 (1)	1 (0.5)

Other adverse experiences occurring in more than 1% of patients treated with UNIRETIC in controlled or uncontrolled trials, some of which were of uncertain drug relationship, listed in decreasing frequency include: upper respiratory infection, headache, pain, flu syndrome, pharyngitis, hyperuricemia, diarrhea, back pain, rhinitis, sinusitis, abnormal ECG, infection, abdominal pain, chest pain, dyspepsia, hyperglycemia, hypokalemia, rash, vertigo, nausea, hypertonia, increased SGPT, urinary tract infection, impotence, peripheral edema, pyuria, bronchitis, and fever. See WARNINGS and PRECAUTIONS for discussion of anaphylactoid reactions, angioedema, hypotension, neutropenia/agranulocytosis, fetal/neonatal morbidity and mortality, serum electrolyte imbalances, and cough.

Continued on next page

Uniretic—Cont.

The following adverse experiences, some of which are of uncertain drug relationship, were reported in UNIRETIC controlled or uncontrolled clinical trials in less than 1% of patients or have been attributed to other ACE inhibitors. Within each organ system, adverse experiences are listed in decreasing frequency.

Cardiovascular: palpitation, flushing, syncope, tachycardia, myocardial infarct, hypotension, postural hypotension, arrhythmia, first degree AV block, ventricular extrasystoles, atrial fibrillation, migraine, hemorrhage, sinus bradycardia, bigeminy, bradycardia, bundle branch block, heart arrest, myocardial ischemia, peripheral vascular disorder, prolonged QT interval, inverted T wave, ventricular fibrillation

Dermatologic: eczema, pruritus, sweating, acne, dry skin, herpes simplex, contact dermatitis, herpes zoster, psoriasis, alopecia, angioedema, erythema nodosum, fungal dermatitis, furunculosis, maculopapular rash, purpuric rash, skin carcinoma, subcutaneous nodule, urticaria, pemphigus

Gastrointestinal: vomiting, constipation, gastroenteritis, periodontal abscess, cholelithiasis, gastritis, gingivitis, esophagitis, flatulence, anorexia, colitis, dysphagia, tooth caries, cheilitis, enteritis, eructation, gastrointestinal carcinoma, gastrointestinal hemorrhage, glossitis, increased appetite, jaundice, melena, rectal hemorrhage, stomatitis, tongue discoloration, tongue edema

Hematologic: anemia, hypochromic anemia, leukopenia, abnormal erythrocytes, ecchymosis, lymphocytosis, hemolysis, lymphadenopathy, eosinophilia, petechia, abnormal WBC, hemolytic anemia

Metabolic: hyperlipemia, increased SGOT, gout, bilirubinemia, increased creatinine, hypercholesterolemia, increased BUN, increased CPK, diabetes mellitus, hyponatremia, thirst, edema, increased alkaline phosphatase, increased amylase, dehydration, decreased glucose tolerance, goiter, hypercalcemia, hyperkalemia, hypocalcemia, hypochloremia, hypoproteinemia, weight gain

Neurologic/Psychiatric: insomnia, postural dizziness, somnolence, dry mouth, anxiety, nervousness, paresthesia, depression, neuritis, hypesthesia, decreased libido, neuralgia, amnesia, ataxia, cerebral infarct, emotional lability, facial paralysis, hypokinesia, neurosis, vocal cord paralysis

Renal: albuminuria, urinary frequency, hematuria, glycosuria, cystitis, dysuria, nocturia, polyuria, kidney calculus, pyelonephritis, urate crystalluria, urinary casts, urinary retention

Respiratory: epistaxis, pneumonia, dyspnea, asthma, lung carcinoma, hemoptysis, laryngitis, voice alteration, eosinophilic pneumonitis

Urogenital: vaginal hemorrhage, breast carcinoma, scrotal edema, vaginitis, breast enlargement, breast pain, dysmenorrhea, leukorrhea

Other: asthenia, conjunctivitis, myalgia, arthralgia, arthrosis, hernia, neck pain, cyst, tenosynovitis, abnormal vision, allergic reaction, arthritis, cataract, cellulitis, moniliasis, otitis media, eye hemorrhage, chills, abscess, bursitis, deafness, ear pain, glaucoma, iritis, neck rigidity, photosensitivity, retinal degeneration, tinnitus

Monotherapy with moexipril has been evaluated for safety in over 3000 patients. In clinical trials, the observed adverse experiences with moexipril were similar to those seen in the UNIRETIC trials.

Hydrochlorothiazide: The following adverse reactions have been reported with hydrochlorothiazide and, within each organ system, are listed by decreasing severity.

Cardiovascular: orthostatic hypotension (may be potentiated by alcohol, barbiturates, or narcotics)

Gastrointestinal: pancreatitis, jaundice (intrahepatic cholestatic, see WARNINGS), sialadenitis, vomiting, diarrhea, cramping, nausea, gastric irritation, constipation, anorexia

Neurologic/Psychiatric: vertigo, dizziness, transient blurred vision, headache, paresthesia, xanthopsia, weakness, restlessness

Musculoskeletal: muscle spasm

Hematologic: aplastic anemia, agranulocytosis, leukopenia, thrombocytopenia

Metabolic: hyperglycemia, glycosuria, hyperuricemia

Hypersensitivity: necrotizing angiitis, Stevens-Johnson syndrome, respiratory distress including pneumonitis and pulmonary edema, purpura, urticaria, rash, photosensitivity

Clinical Laboratory Test Findings

Serum Electrolytes: See PRECAUTIONS, General.

Creatinine and Blood Urea Nitrogen: As with other ACE inhibitors, minor increases in blood urea nitrogen or serum creatinine, reversible upon discontinuation of therapy, were observed in less than 1% of patients with essential hypertension who were treated with UNIRETIC. Increases are more likely to occur in patients with compromised renal function (see PRECAUTIONS, General).

Other (causal relationship unknown): Clinically important changes in standard laboratory tests were rarely associated with UNIRETIC administration.

OVERDOSAGE

No specific information is available on the treatment of overdosage with UNIRETIC. Treatment should be symptomatic and supportive. Therapy with UNIRETIC should be discontinued and the patient observed closely. Suggested measures include induction of emesis and/or gastric lavage and correction of dehydration, electrolyte imbalance and hypotension by established procedures.

Single oral doses of 2 g/kg moexipril were associated with significant lethality in mice. Rats, however, tolerated single oral doses of up to 3 g/kg. The oral LD_{50} of hydrochlorothiazide is greater than 10 g/kg in mice and rats. For the combination of moexipril hydrochloride and hydrochlorothiazide (ratio 7.5:12.5), the approximate LD_{50} was around 10 g/kg for mice and above 10 g/kg for rats. Addition of hydrochlorothiazide to moexipril hydrochloride did not increase the acute toxicity due to moexipril hydrochloride.

Human overdoses of moexipril have not been reported. In case reports of overdoses with other ACE inhibitors, hypotension has been the principal adverse effect noted. The most common signs and symptoms observed with an overdose of hydrochlororthiazide have been those of dehydration and electrolyte depletion (hypokalemia, hypochloremia, hyponatremia). If digitalis has also been administered, hypokalemia may accentuate cardiac arrhythmias.

No data are available to suggest that physiological maneuvers (e.g., maneuvers to change the pH of the urine) would accelerate elimination of moexipril and its metabolites. The dialyzability of moexipril is not known.

Angiotensin II could presumably serve as a specific antagonist-antidote in the setting of moexipril overdose, but angiotensin II is essentially unavailable outside of research facilities. Because the hypotensive effect of moexipril is achieved through vasodilation and effective hypovolemia, it is reasonable to treat moexipril overdose by infusion of normal saline solution. In addition, renal function and serum potassium should be monitored.

DOSAGE AND ADMINISTRATION

Moexipril and hydrochlorothiazide are effective treatments for hypertension. The recommended dosage range of moexipril is 7.5 to 30 mg daily, administered in a single or two divided doses one hour before meals, while hydrochlorothiazide is effective in a dosage of 12.5 to 50 mg daily.

The side effects (see WARNINGS) of moexipril are generally rare and apparently independent of dose; those of hydrochlorothiazide are a mixture of dose-dependent phenomena (primarily hypokalemia) and dose-independent phenomena (e.g., pancreatitis), the former much more common than the latter. Therapy with any combination of moexipril and hydrochlorothiazide will be associated with both sets of dose-independent side effects, but regimens in which moexipril is combined with low doses of hydrochlorothiazide produce minimal effects on serum potassium. In UNIRETIC controlled clinical trials, the average change in serum potassium was near zero in subjects who received 3.75/6.25 mg or 7.5/12.5 mg, but subjects who received 15/25 mg experienced a mild decrease in serum potassium, similar to that experienced by subjects who received hydrochlorothiazide 25 mg monotherapy. To minimize dose-independent side effects, it is usually appropriate to begin combination therapy only after a patient has failed to achieve the desired effect with monotherapy.

Dose Titration Guided by Clinical Effect: A patient whose blood pressure is not adequately controlled with either moexipril or hydrochlorothiazide monotherapy may be given UNIRETIC 7.5/12.5 or UNIRETIC 15/25 one hour before a meal. Further increases of moexipril, hydrochlorothiazide or both depend on clinical response. The hydrochlorothiazide dose should generally not be increased until 2–3 weeks have elapsed.

Total daily doses above 30 mg/50 mg a day have not been studied in hypertensive patients. Patients whose blood pressures are adequately controlled with 25 mg of hydrochlorothiazide daily, but who experience significant potassium loss with this regimen, may achieve blood-pressure control without electrolyte disturbance if they are switched to moexipril 3.75 mg/hydrochlorothiazide 6.25 mg (one-half of the UNIRETIC 7.5/12.5 tablet). For patients who experience an excessive reduction in blood pressure with UNIRETIC 7.5/12.5, the physician may consider prescribing moexipril 3.75 mg/hydrochlorothiazide 6.25 mg.

Replacement Therapy: The combination may be substituted for the titrated individual active ingredients.

Use in Renal Impairment: The usual dosage regimen of UNIRETIC does not need to be adjusted as long as the patient's creatinine clearance is > 40 mL/min/1.73 m^2 (serum creatinine approximately ≤ 3 mg/dL or 265 µmol/L). In patients with more severe renal impairment, loop diuretics are preferred to thiazides, so UNIRETIC is not recommended (see PRECAUTIONS, General).

HOW SUPPLIED

UNIRETIC (moexipril hydrochloride/hydrochlorothiazide) 7.5/12.5 tablets are yellow, oval, film-coated and scored with engraved code 712 on the unscored side and S and P on either side of the score. They are supplied as follows:

Bottles of 100 NDC 0091-3712-01

UNIRETIC (moexipril hydrochloride/hydrochlorothiazide) 15/25 tablets are yellow, oval, film-coated and scored with engraved code 725 on the unscored side and S and P on either side of the score. They are supplied as follows:

Bottles of 100 NDC 0091-3725-01

Store, tightly closed, at controlled room temperature 20°–25°C (68°–77°F). Protect from excessive moisture.

If product package is subdivided, dispense in tight containers as described in USP-NF.

CAUTION: Federal law prohibits dispensing without prescription.

PC2459A Rev. 9/97

Shown in Product Identification Guide, page 337

UNIVASC® Tablets ℞

[*yü-nə-vask*]

(moexipril hydrochloride)

Rx Only

USE IN PREGNANCY

When used in pregnancy during the second and third trimesters, ACE inhibitors can cause injury and even death to the developing fetus. When pregnancy is detected, UNIVASC should be discontinued as soon as possible. **See WARNINGS, Fetal/Neonatal Morbidity and Mortality.**

DESCRIPTION

UNIVASC (moexipril hydrochloride), the hydrochloride salt of moexipril, has the empirical formula $C_{27}H_{34}N_2O_7 \cdot HCl$ and a molecular weight of 535.04. It is chemically described as [3S-[2[R*(R*)], 3R*]]-2-[2-[[1-(ethoxycarbonyl)-3-phenylpropyl]amino] -1- oxopropyl]-1,2,3,4-tetrahydro -6,7- dimethoxy-3-isoquinolinecarboxylic acid, monohydrochloride. It is a non-sulfhydryl containing precursor of the active angiotensin-converting enzyme (ACE) inhibitor moexiprilat and its structural formula is:

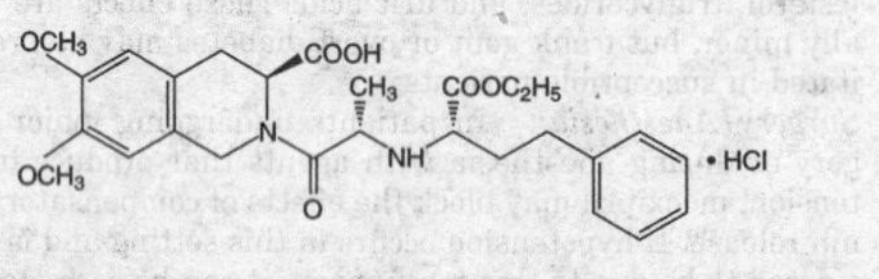

Moexipril hydrochloride is a fine white to off-white powder. It is soluble (about 10% weight-to-volume) in distilled water at room temperature.

UNIVASC is supplied as scored, coated tablets containing 7.5 mg and 15 mg of moexipril hydrochloride for oral administration. In addition to the active ingredient, moexipril hydrochloride, the tablet core contains the following inactive ingredients: lactose, magnesium oxide, crospovidone, magnesium stearate and gelatin. The film coating contains hydroxypropyl methylcellulose, hydroxypropyl cellulose, polyethylene glycol 6000, magnesium stearate, titanium dioxide, and ferric oxide.

CLINICAL PHARMACOLOGY

Mechanism of Action

Moexipril hydrochloride is a prodrug for moexiprilat, which inhibits ACE in humans and animals. The mechanism through which moexiprilat lowers blood pressure is believed to be primarily inhibition of ACE activity. ACE is a peptidyl dipeptidase that catalyzes the conversion of the inactive decapeptide angiotensin I to the vasoconstrictor substance angiotensin II. Angiotensin II is a potent peripheral vasoconstrictor that also stimulates aldosterone secretion by the adrenal cortex and provides negative feedback on renin secretion. ACE is identical to kininase II, an enzyme that degrades bradykinin, an endothelium-dependent vasodilator. Moexiprilat is about 1000 times as potent as moexipril in inhibiting ACE and kininase II. Inhibition of ACE results in decreased angiotensin II formation, leading to decreased vasoconstriction, increased plasma renin activity, and decreased aldosterone secretion. The latter results in diuresis and natriuresis and a small increase in serum potassium concentration (mean increases of about 0.25 mEq/L were seen when moexipril was used alone, see PRECAUTIONS). Whether increased levels of bradykinin, a potent vasodepressor peptide, play a role in the therapeutic effects of moexipril remains to be elucidated. Although the principal mechanism of moexipril in blood pressure reduction is believed to be through the renin-angiotensin-aldosterone system, ACE inhibitors have some effect on blood pressure even in apparent low-renin hypertension. As is the case with other ACE inhibitors, however, the antihypertensive effect of moexipril is considerably smaller in black patients, a predominantly low-renin population, than in non-black hypertensive patients.

Pharmacokinetics and Metabolism

Pharmacokinetics: Moexipril's antihypertensive activity is almost entirely due to its deesterified metabolite, moexiprilat. Bioavailability of oral moexipril is about 13% compared to intravenous (I.V.) moexipril (both measuring the metabolite moexiprilat), and is markedly affected by food, which reduces the peak plasma level (C_{max}) and AUC (see Absorption). Moexipril should therefore be taken in a fasting state. The time of peak plasma concentration (T_{max}) of moexiprilat is about $1^1/_2$ hours and elimination half-life ($t^1/_2$) is estimated at 2 to 9 hours in various studies, the variability reflecting a complex elimination pattern that is not simply exponential. Like all ACE inhibitors, moexiprilat has a prolonged terminal elimination phase, presumably reflecting slow release of drug bound to the ACE. Accumulation of moexiprilat with repeated dosing is minimal, about 30%, compatible with a functional elimination $t^1/_2$ of about 12 hours. Over the dose range of 7.5 to 30 mg, pharmacokinetics are approximately dose proportional.

Absorption: Moexipril is incompletely absorbed, with bioavailability as moexiprilat of about 13%. Bioavailability varies with formulation and food intake which reduces C_{max} and AUC by about 70% and 40% respectively after the ingestion of a low-fat breakfast or by 80% and 50% respectively after the ingestion of a high-fat breakfast.

Distribution: The clearance (CL) for moexipril is 441 mL/min and for moexiprilat 232 mL/min with a $t^1/_2$ of 1.3 and 9.8 hours, respectively. Moexiprilat is about 50% protein bound. The volume of distribution of moexiprilat is about 183 liters.

Metabolism and Excretion: Moexipril is relatively rapidly converted to its active metabolite moexiprilat, but persists longer than some other ACE inhibitor prodrugs, such that its $t^1/_2$ is over one hour and it has a significant AUC. Both moexipril and moexiprilat are converted to diketopiperazine derivatives and unidentified metabolites. After I.V. administration of moexipril, about 40% of the dose appears in urine as moexiprilat, about 26% as moexipril, with small amounts of the metabolites; about 20% of the I.V. dose appears in feces, principally as moexiprilat. After oral administration, only about 7% of the dose appears in urine as moexiprilat, about 1% as moexipril, with about 5% as other metabolites. Fifty-two percent of the dose is recovered in feces as moexiprilat and 1% as moexipril.

Special Populations:

Decreased Renal Function: The effective elimination $t^1/_2$ and AUC of both moexipril and moexiprilat are increased with decreasing renal function. There is insufficient information available to characterize this relationship fully, but at creatinine clearances in the range of 10 to 40 mL/min, the $t^1/_2$ of moexiprilat is increased by a factor of 3 to 4.

Decreased Hepatic Function: In patients with mild to moderate cirrhosis given single 15 mg doses of moexipril, the C_{max} of moexipril was increased by about 50% and the AUC increased by about 120%, while the C_{max} for moexiprilat was decreased by about 50% and the AUC increased by almost 300%.

Elderly Patients: In elderly male subjects (65–80 years old) with clinically normal renal and hepatic function, the AUC and C_{max} of moexiprilat is about 30% greater than those of younger subjects (19–42 years old).

Pharmacokinetic Interactions With Other Drugs:

No clinically important pharmacokinetic interactions occurred when UNIVASC was administered concomitantly with hydrochlorothiazide, digoxin, or cimetidine.

Pharmacodynamics and Clinical Effect

Single and multiple doses of 15 mg or more of UNIVASC gives sustained inhibition of plasma ACE activity of 80–90%, beginning within 2 hours and lasting 24 hours (80%).

In controlled trials, the peak effects of orally administered moexipril increased with the dose administered over a dose range of 7.5 to 60 mg, given once a day. Antihypertensive effects were first detectable about 1 hour after dosing, with a peak effect between 3 and 6 hours after dosing. Just before dosing (i.e., at trough), the antihypertensive effects were less prominently related to dose and the antihypertensive effect tended to diminish during the 24-hour dosing interval when the drug was administered once a day.

In multiple dose studies in the dose range of 7.5 to 30 mg once daily, UNIVASC lowered sitting diastolic and systolic blood pressure effects at trough by 3 to 6 mmHg and 4 to 11 mmHg, more than placebo, respectively. There was a tendency toward increased response with higher doses over this range. These effects are typical of ACE inhibitors but, to date, there are no trials of adequate size comparing moexipril with other antihypertensive agents.

The trough diastolic blood pressure effects of moexipril were approximately 3 to 6 mmHg in various studies. Generally, higher doses of moexipril leave a greater fraction of the peak blood pressure effect still present at trough. During dose titration, any decision as to the adequacy of a dosing regimen should be based on trough blood pressure measurements. If diastolic blood pressure control is not adequate at the end of the dosing interval, the dose can be increased or given as a divided (BID) regimen.

During chronic therapy, the antihypertensive effect of any dose of UNIVASC is generally evident within 2 weeks of treatment, with maximal reduction after 4 weeks. The antihypertensive effects of UNIVASC have been proven to continue during therapy for up to 24 months.

UNIVASC, like other ACE inhibitors, is less effective in decreasing trough blood pressures in blacks than in non-blacks. Placebo-corrected trough group mean diastolic blood pressure effects in blacks in the proposed dose range varied between +1 to −3 mmHg compared with responses in non-blacks of −4 to −6 mmHg.

The effectiveness of UNIVASC was not significantly influenced by patient age, gender, or weight. UNIVASC has been shown to have antihypertensive activity in both pre- and postmenopausal women who have participated in placebo-controlled clinical trials.

Formal interaction studies with moexipril have not been carried out with antihypertensive agents other than thiazide diuretics. In these studies, the added effect of moexipril was similar to its effect as monotherapy. In general, ACE inhibitors have less than additive effects with beta-adrenergic blockers, presumably because both work by inhibiting the renin-angiotensin system.

INDICATIONS AND USAGE

UNIVASC is indicated for treatment of patients with hypertension. It may be used alone or in combination with thiazide diuretics.

In using UNIVASC, consideration should be given to the fact that another ACE inhibitor, captopril, has caused agranulocytosis, particularly in patients with renal impairment or collagen-vascular disease. Available data are insufficient to show that UNIVASC does not have a similar risk (see WARNINGS).

In considering use of UNIVASC, it should be noted that in controlled trials ACE inhibitors have an effect on blood pressure that is less in black patients than in non-blacks. In addition, ACE inhibitors (for which adequate data are available) cause a higher rate of angioedema in black than in non-black patients (see WARNINGS, Angioedema).

CONTRAINDICATIONS

UNIVASC is contraindicated in patients who are hypersensitive to this product and in patients with a history of angioedema related to previous treatment with an ACE inhibitor.

WARNINGS

Anaphylactoid and Possibly Related Reactions

Presumably because angiotensin-converting enzyme inhibitors affect the metabolism of eicosanoids and polypeptides, including endogenous bradykinin, patients recieving ACE inhibitors, including UNIVASC, may be subject to a variety of adverse reactions, some of them serious.

Angioedema: Angioedema involving the face, extremities, lips, tongue, glottis, and/or larynx has been reported in patients treated with ACE inhibitors, including UNIVASC. Symptoms suggestive of angioedema or facial edema occurred in <0.5% of moexipril-treated patients in placebo-controlled trials. None of the cases were considered life-threatening and all resolved either without treatment or with medication (antihistamines or glucocorticoids). One patient treated with hydrochlorothiazide alone experienced laryngeal edema. No instances of angioedema were reported in placebo-treated patients.

In cases of angioedema, treatment should be promptly discontinued and the patient carefully observed until the swelling disappears. In instances where swelling has been confined to the face and lips, the condition has generally resolved without treatment, although antihistamines have been useful in relieving symptoms.

Angioedema associated with involvement of the tongue, glottis, or larynx, may be fatal due to airway obstruction. Appropriate therapy, e.g., subcutaneous epinephrine solution 1:1000 (0.3 to 0.5 mL) and/or measures to ensure a patent airway, should be promptly provided (see ADVERSE REACTIONS).

Anaphylactoid Reactions During Desensitization: Two patients undergoing desensitizing treatment with hymenoptera venom while receiving ACE inhibitors sustained life-threatening anaphylactoid reactions. In the same patients, these reactions did not occur when ACE inhibitors were temporarily withheld, but they reappeared when the ACE inhibitors were inadvertently readministered.

Anaphylactoid Reactions During Membrane Exposure: Anaphylactoid reactions have been reported in patients dialyzed with high-flux membranes and treated concomitantly with an ACE inhibitor. Anaphylactoid reactions have also been reported in patients undergoing low-density lipoprotein apheresis with dextran sulfate absorption.

Hypotension

UNIVASC can cause symptomatic hypotension, although, as with other ACE inhibitors, this is unusual in uncomplicated hypertensive patients treated with UNIVASC alone. Symptomatic hypotension was seen in 0.5% of patients given moexipril and led to discontinuation of therapy in about 0.25%. Symptomatic hypotension is most likely to occur in patients who have been salt- and volume-depleted as a result of prolonged diuretic therapy, dietary salt restriction, dialysis, diarrhea, or vomiting. Volume- and salt-depletion should be corrected and, in general, diuretics stopped, before initiating therapy with UNIVASC (see PRECAUTIONS, Drug Interactions, and ADVERSE REACTIONS).

In patients with congestive heart failure, with or without associated renal insufficiency, ACE inhibitor therapy may cause excessive hypotension, which may be associated with oliguria or progressive azotemia, and rarely, with acute renal failure and death. In these patients, UNIVASC therapy should be started under close medical supervision, and patients should be followed closely for the first two weeks of treatment and whenever the dose of moexipril or an accompanying diuretic is increased. Care in avoiding hypotension should also be taken in patients with ischemic heart disease, aortic stenosis, or cerebrovascular disease, in whom an excessive decrease in blood pressure could result in a myocardial infarction or a cerebrovascular accident.

If hypotension occurs, the patient should be placed in a supine position and, if necessary, treated with an intravenous infusion of normal saline. UNIVASC treatment usually can be continued following restoration of blood pressure and volume.

Neutropenia/Agranulocytosis

Another ACE inhibitor, captopril, has been shown to cause agranulocytosis and bone marrow depression, rarely in patients with uncomplicated hypertension, but more frequently in hypertensive patients with renal impairment, especially if they also have a collagen-vascular disease such as systemic lupus erythematosus or scleroderma. Although there were no instances of severe neutropenia (absolute neutrophil count <500/mm^3) among patients given UNIVASC, as with other ACE inhibitors, monitoring of white blood cell counts should be considered for patients who have collagen-vascular disease, especially if the disease is associated with impaired renal function. Available data from clinical trials of UNIVASC are insufficient to show that UNIVASC does not cause agranulocytosis at rates similar to captopril.

Fetal/Neonatal Morbidity and Mortality

ACE inhibitors can cause fetal and neonatal morbidity and death when administered to pregnant women. Several dozen cases have been reported in the world literature. When pregnancy is detected, ACE inhibitors should be discontinued as soon as possible.

The use of ACE inhibitors during the second and third trimesters of pregnancy has been associated with fetal and neonatal injury, including hypotension, neonatal skull hypoplasia, anuria, reversible or irreversible renal failure, and death. Oligohydramnios has also been reported, presumably resulting from decreased fetal renal function; oligohydramnios in this setting has been associated with fetal limb contractures, craniofacial deformation, and hypoplastic lung development. Prematurity, intrauterine growth retardation, and patent ductus arteriosus have also been reported, although it is not clear whether these were caused by the ACE inhibitor exposure.

Fetal and neonatal morbidity do not appear to have resulted from intrauterine ACE inhibitor exposure limited to the first trimester. Mothers who have used ACE inhibitors only during the first trimester should be informed of this. Nonetheless, when patients become pregnant, physicians should make every effort to discontinue the use of moexipril as soon as possible. Rarely (probably less often than once in every thousand pregnancies), no alternative to ACE inhibitors will be found. In these rare cases, the mothers should be apprised of the potential hazards to their fetuses, and serial ultrasound examinations should be performed to assess the intraamniotic environment.

If oligohydramnios is observed, moexipril should be discontinued unless it is considered life-saving for the mother. Contraction stress testing (CST), a non-stress test (NST), or biophysical profiling (BPP) may be appropriate, depending upon the week of pregnancy. Patients and physicians should be aware, however, that oligohydramnios may not be detected until after the fetus has sustained irreversible injury. Infants with histories of *in utero* exposure to ACE inhibitors should be closely observed for hypotension, oliguria, and hyperakalemia. If oliguria occurs, attention should be directed toward support of blood pressure and renal perfusion. Exchange transfusion or peritoneal dialysis may be required as means of reversing hypotension and/or substituting for disordered renal function.

Theoretically, the ACE inhibitor could be removed from the neonatal circulation by exchange transfusion, but no experience with this procedure has been reported.

No embryotoxic, fetotoxic, or teratogenic effects were seen in rats or in rabbits treated with up to 90.9 and 0.7 times, respectively, the Maximum Recommended Human Dose (MRHD) on a mg/m^2 basis.

Hepatic Failure

Rarely, ACE inhibitors have been associated with a syndrome that starts with cholestatic jaundice and progresses

Continued on next page

Univasc—Cont.

to fulminant hepatic necrosis and sometimes death. The mechanism of this syndrome is not understood. Patients receiving ACE inhibitors who develop jaundice or marked elevations of hepatic enzymes should discontinue the ACE inhibitor and receive appropriate medical follow-up.

PRECAUTIONS

General

Impaired Renal Function: As a consequence of inhibition of the reninangiotensin-aldosterone system, changes in renal function may be anticipated in susceptible individuals. There is no clinical experience of UNIVASC in the treatment of hypertension in patients with renal failure.

Some hypertensive patients with no apparent preexisting renal vascular disease have developed increases in blood urea nitrogen and serum creatinine, usually minor and transient, especially when UNIVASC has been given concomitantly with a thiazide diuretic. This is more likely to occur in patients with preexisting renal impairment. There may be a need for dose adjustment of UNIVASC and/or the discontinuation of the thiazide diuretic.

Evaluation of hypertensive patients should always include assessment of renal function (see DOSAGE AND ADMINISTRATION).

Hypertensive Patients With Congestive Heart Failure: In hypertensive patients with severe congestive heart failure, whose renal function may depend on the activity of the renin-angiotensin-aldosterone system, treatment with ACE inhibitors, including UNIVASC, may be associated with oliguria and/or progressive azotemia and, rarely, acute renal failure and/or death.

Hypertensive Patients With Renal Artery Stenosis: In hypertensive patients with unilateral or bilateral renal artery stenosis, increases in blood urea nitrogen and serum creatinine have been observed in some patients following ACE inhibitor therapy. These increases were almost always reversible upon discontinuation of the ACE inhibitor and/or diuretic therapy. In such patients, renal function should be monitored during the first few weeks of therapy.

Hyperkalemia: In clinical trials, persistent hyperkalemia (serum potassium above 5.4 mEq/L) occurred in approximately 1.3% of hypertensive patients receiving UNIVASC. Risk factors for the development of hyperkalemia with ACE inhibitors include renal insufficiency, diabetes mellitus, and the concomitant use of potassium-sparing diuretics, potassium supplements, and/or potassium-containing salt substitutes, which should be used cautiously, if at all, with UNIVASC (see PRECAUTIONS, Drug Interactions).

Surgery/Anesthesia: In patients undergoing major surgery or during anesthesia with agents that produce hypotension, moexipril may block the effects of compensatory renin release. If hypotension occurs in this setting and is considered to be due to this mechanism, it can be corrected by volume expansion.

Cough: Presumably due to the inhibition of the degradation of endogenous bradykinin, persistent nonproductive cough has been reported with all ACE inhibitors, always resolving after discontinuation of therapy. ACE inhibitor-induced cough should be considered in the differential diagnosis of cough. In controlled trials with moexipril, cough was present in 6.1% of moexipril patients and 2.2% of patients given placebo.

Information for Patients

Food: Patients should be advised to take moexipril one hour before meals. (see CLINICAL PHARMACOLOGY and DOSAGE AND ADMINISTRATION).

Angioedema: Angioedema, including laryngeal edema, may occur with treatment with ACE inhibitors, usually occuring early in therapy (within the first month). Patients should be so advised and told to report immediately any signs or symptoms suggesting angioedema (swelling of the face, extremities, eyes, lips, tongue, difficulty in breathing) and to take no more UNIVASC until they have consulted with the prescribing physician.

Symptomatic Hypotension: Patients should be cautioned that lightheadedness can occur with UNIVASC, especially during the first few days of therapy. If fainting occurs, the patient should stop taking UNIVASC and consult the prescribing physician.

All patients should be cautioned that excessive perspiration and dehydration may lead to an excessive fall in blood pressure because of reduction in fluid volume. Other causes of volume depletion such as vomiting or diarrhea may also lead to a fall in blood pressure; patients should be advised to consult their physician if they develop these conditions.

Hyperkalemia: Patients should be told not to use potassium supplements or salt substitutes containing potassium without consulting their physician.

Neutropenia: Patients should be told to report promptly any indication of infection (e.g., sore throat, fever) that could be a sign of neutropenia.

Pregnancy: Female patients of childbearing age should be told about the consequences of second- and third- trimester exposure to ACE inhibitors and should also be told that these consequences do not appear to have resulted from intrauterine ACE inhibitor exposure that has been limited to the first trimester. Patients should be asked to report pregnancies to their physicians as soon as possible.

Drug Interactions

Diuretics: Excessive reductions in blood pressure may occur in patients on diuretic therapy when ACE inhibitors are started. The possibility of hypotensive effects with UNIVASC can be minimized by discontinuing diuretic therapy for several days or cautiously increasing salt intake before initiation of treatment with UNIVASC. If this is not possible, the starting dose of moexpril should be reduced. (See WARNINGS and DOSAGE AND ADMINISTRATION).

Potassium Supplements and Potassium-Sparing Diuretics: UNIVASC can increase serum potassium because it decreases aldosterone secretion. Use of potassium-sparing diuretics (spironolactone, triamterene, amiloride) or potassium supplements concomitantly with ACE inhibitors can increase the risk of hyperkalemia. Therefore, if concomitant use of such agents is indicated, they should be given with caution and the patient's serum potassium should be monitored.

Oral Anticoagulants: Interaction studies with warfarin failed to identify any clinically important effect on the serum concentrations of the anticogulant or on its anticoagulant effect.

Lithium: Increased serum lithium levels and symptoms of lithium toxicity have been reported in patients receiving ACE inhibitors during therapy with lithium. These drugs should be coadministered with caution, and frequent monitoring of serum lithium levels is recommended. If a diuretic is also used, the risk of lithium toxicity may be increased.

Other Agents: No clinically important pharmacokinetic interactions occured when UNIVASC was administered concomitantly with hydrochlorothiazide, digoxin, or cimetidine. UNIVASC has been used in clinical trails concomitantly with calcium-channel-blocking agents, diuretics, H_2 blockers, digoxin, oral hypoglycemic agents, and cholesterol-lowering agents. There was no evidence of clinically important adverse interactions.

Carcinogenesis, Mutagenesis, Impairment of Fertility

No evidence of carcinogenicity was detected in long-term studies in mice and rats at doses up to 14 or 27.3 times the Maximum Recommended Human Dose (MRHD) on a mg/m^2 basis.

No mutagenicity was detected in the Ames test and microbial reverse mutation assay, with and without metabolic activation, or in an *in vivo* nucleus anomaly test. However, increased chromosomal aberration frequency in Chinese hamster ovary cells was detected under metabolic activation conditions at a 20-hour harvest time.

Reproduction studies have been performed in rabbits at oral doses up to 0.7 times the MRHD on a mg/m^2 basis, and in rats up to 90.9 times the MRHD on a mg/m^2 basis. No indication of impaired fertility, reproductive toxicity, or teratogenicity was observed.

Pregnancy

Pregnancy Categories C (first trimester) and D (second and third trimesters). See WARNINGS, Fetal/Neonatal Morbidity and Mortality.

Nursing Mothers

It is not known whether UNIVASC is excreted in human milk. Because many drugs are excreted in human milk, caution should be exercised when UNIVASC is given to a nursing mother.

Geriatric Use

Of the patients who received UNIVASC in controlled clinical studies, 33% were 65 years of age or older. No overall differences in effectiveness or safety were observed between these patients and younger patients. In elderly patients receiving UNIVASC, plasma levels of drug are slightly higher and renal clearance is reduced when compared to younger patients, but this did not have detectable consequences.

Pediatric Use

Safety and effectiveness of UNIVASC in pediatric patients have not been established.

ADVERSE REACTIONS

UNIVASC has been evaluated for safety in more than 2500 patients with hypertension, more than 250 of these patients were treated for approximately one year. The overall incidence of reported adverse events was only slightly greater in patients treated with UNIVASC than patients treated with placebo.

Reported adverse experiences were usually mild and transient, and there were no differences in adverse reaction rates related to gender, race, age, duration of therapy, or total daily dosage within the range of 3.75 mg to 60 mg. Discontinuation of therapy because of adverse experiences was required in 3.4% of patients treated with UNIVASC and in 1.8% of patients treated with placebo. The most common reasons for discontinutation in patients treated with UNIVASC were cough (0.7%) and dizziness (0.4%).

All adverse experiences considered at least possibly related to treatment that occurred at any dose in placebo-controlled trials of once-daily dosing in more than 1% of patients treated with UNIVASC alone and that were at least as frequent in the UNIVASC group as in the placebo group are shown in the following table:

ADVERSE EVENTS IN PLACEBO-CONTROLLED STUDIES

ADVERSE EVENT	UNIVASC (N=674)		PLACEBO (N=226)	
	N	(%)	N	(%)
Cough Increased	41	(6.1)	5	(2.2)
Dizziness	29	(4.3)	5	(2.2)
Diarrhea	21	(3.1)	5	(2.2)
Flu Syndrome	21	(3.1)	0	(0)
Fatigue	16	(2.4)	4	(1.8)
Pharyngitis	12	(1.8)	2	(0.9)
Flushing	11	(1.6)	0	(0)
Rash	11	(1.6)	2	(0.9)
Myalgia	9	(1.3)	0	(0)

Other adverse events occurring in more than 1% of patients on moexipril that were at least as frequent on placebo include: headache, upper respiratory infection, pain, rhinitis, dyspepsia, nausea, peripheral edema, sinusitis, chest pain, and urinary frequency. See WARNINGS and PRECAUTIONS for discussion of anaphylactoid reactions, angioedema, hypotension, neutropenia/agranulocytosis, second and third trimester fetal/neonatal morbidity and mortality, hyperkalemia, and cough.

Other potentially important adverse experiences reported in controlled or uncontrolled clinical trials in less than 1% of moexipril patients or that have been attributed to other ACE inhibitors include the following:

Cardiovascular: Symptomatic hypotension, postural hypotension, or syncope were seen in 9/1750 (0.51%) patients; these reactions led to discontinuation of therapy in controlled trials in 3/1254 (0.24%) patients who had received UNIVASC monotherapy and in 1/344 (0.3%) patients who had received UNIVASC with hydrochlorothiazide (see PRECAUTIONS and WARNINGS). Other adverse events included angina/myocardial infarction, palpitations, rhythm disturbances, and cerebrovascular accident.

Renal: Of hypertensive patients with no apparent preexisting renal disease, 1% of patients receiving UNIVASC alone and 2% of patients receiving UNIVASC with hydrochlorothiazide experienced increases in serum creatinine to at least 140% of their baseline values (see PRECAUTIONS and DOSAGE AND ADMINISTRATION).

Gastrointestinal: Abdominal pain, constipation, vomiting, appetite/weight change, dry mouth, pancreatitis, hepatitis.

Respiratory: Bronchospasm, dyspnea, eosinophilic pneumonitis.

Urogenital: Renal insufficiency, oliguria.

Dermatologic Apparent hypersensitivity reactions manifested by urticaria, rash, pemphigus, pruritus, photosensitivity.

Neurological and Psychiatric: Drowsiness, sleep disturbances, nervousness, mood changes, anxiety.

Other: Angioedema (see WARNINGS), taste disturbances, tinnitus, sweating, malaise, arthralgia, hemolytic anemia.

Clinical Laboratory Test Findings

Creatinine and Blood Urea Nitrogen: As with other ACE inhibitors, minor increases in blood urea nitrogen or serum creatinine, reversible upon disontinuation of therapy, were observed in approximately 1% of patients with essential hypertension who were treated with UNIVASC. Increases are more likely to occur in patients receiving concomitant diuretics and in patients with compromised renal function (see PRECAUTIONS, General).

Other (causal relationship unknown): Clinically important changes in standard laboratory tests were rarely associated with UNIVASC administration.

Elevations of liver enzymes and uric acid have been reported. In trials, less than 1% of moexipril-treated patients discontinued UNIVASC treatment because of laboratory abnormalities. The incidence of abnormal laboratory values with moexipril was similar to that in the placebo-treated group.

OVERDOSAGE

Human overdoses of moexipril have not been reported. In case reports of overdoses with other ACE inhibitors, hypotension has been the principal adverse effect noted. Single oral doses of 2 g/kg moexipril were associated with significant lethality in mice. Rats, however, tolerated single oral doses of up to 3 g/kg.

No data are available to suggest that physiological maneuvers (e.g., maneuvers to change the pH of the urine) would accelerate elimination of moexipril and its metabolites. The dialyzability of moexipril is not known.

Angiotensin II could presumably serve as a specific antagonist-antidote in the setting of moexipril overdose, but angiotensin II is essentially unavailable outside of research facilities. Because the hypotensive effect of moexipril is achieved through vasodilation and effective hypovolemia, it is reasonable to treat moexipril overdose by infusion of normal saline solution. In addition, renal function and serum potassium should be monitored.

DOSAGE AND ADMINISTRATION

Hypertension

The recommended initial dose of UNIVASC in patients not receiving diuretics is 7.5 mg, one hour prior to meals, once daily. Dosage should be adjusted according to blood pressure response. The antihypertensive effect of UNIVASC may diminish towards the end of the dosing interval. Blood pressure should, therefore, be measured just prior to dosing to determine whether satisfactory blood pressure control is obtained. If control is not adequate, increased dose or divided dosing can be tried. The recommended dose range is 7.5 to 30 mg daily, administered in one or two divided doses one hour before meals. Total daily doses above 60 mg a day have not been studied in hypertensive patients.

In patients who are currently being treated with a diuretic, symptomatic hypotension may occasionally occur following the initial dose of UNIVASC. The diuretic should, if possible, be discontinued for 2 to 3 days before therapy with UNIVASC is begun, to reduce the likelihood of hypotension (see WARNINGS). If the patient's blood pressure is not controlled with UNIVASC alone, diuretic therapy may then be reinstituted. If diuretic therapy cannot be discontinued, an initial dose of 3.75 mg of UNIVASC should be used with medical supervision until blood pressure has stabilized (see WARNINGS and PRECAUTIONS, Drug Interactions).

Dosage Adjustment in Renal Impairment

For patients with a creatinine clearance ≤40 mL/min/1.73 m^2, an initial dose of 3.75 mg once daily should be given cautiously. Doses may be titrated upward to a maximum daily dose of 15 mg.

HOW SUPPLIED

UNIVASC (moexipril hydrochloride) 7.5 mg tablets are pink colored, biconvex, film-coated and scored with engraved code **707** on the unscored side and **SP** above and **7.5** below the score. They are supplied as follows:

Bottles of 90 (Unit-of-Use)	NDC 0091-3707-09
Bottles of 100	NDC 0091-3707-01

UNIVASC (moexipril hydrochloride) 15 mg tablets are salmon colored, biconvex, film-coated, and scored with engraved code **715** on the unscored side and **SP** above and **15** below the score. They are supplied as follows:

Bottles of 90 (Unit-of-Use)	NDC 0091-3715-09
Bottles of 100	NDC 0091-3715-01

Store, tightly closed, at controlled room temperature.

Protect from excessive moisture.

If product package is subdivided, dispense in tight containers as described in USP-NF.

PC1879D Rev. 4/98

Shown in Product Identification Guide, page 337

URSO® ℞

[*ur-sō*]

(ursodiol)

Tablets

250 mg

Direct URSO Inquiries to:

AXCAN PHARMA U.S. INC.
3940 Quebec Avenue North
Minneapolis, MN 55427
(612) 417-0684
(800) 742-6706

DESCRIPTION

URSO® is a bile acid available as 250 mg film-coated tablets for oral administration.

URSO® is ursodiol (ursodeoxycholic acid), a naturally occurring bile acid found in small quantities in normal human bile and in larger quantities in the biles of certain species of bears. It is a bitter-tasting white powder consisting of crystalline particles freely soluble in ethanol and glacial acetic acid, slightly soluble in chloroform, sparingly soluble in ether, and practically insoluble in water. The chemical name of ursodiol is 3α, 7β-dihydroxy-5β-cholan-24-oic ($C_{24}H_{40}O_4$). Ursodiol has a molecular weight of 392.56. Its structure is shown below.

[See chemical structure at top of next column]

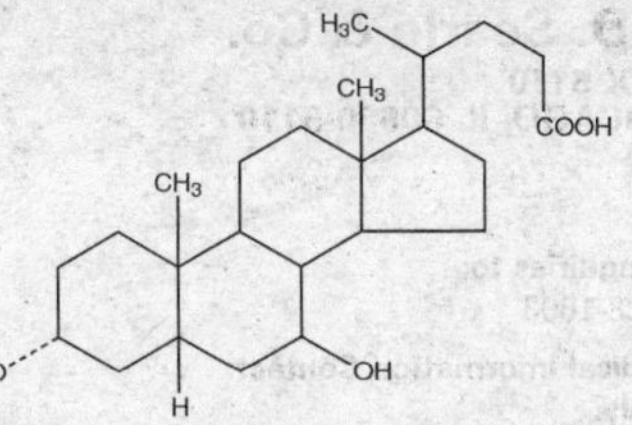

Inactive ingredients: microcrystalline cellulose, povidone, sodium starch glycolate, magnesium stearate, ethylcellulose, dibutyl sebacate, carnauba wax, hydroxypropyl methylcellulose, PEG 3350, PEG 8000, cetyl alcohol, sodium lauryl sulfate and hydrogen peroxide.

CLINICAL PHARMACOLOGY

Ursodiol (UDCA) is normally present as a minor fraction of the total bile acids in humans (about 5%). Following oral administration, the majority of ursodiol is absorbed by passive diffusion and its absorption is incomplete. Once absorbed, ursodiol undergoes hepatic extraction to the extent of about 50% in the absence of liver disease. As the severity of liver disease increases, the extent of extraction decreases. In the liver, ursodiol is conjugated with glycine or taurine, then secreted into bile. These conjugates of ursodiol are absorbed in the small intestine by passive and active mechanisms. The conjugates can also be deconjugated in the ileum by intestinal enzymes, leading to the formation of free ursodiol that can be reabsorbed and reconjugated in the liver. Nonabsorbed ursodiol passes into the colon where it is mostly 7-dehydroxylated to lithocholic acid. Some ursodiol is epimerized to chenodiol (CDCA) via a 7-oxo intermediate. Chenodiol also undergoes 7-dehydroxylation to form lithocholic acid. These metabolites are poorly soluble and excreted in the feces. A small portion of lithocholic acid is reabsorbed, conjugated in the liver with glycine, or taurine and sulfated at the 3 position. The resulting sulfated lithocholic acid conjugates are excreted in bile and then lost in feces.

Lithocholic acid, when administered chronically to animals, causes cholestatic liver injury that may lead to death from liver failure in certain species unable to form sulfate conjugates. Ursodiol is 7-dehydroxylated more slowly than chenodiol. For equimolar doses of ursodiol and chenodiol, steady state levels of ltihocholic acid in biliary bile acids are lower during ursodiol administration than with chenodiol administration. Humans and chimpanzees can sulfate lithocholic acid. Although liver injury has not been associated with ursodiol therapy, a reduced capacity to sulfate may exist in some individuals. Nonetheless, such a deficiency has not yet been clearly demonstrated and must be extremely rare, given the several thousand patient-years of clinical experience with ursodiol.

In healthy subjects, at least 70% of ursodiol (unconjugated) is bound to plasma protein. No information is available on the binding of conjugated ursodiol to plasma protein in healthy subjects or primary biliary cirrhosis (PBC) patients. Its volume of distribution has not been determined, but is expected to be small since the drug is mostly distributed in the bile and small intestine. Ursodiol is excreted primarily in the feces. With treatment, urinary excretion increases, but remains less than 1% except in severe cholestatic liver disease.

During chronic administration of ursodiol, it becomes a major biliary and plasma bile acid. At a chronic dose of 13–15 mg/kg/day, ursodiol constitutes 30–50% of biliary and plasma bile acids.

CLINICAL STUDIES

A U.S., multicenter, randomized, double-blind, placebo-controlled study was conducted to evaluate the efficacy of ursodeoxycholic acid at a dose of 13–15 mg/kg/day, administered in 4 divided doses in 180 patients with PBC. Upon completion of the double-blind portion, all patients entered an open-label active treatment extension phase.

Treatment failure, the main efficacy end point measured during this study, was defined as death, need for liver transplantation, histologic progression by two stages or to cirrhosis, development of varices, ascites or encephalopathy, marked worsening of fatigue or pruritus, inability to tolerate the drug, doubling of serum bilirubin and voluntary withdrawal. After two years of double-blind treatment, the incidence of treatment failure was significantly reduced in the URSO® group (n=89) as compared to the placebo group (n=91). Time to treatment failure was also significantly delayed in the URSO® treated group regardless of either histological stage or baseline bilirubin levels (>1.8 or ≤1.8 mg/dl).

Using a definition of treatment failure which excluded doubling of serum bilirubin and voluntary withdrawal, time to treatment failure was significantly delayed in the URSO® group. In comparison with placebo, treatment with URSO® resulted in a significant improvement in the following serum hepatic biochemistries when compared to baseline: total bilirubin, SGOT, alkaline phosphatase and IgM.

A second study conducted in Canada randomized 222 PBC patients to ursodiol, 14 mg/kg/day or placebo, in a double-blind manner during a two-year period. At two years, a statistically significant difference between the two treatments, in favor of ursodiol, was demonstrated in the following: reduction in the proportion of patients exhibiting a more than 50% increase in serum bilirubin; median percent decrease in bilirubin, transaminases and alkaline phosphatase; incidence of treatment failure; and time to treatment failure. The definition of treatment failure included: discontinuing the study for any reason; a total serum bilirubin level greater than or equal to 1.5 mg/dl or increasing to a level equal to or greater than two times the baseline level; and the development of ascites or encephalopathy.

INDICATIONS AND USAGE

URSO® (ursodiol) tablets are indicated for the treatment of patients with primary biliary cirrhosis.

CONTRAINDICATIONS

Hypersensitivity or intolerance to ursodiol or any of the components of the formulation.

PRECAUTIONS

Patients with variceal bleeding, hepatic encephalopathy, ascites or in need of an urgent liver transplant, should receive appropriate specific treatment.

Drug Interactions

Bile acid sequestering agents such as cholestyramine and colestipol may interfere with the action of **URSO®** by reducing its absorption. Aluminum-based antacids have been shown to adsorb bile acids *in vitro* and may be expected to interfere with **URSO®** in the same manner as the bile acid sequestering agents. Estrogens, oral contraceptives, and clofibrate (and perhaps other lipid-lowering drugs) increase hepatic cholesterol secretion, and encourage cholesterol gallstone formation and hence may counteract the effectiveness of **URSO®**.

Carcinogenicity, Mutagenicity and Impairment of Fertility

In two 24-month oral carcinogenicity studies in mice, ursodiol at doses up to 1,000 mg/kg/day (3,000 mg/m^2/day) was not tumorigenic. Based on body surface area, for a 50 kg person of average height (1.46 m^2 body surface area), this dose represents 5.4 times the recommended maximum clinical dose of 15 mg/kg/day (555 mg/m^2/day).

In a two-year oral carcinogenicity study in Fischer 344 rats, ursodiol at doses up to 300 mg/kg/day (1,800 mg/m^2/day, 3.2 times the recommended maximum human dose based on body surface area) was not tumorigenic.

In a life-span (126–138 weeks) oral carcinogenicity study, Sprague-Dawley rats were treated with doses of 33 to 300 mg/kg/day, 0.4 to 3.2 times the recommended maximum human dose based on body surface area. Ursodiol produced a significantly (p≤0.5, Fisher's exact test) increased incidence of pheochromocytomas of the adrenal medulla in females of the highest dose group.

In 103-week oral carcinogenicity studies of lithocholic acid, a metabolite of ursodiol, doses up to 250 mg/kg/day in mice and 500 mg/kg/day in rats did not produce any tumors. In a 78-week rat study, intrarectal instillation of lithocholic acid (1 mg/kg/day) for 13 months did not produce colorectal tumors. A tumor-promoting effect was observed when it was administered after a single intrarectal dose of a known carcinogen N-methyl-N′-nitro-N-nitrosoguanidine. On the other hand, in a 32-week rat study, ursodiol at a daily dose of 240 mg/kg (1,440 mg/m^2, 2.6 times the maximum recommended human dose based on body surface area) suppressed the colonic carcinogenic effect of another known carcinogen azoxymethane.

Ursodiol was not genotoxic in the Ames test, the mouse lymphoma cell (L5178Y, $TK^{+/-}$) forward mutation test, the human lymphocyte sister chromatid exchange test, the mouse spermatogonia chromosome aberration test, the Chinese hamster micronucleus test and the Chinese hamster bone marrow cell chromosome aberration test.

Ursodiol at oral doses of up to 2,700 mg/kg/day (16,200 mg/m^2/day, 29 times the recommended maximum human dose based on body surface area) was found to have no effect on fertility and reproductive performance of male and female rats.

Pregnancy, Teratogenic Effects. Pregnancy Category B

Teratology studies have been performed in pregnant rats at oral doses up to 2,000 mg/kg/day (12,000 mg/m^2/day, 22 times the recommended maximum human dose based on body surface area) and in pregnant rabbits at oral doses up to 300 mg/kg/day (3,600 mg/m^2/day, 7 times the recommended maximum human dose based on body surface area) and have revealed no evidence of impaired fertility or harm to the fetus due to ursodiol.

There are no adequate or well-controlled studies in pregnant women. Because animal reproduction studies are not always predictive of human response, this drug should be used during pregnancy only if clearly needed.

Nursing Mothers

It is not known whether ursodiol is excreted in human milk. Because many drugs are excreted in human milk, caution should be exercised when **URSO®** is administered to a nursing mother.

Continued on next page

Urso—Cont.

Pediatric Use
The safety and effectiveness of **URSO®** in pediatric patients have not been established.

ADVERSE EVENTS (AEs)

ADVERSE EVENTS	VISIT AT 12 MONTHS		VISIT AT 24 MONTHS	
	UDCA n (%)	Placebo n (%)	UDCA n (%)	Placebo n (%)
Diarrhea	—	—	1 (1.32)	—
Elevated creatinine	—	—	1 (1.32)	—
Elevated blood glucose	1 (1.18)	—	1 (1.32)	—
Leukopenia	—	—	2 (2.63)	—
Peptic ulcer	—	—	1 (1.32)	—
Skin rash	—	—	2 (2.63)	—

Note: Those AEs occurring at the same or higher incidence in the placebo as in the UDCA group have been deleted from this table (this includes diarrhea and thrombocytopenia at 12 months, nausea/vomiting, fever and other toxicity).

UDCA = Ursodeoxycholic acid = Ursodiol

Adverse events are reported regardless of attribution to the test medication.

OVERDOSE
Accidental or intentional overdosage with ursodiol has not been reported. The most severe manifestation of overdosage would likely consist of diarrhea which should be treated symptomatically.

Single oral doses of ursodiol at 10, 5 and 10 g/kg in mice, rats and dogs, respectively were not lethal. A single oral dose of ursodiol at 1.5 g/kg was lethal in hamsters. Symptoms of acute toxicity were salivation and vomiting in dogs, and ataxia, dyspnea, ptosis, agonal convulsions and coma in hamsters.

DOSAGE AND ADMINISTRATION
The recommended adult dosage for **URSO®** in the treatment of PBC is 13–15 mg/kg/day administered in four divided doses with food.

HOW SUPPLIED
Each **URSO®** film-coated tablet, white, engraved with "URS785", contains 250 mg of ursodiol. Available in bottles of 100 tablets (NDC 0091-0785-01). Store at 20°C to 25°C (68°F to 77°F). Dispense in a tight container.

Caution: Federal law prohibits dispensing without a prescription.

Manufactured by:
GLOBAL PHARM INC.
North York, Ontario M3B 1Y5
Canada

for:
AXCAN PHARMA U.S. INC.
3940 Quebec Avenue North
Minneapolis, MN 55427
USA

Distributed by:
SCHWARZ PHARMA
Milwaukee, WI 53201
USA

® Reg. TM of AXCAN PHARMA U.S. INC.
April 1998

Shown in Product Identification Guide, page 337

NOTICE
Before prescribing or administering any product described in PHYSICIANS' DESK REFERENCE check the **PDR Supplements** for revised information.

G.D. Searle & Co.
BOX 5110
CHICAGO, IL 60680-5110

Direct Inquiries to:
(800) 323-1603

For Medical Information Contact:
Generally:
G.D. Searle & Co.
Healthcare Information Services
5200 Old Orchard Road
Skokie, IL 60077
In Emergencies:
Outside IL:
(800) 323-4204 (business hours)
(847) 982-7000 (at other times)
Within IL:
(847) 982-7000

Sales and Ordering:
(800) 323-1603

Alphabetic Product Listing
Product, ID# (NDC*), Form, Strength
Aldactazide, 1011, Tablet, 25 mg/25 mg
Aldactazide, 1021, Tablet, 50 mg/50 mg
Aldactone, 1001, Tablet, 25 mg
Aldactone, 1041, Tablet, 50 mg
Aldactone, 1031, Tablet, 100 mg
Ambien Ⓥ, 5401, Tablet, 5 mg
Ambien Ⓥ, 5421, Tablet, 10 mg
Arthrotec, 1141, Tablet, 50 mg/200 mcg
Arthrotec, 1421, Tablet, 75 mg/200 mcg
Brevicon 21-day, (0108), Wallette, Tablet, 0.5 mg/0.035 mg
Brevicon 28-day, (0254), Wallette, Tablet, 0.5 mg/0.035 mg
Calan, 40 (1771), Tablet, 40 mg
Calan, 80 (1851), Tablet, 80 mg
Calan, 120 (1861), Tablet, 120 mg
Calan SR, 120 (1901), Caplet, 120 mg
Calan SR, 180 (1911), Caplet, 180 mg
Calan SR, 240 (1891), Caplet, 240 mg
Covera-HS 180, (2011), Tablets, 180 mg
Covera-HS 240, (2021), Tablets, 240 mg
Cytotec, 1451, Tablet, 100 mcg
Cytotec, 1461, Tablet, 200 mcg
Daypro, 1381, Caplet, 600 mg
Demulen 1/35-21, Compack, 151, Tablet, 1 mg/35 mcg
Demulen 1/35-28, Compack, 151 (0161), Tablet, 1 mg/35 mcg
Demulen 1/50-21, Compack, 71, Tablet, 1 mg/50 mcg
Demulen 1/50-28, Compack, 71 (0081), Tablet, 1 mg/50 mcg
Flagyl, 1831, Tablet, 250 mg
Flagyl 500 (1821), Tablet, 500 mg
Flagyl 375, (1942), Capsule, 375 mg
Flagyl ER, 1961, Tablet, 750 mg
Kerlone, 10 (5101), Tablet, 10 mg
Kerlone, 20 (5201), Tablet, 20 mg
Lomotil Ⓥ, 61, Tablet, 2.5 mg/0.025 mg
Lomotil Ⓥ, Liquid, 66, 2.5 mg/0.025 mg per 5 ml
Norinyl 1+35 21-day, (0109), Wallette, Tablets, 1 mg/0.035 mg
Norinyl 1+35 28-day, (0259), Wallette, Tablets, 1 mg/0.035 mg
Norinyl 1+50 21-day, (0100), Wallette, Tablets, 1 mg/0.05 mg
Norinyl 1+50 28-day, (0265), Wallette, Tablets, 1 mg/0.05 mg
Norpace, 2752, Capsule, 100 mg
Norpace, 2762, Capsule, 150 mg
Norpace CR, 2732, Capsule, 100 mg
Norpace CR, 2742, Capsule, 150 mg
Synarel, Liquid, (0166), Bottle, 2 mg/ml
Tri-Norinyl 21-day, (0114), Wallette, Tablets, 0.5 mg/0.035 mg
Tri-Norinyl 28-day, (0274), Wallette, Tablets, 0.5 mg/0.035 mg

*When the product ID # is not the same as the NDC #, the NDC # appears in parentheses.

Product Information Available on Request
Flagyl Tablets

Various educational materials are available for physicians, pharmacists, nurses, physicians' assistants, and patients (through the physician). Please ask your Searle representative for information about these materials.

ALDACTAZIDE®
[al-dac 'tuh "zīde]
(spironolactone with hydrochlorothiazide)

℞

> **WARNING**
> Spironolactone, an ingredient of Aldactazide, has been shown to be a tumorigen in chronic toxicity studies in rats (see *Warnings*). Aldactazide should be used only in those conditions described under *Indications and Usage.* Unnecessary use of this drug should be avoided. Fixed-dose combination drugs are not indicated for initial therapy of edema or hypertension. Edema or hypertension requires therapy titrated to the individual patient. If the fixed combination represents the dosage so determined, its use may be more convenient in patient management. The treatment of hypertension and edema is not static but must be reevaluated as conditions in each patient warrant.

DESCRIPTION
Aldactazide oral tablets contain:
spironolactone .... 25 mg
hydrochlorothiazide .... 25 mg
or
spironolactone .... 50 mg
hydrochlorothiazide .... 50 mg
Spironolactone (Aldactone®), an aldosterone antagonist, is 17- hydroxy-7α-mercapto-3-oxo-17α-pregn-4-ene- 21- carboxylic acid γ-lactone acetate and has the following structural formula:

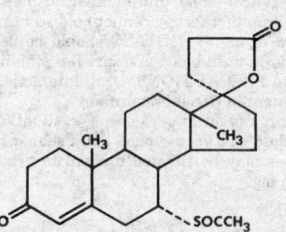

Spironolactone is practically insoluble in water, soluble in alcohol, and freely soluble in benzene and in chloroform. Hydrochlorothiazide, a diuretic and antihypertensive, is 6-chloro-3, 4-dihydro-2H-1,2,4-benzothiadiazine-7-sulfonamide 1,1-dioxide and has the following structural formula:

Hydrochlorothiazide is slightly soluble in water and freely soluble in sodium hydroxide solution.
Inactive ingredients include calcium sulfate, corn starch, flavor, hydroxypropyl cellulose, hydroxypropyl methylcellulose, iron oxide, magnesium stearate, polyethylene glycol, povidone, and titanium dioxide.

CLINICAL PHARMACOLOGY
Mechanism of action: Aldactazide is a combination of two diuretic agents with different but complementary mechanisms and sites of action, thereby providing additive diuretic and antihypertensive effects. Additionally, the spironolactone component helps to minimize the potassium loss characteristically induced by the thiazide component. The diuretic effect of spironolactone is mediated through its action as a specific pharmacologic antagonist of aldosterone, primarily by competitive binding of receptors at the aldosterone-dependent sodium-potassium exchange site in the distal convoluted renal tubule. Hydrochlorothiazide promotes the excretion of sodium and water primarily by inhibiting their reabsorption in the cortical diluting segment of the distal renal tubule.
Aldactazide is effective in significantly lowering the systolic and diastolic blood pressure in many patients with essential hypertension, even when aldosterone secretion is within normal limits.
Both spironolactone and hydrochlorothiazide reduce exchangeable sodium, plasma volume, body weight, and blood pressure. The diuretic and antihypertensive effects of the individual components are potentiated when spironolactone and hydrochlorothiazide are given concurrently.
Pharmacokinetics: Spironolactone is rapidly and extensively metabolized. Sulfur-containing products are the predominant metabolites and are thought to be primarily responsible, together with spironolactone, for the therapeutic effects of the drug. The following pharmacokinetic data

were obtained from 12 healthy volunteers following the administration of 100 mg of spironolactone (Aldactone film-coated tablets) daily for 15 days. On the 15th day, spironolactone was given immediately after a low-fat breakfast and blood was drawn thereafter.

	Accumulation Factor: AUC (0–24 hr, day 15)/AUC (0–24 hr, day 1)	Mean Peak Serum Concentration	Mean (SD) Post-Steady State Half-life
7-α-(thiomethyl) spirolactone (TMS)	1.25	391 ng/mL at 3.2 hr	13.8 hr (6.4) (terminal)
6-β-hydroxy-7-α-(thiomethyl) spirolactone (HTMS)	1.50	125 ng/mL at 5.1 hr	15.0 hr (4.0) (terminal)
Canrenone (C)	1.41	181 ng/mL at 4.3 hr	16.5 hr (6.3) (terminal)
Spironolactone	1.30	80 ng/mL at 2.6 hr	Approximately 1.4 hr (0.5) (β half-life)

The pharmacological activity of spironolactone metabolites in man is not known. However, in the adrenalectomized rat the antimineralocorticoid activities of the metabolites C, TMS, and HTMS, relative to spironolactone, were 1.10, 1.28, and 0.32, respectively. Relative to spironolactone, their binding affinities to the aldosterone receptors in rat kidney slices were 0.19, 0.86, and 0.06, respectively.

In humans the potencies of TMS and 7-α-thiospirolactone in reversing the effects of the synthetic mineralocorticoid, fludrocortisone, on urinary electrolyte composition were 0.33 and 0.26, respectively, relative to spironolactone. However, since the serum concentrations of these steroids were not determined, their incomplete absorption and/or first-pass metabolism could not be ruled out as a reason for their reduced *in vivo* activities.

Both spironolactone and canrenone are more than 90% bound to plasma proteins. The metabolites are excreted primarily in the urine and secondarily in bile.

The effect of food on spironolactone absorption (two 100-mg Aldactone tablets) was assessed in a single dose study of 9 healthy, drug-free volunteers. Food increased the bioavailability of unmetabolized spironolactone by almost 100%. The clinical importance of this finding is not known.

Hydrochlorothiazide is rapidly absorbed following oral administration. Onset of action of hydrochlorothiazide is observed within one hour and persists for 6 to 12 hours. Hydrochlorothiazide plasma concentrations attain peak levels at one to two hours and decline with a half-life of four to five hours. Hydrochlorothiazide undergoes only slight metabolic alteration and is excreted in urine. It is distributed throughout the extracellular space, with essentially no tissue accumulation except in the kidney.

INDICATIONS AND USAGE

Spironolactone, an ingredient of Aldactazide, has been shown to be a tumorigen in chronic toxicity studies in rats (see *Warnings* section). Aldactazide should be used only in those conditions described below. Unnecessary use of this drug should be avoided.

Aldactazide is indicated for:

Edematous conditions for patients with:

Congestive heart failure: For the management of edema and sodium retention when the patient is only partially responsive to, or is intolerant of, other therapeutic measures. The treatment of diuretic-induced hypokalemia in patients with congestive heart failure when other measures are considered inappropriate. The treatment of patients with congestive heart failure taking digitalis when other therapies are considered inadequate or inappropriate.

Cirrhosis of the liver accompanied by edema and/or ascites: Aldosterone levels may be exceptionally high in this condition. Aldactazide is indicated for maintenance therapy together with bed rest and the restriction of fluid and sodium.

The nephrotic syndrome: For nephrotic patients when treatment of the underlying disease, restriction of fluid and sodium intake, and the use of other diuretics do not provide an adequate response.

Essential hypertension

For patients with essential hypertension in whom other measures are considered inadequate or inappropriate. In hypertensive patients for the treatment of a diuretic-induced hypokalemia when other measures are considered inappropriate.

Usage in Pregnancy. The routine use of diuretics in an otherwise healthy woman is inappropriate and exposes mother and fetus to unnecessary hazard. Diuretics do not prevent development of toxemia of pregnancy, and there is no satisfactory evidence that they are useful in the treatment of developing toxemia.

Edema during pregnancy may arise from pathologic causes or from the physiologic and mechanical consequences of pregnancy. Aldactazide is indicated in pregnancy when edema is due to pathologic causes just as it is in the absence of pregnancy (however, see *Warnings* section). Dependent edema in pregnancy, resulting from restriction of venous return by the expanded uterus, is properly treated through elevation of the lower extremities and use of support hose; use of diuretics to lower intravascular volume in this case is unsupported and unnecessary. There is hypervolemia during normal pregnancy which is not harmful to either the fetus or the mother (in the absence of cardiovascular disease), but which is associated with edema, including generalized edema, in the majority of pregnant women. If this edema produces discomfort, increased recumbency will often provide relief. In rare instances, this edema may cause extreme discomfort which is not relieved by rest. In these cases, a short course of diuretics may provide relief and may be appropriate.

CONTRAINDICATIONS

Aldactazide is contraindicated in patients with anuria, acute renal insufficiency, significant impairment of renal excretory function, or hyperkalemia, and in patients who are allergic to thiazide diuretics or to other sulfonamide-derived drugs. Aldactazide may also be contraindicated in acute or severe hepatic failure.

WARNINGS

Potassium supplementation, either in the form of medication or as a diet rich in potassium, should not ordinarily be given in association with Aldactazide therapy. Excessive potassium intake may cause hyperkalemia in patients receiving Aldactazide (see *Precautions* section). Aldactazide should not be administered concurrently with other potassium-sparing diuretics. Spironolactone, when used with ACE inhibitors, even in the presence of a diuretic, has been associated with severe hyperkalemia. Extreme caution should be exercised when Aldactazide is given concomitantly with ACE inhibitors (see *Precautions*).

Sulfonamide derivatives, including thiazides, have been reported to exacerbate or activate systemic lupus erythematosus.

Spironolactone has been shown to be a tumorigen in chronic toxicity studies performed in rats, with its proliferative effects manifested on endocrine organs and the liver. In one study using 25, 75, and 250 times the usual daily human dose (2 mg/kg) there was a statistically significant dose-related increase in benign adenomas of the thyroid and testes. In female rats there was a statistically significant increase in malignant mammary tumors at the mid-dose only. In male rats there was a dose-related increase in proliferative changes in the liver. At the highest dosage level (500 mg/kg), the range of effects included hepatocytomegaly, hyperplastic nodules, and hepatocellular carcinoma; the last was not statistically significant at a value of $p = 0.05$. A dose-related (above 20 mg/kg/day) incidence of myelocytic leukemia was observed in rats fed daily doses of potassium canrenoate for a period of one year. In long-term (two-year) oral carcinogenicity studies of potassium canrenoate in the rat, myelocytic leukemia and hepatic, thyroid, testicular, and mammary tumors were observed. Potassium canrenoate did not produce a mutagenic effect in tests using bacteria or yeast. It did produce a positive mutagenic effect in several *in vitro* tests in mammalian cells following metabolic activation. In an *in vivo* mammalian system potassium canrenoate was not mutagenic. Canrenone and canrenoic acid are the major metabolites of potassium canrenoate. Spironolactone is also metabolized to canrenone. An increased incidence of leukemia was not observed in chronic rat toxicity studies conducted with spironolactone at doses up to 500 mg/kg/day.

PRECAUTIONS

Patients receiving Aldactazide therapy should be carefully evaluated for possible disturbances of fluid and electrolyte balance. Hyperkalemia may occur in patients with impaired renal function or excessive potassium intake and can cause cardiac irregularities, which may be fatal. Consequently, no potassium supplement should ordinarily be given with Aldactazide. Hyperkalemia can be treated promptly by the rapid intravenous administration of glucose (20% to 50%) and regular insulin, using 0.25 to 0.5 units of insulin per gram of glucose. This is a temporary measure to be repeated as required. Aldactazide use should be discontinued and potassium intake (including dietary potassium) restricted.

Hypokalemia may develop as a result of profound diuresis, particularly when Aldactazide is used concomitantly with loop diuretics, glucocorticoids, or ACTH. Hypokalemia may exaggerate the effects of digitalis therapy. Potassium depletion may induce signs of digitalis intoxication at previously tolerated dosage levels.

Concomitant administration of potassium-sparing diuretics and ACE inhibitors or indomethacin has been associated with severe hyperkalemia.

Warning signs of possible fluid and electrolyte imbalance include dryness of the mouth, thirst, weakness, lethargy, drowsiness, restlessness, muscle pains or cramps, muscular fatigue, hypotension, oliguria, tachycardia, and gastrointestinal symptoms.

Aldactazide therapy may cause a transient elevation of BUN. This appears to represent a concentration phenomenon rather than renal toxicity, since the BUN level returns to normal after use of Aldactazide is discontinued. Progressive elevation of BUN is suggestive of the presence of preexisting renal impairment.

Reversible hyperchloremic metabolic acidosis, usually in association with hyperkalemia, has been reported to occur in some patients with decompensated hepatic cirrhosis, even in the presence of normal renal function.

Dilutional hyponatremia, manifested by dryness of the mouth, thirst, lethargy, and drowsiness, and confirmed by a low serum sodium level, may be induced, especially when Aldactazide is administered in combination with other diuretics. A true low-salt syndrome may rarely develop with Aldactazide therapy and may be manifested by increasing mental confusion similar to that observed with hepatic coma. This syndrome is differentiated from dilutional hyponatremia in that it does not occur with obvious fluid retention. Its treatment requires that diuretic therapy be discontinued and sodium administered.

Gynecomastia may develop in association with the use of spironolactone; physicians should be alert to its possible onset. The development of gynecomastia appears to be related to both dosage level and duration of therapy and is normally reversible when Aldactazide is discontinued. In rare instances some breast enlargement may persist when Aldactazide is discontinued.

Thiazides have been demonstrated to alter the metabolism of uric acid and carbohydrates, with possible development of hyperuricemia, gout, and decreased glucose tolerance. Thiazides may temporarily exaggerate abnormalities of glucose metabolism in diabetic patients or cause abnormalities to appear in patients with latent diabetes.

The antihypertensive effects of hydrochlorothiazide may be enhanced in patients who have undergone sympathectomy.

Pathologic changes in the parathyroid gland with hypercalcemia and hypophosphatemia have been observed in patients on prolonged thiazide therapy. Thiazides may also decrease serum PBI levels without evidence of alteration of thyroid function.

A determination of serum electrolytes to detect possible electrolyte imbalance should be performed at periodic intervals.

Both spironolactone and hydrochlorothiazide reduce the vascular responsiveness to norepinephrine. Therefore, caution should be exercised in the management of patients subjected to regional or general anesthesia while they are being treated with Aldactazide. Thiazides may also increase the responsiveness to tubocurarine.

Spironolactone has been shown to increase the half-life of digoxin. This may result in increased serum digoxin levels and subsequent digitalis toxicity. It may be necessary to reduce the maintenance and digitalization doses when spironolactone is administered, and the patient should be carefully monitored to avoid over- or underdigitalization.

Hydrochlorothiazide may raise the concentration of blood uric acid. Dosage adjustment of antigout medications may be necessary. Hydrochlorothiazide may also raise blood glucose concentrations. Dosage adjustments of insulin or hypoglycemic medications may be necessary. Concurrent use of diuretics with lithium is not recommended as it may produce lithium toxicity.

Several reports of possible interference with digoxin radioimmunoassays by spironolactone, or its metabolites, have appeared in the literature. Neither the extent nor the potential clinical significance of its interference (which may be assay-specific) has been fully established.

Usage in Pregnancy. Spironolactone or its metabolites may, and hydrochlorothiazide does, cross the placental barrier. Therefore, the use of Aldactazide in pregnant women requires that the anticipated benefit be weighed against possible hazards to the fetus. These hazards include fetal or neonatal jaundice, thrombocytopenia, and possible other adverse reactions which have been reported in the adult.

Nursing Mothers. Canrenone, a metabolite of spironolactone, and hydrochlorothiazide appear in breast milk. If use of these drugs is deemed essential, an alternative method of infant feeding should be instituted.

ADVERSE REACTIONS

Gynecomastia is observed not infrequently. A few cases of agranulocytosis have been reported in patients taking spironolactone. Other adverse reactions that have been reported in association with the use of spironolactone are: gastrointestinal symptoms including cramping and diarrhea, drowsiness, lethargy, headache, maculopapular or erythematous cutaneous eruptions, urticaria, mental confusion, drug fever, ataxia, inability to achieve or maintain erection, irregular menses or amenorrhea, postmenopausal bleeding, hirsutism, deepening of the voice, gastric bleeding, ulcer-

Continued on next page

Aldactazide—Cont.

ation, gastritis, vomiting, and anaphylactic reactions. Carcinoma of the breast has been reported in patients taking spironolactone, but a cause and effect relationship has not been established. A very few cases of mixed cholestatic/hepatocellular toxicity, with one reported fatality, have been reported with spironolactone administration.
Adverse reactions reported in association with the use of thiazides include: gastrointestinal symptoms (anorexia, nausea, vomiting, diarrhea, abdominal cramps), purpura, thrombocytopenia, leukopenia, agranulocytosis, dermatologic symptoms (cutaneous eruptions, pruritus, erythema multiforme), paresthesia, acute pancreatitis, jaundice, dizziness, vertigo, headache, xanthopsia, photosensitivity, necrotizing angiitis, aplastic anemia, orthostatic hypotension, muscle spasm, weakness, restlessness, hypokalemia, and anaphylactic reactions.
Adverse reactions are usually reversible upon discontinuation of Aldactazide.

DOSAGE AND ADMINISTRATION

Optimal dosage should be established by individual titration of the components (see Box Warning).
Edema in adults (*congestive heart failure, hepatic cirrhosis, or nephrotic syndrome*). The usual maintenance dose of Aldactazide is 100 mg each of spironolactone and hydrochlorothiazide daily, administered in a single dose or in divided doses, but may range from 25 mg to 200 mg of each component daily depending on the response to the initial titration. In some instances it may be desirable to administer separate tablets of either Aldactone (spironolactone) or hydrochlorothiazide in addition to Aldactazide in order to provide optimal individual therapy.
The onset of diuresis with Aldactazide occurs promptly and, due to prolonged effect of the spironolactone component, persists for two to three days after Aldactazide is discontinued.
Edema in children. The usual daily maintenance dose of Aldactazide should be that which provides 0.75 to 1.5 mg of spironolactone per pound of body weight (1.65 to 3.3 mg/kg).
Essential hypertension. Although the dosage will vary depending on the results of titration of the individual ingredients, many patients will be found to have an optimal response to 50 mg to 100 mg each of spironolactone and hydrochlorothiazide daily, given in a single dose or in divided doses.
Concurrent potassium supplementation is not recommended when Aldactazide is used in the long-term management of hypertension or in the treatment of most edematous conditions, since the spironolactone content of Aldactazide is usually sufficient to minimize loss induced by the hydrochlorothiazide component.

HOW SUPPLIED

Aldactazide tablets containing 25 mg of spironolactone (Aldactone) and 25 mg of hydrochlorothiazide are round, tan, film coated, with SEARLE and 1011 debossed on one side and ALDACTAZIDE and 25 on the other side, supplied as:

NDC Number	Size
0025-1011-31	bottle of 100
0025-1011-51	bottle of 500
0025-1011-55	bottle of 2500
0025-1011-34	carton of 100 unit dose

Aldactazide tablets containing 50 mg of spironolactone (Aldactone) and 50 mg of hydrochlorothiazide are oblong, tan, scored, film coated, with SEARLE and 1021 debossed on the scored side and ALDACTAZIDE and 50 on the other side, supplied as:

NDC Number	Size
0025-1021-31	bottle of 100
0025-1021-34	carton of 100 unit dose

Store below 77°F (25°C).
Caution: Federal law prohibits dispensing without prescription.

11/18/96 • A05388-7

Shown in Product Identification Guide, page 337

ALDACTONE® ℞

[*al-dac 'tone*]
(spironolactone)

> **WARNING**
> Spironolactone has been shown to be a tumorigen in chronic toxicity studies in rats (see *Warnings*). Aldactone should be used only in those conditions described under *Indications and Usage.* Unnecessary use of this drug should be avoided.

DESCRIPTION

Aldactone oral tablets contain 25 mg, 50 mg, or 100 mg of the aldosterone antagonist spironolactone, 17-hydroxy-7α-mercapto-3-oxo-17α-pregn-4-ene-21-carboxylic acid γ-lactone acetate, which has the following structural formula:

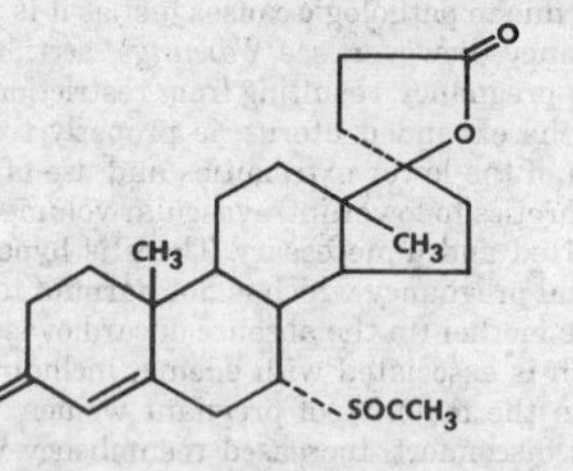

Spironolactone is practically insoluble in water, soluble in alcohol, and freely soluble in benzene and in chloroform.
Inactive ingredients include calcium sulfate, corn starch, flavor, hydroxypropyl methylcellulose, iron oxide, magnesium stearate, polyethylene glycol, povidone, and titanium dioxide.

CLINICAL PHARMACOLOGY

Mechanism of action: Aldactone (spironolactone) is a specific pharmacologic antagonist of aldosterone, acting primarily through competitive binding of receptors at the aldosterone-dependent sodium-potassium exchange site in the distal convoluted renal tubule. Aldactone causes increased amounts of sodium and water to be excreted, while potassium is retained. Aldactone acts both as a diuretic and as an antihypertensive drug by this mechanism. It may be given alone or with other diuretic agents which act more proximally in the renal tubule.
Aldosterone antagonist activity: Increased levels of the mineralocorticoid, aldosterone, are present in primary and secondary hyperaldosteronism. Edematous states in which secondary aldosteronism is usually involved include congestive heart failure, hepatic cirrhosis, and the nephrotic syndrome. By competing with aldosterone for receptor sites, Aldactone provides effective therapy for the edema and ascites in those conditions. Aldactone counteracts secondary aldosteronism induced by the volume depletion and associated sodium loss caused by active diuretic therapy.
Aldactone is effective in lowering the systolic and diastolic blood pressure in patients with primary hyperaldosteronism. It is also effective in most cases of essential hypertension, despite the fact that aldosterone secretion may be within normal limits in benign essential hypertension.
Through its action in antagonizing the effect of aldosterone, Aldactone inhibits the exchange of sodium for potassium in the distal renal tubule and helps to prevent potassium loss. Aldactone has not been demonstrated to elevate serum uric acid, to precipitate gout, or to alter carbohydrate metabolism.
Pharmacokinetics: Spironolactone is rapidly and extensively metabolized. Sulfur-containing products are the predominant metabolites and are thought to be primarily responsible, together with spironolactone, for the therapeutic effects of the drug. The following pharmacokinetic data were obtained from 12 healthy volunteers following the administration of 100 mg of spironolactone (Aldactone film-coated tablets) daily for 15 days. On the 15th day, spironolactone was given immediately after a low-fat breakfast and blood was drawn thereafter.

	Accumulation Factor: AUC (0–24 hr, day 15)/AUC (0–24 hr, day 1)	Mean Peak Serum Concentration	Mean (SD) Post-Steady State Half-life
7-α-(thiomethyl) spirolactone (TMS)	1.25	391 ng/mL at 3.2 hr	13.8 hr (6.4) (terminal)
6-β-hydroxy-7-α-(thiomethyl) spirolactone (HTMS)	1.50	125 ng/mL at 5.1 hr	15.0 hr (4.0) (terminal)
Canrenone (C)	1.41	181 ng/mL at 4.3 hr	16.5 hr (6.3) (terminal)
Spironolactone	1.30	80 ng/mL at 2.6 hr	Approximately 1.4 hr (0.5) (β half-life)

The pharmacological activity of spironolactone metabolites in man is not known. However, in the adrenalectomized rat the antimineralocorticoid activities of the metabolites C, TMS, and HTMS, relative to spironolactone, were 1.10, 1.28, and 0.32, respectively. Relative to spironolactone, their binding affinities to the aldosterone receptors in rat kidney slices were 0.19, 0.86, and 0.06, respectively.
In humans the potencies of TMS and 7-α-thiospirolactone in reversing the effects of the synthetic mineralocorticoid, fludrocortisone, on urinary electrolyte composition were 0.33 and 0.26, respectively, relative to spironolactone. However, since the serum concentrations of these steroids were not determined, their incomplete absorption and/or first-pass metabolism could not be ruled out as a reason for their reduced *in vivo* activities.
Both spironolactone and canrenone are more than 90% bound to plasma proteins. The metabolites are excreted primarily in the urine and secondarily in bile.
The effect of food on spironolactone absorption (two 100-mg Aldactone tablets) was assessed in a single dose study of 9 healthy, drug-free volunteers. Food increased the bioavailability of unmetabolized spironolactone by almost 100%. The clinical importance of this finding is not known.

INDICATIONS AND USAGE

Aldactone (spironolactone) is indicated in the management of:
Primary hyperaldosteronism for:
Establishing the diagnosis of primary hyperaldosteronism by therapeutic trial.
Short-term preoperative treatment of patients with primary hyperaldosteronism.
Long-term maintenance therapy for patients with discrete aldosterone-producing adrenal adenomas who are judged to be poor operative risks or who decline surgery.
Long-term maintenance therapy for patients with bilateral micro- or macronodular adrenal hyperplasia (idiopathic hyperaldosteronism).
Edematous conditions for patients with:
Congestive heart failure: For the management of edema and sodium retention when the patient is only partially responsive to, or is intolerant of, other therapeutic measures. Aldactone is also indicated for patients with congestive heart failure taking digitalis when other therapies are considered inappropriate.
Cirrhosis of the liver accompanied by edema and/or ascites: Aldosterone levels may be exceptionally high in this condition. Aldactone is indicated for maintenance therapy together with bed rest and the restriction of fluid and sodium.
The nephrotic syndrome: For nephrotic patients when treatment of the underlying disease, restriction of fluid and sodium intake, and the use of other diuretics do not provide an adequate response.
Essential hypertension
Usually in combination with other drugs, Aldactone is indicated for patients who cannot be treated adequately with other agents or for whom other agents are considered inappropriate.
Hypokalemia
For the treatment of patients with hypokalemia when other measures are considered inappropriate or inadequate. Aldactone is also indicated for the prophylaxis of hypokalemia in patients taking digitalis when other measures are considered inadequate or inappropriate.
Usage in Pregnancy. The routine use of diuretics in an otherwise healthy woman is inappropriate and exposes mother and fetus to unnecessary hazard. Diuretics do not prevent development of toxemia of pregnancy, and there is no satisfactory evidence that they are useful in the treatment of developing toxemia.
Edema during pregnancy may arise from pathologic causes or from the physiologic and mechanical consequences of pregnancy.
Aldactone is indicated in pregnancy when edema is due to pathologic causes just as it is in the absence of pregnancy (however, see *Warnings* section). Dependent edema in pregnancy, resulting from restriction of venous return by the expanded uterus, is properly treated through elevation of the lower extremities and use of support hose; use of diuretics to lower intravascular volume in this case is unsupported and unnecessary. There is hypervolemia during normal pregnancy which is not harmful to either the fetus or the mother (in the absence of cardiovascular disease), but which is associated with edema, including generalized edema, in the majority of pregnant women. If this edema produces discomfort, increased recumbency will often provide relief. In rare instances, this edema may cause extreme discomfort which is not relieved by rest. In these cases, a short course of diuretics may provide relief and may be appropriate.

CONTRAINDICATIONS

Aldactone is contraindicated for patients with anuria, acute renal insufficiency, significant impairment of renal excretory function, or hyperkalemia.

WARNINGS

Potassium supplementation, either in the form of medication or as a diet rich in potassium, should not ordinarily be given in association with Aldactone therapy. Excessive potassium intake may cause hyperkalemia in patients receiving Aldactone (see *Precautions* section). Aldactone should not be administered concurrently with other potassium-sparing diuretics. Aldactone, when used with ACE inhibitors, even in the presence of a diuretic, has been associated

with severe hyperkalemia. Extreme caution should be exercised when Aldactone is given concomitantly with ACE inhibitors (see *Precautions: Drug interactions*).
Spironolactone has been shown to be a tumorigen in chronic toxicity studies performed in rats, with its proliferative effects manifested on endocrine organs and the liver. In one study using 25, 75, and 250 times the usual daily human dose (2 mg/kg) there was a statistically significant dose-related increase in benign adenomas of the thyroid and testes. In female rats there was a statistically significant increase in malignant mammary tumors at the mid-dose only. In male rats there was a dose-related increase in proliferative changes in the liver. At the highest dosage level (500 mg/kg) the range of effects included hepatocytomegaly, hyperplastic nodules, and hepatocellular carcinoma; the last was not statistically significant at a value of p = 0.05. A dose-related (above 20 mg/kg/day) incidence of myelocytic leukemia was observed in rats fed daily doses of potassium canrenoate for a period of one year. In long-term (two-year) oral carcinogenicity studies of potassium canrenoate in the rat, myelocytic leukemia and hepatic, thyroid, testicular, and mammary tumors were observed. Potassium canrenoate did not produce a mutagenic effect in tests using bacteria or yeast. It did produce a positive mutagenic effect in several *in vitro* tests in mammalian cells following metabolic activation. In an *in vivo* mammalian system potassium canrenoate was not mutagenic. Canrenone and canrenoic acid are the major metabolites of potassium canrenoate. Spironolactone is also metabolized to canrenone. An increased incidence of leukemia was not observed in chronic rat toxicity studies conducted with spironolactone at doses up to 500 mg/kg/day.

PRECAUTIONS

General: Because of the diuretic action of Aldactone (spironolactone), patients should be carefully evaluated for possible disturbances of fluid and electrolyte balance. Hyperkalemia may occur in patients with impaired renal function or excessive potassium intake and can cause cardiac irregularities, which may be fatal. Consequently, no potassium supplement should ordinarily be given with Aldactone. Hyperkalemia can be treated promptly by the rapid intravenous administration of glucose (20% to 50%) and regular insulin, using 0.25 to 0.5 units of insulin per gram of glucose. This is a temporary measure to be repeated as required. Aldactone use should be discontinued and potassium intake (including dietary potassium) restricted.
Reversible hyperchloremic metabolic acidosis, usually in association with hyperkalemia, has been reported to occur in some patients with decompensated hepatic cirrhosis, even in the presence of normal renal function.
Hyponatremia, manifested by dryness of the mouth, thirst, lethargy, and drowsiness, and confirmed by a low serum sodium level, may be caused or aggravated, especially when Aldactone is administered in combination with other diuretics.
Gynecomastia may develop in association with the use of spironolactone; physicians should be alert to its possible onset. The development of gynecomastia appears to be related to both dosage level and duration of therapy and is normally reversible when Aldactone is discontinued. In rare instances some breast enlargement may persist when Aldactone is discontinued.
Aldactone therapy may cause a transient elevation of BUN, especially in patients with preexisting renal impairment. Aldactone may cause mild acidosis.
A determination of serum electrolytes to detect possible electrolyte imbalance should be performed at periodic intervals.
Drug interactions: When used in combination with other diuretics or antihypertensive agents, Aldactone potentiates their effects. Therefore, the dosage of such drugs, particularly the ganglionic blocking agents, should be reduced by at least 50% when Aldactone is added to the regimen.
Concomitant administration of potassium-sparing diuretics with ACE inhibitors or indomethacin has been associated with severe hyperkalemia.
Spironolactone reduces the vascular responsiveness to norepinephrine. Therefore, caution should be exercised in the management of patients subjected to regional or general anesthesia while they are being treated with Aldactone.
Spironolactone has been shown to increase the half-life of digoxin. This may result in increased serum digoxin levels and subsequent digitalis toxicity. It may be necessary to reduce the maintenance and digitalization doses when spironolactone is administered, and the patient should be carefully monitored to avoid over- or underdigitalization.
Drug/Laboratory test interactions: Several reports of possible interference with digoxin radioimmunoassays by spironolactone, or its metabolites, have appeared in the literature. Neither the extent nor the potential clinical significance of its interference (which may be assay-specific) has been fully established.
Usage in pregnancy: Spironolactone or its metabolites may cross the placental barrier. Therefore, the use of Aldactone in pregnant women requires that the anticipated benefit be weighed against possible hazard to the fetus.
Nursing mothers: Canrenone, a metabolite of spironolactone, appears in breast milk. If use of the drug is deemed essential, an alternative method of infant feeding should be instituted.

ADVERSE REACTIONS

Gynecomastia is observed not infrequently. A few cases of agranulocytosis have been reported in patients taking spironolactone. Other adverse reactions that have been reported in association with Aldactone are: gastrointestinal symptoms including cramping and diarrhea, drowsiness, lethargy, headache, maculopapular or erythematous cutaneous eruptions, urticaria, mental confusion, drug fever, ataxia, inability to achieve or maintain erection, irregular menses or amenorrhea, postmenopausal bleeding, hirsutism, deepening of the voice, gastric bleeding, ulceration, gastritis, vomiting, and anaphylactic reactions. Carcinoma of the breast has been reported in patients taking spironolactone, but a cause and effect relationship has not been established. A very few cases of mixed cholestatic/hepatocellular toxicity, with one reported fatality, have been reported with spironolactone administration.
Adverse reactions are usually reversible upon discontinuation of the drug.

DOSAGE AND ADMINISTRATION

Primary hyperaldosteronism. Aldactone may be employed as an initial diagnostic measure to provide presumptive evidence of primary hyperaldosteronism while patients are on normal diets.

Long test: Aldactone is administered at a daily dosage of 400 mg for three to four weeks. Correction of hypokalemia and of hypertension provides presumptive evidence for the diagnosis of primary hyperaldosteronism.

Short test: Aldactone is administered at a daily dosage of 400 mg for four days. If serum potassium increases during Aldactone administration but drops when Aldactone is discontinued, a presumptive diagnosis of primary hyperaldosteronism should be considered.

After the diagnosis of hyperaldosteronism has been established by more definitive testing procedures, Aldactone may be administered in doses of 100 to 400 mg daily in preparation for surgery. For patients who are considered unsuitable for surgery, Aldactone may be employed for long-term maintenance therapy at the lowest effective dosage determined for the individual patient.
Edema in adults *(congestive heart failure, hepatic cirrhosis, or nephrotic syndrome*). An initial daily dosage of 100 mg of Aldactone administered in either single or divided doses is recommended, but may range from 25 to 200 mg daily. When given as the sole agent for diuresis, Aldactone should be continued for at least five days at the initial dosage level, after which it may be adjusted to the optimal therapeutic or maintenance level administered in either single or divided daily doses. If, after five days, an adequate diuretic response to Aldactone has not occurred, a second diuretic which acts more proximally in the renal tubule may be added to the regimen. Because of the additive effect of Aldactone when administered concurrently with such diuretics, an enhanced diuresis usually begins on the first day of combined treatment; combined therapy is indicated when more rapid diuresis is desired. The dosage of Aldactone should remain unchanged when other diuretic therapy is added.
Edema in children. The initial daily dosage should provide approximately 1.5 mg of Aldactone per pound of body weight (3.3 mg/kg) administered in either single or divided doses.
Essential hypertension. For adults, an initial daily dosage of 50 to 100 mg of Aldactone administered in either single or divided doses is recommended. Aldactone may also be given with diuretics which act more proximally in the renal tubule or with other antihypertensive agents. Treatment with Aldactone should be continued for at least two weeks, since the maximum response may not occur before this time. Subsequently, dosage should be adjusted according to the response of the patient.
Hypokalemia. Aldactone in a dosage ranging from 25 mg to 100 mg daily is useful in treating a diuretic-induced hypokalemia, when oral potassium supplements or other potassium-sparing regimens are considered inappropriate.

HOW SUPPLIED

Aldactone 25-mg tablets are round, light yellow, film coated, with SEARLE and 1001 debossed on one side and ALDACTONE and 25 on the other side, supplied as:

NDC Number	Size
0025-1001-31	bottle of 100
0025-1001-51	bottle of 500
0025-1001-52	bottle of 1000
0025-1001-55	bottle of 2500
0025-1001-34	carton of 100 unit dose

Aldactone 50-mg tablets are oval, light orange, scored, film coated, with SEARLE and 1041 debossed on the scored side and ALDACTONE and 50 on the other side, supplied as:

NDC Number	Size
0025-1041-31	bottle of 100
0025-1041-34	carton of 100 unit dose

Aldactone 100-mg tablets are round, peach colored, scored, film coated, with SEARLE and 1031 debossed on the scored side and ALDACTONE and 100 on the other side, supplied as:

NDC Number	Size
0025-1031-31	bottle of 100
0025-1031-34	carton of 100 unit dose

Store below 77°F (25°C).
Caution: Federal law prohibits dispensing without prescription.

11/18/96 • A05449-7

Shown in Product Identification Guide, page 337

AMBIEN® CIV ℞

[*am 'bē-ən*]
(zolpidem tartrate)

DESCRIPTION

Ambien (zolpidem tartrate), is a non-benzodiazepine hypnotic of the imidazopyridine class and is available in 5-mg and 10-mg strength tablets for oral administration.
Chemically, zolpidem is N,N,6-trimethyl-2-p-tolyl-imidazo[1,2-a]pyridine-3-acetamide L-(+)-tartrate (2:1). It has the following structure:

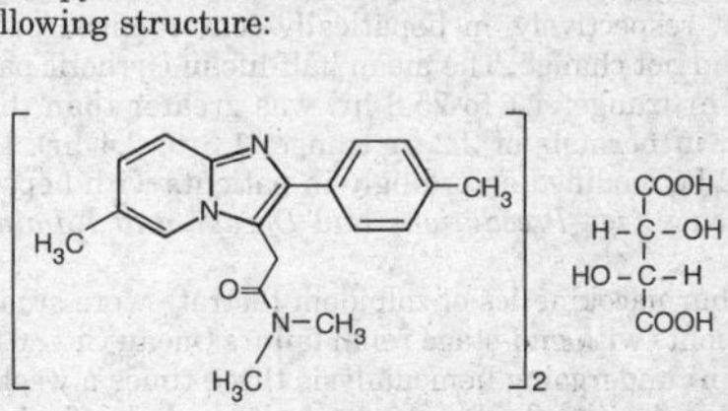

Zolpidem tartrate is a white to off-white crystalline powder that is sparingly soluble in water, alcohol, and propylene glycol. It has a molecular weight of 764.88.
Each Ambien tablet includes the following inactive ingredients: hydroxypropyl methylcellulose, lactose, magnesium stearate, microcrystalline cellulose, polyethylene glycol, sodium starch glycolate, titanium dioxide; the 5-mg tablet also contains FD&C Red No. 40, iron oxide colorant, and polysorbate 80.

CLINICAL PHARMACOLOGY

Pharmacodynamics: Subunit modulation of the $GABA_A$ receptor chloride channel macromolecular complex is hypothesized to be responsible for sedative, anticonvulsant, anxiolytic, and myorelaxant drug properties. The major modulatory site of the $GABA_A$ receptor complex is located on its alpha (α) subunit and is referred to as the benzodiazepine (BZ) or omega (ω) receptor. At least three subtypes of the (ω) receptor have been identified.
While zolpidem is a hypnotic agent with a chemical structure unrelated to benzodiazepines, barbiturates, or other drugs with known hypnotic properties, it interacts with a GABA-BZ receptor complex and shares some of the pharmacological properties of the benzodiazepines. In contrast to the benzodiazepines, which nonselectively bind to and activate all three omega receptor subtypes, zolpidem in vitro binds the (ω_1) receptor preferentially. The (ω_1) receptor is found primarily on the Lamina IV of the sensorimotor cortical regions, substantia nigra (pars reticulata), cerebellum molecular layer, olfactory bulb, ventral thalamic complex, pons, inferior colliculus, and globus pallidus. This selective binding of zolpidem on the (ω_1) receptor is not absolute, but it may explain the relative absence of myorelaxant and anticonvulsant effects in animal studies as well as the preservation of deep sleep (stages 3 and 4) in human studies of zolpidem at hypnotic doses.
Pharmacokinetics: The pharmacokinetic profile of Ambien is characterized by rapid absorption from the GI tract and a short elimination half-life ($T_{1/2}$) in healthy subjects. In a single-dose crossover study in 45 healthy subjects administered 5- and 10-mg zolpidem tartrate tablets, the mean peak concentrations (C_{max}) were 59 (range: 29 to 113) and 121 (range: 58 to 272) ng/mL, respectively, occurring at a mean time (T_{max}) of 1.6 hours for both. The mean Ambien elimination half-life was 2.6 (range: 1.4 to 4.5) and 2.5 (range: 1.4 to 3.8) hours, for the 5- and 10-mg tablets, respectively. Ambien is converted to inactive metabolites that are eliminated primarily by renal excretion. Ambien demonstrated linear kinetics in the dose range of 5 to 20 mg. Total protein binding was found to be 92.5±0.1% and remained constant, independent of concentration between 40 and 790 ng/mL. Zolpidem did not accumulate in young adults following nightly dosing with 20-mg zolpidem tartrate tablets for 2 weeks.
A food-effect study in 30 healthy male volunteers compared the pharmacokinetics of Ambien 10 mg when administered while fasting or 20 minutes after a meal. Results demon-

Continued on next page

Ambien—Cont.

strated that with food, mean AUC and C_{max} were decreased by 15% and 25%, respectively, while mean T_{max} was prolonged by 60% (from 1.4 to 2.2 hr). The half-life remained unchanged. These results suggest that, for faster sleep onset, Ambien should not be administered with or immediately after a meal.

In the elderly, the dose for Ambien should be 5 mg (see *Precautions* and *Dosage and Administration*). This recommendation is based on several studies in which the mean C_{max}, $T_{1/2}$, and AUC were significantly increased when compared to results in young adults. In one study of eight elderly subjects (>70 years), the means for C_{max}, $T_{1/2}$, and AUC significantly increased by 50% (255 vs 384 ng/mL), 32% (2.2 vs 2.9 hr), and 64% (955 vs 1,562 ng·hr/mL), respectively, as compared to younger adults (20 to 40 years) following a single 20-mg oral zolpidem dose. Ambien did not accumulate in elderly subjects following nightly oral dosing of 10 mg for 1 week.

The pharmacokinetics of Ambien in eight patients with chronic hepatic insufficiency were compared to results in healthy subjects. Following a single 20-mg oral zolpidem dose, mean C_{max} and AUC were found to be two times (250 vs 499 ng/mL) and five times (788 vs 4,203 ng·hr/mL) higher, respectively, in hepatically compromised patients. T_{max} did not change. The mean half-life in cirrhotic patients of 9.9 hr (range: 4.1 to 25.8 hr) was greater than that observed in normals of 2.2 hr (range: 1.6 to 2.4 hr). Dosing should be modified accordingly in patients with hepatic insufficiency (see *Precautions* and *Dosage and Administration*).

The pharmacokinetics of zolpidem tartrate were studied in 11 patients with end-stage renal failure (mean Cl_{Cr}=6.5±1.5 mL/min) undergoing hemodialysis three times a week, who were dosed with zolpidem 10 mg orally each day for 14 or 21 days. No statistically significant differences were observed for C_{max}, T_{max}, half-life, and AUC between the first and last day of drug administration when baseline concentration adjustments were made. On day 1, C_{max} was 172±29 ng/mL (range: 46 to 344 ng/mL). After repeated dosing for 14 or 21 days, C_{max} was 203±32 ng/mL (range: 28 to 316 ng/mL). On day 1, T_{max} was 1.7±0.3 hr (range: 0.5 to 3.0 hr); after repeated dosing T_{max} was 0.8±0.2 hr (range: 0.5 to 2.0 hr). This variation is accounted for by noting that last-day serum sampling began 10 hours after the previous dose, rather than after 24 hours. This resulted in residual drug concentration and a shorter period to reach maximal serum concentration. On day 1, $T_{1/2}$ was 2.4±0.4 hr (range 0.4 to 5.1 hr). After repeated dosing, $T_{1/2}$ was 2.5±0.4 hr (range: 0.7 to 4.2 hr). AUC was 796±159 ng·hr/mL after the first dose and 818±170 ng·hr/mL after repeated dosing. Zolpidem was not hemodialyzable. No accumulation of unchanged drug appeared after 14 or 21 days. Ambien pharmacokinetics were not significantly different in renally impaired patients. No dosage adjustment is necessary in patients with compromised renal function. As a general precaution, these patients should be closely monitored.

Postulated relationship between elimination rate of hypnotics and their profile of common untoward effects: The type and duration of hypnotic effects and the profile of unwanted effects during administration of hypnotic drugs may be influenced by the biologic half-life of administered drug and any active metabolites formed. When half-lives are long, drug or metabolites may accumulate during periods of nightly administration and be associated with impairment of cognitive and/or motor performance during waking hours; the possibility of interaction with other psychoactive drugs or alcohol will be enhanced. In contrast, if half-lives, including half-lives of active metabolites, are short, drug and metabolites will be cleared before the next dose is ingested, and carryover effects related to excessive sedation or CNS depression should be minimal or absent. Ambien has a short half-life and no active metabolites. During nightly use for an extended period, pharmacodynamic tolerance or adaptation to some effects of hypnotics may develop. If the drug has a short elimination half-life, it is possible that a relative deficiency of the drug or its active metabolites (ie, in relationship to the receptor site) may occur at some point in the interval between each night's use. This sequence of events may account for two clinical findings reported to occur after several weeks of nightly use of other rapidly eliminated hypnotics, namely, increased wakefulness during the last third of the night, and the appearance of increased signs of daytime anxiety. Increased wakefulness during the last third of the night as measured by polysomnography has not been observed in clinical trials with Ambien.

Controlled trials supporting safety and efficacy

Transient insomnia: Normal adults experiencing transient insomnia (n=462) during the first night in a sleep laboratory were evaluated in a double-blind, parallel group, single-night trial comparing two doses of zolpidem (7.5 and 10 mg) and placebo. Both zolpidem doses were superior to placebo on objective (polysomnographic) measures of sleep latency, sleep duration, and number of awakenings.

Normal elderly adults (mean age 68) experiencing transient insomnia (n = 35) during the first two nights in a sleep laboratory were evaluated in a double-blind, crossover, 2-night trial comparing four doses of zolpidem (5, 10, 15 and 20 mg) and placebo. All zolpidem doses were superior to placebo on the two primary PSG parameters (sleep latency and efficiency) and all four subjective outcome measures (sleep duration, sleep latency, number of awakenings, and sleep quality).

Chronic insomnia: Adult outpatients with chronic insomnia (n=75) were evaluated in a double-blind, parallel group, 5-week trial comparing two doses of zolpidem tartrate (10 and 15 mg) and placebo. On objective (polysomnographic) measures of sleep latency and sleep efficiency, zolpidem 15 mg was superior to placebo for all 5 weeks; zolpidem 10 mg was superior to placebo on sleep latency for the first 4 weeks and on sleep efficiency for weeks 2 and 4. Zolpidem was comparable to placebo on number of awakenings at both doses studied.

Adult outpatients (n=141) with chronic insomnia were evaluated in a double-blind, parallel group, 4-week trial comparing two doses of zolpidem (10 and 15 mg) and placebo. Zolpidem 10 mg was superior to placebo on a subjective measure of sleep latency for all 4 weeks, and on subjective measures of total sleep time, number of awakenings, and sleep quality for the first treatment week. Zolpidem 15 mg was superior to placebo on a subjective measure of sleep latency for the first 3 weeks, on a subjective measure of total sleep time for the first week, and on number of awakenings and sleep quality for the first 2 weeks.

Next-day residual effects: There was no evidence of residual next-day effects seen with Ambien in several studies utilizing the Multiple Sleep Latency Test (MSLT), the Digit Symbol Substitution Test (DSST), and patient ratings of alertness. In one study involving elderly patients, there was a small but statistically significant decrease in one measure of performance, the DSST, but no impairment was seen in the MSLT in this study. In another study involving elderly patients with chronic insomnia, there was no evidence of residual next-day effects utilizing DSST.

Rebound effects: There was no objective (polysomnographic) evidence of rebound insomnia at recommended doses seen in studies evaluating sleep on the nights following discontinuation of Ambien. There was subjective evidence of impaired sleep in the elderly on the first posttreatment night at doses above the recommended elderly dose of 5 mg.

Memory impairment: Controlled studies in adults utilizing objective measures of memory yielded no consistent evidence of next-day memory impairment following the administration of Ambien. However, in one study involving zolpidem doses of 10 and 20 mg, there was a significant decrease in next-morning recall of information presented to subjects during peak drug effect (90 minutes post-dose), ie, these subjects experienced anterograde amnesia. There was also subjective evidence from adverse event data for anterograde amnesia occurring in association with the administration of Ambien, predominantly at doses above 10 mg.

Effects on sleep stages: In studies that measured the percentage of sleep time spent in each sleep stage, Ambien has generally been shown to preserve sleep stages. Sleep time spent in stages 3 and 4 (deep sleep) was found comparable to placebo with only inconsistent, minor changes in REM (paradoxical) sleep at the recommended dose.

INDICATIONS AND USAGE

Ambien (zolpidem tartrate) is indicated for the short-term treatment of insomnia. Hypnotics should generally be limited to 7 to 10 days of use, and reevaluation of the patient is recommended if they are to be taken for more than 2 to 3 weeks.

Ambien should not be prescribed in quantities exceeding a 1-month supply (see *Warnings*).

Ambien has been shown to decrease sleep latency and increase the duration of sleep for up to 5 weeks in controlled clinical studies (see *Clinical Pharmacology*).

CONTRAINDICATIONS

None known.

WARNINGS

Since sleep disturbances may be the presenting manifestation of a physical and/or psychiatric disorder, symptomatic treatment of insomnia should be initiated only after a careful evaluation of the patient. The failure of insomnia to remit after 7 to 10 days of treatment may indicate the presence of a primary psychiatric and/or medical illness which should be evaluated. Worsening of insomnia or the emergence of new thinking or behavior abnormalities may be the consequence of an unrecognized psychiatric or physical disorder. Such findings have emerged during the course of treatment with sedative/hypnotic drugs, including Ambien. Because some of the important adverse effects of Ambien appear to be dose related (see *Precautions* and *Dosage and Administration*), it is important to use the smallest possible effective dose, especially in the elderly.

A variety of abnormal thinking and behavior changes have been reported to occur in association with the use of sedative/hypnotics. Some of these changes may be characterized by decreased inhibition (eg, aggressiveness and extroversion that seemed out of character), similar to effects produced by alcohol and other CNS depressants. Other reported behavioral changes have included bizarre behavior, agitation, hallucinations, and depersonalization. Amnesia and other neuropsychiatric symptoms may occur unpredictably. In primarily depressed patients, worsening of depression, including suicidal thinking, has been reported in association with the use of sedative/hypnotics.

It can rarely be determined with certainty whether a particular instance of the abnormal behaviors listed above are drug induced, spontaneous in origin, or a result of an underlying psychiatric or physical disorder. Nonetheless, the emergence of any new behavioral sign or symptom of concern requires careful and immediate evaluation.

Following the rapid dose decrease or abrupt discontinuation of sedative/hypnotics, there have been reports of signs and symptoms similar to those associated with withdrawal from other CNS-depressant drugs (see *Drug Abuse and Dependence*).

Ambien, like other sedative/hypnotic drugs, has CNS-depressant effects. Due to the rapid onset of action, Ambien should only be ingested immediately prior to going to bed. Patients should be cautioned against engaging in hazardous occupations requiring complete mental alertness or motor coordination such as operating machinery or driving a motor vehicle after ingesting the drug, including potential impairment of the performance of such activities that may occur the day following ingestion of Ambien. Ambien showed additive effects when combined with alcohol and should not be taken with alcohol. Patients should also be cautioned about possible combined effects with other CNS-depressant drugs. Dosage adjustments may be necessary when Ambien is administered with such agents because of the potentially additive effects.

PRECAUTIONS

General

Use in the elderly and/or debilitated patients: Impaired motor and/or cognitive performance after repeated exposure or unusual sensitivity to sedative/hypnotic drugs is a concern in the treatment of elderly and/or debilitated patients. Therefore, the recommended Ambien dosage is 5 mg in such patients (see *Dosage and Administration*) to decrease the possibility of side effects. These patients should be closely monitored.

Use in patients with concomitant illness: Clinical experience with Ambien (zolpidem tartrate) in patients with concomitant systemic illness is limited. Caution is advisable in using Ambien in patients with diseases or conditions that could affect metabolism or hemodynamic responses. Although studies did not reveal respiratory depressant effects at hypnotic doses of Ambien in normals or in patients with mild to moderate chronic obstructive pulmonary disease (COPD), precautions should be observed if Ambien is prescribed to patients with compromised respiratory function, since sedative/hypnotics have the capacity to depress respiratory drive. Post-marketing reports of respiratory insufficiency, most of which involved patients with pre-existing respiratory impairment, have been received. Data in end-stage renal failure patients repeatedly treated with Ambien did not demonstrate drug accumulation or alterations in pharmacokinetic parameters. No dosage adjustment in renally impaired patients is required; however, these patients should be closely monitored (see *Pharmacokinetics*). A study in subjects with hepatic impairment did reveal prolonged elimination in this group; therefore, treatment should be initiated with 5 mg in patients with hepatic compromise, and they should be closely monitored.

Use in depression: As with other sedative/hypnotic drugs, Ambien should be administered with caution to patients exhibiting signs or symptoms of depression. Suicidal tendencies may be present in such patients and protective measures may be required. Intentional overdosage is more common in this group of patients; therefore, the least amount of drug that is feasible should be prescribed for the patient at any one time.

Information for patients: Patient information is printed at the end of this insert. To assure safe and effective use of Ambien, this information and instructions provided in the patient information section should be discussed with patients.

Laboratory tests: There are no specific laboratory tests recommended.

Drug interactions

CNS-active drugs: Ambien was evaluated in healthy volunteers in single-dose interaction studies for several CNS drugs. A study involving haloperidol and zolpidem revealed no effect of haloperidol on the pharmacokinetics or pharmacodynamics of zolpidem. Imipramine in combination with zolpidem produced no pharmacokinetic interaction other than a 20% decrease in peak levels of imipramine, but there was an additive effect of decreased alertness. Similarly,

chlorpromazine in combination with zolpidem produced no pharmacokinetic interaction, but there was an additive effect of decreased alertness and psychomotor performance. The lack of a drug interaction following single-dose administration does not predict a lack following chronic administration.

An additive effect on psychomotor performance between alcohol and zolpidem was demonstrated.

Since the systematic evaluations of Ambien (zolpidem tartrate) in combination with other CNS-active drugs have been limited, careful consideration should be given to the pharmacology of any CNS-active drug to be used with zolpidem. Any drug with CNS-depressant effects could potentially enhance the CNS-depressant effects of zolpidem.

Other drugs: A study involving cimetidine/zolpidem and ranitidine/zolpidem combinations revealed no effect of either drug on the pharmacokinetics or pharmacodynamics of zolpidem. Zolpidem had no effect on digoxin kinetics and did not affect prothrombin time when given with warfarin in normal subjects. Zolpidem's sedative/hypnotic effect was reversed by flumazenil; however, no significant alterations in zolpidem pharmacokinetics were found.

Drug/Laboratory test interactions: Zolpidem is not known to interfere with commonly employed clinical laboratory tests.

Carcinogenesis, mutagenesis, impairment of fertility

Carcinogenesis: Zolpidem was administered to rats and mice for 2 years at dietary dosages of 4, 18, and 80 mg/kg/day. In mice, these doses are 26 to 520 times or 2 to 35 times the maximum 10-mg human dose on a mg/kg or mg/m^2 basis, respectively. In rats these doses are 43 to 876 times or 6 to 115 times the maximum 10-mg human dose on a mg/kg or mg/m^2 basis, respectively. No evidence of carcinogenic potential was observed in mice. Renal liposarcomas were seen in 4/100 rats (3 males, 1 female) receiving 80 mg/kg/day and a renal lipoma was observed in one male rat at the 18 mg/kg/day dose. Incidence rates of lipoma and liposarcoma for zolpidem were comparable to those seen in historical controls and the tumor findings are thought to be a spontaneous occurrence.

Mutagenesis: Zolpidem did not have mutagenic activity in several tests including the Ames test, genotoxicity in mouse lymphoma cells in vitro, chromosomal aberrations in cultured human lymphocytes, unscheduled DNA synthesis in rat hepatocytes in vitro, and the micronucleus test in mice.

Impairment of fertility: In a rat reproduction study, the high dose (100 mg base/kg) of zolpidem resulted in irregular estrus cycles and prolonged precoital intervals, but there was no effect on male or female fertility after daily oral doses of 4 to 100 mg base/kg or 5 to 130 times the recommended human dose in mg/m^2. No effects on any other fertility parameters were noted.

Pregnancy

Teratogenic effects: Pregnancy Category B. Studies to assess the effects of zolpidem on human reproduction and development have not been conducted.

Teratology studies were conducted in rats and rabbits.

In rats, adverse maternal and fetal effects occurred at 20 and 100 mg base/kg and included dose-related maternal lethargy and ataxia and a dose-related trend to incomplete ossification of fetal skull bones. Underossification of various fetal bones indicates a delay in maturation and is often seen in rats treated with sedative/hypnotic drugs. There were no teratogenic effects after zolpidem administration. The no-effect dose for maternal or fetal toxicity was 4 mg base/kg or 5 times the maximum human dose on a mg/m^2 basis.

In rabbits, dose-related maternal sedation and decreased weight gain occurred at all doses tested. At the high dose, 16 mg base/kg, there was an increase in postimplantation fetal loss and underossification of sternebrae in viable fetuses. These fetal findings in rabbits are often secondary to reductions in maternal weight gain. There were no frank teratogenic effects. The no-effect dose for fetal toxicity was 4 mg base/kg or 7 times the maximum human dose on a mg/m^2 basis.

Because animal reproduction studies are not always predictive of human response, this drug should be used during pregnancy only if clearly needed.

Nonteratogenic effects: Studies to assess the effects on children whose mothers took zolpidem during pregnancy have not been conducted. However, children born of mothers taking sedative/hypnotic drugs may be at some risk for withdrawal symptoms from the drug during the postnatal period. In addition, neonatal flaccidity has been reported in infants born of mothers who received sedative/hypnotic drugs during pregnancy.

Labor and delivery: Ambien has no established use in labor and delivery.

Nursing mothers: Studies in lactating mothers indicate that the half-life of zolpidem is similar to that in young normal volunteers (2.6±0.3 hr). Between 0.004 and 0.019% of the total administered dose is excreted into milk, but the effect of zolpidem on the infant is unknown.

In addition, in a rat study, zolpidem inhibited the secretion of milk. The no-effect dose was 4 mg base/kg or 6 times the recommended human dose in mg/m^2.

The use of Ambien in nursing mothers is not recommended.

Pediatric use: Safety and effectiveness in children below the age of 18 have not been established.

Geriatric use: A total of 154 patients in U.S. controlled clinical trials and 897 patients in non-U.S. clinical trials who received zolpidem were ≥60 years of age. For a pool of U.S. patients receiving zolpidem at doses of ≤10 mg or placebo, there were three adverse events occurring at an incidence of at least 3% for zolpidem and for which the zolpidem incidence was at least twice the placebo incidence (ie, they could be considered drug related).

Adverse Event	Zolpidem	Placebo
Dizziness	3%	0%
Drowsiness	5%	2%
Diarrhea	3%	1%

A total of 30/1,959 (1.5%) non-U.S. patients receiving zolpidem reported falls, including 28/30 (93%) who were ≥70 years of age. Of these 28 patients, 23 (82%) were receiving zolpidem doses >10 mg. A total of 24/1,959 (1.2%) non-U.S. patients receiving zolpidem reported confusion, including 18/24 (75%) who were ≥70 years of age. Of these 18 patients, 14 (78%) were receiving zolpidem doses >10 mg.

ADVERSE REACTIONS

Associated with discontinuation of treatment: Approximately 4% of 1,701 patients who received zolpidem at all doses (1.25 to 90 mg) in U.S. premarketing clinical trials discontinued treatment because of an adverse clinical event. Events most commonly associated with discontinuation from U.S. trials were daytime drowsiness (0.5%), dizziness (0.4%), headache (0.5%), nausea (0.6%), and vomiting (0.5%).

Approximately 4% of 1,959 patients who received zolpidem at all doses (1 to 50 mg) in similar foreign trials discontinued treatment because of an adverse event. Events most commonly associated with discontinuation from these trials were daytime drowsiness (1.1%), dizziness/vertigo (0.8%), amnesia (0.5%), nausea (0.5%), headache (0.4%), and falls (0.4%).

Incidence in controlled clinical trials

Most commonly observed adverse events in controlled trials: During short-term treatment (up to 10 nights) with Ambien at doses up to 10 mg, the most commonly observed adverse events associated with the use of zolpidem and seen at statistically significant differences from placebo-treated patients were drowsiness (reported by 2% of zolpidem patients), dizziness (1%), and diarrhea (1%). During longer-term treatment (28 to 35 nights) with zolpidem at doses up to 10 mg, the most commonly observed adverse events associated with the use of zolpidem and seen at statistically significant differences from placebo-treated patients were dizziness (5%) and drugged feelings (3%).

Adverse events observed at an incidence of ≥ 1% in controlled trials: The following tables enumerate treatment-emergent adverse event frequencies that were observed at an incidence equal to 1% or greater among patients with insomnia who received Ambien in U.S. placebo-controlled trials. Events reported by investigators were classified utilizing a modified World Health Organization (WHO) dictionary of preferred terms for the purpose of establishing event frequencies. The prescriber should be aware that these figures cannot be used to predict the incidence of side effects in the course of usual medical practice, in which patient characteristics and other factors differ from those that prevailed in these clinical trials. Similarly, the cited frequencies cannot be compared with figures obtained from other clinical investigators involving related drug products and uses, since each group of drug trials is conducted under a different set of conditions. However, the cited figures provide the physician with a basis for estimating the relative contribution of drug and nondrug factors to the incidence of side effects in the population studied.

The following table was derived from a pool of 11 placebo-controlled short-term U.S. efficacy trials involving zolpidem in doses ranging from 1.25 to 20 mg. The table is limited to data from doses up to and including 10 mg, the highest dose recommended for use.

Incidence of Treatment-Emergent Adverse Experiences in Short-term Placebo-Controlled Clinical Trials
(Percentage of patients reporting)

Body System/ Adverse Event*	Zolpidem (≤10 mg) (N=685)	Placebo (N=473)
Central and Peripheral Nervous System		
Headache	7	6
Drowsiness	2	—
Dizziness	1	—
Gastrointestinal System		
Nausea	2	3
Diarrhea	1	—
Musculoskeletal System		
Myalgia	1	2

* Events reported by at least 1% of Ambien patients are included.

The following table was derived from a pool of three placebo-controlled long-term efficacy trials involving Ambien (zolpidem tartrate). These trials involved patients with chronic insomnia who were treated for 28 to 35 nights with zolpidem at doses of 5, 10, or 15 mg. The table is limited to data from doses up to and including 10 mg, the highest dose recommended for use. The table includes only adverse events occurring at an incidence of at least 1% for zolpidem patients.

Incidence of Treatment-Emergent Adverse Experiences in Long-term Placebo-Controlled Clinical Trials
(Percentage of patients reporting)

Body System/ Adverse Event*	Zolpidem (≤10 mg) (N=152)	Placebo (N=161)
Autonomic Nervous System		
Dry mouth	3	1
Body as a Whole		
Allergy	4	1
Back pain	3	2
Influenza-like symptoms	2	—
Chest pain	1	—
Fatigue	1	2
Cardiovascular System		
Palpitation	2	—
Central and Peripheral Nervous System		
Headache	19	22
Drowsiness	8	5
Dizziness	5	1
Lethargy	3	1
Drugged feeling	3	—
Lightheadedness	2	1
Depression	2	1
Abnormal dreams	1	—
Amnesia	1	—
Anxiety	1	1
Nervousness	1	3
Sleep disorder	1	—
Gastrointestinal System		
Nausea	6	6
Dyspepsia	5	6
Diarrhea	3	2
Abdominal pain	2	2
Constipation	2	1
Anorexia	1	1
Vomiting	1	1
Immunologic System		
Infection	1	1
Musculoskeletal System		
Myalgia	7	7
Arthralgia	4	4
Respiratory System		
Upper respiratory infection	5	6
Sinusitis	4	2
Pharyngitis	3	1
Rhinitis	1	3
Skin and Appendages		
Rash	2	1
Urogenital System		
Urinary tract infection	2	2

* Events reported by at least 1% of patients treated with Ambien.

Dose relationship for adverse events: There is evidence from dose comparison trials suggesting a dose relationship for many of the adverse events associated with zolpidem use, particularly for certain CNS and gastrointestinal adverse events.

Adverse event incidence across the entire preapproval database: Ambien (zolpidem tartrate) was administered to 3,660 subjects in clinical trials throughout the U.S., Canada, and Europe. Treatment-emergent adverse events associated with clinical trial participation were recorded by clinical investigators using terminology of their own choosing. To provide a meaningful estimate of the proportion of individuals experiencing treatment-emergent adverse events, similar types of untoward events were grouped into a smaller number of standardized event categories and classified utilizing a modified World Health Organization (WHO) dictionary of preferred terms. The frequencies presented, therefore, represent the proportions of the 3,660 individuals exposed to zolpidem, at all doses, who experienced

Continued on next page

Ambien—Cont.

an event of the type cited on at least one occasion while receiving zolpidem. All reported treatment-emergent adverse events are included, except those already listed in the table above of adverse events in placebo-controlled studies, those coding terms that are so general as to be uninformative, and those events where a drug cause was remote. It is important to emphasize that, although the events reported did occur during treatment with Ambien, they were not necessarily caused by it.

Adverse events are further classified within body system categories and enumerated in order of decreasing frequency using the following definitions: frequent adverse events are defined as those occurring in greater than 1/100 subjects; infrequent adverse events are those occurring in 1/100 to 1/1,000 patients; rare events are those occurring in less than 1/1,000 patients.

Autonomic nervous system: Infrequent: increased sweating, pallor, postural hypotension, syncope. Rare: abnormal accommodation, altered saliva, flushing, glaucoma, hypotension, impotence, increased saliva, tenesmus.

Body as a whole: Frequent: asthenia. Infrequent: edema, falling, fever, malaise, trauma. Rare: allergic reaction, allergy aggravated, abdominal body sensation, anaphylactic shock, face edema, hot flashes, increased ESR, pain, restless legs, rigors, tolerance increased, weight decrease.

Cardiovascular system: Infrequent: cerebrovascular disorder, hypertension, tachycardia. Rare: angina pectoris, arrhythmia, arteritis, circulatory failure, extrasystoles, hypertension aggravated, myocardial infarction, phlebitis, pulmonary embolism, pulmonary edema, varicose veins, ventricular tachycardia.

Central and peripheral nervous system: Frequent: ataxia, confusion, euphoria, insomnia, vertigo. Infrequent: agitation, decreased cognition, detached, difficulty concentrating, dysarthria, emotional lability, hallucination, hypoesthesia, illusion, leg cramps, migraine, paresthesia, sleeping (after day-time dosing), speech disorder, stupor, tremor. Rare: abnormal gait, abnormal thinking, aggressive reaction, apathy, appetite increased, decreased libido, delusion, dementia, depersonalization, dysphasia, feeling strange, hypokinesia, hypotonia, hysteria, intoxicated feeling, manic reaction, neuralgia, neuritis, neuropathy, neurosis, panic attacks, paresis, personality disorder, somnambulism, suicide attempts, tetany, yawning.

Gastrointestinal system: Frequent: hiccup. Infrequent: constipation, dysphagia, flatulence, gastroenteritis. Rare: enteritis, eructation, esophagospasm, gastritis, hemorrhoids, intestinal obstruction, rectal hemorrhage, tooth caries.

Hematologic and lymphatic system: Rare: anemia, hyperhemoglobinemia, leukopenia, lymphadenopathy, macrocytic anemia, purpura, thrombosis.

Immunologic system: Rare: abscess, herpes simplex, herpes zoster, otitis externa, otitis media.

Liver and biliary system: Infrequent: abnormal hepatic function, increased SGPT. Rare: bilirubinemia, increased SGOT.

Metabolic and nutritional: Infrequent: hyperglycemia, thirst. Rare: gout, hypercholesteremia, hyperlipidemia, increased alkaline phosphatase, increased BUN, periorbital edema.

Musculoskeletal system: Infrequent: arthritis. Rare: arthrosis, muscle weakness, sciatica, tendinitis.

Reproductive system: Infrequent: menstrual disorder, vaginitis. Rare: breast fibroadenosis, breast neoplasm, breast pain.

Respiratory system: Infrequent: bronchitis, coughing, dyspnea. Rare: bronchospasm, epistaxis, hypoxia, laryngitis, pneumonia.

Skin and appendages: Infrequent: pruritus. Rare: acne, bullous eruption, dermatitis, furunculosis, injection-site inflammation, photosensitivity reaction, urticaria.

Special senses: Frequent: diplopia, vision abnormal. Infrequent: eye irritation, eye pain, scleritis, taste perversion, tinnitus. Rare: conjunctivitis, corneal ulceration, lacrimation abnormal, parosmia, photopsia.

Urogenital system: Infrequent: cystitis, urinary incontinence. Rare: acute renal failure, dysuria, micturition frequency, nocturia, polyuria, pyelonephritis, renal pain, urinary retention.

DRUG ABUSE AND DEPENDENCE

Controlled substance: Zolpidem tartrate is classified as a Schedule IV controlled substance by federal regulation.

Abuse and dependence: Studies of abuse potential in former drug abusers found that the effects of single doses of Ambien (zolpidem tartrate) 40 mg were similar, but not identical, to diazepam 20 mg, while zolpidem tartrate 10 mg was difficult to distinguish from placebo.

Sedative/hypnotics have produced withdrawal signs and symptoms following abrupt discontinuation. These reported symptoms range from mild dysphoria and insomnia to a withdrawal syndrome that may include abdominal and muscle cramps, vomiting, sweating, tremors, and convul-

sions. The U.S. clinical trial experience from zolpidem does not reveal any clear evidence for withdrawal syndrome. Nevertheless, the following adverse events included in DSM-III-R criteria for uncomplicated sedative/hypnotic withdrawal were reported during U.S. clinical trials following placebo substitution occurring within 48 hours following last zolpidem treatment: fatigue, nausea, flushing, lightheadedness, uncontrolled crying, emesis, stomach cramps, panic attack, nervousness, and abdominal discomfort. These reported adverse events occurred at an incidence of 1% or less. However, available data cannot provide a reliable estimate of the incidence, if any, of dependence during treatment at recommended doses. Rare post-marketing reports of abuse, dependence and withdrawal have been received.

Because persons with a history of psychiatric disorders or addiction to, or abuse of, drugs or alcohol are at increased risk of habituation and dependence, they should be under careful surveillance when receiving zolpidem or any other hypnotic.

OVERDOSAGE

Signs and symptoms: In European postmarketing reports of overdose with zolpidem alone, impairment of consciousness has ranged from somnolence to light coma. There was one case each of cardiovascular and respiratory compromise. Individuals have fully recovered from zolpidem tartrate overdoses up to 400 mg (40 times the maximum recommended dose). Overdose cases involving multiple CNS-depressant agents, including zolpidem, have resulted in more severe symptomatology, including fatal outcomes.

Recommended treatment: General symptomatic and supportive measures should be used along with immediate gastric lavage where appropriate. Intravenous fluids should be administered as needed. Flumazenil may be useful. As in all cases of drug overdose, respiration, pulse, blood pressure, and other appropriate signs should be monitored and general supportive measures employed. Hypotension and CNS depression should be monitored and treated by appropriate medical intervention. Sedating drugs should be withheld following zolpidem overdosage, even if excitation occurs. The value of dialysis in the treatment of overdosage has not been determined, although hemodialysis studies in patients with renal failure receiving therapeutic doses have demonstrated that zolpidem is not dialyzable.

Poison control center: As with the management of all overdosage, the possibility of multiple drug ingestion should be considered. The physician may wish to consider contacting a poison control center for up-to-date information on the management of hypnotic drug product overdosage.

DOSAGE AND ADMINISTRATION

The dose of Ambien should be individualized.

The recommended dose for adults is 10 mg immediately before bedtime.

Downward dosage adjustment may be necessary when Ambien is administered with agents having known CNS-depressant effects because of the potentially additive effects. Elderly or debilitated patients may be especially sensitive to the effects of Ambien (zolpidem tartrate). Patients with hepatic insufficiency do not clear the drug as rapidly as normals. An initial 5-mg dose is recommended in these patients (see *Precautions*).

The total Ambien dose should not exceed 10 mg.

HOW SUPPLIED

Ambien 5-mg tablets are capsule-shaped, pink, film coated, identified with markings of AMB 5 on one side and 5401 on the other and supplied as:

NDC Number	Size
0025-5401-31	bottle of 100
0025-5401-34	carton of 100 unit dose

Ambien 10-mg tablets are capsule-shaped, white, film coated, identified with markings of AMB 10 on one side and 5421 on the other and supplied as:

NDC Number	Size
0025-5421-31	bottle of 100
0025-5421-34	carton of 100 unit dose

Store at controlled room temperature 20°–25°C (68°–77°F).

Caution: Federal law prohibits dispensing without prescription.

INFORMATION FOR PATIENTS
TAKING AMBIEN

Your doctor has prescribed Ambien to help you sleep. The following information is intended to guide you in the safe use of this medicine. It is not meant to take the place of your doctor's instructions. If you have any questions about Ambien tablets be sure to ask your doctor or pharmacist.

Ambien is used to treat different types of sleep problems, such as:

• trouble falling asleep
• waking up too early in the morning
• waking up often during the night

Some people may have more than one of these problems.

Ambien belongs to a group of medicines known as the "sedative/hypnotics," or simply, sleep medicines. There are

many different sleep medicines available to help people sleep better. Sleep problems are usually temporary, requiring treatment for only a short time, usually 1 or 2 days up to 1 or 2 weeks. Some people have chronic sleep problems that may require more prolonged use of sleep medicine. However, you should not use these medicines for long periods without talking with your doctor about the risks and benefits of prolonged use.

SIDE EFFECTS

Most common side effects: All medicines have side effects. Most common side effects of sleep medicines include:

• drowsiness
• dizziness
• lightheadedness
• difficulty with coordination

You may find that these medicines make you sleepy during the day. How drowsy you feel depends upon how your body reacts to the medicine, which sleep medicine you are taking, and how large a dose your doctor has prescribed. Daytime drowsiness is best avoided by taking the lowest dose possible that will still help you sleep at night. Your doctor will work with you to find the dose of Ambien that is best for you.

To manage these side effects while you are taking this medicine:

• When you first start taking Ambien or any other sleep medicine until you know whether the medicine will still have some carryover effect in you the next day, use extreme care while doing anything that requires complete alertness, such as driving a car, operating machinery, or piloting an aircraft.
• NEVER drink alcohol while you are being treated with Ambien or any sleep medicine. Alcohol can increase the side effects of Ambien or any other sleep medicine.
• Do not take any other medicines without asking your doctor first. This includes medicines you can buy without a prescription. Some medicines can cause drowsiness and are best avoided while taking Ambien.
• Always take the exact dose of Ambien prescribed by your doctor. Never change your dose without talking to your doctor first.

SPECIAL CONCERNS

There are some special problems that may occur while taking sleep medicines.

Memory problems: Sleep medicines may cause a special type of memory loss or "amnesia." When this occurs, a person may not remember what has happened for several hours after taking the medicine. This is usually not a problem since most people fall asleep after taking the medicine. Memory loss can be a problem, however, when sleep medicines are taken while traveling, such as during an airplane flight and the person wakes up before the effect of the medicine is gone. This has been called "traveler's amnesia."

Memory problems are not common while taking Ambien. In most instances memory problems can be avoided if you take Ambien only when you are able to get a full night's sleep (7 to 8 hours) before you need to be active again. Be sure to talk to your doctor if you think you are having memory problems.

Tolerance: When sleep medicines are used every night for more than a few weeks, they may lose their effectiveness to help you sleep. This is known as "tolerance." Sleep medicines should, in most cases, be used only for short periods of time, such as 1 or 2 days and generally no longer than 1 or 2 weeks. If your sleep problems continue, consult your doctor, who will determine whether other measures are needed to overcome your sleep problems.

Dependence: Sleep medicines can cause dependence, especially when these medicines are used regularly for longer than a few weeks or at high doses. Some people develop a need to continue taking their medicines. This is known as dependence or "addiction."

When people develop dependence, they may have difficulty stopping the sleep medicine. If the medicine is suddenly stopped, the body is not able to function normally and unpleasant symptoms (see *Withdrawal*) may occur. They may find they have to keep taking the medicine either at the prescribed dose or at increasing doses just to avoid withdrawal symptoms.

All people taking sleep medicines have some risk of becoming dependent on the medicine. However, people who have been dependent on alcohol or other drugs in the past may have a higher chance of becoming addicted to sleep medicines. This possibility must be considered before using these medicines for more than a few weeks.

If you have been addicted to alcohol or drugs in the past, it is important to tell your doctor before starting Ambien or any sleep medicine.

Withdrawal: Withdrawal symptoms may occur when sleep medicines are stopped suddenly after being used daily for a long time. In some cases, these symptoms can occur even if the medicine has been used for only a week or two.

In mild cases, withdrawal symptoms may include unpleasant feelings. In more severe cases, abdominal and muscle

cramps, vomiting, sweating, shakiness, and rarely, seizures may occur. These more severe withdrawal symptoms are very uncommon.

Another problem that may occur when sleep medicines are stopped is known as "rebound insomnia." This means that a person may have more trouble sleeping the first few nights after the medicine is stopped than before starting the medicine. If you should experience rebound insomnia, do not get discouraged. This problem usually goes away on its own after 1 or 2 nights.

If you have been taking Ambien or any other sleep medicine for more than 1 or 2 weeks, do not stop taking it on your own. Always follow your doctor's directions.

Changes in behavior and thinking: Some people using sleep medicines have experienced unusual changes in their thinking and/or behavior. These effects are not common. However, they have included:

- more outgoing or aggressive behavior than normal
- loss of personal identity
- confusion
- strange behavior
- agitation
- hallucinations
- worsening of depression
- suicidal thoughts

How often these effects occur depends on several factors, such as a person's general health, the use of other medicines, and which sleep medicine is being used. Clinical experience with Ambien suggests that it is uncommonly associated with these behavior changes.

It is also important to realize that it is rarely clear whether these behavior changes are caused by the medicine, an illness, or occur on their own. In fact, sleep problems that do not improve may be due to illnesses that were present before the medicine was used. If you or your family notice any changes in your behavior, or if you have any unusual or disturbing thoughts, call your doctor immediately.

Pregnancy: Sleep medicines may cause sedation of the unborn baby when used during the last weeks of pregnancy. Be sure to tell your doctor if you are pregnant, if you are planning to become pregnant, or if you become pregnant while taking Ambien.

SAFE USE OF SLEEPING MEDICINES

To ensure the safe and effective use of Ambien or any other sleep medicine, you should observe the following cautions:

1. Ambien is a prescription medicine and should be used ONLY as directed by your doctor. Follow your doctor's instructions about how to take, when to take, and how long to take Ambien.
2. Never use Ambien or any other sleep medicine for longer than directed by your doctor.
3. If you notice any unusual and/or disturbing thoughts or behavior during treatment with Ambien or any other sleep medicine, contact your doctor.
4. Tell your doctor about any medicines you may be taking, including medicines you may buy without a prescription. You should also tell your doctor if you drink alcohol. DO NOT use alcohol while taking Ambien or any other sleep medicine.
5. Do not take Ambien or any other sleep medicine unless you are able to get a full night's sleep before you must be active again. For example, Ambien or any other sleep medicine should not be taken on an overnight airplane flight of less than 7 to 8 hours since "traveler's amnesia" may occur.
6. Do not increase the prescribed dose of Ambien or any other sleep medicine unless instructed by your doctor.
7. When you first start taking Ambien or any other sleep medicine until you know whether the medicine will still have some carryover effect in you the next day, use extreme care while doing anything that requires complete alertness, such as driving a car, operating machinery, or piloting an aircraft.
8. Be aware that you may have more sleeping problems the first night or two after stopping Ambien or any other sleep medicine.
9. Be sure to tell your doctor if you are pregnant, if you are planning to become pregnant, or if you become pregnant while taking Ambien.
10. As with all prescription medicines, never share Ambien or any other sleep medicine with anyone else. Always store Ambien or any other sleep medicine in the original container out of reach of children.
11. Ambien works very quickly. You should only take Ambien right before going to bed and are ready to go to sleep.

1/31/97 • A05202-3

Manufactured and distributed by
G.D. Searle & Co.
Chicago, IL 60680
by agreement with
Lorex Pharmaceuticals
Skokie, IL

Address medical inquiries to:
G.D. Searle & Co.
Healthcare Information Services
5200 Old Orchard Road
Skokie, IL 60077

Ambien is a registered trademark of Synthelabo.
Shown in Product Identification Guide, page 337

ARTHROTEC® ℞

[ă 'thrŏ tek]

(diclofenac sodium and misoprostol)
Tablets

CONTRAINDICATIONS AND WARNINGS

ARTHROTEC, because of the abortifacient property of the misoprostol component, is contraindicated in women who are pregnant. (See *PRECAUTIONS*). Reports, primarily from Brazil, of congenital anomalies and reports of fetal death subsequent to misuse of misoprostol alone, as an abortifacient, have been received. Patients must be advised of the abortifacient property and warned not to give the drug to others. ARTHROTEC should not be used in women of childbearing potential unless the patient requires nonsteroidal anti-inflammatory drug (NSAID) therapy and is at high risk of developing gastric or duodenal ulceration or for developing complications from gastric or duodenal ulcers associated with the use of the NSAID. (See *WARNINGS*). In such patients, ARTHROTEC may be prescribed if the patient:

- has had a negative serum pregnancy test within 2 weeks prior to beginning therapy.
- is capable of complying with effective contraceptive measures.
- has received both oral and written warnings of the hazards of misoprostol, the risk of possible contraception failure, and the danger to other women of childbearing potential should the drug be taken by mistake.
- will begin ARTHROTEC only on the second or third day of the next normal menstrual period.

DESCRIPTION

ARTHROTEC is a combination product containing diclofenac sodium, a nonsteroidal anti-inflammatory drug (NSAID) with analgesic properties, and misoprostol, a gastrointestinal (GI) mucosal protective prostaglandin E_1 analog. ARTHROTEC oral tablets are white to off-white, round, biconvex and approximately 11 mm in diameter. Each tablet consists of an enteric-coated core containing 50 mg (ARTHROTEC 50) or 75 mg (ARTHROTEC 75) diclofenac sodium surrounded by an outer mantle containing 200 mcg misoprostol.

Diclofenac sodium is a phenylacetic acid derivative that is a white to off-white, virtually odorless, crystalline powder. Diclofenac sodium is freely soluble in methanol, soluble in ethanol and practically insoluble in chloroform and in dilute acid. Diclofenac sodium is sparingly soluble in water. Its chemical formula and name are:

$C_{14}H_{10}Cl_2NO_2Na$ [M.W. = 318.14] 2-[2,6-dichlorophenyl) amino]benezeneacetic acid, monosodium salt.

Misoprostol is a water-soluble, viscous liquid that contains approximately equal amounts of two diastereomers. Its chemical formula and name are:

$C_{22}H_{38}O_5$ [M.W. = 382.54] (±) methyl 11α, 16-dihydroxy-16-methyl-9-oxoprost-13E-en-1-oate.

Inactive ingredients in ARTHROTEC include: colloidal silicon dioxide; crospovidone; hydrogenated castor oil; hydroxypropyl methylcellulose; lactose; magnesium stearate; methacrylic acid copolymer; microcrystalline cellulose; povidone (polyvidone) K-30; sodium hydroxide; starch (corn); talc; triethyl citrate.

CLINICAL PHARMACOLOGY

Pharmacodynamics and pharmacokinetics of diclofenac sodium

Diclofenac sodium is a nonsteroidal anti-inflammatory drug (NSAID). In pharmacologic studies, diclofenac sodium has shown anti-inflammatory, analgesic and antipyretic properties. The mechanism of action of diclofenac sodium, like other NSAIDs, is not completely understood but may be related to prostaglandin synthetase inhibition.

Diclofenac sodium is completely absorbed from the GI tract after fasting, oral administration. The diclofenac sodium in ARTHROTEC is in a pharmaceutical formulation that resists dissolution in the low pH of gastric fluid but allows a rapid release of drug in the higher pH environment of the duodenum. Only 50% of the absorbed dose is systemically available due to first pass metabolism. Peak plasma levels are achieved in 2 hours (range 1–4 hours), and the area under the plasma concentration curve (AUC) is dose proportional within the range of 25 mg to 150 mg. Peak plasma levels are less than dose proportional and are approximately 1.5 and 2.0 mcg/mL for 50 mg and 75 mg doses, respectively.

Plasma concentrations of diclofenac sodium decline from peak levels in a biexponential fashion, with the terminal phase having a half-life of approximately 2 hours. Clearance and volume of distribution are about 350 mL/min and 550 mL/kg, respectively. More than 99% of diclofenac sodium is reversibly bound to human plasma albumin.

Diclofenac sodium is eliminated through metabolism and subsequent urinary and biliary excretion of the glucuronide and the sulfate conjugates of the metabolites. Approximately 65% of the dose is excreted in the urine and 35% in the bile.

Conjugates of unchanged diclofenac account for 5–10% of the dose excreted in the urine and for less than 5% excreted in the bile. Little or no unchanged unconjugated drug is excreted. Conjugates of the principal metabolite account for 20–30% of the dose excreted in the urine and for 10–20% of the dose excreted in the bile.

Conjugates of three other metabolites together account for 10–20% of the dose excreted in the urine and for small amounts excreted in the bile. The elimination half-life values for these metabolites are shorter than those for the parent drug. Urinary excretion of an additional metabolite (half-life = 80 hours) accounts for only 1.4% of the oral dose. The degree of accumulation of diclofenac metabolites is unknown. Some of the metabolites may have activity.

Pharmacodynamics and pharmacokinetics of misoprostol

Misoprostol is a synthetic prostaglandin E_1 analog with gastric antisecretory and (in animals) muscosal protective properties. NSAIDs inhibit prostaglandin synthesis. A deficiency of prostaglandins within the gastric and duodenal mucosa may lead to diminishing bicarbonate and mucus secretion and may contribute to the mucosal damage caused by NSAIDs.

Misoprostol can increase bicarbonate and mucus production, but in humans this has been shown at doses 200 mcg and above that are also antisecretory. It is therefore not possible to tell whether the ability of misoprostol to prevent gastric and duodenal ulcers is the result of its antisecretory effect, its mucosal protective effect, or both.

In vitro studies on canine parietal cells using tritiated misoprostol acid as the ligand have led to the identification and characterization of specific prostaglandin receptors. Receptor binding is saturable, reversible, and stereospecific. The sites have a high affinity for misoprostol, for its acid metabolite, and for other E type prostaglandins, but not for F or I prostaglandins and other unrelated compounds, such as histamine or cimetidine. Receptor-site affinity for misoprostol correlates well with an indirect index of antisecretory activity. It is likely that these specific receptors allow misoprostol taken with food to be effective topically, despite the lower serum concentrations attained.

Misoprostol produces a moderate decrease in pepsin concentration during basal conditions, but not during histamine stimulation. It has no significant effect on fasting or postprandial gastrin nor intrinsic factor output.

Effects on gastric acid secretion: Misoprostol, over the range of 50–200 mcg, inhibits basal and nocturnal gastric acid secretion, and acid secretion in response to a variety of stimuli, including meals, histamine, pentagastrin, and coffee. Activity is apparent 30 minutes after oral administration and persists for at least 3 hours. In general, the effects of 50 mcg were modest and shorter lived, and only the 200-mcg dose had substantial effects on nocturnal secretion or on histamine- and meal-stimulated secretion.

Orally administered misoprostol is rapidly and extensively absorbed, and it undergoes rapid metabolism to its biologically active metabolite, misoprostol acid. Misoprostol acid in ARTHROTEC reaches a maximum plasma concentration in about 20 minutes and is, thereafter, quickly eliminated with an elimination $t_{1/2}$ of about 30 minutes. There is high variability in plasma levels of misoprostol acid between and within studies, but mean values after single doses show a linear relationship with dose of misoprostol over the range of 200 to 400 mcg. No accumulation of misoprostol acid was found in multiple dose studies, and plasma steady state was achieved within 2 days. The serum protein binding of misoprostol acid is less than 90% and is concentration-independent in the therapeutic range.

After oral administration of radiolabeled misoprostol, about 70% of detected radioactivity appears in the urine. Maximum plasma concentrations of misoprostol acid are diminished when the dose is taken with food, and total availability of misoprostol acid is reduced by use of concomitant antacid. Clinical trials were conducted with concomitant antacid; this effect does not appear to be clinically important.

Pharmacokinetic studies also showed a lack of drug interaction with antipyrine or propranolol given with misoprostol. Misoprostol given for 1 week had no effect on the steady state pharmacokinetics of diazepam when the two drugs were administered 2 hours apart.

Pharmacokinetics of ARTHROTEC

The pharmacokinetics following oral administration of a single dose (see Table 1) or multiple doses of ARTHROTEC

Continued on next page

Arthrotec—Cont.

(diclofenac sodium/misoprostol) to healthy subjects under fasted conditions are similar to the pharmacokinetics of the two individual components.

[See table 1 at right]

The rate and extent of absorption of both diclofenac sodium and misoprostol acid from ARTHROTEC 50 and ARTHROTEC 75 are similar to those from diclofenac sodium and misoprostol formulations each administered alone.

Neither diclofenac sodium nor misoprostol acid accumulated in plasma following repeated doses of ARTHROTEC given every 12 hours under fasted conditions. Food decreases the multiple-dose bioavailability profile of ARTHROTEC 50 and ARTHROTEC 75.

Special populations

A 4-week study, comparing plasma level profiles of diclofenac (50 mg bid) in younger (26–46 years) versus older (66–81 years) adults, did not show differences between age groups (10 patients per age group). In a multiple-dose (bid) crossover study of 24 people aged 65 years or older, the misoprostol contained in ARTHROTEC did not affect the pharmacokinetics of diclofenac sodium.

Differences in the pharmacokinetics of diclofenac have not been detected in studies of patients with renal (50 mg intravenously) or hepatic impairment (100 mg oral solution). In patients with renal impairment (N = 5, creatinine clearance 3 to 42 mL/min), AUC values and elimination rates were comparable to those in healthy people. In patients with biopsy-confirmed cirrhosis or chronic active hepatitis (variably elevated transaminases and mildly elevated bilirubins, N = 10), diclofenac concentrations and urinary elimination values were comparable to those in healthy people.

Pharmacokinetic studies with misoprostol in patients with varying degrees of renal impairment showed an approximate doubling of $t_{1/2}$, C_{max} and AUC compared to healthy people. In people over 64 years of age, the AUC for misoprostol acid is increased.

Misoprostol does not affect the hepatic mixed function oxidase (cytochrome P-450) enzyme system in animals. In a study of people with mild to moderate hepatic impairment, mean misoprostol acid AUC and C_{max} showed approximately double the mean values obtained in healthy people. Three people who had the lowest antipyrine and lowest indocyanine green clearance values had the highest misoprostol acid AUC and C_{max} values.

CLINICAL STUDIES

Osteoarthritis

Diclofenac sodium, as a single ingredient or in combination with misoprostol, has been shown to be effective in the management of the signs and symptoms of osteoarthritis.

Rheumatoid arthritis

Diclofenac sodium, as a single ingredient or in combination with misoprostol, has been shown to be effective in the management of the signs and symptoms of rheumatoid arthritis.

Upper gastrointestinal safety

Diclofenac, and other NSAIDs, have caused serious gastrointestinal toxicity, such as bleeding, ulceration and perforation of the stomach, small intestine or large intestine. Misoprostol has been shown to reduce the incidence of endoscopically diagnosed NSAID-induced gastric and duodenal ulcers. In a 12-week, randomized, double-blind, dose response study, misoprostol 200 mcg administered qid, tid or bid, was significantly more effective than placebo in reducing the incidence of gastric ulcer in OA and RA patients using a variety of NSAIDs. The tid regimen was therapeutically equivalent to misoprostol 200 mcg qid with respect to the prevention of gastric ulcers. Misoprostol 200 mcg given bid was less effective than 200 mcg given tid or qid. The incidence of NSAID-induced duodenal ulcer was also significantly reduced with all three regimens of misoprostol compared to placebo (see Table 2).

Table 2.
Misoprostol 200 mcg Dosage Regimen

	Placebo	bid	tid	qid
Gastric ulcer	11%	6%*	3%*	3%*
Duodenal ulcer	6%	2%*	3%*	1%*

N = 1623; 12 weeks.

* Misoprostol significantly different from placebo (p<0.05)

Results of a study in 572 patients with osteoarthritis demonstrate that patients receiving ARTHROTEC have a lower incidence of gastric ulcers compared to patiens receiving diclofenac sodium (see Table 3).

[See table 3 at right]

INDICATIONS AND USAGE

ARTHROTEC is indicated for treatment of the signs and symptoms of osteoarthritis or rheumatoid arthritis in patients at high risk of developing NSAID-induced gastric and duodenal ulcers and their complications. See *WARNINGS—*

Table 1.

MISOPROSTOL ACID Mean (SD)

Treatment (n=36)	C_{max} (pg/mL)	t_{max} (hr)	AUC (0–4h) (pg·hr/mL)
ARTHROTEC 50	441 (137)	0.30 (0.13)	266 (95)
Cytotec®	478 (201)	0.30 (0.10)	295 (143)
ARTHROTEC 75	304 (110)	0.26 (0.09)	177 (49)
Cytotec	290 (130)	0.35 (0.12)	176 (58)

DICLOFENAC Mean (SD)

Treatment (n=36)	C_{max} (ng/mL)	t_{max} (hr)	AUC (0–12h) (ng·hr/mL)
ARTHROTEC 50	1207 (364)	2.4 (1.0)	1380 (272)
Voltaren®	1298 (441)	2.4 (1.0)	1357 (290)
ARTHROTEC 75	2025 (2005)	2.0 (1.4)	2773 (1347)
Voltaren	2367 (1318)	1.9 (0.7)	2609 (1185)

SD: Standard deviation of the mean
AUC: Area under the curve
C_{max}: Peak concentration
t_{max}: Time to peak concentration

Gastrointestinal effects for a list of factors that may increase the risk of NSAID-induced gastric and duodenal ulcers and their complications.

CONTRAINDICATIONS

See boxed *CONTRAINDICATIONS AND WARNINGS* related to misoprostol.

ARTHROTEC is contraindicated in patients with hypersensitivity to diclofenac or to misoprostol or other prostaglandins. ARTHROTEC should not be given to patients who have experienced asthma, urticaria, or other allergic-type reactions after taking aspirin or other NSAIDs. Severe, rarely fatal, anaphylactic-like reactions to diclofenac sodium have been reported.

WARNINGS

Regarding misoprostol:

See boxed *CONTRAINDICATIONS AND WARNINGS*.

Regarding diclofenac:

Gastrointestinal (GI) effects—risk of GI ulceration, bleeding and perforation

Serious GI toxicity, such as inflammation, bleeding, ulceration and perforation of the stomach, small intestine or large intestine, can occur at any time, with or without warning symptoms, in patients treated with NSAIDs. Minor upper GI problems, such as dyspepsia, are common and may also occur at any time during NSAID therapy. Therefore, physicians and patients should remain alert for ulceration and bleeding, even in the absence of previous GI tract symptoms. Patients should be informed about the signs and/or symptoms and the steps to take if they occur. The utility of periodic laboratory monitoring has not been demonstrated, nor has it been adequately assessed. Only 1 in 5 patients who develop a serious upper GI adverse event on NSAID therapy in symptomatic. It has been demonstrated that upper GI ulcers, gross bleeding, or perforation, caused by NSAIDs, appear to occur in approximately 1% of patients treated for 3–6 months, and in 2–4% of patients treated for 1 year. These trends continue thus, increasing the likelihood of developing a serious GI event at some time during the course of therapy. However, even short-term therapy has risk.

NSAIDs should be prescribed with extreme caution in those with a prior history of ulcer disease or GI bleeding. Most spontaneous reports of fatal GI events are in elderly or debilitated patients and therefore special care should be taken in treating this population. To minimize the potential risk for an adverse event, the lowest effective dose should be used for the shortest possible duration. For very high-risk patients, alternate therapies that do not involve NSAIDs should be considered.

Studies have shown that patients with a history of peptic ulcer disease and/or GI bleeding, and who use NSAIDs, have a greater than 10-fold risk for developing a GI bleed than patients with neither of these risk factors. In addition

to a past history of ulcer disease, pharmacoepidemiological studies have identified several other conditions or co-therapies that may increase the risk for GI bleeding, such as: treatment with oral corticosteroids, treatment with anticoagulants, longer duration of NSAID therapy, older age, smoking, alcoholism, poor general health and *Helicobacter pylori* positive status.

Hepatic effects

Elevations of one or more liver tests may occur during ARTHROTEC therapy. These laboratory abnormalities may progress, may remain unchanged, or may be transient with continued therapy. Borderline elevations (ie, less than 3 times the ULN [ULN = the upper limit of the normal range]), or greater elevations of transaminases occurred in about 15% of diclofenac-treated patients. Of the hepatic enzymes, ALT (SGPT) is the one recommended for the monitoring of liver injury.

In clinical trials, meaningful elevations (ie, more than 3 times the ULN) of AST (SGOT) (ALT was not measured in all studies) occurred in about 2% of approximately 5,700 patients at some time during diclofenac treatment. In a large, open, controlled trial, meaningful elevations of ALT and/or AST occurred in about 4% of 3,700 patients treated for 2–6 months, including marked elevations (ie, more than 8 times the ULN) in about 1% of the 3,700 patients. In that open-label study, a higher incidence of borderline (less than 3 times the ULN), moderate (3–8 times the ULN), and marked (>8 times the ULN) elevations of ALT or AST was observed in patients receiving diclofenac when compared to other NSAIDs. Transaminase elevations were seen more frequently in patients with osteoarthritis than in those with rheumatoid arthritis.

In addition to enzyme elevations seen in clinical trials, post-marketing surveillance has found rare cases of severe hepatic reactions, including liver necrosis, jaundice, and fulminant fatal hepatitis with and without jaundice. Some of these rare reported cases underwent liver transplantation.

Physicians should measure transaminases periodically in patients receiving long-term therapy with diclofenac, because severe hepatotoxicity may develop without a prodrome of distinguishing symptoms. The optimum times for making the first and subsequent transaminase measurements are not known. In the largest U.S. trial (open-label) that involved 3,700 patients monitored first at 8 weeks and 1,200 patients monitored again at 24 weeks, almost all meaningful elevations in transaminases were detected before patients became symptomatic. In 42 of the 51 patients in all trials who developed marked transaminase elevations, abnormal tests occurred during the first 2 months of therapy with diclofenac. Postmarketing experience has shown severe hepatic reactions can occur at any time during treatment with diclofenac. Cases of drug-induced hepatotoxicity have been reported in the first month, and in some cases, the first 2 months of therapy. Based on these experi-

Table 3.

Osteoarthritis patients with a history of ulcer or erosive disease (N=572), 6 weeks	Incidence of ulcers	
	Gastric	Duodenal
ARTHROTEC 50 tid	3%*	6%
ARTHROTEC 75 bid	4%*	3%
diclofenac sodium 75 mg bid	11%	7%
placebo	3%	1%

* Statistically significantly different from diclofenac (p<0.05)

ences, transaminases should be monitored within 4 to 8 weeks after initiating treatment with diclofenac (see *PRECAUTIONS—Laboratory tests*).

In clinical trials with ARTHROTEC, meaningful elevation of ALT (SGPT, more than 3 times the ULN) occurred in 1.6% of 2,184 patients treated with ARTHROTEC, and in 1.4% of 1,691 patients treated with diclofenac sodium. These increases were generally transient, and enzyme levels returned to within the normal range upon discontinuation of ARTHROTEC therapy. The misoprostol component of ARTHROTEC does not appear to exacerbate the hepatic effects caused by the diclofenac sodium component. As with other NSAID containing products, if abnormal liver tests persist or worsen, if clinical signs and/or symptoms consistent with liver disease develop, or if systemic manifestations occur (eg, eosinophilia, rash, etc), ARTHROTEC should be discontinued immediately.

To minimize the possibility that hepatic injury will become severe between transaminase measurements, physicians should inform patients of the warning signs and symptoms of hepatotoxicity (eg, nausea, fatigue, lethargy, pruritus, jaundice, right upper quadrant tenderness, and "flu-like" symptoms), and the appropriate action patients should take if these signs and symptoms appear.

Anaphylactoid reactions

As with other NSAID containing products, anaphylactoid reactions may occur in patients without known prior exposure to ARTHROTEC or its components. ARTHROTEC should not be given to patients with the aspirin triad. The triad typically occurs in asthmatic patients who experience rhinitis with or without nasal polyps, or who exhibit severe, potentially fatal bronchospasm after taking aspirin or other NSAIDs (see *CONTRAINDICATIONS* and *PRECAUTIONS—Preexisting asthma*). Emergency help should be sought in cases where an anaphylactoid reaction occurs. Allergic reactions have been reported by less than 0.1% of patients who received ARTHROTEC in clinical trials, and there have been rare reports of anaphylaxis in the marketed use of ARTHROTEC outside of the United States.

Advanced renal disease

In patients with advanced kidney disease, treatment with ARTHROTEC is not recommended. If NSAID therapy must be initiated however, close monitoring of the patient's kidney function is advisable (see *PRECAUTIONS—Renal effects*).

PRECAUTIONS

Information for patients

See *PATIENT INFORMATION* at the end of this labeling for important information to discuss with the patient.

ARTHROTEC is available only as a unit-of-use package that includes a leaflet containing patient information. The patient should read the leaflet before taking ARTHROTEC and each time the prescription is renewed because the leaflet may have been revised. Keep ARTHROTEC out of the reach of children.

General

ARTHROTEC cannot be used to substitute for corticosteroids or to treat for corticosteroid insufficiency. Abrupt discontinuation of corticosteroids may lead to disease exacerbation. Patients on prolonged corticosteroid therapy should have their therapy tapered slowly if a decision is made to discontinue corticosteroids.

The pharmacological activity of ARTHROTEC in reducing inflammation may diminish the utility of this diagnostic sign in detecting complications of presumed noninfectious, painful conditions.

Renal effects

Caution should be used when initiating treatment with ARTHROTEC in patients with considerable dehydration. It is advisable to rehydrate patients first and then start therapy with ARTHROTEC. Caution is also recommended in patients with preexisting kidney disease (see *WARNINGS—Advanced renal disease*).

As with other NSAIDs, long-term administration of diclofenac has resulted in renal papillary necrosis and other renal medullary changes. Renal toxicity has also been seen in patients in which renal prostaglandins have a compensatory role in the maintenance of renal perfusion. In these patients, administration of an NSAID may cause a dose-dependent reduction in prostaglandin formation and, secondarily, in renal blood flow, which may precipitate overt renal decompensation. Patients at greatest risk of this reaction are those with impaired renal function, heart failure, or liver dysfunction, those taking diuretics and ACE inhibitors, and the elderly. Discontinuation of NSAID therapy is usually followed by recovery to the pretreatment state.

Diclofenac metabolites are eliminated primarily by the kidneys. The extent to which the metabolites may accumulate in patients with renal failure has not been studied. As with other NSAIDs, metabolites of which are excreted by the kidney, patients with significantly impaired renal function should be more closely monitored.

Hematologic effects

Anemia is sometimes seen in patients receiving diclofenac or other NSAIDs. This may be due to fluid retention, GI blood loss, or an incompletely described effect upon erythropoiesis. Patients on long-term treatment with NSAIDs, including ARTHROTEC, should have their hemoglobin or hematocrit checked if they exhibit any signs or symptoms of anemia.

All drugs that inhibit the biosynthesis of prostaglandins may interfere to some extent with platelet function and vascular responses to bleeding.

NSAIDs inhibit platelet aggregation and, unlike aspirin, their effect on platelet function is reversible, quantitatively less, and of shorter duration. ARTHROTEC does not generally affect platelet counts, prothrombin time (PT), or partial thromboplastin time (PTT). Patients receiving ARTHROTEC who may be adversely affected by alterations in platelet function, such as those with coagulation disorders or patients receiving anticoagulants, should be carefully monitored.

Aseptic meningitis

As with other NSAIDs, aseptic meningitis with fever and coma has been observed on rare occasions in patients on diclofenac therapy. Although it is probably more likely to occur in patients with systemic lupus and related connective tissue diseases, it has been reported in patients who do not have an underlying chronic disease. If signs or symptoms of meningitis develop in a patient on diclofenac, the possibility of its being related to diclofenac should be considered.

Fluid retention and edema

Fluid retention and edema have been observed in some patients taking NSAID containing products, including ARTHROTEC. Therefore, as with other NSAID containing products, ARTHROTEC should be used with caution in patients with a history of cardiac decompensation, hypertension, or other conditions predisposing to fluid retention.

Preexisting asthma

Patients with asthma may have aspirin-sensitive asthma. The use of aspirin in patients with aspirin-sensitive asthma has been associated with severe bronchospasm, which can be fatal. Since cross-reactivity, including bronchospasm, between aspirin and other NSAIDs has been reported in such aspirin-sensitive patients. ARTHROTEC should not be administered to patients with this form of aspirin sensitivity and should be used with caution in patients with preexisting asthma.

Porphyria

The use of ARTHROTEC in patients with hepatic porphyria should be avoided. To date, one patient has been described in whom diclofenac sodium probably triggered a clinical attack of porphyria. The postulated mechanism, demonstrated in rats, for causing such attacks by diclofenac sodium, as well as some other NSAIDs, is through stimulation of the porphyrin precursor delta-aminolevulinic acid (ALA).

Laboratory tests

Patients on long-term treatment with NSAIDs should have their CBC and a chemistry profile checked periodically. If clinical signs and symptoms consistent with liver or renal disease develop, systemic manifestations occur (eg, eosinophilia, rash, etc) or if abnormal liver tests persist or worsen, ARTHROTEC should be discontinued.

Effect on blood coagulation: Diclofenac sodium impairs platelet aggregation but does not affect bleeding time, plasma thrombin clotting time, plasma fibrinogen, or factors V and VII to XII. Statistically significant changes in prothrombin and partial thromboplastin times have been reported in normal volunteers. The mean changes were observed to be less than 1 second in both instances, however, and are unlikely to be clinically important. Diclofenac sodium is a prostaglandin synthetase inhibitor, however, and all drugs that inhibit prostaglandin synthesis interfere with platelet function to some degree; therefore, patients who may be adversely affected by such an action should be carefully observed. Misoprostol has not been shown to exacerbate the effects of diclofenac on platelet activity.

Drug interactions

Aspirin: Concomitant administration of ARTHROTEC and aspirin is not recommended because diclofenac sodium is displaced from its binding sites by aspirin, resulting in lower plasma concentrations, peak plasma levels and AUC values.

Digoxin: Elevated digoxin levels have been reported in patients receiving digoxin and diclofenac sodium. Patients receiving digoxin and ARTHROTEC should be monitored for possible digoxin toxicity.

Antihypertensive agents: NSAIDs can inhibit the activity of antihypertensives, including ACE inhibitors. Thus, caution should be taken when administering ARTHROTEC with such agents.

Warfarin: The effects of warfarin and NSAIDs on GI bleeding are synergistic, such that users of both drugs together have a risk of serious bleeding greater than users of either drug alone.

Oral hypoglycemics: Diclofenac sodium does not alter glucose metabolism in healthy people nor does it alter the effects of oral hypoglycemic agents. There are rare reports, however, from marketing experience, of changes in effects of insulin or oral hypoglycemic agents in the presence of diclofenac sodium that necessitated change in the doses of such agents. Both hypo- and hyperglycemic effects have been reported. A direct causal relationship has not been established, but physicians should consider the possibility that diclofenac sodium may alter a diabetic patient's response to insulin or oral hypoglycemic agents.

Methotrexate and cyclosporine: ARTHROTEC, like other NSAID containing products, may affect renal prostaglandins and increase the toxicity of certain drugs. Ingestion of ARTHROTEC may increase serum concentrations of methotrexate and increase cyclosporine nephrotoxicity. Patients who begin taking ARTHROTEC or who increase their dose of ARTHROTEC or any other NSAID containing product while taking methotrexate or cyclosporine may develop toxicity characteristic for these drugs. They should be observed closely, particularly if renal function is impaired.

Lithium: NSAIDs have produced an elevation of plasma lithium levels and a reduction in renal lithium clearance. The mean minimum lithium concentration increased 15% and the renal clearance was decreased by approximately 20%. These effects have been attributed to inhibition of renal prostaglandin synthesis by the NSAID. Thus, when NSAIDs and lithium are administered concurrently, subjects should be observed carefully for signs of lithium toxicity.

Antacids: Antacids reduce the bioavailability of misoprostol acid. Antacids may also delay absorption of diclofenac sodium. Magnesium-containing antacids exacerbate misoprostol-associated diarrhea. Thus, it is not recommended that ARTHROTEC be coadministered with magnesium-containing antacids.

Diuretics: The diclofenac sodium component of ARTHROTEC, like other NSAIDs, can inhibit the activity of diuretics. Concomitant therapy with potassium-sparing diuretics may be associated with increased serum potassium levels.

Other drugs: In small groups of patients (7–10 patients/interaction study), the concomitant administration of azathioprine, gold, chloroquine, D-penicillamine, prednisolone, doxycycline or digitoxin did not significantly affect the peak levels and AUC levels of diclofenac sodium. Phenobarbital toxicity has been reported to have occurred in a patient on chronic phenobarbital treatment following the initiation of diclofenac therapy. *In vitro*, diclofenac interferes minimally with the protein binding of prednisolone (10% decrease in binding). Benzylpenicillin, ampicillin, oxacillin, chlortetracycline, doxycycline, cephalothin, erythromycin, and sulfamethoxazole have no influence, *in vitro*, on the protein binding of diclofenac in human serum.

Animal toxicology

A reversible increase in the number of normal surface gastric epithelial cells occurred in the dog, rat, and mouse during long-term toxicology studies with misoprostol. No such increase has been observed in humans administered misoprostol for up to 1 year. An apparent response of the female mouse to misoprostol in long-term studies at 100 to 1000 times the human dose was hyperostosis, mainly of the medulla of sternebrae. Hyperostosis did not occur in long-term studies in the dog and rat and has not been seen in humans treated with misoprostol.

Carcinogenesis, mutagenesis, impairment of fertility

Long-term animal studies to evaluate the potential for carcinogenesis and animal studies to evaluate the effects on fertility have been performed with each component of ARTHROTEC given alone. ARTHROTEC itself (diclofenac sodium and misoprostol combinations in 250:1 ratio) was not genotoxic in the Ames test, the Chinese hamster ovary cell (CHO/HGPRT) forward mutation test, the rat lymphocyte chromosome aberration test or the mouse micronucleus test.

In a 24-month rat carcinogenicity study, oral misoprostol at doses up to 2.4 mg/kg/day (14.4 mg/m^2/day, 24 times the recommended maximum human dose of 0.6 mg/m^2/day) was not tumorigenic. In a 21-month mouse carcinogenicity study, oral misoprostol at doses up to 16 mg/kg/day (48 mg/m^2/day), 80 times the recommended maximum human dose based on body surface area, was not tumorigenic. Misoprostol, when administered to male and female breeding rats in an oral dose-range of 0.1 to 10 mg/kg/day (0.6 to 60 mg/m^2/day, 1 to 100 times the recommended maximum human dose based on body surface area) produced dose-related pre- and post-implantation losses and a significant decrease in the number of live pups born at the highest dose. These findings suggest the possibility of a general adverse effect on fertility in males and females.

In a 24-month rat carcinogenicity study, oral diclofenac sodium up to 2 mg/kg/day (12 mg/m^2/day) was not tumorigenic. For a 50-kg person of average height (1.46m^2 body surface area), this dose represents 0.08 times the recommended maximum human dose (148 mg/m^2) on a body surface area basis. In a 24-month mouse carcinogenicity study, oral diclofenac sodium at doses up to 0.3 mg/kg/day (0.9 mg/m^2/day, 0.006 times the recommended maximum human dose based on body surface area) in males and 1 mg/kg/day (3 mg/m^2/day, 0.02 times the recommended maximum human dose based on body surface area) in females was not

Continued on next page

Arthrotec—Cont.

tumorigenic. Diclofenac sodium at oral doses up to 4 mg/kg/day (24 mg/m²/day, 0.16 times the recommended maximum human dose based on body surface area) was found to have no effect on fertility and reproductive performance of male and female rats.

Pregnancy

Pregnancy category X: See boxed ***CONTRAINDICATIONS AND WARNINGS*** regarding misoprostol. ARTHROTEC is contraindicated in pregnancy.

Non-teratogenic effects

Misoprostol may endanger pregnancy (may cause miscarriage) and thereby cause harm to the fetus when administered to a pregnant woman. Misoprostol produces uterine contractions, uterine bleeding, and expulsion of the products of conception. Miscarriages caused by misoprostol may be incomplete. In studies in women undergoing elective termination of pregnancy during the first trimester, misoprostol caused partial or complete expulsion of the products of conception in 11% of the subjects and increased uterine bleeding in 41%.

Reports, primarily from Brazil, of congenital anomalies and reports of fetal death subsequent to misuse of misoprostol alone, as an abortifacient, have been received (see boxed ***CONTRAINDICATIONS AND WARNINGS***). If a woman is or becomes pregnant while taking this drug, the drug should be discontinued and the patient apprised of the potential hazard to the fetus.

The diclofenac sodium component of ARTHROTEC, like other NSAIDs which are prostaglandin-inhibiting drugs, may affect the fetal cardiovascular system causing premature closure of the ductus arteriosus. NSAIDs may also inhibit uterine contractions.

Teratogenic effects

An oral teratology study has been performed in pregnant rabbits at dose combinations (250:1 ratio) up to 10 mg/kg/day diclofenac sodium (120 mg/m²/day, 0.8 times the recommended maximum human dose based on body surface area) and 0.04 mg/kg/day misoprostol (0.48 mg/m²/day, 0.8 times the recommended maximum human dose based on body surface area) and has revealed no evidence of teratogenic potential for ARTHROTEC.

Oral teratology studies have been performed in pregnant rats at doses up to 1.6 mg/kg/day (9.6 mg/m²/day, 16 times the recommended maximum human dose based on body surface area) and pregnant rabbits at doses up to 1.0 mg/kg/day (12 mg/m²/day, 20 times the recommended maximum human dose based on body surface area) and have revealed no evidence of teratogenic potential for misoprostol.

Oral teratology studies have been performed in pregnant mice at doses up to 20 mg/kg/day (60 mg/m²/day, 0.4 times the recommended maximum human dose based on body surface area), pregnant rats at doses up to 10 mg/kg/day (60 mg/m²/day. 0.4 times the recommended maximum human dose based on body surface area) and pregnant rabbits at doses up to 10 mg/kg/day (120 mg/m²/day, 0.8 times the recommended maximum human dose based on body surface area) and have revealed no evidence of teratogenic potential for diclofenac sodium.

Nursing mothers

Diclofenac sodium has been found in the milk of nursing mothers. It is unlikely that misoprostol is excreted into milk since the drug is rapidly metabolized throughout the body. Excretion of the active metabolite (misoprostol acid) into milk is possible, but has not been studied. Because of the potential for serious adverse reactions in nursing infants, ARTHROTEC is not recommended for use by nursing mothers.

Pediatric use

Safety and efficacy of ARTHROTEC in patients below the age of 18 years have not been established.

Geriatric use

Approximately 1800 patients treated with diclofenac in U.S. trials and 500 patients treated with ARTHROTEC in multinational trials were older than 65 years of age. No overall differences were observed between efficacy, adverse events or pharmacokinetic profiles of older and younger patients. However, as with any NSAID, the elderly are likely to tolerate adverse events less well than younger patients.

ADVERSE REACTIONS

Adverse reactions associated with ARTHROTEC

Adverse reaction information for ARTHROTEC is derived from Phase III multinational controlled clinical trials in over 2,000 patients receiving ARTHROTEC 50 or ARTHROTEC 75, as well as from blinded, controlled trials of Voltaren® Delayed-Release Tablets (diclofenac) and Cytotec® Tablets (misoprostol).

Gastrointestinal

GI disorders had the highest reported incidence of adverse events for patients receiving ARTHROTEC. These events were generally minor, but let to discontinuation of therapy in 9% of patients on ARTHROTEC and 5% of patients on diclofenac. For GI ulcer rates, see *CLINICAL STUDIES—Upper gastrointestinal safety.*

GI disorder	ARTHROTEC	Diclofenac
Abdominal pain	21%	15%
Diarrhea	19%	11%
Dyspepsia	14%	11%
Nausea	11%	6%
Flatulence	9%	4%

ARTHROTEC can cause more abdominal pain, diarrhea and other GI symptoms than diclofenac alone.

Diarrhea and abdominal pain developed early in the course of therapy, and were usually self-limited (resolved after 2 to 7 days). Rare instances of profound diarrhea leading to severe dehydration have been reported in patients receiving misoprostol. Patients with an underlying condition such as inflammatory bowel disease, or those in whom dehydration, were it to occur, would be dangerous, should be monitored carefully if ARTHROTEC is prescribed. The incidence of diarrhea can be minimized by administering ARTHROTEC with food and by avoiding coadministration with magnesium-containing antacids.

Gynecological

Gynecological disorders previously reported with misoprostol use have also been reported for women receiving ARTHROTEC (see below). Postmenopausal vaginal bleeding may be related to ARTHROTEC administration. If it occurs, diagnostic workup should be undertaken to rule out gynecological pathology.

Elderly

Overall, there were no significant differences in the safety profile of ARTHROTEC in over 500 patients 65 years of age or older compared with younger patients.

Other adverse experiences reported occasionally or rarely with ARTHROTEC, diclofenac or other NSAIDs, or misoprostol are:

Body as a Whole: Asthenia, death, fatigue, fever, infection, malaise, sepsis.

Cardiovascular system: Arrhythmia, atrial fibrillation, congestive heart failure, hypertension, hypotension, increased CPK, increased LDH, myocardial infarction, palpitations, phlebitis, premature ventricular contractions, syncope, tachycardia, vasculitis.

Central and peripheral nervous system: Coma, convulsions, diplopia, drowsiness, hyperesthesia, hypertonia, hypoesthesia, meningitis, migraine, neuralgia, paresthesia, tremor, vertigo.

Digestive: Anorexia, dry mouth, dysphagia, enteritis, esophageal ulceration, gastroesophageal reflux, GI bleeding, GI neoplasm benign, glossitis, hematemesis, hemorrhoids, intestinal perforation, peptic ulcer, stomatitis and ulcerative stomatitis, tenesmus.

Female reproductive disorders: Breast pain, dysmenorrhea, intermenstrual bleeding, leukorrhea, menstrual disorder, menorrhagia, vaginal hemorrhage.

Hemic and lymphatic system: Agranulocytosis, aplastic anemia, coagulation time increased, ecchymosis, eosinophilia, epistaxis, hemolytic anemia, leukocytosis, leukopenia, lymphadenopathy, melena, pulmonary embolism, purpura, pancytopenia, rectal bleeding, thrombocythemia, thrombocytopenia.

Hypersensitivity: Angioedema, laryngeal/pharyngeal edema, urticaria.

Liver and biliary system: Abnormal hepatic function, bilirubinemia, hepatitis, jaundice, liver failure, pancreatitis.

Male reproductive disorders: Impotence, perineal pain.

Metabolic and nutritional: Alkaline phosphatase increased, BUN increased, dehydration, glycosuria, gout, hypercholesterolemia, hyperglycemia, hyperuricemia, hypoglycemia, hyponatremia, periorbital edema, porphyria, weight changes.

Musculoskeletal system: Arthralgia, myalgia.

Psychiatric: Anxiety, asthenia, concentration impaired, confusion, depression, disorientation, dream abnormalities, hallucinations, irritability, malaise, nervousness, paranoia, psychotic reaction, somnolence.

Respiratory system: Asthma, coughing, dyspnea, hyperventilation, pneumonia, respiratory depression.

Skin and appendages: Acne, alopecia, bruising, erythema multiforme, eczema, exfoliative dermatitis, pemphigoid reaction, photosensitivity, pruritus ani, skin ulceration, Stevens-Johnson syndrome, sweating increased, toxic epidermal necrolysis.

Special senses: Hearing impairment, taste loss, taste perversion.

Urinary system: Cystitis, dysuria, hematuria, interstitial nephritis, micturition frequency, nocturia, nephrotic syndrome, oliguria/polyuria, papillary necrosis, proteinuria, renal failure, urinary tract infection.

Vision: Amblyopia, blurred vision, conjunctivitis, glaucoma, iritis, lacrimation abnormal, night blindness, vision abnormal.

OVERDOSAGE

The toxic dose of ARTHROTEC has not been determined. However, signs of overdosage from the components of the product have been described.

Diclofenac sodium

Clinical signs that may suggest diclofenac sodium overdose include GI complaints, confusion, drowsiness or general hypotonia. Reports of overdosage with diclofenac cover 66 cases. In approximately one-half of these reports of overdosage, concomitant medications were also taken. The highest dose of diclofenac was 5.0 g in a 17-year-old man who suffered loss of consciousness, increased intracranial pressure, and aspiration pneumonitis, and died 2 days after overdose. A 24-year-old woman who took 4.0 g and the 28- and 42-year-old women, each of whom took 3.75 g, did not develop any clinically significant signs or symptoms. However, there was a report of a 17-year-old female who experienced vomiting and drowsiness after an overdose of 2.37 g of diclofenac.

Animal studies show a wide range of susceptibilities to acute overdosage, with primates being more resistant to acute toxicity than rodents (LD_{50} in mg/kg: rats, 55; dogs, 500; monkeys, 3200).

Misoprostol

The toxic dose of misoprostol in humans has not been determined. Cumulative total daily doses of 1600 mcg have been tolerated, with only symptoms of GI discomfort being reported. In animals, the acute toxic effects are diarrhea, GI lesions, focal cardiac necrosis, hepatic necrosis, renal tubular necrosis, testicular atrophy, respiratory difficulties, and depression of the central nervous system. Clinical signs that may indicate an overdose are sedation, tremor, convulsions, dyspnea, abdominal pain, diarrhea, fever, palpitations, hypotension, or bradycardia.

ARTHROTEC

Symptoms of ARTHROTEC overdosage should be treated with supportive therapy. In case of acute overdosage, gastric lavage is recommended. Induced diuresis may be beneficial because diclofenac sodium and misoprostol metabolites are excreted in the urine. The effect of dialysis or hemoperfusion on the elimination of diclofenac sodium (99% protein bound) and misoprostol acid remains unproven. The use of oral activated charcoal may help to reduce the absorption of diclofenac sodium and misoprostol.

DOSAGE AND ADMINISTRATION

ARTHROTEC is administered as ARTHROTEC 50 (50 mg diclofenac sodium/200 mcg misoprostol) or as ARTHROTEC 75 (75 mg diclofenac sodium/200 mcg misoprostol).

Note: See *SPECIAL DOSING CONSIDERATIONS* section, below.

Osteoarthritis: The recommended dosage for maximal GI mucosal protection is ARTHROTEC 50 tid. For patients who experience intolerance, ARTHROTEC 75 bid or ARTHROTEC 50 bid can be used, but are less effective in preventing ulcers. This fixed combination product, ARTHROTEC, is not appropriate for patients who would not receive the appropriate dose of both ingredients. Doses of the components delivered with these regimens are as follows:

	OA regimen	Diclofenac sodium (mg/day)	Misoprostol (mcg/day)
ARTHROTEC 50	tid	150	600
	bid	100	400
ARTHROTEC 75	bid	150	400

Rheumatoid Arthritis: The recommended dosage is ARTHROTEC 50 tid or qid. For patients who experience intolerance, ARTHROTEC 75 bid or ARTHROTEC 50 bid can be used, but are less effective in preventing ulcers. This fixed combination product, ARTHROTEC, is not appropriate for patients who would not receive the appropriate dose of both ingredients. Doses of the components delivered with these regimens are as follows:

	RA regimen	Diclofenac sodium (mg/day)	Misoprostol (mcg/day)
ARTHROTEC 50	qid	200	800
	tid	150	600
	bid	100	400
ARTHROTEC 75	bid	150	400

SPECIAL DOSING CONSIDERATIONS: ARTHROTEC contains misoprostol, which provides protection against gastric and duodenal ulcers (see *CLINICAL STUDIES*). For gastric ulcer prevention, the 200 mcg qid and tid regimens are therapeutically equivalent, but more protective than the bid regimen. For duodenal ulcer prevention, the qid regimen is more protective than the tid or bid regimens. However, the

qid regimen is less well tolerated than the tid regimen because of usually self-limited diarrhea related to the misoprostol dose (see *ADVERSE REACTIONS—Gastrointestinal*), and the bid regimen may be better tolerated than tid in some patients.

Dosages may be individualized using the separate products (misoprostol and diclofenac), after which the patient may be changed to the appropriate ARTHROTEC dose. If clinically indicated, misoprostol co-therapy with ARTHROTEC, or use of the individual components to optimize the misoprostol dose and/or frequency of administration, may be appropriate. The total dose of misoprostol should not exceed 800 mcg/day, and no more than 200 mcg of misoprostol should be administered at any one time. Doses of diclofenac higher than 150 mcg/day in osteoarthritis or higher than 225 mg/day in rheumatoid arthritis are not recommended.
For additional information, it may be helpful to refer to the package inserts for Cytotec® tablets and Voltaren® tablets.

HOW SUPPLIED

ARTHROTEC (diclofenac sodium/misoprostol) is supplied as a film-coated tablet in dosage strengths of either 50 mg diclofenac sodium/200 mcg misoprostol or 75 mg diclofenac sodium/200 mcg misoprostol. The 50 mg/200 mcg dosage strength is a round, biconvex, white to off-white tablet imprinted with four "A's" encircling a "50" in the middle on one side and "SEARLE" and "1411" on the other. The 75 mg/200 mcg dosage strength is a round, biconvex, white to off-white tablet imprinted with four "A's" encircling a "75" in the middle on one side and "SEARLE" and "1421" on the other.
The dosage strengths are supplied in:

Strength	NDC Number	Size
50/200	0025-1411-60	bottle of 60
	0025-1411-90	bottle of 90
75/200	0025-1421-60	bottle of 60

Store at or below 25°C (77°F), in a dry area.
Caution: Federal law prohibits dispensing without prescription.

PATIENT INFORMATION

Read this leaflet before taking ARTHROTEC (diclofenac sodium 50 or 75 mg/misoprostol 200 mcg) and each time your prescription is renewed, because the leaflet may be changed.
ARTHROTEC is being prescribed by your doctor for treatment of your arthritis symptoms while at the same time providing protection from the development of stomach and intestinal ulcers due to the arthritis medication. ARTHROTEC contains diclofenac, an arthritis medication. ARTHROTEC also contains misoprostol to decrease the chance of getting stomach and intestinal ulcers that sometimes develop with NSAID medications. Serious side effects are still possible, however, and you should report to your physician any signs or symptoms of gastrointestinal ulceration or bleeding, skin rash, weight gain or swelling. If signs of liver toxicity occur (nausea, fatigue, lethargy, itching, jaundice, right upper quadrant tenderness, and "flu-like" symptoms) you should stop therapy and seek immediate medical attention.
Do not take ARTHROTEC if you are pregnant and do not become pregnant while taking this medication. ARTHROTEC can cause miscarriage, often associated with potentially dangerous bleeding. Such miscarriages may result in hospitalization, surgery, infertility or death.
If you become pregnant during ARTHROTEC therapy, stop taking ARTHROTEC and contact your doctor immediately. Remember that even if you are using a means of birth control, it is still possible to become pregnant. Should this occur, stop taking ARTHROTEC and consult your physician immediately.
ARTHROTEC may cause diarrhea, abdominal pain, upset stomach and/or nausea in some people. In most cases these problems develop during the first few weeks of therapy and stop after about a week with continued treatment. You can minimize possible diarrhea by making sure you take ARTHROTEC with meals and by avoiding the use of antacids containing magnesium (if needed, use one containing aluminum or calcium instead). ARTHROTEC tablets should be swallowed whole, and not chewed, crushed or dissolved.
Because these side effects are usually mild to moderate and usually go away in a matter of days, most patients can continue to take ARTHROTEC. If you have prolonged difficulty (more than 7 days), or if you have severe diarrhea, cramping and/or nausea, call your doctor.
Take ARTHROTEC only according to the directions given by your doctor. Changes in dose should be made only with your doctor's approval.
Do not give ARTHROTEC to anyone else. It has been prescribed for your specific condition, may not be the correct treatment for another person, and could be dangerous for another person, especially a woman who may be, or could become, pregnant.
This information sheet does not cover all possible side effects of ARTHROTEC. See your doctor if you have questions.

Keep out of reach of children.

Revised: Dec. 30, 1997

Packaged by G.D. Searle & Co.
Manufactured by Searle, Morpeth, England
For G.D. Searle Inter-American Co.
Chicago IL 60680 USA

Address medical inquiries to:
G.D. Searle & Co.
Healthcare Information Services
5200 Old Orchard Road
Skokie IL 60077

SEARLE

©1997, G.D. Searle & Co.

A05440-1

Shown in Product Identification Guide, page 337

BREVICON®21-DAY Tablets ℞
(norethindrone and
   ethinyl estradiol)

BREVICON® 28-DAY Tablets ℞
(norethindrone and
   ethinyl estradiol)

NORINYL® 1 + 35 21-DAY Tablets ℞
(norethindrone and
   ethinyl estradiol)

NORINYL® 1 + 35 28-DAY Tablets ℞
(norethindrone and
   ethinyl estradiol))

NORINYL® 1 + 50 21-DAY Tablets ℞
(norethindrone and mestranol)

NORINYL® 1 + 50 28-DAY Tablets ℞
(norethindrone and mestranol)

PHYSICIAN LABELING

Patients should be counseled that this product does not protect against HIV infection (AIDS) and other sexually transmitted diseases.

ORAL CONTRACEPTIVE AGENTS

DESCRIPTION

BREVICON 21-DAY Tablets provide an oral contraceptive regimen consisting of 21 blue tablets containing norethindrone 0.5 mg and ethinyl estradiol 0.035 mg.
BREVICON 28-DAY Tablets provide a continuous oral contraceptive regimen consisting of 21 blue tablets containing norethindrone 0.5 mg and ethinyl estradiol 0.035 mg and 7 orange tablets containing inert ingredients.
NORINYL 1 + 35 21-DAY Tablets provide an oral contraceptive regimen consisting of 21 yellow-green tablets containing norethindrone 1 mg and ethinyl estradiol 0.035 mg.
NORINYL 1 + 35 28-DAY Tablets provide a continuous oral contraceptive regimen consisting of 21 yellow-green tablets containing norethindrone 1 mg and ethinyl estradiol 0.035 mg followed by 7 orange tablets containing inert ingredients.
NORINYL 1 + 50 21-DAY Tablets provide an oral contraceptive regimen consisting of 21 white tablets containing norethindrone 1 mg and mestranol 0.05 mg.
NORINYL 1 + 50 28-DAY Tablets provide a continuous oral contraceptive regimen consisting of 21 white tablets containing norethindrone 1 mg and mestranol 0.05 mg and 7 orange tablets containing inert ingredients.
Norethindrone is a potent progestational agent with the chemical name 17-Hydroxy-19-Nor-17α-pregn-4-en-20-yn-3-one. Ethinyl estradiol is an estrogen with the chemical name 19-nor-17α-pregna-1, 3, 5(10) -trien-20-yne-3, 17-diol. Mestranol is an estrogen with the chemical name 3-Methoxy-19-nor-17α-pregna-1, 3, 5(10) -trien-20-yn-17-ol. Their structural formulae follow:

norethindrone

ethinyl estradiol

[See chemical structure at top of next column]

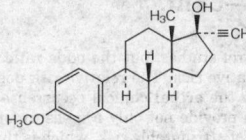

mestranol

The blue BREVICON tablets contain the following inactive ingredients: FD&C Blue No. 1, lactose, magnesium stearate, povidone, and starch.
The yellow-green NORINYL 1 + 35 tablets contain the following inactive ingredients: D&C Green No. 5, D&C Yellow No. 10, lactose, magnesium stearate, povidone, and starch.
The white NORINYL 1 + 50 tablets contain the following inactive ingredients: lactose, magnesium stearate, povidone, and starch.
The inactive orange tablets in the 28-day regimens of BREVICON, NORINYL 1 + 35 and NORINYL 1 + 50 contain the following ingredients: FD&C Yellow No. 6, lactose, magnesium stearate, povidone and starch.

CLINICAL PHARMACOLOGY

Combination oral contraceptives act by suppression of gonadotrophins. Although the primary mechanism of this action is inhibition of ovulation, other alterations include changes in the cervical mucus (which increase the difficulty of sperm entry into the uterus) and the endometrium (which may reduce the likelihood of implantation).

INDICATIONS AND USAGE

Oral contraceptives are indicated for the prevention of pregnancy in women who elect to use these products as a method of contraception.
Oral contraceptives are highly effective. Table I lists the typical accidental pregnancy rates for users of combination oral contraceptives and other methods of contraception.[1] The efficacy of these contraceptive methods, except sterilization, depends upon the reliability with which they are used. Correct and consistent use of methods can result in lower failure rates.
[See table I at top of next page]

CONTRAINDICATIONS

Oral contraceptives should not be used in women who have the following conditions:
• Thrombophlebitis or thromboembolic disorders
• A past history of deep vein thrombophlebitis or thromboembolic disorders
• Cerebral vascular or coronary artery disease
• Known or suspected carcinoma of the breast
• Carcinoma of the endometrium, or other known or suspected estrogen-dependent neoplasia
• Undiagnosed abnormal genital bleeding
• Cholestatic jaundice of pregnancy or jaundice with prior pill use
• Hepatic adenomas, carcinomas or benign liver tumors
• Known or suspected pregnancy

WARNINGS

> **Cigarette smoking increases the risk of serious cardiovascular side effects from oral contraceptive use. This risk increases with age and with heavy smoking (15 or more cigarettes per day) and is quite marked in women over 35 years of age. Women who use oral contraceptives are strongly advised not to smoke.**

The use of oral contraceptives is associated with increased risks of several serious conditions including myocardial infarction, thromboembolism, stroke, hepatic neoplasia and gallbladder disease, although the risk of serious morbidity or mortality is very small in healthy women without underlying risk factors. The risk of morbidity and mortality increases significantly in the presence of other underlying risk factors such as hypertension, hyperlipidemias, hypercholesterolemia, obesity and diabetes.[2-5]

Practitioners prescribing oral contraceptives should be familiar with the following information relating to these risks.

The information contained in this package insert is principally based on studies carried out in patients who used oral contraceptives with higher formulations of both estrogens and progestogens than those in common use today. The effect of long-term use of the oral contraceptives with lower formulations of both estrogens and progestogens remains to be determined.
Throughout this labeling, epidemiological studies reported are of two types: retrospective or case control studies and prospective or cohort studies. Case control studies provide a measure of the relative risk of a disease. Relative risk, the *ratio* of the incidence of a disease among oral contraceptive users to that among non-users, cannot be assessed directly

Continued on next page

Brevicon—Cont.

from case control studies, but the odds ratio obtained is a measure of relative risk. The relative risk does not provide information on the actual clinical occurrence of a disease. Cohort studies provide not only a measure of relative risk but a measure of attributable risk, which is the *difference* in the incidence of disease between oral contraceptive users and non-users. The attributable risk does provide information about the actual occurrence of a disease in the population. (Adapted from ref. 12 and 13 with the author's permission.) For further information, the reader is referred to a text on epidemiological methods.

1. THROMBOEMBOLIC DISORDERS AND OTHER VASCULAR PROBLEMS

a. Myocardial Infarction

An increased risk of myocardial infarction has been attributed to oral contraceptive use. This risk is primarily in smokers or women with other underlying risk factors for coronary artery disease such as hypertension, hypercholesterolemia, morbid obesity and diabetes.[2–5,13] The relative risk of heart attack for current oral contraceptive users has been estimated to be 2 to 6.[2,14–19] The risk is very low under the age of 30. However, there is the possibility of a risk of cardiovascular disease even in very young women who take oral contraceptives.

Smoking in combination with oral contraceptive use has been shown to contribute substantially to the incidence of myocardial infarctions in women in their mid-thirties or older, with smoking accounting for the majority of excess cases.[20]

Mortality rates associated with circulatory disease have been shown to increase substantially in smokers over the age of 35 and non-smokers over the age of 40 among women who use oral contraceptives (see Table II).[16]

TABLE II: CIRCULATORY DISEASE MORTALITY RATES PER 100,000 WOMAN YEARS BY AGE, SMOKING STATUS AND ORAL CONTRACEPTIVE USE

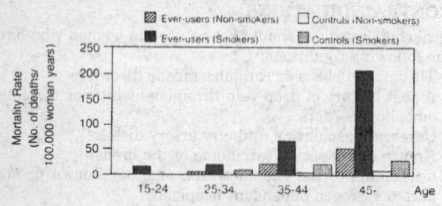

Adapted from P.M. Layde and V. Beral, Table V[16]

Oral contraceptives may compound the effects of well-known risk factors such as hypertension, diabetes, hyperlipidemias, hypercholesterolemia, age and obesity.[3,13,21] In particular, some progestogens are known to decrease HDL cholesterol and cause oral glucose intolerance, while estrogens may create a state of hyperinsulinism.[21–25] Oral contraceptives have been shown to increase blood pressure among users (see **WARNINGS**, section 9). Similar effects on risk factors have been associated with an increased risk of heart disease. Oral contraceptives must be used with caution in women with cardiovascular disease risk factors.

b. Thromboembolism

An increased risk of thromboembolic and thrombotic disease associated with the use of oral contraceptives is well established. Case control studies have found the relative risk of users compared to non-users to be 3 for the first episode of superficial venous thrombosis, 4 to 11 for deep vein thrombosis or pulmonary embolism, and 1.5 to 6 for women with predisposing conditions for venous thromboembolic disease.[12,13,26–31] Cohort studies have shown the relative risk to be somewhat lower, about 3 for new cases and about 4.5 for new cases requiring hospitalization.[32] The risk of thromboembolic disease due to oral contraceptives is not related to length of use and disappears after pill use is stopped.[12]

A 2- to 6-fold increase in relative risk of post-operative thromboembolic complications has been reported with the use of oral contraceptives. The relative risk of venous thrombosis in women who have predisposing conditions is twice that of women without such medical conditions.[83] If feasible, oral contraceptives should be discontinued at least 4 weeks prior to and for 2 weeks after elective surgery and during and following prolonged immobilization. Since the immediate postpartum period also is associated with an increased risk of thromboembolism, oral contraceptives should be started no earlier than 4 to 6 weeks after delivery in women who elect not to breast feed.[33]

TABLE I: PERCENTAGE OF WOMEN EXPERIENCING A CONTRACEPTIVE FAILURE DURING THE FIRST YEAR OF PERFECT USE AND FIRST YEAR OF TYPICAL USE

Method	% of Women Experiencing an Accidental Pregnancy within the First Year of Use	
	Typical Use[a]	Perfect Use[b]
Chance	85	85
Spermicides	21	6
Periodic abstinence	20	1-9
Withdrawal	19	4
Cap		
Parous	36	26
Nulliparous	18	9
Sponge		
Parous	36	20
Nulliparous	18	9
Diaphragm	18	6
Condom		
Female	21	5
Male	12	3
Pill	3	
Progestin only		0.5
Combined		0.1
IUD		
Progesterone	2	1.5
Copper T380A	0.8	0.6
Injection (Depo-Provera)	0.3	0.3
Implants (Norplant)	0.09	0.09
Female sterilization	0.4	0.4
Male sterilization	0.15	0.10

Adapted with permission[1]

[a]Among *typical* couples who initiate use of a method (not necessarily for the first time), the percentage who experience an accidental pregnancy during the first year if they do not stop use for any other reason.

[b]Among couples who initiate use of a method (not necessarily for the first time) and who use it *perfectly* (both consistently and correctly), the percentage who experience an accidental pregnancy during the first year if they do not stop use for any other reason.

c. Cerebrovascular diseases

An increase in both the relative and attributable risks of cerebrovascular events (thrombotic and hemorrhagic strokes) has been shown in users of oral contraceptives. In general, the risk is greatest among older (>35 years), hypertensive women who also smoke. Hypertension was found to be a risk factor for both users and non-users for both types of strokes while smoking interacted to increase the risk for hemorrhagic strokes.[34]

In a large study, the relative risk of thrombotic strokes has been shown to range from 3 for normotensive users to 14 for users with severe hypertension.[35] The relative risk of hemorrhagic stroke is reported to be 1.2 for non-smokers who used oral contraceptives, 2.6 for smokers who did not use oral contraceptives, 7.6 for smokers who used oral contraceptives, 1.8 for normotensive users and 25.7 for users with severe hypertension.[35] The attributable risk also is greater in women in their mid-thirties or older and among smokers.[13]

d. Dose-related risk of vascular disease from oral contraceptives

A positive association has been observed between the amount of estrogen and progestogen in oral contraceptives and the risk of vascular disease.[36–38] A decline in serum high density lipoproteins (HDL) has been reported with many progestational agents.[22–24] A decline in serum high density lipoproteins has been associated with an increased incidence of ischemic heart disease.[39] Because estrogens increase HDL cholesterol, the net effect of an oral contraceptive depends on a balance achieved between doses of estrogen and progestogen and the nature and absolute amount of progestogens used in the contraceptives. The amount of both hormones should be considered in the choice of an oral contraceptive.[37]

Minimizing exposure to estrogen and progestogen is in keeping with good principles of therapeutics. For any particular estrogen/progestogen combination, the dosage regimen prescribed should be one which contains the least amount of estrogen and progestogen that is compatible with a low failure rate and the needs of the individual patient. New acceptors of oral contraceptive agents should be started on preparations containing the lowest estrogen content that produces satisfactory results for the individual.

e. Persistence of risk of vascular disease

There are three studies which have shown persistence of risk of vascular disease for ever-users of oral contraceptives.[17,34,40] In a study in the United States, the risk of developing myocardial infarction after discontinuing oral contraceptives persists for at least 9 years for women 40–49 years who had used oral contraceptives for 5 or more years, but this increased risk was not demonstrated in other age groups.[17] In another study in Great Britain, the risk of developing cerebrovascular disease persisted for at least 6 years after discontinuation of oral contraceptives, although excess risk was very small.[40] There is a significantly in-

creased risk of subarachnoid hemorrhage after termination of use of oral contraceptives.[34] However, these studies were performed with oral contraceptive formulations containing 50 µg or higher of estrogen.

2. ESTIMATES OF MORTALITY FROM CONTRACEPTIVE USE

One study gathered data from a variety of sources which have estimated the mortality rates associated with different methods of contraception at different ages (see Table III).[41] These estimates include the combined risk of death associated with contraceptive methods plus the risk attributable to pregnancy in the event of method failure. Each method of contraception has its specific benefits and risks. The study concluded that with the exception of oral contraceptive users 35 and older who smoke and 40 and older who do not smoke, mortality associated with all methods of birth control is low and below that associated with childbirth. The observation of a possible increase in risk of mortality with age for oral contraceptive users is based on data gathered in the 1970's—but not reported in the U.S. until 1983.[16,41] However, current clinical practice involves the use of lower estrogen dose formulations combined with careful restriction of oral contraceptive use to women who do not have the various risk factors listed in this labeling.

Because of these changes in practice and, also, because of some limited new data which suggest that the risk of cardiovascular disease with the use of oral contraceptives may now be less than previously observed,[78,79] the Fertility and Maternal Health Drugs Advisory Committee was asked to review the topic in 1989. The Committee concluded that although cardiovascular disease risks may be increased with oral contraceptive use after age 40 in healthy non-smoking women (even with the newer low-dose formulations), there are greater potential health risks associated with pregnancy in older women and with the alternative surgical and medical procedures which may be necessary if such women do not have access to effective and acceptable means of contraception.

Therefore, the Committee recommended that the benefits of oral contraceptive use by healthy non-smoking women over 40 may outweigh the possible risks. Of course, older women, as all women who take oral contraceptives, should take the lowest possible dose formulation that is effective.[80]

[See table III at bottom of next page]

3. CARCINOMA OF THE BREAST AND REPRODUCTIVE ORGANS

Numerous epidemiological studies have been performed on the incidence of breast, endometrial, ovarian and cervical cancer in women using oral contraceptives. The overwhelming evidence in the literature suggests that use of oral contraceptives is not associated with an increase in the risk of developing breast cancer, regardless of the age and parity of first use or with most of the marketed brands and doses.[42–44] The Cancer and Steroid Hormone (CASH) study also showed no latent effect on the risk of breast cancer for at least a decade following long-term use.[43] A few studies

have shown a slightly increased relative risk of developing breast cancer,[44–47] although the methodology of these studies, which included differences in examination of users and non-users and differences in age at start of use, has been questioned.[47–49] Some studies have reported an increased relative risk of developing breast cancer, particularly at a younger age. This increased relative risk appears to be related to duration of use.[81,82]

Some studies suggest that oral contraceptive use has been associated with an increase in the risk of cervical intraepithelial neoplasia in some populations of women.[50–53] However, there continues to be controversy about the extent to which such findings may be due to differences in sexual behavior and other factors.

In spite of many studies of the relationship between oral contraceptive use and breast or cervical cancers, a cause and effect relationship has not been established.

4. HEPATIC NEOPLASIA

Benign hepatic adenomas are associated with oral contraceptive use although the incidence of benign tumors is rare in the United States. Indirect calculations have estimated the attributable risk to be in the range of 3.3 cases per 100,000 for users, a risk that increases after 4 or more years of use.[54] Rupture of rare, benign, hepatic adenomas may cause death through intra-abdominal hemorrhage.[55–56]

Studies in the United States and Britain have shown an increased risk of developing hepatocellular carcinoma in long-term (>8 years) oral contraceptive users.[57–59] However, these cancers are extremely rare in the United States and the attributable risk (the excess incidence) of liver cancers in oral contraceptive users is less than 1 per 1,000,000 users.

5. OCULAR LESIONS

There have been clinical case reports of retinal thrombosis associated with the use of oral contraceptives. Oral contraceptives should be discontinued if there is unexplained partial or complete loss of vision; onset of proptosis or diplopia; papilledema; or retinal vascular lesions. Appropriate diagnostic and therapeutic measures should be undertaken immediately.

6. ORAL CONTRACEPTIVE USE BEFORE OR DURING EARLY PREGNANCY

Extensive epidemiological studies have revealed no increased risk of birth defects in women who have used oral contraceptives prior to pregnancy.[60–62] Studies also do not suggest a teratogenic effect, particularly insofar as cardiac anomalies and limb reduction defects are concerned, when taken inadvertently during early pregnancy.[60,61,63,64]

The administration of oral contraceptives to induce withdrawal bleeding should not be used as a test for pregnancy. Oral contraceptives should not be used during pregnancy to treat threatened or habitual abortion.

It is recommended that for any patient who has missed 2 consecutive periods, pregnancy should be ruled out before continuing oral contraceptive use. If the patient has not adhered to the prescribed schedule, the possibility of pregnancy should be considered at the time of the first missed period. Oral contraceptive use should be discontinued if pregnancy is confirmed.

7. GALLBLADDER DISEASE

Earlier studies have reported an increased lifetime relative risk of gallbladder surgery in users of oral contraceptives and estrogens.[65–66] More recent studies, however, have shown that the relative risk of developing gallbladder disease among oral contraceptive users may be minimal.[67] The recent findings of minimal risk may be related to the use of oral contraceptive formulations containing lower hormonal doses of estrogens and progestogens.[68]

8. CARBOHYDRATE AND LIPID METABOLIC EFFECTS

Oral contraceptives have been shown to cause glucose intolerance in a significant percentage of users.[25] Oral contraceptives containing greater than 75 µg of estrogen cause hyperinsulinism, while lower doses of estrogen cause less glucose intolerance.[70] Progestogens increase insulin secretion and create insulin resistance, this effect varying with different progestational agents.[25,71] However, in the non-diabetic woman, oral contraceptives appear to have no effect on fasting blood glucose.[69] Because of these demonstrated effects, prediabetic and diabetic women should be carefully observed while taking oral contraceptives.

Some women may develop persistent hypertriglyceridemia while on the pill.[72] As discussed earlier (see **WARNINGS,** sections 1a. and 1d.), changes in serum triglycerides and lipoprotein levels have been reported in oral contraceptive users.[23]

9. ELEVATED BLOOD PRESSURE

An increase in blood pressure has been reported in women taking oral contraceptives and this increase is more likely in older oral contraceptive users and with continued use.[73,84] Data from the Royal College of General Practitioners and subsequent randomized trials have shown that the incidence of hypertension increases with increasing concentrations of progestogens.

Women with a history of hypertension or hypertension-related diseases or renal disease should be encouraged to use another method of contraception. If women elect to use oral contraceptives, they should be monitored closely and if significant elevation of blood pressure occurs oral contraceptives should be discontinued. For most women, elevated blood pressure will return to normal after stopping oral contraceptives and there is no difference in the occurrence of hypertension among ever- and never-users.[73–75]

10. HEADACHE

The onset or exacerbation of migraine or development of headache with a new pattern which is recurrent, persistent or severe requires discontinuation of oral contraceptives and evaluation of the cause.

11. BLEEDING IRREGULARITIES

Breakthrough bleeding and spotting are sometimes encountered in patients on oral contraceptives, especially during the first 3 months of use. Non-hormonal causes should be considered and adequate diagnostic measures taken to rule out malignancy or pregnancy in the event of breakthrough bleeding, as in the case of any abnormal vaginal bleeding. If pathology has been excluded, time or a change to another formulation may solve the problem. In the event of amenorrhea, pregnancy should be ruled out.

Some women may encounter post-pill amenorrhea or oligomenorrhea, especially when such a condition was pre- existent.

PRECAUTIONS

GENERAL

Patients should be counseled that this product does not protect against HIV infection (AIDS) and other sexually transmitted diseases.

1. PHYSICAL EXAMINATION AND FOLLOW-UP

It is good medical practice for all women to have annual history and physical examinations, including women using oral contraceptives. The physical examination, however, may be deferred until after initiation of oral contraceptives if requested by the woman and judged appropriate by the clinician. The physical examination should include special reference to blood pressure, breasts, abdomen and pelvic organs, including cervical cytology, and relevant laboratory tests. In case of undiagnosed, persistent or recurrent abnormal vaginal bleeding, appropriate measures should be conducted to rule out malignancy. Women with a strong family history of breast cancer or who have breast nodules should be monitored with particular care.

2. LIPID DISORDERS

Women who are being treated for hyperlipidemias should be followed closely if they elect to use oral contraceptives. Some progestogens may elevate LDL levels and may render the control of hyperlipidemias more difficult.

3. LIVER FUNCTION

If jaundice develops in any woman receiving oral contraceptives the medication should be discontinued. Steroid hormones may be poorly metabolized in patients with impaired liver function.

TABLE III: ESTIMATED ANNUAL NUMBER OF BIRTH-RELATED OR METHOD-RELATED DEATHS ASSOCIATED WITH CONTROL OF FERTILITY PER 100,000 NONSTERILE WOMEN, BY FERTILITY CONTROL METHOD ACCORDING TO AGE

Method of control and outcome	15–19	20–24	25–29	30–34	35–39	40–44
No fertility control methods*	7.0	7.4	9.1	14.8	25.7	28.2
Oral contraceptives non-smoker**	0.3	0.5	0.9	1.9	13.8	31.6
Oral contraceptives smoker**	2.2	3.4	6.6	13.5	51.1	117.2
IUD**	0.8	0.8	1.0	1.0	1.4	1.4
Condom*	1.1	1.6	0.7	0.2	0.3	0.4
Diaphragm/Spermicide*	1.9	1.2	1.2	1.3	2.2	2.8
Periodic abstinence*	2.5	1.6	1.6	1.7	2.9	3.6

* Deaths are birth-related

** Deaths are method-related

Estimates adapted from H.W. Ory, Table 3[41]

4. FLUID RETENTION

Oral contraceptives may cause some degree of fluid retention. They should be prescribed with caution, and only with careful monitoring, in patients with conditions which might be aggravated by fluid retention.

5. EMOTIONAL DISORDERS

Women with a history of depression should be carefully observed and the drug discontinued if depression recurs to a serious degree.

6. CONTACT LENSES

Contact lens wearers who develop visual changes or changes in lens tolerance should be assessed by an ophthalmologist.

7. DRUG INTERACTIONS

Reduced efficacy and increased incidence of breakthrough bleeding and menstrual irregularities have been associated with concomitant use of rifampin. A similar association though less marked, has been suggested with barbiturates, phenylbutazone, phenytoin sodium, and possibly with griseofulvin, ampicillin and tetracyclines.[76]

8. INTERACTIONS WITH LABORATORY TESTS

Certain endocrine and liver function tests and blood components may be affected by oral contraceptives:

- **a.** Increased prothrombin and factors VII, VIII, IX, and X; decreased antithrombin 3; increased norepinephrine-induced platelet aggregability.
- **b.** Increased thyroid binding globulin (TBG) leading to increased circulating total thyroid hormone, as measured by protein-bound iodine (PBI), T4 by column or by radioimmunoassay. Free T3 resin uptake is decreased, reflecting the elevated TBG. Free T4 concentration is unaltered.
- **c.** Other binding proteins may be elevated in serum.
- **d.** Sex steroid binding globulins are increased and result in elevated levels of total circulating sex steroids and corticoids; however, free or biologically active levels remain unchanged.
- **e.** Triglycerides may be increased.
- **f.** Glucose tolerance may be decreased.
- **g.** Serum folate levels may be depressed by oral contraceptive therapy. This may be of clinical significance if a woman becomes pregnant shortly after discontinuing oral contraceptives.

9. CARCINOGENESIS

See **WARNINGS** section.

10. PREGNANCY

Pregnancy Category X. See **CONTRAINDICATIONS** and **WARNINGS** sections.

11. NURSING MOTHERS

Small amounts of oral contraceptive steroids have been identified in the milk of nursing mothers and a few adverse effects on the child have been reported, including jaundice and breast enlargement. In addition, oral contraceptives given in the postpartum period may interfere with lactation by decreasing the quantity and quality of breast milk. If possible, the nursing mother should be advised not to use oral contraceptives but to use other forms of contraception until she has completely weaned her child.

INFORMATION FOR THE PATIENT

See **PATIENT LABELING** printed below.

ADVERSE REACTIONS

An increased risk of the following serious adverse reactions has been associated with the use of oral contraceptives (see **WARNINGS** section):

- Thrombophlebitis
- Arterial thromboembolism
- Pulmonary embolism
- Myocardial infarction
- Cerebral hemorrhage
- Cerebral thrombosis
- Hypertension
- Gallbladder disease
- Hepatic adenomas, carcinomas or benign liver tumors

There is evidence of an association between the following conditions and the use of oral contraceptives, although additional confirmatory studies are needed:

- Mesenteric thrombosis
- Retinal thrombosis

The following adverse reactions have been reported in patients receiving oral contraceptives and are believed to be drug-related:

- Nausea
- Vomiting
- Gastrointestinal symptoms (such as abdominal cramps and bloating)
- Breakthrough bleeding
- Spotting
- Change in menstrual flow
- Amenorrhea

Continued on next page

Brevicon—Cont.

- Temporary infertility after discontinuation of treatment
- Edema
- Melasma which may persist
- Breast changes: tenderness, enlargement, secretion
- Change in weight (increase or decrease)
- Change in cervical erosion and secretion
- Diminution in lactation when given immediately post-partum
- Cholestatic jaundice
- Migraine
- Rash (allergic)
- Mental depression
- Reduced tolerance to carbohydrates
- Vaginal candidiasis
- Change in corneal curvature (steepening)
- Intolerance to contact lenses

The following adverse reactions have been reported in users of oral contraceptives and the association has been neither confirmed nor refuted:

- Pre-menstrual syndrome
- Cataracts
- Changes in appetite
- Cystitis-like syndrome
- Headache
- Nervousness
- Dizziness
- Hirsutism
- Loss of scalp hair
- Erythema multiforme
- Erythema nodosum
- Hemorrhagic eruption
- Vaginitis
- Porphyria
- Impaired renal function
- Hemolytic uremic syndrome
- Budd-Chiari syndrome
- Acne
- Changes in libido
- Colitis

OVERDOSAGE

Serious ill effects have not been reported following acute ingestion of large doses of oral contraceptives by young children. Overdosage may cause nausea, and withdrawal bleeding may occur in females.

NON-CONTRACEPTIVE HEALTH BENEFITS

The following non-contraceptive health benefits related to the use of oral contraceptives are supported by epidemiological studies which largely utilized oral contraceptive formulations containing estrogen doses exceeding 0.035 mg of ethinyl estradiol or 0.05 mg of mestranol.[6–11]

Effects on menses:

- Increased menstrual cycle regularity
- Decreased blood loss and decreased incidence of iron deficiency anemia
- Decreased incidence of dysmenorrhea

Effects related to inhibition of ovulation:

- Decreased incidence of functional ovarian cysts
- Decreased incidence of ectopic pregnancies

Effects from long-term use:

- Decreased incidence of fibroadenomas and fibrocystic disease of the breast
- Decreased incidence of acute pelvic inflammatory disease
- Decreased incidence of endometrial cancer
- Decreased incidence of ovarian cancer

DOSAGE AND ADMINISTRATION

To achieve maximum contraceptive effectiveness, oral contraceptives must be taken exactly as directed and at intervals not exceeding 24 hours.

21-Day Schedule: For a DAY 1 START, count the first day of menstrual flow as Day 1 and the first tablet (white or yellow-green or blue) is then taken on Day 1. For a SUNDAY START when menstrual flow begins on or before Sunday, the first tablet (white or yellow-green or blue) is taken on that day. With either a DAY 1 START or SUNDAY START, 1 tablet is taken each day at the same time for 21 days. No tablets are taken for 7 days, then, whether bleeding has stopped or not, a new course is started of 1 tablet a day for 21 days. This institutes a 3 weeks on, 1 week off dosage regimen.

28-Day Schedule: For a DAY 1 START, count the first day of menstrual flow as Day 1 and the first tablet (white or yellow-green or blue) is then taken on Day 1. For a SUNDAY START when menstrual flow begins on or before Sunday, the first tablet (white or yellow-green or blue) is taken on that day. With either a DAY 1 START or SUNDAY START, 1 tablet (white or yellow-green or blue) is taken each day at the same time for 21 days. Then the orange tablets are taken for 7 days, whether bleeding has stopped or not. After all 28 tablets have been taken, whether bleeding has stopped or not, the same dosage schedule is repeated beginning on the following day.

INSTRUCTIONS TO PATIENTS

- To achieve maximum contraceptive effectiveness, the oral contraceptive pill must be taken exactly as directed and at intervals not exceeding 24 hours.
- Important: Women should be instructed to use an additional method of protection until after the first 7 days of administration *in the initial cycle.*
- Due to the normally increased risk of thromboembolism occurring postpartum, women should be instructed not to initiate treatment with oral contraceptives earlier than 4–6 weeks after a full-term delivery. If pregnancy is terminated in the first 12 weeks, the patient should be instructed to start oral contraceptives immediately or within 7 days. If pregnancy is terminated after 12 weeks, the patient should be instructed to start oral contraceptives after 2 weeks.[33,77]
- If spotting or breakthrough bleeding should occur, the patient should continue the medication according to the schedule. Should spotting or breakthrough bleeding persist, the patient should notify her physician.
- If the patient misses 1 pill, she should be instructed to take it as soon as she remembers and then take the next pill at the regular time. The patient should be advised that missing a pill can cause spotting or light bleeding and that she may be a little sick to her stomach on the days she takes the missed pill with her regularly scheduled pill. If the patient has missed more than one pill, see **DETAILED PATIENT LABELING:** HOW TO TAKE THE PILL, WHAT TO DO IF YOU MISS PILLS.
- Use of oral contraceptives in the event of a missed menstrual period:

  1. If the patient has not adhered to the prescribed dosage regimen, the possibility of pregnancy should be considered after the first missed period and oral contraceptives should be withheld until pregnancy has been ruled out.

  2. If the patient has adhered to the prescribed regimen and misses 2 consecutive periods, pregnancy should be ruled out before continuing the contraceptive regimen.

HOW SUPPLIED

BREVICON® 21-DAY Tablets and BREVICON® 28-DAY Tablets (norethindrone and ethinyl estradiol), NORINYL® 1 + 35 21-DAY Tablets and NORINYL® 1 + 35 28-DAY Tablets (norethindrone and ethinyl estradiol), and NORINYL® 1 + 50 21-DAY Tablets and NORINYL® 1 + 50 28-DAY Tablets (norethindrone and mestranol) are available in 21-tablet or 28-tablet blister cards with a WALLETTE® tablet dispenser. Each 28-tablet card contains 7 orange inert tablets.

CAUTION: Federal law prohibits dispensing without prescription.

Store at controlled room temperature 15–25°C (59–77°F).

REFERENCES

1. Hatcher, R.A., Trussell, J., Stewart, F., et al.: *Contraceptive Technology: Sixteenth Revised Edition,* New York, NY, 1994. **2.** Mann, J., et al.: *Br Med J* 2(5956):241–245, 1975. **3.** Knopp, R.H.: *J Reprod Med* 31(9):913–921, 1986. **4.** Mann, J.I., et al.: *Br Med J* 2:445–447, 1976. **5.** Ory, H.: *JAMA* 237: 2619–2622, 1977. **6.** The Cancer and Steroid Hormone Study of the Centers for Disease Control: *JAMA* 249(2): 1596–1599, 1983. **7.** The Cancer and Steroid Hormone Study of the Centers for Disease Control: *JAMA* 257(6):796–800, 1987. **8.** Ory, H.W.: *JAMA* 228(1):68–69, 1974. **9.** Ory, H.W., et al.: *N Engl J Med* 294:419–422, 1976. **10.** Ory, H.W.: *Fam Plann Perspect* 14:182–184, 1982. **11.** Ory, H.W., et al.: *Making Choices,* New York, The Alan Guttmacher Institute, 1983. **12.** Stadel, B.: *N Engl J Med* 305(11):612–618, 1981. **13.** Stadel, B.: *N Engl J Med* 305(12):672–677, 1981. **14.** Adam, S., et al.: *Br J Obstet Gynaecol* 88:838–845, 1981. **15.** Mann, J., et al.: *Br Med J* 2(5965):245–248, 1975. **16.** Royal College of General Practitioners' Oral Contraceptive Study: *Lancet* 1:541–546, 1981. **17.** Slone, D., et al.: *N Engl J Med* 305(8):420–424, 1981. **18.** Vessey, M.P.: *Br J Fam Plann* 6 (Supplement):1–12, 1980. **19.** Russell-Briefel, R., et al.: *Prev Med* 15:352–362, 1986. **20.** Goldbaum, G., et al.: *JAMA* 258(10):1339–1342, 1987. **21.** LaRosa, J.C.: *J Reprod Med* 31(9):906–912, 1986. **22.** Krauss, R.M., et al.: *Am J Obstet Gynecol* 145:446–452, 1983. **23.** Wahl, P., et al.: *N Engl J Med* 308(15):862–867, 1983. **24.** Wynn, V., et al.: *Am J Obstet Gynecol* 142(6):766–771, 1982. **25.** Wynn V., et al.: *J Reprod Med* 31(9):892–897, 1986. **26.** Inman, W.H., et al.: *Br Med J* 2(5599):193–199, 1968. **27.** Maguire, M.G., et al.: *Am J Epidemiol* 110(2):188–195, 1979. **28.** Petitti, D., et al.: *JAMA* 242(11):1150–1154, 1979. **29.** Vessey, M.P., et al.: *Br Med J* 2(5599):199–205, 1968. **30.** Vessey, M.P., et al.: *Br Med J* 2(5658):651–657, 1969. **31.** Porter, J.B., et al.: *Obstet Gynecol* 59(3):299–302, 1982. **32.** Vessey, M.P., et al.: *J Biosoc Sci* 8:373–427, 1976. **33.** Mishell, D.R., et al.: *Reproductive Endocrinology,* Philadelphia, F.A. Davis Co., 1979. **34.** Petitti, D.B., et al.: *Lancet* 2:234–236, 1978. **35.** Collaborative Group for the Study of Stroke in Young Women: *JAMA* 231(7):718–722, 1975. **36.** Inman, W.H., et al.: *Br Med J* 2:203–209, 1970. **37.** Meade, T.W., et al.: *Br Med J* 280 (6224): 1157–1161, 1980. **38.** Kay, C.R.: *Am J Obstet Gynecol* 142(6):762–765, 1982. **39.** Gordon, T., et al.: *Am J Med* 62: 707–714, 1977. **40.** Royal College of General Practitioners' Oral Contraception Study: *J Coll Gen Pract* 33:75–82, 1983. **41.** Ory, H.W.: *Fam Plann Perspect* 15(2):57–63, 1983. **42.** Paul, C., et al.: *Br Med J* 293:723–725, 1986. **43.** The Cancer and Steroid Hormone Study of the Centers for Disease Control: *N Engl J Med* 315(7):405–411, 1986. **44.** Pike, M.C., et al.: *Lancet* 2:926–929, 1983. **45.** Miller, D.R., et al.: *Obstet Gynecol* 68:863–868, 1986. **46.** Olsson, H., et al.: *Lancet* 2:748–749, 1985. **47.** McPherson, K., et al.: *Br J Cancer* 56: 653–660, 1987. **48.** Huggins, G.R., et al.: *Fertil Steril* 47(5): 733–761, 1987. **49.** McPherson, K., et al.: *Br Med J* 293:709–710, 1986. **50.** Ory, H., et al.: *Am J Obstet Gynecol* 124(6): 573–577, 1976. **51.** Vessey, M.P., et al.: *Lancet,* 2:930, 1983. **52.** Brinton, L.A., et al.: *Int J Cancer* 38:339–344, 1986. **53.** WHO Collaborative Study of Neoplasia and Steroid Contraceptives: *Br Med J* 290:961–965, 1985. **54.** Rooks, J.B., et al.: *JAMA* 242(7):644–648, 1979. **55.** Bein, N.N., et al.: *Br J Surg* 64:433–435, 1977. **56.** Klatskin, G.: *Gastroenterology* 73:386–394, 1977. **57.** Henderson, B.E., et al.: *Br J Cancer* 48:437–440, 1983. **58.** Neuberger, J., et al.: *Br Med J* 292: 1355–1357, 1986. **59.** Forman, D., et al.: *Br Med J* 292: 1357–1361, 1986. **60.** Harlap, S., et al.: *Obstet Gynecol* 55(4): 447–452, 1980. **61.** Savolainen, E., et al.: *Am J Obstet Gynecol* 140(5):521–524, 1981. **62.** Janerich, D.T., et al.: *Am J Epidemiol* 112(1):73–79, 1980. **63.** Ferencz, C., et al.: *Teratology* 21:225–239, 1980. **64.** Rothman, K.J., et al.: *Am J Epidemiol* 109(4):433–439, 1979. **65.** Boston Collaborative Drug Surveillance Program: *Lancet* 1:1399–1404, 1973. **66.** Royal College of General Practitioners: *Oral contraceptives and health.* New York, Pittman, 1974. **67.** Rome Group for the Epidemiology and Prevention of Cholelithiasis: *Am J Epidemiol* 119(5):796–805, 1984. **68.** Strom, B.L., et al.: *Clin Pharmacol Ther* 39(3):335–341, 1986. **69.** Perlman, J.A., et al.: *J Chronic Dis* 38(10):857–864, 1985. **70.** Wynn, V., et al.: *Lancet* 1:1045–1049, 1979. **71.** Wynn, V.: *Progesterone and Progestin,* New York, Raven Press, 1983. **72.** Wynn, V., et al.: *Lancet* 2:720–723, 1966. **73.** Fisch, I.R., et al.: *JAMA* 237(23):2499–2503, 1977. **74.** Laragh, J.H.: *Am J Obstet Gynecol* 126(1):141–147, 1976. **75.** Ramcharan, S., et al.: *Pharmacology of Steroid Contraceptive Drugs,* New York, Raven Press, 1977. **76.** Stockley, I.: *Pharm J* 216:140–143, 1976. **77.** Dickey, R.P.: *Managing Contraceptive Pill Patients,* Oklahoma, Creative Informatics Inc., 1984. **78.** Porter J.B., Hunter J., Jick H., et al: *Obstet Gynecol* 1985;66:1–4. **79.** Porter J.B., Hershel J., Walker A.M.: *Obstet Gynecol* 1987;70:29–32. **80.** Fertility and Maternal Health Drugs Advisory Committee, F.D.A., October, 1989. **81.** Schlesselman J., Stadel B.V., Murray P., Lai S.: *Breast cancer in relation to early use of oral contraceptives.* JAMA 1988;259:1828–1833. **82.** Hennekens C.H., Speizer F.E., Lipnick R.J., Rosner B., Bain C., Belanger C., Stampfer M.J., Willett W., Peto R.: *A case-control study of oral contraceptive use and breast cancer.* JNCI 1984:72:39–42. **83.** Royal College of General Practitioners: *Oral contraceptives, venous thrombosis, and varicose veins. J Coll Gen Pract* 28:393–399, 1978. **84.** Royal College of General Practitioners' Oral Contraception Study: *Effect on Hypertension and benign breast disease of progestogen component in combined oral contraceptives. Lancet* 1:624, 1977.

DETAILED PATIENT LABELING

This product (like all oral contraceptives) is intended to prevent pregnancy. It does not protect against HIV infection (AIDS) and other sexually transmitted diseases.

INTRODUCTION

Any woman who considers using oral contraceptives ("birth control pills" or "the pill") should understand the benefits and risks of using this form of birth control. This leaflet will give you much of the information you will need to make this decision and also will help you determine if you are at risk of developing any of the serious side effects of the pill. It will tell you how to use the pill properly so that it will be as effective as possible. However, this leaflet is not a replacement for a careful discussion between you and your health care provider. You should discuss the information provided in this leaflet with him or her, both when you first start taking the pill and during your regular visits. You also should follow the advice of your health care provider with regard to regular checkups while you are on the pill.

EFFECTIVENESS OF ORAL CONTRACEPTIVES

Oral contraceptives are used to prevent pregnancy and are more effective than other non-surgical methods of birth control. When they are taken correctly, without missing any pills, the chance of becoming pregnant is less than 1% (1 pregnancy per 100 women per year of use). Typical failure rates are actually 3% per year. The chance of becoming pregnant increases with each missed pill during a menstrual cycle.

In comparison, typical failure rates for other nonsurgical methods of birth control during the first year are as follows: [See table at top of next page]

Comparison of reversible contraceptive methods: Percentage of women experiencing a contraceptive failure (pregnancy) during the first year of use.

Method	% of Women Experiencing a Pregnancy within the First Year of Use	
	Average Use	Correct Use
No contraception	85	85
Spermicides	21	6
Periodic abstinence	20	1-9[a]
Withdrawal	19	4
Cap		
Given birth	36	26
Never given birth	18	9
Sponge		
Given birth	36	20
Never given birth	18	9
Diaphragm	18	6
Condom		
Female	21	5
Male	12	3
Pill	3	
Progestin only		0.5
Combined		0.1
IUD		
Progesterone	2	1.5
Copper T 380A	0.8	0.6
Injectables	0.3	0.3
Implant	0.09	0.09

Adapted with permission.[1] Hatcher, R.A. Trussell, J. Stewart, F., et al. *Contraceptive Technology: Sixteenth Revised Edition*, New York, NY, 1994.

[a]Depending on method (calendar, ovulation, symptom-thermal)

WHO SHOULD NOT TAKE ORAL CONTRACEPTIVES

Cigarette smoking increases the risk of serious cardiovascular side effects from oral contraceptive use. This risk increases with age and with heavy smoking (15 or more cigarettes per day) and is quite marked in women over 35 years of age. Women who use oral contraceptives are strongly advised not to smoke.

Some women should not use the pill. For example, you should not take the pill if you are pregnant or think you may be pregnant. You also should not use the pill if you have any of the following conditions:
- A history of heart attack or stroke
- Blood clots in the legs (thrombophlebitis), brain (stroke), lungs (pulmonary embolism) or eyes
- A history of blood clots in the deep veins of your legs
- Chest pain (angina pectoris)
- Known or suspected breast cancer or cancer of the lining of the uterus, cervix or vagina
- Unexplained vaginal bleeding (until a diagnosis is reached by your doctor)
- Yellowing of the whites of the eyes or of the skin (jaundice) during pregnancy or during previous use of the pill
- Liver tumor (benign or cancerous)
- Known or suspected pregnancy

Tell your health care provider if you have ever had any of these conditions. Your health care provider can recommend a safer method of birth control.

OTHER CONSIDERATIONS BEFORE TAKING ORAL CONTRACEPTIVES

Tell your health care provider if you have or have had:
- Breast nodules, fibrocystic disease of the breast, an abnormal breast x-ray or mammogram
- Diabetes
- Elevated cholesterol or triglycerides
- High blood pressure
- Migraine or other headaches or epilepsy
- Mental depression
- Gallbladder, heart or kidney disease
- History of scanty or irregular menstrual periods

Women with any of these conditions should be checked often by their health care provider if they choose to use oral contraceptives.

Also, be sure to inform your doctor or health care provider if you smoke or are on any medications.

RISKS OF TAKING ORAL CONTRACEPTIVES

1. Risk of developing blood clots
Blood clots and blockage of blood vessels are the most serious side effects of taking oral contraceptives. In particular, a clot in the legs can cause thrombophlebitis and a clot that travels to the lungs can cause a sudden blocking of the vessel carrying blood to the lungs. Rarely, clots occur in the blood vessels of the eye and may cause blindness, double vision, or impaired vision.

If you take oral contraceptives and need elective surgery, need to stay in bed for a prolonged illness or have recently delivered a baby, you may be at risk of developing blood clots. You should consult your doctor about stopping oral contraceptives three to four weeks before surgery and not taking oral contraceptives for two weeks after surgery or during bed rest. You should also not take oral contraceptives soon after delivery of a baby. It is advisable to wait for at least four weeks after delivery if you are not breast feeding. If you are breast feeding, you should wait until you have weaned your child before using the pill (see **GENERAL PRECAUTIONS, While Breast Feeding**).

2. Heart attacks and strokes
Oral contraceptives may increase the tendency to develop strokes (stoppage or rupture of blood vessels in the brain) and angina pectoris and heart attacks (blockage of blood vessels in the heart). Any of these conditions can cause death or temporary or permanent disability.

Smoking greatly increases the possibility of suffering heart attacks and strokes. Furthermore, smoking and the use of oral contraceptives greatly increase the chances of developing and dying of heart disease.

3. Gallbladder disease
Oral contraceptive users may have a greater risk than non-users of having gallbladder disease, although this risk may be related to pills containing high doses of estrogen.

4. Liver tumors
In rare cases, oral contraceptives can cause benign but dangerous liver tumors. These benign liver tumors can rupture and cause fatal internal bleeding. In addition, a possible but not definite association has been found with the pill and liver cancers in 2 studies in which a few women who developed these very rare cancers were found to have used oral contraceptives for long periods. However, liver cancers are extremely rare. The chance of developing liver cancer from using the pill is thus even rarer.

5. Cancer of the breast and reproductive organs
There is, at present, no confirmed evidence that oral contraceptives increase the risk of cancer of the reproductive organs in human studies. Several studies have found no overall increase in the risk of developing breast cancer. However, women who use oral contraceptives and have a strong family history of breast cancer or who have breast nodules or abnormal mammograms should be followed closely by their doctors. Some studies have reported an increase in the risk of developing breast cancer, particularly at a younger age. This increased risk appears to be related to duration of use.

Some studies have found an increase in the incidence of cancer of the cervix in women who use oral contraceptives. However, this finding may be related to factors other than the use of oral contraceptives.

ESTIMATED RISK OF DEATH FROM A BIRTH CONTROL METHOD OR PREGNANCY

All methods of birth control and pregnancy are associated with a risk of developing certain diseases which may lead to disability or death. An estimate of the number of deaths associated with different methods of birth control and pregnancy has been calculated and is shown in the following table:

[See table below]

In the above table, the risk of death from any birth control method is less than the risk of childbirth except for oral contraceptive users over the age of 35 who smoke and pill users over the age of 40 even if they do not smoke. It can be seen from the table that for women aged 15 to 39 the risk of death is highest with pregnancy (7–26 deaths per 100,000 women, depending on age). Among pill users who do not smoke the risk of death is always lower than that associated with pregnancy for any age group, although over the age of 40 the risk increases to 32 deaths per 100,000 women compared to 28 associated with pregnancy at that age. However, for pill users who smoke and are over the age of 35 the estimated number of deaths exceeds those for other methods of birth control. If a woman is over the age of 40 and smokes, her estimated risk of death is 4 times higher (117/100,000 women) than the estimated risk associated with pregnancy (28/100,000 women) in that age group.

The suggestion that women over 40 who don't smoke should not take oral contraceptives is based on information from older high-dose pills and on less selective use of pills than is practiced today. An Advisory Committee of the FDA discussed this issue in 1989 and recommended that the benefits of oral contraceptive use by healthy, non-smoking women over 40 years of age may outweigh the possible risks. However, all women, especially older women, are cautioned to use the lowest dose pill that is effective.

WARNING SIGNALS

If any of these adverse effects occur while you are taking oral contraceptives, call your doctor immediately:
- Sharp chest pain, coughing of blood or sudden shortness of breath (indicating a possible clot in the lung)
- Pain in the calf (indicating a possible clot in the leg)
- Crushing chest pain or heaviness in the chest (indicating a possible heart attack)
- Sudden severe headache or vomiting, dizziness or fainting, disturbances of vision or speech, weakness or numbness in an arm or leg (indicating a possible stroke)
- Sudden partial or complete loss of vision (indicating a possible clot in the eye)
- Breast lumps (indicating possible breast cancer or fibrocystic disease of the breast: ask your doctor or health care provider to show you how to examine your breasts)
- Severe pain or tenderness in the stomach area (indicating a possible ruptured liver tumor)
- Difficulty in sleeping, weakness, lack of energy, fatigue or change in mood (possibly indicating severe depression)
- Jaundice or a yellowing of the skin or eyeballs, accompanied frequently by fever, fatigue, loss of appetite, dark colored urine or light colored bowel movements (indicating possible liver problems)

SIDE EFFECTS OF ORAL CONTRACEPTIVES

1. Vaginal bleeding
Irregular vaginal bleeding or spotting may occur while you are taking the pill. Irregular bleeding may vary from slight staining between menstrual periods to breakthrough bleeding which is a flow much like a regular period. Irregular

ESTIMATED ANNUAL NUMBER OF BIRTH-RELATED OR METHOD-RELATED DEATHS ASSOCIATED WITH CONTROL OF FERTILITY PER 100,000 NON-STERILE WOMEN, BY FERTILITY CONTROL METHOD ACCORDING TO AGE

Method of control and outcome	15–19	20–24	25–29	30–34	35–39	40–44
No fertility control methods*	7.0	7.4	9.1	14.8	25.7	28.2
Oral contraceptives non-smoker**	0.3	0.5	0.9	1.9	13.8	31.6
Oral contraceptives smoker**	2.2	3.4	6.6	13.5	51.1	117.2
IUD**	0.8	0.8	1.0	1.0	1.4	1.4
Condom*	1.1	1.6	0.7	0.2	0.3	0.4
Diaphragm/Spermicide*	1.9	1.2	1.2	1.3	2.2	2.8
Periodic abstinence*	2.5	1.6	1.6	1.7	2.9	3.6

* Deaths are birth-related
** Deaths are method-related

Continued on next page

Brevicon—Cont.

bleeding occurs most often during the first few months of oral contraceptive use but may also occur after you have been taking the pill for some time. Such bleeding may be temporary and usually does not indicate any serious problem. It is important to continue taking your pills on schedule. If the bleeding occurs in more than 1 cycle or lasts for more than a few days, talk to your doctor or health care provider.

2. Contact lenses
If you wear contact lenses and notice a change in vision or an inability to wear your lenses, contact your doctor or health care provider.

3. Fluid retention
Oral contraceptives may cause edema (fluid retention) with swelling of the fingers or ankles and may raise your blood pressure. If you experience fluid retention, contact your doctor or health care provider.

4. Melasma (Mask of Pregnancy)
A spotty darkening of the skin is possible, particularly of the face.

5. Other side effects
Other side effects may include change in appetite, headache, nervousness, depression, dizziness, loss of scalp hair, rash and vaginal infections.
If any of these side effects occur, contact your doctor or health care provider.

GENERAL PRECAUTIONS

1. Missed periods and use of oral contraceptives before or during early pregnancy
At times you may not menstruate regularly after you have completed taking a cycle of pills. If you have taken your pills regularly and miss 1 menstrual period, continue taking your pills for the next cycle but be sure to inform your health care provider before doing so. If you have not taken the pills daily as instructed and miss 1 menstrual period, or if you miss 2 consecutive menstrual periods, you may be pregnant. You should stop taking oral contraceptives until you are sure you are not pregnant, but continue to use another method of birth control.
There is no conclusive evidence that oral contraceptive use is associated with an increase in birth defects when taken inadvertently during early pregnancy. Previously, a few studies had reported that oral contraceptives might be associated with birth defects but these studies have not been confirmed. Nevertheless, oral contraceptives or any other drugs should not be used during pregnancy unless clearly necessary and prescribed by your doctor. You should check with your doctor about risks to your unborn child from any medication taken during pregnancy.

2. While breast feeding
If you are breast feeding, consult your doctor before starting oral contraceptives. Some of the drug will be passed on to the child in the milk. A few adverse effects on the child have been reported, including yellowing of the skin (jaundice) and breast enlargement. In addition, oral contraceptives may decrease the amount and quality of your milk. If possible, do not use oral contraceptives and use another method of contraception while breast feeding. You should consider starting oral contraceptives only after you have weaned your child completely.

3. Laboratory tests
If you are scheduled for any laboratory tests, tell your doctor you are taking birth control pills. Certain blood tests may be affected by birth control pills.

4. Drug interactions
Certain drugs may interact with birth control pills to make them less effective in preventing pregnancy or cause an increase in breakthrough bleeding. Such drugs include rifampin; drugs used for epilepsy such as barbiturates (for example phenobarbital) and phenytoin (Dilantin is one brand of this drug); phenylbutazone (Butazolidin is one brand of this drug) and possibly certain antibiotics. You may need to use additional contraception when you take drugs which can make oral contraceptives less effective.

5. This product (like all oral contraceptives) is intended to prevent pregnancy. It does not protect against transmission of HIV (AIDS) and other sexually transmitted diseases such as chlamydia, genital herpes, genital warts, gonorrhea, hepatitis B, and syphilis.

HOW TO TAKE ORAL CONTRACEPTIVES

IMPORTANT POINTS TO REMEMBER

BEFORE YOU START TAKING YOUR PILLS:
1. BE SURE TO READ THESE DIRECTIONS:
Before you start taking your pills.
Anytime you are not sure what to do.
2. THE RIGHT WAY TO TAKE THE PILL IS TO TAKE ONE PILL EVERY DAY AT THE SAME TIME.
If you miss pills you could get pregnant. This includes starting the pack late.
The more pills you miss, the more likely you are to get pregnant.

3. MANY WOMEN HAVE SPOTTING OR LIGHT BLEEDING, OR MAY FEEL SICK TO THEIR STOMACH DURING THE FIRST 1–3 PACKS OF PILLS.
If you feel sick to your stomach, do not stop taking the Pill. The problem will usually go away. If it doesn't go away, check with your doctor or clinic.
4. MISSING PILLS CAN ALSO CAUSE SPOTTING OR LIGHT BLEEDING, even when you make up these missed pills.
On the days you take 2 pills to make up for missed pills, you could also feel a little sick to your stomach.
5. IF YOU HAVE VOMITING OR DIARRHEA, for any reason, or IF YOU TAKE SOME MEDICINES, including some antibiotics, your pills may not work as well.
Use a back-up method (such as condoms, foam, or sponge) until you check with your doctor or clinic.
6. IF YOU HAVE TROUBLE REMEMBERING TO TAKE THE PILL, talk to your doctor or clinic about how to make pill-taking easier or about using another method of birth control.
7. IF YOU HAVE ANY QUESTIONS OR ARE UNSURE ABOUT THE INFORMATION IN THIS LEAFLET, call your doctor or clinic.

BEFORE YOU START TAKING YOUR PILLS

1. DECIDE WHAT TIME OF DAY YOU WANT TO TAKE YOUR PILL.
It is important to take it about the same time every day.
2. LOOK AT YOU PILL PACK TO SEE IF IT HAS 21 OR 28 PILLS:
The 21-pill pack has 21 "active" white or yellow-green or blue pills (with hormones) to take for 3 weeks, followed by 1 week without pills.
The 28-pill pack has 21 "active" white or yellow-green or blue pills (with hormones) to take for 3 weeks, followed by 1 week or reminder orange pills (without hormones).
3. ALSO FIND:
1) where on the pack to start taking pills.
2) in what order to take the pills (follow the arrows).

Brevicon, Norinyl 1 + 35, Norinyl 1 + 50
Active Pill Colors: Blue or Yellow-Green or White

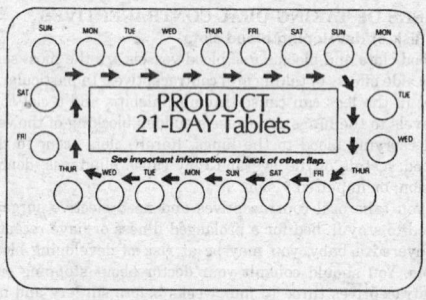

PRODUCT
21-DAY Tablets
See important information on back of other flap.

Brevicon, Norinyl 1 + 35, Norinyl 1 + 50
Active Pill Colors: Blue or Yellow-Green or White
Reminder Pill Color: Orange

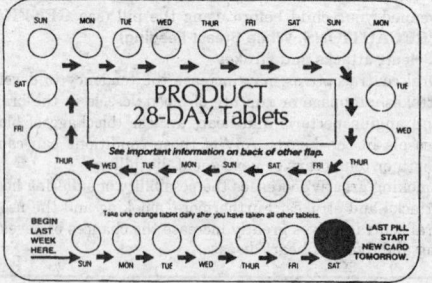

PRODUCT
28-DAY Tablets
See important information on back of other flap.

4. BE SURE YOU HAVE READY AT ALL TIMES:
ANOTHER KIND OF BIRTH CONTROL (such as condoms, foam, or sponge) to use as a back-up in case you miss pills.
AN EXTRA, FULL PILL PACK.

WHEN TO START THE FIRST PACK OF PILLS

You have a choice of which day to start taking you first pack of pills. Decide with your doctor or clinic which is the best day for you. Pick a time of the day which will be easy to remember.
DAY 1 START:
1. Take the first "active" white or yellow-green or blue pill of the first pack during the first 24 hours of your period.
2. You will not need to use a back-up method of birth control, since you are starting the pill at the beginning of your period.

SUNDAY START:
1. Take the first "active" white or yellow-green or blue pill of the first pack on the Sunday after your period starts, even if you are still bleeding. If you period begins on Sunday, start the pack that same day.
2. Use another method of birth control as a back-up method if you have sex anytime from the Sunday you start your first pack until the next Sunday (7 days). Condoms, foam, or the sponge are good back-up methods of birth control.

WHAT TO DO DURING THE MONTH

1. **TAKE ONE PILL AT THE SAME TIME EVERY DAY UNTIL THE PACK IS EMPTY.**
Do not skip pills even if you are spotting or bleeding between your monthly periods or feel sick to your stomach (nausea).
Do not skip pills even if you do not have sex often.
2. **WHEN YOU FINISH A PACK OR SWITCH YOUR BRAND OF PILLS:**
21 pills: Wait 7 days to start the next pack. You will probably have your period during that week. Be sure that no more than 7 days pass between 21-day packs.
28 pills: Start the next pack on the day after your last "reminder" pill. Do not wait any days between packs.

WHAT TO DO IF YOU MISS PILLS

If you **MISS 1** white or yellow-green or blue "active" pill:
1. Take it as soon as you remember. Take the next pill at your regular time. This means you may take 2 pills in 1 day.
2. You do not need to use a back-up birth control method if you have sex.
If you **MISS 2** white or yellow-green or blue "active" pills in a row in **WEEK 1 OR WEEK 2** of your pack:
1. Take 2 pills on the day you remember and 2 pills the next day.
2. Then take 1 pill a day until you finish the pack.
3. You MAY BECOME PREGNANT if you have sex in the 7 days after you miss pills. You MUST use another birth control method (such as condoms, foam, or sponge) as a backup for those 7 days.
If you **MISS 2** white or yellow-green or blue "active" pills in a row in **THE 3rd WEEK:**
1. If you are a Day 1 Starter:
THROW OUT the rest of the pill pack and start a new pack that same day.
If you are a Sunday Starter:
Keep taking 1 pill every day until Sunday.
On Sunday, THROW OUT the rest of the pack and start a new pack of pills that same day.
2. You may not have your period this month but this is expected. However, if you miss your period 2 months in a row, call your doctor or clinic because you might be pregnant.
3. You MAY BECOME PREGNANT if you have sex in the 7 days after you miss pills. You MUST use another birth control method (such as condoms, foam, or sponge) as a backup for those 7 days.
If you **MISS 3 OR MORE** white or yellow-green or blue "active" pills in a row (during the first 3 weeks):
1. If you are a Day 1 Starter:
THROW OUT the rest of the pill pack and start a new pack of pills that same day.
If you are a Sunday Starter:
Keep taking 1 pill every day until Sunday.
On Sunday, THROW OUT the rest of the pack and start a new pack of pills that same day.
2. You may not have your period this month but this is expected. However, if you miss your period 2 months in a row, call your doctor or clinic because you might be pregnant.
3. You MAY BECOME PREGNANT if you have sex in the 7 days after you miss pills. You MUST use another birth control method (such as condoms, foam, or sponge) as a backup for those 7 days.

A REMINDER FOR THOSE ON 28–DAY PACKS:
If you forget any of the 7 orange "reminder" pills in Week 4:
THROW AWAY the pills you missed.
Keep taking 1 pill each day until the pack is empty.
You do not need a back-up method.

FINALLY, IF YOU ARE STILL NOT SURE WHAT TO DO ABOUT THE PILLS YOU HAVE MISSED:
Use a BACK-UP METHOD anytime you have sex.
KEEP TAKING ONE "ACTIVE" PILL EACH DAY until you can reach your doctor or clinic.

6. Missed periods, spotting or light bleeding
At times, you may not have a period after you have completed a pack of pills. If you miss 1 period but you have taken the pills exactly as you were supposed to, continue as usual into the next cycle. If you have not taken the pills correctly, and have missed a period, you may be pregnant and you should stop taking the Pill until your doctor or clinic

determines whether or not you are pregnant. Until you can talk to your doctor or clinic, use an appropriate back-up birth control method. If you miss 2 consecutive periods, you should stop taking the Pill until it is determined that you are not pregnant.

Even if spotting or light bleeding should occur, continue taking the Pill according to the schedule. Should spotting or light bleeding persist, you should notify your doctor or clinic.

7. Stopping the pill before surgery or prolonged bed rest

If you are scheduled for surgery or you need to stay in bed for a long period of time you should tell your doctor that you are on the Pill. You should stop taking the Pill four weeks before your operation to avoid an increased risk of blood clots. Talk to your doctor about when you may start taking the Pill again.

8. Starting the pill after pregnancy

After you have a baby it is advisable to wait 4-6 weeks before starting to take the Pill. Talk to your doctor about when you may start taking the Pill after pregnancy.

9. Pregnancy due to pill failure

When the Pill is taken correctly, the expected pregnancy rate is approximately 1% (i.e., 1 pregnancy per 100 women per year). If pregnancy occurs while taking the Pill, there is little risk to the fetus. The typical failure rate of large numbers of pill users is less than 3% when women who have missed pills are included. If you become pregnant, you should discuss your pregnancy with your doctor.

10. Pregnancy after stopping the pill

There may be some delay in becoming pregnant after you stop taking the Pill, especially if you had irregular periods before you started using the Pill. Your doctor may recommend that you delay becoming pregnant until you have had one or more regular periods.

There does not appear to be any increase in birth defects in newborn babies when pregnancy occurs soon after stopping the Pill.

11. Overdosage

There are no reports of serious illness or side effects in young children who have swallowed a large number of pills. In adults, overdosage may cause nausea and/or bleeding in females. In case of overdosage, contact your doctor, clinic or pharmacist.

12. Other information

Your doctor or clinic will take a medical and family history and will examine you before prescribing the Pill. The physical examination may be delayed to another time if you request it and the health care provider believes that it is a good medical practice to postpone it. You should be reexamined at least once a year. Be sure to inform your doctor or clinic if there is a family history of any of the conditions listed previously in this leaflet. Be sure to keep all appointments with your doctor or clinic because this is a time to determine if there are early signs of side effects from using the Pill.

Do not use the Pill for any condition other than the one for which it was prescribed. The Pill has been prescribed specifically for you, do not give it to others who may want birth control pills.

If you want more information about birth control pills, ask your doctor or clinic. They have a more technical leaflet called **PHYSICIAN LABELING** which you might want to read.

NON-CONTRACEPTIVE HEALTH BENEFITS

In addition to preventing pregnancy, use of oral contraceptives may provide certain non-contraceptive health benefits:

- Menstrual cycles may become more regular
- Blood flow during menstruation may be lighter and less iron may be lost. Therefore, anemia due to iron deficiency is less likely to occur
- Pain or other symptoms during menstruation may be encountered less frequently
- Ectopic (tubal) pregnancy may occur less frequently
- Non-cancerous cysts or lumps in the breast may occur less frequently
- Acute pelvic inflammatory disease may occur less frequently
- Oral contraceptive use may provide some protection against developing two forms of cancer: cancer of the ovaries and cancer of the lining of the uterus
- If you want more information about birth control pills, ask your doctor or pharmacist. They have a more technical leaflet called the Professional Labeling, which you may wish to read.

Store at controlled room temperature 15–25°C (59–77°F).

Keep this and all medications out of the reach of children.

BRIEF SUMMARY

PATIENT PACKAGE INSERT

This product (like all oral contraceptives) is intended to prevent pregnancy. It does not protect against HIV infection (AIDS) and other sexually transmitted diseases.

Oral contraceptives, also known as "birth control pills" or "the pill," are taken to prevent pregnancy and, when taken correctly, have a failure rate of about 1% per year when used without missing any pills. The typical failure rate of large numbers of pill users is less than 3% per year when women who miss pills are included. For most women, oral contraceptives are also free of serious or unpleasant side effects. However, forgetting to take oral contraceptives considerably increases the chances of pregnancy.

For the majority of women, oral contraceptives can be taken safely, but there are some women who are at high risk of developing certain serious diseases that can be life-threatening or may cause temporary or permanent disability. The risks associated with taking oral contraceptives increase significantly if you:

- Smoke
- Have high blood pressure, diabetes or high cholesterol
- Have or have had clotting disorders, heart attack, stroke, angina pectoris, cancer of the breast or sex organs, jaundice or malignant or benign liver tumors

You should not take the pill if you suspect you are pregnant or have unexplained vaginal bleeding.

Cigarette smoking increases the risk of serious cardiovascular side effects from oral contraceptive use. This risk increases with age and with heavy smoking (15 or more cigarettes per day) and is quite marked in women over 35 years of age. Women who use oral contraceptives are strongly advised not to smoke.

Most side effects of the pill are not serious. The most common such effects are nausea, vomiting, bleeding between menstrual periods, weight gain, breast tenderness and difficulty wearing contact lenses. These side effects, especially nausea and vomiting, may subside within the first 3 months of use.

The serious side effects of the pill occur very infrequently, especially if you are in good health and are young. However, you should know that the following medical conditions have been associated with or made worse by the pill:

1. Blood clots in the legs (thrombophlebitis) or lungs (pulmonary embolism), stoppage or rupture of a blood vessel in the brain (stroke), blockage of blood vessels in the heart (heart attack or angina pectoris), eye or other organs of the body. As mentioned above, smoking increases the risk of heart attacks and strokes and subsequent serious medical consequences.
2. Liver tumors, which may rupture and cause severe bleeding. A possible but not definite association has been found with the pill and liver cancer. However, liver cancers are extremely rare. The chance of developing liver cancer from using the pill is thus even rarer.
3. High blood pressure, although blood pressure usually returns to normal when the pill is stopped.

The symptoms associated with these serious side effects are discussed in the detailed leaflet given to you with your supply of pills. Notify your doctor or health care provider if you notice any unusual physical disturbances while taking the pill. In addition, drugs such as rifampin, as well as some anti-convulsants and some antibiotics, may decrease oral contraceptive effectiveness.

Studies to date of women taking the pill have not shown an increase in the incidence of cancer of the breast or cervix. There is, however, insufficient evidence to rule out the possibility that the pill may cause such cancers. Some studies have reported an increase in the risk of developing breast cancer, particularly at a younger age. This increased risk appears to be related to duration of use.

Taking the pill provides some important non-contraceptive health benefits. These include less painful menstruation, less menstrual blood loss and anemia, fewer pelvic infections and fewer cancers of the ovary and the lining of the uterus.

Be sure to discuss any medical condition you may have with your health care provider. Your health care provider will take a medical and family history before prescribing oral contraceptives and will examine you. The physical examination may be delayed to another time if you request it and the health care provider believes that it is a good medical practice to postpone it. You should be reexamined at least once a year while taking oral contraceptives. The detailed patient information leaflet gives you further information which you should read and discuss with your health care provider.

HOW TO TAKE THE PILL

See full text *of HOW TO TAKE THE PILL* which is printed in full in the **DETAILED PATIENT LABELING.**

Keep this and all medications out of the reach of children.

REVISED 10/30/97•A08829

Shown in Product Identification Guide, page 337

CALAN® Tablets ℞

[cal 'an]

(verapamil hydrochloride)

PRODUCT OVERVIEW

KEY FACTS

Calan, a calcium ion antagonist, exerts its pharmacologic effects by modulating the influx of ionic calcium across the cell membrane of the arterial smooth muscle as well as in conductile and contractile myocardial cells. Calan increases myocardial oxygen supply, reduces myocardial oxygen consumption, and is a potent inhibitor of coronary artery spasm, making it an effective antianginal agent. By decreasing the influx of calcium, Calan prolongs the effective refractory period within the AV node and slows AV conduction in a rate-related manner, thereby slowing the ventricular rate in patients with chronic atrial flutter or fibrillation. Calan exerts antihypertensive effects by decreasing systemic vascular resistance, usually without orthostatic decreases in blood pressure or reflex tachycardia.

MAJOR USES

Calan Tablets are indicated for: angina at rest, including vasospastic and unstable angina; chronic stable angina; control (in association with digitalis) of ventricular rate at rest and during stress in patients with chronic atrial flutter and/or atrial fibrillation; prophylaxis of repetitive paroxysmal supraventricular tachycardia; management of essential hypertension.

SAFETY INFORMATION

See complete safety information set forth below.

PRESCRIBING INFORMATION

CALAN® Tablets ℞

[cal 'an]

(verapamil hydrochloride)

DESCRIPTION

Calan (verapamil HCl) is a calcium ion influx inhibitor (slow-channel blocker or calcium ion antagonist) available for oral administration in film-coated tablets containing 40 mg, 80 mg, or 120 mg of verapamil hydrochloride.

The structural formula of verapamil HCl is

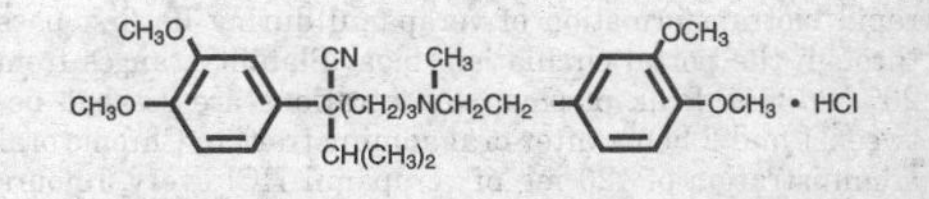

$C_{27}H_{38}N_2O_4 \cdot HCl$ M. W. = 491.08

Benzeneacetonitrile, α-[3-[[2-(3,4-dimethoxyphenyl) ethyl] methylamino]propyl]-3,4-dimethoxy-α-(1-methylethyl) hydrochloride

Verapamil HCl is an almost white, crystalline powder, practically free of odor, with a bitter taste. It is soluble in water, chloroform, and methanol. Verapamil HCl is not chemically related to other cardioactive drugs.

Inactive ingredients include microcrystalline cellulose, corn starch, gelatin, hydroxypropyl cellulose, hydroxypropyl methylcellulose, iron oxide colorant, lactose, magnesium stearate, polyethylene glycol, talc, and titanium dioxide.

CLINICAL PHARMACOLOGY

Calan is a calcium ion influx inhibitor (slow-channel blocker or calcium ion antagonist) that exerts its pharmacologic effects by modulating the influx of ionic calcium across the cell membrane of the arterial smooth muscle as well as in conductile and contractile myocardial cells.

Mechanism of action

Angina: The precise mechanism of action of Calan as an antianginal agent remains to be fully determined, but includes the following two mechanisms:

1. *Relaxation and prevention of coronary artery spasm:* Calan dilates the main coronary arteries and coronary arterioles, both in normal and ischemic regions, and is a potent inhibitor of coronary artery spasm, whether spontaneous or ergonovine-induced. This property increases myocardial oxygen delivery in patients with coronary artery spasm and is responsible for the effectiveness of Calan in vasospastic (Prinzmetal's or variant) as well as unstable angina at rest. Whether this effect plays any role in classical effort angina is not clear, but studies of exercise tolerance have not shown an increase in the maximum exercise rate–pressure product, a widely accepted measure of oxygen utilization. This suggests that, in general, relief of spasm or dilation of coronary arteries is not an important factor in classical angina.
2. *Reduction of oxygen utilization:* Calan regularly reduces the total peripheral resistance (afterload) against which the heart works both at rest and at a given level of exercise by dilating peripheral arterioles. This unloading of the heart reduces myocardial energy consumption and oxygen requirements and probably accounts for the effectiveness of Calan in chronic stable effort angina.

Arrhythmia: Electrical activity through the AV node depends, to a significant degree, upon calcium influx through the slow channel. By decreasing the influx of calcium, Calan prolongs the effective refractory period within the AV node and slows AV conduction in a rate-related manner. This

Continued on next page

Calan—Cont.

property accounts for the ability of Calan to slow the ventricular rate in patients with chronic atrial flutter or atrial fibrillation.

Normal sinus rhythm is usually not affected, but in patients with sick sinus syndrome, Calan may interfere with sinus-node impulse generation and may induce sinus arrest or sino-atrial block. Atrioventricular block can occur in patients without preexisting conduction defects (see *Warnings*). Calan decreases the frequency of episodes of paroxysmal supraventricular tachycardia.

Calan does not alter the normal atrial action potential or intraventricular conduction time, but in depressed atrial fibers it decreases amplitude, velocity of depolarization, and conduction velocity. Calan may shorten the antegrade effective refractory period of the accessory bypass tract. Acceleration of ventricular rate and/or ventricular fibrillation has been reported in patients with atrial flutter or atrial fibrillation and a coexisting accessory AV pathway following administration of verapamil (see *Warnings*).

Calan has a local anesthetic action that is 1.6 times that of procaine on an equimolar basis. It is not known whether this action is important at the doses used in man.

Essential hypertension: Calan exerts antihypertensive effects by decreasing systemic vascular resistance, usually without orthostatic decreases in blood pressure or reflex tachycardia; bradycardia (rate less than 50 beats/min) is uncommon (1.4%). During isometric or dynamic exercise Calan does not alter systolic cardiac function in patients with normal ventricular function.

Calan does not alter total serum calcium levels. However, one report suggested that calcium levels above the normal range may alter the therapeutic effect of Calan.

Pharmacokinetics and metabolism: More than 90% of the orally administered dose of Calan is absorbed. Because of rapid biotransformation of verapamil during its first pass through the portal circulation, bioavailability ranges from 20% to 35%. Peak plasma concentrations are reached between 1 and 2 hours after oral administration. Chronic oral administration of 120 mg of verapamil HCl every 6 hours resulted in plasma levels of verapamil ranging from 125 to 400 ng/ml, with higher values reported occasionally. A non-linear correlation between the verapamil dose administered and verapamil plasma levels does exist. No relationship has been established between the plasma concentration of verapamil and a reduction in blood pressure. In early dose titration with verapamil a relationship exists between verapamil plasma concentration and prolongation of the PR interval. However, during chronic administration this relationship may disappear. The mean elimination half-life in single-dose studies ranged from 2.8 to 7.4 hours. In these same studies, after repetitive dosing, the half-life increased to a range from 4.5 to 12.0 hours (after less than 10 consecutive doses given 6 hours apart). Half-life of verapamil may increase during titration. Aging may affect the pharmacokinetics of verapamil. Elimination half-life may be prolonged in the elderly. In healthy men, orally administered Calan undergoes extensive metabolism in the liver. Twelve metabolites have been identified in plasma; all except norverapamil are present in trace amounts only. Norverapamil can reach steady-state plasma concentrations approximately equal to those of verapamil itself. The cardiovascular activity of norverapamil appears to be approximately 20% that of verapamil. Approximately 70% of an administered dose is excreted as metabolites in the urine and 16% or more in the feces within 5 days. About 3% to 4% is excreted in the urine as unchanged drug. Approximately 90% is bound to plasma proteins. In patients with hepatic insufficiency, metabolism is delayed and elimination half-life prolonged up to 14 to 16 hours (see *Precautions*); the volume of distribution is increased and plasma clearance reduced to about 30% of normal. Verapamil clearance values suggest that patients with liver dysfunction may attain therapeutic verapamil plasma concentrations with one third of the oral daily dose required for patients with normal liver function.

After four weeks of oral dosing (120 mg q.i.d.), verapamil and norverapamil levels were noted in the cerebrospinal fluid with estimated partition coefficient of 0.06 for verapamil and 0.04 for norverapamil.

Hemodynamics and myocardial metabolism: Calan reduces afterload and myocardial contractility. Improved left ventricular diastolic function in patients with IHSS and those with coronary heart disease has also been observed with Calan therapy. In most patients, including those with organic cardiac disease, the negative inotropic action of Calan is countered by reduction of afterload, and cardiac index is usually not reduced. However, in patients with severe left ventricular dysfunction (eg, pulmonary wedge pressure above 20 mm Hg or ejection fraction less than 30%), or in patients taking beta-adrenergic blocking agents or other cardiodepressant drugs, deterioration of ventricular function may occur (see *Drug interactions*).

Pulmonary function: Calan does not induce bronchoconstriction and, hence, does not impair ventilatory function.

INDICATIONS AND USAGE

Calan tablets are indicated for the treatment of the following:

Angina
1. Angina at rest, including:
   — Vasospastic (Prinzmetal's variant) angina
   — Unstable (crescendo, pre-infarction) angina
2. Chronic stable angina (classic effort-associated angina)

Arrhythmias
1. In association with digitalis for the control of ventricular rate at rest and during stress in patients with chronic atrial flutter and/or atrial fibrillation (see *Warnings: Accessory bypass tract*)
2. Prophylaxis of repetitive paroxysmal supraventricular tachycardia

Essential hypertension

CONTRAINDICATIONS

Verapamil HCl tablets are contraindicated in:
1. Severe left ventricular dysfunction (see *Warnings*)
2. Hypotension (systolic pressure less than 90 mm Hg) or cardiogenic shock
3. Sick sinus syndrome (except in patients with a functioning artificial ventricular pacemaker)
4. Second- or third-degree AV block (except in patients with a functioning artificial ventricular pacemaker)
5. Patients with atrial flutter or atrial fibrillation and an accessory bypass tract (eg, Wolff-Parkinson-White, Lown-Ganong-Levine syndromes). (See *Warnings.*)
6. Patients with known hypersensitivity to verapamil hydrochloride.

WARNINGS

Heart failure: Verapamil has a negative inotropic effect, which in most patients is compensated by its afterload reduction (decreased systemic vascular resistance) properties without a net impairment of ventricular performance. In clinical experience with 4,954 patients, 87 (1.8%) developed congestive heart failure or pulmonary edema. Verapamil should be avoided in patients with severe left ventricular dysfunction (eg, ejection fraction less than 30%) or moderate to severe symptoms of cardiac failure and in patients with any degree of ventricular dysfunction if they are receiving a beta-adrenergic blocker (see *Drug interactions*). Patients with milder ventricular dysfunction should, if possible, be controlled with optimum doses of digitalis and/or diuretics before verapamil treatment. **(Note interactions with digoxin under *Precautions*.)**

Hypotension: Occasionally, the pharmacologic action of verapamil may produce a decrease in blood pressure below normal levels, which may result in dizziness or symptomatic hypotension. The incidence of hypotension observed in 4,954 patients enrolled in clinical trials was 2.5%. In hypertensive patients, decreases in blood pressure below normal are unusual. Tilt-table testing (60 degrees) was not able to induce orthostatic hypotension.

Elevated liver enzymes: Elevations of transaminases with and without concomitant elevations in alkaline phosphatase and bilirubin have been reported. Such elevations have sometimes been transient and may disappear even with continued verapamil treatment. Several cases of hepatocellular injury related to verapamil have been proven by rechallenge; half of these had clinical symptoms (malaise, fever, and/or right upper quadrant pain), in addition to elevation of SGOT, SGPT, and alkaline phosphatase. Periodic monitoring of liver function in patients receiving verapamil is therefore prudent.

Accessory bypass tract (Wolff-Parkinson-White or Lown-Ganong-Levine): Some patients with paroxysmal and/or chronic atrial fibrillation or atrial flutter and a coexisting accessory AV pathway have developed increased antegrade conduction across the accessory pathway bypassing the AV node, producing a very rapid ventricular response or ventricular fibrillation after receiving intravenous verapamil (or digitalis). Although a risk of this occurring with oral verapamil has not been established, such patients receiving oral verapamil may be at risk and its use in these patients is contraindicated (see *Contraindications*). Treatment is usually DC-cardioversion. Cardioversion has been used safely and effectively after oral Calan.

Atrioventricular block: The effect of verapamil on AV conduction and the SA node may cause asymptomatic first-degree AV block and transient bradycardia, sometimes accompanied by nodal escape rhythms. PR-interval prolongation is correlated with verapamil plasma concentrations especially during the early titration phase of therapy. Higher degrees of AV block, however, were infrequently (0.8%) observed. Marked first-degree block or progressive development to second- or third-degree AV block requires a reduction in dosage or, in rare instances, discontinuation of verapamil HCl and institution of appropriate therapy, depending on the clinical situation.

Patients with hypertrophic cardiomyopathy (IHSS): In 120 patients with hypertrophic cardiomyopathy (most of them refractory or intolerant to propranolol) who received therapy with verapamil at doses up to 720 mg/day, a variety of

serious adverse effects were seen. Three patients died in pulmonary edema; all had severe left ventricular outflow obstruction and a past history of left ventricular dysfunction. Eight other patients had pulmonary edema and/or severe hypotension; abnormally high (greater than 20 mm Hg) pulmonary wedge pressure and a marked left ventricular outflow obstruction were present in most of these patients. Concomitant administration of quinidine (see *Drug interactions*) preceded the severe hypotension in 3 of the 8 patients (2 of whom developed pulmonary edema). Sinus bradycardia occurred in 11% of the patients, second-degree AV block in 4%, and sinus arrest in 2%. It must be appreciated that this group of patients had a serious disease with a high mortality rate. Most adverse effects responded well to dose reduction, and only rarely did verapamil use have to be discontinued.

PRECAUTIONS

General

Use in patients with impaired hepatic function: Since verapamil is highly metabolized by the liver, it should be administered cautiously to patients with impaired hepatic function. Severe liver dysfunction prolongs the elimination half-life of verapamil to about 14 to 16 hours; hence, approximately 30% of the dose given to patients with normal liver function should be administered to these patients. Careful monitoring for abnormal prolongation of the PR interval or other signs of excessive pharmacologic effects (see *Overdosage*) should be carried out.

Use in patients with attenuated (decreased) neuromuscular transmission: It has been reported that verapamil decreases neuromuscular transmission in patients with Duchenne's muscular dystrophy, and that verapamil prolongs recovery from the neuromuscular blocking agent vecuronium. It may be necessary to decrease the dosage of verapamil when it is administered to patients with attenuated neuromuscular transmission.

Use in patients with impaired renal function: About 70% of an administered dose of verapamil is excreted as metabolites in the urine. Verapamil is not removed by hemodialysis. Until further data are available, verapamil should be administered cautiously to patients with impaired renal function. These patients should be carefully monitored for abnormal prolongation of the PR interval or other signs of overdosage (see *Overdosage*).

Drug interactions

Alcohol: Verapamil may increase blood alcohol concentrations and prolong its effects.

Beta-blockers: Controlled studies in small numbers of patients suggest that the concomitant use of Calan and oral beta-adrenergic blocking agents may be beneficial in certain patients with chronic stable angina or hypertension, but available information is not sufficient to predict with confidence the effects of concurrent treatment in patients with left ventricular dysfunction or cardiac conduction abnormalities. Concomitant therapy with beta-adrenergic blockers and verapamil may result in additive negative effects on heart rate, atrioventricular conduction and/or cardiac contractility.

In one study involving 15 patients treated with high doses of propranolol (median dose, 480 mg/day; range, 160 to 1,280 mg/day) for severe angina, with preserved left ventricular function (ejection fraction greater than 35%), the hemodynamic effects of additional therapy with verapamil HCl were assessed using invasive methods. The addition of verapamil to high-dose beta-blockers induced modest negative inotropic and chronotropic effects that were not severe enough to limit short-term (48 hours) combination therapy in this study. These modest cardiodepressant effects persisted for greater than 6 but less than 30 hours after abrupt withdrawal of beta-blockers and were closely related to plasma levels of propranolol. The primary verapamil/beta-blocker interaction in this study appeared to be hemodynamic rather than electrophysiologic.

In other studies verapamil did not generally induce significant negative inotropic, chronotropic, or dromotropic effects in patients with preserved left ventricular function receiving low or moderate doses of propranolol (less than or equal to 320 mg/day); in some patients, however, combined therapy did produce such effects. Therefore, if combined therapy is used, close surveillance of clinical status should be carried out. Combined therapy should usually be avoided in patients with atrioventricular conduction abnormalities and those with depressed left ventricular function.

Asymptomatic bradycardia (36 beats/min) with a wandering atrial pacemaker has been observed in a patient receiving concomitant timolol (a beta-adrenergic blocker) eyedrops and oral verapamil.

A decrease in metoprolol and propranolol clearance has been observed when either drug is administered concomitantly with verapamil. A variable effect has been seen when verapamil and atenolol were given together.

Digitalis: Clinical use of verapamil in digitalized patients has shown the combination to be well tolerated if digoxin doses are properly adjusted. However, chronic verapamil treatment can increase serum digoxin levels by 50% to 75%

during the first week of therapy, and this can result in digitalis toxicity. In patients with hepatic cirrhosis the influence of verapamil on digoxin kinetics is magnified. Verapamil may reduce total body clearance and extrarenal clearance of digitoxin by 27% and 29%, respectively. Maintenance and digitalization doses should be reduced when verapamil is administered, and the patient should be reassessed to avoid over- or underdigitalization. Whenever overdigitalization is suspected, the daily dose of digitalis should be reduced or temporarily discontinued. On discontinuation of Calan use, the patient should be reassessed to avoid underdigitalization.

Antihypertensive agents: Verapamil administered concomitantly with oral antihypertensive agents (eg, vasodilators, angiotensin-converting enzyme inhibitors, diuretics, beta-blockers) will usually have an additive effect on lowering blood pressure. Patients receiving these combinations should be appropriately monitored. Concomitant use of agents that attenuate alpha-adrenergic function with verapamil may result in a reduction in blood pressure that is excessive in some patients. Such an effect was observed in one study following the concomitant administration of verapamil and prazosin.

Antiarrhythmic agents:

Disopyramide: Until data on possible interactions between verapamil and disopyramide are obtained, disopyramide should not be administered within 48 hours before or 24 hours after verapamil administration.

Flecainide: A study in healthy volunteers showed that the concomitant administration of flecainide and verapamil may have additive effects on myocardial contractility, AV conduction, and repolarization. Concomitant therapy with flecainide and verapamil may result in additive negative inotropic effect and prolongation of atrioventricular conduction.

Quinidine: In a small number of patients with hypertrophic cardiomyopathy (IHSS), concomitant use of verapamil and quinidine resulted in significant hypotension. Until further data are obtained, combined therapy of verapamil and quinidine in patients with hypertrophic cardiomyopathy should probably be avoided.

The electrophysiologic effects of quinidine and verapamil on AV conduction were studied in 8 patients. Verapamil significantly counteracted the effects of quinidine on AV conduction. There has been a report of increased quinidine levels during verapamil therapy.

Other:

Nitrates: Verapamil has been given concomitantly with short- and long-acting nitrates without any undesirable drug interactions. The pharmacologic profile of both drugs and the clinical experience suggest beneficial interactions.

Cimetidine: The interaction between cimetidine and chronically administered verapamil has not been studied. Variable results on clearance have been obtained in acute studies of healthy volunteers; clearance of verapamil was either reduced or unchanged.

Lithium: Increased sensitivity to the effects of lithium (neurotoxicity) has been reported during concomitant verapamil-lithium therapy; lithium levels have been observed sometimes to increase, sometimes to decrease, and sometimes to be unchanged. Patients receiving both drugs must be monitored carefully.

Carbamazepine: Verapamil therapy may increase carbamazepine concentrations during combined therapy. This may produce carbamazepine side effects such as diplopia, headache, ataxia, or dizziness.

Rifampin: Therapy with rifampin may markedly reduce oral verapamil bioavailability.

Phenobarbital: Phenobarbital therapy may increase verapamil clearance.

Cyclosporin: Verapamil therapy may increase serum levels of cyclosporin.

Theophylline: Verapamil may inhibit the clearance and increase the plasma levels of theophylline.

Inhalation anesthetics: Animal experiments have shown that inhalation anesthetics depress cardiovascular activity by decreasing the inward movement of calcium ions. When used concomitantly, inhalation anesthetics and calcium antagonists, such as verapamil, should each be titrated carefully to avoid excessive cardiovascular depression.

Neuromuscular blocking agents: Clinical data and animal studies suggest that verapamil may potentiate the activity of neuromuscular blocking agents (curare-like and depolarizing). It may be necessary to decrease the dose of verapamil and/or the dose of the neuromuscular blocking agent when the drugs are used concomitantly.

Carcinogenesis, mutagenesis, impairment of fertility: An 18-month toxicity study in rats, at a low multiple (6-fold) of the maximum recommended human dose, and not the maximum tolerated dose, did not suggest a tumorigenic potential. There was no evidence of a carcinogenic potential of verapamil administered in the diet of rats for two years at doses of 10, 35, and 120 mg/kg/day or approximately 1, 3.5, and 12 times, respectively, the maximum recommended human daily dose (480 mg/day or 9.6 mg/kg/day).

Verapamil was not mutagenic in the Ames test in 5 test strains at 3 mg per plate with or without metabolic activation.

Studies in female rats at daily dietary doses up to 5.5 times (55 mg/kg/day) the maximum recommended human dose did not show impaired fertility. Effects on male fertility have not been determined.

Pregnancy: Pregnancy Category C. Reproduction studies have been performed in rabbits and rats at oral doses up to 1.5 (15 mg/kg/day) and 6 (60 mg/kg/day) times the human oral daily dose, respectively, and have revealed no evidence of teratogenicity. In the rat, however, this multiple of the human dose was embryocidal and retarded fetal growth and development, probably because of adverse maternal effects reflected in reduced weight gains of the dams. This oral dose has also been shown to cause hypotension in rats. There are no adequate and well-controlled studies in pregnant women. Because animal reproduction studies are not always predictive of human response, this drug should be used during pregnancy only if clearly needed. Verapamil crosses the placental barrier and can be detected in umbilical vein blood at delivery.

Labor and delivery: It is not known whether the use of verapamil during labor or delivery has immediate or delayed adverse effects on the fetus, or whether it prolongs the duration of labor or increases the need for forceps delivery or other obstetric intervention. Such adverse experiences have not been reported in the literature, despite a long history of use of verapamil in Europe in the treatment of cardiac side effects of beta-adrenergic agonist agents used to treat premature labor.

Nursing mothers: Verapamil is excreted in human milk. Because of the potential for adverse reactions in nursing infants from verapamil, nursing should be discontinued while verapamil is administered.

Pediatric use: Safety and effectiveness in pediatric patients have not been established.

Animal pharmacology and/or animal toxicology: In chronic animal toxicology studies verapamil caused lenticular and/or suture line changes at 30 mg/kg/day or greater, and frank cataracts at 62.5 mg/kg/day or greater in the beagle dog but not in the rat. Development of cataracts due to verapamil has not been reported in man.

ADVERSE REACTIONS

Serious adverse reactions are uncommon when Calan therapy is initiated with upward dose titration within the recommended single and total daily dose. See *Warnings* for discussion of heart failure, hypotension, elevated liver enzymes, AV block, and rapid ventricular response. Reversible (upon discontinuation of verapamil) non-obstructive, paralytic ileus has been infrequently reported in association with the use of verapamil. The following reactions to orally administered verapamil occurred at rates greater than 1.0% or occurred at lower rates but appeared clearly drug-related in clinical trials in 4,954 patients:

Constipation	7.3%	Dyspnea	1.4%
Dizziness	3.3%	Bradycardia	
Nausea	2.7%	(HR<50/min)	1.4%
Hypotension	2.5%	AV block	
Headache	2.2%	total (1°, 2°, 3°)	1.2%
Edema	1.9%	2° and 3°	0.8%
CHF/Pulmonary		Rash	1.2%
edema	1.8%	Flushing	0.6%
Fatigue	1.7%		

Elevated liver enzymes (see *Warnings*)

In clinical trials related to the control of ventricular response in digitalized patients who had atrial fibrillation or flutter, ventricular rates below 50 at rest occurred in 15% of patients and asymptomatic hypotension occurred in 5% of patients.

The following reactions, reported in 1.0% or less of patients, occurred under conditions (open trials, marketing experience) where a causal relationship is uncertain; they are listed to alert the physician to a possible relationship:

Cardiovascular: angina pectoris, atrioventricular dissociation, chest pain, claudication, myocardial infarction, palpitations, purpura (vasculitis), syncope.

Digestive system: diarrhea, dry mouth, gastrointestinal distress, gingival hyperplasia.

Hemic and lymphatic: ecchymosis or bruising.

Nervous system: cerebrovascular accident, confusion, equilibrium disorders, insomnia, muscle cramps, paresthesia, psychotic symptoms, shakiness, somnolence.

Skin: arthralgia and rash, exanthema, hair loss, hyperkeratosis, macules, sweating, urticaria, Stevens-Johnson syndrome, erythema multiforme.

Special senses: blurred vision, tinnitus.

Urogenital: gynecomastia, galactorrhea/hyperprolactinemia, increased urination, spotty menstruation, impotence.

Treatment of acute cardiovascular adverse reactions: The frequency of cardiovascular adverse reactions that require therapy is rare; hence, experience with their treatment is limited. Whenever severe hypotension or complete AV block occurs following oral administration of verapamil, the appropriate emergency measures should be applied immediately; eg, intravenously administered norepinephrine bitartrate, atropine sulfate, isoproterenol HCl (all in the usual doses), or calcium gluconate (10% solution). In patients with hypertrophic cardiomyopathy (IHSS), alpha-adrenergic agents (phenylephrine HCl, metaraminol bitartrate, or methoxamine HCl) should be used to maintain blood pressure, and isoproterenol and norepinephrine should be avoided. If further support is necessary, dopamine HCl or dobutamine HCl may be administered. Actual treatment and dosage should depend on the severity of the clinical situation and the judgment and experience of the treating physician.

OVERDOSAGE

Treat all verapamil overdoses as serious and maintain observation for at least 48 hours (especially Calan SR), preferably under continuous hospital care. Delayed pharmacodynamic consequences may occur with the sustained-release formulation. Verapamil is known to decrease gastrointestinal transit time.

Treatment of overdosage should be supportive. Beta adrenergic stimulation or parenteral administration of calcium solutions may increase calcium ion flux across the slow channel, and have been used effectively in treatment of deliberate overdosage with verapamil. In a few reported cases, overdose with calcium channel blockers has been associated with hypotension and bradycardia, initially refractory to atropine but becoming more responsive to this treatment when the patients received large doses (close to 1 gram/hour for more than 24 hours) of calcium chloride. Verapamil cannot be removed by hemodialysis. Clinically significant hypotensive reactions or high degree AV block should be treated with vasopressor agents or cardiac pacing, respectively. Asystole should be handled by the usual measures including cardiopulmonary resuscitation.

DOSAGE AND ADMINISTRATION

The dose of verapamil must be individualized by titration. The usefulness and safety of dosages exceeding 480 mg/day have not been established; therefore, this daily dosage should not be exceeded. Since the half-life of verapamil increases during chronic dosing, maximum response may be delayed.

Angina: Clinical trials show that the usual dose is 80 mg to 120 mg three times a day. However, 40 mg three times a day may be warranted in patients who may have an increased response to verapamil (eg, decreased hepatic function, elderly, etc). Upward titration should be based on therapeutic efficacy and safety evaluated approximately eight hours after dosing. Dosage may be increased at daily (eg, patients with unstable angina) or weekly intervals until optimum clinical response is obtained.

Arrhythmias: The dosage in digitalized patients with chronic atrial fibrillation (see *Precautions*) ranges from 240 to 320 mg/day in divided (t.i.d. or q.i.d.) doses. The dosage for prophylaxis of PSVT (non-digitalized patients) ranges from 240 to 480 mg/day in divided (t.i.d or q.i.d.) doses. In general, maximum effects for any given dosage will be apparent during the first 48 hours of therapy.

Essential hypertension: Dose should be individualized by titration. The usual initial monotherapy dose in clinical trials was 80 mg three times a day (240 mg/day). Daily dosages of 360 and 480 mg have been used but there is no evidence that dosages beyond 360 mg provided added effect. Consideration should be given to beginning titration at 40 mg three times per day in patients who might respond to lower doses, such as the elderly or people of small stature. The antihypertensive effects of Calan are evident within the first week of therapy. Upward titration should be based on therapeutic efficacy, assessed at the end of the dosing interval.

HOW SUPPLIED

Calan 40-mg tablets are round, pink, film coated, with CALAN debossed on one side and 40 on the other, supplied as:

NDC Number	Size
0025-1771-31	bottle of 100

Calan 80-mg tablets are oval, peach colored, scored, film coated, with CALAN debossed on one side and 80 on the other, supplied as:

NDC Number	Size
0025-1851-31	bottle of 100
0025-1851-51	bottle of 500
0025-1851-52	bottle of 1,000

Calan 120-mg tablets are oval, brown, scored, film coated, with CALAN 120 debossed on one side, supplied as:

NDC Number	Size
0025-1861-31	bottle of 100
0025-1861-52	bottle of 1,000

Store at 59° to 77°F (15° to 25°C) and protect from light. Dispense in tight, light-resistant containers.

Continued on next page

Calan—Cont.

Caution: Federal law prohibits dispensing without prescription.

5/1/97 • A05315-2

Shown in Product Identification Guide, page 337

CALAN® SR ℞

[*cal 'an ess ar*]

(verapamil hydrochloride)

Sustained-Release Oral Caplets

PRODUCT OVERVIEW

KEY FACTS

Calan SR, a calcium ion antagonist designed for sustained release in the gastrointestinal tract, exerts an antihypertensive effect by decreasing systemic vascular resistance, usually without orthostatic decreases in blood pressure or reflex tachycardia.

MAJOR USE

Calan SR is indicated for the management of essential hypertension.

SAFETY INFORMATION

See complete safety information set forth below.

PRESCRIBING INFORMATION

CALAN® SR ℞

[*cal 'an ess ar*]

(verapamil hydrochloride)

Sustained-Release Oral Caplets

DESCRIPTION

Calan SR (verapamil hydrochloride) is a calcium ion influx inhibitor (slow-channel blocker or calcium ion antagonist). Calan SR is available for oral administration as light green, capsule-shaped, scored, film-coated tablets (caplets) containing 240 mg of verapamil hydrochloride; as light pink, oval, scored, film-coated tablets (caplets) containing 180 mg of verapamil hydrochloride; and as light violet, oval, film-coated tablets (caplets) containing 120 mg of verapamil hydrochloride. The caplets are designed for sustained release of the drug in the gastrointestinal tract; sustained-release characteristics are not altered when the caplet is divided in half.

The structural formula of verapamil HCl is

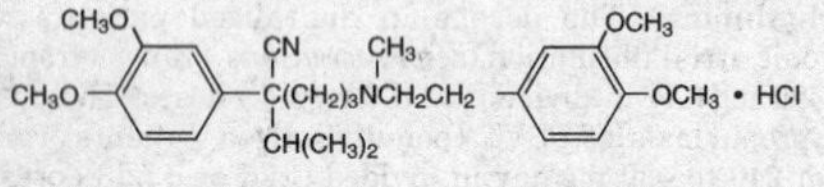

$C_{27}H_{38}N_2O_4$ • HCl M. W. = 491.08

Benzeneacetonitrile, α-[3-[[2-(3, 4-dimethoxyphenyl) ethyl] methylamino]propyl]-3,4-dimethoxy-α- (1-methylethyl) hydrochloride

Verapamil HCl is an almost white, crystalline powder, practically free of odor, with a bitter taste. It is soluble in water, chloroform, and methanol. Verapamil HCl is not chemically related to other cardioactive drugs.

Inactive ingredients include alginate, carnauba wax, hydroxypropyl methylcellulose, magnesium stearate, microcrystalline cellulose, polyethylene glycol, polyvinyl pyrrolidone, talc, titanium dioxide, and coloring agents: 240-mg—D&C Yellow No. 10 Lake and FD&C Blue No. 2 Lake; 120- and 180-mg—iron oxide.

CLINICAL PHARMACOLOGY

Calan (verapamil HCl) is a calcium ion influx inhibitor (slow-channel blocker or calcium ion antagonist) that exerts its pharmacologic effects by modulating the influx of ionic calcium across the cell membrane of the arterial smooth muscle as well as in conductile and contractile myocardial cells.

Mechanism of action

Essential hypertension: Verapamil exerts antihypertensive effects by decreasing systemic vascular resistance, usually without orthostatic decreases in blood pressure or reflex tachycardia; bradycardia (rate less than 50 beats/min) is uncommon (1.4%). During isometric or dynamic exercise Calan does not alter systolic cardiac function in patients with normal ventricular function.

Calan does not alter total serum calcium levels. However, one report suggested that calcium levels above the normal range may alter the therapeutic effect of Calan.

Other pharmacologic actions of Calan include the following:

Calan dilates the main coronary arteries and coronary arterioles, both in normal and ischemic regions, and is a potent inhibitor of coronary artery spasm, whether spontaneous or ergonovine-induced. This property increases myocardial oxygen delivery in patients with coronary artery spasm and is responsible for the effectiveness of Calan in vasospastic (Prinzmetal's or variant) as well as unstable angina at rest. Whether this effect plays any role in classical effort angina is not clear, but studies of exercise tolerance have not shown an increase in the maximum exercise rate–pressure product, a widely accepted measure of oxygen utilization. This suggests that, in general, relief of spasm or dilation of coronary arteries is not an important factor in classical angina.

Calan regularly reduces the total systemic resistance (afterload) against which the heart works both at rest and at a given level of exercise by dilating peripheral arterioles.

Electrical activity through the AV node depends, to a significant degree, upon calcium influx through the slow channel. By decreasing the influx of calcium, Calan prolongs the effective refractory period within the AV node and slows AV conduction in a rate-related manner.

Normal sinus rhythm is usually not affected, but in patients with sick sinus syndrome, Calan may interfere with sinus-node impulse generation and may induce sinus arrest or sinoatrial block. Atrioventricular block can occur in patients without preexisting conduction defects (see *Warnings*).

Calan does not alter the normal atrial action potential or intraventricular conduction time, but depresses amplitude, velocity of depolarization, and conduction in depressed atrial fibers. Calan may shorten the antegrade effective refractory period of the accessory bypass tract. Acceleration of ventricular rate and/or ventricular fibrillation has been reported in patients with atrial flutter or atrial fibrillation and a coexisting accessory AV pathway following administration of verapamil (see *Warnings*).

Calan has a local anesthetic action that is 1.6 times that of procaine on an equimolar basis. It is not known whether this action is important at the doses used in man.

Pharmacokinetics and metabolism: With the immediate-release formulation, more than 90% of the orally administered dose of Calan is absorbed. Because of rapid biotransformation of verapamil during its first pass through the portal circulation, bioavailability ranges from 20% to 35%. Peak plasma concentrations are reached between 1 and 2 hours after oral administration. Chronic oral administration of 120 mg of verapamil HCl every 6 hours resulted in plasma levels of verapamil ranging from 125 to 400 ng/ml, with higher values reported occasionally. A nonlinear correlation between the verapamil dose administered and verapamil plasma level does exist. In early dose titration with verapamil a relationship exists between verapamil plasma concentration and prolongation of the PR interval. However, during chronic administration this relationship may disappear. The mean elimination half-life in single-dose studies ranged from 2.8 to 7.4 hours. In these same studies, after repetitive dosing, the half-life increased to a range from 4.5 to 12.0 hours (after less than 10 consecutive doses given 6 hours apart). Half-life of verapamil may increase during titration. No relationship has been established between the plasma concentraton of verapamil and a reduction in blood pressure.

Aging may affect the pharmacokinetics of verapamil. Elimination half-life may be prolonged in the elderly. In multiple-dose studies under fasting conditions, the bioavailability, measured by AUC, of Calan SR was similar to Calan (immediate release); rates of absorption were of course different.

In a randomized, single-dose, crossover study using healthy volunteers, administration of 240 mg Calan SR with food produced peak plasma verapamil concentrations of 79 ng/ml; time to peak plasma verapamil concentration of 7.71 hours; and AUC (0–24 hr) of 841 ng·hr/ml). When Calan SR was administered to fasting subjects, peak plasma verapamil concentration was 164 ng/ml; time to peak plasma verapamil concentration was 5.21 hours; and AUC (0–24 hr) was 1,478 ng·hr/ml. Similar results were demonstrated for plasma norverapamil. Food thus produces decreased bioavailability (AUC) but a narrower peak-to-trough ratio. Good correlation of dose and response is not available, but controlled studies of Calan SR have shown effectiveness of doses similar to the effective doses of Calan (immediate release).

In healthy men, orally administered Calan undergoes extensive metabolism in the liver. Twelve metabolites have been identified in plasma; all except norverapamil are present in trace amounts only. Norverapamil can reach steady-state plasma concentrations approximately equal to those of verapamil itself. The cardiovascular activity of norverapamil appears to be approximately 20% that of verapamil. Approximately 70% of an administered dose is excreted as metabolites in the urine and 16% or more in the feces within 5 days. About 3% to 4% is excreted in the urine as unchanged drug. Approximately 90% is bound to plasma proteins. In patients with hepatic insufficiency, metabolism of immediate-release verapamil is delayed and elimination half-life prolonged up to 14 to 16 hours (see *Precautions*); the volume of distribution is increased and plasma clearance reduced to about 30% of normal. Verapamil clearance values suggest that patients with liver dysfunction may attain therapeutic verapamil plasma concentrations with one third of the oral daily dose required for patients with normal liver function.

After four weeks of oral dosing (120 mg q.i.d.), verapamil and norverapamil levels were noted in the cerebrospinal fluid with estimated partition coefficient of 0.06 for verapamil and 0.04 for norverapamil.

Hemodynamics and myocardial metabolism: Calan reduces afterload and myocardial contractility. Improved left ventricular diastolic function in patients with IHSS and those with coronary heart disease has also been observed with Calan. In most patients, including those with organic cardiac disease, the negative inotropic action of Calan is countered by reduction of afterload, and cardiac index is usually not reduced. However, in patients with severe left ventricular dysfunction (eg, pulmonary wedge pressure above 20 mm Hg or ejection fraction less than 30%), or in patients taking beta-adrenergic blocking agents or other cardiodepressant drugs, deterioration of ventricular function may occur (see *Drug interactions*).

Pulmonary function: Calan does not induce bronchoconstriction and, hence, does not impair ventilatory function.

INDICATIONS AND USAGE

Calan SR is indicated for the management of essential hypertension.

CONTRAINDICATIONS

Verapamil HCl caplets are contraindicated in:

1. Severe left ventricular dysfunction (see *Warnings*)
2. Hypotension (systolic pressure less than 90 mm Hg) or cardiogenic shock
3. Sick sinus syndrome (except in patients with a functioning artificial ventricular pacemaker)
4. Second- or third-degree AV block (except in patients with a functioning artificial ventricular pacemaker)
5. Patients with atrial flutter or atrial fibrillation and an accessory bypass tract (eg, Wolff-Parkinson-White, Lown-Ganong-Levine syndromes). (See *Warnings.*)
6. Patients with known hypersensitivity to verapamil hydrochloride.

WARNINGS

Heart failure: Verapamil has a negative inotropic effect, which in most patients is compensated by its afterload reduction (decreased systemic vascular resistance) properties without a net impairment of ventricular performance. In clinical experience with 4,954 patients, 87 (1.8%) developed congestive heart failure or pulmonary edema. Verapamil should be avoided in patients with severe left ventricular dysfunction (eg, ejection fraction less than 30%) or moderate to severe symptoms of cardiac failure and in patients with any degree of ventricular dysfunction if they are receiving a beta-adrenergic blocker (see *Drug interactions*). Patients with milder ventricular dysfunction should, if possible, be controlled with optimum doses of digitalis and/or diuretics before verapamil treatment. **(Note interactions with digoxin under *Precautions.*)**

Hypotension: Occasionally, the pharmacologic action of verapamil may produce a decrease in blood pressure below normal levels, which may result in dizziness or symptomatic hypotension. The incidence of hypotension observed in 4,954 patients enrolled in clinical trials was 2.5%. In hypertensive patients, decreases in blood pressure below normal are unusual. Tilt-table testing (60 degrees) was not able to induce orthostatic hypotension.

Elevated liver enzymes: Elevations of transaminases with and without concomitant elevations in alkaline phosphatase and bilirubin have been reported. Such elevations have sometimes been transient and may disappear even in the face of continued verapamil treatment. Several cases of hepatocellular injury related to verapamil have been proven by rechallenge; half of these had clinical symptoms (malaise, fever, and/or right upper quadrant pain) in addition to elevation of SGOT, SGPT, and alkaline phosphatase. Periodic monitoring of liver function in patients receiving verapamil is therefore prudent.

Accessory bypass tract (Wolff-Parkinson-White or Lown-Ganong-Levine): Some patients with paroxysmal and/or chronic atrial fibrillation or atrial flutter and a coexisting accessory AV pathway have developed increased antegrade conduction across the accessory pathway bypassing the AV node, producing a very rapid ventricular response or ventricular fibrillation after receiving intravenous verapamil (or digitalis). Although a risk of this occurring with oral verapamil has not been established, such patients receiving oral verapamil may be at risk and its use in these patients is contraindicated (see *Contraindications*). Treatment is usually DC-cardioversion. Cardioversion has been used safely and effectively after oral Calan.

Atrioventricular block: The effect of verapamil on AV conduction and the SA node may cause asymptomatic first-degree AV block and transient bradycardia, sometimes accompanied by nodal escape rhythms. PR-interval prolongation is correlated with verapamil plasma concentrations,

especially during the early titration phase of therapy. Higher degrees of AV block, however, were infrequently (0.8%) observed. Marked first-degree block or progressive development to second- or third-degree AV block requires a reduction in dosage or, in rare instances, discontinuation of verapamil HCl and institution of appropriate therapy, depending upon the clinical situation.

Patients with hypertrophic cardiomyopathy (IHSS): In 120 patients with hypertrophic cardiomyopathy (most of them refractory or intolerant to propranolol) who received therapy with verapamil at doses up to 720 mg/day, a variety of serious adverse effects were seen. Three patients died in pulmonary edema; all had severe left ventricular outflow obstruction and a past history of left ventricular dysfunction. Eight other patients had pulmonary edema and/or severe hypotension; abnormally high (greater than 20 mm Hg) pulmonary wedge pressure and a marked left ventricular outflow obstruction were present in most of these patients. Concomitant administration of quinidine (see *Drug interactions*) preceded the severe hypotension in 3 of the 8 patients (2 of whom developed pulmonary edema). Sinus bradycardia occurred in 11% of the patients, second-degree AV block in 4%, and sinus arrest in 2%. It must be appreciated that this group of patients had a serious disease with a high mortality rate. Most adverse effects responded well to dose reduction, and only rarely did verapamil use have to be discontinued.

PRECAUTIONS
General
Use in patients with impaired hepatic function: Since verapamil is highly metabolized by the liver, it should be administered cautiously to patients with impaired hepatic function. Severe liver dysfunction prolongs the elimination half-life of immediate-release verapamil to about 14 to 16 hours; hence, approximately 30% of the dose given to patients with normal liver function should be administered to these patients. Careful monitoring for abnormal prolongation of the PR interval or other signs of excessive pharmacologic effects (see *Overdosage*) should be carried out.

Use in patients with attenuated (decreased) neuromuscular transmission: It has been reported that verapamil decreases neuromuscular transmission in patients with Duchenne's muscular dystrophy, and that verapamil prolongs recovery from the neuromuscular blocking agent vecuronium. It may be necessary to decrease the dosage of verapamil when it is administered to patients with attenuated neuromuscular transmission.

Use in patients with impaired renal function: About 70% of an administered dose of verapamil is excreted as metabolites in the urine. Verapamil is not removed by hemodialysis. Until further data are available, verapamil should be administered cautiously to patients with impaired renal function. These patients should be carefully monitored for abnormal prolongation of the PR interval or other signs of overdosage (see *Overdosage*).

Drug interactions
Beta-blockers: Concomitant therapy with beta-adrenergic blockers and verapamil may result in additive negative effects on heart rate, atrioventricular conduction and/or cardiac contractility. The combination of sustained-release verapamil and beta-adrenergic blocking agents has not been studied. However, there have been reports of excessive bradycardia and AV block, including complete heart block, when the combination has been used for the treatment of hypertension. For hypertensive patients, the risks of combined therapy may outweigh the potential benefits. The combination should be used only with caution and close monitoring.

Asymptomatic bradycardia (36 beats/min) with a wandering atrial pacemaker has been observed in a patient receiving concomitant timolol (a beta-adrenergic blocker) eyedrops and oral verapamil.

A decrease in metroprolol and propranolol clearance has been observed when either drug is administered concomitantly with verapamil. A variable effect has been seen when verapamil and atenolol were given together.

Digitalis: Clinical use of verapamil in digitalized patients has shown the combination to be well tolerated if digoxin doses are properly adjusted. However, chronic verapamil treatment can increase serum digoxin levels by 50% to 75% during the first week of therapy, and this can result in digitalis toxicity. In patients with hepatic cirrhosis the influence of verapamil on digoxin kinetics is magnified. Verapamil may reduce total body clearance and extrarenal clearance of digitoxin by 27% and 29%, respectively. Maintenance digitalis doses should be reduced when verapamil is administered, and the patient should be carefully monitored to avoid over- or underdigitalization. Whenever overdigitalization is suspected, the daily dose of digitalis should be reduced or temporarily discontinued. On discontinuation of Calan use, the patient should be reassessed to avoid underdigitalization.

Antihypertensive agents: Verapamil administered concomitantly with oral antihypertensive agents (eg, vasodilators, angiotensin-converting enzyme inhibitors, diuretics,

beta-blockers) will usually have an additive effect on lowering blood pressure. Patients receiving these combinations should be appropriately monitored. Concomitant use of agents that attenuate alpha-adrenergic function with verapamil may result in a reduction in blood pressure that is excessive in some patients. Such an effect was observed in one study following the concomitant administration of verapamil and prazosin.

Antiarrhythmic agents:
Disopyramide: Until data on possible interactions between verapamil and disopyramide phosphate are obtained, disopyramide should not be administered within 48 hours before or 24 hours after verapamil administration.

Flecainide: A study in healthy volunteers showed that the concomitant administration of flecainide and verapamil may have additive effects on myocardial contractility, AV conduction, and repolarization. Concomitant therapy with flecainide and verapamil may result in additive negative inotropic effect and prolongation of atrioventricular conduction.

Quinidine: In a small number of patients with hypertrophic cardiomyopathy (IHSS), concomitant use of verapamil and quinidine resulted in significant hypotension. Until further data are obtained, combined therapy of verapamil and quinidine in patients with hypertrophic cardiomyopathy should probably be avoided.

The electrophysiologic effects of quinidine and verapamil on AV conduction were studied in 8 patients. Verapamil significantly counteracted the effects of quinidine on AV conduction. There has been a report of increased quinidine levels during verapamil therapy.

Other:
Nitrates: Verapamil has been given concomitantly with short- and long-acting nitrates without any undesirable drug interactions. The pharmacologic profile of both drugs and the clinical experience suggest beneficial interactions.

Cimetidine: The interaction between cimetidine and chronically administered verapamil has not been studied. Variable results on clearance have been obtained in acute studies of healthy volunteers; clearance of verapamil was either reduced or unchanged.

Lithium: Increased sensitivity to the effects of lithium (neurotoxicity) has been reported during concomitant verapamil-lithium therapy with either no change or an increase in serum lithium levels. However, the addition of verapamil has also resulted in the lowering of serum lithium levels in patients receiving chronic stable oral lithium. Patients receiving both drugs must be monitored carefully.

Carbamazepine: Verapamil therapy may increase carbamazepine concentrations during combined therapy. This may produce carbamazepine side effects such as diplopia, headache, ataxia, or dizziness.

Rifampin: Therapy with rifampin may markedly reduce oral verapamil bioavailability.

Phenobarbital: Phenobarbital therapy may increase verapamil clearance.

Cyclosporin: Verapamil therapy may increase serum levels of cyclosporin.

Theophylline: Verapamil may inhibit the clearance and increase the plasma levels of theophylline.

Inhalation anesthetics: Animal experiments have shown that inhalation anesthetics depress cardiovascular activity by decreasing the inward movement of calcium ions. When used concomitantly, inhalation anesthetics and calcium antagonists, such as verapamil, should each be titrated carefully to avoid excessive cardiovascular depression.

Neuromuscular blocking agents: Clinical data and animal studies suggest that verapamil may potentiate the activity of neuromuscular blocking agents (curare-like and depolarizing). It may be necessary to decrease the dose of verapamil and/or the dose of the neuromuscular blocking agent when the drugs are used concomitantly.

Carcinogenesis, mutagenesis, impairment of fertility: An 18-month toxicity study in rats, at a low multiple (6-fold) of the maximum recommended human dose, and not the maximum tolerated dose, did not suggest a tumorigenic potential. There was no evidence of a carcinogenic potential of verapamil administered in the diet of rats for two years at doses of 10, 35, and 120 mg/kg/day or approximately 1, 3.5, and 12 times, respectively, the maximum recommended human daily dose (480 mg/day or 9.6 mg/kg/day).

Verapamil was not mutagenic in the Ames test in 5 test strains at 3 mg per plate with or without metabolic activation.

Studies in female rats at daily dietary doses up to 5.5 times (55 mg/kg/day) the maximum recommended human dose did not show impaired fertility. Effects on male fertility have not been determined.

Pregnancy: Pregnancy Category C. Reproduction studies have been performed in rabbits and rats at oral doses up to 1.5 (15 mg/kg/day) and 6 (60 mg/kg/day) times the human oral daily dose, respectively, and have revealed no evidence of teratogenicity. In the rat, however, this multiple of the human dose was embryocidal and retarded fetal growth and development, probably because of adverse maternal effects reflected in reduced weight gains of the dams. This oral dose

has also been shown to cause hypotension in rats. There are no adequate and well-controlled studies in pregnant women. Because animal reproduction studies are not always predictive of human response, this drug should be used during pregnancy only if clearly needed. Verapamil crosses the placental barrier and can be detected in umbilical vein blood at delivery.

Labor and delivery: It is not known whether the use of verapamil during labor or delivery has immediate or delayed adverse effects on the fetus, or whether it prolongs the duration of labor or increases the need for forceps delivery or other obstetric intervention. Such adverse experiences have not been reported in the literature, despite a long history of use of verapamil in Europe in the treatment of cardiac side effects of beta-adrenergic agonist agents used to treat premature labor.

Nursing mothers: Verapamil is excreted in human milk. Because of the potential for adverse reactions in nursing infants from verapamil, nursing should be discontinued while verapamil is administered.

Pediatric use: Safety and efficacy of Calan SR in children below the age of 18 years have not been established.

Animal pharmacology and/or animal toxicology: In chronic animal toxicology studies verapamil caused lenticular and/or suture line changes at 30 mg/kg/day or greater, and frank cataracts at 62.5 mg/kg/day or greater in the beagle dog but not in the rat. Development of cataracts due to verapamil has not been reported in man.

ADVERSE REACTIONS

Serious adverse reactions are uncommon when verapamil therapy is initiated with upward dose titration within the recommended single and total daily dose. See *Warnings* for discussion of heart failure, hypotension, elevated liver enzymes, AV block, and rapid ventricular response. Reversible (upon discontinuation of verapamil) non-obstructive, paralytic ileus has been infrequently reported in association with the use of verapamil. The following reactions to orally administered verapamil occurred at rates greater than 1.0% or occurred at lower rates but appeared clearly drug-related in clinical trials in 4,954 patients:

Constipation	7.3%	Dyspnea	1.4%
Dizziness	3.3%	Bradycardia	
Nausea	2.7%	(HR<50/min)	1.4%
Hypotension	2.5%	AV block	
Headache	2.2%	total (1°, 2°, 3°)	1.2%
Edema	1.9%	2° and 3°	0.8%
CHF, Pulmonary		Rash	1.2%
edema	1.8%	Flushing	0.6%
Fatigue	1.7%		

Elevated liver enzymes (see *Warnings*)

In clinical trials related to the control of ventricular response in digitalized patients who had atrial fibrillation or flutter, ventricular rates below 50/min at rest occurred in 15% of patients and asymptomatic hypotension occurred in 5% of patients.

The following reactions, reported in 1% or less of patients, occurred under conditions (open trials, marketing experience) where a causal relationship is uncertain; they are listed to alert the physician to a possible relationship:

Cardiovascular: angina pectoris, atrioventricular dissociation, chest pain, claudication, myocardial infarction, palpitations, purpura (vasculitis), syncope.

Digestive system: diarrhea, dry mouth, gastrointestinal distress, gingival hyperplasia.

Hemic and lymphatic: ecchymosis or bruising.

Nervous system: cerebrovascular accident, confusion, equilibrium disorders, insomnia, muscle cramps, paresthesia, psychotic symptoms, shakiness, somnolence.

Skin: arthralgia and rash, exanthema, hair loss, hyperkeratosis, macules, sweating, urticaria, Stevens-Johnson syndrome, erythema multiforme.

Special senses: blurred vision.

Urogenital: gynecomastia, galactorrhea/hyperprolactinemia, increased urination, spotty menstruation, impotence.

Treatment of acute cardiovascular adverse reactions: The frequency of cardiovascular adverse reactions that require therapy is rare; hence, experience with their treatment is limited. Whenever severe hypotension or complete AV block occurs following oral administration of verapamil, the appropriate emergency measures should be applied immediately; eg, intravenously administered norepinephrine bitartrate, atropine sulfate, isoproterenol HCl (all in the usual doses), or calcium gluconate (10% solution). In patients with hypertrophic cardiomyopathy (IHSS), alpha-adrenergic agents (phenylephrine HCl, metaraminol bitartrate, or methoxamine HCl) should be used to maintain blood pressure, and isoproterenol and norepinephrine should be avoided. If further support is necessary, dopamine HCl or dobutamine HCl may be administered. Actual treatment and dosage should depend on the severity of the clinical situation and the judgment and experience of the treating physician.

Continued on next page

Calan SR—Cont.

OVERDOSAGE

Treat all verapamil overdoses as serious and maintain observation for at least 48 hours (especially Calan SR), preferably under continuous hospital care. Delayed pharmacodynamic consequences may occur with the sustained-release formulation. Verapamil is known to decrease gastrointestinal transit time.

Treatment of overdosage should be supportive. Beta adrenergic stimulation or parenteral administration of calcium solutions may increase calcium ion flux across the slow channel, and have been used effectively in treatment of deliberate overdosage with verapamil. Verapamil cannot be removed by hemodialysis. Clinically significant hypotensive reactions or high degree AV block should be treated with vasopressor agents or cardiac pacing, respectively. Asystole should be handled by the usual measures including cardiopulmonary resuscitation.

DOSAGE AND ADMINISTRATION

Essential hypertension: The dose of Calan SR should be individualized by titration and the drug should be administered with food. Initiate therapy with 180 mg of sustained-release verapamil HCl, Calan SR, given in the morning. Lower initial doses of 120 mg a day may be warranted in patients who may have an increased response to verapamil (eg, the elderly or small people). Upward titration should be based on therapeutic efficacy and safety evaluated weekly and approximately 24 hours after the previous dose. The antihypertensive effects of Calan SR are evident within the first week of therapy.

If adequate response is not obtained with 180 mg of Calan SR, the dose may be titrated upward in the following manner:

a) 240 mg each morning,
b) 180 mg each morning plus
   180 mg each evening; or
   240 mg each morning plus
   120 mg each evening,
c) 240 mg every 12 hours.

When switching from immediate-release Calan to Calan SR the total daily dose in milligrams may remain the same.

HOW SUPPLIED

Calan SR 240-mg caplets are light green, capsule shaped, scored, film coated, with CALAN debossed on one side and SR 240 on the other, supplied as:

NDC Number	Size
0025-1891-31	bottle of 100
0025-1891-51	bottle of 500
0025-1891-34	carton of 100 unit dose

Calan SR 180-mg caplets are light pink, oval, scored, film coated, with CALAN debossed on one side and SR 180 on the other, supplied as:

NDC Number	Size
0025-1911-31	bottle of 100
0025-1911-34	carton of 100 unit dose

Calan SR 120-mg caplets are light violet, oval, film-coated, with CALAN debossed on one side and SR 120 on the other, supplied as:

NDC Number	Size
0025-1901-31	bottle of 100
0025-1901-34	carton of 100 unit dose

Store at 59° to 77°F (15° to 25°C) and protect from light and moisture. Dispense in tight, light-resistant containers.

Caution: Federal law prohibits dispensing without prescription.

4/25/95 • A05298-3

Shown in Product Identification Guide, page 337

COVERA-HS™ ℞

[*Cō-ver '-ə*]
(verapamil hydrochloride)
Extended-Release Tablets
Controlled-Onset

DESCRIPTION

Covera-HS (verapamil hydrochloride) is a calcium ion influx inhibitor (slow-channel blocker or calcium ion antagonist). Covera-HS is available for oral administration as pale yellow, round, film-coated tablets containing 240 mg of verapamil hydrochloride and as lavender, round, film-coated tablets containing 180 mg of verapamil hydrochloride. Verapamil is administered as a racemic mixture of the R and S enantiomers. The structural formulae of the verapamil HCl enantiomers are:

[See chemical structure at top of next column]

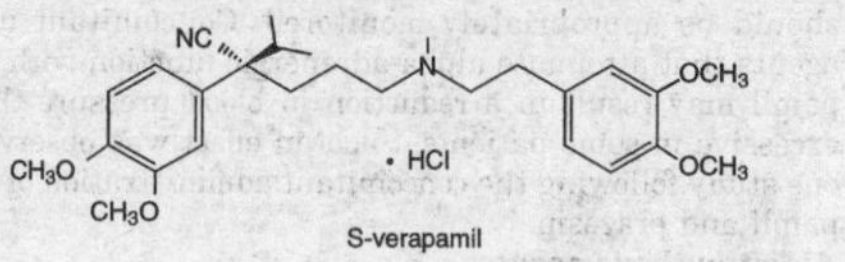

S-verapamil

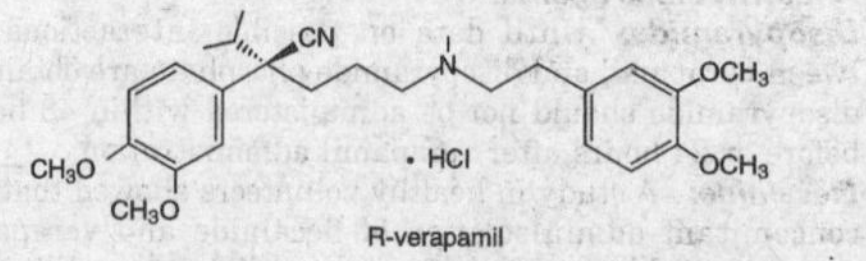

R-verapamil

$C_{27}H_{38}N_2O_4 \cdot HCl$ M.W.=491.07

Benzeneacetonitrile, (±)-α[3[[2-(3,4-dimethoxyphenyl) ethyl]methylamino]propyl]-3,4-dimethoxy-α-(1-methylethyl) hydrochloride

Verapamil HCl is an almost white, crystalline powder, practically free of odor, with a bitter taste. It is soluble in water, chloroform, and methanol. Verapamil HCl is not chemically related to other cardioactive drugs.

Inactive ingredients are black ferric oxide, BHT, cellulose acetate, hydroxyethyl cellulose, hydroxypropyl cellulose, hydroxypropyl methylcellulose, magnesium stearate, polyethylene glycol, polyethylene oxide, polysorbate 80, povidone, sodium chloride, titanium dioxide, and coloring agents: 240-mg—FD&C Blue No. 2 Lake and D&C Yellow No. 10 Lake; 180-mg—FD&C Blue No. 2 Lake and D&C Red No. 30 Lake.

System components and performance: The Covera-HS formulation has been designed to initiate the release of verapamil 4–5 hours after ingestion. This delay is introduced by a layer between the active drug core and outer semipermeable membrane. As water from the gastrointestinal tract enters the tablet, this delay coating is solubilized and released. As tablet hydration continues, the osmotic layer expands and pushes against the drug layer, releasing drug through precision laser-drilled orifices in the outer membrane at a constant rate. This controlled rate of drug delivery in the gastrointestinal lumen is independent of posture, pH, gastrointestinal motility, and fed or fasting conditions.

The biologically inert components of the delivery system remain intact during GI transit and are eliminated in the feces as an insoluble shell.

CLINICAL PHARMACOLOGY

Covera-HS has a unique delivery system, designed for bedtime dosing, incorporating a 4 to 5-hour delay in drug delivery. The unique controlled-onset, extended-release (COER) delivery system, which is designed for bedtime dosing, results in a maximum plasma concentration (C_{max}) of verapamil in the morning hours.

Verapamil is a calcium ion influx inhibitor (L-type calcium channel blocker or calcium channel antagonist). Verapamil exerts its pharmacologic effects by selectively inhibiting the transmembrane influx of ionic calcium into arterial smooth muscle as well as in conductile and contractile myocardial cells without altering serum calcium concentrations.

Mechanism of Action

In vitro: Verapamil binding is voltage-dependent with affinity increasing as the vascular smooth muscle membrane potential is reduced. In addition, verapamil binding is frequency dependent and apparent affinity increases with increased frequency of depolarizing stimulus.

The L-type calcium channel is an oligomeric structure consisting of five putative subunits designated alpha-1, alpha-2, beta, tau, and epsilon. Biochemical evidence points to separate binding sites for 1,4-dihydropyridines, phenylalkylamines, and the benzothiazepines (all located on the alpha-1 subunit). Although they share a similar mechanism of action, calcium channel blockers represent three heterogeneous categories of drugs with differing vascular-cardiac selectivity ratios.

Essential hypertension: Verapamil produces its antihypertensive effect by a combination of vascular and cardiac effects. It acts as a vasodilator with selectivity for the arterial portion of the peripheral vasculature. As a result the systemic vascular resistence is reduced and usually without orthostatic hypotension or reflex tachycardia. Bradycardia (rate less than 50 beats/min) is uncommon (<1% with Covera-HS as assessed by ECG). During isometric or dynamic exercise Covera-HS does not alter systolic cardiac function in patients with normal ventricular function.

Covera-HS does not alter total serum calcium levels. However, one report has suggested that calcium levels above the normal range may alter the therapeutic effect of verapamil.

Covera-HS regularly reduces the total systemic resistance (afterload) against which the heart works both at rest and at a given level of exercise by dilating peripheral arterioles.

Effects in hypertension: Covera-HS was evaluated in two placebo-controlled, parallel design, double-blind studies of 382 patients with mild to moderate hypertension.

In clinical trials 287 patients were randomized to placebo, 120 mg, 180 mg, 360 mg, or 540 mg and treated for 8 weeks (the two higher doses were titrated from low doses and maintained for 6 and 4 weeks, respectively). Covera-HS or placebo was given once daily at 10 pm and blood pressure changes were measured with 36-hour ambulatory blood pressure monitoring (ABPM). The results of these studies demonstrate that Covera-HS, at 180–540 mg, is a consistently and significantly more effective antihypertensive agent than placebo in reducing ambulatory blood pressures. Over this dose range, the placebo-subtracted net decreases in diastolic BP at trough (averaged over 6–10 pm) were dose-related, ranged from 4.5 to 11.2 mm Hg after 4–8 weeks of therapy, and correlated well with sitting cuff blood pressures.

These studies demonstrate that clinically and statistically significant blood pressure reductions are achieved with Covera-HS throughout the 24-hour dosing period.

There were no significant treatment differences between patient subgroups of different age (older or younger than 65 years), sex, race (Caucasian and non-Caucasian) and severity of hypertension at baseline (cuff BP below and above 105 mm Hg).

Angina: Verapamil dilates the main coronary arteries and coronary arterioles, both in normal and ischemic regions, and is a potent inhibitor of coronary artery spasm, whether spontaneous or ergonovine-induced. This property increases myocardial oxygen delivery in patients with coronary artery spasm and is responsible for the effectiveness of verapamil in vasospastic (Prinzmetal's or variant) as well as unstable angina at rest. Whether this effect plays any role in classical effort angina is not clear, but studies of exercise tolerance have not shown an increase in the maximum exercise rate-pressure product, a widely associated measure of oxygen utilization. This suggests that, in general, relief of spasm or dilation of coronary arteries is not an important factor in classical angina.

Verapamil regularly reduces the total systemic resistance (afterload) against which the heart works both at rest and at a given level of exercise by dilating peripheral arterioles.

Effect in chronic stable angina: Covera-HS was evaluated in two placebo-controlled, parallel design, double-blind studies of 453 patients with chronic stable angina.

In the first clinical trial 277 patients were randomized to placebo, 180 mg, 360 mg, or 540 mg and treated for 4 weeks (the two higher doses were titrated from low doses and maintained for 3 and 2 weeks, respectively). A single dose of 240 mg was compared to placebo in a separate study of 176 patients. In these studies Covera-HS was significantly more effective than placebo in improvement of exercise tolerance. Placebo-adjusted net increases in median exercise times at the end of the dosing interval were 0.1 to 1.0 minute for symptom limited duration, 0.3 to 1.4 minutes for time to angina, and 0.1 to 1.1 minutes for time to ST change. Increases in exercise tolerance were in general greater at higher doses, but dose-response relationship was not well defined due to shorter treatment duration for high doses.

In addition, in the first study, 24 to 34% of patients treated with Covera-HS did not experience exercise-limiting angina on exercise treadmill testing (ETT) versus 12% of patients on placebo.

Electrophysiologic effects: Electrical activity through the AV node depends, to a significant degree, upon the transmembrane influx of extracellular calcium through the L-type (slow) channel. By decreasing the influx of calcium, verapamil prolongs the effective refractory period within the AV node and slows AV conduction in a rate-related manner.

Normal sinus rhythm is usually not affected, but in patients with sick sinus syndrome, verapamil may interfere with sinus-node impulse generation and may induce sinus arrest or sinoatrial block. Atrioventricular block can occur in patients without preexisting conduction defects (see *Warnings*).

Covera-HS does not alter the normal atrial action potential or intra-ventricular conduction time, but depresses amplitude, velocity of depolarization, and conduction in depressed atrial fibers. Verapamil may shorten the antegrade effective refractory period of the accessory bypass tract. Acceleration of ventricular rate and/or ventricular fibrillation has been reported in patients with atrial flutter or atrial fibrillation and a coexisting accessory AV pathway following administration of verapamil (see *Warnings).*

Verapamil has a local anesthetic action that is 1.6 times that of procaine on an equimolar basis. It is not known whether this action is important at the doses used in man.

Pharmacokinetics and metabolism: Verapamil is administered as a racemic mixture of the R and S enantiomers. The systemic concentrations of R and S enantiomers, as well as overall bioavailability, are dependent upon the route of administration and the rate and extent of release from the dosage forms. Upon oral administration, there is rapid stereoselective biotransformation during the first pass of verapamil through the portal circulation. In a study in 5 subjects with oral immediate-release verapamil, the systemic bioavailability was from 33% to 65% for the R enantiomer and

from 13% to 34% for the S enantiomer. The R and S enantiomers have differing levels of pharmacologic activity. In studies in animals and humans, the S enantiomer has 8 to 20 times the activity of the R enantiomer in slowing AV conduction. In animal studies, the S enantiomer has 15 and 50 times the activity of the R enantiomer in reducing myocardial contractility in isolated blood-perfused dog papillary muscle and isolated rabbit papillary muscle, respectively, and twice the effect in reducing peripheral resistance. In isolated septal strip preparations from 5 patients, the S enantiomer was 8 times more potent than the R in reducing myocardial contractility. Dose escalation study data indicate that verapamil concentrations increase disproportionally to dose as measured by relative peak plasma concentrations (C_{max}) or areas under the plasma concentration vs time curves (AUC).

Pharmacokinetic Characteristics of Verapamil Enantiomers After Administration of Escalating Doses

		Total Dose of Racemic Verapamil (mg)			
	Isomer	120	180	360	540
Dose Ratio	—	1	1.5	3	4.5
Relative C_{max}	R	1	1.55	4.47	7.06
	S	1	1.62	5.17	9.21
Relative AUC	R	1	1.59	6.14	11.1
	S	1	1.89	8.17	15.9

Pharmacokinetic Characteristics of Verapamil Enantiomers After Administration of a Single 180 mg Dose and at Steady State

	Isomer	First Dose (Verapamil-naive subject)	Steady State (Current verapamil exposure)
C_{max} (ng/ml)	R	59.4	90.5
	S	11.7	21.2
AUC (0–24h) (ng·hr/ml)	R	644	1,223
	S	111	266

Racemic verapamil is released from Covera-HS at a constant rate following solubilization and release of the delay coat through the tablet orifices. This delay coat produces a lag period in drug release for approximately 4–5 hours. The drug release phase is prolonged with the peak plasma concentration (C_{max}) occurring approximately 11 hours after administration. Trough concentrations occur approximately 4 hours after bedtime dosing while the patient is sleeping. Steady-state pharmacokinetics were determined in healthy volunteers. Steady-state concentration is reached by the third or fourth day of dosing.

Steady-State Pharmacokinetics of Verapamil Enantiomers in Healthy Humans

		Verapamil Dose (mg)	
	Isomer	180	240
Mean C_{max} (ng/ml)	R	90.5	120
	S	21.2	28.7
AUC (0–24h) (ng·hr/ml)	R	1,223	1,470
	S	266	322

In general, bioavailability of Covera-HS is higher and half life longer in older (>65 yrs) subjects. Lean body weight also affects its pharmacokinetics inversely, but no gender difference was observed in the clinical trials of Covera-HS. However, there are conflicting data in literature suggesting that verapamil clearance decreased with age in women to a greater degree than in men.

Consumption of a high fat meal just prior to dosing at night had no effect on the pharmacokinetics of Covera-HS. The pharmacokinetics were also not affected by whether the volunteers were supine or ambulatory for the 8 hours following dosing. Administering Covera-HS in the morning led to a slower rate of absorption and/or elimination, but did not affect the extent of absorption or extent of metabolism to norverapamil.

Orally administered verapamil undergoes extensive metabolism in the liver. Thirteen metabolites have been identified in urine. Norverapamil enantiomers can reach steady-state plasma concentrations approximately equal to those of the enantiomers of the parent drug. The cardiovascular activity of norverapamil appears to be approximately 20% that of verapamil. Approximately 70% of an administered dose is

excreted as metabolites in the urine and 16% or more in the feces within 5 days. About 3% to 4% is excreted in the urine as unchanged drug. R-verapamil is 94% bound to plasma albumin, while S-verapamil is 88% bound. In addition, R-verapamil is 92% and S-verapamil 86% bound to alpha-1 acid glycoprotein. In patients with hepatic insufficiency, metabolism of immediate-release verapamil is delayed and elimination half-life prolonged up to 14 to 16 hours because of the extensive hepatic metabolism (see *Precautions*). In addition, in these patients there is a reduced first pass effect, and verapamil is more bioavailable. Verapamil clearance values suggest that patients with liver dysfunction may attain therapeutic verapamil plasma concentrations with one third of the oral daily dose required for patients with normal liver function.

After four weeks of oral dosing of immediate release verapamil (120 mg q.i.d.), verapamil and norverapamil levels were noted in the cerebrospinal fluid with estimated partition coefficient of 0.06 for verapamil and 0.04 for norverapamil.

Hemodynamics: Verapamil reduces afterload and myocardial contractility. In most patients, including those with organic cardiac disease, the negative inotropic action of verapamil is countered by reduction of afterload and cardiac index remains unchanged. During isometric or dynamic exercise, verapamil does not alter systolic cardiac function in patients with normal ventricular function. Improved left ventricular diastolic function in patients with IHSS and those with coronary heart disease has also been observed with verapamil. In patients with severe left ventricular dysfunction (eg, pulmonary wedge pressure above 20 mm Hg or ejection fraction less than 30%), or in patients taking beta-adrenergic blocking agents or other cardio-depressant drugs, deterioration of ventricular function may occur (see *Drug interactions*).

Pulmonary function: Verapamil does not induce bronchoconstriction and, hence, does not impair ventilatory function.

Verapamil has been shown to have either a neutral or relaxant effect on bronchial smooth muscle.

INDICATIONS AND USAGE

Covera-HS is indicated for the management of hypertension and angina.

CONTRAINDICATIONS

Covera-HS is contraindicated in:

1. Severe left ventricular dysfunction (see *Warnings*)

2. Hypotension (systolic pressure less than 90 mm Hg) or cardiogenic shock

3. Sick sinus syndrome (except in patients with a functioning artificial ventricular pacemaker)

4. Second- or third-degree AV block (except in patients with a functioning artificial ventricular pacemaker)

5. Patients with atrial flutter or atrial fibrillation and an accessory bypass tract (eg, Wolff-Parkinson-White, Lown-Ganong-Levine syndromes). (See *Warnings*.)

6. Patients with known hypersensitivity to verapamil hydrochloride.

WARNINGS

Heart failure: Verapamil has a negative inotropic effect, which in most patients is compensated by its afterload reduction (decreased systemic vascular resistance) properties without a net impairment of ventricular performance. In previous clinical experience with 4,954 patients primarily with immediate-release verapamil, 1.8% developed congestive heart failure or pulmonary edema. Verapamil should be avoided in patients with severe left ventricular dysfunction (eg, ejection fraction less than 30%) or moderate to severe symptoms of cardiac failure and in patients with any degree of ventricular dysfunction if they are receiving a beta-adrenergic blocker (see *Drug Interactions*). Patients with milder ventricular dysfunction should, if possible, be controlled with optimum doses of digitalis and/or diuretics before verapamil treatment is started. (**Note interactions with digoxin under *Precautions*.**)

Hypotension: Occasionally, the pharmacologic action of verapamil may produce a decrease in blood pressure below normal levels, which may result in dizziness or symptomatic hypotension. In previous verapamil clinical trials the incidence observed in 4,954 patients was 2.5%. In clinical studies of Covera-HS, 0.4% of hypertensive patients and 1.0% of angina patients developed significant hypotension. In hypertensive patients, decreases in blood pressure below normal are unusual. Tilt-table testing (60 degrees) was not able to induce orthostatic hypotension.

Elevated liver enzymes: Elevations of transaminases with and without concomitant elevations in alkaline phosphatase and bilirubin have been reported. Such elevations have sometimes been transient and may disappear even in the face of continued verapamil treatment. Several cases of hepatocellular injury related to verapamil have been proven by rechallenge; half of these had clinical symptoms (malaise, fever, and/or right upper quadrant pain) in addition to ele-

vation of SGOT, SGPT, and alkaline phosphatase. Periodic monitoring of liver function in patients receiving verapamil is therefore prudent.

Accessory bypass tract (Wolff-Parkinson-White or Lown-Ganong-Levine): Some patients with paroxysmal and/or chronic atrial fibrillation or atrial flutter and a coexisting accessory AV pathway have developed increased antegrade conduction across the accessory pathway bypassing the AV node, producing a very rapid ventricular response or ventricular fibrillation after receiving intravenous verapamil (or digitalis). Although a risk of this occurring with oral verapamil has not been established, such patients receiving oral verapamil may be at risk and its use in these patients is contraindicated (see *Contraindications*). Treatment is usually DC-cardioversion. Cardioversion has been used safely and effectively after oral verapamil.

Atrioventricular block: The effect of verapamil on AV conduction and the SA node may cause asymptomatic first-degree AV block and transient bradycardia, sometimes accompanied by nodal escape rhythms. PR-interval prolongation is correlated with verapamil plasma concentrations, especially during the early titration phase of therapy. Higher degrees of AV block, however, were infrequently (0.8%) observed in previous verapamil clinical trials. Marked first-degree block or progressive development to second- or third-degree AV block requires a reduction in dosage or, in rare instances, discontinuation of verapamil HCl and institution of appropriate therapy, depending upon the clinical situation.

Patients with hypertrophic cardiomopathy (IHSS): In 120 patients with hypertrophic cardiomyopathy (most of them refractory or intolerant to propranolol) who received therapy with verapamil at doses up to 720 mg/day, a variety of serious adverse effects were seen. Three patients died in pulmonary edema; all had severe left ventricular outflow obstruction and a past history of left ventricular dysfunction. Eight other patients had pulmonary edema and/or severe hypotension; abnormally high (greater than 20 mm Hg) pulmonary wedge pressure and a marked left ventricular outflow obstruction were present in most of these patients. Concomitant administration of quinidine (see *Drug interactions*) preceded the severe hypotension in 3 of the 8 patients (2 of whom developed pulmonary edema). Sinus bradycardia occurred in 11% of the patients, second-degree AV block in 4%, and sinus arrest in 2%. It must be appreciated that this group of patients had a serious disease with a high mortality rate. Most adverse efffects responded well to dose reduction, and only rarely did verapamil use have to be discontinued.

PRECAUTIONS
General

Formulation specific: As with any other non-deformable dosage form caution should be used when administering Covera-HS in patients with preexisting severe gastrointestinal narrowing (pathologic or iatrogenic). In patients with extremely short GI transit time (<7 hrs), pharmacokinetic data are not available and dosage adjustment may be required.

Use in patients with impaired hepatic function: Since verapamil is highly metabolized by the liver, it should be administered cautiously to patients with impaired hepatic function. Severe liver dysfunction prolongs the elimination half-life of immediate-release verapamil to about 14 to 16 hours; hence, approximately 30% of the dose given to patients with normal liver function should be administered to these patients. Careful monitoring for abnormal prolongation of the PR interval or other signs of excessive pharmacologic effects (see *Overdosage*) should be carried out.

Use in patients with attenuated (decreased) neuromuscular transmission: It has been reported that verapamil decreases neuromuscular transmission in patients with Duchenne's muscular dystrophy, and that verapamil prolongs recovery from the neuromuscular blocking agent vecuronium. It may be necessary to decrease the dosage of verapamil when it is administered to patients with attenuated neuromuscular transmission.

Use in patients with impaired renal function: About 70% of an administered dose of verapamil is excreted as metabolites in the urine. Verapamil is not removed by hemodialysis. Until further data are available, verapamil should be admiministered cautiously to patients with impaired renal function. These patients should be carefully monitored for abnormal prolongation of the PR interval or other signs of overdosage (see *Overdosage*).

Information for patients: Covera-HS tablets should be swallowed whole; do not break, crush, or chew. The medication in the Covera-HS tablet is released slowly through an outer shell that does not dissolve. The patient should not be concerned if they occasionally observe this outer shell in their stool as it passes from the body.

Drug interactions

Alcohol: Verapamil may increase blood alcohol concentrations and prolong its effects.

Continued on next page

Covera-HS—Cont.

Beta-blockers: Concomitant therapy with beta-adrenergic blockers and verapamil may result in additive negative effects on heart rate, atrioventricular conduction and/or cardiac contractility. The combination of sustained-release verapamil and beta-adrenergic blocking agents has not been studied. However, there have been reports of excessive bradycardia and AV block, including complete heart block, when the combination has been used for the treatment of hypertension. For hypertensive patients, the risks of combined therapy may outweigh the potential benefits. The combination should be used only with caution and close monitoring.

Asymptomatic bradycardia (36 beats/min) with a wandering atrial pacemaker has been observed in a patient receiving concomitant timolol (a beta-adrenergic blocker) eyedrops and oral verapamil.

A decrease in metoprolol and propranolol clearance has been observed when either drug is administered concomitantly with verapamil. A variable effect has been seen when verapamil and atenolol were given together.

Digitalis: Clinical use of verapamil in digitalized patients has shown the combination to be well tolerated if digoxin doses are properly adjusted. However, chronic verapamil treatment can increase serum digoxin levels by 50% to 75% during the first week of therapy, and this can result in digitalis toxicity. In patients with hepatic cirrhosis the influence of verapamil on digoxin kinetics is magnified. Verapamil may reduce total body clearance and extrarenal clearance of digitoxin by 27% and 29%, respectively. Maintenance and digitalization doses should be reduced when verapamil is administered, and the patient should be reassessed to avoid over- to underdigitalization. Whenever overdigitalization is suspected, the daily dose of digitalis should be reduced or temporarily discontinued. On discontinuation of verapamil use, the patient should be reassessed to avoid underdigitalization. In previous clinical trials with other verapamil formulations related to the control of ventricular response in digitalized patients who had atrial fibrillation or atrial flutter, ventricular rates below 50/min at rest occurred in 15% of patients, and asymptomatic hypotension occurred in 5% of patients.

Antihypertensive agents: Verapamil administered concomitantly with oral antihypertensive agents (eg, vasodilators, angiotensin-converting enzyme inhibitors, diuretics, beta-blockers) will usually have an additive effect on lowering blood pressure. Patients receiving these combinations should be appropriately monitored. Concomitant use of agents that attenuate alpha-adrenergic function with verapamil may result in a reduction in blood pressure that is excessive in some patients. Such an effect was observed in one study following the concomitant administration of verapamil and prazosin.

Antiarrhythmic agents:

Disopyramide: Until data on possible interactions between verapamil and disopyramide are obtained, disopyramide should not be administered within 48 hours before or 24 hours after verapamil administration.

Flecainide: A study in healthy volunteers showed that the concomitant administration of flecainide and verapamil may have additive effects on myocardial contractility, AV conduction, and repolarization. Concomitant therapy with flecainide and verapamil may result in additive negative inotropic effect and prolongation of atrioventricular conduction.

Quinidine: In a small number of patients with hypertrophic cardiomyopathy (IHSS), concomitant use of verapamil and quinidine resulted in significant hypotension. Until further data are obtained, combined therapy of verapamil and quinidine in patients with hypertrophic cardiomyopathy should probably be avoided.

The electrophysiologic effects of quinidine and verapamil on AV conduction were studied in 8 patients. Verapamil significantly counteracted the effects of quinidine on AV conduction. There has been a report of increased quinidine levels during verapamil therapy.

Other:

Nitrates: Verapamil has been given concomitantly with short- and long-acting nitrates without any undesirable drug interactions. The pharmacologic profile of both drugs and clinical experience suggest beneficial interactions.

Cimetidine: The interaction between cimetidine and chronically administered verapamil has not been studied. Variable results on clearance have been obtained in acute studies of healthy volunteers; clearance of verapamil was either reduced or unchanged.

Lithium: Increased sensitivity to the effects of lithium (neurotoxicity) has been reported during concomitant verapamil-lithium therapy; lithium levels have been observed sometimes to increase, sometimes to decrease, and sometimes to be unchanged. Patients receiving both drugs must be monitored carefully.

Carbamazepine: Verapamil therapy may increase carbamazepine concentrations during combined therapy. This may produce carbamazepine side effects such as diplopia, headache, ataxia, or dizziness.

Rifampin: Therapy with rifampin may markedly reduce oral verapamil bioavailability.

Phenobarbital: Phenobarbital therapy may increase verapamil clearance.

Cyclosporin: Verapamil therapy may increase serum levels of cyclosporin.

Theophylline: Verapamil may inhibit the clearance and increase the plasma levels of theophylline.

Inhalation anesthetics: Animal experiments have shown that inhalation anesthetics depress cardiovascular activity by decreasing the inward movement of calcium ions. When used concomitantly, inhalation anesthetics and calcium channel blocking agents, such as verapamil, should each be titrated carefully to avoid excessive cardiovascular depression.

Neuromuscular blocking agents: Clinical data and animal studies suggest that verapamil may potentiate the activity of neuromuscular blocking agents (curare-like and depolarizing). It may be necessary to decrease the dose of verapamil and/or the dose of the neuromuscular blocking agent when the drugs are used concomitantly.

Carcinogenesis, mutagenesis, impairment of fertility: An 18-month toxicity study in rats, at a low multiple (6-fold) of the maximum recommended human dose, not the maximum tolerated dose, did not suggest a tumorigenic potential. There was no evidence of a carcinogenic potential of verapamil administered in the diet of rats for two years at doses of 10, 35, and 120 mg/kg/day or approximately 1, 3.5 and 12 times, respectively, the maximum recommended human daily dose (480 mg/day or 9.6 mg/kg/day).

Verapamil was not mutagenic in the Ames test in 5 test strains at 3 mg per plate with or without metabolic activation.

Studies in female rats at daily dietary doses up to 5.5 times (55 mg/kg/day) the maximum recommended human dose did not show impaired fertility. Effects on male fertility have not been determined.

Pregnancy: Pregnancy Category C. Reproduction studies have been performed in rabbits and rats at oral doses up to 1.5 (15 mg/kg/day) and 6 (60 mg/kg/day) times the human oral daily dose, respectively, and have revealed no evidence of teratogenicity. In the rat, however, this multiple of the human dose was embryocidal and retarded fetal growth and development, probably because of adverse maternal effects reflected in reduced weight gains of the dams. This oral dose has also been shown to cause hypotension in rats. There are no adequate and well-controlled studies in pregnant women. Because animal reproduction studies are not always predictive of human response, this drug should be used during pregnancy only if clearly needed. Verapamil crosses the placental barrier and can be detected in umbilical vein blood at delivery.

Labor and delivery: It is not known whether the use of verapamil during labor or delivery has immediate or delayed adverse effects on the fetus, or whether it prolongs the duration of labor or increases the need for forceps delivery or other obstetric intervention. Such adverse experiences have not been reported in the literature, despite a long history of use of verapamil in Europe in the treatment of cardiac side effects of beta-adrenergic agonist agents used to treat premature labor.

Nursing mothers: Verapamil is excreted in human milk. Because of the potential for adverse reactions in nursing infants from verapamil, nursing should be discontinued while verapamil is administered.

Pediatric use: Safety and effectiveness in pediatric patients have not been established.

Elderly use: Dosage adjustment may be required in elderly patients with impaired renal function. Verapamil should be administered cautiously in patients with impaired renal function.

Animal pharmacology and/or animal toxicology: In chronic animal toxicology studies verapamil caused lenticular and/or suture line changes at 30 mg/kg/day or greater, and frank cataracts at 62.5 mg/kg/day or greater in the beagle dog but not in the rat. Development of cataracts due to verapamil has not been reported in man.

ADVERSE REACTIONS

Serious adverse reactions are uncommon when verapamil therapy is initiated with upward dose titration within the recommended single and total daily dose. See *Warnings* for discussion of heart failure, hypotension, elevated liver enzymes, AV block, and rapid ventricular response. Reversible (upon discontinuation of verapamil) non-obstructive, paralytic ileus has been infrequently reported in association with the use of verapamil. The following reactions to orally administered Covera-HS occurred at rates greater than 2.0% or occurred at lower rates but appeared drug-related in clinical trials in hypertension and angina:

	Placebo n=261 %	All doses studied n=572 %
Constipation	2.7	11.7*
Headache	7.3	6.6
Upper respiratory infection	4.6	5.4
Dizziness	2.7	4.7
Fatigue	3.8	4.5
Edema	3.1	3.0
Nausea	1.9	2.1
AV block (1°)	0.0	1.7
Elevated liver enzymes (see *Warnings*)	0.8	1.4
Bradycardia	0.4	1.4
Paresthesia	0.0	1.0
Flushing	0.3	0.8
Hypotension	0.0	0.7
Postural hypotension	0.3	0.4

* Constipation was typically mild, easily manageable, and the incidence usually diminished within about one week. At a typical once-daily dose of 240 mg, the observed incidence was 7.2%.

In previous experience with other formulations of verapamil, the following reactions occurred at rates greater than 1.0% or occurred at lower rates but appeared clearly drug related in clinical trials in 4,954 patients.

Constipation	7.3%
Dizziness	3.3%
Nausea	2.7%
Hypotension	2.5%
Headache	2.2%
Edema	1.9%
CHF/Pulmonary Edema	1.8%
Fatigue	1.7%
Dyspnea	1.4%
Bradycardia (HR<50/min)	1.4%
AV Block (total 1°,2°,3°)	1.2%
AV Block (2° and 3°)	0.8%
Rash	1.2%
Flushing	0.6%
Elevated liver enzymes (see *Warnings*)	

The following reactions, reported with orally administered verapamil in 2% or less of patients, occurred under conditions (open trials, marketing experience) where a causal relationship is uncertain; they are listed to alert the physician to a possible relationship:

Cardiovascular: angina pectoris, AV block (2° & 3°), atrioventricular dissociation, CHF, pulmonary edema, chest pain, claudication, myocardial infarction, palpitations, purpura (vasculitis), syncope.

Digestive system: diarrhea, dry mouth, gastrointestinal distress, gingival hyperplasia.

Hemic and lymphatic: ecchymosis or bruising.

Nervous system: cerebrovascular accident, confusion, equilibrium disorders, insomnia, muscle cramps, psychotic symptoms, shakiness, somnolence.

Skin: arthralgia and rash, exanthema, hair loss, hyperkeratosis, macules, sweating, urticaria, Stevens-Johnson syndrome, erythema multiforme.

Special senses: blurred vision, tinnitus.

Urogenital: gynecomastia, galactorrhea/hyperprolactinemia, increased urination, spotty menstruation, impotence.

Other: allergy aggravated, dyspnea.

Treatment of acute cardiovascular adverse reactions: The frequency of cardiovascular adverse reactions that require therapy is rare; hence, experience with their treatment is limited. Whenever severe hypotension or complete AV block occurs following oral administration of verapamil, the appropriate emergency measures should be applied immediately; eg, intravenously administered norepinephrine bitartrate, atropine sulfate, isoproterenol HCl (all in usual doses), or calcium gluconate (10% solution). In patients with hypertrophic cardiomyopathy (IHSS), alpha-adrenergic agents (phenylephrine HCl, metaraminol bitartrate, or methoxamine HCl) should be used to maintain blood pressure, and isoproterenol and norepinephrine should be avoided. If further support is necessary, dopamine HCl or dobutamine HCl may be administered. Actual treatment and dosage should depend on the severity of the clinical situation and the judgement and experience of the treating physician.

OVERDOSAGE

Treat all verapamil overdoses as serious and maintain observation for at least 48 hours (especially sustained-release verapamil products), preferably under continuous hospital care. Delayed pharmacodynamic consequences may occur with the sustained-release formulations. Verapamil is known to decrease gastrointestinal transit time.

Treatment of overdosage should be supportive. Beta-adrenergic stimulation or parenteral administration of calcium solutions may increase calcium ion flux across the slow channel and have been used effectively in treatment of de-

liberate overdosage with verapamil. In a few reported cases, overdose with calcium channel blockers has been associated with hypotension and bradycardia, initially refractory to atropine but becoming more responsive to this treatment when the patients received large doses (close to 1 gram/hour for more than 24 hours) of calcium chloride. Verapamil cannot be removed by hemodialysis. Clinically significant hypotensive reactions or high degree AV block should be treated with vasopressor agents or cardiac pacing, respectively. Asystole should be handled by the usual measures including cardiopulmonary resuscitation.

DOSAGE AND ADMINISTRATION

Covera-HS should be administered once daily at bedtime. Clinical trials explored dose ranges between 180 mg and 540 mg given at bedtime and found effects to persist throughout the dosing interval.

Covera-HS tablets should be swallowed whole and not chewed, broken, or crushed.

For both hypertension and angina the dose of Covera-HS should be individualized by titration. Initiate therapy with 180 mg of Covera-HS.

If an adequate response is not obtained with 180 mg of Covera-HS, the dose may be titrated upward in the following manner:
a) 240 mg each evening
b) 360 mg each evening (2 × 180 mg)
c) 480 mg each evening (2 × 240 mg)

When Covera-HS is administered at bedtime, office evaluation of blood pressure during morning and early afternoon hours is essentially a measure of peak effect. The usual evaluation of trough effect, which sometimes might be needed to evaluate the appropriateness of any given dose of Covera-HS, would be just prior to bedtime.

HOW SUPPLIED

Covera-HS 240-mg tablets are pale yellow, round, film coated with COVERA-HS 2021 printed on one side, supplied as:

NDC Number	Size
0025-2021-30	bottle of 30
0025-2021-31	bottle of 100
0025-2021-34	carton of 100 unit dose

Covera-HS 180-mg tablets are lavender, round, film coated, with COVERA-HS 2011 printed on one side, supplied as:

NDC Number	Size
0025-2011-30	bottle of 30
0025-2011-31	bottle of 100
0025-2011-34	carton of 100 unit dose

Store at controlled room temperature 20°–25°C (68°–77°F) [see USP]. Dispense in tight, light-resistant containers.

Caution: Federal law prohibits dispensing without prescription.

5/1/97 • A05351-1

Manufactured for
G.D. Searle & Co.
Chicago IL 60680 USA
By Alza Corporation
Palo Alto CA USA
Address medical inquiries to:
G.D. Searle & Co.
Healthcare Information Services
5200 Old Orchard Road
Skokie IL 60077
©1996, G.D. Searle & Co.
Shown in Product Identification Guide, page 337

CYTOTEC®
[sī-tō-těc]
(misoprostol)

℞

tion failure, and the danger to other women of childbearing potential should the drug be taken by mistake.
• will begin Cytotec only on the second or third day of the next normal menstrual period.

DESCRIPTION

Cytotec oral tablets contain either 100 mcg or 200 mcg of misoprostol, a synthetic prostaglandin E_1 analog.

Misoprostol contains approximately equal amounts of the two diastereomers presented below with their enantiomers indicated by (±):

$C_{22}H_{38}O_5$ M.W. = 382.5
(±) methyl 11α, 16-dihydroxy-16-methyl-9-oxoprost-13E-en-1-oate

Misoprostol is a water-soluble, viscous liquid.

Inactive ingredients of tablets are hydrogenated castor oil, hydroxypropyl methylcellulose, microcrystalline cellulose, and sodium starch glycolate.

CLINICAL PHARMACOLOGY

Pharmacokinetics: Misoprostol is extensively absorbed, and undergoes rapid de-esterification to its free acid, which is responsible for its clinical activity and, unlike the parent compound, is detectable in plasma. The alpha side chain undergoes beta oxidation and the beta side chain undergoes omega oxidation followed by reduction of the ketone to give prostaglandin F analogs.

In normal volunteers, Cytotec (misoprostol) is rapidly absorbed after oral administration with a T_{max} of misoprostol acid of 12 ± 3 minutes and a terminal half-life of 20–40 minutes.

There is high variability of plasma levels of misoprostol acid between and within studies but mean values after single doses show a linear relationship with dose over the range of 200–400 mcg. No accumulation of misoprostol acid was noted in multiple dose studies; plasma steady state was achieved within two days.

Maximum plasma concentrations of misoprostol acid are diminished when the dose is taken with food and total availability of misoprostol acid is reduced by use of concomitant antacid. Clinical trials were conducted with concomitant antacid, however, so this effect does not appear to be clinically important.

Mean ± SD	C_{max}(pg/ml)	AUC (0-4) (pg·hr/ml)	T_{max}(min)
Fasting	811 ± 317	417 ± 135	14 ± 8
With Antacid	689 ± 315	349 ± 108*	20 ± 14
With High Fat Breakfast	303 ± 176*	373 ± 111	64 ± 79*

* Comparisons with fasting results statistically significant, $p<0.05$.

After oral administration of radiolabeled misoprostol, about 80% of detected radioactivity appears in urine. Pharmacokinetic studies in patients with varying degrees of renal impairment showed an approximate doubling of $T_{1/2}$, C_{max}, and AUC compared to normals, but no clear correlation between the degree of impairment and AUC. In subjects over 64 years of age, the AUC for misoprostol acid is increased. No routine dosage adjustment is recommended in older patients or patients with renal impairment, but dosage may need to be reduced if the usual dose is not tolerated.

Cytotec does not affect the hepatic mixed function oxidase (cytochrome P-450) enzyme systems in animals.

Drug interaction studies between misoprostol and several nonsteroidal anti-inflammatory drugs showed no effect on the kinetics of ibuprofen or diclofenac, and a 20% decrease in aspirin AUC, not thought to be clinically significant.

Pharmacokinetic studies also showed a lack of drug interaction with antipyrine and propranolol when these drugs were given with misoprostol. Misoprostol given for one week had no effect on the steady state pharmacokinetics of diazepam when the two drugs were administered two hours apart.

The serum protein binding of misoprostol acid is less than 90% and is concentration-independent in the therapeutic range.

Pharmacodynamics: Misoprostol has both antisecretory (inhibiting gastric acid secretion) and (in animals) mucosal protective properties. NSAIDs inhibit prostaglandin synthesis, and a deficiency of prostaglandins within the gastric mucosa may lead to diminishing bicarbonate and mucus secretion and may contribute to the mucosal damage caused by these agents. Misoprostol can increase bicarbonate and mucus production, but in man this has been shown at doses 200 mcg and above that are also antisecretory. It is therefore not possible to tell whether the ability of misoprostol to prevent gastric ulcer is the result of its antisecretory effect, its mucosal protective effect, or both.

In vitro studies on canine parietal cells using tritiated misoprostol acid as the ligand have led to the identification and characterization of specific prostaglandin receptors. Receptor binding is saturable, reversible, and stereospecific. The sites have a high affinity for misoprostol, for its acid metabolite, and for other E type prostaglandins, but not for F or I prostaglandins and other unrelated compounds, such as histamine or cimetidine. Receptor-site affinity for misoprostol correlates well with an indirect index of antisecretory activity. It is likely that these specific receptors allow misoprostol taken with food to be effective topically, despite the lower serum concentrations attained.

Misoprostol produces a moderate decrease in pepsin concentration during basal conditions, but not during histamine stimulation. It has no significant effect on fasting or postprandial gastrin nor on intrinsic factor output.

Effects on gastric acid secretion: Misoprostol, over the range of 50–200 mcg, inhibits basal and nocturnal gastric acid secretion, and acid secretion in response to a variety of stimuli, including meals, histamine, pentagastrin, and coffee. Activity is apparent 30 minutes after oral administration and persists for at least 3 hours. In general, the effects of 50 mcg were modest and shorter lived, and only the 200-mcg dose had substantial effects on nocturnal secretion or on histamine and meal-stimulated secretion.

Uterine effects: Cytotec has been shown to produce uterine contractions that may endanger pregnancy. (See *Contraindications* and *Warnings.*) In studies in women undergoing elective termination of pregnancy during the first trimester, Cytotec caused partial or complete expulsion of the uterine contents in 11% of the subjects and increased uterine bleeding in 41%.

Other pharmacologic effects: Cytotec does not produce clinically significant effects on serum levels of prolactin, gonadotropins, thyroid-stimulating hormone, growth hormone, thyroxine, cortisol, gastrointestinal hormones (somatostatin, gastrin, vasoactive intestinal polypeptide, and motilin), creatinine, or uric acid. Gastric emptying, immunologic competence, platelet aggregation, pulmonary function, or the cardiovascular system are not modified by recommended doses of Cytotec.

Clinical studies: In a series of small short-term (about 1 week) placebo-controlled studies in healthy human volunteers, doses of misoprostol were evaluated for their ability to prevent NSAID-induced mucosal injury. Studies of 200 mcg q.i.d. of misoprostol with tolmetin and naproxen, and of 100 and 200 mcg q.i.d. with ibuprofen, all showed reduction of the rate of significant endoscopic injury from about 70–75% on placebo to 10–30% on misoprostol. Doses of 25–200 mcg q.i.d. reduced aspirin-induced mucosal injury and bleeding.

Preventing gastric ulcers caused by nonsteroidal anti-inflammatory drugs (NSAIDs): Two 12-week, randomized, double-blind trials in osteoarthritic patients who had gastrointestinal symptoms but no ulcer on endoscopy while taking an NSAID compared the ability of 200 mcg of Cytotec, 100 mcg of Cytotec, and placebo to prevent gastric ulcer (GU) formation. Patients were approximately equally divided between ibuprofen, piroxicam, and naproxen, and continued this treatment throughout the 12 weeks. The 200-mcg dose caused a marked, statistically significant reduction in gastric ulcers in both studies. The lower dose was somewhat less effective, with a significant result in only one of the studies.

[See table at top of next page]

In these trials there were no significant differences between Cytotec and placebo in relief of day or night abdominal pain. No effect of Cytotec in preventing duodenal ulcers was demonstrated, but relatively few duodenal lesions were seen.

In another clinical trial, 239 patients receiving aspirin 650–1300 mg q.i.d. for rheumatoid arthritis who had endoscopic evidence of duodenal and/or gastric inflammation were randomized to misoprostol 200 mcg q.i.d. or placebo for eight weeks while continuing to receive aspirin. The study evaluated the possible interference of Cytotec on the efficacy of aspirin in these patients with rheumatoid arthritis by analyzing joint tenderness, joint swelling, physician's clinical assessment, patient's assessment, change in ARA classification, change in handgrip strength, change in duration of morning stiffness, patient's assessment of pain at rest,

Continued on next page

Cytotec—Cont.

movement, interference with daily activity, and ESR. Cytotec did not interfere with the efficacy of aspirin in these patients with rheumatoid arthritis.

INDICATIONS AND USAGE

Cytotec (misoprostol) is indicated for the prevention of NSAID (nonsteroidal anti-inflammatory drugs, including aspirin)-induced gastric ulcers in patients at high risk of complications from gastric ulcer, eg, the elderly and patients with concomitant debilitating disease, as well as patients at high risk of developing gastric ulceration, such as patients with a history of ulcer. Cytotec has not been shown to prevent duodenal ulcers in patients taking NSAIDs. Cytotec should be taken for the duration of NSAID therapy. Cytotec has been shown to prevent gastric ulcers in controlled studies of three months' duration. It had no effect, compared to placebo, on gastrointestinal pain or discomfort associated with NSAID use.

CONTRAINDICATIONS

See boxed *CONTRAINDICATIONS AND WARNINGS.*
Cytotec should not be taken by anyone with a history of allergy to prostaglandins.

WARNINGS

See boxed *CONTRAINDICATIONS AND WARNINGS.*

PRECAUTIONS

Information for patients: Cytotec is contraindicated in women who are pregnant, and should not be used in women of childbearing potential unless the patient requires nonsteroidal anti-inflammatory drug (NSAID) therapy and is at high risk of complications from gastric ulcers associated with the use of the NSAID, or is at high risk of developing gastric ulceration. Women of childbearing potential should be told that they must not be pregnant when Cytotec therapy is initiated, and that they must use an effective contraception method while taking Cytotec.
See boxed *CONTRAINDICATIONS AND WARNINGS.*

Patients should be advised of the following:

Cytotec is intended for administration along with nonsteroidal anti-inflammatory drugs (NSAIDs), including aspirin, to decrease the chance of developing an NSAID-induced gastric ulcer.

Cytotec should be taken only according to the directions given by a physician.

If the patient has questions about or problems with Cytotec, the physician should be contacted promptly.

THE PATIENT SHOULD NOT GIVE CYTOTEC TO ANYONE ELSE. Cytotec has been prescribed for the patient's specific condition, may not be the correct treatment for another person, and may be dangerous to the other person if she were to become pregnant.

The Cytotec package the patient receives from the pharmacist will include a leaflet containing patient information. The patient should read the leaflet before taking Cytotec and each time the prescription is renewed because the leaflet may have been revised.

Keep Cytotec out of the reach of children.

SPECIAL NOTE FOR WOMEN: Cytotec must not be used by pregnant women. Cytotec may cause miscarriage. Miscarriages caused by Cytotec may be incomplete, which could lead to potentially dangerous bleeding, hospitalization, surgery, infertility, or maternal or fetal death.

Cytotec is available only as a unit-of-use package that includes a leaflet containing patient information. See *Patient Information* at the end of this labeling.

Drug interactions: See *Clinical Pharmacology.* Cytotec has not been shown to interfere with the beneficial effects of aspirin on signs and symptoms of rheumatoid arthritis. Cytotec does not exert clinically significant effects on the absorption, blood levels, and antiplatelet effects of therapeutic doses of aspirin. Cytotec has no clinically significant effect on the kinetics of diclofenac or ibuprofen.

Animal toxicology: A reversible increase in the number of normal surface gastric epithelial cells occurred in the dog, rat, and mouse. No such increase has been observed in humans administered Cytotec for up to 1 year.

An apparent response of the female mouse to Cytotec in long-term studies at 100 to 1000 times the human dose was hyperostosis, mainly of the medulla of sternebrae. Hyperostosis did not occur in long-term studies in the dog and rat and has not been seen in humans treated with Cytotec.

Carcinogenesis, mutagenesis, impairment of fertility: There was no evidence of an effect of Cytotec on tumor occurrence or incidence in rats receiving daily doses up to 150 times the human dose for 24 months. Similarly, there was no effect of Cytotec on tumor occurrence or incidence in mice receiving daily doses up to 1000 times the human dose for 21 months. The mutagenic potential of Cytotec was tested in several *in vitro* assays, all of which were negative.

Misoprostol, when administered to breeding male and female rats at doses 6.25 times to 625 times the maximum recommended human therapeutic dose, produced dose-related pre- and post-implantation losses and a significant decrease in the number of live pups born at the highest dose. These findings suggest the possibility of a general adverse effect on fertility in males and females.

Prevention of Gastric Ulcers Induced by Ibuprofen, Piroxicam, or Naproxen
[No. of patients with ulcer(s) (%)]

Therapy	Therapy Duration: 4 weeks	8 weeks	12 weeks	
Study No. 1				
Cytotec 200 mcg q.i.d. (n=74)	1 (1.4)	0	0	1 (1.4)*
Cytotec 100 mcg q.i.d. (n=77)	3 (3.9)	1 (1.3)	1 (1.3)	5 (6.5)*
Placebo (n=76)	11 (14.5)	4 (5.3)	4 (5.3)	19 (25.0)
Study No. 2				
Cytotec 200 mcg q.i.d. (n=65)	1 (1.5)	1 (1.5)	0	2 (3.1)*
Cytotec 100 mcg q.i.d. (n=66)	2 (3.0)	2 (3.0)	1 (1.5)	5 (7.6)
Placebo (n=62)	6 (9.7)	2 (3.2)	3 (4.8)	11 (17.7)
*Studies No. 1 & No. 2***				
Cytotec 200 mcg q.i.d. (n=139)	2 (1.4)	1 (0.7)	0	3 (2.2)*
Cytotec 100 mcg q.i.d. (n=143)	5 (3.5)	3 (2.1)	2 (1.4)	10 (7.0)*
Placebo (n=138)	17 (12.3)	6 (4.3)	7 (5.1)	30 (21.7)

* Statistically significantly different from placebo at the 5% level.
** Combined data from Study No. 1 and Study No. 2.

Pregnancy: Pregnancy Category X. See boxed *CONTRAINDICATIONS AND WARNINGS.*

Nonteratogenic effects: Cytotec may endanger pregnancy (may cause miscarriage) and thereby cause harm to the fetus when administered to a pregnant woman. Cytotec produces uterine contractions, uterine bleeding, and expulsion of the products of conception. Miscarriages caused by Cytotec may be incomplete. In studies in women undergoing elective termination of pregnancy during the first trimester, Cytotec caused partial or complete expulsion of the products of conception in 11% of the subjects and increased uterine bleeding in 41%. Anecdotal reports, primarily from Brazil, of congenital anomalies and reports of fetal death subsequent to misuse of misoprostol as an abortifacient have been received (see *Contraindications and Warnings*). If a woman is or becomes pregnant while taking this drug, the drug should be discontinued and the patient apprised of the potential hazard to the fetus.

Teratogenic effects: Cytotec is not fetotoxic or teratogenic in rats and rabbits at doses 625 and 63 times the human dose, respectively.

Nursing mothers: See *Contraindications.* It is unlikely that Cytotec is excreted in human milk since it is rapidly metabolized throughout the body. However, it is not known if the active metabolite (misoprostol acid) is excreted in human milk. Therefore, Cytotec should not be administered to nursing mothers because the potential excretion of misoprostol acid could cause significant diarrhea in nursing infants.

Pediatric use: Safety and effectiveness in children below the age of 18 years have not been established.

ADVERSE REACTIONS

The following have been reported as adverse events in subjects receiving Cytotec:

Gastrointestinal: In subjects receiving Cytotec 400 or 800 mcg daily in clinical trials, the most frequent gastrointestinal adverse events were diarrhea and abdominal pain. The incidence of diarrhea at 800 mcg in controlled trials in patients on NSAIDs ranged from 14–40% and in all studies (over 5,000 patients) averaged 13%. Abdominal pain occurred in 13–20% of patients in NSAID trials and about 7% in all studies, but there was no consistent difference from placebo.

Diarrhea was dose related and usually developed early in the course of therapy (after 13 days), usually was self-limiting (often resolving after 8 days), but sometimes required discontinuation of Cytotec (2% of the patients). Rare instances of profound diarrhea leading to severe dehydration have been reported. Patients with an underlying condition such as inflammatory bowel disease, or those in whom dehydration, were it to occur, would be dangerous, should be monitored carefully if Cytotec is prescribed. The incidence of diarrhea can be minimized by administering after meals and at bedtime, and by avoiding coadministration of Cytotec with magnesium-containing antacids.

Gynecological: Women who received Cytotec during clinical trials reported the following gynecological disorders: spotting (0.7%), cramps (0.6%), hypermenorrhea (0.5%), menstrual disorder (0.3%) and dysmenorrhea (0.1%). Postmenopausal vaginal bleeding may be related to Cytotec administration. If it occurs, diagnostic workup should be undertaken to rule out gynecological pathology.

Elderly: There were no significant differences in the safety profile of Cytotec in approximately 500 ulcer patients who were 65 years of age or older compared with younger patients.

Additional adverse events which were reported are categorized as follows:

Incidence greater than 1%: In clinical trials, the following adverse reactions were reported by more than 1% of the subjects receiving Cytotec and may be causally related to the drug: nausea (3.2%), flatulence (2.9%), headache (2.4%), dyspepsia (2.0%), vomiting (1.3%), and constipation (1.1%). However, there were no significant differences between the incidences of these events for Cytotec and placebo.

Causal relationship unknown: The following adverse events were infrequently reported. Causal relationships between Cytotec and these events have not been established but cannot be excluded:

Body as a whole: aches/pains, asthenia, fatigue, fever, rigors, weight changes.
Skin: rash, dermatitis, alopecia, pallor, breast pain.
Special senses: abnormal taste, abnormal vision, conjunctivitis, deafness, tinnitus, earache.
Respiratory: upper respiratory tract infection, bronchitis, bronchospasm, dyspnea, pneumonia, epistaxis.
Cardiovascular: chest pain, edema, diaphoresis, hypotension, hypertension, arrhythmia, phlebitis, increased cardiac enzymes, syncope.
Gastrointestinal: Gl bleeding, Gl inflammation/infection, rectal disorder, abnormal hepatobiliary function, gingivitis, reflux, dysphagia, amylase increase.
Hypersensitivity: Anaphylaxis.
Metabolic: glycosuria, gout, increased nitrogen, increased alkaline phosphatase.
Genitourinary: polyuria, dysuria, hematuria, urinary tract infection.
Nervous system/Psychiatric: anxiety, change in appetite, depression, drowsiness, dizziness, thirst, impotence, loss of libido, sweating increase, neuropathy, neurosis, confusion.
Musculoskeletal: arthralgia, myalgia, muscle cramps, stiffness, back pain.
Blood/Coagulation: anemia, abnormal differential, thrombocytopenia, purpura, ESR increased.

OVERDOSAGE

The toxic dose of Cytotec in humans has not been determined. Cumulative total daily doses of 1600 mcg have been tolerated, with only symptoms of gastrointestinal discomfort being reported. In animals, the acute toxic effects are diarrhea, gastrointestinal lesions, focal cardiac necrosis, hepatic necrosis, renal tubular necrosis, testicular atrophy, respiratory difficulties, and depression of the central nervous system. Clinical signs that may indicate an overdose are sedation, tremor, convulsions, dyspnea, abdominal pain, diarrhea, fever, palpitations, hypotension, or bradycardia. Symptoms should be treated with supportive therapy.

It is not known if misoprostol acid is dialyzable. However, because misoprostol is metabolized like a fatty acid, it is unlikely that dialysis would be appropriate treatment for overdosage.

DOSAGE AND ADMINISTRATION

The recommended adult oral dose of Cytotec for the prevention of NSAID-induced gastric ulcers is 200 mcg four times daily with food. If this dose cannot be tolerated, a dose of 100 mcg can be used. (See *Clinical Pharmacology: Clinical studies.*) Cytotec should be taken for the duration of NSAID therapy as prescribed by the physician. Cytotec should be taken with a meal, and the last dose of the day should be at bedtime.

Renal impairment: Adjustment of the dosing schedule in renally impaired patients is not routinely needed, but dosage can be reduced if the 200-mcg dose is not tolerated. (See *Clinical Pharmacology.*)

HOW SUPPLIED

Cytotec 100-mcg tablets are white, round, with SEARLE debossed on one side and 1451 on the other side; supplied as:

NDC Number	Size
0025-1451-60	unit-of-use bottle of 60
0025-1451-20	unit-of-use bottle of 120
0025-1451-34	carton of 100 unit dose

Cytotec 200-mcg tablets are white, hexagonal, with SEARLE debossed above and 1461 debossed below the line on one side and a double stomach debossed on the other side; supplied as:

NDC Number	Size
0025-1461-60	unit-of-use bottle of 60
0025-1461-31	unit-of-use bottle of 100
0025-1461-34	carton of 100 unit dose

Store at or below 25°C (77°F) in a dry area.
Caution: Federal law prohibits dispensing without prescription.

PATIENT INFORMATION

Read this leaflet before taking Cytotec® (misoprostol) and each time your prescription is renewed, because the leaflet may be changed.
Cytotec (misoprostol) is being prescribed by your doctor to decrease the chance of getting stomach ulcers related to the arthritis/pain medication that you take.
Cytotec can cause miscarriage, often associated with potentially dangerous bleeding. This may result in hospitalization, surgery, infertility, or death. **Do not take it if you are pregnant and do not become pregnant while taking this medicine.**
If you become pregnant during Cytotec therapy, stop taking Cytotec and contact your physician immediately. Remember that even if you are on a means of birth control it is still possible to become pregnant. Should this occur, stop taking Cytotec and contact your physician immediately.
Cytotec may cause diarrhea, abdominal cramping, and/or nausea in some people. In most cases these problems develop during the first few weeks of therapy and stop after about a week. You can minimize possible diarrhea by making sure you take Cytotec with food.
Because these side effects are usually mild to moderate and usually go away in a matter of days, most patients can continue to take Cytotec. If you have prolonged difficulty (more than 8 days), or if you have severe diarrhea, cramping and/or nausea, call your doctor.
Take Cytotec only according to the directions given by your physician.
Do not give Cytotec to anyone else. It has been prescribed for your specific condition, may not be the correct treatment for another person, and would be dangerous if the other person were pregnant.
This information sheet does not cover all possible side effects of Cytotec. This patient information leaflet does not address the side effects of your arthritis/pain medication. See your doctor if you have questions.
Keep out of reach of children.

8/8/95 • A05450-1

Shown in Product Identification Guide, page 337

DAYPRO® ℞
[dā-prō]
(oxaprozin)

DESCRIPTION

Daypro (oxaprozin) is a nonsteroidal anti-inflammatory drug (NSAID), chemically designated as 4,5-diphenyl-2-oxazole-propionic acid, and has the following chemical structure:

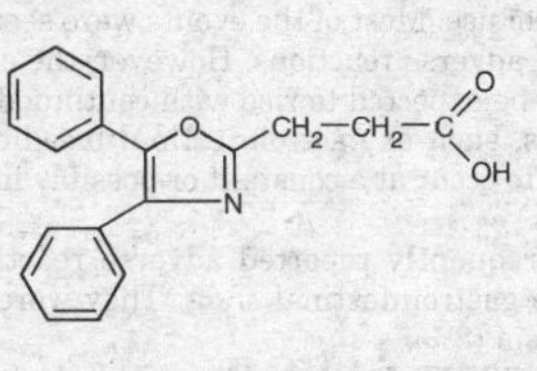

The empirical formula for oxaprozin is $C_{18}H_{15}NO_3$, and the molecular weight is 293. Oxaprozin is a white to off-white powder with a slight odor and a melting point of 162°C to 163°C. It is slightly soluble in alcohol and insoluble in water, with an octanol/water partition coefficient of 4.8 at physiologic pH (7.4). The pK_a in water is 4.3.
Daypro oral caplets contain 600 mg of oxaprozin.
Inactive ingredients in Daypro oral caplets are microcrystalline cellulose, hydroxypropyl methylcellulose, methylcellulose, magnesium stearate, polacrilin potassium, starch, polyethylene glycol, and titanium dioxide.

CLINICAL PHARMACOLOGY

Oxaprozin is a nonsteroidal anti-inflammatory drug (NSAID) that has been shown to have anti-inflammatory, analgesic, and antipyretic properties in animal models. As with other nonsteroidal anti-inflammatory agents, all of the modes of action of oxaprozin are not fully established. Oxaprozin is an inhibitor of several steps along the arachidonic acid pathway of prostaglandin synthesis, and one of its modes of action is presumed to be due to the inhibition of prostaglandin synthesis at the site of inflammation.
Pharmacodynamics: Acute analgesic effects are demonstrable in humans after a single 1200-mg dose of oxaprozin, but anti-inflammatory effects are not reliably achieved after a single dose. Because of the long half-life of oxaprozin, it takes several days of dosing to reach steady state (see *Pharmacokinetics*).
Pharmacokinetics: The pharmacokinetics of oxaprozin have been evaluated in approximately 400 individuals, which have included patients with rheumatoid arthritis, osteoarthritis, healthy elderly volunteers, and patients with cardiac, renal, and hepatic disease.
Oxaprozin demonstrates high oral bioavailability (95%), with peak plasma concentrations occurring between 3 and 5 hours after dosing. Food may reduce the rate of absorption of oxaprozin, but the extent of absorption is unchanged. Antacids have no effect on the rate or extent of oxaprozin absorption.
As is true for most NSAIDs, approximately 99.9% of the oxaprozin present in plasma is bound to albumin. The fraction of the drug present in the tissues across the therapeutic dosage range ranges between 40% and 60% of the total drug in the body and is proportional to dose, since the tissue sites are not saturated with the usual clinical doses.
Figure 1 shows the amount of oxaprozin in the plasma and in the tissue as a function of dose and the concentration of the free drug.

Figure 1.
Amount of oxaprozin in plasma and tissue as a function of dose and free (unbound) oxaprozin concentration.

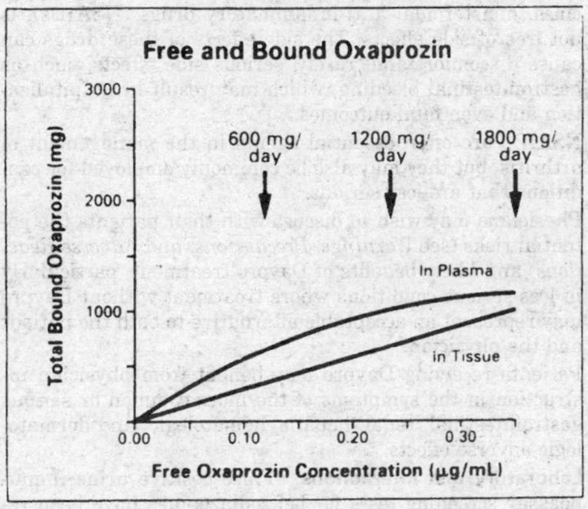

Unbound oxaprozin is the pharmacologically active component; it is able to distribute into tissues and to be cleared from the body. The average unbound concentration is a function of the tissue-bound and plasma-bound drug, and it increases proportionally with dose.
As the amount of oxaprozin in the tissues increases at higher dose, the plasma concentration of oxaprozin is limited by saturation of plasma protein binding. In addition, the increase in free (unbound) oxaprozin results in an increase in clearance. Both of these contribute to the total plasma concentration of oxaprozin increasing less than proportionately with dose.
Oxaprozin kinetics were modeled using a two-compartment model with first-order absorption and protein binding that becomes saturable in the clinical dosage range. As the dose is increased from 600 to 1200 mg daily, the steady state clearance of total oxaprozin increases from 0.25 to 0.34 L/hr, the steady state apparent volume of distribution increases from 10 to 12.5 L, and the accumulation half-life decreases from 25 to 21 hours. The terminal elimination half-life is approximately twice as long as the accumulation half-life because of the increased binding and decreased clearance at lower concentrations. Steady state concentrations in clinical usage are achieved in 4 to 7 days.
Plasma levels of total oxaprozin (free and bound drug) in studies of patients taking 600 to 1200 mg/day for several months ranged from 98 to 230 µg/mL, corresponding to estimated levels of free drug ranging from about 0.10 to 0.40 µg/mL.
Oxaprozin is primarily metabolized in the liver, by both microsomal oxidation (65%) and glucuronic acid conjugation (35%). A small amount (<5%) of active phenolic metabolites is produced, but the contribution to overall activity is minimal. All conjugated metabolites are inactive.
Biliary excretion of unchanged oxaprozin is a minor elimination pathway, and enterohepatic recycling of oxaprozin is insignificant. The glucuronide metabolites can be recovered from the urine (65%) and feces (35%), while unchanged oxaprozin is poorly excreted.
Renal dysfunction appears to alter oxaprozin binding and to reduce unbound clearance and unbound volume of distribution; dosage reductions should be made (see *Precautions: General*).
Age, gender, and well-compensated cardiac failure do not affect the plasma protein binding or the pharmacokinetics of oxaprozin.
Like other NSAIDs exhibiting a high degree of protein binding and a primarily metabolic route of elimination, oxaprozin has the potential for drug-drug interactions (see *Precautions: Drug interactions*).

CLINICAL STUDIES

Rheumatoid arthritis: Daypro was evaluated for managing the signs and symptoms of rheumatoid arthritis in placebo and active controlled clinical trials in a total of 646 patients. Daypro was given in single or divided daily doses of 600 to 1800 mg/day and was found to be comparable to 2600 to 3900 mg/day of aspirin. At these doses there was a trend (over all trials) for oxaprozin to be more effective and cause fewer gastrointestinal side effects than aspirin.
Daypro was given as a once-a-day dose of 1200 mg in most of the clinical trials, but larger doses (up to 26 mg/kg or 1800 mg/day) were used in selected patients. In some patients, Daypro may be better tolerated in divided doses. Due to its long half-life, several days of Daypro therapy were needed for the drug to reach its full effect (see *Individualization of Dosage*).
Osteoarthritis: Daypro was evaluated for the management of the signs and symptoms of osteoarthritis in a total of 616 patients in active controlled clinical trials against aspirin (N=464), piroxicam (N=102), and other NSAIDs. Daypro was given both in variable (600 to 1200 mg/day) and in fixed (1200 mg/day) dosing schedules in either single or divided doses. In these trials, oxaprozin was found to be comparable to 2600 to 3200 mg/day doses of aspirin or 20 mg/day doses of piroxicam. Oxaprozin was effective both in once-daily and in divided dosing schedules. In controlled clinical trials several days of oxaprozin therapy were needed for the drug to reach its full effects (see *Individualization of Dosage*).

INDIVIDUALIZATION OF DOSAGE

Daypro, like other NSAIDs, shows considerable interindividual differences in both pharmacokinetics and clinical response (pharmacodynamics). Therefore, the dosage for each patient should be individualized according to the patient's response to therapy.
The usual starting dose for most normal weight patients with rheumatoid arthritis is 1200 mg, once a day.
The usual starting dose for normal weight patients with mild to moderate osteoarthritis is 600 mg, once a day.
In cases where a quick onset of action is important, the pharmacokinetics of oxaprozin allow therapy to be started with a one-time loading dose of 1200 to 1800 mg (not to exceed 26 mg/kg).
Doses larger than 1200 mg/day should be reserved for patients who weigh more than 50 kg, have normal renal and hepatic function, are at low risk of peptic ulcer, and whose severity of disease justifies maximal therapy. Physicians should ensure that patients are tolerating doses in the 600 to 1200 mg/day range without gastroenterologic, renal, hepatic, or dermatologic adverse effects before advancing to the larger doses.
The maximum recommended total daily dosage is 1800 mg in divided doses.
Most patients will tolerate once-a-day dosing with Daypro, although divided doses may be tried in patients unable to tolerate single doses. As with all drugs of this class, the frequency and severity of adverse events will depend on the dose of the drug, the age and physical condition of the patient, any concurrent medical diagnoses, individual vulnerability, and the duration of therapy. In clinical trials of oxaprozin, no clear dose-response relationship was seen for serious adverse effects, but physicians are cautioned that the reported safety data were developed in patients who had successfully taken lower doses of Daypro before being advanced above 1200 mg/day.
Experience with other NSAIDs has shown that starting therapy with maximal doses in patients at increased risk due to renal or hepatic disease, low body weight, advanced age, a known ulcer diathesis, or known sensitivity to NSAID effects is likely to increase the frequency of adverse events and is not recommended (see *Precautions*).

INDICATIONS AND USAGE

Daypro is indicated for acute and long-term use in the management of the signs and symptoms of osteoarthritis and rheumatoid arthritis.

CONTRAINDICATIONS

Daypro should not be used in patients with previously demonstrated hypersensitivity to oxaprozin or any of its compo-

Continued on next page

Daypro—Cont.

nents or in individuals with the complete or partial syndrome of nasal polyps, angioedema, and bronchospastic reactivity to aspirin or other nonsteroidal anti-inflammatory drugs (NSAIDs).

Severe and occasionally fatal asthmatic and anaphylactic reactions have been reported in patients receiving NSAIDs, and there have been rare reports of anaphylaxis in patients taking oxaprozin.

WARNINGS

RISK OF GASTROINTESTINAL (GI) ULCERATION, BLEEDING, AND PERFORATION WITH NONSTEROIDAL ANTI-INFLAMMATORY DRUG THERAPY: Serious gastrointestinal toxicity, such as bleeding, ulceration, and perforation, can occur at any time, with or without warning symptoms, in patients treated with NSAIDs. Although minor upper gastrointestinal problems, such as dyspepsia, are common, and usually develop early in therapy, physicians should remain alert for ulceration and bleeding in patients treated chronically with NSAIDs, even in the absence of previous GI tract symptoms. In patients observed in clinical trials for several months to 2 years, symptomatic upper GI ulcers, gross bleeding, or perforation appear to occur in approximately 1% of patients treated for 3 to 6 months, and in about 2% to 4% of patients treated for 1 year. Physicians should inform patients about the signs and/or symptoms of serious GI toxicity and what steps to take if they occur.

Patients at risk for developing peptic ulceration and bleeding are those with a prior history of serious GI events, alcoholism, smoking, or other factors known to be associated with peptic ulcer disease. Elderly or debilitated patients seem to tolerate ulceration or bleeding less well than other individuals, and most spontaneous reports of fatal GI events are in these populations. Studies to date are inconclusive concerning the relative risk of various nonsteroidal anti-inflammatory drugs (NSAIDs) in causing such reactions. High doses of any NSAID probably carry a greater risk of these reactions, and substantial benefit should be anticipated to patients prior to prescribing maximal doses of Daypro.

PRECAUTIONS
General

Hepatic effects: As with other nonsteroidal anti-inflammatory drugs, borderline elevations of one or more liver tests may occur in up to 15% of patients. These abnormalities may progress, remain essentially unchanged, or resolve with continued therapy. The SGPT (ALT) test is probably the most sensitive indicator of liver dysfunction. Meaningful (3 times the upper limit of normal) elevations of SGOT (AST) occurred in controlled clinical trials of Daypro in just under 1% of patients. A patient with symptoms and/or signs suggesting liver dysfunction or in whom an abnormal liver test has occurred should be evaluated for evidence of the development of more severe hepatic reaction while on therapy with this drug. Severe hepatic reactions including jaundice have been reported with Daypro, and there may be a risk of fatal hepatitis with oxaprozin, such as has been seen with other NSAIDs. Although such reactions are rare, if abnormal liver tests persist or worsen, clinical signs and symptoms consistent with liver disease develop, or systemic manifestations occur (eosinophilia, rash, fever), Daypro should be discontinued.

Well-compensated hepatic cirrhosis does not appear to alter the disposition of unbound oxaprozin, so dosage adjustment is not necessary. However, the primary route of elimination of oxaprozin is hepatic metabolism, so caution should be observed in patients with severe hepatic dysfunction.

Renal effects: Acute interstitial nephritis, hematuria, and proteinuria have been reported with Daypro as with other NSAIDs. Long-term administration of some nonsteroidal anti-inflammatory drugs to animals has resulted in renal papillary necrosis and other abnormal renal pathology. This was not observed with oxaprozin, but the clinical significance of this difference is unknown.

A second form of renal toxicity has been seen in patients with preexisting conditions leading to a reduction in renal blood flow, where the renal prostaglandins have a supportive role in the maintenance of renal perfusion. In these patients administration of a nonsteroidal anti-inflammatory drug may cause a dose-dependent reduction in prostaglandin formation and may precipitate overt renal decompensation. Patients at greatest risk of this reaction are those with previously impaired renal function, heart failure, or liver dysfunction, those taking diuretics, and the elderly. Discontinuation of nonsteroidal anti-inflammatory drug therapy is often followed by recovery to the pretreatment state. Those patients at high risk who chronically take oxaprozin should have renal function monitored if they have signs or symptoms that may be consistent with mild azotemia, such as malaise, fatigue, or loss of appetite. As with all NSAID therapy, patients may occasionally develop some elevation of serum creatinine and BUN levels without any signs or symptoms.

The pharmacokinetics of oxaprozin may be significantly altered in patients with renal insufficiency or in patients who are undergoing hemodialysis. Such patients should be started on doses of 600 mg/day, with cautious dosage increases if the desired effect is not obtained. Oxaprozin is not dialyzed because of its high degree of protein binding.

Like other NSAIDs, Daypro may worsen fluid retention by the kidneys in patients with uncompensated cardiac failure due to its effect on prostaglandins. It should be used with caution in patients with a history of hypertension, cardiac decompensation, in patients on chronic diuretic therapy, or in those with other conditions predisposing to fluid retention.

Photosensitivity: Oxaprozin has been associated with rash and/or mild photosensitivity in dermatologic testing. An increased incidence of rash on sun-exposed skin was seen in some patients in the clinical trials.

Recommended laboratory testing: Because serious GI tract ulceration and bleeding can occur without warning symptoms, physicians should follow chronically treated patients for the signs and symptoms of ulceration and bleeding and should inform them of the importance of this follow-up (see *Warnings*).

Anemia may occur in patients receiving oxaprozin or other NSAIDs. This may be due to fluid retention, gastrointestinal blood loss, or an incompletely described effect upon erythrogenesis. Patients on long-term treatment with Daypro should have their hemoglobin or hematocrit values determined at appropriate intervals as determined by the clinical situation.

Oxaprozin, like other NSAIDs, can affect platelet aggregation and prolong bleeding time. Daypro should be used with caution in patients with underlying hemostatic defects or in those who are undergoing surgical procedures where a high degree of hemostasis is needed.

Information for patients: Daypro, like other drugs of its class, nonsteroidal anti-inflammatory drugs (NSAIDs), is not free of side effects. The side effects of these drugs can cause discomfort and, rarely, serious side effects, such as gastrointestinal bleeding, which may result in hospitalization and even fatal outcomes.

NSAIDs are often essential agents in the management of arthritis, but they may also be commonly employed for conditions that are less serious.

Physicians may wish to discuss with their patients the potential risks (see *Warnings, Precautions,* and *Adverse Reactions*) and likely benefits of Daypro treatment, particularly in less-serious conditions where treatment without Daypro may represent an acceptable alternative to both the patient and the physician.

Patients receiving Daypro may benefit from physician instruction in the symptoms of the more common or serious gastrointestinal, renal, hepatic, hematologic, and dermatologic adverse effects.

Laboratory test interactions: False-positive urine immunoassay screening tests for benzodiazepines have been reported in patients taking Daypro. This is due to lack of specificity of the screening tests. False-positive test results may be expected for several days following discontinuation of Daypro therapy. Confirmatory tests, such as gas chromatography/mass spectrometry, will distinguish Daypro from benzodiazepines.

Drug interactions

Aspirin: Concomitant administration of Daypro and aspirin is not recommended because oxprozin displaces salicylates from plasma protein binding sites. Coadministration would be expected to increase the risk of salicylate toxicity.

Oral anticoagulants: The anticoagulant effects of warfarin were not affected by the coadministration of 1200 mg/day of Daypro. Nevertheless, caution should be exercised when adding any drug that affects platelet function to the regimen of patients receiving oral anticoagulants.

H_2-receptor antagonists: The total body clearance of oxaprozin was reduced by 20% in subjects who concurrently received therapeutic doses of cimetidine or ranitidine; no other pharmacokinetic parameter was affected. A change of clearance of this magnitude lies within the range of normal variation and is unlikely to produce a clinically detectable difference in the outcome of therapy.

Beta-blockers: Subjects receiving 1200 mg Daypro qd with 100 mg metoprolol bid exhibited statistically significant but transient increases in sitting and standing blood pressures after 14 days. Therefore, as with all NSAIDs, routine blood pressure monitoring should be considered in these patients when starting Daypro therapy.

Other drugs: The coadministration of oxaprozin and antacids, acetaminophen, or conjugated estrogens resulted in no statistically significant changes in pharmacokinetic parameters in single- and/or multiple-dose studies. The interaction of oxaprozin with lithium and cardiac glycosides has not been studied.

Carcinogenesis, mutagenesis, impairment of fertility: In oncogenicity studies, oxaprozin administration for 2 years was associated with the exacerbation of liver neoplasms (he-

patic adenomas and carcinomas) in male CD mice, but not in female CD mice or rats. The significance of this species-specific finding to man is unknown.

Oxaprozin did not display mutagenic potential. Results from the Ames test, forward mutation in yeast and Chinese hamster ovary (CHO) cells, DNA repair testing in CHO cells, micronucleus testing in mouse bone marrow, chromosomal aberration testing in human lymphocytes, and cell transformation testing in mouse fibroblast all showed no evidence of genetic toxicity or cell-transforming ability.

Oxaprozin administration was not associated with impairment of fertility in male and female rats at oral doses up to 200 mg/kg/day (1180 mg/m[2]); the usual human dose is 17 mg/kg/day (629 mg/m[2]). However, testicular degeneration was observed in beagle dogs treated with 37.5 to 150 mg/kg/day (750 to 3000 mg/m[2]) of oxaprozin for 6 months, or 37.5 mg/kg/day for 42 days, a finding not confirmed in other species. The clinical relevance of this finding is not known.

Pregnancy: Teratogenic Effects—Pregnancy Category C. There are no adequate or well-controlled studies in pregnant women. Teratology studies with oxaprozin were performed in mice, rats, and rabbits. In mice and rats, no drug-related developmental abnormalities were observed at 50 to 200 mg/kg/day of oxaprozin (225 to 900 mg/m[2]). However, in rabbits, infrequent malformed fetuses were observed in dams treated with 7.5 to 30 mg/kg/day of oxaprozin (the usual human dosage range). Oxaprozin should be used during pregnancy only if the potential benefits justify the potential risks to the fetus.

Labor and delivery: The effect of oxaprozin in pregnant women is unknown. NSAIDs are known to delay parturition, to accelerate closure of the fetal ductus arteriosus, and to be associated with dystocia. Oxaprozin is known to have caused decreases in pup survival in rat studies. Accordingly, the use of oxaprozin during late pregnancy should be avoided.

Nursing mothers: Studies of oxaprozin excretion in human milk have not been conducted; however, oxaprozin was found in the milk of lactating rats. Since the effects of oxaprozin on infants are not known, caution should be exercised if oxaprozin is administered to nursing women.

Pediatric use: Safety and effectiveness of Daypro in pediatric patients have not been established.

Geriatric use: No adjustment of the dose of Daypro is necessary in the elderly for *pharmacokinetic* reasons, although many elderly may need to receive a reduced dose because of low body weight or disorders associated with aging. No significant differences in the pharmacokinetic profile for oxaprozin were seen in studies in the healthy elderly.

Although selected elderly patients in controlled clinical trials tolerated Daypro as well as younger patients, caution should be exercised in treating the elderly, and extra care should be taken when choosing a dose. As with any NSAID, the elderly are likely to tolerate adverse reactions less well than younger patients.

ADVERSE REACTIONS

Adverse reaction data were derived from patients who received Daypro in multidose, controlled, and open-label clinical trials, and from worldwide marketing experience. Rates for events occurring in more than 1% of patients, and for most of the less common events, are based on 2253 patients who took 1200 to 1800 mg Daypro per day in clinical trials. Of these, 1721 were treated for at least 1 month, 971 for at least 3 months, and 366 for more than 1 year. Rates for the rarer events and for events reported from worldwide marketing experience are difficult to estimate accurately and are only listed as less than 1%.

The adverse event rates below refer to the incidence in the first month of use. Most of the events were seen by this time for common adverse reactions. However, the cumulative incidence can be expected to rise with continued therapy, and some events, such as gastrointestinal bleeding (see *Warnings*), seem to occur at a constant or possibly increasing rate over time.

The most frequently reported adverse reactions were related to the gastrointestinal tract. They were nausea (8%) and dyspepsia (8%).

INCIDENCE GREATER THAN 1%: In clinical trials the following adverse reactions occurred at an incidence greater than 1% and are probably related to treatment. Reactions occurring in 3% to 9% of patients treated with Daypro are indicated by an asterisk(*); those reactions occurring in less than 3% of patients are unmarked.

Digestive system: abdominal pain/distress, anorexia, constipation*, diarrhea*, dyspepsia*, flatulence, nausea*, vomiting.

Nervous system: CNS inhibition (depression, sedation, somnolence, or confusion), disturbance of sleep.

Skin and appendages: rash*.

Special senses: tinnitus.

Urogenital system: dysuria or frequency.

INCIDENCE LESS THAN 1%:

Probable causal relationship: The following adverse reactions were reported in clinical trials or from worldwide marketing experience at an incidence of less than 1%. Those re-

actions reported only from worldwide marketing experience are in *italics*. The probability of a causal relationship exists between the drug and these adverse reactions.

Body as a whole: drug hypersensitivity reactions including anaphylaxis *and serum sickness*.

Cardiovascular system: edema, blood pressure changes.

Digestive system: peptic ulceration and/or GI bleeding (see *Warnings*), liver function abnormalities including *hepatitis* (see *Precautions*), stomatitis, hemorrhoidal or rectal bleeding, *pancreatitis*.

Hematologic system: anemia, thrombocytopenia, leukopenia, ecchymoses, *agranulocytosis, pancytopenia*.

Metabolic system: weight gain, weight loss.

Nervous system: weakness, malaise.

Respiratory system: symptoms of upper respiratory tract infection.

Skin: pruritus, urticaria, photosensitivity, *pseudoporphyria, exfoliative dermatitis, erythema multiforme, Stevens-Johnson syndrome, toxic epidermal necrolysis (Lyell's syndrome)*.

Special senses: blurred vision, conjunctivitis.

Urogenital: *acute interstitial nephritis, nephrotic syndrome*, hematuria, renal insufficiency, *acute renal failure*, decreased menstrual flow.

Causal relationship unknown: The following adverse reactions occurred at an incidence of less than 1% in clinical trials, or were suggested from marketing experience, under circumstances where a causal relationship could not be definitely established. They are listed as alerting information for the physician.

Cardiovascular system: palpitations.

Digestive system: alteration in taste.

Respiratory system: sinusitis, pulmonary infections.

Skin and appendages: alopecia.

Special senses: hearing decrease.

Urogenital system: increase in menstrual flow.

DRUG ABUSE AND DEPENDENCE

Daypro is a non-narcotic drug. Usually reliable animal studies have indicated that Daypro has no known addiction potential in humans.

OVERDOSAGE

No patient experienced either an accidental or intentional overdosage of Daypro in the clinical trials of the drug. Symptoms following acute overdose with other NSAIDs are usually limited to lethargy, drowsiness, nausea, vomiting, and epigastric pain and are generally reversible with supportive care. Gastrointestinal bleeding and coma have occurred following NSAID overdose. Hypertension, acute renal failure, and respiratory depression are rare.

Patients should be managed by symptomatic and supportive care following an NSAID overdose. There are no specific antidotes. Gut decontamination may be indicated in patients seen within 4 hours of ingestion with symptoms or following a large overdose (5 to 10 times the usual dose). This should be accomplished via emesis and/or activated charcoal (60 to 100 g in adults, 1 to 2 g/kg in children) with an osmotic cathartic. Forced diuresis, alkalization of the urine, or hemoperfusion would probably not be useful due to the high degree of protein binding of oxaprozin.

DOSAGE AND ADMINISTRATION

Rheumatoid arthritis: The usual daily dose of Daypro in the management of the signs and symptoms of rheumatoid arthritis is 1200 mg (two 600-mg caplets) once a day. Both smaller and larger doses may be required in individual patients (see *Individualization of Dosage*).

Osteoarthritis: The usual daily dose of Daypro for the management of the signs and symptoms of moderate to severe osteoarthritis is 1200 mg (two 600-mg caplets) once a day. For patients of low body weight or with milder disease, an initial dosage of one 600-mg caplet once a day may be appropriate (see *Individualization of Dosage*).

Regardless of the indication, the dosage should be individualized to the lowest effective dose of Daypro to minimize adverse effects, and the maximum recommended total daily dose is 1800 mg (or 26 mg/kg, whichever is lower) in divided doses.

SAFETY AND HANDLING

Daypro is supplied as a solid dosage form in closed containers, is not known to produce contact dermatitis, and poses no known risk to healthcare workers. It may be disposed of in accordance with applicable local regulations governing the disposal of pharmaceuticals.

HOW SUPPLIED

Daypro 600-mg caplets are white, capsule-shaped, scored, film-coated, with DAYPRO debossed on one side and 1381 on the other side.

NDC Number	Size
0025-1381-31	bottle of 100
0025-1381-34	carton of 100 unit dose

Keep bottles tightly closed and store below 86°F (30°C). Dispense in a tight, light-resistant container with a child-resistant closure. Protect the unit dose from light.

Caution: Federal law prohibits dispensing without prescription.

4/4/97 • A05222-6

Shown in Product Identification Guide, page 337

DEMULEN® 1/35–21 ℞
DEMULEN® 1/35–28 ℞
DEMULEN® 1/50–21 ℞
DEMULEN® 1/50–28 ℞
[dem 'ū-len]
(ethynodiol diacetate with ethinyl estradiol)

PRODUCT OVERVIEW

KEY FACTS

The Searle line of oral contraceptives contains two fixed-dose combination oral contraceptives (DEMULEN 1/35-21 and DEMULEN 1/35-28) containing ethynodiol diacetate (1 mg) with ethinyl estradiol (35 mcg) and two fixed-dose combination oral contraceptives (DEMULEN 1/50-21 and DEMULEN 1/50-28) containing ethinyl estradiol (50 mcg). DEMULEN 1/35-21 and DEMULEN 1/50-21 are 21-day dosage regimens. DEMULEN 1/35-28 and DEMULEN 1/50-28 are 28-day dosage regimens (including 7 days of inert tablets). These forms are packaged in Compack® tablet dispensers.

MAJOR USE

DEMULEN 1/35 and DEMULEN 1/50 are highly effective in preventing pregnancy.

SAFETY INFORMATION

See complete safety information set forth below.

PRESCRIBING INFORMATION

DEMULEN® 1/35–21 ℞
DEMULEN® 1/35–28 ℞
DEMULEN® 1/50–21 ℞
DEMULEN® 1/50–28 ℞
[dem 'ū-len]
(ethynodiol diacetate with ethinyl estradiol)

Patients should be counseled that this product does not protect against HIV infection (AIDS) and other sexually transmitted diseases.

DESCRIPTION

Demulen 1/35-21 and Demulen 1/35-28. Each white tablet contains 1 mg of ethynodiol diacetate and 35 mcg of ethinyl estradiol, and the inactive ingredients include calcium acetate, calcium phosphate, corn starch, hydrogenated castor oil, and povidone. Each blue tablet in the Demulen 1/35-28 package is a placebo containing no active ingredients, and the inactive ingredients include lactose monohydrate, microcrystalline cellulose, anhydrous lactose, FD&C Blue No. 1 Lake, and magnesium stearate.

Demulen 1/50-21 and Demulen 1/50-28. Each white tablet contains 1 mg of ethynodiol diacetate and 50 mcg of ethinyl estradiol, and the inactive ingredients include calcium acetate, calcium phosphate, corn starch, hydrogenated castor oil, and povidone. Each pink tablet in the Demulen 1/50-28 package is a placebo containing no active ingredients, and the inactive ingredients include lactose monohydrate, microcrystalline cellulose, anhydrous lactose, FD&C Yellow No. 6, and magnesium stearate.

The chemical name for ethynodiol diacetate is 19-nor-17α-pregn-4-en-20-yne-3β, 17-diol diacetate, and for ethinyl estradiol it is 19-nor-17α-pregna-1,3,5(10)-trien-20-yne-3, 17-diol. The structural formulas are as follows:

ethynodiol diacetate

ethinyl estradiol

Therapeutic class: Oral contraceptive.

CLINICAL PHARMACOLOGY

Combination oral contraceptives act primarily by suppression of gonadotropins. Although the primary mechanism of

this action is inhibition of ovulation, other alterations in the genital tract, including changes in the cervical mucus (which increase the difficulty of sperm entry into the uterus) and the endometrium (which may reduce the likelihood of implantation) may also contribute to contraceptive effectiveness.

INDICATIONS AND USAGE

Demulen 1/35 and Demulen 1/50 are indicated for the prevention of pregnancy in women who elect to use oral contraceptives as a method of contraception.

Oral contraceptives are highly effective. Table 1 lists the typical accidental pregnancy rates for users of combination oral contraceptives and other methods of contraception. The efficacy of these contraceptive methods, except sterilization and progestogen implants and injections, depends upon the reliability with which they are used. Correct and consistent use of methods can result in lower failure rates.

Table 1. Lowest expected and typical failure rates during the first year of continuous use of a method. Percent of women experiencing an accidental pregnancy in the first year of continuous use.[1,1a]

Method	Lowest Expected*	Typical**
No contraception	85	85
Oral contraceptives		
Combined	0.1	N/A***
Progestogen only	0.5	N/A***
Diaphragm with spermicidal cream or jelly	6	18
Spermicides alone (foam, creams, jellies and vaginal suppositories)	3	21
Vaginal sponge		
Nulliparous	6	18
Parous	9	28
IUD (medicated)		
Progesterone	2	N/A***
Copper T 380A	0.8	N/A***
Condom without spermicides	2	12
Periodic abstinence (all methods)	1–9	20
Progestogen injections	0.3	0.3
Progestogen implants	0.2	0.2
Female sterilization	0.2	0.4
Male sterilization	0.1	0.15

Adapted from Trussell et al.[1]

* The authors' best guess of the percentage of women expected to experience an accidental pregnancy among couples who initiate a method (not necessarily for the first time) and who use it consistently and correctly during the first year if they do not stop for any other reason.

** This term represents "typical" couples who initiate use of a method (not necessarily for the first time), who experience an accidental pregnancy during the first year if they do not stop for any other reason.

*** N/A—Data not available.

CONTRAINDICATIONS

Oral contraceptives should not be used in women who have the following conditions:

• Thrombophlebitis or thromboembolic disorders
• A past history of deep vein thrombophlebitis or thromboembolic disorders
• Cerebral vascular disease, myocardial infarction, or coronary artery disease, or a past history of these conditions
• Known or suspected carcinoma of the breast, or a history of this condition
• Known or suspected carcinoma of the female reproductive organs or suspected estrogen-dependent neoplasia, or a history of these conditions
• Undiagnosed abnormal genital bleeding
• History of cholestatic jaundice of pregnancy or jaundice with prior oral contraceptive use
• Past or present, benign or malignant liver tumors
• Known or suspected pregnancy

WARNINGS

Cigarette smoking increases the risk of serious cardiovascular side effects from oral contraceptive use. This risk increases with age and with heavy smoking (15 or more cigarettes per day) and is quite marked in women over 35 years of age. Women who use oral contraceptives should be strongly advised not to smoke.

The use of oral contraceptives is associated with increased risk of several serious conditions including venous and ar-

Continued on next page

Demulen—Cont.

Table 2. Annual number of birth-related or method-related deaths associated with control of fertility per 100,000 nonsterile women, by fertility control method according to age.[67]

	Age					
Method of control	15–19	20–24	25–29	30–34	35–39	40–44
No fertility control methods*	7.0	7.4	9.1	14.8	25.7	28.2
Oral contraceptives						
nonsmoker**	0.3	0.5	0.9	1.9	13.8	31.6
smoker**	2.2	3.4	6.6	13.5	51.1	117.2
IUD**	0.8	0.8	1.0	1.0	1.4	1.4
Condom*	1.1	1.6	0.7	0.2	0.3	0.4
Diaphragm/ spermicide*	1.9	1.2	1.2	1.3	2.2	2.8
Periodic abstinence*	2.5	1.6	1.6	1.7	2.9	3.6

* Deaths are birth-related
** Deaths are method-related
Adapted from Ory.[67]

terial thromboembolism, thrombotic and hemorrhagic stroke, myocardial infarction, liver tumors or other liver lesions, and gallbladder disease. The risk of morbidity and mortality increases significantly in the presence of other risk factors such as hypertension, hyperlipidemia, obesity, and diabetes mellitus.

Practitioners prescribing oral contraceptives should be familiar with the following information relating to these and other risks.

The information contained herein is principally based on studies carried out in patients who used oral contraceptives with formulations containing higher amounts of estrogens and progestogens than those in common use today. The effect of long-term use of the oral contraceptives with lesser amounts of both estrogens and progestogens remains to be determined.

Throughout this labeling, epidemiological studies reported are of two types: retrospective case-control studies and prospective cohort studies. Case-control studies provide an estimate of the relative risk of a disease, which is defined as the *ratio* of the incidence of a disease among oral contraceptive users to that among nonusers. The relative risk (or odds ratio) does not provide information about the actual clinical occurrence of a disease. Cohort studies provide a measure of both the relative risk and the attributable risk. The latter is the *difference* in the incidence of disease between oral contraceptive users and nonusers. The attributable risk does provide information about the actual occurrence or incidence of a disease in the subject population. For further information, the reader is referred to a text on epidemiological methods.

1. Thromboembolic disorders and other vascular problems.

a. Myocardial infarction. An increased risk of myocardial infarction has been associated with oral contraceptive use.[2–21] This increased risk is primarily in smokers or in women with other underlying risk factors for coronary artery disease such as hypertension, obesity, diabetes, and hypercholesterolemia. The relative risk for myocardial infarction in current oral contraceptive users has been estimated to be 2 to 6. The risk is very low under the age of 30. However, there is the possibility of a risk of cardiovascular disease even in very young women who take oral contraceptives.

Smoking in combination with oral contraceptive use has been reported to contribute substantially to the risk of myocardial infarction in women in their mid-thirties or older, with smoking accounting for the majority of excess cases.[22] Mortality rates associated with circulatory disease have been shown to increase substantially in smokers, especially in those 35 years of age and older among women who use oral contraceptives (see Figure 1, Table 2).

Figure 1. Circulatory disease mortality rates per 100,000 woman-years by age, smoking status, and oral contraceptive use.[14]

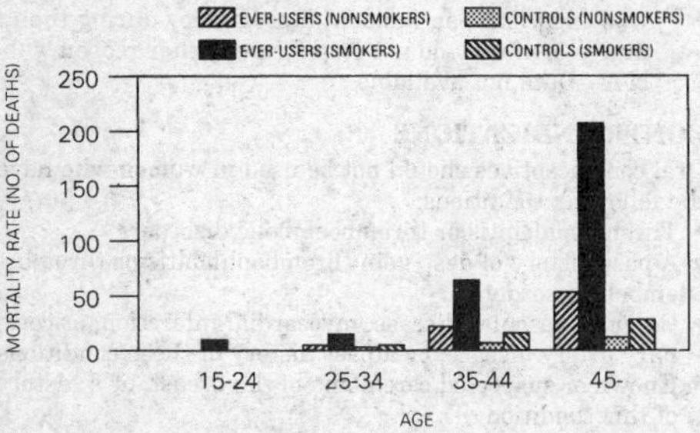

Adapted from Layde and Beral.[14]

Oral contraceptives may compound the effects of well-known cardiovascular risk factors such as hypertension, diabetes, hyperlipidemias, hypercholesterolemia, age, cigarette smoking, and obesity. In particular, some progestogens decrease HDL cholesterol[23–31] and cause glucose intolerance, while estrogens may create a state of hyperinsulinism.[32] Oral contraceptives have been shown to increase blood pressure among some users (see *Warning* No. 9). Similar effects on risk factors have been associated with an increased risk of heart disease.

b. Thromboembolism. An increased risk of thromboembolic and thrombotic disease associated with the use of oral contraceptives is well established.[17,33–51] Case-control studies have estimated the relative risk to be 3 for the first episode of superficial venous thrombosis, 4 to 11 for deep vein thrombosis or pulmonary embolism, and 1.5 to 6 for women with predisposing conditions for venous thromboembolic disease.[34–37,45,46] Cohort studies have shown the relative risk to be somewhat lower, about 3 for new cases (subjects with no past history of venous thrombosis or varicose veins) and about 4.5 for new cases requiring hospitalization.[42,47,48] The risk of venous thromboembolic disease associated with oral contraceptives is not related to duration of use.

A two- to seven-fold increase in relative risk of postoperative thromboembolic complications has been reported with the use of oral contraceptives.[38,39] The relative risk of venous thrombosis in women who have predisposing conditions is about twice that of women without such medical conditions.[43] If feasible, oral contraceptives should be discontinued at least 4 weeks prior to and for 2 weeks after elective surgery of a type associated with an increased risk of thromboembolism, and also during and following prolonged immobilization. Since the immediate postpartum period is also associated with an increased risk of thromboembolism, oral contraceptives should be started no earlier than 4 to 6 weeks after delivery in women who elect not to breast feed.

c. Cerebrovascular diseases. Both the relative and attributable risks of cerebrovascular events (thrombotic and hemorrhagic strokes) have been reported to be increased with oral contraceptive use,[14,17,18,34,42,46,52–59] although, in general, the risk was greatest among older (over 35 years), hypertensive women who also smoked. Hypertension was reported to be a risk factor for both users and nonusers, for both types of strokes, while smoking increased the risk for hemorrhagic strokes.

In one large study,[52] the relative risk for thrombotic stroke was reported as 9.5 times greater in users than in nonusers. It ranged from 3 for normotensive users to 14 for users with severe hypertension.[54] The relative risk for hemorrhagic stroke was reported to be 1.2 for nonsmokers who used oral contraceptives, 1.9 to 2.6 for smokers who did not use oral contraceptives, 6.1 to 7.6 for smokers who used oral contraceptives, 1.8 for normotensive users, and 25.7 for users with severe hypertension. The risk is also greater in older women and among smokers.

d. Dose-related risk of vascular disease with oral contraceptives. A positive association has been reported between the amount of estrogen and progestogen in oral contraceptives and the risk of vascular disease.[41,43,53,59–64] A decline in serum high density lipoproteins (HDL) has been reported with many progestogens.[23–31] A decline in serum high density lipoproteins has been associated with an increased incidence of ischemic heart disease.[65] Because estrogens increase HDL-cholesterol, the net effect of an oral contraceptive depends on the balance achieved between doses of estrogen and progestogen and the nature and absolute amount of progestogens used in the contraceptives. The amount of both steroids should be considered in the choice of an oral contraceptive.

Minimizing exposure to estrogen and progestogen is in keeping with good principles of therapeutics. For any particular estrogen-progestogen combination, the dosage regimen prescribed should be one that contains the least amount of estrogen and progestogen that is compatible with a low failure rate and the needs of the individual patient. New acceptors of oral contraceptives should be started on preparations containing the lowest estrogen content that produces satisfactory results in the individual.

e. Persistence of risk of vascular disease. There are three studies that have shown persistence of risk of vascular disease for users of oral contraceptives. In a study in the United States, the risk of developing myocardial infarction after discontinuing oral contraceptives persisted for at least 9 years for women 40–49 years old who had used oral contraceptives for 5 or more years, but this increased risk was not demonstrated in other age groups.[16] Another American study reported former use of oral contraceptives was significantly associated with increased risk of subarachnoid hemorrhage.[57] In another study, in Great Britain, the risk of developing nonrheumatic heart disease plus hypertension, subarachnoid hemorrhage, cerebral thrombosis, and transient ischemic attacks persisted for at least 6 years after discontinuation of oral contraceptives, although the excess risk was small.[14,18,66] It should be noted that these studies were performed with oral contraceptive formulations containing 50 mcg or more of estrogens.

2. Estimates of mortality from contraceptive use. One study[67] gathered data from a variety of sources that have estimated the mortality rates associated with different methods of contraception at different ages (Table 2). These estimates include the combined risk of death associated with contraceptive methods plus the risk attributable to pregnancy in the event of method failure. Each method of contraception has its specific benefits and risks. The study concluded that, with the exception of oral contraceptive users 35 and older who smoke and 40 or older who do not smoke, mortality associated with all methods of birth control is low and below that associated with childbirth. The observation of a possible increase in risk of mortality with age for oral contraceptive users is based on data gathered in the 1970's, but not reported until 1983.[67] However, current clinical practice involves the use of lower estrogen dose formulations combined with careful restriction of oral contraceptive use to women who do not have the various risk factors listed in this labeling.

Because of these changes in practice and, also, because of some limited new data that suggest that the risk of cardiovascular disease with the use of oral contraceptives may now be less than previously observed,[48,152] the Fertility and Maternal Health Drugs Advisory Committee was asked to review the topic in 1989. The Committee concluded that, although cardiovascular disease risks may be increased with oral contraceptive use after age 40 in healthy nonsmoking women (even with the newer low-dose formulations), there are greater potential health risks associated with pregnancy in older women and with the alternative surgical and medical procedures that may be necessary if such women do not have access to effective and acceptable means of contraception.

Therefore, the Committee recommended that the benefits of oral contraceptive use by healthy nonsmoking women over 40 may outweigh the possible risks. Of course, older women, as all women who take oral contraceptives, should take the lowest dose formulation that is effective.

[See table 2 above]

3. Carcinoma of the breast and reproductive organs. Numerous epidemiological studies have been performed on the incidence of breast, endometrial, ovarian, and cervical cancer in women using oral contraceptives. While there are conflicting reports, most studies suggest that the use of oral contraceptives is not associated with an overall increase in the risk of developing breast cancer.[17,40,68–78] Some studies have reported an increased relative risk of developing breast cancer, particularly at a young age.[79–102,151] This increased relative risk appears to be related to duration of use.

Some studies suggested that oral contraceptive use was associated with an increase in the risk of cervical intraepithelial neoplasia, dysplasia, erosion, carcinoma, or microglandular dysplasia in some populations of women.[17,50,103–115] However, there continues to be controversy about the extent to which such findings may be due to differences in sexual behavior and other factors.

In spite of many studies of the relationship between oral contraceptive use and breast and cervical cancers, a cause and effect relationship has not been established.

4. Hepatic neoplasia. Benign hepatic adenomas and other hepatic lesions have been associated with oral contraceptive use,[116–121] although the incidence of such benign tumors is rare in the United States. Indirect calculations have estimated the attributable risk to be in the range of 3.3 cases per 100,000 for users, a risk that increases after 4 or more years of use.[120] Rupture of benign, hepatic adenomas or other lesions may cause death through intra-abdominal hemorrhage. Therefore, such lesions should be considered in

women presenting with abdominal pain and tenderness, abdominal mass, or shock. About one quarter of the cases presented because of abdominal masses; up to one half had signs and symptoms of acute intraperitoneal hemorrhage.[121] Diagnosis may prove difficult.

Studies from the U.S.,[122,150] Great Britain,[123,124] and Italy[125] have shown an increased risk of hepatocellular carcinoma in long-term (>8 years; relative risk of 7–20) oral contraceptive users. However, these cancers are rare in the United States, and the attributable risk (the excess incidence) of liver cancers in oral contraceptive users approaches less than 1 per 1,000,000 users.

5. Ocular lesions. There have been reports of retinal thrombosis and other ocular lesions associated with the use of oral contraceptives. Oral contraceptives should be discontinued if there is unexplained, gradual or sudden, partial or complete loss of vision; onset of proptosis or diplopia; papilledema; or any evidence of retinal vascular lesions. Appropriate diagnostic and therapeutic measures should be undertaken immediately.

6. Oral contraceptive use before or during pregnancy. Extensive epidemiological studies have revealed no increased risk of birth defects in women who have used oral contraceptives prior to pregnancy.[126,129] The majority of recent studies also do not suggest a teratogenic effect, particularly insofar as cardiac anomalies and limb reduction defects are concerned,[126–129] when the pill is taken inadvertently during early pregnancy.

The administration of oral contraceptives to induce withdrawal bleeding should not be used as a test for pregnancy. Oral contraceptives should not be used during pregnancy to treat threatened or habitual abortion. It is recommended that for any patient who has missed two consecutive periods, pregnancy should be ruled out before continuing oral contraceptive use. If the patient has not adhered to the prescribed schedule, the possibility of pregnancy should be considered at the time of the first missed period and further use of oral contraceptives should be withheld until pregnancy has been ruled out. Oral contraceptive use should be discontinued if pregnancy is confirmed.

7. Gallbladder disease. Earlier studies reported an increased lifetime relative risk of gallbladder surgery in users of oral contraceptives and estrogens.[40,42,53,70] More recent studies, however, have shown that the relative risk of developing gallbladder disease among oral contraceptive users may be minimal.[130–132] The recent findings of minimal risk may be related to the use of oral contraceptive formulations containing lower doses of estrogens and progestogens.

8. Carbohydrate and lipid metabolic effects. Oral contraceptives have been shown to cause a decrease in glucose tolerance in a significant percentage of users.[32] This effect has been shown to be directly related to estrogen dose.[133] Progestogens increase insulin secretion and create insulin resistance, the effect varying with different progestational agents.[32,134] However, in the nondiabetic woman, oral contraceptives appear to have no effect on fasting blood glucose. Because of these demonstrated effects, prediabetic and diabetic women should be carefully observed while taking oral contraceptives.

Some women may have persistent hypertriglyceridemia while on the pill. As discussed earlier (see *Warnings* 1a and 1d), changes in serum triglycerides and lipoprotein levels have been reported in oral contraceptive users.[23–31,135,136]

9. Elevated blood pressure. An increase in blood pressure has been reported in women taking oral contraceptives[50,53,137–139] and this increase is more likely in older oral contraceptive users[137] and with extended duration of use.[53] Data from the Royal College of General Practitioners[138] and subsequent randomized trials have shown that the incidence of hypertension increases with increasing concentrations of progestogens.

Women with a history of hypertension or hypertension-related diseases, or renal disease[139] should be encouraged to use another method of contraception. If such women elect to use oral contraceptives, they should be monitored closely and if significant elevation of blood pressure occurs, oral contraceptives should be discontinued. For most women, elevated blood pressure will return to normal after stopping oral contraceptives,[137] and there is no difference in the occurrence of hypertension among ever- and never-users.[140]

10. Headache. The onset or exacerbation of migraine or the development of headache of a new pattern that is recurrent, persistent, or severe requires discontinuation of oral contraceptives and evaluation of the cause.

11. Bleeding irregularities. Breakthrough bleeding and spotting are sometimes encountered in patients on oral contraceptives, especially during the first three months of use. Nonhormonal causes should be considered and adequate diagnostic measures taken to rule out malignancy or pregnancy in the event of breakthrough bleeding, as in the case of any abnormal vaginal bleeding. If a pathologic basis has been excluded, time alone or a change to another formulation may solve the problem. In the event of amenorrhea, pregnancy should be ruled out.

PRECAUTIONS

1. Physical examination and follow-up. It is good medical practice for all women to have annual history and physical examinations, including women using oral contraceptives. The physical examination, however, may be deferred until after initiation of oral contraceptives if requested by the woman and judged appropriate by the clinician. The physical examination should include special reference to blood pressure, breasts, abdomen, and pelvic organs, including cervical cytology, and relevant laboratory tests. In case of undiagnosed, persistent, or recurrent abnormal vaginal bleeding, appropriate measures should be conducted to rule out malignancy. Women with a strong family history of breast cancer or who have breast nodules should be monitored with particular care.

2. Lipid disorders. Women who are being treated for hyperlipidemias should be followed closely if they elect to use oral contraceptives. Some progestogens may elevate LDL levels and may render the control of hyperlipidemias more difficult.

3. Liver function. If jaundice develops in any woman receiving oral contraceptives, they should be discontinued. Steroids may be poorly metabolized in patients with impaired liver function and should be administered with caution in such patients. Cholestatic jaundice has been reported after combined treatment with oral contraceptives and troleandomycin. Hepatotoxicity following a combination of oral contraceptives and cyclosporine has also been reported.

4. Fluid retention. Oral contraceptives may cause some degree of fluid retention. They should be prescribed with caution, and only with careful monitoring, in patients with conditions that might be aggravated by fluid retention, such as convulsive disorders, migraine syndrome, asthma, or cardiac, hepatic, or renal dysfunction.

5. Emotional disorders. Women with a history of depression should be carefully observed and the drug discontinued if depression recurs to a serious degree.

6. Contact lenses. Contact lens wearers who develop visual changes or changes in lens tolerance should be assessed by an ophthalmologist.

7. Drug interactions. Reduced efficacy and increased incidence of breakthrough bleeding and menstrual irregularities have been associated with concomitant use of rifampin. A similar association, though less marked, has been suggested for barbiturates, phenylbutazone, phenytoin sodium, and possibly with griseofulvin, ampicillin, and tetracyclines.

8. Laboratory test interactions. Certain endocrine and liver function tests and blood components may be affected by oral contraceptives:

a. Increased prothrombin and factors VII, VIII, IX, and X; decreased antithrombin III; increased platelet aggregability.

b. Increased thyroid binding globulin (TBG), leading to increased circulating total thyroid hormone as measured by protein-bound iodine (PBI), T_4 by column or by radioimmunoassay. Free T_3 resin uptake is decreased, reflecting the elevated TBG; free T_4 concentration is unaltered.

c. Other binding proteins may be elevated in the serum.

d. Sex-steroid binding globulins are increased and result in elevated levels of total circulating sex steroids and corticoids; however, free or biologically active levels remain unchanged.

e. Triglycerides and phospholipids may be increased.

f. Glucose tolerance may be decreased.

g. Serum folate levels may be depressed. This may be of clinical significance if a woman becomes pregnant shortly after discontinuing oral contraceptives.

h. Increased sulfobromophthalein and other abnormalities in liver function tests may occur.

i. Plasma levels of trace minerals may be altered.

j. Response to the metyrapone test may be reduced.

9. Carcinogenesis. See *Warnings.*

10. Pregnancy. Pregnancy Category X. See *Contraindications* and *Warnings.*

11. Nursing mothers. Small amounts of oral contraceptive steroids have been identified in the milk of nursing mothers[141–143] and a few adverse effects on the child have been reported, including jaundice and breast enlargement. In addition, oral contraceptives given in the postpartum period may interfere with lactation by decreasing the quantity and quality of breast milk. If possible, the nursing mother should be advised not to use oral contraceptives, but to use other forms of contraception until she has completely weaned her child.

12. Pediatric Use. Safety and effectiveness in pediatric patients have not been established.

13. Venereal diseases. Oral contraceptives are of no value in the prevention or treatment of venereal disease. The prevalence of cervical *Chlamydia trachomatis* and *Neisseria gonorrhoeae* in oral contraceptive users is increased several-fold.[144,145] It should not be assumed that oral contraceptives afford protection against pelvic inflammatory disease from chlamydia.[144] Patients should be counseled that this product does not protect against HIV infection (AIDS) and other sexually transmitted diseases.

14. General.

a. The pathologist should be advised of oral contraceptive therapy when relevant specimens are submitted.

b. Treatment with oral contraceptives may mask the onset of the climacteric. (See *Warnings* regarding risks in this age group.)

INFORMATION FOR THE PATIENT

See patient labeling printed below.

ADVERSE REACTIONS

An increased risk of the following serious adverse reactions has been associated with the use of oral contraceptives (see *Warnings*):

- Thrombophlebitis and thrombosis
- Arterial thromboembolism
- Pulmonary embolism
- Myocardial infarction and coronary thrombosis
- Cerebral hemorrhage
- Cerebral thrombosis
- Hypertension
- Gallbladder disease
- Benign and malignant liver tumors, and other hepatic lesions

There is evidence of an association between the following conditions and the use of oral contraceptives, although additional confirmatory studies are needed:

- Mesenteric thrombosis
- Neuro-ocular lesions (eg, retinal thrombosis and optic neuritis)

The following adverse reactions have been reported in patients receiving oral contraceptives and are believed to be drug-related:

- Nausea
- Vomiting
- Gastrointestinal symptoms (such as abdominal cramps and bloating)
- Breakthrough bleeding
- Spotting
- Change in menstrual flow
- Amenorrhea during or after use
- Temporary infertility after discontinuation of use
- Edema
- Chloasma or melasma, which may persist
- Breast changes: tenderness, enlargement, secretion
- Change in weight (increase or decrease)
- Change in cervical erosion or secretion
- Diminution in lactation when given immediately postpartum
- Cholestatic jaundice
- Migraine
- Rash (allergic)
- Mental depression
- Reduced tolerance to carbohydrates
- Vaginal candidiasis
- Change in corneal curvature (steepening)
- Intolerance to contact lenses

The following adverse reactions or conditions have been reported in users of oral contraceptives and the association has been neither confirmed nor refuted:

- Premenstrual syndrome
- Cataracts
- Changes in appetite
- Cystitis-like syndrome
- Headache
- Nervousness
- Dizziness
- Hirsutism
- Loss of scalp hair
- Erythema multiforme
- Erythema nodosum
- Hemorrhagic eruption
- Vaginitis
- Porphyria
- Impaired renal function
- Hemolytic uremic syndrome
- Acne
- Changes in libido
- Colitis
- Budd-Chiari syndrome
- Endocervical hyperplasia or ectropion

OVERDOSAGE

Serious ill effects have not been reported following acute ingestion of large doses of oral contraceptives by young children.[180,181] Overdosage may cause nausea, and withdrawal bleeding may occur in females.

NON-CONTRACEPTIVE HEALTH BENEFITS

The following non-contraceptive health benefits related to the use of oral contraceptives are supported by epidemiological studies that largely utilized oral contraceptive formulations containing estrogen doses exceeding 35 mcg of ethinyl estradiol or 50 mcg of mestranol.[148,149]

Continued on next page

Demulen—Cont.

Effects on menses:
- Increased menstrual cycle regularity
- Decreased blood loss and decreased risk of iron-deficiency anemia
- Decreased frequency of dysmenorrhea

Effects related to inhibition of ovulation:
- Decreased risk of functional ovarian cysts
- Decreased risk of ectopic pregnancies

Effects from long-term use:
- Decreased risk of fibroadenomas and fibrocystic disease of the breast
- Decreased risk of acute pelvic inflammatory disease
- Decreased risk of endometrial cancer
- Decreased risk of ovarian cancer
- Decreased risk of uterine fibroids

DOSAGE AND ADMINISTRATION

To achieve maximum contraceptive effectiveness, oral contraceptives must be taken exactly as directed and at intervals of 24 hours.

IMPORTANT: If the Sunday start schedule is selected, the patient should be instructed to use an additional method of protection until after the first week of administration *in the initial cycle.* The possibility of ovulation and conception prior to initiation of use should be considered.

Demulen 1/35-21, Demulen 1/35-28, Demulen 1/50-21, and Demulen 1/50-28 Dosage Schedules

The Demulen 1/35-21 and Demulen 1/50-21 Compack® tablet dispensers contain 21 tablets arranged in three numbered rows of 7 tablets each.

The Demulen 1/35-28 and Demulen 1/50-28 tablet dispensers contain 21 white active tablets arranged in three numbered rows of 7 tablets each, followed by a fourth row of 7 pink (blue for Demulen 1/35-28) placebo tablets.

Days of the week are printed above the tablets, starting with Sunday on the left.

Two dosage schedules are described, one of which may be more convenient or suitable than the other for an individual patient.

Schedule #1: Sunday start. The patient begins taking Demulen 1/35-21, Demulen 1/35-28, Demulen 1/50-21, or Demulen 1/50-28 from the first row of her package, one tablet daily, starting on the first Sunday after the onset of menstruation. If the patient's period begins on a Sunday she takes her first tablet that very same day. The 21st tablet or the 28th tablet, depending on whether the patient is taking the 21- or 28-tablet course, will then be taken on a Saturday.

Subsequent cycles:

21-tablet course —The patient begins a new 21-tablet course on the eighth day, Sunday, after taking her last tablet. All subsequent cycles will also begin on Sunday, one tablet being taken each day for 3 weeks followed by a week of no pill-taking.

28-tablet course —The patient begins a new 28-tablet course on the next day, Sunday, and all subsequent cycles will also begin on Sunday, one tablet being taken each and every day.

With a Sunday-start schedule, a woman whose period begins on the day of or 1 to 4 days before taking the first tablet should expect a diminution of flow and fewer menstrual days. The initial cycle will likely be shortened by from 1 to 5 days. Thereafter, cycles should be about 28 days in length.

Schedule #2: Day 1 start. The patient begins taking Demulen 1/35-21 or Demulen 1/50-21 from the first row of her package, one tablet daily, starting with the pill day which corresponds to day 1 of her menstrual cycle; the first day of menstruation is counted as day 1. After the last (Saturday) tablet in row #3 has been taken, if any remain in the first row, the patient completes her 21-tablet schedule starting with Sunday in row #1.

Subsequent cycles: The patient begins a new 21-tablet course on the eighth day after taking her last tablet, again starting the same day of the week on which she began her first course. All subsequent cycles will also begin on that same day, one tablet being taken each day for 3 weeks followed by a week of no pill-taking.

Special notes

Spotting, breakthrough bleeding, or nausea: If spotting (bleeding insufficient to require a pad), breakthrough bleeding (heavier bleeding similar to a menstrual flow), or nausea occurs the patient should continue taking her tablets as directed. The incidence of spotting, breakthrough bleeding, or nausea is minimal, most frequently occurring in the first cycle. Ordinarily spotting or breakthrough bleeding will stop within a week. Usually the patient will begin to cycle regularly within two or three courses of tablet-taking. In the event of spotting or breakthrough bleeding organic causes should be borne in mind. (See *Warning* No. 11.)

Missed menstrual periods. Withdrawal flow will normally occur 2 or 3 days after the last active tablet is taken. Failure of withdrawal bleeding ordinarily does not mean that the patient is pregnant, providing the dosage schedule has been correctly followed. (See *Warning* No. 6.)

If the patient has *not* adhered to the prescribed dosage regimen, the possibility of pregnancy should be considered after the first missed period, and oral contraceptives should be withheld until pregnancy has been ruled out.

If the patient has adhered to the prescribed regimen and misses two consecutive periods, pregnancy should be ruled out before continuing the contraceptive regimen.

The first intermenstrual interval after discontinuing the tablets is usually prolonged; consequently, a patient for whom a 28-day cycle is usual might not begin to menstruate for 35 days or longer. Ovulation in such prolonged cycles will occur correspondingly later in the cycle. Posttreatment cycles after the first one, however, are usually typical for the individual woman prior to taking tablets. (See *Warning* No. 11.)

Missed tablets: If a woman misses taking one active tablet the missed tablet should be taken as soon as it is remembered. In addition, the next tablet should be taken at the usual time. If two consecutive active tablets are missed in week 1 or week 2 of the pack, the dosage should be doubled for the next 2 days. The regular schedule should then be resumed, but an additional method of protection must be used as a backup for the next 7 days if she has sex during that time or she may become pregnant.

If two consecutive active tablets are missed in week 3 of the pack or three consecutive active tablets are missed during any of the first 3 weeks of the pack, direct the patient to do one of the following: Day 1 Starters should discard the rest of the pack and begin a new pack that same day; Sunday Starters should continue to take 1 tablet daily until Sunday, discard the rest of the pack, and begin a new pack that same day. The patient may not have a period this month; however, if she has missed two consecutive periods, pregnancy should be ruled out. An additional method of protection must be used as a backup for the next 7 days after the tablets are missed if she has sex during that time or she may become pregnant.

While there is little likelihood of ovulation if only one active tablet is missed, the possibility of spotting or breakthrough bleeding is increased and should be expected if two or more successive active tablets are missed. However, the possibility of ovulation increases with each successive day that scheduled active tablets are missed.

If one or more placebo tablets of Demulen 1/35-28 or Demulen 1/50-28 are missed, the Demulen 1/35-28 or Demulen 1/50-28 schedule should be resumed on the following Sunday (the eighth day after the last white tablet was taken). Omission of placebo tablets in the 28-tablet courses does not increase the possibility of conception provided that this schedule is followed.

HOW SUPPLIED

Demulen 1/35:

Each white Demulen 1/35 tablet is round in shape, with a debossed SEARLE on one side and 151 and design on the other side, and contains 1 mg of ethynodiol diacetate and 35 mcg of ethinyl estradiol.

Demulen 1/35-21 is packaged in cartons of 6 and 24 Compack tablet dispensers of 21 tablets each.

Demulen 1/35-28 is packaged in cartons of 6 and 24 Compack tablet dispensers. Each Compack contains 21 white Demulen 1/35 tablets and 7 blue placebo tablets. (Placebo tablets have a debossed SEARLE on one side and a "P" on the other side.)

Demulen 1/50:

Each white Demulen 1/50 tablet is round in shape, with a debossed SEARLE on one side and 71 on the other side, and contains 1 mg of ethynodiol diacetate and 50 mcg of ethinyl estradiol.

Demulen 1/50-21 is packaged in cartons of 6 and 24 Compack tablet dispensers of 21 tablets each.

Demulen 1/50-28 is packaged in cartons of 6 and 24 Compack tablet dispensers. Each Compack contains 21 white Demulen 1/50 tablets and 7 pink placebo tablets. (Placebo tablets have a debossed SEARLE on one side and a "P" on the other side.)

Caution: Federal law prohibits dispensing without prescription.

REFERENCES

1. Trussell J, et al. *Stud Fam Plann.* 1987;18(Sept-Oct):237; and 1990;21(Jan-Feb):51. **1a.** *Physicians' Desk Reference.* 47th ed. Oradell, NJ: Medical Economics Co Inc; 1993:2598-2601. **2.** Mann JI, et al. *Br Med J.* 1975;2(May 3):241. **3.** Mann JI, et al. *Br Med J.* 1975;3(Sept 13):631. **4.** Mann JI, et al. *Br Med J.* 1975;2(May 3):245. **5.** Mann JI, et al. *Br Med J.* 1976;2(Aug 21):445. **6.** Arthes FG, et al. *Chest.* 1976;70(Nov):574. **7.** Jain AK. *Am J Obstet Gynecol.* 1976;301(Oct 1):126; and *Stud Fam Plann.* 1977;8(March): 50. **8.** Ory HW. *JAMA.* 1977;237(June 13):2619. **9.** Jick H, et al. *JAMA.* 1978;239(April 3):1403, 1407. **10.** Jick H, et al. *JAMA.* 1978;240(Dec 1):2548. **11.** Shapiro S, et al. *Lancet.* 1979;1(April 7):743. **12.** Rosenberg L, et al. *Am J Epidemiol.* 1980;111(Jan):59. **13.** Krueger DE, et al. *Am J Epidemiol.* 1980;111(June):655. **14.** Layde P, et al. *Lancet.* 1981;1(March 7):541. **15.** Adam SA, et al. *Br J Obstet Gynaecol.* 1981;88(Aug):838. **16.** Slone D, et al. *N Engl J Med.* 1981;305(Aug 20):420. **17.** Ramcharan S, et al. *The Walnut Creek Contraceptive Drug Study.* Vol 3. US Govt Ptg Off; 1981; and *J Reprod Med.* 1980;25(Dec):346. **18.** Layde PM, et al. *J R Coll Gen Pract.* 1983;33(Feb):75. **19.** Rosenberg L, et al. *JAMA.* 1985;253(May 24/31):2965. **20.** Mant D, et al. *J Epidemiol Community Health.* 1987;41(Sept):215. **21.** Croft P, et al. *Br Med J.* 1989;298(Jan 21):165. **22.** Goldbaum GM, et al. *JAMA.* 1987;258(Sept 11):1339. **23.** Bradley DD, et al. *N Engl J Med.* 1978;299(July 6):17. **24.** Tikkanen MJ. *J Reprod Med.* 1986;31(Sept suppl):898. **25.** Lipson A, et al. *Contraception.* 1986;34(Aug):121. **26.** Burkman RT, et al. *Obstet Gynecol.* 1988;71(Jan):33. **27.** Knopp RH, *J Reprod Med.* 1986;31(Sept suppl):913. **28.** Krauss RM, et al. *Am J Obstet Gynecol.* 1983; 145(Feb 15):446. **29.** Wahl P, et al. *N Engl J Med.* 1983;308(April 14):862. **30.** Wynn V, et al. *Am J Obstet Gynecol.* 1982;142(March 15):766. **31.** LaRosa JC. *J Reprod Med.* 1986;31(Sept suppl):906. **32.** Wynn V, et al. *J Reprod Med.* 1986;31(Sept suppl):892. **33.** Royal College of General Practitioners. *J R Coll Gen Pract.* 1967;13(May):267. **34.** Inman WHW, et al. *Br Med J.* 1968;2(April 27):193. **35.** Vessey MP, et al. *Br Med J.* 1968;2(April 27):199. **36.** Vessey MP, et al. *Br Med J.* 1969;2(June 14):651. **37.** Sartwell PE, et al. *Am J Epidemiol.* 1969;90(Nov):365. **38.** Vessey MP, et al. *Br Med J.* 1970;3(July 18):123. **39.** Greene GR, et al. *Am J Public Health.* 1972;62(May):680. **40.** Boston Collaborative Drug Surveillance Programme. *Lancet.* 1973;1(June 23): 1399. **41.** Stolley PD, et al. *Am J Epidemiol.* 1975;102(Sept): 197. **42.** Vessey MP, et al. *J Biosoc Sci.* 1976;8(Oct):373. **43.** Kay CR, *J R Coll Gen Pract.* 1978;28(July):393. **44.** Petitti DB, et al. *Am J Epidemiol.* 1978;108(Dec):480. **45.** Maguire MG, et al. *Am J Epidemiol.* 1979;110(Aug):188. **46.** Petitti DB, et al. *JAMA.* 1979;242(Sept 14):1150. **47.** Porter JB, et al. *Obstet Gynecol.* 1982;59(March):299. **48.** Porter JB, et al. *Obstet Gynecol.* 1985;66(July):1. **49.** Vessey MP, et al. *Br Med J.* 1986;292(Feb 22):526. **50.** Hoover R, et al. *Am J Public Health.* 1978;68(April):335. **51.** Vessey MP. *Br J Fam Plann.* 1980;6(Oct suppl):1. **52.** Collaborative Group for the Study of Stroke in Young Women. *N Engl J Med.* 1973;288(April 26):871. **53.** Royal College of General Practitioners. *Oral Contraceptives and Health.* New York, NY: Pitman Publ Corp; May 1974. **54.** Collaborative Group for the Study of Stroke in Young Women. *JAMA.* 1975;231(Feb 17): 718. **55.** Beral V. *Lancet.* 1976;2(Nov 13):1047. **56.** Vessey MP, et al. *Lancet.* 1977;2(Oct 8):731; and 1981;1(March 7): 549. **57.** Petitti DB, et al. *Lancet.* 1978;2(July 29):234. **58.** Inman WHW. *Br Med J.* 1979;2(Dec 8):1468. **59.** Vessey MP, et al. *Br Med J.* 1984;289(Sept 1):530. **60.** Inman WHW, et al. *Br Med J.* 1970;2(April 25):203. **61.** Meade TW, et al. *Br Med J.* 1980;280(May 10):1157. **62.** Böttiger LE, et al. *Lancet.* 1980;1(May 24):1097. **63.** Kay CR, *Am J Obstet Gynecol.* 1982;142(March 15):762. **64.** Vessey MP, et al. *Br Med J.* 1986;292(Feb 22):526. **65.** Gordon T, et al. *Am J Med.* 1977;62(May): 707. **66.** Beral V, et al. *Lancet.* 1977;2(Oct 8): 727. **67.** Ory H. *Fam Plann Perspect.* 1983;15(March April): 57. **68.** Arthes FG, et al. *Cancer.* 1971;28(Dec):1391. **69.** Vessey MP, et al. *Br Med J.* 1972;3(Sept 23):719. **70.** Boston Collaborative Drug Surveillance Program. *N Engl J Med.* 1974;290(Jan 3):15. **71.** Vessey MP, et al. *Lancet.* 1975; 1(April 26):941. **72.** Casagrande J, et al. *J Natl Cancer Inst.* 1976;56(April):839. **73.** Kelsey JL, et al. *Am J Epidemiol.* 1978;107(March):236. **74.** Kay CR, *Br Med J.* 1981;282(June 27):2089. **75.** Vessey MP, et al. *Br Med J.* 1981;282(June 27): 2093. **76.** The Cancer and Steroid Hormone Study of the Centers for Disease Control and the National Institute of Child Health and Human Development. Oral contraceptive use and the risk of breast cancer. *N Engl J Med.* 1986;315(Aug 14):405. **77.** Paul C, et al. *Br Med J.* 1986;293(Sept 20):723. **78.** Miller DR, et al. *Obstet Gynecol.* 1986;68(Dec):863. **79.** Pike MC, et al. *Lancet.* 1983;2(Oct 22):926. **80.** McPherson K, et al. *Br J Cancer.* 1987;56(Nov): 653. **81.** Hoover R, et al. *N Engl J Med.* 1976;295(Aug 19): 401. **82.** Lees AW, et al. *Int J Cancer.* 1978;22(Dec):700. **83.** Brinton LA, et al. *J Natl Cancer Inst.* 1979;62(Jan):37. **84.** Black MM. *Pathol Res Pract.* 1980;166:491; and *Cancer.* 1980;46(Dec):2747; and *Cancer.* 1983;51(June):2147. **85.** Clavel F, et al. *Bull Cancer (Paris).* 1981;68(Dec):449. **86.** Brinton LA, et al. *Int J Epidemiol.* 1982;11(Dec):316. **87.** Harris NV, et al. *Am J Epidemiol.* 1982;116(Oct):643. **88.** Jick H, et al. *Am J Epidemiol.* 1980;112(Nov):577. **89.** McPherson K, et al. *Lancet.* 1983;2(Dec 17):1414. **90.** Hoover R, et al. *J Natl Cancer Inst.* 1981;67(Oct):815. **91.** Jick H, et al. *Am J Epidemiol.* 1980;112(Nov):586. **92.** Meirik O, et al. *Lancet.* 1986;2(Sept 20):650. **93.** Fasal E, et al. *J Natl Cancer Inst.* 1975;55(Oct):767. **94.** Paffenbarger RS, et al. *Cancer.* 1977;39(April suppl):1887. **95.** Stadel BV, et al. *Contraception.* 1988;38(Sept):287. **96.** Miller DR, et al. *Am J Epidemiol.* 1989;129(Feb):269. **97.** Kay CR, et al. *Br J Cancer.* 1988;58(Nov):675. **98.** Miller DR, et al. *Obstet Gynecol.* 1986;68(Dec):863. **99.** Olsson H, et al. *Lancet.* 1985;1(March 30):748. **100.** Chilvers C, et al. *Lancet.* 1989;1(May 6):973. **101.** Huggins GR, et al. *Fertil Steril.* 1987;47(May):733. **102.** Pike MC, et al. *Br J Cancer.* 1981;43(Jan):72. **103.** Ory H, et al. *Am J Obstet Gynecol.* 1976;124(March 15):573. **104.** Stern E, et al. *Science.* 1977;196(June 24):1460. **105.** Peritz E, et al. *Am J Epidemiol.* 1977;106(Dec):462. **106.** Ory HW, et al. In: Garattini S, Berendes H, eds. *Pharmacology of Steroid Contraceptive Drugs.* New York, NY: Raven Press;

1977:211–224. **107.** Meisels A, et al. *Cancer.* 1977;40(Dec): 3076. **108.** Goldacre MJ, et al. *Br Med J.* 1978;1(March 25): 748. **109.** Swan SH, et al. *Am J Obstet Gynecol.* 1981;139(Jan 1):52. **110.** Vessey MP, et al. *Lancet.* 1983;2(Oct 22):930. **111.** Dallenbach-Hellweg G. *Pathol Res Pract.* 1984;179:38. **112.** Thomas DB, et al. *Br Med J.* 1985;290(March 30):961. **113.** Brinton LA, et al. *Int J Cancer.* 1986;38(Sept):339. **114.** Ebeling K, et al. *Int J Cancer.* 1987;39(April):427. **115.** Beral V. et al. *Lancet.* 1988;2(Dec 10):1331. **116.** Baum JK, et al. *Lancet.* 1973;2(Oct 27):926. **117.** Edmondson HA, et al. *N Engl J Med.* 1976;294(Feb 26): 470. **118.** Bein NN, et al. *Br J Surg.* 1977;64(June):433. **119.** Klatskin G. *Gastroenterology.* 1977;73(Aug):386. **120.** Rooks JB, et al. *JAMA.* 1979;242(Aug 17):644. **121.** Sturtevant FM. In: Moghissi K, ed. *Controversies in Contraception,* Baltimore, MD; Williams & Wilkins; 1979:93–150. **122.** Henderson BE, et al. *Br J Cancer.* 1983;48(July):437. **123.** Neuberger J, et al. *Br Med J.* 1986;292(May 24):1355. **124.** Forman D, et al. *Br Med J.* 1986;292(May 24):1357. **125.** La Vecchia C, et al. *Br J Cancer.* 1989;59(March):460. **126.** Savolainen E, et al. *Am J Obstet Gynecol.* 1981;140(July 1): 521. **127.** Ferencz C, et al. *Teratology.* 1980;21(April):225. **128.** Rothman KJ, et al. *Am J Epidemiol.* 1979;109(April): 433. **129.** Harlap S, et al. *Obstet Gynecol.* 1980;55(April): 447. **130.** Layde PM, et al. *J Epidemiol Community Health.* 1982;36(Dec):274. **131.** Rome Group for the Epidemiology and Prevention of Cholelithiasis (GREPCO). *Am J Epidemiol.* 1984;119(May):796. **132.** Strom BL, et al. *Clin Pharmacol Ther.* 1986;39(March):335. **133.** Wynn V. In: Bardin CE, et al. eds. *Progesterone and Progestins.* New York, NY: Raven Press; 1983:395–410. **134.** Perlman JA, et al. *J Chron Dis.* 1985;38(Oct):857. **135.** Powell MG, et al. *Obstet Gynecol.* 1984;63(June):764. **136.** Wynn V, et al. *Lancet.* 1966;2(Oct 1):720. **137.** Fisch IR, et al. *JAMA.* 1977;237(June 6):2499. **138.** Kay CR, *Lancet.* 1977;1(March 19):624. **139.** Laragh JH. *Am J Obstet Gynecol.* 1976;126(Sept 1):141. **140.** Ramcharan S. In: Garattini S. Berendes HW, eds. *Pharmacology of Steroid Contraceptive Drugs.* New York, NY: Raven Press; 1977:277–288. **141.** Laumas KR, et al. *Am J Obstet Gynecol.* 1967;98(June 1): 411. **142.** Saxena BN, et al. *Contraception.* 1977;16(Dec): 605. **143.** Nilsson S, et al. *Contraception.* 1978;17(Feb):131. **144.** Washington AE, et al. *JAMA.* 1985;253(April 19):2246. **145.** Louv WC, et al. *Am J Obstet Gynecol.* 1989;160(Feb): 396. **146.** Francis WG, et al. *Can Med Assoc J.* 1965;92(Jan 23):191. **147.** Verhulst HL, et al. *J Clin Pharmacol.* 1967;7(Jan-Feb):9. **148.** Ory HW. *Fam Plann Perspect.* 1982;14(July-Aug):182. **149.** Ory HW, et al. *Making Choices: Evaluating the Health Risks and Benefits of Birth Control Methods.* New York, NY: The Alan Guttmacher Institute; 1983. **150.** Palmer JR, et al. *Am J Epidemiol.* 1989;130(Nov):878. **151.** Romieu I, et al. *J Natl Cancer Inst.* 1989;81(Sept):1313. **152.** Porter JB, et al. *Obstet Gynecol.* 1987;70(July):29.

BRIEF SUMMARY OF PATIENT WARNINGS

This product (like all oral contraceptives) is intended to prevent pregnancy. It does not protect against HIV infection (AIDS) and other sexually transmitted diseases.

> **Cigarette smoking increases the risk of serious adverse effects on the heart and blood vessels from oral contraceptive use. This risk increases with age and with heavy smoking (15 or more cigarettes per day) and is quite marked in women over 35 years of age. Women who use oral contraceptives are strongly advised not to smoke.**

In the detailed leaflet, "What You Should Know About Oral Contraceptives," which you have received, the risks and benefits of oral contraceptives are discussed in much more detail. That leaflet also provides information on other forms of contraception. ***Please take time to read it carefully for it may have been recently revised.***

If you have any questions or problems regarding this information, contact your doctor.

Oral contraceptives, also known as "birth control pills" or "the pill," are taken to prevent pregnancy and, when taken correctly, have a failure rate of about 1% per year when used without missing any pills. The typical failure rate of large numbers of pill users is less than 3% per year when women who miss pills are included. However, forgetting to take pills considerably increases the chances of pregnancy.

For most women, oral contraceptives are free of serious or unpleasant side effects. However, oral contraceptive use is associated with certain serious diseases or conditions that can cause severe disability or death, though rarely. There are some women who are at high risk of developing certain serious diseases that can be life-threatening or may cause temporary or permanent disability. The risks associated with taking oral contraceptives increase significantly if you:

- smoke, or
- have high blood pressure, diabetes, high cholesterol, or are overweight, or
- have or have had clotting disorders, heart attack, stroke, angina pectoris (chest pains on exertion), cancer of the breast or sex organs, jaundice (yellowing of the skin or whites of the eyes), or malignant (cancerous) or benign (noncancerous) liver tumors.

Women should not use oral contraceptives if they suspect they are pregnant or if they have unexplained vaginal bleeding.

Most side effects of the pill are not serious. The most common effects are nausea, vomiting, bleeding between menstrual periods, weight gain, breast tenderness, and difficulty wearing contact lenses. These side effects, especially nausea and vomiting, may subside within the first three months of use.

Proper use of oral contraceptives requires that they be taken under your doctor's continuing supervision, because they can be associated with serious side effects. The serious side effects of the pill occur very infrequently, especially if you are in good health and are young. However, you should know that the following medical conditions have been associated with or made worse by the pill, and that certain of the risks may persist after use of the pill has been discontinued:

1. Blood clots in the legs, arms, lungs, heart (heart attack), eyes, abdomen, or elsewhere in the body. As mentioned above, smoking increases the risk of heart attacks and strokes and subsequent serious medical consequences.
2. Stroke, due to a blood clot, or to bleeding in the brain (hemorrhage) as a result of bursting of a blood vessel. Stroke can lead to paralysis in all or part of the body, or to death.
3. Liver tumors, which may rupture and cause severe bleeding and death. A possible, but not definite, association has also been found with the pill and liver cancer. However, with or without use of the pill, liver cancers are extremely rare in the United States.
4. High blood pressure, although blood pressure ordinarily, but not always, returns to original levels when the pill is stopped.
5. Gallbladder disease, which might require surgery.

The symptoms associated with these serious side effects are discussed in the detailed leaflet given to you with your supply of pills. Notify your doctor or health care provider if you notice any unusual physical disturbances while taking the pill. In addition, you should be aware that drugs such as antiepileptics, antibiotics (especially rifampin), as well as certain other drugs, may decrease oral contraceptive effectiveness.

There is a conflict among studies regarding breast cancer and oral contraceptive use. Some studies have reported an increase in the risk of developing breast cancer, particularly at a younger age. This increased risk appears to be related to duration of use. The majority of studies have found no overall increase in the risk of developing breast cancer. Some studies have found an increase in the incidence of cancer of the cervix in women who use oral contraceptives. However, this finding may be related to factors other than the use of oral contraceptives. There is insufficient evidence to rule out the possibility that pills may cause such cancers.

Taking the pill may provide some important non-contraceptive benefits. These include less painful menstruation, less menstrual blood loss and anemia, less risk of fibroids, pelvic infections, and noncancerous breast diseases, and less risk of cancer of the ovary and of the lining of the uterus (womb).

Be sure to discuss any medical condition you may have with your health care provider. He or she will take a medical and family history before prescribing oral contraceptives and will also examine you. The physical examination may be delayed to another time if you request it and the health care provider believes that it is a good medical practice to postpone it. You should be reexamined at least once a year while taking oral contraceptives. The detailed patient information leaflet gives you further information that you should read and discuss with your health care provider.

DETAILED PATIENT LABELING: WHAT YOU SHOULD KNOW ABOUT ORAL CONTRACEPTIVES

This product (like all oral contraceptives) is intended to prevent pregnancy. It does not protect against HIV infection (AIDS) and other sexually transmitted diseases.

INTRODUCTION

It is important that any woman who considers using an oral contraceptive understand the risks involved. Although the oral contraceptives have important advantages over other methods of contraception, they have certain risks that no other method has. Only you and your physician can decide whether the advantages are worth these risks. This leaflet will tell you about the most important risks. It will explain how you can help your doctor prescribe the pill as safely as possible by telling him/her about yourself and being alert for the earliest signs of trouble. And it will tell you how to use the pill properly so that it will be as effective as possible. THERE IS MORE DETAILED INFORMATION AVAILABLE IN THE LEAFLET PREPARED FOR DOCTORS. Your pharmacist can show you a copy or you can request one from the manufacturer by phoning toll-free 1-800-323-4204; you may need your doctor's help in understanding parts of it.

This leaflet is not a replacement for a careful discussion between you and your health care provider. You should discuss the information provided in this leaflet with him or her, both when you first start taking the pill and during your revisits. You should also follow your doctor's advice with regard to regular check-ups while you are on the pill.

If you do not have any of the conditions listed below and are thinking about using oral contraceptives, to help you decide, you need information about the advantages and risks of oral contraceptives and of other contraceptive methods as well. This leaflet describes the advantages and risks of oral contraceptives. Except for sterilization, the intrauterine device (IUD), and abortion, which have their own specific risks, the only risks of other methods are those due to pregnancy should the method fail. Your doctor can answer questions you may have with respect to other methods of contraception, and further questions you may have on oral contraceptives after reading this leaflet.

WHAT ARE ORAL CONTRACEPTIVES?

The most common type of oral contraceptive, often simply called "the pill," is a combination of estrogen and progestogen, the two kinds of female hormones. The amount of estrogen and progestogen can vary, but the amount of estrogen is more important because both the effectiveness and some of the dangers of the pill have been related to the amount of estrogen. The pill works principally by preventing release of an egg from the ovary during the cycle in which the pills are taken.

EFFECTIVENESS OF ORAL CONTRACEPTIVES

The pill is one of the most effective methods of birth control. When they are taken correctly, without missing any pills, the chance of becoming pregnant is less than 1% (1 pregnancy per 100 women per year of use) when used perfectly, without missing any pills. Typical failure rates are actually 3% per year. The chance of becoming pregnant increases with each missed pill during a menstrual cycle.

In comparison, typical failure rates for other methods of birth control during the first year of use are as follows:

Progestogen implants: less than 1%
Progestogen injections: less than 1%
Sterilization: less than 1%
IUD: 3%
Diaphragm with spermicides: 18%
Spermicides alone: 21%
Vaginal sponge: 18% to 28%
Condom alone: 12%
Periodic abstinence (rhythm): 20%
No methods: 85%

WHO SHOULD NOT TAKE ORAL CONTRACEPTIVES

> **Cigarette smoking increases the risk of serious adverse effects on the heart and blood vessels from oral contraceptive use. This risk increases with age and with heavy smoking (15 or more cigarettes per day) and is quite marked in women over 35 years of age. Women who use oral contraceptives are strongly advised not to smoke.**

Some women should not use the pill. For example, you should not take the pill if you are pregnant or think you may be pregnant. You should also not use the pill if you have any of the following conditions:

- Heart attack or stroke (blood clot or hemorrhage in the brain), currently or in the past.
- Blood clots in the legs (thrombophlebitis), lungs (pulmonary embolism), eyes, or elsewhere in the body, currently or in the past.
- Chest pain (angina pectoris), currently or in the past.
- Known or suspected breast cancer or cancer of the lining of the uterus (womb), cervix, or vagina, currently or in the past.
- Unexplained vaginal bleeding (until a diagnosis is reached by your doctor).
- Yellowing of the whites of the eyes or of the skin (jaundice) during pregnancy or during previous use of the pill.
- Liver tumor (whether cancerous or not), currently or in the past.
- Known or suspected pregnancy (one or more menstrual periods missed).

Tell your health care provider if you have ever had any of these conditions. He or she can recommend a safer method of birth control.

OTHER CONSIDERATIONS BEFORE TAKING ORAL CONTRACEPTIVES

Tell your health care provider if you have or have had any of the following conditions, as he or she will want to watch them closely or they might cause him or her to suggest using another method of contraception:

- Breast nodules (lumps), fibrocystic disease (breast cysts), abnormal mammograms (x-ray pictures of the breast), or abnormal Pap smears

Continued on next page

Demulen—Cont.

- Diabetes
- High blood pressure
- High blood cholesterol or triglycerides
- Migraine or other headaches or epilepsy
- Mental depression
- Gallbladder, heart, or kidney disease
- History of scanty or irregular menstrual periods
- Problems during a prior pregnancy
- Fibroid tumors of the womb
- History of jaundice (yellowing of the whites of the eyes or of the skin)
- Varicose veins
- Tuberculosis
- Plans for elective surgery

Women with any of these conditions should be checked often by their health care provider if they choose to use oral contraceptives.

Also, be sure to inform your doctor if you smoke or are on any medications.

RISKS OF TAKING ORAL CONTRACEPTIVES

1. Risk of developing blood clots. Blood clots and blockage of blood vessels are the most serious side effects of taking oral contraceptives. In particular, a clot in the legs can cause thrombophlebitis and a clot that travels to the lungs can cause a sudden blocking of the vessel carrying blood to the lungs. Rarely, clots occur in the blood vessels of the eye and may cause blindness, double vision, or impaired vision.

If you take oral contraceptives and need elective surgery, need to stay in bed for a prolonged illness, or have recently delivered a baby, you may be at risk of developing blood clots. You should consult your doctor about stopping oral contraceptives 3 to 4 weeks before surgery and not taking oral contraceptives for 2 weeks after surgery or during bed rest. You should also not take oral contraceptives soon after delivery of a baby. It is advisable to wait for at least 4 weeks after delivery if you are not breast feeding. If you are breast feeding, you should wait until you have weaned your child before using the pill. (See also the section on Breast feeding in General Precautions.)

The risk of circulatory disease in oral contraceptive users may be higher in users of high-dose pills and may be greater with longer duration of oral contraceptive use. In addition, some of these increased risks may continue for a number of years after stopping oral contraceptives. The risk of abnormal blood clotting increases with age in both users and nonusers of oral contraceptives, but the increased risk from the oral contraceptive appears to be present at all ages. For women aged 20 to 44 it is estimated that about 1 in 2,000 using oral contraceptives will be hospitalized each year because of abnormal clotting. Among nonusers in the same age group, about 1 in 20,000 would be hospitalized each year. For oral contraceptive users in general, it has been estimated that in women between the ages of 15 and 34, the risk of death due to a circulatory disorder is about 1 in 12,000 per year, whereas for nonusers the rate is about 1 in 50,000 per year. In the age group 35 to 44, the risk is estimated to be about 1 in 2,500 per year for oral contraceptive users and about 1 in 10,000 per year for nonusers.

2. Heart attacks and strokes. Oral contraceptives may increase the tendency to develop strokes (stoppage by blood clots or rupture of blood vessels of the brain) and angina pectoris and heart attacks (blockage of blood vessels of the heart). Any of these conditions can cause death or permanent disability.

Smoking greatly increases the possibility of suffering heart attacks and strokes. Furthermore, smoking and the use of oral contraceptives greatly increases the chances of developing and dying of heart disease.

3. Gallbladder disease. Oral contraceptive users probably have a greater risk than nonusers of having gallbladder disease, although this risk may be related to pills containing high doses of estrogens.

4. Liver tumors. In rare cases, oral contraceptives can cause benign but dangerous liver tumors. These benign tumors can rupture and cause fatal internal bleeding. In addition, a possible but not definite association has been found with the pill and liver cancers in several studies, in which a few women who developed these very rare cancers were found to have used oral contraceptives for long periods. However, liver cancers are rare.

5. Cancer of the reproductive organs and breasts. There is conflict among studies regarding breast cancer and oral contraceptive use. Some studies have reported an increase in the risk of developing breast cancer, particularly at a younger age. This increased risk appears to be related to duration of use. The majority of studies have found no overall increase in the risk of developing breast cancer.

Some studies have found an increase in the incidence of cancer of the cervix in women who use oral contraceptives. However, this finding may be related to factors other than the use of oral contraceptives. There is insufficient evidence to rule out the possibility that pills may cause such cancers.

ESTIMATED RISK OF DEATH FROM A BIRTH CONTROL METHOD OR PREGNANCY

All methods of birth control and pregnancy are associated with a risk of developing certain diseases that may lead to disability or death. An estimate of the number of deaths associated with different methods of birth control and pregnancy has been calculated and is shown in the following table.

[See table below]

In the above table, the risk of death from any birth control method is less than the risk of childbirth, except for oral contraceptive users over the age of 35 who smoke and pill users over the age of 40 even if they do not smoke. It can be seen in the table that for women aged 15 to 39, the risk of death was highest with pregnancy (7–26 deaths per 100,000 women, depending on age). Among pill users who do not smoke, the risk of death was always lower than that associated with pregnancy for any age group, although over the age of 40, the risk increases to 32 deaths per 100,000 women, compared to 28 associated with pregnancy at that age. However, for pill users who smoke and are over the age of 35, the estimated number of deaths exceeds those for other methods of birth control. If a woman is over the age of 40 and smokes, her estimated risk of death is four times higher (117/100,000 women) than the estimated risk associated with pregnancy (28/100,000) in that age group.

The suggestion that women over 40 who don't smoke should not take oral contraceptives is based on information from older high-dose pills and on less selective use of pills than is practiced today. An Advisory Committee of the FDA discussed this issue in 1989 and recommended that the benefits of oral contraceptive use by healthy, nonsmoking women over 40 years of age may outweigh the possible risks. However, all women, especially older women, are cautioned to use the lowest dose pill that is effective.

WARNING SIGNALS

If any of these adverse effects occur while you are taking oral contraceptives, call your doctor immediately:

- Sharp chest pain, coughing up of blood, or sudden shortness of breath (indicating a possible blood clot in the lung)
- Pain in the calf (indicating a possible blood clot in the leg)
- Crushing chest pain or heaviness in the chest (indicating a possible heart attack)
- Sudden severe headache or vomiting, dizziness or fainting, disturbances of vision or speech, or numbness in an arm or leg (indicating a possible stroke)
- Sudden partial or complete loss of vision (indicating a possible blood clot in the blood vessels of the eye)
- Breast lumps (indicating possible breast cancer or fibrocystic disease of the breast). Ask your doctor or health care provider to show you how to examine your own breasts
- Severe pain or tenderness or a mass in the stomach area (indicating a possibly ruptured liver tumor)
- Difficulty in sleeping, weakness, lack of energy, fatigue, or change in mood (possibly indicating severe depression)
- Jaundice or a yellowing of the skin or eyeballs, accompanied frequently by fever, fatigue, loss of appetite, dark-colored urine, or light-colored bowel movements (indicating possible liver problems)
- Unusual swelling
- Other unusual conditions

SIDE EFFECTS OF ORAL CONTRACEPTIVES

1. Vaginal bleeding

Spotting. This is a slight staining between your menstrual periods that may not even require a pad. Some women spot even though they take their pills exactly as directed. Many women spot although they have never taken the pills. Spotting does not mean that your ovaries are releasing an egg. Spotting may be the result of irregular pill-taking. Getting back on schedule will usually stop it.

If you should spot while taking the pills, you should not be alarmed, because spotting usually stops by itself within a few days. It seldom occurs after the first pill cycle. Consult your doctor if spotting persists for more than a few days or if it occurs after the second cycle.

Unexpected (breakthrough) bleeding. Unexpected (breakthrough) bleeding does not mean that your ovaries have released an egg. It seldom occurs, but when it does happen it is most common in the first pill cycle. It is a flow much like a regular period, requiring the use of a pad or tampon.

If you experience breakthrough bleeding use a pad or tampon and continue with your schedule. Usually your periods will become regular within a few cycles. Breakthrough bleeding will seldom bother you again.

Consult your doctor if breakthrough bleeding is heavy, does not stop within a week, or if it occurs after the second cycle.

2. Contact lenses. If you wear contact lenses and notice a change in vision or an inability to wear your lenses, contact your doctor or health care provider.

3. Fluid retention or raised blood pressure. Oral contraceptives may cause edema (fluid retention), with swelling of the fingers or ankles. If you experience fluid retention, contact your doctor or health care provider. Some women develop high blood pressure while on the pill, which ordinarily, but not always, returns to the original levels when the pill is stopped. High blood pressure predisposes one to strokes, heart attacks, kidney disease, and other diseases of the blood vessels.

4. Melasma. A spotty darkening of the skin is possible, particularly of the face. This may persist after the pill is discontinued.

5. Other side effects. Other side effects may include nausea and vomiting, change in appetite, headache, nervousness, depression, dizziness, loss of scalp hair, rash, and vaginal infections.

If any of these, or other, side effects occur, call your doctor or health care provider.

GENERAL PRECAUTIONS

1. Missed periods and use of oral contraceptives before or during early pregnancy. Occasionally women who are taking the pill miss periods. It has been reported to occur as frequently as several times each year in some women, depending on various factors such as age and prior history. (Your doctor is the best source of information about this.) The pill should not be used when you are pregnant or suspect you may be pregnant. Very rarely, women who are using the pill as directed become pregnant. The likelihood of becoming pregnant is higher if you occasionally miss one or two pills. Therefore, if you miss a period you should consult your physician before continuing to take the pill. If you miss a period, especially if you have not taken the pill regularly, you should use an alternative method of contraception until pregnancy has been ruled out; if you have missed more than one pill at any time, you should immediately start using an additional method of contraception and complete your pill cycle.

There is no conclusive evidence that oral contraceptive use is associated with an increase in birth defects when taken inadvertently during early pregnancy. Previously, a few studies had reported that oral contraceptives might be associated with birth defects, but these findings have not been seen in more recent studies. Nevertheless, oral contraceptives or any other drugs should not be used during pregnancy unless clearly necessary and prescribed by your doctor. You should check with your doctor about risks to your unborn child of any medication taken during pregnancy.

2. Breast feeding. If you are breast feeding, consult your doctor before starting oral contraceptives. Some of the drug will be passed on to the child in the milk. A few adverse effects on the child have been reported, including yellowing

Annual number of birth-related or method-related deaths associated with control of fertility per 100,000 nonsterile women, by fertility control method according to age.

	Age					
Method of control	15–19	20–24	25–29	30–34	35–39	40–44
No fertility control methods*	7.0	7.4	9.1	14.8	25.7	28.2
Oral contraceptives						
non-smoker**	0.3	0.5	0.9	1.9	13.8	31.6
smoker**	2.2	3.4	6.6	13.5	51.1	117.2
IUD**	0.8	0.8	1.0	1.0	1.4	1.4
Condom*	1.1	1.6	0.7	0.2	0.3	0.4
Diaphragm/ spermicide*	1.9	1.2	1.2	1.3	2.2	2.8
Periodic abstinence*	2.5	1.6	1.6	1.7	2.9	3.6

* Deaths are birth-related
** Deaths are method-related

of the skin (jaundice) and breast enlargement. In addition, oral contraceptives may decrease the amount and quality of your milk. If possible, do not use oral contraceptives while breast feeding. You should use another method of contraception since breast feeding provides only partial protection from becoming pregnant and this partial protection decreases significantly as you breast feed for longer periods of time. You should consider starting oral contraceptives only after you have weaned your child completely.

3. Laboratory tests. If you are scheduled for any laboratory tests, tell your doctor you are taking birth control pills. Certain blood tests may be affected by birth control pills.

4. Drug interactions. Certain drugs may interact with birth control pills to make them less effective in preventing pregnancy or cause an increase in breakthrough bleeding. Such drugs include rifampin, drugs used for epilepsy such as barbiturates (for example, phenobarbital) and phenytoin (Dilantin is one brand of this drug), phenylbutazone (Butazolidin is one brand), and possibly certain antibiotics. You may need to use additional contraception when you take drugs that can make oral contraceptives less effective.

Oral contraceptives may have an influence upon the way other drugs act. Check with your doctor if you are taking *any* other drugs while you are on the pill.

HOW TO TAKE ORAL CONTRACEPTIVES

1. General instructions. You must take your pill every day according to the instructions. Oral contraceptives are most effective if taken 24 hours apart. Take your pill at the same time every day so that you are less likely to forget to take it. You will then maintain an effective dose of the oral contraceptive in your body.

When you first begin to use the pill, you should use an additional method of protection until you have taken your first 7 pills if you are using the Sunday start schedule.

To remove a pill, press down on it. The pill will drop through a hole in the bottom of the Compack.

The two "three weeks on—one week off" schedules. Your Demulen 1/35-21 or Demulen 1/50-21 Compack contains 21 tablets arranged in three numbered rows with the days of the week printed above them.

Day-1 schedule. If you are to begin on day 1, count the day you start to menstruate as day 1 and begin taking your pills that same day. Start in row #1 with the pill under the day that corresponds to the day that your flow began. Continue to take one pill each day on consecutive days of the week.

After the last (Saturday) pill in row #3 has been taken, if any remain in the first row, complete your 21-pill schedule by taking one pill daily starting with Sunday in row #1. Then stop for 1 week before starting to take the pills again. Begin your next pill cycle on the same day of the week that you began the first cycle.

Sunday schedule. Start taking the pills on the first Sunday after your period begins unless your period begins on Sunday. If your period begins on Sunday start taking the pill that very same day.

Begin in row #1 and take your pills, one each day on consecutive days, for 3 weeks (21 days), then stop taking them for 1 week (7 days) before starting to take the pills again on Sunday.

Whether you begin on "day 1" or on Sunday, continue taking your pills as directed, month after month, regardless of whether your flow has or has not ceased, whether you may have experienced spotting or unexpected (breakthrough) bleeding, or whether you feel sick to your stomach during your pill cycle. You will probably have your period about every 28 days.

The "pill-a-day" schedule. Your Demulen 1/35-28 or Demulen 1/50-28 Compack contains 28 pills arranged in four numbered rows of 7 pills each with the days of the week printed above them.

You must take your pills in order, one pill each day. Begin with the Sunday pill in row #1.

1— Start taking the pills on the first Sunday after your period begins unless your period begins on Sunday. *If your period begins on Sunday start taking the pills that very same day.*

2— Continue to take one pill each day on consecutive days of the week.

3— After the Saturday pill in row #1 has been taken begin taking pills in row #2, and so on, until the Saturday pill in row #4 has been taken.

4— Begin a new pill cycle the next day, starting with the Sunday pill in row #1.

You will probably have your period about every 28 days, while you are taking the blue (pink for Demulen 1/50-28) pills.

Continue your pill-a-day schedule, month after month, regardless of whether your flow ceases while you are taking the colored pills, or whether you experience spotting or unexpected (breakthrough) bleeding, or whether you feel sick to your stomach during a cycle.

Take your pill faithfully every "pill day"!

It is important that you take a pill without fail every pill day, at intervals of 24 hours, for two reasons: First, your ovaries may release an egg and therefore you may become pregnant if you do not take your pills regularly. Second, you may spot or start to flow between your periods. This may be inconvenient.

Take your pill at the same time every day!

You are probably wondering why the same time of day is important. By taking your pill at the same time every day it becomes a good habit, and you are much less likely to forget. You may wish to keep your pills in the medicine cabinet near your toothbrush as a reminder to take them when you brush your teeth at night. The best time to take your daily pill may be at bedtime. You may find it helpful to associate your pill-taking with something else you do every day at a particular time.

Another very important reason for you to take your pills as "regular as clockwork" is that you are protected best when you take one every 24 hours; they are made to work that way. Just remember that once every day is not the same as once every 24 hours. Here is why: Suppose you were to take your Monday pill in the morning when you get up, and then not take your Tuesday pill till the evening before you go to bed. True, you will have taken a pill each day, on Monday and on Tuesday—but the time between pill-taking will probably have been more than 36 hours, or more than $1^1/_2$ days! You might spot. Chances are you would still be protected and would not get pregnant, but why risk it when it is so easy to guarantee yourself maximal protection by taking your pill faithfully every pill day and at the same time every pill day?

If you are scheduled for surgery, or you need prolonged bed rest, you should tell your doctor that you are on the pill and stop taking the pill 4 weeks before surgery to avoid an increased risk of blood clots. It is also advisable not to start oral contraceptives sooner than 4 weeks after delivery of a baby.

2. If you forget to take your pill. If you miss only one white (active) pill in a cycle, the chance of becoming pregnant is small. Take the missed pill as soon as you realize that you have forgotten it and continue to take your tablets for the rest of that cycle as directed. Since the risk of pregnancy increases with each additional pill you skip, it is very important that you take one pill a day.

If you forget your pills (except for the inactive colored pills in Demulen 1/35-28 or Demulen 1/50-28) on 2 consecutive days in week 1 or 2 or the pack, do not be surprised if you spot or start to flow. You should take two pills each day for the next 2 days. You may become pregnant if you have sex in the 7 days after you miss pills. You must use another birth control method (such as condoms, foam, or sponge) as a backup for those 7 days.

If you forget two consecutive active pills in week 3 of the pack or if you forget three consecutive active pills in any of the first 3 weeks of the pack, do one of the following: Day 1 Starters should discard the rest of the pack and begin a new pack that same day; Sunday Starters should continue to take 1 pill daily until Sunday, discard the rest of the pack, and begin a new pack that same day. You may not have a period this month but this is expected. However, if you miss your period 2 months in a row, call your doctor or clinic because you might be pregnant. You may become pregnant if you have sex in the 7 days after you miss pills. You must use another method of birth control as a backup for those 7 days.

If you are using Demulen 1/35-28 or Demulen 1/50-28 and forget to take one or more colored pills, begin a new cycle on the next Sunday; use a new package and start taking the white pills. Missing the colored pills does not increase your chances of getting pregnant providing the white pill schedule has been followed.

3. Pregnancy due to pill failure. The incidence of pill failure resulting in pregnancy is approximately 1% (ie, one pregnancy per 100 women per year) if taken every day as directed, but, because some women fail to follow the daily schedule, more typical failure rates are about 3%. If you become pregnant, you should discuss your pregnancy with your doctor.

4. Pregnancy after stopping the pill. There may be some delay in becoming pregnant after you stop using oral contraceptives, especially if you had irregular menstrual cycles before you used oral contraceptives. It may be advisable to postpone conception until you begin menstruating regularly once you have stopped taking the pill and desire pregnancy.

There does not appear to be any increase in birth defects in newborn babies when pregnancy occurs after stopping the pill.

5. Overdosage. Serious ill effects have not been reported following ingestion of large doses of oral contraceptives by young children. Overdosage may cause nausea and withdrawal bleeding in females. In case of overdosage, contact your health care provider, pharmacist, or Poison Control Center.

6. Other information. Your doctor will take a medical and family history before prescribing oral contraceptives and will also examine you. The physical examination may be delayed to another time if you request it and the health care provider believes that it is a good medical practice to postpone it. You should be reexamined at least once a year. Certain health problems or conditions in your medical or family history may require that your doctor see you more frequently while you are taking the pill. Be sure to keep all appointments with your health care provider because this is a time to determine if there are early signs of side effects of oral contraceptive use.

Do not use the drug for any condition other than the one for which it was prescribed. This drug has been prescribed specifically for you; do not give it to others who may want birth control pills.

This product (like all oral contraceptives) is intended to prevent pregnancy. It does not protect against transmission of HIV (AIDS) and other sexually transmitted diseases such as chlamydia, genital herpes, genital warts, gonorrhea, hepatitis B, and syphilis.

HEALTH BENEFITS FROM ORAL CONTRACEPTIVES

In addition to preventing pregnancy, use of oral contraceptives may provide certain benefits. They are:

- Menstrual cycles may become more regular
- Blood flow during menstruation may be lighter and less iron may be lost. Therefore, anemia due to iron deficiency is less likely to occur.
- Pain or other symptoms during menstruation may be encountered less frequently
- Ectopic (tubal) pregnancy may occur less frequently
- Noncancerous cysts or lumps in the breast may occur less frequently
- Acute pelvic inflammatory disease may occur less frequently
- Fibroids of the uterus (womb) may occur less frequently
- Oral contraceptive use may provide some protection against developing two forms of cancer: cancer of the ovaries and cancer of the lining of the uterus (womb)

If you want more information about birth control pills, ask your doctor or pharmacist. They have a more technical leaflet called the Professional Labeling, which you may wish to read. The Professional Labeling is also published in a book entitled *Physicians' Desk Reference,* available in many book stores and public libraries.

Be certain to read new revisions of this leaflet. You may check the date of the most recent revision by phoning the manufacturer toll-free at 1-800-323-4204, or by writing to the address below.

G.D. Searle & Co.
Healthcare Information Services
5200 Old Orchard Road
Skokie, IL 60077

7/15/97 • A05484-5

Shown in Product Identification Guide, page 338

Flagyl® 375 ℞

[flaj 'yl]
(metronidazole capsules)

> **WARNING**
> Metronidazole has been shown to be carcinogenic in mice and rats. (See **PRECAUTIONS.**) Unnecessary use of the drug should be avoided. Its use should be reserved for the conditions described in the **INDICATIONS AND USAGE** section below.

DESCRIPTION

Metronidazole is an oral synthetic antiprotozoal and antibacterial agent, 2-Methyl-5-nitroimidazole-1-ethanol, which has the following structural formula:

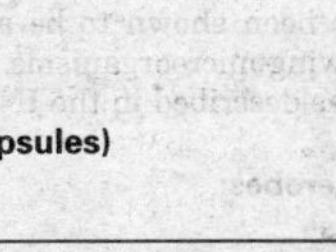

Flagyl® 375 capsules contain 375 mg of metronidazole USP. Inactive ingredients include corn starch, magnesium stearate, gelatin, black iron oxide, titanium dioxide, FD&C Green No. 3, and D&C Yellow No. 10.

CLINICAL PHARMACOLOGY

Disposition of metronidazole in the body is similar for both oral and intravenous dosage forms, with an average elimination half-life in healthy humans of 8 hours.

The major route of elimination of metronidazole and its metabolites is via the urine (60% to 80% of the dose), with fecal excretion accounting for 6% to 15% of the dose. The metabolites that appear in the urine result primarily from side-chain oxidation (1-(β-hydroxyethyl)-2-hydroxymethyl-5-nitroimidazole and 2-methyl-5-nitroimidazole-1-yl-acetic acid] and glucuronide conjugation, with unchanged metronida-

Continued on next page

Flagyl 375—Cont.

zole accounting for approximately 20% of the total. Renal clearance of metronidazole is approximately 10 mL/min/ $1.73m^2$.

Metronidazole is the major component appearing in the plasma, with lesser quantities of the 2-hydroxymethyl metabolite also being present. Less than 20% of the circulating metronidazole is bound to plasma proteins. Both the parent compound and the metabolite possess in vitro bactericidal activity against most strains of anaerobic bacteria and in vitro trichomonacidal activity.

Metronidazole appears in cerebrospinal fluid, saliva, and human milk in concentrations similar to those found in plasma. Bactericidal concentrations of metronidazole have also been detected in pus from hepatic abscesses.

Flagyl® 375 capsules have been shown to have a rate and extent of absorption similar to metronidazole tablets (Flagyl®) and were bioequivalent at an equal single dose of 750 mg. In a study conducted with 23 adult, healthy, female volunteers, oral administration of two 375-mg Flagyl® capsules under fasted conditions produced a mean (± 1 SD) peak plasma concentration (C_{max}) of 21.4 (±2.8) mcg/mL with a mean T_{max} of 1.6 (± 0.7) hours and a mean area under the plasma concentration-time curve (AUC) of 223 (± 44) mcg·hr/mL. In the same study, three 250-mg Flagyl® tablets produced a mean C_{max} of 20.4 (± 3.8) mcg/mL with a mean T_{max} of 1.4 (± 0.4) hours and a mean AUC of 218 (± 50) mcg·hr/mL.

Administration of Flagyl® 375 capsules with food does not affect the extent of absorption of metronidazole; however, the presence of food results in a lower C_{max} and a delayed T_{max} compared to fasted conditions. In a study of 14 healthy, adult, female volunteers, administration of Flagyl® 375 capsules under fasting conditions produced a mean C_{max} of 10.9 (± 1.5) mcg/mL, a mean T_{max} of 1.5 (± 1.4) hours, and a mean AUC of 110 (± 34) mcg·hr/mL compared to a mean C_{max} of 8.6 (± 1.6) mcg/mL, a mean T_{max} of 4.2 (± 1.7) hours, and a mean AUC of 99 (±14) mcg·hr/mL under fed conditions.

Decreased renal function does not alter the single-dose pharmacokinetics of metronidazole. However, plasma clearance of metronidazole is decreased in patients with decreased liver function.

Microbiology:

Metronidazole exerts antimicrobial effects in an anaerobic environment by the following possible mechanism: Once metronidazole enters the organism, the drug is reduced by intracellular electron transport proteins. Because of this alteration to the metronidazole molecule, a concentration gradient is maintained which promotes the drug's intracellular transport. Presumably, free radicals are formed which, in turn, react with cellular components resulting in death of the microorganism.

Metronidazole has been shown to be active against most strains of the following microorganisms both in vitro and in clinical infections as described in the **INDICATIONS AND USAGE** section.

Gram-positive anaerobes:

Clostridium species
Eubacterium species
Peptococcus niger
Peptostreptococcus species

Gram-negative anaerobes:

Bacteroides fragilis group (B. fragilis, B. distasonis, B. ovatus, B. thetaiotaomicron, B. vulgatus)
Fusobacterium species

Protozoal parasites:

Entamoeba histolytica
Trichomonas vaginalis

The following in vitro data are available, **but their clinical significance is unknown:**

Metronidazole exhibits in vitro minimal inhibitory concentrations (MIC's) of 8 µg/mL or less against most (≥90%) strains of the following microorganisms; however, the safety and effectiveness of metronidazole in treating clinical infections due to these microorganisms have not been established in adequate and well-controlled clinical trials.

Gram-negative anaerobes:

Bacteroides fragilis group (B. caccae, B. uniformis)
Prevotella species (P. bivia, P. buccae, P. disiens)

Metronidazole is active against most obligate anaerobes, but does not possess any clinically relevant activity against facultative anaerobes or obligate aerobes.

Susceptibility Tests:

Dilution techniques:

Quantitative methods that are used to determine minimum inhibitory concentrations provide reproducible estimates of the susceptibility of bacteria to antimicrobial compounds. For anaerobic bacteria, the susceptibility to metronidazole can be determined by the reference agar dilution method or by alternate standardized test methods[1]. The MIC values obtained should be interpreted according to the following criteria:

MIC (µg/mL)	Interpretation
≤8	Susceptible (S)
16	Intermediate (I)
≥32	Resistant (R)

For protozoal parasites: Standardized tests do not exist for use in clinical microbiology laboratories.

A report of "Susceptible" indicates that the pathogen is likely to be inhibited by usually achievable concentrations of the antimicrobial compound in the blood. A report of "Intermediate" indicates that the result should be considered equivocal, and, if the microorganism is not fully susceptible to alternative, clinically feasible drugs, the test should be repeated. This category implies possible clinical applicability in body sites where the drug is physiologically concentrated or in situations where high dosage of drug can be used. This category also provides a buffer zone which prevents small uncontrolled technical factors from causing major discrepancies in interpretation. A report of "Resistant" indicates that usually achievable concentrations of the antimicrobial compound in the blood are unlikely to be inhibitory and other therapy should be selected.

Standardized susceptibility test procedures require the use of laboratory control microorganisms that are used to control the technical aspects of the laboratory procedures. Standard metronidazole powder should provide the following MIC values:

Microorganism	MIC (µg/mL)
Bacteroides fragilis ATCC 25285	0.25-1.0
Bacteroides thetaiotaomicron ATCC 29741	0.5-2.0

INDICATIONS AND USAGE

Symptomatic Trichomoniasis. Flagyl® 375 capsules are indicated for the treatment of symptomatic trichomoniasis in females and males when the presence of the trichomonad has been confirmed by appropriate laboratory procedures (wet smears and/or cultures).

Asymptomatic Trichomoniasis. Flagyl® 375 capsules are indicated in the treatment of asymptomatic females when the organism is associated with endocervicitis, cervicitis, or cervical erosion. Since there is evidence that presence of the trichomonad can interfere with accurate assessment of abnormal cytological smears, additional smears should be performed after eradication of the parasite.

Treatment of Asymptomatic Consorts. T. vaginalis infection is a venereal disease. Therefore, asymptomatic sexual partners of treated patients should be treated simultaneously if the organism has been found to be present, in order to prevent reinfection of the partner. The decision as to whether to treat an asymptomatic male partner who has a negative culture or one for whom no culture has been attempted is an individual one. In making this decision, it should be noted that there is evidence that a woman may become reinfected if her consort is not treated. Also, since there can be considerable difficulty in isolating the organism from the asymptomatic male carrier, negative smears and cultures cannot be relied upon in this regard. In any event, the consort should be treated with metronidazole in cases of reinfection.

Amebiasis. Flagyl® 375 capsules are indicated in the treatment of acute intestinal amebiasis (amebic dysentery) and amebic liver abscess.

In amebic liver abscess, metronidazole therapy does not obviate the need for aspiration or drainage of pus.

Anaerobic Bacterial Infections. Flagyl® 375 capsules are indicated in the treatment of serious infections caused by susceptible anaerobic bacteria. Indicated surgical procedures should be performed in conjunction with metronidazole therapy. In a mixed aerobic and anaerobic infection, antimicrobials appropriate for the treatment of the aerobic infection should be used in addition to Flagyl® 375 capsules. In the treatment of most serious anaerobic infections, intravenous metronidazole is usually administered initially. This may be followed by oral therapy with Flagyl® 375 capsules at the discretion of the physician.

INTRA-ABDOMINAL INFECTIONS, including peritonitis, intra-abdominal abscess, and liver abscess, caused by Bacteroides species including the B. fragilis group (B. fragilis, B. distasonis, B. ovatus, B. thetaiotaomicron, B. vulgatus), Clostridium species, Eubacterium species, Peptococcus niger, or Peptostreptococcus species.

SKIN AND SKIN STRUCTURE INFECTIONS caused by Bacteroides species including the B. fragilis group, Clostridium species, Peptococcus niger, Peptostreptococcus species, or Fusobacterium species.

GYNECOLOGIC INFECTIONS, including endometritis, endomyometritis, tubo-ovarian abscess, and postsurgical vaginal cuff infection, caused by Bacteroides species including the B. fragilis group, Clostridium species, Peptococcus niger, or Peptostreptococcus species.

BACTERIAL SEPTICEMIA caused by Bacteroides species including the B. fragilis group or Clostridium species.

BONE AND JOINT INFECTIONS (as adjunctive therapy) caused by Bacteroides species including the B. fragilis group.

CENTRAL NERVOUS SYSTEM (CNS) INFECTIONS, including meningitis and brain abscess, caused by Bacteroides species including the B. fragilis group.

LOWER RESPIRATORY TRACT INFECTIONS, including pneumonia, empyema, and lung abscess, caused by Bacteroides species including the B. fragilis group.

ENDOCARDITIS caused by Bacteroides species including the B. fragilis group.

CONTRAINDICATIONS

Flagyl® 375 capsules are contraindicated in patients with a prior history of hypersensitivity to metronidazole or other nitroimidazole derivatives.

In patients with trichomoniasis, Flagyl® 375 capsules are contraindicated during the first trimester of pregnancy. (See **PRECAUTIONS.**)

WARNINGS

Convulsive seizures and peripheral neuropathy: Convulsive seizures and peripheral neuropathy, the latter characterized mainly by numbness or paresthesia of an extremity, have been reported in patients treated with metronidazole. The appearance of abnormal neurologic signs demands the prompt discontinuation of metronidazole therapy. Metronidazole should be administered with caution to patients with central nervous system diseases.

PRECAUTIONS

General: Patients with severe hepatic disease metabolize metronidazole slowly, with resultant accumulation of metronidazole and its metabolites in the plasma. Accordingly, for such patients, doses below those usually recommended should be administered cautiously. Known or previously unrecognized candidiasis may present more prominent symptoms during therapy with metronidazole and requires treatment with a candidacidal agent.

Information for patients: Alcoholic beverages should be avoided while taking Flagyl® 375 capsules and for at least three days afterward. (See **Drug interactions.**)

Laboratory tests: Metronidazole is a nitroimidazole and should be used with caution in patients with evidence of or history of blood dyscrasia. A mild leukopenia has been observed during its administration; however, no persistent hematologic abnormalities attributable to metronidazole have been observed in clinical studies. Total and differential leukocyte counts are recommended before and after therapy for trichomoniasis and amebiasis, especially if a second course of therapy is necessary, and before and after therapy for anaerobic infections.

Drug interactions: Metronidazole has been reported to potentiate the anticoagulant effect of warfarin and other oral coumarin anticoagulants, resulting in a prolongation of prothrombin time. This possible drug interaction should be considered when metronidazole is prescibed for patients on this type of anticoagulant therapy.

The simultaneous administration of drugs that induce microsomal liver enzymes, such as phenytoin or phenobarbital, may accelerate the elimination of metronidazole, resulting in reduced plasma levels; impaired clearance of phenytoin has also been reported.

The simultaneous administration of drugs that decrease microsomal liver enzyme activity, such as cimetidine, may prolong the half-life and decrease plasma clearance of metronidazole. In patients stabilized on relatively high doses of lithium, short-term metronidazole therapy has been associated with elevation of serum lithium and, in a few cases, signs of lithium toxicity. Serum lithium and serum creatinine levels should be obtained several days after beginning metronidazole to detect any increase that may precede clinical symptoms of lithium intoxication.

Alcoholic beverages should not be consumed during metronidazole therapy and for at least three days afterward because abdominal cramps, nausea, vomiting, headaches, and flushing may occur.

Psychotic reactions have been reported in alcoholic patients who are using metronidazole and disulfiram concurrently. Metronidazole should not be given to patients who have taken disulfiram within the last 2 weeks.

Drug/Laboratory test interactions: Metronidazole may interfere with certain types of determinations of serum chemistry values, such as aspartate aminotransferase (AST, SGOT), alanine aminotransferase (ALT, SGPT), lactate dehydrogenase (LDH), triglycerides, and hexokinase glucose. Values of zero may be observed. All of the assays in which interference has been reported involve enzymatic coupling of the assay to oxidation-reduction of nicotinamide adenine dinucleotide ($NAD^+ \rightleftarrows NADH$). Interference is due to the similarity in absorbance peaks of NADH (340 nm) and metronidazole (322 nm) at pH 7.

Carcinogenesis, mutagenesis, impairment of fertility: Metronidazole has shown evidence of carcinogenic activ-

ity in a number of studies involving chronic, oral administration in mice and rats, but similar studies in the hamster gave negative results.
Prominent among the effects in the mouse was the promotion of pulmonary tumorigenesis. This has been observed in all six reported studies in that species, including one study in which the animals were dosed on an intermittent schedule (administration during every fourth week only). At very high dose levels (approximately 1500 mg/m^2 which is approximately 3 times the most frequently recommended human dose for a 50 kg adult based on mg/m^2) there was a statistically significant increase in the incidence of malignant liver tumors in males. Also, the published results of one of the mouse studies indicate an increase in the incidence of malignant lymphomas as well as pulmonary neoplasms associated with lifetime feeding of the drug. All these effect are statistically significant.
Several long-term, oral-dosing studies in the rat have been completed. There were statistically significant increases in the incidence of various neoplasms, particularly in mammary and hepatic tumors, among female rats administered metronidazole over those noted in the concurrent female control groups.
Two lifetime tumorigenicity studies in hamsters have been performed and reported to be negative.
Metronidazole has shown mutagenic activity in a number of *in vitro* assay systems. *In vivo* studies have failed to demonstrate a potential for genetic damage.
Fertility studies have been performed in mice at doses up to six times the maximum recommended human dose based on mg/m^2 and have revealed no evidence of impaired fertility.

Pregnancy:
Teratogenic effects: Pregnancy Category B. Metronidazole crosses the placental barrier and enters the fetal circulation rapidly. Reproduction studies have been performed in rats at doses up to five times the human dose and have revealed no evidence of impaired fertility or harm to the fetus due to metronidazole. No fetotoxicity was observed when metronidazole was administered orally to pregnant mice at 60 mg/m^2/day, which is approximately 10% of the human dose when expressed as mg/m^2. However, in a single small study where the drug was administered intraperitoneally, some intrauterine deaths were observed. The relationship of these findings to the drug is unknown. There are, however, no adequate and well-controlled studies in pregnant women. Because animal reproduction studies are not always predictive of human response, and because metronidazole is a carcinogen in rodents, this drug should be used during pregnancy only if clearly needed. (See **CONTRAINDICATIONS.**)
Metronidazole use in the second and third trimesters of pregnancy should be restricted to those patients in whom alternative treatment has been inadequate. Use of metronidazole in the first trimester should be carefully evaluated because metronidazole crosses the placental barrier and its effects on human fetal organogenesis are not known. (See above.)
Nursing mothers: Because of the potential for tumorigenicity shown for metronidazole in mouse and rat studies, a decision should be made whether to discontinue nursing or to discontinue the drug, taking into account the importance of the drug to the mother. Metronidazole is secreted in human milk in concentrations similar to those found in plasma.
Geriatric use: Decreased renal function does not alter the single-dose pharmacokinetics of metronidazole. However, plasma clearance of metronidazole is decreased in patients with decreased liver function. Therefore, in elderly patients, monitoring of serum levels may be necessary to adjust the metronidazole dosage accordingly.
Pediatric use: Safety and effectiveness in pediatric patients have not been established, except in the treatment of amebiasis.

ADVERSE REACTIONS

The following reactions have also been reported during treatment with metronidazole:
Central Nervous System: Two serious adverse reactions reported in patients treated with metronidazole have been convulsive seizures and peripheral neuropathy, the latter characterized mainly by numbness or paresthesia of an extremity. Since persistent peripheral neuropathy has been reported in some patients receiving prolonged administration of metronidazole, patients should be specifically warned about these reactions and should be told to stop the drug and report immediately to their physicians if any neurologic symptoms occur. In addition, patients have reported dizziness, vertigo, incoordination, ataxia, confusion, irritability, depression, weakness, and insomnia. (See **WARNINGS.**)
Gastrointestinal: The most common adverse reactions reported have been referable to the gastrointestinal tract, particularly nausea reported by about 12% of patients, sometimes accompanied by headache, anorexia, and occasionally vomiting; diarrhea; epigastric distress; and abdominal cramping. Constipation has also been reported.
A sharp, unpleasant metallic taste is not unusual. Furry tongue, glossitis, and stomatitis have occurred; these may be associated with a sudden overgrowth of *Candida* which may occur during therapy. Rare cases of pancreatitis, which generally abated on withdrawal of the drug, have been reported.
Hematopoietic: Reversible neutropenia (leukopenia); rarely, reversible thrombocytopenia.
Cardiovascular: Flattening of the T-wave may be seen in electrocardiographic tracings.
Hypersensitivity: Urticaria, erythematous rash, flushing, nasal congestion, dryness of the mouth (or vagina or vulva), and fever.
Renal: Dysuria, cystitis, polyuria, incontinence, and a sense of pelvic pressure. Instances of darkened urine have been reported by approximately one patient in 100,000. Although the pigment which is probably responsible for this phenomenon has not been positively identified, it is almost certainly a metabolite of metronidazole and seems to have no clinical significance.
Other: Proliferation of *Candida* in the vagina, dyspareunia, decrease of libido, proctitis, and fleeting joint pains sometimes resembling "serum sickness." If patients receiving metronidazole drink alcoholic beverages, they may experience abdominal distress, nausea, vomiting, flushing, or headache. A modification of the taste of alcoholic beverages has also been reported.
Patients with Crohn's disease are known to have an increased incidence of gastrointestinal and certain extraintestinal cancers. There have been some reports in the medical literature of breast and colon cancer in Crohn's disease patients who have been treated with metronidazole at high doses for extended periods of time. A cause and effect relationship has not been established. Crohn's disease is not an approved indication for Flagyl® 375 capsules.

OVERDOSAGE

Single oral doses of metronidazole, up to 15 g, have been reported in suicide attempts and accidental overdoses. Symptoms reported include nausea, vomiting, and ataxia.
Oral metronidazole has been studied as a radiation sensitizer in the treatment of malignant tumors. Neurotoxic effects, including seizures and peripheral neuropathy, have been reported after 5 to 7 days of doses of 6 to 10.4 g every other day.
Treatment: There is no specific antidote for metronidazole overdose; therefore, management of the patient should consist of symptomatic and supportive therapy.

DOSAGE AND ADMINISTRATION

In elderly patients, the pharmacokinetics of metronidazole may be altered, and, therefore, monitoring of serum levels may be necessary to adjust the metronidazole dosage accordingly.
Trichomoniasis:
In the Female:
Seven-day course of treatment—375 mg two times daily for seven consecutive days.
A seven-day course of treatment may minimize reinfection by protecting the patient long enough for the sexual contacts to obtain treatment. Pregnant patients should not be treated during the first trimester. (See **CONTRAINDICATIONS** and **PRECAUTIONS.**)
When repeat courses of the drug are required, it is recommended that an interval of four to six weeks elapse between courses and that the presence of the trichomonad be reconfirmed by appropriate laboratory measures. Total and differential leukocyte counts should be made before and after re-treatments.
In the Male: Treatment should be individualized as for the female.
Amebiasis:
Adults:
For acute intestinal amebiasis (acute amebic dysentery): 750 mg orally three times daily for 5 to 10 days.
For amebic liver abscess: 750 mg orally three times daily for 5 to 10 days.
Children: 35 to 50 mg/kg/24 hours, divided into three doses, orally for 10 days.
Anaerobic Bacterial Infections: In the treatment of most serious anaerobic infections, intravenous metronidazole is usually administered initially.
The usual adult oral dosage is 7.5 mg/kg every 6 hours. A maximum of 4 g should not be exceeded during a 24-hour period.
The usual duration of therapy is 7 to 10 days; however, infections of the bone and joint, lower respiratory tract, and endocardium may require longer treatment.
Patients with severe hepatic disease metabolize metronidazole slowly, with resultant accumulation of metronidazole and its metabolites in the plasma. Accordingly, for such patients, doses below those usually recommended should be administered cautiously. Close monitoring of plasma metronidazole levels[2] and toxicity is recommended.
The dose of metronidazole should not be specifically reduced in anuric patients because accumulated metabolites may be rapidly removed by dialysis.

HOW SUPPLIED

Flagyl® 375 capsules have an iron gray opaque body imprinted with 375 mg and a light green opaque cap imprinted with FLAGYL, supplied as:

NDC Number	Size
0025-1942-50	Bottle of 50
0025-1942-34	Carton of 100 unit dose

Storage and Stability: Store at controlled room temperature 15–25°C (59–77°F). Dispense in a well-closed container with a child-resistant closure.
Caution: Federal law prohibits dispensing without prescription.

REFERENCES

1. National Committee for Clinical Laboratory Standards, Methods for Antimicrobial Susceptibility Testing of Anaerobic Bacteria—Third Edition. Approved Standard NCCLS Document M11-A3, Vol. 13, No. 26, NCCLS, Villanova, PA, December, 1993.
2. Ralph ED, Kirby WMM. Bioassay of metronidazole with either anaerobic or aerobic incubation, *J. Infect. Dis.* 1975; 132(Nov): 587-591 or Gulaid et al. Determination of metronidazole and its major metabolites in biological fluids by high pressure liquid chromatography, *Br. J. Clin. Pharmacol.* 1978; 6:430-432.

Manufactured by
G.D. Searle & Co.
Box 5110
Chicago IL 60680
Address medical inquiries to:
G.D. Searle & Co.
Healthcare Information Services
5200 Old Orchard Road
Skokie IL 60077
4/16/97 • A05712-3

Shown in Product Identification Guide, page 338

FLAGYL® ER ℞

[flaj 'yl ER]
(metronidazole extended release tablets)
750 mg

> **WARNING**
> Metronidazole has been shown to be carcinogenic in mice and rats. (See PRECAUTIONS.) Unnecessary use of the drug should be avoided. Its use should be reserved for conditions described in the INDICATIONS AND USAGE section below.

DESCRIPTION

Metronidazole is an oral synthetic antiprotozoal and antibacterial agent, 2-methyl-5-nitroimidazole-1-ethanol, which has the following structural formula:

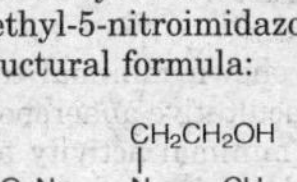

Flagyl ER 750 mg tablets contain 750 mg of metronidazole USP. Inactive ingredients include hydroxypropyl methylcellulose, lactose, magnesium stearate, polyethylene glycol, poly (meth) acrylic acid ester copolymers, polysorbate 80, silicon dioxide, simethicone emulsion, talc, titanium dioxide, FD&C Blue No. 2 Aluminum Lake.

CLINICAL PHARMACOLOGY

Pharmacokinetics: Disposition of metronidazole in the body is similar for both oral and intravenous dosage forms, with an average elimination half-life in healthy humans of 8 hours.
The major route of elimination of metronidazole and its metabolites is via the urine (60% to 80% of the dose), with fecal excretion accounting for 6% to 15% of the dose. The metabolites that appear in the urine result primarily from side-chain oxidation [1-(β-hydroxyethyl)-2-hydroxymethyl-5-nitroimidazole and 2-methyl-5-nitroimidazole-1-yl-acetic acid] and glucuronide conjugation, with unchanged metronidazole accounting for approximately 20% of the total. Renal clearance of metronidazole is approximately 10 mL/min/1.73 m^2.[1]
Flagyl ER 750 mg tablets contain 750 mg of metronidazole in an extended release formulation which allows for once-daily dosing. The steady state pharmacokinetics were determined in 24 healthy adult female subjects with a mean ±

Continued on next page

Flagyl ER—Cont.

SD age of 28.8 ± 8.8 years (range: 19 – 46).[2] The pharmacokinetic parameters of metronidazole after administration of Flagyl ER 750 mg under fed and fasting conditions are summarized in the following table.

Steady State Pharmacokinetic Parameters of Metronidazole after 750 mg of Flagyl ER Given Once a Day for 7 Days

Parameter	Flagyl ER 750 mg daily Mean ± SD (N=24) fed	fasted
$AUC_{(0-24)}$ (μg·hr/mL)	211 ± 60.0	198 ± 75.3
C_{max} (μg/mL)	19.4 ± 4.7	12.5 ± 4.8
C_{min} (μg/mL)	3.4 ± 2.0	4.2 ± 2.2
T_{max} (hrs)	4.6 ± 2.4	6.8 ± 2.8
$T_{1/2}$ (hrs)	7.4 ± 1.6	8.7 ± 2.2

Relative to the fasting state, the rate of metronidazole absorption from the extended release tablet is increased in the fed state resulting in alteration of the extended release characteristics.

Decreased renal function does not alter the single-dose pharmacokinetics of metronidazole. However, plasma clearance of metronidazole is decreased in patients with decreased liver function.

Microbiology: Metronidazole exerts an antimicrobial effect in an anaerobic environment by the following possible mechanism: Once metronidazole enters the organism, the drug is reduced by intracellular electron transport proteins. Because of this alteration to the metronidazole molecule, a concentration gradient is maintained which promotes the drug's intracellular transport. Presumably, free radicals are formed which, in turn, react with cellular components resulting in death of the microorganism.

The following *in vitro* data are available, **but their clinical significance is unknown:**

Metronidazole exhibits *in vitro* minimal inhibitory concentrations (MIC's) of 8 μg/mL or less against most (≥90%) strains of the following microorganisms; however, the safety and effectiveness of metronidazole in treating clinical infections due to these microorganisms have not been established in adequate and well-controlled clinical trials.

Gram-positive anaerobes:
Clostridium species
Eubacterium species
Peptococcus niger
Peptostreptococcus species

Gram-negative anaerobes:
Bacteroides fragilis group (*B. fragilis, B. distasonis, B. ovatus, B. thetaiotaomicron, B. vulgatus*)
Fusobacterium species.
Prevotella species (*P. bivia, P. buccae, P. disiens*)
Porphyromonas species

Protozoal parasites:
Entamoeba histolytica
Trichomonas vaginalis

Metronidazole has shown minimal to no activity against clinically relevant facultative anaerobes or obligate aerobes. Metronidazole has minimal activity against *Lactobacillus* spp and other aerobic microorganisms commonly isolated from the vaginal tract.

Susceptibility Tests:

Dilution techniques:

Quantitative methods that are used to determine minimum inhibitory concentrations provide reproducible estimates of the susceptibility of bacteria to antimicrobial compounds. For anaerobic bacteria, the susceptibility to metronidazole can be determined by the reference agar dilution method or by alternate standardized test methods.[3] The MIC values obtained should be interpreted according to the following criteria:

MIC (μg/mL)	Interpretation
≤ 8	Susceptible (S)
16	Intermediate (I)
≥ 32	Resistant (R)

For protozoal parasites: Standardized tests do not exist for use in clinical microbiology laboratories.

A report of "Susceptible" indicates that the pathogen is likely to be inhibited by usually achievable concentrations of the antimicrobial compound in the blood. A report of "Intermediate" indicates that the result should be considered equivocal, and if the microorganism is not fully susceptible to alternative, clinically feasible drugs, the test should be repeated. This category implies possible clinical applicability in body sites where the drug is physiologically concentrated or in situations where high dosage of drug can be used. This category also provides a buffer zone which prevents small uncontrolled technical factors from causing major discrepancies in interpretation. A report of "Resistant" indicates that usually achievable concentrations of the antimicrobial compound in the blood are unlikely to be inhibitory and other therapy should be selected.

Standardized susceptibility test procedures require the use of laboratory control microorganisms that are used to control the technical aspects of the laboratory procedures. Standard metronidazole powder should provide the following MIC values:

Microorganism	MIC (μg/mL)
Bacteroides fragilis ATCC 25285	0.25–1.0
Bacteroides thetaiotaomicron ATCC 29741	0.5–2.0

INDICATIONS AND USAGE

Bacterial Vaginosis (BV). Flagyl ER 750 mg tablets are indicated in the treatment of women with BV.

CONTRAINDICATIONS

Flagyl ER 750 mg tablets are contraindicated in patients with a prior history of hypersensitivity to metronidazole or other nitroimidazole derivatives.

Flagyl ER, like other formulations of metronidazole-containing products, is contraindicated during the first trimester of pregnancy (See **PRECAUTIONS**.)

WARNINGS

Convulsive seizures and peripheral neuropathy: Convulsive seizures and peripheral neuropathy, the latter characterized mainly by numbness or paresthesia of an extremity, have been reported in patients treated with metronidazole. The appearance of abnormal neurologic signs demands the prompt discontinuation of metronidazole therapy. Metronidazole should be administered with caution to patients with central nervous system diseases.

PRECAUTIONS

General: Patients with severe hepatic disease metabolize metronidazole slowly, with resultant accumulation of metronidazole and its metabolites in the plasma. Accordingly, for such patients, doses below those usually recommended should be administered cautiously. Known or previously unrecognized candidiasis may present more prominent symptoms during therapy with metronidazole and requires treatment with a candidacidal agent.

Information for patients: Alcoholic beverages should be avoided while taking metronidazole and for at least three days afterward. (See **Drug Interactions.**)

Laboratory tests: Metronidazole is a nitroimidazole and should be used with caution in patients with evidence of or history of blood dyscrasia. A mild leukopenia has been observed during its administration; however, no persistent hematologic abnormalities attributable to metronidazole have been observed in clinical studies. Total and differential leukocyte counts should be made before and after re-treatments.

Drug interactions: Metronidazole has been reported to potentiate the anticoagulant effect of warfarin and other oral coumarin anticoagulants, resulting in a prolongation of prothrombin time. This possible drug interaction should be considered when metronidazole is prescribed for patients on this type of anticoagulant therapy.

The simultaneous administration of drugs that induce microsomal liver enzymes, such as phenytoin or phenobarbital, may accelerate the elimination of metronidazole, resulting in reduced plasma levels; impaired clearance of phenytoin has been reported.

The simultaneous administration of drugs that decrease microsomal liver enzyme activity, such as cimetidine, may prolong the half-life and decrease plasma clearance of metronidazole. In patients stabilized on relatively high doses of lithium, short-term metronidazole therapy has been associated with elevation of serum lithium and, in a few cases, signs of lithium toxicity. Serum lithium and serum creatinine levels should be obtained several days after beginning metronidazole to detect any increase that may precede clinical symptoms of lithium intoxication.

Alcoholic beverages should not be consumed during metronidazole therapy and for at least three days afterward because abdominal cramps, nausea, vomiting, headaches, and flushing may occur.

Psychotic reactions have been reported in alcoholic patients who are using metronidazole and disulfiram concurrently. Metronidazole should not be given to patients who have taken disulfiram within the last 2 weeks.

Drug/Laboratory test interactions: Metronidazole may interfere with certain types of determinations of serum chemistry values, such as aspartate aminotransferase (AST, SGOT), alanine aminotransferase (ALT, SGPT), lactate dehydrogenase (LDH), triglycerides, and hexokinase glucose. Values of zero may be observed. All of the assays in which interference has been reported involve enzymatic coupling of the assay to oxidation-reduction of nicotinamide adenine dinucleotide ($NAD^+ \rightleftarrows NADH$). Interference is due to the similarity in absorbance peaks of NADH (340 nm) and metronidazole (322 nm) at pH 7.

Carcinogenesis, mutagenesis, impairment of fertility: Pulmonary tumors have been observed in all six reported studies in the mouse, including one study in which the animals were dosed on an intermittent schedule (administration during every fourth week only).

Malignant liver tumors were increased in male mice treated at approximately 1500 mg/m^2. This dose is approximately 3 times the recommended dose.

Malignant lymphomas and pulmonary neoplasms are also increased with lifetime feeding of the drug to mice (published data).

Mammary and hepatic tumors were increased among female rats administered oral metronidazole compared to concurrent controls.

Two lifetime tumorigenicity studies in hamsters have been performed and reported to be negative.

Metronidazole has shown mutagenic activity in *in vitro* assay systems including the Ames test. Studies in mammals *in vivo* have failed to demonstrate a potential for genetic damage. Fertility studies have been performed in mice at doses up to six times the maximum recommended human dose based on mg/m^2 and have revealed no evidence of impaired fertility.

Pregnancy:

Teratogenic effects: Pregnancy Category B.

Flagyl ER has not been studied in pregnant women. Since metronidazole crosses the placental barrier and enters the fetal circulation rapidly, it should not be administered to pregnant patients during the first trimester. No fetotoxicity was observed when metronidazole was administered orally to pregnant mice at 60 mg/m^2/day, which is approximately 10% of the human dose when expressed as mg/m^2. However, in a single small study where the drug was administered intraperitoneally, some intrauterine deaths were observed. The relationship of these findings to the drug is unknown. There are, however, no adequate and well-controlled studies in pregnant women. (See **CONTRAINDICATIONS**.)

Because animal reproduction studies are not always predictive of human response, and because metronidazole is a carcinogen in rodents, this drug should be used during pregnancy only if clearly needed.

Nursing mothers: Since metronidazole is secreted in human milk in concentrations similar to those found in plasma, and since tumors were increased in rats and mice treated with metronidazole, a decision should be made whether to discontinue nursing or to discontinue the drug, taking into account the importance of the drug to the mother.

Geriatric use: Decreased renal function does not alter the single-dose pharmacokinetics of metronidazole. However, plasma clearance of metronidazole is decreased in patients with decreased liver function. Therefore, in elderly patients, monitoring of serum levels may be necessary to adjust the metronidazole dosage accordingly.

Pediatric use: Safety and effectiveness of this dosage form of metronidazole in pediatric patients have not been established.

ADVERSE REACTIONS

In two multicenter clinical trials, a total of 270 patients received 750 mg Flagyl ER tablets orally once daily for 7 days, and 287 were treated with a comparator agent administered intravaginally once daily for 7 days. (See **CLINICAL STUDIES**.)[4,5]

Most adverse events were described as being of mild or moderate severity. Among patients taking Flagyl ER who reported headaches, 10% considered them severe, and less than 2% of reported episodes of nausea were considered severe. Metallic taste was reported by 9% of patients taking Flagyl ER.

Adverse events reported at ≥2% incidence for either treatment group, irrespective of treatment causality, are summarized in the table below.

[See table at top of next page]

Vulvovaginal candidiasis is a recognized consequence of treatment with many anti-infective agents. In these multicenter clinical trials, there were no statistically significant differences in the incidence rates of yeast vaginitis for groups of patients treated with Flagyl ER or the vaginal comparator.

The following reactions have also been reported during treatment with metronidazole:

Central Nervous System: Two serious adverse reactions reported in patients treated with metronidazole have been convulsive seizures and peripheral neuropathy, the latter characterized mainly by numbness or paresthesia of an extremity. Since persistent peripheral neuropathy has been reported in some patients receiving prolonged administration of metronidazole, patients should be specifically warned about these reactions and should be told to stop the drug and report immediately to their physicians if any neurologic symptoms occur. In addition, patients have reported dizziness, vertigo, incoordination, ataxia, confusion, irrita-

Adverse Events
(≥2% Incidence Rate)—Irrespective of Treatment Causality

	Flagyl ER 7 days (N=267)	Vaginal Preparation (N=285)
Headache	48 (18%)	44 (15%)
Vaginitis	39 (15%)	32 (12%)
Nausea	28 (10%)	8 (3%)
Taste Perversion (metallic taste)	23 (9%)	1 (0%)
Infection Bacterial	19 (7%)	17 (6%)
Influenza-like Symptoms	17 (6%)	20 (7%)
Pruritus Genital	14 (5%)	25 (9%)
Abdominal Pain	10 (4%)	13 (5%)
Dizziness	11 (4%)	3 (1%)
Diarrhea	11 (4%)	3 (1%)
Upper Respiratory Tract Infection	11 (4%)	10 (4%)
Rhinitis	12 (4%)	10 (4%)
Sinusitis	7 (3%)	6 (2%)
Urine Abnormal	7 (3%)	4 (1%)
Pharyngitis	8 (3%)	4 (1%)
Dysmenorrhea	9 (3%)	7 (2%)
Moniliasis	9 (3%)	8 (3%)
Mouth Dry	5 (2%)	2 (1%)
Urinary Tract Infection	6 (2%)	16 (6%)

bility, depression, weakness, and insomnia. (See **WARNINGS.**)

Gastrointestinal: The most common adverse reactions reported have been referable to the gastrointestinal tract, particularly nausea reported by about 12% of patients, sometimes accompanied by headache, anorexia, and occasionally vomiting, diarrhea, epigastric distress, and abdominal cramping. Constipation has also been reported.

Furry tongue, glossitis, and stomatitis have occurred; these may be associated with a sudden overgrowth of *Candida* which may occur during therapy. Rare cases of pancreatitis, which generally abated on withdrawal of the drug, have been reported.

Hematopoietic: Reversible neutropenia (leukopenia); rarely, reversible thrombocytopenia.

Cardiovascular: Flattening of the T-wave may be seen in electrocardiographic tracings.

Hypersensitivity: Urticaria, erythematous rash, flushing, nasal congestion, dryness of the mouth (or vagina or vulva), and fever.

Renal: Dysuria, cystitis, polyuria, incontinence, and a sense of pelvic pressure. Instances of darkened urine have been reported by approximately one patient in 100,000. Although the pigment which is probably responsible for this phenomenon has not been positively identified, it is almost certainly a metabolite of metronidazole and seems to have no clinical significance.

Other: Proliferation of *Candida* in the vagina, dyspareunia, decrease of libido, proctitis, and fleeting joint pains sometimes resembling "serum sickness." If patients receiving metronidazole drink alcoholic beverages, they may experience abdominal distress, nausea, vomiting, flushing, or headache. A modification of the taste of alcoholic beverages has also been reported.

Patients with Crohn's disease are known to have an increased incidence of gastrointestinal and certain extraintestinal cancers. There have been some reports in the medical literature of breast and colon cancer in Crohn's disease patients who have been treated with metronidazole at high doses for extended periods of time. A cause and effect relationship has not been established. Crohn's disease is not an approved indication for Flagyl ER 750 mg tablets.

OVERDOSAGE

Single oral doses of metronidazole, up to 15 g, have been reported in suicide attempts and accidental overdoses. Symptoms reported include nausea, vomiting, and ataxia. Oral metronidazole has been studied as a radiation sensitizer in the treatment of malignant tumors. Neurotoxic effects, including seizures and peripheral neuropathy, have been reported after 5 to 7 days of doses of 6 g to 10.4 g every other day.

Treatment: There is no specific antidote for metronidazole overdose; therefore, management of the patient should consist of symptomatic and supportive therapy.

DOSAGE AND ADMINISTRATION
Bacterial Vaginosis:
Seven-day course of treatment—750 mg once daily by mouth for seven consecutive days.

Flagyl ER 750 mg tablets should be taken under fasting conditions, at least one hour before or two hours after meals. The optimum extended-release characteristics of Flagyl ER 750 mg are obtained when the drug is taken under fasting conditions. (See **CLINICAL PHARMACOLOGY—Pharmacokinetics.**)

Pregnant patients should not be treated during the first trimester. (See **CONTRAINDICATIONS** and **PRECAUTIONS.**)

Patients with severe hepatic disease metabolize metronidazole slowly, with resultant accumulation of metronidazole and its metabolites in the plasma. Accordingly, for such patients, doses below those usually recommended should be administered cautiously. Close monitoring of plasma metronidazole levels[6] and toxicity is recommended.

The dose of metronidazole should not be specifically reduced in anuric patients because accumulated metabolites may be rapidly removed by dialysis.

In elderly patients, the pharmacokinetics of metronidazole may be altered and therefore, monitoring of serum levels may be necessary to adjust the metronidazole dosage accordingly.

HOW SUPPLIED

Flagyl ER 750 mg tablets are oval, blue, film coated, with SEARLE and 1961 embossed on one side and FLAGYL and ER on the other side, supplied as:

NDC Number	Size
0025-1961-30	Bottle of 30

Storage and Stability: Store in a dry place at 25°C (77°F); excursions permitted to 15°–30°C (59°–86°F). [See USP Controlled Room Temperature.] Dispense in a well-closed container with a child-resistant closure.

CLINICAL STUDIES

BV is a clinical syndrome that results from a replacement of the normal, *Lactobacillus*-dominant flora with several other organisms including *Gardnerella vaginalis, Mobiluncus* spp, *Mycoplasma hominis* and anaerobes (*Peptostreptococcus* spp and *Bacteroides* spp).

Flagyl ER was studied in patients with BV in two randomized, multicenter, well-controlled, investigator blind clinical trials.[4,5] A total of 557 otherwise healthy nonpregnant patients with BV were randomized to treatment with Flagyl ER once a day for 7 days (n = 270) or 2% clindamycin vaginal cream one applicator full (5 grams) once a day for 7 days (n = 287).

The primary efficacy endpoint for each treatment regimen was defined as clinical cure assessed at 28–32 days post-therapy. Clinical cure was defined as a return to normal of the vaginal pH (≤4.5), absence of a "fishy" amine odor, and absence of clue cells.

The study results are presented in the table below:
[See table below]

At one month post-therapy the pH of the vagina returned to normal earlier and in a greater percentage of patients in the Flagyl ER treatment group when compared to the 2% clindamycin vaginal cream group; 72% vs 65%, respectively. Likewise, Flagyl ER restored the normal *Lactobacillus*-

predominant vaginal flora in a larger percentage of patients at one month post-therapy when compared to the 2% clindamycin treated group; 74% vs 63%, respectively.

REFERENCES

1. Salas-Herrera IG, Pearson RM, Johnston A, and Turner P. Concentration of metronidazole in cervical mucus and serum after single and repeated oral doses. *J Antimicrobial Chemotherapy* 1991; 28:283–289. **2.** Metronidazole modified-release tablet multiple-dose bioequivalency study (fed/fasting). G.D. Searle & Co., Protocol No. S13-94-02-014; Report No. S13-95-06-014, 11 July 1995. **3.** National Committee for Clinical Laboratory Standards, Methods for Antimicrobial Susceptibility Testing of Anaerobic Bacteria—Third Edition. Approved Standard NCCLS Document M11-A3, Vol. 13, No. 26, NCCLS, Villanova, PA, December, 1993. **4.** Integrated clinical and statistical report for the treatment of bacterial vaginosis with metronidazole modified release tablet—a dose duration study. G.D. Searle & Co., Protocol No. N13-95-02-015; Report No. N13-96-06-015, 19 Nov 1996. **5.** Integrated clinical and statistical report for the treatment of bacterial vaginosis with metronidazole modified release tablet. G.D. Searle & Co., Protocol No. N13-95-02-017; Report No. N13-96-06-017, 11 Nov 1996. **6.** Ralph ED, Kirby WMM. Bioassay of metronidazole with either anaerobic or aerobic incubation. *J Infect Dis* 1975; 132: 587–591 or Gulaid et al. Determination of metronidazole and its major metabolites in biological fluids by high pressure liquid chromatography. *Br J Clin Pharmacol* 1978; 6:430–432.

Rx only   Revised: Mar. 26, 1998

Manufactured by
MOVA Pharmaceuticals, Inc.
P.O. Box 8639
Caguas, Puerto Rico 00726
for G.D. Searle & Co.
Box 5110
Chicago IL 60680 USA

Address medical inquiries to:
G.D. Searle & Co.
Healthcare Information Services
5200 Old Orchard Road
Skokie IL 60077
SEARLE
©1998, G.D. Searle & Co.

633702MV

Shown in Product Identification Guide, page 338

KERLONE®   ℞
[*kur 'lōn*]
(betaxolol hydrochloride)

DESCRIPTION

Kerlone (betaxolol hydrochloride) is a β_1-selective (cardioselective) adrenergic receptor blocking agent available as 10-mg and 20-mg tablets for oral administration. Kerlone is chemically described as 2-propanol, 1-[4-[2-(cyclopropylmethoxy)ethyl]phenoxy]-3-[(1-methylethyl)amino]-, hydrochloride, (±). It has the following chemical structure:

Betaxolol hydrochloride is a water-soluble white crystalline powder with a molecular formula of $C_{18}H_{29}NO_3 \cdot HCl$ and a molecular weight of 343.9. It is freely soluble in water, ethanol, chloroform, and methanol, and has a pKa of 9.4.

The inactive ingredients are hydroxypropyl methylcellulose, lactose, magnesium stearate, polyethylene glycol 400, microcrystalline cellulose, colloidal silicon dioxide, sodium starch glycolate, and titanium dioxide.

CLINICAL PHARMACOLOGY

Kerlone is a β_1-selective (cardioselective) adrenergic receptor blocking agent that has weak membrane-stabilizing activity and no intrinsic sympathomimetic (partial agonist) activity. The preferential effect on β_1 receptors is not absolute, however, and some inhibitory effects on β_2 receptors (found chiefly in the bronchial and vascular musculature) can be expected at higher doses.

Pharmacokinetics and metabolism: In man, absorption of an oral dose is complete. There is a small and consistent first-pass effect resulting in an absolute bioavailability of 89% ± 5% that is unaffected by the concomitant ingestion of food or alcohol. Mean peak blood concentrations of 21.6 ng/ml (range 16.3 to 27.9 ng/ml) are reached between 1.5 and 6 (mean about 3) hours after a single oral dose, in healthy volunteers, of 10 mg of Kerlone. Peak concentrations for 20-mg and 40-mg doses are 2 and 4 times that of a 10-mg dose and have been shown to be linear over the dose range of 5 to 40 mg. The peak to trough ratio of plasma con-

Clinical Cure Rates at One Month

	Flagyl ER % (n/N)	2% clindamycin cream % (n/N)
Study 1	61% (77/126)	59% (80/135)
Study 2	62% (74/119)*	43% (50/117)

* p<0.05 versus clindamycin cream

Continued on next page

Kerlone—Cont.

centrations over 24 hours is 2.7. The mean elimination half-life in various studies in normal volunteers ranged from about 14 to 22 hours after single oral doses and is similar in chronic dosing. Steady state plasma concentrations are attained after 5 to 7 days with once-daily dosing in persons with normal renal function.

Kerlone is approximately 50% bound to plasma proteins. It is eliminated primarily by liver metabolism and secondarily by renal excretion. Following oral administration, greater than 80% of a dose is recovered in the urine as betaxolol and its metabolites. Approximately 15% of the dose administered is excreted as unchanged drug, the remainder being metabolites whose contribution to the clinical effect is negligible.

Steady state studies in normal volunteers and hypertensive patients found no important differences in kinetics. In patients with hepatic disease, elimination half-life was prolonged by about 33%, but clearance was unchanged, leading to little change in AUC. Dosage reductions have not routinely been necessary in these patients. In patients with chronic renal failure undergoing dialysis, mean elimination half-life was approximately doubled, as was AUC, indicating the need for a lower initial dosage (5 mg) in these patients. The clearance of betaxolol by hemodialysis was 0.015 L/h/kg and by peritoneal dialysis, 0.010 L/h/kg. In one study (n=8), patients with stable renal failure, not on dialysis, with mean creatinine clearance of 27 ml/min showed slight increases in elimination half-life and AUC, but no change in C_{max}. In a second study of 30 hypertensive patients with mild to severe renal impairment, there was a reduction in clearance of betaxolol with increasing degrees of renal insufficiency. Inulin clearance (mL/min/1.73 m^2) ranged from 70 to 107 in 7 patients with mild impairment, 41 to 69 in 14 patients with moderate impairment, and 8 to 37 in 9 patients with severe impairment. Clearance following oral dosing was reduced significantly in patients with moderate and severe renal impairment (26% and 35%, respectively) when compared with those with mildly impaired renal function. In the severely impaired group, the mean C_{max} and the mean elimination half-life tended to increase (28% and 24%, respectively) when compared with the mildly impaired group. A starting dose of 5 mg is recommended in patients with severe renal impairment. (See *Dosage and Administration.*)

Studies in elderly patients (n=10) gave inconsistent results but suggest some impairment of elimination, with one small study (n=4) finding a mean half-life of 30 hours. A starting dose of 5 mg is suggested in older patients.

Pharmacodynamics: Clinical pharmacology studies have demonstrated the beta-adrenergic receptor blocking activity of Kerlone by (1) reduction in resting and exercise heart rate, cardiac output, and cardiac work load, (2) reduction of systolic and diastolic blood pressure at rest and during exercise, (3) inhibition of isoproterenol-induced tachycardia, and (4) reduction of reflex orthostatic tachycardia.

The β_1 selectivity of Kerlone in man was shown in three ways: (1) In normal subjects, 10- and 40-mg oral doses of Kerlone, which reduced resting heart rate at least as much as 40 mg of propranolol, produced less inhibition of isoproterenol-induced increases in forearm blood flow and finger tremor than propranolol. In this study, 10 mg of Kerlone was at least comparable to 50 mg of atenolol. Both doses of Kerlone, and the one dose of atenolol, however, had more effect on the isoproterenol-induced changes than placebo (indicating some β_2 effect at clinical doses) and the higher dose of Kerlone was more inhibitory than the lower. (2) In normal subjects, single intravenous doses of betaxolol and propranolol, which produced equal effects on exercise-induced tachycardia, had differing effects on insulin-induced hypoglycemia, with propranolol, but not betaxolol, prolonging the hypoglycemia compared with placebo. Neither drug affected the maximum extent of the hypoglycemic response. (3) In a single-blind crossover study in asthmatics (n=10), intravenous infusion over 30 minutes of low doses of betaxolol (1.5 mg) and propranolol (2 mg) had similar effects on resting heart rate but had differing effects on FEV_1 and forced vital capacity, with propranolol causing statistically significant (10% to 20%) reductions from baseline in mean values for both parameters while betaxolol had no effect on mean values. While blood levels were not measured, the dose of betaxolol used in this study would be expected to produce blood concentrations, at the time of the pulmonary function studies, considerably lower than those achieved during antihypertensive therapy with recommended doses of Kerlone. In a randomized double-blind, placebo-controlled crossover (4×4 Latin Square) study in 10 asthmatics, betaxolol (about 5 or 10 mg IV) had little effect on isoproterenol-induced increases in FEV_1; in contrast, propranolol (about 7 mg IV) inhibited the response.

Consistent with its negative chronotropic effect, due to beta-blockade of the SA node, and lack of intrinsic sympathomimetic activity, Kerlone increases sinus cycle length and sinus node recovery time. Conduction in the AV node is also prolonged.

Significant reductions in blood pressure and heart rate were observed 24 hours after dosing in double-blind, placebo-controlled trials with doses of 5 to 40 mg administered once daily. The antihypertensive response to betaxolol was similar at peak blood levels (3 to 4 hours) and at trough (24 hours). In a large randomized, parallel dose-response study of 5, 10, and 20 mg, the antihypertensive effects of the 5-mg dose were roughly half of the effects of the 20-mg dose (after adjustment for placebo effects) and the 10-mg dose gave more than 80% of the antihypertensive response to the 20-mg dose. The effect of increasing the dose from 10 mg to 20 mg was thus small. In this study, while the antihypertensive response to betaxolol showed a dose-response relationship, the heart rate response (reduction in HR) was not dose related. In other trials, there was little evidence of a greater antihypertensive response to 40 mg than to 20 mg. The maximum effect of each dose was achieved within 1 or 2 weeks. In comparative trials against propranolol, atenolol, and chlorthalidone, betaxolol appeared to be at least as effective as the comparative agent.

Kerlone has been studied in combination with thiazide-type diuretics and the blood pressure effects of the combination appear additive. Kerlone has also been used concurrently with methyldopa, hydralazine, and prazosin.

The mechanism of the antihypertensive effects of beta-adrenergic receptor blocking agents has not been established. Several possible mechanisms have been proposed, however, including: (1) competitive antagonism of catecholamines at peripheral (especially cardiac) adrenergic-neuronal sites, leading to decreased cardiac output, (2) a central effect leading to reduced sympathetic outflow to the periphery, and (3) suppression of renin activity.

The results from long-term studies have not shown any diminution of the antihypertensive effect of Kerlone with prolonged use.

INDICATIONS AND USAGE

Kerlone is indicated in the management of hypertension. It may be used alone or concomitantly with other antihypertensive agents, particularly thiazide-type diuretics.

CONTRAINDICATIONS

Kerlone is contraindicated in patients with known hypersensitivity to the drug.

Kerlone is contraindicated in patients with sinus bradycardia, heart block greater than first degree, cardiogenic shock, and overt cardiac failure (see *Warnings*).

WARNINGS

Cardiac failure: Sympathetic stimulation may be a vital component supporting circulatory function in congestive heart failure, and beta-adrenergic receptor blockade carries the potential hazard of further depressing myocardial contractility and precipitating more severe heart failure. In hypertensive patients who have congestive heart failure controlled by digitalis and diuretics, beta-blockers should be administered cautiously. Both digitalis and beta-adrenergic receptor blocking agents slow AV conduction.

In patients without a history of cardiac failure: Continued depression of the myocardium with beta-blocking agents over a period of time can, in some cases, lead to cardiac failure. Therefore, at the first sign or symptom of cardiac failure, discontinuation of Kerlone should be considered. In some cases beta-blocker therapy can be continued while cardiac failure is treated with cardiac glycosides, diuretics, and other agents, as appropriate.

Exacerbation of angina pectoris upon withdrawal: Abrupt cessation of therapy with certain beta-blocking agents in patients with coronary artery disease has been followed by exacerbations of angina pectoris and, in some cases, myocardial infarction has been reported. Therefore, such patients should be warned against interruption of therapy without the physician's advice. Even in the absence of overt angina pectoris, when discontinuation of Kerlone is planned, the patient should be carefully observed and therapy should be reinstituted, at least temporarily, if withdrawal symptoms occur.

Bronchospastic diseases: PATIENTS WITH BRONCHOSPASTIC DISEASE SHOULD NOT IN GENERAL RECEIVE BETA-BLOCKERS. Because of its relative β_1 selectivity (cardioselectivity), low doses of Kerlone may be used with caution in patients with bronchospastic disease who do not respond to or cannot tolerate alternative treatment. Since β_1 selectivity is not absolute and is inversely related to dose, the lowest possible dose of Kerlone should be used (5 to 10 mg once daily) and a bronchodilator should be made available. If dosage must be increased, divided dosage should be considered to avoid the higher peak blood levels associated with once-daily dosing.

Anesthesia and major surgery: The necessity, or desirability, of withdrawal of a beta-blocking therapy prior to major surgery is controversial. Beta-adrenergic receptor blockade impairs the ability of the heart to respond to beta-adrenergically mediated reflex stimuli. While this might be of benefit in preventing arrhythmic response, the risk of excessive myocardial depression during general anesthesia may be increased and difficulty in restarting and maintaining the heart beat has been reported with beta-blockers. If treatment is continued, particular care should be taken when using anesthetic agents which depress the myocardium, such as ether, cyclopropane, and trichloroethylene, and it is prudent to use the lowest possible dose of Kerlone. Kerlone, like other beta-blockers, is a competitive inhibitor of beta-receptor agonists and its effect on the heart can be reversed by cautious administration of such agents (eg, dobutamine or isoproterenol—see *Overdosage*). Manifestations of excessive vagal tone (eg, profound bradycardia, hypotension) may be corrected with atropine 1 to 3 mg IV in divided doses.

Diabetes and hypoglycemia: Beta-blockers should be used with caution in diabetic patients. Beta-blockers may mask tachycardia occurring with hypoglycemia (patients should be warned of this), although other manifestations such as dizziness and sweating may not be significantly affected. Unlike nonselective beta-blockers, Kerlone does not prolong insulin-induced hypoglycemia.

Thyrotoxicosis: Beta-adrenergic blockade may mask certain clinical signs of hyperthyroidism (eg, tachycardia). Abrupt withdrawal of beta-blockade might precipitate a thyroid storm; therefore, patients known or suspected of being thyrotoxic from whom Kerlone is to be withdrawn should be monitored closely (see *Dosage and Administration: Cessation of therapy*).

PRECAUTIONS

General: Beta-adrenoceptor blockade can cause reduction of intraocular pressure. Since betaxolol hydrochloride is marketed as an ophthalmic solution for treatment of glaucoma, patients should be told that Kerlone may interfere with the glaucoma-screening test. Withdrawal may lead to a return of increased intraocular pressure. Patients receiving beta-adrenergic blocking agents orally and beta-blocking ophthalmic solutions should be observed for potential additive effects either on the intraocular pressure or on the known systemic effects of beta-blockade.

Impaired hepatic or renal function: Kerlone is primarily metabolized in the liver to metabolites that are inactive and then excreted by the kidneys; clearance is somewhat reduced in patients with renal failure but little changed in patients with hepatic disease. Dosage reductions have not routinely been necessary when hepatic insufficiency is present (see *Dosage and Administration*) but patients should be observed. Patients with severe renal impairment and those on dialysis require a reduced dose. (See *Dosage and Administration.*)

Information for patients: Patients, especially those with evidence of coronary artery insufficiency, should be warned against interruption or discontinuation of Kerlone therapy without the physician's advice.

Although cardiac failure rarely occurs in appropriately selected patients, patients being treated with beta-adrenergic blocking agents should be advised to consult a physician at the first sign or symptom of failure.

Patients should know how they react to this medicine before they operate automobiles and machinery or engage in other tasks requiring alertness. Patients should contact their physician if any difficulty in breathing occurs, and before surgery of any type. Patients should inform their physicians or dentists that they are taking Kerlone. Patients with diabetes should be warned that beta-blockers may mask tachycardia occurring with hypoglycemia.

Drug interactions: The following drugs have been coadministered with Kerlone and have not altered its pharmacokinetics: cimetidine, nifedipine, chlorthalidone, and hydrochlorothiazide. Concomitant administration of Kerlone with the oral anticoagulant warfarin has been shown not to potentiate the anticoagulant effect of warfarin.

Catecholamine-depleting drugs (eg, reserpine) may have an additive effect when given with beta-blocking agents. Patients treated with a beta-adrenergic receptor blocking agent plus a catecholamine depletor should therefore be closely observed for evidence of hypotension or marked bradycardia, which may produce vertigo, syncope, or postural hypotension.

Should it be decided to discontinue therapy in patients receiving beta-blockers and clonidine concurrently, the beta-blocker should be discontinued slowly over several days before the gradual withdrawal of clonidine.

Literature reports suggest that oral calcium antagonists may be used in combination with beta-adrenergic blocking agents when heart function is normal, but should be avoided in patients with impaired cardiac function. Hypotension, AV conduction disturbances, and left ventricular failure have been reported in some patients receiving beta-adrenergic blocking agents when an oral calcium antagonist was added to the treatment regimen. Hypotension was more likely to occur if the calcium antagonist were a dihydropyridine derivative, eg, nifedipine, while left ventricular failure and AV conduction disturbances, including complete heart block, were more likely to occur with either verapamil or diltiazem.

Risk of anaphylactic reaction: Although it is known that patients on beta-blockers may be refractory to epinephrine in the treatment of anaphylactic shock, beta-blockers can,

in addition, interfere with the modulation of allergic reaction and lead to an increased severity and/or frequency of attacks. Severe allergic reactions including anaphylaxis have been reported in patients exposed to a variety of allergens either by repeated challenge, or accidental contact, and with diagnostic or therapeutic agents while receiving beta-blockers. Such patients may be unresponsive to the usual doses of epinephrine used to treat allergic reaction.

Carcinogenesis, mutagenesis, impairment of fertility: Lifetime studies with betaxolol HCl in mice at oral dosages of 6, 20, and 60 mg/kg/day (up to 90 × the maximum recommended human dose [MRHD] based on 60-kg body weight) and in rats at 3, 12, or 48 mg/kg/day (up to 72 × MRHD) showed no evidence of a carcinogenic effect. In a variety of *in vitro* and *in vivo* bacterial and mammalian cell assays, betaxolol HCl was nonmutagenic. Betaxolol did not adversely affect fertility or mating performance of male or female rats at doses up to 256 mg/kg/day (380 × MRHD).

Pregnancy: Pregnancy Category C. In a study in which pregnant rats received betaxolol at doses of 4, 40, or 400 mg/kg/day, the highest dose (600 × MRHD) was associated with increased postimplantation loss, reduced litter size and weight, and an increased incidence of skeletal and visceral abnormalities, which may have been a consequence of drug-related maternal toxicity. Other than a possible increased incidence of incomplete descent of testes and sternebral reductions, betaxolol at 4 mg/kg/day and 40 mg/kg/day (6 × MRHD and 60 × MRHD) caused no fetal abnormalities. In a second study with a different strain of rat, 200 mg betaxolol/kg/day (300 × MRHD) was associated with maternal toxicity and an increase in resorptions, but no teratogenicity. In a study in which pregnant rabbits received doses of 1, 4, 12, or 36 mg betaxolol/kg/day (54 × MRHD), a marked increase in postimplantation loss occurred at the highest dose, but no drug-related teratogenicity was observed. The rabbit is more sensitive to betaxolol than other species because of higher bioavailability resulting from saturation of the first-pass effect. In a peri- and postnatal study in rats at doses of 4, 32, and 256 mg betaxolol/kg/day (380 ×MRHD), the highest dose was associated with a marked increase in total litter loss within 4 days postpartum. In surviving offspring, growth and development were also affected.

There are no adequate and well-controlled studies in pregnant women. Kerlone should be used during pregnancy only if the potential benefit justifies the potential risk to the fetus.

Nursing mothers: Since Kerlone is excreted in human milk in sufficient amounts to have pharmacological effects in the infant, caution should be exercised when Kerlone is administered to a nursing mother.

Pediatric use: Safety and effectiveness in pediatric patients have not been established.

Elderly patients: Kerlone may produce bradycardia more frequently in elderly patients. In general, patients 65 years of age and older had a higher incidence rate of bradycardia (heart rate <50 BPM) than younger patients in U.S. clinical trials. In a double-blind study in Europe, 19 elderly patients (mean age = 82) received betaxolol 20 mg daily. Dosage reduction to 10 mg or discontinuation was required for 6 patients due to bradycardia (See *Dosage and Administration*).

ADVERSE REACTIONS

Most adverse reactions have been mild and transient and are typical of beta-adrenergic blocking agents, eg, bradycardia, fatigue, dyspnea, and lethargy. Withdrawal of therapy in U.S. and European controlled clinical trials has been necessary in about 3.5% of patients, principally because of bradycardia, fatigue, dizziness, headache, and impotence. Frequency estimates of adverse events were derived from controlled studies in which adverse reactions were volunteered and elicited in U.S. studies and volunteered and/or elicited in European studies.

In the U.S., the placebo-controlled hypertension studies lasted for 4 weeks, while the active-controlled hypertension studies had a 22- to 24-week double-blind phase. The following doses were studied: betaxolol—5, 10, 20, and 40 mg once daily; atenolol—25, 50, and 100 mg once daily; and propranolol—40, 80, and 160 mg b.i.d.

Kerlone, like other beta-blockers, has been associated with the development of antinuclear antibodies (ANA). In controlled clinical studies, conversion of ANA from negative to positive occurred in 5.3% of the patients treated with betaxolol, 6.3% of the patients treated with atenolol, 4.9% of the patients treated with propranolol, and 3.2% of the patients treated with placebo.

Betaxolol adverse events reported with a 2% or greater frequency, and selected events with lower frequency, in U.S. controlled studies are:

[See table 1 above]

Of the above adverse reactions [listed in Table 1] associated with the use of betaxolol, only bradycardia was clearly dose related, but there was a suggestion of dose relatedness for fatigue, lethargy, and dyspepsia.

In Europe, the placebo-controlled study lasted for 4 weeks, while the comparative studies had a 4- to 52-week double-blind phase. The following doses were studied: betaxolol 20 and 40 mg once daily and atenolol 100 mg once daily.

Table 1

Body System/Adverse Reaction	Betaxolol (N=509) 5–40 mg q.d.* (%)	Propranolol (N=73) 40–160 mg b.i.d. (%)	Atenolol (N=75) 25–100 mg q.d. (%)	Placebo (N=109) (%)
Cardiovascular				
Bradycardia (heart rate <50 BPM)	8.1	4.1	12.0	0
Symptomatic bradycardia	0.8	1.4	0	0
Edema	1.8	0	0	1.8
Central Nervous System				
Headache	6.5	4.1	5.3	15.6
Dizziness	4.5	11.0	2.7	5.5
Fatigue	2.9	9.6	4.0	0
Lethargy	2.8	4.1	2.7	0.9
Psychiatric				
Insomnia	1.2	8.2	2.7	0
Nervousness	0.8	1.4	2.7	0
Bizarre dreams	1.0	2.7	1.3	0
Depression	0.8	2.7	4.0	0
Autonomic				
Impotence	1.2†	0	0	0
Respiratory				
Dyspnea	2.4	2.7	1.3	0.9
Pharyngitis	2.0	0	4.0	0.9
Rhinitis	1.4	0	4.0	0.9
Upper respiratory infection	2.6	0	0	5.5
Gastrointestinal				
Dyspepsia	4.7	6.8	2.7	0.9
Nausea	1.6	1.4	4.0	0
Diarrhea	2.0	6.8	8.0	0.9
Musculoskeletal				
Chest pain	2.4	1.4	2.7	0.9
Arthralgia	3.1	0	4.0	1.8
Skin				
Rash	1.2			

* Five patients received 80 mg q.d.

† N = 336 males; impotence is a known possible adverse effect of this pharmacological class.

Table 2

Body System/Adverse Reaction	Betaxolol (N=155) 20–40 mg q.d. (%)	Atenolol (N=81) 100 mg q.d. (%)	Placebo (N=60) (%)
Cardiovascular			
Bradycardia (heart rate <50 BPM)	5.8	5.0	0
Symptomatic bradycardia	1.9	2.5	0
Palpitation	1.9	3.7	1.7
Edema	1.3	1.2	0
Cold extremities	1.9	0	0
Central Nervous System			
Headache	14.8	9.9	23.3
Dizziness	14.8	17.3	15.0
Fatigue	9.7	18.5	0
Asthenia	7.1	0	16.7
Insomnia	5.0	3.7	3.3
Paresthesia	1.9	2.5	0
Gastrointestinal			
Nausea	5.8	1.2	0
Dyspepsia	3.9	7.4	3.3
Diarrhea	1.9	3.7	0
Musculoskeletal			
Chest pain	7.1	6.2	5.0
Joint pain	5.2	4.9	1.7
Myalgia	3.2	3.7	3.3

From European controlled hypertension clinical trials, the following adverse events reported by 2% or more patients and selected events with lower frequency are presented:

[See table 2 above]

The only adverse event whose frequency clearly rose with increasing dose was bradycardia. Elderly patients were especially susceptible to bradycardia, which in some cases responded to dose-reduction (see *Precautions*).

The following selected (potentially important) adverse events have been reported at an incidence of less than 2% in U.S. controlled and open, long-term clinical studies, European controlled clinical trials, or in marketing experience. It is not known whether a causal relationship exists between betaxolol and these events; they are listed to alert the physician to a possible relationship:

Autonomic: flushing, salivation, sweating.

Body as a whole: allergy, fever, malaise, pain, rigors.

Cardiovascular: angina pectoris, arrhythmia, atrioventricular block, heart failure, hypertension, hypotension, myocardial infarction, thrombosis, syncope.

Central and peripheral nervous system: ataxia, neuralgia, neuropathy, numbness, speech disorder, stupor, tremor, twitching.

Gastrointestinal: anorexia, constipation, dry mouth, increased appetite, mouth ulceration, rectal disorders, vomiting, dysphagia.

Hearing and vestibular: earache, labyrinth disorders, tinnitus, deafness.

Hematologic: anemia, leucocytosis, lymphadenopathy, purpura, thrombocytopenia.

Liver and biliary: increased AST, increased ALT.

Metabolic and nutritional: acidosis, diabetes, hypercholesterolemia, hyperglycemia, hyperkalemia, hyperlipemia, hyperuricemia, hypokalemia, weight gain, weight loss, thirst, increased LDH.

Musculoskeletal: arthropathy, neck pain, muscle cramps, tendonitis.

Psychiatric: abnormal thinking, amnesia, impaired concentration, confusion, emotional lability, hallucinations, decreased libido.

Reproductive disorders: Female: breast pain, breast fibroadenosis, menstrual disorder; Male: Peyronie's disease, prostatitis.

Respiratory: bronchitis, bronchospasm, cough, epistaxis, flu, pneumonia, sinusitis.

Continued on next page

Kerlone—Cont.

Skin: alopecia, eczema, erythematous rash, hypertrichosis, pruritus, skin disorders.
Special senses: abnormal taste, taste loss.
Urinary system: cystitis, dysuria, micturition disorder, oliguria, proteinuria, abnormal renal function, renal pain.
Vascular: cerebrovascular disorder, intermittent claudication, leg cramps, peripheral ischemia, thrombophlebitis.
Vision: abnormal lacrimation, abnormal vision, blepharitis, ocular hemorrhage, conjunctivitis, dry eyes, iritis, cataract, scotoma.

Potential adverse effects: Although not reported in clinical studies with betaxolol, a variety of adverse effects have been reported with other beta-adrenergic blocking agents and may be considered potential adverse effects of betaxolol:
Central nervous system: Reversible mental depression progressing to catatonia, an acute reversible syndrome characterized by disorientation for time and place, short-term memory loss, emotional lability with slightly clouded sensorium, and decreased performance on neuropsychometric tests.
Allergic: Fever combined with aching and sore throat, laryngospasm, respiratory distress.
Hematologic: Agranulocytosis, thrombocytopenic purpura, and nonthrombocytopenic purpura.
Gastrointestinal: Mesenteric arterial thrombosis, ischemic colitis.
Miscellaneous: Raynaud's phenomena. There have been reports of skin rashes and/or dry eyes associated with the use of beta-adrenergic blocking drugs. The reported incidence is small, and in most cases, the symptoms have cleared when treatment was withdrawn. Discontinuation of the drug should be considered if any such reaction is not otherwise explicable. Patients should be closely monitored following cessation of therapy.
The oculomucocutaneous syndrome associated with the beta-blocker practolol has not been reported with Kerlone during investigational use and extensive foreign experience. However, dry eyes have been reported.

OVERDOSAGE

No specific information on emergency treatment of overdosage with Kerlone is available. The most common effects expected are bradycardia, congestive heart failure, hypotension, bronchospasm, and hypoglycemia. In one acute overdosage of betaxolol, a 16-year-old female recovered fully after ingesting 460 mg.
Oral LD_{50}s are 350 to 400 mg betaxolol/kg in mice and 860 to 980 mg/kg in rats.
In the case of overdosage, treatment with Kerlone should be stopped and the patient carefully observed. Hemodialysis or peritoneal dialysis does not remove substantial amounts of the drug. In addition to gastric lavage, the following therapeutic measures are suggested if warranted:
Hypotension: Use sympathomimetic pressor drug therapy, such as dopamine, dobutamine, or norepinephrine. In refractory cases of overdosage of other beta-blockers, the use of glucagon hydrochloride has been reported to be useful.
Bradycardia: Atropine should be administered. If there is no response to vagal blockade, isoproterenol should be administered cautiously. In refractory cases the use of a transvenous cardiac pacemaker may be considered.
Acute cardiac failure: Conventional therapy including digitalis, diuretics, and oxygen should be instituted immediately.
Bronchospasm: Use a β_2-agonist. Additional therapy with aminophylline may be considered.
Heart block (2nd- or 3rd-degree): Use isoproterenol or a transvenous cardiac pacemaker.

DOSAGE AND ADMINISTRATION

The initial dose of Kerlone in hypertension is ordinarily 10 mg once daily either alone or added to diuretic therapy. The full antihypertensive effect is usually seen within 7 to 14 days. If the desired response is not achieved the dose can be doubled after 7 to 14 days. Increasing the dose beyond 20 mg has not been shown to produce a statistically significant additional antihypertensive effect; but the 40-mg dose has been studied and is well tolerated. An increased effect (reduction) on heart rate should be anticipated with increasing dosage. If monotherapy with Kerlone does not produce the desired response, the addition of a diuretic agent or other antihypertensive should be considered (see *Drug interactions*).

Dosage adjustments for specific patients

Patients with renal failure: In patients with renal impairment, clearance of betaxolol declines with decreasing renal function.
In patients with severe renal impairment and those undergoing dialysis the initial dose of Kerlone is 5 mg once daily.
If the desired response is not achieved, dosage may be increased by 5 mg/day increments every 2 weeks to a maximum dose of 20 mg/day.

Patients with hepatic disease: Patients with hepatic disease do not have significantly altered clearance. Dosage adjustments are not routinely needed.
Elderly patients: Consideration should be given to reduction in the starting dose to 5 mg in elderly patients. These patients are especially prone to beta-blocker–induced bradycardia, which appears to be dose related and sometimes responds to reductions in dose.
Cessation of therapy: If withdrawal of Kerlone therapy is planned, it should be achieved gradually over a period of about 2 weeks. Patients should be carefully observed and advised to limit physical activity to a minimum.

HOW SUPPLIED

Kerlone 10-mg tablets are round, white, film coated, with KERLONE 10 debossed on one side and scored on the other, supplied as:

NDC Number	Size
0025-5101-31	bottle of 100

Kerlone 20-mg tablets are round, white, film coated, with KERLONE 20 debossed on one side and β on the other, supplied as:

NDC Number	Size
0025-5201-31	bottle of 100

Store at controlled room temperature 15°-25°C (59°-77°F).

Caution: Federal law prohibits dispensing without prescription.

Manufactured and distributed by
G.D. Searle & Co.
Chicago, IL 60680
by agreement with
Lorex Pharmaceuticals
Skokie, IL

Kerlone is a registered trademark of Synthelabo.

5/8/97 • A05426-2

Shown in Product Identification Guide, page 338

LOMOTIL® Liquid ©V
LOMOTIL® Tablets ©V

[lō-mō ′til]

(diphenoxylate hydrochloride with atropine sulfate)

DESCRIPTION

Each Lomotil tablet and each 5 ml of Lomotil liquid for oral use contains:

diphenoxylate hydrochloride .... 2.5 mg
(Warning—May be habit forming.)
atropine sulfate .... 0.025 mg

Diphenoxylate hydrochloride, an antidiarrheal, is ethyl 1-(3-cyano-3,3-diphenylpropyl)-4-phenylisonipecotate monohydrochloride and has the following structural formula:

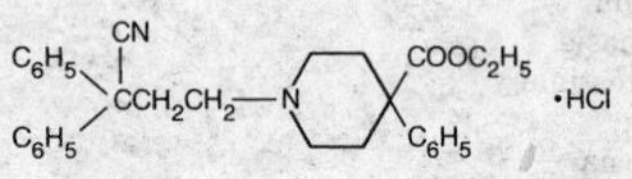

Atropine sulfate, an anticholinergic, is endo-(±)-α-(hydroxymethyl) benzeneacetic acid 8-methyl-8-azabicyclo[3.2.1] oct-3-yl ester sulfate (2:1) (salt) monohydrate and has the following structural formula:

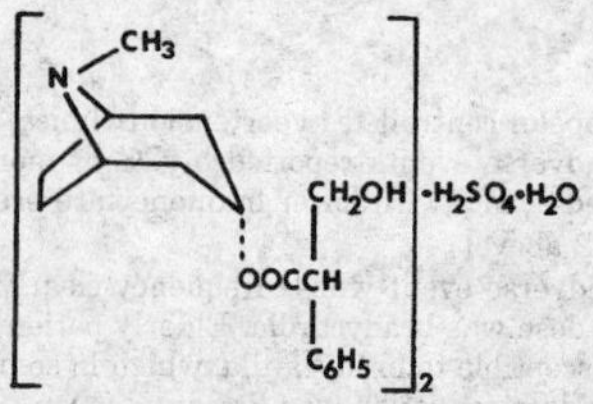

A subtherapeutic amount of atropine sulfate is present to discourage deliberate overdosage.
Inactive ingredients of Lomotil tablets include acacia, corn starch, magnesium stearate, sorbitol, sucrose, and talc. Inactive ingredients of Lomotil liquid include cherry flavor, citric acid, ethyl alcohol 15%, FD&C Yellow No. 6, glycerin, sodium phosphate, sorbitol, and water.

CLINICAL PHARMACOLOGY

Diphenoxylate is rapidly and extensively metabolized in man by ester hydrolysis to diphenoxylic acid (difenoxine), which is biologically active and the major metabolite in the blood. After a 5-mg oral dose of carbon-14 labeled diphenoxylate hydrochloride in ethanolic solution was given to three healthy volunteers, an average of 14% of the drug plus its metabolites was excreted in the urine and 49% in the feces over a four-day period. Urinary excretion of the unmetabolized drug constituted less than 1% of the dose, and diphenoxylic acid plus its glucuronide conjugate constituted about 6% of the dose. In a 16-subject crossover bioavailability study, a linear relationship in the dose range of 2.5 to 10 mg was found between the dose of diphenoxylate hydrochloride (given as Lomotil liquid) and the peak plasma concentration, the area under the plasma concentration-time curve, and the amount of diphenoxylic acid excreted in the urine. In the same study the bioavailability of the tablet compared with an equal dose of the liquid was approximately 90%. The average peak plasma concentration of diphenoxylic acid following ingestion of four 2.5-mg tablets was 163 ng/ml at about 2 hours, and the elimination half-life of diphenoxylic acid was approximately 12 to 14 hours.
In dogs, diphenoxylate hydrochloride has a direct effect on circular smooth muscle of the bowel that conceivably results in segmentation and prolongation of gastrointestinal transit time. The clinical antidiarrheal action of diphenoxylate hydrochloride may thus be a consequence of enhanced segmentation that allows increased contact of the intraluminal contents with the intestinal mucosa.

INDICATIONS AND USAGE

Lomotil is effective as adjunctive therapy in the management of diarrhea.

CONTRAINDICATIONS

Lomotil is contraindicated in patients with
1. Known hypersensitivity to diphenoxylate or atropine.
2. Obstructive jaundice.
3. Diarrhea associated with pseudomembranous enterocolitis or enterotoxin-producing bacteria.

WARNINGS

LOMOTIL IS *NOT* AN INNOCUOUS DRUG AND DOSAGE RECOMMENDATIONS SHOULD BE STRICTLY ADHERED TO, ESPECIALLY IN CHILDREN. LOMOTIL IS NOT RECOMMENDED FOR CHILDREN UNDER 2 YEARS OF AGE. OVERDOSAGE MAY RESULT IN SEVERE RESPIRATORY DEPRESSION AND COMA, POSSIBLY LEADING TO PERMANENT BRAIN DAMAGE OR DEATH (SEE *OVERDOSAGE*). THEREFORE, KEEP THIS MEDICATION OUT OF THE REACH OF CHILDREN.
THE USE OF LOMOTIL SHOULD BE ACCOMPANIED BY APPROPRIATE FLUID AND ELECTROLYTE THERAPY, WHEN INDICATED. IF SEVERE DEHYDRATION OR ELECTROLYTE IMBALANCE IS PRESENT, LOMOTIL SHOULD BE WITHHELD UNTIL APPROPRIATE CORRECTIVE THERAPY HAS BEEN INITIATED. DRUG-INDUCED INHIBITION OF PERISTALSIS MAY RESULT IN FLUID RETENTION IN THE INTESTINE, WHICH MAY FURTHER AGGRAVATE DEHYDRATION AND ELECTROLYTE IMBALANCE.
LOMOTIL SHOULD BE USED WITH SPECIAL CAUTION IN YOUNG CHILDREN BECAUSE THIS AGE GROUP MAY BE PREDISPOSED TO DELAYED DIPHENOXYLATE TOXICITY AND BECAUSE OF THE GREATER VARIABILITY OF RESPONSE IN THIS AGE GROUP.
Antiperistaltic agents may prolong and/or worsen diarrhea associated with organisms that penetrate the intestinal mucosa (toxigenic *E. coli, Salmonella, Shigella*), and pseudomembranous enterocolitis associated with broad-spectrum antibiotics. Antiperistaltic agents should not be used in these conditions.
In some patients with acute ulcerative colitis, agents that inhibit intestinal motility or prolong intestinal transit time have been reported to induce toxic megacolon. Consequently, patients with acute ulcerative colitis should be carefully observed and Lomotil therapy should be discontinued promptly if abdominal distention occurs or if other untoward symptoms develop.
Since the chemical structure of diphenoxylate hydrochloride is similar to that of meperidine hydrochloride, the concurrent use of Lomotil with monoamine oxidase (MAO) inhibitors may, in theory, precipitate hypertensive crisis.
Lomotil should be used with extreme caution in patients with advanced hepatorenal disease and in all patients with abnormal liver function since hepatic coma may be precipitated.
Diphenoxylate hydrochloride may potentiate the action of barbiturates, tranquilizers, and alcohol. Therefore, the patient should be closely observed when any of these are used concomitantly.

PRECAUTIONS

General: Since a subtherapeutic dose of atropine has been added to the diphenoxylate hydrochloride, consideration should be given to the precautions relating to the use of atropine. In children, Lomotil should be used with caution since signs of atropinism may occur even with recommended doses, particularly in patients with Down's syndrome.
Information for patients: INFORM THE PATIENT (PARENT OR GUARDIAN) NOT TO EXCEED THE RECOMMENDED DOSAGE AND TO KEEP LOMOTIL OUT OF THE REACH OF CHILDREN AND IN A CHILD-RESISTANT CONTAINER. INFORM THE PATIENT OF THE CONSEQUENCES OF OVERDOSAGE, INCLUDING SEVERE RESPIRATORY DEPRESSION AND COMA, POSSI-

BLY LEADING TO PERMANENT BRAIN DAMAGE OR DEATH. Lomotil may produce drowsiness or dizziness. The patient should be cautioned regarding activities requiring mental alertness, such as driving or operating dangerous machinery. Potentiation of the action of alcohol, barbiturates, and tranquilizers with concomitant use of Lomotil should be explained to the patient. The physician should also provide the patient with other information in this labeling, as appropriate.

Drug interactions: Known drug interactions include barbiturates, tranquilizers, and alcohol. Lomotil may interact with MAO inhibitors (see *Warnings*).

In studies with male rats, diphenoxylate hydrochloride was found to inhibit the hepatic microsomal enzyme system at a dose of 2 mg/kg/day. Therefore, diphenoxylate has the potential to prolong the biological half-lives of drugs for which the rate of elimination is dependent on the microsomal drug metabolizing enzyme system.

Carcinogenesis, mutagenesis, impairment of fertility: No long-term study in animals has been performed to evaluate carcinogenic potential. Diphenoxylate hydrochloride was administered to male and female rats in their diets to provide dose levels of 4 and 20 mg/kg/day throughout a three-litter reproduction study. At 50 times the human dose (20 mg/kg/day), female weight gain was reduced and there was a marked effect on fertility as only 4 of 27 females became pregnant in three test breedings. The relevance of this finding to usage of Lomotil in humans is unknown.

Pregnancy: Pregnancy Category C. Diphenoxylate hydrochloride has been shown to have an effect on fertility in rats when given in doses 50 times the human dose (see above discussion). Other findings in this study include a decrease in maternal weight gain of 30% at 20 mg/kg/day and of 10% at 4 mg/kg/day. At 10 times the human dose (4 mg/kg/day), average litter size was slightly reduced.

Teratology studies were conducted in rats, rabbits, and mice with diphenoxylate hydrochloride at oral doses of 0.4 to 20 mg/kg/day. Due to experimental design and small numbers of litters, embryotoxic, fetotoxic, or teratogenic effects cannot be adequately assessed. However, examination of the available fetuses did not reveal any indication of teratogenicity.

There are no adequate and well-controlled studies in pregnant women. Lomotil should be used during pregnancy only if the anticipated benefit justifies the potential risk to the fetus.

Nursing mothers: Caution should be exercised when Lomotil is administered to a nursing woman, since the physicochemical characteristics of the major metabolite, diphenoxylic acid, are such that it may be excreted in breast milk and since it is known that atropine is excreted in breast milk.

Pediatric use: Lomotil may be used as an adjunct to the treatment of diarrhea but should be accompanied by appropriate fluid and electrolyte therapy, if needed. LOMOTIL IS NOT RECOMMENDED FOR CHILDREN UNDER 2 YEARS OF AGE. Lomotil should be used with special caution in young children because of the greater variability of response in this age group. See *Warnings* and *Dosage and Administration*. In case of accidental ingestion by children, see *Overdosage* for recommended treatment.

ADVERSE REACTIONS

At *therapeutic* doses, the following have been reported; they are listed in decreasing order of severity, but not of frequency:

Nervous system: numbness of extremities, euphoria, depression, malaise/lethargy, confusion, sedation/drowsiness, dizziness, restlessness, headache.

Allergic: anaphylaxis, angioneurotic edema, urticaria, swelling of the gums, pruritus.

Gastrointestinal system: toxic megacolon, paralytic ileus, pancreatitis, vomiting, nausea, anorexia, abdominal discomfort.

The following atropine sulfate effects are listed in decreasing order of severity, but not of frequency: hyperthermia, tachycardia, urinary retention, flushing, dryness of the skin and mucous membranes. These effects may occur, especially in children.

THIS MEDICATION SHOULD BE KEPT IN A CHILD-RESISTANT CONTAINER AND OUT OF THE REACH OF CHILDREN SINCE AN OVERDOSAGE MAY RESULT IN SEVERE RESPIRATORY DEPRESSION AND COMA, POSSIBLY LEADING TO PERMANENT BRAIN DAMAGE OR DEATH.

DRUG ABUSE AND DEPENDENCE

Controlled substance: Lomotil is classified as a Schedule V controlled substance by federal regulation. Diphenoxylate hydrochloride is chemically related to the narcotic analgesic meperidine.

Drug abuse and dependence: In doses used for the treatment of diarrhea, whether acute or chronic, diphenoxylate has not produced addiction.

Diphenoxylate hydrochloride is devoid of morphine-like subjective effects at therapeutic doses. At high doses it exhibits codeine-like subjective effects. The dose which produces antidiarrheal action is widely separated from the dose which causes central nervous system effects. The insolubility of diphenoxylate hydrochloride in commonly available aqueous media precludes intravenous self-administration. A dose of 100 to 300 mg/day, which is equivalent to 40 to 120 tablets, administered to humans for 40 to 70 days, produced opiate withdrawal symptoms. Since addiction to diphenoxylate hydrochloride is possible at high doses, the recommended dosage should not be exceeded.

OVERDOSAGE

RECOMMENDED DOSAGE SCHEDULES SHOULD BE STRICTLY FOLLOWED. THIS MEDICATION SHOULD BE KEPT IN A CHILD-RESISTANT CONTAINER AND OUT OF THE REACH OF CHILDREN, SINCE AN OVERDOSAGE MAY RESULT IN SEVERE, EVEN FATAL, RESPIRATORY DEPRESSION.

Diagnosis: Initial signs of overdosage may include dryness of the skin and mucous membranes, mydriasis, restlessness, flushing, hyperthermia, and tachycardia followed by lethargy or coma, hypotonic reflexes, nystagmus, pinpoint pupils, and respiratory depression. Respiratory depression may be evidenced as late as 30 hours after ingestion and may recur despite an initial response to narcotic antagonists. TREAT ALL POSSIBLE LOMOTIL OVERDOSAGES AS SERIOUS AND MAINTAIN MEDICAL OBSERVATION FOR AT LEAST 48 HOURS, PREFERABLY UNDER CONTINUOUS HOSPITAL CARE.

Treatment: In the event of overdose, induction of vomiting, gastric lavage, establishment of a patent airway, and possibly mechanically assisted respiration are advised. *In vitro* and animal studies indicate that activated charcoal may significantly decrease the bioavailability of diphenoxylate. In noncomatose patients, a slurry of 100 g of activated charcoal can be administered immediately after the induction of vomiting or gastric lavage.

A pure narcotic antagonist (eg, naloxone) should be used in the treatment of respiratory depression caused by Lomotil. When a narcotic antagonist is administered intravenously, the onset of action is generally apparent within two minutes. It may also be administered subcutaneously or intramuscularly, providing a slightly less rapid onset of action but a more prolonged effect.

To counteract respiratory depression caused by Lomotil overdosage, the following dosage schedule for the narcotic antagonist naloxone hydrochloride should be followed:

Adult dosage: An initial dose of 0.4 mg to 2 mg of naloxone hydrochloride may be administered intravenously. If the desired degree of counteraction and improvement in respiratory function is not obtained, it may be repeated at 2- to 3-minute intervals. If no response is observed after 10 mg of naloxone hydrochloride has been administered, the diagnosis of narcotic-induced or partial narcotic-induced toxicity should be questioned. Intramuscular or subcutaneous administration may be necessary if the intravenous route is not available.

Children: The usual initial dose in children is 0.01 mg/kg body weight given I.V. If this dose does not result in the desired degree of clinical improvement, a subsequent dose of 0.1 mg/kg body weight may be administered. If an I.V. route of administration is not available, naloxone hydrochloride may be administered I.M. or S.C. in divided doses. If necessary, naloxone hydrochloride can be diluted with sterile water for injection.

Following initial improvement of respiratory function, repeated doses of naloxone hydrochloride may be required to counteract recurrent respiratory depression. Supplemental intramuscular doses of naloxone hydrochloride may be utilized to produce a longer-lasting effect.

Since the duration of action of diphenoxylate hydrochloride is longer than that of naloxone hydrochloride, improvement of respiration following administration may be followed by recurrent respiratory depression. Consequently, continuous observation is necessary until the effect of diphenoxylate hydrochloride on respiration has passed. This effect may persist for many hours. The period of observation should extend over at least 48 hours, preferably under continuous hospital care. Although signs of overdosage and respiratory depression may not be evident soon after ingestion of diphenoxylate hydrochloride, respiratory depression may occur from 12 to 30 hours later.

DOSAGE AND ADMINISTRATION

DO NOT EXCEED RECOMMENDED DOSAGE.

Adults: The recommended initial dosage is two Lomotil tablets four times daily or 10 ml (two regular teaspoonfuls) of Lomotil liquid four times daily (20 mg per day). Most patients will require this dosage until initial control has been achieved, after which the dosage may be reduced to meet individual requirements. Control may often be maintained with as little as 5 mg (two tablets or 10 ml of liquid) daily.

Clinical improvement of acute diarrhea is usually observed within 48 hours. If clinical improvement of chronic diarrhea after treatment with a maximum daily dose of 20 mg of diphenoxylate hydrochloride is not observed within 10 days, symptoms are unlikely to be controlled by further administration.

Children: Lomotil is not recommended in children under 2 years of age and should be used with special caution in young children (see *Warnings* and *Precautions*). *The nutritional status and degree of dehydration must be considered. In children under 13 years of age, use Lomotil liquid. Do not use Lomotil tablets for this age group.*

Only the plastic dropper should be used when measuring Lomotil liquid for administration to children.

Dosage schedule for children: The recommended initial total daily dosage of Lomotil liquid for children is 0.3 to 0.4 mg/kg, administered in four divided doses. The following table provides an *approximate* initial daily dosage recommendation for children.

Age (years)	Approximate weight (kg)	(lb)	Dosage in ml (four times daily)
2	11–14	24–31	1.5–3.0
3	12–16	26–35	2.0–3.0
4	14–20	31–44	2.0–4.0
5	16–23	35–51	2.5–4.5
6–8	17–32	38–71	2.5–5.0
9–12	23–55	51–121	3.5–5.0

These pediatric schedules are the best approximation of an average dose recommendation which may be adjusted downward according to the overall nutritional status and degree of dehydration encountered in the sick child. Reduction of dosage may be made as soon as initial control of symptoms has been achieved. Maintenance dosage may be as low as one-fourth of the initial daily dosage. If no response occurs within 48 hours, Lomotil is unlikely to be effective.

KEEP THIS AND ALL MEDICATIONS OUT OF THE REACH OF CHILDREN.

HOW SUPPLIED

Tablets—round, white, with SEARLE debossed on one side and 61 on the other side and containing 2.5 mg of diphenoxylate hydrochloride and 0.025 mg of atropine sulfate, supplied as:

NDC Number	Size
0025-0061-31	bottle of 100
0025-0061-51	bottle of 500
0025-0061-52	bottle of 1,000
0025-0061-55	bottle of 2,500
0025-0061-34	carton of 100 unit dose

Liquid—containing 2.5 mg of diphenoxylate hydrochloride and 0.025 mg of atropine sulfate per 5 ml; bottles of 2 fl oz (NDC Number 0025-0066-02). Dispense only in original container.

A plastic dropper calibrated in increments of $^1/_2$ ml ($^1/_4$ mg) with a capacity of 2 ml (1 mg) accompanies each 2-oz bottle of Lomotil liquid. Only this plastic dropper should be used when measuring Lomotil liquid for administration to children.

12/9/93 • A05758-4

Shown in Product Identification Guide, page 338

NORPACE® Capsules ℞
[*nor 'pāce*]
(disopyramide phosphate)

NORPACE® CR Capsules ℞
(disopyramide phosphate extended-release)

DESCRIPTION

Norpace (disopyramide phosphate) is an antiarrhythmic drug available for oral administration in immediate-release and controlled-release capsules containing 100 mg or 150 mg of disopyramide base, present as the phosphate. The base content of the phosphate salt is 77.6%. The structural formula of Norpace is:

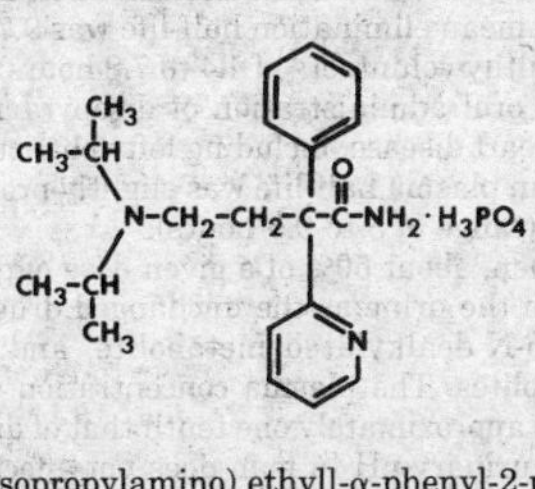

α-[2-(diisopropylamino) ethyl]-α-phenyl-2-pyridine-acetamide phosphate

Norpace is freely soluble in water, and the free base (pKa 10.4) has an aqueous solubility of 1 mg/ml. The chloroform: water partition coefficient of the base is 3.1 at pH 7.2.

Continued on next page

Norpace/Norpace CR—Cont.

Norpace is a racemic mixture of *d* - and *l*-isomers. This drug is not chemically related to other antiarrhythmic drugs.
Norpace CR (controlled-release) capsules are designed to afford a gradual and consistent release of disopyramide. Thus, for maintenance therapy, Norpace CR provides the benefit of less-frequent dosing (every 12 hours) as compared with the every-6-hour dosage schedule of immediate-release Norpace capsules.
Inactive ingredients of Norpace include corn starch, edible ink, FD&C Red No. 3, FD&C Yellow No. 6, gelatin, lactose, talc, and titanium dioxide; the 150-mg capsule also contains FD&C Blue No. 1.
Inactive ingredients of Norpace CR include corn starch, D&C Yellow No. 10, edible ink, ethylcellulose, FD&C Blue No. 1, gelatin, shellac, sucrose, talc, and titanium dioxide; the 150-mg capsule also contains FD&C Red No. 3 and FD&C Yellow No. 6.

CLINICAL PHARMACOLOGY

Mechanisms of Action

Norpace (disopyramide phosphate) is a Type 1 antiarrhythmic drug (ie, similar to procainamide and quinidine). *In animal studies* Norpace decreases the rate of diastolic depolarization (phase 4) in cells with augmented automaticity, decreases the upstroke velocity (phase 0) and increases the action potential duration of normal cardiac cells, decreases the disparity in refractoriness between infarcted and adjacent normally perfused myocardium, and has no effect on alpha- or beta-adrenergic receptors.

Electrophysiology

In man, Norpace at therapeutic plasma levels shortens the sinus node recovery time, lengthens the effective refractory period of the atrium, and has a minimal effect on the effective refractory period of the AV node. Little effect has been shown on AV-nodal and His-Purkinje conduction times or QRS duration. However, prolongation of conduction in accessory pathways occurs.

Hemodynamics

At recommended oral doses, Norpace rarely produces significant alterations of blood pressure in patients without congestive heart failure (see *Warnings*). With intravenous Norpace, either increases in systolic/diastolic or decreases in systolic blood pressure have been reported, depending on the infusion rate and the patient population. Intravenous Norpace may cause cardiac depression with an approximate mean 10% reduction of cardiac output, which is more pronounced in patients with cardiac dysfunction.

Anticholinergic Activity

The *in vitro* anticholinergic activity of Norpace is approximately 0.06% that of atropine; however, the usual dose for Norpace is 150 mg every 6 hours and for Norpace CR 300 mg every 12 hours, compared to 0.4 to 0.6 mg for atropine (see *Warnings* and *Adverse Reactions* for anticholinergic side effects).

Pharmacokinetics

Following oral administration of immediate-release Norpace, disopyramide phosphate is rapidly and almost completely absorbed, and peak plasma levels are usually attained within 2 hours. The usual therapeutic plasma levels of disopyramide base are 2 to 4 mcg/ml, and at these concentrations protein binding varies from 50% to 65%. Because of concentration-dependent protein binding, it is difficult to predict the concentration of the free drug when total drug is measured.
The mean plasma half-life of disopyramide in healthy humans is 6.7 hours (range of 4 to 10 hours). In six patients with impaired renal function (creatinine clearance less than 40 ml/min), disopyramide half-life values were 8 to 18 hours.
After the oral administration of 200 mg of disopyramide to 10 cardiac patients with borderline to moderate heart failure, the time to peak serum concentration of 2.3 ± 1.5 hours (mean ± SD) was increased, and the mean peak serum concentration of 4.8 ± 1.6 mcg/ml was higher than in healthy volunteers. After intravenous administration in these same patients, the mean elimination half-life was 9.7 ± 4.2 hours (range in healthy volunteers of 4.4 to 7.8 hours). In a second study of the oral administration of disopyramide to 7 patients with heart disease, including left ventricular dysfunction, the mean plasma half-life was slightly prolonged to 7.8 ± 1.9 hours (range of 5 to 9.5 hours).
In healthy men, about 50% of a given dose of disopyramide is excreted in the urine as the unchanged drug, about 20% as the mono-N-dealkylated metabolite, and 10% as the other metabolites. The plasma concentration of the major metabolite is approximately one tenth that of disopyramide. Altering the urinary pH in man does not affect the plasma half-life of disopyramide.
In a crossover study in healthy subjects, the bioavailability of disopyramide from Norpace CR capsules was similar to that from the immediate-release capsules. With a single 300-mg oral dose, peak disopyramide plasma concentrations of 3.23 ± 0.75 mcg/ml (mean ± SD) at 2.5 ± 2.3 hours were obtained with two 150-mg immediate-release capsules and 2.22 ± 0.47 mcg/ml at 4.9 ± 1.4 hours with two 150-mg Norpace CR capsules. The elimination half-life of disopyramide was 8.31 ± 1.83 hours with the immediate-release capsules and 11.65 ± 4.72 hours with Norpace CR capsules. The amount of disopyramide and mono-N-dealkylated metabolite excreted in the urine in 48 hours was 128 and 48 mg, respectively, with the immediate-release capsules, and 112 and 33 mg, respectively, with Norpace CR capsules. The differences in the urinary excretion of either constituent were not statistically significant.
Following multiple doses, steady-state plasma levels of between 2 and 4 mcg/ml were attained following either 150 mg every-6-hour dosing with immediate-release capsules or 300 mg every-12-hour dosing with Norpace CR capsules.

INDICATIONS AND USAGE

Norpace and Norpace CR are indicated for the treatment of documented ventricular arrhythmias, such as sustained ventricular tachycardia, that, in the judgment of the physician, are life-threatening. Because of the proarrhythmic effects of Norpace and Norpace CR, their use with lesser arrhythmias is generally not recommended. Treatment of patients with asymptomatic ventricular premature contractions should be avoided.
Initiation of Norpace or Norpace CR treatment, as with other antiarrhythmic agents used to treat life-threatening arrhythmias, should be carried out in the hospital. Norpace CR should not be used initially if rapid establishment of disopyramide plasma levels is desired.
Antiarrhythmic drugs have not been shown to enhance survival in patients with ventricular arrhythmias.

CONTRAINDICATIONS

Norpace and Norpace CR are contraindicated in the presence of cardiogenic shock, preexisting second- or third-degree AV block (if no pacemaker is present), congenital Q-T prolongation, or known hypersensitivity to the drug.

WARNINGS

Mortality

In the National Heart, Lung and Blood Institute's Cardiac Arrhythmia Suppression Trial (CAST), a long-term, multi-center, randomized, double-blind study in patients with asymptomatic non-life-threatening ventricular arrhythmias who had had a myocardial infarction more than 6 days but less than 2 years previously, an excessive mortality or non-fatal cardiac arrest rate (7.7%) was seen in patients treated with encainide or flecainide compared with that seen in patients assigned to carefully matched placebo-treated groups (3.0%). The average duration of treatment with encainide or flecainide in this study was 10 months.
The applicability of the CAST results to other populations (eg, those without recent myocardial infarction) is uncertain. Considering the known proarrhythmic properties of Norpace or Norpace CR and the lack of evidence of improved survival for any antiarrhythmic drug in patients without life-threatening arrhythmias, the use of Norpace or Norpace CR as well as other antiarrhythmic agents should be reserved for patients with life-threatening ventricular arrhythmias.

Negative Inotropic Properties:

Heart Failure/Hypotension

Norpace or Norpace CR may cause or worsen congestive heart failure or produce severe hypotension as a consequence of its negative inotropic properties. Hypotension has been observed primarily in patients with primary cardiomyopathy or inadequately compensated congestive heart failure. Norpace or Norpace CR should not be used in patients with uncompensated or marginally compensated congestive heart failure or hypotension unless the congestive heart failure or hypotension is secondary to cardiac arrhythmia. Patients with a history of heart failure may be treated with Norpace or Norpace CR, but careful attention must be given to the maintenance of cardiac function, including optimal digitalization. If hypotension occurs or congestive heart failure worsens, Norpace or Norpace CR should be discontinued and, if necessary, restarted at a lower dosage only after adequate cardiac compensation has been established.

QRS Widening

Although it is unusual, significant widening (greater than 25%) of the QRS complex may occur during Norpace or Norpace CR administration; in such cases Norpace or Norpace CR should be discontinued.

Q-T Prolongation

As with other Type 1 antiarrhythmic drugs, prolongation of the Q-T interval (corrected) and worsening of the arrhythmia, including ventricular tachycardia and ventricular fibrillation, may occur. Patients who have evidenced prolongation of the Q-T interval in response to quinidine may be at particular risk. As with other Type 1A antiarrhythmics, disopyramide phosphate has been associated with torsade de pointes.
If a Q-T prolongation of greater than 25% is observed and if ectopy continues, the patient should be monitored closely, and consideration be given to discontinuing Norpace or Norpace CR.

Hypoglycemia

In rare instances significant lowering of blood glucose values has been reported during Norpace administration. The physician should be alert to this possibility, especially in patients with congestive heart failure, chronic malnutrition, hepatic, renal, or other diseases, or drugs (eg, beta adrenoceptor blockers, alcohol) which could compromise preservation of the normal glucoregulatory mechanisms in the absence of food. In these patients the blood glucose levels should be carefully followed.

Concomitant Antiarrhythmic Therapy

The concomitant use of Norpace or Norpace CR with other Type 1A antiarrhythmic agents (such as quinidine or procainamide), Type 1C antiarrhythmics (such as encainide, flecainide or propafenone), and/or propranolol should be reserved for patients with life-threatening arrhythmias who are demonstrably unresponsive to single-agent antiarrhythmic therapy. Such use may produce serious negative inotropic effects, or may excessively prolong conduction. This should be considered particularly in patients with any degree of cardiac decompensation or those with a prior history thereof. Patients receiving more than one antiarrhythmic drug must be carefully monitored.

Heart Block

If first-degree heart block develops in a patient receiving Norpace or Norpace CR, the dosage should be reduced. If the block persists despite reduction of dosage, continuation of the drug must depend upon weighing the benefit being obtained against the risk of higher degrees of heart block. Development of second- or third-degree AV block or unifascicular, bifascicular, or trifascicular block requires discontinuation of Norpace or Norpace CR therapy, unless the ventricular rate is adequately controlled by a temporary or implanted ventricular pacemaker.

Anticholinergic Activity

Because of its anticholinergic activity, disopyramide phosphate should not be used in patients with glaucoma, myasthenia gravis, or urinary retention unless adequate overriding measures are taken; these consist of the topical application of potent miotics (eg, pilocarpine) for patients with glaucoma, and catheter drainage or operative relief for patients with urinary retention. Urinary retention may occur in patients of either sex as a consequence of Norpace or Norpace CR administration, but males with benign prostatic hypertrophy are at particular risk. In patients with a family history of glaucoma, intraocular pressure should be measured before initiating Norpace or Norpace CR therapy. Disopyramide phosphate should be used with special care in patients with myasthenia gravis since its anticholinergic properties could precipitate a myasthenic crisis in such patients.

PRECAUTIONS

General

Atrial Tachyarrhythmias

Patients with atrial flutter or fibrillation should be digitalized prior to Norpace or Norpace CR administration to ensure that drug-induced enhancement of AV conduction does not result in an increase of ventricular rate beyond physiologically acceptable limits.

Conduction Abnormalities

Care should be taken when prescribing Norpace or Norpace CR for patients with sick sinus syndrome (bradycardia-tachycardia syndrome), Wolff-Parkinson-White syndrome (WPW), or bundle branch block. The effect of disopyramide phosphate in these conditions is uncertain at present.

Cardiomyopathy

Patients with myocarditis or other cardiomyopathy may develop significant hypotension in response to the usual dosage of disopyramide phosphate, probably due to cardiodepressant mechanisms. Therefore, a loading dose of Norpace should not be given to such patients, and initial dosage and subsequent dosage adjustments should be made under close supervision (see *Dosage and Administration*).

Renal Impairment

More than 50% of disopyramide is excreted in the urine unchanged. Therefore Norpace dosage should be reduced in patients with impaired renal function (see *Dosage and Administration*). The electrocardiogram should be carefully monitored for prolongation of PR interval, evidence of QRS widening, or other signs of overdosage (see *Overdosage*).
Norpace CR is not recommended for patients with severe renal insufficiency (creatinine clearance 40 ml/min or less).

Hepatic Impairment

Hepatic impairment also causes an increase in the plasma half-life of disopyramide. Dosage should be reduced for patients with such impairment. The electrocardiogram should be carefully monitored for signs of overdosage (see *Overdosage*).

Patients with cardiac dysfunction have a higher potential for hepatic impairment; this should be considered when administering Norpace or Norpace CR.

Potassium Imbalance

Antiarrhythmic drugs may be ineffective in patients with hypokalemia, and their toxic effects may be enhanced in patients with hyperkalemia. Therefore, potassium abnormalities should be corrected before starting Norpace or Norpace CR therapy.

Drug Interactions

If phenytoin or other hepatic enzyme inducers are taken concurrently with Norpace or Norpace CR, lower plasma levels of disopyramide may occur. Monitoring of disopyramide plasma levels is recommended in such concurrent use to avoid ineffective therapy. Other antiarrhythmic drugs (eg, quinidine, procainamide, lidocaine, propranolol) have occasionally been used concurrently with Norpace. Excessive widening of the QRS complex and/or prolongation of the Q-T interval may occur in these situations (see *Warnings*). In healthy subjects, no significant drug-drug interaction was observed when Norpace was coadministered with either propranolol or diazepam. Concomitant administration of Norpace and quinidine resulted in slight increases in plasma disopyramide levels and slight decreases in plasma quinidine levels. Norpace does not increase serum digoxin levels.

Patients taking disopyramide phosphate and erythromycin concomitantly may develop increased serum concentrations of disopyramide resulting in excessive widening of the QRS complex and/or prolongation of the Q-T interval (see *Warnings*). Patients taking disopyramide phosphate and hepatic enzyme inhibitors concomitantly should be closely monitored.

Until data on possible interactions between verapamil and disopyramide phosphate are obtained, disopyramide should not be administered within 48 hours before or 24 hours after verapamil administration.

Carcinogenesis, Mutagenesis, Impairment of Fertility

Eighteen months of Norpace administration to rats, at oral doses up to 400 mg/kg/day (about 30 times the usual daily human dose of 600 mg/day, assuming a patient weight of at least 50 kg), revealed no evidence of carcinogenic potential. An evaluation of mutagenic potential by Ames test was negative. Norpace, at doses up to 250 mg/kg/day, did not adversely affect fertility of rats.

Pregnancy

Teratogenic Effects: Pregnancy Category C. Norpace was associated with decreased numbers of implantation sites and decreased growth and survival of pups when administered to pregnant rats at 250 mg/kg/day (20 or more times the usual daily human dose of 12 mg/kg, assuming a patient weight of at least 50 kg), a level at which weight gain and food consumption of dams were also reduced. Increased resorption rates were reported in rabbits at 60 mg/kg/day (5 or more times the usual daily human dose). Effects on implantation, pup growth, and survival were not evaluated in rabbits. There are no adequate and well-controlled studies in pregnant women. Norpace or Norpace CR should be used during pregnancy only if the potential benefit justifies the potential risk to the fetus.

Nonteratogenic Effects: **Norpace has been reported to stimulate contractions of the pregnant uterus.** Disopyramide has been found in human fetal blood.

Labor and Delivery

It is not known whether the use of Norpace or Norpace CR during labor or delivery has immediate or delayed adverse effects on the fetus, or whether it prolongs the duration of labor or increases the need for forceps delivery or other obstetric intervention.

Nursing Mothers

Studies in rats have shown that the concentration of disopyramide and its metabolites is between one and three times greater in milk than it is in plasma. Following oral administration, disopyramide has been detected in human milk at a concentration not exceeding that in plasma. Because of the potential for serious adverse reactions in nursing infants from Norpace or Norpace CR, a decision should be made whether to discontinue nursing or to discontinue the drug, taking into account the importance of the drug to the mother.

Pediatric Use

Safety and effectiveness in pediatric patients have not been established (see *Dosage and Administration*).

ADVERSE REACTIONS

The adverse reactions which were reported in Norpace clinical trials encompass observations in 1,500 patients, including 90 patients studied for at least 4 years. The most serious adverse reactions are hypotension and congestive heart failure. The most common adverse reactions, which are dose dependent, are associated with the anticholinergic properties of the drug. These may be transitory, but may be persistent or can be severe. Urinary retention is the most serious anticholinergic effect.

The following reactions were reported in 10% to 40% of patients:

Anticholinergic: dry mouth (32%), urinary hesitancy (14%), constipation (11%)

The following reactions were reported in 3% to 9% of patients:

Anticholinergic: blurred vision, dry nose/eyes/throat
Genitourinary: urinary retention, urinary frequency and urgency
Gastrointestinal: nausea, pain/bloating/gas
General: dizziness, general fatigue/muscle weakness, headache, malaise, aches/pains

The following reactions were reported in 1% to 3% of patients:

Genitourinary: impotence
Cardiovascular: hypotension with or without congestive heart failure, increased congestive heart failure (see *Warnings*), cardiac conduction disturbances (see *Warnings*), edema/weight gain, shortness of breath, syncope, chest pain
Gastrointestinal: anorexia, diarrhea, vomiting
Dermatologic: generalized rash/dermatoses, itching
Central nervous system: nervousness
Other: hypokalemia, elevated cholesterol/triglycerides

The following reactions were reported in less than 1%:

Depression, insomnia, dysuria, numbness/tingling, elevated liver enzymes, AV block, elevated BUN, elevated creatinine, decreased hemoglobin/hematocrit

Hypoglycemia has been reported in association with Norpace administration (see *Warnings*).

Infrequent occurrences of reversible cholestatic jaundice, fever, and respiratory difficulty have been reported in association with disopyramide therapy, as have rare instances of thrombocytopenia, reversible agranulocytosis, and gynecomastia. Some cases of LE (lupus erythematosus) symptoms have been reported; most cases occurred in patients who had been switched to disopyramide from procainamide following the development of LE symptoms. Rarely, acute psychosis has been reported following Norpace therapy, with prompt return to normal mental status when therapy was stopped. The physician should be aware of these possible reactions and should discontinue Norpace or Norpace CR therapy promptly if they occur.

OVERDOSAGE

Symptoms

Deliberate or accidental overdosage of oral disopyramide may be followed by apnea, loss of consciousness, cardiac arrhythmias, and loss of spontaneous respiration. Death has occurred following overdosage.

Toxic plasma levels of disopyramide produce excessive widening of the QRS complex and Q-T interval, worsening of congestive heart failure, hypotension, varying kinds and degrees of conduction disturbance, bradycardia, and finally asystole. Obvious anticholinergic effects are also observed.

The approximate oral LD_{50} of disopyramide phosphate is 580 and 700 mg/kg for rats and mice, respectively.

Treatment

Experience indicates that prompt and vigorous treatment of overdosage is necessary, even in the absence of symptoms. Such treatment may be lifesaving. No specific antidote for disopyramide phosphate has been identified. Treatment should be symptomatic and may include induction of emesis or gastric lavage, administration of a cathartic followed by activated charcoal by mouth or stomach tube, intravenous administration of isoproterenol and dopamine, insertion of an intra-aortic balloon for counterpulsation, and mechanically assisted ventilation. Hemodialysis or, preferably, hemoperfusion with charcoal may be employed to lower serum concentration of the drug.

The electrocardiogram should be monitored, and supportive therapy with cardiac glycosides and diuretics should be given as required.

If progressive AV block should develop, endocardial pacing should be implemented. In case of any impaired renal function, measures to increase the glomerular filtration rate may reduce the toxicity (disopyramide is excreted primarily by the kidney).

The anticholinergic effects can be reversed with neostigmine at the discretion of the physician.

Altering the urinary pH in humans does not affect the plasma half-life or the amount of disopyramide excreted in the urine.

DOSAGE AND ADMINISTRATION

The dosage of Norpace or Norpace CR must be individualized for each patient on the basis of response and tolerance. The usual adult dosage of Norpace or Norpace CR is 400 to 800 mg per day given in divided doses. The recommended dosage for most adults is 600 mg/day given in divided doses (either 150 mg every 6 hours for immediate-release Norpace or 300 mg every 12 hours for Norpace CR). For patients whose body weight is less than 110 pounds (50 kg), the recommended dosage is 400 mg/day given in divided doses (either 100 mg every 6 hours for immediate-release Norpace or 200 mg every 12 hours for Norpace CR).

For patients with cardiomyopathy or possible cardiac decompensation, a loading dose, as discussed below, should not be given, and initial dosage should be limited to 100 mg of immediate-release Norpace every 6 to 8 hours. Subsequent dosage adjustments should be made gradually, with close monitoring for the possible development of hypotension and/or congestive heart failure (see *Warnings*).

For patients with moderate renal insufficiency (creatinine clearance greater than 40 ml/min) or hepatic insufficiency, the recommended dosage is 400 mg/day given in divided doses (either 100 mg every 6 hours for immediate-release Norpace or 200 mg every 12 hours for Norpace CR).

For patients with severe renal insufficiency (C_{cr} 40 ml/min or less), the recommended dosage regimen of immediate-release Norpace is 100 mg at intervals shown in the table below, with or without an initial loading dose of 150 mg.

IMMEDIATE-RELEASE NORPACE DOSAGE INTERVAL FOR PATIENTS WITH RENAL INSUFFICIENCY

Creatinine clearance (ml/min)	40–30	30–15	less than 15
Approximate maintenance-dosing interval	q 8 hr	q 12 hr	q 24 hr

The above dosing schedules are for Norpace immediate-release capsules; Norpace CR is not recommended for patients with severe renal insufficiency.

For patients in whom rapid control of ventricular arrhythmia is essential, an initial loading dose of 300 mg of immediate-release Norpace (200 mg for patients whose body weight is less than 110 pounds) is recommended, followed by the appropriate maintenance dosage. Therapeutic effects are usually attained 30 minutes to 3 hours after administration of a 300-mg loading dose. If there is no response or evidence of toxicity within 6 hours of the loading dose, 200 mg of immediate-release Norpace every 6 hours may be prescribed instead of the usual 150 mg. If there is no response to this dosage within 48 hours, either Norpace should then be discontinued or the physician should consider hospitalizing the patient for careful monitoring while subsequent immediate-release Norpace doses of 250 mg or 300 mg every 6 hours are given. A limited number of patients with severe refractory ventricular tachycardia have tolerated daily doses of Norpace up to 1600 mg per day (400 mg every 6 hours), resulting in disopyramide plasma levels up to 9 mcg/ml. If such treatment is warranted, it is essential that patients be hospitalized for close evaluation and continuous monitoring.

Norpace CR should not be used initially if rapid establishment of disopyramide plasma levels is desired.

Transferring to Norpace or Norpace CR

The following dosage schedule based on theoretical considerations rather than experimental data is suggested for transferring patients with normal renal function from either quinidine sulfate or procainamide therapy (Type 1 antiarrhythmic agents) to Norpace or Norpace CR therapy:

Norpace or Norpace CR should be started using the regular maintenance schedule **without a loading dose** 6 to 12 hours after the last dose of quinidine sulfate or 3 to 6 hours after the last dose of procainamide.

In patients in whom withdrawal of quinidine sulfate or procainamide is likely to produce life-threatening arrhythmias, the physician should consider hospitalization of the patient.

When transferring a patient from immediate-release Norpace to Norpace CR, the maintenance schedule of Norpace CR may be started 6 hours after the last dose of immediate-release Norpace.

Pediatric Dosage

Controlled clinical studies have not been conducted in pediatric patients; however, the following suggested dosage table is based on published clinical experience.

Total daily dosage should be divided and equal doses administered orally every 6 hours or at intervals according to individual patient needs. Disopyramide plasma levels and therapeutic response must be monitored closely. Patients should be hospitalized during the initial treatment period, and dose titration should start at the lower end of the ranges provided below.

SUGGESTED TOTAL DAILY DOSAGE*

Age (years)	Disopyramide (mg/kg body weight/day)
Under 1	10 to 30
1 to 4	10 to 20

Continued on next page

Norpace/Norpace CR—Cont.

4 to 12	10 to 15
12 to 18	6 to 15

* Dosage is expressed in milligrams of disopyramide base. Since Norpace (disopyramide phosphate) 100-mg capsules contain 100 mg of disopyramide base, the pharmacist can readily prepare a 1-mg/ml to 10-mg/ml liquid suspension by adding the entire contents of Norpace capsules to cherry syrup, NF. The resulting suspension, when refrigerated, is stable for one month and should be thoroughly shaken before the measurement of each dose. The suspension should be dispensed in an amber glass bottle with a child-resistant closure.
Norpace CR capsules should not be used to prepare the above suspension.

HOW SUPPLIED

Norpace (disopyramide phosphate) is supplied in hard gelatin capsules containing either 100 mg or 150 mg of disopyramide base, present as the phosphate.
Norpace 100-mg capsules are white and orange, with markings SEARLE, 2752, NORPACE, and 100 MG.

NDC Number	Size
0025-2752-31	bottle of 100
0025-2752-52	bottle of 1,000

Norpace 150-mg capsules are brown and orange, with markings SEARLE, 2762, NORPACE, and 150 MG.

NDC Number	Size
0025-2762-31	bottle of 100
0025-2762-52	bottle of 1,000

Norpace CR (disopyramide phosphate) Controlled-Release is supplied as specially prepared controlled-release beads in hard gelatin capsules containing either 100 mg or 150 mg of disopyramide base, present as the phosphate.
Norpace CR 100-mg capsules are white and light green, with markings SEARLE, 2732, NORPACE CR, and 100 mg.

NDC Number	Size
0025-2732-31	bottle of 100
0025-2732-51	bottle of 500
0025-2732-34	carton of 100 unit dose

Norpace CR 150-mg capsules are brown and light green, with markings SEARLE, 2742, NORPACE CR, and 150 mg.

NDC Number	Size
0025-2742-31	bottle of 100
0025-2742-51	bottle of 500
0025-2742-34	carton of 100 unit dose

Store at controlled room temperature 20°–25°C (68°–77°F) [see USP].

Caution: Federal law prohibits dispensing without prescription.

4/4/97 • A05855-3

Shown in Product Identification Guide, page 338

SYNAREL® ℞

[sin 'er-el]
(nafarelin acetate)
Nasal Solution 2 mg/mL
(as nafarelin base)

CENTRAL PRECOCIOUS PUBERTY (FOR ENDOMETRIOSIS, SEE ENDOMETRIOSIS SECTION)

DESCRIPTION

SYNAREL (nafarelin acetate) Nasal Solution is intended for administration as a spray to the nasal mucosa. Nafarelin acetate, the active component of SYNAREL Nasal Solution, is a decapeptide with the chemical name: 5-oxo-L-prolyl-L-histidyl-L-tryptophyl-L-seryl-L-tyrosyl -3- (2-naphthyl)-D-alanyl-L-leucyl-L-arginyl-L-prolyl-glycinamide acetate. Nafarelin acetate is a synthetic analog of the naturally occurring gonadotropin-releasing hormone (GnRH).
Nafarelin acetate has the following chemical structure:
[See chemical structure at top of next column]
SYNAREL Nasal Solution contains nafarelin acetate (2 mg/mL, content expressed as nafarelin base) in a solution of benzalkonium chloride, glacial acetic acid, sodium hydroxide or hydrochloric acid (to adjust pH), sorbitol, and purified water.
After priming the pump unit for SYNAREL, each actuation of the unit delivers approximately 100 µL of the spray containing approximately 200 µg nafarelin base. The contents of one spray bottle are intended to deliver at least 60 sprays.

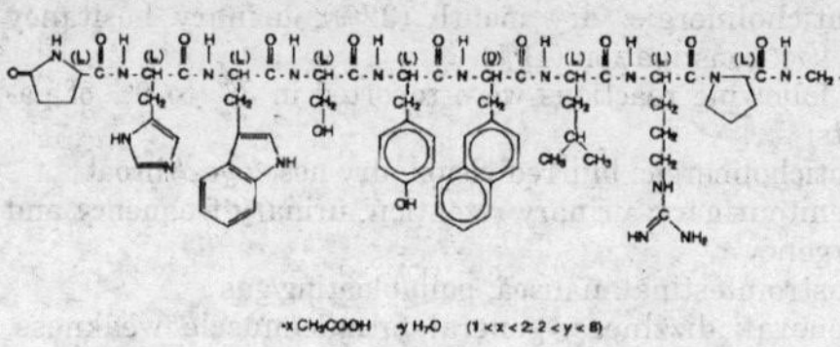

CLINICAL PHARMACOLOGY

Nafarelin acetate is a potent agonistic analog of gonadotropin-releasing hormone (GnRH). At the onset of administration, nafarelin stimulates the release of the pituitary gonadotropins, luteinizing hormone (LH) and follicle stimulating hormone (FSH), resulting in a temporary increase of gonadal steroidogenesis. Repeated dosing abolishes the stimulatory effect on the pituitary gland. Twice daily administration leads to decreased secretion of gonadal steroids by about 4 weeks; consequently, tissues and functions that depend on gonadal steroids for their maintenance become quiescent.
In **children**, nafarelin acetate was rapidly absorbed into the systemic circulation after intranasal administration. Maximum serum concentrations (measured by RIA) were achieved between 10 and 45 minutes. Following a single dose of 400 µg base, the observed peak concentration was 2.2 ng/mL, whereas following a single dose of 600 µg base, the observed peak concentration was 6.6 ng/mL. The average serum half-life of nafarelin following intranasal administration of a 400 µg dose was approximately 2.5 hours. It is not known and cannot be predicted what the pharmacokinetics of nafarelin will be in children given a dose above 600 µg.

In **adult women**, nafarelin acetate was rapidly absorbed into the systemic circulation after intranasal administration. Maximum serum concentrations (measured by RIA) were achieved between 10 and 40 minutes. Following a single dose of 200 µg base, the observed average peak concentration was 0.6 ng/mL (range 0.2 to 1.4 ng/mL), whereas following a single dose of 400 µg base, the observed average peak concentration was 1.8 ng/mL (range 0.5 to 5.3 ng/mL). Bioavailability from a 400 µg dose averaged 2.8% (range 1.2 to 5.6%). The average serum half-life of nafarelin following intranasal administration was approximately 3 hours. About 80% of nafarelin acetate was bound to plasma proteins at 4°C. Twice daily intranasal administration of 200 or 400 µg of SYNAREL in 18 healthy women for 22 days did not lead to significant accumulation of the drug. Based on the mean C_{min} levels on Days 15 and 22, there appeared to be dose proportionality across the two dose levels.
After subcutaneous administration of ^{14}C-nafarelin acetate to men, 44-55% of the dose was recovered in urine and 18.5-44.2% was recovered in feces. Approximately 3% of the administered dose appeared as unchanged nafarelin in urine. The ^{14}C serum half-life of the metabolites was about 85.5 hours. Six metabolites of nafarelin have been identified of which the major metabolite is Tyr-D(2)-Nal-Leu-Arg-Pro-Gly-NH_2(5–10). The activity of the metabolites, the metabolism of nafarelin by nasal mucosa, and the pharmacokinetics of the drug in hepatically- and renally-impaired patients have not been determined.
There appeared to be no significant effect of rhinitis, i.e., nasal congestion, on the systemic bioavailability of SYNAREL; however, if the use of a nasal decongestant for rhinitis is necessary during treatment with SYNAREL, the decongestant should not be used until at least 2 hours following dosing with SYNAREL.
When used regularly in girls and boys with **central precocious puberty (CPP)** at the recommended dose, SYNAREL suppresses LH and sex steroid hormone levels to prepubertal levels, affects a corresponding arrest of secondary sexual development, and slows linear growth and skeletal maturation. In some cases, initial estrogen withdrawal bleeding may occur, generally within 6 weeks after initiation of therapy. Thereafter, menstruation should cease.
In clinical studies the peak response of LH to GnRH stimulation was reduced from a pubertal response to a prepubertal response (<15 mlU/mL) within one month of treatment.
Linear growth velocity, which is commonly pubertal in children with CPP, is reduced in most children within the first year of treatment to values of 5 to 6 cm/year or less. Children with CPP are frequently taller than their chronological age peers; height for chronological age approaches normal in most children during the second or third year of treatment with SYNAREL. Skeletal maturation rate (bone age velocity—change in bone age divided by change in chronological age) is usually abnormal (greater than 1) in children with CPP; in most children, bone age velocity approaches normal (1) during the first year of treatment. This results in a narrowing of the gap between bone age and chronological age, usually by the second or third year of treatment. The mean predicted adult height increases.

In clinical trials, breast development was arrested or regressed in 82% of girls, and genital development was arrested or regressed in 100% of boys. Because pubic hair growth is largely controlled by adrenal androgens, which are unaffected by nafarelin, pubic hair development was arrested or regressed only in 54% of girls and boys.
Reversal of the suppressive effects of SYNAREL has been demonstrated to occur in all children with CPP for whom one-year post- treatment follow-up is available (n=69). This demonstration consisted of the appearance or return of menses, the return of pubertal gonadotropin and gonadal sex steroid levels, and/or the advancement of secondary sexual development. Semen analysis was normal in the two ejaculated specimens obtained thus far from boys who have been taken off therapy to resume puberty. Fertility has not been documented by pregnancies and the effect of long-term use of the drug on fertility is not known.

INDICATIONS AND USAGE FOR CENTRAL PRECOCIOUS PUBERTY
(For Endometriosis, See Endometriosis section)

SYNAREL is indicated for treatment of **central precocious puberty (CPP)** (gonadotropin-dependent precocious puberty) in children of both sexes.
The diagnosis of **central precocious puberty (CPP)** is suspected when premature development of secondary sexual characteristics occurs at or before the age of 8 years in girls and 9 years in boys, and is accompanied by significant advancement of bone age and/or a poor adult height prediction. The diagnosis should be confirmed by pubertal gonadal sex steroid levels and a pubertal LH response to stimulation by native GnRH. Pelvic ultrasound assessment in girls usually reveals enlarged uterus and ovaries, the latter often with multiple cystic formations. Magnetic resonance imaging (MRI) or computed tomography (CT) scanning of the brain is recommended to detect hypothalamic or pituitary tumors, or anatomical changes associated with increased intracranial pressure. Other causes of sexual precocity, such as congenital adrenal hyperplasia, testotoxicosis, testicular tumors and/or other autonomous feminizing or masculinizing disorders, must be excluded by proper clinical hormonal and diagnostic imaging examinations.

CONTRAINDICATIONS

1. Hypersensitivity to GnRH, GnRH agonist analogs or any of the excipients in SYNAREL;
2. Undiagnosed abnormal vaginal bleeding;
3. Use in pregnancy or in women who may become pregnant while receiving the drug. SYNAREL may cause fetal harm when administered to a pregnant woman. Major fetal abnormalities were observed in rats, but not in mice or rabbits, after administration of SYNAREL during the period of organogenesis. There was a dose-related increase in fetal mortality and a decrease in fetal weight in rats (see *Pregnancy* Section). The effects on rat fetal mortality are expected consequences of the alterations in hormonal levels brought about by the drug. If this drug is used during pregnancy or if the patient becomes pregnant while taking this drug, she should be apprised of the potential hazard to the fetus;
4. Use in women who are breast-feeding (see *Nursing Mothers* Section).

WARNINGS

The diagnosis of central precocious puberty (CPP) must be established before treatment is initiated. Regular monitoring of CPP patients is needed to assess both patient response as well as compliance. This is particularly important during the first 6 to 8 weeks of treatment to assure that suppression of pituitary-gonadal function is rapid. Testing may include LH response to GnRH stimulation and circulating gonadal sex steroid levels. Assessment of growth velocity and bone age velocity should begin within 3 to 6 months of treatment initiation.
Some patients may not show suppression of the pituitary-gonadal axis by clinical and/or biochemical parameters. This may be due to lack of compliance with the recommended treatment regimen and may be rectified by recommending that the dosing be done by caregivers. If compliance problems are excluded, the possibility of gonadotropin independent sexual precocity should be reconsidered and appropriate examinations should be conducted. If compliance problems are excluded and if gonadotropin independent sexual precocity is not present, the dose of SYNAREL may be increased to 1800 µg/day administered as 600 µg TID.

PRECAUTIONS

General

As with other drugs that stimulate the release of gonadotropins or that induce ovulation, in adult women with endometriosis ovarian cysts have been reported to occur in the first two months of therapy with SYNAREL. Many, but not all, of these events occurred in women with polycystic ovarian disease. These cystic enlargements may resolve spontaneously, generally by about four to six weeks of therapy, but in some cases may require discontinuation of drug and/or surgical intervention. The relevance, if any, of such events in children is unknown.

Information for Patients, Patients' Parents or Guardians

An information pamphlet for patients is included with the product. Patients and their caregivers should be aware of the following information:

1. Reversibility of the suppressive effects of nafarelin has been demonstrated by the appearance or return of menses, by the return of pubertal gonadotropin and gonadal sex steroid levels, and/or by advancement of secondary sexual development. Semen analysis was normal in the two ejaculated specimens obtained thus far from boys who have been taken off therapy to resume puberty. Fertility has not been documented by pregnancies and the effect of long-term use of the drug on fertility is not known.
2. Patients and their caregivers should be adequately counseled to assure full compliance; irregular or incomplete daily doses may result in stimulation of the pituitary-gonadal axis.
3. During the first month of treatment with SYNAREL, some signs of puberty, e.g., vaginal bleeding or breast enlargement, may occur. This is the expected initial effect of the drug. Such changes should resolve soon after the first month. If such resolution does not occur within the first two months of treatment, this may be due to lack of compliance or the presence of gonadotropin independent sexual precocity. If both possibilities are definitively excluded, the dose of SYNAREL may be increased to 1800 µg/day administered as 600 µg TID.
4. Patients with intercurrent rhinitis should consult their physician for the use of a topical nasal decongestant. If the use of a topical nasal decongestant is required during treatment with SYNAREL, the decongestant should not be used until at least 2 hours following dosing with SYNAREL.
5. Sneezing during or immediately after dosing with SYNAREL should be avoided, if possible, since this may impair drug absorption.

Drug Interactions

No pharmacokinetic-based drug-drug interaction studies have been conducted with SYNAREL. However, because nafarelin acetate is a peptide that is primarily degraded by peptidase and not by cytochrome P-450 enzymes, and the drug is only about 80% bound to plasma proteins at 4°C, drug interactions would not be expected to occur.

Carcinogenesis, Mutagenesis, Impairment of Fertility

Carcinogenicity studies of nafarelin were conducted in rats (24 months) at doses up to 100 µg/kg/day and mice (18 months) at doses up to 500 µg/kg/day using intramuscular doses (up to 110 times and 560 times the maximum recommended human intranasal dose, respectively). These multiples of the human dose are based on the relative bioavailability of the drug by the two routes of administration. As seen with other GnRH agonists, nafarelin acetate given to laboratory rodents at high doses for prolonged periods induced proliferative responses (hyperplasia and/or neoplasia) of endocrine organs. At 24 months, there was an increase in the incidence of pituitary tumors (adenoma/carcinoma) in high-dose female rats and a dose-related increase in male rats. There was an increase in pancreatic islet cell adenomas in both sexes, and in benign testicular and ovarian tumors in the treated groups. There was a dose-related increase in benign adrenal medullary tumors in treated female rats. In mice, there was a dose-related increase in Harderian gland tumors in males and an increase in pituitary adenomas in high-dose females. No metastases of these tumors were observed. It is known that tumorigenicity in rodents is particularly sensitive to hormonal stimulation.

Mutagenicity studies were performed with nafarelin acetate using bacterial, yeast, and mammalian systems. These studies provided no evidence of mutagenic potential.

Reproduction studies in male and female rats have shown full reversibility of fertility suppression when drug treatment was discontinued after continuous administration for up to 6 months. The effect of treatment of prepubertal rats on the subsequent reproductive performance of mature animals has not been investigated.

Pregnancy, Teratogenic Effects

Pregnancy Category X. See *Contraindications* Section. Intramuscular SYNAREL was administered to rats during the period of organogenesis at 0.4, 1.6, and 6.4 µg/kg/day (about 0.5, 2, and 7 times the maximum recommended human intranasal dose based on the relative bioavailability by the two routes of administration). An increase in major fetal abnormalities was observed in 4/80 fetuses at the highest dose. A similar, repeat study at the same doses in rats and studies in mice and rabbits at doses up to 600 µg/kg/day and 0.18 µg/kg/day, respectively, failed to demonstrate an increase in fetal abnormalities after administration during the period of organogenesis. In rats and rabbits, there was a dose-related increase in fetal mortality and a decrease in fetal weight with the highest dose.

Nursing Mothers

It is not known whether SYNAREL is excreted in human milk. Because many drugs are excreted in human milk, and because the effects of SYNAREL on lactation and/or the breastfed child have not been determined, SYNAREL should not be used by nursing mothers.

ADVERSE REACTIONS

In clinical trials of 155 pediatric patients, 2.6% reported symptoms suggestive of drug sensitivity, such as shortness of breath, chest pain, urticaria, rash, and pruritus.

In these 155 patients treated for an average of 41 months and as long as 80 months (6.7 years), adverse events most frequently reported (>3% of patients) consisted largely of episodes occurring during the first 6 weeks of treatment as a result of the transient stimulatory action of nafarelin upon the pituitary-gonadal axis:

acne (10%)
transient breast enlargement (8%)
vaginal bleeding (8%)
emotional lability (6%)
transient increase in pubic hair (5%)
body odor (4%)
seborrhea (3%)

Hot flashes, common in adult women treated for endometriosis, occurred in only 3% of treated children and were transient. Other adverse events thought to be drug-related, and occurring in >3% of patients were rhinitis (5%) and white or brownish vaginal discharge (3%). Approximately 3% of patients withdrew from clinical trials due to adverse events.

In one male patient with concomitant congenital adrenal hyperplasia, and who had discontinued treatment 8 months previously to resume puberty, adrenal rest tumors were found in the left testis. Relationship to SYNAREL is unlikely.

Regular examinations of the pituitary gland by MRI or CT scanning of children during long-term nafarelin therapy as well as during the post-treatment period have occasionally revealed changes in the shape and size of the pituitary gland. These changes include asymmetry and enlargement of the pituitary gland, and a pituitary micro-adenoma has been suspected in a few children. The relationship of these findings to SYNAREL is not known.

OVERDOSAGE

In experimental animals, a single subcutaneous administration of up to 60 times the recommended human dose (on a µg/kg basis, not adjusted for bioavailability) had no adverse effects. At present, there is no clinical evidence of adverse effects following overdosage of GnRH analogs.

Based on studies in monkeys, SYNAREL is not absorbed after oral administration.

DOSAGE AND ADMINISTRATION

For the treatment of **central precocious puberty (CPP)**, the recommended daily dose of SYNAREL is 1600 µg. The dose can be increased to 1800 µg daily if adequate suppression cannot be achieved at 1600 µg/day.

The 1600 µg dose is achieved by two sprays (400 µg) into each nostril in the morning (4 sprays) and two sprays into each nostril in the evening (4 sprays), a total of 8 sprays per day. The 1800 µg dose is achieved by 3 sprays (600 µg) into alternating nostrils three times a day, a total of 9 sprays per day. The patient's head should be tilted back slightly, and 30 seconds should elapse between sprays.

If the prescribed therapy has been well tolerated by the patient, treatment of CPP with SYNAREL should continue until resumption of puberty is desired.

There appeared to be no significant effect of rhinitis, i.e., nasal congestion, on the systemic bioavailability of SYNAREL; however, if the use of a nasal decongestant for rhinitis is necessary during treatment with SYNAREL, the decongestant should not be used until at least 2 hours following dosing with SYNAREL.

Sneezing during or immediately after dosing with SYNAREL should be avoided, if possible, since this may impair drug absorption.

At 1600 µg/day, a bottle of SYNAREL provides about a 7-day supply (about 56 sprays). If the daily dose is increased, increase the supply to the patient to ensure uninterrupted treatment for the duration of therapy.

HOW SUPPLIED

Each 0.5 ounce bottle (NDC 0025-0166-10) contains 10 mL SYNAREL (nafarelin acetate) Nasal Solution 2 mg/mL (as nafarelin base) and is supplied with a metered spray pump that delivers 200 µg of nafarelin per spray. A dust cover and a leaflet of patient instructions are also included.

Store upright at room temperature. Avoid heat above 30°C (86°F). Protect from light. Protect from freezing.

CAUTION: Federal law prohibits dispensing without prescription.

U.S. Patent No. 4,234,571.

SEARLE

Manufactured for
G.D. Searle & Co.
Chicago IL 60680 USA November 1996
By Oread Pharmaceutical Manufacturing, Inc.

Palo Alto CA 94304 02-2260-00-02

SYNAREL® ℞

[*sin 'er-el*]
(nafarelin acetate)
Nasal Solution 2 mg/mL
(as nafarelin base)

ENDOMETRIOSIS
(FOR CENTRAL PRECOCIOUS PUBERTY,
SEE CENTRAL PRECOCIOUS PUBERTY SECTION)

DESCRIPTION

SYNAREL (nafarelin acetate) Nasal Solution is intended for administration as a spray to the nasal mucosa. Nafarelin acetate, the active component of SYNAREL Nasal Solution, is a decapeptide with the chemical name: 5-oxo-L-prolyl-L-histidyl-L-tryptophyl-L-seryl-L-tyrosyl- 3- (2-naphthyl) -D-alanyl-L-leucyl-L-arginyl-L-prolyl-glycinamide acetate. Nafarelin acetate is a synthetic analog of the naturally occurring gonadotropin-releasing hormone (GnRH).

Nafarelin acetate has the following chemical structure:

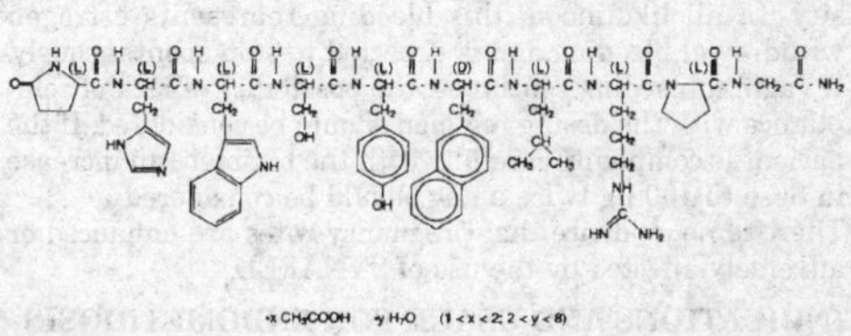

SYNAREL Nasal Solution contains nafarelin acetate (2 mg/mL, content expressed as nafarelin base) in a solution of benzalkonium chloride, glacial acetic acid, sodium hydroxide or hydrochloric acid (to adjust pH), sorbitol, and purified water.

After priming the pump unit for SYNAREL, each actuation of the unit delivers approximately 100 µL of the spray containing approximately 200 µg nafarelin base. The contents of one spray bottle are intended to deliver at least 60 sprays.

CLINICAL PHARMACOLOGY

Nafarelin acetate is a potent agonistic analog of gonadotropin-releasing hormone (GnRH). At the onset of administration, nafarelin stimulates the release of the pituitary gonadotropins, luteinizing hormone (LH) and follicle stimulating hormone (FSH), resulting in a temporary increase of ovarian steroidogenesis. Repeated dosing abolishes the stimulatory effect on the pituitary gland. Twice daily administration leads to decreased secretion of gonadal steroids by about 4 weeks; consequently, tissues and functions that depend on gonadal steroids for their maintenance become quiescent.

In **adult women**, nafarelin acetate is rapidly absorbed into the systemic circulation after intranasal administration. Maximum serum concentrations (measured by RIA) were achieved between 10 and 40 minutes. Following a single dose of 200 µg base, the observed average peak concentration was 0.6 ng/mL (range 0.2 to 1.4 ng/mL), whereas following a single dose of 400 µg base, the observed average peak concentration was 1.8 ng/mL (range 0.5 to 5.3 ng/mL). Bioavailability from a 400 µg dose averaged 2.8% (range 1.2 to 5.6%). The average serum half-life of nafarelin following intranasal administration is approximately 3 hours. About 80% of nafarelin acetate is bound to plasma proteins at 4°C. Twice daily intranasal administration of 200 or 400 µg of SYNAREL in 18 healthy women for 22 days did not lead to significant accumulation of the drug. Based on the mean C_{min} levels on Days 15 and 22, there appeared to be dose proportionality across the two dose levels.

After subcutaneous administration of ^{14}C-nafarelin acetate to men, 44-55% of the dose was recovered in urine and 18.5-44.2% was recovered in feces. Approximately 3% of the administered dose appeared as unchanged nafarelin in urine. The ^{14}C serum half-life of the metabolites was about 85.5 hours. Six metabolites of nafarelin have been identified of which the major metabolite is Tyr-D(2)-Nal-Leu-Arg-Pro-Gly-NH_2(5-10). The activity of the metabolites, the metabolism of nafarelin by nasal mucosa, and the pharmacokinetics of the drug in hepatically- and renally-impaired patients have not been determined.

There appeared to be no significant effect of rhinitis, i.e., nasal congestion, on the systemic bioavailability of SYNAREL; however, if the use of a nasal decongestant for rhinitis is necessary during treatment with SYNAREL, the decongestant should not be used until at least 2 hours following dosing of SYNAREL.

In controlled clinical studies, SYNAREL at doses of 400 and 800 µg/day for 6 months was shown to be comparable to danazol, 800 mg/day, in relieving the clinical symptoms of endometriosis (pelvic pain, dysmenorrhea, and dyspareunia) and in reducing the size of endometrial implants as de-

Continued on next page

Synarel for Endometriosis—Cont.

termined by laparoscopy. The clinical significance of a decrease in endometriotic lesions is not known at this time and, in addition, laparoscopic staging of endometriosis does not necessarily correlate with severity of symptoms.

SYNAREL 400 µg daily induced amenorrhea in approximately 65%, 80%, and 90% of the patients after 60, 90, and 120 days, respectively. In the first, second, and third post-treatment months, normal menstrual cycles resumed in 4%, 82%, and 100%, respectively, of those patients who did not become pregnant.

At the end of treatment, 60% of patients who received SYNAREL, 400 µg/day, were symptom free, 32% had mild symptoms, 7% had moderate symptoms, and 1% had severe symptoms. Of the 60% of patients who had complete relief of symptoms at the end of treatment, 17% had moderate symptoms 6 months after treatment was discontinued, 33% had mild symptoms, 50% remained symptom free, and no patient had severe symptoms.

During the first two months use of SYNAREL, some women experience vaginal bleeding of variable duration and intensity. In all likelihood, this bleeding represents estrogen withdrawal bleeding and is expected to stop spontaneously. If vaginal bleeding continues, the possibility of lack of compliance with the dosing regimen should be considered. If the patient is complying carefully with the regimen, an increase in dose to 400 µg twice a day should be considered.

There is no evidence that pregnancy rates are enhanced or adversely affected by the use of SYNAREL.

INDICATIONS AND USAGE FOR ENDOMETRIOSIS

(For Central Precocious Puberty, See Central Precocious Puberty section)

SYNAREL is indicated for management of endometriosis, including pain relief and reduction of endometriotic lesions. Experience with SYNAREL for the management of endometriosis has been limited to women 18 years of age and older treated for 6 months.

CONTRAINDICATIONS

1. Hypersensitivity to GnRH, GnRH agonist analogs or any of the excipients in SYNAREL;
2. Undiagnosed abnormal vaginal bleeding;
3. Use in pregnancy or in women who may become pregnant while receiving the drug. SYNAREL may cause fetal harm when administered to a pregnant woman. Major fetal abnormalities were observed in rats, but not in mice or rabbits, after administration of SYNAREL during the period of organogenesis. There was a dose-related increase in fetal mortality and a decrease in fetal weight in rats (see *Pregnancy* Section). The effects on rat fetal mortality are expected consequences of the alterations in hormonal levels brought about by the drug. If this drug is used during pregnancy or if the patient becomes pregnant while taking this drug, she should be apprised of the potential hazard to the fetus;
4. Use in women who are breast-feeding (see *Nursing Mothers* Section).

WARNINGS

Safe use of nafarelin acetate in pregnancy has not been established clinically. Before starting treatment with SYNAREL, pregnancy must be excluded.

When used regularly at the recommended dose, SYNAREL usually inhibits ovulation and stops menstruation. Contraception is not insured, however, by taking SYNAREL, particularly if patients miss successive doses. Therefore, patients should use nonhormonal methods of contraception. Patients should be advised to see their physician if they believe they may be pregnant. If a patient becomes pregnant during treatment, the drug must be discontinued and the patient must be apprised of the potential risk to the fetus.

PRECAUTIONS

General

As with other drugs that stimulate the release of gonadotropins or that induce ovulation, ovarian cysts have been reported to occur in the first 2 months of therapy with SYNAREL. Many, but not all, of these events occurred in patients with polycystic ovarian disease. These cystic enlargements may resolve spontaneously, generally by about 4 to 6 weeks of therapy, but in some cases may require discontinuation of drug and/or surgical intervention.

Information for Patients

An information pamphlet for patients is included with the product. Patients should be aware of the following information:

1. Since menstruation should stop with effective doses of SYNAREL, the patient should notify her physician if regular menstruation persists. The cause of vaginal spotting, bleeding or menstruation could be noncompliance with the treatment regimen, or it could be that a higher dose of the drug is required to achieve amenorrhea. The patient should be questioned regarding her compliance. If she is careful and compliant, and menstruation persists to the second month, consideration should be given to

doubling the dose of SYNAREL. If the patient has missed several doses, she should be counseled on the importance of taking SYNAREL regularly as prescribed.

2. Patients should not use SYNAREL if they are pregnant, breast-feeding, have undiagnosed abnormal vaginal bleeding, or are allergic to any of the ingredients in SYNAREL.
3. Safe use of the drug in pregnancy has not been established clinically. Therefore, a nonhormonal method of contraception should be used during treatment. Patients should be advised that if they miss successive doses of SYNAREL, breakthrough bleeding or ovulation may occur with the potential for conception. If a patient becomes pregnant during treatment, she should discontinue treatment and consult her physician.
4. Those adverse events occurring most frequently in clinical studies with SYNAREL are associated with hypoestrogenism; the most frequently reported are hot flashes, headaches, emotional lability, decreased libido, vaginal dryness, acne, myalgia, and reduction in breast size. Estrogen levels returned to normal after treatment was discontinued. Nasal irritation occurred in about 10% of all patients who used intranasal nafarelin.
5. The induced hypoestrogenic state results in a small loss in bone density over the course of treatment, some of which may not be reversible. During one six-month treatment period, this bone loss should not be important. In patients with major risk factors for decreased bone mineral content such as chronic alcohol and/or tobacco use, strong family history of osteoporosis, or chronic use of drugs that can reduce bone mass such as anticonvulsants or corticosteroids, therapy with SYNAREL may pose an additional risk. In these patients the risks and benefits must be weighed carefully before therapy with SYNAREL is instituted. Repeated courses of treatment with gonadotropin-releasing hormone analogs are not advisable in patients with major risk factors for loss of bone mineral content.
6. Patients with intercurrent rhinitis should consult their physician for the use of a topical nasal decongestant. If the use of a topical nasal decongestant is required during treatment with SYNAREL, the decongestant should not be used until at least 2 hours following dosing with SYNAREL.
7. Sneezing during or immediately after dosing with SYNAREL should be avoided, if possible, since this may impair drug absorption.
8. Retreatment cannot be recommended since safety data beyond 6 months are not available.

Drug Interactions

No pharmacokinetic-based drug-drug interaction studies have been conducted with SYNAREL. However, because nafarelin acetate is a peptide that is primarily degraded by peptidase and not by cytochrome P-450 enzymes, and the drug is only about 80% bound to plasma proteins at 4°C, drug interactions would not be expected to occur.

Drug/Laboratory Test Interactions

Administration of SYNAREL in therapeutic doses results in suppression of the pituitary-gonadal system. Normal function is usually restored within 4 to 8 weeks after treatment is discontinued. Therefore, diagnostic tests of pituitary gonadotropic and gonadal functions conducted during treatment and up to 4 to 8 weeks after discontinuation of therapy with SYNAREL may be misleading.

Carcinogenesis, Mutagenesis, Impairment of Fertility

Carcinogenicity studies of nafarelin were conducted in rats (24 months) at doses up to 100 µg/kg/day and mice (18 months) at doses up to 500 µg/kg/day using intramuscular doses (up to 110 times and 560 times the maximum recommended human intranasal dose, respectively). These multiples of the human dose are based on the relative bioavailability of the drug by the two routes of administration. As seen with other GnRH agonists, nafarelin acetate given to laboratory rodents at high doses for prolonged periods induced proliferative responses (hyperplasia and/or neoplasia) of endocrine organs. At 24 months, there was an increase in the incidence of pituitary tumors (adenoma/carcinoma) in high-dose female rats and a dose-related increase in male rats. There was an increase in pancreatic islet cell adenomas in both sexes, and in benign testicular and ovarian tumors in the treated groups. There was a dose-related increase in benign adrenal medullary tumors in treated female rats. In mice, there was a dose-related increase in Harderian gland tumors in males and an increase in pituitary adenomas in high-dose females. No metastases of these tumors were observed. It is known that tumorigenicity in rodents is particularly sensitive to hormonal stimulation. Mutagenicity studies were performed with nafarelin acetate using bacterial, yeast, and mammalian systems. These studies provided no evidence of mutagenic potential.

Reproduction studies in male and female rats have shown full reversibility of fertility suppression when drug treatment was discontinued after continuous administration for up to 6 months. The effect of treatment of prepubertal rats on the subsequent reproductive performance of mature animals has not been investigated.

Pregnancy, Teratogenic Effects

Pregnancy Category X. See Contraindications Section. Intramuscular SYNAREL was administered to rats during the period of organogenesis at 0.4, 1.6, and 6.4 µg/kg/day (about 0.5, 2, and 7 times the maximum recommended human intranasal dose based on the relative bioavailability by the two routes of administration). An increase in major fetal abnormalities was observed in 4/80 fetuses at the highest dose. A similar, repeat study at the same doses in rats and studies in mice and rabbits at doses up to 600 µg/kg/day and 0.18 µg/kg/day, respectively, failed to demonstrate an increase in fetal abnormalities after administration during the period of organogenesis. In rats and rabbits, there was a dose-related increase in fetal mortality and a decrease in fetal weight with the highest dose.

Nursing Mothers

It is not known whether SYNAREL is excreted in human milk. Because many drugs are excreted in human milk, and because the effects of SYNAREL on lactation and/or the breast-fed child have not been determined, SYNAREL should not be used by nursing mothers.

Pediatric Use

Safety and effectiveness of SYNAREL for endometriosis in patients younger than 18 years have not been established.

ADVERSE REACTIONS

As would be expected with a drug which lowers serum estradiol levels, the most frequently reported adverse reactions were those related to hypoestrogenism.

In controlled studies comparing SYNAREL (400 µg/day) and danazol (600 or 800 mg/day), adverse reactions most frequently reported and thought to be drug-related are shown in the figure below.

[See graphic below]

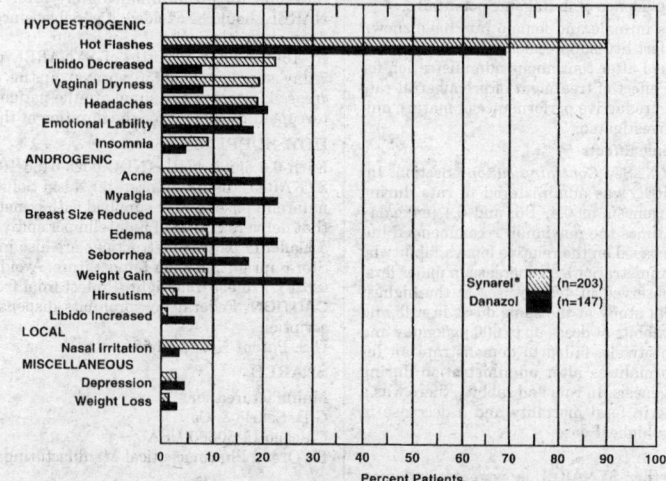

ADVERSE EVENTS DURING 6 MONTHS TREATMENT WITH SYNAREL® 400 µg/day vs DANAZOL 600 OR 800 mg/day

HYPOESTROGENIC
Hot Flashes
Libido Decreased
Vaginal Dryness
Headaches
Emotional Lability
Insomnia
ANDROGENIC
Acne
Myalgia
Breast Size Reduced
Edema
Seborrhea
Weight Gain
Hirsutism
Libido Increased
LOCAL
Nasal Irritation
MISCELLANEOUS
Depression
Weight Loss

Synarel* (n=203)
Danazol (n=147)

Percent Patients
0 10 20 30 40 50 60 70 80 90 100

In addition, less than 1% of patients experienced paresthesia, palpitations, chloasma, maculopapular rash, eye pain, urticaria, asthenia, lactation, breast engorgement, and arthralgia. In formal clinical trials, immediate hypersensitivity thought to be possibly or probably related to nafarelin occurred in 3 (0.2%) of 1509 healthy subjects or patients. During postmarketing surveillance of nafarelin, alopecia has been reported by some patients.

Changes in Bone Density

After six months of treatment with SYNAREL, vertebral trabecular bone density and total vertebral bone mass, measured by quantitative computed tomography (QCT), decreased by an average of 8.7% and 4.3%, respectively, compared to pretreatment levels. There was partial recovery of bone density in the post-treatment period; the average trabecular bone density and total bone mass were 4.9% and 3.3% less than the pretreatment levels, respectively. Total vertebral bone mass, measured by dual photon absorptiometry (DPA), decreased by a mean of 5.9% at the end of treatment. Mean total vertebral mass, re-examined by DPA six months after completion of treatment, was 1.4% below pretreatment levels. There was little, if any, decrease in the mineral content in compact bone of the distal radius and second metacarpal. Use of SYNAREL for longer than the recommended six months or in the presence of other known risk factors for decreased bone mineral content may cause additional bone loss.

Changes in Laboratory Values During Treatment

Plasma enzymes. During clinical trials with SYNAREL, regular laboratory monitoring revealed that SGOT and SGPT levels were more than twice the upper limit of normal in only one patient each. There was no other clinical or laboratory evidence of abnormal liver function and levels returned to normal in both patients after treatment was stopped.

Lipids. At enrollment, 9% of the patients in the group taking SYNAREL 400 µg/day and 2% of the patients in the danazol group had total cholesterol values above 250 mg/dL. These patients also had cholesterol values above 250 mg/dL at the end of treatment.

Of those patients whose pretreatment cholesterol values were below 250 mg/dL, 6% in the group treated with SYNAREL and 18% in the danazol group, had post-treatment values above 250 mg/dL.

The mean ($\pm$ SEM) pretreatment values for total cholesterol from all patients were 191.8 (4.3) mg/dL in the group treated with SYNAREL and 193.1 (4.6) mg/dL in the danazol group. At the end of treatment, the mean values for total cholesterol from all patients were 204.5 (4.8) mg/dL in the group treated with SYNAREL and 207.7 (5.1) mg/dL in the danazol group. These increases from the pretreatment values were statistically significant ($p<0.05$) in both groups.

Triglycerides were increased above the upper limit of 150 mg/dL in 12% of the patients who received SYNAREL and in 7% of the patients who received danazol.

At the end of treatment, no patients receiving SYNAREL had abnormally low HDL cholesterol fractions (less than 30 mg/dL) compared with 43% of patients receiving danazol. None of the patients receiving SYNAREL had abnormally high LDL cholesterol fractions (greater than 190 mg/dL) compared with 15% of those receiving danazol. There was no increase in the LDL/HDL ratio in patients receiving SYNAREL, but there was approximately a 2-fold increase in the LDL/HDL ratio in patients receiving danazol.

Other changes. In comparative studies, the following changes were seen in approximately 10% to 15% of patients. Treatment with SYNAREL was associated with elevations of plasma phosphorus and eosinophil counts, and decreases in serum calcium and WBC counts. Danazol therapy was associated with an increase of hematocrit and WBC.

OVERDOSAGE

In experimental animals, a single subcutaneous administration of up to 60 times the recommended human dose (on a µg/kg basis, not adjusted for bioavailability) had no adverse effects. At present, there is no clinical evidence of adverse effects following overdosage of GnRH analogs. Based on studies in monkeys, SYNAREL is not absorbed after oral administration.

DOSAGE AND ADMINISTRATION

For the management of endometriosis, the recommended daily dose of SYNAREL is 400 µg. This is achieved by one spray (200 µg) into one nostril in the morning and one spray into the other nostril in the evening. Treatment should be started between days 2 and 4 of the menstrual cycle.

In an occasional patient, the 400 µg daily dose may not produce amenorrhea. For these patients with persistent regular menstruation after 2 months of treatment, the dose of SYNAREL may be increased to 800 µg daily. The 800 µg dose is administered as one spray into each nostril in the morning (a total of two sprays) and again in the evening. The recommended duration of administration is six months. Retreatment cannot be recommended since safety data for retreatment are not available. If the symptoms of endometriosis recur after a course of therapy, and further treatment

with SYNAREL is contemplated, it is recommended that bone density be assessed before retreatment begins to ensure that values are within normal limits.

There appeared to be no significant effect of rhinitis, i.e., nasal congestion, on the systemic bioavailability of SYNAREL; however, if the use of a nasal decongestant for rhinitis is necessary during treatment with SYNAREL, the decongestant should not be used until at least 2 hours following dosing with SYNAREL.

Sneezing during or immediately after dosing with SYNAREL should be avoided, if possible, since this may impair drug absorption.

At 400 µg/day, a bottle of SYNAREL provides a 30-day (about 60 sprays) supply. If the daily dose is increased, increase the supply to the patient to ensure uninterrupted treatment for the recommended duration of therapy.

HOW SUPPLIED

Each 0.5 ounce bottle (NDC 0025-0166-10) contains 10 mL SYNAREL (nafarelin acetate) Nasal Solution 2 mg/mL (as nafarelin base) and is supplied with a metered spray pump that delivers 200 µg of nafarelin per spray. A dust cover and a leaflet of patient instructions are also included.

Store upright at room temperature. Avoid heat above 30°C (86°F). Protect from light. Protect from freezing.

CAUTION: Federal law prohibits dispensing without prescription.

U.S. Patent No. 4,234,571.

SEARLE
Manufactured for
G.D. Searle & Co.
Chicago IL 60680 USA   November 1996
by Oread Pharmaceutical Manufacturing, Inc.

©1996, Searle
Palo Alto CA 94304   02-2260-00-02

TRI-NORINYL®-21   ℞
(norethindrone and ethinyl estradiol)
TRI-NORINYL®-28   ℞
(norethindrone and ethinyl estradiol)

PHYSICIAN LABELING

Patients should be counseled that this product does not protect against HIV infection (AIDS) and other sexually transmitted diseases.

ORAL CONTRACEPTIVE AGENTS

DESCRIPTION

TRI-NORINYL 21-DAY Tablets provide an oral contraceptive regimen of 7 blue tablets followed by 9 yellow-green tablets and 5 more blue tablets. Each blue tablet contains norethindrone 0.5 mg and ethinyl estradiol 0.035 mg and each yellow-green tablet contains norethindrone 1 mg and ethinyl estradiol 0.035 mg.

TRI-NORINYL 28-DAY Tablets provide a continuous oral contraceptive regimen of 7 blue tablets, 9 yellow-green tablets, 5 more blue tablets, and then 7 orange tablets. Each blue tablet contains norethindrone 0.5 mg and ethinyl estradiol 0.035 mg, each yellow-green tablet contains norethindrone 1 mg and ethinyl estradiol 0.035 mg, and each orange tablet contains inert ingredients.

Norethindrone is a potent progestational agent with the chemical name 17-Hydroxy-19-nor-17α-pregn-4-en-20-yn-3-one. Ethinyl estradiol is an estrogen with the chemical name 19-Nor-17α-pregna-1, 3, 5(10) -trien-20-yne-3, 17-diol. Their structural formulae follow:

norethindrone

ethinyl estradiol

The yellow-green TRI-NORINYL tablets contain the following inactive ingredients: D&C Green No. 5, D&C Yellow No. 10, lactose, magnesium stearate, povidone, and starch.

The blue TRI-NORINYL tablets contain the following inactive ingredients: FD&C Blue No. 1, lactose, magnesium stearate, povidone, and starch.

The inactive orange tablets in the 28-day regimen contain the following inactive ingredients: FD&C Yellow No. 6, lactose, magnesium stearate, povidone, and starch.

CLINICAL PHARMACOLOGY

Combination oral contraceptives act by suppression of gonadotrophins. Although the primary mechanism of this action is inhibition of ovulation, other alterations include changes in the cervical mucus (which increase the difficulty of sperm entry into the uterus) and the endometrium (which may reduce the likelihood of implantation).

INDICATIONS AND USAGE

Oral contraceptives are indicated for the prevention of pregnancy in women who elect to use these products as a method of contraception.

Oral contraceptives are highly effective. Table I lists the typical accidental pregnancy rates for users of combination oral contraceptives and other methods of contraception.[1] The efficacy of these contraceptive methods, except sterilization, depends upon the reliability with which they are used. Correct and consistent use of methods can result in lower failure rates.

TABLE 1: PERCENTAGE OF WOMEN EXPERIENCING A CONTRACEPTIVE FAILURE DURING THE FIRST YEAR OF PERFECT USE AND FIRST YEAR OF TYPICAL USE

Method	% of Women Experiencing an Accidental Pregnancy within the First Year of Use	
	Typical Use[a]	Perfect Use[b]
Chance	85	85
Spermacides	21	6
Periodic Abstinence	20	1–9
Withdrawal	19	4
Cap		
Parous	36	26
Nulliparous	18	9
Sponge		
Parous	36	20
Nulliparous	18	9
Diaphragm	18	6
Condom		
Female	21	5
Male	12	3
Pill	3	
Progestin only		0.5
Combined		0.1
IUD		
Progesterone	2	1.5
Copper T 380A	0.8	0.6
Injection	0.3	0.3
(Depo-Provera)		
Impants (Norplant)	0.09	0.09
Female sterilization	0.4	0.4
Male sterilization	0.15	0.10

Adapted with permission[1].

---

[a]Among *typical* couples who initiate use of a method (not necessarily for the first time), the percentage who experience an accidental pregnancy during the first year if they do not stop use for any other reason.

[b]Amoung couples who initiate use of a method (not necessarily for the first time) and who use it *perfectly* (both consistently and correctly), the percentage who experience an accidental pregnancy during the first year if they do not stop use for any other reason.

CONTRAINDICATIONS

Oral contraceptives should not be used in women who have the following conditions:

- Thrombophlebitis or thromboembolic disorders
- A past history of deep vein thrombophlebitis or thromboembolic disorders
- Cerebral vascular or coronary artery disease
- Known or suspected carcinoma of the breast
- Carcinoma of the endometrium, or other known or suspected estrogen-dependent neoplasia
- Undiagnosed abnormal genital bleeding
- Cholestatic jaundice of pregnancy or jaundice with prior pill use
- Hepatic adenomas, carcinomas or benign liver tumors
- Known or suspected pregnancy

WARNINGS

Cigarette smoking increases the risk of serious cardiovascular side effects from oral contraceptive use. This risk increases with age and with heavy smoking (15 or more cigarettes per day) and is quite

Continued on next page

Tri-Norinyl—Cont.

marked in women over 35 years of age. Women who use oral contraceptives should be strongly advised not to smoke.

The use of oral contraceptives is associated with increased risks of several serious conditions including myocardial infarction, thromboembolism, stroke, hepatic neoplasia and gallbladder disease, although the risk of serious morbidity or mortality is very small in healthy women without underlying risk factors. The risk of morbidity and mortality increases significantly in the presence of other underlying risk factors such as hypertension, hyperlipidemias, hypercholesterolemia, obesity and diabetes.[2–5]

Practitioners prescribing oral contraceptives should be familiar with the following information relating to these risks.

The information contained in this package insert is principally based on studies carried out in patients who used oral contraceptives with higher formulations of both estrogens and progestogens than those in common use today.[6–11] The effect of long-term use of the oral contraceptives with lower formulations of both estrogens and progestogens remains to be determined.

Throughout this labeling, epidemiological studies reported are of two types: retrospective or case control studies and prospective or cohort studies. Case control studies provide a measure of the relative risk of a disease. Relative risk, the *ratio* of the incidence of a disease among oral contraceptive users to that among non-users, cannot be assessed directly from case control studies, but the odds ratio obtained is a measure of relative risk. The relative risk does not provide information on the actual clinical occurrence of a disease. Cohort studies provide not only a measure of the relative risk but a measure of attributable risk, which is the *difference* in the incidence of disease between oral contraceptive users and non-users. The attributable risk does provide information about the actual occurrence of a disease in the population. (Adapted from ref. 12 and 13 with the author's permission.) For further information, the reader is referred to a text on epidemiological methods.

1. THROMBOEMBOLIC DISORDERS AND OTHER VASCULAR PROBLEMS

a. Myocardial Infarction

An increased risk of myocardial infarction has been attributed to oral contraceptive use. This risk is primarily in smokers or women with other underlying risk factors for coronary artery disease such as hypertension, hypercholesterolemia, morbid obesity and diabetes.[2–5,13] The relative risk of heart attack for current oral contraceptive users has been estimated to be 2 to 6.[2,14–19] The risk is very low under the age of 30. However, there is the possibility of a risk of cardiovascular disease even in very young women who take oral contraceptives.

Smoking in combination with oral contraceptive use has been shown to contribute substantially to the incidence of myocardial infarctions in women in their mid-thirties or older, with smoking accounting for the majority of excess cases.[20]

Mortality rates associated with circulatory disease have been shown to increase substantially in smokers over the age of 35 and non-smokers over the age of 40 among women who use oral contraceptives (see Table II).[16]

TABLE II: CIRCULATORY DISEASE MORTALITY RATES PER 100,000 WOMAN YEARS BY AGE, SMOKING STATUS AND ORAL CONTRACEPTIVE USE

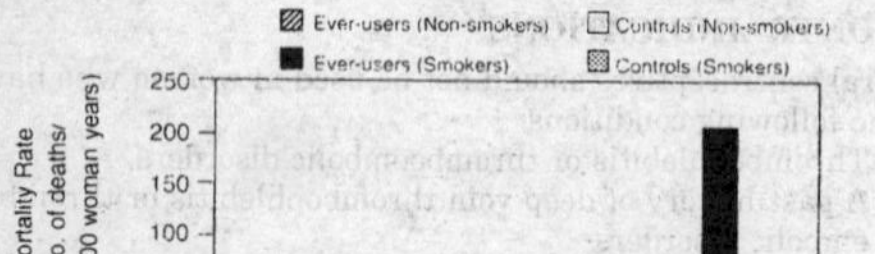

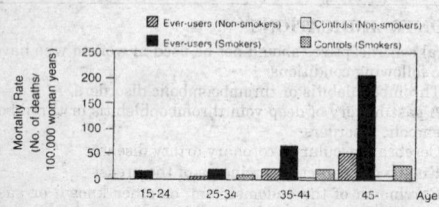

Adapted from P.M. Layde and V. Beral, Table V[16]

Oral contraceptives may compound the effects of well-known risk factors such as hypertension, diabetes, hyperlipidemias, hypercholesterolemia, age and obesity.[3,13,21] In particular, some progestogens are known to decrease HDL cholesterol and cause glucose intolerance, while estrogens may create a state of hyperinsulinism.[21–25] Oral contraceptives have been shown to increase blood pressure among users (see **WARNINGS**, section 9). Similar effects on risk factors have been associated with an increased risk of heart disease. Oral contraceptives must be used with caution in women with cardiovascular disease risk factors.

b. Thromboembolism

An increased risk of thromboembolic and thrombotic disease associated with the use of oral contraceptives is well established. Case control studies have found the relative risk of users compared to non-users to be 3 for the first episode of superficial venous thrombosis, 4 to 11 for deep vein thrombosis or pulmonary embolism, and 1.5 to 6 for women with predisposing conditions for venous thromboembolic disease.[12,13,26–31] Cohort studies have shown the relative risk to be somewhat lower, about 3 for new cases and about 4.5 for new cases requiring hospitalization.[32] The risk of thromboembolic disease due to oral contraceptives is not related to length of use and disappears after pill use is stopped.[12]

A 2-to 6-fold increase in relative risk of post-operative thromboembolic complications has been reported with the use of oral contraceptives. The relative risk of venous thrombosis in women who have predisposing conditions is twice that of women without such medical conditions.[83] If feasible, oral contraceptives should be discontinued at least 4 weeks prior to and for 2 weeks after elective surgery and during and following prolonged immobilization. Since the immediate postpartum period also is associated with an increased risk of thromboembolism, oral contraceptives should be started no earlier than 4 to 6 weeks after delivery in women who elect not to breast feed.[33]

c. Cerebrovascular diseases

An increase in both the relative and attributable risks of cerebrovascular events (thrombotic and hemorrhagic strokes) has been shown in users of oral contraceptives. In general, the risk is greatest among older (>35 years), hypertensive women who also smoke. Hypertension was found to be a risk factor for both users and non-users for both types of strokes while smoking interacted to increase the risk for hemorrhagic strokes.[34]

In a large study, the relative risk of thrombotic strokes has been shown to range from 3 for normotensive users to 14 for users with severe hypertension.[35] The relative risk of hemorrhagic stroke is reported to be 1.2 for non-smokers who used oral contraceptives, 2.6 for smokers who did not use oral contraceptives, 7.6 for smokers who used oral contraceptives, 1.8 for normotensive users and 25.7 for users with severe hypertension.[35] The attributable risk also is greater in women in their mid-thirties or older and among smokers.[13]

d. Dose-related risk of vascular disease from oral contraceptives

A positive association has been observed between the amount of estrogen and progestogen in oral contraceptives and the risk of vascular disease.[36–38] A decline in serum high density lipoproteins (HDL) has been reported with many progestational agents.[22–24] A decline in serum high density lipoproteins has been associated with an increased incidence of ischemic heart disease.[39] Because estrogens increase HDL cholesterol, the net effect of an oral contraceptive depends on a balance achieved between doses of estrogen and progestogen and the nature and absolute amount of progestogens used in the contraceptives. The amount of both hormones should be considered in the choice of an oral contraceptive.[37]

Minimizing exposure to estrogen and progestogen is in keeping with good principles of therapeutics. For any particular estrogen/progestogen combination, the dosage regimen prescribed should be one which contains the least amount of estrogen and progestogen that is compatible with a low failure rate and the needs of the individual patient. New acceptors of oral contraceptive agents should be started on preparations containing the lowest estrogen content that produces satisfactory results for the individual.

e. Persistence of risk of vascular disease

There are three studies which have shown persistence of risk of vascular disease for ever-users of oral contraceptives.[17,34,40] In a study in the United States, the risk of developing myocardial infarction after discontinuing oral contraceptives persists for at least 9 years for women 40–49 years who had used oral contraceptives for 5 or more years, but this increased risk was not demonstrated in other age groups.[17] In another study in Great Britain, the risk of developing cerebrovascular disease persisted for at least 6 years after discontinuation of oral contraceptives, although excess risk was very small.[40] There is a significantly increased relative risk of subarachnoid hemorrhage after termination of use of oral contraceptives.[34] However, these studies were performed with oral contraceptive formulations containing 50 µg or higher of estrogen.

2. ESTIMATES OF MORTALITY FROM CONTRACEPTIVE USE

One study gathered data from a variety of sources which have estimated the mortality rates associated with different methods of contraception at different ages (see Table III).[41] These estimates include the combined risk of death associated with contraceptive methods plus the risk attributable to pregnancy in the event of method failure. Each method of contraception has its specific benefits and risks. The study concluded that with the exception of oral contraceptive users 35 and older who smoke and 40 and older who do not smoke, mortality associated with all methods of birth control is low and below that associated with childbirth. The observation of a possible increase in risk of mortality with age for oral contraceptive users is based on data gathered in the 1970's—but not reported in the U.S. until 1983.[16,41] However, current clinical practice involves the use of lower estrogen dose formulations combined with careful restriction of oral contraceptive use to women who do not have the various risk factors listed in this labeling.

Because of these changes in practice and, also, because of some limited new data which suggest that the risk of cardiovascular disease with the use of oral contraceptives may now be less than previously observed,[78,79] the Fertility and Maternal Health Drugs Advisory Committee was asked to review the topic in 1989. The Committee concluded that although cardiovascular disease risks may be increased with oral contraceptive use after age 40 in healthy non-smoking women (even with the newer low-dose formulations), there are greater potential health risks associated with pregnancy in older women and with the alternative surgical and medical procedures which may be necessary if such women do not have access to effective and acceptable means of contraception.

Therefore, the Committee recommended that the benefits of oral contraceptive use by healthy non-smoking women over 40 may outweigh the possible risks. Of course, older women, as all women who take oral contraceptives, should take the lowest possible dose formulation that is effective.[80]

[See table III below]

3. CARCINOMA OF THE BREAST AND REPRODUCTIVE ORGANS

Numerous epidemiological studies have been performed on the incidence of breast, endometrial, ovarian and cervical cancer in women using oral contraceptives. The overwhelming evidence in the literature suggests that use of oral contraceptives is not associated with an increase in the risk of developing breast cancer, regardless of the age and parity of first use or with most of the marketed brands and doses.[42–44] The Cancer and Steroid Hormone (CASH) study also showed no latent effect on the risk of breast cancer for at least a decade following long-term use.[43] A few studies have shown a slightly increased relative risk of developing breast cancer,[44–47] although the methodology of these studies, which included differences in examination of users and non-users and differences in age at start of use, has been questioned.[47–49] Some studies have reported an increased relative risk of developing breast cancer, particularly at a younger age. This increased relative risk appears to be related to duration of use.[81,82]

Some studies suggest that oral contraceptive use has been associated with an increase in the risk of cervical intraepithelial neoplasia in some populations of women.[50–53] How-

TABLE III: ESTIMATED ANNUAL NUMBER OF BIRTH-RELATED OR METHOD-RELATED DEATHS ASSOCIATED WITH CONTROL OF FERTILITY PER 100,000 NONSTERILE WOMEN, BY FERTILITY CONTROL METHOD ACCORDING TO AGE

Method of control and outcome	15–19	20–24	25–29	30–34	35–39	40–44
No fertility control methods*	7.0	7.4	9.1	14.8	25.7	28.2
Oral contraceptives non-smoker**	0.3	0.5	0.9	1.9	13.8	31.6
Oral contraceptives smoker**	2.2	3.4	6.6	13.5	51.1	117.2
IUD**	0.8	0.8	1.0	1.0	1.4	1.4
Condom*	1.1	1.6	0.7	0.2	0.3	0.4
Diaphragm/Spermicide*	1.9	1.2	1.2	1.3	2.2	2.8
Periodic abstinence*	2.5	1.6	1.6	1.7	2.9	3.6

* Deaths are birth-related
** Deaths are method-related

Estimates adapted from H.W. Ory, Table 3 [41]

ever, there continues to be controversy about the extent to which such findings may be due to differences in sexual behavior and other factors.

In spite of many studies of the relationship between oral contraceptive use and breast or cervical cancers, a cause and effect relationship has not been established.

4. HEPATIC NEOPLASIA

Benign hepatic adenomas are associated with oral contraceptive use although the incidence of benign tumors is rare in the United States. Indirect calculations have estimated the attributable risk to be in the range of 3.3 cases per 100,000 for users, a risk that increases after 4 or more years of use.[54] Rupture of rare, benign, hepatic adenomas may cause death through intra-abdominal hemorrhage.[55–56]

Studies in the United States and Britain have shown an increased risk of developing hepatocellular carcinoma in long-term (>8 years) oral contraceptive users.[57–59] However, these cancers are extremely rare in the United States and the attributable risk (the excess incidence) of liver cancers in oral contraceptive users is less than 1 per 1,000,000 users.

5. OCULAR LESIONS

There have been clinical case reports of retinal thrombosis associated with the use of oral contraceptives. Oral contraceptives should be discontinued if there is unexplained partial or complete loss of vision; onset of proptosis or diplopia; papilledema; or retinal vascular lesions. Appropriate diagnostic and therapeutic measures should be undertaken immediately.

6. ORAL CONTRACEPTIVE USE BEFORE OR DURING EARLY PREGNANCY

Extensive epidemiological studies have revealed no increased risk of birth defects in women who have used oral contraceptives prior to pregnancy.[60–62] Studies also do not suggest a teratogenic effect, particularly insofar as cardiac anomalies and limb reduction defects are concerned, when taken inadvertently during early pregnancy.[60,61,63,64]

The administration of oral contraceptives to induce withdrawal bleeding should not be used as a test for pregnancy. Oral contraceptives should not be used during pregnancy to treat threatened or habitual abortion.

It is recommended that for any patient who has missed 2 consecutive periods, pregnancy should be ruled out before continuing oral contraceptive use. If the patient has not adhered to the prescribed schedule, the possibility of pregnancy should be considered at the time of the first missed period. Oral contraceptive use should be discontinued if pregnancy is confirmed.

7. GALLBLADDER DISEASE

Earlier studies have reported an increased lifetime relative risk of gallbladder surgery in users of oral contraceptives and estrogens.[65–66] More recent studies, however, have shown that the relative risk of developing gallbladder disease among oral contraceptive users may be minimal.[67] The recent findings of minimal risk may be related to the use of oral contraceptive formulations containing lower hormonal doses of estrogens and progestogens.[68]

8. CARBOHYDRATE AND LIPID METABOLIC EFFECTS

Oral contraceptives have been shown to cause glucose intolerance in a significant percentage of users.[25] Oral contraceptives containing greater than 75 µg of estrogen cause hyperinsulinism, while lower doses of estrogen cause produce less glucose intolerance.[70] Progestogens increase insulin secretion and create insulin resistance, this effect varying with different progestational agents.[25,71] However, in the non-diabetic woman, oral contraceptives appear to have no effect on fasting blood glucose.[69] Because of these demonstrated effects, prediabetic and diabetic women should be carefully observed while taking oral contraceptives.

Some women may develop persistent hypertriglyceridemia while on the pill.[72] As discussed earlier (see **WARNINGS**, sections 1a. and 1d.), changes in serum triglycerides and lipoprotein levels have been reported in oral contraceptive users.[23]

9. ELEVATED BLOOD PRESSURE

An increase in blood pressure has been reported in women taking oral contraceptives and this increase is more likely in older oral contraceptive users and with continued use.[73,84] Data from the Royal College of General Practitioners and subsequent randomized trials have shown that the incidence of hypertension increases with increasing concentrations of progestogens.

Women with a history of hypertension or hypertension-related diseases or renal disease should be encouraged to use another method of contraception. If women elect to use oral contraceptives, they should be monitored closely and if significant elevation of blood pressure occurs oral contraceptives should be discontinued. For most women, elevated blood pressure will return to normal after stopping oral contraceptives and there is no difference in the occurrence of hypertension among ever- and never-users.[73–75]

10. HEADACHE

The onset or exacerbation of migraine or development of headache with a new pattern which is recurrent, persistent or severe requires discontinuation of oral contraceptives and evaluation of the cause.

11. BLEEDING IRREGULARITIES

Breakthrough bleeding and spotting are sometimes encountered in patients on oral contraceptives, especially during the first 3 months of use. Non-hormonal causes should be considered and adequate diagnostic measures taken to rule out malignancy or pregnancy in the event of breakthrough bleeding, as in the case of any abnormal vaginal bleeding. If pathology has been excluded, time or a change to another formulation may solve the problem. In the event of amenorrhea, pregnancy should be ruled out.

Some women may encounter post-pill amenorrhea or oligomenorrhea, especially when such a condition was pre-existent.

PRECAUTIONS

GENERAL

Patients Should Be Counseled That This Product Does Not Protect Against HIV infection (AIDS) And Other Sexually Transmitted Diseases.

1. PHYSICAL EXAMINATION AND FOLLOW-UP

It is good medical practice for all women to have annual history and physical examinations, including women using oral contraceptives. The physical examination, however, may be deferred until after initiation of oral contraceptives if requested by the woman and judged appropriate by the clinician. The physical examination should include special reference to blood pressure, breasts, abdomen and pelvic organs, including cervical cytology, and relevant laboratory tests. In case of undiagnosed, persistent or recurrent abnormal vaginal bleeding, appropriate measures should be conducted to rule out malignancy. Women with a strong family history of breast cancer or who have breast nodules should be monitored with particular care.

2. LIPID DISORDERS

Women who are being treated for hyperlipidemias should be followed closely if they elect to use oral contraceptives. Some progestogens may elevate LDL levels and may render the control of hyperlipidemias more difficult.

3. LIVER FUNCTION

If jaundice develops in any woman receiving oral contraceptives the medication should be discontinued. Steroid hormones may be poorly metabolized in patients with impaired liver function.

4. FLUID RETENTION

Oral contraceptives may cause some degree of fluid retention. They should be prescribed with caution, and only with careful monitoring, in patients with conditions which might be aggravated by fluid retention.

5. EMOTIONAL DISORDERS

Women with a history of depression should be carefully observed and the drug discontinued if depression recurs to a serious degree.

6. CONTACT LENSES

Contact lens wearers who develop visual changes or changes in lens tolerance should be assessed by an ophthalmologist.

7. DRUG INTERACTIONS

Reduced efficacy and increased incidence of breakthrough bleeding and menstrual irregularities have been associated with concomitant use of rifampin. A similar association, though less marked, has been suggested with barbiturates, phenylbutazone, phenytoin sodium, and possibly with griseofulvin, ampicillin and tetracyclines.[76]

8. INTERACTIONS WITH LABORATORY TESTS

Certain endocrine and liver function tests and blood components may be affected by oral contraceptives:

a. Increased prothrombin and factors VII, VIII, IX, and X; decreased antithrombin 3; increased norepinephrine-induced platelet aggregability.

b. Increased thyroid binding globulin (TBG) leading to increased circulating total thyroid hormone, as measured by protein-bound iodine (PBI), T4 by column or by radioimmunoassay. Free T3 resin uptake is decreased, reflecting the elevated TBG. Free T4 concentration is unaltered.

c. Other binding proteins may be elevated in serum.

d. Sex steroid binding globulins are increased and result in elevated levels of total circulating sex steroids and corticoids; however, free or biologically active levels remain unchanged.

e. Triglycerides may be increased.

f. Glucose tolerance may be decreased.

g. Serum folate levels may be depressed by oral contraceptive therapy. This may be of clinical significance if a woman becomes pregnant shortly after discontinuing oral contraceptives.

9. CARCINOGENESIS

See **WARNINGS** section.

10. PREGNANCY

Pregnancy Category X. See **CONTRAINDICATIONS** and **WARNINGS** sections.

11. NURSING MOTHERS

Small amounts of oral contraceptive steroids have been identified in the milk of nursing mothers and a few adverse effects on the child have been reported, including jaundice and breast enlargement. In addition, oral contraceptives given in the postpartum period may interfere with lactation by decreasing the quantity and quality of breast milk. If possible, the nursing mother should be advised not to use oral contraceptives but to use other forms of contraception until she has completely weaned her child.

12. PEDIATRIC USE

Safety and effectiveness in pediatric patients have not been established.

INFORMATION FOR THE PATIENT

See **PATIENT LABELING** printed below.

ADVERSE REACTIONS

An increased risk of the following serious adverse reactions has been associated with the use of oral contraceptives (see **WARNINGS** section):

• Thrombophlebitis
• Arterial thromboembolism
• Pulmonary embolism
• Myocardial infarction
• Cerebral hemorrhage
• Cerebral thrombosis
• Hypertension
• Gallbladder disease
• Hepatic adenomas, carcinomas or benign liver tumors

There is evidence of an association between the following conditions and the use of oral contraceptives, although additional confirmatory studies are needed:

• Mesenteric thrombosis
• Retinal thrombosis

The following adverse reactions have been reported in patients receiving oral contraceptives and are believed to be drug-related:

• Nausea
• Vomiting
• Gastrointestinal symptoms (such as abdominal cramps and bloating)
• Breakthrough bleeding
• Spotting
• Change in menstrual flow
• Amenorrhea
• Temporary infertility after discontinuation of treatment
• Edema
• Melasma which may persist
• Breast changes: tenderness, enlargement, secretion
• Change in weight (increase or decrease)
• Change in cervical erosion and secretion
• Diminution in lactation when given immediately postpartum
• Cholestatic jaundice
• Migraine
• Rash (allergic)
• Mental depression
• Reduced tolerance to carbohydrates
• Vaginal candidiasis
• Change in corneal curvature (steepening)
• Intolerance to contact lenses

The following adverse reactions have been reported in users of oral contraceptives and the association has been neither confirmed nor refuted:

• Pre-menstrual syndrome
• Cataracts
• Changes in appetite
• Cystitis-like syndrome
• Headache
• Nervousness
• Dizziness
• Hirsutism
• Loss of scalp hair
• Erythema multiforme
• Erythema nodosum
• Hemorrhagic eruption
• Vaginitis
• Porphyria
• Impaired renal function
• Hemolytic uremic syndrome
• Budd-Chiari syndrome
• Acne
• Changes in libido
• Colitis

OVERDOSAGE

Serious ill effects have not been reported following acute ingestion of large doses of oral contraceptives by young children. Overdosage may cause nausea, and withdrawal bleeding may occur in females.

NON-CONTRACEPTIVE HEALTH BENEFITS

The following non-contraceptive health benefits related to the use of oral contraceptives are supported by epidemiological studies which largely utilized oral contraceptive formulations containing estrogen doses exceeding 0.035 mg of ethinyl estradiol or 0.05 mg of mestranol.[6–11]

Effects on menses:

Continued on next page

Tri-Norinyl—Cont.

- Increased menstrual cycle regularity
- Decreased blood loss and decreased incidence of iron deficiency anemia
- Decreased incidence of dysmenorrhea

Effects related to inhibition of ovulation:
- Decreased incidence of functional ovarian cysts
- Decreased incidence of ectopic pregnancies

Effects from long-term use:
- Decreased incidence of fibroadenomas and fibrocystic disease of the breast
- Decreased incidence of acute pelvic inflammatory disease
- Decreased incidence of endometrial cancer
- Decreased incidence of ovarian cancer

DOSAGE AND ADMINISTRATION

To achieve maximum contraceptive effectiveness, oral contraceptives must be taken exactly as directed and at intervals not exceeding 24 hours.

21-Day Schedule: For a DAY 1 START, count the first day of menstrual flow as Day 1 and the first blue tablet is then taken on Day 1. For a SUNDAY START when menstrual flow begins on or before Sunday, the first blue tablet is taken on that day. With either a DAY 1 START or SUNDAY START, 1 blue tablet is taken for 7 days, then 1 yellow-green tablet for 9 days, then 1 blue tablet for 5 days. With either a DAY 1 START or SUNDAY START 1 tablet is taken each day at the same time for 21 days. No tablets are taken for 7 days, then, whether bleeding has stopped or not, a new course is started of 1 tablet a day for 21 days. This institutes a 3 weeks on, 1 week off dosage regimen.

28-Day Schedule: For a DAY 1 START, count the first day of menstrual flow as Day 1 and the first blue tablet is then taken on Day 1. For a SUNDAY START when menstrual flow begins on or before Sunday, the first blue tablet is taken on that day. With either a DAY 1 START or SUNDAY START, 1 blue tablet is taken for 7 days, then 1 yellow-green tablet for 9 days, then 1 blue tablet for 5 days, then 1 orange tablet (inert) for 7 days, whether bleeding has stopped or not. With either a DAY 1 START or SUNDAY START 1 tablet is taken each day at the same time for 28 days. After all 28 tablets are taken, whether bleeding has stopped or not, the same dosage schedule is repeated beginning on the following day.

INSTRUCTIONS TO PATIENTS

- To achieve maximum contraceptive effectiveness, the oral contraceptive pill must be taken exactly as directed and at intervals not exceeding 24 hours.
- Important: Women should be instructed to use an additional method of protection until after the first 7 days of administration *in the initial cycle.*
- Due to the normally increased risk of thromboembolism occurring postpartum, women should be instructed not to initiate treatment with oral contraceptives earlier than 4 weeks after a full-term delivery. If pregnancy is terminated in the first 12 weeks, the patient should be instructed to start oral contraceptives immediately or within 7 days. If pregnancy is terminated after 12 weeks, the patient should be instructed to start oral contraceptives after 2 weeks.[33,77]
- If spotting or breakthrough bleeding should occur, the patient should continue the medication according to the schedule. Should spotting or breakthrough bleeding persist, the patient should notify her physician.
- If the patient misses 1 pill, she should be instructed to take it as soon as she remembers and then take the next pill at the regular time. The patient should be advised that missing a pill can cause spotting or light bleeding and that she may be a little sick to her stomach on the days she takes the missed pill with her regularly scheduled pill. If the patient has missed more than one pill, see **DETAILED PATIENT LABELING:** HOW TO TAKE THE PILL, WHAT TO DO IF YOU MISS PILLS.
- Use of oral contraceptives in the event of a missed menstrual period:

  1. If the patient has not adhered to the prescribed dosage regimen, the possibility of pregnancy should be considered after the first missed period and oral contraceptives should be withheld until pregnancy has been ruled out.
  2. If the patient has adhered to the prescribed regimen and misses 2 consecutive periods, pregnancy should be ruled out before continuing the contraceptive regimen.

HOW SUPPLIED

TRI-NORINYL®-21 Tablets and TRI-NORINYL®-28 Tablets (norethindrone and ethinyl estradiol) are available in 21-tablet or 28-tablet blister cards with a WALLETTE® tablet dispenser. Each 28-tablet card contains 7 orange inert tablets.

CAUTION: Federal law prohibits dispensing without prescription.

Store at controlled room temperature 15–25°C (59–77°F).

REFERENCES

1. Hatcher, R.A. Trussell, J. Stewart, F., et al.: *Contraceptive Technology: Sixteenth Revised Edition*, New York, NY, 1994. **2.** Mann, J., et al.: *Br Med J* 2(5956):241–245, 1975. **3.** Knopp, R.H.: *J Reprod Med* 31(9):913–921, 1986. **4.** Mann, J.I., et al.: *Br Med J* 2:445–447, 1976. **5.** Ory, H.: *JAMA* 237: 2619–2622, 1977. **6.** The Cancer and Steroid Hormone Study of the Centers for Disease Control: *JAMA* 249(2): 1596–1599, 1983. **7.** The Cancer and Steroid Hormone Study of the Centers for Disease Control: *JAMA* 257(6):796–800, 1987. **8.** Ory, H.W.: *JAMA* 228(1):68–69, 1974. **9.** Ory, H.W., et al.: *N Engl J Med* 294:419–422, 1976. **10.** Ory, H.W.: *Fam Plann Perspect* 14:182–184, 1982. **11.** Ory, H.W., et al.: *Making Choices*, New York, The Alan Guttmacher Institute, 1983. **12.** Stadel, B.: *N Engl J Med* 305(11):612–618, 1981. **13.** Stadel, B: *N Engl J Med* 305(12):672–677, 1981. **14.** Adam, S., et al.: *Br J Obstet Gynaecol* 88:838–845, 1981. **15.** Mann, J., et al.: *Br Med J* 2(5965):245–248, 1975. **16.** Royal College of General Practitioners' Oral Contraceptive Study: *Lancet* 1:541–546, 1981. **17.** Slone, D., et al.: *N Engl J Med* 305(8):420–424, 1981. **18.** Vessey, M.P.: *Br J Fam Plann* 6 (supplement):1–12, 1980. **19.** Russell-Briefel, R., et al.: *Prev Med* 15:352–362, 1986. **20.** Goldbaum, G., et al.: *JAMA* 258(10):1339–1342, 1987. **21.** LaRosa, J.C.: *J Reprod Med* 31(9):906–912, 1986. **22.** Krauss, R.M., et al.: *Am J Obstet Gynecol* 145:446–452, 1983. **23.** Wahl, P., et al.: *N Engl J Med* 308(15):862–867, 1983. **24.** Wynn, V., et al.: *Am J Obstet Gynecol* 142(6):766–771, 1982. **25.** Wynn, V., et al.: *J Reprod Med* 31(9):892–897, 1986. **26.** Inman, W.H., et al.: *Br Med J* 2(5599):193–199, 1968. **27.** Maguire, M.G., et al.: *Am J Epidemiol* 110(2):188–195, 1979. **28.** Petitti, D., et al.: *JAMA* 242(11):1150–1154, 1979. **29.** Vessey, M.P., et al.: *Br Med J* 2(5599):199–205, 1968. **30.** Vessey, M.P., et al.: *Br Med J* 2(5658):651–657, 1969. **31.** Porter, J.B., et al.: *Obstet Gynecol* 59(3):299–302, 1982. **32.** Vessey, M.P., et al.: *J Biosoc Sci* 8:373–427, 1976. **33.** Mishell, D.R., et al.: *Reproductive Endocrinology*, Philadelphia, F.A. Davis Co., 1979. **34.** Petitti, D.B., et al.: *Lancet* 2:234–236, 1978. **35.** Collaborative Group for the Study of Stroke in Young Women: *JAMA* 231(7):718–722, 1975. **36.** Inman, W.H., et al.: *Br Med J* 2:203–209, 1970. **37.** Meade, T.W., et al.: *Br Med J* 280 (6224): 1157–1161, 1980. **38.** Kay, C.R.: *Am J Obstet Gynecol* 142(6):762–765, 1982. **39.** Gordon, T., et al.: *Am J Med* 62: 707–714, 1977. **40.** Royal College of General Practitioners' Oral Contraception Study: *J Coll Gen Pract* 33:75–82, 1983. **41.** Ory, H.W.: *Fam Plann Perspect* 15(2):57–63, 1983. **42.** Paul, C., et al.: *Br Med J* 293:723–725, 1986. **43.** The Cancer and Steroid Hormone Study of the Centers for Disease Control: *N Engl J Med* 315(7):405–411, 1986. **44.** Pike, M.C., et al.: *Lancet* 2:926–929, 1983. **45.** Miller, D.R., et al.: *Obstet Gynecol* 68:863–868, 1986. **46.** Olsson, H., et al.: *Lancet* 2:748–749, 1985. **47.** McPherson, K., et al.: *Br J Cancer* 56: 653–660, 1987. **48.** Huggins, G.R., et al.: *Fertil Steril* 47(5): 733–761, 1987. **49.** McPherson, K., et al.: *Br Med J* 293:709–710, 1986. **50.** Ory, H., et al.: *Am J Obstet Gynecol* 124(6): 573–577, 1976. **51.** Vessey, M.P., et al.: *Lancet*, 2:930, 1983. **52.** Brinton, L.A., et al.: *Int J Cancer* 38:339–344, 1986. **53.** WHO Collaborative Study of Neoplasia and Steroid Contraceptives: *Br Med J* 290:961–965, 1985. **54.** Rooks, J.B., et al.: *JAMA* 242(7):644–648, 1979. **55.** Bein, N.N., et al.: *Br J Surg* 64:433–435, 1977. **56.** Klatskin, G.: *Gastroenterology* 73:386–394, 1977. **57.** Henderson, B.E., et al.: *Br J Cancer* 48:437–440, 1983. **58.** Neuberger, J., et al.: *Br Med J* 292: 1355–1357, 1986. **59.** Forman, D., et al.: *Br Med J* 292: 1357–1361, 1986. **60.** Harlap, S., et al.: *Obstet Gynecol* 55(4): 447–452, 1980. **61.** Savolainen, E., et al.: *Am J Obstet Gynecol* 140(5):521–524, 1981. **62.** Janerich, D.T., et al.: *Am J Epidemiol* 112(1):73–79, 1980. **63.** Ferencz, C., et al.: *Teratology* 21:225–239, 1980. **64.** Rothman, K.J., et al.: *Am J Epidemiol* 109(4):433–439, 1979. **65.** Boston Collaborative Drug Surveillance Program: *Lancet* 1:1399–1404, 1973. **66.** Royal College of General Practitioners: *Oral contraceptives and health.* New York, Pittman, 1974. **67.** Rome Group for the Epidemiology and Prevention of Cholelithiasis: *Am J Epidemiol* 119(5):796–805, 1984. **68.** Strom, B.L., et al.: *Clin Pharmacol Ther* 39(3):335–341, 1986. **69.** Perlman, J.A., et al.: *J Chronic Dis* 38(10):857–864, 1985. **70.** Wynn, V., et al.: *Lancet* 1:1045–1049, 1979. **71.** Wynn, V.: *Progesterone and Progestin*, New York, Raven Press, 1983. **72.** Wynn, V., et al.: *Lancet* 2:720–723, 1966. **73.** Fisch, I.R., et al.: *JAMA* 237(23):2499–2503, 1977. **74.** Laragh, J.H.: *Am J Obstet Gynecol* 126(1):141–147, 1976. **75.** Ramcharan, S., et al.: *Pharmacology of Steroid Contraceptive Drugs*, New York, Raven Press, 1977. **76.** Stockley, I.: *Pharm J* 216:140–143, 1976. **77.** Dickey, R.P.: *Managing Contraceptive Pill Patients*, Oklahoma, Creative Informatics Inc., 1984. **78.** Porter J.B., Hunter J., Jick H., et al: *Obstet Gynecol* 1985;66:1–4. **79.** Porter J.B., Hershel J., Walker A.M.: *Obstet Gynecol* 1987;70:29–32. **80.** Fertility and Maternal Health Drugs Advisory Committee, F.D.A., October, 1989. **81.** Schlesselman J., Stadel B.V., Murray P., Lai S.: *Breast cancer in relation to early use of oral contraceptives.* JAMA 1988;259:1828–1833. **82.** Hennekens C.H., Speizer F.E., Lipnick R.J., Rosner B., Bain C., Belanger C., Stampfer M.J., Willett W., Peto R.: *A case-control study of oral contraceptive use and breast cancer.* JNCI 1984;72:39–42. **83.** Royal College of General Practitioners: *Oral contraceptives, venous thrombosis, and varicose veins. J Coll Gen Pract* 28:393–399, 1978. **84.** Royal College of General Practitioners' Oral Contraceptives Study: *Effect on Hypertension and benign breast disease of progestogen component in combined oral contraceptives. Lancet* 1:624, 1977.

DETAILED PATIENT LABELING

This product (like all oral contraceptives) is intended to prevent pregnancy. It does not protect against HIV infection (AIDS) and other sexually transmitted diseases.

INTRODUCTION

Any woman who considers using oral contraceptives ("birth control pills" or "the pill") should understand the benefits and risks of using this form of birth control. This leaflet will give you much of the information you will need to make this decision and also will help you determine if you are at risk of developing any of the serious side effects of the pill. It will tell you how to use the pill properly so that it will be as effective as possible. However, this leaflet is not a replacement for a careful discussion between you and your health care provider. You should discuss the information provided in this leaflet with him or her, both when you first start taking the pill and during your regular visits. You also should follow the advice of your health care provider with regard to regular checkups while you are on the pill.

EFFECTIVENESS OF ORAL CONTRACEPTIVES

Oral contraceptives are used to prevent pregnancy and are more effective than other non-surgical methods of birth control. When they are taken correctly, without missing any pills, the chance of becoming pregnant is less than 1% (1 pregnancy per 100 women per year of use). Typical failure rates are actually 3% per year. The chance of becoming pregnant increases with each missed pill during a menstrual cycle.

In comparison, typical failure rates for other nonsurgical methods of birth control during the first year are as follows:

Comparison of reversible contraceptive methods: Percentage of women experiencing a contraceptive failure (pregnancy) during the first year of use.

	% of Women Experiencing a Pregnancy within the First Year of Use	
Method	**Average Use**	**Correct Use**
No contraception	85	85
Spermicides	21	6
Periodic abstinence	20	1–9a
Withdrawal	19	4
Cap		
Given birth	36	26
Never given birth	18	9
Sponge		
Given birth	36	20
Never given birth	18	9
Diaphragm	18	6
Condom		
Female	21	5
Male	12	3
Pill	3	
Progestin only		0.5
Combined		0.1
IUD		
Progesterone	2	1.5
Copper T 380A	0.8	0.6
Injectables	0.3	0.3
Implant	0.09	0.09

Adapted with permission—Hatcher, R.A., Trussell, J., Stewart, F., et al: *Contraceptive Technology: Sixteenth Revised Edition*, New York, NY, 1994.

a Depending on method (calendar, ovulation, symptom-thermal)

WHO SHOULD NOT TAKE ORAL CONTRACEPTIVES

Cigarette smoking increases the risk of serious cardiovascular side effects from oral contraceptive use. This risk increases with age and with heavy smoking (15 or more cigarettes per day) and is quite marked in women over 35 years of age. Women who use oral contraceptives are strongly advised not to smoke.

Some women should not use the pill. For example, you should not take the pill if you are pregnant or think you may be pregnant. You also should not use the pill if you have any of the following conditions:

- A history of heart attack or stroke
- Blood clots in the legs (thrombophlebitis), brain (stroke), lungs (pulmonary embolism) or eyes
- A history of blood clots in the deep veins of your legs
- Chest pain (angina pectoris)
- Known or suspected breast cancer or cancer of the lining of the uterus, cervix or vagina
- Unexplained vaginal bleeding (until a diagnosis is reached by your doctor)
- Yellowing of the whites of the eyes or of the skin (jaundice) during pregnancy or during previous use of the pill
- Liver tumor (benign or cancerous)
- Known or suspected pregnancy

Tell your health care provider if you have ever had any of these conditions. Your health care provider can recommend a safer method of birth control.

OTHER CONSIDERATIONS BEFORE TAKING ORAL CONTRACEPTIVES

Tell your health care provider if you have or have had:
- Breast nodules, fibrocystic disease of the breast, an abnormal breast x-ray or mammogram
- Diabetes
- Elevated cholesterol or triglycerides
- High blood pressure
- Migraine or other headaches or epilepsy
- Mental depression
- Gallbladder, heart or kidney disease
- History of scanty or irregular menstrual periods

Women with any of these conditions should be checked often by their health care provider if they choose to use oral contraceptives.

Also, be sure to inform your doctor or health care provider if you smoke or are on any medications.

RISKS OF TAKING ORAL CONTRACEPTIVES

1. Risk of developing blood clots

Blood clots and blockage of blood vessels are the most serious side effects of taking oral contraceptives. In particular, a clot in the legs can cause thrombophlebitis and a clot that travels to the lungs can cause a sudden blocking of the vessel carrying blood to the lungs. Rarely, clots occur in the blood vessels of the eye and may cause blindness, double vision, or impaired vision.

If you take oral contraceptives and need elective surgery, need to stay in bed for a prolonged illness or have recently delivered a baby, you may be at risk of developing blood clots. You should consult your doctor about stopping oral contraceptives three to four weeks before surgery and not taking oral contraceptives for two weeks after surgery or during bed rest. You should also not take oral contraceptives soon after delivery of a baby. It is advisable to wait for at least four weeks after delivery if you are not breast feeding. If you are breast feeding, you should wait until you have weaned your child before using the pill (see **GENERAL PRECAUTIONS, While Breast Feeding**).

2. Heart attacks and strokes

Oral contraceptives may increase the tendency to develop strokes (stoppage or rupture of blood vessels in the brain) and angina pectoris and heart attacks (blockage of blood vessels in the heart). Any of these conditions can cause death or temporary or permanent disability.

Smoking greatly increases the possibility of suffering heart attacks and strokes. Furthermore, smoking and the use of oral contraceptives greatly increase the chances of developing and dying of heart disease.

3. Gallbladder disease

Oral contraceptive users may have a greater risk than non-users of having gallbladder disease, although this risk may be related to pills containing high doses of estrogen.

4. Liver tumors

In rare cases, oral contraceptives can cause benign but dangerous liver tumors. These benign liver tumors can rupture and cause fatal internal bleeding. In addition, a possible but not definite association has been found with the pill and liver cancers in 2 studies in which a few women who developed these very rare cancers were found to have used oral contraceptives for long periods. However, liver cancers are extremely rare. The chance of developing liver cancer from using the pill is thus even rarer.

5. Cancer of the breast and reproductive organs

There is, at present, no confirmed evidence that oral contraceptives increase the risk of cancer of the reproductive organs in human studies. Several studies have found no overall increase in the risk of developing breast cancer. However, women who use oral contraceptives and have a strong family history of breast cancer or who have breast nodules or abnormal mammograms should be followed closely by their doctors. Some studies have reported an increase in the risk of developing breast cancer, particularly at a younger age. This increased risk appears to be related to duration of use.

Some studies have found an increase in the incidence of cancer of the cervix in women who use oral contraceptives. However, this finding may be related to factors other than the use of oral contraceptives.

ESTIMATED ANNUAL NUMBER OF BIRTH-RELATED OR METHOD-RELATED DEATHS ASSOCIATED WITH CONTROL OF FERTILITY PER 100,000 NON-STERILE WOMEN, BY FERTILITY CONTROL METHOD ACCORDING TO AGE

Method of control and outcome	15–19	20–24	25–29	30–34	35–39	40–44
No fertility control methods*	7.0	7.4	9.1	14.8	25.7	28.2
Oral contraceptives non-smoker**	0.3	0.5	0.9	1.9	13.8	31.6
Oral contraceptives smoker**	2.2	3.4	6.6	13.5	51.1	117.2
IUD**	0.8	0.8	1.0	1.0	1.4	1.4
Condom*	1.1	1.6	0.7	0.2	0.3	0.4
Diaphragm/Spermicide*	1.9	1.2	1.2	1.3	2.2	2.8
Periodic abstinence*	2.5	1.6	1.6	1.7	2.9	3.6

* Deaths are birth-related
** Deaths are method-related

ESTIMATED RISK OF DEATH FROM A BIRTH CONTROL METHOD OR PREGNANCY

All methods of birth control and pregnancy are associated with a risk of developing certain diseases which may lead to disability or death. An estimate of the number of deaths associated with different methods of birth control and pregnancy has been calculated and is shown in the following table:

[See table above]

In the above table, the risk of death from any birth control method is less than the risk of childbirth except for oral contraceptive users over the age of 35 who smoke and pill users over the age of 40 even if they do not smoke. It can be seen from the table that for women aged 15 to 39 the risk of death is highest with pregnancy (7–26 deaths per 100,000 women, depending on age). Among pill users who do not smoke the risk of death is always lower than that associated with pregnancy for any age group, although over the age of 40 the risk increases to 32 deaths per 100,000 women compared to 28 associated with pregnancy at that age. However, for pill users who smoke and are over the age of 35 the estimated number of deaths exceeds those for other methods of birth control. If a woman is over the age of 40 and smokes, her estimated risk of death is 4 times higher (117/100,000 women) than the estimated risk associated with pregnancy (28/100,000 women) in that age group.

The suggestion that women over 40 who don't smoke should not take oral contraceptives is based on information from older high-dose pills and on less selective use of pills than is practiced today. An Advisory Committee of the FDA discussed this issue in 1989 and recommended that the benefits of oral contraceptive use by healthy, non-smoking women over 40 years of age may outweigh the possible risks. However, all women, especially older women, are cautioned to use the lowest dose pill that is effective.

WARNING SIGNALS

If any of these adverse effects occur while you are taking oral contraceptives, call your doctor immediately:
- Sharp chest pain, coughing of blood or sudden shortness of breath (indicating a possible clot in the lung)
- Pain in the calf (indicating a possible clot in the leg)
- Crushing chest pain or heaviness in the chest (indicating a possible heart attack)
- Sudden severe headache or vomiting, dizziness or fainting, disturbances of vision or speech, weakness or numbness in an arm or leg (indicating a possible stroke)
- Sudden partial or complete loss of vision (indicating a possible clot in the eye)
- Breast lumps (indicating possible breast cancer or fibrocystic disease of the breast: ask your doctor or health care provider to show you how to examine your breasts)
- Severe pain or tenderness in the stomach area (indicating a possible ruptured liver tumor)
- Difficulty in sleeping, weakness, lack of energy, fatigue or change in mood (possibly indicating severe depression)
- Jaundice or a yellowing of the skin or eyeballs, accompanied frequently by fever, fatigue, loss of appetite, dark colored urine or light colored bowel movements (indicating possible liver problems)

SIDE EFFECTS OF ORAL CONTRACEPTIVES

1. Vaginal bleeding

Irregular vaginal bleeding or spotting may occur while you are taking the pill. Irregular bleeding may vary from slight staining between menstrual periods to breakthrough bleeding which is a flow much like a regular period. Irregular bleeding occurs most often during the first few months of oral contraceptive use but may also occur after you have been taking the pill for some time. Such bleeding may be temporary and usually does not indicate any serious problem. It is important to continue taking your pills on schedule. If the bleeding occurs in more than 1 cycle or lasts for more than a few days, talk to your doctor or health care provider.

2. Contact lenses

If you wear contact lenses and notice a change in vision or an inability to wear your lenses, contact your doctor or health care provider.

3. Fluid retention

Oral contraceptives may cause edema (fluid retention) with swelling of the fingers or ankles and may raise your blood pressure. If you experience fluid retention, contact your doctor or health care provider.

4. Melasma (Mask of Pregnancy)

A spotty darkening of the skin is possible, particularly of the face.

5. Other side effects

Other side effects may include change in appetite, headache, nervousness, depression, dizziness, loss of scalp hair, rash and vaginal infections.

If any of these side effects occurs, contact your doctor or health care provider.

GENERAL PRECAUTIONS

1. Missed periods and use of oral contraceptives before or during early pregnancy

At times you may not menstruate regularly after you have completed taking a cycle of pills. If you have taken your pills regularly and miss 1 menstrual period, continue taking your pills for the next cycle but be sure to inform your health care provider before doing so. If you have not taken the pills daily as instructed and miss 1 menstrual period, or if you miss 2 consecutive menstrual periods, you may be pregnant. You should stop taking oral contraceptives until you are sure you are not pregnant, but continue to use another method of birth control.

There is no conclusive evidence that oral contraceptive use is associated with an increase in birth defects when taken inadvertently during early pregnancy. Previously, a few studies had reported that oral contraceptives might be associated with birth defects but these studies have not been confirmed. Nevertheless, oral contraceptives or any other drugs should not be used during pregnancy unless clearly necessary and prescribed by your doctor. You should check with your doctor about risks to your unborn child from any medication taken during pregnancy.

2. While breast feeding

If you are breast feeding, consult your doctor before starting oral contraceptives. Some of the drug will be passed on to the child in the milk. A few adverse effects on the child have been reported, including yellowing of the skin (jaundice) and breast enlargement. In addition, oral contraceptives may decrease the amount and quality of your milk. If possible, do not use oral contraceptives and use another method of contraception while breast feeding. You should consider starting oral contraceptives only after you have weaned your child completely.

3. Laboratory tests

If you are scheduled for any laboratory tests, tell your doctor you are taking birth control pills. Certain blood tests may be affected by birth control pills.

4. Drug interactions

Certain drugs may interact with birth control pills to make them less effective in preventing pregnancy or cause an increase in breakthrough bleeding. Such drugs include rifampin; drugs used for epilepsy such as barbiturates (for example, phenobarbital) and phenytoin (Dilantin is one brand of this drug); phenylbutazone (Butazolidin is one brand of this drug) and possibly certain antibiotics. You may need to use additional contraception when you take drugs which can make oral contraceptives less effective.

5. This product (like all oral contraceptives) is intended to prevent pregnancy. It does not protect against transmission of HIV (AIDS) and other sexually transmitted diseases such as chlamydia, genital herpes, genital warts, gonorrhea, hepatitis B, and syphilis.

Continued on next page

Tri-Norinyl—Cont.

HOW TO TAKE THE PILL

IMPORTANT POINTS TO REMEMBER

BEFORE YOU START TAKING YOUR PILLS:
1. BE SURE TO READ THESE DIRECTIONS:
   Before you start taking your pills.
   Anytime you are not sure what to do.
2. THE RIGHT WAY TO TAKE THE PILL IS TO TAKE ONE PILL EVERY DAY AT THE SAME TIME. If you miss pills you could get pregnant. This includes starting the pack late.
   The more pills you miss, the more likely you are to get pregnant.
3. MANY WOMEN HAVE SPOTTING OR LIGHT BLEEDING, OR MAY FEEL SICK TO THEIR STOMACH DURING THE FIRST 1–3 PACKS OF PILLS.
   If you feel sick to your stomach, do not stop taking the Pill. The problem will usually go away. It it doesn't go away, check with your doctor or clinic.
4. MISSING PILLS CAN ALSO CAUSE SPOTTING OR LIGHT BLEEDING, even when you make up these missed pills.
   On the days you take 2 pills to make up for missed pills, you could also feel a little sick to your stomach.
5. IF YOU HAVE VOMITING OR DIARRHEA, for any reason, or IF YOU TAKE SOME MEDICINES, including some antibiotics, your pills may not work as well.
   Use a back-up method (such as condoms, foam, or sponge) until you check with your doctor or clinic.
6. IF YOU HAVE TROUBLE REMEMBERING TO TAKE THE PILL, talk to your doctor or clinic about how to make pill-taking easier or about using another method of birth control.
7. IF YOU HAVE ANY QUESTIONS OR ARE UNSURE ABOUT THE INFORMATION IN THIS LEAFLET, call your doctor or clinic.

BEFORE YOU START TAKING YOUR PILLS

1. DECIDE WHAT TIME OF DAY YOU WANT TO TAKE YOUR PILL.
   It is important to take it at about the same time every day.
2. LOOK AT YOUR PILL PACK TO SEE IF IT HAS 21 OR 28 PILLS:
   The 21-pill pack has 21 "active" blue and yellow-green pills (with hormones) to take for 3 weeks, followed by 1 week without pills.
   The 28-pill pack has 21 "active" blue and yellow-green pills (with hormones) to take for 3 weeks, followed by 1 week of reminder orange pills (without hormones).
3. ALSO FIND:
   1) where on the pack to start taking pills.
   2) in what order to take the pills (follow the arrows) and

Active pill colors: blue and yellow-green

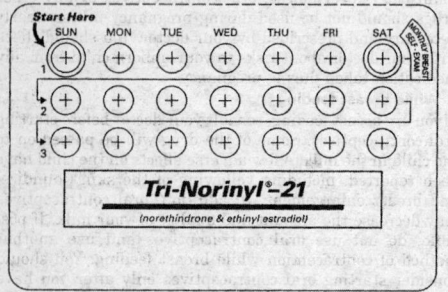

3) the week numbers as shown on the picture below.

Active pill colors: blue and yellow-green
Reminder pill color: orange

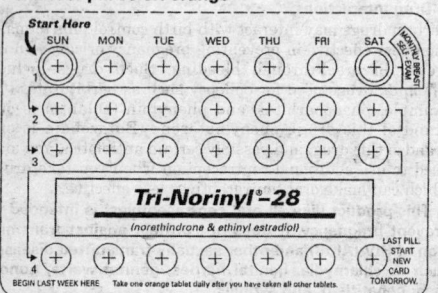

4. BE SURE YOU HAVE READY AT ALL TIMES:
   ANOTHER KIND OF BIRTH CONTROL (such as condoms, foam, or sponge) to use as a back-up in case you miss pills.
   AN EXTRA, FULL PILL PACK.

WHEN TO START THE FIRST PACK OF PILLS

You have a choice of which day to start taking your first pack of pills. Decide with your doctor or clinic which is the best day for you. Pick a time of day which will be easy to remember.

DAY 1 START:
1. Take the first "active" blue pill of the first pack during the first 24 hours of your period.
2. You will not need to use a back-up method of birth control, since you are starting the pill at the beginning of your period.

SUNDAY START:
1. Take the first "active" blue pill of the first pack on the Sunday after your period starts, even if you are still bleeding. If your period begins on Sunday, start the pack that same day.
2. Use another method of birth control as a back-up method if you have sex anytime from the Sunday you start your first pack until the next Sunday (7 days). Condoms, foam, or the sponge are good back-up methods of birth control.

WHAT TO DO DURING THE MONTH

1. **TAKE ONE PILL AT THE SAME TIME EVERY DAY UNTIL THE PACK IS EMPTY.**
   Do not skip pills even if you are spotting or bleeding between monthly periods or feel sick to your stomach (nausea).
   Do not skip pills even if you do not have sex very often.
2. **WHEN YOU FINISH A PACK OR SWITCH YOUR BRAND OF PILLS:**
   21 pills: Wait 7 days to start the next pack. You will probably have your period during that week. Be sure that no more than 7 days pass between 21-pill packs.
   28 pills: Start the next pack on the day after your last "reminder" pill. Do not wait any days between packs.

WHAT TO DO IF YOU MISS PILLS

If you **MISS 1** blue or yellow-green pill "active" pill:
1. Take it as soon as you remember. Take the next pill at your regular time. This means you may take 2 pills in 1 day.
2. You do not need to use a back-up birth control method if you have sex.
   If you **MISS 2** blue or yellow-green "active" pills in a row in **WEEK 1 OR WEEK 2** of your pack:
1. Take 2 pills on the day you remember and 2 pills the next day.
2. Then take 1 pill a day until you finish the pack.
3. You MAY BECOME PREGNANT if you have sex in the 7 days after you miss pills. You MUST use another birth control method (such as condoms, foam, or sponge) as a backup for those 7 days.
   If you **MISS 2** blue or yellow-green "active" pills in a row in **THE 3rd WEEK:**
1. *If you are a Day 1 Starter:*
   THROW OUT the rest of the pill pack and start a new pack that same day.
   If you are a Sunday Starter:
   Keep taking pill every day until Sunday.
   On Sunday, THROW OUT the rest of the pill pack and start a new pack of pills that same day.
2. You may not have your period this month but this is expected. However, if you miss your period 2 months in a row, call your doctor or clinic because you might be pregnant.
3. You MAY BECOME PREGNANT if you have sex in the 7 days after you miss pills. You MUST use another birth control method (such as condoms, foam, or sponge) as a backup for those 7 days.
   If you **MISS 3 OR MORE** blue or yellow-green "active" pills in a row (during the first 3 weeks):
1. *If you are a Day 1 Starter:*
   THROW OUT the rest of the pill pack and start a new pack of pills that same day.
   If you are a Sunday Starter:
   Keep taking 1 pill every day until Sunday.
   On Sunday, THROW OUT the rest of the pill pack and start a new pack of pills that same day.
2. You may not have your period this month but this is expected. However, if you miss your period 2 months in a row, call your doctor or clinic because you might be pregnant.
3. You MAY BECOME PREGNANT if you have sex in the 7 days after you miss pills. You MUST use another birth control method (such as condoms, foam, or sponge) as a backup for those 7 days.

A REMINDER FOR THOSE ON 28-DAY PACKS:
If you forget any of the 7 orange "reminder" pills in Week 4:
THROW AWAY the pills you missed.
Keep taking 1 pill each day until the pack is empty.
You do not need a back-up method.

FINALLY, IF YOU ARE STILL NOT SURE WHAT TO DO ABOUT THE PILLS YOU HAVE MISSED:
Use a BACK-UP METHOD anytime you have sex.
KEEP TAKING ONE "ACTIVE" PILL EACH DAY until you can reach your doctor or clinic.

6. Missed periods, spotting or light bleeding
At times, you may not have a period after you have completed a pack of pills. If you miss 1 period but you have taken the pills exactly as you were supposed to, continue as usual into the next cycle. If you have not taken the pills correctly, and have missed a period, you may be pregnant and you should stop taking the Pill until your doctor or clinic determines whether or not you are pregnant. Until you can talk to your doctor or clinic, use an appropriate back-up birth control method. If you miss 2 consecutive periods, you should stop taking the Pill until it is determined that you are not pregnant.
Even if spotting or light bleeding should occur, continue taking the Pill according to the schedule. Should spotting or light bleeding persist, you should notify your doctor or clinic.

7. Stopping the pill before surgery or prolonged bed rest
If you are scheduled for surgery or you need to stay in bed for a long period of time you should tell your doctor that you are on the Pill. You should stop taking the Pill four weeks before your operation to avoid an increased risk of blood clots. Talk to your doctor about when you may start taking the Pill again.

8. Starting the pill after pregnancy
After you have a baby it is advisable to wait 4–6 weeks before starting to take the Pill. Talk to your doctor about when you may start taking the Pill after pregnancy.

9. Pregnancy due to pill failure
When the Pill is taken correctly, the expected pregnancy rate is approximately 1% (i.e., 1 pregnancy per 100 women per year). If pregnancy occurs while taking the Pill, there is little risk to the fetus. The typical failure rate of large numbers of pill users is less than 3% when women who have missed pills are included. If you become pregnant, you should discuss your pregnancy with your doctor.

10. Pregnancy after stopping the pill
There may be some delay in becoming pregnant after you stop taking the Pill, especially if you had irregular periods before you started using the Pill. Your doctor may recommend that you delay becoming pregnant until you have had one or more regular periods.
There does not appear to be any increase in birth defects in newborn babies when pregnancy occurs soon after stopping the Pill.

11. Overdosage
There are no reports of serious illness or side effects in young children who have swallowed a large number of pills. In adults, overdosage may cause nausea and/or bleeding in females. In case of overdosage, contact your doctor, clinic or pharmacist.

12. Other information
Your doctor or clinic will take a medical and family history and will examine you before prescribing the Pill. The physical examination may be delayed to another time if you request it and the health care provider believes that it is a good medical practice to postpone it. You should be reexamined at least once a year. Be sure to inform your doctor or clinic if there is a family history of any of the conditions listed previously in this leaflet. Be sure to keep all appointments with your doctor or clinic because this is a time to determine if there are early signs of side effects from using the Pill.
Do not use the Pill for any condition other than the one for which it was prescribed. The Pill has been prescribed specifically for you, do not give it to others who may want birth control pills.
If you want more information about birth control pills, ask your doctor or clinic. They have a more technical leaflet called **PHYSICIAN LABELING** which you might want to read.

NON-CONTRACEPTIVE HEALTH BENEFITS

In addition to preventing pregnancy, use of oral contraceptives may provide certain non-contraceptive health benefits:
- Menstrual cycles may become more regular
- Blood flow during menstruation may be lighter and less iron may be lost. Therefore, anemia due to iron deficiency is less likely to occur
- Pain or other symptoms during menstruation may be encountered less frequently
- Ectopic (tubal) pregnancy may occur less frequently
- Non-cancerous cysts or lumps in the breast may occur less frequently
- Acute pelvic inflammatory disease may occur less frequently

• Oral contraceptive use may provide some protection against developing two forms of cancer: cancer of the ovaries and cancer of the lining of the uterus.

Store at controlled room temperature 15–25°C (59–77°F).

BRIEF SUMMARY
PATIENT PACKAGE INSERT

This product (like all oral contraceptives) is intended to prevent pregnancy. It does not protect against HIV infection (AIDS) and other sexually transmitted diseases.

Oral contraceptives, also known as "birth control pills" or "the pill," are taken to prevent pregnancy and, when taken correctly, have a failure rate of about 1% per year when used without missing any pills. The typical failure rate of large numbers of pill users is less than 3% per year when women who miss pills are included. For most women, oral contraceptives are also free of serious or unpleasant side effects. However, forgetting to take oral contraceptives considerably increases the chances of pregnancy.

For the majority of women, oral contraceptives can be taken safely, but there are some women who are at high risk of developing certain serious diseases that can be life-threatening or may cause temporary or permanent disability. The risks associated with taking oral contraceptives increase significantly if you:

- Smoke
- Have high blood pressure diabetes or high cholesterol
- Have or have had clotting disorders, heart attack, stroke, angina pectoris, cancer of the breast or sex organs, jaundice or malignant or benign liver tumors

You should not take the pill if you suspect you are pregnant or have unexplained vaginal bleeding.

Cigarette smoking increases the risk of serious cardiovascular side effects from oral contraceptive use. This risk increases with age and with heavy smoking (15 or more cigarettes per day) and is quite marked in women over 35 years of age. Women who use oral contraceptives are strongly advised not to smoke.

Most side effects of the pill are not serious. The most common such effects are nausea, vomiting, bleeding between menstrual periods, weight gain, breast tenderness and difficulty wearing contact lenses. These side effects, especially nausea and vomiting, may subside within the first 3 months of use.

The serious side effects of the pill occur very infrequently, especially if you are in good health and are young. However, you should know that the following medical conditions have been associated with or made worse by the pill:

1. Blood clots in the legs (thrombophlebitis) or lungs (pulmonary embolism), stoppage or rupture of a blood vessel in the brain (stroke), blockage of blood vessels in the heart (heart attack or angina pectoris), eye or other organs of the body. As mentioned above, smoking increases the risk of heart attacks and strokes and subsequent serious medical consequences.
2. Liver tumors, which may rupture and cause severe bleeding. A possible but not definite association has been found with the pill and liver cancer. However, liver cancers are extremely rare. The chance of developing liver cancer from using the pill is thus even rarer.
3. High blood pressure, although blood pressure usually returns to normal when the pill is stopped.

The symptoms associated with these serious side effects are discussed in the detailed leaflet given to you with your supply of pills. Notify your doctor or health care provider if you notice any unusual physical disturbances while taking the pill. In addition, drugs such as rifampin, as well as some anti-convulsants and some antibiotics, may decrease oral contraceptive effectiveness.

Studies to date of women taking the pill have not shown an increase in the incidence of cancer of the breast or cervix. There is, however, insufficient evidence to rule out the possibility that the pill may cause such cancers. Some studies have reported an increase in the risk of developing breast cancer, particularly at a younger age. This increased risk appears to be related to duration of use.

Taking the pill provides some important non-contraceptive health benefits. These include less painful menstruation, less menstrual blood loss and anemia, fewer pelvic infections and fewer cancers of the ovary and the lining of the uterus.

Be sure to discuss any medical condition you may have with your health care provider. Your health care provider will take a medical and family history before prescribing oral contraceptives and will examine you. The physical examination may be delayed to another time if you request it and the health care provider believes that it is a good medical practice to postpone it. You should be reexamined at least once a year while taking oral contraceptives. The detailed patient information leaflet gives you further information which you should read and discuss with your health care provider.

HOW TO TAKE THE PILL

See full text of HOW TO TAKE THE PILL which is printed in full in the Detailed Patient Labeling.

A08826•7/24/97

Shown in Product Identification Guide, page 338

SEQUUS® Pharmaceuticals, Inc.

960 Hamilton Court
Menlo Park, CA 94025

Direct Inquiries to:
Dept. of Professional Services
800-323-9049
Medical Emergency Contact:
800-323-9049

AMPHOTEC® ℞
(Amphotericin B) Cholesteryl Sulfate Complex for Injection

DESCRIPTION

AMPHOTEC® is a sterile, pyrogen-free, lyophilized powder for reconstitution and intravenous (IV) administration. AMPHOTEC consists of a 1:1 (molar ratio) complex of amphotericin B and cholesteryl sulfate. Upon reconstitution, AMPHOTEC forms a colloidal dispersion of microscopic disc-shaped particles.

Note: Liposomal encapsulation or incorporation into a lipid complex can substantially affect a drug's functional properties relative to those of the unencapsulated drug or nonlipid associated drug. In addition, different liposomal or lipid-complex products with a common active ingredient may vary from one another in the chemical composition and physical form of the lipid component. Such differences may affect the functional properties of these drug products. Amphotericin B is an antifungal polyene antibiotic produced by a strain of *Streptomyces nodosus.*

Amphotericin B, which is the established name for [1R-(1*R**,3*S**,5*R**,6*R**,9*R**,11*R**,15*S**,16*R**,17*R**,18*S**,19*E*,21*E*,23*E*,25*E*,27*E*,29*E*,31*E*,33*R**,35*S**,36*R**,37*S**)]-33-[(3-Amino-3,6-dideoxy-β-D-mannopyranosyl)oxy]-1,3,5,6,9,11,17,37-octahydroxy-15,16,18-trimethyl-13-oxo-14,39-dioxabicyclo-[33.3.1]nonatriaconta-19,21,23,25,27,29,31-heptaene-36-carboxylic acid, has the following structure:

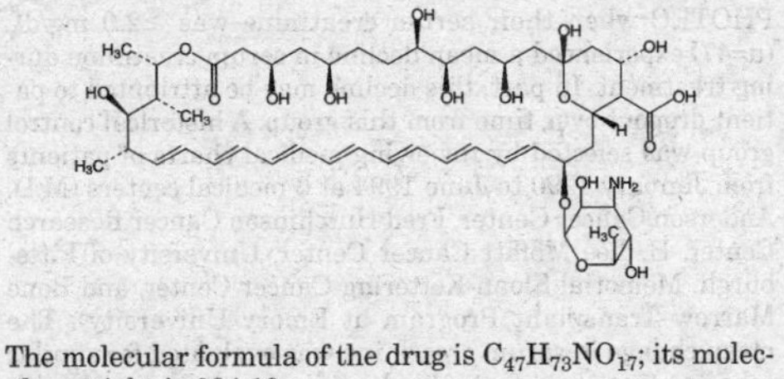

The molecular formula of the drug is $C_{47}H_{73}NO_{17}$; its molecular weight is 924.10.

AMPHOTEC is available in 50 mg and 100 mg single dose vials. Each 50 mg single dose vial contains amphotericin B, 50 mg; sodium cholesteryl sulfate, 26.4 mg; tromethamine, 5.64 mg; disodium edetate dihydrate, 0.372 mg; lactose monohydrate, 950 mg; and hydrochloric acid, qs, as a sterile, nonpyrogenic, lyophilized powder. Each 100 mg single dose vial contains amphotericin B, 100 mg; sodium cholesteryl sulfate, 52.8 mg; tromethamine, 11.28 mg; disodium edetate dihydrate, 0.744 mg; lactose monohydrate, 1900 mg; and hydrochloric acid, qs, as a sterile, nonpyrogenic, lyophilized powder.

MICROBIOLOGY
Mechanism of Action

The active ingredient of AMPHOTEC, amphotericin B, is a polyene antibiotic that acts by binding to sterols (primarily ergosterol) in cell membranes of sensitive fungi, with subsequent leakage of intracellular contents and cell death due to changes in membrane permeability. Amphotericin B also binds to the sterols (primarily cholesterol) in mammalian cell membranes, which is believed to account for its toxicity in animals and humans.

Activity *in vitro* and *in vivo*

AMPHOTEC is active *in vitro* against *Aspergillus* and *Candida* species. One hundred and twelve clinical isolates of four different *Aspergillus* species and 88 clinical isolates of five different *Candida* species were tested, with a majority of MICs <1 μg/mL. AMPHOTEC is also active *in vitro* against other fungi. *In vitro* AMPHOTEC is fungistatic or fungicidal, depending upon the concentration of the drug and the susceptibility of the fungal organism. However, standardized techniques for susceptibility testing for antifungal agents have not been established, and results of susceptibility studies do not necessarily correlate with clinical outcome.

AMPHOTEC is active in murine models against *Aspergillus fumigatus. Candida albicans. Coccidioides immitis* and *Cryptococcus neoformans,* and in an immunosuppressed rabbit model of aspergillosis in which endpoints were prolonged survival of infected animals and clearance of microorganisms from target organ(s). AMPHOTEC also was active in a hamster model of visceral leishmaniasis, a disease caused by infection of macrophages of the mononuclear phagocytic system (MPS) by a protozoal parasite of the genus *Leishmania.* In this hamster model the endpoints were also prolonged survival of infected animals and clearance of microorganisms from target organ(s).

Drug Resistance

Variants with reduced susceptibility to amphotericin B have been isolated from several fungal species after serial passage in cell culture media containing the drug and from some patients receiving prolonged therapy with amphotericin B deoxycholate. Although the relevance of drug resistance to clinical outcome has not been established, fungal organisms that are resistant to amphotericin B may also be resistant to AMPHOTEC.

CLINICAL PHARMACOLOGY
Pharmacokinetics

The pharmacokinetics of amphotericin B, administered as AMPHOTEC, were studied in 51 bone marrow transplant patients with systemic fungal infections. The median (range) age and weight of those patients were 32 (3 to 52) years and 69.5 (14 to 116) kg, respectively. AMPHOTEC doses ranged from 0.5 to 8.0 mg/kg/day. The assay used in this study to measure amphotericin B in plasma does not distinguish amphotericin B that is complexed with cholesteryl sulfate from uncomplexed amphotericin B.

A population modeling approach was used to estimate pharmacokinetic parameters (see table). The pharmacokinetics of amphotericin B, administered as AMPHOTEC, were best described by an open, two-compartment structural model. The pharmacokinetics of amphotericin B, administered as AMPHOTEC, were nonlinear. Steady state volume of distribution (Vss) and total plasma clearance (CLt) increased with escalating doses, resulting in less than proportional increases in plasma concentration over a dose range of 0.5 to 8.0 mg/kg/day. The increased volume of distribution probably reflected uptake by tissues. The covariates of body weight and dose level accounted for a substantial portion of the variability of the pharmacokinetic estimates between patients. The unexplained variability in clearance was 26%. Based on the population model developed for these patients, pharmacokinetic parameters were predicted for two doses of AMPHOTEC and are provided in the following table:

[See first table at top of next page]

In addition, the pharmacokinetics of amphotericin B, administered as amphotericin B deoxycholate, were studied in 15 patients in whom amphotericin B was administered for the treatment of aspergillus infections or empiric therapy. The median (range) age and weight for these patients were 21 (4 to 66) years and 60 (19 to 117) kg, respectively. A population modeling approach was used to estimate the pharmacokinetic parameters. The pharmacokinetics of amphotericin B, administered as amphotericin B deoxycholate, was best described as an open, two-compartment model with linear elimination.

The predicted pharmacokinetic parameters are provided in the following table:

Predicted Pharmacokinetic Parameters of Amphotericin B after Administration of Multiple Doses of 1 mg/kg Amphotericin B Deoxycholate (a)

Mean Pharmacokinetic Parameter (b)	Values
Vss (L/kg)	1.1
CLt (L/h/kg)	0.028
Distribution Half-Life (minutes)	38
Elimination Half-Life (hours)	39
Cmax (μg/mL)	2.9
AUCss (μg/mL·h)	36

[a] Data obtained using population modeling in 15 patients in whom amphotericin B deoxycholate was administered for treatment of aspergillus infection or empiric therapy. The modeling assumes amphotericin B pharmacokinetics after administration of amphotericin B deoxycholate are best described by a 2-compartment model. Infusion rate =0.25 mg/kg/hour.

[b] Definitions: Vss –Volume of distribution at steady state. CLt –Total plasma clearance. Cmax –Maximum plasma concentration achieved at the end of an infusion, AUCss –Area under the plasma concentration time curve at steady-state.

An analytical assay that is able to distinguish between amphotericin B in the AMPHOTEC complex and amphotericin

Continued on next page

Amphotec—Cont.

B which is not complexed to cholesteryl sulfate was used to analyze samples from a study of 25 patients who were either immunocompromised with aspergillosis or both febrile and neutropenic. Following a 1 mg/kg/hour infusion 25 ±18% (mean ±SD) of the total amphotericin B concentration measured in plasma was in the AMPHOTEC complex, dropping to 9.3 ±7.9% at 1 hour and 7.5 ±9.3% at 24 hours after the end of the infusion.

Pharmacokinetics in Special Populations

A population modeling approach was used to assess the effect of renal function, hepatic function, and age on the pharmacokinetics of AMPHOTEC in 51 patients receiving bone marrow transplants as described earlier.

Renal Impairment: The pharmacokinetics of amphotericin B, administered as AMPHOTEC, were not related to baseline serum creatinine clearance in the population studied; the median (range) creatinine clearance for this population was 74.0 (range: 35 −202) mL/min/70 kg. The effect of more severe renal impairment on the pharmacokinetics of AMPHOTEC has not been studied.

Hepatic Impairment: The pharmacokinetics of amphotericin B, administered as AMPHOTEC, were not related to baseline liver function, as determined by liver enzymes and total bilirubin. For the population tested, the mean ±SD values for AST and total bilirubin were 59.4 ±70.0 IU/mL and 3.5 ±3.7 mg/dL, respectively. The effect of more severe hepatic impairment on the pharmacokinetics of AMPHOTEC has not been studied.

Age: The pharmacokinetics of amphotericin B, administered as AMPHOTEC, were not related to the age of the patient. The median (range) age for the population in this study was 32 (3 to 52) years.

INDICATIONS AND USAGE

AMPHOTEC is indicated for the treatment of invasive aspergillosis in patients where renal impairment or unacceptable toxicity precludes the use of amphotericin B deoxycholate in effective doses, and in patients with invasive aspergillosis where prior amphotericin B deoxycholate therapy has failed.

DESCRIPTION OF CLINICAL STUDIES

Clinical Studies in Aspergillosis

Aspergillosis: Data from 161 patients with proven or probable aspergillus infection were pooled from 5 non-comparative open label studies, one of which included emergency-use patients. The patients were treated with AMPHOTEC because of failure to respond to amphotericin B (n=49), development of nephrotoxicity while receiving amphotericin B (n=62), preexisting renal impairment (n=25), or other reasons (n=25).

The median age of these 161 patients (92 males and 69 females) was 41 years (range 2 months —85 years). For the 155 patients with baseline neutrophil data, 33 patients (21%) had neutrophil counts of <500/mm³. The underlying diseases included bone marrow transplant, 69 (43%); hematological malignancy, 51 (32%); solid organ transplant, 25 (15%); solid tumor, 3 (2%); and other diagnoses, 13 (8%) including surgery, 4; HIV infection, 3; immunosuppression for autoimmune disease, 3; diabetes, 2; and no known underlying disease, 1. Pulmonary involvement was the primary infection site, 118 patients (73%), followed by sinus, 14 (9%), CNS, 9 (6%), skin/wound, 9 (6%), and others, 10 (6%) including 3 with bone involvement, 2 with hepatic involvement, 2 with disseminated disease and 1 each with endocarditis, ophthalmitis, ottitis, and involvement of the hard palate. The 49 patients enrolled due to failure to respond to amphotericin B had received amphotericin B deoxycholate prior to AMPHOTEC for ≤7 days (11 patients), 8–14 days (16 patients), and >14 days (22 patients). Patients were defined by their individual physician as being refractory to amphotericin B deoxycholate therapy based on overall clinical judgment after receiving either a minimum of 7 days of amphotericin B or a minimum total dose of 15 mg/kg of amphotericin B. Nephrotoxicity was defined as a serum creatinine that had doubled from baseline, increased by ≥1.5 mg/dL or increased to ≥2.0 mg/dL. Preexisting renal impairment was defined as a serum creatinine that had increased to ≥2.0 mg/dL due to reasons other than amphotericin B.

Classifications of diagnosis and response were based on the definitions previously developed by the Mycoses Study Group.[1] A retrospective response analysis was conducted in which a "complete response" was defined as resolution of all attributable symptoms, signs, and radiographic abnormalities present at enrollment, and a "partial response" was defined as major improvement of the above-mentioned parameters. The total number of responders was the sum of the number of "complete" and "partial" responses.

Of the 161 patients, 80 were considered evaluable for response. Eighty-one (81) were excluded on the basis of inadequate diagnosis, confounding factors, or receiving ≤4 doses of AMPHOTEC. In the 80 evaluable patients the median daily dose was 4 mg/kg/day (range 0.73 −7.5 mg/kg/day)

Predicted Pharmacokinetic Parameters of Amphotericin B after Administration of Multiple Doses of AMPHOTEC

Mean Pharmacokinetic Parameter [a]	AMPHOTEC (mg/kg/day)	
	3	4
Vss (L/kg)	3.8	4.1
CLt (L/h/kg)	0.105	0.112
Distribution Half-Life (minutes)	3.5	3.5
Elimination Half-Life (hours)	27.5	28.2
Cmax (µg/mL)	2.6	2.9
AUCss (µg/mL·h)	29	36

[a] Data obtained using population modeling in 51 bone marrow transplant patients. The modeling assumes amphotericin B pharmacokinetics after administration of AMPHOTEC is best described by a 2-compartment model. Infusion rate =1 mg/kg/hour.

[b] Definitions: Vss −Volume of distribution at steady state, CLt −Total plasma clearance. Cmax −Maximum plasma concentration achieved at the end of an infusion. AUCss −Area under the plasma concentration time curve at steady-state.

Response Rates for Evaluable Patients

Patient Group (n)	Complete Response	Partial Response	Total Responders [a]	Response Rate
Amphotericin B failure (28) [b]	3	9	12	43%
Nephrotoxicity (36) [c]	5	12	17	47%
Preexisting renal Impairment (16) [d]	1	7	8	50%
Total (80)	9	28	37	46%

[a] Total responders = Complete responses + Partial responses.

[b] Defined, based on overall clinical judgment, after receiving a minimum of 7 days of amphotericin B or a minimum of total dose of 15 mg/kg of amphotericin B.

[c] Defined as a serum creatinine that had doubled from baseline or increased by ≥1.5 mg/dL or increased to ≥2.0 mg/dL.

[d] Defined as a serum creatinine that had increased to ≥2.0 mg/dL due to reasons other than amphotericin B deoxycholate.

and the cumulative median dose was 6.3 g (range 0.36 −34.4 grams). Median duration of treatment was 24 days (range 5 −129 days).

[See second table above]

There is no directly comparable control group for the patients described in the above table to be certain whether similar patients would have responded had amphotericin B deoxycholate therapy been continued. A randomized study comparing AMPHOTEC with amphotericin B deoxycholate for therapy of invasive aspergillosis is currently undergoing analysis.

Renal Function

Patients With Renal Dysfunction At Baseline: The subset of patients with aspergillosis from the above five non-comparative open label studies, who initiated treatment with AMPHOTEC when their serum creatinine was ≥2.0 mg/dL (n=47) experienced a mean decline in serum creatinine during treatment. In part, this decline may be attributed to patient dropout over time from this group. A historical control group was selected by reviewing medical charts of patients from January 1990 to June 1994 at 6 medical centers (M.D. Anderson Cancer Center, Fred Hutchinson Cancer Research Center, H. Lee Moffitt Cancer Center, University of Pittsburgh. Memorial Sloan-Kettering Cancer Center, and Bone Marrow Transplant Program at Emory University). The mean change in serum creatinine was evaluated for similar cohorts of patients from this historical control group, with the baseline for assessing change being the day each patient's serum creatinine reached ≥2.0 mg/dL. As shown in the figure, serum creatinine levels were lower during treatment with AMPHOTEC when compared to the serum creatinine levels of amphotericin B deoxycholate patients in the historical control group. There is no directly comparable group to be certain whether this decline is significantly better than the results of serum creatinine levels in patients who had continued on amphotericin B deoxycholate. Since these data were obtained from two separate studies, no statistical testing of the differences between these two groups was performed.

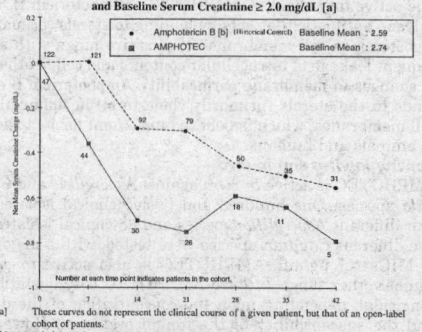

Changes in Mean Serum Creatinine Over Time in Patients with Aspergillosis and Baseline Serum Creatinine ≥ 2.0 mg/dL [a]

[a] These curves do not represent the clinical course of a given patient, but that of an open-label cohort of patients.

[b] Administered as amphotericin B deoxycholate.

Patients with normal renal function at baseline:

In a randomized, double-blind, multicenter study, 213 febrile neutropenic patients were given empirically either 4 mg/kg/day of AMPHOTEC or 0.8 mg/kg/day of amphotericin B deoxycholate for a maximum of 14 days. This study was primarily designed to compare the safety profiles of these two treatments. NOTE: AMPHOTEC is NOT approved for empirical treatment in febrile neutropenic patients.

In the above study, patients had largely normal renal function at baseline; median serum creatinine levels were 0.8 mg/dL for both treatment groups. The mean change in serum creatinine was evaluated for patients with baseline creatinine ≤ 1.5 mg/dL. As shown in the graph, patients in both treatment groups showed an increase in serum creatinine while on study, however AMPHOTEC patients experienced significantly less creatinine increase at each time point.

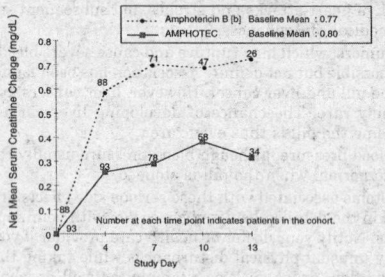

Changes in Mean Serum Creatinine Over Time in Patients with Febrile Neutropenia, and Baseline Serum Creatinine ≤ 1.5 mg/dL [a]

[a] These curves do not represent the clinical course of a given patient, but that of a cohort of patients.

[b] Administered as amphotericin B deoxycholate.

Hypokalemia

In the same empiric study, significantly more amphotericin B deoxycholate patients had at least one laboratory result of serum potassium < 3.0 mEq/L at least one time in the study compared with AMPHOTEC patients (23% vs. 7%), although concomitant supplemental potassium was allowed in the study design. Both groups received approximately equal amounts of potassium supplementation.

Hypomagnesemia

In the same empiric study, there was no overall trend for decreasing serum magnesium in either group.

CONTRAINDICATIONS

AMPHOTEC should not be administered to patients who have documented hypersensitivity to any of its components, unless, in the opinion of the physician, the advantages of using AMPHOTEC outweigh the risks of hypersensitivity.

WARNINGS

Anaphylaxis has been reported with amphotericin B deoxycholate and other amphotericin B-containing drugs. Anaphylactoid reactions require immediate treatment. Epinephrine, oxygen, intravenous steroids, and airway man-

agement should be administered as indicated. If severe respiratory distress occurs, the infusion should be immediately discontinued. The patient should not receive further infusions of AMPHOTEC.

PRECAUTIONS
General
AMPHOTEC should be administered intravenously. Acute infusion-related reactions including fever, chills, hypoxia, hypotension, nausea, or tachypnea usually occur 1 to 3 hours after starting intravenous infusion. These reactions are usually more severe or more frequent after initial doses of AMPHOTEC and usually diminish with subsequent doses. Acute infusion-related reactions can be managed by pretreatment with antihistamines and corticosteroids and/or by reducing the rate of infusion and by prompt administration of antihistamines and corticosteroids. (See **ADVERSE REACTIONS**).
Rapid intravenous infusion should be avoided.
Laboratory Tests, particularly tests of renal and hepatic function, serum electrolytes, complete blood count and prothrombin time should be monitored as medically indicated.
Drug Interactions
No formal drug interaction studies have been conducted with AMPHOTEC. When administered concomitantly, the following drugs are known to interact with amphotericin B; therefore the following drugs may interact with AMPHOTEC.
Antineoplastic agents: Concurrent use of antineoplastic agents and amphotericin B may enhance the potential for renal toxicity, bronchospasm, and hypotension. Caution is urged when antineoplastic agents are given concomitantly with AMPHOTEC.
Corticosteroids and Corticotropin (ACTH): Concurrent use of corticosteroids and corticotropin (ACTH) with amphotericin B may potentiate hypokalemia which could predispose the patient to cardiac dysfunction. If corticosteroids or corticotropin are used concomitantly with AMPHOTEC, serum electrolytes and cardiac function should be monitored.
Cyclosporine and Tacrolimus: In the same randomized, double-blind, empiric trial to compare AMPHOTEC and amphotericin B deoxycholate, patients with normal baseline serum creatinine were prospectively enrolled into four strata: adults receiving cyclosporine or tacrolimus (n=89); or pediatric patients (< 16 years old) receiving cyclosporine or tacrolimus (n=15); adults not receiving cyclosporine or tacrolimus (n=75); or pediatric patients not receiving cyclosporine or tacrolimus (n=34). Patients were assessed for renal toxicity defined as either a doubling or an increase of 1.0 mg/dL or more from baseline serum creatinine, or ≥ 50% decrease from baseline calculated creatinine clearance. Adults and pediatric patients receiving cyclosporine or tacrolimus in addition to AMPHOTEC had a significantly lower rate of renal toxicity (31%, 16/51), compared to the amphotericin B deoxycholate patients receiving cyclosporine or tacrolimus (68%, 34/50). In the adults and pediatric patients not receiving cyclosporine or tacrolimus, only 8% (4/51) of the AMPHOTEC patients experienced renal toxicity compared to 35% (17/49) of the amphotericin B deoxycholate patients.
Digitalis glycosides: Concurrent use of amphotericin B may induce hypokalemia and may potentiate digitalis toxicity. If digitalis glycosides are administered concomitantly with AMPHOTEC, serum potassium levels should be closely monitored.
Flucytosine: Concurrent use of flucytosine with amphotericin B-containing preparations may increase the toxicity of flucytosine by possibly increasing its cellular uptake and/or impairing its renal excretion. Caution is urged when flucytosine is given concomitantly with AMPHOTEC.
Imidazoles (e.g., ketoconazole, miconazole, clotrimazole, fluconazole, etc.): Antagonism between amphotericin B and imidazole derivatives, such as miconazole and ketoconazole which inhibit ergosterol synthesis, has been reported in both *in vitro* and *in vivo* animal studies. The clinical significance of these findings has not been determined.
Other nephrotoxic medications: Concurrent use of amphotericin B and agents such as aminoglycosides and pentamidine may enhance the potential for drug-induced renal toxicity. Caution is urged if aminoglycosides or pentamidine are used concomitantly with AMPHOTEC. Intensive monitoring of renal function is recommended in patients requiring any combination of nephrotoxic medications.
Skeletal muscle relaxants: Amphotericin B-induced hypokalemia may enhance the curariform effect of skeletal muscle relaxants (e.g., tubocurarine) due to hypokalemia. If skeletal muscle relaxants are administered concomitantly with AMPHOTEC, serum potassium levels should be closely monitored.
Carcinogenesis, Mutagenesis and Impairment of Fertility
No long-term studies in animals have been performed with AMPHOTEC or amphotericin B deoxycholate to evaluate carcinogenic potential. AMPHOTEC and/or amphotericin B were not mutagenic *in vitro* with and without an exogenous mammalian microsomal metabolic activation system when assayed in the *Salmonella* reverse mutation assay, the CHO chromosomal aberration assay and the mouse lymphoma forward mutation assay. AMPHOTEC was also negative *in vivo* in the mouse bone marrow micronucleus assay. No

studies have been conducted to determine if AMPHOTEC affects fertility or if it produces adverse effects when administered peri- or postnatally in animals. In multiple dose toxicity studies of up to 13 weeks in rats at doses up to 0.5 times the recommended human dose and in dogs at doses up to 0.4 times the recommended human dose (based on body surface area), ovarian and testicular histology were unaffected.
Pregnancy
Teratogenic Effects. Pregnancy Category B: There are no reports of pregnant women having been treated with AMPHOTEC. Reproduction studies in rats at doses up to 0.4 times the recommended human dose and in rabbits at doses up to 1.1 times the recommended human dose have revealed no evidence of harm to the fetus due to treatment with AMPHOTEC. Because animal reproduction studies are not always predictive of human response and because adequate and well controlled studies have not been conducted in pregnant women, AMPHOTEC should be used during pregnancy only if the anticipated benefit to the patient outweighs the potential risk to the fetus.
Nursing Mothers
It is not known whether AMPHOTEC is excreted in milk. Because of the potential for serious adverse reactions in nursing infants from amphotericin B, a decision should be made to discontinue nursing or discontinue treatment with AMPHOTEC, taking into account the importance of the drug to the mother.
Pediatric Use
Ninety-seven pediatric patients with systemic fungal infections have been treated with AMPHOTEC, at daily doses (mg/kg) similar to those given to adults. No unexpected adverse events have been reported. In the same empiric, multicenter trial, pediatric patients (< 16 years) treated with AMPHOTEC had significantly less renal toxicity than amphotericin B deoxycholate patients. Only 12% (3/25) of pediatric patients treated with AMPHOTEC developed nephrotoxicity compared to 52% (11/21) of pediatric patients receiving amphotericin B deoxycholate. Renal toxicity defined as either a doubling or an increase of 1.0 mg/dL or more from baseline serum creatinine, or ≥ 50% decrease from baseline calculated creatinine clearance.
Geriatric Use
Sixty-one patients at least 65 years of age have been treated with AMPHOTEC. No unexpected adverse events have been reported.

ADVERSE REACTIONS
The following adverse events are based on the experience of 572 AMPHOTEC patients from 5 open studies of patients with systemic fungal infections, of whom 526 were treated with a daily dose of 3–6 mg/kg. Additionally, comparative adverse event data from 150 AMPHOTEC (4 or 6 mg/kg/day) and 146 amphotericin B deoxycholate (0.8 or 1 mg/kg/day) patients in prospectively randomized double-blinded studies of empiric treatment of febrile and neutropenic patients or treatment of aspergillosis are also provided.
Infusion-related adverse events: Infusion-related adverse events (1 to 3 hours after starting intravenous infusion) occurred most frequently in association with the first infusion of AMPHOTEC. Their frequency and severity decreased with subsequent dosing. Based on the combined non-comparative studies, 35% (197/569) of the patients reported chills or chills and fever, possibly or probably related to AMPHOTEC, on the first day of dosing, compared to 14% (58/422) by the seventh dose. In the comparative studies, a similar decreasing trend was noted for AMPHOTEC and amphotericin B deoxycholate. Adverse events that were considered to be possibly or probably related to AMPHOTEC and that occurred in 5% or more of the patients are summarized in the table above:
[See first table above]

Summary of Probably and Possibly Related Adverse Events Reported by ≥5% of AMPHOTEC Patients

Adverse Event	Non-Comparative Studies		Comparative Studies [a]	
	AMPHOTEC (n=572) %	AMPHOTEC Aspergillosis Patients (n=161) %	AMPHOTEC (n=150) %	Amphotericin B Deoxycholate (n=146) %
Body as a Whole				
Chills	50	55	77	53
Fever	33	34	55	47
Headache	5	8	4	3
Chills and fever	3	3	7	2
Cardiovascular System				
Hypotension	10	9	12	6
Tachycardia	10	12	9	5
Hypertension	7	9	7	6
Digestive System				
Nausea	8	12	7	7
Nausea and vomiting	7	11	7	7
Vomiting	6	8	11	8
Liver function test abnormal	4	4	11	8
Hemic and Lymphatic System				
Thrombocytopenia	6	7	1	1
Altered Laboratory Data				
Hypokalemia	8	7	26	29
*Creatinine increased (B)	12	12	21	34
Hypomagnesemia	4	7	6	11
Hyperbilirubinemia	3	2	19	17
Alkaline phosphatase increased	3	3	7	8
Hypocalcemia	1	1	6	9
Hyperglycemia	1	1	6	6
Respiratory System				
Dyspnea	5	4	9	4
Hypoxia	4	6	9	5

[a] From AMPHOTEC (4 or 6 mg/kg/day) and amphotericin B deoxycholate (0.8 or 1 mg/kg/day) patients in prospectively randomized double-blinded studies of empiric treatment of febrile and neutropenic patients or treatment of first-line aspergillosis, respectively.
(b) Includes patients with "kidney function abnormal" which was associated with an increase in creatinine.

Dose of AMPHOTEC	Volume of Reconstituted AMPHOTEC	Infusion Bag Size for 5% Dextrose for Injection
10–35 mg	2–7 mL	50 mL
35–70 mg	7–14 mL	100 mL
70–175 mg	14–35 mL	250 mL
175–350 mg	35–70 mL	500 mL
350–1000 mg	70–200 mL	1000 mL

Continued on next page

Amphotec—Cont.

Additionally, the following adverse events also occurred in 5% or more of AMPHOTEC patients; however, the causal relationship of these adverse events is uncertain:

General (body as a whole): abdomen enlarged, abdominal pain, back pain, chest pain, face edema, injection site inflammation, mucous membrane disorder, pain, sepsis

Cardiovascular system: cardiovascular disorder, hemorrhage, postural hypotension

Digestive system: diarrhea, dry mouth, hematemesis, jaundice, stomatitis

Hemic and lymphatic system: anemia, coagulation disorder, prothrombin decreased

Metabolic and nutritional disorders: edema, generalized edema, hypocalcemia, hypophosphatemia, peripheral edema, weight gain

Nervous system: confusion, dizziness, insomnia, somnolence, thinking abnormal, tremor

Respiratory system: apnea, asthma, cough increased, epistaxis, hyperventilation, lung disorder, rhinitis

Skin and appendages: maculopapular rash, pruritus, rash, sweating

Special Senses: eye hemorrhage

Urogenital: hematuria

The following adverse events occurred in 1% to less than 5% of AMPHOTEC patients.

The causal association between these adverse events and AMPHOTEC is uncertain.

General (body as a whole): accidental injury, allergic reaction, asthenia, death, hypothermia, immune system disorder, infection, injection site pain, injection site reaction, neck pain

Cardiovascular system: arrhythmia, atrial fibrillation, bradycardia, congestive heart failure, heart arrest, phlebitis, shock, supraventricular tachycardia, syncope, vasodilatation, venoocclusive liver disease, ventricular extrasystoles

Digestive system: anorexia, bloody diarrhea, constipation, dyspepsia, fecal incontinence, gamma glutamyl transpeptidase increased, gastrointestinal disorder, gastrointestinal hemorrhage, gingivitis, glossitis, hepatic failure, melena, mouth ulceration, oral moniliasis, rectal disorder

Hemic and lymphatic system: ecchymosis, fibrinogen increased, hypochromic anemia, leukocytosis, leukopenia, petechia, thromboplastin decreased

Metabolic and nutritional disorders: acidosis, BUN increased, dehydration, hyponatremia, hyperkalemia, hyperlipemia, hypernatremia, hypervolemia, hypoglycemia, hypoproteinemia, lactic dehydrogenase increased, AST (SGOT) increased, ALT (SGPT) increased, weight loss

Musculoskeletal system: arthralgia, myalgia

Nervous system: agitation, anxiety, convulsion, depression, hallucinations, hypertonia, nervousness, neuropathy, paresthesia, psychosis, speech disorder, stupor

Respiratory system: hemoptysis, lung edema, pharyngitis, pleural effusion, respiratory disorder, sinusitis

Skin and appendages: acne, alopecia, petechial rash, skin discoloration, skin disorder, skin nodule, skin ulcer, urticaria, vesiculobullous rash

Special senses: amblyopia, deafness, ear disorder, tinnitus

Urogenital system: albuminuria, dysuria, glycosuria, kidney failure, oliguria, urinary incontinence, urinary retention, urinary tract disorder

OVERDOSAGE

AMPHOTEC is not dialyzable. Amphotericin B deoxycholate overdose has been reported to result in cardio-respiratory arrest.

DOSAGE AND ADMINISTRATION

The recommended dose for adults and pediatric patients is 3–4 mg/kg as required, once a day.

AMPHOTEC is administered diluted in 5% Dextrose for Injection by intravenous infusion at a rate of 1 mg/kg/hour. A test dose immediately preceding the first dose is advisable when commencing all new courses of treatment. A small amount of drug (e.g., 10 mL of the final preparation containing between 1.6 to 8.3 mg) should be infused over 15 to 30 minutes and the patient carefully observed for the next 30 minutes.

The infusion time may be shortened to a minimum of 2 hours for patients who show no evidence of intolerance or infusion-related reactions. If the patient experiences acute reactions or cannot tolerate the infusion volume, the infusion time may be extended.

Directions for reconstitution and preparation of infusion admixture

AMPHOTEC must be reconstituted by addition of Sterile Water for Injection. Using sterile syringe and a 20-gauge needle, rapidly add the following volumes to the vial to provide a liquid containing 5 mg of amphotericin B per mL. Shake gently by hand, rotating the vial until all solids have dissolved. Note that the fluid may be opalescent or clear.

50 mg/vial   add   10 mL Sterile Water for Injection
100 mg/vial   add   20 mL Sterile Water for Injection

For infusion, further dilute the reconstituted liquid to a final concentration of approximately 0.6 mg/mL (range 0.16 mg/mL to 0.83 mg/mL). The following table provides dilution recommendations:
[See second table at top of previous page]

Do not reconstitute the lyophilized powder with saline or dextrose solutions, or admix the reconstituted liquid with saline or electrolytes. The use of any solution other than those recommended, or the presence of a bacteriostatic agent (e.g., benzyl alcohol) in the solution may cause precipitation of AMPHOTEC.

Do not filter or use an in-line filter with AMPHOTEC.

Do not mix the infusion admixture with other drugs. If administered through an existing intravenous line, flush with 5% Dextrose for Injection prior to infusion of AMPHOTEC, otherwise administer via a separate line.

Parenteral drug products should be inspected visually for particulate matter and discoloration prior to administration whenever solution and container permit. Do not use if a precipitate or foreign matter is present, or if the seal is not intact. Strict aseptic technique always should be observed during reconstitution and dilution since no preservatives are present in the lyophilized drug or in the solutions used for reconstitution and dilution.

After reconstitution, the drug should be refrigerated at 2–8°C (36–46°F) and used within 24 hours. **Do not freeze.** After further dilution with 5% Dextrose for Injection, the infusion should be stored in a refrigerator (2–8°C) and used within 24 hours. Partially used vials should be discarded.

HOW SUPPLIED

AMPHOTEC® (Amphotericin B Cholesteryl Sulfate Complex for Injection) is a sterile lyophilized powder supplied in single use glass vials. Each vial is individually packaged.
AMPHOTEC 50 mg in 20 mL vial (NDC 61471-115-12)
AMPHOTEC 100 mg in 50 mL vial (NDC 61471-110-12)

STORAGE

Store unopened vials of AMPHOTEC at 15–30°C (59–86°F). AMPHOTEC should be retained in the carton until time of use.

Manufactured by:
Ben Venue Laboratories, Inc., Bedford, OH 44146, USA
Distributed by:
SEQUUS Pharmaceuticals, Inc., Menlo Park, CA 94025, USA
Revision date: October 1997
U.S. Patent Numbers 4,822,777; 5,032,582; 5,194,266; 5,077,057.

REFERENCES
1. [1]Denning DW, LEE JY, Hostetler JS, et al. NIAID Mycoses Study Group multicenter trial of oral itraconazole therapy for invasive aspergillosis. *Am J Med.* 1994;97: 135–144.

Shown in Product Identification Guide, page 338

DOXIL®   ℞
[däk 'sil]
(doxorubicin HCl liposome injection)
FOR INTRAVENOUS INFUSION ONLY
A product of SEQUUS Pharmaceuticals, Inc.

WARNINGS

1. Experience with DOXIL® (doxorubicin HCl liposome injection) at high cumulative doses is too limited to have established its effect on the myocardium. It should therefore be assumed that DOXIL® will have myocardial toxicity similar to conventional formulations of doxorubicin HCl. With these formulations of doxorubicin HCl, serious irreversible myocardial toxicity leading to congestive heart failure often unresponsive to cardiac supportive therapy may be encountered as the total dosage of doxorubicin HCl approaches 550 mg/m^2. Prior use of other anthracyclines or anthracenediones will reduce the total dose of doxorubicin HCl that can be given without cardiac toxicity. Cardiac toxicity also may occur at lower cumulative doses in patients with prior mediastinal irradiation or who are receiving concurrent cyclophosphamide therapy.

   DOXIL® should be administered to patients with a history of cardiovascular disease only when the benefit outweighs the risk to the patient.

2. Acute infusion-associated reactions (flushing, shortness of breath, facial swelling, headache, chills, back pain, tightness in the chest or throat, and/or hypotension) have occurred in about 7% of patients treated with DOXIL®. In most patients, these reactions resolve over the course of several hours to a day once the infusion is terminated. In some patients, the reaction resolves by slowing the infusion rate. (See **WARNINGS—Infusion Reactions.**)

3. Severe myelosuppression may occur.
4. Dosage should be reduced in patients with impaired hepatic function. (See **DOSAGE AND ADMINISTRATION.**)
5. Accidental substitution of DOXIL® for doxorubicin HCl has resulted in severe side effects. DOXIL® exhibits unique pharmacokinetic properties compared to doxorubicin HCl and should not be substituted on a mg per mg basis. (See **DOSAGE AND ADMINISTRATION.**)
6. DOXIL® should be administered only under the supervision of a physician who is experienced in the use of cancer chemotherapeutic agents.

DESCRIPTION

DOXIL® (doxorubicin HCl liposome injection) is doxorubicin hydrochloride (HCl) encapsulated in STEALTH® liposomes for intravenous administration.

Note: Liposomal encapsulation can substantially affect a drug's functional properties relative to those of the unencapsulated drug.

In addition, different liposomal drug products may vary from one another in the chemical composition and physical form of the liposomes. Such differences can substantially affect the functional properties of liposomal drug products. DO NOT SUBSTITUTE.

Doxorubicin is a cytotoxic anthracycline antibiotic isolated from *Streptomyces peucetius* var. *caesius.*

Doxorubicin HCl, which is the established name for (8S,10S)-10-[(3-amino-2,3,6 -trideoxy-α-L-*lyxo*-hexopyranosyl)oxy]-8-glycolyl-7,8,9,10-tetrahydro-6,8,11-trihydroxy-1-methoxy-5,12-naphthacenedione hydrochloride, has the following structure:

The molecular formula of the drug is $C_{27}H_{29}NO_{11} \cdot HCl$; its molecular weight is 579.99.

DOXIL® is provided as a sterile, translucent, red liposomal dispersion in 10-mL glass, single use vials. Each vial contains 20 mg doxorubicin HCl at a concentration of 2 mg/mL and a pH of 6.5. The STEALTH® liposome carriers are composed of N-(carbonyl-methoxypolyethylene glycol 2000)-1,2-distearoyl-*sn*-glycero-3-phosphoethanolamine sodium salt (MPEG-DSPE), 3.19 mg/mL; fully hydrogenated soy phosphatidylcholine (HSPC), 9.58 mg/mL; and cholesterol, 3.19 mg/mL. Each mL also contains ammonium sulfate, approximately 2 mg; histidine as a buffer; hydrochloric acid and/or sodium hydroxide for pH control; and sucrose to maintain isotonicity. Greater than 90% of the drug is encapsulated in the STEALTH® liposomes.

MPEG-DSPE has the following structural formula:

n=ca. 45

HSPC has the following structural formula:

m, n = 14 or 16

CLINICAL PHARMACOLOGY

Mechanism of Action

The active ingredient of DOXIL® is doxorubicin HCl. The mechanism of action of doxorubicin HCl is thought to be related to its ability to bind DNA and inhibit nucleic acid synthesis. Cell structure studies have demonstrated rapid cell penetration and perinuclear chromatin binding, rapid inhibition of mitotic activity and nucleic acid synthesis, and induction of mutagenesis and chromosomal aberrations.

DOXIL® is doxorubicin HCl encapsulated in long-circulating STEALTH® liposomes. Liposomes are microscopic vesicles composed of a phospholipid bilayer that are capable of encapsulating active drugs. The STEALTH® liposomes of DOXIL® are formulated with surface-bound methoxypolyethylene glycol (MPEG), a process often referred to as pegylation, to protect liposomes from detection by the mononuclear phagocyte system (MPS) and to increase blood circulation time.

Representation of a STEALTH® liposome:

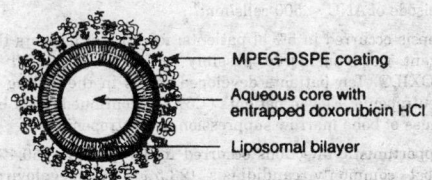

MPEG-DSPE coating

Aqueous core with entrapped doxorubicin HCl

Liposomal bilayer

STEALTH® liposomes have a half-life of approximately 55 hours in humans. They are stable in blood, and direct measurement of liposomal doxorubicin shows that at least 90% of the drug (the assay used cannot quantify less than 5–10% free doxorubicin) remains liposome-encapsulated during circulation.

It is hypothesized that because of their small size (ca. 100 nm) and persistence in the circulation the pegylated DOXIL® liposomes are able to penetrate the altered and often compromised vasculature of tumors. This hypothesis is supported by studies using colloidal gold-containing STEALTH® liposomes, which can be visualized microscopically. Evidence of penetration of STEALTH® liposomes from blood vessels and their entry and accumulation in tumors has been seen in mice with C-26 colon carcinoma tumors and in transgenic mice with Kaposi's sarcoma-like lesions. Once the STEALTH® liposomes distribute to the tissue compartment, the encapsulated doxorubicin HCl becomes available. The exact mechanism of release is not understood.

Pharmacokinetics

The plasma pharmacokinetics of DOXIL® were evaluated in 42 patients with AIDS-related Kaposi's sarcoma (KS) who received single doses of 10 or 20 mg/m² administered by a 30-minute infusion. Twenty-three of these patients received single doses of both 10 and 20 mg/m² with a 3-week washout period between doses. The pharmacokinetic parameter values of DOXIL®, given for total doxorubicin (most liposomally bound), are presented in the following table.

Pharmacokinetic Parameters of DOXIL® in AIDS Patients with Kaposi's Sarcoma

Parameter (units)	Dose 10 mg/m²	Dose 20 mg/m²
Peak Plasma Concentration (µg/mL)	4.12 ± 0.215	8.34 ± 0.49
Plasma Clearance (L/h/m²)	0.056 ± 0.01	0.041 ± 0.004
Steady-State Volume of Distribution (L/m²)	2.83 ± 0.145	2.72 ± 0.120
AUC (µg/mL·h)	277 ± 32.9	590 ± 58.7
First Phase (λ_1) Half-Life (h)	4.7 ± 1.1	5.2 ± 1.4
Second Phase (λ_2) Half-Life (h)	52.3 ± 5.6	55.0 ± 4.8

n=23

Mean ± Standard Error

DOXIL® displayed linear pharmacokinetics. Disposition occurred in two phases after DOXIL® administration, with a relatively short first phase (~5 hours) and a prolonged second phase (~55 hours) that accounted for the majority of the area under the curve (AUC).

Distribution: In contrast to the pharmacokinetics of doxorubicin, which display a large volume of distribution ranging from 700 to 1100 L/m², the steady state volume of distribution of DOXIL® indicated that DOXIL® was confined mostly to the vascular fluid volume. Plasma protein binding of DOXIL® has not been determined; however, the plasma protein binding of doxorubicin is approximately 70%.

Metabolism: Doxorubicinol, the major metabolite of doxorubicin, was detected at very low levels (range: 0.8 to 26.2 ng/mL) in the plasma of patients who received 10 to 20 mg/m² DOXIL®.

Excretion: The plasma clearance of DOXIL® was slow, with a mean clearance value of 0.041 L/h/m² at a dose of 20 mg/m². This is in contrast to doxorubicin, which displays a plasma clearance value ranging from 24 to 35 L/h/m². Because of its slower clearance, the AUC of DOXIL®, primarily representing the circulation of liposome-encapsulated doxorubicin, is approximately two to three orders of magnitude larger than the AUC for a similar dose of conventional doxorubicin HCl as reported in the literature.

Special Populations: The pharmacokinetics of DOXIL® have not been separately evaluated in women, in members of different ethnic groups, or in individuals with renal or hepatic insufficiency.

Drug–Drug Interactions: Although the patient population for the current indication is on various antiviral medications, the drug–drug interactions between DOXIL® and the antiviral drugs have not been evaluated.

Tissue Distribution

Kaposi's sarcoma lesions and normal skin biopsies were obtained at 48 and 96 hours postinfusion of 20 mg/m² DOXIL® in 11 patients. The concentration of DOXIL® in KS lesions was a median of 19 (range, 3–53) times higher than in normal skin at 48 hours posttreatment; however, this was not corrected for likely differences in blood content between KS lesions and normal skin. The corrected ratio may lie between 1 and 22 times. Thus, higher concentrations of DOXIL® are delivered to KS lesions than to normal skin.

Clinical Studies

AIDS-Related Kaposi's Sarcoma

DOXIL® was studied in an open-label, single-arm, multicenter study utilizing DOXIL® at 20 mg/m² by intravenous infusion every three weeks generally until progression or intolerance occurred. In an interim analysis, the treatment history of 383 patients were reviewed, and a cohort of 77 patients was retrospectively identified as having disease progression on prior systemic combination chemotherapy (at least 2 cycles of a regimen containing at least two of three treatments: bleomycin, vincristine or vinblastine, or doxorubicin) or as being intolerant to such therapy. Fortynine of the 77 (64%) patients had received prior doxorubicin HCl.

These 77 patients were predominantly white, homosexual males with a median CD4 count of 10 cells/mm³. Their age ranged from 24 to 54 years, with a mean age of 38 years. Using the ACTG staging criteria,[1] 78% of the patients were at poor risk for tumor burden, 96% at poor risk for immune system, and 58% at poor risk for systemic illness at baseline. Their mean Karnofsky status score was 74%. All 77 patients had cutaneous or subcutaneous lesions, 40% also had oral lesions, 26% pulmonary lesions, and 14% of patients lesions of the stomach/intestine. The majority of these patients had disease progression on prior systemic combination chemotherapy.

The median time on study for these 77 patients was 155 days and ranged from 1 to 456 days. The median cumulative dose was 154 mg/m² and ranged from 20 to 620 mg/m².

Two analyses of tumor response were used to evaluate the effectiveness of DOXIL®: one analysis based on investigator assessment of changes in lesions over the entire body, and one analysis based on changes in indicator lesions.

Investigator Assessment

Investigator response was based on modified ACTG criteria.[1] Partial response was defined as no new lesions, sites of disease, or worsening edema; flattening of ≥50% of previously raised lesions or area of indicator lesions decreasing by ≥50%; and response lasting at least 21 days with no prior progression.

Indicator Lesion Assessment

A retrospectively defined analysis was conducted based on assessment of the response of up to five prospectively identified representative indicator lesions. A partial response was defined as flattening of ≥50% of previously raised indicator lesions, or >50% decrease in the area of indicator lesions and lasting at least 21 days with no prior progression.

Only patients with adequate documentation of baseline status and follow-up assessments were considered evaluable for response. Patients who received concomitant KS treatment during study, who completed local radiotherapy to sites encompassing one or more of the indicator lesions within two months of study entry, who had less than four indicator lesions, or who had less than three raised indicator lesions at baseline (the latter applies solely to indicator lesion assessment) were considered nonevaluable for response. Of the 77 patients who had disease progression on prior systemic combination chemotherapy or who were intolerant to such therapy, 34 were evaluable for investigator assessment and 42 were evaluable for indicator lesion assessment.

Response is summarized in the table below.

Response in Refractory[a] AIDS-KS

Investigator Assessment	All Evaluable Patients (n = 34)	Evaluable Patients Who Received Prior Doxorubicin (n = 20)
Response[b]		
Partial (PR)	27%	30%
Stable	29%	40%
Progression	44%	30%
Duration of PR (days)		
Median	73	89
Range	42+– 210+	42+– 210+
Time to PR (days)		
Median	43	53
Range	15–133	15–109

Indicator Lesion Assessment	All Evaluable Patients (n = 42)	Evaluable Patients Who Received Prior Doxorubicin (n = 23)
Response[b]		
Partial (PR)	48%	52%
Stable	26%	30%
Progression	26%	17%
Duration of PR (days)		
Median	71	79
Range	22+– 210+	35 – 210+
Time to PR (days)		
Median	22	48
Range	15–109	15–109

a Patients with disease that progressed on prior combination chemotherapy or who were intolerant to such therapy.

b There were no complete responses in this population.

Clinical Benefit

Clinical benefit (e.g., decreased pain, disfigurement, pulmonary or gastrointestinal symptoms) was not well evaluated in the open studies carried out to date. A controlled trial with double-blinded assessment of clinical endpoints is ongoing.

INDICATIONS AND USAGE

DOXIL® (doxorubicin HCl liposome injection) is indicated for the treatment of AIDS-related Kaposi's sarcoma in patients with disease that has progressed on prior combination chemotherapy or in patients who are intolerant to such therapy.

CONTRAINDICATIONS

DOXIL® (doxorubicin HCl liposome injection) is contraindicated in patients who have a history of hypersensitivity reactions to a conventional formulation of doxorubicin HCl or the components of DOXIL®.

WARNINGS

Cardiac Toxicity

Experience with DOXIL® (doxorubicin HCl liposome injection) is limited in evaluating cardiac risk. Therefore, warnings related to the use of conventional formulation doxorubicin HCl should be observed.

Special attention must be given to the cardiac toxicity exhibited by doxorubicin HCl. Although uncommon, acute left ventricular failure has occurred, particularly in patients who have received total dosage of the drug exceeding the currently recommended limit of 550 mg/m². This limit appears to be lower (400 mg/m²) in patients who received radiotherapy to the mediastinal area or concomitant therapy with other potentially cardiotoxic agents such as cyclophosphamide.

Caution should be observed in patients who have received other anthracyclines. The total dose of doxorubicin HCl administered to the individual patient should also take into account any previous or concomitant therapy with related compounds such as daunorubicin. Congestive heart failure and/or cardiomyopathy may be encountered after discontinuation of therapy. Patients with a history of cardiovascular disease should be administered DOXIL® only when the potential benefit of treatment outweighs the risk.

The long-term cardiac effects of DOXIL® in patients relative to the conventional formulation of doxorubicin HCl have not been adequately evaluated.

Cardiac function should be carefully monitored in patients treated with DOXIL®. The most definitive test for anthracycline myocardial injury is endomyocardial biopsy. Other methods such as echocardiography or gated radionuclide scans have been used to monitor cardiac function during an-

Continued on next page

Doxil—Cont.

thracycline therapy. Any of these methods should be employed to monitor potential cardiac toxicity during DOXIL® therapy. If these test results indicate possible cardiac injury associated with DOXIL® therapy, the benefit of continued therapy must be carefully weighed against the risk of myocardial injury. (See **ADVERSE REACTIONS—Cardiac Events.**)

Myelosuppression
The majority of experience with DOXIL® has been in AIDS-KS patients who present with baseline myelosuppression due to such factors as their HIV disease or numerous concomitant medications. In this population, myelosuppression appears to be the dose-limiting adverse event. Leukopenia is the most common adverse event (about 60%) experienced in this population; anemia (about 20%) and thrombocytopenia (about 10%) can also be expected.

Because of the potential for bone marrow suppression, careful hematologic monitoring is required during use of DOXIL®, including white blood cell and platelet counts and Hgb/Hct. With the recommended dosage schedule, leukopenia is usually transient. Hematologic toxicity may require dose reduction or suspension or delay of DOXIL® therapy. Persistent severe myelosuppression may result in superinfection or hemorrhage.

DOXIL® may potentiate the toxicity of other anticancer therapies. In particular, hematologic toxicity may be more severe when DOXIL® is administered in combination with other agents that cause bone marrow suppression.

Patients treated with DOXIL® may require G-CSF (or GM-CSF) to support their blood counts. (See **ADVERSE REACTIONS—Hematologic.**)

Infusion Reactions
Acute infusion-associated reactions characterized by flushing, shortness of breath, facial swelling, headache, chills, back pain, tightness in the chest and throat, and/or hypotension have occurred in approximately 6.8% of patients treated with DOXIL®. The reaction appears to occur with the first infusion and does not appear to occur with later infusions if not present initially. In most patients, these reactions resolve over the course of several hours to a day once the infusion is terminated. In some patients, the reaction resolves by slowing the rate of infusion. Similar reactions have not been reported with conventional doxorubicin and they presumably represent a reaction to the DOXIL® liposomes or one of its surface components.

Many patients were able to tolerate further infusions without complications, however, six patients were terminated from DOXIL® therapy because of an infusion reaction.

Palmar-Plantar Erythrodysesthesia
Among 705 patients with AIDS-related Kaposi's sarcoma treated with DOXIL®, 24 (3.4%) developed palmar-plantar skin eruptions characterized by swelling, pain, erythema and, for some patients, desquamation of the skin on the hands and the feet (palmar-plantar erythrodysesthesia). The syndrome was generally seen after six or more weeks of treatment but may occur earlier. The incidence of this reaction may be higher when DOXIL® is administered at doses that are higher or at intervals that are shorter than those recommended. In most patients, the reaction is mild and resolves in one to two weeks so that prolonged delay of therapy need not occur (See **DOSAGE AND ADMINISTRATION**). The reaction can be severe and debilitating in some patients, however, and may require discontinuation of treatment.

Pregnancy Category D
DOXIL® can cause fetal harm when administered to a pregnant woman. DOXIL® is embryotoxic at doses of 1 mg/kg/day (about $^1/_3$ the recommended human dose on a mg/m^2 basis) in rats. DOXIL® is embryotoxic and abortifacient at 0.5 mg/kg/day (about $^1/_4$ the recommended human dose on a mg/m^2 basis) in rabbits. Embryotoxicity was characterized by increased embryo-fetal deaths and reduced live litter sizes.

There are no adequate and well-controlled studies in pregnant women. If DOXIL® is to be used during pregnancy, or if the patient becomes pregnant during therapy, the patient should be apprised of the potential hazard to the fetus. Women of childbearing potential should be advised to avoid pregnancy.

Toxicity Potentiation
The doxorubicin in DOXIL® may potentiate the toxicity of other anticancer therapies. Exacerbation of cyclophosphamide-induced hemorrhagic cystitis and enhancement of the hepatotoxicity of 6-mercaptopurine have been reported with the conventional formulation of doxorubicin HCl. Radiation-induced toxicity to the myocardium, mucosae, skin and liver have been reported to be increased by the administration of doxorubicin HCl.

Injection Site Effects
DOXIL® should be considered an irritant and precautions should be taken to avoid extravasation. On intravenous administration of DOXIL®, extravasation may occur with or without an accompanying stinging or burning sensation and even if blood returns well on aspiration of the infusion needle (See **DOSAGE AND ADMINISTRATION**). If any signs or symptoms of extravasation have occurred, the infusion should be immediately terminated and restarted in another vein. The application of ice over the site of extravasation for approximately 30 minutes may be helpful in alleviating the local reaction. **DOXIL® must not be given by the intramuscular or subcutaneous route.**

In studies with rabbits, lesions that were induced by subcutaneous injection of DOXIL® were minor and reversible compared to more severe and irreversible lesions and tissue necrosis that were induced after subcutaneous injection of conventional doxorubicin HCl.

Hepatic Impairment
The pharmacokinetics of DOXIL® have not been studied in patients with hepatic impairment. Doxorubicin is known to be eliminated in large part by the liver. Thus DOXIL® dosage should be reduced in patients with impaired hepatic function. (See **DOSAGE AND ADMINISTRATION.**)

Prior to DOXIL® administration, evaluation of hepatic function is recommended using conventional clinical laboratory tests such as SGOT, SGPT, alkaline phosphatase and bilirubin. (See **DOSAGE AND ADMINISTRATION.**)

PRECAUTIONS

Laboratory Tests
Complete blood counts, including platelet counts, should be obtained frequently and at a minimum prior to each dose of DOXIL®.

Drug Interactions
No formal drug interaction studies have been conducted with DOXIL®. Until specific compatibility data are available, it is not recommended that DOXIL® be mixed with other drugs. DOXIL® may interact with drugs known to interact with the conventional formulation of doxorubicin HCl.

Carcinogenesis, Mutagenesis, Impairment of Fertility
Although no studies have been conducted with DOXIL®, doxorubicin HCl and related compounds have been shown to have mutagenic and carcinogenic properties when tested in experimental models.

STEALTH® liposomes without drug are negative when tested in Ames, mouse lymphoma and chromosomal aberration assays in vitro, and mammalian micronucleus assay in vivo.

The possible adverse effects on fertility in males and females in humans or experimental animals have not been adequately evaluated. However, DOXIL® resulted in mild to moderate ovarian and testicular atrophy in mice after a single dose of 36 mg/kg (about 5 times the recommended human dose on a mg/m^2 basis). Decreased testicular weights and hypospermia were present in rats after repeat doses of ≥0.25 mg/kg/day (about $^1/_{13}$ the recommended human dose on a mg/m^2 basis), and diffuse degeneration of the seminiferous tubules and a marked decrease in spermatogenesis were observed in dogs after repeat doses of 1 mg/kg/day (equivalent to the recommended human dose on a mg/m^2 basis).

Pregnancy
Pregnancy Category D: (See **WARNINGS.**)

Nursing Mothers
It is not known whether this drug is excreted in human milk. Because many drugs are excreted in human milk and because of the potential for serious adverse reactions in nursing infants from DOXIL®, mothers should discontinue nursing prior to taking this drug.

Pediatric Use
The safety and effectiveness of DOXIL® in pediatric patients have not been established.

Radiation Therapy
Recall of skin reaction due to prior radiotherapy has occurred with DOXIL® administration.

ADVERSE REACTIONS

Information on adverse events is based on the experience reported in 753 patients with AIDS-related KS enrolled in four studies. The majority of patients were treated with 20 mg/m^2 of DOXIL® (doxorubicin HCl liposome injection) every two to three weeks. The median time on study was 127 days and ranged from 1 to 811 days. The median cumulative dose was 120 mg/m^2 and ranged from 3.3 to 798.6 mg/m^2. Twenty-six patients (3.0%) received cumulative doses of greater than 450 mg/m^2.

Of these 753 patients, 61.2% were considered poor risk for KS tumor burden, 91.5% poor for immune system, and 46.9% for systemic illness; 36.2% were poor risk for all three categories. Patients' median CD4 count was 21.0 cells/mm^3, with 50.8% of patients having less than 50 cells/mm^3. The mean absolute neutrophil count at study entry was approximately 3000 cells/mm^3.

Patients received a variety of potentially myelotoxic drugs in combination with DOXIL®. Of the 693 patients with concomitant medication information, 58.7% were on one or more antiretroviral medications; 34.9% patients were on zidovudine (AZT), 20.8% on didanosine (ddl), 16.5% on zalcitabine (ddC), and 9.5% on stavudine (D4T). A total of 85.1% patients were on PCP prophylaxis, most (54.5%) on sulfamethoxazole/trimethoprim. Eighty-five percent of patients were receiving antifungal medications, primarily fluconazole (75.8%). Seventy-two percent of patients were receiving antivirals, 56.3% acyclovir, 29% ganciclovir, and 16% foscarnet. In addition, 47.8% patients received colony stimulating factors (sargramostim/filgrastim) sometime during their course of treatment.

Of the 753 patients enrolled in the DOXIL® clinical trials, adverse event information was available for 705 patients. In many instances it was difficult to determine whether adverse events resulted from DOXIL®, from concomitant therapy, or from the patients' underlying disease(s).

Hematologic
Neutropenia (<1000 neutrophils/mm^3) occurred in 49% of patients on study with 13% of patients having at least one episode of ANC < 500 cells/mm^3.

Sepsis occurred in 5% of patients; for 0.7% of patients the event was considered possibly or probably related to DOXIL®. Ten patients developed sepsis in the setting of neutropenia. Eleven patients (1.6%) discontinued study because of bone marrow suppression or neutropenia.

Opportunistic infections occurred in 355 patients (50.4%), most commonly candidiasis (23.5%), cytomegalovirus (20.1%), herpes simplex (10.5%), Pneumocystis carinii pneumonia (9.2%), and mycobacterium avium (8.4%). Four patients (0.6%) discontinued DOXIL® therapy because of opportunistic infection.

Infusion-Related Reactions (See WARNINGS)
Six patients (0.9%) discontinued DOXIL® therapy because of infusion reactions.

Palmar-Plantar Erythrodysesthesia
Three patients (0.4%) discontinued DOXIL® therapy because of palmar-plantar erythrodysesthesia. (See **WARNINGS.**)

Cardiac Events
Sixty-eight (9.6%) patients experienced cardiac-related adverse events. In 30 patients (4.3%), the event was thought to be possibly or probably related to DOXIL®. Nine cases of possibly or probably related cardiomyopathy and/or congestive heart failure were reported. Seven (1.0%) of the possibly or probably related cardiac events were severe. These severe events included arrhythmia (nonspecific), cardiomyopathy, heart failure, pericardial effusion, and tachycardia. Three patients discontinued study due to cardiac events.

Radiation Therapy
Recall of skin reaction due to prior radiotherapy has occurred with DOXIL® administration.

Eighty-three percent of the patients reported adverse events that were considered to be possibly or probably related to the treatment with DOXIL®. These adverse events are provided below. The table shows all events occurring at ≥5% in the overall treated population that were considered by investigators at least possibly related to DOXIL®. Rates are also given for the subset of refractory/intolerant patients. Adverse reactions only infrequently (5%) led to discontinuation of treatment. Those that did so included bone marrow suppression, cardiac adverse events, infusion-related reactions, toxoplasmosis, palmar-plantar erythrodysesthesia, pneumonia, cough/dyspnea, fatigue, optic neuritis, progression of a non-KS tumor, allergy to penicillin, and unspecified reasons.

Probably and Possibly Drug-Related Adverse Events Reported in ≥ 5% of All Treated Patients

	Refractory or Intolerant AIDS-KS Patients	Total AIDS-KS Patients
Number of Patients	77	705
Number of Patients Reporting Adverse Events	57 (74.0%)	586 (83.1%)
Adverse Event		
Neutropenia (ANC <1000/mm^3)	34 (44.2%)	352 (49.9%)
Anemia	5 (6.5%)	137 (19.4%)
Nausea	14 (18.2%)	119 (16.9%)
Asthenia	5 (6.5%)	70 (9.9%)
Hypochromic Anemia	4 (5.2%)	69 (9.8%)
Thrombocytopenia	5 (6.5%)	65 (9.2%)
Fever	6 (7.8%)	64 (9.1%)
Alopecia	7 (9.1%)	63 (8.9%)

Alkaline Phosphatase Increase	1 (1.3%)	55 (7.8%)	
Vomiting	6 (7.8%)	55 (7.8%)	
Diarrhea	4 (5.2%)	55 (7.8%)	
Stomatitis	4 (5.2%)	48 (6.8%)	
Oral Moniliasis	1 (1.3%)	39 (5.5%)	

Incidence 1% to 5% (Possibly or Probably Related)

Body as a Whole: headache, back pain, infection, allergic reaction, chills.
Cardiovascular: chest pain, hypotension, tachycardia.
Cutaneous: Herpes simplex, rash, itching.
Digestive System: mouth ulceration, glossitis, constipation, aphthous stomatitis, anorexia, dysphagia, abdominal pain.
Hematologic: hemolysis, increased prothrombin time.
Metabolic/Nutritional: SGPT increase, weight loss, hypocalcemia, hyperbilirubinemia, hyperglycemia.
Other: dyspnea, albuminuria, pneumonia, retinitis, emotional lability, dizziness, somnolence.

Incidence Less Than 1% (Possibly or Probably Related)

Body as a Whole: face edema, cellulitis, sepsis, abscess, radiation injury, flu syndrome, moniliasis, hypothermia, injection site hemorrhage, injection site pain, cryptococcosis, ascites.
Cardiovascular System: thrombophlebitis, cardiomyopathy, pericardial effusion, hemorrhage, palpitation, syncope, bundle branch block, congestive heart failure, cardiomegaly, heart arrest, migraine, thrombosis, ventricular arrhythmia.
Digestive System: dyspepsia, cholestatic jaundice, gastritis, gingivitis, ulcerative proctitis, colitis, esophageal ulcer, esophagitis, gastrointestinal hemorrhage, hepatic failure, leukoplakia of mouth, pancreatitis, ulcerative stomatitis, hepatitis, hepatosplenomegaly, increased appetite, jaundice, sclerosing cholangitis, tenesmus, fecal impaction.
Endocrine System: diabetes mellitus.
Hemic and Lymphatic System: eosinophilia, lymphadenopathy, lymphangitis, lymphedema, petechia, thromboplastin decrease.
Metabolic/Nutritional Disorders: lactic dehydrogenase increase, hypernatremia, creatinine increase, BUN increase, dehydration, edema, hypercalcemia, hyperkalemia, hyperlipemia, hyperuricemia, hypoglycemia, hypokalemia, hypolipemia, hypomagnesemia, hyponatremia, hypophosphatemia, hypoproteinemia, ketosis, weight gain.
Musculoskeletal System: myalgia, arthralgia, bone pain, myositis.
Nervous System: paresthesia, insomnia, peripheral neuritis, depression, neuropathy, anxiety, convulsion, hypotonia, acute brain syndrome, confusion, hemiplegia, hypertonia, hypokinesia, vertigo.
Respiratory System: pleural effusion, asthma, bronchitis, cough increase, hyperventilation, pharyngitis, pneumothorax, rhinitis, sinusitis.
Skin and Appendages: maculopapular rash, skin ulcer, exfoliative dermatitis, skin discoloration, herpes zoster, cutaneous moniliasis, erythema multiforme, erythema nodosum, furunculosis, psoriasis, pustular rash, skin necrosis, urticaria, vesiculobullous rash.
Special Senses: otitis media, taste perversion, abnormal vision, blindness, conjunctivitis, eye pain, optic neuritis, tinnitus, visual field defect.
Urogenital System: hematuria, balanitis, cystitis, dysuria, genital edema, glycosuria, kidney failure.

OVERDOSAGE

Acute overdosage with doxorubicin HCl causes increases in mucositis, leukopenia and thrombocytopenia.
Treatment of acute overdosage consists of treatment of the severely myelosuppressed patient with hospitalization, antibiotics, platelet and granulocyte transfusions and symptomatic treatment of mucositis.

DOSAGE AND ADMINISTRATION

AIDS-KS Patients
DOXIL® (doxorubicin HCl liposome injection) should be administered intravenously at a dose of 20 mg/m^2 (doxorubicin HCl equivalent) over 30 minutes, once every three weeks, for as long as patients respond satisfactorily and tolerate treatment.

Do not administer as a bolus injection or an undiluted solution. Rapid infusion may increase the risk of infusion-related reactions. (See **WARNINGS—Infusion Reactions.**)

Each vial contains 20 mg doxorubicin HCl at a concentration of 2 mg/mL.

DOXIL® should be considered an irritant and precautions should be taken to avoid extravasation. On intravenous administration of DOXIL®, extravasation may occur with or without an accompanying stinging or burning sensation and even if blood returns well on aspiration of the infusion needle. If any signs or symptoms of extravasation have occurred the infusion should be immediately terminated and restarted in another vein. The application of ice over the

PALMAR-PLANTAR ERYTHRODYSESTHESIA

Toxicity Grade	Symptoms	Weeks Since Last Dose	
		3	4
0	no symptoms	Redose at 3-week interval	Redose at 3-week interval
1	mild erythema, swelling, or desquamation not interfering with daily activities	Redose unless patient has experienced a previous Grade 3 or 4 skin toxicity in which case wait an additional week	Redose at 25% dose reduction; return to 3-week interval
2	erythema, desquamation, or swelling interfering with, but not precluding normal physical activities; small blisters or ulcerations less than 2 cm in diameter	Wait an additional week	Redose at 50% dose reduction; return to 3-week interval
3	blistering, ulceration, or swelling interfering with walking or normal daily activities; cannot wear regular clothing	Wait an additional week	Discontinue DOXIL®
4	diffuse or local process causing infectious complications, or a bed ridden state or hospitalization	Wait an additional week	Discontinue DOXIL®

site of extravasation for approximately 30 minutes may be helpful in alleviating the local reaction. **DOXIL® must not be given by the intramuscular or subcutaneous route.**

Dose Modifications

The dose modifications shown in the tables below are recommended for managing possible adverse events.
[See table above]

HEMATOLOGICAL TOXICITY

Grade	ANC (cells/mm^3)	Platelets (cells/mm^3)	Modification
1	1500–1900	75,000–150,000	None
2	1000–<1500	50,000–<75,000	None
3	500–999	25,000–<50,000	Wait until ANC ≥1,000 and/or platelets ≥50,000 then redose at 25% dose reduction
4	<500	<25,000	Wait until ANC ≥1,000 and/or platelets ≥50,000 then redose at 50% dose reduction

STOMATITIS

Grade	Symptoms	Modification
1	Painless ulcers, erythema or mild soreness	None
2	Painful erythema, edema or ulcers, but can eat	Wait one week and if symptoms improve redose at 100% dose
3	Painful erythema, edema or ulcers, and cannot eat	Wait one week and if symptoms improve redose at 25% dose reduction
4	Requires parenteral or enteral support	Wait one week and if symptoms improve redose at 50% dose reduction

Patients with Impaired Hepatic Function

Limited clinical experience exists in treating hepatically impaired patients with DOXIL®.

Therefore, based on experience with doxorubicin HCl, it is recommended that DOXIL® dosage be reduced if the bilirubin is elevated as follows: Serum bilirubin 1.2 to 3.0 mg/dL give $^1/_2$ normal dose, >3 mg/dL give $^1/_4$ normal dose.

Preparation for Intravenous Administration

The appropriate dose of DOXIL®, up to a maximum of 90 mg, must be diluted in 250 mL of 5% Dextrose Injection, USP prior to administration. Aseptic technique must be strictly observed since no preservative or bacteriostatic agent is present in DOXIL®. Diluted DOXIL® should be refrigerated at 2°C to 8°C (36°F to 46°F) and administered within 24 hours.

Do not use with in-line filters.

Do not mix with other drugs.

Do not use with any diluent other than 5% Dextrose Injection.

Do not use any bacteriostatic agent, such as benzyl alcohol.

DOXIL® is not a clear solution but a translucent, red liposomal dispersion. **Parenteral drug products should be inspected visually for particulate matter and discoloration prior to administration, whenever solution and container permit. Do not use if a precipitate or foreign matter is present.**

Storage and Stability

Refrigerate unopened vials of DOXIL® at 2°C to 8°C (36°F to 46°F). Avoid freezing. Prolonged freezing may adversely affect liposomal drug products; however, short-term freezing (less than 1 month) does not appear to have a deleterious effect on DOXIL®.

Procedure for Proper Handling and Disposal

Caution should be exercised in the handling and preparation of DOXIL®.

The use of gloves is required.

If DOXIL® comes into contact with skin or mucosa, immediately wash thoroughly with soap and water.

DOXIL® should be considered an irritant and precautions should be taken to avoid extravasation. On intravenous administration of DOXIL®, extravasation may occur with or without an accompanying stinging or burning sensation and even if blood returns well on aspiration of the infusion needle. If any signs or symptoms of extravasation have occurred, the infusion should be immediately terminated and restarted in another vein. DOXIL® must not be given by the intramuscular or subcutaneous route.

DOXIL® should be handled and disposed of in a manner consistent with other anticancer drugs. Several guidelines on this subject exist[2-8] although there is no general agreement that all of the procedures listed in these guidelines are appropriate or necessary.

HOW SUPPLIED

DOXIL® (doxorubicin HCl liposome injection) is supplied as a sterile, translucent, red liposomal dispersion in 10 mL glass, single use vials.

Each vial contains 20 mg doxorubicin HCl at a concentration of 2 mg/mL.

Refrigerate at 2-8°C. Avoid freezing. Prolonged freezing may adversely affect liposomal drug products; however, short-term freezing (less than 1 month) does not appear to have a deleterious affect on DOXIL®.

Continued on next page

Doxil—Cont.

Available as individually cartoned vials in packages of six.
NDC #61471-295-12.

REFERENCES

1. Krown et al. Kaposi's sarcoma in the acquired immune deficiency syndrome: A proposal for uniform evaluation, response, and staging criteria. *J Clin Oncol.* 1989; 7(9): 1201–1207.
2. Recommendations for the safe handling of cytotoxic drugs. NIH Publication No. 92-2621. US Government Printing Office, Washington, DC 20402.
3. OSHA Work-Practice guidelines for personnel dealing with cytotoxic (antineoplastic) drugs. *Am J Hosp Pharm.* 1986; 43:1193–1204.
4. American Society of Hospital Pharmacists Technical Assistance Bulletin on Handling Cytotoxic and Hazardous Drugs. *Am J Hosp Pharm.* 1985; 42:131–137.
5. National Study Commission on Cytotoxic Exposure—Recommendations for Handling Cytotoxic Agents. Available from Louis P. Jeffrey, Sc.D., Chairman, National Study Commission on Cytotoxic Exposure, Massachusetts College of Pharmacy and Allied Health Sciences, 179 Longwood Avenue, Boston, Massachusetts 02115.
6. AMA Council Report. Guidelines for handling parenteral antineoplastics. *JAMA* 1985; 253(11):1590–1592.
7. Clinical Oncologic Society of Australia: Guidelines and recommendation for safe handling of antineoplastic agents. *Med J Australia* 1983; 1:426–428.
8. Jones RB, et al. Safe handling of chemotherapeutic agents: a report from the Mount Sinai Medical Center. *Ca-A Cancer Journal for Clinicians.* 1983; Sept/Oct:258–263.

Manufactured by
Ben Venue Laboratories, Inc., Bedford, Ohio 44146

Distributed by:
SEQUUS® Pharmaceuticals, Inc., Menlo Park, CA 94025
USA
Last Revised: August 4, 1997
Shown in Product Identification Guide, page 338

Serono Laboratories, Inc.
**100 LONGWATER CIRCLE
NORWELL, MA 02061**

Direct Inquiries to:
Customer Service, Sales and Ordering
(888) 398-4567
(781) 982-9000

For Medical Information or to report Adverse Drug Experiences Contact:
Drug Information and Surveillance Group
(888) 275-7376
(781) 982-9000 X 5562

Serono Laboratories, Inc. will be pleased to answer inquiries about the following products:

FERTINEX™
[fĕr 'tĭn-ĕx]
**(urofollitropin for injection, purified)
FOR SUBCUTANEOUS INJECTION**
℞

DESCRIPTION

Fertinex™ (urofollitropin for injection, purified) is a preparation of highly purified Follicle Stimulating Hormone (FSH) extracted from the urine of post-menopausal women. Purification is by immunoaffinity chromatography using murine monoclonal antibody to human FSH. The purification process results in a consistent FSH isoform profile, significantly enhanced specific activity (8,500–13,500 IU FSH/mg protein), and a highly purified preparation. Each ampule of Fertinex™ contains either 75 IU or 150 IU of highly purified FSH and 10 mg lactose in a sterile, lyophilized form. If required, pH is adjusted with 0.1 M hydrochloric acid and/or 0.1 M sodium hydroxide. Fertinex™ is administered by subcutaneous injection.
Fertinex™ contains an acidic, water soluble glycoprotein biologically standardized for FSH gonadotropin activity in terms of the Second International Reference Preparation for Human Menopausal Gonadotropins established in September, 1964 by the Expert Committee on Biological Standards of the World Health Organization. Negligible amounts ($\leq$0.1 IU LH/1000 IU FSH) of luteinizing hormone (LH) activity are contained in Fertinex™.
Therapeutic Class: Infertility.

CLINICAL PHARMACOLOGY

Fertinex™ (urofollitropin for injection, purified) stimulates ovarian follicular growth in women who do not have primary ovarian failure. FSH, the active component of Fertinex™, is the primary hormone responsible for follicular recruitment and development. In order to effect final maturation of the follicle and ovulation in the absence of an endogenous LH surge, human chorionic gonadotropin (hCG) must be given following the administration of Fertinex™ when monitoring of the patient indicates that sufficient follicular development has occurred. There may be a degree of interpatient variability in response to FSH administration.
Pharmacokinetics:
In a comparative, single-dose, double-blind, double-dummy, randomized, cross-over study, Fertinex™ administered subcutaneously demonstrated a similar pharmacokinetic profile to urofollitropin and Fertinex™ administered intramuscularly. No significant differences were found between the treatment groups in AUC/dose and CMAX/dose parameters. A variability in TMAX was observed. Subcutaneous administration of Fertinex™ led to a slower absorption rate resulting in a later TMAX (15±7h) than following IM administration of either Fertinex™ (10±4h) or urofollitropin (9±4h).
Plasma inhibin levels were measured as a pharmacodynamic marker of FSH activity. The inhibin concentration-time profile of inhibin following Fertinex™ administered subcutaneously was found to be similar to that following urofollitropin and Fertinex™ administered intramuscularly.
Special Populations: Safety and efficacy of Fertinex™ in renal or hepatic insufficiency have not been established.
Drug-Drug Interactions: No clinically significant drug-drug interactions have been reported (see PRECAUTIONS).
Clinical Studies:
1. Ovulation Induction:
The safety and efficacy of Fertinex™ administered subcutaneously vs. urofollitropin administered intramuscularly for ovulation induction was assessed in a phase III, open-label, randomized, comparative, multicenter study in oligo-ovulatory infertile women who failed to ovulate or conceive following adequate clomiphene citrate therapy. The purpose of the study was to demonstrate that Fertinex™, a highly purified follicle stimulating hormone (FSH) administered subcutaneously, is clinically not different in terms of safety and efficacy from urofollitropin administered intramuscularly. The principal efficacy parameters recorded were serum estradiol levels, follicular growth, ovulation rate and pregnancy rate. Two hundred eleven patients entered treatment, of whom 108 received Fertinex™ and 103 received urofollitropin. Overall, two hundred and four patients (491 cycles) were considered evaluable. There were no differences between the Fertinex™ administered subcutaneously and the urofollitropin intramuscular treatment groups in serum estradiol levels and follicular growth (follicle number and size) on the day of human chorionic gonadotropin (hCG) administration, nor were there any differences between the treatment groups in ovulation rates or pregnancy rates per patient.
The results of safety and efficacy with Fertinex™ administered subcutaneously for ovulation induction in oligo-ovulatory infertile women are summarized below:
Cumulative Patient Ovulation Rates:
The cumulative patient ovulation rate by cycle is presented for the 102 evaluable patients with documentation of ovulatory status in at least one cycle:

Cycle 1	83%
Cycle 2	97%
Cycle 3	100%

Cumulative Patient Pregnancy Rates:
The cumulative patient pregnancy rate by cycle is presented for 86 evaluable patients who received hCG:

Cycle 1	14%
Cycle 2	21%
Cycle 3	29%

Patients Aborting* 8%
Multiple Births* 21%
Severe Hyperstimulation Syndrome** 0%

* Based upon 25 evaluable clinical pregnancies
** Based upon 108 patients and 266 cycles evaluable for safety

2. Assisted Reproductive Technologies (ART):
The safety and efficacy of Fertinex™ administered subcutaneously for Assisted Reproductive Technologies (ART) were assessed in a phase III, multicenter, non-comparative, clinical trial in ovulatory infertile women undergoing stimulation of multiple follicular development for In Vitro Fertilization and Embryo Transfer (IVF/ET) after pituitary downregulation with a GnRH agonist. The initial and maximal doses of Fertinex™ were 225 and 450 IU, respectively. The principal parameters recorded were serum estradiol on day of hCG administration, the number and maturity of retrieved oocytes, drug therapy and duration, and clinical pregnancy rate per initiated cycle and per retrieval. One

hundred and thirty-nine patients were enrolled in the study; 135 patients were treated with Fertinex™ and 122 patients were considered evaluable for efficacy. The results listed below represent mean data of 118 evaluable patients who received hCG in the 10 study centers:

Total number of oocytes recovered	8.4
Mature oocytes recovered	5.9
Maximum serum E2, day hCG (pg/mL)	1682
Total number of ampules (75 IU)	36
Treatment duration (days)	11.5
Clinical pregnancy attempt	23% (0–60)*
Clinical pregnancy transfer	27% (0–60)*

*reflects range across centers

INDICATIONS AND USAGE

Fertinex™ (urofollitropin for injection, purified) and hCG given in a sequential manner are indicated for the stimulation of follicular recruitment and development and the induction of ovulation in patients with polycystic ovary syndrome and infertility, who have failed to respond or conceive following adequate clomiphene citrate therapy.
Fertinex™ and hCG may also be used to stimulate the development of multiple follicles in ovulatory patients undergoing Assisted Reproductive Technologies (ART) such as in vitro fertilization.
Selection of Patients:
1. Before treatment with Fertinex™ (urofollitropin for injection, purified) is instituted, a thorough gynecologic and endocrinologic evaluation must be performed. This should include an assessment of pelvic anatomy. Patients with tubal obstruction should receive Fertinex™ only if enrolled in an in vitro fertilization program.
2. Primary ovarian failure should be excluded by the determination of gonadotropin levels.
3. Careful examination should be made to rule out the presence of early pregnancy.
4. Patients in late reproductive life have a greater predisposition to endometrial carcinoma as well as a higher incidence of anovulatory disorders. A thorough diagnostic examination should always be performed before starting Fertinex™ therapy in such patients who demonstrate abnormal uterine bleeding or other signs of endometrial abnormalities.
5. Evaluation of the partner's fertility potential should be included in the workup.

CONTRAINDICATIONS

Fertinex™ (urofollitropin for injection, purified) is contraindicated in women who exhibit:
1. High levels of FSH indicating primary ovarian failure.
2. Uncontrolled thyroid or adrenal dysfunction.
3. An organic intracranial lesion such as a pituitary tumor.
4. The presence of any cause of infertility other than anovulation, as stated in the "Indications" unless they are candidates for Assisted Reproductive Technologies.
5. Abnormal bleeding of undetermined origin (see "Selection of Patients").
6. Ovarian cysts or enlargement of undetermined origin.
7. Prior hypersensitivity to urofollitropin.
Fertinex™ is also contraindicated in women who are pregnant and may cause fetal harm when administered to a pregnant woman. There are limited human data on the effects of Fertinex™ when administered during pregnancy.

WARNINGS

Fertinex™ (urofollitropin for injection, purified) should only be used by physicians who are thoroughly familiar with infertility problems and their management. It is a potent gonadotropic substance capable of causing mild to severe adverse reactions. Therefore, the lowest dose consistent with the expectation of good results should be used. Gonadotropin therapy requires a certain time commitment by physicians and supportive health professionals, and its use requires the availability of appropriate monitoring facilities (see "Precautions/Laboratory Tests"). Safe and effective use of Fertinex™ requires monitoring of ovarian response with serum estradiol and vaginal ultrasound, on a regular basis.
Overstimulation of the Ovary During Fertinex™ (urofollitropin for injection, purified) therapy: Ovarian Enlargement: Mild to moderate uncomplicated ovarian enlargement which may be accompanied by abdominal distension and/or abdominal pain occurs in approximately 20% of those treated with urofollitropin and hCG, and generally regresses without treatment within two or three weeks. Careful monitoring of ovarian response can further minimize the risk of overstimulation.
If the ovaries are abnormally enlarged on the last day of Fertinex™ therapy, hCG should not be administered in this course of therapy. This will reduce the chances of development of the Ovarian Hyperstimulation Syndrome.
The Ovarian Hyperstimulation Syndrome (OHSS): OHSS is a medical event distinct from uncomplicated ovarian enlargement. Severe OHSS may progress rapidly (within 24 hours to several days) to become a serious medical event. It is characterized by an apparent dramatic increase in vascular permeability which can result in a rapid accumulation of fluid in the peritoneal cavity, thorax, and potentially, the

pericardium. The early warning signs of development of OHSS are severe pelvic pain, nausea, vomiting, and weight gain. The following symptomatology has been seen with cases of OHSS: abdominal pain, abdominal distension, gastrointestinal symptoms including nausea, vomiting and diarrhea, severe ovarian enlargement, weight gain, dyspnea, and oliguria. Clinical evaluation may reveal hypovolemia, hemoconcentration, electrolyte imbalances, ascites, hemoperitoneum, pleural effusions, hydrothorax, acute pulmonary distress, and thromboembolic events (see "Pulmonary and Vascular Complications"). Transient liver function test abnormalities suggestive of hepatic dysfunction, which may be accompanied by morphologic changes on liver biopsy, have been reported in association with the Ovarian Hyperstimulation Syndrome (OHSS).

Severe OHSS occurred in approximately 6.0% of patients treated with urofollitropin therapy in the initial clinical trials, in patients treated for anovulation due to polycystic ovarian syndrome. In these studies, prospective monitoring of ovarian response using serum estradiol determination or ultrasonographic visualizations was not routinely employed. In more recent clinical trials in oligo-anovulatory and infertile women in which both estradiol and ultrasound measurements were utilized to monitor follicular development, the incidence of severe OHSS was 0.6%. During studies for in vitro fertilization, four cases of OHSS were reported following 1,586 treatment cycles (0.25%). OHSS may be more severe and more protracted if pregnancy occurs. OHSS develops rapidly; therefore, patients should be followed for at least two weeks after hCG administration. Most often, OHSS occurs after treatment has been discontinued and reaches its maximum at about seven to ten days following treatment. Usually, OHSS resolves spontaneously with the onset of menses. If there is evidence that OHSS may be developing prior to hCG administration (see "Precautions/Laboratory Tests"), the hCG must be withheld. If severe OHSS occurs, treatment must be stopped and the patient should be hospitalized.

A physician experienced in the management of this syndrome, or who is experienced in the management in fluid and electrolyte imbalances should be consulted.

Pulmonary and Vascular Complications: The following paragraph describes serious medical events reported following gonadotropin therapy.

Serious pulmonary conditions (e.g., atelectasis, acute respiratory distress syndrome) have been reported. In addition, thromboembolic events both in association with, and separate from the Ovarian Hyperstimulation Syndrome have been reported. Intravascular thrombosis and embolism can result in reduced blood flow to critical organs or the extremities. Sequelae of such events have included venous thrombophlebitis, pulmonary embolism, pulmonary infarction, cerebral vascular occlusion (stroke), and arterial occlusion resulting in loss of limb. In rare cases, pulmonary complications and/or thromboembolic events have resulted in death.

Multiple Births: Reports of multiple births have been associated with urofollitropin-hCG treatment, including triplet and quintuplet gestations. In clinical studies with Fertinex™ 79.2% of the pregnancies following ovulation induction therapy resulted in single births and 20.8% in multiple births. The risk of multiple births in patients undergoing ART procedures is related to the number of embryos replaced. The patient and her partner should be advised of the potential risk of multiple births before starting treatment.

PRECAUTIONS

General: Careful attention should be given to diagnosis in candidates for Fertinex™ (urofollitropin for injection, purified) therapy (see "Indications and Usage/Selection of Patients").

Information for Patients: Prior to the therapy with Fertinex™, patients should be informed of the duration of treatment and monitoring of their condition that will be required. Possible adverse reactions (see "Adverse Reactions") and the risk of multiple births should also be discussed.

Laboratory Tests: In most instances, treatment with Fertinex™ results only in follicular recruitment and development. In order to effect ovulation in the absence of an endogenous LH surge, hCG must be given following the administration of Fertinex™ when monitoring of the patient indicates that sufficient follicular development has occurred. This may be estimated by serum estradiol and vaginal ultrasound. The combination of ultrasound and estradiol is useful for monitoring the development of follicles, timing hCG administration, as well as for detecting ovarian enlargement and minimizing the risk of the Ovarian Hyperstimulation Syndrome and multiple gestation. It is recommended that the number of growing follicles be confirmed using ultrasonography because plasma estrogen alone does not give an indication of the size or number of follicles.

The clinical confirmation of ovulation, with the exception of pregnancy, is obtained by direct and indirect indices of progesterone production. The indices generally used are:
1. A rise in basal body temperature,
2. Increase in serum progesterone, and

3. Menstruation following the shift in basal body temperature.

When used in conjunction with indices of progesterone production, sonographic visualization of the ovaries will assist in determining if ovulation has occurred. Sonographic evidence of ovulation may include the following:
1. Fluid in the cul-de-sac,
2. Ovarian stigmata,
3. Collapsed follicle, and
4. Secretory endometrium.

Accurate interpretation of the indices of follicular development and maturation as well as the determination of ovulation require a physician who is experienced in the interpretation of these tests.

Drug Interactions: No clinically significant drug/drug or drug/food interactions have been reported during Fertinex™ therapy.

Carcinogenesis and Mutagenesis: Carcinogenicity and mutagenicity studies have not been performed.

Pregnancy Category X: See "Contraindications".

Nursing Mothers: It is not known whether this drug is excreted in human milk. Because many drugs are excreted in human milk, caution should be exercised if Fertinex™ is administered to a nursing woman.

ADVERSE REACTIONS

The following adverse reactions reported during urofollitropin therapy are listed in decreasing order of potential severity:
1. Pulmonary and vascular complications (see "Warnings"),
2. Ovarian Hyperstimulation Syndrome (see "Warnings"),
3. Adnexal torsion (as a complication of ovarian enlargement),
4. Mild to moderate ovarian enlargement,
5. Abdominal pain,
6. Sensitivity to urofollitropin
   (Febrile reactions which may be accompanied by chills, musculoskeletal aches, joint pains, malaise, headache, and fatigue have occurred after the administration of urofollitropin. It is not clear whether or not these were pyrogenic responses or possible allergic reactions.)
7. Ovarian cysts,
8. Gastrointestinal symptoms (nausea, vomiting, diarrhea, abdominal cramps, bloating),
9. Pain, rash, swelling, and/or irritation at the site of injection,
10. Breast tenderness,
11. Headache,
12. Dermatological symptoms (dry skin, body rash, hair loss, hives)
13. Hemoperitoneum has been reported during menotropins therapy and, therefore, may also occur during urofollitropin therapy.
14. There have been infrequent reports of ovarian neoplasms, both benign and malignant, in women who have undergone multiple drug regimens for ovulation induction; however, a causal relationship has not been established.

The following medical events have been reported subsequent to pregnancies resulting from urofollitropin therapy:
1. Ectopic Pregnancy
2. Congenital abnormalities
   (Three incidents of chromosomal abnormalities and four birth defects have been reported following urofollitropin-hCG or urofollitropin, Pergonal® (menotropins for injection, USP)-hCG therapy in clinical trials for stimulation prior to in vitro fertilization. The aborted pregnancies included one Trisomy 13, one Trisomy 18, and one fetus with multiple congenital anomalies (hydrocephaly, omphalocele, and meningocele). One meningocele, one external ear defect, one dislocated hip and ankle, and one dilated cardiomyopathy in presence of maternal Systemic Lupus Erythematosis were reported. None of these events were thought to be drug-related. The incidence does not exceed that found in the general population).

DRUG ABUSE AND DEPENDENCE

There have been no reports of abuse or dependence with Fertinex™ (urofollitropin for injection, purified).

OVERDOSAGE

Aside from possible ovarian hyperstimulation and multiple gestations (see "Warnings"), little is known concerning the consequences of acute overdosage with Fertinex™ (urofollitropin for injection, purified).

DOSAGE AND ADMINISTRATION

Dosage:

Polycystic Ovary Syndrome: The dose of Fertinex™ (urofollitropin for injection, purified) to stimulate development of the follicle must be individualized for each patient.

The lowest dose consistent with the expectation of good results should be used. Over the course of treatment, doses of Fertinex™ may range between 75 IU to 300 IU per day depending on the individual patient response. Fertinex™ should be administered until adequate follicular development is indicated by serum estradiol and vaginal ultra-

sonography. A response is generally evident after 5 to 7 days. Subsequent monitoring intervals should be based on individual patient response.

It is recommended that the initial dose of the first cycle be 75 IU of Fertinex™ per day, **ADMINISTERED SUBCUTANEOUSLY.** An adjustment in dose may be considered after 5 to 7 days. An additional dose adjustment may also be considered based on individual patient response. The dose should not be increased more than twice in any cycle or by more than one ampule (75 IU) per adjustment. To complete follicular development and effect ovulation in the absence of an endogenous LH surge, hCG, 5,000 U to 10,000 U, should be given 1 day after the last dose of Fertinex™. Human chorionic gonadotropin should be withheld if the serum estradiol is greater than 2,000 pg/mL. If the ovaries are abnormally enlarged or abdominal pain occurs, Fertinex™ treatment should be discontinued, hCG should not be administered, and the patient should be advised not to have intercourse; this will reduce the chance of development of the Ovarian Hyperstimulation Syndrome and, should spontaneous ovulation occur, reduce the chance of multiple gestation. A follow-up visit should be conducted in the luteal phase.

The initial dose administered in the subsequent cycles should be individualized for each patient based on her response in the preceding cycle. Doses larger than 300 IU of FSH per day are not routinely recommended. As in the initial cycle, 5,000 U to 10,000 U of hCG must be given 1 day after the last dose of Fertinex™ to complete follicular development and induce ovulation. The precautions described above should be followed to minimize the chance of development of the Ovarian Hyperstimulation Syndrome.

The couple should be encouraged to have intercourse daily, beginning on the day prior to the administration of hCG until ovulation becomes apparent from the indices employed for the determination of progestational activity. Care should be taken to ensure insemination. In light of the indices and parameters mentioned, it should become obvious that, unless a physician is willing to devote considerable time to these patients and be familiar with and conduct the necessary laboratory studies, he/she should not use Fertinex™.

Assisted Reproductive Technologies: As in the treatment of patients with polycystic ovary syndrome, the dose of Fertinex™ to stimulate development of the follicle must be individualized for each patient. For Assisted Reproductive Technologies, therapy with Fertinex™ should be initiated in the early follicular phase (cycle day 2 or 3) at a dose of 150 IU per day, until sufficient follicular development is attained. In most cases, therapy should not exceed ten days.

Administration: Dissolve the contents of one or more ampules of Fertinex™ in one-half to one mL of sterile saline (concentration should not exceed 225 IU/0.5 mL) and **ADMINISTER SUBCUTANEOUSLY** immediately. Any unused reconstituted material should be discarded.

Parenteral drug products should be inspected visually, for particulate matter and discoloration prior to administration, whenever solution and container permit.

HOW SUPPLIED

Fertinex™ (urofollitropin for injection, purified) is supplied in a sterile, lyophilized form as a white to off-white powder or pellet in ampules containing 75 IU or 150 IU FSH activity. The following package combinations are available:
— 1 ampule 75 IU Fertinex™ and 1 ampule 2 mL Sodium Chloride Injection (USP), NDC 44087-7075-1
— 1 ampule 150 IU Fertinex™ and 1 ampule 2 mL Sodium Chloride Injection (USP), NDC 44087-7150-1
— 10 ampules 75 IU Fertinex™ and 10 ampules 2 mL Sodium Chloride Injection (USP), NDC 44087-7075-3
— 100 ampules 75 IU Fertinex™ and 100 ampules 2 mL Sodium Chloride Injection (USP), NDC 44087-7075-4

Lyophilized powder may be stored refrigerated or at room temperature (3°–25°C/37°–77°F). Protect from light. Use immediately after reconstitution. Discard unused material.

Caution: Federal law prohibits dispensing without prescription.

Manufactured for: **SERONO LABORATORIES, INC.**, Randolph, MA 02368 U.S.A.
by: Laboratories Serono SA, Aubonne, Switzerland
© Serono Laboratories, Inc., April 1998

GEREF® ℞
[ge ref]
(sermorelin acetate for injection)
For subcutaneous injection only

DESCRIPTION

Sermorelin acetate is the acetate salt of an amidated synthetic 29-amino acid peptide (GRF 1-29 NH₂) that corresponds to the amino-terminal segment of the naturally occurring human growth hormone-releasing hormone (GHRH

Continued on next page

Geref—Cont.

or GRF) consisting of 44 amino acid residues. The structural formula for sermorelin acetate is:

Tyr-Ala-Asp-Ala-Ile-Phe-Thr-Asn-Ser-Tyr-
Arg-Lys-Val-Leu-Gly-Gln-Leu-Ser-Ala-Arg-
Lys-Leu-Leu-Gln-Asp-Ile-Met-Ser-Arg-$NH_2 \cdot (C_2H_4O_2)_{3\text{-}6}$

The free base of sermorelin has the empirical formula $C_{149}H_{246}N_{44}O_{42}S$ and a molecular weight of 3,358 daltons. Geref® is a sterile, non-pyrogenic, lyophilized powder intended for subcutaneous injection after reconstitution with Sodium Chloride Injection, USP. The reconstituted solution has a pH of 5.0 to 5.5.

Geref® is available in vials. The quantitative composition per vial is:

0.5 mg vial: Each vial contains 0.5 mg sermorelin (as the acetate) and 5 mg mannitol. The pH is adjusted with dibasic sodium phosphate and monobasic sodium phosphate buffer.

1.0 mg vial: Each vial contains 1.0 mg sermorelin (as the acetate) and 5 mg mannitol. The pH is adjusted with dibasic sodium phosphate and monobasic sodium phosphate buffer.

CLINICAL PHARMACOLOGY

Geref® (sermorelin acetate for injection) increases plasma growth hormone (GH) concentration by stimulating the pituitary gland to release GH. Geref® is similar to the native hormone (GRF [1-44]-NH_2) in its ability to stimulate GH secretion in humans.

Pharmacokinetics

Absorption

In subcutaneous administration of 2 mg sermorelin to 12 normal volunteers, peak concentrations of sermorelin were reached in 5–20 minutes. the mean absolute bioavailability after SC administration is about 6%.

Distribution

After intravenous administration of 0.24–1.0 mg Geref® to 12 normal volunteeers, the mean volume of distribution ranged between 23.7–25.8 liters.

Metabolism

No metabolism studies have been performed in humans.

Elimination

Sermorelin is rapidly cleared from the circulation, with clearance values in adults ranging between 2.4–2.8 L/min. The half-life of Geref® is short, 11–12 minutes after either intravenous or subcutaneous administration.

Special Populations

Gender/Age: No gender data are available in pediatric patients. In normal adults, the clearance of sermorelin in men and women is similar. No age data are available.

Renal/Hepatic Insufficiency: No data are available.

CLINICAL STUDIES

In one multicenter, open-label clinical study in prepubertal children with idiopathic growth hormone deficiency, 110 children were administered Geref® 0.03 mg (30 mcg) per kg per day by subcutaneous injection. Fifty-six patients were evaluable for efficacy at 12 months. Fifty-four patients were considered unevaluable: 24 for eligibility criteria violations; 10 for protocol discontinuation criteria and 20 for failing to satisfy the efficacy criteria at 6 months for continuing in the study. Fifty-six of all 110 patients and 47 of 56 patients in the evaluable patient subset who initiated and continued with Geref® therapy up to 12 months demonstrated an increase of 2 cm/year or more over the baseline height velocity (HV). For the 56 patients in the evaluable patient subset, mean height velocity (± SD) increased from 4.1 ± 1.0 cm/year at baseline to 8.0 ± 1.5 cm/year at 6 months and 7.2 ± 1.3 cm/year at 12 months, an increase of 3.1 ± 1.4 cm/year (p = 0.0001). Mean height standard deviation score (± SD) increased from −3.71 ± 0.92 at baseline to −3.21 ± 0.91 at 12 months, and increase of 0.50 ± 0.23 over the 12 month period (p = 0.0001). Mean changes in bone age at 12 months were proportional to gains in height (1.04 ± 0.58, ΔBA/ΔHA, n=42).

INDICATIONS AND USAGE

Geref® (sermorelin acetate for injection) is indicated for the treatment of idiopathic growth hormone deficiency in children with growth failure. Most of these short, slowly growing children retain pituitary responsivness to growth hormone releasing hormone.

Selection of Patients and Evaluation of Growth

All children should be pre-pubescent and treatment should be initiated at a bone age of ≤ 7.5 year for females, and ≤ 8 years for males. Prior to initiation of treatment, a growth hormone (GH) stimulation test with Geref® sould be performed in all children. Children who do not adequately respond (i.e., peak GH level ≤ 2 ng/mL) should be excluded from Geref® therapy. The relative growth hormone response to the stimulation test with Geref® is not predictive of the growth response to Geref® therapy. Clinical results are better in children with delayed bone age and in whom treatment is initiated as early as possible in the prepubertal period. Height should be assessed at least every six months during treatment. During Geref® therapy, failure to maintain a pattern of growth consistent with a child's age and stage of development requires investigation. Children should be treated with Geref® for an initial period of 6 months and treatment with growth hormone should be initiated for those children with a poor or waning response to Geref®.

CONTRAINDICATIONS

Geref® (sermorelin acetate for injection) should not be used by patients with a known sensitivity to sermorelin or any of the excipients.

WARNINGS

Following reconstitution of Geref® (sermorelin acetate for injection) with the diluent provided, the solution should be administered immediately. Any unused solution should be discarded.

PRECAUTIONS

General: Geref® (sermorelin acetate for injection) therapy should be carried out under the regular guidance of a physician who is experienced in the diagnosis and management of growth disorders.

The growth response of children treated with Geref® should be evaluated on a periodic basis and children with a poor or waning response should be considered for treatment with growth hormone. The effect of Geref® therapy beyond one year and on final adult height remains to be determined.

In clinical studies, the incidence of hypothyroidism during Geref® therapy was 6.5%. In the largest clinical study, 8 of 110 enrolled patients were on thyroid replacement therapy prior to Geref® therapy and an additional 5 after initiating therapy. Untreated hypothyroidism can jeopardize the response to Geref®. Therefore, thyroid hormone determinations should be performed before the initiation and throughout the duration of Geref® therapy. Thyroid hormone replacement therapy should be initiated when indicated.

Bone age should be monitored periodically during Geref® administration, especially in patients who are pubertal and/or receiving concomitant thyroid replacement therapy. Under these circumstances, epiphyseal maturation may progress rapidly.

Patients with growth hormone deficiency secondary to an intracranial lesion were not studied in clinical trials. It is not recommended that such patients be treated with Geref®.

As with the administration of any peptide, local or systemic allergic reactions may occur. Parents/Patients should be informed that such reactions are possible and that prompt medical attention should be sought if allergic reactions occur.

Laboratory Tests: Serum levels of inorganic phosphorus, alkaline phosphatase, GH and IGF-1 may increase with Geref® therapy.

Drug Interaction: Concomitant glucocorticoid therapy may inhibit the response to Geref®, There was no evidence in the controlled studies of Geref®'s interaction with drugs commonly used in the treatment of routine pediatric problems/illnesses. However, formal drug interactions studies have not been conducted.

Carcinogenesis, Mutagenesis, Impairment of Fertility: Long-term animal studies for carcinogenicity and impairment of fertility have not been performed with Geref®. There has been no evidence from studies to date of Geref®-induced genetic toxicity.

Pregnancy: Pregnancy Category C. During teratology studies Geref® produced minor variations in fetuses of rats and rabbits when given at a dose of 0.5 mg/kg/day. This dose is approximately 3 and 6 times the daily human dose calculated on a body surface area (mg/m^2) basis, for rats and rabbits, respectively. There are no adequate and well controlled studies in pregnant women. Geref® should be used during pregnancy only if the potential benefit justifies the potential risk to the fetus.

Nursing Women: It is not known whether Geref® is excreted in human milk. Because many drugs are excreted in human milk, cautions should be exercised when Geref® is administered to a nursing women.

Information For Patients: Patients being treated with Geref® and/or their parents should be informed of the potential benefits and risks associated with treatment. If home use is determined to be desirable by the physician, instructions on appropriate use should be given, including a review of the contents of the Patient Information Insert. This information is intended to aid in the safe and effective administration of the medication. It is not a disclosure of all possible adverse or intended effects.

If home use is prescribed, a puncture resistant container for the disposal of used syringes and needles should be recommended to the patient. Patients and/or parents should be thoroughly instructed in the importance of proper disposal and cautioned against any reuse of needles and syringes (see Patient Information Insert).

ADVERSE REACTIONS

A large proportion of patients develop anti-GRF antibodies at least once during treatment with Geref® (sermorelin acetate for injection). The significance of these antibodies is not clear and often a positive test at one growth assessment will become negative by the next assessment. The presence of antibodies does not appear to be related to a specific adverse reaction profile. No generalized allergic reactions to Geref® have been reported.

The most common treatment-related adverse event (occurring in about 1 patient in 6) is local injection reaction characterized by pain, swelling or redness. Of 350 patients exposed to Geref® in clinical trials, three discontinued therapy due to injection reactions. Other treatment-related adverse events had individual occurrence rates of less than 6% and include: headache, flushing, dysphagia, dizziness, hyperactivity, somnolence and urticaria.

When administered intravenously for diagnostic use, the following adverse reactions have been noted: flushing of the face, injection site pain, redness and/or swelling, nausea, headache, vomiting, dysgeusia, pallor and tightness in the chest.

DRUG ABUSE AND DEPENDENCE

The clinical pharmacology suggests that Geref® is very unlikely to be associated with drug abuse or dependence and there have been no reports of this from clinical trials.

OVERDOSAGE

The recommended dosage of Geref® (sermorelin acetate for injection) should not be exceeded.

DOSAGE AND ADMINISTRATION

A dosage of 0.03 mg (30 mcg) per kg of body weight once daily at bedtime by subcutaneous injection is recommended. It is also recommended that subcutaneous injection sites be periodically rotated.

Treatment with Geref® should be discontinued when the epiphyses are fused. Patients who fail to respond adequately while on Geref® therapy should be evaluated to determine the cause of unresponsiveness.

Height should be assessed at least every six months during treatment. During Geref® therapy, care shoud be taken to ensure that the child continues to grow at a rate consistent with the child's age and stage of development, and treatment with Geref® should be reevaluated if the response is inadequate. Treatment with growth hormone should be considered for children with a poor or waning response to Geref®.

To prevent possible contamination, wipe the rubber vial stopper with an antiseptic solution before puncturing it with the needle. It is recommended that Geref® be administered using sterile, disposable syringes and needles. The syringes should be of small enough volume that the prescribed dose can be drawn from the vial with reasonable accuracy.

After determining the appropriate patient dose, reconstitute each vial of Geref® with 0.5–1.0 mL of Sodium Chloride Injection, USP.

To reconstitute Geref®, inject the diluent into the vial of Geref® aiming the liquid against the glass vial wall. Swirl the vial with a GENTLE rotary motion until contents are dissolved completely. Do not administer Geref® if particles are visible in the reconstituted solution or if the reconstituted solution is cloudy.

HOW SUPPLIED

Before Reconstitution—Vials of Geref® (sermorelin acetate for injection) should be stored refrigerated (2°–8°C/36°–46°F). Expiration dates are stated on the labels.

After Reconstitution—When reconstituted with Sodium Chloride Injection, USP, the reconstituted solution should be administered immediately. Any unused solution should be discarded.

Geref® (sermorelin acetate for injection) is a sterile, nonpyrogenic, lyophilized powder supplied in packages containing:

1 vial 0.5 mg Geref® and 1 vial 2 mL Sodium Chloride Injection, USP NDC 44087-4005-1

10 vials 0.5 mg Geref® and 10 vials 2 mL Sodium Chloride Injection, USP NDC 44087-4005-3

1 vial 1.0 mg Geref® and 1 vial 2 mL Sodium Chloride Injection, USP NDC 44087-4010-1

10 vials 1.0 mg Geref® and 10 vials 2 mL Sodium Chloride Injection, USP NDC 44087-4010-3

Caution: Federal law prohibits dispensing without prescription.

Product information as of August 1997

Manufactured for:
Serono Laboratories, Inc.
Randolph, MA 02368
By: Laboratories Serono S.A.
Aubonne, Switzerland
® Registered trademark of Serono Laboratories, Inc.
Code N1000101A 10/97

GEREF® DIAGNOSTIC   ℞
[ge ref dī ig nästik]
(sermorelin acetate for injection)
For intravenous injection only
FOR DIAGNOSTIC USE ONLY

DESCRIPTION

Geref® Diagnostic (sermorelin acetate for injection) is a sterile, nonpyrogenic, lyophilized preparation containing 50 mcg sermorelin (as the acetate), 5 mg mannitol, 0.66 mg monobasic sodium phosphate, and 0.04 mg dibasic sodium phosphate. Sermorelin acetate is an acetate salt of a synthetic, 29-amino acid polypeptide that is the amino-terminal segment of the naturally occurring human growth hormone-releasing hormone (GHRH or GRH) consisting of 44 amino acid residues. The structural formula for sermorelin acetate is presented below:

Tyr-Ala-Asp-Ala-Ile-Phe-Thr-Asn-Ser-Tyr-

Arg-Lys-Val-Leu-Gly-Gln-Leu-Ser-Ala-Arg-

Lys-Leu-Leu-Gln-Asp-Ile-Met-Ser-Arg-NH$_2$·(C$_2$H$_4$O$_2$)$_{3-6}$

The free base of sermorelin has the empirical formula C$_{149}$H$_{246}$N$_{44}$O$_{42}$S$_1$ and a molecular weight of 3,358 daltons. Sermorelin appears to be equivalent to GRH (1-44) in its ability to stimulate growth hormone secretion in humans. It has also been called GRH (1-29) and GHRH (1-29).

CLINICAL PHARMACOLOGY

Sermorelin increases plasma growth hormone (GH) concentrations by direct stimulation of the pituitary gland to release GH.

Because baseline GH levels are generally very low (< 4 ng/mL), provocative tests may be useful in determining the functional GH-secreting capability of the pituitary somatotroph. Adults and children with normal responses to standard provocative tests of GH secretion were used to define the range of normal plasma GH-level responses to Geref® Diagnostic. It was found that the absolute peak GH level following Geref® Diagnostic infusion and the time elapsed from infusion to that peak are appropriate measures to evaluate the response to GH infusion. Doses of Geref® Diagnostic used in children and adults in these studies ranged from 0.3 to 6.06 mcg/kg with a majority of patients receiving 1 mcg/kg. Based on these studies and published reports, 1 mcg/kg was chosen as the recommended dose for diagnostic purposes.

A total of 71 Geref® Diagnostic injection tests were performed on 47 boys and 24 girls who showed normal responses to standard, indirect provocative tests such as a clonidine, L-dopa, and arginine. The GH peak plasma response to Geref® Diagnostic was 28 ± 15 ng/mL (average ± S.D.) and the time to this peak was 30 ± 27 minutes (average ± S.D.).

Of all children who had GH responses of >7 ng/mL to standard provocative tests, 96% also had responses to Geref® Diagnostic of >7 ng/mL. In 77 patients who failed to respond to standard provocative tests, mean GH peak responses to Geref® Diagnostic were significantly lower compared to the mean GH peak response of normal control children. However, 53% of the children who failed to respond to standard tests had a GH response to Geref® Diagnostic of more than 7 ng/mL, suggesting that clinical GH deficiency is frequently not due to somatotroph failure.

The following figure shows the time course of average plasma GH-level responses to Geref® Diagnostic injection in normal children and those with subnormal responses to standard provocative tests, i.e., growth hormone-deficient (GHD) children.

Mean (& SD) of GH Response to Geref® Diagnostic in Normal and GHD Children

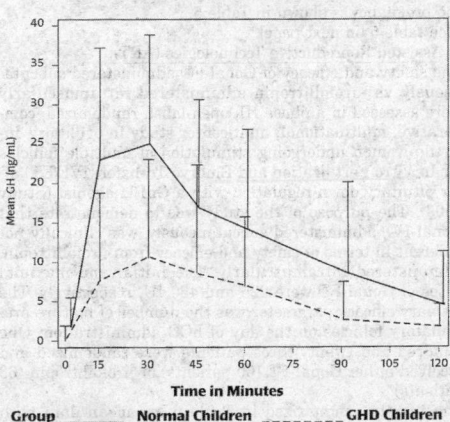

| Group | Normal Children | --- GHD Children |

In 14 published reports that utilized different forms of GRH including GRH (1-44), GRH (1-40), and formulations of GRH (1-29) other than Geref® Diagnostic, 167 normal young adults of both sexes, 19 to 40 years old, were tested with approximately 1 mcg/kg GRH peptide. The data derived from pooling these results are similar to the results obtained from 14 normal male adults, 19 to 30 years old tested with Geref® Diagnostic:

ADULT VOLUNTEERS

Source	N	Age Range	Range of Mean Peak GH (ng/mL)	Mean Peak GH (ng/mL)
14 Studies	167	19–40	10–41	22
Geref® Diagnostic	14	19–30	—	24

In adults, time to peak GH response to Geref® Diagnostic was 35 ± 29 minutes (average ± S.D.).

Preliminary studies have demonstrated a decline in GH responsiveness to GRH with age in persons over 40 years old, but the normal range of GH response to Geref® Diagnostic in older adults has not been established.

INDICATIONS AND USAGE

Geref® Diagnostic as a single intravenous injection is indicated for evaluating the ability of the somatotroph of the pituitary gland to secrete growth hormone (GH). A normal plasma GH response to Geref® Diagnostic demonstrates that the somatotroph is intact. However, a normal response does not exclude GH deficiency because this deficiency is frequently the result of hypothalamic dysfunction in the presence of an intact somatotroph. The Geref® Diagnostic stimulation test is most early interpreted when there is a subnormal response to conventional provocative testing and a normal response to Geref® Diagnostic. Such findings suggest that hypothalamic dysfunction is the cause for the growth hormone deficiency. When both conventional and Geref® Diagnostic testing result in subnormal GH responses, the site of dysfunction cannot be determined with certainty because some patients with GH deficiency due to hypothalamic dysfunction require repeated Geref® Diagnostic administration before demonstrating a normal response.

The Geref® Diagnostic test has not been found useful in the diagnosis of acromegaly.

CONTRAINDICATIONS

Geref® Diagnostic is contraindicated in patients hypersensitive to sermorelin acetate or any of the excipients.

WARNINGS

Although hypersensitivity reactions have been observed with other polypeptide hormones, to date no such reactions have been reported following the administration of a single dose of Geref® Diagnostic. Antibody formation has been reported in humans after chronic subcutaneous administration of large doses of sermorelin (see Adverse Reactions section).

PRECAUTIONS

Drug Interactions: The Geref® Diagnostic test should not be conducted in the presence of drugs that directly affect the pituitary secretion of somatotropin. These include preparations that contain or release somatostatin, insulin, glucocorticoids, or cyclooxygenase inhibitors such as aspirin of indomethacin. Somatotropin levels may be transiently elevated by clonidine, levodopa, and insulin-induced hypoglycemia. Response to Geref® Diagnostic may be blunted in patients who are receiving muscarinic antagonists (atropine) or who are hypothyroid or being treated with antithyroid medication such as propylthiouracil. Obesity, hyperglycemia, and elevated plasma fatty acids generally are associated with subnormal GH responses to Geref® Diagnostic. Exogenous growth hormone therapy should be discontinued at least one week before administering the Geref® Diagnostic test.

Carcinogenesis, Mutagenesis, Impairment of Fertility: Long-term animal studies for carcinogenicity and impairment of fertility have not been performed with Geref® Diagnostic. Geref® Diagnostic was not mutagenic in a battery of *in vivo* and *in vitro* genetic toxicity assays either in the presence or absence of metabolic activator (bacterial mutation tests, gene conversion-DNA repair test, forward mutation test, micronucleus test, chromosome aberration in Chinese hamster bone marrow).

Pregnancy: Pregnancy Category C. During teratology studies, Geref® Diagnostic produced minor variations in fetuses of rats and rabbits when given at a subcutaneous dose of 0.5 mg/kg/day. This subcutaneous dose in approximately 88 and 176 times the single human intravenous dose calculated on a body surface area (mg/m^2) basis, for rats and rabbits, respectively. There are no adequate and well controlled studies in pregnant women. Geref® Diagnostic should be used during pregnancy only if the potential benefit justifies the potential risk to the fetus.

Nursing Mothers: It is not known whether this drug is excreted in human milk. Because many drugs are excreted in human milk, caution should be exercised when Geref® Diagnostic is administered to a nursing woman.

ADVERSE REACTIONS

The following adverse reactions, in decreasing order of frequency, have been reported following sermorelin administration:

Transient warmth and/or flushing of the face
Injection site pain
Redness and/or swelling at injection site
Nausea
Headache
Vomiting
Strange taste in the mouth
Paleness
Tightness in the chest

Approximately one in four patients given repeated doses of one or more of the three forms of GRH (1-29, 1-40, and 1-44) has developed antibodies to GRH. The clinical significance of these antibodies is unknown. One patient who developed antibodies to GRH (1-44) also experienced an allergic reaction described as severe redness, swelling, and urticaria at the injection sites. No long-lasting effects from this reaction were reported. No symptomatic allergic reactions to GRH (1-29) have been reported.

OVERDOSAGE

Changes of heart rate and blood pressure have been reported with the various GRH peptides in intravenous doses exceeding 10 mcg/kg. Cardiovascular collapse in a conceivable, but as of yet, unreported, complication of overdosage with GRH (1-29).

DOSAGE AND ADMINISTRATION

Geref® Diagnostic dosage should be individualized for each patient according to his/her weight. It is recommended that Geref® Diagnostic be administered in a single intravenous dose of 1.0 mcg/kg body weight in the morning following an overnight fast.

Directions:

Children (or subjects less than 50 kg)

1) Reconstitute the contents of one 50 mcg ampule of Geref® Diagnostic with a minimum of 0.5 mL of the accompanying sterile diluent.

2) Venous blood samples for growth hormone determinations should be drawn 15 minutes before and immediately prior to Geref® Diagnostic administration.

3) Administer a bolus of 1 mcg/kg body weight Geref® Diagnostic intravenously followed by a 3 mL normal saline flush.

4) Draw venous blood samples for growth hormone determinations at 15, 30, 45, and 60 minutes after Geref® Diagnostic administration.

Adults (or subjects over 50 kg)

1) Determine the number of ampules needed, based on a dose of 1 mcg/kg body weight.

2) Reconstitute the contents of each ampule with a minimum of 0.5 mL of the accompanying sterile diluent.

3) Follow steps 2–4 above.

Parenteral drug products should be inspected visually for particulate matter and discoloration prior to administration, whenever solution and container permit. The drug should be discarded if not dissolved or if the reconstituted solution is cloudy or discolored.

HOW SUPPLIED

Geref® Diagnostic is supplied in sterile, nonpyrogenic, lyophilized form in ampules containing 50 mcg sermorelin (as the acetate).

The following package combination is available:

NDC 44087-4050-1

1 ampule containing 50 mcg sermorelin (as the acetate) and 1 vial containing 2 mL 0.9% Sodium Chloride Injection, USP

The lyophilized product must be stored refrigerated (2°-8°C/36°-46°F). Use immediately after reconstitution. Discard unused material.

Caution: Federal law prohibits dispensing without prescription.

References available on request.

Manufactured for:
SERONO LABORATORIES, INC.
Randolph, MA 02368 USA
by: Laboratories Serono, SA
Aubonne, Switzerland
Revised March 1998

GONAL-F®   ℞
[gōn al-ĕf]
(follitropin alfa for injection)
For subcutaneous injection

DESCRIPTION

Gonal-F® (follitropin alfa for injection) is a human follicle stimulating hormone (FSH) preparation of recombinant DNA origin, which consists of two non-covalently linked,

Continued on next page

Gonal-F—Cont.

non-identical glycoproteins designated as the α- and β-subunits. The α- and β-subunits have 92 and 111 amino acids, respectively, and their primary and tertiary structure are indistinguishable from those of human follicle stimulating hormone. Recombinant FSH production occurs in genetically modified Chinese Hamster Ovary (CHO) cells cultured in bioreactors. Purification by immunochromatography using an antibody specifically binding FSH results in a highly purified preparation with a consistent FSH isoform profile, and a high specific activity. The biological activity of follitropin alfa is determined by measuring the increase in ovary weight in female rats. The in vivo biological activity of follitropin alfa has been calibrated against the second International Reference Preparation for Human Menopausal Gonadotrophins established in September 1964 by the Expert Committee on Biological Standards of the World Health Organization. Gonal-F® contains no luteinizing hormone (LH) activity. Based on available data derived from physicochemical tests and bioassays follitropin alfa and follitropin beta, another recombinant follicle stimulating hormone product are indistinguishable.

Gonal-F® is a sterile, lyophilized powder intended for subcutaneous injection after reconstitution with Sterile Water for Injection, USP. Each ampule of Gonal-F® contains either 75 IU or 150 IU recombinant FSH, 30 mg sucrose, 1.11 mg dibasic sodium phosphate and 0.45 mg monobasic sodium phosphate monohydrate. O-phosphoric acid and/or sodium hydroxide may be used prior to lyophillization for pH adjustment. Under current storage conditions. Gonal-F® may contain up to 15% of oxidized follitropin alfa.

Therapeutic Class: Infertility

CLINICAL PHARMACOLOGY

Gonal-F® (follitropin alfa for injection) stimulates ovarian follicular growth in women who do not have primary ovarian failure. FSH, the active component of Gonal-F® is the primary hormone responsible for follicular recruitment and development. In order to effect final maturation of the follicle and ovulation in the absence of an endogenous LH surge, human chorionic gonadotropin (hCG) must be given following the administration of Gonal-F® when monitoring of the patient indicates that sufficient follicular development has occurred. There is interpatient variability in response to FSH administration. The physicochemical, immunological, and biological activities of recombinant FSH are comparable to those of pituitary and human menopausal urinederived FSH.

Pharmacokinetics

Single dose pharmacokinetics of r-hFSH were determined following intravenous, subcutaneous and intramuscular administration of 150 IU Gonal-F® to 12 healthy, down-regulated female volunteers. Steady-state pharmacokinetics were also determined in 12 healthy down-regulated female volunteers who were administered a single daily dose of 150 IU for seven days. These pharmacokinetics were confirmed in pituitary down-regulated women undergoing in vitro fertilization and embryo transfer (IVF/ET), treated with FSH doses of up to 450 IU per day. The pharmacokinetic parameters from these studies are included in Table 1.
[See table 1 above]

Absorption

The absorption rate of Gonal-F® following subcutaneous or intramuscular administration was found to be slower than the elimination rate. Hence the pharmacokinetics of Gonal-F® are absorption rate-limited.

Distribution

Human tissue or organ distribution of FSH has not been determined for Gonal-F®.

After intravenous administration, the serum profile of FSH appears to be described by a two compartment open model with a distribution half-life of about 2–2.5 hours. Steady-state serum levels were reached after 4 to 5 days of daily administration.

Metabolism/Excretion

FSH metabolism following administration of Gonal-F® has not been studied in humans. Total clearance after IV administration was 0.6 L/hr; mean residence time was 17-20 hours. FSH renal clearance was 0.07 L/hr after intravenous administration representing approximately 1/8 of total clearance.

Pharmacodynamics

Following daily subcutaneous administration of 150 IU of Gonal-F® for 7 days, serum inhibin and estradiol, and total follicular volume responded as a function of time, with pronounced inter-individual variability. Pharmacodynamic effect lagged behind FSH serum concentration. Of the three pharmacodynamic parameters, serum levels responded with the least delay and declined rapidly after discontinuation of Gonal-F®. Follicular growth was most delayed and continued even after discontinuation of Gonal-F administration, and after serum FSH levels had declined. Maximum follicular volume was better correlated with either inhibin or estradiol peak levels than with FSH concentration. Inhibin rise was an early index of follicular development.

Table 1: Pharmacokinetic parameters (mean ± SD) of FSH following administration of Gonal-F®

Population	Healthy female volunteers			IVF/ET patients
Dose (IU)	Single Dose IM (150)	Single Dose SC (150)	Multiple Dose SC (7 × 150)	Multiple Dose SC (5×225)*
AUC - (IU-hr/L)	206 ± 66	176 ± 87	187 ± 61#	—
C_{max} (IU/L)	3 ± 1	3 ± 1	9 ± 3	—
t_{max} (hr)	25 ± 10	16 ± 10	8 ± 6	—
$t_{1/2}$ terminal (hr)	50 ± 27	24 ± 11	24 ±8	32**
CL/F (L/hr)	—	—	—	0.7 ± 0.2
V_{ss}/F (L)	—	—	—	10 ± 3
F (%)	76 ± 30	66 ± 39	—	—

Abbreviations are: IVF/ET: in vitro fertilization/embryo transfer; C_{max}: peak concentration (above baseline); t_{max}time of C_{max}; CL/F: apparent clearance; V_{ss}/F: apparent steady-state volume of distribution; $t_{1/2}$: absorption half-life; F: biovailability compared to IV

#Steady-state $AUC_{144-168}$ (After the 7th daily SC dose)
*First five days of fixed regimen followed by adjustment of the dose depending on response
**increases with body mass index

Table 2: Cumulative Patient Ovulation and Clinical Pregnancy Rates by Treatment Group in Ovulation Induction

Study 5642	Gonal-F® (n=110)	urofollitropin (n=112)
Cumulative Ovulation Rate		
cycle 1	64%	59%
cycle 2	78%	82%
cycle 3	84%	91%
Cumulative Clinical Pregnancy* Rate		
cycle 1	21%	21%
cycle 2	28%	38%
cycle 3	35%	46%

* A clinical pregnancy was defined as a pregnancy during which a fetal sac (with or without heart activity) was visualized by ultrasound on day 34–36 after hCG administration.

Table 3: Pregnancy Outcome by Treatment Group in Ovulation Induction

Study 5642	Gonal-F® (n=39)	urofollitropin (n=51)
Pregnancies not reaching term	20.5%	13.7%
Single births	74.4%	74.5%
Multiple births	5.1%	11.8%

Population pharmacokinetics and pharmacodynamics

To establish the pharmacokinetics and pharmacodynamics of FSH in a target population, measurements performed during a clinical study of in vitro fertilization/embryo transfer were used in conjunction with pharmacokinetic data from studies in healthy volunteers. The apparent clearance was comparable to that in healthy volunteers. The absorption rate was found to be influenced by the body mass index (BMI), suggesting that the higher the BMI, the lower the rate of absorption. However, FSH serum levels following fixed (during the first five days) and then adjusted doses of Gonal-F® were found to be poor predictors of follicular growth rate. High pre-treatment serum FSH levels may predict lower follicular growth rates.

Special populations: Safety, efficacy, and pharmacokinetics of Gonal-F® in patients with renal or hepatic insufficiency have not been established.

Drug-Drug Interactions: No drug/drug interaction studies have been conducted (see PRECAUTIONS).

Clinical Studies:

The safety and efficacy of Gonal-F® have been examined in four clinical studies two studies for ovulation induction and two studies for assisted reproductive technologies (ART). In these comparative studies there were no clinically significant differences between treatment groups in study outcomes.

1. **Ovulation Induction:**

The safety and efficacy of Gonal-F® administered subcutaneously vs. urofollitropin administered intramuscularly were assessed in a phase III, open-label, randomized, comparative, multinational, multicenter study in oligo-anovulatory infertile women who failed to ovulate or conceive following adequate clomiphene citrate therapy (Study 5642).

The primary efficacy parameter was the ovulation rate. Two hundred and twenty-two patients entered into the first cycle of treatment, of whom 110 received Gonal-F® and 112 received urofollitropin. Ovulation rates were similar between Gonal-F® and urofollitropin treatment groups. The study results for the 222 patients who received treatment in at least one cycle are summarized in table 2.
[See table 2 above]

For the 90 patients who had a clinical pregnancy (39 in Gonal-F® group; 51 in urofollitropin group), the outcome of the pregnancy was:
[See table 3 above]

A second randomized, comparative, open-label, multicenter study was conducted in 23 U.S. centers (Study 5727). The primary efficacy parameter was ovulation rate. Ovulation rates were similar between Gonal-F® and urofollitropin treatment groups. Two hundred and thirty-two patients with oligo-anovulatory infertility received treatment with up to three cycles of Gonal-F® administered subcutaneously (118 patients) or urofollitropin administered intramuscularly (114 patients).

The cumulative patient ovulation rate and clinical pregnancy rates by cycle are presented for the 232 patients who received treatment in at least one cycle.
[See table 4 at top of next page]

For the 85 patients who had a clinical pregnancy (44 in Gonal-F® group; 41 in urofollitropin group), the outcome of the pregnancy is shown in Table 5.
[See table 5 on next page]

2. **Assisted Reproductive Technologies (ART):**

The safety and efficacy of Gonal-F® administered subcutaneously vs. urofollitropin administered intramuscularly were assessed in a phase III, open-label, randomized, comparative, multinational, multicenter study in ovulatory, infertile women undergoing stimulation of multiple follicles for In Vitro Fertilization and Embryo Transfer (IVF/ET) after pituitary down-regulation with a GnRH agonist (Study 5503). The purpose of the study was to demonstrate that Gonal-F®, administered subcutaneously, was clinically not different in terms of safety and efficacy from urofollitropin, administered intramuscularly. The initial and maximal doses of Gonal-F® were 225 and 450 IU, respectively. The primary efficacy parameter was the number of mature preovulatory follicles on the day of hCG administration. One hundred and twenty-three patients were randomized and received either Gonal-F® (60 patients) or urofollitropin (63 patients).

The results summarized in Table 6 are mean data with Gonal-F® and urofollitropin administered to ovulatory infertile women undergoing multiple follicular development for IVF/ET.

[See table 6 below]

For the 22 patients who had a clinical pregnancy (12 in the Gonal-F® group; 10 in the urofollitropin group), the outcome of the pregnancy is shown in Table 7.

[See table 7 below]

A second randomized, comparative, open-label, multicenter study was conducted in 7 U.S. centers (Study 5533). One hundred and fourteen patients with ovulatory infertility undergoing IVF/ET were randomized and received either Gonal-F® by subcutaneous administration (56 patients) or urofollitropin by intramuscular administration (58 patients) following pituitary down-regulation with a GnRH agonist. The primary efficacy parameter was the number of mature pre-ovulatory follicles on the day of hCG administration. Results are summarized in table 8.

[See table 8 at top of next page]

For the 25 patients who had a clinical pregnancy (12 in Gonal-F® group; 13 in urofollitropin group), the outcome of the pregnancy is shown in Table 9.

[See table 9 on next page]

INDICATIONS AND USAGE

Gonal-F® (follitropin alfa for injection) is indicated for the induction of ovulation and pregnancy in anovulatory infertile patients in whom the cause of infertility is functional and not due to primary ovarian failure. Gonal-F® is also indicated for the development of multiple follicles in the ovulatory patient participating in an Assisted Reproductive Technology (ART) program.

Selection of Patients:

1. Before treatment with Gonal-F® is instituted, a thorough gynecologic and endocrinologic evaluation must be performed. This should include an assessment of pelvic anatomy. Patients with tubal obstruction should receive Gonal-F® only if enrolled in an *in vitro* fertilization program.
2. Primary ovarian failure should be excluded by the determination of gonadotropin levels.
3. Appropriate evaluation should be performed to exclude pregnancy.
4. Patients in later reproductive life have a greater predisposition to endometrial carcinoma as well as a higher incidence of anovulatory disorders. A thorough diagnostic evaluation should always be performed in patients who demonstrate abnormal uterine bleeding or other signs of endometrial abnormalities before starting Gonal-F® therapy.
5. Evaluation of the partner's fertility potential should be included in the initial evaluation.

CONTRAINDICATIONS

Gonal-F® (follitropin alfa for injection) is contraindicated in women who exhibit:

1. Prior hypersensitivity to recombinant FSH preparations or one of their excipients.
2. High levels of FSH indicating primary ovarian failure.
3. Uncontrolled thyroid or adrenal dysfunction.
4. An organic intracranial lesion such as a pituitary tumor.
5. Abnormal uterine bleeding of undetermined origin (see "Selection of Patients").
6. Ovarian cyst or enlargement of undetermined origin (see "Selection of Patients").
7. Sex hormone dependent tumors of the reproductive tract and accessory organs.
8. Pregnancy.

WARNINGS

Gonal-F® (follitropin alfa for injection) should only be used by physicians who are thoroughly familiar with infertility problems and their management.

Gonal-F® is a potent gonadotropic substance capable of causing Ovarian Hyperstimulation Syndrome (OHSS) with or without pulmonary or vascular complications. Gonadotropin therapy requires a certain time commitment by physicians and supportive health professionals, and requires the availability of appropriate monitoring facilities (see "Precautions/Laboratory Tests"). Safe and effective use of Gonal-F® requires monitoring of ovarian response with serum estradiol and vaginal ultrasound on a regular basis. The lowest effective dose should be used.

Overstimulation of the Ovary During FSH Therapy:

Ovarian Enlargement: Mild to moderate uncomplicated ovarian enlargement which may be accompanied by abdominal distention and/or abdominal pain occurs in approximately 20% of those treated with urofollitropin and hCG, and generally regresses without treatment within two or three weeks. Careful monitoring of ovarian response can further minimize the risk of overstimulation.

If the ovaries are abnormally enlarged on the last day of Gonal-F® therapy, hCG should not be administered in this course of therapy. This will reduce the chances of development of Ovarian Hyperstimulation Syndrome.

Ovarian Hyperstimulation Syndrome (OHSS): OHSS is a medical event distinct from uncomplicated ovarian enlargement. Severe OHSS may progress rapidly (within 24 hours to several days) to become a serious medical event. It is characterized by an apparent dramatic increase in vascular

Table 4: Cumulative Patient Ovulation and Clinical Pregnancy Rates by Treatment Group in Ovulation Induction

Study 5727	Gonal-F® (n=118)	urofollitropin (n=114)
Cumulative Ovulation Rate		
cycle 1	58%	68%
cycle 2	72%	86%
cycle 3	81%	93%
Cumulative Clinical Pregnancy* Rate		
cycle 1	13%	14%
cycle 2	25%	25%
cycle 3	37%	36%

* A clinical pregnancy was defined as a pregnancy during which a fetal sac (with or without heart activity) was visualized by ultrasound on day 34–36 after hCG administration.

Table 5: Pregnancy Outcome by Treatment Group in Ovulation Induction

Study 5727	Gonal-F® (n=44)	urofollitropin (n=41)
Pregnancies not reaching term	22.7%	22.0%
Single births	63.6%	65.9%
Multiple births	13.7%	12.2%

Table 6: Treatment Outcomes by Treatment Group in ART

Study 5503	Gonal-F® (n=60)	urofollitropin (n=63)
Mean number of follicles ≥ 14mm in diameter on day of hCG	7.8	9.2
Mean number of oocytes recovered per patient	9.3	10.7
Mean Serum E2 (pg/mL) on day of hCG	1576	2193
Mean treatment duration in days (range)	9.9 (5–20)	9.4 (5–14)
Clinical pregnancy* rate per attempt	20%	16%
Clinical pregnancy* rate per embryo transfer	24%	19%

* A clinical pregnancy was defined as a pregnancy during which a fetal sac (with or without heart activity) was visualized by ultrasound on day 34–36 after hCG administration.

Table 7: Pregnancy Outcome by Treatment Group in ART

Study 5503	Gonal-F® (n=12)	urofollitropin (n=10)
Pregnancies not reaching term	25.0%	20.0%
Single births	41.7%	50.0%
Multiple births	33.3%	30.0%

permeability which can result in a rapid accumulation of fluid in the peritoneal cavity, thorax, and potentially, the pericardium. The early warning signs of development of OHSS are severe pelvic pain, nausea, vomiting, and weight gain. The following symptomatology has been seen with cases of OHSS: abdominal pain, abdominal distension, gastrointestinal symptoms including nausea, vomiting and diarrhea, severe ovarian enlargement, weight gain, dyspnea, and oliguria. Clinical evaluation may reveal hypovolemia, hemoconcentration, electrolyte imbalances, ascites, hemoperitoneum, pleural effusions, hydrothorax, acute pulmonary distress, and thromboembolic events (see "Pulmonary and Vascular Complications"). Transient liver function test abnormalities suggestive of hepatic dysfunction, which may be accompanied by morphologic changes on liver biopsy, have been reported in association with Ovarian Hyperstimulation Syndrome (OHSS).

OHSS occurred in 9 of 228 (3.9%) Gonal-F® treated women during ovulation induction clinical trials and of this number, 1 of 228 (0.4%) was classified as severe. In ART clinical studies, OHSS occurred in 0 of 116 (0.0%) Gonal-F® treated women. OHSS may be more severe and more protracted if pregnancy occurs. OHSS develops rapidly; therefore, patients should be followed for at least two weeks after hCG administration. Most often, OHSS occurs after treatment has been discontinued and reaches its maximum at about seven to ten days following treatment. Usually, OHSS resolves spontaneously with the onset of menses. If there is evidence that OHSS may be developing prior to hCG administration (see "Precautions/Laboratory Tests"), the hCG must be withheld.

If severe OHSS occurs, treatment <u>must</u> be stopped and the patient should be hospitalized.

A physician experienced in the management of this syndrome, or who is experienced in the management of fluid and electrolyte imbalances should be consulted.

Pulmonary and Vascular Complications:

Serious pulmonary conditions (e.g., atelectasis, acute respiratory distress syndrome and exacerbation of asthma) have been reported. In addition, thromboembolic events both in association with, and separate from Ovarian Hyperstimulation Syndrome have been reported. Intravascular thrombosis and embolism can result in reduced blood flow to critical

organs or the extremities. Sequelae of such events have included venous thrombophlebitis, pulmonary embolism, pulmonary infarction, cerebral vascular occlusion (stroke), and arterial occlusion resulting in loss of limb. In rare cases, pulmonary complications and/or thromboembolic events have resulted in death.

Multiple Births: Reports of multiple births have been associated with Gonal-F® treatment. In ovulation induction clinical trials, 12.3% of live births were multiple births in women receiving Gonal-F® and 14.5% of live births were multiple births in women receiving urofollitropin. In IVF/ET clinical trials, 44.0% of live births were multiple births in women receiving Gonal-F® and 41.0% of live births were multiple births in women receiving urofollitropin and is dependent on the number of embryos transferred. The patient should be advised of the potential risk of multiple births before starting treatment.

PRECAUTIONS

General: Careful attention should be given to the diagnosis of infertility in candidates for Gonal-F® (follitropin alfa for injection) therapy (see "Indications and Usage/Selection of Patients").

Information for Patients: Prior to therapy with Gonal-F®, patients should be informed of the duration of treatment and monitoring of their condition that will be required. The risks of ovarian hyperstimulation syndrome and multiple births (see **WARNINGS**) and other possible adverse reactions (see "Adverse Reactions") should also be discussed.

Laboratory Tests: In most instances, treatment with Gonal-F® results only in follicular recruitment and development. In the absence of an endogenous LH surge, hCG is given when monitoring of the patient indicates that sufficient follicular development has occurred. This may be estimated by ultrasound alone or in combination with measurement of serum estradiol levels. The combination of both ultrasound and serum estradiol measurement are useful for monitoring the development of follicles, for timing of the ovulatory trigger, as well as for detecting ovarian enlargement and minimizing the risk of the Ovarian Hyperstimulation Syndrome and multiple gestation. It is recommended that

Continued on next page

Gonal-F—Cont.

the number of growing follicles be confirmed using ultrasonography because plasma estrogens do not give an indication of the size or number of follicles.

The clinical confirmation of ovulation, with the exception of pregnancy, is obtained by direct and indirect indices of progesterone production. The indices most generally used are as follows:

1. A rise in basal body temperature;
2. Increase in serum progesterone; and
3. Menstruation following a shift in basal body temperature.

When used in conjuction with the indices of progesterone production, sonographic visualzation of the ovaries will assist in determining if ovulation has occurred. Sonographic evidence of ovulation may include the following:

1. Fluid in the cul-de-sac;
2. Ovarian stigmata;
3. Collapsed follicle; and
4. Secretory endometrium.

Accurate interpretation of the indices of follicle development and maturation require a physician who is experienced in the interpretation of these results.

Drug Interactions: No drug/drug interaction studies have been performed.

Carcinogenesis, Mutagenesis, Impairment of Fertility: Long-term studies in animals have not been performed to evaluate the carcinogenic potential of Gonal-F®. However, r-hFSH showed no mutagenic activity in a series of tests performed to evaluate its potential genetic toxicity including, bacterial and mammalian cell mutation tests, a chromosomal aberration test and a micronucleus test.

Impaired fertility has been reported in rats, exposed to pharmacological doses of r-hFSH (≥40 IU/kg/day) for extended periods, through reduced fecundity.

Pregnancy: Pregnancy Category X. See CONTRAINDICATIONS.

Nursing Mothers: It is not known whether this drug is excreted in human milk. Because many drugs are excreted in human milk and because of the potential for serious adverse reactions in the nursing infant from Gonal-F®, a decision should be made whether to discontinue nursing or to discontinue the drug, taking into account the importance of the drug to the mother.

Pediatric Use: Safety and effectiveness in pediatric patients have not been established.

ADVERSE REACTIONS

The safety of Gonal-F® was examined in four clinical studies that enrolled 691 patients into two studies for ovulation induction (454 patients) and two studies for ART (237 patients).

Adverse events occurring in more than 10% of patients were headache, ovarian cyst, nausea, and upper respiratory tract infection in the US ovulation induction study and headache in the US ART study. Adverse events (without regard to causality assessment) occurring in at least 2% of patients are listed in Table 10 and Table 11.

[See table 10 at right]

Additional adverse events not listed in Table 10 that occurred in 1 to 2% of Gonal-F® treated patients in the US ovulation induction study included the following: leukorrhea, vaginal hemorrhage, migraine, fatigue, asthma, nervousness, somnolence, and hypotension.

[See table 11 at top of next page]

Additional adverse events not listed in Table 11 that occurred in 1 to 2% of Gonal-F® treated patients in the US Assisted Reproductive Technology (ART) study included the following: D&C following delivery or abortion, dysmenorrhea, vaginal hemorrhage, diarrhea, tooth disorder, vomiting, dizziness, paraesthesia, abdomen enlarged, chest pain, fatigue, dyspnea, anorexia, anxiety, somnolence, injection site inflammation, injection site reaction, pruritus, pruritus genital, myalgia thirst and palpitation.

Two additional clinical studies (for ovulation induction and ART, respectively) were conducted in Europe. The safety profiles from these two studies were comparable to that of the data presented above.

The following medical events have been reported subsequent to pregnancies resulting from Gonal-F® therapy in controlled clinical studies:

1. Spontaneous Abortion
2. Ectopic Pregnancy
3. Premature Labor
4. Postpartum Fever
5. Congenital abnormalities

Two incidents of cogenital cardiac malformations have been reported in children born following pregnancies resulting from treatment with Gonal-F® and hCG in Gonal-F® clinical studies 5642 and 5727. In addition, a pregnancy occurring in study 5533 following treatment with Gonal-F® and hCG was complicated by apparent failure of intrauterine growth and terminated for a suspected syndrome of congen-

ital abnormalities. No specific diagnosis was made. The incidence does not exceed that found in the general population.

The following adverse reactions have been previously reported during menotropin therapy:

1. Pulmonary and vascular complications (see "Warnings").
2. Adnexal torsion (as a complication of ovarian enlargement),
3. Mild to moderate ovarian enlargement,
4. Hemoperitoneum

There have been infrequent reports of ovarian neoplasms, both benign and malignant, in women who have undergone multiple drug regimens for ovulation induction; however, a causal relationship has not been established.

Table 8: Treatment Outcomes by Treatment Group in ART

Study 5533	Gonal-F® (n=56)	urofollitropin (n=58)
Mean number of follicles ≥ 14mm in diameter on day of hCG	7.2	8.3
Mean number of oocytes recovered per patient	9.3	12.3
Mean Serum E2 (pg/mL) on day of hCG	1236	1513
Mean treatment duration in days (range)	10.0 (5–15)	9.0 (5–12)
Clinical pregnancy* rate per attempt	21%	22%
Clinical pregnancy* rate per embryo transfer	26%	25%

* A clinical pregnancy was defined as a pregnancy during which a fetal sac (with or without heart activity) was visualized by ultrasound on day 34–36 after hCG administration.

Table 9: Pregnancy Outcome by Treatment Group in ART

Study 5533	Gonal-F® (n=12)	urofollitropin (n=13)
Pregnancies not reaching term	33.3%	30.8%
Single births	41.7%	38.5%
Multiple births	25.0%	30.8%

Table 10: US Controlled Trial in Ovulation Induction, Study 5727

Body System Preferred Term	Gonal-F® Patients (%) Experiencing Events Treatment cycles = 288* n = 118	urofollitropin Patients (%) Experiencing Events Treatment cycles = 277 n = 114
Reproductive, Female		
Intermenstrual Bleeding	9.3%	4.4%
Breast Pain Female	4.2%	6.1%
Ovarian Hyperstimulation**	6.8%	3.5%
Dysmenorrhea	2.5%	6.1%
Ovarian Disorder	1.7%	2.6%
Cervix Lesion	2.5%	0.9%
Menstrual Disorder	2.5%	0.9%
Gastro-intestinal System		
Abdominal Pain	9.3%	12.3%
Nausea	13.6%	3.5%
Flatulence	6.8%	8.8%
Diarrhea	7.6%	3.5%
Vomiting	2.5%	2.6%
Dyspepsia	1.7%	3.5%
Central and Peripheral Nervous System		
Headache	22.0%	20.2%
Dizziness	2.5%	0.0%
Neoplasm		
Ovarian Cyst	15.3%	28.9%
Body as a Whole- General		
Pain	5.9%	6.1%
Back Pain	5.1%	1.8%
Influenza-like Symptoms	4.2%	2.6%
Fever	4.2%	1.8%
Respiratory System		
Upper Respiratory Tract Infection	11.9%	7.9%
Sinusitis	5.1%	5.3%
Pharyngitis	2.5%	3.5%
Coughing	1.7%	2.6%
Rhinitus	0.8%	2.6%
Skin and Appendages		
Acne	4.2%	2.6%
Psychiatric		
Emotional Lability	5.1%	2.6%
Urinary System		
Urinary-Tract Infection	1.7%	4.4%
Resistance Mechanism		
Moniliasis Genital	2.5%	0.9%
Application Site		
Injection Site Pain	2.5%	0.9%

* up to 3 cycles of therapy
** Severe = 0.8% of 118 patients in Study 5727

OVERDOSAGE

Aside from possible ovarian hyperstimulation and multiple gestations (see "Warnings"), there is no information on the consequences of acute overdosage with Gonal-F® (follitropin alfa for injection).

DOSAGE AND ADMINISTRATION

Dosage:

Infertile Patients with oligo-anovulation: The dose of Gonal-F® (follitropin alfa for injection) to stimulate development of the follicle must be individualized for each patients.

The lowest dose consistent with the expectation of good results should be used. Over the course of treatment, doses of Gonal-F® may range up to 300 IU per day depending on the

Table 11: US Controlled Trial in ART, Study 5533

Body System Preferred Term	Gonal-F® Patients (%) Experiencing Events Treatment n = 59	urofollitropin Patients (%) Experiencing Events Treatment n = 61
Reproductive, Female		
Intermenstrual Bleeding	3.6%	5.2%
Leukorrhea	1.7%	3.4%
Vaginal Hemorrhage	3.6%	3.4%
Gastro-intestinal System		
Nausea	5.4%	1.7%
Flatulence	3.6%	0.0%
Central and Peripheral Nervous System		
Headache	12.5%	3.4%
Body as a Whole-General		
Abdominal Pain	8.9%	3.4%
Pelvic Pain Female	7.1%	1.7%
Respiratory System		
Upper Respiratory Tract Infection	3.6%	1.7%
Metabolic and Nutritional		
Weight Increase	3.6%	0.0%

individual patient response. Gonal-F® should be administered until adequate follicular development is indicated by serum estradiol and vaginal ultrasonography. A response is generally evident after 5 to 7 days. Subsequent monitoring intervals should be based on individual patient response.

It is recommended that the initial dose of the first cycle be 75 IU of Gonal-F® per day, ADMINISTERED SUBCUTANEOUSLY. An incremental adjustment in dose of up to 37.5 IU may be considered after 14 days. Further dose increases of the same magnitude could be made, if necessary, every seven days. Treatment duration should not exceed 35 days unless an E2 rise indicates imminent follicular development. To complete follicular development and effect ovulation in the absence of an endogenous LH surge, chorionic gonadotropin, hCG, (5,000 USP units) should be given 1 day after the last dose of Gonal-F®. Chorionic gonadotropin should be withheld if the serum estradiol is greater than 2,000 pg/mL. If the ovaries are abnormally enlarged or abdominal pain occurs, Gonal-F® treatment should be discontinued, hCG should not be administered, and the patient should be advised not to have intercourse; this may reduce the chance of development of the Ovarian Hyperstimulation Syndrome and, should spontaneous ovulation occur, reduce the chance of multiple gestation. A follow-up visit should be conducted in the luteal phase.

The initial dose administered in the subsequent cycles should be individualized for each patient based on her response in the preceding cycle. Doses larger than 300 IU of FSH per day are not routinely recommended. As in the initial cycle, 5,000 USP units of hCG must be given 1 day after the last dose of Gonal-F® to complete follicular development and induce ovulation. The precautions described above should be followed to minimize the chance of development of the Ovarian Hyperstimulation Syndrome.

The couple should be encouraged to have intercourse daily, beginning on the day prior to the administration of hCG until ovulation becomes apparent from the indices employed for the determination of progestational activity. Care should be taken to ensure insemination. In light of the indices and parameters mentioned, it should become obvious that, unless a physician is willing to devote considerable time to these patients and be familiar with and conduct the necessary laboratory studies, he/she should not use Gonal-F®.

Assisted Reproductive Technologies: As in the treatment of patients with oligo-anovulatory infertility, the dose of Gonal-F® to stimulate development of the follicle must be individualized for each patient. For Assisted Reproductive Technologies, therapy with Gonal-F® should be initiated in the early follicular phase (cycle day 2 or 3) at a dose of 150 IU per day, until sufficient follicular development is attained. In most cases, therapy should not exceed ten days. In patients undergoing ART, whose endogenous gonadotropin levels are suppressed, Gonal-F® should be initiated at a dose of 225 IU per day. Treatment should be continued until adequate follicular development is indicated as determined by ultrasound in combination with measurement of serum estradiol levels. Adjustments to dose may be considered after five days based on the patient's response; subsequently dosage should be adjusted no more frequently than every 3–5 days and by no more than 75–150 IU additionally at each adjustment. Doses greater than 450 IU per day are not recommended. Once adequate follicular development is evident, hCG (5,000 to 10,000 USP units) should be administered to induce final follicular maturation in preparation for oocyte retrieval. The administration of hCG must be withheld in cases where the ovaries are abnormally enlarged on the last day of therapy. This should reduce the chance of developing OHSS.

Administration:

Dissolve the contents of one or more ampules of Gonal-F® in one-half to one mL of Sterile Water for Injection, USP (concentration should not exceed 225 IU/0.5 mL) and ADMINISTER SUBCUTANEOUSLY immediately. Any unused reconstituted material should be discarded.

Parenteral drug products should be inspected visually for particulate matter and discoloration prior to administration, whenever solution and container permit.

HOW SUPPLIED

Gonal-F® (follitropin alfa for injection) is supplied in a sterile, lyophilized form in single dose ampules containing 75 or 150 IU FSH activity. The following package combinations are available:

— 1 ampule 75 IU Gonal-F® and 1 ampule 1 mL Sterile Water for Injection, USP, NDC 44087-9075-1
— 10 ampules 75 IU Gonal-F® and 10 ampules 1 mL Sterile Water for Injection USP, NDC 44087-9075-3
— 100 ampules 75 IU Gonal-F® and 100 ampules 1 mL Sterile Water for Injection, USP, NDC 44087-9075-4
— 1 ampule 150 IU Gonal-F® and 1 ampule 1 mL Sterile Water for Injection, USP, NDC 44087-9150-1

Lyophilized ampules may be stored refrigerated or at room temperature (2°-25°C/36°-77°F). Protect from light. Use immediately after reconstitution. Discard unused material.

Caution: Federal law prohibits dispensing without prescription.

Manufactured for:
SERONO LABORATORIES INC.
Randolph, MA 02368 USA

by: Laboratoires Serono SA
Aubonne, Switzerland
Revised: September 1997

PERGONAL®   ℞
[per 'go-nal]
(menotropins for injection, USP)
FOR INTRAMUSCULAR INJECTION

PRODUCT OVERVIEW
KEY FACTS

Pergonal® is a purified, lyophilized preparation of gonadotropins and contains equal amounts of follicle stimulating hormone and luteinizing hormone. Human Chorionic Gonadotropins (hCG), a naturally occurring hormone in postmenopausal urine, is detected in Pergonal®. Pergonal® is administered by intramuscular injection immediately after reconstitution with Sodium Chloride for Injection, USP.

MAJOR USES

Women: Pergonal® is used to stimulate follicular development in hypogonadotropic anovulatory women who do not have primary ovarian failure.

Men: Pergonal® is used concomitantly with Profasi® (hCG) to stimulate spermatogenesis in men with infertility due to primary or secondary hypogonadotropic hypogonadism.

SAFETY INFORMATION

Pergonal® is contraindicated in individuals who have previously demonstrated hypersensitivity to the drug. In rare instances, women may experience excessive ovarian enlargement, ascites, and pleural effusion requiring hospitalization. The risk can be minimized through careful patient

---

monitoring. Multiple births, 75% of which are twins, have been reported in 20% of pregnancies resulting from Pergonal® therapy.

PRESCRIBING INFORMATION
PERGONAL®   ℞
[per 'go-nal]
(menotropins for injection, USP)
FOR INTRAMUSCULAR INJECTION

DESCRIPTION

Pergonal® (menotropins for injection, USP) is a purified preparation of gonadotropins extracted from the urine of postmenopausal women. Each ampule of Pergonal® contains 75 IU or 150 IU of follicle-stimulating hormone (FSH) activity and 75 IU or 150 IU of luteinizing hormone (LH) activity, respectively, plus 10 mg lactose in a sterile, lyophilized form. Human Chorionic Gonadotropins (hCG), a naturally occurring hormone in post-menopausal urine, is detected in Pergonal®. Pergonal® is administered by intramuscular injection.

Pergonal® is biologically standardized for FSH and LH (ICSH) gonadotropin activities in terms of the Second International Reference Preparation for Human Menopausal Gonadotropins established in September, 1964 by the Expert Committee on Biological Standards of the World Health Organization.

Both FSH and LH are glycoproteins that are acidic and water soluble.

Therapeutic class: Infertility.

CLINICAL PHARMACOLOGY
Women:

Pergonal® administered for seven to twelve days produces ovarian follicular growth in women who do not have primary ovarian failure. Treatment with Pergonal® in most instances results only in follicular growth and maturation. In order to effect ovulation, human chorionic gonadotropin (hCG) must be given following the administration of Pergonal® when clinical assessment of the patient indicates that sufficient follicular maturation has occurred.

Men:

Pergonal® administered concomitantly with human chorionic gonadotropin (hCG) for at least three months induces spermatogenesis in men with primary or secondary pituitary hypofunction who have achieved adequate masculinization with prior hCG therapy.

INDICATIONS AND USAGE
Women:

Pergonal® and hCG given in a sequential manner are indicated for the induction of ovulation and pregnancy in the anovulatory infertile patient, in whom the cause of anovulation is functional and is not due to primary ovarian failure.

Pergonal® and hCG may also be used to stimulate the development of multiple follicles in ovulatory patients participating in an in vitro fertilization program.

Men:

Pergonal® with concomitant hCG is indicated for the stimulation of spermatogenesis in men who have primary or secondary hypogonadotropic hypogonadism.

Pergonal® with concomitant hCG has proven effective in inducing spermatogenesis in men with primary hypogonadotropic hypogonadism due to a congenital factor or prepubertal hypophysectomy and in men with secondary hypogonadotropic hypogonadism due to hypophysectomy, craniopharyngioma, cerebral aneurysm or chromophobe adenoma.

SELECTION OF PATIENTS
Women:

1. Before treatment with Pergonal® is instituted, a thorough gynecologic and endocrinologic evaluation must be performed. Except for those patients enrolled in an in vitro fertilization program, this should include a hysterosalpingogram (to rule out uterine and tubal pathology) and documentation of anovulation by means of basal body temperature, serial vaginal smears, examination of cervical mucus, determination of serum (or urinary) progesterone, urinary pregnanediol and endometrial biopsy. Patients with tubal pathology should receive Pergonal® only if enrolled in an in vitro fertilization program.
2. Primary ovarian failure should be excluded by the determination of gonadotropin levels.
3. Careful examination should be made to rule out the presence of an early pregnancy.
4. Patients in late reproductive life have a greater predilection to endometrial carcinoma as well as a higher incidence of anovulatory disorders. Cervical dilation and curettage should always be done for diagnosis before starting Pergonal® therapy in such patients who demonstrate abnormal uterine bleeding or other signs of endometrial abnormalities.
5. Evaluation of the husband's fertility potential should be included in the workup.

Continued on next page

Pergonal—Cont.

Men:
Patient selection should be made based on a documented lack of pituitary function. Prior to hormonal therapy, these patients will have low testosterone levels and low or absent gonadotropin levels. Patients with primary hypogonadotropic hypogonadism will have a subnormal development of masculinization, and those with secondary hypogonadotropic hypogonadism will have decreased masculinization.

CONTRAINDICATIONS
Women:
Pergonal® is contraindicated in women who have:
1. A high FSH level indicating primary ovarian failure.
2. Uncontrolled thyroid and adrenal dysfunction.
3. An organic intracranial lesion such as a pituitary tumor.
4. The presence of any cause of infertility other than anovulation, unless they are candidates for in vitro fertilization.
5. Abnormal bleeding of undetermined origin.
6. Ovarian cysts or enlargement not due to polycystic ovary syndrome.
7. Prior hypersensitivity to menotropins.
8. Pergonal® is contraindicated in women who are pregnant and may cause fetal harm when administered to a pregnant woman. There are limited human data on the effects of Pergonal® when administered during pregnancy.

Men:
Pergonal® is contraindicated in men who have:
1. Normal gonadotropin levels indicating normal pituitary function.
2. Elevated gonadotropin levels indicating primary testicular failure.
3. Infertility disorders other than hypogonadotropic hypogonadism.

WARNINGS
Pergonal® is a drug that should only be used by physicians who are thoroughly familiar with infertility problems. It is a potent gonadotropic substance capable of causing mild to severe adverse reactions in women. Gonadotropin therapy requires a certain time commitment by physicians and supportive health professionals, and its use requires the availability of appropriate monitoring facilities (see "Precautions—Laboratory Tests"). In female patients it must be used with a great deal of care.

Overstimulation of the Ovary During Pergonal® Therapy:
Ovarian Enlargement: Mild to moderate uncomplicated ovarian enlargement which may be accompanied by abdominal distension and/or abdominal pain occurs in approximately 20% of those treated with Pergonal® and hCG, and generally regresses without treatment within two or three weeks.

In order to minimize the hazard associated with the occasional abnormal ovarian enlargement which may occur with Pergonal®-hCG therapy, the lowest dose consistent with expectation of good results should be used. Careful monitoring of ovarian response can further minimize the risk of overstimulation.

If the ovaries are abnormally enlarged on the last day of Pergonal® therapy, hCG should not be administered in this course of therapy; this will reduce the chances of development of the Ovarian Hyperstimulation Syndrome.

The Ovarian Hyperstimulation Syndrome (OHSS): OHSS is a medical event distinct from uncomplicated ovarian enlargement. OHSS may progress rapidly to become a serious medical event. It is characterized by an apparent dramatic increase in vascular permeability which can result in a rapid accumulation of fluid in the peritoneal cavity, thorax, and potentially, the pericardium. The early warning signs of development of OHSS are severe pelvic pain, nausea, vomiting, and weight gain. The following symptomatology has been seen with cases of OHSS: abdominal pain, abdominal distension, gastrointestinal symptoms including nausea, vomiting and diarrhea, severe ovarian enlargement, weight gain, dyspnea, and oliguria. Clinical evaluation may reveal hypovolemia, hemoconcentration, electrolyte imbalances, ascites, hemoperitoneum, pleural effusions, hydrothorax, acute pulmonary distress, and thromboembolic events (see "Pulmonary and Vascular Complications" below). Transient liver function test abnormalities suggestive of hepatic dysfunction, which may be accompanied by morphologic changes on liver biopsy, have been reported in association with the Ovarian Hyperstimulation Syndrome (OHSS).

OHSS occurs in approximately 0.4% of patients when the recommended dose is administered and in 1.3% of patients when higher than recommended doses are administered. Cases of OHSS are more common, more severe and more protracted if pregnancy occurs. OHSS develops rapidly; therefore patients should be followed for at least two weeks after hCG administration. Most often, OHSS occurs after treatment has been discontinued and reaches its maximum at about seven to ten days following treatment. Usually, OHSS resolves spontaneously with the onset of menses. If there is evidence that OHSS may be developing prior to hCG administration (see "Precautions—Laboratory Tests"), the hCG should be withheld.

If OHSS occurs, treatment should be stopped and the patient hospitalized. Treatment is primarily symptomatic, consisting of bed rest, fluid and electrolyte management, and analgesics if needed. The phenomenon of hemoconcentration associated with fluid loss into the peritoneal cavity, pleural cavity, and the pericardial cavity has been seen to occur and should be thoroughly assessed in the following manner: 1) fluid intake and output, 2) weight, 3) hematocrit, 4) serum and urinary electrolytes, 5) urine specific gravity, 6) BUN and creatinine, and 7) abdominal girth. These determinations are to be performed daily or more often if the need arises.

With OHSS there is an increased risk of injury to the ovary. The ascitic, pleural, and pericardial fluid should not be removed unless absolutely necessary to relieve symptoms such as pulmonary distress or cardiac tamponade. Pelvic examination may cause rupture of an ovarian cyst, which may result in hemoperitoneum, and should therefore be avoided. If this does occur, and if bleeding becomes such that surgery is required, the surgical treatment should be designed to control bleeding and to retain as much ovarian tissue as possible. Intercourse should be prohibited in those patients in whom significant ovarian enlargement occurs after ovulation because of the danger of hemoperitoneum resulting from ruptured ovarian cysts.

The management of OHSS may be divided into three phases: the acute, the chronic, and the resolution phases. Because the use of diuretics can accentuate the diminished intravascular volume, diuretics should be avoided except in the late phase of resolution as described below.

Acute Phase: Management during the acute phase should be designed to prevent hemoconcentration due to loss of intravascular volume to the third space and to minimize the risk of thromboembolic phenomena and kidney damage. Treatment is designed to normalize electrolytes while maintaining an acceptable but somewhat reduced intravascular volume. Full correction of the intravascular volume deficit may lead to an unacceptable increase in the amount of third space fluid accumulation. Management includes administration of limited intravenous fluids, electrolytes, and human serum albumin. Monitoring for the development of hyperkalemia is recommended.

Chronic Phase: After stabilizing the patient during the acute phase, excessive fluid accumulation in the third space should be limited by instituting severe potassium, sodium, and fluid restriction.

Resolution Phase: A fall in hematocrit and an increasing urinary output without an increased intake are observed due to the return of third space fluid to the intravascular compartment. Peripheral and/or pulmonary edema may result if the kidneys are unable to excrete third space fluid as rapidly as it is mobilized. Diuretics may be indicated during the resolution phase if necessary to combat pulmonary edema.

Pulmonary and Vascular Complications: Serious pulmonary conditions (e.g., atelectasis, acute respiratory distress syndrome) have been reported. In addition, thromboembolic events both in association with, and separate from, the Ovarian Hyperstimulation Syndrome have been reported following Pergonal® therapy. Intravascular thrombosis and embolism, which may originate in venous or arterial vessels, can result in reduced blood flow to critical organs or the extremities. Sequelae of such events have included venous thrombophlebitis, pulmonary embolism, pulmonary infarction, cerebral vascular occlusion (stroke), and arterial occlusion resulting in loss of limb. In rare cases, pulmonary complications and/or thromboembolic events have resulted in death.

Multiple Births: Data from a clinical trial revealed the following results regarding multiple births: Of the pregnancies following therapy with Pergonal® and hCG, 80% resulted in single births, 15% in twins, and 5% of the total pregnancies resulted in three or more concepti. The patient and her husband should be advised of the frequency and potential hazards of multiple gestation before starting treatment.

Hypersensitivity/Anaphylactic Reactions: Hypersensitivity/ anaphylactic reactions associated with Pergonal® administration have been reported in some patients. These reactions presented as generalized urticaria, facial edema, angioneurotic edema, and/or dyspnea suggestive of laryngeal edema. The relationship of these symptoms to uncharacterized urinary proteins is uncertain.

PRECAUTIONS
General: Careful attention should be given to diagnosis in the selection of candidates for Pergonal® therapy (see "Indications and Usage—Selection of Patients").
Information for Patients: Prior to therapy with Pergonal®, patients should be informed of the duration of treatment and the monitoring of their condition that will be required. Possible adverse reactions (see "Adverse Reactions" section) and the risk of multiple births should also be discussed.
Laboratory Tests:
Women:
Treatment for Induction of Ovulation
In most instances, treatment with Pergonal® results only in follicular growth and maturation. In order to effect ovulation, hCG must be given following the administration of Pergonal® when clinical assessment of the patient indicates that sufficient follicular maturation has occurred. This may be directly estimated by measuring serum (or urinary) estrogen levels and sonographic visualization of the ovaries. The combination of both estradiol levels and ultrasonography are useful for monitoring the growth and development of follicles, timing hCG administration, as well as minimizing the risk of the Ovarian Hyperstimulation Syndrome and multiple gestation.

Other clinical parameters which may have potential use for monitoring menotropins therapy include:
a) Changes in the vaginal cytology;
b) Appearance and volume of the cervical mucus;
c) Spinnbarkeit; and
d) Ferning of the cervical mucus.

The above clinical indices provide an indirect estimate of the estrogenic effect upon the target organs, and therefore should only be used adjunctively with more direct estimates of follicular development, i.e., serum estradiol and ultrasonography.

The clinical confirmation of ovulation, with the exception of pregnancy, is obtained by direct and indirect indices of progesterone production. The indices most generally used are as follows:
a) A rise in basal body temperature;
b) Increase in serum progesterone; and
c) Menstruation following the shift in basal body temperature.

When used in conjunction with indices of progesterone production, sonographic visualization of the ovaries will assist in determining if ovulation has occurred. Sonographic evidence of ovulation may include the following:
a) Fluid in the cul-de-sac;
b) Ovarian stigmata; and
c) Collapsed follicle.

Because of the subjectivity of the various tests for the determination of follicular maturation and ovulation, it cannot be overemphasized that the physician should choose tests with which he/she is thoroughly familiar.

Drug Interactions: No clinically significant drug/drug or drug/food adverse interactions have been reported during Pergonal® therapy.

Carcinogenesis and Mutagenesis: Long-term toxicity studies in animals have not been performed to evaluate the carcinogenic potential of Pergonal®.

Pregnancy: Pregnancy Category X. See "Contraindications" section.

Nursing Mothers: It is not known whether this drug is excreted in human milk. Because many drugs are excreted in human milk, caution should be exercised if Pergonal® is administered to a nursing woman.

ADVERSE REACTIONS
Women:
The following adverse reactions, reported during Pergonal® therapy, are listed in decreasing order of potential severity:
1. Pulmonary and vascular complications (see "Warnings")
2. Ovarian Hyperstimulation Syndrome (see "Warnings")
3. Hemoperitoneum
4. Adnexal torsion (as a complication of ovarian enlargement)
5. Mild to moderate ovarian enlargement
6. Ovarian cysts
7. Abdominal pain
8. Sensitivity to Pergonal® (Febrile reactions suggestive of allergic response have been reported following the administration of Pergonal®. Reports of flu-like symptoms including fever, chills, musculoskeletal aches, joint pains, nausea, headaches and malaise have also been reported).
9. Gastrointestinal symptoms (nausea, vomiting, diarrhea, abdominal cramps, bloating)
10. Pain, rash, swelling and/or irritation at the site of injection
11. Body rashes
12. Dizziness, tachycardia, dyspnea, tachypnea

The following medical events have been reported subsequent to pregnancies resulting from Pergonal® therapy:
1. Ectopic pregnancy
2. Congenital abnormalities
From a study of 287 completed pregnancies following Pergonal®-hCG therapy five incidents of birth defects were reported (1.7%). One infant had multiple congenital anomalies consisting of imperforate anus, aplasia of the sigmoid colon, third degree hypospadias, cecovesicle fistula, bifid scrotum, meningocele, bilateral internal tibial torsion, and right metatarsus adductus. Another infant was born with an imperforate anus and possible congenital heart lesions; another had a supernumerary digit; another was born with hypospadias and exstrophy of the bladder; and the fifth child had Down's syndrome. None of the investigators felt that these defects were drug-related. Subsequently one report of an infant death due to hydrocephalus and cardiac anomalies has been received.

There have been infrequent reports of ovarian neoplasms, both benign and malignant, in women who have undergone multiple drug regimens for ovulation induction; however, a causal relationship has not been established.

	% Pts. Ovul.	% Pts. Preg.	% Abort.	% Multi Preg.	% Twins	% 3 or More Concepti	% Hyperstim. Syndr.
Primary Amenorrhea	62	22	14	25	25	0	0
Secondary Amenorrhea	61	28	24	28	18	10	1.9
Secondary Amen. with Galactorrhea	77	42	21	41	31	10	1.2
Polycystic Ovaries	76	26	39	17	17	0	1.1
Anovulatory Cycles	77	24	15	14	9	5	2.0
Miscellaneous	83	20	36	2	2	0	0.1

Men:

1. Gynecomastia may occur occasionally during Pergonal®-hCG therapy. This is a known effect of hCG treatment.
2. Erythrocytosis (hct 50%, hgb 17.8 g%) was recorded in one patient.

DRUG ABUSE AND DEPENDENCE

There have been no reports of abuse or dependence with Pergonal®.

OVERDOSAGE

Aside from possible ovarian hyperstimulation (see "Warnings"), little is known concerning the consequences of acute overdosage with Pergonal®.

DOSAGE AND ADMINISTRATION

Women:

1. Dosage:

The dose of Pergonal® to produce maturation of the follicle must be individualized for each patient. It is recommended that the initial dose to any patient should be 75 IU of FSH/LH per day, **ADMINISTERED INTRAMUSCULARLY**, for seven to twelve days followed by hCG, 5,000 U to 10,000 U, one day after the last dose of Pergonal®. Administration of Pergonal® should not exceed 12 days in a single course of therapy. The patient should be treated until indices of estrogenic activity, as indicated under "Precautions" above, are equivalent to or greater than those of the normal individual. If serum or urinary estradiol determinations or ultrasonographic visualizations are available, they may be useful as a guide to therapy. If the ovaries are abnormally enlarged on the last day of Pergonal® therapy, hCG should not be administered in this course of therapy; this will reduce the chances of development of the Ovarian Hyperstimulation Syndrome. If there is evidence of ovulation but no pregnancy, repeat this dosage regime for at least two more courses before increasing the dose of Pergonal® to 150 IU of FSH/LH per day for seven to twelve days. As before, this dose should be followed by 5,000 U to 10,000 U of hCG one day after the last dose of Pergonal®. A Pergonal® dose of 150 IU of FSH/ LH per day has proven to be the most effective dose especially for in vitro fertilization. If evidence of ovulation is present, but pregnancy does not ensue, repeat the same dose for two more courses. Doses larger than this are not routinely recommended.

During treatment with both Pergonal® and hCG and during a two-week post-treatment period, patients should be examined at least every other day for signs of excessive ovarian stimulation. It is recommended that Pergonal® administration be stopped if the ovaries become abnormally enlarged or abdominal pain occurs. Most of the Ovarian Hyperstimulation Syndrome occurs after treatment has been discontinued and reaches its maximum at about seven to ten days post-ovulation. Patients should be followed for at least two weeks after hCG administration.

The couple should be encouraged to have intercourse daily, beginning on the day prior to the administration of hCG until ovulation becomes apparent from the indices employed for the determination of progestational activity. Care should be taken to insure insemination. In the light of the foregoing indices and parameters mentioned, it should become obvious that, unless a physician is willing to devote considerable time to these patients and be familiar with and conduct the necessary laboratory studies, he/she should not use Pergonal®.

2. Administration:

Dissolve the contents of one ampule of Pergonal® in one to two ml of sterile saline and **ADMINISTER INTRAMUSCULARLY** immediately. Any unused reconstituted material should be discarded. Parenteral drug products should be inspected visually for particulate matter and discoloration prior to administration, whenever solution and container permit.

Men:

1. Dosage:

Prior to concomitant therapy with Pergonal® and hCG, pretreatment with hCG alone (5,000 U three times a week) is required. Treatment should continue for a period sufficient to achieve serum testosterone levels within the normal range and masculinization as judged by the appearance of secondary sex characteristics. Such pretreatment may require four to six months, then the recommended dose of Pergonal® is 75 IU FSH/LH **ADMINISTERED INTRAMUSCULARLY**, three times a week and the recommended dose of hCG is 2,000 U twice a week. Therapy should be carried on for a minimum of four more months to insure detecting spermatozoa in the ejaculate, as it takes 74± 4 days in the human male for germ cells to reach the spermatozoa stage.

If the patient has not responded with evidence of increased spermatogenesis at the end of four months of therapy, treatment may continue with 75 IU FSH/LH three times a week, or the dose can be increased to 150 IU FSH/LH three times a week, with the hCG dose unchanged.

2. Administration:

Dissolve the contents of one ampule of Pergonal® in one to two ml of sterile saline and **ADMINISTER INTRAMUSCULARLY** immediately. Any unused reconstituted material should be discarded. Parenteral drug products should be inspected visually for particulate matter and discoloration prior to administration, whenever solution and container permit.

HOW SUPPLIED

Pergonal® is supplied in a sterile lyophilized form as a white to off-white powder or pellet in ampules containing 75 IU or 150 IU FSH/LH activity. The following package combinations are available:

— 1 ampule 75 IU Pergonal® and 1 ampule 2 ml Sodium Chloride Injection (USP), NDC 44087-0571-7.
— 10 ampules 75 IU Pergonal® and 10 ampules 2 ml Sodium Chloride Injection (USP), NDC 44087-5075-3.
— 1 ampule 150 IU Pergonal® and 1 ampule 2 ml Sodium Chloride Injection (USP), NDC 44087-5150-1.

By biological assay, one IU of LH for the Second International Reference Preparation (2nd-IRP) for hMG is biologically equivalent to approximately $\frac{1}{2}$ U of hCG.

Lyophilized powder may be stored refrigerated or at room temperature (3°–25°C/37°–77°F). Protect from light. Use immediately after reconstitution. Discard unused material.

CLINICAL STUDIES

Women:

The results of the clinical experience and effectiveness of the administration of Pergonal® to 1,286 patients in 3,002 courses of therapy are summarized below. The values include patients who were treated with other than the recommended dosage regime. The values for the presently recommended dosage regime are essentially the same.

	%
Patients ovulating	75
Patients pregnant	25
Patients aborting	25*
Multiple pregnancies	20†
Twins	15†
Three or more concepti	5†
Fetal abnormalities	1.7†
Hyperstimulation syndrome	1.3

* Based on total pregnancies
† Based on total deliveries

Results by diagnosis group are summarized below (these values include patients who were treated with other than the present recommended dosage regime):

[See table at top of page]

Men:

Clinical results of the treatment of men with primary or secondary hypogonadotropic hypogonadism are as follows:

In the Serono Cooperative study, with an adequate treatment period of 3 to 8 months, 60 of 70 men with primary hypogonadotropic hypogonadism and 8 of 11 men with secondary hypogonadotropic hypogonadism responded with mean increases in their sperm counts from less than 5 to 24 million spermatozoa per milliliter of ejaculate. Forty-one wives of 54 men with primary hypogonadotropic hypogonadism desiring offspring and 7 wives of men with secondary hypogonadotropic hypogonadism conceived. Patients treated with Pergonal® and hCG for less than 3 months or with Pergonal® alone did not respond to therapy.

A world-wide data search revealed that of 160 recorded pregnancies as the result of use of Pergonal®-hCG in men, there were 7 spontaneous abortions, one ectopic pregnancy and 3 congenital anomalies at birth (esophageal atresia in a female infant which was later corrected by surgery, unilateral cryptorchidism, inguinal hernia).

Caution: Federal law prohibits dispensing without prescription.

Manufactured for:
SERONO LABORATORIES, INC.
Randolph, MA 02368 USA
by: Laboratoires Serono, SA
Aubonne, Switzerland
© SERONO LABORATORIES, INC. 1969, 1994
Revised: November 1994

PROFASI® ℞

[*pro 'fah-se*]
(chorionic gonadotropin for injection, USP)

FOR INTRAMUSCULAR INJECTION

DESCRIPTION

Human chorionic gonadotropin (HCG), a polypeptide hormone produced by the human placenta, is composed of an alpha and a beta sub-unit. The alpha sub-unit is essentially identical to the alpha sub-units of the human pituitary gonadotropins, luteinizing hormone (LH) and follicle-stimulating hormone (FSH), as well as to the alpha sub-unit of human thyroid-stimulating hormone (TSH). The beta sub-units of these hormones differ in amino acid sequence.

Chorionic Gonadotropin is a water soluble glycoprotein derived from human pregnancy urine. The sterile lyophilized powder is stable. When reconstituted, the solution should be refrigerated and used within 30 days.

Each vial, when reconstituted with provided diluent, will contain:

Chorionic Gonadotropin **2,000, 5,000 or 10,000** USP Units, Mannitol 100 mg, Dibasic Sodium Phosphate 16 mg, Monobasic Sodium Phosphate 4 mg, with Benzyl Alcohol 0.9% as preservative, in Water for Injection.

CLINICAL PHARMACOLOGY

The action of HCG is virtually identical to that of pituitary LH, although HCG appears to have a small degree of FSH activity as well. It stimulates production of gonadal steroid hormones by stimulating the interstitial cells (Leydig cells) of the testis to produce androgens and the corpus luteum of the ovary to produce progesterone. Androgen stimulation in the male leads to the development of secondary sex characteristics and may stimulate testicular descent when no anatomical impediment to descent is present. This descent is usually reversible when HCG is discontinued. During the normal menstrual cycle, LH participates with FSH in the development and maturation of the normal ovarian follicle, and the mid-cycle LH surge triggers ovulation. HCG can substitute for LH in this function.

During a normal pregnancy, HCG secreted by the placenta maintains the corpus luteum after LH secretion decreases, supporting continued secretion of estrogen and progesterone, and preventing menstruation. HCG HAS NO KNOWN EFFECT ON FAT MOBILIZATION, APPETITE OR SENSE OF HUNGER, OR BODY FAT DISTRIBUTION.

INDICATIONS AND USAGE

HCG HAS NOT BEEN DEMONSTRATED TO BE EFFECTIVE ADJUNCTIVE THERAPY IN THE TREATMENT OF OBESITY. THERE IS NO SUBSTANTIAL EVIDENCE THAT IT INCREASES WEIGHT LOSS BEYOND THAT RESULTING FROM CALORIC RESTRICTION, THAT IT CAUSES A MORE ATTRACTIVE OR "NORMAL" DISTRIBUTION OF FAT, OR THAT IT DECREASES THE HUNGER AND DISCOMFORT ASSOCIATED WITH CALORIE-RESTRICTED DIETS.

1. Prepubertal cryptorchidism not due to anatomic obstruction. In general, HCG is thought to induce testicular descent in situations when descent would have occurred at puberty. HCG thus may help to predict whether or not orchiopexy will be needed in the future. Although, in some cases, descent following HCG administration is permanent, in most cases the response is temporary. Therapy is usually instituted between the ages of 4 and 9.
2. Selected cases of hypogonadotropic hypogonadism (hypogonadism secondary to a pituitary deficiency) in males.
3. Induction of ovulation and pregnancy in the anovulatory, infertile woman in whom the cause of anovulation is secondary and not due to primary ovarian failure, and who has been appropriately pretreated with human menotropins.

Continued on next page

Profasi—Cont.

CONTRAINDICATIONS

Precocious puberty, prostatic carcinoma or other androgen-dependent neoplasm, prior allergic reaction to HCG. HCG may cause fetal harm when administered to a pregnant woman. Combined HCG/PMS (pregnant mare's serum) therapy has been noted to induce high incidences of external congenital anomalies in the offspring of mice, in a dose-dependent manner. The potential extrapolation to humans has not been determined.

WARNINGS

HCG should be used in conjunction with human menopausal gonadotropins only by physicians experienced with infertility problems who are familiar with the criteria for patient selection, contraindications, warnings, precautions, and adverse reactions described in the package insert for menotropins. The principal serious adverse reactions during this use are: (1) Ovarian hyperstimulation, a syndrome of sudden ovarian enlargement, ascites with or without pain, and/or pleural effusion; (2) Enlargement of preexisting ovarian cysts or rupture of ovarian cysts with resultant hemoperitoneum; (3) Multiple births, and (4) Arterial thromboembolism.

The diluent used for reconstitution contains benzyl alcohol. Benzyl alcohol has been reported to be associated with a fatal "Gasping Syndrome" in premature infants.

PRECAUTIONS

General: 1. Induction of androgen secretion by HCG may induce precocious puberty in patients treated for cryptorchidism. Therapy should be discontinued if signs of precocious puberty occur.

2. Since androgens may cause fluid retention, HCG should be used with caution in patients with cardiac or renal disease, epilepsy, migraine, or asthma.

Drug/Laboratory test: HCG can crossreact in the radioimmunoassay of gonadotropins, especially luteinizing hormone. Each individual laboratory should establish the degree of crossreactivity with their gonadotropin assay. Physicians should make the laboratory aware of patients on HCG if gonadotropin levels are requested.

Carcinogenesis, Mutagenesis, Impairment of Fertility: There have been sporadic reports of testicular tumors in otherwise healthy young men receiving HCG for secondary infertility. A causative relationship between HCG and tumor development in these men has not been established. Defects of forelimbs and of the central nervous system, as well as alterations in sex ratio, have been reported in mice on combined gonadotropin and HCG regimens. The dose of gonadotropin used was intended to induce superovulation. No mutagenic effect has been clearly established in humans. Fertility—see "Indications and Usage."

Pregnancy: Teratogenic effects--*Category X:* See "Contraindications" section. Combined HCG/PMS (pregnant mare's serum) therapy has been noted to induce high incidences of external congenital anomalies in the offspring of mice, in a dose-dependent manner. The potential extrapolation to humans has not been determined.

Nursing Mothers: It is not known whether this drug is excreted in human milk. Because many drugs are excreted in human milk, caution should be exercised when HCG is administered to a nursing woman.

Pediatric Use: Safety and effectiveness in children below the age of 4 have not been established.

ADVERSE REACTIONS (See WARNINGS)

Headache, irritability, restlessness, depression, fatigue, edema, precocious puberty, gynecomastia, pain at the site of injection. Hypersensitivity reactions both localized and systemic in nature, including erythema, urticaria, rash, angioedema, dyspnea and shortness of breath, have been reported. The relationship of these allergic-like events to the polypeptide hormone or the diluent containing benzyl alcohol is not clear.

DOSAGE AND ADMINISTRATION (Intramuscular Use Only):

The dosage regimen employed in any particular case will depend upon the indication for use, the age and weight of the patient, and the physician's preference. The following regimens have been advocated by various authorities. Prepubertal cryptorchidism not due to anatomical obstruction:

(1) 4,000 USP Units three times weekly for three weeks.
(2) 5,000 USP Units every second day for four injections.
(3) 15 Injections of 500 to 1,000 USP Units over a period of six weeks.
(4) 500 USP Units three times weekly for four to six weeks. If this course of treatment is not successful, another is begun one month later, giving 1,000 USP Units per injection.

Selected cases of hypogonadotropic hypogonadism in males:
(1) 500 to 1,000 USP Units three times a week for three weeks, followed by the same dose twice a week for three weeks.
(2) 4,000 USP Units three times weekly for six to nine months, following which the dosage may be reduced to 2,000 USP Units three times weekly for an additional three months.

Induction of ovulation and pregnancy in the anovulatory, infertile woman in whom the cause of anovulation is secondary and not due to primary ovarian failure and who has been appropriately pre-treated with human menotropins (See prescribing information for menotropins for dosage and administration for that drug product).

5,000 to 10,000 USP Units one day following the last dose of menotropins. (A dosage of 10,000 USP Units is recommended in the labeling for menotropins.)

Parenteral drug products should be inspected visually for particulate matter and discoloration prior to administration, whenever solution and container permit.

HOW SUPPLIED

Chorionic gonadotropin for injection, USP, is available in 10 mL lyophilized multiple dose vial sets containing either:
5,000 USP Units per Vial-NDC 44087-8005-3
10,000 USP Units per Vial-NDC 44087-8010-3 with 10 mL vial bacteriostatic water for injection, USP (containing benzyl alcohol 0.9% v/v).

Storage: Store dry product at controlled room temperature 15°–30° C (59°–86° F). AFTER RECONSTITUTION, REFRIGERATE THE PRODUCT AT 2°–8° C (36°–46° F) AND USE WITHIN 30 DAYS.

Caution: Federal law prohibits dispensing without prescription.

Manufactured for: SERONO LABORATORIES, INC.
                        Randolph, MA 02368 USA
Manufactured by: Steris Laboratories, Inc.
                        Phoenix, AZ 85043 USA
                        ST-12-90

®Serono Laboratories, Inc. 1984, 1992
Revised June 1993
1-1919-0692
6957012544087F1

SAIZEN®   ℞
[sī- zen]
[somatropin (rDNA origin) for injection]
FOR SUBCUTANEOUS OR INTRAMUSCULAR INJECTION

DESCRIPTION

Saizen® [somatropin (rDNA origin) for injection] is a human growth hormone produced by recombinant DNA technology. Saizen® has 191 amino acid residues and a molecular weight of 22,125 daltons. Its amino acid sequence and structure are identical to the dominant form of human pituitary growth hormone. Saizen® is produced by a mammalian cell line (mouse C127) that has been modified by the addition of the human growth hormone gene. Saizen®, with the correct three-dimensional configuration, is secreted directly through the cell membrane into the cell-culture medium for collection and purification.

Saizen® is a highly purified preparation. Biological potency is determined by measuring the increase in body weight induced in hypophysectomized rats.

Saizen® is a sterile, non-pyrogenic, white, lyophilized powder intended for subcutaneous or intramuscular injection after reconstitution with Bacteriostatic Water for Injection, USP (0.9% Benzyl Alcohol). The reconstituted solution has a pH of 6.5 to 8.5.

Saizen® is available in vials. The quantitative composition per vial is:

5 mg (approximately 15 IU) vial:
Each vial contains 5.0 mg somatropin (approximately 15 IU), 34.2 mg sucrose and 1.165 mg O-phosphoric acid. The pH is adjusted with sodium hydroxide or O-phosphoric acid. The diluent is Bacteriostatic Water for Injection, USP containing 0.9% Benzyl Alcohol added as an antimicrobial preservative.

CLINICAL PHARMACOLOGY

General

In vitro, preclinical, and clinical testing have demonstrated that Saizen® [somatropin (rDNA origin) for injection] is therapeutically equivalent to pituitary-derived human growth hormone. Clinical studies in normal adults also demonstrated equivalent pharmacokinetics.

Actions that have been demonstrated for Saizen®, somatrem, and/or pituitary-derived human growth hormone include:

A. Tissue Growth-
  1. Skeletal Growth: Saizen® stimulates skeletal growth in prepubertal children with pituitary growth hormone deficiency. Skeletal growth is accomplished at the epiphyseal plates at the ends of long bone.

Growth and metabolism of epiphyseal plate cells are directly stimulated by growth hormone and one of its mediators, insulin-like growth factor-I. Serum levels of insulin-like growth factor-I (IGF-I) are low in children and adolescents who are growth hormone deficient, but increase during treatment with Saizen®. Linear growth continues until the growth plates fuse at the end of puberty.

  2. Cell Growth: Treatment with pituitary-derived human growth hormone results in an increase in both the number and the size of skeletal muscle cells.

  3. Organ Growth: Growth hormone of human pituitary origin influences the size and function of internal organs and increases red cell mass. Saizen® has been shown to promote similar organ weight increase to pituitary human growth hormone in an adequate animal model.

B. Protein Metabolism-Linear growth is facilitated in part by growth hormone-stimulated protein synthesis. This is reflected by increased cellular uptake of amino acids and nitrogen retention as demonstrated by a decline in urinary nitrogen excretion and blood urea nitrogen during growth hormone therapy.

C. Carbohydrate Metabolism-Growth hormone is a modulator of carbohydrate metabolism. Children with inadequate secretion of growth hormone sometimes experience fasting hypoglycemia that is improved by treatment with growth hormone. Saizen® therapy may decrease glucose tolerance. Administration of Saizen® to normal adults and patients with growth hormone deficiency resulted in transient increases in mean serum fasting and postprandial insulin levels. However, glucose levels remained in the normal range.

D. Lipid Metabolism-Acute administration of human growth hormone to humans results in lipid mobilization. Nonesterified fatty acids increase in plasma within one hour of Saizen® administration. In growth hormone deficient patients, long-term growth hormone administration often decreases body fat. Mean cholesterol levels decreased in patients treated with Saizen®. The clinical significance of this is unknown.

E. Mineral Metabolism-Growth hormone administration results in the retention of total body potassium, phosphorus, and sodium. Serum calcium levels appear to be unaffected.

F. Connective Tissue/Bone Metabolism-Growth hormone stimulates the synthesis of chondroitin sulfate and collagen as well as the urinary excretion of hydroxyproline.

PHARMACOKINETICS

Absorption—The absolute bioavailability of recombinant growth hormone (r-hGH) after subcutaneous administration ranges between 70–90%.

Distribution—The mean volume of distribution of r-hGH given to healthy volunteers was estimated to be 12.0 ± 1.08 L.

Metabolism—The metabolic fate of somatropin involves classical protein catabolism in both the liver and kidneys. In renal cells, at least a portion of the breakdown products is returned to the systemic circulation. The mean half-life of intravenous somatropin in normal males is 0.6 hours, whereas subcutaneously and intramuscularly administered somatropin has a half-life of 1.75 and 3.4 hours, respectively. The longer half-life observed after subcutaneous or intramuscular administration is due to slow absorption from the injection site.

Excretion—The mean clearance of intravenously administered r-hGH in six normal male volunteers was 14.6 ± 2.8 L/hr.

SPECIAL POPULATIONS

Pediatric—The pharmacokinetics of r-hGH is similar in children and adults.

Gender—No gender studies have been performed in children. In adults, the clearance of r-hGH in both men and women tends to be similar.

Race—No data are available.

Renal Insufficiency—Children and adults with chronic renal failure tend to have decreased clearance of r-hGH as compared to normals.

Hepatic Insufficiency—A reduction in r-hGH clearance has been noted in patients with hepatic dysfunction as compared with normal controls.

INDICATIONS AND USAGE

Saizen® [somatropin (rDNA origin) for injection] is indicated for the long-term treatment of children with growth failure due to inadequate secretion of endogenous growth hormone.

CONTRAINDICATIONS

In general, Saizen® [somatropin (rDNA origin) for injection] is contraindicated in the presence of active neoplasia. Any pre-existing neoplasia should be inactive and its treatment complete prior to instituting therapy with Saizen®. Saizen® should be discontinued if there is evidence of recurrent activity. Since, in rare instances, growth hormone deficiency may be an early sign of the presence of a brain tumor, the presence of such a tumor should be ruled out prior to initi-

ation of treatment. Available information suggests that the rate of tumor recurrence is not increased by growth hormone therapy. Saizen® should not be used for growth promotion in pediatric patients with closed epiphyses.
Saizen® reconstituted with Bacteriostatic Water for Injection, USP (0.9% Benzyl Alcohol) should not be administered to patients with a known sensitivity to Benzyl Alcohol. (See "WARNINGS").

WARNINGS

Benzyl Alcohol as a preservative in Bacteriostatic Water for Injection, USP has been associated with toxicity in newborns. If sensitivity to the diluent occurs, Saizen® [somatropin (rDNA origin) for injection] may be reconstituted with Sterile Water for Injection, USP. When Saizen is reconstituted in this manner, the reconstituted solution should be used immediately and any unused solution should be discarded.

PRECAUTIONS

General: Saizen® [somatropin (rDNA origin) for injection] therapy should be carried out under the regular guidance of a physician who is experienced in the diagnosis and management of growth disorders.
Because human growth hormone may induce a state of insulin resistance, patients should be observed for evidence of glucose intolerance. Human growth hormone should be used with caution in patients with diabetes mellitus or a family history of diabetes mellitus.
Hypothyroidism may develop during Saizen® therapy. Untreated hypothyroidism will jeopardize the response to growth hormone. Therefore, thyroid hormone determinations should be performed periodically during Saizen® administration and thyroid hormone replacement should be initiated when indicated.
Bone age should be monitored periodically during Saizen® administration especially in patients who are pubertal and/or receiving concomitant thyroid replacement therapy. Under these circumstances, epiphyseal maturation may progress rapidly.
Patients with endocrine disorders, including growth hormone deficiency, may have an increased incidence of slipped capital femoral epiphysis. Any child who develops a limp or complains of hip or knee pain during growth hormone therapy should be evaluated.
Intracranial hypertension (IH) with papilledema, visual changes, headache, nausea and/or vomiting has been reported in a small number of patients treated with growth hormone products and it also has been associated more commonly with IGF-I. Symptoms usually occurred within the first eight weeks of the initiation of growth hormone therapy. In all reported cases, IH-associated signs and symptoms resolved after temporary suspension or termination of therapy. Funduscopic examination of patients is recommended at the initiation and periodically during the course of growth hormone therapy.
When growth hormone is administered subcutaneously at the same site over a long period of time, lipodystrophy may result. This can be avoided by rotating the injection site.
As for any protein, local or systemic allergic reactions may occur. Parents/Patient should be informed that such reactions are possible and that prompt medical attention should be sought if allergic reactions occur.
Laboratory Tests: Serum levels of inorganic phosphorus, alkaline phosphatase, and IGF-I may increase with Saizen® therapy.
Drug Interaction: Concomitant glucocorticoid therapy may inhibit the growth promoting effect of Saizen®. There was no evidence in the controlled studies of Saizen® interaction with drugs commonly used in the treatment of routine pediatric problems/illnesses. However, formal drug interaction studies have not been conducted.
Carcinogenesis, Mutagenesis, Impairment of Fertility: Long-term animal studies for carcinogenicity have not been performed with Saizen®. There is no evidence from animal studies to date of Saizen®-induced mutagenicity or impairment of fertility.
Pregnancy: Teratogenic Effects: Pregnancy Category B. Reproduction studies have been performed in rats and rabbits at doses up to 31 and 62 times, respectively, the human (child) weekly dose based on body surface area. The results have revealed no evidence of impaired fertility or harm to the fetus due to Saizen®. There are, however, no adequate and well controlled studies in pregnant women. Because animal reproduction studies are not always predictive of human response, this drug should be used during pregnancy only if clearly needed.
Nursing Women: It is not known whether Saizen® is excreted in human milk. Because many drugs are excreted in human milk, caution should be exercised when Saizen® is administered to a nursing woman.
Information For Patients: Patients being treated with growth hormone and/or their parents should be informed of the potential benefits and risks associated with treatment. If home use is determined to be desirable by the physician, instructions on appropriate use should be given, including a review of the contents of the Patient Information Insert. This information is intended to aid in the safe and effective administration of the medication. It is not a disclosure of all possible adverse or intended effects.
If home use is prescribed, a puncture resistant container for the disposal of used syringes and needles should be recommended to the patient. Patients and/or parents should be thoroughly instructed in the importance of proper disposal and cautioned against any reuse of needles and syringes (see Patient Information Insert).

ADVERSE REACTIONS

As with all protein pharmaceuticals, a small percentage of patients may develop antibodies to the protein. Anti-growth hormone (GH) antibody capacities below 2 mg/L have not been associated with growth attenuation. In some cases when binding capacity exceeds 2 mg/L, growth attenuation has been described. In clinical studies with Saizen® involving 280 patients (204 naive and 76 transfer patients), one patient at 6 months of therapy developed anti-GH antibodies with binding capacities exceeding 2 mg/L. Despite the high binding capacity, these antibodies were not growth attenuating. The patient was subsequently shown to have a hGH-N gene defect. Thus, genetic analysis should be undertaken in any patient in whom anti-GH antibodies with high binding capacities occur. No antibodies against proteins of the host cells were detected in the sera of patients treated up to five years.
Any patient with well-documented growth hormone deficiency who fails to respond to therapy should be tested for antibodies to human growth hormone and for thyroid status.
In clinical studies in which Saizen® was administered to growth hormone deficient children, the following events were infrequently seen: local reactions at the injection site (such as pain, numbness, redness and swelling), hypothyroidism, hypoglycemia, seizures, exacerbation of pre-existing psoriasis and disturbances in fluid balance.
Leukemia has been reported in a small number of growth hormone deficient patients treated with growth hormone. It is uncertain whether this increased risk is related to the pathology of growth hormone deficiency itself, growth hormone therapy, or other associated treatments such as radiation therapy for intracranial tumors. So far, epidemiological data fail to confirm the hypothesis of a relationship between growth hormone therapy and leukemia.

OVERDOSAGE

Long-term overdosage could result in signs and symptoms of gigantism and/or acromegaly consistent with the known effects of excess human growth hormone.

DOSAGE AND ADMINISTRATION

Saizen® [somatropin (rDNA origin) for injection] dosage and schedule of administration should be individualized for each patient. For the treatment of growth hormone inadequacy, a dosage of 0.06 mg/kg (approximately 0.18 IU/kg) administered 3 times per week by subcutaneous or intramuscular injection is recommended.
Treatment with Saizen® of growth failure due to growth hormone deficiency should be discontinued when the epiphyses are fused. Patients who fail to respond adequately while on Saizen® therapy should be evaluated to determine the cause of unresponsiveness.
To prevent possible contamination, wipe the rubber vial stopper with an antiseptic solution before puncturing it with the needle. It is recommended that Saizen® be administered using sterile, disposable syringes and needles. The syringes should be of small enough volume that the prescribed dose can be drawn from the vial with reasonable accuracy.
After determining the appropriate patient dose, reconstitute each 5 mg vial of Saizen® with 1–3 mL of Bacteriostatic Water for Injection, USP (Benzyl Alcohol preserved). For use in patients sensitive to the diluent see "WARNINGS."
To reconstitute Saizen®, inject the diluent into the vial of Saizen® aiming the liquid against the glass vial wall. Swirl the vial with a **GENTLE** rotary motion until contents are dissolved completely. **DO NOT SHAKE**. Because Saizen® growth hormone is a protein, shaking can result in a cloudy solution. The Saizen® solution should be clear immediately after reconstitution. **DO NOT INJECT** Saizen® if the reconstituted product is cloudy immediately after reconstitution or refrigeration. Occasionally, after refrigeration, small colorless particles may be present in the Saizen® solution. This is not unusual for proteins like Saizen®.

STABILITY AND STORAGE

Before Reconstitution—Saizen® [somatropin (rDNA origin) for injection] should be stored at room temperature (15°–30°C/59°–86°F). Expiration dates are stated on the labels.
After Reconstitution—When reconstituted with the diluent provided, the reconstituted solution should be stored under refrigeration (2°–8°C/36°–46°F) for up to 14 days. Avoid freezing reconstituted vials of Saizen®.

HOW SUPPLIED

Saizen® [somatropin (rDNA origin) for injection] is a sterile, non-pyrogenic, white, lyophilized powder supplied in packages containing:
1 vial of 5 mg (approximately 15 IU) Saizen® and 1 vial of 10 mL Bacteriostatic Water for Injection, USP (0.9% Benzyl Alcohol) NDC 44087-1005-2
Product information as of February 1998
Distributed by: Serono Laboratories, Inc., Randolph, MA 02368
®-Registered trademark of Serono Laboratories, Inc., Norwell, MA 02061

SEROPHENE® ℞

[se 'ro-fēn]
(clomiphene citrate tablets, USP)

PRODUCT OVERVIEW

KEY FACTS

Serophene® is an orally administered, non-steroidal compound with some estrogenic activity. The exact mechanism of action is unknown, although it appears to involve the pituitary by stimulating release of pituitary gonadotropins to mediate ovulation.

MAJOR USES

Serophene® is effective in inducing ovulation in infertile women with physiological indications of normal estrogen production. Reduced estrogen levels, while less favorable, do not prevent successful therapy.

SAFETY INFORMATION

Serophene® is contraindicated in patients who have previously experienced hypersensitivity to clomiphene citrate. Visual disturbances, vasomotor flushes, and ovarian enlargement occasionally occur. Because the teratogenic potential of clomiphene citrate is unknown, it should not be administered during pregnancy. Multiple births occur in approximately 10% of pregnancies resulting from clomiphene citrate therapy; the vast majority of these are twins.

PRESCRIBING INFORMATION

SEROPHENE® ℞

[se 'ro-f ēn]
(clomiphene citrate tablets, USP)

DESCRIPTION

Each scored white tablet contains: clomiphene citrate, USP 50 mg. Clomiphene citrate is designated chemically as 2-[p-(2-chloro-1,2-diphenylvinyl) phenoxy] triethylamine dihydrogen citrate and is represented structurally as:

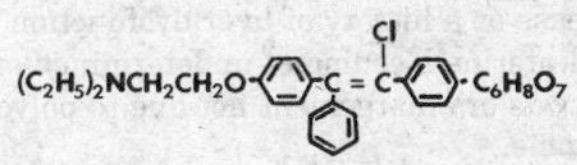

clomiphene citrate, USP (Serophene®)

As shown, one molecule of citric acid is chemically bound with one molecule of the organic base, clomiphene.
Clomiphene citrate is a chemical analog of other triarylethylene compounds such as chlorotrianisene and the cholesterol inhibitor, triparanol.

ACTIONS

Clomiphene citrate, an orally-administered, non-steroidal agent, may induce ovulation in selected anovulatory women. It is a drug of considerable pharmacologic potency. Careful evaluation and selection of the patient and close attention to the timing of the dose is mandatory prior to treatment with clomiphene citrate. Conservative selection and management of the patient contribute to successful therapy of anovulation. Clomiphene citrate induces ovulation in most selected anovulatory patients. The various criteria for ovulation include: an ovulation peak of estrogen excretion followed by a biphasic basal body temperature curve, urinary excretion of pregnanediol at post-ovulatory levels, and endometrial histologic findings characteristic of the luteal phase.
A review of eleven publications appearing between 1964 and 1978 showed that pregnancy occurred in 35% of 5,154 patients with ovulatory dysfunction who received clomiphene citrate.
[See table at top of next page]
Clomiphene citrate therapy appears to mediate ovulation through increased output of pituitary gonadotropins. These stimulate the maturation and endocrine activity of the ovarian follicle which is followed by the development and function of the corpus luteum. Increased urinary excretion of gonadotropins and estrogen suggests involvement of the pituitary.
Studies with ^{14}C labeled clomiphene citrate have shown that it is readily absorbed orally in humans and is excreted principally in the feces. An average of 51% of the administered dose was excreted after 5 days. After intravenous ad-

Continued on next page

Serophene—Cont.

ministration, 37% was excreted in 5 days. The appearance of ^{14}C in the feces six weeks after administration suggests that the remaining drug and/or metabolites are slowly excreted from a sequestered enterohepatic recirculation pool.

INDICATIONS

Clomiphene citrate is indicated for the treatment of ovulatory failure in patients desiring pregnancy and whose husbands are fertile and potent. Impediments to this goal must be excluded or adequately treated before beginning therapy. Administration of clomiphene citrate is indicated only in patients with demonstrated ovulatory dysfunction and in whom the following conditions apply:

1. Normal liver function.
2. Physiologic indications of normal endogenous estrogen (as estimated from vaginal smears, endometrial biopsy, assay of serum [or urinary] estrogen, or from bleeding in response to progesterone). Reduced estrogen levels, while less favorable, do not prevent successful therapy.
3. Clomiphene citrate therapy is not effective for those patients with primary pituitary or ovarian failure. It cannot substitute for appropriate therapy of other disturbances leading to ovulatory dysfunction, e.g., diseases of the thyroid or adrenals.
4. Particularly careful evaluation prior to clomiphene citrate therapy should be done in patients with abnormal uterine bleeding. It is most important that neoplastic lesions are detected.

CONTRAINDICATIONS

Pregnancy:

Although no direct effect of clomiphene citrate therapy on the human fetus has been seen established, clomiphene citrate should not be administered in cases of suspected pregnancy as such effects have been reported in animals. To prevent inadvertent clomiphene citrate administration during early pregnancy, the basal body temperature should be recorded throughout all treatment cycles, and therapy should be discontinued if pregnancy is suspected. If the basal body temperature following clomiphene citrate is biphasic and is not followed by menses, the possibility of an ovarian cyst and/or pregnancy should be excluded. Until the correct diagnosis has been determined, the next course of therapy should be delayed.

Clomiphene citrate is also contraindicated in patients who have:

1. Uncontrolled thyroid or adrenal dysfunction.
2. An organic intracranial lesion such as a pituitary tumor.
3. Liver disease or a history of liver dysfunction.
4. Abnormal uterine bleeding of undetermined origin.
5. Ovarian cysts or enlargement not due to polycystic ovarian syndrome.

WARNINGS

Visual Symptoms:

Patients should be warned that blurring and/or other visual symptoms may occur occasionally with clomiphene citrate therapy. These may make activities such as driving or operating machinery more hazardous than usual, particularly under conditions of variable lighting. While their significance is not yet understood (see "Adverse Reactions"), patients having any visual symptoms should discontinue treatment and have a complete ophthalmologic evaluation.

Ovarian Hyperstimulation Syndrome:

The Ovarian Hyperstimulation Syndrome (OHSS) has been reported to occur in patients receiving drug therapy for ovulation induction, including in rare cases patients receiving clomiphene citrate therapy. OHSS is a medical event distinct from uncomplicated ovarian enlargement. OHSS may progress rapidly (within 24 hours to several days) to become a serious medical event. It is characterized by an apparent dramatic increase in vascular permeability which can result in a rapid accumulation of fluid in the peritoneal cavity, thorax, and potentially, the pericardium. The early warning signs of development of OHSS are severe pelvic pain, nausea, vomiting, and weight gain. The following symptomatology has been seen with cases of OHSS: abdominal pain, abdominal distension, gastrointestinal symptoms including nausea, vomiting and diarrhea, severe ovarian enlargement, weight gain, dyspnea, and oliguria. Clinical evaluation may reveal hypovolemia, hemoconcentration, electrolyte imbalances, ascites, hemoperitoneum, pleural effusions, hydrothorax, acute pulmonary distress, and thromboembolic phenomena. Transient liver function test abnormalities, suggestive of hepatic dysfunction, which may be accompanied by morphologic changes on liver biopsy, have been reported in association with the Ovarian Hyperstimulation Syndrome (OHSS).

PRECAUTIONS

Diagnosis Prior to Clomiphene Citrate Therapy:

Careful evaluation should be given to candidates for clomiphene citrate therapy. A complete pelvic examination should be performed prior to treatment and repeated before each subsequent course. Clomiphene citrate should not be given to patients with an ovarian cyst, as further ovarian enlargement may result.

Since the incidence of endometrial carcinoma and of ovulatory disorders increases with age, endometrial biopsy should always exclude the former as causative in such patients. If abnormal uterine bleeding is present, full diagnostic measures are necessary.

Ovarian Overstimulation During Treatment with Clomiphene Citrate:

To minimize the hazard associated with the occasional abnormal ovarian enlargement during clomiphene citrate therapy (see "Adverse Reactions"), the lowest dose producing good results should be chosen. Some patients with polycystic ovarian syndrome are unusually sensitive to gonadotropins and may have an exaggerated response to usual doses of clomiphene citrate. Maximal enlargement of the ovary, whether abnormal or physiologic, does not occur until several days after discontinuation of clomiphene citrate. The patient complaining of pelvic pains after receiving clomiphene citrate should be examined carefully. If enlargement of the ovary occurs, clomiphene citrate therapy should be withheld until the ovaries have returned to pretreatment size, and the dosage or duration of the next course should be reduced. The ovarian enlargement and cyst formation following clomiphene citrate therapy regress spontaneously within a few days or weeks after discontinuing treatment. Therefore, unless a strong indication for laparoscopy (or laparotomy) exists, such cystic enlargement always should be managed conservatively.

Multiple Pregnancy:

In the reviewed publications, the incidence of multiple pregnancies was increased during those cycles in which clomiphene citrate was given. Among the 1,803 pregnancies on which the outcome was reported, 90% were single and 10% twins. Less than 1% of the reported deliveries resulted in triplets or more.

Of these multiple pregnancies, 96-99% resulted in the births of live infants. The patient and her husband should be advised of the frequency and potential hazards of multiple pregnancy before starting treatment.

Additional Precautions:

Prolonged use of clomiphene may increase the risk of a borderline or invasive ovarian tumor.

ADVERSE REACTIONS

At the recommended dosage of clomiphene citrate, side effects occur infrequently and generally do not interfere with treatment. Adverse reactions tend to occur more frequently at higher doses and in the longer treatment courses used in some early studies.

The most frequent adverse reactions to clomiphene citrate include ovarian enlargement (approximately 1 in 7 patients), vasomotor flushes resembling menopausal symptoms which are not usually severe and promptly disappear after treatment is discontinued (approximately 1 in 10 patients), and abdominal discomfort (approximately 1 in 15 patients). Adverse reactions which occur less frequently (approximately 1 in 50 patients or more) include breast tenderness, nausea and vomiting, nervousness, insomnia, and visual disturbances. Other side effects which occur in less than 1 in 100 patients include headache, dizziness and light-headedness, increased urination, depression, fatigue, urticaria and allergic dermatitis, abnormal uterine bleeding, weight gain, ovarian cysts (ovarian enlargement or cysts could, as such, be complicated by adnexal torsion), and reversible hair loss.

Thromboembolic events, such as pulmonary embolism, arterial occlusion, and phlebitis, have been reported rarely in patients treated with clomiphene citrate. It is not clear what, if any, relationship these events have to clomiphene citrate therapy.

When clomiphene citrate is administered at the recommended dose, abnormal ovarian enlargement (see "Precautions") is infrequent, although the usual cyclic variation in ovarian size may be exaggerated. Similarly, mid-cycle ovarian pain (mittelschmerz) may be accentuated.

PREGNANCIES FOLLOWING CLOMIPHENE CITRATE, USP[a]

			(Range)
Number of Patients	=	5,154	
Percent of Patients Ovulating[b]	=	75	(50-94%)
Percent of Ovulatory Cycles	=	53	(33-69%)
Percent of Patients Pregnant	=	35	(11-52%)
Percent Patients Pregnant / Percent Patients Ovulating	=	46	(22-61%)
Percent Live Births	=	86	(74-99.8%)
Percent Abortions	=	14	(0.2-26%)
Percent of Single Births	=	90	(67-100%)
Percent Surviving	=	99	(98.2-100%)
Percent of Multiple Births	=	10	(0-33%)
Percent Surviving	=	96	(82-100%)

a) includes patients receiving other than recommended dosage regimen.
b) average from studies.

With prolonged or higher dosage, ovarian enlargement and cyst formation (usually luteal) may occur more often, and the luteal phase of the cycle may be prolonged. Patients with polycystic ovarian syndrome may be unusually sensitive to clomiphene therapy. Rare occurrences of massive ovarian enlargement have been reported, for example, in a patient with polycystic ovarian syndrome whose clomiphene citrate therapy consisted of 100 mg daily for 14 days. Since abnormal ovarian enlargement usually regresses spontaneously, most of these patients should be treated conservatively. The Ovarian Hyperstimulation Syndrome has been reported to occur in rare cases in patients receiving clomiphene citrate therapy (see "Warnings").

The incidence of visual symptoms (see "Warnings" for further recommendations), usually described as "blurring" or spots or flashes (scintillating scotomata), correlates with increasing total dose. Other visual symptoms which may occur include diplopia, phosphenes, photophobia, decreased visual acuity, loss of peripheral vision, and spatial distortion. The symptoms disappear usually within a few days or weeks after clomiphene citrate is discontinued. This may be due to intensification and/or prolongation of after-images. Symptoms often appear first, or are accentuated, upon exposure to a more brightly lit environment.

While measured visual acuity generally has not been affected, in one patient taking 200 mg daily, visual blurring developed on the seventh day of treatment and progressed to severe diminution of visual acuity by the tenth day. No other abnormality was coincident, and the visual acuity was normal by the third day after treatment was stopped. Ophthalmologically definable scotomata and electroretinographic retinal function changes have also been reported.

BSP Laboratory Studies:

Greater than 5% retention of sulfobromophthalein (BSP) has been reported in approximately 10% to 20% of patients in whom it was measured. Retention was usually minimal but was elevated during prolonged clomiphene citrate administration or with apparently unrelated liver disease. In some patients, pre-existing BSP retention decreased even though clomiphene citrate therapy was continued. Other liver function tests were usually normal.

Other Laboratory Studies:

Clomiphene citrate has not been reported to cause a significant abnormality in hematologic or renal tests, in protein bound iodine, or in serum cholesterol levels.

Birth Defects:

The following medical events have been reported subsequent to pregnancies following ovulation induction therapy with clomiphene citrate: ectopic pregnancy and congenital abnormalities such as syndactyly, polydactyly, congenital heart defects, retinal aplasia, hypospadias, ovarian dysplasia, cleft lip/palate, microencephaly and neural tube defects, including anencephaly. Some medical literature reports have implied an increased occurrence of neural tube defects, while others indicate that an increased incidence over that found in the general population does not exist. One case of a congenital abnormality (adactyly) in an infant exposed to clomiphene citrate in utero has been reported.

Of 1,803 births following clomiphene citrate administration, 45 infants with birth defects were reported for a cumulative rate of 2.5%.

Six cases of Down's syndrome, one neonatal death with multiple malformations, and one case of each of the following were reported: club-foot, tibial torsion, blocked tear duct, and hemangioma. The other congenital abnormalities were not described. The investigators did not report that these were presumed to be due to therapy. The cumulative rate of congenital abnormalities does not exceed that reported in the general population.

Ovarian cancer has been reported in a very small number of infertile women who have been treated with clomiphene citrate. A causal relationship between treatment with clomiphene citrate and ovarian cancer has not been established.

DOSAGE AND ADMINISTRATION

General Considerations:

Physicians experienced in managing gynecologic or endocrine disorders should supervise the work-up and treatment

of candidate patients for clomiphene citrate therapy. Patients should be chosen for clomiphene citrate therapy only after careful diagnostic evaluation (see "Indications"). The plan of therapy should be outlined in advance. Impediments to achieving the goal of therapy must be excluded or adequately treated before beginning clomiphene citrate.

In determining a starting dose schedule, efficacy must be balanced against potential side effects. For example, the available data so far suggest that ovulation and pregnancy are slightly more attainable with 100 mg/day for 5 days than with 50 mg/day for 5 days. As the dosage is increased, however, ovarian overstimulation and other side effects may be expected to increase. Although the data do not yet establish a relationship between dose level and multiple births, it is reasonable that such a correlation exists on pharmacologic grounds.

For these reasons, treatment of the usual patient should initiate with a 50 mg daily dose for 5 days. The dose may be increased only in those patients who do not respond to the first course (see "Recommended Dosage"). Special treatment with lower dosage over shorter duration is particularly recommended if unusual sensitivity to pituitary gonadotropin is suspected, including patients with polycystic ovarian syndrome (see "Precautions").

Recommended Dosage:

The recommended dosage for the first course of clomiphene citrate is 50 mg (1 tablet) daily for 5 days. Therapy may be started at any time if the patient has had no recent uterine bleeding. If progestin-induced bleeding is intended, or if spontaneous uterine bleeding occurs prior to therapy, the regimen of 50 mg daily for 5 days should be started on or about the fifth day of the cycle. When ovulation occurs at this dosage, there is no advantage to increasing the dose in subsequent cycles of treatment. If ovulation does not appear to have occurred after the first course of therapy, a second course of 100 mg daily (two 50 mg tablets given as a single daily dose) for 5 days may be started. This course may begin as early as 30 days after the previous one. It is recommended that the patient be examined for pregnancy, ovarian enlargement, or cyst formation between each treatment cycle. Increasing the dosage or duration of therapy beyond 100 mg/day for 5 days should not be undertaken.

The majority of patients who respond do so during the first course of therapy, and 3 courses constitute an adequate therapeutic trial. If ovulatory menses do not occur, the diagnosis should be re-evaluated. Treatment beyond this is not recommended in the patient who does not exhibit evidence of ovulation.

Pregnancy:

Properly timed coitus is very important for good results. For regularity of cyclic ovulatory response, it is also important that each course of clomiphene citrate be started on or about the fifth day of the cycle, once ovulation has been established. As with other therapeutic modalities, Serophene® therapy follows the rule of diminishing returns, such that the likelihood of conception diminishes with each succeeding course of therapy. If pregnancy has not been achieved after 3 ovulatory responses to Serophene®, further treatment generally is not recommended. Before starting treatment, patients should be advised of the possibility and potential hazards of multiple pregnancy if conception occurs following clomiphene citrate therapy.

Long-Term Cyclic Therapy —Not Recommended:

Since the relative safety of long-term cyclic therapy has not yet been demonstrated conclusively, and since the majority of patients will ovulate following 3 courses, long-term cyclic therapy is not recommended.

HOW SUPPLIED

Serophene® is available as 50 mg scored white tablets in the following package combinations:

• 1 carton 10 tablets, NDC 44087-8090-6

Each carton contains 2 strips of 5 tablets each.

• 1 carton 30 tablets, NDC 44087-8090-1

Each carton contains 3 strips of 10 tablets, each in a 2 × 5 arrangement.

Protect from light, moisture, and excessive heat. Dispense in well-closed, light resistant container as defined in the USP, with child resistant closure. Store at room temperature (15°–30°C/59°–86°F).

Caution: Federal law prohibits dispensing without prescription.

Manufactured for:
SERONO LABORATORIES, INC.
Randolph, MA 02368 USA
by: TEVA PHARMACEUTICAL INDUSTRIES LTD.
Jerusalem 91010, Israel
©SERONO LABORATORIES, INC. 1982, 1992
Revised: November 1994

SEROSTIM®   ℞

[serō-stim]

[somatropin (rDNA origin) for injection]

DESCRIPTION

Serostim® [somatropin (rDNA origin) for injection] is a human growth hormone produced by recombinant DNA tech-

nology. Serostim® has 191 amino acid residues and a molecular weight of 22,125 daltons. Its amino acid sequence and structure are identical to the dominant form of human pituitary growth hormone. Serostim® is produced by a mammalian cell line (mouse C127) that has been modified by the addition of the human growth hormone gene. Serostim® is secreted directly through the cell membrane into the cell-culture medium for collection and purification.

Serostim® is a highly purified preparation. Biological potency is determined by measuring the increase in the body weight induced in hypophysectomized rats.

Serostim® is available in 4 mg, 5 mg and 6 mg vials for single dose administration. Each 4 mg vial contains 4.0 mg (approximately 12 IU) somatropin, 27.3 mg sucrose, 0.9 mg phosphoric acid. Each 5 mg vial contains 5.0 mg (approximately 15 IU) somatropin, 34.2 mg sucrose and 1.2 mg phosphoric acid. Each 6 mg vial contains 6.0 mg (approximately 18 IU) somatropin, 41.0 mg sucrose and 1.4 mg phosphoric acid. The pH is adjusted with sodium hydroxide or phosphoric acid to give a pH of 7.4 to 8.5 after reconstitution.

CLINICAL PHARMACOLOGY

Serostim® [somatropin (rDNA origin) for injection] is an anabolic and anticatabolic agent which exerts its influence by interacting with specific receptors on a variety of cell types including myocytes, hepatocytes, adipocytes, lymphocytes, and hematopoietic cells. Some, but not all, of its effects are mediated by another class of hormones known as somatomedins (IGF-1 and IGF-2).

AIDS-associated wasting is a metabolic disorder characterized by abnormalities of intermediary metabolism resulting in weight loss, inappropriate depletion of lean body mass (LBM), and paradoxical preservation of body fat. LBM includes primarily skeletal muscle, organ tissue, blood and blood constituents, and both intracellular and extracellular water. Depletion of LBM results in muscle weakness, organ failure, and death. Unlike nutritional intervention for AIDS-associated wasting, in which supplemental calories are converted predominantly to body fat, Serostim® treatment resulted in an increase in LBM and a decrease in body fat with a significant increase in body weight due to the dominant effect of LBM gain.

Effects on Protein, Lipid, and Carbohydrate Metabolism:

A one-week study in 6 patients with HIV associated wasting has shown that treatment with Serostim® improves nitrogen balance, increases protein-sparing lipid oxidation, and has little effect on overall carbohydrate metabolism.

Lean Body Mass Accrual:

In the same study, treatment with Serostim® resulted in the retention of phosphorous, potassium, nitrogen, and sodium. The ratio of retained potassium and nitrogen during Serostim® therapy was consistent with retention of these elements in lean tissue. In clinical studies (12 weeks), Serostim® significantly increased lean body mass. There was also a proportionate increase in intracellular and extracellular fluid during Serostim® therapy suggesting accretion of normally hydrated lean body tissue.

Physical Performance:

Treadmill performance was examined in a 12-week placebo-controlled study. Work output improved significantly in the Serostim® treated group after 12 weeks of therapy and was correlated with LBM. No such correlation was seen with body fat. Isometric muscle performance, as measured by grip strength dynamometry, declined, probably as a result of a transient increase in tissue turgor known to occur with r-hGH therapy.

PHARMACOKINETICS

Subcutaneous Absorption: The absolute bioavailability of Serostim® [somatropin (rDNA origin) for injection] after subcutaneous administration of a formulation not equivalent to the marketed formulation was determined to be 70–90%. The $t^1/_2$ (Mean ±SD) after subcutaneous administration is significantly longer than that seen after intravenous administration to normal male volunteers, down-regulated with somatostatin (3.94 ± 3.44 hrs. vs. 0.58 ± 0.08 hrs.), indicating that the subcutaneous absorption of the clinically tested formulation of the compound is slow and rate-limiting.

Distribution: The steady-state volume of distribution (Mean ± SD) following IV administration of Serostim® in healthy volunteers is 12.0 ± 1.08 L.

Metabolism: Although the liver plays a role in the metabolism of growth hormone, GH is primarily cleaved in the kidney. GH undergoes glomerular filtration and after cleavage within the renal cells, the peptides and amino acids are returned to the systemic circulation.

Elimination: The $t^1/_2$ (Mean ± SD) in nine patients with AIDS related wasting with an average weight of 56.7 ± 6.8 kg, given a fixed dose of 6.0 mg r-hGH subcutaneously was 4.28 ± 2.15 hrs. The renal clearance of r-hGH after subcu-

taneous administration in nine patients with AIDS related wasting was 0.0015 ± 0.0037 L/h. No significant accumulation of r-hGH appears to occur after 6 weeks of dosing as indicated.

Special Populations:

Pediatric: Available evidence suggests that r-hGH clearances are similar in adults and children, but no clinical studies were conducted in children with acquired immune deficiency syndrome or AIDS-related complex.

Gender: Biomedical literature indicates that a gender-related difference in the mean clearance of r-hGH could exist (Clearance of r-hGH in males > Clearance of r-hGH in females). However, no gender-based analysis is available on Serostim® use in normal volunteers or patients infected with HIV.

Race: No data are available.

Renal Insufficiency: It has been reported that individuals with chronic renal failure tend to have decreased hGH clearance compared to normals, but there are no data on Serostim® use in the presence of renal insufficiency.

Hepatic Insufficiency: A reduction in r-hGH clearance has been noted in patients with severe liver dysfunction. However, the clinical significance of this in HIV+ patients is unknown.

CLINICAL STUDIES

The clinical efficacy of Serostim® [somatropin (rDNA origin) for injection] was assessed in two placebo-controlled clinical trials. Of the 205 AIDS subjects exposed to GH, only 5 were women. All study subjects received concomitant anti-HIV therapy.

Clinical Trial 1: A multicenter, double-blind, placebo-controlled study compared Serostim® at an average daily dose of 0.1 mg/kg/day administered subcutaneously to placebo in 178 patients with AIDS wasting. The study participants had unintentional weight loss of at least 10% or weighed less than 90% of the lower limit of ideal body weight. In the 140 evaluable patients (those completing a 12-week course of treatment and who were at least 80% compliant with study drug; Serostim® =69, Placebo = 71), the mean difference in weight increase in the Serostim®- treated group was 1.6 kg (3.5 lb). For those patients that had a week two assessment, 76% had weight gain. After 12 weeks of treatment, 74% of the patients treated with Serostim® gained weight while only 48% of the placebo-treated patients gained weight (p=0.002). Mean differences in lean body mass change between the Serostim® treated group and the placebo treated group was 3.1 kg (6.8 lbs) as measured by DEXA. Significant lean body mass gain (p<0.05) was achieved in 70% of the patients treated with Serostim® after 12 weeks (see Table 1). No change in LBM was observed in placebo-treated patients. Mean increase in weight and lean body mass and mean decrease in body fat (see Figure 1) were significantly greater in the Serostim® treated group than in the placebo group (p=0.011, p<0.001, p<0.001, respectively). While depletion of body weight and lean body mass has been associated with increased morbidity and mortality, the clinical significance of treatment-induced weight gain and LBM accrual has yet to be established.

Treatment with Serostim® resulted in a significant increase of physical function as assessed by treadmill exercise testing. The median treadmill work output increased by 13% (p=0.039) at 12 weeks in the group receiving Serostim® (see Figure 2). There was no improvement in the placebo treated group at 12 weeks. Changes in treadmill performance were significantly correlated with changes of lean body mass.

The most common reason for patient drop-out was concurrent medical events including opportunistic infections. There were decreases in serum albumin in both Serostim® and placebo groups. There was up to a 2.7 fold increase in serum IGF-1 levels. No patients developed antibodies to growth hormone.

Patients completing the 12–week placebo-controlled portion of the study were eligible to receive open-label Serostim® therapy, and 96% (n=136) chose to participate. Since this phase of the trial was open-label, and due to limited numbers of evaluable patients, it is difficult to interpret weight and LBM changes. The patients who initially received placebo had significant increases in median weight (1.4 kg, p=0.012) and lean body mass (2.4 kg, p<0.001) compared to baseline, during their first 12-weeks on Serostim®. These changes were similar in magnitude to those observed in patients initially treated with Serostim®. For those patients who had initially received Serostim® in the placebo-controlled trials, the median weight change during 12-weeks of open label treatment with Serostim® (-0.2 kg) and LBM change (-0.3 kg) were not significant (p=0.700 and p=0.661, respectively), suggesting that the gains of weight and LBM were not lost.

Continued on next page

Serostim—Cont.

Figure 1: Trial 1: Mean Changes in Body Composition

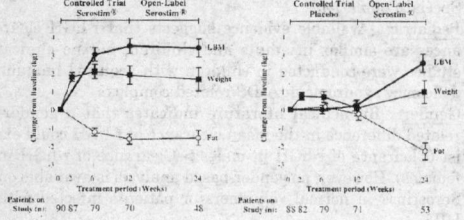

Table 1: Trial 1: Change from Baseline of LBM 12-Week Efficacy Results

	Serostim®		Placebo	
	n	Results	n	Results
Lean Body Mass (kg)	69	+3.1*	69	-0.1
LBM Responders‡	69	70%*	69	12%

‡Major LBM response defined as >4% increase of LBM
*Statistically significantly different from placebo at p<0.05

Figure 2: Median Treadmill Work Output

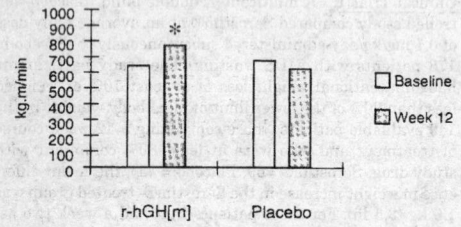

*p = 0.039

Clinical Trial 2: Additional efficacy and safety parameters were evaluated in a second multicenter, double-blind, placebo-controlled study comparing Serostim®, 6 mg/day administered subcutaneously vs. placebo, in AIDS patients with wasting enrolled 177 patients who were randomized in a 2:1 ratio, to receive Serostim® or placebo. In the 78 evaluable patients (those completing a 12-week course of treatment and who were at least 80% compliant with study drug), there was a mean increase in body weight of 1.6 kg, but this change was not significant compared to placebo (p=0.110). The most common reason for patient drop-out was concurrent medical events including opportunistic infections. Patients were asked to respond to a nine item survey that measured subjective assessments of treatment. Positive findings at 6 and 12 weeks were observed in two of the nine items (change in appearance and overall benefit of treatment). Results of other measures were inconclusive.
Survival Analyses: The two placebo-controlled clinical trials of Serostim® in patients with AIDS wasting up to 12 weeks in length found no difference in survival between groups.
Clinical Trial 3: A third open-label, baseline-controlled, multicenter study conducted in Europe administering Serostim®, 6 mg/day subcutaneously, enrolled 24 patients with AIDS wasting. Twenty patients completed the 12-week treatment regimen and had body composition measurements using bioimpedance analysis. The mean increase over baseline for body weight was 1.6 kg (p=0.137, NS) and for lean body mass was 2.3 kg (p=0.037).

INDICATIONS AND USAGE

Serostim® [somatropin (rDNA origin) for injection] is indicated for the treatment of AIDS wasting or cachexia. This indication is based on analyses of surrogate endpoints in studies of up to 12 weeks in duration. Concomitant antiviral therapy is necessary (see PRECAUTIONS: GENERAL). The continued use of Serostim® treatment should be reevaluated in patients who continue to lose weight in the first two weeks of treatment.

CONTRAINDICATIONS

Serostim® [somatropin (rDNA origin) for injection] is contraindicated in patients with a known hypersensitivity to growth hormone.

PRECAUTIONS

General: Serostim® [somatropin (rDNA origin) for injection] therapy should be carried out under the regular guidance of a physician who is experienced in the diagnosis and management of AIDS. Inadequate nutritional intake, mal-

absorption and hypogonadism, which are common in individuals with AIDS and which may contribute to catabolism and weight loss, should also be monitored and treated.
HIV and Growth Hormone Considerations: In some experimental systems, recombinant human Growth Hormone (r-hGH) has been shown to potentiate HIV replication in vitro at concentrations ranging from 50–250 ng/ml. There was no increase in virus production when the antiretroviral agents, zidovudine, didanosine or lamivudine were added to the culture medium. Additional in vitro studies have shown that r-hGH does not interefere with the antiviral activity of zalcitabine or stavudine. In the controlled clinical trials, no significant growth hormone-associated increase in viral burden was observed. However, the protocol required all participants to be on concomitant nucleoside analogue therapy for the duration of the study. In view of the potential for acceleration of virus replication, it is recommended that HIV+ patients be maintained on nucleoside analogue therapy for the duration of Serostim® treatment.
Increased tissue turgor (swelling, particularly in the hands and feet) and musculoskeletal discomfort (pain, swelling and/or stiffness) may occur during treatment with Serostim®, but may resolve spontaneously, with analgesic therapy, or after reducing the frequency of dosing (see Dosage and Administration).
Carpal tunnel syndrome may occur during treatment with Serostim®. If the symptoms of carpal tunnel syndrome do not resolve by decreasing the weekly number of doses of Serostim®, it is recommended that treatment be discontinued. Patients should be informed that allergic reactions are possible and that prompt medical attention should be sought if an allergic reaction occurs. None of the 188 study participants with AIDS wasting who were evaluable for antibody assessments and who were treated with Serostim® for the first time developed detectable antibodies to growth hormone (> 4 pg binding). Patients were not rechallenged.
Recombinant Human Growth Hormone (r-hGH) has been associated with acute pancreatitis.
Hyperglycemia may occur in HIV-infected individuals due to a variety of reasons. Serostim® use was associated with a minimal increase of mean blood glucose concentration. Patients with other risk factors for glucose intolerance should be monitored closely during Serostim® therapy.
No cases of intracranial hypertension (IH) have been observed among patients with AIDS wasting treated with Serostim®. The syndrome of IH, with papilledema, visual changes, headache, and nausea and/or vomiting has been reported in a small number of children with growth failure treated with growth hormone products. Nevertheless, funduscopic evaluation of patients is recommended at the initiation and periodically during the course of Serostim® therapy.
Kaposi's sarcoma, lymphoma, and other malignancies are common in HIV+ individuals. There was no increase in the incidence of Kaposi's sarcoma, lymphoma, or in the progression of cutaneous Kaposi's sarcoma in clinical studies of Serostim®. Patients with internal KS lesions were excluded from the studies. Potential effects on other malignancies are unknown.
Information For Patients: Patients being treated with Serostim® should be informed of the potential benefits and risks associated with treatment. Patients should be instructed to contact their physician should they experience any side effects or discomfort during treatment with Serostim®.
It is recommended that Serostim® be administered using sterile, disposable syringes and needles. Patients should be thoroughly instructed in the importance of proper disposal and cautioned against any reuse of needles and syringes. An appropriate container for the disposal of used syringes and needles should be employed.
Patients should be instructed to rotate injection sites to avoid lipodystrophy.
Drug Interactions: Formal in vitro drug interaction studies have not been conducted. No data are available on drug interactions between Serostim® and HIV protease inhibitors or the non-nucleoside reverse transcriptase inhibitors.
Carcinogenesis, Mutagenesis, Impairment of Fertility:Long-term animal studies for carcinogenicity have not been performed with Serostim®. There is no evidence from animal studies to date of Serostim®-induced mutagenicity or impairment of fertility.
Pregnancy: Pregnancy Category B. Reproduction studies have been performed in rats and rabbits. Doses up to 5 to 10 times the human dose, based on body surface area, have revealed no evidence of impaired fertility or harm to the fetus due to Serostim®. There are, however, no adequate and well controlled studies in pregnant women. Because animal reproduction studies are not always predictive of human response, this drug should be used during pregnancy only if clearly needed.
Nursing Women: It is not known whether Serostim® is excreted in human milk. Because many drugs are excreted in human milk, caution should be exercised when Serostim® is administered to a nursing woman.

Pediatric Use: In two small studies, 11 children with HIV associated failure to thrive were treated subcutaneously with human growth hormone. In one study, five children (age range, 6 to 17 years) were treated with 0.04 mg/kg/day for 26 weeks. In a second study, six children (age range, 8 to 14 years) were treated with 0.07 mg/kg/day for 4 weeks. Treatment appeared to be well tolerated in both studies. These preliminary data collected in a limited number of patients with HIV associated failure to thrive appear to be consistent with safety observations in growth hormone treated adults with AIDS wasting.

ADVERSE REACTIONS

In two placebo-controlled clinical trials in which 205 patients were treated with Serostim® [somatropin (rDNA origin) for injection] the most common adverse reactions judged to be associated with Serostim® were musculoskeletal discomfort and increased tissue turgor (swelling, particularly of the hands or feet) (see PRECAUTIONS: GENERAL). These symptoms were generally rated by investigators as mild to moderate in severity and usually subsided with continued treatment. Discontinuations as a result of these events were rare.
Because of the diverse clinical manifestations of AIDS, and the frequent occurrence of adverse events associated with underlying disease process, it was often difficult to distinguish adverse events possibly associated with the administration of Serostim® from underlying signs or symptoms of AIDS or associated intercurrent illnesses.
Clinical adverse events which occurred during the first 12 weeks of study in at least 10% of those who received Serostim® during the two placebo-controlled trials are listed below by treatment group, without regard to causality assessment.

Table 2: Controlled Trials Adverse Events

Adverse Event	Serostim® (n=205) %	Placebo (n=150) %
Musculoskeletal discomfort	53.7	33.3
Fever	31.2	29.3
Increased tissue turgor	27.3	2.7
Diarrhea	25.9	20.0
Neuropathy	25.9	17.3
Nausea	25.9	16.0
Headache	19.0	20.7
Abdominal pain	17.1	18.7
Fatigue	17.1	16.0
Leukopenia	15.1	24.7
Albuminuria	15.1	9.3
Granulocytopenia	14.1	21.3
Lymphadenopathy	14.1	16.0
Increased sweating	14.1	8.7
Anorexia	12.2	9.3
Anemia	12.2	8.7
Vomiting	11.7	12.0
SGOT increased	11.7	6.0
Insomnia	11.2	9.3
Tachycardia	11.2	6.0
Hyperglycemia	10.2	6.0
SGPT increased	10.2	5.3

Adverse events that occurred in 1% to less than 10% of study participants receiving Serostim® in the two placebo-controlled clinical efficacy studies are listed below by body system. The list of adverse events has been compiled regardless of causal relationship to Serostim®.
Body as a Whole: rigors, flu-like symptoms, back pain, malaise, asthenia, carpal tunnel syndrome (see PRECAUTIONS: GENERAL), chest pain, hot flashes, allergic reaction.
Gastrointestinal System: oral leukoplakia, flatulence, dyspepsia, dry mouth, constipation, ulcerative stomatitis, increased amylase, dysphagia, esophagitis, colitis, pancreatitis, rectal disorder, gastritis, tongue ulceration, gingivitis
Musculoskeletal System: muscle weakness
Central and Peripheral Nervous System: dizziness, convulsions, hypertonia, neuralgia, tremor, encephalopathy, nystagmus, meningism
Respiratory System: dyspnea, coughing, sinusitis, upper respiratory tract infection, pharyngitis, rhinitis, pneumonia, bronchitis, increased sputum, respiratory disorder, bronchospasm, pneumonitis, pleurisy
White Blood Cell and Reticuloendothelial System Disorders: cervical lymphadenopathy, eosinophilia
Skin and appendages: skin disorder, folliculitis, rash, alopecia, photosensitivity reaction, erythematous rash, pruritus, abnormal pigmentation, seborrhea, dermatitis, skin ulceration, acne, skin discoloration, verruca
Psychiatric: depression, anxiety, somnolence, nervousness, appetite increased, amnesia, abnormal thinking
Metabolic and Nutritional: hypertriglyceridemia, increased alkaline phosphatase, dehydration, increased creatinine phosphokinase, increased LDH, glycosuria, hypokalemia, cachexia, thirst, acidosis

Immune System Dysfunction: moniliasis, bacterial infection, Pneumocystis carinii infection, viral infection, infection, Herpes simplex, sepsis, abscess, fungal infection, Herpes zoster
Urinary System: hematuria, urinary tract infection, nocturia
Liver and Biliary System: abnormal hepatic function, hepatomegaly, hepatitis
Vision: retinitis, abnormal vision, photophobia
Platelet, Bleeding and Clotting: thrombocytopenia, purpura
Cardiovascular, General: abnormal ECG, heart murmur, hypertension, hypotension
Application Site: injection site pain, injection site reaction
Neoplasms: Kaposi's sarcoma
Male Reproductive: Epididymitis, penis disorder, inguinal hernia
Hearing and Vestibular: earache, ear disorder, decreasing hearing
Endocrine: gynecomastia, male breast pain
The types and incidence of adverse events reported in an open-label, extension trial and in a single, foreign trial, for up to one year, were not different from, or greater in frequency, than those observed in the primary, placebo-controlled, clinical trials.

OVERDOSAGE

Glucose intolerance can occur with overdosage. Long-term overdosage with growth hormone could result in signs and symptoms of acromegaly.

DOSAGE AND ADMINISTRATION

Serostim® [somatropin (rDNA origin) for injection] should be administered subcutaneously daily at bedtime according to the following dosage recommendations.

Weight Range	Dose*
>55 kg	6 mg SC daily
45–55 kg	5 mg SC daily
35–45 kg	4 mg SC daily

* Based on an approximate daily dosage of 0.1 mg/kg.

In patients who weigh less than 35 kg, Serostim® should be administered at a dose of 0.1 mg/kg subcutaneously daily at bedtime.
Dose reductions for side effects felt to be related to treatment with Serostim®, which are unresponsive to symptomatic treatment, may be affected by reducing the total daily dose or the number of doses given per week.
In patients who continue to lose weight at week 2, reevaluate for concurrent opportunistic infections or other clinical events.
Injection sites should be rotated.
Safety and effectiveness in pediatric patients with AIDS have not been established.
Each vial of Serostim® 4 mg, 5 mg or 6 mg is reconstituted with 1 mL sterile water for injection.
To reconstitute Serostim®, inject the diluent into the vial of Serostim® aiming the liquid against the glass vial wall. Swirl the vial with a gentle rotary motion until contents are dissolved completely. The Serostim® solution should be clear immediately after reconstitution. **DO NOT INJECT** Serostim® if the reconstituted product is cloudy immediately after reconstitution or refrigeration. Occasionally, after refrigeration, small colorless particles may be present in the Serostim® solution. This is not unusual for proteins like Serostim®.

STABILITY AND STORAGE

Before reconstitution: Serostim® [somatropin (rDNA origin) for injection] should be stored at room temperature, 59°–86°F (15°–30°C). Expiration dates are stated on product labels.
After reconstitution: Use within 24 hours after reconstitution with diluent. The reconstituted solution should be stored under refrigerated conditions (36°–46°F/2°–8°C). Sterile Diluent, 1 mL (Sterile Water for Injection, USP) should be stored at room temperature, 59°–86°F (15°–30°C). Avoid freezing vials of Serostim® and Sterile Diluent.

HOW SUPPLIED

Serostim® [somatropin (rDNA origin) for injection] is available in the following forms:
Serostim® vials containing 4 mg (approximately 12 IU) somatropin (mammalian-cell) with Sterile Water for Injection, USP. Package of 7 vials.   NDC 44087-0004-7
Serostim® vials containg 5 mg (approximately 15 IU) somatropin (mammalian-cell) with Sterile Water for Injection, USP. Package of 7 vials.   NDC 44087-0005-7
Serostim® vials containing 6 mg (approximately 18 IU) somatropin (mammalian-cell) with Sterile Water for Injection, USP. Package of 7 vials.   NDC 44087-0006-7
Manufactured for: Serono Laboratories, Inc., Randolph, MA 02368
Caution: Federal law prohibits dispensing without prescription.
February 1998

Shire Richwood Inc.
7900 Tanners Gate Drive, Suite 200
Florence, KY 41042

Direct Inquiries to:
(606) 282-2100
FAX: (606) 282-2118

ADDERALL® TABLETS   ℂ ℞

> AMPHETAMINES HAVE A HIGH POTENTIAL FOR ABUSE. ADMINISTRATION OF AMPHETAMINES FOR PROLONGED PERIODS OF TIME MAY LEAD TO DRUG DEPENDENCE AND MUST BE AVOIDED. PARTICULAR ATTENTION SHOULD BE PAID TO THE POSSIBILITY OF SUBJECTS OBTAINING AMPHETAMINES FOR NON-THERAPEUTIC USE OR DISTRIBUTION TO OTHERS, AND THE DRUGS SHOULD BE PRESCRIBED OR DISPENSED SPARINGLY.

DESCRIPTION

A single entity amphetamine product combining the neutral sulfate salts of dextroamphetamine and amphetamine, with the dextro isomer of amphetamine saccharate and d, l-amphetamine aspartate.
[See table below]
Inactive ingredients: sucrose, lactose, corn starch, acacia and magnesium stearate.
Colors: ADDERALL 5 mg and 10 mg contain FD & C Blue #1
ADDERALL 20 mg and 30 mg contain FD & C Yellow #6 as a color additive.

CLINICAL PHARMACOLOGY

Amphetamines are non-catecholamine sympathomimetic amines with CNS stimulant activity. Peripheral actions include elevation of systolic and diastolic blood pressures and weak bronchodilator and respiratory stimulant action.
There is neither specific evidence which clearly establishes the mechanism whereby amphetamine produces mental and behavioral effects in children, nor conclusive evidence regarding how these effects relate to the condition of the central nervous system.

INDICATIONS

Attention Deficit Disorder with Hyperactivity: Adderall is indicated as an integral part of a total treatment program which typically includes other remedial measures (psychological, educational, social) for a stabilizing effect in children with behavioral syndrome characterized by the following group of developmentally inappropriate symptoms: moderate to severe distractibility, short attention span, hyperactivity, emotional lability, and impulsivity. The diagnosis of this syndrome should not be made with finality when these symptoms are only of comparatively recent origin. Nonlocalizing (soft) neurological signs, learning disability and abnormal EEG may or may not be present, and a diagnosis of central nervous system dysfunction may or may not be warranted.

In Narcolepsy

CONTRAINDICATIONS

Advanced arteriosclerosis, symptomatic cardiovascular disease, moderate to severe hypertension, hyperthyroidism, known hypersensitivity or idiosyncrasy to the sympathomimetic amines, glaucoma.
Agitated states.
Patients with a history of drug abuse.
During or within 14 days following the administration of monoamine oxidase inhibitors (hypertensive crises may result).

WARNINGS

Clinical experience suggests that in psychotic children, administration of amphetamine may exacerbate symptoms of

---

behavior disturbance and thought disorder. Data are inadequate to determine whether chronic administration of amphetamine may be associated with growth inhibition; therefore, growth should be monitored during treatment.
Usage in Nursing Mothers: Amphetamines are excreted in human milk. Mothers taking amphetamines should be advised to refrain from nursing.

PRECAUTIONS

General: Caution is to be exercised in prescribing amphetamines for patients with even mild hypertension.
The least amount feasible should be prescribed or dispensed at one time in order to minimize the possibility of overdosage.
Information for Patients: Amphetamines may impair the ability of the patient to engage in potentially hazardous activities such as operating machinery or vehicles; the patient should therefore be cautioned accordingly.
Drug Interactions: *Acidifying agents*—Gastrointestinal acidifying agents (guanethidine, reserpine, glutamic acid HCl, ascorbic acid, fruit juices, etc.) lower absorption of amphetamines.
Urinary acidifying agents—(ammonium chloride, sodium acid phosphate, etc.) Increase the concentration of the ionized species of the amphetamine molecule, thereby increasing urinary excretion. Both groups of agents lower blood levels and efficacy of amphetamines.
Adrenergic blockers—Adrenergic blockers are inhibited by amphetamines.
Alkalinizing agents—Gastrointestinal alkalinizing agents (sodium bicarbonate, etc.) increase absorption of amphetamines. Urinary alkalinizing agents (acetazolamide, some thiazides) increase the concentration of the non-ionized species of the amphetamine molecule, thereby decreasing urinary excretion. Both groups of agents increase blood levels and therefore potentiate the actions of amphetamines.
Antidepressants, tricyclic—Amphetamines may enhance the activity of tricyclic or sympathomimetic agents; d-amphetamine with desipramine or protriptyline and possibly other tricyclics cause striking and sustained increases in the concentration of d-amphetamine in the brain; cardiovascular effects can be potentiated.
MAO inhibitors—MAOI antidepressants, as well as a metabolite of furazolidone, slow amphetamine metabolism. This slowing potentiates amphetamines, increasing their effect on the release of norepinephrine and other monoamines from adrenergic nerve endings; this can cause headaches and other signs of hypertensive crisis. A variety of neurological toxic effects and malignant hyperpyrexia can occur, sometimes with fatal results.
Antihistamines—Amphetamines may counteract the sedative effect of antihistamines.
Antihypertensives—Amphetamines may antagonize the hypotensive effects of antihypertensives.
Chlorpromazine—Chlorpromazine blocks dopamine and norepinephrine receptors, thus inhibiting the central stimulant effects of amphetamines, and can be used to treat amphetamine poisoning.
Ethosuximide—Amphetamines may delay intestinal absorption of ethosuximide.
Haloperidol—Haloperidol blocks dopamine receptors, thus inhibiting the central stimulant effects of amphetamines.
Lithium carbonate—The anorectic and stimulatory effects of amphetamines may be inhibited by lithium carbonate.
Meperidine—Amphetamines potentiate the analgesic effect of meperidine.
Methenamine therapy—Urinary excretion of amphetamines is increased, and efficacy is reduced, by acidifying agents used in methenamine therapy.
Norepinephrine—Amphetamines enhance the adrenergic effect of norepinephrine.
Phenobarbital—Amphetamines may delay intestinal absorption of phenobarbital; co-administration of phenobarbital may produce a synergistic anticonvulsant action.
Phenytoin—Amphetamines may delay intestinal absorption of phenytoin; co-administration of phenytoin may produce a synergistic anticonvulsant action.
Propoxyphene—In cases of propoxyphene overdosage, amphetamine CNS stimulation is potentiated and fatal convulsions can occur.
Veratrum alkaloids—Amphetamines inhibit the hypotensive effect of veratrum alkaloids.
Drug/Laboratory Test Interactions:
• Amphetamines can cause a significant elevation in plasma corticosteroid levels. This increase is greatest in the evening.

Continued on next page

EACH TABLET CONTAINS:	5 mg	10 mg	20 mg	30 mg
Dextroamphetamine Saccharate	1.25 mg	2.5 mg	5 mg	7.5 mg
Amphetamine Aspartate	1.25 mg	2.5 mg	5 mg	7.5 mg
Dextroamphetamine Sulfate USP	1.25 mg	2.5 mg	5 mg	7.5 mg
Amphetamine Sulfate USP	1.25 mg	2.5 mg	5 mg	7.5 mg
Total amphetamine base equivalence	3.13 mg	6.3 mg	12.6 mg	18.8 mg

Adderall—Cont.

- Amphetamines may interfere with urinary steroid determinations.

Carcinogenesis/Mutagenesis: Mutagenicity studies and long-term studies in animals to determine the carcinogenic potential of amphetamine, have not been performed.

Pregnancy—Teratogenic Effects: Pregnancy Category C. Amphetamine has been shown to have embryotoxic and teratogenic effects when administered to A/Jax mice and C57BL mice in doses approximately 41 times the maximum human dose. Embryotoxic effects were not seen in New Zealand white rabbits given the drug in doses 7 times the human dose nor in rats given 12.5 times the maximum human dose. While there are no adequate and well-controlled studies in pregnant women, there has been one report of severe congenital bony deformity, tracheoesophageal fistula, and anal atresia (vater association) in a baby born to a woman who took dextroamphetamine sulfate with lovastatin during the first trimester of pregnancy. Amphetamines should be used during pregnancy only if the potential benefit justifies the potential risk to the fetus.

Nonteratogenic Effects: Infants born to mothers dependent on amphetamines have an increased risk of premature delivery and low birth weight. Also, these infants may experience symptoms of withdrawal as demonstrated by dysphoria, including agitation, and significant lassitude.

Pediatric Use: Long-term effects of amphetamines in children have not been well established. Amphetamines are not recommended for use in children under 3 years of age with Attention Deficit Disorder with Hyperactivity described under INDICATIONS AND USAGE.

Amphetamines have been reported to exacerbate motor and phonic tics and Tourette's syndrome. Therefore, clinical evaluation for tics and Tourette's syndrome in children and their families should precede use of stimulant medications.

Drug treatment is not indicated in all cases of Attention Deficit Disorder with Hyperactivity and should be considered only in light of the complete history and evaluation of the child. The decision to prescribe amphetamines should depend on the physician's assessment of the chronicity and severity of the child's symptoms and their appropriateness for his/her age. Prescription should not depend solely on the presence of one or more of the behavioral characteristics. When these symptoms are associated with acute stress reactions, treatment with amphetamines is usually not indicated.

ADVERSE REACTIONS

Cardiovascular: Palpitations, tachycardia, elevation of blood pressure. There have been isolated reports of cardiomyopathy associated with chronic amphetamine use.

Central Nervous System: Psychotic episodes at recommended doses (rare), overstimulation, restlessness, dizziness, insomnia, euphoria, dyskinesia, dysphoria, tremor, headache, exacerbation of motor and phonic tics and Tourette's syndrome.

Gastrointestinal: Dryness of the mouth, unpleasant taste, diarrhea, constipation, other gastrointestinal disturbances. Anorexia and weight loss may occur as undesirable effects when amphetamines are used for other than the anorectic effect.

Allergic: Urticaria.

Endocrine: Impotence, changes in libido.

DRUG ABUSE AND DEPENDENCE

Dextroamphetamine sulfate is a Schedule II controlled substance.

Amphetamines have been extensively abused. Tolerance, extreme psychological dependence, and severe social disability have occurred. There are reports of patients who have increased the dosage to many times that recommended. Abrupt cessation following prolonged high dosage administration results in extreme fatigue and mental depression; changes are also noted on the sleep EEG. Manifestations of chronic intoxication with amphetamines include severe dermatoses, marked insomnia, irritability, hyperactivity, and personality changes. The most severe manifestation of chronic intoxication is psychosis, often clinically indistinguishable from schizophrenia. This is rare with oral amphetamines.

OVERDOSAGE

Individual patient response to amphetamines varies widely. While toxic symptoms occasionally occur as an idiosyncrasy at doses as low as 2 mg, they are rare with doses of less than 15 mg; 30 mg can produce severe reactions, yet doses of 400 to 500 mg are not necessarily fatal.

In rats, the oral LD50 of dextroamphetamine sulfate is 96.8 mg/kg.

Symptoms: Manifestations of acute overdosage with amphetamines include restlessness, tremor, hyperreflexia, rapid respiration, confusion, assaultiveness, hallucinations, panic states, hyperpyrexia and rhabdomyolysis.

Fatigue and depression usually follow the central stimulation. Cardiovascular effects include arrhythmias, hypertension or hypotension and circulatory collapse.

Gastrointestinal symptoms include nausea, vomiting, diarrhea, and abdominal cramps. Fatal poisoning is usually preceded by convulsions and coma.

Treatment: Consult with a Certified Poison Control Center for up to date guidance and advice. Management of acute amphetamine intoxication is largely symptomatic and includes gastric lavage, administration of activated charcoal, administration of a cathartic and sedation. Experience with hemodialysis or peritoneal dialysis is inadequate to permit recommendation in this regard. Acidification of the urine increases amphetamine excretion, but is believed to increase risk of acute renal failure if myoglobinuria is present. If acute, severe hypertension complicates amphetamine overdosage, administration of intravenous phentolamine has been suggested. However, a gradual drop in blood pressure will usually result when sufficient sedation has been achieved. Chlorpromazine antagonizes the central stimulant effects of amphetamines and can be used to treat amphetamine intoxication.

DOSAGE AND ADMINISTRATION

Regardless of indication, amphetamines should be administered at the lowest effective dosage and dosage should be individually adjusted. Late evening doses should be avoided because of the resulting insomnia.

Attention Deficit Disorder with Hyperactivity: Not recommended for children under 3 years of age. In children from 3 to 5 years of age, start with 2.5 mg daily; daily dosage may be raised in increments of 2.5 mg at weekly intervals until optimal response is obtained.

In children 6 years of age and older, start with 5 mg once or twice daily; daily dosage may be raised in increments of 5 mg at weekly intervals until optimal response is obtained. Only in rare cases will it be necessary to exceed a total of 40 mg per day. Give first dose on awakening; additional doses (1 or 2) at intervals of 4 to 6 hours.

Where possible, drug administration should be interrupted occasionally to determine if there is a recurrence of behavioral symptoms sufficient to require continued therapy.

Narcolepsy: Usual dose 5 mg to 60 mg per day in divided doses, depending on the individual patient response.

Narcolepsy seldom occurs in children under 12 years of age; however, when it does, dextroamphetamine sulfate, may be used. The suggested initial dose for patients aged 6–12 is 5 mg daily; daily dose may be raised in increments of 5 mg at weekly intervals until optimal response is obtained. In patients 12 years of age and older, start with 10 mg daily; daily dosage may be raised in increments of 10 mg at weekly intervals until optimal response is obtained. If bothersome adverse reactions appear (e.g., insomnia or anorexia), dosage should be reduced. Give first dose on awakening; additional doses (1 or 2) at intervals of 4 to 6 hours.

HOW SUPPLIED

ADDERALL® 5 mg: Blue double-scored tablet, debossed "AD" on one side and "5" on the other side (NDC 58521-031-01)

ADDERALL® 10 mg: Blue double-scored tablet, debossed "AD" on one side and "10" on the other side (NDC 58521-032-01)

ADDERALL® 20 mg: Orange double-scored tablet, debossed "AD" on one side and "20" on the other side (NDC 58521-033-01)

ADDERALL® 30 mg: Orange double-scored tablet, debossed "AD" on one side and "30" on the other side (NDC 58521-034-01)

In bottles of 100 tablets.

Dispense in a tight, light-resistant container as defined in the USP.

Store at controlled room temperature 15°–30°C (59°–86°F).

Rx only

Shire Richwood Inc.
Florence, KY 41042
MG #10185 Revised: June 1998

Shown in Product Identification Guide, page 338

CARBATROL® ℞

[căr-bă 'trōl]

(carbamazepine extended-release capsules)
200 mg and 300 mg

Prescribing information

> **WARNING**
> APLASTIC ANEMIA AND AGRANULOCYTOSIS HAVE BEEN REPORTED IN ASSOCIATION WITH THE USE OF CARBAMAZEPINE. DATA FROM A POPULATION-BASED CASE-CONTROL STUDY DEMONSTRATE THAT THE RISK OF DEVELOPING THESE REACTIONS IS 5–8 TIMES GREATER THAN IN THE GENERAL POPULATION. HOWEVER, THE OVERALL RISK OF THESE REACTIONS IN THE UNTREATED GENERAL POPULATION IS LOW. APPROXIMATELY SIX PATIENTS PER ONE MILLION POPULATION PER YEAR FOR AGRANULOCYTOSIS AND TWO PATIENTS PER ONE MILLION POPULATION PER YEAR FOR APLASTIC ANEMIA.
> ALTHOUGH REPORTS OF TRANSIENT OR PERSISTENT DECREASED PLATELET OR WHITE BLOOD CELL COUNTS ARE NOT UNCOMMON IN ASSOCIATION WITH THE USE OF CARBAMAZEPINE, DATA ARE NOT AVAILABLE TO ESTIMATE ACCURATELY THEIR INCIDENCE OR OUTCOME. HOWEVER, THE VAST MAJORITY OF THE CASES OF LEUKOPENIA HAVE NOT PROGRESSED TO THE MORE SERIOUS CONDITIONS OF APLASTIC ANEMIA OR AGRANULOCYTOSIS.
> BECAUSE OF THE VERY LOW INCIDENCE OF AGRANULOCYTOSIS AND APLASTIC ANEMIA, THE VAST MAJORITY OF MINOR HEMATOLOGIC CHANGES OBSERVED IN MONITORING OF PATIENTS ON CARBAMAZEPINE ARE UNLIKELY TO SIGNAL THE OCCURRENCE OF EITHER ABNORMALITY. NONETHELESS, COMPLETE PRETREATMENT HEMATOLOGICAL TESTING SHOULD BE OBTAINED AS A BASELINE. IF A PATIENT IN THE COURSE OF TREATMENT EXHIBITS LOW OR DECREASED WHITE BLOOD CELL OR PLATELET COUNTS, THE PATIENT SHOULD BE MONITORED CLOSELY. DISCONTINUATION OF THE DRUG SHOULD BE CONSIDERED IF ANY EVIDENCE OF SIGNIFICANT BONE MARROW DEPRESSION DEVELOPS.

Before prescribing Carbatrol, the physician should be thoroughly familiar with the details of this prescribing information, particularly regarding use with other drugs, especially those which accentuate toxicity potential.

DESCRIPTION

CARBATROL* is an anticonvulsant and specific analgesic for trigeminal neuralgia, available for oral administration as 200 mg and 300 mg extended-release capsules of Carbamazepine, USP. Carbamazepine is a white to off-white powder, practically insoluble in water and soluble in alcohol and in acetone. Its molecular weight is 236.27. Its chemical name is 5H-dibenz[b,f]azepine-5-carboxamide, and its structural formula is:

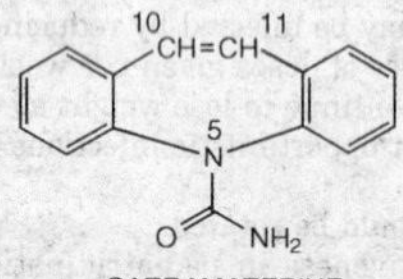

CARBAMAZEPINE

Carbatrol is a multi-component capsule formulation consisting of three different types of beads: immediate-release beads, extended-release beads, and enteric-release beads. The three bead types are combined in a specific ratio to provide twice daily dosing of Carbatrol.

Inactive ingredients: citric acid, colloidal silicon dioxide, lactose monohydrate, microcrystalline cellulose, polyethylene glycol, povidone, sodium lauryl sulfate, talc, triethyl citrate and other ingredients.

The 200 mg capsule shells contain gelatin-NF, FD&C Red #3, FD&C Yellow #6, Yellow Iron Oxide, FD&C Blue #2, and titanium dioxide, and are imprinted with white ink; and the 300 mg capsule shells contain gelatin-NF, FD&C Blue #2, FD&C Yellow #6, Red Iron Oxide, Yellow Iron Oxide, and titanium dioxide, and are imprinted with white ink.

CLINICAL PHARMACOLOGY

In controlled clinical trials, carbamazepine has been shown to be effective in the treatment of psychomotor and grand mal seizures, as well as trigeminal neuralgia.

Mechanism of Action

Carbamazepine has demonstrated anticonvulsant properties in rats and mice with electrically and chemically induced seizures. It appears to act by reducing polysynaptic responses and blocking the post-tetanic potentiation. Carbamazepine greatly reduces or abolishes pain induced by stimulation of the infraorbital nerve in cats and rats. It depresses thalamic potential and bulbar and polysynaptic reflexes, including the inguomandibular reflex in cats. Carbamazepine is chemically unrelated to other anticonvulsants or other drugs used to control the pain of trigeminal neuralgia. The mechanism of action remains unknown.

The principal metabolite of carbamazepine, carbamazepine-10,11-epoxide, has anticonvulsant activity as demonstrated in several *in vivo* animal models of seizures. Though clinical activity for the epoxide has been postulated, the significance of its activity with respect to the safety and efficacy of carbamazepine has not been established.

Pharmacokinetics

Carbamazepine (CBZ): Taken every 12 hours, carbamazepine extended-release capsules provide steady state plasma

levels comparable to immediate-release carbamazepine tablets given every 6 hours, when administered at the same total mg daily dose. Following a single 200 mg oral extended-release dose of carbamazepine, peak plasma concentration was 1.9 ± 0.3 μg/mL and the time to reach the peak was 19 ± 7 hours. Following chronic administration (800 mg every 12 hours), the peak levels were 11.0 ± 2.5 μg/mL and the time to reach the peak was 5.9 ± 1.8 hours. The pharmacokinetics of extended-release carbamazepine is linear over the single dose range of 200–800 mg.

Carbamazepine is 76% bound to plasma proteins. Carbamazepine is primarily metabolized in the liver. Cytochrome P450 3A4 was identified as the major isoform responsible for the formation of carbamazepine-10,11-epoxide. Since carbamazepine induces its own metabolism, the half-life is also variable. Following a single extended-release dose of carbamazepine, the average half-life range from 35–40 hours and 12–17 hours on repeated dosing. The apparent oral clearance following a single dose was 25 ± 5 mL/min and following multiple dosing was 80 ± 30 mL/min.

After oral administration of ^{14}C-carbamazepine, 72% of the administered radioactivity was found in the urine and 28% in the feces. This urinary radioactivity was composed largely of hydroxylated and conjugated metabolites, with only 3% of unchanged carbamazepine.

Carbamazepine-10,11-epoxide (CBZ-E): Carbamazepine-10,11-epoxide is considered to be an active metabolite of carbamazepine. Following a single 200 mg oral extended-release dose of carbamazepine, the peak plasma concentration of carbamazepine-10,11-epoxide was 0.11 ± 0.012 μg/mL and the time to reach the peak was 36 ± 6 hours. Following chronic administration of a extended-release dose of carbamazepine (800 mg every 12 hours), the peak levels of carbamazepine-10,11-epoxide were 2.2 ± 0.9 μg/mL and the time to reach the peak was 14 ± 8 hours. The plasma half-life of carbamazepine-10,11-epoxide following administration of carbamazepine is 34 ± 9 hours. Following a single oral dose of extended-release carbamazepine (200-800 mg) the AUC and C_{max} of carbamazepine-10,11-epoxide were less than 10% of carbamazepine. Following multiple dosing of extended-release carbamazepine (800–1600 mg daily for 14 days), the AUC and C_{max} of carbamazepine-10, 11-epoxide were dose related, ranging from 15.7 μg.hr/mL and 1.5 μg/mL at 800 mg/day to 32.6 μg.hr/mL and 3.2 μg/mL at 1600 mg/day, respectively, and were less than 30% of carbamazepine. Carbamazepine-10,11-epoxide is 50% bound to plasma proteins.

Food Effect: A high fat meal diet increased the rate of absorption of a single 400 mg dose (mean T_{max} was reduced from 24 hours, in the fasting state, to 14 hours and C_{max} increased from 3.2 to 4.3 μg/mL) but not the extent (AUC) of absorption. The elimination half-life remains unchanged between fed and fasting state. The multiple dose study conducted in the fed state showed that the steady-state C_{max} values were within the therapeutic concentration range. The pharmacokinetic profile of extended-release carbamazepine was similar when given by sprinkling the beads over applesauce compared to the intact capsule administered in the fasted state.

* Registered trademark of Shire Richwood Inc.

Special Populations

Hepatic Dysfunction: The effect of hepatic impairment on the pharmacokinetics of carbamazepine is not known. However, given that carbamazepine is primarily metabolized in the liver, it is prudent to proceed with caution in patients with hepatic dysfunction.

Renal Dysfunction: The effect of renal impairment on the pharmacokinetics of carbamazepine is not known.

Gender: No difference in the mean AUC and C_{max} of carbamazepine and carbamazepine-10,11-epoxide was found between males and females.

Age: Carbamazepine is more rapidly metabolized to carbamazepine-10,11-epoxide in young children than adults. In children below the age of 15, there is an inverse relationship between CBZ-E/CBZ ratio and increasing age.

Race: No information is available on the effect of race on the pharmacokinetics of carbamazepine.

INDICATIONS AND USAGE

Epilepsy

Carbatrol is indicated for use as an anticonvulsant drug. Evidence supporting efficacy of carbamazepine as an anticonvulsant was derived from active drug-controlled studies that enrolled patients with the following seizure types:

1. Partial seizures with complex symptomatology (psychomotor, temporal lobe). Patients with these seizures appear to show greater improvements than those with other types.
2. Generalized tonic-clonic seizures (grand mal).
3. Mixed seizure patterns which include the above, or other partial or generalized seizures. Absence seizures (petit mal) do not appear to be controlled by carbamazepine (see PRECAUTIONS, General).

Trigeminal Neuralgia

Carbatrol is indicated in the treatment of the pain associated with true trigeminal neuralgia. Beneficial results have also been reported in glossopharyngeal neuralgia. This drug is not a simple analgesic and should not be used for the relief of trivial aches or pains.

CONTRAINDICATIONS

Carbamazepine should not be used in patients with a history of previous bone marrow depression, hypersensitivity to the drug, or known sensitivity to any of the tricyclic compounds, such as amitriptyline, desipramine, imipramine, protriptyline and nortriptyline. Likewise, on theoretical grounds its use with monoamine oxidase inhibitors is not recommended. Before administration of carbamazepine, MAO inhibitors should be discontinued for a minimum of 14 days, or longer if the clinical situation permits.

WARNINGS

Usage in Pregnancy

Carbamazepine can cause fetal harm when administered to a pregnant women.

Epidemiological data suggest that there may be an association between the use of carbamazepine during pregnancy and congenital malformations, including spina bifida. The prescribing physician will wish to weigh the benefits of therapy against the risks in treating or counseling women of childbearing potential. If this drug is used during pregnancy, or if the patient becomes pregnant while taking this drug, the patient should be apprised of the potential hazard to the fetus.

Retrospective case reviews suggest that, compared with monotherapy, there may be a higher prevalence of teratogenic effects associated with the use of anticonvulsants in combination therapy.

In humans, transplacental passage of carbamazepine is rapid (30–60 minutes), and the drug is accumulated in the fetal tissues, with higher levels found in liver and kidney than in brain and lung.

Carbamazepine has been shown to have adverse effects in reproduction studies in rats when given orally in dosages 10–25 times the maximum human daily dosage (MHDD) of 1200 mg on a mg/kg basis or 1.5–4 times the MHDD on a mg/m^2 basis. In rat teratology studies, 2 of 135 offspring showed kinked ribs at 250 mg/kg and 4 of 119 offspring at 650 mg/kg showed other anomalies (cleft palate, 1; talipes, 1; anophthalmos, 2). In reproduction studies in rats, nursing offspring demonstrated a lack of weight gain and an unkempt appearance at a maternal dosage level of 200 mg/kg.

Antiepileptic drugs should not be discontinued abruptly in patients in whom the drug is administered to prevent major seizures because of the strong possibility of precipitating status epilepticus with attendant hypoxia and threat to life. In individual cases where the severity and frequency of the seizure disorder are such that removal of medication does not pose a serious threat to the patient, discontinuation of the drug may be considered prior to and during pregnancy, although it cannot be said with any confidence that even minor seizures do not pose some hazard to the developing embryo or fetus.

Tests to detect defects using current accepted procedures should be considered a part of routine prenatal care in childbearing women receiving carbamazepine.

General

Patients with a history of adverse hematologic reaction to any drug may be particularly at risk.

Severe dematologic reactions, including toxic epidermal necrolysis (Lyell's syndrome) and Stevens-Johnson syndrome have been reported with carbamazepine. These reactions have been extremely rare. However, a few fatalities have been reported.

Carbamazepine has shown mild anticholinergic activity; therefore, patients with increased intraocular pressure should be closely observed during therapy.

Because of the relationship of the drug to others tricyclic compounds, the possibility of activation of a latent psychosis and, in elderly patients, of confusion or agitation should be considered.

PRECAUTIONS

General

Before initiating therapy, a detailed history and physical examination should be made.

Carbamazepine should be used with caution in patients with a mixed seizure disorder that includes atypical absence seizures, since in these patients carbamazepine has been associated with increased frequency of generalized convulsions (see INDICATIONS AND USAGE).

Therapy should be prescribed only after critical benefit-to-risk appraisal in patients with a history of cardiac, hepatic, or renal damage; adverse hematologic reaction to other drugs; or interrupted courses of therapy with carbamazepine.

Information for Patients

Patients should be made aware of the early toxic signs and symptoms of a potential hematologic problem such as fever, sore throat, rash, ulcers in the mouth, easy bruising, petechial or purpuric hemorrhage, and should be advised to report to the physician immediately if any such signs or symptoms appear.

Since dizziness and drowsiness may occur, patients should be cautioned about the hazards of operating machinery or automobiles or engaging in other potentially dangerous tasks.

If necessary, the Carbatrol capsules can be opened and the contents sprinkled over food, such as a teaspoon of applesauce or other similar food products. Carbatrol capsules or their contents should not be crushed or chewed.

Laboratory Tests

Complete pretreatment blood counts, including platelets and possible reticulocytes and serum iron, should be obtained as a baseline. If a patient in the course of treatment exhibits low or decreased white blood cell or platelet counts, the patient should be monitored closely. Discontinuation of the drug should be considered if any evidence of significant bone marrow depression develops.

Baseline and periodic evaluations of liver function, particularly in patients with a history of liver disease, must be performed during treatment with this drug since liver damage may occur. The drug should be discontinued immediately in cases of aggravated liver dysfunction or active liver disease.

Baseline and periodic eye examinations, including slit-lamp, funduscopy, and tonometry, are recommended since many phenothiazines and related drugs have been shown to cause eye changes.

Baseline and periodic complete urinalysis and BUN determinations are recommended for patients treated with this agent because of observed renal dysfunction.

Monitoring of blood levels (see CLINICAL PHARMACOLOGY) has increased the efficacy and safety of anticonvulsants. This monitoring may be particularly useful in cases of dramatic increase in seizure frequency and for verification of compliance. In addition, measurement of drug serum levels may aid in determining the cause of toxicity when more than one medication is being used.

Thyroid function tests have been reported to show decreased values with carbamazepine administered alone.

Hyponatremia has been reported in association with carbamazepine use, either alone or in combination with other drugs.

Interference with some pregnancy tests has been reported.

Drug Interactions

Clinically meaningful drug interactions have occurred with concomitant medications and include but are not limited to the following:

Agents that may affect carbamazepine plasma levels:

CYP 3A4 inhibitors inhibit carbamazepine metabolism and can thus increase plasma carbamazepine levels. Drugs that have been shown, or would be expected to increase plasma carbamazepine levels include:

cimetidine, danazol, diltiazem, macrolides, erythromycin, troleandomycin, clarithromycin, fluoxetine, loratadine, terfenadine, isoniazid, niacinamide, nicotinamide, propoxyphene, ketoconazole, itraconazole, verapamil, valproate.*

CYP 3A4 inducers can increase the rate of carbamazepine metabolism and can thus decrease plasma carbamazepine levels. Drugs that have been shown, or would be expected, to decrease plasma carbamazepine levels include:

cisplatin, doxorubicin HCL, felbamate, rifampin*, phenobarbital, phenytoin, primidone, theophylline.

*increased levels of the active 10, 11-epoxide

Effect of carbamazepine on plasma levels of concomitant agents:

Carbatrol increases levels of clomipramine HCL, phenytoin and primidone.

Carbatrol induces hepatic CYP activity. Carbatrol causes, or would be expected to cause decreased levels of the following:

acetaminophen, alprazolam, clonazepam, clozapine, dicumarol, doxycycline, ethosuximide, haloperidol, methsuximide, oral contraceptives, phensuximide, phenytoin, theophylline, valproate, warfarin.

The doses of these drugs may therefore have to be increased when carbamazepine is added to the therapeutic regimen.

Concomitant administration of carbamazepine and lithium may increase the risk of neurotoxic side effects. Alterations of thyroid function have been reported in combination therapy with other anticonvulsant medications.

Breakthrough bleeding has been reported among patients receiving concomitant oral contraceptives and their reliability may be adversely affected.

Carcinogenesis, Mutagenesis, Impairment of Fertility

Administration of carbamazepine to Sprague-Dawley rats for two years in the diet at doses of 25, 75, and 250 mg/kg/day (low dose approximately 0.2 times the maximum human daily dose of 1200 mg on a mg/m^2 basis), resulted in a dose-related increase in the incidence of hepatocellular tumors in females and of benign interstitial cell adenomas in the testes of males.

Carbamazepine must, therefore, be considered to be carcinogenic in Sprague-Dawley rats. Bacterial and mammalian mutagenicity studies using carbamazepine produce nega-

Continued on next page

Carbatrol—Cont.

tive results. The significance of these findings relative to the use of carbamazepine in humans is, at present, unknown.

Usage in Pregnancy
Pregnancy Category D (See WARNINGS).

Labor and Delivery
The effect of carbamazepine on human labor and delivery is unknown.

Nursing Mothers
Carbamazepine and its epoxide metabolite are transferred to breast milk and during lactation. The concentrations of carbamazepine and its epoxide metabolite are approximately 50% of the maternal plasma concentration. Because of the potential for serious adverse reactions in nursing infants from carbamazepine, a decision should be made whether to discontinue nursing or to discontinue the drug, taking into account the importance of the drug to the mother.

Pediatric Use
Substantial evidence of carbamazepine effectiveness for use in the management of children with epilepsy (see INDICATIONS for specific seizure types) is derived from clinical investigations performed in adults and from studies in several *in vitro* systems which support the conclusion that (1) the pathogenic mechanisms underlying seizure propagation are essentially identical in adults and children, and (2) the mechanism of action of carbamazepine in treating seizures is essentially identical in adults and children.

Taken as a whole, this information supports a conclusion that the generally acceptable therapeutic range of total carbamazepine in plasma (i.e., 4–12 µg/mL) is the same in children and adults.

The evidence assembled was primarily obtained from short-term use of carbamazepine. The safety of carbamazepine in children has been systematically studied up to 6 months. No longer term data from clinical trials is available.

Geriatric Use
No systematic studies in geriatric patients have been conducted.

ADVERSE REACTIONS

General: If adverse reactions are of such severity that the drug must be discontinued, the physician must be aware that abrupt discontinuation of any anticonvulsant drug in a responsive patient with epilepsy may lead to seizures or even status epilepticus with its life-threatening hazards.

The most severe adverse reactions previously observed with carbamazepine were reported in the hemopoietic system (see BOX WARNING), the skin, and the cardiovascular system.

The most frequently observed adverse reactions, particularly during the initial phases of therapy, are dizziness, drowsiness, unsteadiness, nausea, and vomiting. To minimize the possibility of such reactions, therapy should be initiated at the lowest dosage recommended.

The following additional adverse reactions were previously reported with carbamazepine:

Hemopoietic System: Aplastic anemia, agranulocytosis, pancytopenia, bone marrow depression, thrombocytopenia, leukopenia, leukocytosis, eosinophilia, acute intermittent porphyria.

Skin: Pruritic and erythematous rashes, urticaria, toxic epidermal necrolysis (Lyell's syndrome) (see WARNINGS), Stevens-Johnson syndrome (see WARNINGS), photosensitivity reactions, alterations in skin pigmentation, exfoliative dermatitis, erythema multiforme and nodosum, purpura, aggravation of disseminated lupus erythematosus, alopecia, and diaphoresis. In certain cases, discontinuation of therapy may be necessary. Isolated cases of hirsutism have been reported, but a causal relationship is not clear.

Cardiovascular System: Congestive heart failure, edema, aggravation of hypertension, hypotension, syncope and collapse, aggravation of coronary artery disease, arrhythmias and AV block, thrombophlebitis, thromboembolism, and adenopathy or lymphadenopathy. Some of these cardiovascular complications have resulted in fatalities. Myocardial infarction has been associated with other tricyclic compounds.

Liver: Abnormalities in liver function tests, cholestatic and hepatocellular jaundice, hepatitis.

Respiratory System: Pulmonary hypersensitivity characterized by fever, dyspnea, pneumonitis, or pneumonia.

Genitourinary System: Urinary frequency, acute urinary retention, oliguria with elevated blood pressure, azotemia, renal failure, and impotence. Albuminuria, glycosuria, elevated BUN, and microscopic deposits in the urine have also been reported.

Testicular atrophy occurred in rats receiving carbamazepine orally from 4–52 weeks at dosage levels of 50–400 mg/kg/day. Additionally, rats receiving carbamazepine in the diet for 2 years at dosage levels of 25, 75, and 250 mg/kg/day had a dose-related incidence of testicular atrophy and aspermatogenesis. In dogs, it produced a brownish discoloration, presumably a metabolite, in the urinary bladder at dosage levels of 50 mg/kg/day and higher. Relevance of these findings to humans is unknown.

Nervous System: Dizziness, drowsiness, disturbances of coordination, confusion, headache, fatigue, blurred vision, visual hallucinations, transient diplopia, oculomotor disturbances, nystagmus, speech disturbances, abnormal involuntary movements, peripheral neuritis and paresthesias, depression with agitation, talkativeness, tinnitus, and hyperacusis.

There have been reports of associated paralysis and other symptoms of cerebral arterial insufficiency, but the exact relationship of these reactions to the drug has not been established.

Isolated cases of neuroleptic malignant syndrome have been reported with concomitant use of psychotropic drugs.

Digestive System: Nausea, vomiting, gastric distress and abdominal pain, diarrhea, constipation, anorexia, and dryness of the mouth and pharynx, including glossitis and stomatitis.

Eyes: Scattered punctate cortical lens opacities, as well as conjunctivitis, have been reported. Although a direct causal relationship has not been established, many phenothiazines and related drugs have been shown to cause eye changes.

Musculoskeletal System: Aching joints and muscles, and leg cramps.

Metabolism: Fever and chills, inappropriate antidiuretic hormone (ADH) secretion syndrome has been reported. Cases of frank water intoxication, with decreased serum sodium (hyponatremia) and confusion have been reported in association with carbamazepine use (see PRECAUTIONS, Laboratory Tests). Decreased levels of plasma calcium have been reported.

Other: Isolated cases of a lupus erythematosus-like syndrome have been reported. There have been occasional reports of elevated levels of cholesterol, HDL cholesterol, and triglycerides in patients taking anticonvulsants.

A case of aseptic meningitis, accompanied by myoclonus and peripheral eosinophilia, has been reported in a patient taking carbamazepine in combination with other medications. The patient was successfully dechallenged, and the meningitis reappeared upon rechallenge with carbamazepine.

DRUG ABUSE AND DEPENDENCE

No evidence of abuse potential has been associated with carbamazepine, nor is there evidence of psychological or physical dependence in humans.

OVERDOSAGE

Acute Toxicity
Lowest known lethal dose: adults, >60 g (39-year-old man). Highest known doses survived: adults, 30 g (31-year-old woman); children, 10 g (6-year-old boy); small children, 5 g (3-year-old girl).

Oral LD_{50} in animals (mg/kg): mice, 1100–3750; rats, 3850–4025; rabbits, 1500–2680; guinea pigs, 920.

Signs and Symptoms
The first signs and symptoms appear after 1–3 hours. Neuromuscular disturbances are the most prominent. Cardiovascular disorders are generally milder, and severe cardiac complications occur only when very high doses (>60 g) have been ingested.

Respiration: Irregular breathing, respiratory depression.

Cardiovascular System: Tachycardia, hypotension or hypertension, shock, conduction disorders.

Nervous System and Muscles: Impairment of consciousness ranging in severity to deep coma. Convulsions, especially in small children. Motor restlessness, muscular twitching, tremor, athetoid movements, opisthotonos, ataxia, drowsiness, dizziness, mydriasis, nystagmus, adiadochokinesia, ballism, psychomotor disturbances, dysmetria. Initial hyperreflexia, followed by hyporeflexia.

Gastrointestinal Tract: Nausea, vomiting.

Kidneys and Bladder: Anuria or oliguria, urinary retention.

Laboratory Findings: Isolated instances of overdosage have included leukocytosis, reduced leukocyte count, glycosuria, and acetonuria. EEG may show dysrhythmias.

Combined Poisoning: When alcohol, tricyclic antidepressants, barbiturates, or hydantoins are taken at the same time, the signs and symptoms of acute poisoning with carbamazepine may be aggravated or modified.

Treatment
The prognosis in cases of severe poisoning is critically dependent upon prompt elimination of the drug, which may be achieved by inducing vomiting, irrigating the stomach, and by taking appropriate steps to diminish absorption. If these measures cannot be implemented without risk on the spot, the patient should be transferred at once to a hospital, while ensuring that vital functions are safeguarded. There is no specific antidote.

Elimination of the Drug: Induction of vomiting.
Gastric lavage. Even when more than 4 hours have elapsed following ingestion of the drug, the stomach should be repeatedly irrigated, especially if the patient has also consumed alcohol.

Measures to Reduce Absorption: Activated charcoal, laxatives.

Measures to Accelerate Elimination: Forced diuresis.

Dialysis is indicated only in severe poisoning associated with renal failure. Replacement transfusion is indicated in severe poisoning in small children.

Respiratory Depression: Keep the airways free; resort, if necessary, to endotracheal intubation, artificial respiration, and administration of oxygen.

Hypotension, Shock: Keep the patient's legs raised and administer a plasma expander. If blood pressure fails to rise despite measures taken to increase plasma volume, use of vasoactive substances should be considered.

Convulsions: Diazepam or barbiturates.

Warning: Diazepam or barbiturates may aggravate respiratory depression (especially in children), hypotension, and coma. However, barbiturates should not be used if drugs that inhibit monoamine oxidase have also been taken by the patient either in overdosage or in recent therapy (within 1 week).

Surveillance: Respiration, cardiac function (ECG monitoring), blood pressure, body temperature, pupillary reflexes, and kidney and bladder function should be monitored for several days.

Treatment of Blood Count Abnormalities: If evidence of significant bone marrow depression develops, the following recommendations are suggested: (1) stop the drug, (2) perform daily CBC, platelet, and reticulocyte counts, (3) do a bone marrow aspiration and trephine biopsy immediately and repeat with sufficient frequency to monitor recovery. Special periodic studies might be helpful as follows: (1) white cell and platelet antibodies, (2) ^{59}Fe-ferrokinetic studies, (3) peripheral blood cell typing, (4) cytogenetic studies on marrow and peripheral blood, (5) bone marrow culture studies for colony-forming units, (6) hemoglobin electrophoresis for A_2 and F hemoglobin, and (7) serum folic acid and B_{12} levels.

A fully developed aplastic anemia will require appropriate, intensive monitoring and therapy, for which specialized consultation should be sought.

DOSAGE AND ADMINISTRATION

Monitoring of blood levels has increased the efficacy and safety of anticonvulsants (see PRECAUTIONS, Laboratory Tests). Dosage should be adjusted to the needs of the individual patients. A low initial daily dosage with gradual increase is advised. As soon as adequate control is achieved, the dosage may be reduced very gradually to the minimum effective level. The Carbatrol capsules may be opened and the beads sprinkled over food, such as a teaspoon of applesauce or other similar food products if this method of administration is preferred. Carbatrol capsules or their contents should not be crushed or chewed. Carbatrol can be taken with or without meals.

Carbatrol is an extended-release formulation for twice a day administration. When converting patients from immediate release carbamazepine to Carbatrol extended-release capsules, the same total daily mg dose of carbamazepine should be administered.

Epilepsy (see INDICATIONS AND USAGE)

Adults and children over 12 years of age. Initial: 200 mg twice daily. Increase at weekly intervals by adding up to 200 mg/day until the optimal response is obtained. Dosage generally should not exceed 1000 mg per day in children 12-15 years of age, and 1200 mg daily in patients above 15 years of age. Doses up to 1600 mg daily have been used in adults.

Maintenance: Adjust dosage to the minimum effective level, usually 800–1200 mg daily.

Children under 12 years of age: Children taking total daily dosages of immediate-release carbamazepine of 400 mg or greater may be converted to the same total daily dosage of Carbatrol extended-release capsules, using a twice daily regimen. Ordinarily, optimal clinical response is achieved at daily doses below 35 mg/kg. If satisfactory clinical response has not been achieved, plasma levels should be measured to determine whether or not they are in the therapeutic range. No recommendation regarding the safety of Carbatrol for use at doses above 35 mg/kg/24 hours can be made.

Combination Therapy: Carbatrol may be used alone or with other anticonvulsants. When added to existing anticonvulsant therapy, the drug should be added gradually while the other anticonvulsants are maintained or gradually decreased, except phenytoin, which may have to be increased (see PRECAUTIONS, Drug Interactions and Pregnancy Category D).

Trigeminal Neuralgia (see INDICATIONS AND USAGE)

Initial: On the first day, start with one 200 mg capsule. This daily dose may be increased by up to 200 mg/day every 12 hours only as needed to achieve freedom from pain. Do not exceed 1200 mg daily.

Maintenance: Control of pain can be maintained in most patients with 400–800 mg daily. However, some patients may be maintained on as little as 200 mg daily, while others may require as much as 1200 mg daily. At least once every 3 months throughout the treatment period, attempts should be made to reduce the dose to the minimum effective level or even to discontinue the drug.

HOW SUPPLIED

Carbatrol (carbamazepine extended-release capsules) is supplied in two dosage strengths.

200 mg-Two-piece hard gelatin capsule (light gray opaque body with bluish green opaque cap) printed with the Shire logo in white ink.

Supplied in bottles of 120 .... NDC 58521-172-12

300 mg-Two-piece hard gelatin capsule (black opaque body with bluish green opaque cap) printed with the Shire logo in white ink.

Supplied in bottles of 120 .... NDC 58521-173-12

Store at controlled room temperature 15–25°C (59–77°F). Protect from light and moisture. Dispense in tight, light-resistant container as defined in USP.

Rx only.

Manufactured for:
Shire Richwood Inc.
Florence, KY 41042
1-800-536-7878

B5684 Rev. 7/98

Shown in Product Identification Guide, page 338

DEXTROSTAT® Ⓒ℞

Dextroamphetamine Sulfate Tablets, USP

> **WARNING**
> AMPHETAMINES HAVE A HIGH POTENTIAL FOR ABUSE, ADMINISTRATION OF AMPHETAMINES FOR PROLONGED PERIODS OF TIME MAY LEAD TO DRUG DEPENDENCE AND MUST BE AVOIDED. PARTICULAR ATTENTION SHOULD BE PAID TO THE POSSIBILITY OF SUBJECTS OBTAINING AMPHETAMINES FOR NONTHERAPEUTIC USE OR DISTRIBUTION TO OTHERS, AND THE DRUGS SHOULD BE PRESCRIBED OR DISPENSED SPARINGLY.

DESCRIPTION

DextroStat® (dextroamphetamine sulfate) is the dextro isomer of the compound *d,l*-amphetamine sulfate, a sympathomimetic amine of the amphetamine group. Chemically, dextroamphetamine is *d*-alpha-methylphenethylamine, and is present in all forms of DextroStat® as the neutral sulfate. It has a chemical formula of $(C_9H_{13}N)_2 \cdot H_2SO_4$ and a molecular weight of 368.50.

Structural Formula:

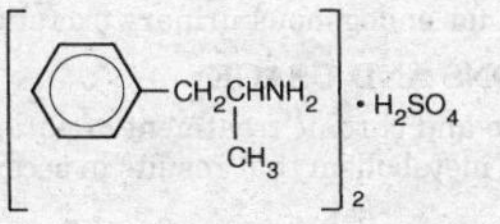

Each round, yellow, scored tablet contains dextroamphetamine sulfate USP, 5 mg or 10 mg. Each tablet also contains the following inactive ingredients: acacia, corn starch, lactose monohydrate, magnesium stearate, sucrose. 10 mg tablet contains sodium starch glycolate. 5 mg and 10 mg tablets contain FD&C Yellow #5 (tartrazine).

CLINICAL PHARMACOLOGY

Amphetamines are non-catecholamine, sympathomimetic amines with CNS stimulant activity. Peripheral actions include elevations of systolic and diastolic blood pressures and weak bronchodilator and respiratory stimulant action.

There is neither specific evidence which clearly establishes the mechanism whereby amphetamines produce mental and behavioral effects in children, nor conclusive evidence regarding how these effects relate to the condition of the central nervous system.

Pharmacokinetics

The single ingestion of two 5 mg tablets by healthy volunteers produced an average peak dextroamphetamine blood level of 29.2 ng/mL at 2 hours post-administration. The average half-life was 10.25 hours. The average urinary recovery was 45% in 48 hours.

INDICATIONS AND USAGE

Dextroamphetamine sulfate tablets are indicated:

1. **In Narcolepsy.**
2. **In Attention Deficit Disorder with Hyperactivity,** as an integral part of a total treatment program which typically includes other remedial measures (psychological, educational, social) for a stabilizing effect in pediatric patients (ages 3 to 16 years) with a behavioral syndrome characterized by the following group of developmentally inappropriate symptoms: moderate to severe distractibility, short attention span, hyperactivity, emotional lability, and impulsivity. The diagnosis of this syndrome should not be made with finality when these symptoms are only of comparatively recent origin. Nonlocalizing (soft) neurological signs, learning disability and abnormal EEG may or may not be present, and a diagnosis of central nervous system dysfunction may or may not be warranted.

CONTRAINDICATIONS

Advanced arteriosclerosis, symptomatic cardiovascular disease, moderate to severe hypertension, hyperthyroidism, known hypersensitivity or idiosyncrasy to the sympathomimetic amines, glaucoma.

Agitated states.

Patients with a history of drug abuse.

During or within 14 days following the administration of monoamine oxidase inhibitors (hypertensive crises may result).

PRECAUTIONS

General: Caution is to be exercised in prescribing amphetamines for patients with even mild hypertension.

The least amount feasible should be prescribed or dispensed at one time in order to minimize the possibility of overdosage.

These products contain FD&C Yellow No. 5 (tartrazine), which may cause allergic-type reactions (including bronchial asthma) in certain susceptible individuals. Although the overall incidence of FD&C Yellow No. 5 (tartrazine) sensitivity in the general population is low, it is frequently seen in patients who also have aspirin hypersensitivity.

Information for Patients: Amphetamines may impair the ability of the patient to engage in potentially hazardous activities such as operating machinery or vehicles; the patient should therefore be cautioned accordingly.

Drug Interactions:

Acidifying agents—Gastrointestinal acidifying agents (guanethidine, reserpine, glutamic acid HCl, ascorbic acid, fruit juices, etc.) lower absorption of amphetamines. Urinary acidifying agents (ammonium chloride, sodium acid phosphate, etc.) increase the concentration of the ionized species of the amphetamine molecule, thereby increasing urinary excretion. Both groups of agents lower blood levels and efficacy of amphetamines.

Adrenergic blockers—Adrenergic blockers are inhibited by amphetamines.

Alkalinizing agents—Gastrointestinal alkalinizing agents (sodium bicarbonate, etc.) increase absorption of amphetamines. Urinary alkalinizing agents (acetazolamide, some thiazides) increase the concentration of the non-ionized species of the amphetamine molecule, thereby decreasing urinary excretion. Both groups of agents increase blood levels and therefore potentiate the actions of amphetamines.

Antidepressants, tricyclic—Amphetamines may enhance the activity of tricyclic or sympathomimetic agents; *d*-amphetamine with desipramine or protriptyline and possibly other tricyclics cause striking and sustained increases in the concentration of *d*-amphetamine in the brain; cardiovascular effects can be potentiated.

MAO inhibitors—MAOI antidepressants, as well as a metabolite of furazolidone, slow amphetamine metabolism. This slowing potentiates amphetamines, increasing their effect on the release of norepinephrine and other monoamines from adrenergic nerve endings; this can cause headaches and other signs of hypertensive crisis. A variety of neurological toxic effects and malignant hyperpyrexia can occur, sometimes with fatal results.

Antihistamines—Amphetamines may counteract the sedative effect of antihistamines.

Antihypertensives—Amphetamines may antagonize the hypotensive effects of antihypertensives.

Chlorpromazine—Chlorpromazine blocks dopamine and norepinephrine reuptake, thus inhibiting the central stimulant effects of amphetamines, and can be used to treat amphetamine poisoning.

Ethosuximide—Amphetamines may delay intestinal absorption of ethosuximide.

Haloperidol—Haloperidol blocks dopamine and norepinephrine reuptake, thus inhibiting the central stimulant effects of amphetamines.

Lithium carbonate—The stimulatory effects of amphetamines may be inhibited by lithium carbonate.

Meperidine—Amphetamines potentiate the analgesic effect of meperidine.

Methenamine therapy—Urinary excretion of amphetamines is increased, and efficacy is reduced, by acidifying agents used in methenamine therapy.

Norepinephrine—Amphetamines enhance the adrenergic effect of norepinephrine.

Phenobarbital—Amphetamines may delay intestinal absorption of phenobarbital; co-administration of phenobarbital may produce a synergistic anticonvulsant action.

Phenytoin-Amphetamines may delay intestinal absorption of phenytoin; co-administration of phenytoin may produce a synergistic anticonvulsant action.

Propoxyphene—In cases of propoxyphene overdosage, amphetamine CNS stimulation is potentiated and fatal convulsions can occur.

Veratrum alkaloids—Amphetamines inhibit the hypotensive effect of veratrum alkaloids.

Drug/Laboratory Test Interactions:

- Amphetamines can cause a significant elevation in plasma corticosteroid levels. This increase is greatest in the evening.
- Amphetamines may interfere with urinary steroid determinations.

Carcinogenesis/Mutagenesis: Mutagenicity studies and long-term studies in animals to determine the carcinogenic potential of DextroStat® (dextroamphetamine sulfate) have not been performed.

Pregnancy-Teratogenic Effects: Pregnancy Category C. Amphetamine has been shown to have embryotoxic and teratogenic effects when administered to A/Jax mice and C57BL mice in doses approximately 41 times the maximum human dose. Embryotoxic effects were not seen in New Zealand white rabbits given the drug in doses 7 times the human dose nor in rats given 12.5 times the maximum human dose. While there are no adequate and well-controlled studies in pregnant women, there has been one report of severe congenital bony deformity, tracheoesophageal fistula, and anal atresia (Vater association) in a baby born to a woman who took dextroamphetamine sulfate with lovastatin during the first trimester of pregnancy. Amphetamines should be used during pregnancy only if the potential benefit justifies the potential risk to the fetus.

Nonteratogenic Effects: Infants born to mothers dependent on amphetamines have an increased risk of premature delivery and low birth weight. Also, these infants may experience symptoms of withdrawal as demonstrated by dysphoria, including agitation, and significant lassitude.

Nursing Mothers: Amphetamines are excreted in human milk. Mothers taking amphetamines should be advised to refrain from nursing.

Pediatric Use: Long-term effects of amphetamines in pediatric patients have not been well established.

Amphetamines are not recommended for use in pediatric patients under 3 years of age with Attention Deficit Disorder with Hyperactivity described under INDICATIONS AND USAGE.

Clinical experience suggests that in psychotic pediatric patients, administration of amphetamines may exacerbate symptoms of behavior disturbance and thought disorder.

Amphetamines have been reported to exacerbate motor and phonic tics and Tourette's syndrome. Therefore, clinical evaluation for tics and Tourette's syndrome in pediatric patients and their families should precede use of stimulant medications.

Data are inadequate to determine whether chronic administration of amphetamines may be associated with growth inhibition; therefore, growth should be monitored during treatment.

Drug treatment is not indicated in all cases of Attention Deficit Disorder with Hyperactivity and should be considered only in light of the complete history and evaluation of the pediatric patient. The decision to prescribe amphetamines should depend on the physician's assessment of the chronicity and severity of the pediatric patient's symptoms and their appropriateness for his/her age.

Prescription should not depend solely on the presence of one or more of the behavioral characteristics.

When these symptoms are associated with acute stress reactions, treatment with amphetamines is usually not indicated.

ADVERSE REACTIONS

Cardiovascular: Palpitations, tachycardia, elevation of blood pressure. There have been isolated reports of cardiomyopathy associated with chronic amphetamine use.

Central Nervous System:

Psychotic episodes at recommended doses (rare), overstimulation, restlessness, dizziness, insomnia, euphoria, dyskinesia, dysphoria, tremor, headache, exacerbation of motor and phonic tics and Tourette's syndrome.

Gastrointestinal: Dryness of the mouth, unpleasant taste, diarrhea, constipation, other gastrointestinal disturbances. Anorexia and weight loss may occur as undesirable effects.

Allergic: Urticaria.

Endocrine: Impotence, changes in libido.

DRUG ABUSE AND DEPENDENCE

Dextroamphetamine sulfate tablets are a Schedule II controlled substance.

Amphetamines have been extensively abused. Tolerance, extreme psychological dependence and severe social disability have occurred. There are reports of patients who have increased the dosage to many times that recommended. Abrupt cessation following prolonged high dosage administration results in extreme fatigue and mental depression; changes are also noted on the sleep EEG.

Manifestation of chronic intoxication with amphetamines include severe dermatoses, marked insomnia, irritability, hyperactivity and personality changes. The most severe

Continued on next page

Dextrostat—Cont.

manifestation of chronic intoxication is psychosis, often clinically indistinguishable from schizophrenia. This is rare with oral amphetamines.

OVERDOSAGE

Individual patient response to amphetamines varies widely. While toxic symptoms occasionally occur as an idiosyncrasy at doses as low as 2 mg, they are rare with doses of less than 15 mg; 30 mg can produce severe reactions, yet doses of 400 to 500 mg are not necessarily fatal.

In rats, the oral LD_{50} of dextroamphetamine sulfate is 96.8 mg/kg.

Manifestations of acute overdosage with amphetamines include restlessness, tremor, hyperreflexia, rhabdomyolysis, rapid respiration, hyperpyrexia, confusion, assultiveness, hallucinations, panic states.

Fatigue and depression usually follow the central stimulation.

Cardiovascular effects include arrhythmias, hypertension or hypotension and circulatory collapse. Gastrointestinal symptoms include nausea, vomiting, diarrhea and abdominal cramps. Fatal poisoning is usually preceded by convulsions and coma.

TREATMENT—Consult with a Certified Poison Control Center for up-to-date guidance and advice. Management of acute amphetamine intoxication is largely symptomatic and includes gastric lavage, administration of activated charcoal, administration of a cathartic, and sedation. Experience with hemodialysis or peritoneal dialysis is inadequate to permit recommendation in this regard. Acidification of the urine increases amphetamine excretion, but is believed to increase risk of acute renal failure if myoglobinuria is present. If acute, severe hypertension complicates amphetamine overdosage, administration of intravenous phentolamine has been suggested. However, a gradual drop in blood pressure will usually result when sufficient sedation has been achieved.

DOSAGE AND ADMINISTRATION

Amphetamines should be administered at the lowest effective dosage and dosage should be individually adjusted. Late evening doses should be avoided because of the resulting insomnia.

Narcolepsy: Usual dose 5 to 60 mg per day in divided doses, depending on the individual patient response.

Narcolepsy seldom occurs in pediatric patients under 12 years of age; however, when it does, DextroStat® (dextroamphetamine sulfate) may be used. The suggested initial dose for patients aged 6 to 12 is 5 mg daily; daily dose may be raised in increments of 5 mg at weekly intervals until optimal response is obtained. In patients 12 years of age and older, start with 10 mg daily; daily dosage may be raised in increments of 10 mg at weekly intervals until optimal response is obtained. If bothersome adverse reactions appear (e.g., insomnia or anorexia), dosage should be reduced. Give first dose on awakening; additional doses (1 or 2) at intervals of 4 to 6 hours.

Attention Deficit Disorder with Hyperactivity: Not recommended for pediatric patients under 3 years of age.

In pediatric patients from 3 to 5 years of age, start with 2.5 mg daily; daily dosage may be raised in increments of 2.5 mg at weekly intervals until optimal response is obtained.

In pediatric patients 6 years of age and older, start with 5 mg once or twice daily; daily dosage may be raised in increments of 5 mg at weekly intervals until optimal response is obtained. Only in rare cases will it be necessary to exceed a total of 40 mg per day.

Give first dose on awakening; additional doses (1 or 2) at intervals of 4 to 6 hours.

When possible, drug administration should be interrupted occasionally to determine if there is a recurrence of behavioral symptoms sufficient to require continued therapy.

HOW SUPPLIED

DextroStat®, (dextroamphetamine sulfate) Tablets are available as follows:

5 mg Yellow, Round, Scored Tablet debossed "RP" on one side and "51" on the other side.
NDC #: 58521-451-01 for 100s
58521-451-05 for 500s
58521-451-10 for 1000s

10 mg Yellow, Round, Double-Scored Tablet debossed "RP" on one side and "52" on the other side.
NDC #: 58521-452-01 for 100s
58521-452-05 for 500s

Dispense in a tight container as defined in the USP. Store at controlled room temperature 15°–30°C (59°–86°F).

DEA Order Form Required.

Rx only.

Shire Richwood Inc.
Florence, KY 41042

MG #9245   Rev 6/98

Shown in Product Identification Guide, page 338

---

sigma-tau Pharmaceuticals, Inc.
**800 SOUTH FREDERICK AVENUE, SUITE 300
GAITHERSBURG, MARYLAND 20877**

Direct Inquiries to:
TEL: (301) 948-1041
800-447-0169
E-mail: info@sigmatau.com
Fax: (301) 948-3194

CARNITOR®   ℞
[car-nĭ-tor]
(Levocarnitine)
**Injection 1 g per 5 mL
and 500 mg per 2.5 mL
FOR INTRAVENOUS USE ONLY**

DESCRIPTION

Levocarnitine is a carrier molecule in the transport of long chain fatty acids across the inner mitochondrial membrane. CARNITOR® (Levocarnitine) Injection is a sterile aqueous solution containing 1 g of levocarnitine per 5 mL ampoule and 500 mg of levocarnitine per 2.5 mL ampoule. The pH is adjusted to 6.0 – 6.5 with hydrochloric acid.

Chemically, levocarnitine is (R)-3-carboxy-2-hydroxy-N,N,N-trimethyl-l-propanaminium hydroxide, inner salt. It is a white powder with a melting point of 196–197°C and is readily soluble in water, hot alcohol, and insoluble in acetone. The pH of a solution (1 in 20) is between 6–8 and its pKa value is 3.8. Its chemical structure is:

$$CH_3-\overset{\overset{\displaystyle CH_3}{|}}{\underset{\underset{\displaystyle CH_3}{|}}{\overset{+}{N}}}-CH_2-\overset{\overset{}{\underset{\underset{\displaystyle OH}{|}}{}}}{CH}-CH_2-COO^-$$

Empirical Formula: $C_7H_{15}NO_3$
Molecular Weight: 161.20

CLINICAL PHARMACOLOGY

CARNITOR® (Levocarnitine) is a naturally occurring substance required in mammalian energy metabolism. It has been shown to facilitate long-chain fatty acid entry into cellular mitochondria, therefore delivering substrate for oxidation and subsequent energy production. Fatty acids are utilized as an energy substrate in all tissues except the brain. In skeletal and cardiac muscle they serve as major fuel. Primary systemic carnitine deficiency is characterized by low plasma, RBC, and/or tissue levels. It has not been possible to determine which symptoms are due to carnitine deficiency and which are due to the underlying organic acidemia, as symptoms of both abnormalities may be expected to improve with carnitine. The literature reports that carnitine can promote the excretion of excess organic or fatty acids in patients with defects in fatty acid metabolism and/or specific organic acidopathies that bioaccumulate acyl CoA esters.[1-6]

Secondary levocarnitine deficiency can be a consequence of inborn errors of metabolism. CARNITOR® may alleviate the metabolic abnormalities of patients with inborn errors that result in accumulation of toxic organic acids. Conditions for which this effect was demonstrated are: glutaric aciduria II, methyl malonic aciduria, propionic acidemia, and medium chain fatty acyl CoA dehydrogenase deficiency.[7,8] Autointoxication occurs in these patients due to the accumulations of acyl CoA compounds that disrupt intermediary metabolism. The subsequent hydrolysis of the acyl CoA compound to its free acid results in acidosis that can be life threatening. Levocarnitine clears the acyl CoA compound by formation of acyl carnitine which is quickly excreted. Levocarnitine deficiency is defined biochemically as abnormally low plasma levels of free carnitine, less than 20 μmol/L at one week post term and may be associated with low tissue and/or urine levels. Further, this condition may be associated with a ratio of plasma ester/free levocarnitine levels greater than 0.4 or abnormally elevated levels of esterified levocarnitine in the urine. In premature infants and newborns, secondary deficiency is defined as plasma free levocarnitine levels below age related normal levels.

BIOAVAILABILITY/PHARMACOKINETICS

In a relative bioavailability study in 15 healthy adult male volunteers CARNITOR® Tablets were found to be bio-equivalent to CARNITOR® Oral Solution. Following the administration of 1980 mg b.i.d., the maximum plasma concentration level (C_{max}) was 80 nmol/mL and the time to maximum concentration (T_{max}) occurred at 3.3 hours. There were no significant differences for AUC and urinary excretion observed between these two formulations.

In the same bioavailability study of 15 healthy adult males, CARNITOR® (Levocarnitine) Injection administered as a slow 3 minute bolus intravenous injection at a dose of 20 mg/Kg showed that free levocarnitine plasma profiles are

---

best fit by a two compartment model. Approximately 76% of free levocarnitine is eliminated in the urine. Using plasma levels uncorrected for endogenous levocarnitine, the mean distribution half life was 0.585 hours and the mean apparent terminal elimination half life was 17.4 hours following a single intravenous dose.

The absolute bioavailability of L-carnitine from CARNITOR® Tablets and Oral Solution was determined compared to the bioavailability of L-carnitine from CARNITOR® (Injection) Intravenous in 15 healthy male volunteers. After correction for circulating endogenous levels of L-carnitine in the plasma, absolute bioavailability was 15.1% ± 5.3% for L-carnitine from CARNITOR® Tablets and 15.9% ± 4.9% from the Oral Solution.

Total body clearance of L-carnitine (Dose/AUC including endogenous baseline levels) was a mean of 4.00 L/hr. Endogenous baseline levels were not subtracted since total body clearance of L-carnitine does not distinguish between exogenous sources of L-carnitine and endogenously synthesized L-carnitine. Volume of distribution of the intravenously administered dose above baseline endogenous levels was calculated to be a mean of 29.0 L ± 7.1 L (approximately 0.39 L/kg) which is an underestimate of the true volume of distribution since plasma L-carnitine is known to equilibrate slowly with, for instance, muscle L-carnitine.

L-carnitine was not bound to plasma protein or albumin when tested at any concentration or with any species including the human.[9]

METABOLISM AND EXCRETION

Five normal adult male volunteers, administered a dose of [³H-methyl]-L-carnitine following 15 days of a high carnitine diet and additional carnitine supplement, excreted 58% to 65% of administered radioactive dose in 5 to 11 days in the urine and feces. Maximum concentration of [³H-methyl]-L-carnitine in serum occurred from 2.0 to 4.5 hr after drug administration. Major metabolites found were trimethylamine N-oxide, primarily in urine (8% to 49% of the administered dose) and [³H]-γ-butyrobetaine, primarily in feces (0.44% to 45% of the administered dose). Urinary excretion of carnitine was 4% to 8% of the dose. Fecal excretion of total carnitine was less than 1% of total carnitine excretion.[10]

After attainment of steady state following 4 days of oral administration of L-carnitine with CARNITOR® Tablets (1980 mg q 12h) or Oral Solution (2000 mg q12h) to 15 healthy male volunteers, urinary excretion of L-carnitine was a mean of 2107 and 2339 μmoles, respectively, equivalent to 8.6% and 9.4%, respectively, of the orally administered doses (uncorrected for endogenous urinary excretion). After a single intravenous dose (20 mg/kg) prior to multiple oral doses, urinary excretion of L-carnitine was 6974 μmoles equivalent to 75.6% of the intravenously administered dose (uncorrected for endogenous urinary excretion).

INDICATIONS AND USAGE

For the acute and chronic treatment of patients with an inborn error of metabolism that results in secondary carnitine deficiency.

CONTRAINDICATIONS

None known.

WARNINGS

None.

PRECAUTIONS

Carcinogenesis, mutagenesis, impairment of fertility

Mutagenicity tests performed in *Salmonella typhimurium*, *Saccharomyces cerevisiae*, and *Schizosaccharomyces pombe* indicate that levocarnitine is not mutagenic. No long-term animal studies have been performed to evaluate the carcinogenic potential of levocarnitine.

Pregnancy

Pregnancy Category B.

Reproductive studies have been performed in rats and rabbits at doses up to 3.8 times the human dose on the basis of surface area and have revealed no evidence of impaired fertility or harm to the fetus due to CARNITOR®. There are, however, no adequate and well controlled studies in pregnant women.

Because animal reproduction studies are not always predictive of human response, this drug should be used during pregnancy only if clearly needed.

Nursing Mothers

It is not known whether this drug is excreted in human milk. Because many drugs are excreted in human milk, a decision should be made whether to discontinue nursing or to discontinue the drug, taking into account the importance of the drug to the mother.

Pediatric use

See Dosage and Administration.

ADVERSE REACTIONS

Transient nausea and vomiting have been observed. Less frequent adverse reactions are body odor, nausea, and gastritis. An incidence for these reactions is difficult to estimate due to the confounding effects of the underlying pathology.

Seizures have been reported to occur in patients with or without pre-existing seizure activity receiving either oral or intravenous levocarnitine. In patients with pre-existing seizure activity, an increase in seizure frequency and/or severity has been reported.

OVERDOSAGE

There have been no reports of toxicity from levocarnitine overdosage. The oral LD_{50} of levocarnitine in mice is 19.2 g/kg. Large doses of levocarnitine may cause diarrhea.

DOSAGE AND ADMINISTRATION

CARNITOR® Injection is administered intravenously. The recommended dose is 50 mg/kg given as a slow 2–3 minute bolus injection or by infusion. Often a loading dose is given in patients with severe metabolic crisis followed by an equivalent dose over the following 24 hours. It should be administered q3h or q4h, and never less than q6h either by infusion or by intravenous injection. All subsequent daily doses are recommended to be in the range of 50 mg/kg or as therapy may require. The highest dose administered has been 300 mg/kg.

It is recommended that a plasma carnitine level be obtained prior to beginning this parenteral therapy. Weekly and monthly monitoring is recommended as well. This monitoring should include blood chemistries, vital signs, plasma carnitine concentrations (the plasma free carnitine level should be between 35 and 60 micromoles/liter) and overall clinical condition.

Parenteral drug products should be inspected visually for particulate matter and discoloration prior to adminstration, whenever solution and container permit.

COMPATIBILITY AND STABILITY

CARNITOR® Injection is compatible and stable when mixed in parenteral solutions of Sodium Chloride 0.9% or Lactated Ringer's in concentrations ranging from 250 mg/500 mL (0.5 mg/mL) to 4200 mg/500 mL (8.0 mg/mL) and stored at room temperature (25°C) for up to 24 hours in PVC plastic bags.

HOW SUPPLIED

CARNITOR® (Levocarnitine) Injection, 200 mg per 1 mL, is available in 5 mL single dose ampoules packaged 5 ampoules per carton (NDC 54482-146-09) and in 2.5 mL single dose ampoules packaged 5 ampoules per carton (NDC 54482-146-10). Made in Italy.

Store ampoules at controlled room temperature (25°C). See USP. Store in carton until their use to protect from light. Discard unused portion of an opened ampoule, as they contain no preservative.

CARNITOR® (Levocarnitine) is also available in the following dosage forms for oral administration:

CARNITOR® (Levocarnitine) Tablets are supplied as 330 mg tablets embossed with "CARNITOR ST" in individual blisters, packaged in boxes of 90 (NDC 54482-144-07). Made in Italy.

CARNITOR® (Levocarnitine) Oral Solution, is supplied in 118 mL (4 FL. OZ.) multiple-unit plastic containers. The multiple-unit containers are packaged 24 per case (NDC 54482-145-08). CARNITOR® (Levocarnitine) Oral Solution is manufactured for Sigma-tau Pharmaceuticals, Inc. By: Alpharma USPD, Inc. Baltimore, MD 21244-2654 and/or for Hi-Tech Pharmacal Co., Inc. Amityville, NY 11701.

Rx only.

REFERENCES

1. Bohmer T, Rynding A, Solberg HE: Carnitine levels in human serum in health and disease. **Clin Chim Acta 57:**55–61, 1974.
2. Brooks H, Goldberg L, Holland R et al: Carnitine-induced effects on cardiac and peripheral hemodynamics. **J Clin Pharmacol 17:**561–578, 1977.
3. Christiansen R, Bremer J: Active transport of butyrobetaine and carnitine into isolated liver cells. **Biochem Biophys Acta 448:**562–577, 1977.
4. Lindstedt S, Lindstedt G: Distribution and excretion of carnitine $^{14}CO_2$ in the rat. **Acta Chim Scand 15:** 701–702, 1961.
5. Rebouche CJ, Engel AG: Carnitine metabolism and deficiency syndromes. **Mayo Clin Proc 58:**533–540, 1983.
6. Rebouche CJ, Paulson DJ: Carnitine metabolism and function in humans. **Ann Rev Nutr 6:**41–68, 1986.
7. Scriver CR, Beaudet AL, Sly WS, Valle D: *The Metabolic Basis of Inherited Disease.* McGraw-Hill, New York, 1989.
8. Schaub J, Van Hoof F, Vis HL: *Inborn Errors of Metabolism.* Raven Press, New York, 1991.
9. Marzo A, Arrigoni Martelli E, Mancinelli A, Cardace G, Corbelletta C, Bassani E, Solbiati M: Protein binding of L-carnitine family components. **Eur J Drug Met Pharmacokin,** Special Issue III: 364–368, 1992.
10. Rebouche C: Quantitative estimation of absorption and degradation of a carnitine supplement by human adults. **Metabolism:** 1305–1310, 1991.

sigma-tau
Pharmaceuticals, Inc.
Gaithersburg, MD 20877
PREVIOUS EDITION IS OBSOLETE
ST-N20-182-06/98

CARNITOR®   ℞
[car-nĭ-tor]
(Levocarnitine)
Tablets (330 mg)

CARNITOR®
(Levocarnitine)
Oral Solution
(1 g per 10 mL multidose)
For oral use only. Not for parenteral use.

DESCRIPTION

CARNITOR® (Levocarnitine) is (R)-3-carboxy-2-hydroxy-N,N,N-trimethyl-1-propanaminium hydroxide, inner salt. Levocarnitine is a carrier molecule in the transport of long chain fatty acids across the inner mitochondrial membrane. As a bulk drug substance it is a white powder with a melting point of 196–197° C and is readily soluble in water, hot alcohol, and insoluble in acetone. The pH of a solution (1 in 20) is between 6–8 and its pKa value is 3.8. Its chemical structure is:

$$CH_3-\overset{\overset{\displaystyle CH_3}{\overset{\displaystyle |}{+}}}{\underset{\underset{\displaystyle CH_3}{\displaystyle |}}{N}}-CH_2-\underset{\underset{\displaystyle OH}{\displaystyle |}}{CH}-CH_2-COO^-$$

Empirical Formula: $C_7H_{15}NO_3$
Molecular Weight: 161.20

Each CARNITOR® (Levocarnitine) Tablet contains 330 mg of levocarnitine and the inactive ingredients magnesium stearate, microcrystalline cellulose and povidone.

Each 118 mL container of the CARNITOR® (Levocarnitine) Oral Solution contains 1 g of levocarnitine/10 mL. Also contains: Artificial Cherry Flavor, D,L-Malic Acid, Purified Water, Sucrose Syrup. Methylparaben NF and Propylparaben NF are added as preservatives. The pH is approximately 5.

CLINICAL PHARMACOLOGY

CARNITOR® (Levocarnitine) is a naturally occurring substance required in mammalian energy metabolism. It has been shown to facilitate long-chain fatty acid entry into cellular mitochondria, therefore delivering substrate for oxidation and subsequent energy production. Fatty acids are utilized as an energy substrate in all tissues except the brain. In skeletal and cardiac muscle they serve as major fuel. Primary systemic carnitine deficiency is characterized by low plasma, RBC, and/or tissue levels. It has not been possible to determine which symptoms are due to carnitine deficiency and which are due to the underlying organic acidemia, as symptoms of both abnormalities may be expected to improve with carnitine. The literature reports that carnitine can promote the excretion of excess organic or fatty acids in patients with defects in fatty acid metabolism and/or specific organic acidopathies that bioaccumulate acyl CoA esters.[1-6]

Secondary levocarnitine deficiency can be a consequence of inborn errors of metabolism. CARNITOR® may alleviate the metabolic abnormalities of patients with inborn errors that result in accumulation of toxic organic acids. Conditions for which this effect was demonstrated are: glutaric aciduria II, methyl malonic, aciduria, propionic acidemia, and medium chain fatty acyl CoA dehydrogenase deficiency.[7,8] Autointoxication occurs in these patients due to the accumulations of acyl CoA compounds that disrupt intermediary metabolism. The subsequent hydrolysis of the acyl CoA compound to its free acid results in acidosis that can be life threatening. Levocarnitine clears the acyl CoA compound by formation of acyl carnitine which is quickly excreted.

Levocarnitine deficiency is defined biochemically as abnormally low plasma levels of free carnitine (less than 20 µmol/L at one week post term) and may be associated with low tissue and/or urine levels. Further, this condition may be associated with a ratio of plasma ester/free levocarnitine levels greater than 0.4 or abnormally elevated levels of esterified levocarnitine in the urine. In premature infants and newborns, secondary deficiency is defined as plasma free levocarnitine levels below age related normal levels.

BIOAVAILABILITY/PHARMACOKINETICS

In a relative bioavailability study in 15 healthy adult male volunteers CARNITOR® Tablets were found to be bio-equivalent to CARNITOR® Oral Solution. Following the administration of 1980 mg b.i.d., the maximum plasma concentration level (C_{max}) was 80 nmol/mL and the time to maximum concentration (T_{max}) occurred at 3.3 hours. There were no significant differences for AUC and urinary excretion observed between these two formulations.

In the same bioavailability study of 15 healthy adult males, CARNITOR® (Levocarnitine) Injection administered as a slow 3 minute bolus intravenous injection at a dose of 20 mg/kg showed that free levocarnitine plasma profiles are best fit by a two compartment model. Approximately 76% of free levocarnitine is eliminated in the urine. Using plasma levels uncorrected for endogenous levocarnitine, the mean distribution half life was 0.585 hours and the mean apparent terminal elimination half life was 17.4 hours following a single intravenous dose.

The absolute bioavailability of L-carnitine from CARNITOR® Tablets and Oral Solution was determined compared to the bioavailability of L-carnitine from CARNITOR® Injection Intravenous in 15 healthy male volunteers. After correction for circulating endogenous levels of L-carnitine in the plasma, absolute bioavailability was 15.1% ± 5.3% for L-carnitine from CARNITOR® Tablets and 15.9% ± 4.9% from the Oral Solution.

Total body clearance of L-carnitine (Dose/AUC including endogenous baseline levels) was a mean of 4.00 L/hr. Endogenous baseline levels were not subtracted since total body clearance of L-carnitine does not distinguish between exogenous sources of L-carnitine and endogenously synthesized L-carnitine. Volume of distribution of the intravenously administered dose above baseline endogenous levels was calculated to be a mean of 29.0 L ± 7.1 L (approximately 0.39 L/kg) which is an underestimate of the true volume of distribution since plasma L-carnitine is known to equilibrate slowly with, for instance, muscle L-carnitine.

L-carnitine was not bound to plasma protein or albumin when tested at any concentration or with any species including the human.[9]

METABOLISM AND EXCRETION

Five normal adult male volunteers, administered a dose of [^{3}H-methyl]-L-carnitine following 15 days of a high carnitine diet and additional carnitine supplement, excreted 58–65% of administered radioactive dose in 5 to 11 days in the urine and feces. Maximum concentration of [^{3}H-methyl]-L-carnitine in serum occurred from 2.0 to 4.5 hr after drug administration. Major metabolites found were trimethylamine N-oxide, primarily in urine (8% to 49% of the administered dose) and [^{3}H]-γ-butyrobetaine, primarily in feces (0.44% to 45% of the administered dose). Urinary excretion of carnitine was 4% to 8% of the dose. Fecal excretion of total carnitine was less than 1% of total carnitine excretion.[10]

After attainment of steady state following 4 days of oral administration of L-carnitine with CARNITOR® Tablets (1980 mg q12h) or Oral Solution (2000 mg q12h) to 15 healthy male volunteers, urinary excretion of L-carnitine was a mean of 2107 and 2339 µmoles, respectively, equivalent to 8.6% and 9.4%, respectively, of the orally administered doses (uncorrected for endogenous urinary excretion). After a single intravenous dose (20 mg/kg) prior to multiple oral doses, urinary excretion of L-carnitine was 6974 µmoles equivalent to 75.6% of the intravenously administered dose (uncorrected for endogenous urinary excretion).

INDICATIONS AND USAGE

CARNITOR® (Levocarnitine) is indicated in the treatment of primary systemic carnitine deficiency. In the reported cases, the clinical presentation consisted of recurrent episodes of Reye-like encephalopathy, hypoketotic hypoglycemia, and/or cardiomyopathy. Associated symptoms included hypotonia, muscle weakness and failure to thrive. A diagnosis of primary carnitine deficiency requires that serum, red cell and/or tissue carnitine levels be low and that the patient does not have a primary defect in fatty acid or organic acid oxidation (see Clinical Pharmacology). In some patients, particularly those presenting with cardiomyopathy, carnitine supplementation rapidly alleviated signs and symptoms. Treatment should include, in addition to carnitine, supportive and other therapy as indicated by the condition of the patient.

CARNITOR® (Levocarnitine) is also indicated for acute and chronic treatment of patients with an inborn error of metabolism that results in a secondary carnitine deficiency.

CONTRAINDICATIONS

None known.

WARNINGS

None.

PRECAUTIONS

General

CARNITOR® (Levocarnitine) Oral Solution is for oral/internal use only.

Not for parenteral use.

Gastrointestinal reactions may result from too rapid consumption of carnitine. CARNITOR® (Levocarnitine) Oral Solution may be consumed alone, or dissolved in drinks or other liquid foods to reduce taste fatigue. It should be consumed slowly and doses should be spaced evenly throughout the day to maximize tolerance.

Carcinogenesis, mutagenesis, impairment of fertility

Mutagenicity tests performed in *Salmonella typhimurium, Saccharomyces cerevisiae,* and *Schizosaccharomyces pombe*

Continued on next page

Carnitor Tablets/Oral Solution—Cont.

indicate that CARNITOR® (Levocarnitine) is not mutagenic. Long-term animal studies have not been conducted to evaluate the carcinogenicity of the compound.

Pregnancy
Pregnancy Category B.
Reproductive studies have been performed in rats and rabbits at doses up to 3.8 times the human dose on the basis of surface area and have revealed no evidence of impaired fertility or harm to the fetus due to CARNITOR®. There are, however, no adequate and well controlled studies in pregnant women. Because animal reproduction studies are not always predictive of human response, this drug should be used during pregnancy only if clearly needed.

Nursing mothers
It is not known whether this drug is excreted in human milk. Because many drugs are excreted in human milk, a decision should be made whether to discontinue nursing or to discontinue the drug, taking into account the importance of the drug to the mother.

Pediatric use
See Dosage and Administration.

ADVERSE REACTIONS
Various mild gastrointestinal complaints have been reported during the long-term administration of oral L- or D,L-carnitine; these include transient nausea and vomiting, abdominal cramps, and diarrhea. Mild myasthenia has been described only in uremic patients receiving D,L-carnitine. Gastrointestinal adverse reactions with CARNITOR® (Levocarnitine) Oral Solution dissolved in liquids might be avoided by a slow consumption of the solution or by a greater dilution. Decreasing the dosage often diminishes or eliminates drug-related patient body odor or gastrointestinal symptoms when present. Tolerance should be monitored very closely during the first week of administration, and after any dosage increases.
Seizures have been reported to occur in patients with or without pre-existing seizure activity receiving either oral or intravenous levocarnitine. In patients with pre-existing seizure activity, an increase in seizure frequency and/or severity has been reported.

OVERDOSAGE
There have been no reports of toxicity from carnitine overdosage. The oral LD_{50} of levocarnitine in mice is 19.2 g/kg. Carnitine may cause diarrhea. Overdosage should be treated with supportive care.

DOSAGE AND ADMINISTRATION
CARNITOR® (Levocarnitine) Tablets.
Adults: The recommended oral dosage for adults is 990 mg two or three times a day using the 330 mg tablets, depending on clinical response.
Infants and children: The recommended oral dosage for infants and children is between 50 and 100 mg/kg/day in divided doses, with a maximum of 3 g/day. Dosage should begin at 50 mg/kg/day. The exact dosage will depend on clinical response.
Monitoring should include periodic blood chemistries, vital signs, plasma carnitine concentrations and overall clinical condition.
CARNITOR® (Levocarnitine) Oral Solution.
For oral use only. **Not for parenteral use.**
Adults: The recommended dosage of levocarnitine is 1 to 3 g/day for a 50 kg subject which is equivalent to 10 to 30 mL/day of CARNITOR® (Levocarnitine) Oral Solution. Higher doses should be administered only with caution and only where clinical and biochemical considerations make it seem likely that higher doses will be of benefit. Dosage should start at 1 g/day, (10 mL/day), and be increased slowly while assessing tolerance and therapeutic response. Monitoring should include periodic blood chemistries, vital signs, plasma carnitine concentrations, and overall clinical condition.
Infants and children: The recommended dosage of levocarnitine is 50 to 100 mg/kg/day which is equivalent to 0.5 mL/kg/day CARNITOR® (Levocarnitine) Oral Solution. Higher doses should be administered only with caution and only where clinical and biochemical considerations make it seem likely that higher doses will be of benefit. Dosage should start at 50 mg/kg/day, and be increased slowly to a maximum of 3 g/day (30 mL/day) while assessing tolerance and therapeutic response. Monitoring should include periodic blood chemistries, vital signs, plasma carnitine concentrations, and overall clinical condition.
CARNITOR® (Levocarnitine) Oral Solution may be consumed alone or dissolved in drink or other liquid food. Doses should be spaced evenly throughout the day (every three or four hours) preferably during or following meals and should be consumed slowly in order to maximize tolerance.

HOW SUPPLIED
CARNITOR® (Levocarnitine) Tablets are supplied as 330 mg tablets embossed with "CARNITOR ST" in individual blisters, packaged in boxes of 90 (NDC 54482-144-07).

Store at controlled room temperature (25°C). See USP.
CARNITOR® (Levocarnitine) Oral Solution is supplied in 118 mL (4 FL. OZ.) multiple-unit plastic containers. The multiple-unit containers are packaged 24 per case (NDC 54482-145-08). Store at controlled room temperature (25°C). See USP.
CARNITOR® (Levocarnitine) Oral Solution is manufactured for Sigma-tau Pharmaceuticals, Inc. By: Alpharma (USPD, Inc. Baltimore, MD 21244-2654 and/or Hi-Tech Pharmacal Co., Inc. Amityville, NY 11701.
CARNITOR® (Levocarnitine) is also available in the following dosage form for intravenous injection:
CARNITOR® (Levocarnitine) Injection, 200 mg per 1 mL, is available in 5 mL single dose ampoules packaged 5 ampoules per carton (NDC 54482-146-09) and 2.5 mL single dose ampoules packaged 5 ampoules per carton (NDC 54482-146-10). Made in Italy.

Rx only

REFERENCES
1. Bohmer T, Rynding A, Solberg HE: Carnitine levels in human serum in health and disease. **Clin Chim Acta 57**:55–61, 1974.
2. Brooks H, Goldberg L, Holland R et al: Carnitine-induced effects on cardiac and peripheral hemodynamics. **J Clin Pharmacol 17**:561–578, 1977.
3. Christiansen R, Bremer J: Active transport of butyrobetaine and carnitine into isolated liver cells. **Biochem Biophys Acta 448**:562–577, 1977.
4. Lindstedt S, Lindstedt G: Distribution and excretion of carnitine $^{14}CO_2$ in the rat. **Acta Chim Scand 15**: 701–702, 1961.
5. Rebouche CJ, Engel AG: Carnitine metabolism and deficiency syndromes. **Mayo Clin Proc 58**:533–540, 1983.
6. Rebouche CJ, Paulson DJ: Carnitine metabolism and function in humans. **Ann Rev Nutr 6**:41–68, 1986.
7. Scriver CR, Beaudet AL, Sly WS, Valle D: *The Metabolic Basis of Inherited Disease.* McGraw-Hill, New York, 1989.
8. Schaub J, Van Hoof F, Vis HL: *Inborn Errors of Metabolism.* Raven Press, New York, 1991.
9. Marzo A, Arrigoni Martelli E, Mancinelli A, Cardace G, Corbelletta C, Bassani E, Solbiati M: Protein binding of L-carnitine family components. **Eur J Drug Met Pharmacokin**, Special Issue III: 364–368, 1992.
10. Rebouche C: Quantitative estimation of absorption and degradation of a carnitine supplement by human adults. **Metabolism**: 1305–1310, 1991.

sigma-tau
Pharmaceuticals, Inc.
Gaithersburg, MD 20877
PREVIOUS EDITION IS OBSOLETE
ST-N18-948-06/98

SmithKline Beecham Consumer Healthcare
Unit of SmithKline Beecham Inc.
POST OFFICE BOX 1467
PITTSBURGH, PA 15230

Direct Inquiries to:
1-800-245-1040 weekdays

DEBROX® Drops   OTC
[de 'brox]
Ear Wax Removal Aid

(See PDR For Nonprescription Drugs.)

DENAVIR™   ℞
brand of
penciclovir cream, 1%
For Dermatologic Use Only

DESCRIPTION
Denavir contains penciclovir, an antiviral agent active against herpes viruses. *Denavir* is available for topical administration as a 1% white cream. Each gram of *Denavir* contains 10 mg of penciclovir and the following inactive ingredients: cetomacrogol 1000 BP, cetostearyl alcohol, mineral oil, propylene glycol, purified water and white petrolatum.
Chemically, penciclovir is known as 9-[4-hydroxy-3-(hydroxymethyl)butyl]guanine. Its molecular formula is $C_{10}H_{15}N_5O_3$; its molecular weight is 253.26. It is a synthetic acyclic guanine derivative and has the following structure:
[See chemical structure at top of next column]

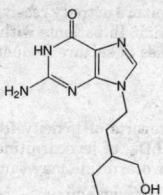

penciclovir

Penciclovir is a white to pale yellow solid. At 20°C it has a solubility of 0.2 mg/mL in methanol, 1.3 mg/mL in propylene glycol, and 1.7 mg/mL in water. In aqueous buffer (pH 2) the solubility is 10.0 mg/mL. Penciclovir is not hygroscopic. Its partition coefficient in n-octanol/water at pH 7.5 is 0.024 (logP=-1.62).

CLINICAL PHARMACOLOGY
Microbiology
Mechanism of Antiviral Activity: The antiviral compound penciclovir has *in vitro* inhibitory activity against herpes simplex virus types 1 (HSV-1) and 2 (HSV-2). In cells infected with HSV-1 or HSV-2, viral thymidine kinase phosphorylates penciclovir to a monophosphate form which, in turn, is converted to penciclovir triphosphate by cellular kinases. *In vitro* studies demonstrate that penciclovir triphosphate inhibits HSV polymerase competitively with deoxyguanosine triphosphate. Consequently, herpes viral DNA synthesis and, therefore, replication are selectively inhibited.
Antiviral Activity *In Vitro* and *in Vivo:* In cell culture studies, penciclovir has antiviral activity against HSV-1 and HSV-2.
Sensitivity test results, expressed as the concentration of the drug required to inhibit growth of the virus by 50% (IC_{50}) or 99% (IC_{99}) in cell culture, vary depending upon a number of factors, including the assay protocols. See Table 1.
[See table at 1 top of next page]
Drug Resistance: Penciclovir-resistant mutants of HSV can result from qualitative changes in viral thymidine kinase or DNA polymerase. The most commonly encountered acyclovir-resistant mutants that are deficient in viral thymidine kinase are also resistant to penciclovir.
Pharmacokinetics
Measurable penciclovir concentrations were not detected in plasma or urine of healthy male volunteers (n=12) following single or repeat application of the 1% cream at a dose of 180 mg penciclovir daily (approximately 67 times the estimated usual clinical dose).
Pediatric Patients: The systemic absorption of penciclovir following topical administration has not been evaluated in patients <18 years of age.

CLINICAL TRIALS
Denavir was studied in two double-blind, placebo (vehicle)-controlled trials for the treatment of recurrent herpes labialis in which otherwise healthy adults were randomized to either *Denavir* or placebo. Therapy was to be initiated by the subjects within 1 hour of noticing signs or symptoms and continued for 4 days, with application of study medication every 2 hours while awake. In both studies, the mean duration of lesions was approximately one-half-day shorter in the subjects treated with *Denavir* (N=1,516) as compared to subjects treated with placebo (N=1,541) (approximately 4.5 days versus 5 days, respectively). The mean duration of lesion pain was also approximately one-half-day shorter in the *Denavir* group compared to the placebo group.

INDICATIONS AND USAGE
Denavir (penciclovir cream) is indicated for the treatment of recurrent herpes labialis (cold sores) in adults.

CONTRAINDICATIONS
Denavir is contraindicated in patients with known hypersensitivity to the product or any of its components.

PRECAUTIONS
General
Denavir should only be used on herpes labialis on the lips and face. Because no data are available, application to human mucous membranes is not recommended. Particular care should be taken to avoid application in or near the eyes since it may cause irritation. The effect of *Denavir* has not been established in immunocompromised patients.
Carcinogenesis, Mutagenesis, Impairment of Fertility
In clinical trials, systemic drug exposure following the topical administration of penciclovir cream was negligible, as the penciclovir content of all plasma and urine samples was below the limit of assay detection (0.1 mcg/mL and 10 mcg/mL, respectively). However, for the purpose of inter-species dose comparisons presented in the following sections, an assumption of 100% absorption of penciclovir from the topi-

Table 1

Method of Assay	Virus Type	Cell Type	IC$_{50}$ (mcg/mL)	IC$_{99}$ (mcg/mL)
Plaque Reduction	HSV-1 (c.i.)	MRC-5	0.2–0.6	
	HSV-1 (c.i.)	WISH	0.04–0.5	
	HSV-2 (c.i.)	MRC-5	0.9–2.1	
	HSV-2 (c.i.)	WISH	0.1–0.8	
Virus Yield Reduction	HSV-1 (c.i.)	MRC-5		0.4–0.5
	HSV-2 (c.i.)	MRC-5		0.6–0.7
DNA Synethesis Inhibition	HSV-1 (SC16)	MRC-5	0.04	
	HSV-2 (MS)	MRC-5	0.05	

(c.i.) =clinical isolates. The latent state of any herpes virus is not known to respond to any antivirial therapy.

cally applied product has been used. Based on use of the maximal recommended topical dose of penciclovir of 0.05 mg/kg/day and an assumption of 100% absorption, the maximum theoretical plasma AUC$_{0-24\ hrs}$ for penciclovir is approximately 0.129 mcg.hr/mL.

Carcinogenesis: Two-year carcinogenicity studies were conducted with famciclovir (the oral prodrug of penciclovir) in rats and mice. An increase in the incidence of mammary adenocarcinoma (a common tumor in female rats of the strain used) was seen in female rats receiving 600 mg/kg/day (approximately 395× the maximum theoretical human exposure to penciclovir following application of the topical product, based on area under the plasma concentration curve comparisons [24 hr. AUC]). No increases in tumor incidence were seen among male rats treated at doses up to 240 mg/kg/day (approximately 190× the maximum theoretical human AUC for penciclovir), or in male and female mice at doses up to 600 mg/kg/day (approximately 100× the maximum theoretical human AUC for penciclovir).

Mutagenesis: When tested *in vitro*, penciclovir did not cause an increase in gene mutation in the Ames assay using multiple strains of *S. typhimurium* or *E. coli* (at up to 20,000 mcg/plate), nor did it cause an increase in unscheduled DNA repair in mammalian HeLa S3 cells (at up to 5,000 mcg/mL). However, an increase in clastogenic responses was seen with penciclovir in the L5178Y mouse lymphoma cell assay at doses ≥1000 mcg/mL) and, in human lymphocytes incubated *in vitro* at doses ≥250 mcg/mL. When tested *in vivo,* penciclovir caused an increase in micronuclei in mouse bone marrow following the intravenous administration of doses ≥500 mg/kg (≥810× the maximum human dose, based on body surface area conversion).

Impairment of Fertility: Testicular toxicity was observed in multiple animal species (rats and dogs) following repeated intravenous administration of penciclovir (160 mg/kg/day and 100 mg/kg/day, respectively, approximately 1155 and 3255× the maximum theoretical human AUC). Testicular changes seen in both species included atrophy of the seminiferous tubules and reductions in epididymal sperm counts and/or an increased incidence of sperm with abnormal morphology or reduced motility. Adverse testicular effects were related to an increasing dose or duration of exposure to penciclovir. No adverse testicular or reproductive effects (fertility and reproductive function) were observed in rats after 10 to 13 weeks dosing at 80 mg/kg/day, or testicular effects in dogs after 13 weeks dosing at 30 mg/kg/day (575 and 845× the maximum theoretical human AUC, respectively). Intravenously administered penciclovir had no effect on fertility or reproductive performance in female rats at doses of up to 80 mg/k/day (260× the maximum human dose [BSA]).

There was no evidence of any clinically significant effects on sperm count, motility or morphology in 2 placebo-controlled clinical trials of Famvir® (famciclovir [the oral prodrug of penciclovir], 250 mg b.i.d.; n=66) in immunocompetent men with recurrent genital herpes, when dosing and follow-up were maintained for 18 and 8 weeks, respectively (approximately 2 and 1 spermatogenic cycles in the human).

Pregnancy
Teratogenic Effects-Pregnancy Category B. No adverse effects on the course and outcome of pregnancy or on fetal development were noted in rats and rabbits following the intravenous administration of penciclovir at doses of 80 and 60 mg/kg/day, respectively (estimated human equivalent doses of 13 and 18 mg/kg/day for the rat and rabbit, respectively, based on body surface area conversion; the body surface area doses being 260 and 355× the maximum recommended dose following topical application of the penciclovir cream). There are, however, no adequate and well-controlled studies in pregnant women. Because animal reproduction studies are not always predictive of human response, penciclovir should be used during pregnancy only if clearly needed.

Nursing Mothers
There is no information on whether penciclovir is excreted in human milk after topical administration. However, following oral administration of famciclovir (the oral prodrug of penciclovir) to lactating rats, penciclovir was excreted in breast milk at concentrations higher than those seen in the plasma. Therefore, a decision should be made whether to

discontinue the drug, taking into account the importance of the drug to the mother. There are no data on the safety of penciclovir in newborns.

Pediatric Use
Safety and effectiveness in pediatric patients have not been established.

Geriatic Use
In 74 patients ≥65 years of age, the adverse events profile was comparable to that observed in younger patients.

ADVERSE REACTIONS
In two double-blind, placebo-controlled trials, 1516 patients were treated with Denavir (penciclovir cream) and 1541 with placebo. The most frequently reported adverse event was headache, which occurred in 5.3% of the patients treated with *Denavir* and 5.8% of the placebo-treated patients. The rates of reported local adverse reactions are shown in Table 2 below. One or more local adverse reactions were reported by 2.7% of the patients treated with *Denavir* and 3.9% of placebo-treated patients.

Table 2—Local Adverse Reactions Reported in Phase III Trials

	Penciclovir n=1516 %	Placebo n=1541 %
Application site reaction	1.3	1.8
Hypesthesia/Local anesthesia	0.9	1.4
Taste perversion	0.2	0.3
Pruritus	0.0	0.3
Pain	0.0	0.1
Rash (erythematous)	0.1	0.1
Allergic reaction	0.0	0.1

Two studies, enrolling 108 healthy subjects, were conducted to evaluate the dermal tolerance of 5% penciclovir cream (a 5-fold higher concentration than the commercial formulation) compared to vehicle using repeated occluded patch testing methodology. The 5% penciclovir cream induced mild erythema in approximately one-half of the subjects exposed, an irritancy profile similar to the vehicle control in terms of severity and proportion of subjects with a response. No evidence of sensitization was observed.

OVERDOSAGE
Since penciclovir is poorly absorbed following oral administration, adverse reactions related to penciclovir ingestion are unlikely.
There is no information on overdose.

DOSAGE AND ADMINISTRATION
Denavir should be applied every 2 hours during waking hours for a period of 4 days. Treatment should be started as early as possible (i.e., during the prodrome or when lesions appear).

HOW SUPPLIED
Denavir is supplied in a 2 gram tube containing 10 mg of penciclovir per gram.
NDC 00135-315-51
Store at or below 30°C (86°F). Do not freeze.
CAUTION: Federal law prohibits dispensing without prescription.
DATE OF ISSUANCE OCTOBER 1996
©SmithKline Beecham, 1996
Comments or questions? Call toll-free 1-800-320-6022.
Manufactured in Crawley, UK by **SmithKline Beecham Pharmaceuticals,** for **SmithKline Beecham Consumer Healthcare, L.P.,** Pittsburgh, PA 15230
DV:L1

OCT 96   50161US1

ECOTRIN®   OTC
Enteric-Coated Aspirin
Antiarthritic, Antiplatelet

DESCRIPTION
'Ecotrin' is enteric-coated aspirin (acetylsalicylic acid, ASA) available in tablet form in 81 mg, 325 mg and 500 mg dosage units.
The enteric coating covers a core of aspirin and is designed to resist disintegration in the stomach, dissolving in the more neutral-to-alkaline environment of the duodenum. Such action helps to protect the stomach from injury that may result from ingestion of plain, buffered or highly buffered aspirin (see SAFETY).

INDICATIONS
'Ecotrin' is indicated for:
• conditions requiring chronic or long-term aspirin therapy for pain and/or inflammation, e.g., rheumatoid arthritis, juvenile rheumatoid arthritis, systemic lupus erythematosus, osteoarthritis (degenerative joint disease), ankylosing spondylitis, psoriatic arthritis, Reiter's syndrome and fibrositis,
• antiplatelet indications of aspirin (see the ANTIPLATELET EFFECT section) and
• situations in which compliance with aspirin therapy may be affected because of the gastrointestinal side effects of plain, i.e., non-enteric-coated, or buffered aspirin.

DOSAGE
For analgesic or anti-inflammatory indications, the OTC maximum dosage for aspirin is 4000 mg per day in divided doses, i.e., up to 650 mg every 4 hours or 1000 mg every 6 hours.
For antiplatelet effect dosage: see the ANTIPLATELET EFFECT section.
Under a physician's direction, the dosage can be increased or otherwise modified as appropriate to the clinical situation. When 'Ecotrin' is used for anti-inflammatory effect, the physician should be attentive to plasma salicylate levels, and may also caution the patient to be alert to the development of tinnitus as an indicator of elevated salicylate levels. It should be noted that patients with a high frequency hearing loss (such as may occur in older individuals) may have difficulty perceiving the tinnitus. Tinnitus would then not be a reliable indicator in such individuals.

INACTIVE INGREDIENTS
81 mg: Carnauba Wax, D&C Yellow 10, FD&C Yellow 6, Hydroxypropyl Methylcellulose, Methacrylic Acid Copolymer, Microcrystalline Cellulose, Polyethylene Glycol, Polysorbate 80, Propylene Glycol, Silicon Dioxide, Starch, Stearic Acid, Talc, Titanium Dioxide, Triethyl Citrate.
325 mg and 500 mg: Carnauba wax, Colloidal Silicon Dioxide, FD&C Yellow #6, Hydroxypropyl Methylcellulose, Maltodextrin, Methacrylic Acid Copolymer, Microcrystalline Cellulose, Pregelatinized Starch, Propylene Glycol, Simethicone, Sodium Hydroxide, Sodium Starch Glycolate, Stearic Acid, Talc, Titanium Dioxide, Triethyl Citrate.

BIOAVAILABILITY
The bioavailability of aspirin from 'Ecotrin' has been demonstrated in a number of salicylate excretion studies. The studies show levels of salicylate (and metabolites) in urine excreted over 48 hours for 'Ecotrin' do not differ statistically from plain, i.e., non-enteric-coated, aspirin.
Plasma studies, in which 'Ecotrin' has been compared with plain aspirin in steady-state studies over eight days, also demonstrate that 'Ecotrin' provides plasma salicylate levels not statistically different from plain aspirin.
Information regarding salicylate levels over a range of doses was generated in a study in which 24 healthy volunteers (12 male and 12 female) took daily (divided) doses of either 2600 mg, 3900 mg, or 5200 mg of 'Ecotrin'. Plasma salicylate levels generally acknowledged to be anti-inflammatory (15 mg/dL) were attained at daily doses of 5200 mg, on Day 2 by females and Day 3 by males. At 3900 mg, anti-inflammatory levels were attained at Day 3 by females and Day 4 by males.
Dissolution of the enteric coating occurs at a neutral-to-basic pH and is therefore dependent on gastric emptying into the duodenum. With continued dosing, appropriate plasma levels are maintained.

SAFETY
The safety of 'Ecotrin' has been demonstrated in a number of endoscopic studies comparing 'Ecotrin', plain aspirin, buffered aspirin, and highly buffered aspirin preparations. In these studies, all forms of aspirin were dosed to the OTC

Continued on next page

Ecotrin—Cont.

maximum (3900–4000 mg per day) for up to 14 days. The normal healthy volunteers participating in these studies were gastroscoped before and after the courses of treatment and 14-day drug-free periods followed active drug. Compared to all the other preparations, there was less gastric damage at a statistically significant level during the 'Ecotrin' courses. There was also statistically less duodenal damage when compared with the plain i.e., non-enteric-coated aspirin.

Details of studies demonstrating the safety and bioavailability of 'Ecotrin' are available to health care professionals. Write: Professional Services Department, SmithKline Beecham Consumer Healthcare, P.O. Box 1467, Pittsburgh, Pa. 15230.

WARNINGS

Children and teenagers should not use this product for chicken pox or flu symptoms before a doctor is consulted about Reye Syndrome, a rare but serious illness reported to be associated with aspirin. Do not take this product for pain for more than 10 days or for fever for more than 3 days, or in conditions affecting children under 12 years of age, unless directed by a doctor. If pain or fever persists or gets worse, if new symptoms occur, or if redness or swelling is present, consult a doctor because these could be signs of a serious condition. Do not take this product if you are allergic to aspirin, have asthma, have stomach problems that persist or recur, or if you have ulcers or bleeding problems unless directed by a doctor. If ringing in the ears or a loss of hearing occurs, consult a doctor before taking any more of this product. **Keep this and all drugs out of the reach of children.** In case of accidental overdose, seek professional assistance or contact a poison control center immediately. As with any medicine, if you are pregnant or nursing a baby, seek the advice of a health professional before using this product. **IT IS ESPECIALLY IMPORTANT NOT TO USE ASPIRIN DURING THE LAST 3 MONTHS OF PREGNANCY UNLESS SPECIFICALLY DIRECTED TO DO SO BY A DOCTOR BECAUSE IT MAY CAUSE PROBLEMS IN THE UNBORN CHILD OR COMPLICATIONS DURING DELIVERY.**

Drug Interaction Precaution: Do not take this product if you are taking a prescription drug for anticoalgulation (thinning of the blood), diabetes, gout, or arthritis unless directed by a doctor.

Professional Warning: There have been occasional reports in the literature concerning individuals with impaired gastric emptying in whom there may be retention of one or more enteric coated aspirin tablets over time. This unusual phenomenon may occur as a result of outlet obstruction from ulcer disease alone or combined with hypotonic gastric peristalsis. Because of the integrity of the enteric coating in an acidic environment, these tablets may accumulate and form a bezoar in the stomach. Individuals with this condition may present with complaints of early satiety or of vague upper abdominal distress. Diagnosis may be made by endoscopy or by abdominal films which show opacities suggestive of a mass of small tablets *(Ref.: Bogacz, K. and Caldron, P.: Enteric-coated Aspirin Bezoar: Elevation of Serum Salicylate Level by Barium Study. Amer. J. Med. 1987:83, 783-6.).* Management may vary according to the condition of the patient. Options include: gastrotomy and alternating slightly basic and neutral lavage (*Ref.: Baum, J.: Enteric-Coated Aspirin and the Problem of Gastric Retention. J. Rheum., 1984:11, 250-1.*). While there have been no clinical reports, it has been suggested that such individuals may also be treated with parenteral cimetidine (to reduce acid secretion) and then given sips of slightly basic liquids to effect gradual dissolution of the enteric coating. Progress may be followed with plasma salicylate levels or via recognition of tinnitus by the patient.

It should be kept in mind that individuals with a history of partial or complete gastrectomy may produce reduced amounts of acid and therefore have less acidic gastric pH. Under these circumstances, the benefits offered by the acid-resistant enteric coating may not exist.

ANTIARTHRITIC AND ANTI-INFLAMMATORY INDICATIONS

For rheumatoid arthritis, juvenile rheumatoid arthritis, systemic lupus erythematosus, osteoarthritis (degenerative joint disease), ankylosing spondylitis, psoriatic arthritis, Reiter's syndrome, and fibrositis.

ANTIPLATELET EFFECT

Aspirin may be recommended to reduce the risk of death and/or nonfatal myocardial infarction (MI) in patients with a previous infarction or unstable angina pectoris and to reduce the risk of transient ischemic attacks in men.

Aspirin is also indicated to reduce the risk of vascular mortality in patients with suspected acute MI. Indications for these conditions follow:

ASPIRIN FOR MYOCARDIAL INFARCTION INDICATIONS

Recurrent Myocardial Infarction (MI) (Reinfarction) or Unstable Angina Pectoris: Aspirin is indicated to reduce the risk of death and/or nonfatal MI in patients with a previous MI or unstable angina pectoris.

Suspected Acute MI: Aspirin is indicated to reduce the risk of vascular mortality in patients with a suspected acute MI.

CLINICAL TRIALS

Recurrent MI (Reinfarction) and Unstable Angina Pectoris: The indication is supported by the results of six large, randomized multicenter, placebo-controlled studies involving 10,816, predominantly male, post-myocardial infarction (MI) patients and one randomized placebo-controlled study of 1,266 men with unstable angina (1–7). Therapy with aspirin was begun at intervals after the onset of acute MI varying from less than 3 days to more than 5 years and continued for periods of from less than 1 year to 4 years. In the unstable angina study, treatment was started within 1 month after the onset of unstable angina and continued for 12 weeks, and congestive heart failure were not included in the study.

Aspirin therapy in MI patients was associated with about a 20-percent reduction in the risk of subsequent death and/or non-fatal reinfarction, a median absolute decrease of 3 percent from the 12- to 22-percent event rates in the placebo groups. In aspirin-treated unstable angina patients the reduction in risk was about 50 percent, a reduction in event rate of 5 percent from the 10-percent rate in the placebo group over the 12-weeks of the study.

Daily dosage of aspirin in the post-myocardial infarction studies was 300 milligrams in one study and 900 to 1,500 milligrams in 5 studies. A dose of 325 milligrams was used in the study of unstable angina.

Suspected Acute MI: The use of aspirin in patients with a suspected acute MI is supported by the results of a large, multicenter 2 × 2 factorial study of 17,187 subjects with suspected acute MI (8). Subjects were randomized within 24 hours of the onset of symptoms so that 8,587 subjects received oral aspirin (162.5 milligrams, enteric-coated) daily for 1 month (the first dose crushed, sucked, or chewed) and 8,600 received oral placebo. Of the subjects, 8,592 were also randomized to receive a single dose of streptokinase (1.5 million units) infused intravenously for about 1 hour, and 8,595 received a placebo infusion. Thus, 4,295 subjects received aspirin plus placebo, 4,300 received streptokinase plus placebo, 4,292 received aspirin plus streptokinase, and 4,300 received double placebo.

Vascular mortality (attributed to cardiac, cerebral, hemorrhagic, other vascular, or unknown causes) occurred in 9.4 percent of the subjects in the aspirin group and in 11.8 percent of the subjects in the oral placebo group in the 35-day followup. This represents an absolute reduction of 2.4 percent in the mean 35-day vascular mortality attributable to aspirin and a 23 percent reduction in the odds of vascular death ($2p < 0.0001$).

Significant absolute reductions in mortality and corresponding reductions in specific clinical events favoring aspirin were found for reinfarction (1.5 percent absolute reduction, 45 percent odds reduction, $2p < 0.0001$), cardiac arrest (1.2 percent absolute reduction, 14.2 percent odds reduction, $2p < 0.01$), and total stroke (0.4 percent absolute reduction, 41.5 percent odds reduction, $2p < 0.01$). The effect of aspirin over and above its effect on mortality was evidenced by small, but significant, reductions in vascular morbidity in those subjects who were discharged.

The beneficial effects of aspirin on mortality were present with or without streptokinase infusion. Aspirin reduced vascular mortality from 10.4 to 8.0 percent for days 0 to 35 in subjects given streptokinase and reduced vascular mortality from 13.2 to 10.7 percent in subjects given no streptokinase. The effects of aspirin and thrombolytic therapy with streptokinase in this study were approximately additive. Subjects who received the combination of streptokinase infusion and daily aspirin had significantly lower vascular mortality at 35 days than those who received either active treatment alone (combination 8.0 percent, aspirin 10.7 percent, streptokinase 10.4 percent, and no treatment 13.2 percent). While this study demonstrated that aspirin has an additive benefit in patients given streptokinase, there is no reason to restrict its use to that specific thrombolytic.

ADVERSE REACTIONS

Gastrointestinal Reactions: Doses of 1,000 milligrams per day of aspirin caused gastrointestinal symptoms and bleeding that in some cases were clinically significant. In the largest post-infarction study (the Aspirin Myocardial Infarction Study (AMIS) with 4,500 people), the percentage incidences of gastrointestinal symptoms for the aspirin (1,000 milligrams of a standard, solid-tablet formulation) and placebo-treated subjects, respectively, were: stomach pain (14.5 percent; 4.4 percent); heartburn (11.9 percent; 4.8 percent); nausea and/or vomiting (7.6 percent; 2.1 percent); hospitalization for gastrointestinal disorder (4.8 percent; 3.5 percent). Symptoms and signs of gastrointestinal irritation were not significantly increased in subjects treated for unstable angina with 325 milligrams buffered aspirin in solution.

Bleeding: In the AMIS and other trials, aspirin-treated subjects had increased rates of gross gastrointestinal bleeding. In the ISIS-2 study (8), there was no significant difference in the incidence of major bleeding (bleeds requiring transfusion) between 8,587 subjects taking 162.5 milligrams aspirin daily and 8,600 subjects taking placebo (31 versus 33 subjects). There were five confirmed cerebral hemorrhages in the aspirin group compared with two in the placebo group, but the incidence of stroke of all causes was significantly reduced from 81 to 47 for the placebo versus aspirin group (0.4 percent absolute change). There was a small and statistically significant excess (0.6 percent) of minor bleeding in people taking aspirin (2.5 percent for aspirin, 1.9 percent for placebo). No other significant adverse effects were reported.

Cardiovascular and Biochemical: In the AMIS trial, the dosage of 1,000 milligrams per day of aspirin was associated with small increases in systolic blood pressure (BP) (average 1.5 to 2.1 millimeters), depending upon whether maximal or last available readings were used. Blood urea nitrogen and uric acid levels were also increased, but by less than 1.0 milligram percent.

Subjects with marked hypertension or renal insufficiency had been excluded from the trial so that the clinical importance of these observations for such subjects or for any subjects treated over more prolonged periods is not known. It is recommended that patients placed on long-term aspirin treatment, even at doses of 300 milligrams per day, be seen at regular intervals to assess changes in these measurements.

Sodium in Buffered Aspirin for Solution Formulations: One tablet daily of buffered aspirin in solutions adds 553 milligrams of sodium to that in the diet and may not be tolerated by patients with active sodium-retaining states such as congestive heart or renal failure. This amount of sodium adds about 30 percent to the 70- to 90-milliequivalents intake suggested as appropriate for dietary treatment of essential hypertension in the "1984 Report of the Joint National Committee on Detection, Evaluation, and Treatment of High Blood Pressure" (9).

DOSAGE AND ADMINISTRATION

Recurrent MI (Reinfarction) and Unstable Angina Pectoris: Although most of the studies used dosages exceeding 300 milligrams, 2 trials used only 300 millgrams and pharmacologic data indicate that this dose inhibits platelet function fully. Therefore, 300 milligrams or a conventional 325 milligram aspirin dose is a reasonable, routine dose that would minimize gastrointestinal adverse reactions. This use of aspirin applies to both solid, oral dosage forms (buffered and plain aspirin) and buffered aspirin in solution.

Suspected Acute MI: The recommended dose of aspirin to treat suspected acute MI is 160 to 162.5 milligrams taken as soon as the infarct is suspected and then daily for at least 30 days. (One-half of a conventional 325-milligram aspirin tablet or two 80- or 81-milligram aspirin tablets may be taken.) This use of aspirin applies to both solid, oral dosage forms buffered, plain, and enteric-coated aspirin and buffered aspirin in solution. If using a solid dosage form, the first dose should be crushed, sucked, or chewed. After the 30-day treatment, physicians should consider further therapy based on the labeling for dosage and administration of aspirin for prevention of recurrent MI (reinfarction).

REFERENCES

(1) Elwood, P.C. et al., "A Randomized Controlled Trial of Acetylsalicylic Acid in the Secondary Prevention of Mortality from Myocardial Infarction," British Medical Journal, 1:436–440, 1974.

(2) The Coronary Drug Project Research Group, "Aspirin in Coronary Heart Disease," Journal of Chronic Diseases, 29: 625–642, 1976.

(3) Breddin, K. et al., "Secondary Prevention of Myocardial Infarction: A Comparison of Acetylsalicylic Acid, Phenprocoumon or Placebo," Homeostasis, 470:263–268, 1979.

(4) Aspirin Myocardial Infarction Study Research Group, "A Randomized, Controlled Trial of Aspirin in Persons Recovered from Myocardial Infarction," Journal of the American Medical Aassociation, 243:661–669, 1980.

(5) Elwood, P.C., and P.M. Sweetnam, "Aspirin and Secondary Mortality After Myocardial Infarction," Lancet, II: 1313–1315, December 22–29, 1979.

(6) The Persantine-Aspirin Reinfarction Study Research Group, "Persantine and Aspirin in Coronary Heart Disease," Circulation, 62:449–461, 1980.

(7) Lewis, H.D. et al., "Protective Effects of Aspirin Against Acute Myocardial Infarction and Death in Men with Unstable Angina, Results of a Veterans Administration Cooperative Study," New England Journal of Medicine, 309:396–403, 1983.

(8) ISIS-2 (Second International Study of Infarct Survival) Collaborative Group, "Randomized Trial of Intravenous

Streptokinase, Oral Aspirin, Both, or Neither Among 17,187 Cases of Suspected Acute Myocardial Infarction: ISIS-2," Lancet, 2:349-360, August 13, 1988.
(9) "1984 Report of the Joint National Committee on Detection, Evaluation, and Treatment of High Blood Pressure," United States Department of Health and Human Services and United States Public Health Service, National Institutes of Health, Publication No. NIH 84-1088, 1984.

"ASPIRIN FOR TRANSIENT ISCHEMIC ATTACKS"

Indication

For reducing the risk of recurrent Transient Ischemic Attacks (TIA's) or stroke in men who have had transient ischemia of the brain due to fibrin platelet emboli. There is inadequate evidence that aspirin or buffered aspirin is effective in reducing TIA's in women at the recommended dosage. There is no evidence that aspirin or buffered aspirin is of benefit in the treatment of completed strokes in men or women.

Clinical Trials

The indication is supported by the results of a Canadian study (1) in which 585 patients with threatened stroke were followed in a randomized clinical trial for an average of 26 months to determine whether aspirin or sulfinpyrazone, singly or in combination, was superior to placebo in preventing transient ischemic attacks, stroke or death. The study showed that, although sulfinpyrazone had no statistically significant effect, aspirin reduced the risk of continuing transient ischemic attacks, stroke or death by 19 percent and reduced the risk of stroke or death by 31 percent. Another aspirin study carried out in the United States with 178 patients, showed a statistically significant number of "favorable outcomes," including reduced transient ischemic attacks, stroke and death (2).

Precautions

Patients presenting with signs and/or symptoms of TIA's should have a complete medical and neurologic evaluation. Consideration should be given to other disorders that resemble TIA's. Attention should be given to risk factors: it is important to evaluate and treat, if appropriate, other diseases associated with TIA's and stroke, such as hypertension and diabetes.

Concurrent administration of absorbable antacids at therapeutic doses may increase the clearance of salicylates in some individuals. The concurrent administration of nonabsorbable antacids may alter the rate of absorption of aspirin, thereby resulting in a decreased acetylsalicylic acid/salicylate ratio in plasma. The clinical significance of these decreases in available aspirin is unknown.

Aspirin at dosages of 1,000 milligrams per day has been associated with small increases in blood pressure, blood urea nitrogen, and serum uric acid levels. It is recommended that patients placed on long-term aspirin treatment be seen at regular intervals to assess changes in these measurements.

Adverse Reactions:

At dosages of 1,000 milligrams or higher of aspirin per day, gastrointestinal side effects include stomach pain, heartburn, nausea and/or vomiting, as well as increased rates of gross gastrointestinal bleeding.

Dosage and Administration

Adult dosage for men is 1,300 mg a day, in divided doses of 650 mg twice a day or 325 mg four times a day.

References

(1) The Canadian Cooperative Study Group, "Randomized Trial of Aspirin and Sulfinpyrazone in Threatened Stroke," New England Journal of Medicine, 299:53–59, 1978.
(2) Fields, W. S., et al., "Controlled Trial of Aspirin in Cerebral Ischemia," Stroke 8:301–316, 1977."

HOW SUPPLIED

'Ecotrin' Tablets
  81 mg in bottle of 36
  325 mg in bottles of 100* and 250
  500 mg in bottles of 60* and 150
  * Without child-resistant caps.

TAMPER-RESISTANT PACKAGE FEATURES FOR YOUR PROTECTION:

• Bottle has imprinted seal under cap.
• The words ECOTRIN LOW or ECOTRIN REG or ECOTRIN MAX appear on each tablet.

• **DO NOT USE THIS PRODUCT IF ANY OF THESE TAMPER-RESISTANT FEATURES ARE MISSING OR BROKEN.**

Comments or Questions? Call Toll-Free 800-245-1040 weekdays.

FEOSOL®Caplets   OTC
Hematinic
Iron Supplement

DESCRIPTION

FEOSOL Caplets contain pure iron micro particles called carbonyl iron. Replacing FEOSOL Capsules, this advanced formula is specially designed to be well absorbed, gentle on the stomach and offers enhanced safety in the event of an accidental overdose. Each FEOSOL carbonyl iron caplet delivers 50 mg of pure elemental iron, the same amount of elemental iron contained in the 250 mg ferrous sulfate capsule. At equivalent doses, carbonyl iron and ferrous sulfate were shown to be equally efficacious in correcting hemoglobin, hematocrit and serum iron levels in iron-deficient patients[1].

SAFETY

According to the American Association of Poison Control Centers, iron containing supplements are the leading cause of pediatric poisoning deaths for children under six in the United States[2]. Widely used as a food additive, carbonyl iron must be gastrically solubilized before it can be absorbed, giving it lower toxicity and enhancing its safety versus any of the ferrous salts[3]. As a result, carbonyl iron presents less chance of harm from accidental overdose. In addition, at equivalent doses, carbonyl iron side effects are no greater than those experienced with ferrous sulfate[4].

WARNINGS

Do not exceed recommended dosage. The treatment of any anemic condition should be under the advice and supervision of a physician. Since oral iron products interfere with absorption of oral tetracycline antibiotics, these products should not be taken within two hours of each other. Occasional gastrointestinal discomfort (such as nausea) may be minimized by taking with meals. Iron containing medication may occasionally cause constipation or diarrhea.
WARNING: Accidental overdose of iron-containing products is a leading cause of fatal poisoning in children under 6. Keep this product out of reach of children. In case of accidental overdose, call a doctor or poison control center immediately.

NUTRITION FACTS

Serving Size: 1 Caplet

Amount per Caplet	% Daily Value
Iron 50 mg	280%

FORMULA
INGREDIENTS

Lactose, Sorbitol, Carbonyl Iron, Crospovidone, Magnesium stearate, Polyethylene Glycol, Stearic Acid, Hydroxypropyl Methylcellulose, Polydextrose, Carnauba Wax, Titanium Dioxide, Triacetin, Blue #2 Al Lake, Red #40 Al Lake, Yellow #6 Al Lake.

DIRECTIONS

Adults—one caplet daily or as directed by a physician. Children under 12 years: Consult a physician.

TAMPER-EVIDENT FEATURE

Each caplet is encased in a plastic cell with a foil back; do not use if cell or foil is broken.

REFERENCES

[1] Devasthali SD, Gordeuk VR, Brittenham GM, et al, "Bioavailability of Carbonyl Iron: A randomized, double-blind study." Eur J Haematology, 1991; 46:272–278.
[2] FDA Consumer; March 1996:7
[3] Heubers, JA, Brittenham GM, Csiba E and Finch CA. "Absorption of carbonyl iron." J Lab Clin Med 1986; 108:473–78.
[4] Devasthali SD, Gordeuk VR, Brittenham GM, et al, "Bioavailability of a Carbonyl Iron: A randomized, double-blind study." Eur J Haematology, 1991; 46:272–278.
Store at room temperature, avoid excessive heat (greater than 100°F) or humidity.

HOW SUPPLIED

Boxes of 30 and 60 caplets in blisters. Also available in single unit packages of 100 caplets intended for institutional use
Comments or Questions? Call Toll-Free 1-800-245-1040 Weekdays.
SmithKline Beecham Consumer Healthcare, L.P.
Pittsburgh, PA 15230   Made in USA

FEOSOL® ELIXIR   OTC
Hematinic
Iron Supplement

DESCRIPTION

'Feosol' Elixir, an unusually palatable iron elixir, provides the body with ferrous sulfate—the standard elixir for simple iron deficiency and iron-deficiency anemia when the need for such therapy has been determined by a physician.

NUTRITION FACTS

Serving Size: 1 teaspoonful
Servings per Container: 94

Amount per teaspoonful	% Daily Value
Iron 44 mg	244%

FORMULA
INGREDIENTS

Purified Water, Sucrose, Glucose, Ferrous Sulfate, Alcohol 5%, Citric Acid, Saccharin Sodium, FD&C Yellow #6, Flavors.

DIRECTIONS

Adults—1 teaspoonful daily or as directed by a doctor. Children under 12 years—Consult a physician. Mix with water or fruit juice to avoid temporary staining of teeth; do not mix with milk or wine-based vehicles.

TAMPER-RESISTANT PACKAGE FEATURE:
IMPRINTED SEAL AROUND BOTTLE CAP: DO NOT USE IF BROKEN.

WARNINGS

Do not exceed recommended dosage. The treatment of any anemic condition should be under the advice and supervision of a physician. Since oral iron products interfere with absorption of oral tetracycline antibiotics, these products should not be taken within two hours of each other. Occasional gastrointestinal discomfort (such as nausea) may be minimized by taking with meals. Iron containing medication may occasionally cause constipation or diarrhea and liquids may cause temporary staining of the teeth (this is less likely when diluted).
WARNING: Accidental overdose of iron-containing products is a leading cause of fatal poisoning in children under 6. Keep this product out of reach of children. In case of accidental overdose, call a doctor or poison control center immediately.
If you are pregnant or nursing a baby, seek the advice of a health professional before using this product.
STORE AT ROOM TEMPERATURE (59–86 F), PROTECT FROM FREEZING.

HOW SUPPLIED

A clear orange liquid in 16 fl. oz. child-resistant bottles.

ALSO AVAILABLE

'Feosol' Tablets, 'Feosol' Caplets.

FEOSOL® TABLETS   OTC
Hematinic
Iron Supplement

DESCRIPTION

Feosol tablets provide the body with ferrous sulfate—an iron supplement for iron deficiency and iron deficiency anemia when the need for such therapy has been determined by a physician.

NUTRITION FACTS

Serving Size: 1 Tablet

Amount per Tablet	% Daily Value
Iron 65 mg	361%

FORMULA
INGREDIENTS

Dried ferrous sulfate 200 mg (65 mg of elemental iron) equivalent to 325 mg of ferrous sulfate USP per tablet. Calcium Sulfate, Starch, Glucose, Hydroxypropyl Methylcellulose, Talc, Stearic Acid, Polyethylene Glycol, Sodium Lauryl Sulfate, Mineral Oil, Titanium Dioxide, D&C Yellow 10, FD&C Blue 2.

DIRECTIONS

Adults and children 12 years and over—One tablet daily or as directed by a physician. Children under 12 years—Consult a physician.

TAMPER-EVIDENT FEATURES:

Each tablet is encased in a plastic cell with a foil back; do not use if cell or foil is broken.

Comments or Questions?
Call toll-free 800-245-1040 weekdays.

WARNINGS

Do not exceed recommended dosage. The treatment of any anemic condition should be under the advice and supervision of a physician. Since oral iron products interfere with absorption of oral tetracycline antibiotics, these products should not be taken within two hours of each other. Occasional gastrointestinal discomfort (such as nausea) may be minimized by taking with meals. Iron containing medication may occasionally cause constipation or diarrhea.
WARNING: Accidental overdose of iron-contraining products is a leading cause of fatal poisoning in children under 6. Keep this product out of reach of children. In case of accidental overdose, call a doctor, or poison control center

Continued on next page

Feosol Tablets—Cont.

immediately. If you are pregnant or nursing a baby, seek the advice of a health professional before using this product.
Store at room temperature (59–86 F).
Not USP for dissolution.

HOW SUPPLIED
Cartons of 100 tablets in child-resistant blisters.
Previously packaged in bottles.
Also available in caplets and elixir.

GAVISCON® REGULAR AND EXTRA STRENGTH TABLETS — OTC
GAVISCON® REGULAR AND EXTRA STRENGTH LIQUID ANTACID
[*gav 'is-kon*]

(See PDR For Nonprescription Drugs.)

GLY-OXIDE® Liquid — OTC
[*gli 'ok-sīd*]

(See PDR For Nonprescription Drugs.)

MASSENGILL® Douches, Towelettes and Cleansing Wash — OTC
[*mas 'sen-gil*]

(See PDR for Nonprescription Drugs)

NICODERM® CQ® — OTC
Nicotine Transdermal System/Stop Smoking Aid

Formerly available only by prescription
Available as:

Step 1 - 21 mg/24 hours
Step 2 - 14 mg/24 hours
Step 3 - 7 mg/24 hours

If you smoke:
Over 10 cigarettes a Day: Start with Step 1
10 Cigarettes a Day or Less: Start with Step 2

WHAT IS THE NICODERM CQ PATCH AND HOW IS IT USED?
NicoDerm CQ is a small, nicotine containing patch. When you put on a NicoDerm CQ patch, nicotine passes through the skin and into your body. NicoDerm CQ is very thin and uses special material to control how fast nicotine passes through the skin. Unlike the sudden jolts of nicotine delivered by cigarettes, the amount of nicotine you receive remains relatively smooth throughout the 24 or 16 hours period you wear the NicoDerm CQ patch. This helps to reduce cravings you may have for nicotine.

Active Ingredient: Nicotine

Purpose: Stop Smoking Aid

Use: To reduce withdrawal symptoms, including nicotine craving, associated with quitting smoking.

Directions:
- Stop smoking completely when you begin using NicoDerm CQ.

STEP 1 (21 mg)	STEP 2 (14 mg)	STEP 3 (7 mg)
Initial Treatment Period	Step Down Treatment Period	Step Down Treatment Period
Weeks 1–6	Weeks 7–8	Weeks 9–10

- Light Smokers (10 cigarettes a day or less): Do not use STEP 1 (21 mg). Use STEP 2 (14 mg) for six weeks and STEP 3 (7 mg) for two weeks and then stop.
- STEPS 2 and 3 allow you to gradually reduce your levels of nicotine. Completing the full program will increase your chances of quitting successfully.
- A the end of 10 weeks (8 weeks for light smokers), stop using NicoDerm CQ. If you still feel the need for NicoDerm CQ, talk with your doctor.
- Each day apply a new patch to a different place on skin that is dry, clean and hairless.
- You may wear the patch for 16 or 24 hours.
- If you crave cigarettes when you wake up, wear the patch for 24 hours.
- If you begin to have vivid dreams or other disruptions of your sleep while wearing the patch for 24 hours, try taking the patch off at bedtime (after about 16 hours) and putting on a new one when you get up the next day.
- Remove the used patch and put on a new patch at the same time every day. Do not leave patch on for more than 24 hours because it may irritate your skin and loses strength after 24 hours.
- Wash your hands after applying or removing NicoDerm QC.

WARNINGS:
- Keep this and all medication away from children and pets. Used patches have enough nicotine to poison children and pets. Fold sticky ends together and insert in the disposal tray in the box. For accidental overdose, seek professional assistance or contact a poison control center immediately.
- Nicotine can increase your baby's heart rate. First try to stop smoking without the nicotine patch. As with any drug, if you are pregnant or nursing a baby, seek the advice of a health professional before using this product.
- Do not smoke even when not wearing the patch. The nicotine in your skin will still be entering your bloodstream for several hours after you take off the patch.

DO NOT USE IF YOU
- Continue to smoke, chew tobacco, use snuff, or use nicotine or other nicotine containing products.

ASK YOUR DOCTOR BEFORE USE IF YOU
- Are under 18 years of age.
- Have heart disease, recent heart attack, or irregular heartbeat. Nicotine can increase your heart rate.
- Have high blood pressure not controlled with medication. Nicotine can increase blood pressure.
- Take prescription medicine for depression or asthma. Your prescription dose may need to be adjusted.
- Are allergic to adhesive tape or have skin problems, because you are more likely to get rashes.

STOP USE AND SEE YOUR DOCTOR IF YOU HAVE
- Skin redness caused by the patch that does not go away after four days, or if your skin swells or you get a rash.
- Irregular heartbeat or palpitations.
- Symptoms of nicotine overdose such as nausea, vomiting, dizziness, weakness and rapid heartbeat.

READ THE LABEL
Read the carton and the User's Guide before using this product. Keep the carton and User's Guide. They contain important information.

Inactive Ingredients: Ethylene vinyl acetate-copolymer, polyisobutylene and high density polyethylene between pigmented and clear polyester backings.
Do not store above 30°C (86°F).

TO INCREASE YOUR SUCCESS IN QUITTING:
1. You must be motivated to quit.
2. Complete the full treatment program, applying a new patch every day.
3. Use with a support program as described in the Users Guide.

USER'S GUIDE:
HOW TO USE NICODERM CQ TO HELP YOU QUIT SMOKING
KEYS TO SUCCESS
1) You must really want to quit smoking for NicoDerm QC to help you.
2) Apply a new patch every day.
3) NicoDerm CQ works best when used together with a support program.
4) If you have trouble using NicoDerm CQ, ask your doctor or pharmacist or call SmithKline Beecham at 1-800-834-5895 weekdays (10:00am - 4:30 pm EST).

SO YOU DECIDED TO QUIT
Congratulations. Your decision to stop smoking is one of the most important things you can do to improve your health. Quitting smoking is a two-part process that involves: overcoming your physical need for nicotine, and breaking your smoking habit. Nico-Derm CQ helps smokers quit by reducing nicotine withdrawal symptoms. Many NicoDerm CQ users will be able to stop smoking for a few days but often will start smoking again. Most smokers try to quit several times before they completely stop. Your own chances of quitting smoking depend how strongly you are addicted to nicotine, how much you want to quit, and how closely you follow a quitting plan like the one that comes with NicoDerm CQ.

QUITTING SMOKING IS HARD!
If you find you cannot stop or if you start smoking again after using NicoDerm CQ please talk to a health care professional who can help you find a program that may work better for you. Breaking this addiction doesn't happen overnight. Because NicoDerm CQ provides some nicotine, the NicoDerm CQ patch will help you stop smoking by reducing nicotine withdrawal symptoms such as nicotine craving, nervousness and irritability. This User's Guide will give you support as you become a non-smoker. It will answer common questions about NicoDerm CQ and give tips to help you stop smoking, and should be referred to often.

WHERE TO GET HELP
You are more likely to stop smoking by using NicoDerm CQ with a support program that helps you break your smoking habit. There may be support groups in your area for people trying to quit. Call your local chapter of the American Lung Association (1-800-586-4872), American Cancer Society (1-800-227-2345) or American Heart Association (1-800-242-8721) for further information. If you find you cannot stop smoking or if you start smoking again after using NicoDerm CQ, remember breaking this addiction doesn't happen overnight. You may want to talk to a health care professional who can help you improve your chances of quitting the next time you try NicoDerm CQ or another method.

LET'S GET ORGANIZED
Your reason for quitting may be a combination of concerns about health, the effect of smoking on your appearance, and pressure from your family and friends to stop smoking. Or maybe you're concerned about the dangerous effect of second-hand smoke on the people you care about. All of these are good reasons. You probably have others. Decide your most important reasons, and write them down on the wallet card inside the back cover of the User's Guide. Carry this card with you. In difficult moments, when you want to smoke, the card will remind you why you are quitting.

WHAT YOU'RE UP AGAINST
Smoking is addictive in two ways. Your need for nicotine has become both physical and mental. You must overcome both addictions to stop smoking. So while NicoDerm CQ will lessen your body's physical addiction to nicotine, you've got to want to quit smoking to overcome the mental dependence on cigarettes. Once you've decided that you're going to quit, it's time to get started. But first, there are some important cautions you should consider.

SOME IMPORTANT CAUTIONS
This product is only for those who want to stop smoking. If you smoke, chew tobacco, use snuff or use nicotine gum or other nicotine containing products while using NicoDerm CQ, you may get a nicotine overdose. Ask your doctor before using NicoDerm CQ if you have heart disease, had a recent heart attack, irregular heartbeat. Nicotine can increase your blood pressure. If you take a prescription medication for asthma or depression, be sure your doctor knows you are quitting smoking. Your prescription medication dose may need to be adjusted. You should ask your doctor before using NicoDerm CQ if you are allergic to adhesive tape or have skin problems, because you are more likely to get rashes.
Nicotine can increase your baby's heart rate. First try to stop smoking without the nicotine patch. As with any drug, if you are pregnant or nursing a baby, seek the advice of a health professional before using this product. Ask your doctor before using NicoDerm CQ if you are under 18 years of age.
You should stop use and see your doctor if you have skin redness caused by the patch that does not go away after four days, or if your skin swells or you get a rash, or if you have irregular heartbeat or palpitations.
Also, stop use if you have symptoms of nicotine overdose. These may include nausea, vomiting, diarrhea, dizziness, weakness and rapid heartbeat. Also, seizures have been seen in children who swallowed cigarettes. They may have a similar reaction to nicotine patches.
Keep this and all drugs out of the reach of children and pets. Even used patches have enough nicotine to poison children and pets. Be sure to fold the sticky ends together and insert in the disposal tray provided in the box. In case of accidental overdose, seek professional assistance or contact a poison control center immediately.

LET'S GET STARTED
Becoming a non-smoker starts today. Your first step is to read through the entire User's Guide carefully.
First, check that you bought the right starting dose. If you smoke more than 10 cigarettes a day, begin with Step 1 (21 mg). As the carton indicates, light smokers should not use Step 1 (21 mg). They should start with Step 2 (14 mg). Light smokers are people who smoke 10 cigarettes or less a day. Throughout this User's Guide we will give specific instructions for light smokers.
Next set your personalized quitting schedule.
Take out a calendar that you can use to track your progress. Pick a quit date, and mark this on your calendar using the stickers in the middle of the User's Guide.
For people who smoke over 10 cigarettes a day:
STEP 1. Initial Treatment Period (weeks 1–6): 21 mg patches. Choose your quit date (it should be soon). This is the day you will quit smoking cigarettes entirely and begin using NicoDerm CQ to reduce your cravings for nicotine. Place the Step 1 sticker on this date. For the first six weeks you'll use the highest-strength (21 mg) NicoDerm CQ patches. Be sure to follow the directions on page 10 of the User's Guide.
Completing the full program will increase your chances of quitting successfully. This is done by changing over to the Step 2 (14 mg) patch for 2 weeks followed by a final 2 weeks with the Step 3 (7mg) patch. The four week step down treatment period allows you to gradually reduce the amount of nicotine you get, rather than stopping suddenly, and will increase your chances of quitting.
STEP 2. First step down treatment period (Weeks 7–8): 14 mg patches. Switching to Step 2 (14 mg) patches after 6

weeks begins to gradually reduce your nicotine usage. Place the Step 2 sticker on this date (the first day of week seven). Use the 14 mg patches for two weeks.

STEP 3. Final step down treatment period (Weeks 9–10): 7 mg patches. After eight weeks, nicotine intake is further reduced by moving down to Step 3 (7 mg) patches. Place the Step 3 sticker on this date (the first day of week nine). Use the 7 mg patches for two weeks.

See the chart in the "DIRECTIONS" section above for the recommended usage schedule for NicoDerm CQ. **Stop using NicoDerm CQ at the end of week 10.** If you still feel the need to use NicoDerm CQ after Week 10, talk with your doctor or health professional.

LIGHT SMOKER DIRECTIONS

Do not use Step 1 (21 mg). You should start with Step 2 (14 mg).

For LIGHT SMOKERS–People who smoke 10 cigarettes or less a day: Begin with STEP 2–Initial Treatment Period (Weeks 1–6): 14 mg patches.

Choose your quit date (it should be soon). This is the day you will quit smoking cigarettes entirely and begin using NicoDerm CQ to reduce your cravings for nicotine. Place the Step 2 sticker on this date. For the first six weeks, you'll use the Step 2 (14 mg) NicoDerm CQ patches. Be sure to follow the directions on page 10.

Continue with STEP 3–Step Down Treatment Period (Weeks 7–8): 7 mg patches.

Completing the full program will increase your chances of quitting successfully. This is done by changing over to the Step 3 (7mg) patches for 2 weeks. The two week step down treatment period allows you to gradually reduce the amount of nicotine you get, rather than stopping suddenly, and will increase your chances of quitting. Place the Step 3 sticker on the first day of week seven. Use the 7 mg patches for two weeks.

Light smokers should not use NicoDerm CQ for longer than 8 weeks. If you still feel the need to use NicoDerm CQ after 8 weeks, talk with your doctor.

PLAN AHEAD

Because smoking is an addiction, it is not easy to stop. After you've given up nicotine, you may still have a strong urge to smoke. Plan ahead NOW for these times, so you're not tempted to start smoking again in a moment of weakness. The following tips may help:

- Keep the phone numbers of supportive friends and family members handy.
- Keep a record of your quitting process. Track when you have a craving for nicotine if it occurs. If you smoke at all, write down what you think caused the slip.
- Put together an Emergency Kit that includes items that will help take your mind off occasional urges to smoke. You might include cinnamon gum or lemon drops to suck on, a relaxing cassette tape and something for your hands to play with, like a smooth rock, rubber band or small metal balls.
- Set aside some small rewards, like a new magazine or a gift certificate from your favorite store, which you'll 'give' yourself after passing difficult hurdles.
- Think now about the times when you most often want a cigarette, and then plan what else you might do instead of smoking. For instance, you might plan to take your coffee break in a new location, or take a walk right after dinner, so you won't be tempted to smoke.

HOW NICODERM CQ WORKS

NicoDerm CQ patches provide nicotine to your system—they work as a temporary aid to help you quit smoking by reducing nicotine withdrawal symptoms, including nicotine craving. NicoDerm CQ provides a lower level of nicotine to your blood than cigarettes, and allows you to gradually do away with your body's need for nicotine. Because NicoDerm CQ does not contain the tar or carbon monoxide of cigarette smoke, it does not have the same health dangers as tobacco. However, it still delivers nicotine, the addictive part of cigarette smoke. Nicotine can cause side effects such as headache, nausea, upset stomach and dizziness.

HOW TO USE NICODERM CQ PATCHES

Read all the following instructions, and the instructions on the outer carton, before using NicoDerm CQ. Refer to them often to make sure your're using NicoDerm CQ correctly. Please refer to the audio tape for additional help.

1. Stop smoking completely before you start using NicoDerm CQ.
2. To reduce craving and other withdrawal symptoms, use NicoDerm CQ according to the dosage schedule in the "directions" section above.

Insert used NicoDerm CQ patches in the child resistant disposal tray provided in the box—safely away from children and pets.

When to apply and remove NicoDerm CQ patches.

Each day apply a new patch to a different place on skin that is dry, clean and hairless. **You can wear a NicoDerm CQ patch for either 16 or 24 hours.** If you crave cigarettes when you wake up, wear the patch for 24 hours. If you begin to have vivid dreams or other disruptions of our sleep while wearing the patch 24 hours, try taking the patch off at bedtime (after about 16 hours) and putting on a new one when you get up the next day. **Do not smoke even when you are not wearing the patch.**

Remove the used patch and put on a new patch at the same time every day. Applying the patch at about the same time each day (first thing in the morning, for instance) will help you remember when to put on a new patch. Do not leave the same NicoDerm CQ patch on for more than 24 hours because it may irritate your skin and because it loses strength after 24 hours. Do not use NicoDerm CQ continuously for more than 10 weeks (8 weeks for light smokers).

How to apply a NicoDerm CQ patch.

1. Do not remove the NicoDerm CQ patch from its sealed protective pouch until you are ready to use it. NicoDerm CQ patches will lose nicotine to the air if you store them out of the pouch.
2. Choose a non-hairy, clean, dry area of skin. Do not put a NicoDerm CQ patch on skin that is burned, broken out, cut or irritated in any way. Make sure your skin is free of lotion and soap before applying a patch.
3. A clear, protective liner covers the sticky silver side of the NicoDerm CQ patch—the side that will be put on your skin. The liner has a slit down the middle to help you remove it from the patch. With the silver side facing you, put half the liner away from the NicoDerm CQ patch starting at the middle slit, as shown in the illustration above. Hold the NicoDerm CQ patch at one of the outside edges (touch the silver side as little as possible), and pull off the other half of the protective liner. Place this liner in the slot in the disposable tray provided in the NicoDerm CQ package where it will be out of reach of children and pets.
4. Immediately apply the sticky side of the NicoDerm CQ patch to your skin. **Press the patch firmly on your skin with the heel of your hand for at least 10 seconds.** Make sure it sticks well to your skin, especially around the edges.
5. Wash your hands when you have finished applying the NicoDerm CQ patch. Nicotine on your hands could get into your eyes and nose, and cause stinging, redness, or more serious problems.
6. After 24 or 16 hours, remove the patch you have been wearing. Fold the used NicoDerm CQ patch in half with the silver side together. Careful dispose of the used patch in the slot of the disposal tray provided in the NicoDerm CQ package where it will be out of the reach of children and pets. Even used patches have enough nicotine to poison children and pets. Wash your hands.
7. Chose a different place on your skin to apply the next NicoDerm CQ patch and repeat Steps 1 to 6. Do not apply a new patch to a previously used skin site for at least one week.

If your NicoDerm CQ patch gets wet during wearing. Water will not harm the NicoDerm CQ patch you are wearing if applied properly. You can bathe, swim or shower for short periods while you are wearing the NicoDerm CQ patch.

If your NicoDerm CQ patch comes off while wearing. NicoDerm CQ patches generally stick well to most people's skin, However, a patch may occasionally come off. If your NicoDerm CQ patch falls off during the day, put on a new patch, making sure you select a non-hairy, non-irritated area of the skin that is clean and dry. If the soap you use has lanolin or moisturizers, the patch may not stick well. Using a different soap may help. Body creams, lotions and sunscreens can also cause problems with keeping your patch on. Do not apply creams or lotions to the place on your skin where you will put the patch. If you have followed the directions and the patch still does not stick to you, try using medical adhesive tape over the patch.

Disposing of NicoDerm CQ patches. Fold the used patch in half with the silver side together. Carefully dispose of the patch in the disposal slot of the tray provided in the NicoDerm CQ package where it will be out of the reach of children and pets. Small amounts of nicotine, even from a used patch can poison children and pets. **Keep all nicotine patches away from children and pets.** Wash. YOUR HANDS AFTER DISPOSING OF THE PATCH.

If your skin reacts to the NicoDerm CQ patch. When you first put on a NicoDerm CQ patch, mild itching, burning or tingling is normal and should go away within an hour. If you remove a NicoDerm CQ patch, the skin under the patch might be somewhat red. Your skin should not stay red for more than a day after removing the patch. **If you get a skin rash after using a NicoDerm CQ patch, or if the skin under the patch becomes swollen or very red, call your doctor. Do not put on a new patch.**

Storage Instructions

Keep each NicoDerm CQ patch in its protective pouch, unopened, until you are ready to use it, because the patch will lose nicotine to the air if it's outside the pouch. Do not store NicoDerm CQ patches above 86°F (30°C) because they are sensitive to heat. Remember, the inside of your car can reach temperatures much higher than this. A slight yellowing of the silver side of the patch is normal. Do not use NicoDerm CQ patches stored in pouches that are damaged or open.

See the chare in the **"DIRECTIONS"** section above for the recommended usage schedule for NicoDerm CQ.

TIPS TO MAKE QUITTING EASIER

Within the first few weeks of giving up smoking, you may be tempted to smoke for pleasure, particularly after completing a difficult task, or at a party or bar. Here are some tips to help get you through the important first stages of becoming a non-smoker:

On Your Quit Date:

- Ask your family, friends and co-workers to support you in your efforts to stop smoking.
- Throw away all your cigarettes, matches, lighters, ashtrays, etc.
- Keep busy on your quit day. Exercise. Go to a movie. Take a walk. Get together with friends.
- Figure out how much money you'll save by not smoking. Most ex-smokers can save more than $1,000 a year on the price of cigarettes alone.
- Write down what you will do with the money you save.
- Know your high risk situations and plan ahead how you will deal with them.
- Visit your dentist and have your teeth cleaned to get rid of the tobacco stains.
- Use a whitening toothpaste to keep your new smile.

Right after Quitting:

- During the first few days after you've stopped smoking, spend as much time as possible at places where smoking is not allowed.
- Drink large quantities of water and fruit juices.
- Try to avoid alcohol, coffee and other beverages you associate with smoking.
- Remember that temporary urges to smoke will pass, even if you don't smoke a cigarette.
- Keep your hands busy with something like a pencil or a paper clip.
- Find other activities which help you relax without cigarettes. Swim, jog, take a walk, play basketball.
- Don't worry too much about gaining weight. Watch what you eat, take time for daily exercise, and change your eating habits if you need to.
- Laughter helps. Watch or read something funny.

WHAT TO EXPECT

Your body is now coming back into balance. During the first few days after you stop smoking, you might feel edgy and nervous and have trouble concentrating. You might get headaches, feel dizzy and a little out of sorts, feel sweaty or have stomach upsets. You might even have trouble sleeping at first. These are typical withdrawal symptoms that will go away with time. Your smoker's cough will get worse before it gets better. But don't worry, that's a good sign. Coughing helps clear the tar deposits out of your lungs.

After a week or two

By now you should be feeling more confident that you can handle those smoking urges. Many of your nicotine withdrawal symptoms have left by now, and you should be noticing some positive signs: less coughing, better breathing and an improved sense of taste and smell, to name a few.

After a month

You probably have the urge to smoke much less often now. But urges may still occur, and when they do, they are likely to be powerful ones that come out of nowhere. Don't let them catch you off guard. Plan ahead for these difficult times. Concentrate on the ways non-smokers are more attractive than smokers. Their skin is less likely to wrinkle. Their teeth are whiter, cleaner. Their breath is fresher. Their hair and clothes smell better. That cough that seems to make even a laugh sound more like a rattle is a thing of the past. Their children and others around them are healthier, too.

What To Do About Relapse.

What should you do if you slip and start smoking again? The answer is simple.

A lapse of one or two or even a few cigarettes should not spoil your efforts! Throw away your cigarettes forgive yourself and continue with the program. Listen to the Audio Tape again and re-read the User's Guide to ensure that you're using NicoDerm CQ correctly and following the other important tips for dealing with the mental and social dependence on nicotine. Your doctor, pharmacist or other health professional can also provide useful counseling on the importance of stopping smoking. You should consider them partners in your quit attempt.

What To Do About Relapse After a Successful Quit Attempt.

If you have taken up regular smoking again, don't be discouraged. Research shows that the best thing you can do is to try again, since several quitting attempts may be needed before your're successful. And your

- Admit that you've slipped, but don't treat yourself as a failure.
- Try to identify the 'trigger' that caused you to slip, and prepare a better plan for dealing with this problem next time.
- Talk positively to yourself—tell yourself that you have learned something from this experience.

Continued on next page

Nicoderm CQ—Cont.

- Make sure you used NicoDerm CQ patches correctly. Remember that it takes practice to do anything and quitting smoking is no exception.

WHEN THE STRUGGLE IS OVER

Once you've stopped smoking, take a second and pat yourself on the back. Now do it again. You deserve it. Remember now why you decided to stop smoking in the first place. Look at your list of reasons. Read them again. And smile. Now think about all the money you are saving and what you'll do with it. All the non-smoking places you can go, and what you might do there. All those years you may have added to your life, and what you'll do with them. Remember that temptation may not be gone forever. However, the hard part is behind you, so look forward with a positive attitude and enjoy your new life as a non-smoker.

QUESTIONS & ANSWERS

1. How will I feel when I stop smoking and start using Nico-Derm CQ?
You'll need to prepare yourself for some nicotine withdrawal symptoms. These begin almost immediately after you stop smoking, and are usually at their worst during the first three or four days. Understand that any of the following is possible
- craving for nicotine
- anxiety, irritability, restlessness, mood changes, nervousness
- drowsiness
- trouble concentrating
- increased appetite and weight gain
- headaches, muscular pain, constipation, fatigue.
NicoDerm CQ reduces nicotine withdrawal symptoms such as irritability and nervousness, as well as the craving for nicotine you used to satisfy by having a cigarette.
2. Is NicoDerm CQ just substituting one form of nicotine for another? NicoDerm CQ does contain nicotine. The purpose of NicoDerm CQ is to provide you with enough nicotine to reduce the physical withdrawal symptoms so you can deal with the mental aspects of quitting.
3. Can I be hurt by using NicoDerm CQ? For most adults, the amount of nicotine in the gum is less than from smoking. If you believe you may be sensitive to even this amount of nicotine, you should not use this product without advice from your doctor (see p. 4 of the User's Guide). There are also some important cautions in the User's Guide (See p. 4).
4. Will I gain weight? Many people do tend to gain a few pounds the first 8–10 weeks after they stop smoking. This is a very small price to pay for the enormous gains that you will make in your overall health and attractiveness. If you continue to gain weight after the first two months, try to analyze what you're doing differently. Reduce your fat intake, choose healthy snacks, and increase your physical activity to burn off the extra calories. Drink lots of water. This is good for your body and skin, and also helps to reduce the amount you eat.
5. Is NicoDerm CQ more expensive than smoking? The total cost of NicoDerm CQ for the twelve week program is similar to what a person who smokes one and a half packs of cigarettes a day would spend on cigarettes for the same period of time. Also use of NicoDerm CQ is only a short-term cost, while the cost of smoking is a long-term cost, because of the health problems smoking causes.
6. What if I slip up? Discard your cigarettes, forgive yourself and then get back on track. Don't consider yourself a failure or punish yourself. In fact, people who have already tried to quit are more likely to be successful the next time.

GOOD LUCK!

Copyright © 1997 SmithKline Beecham
For your family's protection, NicoDerm CQ patches are supplied in child resistant pouches. Do not use if individual pouch is damaged or open.
Manufactured by ALZA Corporation, Palo Alto, CA 94304 for SmithKline Beecham Consumer Healthcare, L.P.
Comments or Questions? Call 1–800–834–5895 Weekdays. (10 a.m.–4:30 p.m. EST).
- **Not for sale to those under 18 years of age.**
- **Proof of age required.**
- **Not for sale in vending machines or from any source where proof of age cannot be verified.**

Available as

NicoDerm CQ Step 1 (21 mg/24 hours)–7 Patches*
NicoDerm CQ Step 1 (21 mg/24 hours)–14 Patches*
NicoDerm CQ Step 2 (14 mg/24 hours)–7 Patches*
NicoDerm CQ Step 3 (7 mg/24 hours)–7 Patches**

*   User's Guide, Audio Tape & Child Resistant Disposal Tray
** User's Guide, & Child Resistant Disposal Tray

NICORETTE®   OTC

Nicotine Polacrilex Gum/Stop Smoking Aid
Available in 2mg and 4mg Strength

If you smoke:
UNDER 25 CIGARETTES A DAY: Use 2 mg
OVER 24 CIGARETTES A DAY: Use 4 mg

Action: **Stop Smoking Aid**
Use:
- To reduce withdrawal symptoms, including nicotine craving, associated with quitting smoking.

Directions:
- Stop smoking completely when you begin using Nicorette.
- Read the enclosed User's Guide before using Nicorette.
- Use properly as directed in the User's Guide.
- Don't eat or drink for 15 minutes before using Nicorette or while chewing a piece.
- Use according to the following 12 week schedule:

Weeks 1 to 6	Weeks 7 to 9	Weeks 10 to 12
1 piece every 1 to 2 hours	1 piece every 2 to 4 hours	1 piece every 4 to 8 hours

- Do not exceed 24 pieces a day.
- Stop using Nicorette at the end of week 12. If you still feel the need for Nicorette, talk with your doctor.

Warnings:
- Keep this and all drugs out of the reach of children and pets. In case of accidental overdose, seek professional assistance or contact a poison control center immediately.
- Nicotine can increase your baby's heart rate; if you are pregnant or nursing a bay, seek the advice of a health professional before using this product.

DO NOT USE IF YOU
- Continue to smoke, chew tobacco, use snuff, or use a nicotine patch or other nicotine containing products.

ASK YOUR DOCTOR BEFORE USE IF YOU
- Are under 18 years of age.
- Have heart disease, recent heart attack, or irregular heartbeat. Nicotine can increase your heart rate.
- Have high blood pressure not controlled with medication. Nicotine can increase blood pressure.
- Have stomach ulcer or take insulin for diabetes.
- Take prescription medicine for depression or asthma. Your prescription dose may need to be adjusted.

STOP USE AND SEE YOUR DOCTOR IF YOU HAVE
- Mouth, teeth or jaw problems.
- Irregular heartbeat, palpitations.
- Symptoms of nicotine overdose such as nausea, vomiting, dizziness, weakness and rapid heartbeat.

READ THE LABEL
Read the carton and the User's Guide before taking this product. Do not discard carton or User's Guide. They contain important information.
[2 mg] Inactive Ingredients: Flavors, glycerin, gum base, sodium carbonate, sorbitol, sodium bicarbonate.
[4 mg] Inactive Ingredients: Flavors, glycerin, gum base, sodium carbonate, sorbitol, D&C Yellow 10.
Do not store above 86°F (30°C). Protect from light.

TO INCREASE YOUR SUCCESS IN QUITTING:
1. **You must be motivated to quit.**
2. **Use Enough** —Chew **at least 9 pieces** of Nicorette per day during the first six weeks.
3. **Use long enough** —Use Nicorette for the full 12 weeks.
4. **Use with a support program** as described in the enclosed User's Guide.

USER'S GUIDE:

HOW TO USE NICORETTE TO HELP YOU QUIT SMOKING
KEYS TO SUCCESS
1) You must really want to quit smoking for Nicorette to help you.
2) You can greatly increase your chances for success by using at least 9 to 12 pieces every day when you start using Nicorette.
3) You should continue to use Nicorette as explained in the User's Guide for 12 full weeks.
4) Nicorette works best when used together with a support program.
5) If you have trouble using Nicorette, ask your doctor or pharmacist or call SmithKline Beecham at 1-800-419-4766 weekdays (10:00am–4:30pm EST).

SO YOU DECIDED TO QUIT
Congratulations. Your decision to stop smoking is an important one. That's why you've made the right choice in choosing Nicorette gum. Your own chances of quitting smoking depend on how much you want to quit, how strongly you are addicted to tobacco, and how closely you follow a quitting program like the one that comes with Nicorette.

QUITTING SMOKING IS HARD!
If you've tried to quit before and haven't succeeded, don't be discouraged! Quitting isn't easy. It takes time, and most people try a few times before they are successful. The important thing is to try again until you succeed. This User's Guide will give you support as you become a non-smoker. It

will answer common questions about Nicorette and give tips to help you stop smoking, and should be referred to often.
WHERE TO GET HELP
You are more likely to stop smoking by using Nicorette with a support program that helps you break your smoking habit. There may be support groups in your area for people trying to quit. Call your local chapter of the American Lung Association (1-800-586-4872), American Cancer Society (1-800-227-2345) or American Heart Association (1-800-242-8721) for further information. If you find you cannot stop smoking or if you start smoking again after using Nicorette, remember breaking this addiction doesn't happen overnight. You may want to talk to a health care professional who can help you improve your chances of quitting the next time you try Nicorette or another method.
LET'S GET ORGANIZED
Your reason for quitting may be a combination of concerns about health, the effect of smoking on your appearance, and pressure from your family and friends to stop smoking. Or maybe you're concerned about the dangerous effect of second-hand smoke on the people you care about. All of these are good reasons. You probably have others. Decide your most important reasons, and write them down on the wallet card inside the back cover of the User's Guide. Carry this card with you. In difficult moments, when you want to smoke, the card will remind you why you are quitting.
WHAT YOU'RE UP AGAINST
Smoking is addictive in two ways. Your need for nicotine has become both physical and mental. You must overcome both addictions to stop smoking. So while Nicorette will lessen your body's physical addition to nicotine, you've got to want to quit smoking to overcome the mental dependence on cigarettes. Once you've decided that you're going to quit, it's time to get started. But first, there are some important cautions you should consider.
SOME IMPORTANT CAUTIONS
This product is only for those who want to stop smoking. Do not smoke, chew tobacco, use snuff or nicotine patches while using Nicorette. If you have heart disease, a recent heart attack, irregular heartbeats, palpitations, high blood pressure not controlled with medication, stomach ulcer, or take insulin for diabetes, ask your doctor whether you should use Nicorette. As with any drug, if you are pregnant or nursing a baby, seek the advice of a health professional before using this product. If you take a prescription medication for asthma or depression, be sure your doctor knows you are quitting smoking. Your prescription medication dose may need to be adjusted. Those under 18 should use this product under a doctor's care. Symptoms of nicotine overdose may include vomiting and diarrhea. Young children are more likely to have additional symptoms, including weakness. Also, seizures have been seen in children who swallowed cigarettes. Keep this and all drugs out of the reach of children. In case of accidental overdose, seek professional assistance or contact a poison control center immediately.
LET'S GET STARTED
Becoming a non-smoker starts today. Your first step is to read through the entire User's Guide carefully. **Next, set your personalized quitting schedule.** Take out a calendar that you can use to track your progress, and identify four dates, using the stickers in the User's Guide.
STEP 1: Your quit date (and the day you'll start using Nicorette gum). Choose your quit date (it should be soon). This is the day you will quit smoking cigarettes entirely and begin using Nicorette to satisfy your craving for nicotine. For the first six weeks, you'll use a piece of Nicorette every hour or two. Be sure to follow the directions on pages 8 and 11 of the User's Guide. Place the Step 1 sticker on this date.
STEP 2: The day you'll start reducing your use of Nicorette. After six weeks, you'll begin gradually reducing your Nicorette usage to one piece every two to four hours. Place the Step 2 sticker on this date (the first day of week seven).
STEP 3: The day you'll further reduce your use of Nicorette. Nine weeks after you begin using Nicorette, you will further reduce your nicotine intake by using one piece every four to eight hours. Place the Step 3 sticker on this date (the first day of week ten). For the next three weeks, you'll use a piece of Nicorette every four to eight hours. **End of treatment: The day you'll complete Nicorette therapy.** Nicorette should not be used for longer than twelve weeks. Identify the date thirteen weeks after the date you chose in Step 1 and place the "EX-Smoker" sticker on your calendar.
PLAN AHEAD
Because smoking is an addiction, it is not easy to stop. After you've given up cigarettes, you will still have a strong urge to smoke. Plan ahead NOW for these times, so you're not defeated in a moment of weakness. The following tips may help:
- Keep the phone numbers of supportive friends and family members handy.
- Keep a record of your quitting process. Track the number of Nicorette pieces you use each day, and whether you feel a craving for cigarettes. If you smoke at all, write down what you think caused the slip.
- Put together an Emergency Kit that includes items that will help take your mind off occasional urges to smoke.

Include cinnamon gum or lemon drops to suck on, a relaxing cassette tape and something for your hands to play with, like a smooth rock, rubber band or small metal balls.

- Set aside some small rewards, like a new magazine or a gift certificate from your favorite store, which you'll 'give' yourself after passing difficult hurdles.

- Think now about the times when you most often want a cigarette, and then plan what else you might do instead of smoking. For instance, you might plan to take your coffee break in a new location, or take a walk right after dinner, so you won't be tempted to smoke.

HOW NICORETTE GUM WORKS

Nicorette's sugar-free chewing pieces provide nicotine to your system—they work as a temporary aid to help you quit smoking by reducing nicotine withdrawal symptoms. Nicorette provides a lower level of nicotine to your blood than cigarettes, and allows you to gradually do away with your body's need for nicotine. Because Nicorette does not contain the tar or carbon monoxide of cigarette smoke, it does not have the same health dangers as tobacco. However, it still delivers nicotine, the addictive part of cigarette smoke. Nicotine can cause side effects such as headache, nausea, upset stomach and dizziness.

HOW TO USE NICORETTE GUM

Before you can use Nicorette correctly, you have to practice! That sounds silly, but it isn't.

Nicorette isn't like ordinary chewing gum. It's a medicine, and must be chewed a certain way to work right. Chewed like ordinary gum, Nicorette won't work well and can cause side effects. An overdose can occur if you chew more than one piece of Nicorette at the same time, or if you chew many pieces one after another. Read all the following instructions before using Nicorette. Refer to them often to make sure you're using Nicorette gum correctly. If you chew too fast, or do not chew correctly, you may get hiccups, heartburn, or other stomach problems.

1. Stop smoking completely before you start using Nicorette.
2. To reduce craving and other withdrawal symptoms, use Nicorette according to the dosage schedule on page 11 of the User's Guide.
3. Chew each Nicorette piece very slowly several times.
4. Stop chewing when you notice a peppery taste, or a slight tingling in your mouth. (This usually happens after about 15 chews, but may vary from person to person.)
5. "PARK" the Nicorette piece between your cheek and gum and leave it there.
6. When the peppery taste or tingle is almost gone (in about a minute), start to chew a few times slowly again. When the taste or tingle returns, stop again.
7. Park the Nicorette piece again (in a different place in your mouth).
8. Repeat steps 3 to 7 (chew, chew, park) until most of the nicotine is gone from the Nicorette piece (usually happens in about half an hour; the peppery taste or tingle won't return).

Throw away the used Nicorette piece, safely away from children and pets.

See the chart in the **"DIRECTIONS"** section above for the recommended usage schedule for Nicorette.

To improve your chances of quitting, use at least 9 pieces of Nicorette a day. Heavier smokers may need more pieces to reduce their cravings. Don't eat or drink for 15 minutes before using Nicorette or while chewing a piece. The effectiveness of Nicorette may be reduced by some foods and drinks, such as coffee, juices, wine or soft drinks.

HOW TO REDUCE YOUR NICORETTE USAGE

The goal of using Nicorette is to slowly reduce your dependence on nicotine. The schedule for using Nicorette will help you reduce your nicotine craving gradually. Here are some tips to help you cut back during each step:

- After a while, start chewing each Nicorette piece for only 10 to 15 minutes, instead of half an hour. Then gradually begin to reduce the number of pieces used.
- Or, try chewing each piece for longer than half an hour, but reduce the number of pieces you use each day.
- Substitute ordinary chewing gum for some of the Nicorette pieces you would normally use. Increase the number of pieces of ordinary gum as you cut back on the Nicorette pieces.

STOP USING NICORETTE AT THE END OF WEEK 12. If you still feel the need to use Nicorette after Week 12, talk with your doctor.

TIPS TO MAKE QUITTING EASIER

Within the first few weeks of giving up smoking, you may be tempted to smoke for pleasure, particularly after completing a difficult task, or at a party or bar. Here are some tips to help get you through the important first stages of becoming a non-smoker:

On your Quit Date:
- Ask your family, friends, and co-workers to support you in your efforts to stop smoking.
- Throw away all your cigarettes, matches, lighters, ashtrays, etc.

- Keep busy on your quit day. Exercise. Go to a movie. Take a walk. Get together with friends.
- Figure out how much money you'll save by not smoking. Most ex-smokers can save more than $1,000 a year.
- Write down what you will do with the money you save.
- Know your high risk situations and plan ahead how you will deal with them.
- Keep Nicorette gum near your bed, so you'll be prepared for any nicotine cravings when you wake up in the morning.
- Visit your dentist and have your teeth cleaned to get rid of the tobacco stains.

Right after Quitting:
- During the first few days after you've stopped smoking, spend as much time as possible at places where smoking is not allowed.
- Drink large quantities of water and fruit juices.
- Try to avoid alcohol, coffee and other beverages you associate with smoking.
- Remember that temporary urges to smoke will pass, even if you don't smoke a cigarette.
- Keep your hands busy with something like a pencil or a paper clip.
- Find other activities which help you relax without cigarettes. Swim, jog, take a walk, play basketball.
- Don't worry too much about gaining weight. Watch what you eat, take time for daily exercise, and change your eating habits if you need to.
- Laughter helps. Watch or read something funny.

WHAT TO EXPECT

Your body is now coming back into balance. During the first few days after you stop smoking, you might feel edgy and nervous and have trouble concentrating. You might get headaches, feel dizzy and a little out of sorts, feel sweaty or have stomach upsets. You might even have trouble sleeping at first. These are typical withdrawal symptoms that will go away with time. Your smoker's cough will get worse before it gets better. But don't worry, that's a good sign. Coughing helps clear the tar deposits out of your lungs.

After a Week or Two.

By now you should be feeling more confident that you can handle those smoking urges. Many of your withdrawal symptoms have left by now, and you should be noticing some positive signs: less coughing, better breathing and an improved sense of taste and smell, to name a few.

After a Month.

You probably have the urge to smoke much less often now. But urges may still occur, and when they do, they are likely to be powerful ones that come out of nowhere. Don't let them catch you off guard. Plan ahead for these difficult times. Concentrate on the ways non-smokers are more attractive than smokers. Their skin is less likely to wrinkle. Their teeth are whiter, cleaner. Their breath is fresher. Their hair and clothes smell better. That cough seems to make even a laugh sound more like a rattle is a thing of the past. Their children and others around them are healthier, too.

What To Do About Relapse.

What should you do if you slip and start smoking again? The answer is simple. A lapse of one or two or even a few cigarettes has not spoiled your efforts! Discard your cigarettes, forgive yourself and try again. If you start smoking again, keep your box of Nicorette for your next quit attempt. If you have taken up regular smoking again, don't be discouraged. Research shows that the best thing you can do is to try again. The important thing is to learn from your last attempt.

- Admit that you've slipped, but don't treat yourself as a failure.
- Try to identify the 'trigger' that caused you to slip, and prepare a better plan for dealing with this problem next time.
- Talk positively to yourself—tell yourself that you have learned something from this experience.
- Make sure you used Nicorette gum correctly over the full 12 weeks to reduce your craving for nicotine.
- Remember that it takes practice to do anything, and quitting smoking is no exception.

WHEN THE STRUGGLE IS OVER

Once you've stopped smoking, take a second and pat yourself on the back. Now do it again. You deserve it. Remember now why you decided to stop smoking in the first place. Look at your list of reasons. Read them again. And smile. Now think about all the money you are saving and what you'll do with it. All the non-smoking places you can go, and what you might do there. All those years you may have added to your life, and what you'll do with them. Remember that temptation may not be gone forever. However, the hard part is behind you, so look forward with a positive attitude and enjoy your new life as a non-smoker.

QUESTIONS & ANSWERS

1. How will I feel when I stop smoking and start using Nicorette? You'll need to prepare yourself for some nicotine withdrawal symptoms. These begin almost immediately after you stop smoking, and are usually at their worst during the first three to four days. Understand that any of the following is possible
- craving for cigarettes
- anxiety, irritability, restlessness, mood changes, nervousness
- drowsiness
- trouble concentrating
- increased appetite and weight gain
- headaches, muscular pain, constipation, fatigue.

Nicorette can help provide relief from withdrawal symptoms such as irritability and nervousness, as well as the craving for nicotine you used to satisfy by having a cigarette.

2. Is Nicorette just substuting one form of nicotine for another? Nicorette does contain nicotine. The purpose of Nicorette is to provide you with enough nicotine to help control the physical withdrawal symptoms so you can deal with the mental aspects of quitting. During the 12 week program, you will gradually reduce your nicotine intake by switching to fewer pieces a day. Remember, don't use Nicorette together with nicotine patches or other nicotine containing products.

3. Can I be hurt by using Nicorette? For most adults, the amount of nicotine in the gum is less than from smoking. Some people will be sensitive to even this amount of nicotine and should not use this product without advice from their doctor. Because Nicorette is a gum-based product, chewing it can cause dental fillings to loosen and aggravate other mouth, tooth and jaw problems. Nicorette can also cause hiccups, heartburn and other stomach problems especially if chewed too quickly or not chewed correctly.

4. Will I gain weight? Many people do tend to gain a few pounds in the first 8–10 weeks after they stop smoking. This is a very small price to pay for the enormous gains that you will make in your overall health and attractiveness. If you continue to gain weight after the first two months, try to analyze what you're doing differently. Reduce your fat intake, choose healthy snacks, and increase your physical activity to burn off the extra calories.

5. Is Nicorette more expensive than smoking? The total cost of Nicorette for the twelve week program is about equal to what a person who smokes one and a half packs of cigarettes a day would spend one cigarettes for the same period of time. Also use of Nicorette is only a short-term cost, while the cost of smoking is a long-term cost, because of the health problems smoking causes.

6. What if I slip up? Discard your cigarettes, forgive yourself and then get back on track. Don't consider a failure or punish yourself. In fact, people who have already tried to quit are more likely to be successful the next time. **GOOD LUCK!**

[End User's Guide]
Copyright © 1997 SmithKline Beecham

To remove the gum, tear off a single unit.
Peel off backing starting at corner with loose edge.
Push gum through foil.
Blister Packaged for your protection. Do not use if individual seals are broken.
Manufactured by Pharmacia & Upjohn AB, Stockholm, Sweden for SmithKline Beecham Consumer Healthcare, LP Pittsburgh, PA 15230
Comments or Questions? Call 1-800-419-4766 weekdays. (10 a.m.–4:30 p.m. EST).
- Not for sale to those under 18 years of age.
- Proof of age required.
- Not for sale in vending machines or from any source where proof of age cannot be verified.

Available as:
Nicorette 2 mg Gum—108 Pieces*
Nicorette 2 mg Gum—48 pieces (refill)
Nicorette 4 mg Gum—108 Pieces*
Nicorette 4 mg Gum—48 pieces (refill)
*User's Guide and Audio Tape included in Kit

OS-CAL® 250+D, 500, 500+D, and 500 Chewable Tablets
OTC
[ahs 'kal]
calcium supplement

(See PDR For Nonprescription Drugs.)

OS-CAL® FORTIFIED Tablets
OTC
[ahs 'kal for 'te-fīd]
multivitamin and minerals supplement
(Formerly marketed as Os-Cal Forte)

(See PDR For Nonprescription Drugs.)

Continued on next page

SINGLET®   OTC
[sĭn ′glĕt]
**Pain Reliever-Fever Reducer/
Nasal Decongestant/Antihistamine**

(See PDR For Nonprescription Drugs.)

TAGAMET HB 200®   OTC
Cimetidine Tablets 200 mg/Acid Reducer

(See PDR For Nonprescription Drugs.)

TUMS®, TUMS E-X®, & TUMS ULTRA®   OTC
Antacid/Calcium Supplement Tablets

TUMS® Anti-gas/Antacid   OTC

(See PDR For Nonprescription Drugs.)

SmithKline Beecham Pharmaceuticals
ONE FRANKLIN PLAZA
P.O. BOX 7929
PHILADELPHIA, PA 19101

For Medical Information Contact:
Medical Department
800-366-8900, ext. 5231

Questions should be directed to Product Information,
1-800-366-8900, ext. 5231.

PRODUCT CODE INDEX

Code	Product, Form and Strength
A30	*Albenza* Tablets 200 mg
A55	*Androderm* Testosterone Transdermal System
189	*Augmentin* 125 mg Chewable Tablets
190	*Augmentin* 250 mg Chewable Tablets
185	*Beepen–VK* Tablets 250 mg
186	*Beepen–VK* Tablets 500 mg
C44	*Compazine* Spansule Capsules 10 mg
C46	*Compazine* Spansule Capsules 15 mg
C60	*Compazine* Suppositories 2½ mg
C61	*Compazine* Suppositories 5 mg
C62	*Compazine* Suppositories 25 mg
C66	*Compazine* Tablets 5 mg
C67	*Compazine* Tablets 10 mg
V39	*Coreg* Tablets 3.125 mg
V40	*Coreg* Tablets 6.25 mg
V41	*Coreg* Tablets 12.5 mg
V42	*Coreg* Tablets 25 mg
E12	*Dexedrine* Spansule Capsules 5 mg
E13	*Dexedrine* Spansule Capsules 10 mg
E14	*Dexedrine* Spansule Capsules 15 mg
E19	*Dexedrine* Tablets 5 mg
E33	*Dibenzyline* Capsules 10 mg
J10	*Eskalith* Controlled Release Tablets 450 mg
H01	*Hycamtin* Injection 4 mg/5 mL
R90	*Requip* Tablets 0.25 mg
R91	*Requip* Tablets 0.5 mg
R92	*Requip* Tablets 1 mg
R93	*Requip* Tablets 2 mg
R94	*Requip* Tablets 5 mg
S03	*Stelazine* Tablets 1 mg
S04	*Stelazine* Tablets 2 mg
S06	*Stelazine* Tablets 5 mg
S07	*Stelazine* Tablets 10 mg
T63	*Thorazine* Spansule Capsules 30 mg
T64	*Thorazine* Spansule Capsules 75 mg
T66	*Thorazine* Spansule Capsules 150 mg
T70	*Thorazine* Suppositories 25 mg
T71	*Thorazine* Suppositories 100 mg
T73	*Thorazine* Tablets 10 mg
T74	*Thorazine* Tablets 25 mg
T76	*Thorazine* Tablets 50 mg
T77	*Thorazine* Tablets 100 mg
T79	*Thorazine* Tablets 200 mg

ALBENZA™   ℞
[al-ben ′-za]
**brand of
albendazole
Tablets**

DESCRIPTION

Albenza (albendazole) is an orally administered broad-spectrum anthelmintic. Chemically it is Methyl 5-(propylthio)-2-benzimidazolecarbamate. Its molecular formula is $C_{12}H_{15}N_3O_2S$. Its molecular weight is 265.34. It has the following chemical structure:

albendazole

Albendazole is a white to off-white powder. It is soluble in dimethylsulfoxide, strong acids and strong bases. It is slightly soluble in methanol, chloroform, ethyl acetate and acetonitrile. Albendazole is practically insoluble in water. Each white to off-white, film-coated tablet contains 200 mg of albendazole.
Inactive ingredients consist of: carnauba wax, hydroxypropyl methylcellulose, lactose monohydrate, magnesium stearate, microcrystalline cellulose, povidone, sodium lauryl sulfate, sodium saccharin, sodium starch glycolate, and starch.

CLINICAL PHARMACOLOGY
Pharmacokinetics
Absorption and Metabolism
Albendazole is poorly absorbed from the gastrointestinal tract due to its low aqueous solubility. Albendazole concentrations are negligible or undetectable in plasma as it is rapidly converted to the sulfoxide metabolite prior to reaching the systemic circulation. The systemic anthelmintic activity has been attributed to the primary metabolite, albendazole sulfoxide. Oral bioavailability appears to be enhanced when albendazole is coadministered with a fatty meal (estimated fat content 40 g) as evidenced by higher (up to 5-fold on average) plasma concentrations of albendazole sulfoxide as compared to the fasted state.
Maximal plasma concentrations of albendazole sulfoxide are typically achieved 2 to 5 hours after dosing and are on average 1.31 mcg/mL (range 0.46 to 1.58 mcg/mL) following oral doses of albendazole (400 mg) in six hydatid disease patients, when administered with a fatty meal. Plasma concentrations of albendazole sulfoxide increase in a dose-proportional manner over the therapeutic dose range following ingestion of a fatty meal (fat content 43.1 g). The mean apparent terminal elimination half-life of albendazole sulfoxide typically ranges from 8 to 12 hours in twenty-five normal subjects, as well as in fourteen hydatid and eight neurocysticercosis patients.
Following 4 weeks of treatment with albendazole (200 mg three times daily), twelve patients' plasma concentrations of albendazole sulfoxide were approximately 20% lower than those observed during the first half of the treatment period, suggesting that albendazole may induce its own metabolism.

Distribution
Albendazole sulfoxide is 70% bound to plasma protein and is widely distributed throughout the body; it has been detected in urine, bile, liver, cyst wall, cyst fluid, and cerebral spinal fluid (CSF). Concentrations in plasma were 3- to 10-fold and 2- to 4-fold higher than those simultaneously determined in cyst fluid and CSF, respectively. Limited *in vitro* and clinical data suggest that albendazole sulfoxide may be eliminated from cysts at a slower rate than observed in plasma.

Metabolism and Excretion
Albendazole is rapidly converted in the liver to the primary metabolite, albendazole sulfoxide, which is further metabolized to albendazole sulfone and other primary oxidative metabolites that have been identified in human urine. Following oral administration, albendazole has not been detected in human urine. Urinary excretion of albendazole sulfoxide is a minor elimination pathway with less than 1% of the dose recovered in the urine. Biliary elimination presumably accounts for a portion of the elimination as evidenced by biliary concentrations of albendazole sulfoxide similar to those achieved in plasma.

Special Populations
Patients with Impaired Renal Function: The pharmacokinetics of albendazole in patients with impaired renal function have not been studied. However, since renal elimination of albendazole and its primary metabolite, albendazole sulfoxide, is negligible, it is unlikely that clearance of these compounds would be altered in these patients.
Biliary Effects: In patients with evidence of extrahepatic obstruction (n=5), the systemic availability of albendazole

---

sulfoxide was increased, as indicated by a 2-fold increase in maximum serum concentration and a 7-fold increase in area under the curve. The rate of absorption/conversion and elimination of albendazole sulfoxide appeared to be prolonged with mean T_{max} and serum elimination half-life values of 10 hours and 31.7 hours, respectively. Plasma concentrations of parent albendazole were measurable in only one of five patients.
Pediatrics: Following single-dose administration of 200 mg to 300 mg (approximately 10 mg/kg) albendazole to three fasted and two fed pediatric patients with hydatid cyst disease (age range 6 to 13 years), albendazole sulfoxide pharmacokinetics were similar to those observed in fed adults.
Elderly Patients: Although no studies have investigated the effect of age on albendazole sulfoxide pharmacokinetics, data in twenty-six hydatid cyst patients (up to 79 years) suggest pharmacokinetics similar to those in young healthy subjects.
Microbiology
The principal mode of action for albendazole is by its inhibitory effect on tubulin polymerization which results in the loss of cytoplasmic microtubules.
In the specified treatment indications albendazole appears to be active against the larval forms of the following organisms:
Echinococcus granulosus
Taenia solium

INDICATIONS AND USAGE
Albenza (albendazole) is indicated for the treatment of the following infections:
Neurocysticercosis. *Albenza* is indicated for the treatment of parenchymal neurocoysticercosis due to active lesions caused by larval forms of the pork tapeworm, *Taenia solium*.
Lesions considered responsive to albendazole therapy appear as nonenhancing cysts with no surrounding edema on contrast-enhanced computerized tomography. Clinical studies in patients with lesions of this type demonstrate a 74% to 88% reduction in number of cysts; 40% to 70% of albendazole-treated patients showed resolution of all active cysts.
Hydatid disease. *Albenza* is indicated for the treatment of cystic hydatid disease of the liver, lung, and peritoneum, caused by the larval form of the dog tapeworm, *Echinococcus granulosus*.
This indication is based on combined clinical studies which demonstrated non-infectious cyst contents in approximately 80–90% of patients given *Albenza* for 3 cycles of therapy of 28 days each. (See **DOSAGE AND ADMINISTRATION**.) Clinical cure (disappearance of cysts) was seen in approximately 30% of these patients, and improvement (reduction in cyst diameter of ≥25%) was seen in an additional 40%.
NOTE: When medically feasible, surgery is considered the treatment of choice for hydatid disease. When administering *Albenza* in the pre- or post-surgical setting, optimal killing of cyst contents is achieved when three courses of therapy have been given.
NOTE: The efficacy of albendazole in the therapy of alveolar hydatid disease caused by *Echinococcus multilocularis* has not been clearly demonstrated in clinical studies.

CONTRAINDICATIONS
Albenza (albendazole) is contraindicated in patients with known hypersensitivity to the benzimidazole class of compounds or any components of *Albenza*.

WARNINGS
Rare fatalities associated with the use of *Albenza* have been reported due to granulocytopenia or pancytopenia. (See **PRECAUTIONS**.) Blood counts should be monitored at the beginning of each 28-day cycle of therapy, and every 2 weeks while on therapy with albendazole. Albendazole may be continued if the total white blood cell count and absolute neutrophil count decrease appear modest and do not progress. Albendazole should not be used in pregnant women except in clinical circumstances where no alternative management is appropriate. Patients should not become pregnant for at least 1 month following cessation of albendazole therapy. If a patient becomes pregnant while taking this drug, albendazole should be discontinued immediately. If pregnancy occurs while taking this drug, the patient should be apprised of the potential hazard to the fetus.

PRECAUTIONS
General: Patients being treated for neurocysticercosis should receive appropriate steroid and anticonvulsant therapy as required. Oral or intravenous corticosteroids should be considered to prevent cerebral hypertensive episodes during the first week of anticysticeral therapy.
Cysticercosis may, in rare cases, involve the retina. Before initiating therapy for neurocysticercosis, the patient should be examined for the presence of retinal lesions. If such lesions are visualized, the need for anticysticeral therapy should be weighed against the possibility of retinal damage caused by albendazole-induced changes to the retinal lesion.
Information for Patients
Patients should be advised that:

- Albendazole may cause fetal harm, therefore, women of childbearing age should begin treatment after a negative pregnancy test.
- Women of childbearing age should be cautioned against becoming pregnant while on albendazole or within 1 month of completing treatment.
- During albendazole therapy, because of the possibility of harm to the liver or bone marrow, routine (every 2 weeks) monitoring of blood counts and liver function tests should take place.
- Albendazole should be taken with food.

Laboratory Tests

White Blood Cell Count: Albendazole has been shown to cause occasional (less than 1% of treated patients) reversible reductions in total white blood cell count. Rarely, more significant reductions may be encountered including granulocytopenia, agranulocytosis, or pancytopenia. Blood counts should be performed at the start of each 28-day treatment cycle and every 2 weeks during each 28-day cycle. Albendazole may be continued if the total white blood cell count decrease appears modest and does not progress.

Liver Function: In clinical trials, treatment with albendazole has been associated with mild to moderate elevations of hepatic enzymes in approximately 16% of patients. These have returned to normal upon discontinuation of therapy. Liver function tests (transaminases) should be performed before the start of each treatment cycle and at least every 2 weeks during treatment. If enzymes are significantly increased, albendazole therapy should be discontinued. Therapy can be reinstituted when liver enzymes have returned to pretreatment levels, but laboratory tests should be performed frequently during repeat therapy.

Patients with abnormal liver function test results prior to commencing albendazole therapy should be carefully evaluated, since the drug is metabolized by the liver and has been associated with hepatotoxicity in a few patients.

Theophylline: Although single doses of albendazole have been shown not to inhibit theophylline metabolism (see **Drug Interactions**), albendazole does induce cytochrome P450 1A in human hepatoma cells. Therefore, it is recommended that plasma concentrations of theophylline be monitored during and after treatment with Albenza (albendazole).

Drug Interactions

Dexamethasone: Steady-state trough concentrations of albendazole sulfoxide were about 56% higher when 8 mg dexamethasone was coadministered with each dose of albendazole (15 mg/kg/day) in eight neurocysticercosis patients.

Praziquantel: In the fed state, praziquantel (40 mg/kg) increased mean maximum plasma concentration and area under the curve of albendazole sulfoxide by about 50% in healthy subjects (n=10) compared with a separate group of subjects (n=6) given albendazole alone. Mean T_{max} and mean plasma elimination half-life of albendazole sulfoxide were unchanged. The pharmacokinetics of praziquantel were unchanged following coadministration with albendazole (400 mg).

Cimetidine: Albendazole sulfoxide concentrations in bile and cystic fluid were increased (about 2-fold) in hydatid cyst patients treated with cimetidine (10 mg/kg/day) (n=7) compared with albendazole (20 mg/kg/day) alone (n=12). Albendazole sulfoxide plasma concentrations were unchanged 4 hours after dosing.

Theophylline: The pharmacokinetics of theophylline (aminophylline 5.8 mg/kg infused over 20 minutes) were unchanged following a single oral dose of albendazole (400 mg) in 6 healthy subjects.

Carcinogenesis, Mutagenesis, Impairment of Fertility

Long-term carcinogenicity studies were conducted in mice and rats. In the mouse study, albendazole was administered in the diet at doses of 25, 100 and 400 mg/kg/day (0.1, 0.5, and 2 times the recommended human dose based on body surface area in mg/m², respectively) for 108 weeks. In the rat study, albendazole was administered in the diet at doses of 3.5, 7, and 20 mg/kg/day (0.04, 0.08, and 0.21 times the recommended human dose based on body surface area in mg/m², respectively) for 117 weeks. There was no evidence of increased incidence of tumors in the treated mice and rats when compared to the control group.

In genotoxicity tests, albendazole was found negative in an Ames Salmonella/Microsome Plate mutation assay with and without metabolic activation or with and without pre-incubation, cell-mediated Chinese Hamster Ovary chromosome aberration test and *in vivo* mouse micronucleus test. In the *in vitro* BALB/3T3 cells transformation assay, albendazole produced weak activity in the presence of metabolic activation while no activity was found in the absence of metabolic activation.

Albendazole did not adversely affect male or female fertility in the rat at an oral dose of 30 mg/kg/day (0.32 times the recommended human dose based on body surface area in mg/m²).

Pregnancy

Teratogenic Effects—Pregnancy Category C: Albendazole has been shown to be teratogenic (to cause embryotoxicity and skeletal malformations) in pregnant rats and rabbits.

Indication	Patient Weight	Dose	Duration
Hydatid Disease	60 kg or greater	400 mg b.i.d., with meals	28-day cycle followed by a 14-day albendazole-free interval, for a total of 3 cycles
	less than 60 kg	15 mg/kg/day given in divided doses b.i.d. with meals (maximum total daily dose 800 mg)	
	NOTE: When administering *Albenza* in the pre- or post-surgical setting, optimal killing of cyst contents is achieved when three courses of therapy have been given.		
Neurocysticercosis	60 kg or greater	400 mg b.i.d., with meals	8–30 days
	less than 60 kg	15 mg/kg/day given in divided doses b.i.d. with meals (maximum total daily dose 800 mg)	

The teratogenic response in the rat was shown at oral doses of 10 and 30 mg/kg/day (0.10 times and 0.32 times the recommended human dose based on body surface area in mg/m², respectively) during gestation days 6 to 15 and in pregnant rabbits at oral doses of 30 mg/kg/day (0.60 times the recommended human dose based on body surface area in mg/m²) administered during gestation days 7 to 19. In the rabbit study, maternal toxicity (33% mortality) was noted at 30 mg/kg/day. In mice, no teratogenic effects were observed at oral doses up to 30 mg/kg/day (0.16 times the recommended human dose based on body surface area in mg/m²), administered during gestation days 6 to 15.

There are no adequate and well-controlled studies of albendazole administration in pregnant women. Albendazole should be used during pregnancy only if the potential benefit justifies the potential risk to the fetus. (See **WARNINGS**.)

Nursing Mothers: Albendazole is excreted in animal milk. It is not known whether it is excreted in human milk. Because many drugs are excreted in human milk, caution should be exercised when albendazole is administered to a nursing woman.

Pediatric Use: Experience in children under the age of 6 years is limited. In hydatid disease, infection in infants and young children is uncommon, but no problems have been encountered in those who have been treated. In neurocysticercosis, infection is more frequently encountered. In five published studies involving pediatric patients as young as 1 year, no significant problems were encountered, and the efficacy appeared similar to the adult population.

Geriatric Use: Experience in patients 65 years of age or older is limited. The number of patients treated for either hydatid disease or neurocysticercosis is limited, but no problems associated with an older population have been observed.

ADVERSE REACTIONS

The adverse event profile of albendazole differs between hydatid disease and neurocysticercosis. Adverse events occurring with a frequency of ≥1% in either disease are described in the table below.

These symptoms were usually mild and resolved without treatment. Treatment discontinuations were predominantly due to leukopenia (0.7%) or hepatic abnormalities (3.8% in hydatid disease). The following incidence reflects events that were reported by investigators to be at least possibly or probably related to albendazole.

Adverse Event Incidence ≥1% in Hydatid Disease and Neurocysticercosis

Adverse Event	Hydatid Disease	Neurocysticercosis
Abnormal Liver Function Tests	15.6	<1.0
Abdominal Pain	6.0	0
Nausea/Vomiting	3.7	6.2
Headache	1.3	11.0
Dizziness/Vertigo	1.2	<1.0
Raised Intracranial Pressure	0	1.5
Meningeal Signs	0	1.0
Reversible Alopecia	1.6	<1.0
Fever	1.0	0

The following adverse events were observed at an incidence of <1%:

Hematologic: Leukopenia. There have been rare reports of granulocytopenia, pancytopenia, agranulocytosis, or thrombocytopenia. (See **WARNINGS**.)

Dermatologic: Rash, urticaria.

Hypersensitivity: Allergic reactions.

Renal: Acute renal failure related to albendazole therapy has been observed.

OVERDOSAGE

Significant toxicity and mortality were shown in male and female mice at doses exceeding 5,000 mg/kg; in rats, at estimated doses between 1,300 and 2,400 mg/kg; in hamsters, at doses exceeding 10,000 mg/kg; and in rabbits, at estimated doses between 500 and 1,250 mg/kg. In the animals, symptoms were demonstrated in a dose-response relationship and included diarrhea, vomiting, tachycardia, and respiratory distress.

One overdosage has been reported with Albenza (albendazole) in a patient who took at least 16 grams over 12 hours. No untoward effects were reported. In case of overdosage, symptomatic therapy (e.g., gastric lavage and activated charcoal) and general supportive measures are recommended.

DOSAGE AND ADMINISTRATION

Dosing of *Albenza* will vary, depending upon which of the following parasitic infections is being treated. [See table above]

Patients being treated for neurocysticercosis should receive appropriate steroid and anticonvulsant therapy as required. Oral or intravenous corticosteroids should be considered to prevent cerebral hypertensive episodes during the first week of treatment.

HOW SUPPLIED

Albenza (albendazole) is supplied as 200 mg, white to off-white, circular, biconvex, bevel-edged, film-coated Tiltab® tablets in bottles of 112.

NDC 0007-5500-40 .... Bottles of 112

Store between 20° and 25°C (68° and 77°F).

Veterans Administration/Military/PHS—Tablets, 200 mg, 12's, 6505-01-447-7334.

AL:L1

Shown in Product Identification Guide, page 338

AMOXIL®   ℞

[ā-mŏx-ĭl]

brand of
amoxicillin
capsules, tablets, chewable
tablets, and powder for
oral suspension

DESCRIPTION

Amoxil formulations contain amoxicillin, a semisynthetic antibiotic, an analog of ampicillin, with a broad spectrum of bactericidal activity against many gram-positive and gram-negative microorganisms. Chemically it is (2S,5R,6R)-6-[(R)-(-)-2-amino-2-(p-hydroxyphenyl)acetamido]-3,3-dimethyl-7-oxo-4-thia-1-azabicyclo[3.2.0]heptane-2-carboxylic acid trihydrate. It may be represented structurally as:

Continued on next page

Amoxil—Cont.

The amoxicillin molecular formula is $C_{16}H_{19}N_3O_5S \cdot 3H_2O$, and the molecular weight is 419.45.

Amoxil capsules, tablets, and powder for oral suspension are intended for oral administration.

Capsules: Each *Amoxil* capsule, with royal blue opaque cap and pink opaque body, contains 250 mg or 500 mg amoxicillin as the trihydrate. The cap and body of the 250-mg capsule are imprinted with the product name AMOXIL and 250; the cap and body of the 500-mg capsule are imprinted with AMOXIL and 500. Inactive ingredients: D&C Red No. 28, FD&C Blue No. 1, FD&C Red No. 40, gelatin, magnesium stearate, and titanium dioxide.

Tablets: Each tablet contains 500 mg or 875 mg amoxicillin as the trihydrate. Each film-coated, capsule-shaped, pink tablet is debossed with AMOXIL centered over 500 or 875, respectively. The 875-mg tablet is scored on the reverse side. Inactive ingredients: colloidal silicon dioxide, crospovidone, FD&C Red No. 30 aluminum lake, hydroxypropyl methylcellulose, magnesium stearate, microcrystalline cellulose, polyethylene glycol, sodium starch glycolate, and titanium dioxide.

Chewable Tablets: Each oval, pink, cherry-banana-peppermint-flavored tablet contains 125 mg or 250 mg amoxicillin as the trihydrate. The tablets are imprinted with the product name AMOXIL on one side and 125 or 250 on the other side. Inactive ingredients: citric acid, corn starch, FD&C Red No. 40, flavorings, glycine, mannitol, magnesium stearate, saccharin sodium, silica gel, and sucrose. Each 125-mg chewable tablet contains 0.0019 mEq (0.044 mg) of sodium; the 250-mg chewable tablet contains 0.0037 mEq (0.085 mg) of sodium.

Powder for Oral Suspension: Each 5 mL of reconstituted suspension contains 125 mg or 250 mg amoxicillin as the trihydrate. Each 5 mL of the 125-mg reconstituted suspension contains 0.12 mEq (2.76 mg) of sodium; each 5 mL of the 250-mg reconstituted suspension contains 0.15 mEq (3.45 mg) of sodium.

Pediatric Drops for Oral Suspension: Each mL of reconstituted suspension contains 50 mg amoxicillin as the trihydrate and 0.03 mEq (0.69 mg) of sodium.

Amoxicillin trihydrate for oral suspension 125 mg/5 mL (reconstituted) is a strawberry-flavored pink suspension; the 250 mg/5 mL or 50 mg/mL is a bubble-gum-flavored pink suspension. Inactive ingredients: FD&C Red No. 3, flavorings, silica gel, sodium benzoate, sodium citrate, sucrose, and xanthan gum.

CLINICAL PHARMACOLOGY

Amoxicillin is stable in the presence of gastric acid and is rapidly absorbed after oral administration. It diffuses readily into most body tissues and fluids, with the exception of brain and spinal fluid, except when meninges are inflamed. The half-life of amoxicillin is 61.3 minutes. Most of the amoxicillin is excreted unchanged in the urine; its excretion can be delayed by concurrent administration of probenecid. In blood serum, amoxicillin is approximately 20% protein-bound.

Orally administered doses of 250-mg and 500-mg amoxicillin capsules result in average peak blood levels 1 to 2 hours after administration in the range of 3.5 µg/mL to 5.0 µg/mL and 5.5 µg/mL to 7.5 µg/mL, respectively.

Mean amoxicillin pharmacokinetic parameters from an open, two-part, single-dose crossover bioequivalence study in 27 adults comparing 875 mg of Amoxil (amoxicillin) with 875 mg of Augmentin® (amoxicillin/clavulanate potassium) showed that the 875-mg tablet of *Amoxil* produces an $AUC_{0-\infty}$ of 35.4 ±8.1 µg.hr/mL and a C_{max} of 13.8 ±4.1 µg/mL. Dosing was at the start of a light meal following an overnight fast.

Amoxicillin chewable tablets, 125 mg and 250 mg, produced blood levels similar to those achieved with the corresponding doses of amoxicillin oral suspensions. Orally administered doses of amoxicillin suspension, 125 mg/ 5 mL and 250 mg/5 mL, result in average peak blood levels 1 to 2 hours after administration in the range of 1.5 µg/mL to 3.0 µg/mL and 3.5 µg/mL to 5.0 µg/mL, respectively.

Detectable serum levels are observed up to 8 hours after an orally administered dose of amoxicillin. Following a 1-gram dose and utilizing a special skin window technique to determine levels of the antibiotic, it was noted that therapeutic levels were found in the interstitial fluid. Approximately 60% of an orally administered dose of amoxicillin is excreted in the urine within 6 to 8 hours.

Microbiology

Amoxicillin is similar to ampicillin in its bactericidal action against susceptible organisms during the stage of active multiplication. It acts through the inhibition of biosynthesis of cell wall mucopeptide. Amoxicillin has been shown to be active against most strains of the following microorganisms, both *in vitro* and in clinical infections as described in the **INDICATIONS AND USAGE** section.

Aerobic gram-positive microorganisms:
Enterococcus faecalis
Staphylococcus spp.[†] (β-lactamase-negative strains only)
Streptococcus pneumoniae
Streptococcus spp. (α- and β-hemolytic strains only)

[†] Staphylococci which are susceptible to amoxicillin but resistant to methicillin/oxacillin should be considered as resistant to amoxicillin.

Aerobic gram-negative microorganisms:
Escherichia coli (β-lactamase-negative strains only)
Haemophilus influenzae (β-lactamase-negative strains only)
Neisseria gonorrhoeae (β-lactamase-negative strains only)
Proteus mirabilis (β-lactamase-negative strains only)

Helicobacter:
Helicobacter pylori

Susceptibility tests

Dilution techniques: Quantitative methods are used to determine antimicrobial minimum inhibitory concentrations (MICs). These MICs provide estimates of the susceptibility of bacteria to antimicrobial compounds. The MICs should be determined using a standardized procedure. Standardized procedures are based on a dilution method[1] (broth or agar) or equivalent with standardized inoculum concentrations and standardized concentrations of **ampicillin** powder. Ampicillin is sometimes used to predict susceptibility of *Streptococcus pneumoniae* to amoxicillin; however, some intermediate strains have been shown to be susceptible to amoxicillin. Therefore, *Streptococcus pneumoniae* susceptibility should be tested using amoxicillin powder. The MIC values should be interpreted according to the following criteria:

For gram-positive aerobes:

Enterococcus

MIC (µg/mL)	Interpretation
≤ 8	Susceptible (S)
≥ 16	Resistant (R)

Staphylococcus[a]

MIC (µg/mL)	Interpretation
≤ 0.25	Susceptible (S)
≥ 0.5	Resistant (R)

Streptococcus (except *S. pneumoniae*)

MIC (µg/mL)	Interpretation
≤ 0.25	Susceptible (S)
0.5 to 4	Intermediate (I)
≥ 8	Resistant (R)

S. pneumoniae[b]
(**Amoxicillin** powder should be used to determine susceptibility.)

MIC (µg/mL)	Interpretation
≤ 0.5	Susceptible (S)
1	Intermediate (I)
≥ 2	Resistant (R)

For gram-negative aerobes:

Enterobacteriaceae

MIC (µg/mL)	Interpretation
≤ 8	Susceptible (S)
16	Intermediate (I)
≥32	Resistant (R)

H. influenzae[c]

MIC (µg/mL)	Interpretation
≤1	Susceptible (S)
2	Intermediate (I)
≥4	Resistant (R)

a. Staphylococci which are susceptible to amoxicillin but resistant to methicillin/oxacillin should be considered as resistant to amoxicillin.

b. These interpretive standards are applicable only to broth microdilution susceptibility tests using cation-adjusted Mueller-Hinton broth with 2-5% lysed horse blood.

c. These interpretive standards are applicable only to broth microdilution test with *Haemophilus influenzae* using *Haemophilus* Test Medium (HTM).[1]

A report of "Susceptible" indicates that the pathogen is likely to be inhibited if the antimicrobial compound in the blood reaches the concentrations usually achievable. A report of "Intermediate" indicates that the result should be considered equivocal, and, if the microorganism is not fully susceptible to alternative, clinically feasible drugs, the test should be repeated. This category implies possible clinical applicability in body sites where the drug is physiologically concentrated or in situations where high dosage of drug can be used. This category also provides a buffer zone which prevents small uncontrolled technical factors from causing major discrepancies in interpretation. A report of "Resistant" indicates that the pathogen is not likely to be inhibited if the antimicrobial compound in the blood reaches the concentrations usually achievable; other therapy should be selected.

Standardized susceptibility test procedures require the use of laboratory control microorganisms to control the techni-

cal aspects of the laboratory procedures. Standard **ampicillin** powder should provide the following MIC values:

Microorganism	MIC (µg/mL)
E. coli ATCC 25922	2 to 8
E. faecalis ATCC 29212	0.5 to 2
H. influenzae ATCC 49247[d]	2 to 8
S. aureus ATCC 29213	0.25 to 1

Using **amoxicillin** to determine susceptibility:

Microorganism	MIC Range (µg/mL)
S. pneumoniae ATCC 49619[e]	0.03 to 0.12

d. This quality control range is applicable to only *H. influenzae* ATCC 49247 tested by a broth microdilution procedure using HTM.[1]

e. This quality control range is applicable to only *S. pneumoniae* ATCC 49619 tested by the broth microdilution procedure using cation-adjusted Mueller-Hinton broth with 2–5% lysed horse blood.

Diffusion techniques: Quantitative methods that require measurement of zone diameters also provide reproducible estimates of the susceptibility of bacteria to antimicrobial compounds. One such standardized procedure[2] requires the use of standardized inoculum concentrations. This procedure uses paper disks impregnated with 10 µg ampicillin to test the susceptibility of microorganisms, except *S. pneumoniae*, to amoxicillin. Interpretation involves correlation of the diameter obtained in the disk test with the MIC for **ampicillin**.

Reports from the laboratory providing results of the standard single-disk susceptibility test with a 10-µg ampicillin disk should be interpreted according to the following criteria:

For gram-positive aerobes:

Enterococcus

Zone Diameter (mm)	Interpretation
≥17	Susceptible (S)
≤16	Resistant (R)

Staphylococcus[f]

Zone Diameter (mm)	Interpretation
≥29	Susceptible (S)
≤28	Resistant (R)

β-hemolytic streptococci

Zone Diameter (mm)	Interpretation
≥26	Susceptible (S)
19 to 25	Intermediate (I)
≤18	Resistant (R)

NOTE: For streptococci (other than β-hemolytic streptococci and *S. pneumoniae*), an ampicillin MIC should be determined.

S. pneumoniae

S. pneumoniae should be tested using a 1-µg oxacillin disk. Isolates with oxacillin zone sizes of ≥20 mm are susceptible to amoxicillin. An amoxicillin MIC should be determined on isolates of *S. pneumoniae* with oxacillin zone sizes of ≤19 mm.

For gram-negative aerobes:

Enterobacteriaceae

Zone Diameter (mm)	Interpretation
≥17	Susceptible (S)
14 to 16	Intermediate (I)
≤13	Resistant (R)

H. influenzae[g]

Zone Diameter (mm)	Interpretation
≥22	Susceptible (S)
19 to 21	Intermediate (I)
≤18	Resistant (R)

f. Staphylococci which are susceptible to amoxicillin but resistant to methicillin/oxacillin should be considered as resistant to amoxicillin.

g. These interpretive standards are applicable only to disk diffusion susceptibility tests with *H. influenzae* using *Haemophilus* Test Medium (HTM).[2]

Interpretation should be as stated above for results using dilution techniques.

As with standard dilution techniques, disk diffusion susceptibility test procedures require the use of laboratory control microorganisms. The 10-µg **ampicillin** disk should provide the following zone diameters in these laboratory test quality control strains:

Microorganism	Zone diameter (mm)
E. coli ATCC 25922	16 to 22
H. influenzae ATCC 49247[h]	13 to 21
S. aureus ATCC 25923	27 to 35

Using 1-µg **oxacillin** disk:

Microorganism	Zone diameter (mm)
S. pneumoniae ATCC 49619[i]	8 to 12

h. This quality control range is applicable to only *H. influenzae* ATCC 49247 tested by a disk diffusion procedure using HTM.[2]

i. This quality control range is applicable to only *S. pneumoniae* ATCC 49619 tested by a disk diffusion procedure using Mueller-Hinton agar supplemented with 5% sheep blood and incubated in 5% CO_2.

Susceptibility testing for *Helicobacter pylori*

In vitro susceptibility testing methods and diagnostic products currently available for determining minimum inhibitory concentrations (MICs) and zone sizes have not been standardized, validated, or approved for testing *H. pylori* microorganisms.

Culture and susceptibility testing should be obtained in patients who fail triple therapy. If clarithromycin resistance is found, a non-clarithromycin-containing regimen should be used.

INDICATIONS AND USAGE

Amoxil (amoxicillin) is indicated in the treatment of infections due to susceptible (ONLY β-lactamase-negative) strains of the designated microorganisms in the conditions listed below:

Infections of the ear, nose, and throat due to *Streptococcus* spp. (α- and β-hemolytic strains only), *Streptococcus pneumoniae*, *Staphylococcus* spp., or *H. influenzae*

Infections of the genitourinary tract due to *E. coli, P. mirabilis,* or *E. faecalis*

Infections of the skin and skin structure due to *Streptococcus* spp. (α- and β-hemolytic strains only), *Staphylococcus* spp., or *E. coli*

Infections of the lower respiratory tract due to *Streptococcus* spp. (α- and β-hemolytic strains only), *Streptococcus pneumoniae*, *Staphylococcus* spp., or *H. influenzae*

Gonorrhea, acute uncomplicated (ano-genital and urethral infections) due to *N. gonorrhoeae* (males and females)

Therapy may be instituted prior to obtaining results from bacteriological and susceptibility studies to determine the causative organisms and their susceptibility to amoxicillin. Indicated surgical procedures should be performed.

H. pylori eradication to reduce the risk of duodenal ulcer recurrence

Triple therapy: *Amoxil*/clarithromycin/lansoprazole

Amoxil, in combination with clarithromycin plus lansoprazole as triple therapy, is indicated for the treatment of patients with *H. pylori* infection and duodenal ulcer disease (active or one-year history of a duodenal ulcer) to eradicate *H. pylori*. Eradication of *H. pylori* has been shown to reduce the risk of duodenal ulcer recurrence. (See **CLINICAL STUDIES** and **DOSAGE AND ADMINISTRATION**.)

Dual therapy: *Amoxil*/lansoprazole

Amoxil (amoxicillin), in combination with lansoprazole delayed-release capsules as dual therapy, is indicated for the treatment of patients with *H. pylori* infection and duodenal ulcer disease (active or one-year history of a duodenal ulcer) **who are either allergic or intolerant to clarithromycin or in whom resistance to clarithromycin is known or suspected.** (See the clarithromycin package insert, **MICROBIOLOGY**.) Eradication of *H. pylori* has been shown to reduce the risk of duodenal ulcer recurrence. (See **CLINICAL STUDIES** and **DOSAGE AND ADMINISTRATION**.)

CONTRAINDICATIONS

A history of allergic reaction to any of the penicillins is a contraindication.

WARNINGS

SERIOUS AND OCCASIONALLY FATAL HYPERSENSITIVITY (ANAPHYLACTIC) REACTIONS HAVE BEEN REPORTED IN PATIENTS ON PENICILLIN THERAPY. ALTHOUGH ANAPHYLAXIS IS MORE FREQUENT FOLLOWING PARENTERAL THERAPY, IT HAS OCCURRED IN PATIENTS ON ORAL PENICILLINS. THESE REACTIONS ARE MORE LIKELY TO OCCUR IN INDIVIDUALS WITH A HISTORY OF PENICILLIN HYPERSENSITIVITY AND/OR A HISTORY OF SENSITIVITY TO MULTIPLE ALLERGENS. THERE HAVE BEEN REPORTS OF INDIVIDUALS WITH A HISTORY OF PENICILLIN HYPERSENSITIVITY WHO HAVE EXPERIENCED SEVERE REACTIONS WHEN TREATED WITH CEPHALOSPORINS. BEFORE INITIATING THERAPY WITH *AMOXIL*, CAREFUL INQUIRY SHOULD BE MADE CONCERNING PREVIOUS HYPERSENSITIVITY REACTIONS TO PENICILLINS, CEPHALOSPORINS, OR OTHER ALLERGENS. IF AN ALLERGIC REACTION OCCURS, *AMOXIL* SHOULD BE DISCONTINUED AND APPROPRIATE THERAPY INSTITUTED. **SERIOUS ANAPHYLACTIC REACTIONS REQUIRE IMMEDIATE EMERGENCY TREATMENT WITH EPINEPHRINE. OXYGEN, INTRAVENOUS STEROIDS, AND AIRWAY MANAGEMENT, INCLUDING INTUBATION, SHOULD ALSO BE ADMINISTERED AS INDICATED.**

Pseudomembranous colitis has been reported with nearly all antibacterial agents, including amoxicillin, and may range in severity from mild to life-threatening. Therefore, it is important to consider this diagnosis in patients who present with diarrhea subsequent to the administration of antibacterial agents.

Treatment with antibacterial agents alters the normal flora of the colon and may permit overgrowth of clostridia. Studies indicate that a toxin produced by *Clostridium difficile* is a primary cause of "antibiotic-associated colitis." After the

Adults and pediatric patients >3 months

Infection	Severity‡	Usual Adult Dose	Usual Dose for Children >3 months§
Ear/nose/throat	Mild/Moderate	500 mg every 12 hours or 250 mg every 8 hours	20 mg/kg/day in divided doses every 8 hours
	Severe	875 mg every 12 hours or 500 mg every 8 hours	40 mg/kg/day in divided doses every 8 hours
Lower respiratory tract	Mild/Moderate or Severe	875 mg every 12 hours or 500 mg every 8 hours	40 mg/kg/day in divided doses every 8 hours
Skin/skin structure	Mild/Moderate	500 mg every 12 hours or 250 mg every 8 hours	20 mg/kg/day in divided doses every 8 hours
	Severe	875 mg every 12 hours or 500 mg every 8 hours	40 mg/kg/day in divided doses every 8 hours
Genitourinary tract	Mild/Moderate	500 mg every 12 hours or 250 mg every 8 hours	20 mg/kg/day in divided doses every 8 hours
	Severe	875 mg every 12 hours or 500 mg every 8 hours	40 mg/kg/day in divided doses every 8 hours
Gonorrhea Acute, uncomplicated ano-genital and urethral infections in males and females		3 grams as single oral dose	Prepubertal children: 50 mg/kg *Amoxil*, combined with 25 mg/kg probenecid as a single dose **NOTE: SINCE PROBENECID IS CONTRAINDICATED IN CHILDREN UNDER 2 YEARS, DO NOT USE THIS REGIMEN IN THESE CASES.**

‡ Dosing for infections caused by less susceptible organisms should follow the recommendations for severe infections.
§ Children weighing 40 kg or more should be dosed according to the adult recommendations.

diagnosis of pseudomembranous colitis has been established, appropriate therapeutic measures should be initiated. Mild cases of pseudomembranous colitis usually respond to drug discontinuation alone. In moderate to severe cases, consideration should be given to management with fluids and electrolytes, protein supplementation, and treatment with an antibacterial drug clinically effective against *Clostridium difficile* colitis.

PRECAUTIONS

General: The possibility of superinfections with mycotic or bacterial pathogens should be kept in mind during therapy. If superinfections occur, amoxicillin should be discontinued and appropriate therapy instituted.

Laboratory Tests: As with any potent drug, periodic assessment of renal, hepatic, and hematopoietic function should be made during prolonged therapy.

All patients with gonorrhea should have a serologic test for syphilis at the time of diagnosis. Patients treated with amoxicillin should have a follow-up serologic test for syphilis after 3 months.

Drug Interactions: Probenecid decreases the renal tubular secretion of amoxicillin. Concurrent use with amoxicillin may result in increased and prolonged blood levels.

Chloramphenicol, erythromycins, sulfonamides, and tetracyclines may interfere with the bactericidal effects of penicillin. This has been demonstrated *in vitro*; however, the clinical significance of this interaction is not well documented.

Drug/Laboratory Test Interactions: High urine concentrations of ampicillin may result in false-positive reactions when testing for the presence of glucose in urine using Clinitest®, Benedict's Solution or Fehling's Solution. Since this effect may also occur with amoxicillin, it is recommended that glucose tests based on enzymatic glucose oxidase reactions (such as Clinistix® or Tes-Tape®) be used.

Following administration of ampicillin to pregnant women, a transient decrease in plasma concentration of total conjugated estriol, estriol-glucuronide, conjugated estrone, and estradiol has been noted. This effect may also occur with amoxicillin.

Carcinogenesis, Mutagenesis, Impairment of Fertility: Long-term studies in animals have not been performed to evaluate carcinogenic potential. Studies to detect mutagenic potential of amoxicillin alone have not been conducted; however, the following information is available from tests on a

4:1 mixture of amoxicillin and potassium clavulanate (*Augmentin*). *Augmentin* was non-mutagenic in the Ames bacterial mutation assay, and the yeast gene conversion assay. *Augmentin* was weakly positive in the mouse lymphoma assay, but the trend toward increased mutation frequencies in this assay occurred at doses that were also associated with decreased cell survival. *Augmentin* was negative in the mouse micronucleus test, and in the dominant lethal assay in mice. Potassium clavulanate alone was tested in the Ames bacterial mutation assay and in the mouse micronucleus test, and was negative in each of these assays. In a multi-generation reproduction study in rats, no impairment of fertility or other adverse reproductive effects were seen at doses up to 500 mg/kg (approximately 3 times the human dose in mg/m²).

Pregnancy: *Teratogenic Effects. Pregnancy Category B.* Reproduction studies have been performed in mice and rats at doses up to ten (10) times the human dose and have revealed no evidence of impaired fertility or harm to the fetus due to amoxicillin. There are, however, no adequate and well-controlled studies in pregnant women. Because animal reproduction studies are not always predictive of human response, this drug should be used during pregnancy only if clearly needed.

Labor and Delivery: Oral ampicillin-class antibiotics are poorly absorbed during labor. Studies in guinea pigs showed that intravenous administration of ampicillin slightly decreased the uterine tone and frequency of contractions but moderately increased the height and duration of contractions. However, it is not known whether use of amoxicillin in humans during labor or delivery has immediate or delayed adverse effects on the fetus, prolongs the duration of labor, or increases the likelihood that forceps delivery or other obstetrical intervention or resuscitation of the newborn will be necessary.

Continued on next page

Information on the SmithKline Beecham Pharmaceuticals products appearing here is based on the labeling in effect on July 31, 1998. Further information on these and other products may be obtained from the Medical Department, SmithKline Beecham Pharmaceuticals, One Franklin Plaza, Philadelphia, PA 19101.

Amoxil—Cont.

Nursing Mothers: Penicillins have been shown to be excreted in human milk. Amoxicillin use by nursing mothers may lead to sensitization of infants. Caution should be exercised when amoxicillin is administered to a nursing woman.

Pediatric Use: Because of incompletely developed renal function in neonates and young infants, the elimination of amoxicillin may be delayed. Dosing of Amoxil (amoxicillin) should be modified in pediatric patients 12 weeks or younger (≤3 months). (See **DOSAGE AND ADMINISTRATION** - Neonates and infants.)

ADVERSE REACTIONS

As with other penicillins, it may be expected that untoward reactions will be essentially limited to sensitivity phenomena. They are more likely to occur in individuals who have previously demonstrated hypersensitivity to penicillins and in those with a history of allergy, asthma, hay fever, or urticaria. The following adverse reactions have been reported as associated with the use of penicillins:

Gastrointestinal: nausea, vomiting, diarrhea, and pseudomembranous colitis

Onset of pseudomembranous colitis symptoms may occur during or after antibiotic treatment. (See **WARNINGS**.)

Hypersensitivity Reactions: Erythematous maculopapular rashes, erythema multiforme, Stevens-Johnson Syndrome, toxic epidermal necrolysis, and urticaria have been reported.

NOTE: These hypersensitivity reactions may be controlled with antihistamines and, if necessary, systemic corticosteroids. Whenever such reactions occur, amoxicillin should be discontinued unless, in the opinion of the physician, the condition being treated is life-threatening and amenable only to amoxicillin therapy.

Liver: A moderate rise in AST (SGOT) has been noted, but the significance of this finding is unknown.

Hemic and Lymphatic Systems: Anemia, thrombocytopenia, thrombocytopenic purpura, eosinophilia, leukopenia, and agranulocytosis have been reported during therapy with penicillins. These reactions are usually reversible on discontinuation of therapy and are believed to be hypersensitivity phenomena.

Central Nervous System: Reversible hyperactivity, agitation, anxiety, insomnia, confusion, behavioral changes, and/or dizziness have been reported rarely.

Combination therapy with clarithromycin and lansoprazole
In clinical trials using combination therapy with amoxicillin plus clarithromycin and lansoprazole, and amoxicillin plus lansoprazole, no adverse reactions peculiar to these drug combinations were observed. Adverse reactions that have occurred have been limited to those that had been previously reported with amoxicillin, clarithromycin, or lansoprazole.

Triple therapy: amoxicillin/clarithromycin/lansoprazole
The most frequently reported adverse events for patients who received triple therapy were diarrhea (7%), headache (6%), and taste perversion (5%). No treatment-emergent adverse events were observed at significantly higher rates with triple therapy than with any dual therapy regimen.

Dual therapy: amoxicillin/lansoprazole
The most frequently reported adverse events for patients who received amoxicillin t.i.d. plus lansoprazole t.i.d. dual therapy were diarrhea (8%) and headache (7%). No treatment-emergent adverse events were observed at significantly higher rates with amoxicillin t.i.d. plus lansoprazole t.i.d. dual therapy than with lansoprazole alone.

For more information on adverse reactions with clarithromycin or lansoprazole, refer to their package inserts, **ADVERSE REACTIONS**.

OVERDOSAGE

In case of overdosage, discontinue medication, treat symptomatically, and institute supportive measures as required. If the overdosage is very recent and there is no contraindication, an attempt at emesis or other means of removal of drug from the stomach may be performed. A prospective study of 51 pediatric patients at a poison-control center suggested that overdosages of less than 250 mg/kg of amoxicillin are not associated with significant clinical symptoms and do not require gastric emptying.[3]

Interstitial nephritis resulting in oliguric renal failure has been reported in a small number of patients after overdosage with amoxicillin. Renal impairment appears to be reversible with cessation of drug administration. High blood levels may occur more readily in patients with impaired renal function because of decreased renal clearance of amoxicillin. Amoxicillin may be removed from circulation by hemodialysis.

DOSAGE AND ADMINISTRATION

Amoxil capsules, chewable tablets and oral suspensions may be given without regard to meals. However, the 875-mg tablet has been studied only when administered at the start of a light meal.

Neonates and infants aged ≤12 weeks (≤3 months)
Due to incompletely developed renal function affecting elimination of amoxicillin in this age group, the recommended upper dose of Amoxil (amoxicillin) is 30 mg/kg/day divided q12h.

[See table at top of previous page]

Dosing recommendations for adults with impaired renal function:
Patients with impaired renal function do not generally require a reduction in dose unless the impairment is severe. Severely impaired patients with a glomerular filtration rate of <30 mL/minute should not receive the 875-mg tablet. Patients with a glomerular filtration rate of 10 to 30 mL/minute should receive 500 mg or 250 mg every 12 hours, depending on the severity of the infection. Patients with a less than 10 mL/minute glomerular filtration rate should receive 500 mg or 250 mg every 24 hours, depending on severity of the infection.

Hemodialysis patients should receive 500 mg or 250 mg every 24 hours, depending on severity of the infection. They should receive an additional dose both during and at the end of dialysis.

There are currently no dosing recommendations for pediatric patients with impaired renal function.

All patients with gonorrhea should be evaluated for syphilis. (See **PRECAUTIONS** - Laboratory Tests.)

Larger doses may be required for stubborn or severe infections.

H. pylori eradication to reduce the risk of duodenal ulcer recurrence
Triple therapy: Amoxil/clarithromycin/lansoprazole
The recommended adult oral dose is 1 gram *Amoxil*, 500 mg clarithromycin, and 30 mg lansoprazole, all given twice daily (q12h) for 14 days. (See **INDICATIONS AND USAGE**.)

Dual therapy: Amoxil/lansoprazole
The recommended adult oral dose is 1 gram Amoxil (amoxicillin) and 30 mg lansoprazole, each given three times daily (q8h) for 14 days. (See **INDICATIONS AND USAGE**.)

Please refer to clarithromycin and lansoprazole full prescribing information for **CONTRAINDICATIONS** and **WARNINGS**, and for information regarding dosing in elderly and renally impaired patients.

General: The children's dosage is intended for individuals whose weight will not cause a dosage to be calculated greater than that recommended for adults.

It should be recognized that in the treatment of chronic urinary tract infections, frequent bacteriological and clinical appraisals are necessary. Smaller doses than those recommended above should not be used. Even higher doses may be needed at times. In stubborn infections, therapy may be required for several weeks. It may be necessary to continue clinical and/or bacteriological follow-up for several months after cessation of therapy. Except for gonorrhea, treatment should be continued for a minimum of 48 to 72 hours beyond the time that the patient becomes asymptomatic or evidence of bacterial eradication has been obtained. It is recommended that there be at least 10 days' treatment for any infection caused by *Streptococcus pyogenes* to prevent the occurrence of acute rheumatic fever.

After reconstitution, the required amount of suspension should be placed directly on the child's tongue for swallowing. Alternate means of administration are to add the required amount of suspension to formula, milk, fruit juice, water, ginger ale, or cold drinks. These preparations should then be taken immediately. To be certain the child is receiving full dosage, such preparations should be consumed in entirety.

Directions For Mixing Oral Suspension
Prepare suspension at time of dispensing as follows: Tap bottle until all powder flows freely. Add approximately $\frac{1}{3}$ of the total amount of water for reconstitution (see table below) and shake vigorously to wet powder. Add remainder of the water and again shake vigorously.

Bottle Size	Amount of Water Required for Reconstitution
125 mg/5 mL	
80 mL	62 mL
100 mL	78 mL
150 mL	116 mL
Each teaspoonful (5 mL) will contain 125 mg amoxicillin.	
125 mg unit dose	5 mL
250 mg/5 mL	
80 mL	59 mL
100 mL	74 mL
150 mL	111 mL
Each teaspoonful (5 mL) with contain 250 mg amoxicillin.	
250 mg unit dose	5 mL

Directions For Mixing Pediatric Drops
Prepare pediatric drops at time of dispensing as follows: Add the required amount of water (see table below) to the bottle and shake vigorously. Each mL of suspension will then contain amoxicillin trihydrate equivalent to 50 mg amoxicillin.

Bottle Size	Amount of Water Required for Reconstitution
15 mL	12 mL
30 mL	23 mL

NOTE: SHAKE BOTH ORAL SUSPENSION AND PEDIATRIC DROPS WELL BEFORE USING. Keep bottle tightly closed. Any unused portion of the reconstituted suspension must be discarded after 14 days. Refrigeration preferable, but not required.

HOW SUPPLIED

Amoxil (amoxicillin) Capsules. Each capsule contains 250 mg or 500 mg amoxicillin as the trihydrate.

250-mg Capsule	
NDC 0029-6006-30	bottles of 100
NDC 0029-6006-32	bottles of 500
500-mg Capsule	
NDC 0029-6007-30	bottles of 100
NDC 0029-6007-32	bottles of 500

Amoxil (amoxicillin) Tablets. Each tablet contains 500 mg or 875 mg amoxicillin as the trihydrate.

500-mg Tablet	
NDC 0029-6046-12	bottles of 20
NDC 0029-6046-20	bottles of 100
NDC 0029-6046-25	bottles of 500
875-mg Tablet	
NDC 0029-6047-12	bottles of 20
NDC 0029-6047-20	bottles of 100
NDC 0029-6047-25	bottles of 500

Amoxil (amoxicillin) Chewable Tablets. Each cherry-banana-peppermint-flavored tablet contains 125 mg or 250 mg amoxicillin as the trihydrate.

125-mg Tablet	
NDC 0029-6004-39	bottles of 60
250-mg Tablet	
NDC 0029-6005-13	bottles of 30
NDC 0029-6005-30	bottles of 100

Amoxil (amoxicillin) for Oral Suspension. Each 5 mL of reconstituted strawberry-flavored suspension contains 125 mg amoxicillin as the trihydrate. Each 5 mL of reconstituted bubble-gum-flavored suspension contains 250 mg amoxicillin as the trihydrate.

125 mg/5 mL	
NDC 0029-6008-21	80-mL bottle
NDC 0029-6008-23	100-mL bottle
NDC 0029-6008-22	150-mL bottle
250 mg/5 mL	
NDC 0029-6009-21	80-mL bottle
NDC 0029-6009-23	100-mL bottle
NDC 0029-6009-22	150-mL bottle
NDC 0029-6008-18	125-mg unit dose bottle
NDC 0029-6009-18	250-mg unit dose bottle

Amoxil (amoxicillin) Pediatric Drops for Oral Suspension. Each mL of bubble-gum-flavored reconstituted suspension contains 50 mg amoxicillin as the trihydrate.

NDC 0029-6035-20	15-mL bottle
NDC 0029-6038-39	30-mL bottle

Store capsules, unreconstituted powder, and chewable tablets at or below 20° C (68° F). Store 500-mg and 875-mg tablets at or below 25° C (77° F). Dispense in a tight container.

CLINICAL STUDIES

H. pylori eradication to reduce the risk of duodenal ulcer recurrence
Randomized, double-blind clinical studies performed in the U.S. in patients with *H. pylori* and duodenal ulcer disease (defined as an active ulcer or history of an ulcer within one year) evaluated the efficacy of lansoprazole in combination with amoxicillin capsules and clarithromycin tablets as triple 14-day therapy, or in combination with amoxicillin capsules as dual 14-day therapy, for the eradication of *H. pylori*. Based on the results of these studies, the safety and efficacy of two different eradication regimens were established:

Triple therapy: amoxicillin 1 gram b.i.d./clarithromycin 500 mg b.i.d./lansoprazole 30 mg b.i.d.

Dual therapy: amoxicillin 1 gram t.i.d./lansoprazole 30 mg t.i.d.

All treatments were for 14 days. *H. pylori* eradication was defined as two negative tests (culture and histology) at 4 to 6 weeks following the end of treatment.

Triple therapy was shown to be more effective than all possible dual therapy combinations. Dual therapy was shown to be more effective than both monotherapies. Eradication of *H. pylori* has been shown to reduce the risk of duodenal ulcer recurrence.

***H. pylori* Eradication Rates – Triple Therapy (amoxicillin/clarithromycin/lansoprazole) Percent of Patients Cured [95% Confidence Interval] (Number of Patients)**

Study	Triple Therapy Evaluable Analysis‖	Triple Therapy Intent-to-Treat Analysis¶
Study 1	92** [80.0–97.7] (n=48)	86** [73.3–93.5] (n=55)
Study 2	86†† [75.7–93.6] (n=66)	83†† [72.0–90.8] (n=70)

‖ This analysis was based on evaluable patients with confirmed duodenal ulcer (active or within one year) and *H. pylori* infection at baseline defined as at least two of three positive endoscopic tests from CLOtest®, (Delta West Ltd., Bentley, Australia), histology and/or culture. Patients were included in the analysis if they completed the study. Additionally, if patients dropped out of the study due to an adverse event related to the study drug, they were included in the analysis as failures of therapy.

¶ Patients were included in the analysis if they had documented *H. pylori* infection at baseline as defined above and had a confirmed duodenal ulcer (active or within one year). All dropouts were included as failures of therapy.

** ($p<0.05$) versus lansoprazole/amoxicillin and lansoprazole/clarithromycin dual therapy.

†† ($p<0.05$) versus clarithromycin/amoxicillin dual therapy.

***H. pylori* Eradication Rates – Dual Therapy (amoxicillin/lansoprazole) Percent of Patients Cured [95% Confidence Interval] (Number of Patients)**

Study	Dual Therapy Evaluable Analysis‡‡	Dual Therapy Intent-to-Treat Analysis§§
Study 1	77‖‖ [62.5–87.2] (n=51)	70‖‖ [56.8–81.2] (n=60)
Study 2	66¶¶ [51.9–77.5] (n=58)	61¶¶ [48.5–72.9] (n=67)

‡‡ This analysis was based on evaluable patients with confirmed duodenal ulcer (active or within one year) and *H. pylori* infection at baseline defined as at least two of three positive endoscopic tests from CLOtest®, histology and/or culture. Patients were included in the analysis if they completed the study. Additionally, if patients dropped out of the study due to an adverse event related to the study drug, they were included in the analysis as failures of therapy.

§§ Patients were included in the analysis if they had documented *H. pylori* infection at baseline as defined above and had a confirmed duodenal ulcer (active or within one year). All dropouts were included as failures of therapy.

‖‖ ($p<0.05$) versus lansoprazole alone.

¶¶ ($p<0.05$) versus lansoprazole alone or amoxicillin alone.

REFERENCES

1. National Committee for Clinical Laboratory Standards. Methods for Dilution Antimicrobial Susceptibility Tests for Bacteria that Grow Aerobically - Fourth Edition; Approved Standard. NCCLS Document M7-A4, Vol. 17, No. 2. NCCLS, Wayne, PA, January 1997.
2. National Committee for Clinical Laboratory Standards. Performance Standards for Antimicrobial Disk Susceptibility Tests - Sixth Edition; Approved Standard. NCCLS Document M2-A6, Vol. 17, No. 1. NCCLS, Wayne, PA, January 1997.
3. Swanson-Biearman B, Dean BS, Lopez G, Krenzelok EP. The effects of penicillin and cephalosporin ingestions in children less than six years of age. *Vet Hum Toxicol* 1988;30:66-67.

Rx only

Veterans Administration/Military/PHS—Chewable Tablets, 125 mg, 60's, 6505-01-159-9245; 250 mg, 100's, 6505-01-253-3834; Capsules, 250 mg, 100's, 6505-01-010-7953; 250 mg, 500's, 6505-01-116-6013; 500 mg, 100's, 6505-01-115-1474; 500 mg, 500's, 6505-01-250-8527; Oral Suspension, 125 mg, 10x5 mL SUP, 6505-01-197-2950; 125 mg/5 mL, 80 mL, 6505-01-412-9703; 125 mg/5 mL, 100 mL, 6505-01-153-3862; 125 mg/5 mL, 150 mL, 6505-01-011-1464; 250 mg, 10x5 mL SUP, 6505-01-160-6013; 250 mg/5 mL, 80 mL, 6505-01-153-3442; 250 mg/5 mL, 100 mL, 6505-01-156-2106; 250 mg/5 mL, 150 mL, 6505-01-066-4195.

AM:L15A

Shown in Product Identification Guide, page 338

ANCEF® ℞

[an-sef′]

(brand of sterile cefazolin for injection and cefazolin injection)

DESCRIPTION

Ancef (cefazolin for injection) is a semi-synthetic cephalosporin for parenteral administration. It is the sodium salt of 3-{[(5-methyl-1, 3, 4-thiadiazol-2-yl) thio]-methyl}-8-oxo-7-[2-(1H-tetrazol-1-yl) acetamido] -5- thia-1-azabicyclo [4.2.0] oct-2-ene-2-carboxylic acid.

The sodium content is 46 mg per gram of cefazolin.

Ancef in lyophilized form is supplied in vials equivalent to 500 mg or 1 gram of cefazolin; in "Piggyback" Vials for intravenous admixture equivalent to 1 gram of cefazolin; and in Pharmacy Bulk Vials equivalent to 5 grams or 10 grams of cefazolin.

Ancef is also supplied as a frozen, sterile, nonpyrogenic solution of cefazolin sodium in an iso-osmotic diluent in plastic containers. After thawing, the solution is intended for intravenous use.

The plastic container is fabricated from a specially designed multilayer plastic, PL 2040. Solutions are in contact with the polyethylene layer of this container and can leach out certain of the chemical components of the plastic in very small amounts within the expiration period. However, the suitability of the plastic has been confirmed in tests in animals according to the USP biological tests for plastic containers as well as by tissue culture toxicity studies.

CLINICAL PHARMACOLOGY

Human Pharmacology: After intramuscular administration of *Ancef* to normal volunteers, the mean serum concentrations were 37 mcg/mL at 1 hour and 3 mcg/mL at 8 hours following a 500 mg dose, and 64 mcg/mL at 1 hour and 7 mcg/mL at 8 hours following a 1 gram dose.

Studies have shown that following intravenous administration of *Ancef* to normal volunteers, mean serum concentrations peaked at approximately 185 mcg/mL and were approximately 4 mcg/mL at 8 hours for a 1 gram dose.

The serum half-life for *Ancef* is approximately 1.8 hours following I.V. administration and approximately 2.0 hours following I.M. administration.

In a study (using normal volunteers) of constant intravenous infusion with dosages of 3.5 mg/kg for 1 hour (approximately 250 mg) and 1.5 mg/kg the next 2 hours (approximately 100 mg), *Ancef* produced a steady serum level at the third hour of approximately 28 mcg/mL.

Studies in patients hospitalized with infections indicate that Ancef (cefazolin for injection) produces mean peak serum levels approximately equivalent to those seen in normal volunteers.

Bile levels in patients without obstructive biliary disease can reach or exceed serum levels by up to five times; however, in patients with obstructive biliary disease, bile levels of *Ancef* are considerably lower than serum levels (< 1.0 mcg/mL).

In synovial fluid, the *Ancef* level becomes comparable to that reached in serum at about 4 hours after drug administration.

Studies of cord blood show prompt transfer of *Ancef* across the placenta. *Ancef* is present in very low concentrations in the milk of nursing mothers.

Ancef is excreted unchanged in the urine. In the first 6 hours approximately 60% of the drug is excreted in the urine and this increases to 70% to 80% within 24 hours. *Ancef* achieves peak urine concentrations of approximately 2400 mcg/mL and 4000 mcg/mL respectively following 500 mg and 1 gram intramuscular doses.

In patients undergoing peritoneal dialysis (2 l/hr.), *Ancef* produced mean serum levels of approximately 10 and 30 mcg/mL after 24 hours' instillation of a dialyzing solution containing 50 mg/l and 150 mg/l, respectively. Mean peak levels were 29 mcg/mL (range 13–44 mcg/mL) with 50 mg/l (three patients), and 72 mcg/mL (range 26–142 mcg/mL) with 150 mg/l (six patients). Intraperitoneal administration of *Ancef* is usually well tolerated.

Controlled studies on adult normal volunteers, receiving 1 gram 4 times a day for 10 days, monitoring CBC, SGOT, SGPT, bilirubin, alkaline phosphatase, BUN, creatinine and urinalysis, indicated no clinically significant changes attributed to *Ancef.*

Microbiology: *In vitro* tests demonstrate that the bactericidal action of cephalosporins results from inhibition of cell wall synthesis. Ancef (cefazolin for injection) is active against the following organisms *in vitro* and in clinical infections:

Staphylococcus aureus (including penicillinase-producing strains)
Staphylococcus epidermidis
Methicillin-resistant staphylococci are uniformly resistant to cefazolin
Group A beta-hemolytic streptococci and other strains of streptococci (many strains of enterococci are resistant)
Streptococcus pneumoniae
Escherichia coli
Proteus mirabilis
Klebsiella species
Enterobacter aerogenes
Haemophilus influenzae

Most strains of indole positive Proteus (*Proteus vulgaris*), *Enterobacter cloacae, Morganella morganii* and *Providencia rettgeri* are resistant. *Serratia, Pseudomonas, Mima, Herellea* species are almost uniformly resistant to cefazolin.

Disk Susceptibility Tests

Disk diffusion technique—Quantitative methods that require measurement of zone diameters give the most precise estimates of antibiotic susceptibility. One such procedure[1] has been recommended for use with disks to test susceptibility to cefazolin.

Reports from a laboratory using the standardized single-disk susceptibility test[1] with a 30 mcg cefazolin disk should be interpreted according to the following criteria:

Susceptible organisms produce zones of 18 mm or greater, indicating that the tested organism is likely to respond to therapy.

Organisms of intermediate susceptibility produce zones 15 to 17 mm, indicating that the tested organism would be susceptible if high dosage is used or if the infection is confined to tissues and fluids (e.g., urine), in which high antibiotic levels are attained.

Resistant organisms produce zones of 14 mm or less, indicating that other therapy should be selected.

1 Bauer, A.W.; Kirby, W.M.M.; Sherris, J.C., and Turck, M.: Antibiotic Testing by a Standardized Single Disc Method, Am. J. Clin. Path. 45:493, 1966. Standardized Disc Susceptibility Test, Federal Register 39:19182-19184, 1974.

For gram-positive isolates, a zone of 18 mm is indicative of a cefazolin-susceptible organism when tested with either the cephalosporin-class disk (30 mcg cephalothin) or the cefazolin disk (30 mcg cefazolin).

Gram-negative organisms should be tested with the cefazolin disk (using the above criteria), since cefazolin has been shown by *in vitro* tests to have activity against certain strains of *Enterobacteriaceae* found resistant when tested with the cephalothin disk. Gram-negative organisms having zones of less than 18 mm around the cephalothin disk may be susceptible to cefazolin.

Standardized procedures require use of control organisms. The 30 mcg cefazolin disk should give zone diameter between 23 and 29 mm for *E. coli* ATCC 25922 and between 29 and 35 mm for *S. aureus* ATCC 25923.

The cefazolin disk should not be used for testing susceptibility to other cephalosporins.

Dilution techniques—A bacterial isolate may be considered susceptible if the minimal inhibitory concentration (MIC) for cefazolin is not more than 16 mcg per mL. Organisms are considered resistant if the MIC is equal to or greater than 64 mcg per mL.

The range of MIC's for the control strains are as follows:

S. aureus ATCC 25923, 0.25 to 1.0 mcg/mL
E. coli ATCC 25922, 1.0 to 4.0 mcg/mL

INDICATIONS AND USAGE

Ancef (cefazolin for injection) is indicated in the treatment of the following serious infections due to susceptible organisms:

RESPIRATORY TRACT INFECTIONS due to *Streptococcus pneumoniae, Klebsiella* species, *Haemophilus influenzae, Staphylococcus aureus* (penicillin-sensitive and penicillin-resistant) and group A beta-hemolytic streptococci.

Injectable benzathine penicillin is considered to be the drug of choice in treatment and prevention of streptococcal infections, including the prophylaxis of rheumatic fever.

Ancef is effective in the eradication of streptococci from the nasopharynx; however, data establishing the efficacy of *Ancef* in the subsequent prevention of rheumatic fever are not available at present.

Continued on next page

Information on the SmithKline Beecham Pharmaceuticals products appearing here is based on the labeling in effect on July 31, 1998. Further information on these and other products may be obtained from the Medical Department, SmithKline Beecham Pharmaceuticals, One Franklin Plaza, Philadelphia, PA 19101.

Ancef—Cont.

URINARY TRACT INFECTIONS due to *Escherichia coli*, *Proteus mirabilis*, *Klebsiella* species and some strains of enterobacter and enterococci.

SKIN AND SKIN STRUCTURE INFECTIONS due to *Staphylococcus aureus* (penicillin-sensitive and penicillin-resistant), group A beta-hemolytic streptococci and other strains of streptococci.

BILIARY TRACT INFECTIONS due to *Escherichia coli*, various strains of streptococci, *Proteus mirabilis*, *Klebsiella* species and *Staphylococcus aureus*.

BONE AND JOINT INFECTIONS due to *Staphylococcus aureus*.

GENITAL INFECTIONS (i.e., prostatitis, epididymitis) due to *Escherichia coli*, *Proteus mirabilis*, *Klebsiella* species and some strains of enterococci.

SEPTICEMIA due to *Streptococcus pneumoniae*, *Staphylococcus aureus* (penicillin-sensitive and penicillin-resistant), *Proteus mirabilis*, *Escherichia coli* and *Klebsiella* species.

ENDOCARDITIS due to *Staphylococcus aureus* (penicillin-sensitive and penicillin-resistant) and group A beta-hemolytic streptococci.

Appropriate culture and susceptibility studies should be performed to determine susceptibility of the causative organism to *Ancef*.

PERIOPERATIVE PROPHYLAXIS: The prophylactic administration of *Ancef* preoperatively, intraoperatively and postoperatively may reduce the incidence of certain postoperative infections in patients undergoing surgical procedures which are classified as contaminated or potentially contaminated (e.g., vaginal hysterectomy, and cholecystectomy in high-risk patients such as those over 70 years of age, with acute cholecystitis, obstructive jaundice or common duct bile stones).

The perioperative use of *Ancef* may also be effective in surgical patients in whom infection at the operative site would present a serious risk (e.g., during open-heart surgery and prosthetic arthroplasty).

The prophylactic administration of *Ancef* should usually be discontinued within a 24-hour period after the surgical procedure. In surgery where the occurrence of infection may be particularly devastating (e.g., open-heart surgery and prosthetic arthroplasty), the prophylactic administration of *Ancef* may be continued for 3 to 5 days following the completion of surgery.

If there are signs of infection, specimens for cultures should be obtained for the identification of the causative organism so that appropriate therapy may be instituted.
(See DOSAGE AND ADMINISTRATION.)

CONTRAINDICATIONS

ANCEF (CEFAZOLIN FOR INJECTION) IS CONTRAINDICATED IN PATIENTS WITH KNOWN ALLERGY TO THE CEPHALOSPORIN GROUP OF ANTIBIOTICS.

WARNINGS

SERIOUS AND OCCASIONALLY FATAL HYPERSENSITIVITY (anaphylactic) REACTIONS HAVE BEEN REPORTED IN PATIENTS ON PENICILLIN THERAPY. THESE REACTIONS ARE MORE LIKELY TO OCCUR IN INDIVIDUALS WITH A HISTORY OF PENICILLIN HYPERSENSITIVITY AND/OR A HISTORY OF SENSITIVITY TO MULTIPLE ALLERGENS. THERE HAVE BEEN REPORTS OF INDIVIDUALS WITH A HISTORY OF PENICILLIN HYPERSENSITIVITY WHO HAVE EXPERIENCED SEVERE REACTIONS WHEN TREATED WITH CEPHALOSPORINS. BEFORE INITIATING THERAPY WITH *ANCEF*, CAREFUL INQUIRY SHOULD BE MADE CONCERNING PREVIOUS HYPERSENSITIVITY REACTIONS TO PENICILLINS, CEPHALOSPORINS OR OTHER ALLERGENS. IF AN ALLERGIC REACTION OCCURS, *ANCEF* SHOULD BE DISCONTINUED AND APPROPRIATE THERAPY SHOULD BE INSTITUTED. **SERIOUS ANAPHYLACTIC REACTIONS REQUIRE IMMEDIATE EMERGENCY TREATMENT WITH EPINEPHRINE. OXYGEN, INTRAVENOUS STEROIDS AND AIRWAY MANAGEMENT, INCLUDING INTUBATION, SHOULD ALSO BE ADMINISTERED AS INDICATED.**

Pseudomembranous colitis has been reported with nearly all antibacterial agents, including *Ancef*, and may range in severity from mild to life-threatening. Therefore, it is important to consider this diagnosis in patients who present with diarrhea subsequent to the administration of antibacterial agents.

Treatment with antibacterial agents alters the normal flora of the colon and may permit overgrowth of clostridia. Studies indicate that a toxin produced by *Clostridium difficile* is one primary cause of "antibiotic-associated colitis."

After the diagnosis of pseudomembranous colitis has been established, therapeutic measures should be initiated. Mild cases of pseudomembranous colitis usually respond to drug discontinuation alone. In moderate to severe cases, consideration should be given to management with fluids and electrolytes, protein supplementation and treatment with an antibacterial drug clinically effective against *C. difficile* colitis.

PRECAUTIONS

General—Prolonged use of Ancef (cefazolin for injection) may result in the overgrowth of nonsusceptible organisms. Careful clinical observation of the patient is essential.

When *Ancef* is administered to patients with low urinary output because of impaired renal function, lower daily dosage is required (see DOSAGE AND ADMINISTRATION). As with other beta-lactam antibiotics, seizures may occur if inappropriately high doses are administered to patients with impaired renal function (see DOSAGE AND ADMINISTRATION).

Ancef, as with all cephalosporins, should be prescribed with caution in individuals with a history of gastrointestinal disease, particularly colitis.

Drug Interactions—Probenecid may decrease renal tubular secretion of cephalosporins when used concurrently, resulting in increased and more prolonged cephalosporin blood levels.

Drug/Laboratory Test Interactions—A false positive reaction for glucose in the urine may occur with Benedict's solution, Fehling's solution or with Clinitest® tablets, but not with enzyme-based tests such as Clinistix® and Tes-Tape®. Positive direct and indirect antiglobulin (Coombs) tests have occurred; these may also occur in neonates whose mothers received cephalosporins before delivery.

Carcinogenesis/Mutagenesis — Mutagenicity studies and long-term studies in animals to determine the carcinogenic potential of Ancef (cefazolin for injection) have not been performed.

Pregnancy — Teratogenic Effects — Pregnancy Category B. Reproduction studies have been performed in rats, mice and rabbits at doses up to 25 times the human dose and have revealed no evidence of impaired fertility or harm to the fetus due to *Ancef*. There are, however, no adequate and well-controlled studies in pregnant women. Because animal reproduction studies are not always predictive of human response, this drug should be used during pregnancy only if clearly needed.

Labor and Delivery—When cefazolin has been administered prior to caesarean section, drug levels in cord blood have been approximately one quarter to one third of maternal drug levels. The drug appears to have no adverse effect on the fetus.

Nursing Mothers—Ancef (cefazolin for injection) is present in very low concentrations in the milk of nursing mothers. Caution should be exercised when *Ancef* is administered to a nursing woman.

Pediatric Use—Safety and effectiveness for use in prematures and infants under 1 month of age have not been established. See DOSAGE AND ADMINISTRATION for recommended dosage in children over 1 month.

The potential for the toxic effect in children from chemicals that may leach from the single-dose I.V. preparation in plastic has not been determined.

ADVERSE REACTIONS

The following reactions have been reported:

Gastrointestinal: Diarrhea, oral candidiasis (oral thrush), vomiting, nausea, stomach cramps, anorexia and pseudomembranous colitis. Onset of pseudomembranous colitis symptoms may occur during or after antibiotic treatment (see WARNINGS). Nausea and vomiting have been reported rarely.

Allergic: Anaphylaxis, eosinophilia, itching, drug fever, skin rash, Stevens-Johnson syndrome.

Hematologic: Neutropenia, leukopenia, thrombocytopenia, thrombocythemia.

Hepatic and Renal: Transient rise in SGOT, SGPT, BUN and alkaline phosphatase levels has been observed without clinical evidence of renal or hepatic impairment.

Local Reactions: Rare instances of phlebitis have been reported at site of injection. Pain at the site of injection after intramuscular administration has occurred infrequently. Some induration has occurred.

Other Reactions: Genital and anal pruritus (including vulvar pruritus, genital moniliasis and vaginitis).

DOSAGE AND ADMINISTRATION
Usual Adult Dosage

Type of Infection	Dose	Frequency
Moderate to severe infections	500 mg to 1 gram	every 6 to 8 hrs.
Mild infections caused by susceptible gram + cocci	250 mg to 500 mg	every 8 hours
Acute, uncomplicated urinary tract infections	1 gram	every 12 hours
Pneumococcal pneumonia	500 mg	every 12 hours
Severe, life-threatening infections (e.g., endocarditis, septicemia)*	1 gram to 1.5 grams	every 6 hours

* In rare instances, doses of up to 12 grams of *Ancef* per day have been used.

Perioperative Prophylactic Use

To prevent postoperative infection in contaminated or potentially contaminated surgery, recommended doses are:
a. 1 gram I.V. or I.M. administered $^{1}/_{2}$ hour to 1 hour prior to the start of surgery.
b. For lengthy operative procedures (e.g., 2 hours or more), 500 mg to 1 gram I.V. or I.M. during surgery (administration modified depending on the duration of the operative procedure).
c. 500 mg to 1 gram I.V. or I.M. every 6 to 8 hours for 24 hours postoperatively.

It is important that (1) the preoperative dose be given just ($^{1}/_{2}$ to 1 hour) prior to the start of surgery so that adequate antibiotic levels are present in the serum and tissues at the time of initial surgical incision; and (2) *Ancef* be administered, if necessary, at appropriate intervals during surgery to provide sufficient levels of the antibiotic at the anticipated moments of greatest exposure to infective organisms. In surgery where the occurrence of infection may be particularly devastating (e.g., open-heart surgery and prosthetic arthroplasty), the prophylactic administration of Ancef (cefazolin for injection) may be continued for 3 to 5 days following the completion of surgery.

Dosage Adjustment for Patients with Reduced Renal Function

Ancef may be used in patients with reduced renal function with the following dosage adjustments: Patients with a creatinine clearance of 55 mL/min. or greater or a serum creatinine of 1.5 mg % or less can be given full doses. Patients with creatinine clearance rates of 35 to 54 mL/min. or serum creatinine of 1.6 to 3.0 mg % can also be given full doses but dosage should be restricted to at least 8 hour intervals. Patients with creatinine clearance rates of 11 to 34 mL/min. or serum creatinine of 3.1 to 4.5 mg % should be given $^{1}/_{2}$ the usual dose every 12 hours. Patients with creatinine clearance rates of 10 mL/min. or less or serum creatinine of 4.6 mg % or greater should be given $^{1}/_{2}$ the usual dose every 18 to 24 hours. All reduced dosage recommendations apply after an initial loading dose appropriate to the severity of the infection. Patients undergoing peritoneal dialysis: See Human Pharmacology.

Pediatric Dosage

In children, a total daily dosage of 25 to 50 mg per kg (approximately 10 to 20 mg per pound) of body weight, divided into three or four equal doses, is effective for most mild to moderately severe infections. Total daily dosage may be increased to 100 mg per kg (45 mg per pound) of body weight for severe infections. Since safety for use in premature infants and in infants under 1 month has not been established, the use of Ancef (cefazolin for injection) in these patients is not recommended.

Pediatric Dosage Guide

Weight		25 mg/kg/Day Divided into 3 Doses		25 mg/kg/Day Divided into 4 Doses	
Lbs	Kg	Approximate Single Dose mg/q8h	Vol. (mL) needed with dilution of 125 mg/mL	Approximate Single Dose mg/q6h	Vol. (mL) needed with dilution of 125 mg/mL
10	4.5	40 mg	0.35 mL	30 mg	0.25 mL
20	9.0	75 mg	0.60 mL	55 mg	0.45 mL
30	13.6	115 mg	0.90 mL	85 mg	0.70 mL
40	18.1	150 mg	1.20 mL	115 mg	0.90 mL
50	22.7	190 mg	1.50 mL	140 mg	1.10 mL

Weight		50 mg/kg/Day Divided into 3 Doses		50 mg/kg/Day Divided into 4 Doses	
Lbs	Kg	Approximate Single Dose mg/q8h	Vol. (mL) needed with dilution of 225 mg/mL	Approximate Single Dose mg/q6h	Vol. (mL) needed with dilution of 225 mg/mL
10	4.5	75 mg	0.35 mL	55 mg	0.25 mL
20	9.0	150 mg	0.70 mL	110 mg	0.50 mL
30	13.6	225 mg	1.00 mL	170 mg	0.75 mL
40	18.1	300 mg	1.35 mL	225 mg	1.00 mL
50	22.7	375 mg	1.70 mL	285 mg	1.25 mL

In children with mild to moderate renal impairment (creatinine clearance of 70 to 40 mL/min.), 60 percent of the normal daily dose given in equally divided doses every 12 hours should be sufficient. In patients with moderate impairment (creatinine clearance of 40 to 20 mL/min.), 25 percent of the normal daily dose given in equally divided doses every 12 hours should be adequate. Children with severe renal impairment (creatinine clearance of 20 to 5 mL/min.) may be given 10 percent of the normal daily dose every 24 hours. All dosage recommendations apply after an initial loading dose.

RECONSTITUTION

Preparation of Parenteral Solution

Parenteral drug products should be SHAKEN WELL when reconstituted, and inspected visually for particulate matter prior to administration. If particulate matter is evident in reconstituted fluids, the drug solutions should be discarded. When reconstituted or diluted according to the instructions below, Ancef (cefazolin for injection) is stable for 24 hours at room temperature or for 10 days if stored under refrigeration (5°C or 41°F). Reconstituted solutions may range in color from pale yellow to yellow without a change in potency.

Single-Dose Vials

For I.M. injection, I.V. direct (bolus) injection or I.V. infusion, reconstitute with Sterile Water for Injection according to the following table. SHAKE WELL.

Vial Size	Amount of Diluent	Approximate Concentration	Approximate Available Volume
500 mg	2.0 mL	225 mg/mL	2.2 mL
1 gram	2.5 mL	330 mg/mL	3.0 mL

Pharmacy Bulk Vials

Add Sterile Water for Injection, Bacteriostatic Water for Injection or Sodium Chloride Injection according to the table below. SHAKE WELL.

Vial Size	Amount of Diluent	Approximate Concentration	Approximate Available Volume
5 grams	23 mL	1 gram/5 mL	26 mL
	48 mL	1 gram/10 mL	51 mL
10 grams	45 mL	1 gram/5 mL	51 mL
	96 mL	1 gram/10 mL	102 mL

"Piggyback" Vials

Reconstitute with 50 to 100 mL of Sodium Chloride Injection or other I.V. solution listed under ADMINISTRATION. When adding diluent to vial, allow air to escape by using a small vent needle or by pumping the syringe. SHAKE WELL. Administer with primary I.V. fluids, as a single dose.

ADMINISTRATION

Intramuscular Administration—Reconstitute vials with Sterile Water for Injection according to the dilution table above. Shake well until dissolved. Ancef should be injected into a large muscle mass. Pain on injection is infrequent with Ancef.

Intravenous Administration—Direct (bolus) injection: Following reconstitution according to the above table, further dilute vials with approximately 5 mL Sterile Water for Injection. Inject the solution slowly over 3 to 5 minutes, directly or through tubing for patients receiving parenteral fluids (see list below).

Intermittent or continuous infusion: Dilute reconstituted Ancef in 50 to 100 mL of one of the following solutions:
Sodium Chloride Injection, USP
5% or 10% Dextrose Injection, USP
5% Dextrose in Lactated Ringer's Injection, USP
5% Dextrose and 0.9% Sodium Chloride Injection, USP
5% Dextrose and 0.45% Sodium Chloride Injection, USP
5% Dextrose and 0.2% Sodium Chloride Injection, USP
Lactated Ringer's Injection, USP
Invert Sugar 5% or 10% in Sterile Water for Injection
Ringer's Injection, USP
5% Sodium Bicarbonate Injection, USP

DIRECTIONS FOR USE OF ANCEF (CEFAZOLIN INJECTION) GALAXY® CONTAINER (PL 2040 PLASTIC)

Ancef in Galaxy® Container (PL 2040 Plastic) is to be administered either as a continuous or intermittent infusion using sterile equipment.

Storage

Store in a freezer capable of maintaining a temperature of −20°C (−4°F).

Thawing of Plastic Container

Thaw frozen container at 25°C or 77°F or under refrigeration (5°C or 41°F). (DO NOT FORCE THAW BY IMMERSION IN WATER BATHS OR BY MICROWAVE IRRADIATION.)
Check for minute leaks by squeezing container firmly. If leaks are detected, discard solution as sterility may be impaired.
Do not add supplementary medication.

The container should be visually inspected. Components of the solution may precipitate in the frozen state and will dissolve upon reaching room temperature with little or no agitation. Potency is not affected. Agitate after solution has reached room temperature. If after visual inspection the solution remains cloudy or if an insoluble precipitate is noted or if any seals or outlet ports are not intact, the container should be discarded.
The thawed solution is stable for 30 days under refrigeration (5°C or 41°F) and 48 hours at 25°C or 77°F. Do not refreeze thawed antibiotics.
Use sterile equipment. It is recommended that the intravenous administration apparatus be replaced at least once every 48 hours.
CAUTION: Do not use plastic containers in series connections. Such use could result in air embolism due to residual air being drawn from the primary container before administration of the fluid from the secondary container is complete.

Preparation for administration:
1. Suspend container from eyelet support.
2. Remove plastic protector from outlet port at bottom of container.
3. Attach administration set. Refer to complete directions accompanying set.

HOW SUPPLIED

Ancef (cefazolin for injection)—supplied in vials equivalent to 500 mg or 1 gram of cefazolin; in "Piggyback" Vials for intravenous admixture equivalent to 1 gram of cefazolin; and in Pharmacy Bulk Vials equivalent to 5 grams or 10 grams of cefazolin.
Ancef (cefazolin injection) as a frozen, iso-osmotic, sterile, nonpyrogenic solution in plastic containers—supplied in 50 mL single-dose containers equivalent to 500 mg or 1 gram of cefazolin. Dextrose Hydrous, USP, has been added to the above dosages to adjust osmolality (approximately 2.4 grams and 2 grams, respectively). Store at or below −20°C (−4°F). (See DIRECTIONS FOR USE OF ANCEF [CEFAZOLIN INJECTION] GALAXY® CONTAINER [PL 2040 PLASTIC].)
As with other cephalosporins, Ancef tends to darken depending on storage conditions; within the stated recommendations, however, product potency is not adversely affected. Before reconstitution protect from light and store between 15° and 30°C (59° and 86°F).
Ancef supplied as a frozen, iso-osmotic, sterile, nonpyrogenic solution in plastic containers is manufactured for SmithKline Beecham Pharmaceuticals by Baxter Healthcare Corporation, Deerfield, IL 60015.
Galaxy is a registered trademark of Baxter International Inc.
Veterans Administration /Military /PHS—500 mg/50 mL, frozen, 24's, 6505-01-274-9683; 1 gram/50 mL, frozen, 24's, 6505-01-237-8453
AF:L51

Shown in Product Identification Guide, page 338

ANDRODERM®
[an-drō-derm]
Testosterone Transdermal System
Controlled Delivery for Once-Daily Application

DESCRIPTION

Androderm (testosterone transdermal system) provides continuous delivery of testosterone (the primary endogenous androgen) for 24 hours following application to intact, nonscrotal skin (e.g., back, abdomen, thighs, upper arms).
Two strengths of *Androderm* are available which deliver *in vivo* 2.5 mg or 5 mg of testosterone per day across skin of average permeability.
Androderm has a central drug delivery reservoir surrounded by a peripheral adhesive area. The *Androderm* 2.5 mg system has a total contact surface area of 37 cm² with a 7.5 cm² central drug delivery reservoir containing 12.2 mg testosterone USP, dissolved in an alcohol-based gel. The *Androderm* 5 mg system has a total contact surface area of 44 cm² with a 15 cm² central drug delivery reservoir containing 24.3 mg testosterone USP, dissolved in an alcohol-based gel. Testosterone USP is a white, or creamy white crystalline powder or crystals chemically described as 17β-hydroxyandrost-4-en-3-one.
[See chemical structure at top of next column]
The *Androderm* systems have six components as shown in Figure 1. Proceeding from the top toward the surface attached to the skin, the system is composed of (1) metallized polyester/Surlyn®* (ethylene-methacrylic acid copolymer)/ethyl vinyl acetate backing film, (2) a drug reservoir of testosterone USP, alcohol USP, glycerin USP, glycerol monooleate, and methyl laurate gelled with an acrylic acid copolymer, (3) a permeable polyethylene microporous membrane, and (4) a peripheral layer of acrylic adhesive surrounding the central, active drug delivery area of the system. Prior to opening of the system and application to

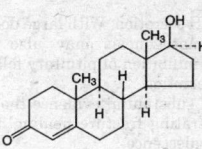

Testosterone
$C_{19}H_{28}O_2$ mw 288.43

the skin, the central delivery surface of the system is sealed with a peelable laminate disc (5) composed of a five-layer laminate containing polyester/polyesterurethane adhesive/aluminum foil/polyesterurethane adhesive polyethylene. The disc is attached to and removed with the release liner (6), a silicone-coated polyester film, which is removed before the system can be used.

*Surlyn is a registered trademark of E.I. DuPont de Nemours & Company.

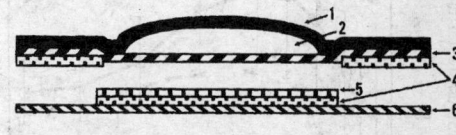

1. Backing Film	3. Microporous Membrane	5. Disc
2. Drug Reservoir	4. Adhesive	6. Release Liner

Figure 1: System Schematic

The active ingredient in the system is testosterone. The remaining components of the system are pharmacologically inactive.

CLINICAL PHARMACOLOGY

Androderm (testosterone transdermal system) delivers physiologic amounts of testosterone producing circulating testosterone concentrations that approximate the normal circadian rhythm of healthy young men.

Testosterone

Androderm (testosterone transdermal system) delivers testosterone, the primary androgenic hormone. Testosterone is responsible for the normal growth and development of the male sex organs and for maintenance of secondary sex characteristics. These effects include the growth and maturation of the prostate, seminal vesicles, penis, and scrotum; development of male hair distribution, such as facial, pubic, chest, and axillary hair; laryngeal enlargement; vocal cord thickening; and alterations in body musculature and fat distribution.
Male hypogonadism results from insufficient secretion of testosterone and is characterized by low serum testosterone concentrations. Symptoms associated with male hypogonadism include the following: impotence and decreased sexual desire; fatigue and loss of energy; mood depression; and regression of secondary sexual characteristics.

General Androgen Effects

Androgens promote retention of nitrogen, sodium, potassium, and phosphorus, and decreased urinary excretion of calcium. Androgens have been reported to increase protein anabolism and decrease protein catabolism. Nitrogen balance is improved only when there is sufficient intake of calories and protein.
Androgens are also responsible for the growth spurt of adolescence and for the eventual termination of linear growth that is brought about by the fusion of the epiphyseal growth centers. In children, exogenous androgens accelerate linear growth rates but may cause disproportionate advancement in bone maturation. Use over long periods may result in fusion of the epiphyseal growth centers and termination of the growth process.
Androgens have been reported to stimulate the production of red blood cells by enhancing erythropoietin production. During exogenous administration of androgens, endogenous testosterone release is inhibited through feedback inhibi-

Continued on next page

Information on the SmithKline Beecham Pharmaceuticals products appearing here is based on the labeling in effect on July 31, 1998. Further information on these and other products may be obtained from the Medical Department, SmithKline Beecham Pharmaceuticals, One Franklin Plaza, Philadelphia, PA 19101.

Androderm—Cont.

tion of pituitary LH secretion. With large doses of exogenous androgens, spermatogenesis may also be suppressed through feedback inhibition of pituitary follicle stimulating hormone (FSH) secretion.

There is a lack of substantial evidence that androgens are effective in accelerating fracture healing or in shortening post-surgical convalescence.

Pharmacokinetics

Absorption

Following Androderm (testosterone transdermal system) application to non-scrotal skin, testosterone is continuously absorbed during the 24-hour dosing period. Daily application of *Androderm* at approximately 10 PM results in a serum testosterone concentration profile that mimics the normal circadian variation observed in healthy young men (Fig. 2 below). Maximum concentrations occur in the early morning hours with minimum concentrations in the evening (Table 1 below).

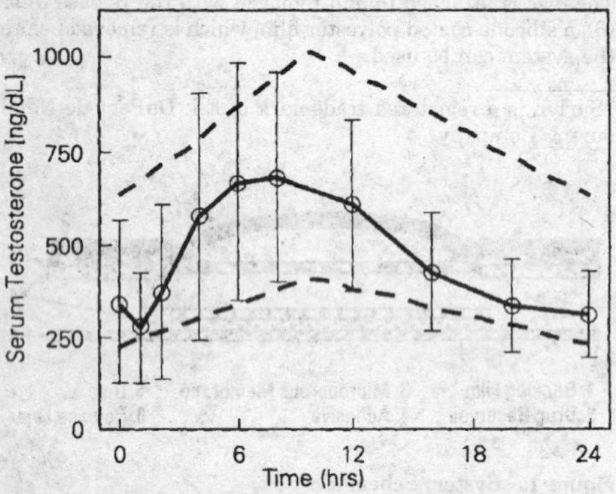

Figure 2: Mean (SD) steady state serum testosterone concentrations during nightly application of *Androderm* 2.5 mg systems in 29 hypogonadal male patients, 27 patients used 2 systems nightly and 2 patients used 3 systems nightly. Area between the dashed lines shows the 95% confidence interval for the circadian variation observed in healthy young men.[1] System application (t=0) at approximately 10 PM.

Table 1: Steady-state serum testosterone pharmacokinetic parameters in hypogonadal men measured during continuous Androderm (testosterone transdermal system) treatment.

Parameter	Units	n	Mean	SD
C_{max}	ng/dL	56	753	276
C_{avg}	ng/dL	56	498	169
C_{min}	ng/dL	56	246	120
T_{max}	hr	56	7.9	2.2
$T_{1/2}$	min	29	71	32
CL	L/day	49	1304	464

C_{max}=maximum serum concentration
C_{avg}=average serum concentration (AUC/24 hr)
C_{min}=minimum serum concentration
T_{max}=time of maximum serum concentration
$T_{1/2}$=elimination half-life
CL=clearance

In a group of 34 hypogonadal men, application of two *Androderm* 2.5 mg systems to the abdomen, back, thighs, or upper arms resulted in average testosterone absorption of 4 to 5 mg over 24 hours. The serum testosterone concentration profiles during application were similar for these sites (Table 2). Applications to the chest and shins resulted in greater inter-individual variability and average 24 hour absorption of 3 to 4 mg.

Table 2: Mean serum testosterone concentrations (ng/dL) measured during single-dose applications of two *Androderm* 2.5 mg systems applied at night to different sites in 34 hypogonadal men.

Sample Time (hr)	Abdomen Mean	Abdomen SD	Back Mean	Back SD	Thigh Mean	Thigh SD	Upper Arm Mean	Upper Arm SD
0	90	82	80	74	85	76	81	69
3	286	201	429	252	271	201	308	226
6	476	236	608	250	489	254	468	245
9	570	234	613	214	592	251	534	204
12	575	244	588	233	594	247	527	199
24	352	164	403	174	367	161	332	124

In a steady-state study of 12 hypogonadal men, nightly application of 1, 2, or 3 *Androderm* 2.5 mg systems resulted in increases in the mean morning serum testosterone concentrations. These concentrations averaged 424, 584, and 766 ng/dL with the application of 1, 2, and 3 systems, respectively. The mean baseline serum testosterone concentration was 76 ng/dL.

Normal range morning serum testosterone concentrations are reached during the first day of dosing. There is no accumulation of testosterone during continuous treatment.

In a study of 20 hypogonadal patients, two *Androderm* 2.5 mg systems and a single *Androderm* 5 mg system produced equivalent serum testosterone concentration profiles. Average steady state concentrations over 24 hours (Cssavg) were 613±169 and 621±176 ng/dL for the two 2.5 mg and single 5 mg systems, respectively. C_{max} values were 925±340 ng/dL for the two 2.5 mg systems and 905±254 ng/dL for the single 5 mg system.

In 16 hypogonadal men, the topical administration of 0.1% triamcinolone cream to the skin under the central drug reservoir prior to application of the *Androderm* system did not significantly alter transdermal absorption of testosterone; however, the rate of complete adherence was lower. In these patients, pretreatment with an ointment formulation significantly reduced testosterone absorption from the system.

Distribution

In serum, testosterone is bound with high affinity to sex hormone binding globulin (SHBG) and with low affinity to albumin. The albumin bound portion easily dissociates and is presumed to be bioactive. The SHBG-bound portion is not considered to be bioactive. The amount of SHBG in serum and the total testosterone concentration determine the distribution of bioactive and non-bioactive androgen.

Bioactive serum testosterone concentrations (BT) measured during Androderm (testosterone transdermal system) treatment paralleled the serum testosterone profile (Figure 2) and remained within the normal reference range.

Metabolism

Inactivation of testosterone occurs primarily in the liver. Testosterone (T) is metabolized to various 17-keto steroids through two different pathways, and the major active metabolites are estradiol (E2) and dihydrotestosterone (DHT). DHT binds with greater affinity to SHBG than does testosterone. In reproductive tissues, DHT is further metabolized to 3-alpha and 3-beta androstanediol.

In many tissues, the activity of testosterone appears to depend on reduction to DHT, which binds to cytosol receptor proteins. The steroid-receptor complex is transported to the nucleus, where it initiates transcription events and cellular changes related to androgen action.

During steady-state pharmacokinetic studies in hypogonadal men treated with *Androderm,* the average DHT:T and E2:T ratios were comparable to those in normal men, approximately 1:10 and 1:200, respectively.

Upon removal of the *Androderm* systems, serum testosterone concentrations decrease with an apparent half-life of approximately 70 minutes. Hypogonadal concentrations are reached within 24 hours following system removal.

Androderm therapy suppresses endogenous testosterone secretion via the pituitary/gonadal axis, resulting in a reduction in baseline serum testosterone concentrations compared to the untreated state.

Excretion

Approximately 90% of a testosterone dose given intramuscularly is excreted in the urine as glucuronide and sulfate conjugates of testosterone and its metabolites; about 6% is excreted in the feces, mostly in unconjugated form.

Special Populations

Geriatric

No age related effects on testosterone pharmacokinetics were observed in clinical trials of *Androderm* in men up to 65 years of age. In a group of 9 elderly testosterone deficient men (65–79 years of age, average baseline testosterone level 184±50 ng/dL), a single application of two *Androderm* 2.5 mg systems to the back resulted in an average testosterone level of 591±121 ng/dL with a T_{max} of 14.2±4.2 hours. The total testosterone delivered over the 24-hour application time was 3.8±0.6 mg, approximately 20% less than the average amount delivered in younger patients.

Race

There is insufficient information available from *Androderm* trials to compare testosterone pharmacokinetics in different racial groups.

Renal Insufficiency

There is no experience with use of *Androderm* in patients with renal insufficiency.

Hepatic Insufficiency

There is no experience with use of *Androderm* in patients with hepatic insufficiency.

Drug-Drug Interactions

See "Precautions" below

Clinical Studies

In clinical studies using the *Androderm* 2.5 mg system, 93% of patients were treated with two systems daily, 6% used three systems daily, and 1% used one system daily.

The hormonal effects of Androderm (testosterone transdermal system) as a treatment for male hypogonadism were demonstrated in four open-label trials that included 94 hypogonadal men, ages 15 to 65 years. In these trials, *Androderm* produced average morning serum testosterone concentrations within the normal reference range in 92% of patients. The mean (SD) serum hormone concentrations and percentage of patients who achieved average concentrations within the normal ranges are shown in Table 3 below.

Table 3: Individual morning serum hormone concentrations (ng/dL) and percent of patients with mean concentrations within the normal range during continuous *Androderm* treatment (n=94).

Normal Range	T (306–1031)	BT (93–420)	DHT (28–85)	E2 (0.9–3.6)
Mean	589	312	47	2.7
SD	209	127	18	1.2
% Normal	92	88	85	77
% High	1	12	2	22
% Low	7	0	13	1

A physiological suppression of the pituitary/gonadal axis occurs during continuous *Androderm* treatment leading to reduced serum LH concentrations. In clinical trials, 10 of 21 (48%) of men with primary (hypergonadotropic) hypogonadism achieved normal range LH concentrations within 6 to 12 months of treatment. LH concentrations may remain elevated in some patients despite serum testosterone concentrations within the normal range.

Twenty-nine patients, previously treated with testosterone, completed 12 months of *Androderm* treatment. Following an 8-week androgen withdrawal period, *Androderm* treatment produced positive effects on fatigue, mood and sexual function. The percent of patients complaining of fatigue decreased from 79% to 10% during treatment ($p<0.001$). The average patient depression score (Beck Depression Inventory) decreased from 6.9 to 3.9 ($p<0.001$). Nocturnal penile tumescence and rigidity monitoring showed an increase in mean duration of erections 0.23 to 0.39 hours per night ($p=0.01$) and an increase in penile tip rigidity from 18% to 50% ($p<0.001$). The total number of self-reported erections reported increased from 2.3 to 7.8 per week ($p<0.001$).

Comparison with intramuscular testosterone: Sixty-six patients, previously treated with testosterone injections, received *Androderm* or intramuscular testosterone enanthate (200 mg every 2 weeks) treatment for 6 months. The percent of time that serum concentrations measured throughout the dosing interval remained within the normal range were as follows:

	Androderm	IM	*p* value
T	82%	72%	0.05
BT	87%	39%	<0.001
DHT	76%	70%	0.06
E2	81%	35%	<0.001

Sexual function was comparable between groups.

Effect on plasma lipids: In 67 men treated for 6 to 12 months, the average (SE) serum total cholesterol and HDL concentrations were 199 (7.6) ng/dL and 46 (2.3) ng/dL. Compared to baseline values during a hypogonadal state achieved by 8 weeks of androgen withdrawal in 29 patients, the following changes in lipids were observed during 1 year of *Androderm* treatment: Cholesterol decreased 1.2%; HDL decreased 8%; Cholesterol/HDL ratio increased 9%. In these patients, lipids measured during *Androderm* treatment were not significantly different from those measured during prior IM injection treatment.

Effects on the prostate: Prostate size and serum prostate specific antigen (PSA) concentrations during treatment were comparable to values reported for eugonadal men. One case of prostate carcinoma occurred during *Androderm* treatment; two cases were detected during IM treatment.

INDICATIONS AND USAGE

Androderm (testosterone transdermal system) is indicated for testosterone replacement therapy in men for conditions associated with a deficiency or absence of endogenous testosterone.

Primary hypogonadism (congenital or acquired)—Testicular failure due to cryptorchidism, bilateral torsion, orchitis, vanishing testis syndrome, or orchidectomy, Klinefelter's syndrome, chemotherapy, or toxic damage from alcohol or heavy metals. These men usually have low serum testosterone concentrations accompanied by gonadotropins (FSH, LH) above the normal range.

Secondary, i.e., hypogonadotropic hypogonadism (congenital or acquired)—idiopathic gonadotropin or luteinizing hormone-releasing hormone (LHRH) deficiency, or pituitary-hypothalamic injury from tumors, trauma, or radiation. These men have low serum testosterone concentrations without associated elevation in gonadotropins. Appropriate adrenal cortical and thyroid hormone replacement therapy may be necessary in patients with multiple pituitary or hypothalamic abnormalities.

CONTRAINDICATIONS

Androgens are contraindicated in men with carcinoma of the breast or known or suspected carcinoma of the prostate. *Androderm* therapy has not been evaluated in women and must not be used in women. Testosterone may cause fetal harm.

Androderm is contraindicated in patients with known hypersensitivity to any of its components.

WARNINGS

Prolonged use of high doses of orally active 17-alpha-alkyl androgens (e.g., methyltestosterone) has been associated with the development of peliosis hepatis, cholestatic jaundice and hepatic neoplasms, including hepatocellular carcinoma (see PRECAUTIONS, Carcinogenesis). Peliosis hepatis can be a life-threatening or fatal complication. Testosterone is not known to produce these adverse effects.

Geriatric patients treated with androgens may be at an increased risk for the development of prostatic hyperplasia. Geriatric patients and other patients with clinical or demographic characteristics that are recognized to be associated with an increased risk of prostate cancer should be evaluated for the presence of subclinical or clinical prostate cancer prior to initiation of testosterone replacement therapy, because testosterone therapy may promote the growth of existing subclinical foci of prostate cancer.[2]

In men receiving testosterone replacement therapy, surveillance for prostate cancer should be consistent with current practices for eugonadal men (see PRECAUTIONS, Carcinogenesis).

Edema, with or without congestive heart failure, may be a serious complication of androgen treatment in patients with preexisting cardiac, renal, or hepatic disease. In addition to discontinuation of the drug, diuretic therapy may be required.

Gynecomastia frequently develops and occasionally persists in patients being treated for hypogonadism.

PRECAUTIONS

General

The physician should instruct patients to report any of the following side effects of androgens:
• Too frequent or persistent erections of the penis
• Any nausea, vomiting, jaundice, or ankle swelling

Virilization of female sexual partners has been reported with male use of a topical testosterone solution. Topically applied creams leave as much as 90 mg residual testosterone on the skin. The occlusive backing film on Androderm (testosterone transdermal system) prevents the partner from coming in contact with the active material in the system. Transfer of the system to the partner is unlikely.

Changes in body hair distribution, significant increase in acne, or other signs of virilization of the female partner should be brought to the attention of a physician.

Information for Patients

An information brochure is available for patients concerning the use of *Androderm*.

Advise patients of the following:

Androderm should not be applied to the scrotum.

Androderm should not be applied over a bony prominence or on a part of the body that could be subject to prolonged pressure during sleep or sitting. Application to these sites has been associated with burn-like blister reactions.

Androderm does not have to be removed during sexual intercourse, nor while taking a shower or bath.

Androderm systems should be applied nightly.

Laboratory Tests

Hemoglobin and hematocrit should be checked periodically to detect polycythemia in patients who are receiving androgen therapy.

Liver function, prostate specific antigen, total cholesterol and HDL cholesterol should be checked periodically.

Drug Interactions

Anticoagulants: C-17 substituted derivatives of testosterone, such as methandrostenolone, have been reported to decrease the anticoagulant requirements of patients receiving oral anticoagulants. Patients receiving oral anticoagulants require close monitoring especially when androgens are started or stopped.

Oxyphenbutazone: Concurrent administration of oxyphenbutazone and androgens may result in elevated serum levels of oxyphenbutazone.

Insulin: In diabetic patients, the metabolic effects of androgens may decrease blood glucose and, therefore, insulin requirements.

Drug/Laboratory Test Interferences

Androgens may decrease levels of thyroxine-binding globulin, resulting in decreased total T_4 serum levels and increased resin uptake of T_3 and T_4. Free thyroid hormone levels remain unchanged, however, and there is no clinical evidence of thyroid dysfunction.

Carcinogenesis, Mutagenesis, Impairment of Fertility

Animal Data: Testosterone has been tested by subcutaneous injection and implantation in mice and rats. The implant induced cervical-uterine tumors in mice, which metastasized in some cases. There is suggestive evidence that injection of testosterone into some strains of female mice increases their susceptibility to hepatoma. Testosterone is also known to increase the number of tumors and decrease the degree of differentiation of chemically induced carcinomas of the liver in rats.

Human Data: There are rare reports of hepatocellular carcinoma in patients receiving long-term therapy with androgens in high doses. Withdrawal of drugs did not lead to regression of the tumors in all cases.

Geriatric patients treated with androgens may be at an increased risk for the development of prostatic hyperplasia. Geriatric patients and other patients with clinical or demographic characteristics that are recognized to be associated with an increased risk of prostate cancer should be evaluated for the presence of subclinical or clinical prostate cancer prior to initiation of testosterone replacement therapy, because testosterone therapy may promote the growth of existing subclinical foci of prostate cancer.[2]

In men receiving testosterone replacement therapy, surveillance for prostate cancer should be consistent with current practices for eugonadal men.

Pregnancy Category X: (See Contraindications).

Teratogenic Effects: *Androderm* must not be used in women.

Nursing Mothers: *Androderm* must not be used in women.

Pediatric Use: *Androderm* has not been evaluated clinically in males under 15 years of age.

ADVERSE REACTIONS

Adverse Events Associated with Androderm (testosterone transdermal system)

In clinical studies of 122 patients treated with *Androderm,* the most common adverse events reported were skin reactions at the site of system application. Transient mild to moderate erythema was observed at the site of application in the majority of patients at some time during treatment. The adverse reactions reported by more than 1% of patients are listed below shown in order of decreasing frequency.

Event	Percent of Patients
pruritus at application site	37%
burn-like blister reaction under system	12%
erythema at application site	7%
vesicles at application site	6%
prostate abnormalities	5%
headache	4%
allergic contact dermatitis to the system	4%
burning at application site	3%
induration at application site	3%
depression	3%
rash	2%
gastrointestinal bleeding	2%

The following reactions occurred in less than 1% of patients: fatigue; body pain; pelvic pain; hypertension; peripheral vascular disease; increased appetite; accelerated growth; anxiety; confusion; decreased libido; paresthesia; thinking abnormalities; vertigo; acne; bullae at application site; mechanical irritation at application site; rash at application site; contamination of application site; prostate carcinoma; dysuria; hematuria; impotence; urinary incontinence; urinary tract infection; testicular abnormalities.

Three types of application site reactions occurred: irritation which included mild to moderate erythema, induration or burning; allergic contact dermatitis; and burn-like blister reactions.

Chronic skin irritation caused 5% of patients to discontinue treatment. Mild skin irritation may be ameliorated by treatment of affected skin with over-the-counter topical hydrocortisone cream applied after system removal.

Applying a small amount of 0.1% triamcinolone acetonide cream (Rx) to the skin under the central drug reservoir of the *Androderm* system has been shown to reduce the incidence and severity of skin irritation. The administration of 0.1% triamcinolone acetonide cream (Rx) does not significantly alter transdermal absorption of testosterone from the system. Ointment formulations should not be used for pretreatment as they may significantly reduce testosterone absorption.

Five patients (4%) developed allergic contact dermatitis after 3 to 8 weeks treatment that required discontinuation. These reactions were characterized by pruritus, erythema, induration and in some instances vesicles or bullae, which recurred with each system application. Rechallenge with components of the system showed ethanol sensitization in 4 patients. One patient's reaction was attributed to testosterone. None of these patients had adverse sequelae related to oral alcohol ingestion or to injectable testosterone use. Older patients may be more prone to develop allergic contact dermatitis.

Fourteen patients (12%) had burn-like blister reactions that involved bullae, epidermal necrosis or the development of ulcerated lesions. These reactions typically occurred once, at a single application site; 5 patients experienced a single recurrence. None withdrew from the clinical trials. These reactions occurred at a rate of approximately 1 in 6,500 system applications (1 in 3,250 treatment days). The majority of these lesions were associated with system application over bony prominences or on parts of the body that may have been subject to prolonged pressure during sleep or sitting (e.g., over the deltoid region of the upper arm, the greater trochanter of the femur, or the ischial tuberosity). The more severe lesions healed over several weeks with scarring in some cases. Such lesions should be treated as burns.

Adverse Events Associated with Injection or Oral Treatments

Skin and Appendages: Hirsutism, male pattern of baldness, seborrhea, and acne.

Endocrine and Urogenital: Gynecomastia and excessive frequency and duration of penile erections. Oligospermia may occur at high dosages (see CLINICAL PHARMACOLOGY).

Fluid and Electrolyte Disturbances: Retention of sodium, chloride, water, potassium, calcium, and inorganic phosphates.

Gastrointestinal: Nausea, cholestatic jaundice, alterations in liver function tests. Rare instances of hepatocellular neoplasms and peliosis hepatis have occurred (see WARNINGS).

Hematologic: Suppression of clotting factors II, V, VII, and X; bleeding in patients on concomitant anticoagulant therapy and polycythemia.

Nervous System: Increased or decreased libido, headache, anxiety, depression and generalized paresthesia.

Metabolic: Increased serum cholesterol.

Miscellaneous: Rarely, anaphylactoid reactions.

DRUG ABUSE AND DEPENDENCE

Androderm (testosterone transdermal system) is a Schedule III controlled substance under the Anabolic Steroids Control Act.

Oral consumption of the *Androderm* system or the gel contents of the system will not result in clinically significant serum testosterone concentrations in the target organs due to extensive first-pass metabolism.

OVERDOSAGE

There is one report of acute overdosage with testosterone enanthate injection: testosterone levels of up to 11,400 ng/dL were implicated in a cerebrovascular accident.

DOSAGE AND ADMINISTRATION

The usual starting dose is one *Androderm* 5 mg system or two *Androderm* 2.5 mg systems applied nightly for 24 hours, providing a total dose of 5 mg/day.

The adhesive side of the *Androderm* system should be applied to a clean, dry area of the skin on the back, abdomen, upper arms, or thighs. Avoid application over bony prominences or on a part of the body that may be subject to prolonged pressure during sleep or sitting (e.g., the deltoid region of the upper arm, the greater trochanter of the femur, and the ischial tuberosity). DO NOT APPLY TO THE SCROTUM. The sites of application should be rotated, with an interval of 7 days between applications to the same site. The area selected should not be oily, damaged, or irritated. (See Table 2.)

The system should be applied immediately after opening the pouch and removing the protective release liner. The system should be pressed firmly in place, making sure there is good contact with the skin, especially around the edges. To ensure proper dosing, the morning serum testosterone concentration may be measured following system application the previous evening. If the serum concentration is outside the normal range, sampling should be repeated with assurance of proper system adhesion as well as appropriate application time. Confirmed serum concentrations outside the normal range may require increasing the daily dose to 7.5 mg (i.e., one 5 mg and one 2.5 mg systems or three 2.5 mg systems) or decreasing the daily dose to 2.5 mg (i.e., one 2.5 mg system), maintaining nightly application. Because of variability in analytical values among diagnostic laboratories, this laboratory work and any later analyses for assessing the effect of *Androderm* therapy, should be performed at the same laboratory so results can be compared.

Mild skin irritation may be ameliorated by treatment of the affected skin with over-the-counter topical hydrocortisone cream applied after system removal.

Applying a small amount of 0.1% triamcinolone acetonide cream (Rx) to the skin under the central drug reservoir of the *Androderm* system has been shown to reduce the incidence and severity of skin irritation. The administration of

Continued on next page

Information on the SmithKline Beecham Pharmaceuticals products appearing here is based on the labeling in effect on July 31, 1998. Further information on these and other products may be obtained from the Medical Department, SmithKline Beecham Pharmaceuticals, One Franklin Plaza, Philadelphia, PA 19101.

Androderm—Cont.

0.1% triamcinolone acetonide cream (Rx) does not significantly alter transdermal absorption of testosterone from the system. **Ointment formulations should not be used for pretreatment as they may significantly reduce testosterone absorption.**

Androderm (testosterone transdermal system) therapy for non-virilized patients may be initiated with one 2.5 mg/day system applied nightly.

HOW SUPPLIED

Androderm (testosterone transdermal system) 2.5 mg/day. Each system contains 12.2 mg testosterone USP for delivery of 2.5 mg of testosterone per day (see DESCRIPTION). Cartons of 60 systems NDC 0007-3155-18

Androderm (testosterone transdermal system) 5 mg/day. Each system contains 24.3 mg testosterone USP for delivery of 5 mg of testosterone per day (see DESCRIPTION). Cartons of 30 systems NDC 0007-3156-13

Storage and Disposal

Store at room temperature, 15° to 30°C (59° to 86°F). Apply to skin immediately upon removal from the protective pouch. Do not store outside the pouch provided. Damaged systems should not be used. The drug reservoir may be burst by excessive pressure or heat. Discard systems in household trash in a manner that prevents accidental application or ingestion by children, pets or others.

REFERENCES

1. Mazer NA, et al. Mimicking the circadian pattern of testosterone and metabolite levels with an enhanced transdermal delivery system. In Gurney, Junjinger, Peppas, eds. *Pulsatile Drug Delivery: Current Applications and Future Trends.* Stuttgart: Wiss. Verl.-Ges.; 1993, 73-97. 2. Schroeder FH. Androgens and carcinoma of the prostate. In Neischlag E, Behre HM, eds. *Testosterone Action, Deficiency, Substitution.* Berlin/Heidelberg: Springer-Verlag; 1990, 245-260.
U.S. Patent Nos. 4,849,224, 4,855,294, 4,863,970, 4,983,395, 5,152,997, and 5,164,190.
Manufactured by:

TheraTech, Inc.　　　　　　　　　　　　　　**Rx only**
Salt Lake City, UT 84108
for **SmithKline Beecham Pharmaceuticals**
Philadelphia, PA
Veterans Administration/Military/PHS—Testosterone Transdermal System, 2.5 mg, 60's, 6505-01-423-4981.
AD:L7

Shown in Product Identification Guide, page 338

AUGMENTIN®　　　　　　　　　　　　　　℞
[og 'men-tin]
amoxicillin/clavulanate potassium
Powder for Oral
Suspension and
Chewable Tablets

DESCRIPTION

Augmentin is an oral antibacterial combination consisting of the semisynthetic antibiotic amoxicillin and the β-lactamase inhibitor, clavulanate potassium (the potassium salt of clavulanic acid). Amoxicillin is an analog of ampicillin, derived from the basic penicillin nucleus, 6-aminopenicillanic acid. The amoxicillin molecular formula is $C_{16}H_{19}N_3O_5S \cdot 3H_2O$ and the molecular weight is 419.46. Chemically, amoxicillin is (2S,5R,6R)-6-[(R)-(-)-2-Amino-2-(p-hydroxyphenyl)acetamido]-3,3-dimethyl-7-oxo-4-thia-1-azabicyclo[3.2.0]heptane-2- carboxylic acid trihydrate and may be represented structurally as:

Clavulanic acid is produced by the fermentation of *Streptomyces clavuligerus*. It is a β-lactam structurally related to

the penicillins and possesses the ability to inactivate a wide variety of β-lactamases by blocking the active sites of these enzymes. Clavulanic acid is particularly active against the clinically important plasmid mediated β-lactamases frequently responsible for transferred drug resistance to penicillins and cephalosporins. The clavulanate potassium molecular formula is $C_8H_8KNO_5$ and the molecular weight is 237.25. Chemically clavulanate potassium is potassium (Z)-(2R,5R)-3-(2-hydroxyethylidene) -7-oxo-4-oxa-1-azabicyclo [3.2.0]-heptane-2-carboxylate and may be represented structurally as:

Inactive Ingredients: Powder for Oral Suspension—Colloidal silicon dioxide, flavorings (See HOW SUPPLIED), succinic acid, xanthan gum, and one or more of the following: aspartame•, hydroxypropyl methylcellulose, mannitol, silica gel, silicon dioxide and sodium saccharin. Chewable Tablets—Colloidal silicon dioxide, flavorings (See HOW SUPPLIED), magnesium stearate, mannitol and one or more of the following: aspartame•, D&C Yellow No. 10, FD&C Red No. 40, glycine, sodium saccharin and succinic acid.
•See PRECAUTIONS—Information for Patients.
Each 125 mg chewable tablet and each 5 mL of reconstituted *Augmentin* 125 mg/5 mL oral suspension contains 0.16 mEq potassium. Each 250 mg chewable tablet and each 5 mL of reconstituted *Augmentin* 250 mg/5 mL oral suspension contains 0.32 mEq potassium. Each 200 mg chewable tablet and each 5 mL of reconstituted *Augmentin* 200 mg/5 mL oral suspension contains 0.14 mEq potassium. Each 400 mg chewable tablet and each 5 mL of reconstituted *Augmentin* 400 mg/5 mL oral suspension contains 0.29 mEq of potassium.

CLINICAL PHARMACOLOGY

Amoxicillin and clavulanate potassium are well absorbed from the gastrointestinal tract after oral administration of *Augmentin*. Dosing in the fasted or fed state has minimal effect on the pharmacokinetics of amoxicillin. While *Augmentin* can be given without regard to meals, absorption of clavulanate potassium when taken with food is greater relative to the fasted state. In one study, the relative bioavailability of clavulanate was reduced when *Augmentin* was dosed at 30 and 150 minutes after the start of a high fat breakfast. The safety and efficacy of *Augmentin* have been established in clinical trials where *Augmentin* was taken without regard to meals.
Oral administration of single doses of 400 mg *Augmentin* chewable tablets and 400 mg/5 mL suspension to 28 adult volunteers yielded comparable pharmacokinetic data:
[See table below]
Oral administration of 5 mL of *Augmentin* 250 mg/5 mL suspension or the equivalent dose of 10 mL *Augmentin* 125 mg/5 mL suspension provides average peak serum concentrations approximately 1 hour after dosing of 6.9 μg/mL for amoxicillin and 1.6 μg/mL for clavulanic acid. The areas under the serum concentration curves obtained during the first 4 hours after dosing were 12.6 μg.hr./mL for amoxicillin and 2.9 μg.hr./mL for clavulanic acid when 5 mL of *Augmentin* 250 mg/5 mL suspension or equivalent dose of 10 mL of *Augmentin* 125 mg/5 mL suspension was administered to adult volunteers. One *Augmentin* 250 mg chewable tablet or 2 *Augmentin* 125 mg chewable tablets are equivalent to 5 mL of *Augmentin* 250 mg/5 mL suspension and provide similar serum levels of amoxicillin and clavulanic acid.
Amoxicillin serum concentrations achieved with *Augmentin* are similar to those produced by the oral administration of equivalent doses of amoxicillin alone. The half-life of amoxicillin after the oral administration of *Augmentin* is 1.3 hours and that of clavulanic acid is 1.0 hour. Time above the minimum inhibitory concentration of 1.0 μg/mL for amoxicillin has been shown to be similar after corresponding q12h and q8h dosing regimens of *Augmentin* in adults and children.

Approximately 50% to 70% of the amoxicillin and approximately 25% to 40% of the clavulanic acid are excreted unchanged in urine during the first 6 hours after administration of 10 mL of *Augmentin* 250 mg/5 mL suspension. Concurrent administration of probenecid delays amoxicillin excretion but does not delay renal excretion of clavulanic acid.

Neither component in *Augmentin* is highly protein-bound; clavulanic acid has been found to be approximately 25% bound to human serum and amoxicillin approximately 18% bound.

Amoxicillin diffuses readily into most body tissues and fluids with the exception of the brain and spinal fluid. The results of experiments involving the administration of clavulanic acid to animals suggest that this compound, like amoxicillin, is well distributed in body tissues.

Two hours after oral administration of a single 35 mg/kg dose of *Augmentin* suspension to fasting children, average concentrations of 3.0 μg/mL of amoxicillin and 0.5 μg/mL of clavulanic acid were detected in middle ear effusions.

Microbiology: Amoxicillin is a semisynthetic antibiotic with a broad spectrum of bactericidal activity against many gram-positive and gram-negative microorganisms. Amoxicillin is, however, susceptible to degradation by β-lactamases and, therefore, the spectrum of activity does not include organisms which produce these enzymes. Clavulanic acid is a β-lactam, structurally related to the penicillins, which possesses the ability to inactivate a wide range of β-lactamase enzymes commonly found in microorganisms resistant to penicillins and cephalosporins. In particular, it has good activity against the clinically important plasmid mediated β-lactamases frequently responsible for transferred drug resistance.

The formulation of amoxicillin and clavulanic acid in *Augmentin* protects amoxicillin from degradation by β-lactamase enzymes and effectively extends the antibiotic spectrum of amoxicillin to include many bacteria normally resistant to amoxicillin and other β-lactam antibiotics. Thus, *Augmentin* possesses the distinctive properties of a broad-spectrum antibiotic and a β-lactamase inhibitor.

Amoxicillin/clavulanic acid has been shown to be active against most strains of the following microorganisms, both *in vitro* and in clinical infections as described in the INDICATIONS AND USAGE section.

GRAM-POSITIVE AEROBES
Staphylococcus aureus (β-lactamase and non-β-lactamase producing)§
§Staphylococci which are resistant to methicillin/oxacillin must be considered resistant to amoxicillin/clavulanic acid.

GRAM-NEGATIVE AEROBES
Enterobacter species (Although most strains of *Enterobacter* species are resistant *in vitro*, clinical efficacy has been demonstrated with *Augmentin* in urinary tract infections caused by these organisms.)
Escherichia coli (β-lactamase and non-β-lactamase producing)
Haemophilus influenzae (β-lactamase and non-β-lactamase producing)
Klebsiella species (All known strains are β-lactamase producing.)
Moraxella catarrhalis (β-lactamase and non-β-lactamase producing)
The following *in vitro* data are available, **but their clinical significance is unknown.**

Amoxicillin/clavulanic acid exhibits *in vitro* minimal inhibitory concentrations (MICs) of 0.5 μg/mL or less against most (≥90%) strains of *Streptococcus pneumoniae* [II]; MICs of 0.06 μg/mL or less against most (≥90%) strains of *Neisseria gonorrhoeae;* MICs of 4 μg/mL or less against most (≥90%) strains of staphylococci and anaerobic bacteria; and MICs of 8 μg/mL or less against most (≥90%) strains of other listed organisms. However, with the exception of organisms shown to respond to amoxicillin alone, the safety and effectiveness of amoxicillin/clavulanic acid in treating clinical infections due to these microorganisms have not been established in adequate and well-controlled clinical trials.

[II]Because amoxicillin has greater *in vitro* activity against *Streptococcus pneumoniae* than does ampicillin or penicillin, the majority of *S. pneumoniae* strains with intermediate susceptibility to ampicillin or penicillin are fully susceptible to amoxicillin.

GRAM-POSITIVE AEROBES
Enterococcus faecalis ¶
Staphylococcus epidermidis (β-lactamase and non-β-lactamase producing)
Staphylococcus saprophyticus (β-lactamase and non-β-lactamase producing)
Streptococcus pneumoniae ¶**
Streptococcus pyogenes ¶**
viridans group *Streptococcus* ¶**
GRAM-NEGATIVE AEROBES
Eikenella corrodens (β-lactamase and non-β-lactamase producing)

Dose†	AUC$_{0-\infty}$ (μg.hr./mL)		C$_{max}$ (μg/mL)‡	
(amoxicillin/clavulanate potassium)	amoxicillin (±S.D.)	clavulanate potassium (±S.D.)	amoxicillin (±S.D.)	clavulanate potassium (±S.D.)
400/57 mg (5 mL of suspension)	17.29 ±2.28	2.34 ±0.94	6.94 ±1.24	1.10 ±0.42
400/57 mg (one chewable tablet)	17.24 ±2.64	2.17 ±0.73	6.67 ±1.37	1.03 ±0.33

† Administered at the start of a light meal.
‡ Mean values of 28 normal volunteers. Peak concentrations occurred approximately 1 hour after the dose.

Neisseria gonorrhoeae ¶ (β-lactamase and non-β-lactamase producing)

Proteus mirabilis ¶ (β-lactamase and non-β-lactamase producing)

ANAEROBIC BACTERIA

Bacteroides species, including *Bacteroides fragilis* (β-lactamase and non-β-lactamase producing)

Fusobacterium species (β-lactamase and non-β-lactamase producing)

Peptostreptococcus species**

¶ Adequate and well-controlled clinical trials have established the effectiveness of amoxicillin alone in treating certain clinical infections due to these organisms.

** These are non-β-lactamase-producing organisms and, therefore, are susceptible to amoxicillin alone.

SUSCEPTIBILITY TESTING

Dilution Techniques: Quantitative methods are used to determine antimicrobial minimal inhibitory concentrations (MICs). These MICs provide estimates of the susceptibility of bacteria to antimicrobial compounds. The MICs should be determined using a standardized procedure. Standardized procedures are based on a dilution method[1] (broth or agar) or equivalent with standardized inoculum concentrations and standardized concentrations of amoxicillin/clavulanate potassium powder.

The recommended dilution pattern utilizes a constant amoxicillin/clavulanate potassium ratio of 2 to 1 in all tubes with varying amounts of amoxicillin. MICs are expressed in terms of the amoxicillin concentration in the presence of clavulanic acid at a constant 2 parts amoxicillin to 1 part clavulanic acid. The MIC values should be interpreted according to the following criteria:

RECOMMENDED RANGES FOR AMOXICILLIN/CLAVULANIC ACID SUSCEPTIBILITY TESTING

For gram-negative enteric aerobes:

MIC (µg/mL)	Interpretation
≤8/4	Susceptible (S)
16/8	Intermediate (I)
≥32/16	Resistant (R)

For *Staphylococcus* †† and *Haemophilus* species:

MIC (µg/mL)	Interpretation
≤4/2	Susceptible (S)
≥8/4	Resistant (R)

†† Staphylococci which are susceptible to amoxicillin/clavulanic acid but resistant to methicillin/oxacillin must be considered as resistant.

For *Streptococcus pneumoniae*: Isolates should be tested using amoxicillin/clavulanic acid and the following criteria should be used:

MIC (µg/mL)	Interpretation
≤0.5/0.25	Susceptible (S)
1/0.5	Intermediate (I)
≥2/1	Resistant (R)

A report of "Susceptible" indicates that the pathogen is likely to be inhibited if the antimicrobial compound in the blood reaches the concentration usually achievable. A report of "Intermediate" indicates that the result should be considered equivocal, and, if the microorganism is not fully susceptible to alternative, clinically feasible drugs, the test should be repeated. This category implies possible clinical applicability in body sites where the drug is physiologically concentrated or in situations where high dosage of drug can be used. This category also provides a buffer zone that prevents small uncontrolled technical factors from causing major discrepancies in interpretation. A report of "Resistant" indicates that the pathogen is not likely to be inhibited if the antimicrobial compound in the blood reaches the concentrations usually achievable; other therapy should be selected.

Standardized susceptibility test procedures require the use of laboratory control microorganisms to control the technical aspects of the laboratory procedures. Standard amoxicillin/clavulanate potassium powder should provide the following MIC values:

Microorganism	MIC Range (µg/mL)‡‡
Escherichia coli ATCC 25922	2 to 8
Escherichia coli ATCC 35218	4 to 16
Enterococcus faecalis ATCC 29212	0.25 to 1.0
Haemophilus influenzae ATCC 49247	2 to 16
Staphylococcus aureus ATCC 29213	0.12 to 0.5
Streptococcus pneumoniae ATCC 49619	0.03 to 0.12

‡‡ Expressed as concentration of amoxicillin in the presence of clavulanic acid at a constant 2 parts amoxicillin to 1 part clavulanic acid.

Diffusion Techniques: Quantitative methods that require measurement of zone diameters also provide reproducible estimates of the susceptibility of bacteria to antimicrobial compounds. One such standardized procedure[2] requires the use of standardized inoculum concentrations. This procedure uses paper disks impregnated with 30 µg of amoxicillin/clavulanate potassium (20 µg amoxicillin plus 10 µg clavulanate potassium) to test the susceptibility of microorganisms to amoxicillin/clavulanic acid.

Reports from the laboratory providing results of the standard single-disk susceptibility test with a 30 µg amoxicillin/clavulanate potassium (20 µg amoxicillin plus 10 µg clavulanate potassium) disk should be interpreted according to the following criteria:

RECOMMENDED RANGES FOR AMOXICILLIN/CLAVULANIC ACID SUSCEPTIBILITY TESTING

For *Staphylococcus* §§ species and *H. influenzae*[a]:

Zone Diameter (mm)	Interpretation
≥20	Susceptible (S)
≤19	Resistant (R)

For other organisms except *S. pneumoniae*[b] and *N. gonorrhoeae*[c]:

Zone Diameter (mm)	Interpretation
≥18	Susceptible (S)
14 to 17	Intermediate (I)
≤13	Resistant (R)

§§ Staphylococci which are resistant to methicillin/oxacillin must be considered as resistant to amoxicillin/clavulanic acid.

[a] A broth microdilution method should be used for testing *H. influenzae*. Beta-lactamase negative, ampicillin-resistant strains must be considered resistant to amoxicillin/clavulanic acid.

[b] Susceptibility of *S. pneumoniae* should be determined using a 1 µg oxacillin disk. Isolates with oxacillin zone sizes of ≥20 mm are susceptible to amoxicillin/clavulanic acid. An amoxicillin/clavulanic acid MIC should be determined on isolates of *S. pneumoniae* with oxacillin zone sizes of ≤19 mm.

[c] A broth microdilution method should be used for testing *N. gonorrhoeae* and interpreted according to penicillin breakpoints.

Interpretation should be as stated above for results using dilution techniques. Interpretation involves correlation of the diameter obtained in the disk test with the MIC for amoxicillin/clavulanic acid.

As with standardized dilution techniques, diffusion methods require the use of laboratory control microorganisms that are used to control the technical aspects of the laboratory procedures. For the diffusion technique, the 30 µg amoxicillin/clavulanate potassium (20 µg amoxicillin plus 10 µg clavulanate potassium) disk should provide the following zone diameters in these laboratory quality control strains:

Microorganism	Zone Diameter (mm)
Escherichia coli ATCC 25922	19 to 25 mm
Escherichia coli ATCC 35218	18 to 22 mm
Staphylococcus aureus ATCC 25923	28 to 36 mm

INDICATIONS AND USAGE

Augmentin is indicated in the treatment of infections caused by susceptible strains of the designated organisms in the conditions listed below:

Lower Respiratory Tract Infections—caused by β-lactamase-producing strains of *Haemophilus influenzae* and *Moraxella (Branhamella) catarrhalis.*

Otitis Media—caused by β-lactamase-producing strains of *Haemophilus influenzae* and *Moraxella (Branhamella) catarrhalis.*

Sinusitis—caused by β-lactamase-producing strains of *Haemophilus influenzae* and *Moraxella (Branhamella) catarrhalis.*

Skin and Skin Structure Infections—caused by β-lactamase-producing strains of *Staphylococcus aureus, Escherichia coli* and *Klebsiella* spp.

Urinary Tract Infections—caused by β-lactamase-producing strains of *Escherichia coli, Klebsiella* spp. and *Enterobacter* spp.

While *Augmentin* is indicated only for the conditions listed above, infections caused by ampicillin-susceptible organisms are also amenable to *Augmentin* treatment due to its amoxicillin content. Therefore, mixed infections caused by ampicillin-susceptible organisms and β-lactamase-producing organisms susceptible to *Augmentin* should not require the addition of another antibiotic. Because amoxicillin has greater *in vitro* activity against *Streptococcus pneumoniae* than does ampicillin or penicillin, the majority of *S. pneumoniae* strains with intermediate susceptibility to ampicillin or penicillin are fully susceptible to amoxicillin and *Augmentin.* (See Microbiology subsection.)

Bacteriological studies, to determine the causative organisms and their susceptibility to *Augmentin*, should be performed together with any indicated surgical procedures. Therapy may be instituted prior to obtaining the results from bacteriological and susceptibility studies to determine the causative organisms and their susceptibility to *Augmentin* when there is reason to believe the infection may involve any of the β-lactamase-producing organisms listed above. Once the results are known, therapy should be adjusted, if appropriate.

CONTRAINDICATIONS

Augmentin is contraindicated in patients with a history of allergic reactions to any penicillin. It is also contraindicated in patients with a previous history of *Augmentin*-associated cholestatic jaundice/hepatic dysfunction.

WARNINGS

SERIOUS AND OCCASIONALLY FATAL HYPERSENSITIVITY (ANAPHYLACTIC) REACTIONS HAVE BEEN REPORTED IN PATIENTS ON PENICILLIN THERAPY. THESE REACTIONS ARE MORE LIKELY TO OCCUR IN INDIVIDUALS WITH A HISTORY OF PENICILLIN HYPERSENSITIVITY AND/OR A HISTORY OF SENSITIVITY TO MULTIPLE ALLERGENS. THERE HAVE BEEN REPORTS OF INDIVIDUALS WITH A HISTORY OF PENICILLIN HYPERSENSITIVITY WHO HAVE EXPERIENCED SEVERE REACTIONS WHEN TREATED WITH CEPHALOSPORINS. BEFORE INITIATING THERAPY WITH *AUGMENTIN*, CAREFUL INQUIRY SHOULD BE MADE CONCERNING PREVIOUS HYPERSENSITIVITY REACTIONS TO PENICILLINS, CEPHALOSPORINS OR OTHER ALLERGENS. IF AN ALLERGIC REACTION OCCURS, *AUGMENTIN* SHOULD BE DISCONTINUED AND THE APPROPRIATE THERAPY INSTITUTED. **SERIOUS ANAPHYLACTIC REACTIONS REQUIRE IMMEDIATE EMERGENCY TREATMENT WITH EPINEPHRINE. OXYGEN, INTRAVENOUS STEROIDS AND AIRWAY MANAGEMENT, INCLUDING INTUBATION, SHOULD ALSO BE ADMINISTERED AS INDICATED.**

Pseudomembranous colitis has been reported with nearly all antibacterial agents, including *Augmentin*, and has ranged in severity from mild to life-threatening. Therefore, it is important to consider this diagnosis in patients who present with diarrhea subsequent to the administration of antibacterial agents.

Treatment with antibacterial agents alters the normal flora of the colon and may permit overgrowth of clostridia. Studies indicate that a toxin produced by *Clostridium difficile* is one primary cause of "antibiotic associated colitis."

After the diagnosis of pseudomembranous colitis has been established, appropriate therapeutic measures should be initiated. Mild cases of pseudomembranous colitis usually respond to drug discontinuation alone. In moderate to severe cases, consideration should be given to management with fluids and electrolytes, protein supplementation and treatment with an antibacterial drug clinically effective against *Clostridium difficile* colitis.

Augmentin should be used with caution in patients with evidence of hepatic dysfunction. Hepatic toxicity associated with the use of *Augmentin* is usually reversible. On rare occasions, deaths have been reported (less than 1 death reported per estimated 4 million prescriptions worldwide). These have generally been cases associated with serious underlying diseases or concomitant medications. (See CONTRAINDICATIONS and ADVERSE REACTIONS—*Liver.*)

PRECAUTIONS

General: While *Augmentin* possesses the characteristic low toxicity of the penicillin group of antibiotics, periodic assessment of organ system functions, including renal, hepatic and hematopoietic function, is advisable during prolonged therapy.

A high percentage of patients with mononucleosis who receive ampicillin develop an erythematous skin rash. Thus, ampicillin class antibiotics should not be administered to patients with mononucleosis.

The possibility of superinfections with mycotic or bacterial pathogens should be kept in mind during therapy. If superinfections occur (usually involving *Pseudomonas* or *Candida*), the drug should be discontinued and/or appropriate therapy instituted.

Information for the Patient: Augmentin may be taken every 8 hours or every 12 hours, depending on the strength of the product prescribed. Each dose should be taken with a meal or snack to reduce the possibility of gastrointestinal upset. Many antibiotics can cause diarrhea. If diarrhea is severe or lasts more than 2 or 3 days, call your doctor.

Make sure your child completes the entire prescribed course of treatment, even if he/she begins to feel better after a few days. Keep suspension refrigerated. Shake well before using. When dosing a child with *Augmentin* suspension (liq-

Continued on next page

Information on the SmithKline Beecham Pharmaceuticals products appearing here is based on the labeling in effect on July 31, 1998. Further information on these and other products may be obtained from the Medical Department, SmithKline Beecham Pharmaceuticals, One Franklin Plaza, Philadelphia, PA 19101.

Augmentin Powder/Chewable—Cont.

uid), use a dosing spoon or medicine dropper. Be sure to rinse the spoon or dropper after each use. Bottles of *Augmentin* suspension may contain more liquid than required. Follow your doctor's instructions about the amount to use and the days of treatment your child requires. Discard any unused medicine.

Phenylketonurics: Each 200 mg *Augmentin* chewable tablet contains 2.1 mg phenylalanine; each 400 mg chewable tablet contains 4.2 mg phenylalanine; each 5 mL of either the 200 mg/5 mL or 400 mg/5 mL oral suspension contains 7 mg phenylalanine. The other *Augmentin* products do not contain phenylalanine and can be used by phenylketonurics. Contact your physician or pharmacist.

Drug Interactions: Probenecid decreases the renal tubular secretion of amoxicillin. Concurrent use with *Augmentin* may result in increased and prolonged blood levels of amoxicillin. Co-administration of probenecid cannot be recommended.

The concurrent administration of allopurinol and ampicillin increases substantially the incidence of rashes in patients receiving both drugs as compared to patients receiving ampicillin alone. It is not known whether this potentiation of ampicillin rashes is due to allopurinol or the hyperuricemia present in these patients. There are no data with *Augmentin* and allopurinol administered concurrently.

In common with other broad-spectrum antibiotics, *Augmentin* may reduce the efficacy of oral contraceptives.

Drug/Laboratory Test Interactions: Oral administration of *Augmentin* will result in high urine concentrations of amoxicillin. High urine concentrations of ampicillin may result in false-positive reactions when testing for the presence of glucose in urine using Clinitest®, Benedict's Solution or Fehling's Solution. Since this effect may also occur with amoxicillin and therefore *Augmentin,* it is recommended that glucose tests based on enzymatic glucose oxidase reactions (such as Clinistix® or Tes-Tape®) be used.

Following administration of ampicillin to pregnant women a transient decrease in plasma concentration of total conjugated estriol, estriol-glucuronide, conjugated estrone and estradiol has been noted. This effect may also occur with amoxicillin and therefore *Augmentin.*

Carcinogenesis, Mutagenesis, Impairment of Fertility: Long-term studies in animals have not been performed to evaluate carcinogenic potential.

Mutagenesis: The mutagenic potential of *Augmentin* was investigated *in vitro* with an Ames test, a human lymphocyte cytogenetic assay, a yeast test and a mouse lymphoma forward mutation assay, and *in vivo* with mouse micronucleus tests and a dominant lethal test. All were negative apart from the *in vitro* mouse lymphoma assay where weak activity was found at very high, cytotoxic concentrations.

Impairment of Fertility: Augmentin at oral doses of up to 1200 mg/kg/day (5.7 times the maximum human dose, 1480 mg/m^2/day, based on body surface area) was found to have no effect on fertility and reproductive performance in rats, dosed with a 2:1 ratio formulation of amoxicillin:clavulanate.

Teratogenic effects. Pregnancy (Category B): Reproduction studies performed in pregnant rats and mice given *Augmentin* at oral dosages up to 1200 mg/kg/day, equivalent to 7200 and 4080 mg/m^2/day, respectively (4.9 and 2.8 times the maximum human oral dose based on body surface area), revealed no evidence of harm to the fetus due to *Augmentin.* There are, however, no adequate and well-controlled studies in pregnant women. Because animal reproduction studies are not always predictive of human response, this drug should be used during pregnancy only if clearly needed.

Labor and Delivery: Oral ampicillin class antibiotics are generally poorly absorbed during labor. Studies in guinea pigs have shown that intravenous administration of ampicillin decreased the uterine tone, frequency of contractions, height of contractions and duration of contractions. However, it is not known whether the use of *Augmentin* in humans during labor or delivery has immediate or delayed adverse effects on the fetus, prolongs the duration of labor, or increases the likelihood that forceps delivery or other obstetrical intervention or resuscitation of the newborn will be necessary.

Nursing Mothers: Ampicillin class antibiotics are excreted in the milk; therefore, caution should be exercised when *Augmentin* is administered to a nursing woman.

Pediatric Use: Because of incompletely developed renal function in neonates and young infants, the elimination of amoxicillin may be delayed. Dosing of *Augmentin* should be modified in pediatric patients younger than 12 weeks (3 months). (See DOSAGE AND ADMINISTRATION–Pediatric.)

ADVERSE REACTIONS

Augmentin is generally well tolerated. The majority of side effects observed in clinical trials were of a mild and transient nature and less than 3% of patients discontinued therapy because of drug-related side effects. From the original premarketing studies, where both pediatric and adult patients were enrolled, the most frequently reported adverse effects were diarrhea/loose stools (9%), nausea (3%), skin rashes and urticaria (3%), vomiting (1%) and vaginitis (1%). The overall incidence of side effects, and in particular diarrhea, increased with the higher recommended dose. Other less frequently reported reactions include: abdominal discomfort, flatulence and headache.

In pediatric patients (aged 2 months to 12 years), one U.S./Canadian clinical trial was conducted which compared *Augmentin* 45/6.4 mg/kg/day (divided q12h) for 10 days versus *Augmentin* 40/10 mg/kg/day (divided q8h) for 10 days in the treatment of acute otitis media. A total of 575 patients were enrolled, and only the suspension formulations were used in this trial. Overall, the adverse event profile seen was comparable to that noted above. However, there were differences in the rates of diarrhea, skin rashes/urticaria, and diaper area rashes. (See CLINICAL STUDIES.)

The following adverse reactions have been reported for ampicillin class antibiotics:

Gastrointestinal: Diarrhea, nausea, vomiting, indigestion, gastritis, stomatitis, glossitis, black "hairy" tongue, mucocutaneous candidiasis, enterocolitis, and hemorrhagic/pseudomembranous colitis. Onset of pseudomembranous colitis symptoms may occur during or after antibiotic treatment. (See WARNINGS.)

Hypersensitivity Reactions: Skin rashes, pruritus, urticaria, angioedema, serum sickness-like reactions (urticaria or skin rash accompanied by arthritis, arthralgia, myalgia and frequently fever), erythema multiforme (rarely Stevens-Johnson Syndrome) and an occasional case of exfoliative dermatitis (including toxic epidermal necrolysis) have been reported. These reactions may be controlled with antihistamines and, if necessary, systemic corticosteroids. Whenever such reactions occur, the drug should be discontinued, unless the opinion of the physician dictates otherwise. Serious and occasional fatal hypersensitivity (anaphylactic) reactions can occur with oral penicillin. (See WARNINGS.)

Liver: A moderate rise in AST (SGOT) and/or ALT (SGPT) has been noted in patients treated with ampicillin class antibiotics but the significance of these findings is unknown. Hepatic dysfunction, including increases in serum transaminases (AST and/or ALT), serum bilirubin and/or alkaline phosphatase, has been infrequently reported with *Augmentin.* It has been reported more commonly in the elderly, in males, or in patients on prolonged treatment. The histologic findings on liver biopsy have consisted of predominantly cholestatic, hepatocellular, or mixed cholestatic-hepatocellular changes. The onset of signs/symptoms of hepatic dysfunction may occur during or several weeks after therapy has been discontinued. The hepatic dysfunction, which may be severe, is usually reversible. On rare occasions, deaths have been reported (less than 1 death reported per estimated 4 million prescriptions worldwide). These have generally been cases associated with serious underlying diseases or concomitant medications.

Renal: Interstitial nephritis and hematuria have been reported rarely.

Hemic and Lymphatic Systems: Anemia, including hemolytic anemia, thrombocytopenia, thrombocytopenic purpura, eosinophilia, leukopenia and agranulocytosis have been reported during therapy with penicillins. These reactions are usually reversible on discontinuation of therapy and are believed to be hypersensitivity phenomena. A slight thrombocytosis was noted in less than 1% of the patients treated with *Augmentin.* There have been reports of increased prothrombin time in patients receiving *Augmentin* and anticoagulant therapy concomitantly.

Central Nervous System: Agitation, anxiety, behavioral changes, confusion, convulsions, dizziness, insomnia, and reversible hyperactivity have been reported rarely.

OVERDOSAGE

Most patients have been asymptomatic following overdosage or have experienced primarily gastrointestinal symptoms including stomach and abdominal pain, vomiting, and diarrhea. Rash, hyperactivity, or drowsiness have also been observed in a small number of patients.

In the case of overdosage, discontinue *Augmentin*, treat symptomatically, and institute supportive measures as required. If the overdosage is very recent and there is no contraindication, an attempt at emesis or other means of removal of drug from the stomach may be performed. A prospective study of 51 pediatric patients at a poison center suggested that overdosages of less than 250 mg/kg of amoxicillin are not associated with significant clinical symptoms and do not require gastric emptying.[3]

Interstitial nephritis resulting in oliguric renal failure has been reported in a small number of patients after overdosage with amoxicillin. Renal impairment appears to be reversible with cessation of drug administration. High blood levels may occur more readily in patients with impaired renal function because of decreased renal clearance of both amoxicillin and clavulanate. Both amoxicillin and clavulanate are removed from the circulation by hemodialysis.

DOSAGE AND ADMINISTRATION

Dosage:

Pediatric Patients: Based on the amoxicillin component, *Augmentin* should be dosed as follows:

Neonates and infants aged < 12 weeks (3 months)

Due to incompletely developed renal function affecting elimination of amoxicillin in this age group, the recommended dose of *Augmentin* is 30 mg/kg/day divided q12h, based on the amoxicillin component. Clavulanate elimination is unaltered in this age group. Experience with the 200 mg/5 mL formulation in this age group is limited and, thus, use of the 125 mg/5 mL oral suspension is recommended.

Patients aged 12 weeks (3 months) and older

INFECTIONS	DOSING REGIMEN	
	q12h‖	q8h
	200 mg/5 mL or 400 mg/5 mL oral suspension¶¶	125 mg/5 mL or 250 mg/5 mL oral suspension¶¶
Otitis media***, sinusitis, lower respiratory tract infections, and more severe infections	45 mg/kg/day q12h	40 mg/kg/day q8h
Less severe infections	25 mg/kg/day q12h	20 mg/kg/day q8h

‖ The q12h regimen is recommended as it is associated with significantly less diarrhea. (See CLINICAL STUDIES.) However, the q12h formulations (200 mg and 400 mg) contain aspartame and should not be used by phenylketonurics.

¶¶ Each strength of *Augmentin* suspension is available as a chewable tablet for use by older children.

*** Duration of therapy studied and recommended for acute otitis media is 10 days.

Pediatric patients weighing 40 kg and more should be dosed according to the following adult recommendations: The usual adult dose is 1 *Augmentin* 500 mg tablet every 12 hours or 1 *Augmentin* 250 mg tablet every 8 hours. For more severe infections and infections of the respiratory tract, the dose should be 1 *Augmentin* 875 mg tablet every 12 hours or 1 *Augmentin* 500 mg tablet every 8 hours. Among adults treated with 875 mg every 12 hours, significantly fewer experienced severe diarrhea or withdrawals with diarrhea vs. adults treated with 500 mg every 8 hours. For detailed adult dosage recommendations, please see complete prescribing information for *Augmentin* Tablets.

Hepatically impaired patients should be dosed with caution and hepatic function monitored at regular intervals. (See WARNINGS.)

Adults: Adults who have difficulty swallowing may be given the 125 mg/5 mL or 250 mg/5 mL suspension in place of the 500 mg tablet. The 200 mg/5 mL suspension or the 400 mg/5 mL suspension may be used in place of the 875 mg tablet. See dosage recommendations above for children weighing 40 kg or more.

The *Augmentin* 250 mg tablet and the 250 mg chewable tablet do *not* contain the same amount of clavulanic acid (as the potassium salt). The *Augmentin* 250 mg tablet contains 125 mg of clavulanic acid, whereas the 250 mg chewable tablet contains 62.5 mg of clavulanic acid. Therefore, the *Augmentin* 250 mg tablet and the 250 mg chewable tablet should *not* be substituted for each other, as they are not interchangeable.

Due to the different amoxicillin to clavulanic acid ratios in the *Augmentin* 250 mg tablet (250/125) versus the *Augmentin* 250 mg chewable tablet (250/62.5), the *Augmentin* 250 mg tablet should not be used until the child weighs at least 40 kg and more.

DIRECTIONS FOR MIXING ORAL SUSPENSION

Prepare a suspension at time of dispensing as follows: Tap bottle until all the powder flows freely. Add approximately $^2/_3$ of the total amount of water for reconstitution (see table below) and shake vigorously to suspend powder. Add remainder of the water and again shake vigorously.

***Augmentin* 125 mg/5 mL Suspension**

Bottle Size	Amount of Water Required for Reconstitution
75 mL	67 mL
100 mL	90 mL
150 mL	134 mL

Each teaspoonful (5 mL) will contain 125 mg amoxicillin and 31.25 mg of clavulanic acid as the potassium salt.

***Augmentin* 200 mg/5 mL Suspension**

Bottle Size	Amount of Water Required for Suspension
50 mL	47 mL
75 mL	69 mL
100 mL	91 mL

Each teaspoonful (5 mL) will contain 200 mg amoxicillin and 28.5 mg of clavulanic acid as the potassium salt.

***Augmentin* 250 mg/5 mL Suspension**

Bottle Size	Amount of Water Required for Reconstitution
75 mL	65 mL
100 mL	87 mL
150 mL	130 mL

Each teaspoonful (5 mL) will contain 250 mg amoxicillin and 62.5 mg of clavulanic acid as the potassium salt.

***Augmentin* 400 mg/5 mL Suspension**

Bottle Size	Amount of Water Required for Suspension
50 mL	44 mL
75 mL	66 mL
100 mL	87 mL

Each teaspoonful (5 mL) will contain 400 mg amoxicillin and 57.0 mg of clavulanic acid as the potassium salt.

Note: SHAKE ORAL SUSPENSION WELL BEFORE USING.

Reconstituted suspension must be stored under refrigeration and discarded after 10 days.

Administration: *Augmentin* may be taken without regard to meals; however, absorption of clavulanate potassium is enhanced when *Augmentin* is administered at the start of a meal. To minimize the potential for gastrointestinal intolerance, *Augmentin* should be taken at the start of a meal.

HOW SUPPLIED

***AUGMENTIN* 125 MG/5 ML FOR ORAL SUSPENSION:** Each 5 mL of reconstituted banana-flavored suspension contains 125 mg amoxicillin and 31.25 mg clavulanic acid as the potassium salt.

NDC 0029-6085-39 .... 75 mL bottle
NDC 0029-6085-23 .... 100 mL bottle
NDC 0029-6085-22 .... 150 mL bottle

***AUGMENTIN* 200 MG/5 ML FOR ORAL SUSPENSION:** Each 5 mL of reconstituted orange-raspberry-flavored suspension contains 200 mg amoxicillin and 28.5 mg clavulanic acid as the potassium salt.

NDC 0029-6087-29 .... 50 mL bottle
NDC 0029-6087-39 .... 75 mL bottle
NDC 0029-6087-51 .... 100 mL bottle

***AUGMENTIN* 250 MG/5 ML FOR ORAL SUSPENSION:** Each 5 mL of reconstituted orange-flavored suspension contains 250 mg amoxicillin and 62.5 mg clavulanic acid as the potassium salt.

NDC 0029-6090-39 .... 75 mL bottle
NDC 0029-6090-23 .... 100 mL bottle
NDC 0029-6090-22 .... 150 mL bottle

***AUGMENTIN* 400 MG/5 ML FOR ORAL SUSPENSION:** Each 5 mL of reconstituted orange-raspberry-flavored suspension contains 400 mg amoxicillin and 57 mg clavulanic acid as the potassium salt.

NDC 0029-6092-29 .... 50 mL bottle
NDC 0029-6092-39 .... 75 mL bottle
NDC 0029-6092-51 .... 100 mL bottle

***AUGMENTIN* 125 MG CHEWABLE TABLETS:** Each mottled yellow, round, lemon-lime-flavored tablet, debossed with BMP 189, contains 125 mg amoxicillin as the trihydrate and 31.25 mg clavulanic acid as the potassium salt.

NDC 0029-6073-47 .... carton of 30 tablets

***AUGMENTIN* 200 MG CHEWABLE TABLETS:** Each mottled pink, round, biconvex, cherry-banana-flavored tablet contains 200 mg amoxicillin as the trihydrate and 28.5 mg clavulanic acid as the potassium salt.

NDC 0029-6071-12 .... carton of 20 tablets

***AUGMENTIN* 250 MG CHEWABLE TABLETS:** Each mottled yellow, round, lemon-lime-flavored tablet, debossed with BMP 190, contains 250 mg amoxicillin as the trihydrate and 62.5 mg clavulanic acid as the potassium salt.

NDC 0029-6074-47 .... carton of 30 tablets

***AUGMENTIN* 400 MG CHEWABLE TABLETS:** Each mottled pink, round, biconvex, cherry-banana-flavored tablet contains 400 mg amoxicillin as the trihydrate and 57.0 mg clavulanic acid as the potassium salt.

NDC 0029-6072-12 .... carton of 20 tablets

***AUGMENTIN* is also supplied as:**

***AUGMENTIN* 250 MG TABLETS** (250 mg amoxicillin/125 mg clavulanic acid):

NDC 0029-6075-27 .... bottles of 30
NDC 0029-6075-31 .... 100 Unit Dose tablets

***AUGMENTIN* 500 MG TABLETS** (500 mg amoxicillin/125 mg clavulanic acid):

NDC 0029-6080-12 .... bottles of 20
NDC 0029-6080-31 .... 100 Unit Dose tablets

***AUGMENTIN* 875 MG TABLETS** (875 mg amoxicillin/125 mg clavulanic acid):

NDC 0029-6086-12 .... bottles of 20
NDC 0029-6086-21 .... 100 Unit Dose tablets

Store tablets and dry powder at or below 25°C (77°F). Dispense in tightly closed, moisture-proof containers. Store reconstituted suspension under refrigeration. Discard unused suspension after 10 days.

CLINICAL STUDIES

In pediatric patients (aged 2 months to 12 years), one U.S./Canadian clinical trial was conducted which compared *Augmentin* 45/6.4 mg/kg/day (divided q12h) for 10 days versus *Augmentin* 40/10 mg/kg/day (divided q8h) for 10 days in the treatment of acute otitis media. Only the suspension formulations were used in this trial. A total of 575 patients were enrolled, with an even distribution among the two treatment groups and a comparable number of patients were evaluable (i.e., ≥84%) per treatment group. Strict otitis media-specific criteria were required for eligibility and a strong correlation was found at the end of therapy and follow-up between these criteria and physician assessment of clinical response. The clinical efficacy rates at the end of therapy visit (defined as 2–4 days after the completion of therapy) and at the follow-up visit (defined as 22–28 days post-completion of therapy) were comparable for the two treatment groups, with the following cure rates obtained for the evaluable patients: At end of therapy, 87.2% (n=265) and 82.3% (n=260) for 45 mg/kg/day q12h and 40 mg/kg/day q8h, respectively. At follow-up, 67.1% (n=249) and 68.7% (n=243) for 45 mg/kg/day q12h and 40 mg/kg/day q8h, respectively. The incidence of diarrhea††† was significantly lower in patients in the q12h treatment group compared to patients who received the q8h regimen (14.3% and 34.3%, respectively). In addition, the number of patients with either severe diarrhea or who were withdrawn with diarrhea was significantly lower in the q12h treatment group (3.1% and 7.6% for the q12h/10 day and q8h/10 day, respectively). In the q12h treatment group, 3 patients (1.0%) were withdrawn with an allergic reaction, while 1 patient (0.3%) in the q8h group was withdrawn for this reason. The number of patients with a candidal infection of the diaper area was 3.8% and 6.2% for the q12h and q8h groups, respectively.

It is not known if the finding of a statistically significant reduction in diarrhea with the oral suspensions dosed q12h, versus suspensions dosed q8h, can be extrapolated to the chewable tablets. The presence of mannitol in the chewable tablets may contribute to a different diarrhea profile. The q12h oral suspensions are sweetened with aspartame only.

††† Diarrhea was defined as either: (a) three or more watery or four or more loose/watery stools in one day; OR (b) two watery stools per day or three loose/watery stools per day for two consecutive days.

REFERENCES

1. National Committee for Clinical Laboratory Standards. Methods for Dilution Antimicrobial Susceptibility Tests for Bacteria That Grow Aerobically — Third Edition. Approved Standard NCCLS Document M7-A3, Vol. 13, No. 25. NCCLS, Villanova, PA, Dec. 1993.
2. National Committee for Clinical Laboratory Standards. Performance Standard for Antimicrobial Disk Susceptibility Tests — Fifth Edition. Approved Standard NCCLS Document M2-A5, Vol. 13, No. 24. NCCLS, Villanova, PA, Dec. 1993.
3. Swanson-Biearman B, Dean BS, Lopez G, Krenzelok EP. The effects of penicillin and cephalosporin ingestions in children less than six years of age. *Vet Hum Toxicol* 1988; 30:66–67.

Veterans Administration/Military/PHS—Chewable Tablets, 125 mg, 30's, 6505-01-282-6332; 250 mg, 30's, 6505-01-264-2366; Tablets, 250 mg, 30's, 6505-01-203-6259; 250 mg, 100's SUP, 6505-01-339-6919; 500 mg, 20's 6505-01-431-0403; 500 mg, 100's SUP, 6505-01-303-8962; 875 mg, 20's, 6505-01-430-9740; 875 mg, 100's SUP, 6505-01-431-0402; Oral Suspension, 125 mg/5 mL, 75 mL, 6505-01-340-0847; 125 mg/5 mL, 100 mL, 6505-01-408-8181; 125 mg/5 mL, 150 mL, 6505-01-204-5388; 250 mg/5 mL, 75 mL, 6505-01-207-8205; 250 mg/5 mL, 100 mL, 6505-01-408-8352; 250 mg/5 mL, 150 mL, 6505-01-207-0795.

AG:PL5A

Shown in Product Identification Guide, page 338

AUGMENTIN® ℞

[og' men-tin]

amoxicillin/clavulanate potassium
Tablets

DESCRIPTION

Augmentin is an oral antibacterial combination consisting of the semisynthetic antibiotic amoxicillin and the β-lactamase inhibitor, clavulanate potassium (the potassium salt of clavulanic acid). Amoxicillin is an analog of ampicillin, derived from the basic penicillin nucleus, 6-aminopenicillanic acid. The amoxicillin molecular formula is $C_{16}H_{19}N_3O_5S \cdot 3H_2O$ and the molecular weight is 419.46. Chemically, amoxicillin is (2*S*,5*R*,6*R*)-6-[(*R*)-(-)-2-Amino-2-(*p*-hydroxyphenyl)acetamido] -3,3- dimethyl -7-oxo-4-thia -1- azabicyclo[3.2.0]heptane-2-carboxylic acid trihydrate and may be represented structurally as:

[See chemical structure at top of next column]

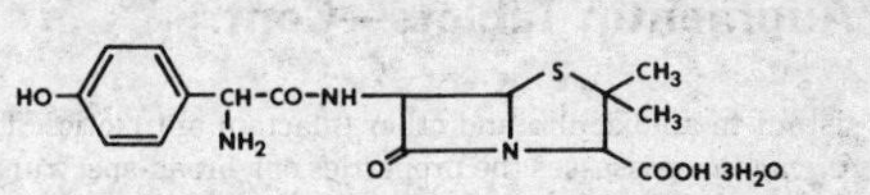

Clavulanic acid is produced by the fermentation of *Streptomyces clavuligerus*. It is a β-lactam structurally related to the penicillins and possesses the ability to inactivate a wide variety of β-lactamases by blocking the active sites of these enzymes. Clavulanic acid is particularly active against the clinically important plasmid mediated β-lactamases frequently responsible for transferred drug resistance to penicillins and cephalosporins. The clavulanate potassium molecular formula is $C_8H_8KNO_5$ and the molecular weight is 237.25. Chemically clavulanate potassium is potassium (*Z*)-(2*R*, 5*R*)-3-(2-hydroxyethylidene)-7-oxo-4-oxa-1-azabicyclo[3.2.0]-heptane-2-carboxylate, and may be represented structurally as:

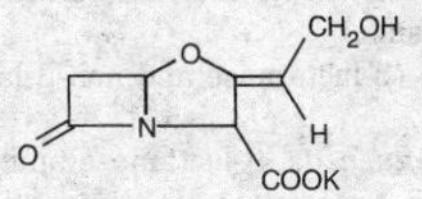

Inactive Ingredients: Colloidal silicon dioxide, hydroxypropyl methylcellulose, magnesium stearate, microcrystalline cellulose, polyethylene glycol, sodium starch glycolate and titanium dioxide.

Each *Augmentin* tablet contains 0.63 mEq potassium.

CLINICAL PHARMACOLOGY

Amoxicillin and clavulanate potassium are well absorbed from the gastrointestinal tract after oral administration of *Augmentin*. Dosing in the fasted or fed state has minimal effect on the pharmacokinetics of amoxicillin. While *Augmentin* can be given without regard to meals, absorption of clavulanate potassium when taken with food is greater relative to the fasted state. In one study, the relative bioavailability of clavulanate was reduced when *Augmentin* was dosed at 30 and 150 minutes after the start of a high fat breakfast. The safety and efficacy of *Augmentin* have been established in clinical trials where *Augmentin* was taken without regard to meals.

Mean* amoxicillin and clavulanate potassium pharmacokinetic parameters are shown in the table below:

[See table at top of next page]

Amoxicillin serum concentrations achieved with *Augmentin* are similar to those produced by the oral administration of equivalent doses of amoxicillin alone. The half-life of amoxicillin after the oral administration of *Augmentin* is 1.3 hours and that of clavulanic acid is 1.0 hour.

Approximately 50% to 70% of the amoxicillin and approximately 25% to 40% of the clavulanic acid are excreted unchanged in urine during the first 6 hours after administration of a single *Augmentin* 250 mg or 500 mg tablet.

Concurrent administration of probenecid delays amoxicillin excretion but does not delay renal excretion of clavulanic acid.

Neither component in *Augmentin* is highly protein-bound; clavulanic acid has been found to be approximately 25% bound to human serum and amoxicillin approximately 18% bound.

Amoxicillin diffuses readily into most body tissues and fluids with the exception of the brain and spinal fluid. The results of experiments involving the administration of clavulanic acid to animals suggest that this compound, like amoxicillin, is well distributed in body tissues.

Microbiology: Amoxicillin is a semisynthetic antibiotic with a broad spectrum of bactericidal activity against many gram-positive and gram-negative microorganisms. Amoxicillin is, however, susceptible to degradation by β-lactamases and, therefore, the spectrum of activity does not include organisms which produce these enzymes. Clavulanic acid is a β-lactam, structurally related to the penicillins, which possesses the ability to inactivate a wide range of β-lactamase enzymes commonly found in microorganisms resistant to penicillins and cephalosporins. In particular, it has good activity against the clinically important plasmid mediated β-lactamases frequently responsible for transferred drug resistance.

The formulation of amoxicillin and clavulanic acid in *Augmentin* protects amoxicillin from degradation by β-lactamase enzymes and effectively extends the antibiotic spectrum of amoxicillin to include many bacteria normally re-

Continued on next page

Information on the SmithKline Beecham Pharmaceuticals products appearing here is based on the labeling in effect on July 31, 1998. Further information on these and other products may be obtained from the Medical Department, SmithKline Beecham Pharmaceuticals, One Franklin Plaza, Philadelphia, PA 19101.

Augmentin Tablets—Cont.

sistant to amoxicillin and other β-lactam antibiotics. Thus, *Augmentin* possesses the properties of a broad-spectrum antibiotic and a β-lactamase inhibitor.

Amoxicillin/clavulanic acid has been shown to be active against most strains of the following microorganisms, both *in vitro* and in clinical infections as described in the INDICATIONS AND USAGE section.

GRAM-POSITIVE AEROBES

Staphylococcus aureus (β-lactamase and non-β-lactamase producing)[‡]

‡Staphylococci which are resistant to methicillin/oxacillin must be considered resistant to amoxicillin/clavulanic acid.

GRAM-NEGATIVE AEROBES

Enterobacter species (Although most strains of *Enterobacter* species are resistant *in vitro*, clinical efficacy has been demonstrated with *Augmentin* in urinary tract infections caused by these organisms.)

Escherichia coli (β-lactamase and non-β-lactamase producing)

Haemophilus influenzae (β-lactamase and non-β-lactamase producing)

Klebsiella species (All known strains are β-lactamase producing.)

Moraxella catarrhalis (β-lactamase and non-β-lactamase producing)

The following *in vitro* data are available, **but their clinical significance is unknown.**

Amoxicillin/clavulanic acid exhibits *in vitro* minimal inhibitory concentrations (MICs) of 0.5 µg/mL or less against most (≥90%) strains of *Streptococcus pneumoniae*§; MICs of 0.06 µg/mL or less against most (≥90%) strains of *Neisseria gonorrhoeae*; MICs of 4 µg/mL or less against most (≥90%) strains of staphylococci and anaerobic bacteria; and MICs of 8 µg/mL or less against most (≥90%) strains of other listed organisms. However, with the exception of organisms shown to respond to amoxicillin alone, the safety and effectiveness of amoxicillin/clavulanic acid in treating clinical infections due to these microorganisms have not been established in adequate and well-controlled clinical trials.

§ Because amoxicillin has greater *in vitro* activity against *Streptococcus pneumoniae* than does ampicillin or penicillin, the majority of *S. pneumoniae* strains with intermediate susceptibility to amipicillin or penicillin are fully susceptible to amoxicillin.

GRAM-POSITIVE AEROBES

Enterococcus faecalis[‖]

Staphylococcus epidermidis (β-lactamase and non-β-lactamase producing)

Staphylococcus saprophyticus (β-lactamase and non-β-lactamase producing)

Streptococcus pneumoniae[‖ ¶]

Streptococcus pyogenes[‖ ¶]

viridans group *Streptococcus*[‖ ¶]

GRAM-NEGATIVE AEROBES

Eikenella corrodens (β-lactamase and non-β-lactamase producing)

Neisseria gonorrhoeae[‖] (β-lactamase and non-β-lactamase producing)

Proteus mirabilis[‖] (β-lactamase and non-β-lactamase producing)

ANAEROBIC BACTERIA

Bacteroides species, including *Bacteroides fragilis* (β-lactamase and non-β-lactamase producing)

Fusobacterium species (β-lactamase and non-β-lactamase producing)

Peptostreptococcus species¶

‖Adequate and well-controlled clinical trials have established the effectiveness of amoxicillin alone in treating certain clinical infections due to these organisms.

¶These are non-β-lactamase-producing organisms and, therefore, are susceptible to amoxicillin alone.

SUSCEPTIBILITY TESTING

Dilution Techniques: Quantitative methods are used to determine antimicrobial minimal inhibitory concentrations (MICs). These MICs provide estimates of the susceptibility of bacteria to antimicrobial compounds. The MICs should be determined using a standardized procedure. Standardized procedures are based on a dilution method[1] (broth or agar) or equivalent with standardized inoculum concentrations and standardized concentrations of amoxicillin/clavulanate potassium powder.

The recommended dilution pattern utilizes a constant amoxicillin/clavulanate potassium ratio of 2 to 1 in all tubes with varying amounts of amoxicillin. MICs are expressed in terms of the amoxicillin concentration in the presence of clavulanic acid at a constant 2 parts amoxicillin to 1 part clavulanic acid. The MIC values should be interpreted according to the following criteria:

Dose† and regimen amoxicillin/ clavulanate potassium	AUC$_{0-24}$ (µg.hr/mL) amoxicillin (±S.D.)	AUC$_{0-24}$ (µg.hr/mL) clavulanate potassium (±S.D.)	C$_{max}$ (µg/mL) amoxicillin (±S.D.)	C$_{max}$ (µg/mL) clavulanate potassium (±S.D.)
250/125 mg q8h	26.7 ± 4.56	12.6 ± 3.25	3.3 ± 1.12	1.5 ± 0.70
500/125 mg q12h	33.4 ± 6.76	8.6 ± 1.95	6.5 ± 1.41	1.8 ± 0.61
500/125 mg q8h	53.4 ± 8.87	15.7 ± 3.86	7.2 ± 2.26	2.4 ± 0.83
875/125 mg q12h	53.5 ± 12.31	10.2 ± 3.04	11.6 ± 2.78	2.2 ± 0.99

* Mean values of 14 normal volunteers (n=15 for clavulanate potassium in the low-dose regimens). Peak concentrations occurred approximately 1.5 hours after the dose.

† Administered at the start of a light meal.

RECOMMENDED RANGES FOR AMOXICILLIN/CLAVULANIC ACID SUSCEPTIBILITY TESTING

For gram-negative enteric aerobes:

MIC (µg/mL)	Interpretation
≤8/4	Susceptible (S)
16/8	Intermediate (I)
≥32/16	Resistant (R)

For *Staphylococcus*** and *Haemophilus* species:

MIC (µg/mL)	Interpretation
≤4/2	Susceptible (S)
≥8/4	Resistant (R)

** Staphylococci which are susceptible to amoxicillin/clavulanic acid but resistant to methicillin/oxacillin must be considered as resistant.

For *Streptococcus pneumoniae*: Isolates should be tested using amoxicillin/clavulanic acid and the following criteria should be used:

MIC (µg/mL)	Interpretation
≤0.5/0.25	Susceptible (S)
1/0.5	Intermediate (I)
≥2/1	Resistant (R)

A report of "Susceptible" indicates that the pathogen is likely to be inhibited if the antimicrobial compound in the blood reaches the concentration usually achievable. A report of "Intermediate" indicates that the result should be considered equivocal, and, if the microorganism is not fully susceptible to alternative, clinically feasible drugs, the test should be repeated. This category implies possible clinical applicability in body sites where the drug is physiologically concentrated or in situations where high dosage of drug can be used. This category also provides a buffer zone which prevents small uncontrolled technical factors from causing major discrepancies in interpretation. A report of "Resistant" indicates that the pathogen is not likely to be inhibited if the antimicrobial compound in the blood reaches the concentrations usually achievable; other therapy should be selected.

Standardized susceptibility test procedures require the use of laboratory control microorganisms to control the technical aspects of the laboratory procedures. Standard amoxicillin/clavulanate potassium powder should provide the following MIC values:

Microorganism	MIC Range (µg/mL) ††
Escherichia coli ATCC 25922	2 to 8
Escherichia coli ATCC 35218	4 to 16
Enterococcus faecalis ATCC 29212	0.25 to 1.0
Haemophilus influenzae ATCC 49247	2 to 16
Staphylococcus aureus ATCC 29213	0.12 to 0.5
Streptococcus pneumoniae ATCC 49619	0.03 to 0.12

†† Expressed as concentration of amoxicillin in the presence of clavulanic acid at a constant 2 parts amoxicillin to 1 part clavulanic acid.

Diffusion Techniques: Quantitative methods that require measurement of zone diameters also provide reproducible estimates of the susceptibility of bacteria to antimicrobial compounds. One such standardized procedure[2] requires the use of standardized inoculum concentrations. This procedure uses paper disks impregnated with 30 µg of amoxicillin/clavulanate potassium (20 µg amoxicillin plus 10 µg clavulanate potassium) to test the susceptibility of microorganisms to amoxicillin/clavulanic acid.

Reports from the laboratory providing results of the standard single-disk susceptibility test with a 30 µg amoxicillin/clavulanate acid (20 µg amoxicillin plus 10 µg clavulanate potassium) disk should be interpreted according to the following criteria:

RECOMMENDED RANGES FOR AMOXICILLIN/CLAVULANIC ACID SUSCEPTIBILITY TESTING

For *Staphylococcus*‡‡ species and *H. influenzae*[a]:

Zone Diameter (mm)	Interpretation
≥20	Susceptible (S)
≤19	Resistant (R)

For other organisms except *S. pneumoniae*[b] and *N. gonorrhoeae*[c]:

Zone Diameter (mm)	Interpretation
≥18	Susceptible (S)
14 to 17	Intermediate (I)
≤13	Resistant (R)

‡‡ Staphylococci which are resistant to methicillin/oxacillin must be considered as resistant to amoxicillin/clavulanic acid.

[a] A broth microdilution method should be used for testing *H. influenzae*. Beta-lactamase negative, ampicillin-resistant strains must be considered resistant to amoxicillin/clavulanic acid.

[b] Susceptibility of *S. pneumoniae* should be determined using a 1 µg oxacillin disk. Isolates with oxacillin zone sizes of ≥20 mm are susceptible to amoxicillin/clavulanic acid. An amoxicillin/clavulanic acid MIC should be determined on isolates of *S. pneumoniae* with oxacillin zone sizes of ≤19 mm.

[c] A broth microdilution method should be used for testing *N. gonorrhoeae* and interpreted according to penicillin breakpoints.

Interpretation should be as stated above for results using dilution techniques. Interpretation involves correlation of the diameter obtained in the disk test with the MIC for amoxicillin/clavulanic acid.

As with standardized dilution techniques, diffusion methods require the use of laboratory control microorganisms that are used to control the technical aspects of the laboratory procedures. For the diffusion technique, the 30 µg amoxicillin/clavulanate potassium (20 µg amoxicillin plus 10 µg clavulanate potassium) disk should provide the following zone diameters in these laboratory quality control strains:

Microorganism	Zone Diameter (mm)
Escherichia coli ATCC 25922	19 to 25
Escherichia coli ATCC 35218	18 to 22
Staphylococcus aureus ATCC 25923	28 to 36

INDICATIONS AND USAGE

Augmentin is indicated in the treatment of infections caused by susceptible strains of the designated organisms in the conditions listed below:

Lower Respiratory Tract Infections—caused by β-lactamase-producing strains of *Haemophilus influenzae* and *Moraxella (Branhamella) catarrhalis.*

Otitis Media—caused by β-lactamase-producing strains of *Haemophilus influenzae* and *Moraxella (Branhamella) catarrhalis.*

Sinusitis—caused by β-lactamase-producing strains of *Haemophilus influenzae* and *Moraxella (Branhamella) catarrhalis.*

Skin and Skin Structure Infections—caused by β-lactamase-producing strains of *Staphylococcus aureus, Escherichia coli* and *Klebsiella* spp.

Urinary Tract Infections—caused by β-lactamase-producing strains of *Escherichia coli, Klebsiella* spp. and *Enterobacter* spp.

While *Augmentin* is indicated only for the conditions listed above, infections caused by ampicillin-susceptible organisms are also amenable to *Augmentin* treatment due to its amoxicillin content. Therefore, mixed infections caused by ampicillin-susceptible organisms and β-lactamase-producing organisms susceptible to *Augmentin* should not require the addition of another antibiotic. Because amoxicillin has greater *in vitro* activity against *Streptococcus pneumoniae* than does ampicillin or penicillin, the majority of *S. pneumoniae* strains with intermediate susceptibility to ampicillin or penicillin are fully susceptible to amoxicillin and *Augmentin.* (See Microbiology subsection.)

Bacteriological studies, to determine the causative organisms and their susceptibility to *Augmentin,* should be performed together with any indicated surgical procedures.

Therapy may be instituted prior to obtaining the results from bacteriological and susceptibility studies to determine the causative organisms and their susceptibility to *Augmentin* when there is reason to believe the infection may involve any of the β-lactamase-producing organisms listed above. Once the results are known, therapy should be adjusted, if appropriate.

CONTRAINDICATIONS

Augmentin is contraindicated in patients with a history of allergic reactions to any penicillin. It is also contraindicated in patients with a previous history of *Augmentin*-associated cholestatic jaundice/hepatic dysfunction.

WARNINGS

SERIOUS AND OCCASIONALLY FATAL HYPERSENSITIVITY (ANAPHYLACTIC) REACTIONS HAVE BEEN REPORTED IN PATIENTS ON PENICILLIN THERAPY. THESE REACTIONS ARE MORE LIKELY TO OCCUR IN INDIVIDUALS WITH A HISTORY OF PENICILLIN HYPERSENSITIVITY AND/OR A HISTORY OF SENSITIVITY TO MULTIPLE ALLERGENS. THERE HAVE BEEN REPORTS OF INDIVIDUALS WITH A HISTORY OF PENICILLIN HYPERSENSITIVITY WHO HAVE EXPERIENCED SEVERE REACTIONS WHEN TREATED WITH CEPHALOSPORINS. BEFORE INITIATING THERAPY WITH *AUGMENTIN*, CAREFUL INQUIRY SHOULD BE MADE CONCERNING PREVIOUS HYPERSENSITIVITY REACTIONS TO PENICILLINS, CEPHALOSPORINS OR OTHER ALLERGENS. IF AN ALLERGIC REACTION OCCURS, *AUGMENTIN* SHOULD BE DISCONTINUED AND THE APPROPRIATE THERAPY INSTITUTED. **SERIOUS ANAPHYLACTIC REACTIONS REQUIRE IMMEDIATE EMERGENCY TREATMENT WITH EPINEPHRINE. OXYGEN, INTRAVENOUS STEROIDS AND AIRWAY MANAGEMENT, INCLUDING INTUBATION, SHOULD ALSO BE ADMINISTERED AS INDICATED.**

Pseudomembranous colitis has been reported with nearly all antibacterial agents, including *Augmentin*, and has ranged in severity from mild to life-threatening. Therefore, it is important to consider this diagnosis in patients who present with diarrhea subsequent to the administration of antibacterial agents.

Treatment with antibacterial agents alters the normal flora of the colon and may permit overgrowth of clostridia. Studies indicate that a toxin produced by *Clostridium difficile* is one primary cause of "antibiotic associated colitis."

After the diagnosis of pseudomembranous colitis has been established, appropriate therapeutic measures should be initiated. Mild cases of pseudomembranous colitis usually respond to drug discontinuation alone. In moderate to severe cases, consideration should be given to management with fluids and electrolytes, protein supplementation and treatment with an antibacterial drug clinically effective against *Clostridium difficile* colitis.

Augmentin should be used with caution in patients with evidence of hepatic dysfunction. Hepatic toxicity associated with the use of *Augmentin* is usually reversible. On rare occasions, deaths have been reported (less than 1 death reported per estimated 4 million prescriptions worldwide). These have generally been cases associated with serious underlying diseases or concomitant medications. (See CONTRAINDICATIONS and ADVERSE REACTIONS—*Liver*.)

PRECAUTIONS

General: While *Augmentin* possesses the characteristic low toxicity of the penicillin group of antibiotics, periodic assessment of organ system functions, including renal, hepatic and hematopoietic function, is advisable during prolonged therapy.

A high percentage of patients with mononucleosis who receive ampicillin develop an erythematous skin rash. Thus, ampicillin class antibiotics should not be administered to patients with mononucleosis.

The possibility of superinfections with mycotic or bacterial pathogens should be kept in mind during therapy. If superinfections occur (usually involving *Pseudomonas* or *Candida*), the drug should be discontinued and/or appropriate therapy instituted.

Drug Interactions: Probenecid decreases the renal tubular secretion of amoxicillin. Concurrent use with *Augmentin* may result in increased and prolonged blood levels of amoxicillin. Co-administration of probenecid cannot be recommended.

The concurrent administration of allopurinol and ampicillin increases substantially the incidence of rashes in patients receiving both drugs as compared to patients receiving ampicillin alone. It is not known whether this potentiation of ampicillin rashes is due to allopurinol or the hyperuricemia present in these patients. There are no data with *Augmentin* and allopurinol administered concurrently.

In common with other broad-spectrum antibiotics, *Augmentin* may reduce the efficacy of oral contraceptives.

Drug/Laboratory Test Interactions: Oral administration of *Augmentin* will result in high urine concentrations of amoxicillin. High urine concentrations of ampicillin may result in false-positive reactions when testing for the presence of glucose in urine using Clinitest®, Benedict's Solution or Fehling's Solution. Since this effect may also occur with amoxicillin and therefore *Augmentin*, it is recommended that glucose tests based on enzymatic glucose oxidase reactions (such as Clinistix® or Tes-Tape®) be used.

Following administration of ampicillin to pregnant women a transient decrease in plasma concentration of total conjugated estriol, estriol-glucuronide, conjugated estrone and estradiol has been noted. This effect may also occur with amoxicillin and therefore *Augmentin*.

Carcinogenesis, Mutagenesis, Impairment of Fertility: Long-term studies in animals have not been performed to evaluate carcinogenic potential.

Mutagenesis: The mutagenic potential of *Augmentin* was investigated *in vitro* with an Ames test, a human lymphocyte cytogenetic assay, a yeast test and a mouse lymphoma forward mutation assay, and *in vivo* with mouse micronucleus tests and a dominant lethal test. All were negative apart from the *in vitro* mouse lymphoma assay where weak activity was found at very high, cytotoxic concentrations.

Impairment of Fertility: *Augmentin* at oral doses of up to 1200 mg/kg/day (5.7 times the maximum human dose, 1480 mg/m^2/day, based on body surface area) was found to have no effect on fertility and reproductive performance in rats, dosed with a 2:1 ratio formulation of amoxicillin:clavulanate.

Teratogenic effects. Pregnancy (Category B): Reproduction studies performed in pregnant rats and mice given *Augmentin* at oral dosages up to 1200 mg/kg/day, equivalent to 7200 and 4080 mg/m^2/day, respectively (4.9 and 2.8 times the maximum human oral dose based on body surface area), revealed no evidence of harm to the fetus due to *Augmentin*. There are, however, no adequate and well-controlled studies in pregnant women. Because animal reproduction studies are not always predictive of human response, this drug should be used during pregnancy only if clearly needed.

Labor and Delivery: Oral ampicillin class antibiotics are generally poorly absorbed during labor. Studies in guinea pigs have shown that intravenous administration of ampicillin decreased the uterine tone, frequency of contractions, height of contractions and duration of contractions. However, it is not known whether the use of *Augmentin* in humans during labor or delivery has immediate or delayed adverse effects on the fetus, prolongs the duration of labor, or increases the likelihood that forceps delivery or other obstetrical intervention or resuscitation of the newborn will be necessary.

Nursing Mothers: Ampicillin class antibiotics are excreted in the milk; therefore, caution should be exercised when *Augmentin* is administered to a nursing woman.

ADVERSE REACTIONS

Augmentin is generally well tolerated. The majority of side effects observed in clinical trials were of a mild and transient nature and less than 3% of patients discontinued therapy because of drug-related side effects. The most frequently reported adverse effects were diarrhea/loose stools (9%), nausea (3%), skin rashes and urticaria (3%), vomiting (1%) and vaginitis (1%). The overall incidence of side effects, and in particular diarrhea, increased with the higher recommended dose. Other less frequently reported reactions include: abdominal discomfort, flatulence and headache.

The following adverse reactions have been reported for ampicillin class antibiotics:

Gastrointestinal: Diarrhea, nausea, vomiting, indigestion, gastritis, stomatitis, glossitis, black "hairy" tongue, mucocutaneous candidiasis, enterocolitis, and hemorrhagic/pseudomembranous colitis. Onset of pseudomembranous colitis symptoms may occur during or after antibiotic treatment. (See WARNINGS.)

Hypersensitivity Reactions: Skin rashes, pruritus, urticaria, angioedema, serum sickness-like reactions (urticaria or skin rash accompanied by arthritis, arthralgia, myalgia and frequently fever), erythema multiforme (rarely Stevens-Johnson Syndrome) and an occasional case of exfoliative dermatitis (including toxic epidermal necrolysis) have been reported. These reactions may be controlled with antihistamines and, if necessary, systemic corticosteroids. Whenever such reactions occur, the drug should be discontinued, unless the opinion of the physician dictates otherwise. Serious and occasional fatal hypersensitivity (anaphylactic) reactions can occur with oral penicillin. (See WARNINGS.)

Liver: A moderate rise in AST (SGOT) and/or ALT (SGPT) has been noted in patients treated with ampicillin class antibiotics but the significance of these findings is unknown. Hepatic dysfunction, including increases in serum transaminases (AST and/or ALT), serum bilirubin and/or alkaline phosphatase, has been infrequently reported with *Augmentin*. It has been reported more commonly in the elderly, in males, or in patients on prolonged treatment. The histologic findings on liver biopsy have consisted of predominantly cholestatic, hepatocellular, or mixed cholestatic-hepatocellular changes. The onset of signs/symptoms of hepatic dysfunction may occur during or several weeks after therapy has been discontinued. The hepatic dysfunction, which may be severe, is usually reversible. On rare occasions, deaths have been reported (less than 1 death reported per estimated 4 million prescriptions worldwide). These have generally been cases associated with serious underlying diseases or concomitant medications.

Renal: Interstitial nephritis and hematuria have been reported rarely.

Hemic and Lymphatic Systems: Anemia, including hemolytic anemia, thrombocytopenia, thrombocytopenic purpura, eosinophilia, leukopenia and agranulocytosis have been reported during therapy with penicillins. These reactions are usually reversible on discontinuation of therapy and are believed to be hypersensitivity phenomena. A slight thrombocytosis was noted in less than 1% of the patients treated with *Augmentin*. There have been reports of increased prothrombin time in patients receiving *Augmentin* and anticoagulant therapy concomitantly.

Central Nervous System: Agitation, anxiety, behavioral changes, confusion, convulsions, dizziness, insomnia, and reversible hyperactivity have been reported rarely.

OVERDOSAGE

Most patients have been asymptomatic following overdosage or have experienced primarily gastrointestinal symptoms including stomach and abdominal pain, vomiting, and diarrhea. Rash, hyperactivity, or drowsiness have also been observed in a small number of patients.

In the case of overdosage, discontinue *Augmentin*, treat symptomatically, and institute supportive measures as required. If the overdosage is very recent and there is no contraindication, an attempt at emesis or other means of removal of drug from the stomach may be performed. A prospective study of 51 pediatric patients at a poison center suggested that overdosages of less than 250 mg/kg of amoxicillin are not associated with significant clinical symptoms and do not require gastric emptying.[3]

Interstitial nephritis resulting in oliguric renal failure has been reported in a small number of patients after overdosage with amoxicillin. Renal impairment appears to be reversible with cessation of drug administration. High blood levels may occur more readily in patients with impaired renal function because of decreased renal clearance of both amoxicillin and clavulanate. Both amoxicillin and clavulanate are removed from the circulation by hemodialysis. (See DOSAGE AND ADMINISTRATION for recommended dosing for patients with impaired renal function.)

DOSAGE AND ADMINISTRATION

Since both the *Augmentin* 250 mg and 500 mg tablets contain the same amount of clavulanic acid (125 mg, as the potassium salt), 2 *Augmentin* 250 mg tablets are not equivalent to 1 *Augmentin* 500 mg tablet. Therefore, 2 *Augmentin* 250 mg tablets should not be substituted for 1 *Augmentin* 500 mg tablet.

Dosage:

Adults: The usual adult dose is 1 *Augmentin* 500 mg tablet every 12 hours or 1 *Augmentin* 250 mg tablet every 8 hours. For more severe infections and infections of the respiratory tract, the dose should be 1 *Augmentin* 875 mg tablet every 12 hours or 1 *Augmentin* 500 mg tablet every 8 hours. Patients with impaired renal function do not generally require a reduction in dose unless the impairment is severe. Severely impaired patients with a glomerular filtration rate of <30 mL/minute should not receive the 875 mg tablet. Patients with a glomerular filtration rate of 10 to 30 mL/minute should receive 500 mg or 250 mg every 12 hours, depending on the severity of the infection. Patients with a less than 10 mL/minute glomerular filtration rate should receive 500 mg or 250 mg every 24 hours, depending on severity of the infection.

Hemodialysis patients should receive 500 mg or 250 mg every 24 hours, depending on severity of the infection. They should receive an additional dose both during and at the end of dialysis.

Hepatically impaired patients should be dosed with caution and hepatic function monitored at regular intervals. (See WARNINGS.)

Pediatric Patients: Pediatric patients weighing 40 kg or more should be dosed according to the adult recommendations.

Due to the different amoxicillin to clavulanic acid ratios in the *Augmentin* 250 mg tablet (250/125) versus the *Augmentin* 250 mg chewable tablet (250/62.5), the *Augmentin* 250 mg tablet should not be used until the pediatric patient weighs at least 40 kg or more.

Administration: *Augmentin* may be taken without regard to meals; however, absorption of clavulanate potassium is enhanced when *Augmentin* is administered at the start of a meal. To minimize the potential for gastrointestinal intolerance, *Augmentin* should be taken at the start of a meal.

HOW SUPPLIED

AUGMENTIN 250 MG TABLETS: Each white oval film-coated tablet, debossed with AUGMENTIN on 1 side and

Continued on next page

Information on the SmithKline Beecham Pharmaceuticals products appearing here is based on the labeling in effect on July 31, 1998. Further information on these and other products may be obtained from the Medical Department, SmithKline Beecham Pharmaceuticals, One Franklin Plaza, Philadelphia, PA 19101.

Augmentin Tablets—Cont.

250/125 on the other side, contains 250 mg amoxicillin as the trihydrate and 125 mg clavulanic acid as the potassium salt.
NDC 0029-6075-27 .... bottles of 30
NDC 0029-6075-31 .... Unit Dose (10×10) 100 tablets
***AUGMENTIN* 500 MG TABLETS:** Each white oval film-coated tablet, debossed with AUGMENTIN on 1 side and 500/125 on the other side, contains 500 mg amoxicillin as the trihydrate and 125 mg clavulanic acid as the potassium salt.
NDC 0029-6080-12 .... bottles of 20
NDC 0029-6080-31 .... Unit Dose (10×10) 100 tablets
***AUGMENTIN* 875 MG TABLETS:** Each scored white capsule-shaped tablet, debossed with AUGMENTIN 875 on 1 side and *SB* on the other side, contains 875 mg amoxicillin as the trihydrate and 125 mg clavulanic acid as the potassium salt.
NDC 0029-6086-12 .... bottles of 20
NDC 0029-6086-21 .... Unit Dose (10×10) 100 tablets
***AUGMENTIN* is also supplied as:**
AUGMENTIN 125 MG/5 ML (125 mg amoxicillin/31.25 mg clavulanic acid) FOR ORAL SUSPENSION:
NDC 0029-6085-39 .... 75 mL bottle
NDC 0029-6085-23 .... 100 mL bottle
NDC 0029-6085-22 .... 150 mL bottle
AUGMENTIN 200 MG/5 ML (200 mg amoxicillin/28.5 mg clavulanic acid) FOR ORAL SUSPENSION:
NDC 0029-6087-29 .... 50 mL bottle
NDC 0029-6087-39 .... 75 mL bottle
NDC 0029-6087-51 .... 100 mL bottle
AUGMENTIN 250 MG/5 ML (250 mg amoxicillin/62.5 mg clavulanic acid) FOR ORAL SUSPENSION:
NDC 0029-6090-39 .... 75 mL bottles
NDC 0029-6090-23 .... 100 mL bottle
NDC 0029-6090-22 .... 150 mL bottle
AUGMENTIN 400 MG/5 ML (400 mg amoxicillin/57 mg clavulanic acid) FOR ORAL SUSPENSION:
NDC 0029-6092-29 .... 50 mL bottle
NDC 0029-6092-39 .... 75 mL bottle
NDC 0029-6092-51 .... 100 mL bottle
AUGMENTIN 125 MG (125 mg amoxicillin/31.25 mg clavulanic acid) CHEWABLE TABLETS:
NDC 0029-6073-47 .... carton of 30 (5×6) tablets
AUGMENTIN 200 MG (200 mg amoxicillin/28.5 mg clavulanic acid) CHEWABLE TABLETS:
NDC 0029-6071-12 .... carton of 20 tablets
AUGMENTIN 250 MG (250 mg amoxicillin/62.5 mg clavulanic acid) CHEWABLE TABLETS:
NDC 0029-6074-47 .... carton of 30 (5×6) tablets
AUGMENTIN 400 MG (400 mg amoxicillin/57.0 mg clavulanic acid) CHEWABLE TABLETS:
NDC 0029-6072-12 .... carton of 20 tablets
Store tablets and dry powder at or below 25°C (77°F). Dispense in tightly closed, moisture-proof containers.

CLINICAL STUDIES

Data from two pivotal studies in 1,191 patients treated for either lower respiratory tract infections or complicated urinary tract infections compared a regimen of 875 mg *Augmentin* tablets q12h to 500 mg *Augmentin* tablets dosed q8h (584 and 607 patients, respectively). Comparable efficacy was demonstrated between the q12h and q8h dosing regimens. There was no significant difference in the percentage of adverse events in each group. The most frequently reported adverse event was diarrhea; incidence rates were similar for the 875 mg q12h and 500 mg q8h dosing regimens (14.9% and 14.3%, respectively). However, there was a statistically significant difference ($p<0.05$) in rates of severe diarrhea or withdrawals with diarrhea between the regimens: 1.0% for 875 mg q12h dosing versus 2.5% for the 500 mg q8h dosing.
In one of these pivotal studies, 629 patients with either pyelonephritis or a complicated urinary tract infection (i.e., patients with abnormalities of the urinary tract that predispose to relapse of bacteriuria following eradication) were randomized to receive either 875 mg *Augmentin* tablets q12h or 500 mg *Augmentin* tablets q8h in the following distribution:

	875 mg q12h	500 mg q8h
Pyelonephritis	173 patients	188 patients
Complicated UTI	135 patients	133 patients
Total patients	308	321

The number of bacteriologically evaluable patients was comparable between the two dosing regimens. *Augmentin* produced comparable bacteriological success rates in patients assessed 2 to 4 days immediately following end of therapy. The bacteriologic efficacy rates were comparable at one of the follow-up visits (5 to 9 days post-therapy) and at a late post-therapy visit (in the majority of cases, this was 2 to 4 weeks post-therapy), as seen in the table below:

	875 mg q12h	500 mg q8h
2 to 4 days	81%, n=58	80%, n=54
5 to 9 days	58.5%, n=41	51.9%, n=52
2 to 4 weeks	52.5%, n=101	54.8%, n=104

As noted before, though there was no significant difference in the percentage of adverse events in each group, there was a statistically significant difference in rates of severe diarrhea or withdrawals with diarrhea between the regimens.

REFERENCES

1. National Committee for Clinical Laboratory Standards. Methods for Dilution Antimicrobial Susceptibility Tests for Bacteria that Grow Aerobically—Third Edition. Approved Standard NCCLS Document M7-A3, Vol. 13, No. 25. NCCLS, Villanova, PA, December 1993.
2. National Committee for Clinical Laboratory Standards. Performance Standards for Antimicrobial Disk Susceptibility Tests—Fifth Edition. Approved Standard NCCLS Document M2-A5, Vol. 13, No. 24. NCCLS, Villanova, PA, December 1993.
3. Swanson-Biearman B, Dean BS, Lopez G, Krenzelok EP. The effects of penicillin and cephalosporin ingestions in children less than six years of age. *Vet Hum Toxicol* 1988; 30:66–67.

Veterans Administration/Military/PHS—Chewable Tablets, 125 mg, 30's 6505-01-282-6332; 250 mg, 30's, 6505-01-264-2366; Tablets, 250 mg, 30's, 6505-01-203-6259; 250 mg, 100's SUP, 6505-01-339-6919; 500 mg, 20's, 6505-01-431-0403; 500 mg, 100's SUP, 6505-01-303-8962; 875 mg, 20's, 6505-01-430-9740; 875 mg, 100's SUP, 6505-01-431-0402; Oral Suspension, 125 mg/5 mL, 75 mL, 6505-01-340-0847; 125 mg/5 mL, 100 mL, 6505-01-408-8181; 125 mg/5 mL, 150 mL, 6505-01-204-5388; 250 mg/5 mL, 75 mL, 6505-01-207-8205; 250 mg/5 mL, 100 mL, 6505-01-408-8352; 250 mg/5 mL, 150 mL, 6505-01-207-0795.
AG:AL5
Shown in Product Identification Guide, page 339

BACTROBAN® ℞

[back 'tro-ban]
(mupirocin)
Ointment 2%
For Dermatologic Use

DESCRIPTION

Each gram of *Bactroban* Ointment 2% contains 20 mg mupirocin in a bland water miscible ointment base (polyethylene glycol ointment, N.F.) consisting of polyethylene glycol 400 and polyethylene glycol 3350. Mupirocin is a naturally occurring antibiotic. The chemical name is (*E*)-(2*S* ,3*R* , 4*R* , 5*S*)-5-[(2*S* , 3*S* , 4*S* , 5*S*)-2,3-Epoxy-5-hydroxy-4-methylhexyl] tetrahydro -3,4- dihydroxy-β-methyl -2*H* -pyran-2-crotonic acid, ester with 9-hydroxynonanoic acid. The chemical structure is:

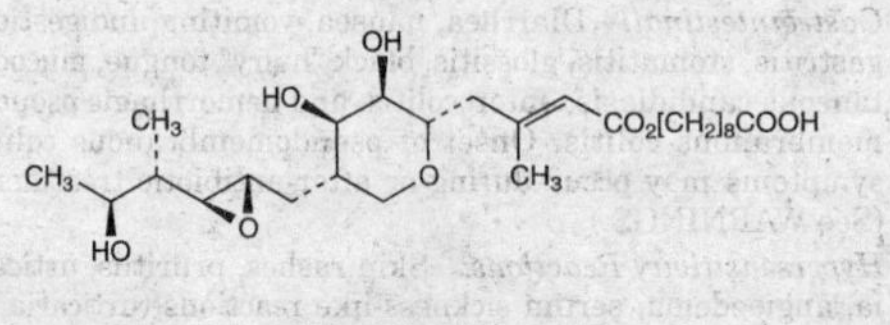

mupirocin

CLINICAL PHARMACOLOGY

Mupirocin is produced by fermentation of the organism *Pseudomonas fluorescens.* Mupirocin inhibits bacterial protein synthesis by reversibly and specifically binding to bacterial isoleucyl transfer-RNA synthetase. Due to this mode of action, mupirocin shows no cross resistance with chloramphenicol, erythromycin, fusidic acid, gentamicin, lincomycin, methicillin, neomycin, novobiocin, penicillin, streptomycin, and tetracycline.
Application of ^{14}C-labeled mupirocin ointment to the lower arm of normal male subjects followed by occlusion for 24 hours showed no measurable systemic absorption (<1.1 nanogram mupirocin per milliliter of whole blood). Measurable radioactivity was present in the stratum corneum of these subjects 72 hours after application.
Microbiology: The following bacteria are susceptible to the action of mupirocin *in vitro:* the aerobic isolates of *Staphylococcus aureus* (including methicillin-resistant and β-lactamase producing strains), *Staphylococcus epidermidis, Staphylococcus saprophyticus,* and *Streptococcus pyogenes.*
Only the organisms listed in the INDICATIONS AND USAGE section have been shown to be clinically susceptible to mupirocin.

INDICATIONS AND USAGE

Bactroban (mupirocin) Ointment is indicated for the topical treatment of impetigo due to: *Staphylococcus aureus,* beta-hemolytic *Streptococcus**, and *Streptococcus pyogenes.*

*Efficacy for this organism in this organ system was studied in fewer than ten infections.

CONTRAINDICATIONS

This drug is contraindicated in individuals with a history of sensitivity reactions to any of its components.

WARNINGS

Bactroban Ointment is not for ophthalmic use.

PRECAUTIONS

If a reaction suggesting sensitivity or chemical irritation should occur with the use of *Bactroban* Ointment, treatment should be discontinued and appropriate alternative therapy for the infection instituted.
As with other antibacterial products prolonged use may result in overgrowth of nonsusceptible organisms, including fungi.
Bactroban is not formulated for use on mucosal surfaces. Intranasal use has been associated with isolated reports of stinging and drying.
Polyethylene glycol can be absorbed from open wounds and damaged skin and is excreted by the kidneys. In common with other polyethylene glycol-based ointments, *Bactroban* should not be used in conditions where absorption of large quantities of polyethylene glycol is possible, especially if there is evidence of moderate or severe renal impairment.
Pregnancy Category B: Reproduction studies have been performed in rats and rabbits at systemic doses, i.e., orally, subcutaneously, and intramuscularly, up to 100 times the human topical dose and have revealed no evidence of impaired fertility or harm to the fetus due to mupirocin. There are, however, no adequate and well-controlled studies in pregnant women. Because animal studies are not always predictive of human response, this drug should be used during pregnancy only if clearly needed.
Nursing Mothers: It is not known whether *Bactroban* is present in breast milk. Nursing should be temporarily discontinued while using *Bactroban.*

ADVERSE REACTIONS

The following local adverse reactions have been reported in connection with the use of *Bactroban* Ointment: burning, stinging, or pain in 1.5% of patients; itching in 1% of patients; rash, nausea, erythema, dry skin, tenderness, swelling, contact dermatitis, and increased exudate in less than 1% of patients.

DOSAGE AND ADMINISTRATION

A small amount of *Bactroban* Ointment should be applied to the affected area three times daily. The area treated may be covered with a gauze dressing if desired. Patients not showing a clinical response within 3 to 5 days should be re-evaluated.

HOW SUPPLIED

Bactroban (mupirocin) Ointment 2% is supplied in 15 gram and 30 gram tubes.
NDC 0029-1525-22 (15 gram tube)
NDC 0029-1525-25 (30 gram tube)
Store between 15° and 30°C (59° and 86°F).
Veterans Administration/Military/PHS—15 gram, 6505-01-375-5686, 30 gram, 6505-01-352-3658.
BC:L6C

BACTROBAN® CREAM ℞

[back- 'trō-ban]
brand of
mupirocin calcium cream, 2%
For Dermatologic Use

DESCRIPTION

Bactroban Cream (mupirocin calcium cream), 2% contains the dihydrate crystalline calcium hemi-salt of the antibiotic mupirocin. Chemically, it is (α*E*,2*S*,3*R*,4*R*,5*S*)-5-[(2*S*,3*S*,4*S*,5*S*)-2,3-Epoxy-5-hydroxy-4-methylhexyl]tetrahydro-3,4-dihydroxy-β-methyl-2*H*-pyran-2-crotonic acid, ester with 9-hydroxynonanoic acid, calcium salt (2:1), dihydrate.
The molecular formula of mupirocin calcium is $(C_{26}H_{43}O_9)_2Ca \cdot 2H_2O$, and the molecular weight is 1075.3. The molecular weight of mupirocin free acid is 500.6. The structural formula of mupirocin calcium is:

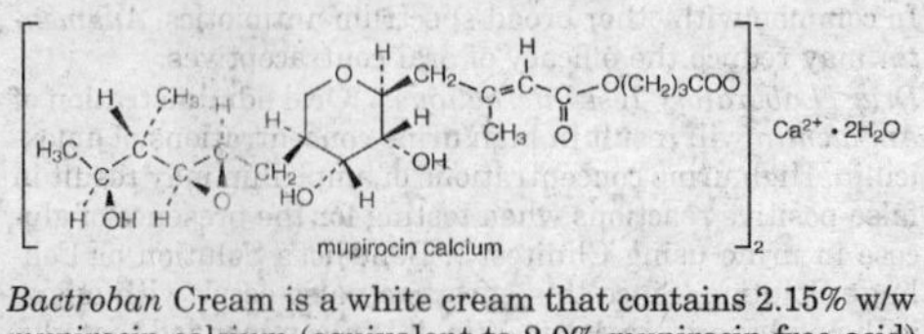

Bactroban Cream is a white cream that contains 2.15% w/w mupirocin calcium (equivalent to 2.0% mupirocin free acid) in an oil and water-based emulsion. The inactive ingredients are benzyl alcohol, cetomacrogol 1000, cetyl alcohol, mineral oil, phenoxyethanol, purified water, stearyl alcohol and xanthan gum.

CLINICAL PHARMACOLOGY

Pharmacokinetics

Systemic absorption of mupirocin through intact human skin is minimal. The systemic absorption of mupirocin was studied following application of *Bactroban* Cream three times a day for 5 days to various skin lesions (greater than 10 cm in length or 100 cm^2 in area) in 16 adults (aged 29 to 60 years) and 10 children (aged 3 to 12 years). Some systemic absorption was observed as evidenced by the detection of the metabolite, monic acid, in urine. Data from this study indicated more frequent occurrence of percutaneous absorption in children (90% of patients) compared to adults (44% of patients). However, the observed urinary concentrations in children (0.07 – 1.3 µg/mL [1 pediatric patient had no detectable level]) are within the observed range (0.08 – 10.03 µg/mL [9 adults had no detectable level]) in the adult population. In general, the degree of percutaneous absorption following multiple dosing appears to be minimal in adults and children. Any mupirocin reaching the systemic circulation is rapidly metabolized, predominantly to inactive monic acid, which is eliminated by renal excretion.

Microbiology

Mupirocin is an antibacterial agent produced by fermentation using the organism *Pseudomonas fluorescens*. It is active against a wide range of gram-positive bacteria including methicillin-resistant *Staphylococcus aureus* (MRSA). It is also active against certain gram-negative bacteria. Mupirocin inhibits bacterial protein synthesis by reversibly and specifically binding to bacterial isoleucyl transfer-RNA synthetase. Due to this unique mode of action, mupirocin demonstrates no *in vitro* cross-resistance with other classes of antimicrobial agents.

Resistance occurs rarely. However, when mupirocin resistance does occur, it appears to result from the production of a modified isoleucyl-tRNA synthetase. High-level plasmid-mediated resistance (MIC >1024 mcg/mL) has been reported in some strains of *S. aureus* and coagulase-negative staphylococci.

Mupirocin is bactericidal at concentrations achieved by topical application. However, the minimum bactericidal concentration (MBC) against relevant pathogens is generally eight-fold to thirty-fold higher than the minimum inhibitory concentration (MIC). In addition, mupirocin is highly protein bound (>97%), and the effect of wound secretions on the MICs of mupirocin has not been determined.

Mupirocin has been shown to be active against most strains of *Staphylococcus aureus* and *Streptococcus pyogenes*, both *in vitro* and in clinical studies. (See **INDICATIONS AND USAGE** section.) The following *in vitro* data are available, BUT THEIR CLINICAL SIGNIFICANCE IS UNKNOWN. Mupirocin is active against most strains of *Staphylococcus epidermidis* and *Staphylococcus saprophyticus*.

INDICATIONS AND USAGE

Bactroban Cream (mupirocin calcium cream), 2% is indicated for the treatment of secondarily infected traumatic skin lesions (up to 10 cm in length or 100 cm^2 in area) due to susceptible strains of *Staphylococcus aureus* and *Streptococcus pyogenes*.

CONTRAINDICATIONS

Bactroban Cream is contraindicated in patients with known hypersensitivity to any of the constituents of the product.

WARNINGS

Avoid contact with the eyes.

In the event of a sensitization or severe local irritation from *Bactroban* Cream, usage should be discontinued, and appropriate alternative therapy for the infection instituted.

PRECAUTIONS

General

As with other antibacterial products, prolonged use may result in overgrowth of nonsusceptible microorganisms, including fungi. (See **DOSAGE AND ADMINISTRATION**.)

Bactroban Cream is not formulated for use on mucosal surfaces.

Information for Patients

- Use this medication only as directed by your healthcare provider. It is for external use only. Avoid contact with the eyes.
- The treated area may be covered by gauze dressing if desired.
- Report to your healthcare provider any signs of local adverse reactions. The medication should be stopped and your healthcare provider contacted if irritation, severe itching or rash occurs.
- If no improvement is seen in 3 to 5 days, contact your healthcare provider.

Drug Interactions

The effect of the concurrent application of topical mupirocin calcium cream and other topical products has not been studied.

Carcinogenesis, Mutagenesis, Impairment of Fertility

Long-term studies in animals to evaluate carcinogenic potential of mupirocin calcium have not been conducted.

Results of the following studies performed with mupirocin calcium or mupirocin sodium *in vitro* and *in vivo* did not indicate a potential for mutagenicity: rat primary hepatocyte unscheduled DNA synthesis, sediment analysis for DNA strand breaks, *Salmonella* reversion test (Ames), *Escherichia coli* mutation assay, metaphase analysis of human lymphocytes, mouse lymphoma assay, and bone marrow micronuclei assay in mice.

Fertility studies were performed in rats with mupirocin administered subcutaneously at doses up to 49 times a human topical dose of 1 gram/day (approximately 20 mg mupirocin per day) on a mg/m^2 basis and revealed no evidence of impaired fertility from mupirocin sodium.

Pregnancy

Teratogenic Effects. Pregnancy Category B. Teratology studies have been performed in rats and rabbits with mupirocin administered subcutaneously at doses up to 78 and 154 times, respectively, a human topical dose of 1 gram/day (approximately 20 mg mupirocin per day) on a mg/m^2 basis and revealed no evidence of harm to the fetus due to mupirocin. There are, however, no adequate and well-controlled studies in pregnant women. Because animal reproduction studies are not always predictive of human response, this drug should be used during pregnancy only if clearly needed.

Nursing Mothers

It is not known whether this drug is excreted in human milk. Because many drugs are excreted in human milk, caution should be exercised when *Bactroban* Cream is administered to a nursing woman.

Pediatric Use

The safety and effectiveness of *Bactroban* Cream have been established in the age groups 3 months to 16 years. Use of *Bactroban* Cream in these age groups is supported by evidence from adequate and well-controlled studies of *Bactroban* Cream in adults with additional data from 93 pediatric patients studied as part of the pivotal trials in adults. (See **CLINICAL STUDIES** section.)

Geriatric Use

In two well-controlled studies, 30 patients over 65 years old were treated with *Bactroban* Cream. No overall difference in the efficacy or safety of *Bactroban* Cream was observed in this patient population when compared to that observed in younger patients.

ADVERSE REACTIONS

In two randomized, double-blind, double-dummy trials, 339 patients were treated with topical *Bactroban* Cream plus oral placebo. Adverse events thought to be possibly or probably drug-related occurred in 28 (8.3%) patients. The incidence of those events that were reported in at least 1% of patients enrolled in these trials were: headache (1.7%), rash and nausea (1.1% each).

Other adverse events thought to be possibly or probably drug-related which occurred in less than 1% of patients were: abdominal pain, burning at application site, cellulitis, dermatitis, dizziness, pruritus, secondary wound infection, and ulcerative stomatitis.

In a supportive study in the treatment of secondarily infected eczema, 82 patients were treated with *Bactroban* Cream. The incidence of adverse events thought to be possibly or probably drug-related was as follows: nausea (4.9%), headache and burning at application site (3.6% each), pruritus (2.4%) and one report each of abdominal pain, bleeding secondary to eczema, pain secondary to eczema, hives, dry skin and rash.

OVERDOSAGE

Intravenous infusions of 252 mg, as well as single oral doses of 500 mg of mupirocin, have been well tolerated in healthy adult subjects. There is no information regarding overdose of *Bactroban* Cream.

DOSAGE AND ADMINISTRATION

A small amount of *Bactroban* Cream should be applied to the affected area three times daily for 10 days. The area treated may be covered with gauze dressing if desired. Patients not showing a clinical response within 3 to 5 days should be re-evaluated.

CLINICAL STUDIES

The efficacy of topical *Bactroban* Cream for the treatment of secondarily infected traumatic skin lesions (e.g., lacerations, sutured wounds and abrasions not more than 10 cm in length or 100 cm^2 in total area) was compared to that of oral cephalexin in two randomized, double-blind, double-dummy clinical trials. Clinical efficacy rates at follow-up in the per protocol populations (adults and pediatric patients included) were 96.1% for *Bactroban* Cream (n=231) and 93.1% for oral cephalexin (n=219). Pathogen eradication rates at follow-up in the per protocol populations were 100% for both *Bactroban* Cream and oral cephalexin.

Pediatrics

There were 93 pediatric patients aged 2 weeks to 16 years enrolled per protocol in the secondarily infected skin lesion studies, although only 3 were less than 2 years of age in the *Bactroban* Cream treated population. Patients were randomized to either 10 days of topical *Bactroban* Cream t.i.d. or 10 days of oral cephalexin (250 mg q.i.d. for patients >40 kg or 25 mg/kg/day oral suspension in four divided doses for patients ≤40 kg). Clinical efficacy at follow-up (7 to 12 days post-therapy) in the per protocol populations was 97.7% (43/44) for *Bactroban* Cream and 93.9% (46/49) for cephalexin. Only one adverse event (headache) was thought to be possibly or probably related to drug therapy in the *Bactroban* Cream intent-to-treat pediatric population of 70 children (1.4%).

HOW SUPPLIED

Bactroban Cream (mupirocin calcium cream), 2% is supplied in 15 gram and 30 gram tubes.

NDC 0029-1527-22 (15 gram tube)

NDC 0029-1527-25 (30 gram tube)

Store at or below 25°C (77°F). Do not freeze.

Manufactured by **DPT Laboratories**
San Antonio, TX 78215

Distributed by
SmithKline Beecham Pharmaceuticals
Philadelphia, PA 19101

BB:L2

BACTROBAN® NASAL ℞

[*back 'tro-ban*]

brand of mupirocin calcium ointment, 2% for intranasal use only

DESCRIPTION

Bactroban Nasal (mupirocin calcium ointment), 2% contains the dihydrate crystalline calcium hemi-salt of the antibiotic mupirocin. Chemically, it is (α *E*,2*S*,3*R*,4*R*,5*S*)-5-[(2*S*,3*S*,4*S*,5*S*)-2,3-epoxy-5-hydroxy-4-methylhexyl] tetrahydro-3,4-dihydroxy-β-methyl-2*H*-pyran-2-crotonic acid, ester with 9-hydroxynonanoic acid, calcium salt (2:1), dihydrate.

The molecular formula of mupirocin calcium is $(C_{52}H_{86}O_{18})_2Ca{\cdot}2H_2O$, and the molecular weight is 1075.3. The molecular weight of mupirocin free acid is 500.6. The structural formula of mupirocin calcium is:

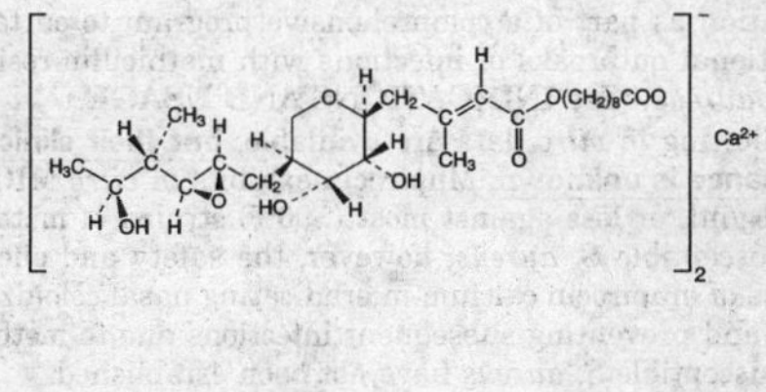

Bactroban Nasal is a white to off-white ointment that contains 2.15% w/w mupirocin calcium (equivalent to 2.0% pure mupirocin free acid) in a soft white ointment base. The inactive ingredients are paraffin and a mixture of glycerin esters (Softisan® 649).

CLINICAL PHARMACOLOGY

Pharmacokinetics

Following single or repeated intranasal applications of 0.2 gram of *Bactroban* Nasal t.i.d. for 3 days to five healthy **adult** male subjects, no evidence of systemic absorption of mupirocin was demonstrated. The dosage regimen used in this study was for pharmacokinetic characterization only. (See **DOSAGE AND ADMINISTRATION** for proper clinical dosing information.)

In this study, the concentrations of mupirocin in urine and of monic acid in urine and serum were below the limit of determination of the assay for up to 72 hours after the applications. The lowest levels of determination of the assay used were 50 ng/mL of mupirocin in urine, 75 ng/mL of monic acid in urine, and 10 ng/mL of monic acid in serum. Based on the detectable limit of the urine assay for monic acid, one can extrapolate that a mean of 3.3% (range: 1.2–5.1%) of the applied dose could be systemically absorbed from the nasal mucosa of **adults**.

Data from a report of a pharmacokinetic study in neonates and premature infants indicate that, unlike in adults, significant systemic absorption occurred following intranasal administration of *Bactroban* Nasal in this population. **At this time, the pharmacokinetic properties of mupirocin following intranasal application of *Bactroban* Nasal have not**

Continued on next page

Information on the SmithKline Beecham Pharmaceuticals products appearing here is based on the labeling in effect on July 31, 1998. Further information on these and other products may be obtained from the Medical Department, SmithKline Beecham Pharmaceuticals, One Franklin Plaza, Philadelphia, PA 19101.

Bactroban Nasal—Cont.

been adequately characterized in neonates or other children less than 12 years of age, and in addition, the safety of the product in children less than 12 years of age has not been established.

The effect of the concurrent application of intranasal mupirocin calcium ointment, 2% with other intranasal products has not been studied. (See **PRECAUTIONS, Drug Interactions.**)

Following intravenous or oral administration, mupirocin is rapidly metabolized. The principal metabolite, monic acid, demonstrates no antibacterial activity. In a study conducted in seven healthy adult male subjects, the elimination half-life after intravenous administration of mupirocin was 20 to 40 minutes for mupirocin and 30 to 80 minutes for monic acid. Monic acid is predominantly eliminated by renal excretion. The pharmacokinetics of mupirocin has not been studied in individuals with renal insufficiency.

Microbiology

Mupirocin is an antibacterial agent produced by fermentation using the microorganism *Pseudomonas fluorescens.* Mupirocin inhibits bacterial protein synthesis by reversibly and specifically binding to bacterial isoleucyl transfer-RNA synthetase. Due to this mode of action, mupirocin demonstrates no *in vitro* cross-resistance with other classes of antimicrobial agents.

When mupirocin resistance does occur, it appears to result from the production of a modified isoleucyl-tRNA synthetase. High-level plasmid-mediated resistance (MIC >1024 mcg/mL) has been reported in some strains of *S. aureus* and coagulase-negative staphylococci.

Mupirocin is bactericidal at concentrations achieved topically by intranasal administration. However, the minimum bactericidal concentration (MBC) against relevant intranasal pathogens is generally eight-fold to thirty-fold higher than the minimum inhibitory concentration (MIC). In addition, mupirocin is highly protein bound (>97%), and the effect of nasal secretions on the MIC's of intranasally applied mupirocin has not been determined.

Mupirocin has been shown to be active against most strains of methicillin-resistant *S. aureus*, both *in vitro* and in clinical studies of the eradication of nasal colonization. *Bactroban* Nasal has only established clinical utility in nasal eradication as part of a comprehensive program to curtail institutional outbreaks of infections with methicillin-resistant *S. aureus*. (See **INDICATIONS AND USAGE.**)

The following *in vitro* data are available, **but their clinical significance is unknown.** Mupirocin exhibits *in vitro* MIC's of 1 mcg/mL or less against most (>90%) strains of methicillin-susceptible *S. aureus*; however, the safety and effectiveness of mupirocin calcium in eradicating nasal colonization of and preventing subsequent infections due to methicillin-susceptible *S. aureus* have not been established.

INDICATIONS AND USAGE

Bactroban Nasal (mupirocin calcium ointment), 2% is indicated for the eradication of nasal colonization with methicillin-resistant *Staphylococcus aureus* in adult patients and health care workers as part of a comprehensive infection control program to reduce the risk of infection among patients at high risk of methicillin-resistant *S. aureus* infection during institutional outbreaks of infections with this pathogen.

NOTE:

(1) There are insufficient data at this time to establish that this product is safe and effective as part of an intervention program to prevent autoinfection of high-risk patients from their own nasal colonization with *S. aureus*.

(2) There are insufficient data at this time to recommend use of *Bactroban* Nasal for general prophylaxis of any infection in any patient population.

(3) Greater than 90% of subjects/patients in clinical trials had eradication of nasal colonization 2 to 4 days after therapy was completed. Approximately 30% recolonization was reported in one domestic study within 4 weeks after completion of therapy. These eradication rates were clinically and statistically superior to those reported in subjects/patients in the vehicle-treated arms of the adequate and well-controlled studies. Those treated with vehicle had eradication rates of 5% to 30% at 2 to 4 days post-therapy with 85% to 100% recolonization within 4 weeks.

All adequate and well-controlled trials of this product were vehicle-controlled; therefore, no data from direct, head-to-head comparisons with other products are available at this time.

CONTRAINDICATIONS

Bactroban Nasal is contraindicated in patients with known hypersensitivity to any of the constituents of the product.

WARNINGS

AVOID CONTACT WITH THE EYES. Application of *Bactroban* Nasal to the eye under testing conditions has caused severe symptoms such as burning and tearing. These symptoms resolved within days to weeks after discontinuation of the ointment.

In the event of a sensitization or severe local irritation from *Bactroban* Nasal, usage should be discontinued.

PRECAUTIONS

General

As with other antibacterial products, prolonged use may result in overgrowth of nonsusceptible microorganisms, including fungi. (See **DOSAGE AND ADMINISTRATION.**)

Information for Patients

Patients should be given the following instructions:

— Apply approximately one-half of the ointment from the single-use tube directly into one nostril and the other half into the other nostril;
— Avoid contact of the medication with the eyes;
— Discard the tube after using, do not re-use;
— Press the sides of the nose together and gently massage after application to spread the ointment throughout the inside of the nostrils; and
— Discontinue usage of the medication and call your health care practitioner if sensitization or severe local irritation occurs.

Drug Interactions

The effect of the concurrent application of intranasal mupirocin calcium and other intranasal products has not been studied. Until further information is known, mupirocin calcium ointment, 2% should not be applied concurrently with any other intranasal products.

Carcinogenesis, Mutagenesis, Impairment of Fertility

Long-term studies in animals to evaluate carcinogenic potential of mupirocin calcium have not been conducted.

Results of the following studies performed with mupirocin calcium or mupirocin sodium *in vitro* and *in vivo* did not indicate a potential for mutagenicity: rat primary hepatocyte unscheduled DNA synthesis, sediment analysis for DNA strand breaks, *Salmonella* reversion test (Ames), *Escherichia coli* mutation assay, metaphase analysis of human lymphocytes, mouse lymphoma assay, and bone marrow micronuclei assay in mice.

Reproduction studies were performed in rats with mupirocin administered subcutaneously at doses up to **40** times the human intranasal dose (approximately 20 mg mupirocin per day) on a mg/m^2 basis and revealed no evidence of impaired fertility from mupirocin sodium.

Pregnancy

Teratogenic Effects. Pregnancy Category B. Reproduction studies have been performed in rats and rabbits with mupirocin administered subcutaneously at doses up to 65 and 130 times, respectively, the human intranasal dose (approximately 20 mg mupirocin per day) on a mg/m^2 basis and revealed no evidence of harm to the fetus due to mupirocin. There are, however, no adequate and well-controlled studies in pregnant women. Because animal reproduction studies are not always predictive of human response, this drug should be used during pregnancy only if clearly needed.

Nursing Mothers

It is not known whether this drug is excreted in human milk. Because many drugs are excreted in human milk, caution should be exercised when *Bactroban* Nasal is administered to a nursing woman.

Pediatric Use

Safety in children under the age of 12 years has not been established. (See **CLINICAL PHARMACOLOGY.**)

ADVERSE REACTIONS

Clinical Trials

In clinical trials, 210 domestic and 2,130 foreign adult subjects/patients received *Bactroban* Nasal ointment. Less than 1% of domestic or foreign subjects and patients in clinical trials were withdrawn due to adverse events.

The most frequently reported adverse events in foreign clinical trials were as follows: rhinitis (1.0%), taste perversion (0.8%), pharyngitis (0.5%).

In domestic clinical trials, 17% (36/210) of adults treated with *Bactroban* Nasal ointment reported adverse events thought to be at least possibly drug-related. The incidence of adverse events that were reported in at least 1% of adults enrolled in domestic clinical trials were as follows:

ADVERSE EVENTS (≥1% INCIDENCE)-ADULTS IN U.S. TRIALS

	% of Subjects/Patients Experiencing Event *Bactroban* Nasal 2% (n=210)
Headache	9%
Rhinitis	6%
Respiratory disorder, including upper respiratory tract congestion	5%
Pharyngitis	4%
Taste perversion	3%
Burning/Stinging	2%
Cough	2%
Pruritus	1%

The following events thought possibly drug-related were reported in less than 1% of adults enrolled in domestic clinical trials: blepharitis, diarrhea, dry mouth, ear pain, epistaxis, nausea and rash.

All adequate and well-controlled clinical trials have been performed using *Bactroban* Nasal ointment, 2% in one arm and the vehicle ointment in the other arm of the study. No adequate and well-controlled safety data are available from direct, head-to-head comparative studies of this product and other products for this indication.

OVERDOSAGE

Following single or repeated intranasal applications of *Bactroban* Nasal to adults, no evidence for systemic absorption of mupirocin was obtained. Intravenous infusions of 252 mg, as well as single oral doses of 500 mg of mupirocin, have been well tolerated in healthy adult subjects. There is no information regarding local overdose of *Bactroban* Nasal or regarding oral ingestion of the nasal ointment formulation.

DOSAGE AND ADMINISTRATION

(See **INDICATIONS AND USAGE.**)

Adults (12 years of age and older): Approximately one-half of the ointment from the single-use tube should be applied into one nostril and the other half into the other nostril twice daily (morning and evening) for 5 days.

After application, the nostrils should be closed by pressing together and releasing the sides of the nose repetitively for approximately 1 minute. This will spread the ointment throughout the nares.

The single-use 1.0 gram tube will deliver a total of approximately 0.5 grams of the ointment (approximately 0.25 grams/nostril).

The tube should be discarded after usage; it should not be re-used.

The safety and effectiveness of applications of this medication for greater than 5 days have not been established. There are no human clinical or pre-clinical animal data to support the use of this product in a chronic manner or in manners other than those described in this package insert. Until further information is known, *Bactroban* Nasal should not be applied concurrently with any other intranasal products.

HOW SUPPLIED

Bactroban Nasal (mupirocin calcium ointment), 2% is supplied in 1.0 gram tubes packaged in cartons of 10.

NDC 0029-1526-11 (1.0 gram tubes in packages of 10).

Store at or below 25°C (77°F).

REFERENCE

1. National Committee for Clinical Laboratory Standards. Methods for Dilution Antimicrobial Susceptibility Tests for Bacteria That Grow Aerobically—Third Edition; Approved Standard NCCLS Document M7-A3. Vol. 12, No. 25, NCCLS, Villanova, PA, December 1993.

Manufactured by **DPT Laboratories**
San Antonio, TX 78215
Distributed by **SmithKline Beecham Pharmaceuticals**
Philadelphia, PA 19101
BN:L2

COMPAZINE® ℞

[komp 'ah-zeen]
(brand of prochlorperazine)

DESCRIPTION

Tablets—Each round, yellow-green, coated tablet contains prochlorperazine maleate equivalent to prochlorperazine as follows: 5 mg imprinted SKF and C66; 10 mg imprinted SKF and C67.

5 mg and 10 mg Tablets —Inactive ingredients consist of cellulose, lactose, magnesium stearate, polyethylene glycol, sodium croscarmellose, titanium dioxide, D&C Yellow No. 10, FD&C Blue No. 2, FD&C Yellow No. 6, FD&C Red No. 40, iron oxide, starch, stearic acid and trace amounts of other inactive ingredients including aluminum lake dyes.

Spansule® sustained release capsules—Each Compazine® *Spansule* capsule is so prepared that an initial dose is released promptly and the remaining medication is released gradually over a prolonged period.

Each capsule, with black cap and natural body, contains prochlorperazine maleate equivalent to prochlorperazine. The 10 mg capsule is imprinted 10 mg and 3344 on the black cap and is imprinted 10 mg and SB on the natural body. The 15 mg capsule is imprinted 15 mg and 3346 on the black cap and is imprinted 15 mg and SB on the natural body. Inactive ingredients consist of benzyl alcohol, cetylpyridinium chloride, D&C Green No. 5, D&C Yellow No. 10, FD&C Blue No. 1, aluminum lake, FD&C Red No. 40,

FD&C Yellow No. 6, gelatin, glyceryl monostearate, sodium lauryl sulfate, starch, sucrose, wax and trace amounts of other inactive ingredients.

Vials, 2 mL (5 mg/mL) and 10 mL (5 mg/mL)—Each mL contains, in aqueous solution, 5 mg prochlorperazine as the edisylate, 5 mg sodium biphosphate, 12 mg sodium tartrate, 0.9 mg sodium saccharin and 0.75% benzyl alcohol as preservative.

Suppositories—Each suppository contains $2^1/_2$ mg, 5 mg or 25 mg of prochlorperazine; with glycerin, glyceryl monopalmitate, glyceryl monostearate, hydrogenated cocoanut oil fatty acids and hydrogenated palm kernel oil fatty acids.

Syrup—Each 5 mL (1 teaspoonful) of clear, yellow-orange, fruit-flavored liquid contains 5 mg of prochlorperazine as the edisylate. Inactive ingredients consist of FD&C Yellow No. 6, flavors, polyoxyethylene polyoxypropylene glycol, sodium benzoate, sodium citrate, sucrose and water.

INDICATIONS

For control of severe nausea and vomiting.

For management of the manifestations of psychotic disorders.

Compazine (prochlorperazine) is effective for the short-term treatment of generalized non-psychotic anxiety. However, *Compazine* is not the first drug to be used in therapy for most patients with non-psychotic anxiety, because certain risks associated with its use are not shared by common alternative treatments (e.g., benzodiazepines).

When used in the treatment of non-psychotic anxiety, *Compazine* should not be administered at doses of more than 20 mg per day or for longer than 12 weeks, because the use of *Compazine* at higher doses or for longer intervals may cause persistent tardive dyskinesia that may prove irreversible (see WARNINGS).

The effectiveness of *Compazine* as treatment for non-psychotic anxiety was established in 4-week clinical studies of outpatients with generalized anxiety disorder. This evidence does not predict that *Compazine* will be useful in patients with other non-psychotic conditions in which anxiety, or signs that mimic anxiety, are found (e.g., physical illness, organic mental conditions, agitated depression, character pathologies, etc.).

Compazine has not been shown effective in the management of behavioral complications in patients with mental retardation.

CONTRAINDICATIONS

Do not use in patients with known hypersensitivity to phenothiazines.

Do not use in comatose states or in the presence of large amounts of central nervous system depressants (alcohol, barbiturates, narcotics, etc.).

Do not use in pediatric surgery.

Do not use in pediatric patients under 2 years of age or under 20 lbs. Do not use in children for conditions for which dosage has not been established.

WARNINGS

The extrapyramidal symptoms which can occur secondary to Compazine (prochlorperazine) may be confused with the central nervous system signs of an undiagnosed primary disease responsible for the vomiting, e.g., Reye's syndrome or other encephalopathy. The use of Compazine (prochlorperazine) and other potential hepatotoxins should be avoided in children and adolescents whose signs and symptoms suggest Reye's syndrome.

Tardive Dyskinesia: Tardive dyskinesia, a syndrome consisting of potentially irreversible, involuntary, dyskinetic movements, may develop in patients treated with neuroleptic (antipsychotic) drugs. Although the prevalence of the syndrome appears to be highest among the elderly, especially elderly women, it is impossible to rely upon prevalence estimates to predict, at the inception of neuroleptic treatment, which patients are likely to develop the syndrome. Whether neuroleptic drug products differ in their potential to cause tardive dyskinesia is unknown.

Both the risk of developing the syndrome and the likelihood that it will become irreversible are believed to increase as the duration of treatment and the total cumulative dose of neuroleptic drugs administered to the patient increase. However, the syndrome can develop, although much less commonly, after relatively brief treatment periods at low doses.

There is no known treatment for established cases of tardive dyskinesia, although the syndrome may remit, partially or completely, if neuroleptic treatment is withdrawn. Neuroleptic treatment itself, however, may suppress (or partially suppress) the signs and symptoms of the syndrome and thereby may possibly mask the underlying disease process.

The effect that symptomatic suppression has upon the long-term course of the syndrome is unknown.

Given these considerations, neuroleptics should be prescribed in a manner that is most likely to minimize the occurrence of tardive dyskinesia. Chronic neuroleptic treatment should generally be reserved for patients who suffer from a chronic illness that, 1) is known to respond to neu-

roleptic drugs, and 2) for whom alternative, equally effective, but potentially less harmful treatments are *not* available or appropriate. In patients who do require chronic treatment, the smallest dose and the shortest duration of treatment producing a satisfactory clinical response should be sought. The need for continued treatment should be reassessed periodically.

If signs and symptoms of tardive dyskinesia appear in a patient on neuroleptics, drug discontinuation should be considered. However, some patients may require treatment despite the presence of the syndrome.

For further information about the description of tardive dyskinesia and its clinical detection, please refer to the sections on PRECAUTIONS and ADVERSE REACTIONS.

Neuroleptic Malignant Syndrome (NMS): A potentially fatal symptom complex sometimes referred to as Neuroleptic Malignant Syndrome (NMS) has been reported in association with antipsychotic drugs. Clinical manifestations of NMS are hyperpyrexia, muscle rigidity, altered mental status and evidence of autonomic instability (irregular pulse or blood pressure, tachycardia, diaphoresis and cardiac dysrhythmias).

The diagnostic evaluation of patients with this syndrome is complicated. In arriving at a diagnosis, it is important to identify cases where the clinical presentation includes both serious medical illness (e.g., pneumonia, systemic infection, etc.) and untreated or inadequately treated extrapyramidal signs and symptoms (EPS). Other important considerations in the differential diagnosis include central anticholinergic toxicity, heat stroke, drug fever and primary central nervous system (CNS) pathology.

The management of NMS should include 1) immediate discontinuation of antipsychotic drugs and other drugs not essential to concurrent therapy, 2) intensive symptomatic treatment and medical monitoring, and 3) treatment of any concomitant serious medical problems for which specific treatments are available. There is no general agreement about specific pharmacological treatment regimens for uncomplicated NMS.

If a patient requires antipsychotic drug treatment after recovery from NMS, the potential reintroduction of drug therapy should be carefully considered. The patient should be carefully monitored, since recurrences of NMS have been reported.

An encephalopathic syndrome (characterized by weakness, lethargy, fever, tremulousness and confusion, extrapyramidal symptoms, leukocytosis, elevated serum enzymes, BUN and FBS) has occurred in a few patients treated with lithium plus a neuroleptic. In some instances, the syndrome was followed by irreversible brain damage. Because of a possible causal relationship between these events and the concomitant administration of lithium and neuroleptics, patients receiving such combined therapy should be monitored closely for early evidence of neurologic toxicity and treatment discontinued promptly if such signs appear. This encephalopathic syndrome may be similar to or the same as neuroleptic malignant syndrome (NMS).

Patients with bone marrow depression or who have previously demonstrated a hypersensitivity reaction (e.g., blood dyscrasias, jaundice) with a phenothiazine should not receive any phenothiazine, including *Compazine*, unless in the judgment of the physician the potential benefits of treatment outweigh the possible hazards.

Compazine (prochlorperazine) may impair mental and/or physical abilities, especially during the first few days of therapy. Therefore, caution patients about activities requiring alertness (e.g., operating vehicles or machinery).

Phenothiazines may intensify or prolong the action of central nervous system depressants (e.g., alcohol, anesthetics, narcotics).

Usage in Pregnancy: Safety for the use of *Compazine* during pregnancy has not been established. Therefore, *Compazine* is not recommended for use in pregnant patients except in cases of severe nausea and vomiting that are so serious and intractable that, in the judgment of the physician, drug intervention is required and potential benefits outweigh possible hazards.

There have been reported instances of prolonged jaundice, extrapyramidal signs, hyperreflexia or hyporeflexia in newborn infants whose mothers received phenothiazines.

Nursing Mothers: There is evidence that phenothiazines are excreted in the breast milk of nursing mothers. Caution should be exercised when *Compazine* is administered to a nursing woman.

PRECAUTIONS

The antiemetic action of Compazine (prochlorperazine) may mask the signs and symptoms of overdosage of other drugs and may obscure the diagnosis and treatment of other conditions such as intestinal obstruction, brain tumor and Reye's syndrome (see WARNINGS).

When *Compazine* is used with cancer chemotherapeutic drugs, vomiting as a sign of the toxicity of these agents may be obscured by the antiemetic effect of *Compazine*.

Because hypotension may occur, large doses and parenteral administration should be used cautiously in patients with

impaired cardiovascular systems. To minimize the occurrence of hypotension after injection, keep patient lying down and observe for at least $^1/_2$ hour. If hypotension occurs after parenteral or oral dosing, place patient in head-low position with legs raised. If a vasoconstrictor is required, Levophed®* and Neo-Synephrine®† are suitable. Other pressor agents, including epinephrine, should not be used because they may cause a paradoxical further lowering of blood pressure.

Aspiration of vomitus has occurred in a few post-surgical patients who have received Compazine (prochlorperazine) as an antiemetic. Although no causal relationship has been established, this possibility should be borne in mind during surgical aftercare.

Deep sleep, from which patients can be aroused, and coma have been reported, usually with overdosage.

Neuroleptic drugs elevate prolactin levels; the elevation persists during chronic administration. Tissue culture experiments indicate that approximately one third of human breast cancers are prolactin-dependent *in vitro*, a factor of potential importance if the prescribing of these drugs is contemplated in a patient with a previously detected breast cancer. Although disturbances such as galactorrhea, amenorrhea, gynecomastia and impotence have been reported, the clinical significance of elevated serum prolactin levels is unknown for most patients. An increase in mammary neoplasms has been found in rodents after chronic administration of neuroleptic drugs. Neither clinical nor epidemiologic studies conducted to date, however, have shown an association between chronic administration of these drugs and mammary tumorigenesis; the available evidence is considered too limited to be conclusive at this time.

Chromosomal aberrations in spermatocytes and abnormal sperm have been demonstrated in rodents treated with certain neuroleptics.

As with all drugs which exert an anticholinergic effect, and/or cause mydriasis, prochlorperazine should be used with caution in patients with glaucoma.

Because phenothiazines may interfere with thermoregulatory mechanisms, use with caution in persons who will be exposed to extreme heat.

Phenothiazines can diminish the effect of oral anticoagulants.

Phenothiazines can produce alpha-adrenergic blockade.

Thiazide diuretics may accentuate the orthostatic hypotension that may occur with phenothiazines.

Antihypertensive effects of guanethidine and related compounds may be counteracted when phenothiazines are used concomitantly.

Concomitant administration of propranolol with phenothiazines results in increased plasma levels of both drugs.

Phenothiazines may lower the convulsive threshold; dosage adjustments of anticonvulsants may be necessary. Potentiation of anticonvulsant effects does not occur. However, it has been reported that phenothiazines may interfere with the metabolism of Dilantin®‡ and thus precipitate *Dilantin* toxicity.

The presence of phenothiazines may produce false-positive phenylketonuria (PKU) test results.

Long-Term Therapy: Given the likelihood that some patients exposed chronically to neuroleptics will develop tardive dyskinesia, it is advised that all patients in whom chronic use is contemplated be given, if possible, full information about this risk. The decision to inform patients and/or their guardians must obviously take into account the clinical circumstances and the competency of the patient to understand the information provided.

To lessen the likelihood of adverse reactions related to cumulative drug effect, patients with a history of long-term therapy with Compazine (prochlorperazine) and/or other neuroleptics should be evaluated periodically to decide whether the maintenance dosage could be lowered or drug therapy discontinued.

Children with acute illnesses (e.g., chickenpox, CNS infections, measles, gastroenteritis) or dehydration seem to be much more susceptible to neuromuscular reactions, particularly dystonias, than are adults. In such patients, the drug should be used only under close supervision.

Drugs which lower the seizure threshold, including phenothiazine derivatives, should not be used with Amipaque®§. As with other phenothiazine derivatives, Compazine (prochlorperazine) should be discontinued at least 48 hours before myelography, should not be resumed for at least 24 hours postprocedure, and should not be used for the control of nausea and vomiting occurring either prior to myelography with *Amipaque*, or postprocedure.

Continued on next page

Information on the SmithKline Beecham Pharmaceuticals products appearing here is based on the labeling in effect on July 31, 1998. Further information on these and other products may be obtained from the Medical Department, SmithKline Beecham Pharmaceuticals, One Franklin Plaza, Philadelphia, PA 19101.

Compazine—Cont.

ADVERSE REACTIONS

Drowsiness, dizziness, amenorrhea, blurred vision, skin reactions and hypotension may occur. Neuroleptic Malignant Syndrome (NMS) has been reported in association with antipsychotic drugs (see WARNINGS).

Cholestatic jaundice has occurred. If fever with grippe-like symptoms occurs, appropriate liver studies should be conducted. If tests indicate an abnormality, stop treatment. There have been a few observations of fatty changes in the livers of patients who have died while receiving the drug. No causal relationship has been established.

Leukopenia and agranulocytosis have occurred. Warn patients to report the sudden appearance of sore throat or other signs of infection. If white blood cell and differential counts indicate leukocyte depression, stop treatment and start antibiotic and other suitable therapy.

Neuromuscular (Extrapyramidal) Reactions

These symptoms are seen in a significant number of hospitalized mental patients. They may be characterized by motor restlessness, be of the dystonic type, or they may resemble parkinsonism.

Depending on the severity of symptoms, dosage should be reduced or discontinued. If therapy is reinstituted, it should be at a lower dosage. Should these symptoms occur in children or pregnant patients, the drug should be stopped and not reinstituted. In most cases barbiturates by suitable route of administration will suffice. (Or, injectable Benadryl® may be useful). In more severe cases, the administration of an anti-parkinsonism agent, except levodopa, usually produces rapid reversal of symptoms. Suitable supportive measures such as maintaining a clear airway and adequate hydration should be employed.

Motor Restlessness: Symptoms may include agitation or jitteriness and sometimes insomnia. These symptoms often disappear spontaneously. At times these symptoms may be similar to the original neurotic or psychotic symptoms. Dosage should not be increased until these side effects have subsided.

If these symptoms become too troublesome, they can usually be controlled by a reduction of dosage or change of drug. Treatment with anti-parkinsonian agents, benzodiazepines or propranolol may be helpful.

Dystonias: Symptoms may include: spasm of the neck muscles, sometimes progressing to torticollis; extensor rigidity of back muscles, sometimes progressing to opisthotonos; carpopedal spasm, trismus, swallowing difficulty, oculogyric crisis and protrusion of the tongue.

These usually subside within a few hours, and almost always within 24 to 48 hours, after the drug has been discontinued.

In mild cases, reassurance or a barbiturate is often sufficient. In moderate cases, barbiturates will usually bring rapid relief. In more severe adult cases, the administration of an anti-parkinsonism agent, except levodopa, usually produces rapid reversal of symptoms. In children, reassurance and barbiturates will usually control symptoms. (Or, injectable Benadryl may be useful. Note: See Benadryl prescribing information for appropriate children's dosage.) If appropriate treatment with anti-parkinsonism agents or Benadryl fails to reverse the signs and symptoms, the diagnosis should be reevaluated.

Pseudo-parkinsonism: Symptoms may include: mask-like facies; drooling; tremors; pillrolling motion; cogwheel rigidity; and shuffling gait. Reassurance and sedation are important. In most cases these symptoms are readily controlled when an anti-parkinsonism agent is administered concomitantly. Anti-parkinsonism agents should be used only when required. Generally, therapy of a few weeks to 2 or 3 months will suffice. After this time patients should be evaluated to determine their need for continued treatment. (Note: Levodopa has not been found effective in pseudo-parkinsonism.) Occasionally it is necessary to lower the dosage of Compazine (prochlorperazine) or to discontinue the drug.

Tardive Dyskinesia: As with all antipsychotic agents, tardive dyskinesia may appear in some patients on long-term therapy or may appear after drug therapy has been discontinued. The syndrome can also develop, although much less frequently, after relatively brief treatment periods at low doses. This syndrome appears in all age groups. Although its prevalence appears to be highest among elderly patients, especially elderly women, it is impossible to rely upon prevalence estimates to predict at the inception of neuroleptic treatment which patients are likely to develop the syndrome. The symptoms are persistent and in some patients appear to be irreversible. The syndrome is characterized by rhythmical involuntary movements of the tongue, face, mouth or jaw (e.g., protrusion of tongue, puffing of cheeks, puckering of mouth, chewing movements). Sometimes these may be accompanied by involuntary movements of extremities. In rare instances, these involuntary movements of the extremities are the only manifestations of tardive dyskinesia. A variant of tardive dyskinesia, tardive dystonia, has also been described.

There is no known effective treatment for tardive dyskinesia; anti-parkinsonism agents do not alleviate the symptoms of this syndrome. It is suggested that all antipsychotic agents be discontinued if these symptoms appear.

Should it be necessary to reinstitute treatment, or increase the dosage of the agent, or switch to a different antipsychotic agent, the syndrome may be masked.

It has been reported that fine vermicular movements of the tongue may be an early sign of the syndrome and if the medication is stopped at that time the syndrome may not develop.

Contact Dermatitis: Avoid getting the Injection solution on hands or clothing because of the possibility of contact dermatitis.

Adverse Reactions Reported with Compazine (prochlorperazine) or Other Phenothiazine Derivatives: Adverse reactions with different phenothiazines vary in type, frequency and mechanism of occurrence, i.e., some are dose-related, while others involve individual patient sensitivity. Some adverse reactions may be more likely to occur, or occur with greater intensity, in patients with special medical problems, e.g., patients with mitral insufficiency or pheochromocytoma have experienced severe hypotension following recommended doses of certain phenothiazines.

Not all of the following adverse reactions have been observed with every phenothiazine derivative, but they have been reported with 1 or more and should be borne in mind when drugs of this class are administered: extrapyramidal symptoms (opisthotonos, oculogyric crisis, hyperreflexia, dystonia, akathisia, dyskinesia, parkinsonism) some of which have lasted months and even years—particularly in elderly patients with previous brain damage; grand mal and petit mal convulsions, particularly in patients with EEG abnormalities or history of such disorders; altered cerebrospinal fluid proteins; cerebral edema; intensification and prolongation of the action of central nervous system depressants (opiates, analgesics, antihistamines, barbiturates, alcohol), atropine, heat, organophosphorus insecticides; autonomic reactions (dryness of mouth, nasal congestion, headache, nausea, constipation, obstipation, adynamic ileus, ejaculatory disorders/impotence, priapism, atonic colon, urinary retention, miosis and mydriasis); reactivation of psychotic processes, catatonic-like states; hypotension (sometimes fatal); cardiac arrest; blood dyscrasias (pancytopenia, thrombocytopenic purpura, leukopenia, agranulocytosis, eosinophilia, hemolytic anemia, aplastic anemia); liver damage (jaundice, biliary stasis); endocrine disturbances (hyperglycemia, hypoglycemia, glycosuria, lactation, galactorrhea, gynecomastia, menstrual irregularities, false-positive pregnancy tests); skin disorders (photosensitivity, itching, erythema, urticaria, eczema up to exfoliative dermatitis); other allergic reactions (asthma, laryngeal edema, angioneurotic edema, anaphylactoid reactions); peripheral edema; reversed epinephrine effect; hyperpyrexia; mild fever after large I.M. doses; increased appetite; increased weight; a systemic lupus erythematosus-like syndrome; pigmentary retinopathy; with prolonged administration of substantial doses, skin pigmentation, epithelial keratopathy, and lenticular and corneal deposits.

EKG changes—particularly nonspecific, usually reversible Q and T wave distortions—have been observed in some patients receiving phenothiazine tranquilizers.

Although phenothiazines cause neither psychic nor physical dependence, sudden discontinuance in long-term psychiatric patients may cause temporary symptoms, e.g., nausea and vomiting, dizziness, tremulousness.

Note: There have been occasional reports of sudden death in patients receiving phenothiazines. In some cases, the cause appeared to be cardiac arrest or asphyxia due to failure of the cough reflex.

DOSAGE AND ADMINISTRATION

Notes on Injection: Stability—This solution should be protected from light. This is a clear, colorless to pale yellow solution; a slight yellowish discoloration will not alter potency. If markedly discolored, solution should be discarded.

Compatibility—It is recommended that Compazine (prochlorperazine) Injection not be mixed with other agents in the syringe.

DOSAGE AND ADMINISTRATION—ADULTS

(For children's dosage and administration, see below.) Dosage should be increased more gradually in debilitated or emaciated patients.

Elderly Patients: In general, dosages in the lower range are sufficient for most elderly patients. Since they appear to be more susceptible to hypotension and neuromuscular reactions, such patients should be observed closely. Dosage should be tailored to the individual, response carefully monitored and dosage adjusted accordingly. Dosage should be increased more gradually in elderly patients.

1. To Control Severe Nausea and Vomiting: Adjust dosage to the response of the individual. Begin with the lowest recommended dosage.

Oral Dosage—Tablets: Usually one 5 mg or 10 mg tablet 3 or 4 times daily. Daily dosages above 40 mg should be used only in resistant cases.

Spansule capsules: Initially, usually one 15 mg capsule on arising or one 10 mg capsule q12h. Daily doses above 40 mg should be used only in resistant cases.

Rectal Dosage: 25 mg twice daily.

I.M. Dosage: Initially 5 to 10 mg (1 to 2 mL) injected deeply into the upper outer quadrant of the buttock. If necessary, repeat every 3 or 4 hours. Total I.M. dosage should not exceed 40 mg per day.

I.V. Dosage: $2\frac{1}{2}$ to 10 mg ($\frac{1}{2}$ to 2 mL) by slow I.V. injection or infusion at a rate not to exceed 5 mg per minute. Compazine Injection may be administered either undiluted or diluted in isotonic solution. A single dose of the drug should not exceed 10 mg; total I.V. dosage should not exceed 40 mg per day. When administered I.V., do not use bolus injection. Hypotension is a possibility if the drug is given by I.V. injection or infusion.

Subcutaneous administration is not advisable because of local irritation.

2. Adult Surgery (for severe nausea and vomiting): Total parenteral dosage should not exceed 40 mg per day. Hypotension is a possibility if the drug is given by I.V. injection or infusion.

I.M. Dosage: 5 to 10 mg (1 to 2 mL) 1 to 2 hours before induction of anesthesia (repeat once in 30 minutes, if necessary), or to control acute symptoms during and after surgery (repeat once if necessary).

I.V. Dosage: 5 to 10 mg (1 to 2 mL) as a slow I.V. injection or infusion 15 to 30 minutes before induction of anesthesia, or to control acute symptoms during or after surgery. Repeat once if necessary. Compazine (prochlorperazine) may be administered either undiluted or diluted in isotonic solution, but a single dose of the drug should not exceed 10 mg. The rate of administration should not exceed 5 mg per minute. When administered I.V., do not use bolus injection.

3. In Adult Psychiatric Disorders: Adjust dosage to the response of the individual and according to the severity of the condition. Begin with the lowest recommended dose. Although response ordinarily is seen within a day or 2, longer treatment is usually required before maximal improvement is seen.

Oral Dosage: Non-Psychotic Anxiety—Usual dosage is 5 mg 3 or 4 times daily; by Spansule capsule, usually one 15 mg capsule on arising or one 10 mg capsule q12h. Do not administer in doses of more than 20 mg per day or for longer than 12 weeks.

Psychotic Disorders—In relatively mild conditions, as seen in private psychiatric practice or in outpatient clinics, dosage is 5 or 10 mg 3 or 4 times daily.

In moderate to severe conditions, for hospitalized or adequately supervised patients, usual starting dosage is 10 mg 3 or 4 times daily. Increase dosage gradually until symptoms are controlled or side effects become bothersome. When dosage is increased by small increments every 2 or 3 days, side effects either do not occur or are easily controlled. Some patients respond satisfactorily on 50 to 75 mg daily. In more severe disturbances, optimum dosage is usually 100 to 150 mg daily.

I.M. Dosage: For immediate control of severely disturbed adults, inject an initial dose of 10 to 20 mg (2 to 4 mL) deeply into the upper outer quadrant of the buttock. Many patients respond shortly after the first injection. If necessary, however, repeat the initial dose every 2 to 4 hours (or, in resistant cases, every hour) to gain control of the patient. More than three or four doses are seldom necessary. After control is achieved, switch patient to an oral form of the drug at the same dosage level or higher. If, in rare cases, parenteral therapy is needed for a prolonged period, give 10 to 20 mg (2 to 4 mL) every 4 to 6 hours. Pain and irritation at the site of injection have seldom occurred.

Subcutaneous administration is not advisable because of local irritation.

DOSAGE AND ADMINISTRATION—CHILDREN

Do not use in pediatric surgery.

Children seem more prone to develop extrapyramidal reactions, even on moderate doses. Therefore, use lowest effective dosage. Tell parents not to exceed prescribed dosage, since the possibility of adverse reactions increases as dosage rises.

Occasionally the patient may react to the drug with signs of restlessness and excitement; if this occurs, do not administer additional doses. Take particular precaution in administering the drug to children with acute illnesses or dehydration (see under Dystonias).

When writing a prescription for the $2\frac{1}{2}$ mg size suppository, write "$2\frac{1}{2}$," not "2.5"; this will help avoid confusion with the 25 mg adult size.

1. Severe Nausea and Vomiting in Children: Compazine (prochlorperazine) should not be used in pediatric patients under 20 pounds in weight or 2 years of age. It should not be used in conditions for which children's dosages have not been established. Dosage and frequency of administration should be adjusted according to the severity of the symptoms and the response of the patient. The duration of activity following intramuscular administration may last up to 12 hours. Subsequent doses may be given by the same route if necessary.

Oral or Rectal Dosage: More than 1 day's therapy is seldom necessary.

Weight	Usual Dosage	Not to Exceed
under 20 lbs not recommended		
20 to 29 lbs	$2^1/_2$ mg 1 or 2 times a day	7.5 mg per day
30 to 39 lbs	$2^1/_2$ mg 2 or 3 times a day	10 mg per day
40 to 85 lbs	$2^1/_2$ mg 3 times a day or 5 mg 2 times a day	15 mg per day

I.M. Dosage: Calculate each dose on the basis of 0.06 mg of the drug per lb of body weight; give by deep I.M. injection. Control is usually obtained with one dose.

2. **In Psychotic Children:**

Oral or Rectal Dosage: For children 2 to 12 years, starting dosage is $2^1/_2$ mg 2 or 3 times daily. Do not give more than 10 mg the first day. Then increase dosage according to patient's response.

FOR AGES 2 to 5, total daily dosage usually does not exceed 20 mg.

FOR AGES 6 to 12, total daily dosage usually does not exceed 25 mg.

I.M. Dosage: For ages under 12, calculate each dose on the basis of 0.06 mg of Compazine (prochlorperazine) per lb of body weight; give by deep I.M. injection. Control is usually obtained with one dose. After control is achieved, switch the patient to an oral form of the drug at the same dosage level or higher.

OVERDOSAGE

(See also ADVERSE REACTIONS.)

SYMPTOMS—Primarily involvement of the extrapyramidal mechanism producing some of the dystonic reactions described above.

Symptoms of central nervous system depression to the point of somnolence or coma. Agitation and restlessness may also occur. Other possible manifestations include convulsions, EKG changes and cardiac arrhythmias, fever and autonomic reactions such as hypotension, dry mouth and ileus.

TREATMENT—It is important to determine other medications taken by the patient since multiple-dose therapy is common in overdosage situations. Treatment is essentially symptomatic and supportive. Early gastric lavage is helpful. Keep patient under observation and maintain an open airway, since involvement of the extrapyramidal mechanism may produce dysphagia and respiratory difficulty in severe overdosage. **Do not attempt to induce emesis because a dystonic reaction of the head or neck may develop that could result in aspiration of vomitus.** Extrapyramidal symptoms may be treated with anti-parkinsonism drugs, barbiturates or *Benadryl*. See prescribing information for these products. Care should be taken to avoid increasing respiratory depression.

If administration of a stimulant is desirable, amphetamine, dextroamphetamine or caffeine with sodium benzoate is recommended.

Stimulants that may cause convulsions (e.g., picrotoxin or pentylenetetrazol) should be avoided.

If hypotension occurs, the standard measures for managing circulatory shock should be initiated. If it is desirable to administer a vasoconstrictor, *Levophed* and *Neo-Synephrine* are most suitable. Other pressor agents, including epinephrine, are not recommended because phenothiazine derivatives may reverse the usual elevating action of these agents and cause a further lowering of blood pressure.

Limited experience indicates that phenothiazines are *not* dialyzable.

Special note on Spansule *capsules* —Since much of the *Spansule* capsule medication is coated for gradual release, therapy directed at reversing the effects of the ingested drug and at supporting the patient should be continued for as long as overdosage symptoms remain. Saline cathartics are useful for hastening evacuation of pellets that have not already released medication.

HOW SUPPLIED

Tablets—5 and 10 mg, in bottles of 100; in Single Unit Packages of 100 (intended for institutional use only).
5 mg 100's: NDC 0007-3366-20
5 mg SUP 100's: NDC 0007-3366-21
10 mg 100's: NDC 0007-3367-20
10 mg SUP 100's: NDC 0007-3367-21

***Spansule* capsules**—10 and 15 mg, in bottles of 50.
10 mg 50's: NDC 0007-3344-15
15 mg 50's: NDC 0007-3346-15

Vials—2 mL (5 mg/mL), in boxes of 25 and 10 mL (5 mg/mL), in boxes of 1.
2 mL (5 mg/mL), in boxes of 25: NDC 0007-3352-16
10 mL (5 mg/mL), in boxes of 1: NDC 0007-3343-01

Suppositories—$2^1/_2$ mg (for young children), 5 mg (for older children) and 25 mg (for adults), in boxes of 12.
$2^1/_2$ mg, in boxes of 12: NDC 0007-3360-03
5 mg, in boxes of 12: NDC 0007-3361-03
25 mg, in boxes of 12: NDC 0007-3362-03

Syrup—5 mg/5 mL (1 teaspoonful) in 4 fl oz bottles.
5 mg/5 mL, 4 fl oz: NDC 0007-3363-44

Store Compazine (prochlorperazine) vials below 30°C (86°F). Do not freeze. Other dosage forms can be stored between 15° and 30°C (59° and 86°F). Protect from light.

* norepinephrine bitartrate, Sanofi Winthrop Pharmaceuticals.
† phenylephrine hydrochloride, Sanofi Winthrop Pharmaceuticals.
‡ phenytoin, Parke-Davis.
§ metrizamide, Sanofi Winthrop Pharmaceuticals.
‖ diphenhydramine hydrochloride, Parke-Davis.

Veterans Administration/Military/PHS—Vials, 2 mL, 25's, 6505-01-230-3931; 10 mL, 1's, 6505-00-684-9630; Suppositories, $2^1/_2$ mg, 12's, 6505-00-133-5213; 5 mg, 12's, 6505-01-153-2894; 25 mg, 12's, 6505-00-133-5214; Syrup, 5 mg/5 mL, 4 fl oz, 6505-01-039-5849; Tablets, 5 mg, 100's, 6505-00-761-5640; 5 mg, 100's (SUP), 6505-00-118-2563; 10 mg, 100's, 6505-01-354-1042; 10 mg, 100's (SUP), 6505-00-092-3139.
CZ:L90

Shown in Product Identification Guide, page 339

COREG® ℞

[kō-reg]
brand of carvedilol Tablets

DESCRIPTION

Carvedilol is a nonselective β-adrenergic blocking agent with α_1-blocking activity. It is (±)-1-(Carbazol-4-yloxy)-3-[[2-(o-methoxyphenoxy)ethyl]amino]-2-propanol. It is a racemic mixture with the following structure:

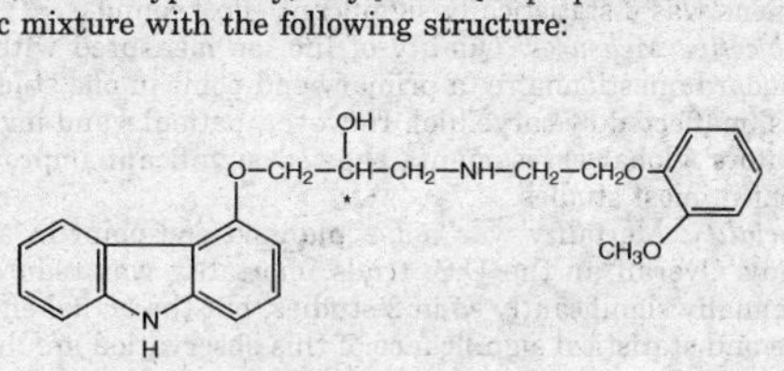

carvedilol

Tablets for Oral Administration:

Coreg (carvedilol) is a white, oval, film-coated tablet containing 3.125 mg, 6.25 mg, 12.5 mg or 25 mg of carvedilol. The 6.25 mg, 12.5 mg and 25 mg tablets are Tiltab® tablets. Inactive ingredients consist of colloidal silicon dioxide, crospovidone, hydroxypropyl methylcellulose, lactose, magnesium stearate, polyethylene glycol, polysorbate 80, povidone, sucrose and titanium dioxide.

Carvedilol is a white to off-white powder with a molecular weight of 406.5 and a molecular formula of $C_{24}H_{26}N_2O_4$. It is freely soluble in dimethylsulfoxide; soluble in methylene chloride and methanol; sparingly soluble in 95% ethanol and isopropanol; slightly soluble in ethyl ether; and practically insoluble in water, gastric fluid (simulated, TS, pH 1.1) and intestinal fluid (simulated, TS without pancreatin, pH 7.5).

CLINICAL PHARMACOLOGY

Coreg is a racemic mixture in which nonselective β-adrenoreceptor blocking activity is present in the S(-) enantiomer and α-adrenergic blocking activity is present in both R(+) and S(-) enantiomers at equal potency. *Coreg* has no intrinsic sympathomimetic activity.

Pharmacokinetics

Coreg is rapidly and extensively absorbed following oral administration, with absolute bioavailability of approximately 25% to 35% due to a significant degree of first-pass metabolism. Following oral administration, the apparent mean terminal elimination half-life of carvedilol generally ranges from 7 to 10 hours. Plasma concentrations achieved are proportional to the oral dose administered. When administered with food, the rate of absorption is slowed, as evidenced by a delay in the time to reach peak plasma levels, with no significant difference in extent of bioavailability. Taking *Coreg* with food should minimize the risk of orthostatic hypotension.

Carvedilol is extensively metabolized. Following oral administration of radiolabelled carvedilol to healthy volunteers, carvedilol accounted for only about 7% of the total radioactivity in plasma as measured by area under the curve (AUC). Less than 2% of the dose was excreted unchanged in the urine. Carvedilol is metabolized primarily by aromatic ring oxidation and glucuronidation. The oxidative metabolites are further metabolized by conjugation via glucuronidation and sulfation. The metabolites of carvedilol are excreted primarily via the bile into the feces. Demethylation and hydroxylation at the phenol ring produce three active metabolites with β-receptor blocking activity. Based on preclinical studies, the 4'-hydroxyphenyl metabolite is approximately 13 times more potent than carvedilol for β-blockade. Compared to carvedilol, the three active metabolites exhibit weak vasodilating activity. Plasma concentrations of the active metabolites are about one-tenth of those observed for carvedilol and have pharmacokinetics similar to the parent.

Carvedilol undergoes stereoselective first-pass metabolism with plasma levels of R(+)-carvedilol approximately 2 to 3 times higher than S(-)-carvedilol following oral administration in healthy subjects. The mean apparent terminal elimination half-lives for R(+)-carvedilol range from 5 to 9 hours compared with 7 to 11 hours for the S(-)-enantiomer.

The primary P450 enzymes responsible for the metabolism of both R(+) and S(-)-carvedilol in human liver microsomes were CYP2D6 and CYP2C9 and to a lesser extent CYP3A4, 2C19, 1A2, and 2E1. CYP2D6 is thought to be the major enzyme in the 4'- and 5'-hydroxylation of carvedilol, with a potential contribution from 3A4. CYP2C9 is thought to be of primary importance in the O-methylation pathway of S(-)-carvedilol.

Carvedilol is subject to the effects of genetic polymorphism with poor metabolizers of debrisoquin (a marker for cytochrome P450 2D6) exhibiting 2- to 3-fold higher plasma concentrations of R(+)-carvedilol compared to extensive metabolizers. In contrast, plasma levels of S(-)- carvedilol are increased only about 20% to 25% in poor metabolizers, indicating this enantiomer is metabolized to a lesser extent by cytochrome P450 2D6 than R(+)-carvedilol. The pharmacokinetics of carvedilol do not appear to be different in poor metabolizers of S-mephenytoin (patients deficient in cytochrome P450 2C19).

Carvedilol is more than 98% bound to plasma proteins, primarily with albumin. The plasma-protein binding is independent of concentration over the therapeutic range. Carvedilol is a basic, lipophilic compound with a steady-state volume of distribution of approximately 115 L, indicating substantial distribution into extravascular tissues. Plasma clearance ranges from 500 to 700 mL/min.

Congestive Heart Failure: Steady-state plasma concentrations of carvedilol and its enantiomers increased proportionally over the 6.25 to 50 mg dose range in patients with congestive heart failure. Compared to healthy subjects, congestive heart failure patients had increased mean AUC and C_{max} values for carvedilol and its enantiomers, with up to 50% to 100% higher values observed in 6 patients with NYHA class IV heart failure. The mean apparent terminal elimination half-life for carvedilol was similar to that observed in healthy subjects.

Pharmacokinetic Drug-Drug Interactions: Since carvedilol undergoes substantial oxidative metabolism, the metabolism and pharmacokinetics of carvedilol may be affected by induction or inhibition of cytochrome P450 enzymes.

Rifampin: In a pharmacokinetic study conducted in 8 healthy male subjects, rifampin (600 mg daily for 12 days) decreased the AUC and C_{max} of carvedilol by about 70%.

Cimetidine: In a pharmacokinetic study conducted in 10 healthy male subjects, cimetidine (1000 mg/day) increased the steady-state AUC of carvedilol by 30% with no change in C_{max}.

Glyburide: In 12 healthy subjects, combined administration of carvedilol (25 mg once daily) and a single dose of glyburide did not result in a clinically relevant pharmacokinetic interaction for either compound.

Hydrochlorothiazide: A single oral dose of carvedilol 25 mg did not alter the pharmacokinetics of a single oral dose of hydrochlorothiazide 25 mg in 12 patients with hypertension. Likewise, hydrochlorothiazide had no effect on the pharmacokinetics of carvedilol.

Digoxin: Following concomitant administration of carvedilol (25 mg once daily) and digoxin (0.25 mg once daily) for 14 days, steady-state AUC and trough concentrations of digoxin were increased by 14% and 16%, respectively, in 12 hypertensive patients.

Torsemide: In a study of 12 healthy subjects, combined oral administration of carvedilol 25 mg once daily and torsemide 5 mg once daily for 5 days did not result in any significant differences in their pharmacokinetics compared with administration of the drugs alone.

Warfarin: Carvedilol (12.5 mg twice daily) did not have an effect on the steady-state prothrombin time ratios and did not alter the pharmacokinetics of R(+)- and S(-)-warfarin following concomitant administration with warfarin in 9 healthy volunteers.

Continued on next page

Information on the SmithKline Beecham Pharmaceuticals products appearing here is based on the labeling in effect on July 31, 1998. Further information on these and other products may be obtained from the Medical Department, SmithKline Beecham Pharmaceuticals, One Franklin Plaza, Philadelphia, PA 19101.

Consult 1999 PDR® supplements and future editions for revisions

Coreg—Cont.

Special Populations

Elderly: Plasma levels of carvedilol average about 50% higher in the elderly compared to young subjects.

Hepatic Impairment: Compared to healthy subjects, patients with cirrhotic liver disease exhibit significantly higher concentrations of carvedilol (approximately 4- to 7-fold) following single-dose therapy (see WARNINGS, Hepatic Injury).

Renal Insufficiency: Although carvedilol is metabolized primarily by the liver, plasma concentrations of carvedilol have been reported to be increased in patients with renal impairment. Based on mean AUC data, approximately 40% to 50% higher plasma concentrations of carvedilol were observed in hypertensive patients with moderate to severe renal impairment compared to a control group of hypertensive patients with normal renal function. However, the ranges of AUC values were similar for both groups. Changes in mean peak plasma levels were less pronounced, approximately 12% to 26% higher in patients with impaired renal function. Consistent with its high degree of plasma protein-binding, carvedilol does not appear to be cleared significantly by hemodialysis.

Pharmacodynamics and Clinical Trials
Congestive Heart Failure
Pharmacodynamics

The basis for the beneficial effects of Coreg (carvedilol) in congestive heart failure is not established.

Two placebo-controlled studies compared the acute hemodynamic effects of *Coreg* to baseline measurements in 59 and 49 patients with NYHA class II-IV heart failure receiving diuretics, ACE inhibitors, and digitalis. There were significant reductions in systemic blood pressure, pulmonary artery pressure, pulmonary capillary wedge pressure, and heart rate. Initial effects on cardiac output, stroke volume index, and systemic vascular resistance were small and variable.

These studies measured hemodynamic effects again at 12 to 14 weeks. *Coreg* significantly reduced systemic blood pressure, pulmonary artery pressure, right atrial pressure, systemic vascular resistance, and heart rate, while stroke volume index was increased.

Among 839 patients with NYHA class II-III heart failure treated for 26 to 52 weeks in 4 U.S. placebo-controlled trials, average left ventricular ejection fraction (EF) measured by radionuclide ventriculography increased by 8 EF units (%) in *Coreg* patients and by 2 EF units in placebo patients (between-group difference of 6 EF units). This treatment effect was nominally statistically significant in each trial.

Hypertension
Pharmacodynamics

The mechanism by which β-blockade produces an antihypertensive effect has not been established.

β-adrenoreceptor blocking activity has been demonstrated in animal and human studies showing that carvedilol (1) reduces cardiac output in normal subjects; (2) reduces exercise- and/or isoproterenol-induced tachycardia and (3) reduces reflex orthostatic tachycardia. Significant β-adrenoreceptor blocking effect is usually seen within 1 hour of drug administration.

α_1-adrenoreceptor blocking activity has been demonstrated in human and animal studies, showing that carvedilol (1) attenuates the pressor effects of phenylephrine; (2) causes vasodilation and (3) reduces peripheral vascular resistance. These effects contribute to the reduction of blood pressure and usually are seen within 30 minutes of drug administration.

Due to the α_1-receptor blocking activity of carvedilol, blood pressure is lowered more in the standing than in the supine position, and symptoms of postural hypotension (1.8%), including rare instances of syncope, can occur. Following oral administration, when postural hypotension has occurred, it has been transient and is uncommon when Coreg (carvedilol) is administered with food at the recommended starting dose and titration increments are closely followed (see DOSAGE AND ADMINISTRATION).

In hypertensive patients with normal renal function, therapeutic doses of *Coreg* decreased renal vascular resistance with no change in glomerular filtration rate or renal plasma flow. Changes in excretion of sodium, potassium, uric acid and phosphorus in hypertensive patients with normal renal function were similar after *Coreg* and placebo. *Coreg* has little effect on plasma catecholamines, plasma aldosterone or electrolyte levels, but it does significantly reduce plasma renin activity when given for at least 4 weeks. It also increases levels of atrial natriuretic peptide.

CLINICAL TRIALS
Congestive Heart Failure

Four U.S. multicenter, double-blind, placebo-controlled studies enrolled 1094 patients (696 randomized to carvedilol) with NYHA class II-III heart failure and ejection fraction <0.35. The vast majority were on digitalis, diuretics, and an ACE inhibitor at study entry. Patients were assigned to the studies based upon exercise ability. An Austra-

lia-New Zealand double-blind, placebo-controlled study enrolled 415 patients (half randomized to carvedilol) with less severe heart failure. All protocols excluded patients expected to undergo cardiac surgery during the 6 to 12 months of double-blind follow-up. All randomized patients had tolerated a 2-week course on carvedilol 6.25 mg b.i.d.

In each study, there was a primary end-point, either progression of heart failure (one U.S. study) or exercise tolerance (2 U.S. studies meeting enrollment goals and the Australia-New Zealand study). There were many secondary end-points specified in these studies, including NYHA classification, patient and physician global assessments, and cardiovascular hospitalization. Death was not a specified end-point in any study, but it was analyzed in all studies. Other analyses not prospectively planned included the sum of deaths and total or cardiovascular hospitalizations. In situations where the primary end-points of a trial do not show a significant benefit of treatment, assignment of significance values to the other results is complex, and such values need to be interpreted cautiously.

The results of the U.S. and Australia-New Zealand trials were as follows:

Slowing Progression of Heart Failure: One U.S. multicenter study (366 subjects) had as its primary end-point the sum of cardiovascular mortality, cardiovascular hospitalization, and sustained increase in heart failure medications. Heart failure progression was reduced, during an average follow-up of 7 months, by 48% (p=0.008).

In the Australia-New Zealand study, death and total hospitalizations were reduced by about 25% over 18 to 24 months. In the three largest U.S. studies, death and total hospitalizations were reduced by 19%, 39% and 49%, nominally statistically significant in the last two studies. The Australia-New Zealand results were statistically borderline.

Functional Measures: None of the multicenter studies had NYHA classification as a primary end-point, but all such studies had it as a secondary end-point. There was at least a trend toward improvement in NYHA class in all studies. Exercise tolerance was the primary end-point in 3 studies; in none was a statistically significant effect found.

Subjective Measures: Quality of life, as measured with a standard questionnaire (a primary end-point in one study), was unaffected by carvedilol. However, patients' and investigators' global assessments showed significant improvement in most studies.

Mortality: Mortality was not a planned end-point in any study. Overall, in the U.S. trials, mortality was reduced, nominally significantly so in 2 studies, but the actual effect size and statistical significance of this observation are difficult to define.

Hypertension

Coreg was studied in two placebo-controlled trials that utilized twice-daily dosing, at total daily doses of 12.5 to 50 mg. In these and other studies, the starting dose did not exceed 12.5 mg. At 50 mg per day, *Coreg* reduced sitting trough (12-hour) blood pressure by about 9/5.5 mm Hg; at 25 mg/day the effect was about 7.5/3.5 mm Hg. Comparisons of trough to peak blood pressure showed a trough to peak ratio for blood pressure response of about 65%. Heart rate fell by about 7.5 beats per minute at 50 mg/day. In general, as is true for other β-blockers, responses were smaller in black than non-black patients. There were no age- or gender-related differences in response.

The peak antihypertensive effect occurred 1 to 2 hours after a dose. The dose-related blood pressure response was accompanied by a dose-related increase in adverse effects (see ADVERSE REACTIONS).

INDICATIONS AND USAGE
Congestive Heart Failure

Coreg is indicated for the treatment of mild or moderate (NYHA class II or III) heart failure of ischemic or cardiomyopathic origin, in conjunction with digitalis, diuretics, and ACE inhibitor, to reduce the progression of disease as evidenced by cardiovascular death, cardiovascular hospitalization, or the need to adjust other heart failure medications.

Coreg may be used in patients unable to tolerate an ACE inhibitor. *Coreg* may be used in patients who are or are not receiving digitalis, hydralazine or nitrate therapy.

Hypertension

Coreg (carvedilol) is also indicated for the management of essential hypertension. It can be used alone or in combination with other antihypertensive agents, especially thiazide-type diuretics (see PRECAUTIONS, Drug Interactions).

CONTRAINDICATIONS

Coreg is contraindicated in patients with NYHA class IV decompensated cardiac failure requiring intravenous inotropic therapy, bronchial asthma (two cases of death from status asthmaticus have been reported in patients receiving single doses of *Coreg*) or related bronchospastic conditions, second- or third-degree AV block, sick sinus syndrome (unless a permanent pacemaker is in place), cardiogenic shock or severe bradycardia.

Use of *Coreg* in patients with clinically manifest hepatic impairment is not recommended.

Coreg is contraindicated in patients with hypersensitivity to the drug.

WARNINGS

Hepatic Injury: Mild hepatocellular injury, confirmed by rechallenge, has occurred rarely with *Coreg* therapy. In controlled studies of hypertensive patients, the incidence of liver function abnormalities reported as adverse experiences was 1.1% (13 of 1,142 patients) in patients receiving *Coreg* and 0.9% (4 of 462 patients) in those receiving placebo. One patient receiving carvedilol in a placebo-controlled trial withdrew for abnormal hepatic function.

In controlled studies of congestive heart failure, the incidence of liver function abnormalities reported as adverse experiences was 5.0% (38 of 765 patients) in patients receiving *Coreg* and 4.6% (20 of 437 patients) in those receiving placebo. Three patients receiving carvedilol (0.4%) and two patients receiving placebo (0.5%) in placebo-controlled trials withdrew for abnormal hepatic function.

Hepatic injury has been reversible and has occurred after short- and/or long-term therapy with minimal clinical symptomatology. No deaths due to liver function abnormalities have been reported.

At the first symptom/sign of liver dysfunction (e.g., pruritus, dark urine, persistent anorexia, jaundice, right upper quadrant tenderness or unexplained "flu-like" symptoms), laboratory testing should be performed. If the patient has laboratory evidence of liver injury or jaundice, carvedilol should be stopped and not restarted.

Peripheral Vascular Disease: β-blockers can precipitate or aggravate symptoms of arterial insufficiency in patients with peripheral vascular disease. Caution should be exercised in such individuals.

Anesthesia and Major Surgery: If *Coreg* treatment is to be continued perioperatively, particular care should be taken when anesthetic agents which depress myocardial function, such as ether, cyclopropane and trichloroethylene, are used. See OVERDOSAGE for information on treatment of bradycardia and hypertension.

Diabetes and Hypoglycemia: β-blockers may mask some of the manifestations of hypoglycemia, particularly tachycardia. Nonselective β-blockers may potentiate insulin-induced hypoglycemia and delay recovery of serum glucose levels. Patients subject to spontaneous hypoglycemia, or diabetic patients receiving insulin or oral hypoglycemic agents, should be cautioned about these possibilities and carvedilol should be used with caution. In congestive heart failure patients, there is a risk of worsening hyperglycemia (see PRECAUTIONS).

Thyrotoxicosis: β-adrenergic blockade may mask clinical signs of hyperthyroidism, such as tachycardia. Abrupt withdrawal of β-blockade may be followed by an exacerbation of the symptoms of hyperthyroidism or may precipitate thyroid storm.

PRECAUTIONS
General

Since Coreg (carvedilol) has β-blocking activity, it should not be discontinued abruptly, particularly in patients with ischemic heart disease. Instead, it should be discontinued over 1 to 2 weeks.

In clinical trials, *Coreg* caused bradycardia in about 2% of hypertensive patients and 9% of congestive heart failure patients. If pulse rate drops below 55 beats/min., the dosage should be reduced.

Hypotension and postural hypotension occurred in 9.7% and syncope in 3.4% of congestive heart failure patients receiving carvedilol compared to 3.6% and 2.5% of placebo patients, respectively. The risk for these events was highest during the first 30 days of dosing, corresponding to the up-titration period and was a cause for discontinuation of therapy in 0.7% of carvedilol patients, compared to 0.4% of placebo patients.

Postural hypotension occurred in 1.8% and syncope in 0.1% of hypertensive patients, primarily following the initial dose or at the time of dose increase and was a cause for discontinuation of therapy in 1% of patients.

To decrease the likelihood of syncope or excessive hypotension, treatment should be initiated with 3.125 mg b.i.d. for congestive heart failure patients and 6.25 mg b.i.d. for hypertensive patients. Dosage should then be increased slowly, according to recommendations in the DOSAGE AND ADMINISTRATION section, and the drug should be taken with food. During initiation of therapy, the patient should be cautioned to avoid situations such as driving or hazardous tasks, where injury could result should syncope occur.

Rarely, use of carvedilol in patients with congestive heart failure has resulted in deterioration of renal function. Patients at risk appear to be those with low blood pressure (systolic BP<100 mm Hg), ischemic heart disease and diffuse vascular disease, and/or underlying renal insufficiency. Renal function has returned to baseline when carvedilol was stopped. In patients with these risk factors it is recommended that renal function be monitored during up-titration of carvedilol and the drug discontinued or dosage reduced if worsening of renal function occurs.

Worsening cardiac failure or fluid retention may occur during up-titration of carvedilol. If such symptoms occur, diuretics should be increased and the carvedilol dose should not be advanced until clinical stability resumes (see DOSAGE AND ADMINISTRATION). Occasionally it is necessary to lower the carvedilol dose or temporarily discontinue it. Such episodes do not preclude subsequent successful titration of carvedilol.

In patients with pheochromocytoma, an α-blocking agent should be initiated prior to the use of any β-blocking agent. Although carvedilol has both α- and β-blocking pharmacologic activities, there has been no experience with its use in this condition. Therefore, caution should be taken in the administration of carvedilol to patients suspected of having pheochromocytoma.

Agents with non-selective β-blocking activity may provoke chest pain in patients with Prinzmetal's variant angina. There has been no clinical experience with carvedilol in these patients although the α-blocking activity may prevent such symptoms. However, caution should be taken in the administration of carvedilol to patients suspected of having Prinzmetal's variant angina.

Risk of Anaphylactic Reaction
While taking β-blockers, patients with a history of severe anaphylactic reaction to a variety of allergens may be more reactive to repeated challenge, either accidental, diagnostic or therapeutic. Such patients may be unresponsive to the usual doses of epinephrine used to treat allergic reaction.

Nonallergic Bronchospasm (e.g., chronic bronchitis and emphysema)
Patients with bronchospastic disease should, in general, not receive β-blockers. *Coreg* may be used with caution, however, in patients who do not respond to, or cannot tolerate, other antihypertensive agents. It is prudent, if Coreg (carvedilol) is used, to use the smallest effective dose, so that inhibition of endogenous or exogenous β-agonists is minimized.

In clinical trials of patients with congestive heart failure, patients with bronchospastic disease were enrolled if they did not require oral or inhaled medication to treat their bronchospastic disease. In such patients, it is recommended that carvedilol be used with caution. The dosing recommendations should be followed closely and the dose should be lowered if any evidence of bronchospasm is observed during up-titration.

Hypertensive Patients with Left Ventricular Failure: In hypertensive patients who have congestive heart failure controlled with digitalis, diuretics and/or an angiotensin-converting enzyme inhibitor, Coreg (carvedilol) may be used. However, since it is likely that such patients are dependent, in part, on sympathetic stimulation for circulatory support, it is recommended that dosing follow the instructions for patients with congestive heart failure.

In congestive heart failure patients with diabetes, carvedilol therapy may lead to worsening hyperglycemia, which responds to intensification of hypoglycemic therapy. It is recommended that blood glucose be monitored when carvedilol dosing is initiated, adjusted, or discontinued.

Information for Patients
Patients taking *Coreg* should be advised of the following:
— they should not interrupt or discontinue using *Coreg* without a physician's advice.
— congestive heart failure patients should consult their physician if they experience signs or symptoms of worsening heart failure such as weight gain or increasing shortness of breath.
— they may experience a drop in blood pressure when standing, resulting in dizziness and, rarely, fainting. Patients should sit or lie down when these symptoms of lowered blood pressure occur.
— if patients experience dizziness or fatigue, they should avoid driving or hazardous tasks.
— they should consult a physician if they experience dizziness or faintness, in case the dosage should be adjusted.
— they should take *Coreg* with food.
— diabetic patients should report any changes in blood sugar levels to their physician.
— contact lens wearers may experience decreased lacrimation.

Drug Interactions
(Also see CLINICAL PHARMACOLOGY, Pharmacokinetic Drug-Drug Interactions.)

Inhibitors of CYP2D6; poor metabolizers of debrisoquin: Interactions of carvedilol with strong inhibitors of CYP2D6 (such as quinidine, fluoxetine, paroxetine, and propafenone) have not been studied, but these drugs would be expected to increase blood levels of the R(+) enantiomer of carvedilol (see CLINICAL PHARMACOLOGY). Retrospective analysis of side effects in clinical trials showed that poor 2D6 metabolizers had a higher rate of dizziness during up-titration, presumably resulting from vasodilating effects of the higher concentrations of the α-blocking R(+) enantiomer.

Catecholamine-depleting agents: Patients taking both agents with β-blocking properties and a drug that can deplete catecholamines (e.g., reserpine and monoamine oxidase inhibitors) should be observed closely for signs of hypotension and/or severe bradycardia.

Clonidine: Concomitant administration of clonidine with agents with β-blocking properties may potentiate blood-pressure- and heart-rate-lowering effects. When concomitant treatment with agents with β-blocking properties and clonidine is to be terminated, the β-blocking agent should be discontinued first. Clonidine therapy can then be discontinued several days later by gradually decreasing the dosage.

Digoxin: Digoxin concentrations are increased by about 15% when digoxin and carvedilol are administered concomitantly. Both digoxin and *Coreg* slow AV conduction. Therefore, increased monitoring of digoxin is recommended when initiating, adjusting or discontinuing *Coreg*.

Inducers and inhibitors of hepatic metabolism: Rifampin reduced plasma concentrations of carvedilol by about 70%. Cimetidine increased AUC by about 30% but caused no change in C_{max}.

Calcium channel blockers: Isolated cases of conduction disturbance (rarely with hemodynamic compromise) have been observed when *Coreg* is co-administered with diltiazem. As with other agents with β-blocking properties, if Coreg (carvedilol) is to be administered orally with calcium channel blockers of the verapamil or diltiazem type, it is recommended that ECG and blood pressure be monitored.

Insulin or oral hypoglycemics: Agents with β-blocking properties may enhance the blood-sugar-reducing effect of insulin and oral hypoglycemics. Therefore, in patients taking insulin or oral hypoglycemics, regular monitoring of blood glucose is recommended.

Carcinogenesis, Mutagenesis, Impairment of Fertility
In 2-year studies conducted in rats given carvedilol at doses up to 75 mg/kg/day (12 times the maximum recommended human dose [MRHD] when compared on a mg/m² basis) or in mice given up to 200 mg/kg/day (16 times the MRHD on a mg/m² basis), carvedilol had no carcinogenic effect.

Carvedilol was negative when tested in a battery of genotoxicity assays, including the Ames and the CHO/HGPRT assays for mutagenicity and the *in vitro* hamster micronucleus and *in vivo* human lymphocyte cell tests for clastogenicity.

Continued on next page

Information on the SmithKline Beecham Pharmaceuticals products appearing here is based on the labeling in effect on July 31, 1998. Further information on these and other products may be obtained from the Medical Department, SmithKline Beecham Pharmaceuticals, One Franklin Plaza, Philadelphia, PA 19101.

Table 1

Adverse Events in U.S. Placebo-Controlled Congestive Heart Failure Trials Incidence >2%, Regardless of Causality; Withdrawal Rates due to Adverse Events

	Adverse Reactions		Withdrawals	
	Coreg (n=765) % occurrence	Placebo (n=437) % occurrence	*Coreg* (n=765) % withdrawals	Placebo (n=437) % withdrawals
Autonomic Nervous System				
Sweating increased	2.9	2.1	—	—
Body as a Whole				
Fatigue	23.9	22.4	0.7	0.7
Chest pain	14.4	14.2	0.1	—
Pain	8.6	7.6	—	0.2
Injury	5.9	5.5	—	—
Drug level increased	5.1	3.7	—	0.2
Edema generalized	5.1	2.5	—	—
Edema dependent	3.7	1.8	—	—
Fever	3.1	2.3	—	—
Edema legs	2.2	0.2	0.1	0.2
Cardiovascular				
Bradycardia	8.8	0.9	0.8	—
Hypotension	8.5	3.4	0.4	0.2
Syncope	3.4	2.5	0.3	0.2
Hypertension	2.9	2.5	0.1	—
AV block	2.9	0.5	—	—
Angina pectoris aggravated	2.0	1.1	—	—
Central Nervous System				
Dizziness	32.4	19.2	0.4	—
Headache	8.1	7.1	0.3	—
Paresthesia	2.0	1.8	0.1	—
Gastrointestinal				
Diarrhea	11.8	5.9	0.3	—
Nausea	8.5	4.8	—	—
Abdominal Pain	7.2	7.1	0.3	—
Vomiting	6.3	4.3	0.1	—
Hematologic				
Thrombocytopenia	2.0	0.5	0.1	—
Metabolic				
Hyperglycemia	12.2	7.8	0.1	—
Weight increase	9.7	6.9	0.1	0.5
Gout	6.3	6.2	—	—
BUN increased	6.0	4.6	0.3	0.2
NPN increased	5.8	4.6	0.3	0.2
Hypercholesterolemia	4.1	2.5	—	—
Dehydration	2.1	1.6	—	—
Hypervolemia	2.0	0.9	—	—
Musculoskeletal				
Back pain	6.9	6.6	—	—
Arthralgia	6.4	4.8	0.1	0.2
Myalgia	3.4	2.7	—	—
Resistance Mechanism				
Upper respiratory tract infection	18.3	17.6	—	—
Infection	2.2	0.9	—	—
Respiratory				
Sinusitis	5.4	4.3	—	—
Bronchitis	5.4	3.4	—	0.2
Pharyngitis	3.1	2.7	—	—
Urinary/Renal				
Urinary tract infection	3.1	2.7	—	—
Hematuria	2.9	2.1	—	—
Vision				
Vision abnormal	5.0	1.8	0.1	—

Coreg—Cont.

At doses ≥ 200 mg/kg/day (≥ 32 times the MRHD as mg/m^2) carvedilol was toxic to adult rats (sedation, reduced weight gain) and was associated with a reduced number of successful matings, prolonged mating time, significantly fewer corpora lutea and implants per dam and complete resorption of 18% of the litters. The no-observed-effect dose level for overt toxicity and impairment of fertility was 60 mg/kg/day (10 times the MRHD as mg/m^2).

Pregnancy: Teratogenic Effects. Pregnancy Category C.
Studies performed in pregnant rats and rabbits given carvedilol revealed increased post-implantation loss in rats at doses of 300 mg/kg/day (50 times the MRHD as mg/m^2) and in rabbits at doses of 75 mg/kg/day (25 times the MRHD as mg/m^2). In the rats, there was also a decrease in fetal body weight at the maternally toxic dose of 300 mg/kg/day (50 times the MRHD as mg/m^2), which was accompanied by an elevation in the frequency of fetuses with delayed skeletal development (missing or stunted 13th rib). In rats the no-observed-effect level for developmental toxicity was 60 mg/kg/day (10 times the MRHD as mg/m^2); in rabbits it was 15 mg/kg/day (5 times the MRHD as mg/m^2). There are no adequate and well-controlled studies in pregnant women. *Coreg* should be used during pregnancy only if the potential benefit justifies the potential risk to the fetus.

Nursing Mothers
It is not known whether this drug is excreted in human milk. Studies in rats have shown that carvedilol and/or its metabolites (as well as other β-blockers) cross the placental barrier and are excreted in breast milk. There was increased mortality at one week post-partum in neonates from rats treated with 60 mg/kg/day (10 times the MRHD as mg/m^2) and above during the last trimester through day 22 of lactation. Because many drugs are excreted in human milk and because of the potential for serious adverse reactions in nursing infants from β-blockers, especially bradycardia, a decision should be made whether to discontinue nursing or to discontinue the drug, taking into account the importance of the drug to the mother. The effects of other α- and β-blocking agents have included perinatal and neonatal distress.

Pediatric Use
Safety and efficacy in patients younger than 18 years of age have not been established.

Geriatric Use
Of the 765 patients with congestive heart failure randomized to *Coreg* in U.S. clinical trials, 31% (235) were 65 years of age or older. Of 1,869 patients receiving *Coreg* in congestive heart failure trials worldwide, 39% were 65 years of age or older. There were no notable differences in efficacy or the incidence of adverse events between older and younger patients.

Of the 2,065 hypertensive patients in U.S. clinical trials of efficacy or safety who were treated with Coreg (carvedilol), 21% (436) were 65 years of age or older. Of 3,722 patients receiving *Coreg* in hypertension clinical trials conducted worldwide, 24% were 65 years of age or older. There were no notable differences in efficacy or the incidence of adverse events between older and younger patients. With the exception of dizziness (incidence 8.8% in the elderly vs. 6% in younger patients), there were no events for which the incidence in the elderly exceeded that in the younger population by greater than 2.0%.

Similar results were observed in a postmarketing surveillance study of 3,328 *Coreg* patients, of whom approximately 20% were 65 years of age or older.

ADVERSE REACTIONS
Congestive Heart Failure
Coreg has been evaluated for safety in congestive heart failure in more than 1,900 patients worldwide of whom 1,300 participated in U.S. clinical trials. Approximately 54% of the total treated population received *Coreg* for at least 6 months and 20% received *Coreg* for at least 12 months. The adverse experience profile of *Coreg* in congestive heart failure patients was consistent with the pharmacology of the drug and the health status of the patients. In U.S. clinical trials comparing *Coreg* in daily doses up to 100 mg (n=765) to placebo (n=437), 5.4% of *Coreg* patients discontinued for adverse experiences vs. 8.0% of placebo patients.

Table 1 shows adverse events in U.S. placebo-controlled clinical trials of congestive heart failure patients that occurred with an incidence of greater than 2% regardless of causality and were more frequent in drug-treated patients than placebo-treated patients. Median study medication exposure was 6.33 months for both Coreg (carvedilol) and placebo patients.

[See table 1 at top of previous page]

Incidence >2%, Regardless of Causality; Withdrawal Rates due to Adverse Events
In addition to the events in Table 1, asthenia, cardiac failure, flatulence, anorexia, dyspepsia, palpitation, extrasystoles, hyperkalemia, arthritis, angina pectoris, insomnia, depression, anemia, viral infection, dyspnea, coughing, respiratory disorder, rhinitis, rash, and leg cramps were also reported, but rates were equal to, or more common in, placebo-treated patients.

The following adverse events were reported more frequently with *Coreg* in U.S. placebo-controlled trials in patients with congestive heart failure:

Incidence >1% to <2%
Body as a Whole: Peripheral edema, allergy, sudden death, malaise, hypovolemia.
Cardiovascular: Fluid overload, postural hypotension.
Central and Peripheral Nervous System: Hypesthesia, vertigo.

Gastrointestinal: Melena, periodontitis.
Liver and Biliary System: SGPT increased, SGOT increased.
Metabolic and Nutritional: Hyperuricemia, hypoglycemia, hyponatremia, increased alkaline phosphatase, glycosuria.
Platelet, Bleeding and Clotting: Prothrombin decreased, purpura.
Psychiatric: Somnolence.
Reproductive, male: Impotence.
Urinary System: Abnormal renal function, albuminuria.
POSTMARKETING EXPERIENCE
The following adverse reaction has been reported in postmarketing experience: reports of aplastic anemia have been rare and received only when carvedilol was administered concomitantly with other medications associated with the event.

Hypertension
Coreg (carvedilol) has been evaluated for safety in hypertension in more than 2,193 patients in U.S. clinical trials and in 2,976 patients in international clinical trials. Approximately 36% of the total treated population received *Coreg* for at least 6 months. In general, *Coreg* was well tolerated at doses up to 50 mg daily. Most adverse events reported during *Coreg* therapy were of mild to moderate severity. In U.S. controlled clinical trials directly comparing *Coreg* monotherapy in doses up to 50 mg (n=1,142) to placebo (n=462), 4.9% of *Coreg* patients discontinued for adverse events vs. 5.2% of placebo patients. Although there was no overall difference in discontinuation rates, discontinuations were more common in the carvedilol group for postural hypotension (1% vs. 0). The overall incidence of adverse events in U.S. placebo-controlled trials was found to increase with increasing dose of *Coreg*. For individual adverse events this could only be distinguished for dizziness, which increased in frequency from 2% to 5% as total daily dose increased from 6.25 mg to 50 mg.

Table 2 shows adverse events in U.S. placebo-controlled clinical trials for hypertension that occurred with an incidence of greater than 1% regardless of causality, and that were more frequent in drug-treated patients than placebo-treated patients.

[See table 2 below]

In addition to the events in Table 2, chest pain, dyspepsia, headache, nausea, pain, sinusitis and upper respiratory tract infection were also reported, but rates were at least as great in placebo-treated patients.

The following adverse events were reported as possibly or probably related in worldwide open or controlled trials with Coreg (carvedilol) in patients with hypertension or congestive heart failure.

Incidence >0.1% to ≤1%
Cardiovascular: Peripheral ischemia, tachycardia.
Central and Peripheral Nervous System: Hypokinesia.
Gastrointestinal: Bilirubinemia, increased hepatic enzymes (0.2% of hypertension patients and 0.4% of congestive heart failure patients were discontinued from therapy because of increases in hepatic enzymes; see WARNINGS, Hepatic Injury).
General: Substernal chest pain, edema.
Psychiatric: Nervousness, sleep disorder, aggravated depression, impaired concentration, abnormal thinking, paroniria, emotional lability.
Respiratory System: Asthma (see CONTRAINDICATIONS).
Reproductive: Male: decreased libido.
Skin and Appendages: Pruritus, rash erythematous, rash maculopapular, rash psoriaform, photosensitivity reaction.
Special Senses: Tinnitus.
Urinary System: Micturition frequency.
Autonomic Nervous System: Dry mouth, sweating increased.
Metabolic and Nutritional: Hypokalemia, diabetes mellitus, hypertriglyceridemia.
Hematologic: Anemia, leukopenia.
The following events were reported in ≤0.1% of patients and are potentially important: complete AV block, bundle branch block, myocardial ischemia, cerebrovascular disorder, convulsions, migraine, neuralgia, paresis, anaphylactoid reaction, alopecia, exfoliative dermatitis, amnesia, GI hemorrhage, bronchospasm, pulmonary edema, decreased hearing, respiratory alkalosis, increased BUN, decreased HDL, pancytopenia and atypical lymphocytes.
Other adverse events occurred sporadically in single patients and cannot be distinguished from concurrent disease states or medications.
Coreg therapy has not been associated with clinically significant changes in routine laboratory tests in hypertensive patients. No clinically relevant changes were noted in serum potassium, fasting serum glucose, total triglycerides, total cholesterol, HDL cholesterol, uric acid, blood urea nitrogen or creatinine.

OVERDOSAGE
The acute oral LD$_{50}$ doses in male and female mice and male and female rats are over 8000 mg/kg.

Table 2

Adverse Events in U.S. Placebo-Controlled Hypertension Trials
Incidence ≥1%, Regardless of Causality; Withdrawal Rates due to Adverse Events

	Adverse Reactions		Withdrawals	
	Coreg (n=1,142) % occurrence	**Placebo** (n=462) % occurrence	**Coreg** (n=1,142) % withdrawals	**Placebo** (n=462) % withdrawals
Body as a Whole				
Fatigue	4.3	3.9	0.3	0.2
Injury	2.9	2.6	0.1	—
Cardiovascular				
Bradycardia	2.1	0.2	0.4	—
Postural hypotension	1.8	—	1.0	—
Dependent edema	1.7	1.5	0.1	0.4
Peripheral edema	1.4	0.4	0.2	—
Central Nervous System				
Dizziness	6.2	5.4	0.4	1.3
Insomnia	1.6	0.6	—	0.2
Somnolence	1.8	1.5	—	—
Gastrointestinal				
Abdominal pain	1.4	1.3	0.1	—
Diarrhea	2.2	1.3	0.1	—
Hematologic				
Thrombocytopenia	1.1	0.2	—	—
Metabolic				
Hypertriglyceridemia	1.2	0.2	—	—
Musculoskeletal				
Back pain	2.3	1.5	0.1	—
Resistance Mechanism				
Viral infection	1.8	1.3	—	—
Respiratory				
Rhinitis	2.1	1.9	—	—
Pharyngitis	1.5	0.6	—	—
Dyspnea	1.4	0.9	0.4	0.2
Urinary/Renal				
Urinary tract infection	1.8	0.6	—	—

Overdosage may cause severe hypotension, bradycardia, cardiac insufficiency, cardiogenic shock and cardiac arrest. Respiratory problems, bronchospasms, vomiting, lapses of consciousness and generalized seizures may also occur.

The patient should be placed in a supine position and, where necessary, kept under observation and treated under intensive-care conditions. Gastric lavage or pharmacologically induced emesis may be used shortly after ingestion.

The following agents may be administered:

for excessive bradycardia: atropine, 2 mg IV.

to support cardiovascular function: glucagon, 5 to 10 mg IV rapidly over 30 seconds, followed by a continuous infusion of 5 mg/hour; sympathomimetics (dobutamine, isoprenaline, adrenaline) at doses according to body weight and effect.

If peripheral vasodilation dominates, it may be necessary to administer adrenaline or noradrenaline with continuous monitoring of circulatory conditions. For therapy-resistant bradycardia, pacemaker therapy should be performed. For bronchospasm, β-sympathomimetics (as aerosol or IV) or aminophylline IV should be given. In the event of seizures, slow IV injection of diazepam or clonazepam is recommended.

NOTE: In the event of severe intoxication where there are symptoms of shock, treatment with antidotes must be continued for a sufficiently long period of time consistent with the 7- to 10-hour half-life of carvedilol.

Cases of overdosage with *Coreg* alone or in combination with other drugs have been reported. Quantities ingested in some cases exceeded 1000 milligrams. Symptoms experienced included low blood pressure and heart rate. Standard supportive treatment was provided and individuals recovered.

DOSAGE AND ADMINISTRATION

Congestive Heart Failure

DOSAGE MUST BE INDIVIDUALIZED AND CLOSELY MONITORED BY A PHYSICIAN DURING UP-TITRATION. Prior to initiation of *Coreg,* the dosing of digitalis, diuretics and ACE inhibitors (if used) should be stabilized. The recommended starting dose of *Coreg* is 3.125 mg twice daily for two weeks. If this dose is tolerated, it can then be increased to 6.25 mg twice daily. Dosing should then be doubled every 2 weeks to the highest level tolerated by the patient. At initiation of each new dose, patients should be observed for signs of dizziness or light-headedness for one hour. The maximum recommended dose is 25 mg twice daily in patients weighing less than 85 kg (187 lbs) and 50 mg twice daily in patients weighing more than 85 kg. Coreg (carvedilol) should be taken with food to slow the rate of absorption and reduce the incidence of orthostatic effects.

Before each dose increase the patient should be seen in the office and evaluated for symptoms of worsening heart failure, vasodilation (dizziness, light-headedness, symptomatic hypotension) or bradycardia, in order to determine tolerability of *Coreg.* Transient worsening of heart failure may be treated with increased doses of diuretics although occasionally it is necessary to lower the dose of *Coreg* or temporarily discontinue it. Symptoms of vasodilation often respond to a reduction in the dose of diuretics or ACE inhibitor. If these changes do not relieve symptoms, the dose of *Coreg* may be decreased. The dose of *Coreg* should not be increased until symptoms of worsening heart failure or vasodilation have been stabilized. Initial difficulty with titration should not preclude later attempts to introduce *Coreg*. If congestive heart failure patients experience bradycardia (pulse rate below 55 beats/min.), the dose of *Coreg* should be reduced.

Hypertension

DOSAGE MUST BE INDIVIDUALIZED. The recommended starting dose of *Coreg* is 6.25 mg twice daily. If this dose is tolerated, using standing systolic pressure measured about 1 hour after dosing as a guide, the dose should be maintained for 7 to 14 days, and then increased to 12.5 mg twice daily if needed, based on trough blood pressure, again using standing systolic pressure one hour after dosing as a guide for tolerance. This dose should also be maintained for 7 to 14 days and can then be adjusted upward to 25 mg twice daily if tolerated and needed. The full antihypertensive effect of *Coreg* is seen within 7 to 14 days. Total daily dose should not exceed 50 mg. *Coreg* should be taken with food to slow the rate of absorption and reduce the incidence of orthostatic effects.

Addition of a diuretic to *Coreg*, or *Coreg* to a diuretic can be expected to produce additive effects and exaggerate the orthostatic component of *Coreg* action.

Coreg (carvedilol) should not be given to patients with severe hepatic impairment (see CONTRAINDICATIONS).

HOW SUPPLIED

Tablets: White, oval, film-coated tablets: 3.125 mg-engraved with 39 and SB, in bottles of 100; 6.25 mg-engraved with 4140 and SB, in bottles of 100; 12.5 mg-engraved with 4141 and SB, in bottles of 100; 25 mg-engraved with 4142 and SB, in bottles of 100. The 6.25 mg, 12.5 mg and 25 mg tablets are Tiltab® tablets.

Store below 30°C (86°F). Protect from moisture. Dispense in a tight, light-resistant container.

3.125 mg 100's: NDC 0007-4139-20
6.25 mg 100's: NDC 0007-4140-20
12.5 mg 100's: NDC 0007-4141-20
25 mg 100's: NDC 0007-4142-20

Coreg is a registered trademark.

Coreg is copromoted by SmithKline Beecham Pharmaceuticals and Roche Laboratories Inc.

Manufactured and distributed by
SmithKline Beecham Pharmaceuticals
Philadelphia, PA 19101

Veterans Administration/Military/PHS—Tablets, 3.125 mg, 100's, 6505-01-449-2168; 6.25 mg, 100's, 6505-01-449-2161; 12.5 mg, 100's 6505-01-449-2155; 25 mg, 100's, 6505-01-449-2148.

CO:L4B

Shown in Product Identification Guide, page 339

DEXEDRINE® Ⓒ

[dex 'eh-dreen]
(brand of dextroamphetamine sulfate)
SPANSULE® CAPSULES
brand of sustained release capsules
and TABLETS

WARNING

AMPHETAMINES HAVE A HIGH POTENTIAL FOR ABUSE. ADMINISTRATION OF AMPHETAMINES FOR PROLONGED PERIODS OF TIME MAY LEAD TO DRUG DEPENDENCE AND MUST BE AVOIDED. PARTICULAR ATTENTION SHOULD BE PAID TO THE POSSIBILITY OF SUBJECTS OBTAINING AMPHETAMINES FOR NON-THERAPEUTIC USE OR DISTRIBUTION TO OTHERS, AND THE DRUGS SHOULD BE PRESCRIBED OR DISPENSED SPARINGLY.

DESCRIPTION

Dexedrine (dextroamphetamine sulfate) is the dextro isomer of the compound *d,l*-amphetamine sulfate, a sympathomimetic amine of the amphetamine group. Chemically, dextroamphetamine is *d*-alpha-methylphenethylamine, and is present in all forms of *Dexedrine* as the neutral sulfate.

Spansule® capsules

Each *Spansule* sustained release capsule is so prepared that an initial dose is released promptly and the remaining medication is released gradually over a prolonged period.

Each capsule, with brown cap and clear body, contains dextroamphetamine sulfate. The 5 mg capsule is imprinted 5 mg and 3512 on the brown cap and is imprinted 5 mg and SB on the clear body. The 10 mg capsule is imprinted 10 mg and 3513 on the brown cap and is imprinted 10 mg and SB on the clear body. The 15 mg capsule is imprinted 15 mg and 3514 on the brown cap and is imprinted 15 mg and SB on the clear body. Inactive ingredients consist of acacia, benzyl alcohol, calcium sulfate, cetylpyridinium chloride, FD&C Blue No. 1, FD&C Red No. 40, FD&C Yellow No. 5 (tartrazine), FD&C Yellow No. 6, gelatin, glyceryl distearate, glyceryl monostearate, sodium lauryl sulfate, starch, sucrose, wax and trace amounts of other inactive ingredients.

Tablets

Each triangular, orange, scored tablet is debossed SKF and E19 and contains dextroamphetamine sulfate, 5 mg. Inactive ingredients consist of calcium sulfate, FD&C Yellow No. 5 (tartrazine), FD&C Yellow No. 6, gelatin, lactose, mineral oil, starch, stearic acid, sucrose, talc and trace amounts of other inactive ingredients.

CLINICAL PHARMACOLOGY

Amphetamines are non-catecholamine, sympathomimetic amines with CNS stimulant activity. Peripheral actions include elevations of systolic and diastolic blood pressures and weak bronchodilator and respiratory stimulant action.

There is neither specific evidence which clearly establishes the mechanism whereby amphetamines produce mental and behavioral effects in children, nor conclusive evidence regarding how these effects relate to the condition of the central nervous system.

Dexedrine (dextroamphetamine sulfate) *Spansule* capsules are formulated to release the active drug substance *in vivo* in a more gradual fashion than the standard formulation, as demonstrated by blood levels. The formulation has not been shown superior in effectiveness over the same dosage of the standard, noncontrolled-release formulations given in divided doses.

Pharmacokinetics

Tablet—The single ingestion of two 5 mg tablets by healthy volunteers produced an average peak dextroamphetamine blood level of 29.2 ng/mL at 2 hours post-administration. The average half-life was 10.25 hours. The average urinary recovery was 45% in 48 hours.

Spansule capsule—Ingestion of a *Spansule* capsule containing 15 mg radiolabeled dextroamphetamine sulfate by healthy volunteers produced a peak blood level of radioactivity, on the average, at 8 to 10 hours post-administration with peak urinary recovery seen at 12 to 24 hours.

INDICATIONS AND USAGE

Dexedrine (dextroamphetamine sulfate) is indicated:

1. In Narcolepsy.

2. In Attention Deficit Disorder with Hyperactivity, as an integral part of a total treatment program which typically includes other remedial measures (psychological, educational, social) for a stabilizing effect in pediatric patients (ages 3 years to 16 years) with a behavioral syndrome characterized by the following group of developmentally inappropriate symptoms: moderate to severe distractibility, short attention span, hyperactivity, emotional lability, and impulsivity. The diagnosis of this syndrome should not be made with finality when these symptoms are only of comparatively recent origin. Nonlocalizing (soft) neurological signs, learning disability, and abnormal EEG may or may not be present, and a diagnosis of central nervous system dysfunction may or may not be warranted.

CONTRAINDICATIONS

Advanced arteriosclerosis, symptomatic cardiovascular disease, moderate to severe hypertension, hyperthyroidism, known hypersensitivity or idiosyncrasy to the sympathomimetic amines, glaucoma.

Agitated states.

Patients with a history of drug abuse.

During or within 14 days following the administration of monoamine oxidase inhibitors (hypertensive crises may result).

PRECAUTIONS

General: Caution is to be exercised in prescribing amphetamines for patients with even mild hypertension.

The least amount feasible should be prescribed or dispensed at one time in order to minimize the possibility of overdosage.

These products contain FD&C Yellow No. 5 (tartrazine), which may cause allergic-type reactions (including bronchial asthma) in certain susceptible individuals. Although the overall incidence of FD&C Yellow No. 5 (tartrazine) sensitivity in the general population is low, it is frequently seen in patients who also have aspirin hypersensitivity.

Information for Patients: Amphetamines may impair the ability of the patient to engage in potentially hazardous activities such as operating machinery or vehicles; the patient should therefore be cautioned accordingly.

Drug Interactions

Acidifying agents—Gastrointestinal acidifying agents (guanethidine, reserpine, glutamic acid HCl, ascorbic acid, fruit juices, etc.) lower absorption of amphetamines. Urinary acidifying agents (ammonium chloride, sodium acid phosphate, etc.) increase the concentration of the ionized species of the amphetamine molecule, thereby increasing urinary excretion. Both groups of agents lower blood levels and efficacy of amphetamines.

Adrenergic blockers—Adrenergic blockers are inhibited by amphetamines.

Alkalinizing agents—Gastrointestinal alkalinizing agents (sodium bicarbonate, etc.) increase absorption of amphetamines. Urinary alkalinizing agents (acetazolamide, some thiazides) increase the concentration of the non-ionized species of the amphetamine molecule, thereby decreasing urinary excretion. Both groups of agents increase blood levels and therefore potentiate the actions of amphetamines.

Antidepressants, tricyclic—Amphetamines may enhance the activity of tricyclic or sympathomimetic agents; d-amphetamine with desipramine or protriptyline and possibly other tricyclics cause striking and sustained increases in the concentration of d-amphetamine in the brain; cardiovascular effects can be potentiated.

MAO inhibitors—MAOI antidepressants, as well as a metabolite of furazolidone, slow amphetamine metabolism. This slowing potentiates amphetamines, increasing their effect on the release of norepinephrine and other monoamines from adrenergic nerve endings; this can cause headaches and other signs of hypertensive crisis. A variety of neurological toxic effects and malignant hyperpyrexia can occur, sometimes with fatal results.

Antihistamines—Amphetamines may counteract the sedative effect of antihistamines.

Antihypertensives—Amphetamines may antagonize the hypotensive effects of antihypertensives.

Chlorpromazine—Chlorpromazine blocks dopamine and norepinephrine reuptake, thus inhibiting the central stimulant effects of amphetamines, and can be used to treat amphetamine poisoning.

Continued on next page

Information on the SmithKline Beecham Pharmaceuticals products appearing here is based on the labeling in effect on July 31, 1998. Further information on these and other products may be obtained from the Medical Department, SmithKline Beecham Pharmaceuticals, One Franklin Plaza, Philadelphia, PA 19101.

Dexedrine Spansule—Cont.

Ethosuximide—Amphetamines may delay intestinal absorption of ethosuximide.

Haloperidol—Haloperidol blocks dopamine and norepinephrine reuptake, thus inhibiting the central stimulant effects of amphetamines.

Lithium carbonate—The stimulatory effects of amphetamines may be inhibited by lithium carbonate.

Meperidine—Amphetamines potentiate the analgesic effect of meperidine.

Methenamine therapy—Urinary excretion of amphetamines is increased, and efficacy is reduced, by acidifying agents used in methenamine therapy.

Norepinephrine—Amphetamines enhance the adrenergic effect of norepinephrine.

Phenobarbital—Amphetamines may delay intestinal absorption of phenobarbital; co-administration of phenobarbital may produce a synergistic anticonvulsant action.

Phenytoin—Amphetamines may delay intestinal absorption of phenytoin; co-administration of phenytoin may produce a synergistic anticonvulsant action.

Propoxyphene—In cases of propoxyphene overdosage, amphetamine CNS stimulation is potentiated and fatal convulsions can occur.

Veratrum alkaloids—Amphetamines inhibit the hypotensive effect of veratrum alkaloids.

Drug/Laboratory Test Interactions

- Amphetamines can cause a significant elevation in plasma corticosteroid levels. This increase is greatest in the evening.
- Amphetamines may interfere with urinary steroid determinations.

Carcinogenesis/Mutagenesis: Mutagenicity studies and long-term studies in animals to determine the carcinogenic potential of Dexedrine (dextroamphetamine sulfate) have not been performed.

Pregnancy—Teratogenic Effects: Pregnancy Category C. *Dexedrine* has been shown to have embryotoxic and teratogenic effects when administered to A/Jax mice and C57BL mice in doses approximately 41 times the maximum human dose. Embryotoxic effects were not seen in New Zealand white rabbits given the drug in doses 7 times the human dose nor in rats given 12.5 times the maximum human dose. While there are no adequate and well-controlled studies in pregnant women, there has been one report of severe congenital bony deformity, tracheoesophageal fistula, and anal atresia (Vater association) in a baby born to a woman who took dextroamphetamine sulfate with lovastatin during the first trimester of pregnancy. *Dexedrine* should be used during pregnancy only if the potential benefit justifies the potential risk to the fetus.

Nonteratogenic Effects: Infants born to mothers dependent on amphetamines have an increased risk of premature delivery and low birth weight. Also, these infants may experience symptoms of withdrawal as demonstrated by dysphoria, including agitation, and significant lassitude.

Nursing Mothers: Amphetamines are excreted in human milk. Mothers taking amphetamines should be advised to refrain from nursing.

Pediatric Use: Long-term effects of amphetamines in pediatric patients have not been well established.

Amphetamines are not recommended for use in pediatric patients under 3 years of age with Attention Deficit Disorder with Hyperactivity described under INDICATIONS AND USAGE.

Clinical experience suggests that in psychotic children, administration of amphetamines may exacerbate symptoms of behavior disturbance and thought disorder.

Amphetamines have been reported to exacerbate motor and phonic tics and Tourette's syndrome. Therefore, clinical evaluation for tics and Tourette's syndrome in children and their families should precede use of stimulant medications.

Data are inadequate to determine whether chronic administration of amphetamines may be associated with growth inhibition; therefore, growth should be monitored during treatment.

Drug treatment is not indicated in all cases of Attention Deficit Disorder with Hyperactivity and should be considered only in light of the complete history and evaluation of the child. The decision to prescribe amphetamines should depend on the physician's assessment of the chronicity and severity of the child's symptoms and their appropriateness for his/her age. Prescription should not depend solely on the presence of one or more of the behavioral characteristics. When these symptoms are associated with acute stress reactions, treatment with amphetamines is usually not indicated.

ADVERSE REACTIONS

Cardiovascular: Palpitations, tachycardia, elevation of blood pressure. There have been isolated reports of cardiomyopathy associated with chronic amphetamine use.

Central Nervous System: Psychotic episodes at recommended doses (rare), overstimulation, restlessness, dizzi-ness, insomnia, euphoria, dyskinesia, dysphoria, tremor, headache, exacerbation of motor and phonic tics and Tourette's syndrome.

Gastrointestinal: Dryness of the mouth, unpleasant taste, diarrhea, constipation, other gastrointestinal disturbances. Anorexia and weight loss may occur as undesirable effects.

Allergic: Urticaria.

Endocrine: Impotence, changes in libido.

DRUG ABUSE AND DEPENDENCE

Dextroamphetamine sulfate is a Schedule II controlled substance.

Amphetamines have been extensively abused. Tolerance, extreme psychological dependence and severe social disability have occurred. There are reports of patients who have increased the dosage to many times that recommended. Abrupt cessation following prolonged high dosage administration results in extreme fatigue and mental depression; changes are also noted on the sleep EEG.

Manifestations of chronic intoxication with amphetamines include severe dermatoses, marked insomnia, irritability, hyperactivity and personality changes. The most severe manifestation of chronic intoxication is psychosis, often clinically indistinguishable from schizophrenia. This is rare with oral amphetamines.

OVERDOSAGE

Individual patient response to amphetamines varies widely. While toxic symptoms occasionally occur as an idiosyncrasy at doses as low as 2 mg, they are rare with doses of less than 15 mg; 30 mg can produce severe reactions, yet doses of 400 to 500 mg are not necessarily fatal.

In rats, the oral LD_{50} of dextroamphetamine sulfate is 96.8 mg/kg.

Manifestations of acute overdosage with amphetamines include restlessness, tremor, hyperreflexia, rhabdomyolysis, rapid respiration, hyperpyrexia, confusion, assaultiveness, hallucinations, panic states.

Fatigue and depression usually follow the central stimulation.

Cardiovascular effects include arrhythmias, hypertension or hypotension and circulatory collapse. Gastrointestinal symptoms include nausea, vomiting, diarrhea and abdominal cramps. Fatal poisoning is usually preceded by convulsions and coma.

TREATMENT—Consult with a Certified Poison Control Center for up-to-date guidance and advice. Management of acute amphetamine intoxication is largely symptomatic and includes gastric lavage, administration of activated charcoal, administration of a cathartic, and sedation. Experience with hemodialysis or peritoneal dialysis is inadequate to permit recommendation in this regard. Acidification of the urine increases amphetamine excretion, but is believed to increase risk of acute renal failure if myoglobinuria is present. If acute, severe hypertension complicates amphetamine overdosage, administration of intravenous phentolamine (Regitine®, CIBA) has been suggested. However, a gradual drop in blood pressure will usually result when sufficient sedation has been achieved.

Chlorpromazine antagonizes the central stimulant effects of amphetamines and can be used to treat amphetamine intoxication.

Since much of the *Spansule* capsule medication is coated for gradual release, therapy directed at reversing the effects of the ingested drug and at supporting the patient should be continued for as long as overdosage symptoms remain. Saline cathartics are useful for hastening the evacuation of pellets that have not already released medication.

DOSAGE AND ADMINISTRATION

Amphetamines should be administered at the lowest effective dosage and dosage should be individually adjusted. Late evening doses—particularly with the *Spansule* capsule form—should be avoided because of the resulting insomnia.

Narcolepsy: Usual dose 5 to 60 mg per day in divided doses, depending on the individual patient response.

Narcolepsy seldom occurs in children under 12 years of age; however, when it does, Dexedrine (dextroamphetamine sulfate) may be used. The suggested initial dose for patients aged 6 to 12 is 5 mg daily; daily dose may be raised in increments of 5 mg at weekly intervals until optimal response is obtained. In patients 12 years of age and older, start with 10 mg daily; daily dosage may be raised in increments of 10 mg at weekly intervals until optimal response is obtained. If bothersome adverse reactions appear (e.g., insomnia or anorexia), dosage should be reduced. *Spansule* capsules may be used for once-a-day dosage wherever appropriate. With tablets, give first dose on awakening; additional doses (1 or 2) at intervals of 4 to 6 hours.

Attention Deficit Disorder with Hyperactivity: Not recommended for pediatric patients under 3 years of age.

In pediatric patients from 3 to 5 years of age, start with 2.5 mg daily, by tablet; daily dosage may be raised in increments of 2.5 mg at weekly intervals until optimal response is obtained.

In pediatric patients 6 years of age and older, start with 5 mg once or twice daily; daily dosage may be raised in incre-ments of 5 mg at weekly intervals until optimal response is obtained. Only in rare cases will it be necessary to exceed a total of 40 mg per day.

Spansule capsules may be used for once-a-day dosage wherever appropriate.

With tablets, give first dose on awakening; additional doses (1 or 2) at intervals of 4 to 6 hours.

Where possible, drug administration should be interrupted occasionally to determine if there is a recurrence of behavioral symptoms sufficient to require continued therapy.

HOW SUPPLIED

Dexedrine **Spansule capsules:** Each capsule, with brown cap and clear body, contains dextroamphetamine sulfate. The 5 mg capsule is imprinted 5 mg and 3512 on the brown cap and is imprinted 5 mg and SB on the clear body. The 10 mg capsule is imprinted 10 mg and 3513 on the brown cap and is imprinted 10 mg and SB on the clear body. The 15 mg capsule is imprinted 15 mg and 3514 on the brown cap and is imprinted 15 mg and SB on the clear body. Available: 5 mg, 10 mg, and 15 mg in bottles of 50.

Store between 15° and 30°C (59° and 86°F). Dispense in a tight, light-resistant container.

5 mg 50's: NDC 0007-3512-15

10 mg 50's: NDC 0007-3513-15

15 mg 50's: NDC 0007-3514-15

Dexedrine (dextroamphetamine sulfate) Tablets: Triangular, orange, scored, debossed SKF and E19. Available: 5 mg in bottles of 100.

Store between 15° and 30°C (59° and 86°F). Dispense in a tight, light-resistant container.

5 mg 100's: NDC 0007-3519-20

Veterans Administration/Military/PHS—Spansule Capsules, 5 mg, 50's, 6505-01-153-4029; 10 mg, 50's, 6505-01-153-3038; 15 mg, 50's, 6505-00-769-2090; Tablets, 5 mg, 100's, 6505-00-106-8715.

DX:L47A

Shown in Product Identification Guide, page 339

DIBENZYLINE® Capsules ℞
[di-benz 'eh-leen]
brand of phenoxybenzamine hydrochloride

DESCRIPTION

Each *Dibenzyline* capsule, with red cap and red body, is imprinted SKF and E33 and contains phenoxybenzamine hydrochloride, 10 mg. Inactive ingredients consist of benzyl alcohol, cetylpyridinium chloride, D&C Red No. 33, FD&C Red No. 3, FD&C Yellow No. 6, gelatin, lactose, sodium lauryl sulfate and trace amounts of other inactive ingredients. *Dibenzyline* is N -(2-Chloroethyl)-N -(1-methyl-2-phenoxyethyl)benzylamine hydrochloride.

Phenoxybenzamine hydrochloride is a colorless, crystalline powder with a molecular weight of 340.3 which melts between 136° and 141°C. It is soluble in water, alcohol and chloroform; insoluble in ether.

CLINICAL PHARMACOLOGY

Dibenzyline (phenoxybenzamine hydrochloride) is a long-acting, adrenergic, *alpha* -receptor blocking agent which can produce and maintain "chemical sympathectomy" by oral administration. It increases blood flow to the skin, mucosa and abdominal viscera, and lowers both supine and erect blood pressures. It has no effect on the parasympathetic system.

Twenty to 30 percent of orally administered phenoxybenzamine appears to be absorbed in the active form.[1]

The half-life of orally administered phenoxybenzamine hydrochloride is not known; however, the half-life of intravenously administered drug is approximately 24 hours. Demonstrable effects with intravenous administration persist for at least 3 to 4 days, and the effects of daily administration are cumulative for nearly a week.[1]

INDICATION AND USAGE

Pheochromocytoma, to control episodes of hypertension and sweating. If tachycardia is excessive, it may be necessary to use a beta-blocking agent concomitantly.

CONTRAINDICATIONS

Conditions where a fall in blood pressure may be undesirable.

WARNING

Dibenzyline-induced *alpha* -adrenergic blockade leaves *beta* -adrenergic receptors unopposed. Compounds that stimulate both types of receptors may therefore produce an exaggerated hypotensive response and tachycardia.

PRECAUTIONS

General—Administer with caution in patients with marked cerebral or coronary arteriosclerosis or renal damage. Adrenergic blocking effect may aggravate symptoms of respiratory infections.

Drug Interactions[2]—Dibenzyline (phenoxybenzamine hydrochloride) may interact with compounds that stimulate

both *alpha* - and *beta* -adrenergic receptors (i.e., epinephrine) to produce an exaggerated hypotensive response and tachycardia. (See WARNING.)

Dibenzyline blocks hyperthermia production by levarterenol, and blocks hypothermia production by reserpine.

Carcinogenesis, Mutagenesis, Impairment of Fertility—Phenoxybenzamine hydrochloride has shown *in vitro* mutagenic activity in the Ames test and in the mouse lymphoma assay; it has not shown mutagenic activity in the micronucleus test in mice. In rats and mice repeated intraperitoneal administration of phenoxybenzamine hydrochloride resulted in peritoneal sarcomas. Chronic oral dosing in rats has produced malignant tumors in the gastrointestinal tract. The majority of these tumors were found in the nonglandular stomach of the rats.

In chronic oral studies in rats, ulcerative and/or erosive gastritis of the glandular stomach occurred which was probably drug related.

Pregnancy-Teratogenic Effects—Pregnancy Category C. Adequate reproductive studies have not been performed with Dibenzyline (phenoxybenzamine hydrochloride). It is also not known whether *Dibenzyline* can cause fetal harm when administered to a pregnant woman. *Dibenzyline* should be given to a pregnant woman only if clearly needed.

Nursing Mothers—It is not known whether this drug is excreted in human milk. Because many drugs are excreted in human milk, and because of the potential for serious adverse reactions from phenoxybenzamine hydrochloride, a decision should be made whether to discontinue nursing or to discontinue the drug, taking into account the importance of the drug to the mother.

Pediatric Use—Safety and effectiveness in pediatric patients have not been established.

ADVERSE REACTIONS

The following adverse reactions have been observed, but there are insufficient data to support an estimate of their frequency.

Autonomic Nervous System*: Postural hypotension, tachycardia, inhibition of ejaculation, nasal congestion, miosis.

Miscellaneous: Gastrointestinal irritation, drowsiness, fatigue.

---

*These so-called "side effects" are actually evidence of adrenergic blockade and vary according to the degree of blockade.

OVERDOSAGE

SYMPTOMS—These are largely the result of block of the sympathetic nervous system and of the circulating epinephrine. They may include postural hypotension resulting in dizziness or fainting; tachycardia, particularly postural; vomiting; lethargy; shock.

TREATMENT—When symptoms and signs of overdosage exist, discontinue the drug. Treatment of circulatory failure, if present, is a prime consideration. In cases of mild overdosage, recumbent position with legs elevated usually restores cerebral circulation. In the more severe cases, the usual measures to combat shock should be instituted. Usual pressor agents are *not* effective. Epinephrine is contraindicated because it stimulates both *alpha* and *beta* receptors; since *alpha* receptors are blocked, the net effect of epinephrine administration is vasodilation and a further drop in blood pressure (epinephrine reversal).

The patient may have to be kept flat for 24 hours or more in the case of overdose, as the effect of the drug is prolonged. Leg bandages and an abdominal binder may shorten the period of disability.

I.V. infusion of levarterenol bitartrate* may be used to combat severe hypotensive reactions, because it stimulates *alpha* receptors primarily. Although Dibenzyline (phenoxybenzamine hydrochloride) is an *alpha*-adrenergic blocking agent, a sufficient dose of levarterenol bitartrate will overcome this effect.

The oral LD_{50} for phenoxybenzamine hydrochloride is approximately 2000 mg/kg in rats and approximately 500 mg/kg in guinea pigs.

DOSAGE AND ADMINISTRATION

The dosage should be adjusted to fit the needs of each patient. Small initial doses should be *slowly* increased until the desired effect is obtained or the side effects from blockade become troublesome. *After each increase, the patient should be observed on that level before instituting another increase.* The dosage should be carried to a point where symptomatic relief and/or objective improvement are obtained, but not so high that the side effects from blockade become troublesome.

Initially, 10 mg of Dibenzyline (phenoxybenzamine hydrochloride) twice a day. Dosage should be increased every other day, usually to 20 to 40 mg 2 or 3 times a day, until an optimal dosage is obtained, as judged by blood pressure control.

STORAGE

Store between 15° and 30°C(59° and 86°F).

HOW SUPPLIED

Dibenzyline (phenoxybenzamine hydrochloride) capsules, 10 mg, in bottles of 100 (*NDC* 0007-3533-20).

REFERENCES

1. Weiner, N.: Drugs That Inhibit Adrenergic Nerves and Block Adrenergic Receptors, in Goodman, L., and Gilman, A., *The Pharmacological Basis of Therapeutics,* ed. 6, New York, Macmillan Publishing Co., 1980, p. 179; p. 182.
2. Martin, E.W.: *Drug Interactions Index 1978/1979,* Philadelphia, J.B. Lippincott Co., 1978, pp. 209–210.

---

*Available as Levophed® Bitartrate (brand of norepinephrine bitartrate) from Sanofi Winthrop Pharmaceuticals.

Veterans Administration/Military/PHS—Capsules, 10 mg, 100's, 6505-00-890-1193.

DI:L26

Shown in Product Identification Guide, page 339

DYAZIDE® ℞

[*dye-uh-zide '*]

capsules

diuretic • antihypertensive

DESCRIPTION

Each *Dyazide* capsule for oral use, with opaque red cap and opaque white body, contains hydrochlorothiazide 25 mg and triamterene 37.5 mg, and is imprinted with the product name DYAZIDE and SB. Hydrochlorothiazide is a diuretic/antihypertensive agent and triamterene is an antikaliuretic agent.

Hydrochlorothiazide is slightly soluble in water. It is soluble in dilute ammonia, dilute aqueous sodium hydroxide and dimethylformamide. It is sparingly soluble in methanol.

Hydrochlorothiazide is 6-chloro-3,4-dihydro-2H -1,2,4-benzothiadiazine-7-sulfonamide 1,1-dioxide and its structural formula is:

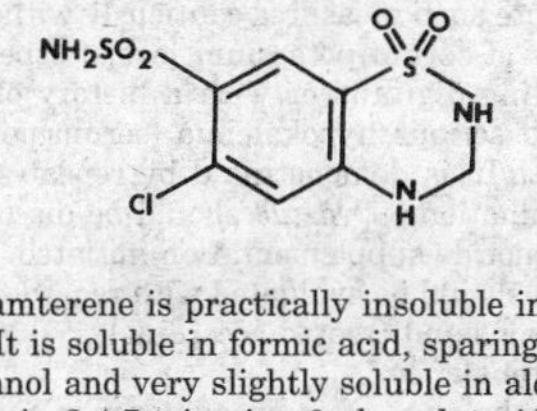

At 50°C, triamterene is practically insoluble in water (less than 0.1%). It is soluble in formic acid, sparingly soluble in methoxyethanol and very slightly soluble in alcohol.

Triamterene is 2,4,7-triamino-6-phenylpteridine and its structural formula is:

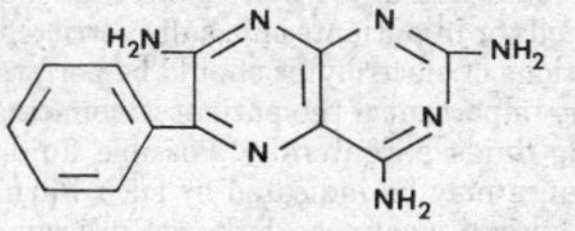

Inactive ingredients consist of benzyl alcohol, cetylpyridinium chloride, D&C Red No. 33, FD&C Yellow No. 6, gelatin, glycine, lactose, magnesium stearate, microcrystalline cellulose, povidone, polysorbate 80, sodium starch glycolate, titanium dioxide and trace amounts of other inactive ingredients.

CLINICAL PHARMACOLOGY

Dyazide is a diuretic/antihypertensive drug product that combines natriuretic and antikaliuretic effects. Each component complements the action of the other. The hydrochlorothiazide component blocks the reabsorption of sodium and chloride ions, and thereby increases the quantity of sodium traversing the distal tubule and the volume of water excreted. A portion of the additional sodium presented to the distal tubule is exchanged there for potassium and hydrogen ions. With continued use of hydrochlorothiazide and depletion of sodium, compensatory mechanisms tend to increase this exchange and may produce excessive loss of potassium, hydrogen and chloride ions. Hydrochlorothiazide also decreases the excretion of calcium and uric acid, may increase the excretion of iodide and may reduce glomerular filtration rate. The exact mechanism of the antihypertensive effect of hydrochlorothiazide is not known.

The triamterene component of *Dyazide* exerts its diuretic effect on the distal renal tubule to inhibit the reabsorption of sodium in exchange for potassium and hydrogen ions. Its natriuretic activity is limited by the amount of sodium reaching its site of action. Although it blocks the increase in this exchange that is stimulated by mineralocorticoids (chiefly aldosterone) it is not a competitive antagonist of aldosterone and its activity can be demonstrated in adrenalectomized rats and patients with Addison's disease. As a result, the dose of triamterene required is not proportionally related to the level of mineralocorticoid activity, but is dictated by the response of the individual patients, and the kaliuretic effect of concomitantly administered drugs. By inhibiting the distal tubular exchange mechanism, triamterene maintains or increases the sodium excretion and reduces the excess loss of potassium, hydrogen and chloride ions induced by hydrochlorothiazide. As with hydrochlorothiazide, triamterene may reduce glomerular filtration and renal plasma flow. Via this mechanism it may reduce uric acid excretion although it has no tubular effect on uric acid reabsorption or secretion. Triamterene does not affect calcium excretion. No predictable antihypertensive effect has been demonstrated for triamterene.

Duration of diuretic activity and effective dosage range of the hydrochlorothiazide and triamterene components of *Dyazide* are similar. Onset of diuresis with *Dyazide* takes place within 1 hour, peaks at 2 to 3 hours and tapers off during the subsequent 7 to 9 hours.

Dyazide capsule is well absorbed.

Upon administration of a single oral dose to fasted normal male volunteers, the following mean pharmacokinetic parameters were determined:

[See table at top of next page]

where AUC(0–48), Cmax, Tmax and Ae represent area under the plasma concentration versus time plot, maximum plasma concentration, time to reach Cmax and amount excreted in urine over 48 hours.

Dyazide capsule is bioequivalent to a single-entity 25 mg hydrochlorothiazide tablet and 37.5 mg triamterene capsule used in the double-blind clinical trial below. (See Clinical Trials.)

In a limited study involving 12 subjects, coadministration of *Dyazide* with a high-fat meal resulted in: (1) an increase in the mean bioavailability of triamterene by about 67% (90% confidence interval = 0.99, 1.90), p-hydroxytriamterene sulfate by about 50% (90% confidence interval = 1.06, 1.77), hydrochlorothiazide by about 17% (90% confidence interval = 0.90, 1.34); (2) increases in the peak concentrations of triamterene and p-hydroxytriamterene; and (3) a delay of up to 2 hours in the absorption of the active constituents.

Clinical Trials

A placebo-controlled, double-blind trial was conducted to evaluate the efficacy of *Dyazide* capsules. This trial demonstrated that *Dyazide* (25 mg hydrochlorothiazide/37.5 mg triamterene) was effective in controlling blood pressure while reducing the incidence of hydrochlorothiazide-induced hypokalemia. This trial involved 636 patients with mild to moderate hypertension controlled by hydrochlorothiazide 25 mg daily and who had hypokalemia (serum potassium <3.5 mEq/L) secondary to the hydrochlorothiazide. Patients were randomly assigned to 4 weeks' treatment with once-daily regimens of 25 mg hydrochlorothiazide plus placebo, or 25 mg hydrochlorothiazide combined with one of the following doses of triamterene: 25 mg, 37.5 mg, 50 mg or 75 mg.

Blood pressure and serum potassium were monitored at baseline and throughout the trial. All five treatment groups had similar mean blood pressure and serum potassium concentrations at baseline (mean systolic blood pressure range: 137±14 mmHg to 140±16 mmHg; mean diastolic blood pressure range: 86±9 mmHg to 88±8 mmHg; mean serum potassium range: 2.3 to 3.4 mEq/L with the majority of patients having values between 3.1 and 3.4 mEq/L).

While all triamterene regimens reversed hypokalemia, at week 4 the 37.5 mg regimen proved optimal compared with the other tested regimens. On this regimen, 81% of the patients had a significant ($p<0.05$) reversal of hypokalemia vs. 59% of patients on the placebo/hydrochlorothiazide regimen. The mean serum potassium concentration on 37.5 mg triamterene went from 3.2±0.2 mEq/L at baseline to 3.7±0.3 mEq/L at week 4, a significantly greater ($p<0.05$) improvement than that achieved with placebo/hydrochlorothiazide (i.e., 3.2±0.2 mEq/L at baseline and 3.5±0.4 mEq/L at week 4). Also, 51% of patients in the 37.5 mg triamterene group had an increase in serum potassium of ≥0.5 mEq/L at week 4 vs. 33% in the placebo group. The 37.5 mg triamterene/25 mg hydrochlorothiazide regimen also maintained control of blood pressure; mean supine systolic blood pressure at week 4 was 138±21 mmHg while mean supine diastolic blood pressure was 87±13 mmHg.

INDICATIONS AND USAGE

This fixed combination drug is not indicated for the initial therapy of edema or hypertension except in individuals in whom the development of hypokalemia cannot be risked.

Dyazide is indicated for the treatment of hypertension or edema in patients who develop hypokalemia on hydrochlorothiazide alone.

Continued on next page

Information on the SmithKline Beecham Pharmaceuticals products appearing here is based on the labeling in effect on July 31, 1998. Further information on these and other products may be obtained from the Medical Department, SmithKline Beecham Pharmaceuticals, One Franklin Plaza, Philadelphia, PA 19101.

Dyazide—Cont.

Dyazide is also indicated for those patients who require a thiazide diuretic and in whom the development of hypokalemia cannot be risked.
Dyazide may be used alone or as an adjunct to other antihypertensive drugs, such as beta-blockers. Since *Dyazide* may enhance the action of these agents, dosage adjustments may be necessary.
Usage in Pregnancy: The routine use of diuretics in an otherwise healthy woman is inappropriate and exposes mother and fetus to unnecessary hazard. Diuretics do not prevent development of toxemia of pregnancy, and there is no satisfactory evidence that they are useful in the treatment of developed toxemia.
Edema during pregnancy may arise from pathological causes or from the physiologic and mechanical consequences of pregnancy. Diuretics are indicated in pregnancy when edema is due to pathologic causes, just as they are in the absence of pregnancy. Dependent edema in pregnancy resulting from restriction of venous return by the expanded uterus is properly treated through elevation of the lower extremities and use of support hose; use of diuretics to lower intravascular volume in this case is illogical and unnecessary. There is hypervolemia during normal pregnancy which is harmful to neither the fetus nor the mother (in the absence of cardiovascular disease), but which is associated with edema, including generalized edema in the majority of pregnant women. If this edema produces discomfort, increased recumbency will often provide relief. In rare instances this edema may cause extreme discomfort which is not relieved by rest. In these cases a short course of diuretics may provide relief and may be appropriate.

CONTRAINDICATIONS

Antikaliuretic Therapy and Potassium Supplementation
Dyazide should not be given to patients receiving other potassium-sparing agents such as spironolactone, amiloride or other formulations containing triamterene. Concomitant potassium-containing salt substitutes should also not be used. Potassium supplementation should not be used with *Dyazide* except in severe cases of hypokalemia. Such concomitant therapy can be associated with rapid increases in serum potassium levels. If potassium supplementation is used, careful monitoring of the serum potassium level is necessary.
Impaired Renal Function
Dyazide is contraindicated in patients with anuria, acute and chronic renal insufficiency or significant renal impairment.
Hypersensitivity
Hypersensitivity to either drug in the preparation or to other sulfonamide-derived drugs is a contraindication.
Hyperkalemia
Dyazide should not be used in patients with preexisting elevated serum potassium.

WARNINGS: Hyperkalemia

Abnormal elevation of serum potassium levels (greater than or equal to 5.5 mEq/liter) can occur with all potassium-sparing diuretic combinations, including *Dyazide*. Hyperkalemia is more likely to occur in patients with renal impairment and diabetes (even without evidence of renal impairment), and in the elderly or severely ill. Since uncorrected hyperkalemia may be fatal, serum potassium levels must be monitored at frequent intervals especially in patients first receiving *Dyazide*, when dosages are changed or with any illness that may influence renal function.

If hyperkalemia is suspected (warning signs include paresthesias, muscular weakness, fatigue, flaccid paralysis of the extremities, bradycardia and shock), an electrocardiogram (ECG) should be obtained. However, it is important to monitor serum potassium levels because hyperkalemia may not be associated with ECG changes.
If hyperkalemia is present, *Dyazide* should be discontinued immediately and a thiazide alone should be substituted. If the serum potassium exceeds 6.5 mEq/liter more vigorous therapy is required. The clinical situation dictates the procedures to be employed. These include the intravenous administration of calcium chloride solution, sodium bicarbonate solution and/or the oral or parenteral administration of glucose with a rapid-acting insulin preparation. Cationic exchange resins such as sodium polystyrene sulfonate may be orally or rectally administered. Persistent hyperkalemia may require dialysis.
The development of hyperkalemia associated with potassium-sparing diuretics is accentuated in the presence of renal impairment (see CONTRAINDICATIONS section). Patients with mild renal functional impairment should not receive this drug without frequent and continuing monitoring of serum electrolytes. Cumulative drug effects may be observed in patients with impaired renal function. The renal clearances of hydrochlorothiazide and the pharmacologically active metabolite of triamterene, the sulfate ester of hydroxytriamterene, have been shown to be reduced and the plasma levels increased following *Dyazide* administration to elderly patients and patients with impaired renal function.

	AUC(0–48) ng*hrs/mL (±SD)	Cmax ng/mL (±SD)	Median Tmax hrs	Ae mg (±SD)
triamterene	148.7 (87.9)	46.4 (29.4)	1.1	2.7 (1.4)
hydroxytriamterene sulfate	1865 (471)	720 (364)	1.3	19.7 (6.1)
hydrochlorothiazide	834 (177)	135.1 (35.7)	2.0	14.3 (3.8)

Hyperkalemia has been reported in diabetic patients with the use of potassium-sparing agents even in the absence of apparent renal impairment. Accordingly, serum electrolytes must be frequently monitored if *Dyazide* is used in diabetic patients.
Metabolic or Respiratory Acidosis
Potassium-sparing therapy should also be avoided in severely ill patients in whom respiratory or metabolic acidosis may occur. Acidosis may be associated with rapid elevations in serum potassium levels. If *Dyazide* is employed, frequent evaluations of acid/base balance and serum electrolytes are necessary.

PRECAUTIONS

Impaired Hepatic Function
Thiazides should be used with caution in patients with impaired hepatic function. They can precipitate hepatic coma in patients with severe liver disease. Potassium depletion induced by the thiazide may be important in this connection. Administer *Dyazide* cautiously and be alert for such early signs of impending coma as confusion, drowsiness and tremor; if mental confusion increases discontinue *Dyazide* for a few days. Attention must be given to other factors that may precipitate hepatic coma, such as blood in the gastrointestinal tract or preexisting potassium depletion.
Hypokalemia
Hypokalemia is uncommon with *Dyazide*; but, should it develop, corrective measures should be taken such as potassium supplementation or increased intake of potassium-rich foods. Institute such measures cautiously with frequent determinations of serum potassium levels, especially in patients receiving digitalis or with a history of cardiac arrhythmias. If serious hypokalemia (serum potassium less than 3.0 mEq/L) is demonstrated by repeat serum potassium determinations, *Dyazide* should be discontinued and potassium chloride supplementation initiated. Less serious hypokalemia should be evaluated with regard to other coexisting conditions and treated accordingly.
Electrolyte Imbalance
Electrolyte imbalance, often encountered in such conditions as heart failure, renal disease or cirrhosis of the liver, may also be aggravated by diuretics and should be considered during *Dyazide* therapy when using high doses for prolonged periods or in patients on a salt-restricted diet. Serum determinations of electrolytes should be performed, and are particularly important if the patient is vomiting excessively or receiving fluids parenterally. Possible fluid and electrolyte imbalance may be indicated by such warning signs as: dry mouth, thirst, weakness, lethargy, drowsiness, restlessness, muscle pain or cramps, muscular fatigue, hypotension, oliguria, tachycardia and gastrointestinal symptoms.
Hypochloremia
Although any chloride deficit is generally mild and usually does not require specific treatment except under extraordinary circumstances (as in liver disease or renal disease), chloride replacement may be required in the treatment of metabolic alkalosis. Dilutional hyponatremia may occur in edematous patients in hot weather; appropriate therapy is water restriction, rather than administration of salt, except in rare instances when the hyponatremia is life threatening. In actual salt depletion, appropriate replacement is the therapy of choice.
Renal Stones
Triamterene has been found in renal stones in association with the other usual calculus components. *Dyazide* should be used with caution in patients with a history of renal stones.
Laboratory Tests
Serum Potassium: The normal adult range of serum potassium is 3.5 to 5.0 mEq per liter with 4.5 mEq often being used for a reference point. If hypokalemia should develop, corrective measures should be taken such as potassium supplementation or increased dietary intake of potassium-rich foods.
Institute such measures cautiously with frequent determinations of serum potassium levels. Potassium levels persistently above 6 mEq per liter require careful observation and treatment. Serum potassium levels do not necessarily indicate true body potassium concentration. A rise in plasma pH may cause a decrease in plasma potassium concentration and an increase in the intracellular potassium concentration. Discontinue corrective measures for hypokalemia immediately if laboratory determinations reveal an abnormal elevation of serum potassium. Discontinue *Dyazide* and substitute a thiazide diuretic alone until potassium levels return to normal.
Serum Creatinine and BUN: *Dyazide* may produce an elevated blood urea nitrogen level, creatinine level or both. This apparently is secondary to a reversible reduction of glomerular filtration rate or a depletion of intravascular fluid volume (prerenal azotemia) rather than renal toxicity; levels usually return to normal when *Dyazide* is discontinued. If azotemia increases, discontinue *Dyazide*. Periodic BUN or serum creatinine determinations should be made, especially in elderly patients and in patients with suspected or confirmed renal insufficiency.
Serum PBI: Thiazide may decrease serum PBI levels without sign of thyroid disturbance.
Parathyroid Function: Thiazides should be discontinued before carrying out tests for parathyroid function. Calcium excretion is decreased by thiazides. Pathologic changes in the parathyroid glands with hypercalcemia and hypophosphatemia have been observed in a few patients on prolonged thiazide therapy. The common complications of hyperparathyroidism such as bone resorption and peptic ulceration have not been seen.
Drug Interactions
Angiotensin-converting enzyme inhibitors: Potassium-sparing agents should be used with caution in conjunction with angiotensin-converting enzyme (ACE) inhibitors due to an increased risk of hyperkalemia.
Oral hypoglycemic drugs: Concurrent use with chlorpropamide may increase the risk of severe hyponatremia.
Nonsteroidal anti-inflammatory drugs: A possible interaction resulting in acute renal failure has been reported in a few patients on *Dyazide* when treated with indomethacin, a nonsteroidal anti-inflammatory agent. Caution is advised in administering nonsteroidal anti-inflammatory agents with *Dyazide*.
Lithium: Lithium generally should not be given with diuretics because they reduce its renal clearance and increase the risk of lithium toxicity. Read circulars for lithium preparations before use of such concomitant therapy with *Dyazide*.
Surgical considerations: Thiazides have been shown to decrease arterial responsiveness to norepinephrine (an effect attributed to loss of sodium). This diminution is not sufficient to preclude effectiveness of the pressor agent for therapeutic use. Thiazides have also been shown to increase the paralyzing effect of nondepolarizing muscle relaxants such as tubocurarine (an effect attributed to potassium loss); consequently caution should be observed in patients undergoing surgery.
Other Considerations: Concurrent use of hydrochlorothiazide with amphotericin B or corticosteroids or corticotropin (ACTH) may intensify electrolyte imbalance, particularly hypokalemia, although the presence of triamterene minimizes the hypokalemic effect.
Thiazides may add to or potentiate the action of other antihypertensive drugs. See INDICATIONS AND USAGE for concomitant use with other antihypertensive drugs.
The effect of oral anticoagulants may be decreased when used concurrently with hydrochlorothiazide; dosage adjustments may be necessary.
Dyazide may raise the level of blood uric acid; dosage adjustments of antigout medication may be necessary to control hyperuricemia and gout.
The following agents given together with triamterene may promote serum potassium accumulation and possibly result in hyperkalemia because of the potassium-sparing nature of triamterene, especially in patients with renal insufficiency: blood from blood bank (may contain up to 30 mEq of potassium per liter of plasma or up to 65 mEq per liter of whole blood when stored for more than 10 days); low-salt milk (may contain up to 60 mEq of potassium per liter); potassium-containing medications (such as parenteral penicillin G potassium); salt substitutes (most contain substantial amounts of potassium).
Exchange resins, such as sodium polystyrene sulfonate, whether administered orally or rectally, reduce serum potassium levels by sodium replacement of the potassium; fluid retention may occur in some patients because of the increased sodium intake.
Chronic or overuse of laxatives may reduce serum potassium levels by promoting excessive potassium loss from the intestinal tract; laxatives may interfere with the potassium-retaining effects of triamterene.
The effectiveness of methenamine may be decreased when used concurrently with hydrochlorothiazide because of alkalinization of the urine.

Drug/Laboratory Test Interactions
Triamterene and quinidine have similar fluorescence spectra; thus, *Dyazide* will interfere with the fluorescent measurement of quinidine.

Carcinogenesis, Mutagenesis, Impairment of Fertility

Carcinogenesis
Long-term studies have not been conducted with *Dyazide* (the triamterene/hydrochlorothiazide combination), or with triamterene alone.
Hydrochlorothiazide: Two-year feeding studies in mice and rats, conducted under the auspices of the National Toxicology Program (NTP), treated mice and rats with doses of hydrochlorothiazide up to 600 and 100 mg/kg/day, respectively. On a body-weight basis, these doses are 600 times (in mice) and 100 times (in rats) the Maximum Recommended Human Dose (MRHD) for the hydrochlorothiazide component of *Dyazide* at 50 mg/day (or 1.0 mg/kg/day based on 50 kg individuals). On the basis of body-surface area, these doses are 56 times (in mice) and 21 times (in rats) the MRHD. These studies uncovered no evidence of carcinogenic potential of hydrochlorothiazide in rats or female mice, but there was equivocal evidence of hepatocarcinogenicity in male mice.

Mutagenesis
Studies of the mutagenic potential of *Dyazide* (the triamterene/hydrochlorothiazide combination), or of triamterene alone have not been performed.
Hydrochlorothiazide: Hydrochlorothiazide was not genotoxic in *in vitro* assays using strains TA 98, TA 100, TA 1535, TA 1537 and TA 1538 of *Salmonella typhimurium* (the Ames test); in the Chinese Hamster Ovary (CHO) test for chromosomal aberrations; or in *in vivo* assays using mouse germinal cell chromosomes, Chinese hamster bone marrow chromosomes, and the *Drosophila* sex-linked recessive lethal trait gene. Positive test results were obtained in the *in vitro* CHO Sister Chromatid Exchange (clastogenicity) test, and in the mouse Lymphoma Cell (mutagenicity) assays, using concentrations of hydrochlorothiazide of 43 to 1300 mcg/mL. Positive test results were also obtained in the *Aspergillus nidulans* nondisjunction assay, using an unspecified concentration of hydrochlorothiazide.

Impairment of Fertility
Studies of the effects of *Dyazide* (the triamterene/hydrochlorothiazide combination), or of triamterene alone on animal reproductive function have not been conducted.
Hydrochlorothiazide: Hydrochlorothiazide had no adverse effects on the fertility of mice and rats of either sex in studies wherein these species were exposed, via their diet, to doses of up to 100 and 4 mg/kg/day, respectively, prior to mating and throughout gestation. Corresponding multiples of the MRHD are 100 (mice) and 4 (rats) on the basis of body-weight and 9.4 (mice) and 0.8 (rats) on the basis of body-surface area.

Pregnancy: Category C
Teratogenic Effects
Dyazide: Animal reproduction studies to determine the potential for fetal harm by *Dyazide* have not been conducted. However, a One Generation Study in the rat approximated *Dyazide* composition by using a 1:1 ratio of triamterene to hydrochlorothiazide (30:30 mg/kg/day); there was no evidence of teratogenicity at those doses which were, on a body-weight basis, 15 and 30 times, respectively, the MRHD, and on the basis of body-surface area, 3.1 and 6.2 times, respectively, the MRHD.
The safe use of *Dyazide* in pregnancy has not been established since there are no adequate and well-controlled studies with *Dyazide* in pregnant women. *Dyazide* should be used during pregnancy only if the potential benefit justifies the risk to the fetus.
Triamterene: Reproduction studies have been performed in rats at doses as high as 20 times the MRHD on the basis of body-weight, and 6 times the human dose on the basis of body-surface area without evidence of harm to the fetus due to triamterene.
Because animal reproduction studies are not always predictive of human response, this drug should be used during pregnancy only if clearly needed.
Hydrochlorothiazide: Hydrochlorothiazide was orally administered to pregnant mice and rats during respective periods of major organogenesis at doses up to 3000 and 1000 mg/kg/day, respectively. At these doses, which are multiples of the MRHD equal to 3000 for mice and 1000 for rats, based on body-weight, and equal to 282 for mice and 206 for rats, based on body-surface area, there was no evidence of harm to the fetus.
There are, however, no adequate and well-controlled studies in pregnant women. Because animal reproduction studies are not always predictive of human response, this drug should be used during pregnancy only if clearly needed.
Nonteratogenic Effects—Thiazides and triamterene have been shown to cross the placental barrier and appear in cord blood. The use of thiazides and triamterene in pregnant women requires that the anticipated benefit be weighed against possible hazards to the fetus. These hazards include fetal or neonatal jaundice, pancreatitis, thrombocytopenia and possible other adverse reactions which have occurred in the adult.
Nursing Mothers—Thiazides and triamterene in combination have not been studied in nursing mothers. Triamterene appears in animal milk; this may occur in humans. Thiazides are excreted in human breast milk. If use of the combination drug product is deemed essential, the patient should stop nursing.
Pediatric Use—Safety and effectiveness in children have not been established.

ADVERSE REACTIONS
Adverse effects are listed in decreasing order of frequency; however, the most serious adverse effects are listed first regardless of frequency. The serious adverse effects associated with *Dyazide* have commonly occurred in less than 0.1% of patients treated with this product.
Hypersensitivity: anaphylaxis, rash, urticaria, photosensitivity.
Cardiovascular: arrhythmia, postural hypotension.
Metabolic: diabetes mellitus, hyperkalemia, hyperglycemia, glycosuria, hyperuricemia, hypokalemia, hyponatremia, acidosis, hypochloremia.
Gastrointestinal: jaundice and/or liver enzyme abnormalities, pancreatitis, nausea and vomiting, diarrhea, constipation, abdominal pain.
Renal: acute renal failure (one case of irreversible renal failure has been reported), interstitial nephritis, renal stones composed primarily of triamterene, elevated BUN and serum creatinine, abnormal urinary sediment.
Hematologic: leukopenia, thrombocytopenia and purpura, megaloblastic anemia.
Musculoskeletal: muscle cramps.
Central Nervous System: weakness, fatigue, dizziness, headache, dry mouth.
Miscellaneous: impotence, sialadenitis.
Thiazides alone have been shown to cause the following additional adverse reactions:
Central Nervous System: paresthesias, vertigo.
Ophthalmic: xanthopsia, transient blurred vision.
Respiratory: allergic pneumonitis, pulmonary edema, respiratory distress.
Other: necrotizing vasculitis, exacerbation of lupus.
Hematologic: aplastic anemia, agranulocytosis, hemolytic anemia.
Neonate and infancy: thrombocytopenia and pancreatitis—rarely, in newborns whose mothers have received thiazides during pregnancy.

DOSAGE AND ADMINISTRATION
The usual dose of *Dyazide* is one or two capsules given once daily, with appropriate monitoring of serum potassium and of the clinical effect. (See WARNINGS, Hyperkalemia.)

OVERDOSAGE
Electrolyte imbalance is the major concern (see WARNINGS section). Symptoms reported include: polyuria, nausea, vomiting, weakness, lassitude, fever, flushed face and hyperactive deep tendon reflexes. If hypotension occurs, it may be treated with pressor agents such as levarterenol to maintain blood pressure. Carefully evaluate the electrolyte pattern and fluid balance. Induce immediate evacuation of the stomach through emesis or gastric lavage. There is no specific antidote.
Reversible acute renal failure following ingestion of 50 tablets of a product containing a combination of 50 mg triamterene and 25 mg hydrochlorothiazide has been reported.
Although triamterene is largely protein-bound (approximately 67%), there may be some benefit to dialysis in cases of overdosage.

HOW SUPPLIED
Capsules containing 25 mg hydrochlorothiazide and 37.5 mg triamterene, in bottles of 1000 capsules; in Single Unit Packages (unit-dose) of 100 (intended for institutional use only); in Patient-Pak™ unit-of-use bottles of 100.
They are supplied as follows:
NDC 0007-3650-21—Single Unit Packages (unit-dose) of 100 (intended for institutional use only).
NDC 0007-3650-22—in Patient-Pak™ unit-of-use bottles of 100.
NDC 0007-3650-30—bottles of 1000.
Store between 15° and 30°C (59° and 86°F). Protect from light. Dispense in a tight, light-resistant container.
Veterans Administration/Military/PHS—Capsules, 100's (SUP), 6505-01-390-0308; 100's, 6505-01-390-0348; 1000's, 6505-01-390-0358.
DZ:L65A

Shown in Product Identification Guide, page 339

DYRENIUM® ℞
[*di-ren 'ee-um*]
brand of triamterene
Capsules
50 mg and 100 mg
potassium-sparing diuretic

DESCRIPTION
Dyrenium (triamterene) is a potassium-sparing diuretic.
Triamterene is 2,4,7-triamino-6-phenyl-pteridine. Its molecular weight is 253.27. At 50°C, triamterene is slightly soluble in water. It is soluble in dilute ammonia, dilute aqueous sodium hydroxide and dimethylformamide. It is sparingly soluble in methanol.
Each capsule for oral use, with opaque red cap and body, contains triamterene, 50 or 100 mg, and is imprinted with the product name DYRENIUM, strength (50 or 100) and SKF. Inactive ingredients consist of benzyl alcohol, cetylpyridinium chloride, D&C Red No. 33, FD&C Yellow No. 6, gelatin, lactose, magnesium stearate, povidone, sodium lauryl sulfate, titanium dioxide and trace amounts of other inactive ingredients.

CLINICAL PHARMACOLOGY
Triamterene has a unique mode of action; it inhibits the reabsorption of sodium ions in exchange for potassium and hydrogen ions at that segment of the distal tubule under the control of adrenal mineralocorticoids (especially aldosterone). This activity is not directly related to aldosterone secretion or antagonism; it is a result of a direct effect on the renal tubule.
The fraction of filtered sodium reaching this distal tubular exchange site is relatively small, and the amount which is exchanged depends on the level of mineralocorticoid activity. Thus, the degree of natriuresis and diuresis produced by inhibition of the exchange mechanism is necessarily limited. Increasing the amount of available sodium and the level of mineralocorticoid activity by the use of more proximally acting diuretics will increase the degree of diuresis and potassium conservation.
Triamterene occasionally causes increases in serum potassium which can result in hyperkalemia. It does not produce alkalosis because it does not cause excessive excretion of titratable acid and ammonium.
Triamterene has been shown to cross the placental barrier and appear in the cord blood of animals.

Pharmacokinetics
Onset of action is 2 to 4 hours after ingestion. In normal volunteers the mean peak serum levels were 30 ng/mL at 3 hours. The average percent of drug recovered in the urine (0 to 48 hours) was 21%. Triamterene is primarily metabolized to the sulfate conjugate of hydroxytriamterene. Both the plasma and urine levels of this metabolite greatly exceed triamterene levels. Triamterene is rapidly absorbed, with somewhat less than 50% of the oral dose reaching the urine. Most patients will respond to Dyrenium (triamterene) during the first day of treatment. Maximum therapeutic effect, however, may not be seen for several days. Duration of diuresis depends on several factors, especially renal function, but it generally tapers off 7 to 9 hours after administration.

INDICATIONS AND USAGE
Dyrenium (triamterene) is indicated in the treatment of edema associated with congestive heart failure, cirrhosis of the liver, and the nephrotic syndrome; also in steroid-induced edema, idiopathic edema and edema due to secondary hyperaldosteronism.
Dyrenium may be used alone or with other diuretics either for its added diuretic effect or its potassium-sparing potential. It also promotes increased diuresis when patients prove resistant or only partially responsive to thiazides or other diuretics because of secondary hyperaldosteronism.
Usage in Pregnancy. The routine use of diuretics in an otherwise healthy woman is inappropriate and exposes mother and fetus to unnecessary hazard. Diuretics do not prevent development of toxemia of pregnancy, and there is no satisfactory evidence that they are useful in the treatment of developed toxemia.
Edema during pregnancy may arise from pathological causes or from the physiologic and mechanical consequences of pregnancy. Diuretics are indicated in pregnancy when edema is due to pathologic causes, just as they are in the absence of pregnancy (however, see PRECAUTIONS below). Dependent edema in pregnancy, resulting from restriction of venous return by the expanded uterus, is properly treated through elevation of the lower extremities and use of support hose; use of diuretics to lower intravascular volume in this case is illogical and unnecessary. There is hypervolemia during normal pregnancy which is harmful to neither the fetus nor the mother (in the absence of cardiovascular disease), but which is associated with edema, including generalized edema, in the majority of pregnant women. If this edema produces discomfort, increased recumbency will often provide relief. In rare instances, this edema may cause extreme discomfort which is not relieved by rest. In these cases, a short course of diuretics may provide relief and may be appropriate.

Continued on next page

Information on the SmithKline Beecham Pharmaceuticals products appearing here is based on the labeling in effect on July 31, 1998. Further information on these and other products may be obtained from the Medical Department, SmithKline Beecham Pharmaceuticals, One Franklin Plaza, Philadelphia, PA 19101.

Dyrenium—Cont.

CONTRAINDICATIONS

Anuria. Severe or progressive kidney disease or dysfunction with the possible exception of nephrosis. Severe hepatic disease. Hypersensitivity to the drug.

Dyrenium (triamterene) should not be used in patients with pre-existing elevated serum potassium, as is sometimes seen in patients with impaired renal function or azotemia, or in patients who develop hyperkalemia while on the drug. Patients should not be placed on dietary potassium supplements, potassium salts or potassium-containing salt substitutes in conjunction with *Dyrenium*.

Dyrenium should not be given to patients receiving other potassium-sparing agents such as spironolactone, amiloride hydrochloride or other formulations containing triamterene. Two deaths have been reported in patients receiving concomitant spironolactone and *Dyrenium* or Dyazide®. Although dosage recommendations were exceeded in one case and in the other serum electrolytes were not properly monitored, these two drugs should not be given concomitantly.

WARNINGS

> Abnormal elevation of serum potassium levels (greater than or equal to 5.5 mEq/liter) can occur with all potassium-sparing agents, including *Dyrenium*. Hyperkalemia is more likely to occur in patients with renal impairment and diabetes (even without evidence of renal impairment), and in the elderly or severely ill. Since uncorrected hyperkalemia may be fatal, serum potassium levels must be monitored at frequent intervals especially in patients receiving *Dyrenium*, when dosages are changed or with any illness that may influence renal function.

There have been isolated reports of hypersensitivity reactions; therefore, patients should be observed regularly for the possible occurrence of blood dyscrasias, liver damage or other idiosyncratic reactions.

Periodic BUN and serum potassium determinations should be made to check kidney function, especially in patients with suspected or confirmed renal insufficiency. It is particularly important to make serum potassium determinations in elderly or diabetic patients receiving the drug; these patients should be observed carefully for possible serum potassium increases.

If hyperkalemia is present or suspected, an electrocardiogram should be obtained. If the ECG shows no widening of the QRS or arrhythmia in the presence of hyperkalemia, it is usually sufficient to discontinue Dyrenium (triamterene) and any potassium supplementation and substitute a thiazide alone. Sodium polystyrene sulfonate (Kayexalate®, Winthrop) may be administered to enhance the excretion of excess potassium. **The presence of a widened QRS complex or arrhythmia in association with hyperkalemia requires prompt additional therapy.** For tachyarrhythmia, infuse 44 mEq of sodium bicarbonate or 10 mL of 10% calcium gluconate or calcium chloride over several minutes. For asystole, bradycardia or A-V block transvenous pacing is also recommended.

The effect of calcium and sodium bicarbonate is transient and repeated administration may be required. When indicated by the clinical situation, excess K^+ may be removed by dialysis or oral or rectal administration of Kayexalate®. Infusion of glucose and insulin has also been used to treat hyperkalemia.

PRECAUTIONS

General

Dyrenium (triamterene) tends to conserve potassium rather than to promote the excretion as do many diuretics and, occasionally, can cause increases in serum potassium which, in some instances, can result in hyperkalemia. In rare instances, hyperkalemia has been associated with cardiac irregularities.

Electrolyte imbalance often encountered in such diseases as congestive heart failure, renal disease or cirrhosis may be aggravated or caused independently by any effective diuretic agent including *Dyrenium*. The use of full doses of a diuretic when salt intake is restricted can result in a low-salt syndrome.

Triamterene can cause mild nitrogen retention which is reversible upon withdrawal of the drug and is seldom observed with intermittent (every-other-day) therapy.

Triamterene may cause a decreasing alkali reserve with the possibility of metabolic acidosis.

By the very nature of their illness, cirrhotics with splenomegaly sometimes have marked variations in their blood pictures. Since triamterene is a weak folic acid antagonist, it may contribute to the appearance of megaloblastosis in cases where folic acid stores have been depleted. Therefore, periodic blood studies in these patients are recommended. They should also be observed for exacerbations of underlying liver disease.

Triamterene has elevated uric acid, especially in persons predisposed to gouty arthritis.

Triamterene has been reported in renal stones in association with other calculus components. *Dyrenium* should be used with caution in patients with histories of renal stones.

Information for Patients

To help avoid stomach upset, it is recommended that the drug be taken after meals.

If a single daily dose is prescribed, it may be preferable to take it in the morning to minimize the effect of increased frequency of urination on nighttime sleep.

If a dose is missed, the patient should not take more than the prescribed dose at the next dosing interval.

Laboratory Tests

Hyperkalemia will rarely occur in patients with adequate urinary output, but it is a possibility if large doses are used for considerable periods of time. If hyperkalemia is observed, Dyrenium (triamterene) should be withdrawn. The normal adult range of serum potassium is 3.5 to 5.0 mEq per liter with 4.5 mEq often being used for a reference point. Potassium levels persistently above 6 mEq per liter require careful observation and treatment. Normal potassium levels tend to be higher in neonates (7.7 mEq per liter) than in adults.

Serum potassium levels do not necessarily indicate true body potassium concentration. A rise in plasma pH may cause a decrease in plasma potassium concentration and an increase in the intracellular potassium concentration. Because *Dyrenium* conserves potassium, it has been theorized that in patients who have received intensive therapy or been given the drug for prolonged periods, a rebound kaliuresis could occur upon abrupt withdrawal. In such patients withdrawal of *Dyrenium* should be gradual.

Drug Interactions

Caution should be used when lithium and diuretics are used concomitantly because diuretic-induced sodium loss may reduce the renal clearance of lithium and increase serum lithium levels with risk of lithium toxicity. Patients receiving such combined therapy should have serum lithium levels monitored closely and the lithium dosage adjusted if necessary.

A possible interaction resulting in acute renal failure has been reported in a few subjects when indomethacin, a nonsteroidal anti-inflammatory agent, was given with triamterene. Caution is advised in administering nonsteroidal anti-inflammatory agents with triamterene.

The effects of the following drugs may be potentiated when given together with triamterene: antihypertensive medication, other diuretics, preanesthetic and anesthetic agents, skeletal muscle relaxants (nondepolarizing).

Potassium-sparing agents should be used with caution in conjunction with angiotensin-converting enzyme (ACE) inhibitors due to an increased risk of hyperkalemia.

The following agents, given together with triamterene, may promote serum potassium accumulation and possibly result in hyperkalemia because of the potassium-sparing nature of triamterene, especially in patients with renal insufficiency: blood from blood bank (may contain up to 30 mEq of potassium per liter of plasma or up to 65 mEq per liter of whole blood when stored for more than 10 days); low-salt milk (may contain up to 60 mEq of potassium per liter); potassium-containing medications (such as parenteral penicillin G potassium); salt substitutes (most contain substantial amounts of potassium).

Dyrenium (triamterene) may raise blood glucose levels; for adult-onset diabetes, dosage adjustments of hypoglycemic agents may be necessary during and after therapy; concurrent use with chlorpropamide may increase the risk of severe hyponatremia.

Drug/Laboratory Test Interactions

Triamterene and quinidine have similar fluorescence spectra; thus, triamterene will interfere with the fluorescent measurement of quinidine.

Carcinogenesis, Mutagenesis, Impairment of Fertility

Long-term studies to determine the carcinogenic potential of triamterene are not available. Studies to determine the mutagenic potential of triamterene are not available. Reproductive studies have been performed in rats at doses up to 30 times the human dose and have revealed no evidence of impaired fertility.

Pregnancy

Teratogenic Effects: Pregnancy Category B: Reproduction studies have been performed in rats at doses up to 30 times the human dose and have revealed no evidence of impaired fertility or harm to the fetus due to triamterene. There are, however, no adequate and well-controlled studies in pregnant women. Because animal reproductive studies are not always predictive of human response, this drug should be used during pregnancy only if clearly needed.

Nonteratogenic Effects: Triamterene has been shown to cross the placental barrier and appear in the cord blood of animals; this may occur in humans. The use of *Dyrenium* in pregnant women requires that the anticipated benefit be weighed against possible hazards to the fetus. These possible hazards include adverse reactions which have occurred in the adult.

Nursing Mothers: Triamterene appears in animal milk; this may occur in humans. If use of the drug is deemed essential, the patient should stop nursing.

Pediatric Use: Safety and effectiveness in children have not been established.

ADVERSE REACTIONS

Adverse effects are listed in decreasing order of frequency; however, the most serious adverse effects are listed first regardless of frequency. All adverse effects occur rarely (that is, 1 in 1000, or less).

Hypersensitivity: anaphylaxis, rash, photosensitivity.

Metabolic: hyperkalemia, hypokalemia.

Renal: azotemia, elevated BUN and creatinine, renal stones, acute interstitial nephritis (rare), acute renal failure (one case of irreversible renal failure has been reported).

Gastrointestinal: jaundice and/or liver enzyme abnormalities, nausea and vomiting, diarrhea.

Hematologic: thrombocytopenia, megaloblastic anemia.

Central Nervous System: weakness, fatigue, dizziness, headache, dry mouth.

OVERDOSAGE

In the event of overdosage it can be theorized that electrolyte imbalance would be the major concern, with particular attention to possible hyperkalemia. Other symptoms that might be seen would be nausea and vomiting, other G.I. disturbances and weakness. It is conceivable that some hypotension could occur. As with an overdose of any drug, immediate evacuation of the stomach should be induced through emesis and gastric lavage. Careful evaluation of the electrolyte pattern and fluid balance should be made. There is no specific antidote.

Reversible acute renal failure following ingestion of 50 tablets of a product containing a combination of 50 mg triamterene and 25 mg hydrochlorothiazide has been reported. The oral LD_{50} in mice is 380 mg/kg. The amount of drug in a single dose ordinarily associated with symptoms of overdose or likely to be life-threatening is not known.

Although triamterene is 67% protein-bound, there may be some benefit to dialysis in cases of overdosage.

DOSAGE AND ADMINISTRATION

Adult Dosage

Dosage should be titrated to the needs of the individual patient. When used alone, the usual starting dose is 100 mg twice daily after meals. When combined with another diuretic or antihypertensive agent, the total daily dosage of each agent should usually be lowered initially and then adjusted to the patient's needs. The total daily dosage should not exceed 300 mg. Please refer to PRECAUTIONS-General.

When Dyrenium (triamterene) is added to other diuretic therapy or when patients are switched to *Dyrenium* from other diuretics, all potassium supplementation should be discontinued.

HOW SUPPLIED

Capsules: 50 mg in bottles of 100 and 100 mg in bottles of 100.

Store between 15° and 30°C (59° and 86°F). Protect from light.

50 mg 100's: NDC 0108-3806-20

100 mg 100's: NDC 0108-3807-20

Veterans Administration/Military/PHS—Capsules, 50 mg, 100's, 6505-01-058-5726; 100 mg, 100's, 6505-00-982-9143. DY:L42

Shown in Product Identification Guide, page 339

ENGERIX–B®   ℞

[en 'jur-ix bee]

Hepatitis B Vaccine (Recombinant)

DESCRIPTION

Engerix-B [Hepatitis B Vaccine (Recombinant)] is a noninfectious recombinant DNA hepatitis B vaccine developed and manufactured by SmithKline Beecham Biologicals. It contains purified surface antigen of the virus obtained by culturing genetically engineered *Saccharomyces cerevisiae* cells, which carry the surface antigen gene of the hepatitis B virus. The surface antigen expressed in *Saccharomyces cerevisiae* cells is purified by several physicochemical steps and formulated as a suspension of the antigen adsorbed on aluminum hydroxide. The procedures used to manufacture *Engerix-B* result in a product that contains no more than 5% yeast protein. No substances of human origin are used in its manufacture.

Engerix-B is supplied as a sterile suspension for intramuscular administration. The vaccine is ready for use without reconstitution; it must be shaken before administration since a fine white deposit with a clear colorless supernatant may form on storage.

Each 1 mL of vaccine consists of 20 mcg of hepatitis B surface antigen adsorbed on 0.5 mg aluminum as aluminum hydroxide. Each 0.5 mL of vaccine consists of 10 mcg of hepatitis B surface antigen adsorbed on 0.25 mg aluminum as

aluminum hydroxide. Both formulations contain 1:20,000 thimerosal (mercury derivative) as a preservative, sodium chloride (9 mg/mL) and phosphate buffers (disodium phosphate dihydrate, 0.98 mg/mL; sodium dihydrogen phosphate dihydrate, 0.71 mg/mL).

CLINICAL PHARMACOLOGY

Several hepatitis viruses are known to cause a systemic infection resulting in major pathologic changes in the liver (e.g., A, B, C, D, E). The estimated lifetime risk of HBV infection in the United States varies from almost 100% for the highest-risk groups to approximately 5% for the population as a whole.[1] Hepatitis B infection can have serious consequences including acute massive hepatic necrosis, chronic active hepatitis and cirrhosis of the liver. Sixty to 80% of neonates and 6 to 10% of adults who are infected in the United States will become hepatitis B virus carriers.[1] It has been estimated that more than 170 million people in the world today are persistently infected with hepatitis B virus.[2] The Centers for Disease Control (CDC) estimates that there are approximately 0.75 to 1.0 million chronic carriers of hepatitis B virus in the United States.[1] Those patients who become chronic carriers can infect others and are at increased risk of developing primary hepatocellular carcinoma. Among other factors, infection with hepatitis B may be the single most important factor for development of this carcinoma.[1,3] Considering the serious consequences of infection, immunization should be considered for all persons at potential risk of exposure to the hepatitis B virus. Mothers infected with hepatitis B virus can infect their infants at, or shortly after, birth if they are carriers of the HBsAg antigen or develop an active infection during the third trimester of pregnancy. Infected infants usually become chronic carriers. Therefore, screening of pregnant women for hepatitis B is recommended.[1] Because a vaccination strategy limited to high-risk individuals has failed to substantially lower the overall incidence of hepatitis B infection, both the Immunization Practices Advisory Committee (ACIP) and the Committee on Infectious Diseases of the American Academy of Pediatrics (AAP) have endorsed universal infant immunization as part of a comprehensive strategy for the control of hepatitis B infection.[4,5] The ACIP, AAP, American Academy of Family Physicians (AAFP) and American Medical Association (AMA) recommend routine vaccination of adolescents 11 to 12 years of age who have not been vaccinated previously.[6] The AAP further recommends that providers administer hepatitis B vaccine to all previously unvaccinated adolescents.[7] (See INDICATIONS AND USAGE.) There is no specific treatment for acute hepatitis B infection. However, those who develop anti-HBs antibodies after active infection are usually protected against subsequent infection. Antibody titers ≥10 mIU/mL against HBsAg are recognized as conferring protection against hepatitis B.[8] Seroconversion is defined as antibody titers ≥1 mIU/mL.

Immunogenicity in Healthy Adults and Adolescents: Clinical trials in healthy adult and adolescent subjects have shown that following a course of three doses of 20 mcg *Engerix-B* given according to the ACIP recommended schedule of injections at months 0, 1 and 6, the seroprotection (antibody titers ≥10 mIU/mL) rate for all individuals was 79% at month 6 and 96% at month 7; the geometric mean antibody titer (GMT) for seroconverters at month 7 was 2,204 mIU/mL. On an alternate schedule (injections at months 0, 1 and 2) designed for certain populations (e.g., neonates born of hepatitis B infected mothers, individuals who have or might have been recently exposed to the virus, and certain travelers to high-risk areas. See INDICATIONS AND USAGE.), 99% of all individuals were seroprotected at month 3 and remained protected through month 12. On the alternate schedule, an additional dose at 12 months produced a GMT for seroconverters at month 13 of 9,163 mIU/mL.

Immunogenicity in Adolescents: In clinical trials with healthy adolescent subjects 11 through 19 years of age, immunization with 10 mcg using a 0, 1, 6-month schedule produced a seroprotection rate of 97% at month 8 (N=119) with a GMT of 1,989 mIU/mL (N=118, 95% confidence intervals=1,318–3,020). Immunization with 20 mcg using a 0, 1, 6-month schedule produced a seroprotection rate of 99% at month 8 (N=122) with a GMT of 7,672 mIU/mL (N=122, 95% confidence intervals=5,248–10,965).

Immunogenicity in Neonates: Immunization with 10 mcg at 0, 1 and 2 months of age produced a seroprotection rate of 96% in infants by month 4, with a GMT among seroconverters of 210 mIU/mL (N=311); an additional dose at month 12 produced a GMT among seroconverters of 2,941 mIU/mL at month 13 (N=126).
Immunization with 10 mcg at 0, 1 and 6 months of age produced seroconversion in 100% of infants by month 7 with a GMT of 713 mIU/mL (N=52), and the seroprotection rate was 97%.
Clinical trials indicate that administration of hepatitis B immune globulin at birth does not alter the response to *Engerix-B*.

Immunogenicity in Children: In clinical trials with 242 children ages 6 months to, and including, 10 years given 10 mcg at months 0, 1 and 6, the seroprotection rate was 98% 1 to 2 months after the third dose; the GMT of seroconverters was 4,023 mIU/mL.

Immunogenicity in Older Subjects: Among older subjects given 20 mcg at months 0, 1 and 6, the seroprotection rate 1 month after the third dose was 88%. However, as with other hepatitis B vaccines, in adults over 40 years of age, *Engerix-B* vaccine produced anti-HBs titers that were lower than those in younger adults (GMT among seroconverters 1 month after the third 20 mcg dose with a 0, 1, 6-month schedule: 610 mIU/mL for individuals over 40 years of age, N=50).

Immunogenicity in Subjects with Chronic Hepatitis C: In a clinical trial of subjects with chronic hepatitis C, 31 subjects received *Engerix-B* on the usual 0, 1, 6-month schedule. All subjects responded with seroprotective titers. The GMT of anti-HBs was 1,260 mIU/mL (95% CI:709-2237).

Hemodialysis Patients: Hemodialysis patients given hepatitis B vaccines respond with lower titers,[9] which remain at protective levels for shorter durations than in normal subjects. In a study in which patients on chronic hemodialysis (mean time on dialysis was 24 months; N=562) received 40 mcg of the plasma-derived vaccine at months 0, 1 and 6, approximately 50% of patients achieved antibody titers ≥10 mIU/mL.[9] Since a fourth dose of *Engerix-B* given to healthy adults at month 12 following the 0, 1, 2-month schedule resulted in a substantial increase in the GMT (see above), a four-dose regimen was studied in hemodialysis patients. In a clinical trial of adults who had been on hemodialysis for a mean of 56 months (N=43), 67% of patients were seroprotected 2 months after the last dose of 40 mcg of *Engerix-B* (two × 20 mcg) given on a 0, 1, 2, 6-month schedule; the GMT among seroconverters was 93 mIU/mL.

Protective Efficacy: Protective efficacy with *Engerix-B* has been demonstrated in a clinical trial in neonates at high risk of hepatitis B infection.[10,11] Fifty-eight neonates born of mothers who were both HBsAg and HBeAg positive were given *Engerix-B* (10 mcg at 0, 1 and 2 months) without concomitant hepatitis B immune globulin. Two infants became chronic carriers in the 12-month follow-up period after initial inoculation. Assuming an expected carrier rate of 70%,[1] the protective efficacy rate against the chronic carrier state during the first 12 months of life was 95%.

Other Clinical Studies: In one study,[12] four of 244 (1.6%) adults (homosexual men) at high risk of contracting hepatitis B virus became infected during the period prior to completion of three doses of *Engerix-B* (20 mcg at 0, 1, 6 months). No additional patients became infected during the 18-month follow-up period after completion of the immunization course.

Interchangeability with Other Hepatitis B Vaccines: Recombinant DNA vaccines are produced in yeast by expression of a hepatitis B virus gene sequence that codes for the hepatitis B surface antigen. Like plasma-derived vaccine, the yeast-derived vaccines are protein particles visible by electron microscopy and have hepatitis B surface antigen epitopes as determined by monoclonal antibody analyses. Yeast-derived vaccines have been shown by *in vitro* analyses to induce antibodies (anti-HBs) which are immunologically comparable by epitope specificity and binding affinity to antibodies induced by plasma-derived vaccine.[13] In cross absorption studies, no differences were detected in the spectra of antibodies induced in man to plasma-derived or to yeast-derived hepatitis B vaccines.[13]
Additionally, patients immunized approximately 3 years previously with plasma-derived vaccine and whose antibody titers were <100 mIU/mL (GMT: 35 mIU/mL; range: 9–94) were given a 20 mcg dose of *Engerix-B*. All patients, including two who had not responded to the plasma-derived vaccine, showed a response to *Engerix-B* (GMT: 5,069 mIU/mL; range: 624–15,019). There have been no clinical studies in which a three-dose vaccine series was initiated with a plasma-derived hepatitis B vaccine and completed with *Engerix-B*, or vice versa. However, because the *in vitro* and *in vivo* studies described above indicate the comparability of the antibody produced in response to plasma-derived vaccine and *Engerix-B*, it should be possible to interchange the use of *Engerix-B* and plasma-derived vaccines (but see CONTRAINDICATIONS).
A controlled study (N=48) demonstrated that completion of a course of immunization with one dose of *Engerix-B* (20 mcg, month 6) following two doses of Recombivax HB® (10 mcg, months 0 and 1) produced a similar GMT (4,077 mIU/mL) to immunization with three doses of *Recombivax HB* (10 mcg, months 0, 1 and 6; 2,654 mIU/mL). Thus, *Engerix-B* can be used to complete a vaccination course initiated with *Recombivax HB*.

INDICATIONS AND USAGE

Engerix-B is indicated for immunization against infection caused by all known subtypes of hepatitis B virus. As hepatitis D (caused by the delta virus) does not occur in the absence of hepatitis B infection, it can be expected that hepatitis D will also be prevented by *Engerix-B* vaccination.
Engerix-B will not prevent hepatitis caused by other agents, such as hepatitis A, C and E viruses, or other pathogens known to infect the liver.
Immunization is recommended in persons of all ages, especially those who are, or will be, at increased risk of exposure to hepatitis B virus,[1] for example:

Health Care Personnel: Dentists and oral surgeons. Dental, medical and nursing students. Physicians, surgeons and podiatrists. Nurses. Paramedical and ambulance personnel and custodial staff who may be exposed to the virus via blood or other patient specimens. Dental hygienists and dental nurses. Laboratory and blood-bank personnel handling blood, blood products, and other patient specimens. Hospital cleaning staff who handle waste.
Selected Patients and Patient Contacts: Patients and staff in hemodialysis units and hematology/oncology units. Patients requiring frequent and/or large volume blood transfusions or clotting factor concentrates (e.g., persons with hemophilia, thalassemia, sickle-cell anemia, cirrhosis). Clients (residents) and staff of institutions for the mentally handicapped. Classroom contacts of deinstitutionalized mentally handicapped persons who have persistent hepatitis B surface antigenemia and who show aggressive behavior. Household and other intimate contacts of persons with persistent hepatitis B surface antigenemia.
Infants, Including Those Born of HBsAG-Positive Mothers Whether HBeAg Positive or Negative (See DOSAGE AND ADMINISTRATION.)
Adolescents (See CLINICAL PHARMACOLOGY.)
Subpopulations with a Known High Incidence of the Disease, such as: Alaskan Eskimos. Pacific Islanders. Indochinese immigrants. Haitian immigrants. Refugees from other HBV endemic areas. All infants of women born in areas where the infection is highly endemic.
Individuals with Chronic Hepatits C: Risk factors for hepatitis C are similar to those for hepatitis B. Consequently, immunization with hepatitis B vaccine is recommended for individuals with chronic hepatitis C.
Persons Who May Be Exposed to the Hepatitis B Virus by Travel to High-Risk Areas (See ACIP Guidelines, 1990.)
Military Personnel Identified as Being at Increased Risk
Morticians and Embalmers
Persons at Increased Risk of the Disease Due to Their Sexual Practices,[14] such as: Persons with more than one sexual partner in a 6-month period. Persons who have contracted a sexually transmitted disease. Homosexually active males. Female prostitutes.
Prisoners
Users of Illicit Injectable Drugs
Others: Police and fire department personnel who render first aid or medical assistance, and any others who, through their work or personal life-style, may be exposed to the hepatitis B virus. Adoptees from countries of high HBV endemicity.
Use with Other Vaccines: The Immunization Practices Advisory Committee states that, in general, simultaneous administration of certain live and inactivated pediatric vaccines has not resulted in impaired antibody responses or increased rates of adverse reactions.[15] Separate sites and syringes should be used for simultaneous administration of injectable vaccines.

CONTRAINDICATIONS

Hypersensitivity to yeast or any other component of the vaccine is a contraindication for use of the vaccine. Patients experiencing hypersensitivity after an Engerix-B [Hepatitis B Vaccine (Recombinant)] injection should not receive further injections of *Engerix-B*.

WARNINGS

Hepatitis B has a long incubation period. Hepatitis B vaccination may not prevent hepatitis B infection in individuals who had an unrecognized hepatitis B infection at the time of vaccine administration. Additionally, it may not prevent infection in individuals who do not achieve protective antibody titers.

PRECAUTIONS

General As with any percutaneous vaccine, epinephrine should be available for use in case of anaphylaxis or anaphylactoid reaction.
As with any vaccine, administration of *Engerix-B* should be delayed, if possible, in persons with any febrile illness or active infection.
Multiple Sclerosis: Although no causal relationship has been established, rare instances of exacerbation of multiple sclerosis have been reported following administration of hepatitis B vaccines and other vaccines. In persons with multiple sclerosis, the benefit of immunization for prevention of hepatitis B infection and sequelae must be weighed against the risk of exacerbation of the disease.
Pregnancy Pregnancy Category C: Animal reproduction studies have not been conducted with *Engerix-B*. It is also

Continued on next page

Information on the SmithKline Beecham Pharmaceuticals products appearing here is based on the labeling in effect on July 31, 1998. Further information on these and other products may be obtained from the Medical Department, SmithKline Beecham Pharmaceuticals, One Franklin Plaza, Philadelphia, PA 19101.

Engerix-B—Cont.

not known whether *Engerix-B* can cause fetal harm when administered to a pregnant woman or can affect reproduction capacity. *Engerix-B* should be given to a pregnant woman only if clearly needed.

Nursing Mothers It is not known whether *Engerix-B* is excreted in human milk. Because many drugs are excreted in human milk, caution should be exercised when *Engerix-B* is administered to a nursing woman.

Pediatric Use *Engerix-B* has been shown to be well tolerated and highly immunogenic in infants and children of all ages. Newborns also respond well; maternally transferred antibodies do not interfere with the active immune response to the vaccine. (See CLINICAL PHARMACOLOGY for seroconversion rates and titers in neonates and children. See DOSAGE AND ADMINISTRATION for recommended pediatric dosage and for recommended dosage for infants born of HBsAg-positive mothers.)

ADVERSE REACTIONS

Engerix-B [Hepatitis B Vaccine (Recombinant)] is generally well tolerated. As with any vaccine, however, it is possible that expanded commercial use of the vaccine could reveal rare adverse reactions.

Ten double-blind studies involving 2,252 subjects showed no significant difference in the frequency or severity of adverse experiences between *Engerix-B* and plasma-derived vaccines. In 36 clinical studies a total of 13,495 doses of *Engerix-B* were administered to 5,071 healthy adults and children who were initially seronegative for hepatitis B markers, and healthy neonates. All subjects were monitored for 4 days post-administration. Frequency of adverse experiences tended to decrease with successive doses of *Engerix-B*. Using a symptom checklist,‡ the most frequently reported adverse reactions were injection site soreness (22%) and fatigue‡ (14%). Other reactions are listed below.

Incidence 1% to 10% of Injections

Local reactions at injection site: Induration; erythema; swelling.

Body as a whole: Fever (>37.5°C).

Nervous system: Headache‡; dizziness.‡

‡ Parent or guardian completed forms for children and neonates. Neonatal checklist did not include headache, fatigue or dizziness.

Incidence <1% of Injections

Local reactions at injection site: Pain; pruritus; ecchymosis.

Body as a whole: Sweating; malaise; chills; weakness; flushing; tingling.

Cardiovascular system: Hypotension.

Respiratory system: Influenza-like symptoms; upper respiratory tract illnesses.

Gastrointestinal system: Nausea; anorexia; abdominal pain/cramps; vomiting; constipation; diarrhea.

Lymphatic system: Lymphadenopathy.

Musculoskeletal system: Pain/stiffness in arm, shoulder or neck; arthralgia; myalgia; back pain.

Skin and appendages: Rash; urticaria; petechiae; pruritus; erythema.

Nervous system: Somnolence; insomnia; irritability; agitation.

Additional adverse experiences have been reported with the commercial use of *Engerix-B*. Those listed below are to serve as alerting information to physicians.

Hypersensitivity: Anaphylaxis; erythema multiforme including Stevens-Johnson syndrome; angioedema; arthritis. An apparent hypersensitivity syndrome (serum-sickness-like) of delayed onset has been reported days to weeks after vaccination, including: arthralgia/arthritis (usually transient), fever and dermatologic reactions such as urticaria, erythema multiforme, ecchymoses and erythema nodosum (see CONTRAINDICATIONS).

Cardiovascular system: Tachycardia/palpitations.

Respiratory system: Bronchospasm including asthma-like symptoms.

Gastrointestinal system: Abnormal liver function tests; dyspepsia.

Nervous system: Migraine; syncope; paresis; neuropathy including hypoesthesia, paresthesia, Guillain-Barré syndrome and Bell's palsy, transverse myelitis; optic neuritis; multiple sclerosis; seizures.

Hematologic: Thrombocytopenia.

Skin and appendages: Eczema; purpura; herpes zoster; erythema nodosum; alopecia.

Special senses: Conjunctivitis; keratitis; visual disturbances; vertigo; tinnitus; earache.

Potential Adverse Experiences: In addition, certain other adverse experiences not observed with *Engerix-B* have been reported with Heptavax-B®† and/or *Recombivax HB*. Those listed below are to serve as alerting information to physicians:

Urogenital system: Dysuria.

DOSAGE AND ADMINISTRATION

Injection: Engerix-B should be administered by intramuscular injection. *Do not inject intravenously or intradermally.* In adults, the injection should be given in the deltoid region but it may be preferable to inject in the anterolateral thigh in neonates and infants, who have smaller deltoid muscles. *Engerix-B* should not be administered in the gluteal region; such injections may result in suboptimal response. The attending physician should determine final selection of the injection site and needle size, depending upon the patient's age and the size of the target muscle. A 1–inch 23–gauge needle is sufficient to penetrate the anterolateral thigh in infants younger than 12 months of age. A 5/8–inch 25–gauge needle may be used to administer the vaccine in the deltoid region of toddlers and children up to, and including, 10 years of age. The 1–inch 23–gauge needle is appropriate for use in older children and adults.[16]

Engerix-B may be administered subcutaneously to persons at risk of hemorrhage (e.g., hemophiliacs). However, hepatitis B vaccines administered subcutaneously are known to result in lower GMTs. Additionally, when other aluminum-adsorbed vaccines have been administered subcutaneously, an increased incidence of local reactions including subcutaneous nodules has been observed. Therefore, subcutaneous administration should be used only in persons who are at risk of hemorrhage with intramuscular injections.

Preparation for Administration: Shake well before withdrawal and use. Parenteral drug products should be inspected visually for particulate matter or discoloration prior to administration. With thorough agitation, *Engerix-B* is a slightly turbid white suspension. Discard if it appears otherwise. The vaccine should be used as supplied; no dilution is necessary. The full recommended dose of the vaccine should be used. Any vaccine remaining in a single-dose vial should be discarded.

Dosing Schedules: The usual immunization regimen (see Table 1) consists of three doses of vaccine given according to the following schedule: 1st dose: at elected date; 2nd dose: 1 month later; 3rd dose: 6 months after first dose.

There is an alternate schedule with injections at 0, 1 and 2 months designed for certain populations (e.g., neonates born of hepatitis B infected mothers, others who have or might have been recently exposed to the virus, certain travelers to high-risk areas. See INDICATIONS AND USAGE.). On this alternate schedule, an additional dose at 12 months is recommended for infants born of infected mothers and for others for whom prolonged maintenance of protective titers is desired.

In infants born of mothers who are not hepatitis B infected, *Engerix-B* may be administered at birth, 1 month of age and 6 months of age.

Table 1

Group	Dose	Schedule §
Infants born of:		
HBsAg-negative mothers	10 mcg/0.5 mL	Usual
HBsAg-positive mothers	10 mcg/0.5 mL	Either
Children:		
0 through 10 years of age	10 mcg/0.5 mL	Either
Adolescents:		
11 through 19 years of age	10 mcg/0.5 mL	Usual
	20 mcg/1.0 mL	Either
Adults (>19 years)	20 mcg/1.0 mL	Either
Adult hemodialysis	40 mcg/2.0 mL[II]	0, 1, 2, 6 months

§ Usual dosing schedule is 0, 1, 6 months; alternate dosing schedule is 0, 1, 2, 12 months. When the alternate schedule is used for adolescents, the 20 mcg/1.0 mL dose should be used.

II Two × 20 mcg in one or two injections.

For hemodialysis patients, in whom vaccine-induced protection is less complete and may persist only as long as antibody levels remain above 10 mIU/mL, the need for booster doses should be assessed by annual antibody testing. 40 mcg (two × 20 mcg) booster doses with *Engerix-B* should be given when antibody levels decline below 10 mIU/mL.[1] Data show individuals given a booster with *Engerix-B* achieve high antibody titers. (See CLINICAL PHARMACOLOGY.)

booster vaccinations: Whenever administration of a booster dose is appropriate, the dose of *Engerix-B* is 10 mcg for children 10 years of age and under; 20 mcg for adolescents 11 through 19 years of age and 20 mcg for adults. Studies have demonstrated a substantial increase in antibody titers after Engerix-B [Hepatitis B Vaccine (Recombinant)] booster vaccination following an initial course with both plasma- and yeast-derived vaccines. (See CLINICAL PHARMACOLOGY.)

See previous section for discussion on booster vaccination for adult hemodialysis patients.

Known or presumed exposure to hepatitis B virus: Unprotected individuals with known or presumed exposure to the hepatitis B virus (e.g., neonates born of infected mothers, others experiencing percutaneous or permucosal exposure) should be given hepatitis B immune globulin (HBIG) in addition to *Engerix-B* in accordance with ACIP recommendations[1] and with the package insert for HBIG. *Engerix-B* can be given on either dosing schedule (see above).

STORAGE

Store between 2° and 8°C (35° and 46°F). *Do not freeze;* discard if product has been frozen. Do not dilute to administer.

HOW SUPPLIED

Adult Dose

20 mcg/mL in Single-Dose Vials in packages of 1 and 25 vials.
NDC 58160-860-01 (package of 1)
NDC 58160-860-16 (package of 25)

20 mcg/mL in Single-Dose Prefilled Disposable Syringes.
NDC 58160-861-05 (package of 5)

20 mcg/mL in 10 mL Multi-Dose Vials.
NDC 58160-862-01 (package of 1)

20 mcg/mL in Single-Dose Prefilled Disposable Tip-Lok™ Syringes with 1-inch 23-gauge needles.
NDC 58160-861-35 (package of 5)

Pediatric/Adolescent Doses

10 mcg/0.5 mL in Single-Dose Vials in packages of 1 and 10 vials.
NDC 58160-859-01 (package of 1)
NDC 58160-859-11 (package of 10)

10 mcg/0.5 mL in Single-Dose Prefilled Disposable Syringes with 1-inch 23-gauge needles.
NDC 58160-859-05 (package of 5)

10 mcg/0.5 mL in Single-Dose Prefilled Disposable Tip-Lok™ Syringes with 1-inch 23-gauge needles.
NDC 58160-859-35 (package of 5)

10 mcg/0.5 mL in Single-Dose Prefilled Disposable Syringes with 5/8-inch 25-gauge needles.
NDC 58160-859-06 (package of 5)

10 mcg/0.5 mL in Single-Dose Prefilled Disposable Tip-Lok™ Syringes with 5/8-inch 25-gauge needles.
NDC 58160-859-36 (package of 5)

REFERENCES

1. Centers for Disease Control: Protection against viral hepatitis: recommendations of the Immunization Practices Advisory Committee (ACIP). *MMWR.* 39(No. RR-2), 1990. 2. Robinson, W.S.: Hepatitis B virus and the delta virus. In Mandell, G.L., Douglas, R.G., Bennett, J.E. (eds): *Principles and practice of infectious diseases,* vol. 3, New York, John Wiley & Sons, 1990, pp. 1204-1231. 3. Beasley, R.P., et al.: Efficacy of hepatitis B immune globulin for prevention of perinatal transmission of hepatitis B virus carrier state: final report of a randomized double-blind, placebo-controlled trial. *Hepatology* 3:135-141, 1983. 4. Centers for Disease Control: Hepatitis B virus: a comprehensive strategy for eliminating transmission in the United States through universal childhood vaccination: recommendations of the Immunization Practices Advisory Committee (ACIP). *MMWR.* 40(No. RR-13):1-25, 1991. 5. Committee on Infectious Diseases: Universal hepatitis B immunization. *Pediatrics.* 89(4):795-800, 1992. 6. Centers for Disease Control: Immunization of adolescents: recommendations of the Advisory Committee on Immunization Practices, the American Academy of Pediatrics, the American Academy of Family Physicians, and the American Medical Association. *MMWR.* 45(No. RR-13), 1996. 7. American Academy of Pediatrics: Immunization in special clinical circumstances: adolescents and college populations and hepatitis vaccines. In Peter, G. (ed): *1994 Redbook: Report of the Committee on Infectious Diseases.* 23rd ed. Elk Grove Village, IL, American Academy of Pediatrics, 1994, pp 64–65, 224–237. 8. Ambrosch, F.: Persistence of vaccine-induced antibodies to hepatitis B surface antigen–the need for booster vaccination in adult subjects. *Postgrad. Med. J.* 63(Suppl. 2):129-135, 1987. 9. Stevens, C.E., et al.: Hepatitis B vaccine in patients receiving hemodialysis. *N. Engl. J. Med.* 311:496-501, 1984. 10. Andre, F.E., and Safary, A.: Clinical experience with a yeast-derived hepatitis B vaccine. In Zuckerman, A.J.(ed): *Viral hepatitis and liver disease,* Alan R. Liss, Inc., 1988, pp. 1025-1030. 11. Poovorawan, Y., et al.: Protective efficacy of a recombinant DNA hepatitis B vaccine in neonates of HBe antigen-positive mothers. *JAMA.* 261(22):3278-3281, June 9, 1989. 12. Goilav, C., et al.: Immunization of homosexual men with a recombinant DNA vaccine against hepatitis B: immunogenicity and protection. In Zuckerman, A.J. (ed): *Viral hepatitis and liver disease,* Alan R. Liss, Inc., 1988, pp. 1057-1058. 13. Hauser, P., et al.: Immunological properties of recombinant HBsAg produced in yeast. *Postgrad. Med. J.* 63(Suppl. 2):83-91, 1987. 14. Centers for Disease Control and Prevention. 1998 Guidelines for treatment of sexually transmitted diseases. *MMWR.* 1998;47 (RR-1):102. 15. Centers for Disease Control: Recommendations of the Immunization Practices Advisory Committee (ACIP): General Rec-

ommendations on Immunization. *MMWR.* 38(13): April 7, 1989. 16. Centers for Disease Control and Prevention: General Recommendations on Immunization: Recommendations of the Advisory Committee on Immunization Practices (ACIP). *MMWR.* 1994;43(RR-1):6.

---

* yeast-derived, Hepatitis B Vaccine, MSD.
† plasma-derived, Hepatitis B Vaccine, MSD.
Rx only
U.S. License No. 1090

Manufactured by **SmithKline Beecham Biologicals**
Rixensart, Belgium
Distributed by **SmithKline Beecham Pharmaceuticals**
Philadelphia, PA 19101
Engerix-B is a registered trademark and *Tip-Lok* is a trademark of SmithKline Beecham.
Veterans Administration/Military/PHS—Vial, 10 mcg/0.5 mL, 1's, 6505-01-311-5220; Prefilled Syringe, 10 mcg/0.5 mL, 6505-01-392-6766; Vial, 20 mcg/mL, 1's, 6505-01-311-5221; 20 mcg/mL, 25's, 6505-01-311-5222; Prefilled Syringe, 20 mcg/mL, 5's, 6505-01-392-6768; 10 mL Multi-Dose Vial, 20 mcg/mL, 1's, 6505-01-428-3900.

EB:L24

Shown in Product Identification Guide, page 339

ESKALITH® ℞
[ess-kah 'lith]
(brand of lithium carbonate)
Capsules, 300 mg
ESKALITH CR® ℞
(brand of lithium carbonate)
Controlled Release Tablets, 450 mg

WARNING
Lithium toxicity is closely related to serum lithium levels, and can occur at doses close to therapeutic levels. Facilities for prompt and accurate serum lithium determinations should be available before initiating therapy (see DOSAGE AND ADMINISTRATION).

DESCRIPTION
Eskalith contains lithium carbonate, a white, light alkaline powder with molecular formula Li_2CO_3 and molecular weight 73.89. Lithium is an element of the alkali-metal group with atomic number 3, atomic weight 6.94 and an emission line at 671 nm on the flame photometer.
***Eskalith* Capsules:** Each capsule, with opaque gray cap and opaque yellow body, is imprinted with the product name ESKALITH and SB and contains lithium carbonate, 300 mg. Inactive ingredients consist of benzyl alcohol, cetylpyridinium chloride, D&C Yellow No. 10, FD&C Green No. 3, FD&C Red No. 40, FD&C Yellow No. 6, gelatin, lactose, magnesium stearate, povidone, sodium lauryl sulfate, titanium dioxide and trace amounts of other inactive ingredients.
***Eskalith CR* Controlled Release Tablets:** Each round, buff, scored tablet is debossed SKF and J10 and contains lithium carbonate, 450 mg. Inactive ingredients consist of alginic acid, gelatin, iron oxide, magnesium stearate and sodium starch glycolate.
Eskalith CR tablets 450 mg are designed to release a portion of the dose initially and the remainder gradually; the release pattern of the controlled release tablets reduces the variability in lithium blood levels seen with the immediate release dosage forms.

ACTIONS
Preclinical studies have shown that lithium alters sodium transport in nerve and muscle cells and effects a shift toward intraneuronal metabolism of catecholamines, but the specific biochemical mechanism of lithium action in mania is unknown.

INDICATIONS
Eskalith (lithium carbonate) is indicated in the treatment of manic episodes of manic-depressive illness. Maintenance therapy prevents or diminishes the intensity of subsequent episodes in those manic-depressive patients with a history of mania.
Typical symptoms of mania include pressure of speech, motor hyperactivity, reduced need for sleep, flight of ideas, grandiosity, elation, poor judgment, aggressiveness and possibly hostility. When given to a patient experiencing a manic episode, *Eskalith* may produce a normalization of symptomatology within 1 to 3 weeks.

WARNINGS
Lithium should generally not be given to patients with significant renal or cardiovascular disease, severe debilitation or dehydration, or sodium depletion, since the risk of lithium toxicity is very high in such patients. If the psychiatric indication is life-threatening, and if such a patient fails to respond to other measures, lithium treatment may be un-

dertaken with extreme caution, including daily serum lithium determinations and adjustment to the usually low doses ordinarily tolerated by these individuals. In such instances, hospitalization is a necessity.
Chronic lithium therapy may be associated with diminution of renal concentrating ability, occasionally presenting as nephrogenic diabetes insipidus, with polyuria and polydipsia. Such patients should be carefully managed to avoid dehydration with resulting lithium retention and toxicity. This condition is usually reversible when lithium is discontinued. Morphologic changes with glomerular and interstitial fibrosis and nephron atrophy have been reported in patients on chronic lithium therapy. Morphologic changes have also been seen in manic-depressive patients never exposed to lithium. The relationship between renal functional and morphologic changes and their association with lithium therapy have not been established.
When kidney function is assessed, for baseline data prior to starting lithium therapy or thereafter, routine urinalysis and other tests may be used to evaluate tubular function (e.g., urine specific gravity or osmolality following a period of water deprivation, or 24-hour urine volume) and glomerular function (e.g., serum creatinine or creatinine clearance). During lithium therapy, progressive or sudden changes in renal function, even within the normal range, indicate the need for reevaluation of treatment.
An encephalopathic syndrome (characterized by weakness, lethargy, fever, tremulousness and confusion, extrapyramidal symptoms, leukocytosis, elevated serum enzymes, BUN and FBS) has occurred in a few patients treated with lithium plus a neuroleptic. In some instances, the syndrome was followed by irreversible brain damage. Because of a possible causal relationship between these events and the concomitant administration of lithium and neuroleptics, patients receiving such combined therapy should be monitored closely for early evidence of neurologic toxicity and treatment discontinued promptly if such signs appear. This encephalopathic syndrome may be similar to or the same as neuroleptic malignant syndrome (NMS).
Lithium toxicity is closely related to serum lithium levels, and can occur at doses close to therapeutic levels (see DOSAGE AND ADMINISTRATION).
Outpatients and their families should be warned that the patient must discontinue lithium carbonate therapy and contact his physician if such clinical signs of lithium toxicity as diarrhea, vomiting, tremor, mild ataxia, drowsiness or muscular weakness occur.
Lithium carbonate may impair mental and/or physical abilities. Caution patients about activities requiring alertness (e.g., operating vehicles or machinery).
Lithium may prolong the effects of neuromuscular blocking agents. Therefore, neuromuscular blocking agents should be given with caution to patients receiving lithium.
Usage in Pregnancy: Adverse effects on implantation in rats, embryo viability in mice and metabolism *in vitro* of rat testes and human spermatozoa have been attributed to lithium, as have teratogenicity in submammalian species and cleft palates in mice.
In humans, lithium carbonate may cause fetal harm when administered to a pregnant woman. Data from lithium birth registries suggest an increase in cardiac and other anomalies, especially Ebstein's anomaly. If this drug is used in women of childbearing potential, or during pregnancy, or if a patient becomes pregnant while taking this drug, the patient should be apprised of the potential hazard to the fetus.
Usage in Nursing Mothers: Lithium is excreted in human milk. Nursing should not be undertaken during lithium therapy except in rare and unusual circumstances where, in the view of the physician, the potential benefits to the mother outweigh possible hazards to the child.
Usage in Pediatric Patients: Since information regarding the safety and effectiveness of lithium carbonate in children under 12 years of age is not available, its use in such patients is not recommended.
There has been a report of a transient syndrome of acute dystonia and hyperreflexia occurring in a 15 kg child who ingested 300 mg of lithium carbonate.
Usage in the Elderly: Elderly patients often require lower lithium dosages to achieve therapeutic serum levels. They may also exhibit adverse reactions at serum levels ordinarily tolerated by younger patients.

PRECAUTIONS
The ability to tolerate lithium is greater during the acute manic phase and decreases when manic symptoms subside (see DOSAGE AND ADMINISTRATION).
Caution should be used when lithium and diuretics are used concomitantly because diuretic-induced sodium loss may reduce the renal clearance of lithium and increase serum lithium levels with risk of lithium toxicity. Patients receiving such combined therapy should have serum lithium levels monitored closely and the lithium dosage adjusted if necessary.
The distribution space of lithium approximates that of total body water. Lithium is primarily excreted in urine with insignificant excretion in feces. Renal excretion of lithium is

proportional to its plasma concentration. The half-life of elimination of lithium is approximately 24 hours. Lithium decreases sodium reabsorption by the renal tubules which could lead to sodium depletion. Therefore, it is essential for the patient to maintain a normal diet, including salt, and an adequate fluid intake (2500 to 3000 mL) at least during the initial stabilization period. Decreased tolerance to lithium has been reported to ensue from protracted sweating or diarrhea and, if such occur, supplemental fluid and salt should be administered under careful medical supervision and lithium intake reduced or suspended until the condition is resolved.
In addition to sweating and diarrhea, concomitant infection with elevated temperatures may also necessitate a temporary reduction or cessation of medication.
Previously existing underlying thyroid disorders do not necessarily constitute a contraindication to lithium treatment; where hypothyroidism exists, careful monitoring of thyroid function during lithium stabilization and maintenance allows for correction of changing thyroid parameters, if any; where hypothyroidism occurs during lithium stabilization and maintenance, supplemental thyroid treatment may be used.
Indomethacin and piroxicam have been reported to increase significantly, steady-state plasma lithium levels. In some cases, lithium toxicity has resulted from such interactions. There is also some evidence that other nonsteroidal antiinflammatory agents may have a similar effect. When such combinations are used, increased plasma lithium level monitoring is recommended. Concurrent use of metronidazole with lithium may provoke lithium toxicity due to reduced renal clearance. Patients receiving such combined therapy should be monitored closely.
There is evidence that angiotensin-converting enzyme inhibitors, such as enalapril and captopril, may substantially increase steady-state plasma lithium levels, sometimes resulting in lithium toxicity. When such combinations are used, lithium dosage may need to be decreased, and plasma lithium levels should be measured more often.
Concurrent use of calcium channel blocking agents with lithium may increase the risk of neurotoxicity in the form of ataxia, tremors, nausea, vomiting, diarrhea and/or tinnitus. Caution is recommended.
The concomitant administration of lithium with selective serotonin reuptake inhibitors should be undertaken with caution as this combination has been reported to result in symptoms such as diarrhea, confusion, tremor, dizziness and agitation.
The following drugs can lower serum lithium concentrations by increasing urinary lithium excretion: acetazolamide, urea, xanthine preparations and alkalinizing agents such as sodium bicarbonate.
The following have also been shown to interact with lithium: methyldopa, phenytoin and carbamazepine.

ADVERSE REACTIONS
The occurrence and severity of adverse reactions are generally directly related to serum lithium concentrations as well as to individual patient sensitivity to lithium, and generally occur more frequently and with greater severity at higher concentrations.
Adverse reactions may be encountered at serum lithium levels below 1.5 mEq/L. Mild to moderate adverse reactions may occur at levels from 1.5 to 2.5 mEq/L, and moderate to severe reactions may be seen at levels of 2.0 mEq/L and above.
Fine hand tremor, polyuria and mild thirst may occur during initial therapy for the acute manic phase, and may persist throughout treatment. Transient and mild nausea and general discomfort may also appear during the first few days of lithium administration.
These side effects usually subside with continued treatment or a temporary reduction or cessation of dosage. If persistent, cessation of lithium therapy may be required.
Diarrhea, vomiting, drowsiness, muscular weakness and lack of coordination may be early signs of lithium intoxication, and can occur at lithium levels below 2.0 mEq/L. At higher levels, ataxia, giddiness, tinnitus, blurred vision and a large output of dilute urine may be seen. Serum lithium levels above 3.0 mEq/L may produce a complex clinical picture, involving multiple organs and organ systems. Serum lithium levels should not be permitted to exceed 2.0 mEq/L during the acute treatment phase.
The following reactions have been reported and appear to be related to serum lithium levels, including levels within the therapeutic range: **Neuromuscular/Central Nervous Sys-**

Continued on next page

Information on the SmithKline Beecham Pharmaceuticals products appearing here is based on the labeling in effect on July 31, 1998. Further information on these and other products may be obtained from the Medical Department, SmithKline Beecham Pharmaceuticals, One Franklin Plaza, Philadelphia, PA 19101.

Eskalith/Eskalith CR—Cont.

tem—tremor, muscle hyperirritability (fasciculations, twitching, clonic movements of whole limbs), hypertonicity, ataxia, choreo-athetotic movements, hyperactive deep tendon reflex, extrapyramidal symptoms including acute dystonia, cogwheel rigidity, blackout spells, epileptiform seizures, slurred speech, dizziness, vertigo, downbeat nystagmus, incontinence of urine or feces, somnolence, psychomotor retardation, restlessness, confusion, stupor, coma, tongue movements, tics, tinnitus, hallucinations, poor memory, slowed intellectual functioning, startled response, worsening of organic brain syndromes, myasthenia gravis (rarely); **Cardiovascular**—cardiac arrhythmia, hypotension, peripheral circulatory collapse, bradycardia, sinus node dysfunction with severe bradycardia (which may result in syncope); **Gastrointestinal**—anorexia, nausea, vomiting, diarrhea, gastritis, salivary gland swelling, abdominal pain, excessive salivation, flatulence, indigestion; **Genitourinary**—glycosuria, decreased creatinine clearance, albuminuria, oliguria, and symptoms of nephrogenic diabetes insipidus including polyuria, thirst and polydipsia; **Dermatologic**—drying and thinning of hair, alopecia, anesthesia of skin, acne, chronic folliculitis, xerosis cutis, psoriasis or its exacerbation, generalized pruritus with or without rash, cutaneous ulcers, angioedema; **Autonomic**—blurred vision, dry mouth, impotence/sexual dysfunction; **Thyroid Abnormalities**—euthyroid goiter and/or hypothyroidism (including myxedema) accompanied by lower T_3 and T_4. I^{131} uptake may be elevated. (See PRECAUTIONS.) Paradoxically, rare cases of hyperthyroidism have been reported; **EEG Changes**—diffuse slowing, widening of the frequency spectrum, potentiation and disorganization of background rhythm; **EKG Changes**—reversible flattening, isoelectricity or inversion of T-waves; **Miscellaneous**—fatigue, lethargy, transient scotomata, exophthalmos, dehydration, weight loss, leukocytosis, headache, transient hyperglycemia, hypercalcemia, hyperparathyroidism, excessive weight gain, edematous swelling of ankles or wrists, metallic taste, dysgeusia/taste distortion, salty taste, thirst, swollen lips, tightness in chest, swollen and/or painful joints, fever, polyarthralgia, dental caries.

Some reports of nephrogenic diabetes insipidus, hyperparathyroidism and hypothyroidism which persist after lithium discontinuation have been received.

A few reports have been received of the development of painful discoloration of fingers and toes and coldness of the extremities within one day of the starting of treatment with lithium. The mechanism through which these symptoms (resembling Raynaud's syndrome) developed is not known. Recovery followed discontinuance.

Cases of pseudotumor cerebri (increased intracranial pressure and papilledema) have been reported with lithium use. If undetected, this condition may result in enlargement of the blind spot, constriction of visual fields and eventual blindness due to optic atrophy.

Lithium should be discontinued, if clinically possible, if this syndrome occurs.

DOSAGE AND ADMINISTRATION

Immediate release capsules are usually given t.i.d. or q.i.d. Doses of controlled release tablets are usually given b.i.d. (approximately 12-hour intervals). When initiating therapy with immediate release or controlled release lithium, dosage must be individualized according to serum levels and clinical response.

When switching a patient from immediate release capsules to the Eskalith CR (lithium carbonate) Controlled Release Tablets, give the same total daily dose when possible. Most patients on maintenance therapy are stabilized on 900 mg daily, e.g., 450 mg *Eskalith CR* b.i.d. When the previous dosage of immediate release lithium is not a multiple of 450 mg, for example, 1500 mg, initiate *Eskalith CR* dosage at the multiple of 450 mg nearest to, but *below,* the original daily dose, i.e., 1350 mg. When the two doses are unequal, give the larger dose in the evening. In the above example, with a total daily dosage of 1350 mg, generally 450 mg *Eskalith CR* should be given in the morning and 900 mg *Eskalith CR* in the evening. If desired, the total daily dosage of 1350 mg can be given in three equal 450 mg *Eskalith CR* doses. These patients should be monitored at 1 to 2 week intervals, and dosage adjusted if necessary, until stable and satisfactory serum levels and clinical state are achieved.

When patients require closer titration than that available with *Eskalith CR* doses in increments of 450 mg, immediate release capsules should be used.

Acute Mania—Optimal patient response to Eskalith (lithium carbonate) can usually be established and maintained with 1800 mg per day in divided doses. Such doses will normally produce the desired serum lithium level ranging between 1.0 and 1.5 mEq/L.

Dosage must be individualized according to serum levels and clinical response. Regular monitoring of the patient's clinical state and serum lithium levels is necessary. Serum levels should be determined twice per week during the acute phase, and until the serum level and clinical condition of the patient have been stabilized.

Long-Term Control—The desirable serum lithium levels are 0.6 to 1.2 mEq/L. Dosage will vary from one individual to another, but usually 900 mg to 1200 mg per day in divided doses will maintain this level. Serum lithium levels in uncomplicated cases receiving maintenance therapy during remission should be monitored at least every two months.

Patients unusually sensitive to lithium may exhibit toxic signs at serum levels below 1.0 mEq/L.

N.B.: Blood samples for serum lithium determinations should be drawn immediately prior to the next dose when lithium concentrations are relatively stable (i.e., 8 to 12 hours after the previous dose). Total reliance must not be placed on serum levels alone. Accurate patient evaluation requires both clinical and laboratory analysis.

Elderly patients often respond to reduced dosage, and may exhibit signs of toxicity at serum levels ordinarily tolerated by younger patients.

OVERDOSAGE

The toxic levels for lithium are close to the therapeutic levels. It is therefore important that patients and their families be cautioned to watch for early toxic symptoms and to discontinue the drug and inform the physician should they occur. Toxic symptoms are listed in detail under ADVERSE REACTIONS.

Treatment

No specific antidote for lithium poisoning is known. Early symptoms of lithium toxicity can usually be treated by reduction or cessation of dosage of the drug and resumption of the treatment at a lower dose after 24 to 48 hours. In severe cases of lithium poisoning, the first and foremost goal of treatment consists of elimination of this ion from the patient. Treatment is essentially the same as that used in barbiturate poisoning: 1) gastric lavage, 2) correction of fluid and electrolyte imbalance, and 3) regulation of kidney function. Urea, mannitol and aminophylline all produce significant increases in lithium excretion. Hemodialysis is an effective and rapid means of removing the ion from the severely toxic patient. Infection prophylaxis, regular chest X-rays and preservation of adequate respiration are essential.

HOW SUPPLIED

Capsules: gray and yellow, imprinted with the product name ESKALITH and SB, in bottles of 100 and 500.
300 mg 100's: NDC 0007-4007-20
300 mg 500's: NDC 0007-4007-25
Controlled Release Tablets: round, buff, scored, debossed SKF and J10, in bottles of 100.
450 mg 100's: NDC 0007-4010-20
STORAGE CONDITIONS: Store between 15° and 30°C (59° and 86°F).
Veterans Administration/Military/PHS—Capsules, 300 mg, 100's, 6505-00-482-8058; 300 mg, 500's, 6505-01-016-7746; CR Tablets, 450 mg, 100's, 6505-01-170-2364.
EL:L42

Shown in Product Identification Guide, page 339

FAMVIR® ℞

[fam'-vir]
(brand of famciclovir)
Tablets

DESCRIPTION

Famvir contains famciclovir, an orally administered prodrug of the antiviral agent penciclovir. Chemically, famciclovir is known as 2-[2-(2-amino-9*H*-purin-9-yl)ethyl]-1,3-propanediol diacetate. Its molecular formula is $C_{14}H_{19}N_5O_4$; its molecular weight is 321.3. It is a synthetic acyclic guanine derivative and has the following structure:

[See chemical structure at top of next column]

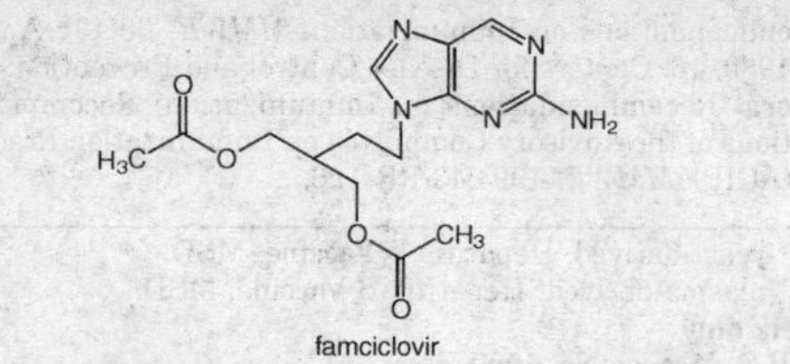

famciclovir

Famciclovir is a white to pale yellow solid. It is freely soluble in acetone and methanol, and sparingly soluble in ethanol and isopropanol. At 25° C famciclovir is freely soluble (>25% w/v) in water initially, but rapidly precipitates as the sparingly soluble (2–3% w/v) monohydrate. Famciclovir is not hygroscopic below 85% relative humidity. Partition coefficients are: octanol/water (pH 4.8) P=1.09 and octanol/phosphate buffer (pH 7.4) P=2.08.

Tablets for Oral Administration: Each white, film-coated tablet contains famciclovir. The 125 mg and 250 mg tablets are round; the 500 mg tablets are oval. Inactive ingredients consist of hydroxypropyl cellulose, hydroxypropyl methylcellulose, lactose, magnesium stearate, polyethylene glycols, sodium starch glycolate and titanium dioxide.

MICROBIOLOGY

Mechanism of Antiviral Activity: Famciclovir undergoes rapid biotransformation to the active antiviral compound penciclovir, which has inhibitory activity against herpes simplex virus types 1 (HSV-1) and 2 (HSV-2) and varicella zoster virus (VZV). In cells infected with HSV-1, HSV-2 or VZV, viral thymidine kinase phosphorylates penciclovir to a monophosphate form that, in turn, is converted to penciclovir triphosphate by cellular kinases. *In vitro* studies demonstrate that penciclovir triphosphate inhibits HSV-2 DNA polymerase competitively with deoxyguanosine triphosphate. Consequently, herpes viral DNA synthesis and, therefore, replication are selectively inhibited.

Penciclovir triphosphate has an intracellular half-life of 10 hours in HSV-1-, 20 hours in HSV-2- and 7 hours in VZV-infected cells cultured *in vitro*; however, the clinical significance is unknown.

Antiviral Activity *In Vitro* and *In Vivo*: In cell culture studies, penciclovir has antiviral activity against the following herpesviruses (listed in decreasing order of potency): HSV-1, HSV-2 and VZV. Sensitivity test results, expressed as the concentration of the drug required to inhibit the growth of the virus by 50% (IC_{50}) or 99% (IC_{99}) in cell culture, vary greatly depending upon a number of factors, including the assay protocols, and in particular the cell type used. See Table 1.

[See table 1 below]

Drug Resistance: Penciclovir-resistant mutants of HSV and VZV can result from complete loss of viral thymidine kinase activity (TK negative), reduced TK activity (TK altered) or DNA polymerase mutations. The most commonly encountered acyclovir-resistant mutants that are TK negative are also resistant to penciclovir. The possibility of viral resistance to penciclovir should be considered in patients who fail to respond or experience recurrent viral infections during therapy.

CLINICAL PHARMACOLOGY

Pharmacokinetics

Absorption and Bioavailability: Famciclovir is the diacetyl 6-deoxy analog of the active antiviral compound penciclovir. Following oral administration, little or no famciclovir is detected in plasma or urine.

The absolute bioavailability of famciclovir is 77±8% as determined following the administration of a 500 mg famciclovir oral dose and a 400 mg penciclovir intravenous dose to 12 healthy male subjects.

Penciclovir concentrations increased in proportion to dose over a famciclovir dose range of 125 mg to 750 mg administered as a single dose. Single oral dose administration of 125 mg, 250 mg or 500 mg famciclovir to healthy male volunteers across 17 studies gave the following pharmacokinetic parameters:

Table 1

Method of Assay	Virus Type	Cell Type	IC_{50} (mcg/mL)	IC_{99}
Plaque Reduction	VZV (c.i.)	MRC-5	5.0 ± 3.0	
	VZV (c.i.)	Hs68	0.9 ± 0.4	
	HSV-1 (c.i.)	MRC-5	0.2 – 0.6	
	HSV-1 (c.i.)	WISH	0.04 – 0.5	
	HSV-2 (c.i.)	MRC-5	0.9 – 2.1	
	HSV-2 (c.i.)	WISH	0.1 – 0.8	
Virus Yield	HSV-1 (c.i.)	MRC-5		0.4 – 0.5
Reduction	HSV-2 (c.i.)	MRC-5		0.6 – 0.7
DNA Synthesis	VZV (Ellen)	MRC-5	0.1	
Inhibition	HSV-1 (SC16)	MRC-5	0.04	
	HSV-2 (MS)	MRC-5	0.05	

(c.i.) = clinical isolates.

Table 2

Dose	AUC (0–inf)[†] (mcg.hr./mL)	C_{max}[‡] (mcg/mL)	T_{max}[§] (h)
125 mg	2.24	0.8	0.9
250 mg	4.48	1.6	0.9
500 mg	8.95	3.3	0.9

† AUC (0–inf) (mcg.hr./mL)=area under the plasma concentration-time profile extrapolated to infinity.
‡ C_{max} (mcg/mL)=maximum observed plasma concentration.
§ T_{max} (h)=time to C_{max}.

Following single oral-dose administration of 500 mg famciclovir to seven patients with herpes zoster, the mean ± SD AUC, C_{max}, and T_{max} were 12.1±1.7 mcg.hr./mL, 4.0±0.7 mcg/mL, and 0.7±0.2 hours, respectively. The AUC of penciclovir was approximately 35% greater in patients with herpes zoster as compared to healthy volunteers. Some of this difference may be due to differences in renal function between the two groups.

There is no accumulation of penciclovir after the administration of 500 mg famciclovir t.i.d. for 7 days.

Penciclovir C_{max} decreased approximately 50% and T_{max} was delayed by 1.5 hours when a capsule formulation of famciclovir was administered with food (nutritional content was approximately 910 Kcal and 26% fat). There was no effect on the extent of availability (AUC) of penciclovir. There was an 18% decrease in C_{max} and a delay in T_{max} of about 1 hour when famciclovir was given 2 hours after a meal as compared to its administration 2 hours before a meal. Because there was no effect on the extent of systemic availability of penciclovir, it appears that *Famvir* can be taken without regard to meals.

Distribution: The volume of distribution (Vd_β) was 1.08±0.17 L/kg in 12 healthy male subjects following a single intravenous dose of penciclovir at 400 mg administered as a 1-hour intravenous infusion.

Penciclovir is <20% bound to plasma proteins over the concentration range of 0.1 to 20 mcg/mL. The blood/plasma ratio of penciclovir is approximately 1.

Metabolism: Following oral administration, famciclovir is deacetylated and oxidized to form penciclovir. Metabolites that are inactive include 6-deoxy penciclovir, monoacetylated penciclovir, and 6-deoxy monoacetylated penciclovir (5%, <0.5% and <0.5% of the dose in the urine, respectively). Little or no famciclovir is detected in plasma or urine. An *in vitro* study using human liver microsomes demonstrated that cytochrome P450 does not play an important role in famciclovir metabolism. The conversion of 6-deoxy penciclovir to penciclovir is catalyzed by aldehyde oxidase.

Elimination: Approximately 94% of administered radioactivity was recovered in urine over 24 hours (83% of the dose was excreted in the first 6 hours) after the administration of 5 mg/kg radiolabeled penciclovir as a 1-hour infusion to three healthy male volunteers. Penciclovir accounted for 91% of the radioactivity excreted in the urine.

Following the oral administration of a single 500 mg dose of radiolabeled famciclovir to three healthy male volunteers, 73% and 27% of administered radioactivity were recovered in urine and feces over 72 hours, respectively. Penciclovir accounted for 82% and 6-deoxy penciclovir accounted for 7% of the radioactivity excreted in the urine. Approximately 60% of the administered radiolabeled dose was collected in urine in the first 6 hours.

After intravenous administration of penciclovir in 48 healthy male volunteers, mean ± S.D. total plasma clearance of penciclovir was 36.6±6.3 L/hr (0.48±0.09 L/hr/kg). Penciclovir renal clearance accounted for 74.5±8.8% of total plasma clearance.

Renal clearance of penciclovir following the oral administration of a single 500 mg dose of famciclovir to 109 healthy male volunteers was 27.7±7.6 L/hr.

The plasma elimination half-life of penciclovir was 2.0±0.3 hours after intravenous administration of penciclovir to 48 healthy male volunteers and 2.3±0.4 hours after oral administration of 500 mg famciclovir to 124 healthy male volunteers. The half-life in seven patients with herpes zoster was 3.0±1.1 hours.

HIV-Infected Patients: Following oral administration of a single dose of 500 mg famciclovir (the oral prodrug of penciclovir) to HIV-positive patients, the pharmacokinetic parameters of penciclovir were comparable to those observed in healthy subjects.

Renal Insufficiency: Apparent plasma clearance, renal clearance, and the plasma-elimination rate constant of penciclovir decreased linearly with reductions in renal function. After the administration of a single 500 mg famciclovir oral dose (n=27) to healthy volunteers and to volunteers with varying degrees of renal insufficiency (CL_{CR} ranged from 6.4 to 138.8 mL/min.), the following results were obtained (Table 3):
[See table 3 above]

In a multiple dose study of famciclovir conducted in subjects with varying degrees of renal impairment (n=18), the pharmacokinetics of penciclovir were comparable to those after single doses.

Table 3

Parameter (mean ± S.D.)	CL_{CR}[†] ≥60 (mL/min.)	CL_{CR} 40–59 (mL/min.)	CL_{CR} 20–39 (mL/min.)	CL_{CR} <20 (mL/min.)
CL_{CR} (mL/min)	88.1 ± 20.6	49.3 ± 5.9	26.5 ± 5.3	12.7 ± 5.9
CL_R (L/hr)	30.1 ± 10.6	13.0 ± 1.3‡	4.2 ± 0.9	1.6 ± 1.0
CL/F§ (L/hr)	66.9 ± 27.5	27.3 ± 2.8	12.8 ± 1.3	5.8 ± 2.8
Half-life (hr)	2.3 ± 0.5	3.4 ± 0.7	6.2 ± 1.6	13.4 ± 10.2
n	15	5	4	3

† CL_{CR} is measured creatinine clearance.
‡ n=4.
§ CL/F consists of bioavailability factor and famciclovir to penciclovir conversion factor.

Table 4

	Recurrence Rates at 6 Months		Recurrence Rates at 12 Months	
	Famvir 250 mg b.i.d.	Placebo	*Famvir* 250 mg b.i.d.	Placebo
n	236	233	236	233
Recurrence-free	39%	10%	29%	6%
Recurrences†	47%	74%	53%	78%
Lost to Follow-up‡	14%	16%	17%	16%

† Based on patient reported data; not necessarily confirmed by a physician.
‡ Patients recurrence-free at time of last contact prior to withdrawal.

A dosage adjustment is recommended for patients with renal insufficiency (see DOSAGE AND ADMINISTRATION).

Hepatic Insufficiency: Well-compensated chronic liver disease (chronic hepatitis [n=6], chronic ethanol abuse [n=8], or primary biliary cirrhosis [n=1]) had no effect on the extent of availability (AUC) of penciclovir following a single dose of 500 mg famciclovir. However, there was a 44% decrease in penciclovir mean maximum plasma concentration and the time to maximum plasma concentration was increased by 0.75 hours in patients with hepatic insufficiency compared to normal volunteers. No dosage adjustment is recommended for patients with well-compensated hepatic impairment. The pharmacokinetics of penciclovir have not been evaluated in patients with severe uncompensated hepatic impairment.

Elderly Subjects: Based on cross-study comparisons, mean penciclovir AUC was 40% larger and penciclovir renal clearance was 22% lower after the oral administration of famciclovir in elderly volunteers (n=18, age 65 to 79 years) compared to younger volunteers. Some of this difference may be due to differences in renal function between the two groups.

Gender: The pharmacokinetics of penciclovir were evaluated in 18 healthy male and 18 healthy female volunteers after single-dose oral administration of 500 mg famciclovir. AUC of penciclovir was 9.3±1.9 mcg.hr./mL and 11.1±2.1 mcg.hr./mL in males and females, respectively. Penciclovir renal clearance was 28.5±8.9 L/hr and 21.8±4.3 L/hr, respectively. These differences were attributed to differences in renal function between the two groups. No famciclovir dosage adjustment based on gender is recommended.

Pediatric Patients: The pharmacokinetics of famciclovir or penciclovir have not been evaluated in patients <18 years of age.

Race: The pharmacokinetics of famciclovir or penciclovir with respect to race have not been evaluated.

Drug Interactions

Effects on penciclovir

No clinically significant alterations in penciclovir pharmacokinetics were observed following single-dose administration of 500 mg famciclovir after pre-treatment with multiple doses of allopurinol, cimetidine, theophylline, or zidovudine. No clinically significant effect on penciclovir pharmacokinetics was observed following multiple-dose (t.i.d.) administration of famciclovir (500 mg) with multiple doses of digoxin.

Effects of famciclovir on co-administered drugs

The steady-state pharmacokinetics of digoxin were not altered by concomitant administration of multiple doses of famciclovir (500 mg t.i.d.). No clinically significant effect on the pharmacokinetics of zidovudine or zidovudine glucuronide was observed following a single oral dose of 500 mg famciclovir.

CLINICAL TRIALS

Herpes Zoster

Famvir (famciclovir) was studied in a placebo-controlled, double-blind trial of 419 immunocompetent adults with uncomplicated herpes zoster. Comparisons included *Famvir* 500 mg t.i.d., *Famvir* 750 mg t.i.d., or placebo. Treatment was begun within 72 hours of initial lesion appearance and therapy was continued for 7 days.

The median time to full crusting in *Famvir*-treated patients was 5 days compared to 7 days in placebo-treated patients. The times to full crusting, loss of vesicles, loss of ulcers, and loss of crusts were shorter for *Famvir* 500 mg-treated patients than for placebo-treated patients in the overall study population. The effects of *Famvir* were greater when therapy was initiated within 48 hours of rash onset; it was also more pronounced in patients 50 years of age or older. Among the 65.2% of patients with at least one positive viral culture, *Famvir*-treated patients had a shorter median duration of viral shedding than placebo-treated patients (1 day and 2 days, respectively).

There were no overall differences in the duration of pain before rash healing between *Famvir* and placebo-treated groups. In addition, there was no difference in the incidence of pain after rash healing (postherpetic neuralgia) between the treatment groups. In the 186 patients (44.4% of total study population) who did develop post herpetic neuralgia, the median duration of postherpetic neuralgia was shorter in patients treated with *Famvir* 500 mg than in those treated with placebo (63 days and 119 days, respectively). No additional efficacy was demonstrated with higher doses of *Famvir*.

A double-blind controlled trial in 545 immunocompetent adults with uncomplicated herpes zoster treated within 72 hours of initial lesion appearance compared three doses of *Famvir* to acyclovir 800 mg 5 times per day. Times to full lesion crusting and times to loss of acute pain were comparable for all groups and there were no statistically significant differences in the time to loss of postherpetic neuralgia between *Famvir* and acyclovir-treated groups.

Herpes Simplex Infections

Recurrent Genital Herpes: In two placebo-controlled trials, 626 immunocompetent adults with a recurrence of genital herpes were treated with *Famvir* 125 mg b.i.d. (n=160), *Famvir* 250 mg b.i.d. (n=169), *Famvir* 500 mg b.i.d. (n=154) or placebo (n=143) for 5 days. Treatment was initiated within 6 hours of either symptom onset or lesion appearance. In the two studies combined, the median time to healing in *Famvir* 125 mg-treated patients was 4 days compared to 5 days in placebo-treated patients and the median time to cessation of viral shedding was 1.8 vs. 3.4 days in *Famvir* 125 mg and placebo recipients, respectively. The median time to loss of all symptoms was 3.2 days in *Famvir* 125 mg-treated patients vs. 3.8 days in placebo-treated patients. No additional efficacy was demonstrated with higher doses of *Famvir*.

Suppression of Recurrent Genital Herpes: 934 immunocompetent adults with a history of 6 or more recurrences per year were randomized into two double-blind, 1-year, placebo-controlled trials. Comparisons included *Famvir* 125 mg t.i.d., 250 mg b.i.d., 250 mg t.i.d. and placebo. At one-year, 60% to 65% of patients were still receiving *Famvir* and 25% were receiving placebo treatment. Patient reported recurrence rates for the 250 mg b.i.d. dose at 6 and 12 months are shown in Table 4.
[See table 4 above]

Famvir-treated patients had approximately 1/5 the median number of recurrences as compared to placebo-treated patients.

Higher doses of *Famvir* were not associated with an increase in efficacy.

Continued on next page

Information on the SmithKline Beecham Pharmaceuticals products appearing here is based on the labeling in effect on July 31, 1998. Further information on these and other products may be obtained from the Medical Department, SmithKline Beecham Pharmaceuticals, One Franklin Plaza, Philadelphia, PA 19101.

Famvir—Cont.

Recurrent Mucocutaneous Herpes Simplex Infection in HIV-Infected Patients
A randomized, double-blind, multicenter study compared famciclovir 500 mg twice daily for 7 days (n=150) with oral acyclovir 400 mg 5 times daily for 7 days (n=143) in HIV-infected patients with recurrent mucocutaneous HSV infection treated within 48 hours of lesion onset. Approximately 40% of patients had a CD_4 count below 200 cells/mm^3, 54% of patients had anogenital lesions and 35% had orolabial lesions. Famciclovir therapy was comparable to oral acyclovir in reducing new lesion formation and in time to complete healing.

INDICATIONS AND USAGE
Herpes Zoster: Famvir (famciclovir) is indicated for the treatment of acute herpes zoster (shingles).
Herpes Simplex Infections: Famvir is indicated for:
• treatment or suppression of recurrent genital herpes in immunocompetent patients
• treatment of recurrent mucocutaneous herpes simplex infections in HIV-infected patients.

CONTRAINDICATIONS
Famvir (famciclovir) is contraindicated in patients with known hypersensitivity to the product, its components, and Denavir® (penciclovir cream).

PRECAUTIONS
General
The efficacy of Famvir has not been established for initial episode genital herpes infection, ophthalmic zoster, disseminated zoster or in immunocompromised patients with herpes zoster.
Dosage adjustment is recommended when administering Famvir to patients with creatinine clearance values <60 mL/min. (see DOSAGE AND ADMINISTRATION). In patients with underlying renal disease who have received inappropriately high doses of Famvir for their level of renal function, acute renal failure has been reported.
Information for Patients
Patients should be informed that Famvir is not a cure for genital herpes. There are no data evaluating whether Famvir will prevent transmission of infection to others. As genital herpes is a sexually transmitted disease, patients should avoid contact with lesions or intercourse when lesions and/or symptoms are present to avoid infecting partners. Genital herpes can also be transmitted in the absence of symptoms through asymptomatic viral shedding. If medical management of recurrent episodes is indicated, patients should be advised to initiate therapy at the first sign or symptom.
Drug Interactions
Concurrent use with probenecid or other drugs significantly eliminated by active renal tubular secretion may result in increased plasma concentrations of penciclovir.
The conversion of 6-deoxy penciclovir to penciclovir is catalyzed by aldehyde oxidase. Interactions with other drugs metabolized by this enzyme could potentially occur.
Carcinogenesis, Mutagenesis, Impairment of Fertility
Famciclovir was administered orally unless otherwise stated.
Carcinogenesis: Two-year dietary carcinogenicity studies with famciclovir were conducted in rats and mice. An increase in the incidence of mammary adenocarcinoma (a common tumor in animals of this strain) was seen in female rats receiving the high dose of 600 mg/kg/day (1.5 to 9.0x the human systemic exposure at the recommended daily oral doses of 500 mg t.i.d., 250 mg b.i.d., or 125 mg b.i.d. based on area under the plasma concentration curve comparisons [24 hr AUC] for penciclovir). No increases in tumor incidence were reported in male rats treated at doses up to 240 mg/kg/day (0.9 to 5.4x the human AUC), or in male and female mice at doses up to 600 mg/kg/day (0.4 to 2.4x the human AUC).
Mutagenesis: Famciclovir and penciclovir (the active metabolite of famciclovir) were tested for genotoxic potential in a battery of in vitro and in vivo assays. Famciclovir and penciclovir were negative in in vitro tests for gene mutations in bacteria (S. typhimurium and E. coli) and unscheduled DNA synthesis in mammalian HeLa 83 cells (at doses up to 10,000 and 5000 mcg/plate, respectively). Famciclovir was also negative in the L5178Y mouse lymphoma assay (5000 mcg/mL), the in vivo mouse micronucleus test (4800 mg/kg), and rat dominant lethal study (5000 mg/kg). Famciclovir induced increases in polyploidy in human lymphocytes in vitro in the absence of chromosomal damage (1200 mcg/mL). Penciclovir was positive in the L5178Y mouse lymphoma assay for gene mutation/chromosomal aberrations, with and without metabolic activation (1000 mcg/mL). In human lymphocytes, penciclovir caused chromosomal aberrations in the absence of metabolic activation (250 mcg/mL). Penciclovir caused an increased incidence of micronuclei in mouse bone marrow in vivo when administered intravenously at doses highly toxic to bone marrow (500 mg/kg), but not when administered orally.

Table 5
Selected Adverse Events Reported by ≥2% of Patients in Placebo-controlled Famvir (famciclovir) Trials*

Event	Herpes Zoster		Recurrent Genital Herpes		Genital Herpes-Suppression	
	Famvir (n=273) %	Placebo (n=146) %	Famvir (n=640) %	Placebo (n=225) %	Famvir (n=458) %	Placebo (n=63) %
Nervous System						
Headache	22.7	17.8	23.6	16.4	39.3	42.9
Paresthesia	2.6	0.0	1.3	0.0	0.9	0.0
Migraine	0.7	0.7	1.3	0.4	3.1	0.0
Gastrointestinal						
Nausea	12.5	11.6	10.0	8.0	7.2	9.5
Diarrhea	7.7	4.8	4.5	7.6	9.0	9.5
Vomiting	4.8	3.4	1.3	0.9	3.1	1.6
Flatulence	1.5	0.7	1.9	2.2	4.8	1.6
Abdominal Pain	1.1	3.4	3.9	5.8	7.9	7.9
Body as a Whole						
Fatigue	4.4	3.4	6.3	4.4	4.8	3.2
Skin and Appendages						
Pruritus	3.7	2.7	0.9	0.0	2.2	0.0
Rash	0.4	0.7	0.6	0.4	3.3	1.6
Reproductive Female						
Dysmenorrhea	0.0	0.7	2.2	1.3	7.6	6.3

*Patients may have entered into more than one clinical trial.

Table 6
Selected Laboratory Abnormalities in Genital Herpes Suppression Studies*

Parameter	Famvir (n = 660)† %	Placebo (n = 210)† %
Anemia (<0.8 × NRL)	0.1	0.0
Leukopenia (<0.75 × NRL)	1.3	0.9
Neutropenia (<0.8 × NRL)	3.2	1.5
AST (SGOT) (>2 × NRH)	2.3	1.2
ALT (SGPT) (>2 × NRH)	3.2	1.5
Total Bilirubin (>1.5 × NRH)	1.9	1.2
Serum Creatinine (>1.5 × NRH)	0.2	0.3
Amylase (>1.5 × NRH)	1.5	1.9
Lipase (>1.5 × NRH)	4.9	4.7

* Percentage of patients with laboratory abnormalities that were increased or decreased from baseline and were outside of specified ranges.
†n values represent the minimum number of patients assessed for each laboratory parameter.
NRH = Normal Range High.
NRL = Normal Range Low.

Table 7

Indication and Normal Dosage Regimen	Creatinine Clearance (mL/min.)	Adjusted Dosage Regimen Dose (mg)	Dosing Interval
Herpes Zoster			
500 mg every 8 hours	>60	500	every 8 hours
	40–59	500	every 12 hours
	20–39	500	every 24 hours
	<20	250	every 24 hours
	HD*	250	following each dialysis
Recurrent Genital Herpes			
125 mg every 12 hours	≥40	125	every 12 hours
	20–39	125	every 24 hours
	<20	125	every 24 hours
	HD*	125	following each dialysis
Suppression of Recurrent Genital Herpes			
250 mg every 12 hours	≥40	250	every 12 hours
	20–39	125	every 12 hours
	<20	125	every 24 hours
	HD*	125	following each dialysis
Recurrent Orolabial and Genital Herpes Simplex Infection in HIV-Infected Patients			
500 mg every 12 hours	≥40	500	every 12 hours
	20–39	500	every 24 hours
	<20	250	every 24 hours
	HD*	250	following each dialysis

* Hemodialysis

Impairment of Fertility: Testicular toxicity was observed in rats, mice, and dogs following repeated administration of famciclovir or penciclovir. Testicular changes included atrophy of the seminiferous tubules, reduction in sperm count, and/or increased incidence of sperm with abnormal morphology or reduced motility. The degree of toxicity to male

reproduction was related to dose and duration of exposure. In male rats, decreased fertility was observed after 10 weeks of dosing at 500 mg/kg/day (1.9 to 11.4x the human AUC). The no observable effect level for sperm and testicular toxicity in rats following chronic administration (26 weeks) was 50 mg/kg/day (0.2 to 1.2x the human systemic exposure based on AUC comparisons). Testicular toxicity was observed following chronic administration to mice (104 weeks) and dogs (26 weeks) at doses of 600 mg/kg/day (0.4 to 2.4x the human AUC) and 150 mg/kg/day (1.7 to 10.2x the human AUC), respectively.
Famciclovir had no effect on general reproductive performance or fertility in female rats at doses up to 1000 mg/kg/day (3.6 to 21.6x the human AUC).
Two placebo-controlled studies in a total of 130 otherwise healthy men with a normal sperm profile over an 8-week baseline period and recurrent genital herpes receiving oral *Famvir* (250 mg b.i.d.) (n=66) or placebo (n=64) therapy for 18 weeks showed no evidence of significant effects on sperm count, motility or morphology during treatment or during an 8-week follow-up.

Pregnancy

Teratogenic Effects—Pregnancy Category B. Famciclovir was tested for effects on embryo-fetal development in rats and rabbits at oral doses up to 1000 mg/kg/day (approximately 3.6 to 21.6x and 1.8 to 10.8x the human systemic exposure to penciclovir based on AUC comparisons for the rat and rabbit, respectively) and intravenous doses of 360 mg/kg/day in rats (2 to 12x the human dose based on body surface area [BSA] comparisons) or 120 mg/kg/day in rabbits (1.5 to 9.0x the human dose [BSA]). No adverse effects were observed on embryo-fetal development. Similarly, no adverse effects were observed following intravenous administration of penciclovir to rats (80 mg/kg/day, 0.4 to 2.6x the human dose [BSA]) or rabbits (60 mg/kg/day, 0.7 to 4.2x the human dose [BSA]). There are, however, no adequate and well-controlled studies in pregnant women. Because animal reproduction studies are not always predictive of human response, famciclovir should be used during pregnancy only if the benefit to the patient clearly exceeds the potential risk to the fetus.

Pregnancy Exposure Registry: To monitor maternal-fetal outcomes of pregnant women exposed to *Famvir*, SmithKline Beecham maintains a *Famvir* Pregnancy Registry. Physicians are encouraged to register their patients by calling (800) 366-8900, ext. 5231.

Nursing Mothers

Following oral administration of famciclovir to lactating rats, penciclovir was excreted in breast milk at concentrations higher than those seen in the plasma. It is not known whether it is excreted in human milk. There are no data on the safety of *Famvir* in infants.

Usage in Children

Safety and efficacy in children under the age of 18 years have not been established.

Geriatric Use

Of 816 patients with herpes zoster in clinical studies who were treated with *Famvir*, 248 (30.4%) were ≥65 years of age and 103 (13%) were ≥75 years of age. No overall differences were observed in the incidence or types of adverse events between younger and older patients.

ADVERSE REACTIONS

Immunocompetent Patients

The safety of *Famvir* has been evaluated in clinical studies involving 816 *Famvir*-treated patients with herpes zoster (*Famvir*, 250 mg t.i.d. to 750 mg t.i.d.); 528 *Famvir*-treated patients with recurrent genital herpes (*Famvir*, 125 mg b.i.d. to 500 mg t.i.d.); and 1,197 patients with recurrent genital herpes treated with *Famvir* as suppressive therapy (125 mg q.d. to 250 mg t.i.d.) of which 570 patients received *Famvir* (open-labeled and/or double-blind) for at least 10 months. Table 5 lists selected adverse events.

[See table 5 on top of previous page]

The following adverse events have been reported during post-approval use of *Famvir:* urticaria, hallucinations and confusion (including delirium, disorientation, confusional state, occurring predominantly in the elderly). Because these adverse events are reported voluntarily from a population of unknown size, estimates of frequency cannot be made. Table 6 lists selected laboratory abnormalities in genital herpes suppression trials.

[See table 6 on previous page]

HIV-Infected Patients

In HIV-infected patients, the most frequently reported adverse events for famciclovir (500 mg twice daily; n=150) and acyclovir (400 mg, 5x/day; n=143), respectively, were headache (16.0 vs 15.4%), nausea (10.7 vs 12.6%), diarrhea (6.7 vs 10.5%), vomiting (4.7 vs 3.5%), fatigue (4.0 vs 2.1%), and abdominal pain (3.3 vs 5.6%).

OVERDOSAGE

Appropriate symptomatic and supportive therapy should be given. Penciclovir is removed by hemodialysis (see PRECAUTIONS, General).

DOSAGE AND ADMINISTRATION

Herpes Zoster

The recommended dosage is 500 mg every 8 hours for 7 days. Therapy should be initiated promptly as soon as herpes zoster is diagnosed. No data are available on efficacy of treatment started greater than 72 hours after rash onset.

Herpes Simplex Infections

Recurrent genital herpes: The recommended dosage is 125 mg twice daily for 5 days. Initiate therapy at the first sign or symptom if medical management of a genital herpes recurrence is indicated. The efficacy of *Famvir* has not been established when treatment is initiated more than 6 hours after onset of symptoms or lesions.

Suppression of recurrent genital herpes: The recommended dosage is 250 mg twice daily for up to 1 year. The safety and efficacy of *Famvir* therapy beyond 1 year of treatment have not been established.

HIV-Infected Patients

For recurrent orolabial or genital herpes simplex infection, the recommended dosage is 500 mg twice daily for 7 days. In patients with reduced renal function, dosage reduction is recommended (see PRECAUTIONS, General).

[See table 7 on previous page]

Administration with Food

When famciclovir was administered with food, penciclovir C_{max} decreased approximately 50%. Because the systemic availability of penciclovir (AUC) was not altered, it appears that *Famvir* may be taken without regard to meals.

HOW SUPPLIED

Famvir is supplied as film-coated tablets as follows: 125 mg in bottles of 30; 250 mg in bottles of 30; and 500 mg in bottles of 30 and Single Unit Packages of 50 (intended for institutional use only).
Famvir 125 mg tablets are white, round, debossed with FAMVIR on one side and 125 on the other.
125 mg 30's: NDC 0007-4115-13
Famvir 250 mg tablets are white, round, debossed with FAMVIR on one side and 250 on the other.
250 mg 30's: NDC 0007-4116-13
Famvir 500 mg tablets are white, oval, debossed with FAMVIR on one side and 500 on the other.
500 mg 30's: NDC 0007-4117-13
500 mg SUP 50's: NDC 0007-4117-19
Store between 15° and 30° C (59° and 86° F).

Rx only

Manufactured in Crawley, UK
by **SmithKline Beecham Pharmaceuticals**
for **SmithKline Beecham Pharmaceuticals**
Philadelphia, PA 19101

Veterans Administration/Military/PHS—Tablets, 125 mg, 30's, 6505-01-425-3169; 250 mg, 30's, 6505-01-425-3166; 500 mg, 30's, 6505-01-395-0397; 500 mg, SUP 50's, 6505-01-395-0399.
FV:L16A

Shown in Product Identification Guide, page 339

FASTIN® ℂⅣ

[făs 'tĭn]
(brand of phentermine hydrochloride)
Capsules

DESCRIPTION

Each Fastin (phentermine hydrochloride) capsule contains phentermine hydrochloride, 30 mg (equivalent to 24 mg phentermine).
Phentermine hydrochloride is a white crystalline powder, very soluble in water and alcohol. Chemically, the product is phenyl-tertiary-butylamine hydrochloride. **Inactive Ingredients:** FD&C Blue No. 1, invert sugar, methylcellulose, polyethylene glycol, starch, sucrose and titanium dioxide. The branding ink used on the gelatin capsules contains: aluminum lake, ethyl alcohol, FD&C Blue No. 1, isopropyl alcohol, n-butyl alcohol, pharmaceutical shellac (modified) or refined shellac (food grade) and propylene glycol.

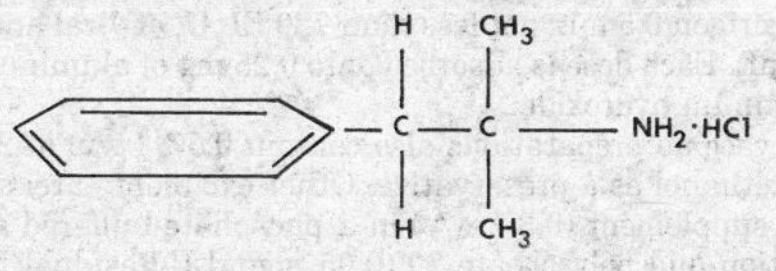

ACTIONS

Fastin is a sympathomimetic amine with pharmacologic activity similar to the prototype drugs of this class used in obesity, the amphetamines. Actions include central nervous system stimulation and elevation of blood pressure. Tachyphylaxis and tolerance have been demonstrated with all drugs of this class in which these phenomena have been looked for.
Drugs of this class used in obesity are commonly known as "anorectics" or "anorexigenics." It has not been established that the action of such drugs in treating obesity is primarily one of appetite suppression. Other central nervous system actions, or metabolic effects, may be involved, for example.
Adult obese subjects instructed in dietary management and treated with "anorectic" drugs lose more weight on the average than those treated with placebo and diet, as determined in relatively short-term clinical trials.
The magnitude of increased weight loss of drug-treated patients over placebo-treated patients is only a fraction of a pound a week. The rate of weight loss is greatest in the first weeks of therapy for both drug and placebo subjects and tends to decrease in succeeding weeks. The possible origins of the increased weight loss due to the various drug effects are not established. The amount of weight loss associated with the use of an "anorectic" drug varies from trial to trial, and the increased weight loss appears to be related in part to variables other than the drugs prescribed, such as the physician-investigator, the population treated and the diet prescribed. Studies do not permit conclusions as to the relative importance of the drug and non-drug factors on weight loss.
The natural history of obesity is measured in years, whereas the studies cited are restricted to a few weeks' duration; thus, the total impact of drug-induced weight loss over that of diet alone must be considered clinically limited.

INDICATION

Fastin is indicated as a short-term (a few weeks) adjunct in a regimen of weight reduction based on exercise, behavioral modification and caloric restriction in the management of exogenous obesity for patients with an initial body mass index ≥30 kg/m^2, or ≥27 kg/m^2 in the presence of other risk factors (e.g., hypertension, diabetes, hyperlipidemia).
Below is a chart of Body Mass Index (BMI) based on various heights and weights.
BMI is calculated by taking the patient's weight, in kilograms (kg), divided by the patient's height, in meters (m), squared. Metric conversions are as follows: pounds ÷ 2.2=kg; inches × 0.0254=meters.

BODY MASS INDEX (BMI), kg/m^2

	Height (feet, inches)					
Weight (pounds)	5'0"	5'3"	5'6"	5'9"	6'0"	6'3"
140	27	25	23	21	19	18
150	29	27	24	22	20	19
160	31	28	26	24	22	20
170	33	30	28	25	23	21
180	35	32	29	27	25	23
190	37	34	31	28	26	24
200	39	36	32	30	27	25
210	41	37	34	31	29	26
220	43	39	36	33	30	28
230	45	41	37	34	31	29
240	47	43	39	36	33	30
250	49	44	40	37	34	31

The limited usefulness of agents of this class (see ACTIONS) should be measured against possible risk factors inherent in their use such as those described below.

CONTRAINDICATIONS

Advanced arteriosclerosis, cardiovascular disease, moderate to severe hypertension, hyperthyroidism, known hypersensitivity or idiosyncrasy to the sympathomimetic amines, glaucoma.
Agitated states.
Patients with a history of drug abuse.
During or within 14 days following the administration of monoamine oxidase inhibitors (hypertensive crises may result).

WARNINGS

Fastin (phentermine hydrochloride) capsules are indicated only as short-term monotherapy for the management of exogenous obesity. The safety and efficacy of combination therapy with phentermine and any other drug products for weight loss, including selective serotonin reuptake inhibitors (e.g., fluoxetine, sertraline, fluvoxamine, paroxetine), have not been established. Therefore, coadministration of these drug products for weight loss is not recommended.

Continued on next page

Information on the SmithKline Beecham Pharmaceuticals products appearing here is based on the labeling in effect on July 31, 1998. Further information on these and other products may be obtained from the Medical Department, SmithKline Beecham Pharmaceuticals, One Franklin Plaza, Philadelphia, PA 19101.

Fastin—Cont.

Primary Pulmonary Hypertension (PPH) – a rare, frequently fatal disease of the lungs – has been reported to occur in patients receiving a combination of phentermine with fenfluramine or dexfenfluramine. The possibility of an association between PPH and the use of phentermine alone cannot be ruled out; there have been rare cases of PPH in patients who reportedly have taken phentermine alone. The initial symptom of PPH is usually dyspnea. Other initial symptoms include: angina pectoris, syncope or lower extremity edema. Patients should be advised to report immediately any deterioration in exercise tolerance. Treatment should be discontinued in patients who develop new, unexplained symptoms of dyspnea, angina pectoris, syncope or lower extremity edema.

Valvular Heart Disease: Serious, regurgitant cardiac valvular disease, primarily affecting the mitral, aortic and/or tricuspid valves, has been reported in otherwise healthy persons who had taken a combination of phentermine with fenfluramine or dexfenfluramine for weight loss. The etiology of these valvulopathies has not been established and their course in individuals after the drugs are stopped is not known. The possibility of an association between valvular heart disease and the use of phentermine alone cannot be ruled out; there have been rare cases of valvular heart disease in patients who reportedly have taken phentermine alone.

Tolerance to the anorectic effect usually develops within a few weeks. When this occurs, the recommended dose should not be exceeded in an attempt to increase the effect; rather, the drug should be discontinued.

Fastin may impair the ability of the patient to engage in potentially hazardous activities such as operating machinery or driving a motor vehicle; the patient should therefore be cautioned accordingly.

Drug Dependence: *Fastin* is related chemically and pharmacologically to the amphetamines. Amphetamines and related stimulant drugs have been extensively abused, and the possibility of abuse of *Fastin* should be kept in mind when evaluating the desirability of including a drug as part of a weight reduction program. Abuse of amphetamines and related drugs may be associated with intense psychological dependence and severe social dysfunction. There are reports of patients who have increased the dosage to many times that recommended. Abrupt cessation following prolonged high dosage administration results in extreme fatigue and mental depression; changes are also noted on the sleep EEG. Manifestations of chronic intoxication with anorectic drugs include severe dermatoses, marked insomnia, irritability, hyperactivity and personality changes. The most severe manifestation of chronic intoxications is psychosis, often clinically indistinguishable from schizophrenia.

Usage with Alcohol: Concomitant use of alcohol with *Fastin* may result in an adverse drug interaction.

PRECAUTIONS

General

Caution is to be exercised in prescribing Fastin (phentermine hydrochloride) for patients with even mild hypertension.

Insulin requirements in diabetes mellitus may be altered in association with the use of *Fastin* and the concomitant dietary regimen.

Fastin may decrease the hypotensive effect of guanethidine.

The least amount feasible should be prescribed or dispensed at one time in order to minimize the possibility of overdosage.

Carcinogenesis, Mutagenesis, Impairment of Fertility: Studies have not been performed with Fastin (phentermine hydrochloride) to determine the potential for carcinogenesis, mutagenesis or impairment of fertility.

Pregnancy—Teratogenic Effects: Pregnancy Category C. Animal reproduction studies have not been conducted with *Fastin*. It is also not known whether *Fastin* can cause fetal harm when administered to a pregnant woman or can affect reproductive capacity. *Fastin* should be given to a pregnant woman only if clearly needed.

Nursing Mothers

Because of the potential for serious adverse reactions in nursing infants, a decision should be made whether to discontinue nursing or to discontinue the drug, taking into account the importance of the drug to the mother.

Pediatric Use

Safety and effectiveness in pediatric patients have not been established.

ADVERSE REACTIONS

Cardiovascular: Primary pulmonary hypertension and/or regurgitant cardiac valvular disease (see WARNINGS), palpitation, tachycardia, elevation of blood pressure.

Central Nervous System: Overstimulation, restlessness, dizziness, insomnia, euphoria, dysphoria, tremor, headache; rarely psychotic episodes at recommended doses.

Gastrointestinal: Dryness of the mouth, unpleasant taste, diarrhea, constipation, other gastrointestinal disturbances.

Allergic: Urticaria.

Endocrine: Impotence, changes in libido.

DOSAGE AND ADMINISTRATION

Exogenous Obesity: One capsule at approximately 2 hours after breakfast for appetite control. Late evening medication should be avoided because of the possibility of resulting insomnia.

Administration of one capsule (30 mg) daily has been found to be adequate in depression of the appetite for 12 to 14 hours.

Fastin is not recommended for use in patients 16 years of age and under.

OVERDOSAGE

Manifestations of acute overdosage with phentermine include restlessness, tremor, hyperreflexia, rapid respiration, confusion, assaultiveness, hallucinations, panic states. Fatigue and depression usually follow the central stimulation. Cardiovascular effects include arrhythmias, hypertension or hypotension, and circulatory collapse. Gastrointestinal symptoms include nausea, vomiting, diarrhea and abdominal cramps. Fatal poisoning usually terminates in convulsions and coma.

Management of acute phentermine intoxication is largely symptomatic and includes lavage and sedation with a barbiturate. Experience with hemodialysis or peritoneal dialysis is inadequate to permit recommendations in this regard. Acidification of the urine increases phentermine excretion. Intravenous phentolamine (Regitine®, CIBA) has been suggested for possible acute, severe hypertension, if this complicates phentermine overdosage.

HOW SUPPLIED

Blue and clear capsules with blue and white beads containing 30 mg phentermine hydrochloride (equivalent to 24 mg phentermine) imprinted with BEECHAM on cap and product name FASTIN® on body.

NDC 0029-2205-30 .... bottles of 100
NDC 0029-2205-39 .... bottles of 450

Store at room temperature.

Manufactured by
King Pharmaceuticals, Inc.
Bristol, TN 37620 for
SmithKline Beecham Pharmaceuticals
Philadelphia, PA 19101

FA:L5

Shown in Product Identification Guide, page 339

HEPATITIS A VACCINE, INACTIVATED ℞
HAVRIX®

[have 'rix]

DESCRIPTION

Havrix (Hepatitis A Vaccine, Inactivated) is a noninfectious hepatitis A vaccine developed and manufactured by SmithKline Beecham Biologicals. The virus (strain HM175) is propagated in MRC_5 human diploid cells. After removal of the cell culture medium, the cells are lysed to form a suspension. This suspension is purified through ultrafiltration and gel permeation chromatography procedures. Treatment of this lysate with formalin ensures viral inactivation.

Havrix contains a sterile suspension of inactivated virus; viral antigen activity is referenced to a standard using an enzyme linked immunosorbent assay (ELISA), and is therefore expressed in terms of ELISA Units (EL.U.).

Havrix is supplied as a sterile suspension for intramuscular administration. The vaccine is ready for use without reconstitution; it must be shaken before administration to assure a uniform suspension. After shaking, the vaccine is a homogenous white turbid suspension.

Each 1 mL adult dose of vaccine consists of not less than 1440 EL.U. of viral antigen, adsorbed on 0.5 mg of aluminum, as aluminum hydroxide.

There are two pediatric dose formulations, each with its own dosing schedule (see DOSAGE AND ADMINISTRATION). The formulations are: not less than 360 EL.U. of viral antigen/0.5 mL; not less than 720 EL.U. of viral antigen/0.5 mL. Each dose is adsorbed onto 0.25 mg of aluminum, as aluminum hydroxide.

The vaccine preparations also contain 0.5% (w/v) of 2-phenoxyethanol as a preservative. Other excipients are: amino acid supplement (0.3% w/v) in a phosphate-buffered saline solution and polysorbate 20 (0.05 mg/mL). Residual MRC_5 cellular proteins (not more than 5 mcg/adult dose) and traces of formalin (not more than 0.1 mg/mL) are present.

CLINICAL PHARMACOLOGY

The hepatitis A virus (HAV) belongs to the picornavirus family. Only one serotype of HAV has been described.[1]

Hepatitis A is highly contagious with the predominant mode of transmission being person-to-person via the fecal-oral route. Infection has been shown to be spread (1) by contaminated water or food; (2) by infected food handlers[2]; (3) after breakdown in usual sanitary conditions or after floods or natural disasters; (4) by ingestion of raw or undercooked shellfish (oysters, clams, mussels) from contaminated waters[3]; (5) during travel to areas of the world with poor hygienic conditions[4,5]; (6) among institutionalized children and adults[6]; (7) in day-care centers where children have not been toilet trained[7]; (8) by parenteral transmission, either blood transfusions or sharing needles with infected people.[1]

The level of economic development influences the prevalence of hepatitis A and the age at which it is most likely to occur. In developing countries with poor hygiene and sanitation, about 90% of children are infected by age 5 years.[1]

As conditions improve, the prevalence decreases and the age at which infection occurs increases. Hence it is more likely to occur in adulthood, when disease is generally more severe and more likely to be fatal.[1] In the United States, attack rates for hepatitis A infection are cyclical and vary by population. The rates have increased gradually from 9.2 per 100,000 in 1983 to 14.6 per 100,000 in 1989.[8]

The incubation period for hepatitis A averages 28 days (range: 15 to 50 days).[9] The course of hepatitis A infection is extremely variable, ranging from asymptomatic infection to icteric hepatitis. However, most adults (76% to 97%)[10] become symptomatic. Symptoms range from mild and transient to severe and prolonged and may include fever, nausea, vomiting and diarrhea in the prodromal phase, followed by jaundice in up to 88% of adults, as well as hepatomegaly and biochemical evidence of hepatocellular damage.[10] Recovery is generally complete and followed by protection against HAV infection. However, illness may be prolonged, and relapse of clinical illness and viral shedding have been described.[11]

Hepatitis A infection is often asymptomatic in children under 2 years of age, who nonetheless excrete the virus in their stool and thereby serve as a source of infection.[10] In older patients and persons with underlying liver disease,[1] it is generally much more severe. This is reflected in mortality rates. While an overall case fatality rate of 0.6% has been reported, a case fatality rate of 2.7% has been reported in patients ≥49 years of age.[1] Indeed, while 67% of cases occur in children, over 70% of deaths occur in those over the age of 49 years.[1]

There is no chronic carrier state. The virus replicates in the liver and is excreted in bile. The highest concentrations of HAV are found in stools of infected persons during the 2-week period immediately before the onset of jaundice and decline after jaundice appears.[12] Children and infants may shed HAV for longer periods than adults, possibly lasting as long as several weeks after the onset of clinical illness.[13]

Chronic shedding of HAV in feces has not been demonstrated, but relapses of hepatitis A can occur in as many as 20% of patients[1,14] and fecal shedding of HAV may recur at this time.[11]

The presence of antibodies to HAV (anti-HAV) confers protection against hepatitis A infection. However, the lowest titer needed to confer protection has not been determined.

In a chimpanzee challenge study, the quality of protection afforded by immune globulin (IG) prepared from initially seronegative human volunteers vaccinated with *Havrix* was comparable to that afforded by commercial IG. In this experiment chimpanzees immunized with either preparation developed passive-active immunity, when challenged with wild-type HAV. No animal in either group developed clinical illness.

In vitro studies in a randomly selected subset of human subjects (n=80) showed anti-HAV induced by *Havrix* to have functional activity. This was demonstrated by a neutralization assay and a competitive inhibition assay using a panel of monoclonal antibodies known to have neutralizing activity.

Immunogenicity in Adults: In three clinical studies involving over 400 healthy adult volunteers given a single 1440 EL.U. dose of *Havrix*, specific humoral antibodies against HAV were elicited in more than 96% of subjects when measured 1 month after vaccination. By day 15, 80% to 98% of vaccinees had already seroconverted (anti-HAV ≥20 mIU/mL [the lower limit of antibody measurement by current assay]). Geometric mean titers (GMTs) of seroconverters ranged from 264 to 339 mIU/mL at day 15 and increased to a range of 335 to 637 mIU/mL by 1 month following vaccination.[15]

The GMTs obtained following a single dose of *Havrix* are at least several times higher than that expected following receipt of IG.

In a clinical study using 2.5 to 5 times the standard dose of IG (standard dose=0.02 to 0.06 mL/kg), the GMT in recipients was 146 mIU/mL at 5 days post-administration, 77 mIU/mL at month 1 and 63 mIU/mL at month 2.[15]

In two clinical trials in which a booster dose of 1440 EL.U. was given 6 months following the initial dose, 100% of vaccinees (n=269) were seropositive 1 month after the booster dose, with GMTs ranging from 3318 mIU/mL to 5925 mIU/mL. The titers obtained from this additional dose approximate those observed several years after natural infection.

In a subset of vaccinees (n=89), a single dose of *Havrix* 1440 EL.U. elicited specific anti-HAV neutralizing antibodies in more than 94% of vaccinees when measured 1 month after

vaccination. These neutralizing antibodies persisted until month 6. One hundred percent of vaccinees had neutralizing antibodies when measured 1 month after a booster dose given at month 6.

Immunogenicity of *Havrix* was studied in subjects with chronic liver disease of various etiologies. 189 healthy adults and 220 adults with either chronic hepatitis B (n=46), chronic hepatitis C (n=104) or moderate chronic liver disease of other etiology (n=70) were vaccinated with *Havrix* 1440 EL.U. on a 0, 6 month schedule. The last group consisted of alcoholic cirrhosis (n=17), autoimmune hepatitis (n=10), chronic hepatitis/cryptogenic cirrhosis (n=9), hemochromatosis (n=2), primary biliary cirrhosis (n=15), primary sclerosing cholangitis (n=4) and unspecified (n=13). At each time point, GMTs were lower for subjects with chronic liver disease than for healthy subjects. At month 7, the GMTs ranged from 478 mIU/mL (chronic hepatitis C) to 1245 mIU/mL (healthy), as determined by a commercial ELISA. The relevance of these data to the duration of protection afforded by *Havrix* is unknown. One month after the first dose, seroconversion rates in adults with chronic liver disease were lower than in healthy adults. However, 1 month after the booster dose at month 6, seroconversion rates were similar in all groups; rates ranged from 94.7% to 98.1%.

Immunogenicity in Children and Adolescents: In six clinical studies involving pediatric vaccinees (n=762) ranging from 1 to 18 years of age, the GMT following two doses of *Havrix* 360 EL.U. given 1 month apart ranged from 197 to 660 mIU/mL. Ninety-nine percent of subjects seroconverted following two doses. When a booster (third) dose of *Havrix* 360 EL.U. was administered 6 months following the initial dose, all subjects were seropositive 1 month following the booster dose with GMTs rising to a range of 3388 to 4643 mIU/mL. In one study in which children were followed for an additional 6 months, all subjects remained seropositive. Solicited adverse effects were similar in frequency and nature to those seen following administration of Engerix-B® [Hepatitis B Vaccine (Recombinant)].

In four clinical studies, children and adolescents (n=314), ranging from 2 to 19 years of age, were immunized with two doses of *Havrix* 720 EL.U./0.5 mL given six months apart. One month after the first dose, seroconversion ranged from 96.8% to 100%, with GMTs of 194 mIU/mL to 305 mIU/mL. In studies in which sera were obtained 2 weeks following the initial dose, seroconversion ranged from 91.6% to 96.1%. One month following a booster dose at month 6, all subjects were seropositive with GMTs ranging from 2495 mIU/mL to 3644 mIU/mL.[15]

In one additional study in which the booster dose was delayed until 1 year following the initial dose, 95.2% of the subjects were seropositive just prior to administration of the booster dose. One month later, all subjects were seropositive with a GMT of 2657 mIU/mL.[15]

Also, *Havrix* has been found to be highly efficacious in a clinical study of children at high risk of HAV infection (see below).

At present, the duration of protection afforded by *Havrix* has not been established. Therefore it is unknown if the protection provided to immunized children will last until adulthood.

Protective Efficacy: Protective efficacy with *Havrix* has been demonstrated in a double-blind, randomized controlled study in school children (age 1 to 16 years) in Thailand who were at high risk of HAV infection. A total of 40,119 children were randomized to be vaccinated with either *Havrix* 360 EL.U. or *Engerix-B* at 0, 1, 12 months. 19,037 children received a primary course (0, 1 months) of *Havrix* and 19,120 children received a primary course (0, 1 months) of *Engerix-B*. 38,157 children entered surveillance at day 138 and were observed for an additional 8 months. Using the protocol-defined endpoint (≥2 days absence from school, ALT level >45 U/mL, and a positive result in the HAVAB-M test), 32 cases of clinical hepatitis A occurred in the control group; in the *Havrix* group, two cases were identified. These two cases were mild both in terms of biochemical and clinical indices of hepatitis A disease. Thus the calculated efficacy rate for prevention of clinical hepatitis A was 94% (95% confidence intervals 74% to 98%).[16]

In outbreak investigations occurring in the trial, 26 clinical cases of hepatitis A (of a total of 34 occurring in the trial) occurred. No cases occurred in *Havrix* vaccinees.

Using additional virological and serological analyses post hoc, the efficacy of *Havrix* was confirmed. Up to three additional cases of very mild clinical illness may have occurred in vaccinees. Using available testing, these illnesses could neither be proven nor disproven to have been caused by HAV. By including these as cases, the calculated efficacy rate for prevention of clinical hepatitis A would be 84% (95% confidence intervals 60% to 94%).

In a study designed to interrupt an epidemic of hepatitis A among Native Americans in Alaska, vaccination with a single dose of *Havrix* (1440 EL.U./mL in adults, 720 EL.U./0.5 mL in children and adolescents), appeared to be efficacious.[15]

INDICATIONS AND USAGE

Havrix is indicated for active immunization of persons ≥2 years of age against disease caused by hepatitis A virus (HAV).

Havrix will not prevent hepatitis caused by other agents such as hepatitis B virus, hepatitis C virus, hepatitis E virus or other pathogens known to infect the liver.

Immunization with *Havrix* is indicated for those people desiring protection against hepatitis A. Primary immunization should be completed at least 2 weeks prior to expected exposure to HAV. Individuals who are, or will be, at increased risk of infection by HAV include:

Travelers.

Persons traveling to areas of higher endemicity for hepatitis A. These areas include, but are not limited to, Africa, Asia (except Japan), the Mediterranean basin, eastern Europe, the Middle East, Central and South America, Mexico, and parts of the Caribbean. Current CDC advisories should be consulted with regard to specific locales.

Military personnel.

People living in, or relocating to, areas of high endemicity.

Certain ethnic and geographic populations that experience cyclic hepatitis A epidemics such as:

Native peoples of Alaska and the Americas.

People with chronic liver disease including:

—Alcoholic cirrhosis
—Chronic hepatitis B
—Chronic hepatitis C
—Autoimmune hepatitis
—Primary biliary cirrhosis

Others.

—Persons engaging in high-risk sexual activity (such as men having sex with men)
—Residents of a community experiencing an outbreak of hepatitis A
—Users of illicit injectable drugs
—Persons who have clotting-factor disorders (hemophiliacs and other recipients of therapeutic blood products)

Hepatitis A transmission has been documented in persons with clotting disorders. Susceptible persons in this category, especially those who receive solvent-detergent-treated clotting-factor concentrates, should be vaccinated against hepatitis A[17] (see PRECAUTIONS and DOSAGE AND ADMINISTRATION).

Although the epidemiology of hepatitis A does not permit the identification of other specific populations at high risk of disease, outbreaks of hepatitis A or exposure to hepatitis A virus have been described in a variety of populations in which *Havrix* may be useful:

—Certain institutional workers (e.g., caretakers for the developmentally challenged)
—Employees of child day-care centers
—Laboratory workers who handle live hepatitis A virus
—Handlers of primate animals that may be harboring HAV

People exposed to hepatitis A.

For those requiring both immediate and long-term protection, *Havrix* may be administered concomitantly with IG.

The ACIP has issued the following recommendations regarding food handlers: "Persons who work as food handlers can contract hepatitis A and transmit HAV to others. To decrease the frequency of evaluations of food handlers with hepatitis A and the need for postexposure prophylaxis of patrons, vaccination may be considered where state or local health authorities or private employers determine that such vaccination is cost-effective."[17]

CONTRAINDICATIONS

Havrix is contraindicated in people with known hypersensitivity to any component of the vaccine.

WARNINGS

There have been rare reports of anaphylaxis/anaphylactoid reactions following commercial use of the vaccine in other countries. Patients experiencing hypersensitivity reactions after a *Havrix* injection should not receive further *Havrix* injections. (See CONTRAINDICATIONS.)

Hepatitis A has a relatively long incubation period (15 to 50 days). Hepatitis A vaccine may not prevent hepatitis A infection in individuals who have an unrecognized hepatitis A infection at the time of vaccination. Additionally, it may not prevent infection in individuals who do not achieve protective antibody titers (although the lowest titer needed to confer protection has not been determined).

PRECAUTIONS

General

As with any parenteral vaccine, epinephrine should be available for use in case of anaphylaxis or anaphylactoid reaction.

As with any vaccine, administration of *Havrix* should be delayed, if possible, in people with any febrile illness, except when, in the opinion of the physician, withholding vaccine entails the greater risk.

Havrix should be administered with caution to people with thrombocytopenia or a bleeding disorder since bleeding may occur following an intramuscular administration to these subjects.

As with any vaccine, if administered to immunosuppressed persons or persons receiving immunosuppressive therapy, the expected immune response may not be obtained.[18]

Care is to be taken by the health-care provider for the safe and effective use of *Havrix*.

Prior to an injection of any vaccine, all known precautions should be taken to prevent adverse reactions. This includes a review of the patient's history with respect to possible hypersensitivity to the vaccine or similar vaccines.

A separate sterile syringe and needle (for single-dose vial) or a sterile disposable unit (prefilled syringe) must be used for each patient to prevent the transmission of infectious agents from person to person. Needles should not be recapped and should be properly disposed.

Special care should be taken to ensure that *Havrix* is not injected into a blood vessel.

Information for Patients

Patients, parents or guardians should be fully informed of the benefits and risks of immunization with *Havrix*.

Havrix is indicated in a variety of situations (see INDICATIONS AND USAGE). For persons traveling to endemic or epidemic areas, current CDC advisories should be consulted with regard to specific locales.

Travelers should take all necessary precautions to avoid contact with or ingestion of contaminated food or water.

The duration of immunity following a complete schedule of immunization with *Havrix* has not been established.

Drug Interactions

Preliminary results suggest that the concomitant administration of a wide variety of other vaccines is unlikely to interfere with the immune response to *Havrix*.

As with other intramuscular injections, *Havrix* should be given with caution to individuals on anticoagulant therapy.

When concomitant administration of other vaccines or IG is required, they should be given with different syringes and at different injection sites.

Carcinogenesis, Mutagenesis, Impairment of Fertility

Havrix has not been evaluated for its carcinogenic potential, mutagenic potential or potential for impairment of fertility.

Pregnancy: Pregnancy Category C.

Animal reproduction studies have not been conducted with *Havrix*. It is also not known whether *Havrix* can cause fetal harm when administered to a pregnant woman or can affect reproduction capacity. *Havrix* should be given to a pregnant woman only if clearly needed.

Nursing Mothers

It is not known whether *Havrix* is excreted in human milk. Because many drugs are excreted in human milk, caution should be exercised when *Havrix* is administered to a nursing woman.

Pediatric Use

Havrix is well tolerated and highly immunogenic and effective in children ≥2 years of age. (See CLINICAL PHARMACOLOGY for immunogenicity and efficacy data. See DOSAGE AND ADMINISTRATION for recommended dosage.)

ADVERSE REACTIONS

During clinical trials involving more than 31,000 individuals receiving doses ranging from 360 EL.U. to 1440 EL.U. and during extensive postmarketing experience in Europe, Havrix (Hepatitis A Vaccine, Inactivated) has been generally well tolerated. As with all pharmaceuticals, however, it is possible that expanded commercial use of the vaccine could reveal rare adverse events not observed in clinical studies.

The frequency of solicited adverse events tended to decrease with successive doses of *Havrix*. Most events reported were considered by the subjects as mild and did not last for more than 24 hours.

Of solicited adverse events in clinical trials, the most frequently reported by volunteers was injection-site soreness (56% of adults and 21% of children); however, less than 0.5% of soreness was reported as severe. Headache was reported by 14% of adults and less than 9% of children. Other solicited and unsolicited events occurring during clinical trials are listed below:

Incidence 1% to 10% of Injections

Local reactions at injection site: induration, redness, swelling.

Body as a whole: fatigue, fever (>37.5°C), malaise.

Gastrointestinal: anorexia, nausea.

Incidence <1% of Injections

Local reaction at injection site: hematoma.

Dermatologic: pruritus, rash, urticaria.

Respiratory: pharyngitis, other upper respiratory tract infections.

Continued on next page

Information on the SmithKline Beecham Pharmaceuticals products appearing here is based on the labeling in effect on July 31, 1998. Further information on these and other products may be obtained from the Medical Department, SmithKline Beecham Pharmaceuticals, One Franklin Plaza, Philadelphia, PA 19101.

Havrix—Cont.

Gastrointestinal: abdominal pain, diarrhea, dysgeusia, vomiting.
Musculoskeletal: arthralgia, elevation of creatine phosphokinase, myalgia.
Hematologic: lymphadenopathy.
Central nervous system: hypertonic episode, insomnia, photophobia, vertigo.

Additional Safety Data

Safety data were obtained from two additional sources in which large populations were vaccinated. In an outbreak setting in which 4,930 individuals were immunized with a single dose of either 720 EL.U. or 1440 EL.U. of *Havrix*, the vaccine was well-tolerated and no serious adverse events due to vaccination were reported. Overall, less than 10% of vaccinees reported solicited general adverse events following the vaccine. The most common solicited local adverse event was pain at the injection site, reported in 22.3% of subjects at 24 hours and decreasing to 2.4% by 72 hours.
In a field efficacy trial, 19,037 children received the 360 EL.U. dose of *Havrix*. The most commonly reported adverse events following administration of *Havrix* were injection-site pain (9.5%) and tenderness (8.1%), which were reported following first doses of *Havrix*. Other adverse events were infrequent and comparable to the control vaccine *Engerix-B*. Additionally, no serious adverse events due to the vaccine were reported. The large trial further allowed for analysis of rare adverse events, including hospitalization and death. No significant differences were found between the cohorts. In subjects with chronic liver disease, *Havrix* was safe and well-tolerated. Local injection site reactions were similar among all four groups and no serious adverse reactions attributed to the vaccine were reported in subjects with chronic liver disease.

Postmarketing Reports

Rare voluntary reports of adverse events in people receiving *Havrix* that have been reported since market introduction of the vaccine include the following:
Local: localized edema.
While no causal relationship has been established, the following rare events have been reported:
Body as a whole: anaphylaxis/anaphylactoid reactions, somnolence.
Cardiovascular: syncope.
Hepatobiliary: jaundice, hepatitis.
Dermatologic: erythema multiforme, hyperhydrosis, angioedema.
Respiratory: dyspnea.
Hematologic: lymphadenopathy.
Central nervous system: convulsions, encephalopathy, dizziness, neuropathy, myelitis, paresthesia, Guillain-Barré syndrome, multiple sclerosis.
Other: congenital abnormality.

Reporting of Adverse Events

The U.S. Department of Health and Human Services has established the Vaccine Adverse Events Reporting System (VAERS) to accept reports of suspected adverse events after the administration of any vaccine, including, but not limited to, the reporting of events required by the National Childhood Vaccine Injury Act of 1986. The toll-free number for VAERS forms and information is 1-800-822-7967.[19]

DOSAGE AND ADMINISTRATION

Havrix should be administered by intramuscular injection. *Do not inject intravenously, intradermally or subcutaneously.* In adults, the injection should be given in the deltoid region. *Havrix* should not be administered in the gluteal region; such injections may result in suboptimal response.
Havrix may be administered concomitantly with IG, although the ultimate antibody titer obtained is likely to be lower than when the vaccine is given alone. *Havrix* has been administered simultaneously with *Engerix-B* without interference with their respective immune responses.
For individuals with clotting-factor disorders who are at risk of hemorrhage following intramuscular injection, the ACIP recommends that when any intramuscular vaccine is indicated for such patients, "...it should be administered intramuscularly if, in the opinion of a physician familiar with the patient's bleeding risk, the vaccine can be administered with reasonable safety by this route. If the patient receives antihemophilia or other similar therapy, intramuscular vaccination can be scheduled shortly after such therapy is administered. A fine needle (≤23 gauge) can be used for the vaccination and firm pressure applied to the site (without rubbing) for at least two minutes. The patient or family should be instructed concerning the risk of hematoma from the injection."[20]
When concomitant administration of other vaccines or IG is required, they should be given with different syringes and at different injection sites.
Preparation for Administration: Shake vial or syringe well before withdrawal and use. Parenteral drug products should be inspected visually for particulate matter or discol-

oration prior to administration. With thorough agitation, *Havrix* is a turbid white suspension. Discard if it appears otherwise.
The vaccine should be used as supplied; no dilution or reconstitution is necessary. The full recommended dose of the vaccine should be used. After removal of the appropriate volume from a single-dose vial, any vaccine remaining in the vial should be discarded.
Primary immunization for adults consists of a single dose of 1440 EL.U. in 1 mL. Primary immunization for children and adolescents (2 through 18 years of age) may follow either of these two schedules:

Group	Dose	Schedule
Children and adolescents (2 through 18 years of age)	Primary course: 360 EL.U./0.5 mL	two doses, given 1 month apart (month 0 and month 1)
	Booster: 360 EL.U./0.5 mL	6 to 12 months after primary course
OR		
	Primary course: 720 EL.U./0.5 mL	one dose (month 0)
	Booster: 720 EL.U./0.5 mL	6 to 12 months after primary course

Individuals should not be alternated between the 360 EL.U. and 720 EL.U. doses. Those who receive an initial 360 EL.U. dose should continue on the 360 EL.U. dosing schedule. Likewise, those individuals who receive a single 720 EL.U. primary dose should receive a 720 EL.U. booster dose.
For all age groups, a booster dose is recommended anytime between 6 and 12 months after the initiation of the primary dose in order to ensure the highest antibody titers.
In those with an impaired immune system, adequate anti-HAV response may not be obtained after the primary immunization course. Such patients may therefore require administration of additional doses of vaccine.

STORAGE

Store between 2° and 8°C (36° and 46°F). Do not freeze; discard if product has been frozen. Do not dilute to administer.

HOW SUPPLIED

360 EL.U./0.5 mL in Single-Dose Vials
NDC 58160-836-01 Package of 1
720 EL.U./0.5 mL in Single-Dose Vials and Prefilled Syringes
NDC 58160-837-01 Package of 1 Single-Dose Vial
NDC 58160-837-02 Package of 1 Prefilled Syringe
NDC 58160-837-05 Package of 5 Prefilled Syringes with 5/8-inch 25-gauge needles
NDC 58160-837-35 Package of 5 Prefilled Disposable Tip-Lok™ Syringes with 5/8-inch 25-gauge needles
1440 EL.U./mL in Single-Dose Vials, Prefilled Syringes and Multi-Dose Vials
NDC 58160-835-01 Package of 1 Single-Dose Vial
NDC 58160-835-02 Package of 1 Prefilled Syringe
NDC 58160-835-05 Package of 5 Prefilled Syringes with 1-inch 23-gauge needles
NDC 58160-835-07 Package of 1 Multi-Dose Vial, containing 10 doses
NDC 58160-835-35 Package of 5 Prefilled Disposable Tip-Lok™ Syringes with 1-inch 23-gauge needles

REFERENCES

1. Hadler SC: Global impact of hepatitis A virus infection changing patterns. In Hollinger FB, Lemon SM, Margolis H (eds): *Viral Hepatitis and Liver Disease.* Baltimore, Williams & Wilkins, 1991, pp. 14-20. **2.** Dienstag JL, Routenberg JA, Purcell RH, et al: Foodhandler-associated outbreak of hepatitis type A. An immune electron microscopic study. *Ann Intern Med.* 1975;83:647. **3.** Mackowiak PA, Caraway CT, Portnoy BL: Oyster-associated hepatitis. Lessons from the Louisiana experience. *Am J Epidemiol.* 1976;103:181. **4.** Woodson RD, Clinton JJ: Hepatitis prophylaxis abroad. Effectiveness of immune serum globulin in protecting Peace Corps volunteers. *JAMA.* 1969;1009:1053. **5.** Krugman S, Giles JP: Viral hepatitis. New light on an old disease. *JAMA.* 1970;212:1019. **6.** Mosley JW: Hepatitis types B and non-B. Epidemiologic background. *JAMA.* 1975;233:967. **7.** Hadler SC, Erben JJ, Francis DP, et al: Risk factors for hepatitis A in daycare centers. *J Infect Dis.* 1982;145:255. **8.** Shapiro CN, Shaw SE, Mandel EJ, Hadler SC: Epidemiology of hepatitis A in the United States. In Hollinger FB, Lemon SM, Margolis H (eds): *Viral Hepatitis and Liver Disease.* Baltimore, Williams & Wilkins, 1991, pp. 71-76. **9.** Centers for Disease Control: Protection against viral hepatitis: Recommendations of the Immunization Practices Advisory Committee (ACIP). *MMWR.* 1990;39(No. RR-2):1-26.
10. Lemon SM: Type A viral hepatitis: new developments in an old disease. *N Engl J Med.* Oct. 24, 1985;313(17):1059-1067. **11.** Sjogren MH, Tanno H, Fay O, et al: Hepatitis A virus in stool during clinical relapse. *Ann Intern Med.* 1987;106:221-226. **12.** Hollinger FB, Ticehurst J: Hepatitis A Virus. In Hollinger FB, Robinson WS, Purcell RH, et al (eds): *Viral Hepatitis.* New York, Raven Press, 1990, pp. 1-37. **13.** Tassopoulos NC, Papaevangelou GJ, Ticehurst JR, et al: Fecal excretion of Greek strains of hepatitis A virus in patients with hepatitis A and in experimentally infected chimpanzees. *J Infect Dis.* 1986; 154:231-237. **14.** Chiriaco P, Gaudalupi C, Armigliato MK, et al: Polyphasic course of hepatitis type A in children. *J Infect Dis.* 1986; 153:378. **15.** Data on file, SmithKline Beecham Pharmaceuticals. **16.** Innis BL, Snitbhan R, Kunasol P, et al: Protection against hepatitis A by an inactivated vaccine. *JAMA.* 1994;271(17): 1328-1364. **17.** Centers for Disease Control and Prevention: Prevention of hepatitis A through active or passive immunization. Recommendations of the Advisory Committee on Immunization Practices (ACIP). *MMWR.* 1996; 45(No. RR-15): 21-23. **18.** ACIP: Use of vaccines and immune globulins in persons with altered immunocompetence. *MMWR.* 1993;42 (No. RR-4). **19.** Centers for Disease Control: Vaccine Adverse Event Reporting System—United States. *MMWR.* 1990;39: 730-733. **20.** Centers for Disease Control and Prevention: General recommendations on immunization. Recommendations of the Advisory Committee on Immunization Practices (ACIP). *MMWR.* 1994;43(No. RR-1):23.

U.S. License No. 1090
Manufactured by **SmithKline Beecham Biologicals**
Rixensart, Belgium
Distributed by **SmithKline Beecham Pharmaceuticals**
Philadelphia, PA 19101
Havrix is a registered trademark of SmithKline Beecham.
Veterans Administration/Military/PHS—1440 EL.U./mL single dose, 1's, 6505-01-398-3329; 1440 EL.U./mL prefilled syringe, 1's, 6505-01-397-6045; 1440 EL.U./mL prefilled syringe, 5's, 6505-01-442-7289; 360 EL.U./0.5 mL, single dose, 1's, 6505-01-413-1330; 720 EL.U./0.5 mL, single dose, 1's 6505-01-431-9404; 720 EL.U./0.5 mL, prefilled syringe, 1's, 6505-01-431-9401.
HA:L10

Shown in Product Identification Guide, page 339

HYCAMTIN™ ℞
[hī-kam′-tin]
brand of topotecan hydrochloride for Injection (for intravenous use)

WARNING

Hycamtin (topotecan hydrochloride) for Injection should be administered under the supervision of a physician experienced in the use of cancer chemotherapeutic agents. Appropriate management of complications is possible only when adequate diagnostic and treatment facilities are readily available.
Therapy with *Hycamtin* should not be given to patients with baseline neutrophil counts of less than 1500 cells/mm³. In order to monitor the occurrence of bone marrow suppression, primarily neutropenia, which may be severe and result in infection and death, frequent peripheral blood cell counts should be performed on all patients receiving *Hycamtin*.

DESCRIPTION

Hycamtin (topotecan hydrochloride) is a semi-synthetic derivative of camptothecin and is an anti-tumor drug with topoisomerase I-inhibitory activity.
Hycamtin (topotecan hydrochloride) for Injection is supplied as a sterile lyophilized, buffered, light yellow to greenish powder available in single-dose vials. Each vial contains topotecan hydrochloride equivalent to 4 mg of topotecan as free base. The reconstituted solution ranges in color from yellow to yellow-green and is intended for administration by intravenous infusion.
Inactive ingredients are mannitol, 48 mg, and tartaric acid, 20 mg. Hydrochloric acid and sodium hydroxide may be used to adjust the pH. The solution pH ranges from 2.5 to 3.5. The chemical name for topotecan hydrochloride is (S)-10-[(dimethylamino)methyl]-4-ethyl-4,9-dihydroxy-1H-pyrano [3′,4′:6,7]indolizino[1,2-b]quinoline-3,14-(4H,12H)-dione monohydrochloride. It has the molecular formula $C_{23}H_{23}N_3O_5$•HCl and a molecular weight of 457.9.
Topotecan hydrochloride has the following structural formula:
[See chemical structure at top of next column]
It is soluble in water and melts with decomposition at 213° to 218°C.

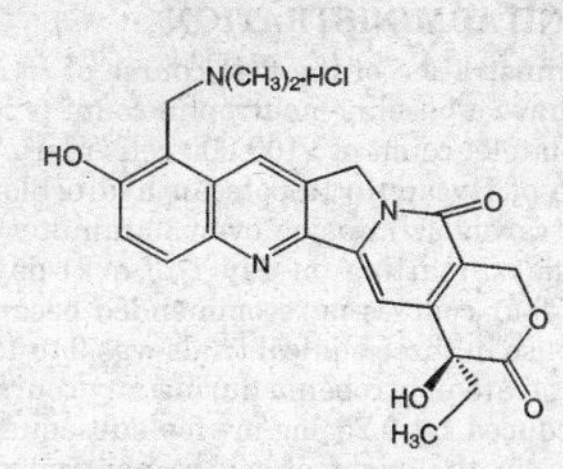

CLINICAL PHARMACOLOGY

Mechanism of Action

Topoisomerase I relieves torsional strain in DNA by inducing reversible single strand breaks. Topotecan binds to the topoisomerase I-DNA complex and prevents religation of these single strand breaks. The cytotoxicity of topotecan is thought to be due to double strand DNA damage produced during DNA synthesis when replication enzymes interact with the ternary complex formed by topotecan, topoisomerase I and DNA. Mammalian cells cannot efficiently repair these double strand breaks.

Pharmacokinetics

The pharmacokinetics of topotecan have been evaluated in cancer patients following doses of 0.5 to 1.5 mg/m^2 administered as a 30-minute infusion. Topotecan exhibits multiexponential pharmacokinetics with a terminal half-life of 2 to 3 hours. Total exposure (AUC) is approximately dose-proportional. Binding of topotecan to plasma proteins is about 35%.

Metabolism and Elimination: Topotecan undergoes a reversible pH dependent hydrolysis of its lactone moiety; it is the lactone form that is pharmacologically active. At pH≤4 the lactone is exclusively present whereas the ring-opened hydroxy-acid form predominates at physiologic pH. *In vitro* studies in human liver microsomes indicate that metabolism of topotecan to an N-demethylated metabolite represents a minor metabolic pathway.

In humans, about 30% of the dose is excreted in the urine and renal clearance is an important determinant of topotecan elimination (see Special Populations).

Special Populations

Gender: The overall mean topotecan plasma clearance in male patients was approximately 24% higher than in female patients, largely reflecting difference in body size.

Geriatrics: Topotecan pharmacokinetics have not been specifically studied in an elderly population, but population pharmacokinetic analysis in female patients did not identify age as a significant factor. Decreased renal clearance, common in the elderly, is a more important determinant of topotecan clearance.

Race: The effect of race on topotecan pharmacokinetics has not been studied.

Renal Impairment: In patients with mild renal impairment (creatinine clearance of 40 to 60 mL/min.), topotecan plasma clearance was decreased to about 67% of the value in patients with normal renal function. In patients with moderate renal impairment (Cl_{cr} of 20 to 39 mL/min.), topotecan plasma clearance was reduced to about 34% of the value in control patients, with an increase in half-life. Mean half-life, estimated in three renally impaired patients, was about 5.0 hours. Dosage adjustment is recommended for these patients (see DOSAGE AND ADMINISTRATION).

Hepatic Impairment: Plasma clearance in patients with hepatic impairment (serum bilirubin levels between 1.7 and 15.0 mg/dL) was decreased to about 67% of the value in patients without hepatic impairment. Topotecan half-life increased slightly, from 2.0 hours to 2.5 hours, but these hepatically impaired patients tolerated the usual recommended topotecan dosage regimen (see DOSAGE AND ADMINISTRATION).

Drug Interactions: Pharmacokinetic studies of the interaction of topotecan with concomitantly administered medications have not been formally investigated. *In vitro* inhibition studies using marker substrates known to be metabolized by human P450 CYP1A2, CYP2A6, CYP2C8/9, CYP2C19, CYP2D6, CYP2E, CYP3A or CYP4A or dihydropyrimidine dehydrogenase indicate that the activities of these enzymes were not altered by topotecan. Enzyme inhibition by topotecan has not been evaluated *in vivo.*

Pharmacodynamics: The dose-limiting toxicity of topotecan is leukopenia. White blood cell count decreases with increasing topotecan dose or topotecan AUC. When topotecan is administered at a dose of 1.5 mg/m^2/day for 5 days, an 80% to 90% decrease in white blood cell count at nadir is typically observed after the first cycle of therapy.

CLINICAL STUDIES

Hycamtin (topotecan hydrochloride) was studied in four clinical trials of 452 patients with metastatic ovarian carcinoma. All patients had disease that had recurred on, or was unresponsive to, a platinum-containing regimen. Patients in these four studies received an initial dose of 1.5 mg/m^2 given by intravenous infusion over 30 minutes for 5 consecutive days, starting on day 1 of a 21-day course.

Two of the studies, involving 223 patients given topotecan, are mature enough for evaluation (although survival results are incomplete). *Hycamtin* was compared with paclitaxel in a randomized trial involving 112 patients treated with *Hycamtin* (1.5 mg/m^2/day x 5 days starting on day 1 of a 21-day course) and 114 patients treated with paclitaxel (175 mg/m^2 over 3 hours on day 1 of a 21-day course). All patients had recurrent ovarian cancer after a platinum-containing regimen or had not responded to at least one prior platinum-containing regimen. Patients who did not respond to the study therapy, or who progressed, could be given the alternative treatment.

Response rates, response duration and time to progression are shown in Table 1.

Table 1. Efficacy of Hycamtin (topotecan hydrochloride) vs. Paclitaxel in Ovarian Cancer

Parameter	*Hycamtin* (n=112)	Paclitaxel (n=114)
Complete Response Rate	5.4%	3.5%
Partial Response Rate	14.3%	8.8%
Overall Response Rate	19.6%	12.3%
95% Confidence Interval	12.8 to 28.2%	6.9 to 19.7%
(p-value)	(0.092)	
Response Duration (weeks) Median	32.1	23.1
95% Confidence Interval	24.1† to ∞	23.1† to 24.4†
hazard-ratio (*Hycamtin*:paclitaxel)	0.424	
(p-value)	(0.224)	
Time to Progression (weeks) Median	23.1	14.0
95% Confidence Interval	17.1† to 29.6†	11.9† to 18.3†
hazard-ratio (*Hycamtin*:paclitaxel)	0.578	
(p-value)	(0.002)	

The calculation for duration of response was based on the interval between first response and time to progression.

† Value corresponds to a censored event; i.e., patient had not yet progressed.

The time to response was longer with *Hycamtin* compared to paclitaxel with a mean of 10 weeks (range 3.1 to 24.1) vs 7 weeks (range 2.4 to 12.3). Consequently, the efficacy of *Hycamtin* may not be achieved if patients are withdrawn from treatment prematurely.

In the crossover phase, 5 of 53 (9.4%) patients who received *Hycamtin* after paclitaxel had a partial response and 1 of 37 (2.7%) patients who received paclitaxel after *Hycamtin* had a complete response.

Hycamtin was active in patients who had developed resistance to platinum-containing therapy, defined as tumor progression while on, or tumor relapse within 6 months after completion of, a platinum-containing regimen. One complete and seven partial responses were seen in 60 patients, for a response rate of 13%. In the same study, there were no complete responders and four partial responders on the paclitaxel arm, for a response rate of 7%.

The adverse reaction profile for paclitaxel in this study was consistent with the product's approved labeling; the adverse reaction profile for *Hycamtin* in this study was consistent with that observed in all 452 patients from the four ovarian cancer clinical trials (see ADVERSE REACTIONS).

Hycamtin was also studied in an open-label, non-comparative trial in 111 patients with recurrent ovarian cancer after treatment with a platinum-containing regimen, or who had not responded to one prior platinum-containing regimen. The response rate was 14% (95% CI=7.9% to 20.9%). The median duration of response was 18 weeks (range 5 to 42 weeks). The time to progression was 8.4 weeks (range: 0.7 to 72.1 weeks).

INDICATIONS AND USAGE

Hycamtin (topotecan hydrochloride) is indicated for the treatment of patients with metastatic carcinoma of the ovary after failure of initial or subsequent chemotherapy.

CONTRAINDICATIONS

Hycamtin is contraindicated in patients who have a history of hypersensitivity reactions to topotecan or to any of its ingredients. *Hycamtin* should not be used in patients who are pregnant or breast-feeding, or those with severe bone marrow depression.

WARNINGS

Bone marrow suppression (primarily neutropenia) is the dose-limiting toxicity of topotecan. Neutropenia is not cumulative over time.

Neutropenia: Severe (grade 4, <500 cells/mm^3) neutropenia was most common during course 1 of treatment (60% of patients) and occurred in 40% of all courses, with a median duration of 7 days. The nadir neutrophil count occurred at a median of 11 days. Prophylactic G-CSF was given in 27% of courses after the first cycle. Therapy-related sepsis or febrile neutropenia occurred in 26% of patients and sepsis was fatal in 0.7%.

Thrombocytopenia: Grade 4 thrombocytopenia (<25,000/mm^3) occurred in 26% of patients and in 9% of courses, with a median duration of 5 days and platelet nadir at a median of 15 days. Platelet transfusions were given to 13% of patients and in 4% of courses.

Anemia: Severe anemia (grade 3/4, <8 gm/dL) occurred in 40% of patients and in 16% of courses. Median nadir was at day 15. Transfusions were needed in 56% of patients and in 23% of courses.

Monitoring of Bone Marrow Function: *Hycamtin* should only be administered in patients with adequate bone marrow reserves, including baseline neutrophil counts of at least 1,500 cells/mm^3 and platelet count at least 100,000/mm^3. Frequent monitoring of peripheral blood cell counts should be instituted during treatment with *Hycamtin*. Patients should not be treated with subsequent courses of *Hycamtin* until neutrophils recover to >1,000 cells/mm^3, platelets recover to >100,000 cells/mm^3 and hemoglobin levels recover to 9.0 g/dL (with transfusion if necessary). Severe myelotoxicity has been reported when *Hycamtin* is used in combination with cisplatin (see Drug Interactions).

Pregnancy: *Hycamtin* may cause fetal harm when administered to a pregnant woman. The effects of topotecan on pregnant women have not been studied. If topotecan is used during a patient's pregnancy, or if a patient becomes pregnant while taking topotecan, she should be warned of the potential hazard to the fetus. Fecund women should be warned to avoid becoming pregnant. In rabbits, a dose of 0.10 mg/kg/day (about equal to the clinical dose on a mg/m^2 basis) given on days 6 through 20 of gestation caused maternal toxicity, embryolethality, and reduced fetal body weight. In the rat, a dose of 0.23 mg/kg/day (about equal to the clinical dose on a mg/m^2 basis) given for 14 days before mating through gestation day 6 caused fetal resorption, microphthalmia, pre-implant loss, and mild maternal toxicity. A dose of 0.10 mg/kg/day (about half the clinical dose on a mg/m^2 basis) given to rats on days 6 through 17 of gestation caused an increase in post-implantation mortality. This dose also caused an increase in total fetal malformations. The most frequent malformations were of the eye (microphthalmia, anophthalmia, rosette formation of the retina, coloboma of the retina, ectopic orbit), brain (dilated lateral and third ventricles), skull and vertebrae.

PRECAUTIONS

General: Inadvertent extravasation with Hycamtin (topotecan hydrochloride) has been associated with only mild local reactions such as erythema and bruising.

Hematology: Monitoring of bone marrow function is essential (see WARNINGS and DOSAGE AND ADMINISTRATION).

Carcinogenesis, Mutagenesis, Impairment of Fertility: Carcinogenicity testing of topotecan has not been performed. Topotecan, however, is known to be genotoxic to mammalian cells and is a probable carcinogen. Topotecan was mutagenic to L5178Y mouse lymphoma cells and clastogenic to cultured human lymphocytes with and without metabolic activation. It was also clastogenic to mouse bone marrow. Topotecan did not cause mutations in bacterial cells.

Drug Interactions: Concomitant administration of G-CSF can prolong the duration of neutropenia, so if G-CSF is to be used, it should not be initiated until day 6 of the course of therapy, 24 hours after completion of treatment with *Hycamtin.*[1]

Myelosuppression was more severe when *Hycamtin* was given in combination with cisplatin in Phase I studies. In a

Continued on next page

Information on the SmithKline Beecham Pharmaceuticals products appearing here is based on the labeling in effect on July 31, 1998. Further information on these and other products may be obtained from the Medical Department, SmithKline Beecham Pharmaceuticals, One Franklin Plaza, Philadelphia, PA 19101.

Hycamtin—Cont.

reported study on concomitant administration of cisplatin 50 mg/m^2 and *Hycamtin* at a dose of 1.25 mg/m^2/day ×5 days, one of three patients had neutropenia for 12 days and a second patient died with neutropenic sepsis. There are no adequate data to define a safe and effective regimen for *Hycamtin* and cisplatin in combination.

Pregnancy: Pregnancy Category D. (See WARNINGS section.)

Nursing Mothers: It is not known whether the drug is excreted in human milk. Breast-feeding should be discontinued when women are receiving *Hycamtin* (see CONTRAINDICATIONS).

Pediatric Use: Safety and effectiveness in pediatric patients have not been established.

ADVERSE REACTIONS

Data in the following section are based on the experience of 452 patients with metastatic ovarian carcinoma treated with *Hycamtin*. Table 2 lists the principal hematologic toxicities and Table 3 lists non-hematologic toxicities occurring in at least 19% of patients.

Table 2. Summary of Hematologic Adverse Events in Patients Receiving *Hycamtin*

Hematologic Adverse Events	Patients n=452 % Incidence	Courses n=2375 % Incidence
Neutropenia		
<1,500 cells/mm^3	98	78
<500 cells/mm^3	81	40
Leukopenia		
<3,000 cells/mm^3	98	77
<1,000 cells/mm^3	32	11
Thrombocytopenia		
<75,000/mm^3	63	39
<25,000/mm^3	26	9
Anemia		
<10 g/dL	95	76
<8 g/dL	40	16
Sepsis or fever/infection with Grade 4 neutropenia	26	7
Platelet transfusions	13	4
RBC transfusions	56	23

[See table 3 below]
Premedications were not routinely used in these clinical studies.

Hematologic: (See WARNINGS)

Gastrointestinal: The incidence of nausea was 77% (10% grade 3/4) and vomiting occurred in 58% (9% grade 3/4) of patients (see Table 3). The prophylactic use of antiemetics was not routine in patients treated with *Hycamtin*. Forty-two percent of patients had diarrhea (5% grade 3/4), 39% constipation (3% grade 3/4) and 33% had abdominal pain (6% grade 3/4).

Skin/Appendages: Total alopecia (grade 2) occurred in 42% of patients.

Central and Peripheral Nervous System: Headache (21%) was the most frequently reported neurologic toxicity. Paresthesia occurred in 9% of patients but was generally grade 1.

Liver/Biliary: Grade 1 transient elevations in SGOT/AST and SGPT/ALT occurred in 5% of patients. Greater elevations, grade 3/4, occurred in <1%. Grade 3/4 elevated bilirubin occurred in <3% of patients.

Respiratory: Dyspnea (20%); grade 3/4 dyspnea (4%).
Table 4 shows the grade 3/4 hematologic and major non-hematologic adverse events in the topotecan/paclitaxel comparator trial.

Table 4. Comparative Toxicity Profiles for Ovarian Cancer Patients Randomized to Receive *Hycamtin* or Paclitaxel

Adverse Event	Hycamtin Pts	Hycamtin Courses	Paclitaxel Pts	Paclitaxel Courses
	n=112	n=555	n=114	n=550
Hematologic Grade 3/4	%	%	%	%
Grade 4 neutropenia (<500 cells/mL)	79.5	36.7	21.9	8.5
Grade 3/4 Anemia (Hgb <8 g/dL)	40.5	16.0	6.3	2.0
Grade 4 Thrombocytopenia (<25,000 plts/mL)	25.3	9.6	1.8	0.4
Fever/Grade 4 neutropenia	23.2	5.4	2.6	0.5
Documented Sepsis	5.4	1.1	1.8	0.4
Death related to Sepsis	1.8	0.4	0.0	0.0
Non-hematologic Grade 3/4				
Gastrointestinal				
Abdominal pain	5.4	1.1	3.5	0.9
Constipation	5.4	1.1	0.0	0.0
Diarrhea	6.3	1.6	0.9	0.2
Intestinal Obstruction	4.5	1.1	4.4	0.9
Nausea	8.9	3.1	1.8	0.4
Stomatitis	0.9	0.2	0.9	0.2
Vomiting	9.8	2.0	2.6	0.5
Constitutional				
Anorexia	3.6	0.2	0.0	0.0
Dyspnea	6.3	1.8	5.3	1.3
Fatigue	8.0	2.2	5.3	2.0
Malaise	1.8	0.5	1.8	0.4
Neuromuscular				
Arthralgia	0.9	0.2	3.5	0.5
Asthenia	5.4	1.8	3.5	1.3
Headache	0.9	0.2	1.8	0.9
Myalgia	0.0	0.0	2.6	1.6
Pain	5.4	1.1	10.5	2.2

Premedications were not routinely used in patients randomized to *Hycamtin*, while patients receiving paclitaxel received routine pretreatment with corticosteroids, diphenhydramine, and histamine receptor type 2 blockers.

Postmarketing Reports of Adverse Events. Reports of adverse events in patients taking Hycamtin (topotecan hydrochloride) received after market introduction, which are not listed above, include the following:

Hematologic: *Rare*—severe bleeding (in association with thrombocytopenia).

Skin/Appendages: *Rare*—severe dermatitis, severe pruritus.

Body as a Whole: *Infrequent*—allergic manifestations; *rare*—anaphylactoid reactions, angioedema.

OVERDOSAGE

There is no known antidote for overdosage with *Hycamtin*. The primary anticipated complication of overdosage would consist of bone marrow suppression.
The LD$_{10}$ in mice receiving single intravenous infusions of *Hycamtin* was 75 mg/m^2 (CI 95%: 47 to 97).

DOSAGE AND ADMINISTRATION

Prior to administration of the first course of *Hycamtin*, patients must have a baseline neutrophil count of >1500 cells/mm^3 and a platelet count of >100,000 cells/mm^3. The recommended dose of Hycamtin (topotecan hydrochloride) is 1.5 mg/m^2 by intravenous infusion over 30 minutes daily for 5 consecutive days, starting on day 1 of a 21-day course. A minimum of four courses is recommended because median time to response in three clinical trials was 9 to 12 weeks. In the event of severe neutropenia during any course, the dose should be reduced by 0.25 mg/m^2 for subsequent courses. Alternatively, in the event of severe neutropenia, G-CSF may be administered following the subsequent course (before resorting to dose reduction) starting from day 6 of the course (24 hours after completion of topotecan administration).

Adjustment of Dose in Special Populations

Hepatic Impairment: No dosage adjustment appears to be required for treating patients with impaired hepatic function (plasma bilirubin >1.5 to <10 mg/dL).

Renal Functional Impairment: No dosage adjustment appears to be required for treating patients with mild renal impairment (Cl$_{cr}$ 40 to 60 mL/min). Dosage adjustment to 0.75 mg/m^2 is recommended for patients with moderate renal impairment (20 to 39 mL/min). Insufficient data are available in patients with severe renal impairment to provide a dosage recommendation.

Elderly Patients: No dosage adjustment appears to be needed in the elderly, other than adjustments related to renal function.

PREPARATION FOR ADMINISTRATION

Precautions: *Hycamtin* is a cytotoxic anticancer drug. As with other potentially toxic compounds, *Hycamtin* should be prepared under a vertical laminar flow hood while wearing gloves and protective clothing. If *Hycamtin* solution contacts the skin, wash the skin immediately and thoroughly with soap and water. If *Hycamtin* contacts mucous membranes, flush thoroughly with water.

Preparation for Intravenous Administration: Each *Hycamtin* 4 mg vial is reconstituted with 4 mL Sterile Water for Injection. Then the appropriate volume of the reconstituted solution is diluted in either 0.9% Sodium Chloride Intravenous Infusion or 5% Dextrose Intravenous Infusion prior to administration.
Because the lyophilized dosage form contains no antibacterial preservative, the reconstituted product should be used immediately.

STABILITY

Unopened vials of Hycamtin (topotecan hydrochloride) are stable until the date indicated on the package when stored between 20° and 25°C (68°and 77°F) [see USP] and protected from light in the original package. Because the vials contain no preservative, contents should be used immediately after reconstitution.
Reconstituted vials of *Hycamtin* diluted for infusion are stable at approximately 20° to 25°C (68° to 77°F) and ambient lighting conditions for 24 hours.

HOW SUPPLIED

Hycamtin (topotecan hydrochloride) for Injection is supplied in 4 mg (free base) single-dose vials.
NDC 0007-4201-01 (package of 1)
NDC 0007-4201-05 (package of 5)
Storage: Store the vials protected from light in the original cartons at controlled room temperature between 20° and 25°C (68° and 77°F) [see USP].
Handling and Disposal: Procedures for proper handling and disposal of anticancer drugs should be used. Several guidelines on this subject have been published.[2-8] There is no general agreement that all of the procedures recommended in the guidelines are necessary or appropriate.

REFERENCES

1. Rowinsky, et al. Phase 1 and pharmacologic study of high doses of the topoisomerase I inhibitor topotecan with granulocyte colony-stimulating factor in patients with solid tumors. J Clin Oncol. 1996;14:1224-1235.
2. Recommendations for the safe handling of parenteral antineoplastic drugs. NIH Publication No. 83-2621. For sale by the Superintendent of Documents, US Government Printing Office, Washington, DC 20402.
3. AMA Council Report. Guidelines for handling parenteral antineoplastics. JAMA 1985;253(11):1590-1592.
4. National Study Commission on Cytotoxic Exposure-recommendations for handling cytotoxic agents. Available from Louis P. Jeffry, Chairman, National Study Commission on Cytotoxic Exposure. Massachusetts College of Pharmacy and Allied Health Sciences, 179 Longwood Avenue, Boston, Massachusetts, 02115.
5. Clinical Oncological Society of Australia. Guidelines and recommendations for safe handling of antineoplastic agents. Med J Austr. 1983;1:426-428.
6. Jones RB, et al. Safe handling of chemotherapeutic agents: A report from the Mount Sinai Medical Center. CA-A Cancer Journal for Clinicians 1983;Sept./Oct.:258-263.

Table 3. Summary of Non-hematologic Adverse Events in Patients Receiving Hycamtin (topotecan hydrochloride)

Non-hematologic Adverse Events	All Grades % Incidence n=452 Patients	All Grades % Incidence n=2375 Courses	Grade 3 % Incidence n=452 Patients	Grade 3 % Incidence n=2375 Courses	Grade 4 % Incidence n=452 Patients	Grade 4 % Incidence n=2375 Courses
Gastrointestinal						
Nausea	77	50	10	3	<1	<1
Vomiting	58	26	6	3	3	<1
Diarrhea	42	19	4	1	<1	<1
Constipation	39	18	2	<1	1	<1
Abdominal Pain	33	13	4	<1	2	<1
Stomatitis	24	9	2	<1	<1	<1
Anorexia	19	8	2	<1	0	0
Body as a Whole						
Fatigue	37	25	6	2	0	0
Fever	34	13	1	<1	<1	<1
Asthenia	21	10	3	<1	1	<1
Skin/Appendages						
Alopecia	59	62	NA	NA	NA	NA

7. American Society of Hospital Pharmacists Technical Assistance Bulletin on Handling Cytotoxic and Hazardous Drugs. Am J Hos Pharm 1990;47:1033-1049.
8. OSHA Work-Practice guidelines for personnel dealing with cytotoxic (antineoplastic) drugs. Am J Hosp Pharm 1986;43:1193-1204.

HY:L8

Shown in Product Identification Guide, page 339

INFANRIX™ Diphtheria and Tetanus Toxoids and Acellular Pertussis Vaccine Adsorbed ℞

CAUTION: Federal (USA) law prohibits dispensing without prescription.

DESCRIPTION

Infanrix (Diphtheria and Tetanus Toxoids and Acellular Pertussis Vaccine Adsorbed) is a sterile combination of diphtheria and tetanus toxoids and three pertussis antigens [inactivated pertussis toxin (PT), filamentous hemagglutinin (FHA) and pertactin (69 kiloDalton outer membrane protein)] adsorbed onto aluminum hydroxide. *Infanrix* is intended for intramuscular injection only. After shaking, the vaccine is a homogeneous white turbid suspension.

Three acellular pertussis antigens (pertussis toxin [PT], filamentous hemagglutinin [FHA] and pertactin) are isolated from phase 1 *Bordetella pertussis* culture grown in modified Stainer-Scholte liquid medium. PT and FHA are extracted from the fermentation broth by adsorption on hydroxyapatite gel; pertactin is extracted from the cells by heat treatment and flocculation using barium chloride. These antigens are purified in successive chromatographic steps: PT and FHA by hydrophobic, affinity and size exclusion; pertactin by ion exchange, hydrophobic and size exclusion processes. PT is detoxified using formaldehyde and glutaraldehyde. FHA and pertactin are treated with formaldehyde.

Diphtheria toxin is produced by growing *Corynebacterium diphtheriae* in Linggoud and Fenton medium containing a bovine extract. Tetanus toxin is produced by growing *Clostridium tetani* in a modified Latham medium. Both toxins are detoxified with formaldehyde, concentrated by ultrafiltration, and purified by precipitation, sterile filtration and dialysis.

Each antigen is individually adsorbed onto aluminum hydroxide. Each 0.5 mL dose contains, by assay, not more than 0.625 mg aluminum. Each 0.5 mL dose is formulated to contain 25 Lf diphtheria toxoid, 10 Lf tetanus toxoid (both toxoids induce at least 2 antitoxin units/mL of serum in the guinea pig potency test), 25 mcg PT, 25 mcg FHA and 8 mcg pertactin. The potency of the pertussis component is evaluated by measurement of the antibody response to PT, FHA and pertactin in immunized mice using an ELISA.

Each 0.5 mL dose also contains 2.5 mg 2-phenoxyethanol as a preservative, 4.5 mg sodium chloride, water for injection and not more than 0.02% (w/v) residual formaldehyde. The vaccine contains polysorbate 80 (Tween 80) which is used in the production of the pertussis concentrate. The inactivated acellular pertussis components contribute less than 5 endotoxin units (EU) per 0.5 mL dose.

Diphtheria and Tetanus Toxoids adsorbed bulk concentrates for further manufacturing use are produced by Chiron Behring GmbH & Co, Marburg, Germany. The acellular pertussis antigens are manufactured by SmithKline Beecham Biologicals S.A., Rixensart, Belgium. Formulation, filling, testing, packaging and release of the vaccine are conducted by SmithKline Beecham Biologicals S.A.

CLINICAL PHARMACOLOGY

Simultaneous immunization against diphtheria, tetanus and pertussis during infancy and childhood using a conventional whole-cell DTP vaccine has been a routine practice in the United States since the late 1940s. It has played a major role in markedly reducing the incidence of, and deaths from, each of these diseases.

Diphtheria

Diphtheria is primarily a localized and generalized intoxication caused by diphtheria toxin, an extracellular protein metabolite of toxigenic strains of *Corynebacterium diphtheriae*. While the incidence of diphtheria in the United States has decreased from over 200,000 cases reported in 1921,[1] before the general use of diphtheria toxoid, to only 30 cases of respiratory diphtheria reported from 1983 to 1993,[2] the ratio of fatalities to attack rate has remained constant at about 5% to 10%. The highest case fatality rates are in the very young and in the elderly. Diphtheria remains a serious disease in some areas of the world as evidenced by the recent outbreak in the former Soviet Union.[3] Protection against disease is due to the development of neutralizing antibodies to the diphtheria toxin. Following adequate immunization with diphtheria toxoid, it is thought that protection lasts for at least 10 years.[1] Serum antitoxin levels of at least 0.01 antitoxin units per mL are generally regarded as protective.[4] This significantly reduces both the risk of developing diphtheria and the severity of clinical illness. Immunization with diphtheria toxoid does not, however, eliminate carriage of *C. diphtheriae* in the pharynx or nose or on the skin.[1] Efficacy of the diphtheria toxoid used in Infanrix (Diphtheria and Tetanus Toxoids and Acellular Pertussis Vaccine Adsorbed) was determined on the basis of immunogenicity studies, with a comparison to a serological correlate of protection (0.01 antitoxin units/mL) established by the Panel on Review of Bacterial Vaccines and Toxoids.[4] A Vero cell toxin neutralizing test confirmed the ability of infant sera (N=45), obtained 1 month after the primary course, to neutralize diphtheria toxin. Protective titers (≥0.01 antitoxin units/mL of serum) were achieved in 100% of the sera tested.

Tetanus

Tetanus is an intoxication manifested primarily by neuromuscular dysfunction caused by a potent exotoxin released by *Clostridium tetani*. The incidence of tetanus in the United States has dropped dramatically with the routine use of tetanus toxoid to a record low of 45 cases in 1992.[2] Tetanus in the U.S. is primarily a disease of older adults. Of 99 tetanus patients with complete information reported to the Centers for Disease Control and Prevention during 1987 and 1988, 68% were ≥50 years of age, while only 6 were <20 years of age. No cases of neonatal tetanus were reported. Overall, the case-fatality rate was 21%. The disease continues to occur almost exclusively among persons who are unvaccinated or inadequately vaccinated or whose vaccination histories are unknown or uncertain.[5]

Spores of *C. tetani* are ubiquitous. Serological tests indicate that naturally acquired immunity to tetanus toxin does not occur in the U.S. Thus, universal primary immunization with tetanus toxoid, with subsequent maintenance of adequate antitoxin levels by means of timed boosters, is necessary to protect all age groups.[1] Protection against disease is due to the development of neutralizing antibodies to the tetanus toxin. Tetanus toxoid is a highly effective antigen and a completed primary series generally induces serum antitoxin levels of at least 0.01 antitoxin units per mL, a level which has been reported to be protective.[4] It is thought that protection persists for at least 10 years.[1] Efficacy of the tetanus toxoid used in *Infanrix* was determined on the basis of immunogenicity studies with a comparison to a serological correlate of protection (0.01 antitoxin units per mL) established by the Panel on Review of Bacterial Vaccines and Toxoids.[4] An *in vivo* mouse toxin neutralizing test confirmed the ability of infant sera (N=45), obtained 1 month after the primary course, to neutralize tetanus toxin. Protective titers (≥0.01 antitoxin units/mL of serum) were achieved in 100% of the sera tested.

Pertussis

Pertussis (whooping cough) is a disease of the respiratory tract caused by *Bordetella pertussis*. Pertussis is highly communicable (attack rates in unimmunized household contacts of up to 90% have been reported[6]) and can cause severe disease, particularly among the very young.[1] Since immunization against pertussis became widespread, the number of reported cases and associated mortality in the United States have declined from an average annual incidence and mortality of 150 cases and 6 deaths per 100,000 population, respectively, in the early 1940s, to annual reported incidences of 1.6, 2.6 and 1.8 cases per 100,000 population in 1992, 1993 and 1994, respectively.[2,7] Precise epidemiologic data do not exist, since bacteriological confirmation of pertussis can be obtained in less than half of the suspected cases. Most reported illness from *B. pertussis* occurs in infants and young children in whom complications can be severe. From 1980 to 1989, of 10,749 pertussis cases reported nationally in infants less than 1 year of age, 69% were hospitalized, 22% had pneumonia, 3.0% had seizures, 0.9% had encephalopathy and 0.6% died.[8] Older children and adults, in whom classic signs are often absent, may go undiagnosed and may serve as reservoirs of disease.[9]

Routine vaccination with whole-cell DTP vaccine has significantly reduced pertussis-related morbidity and mortality. However, concerns regarding reactogenicity of whole-cell DTP vaccine have spurred development of safer pertussis vaccines with high efficacy. The role of the different components produced by *B. pertussis* in either the pathogenesis of, or the immunity to, pertussis is not well understood.

Antigenic components of *B. pertussis* believed to contribute to protective immunity include: pertussis toxin; filamentous hemagglutinin; and pertactin.[10,11] Although the role of these antigens in providing protective immunity in humans is not well understood, clinical trials which evaluated candidate acellular DTP vaccines manufactured by SmithKline Beecham Biologicals supported the efficacy of three-component *Infanrix*.[12-14]

Infanrix, which contains three pertussis antigens (PT, FHA and pertactin), has been shown to be effective in preventing WHO-defined pertussis in two published clinical trials when administered as a primary series.[13,14]

A double-blind, randomized, placebo-controlled (DT) trial conducted in Italy, sponsored by the National Institutes of Health (NIH), assessed the absolute protective efficacy of *Infanrix* when administered at 2, 4 and 6 months of age.[13] A total of 15,601 infants were immunized with one of two tricomponent acellular DTP vaccines (containing inactivated PT, FHA and pertactin), or with a U.S.-licensed whole-cell DTP vaccine manufactured by Connaught Laboratories, Inc., or with DT vaccine alone. The mean length of follow-up was 17 months, beginning 30 days after the third dose of vaccine. The population used in the primary analysis of vaccine efficacy included 4,481 *Infanrix* vaccinees, 4,348 whole-cell DTP vaccinees and 1,470 DT vaccinees. After three doses, the protective efficacy of *Infanrix* against WHO-defined typical pertussis (21 days or more of paroxysmal cough with infection confirmed by culture and/or serologic testing) was 84% (95% CI: 76% to 89%) while the efficacy of the whole-cell DTP vaccine was 36% (95% CI: 14% to 52%). When the definition of pertussis was expanded to include clinically milder disease with respect to type and duration of cough, with infection confirmed by culture and/or serologic testing, the efficacy of *Infanrix* was calculated to be 71% (95% CI: 60% to 78%) against >7 days of any cough and 73% (95% CI: 63% to 80%) against ≥14 days of any cough. A longer follow-up of the Italian trial showed that after three doses, the absolute efficacy of *Infanrix* remained high against WHO-defined pertussis at 78% (95% CI: 62% to 87%) in children whose average age was then 33 months (20-39 months).[15]

A prospective, blinded efficacy trial was also conducted in Germany employing a household contact study design.[14] In preparation for this study, three doses of Infanrix (Diphtheria and Tetanus Toxoids and Acellular Pertussis Vaccine Adsorbed) were administered at 3, 4 and 5 months of age to more than 22,000 children living in six areas of Germany in a large safety and immunogenicity trial. Infants who did not participate in this trial could have received whole-cell DTP vaccine (manufactured by Behringwerke A.G., Germany) or DT vaccine. Pediatricians were asked to monitor households with a first potential case (index case) of typical pertussis which was identified by spontaneous presentation to a physician. Households were enrolled in the study if there was at least one other household member (a household contact) 6 to 47 months of age. Prospective follow-up of household contacts of index cases for the incidence and progression of pertussis was performed by a separate physician who was blinded to the vaccination status of the household. Calculation of vaccine efficacy was based on attack rates of pertussis in household contacts classified by vaccination status. Of the 173 unvaccinated household contacts, 96 developed WHO-defined pertussis (21 days or more of paroxysmal cough with infection confirmed by culture and/or serologic testing), as compared to 7 of 112 contacts vaccinated with *Infanrix* and 1 of 75 contacts vaccinated with whole-cell DTP vaccine. The protective efficacy of *Infanrix* was calculated to be 89% (95% CI: 77% to 95%), with no indication of waning of protection up until the time of the booster. The protective efficacy of the whole-cell DTP vaccine was calculated to be 98% (95% CI: 83% to 100%). The average age of *Infanrix* vaccinees at the time of follow-up in this trial was 13 months (range 6-25 months). When the definition of pertussis was expanded to include clinically milder disease, with infection confirmed by culture and/or serologic testing, the efficacy of *Infanrix* against ≥7 days of any cough was 67% (95% CI: 52% to 78%) and against ≥7 days of paroxysmal cough was 81% (95% CI: 68% to 89%). The corresponding efficacy rates of *Infanrix* against ≥14 days of any cough or paroxysmal cough were 73% (95% CI: 59% to 82%) and 84% (95% CI: 71% to 91%), respectively.

Immune Response to Infanrix *Administered as a Three-Dose Primary Series*

The immune responses to each of the three pertussis antigens contained in *Infanrix* were evaluated in sera obtained 1 month after the third dose of vaccine in each of three studies (schedule of administration: 2, 4 and 6 months of age in the Italian efficacy study and one U.S. study; 3, 4 and 5 months of age in the German efficacy study). One month after the third dose of *Infanrix*, the response rates to each pertussis antigen were similar in all three studies. Thus, although a serologic correlate of protection for pertussis has not been established, the antibody responses to these three pertussis antigens (PT, FHA and pertactin) in a U.S. population were similar to those achieved in two populations in which efficacy of *Infanrix* was demonstrated.

Immune Response to Simultaneously Administered Vaccines

In a small clinical trial in the United States, *Infanrix* was given simultaneously, at separate sites, with hepatitis B vaccine, *Haemophilus influenzae* type b vaccine (Hib) and poliovirus vaccine live oral (OPV), at 2, 4 and 6 months of

Continued on next page

Information on the SmithKline Beecham Pharmaceuticals products appearing here is based on the labeling in effect on July 31, 1998. Further information on these and other products may be obtained from the Medical Department, SmithKline Beecham Pharmaceuticals, One Franklin Plaza, Philadelphia, PA 19101.

Infanrix—Cont.

age. One month after the third dose of hepatitis B vaccine given simultaneously with *Infanrix*, 100% of infants demonstrated anti-HBs antibodies ≥10 mIU/mL (N=64). Ninety percent of infants who received Hib simultaneously with *Infanrix* achieved anti-PRP antibodies ≥1 mcg/mL (N=72), and 96% to 100% of infants who received OPV simultaneously with *Infanrix* showed protective neutralizing antibody to poliovirus types 1, 2 and 3 (N=60–61).[16]

In the Italian efficacy trial, 92% of infants received hepatitis B vaccine with the first and second dose of *Infanrix*. Ninety-four percent of infants received OPV with the first and second dose of *Infanrix*.[13]

INDICATIONS AND USAGE

Infanrix is indicated for active immunization against diphtheria, tetanus and pertussis (whooping cough) in infants and children 6 weeks to 7 years of age (prior to seventh birthday). Because of the substantial risks of complications from pertussis disease, completion of a primary series of vaccine early in life is strongly recommended.[1]

Individuals 7 years of age or older should not receive this vaccine. In such individuals, Tetanus and Diphtheria Toxoids Adsorbed For Adult Use (Td) is preferable to use of either tetanus or diphtheria vaccines alone.

Children who have recovered from culture-confirmed pertussis need not receive further doses of a pertussis-containing vaccine, but should receive additional doses of Diphtheria and Tetanus Toxoids Adsorbed (DT) for pediatric use to complete the series in accordance with ACIP recommendations.[1]

In instances where the pertussis vaccine component is contraindicated, Diphtheria and Tetanus Toxoids Adsorbed (DT) for pediatric use may be substituted for each of the remaining doses[1] (see CONTRAINDICATIONS).

The decision to administer or delay vaccination because of a current or recent febrile illness depends on the severity of symptoms and on the etiology of the disease. All vaccines can be administered to persons with minor illness such as diarrhea, mild upper respiratory infections with or without low-grade fever or other low-grade febrile illness.[17,18]

Where passive protection is required, Tetanus Immune Globulin and/or Diphtheria Antitoxin may also be administered at separate sites.[1,17]

As with any vaccine, *Infanrix* may not protect 100% of individuals receiving the vaccine.

This product is not recommended for treatment of actual infections.

CONTRAINDICATIONS

Hypersensitivity to any component of the vaccine is a contraindication (see DESCRIPTION).

It is a contraindication to use this vaccine after an immediate anaphylactic reaction temporally associated with a previous dose. Because of the uncertainty as to which component of the vaccine might be responsible, no further vaccination with diphtheria, tetanus or pertussis should be given. Alternatively, because of the importance of tetanus vaccination, such individuals may be referred to an allergist for evaluation.[1]

Immunization should be deferred during the course of a moderate or severe febrile illness or acute infection (see PRECAUTIONS).[1,17,18]

Elective immunization should be deferred during an outbreak of poliomyelitis.[19]

Safety data on the use of Infanrix (Diphtheria and Tetanus Toxoids and Acellular Pertussis Vaccine Adsorbed) in children for whom whole-cell pertussis vaccine is contraindicated are not available. Until such data are available, it would be prudent to consider Advisory Committee on Immunization Practices (ACIP) and American Academy of Pediatrics (AAP) contraindications to whole-cell DTP vaccine as contraindications to *Infanrix*.[1,18,20]

The ACIP states that "if any of the following events occur in temporal relationship to the administration of DTP, further vaccination with DTP is contraindicated":

1. An immediate anaphylactic reaction.
2. Encephalopathy (not due to another identifiable cause). This is defined as an acute, severe central nervous system disorder occurring within 7 days following vaccination (with whole-cell DTP or acellular DTP), and generally consisting of major alterations in consciousness, unresponsiveness, generalized or focal seizures that persist more than a few hours, with failure to recover within 24 hours. Even though causation by DTP vaccine cannot be established, no subsequent doses of pertussis vaccine should be given.

WARNINGS

If any of the following events occur in temporal relation to receipt of whole-cell DTP or acellular DTP vaccine, the decision to give subsequent doses of vaccine containing the pertussis component should be carefully considered. There may be circumstances, such as high incidence of pertussis, in which the potential benefits outweigh possible risks, par-

ticularly since these events have not been proven to cause permanent sequelae.[1,18] The following events were previously considered contraindications and are now considered precautions by the ACIP:

- **Temperature of ≥40.5°C (105°F) within 48 hours not due to another identifiable cause**
- **Collapse or shock-like state (hypotonic-hyporesponsive episode) within 48 hours**
- **Persistent, inconsolable crying lasting ≥3 hours, occurring within 48 hours**
- **Convulsions with or without fever occurring within 3 days**

In the Italian efficacy trial, the incidence of temperature ≥104°F, crying for 3 hours or more and seizures within 48 hours of vaccination was less than that following administration of whole-cell DTP vaccine manufactured by Connaught Laboratories, Inc. No hypotonic-hyporesponsive episodes were reported after administration of *Infanrix* in this trial[13] (see ADVERSE EVENTS–Table 7).

A committee of the Institute of Medicine (IOM) has concluded that evidence is consistent with a causal relationship between whole-cell DTP vaccine and acute neurologic illness, and under special circumstances, between whole-cell DTP vaccine and chronic neurologic disease in the context of the National Childhood Encephalopathy Study (NCES) report.[21,22] However, the IOM committee concluded that the evidence was insufficient to indicate whether or not whole-cell DTP vaccine increased the overall risk of chronic neurologic disease.[22] While acute encephalopathy and permanent neurologic damage have not been reported in temporal association after administration of *Infanrix*, the data at this time are insufficient to rule this out.

The ACIP and the AAP recognize certain circumstances in which children with stable central nervous system disorders, such as well-controlled seizures or satisfactorily explained single seizures, may receive pertussis vaccine. The decision to administer a pertussis-containing vaccine to such children must be made by the physician on an individual basis, with consideration of all relevant factors, and assessment of potential risks and benefits for that individual. ACIP and AAP have issued guidelines for such children.[1,18,20] The parent or guardian should be advised of the potential increased risk involved (see Information for the Patient).

Studies suggest that, when given whole-cell DTP vaccine, infants and children with a history of convulsions in first-degree family members (i.e., siblings and parents) have a 2.4-fold increased risk for neurologic events compared with those without such histories.[23] However, the ACIP has concluded that a history of convulsions or other central nervous system disorders in parents or siblings is not a contraindication to pertussis vaccine and that children with such family histories should receive pertussis vaccine according to the recommended schedule.[1,17,18,24]

For children at higher risk for seizures than the general population, it may be prudent to extend the ACIP and AAP recommendations for whole-cell DTP vaccine to *Infanrix*: that acetaminophen be administered at age-appropriate doses at the time of DTP vaccination and every 4 to 6 hours for 24 hours.[1,18,20]

Infanrix should not be given to infants or children with any coagulation disorder, including thrombocytopenia, that would contraindicate intramuscular injection unless the potential benefit clearly outweighs the risk of administration.

PRECAUTIONS

Although a moderate or severe febrile illness is sufficient reason to postpone vaccination, minor illnesses such as mild upper respiratory infections with or without low-grade fever are not contraindications.[1,18]

Before the injection of any biological, the physician should take all reasonable precautions to prevent allergic or other adverse reactions, including understanding the use of the biological concerned, and the nature of the side effects and adverse reactions that may follow its use.

Prior to immunization, the patient's medical history should be reviewed. The physician should review the patient's immunization history for possible vaccine sensitivity, previous vaccination-related adverse reactions and occurrence of any adverse-event-related symptoms and/or signs, in order to determine the existence of any contraindication to immunization with *Infanrix* and to allow an assessment of benefits and risks. Epinephrine injection (1:1000) and other appropriate agents used for the control of immediate allergic reactions must be immediately available should an acute anaphylactic reaction occur.

A separate sterile syringe and needle or a sterile disposable unit should be used for each individual patient to prevent transmission of hepatitis or other infectious agents from one person to another. Needles should be disposed of properly and should not be recapped.

Special care should be taken to prevent injection into a blood vessel.

Infanrix (Diphtheria and Tetanus Toxoids and Acellular Pertussis Vaccine Adsorbed) is not contraindicated for use in individuals with HIV infection.[17,25]

As with any vaccine, if administered to immunosuppressed persons, including individuals receiving immunosuppressive therapy, the expected immune response may not be obtained.[25]

Information for the Patient

Parents or guardians should be informed of the potential benefits and risks of the vaccine, and of the importance of completing the immunization series. It is important when a child returns for the next dose in a series that the parent/guardian be questioned concerning occurrence of any symptoms and/or signs of an adverse reaction after a previous dose of the same vaccine. The physician should inform the parents or guardians about the potential for adverse reactions that have been temporally associated with administration of *Infanrix* or other pertussis-containing vaccines. The parents or guardians of infants and children with a family history of convulsions should be advised of the potential increased risk of seizures following DTP vaccination. In particular, they should be told, before the child is vaccinated, to seek immediate medical evaluation in the unlikely event of a seizure.[24] The adult accompanying the recipient should be told to report severe or unusual adverse reactions to the physician or clinic where the vaccine was administered.

The parent or guardian should be given the Vaccine Information Materials, which are required by the National Childhood Vaccine Injury Act of 1986 to be given prior to immunization.

The U.S. Department of Health and Human Services has established a Vaccine Adverse Event Reporting System (VAERS) to accept all reports of suspected adverse events after the administration of any vaccine, including but not limited to the reporting of events required by the National Childhood Vaccine Injury Act of 1986.[26] The VAERS toll-free number is 1-800-822-7967.

Drug Interactions

For information regarding simultaneous administration with other vaccines, refer to DOSAGE AND ADMINISTRATION and CLINICAL PHARMACOLOGY.

As with other intramuscular injections, *Infanrix* should not be given to infants or children on anticoagulant therapy unless the potential benefit clearly outweighs the risk of administration (see WARNINGS).

Immunosuppressive therapies, including irradiation, antimetabolites, alkylating agents, cytotoxic drugs and corticosteroids (used in greater than physiologic doses), may reduce the immune response to vaccines. Although no specific data from studies with pertussis vaccine under these conditions are available, if immunosuppressive therapy will be discontinued shortly, it would be reasonable to defer immunization until the patient has been off therapy for 1 month; otherwise, the patient should be vaccinated while still on therapy (see PRECAUTIONS).[1] If *Infanrix* is administered to a person receiving immunosuppressive therapy, or a recent injection of immune globulin, or who has an immunodeficiency disorder, an adequate immunologic response may not be obtained.

Tetanus Immune Globulin or Diphtheria Antitoxin, if used, should be given at a separate site, with a separate needle and syringe.

Carcinogenesis, Mutagenesis, Impairment of Fertility

Infanrix has not been evaluated for carcinogenic or mutagenic potential, or for impairment of fertility.

Pregnancy: Pregnancy Category C

Animal reproduction studies have not been conducted with *Infanrix*. It is not known whether *Infanrix* can cause fetal harm when administered to a pregnant woman or if *Infanrix* can affect reproductive capacity. *Infanrix* is not recommended for use in a pregnant woman. *Infanrix* is not recommended for persons 7 years of age or older (see WARNINGS).

Pediatric Use

Safety and effectiveness of *Infanrix* in infants below the age of 6 weeks have not been established (see DOSAGE AND ADMINISTRATION). *Infanrix* is not recommended for individuals 7 years of age or older (see WARNINGS). Tetanus and Diphtheria Adsorbed For Adult Use (Td) is to be used in individuals 7 years of age or older.

ADVERSE REACTIONS

A total of 92,502 doses of *Infanrix* has been administered in clinical studies. In these studies, 28,749 infants have received *Infanrix* as a three-dose primary series, 5,830 children have received *Infanrix* as a fourth dose following three doses of *Infanrix*, and 22 children have received *Infanrix* as a fifth dose following four doses of *Infanrix*. In addition, 439 children and 169 children have received *Infanrix* as a fourth or fifth dose following three or four doses of whole-cell DTP vaccine, respectively. In comparative studies, *Infanrix* has been shown to be followed by fewer of the local and systemic adverse reactions commonly associated with whole-cell DTP vaccination. However, studies have shown that the rate of erythema, swelling and fever increased with successive doses of *Infanrix*.

In the double-blind, randomized comparative trial in Italy, safety data in a three-dose primary series are available for 4,696 infants who received at least one dose of *Infanrix* and

4,678 infants who received at least one dose of U.S.-licensed whole-cell DTP vaccine manufactured by Connaught Laboratories, Inc.[13,15] Data were actively collected by parents using standardized diaries for eight consecutive evenings after each vaccine dose with follow-up telephone calls made by nurses after the eighth day. Table 1 lists adverse events reported during the three days after each dose. All common solicited adverse events were less frequent following vaccination with *Infanrix* as compared to whole-cell DTP after each one of the three doses.

[See table 1 above]

Table 1.[13] Adverse Events (%) Occurring Within the 3 Days Following Vaccination of Italian Infants with Either *Infanrix* or Whole-Cell DTP at 2, 4 and 6 Months of Age

	Infanrix			Whole-Cell DTP Vaccine		
	Dose 1	Dose 2	Dose 3	Dose 1	Dose 2	Dose 3
No. of infants	4,696	4,560	4,505	4,678	4,474	4,368
Local						
Redness	4.8	8.6	16.0	27.1	24.2	28.0
Redness ≥2.4 cm	1.0	1.3	3.5	12.4	7.3	7.7
Swelling	5.2	8.2	14.5	28.9	23.5	25.8
Swelling ≥2.4 cm	0.7	1.2	2.9	13.1	7.4	8.0
Tenderness	4.7	4.0	5.2	36.0	26.8	25.9
Systemic						
Fever ≥100.4°F*	7.1	7.9	9.0	46.8	36.1	39.8
Irritability	36.3	4.9	28.8	57.2	50.1	47.2
Drowsiness	34.9	18.8	11.4	54.0	34.1	23.0
Loss of Appetite	16.5	13.9	11.5	31.2	22.8	19.1
Vomiting	5.8†	4.1†	3.3	6.7	4.7	4.8
Crying ≥1 Hour	3.9	3.3	2.2	17.3	11.1	8.2

*Rectal temperatures.
†For the comparison of *Infanrix* and whole-cell DTP vaccine, all adverse events reached statistical significance ($p<0.001$) at all doses except vomiting at doses 1 and 2, which was not statistically significant at $p<0.05$.

A similar reduction in adverse events was seen in a randomized, double-blind, comparative trial conducted in the U.S. when Infanrix (Diphtheria and Tetanus Toxoids and Acellular Pertussis Vaccine Adsorbed) was compared to two U.S.-licensed whole-cell DTP vaccines. Adverse events were actively solicited using standardized diaries with follow-up telephone calls made at days 1, 4 and 8 by blinded study personnel. Table 2 summarizes the frequency of adverse events within 3 days of the three primary immunizing doses. The incidence of redness, swelling, pain, fever (rectal temperature >101°F), fussiness, drowsiness and poor appetite, were lower following *Infanrix* than following either whole-cell DTP vaccine.

[See table 2 at top of next page]

The frequencies of adverse reactions following each dose in children who received *Infanrix* at 2, 4 and 6 months of age in a U.S. NIH-sponsored trial are shown in Table 3. Of the 120 infants who received the three-dose primary series, a subset of 76 received a fourth dose of *Infanrix* at 15 to 20 months of age. Adverse events were actively solicited using standardized diaries with follow-up telephone calls made at day 3 by blinded study personnel.

[See table 3 on next page]

Of 22,505 children who had previously received three doses of *Infanrix* at 3, 4 and 5 months of age in the large German safety study, 5,361 received a fourth dose at 10 to 36 (mean 20) months of age. Standardized diaries were available on 2,457 children receiving the primary series and 1,809 children receiving the fourth dose. Local and systemic reaction rates within 3 days of vaccination for each dose are reported in Table 4. In this study, the rate of erythema, swelling, pain and fever increased with successive doses of *Infanrix*.

[See table 4 on next page]

In another study conducted in Germany, which was double-blinded and randomized, additional safety data are available from 13- to 27-month-old children who received Infanrix (Diphtheria and Tetanus Toxoids and Acellular Pertussis Vaccine Adsorbed) or whole-cell DTP vaccine, manufactured by Behringwerke, A.G., as a fourth dose. These children had previously received three doses of the same vaccine. The rates of adverse events, which were actively solicited using standardized diaries, are presented in Table 5. The incidence of redness, swelling, severe swelling (greater than 2 cm), pain, fever, severe fever (rectal temperature >103.1°F), restlessness, loss of appetite, vomiting, drowsiness and unusual crying was lower following vaccination with *Infanrix* compared to whole-cell DTP vaccine.

[See table 5 on page 3065]

Cases of edematous swelling, generally beginning within 48 hours of vaccination and resolving spontaneously over an average of 4 days without sequelae, have been reported with *Infanrix*.[15] In the German study in which 5,361 children received a fourth dose of *Infanrix* after three doses of the same vaccine, swelling of the injected thigh was reported spontaneously in 62 vaccinees (1.2%). This swelling was associated with pain upon digital pressure in 53% of cases, with rectal temperature ≥100.4°F in 45% of cases, and with injection site redness in 71% of cases (redness of the entire thigh was reported in 17% of such cases). The mean difference in the circumference of the thighs in those subjects in whom this was measured (N=17) was 2.2 cm (range: 0.5 to 5 cm). In 1,809 children for whom standardized diaries were available, edematous swelling was observed in 2.5% of vaccinees. In clinical studies of *Infanrix* to date, edematous swelling has been seen only with *Infanrix* as a fourth dose in *Infanrix*-primed individuals. In other countries where *Infanrix* has been licensed, limb swelling has been reported rarely following administration of *Infanrix* at any dose, including the primary series. Edematous swelling has also been reported following administration of other acellular DTP vaccines,[29] acellular pertussis vaccine alone (without DT),[30] whole-cell DTP vaccine[31] and other vaccines.[32]

Table 6 lists the frequency of adverse events in U.S. children who received *Infanrix* (N=110) or U.S.-licensed whole-cell DTP vaccine (N=55) manufactured by Lederle Laboratories at 15 to 20 months of age[33] and in U.S. children who received *Infanrix* (N=115) or U.S.-licensed whole-cell DTP vaccine (N=57) manufactured by Lederle Laboratories at 4 to 6 years of age.[34] All children had previously received three or four doses of whole-cell DTP vaccine at approximately 2, 4, 6 and 15–18 months of age. Adverse events were actively solicited using standardized diaries with follow-up telephone calls made at days 1, 4 and 8 by blinded study personnel. Significantly fewer solicited local and general adverse events were reported following *Infanrix* than following whole-cell DTP vaccine when administered as the fourth or fifth dose in those previously primed with three or four doses of whole-cell DTP vaccine.

[See table 6 on page 3065]

Severe adverse events reported from the double-blind, randomized comparative Italian study involving 4,696 children administered Infanrix (Diphtheria and Tetanus Toxoids and Acellular Pertussis Vaccine Adsorbed) or 4,678 children administered whole-cell DTP vaccine (manufactured by Connaught Laboratories, Inc.) as a three-dose primary series are shown in Table 7. The incidence of rectal temperature ≥104°F, hypotonic-hyporesponsive episodes and persistent crying ≥3 hours following administration of *Infanrix* was significantly less than that following administration of whole-cell DTP vaccine.[13] Hospitalization rates and death rates within 7 days of vaccination were similar between *Infanrix* and DT vaccine recipients.[15]

[See table 7 on page 3065]

In the large German safety trial that enrolled 22,505 infants (66,867 doses of *Infanrix* administered as a three-dose primary series), all subjects were monitored for unsolicited adverse events that occurred within 28 days following vaccination using report cards. In a subset of subjects (N=2,457), these cards were standardized diaries which solicited specific adverse events that occurred within 8 days of each vaccination in addition to unsolicited adverse events which occurred throughout the course of the entire trial (from study enrollment until approximately 30 days following the third vaccination). Cards from the whole cohort were returned at subsequent visits and were supplemented by spontaneous reporting by parents and a medical history after the first and second doses of vaccine. In the subset of 2,457, adverse events following the third dose of vaccine were reported via standardized diaries and spontaneous reporting at a follow-up visit. Adverse events in the remainder of the cohort were reported via report cards which were returned by mail approximately 28 days after the third dose of vaccine. Adverse events (rates per 1,000 doses) occurring within 7 days including those events deemed by investigators as related as well as those felt to be unrelated to vaccination included: unusual crying (0.09), febrile seizure (0.0), afebrile seizure (0.13) and hypotonic-hyporesponsive episodes (0.01).

Rates of serious adverse experiences that are less common than those reported in the German safety trial are not known at this time.

In clinical trials involving more than 29,000 infants and children, 14 deaths in Infanrix (Diphtheria and Tetanus Toxoids and Acellular Pertussis Vaccine Adsorbed) recipients were reported. Causes of deaths included nine cases of Sudden Infant Death Syndrome (SIDS) and one of each of the following: meal aspiration, hepatoblastoma, neuroblastoma, invasive bacterial infection and sudden death in a child greater than 1 year of age. None of these events was determined to be vaccine-related. The rate of SIDS observed in the large German safety study was 0.3/1000 vaccinated infants. The rate of SIDS in the Italian efficacy trial was 0.4/1000 *Infanrix*-vaccinated infants. The reported rate of SIDS in the U.S. from 1985 to 1991 was 1.5/1000 live births.[35] By chance alone, some cases of SIDS can be expected to follow receipt of whole-cell DTP or acellular DTP vaccine.[18]

Rarely, an anaphylactic reaction (i.e., hives, swelling of the mouth, difficulty breathing, hypotension, shock) has been reported after receiving preparations containing diphtheria, tetanus and/or pertussis antigens.[1,18] Arthus-type hypersensitivity reactions, characterized by severe local reactions, may follow receipt of tetanus toxoid. A few cases of peripheral mono-neuropathy have been reported following tetanus toxoid administration, although the IOM concluded that the evidence was inadequate to accept or reject a causal relationship.[36]

A review by the IOM found evidence for a causal relationship between receipt of tetanus toxoid and both brachial neuritis and Guillain-Barré Syndrome.[36]

Additional Adverse Reactions Evaluated in Conjunction with Whole-Cell DTP Vaccination

Whole-cell DTP vaccine has been associated with acute encephalopathy.[21] In the National Childhood Encephalopathy Study (NCES), a large, case-control study in England, children 2 to 35 months of age with serious, acute neurologic disorders, such as encephalopathy or complicated convulsion(s), were more likely to have received DTP vaccine in the 7 days preceding onset than their age-matched controls. Among children presumed to be neurologically normal before entering the study, the relative risk (estimated by odds ratio) of a neurologic illness occurring within the 7-day period following receipt of DTP dose, compared to children not receiving DTP vaccine in the 7-day period before onset of their illness, was 3.3 ($p<0.001$). The attributable risk for all neurologic events was estimated to be 1:140,000 doses of DTP vaccine administered. In this study, a causal relationship between receipt of DTP vaccine and permanent neurologic injury was suggested.[1,37–40]

A 10-year follow-up to the NCES demonstrated that children who experience a serious acute neurologic illness following whole-cell DTP vaccine are at increased risk for chronic nervous system dysfunction or death.[41] However, the IOM concluded that the results were insufficient to determine whether DTP vaccine increases the overall risk for chronic nervous system dysfunction in children.[18,22]

Subsequent studies have failed to provide evidence in support of a causal relationship between DTP vaccination and either serious acute neurologic illness or permanent neurologic injury.[42–45] The ACIP and AAP continue to recommend the use of DTP vaccine.

Among a subset of children who were participating in the NCES and who had infantile spasms, both DTP and DT vaccination appeared either to precipitate early manifestations of the condition or to lead to its identification by parents.[46] IOM reviewed this and other studies and concluded that neither vaccine causes the illness.[18,21,45,47] The incidence of onset of infantile spasms increases at 3 to 9 months of age, the time period in which the second and third doses of DTP vaccine are generally given. Therefore, some cases of infantile spasms can be expected to be temporally associated with receipt of whole-cell DTP or acellular DTP vaccine by chance alone.

SIDS has occurred in infants following administration of whole-cell DTP and acellular DTP vaccine. Large case-control studies of SIDS in the United States have shown that SIDS was not causally related to receipt of DTP vaccine.[48,49] It should be recognized that the first three primary immunizing doses of DTP vaccine are usually administered to infants 2 to 6 months old and that approximately 85% of SIDS cases occur between the ages of 1 and 6 months, with the peak incidence occurring at 6 weeks to 4 months of age. By

Continued on next page

Information on the SmithKline Beecham Pharmaceuticals products appearing here is based on the labeling in effect on July 31, 1998. Further information on these and other products may be obtained from the Medical Department, SmithKline Beecham Pharmaceuticals, One Franklin Plaza, Philadelphia, PA 19101.

Infanrix—Cont.

chance alone, some cases of SIDS can be expected to be temporally related to recent receipt of whole-cell DTP or acellular DTP vaccine. A review by the committee of the IOM concluded that available evidence did not indicate a causal relation between DTP vaccine and SIDS.[18,21]

A bulging fontanelle associated with increased intracranial pressure, which occurred within 24 hours following DTP immunization, has been reported, although a causal relationship has not been established.[50-52]

As with any vaccine, there is the possibility that broad use of Infanrix (Diphtheria and Tetanus Toxoids and Acellular Pertussis Vaccine Adsorbed) could reveal adverse reactions not observed in clinical trials.

Reporting Adverse Events

The National Childhood Vaccine Injury Act requires that the manufacturer and lot number of the vaccine administered be recorded by the healthcare provider in the vaccine recipient's permanent medical record, along with the date of administration of the vaccine and the name, address and title of the person administering the vaccine.[53] The Act further requires the healthcare provider to report to the U.S. Department of Health and Human Services via VAERS the occurrence following immunization of any event set forth in the Vaccine Injury Table including: anaphylaxis or anaphylactic shock within 4 hours, encephalopathy or encephalitis within 72 hours, or any sequelae thereof (including death).[53,54] In addition, any event considered a contraindication to further doses should be reported.

DOSAGE AND ADMINISTRATION

Preparation for Administration

Shake the vial well before withdrawal and use. The vaccine is ready to use without reconstitution. Parenteral drug products should be inspected visually for particulate matter or discoloration prior to administration, whenever solution and container permit. With thorough agitation, Infanrix is a homogeneous white turbid suspension. Discard if it appears otherwise. Since this product is a suspension containing an adjuvant, shake vigorously to obtain a uniform suspension prior to withdrawal from the vial. DO NOT USE IF RESUSPENSION DOES NOT OCCUR WITH VIGOROUS SHAKING. After removal of the 0.5 mL dose, any vaccine remaining in the vial should be discarded.

Infanrix should be administered by intramuscular injection. The preferred sites are the anterolateral aspects of the thigh or the deltoid muscle of the upper arm. The vaccine should not be injected in the gluteal area or areas where there may be a major nerve trunk. Before injection, the skin at the injection site should be cleaned and prepared with a suitable germicide. After insertion of the needle, aspirate to ensure that the needle has not entered a blood vessel.

Do not administer this product subcutaneously.

Primary Immunization

The primary immunization course for children less than 7 years of age is three doses of 0.5 mL, given intramuscularly, at 4- to 8-week intervals (preferably 8 weeks). The customary age for the first dose is 2 months of age, but it may be given starting at 6 weeks of age and up to the seventh birthday. It is recommended that Infanrix be given for all three doses since no interchangeability data on acellular DTP vaccines exist for the primary series. Infanrix may be used to complete the primary series in infants who have received one or two doses of whole-cell DTP vaccine. However, the safety and efficacy of Infanrix in such infants have not been evaluated.

Booster Immunization

When Infanrix is given for the primary series, a fourth dose is recommended at 15 to 20 months of age. The interval between the third and fourth dose should be at least 6 months. At this time, data are insufficient to establish the frequency of adverse events following a fifth dose of Infanrix in children who have previously received four doses of Infanrix.

If a child has received whole-cell DTP vaccine for one or more doses, Infanrix may be given to complete the five-dose series. A fourth dose is recommended at 15 to 20 months of age. The interval between the third and fourth dose should be at least 6 months. Children 4 to 6 years of age (up to the seventh birthday) who received all four doses by the fourth birthday, including one or more doses of whole-cell DTP vaccine, should receive a single dose of Infanrix before entering kindergarten or elementary school. This dose is not needed if the fourth dose was given on or after the fourth birthday.

Additional Dosing Information

If any recommended dose of pertussis vaccine cannot be given, DT (For Pediatric Use) should be given as needed to complete the series.

Interruption of the recommended schedule with a delay between doses should not interfere with the final immunity achieved with Infanrix. There is no need to start the series over again, regardless of the time elapsed between doses. The use of reduced volume (fractional doses) is not recommended. The effect of such practices on the frequency of serious adverse events and on protection against disease has not been determined.[17]

Preterm infants should be vaccinated according to their chronological age from birth.[17]

For persons 7 years of age or older, Tetanus and Diphtheria Toxoids (Td) for adult use should be given for routine booster immunization against tetanus and diphtheria.

Simultaneous Vaccine Administration

In clinical trials, Infanrix was routinely administered, at separate sites, concomitantly with one or more of the following vaccines: poliovirus vaccine live oral (OPV), hepatitis B vaccine, and Haemophilus influenzae type b vaccine (Hib) (see CLINICAL PHARMACOLOGY).

No data are available on the simultaneous administration of measles, mumps and rubella vaccine (MMR), varicella vaccine or inactivated polio virus (IPV) with Infanrix.

When concomitant administration of other vaccines is required, they should be given with different syringes and at different injection sites.

The ACIP encourages routine simultaneous administration of acellular DTP, OPV (or IPV), Hib, MMR and hepatitis B vaccine for children who are at the recommended age to receive these vaccines and for whom no specific contraindications exist at the time of the visit, unless, in the judgment of

Table 2.[27] Adverse Events (%) Occurring Within the 3 Days Following Vaccination of U.S. Infants with Either Infanrix or Whole-Cell DTP at 2, 4 and 6 Months of Age

	Infanrix			Whole-Cell DTP Vaccine-Lederle			Whole-Cell DTP Vaccine-Connaught		
	Dose 1	Dose 2	Dose 3	Dose 1	Dose 2	Dose 3	Dose 1	Dose 2	Dose 3
No. of infants	407	402	395	74	73	73	76	75	74
Local									
Redness*	10.6	19.4	25.8	28.4	42.5	39.7	35.5	50.7	50.0
Swelling	7.4†¶	12.2†¶	17.5¶	23.0†	26.0†	27.4	30.3¶	37.3¶	31.1¶
Pain*‡	2.7	2.0	1.5	17.6	15.1	9.6	38.2	17.3	14.9
Systemic									
Fever									
>101°F§	0.5†¶	0.7†¶	5.1	12.2†	8.2†	6.8	14.5¶	18.7¶	8.1
Fussiness**	3.9†¶	3.5†¶	4.1	25.7†	13.7†	6.8	21.1¶	16.0¶	8.1
Drowsiness	26.3†¶	16.4†¶	12.9†	51.4†	34.2†	23.3†	52.6¶	28.0¶	18.9
Poor Appetite	8.1†¶	7.7	6.6	31.1†	15.1	9.6	19.7¶	14.7	9.5
Vomiting	6.6	3.7	3.8	8.1	4.1	2.7	7.9	2.7	2.7

‡ Moderate or severe = cried or protested to touch or cried when leg moved.
** Moderate or severe = prolonged crying and refusal to play or persistent crying that could not be comforted.
§ Rectal temperatures.
* p<0.05 for the comparison of Infanrix and both whole-cell DTP vaccines.
† p<0.05 for the comparison of Infanrix and whole-cell DTP vaccine-Lederle.
¶ p<0.05 for the comparison of Infanrix and whole-cell DTP vaccine-Connaught.

Table 3.[15,28] Adverse Events (%) Occurring Within the 3 Days Following Vaccination with Infanrix in U.S. Infants and Children in Which All Doses Were Infanrix

Event	Primary (N = 120 infants)			Booster (N = 76 children)
	Dose 1 (2 months)	Dose 2 (4 months)	Dose 3 (6 months)	Dose 4 (15 to 20 months)
Local				
Redness	16.6	15.4	26.3	39.5
Swelling	12.5	15.4	21.0	32.9
Pain*	5.0	5.1	0.9	10.5
Systemic				
Fever (>101°F)†	0.0	0.9	3.5	6.6
Anorexia	7.5	6.0	9.6	11.8
Vomiting	5.8	6.8	3.5	2.6
Drowsiness	37.5	19.7	13.2	6.6
Fussiness‡	3.3	7.7	8.8	9.2

* Moderate or severe = cried or protested to touch or cried when limb moved.
† Rectal temperatures for primary series; oral temperatures for booster.
‡ Moderate or severe = prolonged crying and refusal to play or persistent crying that could not be comforted.

Table 4.[15] Adverse Events (%) Occurring Within the 3 Days Following Vaccination with Infanrix in German Infants and Children in Which All Doses Were Infanrix

Event	Primary (N=2,457 infants)			Booster (N=1,809 children)*
	Dose 1 (3 months)	Dose 2 (4 months)	Dose 3 (5 months)	Dose 4 (10 to 36 months†)
Local				
Redness	8.9	23.6	26.6	45.9
Redness >2 cm	0.0	0.5	1.3	13.8
Swelling	3.9	14.1	18.5	35.4
Swelling >2 cm	0.0	0.3	1.3	11.4
Pain	2.0	2.6	3.7	26.3
Systemic				
Fever (≥100.4°F)‡	6.3	8.3	13.3	26.4
Fever (>103.1°F)‡	0.0	0.1	0.1	1.1
Loss of Appetite	8.0	7.4	6.5	11.6
Vomiting	4.3	3.9	3.4	2.9
Restlessness	10.3	9.5	8.6	15.9
Unusual Crying	3.9	4.3	4.1	6.4
Diarrhea	6.0	4.9	4.0	11.0

* May not be same children as in primary series.
† Mean = 20 months.
‡ Rectal temperatures.

the provider, complete vaccination of the child will not be compromised by administering vaccines at different visits. Simultaneous administration is particularly important if the child might not return for subsequent vaccinations.[17]

STORAGE

Store *Infanrix* between 2° and 8°C (36° and 46°F). **Do not freeze.** Discard if the vaccine has been frozen. Do not use after expiration date shown on the label.

HOW SUPPLIED

Infanrix (Diphtheria and Tetanus Toxoids and Acellular Pertussis Vaccine Adsorbed) is supplied as a turbid white suspension in vials containing a 0.5 mL single dose, in packages of 10 vials.
NDC 58160-840-11 (package of 10)

References

1. Centers for Disease Control. Diphtheria, tetanus and pertussis: Recommendations for vaccine use and other preventive measures. Recommendations of the Immunization Practices Advisory Committee (ACIP). *MMWR.* 1991;Vol. 40 (No. RR-10):1–28.
2. Centers for Disease Control and Prevention. Summary of Notifiable Diseases, United States, 1993. *MMWR.* 1994;Vol. 42 (No. 53):1–28.
3. Centers for Disease Control and Prevention. Diphtheria Epidemic-New independent states of the former Soviet Union, 1990-1994. *MMWR.* 1995;44 (No.10):177–181.
4. Biological products; bacterial vaccines and toxoids; implementation of efficacy review. *Federal Register.* Friday, December 13, 1985; Vol. 50 (No. 240):51002–51117.
5. Centers for Disease Control. Tetanus—United States, 1987 and 1988. *MMWR.* 1990;Vol. 39 (No. 3):37–44.
6. Kendrick PL. Secondary familial attack rates from pertussis in vaccinated and unvaccinated children. *Am J Hygiene.* 1940;32:89–91.
7. Centers for Disease Control. Pertussis—United States, January 1994-June 1995. *MMWR.* 1995; Vol. 44 (No. 28):525–529.
8. Farizo KM, et al. Epidemiologic features of pertussis in the United States, 1980-1989. *Clin Infect Dis.* 1992;14: 708–719.
9. Nennig ME, et al. Prevalence and incidence of adult pertussis in an urban population. *JAMA.* 1996; Vol. 275 (No. 21):1672–1674.
10. Cowell JL, et al. Prospective protective antigens and animal models for pertussis. In: Leive L and Schlessinger D, eds. *Microbiology-1984.* Washington, DC: American Society for Microbiology, 1984, pp. 172–175.
11. Shahin RD, et al. Characterization of the protective capacity and immunogenicity of the 69-kD outer membrane protein of *Bordetella pertussis. J Exper Med.* 1990;171(1):63–73.
12. Gustafsson L, et al. A controlled trial of a two-component acellular, a five-component acellular, and a whole-cell pertussis vaccine. *N Engl J Med.* 1996;334(6):349–355.
13. Greco D, et al. A controlled trial of two acellular vaccines and one whole-cell vaccine against pertussis. *N Engl J Med.* 1996;334(6):341–348.
14. Schmitt H-J, et al. Efficacy of acellular pertussis vaccine in early childhood after household exposure. *JAMA.* 1996;275(1):37–41.
15. Data on file, SmithKline Beecham Pharmaceuticals, Philadelphia, PA.
16. Blatter M, et al. Immunogenicity of diphtheria-tetanus-acellular pertussis (DT-tricomponent Pa), hepatitis B (HB) and *Haemophilus influenzae* type b (Hib) vaccines administered concomitantly at separate sites along with oral poliovirus vaccine (OPV) in infants. Abstract G102, Interscience Conference on Antimicrobial Agents and Chemotherapy, 1996.
17. Centers for Disease Control and Prevention. General recommendations on immunization. Recommendations of the Advisory Committee on Immunization Practices (ACIP). *MMWR.* 1994; Vol. 43 (No. RR-1):1–38.
18. Centers for Disease Control and Prevention. Update: Vaccine side effects, adverse reactions, contraindications, and precautions—recommendations of the Advisory Committee on Immunization Practices (ACIP). *MMWR.* 1996;Vol. 45 (No. RR-12):1–35.
19. Wilson GS. The hazards of immunization. Provocation poliomyelitis. 1967, pp. 270–274.
20. American Academy of Pediatrics. Pertussis. *Report of the Committee on Infectious Diseases.* 23rd ed. Elk Grove Village, IL: American Academy of Pediatrics, 1994.
21. Howson CP, et al. Adverse effects of pertussis and rubella vaccines. Institute of Medicine (IOM). Washington, DC: National Academy Press, 1991.
22. Stratton KR, et al. DPT vaccine and chronic nervous system dysfunction: a new analysis. Institute of Medicine (IOM). Washington, DC: National Academy Press, 1994 (Supplement).
23. Livengood JR, et al. Family history of convulsions and use of pertussis vaccine. *J Pediatr.* 1989;115(4):527–531.
24. Centers for Disease Control. Pertussis immunization: family history of convulsions and use of antipyretics-supplementary ACIP statement. Recommendations of the Immunization Practices Advisory Committee (ACIP). *MMWR.* 1987;Vol. 36 (No. 18):281–282.
25. Centers for Disease Control and Prevention. Use of vaccines and immune globulins for persons with altered immunocompetence. Recommendations of the Advisory Committee on Immunization Practices (ACIP). *MMWR.* 1993;Vol. 42 (No. RR-4):1–3.
26. Centers for Disease Control. Vaccine Adverse Event Reporting System-United States. *MMWR.* 1990;Vol. 39 (No. 41):730–733.

Table 5.[15] Adverse Events (%) Occurring Within the 3 Days Following Vaccination with *Infanrix* or Whole-Cell DTP (Fourth Dose) in German Children Who Had Received Three Previous Doses of the Same Vaccine

Event	*Infanrix* After *Infanrix* Primary (N=268)	Whole-Cell DTP Vaccine After Whole-Cell DTP Vaccine Primary (N=92)
Local		
Redness	32.8	43.5
Redness >2 cm	4.5	3.3
Swelling	22.4	31.5
Swelling >2 cm	3.0	7.6
Pain*	15.7	55.4
Systemic		
Fever (≥100.4°F)*†	26.9	64.1
Fever (>103.1°F)†‡	0.4	4.3
Restlessness*	12.3	32.6
Loss of Appetite*	10.8	43.5
Vomiting	3.4	7.6
Drowsiness*	10.4	31.5
Unusual Crying*	7.8	33.7

* $p<0.0001$.
† Rectal temperatures.
‡ $p<0.05$.

Table 6.[33,34] Adverse Events (%) Occurring Within the 3 Days Following Vaccination with *Infanrix* Administered at 15 to 20 Months and 4 to 6 Years of Age in U.S. Children Who Had Previously Received Three or Four Doses of Whole-Cell DTP Vaccine

Event	15 to 20 months Three Previous Doses of Whole-Cell DTP Vaccine		4 to 6 years Four Previous Doses of Whole-Cell DTP Vaccine	
	Infanrix (N=110)	Whole-Cell DTP Vaccine (N=55)	*Infanrix* (N=115)	Whole-Cell DTP Vaccine (N=57)
Local				
Redness*	23	45	19	40
Redness† >10 mm	5	31	7	26
Swelling	14	24	15*	33*
Swelling >10 mm	7	15	8	18
Pain†§	5	38	12	40
Systemic				
Fever* ≥99.4°F‡	25	42	23	47
Fever† >100.5°F‡	2	20	1	12
Fussiness	34†	69†	20	30
Drowsiness	9*	24*	11	18
Poor Appetite*	9	20	6	16
Vomiting	2	0	1	4

* $p<0.05$.
† $p<0.0001$.
‡ Oral temperatures.
§ Moderate or severe = cried or protested to touch or cried when arm moved.

Table 7.[13] Severe Adverse Events Occurring Within 48 Hours Following Vaccination with *Infanrix* or Whole-Cell DTP in Italian Infants at 2, 4 or 6 Months of Age

Event	*Infanrix* (N=13,761 doses)		Whole-Cell DTP Vaccine (N=13,520 Doses)	
	Number	Rate/ 1,000 Doses	Number	Rate/ 1,000 Doses
Fever ≥104°F*†	5	0.36	32	2.4
Hypotonic-Hyporesponsive Episode‡	0	0	9	0.67
Persistent crying ≥3 hours*	6	0.44	54	4.0
Seizures**	1§	0.07	3¶	0.22

* $p<0.001$.
† Rectal temperatures.
‡ $p = 0.002$.
§ Maximum rectal temperature within 72 hours of vaccination = 103.1°F.
¶ Maximum rectal temperature within 72 hours of vaccination = 99.5°F, 101.3°F and 102.2°F.
** Not statistically significant at $p<0.05$.

Continued on next page

Information on the SmithKline Beecham Pharmaceuticals products appearing here is based on the labeling in effect on July 31, 1998. Further information on these and other products may be obtained from the Medical Department, SmithKline Beecham Pharmaceuticals, One Franklin Plaza, Philadelphia, PA 19101.

Infarix—Cont.

27. Bernstein HH, et al. Reactogenicity and immunogenicity of a three-component acellular pertussis vaccine administered as the primary series to 2, 4 and 6 month-old infants in the United States. *Vaccine.* 1995;Vol. 13(17): 1631–1635.

28. Decker MD, et al. Comparison of 13 acellular pertussis vaccines: adverse reactions. *Pediatrics.* 1995;96:557–566.

29. Noble GR, et al. Acellular and whole-cell pertussis vaccines in Japan. Report of a visit by US scientists. *JAMA.* 1987;257(10):1351–1356.

30. Blennow M, et al. Adverse reactions and serologic response to a booster dose of acellular pertussis vaccine in children immunized with acellular or whole-cell vaccine as infants. *Pediatrics.* 1989;84(1):62–67.

31. Pim C, et al. Local reactions to kindergarten DPT boosters—Cranbrook. *Dis Surveill.* 1988; 9:230–239.

32. Gold R, et al. Safety and immunogenicity of *Haemophilus influenzae* vaccine (tetanus toxoid conjugate) administered concurrently or combined with diphtheria and tetanus toxoids, pertussis vaccine and inactivated poliomyelitis vaccine to healthy infants at two, four and six months of age. *Pediatr Infect Dis J.* 1994;13:348–355.

33. Bernstein HH, et al. Comparison of a three-component acellular pertussis vaccine with a whole-cell pertussis vaccine in 15- through 20-month-old infants. *Pediatrics.* 1994;93(4):656–659.

34. Annunziato PW, et al. Comparison of a three-component acellular pertussis vaccine with a whole-cell pertussis vaccine in 4- through 6-year-old children. *Arch Pediatr Adolesc Med.* 1994;148:503–507.

35. Willinger M, et al. Infant sleep position and risk for Sudden Infant Death Syndrome: Report of meeting held January 13 and 14, 1994, National Institutes of Health, Bethesda, MD. *Pediatrics.* 1994;93:814–819.

36. Stratton KR, et al. Adverse events associated with childhood vaccines. Evidence bearing on causality. Institute of Medicine (IOM). Washington, DC: National Academy Press, 1994.

37. Miller D, et al. Pertussis vaccine and whooping cough as risk factors for acute neurological illness and death in young children. *Dev Biol Stand.* 1985;61:389–394.

38. Miller DL, et al. Pertussis immunization and serious acute neurological illness in children. *Br Med J.* 1981;282:1595–1599.

39. Ross E, et al. Risk and pertussis vaccine (letter). *Arch Dis Child.* 1986;61:98–99.

40. Miller D, et al. Severe neurological illness: further analyses of the British National Childhood Encephalopathy Study. *Tokai J Exp Clin Med.* 1988;13(suppl):145–155.

41. Miller DL, et al. Pertussis immunization and serious acute neurological illnesses in children. *Br Med J.* 1993;307:1171–1176.

42. Pollock TM, et al. A 7-year survey of disorders attributed to vaccination in North West Thames region. *Lancet.* 1983;1:753–757.

43. Walker AM, et al. Neurologic events following diphtheria-tetanus-pertussis immunization. *Pediatrics.* 1988;81(3):345–349.

44. Griffin MR, et al. Risk of seizures and encephalopathy after immunization with the diphtheria-tetanus-pertussis vaccine. *JAMA.* 1990;263(12):1641–1645.

45. Shields WD, et al. Relationship of pertussis immunization to the onset of neurologic disorders: a retrospective epidemiologic study. *J Pediatr.* 1988;113:801–805.

46. Bellman MH, et al. Infantile spasms and pertussis immunization. *Lancet.* 1983;(1):1031–1034.

47. Melchior JC. Infantile spasms and early immunization against whooping cough: Danish survey from 1970 to 1975. *Arch Dis Child.* 1977;52:134–137.

48. Griffin MR, et al. Risk of Sudden Infant Death Syndrome after immunization with the diphtheria-tetanus-pertussis vaccine. *N Engl J Med.* 1988; Vol. 319 (10): 618–623.

49. Hoffman HJ, et al. Diphtheria-tetanus-pertussis immunization and sudden infant death: Results of the National Institute of Child Health and Human Development Cooperative Epidemiological Study of Sudden Infant Death Syndrome Risk Factors. *Pediatrics.* 1987; 79(4):598–611.

50. Jacob J, et al. Increased intracranial pressure after diphtheria, tetanus and pertussis immunization. *Am J Dis Child.* 1979;133(2):217–218.

51. Mathur R, et al. Bulging fontanel following triple vaccine. *Indian Pediatr.* 1981;18(6):417–418.

52. Shendurnikar N, et al. Bulging fontanel following DPT vaccine. *Indian Pediatr.* 1986; 23(11):960.

53. Centers for Disease Control. National Childhood Vaccine Injury Act: Requirements for permanent vaccination records and for reporting of selected events after vaccination. *MMWR.* 1988;Vol. 37 (No. 13):197–200.

54. National Vaccine Injury Compensation Program: Revision of the vaccine injury table. *Federal Register.* Wednesday, February 8, 1995; Vol. 60 (No. 26):7694.

Manufactured by **SmithKline Beecham Biologicals**
Rixensart, Belgium, U.S. License 1090, and
Chiron Behring GmbH & Co
Marburg, Germany, U.S. License 0097
Distributed by **SmithKline Beecham Pharmaceuticals**
Philadelphia, PA 19101
DATE OF ISSUANCE JAN. 1997
©SmithKline Beecham, 1997
Infarix is a trademark of SmithKline Beecham.
IN:L2

Shown in Product Identification Guide, page 339

KYTRIL® ℞
[kī '-tril]
granisetron
hydrochloride
Injection

DESCRIPTION

Kytril (granisetron hydrochloride) Injection is an antinauseant and antiemetic agent. Chemically it is *endo*-N-(9-methyl-9-azabicyclo [3.3.1] non-3-yl)-1-methyl-1H-indazole-3-carboxamide hydrochloride with a molecular weight of 348.9 (312.4 free base). Its empirical formula is $C_{18}H_{24}N_4O\cdot HCl$ while its chemical structure is:

granisetron hydrochloride

Granisetron hydrochloride is a white to off-white solid that is readily soluble in water and normal saline at 20°C. *Kytril* Injection is a clear, colorless, sterile, nonpyrogenic, aqueous solution for intravenous administration.

Kytril is available in 1 mL single-dose and 4 mL multi-dose vials.

Single-Dose Vials: Each 1 mL of preservative-free aqueous solution contains 1.12 mg granisetron hydrochloride equivalent to granisetron, 1.0 mg and sodium chloride, 9.0 mg. The solution's pH ranges from 4.7 to 7.3.

Multi-Dose Vials: Each 1 mL contains 1.12 mg granisetron hydrochloride equivalent to granisetron, 1.0 mg; sodium chloride, 9 mg; citric acid, 2 mg; benzyl alcohol, 10 mg, as a preservative. The solution's pH ranges from 4.0 to 6.0.

CLINICAL PHARMACOLOGY

Granisetron is a selective 5-hydroxytryptamine₃ (5-HT₃) receptor antagonist with little or no affinity for other serotonin receptors, including 5-HT₁; 5-HT₁ₐ; 5-HT₁ᵦ/c; 5-HT₂; for alpha₁-, alpha₂- or beta-adrenoreceptors; for dopamine-D₂; or for histamine-H₁; benzodiazepine; picrotoxin, or opioid receptors.

Serotonin receptors of the 5-HT₃ type are located peripherally on vagal nerve terminals and centrally in the chemoreceptor trigger zone of the area postrema. During chemotherapy-induced vomiting, mucosal enterochromaffin cells release serotonin, which stimulates 5-HT₃ receptors. This evokes vagal afferent discharge, inducing vomiting. Animal studies demonstrate that, in binding to 5-HT₃ receptors, granisetron blocks serotonin stimulation and subsequent vomiting after emetogenic stimuli such as cisplatin. In the ferret animal model, a single granisetron injection prevented vomiting due to high-dose cisplatin or arrested vomiting within 5 to 30 seconds.

In most human studies, granisetron has had little effect on blood pressure, heart rate or ECG. No evidence of an effect on plasma prolactin or aldosterone concentrations has been found in other studies.

Kytril Injection exhibited no effect on oro-cecal transit time in normal volunteers given a single intravenous infusion of 50 mcg/kg or 200 mcg/kg. Single and multiple oral doses slowed colonic transit in normal volunteers.

Pharmacokinetics
In adult cancer patients undergoing chemotherapy and in volunteers, infusion of a single 40 mcg/kg dose of *Kytril* Injection produced the following mean pharmacokinetic data: [See table 1 below]

There was high inter and intrasubject variability noted in these studies. No difference in mean AUC was found between males and females, although males had a higher C_{max} generally.

Granisetron metabolism involves N-demethylation and aromatic ring oxidation followed by conjugation. Animal studies suggest that some of the metabolites may also have 5-HT₃ receptor antagonist activity.

Clearance is predominantly by hepatic metabolism. In normal volunteers, approximately 12% of the administered dose is eliminated unchanged in the urine in 48 hours. The remainder of the dose is excreted as metabolites, 49% in the urine and 34% in the feces.

In vitro liver microsomal studies show that granisetron's major route of metabolism is inhibited by ketoconazole, suggestive of metabolism mediated by the cytochrome P-450 3A subfamily.

Plasma protein binding is approximately 65% and granisetron distributes freely between plasma and red blood cells.

Elderly: The ranges of the pharmacokinetic parameters in elderly volunteers (mean age 71 years), given a single 40 mcg/kg intravenous dose of *Kytril* Injection, were generally similar to those in younger healthy volunteers; mean values were lower for clearance and longer for half-life in the elderly (see Table 1).

Pediatric Patients: A pharmacokinetic study in pediatric cancer patients (2 to 16 years of age), given a single 40 mcg/kg intravenous dose of *Kytril* Injection, showed that volume of distribution and total clearance increased with age. No relationship with age was observed for peak plasma concentration or terminal phase plasma half-life. When volume of distribution and total clearance are adjusted for body weight, the pharmacokinetics of granisetron are similar in pediatric and adult cancer patients.

Renal Failure Patients: Total clearance of granisetron was not affected in patients with severe renal failure who received a single 40 mcg/kg intravenous dose of *Kytril* Injection.

Hepatically Impaired Patients: A pharmacokinetic study in patients with hepatic impairment due to neoplastic liver involvement showed that total clearance was approximately halved compared to patients without hepatic impairment. Given the wide variability in pharmacokinetic parameters noted in patients and the good tolerance of doses well above the recommended 10 mcg/kg dose, dosage adjustment in patients with possible hepatic functional impairment is not necessary.

CLINICAL TRIALS

Kytril Injection has been shown to prevent nausea and vomiting associated with single-day and repeat cycle cancer chemotherapy.

Single-Day Chemotherapy

Cisplatin-Based Chemotherapy: In a double-blind, placebo-controlled study in 28 cancer patients, *Kytril* Injection, administered as a single intravenous infusion of 40 mcg/kg, was significantly more effective than placebo in preventing nausea and vomiting induced by cisplatin chemotherapy. See Table 2.

Table 1. Pharmacokinetic Parameters in Adult Cancer Patients Undergoing Chemotherapy and in Volunteers, Following a Single Intravenous 40 mcg/kg Dose of Kytril (granisetron hydrochloride) Injection

	Peak Plasma Concentration (ng/mL)	Terminal Phase Plasma Half-Life (h)	Total Clearance (L/h/kg)	Volume of Distribution (L/kg)
Cancer Patients				
Mean	63.8*	8.95*	0.38*	3.07*
Range	18.0 to 176	0.90 to 31.1	0.14 to 1.54	0.85 to 10.4
Volunteers				
21 to 42 years				
Mean	64.3†	4.91†	0.79†	3.04†
Range	11.2 to 182	0.88 to 15.2	0.20 to 2.56	1.68 to 6.13
65 to 81 years				
Mean	57.0†	7.69†	0.44†	3.97†
Range	14.6 to 153	2.65 to 17.7	0.17 to 1.06	1.75 to 7.01

* 5-minute infusion.
† 3-minute infusion.

Table 2. Prevention of Chemotherapy-Induced Nausea and Vomiting—Single-Day Cisplatin Therapy [1]

	Kytril Injection	Placebo	P-Value
Number of Patients	14	14	
Response Over 24 Hours			
Complete Response[2]	93%	7%	<0.001
No Vomiting	93%	14%	<0.001
No More Than Mild Nausea	93%	7%	<0.001

1. Cisplatin administration began within 10 minutes of Kytril Injection infusion and continued for 1.5 to 3.0 hours. Mean cisplatin dose was 86 mg/m^2 in the Kytril Injection group and 80 mg/m^2 in the placebo group.
2. No vomiting and no moderate or severe nausea.

Kytril Injection was also evaluated in a randomized dose response study of cancer patients receiving cisplatin ≥75 mg/m^2. Additional chemotherapeutic agents included: anthracyclines, carboplatin, cytostatic antibiotics, folic acid derivatives, methylhydrazine, nitrogen mustard analogs, podophyllotoxin derivatives, pyrimidine analogs and vinca alkaloids. Kytril Injection doses of 10 and 40 mcg/kg were superior to 2 mcg/kg in preventing cisplatin-induced nausea and vomiting, but 40 mcg/kg was not significantly superior to 10 mcg/kg. See Table 3.
[See table 3 above]

Kytril (granisetron hydrochloride) Injection was also evaluated in a double-blind, randomized dose response study of 353 patients stratified for high (≥80 to 120 mg/m^2) or low (50 to 79 mg/m^2) cisplatin dose. Response rates of patients for both cisplatin strata are given in Table 4.
[See table 4 above]
For both the low and high cisplatin strata, the 10, 20 and 40 mcg/kg doses were more effective than the 5 mcg/kg dose in preventing nausea and vomiting within 24 hours of chemotherapy administration. The 10 mcg/kg dose was at least as effective as the higher doses.

Moderately Emetogenic Chemotherapy: Kytril Injection, 40 mcg/kg, was compared with the combination of chlorpromazine (50 to 200 mg/24 hours) and dexamethasone (12 mg) in patients treated with moderately emetogenic chemotherapy, including primarily carboplatin >300 mg/m^2, cisplatin 20 to 50 mg/m^2 and cyclophosphamide >600 mg/m^2. Kytril Injection was superior to the chlorpromazine regimen in preventing nausea and vomiting. See Table 5.

Table 5. Prevention of Chemotherapy-Induced Nausea and Vomiting—Single-Day Moderately Emetogenic Chemotherapy

	Kytril Injection	Chlorpromazine [1]	P-Value
Number of Patients	133	133	
Response Over 24 Hours			
Complete Response[2]	68%	47%	<0.001
No Vomiting	73%	53%	<0.001
No More Than Mild Nausea	77%	59%	<0.001

1. Patients also received dexamethasone, 12 mg.
2. No vomiting and no moderate or severe nausea.

In other studies of moderately emetogenic chemotherapy, no significant difference in efficacy was found between Kytril doses of 40 mcg/kg and 160 mcg/kg doses.

Repeat-Cycle Chemotherapy
In an uncontrolled trial, 512 cancer patients received Kytril Injection, 40 mcg/kg, prophylactically, for two cycles of chemotherapy, 224 patients received it for at least four cycles and 108 patients received it for at least six cycles. Kytril Injection efficacy remained relatively constant over the first six repeat cycles, with complete response rates (no vomiting and no moderate or severe nausea in 24 hours) of 60% to 69%. No patients were studied for more than 15 cycles.

Pediatric Studies
A randomized double-blind study evaluated the 24-hour response of 80 pediatric cancer patients (age 2 to 16 years) to Kytril Injection 10, 20 or 40 mcg/kg. Patients were treated with cisplatin ≥60 mg/m^2, cytarabine ≥3 g/m^2, cyclophosphamide ≥1 g/m^2 or nitrogen mustard ≥6 mg/m^2. See Table 6.

Table 3. Prevention of Chemotherapy-Induced Nausea and Vomiting—Single-Day High-Dose Cisplatin Therapy [1]

	Kytril Injection (mcg/kg)			P-Value (vs. 2 mcg/kg)	
	2	10	40	10	40
Number of Patients	52	52	53		
Response Over 24 Hours					
Complete Response[2]	31%	62%	68%	<0.002	<0.001
No Vomiting	38%	65%	74%	<0.001	<0.001
No More Than Mild Nausea	58%	75%	79%	NS	0.007

1. Cisplatin administration began within 10 minutes of Kytril Injection infusion and continued for 2.6 hours (mean). Mean cisplatin doses were 96 to 99 mg/m^2.
2. No vomiting and no moderate or severe nausea.

Table 4. Prevention of Chemotherapy-Induced Nausea and Vomiting—Single-Day High-Dose and Low-Dose Cisplatin Therapy[1]

	Kytril Injection (mcg/kg)				P-Value (vs. 5 mcg/kg)		
	5	10	20	40	10	20	40
High-Dose Cisplatin							
Number of Patients	40	49	48	47			
Response Over 24 Hours							
Complete Response[2]	18%	41%	40%	47%	0.018	0.025	0.004
No Vomiting	28%	47%	44%	53%	NS	NS	0.016
No Nausea	15%	35%	38%	43%	0.036	0.019	0.005
Low-Dose Cisplatin							
Number of Patients	42	41	40	46			
Response Over 24 Hours							
Complete Response[2]	29%	56%	58%	41%	0.012	0.009	NS
No Vomiting	36%	63%	65%	43%	0.012	0.008	NS
No Nausea	29%	56%	38%	33%	0.012	NS	NS

1. Cisplatin administration began within 10 minutes of Kytril Injection infusion and continued for 2 hours (mean). Mean cisplatin doses were 64 and 98 mg/m^2 for low and high strata.
2. No vomiting and no use of rescue antiemetic.

Table 6. Prevention of Chemotherapy-Induced Nausea and Vomiting in Pediatric Patients

	Kytril Injection Dose (mcg/kg)		
	10	20	40
Number of Patients	29	26	25
Median Number of Vomiting Episodes	2	3	1
Complete Response Over 24 Hours[1]	21%	31%	32%

1. No vomiting and no moderate or severe nausea.

A second pediatric study compared Kytril Injection 20 mcg/kg to chlorpromazine plus dexamethasone in 88 patients treated with ifosfamide ≥3 g/m^2/day for two or three days. Kytril Injection was administered on each day of ifosfamide treatment. At 24 hours, 22% of Kytril Injection patients achieved complete response (no vomiting and no moderate or severe nausea in 24 hours) compared with 10% on the chlorpromazine regimen. The median number of vomiting episodes with Kytril Injection was 1.5; with chlorpromazine it was 7.0.

INDICATIONS AND USAGE
Kytril (granisetron hydrochloride) Injection is indicated for the prevention of nausea and vomiting associated with initial and repeat courses of emetogenic cancer therapy, including high-dose cisplatin.

CONTRAINDICATIONS
Kytril Injection is contraindicated in patients with known hypersensitivity to the drug or to any of its components.

PRECAUTIONS
Drug Interactions
Granisetron does not induce or inhibit the cytochrome P-450 drug-metabolizing enzyme system. There have been no definitive drug-drug interaction studies to examine pharmacokinetic or pharmacodynamic interaction with other drugs, but in humans, Kytril Injection has been safely administered with drugs representing benzodiazepines, neuroleptics and anti-ulcer medications commonly prescribed with antiemetic treatments. Kytril Injection also does not appear to interact with emetogenic cancer chemotherapies. Because granisetron is metabolized by hepatic cytochrome P-450 drug-metabolizing enzymes, inducers or inhibitors of these enzymes may change the clearance and, hence, the half-life of granisetron.

Carcinogenesis, Mutagenesis, Impairment of Fertility
In a 24-month carcinogenicity study, rats were treated orally with granisetron 1, 5 or 50 mg/kg/day (6, 30 or 300 mg/m^2/day). The 50 mg/kg/day dose was reduced to 25 mg/

kg/day (150 mg/m^2/day) during week 59 due to toxicity. For a 50 kg person of average height (1.46m^2 body surface area), these doses represent 16, 81 and 405 times the recommended clinical dose (0.37 mg/m^2, i.v.) on a body surface area basis. There was a statistically significant increase in the incidence of hepatocellular carcinomas and adenomas in males treated with 5 mg/kg/day (30 mg/m^2/day, 81 times the recommended human dose based on body surface area) and above, and in females treated with 25 mg/kg/day (150 mg/m^2/day, 405 times the recommended human dose based on body surface area). No increase in liver tumors was observed at a dose of 1 mg/kg/day (6 mg/m^2/day, 16 times the recommended human dose based on body surface area) in males and 5 mg/kg/day (30 mg/m^2/day, 81 times the recommended human dose based on body surface area) in females. In a 12-month oral toxicity study, treatment with granisetron 100 mg/kg/day (600 mg/m^2/day, 1622 times the recommended human dose based on body surface area) produced hepatocellular adenomas in male and female rats while no such tumors were found in the control rats. A 24-month mouse carcinogenicity study of granisetron did not show a statistically significant increase in tumor incidence, but the study was not conclusive.
Because of the tumor findings in rat studies, Kytril (granisetron hydrochloride) Injection should be prescribed only at the dose and for the indication recommended (see INDICATIONS AND USAGE, and DOSAGE AND ADMINISTRATION).
Granisetron was not mutagenic in *in vitro* Ames test and mouse lymphoma cell forward mutation assay, and *in vivo* mouse micronucleus test and *in vitro* and *ex vivo* rat hepatocyte UDS assays. It, however, produced a significant increase in UDS in HeLa cells *in vitro* and a significant increased incidence of cells with polyploidy in an *in vitro* human lymphocyte chromosomal aberration test.
Granisetron at subcutaneous doses up to 6 mg/kg/day (36 mg/m^2/day, 97 times the recommended human dose based on body surface area) was found to have no effect on fertility and reproductive performance of male and female rats.

Pregnancy
Teratogenic Effects. Pregnancy Category B. Reproduction studies have been performed in pregnant rats at intravenous doses up to 9 mg/kg/day (54 mg/m^2/day, 146 times the recommended human dose based on body surface area) and pregnant rabbits at intravenous doses up to 3 mg/kg/day (35.4 mg/m^2/day, 96 times the recommended human dose

Continued on next page

Information on the SmithKline Beecham Pharmaceuticals products appearing here is based on the labeling in effect on July 31, 1998. Further information on these and other products may be obtained from the Medical Department, SmithKline Beecham Pharmaceuticals, One Franklin Plaza, Philadelphia, PA 19101.

Kytril Injection—Cont.

based on body surface area) and have revealed no evidence of impaired fertility or harm to the fetus due to granisetron. There are, however, no adequate and well-controlled studies in pregnant women. Because animal reproduction studies are not always predictive of human response, this drug should be used during pregnancy only if clearly needed.

Nursing Mothers

It is not known whether granisetron is excreted in human milk. Because many drugs are excreted in human milk, caution should be exercised when *Kytril* Injection is administered to a nursing woman.

Pediatric Use

See DOSAGE AND ADMINISTRATION for use in children 2 to 16 years of age. Safety and effectiveness in children under 2 years of age have not been established.

Geriatric Use

During clinical trials, 713 patients 65 years of age or older received Kytril (granisetron HCl) Injection. Effectiveness and safety were similar in patients of various ages.

ADVERSE REACTIONS

The following have been reported during controlled clinical trials or in the routine management of patients. The percentage figures are based on clinical trial experience only. Table 7 gives the comparative frequencies of the five most commonly reported adverse events (≥3%) in patients receiving *Kytril* Injection, in single-day chemotherapy trials. These patients received chemotherapy, primarily cisplatin, and intravenous fluids during the 24-hour period following *Kytril* Injection administration. Events were generally recorded over seven days post-*Kytril* Injection administration. In the absence of a placebo group, there is uncertainty as to how many of these events should be attributed to *Kytril*, except for headache, which was clearly more frequent than in comparison groups.

Table 7. Principal Adverse Events in Clinical Trials—Single-Day Chemotherapy

	Percent of Patients with Event	
	Kytril Injection 40 mcg/kg (n=1,268)	Comparator[1] (n=422)
Headache	14%	6%
Asthenia	5%	6%
Somnolence	4%	15%
Diarrhea	4%	6%
Constipation	3%	3%

1. Metoclopramide/dexamethasone and phenothiazines/dexamethasone.

In over 3,000 patients receiving *Kytril* Injection (2 to 160 mcg/kg) in single-day and multiple-day clinical trials with emetogenic cancer therapies, adverse events, other than those in Table 7, were observed; attribution of many of these events to *Kytril* is uncertain.

Hepatic: In comparative trials, mainly with cisplatin regimens, elevations of AST and ALT (>2 times the upper limit of normal) following administration of *Kytril* Injection occurred in 2.8% and 3.3% of patients, respectively. These frequencies were not significantly different from those seen with comparators (AST: 2.1%; ALT: 2.4%).

Cardiovascular: Hypertension (2%); hypotension, arrhythmias such as sinus bradycardia, atrial fibrillation, varying degrees of A-V block, ventricular ectopy including nonsustained tachycardia, and ECG abnormalities have been observed rarely.

Central Nervous System: Agitation, anxiety, CNS stimulation and insomnia were seen in less than 2% of patients. Extrapyramidal syndrome occurred rarely and only in the presence of other drugs associated with this syndrome.

Hypersensitivity: Rare cases of hypersensitivity reactions, sometimes severe (e.g., anaphylaxis, shortness of breath, hypotension, urticaria) have been reported.

Other: Fever (3%), taste disorder (2%), skin rashes (1%). In multiple-day comparative studies, fever occurred more frequently with *Kytril* Injection (8.6%) than with comparative drugs (3.4%, $P < 0.014$), which usually included dexamethasone.

OVERDOSAGE

There is no specific antidote for Kytril (granisetron hydrochloride) Injection overdosage. In case of overdosage, symptomatic treatment should be given. Overdosage of up to 38.5 mg of granisetron hydrochloride injection has been reported without symptoms or only the occurrence of a slight headache.

DOSAGE AND ADMINISTRATION

The recommended dosage for *Kytril* Injection is 10 mcg/kg administered intravenously within 30 minutes before initiation of chemotherapy, and only on the day(s) chemotherapy is given. *Kytril* Injection may be administered intravenously

either undiluted over 30 seconds, or diluted with 0.9% Sodium Chloride or 5% Dextrose and infused over 5 minutes.

Pediatric Use: The recommended dose in children 2 to 16 years of age is 10 mcg/kg (see CLINICAL TRIALS). Children under 2 years of age have not been studied.

Use in the Elderly, Renal Failure Patients or Hepatically Impaired Patients: No dosage adjustment is recommended. (See CLINICAL PHARMACOLOGY, Pharmacokinetics.)

Infusion Preparation

Kytril Injection, administered as a 5–minute infusion, should be diluted in 0.9% Sodium Chloride or 5% Dextrose to a total volume of 20 to 50 mL.

Stability

Intravenous infusion of *Kytril* Injection should be prepared at the time of administration. However, *Kytril* Injection has been shown to be stable for at least 24 hours when diluted in 0.9% Sodium Chloride or 5% Dextrose and stored at room temperature under normal lighting conditions.

As a general precaution, *Kytril* Injection should not be mixed in solution with other drugs. Parenteral drug products should be inspected visually for particulate matter and discoloration before administration whenever solution and container permit.

HOW SUPPLIED

Kytril (granisetron hydrochloride) Injection, 1 mg/mL (free base), is supplied in 1 mL Single-Use Vials and 4 mL Multi-Dose Vials.

NDC 0029-4149-01 (package of 1 Single-Dose Vial)

NDC 0029-4152-01 (package of 1 Multi-Dose Vial)

Store single-dose vials at 30°C (86°F) or below, and multi-dose vials between 20° and 25°C (68° and 77°F) [see USP]. Once the multi-dose vial is penetrated, its contents should be used within 30 days.

Do not freeze. Protect from light.

Veterans Administration/Military/PHS—Vial, 1 mg/mL, 1's (multiples of 6), 6505-01-391-6108.

KY:L10

Shown in Product Identification Guide, page 339

KYTRIL®

℞

[kī '-tril]

granisetron hydrochloride

Tablets

DESCRIPTION

Kytril Tablets contain granisetron hydrochloride, an antinauseant and antiemetic agent. Chemically it is *endo*-N-(9-methyl-9-azabicyclo [3.3.1] non-3-yl)-1-methyl-1H-indazole-3-carboxamide hydrochloride with a molecular weight of 348.9 (312.4 free base). Its empirical formula is $C_{18}H_{24}N_4O \bullet HCl$, while its chemical structure is:

granisetron hydrochloride

Granisetron hydrochloride is a white to off-white solid that is readily soluble in water and normal saline at 20°C.

Tablets for Oral Administration: Each white, triangular, biconvex, film-coated *Kytril* Tablet contains 1.12 mg granisetron hydrochloride equivalent to granisetron, 1.0 mg. Inactive ingredients are: hydroxypropyl methylcellulose, lactose, magnesium stearate, microcrystalline cellulose, polyethylene glycol, polysorbate 80, sodium starch glycolate and titanium dioxide.

CLINICAL PHARMACOLOGY

Granisetron is a selective 5-hydroxytryptamine$_3$ (5-HT$_3$) receptor antagonist with little or no affinity for other serotonin receptors, including 5-HT$_1$; 5-HT$_{1A}$; 5-HT$_{1B/C}$; 5-HT$_2$; for alpha$_1$-, alpha$_2$-, or beta-adrenoreceptors; for dopamine-D$_2$; or for histamine-H$_1$; benzodiazepine; picrotoxin; or opioid receptors.

Serotonin receptors of the 5-HT$_3$ type are located peripherally on vagal nerve terminals and centrally in the chemoreceptor trigger zone of the area postrema. During chemotherapy that induces vomiting, mucosal enterochromaffin cells release serotonin, which stimulates 5-HT$_3$ receptors. This evokes vagal afferent discharge, inducing vomiting. Animal studies demonstrate that, in binding to 5-HT$_3$ receptors, granisetron blocks serotonin stimulation and subsequent vomiting after emetogenic stimuli such as cisplatin. In the ferret animal model, a single granisetron injection prevented vomiting due to high-dose cisplatin or arrested vomiting within 5 to 30 seconds.

In most human studies, granisetron has had little effect on blood pressure, heart rate or ECG. No evidence of an effect on plasma prolactin or aldosterone concentrations has been found in other studies.

Following single and multiple oral doses, *Kytril* slowed colonic transit in normal volunteers. However, *Kytril* had no effect on oro-cecal transit time in normal volunteers when given as a single intravenous (IV) infusion of 50 mcg/kg or 200 mcg/kg.

Pharmacokinetics

In healthy volunteers and adult cancer patients undergoing chemotherapy, administration of oral *Kytril* produced the following mean pharmacokinetic data:

[See table 1 below]

The effects of gender on the pharmacokinetics of oral *Kytril* have not been studied. However, after intravenous infusion of *Kytril*, no difference in mean AUC was found between males and females, although males had a higher C$_{max}$ generally.

When oral *Kytril* was administered with food, AUC was decreased by 5% and C$_{max}$ increased by 30% in non-fasted healthy volunteers who received a single dose of 10 mg.

Granisetron metabolism involves N-demethylation and aromatic ring oxidation followed by conjugation. Animal studies suggest that some of the metabolites may also have 5-HT$_3$ receptor antagonist activity.

Clearance is predominantly by hepatic metabolism. In normal volunteers, approximately 11% of the orally administered dose is eliminated unchanged in the urine in 48 hours. The remainder of the dose is excreted as metabolites, 48% in the urine and 38% in the feces.

In vitro liver microsomal studies show that granisetron's major route of metabolism is inhibited by ketoconazole, suggestive of metabolism mediated by the cytochrome P-450 3A subfamily.

Plasma protein binding is approximately 65% and granisetron distributes freely between plasma and red blood cells. In the elderly and in patients with renal failure or hepatic impairment, the pharmacokinetics of granisetron was determined following administration of intravenous *Kytril*:

Elderly: The ranges of the pharmacokinetic parameters in elderly volunteers (mean age 71 years), given a single 40 mcg/kg intravenous dose of *Kytril* Injection, were generally similar to those in younger healthy volunteers; mean values were lower for clearance and longer for half-life in the elderly.

Renal Failure Patients: Total clearance of granisetron was not affected in patients with severe renal failure who received a single 40 mcg/kg intravenous dose of *Kytril* Injection.

Hepatically Impaired Patients: A pharmacokinetic study with intravenous *Kytril* in patients with hepatic impairment due to neoplastic liver involvement showed that total clearance was approximately halved compared to patients without hepatic impairment. Given the wide variability in pharmacokinetic parameters noted in patients and the good tolerance of doses well above the recommended 1.0 mg b.i.d. dose, dosage adjustment in patients with possible hepatic functional impairment is not necessary.

Table 1. Pharmacokinetic Parameters (Median [range]) Following Oral Kytril (granisetron hydrochloride)

	Peak Plasma Concentration (ng/mL)	Terminal Phase Plasma Half-Life (h)	Volume of Distribution (L/kg)	Total Clearance (L/h/kg)
Cancer Patients 1.0 mg b.i.d., 7 days (n=27)	5.99 [0.63 to 30.9]	N.D.*	N.D.	0.52 [0.09 to 7.37]
Volunteers single 1.0 mg dose (n=39)	3.63 [0.27 to 9.14]	6.23 [0.96 to 19.9]	3.94 [1.89 to 39.4]	0.41 [0.11 to 24.6]

* Not determined after oral administration; following a single intravenous dose of 40 mcg/kg, terminal phase half-life was determined to be 8.95 hours.

N.D. Not determined

Pediatric Patients: A pharmacokinetic study in pediatric cancer patients (2 to 16 years of age), given a single 40 mcg/kg intravenous dose of *Kytril* Injection, showed that volume of distribution and total clearance increased with age. No relationship with age was observed for peak plasma concentration or terminal phase plasma half-life. When volume of distribution and total clearance are adjusted for body weight, the pharmacokinetics of granisetron are similar in pediatric and adult cancer patients.

CLINICAL TRIALS

Oral *Kytril* prevents nausea and vomiting associated with initial and repeat courses of emetogenic cancer therapy, as shown by 24-hour efficacy data from studies using both moderately- and highly-emetogenic chemotherapy.

Moderately Emetogenic Chemotherapy: The first trial compared oral *Kytril* doses of 0.25 to 2.0 mg b.i.d., in 930 cancer patients receiving, principally, cyclophosphamide, carboplatin and cisplatin (20 mg/m^2 to 50 mg/m^2). Efficacy was based on: complete response (i.e., no vomiting, no moderate or severe nausea, no rescue medication), no vomiting and no nausea. Table 2 summarizes the results of this study.
[See table 2 above]

Results from a second double-blind, randomized trial evaluating *Kytril* 2.0 mg q.d. and *Kytril* 1.0 mg b.i.d. were compared to prochlorperazine 10 mg b.i.d. derived from a historical control. At 24 hours, there was no statistically significant difference in efficacy between the two oral *Kytril* regimens. Both regimens were statistically superior to the prochlorperazine control regimen (See Table 3).
[See table 3 above]

Results from a *Kytril* 2.0 mg q.d. alone treatment arm in a third double-blind, randomized trial, were compared to prochlorperazine (PCPZ), 10 mg b.i.d., derived from a historical control. The 24-hour results for *Kytril* 2.0 mg q.d. were statistically superior to PCPZ for all efficacy parameters: complete response (58%), no vomiting (79%), no nausea (51%), total control (49%). The PCPZ rates are shown in Table 3.

Cisplatin-based Chemotherapy: The first double-blind trial compared oral *Kytril* 1.0 mg b.i.d., relative to placebo (historical control), in 119 cancer patients receiving high-dose cisplatin (mean dose 80 mg/m^2). At 24 hours, oral *Kytril* 1.0 mg b.i.d. was significantly ($P<0.001$) superior to placebo (historical control) in all efficacy parameters: complete response (52%), no vomiting (56%) and no nausea (45%). The placebo rates were 7%, 14%, and 7%, respectively, for the three efficacy parameters.

Results from a *Kytril* 2.0 q.d. alone treatment arm in a second double-blind, randomized trial, were compared to both *Kytril* 1.0 mg b.i.d. and placebo historical controls. The 24-hour results for *Kytril* 2.0 mg q.d. were: complete response (44%), no vomiting (58%), no nausea (46%), total control (40%). The efficacy of *Kytril* 2.0 mg q.d. was comparable to *Kytril* 1.0 mg b.i.d. and statistically superior to placebo. The placebo rates were 7%, 14%, 7%, 7%, respectively, for the four parameters.

No controlled study comparing granisetron injection with the oral formulation to prevent chemotherapy-induced nausea and vomiting has been performed.

INDICATIONS AND USAGE

Kytril (granisetron hydrochloride) is indicated for the prevention of nausea and vomiting associated with initial and repeat courses of emetogenic cancer therapy, including high-dose cisplatin.

CONTRAINDICATIONS

Kytril is contraindicated in patients with known hypersensitivity to the drug or any of its components.

PRECAUTIONS
Drug Interactions

Granisetron does not induce or inhibit the cytochrome P-450 drug-metabolizing enzyme system. There have been no definitive drug-drug interaction studies to examine pharmacokinetic or pharmacodynamic interaction with other drugs but, in humans, *Kytril* Injection has been safely administered with drugs representing benzodiazepines, neuroleptics and anti-ulcer medications commonly prescribed with antiemetic treatments. *Kytril* Injection also does not appear to interact with emetogenic cancer chemotherapies. Because granisetron is metabolized by hepatic cytochrome P-450 drug-metabolizing enzymes, inducers or inhibitors of these enzymes may change the clearance and, hence, the half-life of granisetron.

Carcinogenesis, Mutagenesis, Impairment of Fertility

In a 24-month carcinogenicity study, rats were treated orally with granisetron 1, 5 or 50 mg/kg/day (6, 30 or 300 mg/m^2/day). The 50 mg/kg/day dose was reduced to 25 mg/kg/day (150 mg/m^2/day) during week 59 due to toxicity. For a 50 kg person of average height (1.46m^2 body surface area), these doses represent 4, 20 and 101 times the recommended clinical dose (1.48 mg/m^2, oral) on a body surface area basis. There was a statistically significant increase in the incidence of hepatocellular carcinomas and adenomas in males treated with 5 mg/kg/day (30 mg/m^2/day, 20 times the recommended human dose based on body surface area) and above, and in females treated with 25 mg/kg/day (150 mg/

m^2/day, 101 times the recommended human dose based on body surface area). No increase in liver tumors was observed at a dose of 1 mg/kg/day (6 mg/m^2/day, 4 times the recommended human dose based on body surface area in males and 5 mg/kg/day (30 mg/m^2/day, 20 times the recommended human dose based on body surface area) in females. In a 12-month oral toxicity study, treatment with granisetron 100 mg/kg/day (600 mg/m^2/day, 405 times the recommended human dose based on body surface area) produced hepatocellular adenomas in male and female rats while no such tumors were found in the control animals. A 24-month mouse carcinogenicity study of granisetron did not show a statistically significant increase in tumor incidence, but the study was not conclusive.

Because of the tumor findings in rat studies, Kytril (granisetron hydrochloride) Tablets should be prescribed only at the dose and for the indication recommended (see INDICATIONS AND USAGE, and DOSAGE AND ADMINISTRATION).

Granisetron was not mutagenic in *in vitro* Ames test and mouse lymphoma cell forward mutation assay, and *in vivo* mouse micronucleus test and *in vitro* and *ex vivo* rat hepatocyte UDS assays. It, however, produced a significant increase in UDS in HeLa cells *in vitro* and a significant increased incidence of cells with polyploidy in an *in vitro* human lymphocyte chromosomal aberration test.

Granisetron at oral doses up to 100 mg/kg/day (600 mg/m^2/day, 405 times the recommended human dose based on body surface area) was found to have no effect on fertility and reproductive performance of male and female rats.

Pregnancy

Teratogenic Effects. Pregnancy Category B. Reproduction studies have been performed in pregnant rats at oral doses up to 125 mg/kg/day (750 mg/m^2/day, 507 times the recommended human dose based on body surface area) and preg-

nant rabbits at oral doses up to 32 mg/kg/day (378 mg/m^2/day, 255 times the recommended human dose based on body surface area) and have revealed no evidence of impaired fertility or harm to the fetus due to granisetron. There are, however, no adequate and well-controlled studies in pregnant women. Because animal reproduction studies are not always predictive of human response, this drug should be used during pregnancy only if clearly needed.

Nursing Mothers

It is not known whether granisetron is excreted in human milk. Because many drugs are excreted in human milk, caution should be exercised when *Kytril* is administered to a nursing woman.

Pediatric Use

Safety and effectiveness in children have not been established.

Geriatric Use

During clinical trials, 325 patients 65 years of age or older received oral *Kytril*; 298 were 65 to 74 years of age and 27 were 75 years of age or older. Efficacy and safety were maintained with increasing age.

ADVERSE REACTIONS

Over 3,700 patients have received oral *Kytril* in clinical trials with emetogenic cancer therapies consisting primarily of cyclophosphamide or cisplatin regimens.

Continued on next page

Information on the SmithKline Beecham Pharmaceuticals products appearing here is based on the labeling in effect on July 31, 1998. Further information on these and other products may be obtained from the Medical Department, SmithKline Beecham Pharmaceuticals, One Franklin Plaza, Philadelphia, PA 19101.

Table 2. Prevention of Nausea and Vomiting 24 Hours Post-Chemotherapy[1]

	Percentages of Patients Oral *Kytril* Dose			
Efficacy Measures	0.25 mg b.i.d. (n=229) %	0.5 mg b.i.d. (n=235) %	1.0 mg b.i.d. (n=233) %	2.0 mg b.i.d. (n=233) %
Complete Response[2]	61	70*	81*†	72*
No Vomiting	66	77*	88*	79*
No Nausea	48	57	63*	54

1. Chemotherapy included oral and injectable cyclophosphamide, carboplatin, cisplatin (20 mg/m^2 to 50 mg/m^2), dacarbazine, doxorubicin, epirubicin.
2. No vomiting, no moderate or severe nausea, no rescue medication.
* Statistically significant ($P<0.01$) vs. 0.25 mg b.i.d.
† Statistically significant ($P<0.01$) vs. 0.5 mg b.i.d.

Table 3. Prevention of Nausea and Vomiting 24 Hours Post-Chemotherapy[1]

	Percentages of Patients		
Efficacy Measures	Oral *Kytril* 1.0 mg b.i.d. (n=354) %	Oral *Kytril* 2.0 mg q.d. (n=343) %	Prochlorperazine[2] 10.0 mg b.i.d. (n=111) %
Complete Response[3]	69*	64*	41
No Vomiting	82*	77*	48
No Nausea	51*	53*	35
Total Control[4]	51*	50*	33

1. Moderately emetogenic chemotherapeutic agents included cisplatin (20 mg/m^2 to 50 mg/m^2), oral and intravenous cyclophosphamide, carboplatin, dacarbazine, doxorubicin.
2. Historical control from a previous double-blind *Kytril* trial.
3. No vomiting, no moderate or severe nausea, no rescue medication.
4. No vomiting, no nausea, no rescue medication.
* Statistically significant ($P<0.05$) vs. prochlorperazine historical control.

Table 4. Principal Adverse Events in Clinical Trials

	Percent of Patients with Event			
	Oral *Kytril*[1] 1.0 mg b.i.d. (n=978)	Oral *Kytril*[1] 2.0 mg q.d. (n=1450)	Comparator[2] (n=599)	Placebo (n=185)
Headache[3]	21%	20%	13%	12%
Constipation	18%	14%	16%	8%
Asthenia	14%	18%	10%	4%
Diarrhea	8%	9%	10%	4%
Abdominal pain	6%	4%	6%	3%
Dyspepsia	4%	6%	5%	4%

1. Adverse events were recorded for 7 days when oral *Kytril* was given on a single day and for up to 28 days when oral *Kytril* was administered for 7 or 14 days.
2. Metoclopramide/dexamethasone; phenothiazines/dexamethasone; dexamethasone alone; prochlorperazine.
3. Usually mild to moderate in severity.

Kytril Tablets—Cont.

In patients receiving oral *Kytril* 1.0 mg b.i.d. for 1, 7 or 14 days, 2.0 mg q.d. for 1 day, the following table lists adverse experiences reported in more than 5% of the patients with comparator and placebo incidences.

[See table 4 on previous page]

Other adverse events reported in clinical trials were:

Gastrointestinal: In single-day dosing studies in which adverse events were collected for 7 days, nausea (20%) and vomiting (12%) were recorded as adverse events after the 24-hour efficacy assessment period.

Hepatic: In comparative trials, elevation of AST and ALT (>2 times the upper limit of normal) following the administration of oral *Kytril* occurred in 5% and 6% of patients, respectively. These frequencies were not significantly different from those seen with comparators (AST: 2%; ALT: 9%).

Cardiovascular: Hypertension (1%); hypotension, angina pectoris, atrial fibrillation and syncope have been observed rarely.

Central Nervous System: Dizziness (5%), insomnia (5%), anxiety (2%), somnolence (1%). One case compatible with but not diagnostic of extrapyramidal symptoms has been reported in a patient treated with oral *Kytril*.

Hypersensitivity: Rare cases of hypersensitivity reactions, sometimes severe (e.g., anaphylaxis, shortness of breath, hypotension, urticaria) have been reported.

Other: Fever (5%). Events often associated with chemotherapy also have been reported: leukopenia (9%), decreased appetite (6%), anemia (4%), alopecia (3%), thrombocytopenia (2%).

Over 5,000 patients have received injectable *Kytril* in clinical trials.

Table 5 gives the comparative frequencies of the five commonly reported adverse events (≥3%) in patients receiving *Kytril* Injection, 40 mcg/kg, in single-day chemotherapy trials. These patients received chemotherapy, primarily cisplatin, and intravenous fluids during the 24-hour period following *Kytril* Injection administration.

Table 5. Principal Adverse Events in Clinical Trials—Single-Day Chemotherapy

	Percent of Patients with Event	
	Kytril Injection[1] 40 mcg/kg (n=1,268)	Comparator[2] (n=422)
Headache	14%	6%
Asthenia	5%	6%
Somnolence	4%	15%
Diarrhea	4%	6%
Constipation	3%	3%

1. Adverse events were generally recorded over 7 days post-*Kytril* Injection administration.
2. Metoclopramide/dexamethasone and phenothiazines/dexamethasone.

In the absence of a placebo group, there is uncertainty as to how many of these events should be attributed to *Kytril*, except for headache, which was clearly more frequent than in comparison groups.

OVERDOSAGE

There is no specific treatment for granisetron hydrochloride overdosage. In case of overdosage, symptomatic treatment should be given. Overdosage of up to 38.5 mg of granisetron hydrochloride injection has been reported without symptoms or only the occurrence of a slight headache.

DOSAGE AND ADMINISTRATION

The recommended adult dosage of oral Kytril (granisetron hydrochloride) is 2 mg once daily or 1 mg twice daily. In the 2 mg once-daily regimen, two 1 mg tablets are given up to 1 hour before chemotherapy. In the 1 mg twice-daily regimen, the first 1 mg tablet is given up to 1 hour before chemotherapy, and the second tablet, 12 hours after the first. Either regimen is administered only on the day(s) chemotherapy is given. Continued treatment, while not on chemotherapy, has not been found to be useful.

Use in the Elderly, Pediatric Patients, Renal Failure Patients or Hepatically Impaired Patients: No dosage adjustment is recommended. (See CLINICAL PHARMACOLOGY, Pharmacokinetics.)

HOW SUPPLIED

Tablets: White, triangular, biconvex, film-coated tablets debossed K1 on one face: 1 mg in Unit-of-Use Packages of 2; in Single Unit Packages of 20 (intended for institutional use only).

1 mg Unit-of-Use 2's: NDC 0029-4151-39
1 mg SUP 20's: NDC 0029-4151-05
Store between 15° and 30°C (59° and 86°F). Protect from light.

Manufactured in Crawley, UK, by
SmithKline Beecham Pharmaceuticals
for **SmithKline Beecham Pharmaceuticals**
Philadelphia, PA 19101
Veterans Administration/Military/PHS—Tablets, 1 mg, 2's, 6505-01-412-0329; 1 mg, 20's, 6505-01-412-0324.
KY:L4T

Shown in Product Identification Guide, page 339

MONOCID® ℞
[mon 'oh-sid]
brand of sterile cefonicid sodium
(lyophilized)

DESCRIPTION

Monocid (sterile cefonicid sodium), a sterile, lyophilized, semi-synthetic, broad-spectrum cephalosporin antibiotic for intravenous and intramuscular administration, is 5-Thia-1-azabicyclo[4.2.0]oct-2-ene-2-carboxylic acid, 7-[(hydroxyphenyl-acetyl)-amino]-8-oxo-3-[[[1-(sulfomethyl)-1*H*-tetrazol-5-yl]thio]methyl]-disodium salt, [6*R*-[6α, 7β(*R**)]]. Cefonicid sodium contains 85 mg (3.7 mEq) sodium per gram of cefonicid activity.

CLINICAL PHARMACOLOGY

Human Pharmacology

The table below demonstrates the levels and duration of Monocid (sterile cefonicid sodium) in serum following intravenous and intramuscular administration of 1 gram to normal volunteers.

[See table below]

Serum half-life is approximately 4.5 hours with intravenous and intramuscular administration. *Monocid* is highly (greater than 90%) and reversibly protein bound.

Monocid is not metabolized; 99% is excreted unchanged in the urine in 24 hours. A 500 mg IM dose provides a high (384 mcg/mL) urinary concentration at 6 to 8 hours. Probenecid, given concurrently with *Monocid*, slows renal excretion, produces higher peak serum levels and significantly increases the serum half-life of the drug (8.2 hours).

Monocid reaches therapeutic levels in the following tissues and fluids:

[See table at bottom of next page]

Note: Although *Monocid* reaches therapeutic levels in bile, those levels are lower than those seen with other cephalosporins, and amounts of *Monocid* released into the gastrointestinal tract are minute. This small amount of *Monocid* in the gastrointestinal tract is thought to be the reason for the low incidence of gastrointestinal reactions following therapy with *Monocid*.

No disulfiram-like reactions were reported in a crossover study conducted in healthy volunteers receiving *Monocid* and alcohol.

Microbiology

The bactericidal action of Monocid (sterile cefonicid sodium) results from inhibition of cell-wall synthesis. *Monocid* is highly resistant to beta-lactamases produced by *Staphylococcus aureus*, *Haemophilus influenzae*, *Neisseria gonorrhoeae* and Richmond type I beta-lactamases. *Monocid* is resistant to degradation by beta-lactamases from certain members of *Enterobacteriaceae*. Active against a wide range of gram-positive and gram-negative organisms, *Monocid* is usually active against the following organisms *in vitro* and in clinical situations:

Gram-Positive Aerobes: *Staphylococcus aureus* (beta-lactamase producing and non-beta-lactamase producing) and *S. epidermidis* (Note: Methicillin-resistant staphylococci are resistant to cephalosporins, including cefonicid.); *Streptococcus pneumoniae*, *S. pyogenes* (Group A beta-hemolytic *Streptococcus*), and *S. agalactiae* (Group B *Streptococcus*).

Gram-Negative Aerobes: *Escherichia coli*; *Klebsiella pneumoniae*; *Providencia rettgeri* (formerly *Proteus rettgeri*); *Proteus vulgaris*; *Morganella morganii* (formerly *Proteus morganii*); *Proteus mirabilis*; and *Haemophilus influenzae* (ampicillin-sensitive and -resistant).

The following *in vitro* data are available but their clinical significance is unknown. *Monocid* is usually active against the following organisms *in vitro*:

Gram-Negative Aerobes: *Moraxella* (formerly *Branhamella) catarrhalis*; *Klebsiella oxytoca*; *Enterobacter aerogenes*; *Neisseria gonorrhoeae* (penicillin-sensitive and -resistant); *Citrobacter freundii* and *C. diversus*.

Gram-Positive Anaerobes: *Clostridium perfringens*; *Peptostreptococcus anaerobius*; *Peptococcus magnus*; *P. prevotii*; and *Propionibacterium acnes*.

Gram-Negative Anaerobes: *Fusobacterium nucleatum*.

Monocid (sterile cefonicid sodium) is usually inactive *in vitro* against most strains of *Pseudomonas*, *Serratia*, *Enterococcus* and *Acinetobacter*. Most strains of *B. fragilis* are resistant.

Susceptibility Testing

Results from standardized single-disk susceptibility tests using a 30 mcg *Monocid* disk should be interpreted according to the following criteria:

Zones of 18 mm or greater indicate that the tested organism is susceptible to *Monocid* and is likely to respond to therapy.

Zones from 15 to 17 mm indicate that the tested organism is of intermediate (moderate) susceptibility, and is likely to respond to therapy if a higher dosage is used or if the infection is confined to tissues and fluids in which high antibiotic levels are attained.

Zones of 14 mm or less indicate that the organism is resistant.

Only the *Monocid* disk should be used to determine susceptibility, since *in vitro* tests show that *Monocid* has activity against certain strains not susceptible to other cephalosporins. The *Monocid* disk should not be used for testing susceptibility to other cephalosporins.

A bacterial isolate may be considered susceptible if the MIC value for *Monocid* is equal to or less than 8 mcg/mL in accordance with the National Committee for Clinical Laboratory Standards (NCCLS) guidelines. Organisms are considered resistant if the MIC is equal to or greater than 32 mcg/mL. For most organisms the MBC value for *Monocid* is the same as the MIC value.

The standardized quality control procedure requires use of control organisms. The 30 mcg *Monocid* disk should give the zone diameters listed below for the quality control strains.

Organism	ATCC	Zone Size Range
E. coli	25922	25 to 29 mm
S. aureus	25923	22 to 28 mm

INDICATIONS AND USAGE

Due to the long half-life of *Monocid*, a 1 gram dose results in therapeutic serum levels which provide coverage against susceptible organisms (listed below) for 24 hours.

Studies on specimens obtained prior to therapy should be used to determine the susceptibility of the causative organisms to *Monocid*. Therapy with *Monocid* may be initiated pending results of the studies; however, treatment should be adjusted according to study findings.

Treatment

Monocid (sterile cefonicid sodium) is indicated in the treatment of infections due to susceptible strains of the microorganisms listed below:

LOWER RESPIRATORY TRACT INFECTIONS, due to *Streptococcus pneumoniae*; *Klebsiella pneumoniae**; *Escherichia coli*; and *Haemophilus influenzae* (ampicillin-resistant and ampicillin-sensitive).

URINARY TRACT INFECTIONS, due to *Escherichia coli*; *Proteus mirabilis* and *Proteus* spp. (which may include the organisms now called *Proteus vulgaris*,* *Providencia rettgeri* and *Morganella morganii*); and *Klebsiella pneumoniae*.*

SKIN AND SKIN STRUCTURE INFECTIONS, due to *Staphylococcus aureus* and *S. epidermidis*; *Streptococcus pyogenes* (Group A *Streptococcus*) and *S. agalactiae* (Group B *Streptococcus*).

SEPTICEMIA, due to *Streptococcus pneumoniae* and *Escherichia coli*.*

BONE AND JOINT INFECTIONS, due to *Staphylococcus aureus*.

* Efficacy for this organism in this organ system has been demonstrated in fewer than 10 infections.

Surgical Prophylaxis

Administration of a single 1 gram dose of *Monocid* before surgery may reduce the incidence of postoperative infections in patients undergoing surgical procedures classified as contaminated or potentially contaminated (e.g., colorectal surgery, vaginal hysterectomy, or cholecystectomy in high-risk patients), or in patients in whom infection at the operative site would present a serious risk (e.g., prosthetic arthroplasty, open heart surgery). Although cefonicid has been shown to be as effective as cefazolin in prevention of infection following coronary artery bypass surgery, no placebo-controlled trials have been conducted to evaluate any cephalosporin antibiotic in the prevention of infection following coronary artery bypass surgery or prosthetic heart valve replacement.

In cesarean section, the use of *Monocid* (after the umbilical cord has been clamped) may reduce the incidence of certain postoperative infections.

Serum Concentrations After 1 Gram Administration (mcg/mL)

Interval	5 min.	15 min.	30 min.	1 hr.	2 hr.	4 hr.	6 hr.	8 hr.	10 hr.	12 hr.	24 hr.
IV	221.3	176.4	147.6	124.2	88.9	61.4	40.0	29.3	20.6	15.2	2.6
IM	13.5	45.9	73.1	98.6	97.1	77.8	54.9	38.5	28.9	20.6	4.5

When administered 1 hour prior to surgical procedures for which it is indicated, a single 1 gram dose of *Monocid* provides protection from most infections due to susceptible organisms throughout the course of the procedure. Intraoperative and/or postoperative administrations of *Monocid* are not necessary. Daily doses of *Monocid* may be administered for 2 additional days in patients undergoing prosthetic arthroplasty or open heart surgery.

If there are signs of infection, the causative organisms should be identified and appropriate therapy determined through susceptibility testing.

Before using *Monocid* concomitantly with other antibiotics, the prescribing information for those agents should be reviewed for contraindications, warnings, precautions and adverse reactions. Renal function should be carefully monitored.

CONTRAINDICATIONS

Monocid (sterile cefonicid sodium) is contraindicated in persons who have shown hypersensitivity to cephalosporin antibiotics.

WARNINGS

BEFORE THERAPY WITH MONOCID (STERILE CEFONICID SODIUM) IS INSTITUTED, CAREFUL INQUIRY SHOULD BE MADE TO DETERMINE WHETHER THE PATIENT HAS HAD PREVIOUS HYPERSENSITIVITY REACTIONS TO CEPHALOSPORINS, PENICILLINS OR OTHER DRUGS. THIS PRODUCT SHOULD BE GIVEN CAUTIOUSLY TO PENICILLIN-SENSITIVE PATIENTS. ANTIBIOTICS SHOULD BE ADMINISTERED WITH CAUTION TO ANY PATIENT WHO HAS DEMONSTRATED SOME FORM OF ALLERGY, PARTICULARLY TO DRUGS. SERIOUS ACUTE HYPERSENSITIVITY REACTIONS MAY REQUIRE EPINEPHRINE AND OTHER EMERGENCY MEASURES.

Pseudomembranous colitis has been reported with nearly all antibacterial agents, including *Monocid*, and has ranged in severity from mild to life-threatening. Therefore, it is important to consider this diagnosis in patients who present with diarrhea subsequent to the administration of antibacterial agents.

Treatment with antibacterial agents alters the normal flora of the colon and may permit overgrowth of clostridia. Studies indicate that a toxin produced by *Clostridium difficile* is one primary cause of "antibiotic-associated colitis."

Mild cases of pseudomembranous colitis usually respond to drug discontinuation alone. In moderate to severe cases, consideration should be given to management with fluids and electrolytes, protein supplementation and treatment with an antibacterial drug clinically effective against *C. difficile* colitis.

PRECAUTIONS

General: With any antibiotic, prolonged use may result in overgrowth of nonsusceptible organisms. Careful observation is essential, and appropriate measures should be taken if superinfection occurs.

Drug Interactions: Nephrotoxicity has been reported following concomitant administration of other cephalosporins and aminoglycosides.

Carcinogenesis, Mutagenesis, Impairment of Fertility: Beta-lactam antibiotics with methyl-thio-tetrazole side chains have been shown to cause testicular atrophy in prepubertal rats, which persisted into adulthood and resulted in decreased spermatogenesis and decreased fertility. Cefonicid, which contains a methylsulfonic-thio-tetrazole moiety, has no adverse effect on the male reproductive system of prepubertal, juvenile or adult rats when given under identical conditions.

Carcinogenicity studies of cefonicid have not been conducted; however, results of mutagenicity studies (i.e., Ames/Salmonella/microsome plate assay and the micronucleus test in mice) were negative.

Pregnancy: (Category B.) Reproduction studies have been performed in mice, rabbits and rats at doses up to an equivalent of 40 times the usual adult human dose and have revealed no evidence of impaired fertility or harm to the fetus due to Monocid (sterile cefonicid sodium). There are, however, no adequate and well-controlled studies in pregnant women. Because animal reproduction studies are not always predictive of human response, this drug should be used in pregnancy only if clearly needed.

Labor and Delivery: In cesarean section, *Monocid* should be administered only after the umbilical cord has been clamped.

Nursing Mothers: *Monocid* is excreted in human milk in low concentrations. Caution should be exercised when *Monocid* is administered to a nursing woman.

Pediatric Use: Safety and effectiveness in children have not been established.

ADVERSE REACTIONS

Monocid (sterile cefonicid sodium) is generally well tolerated and adverse reactions have occurred infrequently. The most common adverse reaction has been pain on IM injection. On-therapy conditions occurring in greater than 1% of *Monocid*-treated patients were:

Injection Site Phenomena (5.7%): Pain and/or discomfort on injection; less often, burning, phlebitis at IV site.
Increased Platelets (1.7%).
Increased Eosinophils (2.9%).
Liver Function Test Alterations (1.6%): Increased alkaline phosphatase, increased SGOT, increased SGPT, increased GGTP, increased LDH.

Less frequent on-therapy conditions occurring in less than 1% of *Monocid*-treated patients were:

Hypersensitivity Reactions: Fever, rash, pruritus, erythema, myalgia and anaphylactoid-type reactions have been reported.
Hematology: Decreased WBC, neutropenia, thrombocytopenia, positive Coombs' test.
Renal: Increased BUN and creatinine levels have occasionally been seen. Rare reports of acute renal failure associated with interstitial nephritis, observed with other beta-lactam antibiotics, have also occurred with *Monocid*.
Gastrointestinal: Diarrhea and pseudomembranous colitis. Onset of pseudomembranous colitis symptoms may occur during or after antibiotic treatment (see WARNINGS).

DOSAGE AND ADMINISTRATION

General

The usual adult dosage is 1 gram of Monocid (sterile cefonicid sodium) given once every 24 hours, intravenously or by deep intramuscular injection. Doses in excess of 1 gram daily are rarely necessary; however, in exceptional cases dosage of up to 2 grams given once daily have been well tolerated. When administering 2 gram IM doses once daily, $\frac{1}{2}$ the dose should be administered in different large muscle masses.

Outpatient Use

Monocid has been used (once daily IM or IV) on an outpatient basis. Individuals responsible for outpatient administration of *Monocid* should be instructed thoroughly in appropriate procedures for storage, reconstitution and administration.

Surgical Prophylaxis

When administered 1 hour prior to appropriate surgical procedures (see INDICATIONS AND USAGE), a 1 gram dose of *Monocid* provides protection from most infections due to susceptible organisms throughout the course of the procedure. Intraoperative and/or postoperative administrations of *Monocid* are not necessary. Daily doses of *Monocid* may be administered for 2 additional days in patients undergoing prosthetic arthroplasty or open heart surgery.

In cesarean section *Monocid* should be administered only after the umbilical cord has been clamped.

Dosage of Monocid® in Adults with Reduced Renal Function

(Monitor renal function and adjust accordingly.)

Creatinine Clearance (mL/min per 1.73 M²)	Dosage Regimen	
	Mild to Moderate Infections	Severe Infections
79 to 60	10 mg/kg (every 24 hours)	25 mg/kg (every 24 hours)
59 to 40	8 mg/kg (every 24 hours)	20 mg/kg (every 24 hours)
39 to 20	4 mg/kg (every 24 hours)	15 mg/kg (every 24 hours)
19 to 10	4 mg/kg (every 48 hours)	15 mg/kg (every 48 hours)
9 to 5	4 mg/kg (every 3 to 5 days)	15 mg/kg (every 3 to 5 days)
<5	3 mg/kg (every 3 to 5 days)	4 mg/kg (every 3 to 5 days)

General Guidelines for Dosage of Monocid®, IV or IM

Type of Infection	Daily Dose (grams)	Frequency
Uncomplicated Urinary Tract	0.5	once every 24 hours
Mild to Moderate	1	once every 24 hours
Severe or Life-Threatening	2*	once every 24 hours
Surgical Prophylaxis	1	1 hour preoperatively

* When administering 2 gram IM doses once daily, $\frac{1}{2}$ the dose should be administered in different large muscle masses.

Impaired Renal Function

Modification of Monocid (sterile cefonicid sodium) dosage is necessary in patients with impaired renal function. Following an initial loading dosage of 7.5 mg/kg IM or IV, the maintenance dosing schedule shown below should be followed. Further dosing should be determined by severity of the infection and susceptibility of the causative organism. [See table at top of page]

Note: It is not necessary to administer additional dosage following dialysis.

Preparation of Parenteral Solution

Parenteral drug products should be SHAKEN WELL when reconstituted, and inspected visually for particulate matter prior to administration. If particulate matter is evident in reconstituted fluids, the drug solutions should be discarded.

RECONSTITUTION

Single-Dose Vials

For IM injection, IV direct (bolus) injection or IV infusion, reconstitute with Sterile Water for Injection according to the following table. SHAKE WELL.

Vial Size	Diluent to Be Added	Approx. Avail. Volume	Approx. Avg. Concentration
500 mg	2.0 mL	2.2 mL	225 mg/mL
1 gram	2.5 mL	3.1 mL	325 mg/mL

These solutions of Monocid (sterile cefonicid sodium) are stable 24 hours at room temperature or 72 hours if refrigerated (5°C). Slight yellowing does not affect potency.

Continued on next page

Information on the SmithKline Beecham Pharmaceuticals products appearing here is based on the labeling in effect on July 31, 1998. Further information on these and other products may be obtained from the Medical Department, SmithKline Beecham Pharmaceuticals, One Franklin Plaza, Philadelphia, PA 19101.

Tissue and Body Fluid Levels

Tissue or Body Fluid	Dosage and Route (No. of Patients Sampled)	Time of Sampling After Dose	Average Tissue or Fluid Levels (mcg/g or/mL)
Bone	1 g IM (7)	60 to 90 min.	6.8
	1 g IV (10)	44 to 99 min.	14.0
Gallbladder	1 g IM (10)	60 to 70 min.	15.5
Bile	1 g IM (10)	60 to 70 min.	7.5
Prostate	1 g IM (10)	50 to 115 min.	13.0
Uterine Tissue	1 g IM (6)	60 to 90 min.	17.5
Wound Fluid	1 g IM (10)	60 to 75 min.	37.7
Purulent Wound	1 g IM (9)	60 min.	11.5
Adipose Tissue	1 g IM (5)	60 min.	4.0
Atrial Appendage	1 g IM (7)	77 to 170 min.	7.5
	2 g IM (7)	105 to 170 min.	8.7
	15 mg/kg IV (10)	53 to 160 min.	15.4

Monocid—Cont.

For IV infusion, dilute reconstituted solution in 50 to 100 mL of the parenteral fluids listed under ADMINISTRATION.

Pharmacy Bulk Vials (10 grams)

For IM injection, IV direct (bolus) injection or IV infusion, reconstitute with Sterile Water for Injection, Bacteriostatic Water for Injection or Sodium Chloride Injection according to the following table:

Amount of Diluent	Approx. Concentration	Approx. Avail. Volume
25 mL	1 gram/3 mL	31 mL
45 mL	1 gram/5 mL	51 mL

These solutions of *Monocid* are stable 24 hours at room temperature or 72 hours if refrigerated (5°C). Slight yellowing does not affect potency.

For IV infusion add to parenteral fluids listed under ADMINISTRATION.

"Piggyback" Vials

Reconstitute with 50 to 100 mL of Sodium Chloride Injection or other IV solution listed under ADMINISTRATION. Administer with primary IV fluids, as a single dose. These solutions of *Monocid* are stable 24 hours at room temperature or 72 hours if refrigerated (5°C). Slight yellowing does not affect potency.

A solution of 1 gram of *Monocid* in 18 mL of Sterile Water for Injection is isotonic.

ADMINISTRATION

IM Injection: Inject well within the body of a relatively large muscle. Aspiration is necessary to avoid inadvertent injection into a blood vessel. When administering 2 gram IM doses once daily, $\frac{1}{2}$ the dose should be given in different large muscle masses.

IV Administration: For direct (bolus) injection, administer reconstituted *Monocid* slowly over 3 to 5 minutes, directly or through tubing for patients receiving parenteral fluids (see list below). For infusion, dilute reconstituted *Monocid* in 50 to 100 mL of 1 of the following solutions:

0.9% Sodium Chloride Injection, USP
5% Dextrose Injection, USP
5% Dextrose and 0.9% Sodium Chloride Injection, USP
5% Dextrose and 0.45% Sodium Chloride Injection, USP
5% Dextrose and 0.2% Sodium Chloride Injection, USP
10% Dextrose Injection, USP
Ringer's Injection, USP
Lactated Ringer's Injection, USP
5% Dextrose and Lactated Ringer's Injection
10% Invert Sugar in Sterile Water for Injection
5% Dextrose and 0.15% Potassium Chloride Injection
Sodium Lactate Injection, USP

In these fluids *Monocid* is stable 24 hours at room temperature or 72 hours if refrigerated (5°C). Slight yellowing does not affect potency.

HOW SUPPLIED

Monocid (sterile cefonicid sodium) is supplied in vials equivalent to 1 gram of cefonicid and in "Piggyback" Vials for IV admixture equivalent to 1 gram of cefonicid.
1 gram vial: NDC 0007-4353-01
1 gram "Piggyback" Vial (pack of 10): NDC 0007-4354-11
As with other cephalosporins, *Monocid* may darken on storage. However, if stored as recommended, this color change does not affect potency.
Before reconstitution, *Monocid* should be protected from light and refrigerated (2° to 8°C).

Veterans Administration/Military/PHS—Vial, 1 gram/10 mL, 1's, 6505-01-189-4698.

MC:L27

Shown in Product Identification Guide, page 339

OmniHIB™
[ahm-nee-hib]

Haemophilus b Conjugate Vaccine
(Tetanus Toxoid Conjugate)

℞

Caution: Federal (U.S.A.) law prohibits dispensing without prescription.
NOTE: Haemophilus b Conjugate Vaccine (Tetanus Toxoid Conjugate)—OmniHIB™ (distributed by SmithKline Beecham Pharmaceuticals) is identical to Haemophilus b Conjugate Vaccine (Tetanus Toxoid Conjugate)—ActHIB™; both products are manufactured by Pasteur Mérieux Sérums & Vaccins S.A.

DESCRIPTION

OmniHIB™, Haemophilus b Conjugate Vaccine (Tetanus Toxoid Conjugate), produced by Pasteur Mérieux Sérums & Vaccins S.A., for intramuscular use, is a sterile, lyophilized powder which is reconstituted at the time of use with saline diluent (0.4% Sodium Chloride). The vaccine consists of the Haemophilus b polysaccharide, a high molecular weight polymer prepared from the *Haemophilus influenzae* type b strain 1482 grown in a semi-synthetic medium, covalently bound to tetanus toxoid.[1] The lyophilized powder and saline diluent contain no preservatives. Each single dose of 0.5 mL is formulated to contain 10 µg of purified capsular polysaccharide, 24 µg of tetanus toxoid and 8.5% of sucrose. The tetanus toxoid is prepared by extraction, ammonium sulfate purification, and formalin inactivation of the toxin from cultures of *Clostridium tetani* (Harvard strain) grown in a modified Mueller and Miller medium.[2] The toxoid is filter sterilized prior to the conjugation process. Potency of OmniHIB is specified on each lot by limits on the content of PRP polysaccharide and protein in each dose and the proportion of polysaccharide and protein in the vaccine which is characterized as high molecular weight conjugate. The reconstituted vaccine is clear and colorless.

CLINICAL PHARMACOLOGY

NOTE: Haemophilus b Conjugate Vaccine (Tetanus Toxoid Conjugate)—OmniHIB (distributed by SmithKline Beecham Pharmaceuticals) is identical to Haemophilus b Conjugate Vaccine (Tetanus Toxoid Conjugate)—ActHIB; both products are manufactured by Pasteur Mérieux Sérums & Vaccins S.A.

H influenzae type b was the leading cause of invasive bacterial disease among children in the United States prior to licensing of Haemophilus b conjugate vaccines. Based on its active surveillance areas, the Centers for Disease Control and Prevention (CDC) now estimate that *H influenzae* type b disease in children under the age of 5 years has been reduced by 95%.[3] Before effective vaccines were introduced, it was estimated that one in 200 children developed invasive *H influenzae* type b disease by the age of 5 years. In children less than 5 years of age, the mortality rate for invasive *H influenzae* type b disease ranged between 3% and 6%.[3] In more than 60% of these children, meningitis was the clinical syndrome and permanent sequelae ranging from mild hearing loss to mental retardation affecting 20% to 30% of all survivors.[3] Ninety-five percent of the cases of invasive *H influenzae* disease among children <5 years of age were caused by organisms with the type b polysaccharide capsule. Approximately two-thirds of all cases of invasive *H influenzae* type b disease affected infants and children <15 months of age, a group for which a vaccine was not available until late 1990.[4,5]

Incidence rates of invasive *H influenzae* type b disease have been shown to be increased in certain high-risk groups, such as native Americans (both American Indians and Eskimos), blacks, individuals of lower socioeconomic status, and patients with asplenia, sickle cell disease, Hodgkin's disease, and antibody deficiency syndromes.[5,6] Studies also have suggested that the risk of acquiring primary invasive *H influenzae* type b disease for children under 5 years of age appears to be greater for those who attend day-care facilities.[7,8,9,10]

The potential for person to person transmission of the organism among susceptible individuals has been recognized. Studies of secondary spread of disease in household contacts of index patients have shown a substantially increased risk among exposed household contacts under 4 years of age.[11] Adults can be colonized with *H influenzae* type b from children infected with the organism.[12]

The response to OmniHIB is typical of a T-dependent immune response to antigen. The predominant isotype of anticapsular polysaccharide (polyribosyl-ribitol-phosphate or PRP) antibody induced by OmniHIB is IgG.[13] A substantial booster response has been demonstrated in children 12 months of age or older who previously received two or three doses. Bactericidal activity against *H influenzae* type b is demonstrated in serum after immunization and statistically correlates with the anti-PRP antibody response induced by OmniHIB.[14]

Antibody to *H influenzae* capsular polysaccharide (anti-PRP) titers of >1.0 µg/mL following vaccination with unconjugated PRP vaccine correlated with long-term protection against invasive *H influenzae* type b disease in children older than 24 months of age.[15] Although the relevance of this threshold to clinical protection after immunization with conjugate vaccines is not known, particularly in light of the induced, immunologic memory, this level continues to be considered as indicative of long-term protection.[4] The immunogenicity and safety of OmniHIB has been demonstrated in the United States and worldwide. OmniHIB induced, on average anti-PRP levels ≥1.0 µg/mL in 90% of infants after the primary series and in more than 98% of infants after a booster dose.[14]

Two clinical trials supported by the National Institutes of Health (NIH) have compared the anti-PRP antibody responses to three Haemophilus b conjugate vaccines in a racially mixed population of children. These studies were done in Tennessee[16] (Table 1) and in Minnesota, Missouri and Texas[17] (Table 2) in infants immunized with OmniHIB and other Haemophilus b conjugate vaccines at 2, 4 and 6 months of age. All Haemophilus b conjugate vaccines were administered concomitantly with Poliovirus Vaccine Live Oral and DTP vaccines at separate sites.
[See tables 1 and 2 below]

TABLE 1[16] ANTI-PRP ANTIBODY RESPONSES IN 2-MONTH-OLD INFANTS NIH TRIAL IN TENNESSEE

VACCINE	N*	GEOMETRIC MEAN TITER (GMT) (µg/mL)			POST THIRD IMMUNIZATION
		Pre-Immunization	Post Second Immunization	Post Third Immunization	% ≥1.0 µg/mL
PRP-T† (OmniHIB™)	65	0.10	0.30	3.64	83%
PRP-OMP¶ (PedvaxHIB®)	64	0.11	0.84	N/A	50%**
HbOC‡ (HibTITER®)	61	0.07	0.13	3.08	75%

TABLE 2[17] ANTI-PRP ANTIBODY RESPONSES IN 2-MONTH-OLD INFANTS NIH TRIAL IN MINNESOTA, MISSOURI AND TEXAS

VACCINE	N*	GEOMETRIC MEAN TITER (GMT) (µg/mL)			POST THIRD§ IMMUNIZATION
		Pre-Immunization	Post Second Immunization	Post Third§ Immunization	% ≥1.0 µg/mL
PRP-T† (OmniHIB™)	142	0.25	1.25	6.37	97%
PRP-OMP¶ (PedvaxHIB®)	149	0.18	4.00	N/A	85%**
HbOC‡ (HibTITER®)	167	0.17	0.45	6.31	90%

* N = Number of Children
§ Sera were obtained after the third dose from 86 and 110 infants, in PRP-T and HbOC vaccine groups, respectively.
† Haemophilus b Conjugate Vaccine (Tetanus Toxoid Conjugate)
¶ Haemophilus b Conjugate Vaccine (Meningococcal Protein Conjugate)
** Seroconversion after the recommended 2-dose primary immunization series is shown.
‡ Haemophilus b Conjugate Vaccine (Diphtheria CRM197 Protein Conjugate)
N/A Not applicable in this comparison trial although third dose data have been published.[16,17]

Native American populations have high rates of *H influenzae* type b disease and have been observed to have low immune responses to Haemophilus b conjugate vaccines. Following three doses of OmniHIB at six weeks, four and six months of age, 75% of Native Americans in Alaska showed an anti-PRP antibody titer of ≥1.0 µg/mL.[18]

In three U.S. trials in 12- to 15-month-old children and one trial in 17- to 24-month-old children who had not previously received Haemophilus b conjugate vaccination, a single dose of OmniHIB produced an anti-PRP antibody response comparable to those seen after three doses were administered in infants (Table 3).[18]

TABLE 3 [18] ANTI-PRP ANTIBODY RESPONSES IN
12- TO 24-MONTH-OLD CHILDREN IMMUNIZED
WITH A SINGLE DOSE OF OmniHIB

AGE GROUP	N	GMT (µg/mL)		% SUBJECTS RESPONDING WITH ≥1.0 µg/mL	
		Pre	Post	Pre	Post
12 to 15 months	256	0.06	5.12	1.6	90.2
17 to 24 months	81	0.10	4.4	3.7	81.5

These trials demonstrated that OmniHIB consistently conferred an anti-PRP antibody response previously shown to correlate with protection, when administered either as a regimen of three doses at least four to eight weeks apart in infants 2 to 6 months of age or as a single dose in children 12 months of age and older.[18]

OmniHIB has been found to be immunogenic in children with sickle cell anemia, a condition which may cause increased susceptibility to Haemophilus b disease. Two doses of OmniHIB given at two month intervals induced anti-PRP antibody titers of >1.0 µg/mL in 89% of these children with a mean age of 11 months. This is comparable to anti-PRP antibody levels demonstrated in normal children of similar age following two doses of OmniHIB.[19]

Although OmniHIB produces an antibody response to tetanus toxoid, data do not exist to substantiate the correlation of this response with protection against tetanus.
IMMUNIZATION WITH OmniHIB ALONE DOES NOT SUBSTITUTE FOR ROUTINE TETANUS IMMUNIZATION.

INDICATIONS AND USAGE

NOTE: Haemophilus b Conjugate Vaccine (Tetanus Toxoid Conjugate)—OmniHIB (distributed by SmithKline Beecham Pharmaceuticals) is identical to Haemophilus b Conjugate Vaccine (Tetanus Toxoid Conjugate)—ActHIB; both products are manufactured by Pasteur Mérieux Sérums & Vaccins S.A.

OmniHIB is indicated for the active immunization of infants and children 2 months through 5 years of age for the prevention of invasive disease caused by *H influenzae* type b.

Antibody levels associated with protection may not be achieved earlier than two weeks following the last recommended dose.
As with any vaccine, vaccination with OmniHIB may not protect 100% of susceptible individuals.

CONTRAINDICATIONS

OmniHIB IS CONTRAINDICATED IN CHILDREN WITH A HISTORY OF HYPERSENSITIVITY TO ANY COMPONENT OF THIS VACCINE, INCLUDING TETANUS TOXOID.

WARNINGS

If OmniHIB is administered to immunosuppressed persons or persons receiving immunosuppressive therapy, the expected antibody response may not be obtained. This includes patients with asymptomatic or symptomatic HIV-infection,[20] severe combined immunodeficiency, hypogammaglobulinemia, or agammaglobulinemia; altered immune states due to diseases such as leukemia, lymphoma, or generalized malignancy; or an immune system compromised by treatment with corticosteroids, alkylating drugs, antimetabolites or radiation.[21]
IMMUNIZATION WITH OmniHIB ALONE DOES NOT SUBSTITUTE FOR ROUTINE TETANUS IMMUNIZATION.

PRECAUTIONS

GENERAL
EPINEPHRINE INJECTION (1:1000) MUST BE IMMEDIATELY AVAILABLE SHOULD AN ANAPHYLACTIC OR OTHER ALLERGIC REACTION OCCUR DUE TO ANY COMPONENT OF THE VACCINE.
Prior to an injection of any vaccine, all known precautions should be taken to prevent adverse reactions. This includes a review of the patient's history with respect to possible hypersensitivity to this vaccine or similar vaccines. The

health-care provider should ask the parent or guardian about the recent health status of the infant or child to be immunized including the infant's or child's previous immunization history prior to administration of OmniHIB.
Any acute infection or febrile illness is reason for delaying use of OmniHIB except when in the opinion of the physician, withholding the vaccine entails a greater risk.
As reported with Haemophilus b polysaccharide vaccines,[22] cases of *H influenzae* type b disease may occur subsequent to vaccination and prior to the onset of protective effects of the vaccine.[18] (See INDICATIONS AND USAGE section)
Antigenuria has been detected in some instances following receipt of OmniHIB; therefore, urine antigen detection may not have definitive diagnostic value in suspected *H influenzae* type b disease within one week of immunization.[23]
Special care should be taken to ensure that OminHIB is not injected into a blood vessel.
Administration of OmniHIB is not contraindicated in individuals with an HIV infection.[21]
A separate, sterile syringe and needle or a sterile disposable unit should be used for each patient to prevent transmission of hepatitis or other infectious agents from person to person. Needles should not be recapped and should be properly disposed.

INFORMATION FOR PATIENT
The health-care provider should inform the parent or guardian of the benefits and risks of the vaccine.
The physician should inform the parent or guardian about the significant adverse reactions that have been temporally associated with OmniHIB administration. The parent or guardian should be instructed to report any serious adverse reactions to the health-care provider.
As part of the child's immunization record, the date, lot number and manufacturer of the vaccine administered should be recorded.[24,25,26]
The U.S. Department of Health and Human Services has established a new Vaccine Adverse Event Reporting System (VAERS) to accept all reports of suspected adverse events after the administration of any vaccine, including but not limited to the reporting of events required by the National Childhood Vaccine Injury Act of 1986.[24] The toll-free number for VAERS forms and information is 1-800-822-7967.
The National Vaccine Injury Compensation Program, established by the National Childhood Vaccine Injury Act of 1986, requires physicians and other health-care providers who administer vaccines to maintain permanent vaccination records and to report occurrences of certain adverse events to the U.S. Department of Health and Human Services. Reportable events include those listed in the Act for each vaccine and events specified in the package insert as contraindications to further doses of the vaccine.[25,26]
The health-care provider should inform the parent or guardian of the importance of completing the immunization series.
The health-care provider should provide the Vaccine Information Materials (VIMs) which are required to be given with each immunization.

DRUG INTERACTIONS
There are no known interactions of OmniHIB with drugs or foods.
In clinical trials, OmniHIB was routinely administered, at separate sites, concomitantly with one or more of the following vaccines: DTP vaccine, Poliovirus Vaccine Live Oral, Measles, Mumps and Rubella vaccine (MMR), Hepatitis B vaccine and occasionally Inactivated Polio Vaccine (IPV). No significant impairment of the antibody response to any antigen was observed in three clinical trials when Connaught Laboratories, Inc. (CLI) DTP vaccine was given concurrently with OmniHIB at separate sites.[18] Interference with the antibody response to the pertussis component has been suggested with a DTP vaccine unlicensed in the U.S.[27] No impairment of the antibody response to the individual antigens was demonstrated when OmniHIB was given at the same time, at separate sites, with Inactivated Polio Vaccine (IPV) or Measles, Mumps and Rubella vaccine (MMR).[18] In addition, more than 47,000 infants in Finland have received a third dose of OmniHIB concomitantly with MMR vaccine.[18]
No data are available on the antibody response to OPV or Hepatitis B vaccines when given concurrently with OmniHIB.

CARCINOGENESIS, MUTAGENESIS, IMPAIRMENT OF FERTILITY
OmniHIB has not been evaluated for its carcinogenic, mutagenic potential or impairment of fertility.

PREGNANCY
REPRODUCTIVE STUDIES—PREGNANCY CATEGORY C
Animal reproduction studies have not been conducted with OmniHIB. It is also not known whether OmniHIB can cause fetal harm when administered to a pregnant woman or can affect reproduction capacity. OmniHIB is NOT recommended for use in a pregnant woman.

PEDIATRIC USE
SAFETY AND EFFECTIVENESS OF OmniHIB IN INFANTS BELOW THE AGE OF SIX WEEKS HAVE NOT BEEN ESTABLISHED. (See DOSAGE AND ADMINISTRATION section.)

ADVERSE REACTIONS

NOTE: Haemophilus b Conjugate Vaccine (Tetanus Toxoid Conjugate)—OmniHIB (distributed by SmithKline Beecham Pharmaceuticals) is identical to Haemophilus b Conjugate Vaccine (Tetanus Toxoid Conjugate)—ActHIB; both products are manufactured by Pasteur Mérieux Sérums & Vaccins S.A.
More than 7,000 infants and young children (≤2 years of age) have received at least one dose of OmniHIB during U.S. clinical trials. Of these, 1,064 subjects 12 to 24 months of age who received OmniHIB alone reported no serious or life threatening adverse reactions.
Summarized in Table 4 are adverse reactions temporally associated with OmniHIB immunization in 188 subjects 12 to 15 months of age.[18]

TABLE 4 [18] PERCENTAGE OF 12- TO 15-MONTH-OLD
CHILDREN PRESENTING
WITH LOCAL OR SYSTEMIC
REACTIONS WITHIN THE FIRST 24 HOURS OF
IMMUNIZATION WITH OmniHIB (n=188)

REACTIONS	DOSE 1*	DOSE 2*
Local		
Pain	9.0%	6.4%
Erythema (1 to 5 cm)	24.0%	18.6%
Induration	9.6%	9.0%
Systemic		
Fever (>100.6°F)	7.4%	6.4%
Irritability	30.9%	28.2%
Lethargy	18.6%	17.0%
Anorexia	9.0%	8.5%
Rhinorrhea	24.5%	21.3%
Diarrhea	5.8%	8.5%
Vomiting	4.3%	3.7%
Cough	9.6%	4.3%

*DTP was not administered concomitantly with OmniHIB.

When OmniHIB was administered to infants at 2, 4, and 6 months of age concomitantly, at separate sites, with CLI DTP vaccine, the systemic adverse experience profile was not different from that seen when CLI DTP vaccine was administered alone.[18] *Refer to product insert for CLI whole-cell DTP.*
Adverse reactions from a U.S. multicenter trial in 2-, 4- and 6-month-old infants are summarized in Table 5. Systemic adverse reactions listed in Table 5 are more prominent than those in Table 4 because infants also received concomitant immunization with DTP.[14,18]
[See table 5 at top of next page]
In general, the rates of minor systemic reactions after OmniHIB and DTP immunization were comparable to those usually reported after DTP vaccine alone.[28,29,30,31]
Adverse reactions associated with OmniHIB generally subsided after 24 hours and usually do not persist beyond 48 hours after immunization.
In a randomized, double-blind U.S. clinical trial, OmniHIB was given concomitantly with DTP to more than 5,000 infants and hepatitis B vaccine was given with DTP to a similar number. In this large study, deaths due to sudden infant death syndrome (SIDS) and other causes were observed but were not different in the two groups. In the first 48 hours following immunization, two definite and three possible seizures were observed after OmniHIB and DTP in comparison with none after hepatitis B vaccine and DTP.[18] This rate of seizures following OmniHIB and DTP was not greater than previously reported in infants receiving DTP alone. Other adverse reactions reported with administration of other Haemophilus b conjugate vaccines include urticaria, seizures, hives, renal failure and Guillain-Barré syndrome (GBS).[18,32] A cause and effect relationship among any of these events and the vaccination has not been established.
When OmniHIB was given with DTP and inactivated poliovirus vaccine to more than 100,000 Finnish infants, the rate and extent of serious adverse reactions were not different from those seen when other Haemophilus b conjugate vaccines were evaluated in Finland (i.e. HibTITER®, ProHIBiT®).[18]

Continued on next page

Information on the SmithKline Beecham Pharmaceuticals products appearing here is based on the labeling in effect on July 31, 1998. Further information on these and other products may be obtained from the Medical Department, SmithKline Beecham Pharmaceuticals, One Franklin Plaza, Philadelphia, PA 19101.

OmniHIB—Cont.

Reporting of Adverse Events

Reporting by the parent or guardian of all adverse events occurring after vaccine administration should be encouraged. Adverse events following immunization with vaccine should be reported by the health-care provider to the U.S. Department of Health and Human Services (DHHS) Vaccine Adverse Event Reporting System (VAERS). Reporting forms and information about reporting requirements or completion of the form can be obtained from VAERS through a toll-free number 1-800-822-7967.[24,25,26]

Health-care providers also should report these events to the Director of Medical Affairs, Connaught Laboratories, Inc., Route 611, P.O. Box 187, Swiftwater, PA 18370 or call 1-800-822-2463.

DOSAGE AND ADMINISTRATION

NOTE: Haemophilus b Conjugate Vaccine (Tetanus Toxoid Conjugate)—OmniHIB (distributed by SmithKline Beecham Pharmaceuticals) is identical to Haemophilus b Conjugate Vaccine (Tetanus Toxoid Conjugate)—ActHIB; both products are manufactured by Pasteur Mérieux Sérums & Vaccins S.A.

Parenteral drug products should be inspected visually for particulate matter and/or discoloration prior to administration, whenever solution and container permit. If these conditions exist, the vaccine should not be administered.

RECONSTITUTION:

WITH DILUENT SUPPLIED: Prior to reconstitution, cleanse the vaccine vial rubber barrier with a suitable germicide and inject the entire volume of diluent contained in the syringe into the vial of lyophilized vaccine. Thorough agitation is advised to ensure complete rehydration. The entire volume of reconstituted vaccine is then drawn back into a new syringe before injection of one 0.5 mL dose. The vaccine will appear clear and colorless.

Reconstitution instructions for diluent supplied: see Figures 1, 2, and 3 below.

Administer OmniHIB intramuscularly after reconstitution with diluent supplied. (In the event of coagulation disorders, OmniHIB may be given subcutaneously in the mid-lateral aspect of the thigh.[14]) **Vaccine should be used immediately after reconstitution.**

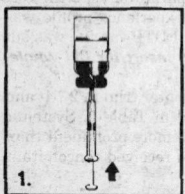

Figure 1. Insert syringe needle through the rubber barrier into the OmniHIB vial and inject 0.6 mL of diluent supplied.

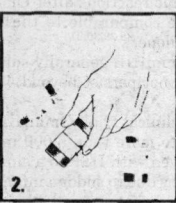

Figure 2. Agitate vial thoroughly to ensure complete reconstitution.

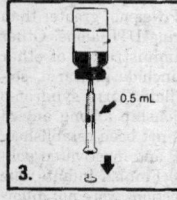

Figure 3. After reconstitution, discard syringe and withdraw total volume of reconstituted vaccine in a new syringe and administer 0.5 mL intramuscularly (or subcutaneously if coagulation disorders exist).

Each 0.5 mL dose is formulated to contain 10 µg of purified capsular polysaccharide conjugated to 24 µg of inactivated tetanus toxoid and 8.5% of sucrose.

Before injection, the skin over the site to be injected should be cleansed with a suitable germicide. After insertion of the needle, aspirate to ensure that the needle has not entered a blood vessel.

DO NOT INJECT INTRAVENOUSLY.

Each dose of OmniHIB is administered intramuscularly in the outer aspect of the vastus lateralis (mid-thigh) or deltoid. The vaccine should not be injected into the gluteal area

or areas where there may be a nerve trunk. During the course of primary immunizations, injections should not be made more than once at the same site.

OmniHIB is indicated for infants and children 2 months through 5 years of age for intramuscular administration in accordance with the schedule indicated in Table 6.[14,16]

Infants between 2 and 6 months of age should receive three 0.5 mL doses at eight week intervals, followed by a booster dose at 15 to 18 months of age. Infants 7 to 11 months of age who have not been previously immunized should receive two 0.5 mL doses at eight week intervals, followed by a booster dose at 15 to 18 months of age; children 12 to 14 months of age who have not been previously immunized should receive one 0.5 mL dose, followed by a booster dose at 15 to 18 months of age; and children 15 to 60 months of age who have not been previously immunized should receive a single 0.5 mL dose.

TABLE 6[14,16,33]

IMMUNIZATION SCHEDULE

AGE AT FIRST DOSE	PRIMARY SERIES	BOOSTER
2 to 6 months	3 Doses, 8 weeks apart	1 Dose, 15 to 18 months
7 to 11 months	2 Doses, 8 weeks apart	1 Dose, 15 to 18 months
12 to 14 months	1 Dose	1 Dose, 15 to 18 months*
15 to 60 months	1 Dose	None

* Administer vaccine not earlier than 2 months after the previous dose.

Preterm infants should be vaccinated according to their chronological age from birth.[33]

Interruption of the recommended schedule with a delay between doses should not interfere with the final immunity achieved with OmniHIB. There is no need to start the series over again, regardless of the time elapsed between doses.

No data are available to support the interchangeably of OmniHIB and ActHIB with other Haemophilus b conjugate vaccines. Therefore, it is recommended that the same conjugate vaccine be used throughout each immunization schedule, consistent with the data supporting approval and licensure of the vaccine. Since OmniHIB and ActHIB are the same vaccine these may be used interchangeably.

HOW SUPPLIED

Vial, 1 Dose, lyophilized vaccine (5 × 1 Dose vials per package), packaged with prefilled 0.6 mL Syringe containing diluent (5 × 0.6 mL syringes per package)–Product No. 0007-4408-05

Administer vaccine immediately after reconstitution.

STORAGE

Store lyophilized vaccine and prefilled syringe containing diluent between 2°-8°C (35°-46°F). DO NOT FREEZE.

REFERENCES

1. Chu CY, et al. Further studies on the immunogenicity of *Haemophilus influenzae* type b and pneumococcal type 6A polysaccharide-protein conjugate. Infect Immun 40: 245-246, 1983
2. Mueller JH, et al. Production of diphtheria toxin of high potency (100 Lf) on a reproducible medium. J Immunol 40:21-32, 1941
3. Adams WG, et al. Decline of Childhood *Haemophilus influenzae* Type b (Hib) Disease in the Hib Vaccine Era. JAMA 269: 221-226, 1993
4. Recommendations of the Immunization Practices Advisory Committee (ACIP). Haemophilus b conjugate vaccines for prevention of *Haemophilus influenzae* type b disease among infants and children two months of age and older. MMWR 40: No. RR-1, 1991
5. Broome CV. Epidemiology of *Haemophilus influenzae* type b infections in the United States. Pediatr Infect Dis J 6: 779-782, 1987
6. ACIP. Polysaccharide vaccine for prevention of *Haemophilus influenzae* type b disease. MMWR 34:201-205, 1985
7. Istre GR, et al. Risk factors for primary invasive *Haemophilus influenzae* disease: Increased risk from day care attendance and school-aged household members. J Pediatr 106:190-195, 1985
8. Redmond SR, et al. *Haemophilus influenzae* type b disease. An epidemiologic study with special reference to day-care centers. JAMA 252: 2581-2584, 1984
9. Murphy TV, et al. County-wide surveillance of invasive Haemophilus infections: Risk of associated cases in Child Care Programs (CCPs). Twenty-third Interscience Conference on Antimicrobial Agents and Chemotherapy (Abstract #788) 229, 1983
10. Fleming D, et al. *Haemophilus influenzae* b (Hib) disease-secondary spread in day care. Twenty-fourth Interscience Conference on Antimicrobial Agents and Chemotherapy (Abstract #967) 261, 1984
11. CDC. Prevention of secondary cases of *Haemophilus influenzae* type b disease. MMWR 31: 672-680, 1982
12. Michaels RH, et al. Pharyngeal colonization with *Haemophilus influenzae* type b: A longitudinal study of families with a child with meningitis or epiglottitis due to *H. influenzae* type b. J Infec Dis 136: 222-227, 1977
13. Holmes SJ, et al. Immunogenicity of four *Haemophilus influenzae* type b conjugate vaccines in 17- to 19-month-old children. J Pediatr 118: 364-371, 1991
14. Data on file, Pasteur Mérieux Sérums & Vaccins S.A.
15. Peltola H, et al. Prevention of *Haemophilus influenzae* type b bacteremic infections with the capsular polysaccharide vaccine. N Engl J Med 310: 1561-1566, 1984
16. Decker MD, et al. Comparative trial in infants of four conjugate *Haemophilus influenzae* type b vaccines. J Pediatr 120:184-189, 1992
17. Granoff DM, et al. Differences in the immunogenicity of three *Haemophilus influenzae* type b conjugate vaccines in infants. J Pediatr 121:187-194, 1992
18. Data on file, Connaught Laboratories, Inc.
19. Kaplan SL, et al. Immunogenicity of *Haemophilus influenzae* type b, polysaccharide-tetanus protein conjugate vaccine in children with sickle hemoglobinopathy or malignancies, and after systemic *Haemophilus influenzae* type b infection. J Pediatr 120:367-370, 1992
20. Steinhoff MC, et al. Antibody responses to *Haemophilus influenzae* type b vaccines in men with human immuno-deficiency virus infection. N Engl J Med 325 (26): 1837-1842, 1991
21. ACIP. General recommendations on immunization. MMWR 38: 205-227, 1989

TABLE 5[14] PERCENTAGE OF INFANTS PRESENTING WITH LOCAL OR SYSTEMIC REACTIONS AT 6, 24, AND 48 HOURS OF IMMUNIZATION WITH OmniHIB ADMINISTERED SIMULTANEOUSLY, AT SEPARATE SITES, WITH CLI DTP VACCINE

REACTION	2 Months (n=365) 6 Hrs.	24 Hrs.	48 Hrs.	4 Months (n=364) 6 Hrs.	24 Hrs.	48 Hrs.	6 Months (n=365) 6 Hrs.	24 Hrs.	48 Hrs.
Local§									
Tenderness	46.3%	11.5%	2.2%	23.4%	7.4%	1.1%	19.2%	6.0%	1.1%
Erythema	14.3%	4.1%	0.3%@	8.8%	5.8%	0.6%	11.5%	6.9%	1.6%
Induration	22.5%	6.3%	1.9%	12.4%	4.7%	0.8%	9.6%	3.8%	1.1%
Systemic*									
Fever >100.8°F†	20.1%	1.3%	0.6%	14.6%	6.6%	1.4%	15.7%	8.8%	0.8%
Irritability	72.6%	21.9%	12.6%	48.4%	25.0%	13.2%	44.1%	25.2%	10.1%
Drowsiness	57.5%	29.9%	10.4%	44.2%	18.1%	7.4%	32.6%	13.4%	2.5%
Anorexia	15.3%	5.8%	4.9%	8.0%	5.0%	3.0%	5.5%	4.9%	2.2%
Diarrhea	4.4%	6.6%	5.2%	5.0%	4.7%	4.7%	4.7%	6.3%	3.6%
Vomiting	2.7%	4.1%	2.7%	2.5%	3.3%	2.8%	2.2%	2.7%	1.9%
Persistent Crying	Percentage of infants within 72 hours after immunization was 1.6% after dose one, 0.6% after dose two, and 0.3% after dose three.								

§ Local reactions were evaluated at the OmniHIB injection site.
* The adverse reaction profile is defined by the concomitant use of CLI DTP vaccine.
† The number of individuals observed at each time point for fever varied from 357 to 363.

22. FDA Workshop on Haemophilus b Polysaccharide Vaccine-A Preliminary Report. MMWR 36: 529-531, 1987
23. Rothstein EP, et al. Comparison of antigenuria after immunization with three *Haemophilus influenzae* type b conjugate vaccines. Pediatr Infect Dis J 10: 311-314, 1991
24. Vaccine Adverse Event Reporting System-United States. MMWR 39: 730-733, 1990
25. CDC. National Childhood Vaccine Injury Act: Requirements for permanent vaccination records and for reporting of selected events after vaccination. MMWR 37: 197-200, 1988
26. National Childhood Vaccine Injury Act of 1986 (Amended 1987)
27. Clemens JD, et al. Impact of *Haemophilus influenzae* Type b Polysaccharide-Tetanus Protein Conjugate Vaccine on responses to concurrently administered Diphtheria-Tetanus-Pertussis Vaccine. JAMA 267: 673-678, 1992
28. Cody CL, et al. Nature and rates of adverse reactions associated with DTP and DT immunizations in infants and children. Pediatr 68: 650-660, 1981
29. Barkin RM, et al. Diphtheria-tetanus-pertussis vaccine: reactogenicity of commercial products. Pediatr 63: 256-260, 1979
30. Baraff LJ, et al. DTP-associated reactions: an analysis by injection site, manufacturer, prior reactions and dose. Pediatr 73: 31-39, 1984
31. Long SS, et al. Longitudinal study of adverse reactions following diphtheria-tetanus-pertussis vaccine in infancy. Pediatr 85: 294-302, 1990
32. D'Cruz OF, et al. Acute inflammatory demyelinating polyradiculoneuropathy (Guillain-Barré Syndrome) after immunization with *Haemophilus influenzae* type b conjugate vaccine. J Pediatr 115: 743-746, 1989
33. Report on the Committee on Infectious Diseases. American Academy of Pediatrics. Twenty-second Edition, 1991

A.H.F.S. Category 80:12
Manufactured by
PASTEUR MÉRIEUX Sérums & Vaccins S.A.
Lyon, France U.S. License No. 384
Distributed by
SmithKline Beecham Pharmaceuticals
Philadelphia, PA 19101
Veterans Administration/Military/PHS—Vial, 0.5 mL, 5's, 6505-01-371-1161.
OM:L1

Shown in Product Identification Guide, page 339

ORNADE® SPANSULE® CAPSULES ℞

[*or 'naid*]
brand of sustained release capsules

DESCRIPTION

Ornade is a combination of an oral nasal decongestant and an antihistamine.

Each *Ornade* Spansule capsule contains phenylpropanolamine hydrochloride, 75 mg and chlorpheniramine maleate, 12 mg. Inactive ingredients consist of benzyl alcohol, cetylpyridinium chloride, FD&C Blue No. 1, FD&C Red No. 3, FD&C Yellow No. 6, D&C Red No. 27, D&C Red No. 30, gelatin, glyceryl distearate, iron oxide, polyethylene glycol, povidone, silicon dioxide, sodium lauryl sulfate, starch, sucrose, titanium dioxide, wax and trace amounts of other inactive ingredients.

Each *Ornade* Spansule capsule is so prepared that an initial dose is released promptly and the remaining medication is released gradually over a prolonged period.

CLINICAL PHARMACOLOGY

Phenylpropanolamine Hydrochloride

Phenylpropanolamine hydrochloride is a sympathomimetic agent which is closely related to ephedrine in chemical structure and pharmacologic action, but produces less central nervous system stimulation than ephedrine. It is a vasoconstrictor with decongestant action on nasal and upper respiratory tract mucosal membranes.

Chlorpheniramine Maleate

Chlorpheniramine maleate is an antihistamine with anticholinergic (drying) and sedative side effects. Antihistamines appear to compete with histamine for H_1 cell receptor sites on effector cells.

Pharmacokinetics

A single *Ornade* Spansule capsule produces blood levels comparable to those produced by administration of three 25 mg doses of phenylpropanolamine hydrochloride and three 4 mg doses of chlorpheniramine maleate in conventional release form given at 4-hour intervals. At steady-state conditions, the following peak levels are reached after the oral administration of an *Ornade* Spansule capsule: 21 ng/mL chlorpheniramine maleate in 7.7 hours; 173 ng/mL phenylpropanolamine hydrochloride in 6.1 hours; under these circumstances, the half-lives are approximately 21 and 7 hours, respectively.

INDICATIONS AND USAGE

For the treatment of the symptoms of seasonal and perennial allergic rhinitis and vasomotor rhinitis, including nasal obstruction (congestion); also for the treatment of runny nose, sneezing and nasal congestion associated with the common cold.

CONTRAINDICATIONS

Hypersensitivity to either phenylpropanolamine hydrochloride or chlorpheniramine maleate and other antihistamines of similar chemical structure; severe hypertension; coronary artery disease.

This drug should NOT be used in newborn or premature infants.

Because of the higher risk of antihistamines for infants generally, and for newborns and prematures in particular, antihistamine therapy is contraindicated in nursing mothers.

As with any product containing a sympathomimetic, *Ornade* Spansule capsules should NOT be used in patients taking monoamine oxidase (MAO) inhibitors.

WARNINGS

Ornade Spansule capsules may potentiate the effects of alcohol and other CNS depressants. Also, this product should not be taken simultaneously with other products containing phenylpropanolamine hydrochloride or amphetamines.

Ornade Spansule capsules should be used with considerable caution in patients with narrow-angle glaucoma, stenosing peptic ulcer, pyloroduodenal obstruction, symptomatic prostatic hypertrophy, or bladder neck obstruction.

Use in Children: In infants and children, especially, antihistamines in *overdosage* may cause hallucinations, convulsions, or death. As in adults, antihistamines may diminish mental alertness in children. In the young child, particularly, they may produce excitation.

Use in the Elderly (approximately 60 years or older): Antihistamines are more likely to cause dizziness, sedation and hypotension in elderly patients.

PRECAUTIONS

General: Use with caution in patients with lower respiratory disease including asthma, hypertension, cardiovascular disease, hyperthyroidism, increased intraocular pressure, or diabetes.

Information for Patients: Caution patients about activities requiring alertness (e.g., operating vehicles or machinery). Also caution patients about the possible additive effects of alcohol and other CNS depressants (hypnotics, sedatives, tranquilizers, etc.), and not to take simultaneously other products containing phenylpropanolamine hydrochloride or amphetamines. Patients should not take *Ornade* Spansule capsules in conjunction with a monoamine oxidase inhibitor or an oral anticoagulant.

Drug Interactions: *Ornade* Spansule capsules may interact with alcohol and other CNS depressants to potentiate their effects.

This product may have additive effects when taken simultaneously with other products containing phenylpropanolamine hydrochloride or amphetamines.

MAO inhibitors prolong and intensify the anticholinergic (drying) effects of antihistamines and potentiate the pressor effects of sympathomimetics such as phenylpropanolamine hydrochloride (see CONTRAINDICATIONS).

Phenylpropanolamine hydrochloride should not be used with ganglionic blocking drugs—such as mecamylamine—which potentiate reactions of sympathomimetics. It also should not be used with adrenergic blocking drugs, such as guanethidine sulfate or bethanidine, since it antagonizes the hypotensive action of these drugs.

The action of oral anticoagulants may be inhibited by antihistamines.

The CNS depressant and atropine-like effects of anticholinergics may be potentiated by concomitant administration of antihistamines. Concomitant administration of anticholinergics such as trihexyphenidyl, and other drugs with anticholinergic action (such as imipramine), with antihistamines may result in xerostomia.

β-adrenergic blockers may be antagonized by antihistamines.

Concomitant administration of corticosteroids and antihistamines may decrease the effects of the corticosteroids by enzyme induction.

Antihistamines inhibit norepinephrine reuptake by tissues and therefore potentiate the cardiovascular effects of norepinephrine.

Concomitant use of antihistamines with phenothiazines may produce an additive CNS depressant effect; concomitant use also may cause urinary retention or glaucoma.

Carcinogenesis, Mutagenesis, Impairment of Fertility: A long-term oncogenic study in rats with the chlorpheniramine maleate component of *Ornade* Spansule capsules did not produce an increase in the incidence of tumors in the drug-treated groups, as compared with the controls. No evidence of mutagenicity was found when chlorpheniramine maleate was evaluated in a battery of mutagenic studies, including the Ames test.

In an early study in rats with chlorpheniramine maleate a reduction in fertility was observed in female rats at doses approximately 67 times the human dose. More recent studies in rabbits and rats, using more appropriate methodology and doses up to approximately 50 and 85 times the human dose, showed no reduction in fertility.

There are no studies available which indicate whether phenylpropanolamine hydrochloride has carcinogenic or mutagenic effects or impairs fertility.

Pregnancy, Teratogenic Effects, Pregnancy Category B: Reproduction studies have been performed with the components of *Ornade* Spansule capsules. Studies with chlorpheniramine maleate in rabbits and rats at doses up to 50 times and 85 times the human dose, respectively, revealed no evidence of harm to the fetus. A study with phenylpropanolamine hydrochloride in rats at doses up to 7 times the human dose revealed no evidence of harm to the fetus. There are, however, no adequate and well-controlled studies in pregnant women. Because animal reproduction studies are not always predictive of human response, *Ornade* Spansule capsules should be used during pregnancy only if clearly needed.

Nonteratogenic Effects: Studies of chlorpheniramine maleate in rats showed a decrease in the postnatal survival rate of offspring of animals dosed with 33 and 67 times the human dose.

Nursing Mothers: Small amounts of antihistamines are excreted in breast milk. Because of the higher risk with antihistamines in infants generally, and for newborns and prematures in particular, *Ornade* Spansule capsules should not be administered to a nursing mother (see CONTRAINDICATIONS).

Pediatric Use: The safety and effectiveness of *Ornade* Spansule capsules in children under 12 years of age have not been established.

In infants and children, especially, antihistamines in *overdosage* may cause hallucinations, convulsions, or death.

As in adults, antihistamines may diminish mental alertness in children. In the young child, particularly, they may produce excitation. (See WARNINGS.)

ADVERSE REACTIONS

The following adverse reactions have been reported following the use of antihistamines and/or sympathomimetic amines:

General: Anaphylactic shock; chills; drug rash; excessive dryness of mouth, nose and throat; increased intraocular pressure; excessive perspiration; photosensitivity; urticaria; weakness.

Cardiovascular System: Angina pain; extrasystoles; headache; hypertension; hypotension; palpitations; tachycardia.

Hematologic: Agranulocytosis; hemolytic anemia; leukopenia; thrombocytopenia.

Nervous System: Blurred vision; confusion; convulsions; diplopia; disturbed coordination; dizziness; drowsiness; euphoria; excitation; fatigue; hysteria; insomnia; irritability; acute labyrinthitis; nervousness; neuritis; paresthesia; restlessness; sedation; tinnitus; tremor; vertigo.

GI System: Abdominal pain; anorexia; constipation; diarrhea; epigastric distress; nausea; vomiting.

GU System: Dysuria; early menses; urinary frequency; urinary retention.

Respiratory System: Thickening of bronchial secretions; tightness of chest and wheezing; nasal stuffiness.

OVERDOSAGE

In the event of overdosage, emergency treatment should be started immediately.

Symptoms: Effects of antihistamine overdosage may vary from central nervous system depression (sedation, apnea, diminished mental alertness, cardiovascular collapse) to stimulation (insomnia, hallucinations, tremors, or convulsions) to death.

Other signs and symptoms may be dizziness, tinnitus, ataxia, blurred vision and hypotension. Stimulation is particularly likely in children, as are atropine-like signs and symptoms (dry mouth; fixed, dilated pupils; flushing; hyperthermia; and gastrointestinal symptoms). In large doses, sympathomimetics may cause giddiness, headache, nausea, vomiting, sweating, thirst, tachycardia, precordial pain, palpitations, difficulty in micturition, muscular weakness and tenseness, anxiety, restlessness and insomnia. Many patients can present a toxic psychosis with delusions and hal-

Continued on next page

Information on the SmithKline Beecham Pharmaceuticals products appearing here is based on the labeling in effect on July 31, 1998. Further information on these and other products may be obtained from the Medical Department, SmithKline Beecham Pharmaceuticals, One Franklin Plaza, Philadelphia, PA 19101.

Ornade Spansule—Cont.

lucinations. Some may develop cardiac arrhythmias, circulatory collapse, convulsions, coma and respiratory failure.

Toxicity: In acute oral toxicity tests in rats, the LD_{50} for the ratio of 75 mg phenylpropanolamine hydrochloride and 12 mg chlorpheniramine maleate was 774.2 mg/kg; in mice, the LD_{50} for the formulation was 757.4 mg/kg.

Treatment: The patient should be induced to vomit even if emesis has occurred spontaneously. Pharmacologically induced vomiting by the administration of ipecac syrup is a preferred method. But vomiting should not be induced in patients with impaired consciousness. The action of ipecac is facilitated by physical activity and by the administration of 8 to 12 fluid ounces of water. If emesis does not occur within 15 minutes, the dose of ipecac should be repeated. Precautions against aspiration must be taken, especially in infants and children.

Following emesis, any drug remaining in the stomach may be adsorbed by activated charcoal administered as a slurry with water. If vomiting is unsuccessful or contraindicated, gastric lavage should be performed. Isotonic and one-half isotonic saline are the lavage solutions of choice. Since much of the *Spansule* capsule medication is coated for gradual release, saline cathartics should be administered to hasten evacuation of pellets that have not already released medication. Saline cathartics, such as milk of magnesia, draw water into the bowel by osmosis and therefore may be valuable for their action in rapid dilution of bowel content. Dialysis has not been reported to be effective in the treatment of phenylpropanolamine hydrochloride and chlorpheniramine maleate overdosage. After emergency treatment, the patient should continue to be medically monitored.

Treatment of the signs and symptoms of overdosage is symptomatic and supportive. *Stimulants* (analeptic agents) should *not* be used. Vasopressors may be used to treat hypotension. Short-acting barbiturates, diazepam, or paraldehyde may be administered to control seizures. Hyperpyrexia, especially in children, may require treatment with tepid water sponge baths or a hypothermic blanket. Apnea is treated with ventilatory support.

DOSAGE AND ADMINISTRATION

Adults and children 12 years of age and over—one capsule every 12 hours.

Ornade Spansule capsules are not recommended in children under 12.

HOW SUPPLIED

In gelatin capsules with opaque red cap and natural body. Each capsule is imprinted with the product name ORNADE and SB, and filled with small red, white and gray pellets; in bottles of 50 and 500 capsules, and in Single Unit Packages of 100 capsules (intended for institutional use only). Each capsule contains 75 mg phenylpropanolamine hydrochloride and 12 mg chlorpheniramine maleate. Capsules should be stored between 15° and 30°C (59° and 86°F).

NDC 0007-4421-15 50's

NDC 0007-4421-25 500's

WARNING: Manufactured with carbon tetrachloride and methyl chloroform, substances which harm public health and environment by destroying ozone in the upper atmosphere.

Veterans Administration/Military/PHS—*Spansule* capsules, 500's, 6505-01-108-9574.

OR:L42

Shown in Product Identification Guide, page 339

PARNATE® ℞

[pahr 'naight]

brand of tranylcypromine sulfate

Tablets 10 mg

Before prescribing, the physician should be familiar with the entire contents of this prescribing information.

DESCRIPTION

Chemically, tranylcypromine sulfate is (±)-*trans* -2-phenylcyclopropylamine sulfate (2:1).

Each round, rose-red, film-coated tablet is imprinted with the product name PARNATE and SKF and contains tranylcypromine sulfate equivalent to 10 mg of tranylcypromine. Inactive ingredients consist of cellulose, citric acid, croscarmellose sodium, D&C Red No. 7, FD&C Blue No. 2, FD&C Red No. 40, FD&C Yellow No. 6, gelatin, iron oxide, lactose, magnesium stearate, talc, titanium dioxide and trace amounts of other inactive ingredients.

NOTE: Parnate (tranylcypromine sulfate) tablets have been changed from rose-red sugar-coated tablets to rose-red film-coated tablets. The film-coated tablets differ in size from the sugar-coated tablets, but the drug content remains unchanged.

ACTION

Tranylcypromine is a non-hydrazine monoamine oxidase inhibitor with a rapid onset of activity. It increases the concentration of epinephrine, norepinephrine, and serotonin in storage sites throughout the nervous system and, in theory, this increased concentration of monoamines in the brain stem is the basis for its antidepressant activity. When tranylcypromine is withdrawn, monoamine oxidase activity is recovered in 3 to 5 days, although the drug is excreted in 24 hours.

INDICATIONS

For the treatment of Major Depressive Episode Without Melancholia.

Parnate (tranylcypromine sulfate) should be used in adult patients who can be closely supervised. It should rarely be the first antidepressant drug given. Rather, the drug is suited for patients who have failed to respond to the drugs more commonly administered for depression.

The effectiveness of *Parnate* has been established in adult outpatients, most of whom had a depressive illness which would correspond to a diagnosis of Major Depressive Episode Without Melancholia. As described in the American Psychiatric Association's Diagnostic and Statistical Manual, third edition (DSM III), Major Depressive Episode implies a prominent and relatively persistent (nearly every day for at least 2 weeks) depressed or dysphoric mood that usually interferes with daily functioning and includes at least 4 of the following 8 symptoms: change in appetite, change in sleep, psychomotor agitation or retardation, loss of interest in usual activities or decrease in sexual drive, increased fatigability, feelings of guilt or worthlessness, slowed thinking or impaired concentration and suicidal ideation or attempts.

The effectiveness of *Parnate* in patients who meet the criteria for Major Depressive Episode with Melancholia (endogenous features) has not been established.

SUMMARY OF CONTRAINDICATIONS

Parnate (tranylcypromine sulfate) should not be administered in combination with any of the following: MAO inhibitors or dibenzazepine derivatives; sympathomimetics (including amphetamines); some central nervous system depressants (including narcotics and alcohol); antihypertensive, diuretic, antihistaminic, sedative or anesthetic drugs; bupropion HCl; buspirone HCl; dextromethorphan; cheese or other foods with a high tyramine content; or excessive quantities of caffeine.

Parnate (tranylcypromine sulfate) should not be administered to any patient with a confirmed or suspected cerebrovascular defect or to any patient with cardiovascular disease, hypertension or history of headache.

(For complete discussion of contraindications and warnings, see below.)

CONTRAINDICATIONS

Parnate (tranylcypromine sulfate) is contraindicated:

1. In patients with cerebrovascular defects or cardiovascular disorders

Parnate should not be administered to any patient with a confirmed or suspected cerebrovascular defect or to any patient with cardiovascular disease or hypertension.

2. In the presence of pheochromocytoma

Parnate should not be used in the presence of pheochromocytoma since such tumors secrete pressor substances.

3. In combination with MAO inhibitors or with dibenzazepine-related entities

Parnate (tranylcypromine sulfate) should not be administered together or in rapid succession with other MAO inhibitors or with dibenzazepine-related entities. Hypertensive crises or severe convulsive seizures may occur in patients receiving such combinations.

In patients being transferred to *Parnate* from another MAO inhibitor or from a dibenzazepine-related entity, allow a medication-free interval of at least a week, then initiate *Parnate* using half the normal starting dosage for at least the first week of therapy. Similarly, at least a week should elapse between the discontinuance of *Parnate* and the administration of another MAO inhibitor or a dibenzazepine-related entity, or the readministration of *Parnate*.

The following list includes some other MAO inhibitors, dibenzazepine-related entities and tricyclic antidepressants, and the companies which market them.

Other MAO Inhibitors

Generic Name	Trademark
Furazolidone	Furoxone® (Roberts Laboratories)
Isocarboxazid	Marplan® (Roche Laboratories)
Pargyline HCl	Eutonyl® (Abbott Laboratories)
Pargyline HCl and methyclothiazide	Eutron® (Abbott Laboratories)
Phenelzine sulfate	Nardil® (Parke-Davis)
Procarbazine HCl	Matulane® (Roche Laboratories)

Dibenzazepine-Related and Other Tricyclics

Generic Name	Trademark
Amitriptyline HCl	Elavil® (Zeneca)
	Endep® (Roche Products)
Perphenazine and amitriptyline HCl	Etrafon® (Schering)
	Triavil® (Merck and Co.)
Clomipramine hydrochloride	Anafranil® (CibaGeneva)
Desipramine HCl	Norpramin® (Marion Merrell Dow)
	Pertofrane® (Rhône-Poulenc Rorer Pharmaceuticals)
Imipramine HCl	Janimine® (Abbott Laboratories)
	Tofranil® (CibaGeneva)
Nortriptyline HCl	Aventyl® (Eli Lilly & Co.)
	Pamelor® (Sandoz)
Protriptyline HCl	Vivactil® (Merck and Co.)
Doxepin HCl	Adapin® (Fisons)
	Sinequan® (Roerig)
Carbamazepine	Tegretol® (CibaGeneva)
Cyclobenzaprine HCl	Flexeril® (Merck and Co.)
Amoxapine	Asendin™ (Lederle)
Maprotiline HCl	Ludiomil® (CibaGeneva)
Trimipramine maleate	Surmontil® (Wyeth-Ayerst Laboratories)

4. In combination with bupropion

The concurrent administration of a MAO inhibitor and bupropion hydrochloride (Wellbutrin®, Burroughs Wellcome) is contraindicated. At least 14 days should elapse between discontinuation of a MAO inhibitor and initiation of treatment with bupropion hydrochloride.

5. In combination with dexfenfluramine hydrochloride

Because Redux (dexfenfluramine hydrochloride, Wyeth) is a serotonin releaser and reuptake inhibitor, it should not be used concomitantly with Parnate (tranylcypromine sulfate).

6. In combination with selective serotonin reuptake inhibitors (SSRIs)

As a general rule, *Parnate* should not be administered in combination with any SSRI. There have been reports of serious, sometimes fatal, reactions (including hyperthermia, rigidity, myoclonus, autonomic instability with possible rapid fluctuations of vital signs, and mental status changes that include extreme agitation progressing to delirium and coma) in patients receiving fluoxetine (Prozac®, Lilly) in combination with a monoamine oxidase inhibitor (MAOI), and in patients who have recently discontinued fluoxetine and are then started on a MAOI. Some cases presented with features resembling neuroleptic malignant syndrome. Therefore, fluoxetine and other SSRIs should not be used in combination with a MAOI, or within 14 days of discontinuing therapy with a MAOI. Since fluoxetine and its major metabolite have very long elimination half-lives, at least 5 weeks should be allowed after stopping fluoxetine before starting a MAOI.

At least 2 weeks should be allowed after stopping sertraline (Zoloft®, Roerig) or paroxetine (Paxil®, SmithKline Beecham Pharmaceuticals) before starting a MAOI.

7. In combination with buspirone

Parnate (tranylcypromine sulfate) should not be used in combination with buspirone HCl (BuSpar®, Bristol-Myers Squibb), since several cases of elevated blood pressure have been reported in patients taking MAO inhibitors who were then given buspirone HCl. At least 10 days should elapse between the discontinuation of *Parnate* and the institution of buspirone HCl.

8. In combination with sympathomimetics

Parnate (tranylcypromine sulfate) should not be administered in combination with sympathomimetics, including amphetamines, and over-the-counter drugs such as cold, hay fever or weight-reducing preparations that contain vasoconstrictors.

During *Parnate* therapy, it appears that certain patients are particularly vulnerable to the effects of sympathomimetics when the activity of certain enzymes is inhibited. Use of sympathomimetics and compounds such as guanethidine, methyldopa, reserpine, dopamine, levodopa and tryptophan with *Parnate* may precipitate hypertension, headache and related symptoms. In addition, use with tryptophan may precipitate disorientation, memory impairment and other neurologic and behavioral signs.

9. In combination with meperidine

Do not use meperidine concomitantly with MAO inhibitors or within 2 or 3 weeks following MAOI therapy. Serious reactions have been precipitated with concomitant use, including coma, severe hypertension or hypotension, severe respiratory depression, convulsions, malignant hyperpyrexia, excitation, peripheral vascular collapse and death. It is thought that these reactions may be mediated by accumulation of 5-HT (serotonin) consequent to MAO inhibition.

10. In combination with dextromethorphan

The combination of MAO inhibitors and dextromethorphan has been reported to cause brief episodes of psychosis or bizarre behavior.

11. In combination with cheese or other foods with a high tyramine content

Hypertensive crises have sometimes occurred during *Parnate* therapy after ingestion of foods with a high tyramine content. In general, the patient should avoid protein foods in which aging or protein breakdown is used to increase flavor. In particular, patients should be instructed not to take foods such as cheese (particularly strong or aged varieties), sour cream, Chianti wine, sherry, beer (including nonalcoholic beer), liqueurs, pickled herring, anchovies, caviar, liver, canned figs, dried fruits (raisins, prunes, etc.) bananas, raspberries, avocados, overripe fruit, chocolate, soy sauce, sauerkraut, the pods of broad beans (fava beans), yeast extracts, yogurt, meat extracts or meat prepared with tenderizers.

12. In patients undergoing elective surgery

Patients taking *Parnate* should not undergo elective surgery requiring general anesthesia. Also, they should not be given cocaine or local anesthesia containing sympathomimetic vasoconstrictors. The possible combined hypotensive effects of *Parnate* and spinal anesthesia should be kept in mind. *Parnate* should be discontinued at least 10 days prior to elective surgery.

ADDITIONAL CONTRAINDICATIONS

In general, the physician should bear in mind the possibility of a lowered margin of safety when Parnate (tranylcypromine sulfate) is administered in combination with potent drugs.

1. *Parnate* should not be used in combination with some central nervous system depressants such as narcotics and alcohol, or with hypotensive agents. A marked potentiating effect on these classes of drugs has been reported.

2. Anti-parkinsonism drugs should be used with caution in patients receiving *Parnate* since severe reactions have been reported.

3. *Parnate* should not be used in patients with a history of liver disease or in those with abnormal liver function tests.

4. Excessive use of caffeine in any form should be avoided in patients receiving *Parnate*.

WARNING TO PHYSICIANS

Parnate (tranylcypromine sulfate) is a potent agent with the capability of producing serious side effects. *Parnate* is not recommended in those depressive reactions where other antidepressant drugs may be effective. **It should be reserved for patients who can be closely supervised and who have not responded satisfactorily to the drugs more commonly administered for depression.**

Before prescribing, the physician should be completely familiar with the full material on dosage, side effects and contraindications on these pages, with the principles of MAO inhibitor therapy and the side effects of this class of drugs. Also, the physician should be familiar with the symptomatology of mental depressions and alternate methods of treatment to aid in the careful selection of patients for *Parnate* therapy. In depressed patients, the possibility of suicide should always be considered and adequate precautions taken.

Pregnancy Warning: Use of any drug in pregnancy, during lactation or in women of childbearing age requires that the potential benefits of the drug be weighed against its possible hazards to mother and child.

Animal reproductive studies show that *Parnate* passes through the placental barrier into the fetus of the rat, and into the milk of the lactating dog. The absence of a harmful action of *Parnate* on fertility or on postnatal development by either prenatal treatment or from the milk of treated animals has not been demonstrated. Tranylcypromine is excreted in human milk.

WARNING TO THE PATIENT

Patients should be instructed to report promptly the occurrence of headache or other unusual symptoms, i.e., palpitation and/or tachycardia, a sense of constriction in the throat or chest, sweating, dizziness, neck stiffness, nausea or vomiting.

Patients should be warned against eating the foods listed in Section 11 under Contraindications while on Parnate (tranylcypromine sulfate) therapy. Also, they should be told not to drink alcoholic beverages. The patient should also be warned about the possibility of hypotension and faintness, as well as drowsiness sufficient to impair performance of potentially hazardous tasks such as driving a car or operating machinery.

Patients should also be cautioned not to take concomitant medications, whether prescription or over-the-counter drugs such as cold, hay fever or weight-reducing preparations, without the advice of a physician. They should be advised not to consume excessive amounts of caffeine in any form. Likewise, they should inform other physicians, and their dentist, about their use of *Parnate*.

WARNINGS

HYPERTENSIVE CRISES: The most important reaction associated with Parnate (tranylcypromine sulfate) is the occurrence of hypertensive crises which have sometimes been fatal.

These crises are characterized by some or all of the following symptoms: occipital headache which may radiate frontally, palpitation, neck stiffness or soreness, nausea or vomiting, sweating (sometimes with fever and sometimes with cold, clammy skin) and photophobia. Either tachycardia or bradycardia may be present, and associated constricting chest pain and dilated pupils may occur. **Intracranial bleeding, sometimes fatal in outcome, has been reported in association with the paradoxical increase in blood pressure.** In all patients taking *Parnate* blood pressure should be followed closely to detect evidence of any pressor response. It is emphasized that full reliance should not be placed on blood pressure readings, but that the patient should also be observed frequently.

Therapy should be discontinued immediately upon the occurrence of palpitation or frequent headaches during *Parnate* therapy. These signs may be prodromal of a hypertensive crisis.

Important:
Recommended treatment in
hypertensive crises

If a hypertensive crisis occurs, Parnate (tranylcypromine sulfate) should be discontinued and therapy to lower blood pressure should be instituted immediately. Headache tends to abate as blood pressure is lowered. On the basis of present evidence, phentolamine (available as Regitine®*) is recommended. (The dosage reported for phentolamine is 5 mg I.V.) Care should be taken to administer this drug slowly in order to avoid producing an excessive hypotensive effect. Fever should be managed by means of external cooling. Other symptomatic and supportive measures may be desirable in particular cases. Do not use parenteral reserpine.

PRECAUTIONS
Hypotension

Hypotension has been observed during Parnate (tranylcypromine sulfate) therapy. Symptoms of postural hypotension are seen most commonly but not exclusively in patients with pre-existent hypertension; blood pressure usually returns rapidly to pretreatment levels upon discontinuation of the drug. At doses above 30 mg daily, postural hypotension is a major side effect and may result in syncope. Dosage increases should be made more gradually in patients showing a tendency toward hypotension at the beginning of therapy. Postural hypotension may be relieved by having the patient lie down until blood pressure returns to normal.

Also, when *Parnate* is combined with those phenothiazine derivatives or other compounds known to cause hypotension, the possibility of additive hypotensive effects should be considered.

OTHER PRECAUTIONS

There have been reports of drug dependency in patients using doses of tranylcypromine significantly in excess of the therapeutic range. Some of these patients had a history of previous substance abuse. The following withdrawal symptoms have been reported: restlessness, anxiety, depression, confusion, hallucinations, headache, weakness and diarrhea.

Drugs which lower the seizure threshold, including MAO inhibitors, should not be used with Amipaque®†. As with other MAO inhibitors, Parnate (tranylcypromine sulfate) should be discontinued at least 48 hours before myelography and should not be resumed for at least 24 hours postprocedure.

In depressed patients, the possibility of suicide should always be considered and adequate precautions taken. Exclusive reliance on drug therapy to prevent suicidal attempts is unwarranted, as there may be a delay in the onset of therapeutic effect or an increase in anxiety and agitation. Also, some patients fail to respond to drug therapy or may respond only temporarily.

MAO inhibitors may have the capacity to suppress anginal pain that would otherwise serve as a warning of myocardial ischemia.

The usual precautions should be observed in patients with impaired renal function since there is a possibility of cumulative effects in such patients.

Older patients may suffer more morbidity than younger patients during and following an episode of hypertension or malignant hyperthermia. Older patients have less compensatory reserve to cope with any serious adverse reaction. Therefore, *Parnate* should be used with caution in the elderly population.

Although excretion of *Parnate* is rapid, inhibition of MAO may persist up to 10 days following discontinuation.

Because the influence of *Parnate* on the convulsive threshold is variable in animal experiments, suitable precautions should be taken if epileptic patients are treated.

Some MAO inhibitors have contributed to hypoglycemic episodes in diabetic patients receiving insulin or oral hypoglycemic agents. Therefore, *Parnate* should be used with caution in diabetics using these drugs.

Parnate may aggravate coexisting symptoms in depression, such as anxiety and agitation.

Use Parnate (tranylcypromine sulfate) with caution in hyperthyroid patients because of their increased sensitivity to pressor amines.

Parnate should be administered with caution to patients receiving Antabuse®‡. In a single study, rats given high intraperitoneal doses of *d* or *l* isomers of tranylcypromine sulfate plus disulfiram experienced severe toxicity including convulsions and death. Additional studies in rats given high oral doses of racemic tranylcypromine sulfate (*Parnate*) and disulfiram produced no adverse interaction.

ADVERSE REACTIONS

Overstimulation which may include increased anxiety, agitation and manic symptoms is usually evidence of excessive therapeutic action. Dosage should be reduced, or a phenothiazine tranquilizer should be administered concomitantly. Patients may experience restlessness or insomnia; may notice some weakness, drowsiness, episodes of dizziness or dry mouth; or may report nausea, diarrhea, abdominal pain or constipation. Most of these effects can be relieved by lowering the dosage or by giving suitable concomitant medication.

Tachycardia, significant anorexia, edema, palpitation, blurred vision, chills and impotence have each been reported.

Headaches without blood pressure elevation have occurred. Rare instances of hepatitis and skin rash have been reported.

Impaired water excretion compatible with the syndrome of inappropriate secretion of antidiuretic hormone (SIADH) has been reported.

Tinnitus, muscle spasm, tremors, myoclonic jerks, numbness, paresthesia, urinary retention and retarded ejaculation have been reported.

Hematologic disorders including anemia, leukopenia, agranulocytosis and thrombocytopenia have been reported.

Post-Introduction Reports

The following are spontaneously reported adverse events temporally associated with *Parnate* therapy. No clear relationship between *Parnate* and these events has been established. Localized scleroderma, flare-up of cystic acne, ataxia, confusion, disorientation, memory loss, urinary frequency, urinary incontinence, urticaria, fissuring in corner of mouth, akinesia.

DOSAGE AND ADMINISTRATION

Dosage should be adjusted to the requirements of the individual patient. Improvement should be seen within 48 hours to 3 weeks after starting therapy.

The usual effective dosage is 30 mg per day, usually given in divided doses. If there are no signs of improvement after a reasonable period (up to 2 weeks), then the dosage may be increased in 10 mg per day increments at intervals of 1 to 3 weeks; the dosage range may be extended to a maximum of 60 mg per day from the usual 30 mg per day.

OVERDOSAGE

SYMPTOMS: The characteristic symptoms that may be caused by overdosage are usually those described above. However, an intensification of these symptoms and sometimes severe additional manifestations may be seen, depending on the degree of overdosage and on individual susceptibility. Some patients exhibit insomnia, restlessness and anxiety, progressing in severe cases to agitation, mental confusion and incoherence. Hypotension, dizziness, weakness and drowsiness may occur, progressing in severe cases to extreme dizziness and shock. A few patients have displayed hypertension with severe headache and other symptoms. Rare instances have been reported in which hypertension was accompanied by twitching or myoclonic fibrillation of skeletal muscles with hyperpyrexia, sometimes progressing to generalized rigidity and coma.

TREATMENT: Gastric lavage is helpful if performed early. Treatment should normally consist of general supportive measures, close observation of vital signs and steps to counteract specific symptoms as they occur, since MAO

Continued on next page

Information on the SmithKline Beecham Pharmaceuticals products appearing here is based on the labeling in effect on July 31, 1998. Further information on these and other products may be obtained from the Medical Department, SmithKline Beecham Pharmaceuticals, One Franklin Plaza, Philadelphia, PA 19101.

Parnate—Cont.

inhibition may persist. The management of hypertensive crises is described under WARNINGS in the HYPERTENSIVE CRISES section.
External cooling is recommended if hyperpyrexia occurs. Barbiturates have been reported to help relieve myoclonic reactions, but frequency of administration should be controlled carefully because Parnate (tranylcypromine sulfate) may prolong barbiturate activity. When hypotension requires treatment, the standard measures for managing circulatory shock should be initiated. If pressor agents are used, the rate of infusion should be regulated by careful observation of the patient because an exaggerated pressor response sometimes occurs in the presence of MAO inhibition. Remember that the toxic effect of *Parnate* may be delayed or prolonged following the last dose of the drug. Therefore, the patient should be closely observed for at least a week. It is not known if tranylcypromine is dialyzable.

HOW SUPPLIED

Parnate is supplied as round, rose-red, film-coated tablets imprinted with the product name PARNATE and SKF and contains tranylcypromine sulfate equivalent to 10 mg of tranylcypromine, in bottles of 100 with a desiccant.
10 mg 100's: NDC 0007-4471-20
Store between 15° and 30°C (59° to 86°F).

---

*phentolamine mesylate USP, Ciba Geneva.
†metrizamide, Sanofi Winthrop Pharmaceuticals.
‡disulfiram, Wyeth-Ayerst Laboratories.

Veterans Administration/Military/PHS—Tablets, 10 mg, 100's, 6505-01-211-9008.
PT:L64

Shown in Product Identification Guide, page 339

PAXIL® ℞
[*packs 'ill*]
brand of paroxetine hydrochloride tablets and oral suspension

DESCRIPTION

Paxil (paroxetine hydrochloride) is an orally administered antidepressant with a chemical structure unrelated to other selective serotonin reuptake inhibitors or to tricyclic, tetracyclic or other available antidepressant agents. It is the hydrochloride salt of a phenylpiperidine compound identified chemically as (-)-*trans*-4*R*-(4'-fluorophenyl)-3*S*-[(3',4'-methylenedioxyphenoxy) methyl] piperidine hydrochloride hemihydrate and has the empirical formula of $C_{19}H_{20}FNO_3 \cdot HCl \cdot 1/2H_2O$. The molecular weight is 374.8 (329.4 as free base). The structural formula is:

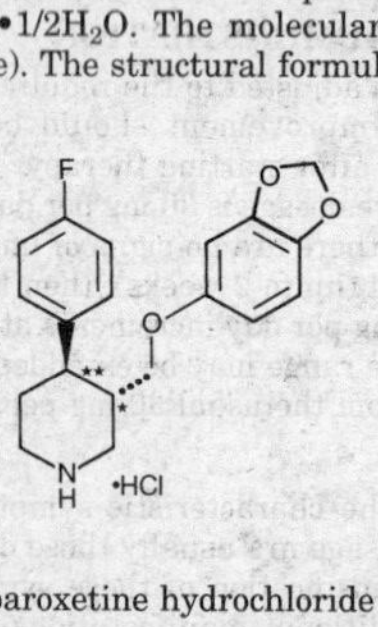

paroxetine hydrochloride

Paroxetine hydrochloride is an odorless, off-white powder, having a melting point range of 120° to 138°C and a solubility of 5.4 mg/mL in water.
Each film-coated tablet contains paroxetine hydrochloride equivalent to paroxetine as follows: 10 mg-yellow; 20 mg-pink (scored); 30 mg-blue, 40 mg-green. Inactive ingredients consist of dibasic calcium phosphate dihydrate, hydroxypropyl methylcellulose, magnesium stearate, polyethylene glycols, polysorbate 80, sodium starch glycolate, titanium dioxide and one or more of the following: D&C Red No. 30, D&C Yellow No. 10, FD&C Blue No. 2, FD&C Yellow No. 6.

Suspension for Oral Administration

Each 5 mL or orange-colored, orange-flavored liquid contains paroxetine hydrochloride equivalent to paroxetine, 10 mg. Inactive ingredients consist of polacrilin potassium, microcrystalline cellulose, propylene glycol, glycerin, sorbitol, methyl paraben, propyl paraben, sodium citrate dihydrate, citric acid anhydrate, sodium saccharin, flavorings, FD&C Yellow No. 6 and simethicone emulsion, USP.

CLINICAL PHARMACOLOGY

Pharmacodynamics

The antidepressant action of paroxetine and its efficacy in the treatment of obsessive compulsive disorder (OCD) and panic disorder (PD) is presumed to be linked to potentiation of serotonergic activity in the central nervous system resulting from inhibition of neuronal reuptake of serotonin (5-hydroxy-tryptamine, 5-HT). Studies at clinically relevant doses in humans have demonstrated that paroxetine blocks the uptake of serotonin into human platelets. *In vitro* studies in animals also suggest that paroxetine is a potent and highly selective inhibitor of neuronal serotonin reuptake and has only very weak effects on norepinephrine and dopamine neuronal reuptake. *In vitro* radioligand binding studies indicate that paroxetine has little affinity for muscarinic, $alpha_1$-, $alpha_2$-, beta-adrenergic-, dopamine (D_2)-, $5\text{-}HT_1$-, $5\text{-}HT_2$- and histamine (H_1)-receptors; antagonism of muscarinic, histaminergic and $alpha_1$-adrenergic receptors has been associated with various anticholinergic, sedative and cardiovascular effects for other psychotropic drugs.
Because the relative potencies of paroxetine's major metabolites are at most 1/50 of the parent compound, they are essentially inactive.

Pharmacokinetics

Paroxetine is equally bioavailable from oral suspension and tablet.
Paroxetine hydrochloride is completely absorbed after oral dosing of a solution of the hydrochloride salt. In a study in which normal male subjects (n=15) received 30 mg tablets daily for 30 days, steady-state paroxetine concentrations were achieved by approximately 10 days for most subjects, although it may take substantially longer in an occasional patient. At steady state, mean values of C_{max}, T_{max}, C_{min} and $T_{1/2}$ were 61.7 ng/mL (CV 45%), 5.2 hr. (CV 10%), 30.7 ng/mL (CV 67%) and 21.0 hr. (CV 32%), respectively. The steady-state C_{max} and C_{min} values were about 6 and 14 times what would be predicted from single-dose studies. Steady-state drug exposure based on AUC_{0-24} was about 8 times greater than would have been predicted from single-dose data in these subjects. The excess accumulation is a consequence of the fact that one of the enzymes that metabolizes paroxetine is readily saturable.
In steady-state dose proportionality studies involving elderly and nonelderly patients, at doses of 20 to 40 mg daily for the elderly and 20 to 50 mg daily for the nonelderly, some nonlinearity was observed in both populations, again reflecting a saturable metabolic pathway. In comparison to C_{min} values after 20 mg daily, values after 40 mg daily were only about 2 to 3 times greater than doubled.
Paroxetine is extensively metabolized after oral administration. The principal metabolites are polar and conjugated products of oxidation and methylation, which are readily cleared. Conjugates with glucuronic acid and sulfate predominate, and major metabolites have been isolated and identified. Data indicate that the metabolites have no more than 1/50 the potency of the parent compound at inhibiting serotonin uptake. The metabolism of paroxetine is accomplished in part by cytochrome $P_{450}IID_6$. Saturation of this enzyme at clinical doses appears to account for the nonlinearity of paroxetine kinetics with increasing dose and increasing duration of treatment. The role of this enzyme in paroxetine metabolism also suggests potential drug-drug interactions (see PRECAUTIONS).
Approximately 64% of a 30 mg oral solution dose of paroxetine was excreted in the urine with 2% as the parent compound and 62% as metabolites over a 10-day post-dosing period. About 36% was excreted in the feces (probably via the bile), mostly as metabolites and less than 1% as the parent compound over the 10-day post-dosing period.
Distribution: Paroxetine distributes throughout the body, including the CNS, with only 1% remaining in the plasma.
Protein Binding: Approximately 95% and 93% of paroxetine is bound to plasma protein at 100 ng/mL and 400 ng/mL, respectively. Under clinical conditions, paroxetine concentrations would normally be less than 400 ng/mL. Paroxetine does not alter the *in vitro* protein binding of phenytoin or warfarin.
Renal and Liver Disease: Increased plasma concentrations of paroxetine occur in subjects with renal and hepatic impairment. The mean plasma concentrations in patients with creatinine clearance below 30 mL/min was approximately 4 times greater than seen in normal volunteers. Patients with creatinine clearance of 30 to 60 mL/min and patients with hepatic functional impairment had about a 2-fold increase in plasma concentrations (AUC, C_{max}).
The initial dosage should therefore be reduced in patients with severe renal or hepatic impairment, and upward titration, if necessary, should be at increased intervals (see DOSAGE AND ADMINISTRATION).
Elderly Patients: In a multiple-dose study in the elderly at daily paroxetine doses of 20, 30 and 40 mg, C_{min} concentrations were about 70% to 80% greater than the respective C_{min} concentrations in nonelderly subjects. Therefore the initial dosage in the elderly should be reduced (see DOSAGE AND ADMINISTRATION).

Clinical Trials

Depression

The efficacy of *Paxil* as a treatment for depression has been established in 6 placebo-controlled studies of patients with depression (ages 18 to 73). In these studies *Paxil* was shown to be significantly more effective than placebo in treating depression by at least 2 of the following measures: Hamilton Depression Rating Scale (HDRS), the Hamilton depressed mood item, and the Clinical Global Impression (CGI)-Severity of Illness. *Paxil* was significantly better than placebo in improvement of the HDRS sub-factor scores, including the depressed mood item, sleep disturbance factor and anxiety factor.
A study of depressed outpatients who had responded to *Paxil* (HDRS total score <8) during an initial 8-week open-treatment phase and were then randomized to continuation on *Paxil* or placebo for 1 year demonstrated a significantly lower relapse rate for patients taking *Paxil* (15%) compared to those on placebo (39%). Effectiveness was similar for male and female patients.

Obsessive Compulsive Disorder

The effectiveness of *Paxil* in the treatment of obsessive compulsive disorder (OCD) was demonstrated in two 12-week multicenter placebo-controlled studies of adult outpatients (Studies 1 and 2). Patients in all studies had moderate to severe OCD (DSM-IIIR) with mean baseline ratings on the Yale Brown Obsessive Compulsive Scale (YBOCS) total score ranging from 23 to 26. Study 1, a dose-range finding study where patients were treated with fixed doses of 20, 40 or 60 mg of paroxetine/day demonstrated that daily doses of paroxetine 40 and 60 mg are effective in the treatment of OCD. Patients receiving doses of 40 and 60 mg paroxetine experienced a mean reduction of approximately 6 and 7 points respectively on the YBOCS total score which was significantly greater than the approximate 4 point reduction at 20 mg and a 3 point reduction in the placebo-treated patients. Study 2 was a flexible dose study comparing paroxetine (20 to 60 mg daily) with clomipramine (25 to 250 mg daily). In this study, patients receiving paroxetine experienced a mean reduction of approximately 7 points on the YBOCS total score which was significantly greater than the mean reduction of approximately 4 points in placebo-treated patients.
The following table provides the outcome classification by treatment group on Global Improvement items of the Clinical Global Impressions (CGI) scale for Study 1.

Outcome Classification (%) on CGI-Global Improvement Item for Completers in Study 1

Outcome Classification	Placebo (N=74)	*Paxil* 20 mg (N=75)	*Paxil* 40 mg (N=66)	*Paxil* 60 mg (N=66)
Worse	14%	7%	7%	3%
No Change	44%	35%	22%	19%
Minimally Improved	24%	33%	29%	34%
Much Improved	11%	18%	22%	24%
Very Much Improved	7%	7%	20%	20%

Subgroup analyses did not indicate that there were any differences in treatment outcomes as a function of age or gender.
The long-term maintenance effects of *Paxil* in OCD were demonstrated in a long-term extension to Study 1. Patients who were responders on paroxetine during the 3-month double-blind phase and a 6-month extension on open-label paroxetine (20 to 60 mg/day) were randomized to either paroxetine or placebo in a 6-month double-blind relapse prevention phase. Patients randomized to paroxetine were significantly less likely to relapse than comparably treated patients who were randomized to placebo.

Panic Disorder

The effectiveness of *Paxil* in the treatment of panic disorder was demonstrated in three 10 to 12 week multicenter, placebo-controlled studies of adult outpatients (Studies 1–3). Patients in all studies had panic disorder (DSM-IIIR), with or without agoraphobia. In these studies, *Paxil* was shown to be significantly more effective than placebo in treating panic disorder by at least 2 out of 3 measures of panic attack frequency and on the Clinical Global Impression Severity of Illness score.
Study 1 was a 10-week dose-range finding study; patients were treated with fixed paroxetine doses of 10, 20, or 40 mg/day or placebo. A significant difference from placebo was observed only for the 40 mg/day group. At endpoint, 76% of patients receiving paroxetine 40 mg/day were free of panic attacks, compared to 44% of placebo-treated patients.
Study 2 was a 12-week flexible-dose study comparing paroxetine (10 to 60 mg daily) and placebo. At endpoint, 51% of paroxetine patients were free of panic attacks compared to 32% of placebo-treated patients.
Study 3 was a 12-week flexible-dose study comparing paroxetine (10 to 60 mg daily) to placebo in patients concurrently receiving standardized cognitive behavioral therapy. At endpoint, 33% of the paroxetine-treated patients showed a reduction to 0 or 1 panic attacks compared to 14% of placebo patients.
In both Studies 2 and 3, the mean paroxetine dose for completers at endpoint was approximately 40 mg/day of paroxetine.
Long-term maintenance effects of *Paxil* in panic disorder were demonstrated in an extension to Study 1. Patients who

were responders during the 10-week double-blind phase and during a 3-month double-blind extension phase were randomized to either paroxetine (10, 20, or 40 mg/day) or placebo in a 3-month double-blind relapse prevention phase. Patients randomized to paroxetine were significantly less likely to relapse than comparably treated patients who were randomized to placebo.

Subgroup analyses did not indicate that there were any differences in treatment outcomes as a function of age or gender.

INDICATIONS AND USAGE

Depression

Paxil (paroxetine hydrochloride) is indicated for the treatment of depression.

The efficacy of *Paxil* in the treatment of a major depressive episode was established in 6-week controlled trials of outpatients whose diagnoses corresponded most closely to the DSM-III category of major depressive disorder (see CLINICAL PHARMACOLOGY). A major depressive episode implies a prominent and relatively persistent depressed or dysphoric mood that usually interferes with daily functioning (nearly every day for at least 2 weeks); it should include at least 4 of the following 8 symptoms: change in appetite, change in sleep, psychomotor agitation or retardation, loss of interest in usual activities or decrease in sexual drive, increased fatigue, feelings of guilt or worthlessness, slowed thinking or impaired concentration, and a suicide attempt or suicidal ideation.

The antidepressant action of *Paxil* in hospitalized depressed patients has not been adequately studied.

The efficacy of *Paxil* in maintaining an antidepressant response for up to 1 year was demonstrated in a placebo-controlled trial (see CLINICAL PHARMACOLOGY). Nevertheless, the physician who elects to use *Paxil* for extended periods should periodically re-evaluate the long-term usefulness of the drug for the individual patient.

Obsessive Compulsive Disorder

Paxil is indicated for the treatment of obsessions and compulsions in patients with obsessive compulsive disorder (OCD) as defined in the DSM-IV. The obsessions or compulsions cause marked distress, are time-consuming, or significantly interfere with social or occupational functioning.

The efficacy of *Paxil* was established in two 12 week trials with obsessive compulsive outpatients whose diagnoses corresponded most closely to the DSM-IIIR category of obsessive compulsive disorder (see CLINICAL PHARMACOLOGY—Clinical Trials).

Obsessive compulsive disorder is characterized by recurrent and persistent ideas, thoughts, impulses or images (obsessions) that are ego-dystonic and/or repetitive, purposeful and intentional behaviors (compulsions) that are recognized by the person as excessive or unreasonable.

Long-term maintenance of efficacy was demonstrated in a 6-month relapse prevention trial. In this trial, patients assigned to paroxetine showed a lower relapse rate compared to patients on placebo (see CLINICAL PHARMACOLOGY). Nevertheless, the physician who elects to use *Paxil* for extended periods should periodically reevaluate the long-term usefulness of the drug for the individual patient (see DOSAGE AND ADMINISTRATION).

Panic Disorder

Paxil is indicated for the treatment of panic disorder, with or without agoraphobia, as defined in DSM-IV. Panic disorder is characterized by the occurrence of unexpected panic attacks and associated concern about having additional attacks, worry about the implications or consequences of the attacks, and/or a significant change in behavior related to the attacks.

The efficacy of Paxil (paroxetine hydrochloride) was established in three 10 to 12 week trials in panic disorder patients whose diagnoses corresponded to the DSM-IIIR category of panic disorder (see Clinical Pharmacology—Clinical Trials).

Panic disorder (DSM-IV) is characterized by recurrent unexpected panic attacks, i.e., a discrete period of intense fear or discomfort in which four (or more) of the following symptoms develop abruptly and reach a peak within 10 minutes: (1) palpitations, pounding heart, or accelerated heart rate; (2) sweating; (3) trembling or shaking; (4) sensations of shortness of breath or smothering; (5) feeling of choking; (6) chest pain or discomfort; (7) nausea or abdominal distress; (8) feeling dizzy, unsteady, lightheaded, or faint; (9) derealization (feelings of unreality) or depersonalization (being detached from oneself); (10) fear of losing control; (11) fear of dying; (12) paresthesias (numbness or tingling sensations); (13) chills or hot flushes.

Long-term maintenance of efficacy was demonstrated in a 3-month relapse prevention trial. In this trial, patients with panic disorder assigned to paroxetine demonstrated a lower relapse rate compared to patients on placebo (see CLINICAL PHARMACOLOGY). Nevertheless, the physician who prescribes *Paxil* for extended periods should periodically reevaluate the long-term usefulness of the drug for the individual patient.

CONTRAINDICATIONS

Concomitant use in patients taking monoamine oxidase inhibitors (MAOIs) is contraindicated (see WARNINGS and PRECAUTIONS).

WARNINGS

Potential for Interaction with Monoamine Oxidase Inhibitors

In patients receiving another serotonin reuptake inhibitor drug in combination with a monoamine oxidase inhibitor (MAOI), there have been reports of serious, sometimes fatal, reactions including hyperthermia, rigidity, myoclonus, autonomic instability with possible rapid fluctuations of vital signs, and mental status changes that include extreme agitation progressing to delirium and coma. These reactions have also been reported in patients who have recently discontinued that drug and have been started on a MAOI. Some cases presented with features resembling neuroleptic malignant syndrome. While there are no human data showing such an interaction with *Paxil*, limited animal data on the effects of combined use of paroxetine and MAOIs suggest that these drugs may act synergistically to elevate blood pressure and evoke behavioral excitation. Therefore, it is recommended that Paxil (paroxetine hydrochloride) not be used in combination with a MAOI, or within 14 days of discontinuing treatment with a MAOI. At least 2 weeks should be allowed after stopping *Paxil* before starting a MAOI.

PRECAUTIONS

General

Activation of Mania/Hypomania: During premarketing testing, hypomania or mania occurred in approximately 1.0% of *Paxil*-treated unipolar patients compared to 1.1% of active-control and 0.3% of placebo-treated unipolar patients. In a subset of patients classified as bipolar, the rate of manic episodes was 2.2% for *Paxil* and 11.6% for the combined active-control groups. As with all antidepressants, *Paxil* should be used cautiously in patients with a history of mania.

Seizures: During premarketing testing, seizures occurred in 0.1% of *Paxil*-treated patients, a rate similar to that associated with other antidepressants. *Paxil* should be used cautiously in patients with a history of seizures. It should be discontinued in any patient who develops seizures.

Suicide: The possibility of a suicide attempt is inherent in depression and may persist until significant remission occurs. Close supervision of high-risk patients should accompany initial drug therapy. Prescriptions for *Paxil* should be written for the smallest quantity of tablets consistent with good patient management, in order to reduce the risk of overdose.

Hyponatremia: Several cases of hyponatremia have been reported. The hyponatremia appeared to be reversible when *Paxil* was discontinued. The majority of these occurrences have been in elderly individuals, some in patients taking diuretics or who were otherwise volume depleted.

Abnormal Bleeding: There have been several reports of abnormal bleeding (mostly ecchymosis and purpura) associated with paroxetine treatment, including a report of impaired platelet aggregation. While a causal relationship to paroxetine is unclear, impaired platelet aggregation may result from platelet serotonin depletion and contribute to such occurrences.

Use in Patients with Concomitant Illness: Clinical experience with *Paxil* in patients with certain concomitant systemic illness is limited. Caution is advisable in using *Paxil* in patients with diseases or conditions that could affect metabolism or hemodynamic responses.

Paxil has not been evaluated or used to any appreciable extent in patients with a recent history of myocardial infarction or unstable heart disease. Patients with these diagnoses were excluded from clinical studies during the product's premarket testing. Evaluation of electrocardiograms of 682 patients who received *Paxil* in double-blind, placebo-controlled trials, however, did not indicate that *Paxil* is associated with the development of significant ECG abnormalities. Similarly, Paxil (paroxetine hydrochloride) does not cause any clinically important changes in heart rate or blood pressure.

Increased plasma concentrations of paroxetine occur in patients with severe renal impairment (creatinine clearance <30 mL/min.) or severe hepatic impairment. A lower starting dose should be used in such patients (see DOSAGE AND ADMINISTRATION).

Information for Patients

Physicians are advised to discuss the following issues with patients for whom they prescribe *Paxil:*

Interference with Cognitive and Motor Performance: Any psychoactive drug may impair judgment, thinking or motor skills. Although in controlled studies *Paxil* has not been shown to impair psychomotor performance, patients should be cautioned about operating hazardous machinery, including automobiles, until they are reasonably certain that *Paxil* therapy does not affect their ability to engage in such activities.

Completing Course of Therapy: While patients may notice improvement with *Paxil* therapy in 1 to 4 weeks, they should be advised to continue therapy as directed.

Concomitant Medication: Patients should be advised to inform their physician if they are taking, or plan to take, any prescription or over-the-counter drugs, since there is a potential for interactions.

Alcohol: Although *Paxil* has not been shown to increase the impairment of mental and motor skills caused by alcohol, patients should be advised to avoid alcohol while taking *Paxil*.

Pregnancy: Patients should be advised to notify their physician if they become pregnant or intend to become pregnant during therapy.

Nursing: Patients should be advised to notify their physician if they are breast-feeding an infant (see PRECAUTIONS-Nursing Mothers).

Laboratory Tests

There are no specific laboratory tests recommended.

Drug Interactions

Tryptophan: As with other serotonin reuptake inhibitors, an interaction between paroxetine and tryptophan may occur when they are co-administered. Adverse experiences, consisting primarily of headache, nausea, sweating and dizziness, have been reported when tryptophan was administered to patients taking Paxil (paroxetine hydrochloride). Consequently, concomitant use of *Paxil* with tryptophan is not recommended.

Monoamine Oxidase Inhibitors: See CONTRAINDICATIONS and WARNINGS.

Warfarin: Preliminary data suggest that there may be a pharmacodynamic interaction (that causes an increased bleeding diathesis in the face of unaltered prothrombin time) between paroxetine and warfarin. Since there is little clinical experience, the concomitant administration of *Paxil* and warfarin should be undertaken with caution.

Sumatriptan: There have been rare postmarketing reports describing patients with weakness, hyperreflexia, and incoordination following the use of a selective serotonin reuptake inhibitor (SSRI) and sumatriptan. If concomitant treatment with sumatriptan and an SSRI (e.g., fluoxetine, fluvoxamine, paroxetine, sertraline) is clinically warranted, appropriate observation of the patient is advised.

Drugs Affecting Hepatic Metabolism: The metabolism and pharmacokinetics of paroxetine may be affected by the induction or inhibition of drug-metabolizing enzymes.

Cimetidine—Cimetidine inhibits many cytochrome P_{450} (oxidative) enzymes. In a study where *Paxil* (30 mg q.d.) was dosed orally for 4 weeks, steady-state plasma concentrations of paroxetine were increased by approximately 50% during co-administration with oral cimetidine (300 mg t.i.d.) for the final week. Therefore, when these drugs are administered concurrently, dosage adjustment of *Paxil* after the 20 mg starting dose should be guided by clinical effect. The effect of paroxetine on cimetidine's pharmacokinetics was not studied.

Phenobarbital—Phenobarbital induces many cytochrome P_{450} (oxidative) enzymes. When a single oral 30 mg dose of *Paxil* was administered at phenobarbital steady state (100 mg q.d. for 14 days), paroxetine AUC and $T_{1/2}$ were reduced (by an average of 25% and 38%, respectively) compared to paroxetine administered alone. The effect of paroxetine on phenobarbital pharmacokinetics was not studied. Since *Paxil* exhibits nonlinear pharmacokinetics, the results of this study may not address the case where the two drugs are both being chronically dosed. No initial *Paxil* dosage adjustment is considered necessary when co-administered with phenobarbital; any subsequent adjustment should be guided by clinical effect.

Phenytoin—When a single oral 30 mg dose of *Paxil* was administered at phenytoin steady state (300 mg q.d. for 14 days), paroxetine AUC and $T_{1/2}$ were reduced (by an average of 50% and 35%, respectively) compared to *Paxil* administered alone. In a separate study, when a single oral 300 mg dose of phenytoin was administered at paroxetine steady state (30 mg q.d. for 14 days), phenytoin AUC was slightly reduced (12% on average) compared to phenytoin administered alone. Since both drugs exhibit nonlinear pharmacokinetics, the above studies may not address the case where the two drugs are both being chronically dosed. No initial dosage adjustments are considered necessary when these drugs are co-administered; any subsequent adjustments should be guided by clinical effect (see ADVERSE REACTIONS-Postmarketing Reports).

Continued on next page

Information on the SmithKline Beecham Pharmaceuticals products appearing here is based on the labeling in effect on July 31, 1998. Further information on these and other products may be obtained from the Medical Department, SmithKline Beecham Pharmaceuticals, One Franklin Plaza, Philadelphia, PA 19101.

Paxil—Cont.

Drugs Metabolized by Cytochrome $P_{450}IID_6$: Many drugs, including most antidepressants (paroxetine, other SSRIs and many tricyclics), are metabolized by the cytochrome P_{450} isozyme $P_{450}IID_6$. Like other agents that are metabolized by $P_{450}IID_6$, paroxetine may significantly inhibit the activity of this isozyme. In most patients (>90%), this $P_{450}IID_6$ isozyme is saturated early during *Paxil* dosing. In one study, daily dosing of *Paxil* (20 mg q.d.) under steady-state conditions increased single dose desipramine (100 mg) C_{max}, AUC and $T_{1/2}$ by an average of approximately two-, five- and three-fold, respectively. Concomitant use of *Paxil* with other drugs metabolized by cytochrome $P_{450}IID_6$ has not been formally studied but may require lower doses than usually prescribed for either *Paxil* or the other drug.

Therefore, co-administration of *Paxil* with other drugs that are metabolized by this isozyme, including certain antidepressants (e.g., nortriptyline, amitriptyline, imipramine, desipramine and fluoxetine), phenothiazines (e.g., thioridazine) and Type 1C antiarrhythmics (e.g., propafenone, flecainide and encainide), or that inhibit this enzyme (e.g., quinidine), should be approached with caution.

At steady state, when the $P_{450}IID_6$ pathway is essentially saturated, paroxetine clearance is governed by alternative P_{450} isozymes which, unlike $P_{450}IID_6$, show no evidence of saturation (see PRECAUTIONS-Tricyclic Antidepressants).

Drugs Metabolized by Cytochrome $P_{450}IIIA_4$: An *in vivo* interaction study involving the co-administration under steady-state conditions of paroxetine and terfenadine, a substrate for cytochrome $P_{450}IIIA_4$, revealed no effect of paroxetine on terfenadine pharmacokinetics. In addition, *in vitro* studies have shown ketoconazole, a potent inhibitor of $P_{450}IIIA_4$ activity, to be at least 100 times more potent than paroxetine as an inhibitor of the metabolism of several substrates for this enzyme, including terfenadine, astemizole, cisapride, triazolam, and cyclosporin. Based on the assumption that the relationship between paroxetine's *in vitro* Ki and its lack of effect on terfenadine's *in vivo* clearance predicts its effect on other $IIIA_4$ substrates, paroxetine's extent of inhibition of $IIIA_4$ activity is not likely to be of clinical significance.

Tricyclic Antidepressants (TCA): Caution is indicated in the co-administration of tricyclic antidepressants (TCAs) with *Paxil,* because paroxetine may inhibit TCA metabolism. Plasma TCA concentrations may need to be monitored, and the dose of TCA may need to be reduced, if a TCA is co-administered with *Paxil* (see PRECAUTIONS-Drugs Metabolized by Cytochrome $P_{450}IID_6$).

Drugs Highly Bound to Plasma Protein: Because paroxetine is highly bound to plasma protein, administration of *Paxil* to a patient taking another drug that is highly protein bound may cause increased free concentrations of the other drug, potentially resulting in adverse events. Conversely, adverse effects could result from displacement of paroxetine by other highly bound drugs.

Alcohol: Although *Paxil* does not increase the impairment of mental and motor skills caused by alcohol, patients should be advised to avoid alcohol while taking Paxil (paroxetine hydrochloride).

Lithium: A multiple-dose study has shown that there is no pharmacokinetic interaction between *Paxil* and lithium carbonate. However, since there is little clinical experience, the concurrent administration of paroxetine and lithium should be undertaken with caution.

Digoxin: The steady-state pharmacokinetics of paroxetine was not altered when administered with digoxin at steady state. Mean digoxin AUC at steady state decreased by 15% in the presence of paroxetine. Since there is little clinical experience, the concurrent administration of paroxetine and digoxin should be undertaken with caution.

Diazepam: Under steady-state conditions, diazepam does not appear to affect paroxetine kinetics. The effects of paroxetine on diazepam were not evaluated.

Procyclidine: Daily oral dosing of *Paxil* (30 mg q.d.) increased steady-state AUC_{0-24}, C_{max} and C_{min} values of procyclidine (5 mg oral q.d.) by 35%, 37% and 67%, respectively, compared to procyclidine alone at steady state. If anticholinergic effects are seen, the dose of procyclidine should be reduced.

Beta-Blockers: In a study where propranolol (80 mg b.i.d.) was dosed orally for 18 days, the established steady-state plasma concentrations of propranolol were unaltered during co-administration with *Paxil* (30 mg q.d.) for the final 10 days. The effects of propranolol on paroxetine have not been evaluated (see ADVERSE REACTIONS-Postmarketing Reports).

Theophylline: Reports of elevated theophylline levels associated with *Paxil* treatment have been reported. While this interaction has not been formally studied, it is recommended that theophylline levels be monitored when these drugs are concurrently administered.

Electroconvulsive Therapy (ECT): There are no clinical studies of the combined use of ECT and *Paxil.*

Carcinogenesis, Mutagenesis, Impairment of Fertility

Carcinogenesis: Two-year carcinogenicity studies were conducted in rodents given paroxetine in the diet at 1, 5, and 25 mg/kg/day (mice) and 1, 5, and 20 mg/kg/day (rats). These doses are up to 2.4 (mouse) and 3.9 (rat) times the maximum recommended human dose (MRHD) for depression on a mg/m² basis. Because the MRHD for depression is slightly less than that for OCD (50 mg vs. 60 mg), the doses used in these carcinogenicity studies were only 2.0 (mouse) and 3.2 (rat) times the MRHD for OCD. There was a significantly greater number of male rats in the high-dose group with reticulum cell sarcomas (1/100, 0/50, 0/50 and 4/50 for control, low-, middle- and high-dose groups, respectively) and a significantly increased linear trend across dose groups for the occurrence of lymphoreticular tumors in male rats. Female rats were not affected. Although there was a dose-related increase in the number of tumors in mice, there was no drug-related increase in the number of mice with tumors. The relevance of these findings to humans is unknown.

Mutagenesis: Paroxetine produced no genotoxic effects in a battery of 5 *in vitro* and 2 *in vivo* assays that included the following: bacterial mutation assay, mouse lymphoma mutation assay, unscheduled DNA synthesis assay, and tests for cytogenetic aberrations *in vivo* in mouse bone marrow and *in vitro* in human lymphocytes and in a dominant lethal test in rats.

Impairment of Fertility: A reduced pregnancy rate was found in reproduction studies in rats at a dose of paroxetine of 15 mg/kg/day which is 2.9 times the MRHD for depression or 2.4 times the MRHD for OCD on a mg/m² basis. Irreversible lesions occurred in the reproductive tract of male rats after dosing in toxicity studies for 2 to 52 weeks. These lesions consisted of vacuolation of epididymal tubular epithelium at 50 mg/kg/day and atrophic changes in the seminiferous tubules of the testes with arrested spermatogenesis at 25 mg/kg/day (9.8 and 4.9 times the MRHD for depression; 8.2 and 4.1 times the MRHD for OCD and PD on a mg/m² basis).

Pregnancy

Teratogenic Effects–Pregnancy Category C

Reproduction studies were performed at doses up to 50 mg/kg/day in rats and 6 mg/kg/day in rabbits administered during organogenesis. These doses are equivalent to 9.7 (rat) and 2.2 (rabbit) times the maximum recommended human dose (MRHD) for depression (50 mg) and 8.1 (rat) and 1.9 (rabbit) times the MRHD for OCD, on a mg/m² basis. These studies have revealed no evidence of teratogenic effects. However, in rats, there was an increase in pup deaths during the first 4 days of lactation when dosing occurred during the last trimester of gestation and continued throughout lactation. This effect occurred at a dose of 1 mg/kg/day or 0.19 times (mg/m²) the MRHD for depression and at 0.16 times (mg/m²) the MRHD for OCD. The no-effect dose for rat pup mortality was not determined. The cause of these deaths is not known. There are no adequate and well-controlled studies in pregnant women. Because animal reproduction studies are not always predictive of human response, this drug should be used during pregnancy only if the potential benefit justifies the potential risk to the fetus.

Labor and Delivery

The effect of paroxetine on labor and delivery in humans is unknown.

Nursing Mothers

Like many other drugs, paroxetine is secreted in human milk, and caution should be exercised when Paxil (paroxetine hydrochloride) is administered to a nursing woman.

Pediatric Use

Safety and effectiveness in the pediatric population have not been established.

Geriatric Use

In worldwide premarketing *Paxil* clinical trials, 17% of *Paxil*-treated patients (approximately 700) were 65 years of age or older. Pharmacokinetic studies revealed a decreased clearance in the elderly, and a lower starting dose is recommended; there were, however, no overall differences in the adverse event profile between elderly and younger patients, and effectiveness was similar in younger and older patients (see CLINICAL PHARMACOLOGY and DOSAGE AND ADMINISTRATION).

ADVERSE REACTIONS

Associated with Discontinuation of Treatment

Twenty percent (1,199/6,145) of *Paxil* patients in worldwide clinical trials in depression and 11.8% (64/542) and 9.4% (44/469) of *Paxil* patients in worldwide trials in OCD and panic disorder, respectively, discontinued treatment due to an adverse event. The most common events (≥1%) associated with discontinuation and considered to be drug related (i.e., those events associated with dropout at a rate approximately twice or greater for *Paxil* compared to placebo) included the following:

[See table below]

Where numbers are not provided the incidence of the adverse events in Paxil (paroxetine hydrochloride) patients was not >1% or was not greater than or equal to two times the incidence of placebo.

1. Incidence corrected for gender.

Commonly Observed Adverse Events

Depression

The most commonly observed adverse events associated with the use of paroxetine (incidence of 5% or greater and incidence for *Paxil* at least twice that for placebo, derived from Table 1 below) were: asthenia, sweating, nausea, decreased appetite, somnolence, dizziness, insomnia, tremor, nervousness, ejaculatory disturbance and other male genital disorders.

Obsessive Compulsive Disorder

The most commonly observed adverse events associated with the use of paroxetine (incidence of 5% or greater and incidence for *Paxil* at least twice that of placebo, derived from Table 2 below) were: nausea, dry mouth, decreased appetite, constipation, dizziness, somnolence, tremor, sweating, impotence and abnormal ejaculation.

Panic Disorder

The most commonly observed adverse events associated with the use of paroxetine (incidence of 5% or greater and incidence for *Paxil* at least twice that for placebo, derived from Table 2 below) were: asthenia, sweating, decreased appetite, libido decreased, tremor, abnormal ejaculation, female genital disorders and impotence.

Incidence in Controlled Clinical Trials

Depression

Table 1 enumerates adverse events that occurred at an incidence of 1% or more among paroxetine-treated patients who participated in short term (6-week) placebo-controlled trials in which patients were dosed in a range of 20 to 50 mg/day. Reported adverse events were classified using a standard COSTART-based Dictionary terminology.

The prescriber should be aware that these figures cannot be used to predict the incidence of side effects in the course of usual medical practice where patient characteristics and other factors differ from those which prevailed in the clinical trials. Similarly, the cited frequencies cannot be compared with figures obtained from other clinical investigations involving different treatments, uses and investigators. The cited figures, however, do provide the prescribing physician with some basis for estimating the relative contribution of drug and nondrug factors to the side effect incidence rate in the population studied.

[See table 1 at top of next page]

Obsessive Compulsive Disorder and Panic Disorder

Table 2 enumerates adverse events that occurred at a frequency of 2% or more among OCD patients on *Paxil* who participated in placebo-controlled trials of 12-weeks dura-

	Depression		OCD		Panic Disorder	
	Paxil	Placebo	*Paxil*	Placebo	*Paxil*	Placebo
CNS						
Somnolence	2.3%	0.7%	—		1.9%	0.3%
Insomnia	—	—	1.7%	0%	1.3%	0.3%
Agitation	1.1%	0.5%	—			
Tremor	1.1%	0.3%	—			
Dizziness	—	—	1.5%	0%		
Gastrointestinal						
Constipation	—		1.1%	0%		
Nausea	3.2%	1.1%	1.9%	0%	3.2%	1.2%
Diarrhea	1.0%	0.3%	—			
Dry mouth	1.0%	0.3%	—			
Vomiting	1.0%	0.3%	—			
Other						
Asthenia	1.6%	0.4%	1.9%	0.4%		
Abnormal ejaculation[1]	1.6%	0%	2.1%	0%		
Sweating	1.0%	0.3%	—			
Impotence[1]	—		1.5%	0%		

tion in which patients were dosed in a range of 20 to 60 mg/day or among patients with panic disorder on *Paxil* who participated in placebo-controlled trials of 10 to 12 weeks duration in which patients were dosed in a range of 10 to 60 mg/day.

[See table 2 at top of next page]

Dose Dependency of Adverse Events: A comparison of adverse event rates in a fixed-dose study comparing *Paxil* 10, 20, 30 and 40 mg/day with placebo in the treatment of depression revealed a clear dose dependency for some of the more common adverse events associated with *Paxil* use, as shown in the following table:

Table 3. Treatment-Emergent Adverse Experience Incidence in a Depression Dose-Comparison Trial*

Body System/ Preferred Term	Placebo n=51	Paxil 10 mg n=102	20 mg n=104	30 mg n=101	40 mg n=102
Body as a Whole					
Asthenia	0.0%	2.9%	10.6%	13.9%	12.7%
Dermatology					
Sweating	2.0%	1.0%	6.7%	8.9%	11.8%
Gastrointestinal					
Constipation	5.9%	4.9%	7.7%	9.9%	12.7%
Decreased Appetite	2.0%	2.0%	5.8%	4.0%	4.9%
Diarrhea	7.8%	9.8%	19.2%	7.9%	14.7%
Dry Mouth	2.0%	10.8%	18.3%	15.8%	20.6%
Nausea	13.7%	14.7%	26.9%	34.7%	36.3%
Nervous System					
Anxiety	0.0%	2.0%	5.8%	5.9%	5.9%
Dizziness	3.9%	6.9%	6.7%	8.9%	12.7%
Nervousness	0.0%	5.9%	5.8%	4.0%	2.9%
Paresthesia	0.0%	2.9%	1.0%	5.0%	5.9%
Somnolence	7.8%	12.7%	18.3%	20.8%	21.6%
Tremor	0.0%	0.0%	7.7%	7.9%	14.7%
Special Senses					
Blurred Vision	2.0%	2.9%	2.9%	2.0%	7.8%
Urogenital System					
Abnormal Ejaculation	0.0%	5.8%	6.5%	10.6%	13.0%
Impotence	0.0%	1.9%	4.3%	6.4%	1.9%
Male Genital Disorders	0.0%	3.8%	8.7%	6.4%	3.7%

*   Rule for including adverse events in table: incidence at least 5% for one of paroxetine groups and ≥ twice the placebo incidence for at least one paroxetine group.

In a fixed-dose study comparing placebo and *Paxil* 20, 40 and 60 mg in the treatment of OCD, there was no clear relationship between adverse events and the dose of *Paxil* to which patients were assigned. No new adverse events were observed in the *Paxil* 60 mg dose group compared to any of the other treatment groups.

In a fixed-dose study comparing placebo and *Paxil* 10, 20 and 40 mg in the treatment of panic disorder, there was no clear relationship between adverse events and the dose of *Paxil* to which patients were assigned, except for asthenia, dry mouth, anxiety, libido decreased, tremor and abnormal ejaculation. In flexible dose studies, no new adverse events were observed in patients receiving *Paxil* 60 mg compared to any of the other treatment groups.

Adaptation to Certain Adverse Events: Over a 4- to 6-week period, there was evidence of adaptation to some adverse events with continued therapy (e.g., nausea and dizziness), but less to other effects (e.g., dry mouth, somnolence and asthenia).

Weight and Vital Sign Changes: Significant weight loss may be an undesirable result of treatment with *Paxil* for some patients but, on average, patients in controlled trials had minimal (about 1 pound) weight loss vs. smaller changes on placebo and active control. No significant changes in vital signs (systolic and diastolic blood pressure, pulse and temperature) were observed in patients treated with *Paxil* in controlled clinical trials.

ECG Changes: In an analysis of ECGs obtained in 682 patients treated with *Paxil* and 415 treated with placebo in controlled clinical trials, no clinically significant changes were seen in the ECGs of either group.

Liver Function Tests: In placebo-controlled clinical trials, patients treated with *Paxil* exhibited abnormal values on liver function tests at no greater rate than that seen in placebo-treated patients. In particular, the *Paxil*-vs.-placebo comparisons for alkaline phosphatase, SGOT, SGPT and bilirubin revealed no differences in the percentage of patients with marked abnormalities.

Other Events Observed During the Premarketing Evaluation of Paxil (paroxetine hydrochloride)

During its premarketing assessment in depression, multiple doses of *Paxil* were administered to 6,145 patients in phase

Table 1. Treatment-Emergent Adverse Experience Incidence in Placebo-Controlled Clinical Trials for Depression[1]

Body System	Preferred Term	Paxil (n=421)	Placebo (n= 421)
Body as a Whole	Headache	18%	17%
	Asthenia	15%	6%
Cardiovascular	Palpitation	3%	1%
	Vasodilation	3%	1%
Dermatologic	Sweating	11%	2%
	Rash	2%	1%
Gastrointestinal	Nausea	26%	9%
	Dry Mouth	18%	12%
	Constipation	14%	9%
	Diarrhea	12%	8%
	Decreased Appetite	6%	2%
	Flatulence	4%	2%
	Oropharynx Disorder [2]	2%	0%
	Dyspepsia	2%	1%
Musculoskeletal	Myopathy	2%	1%
	Myalgia	2%	1%
	Myasthenia	1%	0%
Nervous System	Somnolence	23%	9%
	Dizziness	13%	6%
	Insomnia	13%	6%
	Tremor	8%	2%
	Nervousness	5%	3%
	Anxiety	5%	3%
	Paresthesia	4%	2%
	Libido Decreased	3%	0%
	Drugged Feeling	2%	1%
	Confusion	1%	0%
Respiration	Yawn	4%	0%
Special Senses	Blurred Vision	4%	1%
	Taste Perversion	2%	0%
Urogenital System	Ejaculatory Disturbance[3,4]	13%	0%
	Other Male Genital Disorders[3,5]	10%	0%
	Urinary Frequency	3%	1%
	Urination Disorder [6]	3%	0%
	Female Genital Disorders[3,7]	2%	0%

1. Events reported by at least 1% of patients treated with Paxil (paroxetine hydrochloride) are included, except the following events which had an incidence on placebo ≥ *Paxil*: abdominal pain, agitation, back pain, chest pain, CNS stimulation, fever, increased appetite, myoclonus, pharyngitis, postural hypotension, respiratory disorder (includes mostly "cold symptoms" or "URI"), trauma and vomiting.
2. Includes mostly "lump in throat" and "tightness in throat."
3. Percentage corrected for gender.
4. Mostly "ejaculatory delay."
5. Includes "anorgasmia," "erectile difficulties," "delayed ejaculation/orgasm," and "sexual dysfunction," and "impotence."
6. Includes mostly "difficulty with micturition" and "urinary hesitancy."
7. Includes mostly "anorgasmia" and "difficulty reaching climax/orgasm."

2 and 3 studies. The conditions and duration of exposure to *Paxil* varied greatly and included (in overlapping categories) open and double-blind studies, uncontrolled and controlled studies, inpatient and outpatient studies, and fixed-dose and titration studies. During premarketing clinical trials in OCD and panic disorder, 542 and 469 patients, respectively, received multiple doses of *Paxil*. Untoward events associated with this exposure were recorded by clinical investigators using terminology of their own choosing. Consequently, it is not possible to provide a meaningful estimate of the proportion of individuals experiencing adverse events without first grouping similar types of untoward events into a smaller number of standardized event categories.

In the tabulations that follow, reported adverse events were classified using a standard COSTART-based Dictionary terminology. The frequencies presented, therefore, represent the proportion of the 7,156 patients exposed to multiple doses of Paxil (paroxetine hydrochloride) who experienced an event of the type cited on at least one occasion while receiving *Paxil*. All reported events are included except those already listed in Tables 1 and 2, those reported in terms so general as to be uninformative and those events where a drug cause was remote. It is important to emphasize that although the events reported occurred during treatment with paroxetine, they were not necessarily caused by it.

Events are further categorized by body system and listed in order of decreasing frequency according to the following definitions: frequent adverse events are those occurring on one or more occasions in at least 1/100 patients (only those not already listed in the tabulated results from placebo-controlled trials appear in this listing); infrequent adverse events are those occurring in 1/100 to 1/1000 patients; rare events are those occurring in fewer than 1/1000 patients. Events of major clinical importance are also described in the PRECAUTIONS section.

Body as a Whole: *frequent:* chills, malaise; *infrequent:* allergic reaction, carcinoma, face edema, moniliasis, neck pain; *rare:* abscess, adrenergic syndrome, cellulitis, neck rigidity, pelvic pain, peritonitis, ulcer.

Cardiovascular System: *frequent:* hypertension, syncope, tachycardia; *infrequent:* bradycardia, conduction abnormalities, electrocardiogram abnormal, hematoma, hypotension, migraine, peripheral vascular disorder; *rare:* angina pectoris, arrhythmia, atrial fibrillation, bundle branch block, cerebral ischemia, cerebrovascular accident, congestive heart failure, heart block, low cardiac output, myocardial infarct, myocardial ischemia, pallor, phlebitis, pulmonary embolus, supraventricular extrasystoles, thrombophlebitis, thrombosis, varicose vein, vascular headache, ventricular extrasystoles.

Digestive System: *infrequent:* bruxism, colitis, dysphagia, eructation, gastroenteritis, gingivitis, glossitis, increased salivation, liver function tests abnormal, mouth ulceration, rectal hemorrhage, ulcerative stomatitis; *rare:* aphthous stomatitis, bloody diarrhea, bulimia, cholelithiasis, duodenitis, enteritis, esophagitis, fecal impactions, fecal incontinence, gastritis, gum hemorrhage, hematemesis, hepatitis, ileus, intestinal obstruction, jaundice, melena, peptic ulcer, salivary gland enlargement, stomach ulcer, stomatitis, tongue discoloration, tongue edema, tooth caries, tooth malformation.

Endocrine System: *rare:* diabetes mellitus, hyperthyroidism, hypothyroidism, thyroiditis.

Hemic and Lymphatic Systems: *infrequent:* anemia, leukopenia, lymphadenopathy, purpura; *rare:* abnormal erythrocytes, basophilia, eosinophilia, hypochromic anemia, iron deficiency anemia, leukocytosis, lymphedema, abnormal lymphocytes, lymphocytosis, microcytic anemia, monocytosis, normocytic anemia, thrombocythemia.

Continued on next page

Information on the SmithKline Beecham Pharmaceuticals products appearing here is based on the labeling in effect on July 31, 1998. Further information on these and other products may be obtained from the Medical Department, SmithKline Beecham Pharmaceuticals, One Franklin Plaza, Philadelphia, PA 19101.

Paxil—Cont.

Metabolic and Nutritional: *frequent:* edema, weight gain, weight loss; *infrequent:* hyperglycemia, peripheral edema, SGOT increased, SGPT increased, thirst; *rare:* alkaline phosphatase increased, bilirubinemia, BUN increased, creatinine phosphokinase increased, dehydration, gamma globulins increased, gout, hypercalcemia, hypercholesteremia, hyperkalemia, hyperphosphatemia, hypocalcemia, hypoglycemia, hypokalemia, hyponatremia, ketosis, lactic dehydrogenase increased.

Musculoskeletal System: *frequent:* arthralgia; *infrequent:* arthritis; *rare:* arthrosis, bursitis, myositis, osteoporosis, generalized spasm, tenosynovitis, tetany.

Nervous System: *frequent:* amnesia, CNS stimulation, concentration impaired, depression, emotional lability, vertigo; *infrequent:* abnormal thinking, akinesia, alcohol abuse, ataxia, convulsion, depersonalization, dystonia, hallucinations, hostility, hyperkinesia, hypertonia, hypesthesia, incoordination, lack of emotion, manic reaction, neurosis, paralysis, paranoid reaction; *rare:* abnormal electroencephalogram, abnormal gait, antisocial reaction, aphasia, choreoathetosis, circumoral paresthesias, delirium, delusions, diplopia, drug dependence, dysarthria, dyskinesia, euphoria, extrapyramidal syndrome, fasciculations, grand mal convulsion, hyperalgesia, hypokinesia, hysteria, libido increased, manic-depressive reaction, meningitis, myelitis, neuralgia, neuropathy, nystagmus, peripheral neuritis, psychosis, psychotic depression, reflexes decreased, reflexes increased, stupor, trismus, withdrawal syndrome.

Respiratory System: *frequent:* cough increased, rhinitis; *infrequent:* asthma, bronchitis, dyspnea, epistaxis, hyperventilation, pneumonia, respiratory flu, sinusitis, voice alteration; *rare:* emphysema, hemoptysis, hiccups, lung fibrosis, pulmonary edema, sputum increased.

Skin and Appendages: *frequent:* pruritus; *infrequent:* acne, alopecia, dry skin, ecchymosis, eczema, furunculosis, urticaria; *rare:* angioedema, contact dermatitis, erythema nodosum, erythema multiforme, fungal dermatitis, herpes simplex, herpes zoster, hirsutism, maculopapular rash, photosensitivity, seborrhea, skin discoloration, skin hypertrophy, skin melanoma, skin ulcer, vesiculobullous rash.

Special Senses: *frequent:* tinnitus; *infrequent:* abnormality of accommodation, conjunctivitis, ear pain, eye pain, mydriasis, otitis media, taste loss, visual field defect; *rare:* amblyopia, anisocoria, blepharitis, cataract, conjunctival edema, corneal ulcer, deafness, exophthalmos, eye hemorrhage, glaucoma, hyperacusis, keratoconjunctivitis, night blindness, otitis externa, parosmia, photophobia, ptosis, retinal hemorrhage.

Urogenital System: *infrequent:* abortion, amenorrhea, breast pain, cystitis, dysmenorrhea, dysuria, hematuria, menorrhagia, nocturia, polyuria, urethritis, urinary incontinence, urinary retention, urinary urgency, vaginitis; *rare:* breast atrophy, breast carcinoma, breast enlargement, breast neoplasm, epididymitis, female lactation, fibrocystic breast, kidney calculus, kidney function abnormal, kidney pain, leukorrhea, mastitis, metrorrhagia, nephritis, oliguria, prostatic carcinoma, pyuria, urethritis, uterine spasm, urolith, vaginal hemorrhage, vaginal moniliasis.

Table 2. Treatment Emergent Adverse Experience Incidence in Placebo-Controlled Clinical Trials for Obsessive Compulsive Disorder and Panic Disorder [1]

Body System	Preferred Term	Obsessive Compulsive Disorder: Paxil (n=542)	Obsessive Compulsive Disorder: Placebo (n=265)	Panic Disorder: Paxil (n=469)	Panic Disorder: Placebo (n=324)
Body as a Whole	Asthenia	22%	14%	14%	5%
	Abdominal Pain	—	—	4%	3%
	Chest Pain	3%	2%	—	—
	Back Pain	—	—	3%	2%
	Chills	2%	1%	2%	1%
Cardiovascular	Vasodilation	4%	1%	—	—
	Palpitation	2%	0%	—	—
Dermatologic	Sweating	9%	3%	14%	6%
	Rash	3%	2%	—	—
Gastrointestinal	Nausea	23%	10%	23%	17%
	Dry Mouth	18%	9%	18%	11%
	Constipation	16%	6%	8%	5%
	Diarrhea	10%	10%	12%	7%
	Decreased Appetite	9%	3%	7%	3%
	Increased Appetite	4%	3%	2%	1%
Nervous System	Insomnia	24%	13%	18%	10%
	Somnolence	24%	7%	19%	11%
	Dizziness	12%	6%	14%	10%
	Tremor	11%	1%	9%	1%
	Nervousness	9%	8%	—	—
	Libido Decreased	7%	4%	9%	1%
	Agitation	—	—	5%	4%
	Anxiety	—	—	5%	4%
	Abnormal Dreams	4%	1%	—	—
	Concentration Impaired	3%	2%	—	—
	Depersonalization	3%	0%	—	—
	Myoclonus	3%	0%	3%	2%
	Amnesia	2%	1%	—	—
Respiratory System	Rhinitis	—	—	3%	0%
Special Senses	Abnormal Vision	4%	2%	—	—
	Taste Perversion	2%	0%	—	—
Urogenital System	Abnormal Ejaculation[2]	23%	1%	21%	1%
	Female Genital Disorder[2]	3%	0%	9%	1%
	Impotence [2]	8%	1%	5%	0%
	Urinary Frequency	3%	1%	2%	0%
	Urination Impaired	3%	0%	—	—
	Urinary Tract Infection	2%	1%	2%	1%

1. Events reported by at least 2% of OCD or panic disorder *Paxil*-treated patients are included, except the following events which had an incidence on placebo ≥ *Paxil:* [OCD]: abdominal pain, agitation, anxiety, back pain, cough increased, depression, headache, hyperkinesia, infection, paresthesia, pharyngitis, respiratory disorder, rhinitis and sinusitis. [panic disorder]: abnormal dreams, abnormal vision, chest pain, cough increased, depersonalization, depression, dysmenorrhea, dyspepsia, flu syndrome, headache, infection, myalgia, nervousness, palpitation, paresthesia, pharyngitis, rash, respiratory disorder, sinusitis, taste perversion, trauma, urination impaired and vasodilation.
2. Percentage corrected for gender.

Postmarketing Reports

Voluntary reports of adverse events in patients taking Paxil (paroxetine hydrochloride) that have been received since market introduction and not listed above that may have no causal relationship with the drug include acute pancreatitis, elevated liver function tests (the most severe cases were deaths due to liver necrosis, and grossly elevated transaminases associated with severe liver dysfunction), Guillain-Barré syndrome, toxic epidermal necrolysis, priapism, thrombocytopenia, syndrome of inappropriate ADH secretion, symptoms suggestive of prolactinemia and galactorrhea, neuroleptic malignant syndrome-like events; extrapyramidal symptoms which have included akathisia, bradykinesia, cogwheel rigidity, dystonia, hypertonia, oculogyric crisis which has been associated with concomitant use of pimozide, tremor and trismus; and serotonin syndrome, associated in some cases with concomitant use of serotonergic drugs and with drugs which may have impaired *Paxil* metabolism (symptoms have included agitation, confusion, diaphoresis, hallucinations, hyperreflexia, myoclonus, shivering, tachycardia and tremor). There have been spontaneous reports that abrupt discontinuation may lead to symptoms such as dizziness, sensory disturbances, agitation or anxiety, nausea and sweating; these events are generally self-limiting. There has been a case report of an elevated phenytoin level after 4 weeks of *Paxil* and phenytoin co-administration. There has been a case report of severe hypotension when *Paxil* was added to chronic metoprolol treatment.

DRUG ABUSE AND DEPENDENCE

Controlled Substance Class: Paxil (paroxetine hydrochloride) is not a controlled substance.

Physical and Psychologic Dependence: *Paxil* has not been systematically studied in animals or humans for its potential for abuse, tolerance or physical dependence. While the clinical trials did not reveal any tendency for any drug-seeking behavior, these observations were not systematic and it is not possible to predict on the basis of this limited experience the extent to which a CNS-active drug will be misused, diverted and/or abused once marketed. Consequently, patients should be evaluated carefully for history of drug abuse, and such patients should be observed closely for signs of *Paxil* misuse or abuse (e.g., development of tolerance, incrementations of dose, drug-seeking behavior).

OVERDOSAGE

Human Experience: Overdose with *Paxil* (up to 2000 mg) alone and in combination with other drugs has been reported. Signs and symptoms of overdose with *Paxil* include nausea, vomiting, sedation, dizziness, sweating, and facial flush. There are no reports of coma or convulsions following overdosage with *Paxil* alone. A fatal outcome has been reported rarely when *Paxil* was taken in combination with other agents, or when taken alone.

Overdosage Management: Treatment should consist of those general measures employed in the management of overdosage with any antidepressant. There are no specific antidotes for *Paxil.* Establish and maintain an airway; ensure adequate oxygenation and ventilation. Gastric evacuation either by the induction of emesis or lavage or both should be performed. In most cases, following evacuation, 20 to 30 grams of activated charcoal may be administered every 4 to 6 hours during the first 24 to 48 hours after ingestion. An ECG should be taken and monitoring of cardiac function instituted if there is any evidence of abnormality. Supportive care with frequent monitoring of vital signs and careful observation is indicated. Due to the large volume of distribution of *Paxil,* forced diuresis, dialysis, hemoperfusion and exchange transfusion are unlikely to be of benefit. A specific caution involves patients taking or recently having taken paroxetine who might ingest by accident or intent excessive quantities of a tricyclic antidepressant. In such a case, accumulation of the parent tricyclic and its active metabolite may increase the possibility of clinically significant sequelae and extend the time needed for close medical observation.

In managing overdosage, consider the possibility of multiple-drug involvement. The physician should consider contacting a poison control center for additional information on the treatment of any overdose. Telephone numbers for certified poison control centers are listed in the *Physicians' Desk Reference* (PDR).

DOSAGE AND ADMINISTRATION

Depression

Usual Initial Dosage: Paxil (paroxetine hydrochloride) should be administered as a single daily dose, usually in the morning. The recommended initial dose is 20 mg/day. Patients were dosed in a range of 20 to 50 mg/day in the clinical trials demonstrating the antidepressant effectiveness of *Paxil.* As with all antidepressants, the full antidepressant effect may be delayed. Some patients not responding to a 20 mg dose may benefit from dose increases, in 10 mg/day increments, up to a maximum of 50 mg/day. Dose changes should occur at intervals of at least 1 week.

Maintenance Therapy: There is no body of evidence available to answer the question of how long the patient treated with *Paxil* should remain on it. It is generally agreed that acute episodes of depression require several months or longer of sustained pharmacologic therapy. Whether the dose of an antidepressant needed to induce remission is identical to the dose needed to maintain and/or sustain euthymia is unknown.

Systematic evaluation of the efficacy of Paxil (paroxetine hydrochloride) has shown that efficacy is maintained for periods of up to 1 year with doses that averaged about 30 mg.

Obsessive Compulsive Disorder

Usual Initial Dosage: Paxil (paroxetine hydrochloride) should be administered as a single daily dose, usually in the morning. The recommended dose of *Paxil* in the treatment of OCD is 40 mg daily. Patients should be started on 20 mg/day and the dose can be increased in 10 mg/day increments. Dose changes should occur at intervals of at least 1 week. Patients were dosed in a range of 20 to 60 mg/day in the clinical trials demonstrating the effectiveness of *Paxil* in the treatment of OCD. The maximum dosage should not exceed 60 mg/day.

Maintenance Therapy: Long-term maintenance of efficacy was demonstrated in a 6-month relapse prevention trial. In this trial, patients with OCD assigned to paroxetine demonstrated a lower relapse rate compared to patients on placebo (see CLINICAL PHARMACOLOGY). OCD is a chronic condition, and it is reasonable to consider continuation for a responding patient. Dosage adjustments should be made to maintain the patient on the lowest effective dosage, and patients should be periodically reassessed to determine the need for continued treatment.

Panic Disorder

Usual Initial Dosage: Paxil should be administered as a single daily dose, usually in the morning. The target dose of *Paxil* in the treatment of panic disorder is 40 mg/day. Patients should be started on 10 mg/day. Dose changes should occur in 10 mg/week increments and at intervals of at least 1 week. Patients were dosed in a range of 10 to 60 mg/day in the clinical trials demonstrating the effectiveness of *Paxil*. The maximum dosage should not exceed 60 mg/day.

Maintenance Therapy: Long-term maintenance of efficacy was demonstrated in a 3-month relapse prevention trial. In this trial, patients with panic disorder assigned to paroxetine demonstrated a lower relapse rate compared to patients on placebo (see CLINICAL PHARMACOLOGY). Panic disorder is a chronic condition, and it is reasonable to consider continuation for a responding patient. Dosage adjustments should be made to maintain the patient on the lowest effective dosage, and patients should be periodically reassessed to determine the need for continued treatment.

Dosage for Elderly or Debilitated, and Patients with Severe Renal or Hepatic Impairment: The recommended initial dose is 10 mg/day for elderly patients, debilitated patients, and/or patients with severe renal or hepatic impairment. Increases may be made if indicated. Dosage should not exceed 40 mg/day.

Switching Patients to or from a Monoamine Oxidase Inhibitor: At least 14 days should elapse between discontinuation of a MAOI and initiation of *Paxil* therapy. Similarly, at least 14 days should be allowed after stopping *Paxil* before starting a MAOI.

NOTE: SHAKE SUSPENSION WELL BEFORE USING.

HOW SUPPLIED

Tablets: Film-coated, modified-oval as follows:

10 mg yellow tablets engraved on the front with PAXIL and on the back with 10.

NDC 0029-3210-13 Bottles of 30

20 mg pink, scored tablets engraved on the front with PAXIL and on the back with 20.

NDC 0029-3211-13 Bottles of 30
NDC 0029-3211-20 Bottles of 100
NDC 0029-3211-21 SUP 100's (intended for institutional use only)

30 mg blue tablets engraved on the front with PAXIL and on the back with 30.

NDC 0029-3212-13 Bottles of 30

40 mg green tablets engraved on the front with PAXIL and on the back with 40.

NDC 0029-3213-13 Bottles of 30

Store between 15° and 30°C (59° and 86°F).

Oral Suspension: Orange-colored, orange-flavored, 10 mg/5 mL, in 250 mL white bottles. Manufactured in Crawley, UK, by SmithKline Beecham Pharmaceuticals.

NDC 0029-3215-48

Store suspension at or below 25°C (77°F).

Veterans Administration/Military/PHS—Tablets,10 mg, 30's, 6505–01–431–5699; 20 mg, 30's, 6505-01-371-8323; 20 mg, 100's, 6505-01-371-8322; 20 mg, SUP, 100's, 6505-01-371-8321; 30 mg, 30's, 6505-01-371-8320; 40 mg, 30's, 6505–01–431–5702.

PX:L14

Shown in Product Identification Guide, page 339

RABIES VACCINE ADSORBED ℞

DESCRIPTION

Rabies Vaccine Adsorbed is a sterile, cell-culture derived rabies vaccine for pre- and post-exposure prophylaxis in humans. It is prepared with the CVS Kissling/MDPH strain of rabies virus. The virus is propagated in a diploid cell line derived from fetal rhesus lung cells (FRhL-2 cell line) in a serum-free, chemically defined, antibiotic-free medium. The virus harvest, which is clarified by centrifugation and filtration, is inactivated with betapropiolactone. After inactivation, the virus is adsorbed to aluminum phosphate.

The final vaccine is a suspension containing 2.5 international units or more of rabies antigen per 1.0 mL dose. It contains no more than 2.0 mg aluminum phosphate per mL and also contains 0.01% sodium ethylmercurithiosalicylate (thimerosal) as a preservative. The solution is a light pink color due to the presence of phenol red.

Rabies Vaccine Adsorbed is intended for intramuscular (IM) injection. CAUTION: THIS VACCINE IS NOT FOR USE BY THE INTRADERMAL (ID) ROUTE.

CLINICAL PHARMACOLOGY

The immune response to rabies vaccines can be ascertained by measuring antibody directed against rabies virus by means of the rapid fluorescent focus inhibition test (RFFIT). Serum antibody levels against rabies virus are usually expressed in terms of international units or serum titers. The definition of a minimally acceptable antibody titer in vaccinees varies among laboratories and is dependent on the type of test performed. The Centers for Disease Control considers complete virus neutralization at a 1:5 serum dilution by the RFFIT a minimally acceptable response to pre-exposure vaccination. The World Health Organization specifies that a minimum titer of 0.5 international units is an adequate response to vaccination.

In field trials of Rabies Vaccine Adsorbed, 99% or greater of 1,567 persons who had not been immunized previously against rabies responded with serum titers of 0.5 international units (a dilution titer of approximately 1:25) or greater by 2 weeks after the last of 3 IM injections of Rabies Vaccine Adsorbed given over a 3- or 4-week period. At 9 to 12 months post-immunization, 97% of 605 persons had antibody titers at or above a level of 0.1 international units (a 1:5 dilution of serum). In addition, 97% or more of 2,148 persons previously immunized with Duck Embryo Rabies Vaccine, Human Diploid Rabies Vaccine or Rabies Vaccine Adsorbed showed 4-fold increased antibody titers following a single booster injection of Rabies Vaccine Adsorbed.

In post-exposure field trials and clinical simulations of post-exposure prophylaxis, 5 doses of Rabies Vaccine Adsorbed, in conjunction with Rabies Immune Globulin, induced active antibody production in all previously unvaccinated persons between the seventh and fourteenth day following initiation of treatment. In post-exposure rabies prophylaxis, Rabies Immune Globulin is given concomitantly with the first injection of rabies vaccine to provide immediate passive immunoprophylaxis. If not given when vaccination was begun, Rabies Immune Globulin may be given up to 7 days after administration of the first dose of vaccine.

Rabies Vaccine Adsorbed has been used successfully to immunize both adults and children 6 years of age and older. There have been reports of possible vaccine failures when human diploid cell rabies vaccine (HDCV) has been administered in the gluteal area. Subcutaneous fat in the gluteal area may interfere with the immunogenicity of HDCV.[1-3] It is not known if an adequate response would be obtained after gluteal administration of Rabies Vaccine Adsorbed. Therefore, adults and older children should receive this vaccine in the deltoid muscle. For younger children the anterolateral aspect of the thigh is also acceptable.

INDICATIONS AND USAGE

Rabies Vaccine Adsorbed is indicated for immunization against rabies in the following circumstances: primary pre-exposure immunization which is intended to induce immunity before exposure to the virus; pre-exposure booster immunization which is intended to augment or reinforce the level of immunity induced by previous immunization against rabies; or post-exposure prophylaxis which is given to persons who, in the judgment of the treating physician, may have been exposed to rabies virus. Each circumstance requires a different schedule of injections.

A. **Primary Pre-Exposure Vaccination** (see Table 1): Pre-exposure vaccination is given to persons who are at greater than usual risk of possible rabies exposure by reason of occupation or avocation. The list of such persons includes, but is not limited to, veterinarians and staff, certain laboratory workers, animal handlers and persons spending time (e.g., 1 month or more) in foreign countries where canine rabies is enzootic. Persons whose vocational or avocational pursuits bring them into contact with potentially rabid dogs, cats, foxes, skunks, raccoons, bats or other species at risk of having rabies should also be considered for pre-exposure prophylaxis.

Pre-exposure vaccination is given as a series of 3 individual injections of Rabies Vaccine Adsorbed with the second and third injections being given 7 and 21 or 28 days after the first injection, respectively. Pre-exposure vaccination does not eliminate the need for prompt post-exposure prophylaxis following an exposure; it only eliminates the need for Rabies Immune Globulin and reduces the number of injections of rabies vaccine needed for post-exposure prophylaxis. Criteria for pre-exposure vaccination are summarized in Table 1.

B. **Pre-Exposure Booster Vaccination** (see Table 1): Pre-exposure booster vaccination is given to persons who have received previous rabies vaccination and remain at increased risk of rabies exposure by reasons of occupation or avocation. Persons who work with live rabies virus in research laboratories or vaccine production facilities (continuous-risk category; see Table 1) should have a serum sample tested for rabies antibody every 6 months. Booster doses of vaccine should be given to maintain a serum titer corresponding to at least complete neutralization at a 1:5 serum dilution by the RFFIT. The frequent-risk category includes other laboratory workers, such as those doing rabies diagnostic testing, spelunkers,

veterinarians and staff, animal-control and wildlife officers in areas where animal rabies is epizootic, and international travelers living or visiting (for >30 days) in areas where canine rabies is endemic. Persons among this group should have a serum sample tested for rabies antibody every 2 years and, if the titer is less than complete neutralization at a 1:5 serum dilution by the RFFIT, should have a booster dose of vaccine. Alternatively, a booster can be administered in lieu of a titer determination. Veterinarians and animal-control and wildlife officers working in areas of low rabies enzooticity (infrequent-exposure group) do not require routine pre-exposure booster doses of Rabies Vaccine Adsorbed after completion of primary pre-exposure vaccination (Table 1).

A single booster injection of Rabies Vaccine Adsorbed has been shown to increase antibody titers in persons who have previously been immunized with Rabies Vaccine Adsorbed or Human Diploid Cell Rabies Vaccine. Persons who have been shown to have developed antibody responses to a previous series of injections of Duck Embryo Rabies Vaccine also respond to a single booster dose of Rabies Vaccine Adsorbed.

[See tables 1 & 2 at top of next page]

C. **Post-Exposure Prophylaxis:** Factors to be considered for appropriate post-exposure antirabies treatment are given in Table 2.[4,5] These include the species of animal with which the person has had contact, the circumstances of the biting incident and vaccination status of the exposing animal, the type of exposure and the previous rabies immunization history of the person exposed. Carnivorous wild animals (especially skunks, raccoons and foxes) and bats are the animals most commonly infected with rabies and the cause of most of the indigenous cases of human rabies in the United States since 1960. In contrast, with the exception of woodchucks, rodents (such as squirrels, hamsters, guinea pigs, gerbils, chipmunks, rats and mice) and lagomorphs (including rabbits and hares) are rarely found to be infected with rabies and have not been known to cause human rabies in the United States. The likelihood that a domestic dog or cat is infected with rabies varies from region to region and depends, in part, on the vaccination history of the animal. In addition, an unprovoked attack is more likely than a provoked attack to indicate that an animal is rabid. Moreover, rabies is transmitted by introducing the virus into open wounds or mucous membranes. Thus, the likelihood of rabies infection depends, in part, on whether the exposure occurred by penetrating the skin or by contamination of mucous membranes by saliva or other potentially infectious material. Physicians should evaluate each possible exposure to rabies and, if necessary, consult with their state or local public health officials regarding the need for rabies prophylaxis.

1. Local Treatment of Wounds: Immediate and thorough washing of all bite wounds and scratches with soap and water is perhaps the most effective measure for preventing rabies. In experimental animals, simple local wound cleaning has been shown to reduce markedly the likelihood of rabies. Tetanus prophylaxis and measures to control bacterial infection should be given as indicated.

2. Specific Treatment: RABIES VACCINE ADSORBED IS NOT INTENDED FOR USE IN PATIENTS KNOWN TO HAVE CLINICAL MANIFESTATION OF RABIES. The injection schedule for post-exposure prophylaxis depends on whether the patient has had or has not had previous vaccination against rabies. For persons who have not previously been vaccinated against rabies, the schedule consists of an initial injection IM of Rabies Immune Globulin (Human) (HRIG), 20 international units per kilogram body weight in total. If anatomically feasible, up to half the dose of HRIG should be thoroughly infiltrated around the wound(s) and the remainder should be administered IM in the gluteal region (for specific instructions for HRIG use, see the product package insert). The HRIG injection is followed by a series of 5 individual injections of Rabies Vaccine Adsorbed given IM on days 0, 3, 7, 14 and 28. The HRIG and Rabies Vaccine Adsorbed should be given at separate sites using separate syringes. Post-exposure rabies prophylaxis should begin the same day exposure occurred or as soon after exposure as possible. The combined use of HRIG and Rabies Vaccine Adsorbed is recommended for both bite and non-bite exposures, regardless of the interval between exposure and initiation of treatment. The sooner treatment is begun after expo-

Continued on next page

Information on the SmithKline Beecham Pharmaceuticals products appearing here is based on the labeling in effect on July 31, 1998. Further information on these and other products may be obtained from the Medical Department, SmithKline Beecham Pharmaceuticals, One Franklin Plaza, Philadelphia, PA 19101.

Rabies Vaccine Adsorbed—Cont.

sure, the better. However, there have been instances in which the decision to begin treatment was made as late as 6 months or longer after exposure due to delay in recognition that an exposure had occurred. Post-exposure antirabies vaccine should always include administration of both passive antibody and vaccination with the exception of persons who have previously received complete vaccination regimens (pre-exposure or post-exposure) with a cell culture vaccine, or persons who have been vaccinated with other types of vaccines and have had documented rabies antibody titers. Persons who have previously received rabies vaccination are given 2 IM doses of Rabies Vaccine Adsorbed: 1 on day 0 and another on day 3. They should not be given HRIG.

3. Treatment Outside the United States: If post-exposure prophylaxis is begun outside the United States with locally produced biologics, it may be desirable to provide additional treatment when the patient reaches the United States. State health departments should be contacted for specific advice in each case.[4]

CONTRAINDICATIONS

Rabies Vaccine Adsorbed is contraindicated in persons who have had life-threatening allergic reactions to previous injections of this vaccine or to components of this vaccine, including thimerosal. No such reactions have been seen to date but are theoretically possible since less severe allergic reactions have been observed. Persons who have experienced non-life-threatening allergic reactions to Rabies Vaccine Adsorbed may receive additional injections under appropriate medical supervision, if the indications for vaccination justify the risk and vaccines are not available to which the patient has not had a reaction.

WARNINGS

Pre-exposure immunization should be delayed in persons with an acute intercurrent illness.

Rabies Vaccine Adsorbed should be injected into the deltoid muscle unless the use of that muscle is contraindicated. As is the case in giving any adsorbed vaccine, care should be taken to avoid accidently depositing Rabies Vaccine Adsorbed in close approximation to a peripheral nerve or in adipose and subcutaneous tissue.

PRECAUTIONS

General: In adults and children, the vaccine should be injected into the deltoid muscle. In small children, the mid-lateral aspect of the thigh area may be preferable.

As with the injection of any biologic material that may induce an allergic reaction, epinephrine injection (1:1,000) should be available for immediate use should an anaphylactic reaction occur.

This vaccine should be given with caution to persons who are known to be sensitive to or allergic to monkey proteins. If a patient known to be allergic to monkey proteins has been exposed to a known rabid animal, and if no other rabies vaccine is available, then administration of Rabies Vaccine Adsorbed to the allergic patient should be done under the supervision of a physician qualified in the management of allergic reactions. Local or mild post-vaccination reactions are not a contraindication to continuing immunization.

Drug Interactions: Immunosuppressive agents, antimalarials and immunosuppressive diseases can interfere with development of active immunity after vaccination and may reduce the effectiveness of rabies vaccine. Immunosuppressive agents should not be given during post-exposure therapy unless essential for treatment of other conditions. When post-exposure prophylaxis is given to immunosuppressed persons, it is important that serum be tested for rabies antibody to ensure that an adequate response occurred.

Laboratory Tests: Routine testing for rabies antibody response to vaccination is not necessary. Experience from clinical trials documented that antibodies can be detected consistently in serum samples obtained approximately 2 weeks after the last injection. For immunosuppressed persons see Drug Interactions.

Pregnancy Category C: Animal reproduction studies have not been conducted with Rabies Vaccine Adsorbed. It is also not known whether Rabies Vaccine Adsorbed can cause fetal harm when administered to a pregnant woman or can affect reproductive capacity. Rabies Vaccine Adsorbed should be given to a pregnant woman only if clearly needed.

Pediatric Use: Rabies Vaccine Adsorbed has been administered to children as young as 6 years old without noticeable difference in effects from its administration to adults. All children from whom post-vaccination serum was obtained showed rabies antibody titers greater than 1:5. However, because of the limited experience with this vaccine in children, special precautions should be taken for unexpected adverse events.

ADVERSE REACTIONS

Once initiated, rabies prophylaxis should not be interrupted due to mild local or systemic reactions.

Table 1. Pre-Exposure Vaccination Criteria*

PRE-EXPOSURE VACCINATION. Primary pre-exposure vaccination consists of 3 doses of Rabies Vaccine Adsorbed, 1.0 mL, IM (i.e., deltoid area), 1 each on days 0, 7 and 21 or 28. Administration of routine booster doses of vaccine depends on exposure risk category as noted below.

Criteria for Pre-Exposure Vaccination

Risk Category	Nature of Risk	Typical Populations	Pre-Exposure Regimen
Continuous	Virus present continuously, often in high concentrations. Aerosol, mucous membrane, bite or non-bite exposure possible. Exposure may go unrecognized.	Rabies research laboratory workers[†]; rabies biologics production workers.	Primary course. Serology every 6 months; booster vaccination when antibody level falls below acceptable level.[‡]
Frequent	Exposure usually episodic, with source recognized, but exposure may also be unrecognized. Aerosol, mucous membrane, bite or non-bite exposure.	Rabies diagnostic laboratory workers,[†] spelunkers, veterinarians and staff, and animal-control and wildlife workers in rabies enzootic areas; travelers visiting foreign areas of enzootic rabies for more than 30 days.	Primary course. Serologic testing or booster vaccination every 2 years.[‡]
Infrequent (greater than population at large)	Exposure nearly always episodic with source recognized. Mucous membrane, bite or non-bite exposure.	Veterinarians and animal-control and wildlife workers in areas of low rabies enzooticity. Veterinary students.	Primary course. No serologic testing or booster vaccination.
Rare (population at large)	Exposure always episodic. Mucous membrane or bite with source recognized.	U.S. population at large, including individuals in rabies enzootic areas.	No vaccination necessary.

* References 4 and 5.
†Judgment of relative risk and extra monitoring of immunization status is the responsibility of the laboratory supervisor (see U.S. Department of Health and Human Services' Biosafety in *Microbiological and Biomedical Laboratories*, 1984).
‡Pre-exposure booster vaccination consists of 1 dose of Rabies Vaccine Adsorbed, 1.0 mL dose intramuscular (deltoid muscle). Minimum acceptable antibody level is complete virus neutralization at a 1:5 serum dilution by RFFIT. Administer booster dose if titer falls below 1:5.

Table 2. Rabies Post-Exposure Prophylaxis Guide*

Animal Type	Evaluation and Disposition of Animal	Post-Exposure Prophylaxis Recommendations
Dogs and cats	Healthy and available for 10 days' observation	Should not begin prophylaxis unless animal develops symptoms of rabies[†]
	Rabid or suspected rabid Unknown (escaped)	Immediate vaccination Consult public health officials
Skunks, raccoons, bats, foxes and most other carnivores; woodchucks	Regarded as rabid unless geographic area is known to be free of rabies or until animal proven negative by laboratory tests[‡]	Immediate vaccination
Livestock, rodents and lagomorphs (rabbits and hares)	Consider individually	Consult public health officials. Bites of squirrels, hamsters, guinea pigs, gerbils, chipmunks, rats, mice, other rodents, rabbits and hares almost never require antirabies treatment.

* References 4 and 5.
†During the 10-day holding period, begin treatment with Rabies Vaccine Adsorbed with or without Rabies Immune Globulin (Human) at first sign of rabies in a dog or cat that has bitten someone (see Post-Exposure Prophylaxis below). The symptomatic animal should be killed immediately and tested.
‡The animal should be killed and tested as soon as possible. Holding for observation is not recommended. Discontinue vaccine if immunofluorescence test results of the animal are negative.

Local: Approximately 65% to 70% of persons given IM injections of Rabies Vaccine Adsorbed reported subjective mild, transient discomfort localized to the injection site. In a few, aching of the injected muscle and a mild local inflammatory reaction consisting of swelling, induration or erythema were present for 48 hours. These local complaints can usually be successfully treated with simple analgesics.
Systemic: Mild, transient constitutional reactions have been reported by 8% to 10% of Rabies Vaccine Adsorbed recipients. These consisted chiefly of headache, nausea, slight fever or fatigue. Also, serum-sickness-like reactions, some with arthralgia, suggestive of hypersensitivity to Rabies Vaccine Adsorbed, have been reported in less than 1% of vaccinees between 7 and 14 days after vaccination. These hypersensitivity reactions have occurred after booster vaccination, but have not been seen following primary immunization with Rabies Vaccine Adsorbed.
The occurrence of allergic reactions in patients receiving either Rabies Vaccine Adsorbed or Human Diploid Cell Rabies Vaccine raises special difficulties for the managing physician. The use of pre-exposure booster doses of Human Diploid Cell Rabies Vaccine has been limited by the observation of serum-sickness-like allergic reactions that occur in approximately 6% of individuals who receive boosters with that vaccine.[5] These reactions are thought to be due to small

amounts of human serum albumin that have been rendered allergenic by betapropiolactone. Human serum albumin is not used in the medium used to grow the rabies virus for Rabies Vaccine Adsorbed and therefore is not present when betapropiolactone is added to inactivate the virus. Nevertheless, systemic allergic reactions have also occurred in some individuals following booster doses of Rabies Vaccine Adsorbed at a rate of less than 1%. However, it is not known whether patients who are allergic to Rabies Vaccine Adsorbed are also allergic to Human Diploid Cell Rabies Vaccine and vice versa. Thus, judgments must be made regarding whether or not to continue the vaccination schedule and whether or not to change the vaccines.
Other: Neurologic reactions such as those reported to be temporally associated with the administration of other viral vaccines, including Human Diploid Cell Rabies Vaccine, for example, allergic peripheral neuritis, encephalomyelitis or transverse myelitis, have not been reported in recipients of Rabies Vaccine Adsorbed.
If serious adverse reactions are noted, report them promptly to the manufacturer: Michigan Department of Public Health, 517-335-8050 during working hours or 517-335-9030 at other times. Reports may also be submitted directly to the FDA on form FDA-1639, single copies of which may be obtained from the Division of Epidemiology and Surveillance (HFN-730), 5600 Fishers Lane, Rockville, MD 20857.

DOSAGE AND ADMINISTRATION

Each vial of Rabies Vaccine Adsorbed contains a sufficient volume of vaccine to enable withdrawing a full dose of 1.0 mL. The vial should be shaken gently before withdrawing the vaccine to ensure complete suspension of the aluminum phosphate adjuvant. The vaccine should be given IM. THIS VACCINE IS NOT FOR USE BY THE ID ROUTE. Before injecting the vaccine, the syringe barrel should be retracted sufficiently to create a back-pressure to ascertain whether the needle is in the lumen of a blood vessel.

In adults and children, the site of the injection is the deltoid muscle. Administration into the buttock is not recommended since experience with other vaccines has shown that acceptable antibody titers may not be obtained.[3] In small children, who may have insufficient deltoid muscle mass, the anterolateral aspect of the thigh is an acceptable injection site.

Pre-Exposure Vaccination: Pre-exposure vaccination consists of three 1.0 mL IM injections of rabies vaccine, 1 each given at 0, 7 and 21 or 28 days. (Also see Table 1.)

Booster Vaccination: Booster vaccination consists of a single 1.0 mL IM injection of vaccine.

Post-Exposure Prophylaxis: Post-exposure prophylaxis for persons not previously vaccinated against rabies consists of an injection of HRIG, 20 international units per kilogram body weight, and five 1.0 mL injections of Rabies Vaccine Adsorbed, intramuscularly, 1 each to be given on days 0, 3, 7, 14 and 28. The amount of HRIG administered should not exceed the recommended amount. Post-exposure prophylaxis for persons who have been previously vaccinated against rabies consists of two 1.0 mL IM injections of Rabies Vaccine Adsorbed: 1 at day 0 and the second on day 3. HRIG should not be given. Persons should be considered to have been immunized previously if they received pre- or post-exposure prophylaxis with Rabies Vaccine Adsorbed or Human Diploid Cell Rabies Vaccine or have been documented to have had an adequate antibody response to Duck Embryo Rabies Vaccine. (Also see Table 2.)

Parenteral drug products should be inspected for particulate matter and discoloration prior to administration, whenever solution and container permit. This vaccine should have a light pink color due to the presence of phenol red in a neutral solution. Do not use vials that are discolored or contain particulate matter.

HOW SUPPLIED

Rabies Vaccine Adsorbed is supplied in a single-dose, rubber-stoppered vial which contains sufficient volume to enable withdrawing a full 1.0 mL dose.

Package of 1: NDC 0007-4840-01

STORAGE

Rabies Vaccine Adsorbed should be stored at 2° to 8°C (35° to 46°F). Do not freeze; discard if product has been frozen.

REFERENCES

1. Shill, M., Baynes, R.D., and Miller, S.D.: Fatal Rabies Encephalitis Despite Appropriate Post-Exposure Prophylaxis. *N. Engl. J. Med.* 316:1257–1258, 1987.
2. Baer, G.M., and Fishbein, D.B.: Rabies Post-Exposure Prophylaxis. *N. Engl. J. Med.* 316:1270–1272, 1987.
3. Centers for Disease Control: Human Rabies Despite Treatment with Rabies Immune Globulin and Human Diploid Cell Rabies Vaccine—Thailand. *MMWR.* 36:(November 27) 757–760, 765, 1987.
4. Centers for Disease Control: Rabies Prevention—United States, 1991: Recommendations of the Immunization Practices Advisory Committee (ACIP). *MMWR.* 40 (No. RR-3): 1–19, 1991.
5. Centers for Disease Control: Rabies Vaccine Adsorbed: A New Rabies Vaccine for Use in Humans. *MMWR.* April 1988.

Additional References

6. Corey, L., and Hattwick, M.A.W.: Treatment of Persons Exposed to Rabies. *JAMA.* 232:272–276, 1975.
7. Burgoyne, G.H., Kajiya, K.D., Brown, D.W., and Mitchell, J.R.: Rhesus Diploid Rabies Vaccine (Adsorbed): A New Rabies Vaccine Using FRhL-2 Cells. *J. Infect. Dis.* 152:204–210, 1985.
8. Berlin, B.S., Mitchell, J.R., Burgoyne, G.H., et al.: Rhesus Diploid Rabies Vaccine (Adsorbed), A New Rabies Vaccine: Results of Initial Clinical Studies of Pre-Exposure Vaccination. *JAMA.* 247:1726–1728, 1982.
9. Berlin, B.S., Mitchell, J.R., Burgoyne, G.H., et al.: Rhesus Diploid Rabies Vaccine (Adsorbed), A New Rabies Vaccine II. Results of Clinical Studies Simulating Prophylactic Therapy for Rabies Exposure. *JAMA.* 249: 2663–2665, 1983.
10. Bahmanyar, M., Fayaz, A., Nour-Salehi, S., et al.: Successful Protection of Humans Exposed to Rabies Infection. *JAMA.* 236:2751–2754, 1976.

Manufactured by
Michigan Department of Public Health
Lansing, MI 48909
U.S. License No. 99
Distributed by
SmithKline Beecham Pharmaceuticals
Philadelphia, PA 19101
Veterans Administration/Military/PHS—Vial, 1 mL, 1's, 6505-01-378-0232.
RV:L3

Shown in Product Identification Guide, page 340

RELAFEN® ℞

[*rel 'ah-fen*]
brand of nabumetone tablets

DESCRIPTION

Relafen (nabumetone) is a naphthylalkanone designated chemically as 4-(6-methoxy-2-naphthalenyl)-2-butanone. It has the following structure:

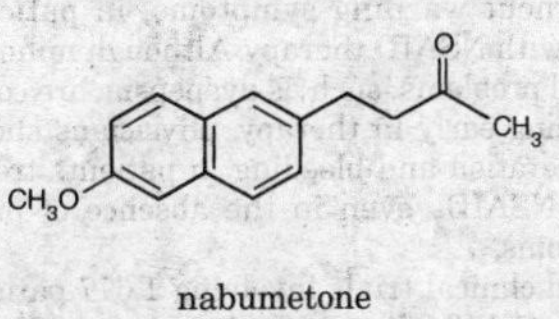

nabumetone

Nabumetone is a white to off-white crystalline substance with a molecular weight of 228.3. It is nonacidic and practically insoluble in water, but soluble in alcohol and most organic solvents. It has an n-octanol:phosphate buffer partition coefficient of 2400 at pH 7.4.

Tablets for Oral Administration: Each oval-shaped, film-coated tablet contains 500 mg or 750 mg of nabumetone. Inactive ingredients consist of hydroxypropyl methylcellulose, microcrystalline cellulose, polyethylene glycol, polysorbate 80, sodium lauryl sulfate, sodium starch glycolate and titanium dioxide. The 750 mg tablets also contain iron oxides.

CLINICAL PHARMACOLOGY

Relafen is a nonsteroidal anti-inflammatory drug (NSAID) that exhibits anti-inflammatory, analgesic and antipyretic properties in pharmacologic studies. As with other nonsteroidal anti-inflammatory agents, its mode of action is not known. However, the ability to inhibit prostaglandin synthesis may be involved in the anti-inflammatory effect.

The parent compound is a prodrug, which undergoes hepatic biotransformation to the active component, 6-methoxy-2-naphthylacetic acid (6MNA), that is a potent inhibitor of prostaglandin synthesis.

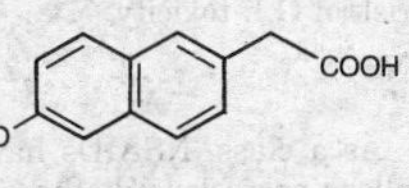

6-methoxy-2-naphthylacetic acid (6MNA)

It is acidic and has an n-octanol:phosphate buffer partition coefficient of 0.5 at pH 7.4.

Pharmacokinetics

After oral administration, approximately 80% of a radiolabelled dose of nabumetone is found in the urine, indicating that nabumetone is well absorbed from the gastrointestinal tract. Nabumetone itself is not detected in the plasma because, after absorption, it undergoes rapid biotransformation to the principal active metabolite, 6-methoxy-2-naphthylacetic acid (6MNA). Approximately 35% of a 1000 mg oral dose of nabumetone is converted to 6MNA and 50% is converted into unidentified metabolites which are subsequently excreted in the urine. Following oral administration of *Relafen,* 6MNA exhibits pharmacokinetic characteristics that generally follow a one-compartment model with first order input and first order elimination.

6MNA is more than 99% bound to plasma proteins. The free fraction is dependent on total concentration of 6MNA and is proportional to dose over the range of 1000 mg to 2000 mg. It is 0.2% to 0.3% at concentrations typically achieved following administration of *Relafen* 1000 mg and is approximately 0.6% to 0.8% of the total concentrations at steady state following daily administration of 2000 mg.

Steady-state plasma concentrations of 6MNA are slightly lower than predicted from single-dose data. This may result from the higher fraction of unbound 6MNA which undergoes greater hepatic clearance.

Coadministration of food increases the rate of absorption and subsequent appearance of 6MNA in the plasma but does not affect the extent of conversion of nabumetone into 6MNA. Peak plasma concentrations of 6MNA are increased by approximately one third.

Coadministration with an aluminum-containing antacid had no significant effect on the bioavailability of 6MNA.

[See table 1 at bottom of next page]

The simulated curves in the graph below illustrate the range of active metabolite plasma concentrations that would be expected from 95% of patients following 1000 mg to 2000 mg doses to steady state. The cross-hatched area represents the expected overlap in plasma concentrations due to intersubject variation following oral administration of 1000 mg to 2000 mg of *Relafen.*

Nabumetone Active Metabolite (6MNA) Plasma Concentrations at Steady State Following Once-Daily Dosing of Nabumetone
1000 mg (n=31) 2000 mg (n=12)

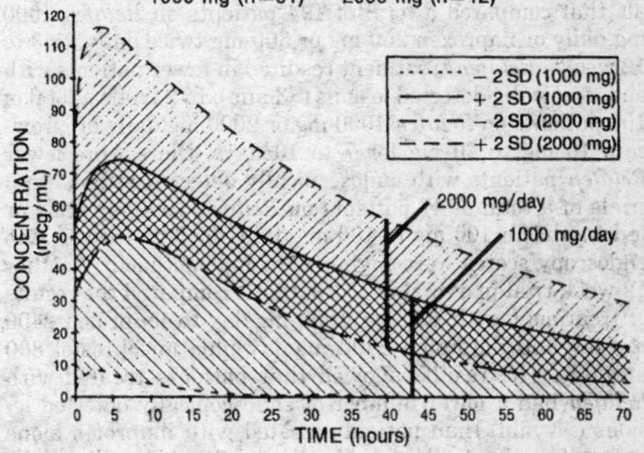

6MNA undergoes biotransformation in the liver, producing inactive metabolites that are eliminated as both free metabolites and conjugates. None of the known metabolites of 6MNA has been detected in plasma. Preliminary *in vivo* and *in vitro* studies suggest that unlike other NSAIDs, there is no evidence of enterohepatic recirculation of the active metabolite. Approximately 75% of a radiolabelled dose was recovered in urine in 48 hours. Approximately 80% was recovered in 168 hours. A further 9% appeared in the feces. In the first 48 hours, metabolites consisted of:

—nabumetone, unchanged	not detectable
—6-methoxy-2-naphthylacetic acid (6MNA), unchanged	<1%
—6MNA, conjugated	11%
—6-hydroxy-2-naphthylacetic acid (6HNA), unchanged	5%
—6HNA, conjugated	7%
—4-(6-hydroxy-2-naphthyl)-butan-2-ol, conjugated	9%
—*O*-desmethyl-nabumetone, conjugated	7%
—unidentified minor metabolites	34%
Total % Dose:	73%

Following oral administration of dosages of 1000 mg to 2000 mg to steady state, the mean plasma clearance of 6MNA is 20 to 30 mL/min. and the elimination half-life is approximately 24 hours.

Elderly Patients: Steady-state plasma concentrations in elderly patients were generally higher than in young healthy subjects. (See Table 1 for summary of pharmacokinetic parameters.)

Renal Insufficiency: In studies of patients with renal insufficiency, the mean terminal half-life of 6MNA was increased in patients with severe renal dysfunction (creatinine clearance <30 mL/min./1.73 m^2). In patients undergoing hemodialysis, steady-state plasma concentrations of the active metabolite were similar to those observed in healthy subjects. Due to extensive protein-binding, 6MNA is not dialyzable.

Hepatic Impairment: Data in patients with severe hepatic impairment are limited. Biotransformation of nabumetone to 6MNA and the further metabolism of 6MNA to inactive metabolites is dependent on hepatic function and could be reduced in patients with severe hepatic impairment (history of or biopsy-proven cirrhosis).

Special Studies

Gastrointestinal: Relafen (nabumetone) was compared to aspirin in inducing gastrointestinal blood loss. Food intake was not monitored. Studies utilizing ^{51}Cr-tagged red blood cells in healthy males showed no difference in fecal blood loss after 3 or 4 weeks' administration of *Relafen* 1000 mg or 2000 mg daily when compared to either placebo-treated or nontreated subjects. In contrast, aspirin 3600 mg daily produced an increase in fecal blood loss when compared to the *Relafen*-treated, placebo-treated or nontreated subjects. The clinical relevance of the data is unknown.

The following endoscopy trials entered patients who had been previously treated with NSAIDs. These patients had varying baseline scores and different courses of treatment. The trials were not designed to correlate symptoms and en-

Continued on next page

Information on the SmithKline Beecham Pharmaceuticals products appearing here is based on the labeling in effect on July 31, 1998. Further information on these and other products may be obtained from the Medical Department, SmithKline Beecham Pharmaceuticals, One Franklin Plaza, Philadelphia, PA 19101.

Relafen—Cont.

doscopy scores. The clinical relevance of these endoscopy trials, i.e., either G.I. symptoms or serious G.I. events, is not known.

Ten endoscopy studies were conducted in 488 patients who had baseline and post-treatment endoscopy. In 5 clinical trials that compared a total of 194 patients on *Relafen* 1000 mg daily or naproxen 250 mg or 500 mg twice daily for 3 to 12 weeks, *Relafen* treatment resulted in fewer patients with endoscopically detected lesions (>3 mm). In 2 trials a total of 101 patients on *Relafen* 1000 mg or 2000 mg daily or piroxicam 10 mg to 20 mg for 7 to 10 days, there were fewer *Relafen* patients with endoscopically detected lesions. In 3 trials of a total of 47 patients on *Relafen* 1000 mg daily or indomethacin 100 mg to 150 mg daily for 3 to 4 weeks, the endoscopy scores were higher with indomethacin. Another 12-week trial in a total of 171 patients compared the results of treatment with *Relafen* 1000 mg/day to ibuprofen 2400 mg/day and ibuprofen 2400 mg/day plus misoprostol 800 mcg/day. The results showed that patients treated with *Relafen* had a lower number of endoscopically detected lesions (>5 mm) than patients treated with ibuprofen alone but comparable to the combination of ibuprofen plus misoprostol. The results did not correlate with abdominal pain.

Other: In 1-week repeat-dose studies in healthy volunteers, *Relafen* 1000 mg daily had little effect on collagen-induced platelet aggregation and no effect on bleeding time. In comparison, naproxen 500 mg daily suppressed collagen-induced platelet aggregation and significantly increased bleeding time.

CLINICAL TRIALS

Osteoarthritis: The use of *Relafen* in relieving the signs and symptoms of osteoarthritis was assessed in double-blind controlled trials in which 1,047 patients were treated for 6 weeks to 6 months. In these trials, *Relafen* in a dose of 1000 mg/day administered at night was comparable to naproxen 500 mg/day and to aspirin 3600 mg/day.

Rheumatoid Arthritis: The use of *Relafen* in relieving the signs and symptoms of rheumatoid arthritis was assessed in double-blind, randomized, controlled trials in which 770 patients were treated for 3 weeks to 6 months. *Relafen*, in a dose of 1000 mg/day administered at night was comparable to naproxen 500 mg/day and to aspirin 3600 mg/day.

In controlled clinical trials of rheumatoid arthritis patients, *Relafen* has been used in combination with gold, d-penicillamine and corticosteroids.

INDIVIDUALIZATION OF DOSING

There is considerable interpatient variation in response to *Relafen*. Therapy is usually initiated at a *Relafen* dose of 1000 mg daily, then adjusted, if needed, based on clinical response.

In clinical trials with osteoarthritis and rheumatoid arthritis patients, most patients responded to *Relafen* in doses of 1000 mg/day administered nightly; total daily dosages up to 2000 mg were used. In open-labelled studies, 1,490 patients were permitted dosage increases and were followed for approximately 1 year (mode). Twenty percent of patients (n=294) were withdrawn for lack of effectiveness during the first year of these open-labelled studies. The following table provides patient-exposure to doses used in the U.S. clinical trials:

Table 2. Clinical double-blind and open-labelled trials of Relafen (nabumetone) in osteoarthritis and rheumatoid arthritis

Relafen Dose	Number of Patients OA	Number of Patients RA	Mean/Mode Duration of Treatment (yrs.) OA	Mean/Mode Duration of Treatment (yrs.) RA
500 mg	17	6	0.4/–	0.2/–
1000 mg	917	701	1.2/1	1.4/1
1500 mg	645	224	2.3/1	1.7/1
2000 mg	15	100	0.6/1	1.3/1

As with other NSAIDs, the lowest dose should be sought for each patient. Patients weighing under 50 kg may be less likely to require dosages beyond 1000 mg. Therefore, after observing the response to initial therapy, the dose should be adjusted to meet individual patients' requirements.

INDICATIONS AND USAGE

Relafen is indicated for acute and chronic treatment of signs and symptoms of osteoarthritis and rheumatoid arthritis.

CONTRAINDICATIONS

Relafen is contraindicated in patients who have previously exhibited hypersensitivity to it.

Relafen is contraindicated in patients in whom *Relafen*, aspirin or other NSAIDs induce asthma, urticaria or other allergic-type reactions. Fatal asthmatic reactions have been reported in such patients receiving NSAIDs.

WARNINGS

Risk of G.I. Ulceration, Bleeding and Perforation with NSAID Therapy: Serious gastrointestinal toxicity such as bleeding, ulceration and perforation can occur at any time, with or without warning symptoms, in patients treated chronically with NSAID therapy. Although minor upper gastrointestinal problems, such as dyspepsia, are common, usually developing early in therapy, physicians should remain alert for ulceration and bleeding in patients treated chronically with NSAIDs even in the absence of previous G.I. tract symptoms.

In controlled clinical trials involving 1,677 patients treated with *Relafen* (1,140 followed for 1 year and 927 for 2 years), the cumulative incidence of peptic ulcers was 0.3% (95% Cl; 0%, 0.6%) at 3 to 6 months, 0.5% (95% Cl; 0.1%, 0.9%) at 1 year and 0.8% (95% Cl; 0.3%, 1.3%) at 2 years. Physicians should inform patients about the signs and symptoms of serious G.I. toxicity and what steps to take if they occur. In patients with active peptic ulcer, physicians must weigh the benefits of Relafen (nabumetone) therapy against possible hazards, institute an appropriate ulcer treatment regimen and monitor the patients' progress carefully.

Studies to date have not identified any subset of patients not at risk of developing peptic ulceration and bleeding. Except for a prior history of serious G.I. events and other risk factors known to be associated with peptic ulcer disease, such as alcoholism, smoking, etc., no risk factors (e.g., age, sex) have been associated with increased risk. Elderly or debilitated patients seem to tolerate ulceration or bleeding less well than other individuals and most spontaneous reports of fatal G.I. events are in this population.

High doses of any NSAID probably carry a greater risk of these reactions, although controlled clinical trials showing this do not exist in most cases. In considering the use of relatively large doses (within the recommended dosage range), sufficient benefit should be anticipated to offset the potential increased risk of G.I. toxicity.

PRECAUTIONS

General

Renal Effects: As a class, NSAIDs have been associated with renal papillary necrosis and other abnormal renal pathology during long-term administration to animals.

A second form of renal toxicity often associated with NSAIDs is seen in patients with conditions leading to a reduction in renal blood flow or blood volume, where renal prostaglandins have a supportive role in the maintenance of renal perfusion. In these patients, administration of an NSAID results in a dose-dependent decrease in prostaglandin synthesis and, secondarily, in a reduction of renal blood flow, which may precipitate overt renal decompensation. Patients at greatest risk of this reaction are those with impaired renal function, heart failure, liver dysfunction, those taking diuretics, and the elderly. Discontinuation of NSAID therapy is typically followed by recovery to the pretreatment state.

Because nabumetone undergoes extensive hepatic metabolism, no adjustment of *Relafen* dosage is generally necessary in patients with renal insufficiency. However, as with all NSAIDs, patients with impaired renal function should be monitored more closely than patients with normal renal function (see CLINICAL PHARMACOLOGY, Special Studies). The oxidized and conjugated metabolites of 6MNA are eliminated primarily by the kidneys. The extent to which these largely inactive metabolites may accumulate in patients with renal failure has not been studied. As with other drugs whose metabolites are excreted by the kidneys, the possibility that adverse reactions (not listed in ADVERSE REACTIONS) may be attributable to these metabolites should be considered.

Table 1. Mean pharmacokinetic parameters of nabumetone active metabolite (6MNA) at steady state following oral administration of 1000 mg or 2000 mg doses of Relafen (nabumetone)

Abbreviation (units)	Young Adults Mean ± SD 1000 mg n=31	Young Adults Mean ± SD 2000 mg n=12	Elderly Mean± SD 1000 mg n=27
t_{max} (hours)	3.0 (1.0 to 12.0)	2.5 (1.0 to 8.0)	4.0 (1.0 to 10.0)
$t^1/_2$ (hours)	22.5 ± 3.7	26.2 ± 3.7	29.8 ± 8.1
CL_{SS}/F (mL/min.)	26.1 ± 17.3	21.0 ± 4.0	18.6 ± 13.4
Vd_{SS}/F (L)	55.4 ± 26.4	53.4 ± 11.3	50.2 ± 25.3

Hepatic Function: As with other NSAIDs, borderline elevations of one or more liver function tests may occur in up to 15% of patients. These abnormalities may progress, may remain essentially unchanged, or may return to normal with continued therapy. The ALT (SGPT) test is probably the most sensitive indicator of liver dysfunction. Meaningful (3 times the upper limit of normal) elevations of ALT (SGPT) or AST (SGOT) have occurred in controlled clinical trials of Relafen (nabumetone) in less than 1% of patients. A patient with symptoms and/or signs suggesting liver dysfunction, or in whom an abnormal liver test has occurred, should be evaluated for evidence of the development of a more severe hepatic reaction while on *Relafen* therapy. Severe hepatic reactions, including jaundice and fatal hepatitis, have been reported with other NSAIDs. Although such reactions are rare, if abnormal liver tests persist or worsen, if clinical signs and symptoms consistent with liver disease develop, or if systemic manifestations occur (e.g., eosinophilia, rash, etc.), *Relafen* should be discontinued. Because nabumetone's biotransformation to 6MNA is dependent upon hepatic function, the biotransformation could be decreased in patients with severe hepatic dysfunction. Therefore, *Relafen* should be used with caution in patients with severe hepatic impairment (see Pharmacokinetics, *Hepatic Impairment*).

Fluid Retention and Edema: Fluid retention and edema have been observed in some patients taking *Relafen*. Therefore, as with other NSAIDs, *Relafen* should be used cautiously in patients with a history of congestive heart failure, hypertension or other conditions predisposing to fluid retention.

Photosensitivity: Based on U.V. light photosensitivity testing, *Relafen* may be associated with more reactions to sun exposure than might be expected based on skin tanning types.

Information for Patients: *Relafen*, like other drugs of its class, is not free of side effects. The side effects of these drugs can cause discomfort and, rarely, there are more serious side effects, such as gastrointestinal bleeding, which may result in hospitalization and even fatal outcome.

NSAIDs are often essential agents in the management of arthritis, but they also may be commonly employed for conditions which are less serious. Physicians may wish to discuss with their patients the potential risks (see WARNINGS, PRECAUTIONS and ADVERSE REACTIONS) and likely benefits of NSAID treatment, particularly when the drugs are used for less serious conditions where treatment without NSAIDs may represent an acceptable alternative to both the patient and the physician.

Laboratory Tests: Because severe G.I. tract ulceration and bleeding can occur without warning symptoms, physicians should follow chronically treated patients for signs and symptoms of ulceration and bleeding, and should inform them of the importance of this follow-up (see WARNINGS, Risk of G.I. Ulceration, Bleeding and Perforation with NSAID Therapy).

Drug Interactions: *In vitro* studies have shown that, because of its affinity for protein, 6MNA may displace other protein-bound drugs from their binding site. Caution should be exercised when administering *Relafen* with warfarin since interactions have been seen with other NSAIDs.

Concomitant administration of an aluminum-containing antacid had no significant effect on the bioavailability of 6MNA. When administered with food or milk, there is more rapid absorption; however, the total amount of 6MNA in the plasma is unchanged (see Pharmacokinetics).

Carcinogenesis, Mutagenesis: In two-year studies conducted in mice and rats, nabumetone had no statistically significant tumorigenic effect. Nabumetone did not show mutagenic potential in the Ames test and mouse micronucleus test *in vivo*. However, nabumetone- and 6MNA-treated lymphocytes in culture showed chromosomal aberrations at 80 mcg/mL and higher concentrations (equal to the average human exposure to *Relafen* at the maximum recommended dose).

Impairment of Fertility: Nabumetone did not impair fertility of male or female rats treated orally at doses of 320 mg/kg/day (1888 mg/m^2) before mating.

Pregnancy: Teratogenic Effects. Pregnancy Category C. Nabumetone did not cause any teratogenic effect in rats given up to 400 mg/kg (2360 mg/m^2) and in rabbits up to 300 mg/kg (3540 mg/m^2) orally. However, increased post-implantation loss was observed in rats at 100 mg/kg (590 mg/m^2) orally and at higher doses (equal to the average human exposure to 6MNA at the maximum recommended human dose). There are no adequate, well-controlled studies in pregnant women. This drug should be used during pregnancy only if clearly needed.

Because of the known effect of prostaglandin-synthesis-inhibiting drugs on the human fetal cardiovascular system

(closure of ductus arteriosus), use of Relafen (nabumetone) during the third trimester of pregnancy is not recommended.

Labor and Delivery: The effects of *Relafen* on labor and delivery in women are not known. As with other drugs known to inhibit prostaglandin synthesis, an increased incidence of dystocia and delayed parturition occurred in rats treated throughout pregnancy.

Nursing Mothers: *Relafen* is not recommended for use in nursing mothers because of the possible adverse effects of prostaglandin-synthesis-inhibiting drugs on neonates. It is not known whether nabumetone or its metabolites are excreted in human milk; however, 6MNA is excreted in the milk of lactating rats.

Pediatric Use: *Relafen* is not recommended for use in children because the safety and efficacy in children have not been established.

Geriatric Use: Of the 1,677 patients in U.S. clinical studies who were treated with *Relafen,* 411 patients (24%) were 65 years of age or older; 22 patients (1%) were 75 years of age or older. No overall differences in efficacy or safety were observed between these older patients and younger ones. Similar results were observed in a 1-year, non-U.S. postmarketing surveillance study of 10,800 *Relafen* patients, of whom 4,577 patients (42%) were 65 years of age or older.

ADVERSE REACTIONS

Adverse reaction information was derived from blinded-controlled and open-labelled clinical trials and from worldwide marketing experience. In the description below, rates of the more common events (greater than 1%) and many of the less common events (less than 1%) represent results of U.S. clinical studies.

Of the 1,677 patients who received *Relafen* during U.S. clinical trials, 1,524 were treated for at least 1 month, 1,327 for at least 3 months, 929 for at least a year and 750 for at least 2 years. Over 300 patients have been treated for 5 years or longer.

The most frequently reported adverse reactions were related to the gastrointestinal tract. They were diarrhea, dyspepsia and abdominal pain.

Incidence ≥1% — Probably Causally Related

Gastrointestinal: Diarrhea (14%), dyspepsia (13%), abdominal pain (12%), constipation*, flatulence*, nausea*, positive stool guaiac*, dry mouth, gastritis, stomatitis, vomiting.

Central Nervous System: Dizziness*, headache*, fatigue, increased sweating, insomnia, nervousness, somnolence.

Dermatologic: Pruritus*, rash*.

Special Senses: Tinnitus*.

Miscellaneous: Edema*.

*Incidence of reported reaction between 3% and 9%. Reactions occurring in 1% to 3% of the patients are unmarked.

Incidence <1% — Probably Causally Related†

Gastrointestinal: Anorexia, cholestatic jaundice, duodenal ulcer, dysphagia, gastric ulcer, gastroenteritis, gastrointestinal bleeding, increased appetite, liver function abnormalities, melena.

Central Nervous System: Asthenia, agitation, anxiety, confusion, depression, malaise, paresthesia, tremor, vertigo.

Dermatologic: Bullous eruptions, photosensitivity, urticaria, pseudoporphyria cutanea tarda, *toxic epidermal necrolysis.*

Cardiovascular: Vasculitis.

Metabolic: Weight gain.

Respiratory: Dyspnea, *eosinophilic pneumonia, hypersensitivity pneumonitis.*

Genitourinary: Albuminuria, azotemia, *hyperuricemia, interstitial nephritis, nephrotic syndrome, vaginal bleeding.*

Special Senses: Abnormal vision.

Hypersensitivity: *Anaphylactoid reaction, anaphylaxis,* angioneurotic edema.

† Adverse reactions reported only in worldwide postmarketing experience or in the literature, not seen in clinical trials, are considered rarer and are italicized.

Incidence <1% — Causal Relationship Unknown‡

Gastrointestinal: Bilirubinuria, duodenitis, eructation, gallstones, gingivitis, glossitis, pancreatitis, rectal bleeding.

Central Nervous System: Nightmares.

Dermatologic: Acne, alopecia, *erythema multiforme, Stevens-Johnson Syndrome.*

Cardiovascular: Angina, arrhythmia, hypertension, myocardial infarction, palpitations, syncope, thrombophlebitis.

Respiratory: Asthma, cough.

Genitourinary: Dysuria, hematuria, impotence, renal stones.

Special Senses: Taste disorder.

Body as a Whole: Fever, chills.

Hematologic/Lymphatic: Anemia, leukopenia, granulocytopenia, thrombocytopenia.

Metabolic/Nutritional: Hyperglycemia, hypokalemia, weight loss.

‡ Adverse reactions reported only in worldwide postmarketing experience or in the literature, not seen in clinical trials, are considered rarer and are italicized.

OVERDOSAGE

Since only 1 case of Relafen (nabumetone) overdose has been reported, the experience is limited. If acute overdose occurs, it is recommended that the stomach be emptied by vomiting or lavage and general supportive measures be instituted, as necessary. In addition, the use of activated charcoal, up to 60 grams, may effectively reduce nabumetone absorption. Coadministration of nabumetone with charcoal to man has resulted in an 80% decrease in maximum plasma concentrations of the active metabolite.

The 1 overdose occurred in a 17-year-old female patient who had a history of abdominal pain and was hospitalized for increased abdominal pain following ingestion of 30 *Relafen* tablets (15 grams total). Stools were negative for occult blood and there was no fall in serum hemoglobin concentration. The patient had no other symptoms. She was given an H_2-receptor antagonist and discharged from the hospital without sequelae.

DOSAGE AND ADMINISTRATION

Osteoarthritis and Rheumatoid Arthritis

The recommended starting dose is 1000 mg taken as a single dose with or without food. Some patients may obtain more symptomatic relief from 1500 mg to 2000 mg per day. Relafen (nabumetone) can be given in either a single or twice-daily dose. Dosages over 2000 mg per day have not been studied. The lowest effective dose should be used for chronic treatment.

HOW SUPPLIED

Tablets: Oval-shaped, film-coated: 500 mg—white, imprinted with the product name RELAFEN and 500, in bottles of 100 and 500, and in Single Unit Packages of 100 (intended for institutional use only). 750 mg—beige, imprinted with the product name RELAFEN and 750, in bottles of 100 and 500, and in Single Unit Packages of 100 (intended for institutional use only).

Store at controlled room temperature (59° to 86°F) in well-closed container; dispense in light-resistant container.

500 mg 100's: NDC 0029-4851-20
500 mg 500's: NDC 0029-4851-25
500 mg SUP 100's: NDC 0029-4851-21

750 mg 100's: NDC 0029-4852-20
750 mg 500's: NDC 0029-4852-25
750 mg SUP 100's: NDC 0029-4852-21

Veterans Administration/Military/PHS—Tablets, 500 mg, 100's, 6505-01-352-9299; 500 mg, 100's (SUP), 6505-01-352-9300; 750 mg, 100's, 6505-01-377-1644.

RL:L7

Shown in Product Identification Guide, page 340

REQUIP™ ℞

[ri-'kwip]

brand of ropinirole hydrochloride Tablets

DESCRIPTION

Requip (ropinirole hydrochloride), an orally administered anti-Parkinsonian drug, is a non-ergoline dopamine agonist. It is the hydrochloride salt of 4-[2-(dipropylamino)-ethyl]-1,3-dihydro-2H-indol-2-one monohydrochloride and has an empirical formula of $C_{16}H_{24}N_2O \bullet HCl$. The molecular weight is 296.84 (260.38 as the free base).

The structural formula is:

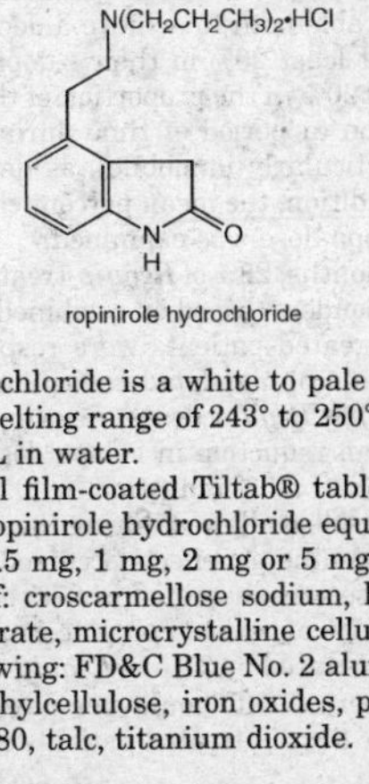

ropinirole hydrochloride

Ropinirole hydrochloride is a white to pale greenish-yellow powder with a melting range of 243° to 250°C and a solubility of 133 mg/mL in water.

Each pentagonal film-coated Tiltab® tablet with beveled edges contains ropinirole hydrochloride equivalent to ropinirole, 0.25 mg, 0.5 mg, 1 mg, 2 mg or 5 mg. Inactive ingredients consist of: croscarmellose sodium, hydrous lactose, magnesium stearate, microcrystalline cellulose, and one or more of the following: FD&C Blue No. 2 aluminum lake, hydroxypropyl methylcellulose, iron oxides, polyethylene glycol, polysorbate 80, talc, titanium dioxide.

CLINICAL PHARMACOLOGY

Mechanism of Action

Requip is a non-ergoline dopamine agonist with high relative *in vitro* specificity and full intrinsic activity at the D_2 and D_3 dopamine receptor subtypes, binding with higher affinity to D_3 than to D_2 or D_4 receptor subtypes. The relevance of D_3 receptor binding in Parkinson's disease is unknown.

Ropinirole has moderate *in vitro* affinity for opioid receptors. Ropinirole and its metabolites have negligible *in vitro* affinity for dopamine D_1, 5-HT_1, 5-HT_2, benzodiazepine, GABA, muscarinic, alpha$_1$-, alpha$_2$-, and beta-adrenoreceptors.

The precise mechanism of action of *Requip* as a treatment for Parkinson's disease is unknown, although it is believed to be due to stimulation of post-synaptic dopamine D_2-type receptors within the caudate-putamen in the brain. This conclusion is supported by studies that show that ropinirole improves motor function in various animal models of Parkinson's disease. In particular, ropinirole attenuates the motor deficits induced by lesioning the ascending nigrostriatal dopaminergic pathway with the neurotoxin 1-methyl-4-phenyl-1,2,3,6-tetrahydropyridine (MPTP) in primates.

Clinical Pharmacology Studies

In healthy normotensive subjects, single oral doses of *Requip* in the range 0.01 to 2.5 mg had little or no effect on supine blood pressure and pulse rates. Upon standing, *Requip* caused decreases in systolic and diastolic blood pressure at doses above 0.25 mg. In some subjects, these changes were associated with the emergence of orthostatic symptoms, bradycardia and, in one case, transient sinus arrest with syncope. The effect of repeat dosing and slow titration of *Requip* was not studied in healthy volunteers.

The mechanism of *Requip*-induced postural hypotension is presumed to be due to a D_2-mediated blunting of the noradrenergic response to standing and subsequent decrease in peripheral vascular resistance. Nausea is a common concomitant of orthostatic signs and symptoms.

At oral doses as low as 0.2 mg, *Requip* suppressed serum prolactin concentrations in healthy male volunteers.

Requip had no dose-related effect on ECG wave form and rhythm in young healthy male volunteers in the range of 0.01 to 2.5 mg.

Pharmacokinetics

Absorption, Distribution, Metabolism and Elimination

Ropinirole is rapidly absorbed after oral administration, reaching peak concentration in approximately 1-2 hours. In clinical studies, over 88% of a radiolabeled dose was recovered in urine and the absolute bioavailability was 55%, indicating a first pass effect. Relative bioavailability from a tablet compared to an oral solution is 85%. Food does not affect the extent of absorption of ropinirole, although its T_{max} is increased by 2.5 hours when the drug is taken with a meal. The clearance of ropinirole after oral administration to patients is 47 L/hr (cv=45%) and its elimination half-life is approximately 6 hours. Ropinirole is extensively metabolized by the liver to inactive metabolites and displays linear kinetics over the therapeutic dosing range of 1 mg to 8 mg t.i.d. Steady-state concentrations are expected to be achieved within 2 days of dosing. Accumulation upon multiple dosing is predictive from single dosing.

Ropinirole is widely distributed throughout the body, with an apparent volume of distribution of 7.5 L/kg (cv=32%). It is up to 40% bound to plasma proteins and has a blood-to-plasma ratio of 1:1.

The major metabolic pathways are N-despropylation and hydroxylation to form the inactive N-despropyl and hydroxy metabolites. *In vitro* studies indicate that the major cytochrome P_{450} isozyme involved in the metabolism of ropinirole is CYP1A2, an enzyme known to be stimulated by smoking and omeprazole, and inhibited by, for example, fluvoxamine, mexiletine, and the older fluoroquinolones, such as ciprofloxacin and norfloxacin. The N-despropyl metabolite is converted to carbamyl glucuronide, carboxylic acid, and N-despropyl hydroxy metabolites. The hydroxy metabolite of ropinirole is rapidly glucuronidated. Less than 10% of the administered dose is excreted as unchanged drug in urine. N-despropyl ropinirole is the predominant metabolite found in urine (40%), followed by the carboxylic acid metabolite (10%), and the glucuronide of the hydroxy metabolite (10%).

P_{450} Interaction: *In vitro* metabolism studies showed that CYP1A2 was the major enzyme responsible for the metabolism of ropinirole. There is thus the potential for inhibitors or substrates of this enzyme to alter its clearance when coadministered with ropinirole. Therefore, if therapy with a drug known to be a potent inhibitor of CYP1A2 is stopped or started during treatment with *Requip*, adjustment of the *Requip* dose may be required.

Continued on next page

Information on the SmithKline Beecham Pharmaceuticals products appearing here is based on the labeling in effect on July 31, 1998. Further information on these and other products may be obtained from the Medical Department, SmithKline Beecham Pharmaceuticals, One Franklin Plaza, Philadelphia, PA 19101.

Requip—Cont.

Population Subgroups
Because therapy with *Requip* is initiated at a subtherapeutic dosage and gradually titrated upward according to clinical tolerability to obtain the optimum therapeutic effect, adjustment of the initial dose based on gender, weight or age is not necessary.
Age: Oral clearance of ropinirole is reduced by 30% in patients above 65 years of age compared to younger patients. Dosage adjustment is not necessary in the elderly (above 65 years) as the dose of ropinirole is to be individually titrated to clinical response.
Gender: Female and male patients showed similar oral clearance.
Race: The influence of race on the pharmacokinetics of ropinirole has not been evaluated.
Cigarette Smoking: The effect of smoking on the oral clearance of ropinirole has not been evaluated. Smoking is expected to increase the clearance of ropinirole since CYP1A2 is known to be induced by smoking.
Renal Impairment: Based on population pharmacokinetic analysis, no difference was observed in the pharmacokinetics of ropinirole in patients with moderate renal impairment (creatinine clearance between 30 to 50 mL/min.) compared to an age-matched population with creatinine clearance above 50 mL/min. Therefore, no dosage adjustment is necessary in moderately renally impaired patients. The use of Requip (ropinirole hydrochloride) in patients with severe renal impairment has not been studied.
The effect of hemodialysis on drug removal is not known, but because of the relatively high apparent volume of distribution of ropinirole (525 L), the removal of the drug by hemodialysis is unlikely.
Hepatic Impairment: The pharmacokinetics of ropinirole have not been studied in hepatically impaired patients. These patients may have higher plasma levels and lower clearance of the drug than patients with normal hepatic function. The drug should be titrated with caution in this population.
Other Diseases: Population pharmacokinetic analysis revealed no change in the oral clearance of ropinirole in patients with concomitant diseases, such as hypertension, depression, osteoporosis/arthritis, and insomnia, compared to patients with Parkinson's disease only.
Clinical Trials
The effectiveness of *Requip* in the treatment of Parkinson's disease was evaluated in a multi-national drug development program consisting of 11 randomized, controlled trials. Four were conducted in patients with early Parkinson's disease and no concomitant L-dopa and 7 were conducted in patients with advanced Parkinson's disease with concomitant L-dopa.
Among these 11 studies, three placebo-controlled studies provide the most persuasive evidence of ropinirole's effectiveness in the management of patients with Parkinson's disease who were and were not receiving concomitant L-dopa. Two of these three trials enrolled patients with early Parkinson's disease (without L-dopa) and one enrolled patients receiving L-dopa.
In these studies a variety of measures were used to assess the effects of treatment (e.g., the Unified Parkinson's Disease Rating Scale [UPDRS], Clinical Global Impression scores, patient diaries recording time "on" and "off," and tolerability of L-dopa dose reductions).
In both studies of early Parkinson's disease (without L-dopa) patients, the motor component (Part III) of the UPDRS was the primary outcome assessment. The UPDRS is a four-part multi-item rating scale intended to evaluate mentation (Part I), activities of daily living (Part II), motor performance (Part III), and complications of therapy (Part IV). Part III of the UPDRS contains 14 items designed to assess the severity of the cardinal motor findings in patients with Parkinson's disease (e.g., tremor, rigidity, bradykinesia, postural instability, etc.) scored for different body regions and has a maximum (worst) score of 108. Responders were defined as patients with at least a 30% reduction in the Part III score.
In the study of advanced Parkinson's disease (with L-dopa) patients, both reduction in percent awake time spent "off" and the ability to reduce the daily use of L-dopa were assessed as a combined endpoint and individually.
Studies in Patients with Early Parkinson's Disease (without L-dopa)
One early therapy study was a 12-week multicenter study in which 63 patients (41 on *Requip*) with idiopathic Parkinson's disease receiving concomitant anti-Parkinson medication (but not L-dopa) were randomized to either *Requip* or placebo. Patients had a mean disease duration of approximately 2 years. Patients were eligible for enrollment if they presented with bradykinesia and at least tremor, rigidity, or postural instability. In addition, they must have been classified as Hoehn & Yahr Stage I-IV. This scale, ranging from I=unilateral involvement with minimal impairment to V=confined to wheelchair or bed, is a standard instrument used for staging patients with Parkinson's disease. The primary outcome measure in this trial was the proportion of patients experiencing a decrease (compared to baseline) of at least 30% in the UPDRS motor score.
Patients were titrated for up to 10 weeks, starting at 0.5 mg b.i.d., with weekly increments of 0.5 mg b.i.d. to a maximum of 5 mg b.i.d. Once patients reached their maximally tolerated dose (or 5 mg b.i.d.), they were maintained on that dose through 12 weeks. The mean dose achieved by patients at study endpoint was 7.4 mg/day. At the end of 12 weeks, 71% of *Requip*-treated patients were responders, compared with 41% of patients in the placebo group (p=0.021).
Statistically significant differences between the percentage of responders on *Requip* compared to placebo were seen after 8 weeks of treatment.
In addition, the mean percentage improvement from baseline in the Total Motor Score was 43% in *Requip*-treated patients compared with 21% in placebo-treated patients (p=0.018).
Statistically significant differences in UPDRS motor score between *Requip* and placebo were seen after 2 weeks of treatment.
The median daily dose at which a 30% reduction in UPDRS motor score was sustained was 4 mg.
The second trial in early Parkinson's disease (without L-dopa) patients was a double-blind, randomized, placebo-controlled 6-month study. Patients were essentially similar to those in the study described above; concomitant use of selegiline was allowed, but patients were not permitted to use anticholinergics or amantadine during the study. Patients had a mean disease duration of 2 years and limited (not more than a 6-week period) or no prior exposure to L-dopa. The starting dose of *Requip* in this trial was 0.25 mg t.i.d. The dose was titrated at weekly intervals by increments of 0.25 mg t.i.d. to a dose of 1.0 mg t.i.d. Further titrations at weekly intervals were at increments of 0.5 mg t.i.d. up to a dose of 3.0 mg t.i.d and then weekly at increments of 1.0 mg t.i.d. Patients were to be titrated to a dose of at least 1.5 mg t.i.d. and then to their maximally tolerated dose, up to a maximum of 8.0 mg t.i.d. The mean dose attained in patients at study endpoint was 15.7 mg/day.
The primary measure of effectiveness was the mean percent reduction (improvement) from baseline in the UPDRS Motor Score. In this study 241 patients were enrolled. At the end of the 6-month study, *Requip*-treated patients had 22% improvement in motor score, compared with a 4% worsening in the placebo group (p<0.001).
Statistically significant differences in UPDRS motor score improvement between *Requip* and placebo were seen after 12 weeks of treatment.
Study in Patients with Advanced Parkinson's Disease (with L-dopa)
This double-blind, randomized, placebo-controlled 6-month trial evaluated 148 patients (Hoehn & Yahr II-IV) who were not adequately controlled on L-dopa. Patients in this study had a mean disease duration of approximately 9 years, had been exposed to L-dopa for approximately 7 years, and had experienced "on-off" periods with L-dopa therapy. Patients previously receiving stable doses of selegiline, amantadine and/or anticholinergic agents could continue on these agents during the study. Patients were started at a *Requip* dose of 0.25 mg t.i.d. and titrated upward by weekly intervals until an optimal therapeutic response was achieved. The maximum dose of study medication was 8 mg t.i.d. All patients had to be titrated to at least a dose of 2.5 mg t.i.d. Patients could then be maintained on this dose level or higher for the remainder of the study. Once a dose of 2.5 mg t.i.d. was achieved, patients underwent a mandatory reduction in their L-dopa dose, to be followed by additional mandatory reductions with continued escalation of the *Requip* dose. Reductions in the dosage of L-dopa were also allowed if patients experienced adverse events that the investigator considered related to dopaminergic therapy. The mean dose attained at study endpoint was 16.3 mg/day. The primary outcome was the proportion of responders, defined as patients who were able both to achieve a decrease (compared to baseline) of at least 20% in their L-dopa dose and a decrease of at least 20% in the proportion of the time awake in the "off" condition (a period of time during the day when patients are particularly immobile), as determined by patient diary. In addition, the mean percent change from baseline in daily L-dopa dose was examined.
At the end of 6 months, 28% of *Requip*-treated patients were classified as responders (based on combined endpoint) while 11% of placebo-treated patients were responders (p=0.02).
Based on the protocol-mandated reductions in L-dopa dosage with escalating *Requip* doses, *Requip*-treated patients had a 19.4% mean reduction in L-dopa dose while placebo-treated patients had a 3% reduction (p<0.001). L-dopa dosage reduction was also allowed during the study if dyskinesias or other dopaminergic effects occurred. Overall, reduction of L-dopa dose was sustained in 87% of *Requip*-treated patients and in 57% of patients on placebo. On average, the L-dopa dose was reduced by 31% in *Requip*-treated patients.
The mean number of "off" hours per day during baseline was 6.4 hours for *Requip*-treated patients and 7.3 hours for patients treated with placebo. At the end of the 6-month study, patients treated with *Requip* had a mean of 4.9 hours per day of "off" time, while placebo-treated patients had a mean of 6.4 hours per day of "off" time.

INDICATIONS AND USAGE
Requip (ropinirole hydrochloride) is indicated for the treatment of the signs and symptoms of idiopathic Parkinson's disease.
The effectiveness of *Requip* was demonstrated in randomized, controlled trials in patients with early Parkinson's disease who were not receiving concomitant L-dopa therapy as well as in patients with advanced disease on concomitant L-dopa (see CLINICAL PHARMACOLOGY, Clinical Trials).

CONTRAINDICATIONS
Requip is contraindicated for patients known to have hypersensitivity to the product.

WARNINGS
Syncope
Syncope, sometimes associated with bradycardia, was observed in association with ropinirole in both early Parkinson's disease (without L-dopa) patients and advanced Parkinson's disease (with L-dopa) patients. In the two double-blind placebo-controlled studies of *Requip* in patients with Parkinson's disease who were not being treated with L-dopa, 11.5% (18 of 157) of patients on *Requip* had syncope compared to 1.4% (2 of 147) of patients on placebo. Most of these cases occurred more than 4 weeks after initiation of therapy with *Requip*, and were usually associated with a recent increase in dose.
Of 208 patients being treated with both L-dopa and *Requip*, in placebo-controlled advanced Parkinson's disease trials, there were reports of syncope in 6 (2.9%) compared to 2 of 120 (1.7%) of placebo/L-dopa patients.
Because the studies of *Requip* excluded patients with significant cardiovascular disease, it is not known to what extent the estimated incidence figures apply to Parkinson's disease patients as a whole.
Two of 47 Parkinson's disease patient volunteers enrolled in phase 1 studies had syncope following a 1 mg dose. In phase 1 studies including 110 healthy volunteers, one patient developed hypotension, bradycardia, and sinus arrest of 26 seconds accompanied by syncope; the patient recovered spontaneously without intervention. One other healthy volunteer reported syncope.
Symptomatic Hypotension
Dopamine agonists, in clinical studies and clinical experience, appear to impair the systemic regulation of blood pressure, with resulting postural hypotension, especially during dose escalation. Parkinson's disease patients, in addition, appear to have an impaired capacity to respond to a postural challenge. For these reasons, Parkinson's patients being treated with dopaminergic agonists ordinarily (1) require careful monitoring for signs and symptoms of postural hypotension, especially during dose escalation, and (2) should be informed of this risk (see PRECAUTIONS, Information for Patients).
Although the clinical trials were not designed to systematically monitor blood pressure, there were individual reported cases of postural hypotension in early Parkinson's disease (without L-dopa) *Requip*-treated patients. Most of these cases occurred more than 4 weeks after initiation of therapy with *Requip*, and were usually associated with a recent increase in dose.
In phase 1 studies of *Requip* that included 110 healthy volunteers, nine subjects had documented symptomatic postural hypotension. These episodes appeared mainly at doses above 0.8 mg and these doses are higher than the starting doses recommended for Parkinson's disease patients. In eight of these nine individuals, the hypotension was accompanied by bradycardia, but did not develop into syncope. (See Syncope above.) None of these events resulted in death or hospitalization.
One of 47 Parkinson's disease patient volunteers enrolled in phase 1 studies had documented hypotension following a 2 mg dose on two occasions.
Hallucinations
In double-blind, placebo-controlled, early therapy studies in patients with Parkinson's disease who were not treated with L-dopa, 5.2% (8 of 157) of patients treated with *Requip* reported hallucinations, compared to 1.4% of patients on placebo (2 of 147). Among those patients receiving both *Requip* and L-dopa, in advanced Parkinson's disease (with L-dopa) studies, 10.1% (21 of 208) were reported to experience hallucinations, compared to 4.2% (5 of 120) of patients treated with placebo and L-dopa.
Hallucinations were of sufficient severity to cause discontinuation of treatment in 1.3% of the early Parkinson's disease (without L-dopa) patients and 1.9% of the advanced Parkinson's disease (with L-dopa) patients compared to 0% and 1.7% of placebo patients, respectively.

PRECAUTIONS
General
Dyskinesia: *Requip* may potentiate the dopaminergic side effects of L-dopa and may cause and/or exacerbate pre-exist-

Table 1: Treatment-Emergent Adverse Event[1] Incidence in Double-blind, Placebo-controlled Early Parkinson's Disease (without L-dopa) Trials (Events ≥2% of Patients Treated with *Requip* and Numerically More Frequent than the Placebo Group)

	Requip N = 157 (%)	Placebo N = 147 (%)
Autonomic Nervous System		
Flushing	3	1
Dry Mouth	5	3
Increased Sweating	6	4
Body as a Whole		
Asthenia	6	1
Chest Pain	4	2
Dependent Edema	6	3
Leg Edema	7	1
Fatigue	11	4
Malaise	3	1
Pain	8	4
Cardiovascular General		
Hypertension	5	3
Hypotension	2	0
Orthostatic Symptoms	6	5
Syncope	12	1
Central/Peripheral Nervous System		
Dizziness	40	22
Hyperkinesia	2	1
Hypesthesia	4	2
Vertigo	2	0
Gastrointestinal System		
Abdominal Pain	6	3
Anorexia	4	1
Dyspepsia	10	5
Flatulence	3	1
Nausea	60	22
Vomiting	12	7
Heart Rate/Rhythm		
Extrasystoles	2	1
Atrial Fibrillation	2	0
Palpitation	3	2
Tachycardia	2	0
Metabolic/Nutritional		
Increased Alkaline Phosphatase	3	1
Psychiatric		
Amnesia	3	1
Impaired Concentration	2	0
Confusion	5	1
Hallucination	5	1
Somnolence	40	6
Yawning	3	0

Continued

ing dyskinesia. Decreasing the dose of L-dopa may ameliorate this side effect.

Renal and Hepatic: No dosage adjustment is needed in patients with mild to moderate renal impairment (creatinine clearance of 30 to 50 mL/min.). Because the use of *Requip* in patients with severe renal or hepatic impairment has not been studied, administration of *Requip* to such patients should be carried out with caution.

Events Reported with Dopaminergic Therapy:

Withdrawal Emergent Hyperpyrexia and Confusion: Although not reported with *Requip*, a symptom complex resembling the neuroleptic malignant syndrome (characterized by elevated temperature, muscular rigidity, altered consciousness, and autonomic instability), with no other obvious etiology, has been reported in association with rapid dose reduction, withdrawal of, or changes in anti-Parkinsonian therapy.

Fibrotic Complications: Cases of retroperitoneal fibrosis, pulmonary infiltrates, pleural effusion, and pleural thickening have been reported in some patients treated with ergot-derived dopaminergic agents. While these complications may resolve when the drug is discontinued, complete resolution does not always occur.

Although these adverse events are believed to be related to the ergoline structure of these compounds, whether other, nonergot derived dopamine agonists can cause them is unknown.

In the *Requip* development program, a 69-year-old man with obstructive lung disease was treated with *Requip* for 16 months and developed pleural thickening and effusion accompanied by lower extremity edema, cardiomegaly, pleuritic pain, and shortness of breath. Pleural biopsy demonstrated chronic inflammation and sclerosis. The effusion resolved after medical therapy and discontinuation of *Requip*. The patient was lost to follow-up. The relationship of these events to Requip (ropinirole hydrochloride) cannot be established.

Retinal pathology in albino rats: Retinal degeneration was observed in albino rats in the 2-year carcinogenicity study at all doses tested (equivalent to 0.6 to 20 times the maximum recommended human dose on a mg/m² basis), but was statistically significant at the highest dose (50 mg/kg/day). Additional studies to further evaluate the specific pathology (e.g., loss of photoreceptor cells) have not been performed. Similar changes were not observed in a 2-year carcinogenicity study in albino mice or in rats or monkeys treated for 1 year.

The potential significance of this effect in humans has not been established, but cannot be disregarded because disruption of a mechanism that is universally present in vertebrates (e.g., disk shedding) may be involved.

Binding to melanin: *Requip* binds to melanin-containing tissues (i.e., eyes, skin) in pigmented rats. After a single dose, long-term retention of drug was demonstrated, with a half-life in the eye of 20 days. It is not known if *Requip* accumulates in these tissues over time.

Information for Patients

Patients should be instructed to take *Requip* only as prescribed.

Requip can be taken with or without food. Since ingestion with food reduces the maximum concentration (C_{max}) of *Requip*, patients should be advised that taking *Requip* with food may reduce the occurrence of nausea. However, this has not been established in controlled clinical trials.

Patients should be informed that hallucinations can occur, and that the elderly are at a higher risk than younger patients with Parkinson's disease.

Patients should be advised that they may develop postural (orthostatic) hypotension with or without symptoms such as dizziness, nausea, syncope, and sometimes sweating. Hypotension and/or orthostatic symptoms may occur more frequently during initial therapy or with an increase in dose at any time (cases have been seen after weeks of treatment). Accordingly, patients should be cautioned against rising rapidly after sitting or lying down, especially if they have been doing so for prolonged periods, and especially at the initiation of treatment with *Requip*.

Patients should be advised that *Requip* may cause somnolence. Accordingly, they should be advised neither to drive a car nor to operate other complex machinery, until they have gained sufficient experience on *Requip* to gauge whether or not it affects their mental and/or motor performance adversely.

Because of the possible additive sedative effects, caution should also be used when patients are taking alcohol or other CNS depressants (e.g., benzodiazepines, antipsychotics, antidepressants, etc.) in combination with *Requip*.

Continued on next page

Information on the SmithKline Beecham Pharmaceuticals products appearing here is based on the labeling in effect on July 31, 1998. Further information on these and other products may be obtained from the Medical Department, SmithKline Beecham Pharmaceuticals, One Franklin Plaza, Philadelphia, PA 19101.

Requip—Cont.

Because of the possibility that ropinirole may be excreted in breast milk, patients should be advised to notify their physicians if they intend to breast-feed or are breast-feeding an infant.

Because ropinirole has been shown to have adverse effects on embryo-fetal development, including teratogenic effects, in animals, and because experience in humans is limited, patients should be advised to notify their physician if they become pregnant or intend to become pregnant during therapy (see PRECAUTIONS, Pregnancy).

Drug Interactions

P_{450} Interaction: *In vitro* metabolism studies showed that CYP1A2 was the major enzyme responsible for the metabolism of ropinirole. There is thus the potential for substrates or inhibitors of this enzyme when coadministered with ropinirole to alter its clearance. Therefore, if therapy with a drug known to be a potent inhibitor of CYP1A2 is stopped or started during treatment with *Requip*, adjustment of the *Requip* dose may be required.

L-dopa: Co-administration of carbidopa + L-dopa (Sinemet® 10/100 mg b.i.d.) with ropinirole (2.0 mg t.i.d.) had no effect on the steady-state pharmacokinetics of ropinirole (n=28 patients). Oral administration of *Requip* 2.0 mg t.i.d. increased mean steady state C_{max} of L-dopa by 20% but its AUC was unaffected (n=23 patients).

Digoxin: Co-administration of *Requip* (2.0 mg t.i.d.) with digoxin (0.125–0.25 mg q.d.) did not alter the steady-state pharmacokinetics of digoxin in 10 patients.

Theophylline: Administration of theophylline (300 mg b.i.d., a substrate of CYP1A2) did not alter the steady-state pharmacokinetics of ropinirole (2 mg t.i.d.) in 12 patients with Parkinson's disease. Ropinirole (2 mg t.i.d.) did not alter the pharmacokinetics of theophylline (5 mg/kg i.v.) in 12 patients with Parkinson's disease.

Ciprofloxacin: Co-administration of ciprofloxacin (500 mg b.i.d.), an inhibitor of CYP1A2, with ropinirole (2 mg t.i.d.) increased ropinirole AUC by 84% on average, and C_{max} by 60% (n=12 patients).

Estrogens: Population pharmacokinetic analysis revealed that estrogens (mainly ethinylestradiol: intake 0.6–3 mg over 4-month to 23-year period) reduced the oral clearance of ropinirole by 36% in 16 patients. Dosage adjustment may not be needed for *Requip* in patients on estrogen therapy because patients must be carefully titrated with ropinirole to tolerance or adequate effect. However, if estrogen therapy is stopped or started during treatment with *Requip*, then adjustment of the Requip (ropinirole hydrochloride) dose may be required.

Dopamine Antagonists: Since ropinirole is a dopamine agonist, it is possible that dopamine antagonists, such as neuroleptics (phenothiazines, butyrophenones, thioxanthenes) or metoclopramide, may diminish the effectiveness of *Requip*.

Population analysis showed that commonly administered drugs, e.g., selegiline, amantadine, tricyclic antidepressants, benzodiazepines, ibuprofen, thiazides, antihistamines, and anticholinergics did not affect the oral clearance of ropinirole.

Carcinogenesis, Mutagenesis, Impairment of Fertility

Two-year carcinogenicity studies were conducted in Charles River CD-1 mice at doses of 5, 15, and 50 mg/kg/day and in Sprague-Dawley rats at doses of 1.5, 15, and 50 mg/kg/day (top doses equivalent to 10 times and 20 times, respectively, the maximum recommended human dose of 24 mg/day on a mg/m^2 basis). In the male rat, there was a significant increase in testicular Leydig cell adenomas at all doses tested, i.e., ≥1.5 mg/kg (0.6 times the maximum recommended human dose on a mg/m^2 basis). This finding is of questionable significance because the endocrine mechanisms believed to be involved in the production of Leydig cell hyperplasia and adenomas in rats are not relevant to humans. In the female mouse, there was an increase in benign uterine endometrial polyps at a dose of 50 mg/kg/day (10 times the maximum recommended human dose on a mg/m^2 basis).

Ropinirole was not mutagenic or clastogenic in the *in vitro* Ames test, the *in vitro* chromosome aberration test in human lymphocytes, the *in vitro* mouse lymphoma (L1578Y cells) assay, and the *in vivo* mouse micronucleus test.

When administered to female rats prior to and during mating and throughout pregnancy, ropinirole caused disruption of implantation at doses of 20 mg/kg/day (8 times the maximum recommended human dose on a mg/m^2 basis) or greater. This effect is thought to be due to the prolactin-lowering effect of ropinirole. In humans, chorionic gonadotropin, not prolactin, is essential for implantation. In rat studies using low doses (5 mg/kg) during the prolactin-dependent phase of early pregnancy (gestation days 0–8), ropinirole did not affect female fertility at dosages up to 100 mg/kg/day (40 times the maximum recommended human dose on a mg/m^2 basis). No effect on male fertility was observed in rats at dosages up to 125 mg/kg/day (50 times the maximum recommended human dose on a mg/m^2 basis).

Table 1: (Continued) Treatment-Emergent Adverse Event[1] Incidence in Double-blind, Placebo-controlled Early Parkinson's Disease (without L-dopa) Trials (Events ≥2% of Patients Treated with *Requip* and Numerically More Frequent than the Placebo Group)

	Requip N = 157 (%)	Placebo N = 147 (%)
Reproductive Male		
Impotence	3	1
Resistance Mechanism		
Viral Infection	11	3
Respiratory System		
Bronchitis	3	1
Dyspnea	3	0
Pharyngitis	6	4
Rhinitis	4	3
Sinusitis	4	3
Urinary System		
Urinary Tract Infection	5	4
Vascular Extracardiac		
Peripheral Ischemia	3	0
Vision		
Eye Abnormality	3	1
Abnormal Vision	6	3
Xerophthalmia	2	0

1. Patients have reported multiple adverse experiences during the study or at discontinuation; thus, patients may be included in more than one category.

Pregnancy

Pregnancy Category C: In animal reproduction studies, ropinirole has been shown to have adverse effects on embryo-fetal development, including teratogenic effects. Ropinirole given to pregnant rats during organogenesis (20 mg/kg on gestation days 6 and 7 followed by 20, 60, 90, 120 or 150 mg/kg on gestation days 8 through 15) resulted in decreased fetal body weight at 60 mg/kg/day, increased fetal death at 90 mg/kg/day, and digital malformations at 150 mg/kg/day (24, 36 and 60 times the maximum recommended clinical dose on a mg/m^2 basis, respectively). The combined administration of ropinirole (10 mg/kg/day; 8 times the maximum recommended human dose on a mg/m^2 basis) and L-dopa (250 mg/kg/day) to pregnant rabbits during organogenesis produced a greater incidence and severity of fetal malformations (primarily digit defects) than were seen in the offspring of rabbits treated with L-dopa alone. No indication of an effect on development of the conceptus was observed in rabbits when a maternally toxic dose of ropinirole was administered alone (20 mg/kg/day: 16 times the maximum recommended human dose on a mg/m^2 basis). In a perinatal-postnatal study in rats, 10 mg/kg/day (4 times the maximum recommended human dose on a mg/m^2 basis) of ropinirole impaired growth and development of nursing offspring and altered neurological development of female offspring.

There are no adequate and well-controlled studies using *Requip* in pregnant women. *Requip* should be used during pregnancy only if the potential benefit outweighs the potential risk to the fetus.

Nursing Mothers

Requip inhibits prolactin secretion in humans and could potentially inhibit lactation.

Studies in rats have shown that *Requip* and/or its metabolite(s) is excreted in breast milk. It is not known whether this drug is excreted in human milk. Because many drugs are excreted in human milk and because of the potential for serious adverse reactions in nursing infants from *Requip*, a decision should be made whether to discontinue nursing or to discontinue the drug, taking into account the importance of the drug to the mother.

Pediatric Use

Safety and effectiveness in the pediatric population have not been established.

ADVERSE REACTIONS

During the pre-marketing development of *Requip*, patients received *Requip* either without L-dopa (early Parkinson's disease studies) or as concomitant therapy with L-dopa (advanced Parkinson's disease studies). Because these 2 populations may have differential risks for various adverse events, this section will, in general, present adverse event data for these 2 populations separately.

Early Parkinson's Disease (without L-dopa)

The most commonly observed adverse events (>5%) in the double-blind, placebo-controlled early Parkinson's disease trials associated with the use of *Requip* (n=157) not seen at an equivalent frequency among the placebo-treated patients (n=147) were, in order of decreasing incidence: nausea, dizziness, somnolence, headache, vomiting, syncope, fatigue, dyspepsia, viral infection, constipation, pain, increased sweating, asthenia, dependent/leg edema, orthostatic symptoms, abdominal pain, pharyngitis, confusion, hallucinations, urinary tract infections, and abnormal vision.

Approximately 24% of 157 *Requip*-treated patients who participated in the double-blind, placebo-controlled early Parkinson's disease (without L-dopa) trials discontinued treatment due to adverse events compared to 13% of 147 patients who received placebo. The adverse events most commonly causing discontinuation of treatment by *Requip*-treated patients were: nausea (6.4%), dizziness (3.8%), aggravated Parkinson's disease (1.3%), hallucinations (1.3%), somnolence (1.3%), vomiting (1.3%) and headache (1.3%). Of these, hallucinations appear to be dose-related. While other adverse events leading to discontinuation may be dose-related, the titration design utilized in these trials precluded an adequate assessment of the dose response. For example, in the larger of the 2 trials described in CLINICAL PHARMACOLOGY, Clinical Trials, the difference in the rate of discontinuations emerged only after 10 weeks of treatment, suggesting, although not proving, that the effect could be related to dose.

Adverse Event Incidence in Controlled Clinical Studies

Table 1 lists treatment-emergent adverse events that occurred in ≥2% of patients with early Parkinson's disease (without L-dopa) treated with *Requip* participating in the double-blind, placebo-controlled studies and were numerically more common in the *Requip* group. In these studies, either Requip (ropinirole hydrochloride) or placebo was used as early therapy (i.e., without L-dopa).

The prescriber should be aware that these figures cannot be used to predict the incidence of adverse events in the course of usual medical practice where patient characteristics and other factors differ from those that prevailed in the clinical studies. Similarly, the cited frequencies cannot be compared with figures obtained from other clinical investigations involving different treatments, uses and investigators. However, the cited figures do provide the prescribing physician with some basis for estimating the relative contribution of drug and non-drug factors to the adverse-events incidence rate in the population studied.

[See table 1 at top of previous page and above]

Table 2: Treatment-Emergent Adverse Event[1] Incidence in Double-blind, Placebo-controlled Advanced Parkinson's Disease (with L-dopa) Trials (Events ≥2% of Patients Treated with *Requip* and Numerically More Frequent than the Placebo Group)

	Requip N = 208 (%)	Placebo N = 120 (%)
Autonomic Nervous System		
Dry Mouth	5	1
Increased Sweating	7	2
Body as a Whole		
Increased Drug Level	7	3
Pain	5	3
Cardiovascular General		
Hypotension	2	1
Syncope	3	2
Central/Peripheral Nervous System		
Dizziness	26	16
Dyskinesia	34	13
Falls	10	7
Headache	17	12
Hypokinesia	5	4
Paresis	3	0
Paresthesia	5	3
Tremor	6	3
Gastrointestinal System		
Abdominal Pain	9	8
Constipation	6	3
Diarrhea	5	3
Dysphagia	2	1
Flatulence	2	1
Nausea	30	18
Increased Saliva	2	1
Vomiting	7	4
Metabolic/Nutritional		
Weight Decrease	2	1
Musculoskeletal System		
Arthralgia	7	5
Arthritis	3	1
Psychiatric		
Amnesia	5	1
Anxiety	6	3
Confusion	9	2
Abnormal Dreaming	3	2
Hallucination	10	4
Nervousness	5	3
Somnolence	20	8
Red Blood Cell		
Anemia	2	0
Resistance Mechanism		
Upper Repiratory Tract Infection	9	8

Continued

Other events reported by 1% or more of early Parkinson's disease (without L-dopa) patients treated with *Requip*, but that were equally or more frequent in the placebo group were: headache, upper respiratory infection, insomnia, arthralgia, tremor, back pain, anxiety, dyskinesias, aggravated Parkinsonism, depression, falls, myalgia, leg cramps, paresthesias, nervousness, diarrhea, arthritis, hot flushes, weight loss, rash, cough, hyperglycemia, muscle spasm, arthrosis, abnormal dreams, dystonia, increased salivation, bradycardia, gout, basal cell carcinoma, gingivitis, hematuria, and rigors.

Among the treatment-emergent adverse events in patients treated with *Requip*, hallucinations appear to be dose-related.

The incidence of adverse events was not materially different between women and men.

Advanced Parkinson's Disease (with L-dopa)

The most commonly observed adverse events (>5%), in the double-blind, placebo-controlled advanced Parkinson's disease (with L-dopa) trials associated with the use of *Requip* (n = 208) as an adjunct to L-dopa not seen at an equivalent frequency among the placebo-treated patients (n = 120) were, in order of decreasing incidence: dyskinesias, nausea, dizziness, aggravated Parkinsonism, somnolence, headache, insomnia, injury, hallucinations, falls, abdominal pain, upper respiratory infection, confusion, increased sweating, vomiting, viral infection, increased drug level, arthralgia, tremor, anxiety, urinary tract infection, constipation, dry mouth, pain, hypokinesia, and paresthesia.

Approximately 24% of 208 patients who received Requip (ropinirole hydrochloride) in the double-blind, placebo-controlled advanced Parkinson's disease (with L-dopa) trials discontinued treatment due to adverse events compared to 18% of 120 patients who received placebo. The events most commonly (≥1%) causing discontinuation of treatment by *Requip*-treated patients were: dizziness (2.9%), dyskinesias (2.4%), vomiting (2.4%), confusion (2.4%), nausea (1.9%), hallucinations (1.9%), anxiety (1.9%), and increased sweating (1.4%). Of these, hallucinations and dyskinesias appear to be dose-related.

Adverse Event Incidence in Controlled Clinical Studies

Table 2 lists treatment-emergent adverse events that occurred in ≥2% of patients with advanced Parkinson's disease (with L-dopa) treated with *Requip* who participated in the double-blind, placebo-controlled studies and were numerically more common in the *Requip* group. In these studies, either *Requip* or placebo was used as an adjunct to L-dopa. Adverse events were usually mild or moderate in intensity.

The prescriber should be aware that these figures cannot be used to predict the incidence of adverse events in the course of usual medical practice where patient characteristics and other factors differ from those that prevailed in the clinical studies. Similarly, the cited frequencies cannot be compared with figures obtained from other clinical investigations involving different treatments, uses, and investigators. However, the cited figures do provide the prescribing physician with some basis for estimating the relative contribution of drug and non-drug factors to the adverse-events incidence rate in the population studied.

[See table 2 above and on next page]

Other events reported by 1% or more of patients treated with both *Requip* and L-dopa, but equally or more frequent in the placebo/L-dopa group were: myocardial infarction, orthostatic symptoms, virus infections, asthenia, dyspepsia, myalgia, back pain, depression, leg cramps, fatigue, rhinitis, chest pain, hematuria, vertigo, tinnitus, leg edema, hot flushes, abnormal gait, hyperkinesia, and pharyngitis.

Among the treatment-emergent adverse events in patients treated with *Requip*, hallucinations and dyskinesias appear to be dose-related.

Other Adverse Events Observed During All Phase 2/3 Clinical Trials: *Requip* has been administered to 1,599 individuals in clinical trials. During these trials, all adverse events were recorded by the clinical investigators using terminology of their own choosing. To provide a meaningful estimate of the proportion of individuals having adverse events, similar types of events were grouped into a smaller number of standardized categories using modified WHOART dictionary terminology. These categories are used in the listing below. The frequencies presented represent the proportion of the 1,599 individuals exposed to *Requip* who experienced events of the type cited on at least one occasion while receiving *Requip*. All reported events that occurred at least twice (or once for serious or potentially seri-

Continued on next page

Information on the SmithKline Beecham Pharmaceuticals products appearing here is based on the labeling in effect on July 31, 1998. Further information on these and other products may be obtained from the Medical Department, SmithKline Beecham Pharmaceuticals, One Franklin Plaza, Philadelphia, PA 19101.

Requip—Cont.

ous events), except those already listed above, trivial events, and terms too vague to be meaningful are included, without regard to determination of a causal relationship to Requip (ropinirole hydrochloride), except that events very unlikely to be drug-related have been deleted.

Events are further classified within body system categories and enumerated in order of decreasing frequency using the following definitions: frequent adverse events are defined as those occurring in at least 1/100 patients and infrequent adverse events are those occurring in 1/100 to 1/1000 patients and rare events are those occurring in fewer than 1/1000 patients.

Body as a Whole: *infrequent* — cellulitis, peripheral edema, fever, influenza-like symptoms, enlarged abdomen, precordial chest pain, and generalized edema; *rare* — ascites.

Cardiovascular: *infrequent* — cardiac failure, bradycardia, tachycardia, supraventricular tachycardia, angina pectoris, bundle branch block, cardiac arrest, cardiomegaly, aneurysm, mitral insufficiency; *rare* — ventricular tachycardia.

Central/Peripheral Nervous System: *frequent* — neuralgia; *infrequent* — involuntary muscle contractions, hypertonia, dysphonia, abnormal coordination, extrapyramidal disorder, migraine, choreoathetosis, coma, stupor, aphasia, convulsions, hypotonia, peripheral neuropathy, paralysis; *rare* — grand mal convulsions, hemiparesis, hemiplegia.

Endocrine: *infrequent* — hypothyroidism, gynecomastia, hyperthyroidism; *rare* — goiter, SIADH.

Gastrointestinal: *infrequent* — increased hepatic enzymes, bilirubinemia, cholecystitis, cholelithiasis colitis, dysphagia, periodontitis, fecal incontinence, gastroesophageal reflux, hemorrhoids, toothache, eructation, gastritis, esophagitis, hiccups, diverticulitis, duodenal ulcer, gastric ulcer, melena, duodenitis, gastrointestinal hemorrhage, glossitis, rectal hemorrhage, pancreatitis, stomatitis and ulcerative stomatitis, tongue edema; *rare* — biliary pain, hemorrhagic gastritis, hematemesis, salivary duct obstruction.

Hematologic: *infrequent* — purpura, thrombocytopenia, hematoma, Vitamin B12 deficiency, hypochromic anemia, eosinophilia, leukocytosis, leukopenia, lymphocytosis, lymphopenia, lymphedema.

Metabolic/Nutritional: *frequent* — increased BUN; *infrequent* — hypoglycemia, increased alkaline phosphatase, increased LDH, weight increase, hyperphosphatemia, hyperuricemia, diabetes mellitus, glycosuria, hypokalemia, hypercholesterolemia, hyperkalemia, acidosis, hyponatremia, thirst, increased CPK, dehydration; *rare* — hypochloremia.

Musculoskeletal: *infrequent* — aggravated arthritis, tendinitis, osteoporosis, bursitis, polymyalgia rheumatica, muscle weakness, skeletal pain, torticollis; *rare* — Dupuytren's contracture requiring surgery.

Neoplasm: *infrequent* — malignant breast neoplasm; *rare* — bladder carcinoma, benign brain neoplasm, esophageal carcinoma, malignant laryngeal neoplasm, lipoma, rectal carcinoma, uterine neoplasm.

Psychiatric: *infrequent* — increased libido, agitation, apathy, impaired concentration, depersonalization, paranoid reaction, personality disorder, euphoria, delirium, dementia, delusion, emotional lability, decreased libido, manic reaction, somnambulism, aggressive reaction, neurosis; *rare* — suicide attempt.

Genito-urinary: *infrequent* — amenorrhea, vaginal hemorrhage, penile disorder, prostatic disorder, balanoposthitis, epididymitis, perineal pain, dysuria, micturition frequency, albuminuria, nocturia, polyuria, renal calculus; *rare* — breast enlargement, mastitis, uterine hemorrhage, ejaculation disorder, Peyronie's Disease, pyelonephritis, acute renal failure, uremia.

Resistance Mechanism: *infrequent* — herpes zoster, otitis media, sepsis, abscess, herpes simplex, fungal infection, genital moniliasis.

Respiratory: *infrequent* — asthma, epistaxis, laryngitis, pleurisy, pulmonary edema.

Skin/Appendage: *infrequent* — pruritis, dermatitis, eczema, skin ulceration, alopecia, skin hypertrophy, skin discoloration, urticaria, fungal dermatitis, furunculosis, hyperkeratosis, photosensitivity reaction, psoriasis, maculopapular rash, psoriaform rash, seborrhea.

Special Senses: *infrequent* — tinnitus, earache, decreased hearing, abnormal lacrimation, conjunctivitis, blepharitis, glaucoma, abnormal accommodation, blepharospasm, eye pain, photophobia; *rare* — scotoma.

Vascular Extracardiac: *infrequent* — varicose veins, phlebitis, peripheral gangrene; *rare* — limb embolism, pulmonary embolism, gangrene, subarachnoid hemorrhage, deep thrombophlebitis, leg thrombophlebitis, thrombosis.

DRUG ABUSE AND DEPENDENCE
Controlled Substance Class
Requip is not a controlled substance.
Physical and Psychological Dependence
Animal studies and human clinical trials with Requip (ropinirole hydrochloride) did not reveal any potential for drug-seeking behavior or physical dependence.

Table 2: (Continued) Treatment-Emergent Adverse Event[1] Incidence in Double-blind, Placebo-controlled Advanced Parkinson's Disease (with L-dopa) Trials (Events ≥2% of Patients Treated with Requip and Numerically More Frequent than the Placebo Group)

	Requip N = 208 (%)	Placebo N = 120 (%)
Respiratory System		
Dyspnea	3	2
Urinary System		
Pyuria	2	1
Urinary Incontinence	2	1
Urinary Tract Infection	6	3
Vision		
Diplopia	2	1

1. Patients may have reported multiple adverse experiences during the study or at discontinuation; thus, patients must be included in more than one category.

OVERDOSAGE
There were no reports of intentional overdose of *Requip* in the premarketing clinical trials. A total of 27 patients accidentally took more than their prescribed dose of *Requip*, with 10 patients ingesting more than 24 mg/day. The largest overdose reported in premarketing clinical trials was 435 mg taken over a 7-day period (62.1 mg/day). Of patients who received a dose greater than 24 mg/day, one experienced mild oro-facial dyskinesia, another patient experienced intermittent nausea. Other symptoms reported with accidental overdoses were: agitation, increased dyskinesia, grogginess, sedation, orthostatic hypotension, chest pain, confusion, vomiting and nausea.

Overdose Management
It is anticipated that the symptoms of *Requip* overdose will be related to its dopaminergic activity. General supportive measures are recommended. Vital signs should be maintained, if necessary. Removal of any unabsorbed material (e.g., by gastric lavage) should be considered.

DOSAGE AND ADMINISTRATION
In all clinical studies, dosage was initiated at a subtherapeutic level and gradually titrated to therapeutic response. The dosage should be increased to achieve a maximum therapeutic effect, balanced against the principal side effects of nausea, dizziness, somnolence and dyskinesia.

Requip should be taken three times daily. *Requip* can be taken with or without food. Since ingestion with food reduces the maximum concentration (C_{max}) of *Requip*, patients should be advised that taking with food may reduce the occurrence of nausea. However, this has not been established in controlled clinical trials.

The recommended starting dose is 0.25 mg three times daily. Based on individual patient response, dosage should then be titrated with weekly increments as described in the table below. After week 4, if necessary, daily dosage may be increased by 1.5 mg per day on a weekly basis up to a dose of 9 mg per day, and then by up to 3 mg per day weekly to a total dose of 24 mg per day.

Ascending-Dose Schedule of Requip

Week	Dosage	Total Daily Dose
1	0.25 mg three times daily	0.75 mg
2	0.5 mg three times daily	1.5 mg
3	0.75 mg three times daily	2.25 mg
4	1.0 mg three times daily	3.0 mg

Doses greater than 24 mg/day have not been tested in clinical trials.

When *Requip* is administered as adjunct therapy to L-dopa, the concurrent dose of L-dopa may be decreased gradually as tolerated. L-dopa dosage reduction was allowed during the advanced Parkinson's disease (with L-dopa) study if dyskinesias or other dopaminergic effects occurred. Overall, reduction of L-dopa dose was sustained in 87% of *Requip*-treated patients and in 57% of patients on placebo. On average the L-dopa dose was reduced by 31% in *Requip*-treated patients.

Requip should be discontinued gradually over a 7-day period. The frequency of administration should be reduced from three times daily to twice daily for 4 days. For the remaining 3 days, the frequency should be reduced to once daily prior to complete withdrawal of Requip (ropinirole hydrochloride).

HOW SUPPLIED
Tablets: Each pentagonal film-coated Tiltab® tablet with beveled edges contains ropinirole hydrochloride as follows: 0.25 mg – white imprinted with SB and 4890; 0.5 mg – yellow imprinted with SB and 4891; 1.0 mg – pale green imprinted with SB and 4892; 2.0 mg – pale yellowish pink imprinted with SB and 4893; 5.0 mg – pale blue imprinted with SB and 4894.

0.25 mg SUP 30's: NDC 0007-4890-14
0.25 mg bottles of 100: NDC 0007-4890-20
0.5 mg SUP 30's: NDC 0007-4891-14
0.5 mg bottles of 100: NDC 0007-4891-20
1 mg SUP 30's: NDC 0007-4892-14
1 mg bottles of 100: NDC 0007-4892-20
2 mg SUP 30's: NDC 0007-4893-14
2 mg bottles of 100: NDC 0007-4893-20
5 mg SUP 30's: NDC 0007-4894-14
5 mg bottles of 100: NDC 0007-4894-20
STORAGE
Protect from light.
Store at controlled room temperature 20°-25°C (68°-77°F) [see USP].
Manufactured by **SmithKline Beecham Pharmaceuticals**, Crawley, UK for
SmithKline Beecham Pharmaceuticals, Philadelphia, PA 19101
RQ:L1B

Shown in Product Identification Guide, page 340

STELAZINE®
[stel 'ah-zeen]
brand of trifluoperazine hydrochloride
Antianxiety/Antipsychotic

℞

DESCRIPTION
Tablets: Each round, blue, film-coated tablet contains trifluoperazine hydrochloride equivalent to trifluoperazine as follows: 1 mg imprinted SKF and S03; 2 mg imprinted SKF and S04; 5 mg imprinted SKF and S06; 10 mg imprinted SKF and S07. Inactive ingredients consist of cellulose, croscarmellose sodium, FD&C Blue No. 2, FD&C Yellow No. 6, FD&C Red No. 40, gelatin, iron oxide, lactose, magnesium stearate, talc, titanium dioxide and trace amounts of other inactive ingredients.

Multi-Dose Vials, 10 mL (2 mg/mL)—Each mL contains, in aqueous solution, trifluoperazine, 2 mg, as the hydrochloride; sodium tartrate, 4.75 mg; sodium biphosphate, 11.6 mg; sodium saccharin, 0.3 mg; benzyl alcohol, 0.75%, as preservative.

Concentrate—Each mL of clear, yellow, banana-vanilla-flavored liquid contains 10 mg of trifluoperazine as the hydrochloride. Inactive ingredients consist of D&C Yellow No. 10, FD&C Yellow No. 6, flavor, sodium benzoate, sodium bisulfite, sucrose and water.

N.B.: The Concentrate is for use in severe neuropsychiatric conditions when oral medication is preferred and other oral forms are considered impractical.

INDICATIONS
For the management of the manifestations of psychotic disorders.

Stelazine (trifluoperazine HCl) is effective for the short-term treatment of generalized non-psychotic anxiety. However, *Stelazine* is not the first drug to be used in therapy for most patients with non-psychotic anxiety because certain risks associated with its use are not shared by common alternative treatments (i.e., benzodiazepines).

When used in the treatment of non-psychotic anxiety, *Stelazine* should not be administered at doses of more than 6 mg per day or for longer than 12 weeks because the use of *Stelazine* at higher doses or for longer intervals may cause persistent tardive dyskinesia that may prove irreversible (see WARNINGS).

The effectiveness of *Stelazine* as a treatment for non-psychotic anxiety was established in a 4-week clinical multicenter study of outpatients with generalized anxiety disorder (DSM-III). This evidence does not predict that *Stelazine* will be useful in patients with other non-psychotic conditions in which anxiety, or signs that mimic anxiety, are found (i.e., physical illness, organic mental conditions, agitated depression, character pathologies, etc.).
Stelazine (trifluoperazine HCl) has not been shown effective in the management of behavioral complications in patients with mental retardation.

CONTRAINDICATIONS

A known hypersensitivity to phenothiazines, comatose or greatly depressed states due to central nervous system depressants and, in cases of existing blood dyscrasias, bone marrow depression and pre-existing liver damage.

WARNINGS

Tardive Dyskinesia: Tardive dyskinesia, a syndrome consisting of potentially irreversible, involuntary, dyskinetic movements, may develop in patients treated with neuroleptic (antipsychotic) drugs. Although the prevalence of the syndrome appears to be highest among the elderly, especially elderly women, it is impossible to rely upon prevalence estimates to predict, at the inception of neuroleptic treatment, which patients are likely to develop the syndrome. Whether neuroleptic drug products differ in their potential to cause tardive dyskinesia is unknown.
Both the risk of developing the syndrome and the likelihood that it will become irreversible are believed to increase as the duration of treatment and the total cumulative dose of neuroleptic drugs administered to the patient increase. However, the syndrome can develop, although much less commonly, after relatively brief treatment periods at low doses.
There is no known treatment for established cases of tardive dyskinesia, although the syndrome may remit, partially or completely, if neuroleptic treatment is withdrawn. Neuroleptic treatment itself, however, may suppress (or partially suppress) the signs and symptoms of the syndrome and thereby may possibly mask the underlying disease process. The effect that symptomatic suppression has upon the long-term course of the syndrome is unknown.
Given these considerations, neuroleptics should be prescribed in a manner that is most likely to minimize the occurrence of tardive dyskinesia. Chronic neuroleptic treatment should generally be reserved for patients who suffer from a chronic illness that 1) is known to respond to neuroleptic drugs, and, 2) for whom alternative, equally effective, but potentially less harmful treatments are *not* available or appropriate. In patients who do require chronic treatment, the smallest dose and the shortest duration of treatment producing a satisfactory clinical response should be sought. The need for continued treatment should be reassessed periodically.
If signs and symptoms of tardive dyskinesia appear in a patient on neuroleptics, drug discontinuation should be considered. However, some patients may require treatment despite the presence of the syndrome.
For further information about the description of tardive dyskinesia and its clinical detection, please refer to the sections on PRECAUTIONS and ADVERSE REACTIONS.

Neuroleptic Malignant Syndrome (NMS)

A potentially fatal symptom complex sometimes referred to as Neuroleptic Malignant Syndrome (NMS) has been reported in association with antipsychotic drugs. Clinical manifestations of NMS are hyperpyrexia, muscle rigidity, altered mental status and evidence of autonomic instability (irregular pulse or blood pressure, tachycardia, diaphoresis, and cardiac dysrhythmias).
The diagnostic evaluation of patients with this syndrome is complicated. In arriving at a diagnosis, it is important to identify cases where the clinical presentation includes both serious medical illness (e.g., pneumonia, systemic infection, etc.) and untreated or inadequately treated extrapyramidal signs and symptoms (EPS). Other important considerations in the differential diagnosis include central anticholinergic toxicity, heat stroke, drug fever and primary central nervous system (CNS) pathology.
The management of NMS should include 1) immediate discontinuation of antipsychotic drugs and other drugs not essential to concurrent therapy, 2) intensive symptomatic treatment and medical monitoring, and 3) treatment of any concomitant serious medical problems for which specific treatments are available. There is no general agreement about specific pharmacological treatment regimens for uncomplicated NMS.
If a patient requires antipsychotic drug treatment after recovery from NMS, the potential reintroduction of drug therapy should be carefully considered. The patient should be carefully monitored, since recurrences of NMS have been reported.
An encephalopathic syndrome (characterized by weakness, lethargy, fever, tremulousness and confusion, extrapyramidal symptoms, leukocytosis, elevated serum enzymes, BUN and FBS) has occurred in a few patients treated with lithium plus a neuroleptic. In some instances, the syndrome was followed by irreversible brain damage. Because of a possible causal relationship between these events and the concomitant administration of lithium and neuroleptics, patients receiving such combined therapy should be monitored closely for early evidence of neurologic toxicity and treatment discontinued promptly if such signs appear. This encephalopathic syndrome may be similar to or the same as neuroleptic malignant syndrome (NMS).
Patients who have demonstrated a hypersensitivity reaction (e.g., blood dyscrasias, jaundice) with a phenothiazine should not be re-exposed to any phenothiazine, including Stelazine (trifluoperazine HCl), unless in the judgment of the physician the potential benefits of treatment outweigh the possible hazard.
Stelazine Concentrate contains sodium bisulfite, a sulfite that may cause allergic-type reactions including anaphylactic symptoms and life-threatening or less severe asthmatic episodes in certain susceptible people. The overall prevalence of sulfite sensitivity in the general population is unknown and probably low. Sulfite sensitivity is seen more frequently in asthmatic than in non-asthmatic people.
Stelazine (trifluoperazine HCl) may impair mental and/or physical abilities, especially during the first few days of therapy. Therefore, caution patients about activities requiring alertness (e.g., operating vehicles or machinery).
If agents such as sedatives, narcotics, anesthetics, tranquilizers or alcohol are used either simultaneously or successively with the drug, the possibility of an undesirable additive depressant effect should be considered.
Usage in Pregnancy: Safety for the use of *Stelazine* during pregnancy has not been established. Therefore, it is not recommended that the drug be given to pregnant patients except when, in the judgment of the physician, it is essential. The potential benefits should clearly outweigh possible hazards. There are reported instances of prolonged jaundice, extrapyramidal signs, hyperreflexia or hyporeflexia in newborn infants whose mothers received phenothiazines.
Reproductive studies in rats given over 600 times the human dose showed an increased incidence of malformations above controls and reduced litter size and weight linked to maternal toxicity. These effects were not observed at half this dosage. No adverse effect on fetal development was observed in rabbits given 700 times the human dose nor in monkeys given 25 times the human dose.
Nursing Mothers: There is evidence that phenothiazines are excreted in the breast milk of nursing mothers. Because of the potential for serious adverse reactions in nursing infants from trifluoperazine, a decision should be made whether to discontinue nursing or to discontinue the drug, taking into account the importance of the drug to the mother.

PRECAUTIONS

General

Given the likelihood that some patients exposed chronically to neuroleptics will develop tardive dyskinesia, it is advised that all patients in whom chronic use is contemplated be given, if possible, full information about this risk. The decision to inform patients and/or their guardians must obviously take into account the clinical circumstances and the competency of the patient to understand the information provided.
Thrombocytopenia and anemia have been reported in patients receiving the drug. Agranulocytosis and pancytopenia have also been reported—warn patients to report the sudden appearance of sore throat or other signs of infection. If white blood cell and differential counts indicate cellular depression, stop treatment and start antibiotic and other suitable therapy.
Jaundice of the cholestatic type of hepatitis or liver damage has been reported. If fever with grippe-like symptoms occurs, appropriate liver studies should be conducted. If tests indicate an abnormality, stop treatment.
One result of therapy may be an increase in mental and physical activity. For example, a few patients with angina pectoris have complained of increased pain while taking the drug. Therefore, angina patients should be observed carefully and, if an unfavorable response is noted, the drug should be withdrawn.
Because hypotension has occurred, large doses and parenteral administration should be avoided in patients with impaired cardiovascular systems. To minimize the occurrence of hypotension after injection, keep patient lying down and observe for at least $^1/_2$ hour. If hypotension occurs from parenteral or oral dosing, place patient in head-low position with legs raised. If a vasoconstrictor is required, Levophed®* and Neo-Synephrine®† are suitable. Other pressor agents, including epinephrine, should not be used as they may cause a paradoxical further lowering of blood pressure.
Since certain phenothiazines have been reported to produce retinopathy, the drug should be discontinued if ophthalmoscopic examination or visual field studies should demonstrate retinal changes.
An antiemetic action of Stelazine (trifluoperazine HCl) may mask the signs and symptoms of toxicity or overdosage of other drugs and may obscure the diagnosis and treatment of other conditions such as intestinal obstruction, brain tumor and Reye's syndrome.
With prolonged administration at high dosages, the possibility of cumulative effects, with sudden onset of severe central nervous system or vasomotor symptoms, should be kept in mind.
Neuroleptic drugs elevate prolactin levels; the elevation persists during chronic administration. Tissue culture experiments indicate that approximately $^1/_3$ of human breast cancers are prolactin-dependent in vitro, a factor of potential importance if the prescribing of these drugs is contemplated in a patient with a previously detected breast cancer. Although disturbances such as galactorrhea, amenorrhea, gynecomastia and impotence have been reported, the clinical significance of elevated serum prolactin levels is unknown for most patients. An increase in mammary neoplasms has been found in rodents after chronic administration of neuroleptic drugs. Neither clinical nor epidemiologic studies conducted to date, however, have shown an association between chronic administration of these drugs and mammary tumorigenesis; the available evidence is considered too limited to be conclusive at this time.
Chromosomal aberrations in spermatocytes and abnormal sperm have been demonstrated in rodents treated with certain neuroleptics.
Because phenothiazines may interfere with thermoregulatory mechanisms, use with caution in persons who will be exposed to extreme heat.
As with all drugs which exert an anticholinergic effect, and/or cause mydriasis, trifluoperazine should be used with caution in patients with glaucoma.
Phenothiazines may diminish the effect of oral anticoagulants.
Phenothiazines can produce alpha-adrenergic blockade.
Concomitant administration of propranolol with phenothiazines results in increased plasma levels of both drugs.
Antihypertensive effects of guanethidine and related compounds may be counteracted when phenothiazines are used concurrently.
Thiazide diuretics may accentuate the orthostatic hypotension that may occur with phenothiazines.
Phenothiazines may lower the convulsive threshold; dosage adjustments of anticonvulsants may be necessary. Potentiation of anticonvulsant effects does not occur. However, it has been reported that phenothiazines may interfere with the metabolism of Dilantin®‡ and thus precipitate *Dilantin* toxicity.
Drugs which lower the seizure threshold, including phenothiazine derivatives, should not be used with Amipaque®§.
As with other phenothiazine derivatives, *Stelazine* should be discontinued at least 48 hours before myelography, should not be resumed for at least 24 hours postprocedure and should not be used for the control of nausea and vomiting occurring either prior to myelography or postprocedure with *Amipaque*.
The presence of phenothiazines may produce false-positive phenylketonuria (PKU) test results.
Long-Term Therapy: To lessen the likelihood of adverse reactions related to cumulative drug effect, patients with a history of long-term therapy with Stelazine (trifluoperazine HCl) and/or other neuroleptics should be evaluated periodically to decide whether the maintenance dosage could be lowered or drug therapy discontinued.

ADVERSE REACTIONS

Drowsiness, dizziness, skin reactions, rash, dry mouth, insomnia, amenorrhea, fatigue, muscular weakness, anorexia, lactation, blurred vision and neuromuscular (extrapyramidal) reactions.

Neuromuscular (Extrapyramidal) Reactions

These symptoms are seen in a significant number of hospitalized mental patients. They may be characterized by motor restlessness, be of the dystonic type, or they may resemble parkinsonism.
Depending on the severity of symptoms, dosage should be reduced or discontinued. If therapy is reinstituted, it should be at a lower dosage. Should these symptoms occur in children or pregnant patients, the drug should be stopped and not reinstituted. In most cases barbiturates by suitable route of administration will suffice. (Or, injectable Benadryl®‖ may be useful.) In more severe cases, the administration of an anti-parkinsonism agent, except levodopa, usually produces rapid reversal of symptoms. Suitable supportive measures such as maintaining a clear airway and adequate hydration should be employed.

Continued on next page

Information on the SmithKline Beecham Pharmaceuticals products appearing here is based on the labeling in effect on July 31, 1998. Further information on these and other products may be obtained from the Medical Department, SmithKline Beecham Pharmaceuticals, One Franklin Plaza, Philadelphia, PA 19101.

Stelazine—Cont.

Motor Restlessness: Symptoms may include agitation or jitteriness and sometimes insomnia. These symptoms often disappear spontaneously. At times these symptoms may be similar to the original neurotic or psychotic symptoms. Dosage should not be increased until these side effects have subsided.

If this phase becomes too troublesome, the symptoms can usually be controlled by a reduction of dosage or change of drug. Treatment with anti-parkinsonian agents, benzodiazepines or propranolol may be helpful.

Dystonias: Symptoms may include: spasm of the neck muscles, sometimes progressing to torticollis; extensor rigidity of back muscles, sometimes progressing to opisthotonos; carpopedal spasm, trismus, swallowing difficulty, oculogyric crisis and protrusion of the tongue.

These usually subside within a few hours, and almost always within 24 to 48 hours, after the drug has been discontinued.

In mild cases, reassurance or a barbiturate is often sufficient. *In moderate cases,* barbiturates will usually bring rapid relief. *In more severe adult cases,* the administration of an anti-parkinsonism agent, except levodopa, usually produces rapid reversal of symptoms. Also, intravenous caffeine with sodium benzoate seems to be effective. *In children,* reassurance and barbiturates will usually control symptoms. (Or, injectable *Benadryl* may be useful.) Note: See *Benadryl* prescribing information for appropriate children's dosage. If appropriate treatment with anti-parkinsonism agents or *Benadryl* fails to reverse the signs and symptoms, the diagnosis should be reevaluated.

Pseudo-parkinsonism: Symptoms may include: mask-like facies; drooling; tremors; pill-rolling motion; cogwheel rigidity; and shuffling gait. Reassurance and sedation are important. In most cases these symptoms are readily controlled when an anti-parkinsonism agent is administered concomitantly. Anti-parkinsonism agents should be used only when required. Generally, therapy of a few weeks to 2 to 3 months will suffice. After this time patients should be evaluated to determine their need for continued treatment. (Note: Levodopa has not been found effective in pseudo-parkinsonism.) Occasionally it is necessary to lower the dosage of Stelazine (trifluoperazine HCl) or to discontinue the drug.

Tardive Dyskinesia: As with all antipsychotic agents, tardive dyskinesia may appear in some patients on long-term therapy or may appear after drug therapy has been discontinued. The syndrome can also develop, although much less frequently, after relatively brief treatment periods at low doses. This syndrome appears in all age groups. Although its prevalence appears to be highest among elderly patients, especially elderly women, it is impossible to rely upon prevalence estimates to predict at the inception of neuroleptic treatment which patients are likely to develop the syndrome. The symptoms are persistent and in some patients appear to be irreversible. The syndrome is characterized by rhythmical involuntary movements of the tongue, face, mouth or jaw (e.g., protrusion of tongue, puffing of cheeks, puckering of mouth, chewing movements). Sometimes these may be accompanied by involuntary movements of extremities. In rare instances, these involuntary movements of the extremities are the only manifestations of tardive dyskinesia. A variant of tardive dyskinesia, tardive dystonia, has also been described.

There is no known effective treatment for tardive dyskinesia; anti-parkinsonism agents do not alleviate the symptoms of this syndrome. If clinically feasible, it is suggested that all antipsychotic agents be discontinued if these symptoms appear. Should it be necessary to reinstitute treatment, or increase the dosage of the agent, or switch to a different antipsychotic agent, the syndrome may be masked.

It has been reported that fine vermicular movements of the tongue may be an early sign of the syndrome and if the medication is stopped at that time the syndrome may not develop.

Adverse Reactions Reported with Stelazine (trifluoperazine HCl) or Other Phenothiazine Derivatives: Adverse effects with different phenothiazines vary in type, frequency, and mechanism of occurrence, i.e., some are dose-related, while others involve individual patient sensitivity. Some adverse effects may be more likely to occur, or occur with greater intensity, in patients with special medical problems, e.g., patients with mitral insufficiency or pheochromocytoma have experienced severe hypotension following recommended doses of certain phenothiazines.

Neuroleptic Malignant Syndrome (NMS) has been reported in association with antipsychotic drugs. (See WARNINGS.)

Not all of the following adverse reactions have been observed with every phenothiazine derivative, but they have been reported with one or more and should be borne in mind when drugs of this class are administered: extrapyramidal symptoms (opisthotonos, oculogyric crisis, hyperreflexia, dystonia, akathisia, dyskinesia, parkinsonism) some of which have lasted months and even years—particularly in elderly patients with previous brain damage; grand mal and

petit mal convulsions, particularly in patients with EEG abnormalities or history of such disorders; altered cerebrospinal fluid proteins; cerebral edema; intensification and prolongation of the action of central nervous system depressants (opiates, analgesics, antihistamines, barbiturates, alcohol); atropine, heat, organophosphorus insecticides; autonomic reactions (dryness of mouth, nasal congestion, headache, nausea, constipation, obstipation, adynamic ileus, ejaculatory disorders/impotence, priapism, atonic colon, urinary retention, miosis and mydriasis); reactivation of psychotic processes, catatonic-like states; hypotension (sometimes fatal); cardiac arrest; blood dyscrasias (pancytopenia, thrombocytopenic purpura, leukopenia, agranulocytosis, eosinophilia, hemolytic anemia, aplastic anemia); liver damage (jaundice, biliary stasis); endocrine disturbances (hyperglycemia, hypoglycemia, glycosuria, lactation, galactorrhea, gynecomastia, menstrual irregularities, false-positive pregnancy tests); skin disorders (photosensitivity, itching, erythema, urticaria, eczema up to exfoliative dermatitis); other allergic reactions (asthma, laryngeal edema, angioneurotic edema, anaphylactoid reactions); peripheral edema; reversed epinephrine effect; hyperpyrexia; mild fever after large I.M. doses; increased appetite; increased weight; a systemic lupus erythematosus-like syndrome; pigmentary retinopathy; with prolonged administration of substantial doses, skin pigmentation, epithelial keratopathy, and lenticular and corneal deposits.

EKG changes—particularly nonspecific, usually reversible Q and T wave distortions—have been observed in some patients receiving phenothiazine tranquilizers. Although phenothiazines cause neither psychic nor physical dependence, sudden discontinuance in long-term psychiatric patients may cause temporary symptoms, e.g., nausea and vomiting, dizziness, tremulousness.

Note: There have been occasional reports of sudden death in patients receiving phenothiazines. In some cases, the cause appeared to be cardiac arrest or asphyxia due to failure of the cough reflex.

DOSAGE AND ADMINISTRATION—ADULTS

Dosage should be adjusted to the needs of the individual. The lowest effective dosage should always be used. Dosage should be increased more gradually in debilitated or emaciated patients. When maximum response is achieved, dosage may be reduced gradually to a maintenance level. Because of the inherent long action of the drug, patients may be controlled on convenient b.i.d. administration; some patients may be maintained on once-a-day administration.

When Stelazine (trifluoperazine HCl) is administered by intramuscular injection, equivalent oral dosage may be substituted once symptoms have been controlled.

Note: Although there is little likelihood of contact dermatitis due to the drug, persons with known sensitivity to phenothiazine drugs should avoid direct contact.

Elderly Patients: In general, dosages in the lower range are sufficient for most elderly patients. Since they appear to be more susceptible to hypotension and neuromuscular reactions, such patients should be observed closely. Dosage should be tailored to the individual, response carefully monitored, and dosage adjusted accordingly. Dosage should be increased more gradually in elderly patients.

Non-psychotic Anxiety

Usual dosage is 1 or 2 mg twice daily. Do not administer at doses of more than 6 mg per day or for longer than 12 weeks.

Psychotic Disorders

Oral: Usual starting dosage is 2 mg to 5 mg b.i.d. (Small or emaciated patients should always be started on the lower dosage.)

Most patients will show optimum response on 15 mg or 20 mg daily, although a few may require 40 mg a day or more. Optimum therapeutic dosage levels should be reached within 2 or 3 weeks.

When the Concentrate dosage form is to be used, it should be added to 60 mL (2 fl oz) or more of diluent *just prior to administration* to insure palatability and stability. Vehicles suggested for dilution are: tomato or fruit juice, milk, simple syrup, orange syrup, carbonated beverages, coffee, tea or water. Semisolid foods (soup, puddings, etc.) may also be used.

Intramuscular (for prompt control of severe symptoms): Usual dosage is 1 mg to 2 mg ($\frac{1}{2}$ to 1 mL) by deep intramuscular injection q4 to 6h, p.r.n. More than 6 mg within 24 hours is rarely necessary.

Only in very exceptional cases should intramuscular dosage exceed 10 mg within 24 hours. Injections should not be given at intervals of less than 4 hours because of a possible cumulative effect.

Note: Stelazine (trifluoperazine HCl) Injection has been usually well tolerated and there is little, if any, pain and irritation at the site of injection.

This solution should be protected from light. This is a clear, colorless to pale yellow solution; a slight yellowish discoloration will not alter potency. If markedly discolored, solution should be discarded.

DOSAGE AND ADMINISTRATION—PSYCHOTIC CHILDREN

Dosage should be adjusted to the weight of the child and severity of the symptoms. These dosages are for children, ages 6 to 12, who are hospitalized or under close supervision.

Oral: The starting dosage is 1 mg administered once a day or b.i.d. Dosage may be increased gradually until symptoms are controlled or until side effects become troublesome. While it is usually not necessary to exceed dosages of 15 mg daily, some older children with severe symptoms may require higher dosages.

Intramuscular: There has been little experience with the use of Stelazine (trifluoperazine HCl) Injection in children. However, if it is necessary to achieve rapid control of severe symptoms, 1 mg ($\frac{1}{2}$ mL) of the drug may be administered intramuscularly once or twice a day.

OVERDOSAGE

(See also under ADVERSE REACTIONS.) SYMPTOMS—Primarily involvement of the extrapyramidal mechanism producing some of the dystonic reactions described above. Symptoms of central nervous system depression to the point of somnolence or coma. Agitation and restlessness may also occur. Other possible manifestations include convulsions, EKG changes and cardiac arrhythmias, fever and autonomic reactions such as hypotension, dry mouth and ileus. TREATMENT—It is important to determine other medications taken by the patient since multiple dose therapy is common in overdosage situations. Treatment is essentially symptomatic and supportive. Early gastric lavage is helpful. Keep patient under observation and maintain an open airway, since involvement of the extrapyramidal mechanism may produce dysphagia and respiratory difficulty in severe overdosage. **Do not attempt to induce emesis because a dystonic reaction of the head or neck may develop that could result in aspiration of vomitus.** Extrapyramidal symptoms may be treated with anti-parkinsonism drugs, barbiturates, or *Benadryl.* See prescribing information for these products. Care should be taken to avoid increasing respiratory depression. If administration of a stimulant is desirable, amphetamine, dextroamphetamine or caffeine with sodium benzoate is recommended. Stimulants that may cause convulsions (e.g., picrotoxin or pentylenetetrazol) should be avoided.

If hypotension occurs, the standard measures for managing circulatory shock should be initiated. If it is desirable to administer a vasoconstrictor, *Levophed* and *Neo-Synephrine* are most suitable. Other pressor agents, including epinephrine, are not recommended because phenothiazine derivatives may reverse the usual elevating action of these agents and cause a further lowering of blood pressure.

Limited experience indicates that phenothiazines are *not* dialyzable.

HOW SUPPLIED

Tablets, 1 mg, 2 mg, 5 mg and 10 mg in bottles of 100.
1 mg 100's: NDC 0108-4903-20
2 mg 100's: NDC 0108-4904-20
5 mg 100's: NDC 0108-4906-20
10 mg 100's: NDC 0108-4907-20
Multi-Dose Vials, 10 mL (2 mg/mL), in 1's:
NDC 0108-4902-01
Concentrate (for institutional use), 10 mg/mL, in 2 fl oz bottles and in cartons of 12 bottles.
The Concentrate form is light-sensitive. For this reason, it should be protected from light and dispensed in amber bottles. *Refrigeration is not required.*
10 mg/mL 2 fl oz (carton of 12): NDC 0108-4901-42
Store all Stelazine (trifluoperazine HCl) formulations between 15° and 30°C (59° and 86°F).

---

* norepinephrine bitartrate, Sanofi Winthrop Pharmaceuticals.
† phenylephrine hydrochloride, Sanofi Winthrop Pharmaceuticals.
‡ phenytoin, Parke-Davis.
§ metrizamide, Sanofi Winthrop Pharmaceuticals.
‖ diphenhydramine hydrochloride, Parke-Davis.
Veterans Administration/Military/PHS—Injection, 2 mg/mL, 10 mL, 1's, 6505-01-220-1479; Tablets, 1 mg, 100's, 6505-00-761-5658; 2 mg, 100's, 6505-01-361-5235; 5 mg, 100's, 6505-01-311-3784; 10 mg, 100's, 6505-01-246-1918.

SZ:L70

Shown in Product Identification Guide, page 340

TAGAMET®   ℞

[tag 'ah-met]
brand of cimetidine tablets
cimetidine hydrochloride liquid and
cimetidine hydrochloride injection

DESCRIPTION

Tagamet (cimetidine) is a histamine H_2-receptor antagonist. Chemically it is N''-cyano-N-methyl-N'-[2-[[(5-methyl-1H-imidazol-4-yl) methyl] thio]-ethyl]-guanidine.

The empirical formula for cimetidine is $C_{10}H_{16}N_6S$ and for cimetidine hydrochloride, $C_{10}H_{16}N_6SHCl$; these represent molecular weights of 252.34 and 288.80, respectively.

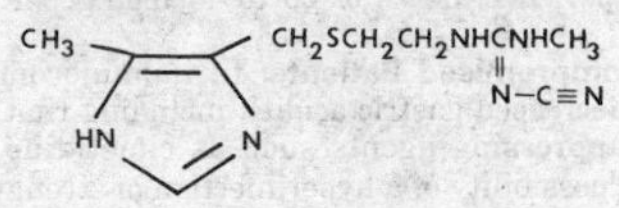

Cimetidine

Cimetidine contains an imidazole ring, and is chemically related to histamine.
(The liquid and injection dosage forms contain cimetidine as the hydrochloride.)
Cimetidine has a bitter taste and characteristic odor.
Solubility Characteristics: Cimetidine is soluble in alcohol, slightly soluble in water, very slightly soluble in chloroform and insoluble in ether. Cimetidine hydrochloride is freely soluble in water, soluble in alcohol, very slightly soluble in chloroform and practically insoluble in ether.
Tablets for Oral Administration: Each light green, film-coated tablet contains cimetidine as follows: 200 mg—round, imprinted with the product name TAGAMET, SKF and 200; 300 mg—round, debossed with the product name TAGAMET, SB and 300; 400 mg—oval Tiltab® tablets, debossed with the product name TAGAMET, SB and 400; 800 mg—oval Tiltab® tablets, debossed with the product name TAGAMET, SB and 800. Inactive ingredients consist of cellulose, D&C Yellow No. 10, FD&C Blue No. 2, FD&C Red No. 40, FD&C Yellow No. 6, hydroxypropyl methylcellulose, iron oxides, magnesium stearate, povidone, propylene glycol, sodium lauryl sulfate, sodium starch glycolate, starch, titanium dioxide and trace amounts of other inactive ingredients.
Liquid for Oral Administration: Each 5 mL (1 teaspoonful) of clear, light orange, mint-peach flavored liquid contains cimetidine hydrochloride equivalent to cimetidine, 300 mg; alcohol, 2.8%. Inactive ingredients consist of FD&C Yellow No. 6, flavors, methylparaben, polyoxyethylene polyoxypropylene glycol, propylene glycol, propylparaben, saccharin sodium, sodium chloride, sodium phosphate, sorbitol and water.
Injection:
Single-Dose Vials for Intramuscular or Intravenous Administration: Each 2 mL contains, in sterile aqueous solution (pH range 3.8 to 6), cimetidine hydrochloride equivalent to cimetidine, 300 mg; phenol, 10 mg.
Multi-Dose Vials for Intramuscular or Intravenous Administration: 8 mL (300 mg/2 mL): Each 2 mL contains, in sterile aqueous solution (pH range 3.8 to 6), cimetidine hydrochloride equivalent to cimetidine, 300 mg; phenol, 10 mg.
Single-Dose Premixed Plastic Containers for Intravenous Administration: Each 50 mL of sterile aqueous solution (pH range 5 to 7) contains cimetidine hydrochloride equivalent to 300 mg cimetidine and 0.45 grams sodium chloride. No preservative has been added.
The plastic container is fabricated from specially formulated polyvinyl chloride. The amount of water that can permeate from inside the container into the overwrap is insufficient to affect the solution significantly. Solutions in contact with the plastic container can leach out certain of its chemical components in very small amounts within the expiration period, e.g., di 2-ethylhexyl phthalate (DEHP), up to 5 parts per million. However, the safety of the plastic has been confirmed in tests in animals according to the USP biological tests for plastic containers as well as by tissue culture toxicity studies.
ADD-Vantage®* Vials for Intravenous Administration: Each 2 mL contains, in sterile aqueous solution (pH range 3.8 to 6), cimetidine hydrochloride equivalent to cimetidine, 300 mg; phenol, 10 mg.
All of the above injection formulations are pyrogen free, and sodium hydroxide N.F. is used as an ingredient to adjust the pH.

CLINICAL PHARMACOLOGY

Tagamet (cimetidine) competitively inhibits the action of histamine at the histamine H_2 receptors of the parietal cells and thus is a histamine H_2-receptor antagonist.
Tagamet is not an anticholinergic agent. Studies have shown that *Tagamet* inhibits both daytime and nocturnal basal gastric acid secretion. *Tagamet* also inhibits gastric acid secretion stimulated by food, histamine, pentagastrin, caffeine and insulin.

Antisecretory Activity

1) **Acid Secretion:** *Nocturnal: Tagamet* 800 mg orally at bedtime reduces mean hourly H^+ activity by greater than 85% over an 8-hour period in duodenal ulcer patients, with no effect on daytime acid secretion. *Tagamet* 1600 mg orally h.s. produces 100% inhibition of mean hourly H^+ activity over an 8-hour period in duodenal ulcer patients, but also reduces H^+ activity by 35% for an additional 5 hours into the following morning. *Tagamet* 400 mg b.i.d. and 300 mg q.i.d. decrease nocturnal acid secretion in a dose-related manner, i.e., 47% to 83% over a 6- to 8-hour period and 54% over a 9-hour period, respectively.
Food Stimulated: During the first hour after a standard experimental meal, oral *Tagamet* 300 mg inhibited gastric acid secretion in duodenal ulcer patients by at least 50%. During the subsequent 2 hours *Tagamet* inhibited gastric acid secretion by at least 75%.
The effect of a 300 mg breakfast dose of *Tagamet* continued for at least 4 hours and there was partial suppression of the rise in gastric acid secretion following the luncheon meal in duodenal ulcer patients. This suppression of gastric acid output was enhanced and could be maintained by another 300 mg dose of *Tagamet* given with lunch.
In another study, *Tagamet* 300 mg given with the meal increased gastric pH as compared with placebo.

Mean Gastric pH

	Tagamet	Placebo
1 hour	3.5	2.6
2 hours	3.1	1.6
3 hours	3.8	1.9
4 hours	6.1	2.2

24-Hour Mean H^+ Activity: *Tagamet* 800 mg h.s., 400 mg b.i.d. and 300 mg q.i.d. all provide a similar, moderate (less than 60%) level of 24-hour acid suppression. However, the 800 mg h.s. regimen exerts its entire effect on nocturnal acid, and does not affect daytime gastric physiology.
Chemically Stimulated: Oral Tagamet (cimetidine) significantly inhibited gastric acid secretion stimulated by betazole (an isomer of histamine), pentagastrin, caffeine and insulin as follows:

Stimulant	Stimulant Dose	*Tagamet*	% Inhibition
Betazole	1.5mg/kg (sc)	300mg (po)	85% at $2^1/_2$ hours
Pentagastrin	6mcg/kg/hr (iv)	100mg/hr (iv)	60% at 1 hour
Caffeine	5mg/kg/hr (iv)	300mg (po)	100% at 1 hour
Insulin	0.03 units/kg/hr (iv)	100mg/hr (iv)	82% at 1 hour

When food and betazole were used to stimulate secretion, inhibition of hydrogen ion concentration usually ranged from 45% to 75% and the inhibition of volume ranged from 30% to 65%.
Parenteral administration also significantly inhibits gastric acid secretion. In a crossover study involving patients with active or healed duodenal or gastric ulcers, either continuous I.V. infusion of *Tagamet* 37.5 mg/hour (900 mg/day) or intermittent injection of *Tagamet* 300 mg q6h (1200 mg/day) maintained gastric pH above 4.0 for more than 50% of the time under steady-state conditions.

2) **Pepsin:** Oral *Tagamet* 300 mg reduced total pepsin output as a result of the decrease in volume of gastric juice.
3) **Intrinsic Factor:** Intrinsic factor secretion was studied with betazole as a stimulant. Oral *Tagamet* 300 mg inhibited the rise in intrinsic factor concentration produced by betazole, but some intrinsic factor was secreted at all times.

*ADD-Vantage® is a trademark of Abbott Laboratories.

Other

Lower Esophageal Sphincter Pressure and Gastric Emptying
Tagamet has no effect on lower esophageal sphincter (LES) pressure or the rate of gastric emptying.

Pharmacokinetics

Tagamet is rapidly absorbed after oral administration and peak levels occur in 45 to 90 minutes. The half-life of *Tagamet* is approximately 2 hours. Both oral and parenteral (I.V. or I.M.) administration provide comparable periods of therapeutically effective blood levels; blood concentrations remain above that required to provide 80% inhibition of basal gastric acid secretion for 4 to 5 hours following a dose of 300 mg.
Steady-state blood concentrations of cimetidine with continuous infusion of *Tagamet* are determined by the infusion rate and clearance of the drug in the individual patient. In a study of peptic ulcer patients with normal renal function, an infusion rate of 37.5 mg/hour produced average steady-state plasma cimetidine concentrations of about 0.9 mcg/mL. Blood levels with other infusion rates will vary in direct proportion to the infusion rate.
The principal route of excretion of *Tagamet* is the urine. Following parenteral administration, most of the drug is excreted as the parent compound; following oral administration, the drug is more extensively metabolized, the sulfoxide being the major metabolite. Following a single oral dose, 48% of the drug is recovered from the urine after 24 hours as the parent compound. Following I.V. or I.M. administration, approximately 75% of the drug is recovered from the urine after 24 hours as the parent compound.

CLINICAL TRIALS

Duodenal Ulcer

Tagamet (cimetidine) has been shown to be effective in the treatment of active duodenal ulcer and, at reduced dosage, in maintenance therapy following healing of active ulcers.
Active Duodenal Ulcer: *Tagamet* accelerates the rate of duodenal ulcer healing. Healing rates reported in U.S. and foreign controlled trials with *Tagamet* are summarized below, beginning with the regimen providing the lowest nocturnal dose.

Duodenal Ulcer Healing Rates with Various *Tagamet* Dosage Regimens*

Regimen	300 mg q.i.d.	400 mg b.i.d.	800 mg h.s.	1600 mg h.s.
week 4	68%	73%	80%	86%
week 6	80%	80%	89%	—
week 8	—	92%	94%	—

* Averages from controlled clinical trials.

A U.S., double-blind, placebo-controlled, dose-ranging study demonstrated that all once-daily at bedtime (h.s.) *Tagamet* regimens were superior to placebo in ulcer healing and that *Tagamet* 800 mg h.s. healed 75% of patients at 4 weeks. The healing rate with 800 mg h.s. was significantly superior to 400 mg h.s. (66%) and not significantly different from 1600 mg h.s. (81%).
In the U.S. dose-ranging trial, over 80% of patients receiving *Tagamet* 800 mg h.s. experienced nocturnal pain relief after 1 day. Relief from daytime pain was reported in approximately 70% of patients after 2 days. As with ulcer healing, the 800 mg h.s. dose was superior to 400 mg h.s. and not different from 1600 mg h.s.
In foreign, double-blind studies with *Tagamet* 800 mg h.s., 79% to 85% of patients were healed at 4 weeks.
While short-term treatment with Tagamet (cimetidine) can result in complete healing of the duodenal ulcer, acute therapy will not prevent ulcer recurrence after *Tagamet* has been discontinued. Some follow-up studies have reported that the rate of recurrence once therapy was discontinued was slightly higher for patients healed on *Tagamet* than for patients healed on other forms of therapy; however, the *Tagamet*-treated patients generally had more severe disease.
Maintenance Therapy in Duodenal Ulcer: Treatment with a reduced dose of *Tagamet* has been proven effective as maintenance therapy following healing of active duodenal ulcers.
In numerous placebo-controlled studies conducted worldwide, the percent of patients with observed ulcers at the end of 1 year's therapy with *Tagamet* 400 mg h.s. was significantly lower (10% to 45%) than in patients receiving placebo (44% to 70%). Thus, from 55% to 90% of patients were maintained free of observed ulcers at the end of 1 year with *Tagamet* 400 mg h.s.
Factors such as smoking, duration and severity of disease, gender, and genetic traits may contribute to variations in actual percentages.
Trials of other anti-ulcer therapy, whether placebo-controlled, positive-controlled or open, have demonstrated a range of results similar to that seen with *Tagamet*.

Active Benign Gastric Ulcer

Tagamet has been shown to be effective in the short-term treatment of active benign gastric ulcer.
In a multicenter, double-blind U.S. study, patients with endoscopically confirmed benign gastric ulcer were treated with *Tagamet* 300 mg four times a day or with placebo for 6 weeks. Patients were limited to those with ulcers ranging from 0.5 to 2.5 cm in size. Endoscopically confirmed healing at 6 weeks was seen in significantly* more *Tagamet*-treated patients than in patients receiving placebo, as shown below:

	Tagamet	Placebo
week 2	14/63 (22%)	7/63 (11%)
total at week 6	43/65 (66%) *	30/67 (45%)

$^*p<0.05$

Continued on next page

Information on the SmithKline Beecham Pharmaceuticals products appearing here is based on the labeling in effect on July 31, 1998. Further information on these and other products may be obtained from the Medical Department, SmithKline Beecham Pharmaceuticals, One Franklin Plaza, Philadelphia, PA 19101.

Tagamet—Cont.

In a similar multicenter U.S. study of the 800 mg h.s. oral regimen, the endoscopically confirmed healing rates were:

	Tagamet	Placebo
total at week 6	63/83 (76%) *	44/80 (55%)

*p = 0.005

Similarly, in worldwide double-blind clinical studies, endoscopically evaluated benign gastric ulcer healing rates were consistently higher with *Tagamet* than with placebo.

Gastroesophageal Reflux Disease

In two multicenter, double-blind, placebo-controlled studies in patients with gastroesophageal reflux disease (GERD) and endoscopically proven erosions and/or ulcers, *Tagamet* was significantly more effective than placebo in healing lesions. The endoscopically confirmed healing rates were:

Trial		*Tagamet* (800 mg b.i.d.)	*Tagamet* (400 mg q.i.d.)	Placebo	p-Value (800 mg b.i.d. vs. placebo)
1	Week 6	45%	52%	26%	0.02
	Week 12	60%	66%	42%	0.02
2	Week 6	50%		20%	<0.01
	Week 12	67%		36%	<0.01

In these trials *Tagamet* was superior to placebo by most measures in improving symptoms of day- and night-time heartburn, with many of the differences statistically significant. The q.i.d. regimen was generally somewhat better than the b.i.d. regimen where these were compared.

Prevention of Upper Gastrointestinal Bleeding in Critically Ill Patients

A double-blind, placebo-controlled randomized study of continuous infusion cimetidine was performed in 131 critically ill patients (mean APACHE II score = 15.99) to compare the incidence of upper gastrointestinal bleeding, manifested as hematemesis or bright red blood which did not clear after adjustment of the nasogastric tube and a 5 to 10 minute lavage, persistent Gastroccult® positive coffee grounds for 8 consecutive hours which did not clear with 100 cc lavage and/or which were accompanied by a drop in hematocrit of 5 percentage points, or melena, with an endoscopically documented upper gastrointestinal source of bleed. 14% (9/65) of patients treated with cimetidine continuous infusion developed bleeding compared to 33% (22/66) of the placebo group. Coffee grounds was the manifestation of bleeding that accounted for the difference between groups. Another randomized, double-blind placebo-controlled study confirmed these results for an end point of upper gastrointestinal bleeding with a confirmed upper gastrointestinal source noted on endoscopy, and by post hoc analyses of bleeding episodes between groups.

Pathological Hypersecretory Conditions
(such as Zollinger-Ellison Syndrome)

Tagamet significantly inhibited gastric acid secretion and reduced occurrence of diarrhea, anorexia and pain in patients with pathological hypersecretion associated with Zollinger-Ellison Syndrome, systemic mastocytosis and multiple endocrine adenomas. Use of *Tagamet* was also followed by healing of intractable ulcers.

INDICATIONS AND USAGE

Tagamet (cimetidine) is indicated in:

(1) **Short-term treatment of active duodenal ulcer.** Most patients heal within 4 weeks and there is rarely reason to use *Tagamet* at full dosage for longer than 6 to 8 weeks (see Dosage and Administration–Duodenal Ulcer). Concomitant antacids should be given as needed for relief of pain. However, simultaneous administration of *Tagamet* and antacids is not recommended, since antacids have been reported to interfere with the absorption of *Tagamet.*

(2) **Maintenance therapy for duodenal ulcer patients at reduced dosage after healing of active ulcer.** Patients have been maintained on continued treatment with *Tagamet* 400 mg h.s. for periods of up to 5 years.

(3) **Short-term treatment of active benign gastric ulcer.** There is no information concerning usefulness of treatment periods of longer than 8 weeks.

(4) **Erosive gastroesophageal reflux disease (GERD).** Erosive esophagitis diagnosed by endoscopy. Treatment is indicated for 12 weeks for healing of lesions and control of symptoms. The use of *Tagamet* beyond 12 weeks has not been established (see Dosage and Administration—GERD).

(5) **Prevention of upper gastrointestinal bleeding in critically ill patients.**

(6) **The treatment of pathological hypersecretory conditions** (i.e., Zollinger-Ellison Syndrome, systemic mastocytosis, multiple endocrine adenomas).

CONTRAINDICATIONS

Tagamet is contraindicated for patients known to have hypersensitivity to the product.

PRECAUTIONS

General: Rare instances of cardiac arrhythmias and hypotension have been reported following the rapid administration of Tagamet (cimetidine hydrochloride) Injection by intravenous bolus.

Symptomatic response to *Tagamet* therapy does not preclude the presence of a gastric malignancy. There have been rare reports of transient healing of gastric ulcers despite subsequently documented malignancy.

Reversible confusional states (see Adverse Reactions) have been observed on occasion, predominantly, but not exclusively, in severely ill patients. Advancing age (50 or more years) and preexisting liver and/or renal disease appear to be contributing factors. In some patients these confusional states have been mild and have not required discontinuation of *Tagamet* therapy. In cases where discontinuation was judged necessary, the condition usually cleared within 3 to 4 days of drug withdrawal.

Drug Interactions: *Tagamet,* apparently through an effect on certain microsomal enzyme systems, has been reported to reduce the hepatic metabolism of warfarin-type anticoagulants, phenytoin, propranolol, nifedipine, chlordiazepoxide, diazepam, certain tricyclic antidepressants, lidocaine, theophylline and metronidazole, thereby delaying elimination and increasing blood levels of these drugs.

Clinically significant effects have been reported with the warfarin anticoagulants; therefore, close monitoring of prothrombin time is recommended, and adjustment of the anticoagulant dose may be necessary when *Tagamet* is administered concomitantly. Interaction with phenytoin, lidocaine and theophylline has also been reported to produce adverse clinical effects.

However, a crossover study in healthy subjects receiving either *Tagamet* 300 mg q.i.d. or 800 mg h.s. concomitantly with a 300 mg b.i.d. dosage of theophylline (Theo-Dur®, Key Pharmaceuticals, Inc.) demonstrated less alteration in steady-state theophylline peak serum levels with the 800 mg h.s. regimen, particularly in subjects aged 54 years and older. Data beyond 10 days are not available. (Note: All patients receiving theophylline should be monitored appropriately, regardless of concomitant drug therapy.)

Dosage of the drugs mentioned above and other similarly metabolized drugs, particularly those of low therapeutic ratio or in patients with renal and/or hepatic impairment, may require adjustment when starting or stopping concomitantly administered *Tagamet* to maintain optimum therapeutic blood levels.

Alteration of pH may affect absorption of certain drugs (e.g., ketoconazole). If these products are needed, they should be given at least 2 hours before cimetidine administration.

Additional clinical experience may reveal other drugs affected by the concomitant administration of *Tagamet.*

Carcinogenesis, Mutagenesis, Impairment of Fertility: In a 24-month toxicity study conducted in rats, at dose levels of 150, 378 and 950 mg/kg/day (approximately 8 to 48 times the recommended human dose), there was a small increase in the incidence of benign Leydig cell tumors in each dose group; when the combined drug-treated groups and control groups were compared, this increase reached statistical significance. In a subsequent 24-month study, there were no differences between the rats receiving 150 mg/kg/day and the untreated controls. However, a statistically significant increase in benign Leydig cell tumor incidence was seen in the rats that received 378 and 950 mg/kg/day. These tumors were common in control groups as well as treated groups and the difference became apparent only in aged rats.

Tagamet (cimetidine) has demonstrated a weak antiandrogenic effect. In animal studies this was manifested as reduced prostate and seminal vesicle weights. However, there was no impairment of mating performance or fertility, nor any harm to the fetus in these animals at doses 8 to 48 times the full therapeutic dose of *Tagamet,* as compared with controls. The cases of gynecomastia seen in patients treated for 1 month or longer may be related to this effect. In human studies, *Tagamet* has been shown to have no effect on spermatogenesis, sperm count, motility, morphology or *in vitro* fertilizing capacity.

Pregnancy: Teratogenic Effects. Pregnancy Category B: Reproduction studies have been performed in rats, rabbits and mice at doses up to 40 times the normal human dose and have revealed no evidence of impaired fertility or harm to the fetus due to *Tagamet.* There are, however, no adequate and well-controlled studies in pregnant women. Because animal reproductive studies are not always predictive of human response, this drug should be used during pregnancy only if clearly needed.

Nursing Mothers: Cimetidine is secreted in human milk and, as a general rule, nursing should not be undertaken while a patient is on a drug.

Pediatric Use: Clinical experience in children is limited. Therefore, *Tagamet* therapy cannot be recommended for children under 16, unless, in the judgment of the physician, anticipated benefits outweigh the potential risks. In very limited experience, doses of 20 to 40 mg/kg per day have been used.

Immunocompromised Patients: In immunocompromised patients, decreased gastric acidity, including that produced by acid-suppressing agents such as cimetidine, may increase the possibility of a hyperinfection of strongyloidiasis.

ADVERSE REACTIONS

Adverse effects reported in patients taking *Tagamet* are described below by body system. Incidence figures of 1 in 100 and greater are generally derived from controlled clinical studies.

Gastrointestinal: Diarrhea (usually mild) has been reported in approximately 1 in 100 patients.

CNS: Headaches, ranging from mild to severe, have been reported in 3.5% of 924 patients taking 1600 mg/day, 2.1% of 2,225 patients taking 800 mg/day and 2.3% of 1,897 patients taking placebo. Dizziness and somnolence (usually mild) have been reported in approximately 1 in 100 patients on either 1600 mg/day or 800 mg/day.

Reversible confusional states, e.g., mental confusion, agitation, psychosis, depression, anxiety, hallucinations, disorientation, have been reported predominantly, but not exclusively, in severely ill patients. They have usually developed within 2 to 3 days of initiation of *Tagamet* therapy and have cleared within 3 to 4 days of discontinuation of the drug.

Endocrine: Gynecomastia has been reported in patients treated for 1 month or longer. In patients being treated for pathological hypersecretory states, this occurred in about 4% of cases while in all others the incidence was 0.3% to 1% in various studies. No evidence of induced endocrine dysfunction was found, and the condition remained unchanged or returned toward normal with continuing Tagamet (cimetidine) treatment.

Reversible impotence has been reported in patients with pathological hypersecretory disorders, e.g., Zollinger-Ellison Syndrome, receiving *Tagamet,* particularly in high doses, for at least 12 months (range 12 to 79 months, mean 38 months). However, in large-scale surveillance studies at regular dosage, the incidence has not exceeded that commonly reported in the general population.

Hematologic: Decreased white blood cell counts in *Tagamet*-treated patients (approximately 1 per 100,000 patients), including agranulocytosis (approximately 3 per million patients), have been reported, including a few reports of recurrence on rechallenge. Most of these reports were in patients who had serious concomitant illnesses and received drugs and/or treatment known to produce neutropenia. Thrombocytopenia (approximately 3 per million patients) and, very rarely, cases of pancytopenia or aplastic anemia have also been reported. As with some other H_2-receptor antagonists, there have been extremely rare reports of immune hemolytic anemia.

Hepatobiliary: Dose-related increases in serum transaminase have been reported. In most cases they did not progress with continued therapy and returned to normal at the end of therapy. There have been rare reports of cholestatic or mixed cholestatic-hepatocellular effects. These were usually reversible. Because of the predominance of cholestatic features, severe parenchymal injury is considered highly unlikely. However, as in the occasional liver injury with other H_2-receptor antagonists, in exceedingly rare circumstances fatal outcomes have been reported.

There has been reported a single case of biopsy-proven periportal hepatic fibrosis in a patient receiving *Tagamet.*

Rare cases of pancreatitis, which cleared on withdrawal of the drug, have been reported.

Hypersensitivity: Rare cases of fever and allergic reactions including anaphylaxis and hypersensitivity vasculitis, which cleared on withdrawal of the drug, have been reported.

Renal: Small, possibly dose-related increases in plasma creatinine, presumably due to competition for renal tubular secretion, are not uncommon and do not signify deteriorating renal function. Rare cases of interstitial nephritis and urinary retention, which cleared on withdrawal of the drug, have been reported.

Cardiovascular: Rare cases of bradycardia, tachycardia and A-V heart block have been reported with H_2-receptor antagonists.

Musculoskeletal: There have been rare reports of reversible arthralgia and myalgia; exacerbation of joint symptoms in patients with preexisting arthritis has also been reported. Such symptoms have usually been alleviated by a reduction in Tagamet (cimetidine) dosage. Rare cases of polymyositis have been reported, but no causal relationship has been established.

Integumental: Mild rash and, very rarely, cases of severe generalized skin reactions including Stevens-Johnson syndrome, epidermal necrolysis, erythema multiforme, exfoliative dermatitis and generalized exfoliative erythroderma have been reported with H_2-receptor antagonists. Reversible alopecia has been reported very rarely.

Immune Function: There have been extremely rare reports of strongyloidiasis hyperinfection in immunocompromised patients.

OVERDOSAGE

Studies in animals indicate that toxic doses are associated with respiratory failure and tachycardia that may be controlled by assisted respiration and the administration of a beta-blocker.

Reported acute ingestions orally of up to 20 grams have been associated with transient adverse effects similar to those encountered in normal clinical experience. The usual measures to remove unabsorbed material from the gastrointestinal tract, clinical monitoring and supportive therapy should be employed.

There have been reports of severe CNS symptoms, including unresponsiveness, following ingestion of between 20 and 40 grams of cimetidine, and extremely rare reports following concomitant use of multiple CNS-active medications and ingestion of cimetidine at doses less than 20 grams. An elderly, terminally ill dehydrated patient with organic brain syndrome receiving concomitant antipsychotic agents and *Tagamet* 4800 mg intravenously over a 24-hour period experienced mental deterioration with reversal on *Tagamet* discontinuation.

There have been two deaths in adults who were reported to have ingested over 40 grams orally on a single occasion.

DOSAGE AND ADMINISTRATION

Duodenal Ulcer

Active Duodenal Ulcer: Clinical studies have indicated that suppression of nocturnal acid is the most important factor in duodenal ulcer healing (see Clinical Pharmacology—Acid Secretion). This is supported by recent clinical trials (see Clinical Trials—Active Duodenal Ulcer). Therefore, there is no apparent rationale, except for familiarity with use, for treating with anything other than a once-daily at bedtime dosage regimen (h.s.).

In a U.S. dose-ranging study of 400 mg h.s., 800 mg h.s. and 1600 mg h.s., a continuous dose response relationship for ulcer healing was demonstrated.

However, 800 mg h.s. is the dose of choice for most patients, as it provides a high healing rate (the difference between 800 mg h.s. and 1600 mg h.s. being small), maximal pain relief, a decreased potential for drug interactions (see Precautions—Drug Interactions) and maximal patient convenience. Patients unhealed at 4 weeks, or those with persistent symptoms, have been shown to benefit from 2 to 4 weeks of continued therapy.

It has been shown that patients who both have an endoscopically demonstrated ulcer larger than 1.0 cm and are also heavy smokers (i.e., smoke one pack of cigarettes or more per day) are more difficult to heal. There is some evidence which suggests that more rapid healing can be achieved in this subpopulation with *Tagamet* 1600 mg at bedtime. While early pain relief with either 800 mg h.s. or 1600 mg h.s. is equivalent in all patients, 1600 mg h.s. provides an appropriate alternative when it is important to ensure healing within 4 weeks for this subpopulation. Alternatively, approximately 94% of all patients will also heal in 8 weeks with *Tagamet* 800 mg h.s.

Other *Tagamet* regimens in the U.S. which have been shown to be effective are: 300 mg four times daily, with meals and at bedtime, the original regimen with which U.S. physicians have the most experience, and 400 mg twice daily, in the morning and at bedtime (see Clinical Trials—Active Duodenal Ulcer).

Concomitant antacids should be given as needed for relief of pain. However, simultaneous administration of *Tagamet* and antacids is not recommended, since antacids have been reported to interfere with the absorption of Tagamet (cimetidine).

While healing with *Tagamet* often occurs during the first week or two, treatment should be continued for 4 to 6 weeks unless healing has been demonstrated by endoscopic examination.

Maintenance Therapy for Duodenal Ulcer: In those patients requiring maintenance therapy, the recommended adult oral dose is 400 mg at bedtime.

Active Benign Gastric Ulcer

The recommended adult oral dosage for short-term treatment of active benign gastric ulcer is 800 mg h.s., or 300 mg four times a day with meals and at bedtime. Controlled clinical studies were limited to 6 weeks of treatment (see Clinical Trials). 800 mg h.s. is the preferred regimen for most patients based upon convenience and reduced potential for drug interactions. Symptomatic response to *Tagamet* does not preclude the presence of a gastric malignancy. It is important to follow gastric ulcer patients to assure rapid progress to complete healing.

Erosive Gastroesophageal Reflux Disease (GERD)

The recommended adult oral dosage for the treatment of erosive esophagitis that has been diagnosed by endoscopy is 1600 mg daily in divided doses (800 mg b.i.d. or 400 mg q.i.d.) for 12 weeks. The use of *Tagamet* beyond 12 weeks has not been established.

Prevention of Upper Gastrointestinal Bleeding

The recommended adult dosing regimen is continuous I.V. infusion of 50 mg/hour. Patients with creatinine clearance less than 30 cc/min. should receive half the recommended dose. Treatment beyond 7 days has not been studied.

Pathological Hypersecretory Conditions
(such as Zollinger-Ellison Syndrome)

Recommended adult oral dosage: 300 mg four times a day with meals and at bedtime. In some patients it may be necessary to administer higher doses more frequently. Doses should be adjusted to individual patient needs, but should not usually exceed 2400 mg per day and should continue as long as clinically indicated.

Parenteral Administration

In hospitalized patients with pathological hypersecretory conditions or intractable ulcers, or in patients who are unable to take oral medication, *Tagamet* may be administered parenterally.

The doses and regimen for parenteral administration in patients with GERD have not been established.

All parenteral drug products should be inspected visually for particulate matter and discoloration prior to administration.

Recommendations for parenteral administration:

Intramuscular injection: 300 mg q 6 to 8 hours (no dilution necessary). Transient pain at the site of injection has been reported.

Intravenous injection: 300 mg q 6 to 8 hours. In some patients it may be necessary to increase dosage. When this is necessary, the increases should be made by more frequent administration of a 300 mg dose, but should not exceed 2400 mg per day. Dilute Tagamet (cimetidine hydrochloride) Injection, 300 mg, in Sodium Chloride Injection (0.9%) or another compatible I.V. solution (see Stability of *Tagamet* Injection) to a total volume of 20 mL and inject over a period of not less than 5 minutes (see Precautions).

Intermittent intravenous infusion: 300 mg q 6 to 8 hours, infused over 15 to 20 minutes. In some patients it may be necessary to increase dosage. When this is necessary, the increases should be made by more frequent administration of a 300 mg dose, but should not exceed 2400 mg per day. **Vials:** Dilute *Tagamet* Injection, 300 mg, in at least 50 mL of 5% Dextrose Injection, or another compatible I.V. solution (see Stability of *Tagamet* Injection). **Plastic containers:** Use premixed *Tagamet* Injection, 300 mg, in 0.9% Sodium Chloride in 50 mL plastic containers. **ADD-Vantage® Vials:** Dilute contents of one vial in an ADD-Vantage® Diluent Container, available in 50 mL and 100 mL sizes of 0.9% Sodium Chloride Injection, and 5% Dextrose Injection.

Continuous intravenous infusion: 37.5 mg/hour (900 mg/day). For patients requiring a more rapid elevation of gastric pH, continuous infusion may be preceded by a 150 mg loading dose administered by I.V. infusion as described above. Dilute 900 mg *Tagamet* Injection in a compatible I.V. fluid (see Stability of *Tagamet* Injection) for constant rate infusion over a 24-hour period. Note: *Tagamet* may be diluted in 100 to 1000 mL; however, a volumetric pump is recommended if the volume for 24-hour infusion is less than 250 mL. In one study in patients with pathological hypersecretory states, the mean infused dose of cimetidine was 160 mg/hour with a range of 40 to 600 mg/hour. These doses maintained the intragastric acid secretory rate at 10 mEq/hour or less. The infusion rate should be adjusted to individual patient requirements.

DIRECTIONS FOR USE OF TAGAMET (cimetidine hydrochloride) INJECTION IN PLASTIC CONTAINERS

To open: Tear overwrap down side at slit and remove solution containers.

Some opacity of the plastic due to moisture absorption during the sterilization process may be observed. This is normal and does not affect solution quality or safety. The opacity will diminish gradually.

Do not add other drugs to premixed *Tagamet* Injection in plastic containers.

CAUTION: Check for minute leaks by squeezing inner bag firmly. If leaks are found, discard solution as sterility may be impaired. Additives should not be introduced into this solution. Do not use if the solution is cloudy or precipitated or if the seal is not intact.

Do not use plastic containers in series connections. Such use could result in air embolism due to residual air being drawn from the primary container before administration of the fluid from the secondary container is complete.

Use sterile equipment.

Preparation for administration:

1. Suspend container from eyelet support.
2. Remove plastic protector from outlet port at bottom of container.
3. Attach administration set. Refer to complete directions accompanying set.

DIRECTIONS FOR USE OF TAGAMET® INJECTION IN ADD-VANTAGE® VIALS are enclosed in ADD-Vantage® Vial packaging.

Stability of *Tagamet* Injection

When added to or diluted with most commonly used intravenous solutions, e.g., Sodium Chloride Injection (0.9%), Dextrose Injection (5% or 10%), Lactated Ringer's Solution, 5% Sodium Bicarbonate Injection, Tagamet (cimetidine hydrochloride) Injection should not be used after more than 48 hours of storage at room temperature.

Tagamet Injection premixed in plastic containers is stable through the labeled expiration date when stored under the recommended conditions.

Dosage Adjustment for Patients with Impaired Renal Function

Patients with severely impaired renal function have been treated with *Tagamet*. However, such usage has been very limited. On the basis of this experience the recommended dosage is 300 mg q 12 hours orally or by intravenous injection. Should the patient's condition require, the frequency of dosing may be increased to q 8 hours or even further with caution. In severe renal failure, accumulation may occur and the lowest frequency of dosing compatible with an adequate patient response should be used. When liver impairment is also present, further reductions in dosage may be necessary. Hemodialysis reduces the level of circulating *Tagamet*. Ideally, the dosage schedule should be adjusted so that the timing of a scheduled dose coincides with the end of hemodialysis.

Patients with creatinine clearance less than 30 cc/min. who are being treated for prevention of upper gastrointestinal bleeding should receive half the recommended dose.

HOW SUPPLIED

Tablets: Light green, film-coated as follows: 200 mg—round, imprinted with the product name TAGAMET, SKF and 200—tablets in bottles of 100; 300 mg—round, debossed with the product name TAGAMET, SB and 300—tablets in bottles of 100 and Single Unit Packages of 100 (intended for institutional use only); 400 mg—oval-shaped Tiltab®, debossed with the product name, TAGAMET, SB and 400—tablets in bottles of 60 and Single Unit Packages of 100 (intended for institutional use only); 800 mg—oval-shaped Tiltab®, debossed with the product name TAGAMET, SB and 800—tablets in bottles of 30 and Single Unit Packages of 100 (intended for institutional use only).

Store between 15° and 30°C (59° and 86°F); dispense in a tight light-resistant container.

200 mg 100's: NDC 0108-5012-20
300 mg 100's: NDC 0108-5013-20
300 mg SUP 100's: NDC 0108-5013-21
400 mg 60's: NDC 0108-5026-18
400 mg SUP 100's: NDC 0108-5026-21
800 mg 30's: NDC 0108-5027-13
800 mg SUP 100's: NDC 0108-5027-21

Liquid: Clear, light orange, mint-peach flavored, as follows: 300 mg/5 mL in 8 fl oz (237 mL) amber glass bottles; 300 mg/5 mL in single-dose units in packages of 10 (intended for institutional use only).

Store between 15° and 30°C (59° and 86°F); dispense in a tight light-resistant container.

300 mg/5 mL 8 fl oz: NDC 0108-5014-48
300 mg/5 mL SUP 10's: NDC 0108-5014-10

Injection:

Vials: 300 mg/2 mL in single-dose vials, in packages of 25, and in 8 mL multi-dose vials, in packages of 10 and 25.

Store between 15° and 30°C (59° and 86°F); do not refrigerate.

300 mg/2 mL Single-Dose Vials: NDC 0108-5017-16 (package of 25 vials)

300 mg/2 mL in 8 mL Multi-Dose Vials:
NDC 0108-5022-11 (package of 10 vials)
NDC 0108-5022-16 (package of 25 vials)

Single-Dose Premixed Plastic Containers: 300 mg in 50 mL of 0.9% Sodium Chloride in single-dose plastic containers, in packages of 4 units. No preservative has been added.

Exposure of the premixed product to excessive heat should be avoided. It is recommended the product be stored between 15° and 30°C (59° and 86°F). Brief exposure up to 40°C does not adversely affect the premixed product.

300 mg/50 mL SUP's: NDC 0108-5029-04

ADD-Vantage® Vials: 300 mg/2 mL in single-dose ADD-Vantage® Vials, in packages of 25.

Store between 15° and 30°C (59° and 86°F); do not refrigerate.

300 mg/2 mL: NDC 0108-5031-16 (package of 25 vials)

Continued on next page

Information on the SmithKline Beecham Pharmaceuticals products appearing here is based on the labeling in effect on July 31, 1998. Further information on these and other products may be obtained from the Medical Department, SmithKline Beecham Pharmaceuticals, One Franklin Plaza, Philadelphia, PA 19101.

Tagamet—Cont.

Tagamet (cimetidine hydrochloride) Injection premixed in single-dose plastic containers is manufactured for SmithKline Beecham Pharmaceuticals by Baxter Healthcare Corporation, Deerfield, IL 60015.

Veterans Administration/Military/PHS—Tablets, 300 mg, 100's, 6505–01–050–3547; 300 mg, SUP, 100's, 6505-01-050-3546; 300 mg, 100's, 6505-01-050-3547; 300 mg, 500's, 6505-01-323-5256; 300 mg, 500's BULK, 6505-01-388-1904; 400 mg, 60's, 6505-01-176-0712; 400 mg, 500's, 6505-01-323-5255; 400 mg, 500's BULK, 6505-01-388-1901; 800 mg, 30's, 6505-01-291-8374; 800 mg, SUP, 100's, 6505-01-339-1872; 800 mg, 500's BULK, 6505-01-388-1022; Injection, 300 mg/2 mL, 25's, 6505-01-351-9271; 8 mL, 300 mg/2 mL, 10's, 6505-01-069-1661; 8 mL, 300 mg/2 mL, 25's, 6505-01-282-2970; 300 mg/50 mL, MINI-BAG, 48's, 6505-01-242-8865; 300 mg/2 mL, ADD-Vantage, 25's, 6505-01-307-8201; Liquid, 300 mg/5 mL, SUP, 10's, 6505-01-222-3560.

TG:L92A

Shown in Product Identification Guide, page 340

TAZICEF® ℞

[taz 'i-sef]

brand of ceftazidime for injection
for intravenous or intramuscular use

DESCRIPTION

Ceftazidime is a semisynthetic, broad-spectrum, beta-lactam antibiotic for intravenous or intramuscular administration. It is the pentahydrate of Pyridinium, 1-[[7- [[(2- amino-4-thiazolyl) [(1-carboxy-1-methylethoxy) imino]acetyl] amino]-2-carboxy -8- oxo -5- thia-1-azabicyclo (4.2.0.) oct -2-en -3- yl] methyl]-,hydroxide,inner salt, [6R-[6α,7β(Z)]].

Its molecular formula is $C_{22}H_{22}N_6O_7S_2{\cdot}5H_20$ and the molecular weight is 636.65.

Tazicef (ceftazidime for injection) is a sterile, dry, powdered mixture of ceftazidime pentahydrate and sodium carbonate. The sodium carbonate at a concentration of 118 mg/gram of ceftazidime activity has been admixed to facilitate dissolution. The total sodium content of the mixture is approximately 54 mg (2.3 mEq)/gram of ceftazidime activity.

Tazicef in sterile crystalline form is supplied in vials equivalent to 1 gram or 2 grams of anhydrous ceftazidime, in piggyback vials equivalent to 1 gram or 2 grams of anhydrous ceftazidime and ADD-Vantage® vials equivalent to 1 gram or 2 grams of anhydrous ceftazidime. Solutions of *Tazicef* range in color from light yellow to amber, depending upon the diluent and volume used. The pH of freshly reconstituted solutions usually ranges from 5.0 to 8.0.

CLINICAL PHARMACOLOGY

After intravenous administration of 500 mg and 1 gram doses of ceftazidime over 5 minutes to normal adult male volunteers, mean peak serum concentrations of 45 mcg/mL and 90 mcg/mL, respectively, were achieved. After intravenous infusion of 500 mg, 1 gram and 2 gram doses of ceftazidime over 20 to 30 minutes to normal adult male volunteers, mean peak serum concentrations of 42 mcg/mL, 69 mcg/mL and 170 mcg/mL, respectively, were achieved. The average serum concentrations following intravenous infusion of 500 mg, 1 gram and 2 gram doses to these volunteers over an 8-hour interval are given in Table 1.

Table 1

Ceftazidime IV Dosage	Serum Concentrations (mcg/mL)				
	0.5 hr.	1 hr.	2 hr.	4 hr.	8 hr.
500 mg	42	25	12	6	2
1 gram	60	39	23	11	3
2 grams	129	75	42	13	5

The absorption and elimination of ceftazidime were directly proportional to the size of the dose. The half-life following intravenous administration was approximately 1.9 hours. Less than 10% of ceftazidime was protein bound. The degree of protein binding was independent of concentration. There was no evidence of accumulation of ceftazidime in the serum in individuals with normal renal function following multiple intravenous doses of 1 gram and 2 grams every 8 hours for 10 days.

Following intramuscular administration of 500 mg and 1 gram doses of ceftazidime to normal adult volunteers, the mean peak serum concentrations were 17 mcg/mL and 39 mcg/mL, respectively, at approximately 1 hour. Serum concentrations remained above 4 mcg/mL for 6 and 8 hours after the intramuscular administration of 500 mg and 1 gram doses, respectively. The half-life of ceftazidime in these volunteers was approximately 2 hours.

Table 2. Ceftazidime Concentrations in Body Tissues and Fluids

Tissue or Fluid	Dose/ Route	No. Patients	Time of Sample Post-Dose	Average Tissue or Fluid Level (mcg/mL or mcg/g)
Urine	500 mg IM	6	0 to 2 hours	2,100
	2 grams IV	6	0 to 2 hours	12,000
Bile	2 grams IV	3	90 min.	36.4
Synovial fluid	2 grams IV	13	2 hours	25.6
Peritoneal fluid	2 grams IV	8	2 hours	48.6
Sputum	1 gram IV	8	1 hour	9
Cerebrospinal fluid	2 grams q8h IV	5	120 min.	9.8
(inflamed meninges)	2 grams q8h IV	6	180 min.	9.4
Aqueous humor	2 grams IV	13	1 to 3 hours	11
Blister fluid	1 gram IV	7	2 to 3 hours	19.7
Lymphatic fluid	1 gram IV	7	2 to 3 hours	23.4
Bone	2 grams IV	8	0.67 hour	31.1
Heart muscle	2 grams IV	35	30 to 280 min.	12.7
Skin	2 grams IV	22	30 to 180 min.	6.6
Skeletal muscle	2 grams IV	35	30 to 280 min.	9.4
Myometrium	2 grams IV	31	1 to 2 hours	18.7

The presence of hepatic dysfunction had no effect on the pharmacokinetics of ceftazidime in individuals administered 2 grams intravenously every 8 hours for 5 days. Therefore, a dosage adjustment from the normal recommended dosage is not required for patients with hepatic dysfunction, provided renal function is not impaired.

Approximately 80% to 90% of an intramuscular or intravenous dose of ceftazidime is excreted unchanged by the kidneys over a 24-hour period. After the intravenous administration of single 500 mg or 1 gram doses, approximately 50% of the dose appeared in the urine in the first 2 hours. An additional 20% was excreted between 2 and 4 hours after dosing, and approximately another 12% of the dose appeared in the urine between 4 and 8 hours later. The elimination of ceftazidime by the kidneys resulted in high therapeutic concentrations in the urine.

The mean renal clearance of ceftazidime was approximately 100 mL/min. The calculated plasma clearance of approximately 115 mL/min. indicated nearly complete elimination of ceftazidime by the renal route. Administration of probenecid prior to dosing had no effect on the elimination kinetics of ceftazidime. This suggests that ceftazidime is eliminated by glomerular filtration and is not actively secreted by renal tubular mechanisms.

Since ceftazidime is eliminated almost solely by the kidneys, its serum half-life is significantly prolonged in patients with impaired renal function. Consequently, dosage adjustments in such patients as described in the DOSAGE AND ADMINISTRATION section are suggested.

Therapeutic concentrations of ceftazidime are achieved in the following body tissues and fluid.

[See table 2 above]

Microbiology

Ceftazidime is bactericidal in action, exerting its effect by inhibition of enzymes responsible for cell-wall synthesis. A wide range of gram-negative organisms is susceptible to ceftazidime *in vitro*, including strains resistant to gentamicin and other aminoglycosides. In addition, ceftazidime has been shown to be active against gram-positive organisms. It is highly stable to most clinically important beta-lactamases, plasmid or chromosomal, which are produced by both gram-negative and gram-positive organisms and, consequently, is active against many strains resistant to ampicillin and other cephalosporins.

Ceftazidime has been shown to be active against the following organisms both *in vitro* and in clinical infections (see INDICATIONS AND USAGE).

Aerobes, Gram-Negative: *Citrobacter* species (including *Citrobacter freundii* and *Citrobacter diversus*): *Enterobacter* species (including *Enterobacter cloacae* and *Enterobacter aerogenes*); *Escherichia coli; Haemophilus influenzae*, including ampicillin-resistant strains; *Klebsiella* species (including *Klebsiella pneumoniae*); *Neisseria meningitidis; Proteus mirabilis; Proteus vulgaris; Pseudomonas* species (including *Pseudomonas aeruginosa*); and *Serratia* species.

Aerobes, Gram-Positive: *Staphylococcus aureus,* including penicillinase- and non-penicillinase-producing strains; *Streptococcus agalactiae* (group B streptococci); and *Streptococcus pneumoniae*; and *Streptococcus pyogenes* (group A beta-hemolytic streptococci).

Anaerobes: *Bacteroides* species (NOTE: Many strains of *Bacteroides fragilis* are resistant).

Ceftazidime has been shown to be active *in vitro* against most strains of the following organisms; however, the clinical significance of these data is unknown: *Acinetobacter* species; *Clostridium* species (not including *Clostridium difficile*); *Haemophilus parainfluenzae; Morganella morganii* (formerly *Proteus morganii*); *Neisseria gonorrhoeae; Peptococcus* species; *Peptostreptococcus* species; *Providencia* species (including *Providencia rettgeri,* formerly *Proteus rettgeri*); *Salmonella* species; *Shigella* species; *Staphylococcus epidermidis*; and *Yersinia enterocolitica.*

Ceftazidime and the aminoglycosides have been shown to be synergistic *in vitro* against Enterobacteriaceae and *Pseudomonas aeruginosa.* Ceftazidime and carbenicillin have also been shown to be synergistic *in vitro* against *P. aeruginosa.*

Ceftazidime is not active *in vitro* against: *Campylobacter* species; *Clostridium difficile; Listeria monocytogenes;* methicillin-resistant staphylococci; or *Streptococcus faecalis* and many other enterococci.

Susceptibility Tests

Diffusion Techniques

Quantitative methods that require measurement of zone diameters give an estimate of antibiotic susceptibility. One such procedure[1–3] has been recommended for use with disks to test susceptibility to ceftazidime.

Reports from the laboratory giving results of the standard single-disk susceptibility test with a 30 mcg ceftazidime disk should be interpreted according to the following criteria:

Susceptible organisms produce zones of 18 mm or greater, indicating that the test organism is likely to respond to therapy.

Organisms that produce zones of 15 mm to 17 mm are expected to be susceptible if high dosage is used or if the infection is confined to tissues and fluids (e.g., urine) in which high antibiotic levels are attained.

Resistant organisms produce zones of 14 mm or less, indicating that other therapy should be selected.

Organisms should be tested with the ceftazidime disk, since ceftazidime has been shown by *in vitro* tests to be active against certain strains found resistant when other beta-lactam disks are used.

Standardized procedures require the use of laboratory control organisms. The 30 mcg ceftazidime disk should give zone diameters between 25 mm and 32 mm for *E. coli* ATCC 25922. For *P. aeruginosa* ATCC 27853, the zone diameters should be between 22 mm and 29 mm. For *S. aureus* ATCC 25923, the zone diameters should be between 16 mm and 20 mm.

Dilution Techniques

In other susceptibility testing procedures, e.g., ICS agar dilution or the equivalent, a bacterial isolate may be considered susceptible if the MIC value for ceftazidime is not more than 16 mcg/mL. Organisms are considered resistant to ceftazidime if the MIC is equal to or greater than 64 mcg/mL. Organisms having an MIC value of less than 64 mcg/mL but greater than 16 mcg/mL are expected to be susceptible if high dosage is used or if the infection is confined to tissues and fluids (e.g., urine) in which high antibiotic levels are attained.

As with standard diffusion methods, dilution procedures require the use of laboratory control organisms. Standard ceftazidime powder should give MIC values in the range of 4 mcg/mL and 16 mcg/mL for *S. aureus* ATCC 25923. For *E. coli* ATCC 25922, the MIC range should be between 0.125 mcg/mL and 0.5 mcg/mL. For *P. aeruginosa* ATCC 27853, the MIC range should be between 0.5 mcg/mL and 2 mcg/mL.

INDICATIONS AND USAGE

Tazicef (ceftazidime for injection) is indicated for the treatment of patients with infections caused by susceptible strains of the designated organisms in the diseases listed below:

LOWER RESPIRATORY TRACT INFECTIONS, including pneumonia, caused by *P. aeruginosa* and other *Pseudomonas* species; *H. influenzae*, including ampicillin-resistant strains; *Klebsiella* species; *Enterobacter* species, *P. mirabilis; E. coli; Serratia* species; *Citrobacter* species; *S. pneumoniae;* and *S. aureus* (methicillin-susceptible strains).
SKIN AND SKIN STRUCTURE INFECTIONS, caused by *P. aeruginosa, Klebsiella* species; *E. coli; Proteus* species including *P. mirabilis* and indole-positive *Proteus, Enterobacter* species; *Serratia* species; *S. aureus* (methicillin-susceptible strains) and *S. pyogenes* (group A beta-hemolytic streptococci).
URINARY TRACT INFECTIONS, both complicated and uncomplicated, caused by *P. aeruginosa; Enterobacter* species; *Proteus* species, including *P. mirabilis* and indole-positive *Proteus; Klebsiella* species and *E. coli.*
BACTERIAL SEPTICEMIA, caused by *P. aeruginosa, Klebsiella* species; *H. influenzae; E. coli, Serratia* species, *S. pneumoniae* and *S. aureus* (methicillin-susceptible strains).
BONE AND JOINT INFECTIONS, caused by *P. aeruginosa; Klebsiella* species; *Enterobacter* species; and *S. aureus* (methicillin-susceptible strains).
GYNECOLOGIC INFECTIONS, including endometritis, pelvic cellulitis and other infections of the female genital tract caused by *E. coli.*
INTRA-ABDOMINAL INFECTIONS, including peritonitis caused by *E. coli, Klebsiella* species; *S. aureus* (methicillin-susceptible strains), and polymicrobial infections caused by aerobic and anaerobic organisms, and *Bacteroides* species (many strains of *B. fragilis* are resistant).
CENTRAL NERVOUS SYSTEM INFECTIONS, including meningitis caused by *H. influenzae* and *Neisseria meningitidis.* Ceftazidime has also been used successfully in a limited number of cases of meningitis due to *P. aeruginosa* and *S. pneumoniae.*
Specimens for bacterial cultures should be obtained prior to therapy in order to isolate and identify causative organisms and to determine their susceptibility to ceftazidime. Therapy may be instituted before results of susceptibility studies are known; however, once these results become available, the antibiotic treatment should be adjusted accordingly.
Tazicef (ceftazidime for injection) may be used alone in cases of confirmed or suspected sepsis. Ceftazidime has been used successfully in clinical trials as empiric therapy in cases where various concomitant therapies with other antibiotics have been used.
Tazicef may also be used concomitantly with other antibiotics, such as aminoglycosides, vancomycin and clindamycin, in severe and life-threatening infections and in the immunocompromised patient. When such concomitant treatment is appropriate, prescribing information in the labeling for the other antibiotics should be followed. The dose depends on the severity of the infection and the patient's condition.

CONTRAINDICATIONS

Tazicef is contraindicated in patients who have shown hypersensitivity to ceftazidime or the cephalosporin group of antibiotics.

WARNINGS

SERIOUS AND OCCASIONALLY FATAL HYPERSENSITIVITY (anaphylactic) REACTIONS HAVE BEEN REPORTED IN PATIENTS ON PENICILLIN THERAPY. THESE REACTIONS ARE MORE LIKELY TO OCCUR IN INDIVIDUALS WITH A HISTORY OF PENICILLIN HYPERSENSITIVITY AND/OR A HISTORY OF SENSITIVITY TO MULTIPLE ALLERGENS. THERE HAVE BEEN REPORTS OF INDIVIDUALS WITH A HISTORY OF PENICILLIN HYPERSENSITIVITY WHO HAVE EXPERIENCED SEVERE REACTIONS WHEN TREATED WITH CEPHALOSPORINS. BEFORE INITIATING THERAPY WITH *TAZICEF*, CAREFUL INQUIRY SHOULD BE MADE CONCERNING PREVIOUS HYPERSENSITIVITY REACTIONS TO PENICILLINS, CEPHALOSPORINS OR OTHER ALLERGENS. IF AN ALLERGIC REACTION OCCURS, *TAZICEF* SHOULD BE DISCONTINUED AND APPROPRIATE THERAPY SHOULD BE INSTITUTED. SERIOUS ANAPHYLACTIC REACTIONS REQUIRE IMMEDIATE EMERGENCY TREATMENT WITH EPINEPHRINE. OXYGEN, INTRAVENOUS STEROIDS AND AIRWAY MANAGEMENT, INCLUDING INTUBATION, SHOULD ALSO BE ADMINISTERED AS INDICATED.

Pseudomembranous colitis has been reported with nearly all antibacterial agents, including *Tazicef*, and may range in severity from mild to life-threatening. Therefore, it is important to consider this diagnosis in patients who present with diarrhea subsequent to the administration of antibacterial agents.

Treatment with antibacterial agents alters the normal flora of the colon and may permit overgrowth of clostridia. Studies indicate that a toxin produced by *Clostridium difficile* is one primary cause of "antibiotic-associated colitis."
After the diagnosis of pseudomembranous colitis has been established, therapeutic measures should be initiated. Mild cases of pseudomembranous colitis usually respond to drug discontinuation alone. In moderate to severe cases, consideration should be given to management with fluids and electrolytes, protein supplementation and treatment with an antibacterial drug clinically effective against *C. difficile* colitis.
Elevated levels of ceftazidime in patients with renal insufficiency can lead to seizures, encephalopathy, asterixis and neuromuscular excitability (see PRECAUTIONS).

Table 3. Recommended Dosage Schedule

	Dose	Frequency
Adults		
Usual recommended dose	**1 gram IV or IM**	**q8 to 12h**
Uncomplicated urinary tract infections	250 mg IV or IM	q12h
Bone and joint infections	2 grams IV	q12h
Complicated urinary tract infections	500 mg IV or IM	q8 to 12h
Uncomplicated pneumonia; mild skin and skin structure infections	500 mg to 1 gram IV or IM	q8h
Serious gynecological and intra-abdominal infections	2 grams IV	q8h
Meningitis	2 grams IV	q8h
Very severe life-threatening infections, especially in immunocompromised patients	2 grams IV	q8h
Lung infections caused by *Pseudomonas* species in patients with cystic fibrosis with normal renal function*	30 to 50 mg/kg IV to a maximum of 6 grams/day	q8h
Neonates (0 to 4 weeks)	30 mg/kg IV	q12h
Infants and children (1 month to 12 years)	30 to 50 mg/kg IV to a maximum of 6 grams/day†	q8h

* Although clinical improvement has been shown, bacteriological cures cannot be expected in patients with chronic respiratory disease and cystic fibrosis.
† The higher dose should be reserved for immunocompromised children or children with cystic fibrosis or meningitis.

PRECAUTIONS

General: Ceftazidime has not been shown to be nephrotoxic; however, high and prolonged serum antibiotic concentrations can occur from usual doses in patients with transient or persistent reduction of urinary output because of renal insufficiency. The total daily dosage should be reduced when ceftazidime is administered to patients with renal insufficiency (see DOSAGE AND ADMINISTRATION). In these patients, elevated levels of ceftazidime can lead to seizures, encephalopathy, asterixis and neuromuscular excitability. Continued dosage should be determined by degree of renal impairment, severity of infection and susceptibility of the causative organisms.
As with other antibiotics, prolonged use of Tazicef (ceftazidime for injection) may result in overgrowth of nonsusceptible organisms. Repeated evaluation of the patient's condition is essential. If superinfection occurs during therapy, appropriate measures should be taken.
Cephalosporins may be associated with a fall in prothrombin activity. Those at risk include patients with renal or hepatic impairment, or poor nutritional state, as well as patients receiving a protracted course of antimicrobial therapy. Prothrombin time should be monitored in patients at risk and exogenous vitamin K administered as indicated.
Tazicef should be prescribed with caution in individuals with a history of gastrointestinal disease, particularly colitis.
Drug Interactions: Nephrotoxicity has been reported following concomitant administration of cephalosporins with aminoglycoside antibiotics or potent diuretics, such as furosemide. Renal function should be carefully monitored, especially if higher dosages of the aminoglycosides are to be administered or if therapy is prolonged, because of the potential nephrotoxicity and ototoxicity of aminoglycoside antibiotics. Nephrotoxicity and ototoxicity were not noted when ceftazidime was given alone in clinical trials.
Chloramphenicol in combination with cephalosporins, including ceftazidime, has been shown to be antagonistic *in vitro*. Due to the possibility of antagonism *in vivo*, this combination should be avoided.
Drug/Laboratory Test Interactions: The administration of ceftazidime may result in a false-positive reaction for glucose in the urine when using Clinitest® tablets, Benedict's solution or Fehling's solution. It is recommended that glucose tests based on enzymatic glucose oxidase reactions (such as Clinistix® or Tes-Tape® [Glucose Enzymatic Test Strip USP]) be used.
Carcinogenesis, Mutagenesis, Impairment of Fertility: Long-term studies in animals have not been performed to evaluate carcinogenic potential. However, a mouse micronucleus test and an Ames test were both negative for mutagenic effects.
Pregnancy: Teratogenic Effects: **Pregnancy Category B.** Reproduction studies have been performed in mice and rats at doses up to 40 times the human dose and have revealed no evidence of impaired fertility or harm to the fetus due to *Tazicef*. There are, however, no adequate and well-controlled studies in pregnant women. Because animal reproduction studies are not always predictive of human response, this drug should be used during pregnancy only if clearly needed.
Nursing Mothers: Ceftazidime is excreted in human milk in low concentrations. Caution should be exercised when *Tazicef* is administered to a nursing woman.
Pediatric Use: See DOSAGE AND ADMINISTRATION.

ADVERSE REACTIONS

Ceftazidime is generally well-tolerated. The incidence of adverse reactions associated with the administration of ceftazidime was low in clinical trials. The most common were local reactions following IV injection and allergic and gastrointestinal reactions. Other adverse reactions were encountered infrequently. No disulfiram-like reactions were reported.
The following adverse effects from clinical trials were considered to be either related to ceftazidime therapy or were of uncertain etiology:
Local Effects, reported in less than 2% of patients, were phlebitis and inflammation at the site of injection (1 in 69 patients).
Hypersensitivity Reactions, reported in 2% of patients, were pruritus, rash and fever. Immediate reactions, generally manifested by rash and/or pruritus, occurred in 1 in 285 patients. Angioedema and anaphylaxis (bronchospasm and/or hypotension) have been reported very rarely.
Gastrointestinal Symptoms, reported in less than 2% of patients, were diarrhea (1 in 78), nausea (1 in 156), vomiting (1 in 500) and abdominal pain (1 in 416). The onset of pseudomembranous colitis symptoms may occur during or after treatment (see WARNINGS).
Central Nervous System Reactions (fewer than 1%) include headache, dizziness and paresthesia. Seizures have been reported with several cephalosporins, including ceftazidime. In addition, encephalopathy, asterixis and neuromuscular excitability have been reported in renally impaired patients treated with unadjusted dosage regimens of ceftazidime (see PRECAUTIONS: General).
Less Frequent Adverse Events (less than 1%) were candidiasis (including oral thrush) and vaginitis.
Laboratory Test Changes noted during Tazicef (ceftazidime for injection) clinical trials were transient and included: eosinophilia (1 in 13), positive Coombs' test without hemolysis (1 in 23), thrombocytosis (1 in 45), and slight elevations in one or more of the hepatic enzymes, aspartate aminotransferase (AST, SGOT) (1 in 16), alanine aminotransferase (ALT, SGPT) (1 in 15), LDH (1 in 18), GGT (1 in 19) and alkaline phosphatase (1 in 23). As with some other cephalosporins, transient elevations of blood urea, blood urea nitrogen and/or serum creatinine were observed occasionally. Transient leukopenia, neutropenia, agranulocytosis, thrombocytopenia and lymphocytosis were seen very rarely.

Continued on next page

Information on the SmithKline Beecham Pharmaceuticals products appearing here is based on the labeling in effect on July 31, 1998. Further information on these and other products may be obtained from the Medical Department, SmithKline Beecham Pharmaceuticals, One Franklin Plaza, Philadelphia, PA 19101.

Consult 1999 PDR® supplements and future editions for revisions

Tazicef—Cont.

In addition to the adverse reactions listed above that have been observed with ceftazidime, the following adverse reactions and altered laboratory tests have been reported for cephalosporin-class antibiotics:

Adverse Reactions: Urticaria, Stevens-Johnson syndrome, erythema multiforme, toxic epidermal necrolysis, colitis, renal dysfunction, toxic nephropathy, hepatic dysfunction including cholestasis, aplastic anemia, hemolytic anemia, hemorrhage.

Altered Laboratory Tests: Prolonged prothrombin time, false-positive test for urinary glucose, elevated bilirubin, pancytopenia.

OVERDOSAGE

Ceftazidime overdosage has occurred in patients with renal failure. Reactions have included seizure activity, encephalopathy, asterixis and neuromuscular excitability. Patients who receive an acute overdosage should be carefully observed and given supportive treatment. In the presence of renal insufficiency, hemodialysis or peritoneal dialysis may aid in the removal of ceftazidime from the body.

DOSAGE AND ADMINISTRATION

Dosage: The usual adult dosage is 1 gram administered intravenously or intramuscularly every 8 or 12 hours. The dosage and route should be determined by the susceptibility of the causative organisms, the severity of infection and the condition and renal function of the patient.

The guidelines for dosage of *Tazicef* are listed in Table 3. The following dosage schedule is recommended.

[See table 3 at top of previous page]

Impaired Hepatic Function: No adjustment in dosage is required for patients with hepatic dysfunction.

Impaired Renal Function: Ceftazidime is excreted by the kidneys, almost exclusively by glomerular filtration. Therefore, in patients with impaired renal function (GFR <50 mL/min.), it is recommended that the dosage of ceftazidime be reduced to compensate for its slower excretion. In patients with suspected renal insufficiency, an initial loading dose of 1 gram of ceftazidime may be given. An estimate of GFR should be made to determine the appropriate maintenance dose. The recommended dosage is presented in Table 4.

Table 4. Recommended Maintenance Doses of Tazicef (ceftazidime for injection) in Renal Insufficiency

NOTE: IF THE DOSE RECOMMENDED IN TABLE 3 ABOVE IS LOWER THAN THAT RECOMMENDED FOR PATIENTS WITH RENAL INSUFFICIENCY AS OUTLINED IN TABLE 4, THE LOWER DOSE SHOULD BE USED.

Creatinine Clearance (mL/min.)	Recommended Unit Dose of Ceftazidime	Frequency of Dosing
50 to 31	1 gram	q12h
30 to 16	1 gram	q24h
15 to 6	500 mg	q24h
<5	500 mg	q48h

When only serum creatinine is available, the following formula (Cockcroft's equation)[4] may be used to estimate creatinine clearance. The serum creatinine should represent a steady state of renal function:

Males:
$$\text{Creatinine clearance (mL/min.)} = \frac{\text{Weight (kg)} \times (140 - \text{age})}{72 \times \text{serum creatinine (mg/dL)}}$$

Females:
$0.85 \times$ male value

In patients with severe infections who would normally receive 6 grams of ceftazidime daily were it not for renal insufficiency, the unit dose given in the table above may be increased by 50% or the dosing frequency increased appropriately. Further dosing should be determined by therapeutic monitoring, severity of the infection and susceptibility of the causative organism.

In children as for adults, the creatinine clearance should be adjusted for body surface area or lean body mass and the dosing frequency reduced in cases of renal insufficiency.

In patients undergoing hemodialysis, a loading dose of 1 gram is recommended, followed by 1 gram after each hemodialysis period.

Tazicef (ceftazidime for injection) can also be used in patients undergoing intra-peritoneal dialysis (IPD) and continuous ambulatory peritoneal dialysis (CAPD). In such patients, a loading dose of *Tazicef* 1 gram may be given, followed by 500 mg every 24 hours. In addition to intravenous use, *Tazicef* can be incorporated in the dialysis fluid at a concentration of 250 mg for 2 liters of dialysis fluid.

NOTE: Generally, *Tazicef* should be continued for 2 days after the signs and symptoms of infection have disappeared, but in complicated infections longer therapy may be required.

Administration: *Tazicef* may be given intravenously or by deep intramuscular injection into a large muscle mass such as the upper outer quadrant of the gluteus maximus or lateral part of the thigh.

NOTE: Ceftazidime for injection in ADD-Vantage® vials is not intended for direct intravenous or intramuscular injection.

Intramuscular Administration: For intramuscular administration, *Tazicef* should be reconstituted with Sterile Water for Injection. Refer to Table 5.

Intravenous Administration: The IV route is preferable for patients with bacterial septicemia, bacterial meningitis, peritonitis, or other severe or life-threatening infections, or for patients who may be poor risks because of lowered resistance resulting from such debilitating conditions as malnutrition, trauma, surgery, diabetes, heart failure or malignancy, particularly if shock is present or pending.

For direct intermittent intravenous administration, reconstitute *Tazicef* as directed in Table 5 with Sterile Water for Injection. Slowly inject directly into the vein over a period of 3 to 5 minutes or give through the tubing of an administration set while the patient is also receiving one of the compatible intravenous fluids (see COMPATIBILITY AND STABILITY).

For intravenous infusion, reconstitute the 1 or 2 gram piggyback vial with 100 mL of Sodium Chloride Injection or one of the compatible intravenous fluids listed under the COMPATIBILITY AND STABILITY section. Alternatively, reconstitute the 1 gram or 2 gram vial and add an appropriate quantity of the resulting solution to an IV container with one of the compatible intravenous fluids.

Intermittent intravenous infusion with a Y-type administration set can be accomplished with compatible solutions. However, during infusion of a solution containing *Tazicef* it is advisable to discontinue the other solution.

All vials of *Tazicef* as supplied are under reduced pressure. When *Tazicef* is dissolved, carbon dioxide is released and a positive pressure develops. See RECONSTITUTION.

Solutions of *Tazicef*, like those of most beta-lactam antibiotics, should not be added to solutions of aminoglycoside antibiotics because of potential interaction.

However, if concurrent therapy with *Tazicef* and an aminoglycoside is indicated, each of these antibiotics can be administered separately to the same patient.

TAZICEF INJECTION IN ADD-VANTAGE® VIALS

NOTE: Tazicef (ceftazidime for injection) in the ADD-Vantage® vial is intended to be administered as a single-dose intravenous infusion with the ADD-Vantage® flexible diluent container.

Tazicef in single-dose ADD-Vantage® vials should be prepared as directed (see RECONSTITUTION, for ADD-Vantage® Vials) with either 0.9% Sodium Chloride Injection in the 50 mL or 100 mL flexible diluent containers, 0.45% Sodium Chloride Injection in the 50 mL container or 5% Dextrose Injection in the 50 mL or 100 mL containers.

RECONSTITUTION

Single-Dose Vials:

For IM injection, IV direct (bolus) injection or IV infusion, reconstitute with Sterile Water for Injection according to the following table. The vacuum may assist entry of the diluent. SHAKE WELL.

Table 5

Vial Size	Diluent to Be Added	Approx. Avail. Volume	Average Concentration
Intramuscular or Intravenous Direct (bolus) Injection			
1 gram	3.0 mL	3.6 mL	280 mg/mL
Intravenous Infusion			
1 gram	10 mL	10.6 mL	95 mg/mL
2 gram	10 mL	11.2 mL	180 mg/mL

Withdraw the total volume of solution into the syringe (the pressure in the vial may aid withdrawal). The withdrawn solution may contain some bubbles of carbon dioxide.

NOTE: **As with the administration of all parenteral products, accumulated gases should be expressed from the syringe immediately before injection of *Tazicef*.**

These solutions of *Tazicef* are stable for 24 hours at room temperature or 7 days if refrigerated (5°C). Slight yellowing does not affect potency.

For IV infusion, dilute reconstituted solution in 50 to 100 mL of one of the parenteral fluids listed under COMPATIBILITY AND STABILITY.

"Piggyback" Vials:

For IV infusion, reconstitute with 10 mL of Sodium Chloride Injection according to the following table. The vacuum may assist entry of the diluent. SHAKE WELL.

Table 6

Vial Size	Diluent to Be Added	Approx. Avail. Volume	Approx. Avg. Concentration
1 gram	100 mL*	100 mL	10 mg/mL
2 gram	100 mL*	100 mL	20 mg/mL

* Addition should be in two stages.

Insert a gas relief needle through the vial closure to relieve the internal pressure. With the gas relief needle in position, add the remaining 90 mL of Sodium Chloride Injection. Remove the gas relief needle and syringe needle; shake the vial and set up for infusion in the normal way.

NOTE: **To preserve product sterility, it is important that a gas relief needle is not inserted through the vial closure before the product has dissolved.**

These solutions of Tazicef (ceftazidime for injection) are stable for 24 hours at room temperature or 7 days if refrigerated (5°C). Slight yellowing does not affect potency.

ADD-Vantage® Vials: ADD-Vantage® vials of Tazicef (ceftazidime for injection) are to be reconstituted only with 0.9% Sodium Chloride Injection or 5% Dextrose Injection in the 50 mL or 100 mL flexible diluent containers, or with 0.45% Sodium Chloride Injection in the 50 mL container.

DIRECTIONS FOR USE OF TAZICEF® INJECTION IN ADD-VANTAGE® VIALS

To Open Diluent Container:

Peel overwrap at corner and remove solution container. Some opacity of the plastic due to moisture absorption during the sterilization process may be observed. This is normal and does not affect the solution quality or safety. The opacity will diminish gradually.

To Assemble Vial and Flexible Diluent Container: (Use Aseptic Technique)

1. Remove the protective covers from the top of the vial and the vial port on the diluent container as follows:
   a. To remove the breakaway vial cap, swing the pull ring over the top of the vial and pull down far enough to start the opening (SEE FIGURE 1), then pull straight up to remove the cap. (SEE FIGURE 2.)
   NOTE: Do not access vial with syringe.

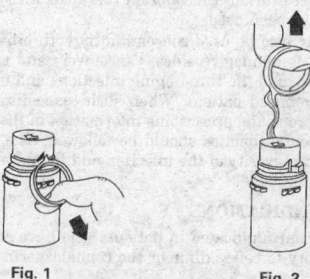

Fig. 1   Fig. 2

   b. To remove the vial port cover, grasp the tab on the pull ring, pull up to break the three tie strings, then pull back to remove the cover. (SEE FIGURE 3.)
2. Screw the vial into the vial port until it will go no further. THE VIAL MUST BE SCREWED IN TIGHTLY TO ASSURE A SEAL. This occurs approximately $1/2$ turn (180°) after the first audible click. (SEE FIGURE 4.) The clicking sound does not assure a seal; the vial must be turned as far as it will go.
   NOTE: Once vial is sealed, do not attempt to remove. (SEE FIGURE 4.)
3. Recheck the vial to assure that it is tight by trying to turn it further in the direction of assembly.
4. Label appropriately.

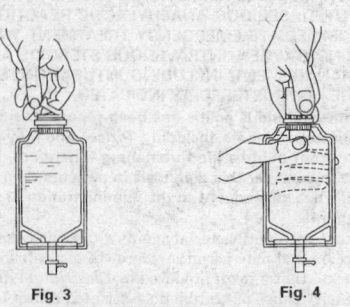

Fig. 3   Fig. 4

To Reconstitute the Drug:

1. Squeeze the bottom of the diluent container gently to inflate the portion of the container surrounding the end of the drug vial.

2. With the other hand, push the drug vial down into the container telescoping the walls of the container. Grasp the inner cap of the vial through the walls of the container. (SEE FIGURE 5.)
3. Pull the inner cap from the drug vial. (SEE FIGURE 6.) Verify that the rubber stopper has been pulled out, allowing the drug and diluent to mix.
4. Mix container contents thoroughly and use within the specified time.

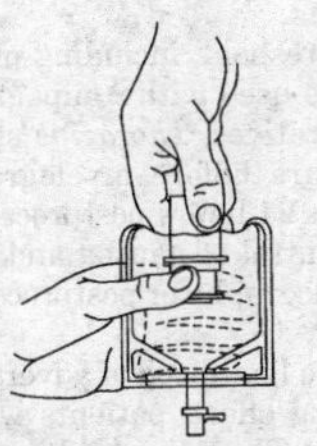

Fig. 5

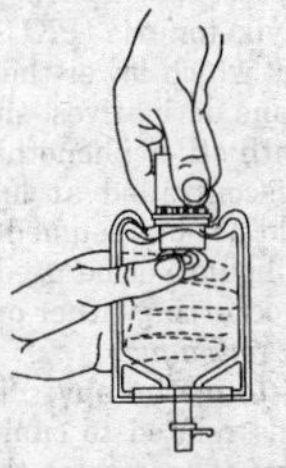

Fig. 6

Preparation for Administration:
(Use Aseptic Technique)

1. Confirm the activation and admixture of vial contents.
2. Check for leaks by squeezing container firmly. If leaks are found discard unit as sterility may be impaired.
3. Close flow control clamp of administration set.
4. Remove cover from outlet port at bottom of container.
5. Insert piercing pin of administration set into port with a twisting motion until the pin is firmly seated. **NOTE:** See full directions on administration set carton.
6. Lift the free end of the hanger loop on the bottom of the vial, breaking the two tie strings. Bend the loop outward to lock it in the upright position, then suspend container from hanger.
7. Squeeze and release drip chamber to establish proper fluid level in chamber.
8. Open flow control clamp and clear air from set. Close clamp.
9. Attach set to venipuncture device. If device is not indwelling, prime and make venipuncture.
10. Regulate rate of administration with flow control clamp.

WARNING: Do not use flexible container in series connections.

COMPATIBILITY AND STABILITY

Intramuscular: Tazicef (ceftazidime for injection) when reconstituted as directed with Sterile Water for Injection, maintains satisfactory potency for 24 hours at room temperature or for 7 days under refrigeration (5°C). Solutions in Sterile Water for Injection that are frozen immediately after reconstitution in the original container are stable for 3 months when stored at −20°C. Once thawed, solutions should not be refrozen. Thawed solutions may be stored for up to 8 hours at room temperature or for 4 days in a refrigerator (5°C).

Intravenous: Tazicef (ceftazidime for injection) when reconstituted as directed with Sterile Water for Injection, maintains satisfactory potency for 24 hours at room temperature or for 7 days under refrigeration (5°C). Solutions in Sterile Water for Injection in the original container or in 0.9% Sodium Chloride Injection in Viaflex® small volume containers that are frozen immediately after reconstitution are stable for 3 months when stored at −20°C. For larger volumes where it may be necessary to warm the frozen product (to a maximum of 40°C), care should be taken to avoid heating after thawing is complete. Once thawed, solutions should not be refrozen. Thawed solutions may be stored for up to 8 hours at room temperature or for 4 days in a refrigerator (5°C).

Tazicef is compatible with the more commonly used intravenous infusion fluids. Solutions at concentrations between 1 mg/mL and 40 mg/mL in the following infusion fluids may be stored for up to 24 hours at room temperature or 7 days if refrigerated: 0.9% Sodium Chloride Injection; Ringer's Injection USP; Lactated Ringer's Injection USP; 5% Dextrose Injection; 5% Dextrose and 0.225% Sodium Chloride Injection; 5% Dextrose and 0.45% Sodium Chloride Injection; 5% Dextrose and 0.9% Sodium Chloride Injection; 10% Dextrose Injection.

Tazicef is less stable in Sodium Bicarbonate Injection than in other intravenous fluids. It is not recommended as a diluent. Solutions of *Tazicef* in 5% Dextrose and 0.9% Sodium Chloride Injection are stable for at least 6 hours at room temperature in plastic tubing, drip chambers and volume control devices of common intravenous infusion sets.

Ceftazidime at a concentration of 20 mg/mL has been found physically compatible for 24 hours at room temperature or 7 days under refrigeration in Sterile Water for Injection when admixed with: cefazolin sodium (Ancef®) 330 mg/mL; heparin 1000 units/mL; and cimetidine HCl (Tagamet®) 150 mg/mL.

Ceftazidime at a concentration of 20 mg/mL has been found physically compatible for 24 hours at room temperature or 7 days under refrigeration in 5% Dextrose Injection when admixed with potassium chloride 40 mEq/L.

Vancomycin solution exhibits a physical incompatibility when mixed with a number of drugs, including ceftazidime. The likelihood of precipitation with ceftazidime is dependent on the concentrations of vancomycin and ceftazidime present. It is therefore recommended, when both drugs are to be administered by intermittent IV infusion, that they be given separately, flushing the IV lines (with one of the compatible IV fluids) between the administration of these two agents.

ADD-Vantage®* Vials: Ordinarily, ADD-Advantage® vials should be reconstituted only when it is certain that the patient is ready to receive the drug. However, *Tazicef* in ADD-Vantage® vials is stable for 24 hours at room temperature when reconstituted as directed (see RECONSTITUTION, ADD-Vantage® Vials and DIRECTIONS FOR USE OF TAZICEF® INJECTION IN ADD-VANTAGE® VIALS).

Note: Parenteral drug products should be inspected visually for particulate matter prior to administration wherever solution and container permit.

As with other cephalosporins, *Tazicef* powder, as well as solutions, tends to darken depending on storage conditions; within the stated recommendations, however, product potency is not adversely affected.

HOW SUPPLIED

Tazicef in the dry state should be stored between 15° and 30°C (59° and 86°F) and protected from light. Tazicef (ceftazidime for injection) is a dry, white to off-white powder supplied in vials as follows:

Vials: equivalent to 1 gram and 2 grams of ceftazidime.
1 gram (tray of 25): NDC 0007-5082-16
2 gram (tray of 10): NDC 0007-5084-11
"Piggyback" Vials for IV admixture: equivalent to 1 gram and 2 grams of ceftazidime.
1 gram (tray of 10): NDC 0007-5083-11
2 gram (tray of 10): NDC 0007-5085-11
ADD-Vantage® Vials: equivalent to 1 gram and 2 grams of ceftazidime.
1 gram: NDC 0007-5090-16
2 gram: NDC 0007-5091-11
Also available as:
Pharmacy Bulk Vials: equivalent to 6 grams of ceftazidime.
6 gram (tray of 10): NDC 0007-5086-11
Galaxy® Containers (PL 2040 Plastic): equivalent to 1 gram and 2 grams of ceftazidime.
1 gram 1's: NDC 0007-5088-04
2 gram 1's: NDC 0007-5089-04
* ADD-Vantage® is a trademark of Abbott Laboratories.

REFERENCES

1. Bauer, A.W.; Kirby, W.M.M., and Sherris, J.C., et al.: Antibiotic susceptibility testing by a standardized single disc method, Am. J. Clin. Pathol. 45:493, 1966.
2. National Committee for Clinical Laboratory Standards, Approved Standard: Performance Standards for Antimicrobial Disc Susceptibility Tests (M2-A3), December, 1984.
3. Standardized disc susceptibility test, Federal Register 39: 19182–19184, 1974.
4. Cockcroft, D.W., and Gault, M.H.: Prediction of creatinine clearance from serum creatinine, Nephron 16:31–41, 1976.

Jointly manufactured by
SmithKline Beecham Pharmaceuticals
Philadelphia, PA 19101 and
Bristol-Myers Squibb Co.
New York, NY 10154
TF:L16

THORAZINE® ℞

[thor 'ah-zeen]
brand of chlorpromazine
tranquilizer · antiemetic

DESCRIPTION

Thorazine (chlorpromazine) is 10-(3-dimethylaminopropyl)-2-chlorphenothiazine, a dimethylamine derivative of phenothiazine. It is present in oral and injectable forms as the hydrochloride salt, and in the suppositories as the base.

Tablets—Each round, orange, coated tablet contains chlorpromazine hydrochloride as follows: 10 mg imprinted SKF and T73; 25 mg imprinted SKF and T74; 50 mg imprinted SKF and T76; 100 mg imprinted SKF and T77; 200 mg imprinted SKF and T79. Inactive ingredients consist of benzoic acid, croscarmellose sodium, D&C Yellow No. 10, FD&C Blue No. 2, FD&C Yellow No. 6, gelatin, hydroxypropyl methylcellulose, lactose, magnesium stearate, methylparaben, polyethylene glycol, propylparaben, talc, titanium dioxide and trace amounts of other inactive ingredients.

Spansule® sustained release capsules—Each *Thorazine* Spansule® capsule is so prepared that an initial dose is released promptly and the remaining medication is released gradually over a prolonged period.

Each capsule, with opaque orange cap and natural body, contains chlorpromazine hydrochloride as follows: 30 mg imprinted SKF and T63; 75 mg imprinted SKF and T64; 150 mg imprinted SKF and T66. Inactive ingredients consist of benzyl alcohol, calcium sulfate, cetylpyridinium chloride, FD&C Yellow No. 6, gelatin, glyceryl distearate, glyceryl monostearate, iron oxide, povidone, silicon dioxide, sodium lauryl sulfate, starch, sucrose, titanium dioxide, wax and trace amounts of other inactive ingredients.

Ampuls—Each mL contains, in aqueous solution, chlorpromazine hydrochloride, 25 mg; ascorbic acid, 2 mg; sodium bisulfite, 1 mg; sodium chloride, 6 mg; sodium sulfite, 1 mg.

Multi-Dose Vials—Each mL contains, in aqueous solution, chlorpromazine hydrochloride, 25 mg; ascorbic acid, 2 mg; sodium bisulfite, 1 mg; sodium chloride, 1 mg; sodium sulfite, 1 mg; benzyl alcohol, 2%, as a preservative.

Syrup—Each 5 mL (1 teaspoonful) of clear, orange-custard flavored liquid contains chlorpromazine hydrochloride, 10 mg. Inactive ingredients consist of citric acid, flavors, sodium benzoate, sodium citrate, sucrose and water.

Suppositories—Each suppository contains chlorpromazine, 25 or 100 mg, glycerin, glyceryl monopalmitate, glyceryl monostearate, hydrogenated coconut oil fatty acids and hydrogenated palm kernel oil fatty acids.

Concentrate—Each mL of clear, custard flavored liquid contains chlorpromazine hydrochloride, 30 or 100 mg. Inactive ingredients consist of calcium disodium edetate, citric acid, flavors, hydroxypropyl methylcellulose, propylene glycol, saccharin sodium, sodium benzoate, water and trace amounts of other inactive ingredients.

ACTIONS

The precise mechanism whereby the therapeutic effects of chlorpromazine are produced is not known. The principal pharmacological actions are psychotropic. It also exerts sedative and antiemetic activity. Chlorpromazine has actions at all levels of the central nervous system—primarily at subcortical levels—as well as on multiple organ systems. Chlorpromazine has strong antiadrenergic and weaker peripheral anticholinergic activity; ganglionic blocking action is relatively slight. It also possesses slight antihistaminic and antiserotonin activity.

INDICATIONS

For the management of manifestations of psychotic disorders.

To control nausea and vomiting.

For relief of restlessness and apprehension before surgery.

For acute intermittent porphyria.

As an adjunct in the treatment of tetanus.

To control the manifestations of the manic type of manic-depressive illness.

For relief of intractable hiccups.

For the treatment of severe behavioral problems in children (1 to 12 years of age) marked by combativeness and/or explosive hyperexcitable behavior (out of proportion to immediate provocations), and in the short-term treatment of hyperactive children who show excessive motor activity with accompanying conduct disorders consisting of some or all of the following symptoms: impulsivity, difficulty sustaining attention, aggressivity, mood lability and poor frustration tolerance.

CONTRAINDICATIONS

Do not use in patients with known hypersensitivity to phenothiazines.

Do not use in comatose states or in the presence of large amounts of central nervous system depressants (alcohol, barbiturates, narcotics, etc.).

WARNINGS

The extrapyramidal symptoms which can occur secondary to Thorazine (chlorpromazine) may be confused with the central nervous system signs of an undiagnosed primary disease responsible for the vomiting, e.g., Reye's syndrome or other encephalopathy. The use of *Thorazine* and other potential hepatotoxins should be avoided in children and adolescents whose signs and symptoms suggest Reye's syndrome.

Tardive Dyskinesia: Tardive dyskinesia, a syndrome consisting of potentially irreversible, involuntary, dyskinetic movements, may develop in patients treated with neuroleptic (antipsychotic) drugs. Although the prevalence of the syndrome appears to be highest among the elderly, especially elderly women, it is impossible to rely upon prevalence estimates to predict, at the inception of neuroleptic

Continued on next page

Information on the SmithKline Beecham Pharmaceuticals products appearing here is based on the labeling in effect on July 31, 1998. Further information on these and other products may be obtained from the Medical Department, SmithKline Beecham Pharmaceuticals, One Franklin Plaza, Philadelphia, PA 19101.

Thorazine—Cont.

treatment, which patients are likely to develop the syndrome. Whether neuroleptic drug products differ in their potential to cause tardive dyskinesia is unknown.

Both the risk of developing the syndrome and the likelihood that it will become irreversible are believed to increase as the duration of treatment and the total cumulative dose of neuroleptic drugs administered to the patient increase. However, the syndrome can develop, although much less commonly, after relatively brief treatment periods at low doses.

There is no known treatment for established cases of tardive dyskinesia, although the syndrome may remit, partially or completely, if neuroleptic treatment is withdrawn. Neuroleptic treatment itself, however, may suppress (or partially suppress) the signs and symptoms of the syndrome and thereby may possibly mask the underlying disease process. The effect that symptomatic suppression has upon the long-term course of the syndrome is unknown.

Given these considerations, neuroleptics should be prescribed in a manner that is most likely to minimize the occurrence of tardive dyskinesia. Chronic neuroleptic treatment should generally be reserved for patients who suffer from a chronic illness that, 1) is known to respond to neuroleptic drugs, and, 2) for whom alternative, equally effective, but potentially less harmful treatments are *not* available or appropriate. In patients who do require chronic treatment, the smallest dose and the shortest duration of treatment producing a satisfactory clinical response should be sought. The need for continued treatment should be reassessed periodically.

If signs and symptoms of tardive dyskinesia appear in a patient on neuroleptics, drug discontinuation should be considered. However, some patients may require treatment despite the presence of the syndrome.

For further information about the description of tardive dyskinesia and its clinical detection, please refer to the sections on PRECAUTIONS and ADVERSE REACTIONS.

Neuroleptic Malignant Syndrome (NMS): A potentially fatal symptom complex sometimes referred to as Neuroleptic Malignant Syndrome (NMS) has been reported in association with antipsychotic drugs. Clinical manifestations of NMS are hyperpyrexia, muscle rigidity, altered mental status and evidence of autonomic instability (irregular pulse or blood pressure, tachycardia, diaphoresis and cardiac dysrhythmias).

The diagnostic evaluation of patients with this syndrome is complicated. In arriving at a diagnosis, it is important to identify cases where the clinical presentation includes both serious medical illness (e.g., pneumonia, systemic infection, etc.) and untreated or inadequately treated extrapyramidal signs and symptoms (EPS). Other important considerations in the differential diagnosis include central anticholinergic toxicity, heat stroke, drug fever and primary central nervous system (CNS) pathology.

The management of NMS should include 1) immediate discontinuation of antipsychotic drugs and other drugs not essential to concurrent therapy, 2) intensive symptomatic treatment and medical monitoring, and 3) treatment of any concomitant serious medical problems for which specific treatments are available. There is no general agreement about specific pharmacological treatment regimens for uncomplicated NMS.

If a patient requires antipsychotic drug treatment after recovery from NMS, the potential reintroduction of drug therapy should be carefully considered. The patient should be carefully monitored, since recurrences of NMS have been reported.

An encephalopathic syndrome (characterized by weakness, lethargy, fever, tremulousness and confusion, extrapyramidal symptoms, leukocytosis, elevated serum enzymes, BUN and FBS) has occurred in a few patients treated with lithium plus a neuroleptic. In some instances, the syndrome was followed by irreversible brain damage. Because of a possible causal relationship between these events and the concomitant administration of lithium and neuroleptics, patients receiving such combined therapy should be monitored closely for early evidence of neurologic toxicity and treatment discontinued promptly if such signs appear. This encephalopathic syndrome may be similar to or the same as neuroleptic malignant syndrome (NMS).

Thorazine (chlorpromazine) ampuls and multi-dose vials contain sodium bisulfite and sodium sulfite, sulfites that may cause allergic-type reactions including anaphylactic symptoms and life-threatening or less severe asthmatic episodes in certain susceptible people. The overall prevalence of sulfite sensitivity in the general population is unknown and probably low. Sulfite sensitivity is seen more frequently in asthmatic than in nonasthmatic people.

Patients with bone marrow depression or who have previously demonstrated a hypersensitivity reaction (e.g., blood dyscrasias, jaundice) with a phenothiazine should not receive any phenothiazine, including *Thorazine*, unless in the judgment of the physician the potential benefits of treatment outweigh the possible hazard.

Thorazine may impair mental and/or physical abilities, especially during the first few days of therapy. Therefore, caution patients about activities requiring alertness (e.g., operating vehicles or machinery).

The use of alcohol with this drug should be avoided due to possible additive effects and hypotension.

Thorazine may counteract the antihypertensive effect of guanethidine and related compounds.

Usage in Pregnancy: Safety for the use of Thorazine (chlorpromazine) during pregnancy has not been established. Therefore, it is not recommended that the drug be given to pregnant patients except when, in the judgment of the physician, it is essential. The potential benefits should clearly outweigh possible hazards. There are reported instances of prolonged jaundice, extrapyramidal signs, hyperreflexia or hyporeflexia in newborn infants whose mothers received phenothiazines.

Reproductive studies in rodents have demonstrated potential for embryotoxicity, increased neonatal mortality and nursing transfer of the drug. Tests in the offspring of the drug-treated rodents demonstrate decreased performance. The possibility of permanent neurological damage cannot be excluded.

Nursing Mothers: There is evidence that chlorpromazine is excreted in the breast milk of nursing mothers. Because of the potential for serious adverse reactions in nursing infants from chlorpromazine, a decision should be made whether to discontinue nursing or to discontinue the drug, taking into account the importance of the drug to the mother.

PRECAUTIONS
General
Given the likelihood that some patients exposed chronically to neuroleptics will develop tardive dyskinesia, it is advised that all patients in whom chronic use is contemplated be given, if possible, full information about this risk. The decision to inform patients and/or their guardians must obviously take into account the clinical circumstances and the competency of the patient to understand the information provided.

Thorazine (chlorpromazine) should be administered cautiously to persons with cardiovascular, liver or renal disease. There is evidence that patients with a history of hepatic encephalopathy due to cirrhosis have increased sensitivity to the CNS effects of *Thorazine* (i.e., impaired cerebration and abnormal slowing of the EEG).

Because of its CNS depressant effect, *Thorazine* should be used with caution in patients with chronic respiratory disorders such as severe asthma, emphysema and acute respiratory infections, particularly in children (1 to 12 years of age).

Because *Thorazine* can suppress the cough reflex, aspiration of vomitus is possible.

Thorazine (chlorpromazine) prolongs and intensifies the action of CNS depressants such as anesthetics, barbiturates and narcotics. When *Thorazine* is administered concomitantly, about $1/4$ to $1/2$ the usual dosage of such agents is required. When *Thorazine* is not being administered to reduce requirements of CNS depressants, it is best to stop such depressants before starting *Thorazine* treatment. These agents may subsequently be reinstated at low doses and increased as needed.

Note: *Thorazine* does *not* intensify the anticonvulsant action of barbiturates. Therefore, dosage of anticonvulsants, including barbiturates, should *not* be reduced if *Thorazine* is started. Instead, start *Thorazine* at low doses and increase as needed.

Use with caution in persons who will be exposed to extreme heat, organophosphorus insecticides, and in persons receiving atropine or related drugs.

Neuroleptic drugs elevate prolactin levels; the elevation persists during chronic administration. Tissue culture experiments indicate that approximately $1/3$ of human breast cancers are prolactin-dependent *in vitro*, a factor of potential importance if the prescribing of these drugs is contemplated in a patient with a previously detected breast cancer. Although disturbances such as galactorrhea, amenorrhea, gynecomastia and impotence have been reported, the clinical significance of elevated serum prolactin levels is unknown for most patients. An increase in mammary neoplasms has been found in rodents after chronic administration of neuroleptic drugs. Neither clinical nor epidemiologic studies conducted to date, however, have shown an association between chronic administration of these drugs and mammary tumorigenesis; the available evidence is considered too limited to be conclusive at this time.

Chromosomal aberrations in spermatocytes and abnormal sperm have been demonstrated in rodents treated with certain neuroleptics.

As with all drugs which exert an anticholinergic effect, and/or cause mydriasis, chlorpromazine should be used with caution in patients with glaucoma.

Chlorpromazine diminishes the effect of oral anticoagulants.

Phenothiazines can produce alpha-adrenergic blockade.

Chlorpromazine may lower the convulsive threshold; dosage adjustments of anticonvulsants may be necessary. Potentiation of anticonvulsant effects does not occur. However, it has been reported that chlorpromazine may interfere with the metabolism of Dilantin®* and thus precipitate *Dilantin* toxicity.

Concomitant administration with propranolol results in increased plasma levels of both drugs.

Thiazide diuretics may accentuate the orthostatic hypotension that may occur with phenothiazines.

The presence of phenothiazines may produce false-positive phenylketonuria (PKU) test results.

Drugs which lower the seizure threshold, including phenothiazine derivatives, should not be used with Amipaque®†. As with other phenothiazine derivatives, *Thorazine* should be discontinued at least 48 hours before myelography, should not be resumed for at least 24 hours postprocedure, and should not be used for the control of nausea and vomiting occurring either prior to myelography or postprocedure with *Amipaque*.

Long-Term Therapy: To lessen the likelihood of adverse reactions related to cumulative drug effect, patients with a history of long-term therapy with *Thorazine* and/or other neuroleptics should be evaluated periodically to decide whether the maintenance dosage could be lowered or drug therapy discontinued.

Antiemetic Effect: The antiemetic action of *Thorazine* may mask the signs and symptoms of overdosage of other drugs and may obscure the diagnosis and treatment of other conditions such as intestinal obstruction, brain tumor and Reye's syndrome. (See WARNINGS.)

When *Thorazine* is used with cancer chemotherapeutic drugs, vomiting as a sign of the toxicity of these agents may be obscured by the antiemetic effect of *Thorazine*.

Abrupt Withdrawal: Like other phenothiazines, Thorazine (chlorpromazine) is not known to cause psychic dependence and does not produce tolerance or addiction. There may be, however, following abrupt withdrawal of high-dose therapy, some symptoms resembling those of physical dependence such as gastritis, nausea and vomiting, dizziness and tremulousness. These symptoms can usually be avoided or reduced by gradual reduction of the dosage or by continuing concomitant anti-parkinsonism agents for several weeks after *Thorazine* is withdrawn.

ADVERSE REACTIONS
Note: Some adverse effects of *Thorazine* may be more likely to occur, or occur with greater intensity, in patients with special medical problems, e.g., patients with mitral insufficiency or pheochromocytoma have experienced severe hypotension following recommended doses.

Drowsiness, usually mild to moderate, may occur, particularly during the first or second week, after which it generally disappears. If troublesome, dosage may be lowered.

Jaundice: Overall incidence has been low, regardless of indication or dosage. Most investigators conclude it is a sensitivity reaction. Most cases occur between the second and fourth weeks of therapy. The clinical picture resembles infectious hepatitis, with laboratory features of obstructive jaundice, rather than those of parenchymal damage. It is usually promptly reversible on withdrawal of the medication; however, chronic jaundice has been reported.

There is no conclusive evidence that preexisting liver disease makes patients more susceptible to jaundice. Alcoholics with cirrhosis have been successfully treated with Thorazine (chlorpromazine) without complications. Nevertheless, the medication should be used cautiously in patients with liver disease. Patients who have experienced jaundice with a phenothiazine should not, if possible, be reexposed to *Thorazine* or other phenothiazines.

If fever with grippe-like symptoms occurs, appropriate liver studies should be conducted. If tests indicate an abnormality, stop treatment.

Liver function tests in jaundice induced by the drug may mimic extrahepatic obstruction; withhold exploratory laparotomy until extrahepatic obstruction is confirmed.

Hematological Disorders, including agranulocytosis, eosinophilia, leukopenia, hemolytic anemia, aplastic anemia, thrombocytopenic purpura and pancytopenia have been reported.

Agranulocytosis—Warn patients to report the sudden appearance of sore throat or other signs of infection. If white blood cell and differential counts indicate cellular depression, stop treatment and start antibiotic and other suitable therapy.

Most cases have occurred between the fourth and tenth weeks of therapy; patients should be watched closely during that period.

Moderate suppression of white blood cells is not an indication for stopping treatment unless accompanied by the symptoms described above.

Cardiovascular:

Hypotensive Effects—Postural hypotension, simple tachycardia, momentary fainting and dizziness may occur after the first injection; occasionally after subsequent injections; rarely, after the first oral dose. Usually recovery is sponta-

neous and symptoms disappear within 1/2 to 2 hours. Occasionally, these effects may be more severe and prolonged, producing a shock-like condition.

To minimize hypotension after injection, keep patient lying down and observe for at least 1/2 hour. To control hypotension, place patient in head-low position with legs raised. If a vasoconstrictor is required, Levophed®‡ and Neo-Synephrine®§ are the most suitable. Other pressor agents, including epinephrine, should not be used as they may cause a paradoxical further lowering of blood pressure.

EKG Changes—particularly nonspecific, usually reversible Q and T wave distortions—have been observed in some patients receiving phenothiazine tranquilizers, including Thorazine (chlorpromazine).

Note: Sudden death, apparently due to cardiac arrest, has been reported.

CNS Reactions:

Neuromuscular (Extrapyramidal) Reactions—Neuromuscular reactions include dystonias, motor restlessness, pseudo-parkinsonism and tardive dyskinesia, and appear to be dose-related. They are discussed in the following paragraphs:

Dystonias: Symptoms may include spasm of the neck muscles, sometimes progressing to acute, reversible torticollis; extensor rigidity of back muscles, sometimes progressing to opisthotonos; carpopedal spasm, trismus, swallowing difficulty, oculogyric crisis and protrusion of the tongue. These usually subside within a few hours, and almost always within 24 to 48 hours after the drug has been discontinued.

In mild cases, reassurance or a barbiturate is often sufficient. *In moderate cases,* barbiturates will usually bring rapid relief. *In more severe adult cases,* the administration of an anti-parkinsonism agent, except levodopa, usually produces rapid reversal of symptoms. *In children (1 to 12 years of age),* reassurance and barbiturates will usually control symptoms. (Or, parenteral Benadryl®‖ may be useful. See *Benadryl* prescribing information for appropriate children's dosage.) If appropriate treatment with anti-parkinsonism agents or *Benadryl* fails to reverse the signs and symptoms, the diagnosis should be reevaluated.

Suitable supportive measures such as maintaining a clear airway and adequate hydration should be employed when needed. If therapy is reinstituted, it should be at a lower dosage. Should these symptoms occur in children or pregnant patients, the drug should not be reinstituted.

Motor Restlessness: Symptoms may include agitation or jitteriness and sometimes insomnia. These symptoms often disappear spontaneously. At times these symptoms may be similar to the original neurotic or psychotic symptoms. Dosage should not be increased until these side effects have subsided.

If these symptoms become too troublesome, they can usually be controlled by a reduction of dosage or change of drug. Treatment with anti-parkinsonian agents, benzodiazepines or propranolol may be helpful.

Pseudo-parkinsonism: Symptoms may include: mask-like facies, drooling, tremors, pillrolling motion, cogwheel rigidity and shuffling gait. In most cases these symptoms are readily controlled when an anti-parkinsonism agent is administered concomitantly. Anti-parkinsonism agents should be used only when required. Generally, therapy of a few weeks to 2 or 3 months will suffice. After this time patients should be evaluated to determine their need for continued treatment. (Note: Levodopa has not been found effective in neuroleptic-induced pseudo-parkinsonism.) Occasionally it is necessary to lower the dosage of Thorazine (chlorpromazine) or to discontinue the drug.

Tardive Dyskinesia: As with all antipsychotic agents, tardive dyskinesia may appear in some patients on long-term therapy or may appear after drug therapy has been discontinued. The syndrome can also develop, although much less frequently, after relatively brief treatment periods at low doses. This syndrome appears in all age groups. Although its prevalence appears to be highest among elderly patients, especially elderly women, it is impossible to rely upon prevalence estimates to predict at the inception of neuroleptic treatment which patients are likely to develop the syndrome. The symptoms are persistent and in some patients appear to be irreversible. The syndrome is characterized by rhythmical involuntary movements of the tongue, face, mouth or jaw (e.g., protrusion of tongue, puffing of cheeks, puckering of mouth, chewing movements). Sometimes these may be accompanied by involuntary movements of extremities. In rare instances, these involuntary movements of the extremities are the only manifestations of tardive dyskinesia. A variant of tardive dyskinesia, tardive dystonia, has also been described.

There is no known effective treatment for tardive dyskinesia; anti-parkinsonism agents do not alleviate the symptoms of this syndrome. If clinically feasible, it is suggested that all antipsychotic agents be discontinued if these symptoms appear. Should it be necessary to reinstitute treatment, or increase the dosage of the agent, or switch to a different antipsychotic agent, the syndrome may be masked.

It has been reported that fine vermicular movements of the tongue may be an early sign of the syndrome and if the medication is stopped at that time the syndrome may not develop.

Adverse Behavioral Effects—Psychotic symptoms and catatonic-like states have been reported rarely.

Other CNS Effects—Neuroleptic Malignant Syndrome (NMS) has been reported in association with antipsychotic drugs. (See WARNINGS.)

Cerebral edema has been reported.

Convulsive seizures *(petit mal* and *grand mal)* have been reported, particularly in patients with EEG abnormalities or history of such disorders.

Abnormality of the cerebrospinal fluid proteins has also been reported.

Allergic Reactions of a mild urticarial type or photosensitivity are seen. Avoid undue exposure to sun. More severe reactions, including exfoliative dermatitis, have been reported occasionally.

Contact dermatitis has been reported in nursing personnel; accordingly, the use of rubber gloves when administering *Thorazine* liquid or injectable is recommended.

In addition, asthma, laryngeal edema, angioneurotic edema and anaphylactoid reactions have been reported.

Endocrine Disorders: Lactation and moderate breast engorgement may occur in females on large doses. If persistent, lower dosage or withdraw drug. False-positive pregnancy tests have been reported, but are less likely to occur when a serum test is used. Amenorrhea and gynecomastia have also been reported. Hyperglycemia, hypoglycemia and glycosuria have been reported.

Autonomic Reactions: Occasional dry mouth; nasal congestion; nausea; obstipation; constipation; adynamic ileus; urinary retention; priapism; miosis and mydriasis, atonic colon, ejaculatory disorders/impotence.

Special Considerations in Long-Term Therapy: Skin pigmentation and ocular changes have occurred in some patients taking substantial doses of Thorazine (chlorpromazine) for prolonged periods.

Skin Pigmentation—Rare instances of skin pigmentation have been observed in hospitalized mental patients, primarily females who have received the drug usually for 3 years or more in dosages ranging from 500 mg to 1500 mg daily. The pigmentary changes, restricted to exposed areas of the body, range from an almost imperceptible darkening of the skin to a slate gray color, sometimes with a violet hue. Histological examination reveals a pigment, chiefly in the dermis, which is probably a melanin-like complex. The pigmentation may fade following discontinuance of the drug.

Ocular Changes—Ocular changes have occurred more frequently than skin pigmentation and have been observed both in pigmented and nonpigmented patients receiving Thorazine (chlorpromazine) usually for 2 years or more in dosages of 300 mg daily and higher. Eye changes are characterized by deposition of fine particulate matter in the lens and cornea. In more advanced cases, star-shaped opacities have also been observed in the anterior portion of the lens. The nature of the eye deposits has not yet been determined. A small number of patients with more severe ocular changes have had some visual impairment. In addition to these corneal and lenticular changes, epithelial keratopathy and pigmentary retinopathy have been reported. Reports suggest that the eye lesions may regress after withdrawal of the drug.

Since the occurrence of eye changes seems to be related to dosage levels and/or duration of therapy, it is suggested that long-term patients on moderate to high dosage levels have periodic ocular examinations.

Etiology—The etiology of both of these reactions is not clear, but exposure to light, along with dosage/duration of therapy, appears to be the most significant factor. If either of these reactions is observed, the physician should weigh the benefits of continued therapy against the possible risks and, on the merits of the individual case, determine whether or not to continue present therapy, lower the dosage, or withdraw the drug.

Other Adverse Reactions: Mild fever may occur after large I.M. doses. Hyperpyrexia has been reported. Increases in appetite and weight sometimes occur. Peripheral edema and a systemic lupus erythematosus-like syndrome have been reported.

Note: There have been occasional reports of sudden death in patients receiving phenothiazines. In some cases, the cause appeared to be cardiac arrest or asphyxia due to failure of the cough reflex.

DOSAGE AND ADMINISTRATION—ADULTS

Adjust dosage to individual and the severity of his condition, recognizing that the milligram for milligram potency relationship among all dosage forms has not been precisely established clinically. It is important to increase dosage until symptoms are controlled. Dosage should be increased more gradually in debilitated or emaciated patients. In continued therapy, gradually reduce dosage to the lowest effective maintenance level, after symptoms have been controlled for a reasonable period.

In general, dosage recommendations for other oral forms of the drug may be applied to Spansule® brand sustained release capsules on the basis of total daily dosage in milligrams.

The 100 mg and 200 mg tablets are for use in severe neuropsychiatric conditions.

Increase parenteral dosage only if hypotension has not occurred. Before using I.M., see IMPORTANT NOTES ON INJECTION.

Elderly Patients—In general, dosages in the lower range are sufficient for most elderly patients. Since they appear to be more susceptible to hypotension and neuromuscular reactions, such patients should be observed closely. Dosage should be tailored to the individual, response carefully monitored, and dosage adjusted accordingly. Dosage should be increased more gradually in elderly patients.

Psychotic Disorders—Increase dosage gradually until symptoms are controlled. Maximum improvement may not be seen for weeks or even months. Continue optimum dosage for 2 weeks; then gradually reduce dosage to the lowest effective maintenance level. Daily dosage of 200 mg is not unusual. Some patients require higher dosages (e.g., 800 mg daily is not uncommon in discharged mental patients).

HOSPITALIZED PATIENTS: ACUTELY DISTURBED OR MANIC—*I.M.:* 25 mg (1 mL). If necessary, give additional 25 to 50 mg injection in 1 hour. Increase subsequent I.M. doses gradually over several days—up to 400 mg q4 to 6h in exceptionally severe cases—until patient is controlled. Usually patient becomes quiet and cooperative within 24 to 48 hours and oral doses may be substituted and increased until the patient is calm. 500 mg a day is generally sufficient. While gradual increases to 2,000 mg a day or more may be necessary, there is usually little therapeutic gain to be achieved by exceeding 1,000 mg a day for extended periods. In general, dosage levels should be lower in the elderly, the emaciated and the debilitated. LESS ACUTELY DISTURBED—*Oral:* 25 mg t.i.d. Increase gradually until effective dose is reached—usually 400 mg daily. OUTPATIENTS—*Oral:* 10 mg t.i.d. or q.i.d., or 25 mg b.i.d. or t.i.d. MORE SEVERE CASES—*Oral:* 25 mg t.i.d. After 1 or 2 days, daily dosage may be increased by 20 to 50 mg at semiweekly intervals until patient becomes calm and cooperative. PROMPT CONTROL OF SEVERE SYMPTOMS—*I.M.:* 25 mg (1 mL). If necessary, repeat in 1 hour. Subsequent doses should be oral, 25 to 50 mg t.i.d.

Nausea and Vomiting—*Oral:* 10 to 25 mg q4 to 6h, p.r.n., increased, if necessary. *I.M.:* 25 mg (1 mL). If no hypotension occurs, give 25 to 50 mg q3 to 4h, p.r.n., until vomiting stops. Then switch to oral dosage. *Rectal:* One 100 mg suppository q6 to 8h, p.r.n. In some patients, half this dose will do.

DURING SURGERY—*I.M.:* 12.5 mg (0.5 mL). Repeat in 1/2 hour if necessary and if no hypotension occurs. *I.V.:* 2 mg per fractional injection, at 2-minute intervals. Do not exceed 25 mg. Dilute to 1 mg/mL, i.e., 1 mL (25 mg) mixed with 24 mL of saline.

Presurgical Apprehension—*Oral:* 25 to 50 mg, 2 to 3 hours before the operation. *I.M.:* 12.5 to 25 mg (0.5 to 1 mL), 1 to 2 hours before operation.

Intractable Hiccups—*Oral:* 25 to 50 mg t.i.d. or q.i.d. If symptoms persist for 2 to 3 days, give 25 to 50 mg (1 to 2 mL) I.M. Should symptoms persist, use *slow* I.V. infusion with patient flat in bed: 25 to 50 mg (1 to 2 mL) in 500 to 1,000 mL of saline. Follow blood pressure closely.

Acute Intermittent Porphyria—*Oral:* 25 to 50 mg t.i.d. or q.i.d. Can usually be discontinued after several weeks, but maintenance therapy may be necessary for some patients. *I.M.:* 25 mg (1 mL) t.i.d. or q.i.d. until patient can take oral therapy.

Tetanus—*I.M.:* 25 to 50 mg (1 to 2 mL) given 3 or 4 times daily, usually in conjunction with barbiturates. Total doses and frequency of administration must be determined by the patient's response, starting with low doses and increasing gradually. *I.V.:* 25 to 50 mg (1 to 2 mL). Dilute to at least 1 mg per mL and administer at a rate of 1 mg per minute.

DOSAGE AND ADMINISTRATION—PEDIATRIC PATIENTS (6 months to 12 years of age)

Thorazine (chlorpromazine) should generally not be used in pediatric patients under 6 months of age except where potentially lifesaving. It should not be used in conditions for which specific pediatric dosages have not been established.

Severe Behavioral Problems—OUTPATIENTS—Select route of administration according to severity of patient's condition and increase dosage gradually as required. *Oral:* 1/4 mg/lb body weight q4 to 6h, p.r.n. (e.g., for 40 lb child—10

Continued on next page

Information on the SmithKline Beecham Pharmaceuticals products appearing here is based on the labeling in effect on July 31, 1998. Further information on these and other products may be obtained from the Medical Department, SmithKline Beecham Pharmaceuticals, One Franklin Plaza, Philadelphia, PA 19101.

Consult 1999 PDR® supplements and future editions for revisions

Thorazine—Cont.

mg q4 to 6h). *Rectal:* 1/2 mg/lb body weight q6 to 8h, p.r.n. (e.g., for 20 to 30 lb child—half a 25 mg suppository q6 to 8h). *I.M.:* 1/4 mg/lb body weight q6 to 8h, p.r.n.

HOSPITALIZED PATIENTS—As with outpatients, start with low doses and increase dosage gradually. In severe behavior disorders or psychotic conditions, higher dosages (50 to 100 mg daily, and in older children, 200 mg daily or more) may be necessary. There is little evidence that behavior improvement in severely disturbed mentally retarded patients is further enhanced by doses beyond 500 mg per day. *Maximum I.M. Dosage:* Children up to 5 years (or 50 lbs), not over 40 mg/day; 5 to 12 years (or 50 to 100 lbs), not over 75 mg/day except in unmanageable cases.

Nausea and Vomiting—Dosage and frequency of administration should be adjusted according to the severity of the symptoms and response of the patient. The duration of activity following intramuscular administration may last up to 12 hours. Subsequent doses may be given by the same route if necessary. *Oral:* 1/4 mg/lb body weight (e.g., 40 lb child—10 mg q4 to 6h). *Rectal:* 1/2 mg/lb body weight q6 to 8h, p.r.n. (e.g., 20 to 30 lb child—half of a 25 mg suppository q6 to 8h). *I.M.:* 1/4 mg/lb body weight q6 to 8h, p.r.n. *Maximum I.M. Dosage:* Pediatric patients 6 months to 5 yrs. (or 50 lbs), not over 40 mg/day; 5 to 12 yrs. (or 50 to 100 lbs), not over 75 mg/day except in severe cases. DURING SURGERY—*I.M.:* 1/8 mg/lb body weight. Repeat in 1/2 hour if necessary and if no hypotension occurs. *I.V.:*1 mg per fractional injection at 2-minute intervals and not exceeding recommended I.M. dosage. Always dilute to 1 mg/ mL, i.e., 1 mL (25 mg) mixed with 24 mL of saline.

Presurgical Apprehension—1/4 mg/lb body weight, either *orally* 2 to 3 hours before operation, or *I.M.* 1 to 2 hours before.

Tetanus—*I.M.* or *I.V.:* 1/4 mg/lb body weight q6 to 8h. When given I.V., dilute to at least 1 mg/mL and administer at rate of 1 mg per 2 minutes. In patients up to 50 lbs, do not exceed 40 mg daily; 50 to 100 lbs, do not exceed 75 mg, except in severe cases.

IMPORTANT NOTES ON INJECTION

Inject slowly, deep into upper outer quadrant of buttock.

Because of possible hypotensive effects, reserve parenteral administration for bedfast patients or for acute ambulatory cases, and keep patient lying down for at least 1/2 hour after injection. If irritation is a problem, dilute Injection with saline or 2% procaine; mixing with other agents in the syringe is not recommended. Subcutaneous injection is not advised. Avoid injecting undiluted Thorazine (chlorpromazine) into vein. I.V. route is only for severe hiccups, surgery and tetanus.

Because of the possibility of contact dermatitis, avoid getting solution on hands or clothing. This solution should be protected from light. This is a clear, colorless to pale yellow solution; a slight yellowish discoloration will not alter potency. If markedly discolored, solution should be discarded. For information on sulfite sensitivity, see the WARNINGS section of this labeling.

Note on Concentrate: When the Concentrate is to be used, add the desired dosage of Concentrate to 60 mL (2 fl oz) or more of diluent *just prior to administration.* This will insure palatability and stability. Vehicles suggested for dilution are: tomato or fruit juice, milk, simple syrup, orange syrup, carbonated beverages, coffee, tea or water. Semisolid foods (soups, puddings, etc.) may also be used. The Concentrate is light sensitive; it should be protected from light and dispensed in amber glass bottles. *Refrigeration is not required.*

OVERDOSAGE

(See also ADVERSE REACTIONS.)

SYMPTOMS—Primarily symptoms of central nervous system depression to the point of somnolence or coma. Hypotension and extrapyramidal symptoms.

Other possible manifestations include agitation and restlessness, convulsions, fever, autonomic reactions such as dry mouth and ileus, EKG changes and cardiac arrhythmias.

TREATMENT—It is important to determine other medications taken by the patient since multiple drug therapy is common in overdosage situations. Treatment is essentially symptomatic and supportive. Early gastric lavage is helpful. Keep patient under observation and maintain an open airway, since involvement of the extrapyramidal mechanism may produce dysphagia and respiratory difficulty in severe overdosage. **Do not attempt to induce emesis because a dystonic reaction of the head or neck may develop that could result in aspiration of vomitus.** Extrapyramidal symptoms may be treated with anti-parkinsonism drugs, barbiturates, or *Benadryl*. See prescribing information for these products. Care should be taken to avoid increasing respiratory depression.

If administration of a stimulant is desirable, amphetamine, dextroamphetamine, or caffeine with sodium benzoate is recommended. Stimulants that may cause convulsions (e.g., picrotoxin or pentylenetetrazol) should be avoided.

If hypotension occurs, the standard measures for managing circulatory shock should be initiated. If it is desirable to administer a vasoconstrictor, *Levophed* and *Neo-Synephrine* are most suitable. Other pressor agents, including epinephrine, are not recommended because phenothiazine derivatives may reverse the usual elevating action of these agents and cause a further lowering of blood pressure.

Limited experience indicates that phenothiazines are *not* dialyzable.

Special note on Spansule® capsules—Since much of the *Spansule* capsule medication is coated for gradual release, therapy directed at reversing the effects of the ingested drug and at supporting the patient should be continued for as long as overdosage symptoms remain. Saline cathartics are useful for hastening evacuation of pellets that have not already released medication.

HOW SUPPLIED

Tablets: 10 mg, in bottles of 100; 25 mg or 50 mg, in bottles of 100 and 1000. For use in severe neuropsychiatric conditions, 100 mg and 200 mg, in bottles of 100 and 1000.

NDC 0007-5073-20 10 mg 100's
NDC 0007-5074-20 25 mg 100's
NDC 0007-5074-30 25 mg 1000's
NDC 0007-5076-20 50 mg 100's
NDC 0007-5076-30 50 mg 1000's
NDC 0007-5077-20 100 mg 100's
NDC 0007-5077-30 100 mg 1000's
NDC 0007-5079-20 200 mg 100's
NDC 0007-5079-30 200 mg 1000's

Spansule® brand of sustained release capsules: 30 mg, 75 mg or 150 mg, in bottles of 50.

NDC 0007-5063-15 30 mg 50's
NDC 0007-5064-15 75 mg 50's
NDC 0007-5066-15 150 mg 50's

Ampuls: 1 mL and 2 mL (25 mg/mL), in boxes of 10.

NDC 0007-5060-11 25 mg/mL in 1 mL Ampuls (box of 10)
NDC 0007-5061-11 25 mg/mL in 2 mL Ampuls (box of 10)

Multi-Dose Vials: 10 mL (25 mg/mL), in boxes of 1.

NDC 0007-5062-01 25 mg/mL in 10 mL Multi-Dose Vials (box of 1)

Syrup: 10 mg/5 mL, in 4 fl oz bottles.

NDC 0007-5072-44 10 mg/5 mL 4 fl oz

Suppositories: 25 mg or 100 mg, in boxes of 12.

NDC 0007-5070-03 25 mg (box of 12)
NDC 0007-5071-03 100 mg (box of 12)

Concentrate: Intended for institutional use. 30 mg/mL, in 4 fl oz bottles, and 100 mg/mL, in 8 fl oz bottles, in cartons of 12.

The Concentrate form is light-sensitive. For this reason, it should be protected from light and dispensed in amber bottles. *Refrigeration is not required.*

NDC 0007-5047-44 30 mg/mL 4 fl oz (carton of 12)
NDC 0007-5049-48 100 mg/mL 8 fl oz (carton of 12)

All dosage forms except Syrup should be stored between 15° and 30°C (59° and 86°F). Syrup should be stored below 25°C (77°F).

---

* phenytoin, Parke-Davis.
† metrizamide, Sanofi Winthrop Pharmaceuticals.
‡ norepinephrine bitartrate, Sanofi Winthrop Pharmaceuticals.
§ phenylephrine hydrochloride, Sanofi Winthrop Pharmaceuticals.
‖ diphenhydramine hydrochloride, Parke-Davis.

WARNING: Thorazine® *Spansule* capsules are manufactured with carbon tetrachloride and methyl chloroform, substances which harm public health and environment by destroying ozone in the upper atmosphere.

Veterans Administration/Military/PHS—Concentrate, 30 mg/mL, 4 oz, 6505-00-660-1664; 100 mg/mL, 8 oz, 6505-00-126-2044; Ampuls, 25 mg/mL, 1 mL, 10's, 6505-01-196-6216; 25 mg/mL, 2 mL, 10's, 6505-00-129-6709; *Spansule* capsules, 30 mg, 50's, 6505-01-343-3074; 75 mg, 50's, 6505-00-684-8672; Suppositories, 25 mg, 12's, 6505-01-153-3217; 100 mg, 12's, 6505-01-142-6379; Syrup, 10 mg/5 mL, 4 oz, 6505-01-156-1640; Tablets, 10 mg, 100's, 6505-00-763-5750; 25 mg, 1000's, 6505-00-022-1326; 50 mg, 1000's, 6505-00-022-1327; 100 mg, 100's, 6505-00-763-5748; 100 mg, 1000's, 6505-00-014-1182; 200 mg, 100's, 6505-00-014-1183; 200 mg, 1000's, 6505-00-014-1186.

TZ:L82

Shown in Product Identification Guide, page 340

TICAR® ℞

[*ti 'kar*]

brand of sterile ticarcillin disodium
for Intramuscular or Intravenous Administration

DESCRIPTION

Ticar is a semisynthetic injectable penicillin derived from the penicillin nucleus, 6-aminopenicillanic acid. Chemically, it is *N*-(2-Carboxy-3,3-dimethyl-7-oxo-4-thia-1-azabicyclo [3.2.0]hept-6-yl)-3-thiophenemalonamic acid disodium salt.

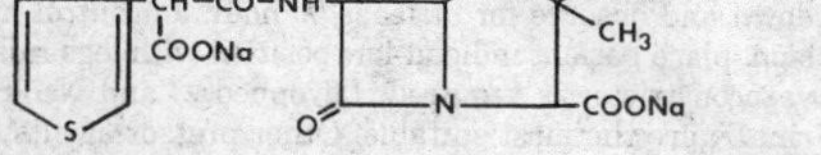

It is supplied as a white to pale yellow powder for reconstitution. The reconstituted solution is clear, colorless or pale yellow, having a pH of 6.0 to 8.0. Ticarcillin is very soluble in water; its solubility is greater than 600 mg/mL.

ACTIONS

Pharmacology

Ticarcillin is not absorbed orally; therefore, it must be given intravenously or intramuscularly. Following intramuscular administration, peak serum concentrations occur within 1/2 to 1 hour. Somewhat higher and more prolonged serum levels can be achieved with the concurrent administration of probenecid.

The minimum inhibitory concentrations (MICs) for many strains of *Pseudomonas* are relatively high by usual standards; serum levels of 60 mcg/mL or greater are required. However, the low degree of toxicity of ticarcillin permits the use of doses large enough to achieve inhibitory levels for these strains in serum or tissues. Other susceptible organisms usually require serum levels in the 10 to 25 mcg/mL range.

[See first table at bottom of next page]

As with other penicillins, ticarcillin is eliminated by glomerular filtration and tubular secretion. It is not highly bound to serum protein (approximately 45%) and is excreted unchanged in high concentrations in the urine. After the administration of a 1 to 2 gram I.M. dose, a urine concentration of 2000 to 4000 mcg/mL may be obtained in patients with normal renal function. The serum half-life of ticarcillin in normal individuals is approximately 70 minutes.

An inverse relationship exists between serum half-life and creatinine clearance, but the dosage of *Ticar* need only be adjusted in cases of severe renal impairment (see DOSAGE AND ADMINISTRATION). The administered ticarcillin may be removed from patients undergoing dialysis; the actual amount removed depends on the duration and type of dialysis.

Ticarcillin can be detected in tissues and interstitial fluid following parenteral administration. Penetration into the cerebrospinal fluid, bile and pleural fluid has been demonstrated.

Microbiology

Ticarcillin is bactericidal and demonstrates substantial *in vitro* activity against both gram-positive and gram-negative organisms. Many strains of the following organisms were found to be susceptible to ticarcillin *in vitro*:

Pseudomonas aeruginosa (and other species)
Escherichia coli
Proteus mirabilis
Morganella morganii (formerly *Proteus morganii)*
Providencia rettgeri (formerly *Proteus rettgeri)*
Proteus vulgaris
Enterobacter species
Haemophilus influenzae
Neisseria species
Salmonella species
Staphylococcus aureus (non-penicillinase producing)
Staphylococcus epidermidis
Beta-hemolytic streptococci (Group A)
Streptococcus faecalis (Enterococcus)
Streptococcus pneumoniae
Anaerobic bacteria, including:
Bacteroides species including *B. fragilis*
Fusobacterium species
Veillonella species
Clostridium species
Eubacterium species
Peptococcus species
Peptostreptococcus species

In vitro synergism between ticarcillin and gentamicin sulfate, tobramycin sulfate or amikacin sulfate against certain strains of *Pseudomonas aeruginosa* has been demonstrated.

Some strains of such microorganisms as *Mima-Herellea (Acinetobacter), Citrobacter* and *Serratia* have shown susceptibility.

Ticarcillin is not stable in the presence of penicillinase.

Some strains of *Pseudomonas* have developed resistance fairly rapidly.

DISK SUSCEPTIBILITY TESTS

Susceptibility Tests: Ticarcillin disks or powders should be used for testing susceptibility to ticarcillin. However, organisms reportedly susceptible to carbenicillin are susceptible to ticarcillin.

Diffusion Techniques: For the disk diffusion method of susceptibility testing a 75 mcg *Ticar* disk should be used. The method for this test is the one outlined in NCCLS publication M2-A3* with the following interpretative criteria:

[See second table at bottom of next page]

Adults:

Bacterial septicemia Respiratory tract infections Skin and soft-tissue infections Intra-abdominal infections Infections of the female pelvis and genital tract	200 to 300 mg/kg/day by I.V. infusion in divided doses every 4 or 6 hours. (The usual dose is 3 grams given every 4 hours [18 grams/day] or 4 grams given every 6 hours [16 grams/day] depending on weight and the severity of the infection.)

Urinary tract infections
Complicated: 150 to 200 mg/kg/day by I.V. infusion in divided doses every 4 or 6 hours.
                 (Usual recommended dosage for average [70 kg] adults: 3 grams q.i.d.)
Uncomplicated: 1 gram I.M. or direct I.V. every 6 hours.

Infections complicated by renal insufficiency*:   Initial loading dose of 3 grams I.V. followed by I.V. doses, based on creatinine clearance and type of dialysis, as indicated below:

Creatinine clearance mL/min.:	
over 60	3 grams every 4 hours
30 to 60	2 grams every 4 hours
10 to 30	2 grams every 8 hours
less than 10	2 grams every 12 hours (or 1 gram I.M. every 6 hours)
less than 10 with hepatic dysfunction	2 grams every 24 hours (or 1 gram I.M. every 12 hours)
patients on peritoneal dialysis	3 grams every 12 hours
patients on hemodialysis	2 grams every 12 hours supplemented with 3 grams after each dialysis

> To calculate creatinine clearance† from a serum creatinine value use the following formula:
>
> $$C_{cr} = \frac{(140 - Age)\ (wt.\ in\ kg)}{72 \times S_{cr}(mg/100\ mL)}$$
>
> This is the calculated creatinine clearance for adult males; for females it is 15% less.

†Cockcroft, D.W., et al: Prediction of Creatinine Clearance from Serum Creatinine. Nephron 16:31–41, 1976.

* The half-life of ticarcillin in patients with renal failure is approximately 13 hours.

Children under 40 kg (88 lbs):

The daily dose for children should not exceed the adult dosage.

Bacterial septicemia Respiratory tract infections Skin and soft-tissue infections Intra-abdominal infections Infections of the female pelvis and genital tract	200 to 300 mg/kg/day by I.V. infusion in divided doses every 4 or 6 hours.

Urinary tract infections
Complicated: 150 to 200 mg/kg/day by I.V. infusion in divided doses every 4 or 6 hours.
Uncomplicated: 50 to 100 mg/kg/day I.M. or direct I.V. in divided doses every 6 or 8 hours.

Infections complicated by renal insufficiency: Clinical data are insufficient to recommend an optimum dose.

Children weighing more than 40 kg (88 lbs) should receive adult dosages.

Neonates: In the neonate, for severe infections (sepsis) due to susceptible strains of *Pseudomonas*, *Proteus* and *E. coli*, the following ticarcillin dosages may be given I.M. or by 10 to 20 minute I.V. infusion:

Infants under 2000 grams body weight:
   Aged 0 to 7 days 75 mg/kg/12 hours
         (150 mg/kg/day)
   Aged over 7 days 75 mg/kg/8 hours
         (225 mg/kg/day)

Infants over 2000 grams body weight:
   Aged 0 to 7 days 75 mg/kg/8 hours
         (225 mg/kg/day)
   Aged over 7 days 100 mg/kg/8 hours
         (300 mg/kg/day)

This dosage schedule is intended to produce peak serum concentrations of 125 to 150 mcg/mL 1 hour after a dose of ticarcillin and trough concentrations of 25 to 50 mcg/mL immediately before the next dose.

NOTE: Gentamicin, tobramycin or amikacin may be used concurrently with ticarcillin for initial therapy until results of culture and susceptibility studies are known.
Seriously ill patients should receive the higher doses. *Ticar* has proved to be useful in infections in which protective mechanisms are impaired, such as in acute leukemia and during therapy with immunosuppressive or oncolytic drugs.

Dilution Techniques: Dilution techniques for determining the MIC (minimum inhibitory concentration) are published by NCCLS for the broth and agar dilution procedures. The MIC data should be interpreted in light of the concentrations present in serum, tissue and body fluids. Organisms with MIC ≤64 are considered susceptible when they are in tissue but organisms with MIC ≤128 would be susceptible in urine where the *Ticar* concentrations are much greater. At present, only dilution methods can be recommended for testing antibiotic susceptibility of obligate anaerobes. Susceptibility testing methods require the use of control organisms. The 75 mcg ticarcillin disk should give zone diameters between 22 and 28 mm for *P. aeruginosa* ATCC 27853 and 24 and 30 mm for *E. coli* ATCC 25922. Reference strains are available for dilution testing of ticarcillin. 95% of the MICs should fall within the following MIC ranges and the majority of MICs should be at values close to the center of the pertinent range (reference NCCLS publication M7-A†).

   S. aureus ATCC 29213, 2.0 to 8.0 mcg/mL; *S. faecalis* ATCC 29212, 16 to 64 mcg/mL; *E. coli* ATCC 25922, 2.0 to 8.0 mcg/mL; *P. aeruginosa* ATCC 27853, 8.0 to 32 mcg/mL.

*Performance Standards for Antimicrobial Disc Susceptibility Tests, National Committee for Clinical Laboratory Standards, Vol. 4, No. 16, pp. 369–402, 1984.
†Methods for Dilution Antimicrobial Susceptibility Tests for Bacteria That Grow Aerobically, Vol. 5, No. 22, pp. 579–618, 1985.

INDICATIONS

Ticar is indicated for the treatment of the following infections:
   Bacterial septicemia‡
   Skin and soft-tissue infections‡
   Acute and chronic respiratory tract infections‡§
   ‡Caused by susceptible strains of *Pseudomonas aeruginosa*, *Proteus* species (both indole-positive and indole-negative) and *Escherichia coli*.

TICARCILLIN SERUM LEVELS
mcg/mL

Dosage	Route	1/4 hr.	1/2 hr.	1 hr.	2 hr.	3 hr.	4 hr.	6 hr.
Adults:								
500 mg	I.M.	—	7.7	8.6	6.0	4.0	—	2.9
1 gram	I.M.	—	31.0	18.7	15.7	9.7	—	3.4
2 grams	I.M.	—	63.6	39.7	32.3	18.9	—	3.4
3 grams	I.V.	190.0	140.0	107.0	52.2	31.3	13.8	4.2
5 grams	I.V.	327.0	280.0	175.0	106.0	63.0	28.5	9.6
3 grams + 1 gram probenecid	I.V. Oral	223.0	166.0	123.0	78.0	54.0	35.4	17.1

Neonates:		1/2 hr.	1 hr.	1 1/2 hr.	2 hr.	4 hr.	8 hr.
50 mg/kg	I.M.	64.0	70.7	63.7	60.1	33.2	11.6

Culture	Susceptible	Intermediate	Resistant
P. aeruginosa and *Enterobacteriaceae*	≥15 mm	12 to 14 mm	≤11 mm
The MIC correlates are:	Resistant >128 mcg/mL Susceptible ≤64 mcg/mL		

Continued on next page

Information on the SmithKline Beecham Pharmaceuticals products appearing here is based on the labeling in effect on July 31, 1998. Further information on these and other products may be obtained from the Medical Department, SmithKline Beecham Pharmaceuticals, One Franklin Plaza, Philadelphia, PA 19101.

Consult 1999 PDR® supplements and future editions for revisions

Ticar—Cont.

§Though clinical improvement has been shown, bacteriological cures cannot be expected in patients with chronic respiratory disease or cystic fibrosis.

Genitourinary tract infections (complicated and uncomplicated) due to susceptible strains of *Pseudomonas aeruginosa, Proteus* species (both indole-positive and indole-negative), *Escherichia coli, Enterobacter* and *Streptococcus faecalis* (enterococcus).

Ticarcillin is also indicated in the treatment of the following infections due to susceptible anaerobic bacteria:

1. Bacterial septicemia.
2. Lower respiratory tract infections such as empyema, anaerobic pneumonitis and lung abscess.
3. Intra-abdominal infections such as peritonitis and intra-abdominal abscess (typically resulting from anaerobic organisms resident in the normal gastrointestinal tract).
4. Infections of the female pelvis and genital tract, such as endometritis, pelvic inflammatory disease, pelvic abscess and salpingitis.
5. Skin and soft-tissue infections.

Although ticarcillin is primarily indicated in gram-negative infections, its *in vitro* activity against gram-positive organisms should be considered in treating infections caused by both gram-negative and gram-positive organisms (see Microbiology).

Based on the *in vitro* synergism between ticarcillin and gentamicin sulfate, tobramycin sulfate or amikacin sulfate against certain strains of *Pseudomonas aeruginosa,* combined therapy has been successful, using full therapeutic dosages. (For additional prescribing information, see the gentamicin sulfate, tobramycin sulfate and amikacin sulfate package inserts.)

NOTE: Culturing and susceptibility testing should be performed initially and during treatment to monitor the effectiveness of therapy and the susceptibility of the bacteria.

CONTRAINDICATIONS

A history of allergic reaction to any of the penicillins is a contraindication.

WARNINGS

Serious and occasionally fatal hypersensitivity (anaphylactoid) reactions have been reported in patients receiving penicillin. These reactions are more likely to occur in persons with a history of sensitivity to multiple allergens.

There are reports of patients with a history of penicillin hypersensitivity reactions who experience severe hypersensitivity reactions when treated with a cephalosporin. Before therapy with a penicillin, careful inquiry should be made about previous hypersensitivity reactions to penicillins, cephalosporins and other allergens. If a reaction occurs, the drug should be discontinued unless, in the opinion of the physician, the condition being treated is life-threatening and amenable only to ticarcillin therapy. **Serious anaphylactoid reactions require immediate emergency treatment with epinephrine. Oxygen, intravenous steroids and airway management, including intubation, should also be administered as indicated.**

Some patients receiving high doses of ticarcillin may develop hemorrhagic manifestations associated with abnormalities of coagulation tests, such as bleeding time and platelet aggregation. On withdrawal of the drug, the bleeding should cease and coagulation abnormalities revert to normal. Other causes of abnormal bleeding should also be considered. Patients with renal impairment, in whom excretion of ticarcillin is delayed, should be observed for bleeding manifestations. Such patients should be dosed strictly according to recommendations (see DOSAGE AND ADMINISTRATION). If bleeding manifestations appear, ticarcillin treatment should be discontinued and appropriate therapy instituted.

Pseudomembranous colitis has been reported with nearly all antibacterial agents, including *Ticar,* and has ranged in severity from mild to life-threatening. Therefore, it is important to consider this diagnosis in patients who present with diarrhea subsequent to the administration of antibacterial agents.

Treatment with antibacterial agents alters the normal flora of the colon and may permit overgrowth of clostridia. Studies indicate that a toxin produced by *Clostridium difficile* is 1 primary cause of "antibiotic-associated colitis."

Mild cases of pseudomembranous colitis usually respond to drug discontinuation alone. In moderate to severe cases, consideration should be given to management with fluids and electrolytes, protein supplementation and treatment with an antibacterial drug effective against *C. difficile.*

PRECAUTIONS

Although *Ticar* exhibits the characteristic low toxicity of the penicillins, as with any other potent agent, it is advisable to check periodically for organ system dysfunction (including renal, hepatic and hematopoietic) during prolonged treatment. If overgrowth of resistant organisms occurs, the appropriate therapy should be initiated.

Since the theoretical sodium content is 5.2 mEq (120 mg) per gram of ticarcillin, and the actual vial content can be as high as 6.5 mEq/gram, electrolyte and cardiac status should be monitored carefully.

In a few patients receiving intravenous ticarcillin, hypokalemia has been reported. Serum potassium should be measured periodically, and, if necessary, corrective therapy should be implemented.

As with any penicillin, the possibility of an allergic response, including anaphylaxis, exists, particularly in hypersensitive patients.

Usage During Pregnancy

Reproduction studies have been performed in mice and rats and have revealed no evidence of impaired fertility or harm to the fetus due to ticarcillin. There are no well-controlled studies in pregnant women, but investigational experience does not include any positive evidence of adverse effects on the fetus. Although there is no clearly defined risk, such experience cannot exclude the possibility of infrequent or subtle damage to the fetus. Ticarcillin should be used in pregnant women only when clearly needed.

ADVERSE REACTIONS

The following adverse reactions may occur:

Hypersensitivity Reactions: Skin rashes, pruritus, urticaria, drug fever.

Gastrointestinal Disturbances: Nausea and vomiting, pseudomembranous colitis. Onset of pseudomembranous colitis symptoms may occur during or after antibiotic treatment. (See WARNINGS.)

Hemic and Lymphatic Systems: As with other penicillins, anemia, thrombocytopenia, leukopenia, neutropenia and eosinophilia.

Abnormalities of Blood, Hepatic and Renal Laboratory Studies: As with other semisynthetic penicillins, SGOT and SGPT elevations have been reported. To date, clinical manifestations of hepatic or renal disorders have not been observed which could be ascribed solely to ticarcillin.

CNS: Patients, especially those with impaired renal function, may experience convulsions or neuromuscular excitability when very high doses of the drug are administered.

Other: Local reactions such as pain (rarely accompanied by induration) at the site of the injection have been reported. Vein irritation and phlebitis can occur, particularly when undiluted solution is directly injected into the vein.

DOSAGE AND ADMINISTRATION

Clinical experience indicates that in serious urinary tract and systemic infections, intravenous therapy in the higher doses should be used. Intramuscular injections should not exceed 2 grams per injection.

[See table at top of previous page]

DIRECTIONS FOR USE

1 gram, 3 gram and 6 gram Standard Vials

Intramuscular Use (concentration of approximately 385 mg/mL): For initial reconstitution use Sterile Water for Injection, USP, Sodium Chloride Injection, USP, or 1% Lidocaine Hydrochloride solution‡ (without epinephrine).

Each gram of ticarcillin should be reconstituted with 2 mL of Sterile Water for Injection, USP, Sodium Chloride Injection, USP, or 1% Lidocaine Hydrochloride solution‡ (without epinephrine) and **used promptly.** Each 2.6 mL of the resulting solution will then contain 1 gram of ticarcillin.

‡For full product information, refer to manufacturer's package insert for Lidocaine Hydrochloride.

Only the 1 gram vial should be used for intramuscular administration. As with all intramuscular preparations, Ticar (ticarcillin disodium) should be injected well within the body of a relatively large muscle using usual techniques and precautions.

Intravenous Administration (concentration of approximately 200 mg/mL): For initial reconstitution use Sodium Chloride Injection, USP, Dextrose Injection 5% or Lactated Ringer's Injection.

Reconstitute each gram of ticarcillin with 4 mL of the appropriate diluent. After the addition of 4 mL of diluent per gram of ticarcillin, each 1.0 mL of the resulting solution will have an approximate concentration of 200 mg. Once dissolved, further dilute if desired.

Direct Intravenous Injection: In order to avoid vein irritation, administer solution as slowly as possible.

Intravenous Infusion: Administer by continuous or intermittent intravenous drip. Intermittent infusion should be administered over a 30 minute to 2-hour period in equally divided doses.

3 gram Piggyback Bottle

Intravenous Infusion (concentrations of approximately 29 mg/mL to 100 mg/mL): The 3 gram bottle should be reconstituted with a minimum of 30 mL of the desired intravenous solution listed below.

Amount of Diluent	Concentration of Solution
100 mL	1 gram/34 mL (~29 mg/mL)
60 mL	1 gram/20 mL (50 mg/mL)
30 mL	1 gram/10 mL (100 mg/mL)

In order to avoid vein irritation, the solution should be administered as slowly as possible. A dilution of approximately 50 mg/mL or more will further reduce the incidence of vein irritation.

Intravenous Infusion: Stability studies in the intravenous solutions listed below indicate that ticarcillin disodium will provide sufficient activity between 21° and 24°C (70° and 75°F) within the stated time periods at concentrations between 10 mg/mL and 50 mg/mL — see Stability Period section below.

After reconstitution and prior to administration *Ticar* as with other parenteral drugs should be inspected visually for particulate matter and discoloration.

[See table below]

Refrigerated solutions stored longer than 72 hours should not be used for multidose purposes.

After reconstitution and dilution to a concentration of 10 mg/mL to 100 mg/mL, this solution can be frozen −18°C (0°F) and stored for up to 30 days. The thawed solution must be used within 24 hours.

Unused solutions should be discarded after the time periods mentioned above.

It is recommended that *Ticar* and gentamicin sulfate, tobramycin sulfate or amikacin sulfate not be mixed together in the same I.V. solution due to the gradual inactivation of gentamicin sulfate, tobramycin sulfate or amikacin sulfate under these circumstances. The therapeutic effect of *Ticar* and these aminoglycoside drugs remains unimpaired when administered separately.

HOW SUPPLIED

Ticar (sterile ticarcillin disodium). Each vial contains ticarcillin disodium equivalent to 1 gram, 3 grams, 6 grams of ticarcillin.

NDC 0029-6550-22 .... 1 gram Vial
NDC 0029-6552-26 .... 3 gram Vial
NDC 0029-6555-26 .... 6 gram Vial
NDC 0029-6552-21 .... 3 gram Piggyback Bottle

Ticar is also supplied as:

NDC 0029-6558-21 ...... 20 gram Pharmacy Bulk Package
NDC 0029-6559-21 ...... 30 gram Pharmacy Bulk Package
NDC 0029-6552-40 ..... 3 gram ADD-Vantage®§ Antibiotic Vial

Ticar (sterile ticarcillin disodium). Each vial contains ticarcillin disodium equivalent to 20 grams, 30 grams, 3 grams of ticarcillin.

Store dry powder at room temperature or below.

§ADD-Vantage® is a trademark of Abbott Laboratories.

TR:L4IV

TIMENTIN® ℞

[*tī ′mĕn-tĭn*]

brand of sterile ticarcillin disodium and clavulanate potassium for Intravenous Administration

DESCRIPTION

Timentin is a sterile injectable antibacterial combination consisting of the semisynthetic antibiotic, ticarcillin disodium, and the β-lactamase inhibitor, clavulanate potassium (the potassium salt of clavulanic acid), for intravenous administration. Ticarcillin is derived from the basic penicillin nucleus, 6-amino-penicillanic acid.

Chemically, ticarcillin disodium is *N*-(2-Carboxy-3,3-dimethyl -7-oxo-4-thia-1-azabicyclo[3.2.0] hept-6-yl)-3-thiophenemalonamic acid disodium salt and may be represented as:

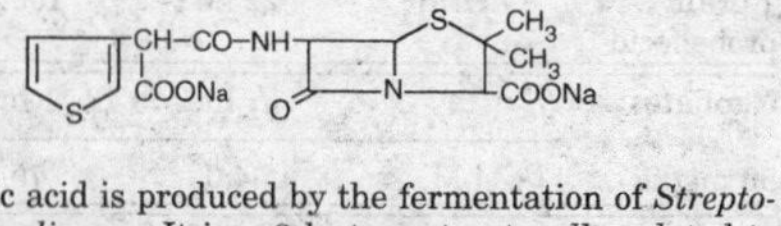

Clavulanic acid is produced by the fermentation of *Streptomyces clavuligerus.* It is a β-lactam structurally related to the penicillins and possesses the ability to inactivate a wide variety of β-lactamases by blocking the active sites of these enzymes. Clavulanic acid is particularly active against the clinically important plasmid-mediated β-lactamases frequently responsible for transferred drug resistance to penicillins and cephalosporins.

STABILITY PERIOD

Intravenous Solution (concentration of 10 mg/mL to 100 mg/mL)	Room Temperature 21° to 24°C (70° to 75°F)	Refrigeration 4°C (40°F)
Sodium Chloride Injection, USP	72 hours	14 days
Dextrose Injection 5%	72 hours	14 days
Lactated Ringer's Injection	48 hours	14 days

Chemically, clavulanate potassium is potassium (Z)-(2*R*,5*R*)-3-(2-hydroxyethylidene)-7-oxo-4-oxa-1-azabicyclo [3.2.0]heptane-2-carboxylate and may be represented structurally as:

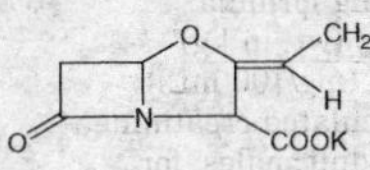

Timentin is supplied as a white to pale yellow powder for reconstitution. *Timentin* is very soluble in water, its solubility being greater than 600 mg/mL. The reconstituted solution is clear, colorless or pale yellow, having a pH of 5.5 to 7.5.

For the *Timentin* 3.1 gram and 3.2 gram dosages, the theoretical sodium content is 4.75 mEq (109 mg) per gram of *Timentin*. The theoretical potassium content is 0.15 mEq (6 mg) and 0.3 mEq (11.9 mg) per gram of *Timentin* for the 3.1 gram and 3.2 gram dosages, respectively.

CLINICAL PHARMACOLOGY

After an intravenous infusion (30 min.) of 3.1 grams or 3.2 grams *Timentin*, peak serum concentrations of both ticarcillin and clavulanic acid are attained immediately after completion of infusion. Ticarcillin serum levels are similar to those produced by the administration of equivalent amounts of ticarcillin alone with a mean peak serum level of 330 μg/mL for the 3.1 gram and 3.2 gram formulations. The corresponding mean peak serum levels for clavulanic acid were 8 μg/mL and 16 μg/mL for the 3.1 gram and 3.2 gram formulations, respectively. (See following table.)

[See first table above]

The mean area under the serum concentration curves for ticarcillin was 485 μg.hr./mL for the *Timentin* 3.1 gram and 3.2 gram formulations. The corresponding areas under the serum concentration curves for clavulanic acid were 8.2 μg.hr./mL and 15.6 μg.hr./mL for the *Timentin* 3.1 gram and 3.2 gram formulations, respectively.

The mean serum half-lives of ticarcillin and clavulanic acid in healthy volunteers are 1.1 hours and 1.1 hours, respectively, following administration of 3.1 grams or 3.2 grams of *Timentin*.

In pediatric patients receiving approximately 50 mg/kg *Timentin* (30:1 ratio ticarcillin to clavulanate), mean ticarcillin serum half-lives were 4.4 hours in neonates (n=18) and 1.0 hour in infants and children (n=41). The corresponding clavulanate serum half-lives averaged 1.9 hours in neonates (n=14) and 0.9 hour in infants and children (n=40). Area under the serum concentration time curves averaged 339 μg.hr./mL in infants and children (n=41), whereas the corresponding mean clavulanate area under the serum concentration time curves was approximately 7 μg.hr./mL in the same population (n=40).

Approximately 60% to 70% of ticarcillin and approximately 35% to 45% of clavulanic acid are excreted unchanged in urine during the first 6 hours after administration of a single dose of *Timentin* to normal volunteers with normal renal function. Two hours after an intravenous injection of 3.1 grams or 3.2 grams *Timentin*, concentrations of ticarcillin in urine generally exceed 1500 μg/mL. The corresponding concentrations of clavulanic acid in urine generally exceed 40 μg/mL and 70 μg/mL following administration of the 3.1 gram and 3.2 gram doses, respectively. By 4 to 6 hours after injection, the urine concentrations of ticarcillin and clavulanic acid usually decline to approximately 190 μg/mL and 2 μg/mL, respectively, for both doses. Neither component of *Timentin* is highly protein bound; ticarcillin has been found to be approximately 45% bound to human serum protein and clavulanic acid approximately 9% bound.

Somewhat higher and more prolonged serum levels of ticarcillin can be achieved with the concurrent administration of probenecid; however, probenecid does not enhance the serum levels of clavulanic acid.

Ticarcillin can be detected in tissues and interstitial fluid following parenteral administration.

Penetration of ticarcillin into bile and pleural fluid has been demonstrated. The results of experiments involving the administration of clavulanic acid to animals suggest that this compound, like ticarcillin, is well distributed in body tissues.

An inverse relationship exists between the serum half-life of ticarcillin and creatinine clearance. The dosage of *Timentin* need only be adjusted in cases of severe renal impairment. (See **DOSAGE AND ADMINISTRATION.**)

Ticarcillin may be removed from patients undergoing dialysis; the actual amount removed depends on the duration and type of dialysis.

MICROBIOLOGY: Ticarcillin is a semisynthetic antibiotic with a broad spectrum of bactericidal activity against many gram-positive and gram-negative aerobic and anaerobic bacteria.

Ticarcillin is, however, susceptible to degradation by β-lactamases and, therefore, the spectrum of activity does not normally include organisms which produce these enzymes. Clavulanic acid is a β-lactam, structurally related to the penicillins, which possesses the ability to inactivate a wide range of β-lactamase enzymes commonly found in microorganisms resistant to penicillins and cephalosporins. In particular, it has good activity against the clinically important plasmid-mediated β-lactamases frequently responsible for transferred drug resistance.

SERUM LEVELS IN ADULTS
AFTER A 30-MINUTE I.V. INFUSION OF TIMENTIN®

TICARCILLIN SERUM LEVELS (μg/mL)

Dose	0	15 min.	30 min.	1 hr.	1.5 hr.	3.5 hr.	5.5 hr.
3.1 gram	324	223	176	131	90	27	6
	(293 to 388)	(184 to 293)	(135 to 235)	(102 to 195)	(65 to 119)	(19 to 37)	(5 to 7)
3.2 gram	336	214	186	122	78	29	10
	(301 to 386)	(180 to 258)	(160 to 218)	(108 to 136)	(33 to 113)	(19 to 44)	(5 to 15)

CLAVULANIC ACID SERUM LEVELS (μg/mL)

Dose	0	15 min.	30 min.	1 hr.	1.5 hr.	3.5 hr.	5.5 hr.
3.1 gram	8.0	4.6	2.6	1.8	1.2	0.3	0
	(5.3 to 10.3)	(3.0 to 7.6)	(1.8 to 3.4)	(1.6 to 2.2)	(0.8 to 1.6)	(0.2 to 0.3)	
3.2 gram	15.8	8.3	5.2	3.4	2.5	0.5	0
	(11.7 to 21.0)	(6.4 to 10.0)	(3.5 to 6.3)	(1.9 to 4.0)	(1.3 to 3.4)	(0.2 to 0.8)	

RECOMMENDED RANGES FOR *TIMENTIN* SUSCEPTIBILITY TESTING[1–3]

Diffusion Method Disk Zone Size, mm: Res.	Inter.	Susc.	Dilution Method MIC Correlates[4], mcg/mL: Res.	Susc.
≤11	12 to 14	≥15	≥128	≤64

[1] The non-β-lactamase-producing organisms which are normally susceptible to ticarcillin will have similar zone sizes as for ticarcillin.

[2] Staphylococci which are susceptible to *Timentin* but resistant to methicillin, oxacillin or nafcillin must be considered as resistant.

[3] The quality control cultures should have the following assigned daily ranges for *Timentin*:

		Disks	MIC Range (mcg/mL)
E. coli	(ATCC 25922)	24 to 30 mm	2/2 to 8/2
S. aureus	(ATCC 25923)	32 to 40 mm	—
Ps. aeruginosa	(ATCC 27853)	20 to 28 mm	8/2 to 32/2
E. coli	(ATCC 35218)	21 to 25 mm	4/2 to 16/2
S. aureus	(ATCC 29213)	—	0.5/2 to 2/2

[4] Expressed as concentration of ticarcillin in the presence of a constant 2.0 mcg/mL concentration of clavulanic acid.

The formulation of ticarcillin with clavulanic acid in *Timentin* protects ticarcillin from degradation by β-lactamase enzymes and effectively extends the antibiotic spectrum of ticarcillin to include many bacteria normally resistant to ticarcillin and other β-lactam antibiotics. Thus *Timentin* possesses the distinctive properties of a broad-spectrum antibiotic and a β-lactamase inhibitor.

While *in vitro* studies have demonstrated the susceptibility of most strains of the following organisms, clinical efficacy for infections other than those included in the INDICATIONS AND USAGE section has not been documented:

GRAM-NEGATIVE BACTERIA: *Pseudomonas aeruginosa* (β-lactamase and non-β-lactamase producing), *Pseudomonas* species including *P. maltophilia* (β-lactamase and non-β-lactamase producing), *Escherichia coli* (β-lactamase and non-β-lactamase producing), *Proteus mirabilis* (β-lactamase and non-β-lactamase producing), *Proteus vulgaris* (β-lactamase and non-β-lactamase producing), *Providencia rettgeri* (formerly *Proteus rettgeri*) (β-lactamase and non-β-lactamase producing), *Providencia stuartii* (β-lactamase and non-β-lactamase producing), *Morganella morganii* (formerly *Proteus morganii*) (β-lactamase and non-β-lactamase producing), *Enterobacter* species (Although most strains of *Enterobacter* species are resistant *in vitro*, clinical efficacy has been demonstrated with *Timentin* in urinary tract infections caused by these organisms.), *Acinetobacter* species (β-lactamase and non-β-lactamase producing), *Hemophilus influenzae* (β-lactamase and non-β-lactamase producing), *Branhamella catarrhalis* (β-lactamase and non-β-lactamase producing), *Serratia* species including *S. marcescens* (β-lactamase and non-β-lactamase producing), *Neisseria gonorrhoeae* (β-lactamase and non-β-lactamase producing), *Neisseria meningitidis**, *Salmonella* species (β-lactamase and non-β-lactamase producing), *Klebsiella* species including *K. pneumoniae* (β-lactamase and non-β-lactamase producing), *Citrobacter* species including *C. freundii, C. diversus* and *C. amalonaticus* (β-lactamase and non-β-lactamase producing).

GRAM-POSITIVE BACTERIA: *Staphylococcus aureus* (β-lactamase and non-β-lactamase producing), *Staphylococcus saprophyticus, Staphylococcus epidermidis* (coagulase-negative staphylococci) (β-lactamase and non-β-lactamase producing), *Streptococcus pneumoniae** (*D. pneumoniae*), *Streptococcus bovis**, *Streptococcus agalactiae** (Group B), *Streptococcus faecalis** (*Enterococcus*), *Streptococcus pyogenes** (Group A, β-hemolytic), Viridans group streptococci*.

ANAEROBIC BACTERIA: *Bacteroides* species, including *B. fragilis* group (*B. fragilis, B. vulgatus*) (β-lactamase and non-β-lactamase producing), non-*B. fragilis* (*B. melaninogenicus*) (β-lactamase and non-β-lactamase producing), *B. thetaiotaomicron, B. ovatus, B. distasonis* (β-lactamase and non-β-lactamase-producing), *Clostridium* species including *C. perfringens, C. difficile, C. sporogenes, C. ramosum* and *C. bifermentans**, *Eubacterium* species, *Fusobacterium* species including *F. nucleatum* and *F. necrophorum**, *Peptococcus* species*, *Peptostreptococcus* species*, *Veillonella* species.

*These are non-β-lactamase-producing strains and therefore are susceptible to ticarcillin alone. Some of the β-lactamase-producing strains are also susceptible to ticarcillin alone.

In vitro synergism between *Timentin* and gentamicin, tobramycin or amikacin against multiresistant strains of *Pseudomonas aeruginosa* has been demonstrated.

SUSCEPTIBILITY TESTING:

Diffusion Technique: An 85 mcg *Timentin* (75 mcg ticarcillin plus 10 mcg clavulanic acid) diffusion disk is available for use with the Kirby-Bauer method. Based on the zone sizes given below, a report of "Susceptible" indicates that the infecting organism is likely to respond to *Timentin* therapy, while a report of "Resistant" indicates that the organism is not likely to respond to therapy with this antibiotic. A report of "Intermediate" susceptibility indicates that the organism would be susceptible to *Timentin* at a higher dosage or if the infection is confined to tissues or fluids (e.g., urine) in which high antibiotic levels are attained.

Dilution Technique: Broth or agar dilution methods may be used to determine the minimal inhibitory concentration (MIC) values for bacterial isolates to *Timentin*. Tubes should be inoculated with the test culture containing 10^4 to 10^5 CFU/mL or plates spotted with a test solution containing 10^3 to 10^4 CFU/mL.

The recommended dilution pattern utilizes a constant level of clavulanic acid, 2 mcg/mL, in all tubes together with varying amounts of ticarcillin. MICs are expressed in terms of the ticarcillin concentration in the presence of 2 mcg/mL clavulanic acid.

[See second table above]

INDICATIONS AND USAGE

Timentin is indicated in the treatment of infections caused by susceptible strains of the designated microorganisms in the conditions listed below:

Septicemia, including bacteremia, caused by β-lactamase-producing strains of *Klebsiella* spp.*, *E. coli**, *Staphylococcus aureus**, or *Pseudomonas aeruginosa** (or other *Pseudomonas* species*)

Lower Respiratory Infections caused by β-lactamase-producing strains of *Staphylococcus aureus, Hemophilus influenzae**, or *Klebsiella* spp.*

Bone and Joint Infections caused by β-lactamase-producing strains of *Staphylococcus aureus*

Continued on next page

Information on the SmithKline Beecham Pharmaceuticals products appearing here is based on the labeling in effect on July 31, 1998. Further information on these and other products may be obtained from the Medical Department, SmithKline Beecham Pharmaceuticals, One Franklin Plaza, Philadelphia, PA 19101.

Timentin—Cont.

Skin and Skin Structure Infections caused by β-lactamase-producing strains of *Staphylococcus aureus, Klebsiella* spp.*, or *E. coli**

Urinary Tract Infections (complicated and uncomplicated) caused by β-lactamase-producing strains of *E. coli, Klebsiella* spp., *Pseudomonas aeruginosa** (or other *Pseudomonas* spp.*), *Citrobacter* spp.*, *Enterobacter cloacae**, *Serratia marcescens**, or *Staphylococcus aureus**

Gynecologic Infections endometritis caused by β-lactamase-producing strains of *B. melaninogenicus**, *Enterobacter* spp. (including *E. cloacae**), *Escherichia coli, Klebsiella pneumoniae**, *Staphylococcus aureus*, or *Staphylococcus epidermidis*

Intra-abdominal Infections peritonitis caused by β-lactamase-producing strains of *Escherichia coli, Klebsiella pneumoniae*, or *Bacteroides fragilis** group

*Efficacy for this organism in this organ system was studied in fewer than 10 infections.

NOTE: For information on use in pediatric patients (≥3 months of age) see PRECAUTIONS–Pediatric Use and CLINICAL STUDIES sections. There are insufficient data to support the use of *Timentin* in pediatric patients under 3 months of age or for the treatment of septicemia and/or infections in the pediatric population where the suspected or proven pathogen is *Haemophilus influenzae* type b.

While *Timentin* is indicated only for the conditions listed above, infections caused by ticarcillin-susceptible organisms are also amenable to *Timentin* treatment due to its ticarcillin content. Therefore, mixed infections caused by ticarcillin-susceptible organisms and β-lactamase-producing organisms susceptible to ticarcillin/clavulanic acid should not require the addition of another antibiotic.

Appropriate culture and susceptibility tests should be performed before treatment in order to isolate and identify organisms causing infection and to determine their susceptibility to ticarcillin/clavulanic acid. Because of its broad spectrum of bactericidal activity against gram-positive and gram-negative bacteria, *Timentin* is particularly useful for the treatment of mixed infections and for presumptive therapy prior to the identification of the causative organisms. *Timentin* has been shown to be effective as single drug therapy in the treatment of some serious infections where normally combination antibiotic therapy might be employed. Therapy with *Timentin* may be initiated before results of such tests are known when there is reason to believe the infection may involve any of the β-lactamase-producing organisms listed above; however, once these results become available, appropriate therapy should be continued.

Based on the *in vitro* synergism between ticarcillin/clavulanic acid and aminoglycosides against certain strains of *Pseudomonas aeruginosa*, combined therapy has been successful, especially in patients with impaired host defenses. Both drugs should be used in full therapeutic doses. As soon as results of culture and susceptibility tests become available, antimicrobial therapy should be adjusted as indicated.

CONTRAINDICATIONS

Timentin is contraindicated in patients with a history of hypersensitivity reactions to any of the penicillins.

WARNINGS

SERIOUS AND OCCASIONALLY FATAL HYPERSENSITIVITY (ANAPHYLACTIC) REACTIONS HAVE BEEN REPORTED IN PATIENTS ON PENICILLIN THERAPY. THESE REACTIONS ARE MORE LIKELY TO OCCUR IN INDIVIDUALS WITH A HISTORY OF PENICILLIN HYPERSENSITIVITY AND/OR A HISTORY OF SENSITIVITY TO MULTIPLE ALLERGENS. THERE HAVE BEEN REPORTS OF INDIVIDUALS WITH A HISTORY OF PENICILLIN HYPERSENSITIVITY WHO HAVE EXPERIENCED SEVERE REACTIONS WHEN TREATED WITH CEPHALOSPORINS. BEFORE INITIATING THERAPY WITH *TIMENTIN*, CAREFUL INQUIRY SHOULD BE MADE CONCERNING PREVIOUS HYPERSENSITIVITY REACTIONS TO PENICILLINS, CEPHALOSPORINS, OR OTHER ALLERGENS. IF AN ALLERGIC REACTION OCCURS, *TIMENTIN* SHOULD BE DISCONTINUED AND THE APPROPRIATE THERAPY INSTITUTED. **SERIOUS ANAPHYLACTIC REACTIONS REQUIRE IMMEDIATE EMERGENCY TREATMENT WITH EPINEPHRINE. OXYGEN, INTRAVENOUS STEROIDS AND AIRWAY MANAGEMENT, INCLUDING INTUBATION, SHOULD ALSO BE PROVIDED AS INDICATED.**

Pseudomembranous colitis has been reported with nearly all antibacterial agents, including *Timentin*, and may range in severity from mild to life-threatening. Therefore, it is important to consider this diagnosis in patients who present with diarrhea subsequent to the administration of antibacterial agents.

Treatment with antibacterial agents alters the normal flora of the colon and may permit overgrowth of clostridia. Studies indicate that a toxin produced by *Clostridium difficile* is a primary cause of "antibiotic-associated colitis."

Creatinine clearance mL/min.	Dosage
over 60	3.1 grams every 4 hrs.
30 to 60	2 grams every 4 hrs.
10 to 30	2 grams every 8 hrs.
less than 10	2 grams every 12 hrs.
less than 10 with hepatic dysfunction	2 grams every 24 hrs.
patients on peritoneal dialysis	3.1 grams every 12 hrs.
patients on hemodialysis	2 grams every 12 hrs. supplemented with 3.1 grams after each dialysis

To calculate creatinine clearance‡ from a serum creatinine value use the following formula.

$$C_{cr} = \frac{(140 - Age)(wt. \text{ in kg})}{72 \times S_{cr} \text{ (mg/100 mL)}}$$

This is the calculated creatinine clearance for adult males; for females it is 15% less.

‡Cockcroft, D.W., et al: Prediction of Creatinine Clearance from Serum Creatinine. Nephron 16:31–41, 1976.

†The half-life of ticarcillin in patients with renal failure is approximately 13 hours.

STABILITY PERIOD
(3.1 gram and 3.2 gram Vials and Piggyback Bottles)

Intravenous Solution (ticarcillin concentrations of 10 mg/mL to 100 mg/mL)	Room Temperature 21° to 24°C (70° to 75°F)	Refrigerated 4°C (40°F)
Dextrose Injection 5%, USP	24 hours	3 days
Sodium Chloride Injection, USP	24 hours	7 days
Lactated Ringer's Injection, USP	24 hours	7 days

After the diagnosis of pseudomembranous colitis has been established, appropriate therapeutic measures should be initiated. Mild cases of pseudomembranous colitis usually respond to drug discontinuation alone. In moderate to severe cases, consideration should be given to management with fluids and electrolytes, protein supplementation and treatment with an antibacterial drug clinically effective against *Clostridium difficile* colitis.

When very high doses of *Timentin* are administered, especially in the presence of impaired renal function, patients may experience convulsions. (See **ADVERSE REACTIONS** and **OVERDOSAGE**.)

PRECAUTIONS

General: While *Timentin* possesses the characteristic low toxicity of the penicillin group of antibiotics, periodic assessment of organ system functions, including renal, hepatic, and hematopoietic function, is advisable during prolonged therapy.

Bleeding manifestations have occurred in some patients receiving β-lactam antibiotics. These reactions have been associated with abnormalities of coagulation tests such as clotting time, platelet aggregation, and prothrombin time and are more likely to occur in patients with renal impairment.

If bleeding manifestations appear, *Timentin* treatment should be discontinued and appropriate therapy instituted.

Timentin has only rarely been reported to cause hypokalemia; however, the possibility of this occurring should be kept in mind particularly when treating patients with fluid and electrolyte imbalance. Periodic monitoring of serum potassium may be advisable in patients receiving prolonged therapy.

The theoretical sodium content is 4.75 mEq (109 mg) per gram of *Timentin*. This should be considered when treating patients requiring restricted salt intake.

As with any penicillin, an allergic reaction, including anaphylaxis, may occur during *Timentin* administration, particularly in a hypersensitive individual.

The possibility of superinfections with mycotic or bacterial pathogens should be kept in mind, particularly during prolonged treatment. If superinfections occur, appropriate measures should be taken.

Drug/Laboratory Test Interactions: As with other penicillins, the mixing of *Timentin* with an aminoglycoside in solutions for parenteral administration can result in substantial inactivation of the aminoglycoside.

Probenecid interferes with the renal tubular secretion of ticarcillin, thereby increasing serum concentrations and prolonging serum half-life of the antibiotic.

High urine concentrations of ticarcillin may produce false-positive protein reactions (pseudoproteinuria) with the following methods: sulfosalicylic acid and boiling test, acetic acid test, biuret reaction and nitric acid test. The bromphenol blue (Multi-stix®) reagent strip test has been reported to be reliable.

The presence of clavulanic acid in *Timentin* may cause a nonspecific binding of IgG and albumin by red cell membranes leading to a false-positive Coombs test.

Carcinogenesis, Mutagenesis, Impairment of Fertility: Long-term studies in animals have not been performed to evaluate carcinogenic potential. However, results from assays for gene mutation *in vitro* using bacteria (Ames tests) and yeast, and for chromosomal effects *in vitro* in human lymphocytes, and *in vivo* in mouse bone marrow (micronucleus test) indicate that *Timentin* is without any mutagenic potential.

Pregnancy (Category B): Reproduction studies have been performed in rats given doses up to 1050 mg/kg/day and have revealed no evidence of impaired fertility or harm to the fetus due to *Timentin*. There are, however, no adequate and well-controlled studies in pregnant women. Because animal reproduction studies are not always predictive of human response, this drug should be used during pregnancy only if clearly needed.

Nursing Mothers: It is not known whether this drug is excreted in human milk. Because many drugs are excreted in human milk, caution should be exercised when *Timentin* is administered to a nursing woman.

Pediatric Use: The safety and effectiveness of *Timentin* have been established in the age group of 3 months to 16 years. Use of *Timentin* in these age groups is supported by evidence from adequate and well-controlled studies of *Timentin* in adults with additional efficacy, safety, and pharmacokinetic data from both comparative and non-comparative studies in pediatric patients. There are insufficient data to support the use of *Timentin* in pediatric patients under 3 months of age or for the treatment of septicemia and/or infections in the pediatric population where the suspected or proven pathogen is *Haemophilus influenzae* type b.

In those patients in whom meningeal seeding from a distant infection site or in whom meningitis is suspected or documented, or in patients who require prophylaxis against central nervous system infection, an alternate agent with demonstrated clinical efficacy in this setting should be used.

ADVERSE REACTIONS

As with other penicillins, the following adverse reactions may occur:

Hypersensitivity reactions: skin rash, pruritus, urticaria, arthralgia, myalgia, drug fever, chills, chest discomfort, and anaphylactic reactions

Central nervous system: headache, giddiness, neuromuscular hyperirritability, or convulsive seizures

Gastrointestinal disturbances: disturbances of taste and smell, stomatitis, flatulence, nausea, vomiting and diarrhea, epigastric pain, and pseudomembranous colitis have been reported. Onset of pseudomembranous colitis symptoms may occur during or after antibiotic treatment. (See **WARNINGS**.)

Hemic and lymphatic systems: thrombocytopenia, leukopenia, neutropenia, eosinophilia, reduction of hemoglobin or hematocrit, and prolongation of prothrombin time and bleeding time

Abnormalities of hepatic and renal function tests: elevation of serum aspartate aminotransferase (SGOT), serum alanine aminotransferase (SGPT), serum alkaline phosphatase, serum LDH, serum bilirubin. There have been reports of transient hepatitis and cholestatic jaundice—as with some other penicillins and some cephalosporins. Elevation of serum creatinine and/or BUN, hypernatremia, reduction in serum potassium and uric acid

Local reactions: pain, burning, swelling, and induration at the injection site and thrombophlebitis with intravenous administration

Available safety data for pediatric patients treated with *Timentin* demonstrate a similar adverse event profile to that observed in adult patients.

DRUG ABUSE AND DEPENDENCE

Neither *Timentin* abuse nor *Timentin* dependence has been reported.

OVERDOSAGE

As with other penicillins, neurotoxic reactions may arise when very high doses of *Timentin* are administered, especially in patients with impaired renal function. (See **WARNINGS** and **ADVERSE REACTIONS**—*Central nervous system.*)

In case of overdosage, discontinue *Timentin*, treat symptomatically, and institute supportive measures as required. Ticarcillin may be removed from circulation by hemodialysis. The molecular weight, degree of protein binding, and pharmacokinetic profile of clavulanic acid together with information from a single patient with renal insufficiency all suggest that this compound may also be removed by hemodialysis.

DOSAGE AND ADMINISTRATION

Timentin should be administered by intravenous infusion (30 min.).

Adults: The usual recommended dosage for systemic and urinary tract infections for average (60 kg) adults is 3.1 grams *Timentin* (3.1 gram vial containing 3 grams ticarcillin and 100 mg clavulanic acid) given every 4 to 6 hours. For gynecologic infections, *Timentin* should be administered as follows: Moderate infections 200 mg/kg/day in divided doses every 6 hours and for severe infections 300 mg/kg/day in divided doses every 4 hours. For patients weighing less than 60 kg, the recommended dosage is 200 to 300 mg/kg/day, based on ticarcillin content, given in divided doses every 4 to 6 hours.

In urinary tract infections, a dosage of 3.2 grams *Timentin* (3.2 gram vial containing 3 grams ticarcillin and 200 mg clavulanic acid) given every 8 hours is adequate.

Pediatric Patients (≥3 months):

For patients <60 kg:

In patients <60 kg, *Timentin* is dosed at 50 mg/kg/dose based on the ticarcillin component. *Timentin* should be administered as follows: Mild to moderate infections 200 mg/kg/day in divided doses every 6 hours; for severe infections, 300 mg/kg/day in divided doses every 4 hours.

For patients ≥60 kg:

For mild to moderate infections, 3.1 grams *Timentin* (3 grams of ticarcillin and 100 mg of clavulanic acid) administered every 6 hours; for severe infections, 3.1 grams every 4 hours.

Renal impairment:

For infections complicated by renal insufficiency†, an initial loading dose of 3.1 grams should be followed by doses based on creatinine clearance and type of dialysis as indicated below:

[See first table at top of previous page]

Dosage for any individual patient must take into consideration the site and severity of infection, the susceptibility of the organisms causing infection, and the status of the patient's host defense mechanisms.

The duration of therapy depends upon the severity of infection. Generally, *Timentin* should be continued for at least 2 days after the signs and symptoms of infection have disappeared. The usual duration is 10 to 14 days; however, in difficult and complicated infections, more prolonged therapy may be required.

Frequent bacteriologic and clinical appraisals are necessary during therapy of chronic urinary tract infection and may be required for several months after therapy has been completed; persistent infections may require treatment for several weeks, and doses smaller than those indicated above should not be used.

In certain infections, involving abscess formation, appropriate surgical drainage should be performed in conjunction with antimicrobial therapy.

INTRAVENOUS ADMINISTRATION
DIRECTIONS FOR USE
3.1 gram and 3.2 gram Vials and Piggyback Bottles

The 3.1 gram or 3.2 gram vial should be reconstituted by adding approximately 13 mL of Sterile Water for Injection, USP, or Sodium Chloride Injection, USP, and shaking well. When dissolved, the concentration of ticarcillin will be approximately 200 mg/mL with corresponding concentrations of 6.7 mg/mL and 13.4 mg/mL clavulanic acid for the 3.1 gram and 3.2 gram respective doses. Conversely, each 5.0 mL of the 3.1 gram dose reconstituted with approximately 13 mL of diluent will contain approximately 1 gram of ticarcillin and 33 mg of clavulanic acid. For the 3.2 gram dose reconstituted with 13 mL of diluent, each 5.0 mL will contain 1 gram of ticarcillin and 66 mg of clavulanic acid.

INTRAVENOUS INFUSION: The dissolved drug should be further diluted to desired volume using the recommended solution listed in the COMPATIBILITY AND STABILITY Section (STABILITY PERIOD) to a concentration between 10 mg/mL to 100 mg/mL. The solution of reconstituted drug may then be administered over a period of 30 minutes by direct infusion or through a Y-type intravenous infusion set. If this method or the "piggyback" method of administration is used, it is advisable to discontinue temporarily the administration of any other solutions during the infusion of *Timentin*.

Stability—For I.V. solutions, see STABILITY PERIOD below.

When *Timentin* is given in combination with another antimicrobial, such as an aminoglycoside, each drug should be given separately in accordance with the recommended dosage and routes of administration for each drug.

After reconstitution and prior to administration, *Timentin*, as with other parenteral drugs, should be inspected visually for particulate matter. If this condition is evident, the solution should be discarded.

The color of reconstituted solutions of *Timentin* normally ranges from light to dark yellow depending on concentration, duration and temperature of storage while maintaining label claim characteristics.

COMPATIBILITY AND STABILITY
3.1 gram and 3.2 gram Vials and Piggyback Bottles
(Dilutions derived from a stock solution of 200 mg/mL)

The concentrated stock solution at 200 mg/mL is stable for up to 6 hours at room temperature 21° to 24°C (70° to 75°F) or up to 72 hours under refrigeration 4°C (40°F).

If the concentrated stock solution (200 mg/mL) is held for up to 6 hours at room temperature 21° to 24°C (70° to 75°F) or up to 72 hours under refrigeration 4°C (40°F) and further diluted to a concentration between 10 mg/mL and 100 mg/mL with any of the diluents listed below, then the following stability periods apply.

[See second table at top of previous page]

If the concentrated stock solution (200 mg/mL) is stored for up to 6 hours at room temperature and then further diluted to a concentration between 10 mg/mL and 100 mg/mL, solutions of Sodium Chloride Injection, USP, and Lactated Ringer's Injection, USP, may be stored frozen −18°C (0°F) for up to 30 days. Solutions prepared with Dextrose Injection 5%, USP, may be stored frozen −18°C (0°F) for up to 7 days. All thawed solutions should be used within 8 hours or discarded. Once thawed, solutions should not be refrozen.

NOTE: *Timentin* is incompatible with Sodium Bicarbonate. Unused solutions must be discarded after the time periods listed above.

HOW SUPPLIED

Timentin (sterile ticarcillin disodium and clavulanate potassium).

Each 3.1 gram vial contains sterile ticarcillin disodium equivalent to 3 grams ticarcillin and sterile clavulanate potassium equivalent to 0.1 gram clavulanic acid.

NDC 0029-6571-26 .... 3.1 gram Vial
NDC 0029-6571-21 .... 3.1 gram Piggyback Bottle

Timentin is also supplied as:

NDC 0029-6571-40 .... 3.1 gram ADD-Vantage®§ Antibiotic Vial

Each 31 gram Pharmacy Bulk Package contains sterile ticarcillin disodium equivalent to 30 grams ticarcillin and sterile clavulanate potassium equivalent to 1 gram clavulanic acid.

NDC 0029-6579-21 .... 31 gram Pharmacy Bulk Package

Timentin vials should be stored at or below 24°C (75°F).

NDC 0029-6571-31 ...... *Timentin* as an iso-osmotic, sterile, nonpyrogenic, frozen solution in Galaxy®[II] (PL 2040) Plastic Containers—supplied in 100 mL single-dose containers equivalent to 3 grams ticarcillin and clavulanate potassium equivalent to 0.1 gram clavulanic acid.

CLINICAL STUDIES

Timentin has been studied in a total of 296 pediatric patients (excluding neonates and infants less than 3 months) in six controlled clinical trials. The majority of patients studied had intra-abdominal infections, and the primary comparator was clindamycin and gentamicin with or without ampicillin. At the end-of-therapy visit, comparable efficacy was reported in the *Timentin* and appropriate comparator arms.

Timentin was also evaluated in an additional 408 pediatric patients (excluding neonates and infants less than 3 months) in three uncontrolled U.S. clinical trials. Patients were treated across a broad range of presenting diagnoses including: infections in bone and joint, skin and skin structure, lower respiratory tract, urinary tract, as well as intra-abdominal and gynecologic infections. Patients received *Timentin* either 300 mg/kg/day (based on the ticarcillin component) divided q4h for severe infection or 200 mg/kg/day (based on the ticarcillin component) divided q6h for mild to moderate infections. The efficacy rates were comparable to those obtained in the controlled trials.

The adverse event profile in these 704 *Timentin*-treated pediatric patients was comparable to that seen in adult patients.

§ADD-Vantage® is a trademark of Abbott Laboratories.

[II]Galaxy® is a trademark of Baxter International Inc.

Veterans Administration/Military/PHS—Injection, 3.1 gram, 50 mL, 1's 6505-01-312-9086; 3.1 gram, 100 mL Pharmacy Bulk, 1's 6505-01-231-9930; 3.1 gram, ADD-Vantage, 1's 6505-01-283-0066; 31.0 gram, 100 mL Bulk, 1's 6505-01-267-7965; 3.1 gram, frozen bag, 12's, 6505-01-344-1132.

TI:L7IV

Shown in Product Identification Guide, page 340

URISPAS® ℞

[*yore 'eh-spaz*]
brand of flavoxate HCl
100 mg tablets

DESCRIPTION

Urispas (flavoxate HCl) tablets contain flavoxate hydrochloride, a synthetic urinary tract spasmolytic.

Chemically, flavoxate hydrochloride is 2-piperidinoethyl 3-methyl -4- oxo-2- phenyl -4H- 1-benzopyran -8- carboxylate hydrochloride. The empirical formula of flavoxate hydrochloride is $C_{24}H_{25}NO_4 \cdot HCl$. The molecular weight is 427.94.

Urispas is supplied in tablets for oral administration. Each round, white, film-coated *Urispas* tablet is debossed URISPAS SKF and contains flavoxate hydrochloride, 100 mg. Inactive ingredients consist of calcium phosphate, castor oil, cellulose acetate phthalate, magnesium stearate, polyethylene glycol, starch and talc.

CLINICAL PHARMACOLOGY

Flavoxate hydrochloride counteracts smooth muscle spasm of the urinary tract and exerts its effect directly on the muscle.

In a single study of 11 normal male subjects, the time to onset of action was 55 minutes. The peak effect was observed at 112 minutes. 57% of the flavoxate HCl was excreted in the urine within 24 hours.

INDICATIONS AND USAGE

Urispas (flavoxate HCl) is indicated for symptomatic relief of dysuria, urgency, nocturia, suprapubic pain, frequency and incontinence as may occur in cystitis, prostatitis, urethritis, urethrocystitis/urethrotrigonitis. *Urispas* is not indicated for definitive treatment, but is compatible with drugs used for the treatment of urinary tract infections.

CONTRAINDICATIONS

Urispas (flavoxate HCl) is contraindicated in patients who have any of the following obstructive conditions: pyloric or duodenal obstruction, obstructive intestinal lesions or ileus, achalasia, gastrointestinal hemorrhage and obstructive uropathies of the lower urinary tract.

WARNINGS

Urispas (flavoxate HCl) should be given cautiously in patients with suspected glaucoma.

PRECAUTIONS

Information for Patients: Patients should be informed that if drowsiness and blurred vision occur, they should not operate a motor vehicle or machinery or participate in activities where alertness is required.

Carcinogenesis, Mutagenesis, Impairment of Fertility: Mutagenicity studies and long-term studies in animals to determine the carcinogenic potential of Urispas (flavoxate HCl) have not been performed.

Pregnancy: Teratogenic Effects—Pregnancy Category B. Reproduction studies have been performed in rats and rabbits at doses up to 34 times the human dose and revealed no evidence of impaired fertility or harm to the fetus due to flavoxate HCl. There are, however, no well-controlled studies in pregnant women. Because animal reproduction studies are not always predictive of human response, this drug should be used during pregnancy only if clearly needed.

Nursing Mothers: It is not known whether this drug is excreted in human milk. Because many drugs are excreted in human milk, caution should be exercised when *Urispas* is administered to a nursing woman.

Pediatric Use: Safety and effectiveness in children below the age of 12 years have not been established.

ADVERSE REACTIONS

The following adverse reactions have been observed, but there are not enough data to support an estimate of their frequency.

Gastrointestinal: Nausea, vomiting, dry mouth.

CNS: Vertigo, headache, mental confusion, especially in the elderly, drowsiness, nervousness.

Hematologic: Leukopenia (one case which was reversible upon discontinuation of the drug).

Cardiovascular: Tachycardia and palpitation.

Allergic: Urticaria and other dermatoses, eosinophilia and hyperpyrexia.

Ophthalmic: Increased ocular tension, blurred vision, disturbance in eye accommodation.

Renal: Dysuria.

Continued on next page

Information on the SmithKline Beecham Pharmaceuticals products appearing here is based on the labeling in effect on July 31, 1998. Further information on these and other products may be obtained from the Medical Department, SmithKline Beecham Pharmaceuticals, One Franklin Plaza, Philadelphia, PA 19101.

Urispas—Cont.

OVERDOSAGE

The oral LD_{50} for flavoxate HCl in rats is 4273 mg/kg. The oral LD_{50} for flavoxate HCl in mice is 1837 mg/kg.
It is not known whether flavoxate HCl is dialyzable.

DOSAGE AND ADMINISTRATION

Adults and children over 12 years of age: One or two 100 mg tablets 3 or 4 times a day. With improvement of symptoms, the dose may be reduced. This drug cannot be recommended for infants and children under 12 years of age because safety and efficacy have not been demonstrated in this age group.

HOW SUPPLIED

Urispas (flavoxate HCl), 100 mg, is supplied as round, white, film-coated tablets debossed with the product name URISPAS and SKF, in bottles of 100 and in Single Unit Packages of 100 (intended for institutional use only).
100 mg 100's: NDC 0007-5290-20
100 mg SUP 100's: NDC 0007-5290-21
Store between 15° and 30°C (59° and 86°F).
Veterans Administration/Military/PHS—Tablets, 100 mg, 100's, 6505-00-172-3420; 100 mg, 100's SUP, 6505-01-156-1935.
UR:L18

Shown in Product Identification Guide, page 340

Solvay Pharmaceuticals, Inc.
901 SAWYER ROAD
MARIETTA, GA 30062

For Medical Information Contact:
Generally:
Medical Services Department
(770) 578-9000
FAX: (770) 578-5586
In Emergencies:
770 429-7110

Sales and Ordering:
Orders may be placed by calling this toll free number:
(800) 241-1643
Mail orders should be sent to:
Solvay Pharmaceuticals
Order Entry Department
901 Sawyer Road
Marietta, GA 30062

CORTENEMA®
(Hydrocortisone Retention Enema)
100 mg/60 mL
Disposable Unit for Rectal Use Only

℞

DESCRIPTION

Each disposable unit (60 mL) contains:
Hydrocortisone, 100 mg in an aqueous solution containing carbomer 934P, polysorbate 80, purified water, sodium hydroxide and methylparaben, 0.18% as a preservative.
CORTENEMA® is a convenient disposable single-dose hydrocortisone enema designed for ease of self-administration. Hydrocortisone is a naturally occurring glucocorticoid (adrenal corticosteroid), which similarly as its acetate and sodium hemisuccinate derivatives, is partially absorbed following rectal administration. Absorption studies in ulcerative colitis patients have shown up to 50% absorption of hydrocortisone administered as CORTENEMA® and up to 30% of hydrocortisone acetate administered in an identical vehicle.

ACTIONS

CORTENEMA® provides the potent anti-inflammatory effect of hydrocortisone. Because this drug is absorbed from the colon, it acts both topically and systemically. Although rectal hydrocortisone, used as recommended for CORTENEMA®, has a low incidence of reported adverse reactions, prolonged use presumably may cause systemic reactions associated with oral dosage forms.

INDICATIONS AND USAGE

CORTENEMA® is indicated as adjunctive therapy in the treatment of ulcerative colitis, especially distal forms, including ulcerative proctitis, ulcerative proctosigmoiditis, and left-sided ulcerative colitis. It has proved useful also in some cases involving the transverse and ascending colons.

CONTRAINDICATIONS

Systemic fungal infections; and ileocolostomy during the immediate or early post-operative period.

WARNINGS

In severe ulcerative colitis, it is hazardous to delay needed surgery while awaiting response to medical treatment.

Damage to the rectal wall can result from careless or improper insertion of an enema tip.
In patients on corticosteroid therapy subjected to unusual stress, increased dosage of rapidly acting corticosteroids before, during, and after the stressful situation is indicated.
Corticosteroids may mask some signs of infection, and new infections may appear during their use. There may be decreased resistance and inability to localize infection when corticosteroids are used.
Prolonged use of corticosteroids may produce posterior subcapsular cataracts, glaucoma with possible damage to the optic nerves, and may enhance the establishment of secondary ocular infections due to fungi or viruses.
Usage in pregnancy: Since adequate human reproduction studies have not been done with corticosteroids, the use of these drugs in pregnancy, nursing mothers or women of childbearing potential requires that the possible benefits of the drug be weighed against the potential hazards to the mother and embryo or fetus. Neonates born of mothers who have received substantial doses of corticosteroids during pregnancy should be carefully observed for signs of hypoadrenalism.
Average and large doses of hydrocortisone or cortisone can cause elevation of blood pressure, salt and water retention, and increased excretion of potassium. These effects are less likely to occur with the synthetic derivatives except when used in large doses. Dietary salt restriction and potassium supplementation may be necessary. All corticosteroids increase calcium excretion.
While on corticosteroid therapy patients should not be vaccinated against smallpox. Other immunization procedures should not be undertaken in patients who are on corticosteroids, especially on high dose, because of possible hazards of neurological complications and a lack of antibody response.
If corticosteroids are indicated in patients with latent tuberculosis or tuberculin reactivity, close observation is necessary as reactivation of the disease may occur. During prolonged corticosteroid therapy, these patients should receive chemoprophylaxis.

PRECAUTIONS

CORTENEMA® hydrocortisone retention enema should be used with caution where there is a probability of impending perforation, abscess or other pyogenic infection; fresh intestinal anastomoses; obstruction; or extensive fistulas and sinus tracts. Use with caution in presence of active or latent peptic ulcer; diverticulitis; renal insufficiency; hypertension; osteoporosis; and myasthenia gravis.
Steroid therapy might impair prognosis in surgery by increasing the hazard of infection. If infection is suspected, appropriate antibiotic therapy must be administered, usually in larger than ordinary doses.
Drug-induced secondary adrenocortical insufficiency may occur with prolonged CORTENEMA® therapy. This is minimized by gradual reduction of dosage. This type of relative insufficiency may persist for months after discontinuation of therapy; therefore, in any situation of stress occurring during that period, hormone therapy should be reinstituted. Since mineralocorticoid secretion may be impaired, salt and/or a mineralocorticoid should be administered concurrently.
There is an enhanced effect of corticosteroids on patients with hypothyroidism and in those with cirrhosis.
Corticosteroid should be used cautiously in patients with ocular herpes simplex because of possible corneal perforation. The lowest possible dose of corticosteroid should be used to control the conditions under treatment, and when reduction in dosage is possible, the reduction should be gradual.
Psychic derangement may appear when corticosteroids are used, ranging from euphoria, insomnia, mood swings, personality changes, and severe depression, to frank psychotic manifestations. Also, existing emotional instability or psychotic tendencies may be aggravated by corticosteroids.
Aspirin should be used cautiously in conjunction with corticosteroids in hypoprothrombinemia.
Pediatric Use
Safety and effectiveness in pediatric patients have not been established.
Growth and development of pediatric patients on prolonged corticosteroid therapy should be carefully observed.

ADVERSE REACTIONS

Local pain or burning, and rectal bleeding attributed to CORTENEMA® have been reported rarely. Apparent exacerbations or sensitivity reactions also occur rarely. The following adverse reactions should be kept in mind whenever corticosteroids are given by rectal administration.
Fluid and Electrolyte Disturbances: Sodium retention; fluid retention; congestive heart failure in susceptible patients; potassium loss; hypokalemic alkalosis; hypertension. **Musculoskeletal:** Muscle weakness; steroid myopathy; loss of muscle mass; osteoporosis; vertebral compression fractures; aseptic necrosis of femoral and humeral heads; pathologic fracture of long bones. **Gastrointestinal:** Peptic ulcer with possible perforation and hemorrhage; pancreatitis; abdominal distention; ulcerative esophagitis. **Dermatologic:** Impaired wound healing; thin fragile skin; petechiae and ecchymoses; facial erythema; increased sweating; may suppress reactions to skin tests. **Neurological:** Convulsions; increased intracranial pressure with papilledema (pseudotumor cerebri) usually after treatment; vertigo; headache. **Endocrine:** Menstrual irregularities; development of Cushingoid state; suppression of growth in pediatric patients; secondary adrenocortical and pituitary unresponsiveness, particularly in times of stress, as in trauma, surgery or illness; decreased carbohydrate tolerance; manifestations of latent diabetes requirements for insulin or oral hypoglycemic agents in diabetics. **Ophthalmic:** Posterior subcapsular cataracts; increased intraocular pressure; glaucoma; exophthalmos. **Metabolic:** Negative nitrogen balance due to protein catabolism.

DOSAGE AND ADMINISTRATION

The use of CORTENEMA® hydrocortisone retention enema is predicated upon the concomitant use of modern supportive measures such as rational dietary control, sedatives, antidiarrheal agents, antibacterial therapy, blood replacement if necessary, etc.
The usual course of therapy is one CORTENEMA® nightly for 21 days, or until the patient comes into remission both clinically and proctologically. Clinical symptoms usually subside promptly within 3 to 5 days. Improvement in the appearance of the mucosa, as seen by sigmoidoscopic examination, may lag somewhat behind clinical improvement. Difficult cases may require as long as 2 or 3 months of CORTENEMA® treatment. Where the course of therapy extends beyond 21 days, CORTENEMA® should be discontinued gradually by reducing administration to every other night for 2 or 3 weeks.
If clinical or proctologic improvement fails to occur within 2 or 3 weeks after starting CORTENEMA®, discontinue its use.
Symptomatic improvement, evidenced by decreased diarrhea and bleeding; weight gain; improved appetite; lessened fever; and decreased leukocytosis, may be misleading and should not be used as the sole criterion in judging efficacy. Sigmoidoscopic examination and X-ray visualization are essential for adequate monitoring of ulcerative colitis. Biopsy is useful for differential diagnosis.
Patient instructions for administering CORTENEMA® are enclosed in each box of seven units. We recommend that the patient lie on his left side during administration and for 30 minutes thereafter, so that the fluid will distribute throughout the left colon. Every effort should be made to retain the enema for at least an hour and preferably, all night. This may be facilitated by prior sedation and/or antidiarrheal medication, especially early in therapy, when the urge to evacuate is great.

HOW SUPPLIED

CORTENEMA®, hydrocortisone 100 mg retention enema, is supplied as disposable single-dose bottles with lubricated rectal applicator tips, in boxes of seven × 60 mL (NDC 0032-1904-82) and boxes of one × 60 mL (NDC 0032-1904-73).
Store at controlled room temperature, 15°–30°C (59°–86°F).
Rx Only

0638
7E Rev 2/98

Solvay
Pharmaceuticals
Marietta, GA 30062
©1998 Solvay Pharmaceuticals, Inc.

CREON® 5
CREON® 10
CREON® 20
MINIMICROSPHERES®
(Pancrelipase Delayed-release Capsules, USP)

℞

PRESCRIBING INFORMATION

DESCRIPTION

CREON® 5, CREON® 10, and CREON® 20 Capsules are orally administered and contain delayed-release MINIMICROSPHERES® of pancrelipase, which is of porcine pancreatic origin. Each CREON 5 Capsule contains lipase 5,000 USP Units, protease 18,750 USP Units and amylase 16,600 USP Units. Each CREON 10 Capsule contains lipase 10,000 USP Units, protease 37,500 USP Units and amylase 33,200 USP Units. Each CREON 20 Capsule contains lipase 20,000 USP Units, protease 75,000 USP Units and amylase 66,400 USP Units.
Inactive ingredients include dibutyl phthalate, dimethicone, hydroxypropylmethylcellulose phthalate, light mineral oil and polyethylene glycol. The capsule shells contain gelatin, red iron oxide, titanium dioxide, yellow iron oxide. The CREON 5 capsule shell contains FD & C blue No. 2. In addition, the CREON 10 capsule shell contains black iron oxide and the CREON® 5, CREON¹⁰, and CREON²⁰ Capsules imprinting ink contains dimethicone, 2-ethoxyethanol, shellac, soya lecithin and titanium dioxide.

CLINICAL PHARMACOLOGY

The pancreatic enzymes in CREON 5, CREON 10, and CREON 20 Capsules are enteric-coated to resist gastric destruction or inactivation. The pancreatic enzymes catalyze the hydrolysis of fats to glycerol and fatty acids, protein into proteases and derived substances and starch into dextrins and short chain sugars.

INDICATIONS

CREON 5, CREON 10, and CREON 20 Capsules are indicated for patients with pancreatic exocrine insufficiency as is often associated with:

- cystic fibrosis
- chronic pancreatitis
- post-pancreatectomy
- post-gastrointestinal bypass surgery (e.g., Billroth II gastroenterostomy)
- ductal obstruction from neoplasm (e.g., of the pancreas or common bile duct)

CONTRAINDICATIONS

CREON 5, CREON 10, and CREON 20 Capsules are contraindicated in the early stages of acute pancreatitis or in patients who are known to be hypersensitive to pork protein.

WARNINGS

Should symptoms of hypersensitivity appear, discontinue medication and initiate symptomatic and supportive therapy if necessary.

Strictures in the ileo-cecal region and/or ascending colon have been reported in cystic fibrosis patients treated with high doses of high-potency pancreatic enzyme supplements containing 20,000 or greater USP units of lipase per capsule. The underlying mechanism is unknown, but caution should be exercised when doses in excess of 6,000 USP units per kg per meal fail to resolve symptoms, especially in patients with a history of intestinal complications such as meconium ileus equivalent, short bowel syndrome, surgery or Crohn's disease. If symptoms suggestive of gastrointestinal obstruction occur, the possibility of bowel stricture should be investigated including evaluation of pancreatic enzyme therapy.

PRECAUTIONS

CREON 5, CREON 10, and CREON 20 Capsules MINIMICROSPHERES® SHOULD NOT BE CRUSHED OR CHEWED or placed on foods having a pH greater than 5.5. These can dissolve the protective enteric coating resulting in early release of enzymes, irritation of oral mucosa, and/or loss of enzyme activity.

Information for Patients: CREON 5, CREON 10, and CREON 20 Capsules are a pancreatic enzyme product prescribed to promote improved digestion of foods, especially fat. The prescribed dosage should be taken with each meal and snack or as directed by the physician. The capsules can be swallowed whole, or the contents poured on soft, bland food. Care should be taken to avoid chewing or crushing of the capsule contents, which can result in early release of enzymes, irritation of oral mucosa, and/or loss of enzyme activity. Patients should maintain adequate fluid intake. The prescribed dose range should not be exceeded without calling your doctor.

The most common adverse reactions involve the stomach and intestine including diarrhea, nausea, vomiting, bloating, constipation, stomach cramps or pain. If these symptoms are persistent, contact your doctor.

Carcinogenesis, Mutagenesis, Impairment of Fertility: Long-term studies in animals have not been performed to evaluate carcinogenic potential.

Pregnancy, Category C: Animal reproduction studies have not been conducted with pancrelipase. It is also not known whether pancrelipase can cause fetal harm when administered to a pregnant woman or can affect reproduction capacity. CREON 5, CREON 10, and CREON 20 Capsules should be given to a pregnant woman only if clearly needed.

Nursing Mothers: It is not known whether this drug is excreted in human milk. Because many drugs are excreted in human milk, caution should be exercised when CREON 5, CREON 10, and CREON 20 Capsules are administered to a nursing mother.

ADVERSE REACTIONS

The most frequently reported adverse reactions to pancreatic enzyme-containing products are gastrointestinal in nature which may include nausea, vomiting, bloating, cramping, constipation or diarrhea. Less frequently, allergic-type reactions have also been observed. Very high doses of pancreatin have been associated with hyperuricosuria and hyperuricemia.

DOSAGE AND ADMINISTRATION

Clinical experience should dictate initial starting dose. Doses should be taken during meals or snacks, not before or after. Do not take without food.

Adults and Children Over 6 Years Old:

CREON 5: Usual initial starting dosage is two to four CREON 5 Capsules per meal or snack.

CREON 10: Usual initial starting dosage is one to two CREON 10 Capsules per meal or snack.

CREON 20: Usual initial starting dosage is one CREON 20 capsule per meal or snack.

Children Under 6 Years Old:

CREON 5: The exact dosage of CREON 5 Capsules should be selected based on clinical experience for this age group. Patients can be started on one to two capsules per meal or snack.

CREON 10: Usual initial starting dosage is up to one CREON 10 Capsule per meal or snack.

CREON 20: The exact dosage of CREON 20 Capsules should be selected based on clinical experience for this age group.

For cystic fibrosis patients typical doses are 1,500–3,000 USP lipase units/kg/meal.

Dosage should be adjusted according to the severity of the disease, control of steatorrhea and maintenance of good nutritional status. Doses in excess of 6,000 USP lipase units/kg/meal are not recommended.

Dose increases, if required, should occur with careful monitoring of body weight and stool fat content. When changing strengths of pancreatic enzyme products, care should be taken to maintain equivalent lipase units for each divided dosage.

It is important to ensure adequate hydration of patients at all times while taking pancreatic enzymes.

Where swallowing of capsules is difficult, the capsules may be carefully opened and the MINIMICROSPHERES® added to a small amount of soft food, with a pH less than 5.5. The soft food should be swallowed immediately without chewing and followed with a glass of water or juice to insure swallowing.

HOW SUPPLIED

CREON® 5 MINIMICROSPHERES® (Pancrelipase Delayed-release Capsules, USP) are available in a two-piece gelatin capsule (orange opaque top half, blue opaque bottom half) imprinted in white with "SOLVAY" and "1205". Each capsule contains tan-colored delayed-release MINIMICROSPHERES® of pancrelipase supplied in bottles of:

100	NDC 0032-1205-01
250	NDC 0032-1205-07

CREON® 10 MINIMICROSPHERES® (Pancrelipase Delayed-release Capsules, USP) are available in a two-piece gelatin capsule (brown opaque top half, natural transparent bottom half) imprinted in white with "SOLVAY" and "1210". Each capsule contains tan-colored delayed-release MINIMICROSPHERES® of pancrelipase supplied in bottles of:

100	NDC 0032-1210-01
250	NDC 0032-1210-07

CREON® 20 MINIMICROSPHERES® (Pancrelipase Delayed-release Capsules, USP) are available in a two-piece gelatin capsule (orange opaque top half, natural transparent bottom half) imprinted in white with "SOLVAY" and "1220". Each capsule contains tan-colored delayed release MINIMICROSPHERES® of pancrelipase supplied in bottles of:

100	NDC 0032-1220-01
250	NDC 0032-1220-07

CREON 5, CREON 10, and CREON 20 Capsules must be stored at 25°C (77°F); excursions permitted to 15°–30°C (59°–86°F). [see USP Controlled Room Temperature.] PROTECT FROM MOISTURE. DO NOT REFRIGERATE. Dispense in tight, light-resistant containers. For human consumption only.

CAUTION: Federal law prohibits dispensing without prescription.

Manufactured By:
Solvay Pharmaceuticals GmbH
Hannover, Germany

Marketed by:
SOLVAY
PHARMACEUTICALS
Marietta, GA 30062
Rev 7/97
©1997
Solvay Pharmaceuticals, Inc.

Shown in Product Identification Guide, page 340

DUPHALAC®
(Lactulose Solution, USP)
10 g/15 mL

℞

DESCRIPTION

DUPHALAC® (lactulose solution, USP) is a synthetic disaccharide in solution form for oral administration.

Each 15 mL of DUPHALAC Solution contains: 10 g lactulose (and less than 1.6 g galactose less than 1.2 g lactose, and 1.2 g or less of other sugars).

DUPHALAC Solution is a colonic acidifier which promotes laxation.

The chemical name for lactulose is 4-O-β-D-galactopyranosyl-D-fructofuranose. It has the following structural formula:

Its empirical formula is $C_{12}H_{22}O_{11}$ and its molecular weight is 342.30. It is freely soluble in water.

CLINICAL PHARMACOLOGY

DUPHALAC Solution is poorly absorbed from the gastrointestinal tract and no enzyme capable of hydrolysis of this disaccharide is present in human gastrointestinal tissue. As a result, oral doses of DUPHALAC Solution reach the colon virtually unchanged. In the colon, DUPHALAC Solution is broken down primarily to lactic acid, and also to small amounts of formic and acetic acids, by the action of colonic bacteria, which results in an increase in osmotic pressure and slight acidification of the colonic contents. This in turn causes an increase in stool water content and softens the stool.

Since DUPHALAC Solution does not exert its effect until it reaches the colon, and since transit time through the colon may be slow, 24 to 48 hours may be required to produce the desired bowel movement.

DUPHALAC Solution given orally to man and experimental animals resulted in only small amounts reaching the blood. Urinary excretion has been determined to be 3% or less and is essentially complete within 24 hours.

INDICATIONS AND USAGE

For the treatment of constipation. In patients with a history of chronic constipation, DUPHALAC (lactulose solution) therapy increases the number of bowel movements per day and the number of days on which bowel movements occur.

CONTRAINDICATIONS

Since DUPHALAC Solution contains galactose (less than 1.6 g/15 mL), it is contraindicated in patients who require a low galactose diet.

WARNINGS

A theoretical hazard may exist for patients being treated with lactulose solution who may be required to undergo electrocautery procedures during proctoscopy or colon-oscopy. Accumulation of H_2 gas in significant concentration in the presence of an electrical spark may result in an explosive reaction. Although this complication has not been reported with lactulose, patients on lactulose therapy undergoing such procedures should have a thorough bowel cleansing with a non-fermentable solution. Insufflation of CO_2 as an additional safeguard may be pursued but is considered to be a redundant measure.

PRECAUTIONS

General: Since DUPHALAC Solution contains galactose (less than 1.6 g/15 mL and lactose (less than 1.2 g/15 mL), it should be used with caution in diabetics.

Information for Patients: In the event that an unusual diarrheal condition occurs, contact your physician.

Laboratory Tests: Elderly, debilitated patients who receive DUPHALAC Solution for more than six months should have serum electrolytes (potassium, chloride, carbon dioxide) measured periodically.

Drug Interaction: Results of preliminary studies in humans and rats suggest that nonabsorbable antacids given concurrently with lactulose may inhibit the desired lactulose-induced drop in colonic pH. Therefore, a possible lack of desired effect of treatment should be taken into consideration before such drugs are given concomitantly with DUPHALAC Solution.

Carcinogenesis, Mutagenesis, Impairment of Fertility: There are no known human data on long-term potential for carcinogenicity, mutagenicity, or impairment of fertility.

There are no known animal data on long-term potential for mutagenicity.

Administration of lactulose solution in the diet of mice for 18 months in concentrations of 3 and 10 percent (V/W) did not produce any evidence of carcinogenicity.

In studies in mice, rats and rabbits doses of lactulose solution up to 6 or 12 mL/kg/day produced no deleterious effects in breeding, conception, or parturition.

Pregnancy:

Teratogenic Effects:

Pregnancy Category B: Reproduction studies have been performed in mice, rats, and rabbits at doses up to 3 or 6

Continued on next page

Duphalac—Cont.

times the usual human oral dose and have revealed no evidence of impaired fertility or harm to the fetus due to lactulose. There are, however, no adequate and well-controlled studies in pregnant women. Because animal reproduction studies are not always predictive of human response, this drug should be used during pregnancy only if clearly needed.

Nursing Mothers: It is not known whether this drug is excreted in human milk. Because many drugs are excreted in human milk, caution should be exercised when DUPHALAC® (Lactulose Solution) is administered to a nursing woman.

Pediatric Use: Safety and effectiveness in children have not been established.

ADVERSE REACTIONS

Precise frequency data are not available.
Initial dosing may produce flatulence and intestinal cramps, which are usually transient. Excessive dosage can lead to diarrhea with potential complications such as loss of fluids, hypokalemia and hypernatremia.
Nausea and vomiting have been reported.

OVERDOSAGE

Signs and Symptoms: There have been no reports of accidental overdosage. In the event of overdosage, it is expected that diarrhea and abdominal cramps would be the major symptoms. Medication should be terminated.

Oral LD_{50}: The acute oral LD_{50} of the drug is 48.8 mL/kg in mice and greater than 30 mL/kg in rats.

Dialysis: Dialysis data are not available for lactulose. Its molecular similarity to sucrose, however, would suggest that it should be dialyzable.

DOSAGE AND ADMINISTRATION

The usual dose is 1 to 2 tablespoonfuls (15 to 30 mL. containing 10 g to 20 g of lactulose) daily. The dose may be increased to 60 mL daily if necessary. Twenty-four to 48 hours may be required to produce a normal bowel movement.
Note: Some patients have found that DUPHALAC Solution may be more acceptable when mixed with fruit juice, water or milk.

HOW SUPPLIED

DUPHALAC (lactulose solution) is a colorless to yellow color + solution that may darken on standing, for oral administration, containing 10 g/15 mL lactulose (667 mg/mL).
It is available as:
NDC 0032-1602-08
8 fl oz bottles
NDC 0032-1602-78
16 fl oz bottles
NDC 0032-1602-80
32 fl oz bottles
NDC 0032-1602-84
30 mL unit dose cups in trays of 10 cups.
Store at controlled room temperature, 15°–30°C (59°–86°F). Do not freeze.
+Under recommended storage conditions, a normal darkening of color may occur. Such darkening is characteristic of sugar solutions and does not affect therapeutic action. Prolonged exposure to temperatures above 30°C (86°F) or to direct light may cause extreme darkening and turbidity which may be pharmaceutically objectionable. If this condition develops, do not use.
Prolonged exposure to freezing temperatures may cause change to a semisolid, too viscous to pour. Viscosity will return to normal upon warming to room temperature.
CAUTION: Federal law prohibits dispensing without prescription.
DUPHALAC is a registered trademark of Solvay Duphar B.V.
Manufactured By:
Solvay Duphar B.V.
Weesp, The Netherlands
Marketed by:
SOLVAY PHARMACEUTICALS
MARIETTA, GA 30062
6E1379 Rev 11/94
©1994
SOLVAY PHARMACEUTICALS, INC.

ESTRATAB®

℞

(Esterified Estrogens Tablets, USP)
0.3 mg, 0.625 mg, 2.5 mg
Physician Labeling

1. ESTROGENS HAVE BEEN REPORTED TO INCREASE THE RISK OF ENDOMETRIAL CARCINOMA IN POST-MENOPAUSAL WOMEN.
Close clinical surveillance of all women taking estrogens is important. Adequate diagnostic measures, including endometrial sampling when indicated, should be undertaken to rule out malignancy in all cases of undiagnosed persistent or recurring abnormal vaginal bleeding. There is no evidence that "natural" estrogens are more or less hazardous than "synthetic" estrogens at equi-estrogenic doses.

2. ESTROGENS SHOULD NOT BE USED DURING PREGNANCY.
There is no indication for estrogen therapy during pregnancy or during the immediate postpartum period. Estrogens are ineffective for the prevention or treatment of threatened or habitual abortion. Estrogens are not indicated for the prevention of postpartum breast engorgement.
Estrogen therapy during pregnancy is associated with an increased risk of congenital defects in the reproductive organs of the fetus, and possibly other birth defects. Studies of women who received diethylstilbestrol (DES) during pregnancy have shown that female offspring have an increased risk of vaginal adenosis, squamous-cell dysplasia of the uterine cervix, and clear cell vaginal cancer later in life; male offspring have an increased risk of urogenital abnormalities and possibly testicular cancer later in life. The 1985 DES Task Force concluded that use of DES during pregnancy is associated with a subsequent increased risk of breast cancer in the mothers, although a causal relationship is still unproven and the observed level of excess risk is similar to that for a number of other breast cancer risk factors.

DESCRIPTION

ESTRATAB® (Esterified Estrogens Tablets, USP)
Each blue, sugarcoated tablet contains 0.3 mg. Each yellow, sugarcoated tablet contains 0.625 mg. Each light purple, sugarcoated tablet contains 2.5 mg.
ESTRATAB® Tablets for oral administration is a mixture of the sodium salts of the sulfate esters of the estrogenic substances, principally estrone, that are prepared synthetically from plant sterol precursors. Esterified Estrogens, USP contain not less than 75.0 percent and not more than 85.0 percent of sodium estrone sulfate, and not less than 6.0 percent and not more than 15.0 percent of sodium equilin sulfate, in such proportion that the total of these two components is not less than 90.0 percent.
Inactive Ingredients: Acacia, calcium carbonate, carnauba wax, carboxymethylcellulose sodium, citric acid, colloidal silicon dioxide, diacetylated monoglyceride, gelatin, anhydrous lactose, magnesium stearate, methylparaben, microcrystalline cellulose, pharmaceutical glaze, povidone, propylparaben, shellac, sodium benzoate, sodium bicarbonate, sorbic acid, sucrose, corn starch, talc, titanium dioxide and tribasic calcium phosphate. The 0.3 mg tablet coating contains FD&C Blue #1 Lake; the 0.625 mg tablet coating contains D&C Yellow #10 Lake, FD&C Yellow #6 Lake and FD&C Blue #2 Lake; and the 2.5 mg tablet coating contains FD&C Red #40 Lake and FD&C Blue #2 Lake. In addition, the tablet imprinting ink for the 0.3 mg and 0.625 mg tablets contains black iron oxide, FD&C Blue #2 Lake, FD&C Red #40 Lake and FD&C Yellow #6 Lake. The 2.5 mg imprinting ink contains Soya lecithin, dimethyl polysiloxane, pharmaceutical shellac and titanium dioxide.

ACTIONS/CLINICAL PHARMACOLOGY

Estrogen drug products act by regulating the transcription of a limited number of genes. Estrogens diffuse through cell membranes, distribute themselves throughout the cell, and bind to and activate the nuclear estrogen receptor, a DNA-binding protein which is found in estrogen-responsive tissues. The activated estrogen receptor binds to specific DNA sequences, or hormone response elements, which enhance the transcription of adjacent genes and in turn lead to the observed effects. Estrogen receptors have been identified in tissues of the reproductive tract, breast, pituitary, hypothalamus, liver, and bone of women.
Estrogens are important in the development and maintenance of the female reproductive system and secondary sex characteristics. By direct action, they cause growth and development of the uterus, Fallopian tubes, and vagina. With other hormones, such as pituitary hormones and progesterone, they cause enlargement of the breasts through promotion of ductal growth, stromal development, and the accretion of fat. Estrogens are intricately involved with other hormones, especially progesterone, in the processes of the ovulatory menstrual cycle and pregnancy, and affect the release of pituitary gonadotropins. They also contribute to the shaping of the skeleton, maintenance of tone and elasticity of urogenital structures, changes in epiphyses of the long bones that allow for the pubertal growth spurt and its termination, and pigmentation of the nipples and genitals.
Estrogens occur naturally in several forms. The primary source of estrogen in normally cycling adult women is the ovarian follicle, which secretes 70 to 500 micrograms of estradiol daily, depending on the phase of the menstrual cycle. This is converted primarily to estrone, which circulates in roughly equal proportion to estradiol, and to small amounts of estriol. After menopause, most endogenous estrogen is produced by conversion of androstenedione, secreted by the adrenal cortex, to estrone by peripheral tissues. Thus, estrone – – especially in its sulfate ester form – – is the most abundant circulating estrogen in postmenopausal women. Although circulating estrogens exist in a dynamic equilibrium of metabolic interconversions, estradiol is the principle intracellular human estrogen and is substantially more potent than estrone or estriol at the receptor.
Estrogens used in therapy are well absorbed through the skin, mucous membranes, and gastrointestinal tract. When applied for a local action, absorption is usually sufficient to cause systemic effects. When conjugated with aryl and alkyl groups for parenteral administration, the rate of absorption of oily preparations is slowed with a prolonged duration of action, such that a single intramuscular injection of estradiol valerate or estradiol cypionate is absorbed over several weeks.
Administered estrogens and their esters are handled within the body essentially the same as the endogenous hormones. Metabolic conversion of estrogens occurs primarily in the liver (first pass effect), but also at local target tissue sites. Complex metabolic processes result in a dynamic equilibrium of circulating conjugated and unconjugated estrogenic forms which are continually interconverted, especially between estrone and estradiol and between esterified and nonesterified forms. Although naturally-occurring estrogens circulate in the blood largely bound to sex hormone-binding globulin and albumin, only unbound estrogens enter target tissue cells. A significant proportion of the circulating estrogen exists as sulfate conjugates, especially estrone sulfate, which serves as a circulating reservoir for the formation of more active estrogenic species. A certain proportion of the estrogen is excreted into the bile and then reabsorbed from the intestine. During this enterohepatic recirculation, estrogens are desulfated and resulfated and undergo degradation through conversion to less active estrogens (estriol and other estrogens), oxidation to nonestrogenic substances (catecholestrogens, which interact with catecholamine metabolism, especially in the central nervous system), and conjugation with glucuronic acids (which are then rapidly excreted in the urine).
When given orally, naturally-occurring estrogens and their esters are extensively metabolized (first pass effect) and circulate primarily as estrone sulfate, with smaller amounts of other conjugated and unconjugated estrogenic species. This results in limited oral potency. By contrast, synthetic estrogens, such as ethinyl estradiol and the nonsteroidal estrogens, are degraded very slowly in the liver and other tissues, which results in their high intrinsic potency. Estrogen drug products administered by non-oral routes are not subject to first-pass metabolism, but also undergo significant hepatic uptake, metabolism, and enterohepatic recycling.

Clinical Studies
A two-year, double-blind, placebo-controlled, randomized study was conducted in 406 postmenopausal women to determine the efficacy of continuously administered ESTRATAB® Tablets (0.3 mg, 0.625 mg, and 1.25 mg), unopposed by a progestin, on the prevention of postmenopausal osteoporosis. Efficacy was evaluated by semi-annual determination of lumbar spine (L1-L4) BMD and hip BMD changes (DXA). The results (see Tables 1, 2 and Figures 1,2) of this study demonstrate that ESTRATAB® Tablets, at doses of 0.3 mg, 0.625 mg, and 1.25 mg, is effective in the prevention of postmenopausal osteoporosis. Compared to placebo, patients treated with ESTRATAB® Tablets had significant increases in lumbar BMD and hip BMD.
[See table 1 below]
[See table 2 at top of next page]
[See figures 1 & 2 in next column]

Table 1. Mean Percent Change From Baseline in Lumbar Spine (L1-L4) BMD

| | Mean Percent Change in Lumbar Spine BMD | | | |
	6 Mos.	12 Mos.	18 Mos.	24 Mos.
Placebo	-0.25	-1.04[a]	-1.65[a]	-1.97[a]
ESTRATAB® 0.3 mg	0.81[a,b]	1.32[a,b]	1.47[a,b]	1.42[a,b]
ESTRATAB® 0.625 mg	1.32[a,b]	2.17[a,b]	2.13[a,b]	2.29[a,b]
ESTRATAB® 1.25 mg	2.98[a,b]	3.69[a,b]	4.11[a,b]	4.36[a,b]

[a] $p < 0.05$ compared to baseline
[b] $p < 0.05$ compared to placebo

Table 2. Mean Percent Change From Baseline in Hip BMD

| | Mean Percent Change in Hip BMD | | | |
	6 Mos.	12 Mos.	18 Mos.	24 Mos.
Placebo	-0.06	-0.48	-0.48	-0.82
ESTRATAB® 0.3 mg	1.09[a,b]	1.21[a,b]	1.71[a,b]	1.59[a,b]
ESTRATAB® 0.625 mg	0.73	1.71[a,b]	2.25[a,b]	2.28[a,b]
ESTRATAB® 1.25 mg	1.46[a,b]	1.55[a,b]	1.72[a,b]	2.06[a,b]

[a] $p < 0.05$ compared to baseline
[b] $p < 0.05$ compared to placebo

Table 3. Incidence of Endometrial Hyperplasia After 1 and 2 Years

| | | Incidence of Hyperplasia | | | |
| | | 1 Year | | 2 Years | |
	No. Pat.	N	%	N	%
Placebo	60	1	1.67	1	1.67
ESTRATAB® 0.3 mg	59	1	1.69	1	1.69
ESTRATAB® 0.625 mg	59	12	20.3[a,b]	17	28.8[a,b]
ESTRATAB® 1.25 mg	60	26	43.3[a,b]	32	53.3[a,b]

[a] $p < 0.05$ compared to baseline
[b] $p <$ compared to ESTRATAB® 0.3 mg

Table 4. Mean Percent Change From Baseline in Lipid Parameters After Two Years

| | Lipid Parameters | | | |
	HDL Cholesterol	LDL Cholesterol	Triglycerides	Total Cholesterol
Placebo	2.64	1.22	17.34[a]	1.98
ESTRATAB® 0.3 mg	5.59[a]	-4.62[a,b]	15.02[a]	-1.89
ESTRATAB® 0.625 mg	10.54[a,b]	-3.71	16.03[a]	0.09
ESTRATAB® 1.25 mg	12.31[a,b]	-14.71[a,b]	28.77[a]	5.15[a,b]

[a] $p < 0.05$ compared to baseline
[b] $p < 0.05$ compared to placebo

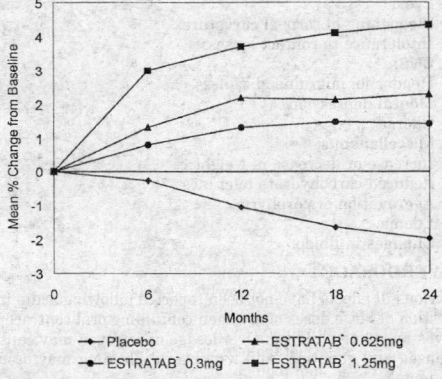

Figure 1. Percent Change From Baseline in Lumbar Spine (L1-L4) BMD Over 24 Months

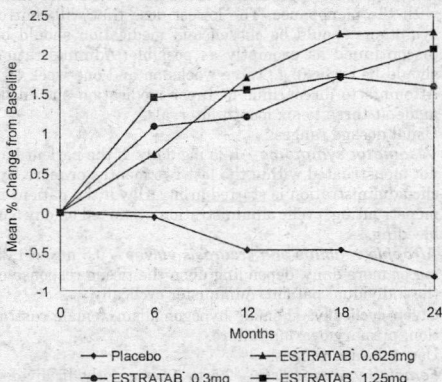

Figure 2. Percent Change From Baseline in Hip BMD Over 24 Months

INFORMATION REGARDING ENDOMETRIAL EFFECTS. As shown in Table 3, only one case of endometrial hyperplasia occurred in the groups treated with placebo or unopposed 0.3-mg ESTRATAB® Tablets. The incidence of endometrial hyperplasia was significantly greater with un-

opposed ESTRATAB® Tablets in doses of 0.625 mg and 1.25 mg.
[See table 3 above]
INFORMATION REGARDING LIPID EFFECTS. As shown in Table 4, ESTRATAB® Tablets increase HDL-Cholesterol and decrease LDL-Cholesterol. The following table summarizes mean percent changes from baseline values after 2 years of treatment.
[See table 4 above]

INDICATIONS AND USAGE

ESTRATAB® Tablets are indicated in the:
1. Treatment of moderate to severe vasomotor symptoms associated with the menopause. (There is no adequate evidence that estrogens are effective for nervous symptoms or depression which might occur during menopause, and they should not be used to treat these conditions).
2. Treatment of vulval and vaginal atrophy.
3. Treatment of hypoestrogenism due to hypogonadism, castration, or primary ovarian failure.
4. Treatment of breast cancer (for palliation only) in appropriately selected women and men with metastatic disease.
5. Treatment of advanced androgen - dependent carcinoma of the prostate (for palliation only).
6. Prevention of osteoporosis.
Since estrogen administration is associated with risk as well as benefit, selection of patients should ideally be based on prospective identification of risk factors for developing osteoporosis. Unfortunately, there is no certain way to identify those women who will develop osteoporotic fractures. Most prospective studies of efficacy for this indication have been carried out in white menopausal women, without stratification by other risk factors, and tend to show a universally salutary effect on bone. Thus, patient selection must be individualized based on the balance of risks and benefits. A more favorable risk/benefit ratio exists in a hysterectomized woman because she has no risk of endometrial cancer (see Boxed Warning).
Estrogen replacement therapy reduces bone resorption and retards or halts postmenopausal bone loss. Case-control studies have shown an approximately 60 percent reduction in hip and wrist fractures in women whose estrogen replacement was begun within a few years of menopause. Studies also suggest that estrogen reduces the rate of vertebral fractures. Even when started as late as 6 years after menopause, estrogen prevents further loss of bone mass for as long as the treatment is continued.
The results of a two-year, randomized, placebo-controlled, double-blind dose-ranging study have shown that daily continuous treatment with 0.3, 0.625, or 1.25 mg esterified estrogens prevents vertebral bone mass loss in postmeno-

pausal women (See ACTIONS/CLINICAL PHARMACOLOGY). When estrogen therapy is discontinued, bone mass declines at a rate comparable to the immediate postmenopausal period. There is no evidence that estrogen replacement restores bone mass to premenopausal levels.
At skeletal maturity there are sex and race differences in both the total amount of bone present and its density, in favor of men and blacks. Thus, women are at higher risk than men because they start with less bone mass and, for several years following natural or induced menopause, the rate of mass decline is accelerated. White and Asian women are at higher risk than black women.
Early menopause is one of the strongest predictors for the development of osteoporosis. In addition, other factors affecting the skeleton which are associated with osteoporosis include genetic factors (small build, family history), endocrine factors (nulliparity, thyrotoxicosis, hyperparathyroidism, Cushing's syndrome, hyperprolactinemia, Type I diabetes), lifestyle (cigarette smoking, alcohol abuse, sedentary exercise habits) and nutrition (below average body weight, dietary calcium intake).
The mainstays of prevention and management of osteoporosis are estrogen, an adequate lifetime calcium intake, and exercise. Postmenopausal women absorb dietary calcium less efficiently than premenopausal women and require an average of 1500 mg/day of elemental calcium to remain in neutral calcium balance. By comparison, premenopausal women require about 1000 mg/day and the average calcium intake in the USA is 400–600 mg/day. Therefore, when not contraindicated, calcium supplementation may be helpful.
Weight-bearing exercise and nutrition may be important adjuncts to the prevention and management of osteoporosis. Immobilization and prolonged bed rest produce rapid bone loss, while weight-bearing exercise has been shown both to reduce bone loss and to increase bone mass. The optimal type and amount of physical activity that would prevent osteoporosis have not been established. However, in two studies, an hour of walking and running exercises twice or three times weekly significantly increased lumbar spine bone mass.

CONTRAINDICATIONS

Estrogens should not be used in individuals with any of the following conditions:
1. Known or suspected pregnancy (See Boxed Warning). Estrogens may cause fetal harm when administered to a pregnant woman.
2. Known or suspected cancer of the breast except in appropriately selected patients being treated for metastatic disease.
3. Known or suspected estrogen-dependent neoplasia.
4. Undiagnosed abnormal genital bleeding.
5. Active thrombophlebitis or thromboembolic disorders.

WARNINGS

1. **Induction of malignant neoplasms**
   Endometrial Cancer: The reported endometrial cancer risk among unopposed estrogen users is about 2- to 12-fold greater than in non-users, and appears dependent on duration of treatment and on estrogen dose. Most studies show no significant increased risk associated with use of estrogens for less than one year. The greatest risk appears associated with prolonged use – – with increased risks of 15- to 24-fold for five to ten years or more. In three studies, persistence of risk was demonstrated for 8 to over 15 years after cessation of estrogen treatment. In one study a significant decrease in the incidence of endometrial cancer occurred six months after estrogen withdrawal. Concurrent progestin therapy may offset this risk but the overall health impact in postmenopausal women is not known (see **PRECAUTIONS**).
   Breast Cancer: While the majority of studies have not shown an increased risk of breast cancer in women who have ever used estrogen replacement therapy, some have reported a moderately increased risk (relative risks of 1.3–2.0) in those taking higher doses or those taking lower doses for prolonged periods of time, especially in excess of 10 years. Other studies have not shown this relationship.
   Congenital lesions with malignant potential: Estrogen therapy during pregnancy is associated with an increased risk of fetal congenital reproductive tract disorders, and possibly other birth defects. Studies of women who received DES during pregnancy have shown that female offspring have an increased risk of vaginal adenosis, squamous cell dysplasia of the uterine cervix, and clear cell vaginal cancer later in life; male offspring have an increased risk of urogenital abnormalities and possibly testicular cancer later in life. Although some of these changes are benign, others are precursors of malignancy.
2. **Gallbladder disease**
   Two studies have reported a 2- to 4-fold increase in the risk of gallbladder disease requiring surgery in women receiving postmenopausal estrogens.

Continued on next page

Estratab—Cont.

3. Cardiovascular disease

Large doses of estrogen (5 mg conjugated estrogens per day), comparable to those used to treat cancer of the prostate and breast, have been shown in a large prospective clinical trial in men to increase the risks of nonfatal myocardial infarction, pulmonary embolism, and thrombophlebitis. These risks cannot necessarily be extrapolated from men to women. However, to avoid the theoretical cardiovascular risk caused by high estrogen doses, the dose for estrogen replacement therapy should not exceed the lowest effective dose.

4. Elevated Blood Pressure

Occasional blood pressure increases during estrogen replacement therapy have been attributed to idiosyncratic reactions to estrogens. More often, blood pressure has remained the same or has dropped. One study showed that postmenopausal estrogen users have higher blood pressure than nonusers. Two other studies showed slightly lower blood pressure among estrogen users compared to nonusers. Postmenopausal estrogen use does not increase the risk of stroke. Nonetheless, blood pressure should be monitored at regular intervals with estrogen use.

5. Hypercalcemia

Administration of estrogens may lead to severe hypercalcemia in patients with breast cancer and bone metastases. If this occurs, the drug should be stopped and appropriate measures taken to reduce the serum calcium level.

PRECAUTIONS
General

1. *Addition of a progestin:* Studies of the addition of a progestin for ten or more days of a cycle of estrogen administration have reported a lowered incidence of endometrial hyperplasia than would be induced by estrogen treatment alone. Morphological and biochemical studies of endometria suggest that 10 to 14 days of progestin are needed to provide maximal maturation of the endometrium and to reduce the likelihood of hyperplastic changes.

There are, however, possible risks which may be associated with the use of progestins in estrogen replacement regimens. These include:

(a) adverse effects on lipoprotein metabolism (lowering HDL and raising LDL) which could diminish the purported cardioprotective effects of estrogen therapy (see **PRECAUTIONS** below);

(b) impairment of glucose tolerance; and

(c) possible enhancement of mitotic activity in breast epithelial tissue, although few epidemiological data are available to address this point (see **PRECAUTIONS** below).

The choice of progestin, its dose, and its regimen may be important in minimizing these adverse effects, but these issues will require further study before they are clarified.

2. *Cardiovascular risk:* **A causal relationship between estrogen replacement therapy and reduction of cardiovascular disease in postmenopausal women has not been proven. Furthermore, the effect of added progestins on this putative benefit is not yet known.**

In recent years many published studies have suggested that there may be a cause-effect relationship between postmenopausal oral estrogen replacement therapy **without added progestins** and a decrease in cardiovascular disease in women. Although most of the observational studies which assessed this statistical association have reported a 20% to 50% reduction in coronary heart disease risk and associated mortality in estrogen takers, the following should be considered when interpreting these reports:

(a) Because only one of these studies was randomized and it was too small to yield statistically significant results, all relevant studies were subject to selection bias. Thus, the apparently reduced risk of coronary artery disease cannot be attributed with certainty to estrogen replacement therapy. It may instead have been caused by life-style and medical characteristics of the women studied with the result that healthier women were selected for estrogen therapy. In general, treated women were of higher socioeconomic and educational status, more slender, more physically active, more likely to have undergone surgical menopause, and less likely to have diabetes than the untreated women. Although some studies attempted to control for these selection factors, it is common for properly designed randomized trials to fail to confirm benefits suggested by less rigorous study designs. Thus, ongoing and future large-scale randomized trials may fail to confirm this apparent benefit.

(b) Current medical practice often includes the use of concomitant progestin therapy in women with intact uteri (see **PRECAUTIONS** and **WARNINGS**). While the effects of added progestins on the risk of ischemic

heart disease are not known, all available progestins reverse at least some of the favorable effects of estrogens on HDL and LDL levels.

(c) While the effects of added progestins on the risk of breast cancer are also unknown, available epidemiological evidence suggests that progestins do not reduce, and may enhance, the moderately increased breast cancer incidence that has been reported with prolonged estrogen replacement therapy (see **WARNINGS** above).

Because relatively long-term use of estrogens by a woman with a uterus has been shown to induce endometrial cancer, physicians often recommend that women who are deemed candidates for hormone replacement should take progestins as well as estrogens. When considering prescribing concomitant estrogens and progestins for hormone replacement therapy, physicians and patients are advised to carefully weigh the potential benefits and risks of the added progestin. Large-scale randomized, placebo-controlled, prospective clinical trials are required to clarify these issues.

3. *Physical Examination:* A complete medical and family history should be taken prior to the initiation of any estrogen therapy. The pretreatment and periodic physical examinations should include special reference to blood pressure, breasts, abdomen, and pelvic organs, and should include a Papanicolaou smear. As a general rule, estrogen should not be prescribed for longer than one year without reexamining the patient.

4. *Hypercoagulability:* Some studies have shown that women taking estrogen replacement therapy have hypercoagulability, primarily related to decreased antithrombin activity. This effect appears dose- and duration-dependent and is less pronounced than that associated with oral contraceptive use. Also, postmenopausal women tend to have increased coagulation parameters at baseline compared to premenopausal women. There is some suggestion that low dose postmenopausal mestranol may increase the risk of thromboembolism, although the majority of studies (of primarily conjugated estrogen users) reports no such increase. There is insufficient information on hypercoagulability in women who have had previous thromboembolic disease.

5. *Familial hyperlipoproteinemia:* Estrogen therapy may be associated with massive elevations of plasma triglycerides leading to pancreatitis and other complications in patients with familial defects of lipoprotein metabolism.

6. *Fluid retention:* Because estrogen may cause some degree of fluid retention, conditions which might be exacerbated by this factor such as asthma, epilepsy, migraine, and cardiac or renal dysfunction, require careful observation.

7. *Uterine bleeding and mastodynia:* Certain patients may develop undesirable manifestations of estrogenic stimulation, such as abnormal uterine bleeding, and mastodynia.

8. *Impaired liver function:* Estrogens may be poorly metabolized in patients with impaired liver function and should be administered with caution.

Information for the Patient

See text of Patient Package Insert below which appears after the **HOW SUPPLIED** section.

Laboratory Tests

Estrogen administration should generally be guided by clinical response at the smallest dose, rather than laboratory monitoring, for relief of symptoms for those indications in which symptoms are observable. For prevention of osteoporosis, however, see **DOSAGE AND ADMINISTRATION** section.

Drug/Laboratory Test Interactions

1. Accelerated prothrombin time, partial thromboplastin time, and platelet aggregation time; increased platelet count; increased factors II, VII antigen, VIII antigen, VIII coagulant activity, IX, X, XII, VII-X complex, II-VII-X complex, and beta-thromboglobulin; decreased levels of anti-factor Xa and antithrombin III, decreased antithrombin III activity; increased levels of fibrinogen and fibrinogen activity; increased plasminogen antigen and activity.

2. Increased thyroid-binding globulin (TBG) leading to increased circulating total thyroid hormone, as measured by protein-bound iodine (PBI), T4 levels (by column or by radioimmunoassay) or T3 levels by radioimmunoassay. T3 resin uptake is decreased, reflecting the elevated TBG. Free T4 and T3 concentrations are unaltered.

3. Other binding proteins may be elevated in serum, i.e., corticosteroid binding globulin (CBG), sex hormone-binding globulin (SHBG), leading to increased circulating corticosteroids and sex steroids respectively. Free or biologically active hormone concentrations are unchanged. Other plasma proteins may be increased (angiotensinogen/renin substrate, alpha-1-antitrypsin, ceruloplasmin).

4. Increased plasma HDL and HDL-2 subfraction concentrations, reduced LDL cholesterol concentration, increased triglyceride levels.

5. Impaired glucose tolerance.

6. Reduced response to metyrapone test.

7. Reduced serum folate concentration.

Carcinogenesis, Mutagenesis, Impairment of Fertility

Long-term, continuous administration of natural and synthetic estrogens in certain animal species increases the frequency of carcinomas of the breast, uterus, cervix, vagina, testis and liver. See **CONTRAINDICATIONS** and **WARNINGS**.

Pregnancy Category X

Estrogens should not be used during pregnancy. See **CONTRAINDICATIONS** and Boxed Warning.

Nursing Mothers

As a general principle, the administration of any drug to nursing mothers should be done only when clearly necessary since many drugs are excreted in human milk. In addition, estrogen administration to nursing mothers has been shown to decrease the quantity and quality of the milk.

ADVERSE REACTIONS

The following additional adverse reactions have been reported with estrogen therapy (See **WARNINGS** regarding induction of neoplasia, adverse effects on the fetus, increased incidence of gallbladder disease, cardiovascular disease, elevated blood pressure, and hypercalcemia.)

1. Genitourinary system:
   Changes in vaginal bleeding pattern and abnormal withdrawal bleeding or flow.
   Breakthrough bleeding, spotting.
   Increase in size of uterine leiomyomata.
   Vaginal candidiasis.
   Change in amount of cervical secretion.
2. Breasts:
   Tenderness, enlargement.
3. Gastrointestinal:
   Nausea, vomiting.
   Abdominal cramps, bloating.
   Cholestatic jaundice.
   Increased incidence of gallbladder disease.
4. Skin:
   Chloasma or melasma which may persist when drug is discontinued.
   Erythema multiforme.
   Erythema nodosum.
   Hemorrhagic eruption.
   Loss of scalp hair.
   Hirsutism.
5. Eyes:
   Steepening of corneal curvature.
   Intolerance to contact lenses.
6. CNS:
   Headache, migraine, dizziness.
   Mental depression.
   Chorea
7. Miscellaneous:
   Increase or decrease in weight.
   Reduced carbohydrate tolerance.
   Aggravation of porphyria.
   Edema.
   Changes in libido.

OVERDOSAGE

Serious ill effects have not been reported following acute ingestion of large doses of estrogen-containing oral contraceptives by young children. Overdosage of estrogen may cause nausea and vomiting, and withdrawal bleeding may occur in females.

DOSAGE AND ADMINISTRATION

1. **Given cyclically for short term use only:**
   For treatment of moderate to severe *vasomotor* symptoms, atrophic vaginitis, or kraurosis vulvae associated with the menopause. The lowest dose that will control symptoms should be chosen and medication should be discontinued as promptly as possible. Administration should be cyclic (e.g., three weeks on and one week off). Attempts to discontinue or taper medication should be made at three to six month intervals.
   Usual dosage ranges:
   Vasomotor symptoms – 1.25 mg daily. If the patient has not menstruated within the last two months or more, cyclic administration is started arbitrarily. If the patient is menstruating, cyclic administration is started on day 5 of bleeding.
   Atrophic vaginitis and kraurosis vulvae – 0.3 mg to 1.25 mg or more daily, depending upon the tissue response of the individual patient. Administer cyclically.
2. **Given cyclically:** Female hypogonadism; female castration; primary ovarian failure.
   Usual dosage ranges:
   Female hypogonadism – 2.5 to 7.5 mg daily, in divided doses for 20 days, followed by a rest period of 10 days' duration. If bleeding does not occur by the end of this period, the same dosage schedule is repeated. The number of courses of estrogen therapy necessary to produce bleeding may vary depending on the responsiveness of the endometrium.

If bleeding occurs before the end of the 10 day period, begin a 20 day estrogen-progestin cyclic regimen with ESTRATAB® (Esterified Estrogens Tablets, USP), 2.5 to 7.5 mg daily in divided doses, for 20 days. During the last five days of estrogen therapy, give an oral progestin. If bleeding occurs before this regimen is concluded, therapy is discontinued and may be resumed on the fifth day of bleeding.

Female castration, and primary ovarian failure – 1.25 mg daily, cyclically. Adjust dosage upward or downward according to severity of symptoms and response of the patient. For maintenance, adjust dosage to lowest level that will provide effective control.

3. **Given chronically:** Inoperable progressing prostatic cancer – 1.25 to 2.5 mg three times daily. The effectiveness of therapy can be judged by phosphatase determinations as well as by symptomatic improvement of the patient. Inoperable progressing breast cancer in appropriately selected men and postmenopausal women. (See **INDICATIONS**) - - Suggested dosage is 10 mg three times daily for a period of at least three months.

4. **For prevention of osteoporosis** – – therapy with ESTRATAB® Tablets to prevent postmenopausal bone loss should be initiated as soon as possible after menopause. Therapy should be initiated at a daily dose of 0.3 mg and may be increased to a maximum daily dose of 1.25 mg if necessary to control concurrent menopausal symptoms.

Discontinuation of estrogen replacement therapy may re-establish the natural rate of bone loss.

Treated patients with an intact uterus should be monitored closely for signs of endometrial cancer, and appropriate diagnostic measures should be taken to rule out malignancy in the event of persistent or recurring abnormal vaginal bleeding.

HOW SUPPLIED

ESTRATAB® (Esterified Estrogens Tablets, USP) are available in the following strengths and package sizes:
— Each blue tablet with black imprint "SOLVAY 1014" contains 0.3 mg, in bottles of 100 (NDC 0032-1014-01).
— Each yellow tablet with black imprint "SOLVAY 1022" contains 0.625 mg, in bottles of 100 (NDC 0032-1022-01) and 1000 (NDC 0032-1022-10).
— Each light purple tablet with white imprint "SOLVAY 1025" contains 2.5 mg, in bottles of 100 (NDC 0032-1025-01).

Storage

Store and dispense in tight, light-resistant containers as defined in the USP. Store below 30°C (86°F). Protect from moisture.

℞ only

Manufactured by:

Solvay
Pharmaceuticals, Inc.
Marietta, GA 30062

INFORMATION FOR THE PATIENT

This leaflet describes when and how to use estrogens and the risks of estrogen treatment.

Estrogens have important benefits but also some risks. You must decide, with your doctor, whether the risks to you of estrogen use are acceptable because of their benefits. If you use estrogens, check with your doctor to make sure you are using the lowest possible dose that works, and that you don't use them for longer than necessary. How long you need to use estrogens will depend on the reason for use.

1. **ESTROGENS INCREASE THE RISK OF CANCER OF THE UTERUS IN WOMEN WHO HAVE HAD THEIR MENOPAUSE ("CHANGE OF LIFE")**

If you use any estrogen-containing drug, it is important to visit your doctor regularly and report any unusual vaginal bleeding right away. Vaginal bleeding after menopause may be a warning sign of uterine cancer. Your doctor should evaluate any unusual vaginal bleeding to find out the cause.

2. **ESTROGENS SHOULD NOT BE USED DURING PREGNANCY.**

Estrogens do not prevent miscarriage (spontaneous abortion) and are not needed in the days following childbirth. If you take estrogens during pregnancy, your unborn child has a greater than usual chance of having birth defects. The risk of developing these defects is small, but clearly larger than the risk in children whose mothers did not take estrogen during pregnancy. These birth defects may affect the baby's urinary system and sex organs. Daughters born to mothers who took DES (an estrogen drug) have a higher than usual chance of developing cancer of the vagina or cervix when they become teenagers or young adults. Sons may have a higher than usual chance of developing cancer of the testicles when they become teenagers or young adults.

USES OF ESTROGEN

(NOT EVERY ESTROGEN DRUG IS APPROVED FOR EVERY USE LISTED IN THIS SECTION). If you want to know which of these possible uses are approved for the medicine prescribed for you, ask your doctor or pharmacist to show you the professional labeling.

You can also look up the specific estrogen product in a book called the "Physicians' Desk Reference", which is available in many book stores and public libraries. (Generic drugs carry virtually the same labeling information as their brand name versions).

To reduce moderate or severe menopausal symptoms.

Estrogens are hormones made by the ovaries of normal women. Between ages 45 and 55, the ovaries normally stop making estrogens. This leads to a drop in body estrogen levels which causes the "change of life" or menopause (the end of monthly menstrual periods). If both ovaries are removed during an operation before natural menopause takes place, the sudden drop in estrogen levels causes "surgical menopause."

When the estrogen levels begin dropping, some women develop very uncomfortable symptoms, such as feelings of warmth in the face, neck, and chest, or sudden intense episodes of heat and sweating ("hot flashes" or "hot flushes"). Using estrogen drugs can help the body adjust to lower estrogen levels and reduce these symptoms. Most women have only mild menopausal symptoms or none at all and do not need to use estrogen drugs for these symptoms. Others may need to take estrogens for a few months while their bodies adjust to lower estrogen levels. The majority of women do not need estrogen replacement for longer than six months for these symptoms.

To treat vulval and vaginal atrophy (itching, burning, dryness in or around the vagina, difficulty or burning on urination) associated with menopause.

To treat certain conditions in which a young woman's ovaries do not produce enough estrogen naturally.

To treat certain types of abnormal vaginal bleeding due to hormonal imbalance when your doctor has found no serious cause of the bleeding.

To treat certain cancers in special situations, in men and women.

To prevent thinning of bones. Osteoporosis is a thinning of the bones that makes them weaker and allows them to break more easily. The bones of the spine, wrists and hips break most often in osteoporosis. Both men and women start to lose bone mass after about age 40, but women lose bone mass faster after the menopause. Using estrogens after the menopause slows down bone thinning and may prevent bones from breaking. Lifelong adequate calcium intake, either in the diet (such as dairy products) or by calcium supplements (to reach a total daily intake of 1000 milligrams per day before menopause or 1500 milligrams per day after menopause), may help to prevent osteoporosis. Regular weight-bearing exercise (like walking and running for an hour, two or three times a week) may also help to prevent osteoporosis. Before you change your calcium intake or exercise habits, it is important to discuss these lifestyle changes with your doctor to find out if they are safe for you.

Since estrogen use has some risks, only women who are likely to develop osteoporosis should use estrogens for prevention. Women who are likely to develop osteoporosis often have the following characteristics: white or Asian race, slim, cigarette smokers, and a family history of osteoporosis in a mother, sister, or aunt. Women who have relatively early menopause, often because their ovaries were removed during an operation ("surgical menopause"), are more likely to develop osteoporosis than women whose menopause happens at the average age.

WHO SHOULD NOT USE ESTROGENS

Estrogens should not be used:

During pregnancy (see Boxed Warning). If you think you may be pregnant, do not use any form of estrogen-containing drug. Using estrogens while you are pregnant may cause your unborn child to have birth defects. Estrogens do not prevent miscarriage.

If you have unusual vaginal bleeding which has not been evaluated by your doctor (see Boxed Warning). Unusual vaginal bleeding can be a warning sign of cancer of the uterus, especially if it happens after menopause. Your doctor must find out the cause of the bleeding so that he or she can recommend the proper treatment. Taking estrogens without visiting your doctor can cause you serious harm if your vaginal bleeding is caused by cancer of the uterus.

If you have had cancer. Since estrogens increase the risk of certain types of cancers, you should not use estrogens if you have ever had cancer of the breast or uterus, unless your doctor recommends that the drug may help in the cancer treatment. (For certain patients with breast or prostate cancer, estrogens may help.)

If you have any circulation problems. Estrogen drugs should not be used except in unusually special situations in which your doctor judges that you need estrogen therapy so much

that the risks are acceptable. Men and women with abnormal blood clotting conditions should avoid estrogen use (see **DANGERS OF ESTROGENS**, below).

When they do not work. During menopause, some women develop nervous symptoms or depression. Estrogens do not relieve these symptoms. You may have heard that taking estrogens for years after menopause will keep your skin soft and supple and keep you feeling young. There is no evidence for these claims and such long-term estrogen use may have serious risks.

After childbirth or when breastfeeding a baby. Estrogens should not be used to try to stop the breasts from filling with milk after a baby is born. Such treatment may increase the risk of developing blood clots (see **DANGERS OF ESTROGENS**, below).

If you are breastfeeding, you should avoid using any drugs because many drugs pass through to the baby in the milk. While nursing a baby, you should take drugs only on the advice of your health care provider.

DANGERS OF ESTROGENS

Cancer of the uterus. Your risk of developing cancer of the uterus gets higher the longer you use estrogens and the larger doses you use. One study showed that after women stop taking estrogens, this higher cancer risk quickly returns to the usual level of risk (as if you had never used estrogen therapy). Three other studies showed that the cancer risk stayed high for 8 to more than 15 years after stopping estrogen treatment. **Because of this risk, IT IS IMPORTANT TO TAKE THE LOWEST DOSE THAT WORKS AND TO TAKE IT ONLY AS LONG AS YOU NEED IT.**

Using progestin therapy together with estrogen therapy may reduce the higher risk of uterine cancer related to estrogen use (but see **OTHER INFORMATION**, below).

If you have had your uterus removed (total hysterectomy), there is no danger of developing cancer of the uterus.

Cancer of the breast. Most studies have not shown a higher risk of breast cancer in women who have ever used estrogens. However, some studies have reported that breast cancer developed more often (up to twice the usual rate) in women who used estrogens for long periods of time (especially more than 10 years), or who used higher doses for shorter time periods.

Regular breast examinations by a health professional and monthly self-examination are recommended for all women.

Gallbladder disease. Women who use estrogens after menopause are more likely to develop gallbladder disease needing surgery than women who do not use estrogens.

Abnormal blood clotting. Taking estrogens may cause changes in your blood clotting system. These changes allow the blood to clot more easily, possibly allowing clots to form in your bloodstream. If blood clots do form in your bloodstream, they can cut off the blood supply to vital organs, causing serious problems. These problems may include a stroke (by cutting off blood to the brain), a heart attack (by cutting off blood to the heart), a pulmonary embolus (by cutting off blood to the lungs), or other problems. Any of these conditions may cause death or serious long term disability. However, most studies of low dose estrogen usage by women do not show an increased risk of these complications.

SIDE EFFECTS

In addition to the risks listed above, the following side effects have been reported with estrogen use:

• Nausea, vomiting.
• Breast tenderness or enlargement.
• Enlargement of benign tumors ("fibroids") of the uterus.
• Retention of excess fluid. This may make some conditions worsen, such as asthma, epilepsy, migraine, heart disease, or kidney disease.
• A spotty darkening of the skin, particularly on the face.

REDUCING RISK OF ESTROGEN USE

If you use estrogens, you can reduce your risks by doing these things:

See your doctor regularly. While you are using estrogens, it is important to visit your doctor at least once a year for a check-up. If you develop vaginal bleeding while taking estrogens, you may need further evaluation. If members of your family have had breast cancer or if you have ever had breast lumps or an abnormal mammogram (breast x-ray), you may need to have more frequent breast examinations.

Reassess your need for estrogens. You and your doctor should reevaluate whether or not you still need estrogens at least every six months.

Be alert for signs of trouble. If any of these warning signals (or any other unusual symptoms) happen while you are using estrogens, call your doctor immediately:

• Abnormal bleeding from the vagina (possible uterine cancer).
• Pains in the calves or chest, sudden shortness of breath, or coughing blood (possible clot in the legs, heart, or lungs).
• Severe headache or vomiting, dizziness, faintness, changes in vision or speech, weakness or numbness of an arm or leg (possible clots in the brain or eye).

Continued on next page

Estratab—Cont.

- Breast lumps (possible breast cancer; ask your doctor or health professional to show you how to examine your breasts monthly).
- Yellowing of the skin or eyes (possible liver problem).
- Pain, swelling, or tenderness in the abdomen (possible gallbladder problem).

OTHER INFORMATION

Estrogens increase the risk of developing a condition (endometrial hyperplasia) that may lead to cancer of the lining of the uterus. Taking progestins, another hormone drug, with estrogens lowers the risk of developing this condition. Therefore, if your uterus has not been removed, your doctor may prescribe a progestin for you to take together with the estrogen.

You should know, however, that taking estrogens with progestins may have additional risks. These include:

— unhealthy effects on blood fats (especially the lowering of HDL blood cholesterol, the "good" blood fat which protects against heart disease);

— unhealthy effects on blood sugar (which might make a diabetic condition worse); and

— a possible further increase in breast cancer risk which may be associated with long-term estrogen use.

Some research had shown that estrogens taken **without** progestins may protect women against developing heart disease. However, this is not certain. The protection shown may have been caused by the characteristics of the estrogen-treated women, and not by the estrogen treatment itself. In general, treated women were slimmer, more physically active, and were less likely to have diabetes than the untreated women. These characteristics are known to protect against heart disease.

You are cautioned to discuss very carefully with your doctor or health care provider all the possible risks and benefits of long-term estrogen and progestin treatment as they affect you personally.

Your doctor has prescribed this drug for you and you alone. Do not give the drug to anyone else.

If you will be taking calcium supplements as part of the treatment to help prevent osteoporosis, check with your doctor about how much to take.

Keep this and all drugs out of the reach of children. In case of overdose, call your doctor, hospital, or poison control center immediately.

This leaflet provides a summary of the most important information about estrogens. If you want more information, ask your doctor or pharmacist to show you the professional labeling. The professional labeling is also published in a book called the "Physicians' Desk Reference," which is available in book stores and public libraries. Generic drugs carry virtually the same labeling information as their brand name versions.

HOW SUPPLIED

ESTRATAB® (Esterified Estrogens Tablets, USP) for oral administration.

Each blue tablet contains 0.3 mg.

Each yellow tablet contains 0.625 mg.

Each light purple tablet contains 2.5 mg.

℞ only

The appearance of ESTRATAB® Tablets is a trademark of Solvay Pharmaceuticals, Inc.

1222

7E Rev 2/98

Solvay
Pharmaceuticals, Inc.
Marietta, GA 30062

Shown in Product Identification Guide, page 340

ESTRATEST® ℞

[*es 'trah-test*]

ESTRATEST® H.S. ℞

(Esterified Estrogens and Methyltestosterone) Tablets

WARNING

1. ESTROGENS HAVE BEEN REPORTED TO INCREASE THE RISK OF ENDOMETRIAL CARCINOMA.

Three independent case control studies have reported an increased risk of endometrial cancer in postmenopausal women exposed to exogenous estrogens for prolonged periods.[1–3] This risk was independent of the other known risk factors for endometrial cancer. These studies are further supported by the finding that incidence rates of endometrial cancer have increased sharply since 1969 in eight different areas of the United States with population-based cancer reporting systems, an increase which may be related to the rapidly expanding use of estrogens during the last decade.[4]

The three case control studies reported that the risk of endometrial cancer in estrogen users was about 4.5 to 13.9 times greater than in nonusers. The risk appears to depend on both duration of treatment[1] and on estrogen dose.[3] In view of these findings, when estrogens are used for the treatment of menopausal symptoms, the lowest dose that will control symptoms should be utilized and medication should be discontinued as soon as possible. When prolonged treatment is medically indicated, the patient should be reassessed on at least a semiannual basis to determine the need for continued therapy. Although the evidence must be considered preliminary, one study suggests that cyclic administration of low doses of estrogen may carry less risk than continuous administration;[3] it therefore appears prudent to utilize such a regimen.

Close clinical surveillance of all women taking estrogens is important. In all cases of undiagnosed persistent or recurring abnormal vaginal bleeding, adequate diagnostic measures should be undertaken to rule out malignancy.

There is no evidence at present that "natural" estrogens are more or less hazardous than "synthetic" estrogens at equiestrogenic doses.

2. ESTROGENS SHOULD NOT BE USED DURING PREGNANCY.

The use of female sex hormones, both estrogens and progestogens, during early pregnancy may seriously damage the offspring. It has been shown that females exposed in utero to diethylstilbestrol, a non-steroidal estrogen, have an increased risk of developing in later life a form of vaginal or cervical cancer that is ordinarily extremely rare.[5,6] This risk has been estimated as not greater than 4 per 1000 exposures.[7] Furthermore, a high percentage of such exposed women (from 30 to 90 percent) have been found to have vaginal adenosis,[8–12] epithelial changes of the vagina and cervix. Although these changes are histologically benign, it is not known whether they are precursors of malignancy. Although similar data are not available with the use of other estrogens, it cannot be presumed they would not induce similar changes.

Several reports suggest an association between intrauterine exposure to female sex hormones and congenital anomalies, including congenital heart defects and limb reduction defects.[13–16] One case control study[16] estimated a 4.7 fold increased risk of limb reduction defects in infants exposed in utero to sex hormones (oral contraceptives, hormone withdrawal tests for pregnancy, or attempted treatment for threatened abortion). Some of these exposures were very short and involved only a few days of treatment. The data suggest that the risk of limb reduction defects in exposed fetuses is somewhat less than 1 per 1000.

In the past, female sex hormones have been used during pregnancy in an attempt to treat threatened or habitual abortion. There is considerable evidence that estrogens are ineffective for these indications, and there is no evidence from well controlled studies that progestogens are effective for these uses.

If ESTRATEST® or ESTRATEST® H.S. is used during pregnancy, or if the patient becomes pregnant while taking this drug, she should be apprised of the potential risks to the fetus, and the advisability of pregnancy continuation.

DESCRIPTION

ESTRATEST®: Each dark green, capsule shaped, sugar-coated oral tablet contains: 1.25 mg of Esterified Estrogens, USP and 2.5 mg of Methyltestosterone.

ESTRATEST® H.S. (Half-Strength): Each light green, capsule shaped, sugar-coated oral tablet contains: 0.625 mg of Esterified Estrogens, USP and 1.25 mg of Methyltestosterone.

ESTERIFIED ESTROGENS: Esterified Estrogens, USP is a mixture of the sodium salts of the sulfate esters of the estrogenic substances, principally estrone, that are of the type excreted by pregnant mares. Esterified Estrogens contain not less than 75.0 percent and not more than 85.0 percent of sodium estrone sulfate, and not less than 6.0 percent and not more than 15.0 percent of sodium equilin sulfate, in such proportion that the total of these two components is not less than 90.0 percent.

Category: Estrogens

METHYLTESTOSTERONE: Methyltestosterone is an androgen. Androgens are derivatives of cyclopentano-perhydrophenanthrene. Endogenous androgens are C-19 steroids with a side chain at C-17, and with two angular methyl groups. Testosterone is the primary endogenous androgen. Fluoxymesterone and methyltestosterone are synthetic derivatives of testosterone.

Methyltestosterone is a white to light yellow crystalline substance that is virtually insoluble in water but soluble in organic solvents. It is stable in air but decomposes in light.

Methyltestosterone structural formula:

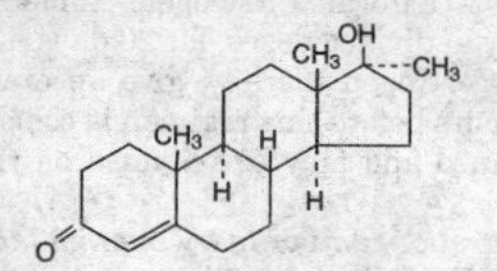

$C_{20}H_{30}O_2$, 302.46

Androst-4-en-3-one, 17-hydroxy-17-methyl-, (17B)-

Category: Androgen.

ESTRATEST® and ESTRATEST® H.S. Tablets contain the following inactive ingredients: acacia, calcium carbonate, citric acid, gelatin, lactose (anhydrous), magnesium stearate, methylparaben, microcrystalline cellulose, pharmaceutical glaze, povidone, propylparaben, sodium benzoate, sodium bicarbonate, sodium carboxymethylcellulose, sorbic acid, sucrose, starch (corn), talc, titanium dioxide, tribasic calcium phosphate, and other minor ingredients.

ESTRATEST® Tablets also contain: FD&C Blue No. 1 Lake, FD&C Yellow No. 6 Lake, and FD&C Yellow No. 10 Lake.

ESTRATEST® H.S. Tablets also contain: FD&C Yellow No. 10 Lake, FD&C Blue No. 1 Lake, and FD&C Blue No. 2 Lake.

CLINICAL PHARMACOLOGY

Estrogens: Estrogens are important in the development and maintenance of the female reproductive system and secondary sex characteristics. They promote growth and development of the vagina, uterus, and fallopian tubes, and enlargement of the breasts. Indirectly, they contribute to the shaping of the skeleton, maintenance of tone and elasticity of urogenital structures, changes in the epiphyses of the long bones that allow for the pubertal growth spurt and its termination, growth of axillary and pubic hair, and pigmentation of the nipples and genitals. Decline of estrogenic activity at the end of the menstrual cycle can bring on menstruation, although the cessation of progesterone secretion is the most important factor in the mature ovulatory cycle. However, in the preovulatory or nonovulatory cycle, estrogen is the primary determinant in the onset of menstruation. Estrogens also affect the release of pituitary gonadotropins.

The pharmacologic effects of esterified estrogens are similar to those of endogenous estrogens. They are soluble in water and are well absorbed from the gastrointestinal tract.

In responsive tissues (female genital organs, breasts, hypothalamus, pituitary) estrogens enter the cell and are transported into the nucleus. As a result of estrogen action, specific RNA and protein synthesis occurs.

Estrogen Pharmacokinetics

Metabolism and inactivation occur primarily in the liver. Some estrogens are excreted into the bile; however they are reabsorbed from the intestine and returned to the liver through the portal venous system. Water soluble esterified estrogens are strongly acidic and are ionized in body fluids, which favor excretion through the kidneys since tubular reabsorption is minimal.

Androgens Endogenous androgens are responsible for the normal growth and development of the male sex organs and for maintenance of secondary sex characteristics. These effects include the growth and maturation of prostate, seminal vesicles, penis, and scrotum; the development of male hair distribution, such as beard, pubic, chest, and axillary hair, laryngeal enlargement, vocal cord thickening, alterations in body musculature, and fat distribution. Drugs in this class also cause retention of nitrogen, sodium, potassium, phosphorus, and decreased urinary excretion of calcium. Androgens have been reported to increase protein anabolism and decrease protein catabolism. Nitrogen balance is improved only when there is sufficient intake of calories and protein. Androgens are responsible for the growth spurt of adolescence and for the eventual termination of linear growth which is brought about by fusion of the epiphyseal growth centers. In children, exogenous androgens accelerate linear growth rates, but may cause a disproportionate advancement in bone maturation. Use over long periods may result in fusion of the epiphyseal growth centers and termination of growth process. Androgens have been reported to stimulate the production of red blood cells by enhancing the production of erythropoietic stimulating factor.

Androgen Pharmacokinetics

Testosterone given orally is metabolized by the gut and 44 percent is cleared by the liver in the first pass. Oral doses as high as 400 mg per day are needed to achieve clinically effective blood levels for full replacement therapy. The synthetic androgens (methyltestosterone and fluoxymesterone) are less extensively metabolized by the liver and have longer half-lives. They are more suitable than testosterone for oral administration.

Testosterone in plasma is 98 percent bound to a specific testosterone-estradiol binding globulin, and about 2 percent is free. Generally, the amount of this sex-hormone binding

globulin in the plasma will determine the distribution of testosterone between free and bound forms, and the free testosterone concentration will determine its half-life.

About 90 percent of a dose of testosterone is excreted in the urine as glucuronic and sulfuric acid conjugates of testosterone and its metabolites; about 6 percent of a dose is excreted in the feces, mostly in the unconjugated form. Inactivation of testosterone occurs primarily in the liver. Testosterone is metabolized to various 17-keto steroids through two different pathways. There are considerable variations of the half-life of testosterone as reported in the literature, ranging from 10 to 100 minutes.

In many tissues the activity of testosterone appears to depend on reduction to dihydrotestosterone, which binds to cytosol receptor proteins. The steroid-receptor complex is transported to the nucleus where it initiates transcription events and cellular changes related to androgen action.

INDICATIONS AND USAGE

ESTRATEST® and ESTRATEST® H.S. are indicated in the treatment of:

Moderate to severe *vasomotor* symptoms associated with the menopause in those patients not improved by estrogens alone. (There is no evidence that estrogens are effective for nervous symptoms or depression without associated vasomotor symptoms, and they should not be used to treat such conditions.)

ESTRATEST® AND ESTRATEST® H.S. HAVE NOT BEEN SHOWN TO BE EFFECTIVE FOR ANY PURPOSE DURING PREGNANCY AND ITS USE MAY CAUSE SEVERE HARM TO THE FETUS (SEE BOXED WARNING).

CONTRAINDICATIONS

Estrogens should not be used in women with any of the following conditions:

1. Known or suspected cancer of the breast except in appropriately selected patients being treated for metastatic disease.
2. Known or suspected estrogen-dependent neoplasia.
3. Known or suspected pregnancy (See Boxed Warning).
4. Undiagnosed abnormal genital bleeding.
5. Active thrombophlebitis or thromboembolic disorders.
6. A past history of thrombophlebitis, thrombosis, or thromboembolic disorders associated with previous estrogen use (except when used in treatment of breast malignancy).

Methyltestosterone should not be used in:

1. The presence of severe liver damage.
2. Pregnancy and in breast-feeding mothers because of the possibility of masculinization of the female fetus or breast-fed infant.

WARNINGS

Associated with Estrogens:

1. **Induction of malignant neoplasms.** Long term continuous administration of natural and synthetic estrogens in certain animal species increases the frequency of carcinomas of the breast, cervix, vagina, and liver. There is now evidence that estrogens increase the risk of carcinoma of the endometrium in humans (See Boxed Warning).

   At the present time there is no satisfactory evidence that estrogens given to postmenopausal women increase the risk of cancer of the breast,[18] although a recent long-term follow-up of a single physician's practice has raised this possibility.[18a] Because of the animal data, there is a need for caution in prescribing estrogens for women with a strong family history of breast cancer or who have breast nodules, fibrocystic disease, or abnormal mammograms.

2. **Gallbladder disease.** A recent study has reported a 2 to 3-fold increase in the risk of surgically confirmed gallbladder disease in women receiving postmenopausal estrogens,[18] similar to the 2-fold increase previously noted in users of oral contraceptives.[19–24a] In the case of oral contraceptives the increased risk appeared after two years of use.[24]

3. **Effects similar to those caused by estrogen-progestogen oral contraceptives.** There are several serious adverse effects of oral contraceptives, most of which have not, up to now, been documented as consequences of postmenopausal estrogen therapy. This may reflect the comparatively low doses of estrogen used in postmenopausal women. It would be expected that the larger doses of estrogen used to treat prostatic or breast cancer or postpartum breast engorgement are more likely to result in these adverse effects, and, in fact, it has been shown that there is an increased risk of thrombosis in men receiving estrogens for prostatic cancer and women for postpartum breast engorgement.[20–23]

   a. **Thromboembolic disease.** It is now well established that users of oral contraceptives have an increased risk of various thromboembolic and thrombotic vascular diseases, such as thrombophlebitis, pulmonary embolism, stroke, and myocardial infarction.[24–31] Cases of retinal thrombosis, mesenteric thrombosis, and optic neuritis have been reported in oral contraceptive users. There is evidence that the risk of several of these adverse reactions is related to the dose of the drug.[32,33]

An increased risk of postsurgery thromboembolic complications has also been reported in users of oral contraceptives.[34,35] If feasible, estrogen should be discontinued at least 4 weeks before surgery of the type associated with an increased risk of thromboembolism, or during periods of prolonged immobilization.

While an increased rate of thromboembolic and thrombotic disease in postmenopausal users of estrogens has not been found,[18–36] this does not rule out the possibility that such an increase may be present or that subgroups of women who have underlying risk factors or who are receiving relatively large doses of estrogens may have increased risk. Therefore estrogens should not be used in persons with active thrombophlebitis or thromboembolic disorders, and they should not be used (except in treatment of malignancy) in persons with a history of such disorders in association with estrogen use. They should be used with caution in patients with cerebral vascular or coronary artery disease and only for those in whom estrogens are clearly needed.

Large doses of estrogen (5 mg esterified estrogens per day), comparable to those used to treat cancer of the prostate and breast, have been shown in a large prospective clinical trial in men[37] to increase the risk of nonfatal myocardial infarction, pulmonary embolism and thrombophlebitis. When estrogen doses of this size are used, any of the thromboembolic and thrombotic adverse effects associated with oral contraceptive use should be considered a clear risk.

b. **Hepatic adenoma.** Benign hepatic adenomas appear to be associated with the use of oral contraceptives.[38–40] Although benign and rare, these may rupture and may cause death through intra-abdominal hemorrhage. Such lesions have not yet been reported in association with other estrogen or progestogen preparations but should be considered in estrogen users having abdominal pain and tenderness, abdominal mass, or hypovolemic shock. Hepatocellular carcinoma has also been reported in women taking estrogen-containing oral contraceptives.[39] The relationship of this malignancy to these drugs is not known at this time.

c. **Elevated blood pressure.** Increased blood pressure is not uncommon in women using oral contraceptives. There is now a report that this may occur with use of estrogens in the menopause[41] and blood pressure should be monitored with estrogen use, especially if high doses are used.

d. **Glucose tolerance.** A worsening of glucose tolerance has been observed in a significant percentage of patients on estrogen-containing oral contraceptives. For this reason, diabetic patients should be carefully observed while receiving estrogens.

4. **Hypercalcemia.** Administration of estrogens may lead to severe hypercalcemia in patients with breast cancer and bone metastases. If this occurs, the drug should be stopped and appropriate measures taken to reduce the serum calcium level.

Associated with Methyltestosterone

In patients with breast cancer, androgen therapy may cause hypercalcemia by stimulating osteolysis. In this case, the drug should be discontinued.

Prolonged use of high doses of androgens has been associated with the development of peliosis hepatis and hepatic neoplasms including hepatocellular carcinoma. (See PRECAUTIONS—*Carcinogenesis*). Peliosis hepatis can be a life-threatening or fatal complication.

Cholestatic hepatitis and jaundice occur with 17-alpha-alkylandrogens at a relatively low dose. If cholestatic hepatitis with jaundice appears or if liver function tests become abnormal, the androgen should be discontinued and the etiology should be determined. Drug-induced jaundice is reversible when the medication is discontinued.

Edema with or without heart failure may be a serious complication in patients with preexisting cardiac, renal, or hepatic disease. In addition to discontinuation of the drug, diuretic therapy may be required.

PRECAUTIONS

Associated with Estrogens
A. General Precautions.

1. A complete medical and family history should be taken prior to the initiation of any estrogen therapy. The pretreatment and periodic physical examinations should include special reference to blood pressure, breasts, abdomen, and pelvic organs, and should include a Papanicolaou smear. As a general rule, estrogen should not be prescribed for longer than one year without another physical examination being performed.

2. Fluid retention—Because estrogens may cause some degree of fluid retention, conditions which might be influenced by this factor such as asthma, epilepsy, migraine, and cardiac or renal dysfunction, require careful observation.

3. Certain patients may develop undesirable manifestations of excessive estrogenic stimulation, such as abnormal or excessive uterine bleeding, mastodynia, etc.

4. Oral contraceptives appear to be associated with an increased incidence of mental depression.[24] Although it is not clear whether this is due to the estrogenic or progestogenic component of the contraceptive, patients with a history of depression should be carefully observed.

5. Preexisting uterine leiomyomata may increase in size during estrogen use.

6. The pathologist should be advised of estrogen therapy when relevant specimens are submitted.

7. Patients with a past history of jaundice during pregnancy have an increased risk of recurrence of jaundice while receiving estrogen-containing oral contraceptive therapy. If jaundice develops in any patient receiving estrogen, the medication should be discontinued while the cause is investigated.

8. Estrogens may be poorly metabolized in patients with impaired liver function and they should be administered with caution in such patients.

9. Because estrogens influence the metabolism of calcium and phosphorus, they should be used with caution in patients with metabolic bone diseases that are associated with hypercalcemia or in patients with renal insufficiency.

10. Because of the effects of estrogens on epiphyseal closure, they should be used judiciously in young patients in whom bone growth is not complete.

11. Certain endocrine and liver function tests may be affected by estrogen-containing oral contraceptives. The following similar changes may be expected with larger doses of estrogen:

a. Increased sulfobromophthalein retention.

b. b. Increased prothrombin and factors VII, VIII, IX and X; decreased antithrombin 3; increased norepinephrine-induced platelet aggregability.

c. c. Increased thyroid binding globulin (TBG) leading to increased circulating total thyroid hormone, as measured by PBI, T4 by column, or T4 by radioimmunoassay. Free T3 resin uptake is decreased, reflecting the elevated TBG; free T4 concentration is unaltered.

d. Impaired glucose tolerance.

e. Decreased pregnanediol excretion.

f. Reduced response to metyrapone test.

g. Reduced serum folate concentration.

h. Increased serum triglyceride and phospholipid concentration.

B. Information for the Patient. See text of Patient Package Insert which appears after the REFERENCES.

C. Pregnancy Category X. See CONTRAINDICATIONS and Boxed WARNING.

D. Nursing Mothers. As a general principle, the administration of any drug to nursing mothers should be done only when clearly necessary since many drugs are excreted in human milk.

Associated with Methyltestosterone:
A. General Precautions

1. Women should be observed for signs of virilization (deepening of the voice, hirsutism, acne, clitoromegaly, and menstrual irregularities). Discontinuation of drug therapy at the time of evidence of mild virilism is necessary to prevent irreversible virilization. Such virilization is usual following androgen use at high doses.

2. Prolonged dosage of androgen may result in sodium and fluid retention. This may present a problem, especially in patients with compromised cardiac reserve or renal disease.

3. Hypersensitivity may occur rarely.

4. PBI may be decreased in patients taking androgens.

5. Hypercalcemia may occur. If this does occur, the drug should be discontinued.

B. Information for the Patient

The physician should instruct patients to report any of the following side effects of androgens:

Women: Hoarseness, acne, changes in menstrual periods, or more hair on the face.

All Patients: Any nausea, vomiting, changes in skin color or ankle swelling.

C. Laboratory tests

1. Women with disseminated breast carcinoma should have frequent determination of urine and serum calcium levels during the course of androgen therapy (See WARNINGS).

2. Because of the hepatotoxicity associated with the use of 17-alpha-alkylated androgens, liver function tests should be obtained periodically.

3. Hemoglobin and hematocrit should be checked periodically for polycythemia in patients who are receiving high doses of androgens.

D. Drug Interactions

1. *Anticoagulants* C-17 substituted derivatives of testosterone, such as methandrostenolone, have been reported

Continued on next page

Estratest/Estratest H.S.—Cont.

to decrease the anticoagulant requirements of patients receiving oral anticoagulants. Patients receiving oral anticoagulant therapy require close monitoring, especially when androgens are started or stopped.

2. *Oxyphenbutazone.* Concurrent administration of oxyphenbutazone and androgens may result in elevated serum levels of oxyphenbutazone.

3. *Insulin.* In diabetic patients the metabolic effects of androgens may decrease blood glucose and insulin requirements.

E. Drug/Laboratory Test Interferences

Androgens may decrease levels of thyroxine-binding globulin, resulting in decreased T_4 serum levels and increased resin uptake of T_3 and T_4. Free thyroid hormone levels remain unchanged, however, and there is no clinical evidence of thyroid dysfunction.

F. Carcinogenesis

Animal Data. Testosterone has been tested by subcutaneous injection and implantation in mice and rats. The implant induced cervical-uterine tumors in mice, which metastasized in some cases. There is suggestive evidence that injection of testosterone into some strains of female mice increases their susceptibility to hepatoma. Testosterone is also known to increase the number of tumors and decrease the degree of differentiation of chemically induced carcinomas of the liver in rats.

Human Data. There are rare reports of hepatocellular carcinoma in patients receiving long-term therapy with androgens in high doses. Withdrawal of the drugs did not lead to regression of the tumors in all cases.

Geriatric patients treated with androgens may be at an increased risk for the development of prostatic hypertrophy and prostatic carcinoma.

G. Pregnancy

Teratogenic Effects. Pregnancy Category X (see CONTRAINDICATIONS).

H. Nursing Mothers

It is not known whether androgens are excreted in human milk. Because many drugs are excreted in human milk and because of the potential for serious adverse reactions in nursing infants from androgens, a decision should be made whether to discontinue nursing or to discontinue the drug, taking into account the importance of the drug to the mother.

ADVERSE REACTIONS

Associated with Estrogens (See Warnings regarding induction of neoplasia, adverse effects on the fetus, increased incidence of gallbladder disease, and adverse effects similar to those of oral contraceptives, including thromboembolism). The following additional adverse reactions have been reported with estrogenic therapy, including oral contraceptives:

1. Genitourinary system.
Breakthrough bleeding, spotting, change in menstrual flow.
Dysmenorrhea.
Premenstrual-like syndrome.
Amenorrhea during and after treatment.
Increase in size of uterine fibromyomata.
Vaginal candidiasis.
Change in cervical erosion and in degree of cervical secretion.
Cystitis-like syndrome.

2. Breasts.
Tenderness, enlargement, secretion.

3. Gastrointestinal.
Nausea, vomiting.
Abdominal cramps, bloating.
Cholestatic jaundice.

4. Skin.
Chloasma or melasma which may persist when drug is discontinued.
Erythema multiforme.
Erythema nodosum.
Hemorrhagic eruption.
Loss of scalp hair.
Hirsutism.

5. Eyes.
Steepening of corneal curvature.
Intolerance to contact lenses.

6. CNS.
Headache, migraine, dizziness.
Mental depression.
Chorea.

7. Miscellaneous.
Increase or decrease in weight.
Reduced carbohydrate tolerance.
Aggravation of porphyria.
Edema.
Changes in libido.

Associated with Methyltestosterone

A. Endocrine and Urogenital

1. *Female:* The most common side effects of androgen therapy are amenorrhea and other menstrual irregulari-

ties, inhibition of gonadotropin secretion, and virilization, including deepening of the voice and clitoral enlargement. The latter usually is not reversible after androgens are discontinued. When administered to a pregnant woman androgens cause virilization of external genitalia of the female fetus.

2. *Skin and Appendages:* Hirsutism, male pattern of baldness, and acne.

3. *Fluid and Electrolyte Disturbances:* Retention of sodium, chloride, water, potassium, calcium, and inorganic phosphates.

4. *Gastrointestinal:* Nausea, cholestatic jaundice, alterations in liver function test, rarely hepatocellular neoplasms, and peliosis hepatis (see WARNINGS).

5. *Hematologic:* Suppression of clotting factors II, V, VII, and X, bleeding in patients on concomitant anticoagulant therapy, and polycythemia.

6. *Nervous System:* Increased or decreased libido, headache, anxiety, depression, and generalized paresthesia.

7. *Metabolic:* Increased serum cholesterol.

8. *Miscellaneous:* Inflammation and pain at the site of intramuscular injection or subcutaneous implantation of testosterone containing pellets, stomatitis with buccal preparations, and rarely anaphylactoid reactions.

OVERDOSAGE

Numerous reports of ingestion of large doses of estrogen-containing oral contraceptives by young children indicate that serious ill effects do not occur. Overdosage of estrogen may cause nausea, and withdrawal bleeding may occur in females.

There have been no reports of acute overdosage with the androgens.

DOSAGE AND ADMINISTRATION

1. *Given cyclically for short-term use only:*

For treatment of moderate to severe *vasomotor* symptoms associated with the menopause in patients not improved by estrogen alone.

The lowest dose that will control symptoms should be chosen and medication should be discontinued as promptly as possible.

Administration should be cyclic (e.g., three weeks on and one week off).

Attempts to discontinue or taper medication should be made at three to six month intervals.

Usual Dosage Range: 1 tablet of ESTRATEST or 1 to 2 tablets of ESTRATEST H.S. daily as recommended by the physician.

Treated patients with an intact uterus should be monitored closely for signs of endometrial cancer and appropriate diagnostic measures should be taken to rule out malignancy in the event of persistent or recurring abnormal vaginal bleeding.

HOW SUPPLIED

ESTRATEST® (Imprinted "SOLVAY 1026") in bottles of 100—NDC 0032-1026-01 and 1000—NDC 0032-1026-10.
ESTRATEST® (Dark green, capsule shaped, sugar-coated oral tablets) contains: 1.25 mg of Esterified Estrogens, USP and 2.5 mg of Methyltestosterone, USP.
ESTRATEST® H.S. (Imprinted "SOLVAY 1023") in bottles of 100—NDC 0032-1023-01.
ESTRATEST® H.S. "Half-Strength" (Light green, capsule shaped, sugar-coated oral tablets) contains: 0.625 mg of Esterified Estrogens, USP and 1.25 mg of Methyltestosterone, USP.
Store at controlled room temperature, 15°–30°C (59°–86°F).

REFERENCES

1. Ziel, H.K., *et al.:* N. Engl. J. Med. *293* :1167–1170, 1975.
2. Smith, D.C., *et al.:* N. Engl. J. Med. *293* :1164–1167, 1975.
3. Mack, T.M., *et al.:* N. Engl. J. Med. *294* :1262–1267, 1976.
4. Weiss, N.S., *et al.:* N. Engl. J. Med. *294* :1259–1262, 1976.
5. Herbst, A.L., *et al.:* N. Engl. J. Med. *284* :878–881, 1971.
6. Greenwald, P., *et al.:* N. Engl. J. Med. *285* :390–392, 1971.
7. Lanier, A., *et al.:* Mayo Clin. Proc. *48* :793–799, 1973.
8. Herbst, A., *et al.:* Obstet. Gynecol. *40* :287–298, 1972.
9. Herbst, A., *et al.:* Am. J. Obstet. Gynecol. *118* :607–615, 1974.
10. Herbst, A., *et al.:* N. Engl. J. Med. *292* :334–339, 1975.
11. Stafl, A., *et al.:* Obstet. Gynecol. *43* –128, 1974.
12. Sherman, A.I., *et al.:* Obstet. Gynecol. *44* :531–545, 1974.
13. Gal, I., *et al.:* Nature *216* :83, 1967.
14. Levy, E.P., *et al.:* Lancet *1* :611, 1973.
15. Nora, J., *et al.:* Lancet *1* :941–942, 1973.
16. Janerich, D.T., *et al.:* N. Engl. J. Med. *291* :697–700, 1974.
17. Estrogens for Oral or Parenteral Use: Federal Register *40* :8212, 1975.
18. Boston Collaborative Drug Surveillance Program: N. Engl. J. Med. *290* :15–19, 1974.
18a.Hoover, R., *et al.:* N. Engl. J. Med. *295* :401–405, 1976.
19. Boston Collaborative Drug Surveillance Program: Lancet *1* :1399–1404, 1973.
20. Daniel, D.G., *et al.:* Lancet *2* :287–289, 1967.
21. The Veterans Administration Cooperative Urological Research Group: J. Urol. *98* :516–522, 1967.
22. Bailar, J. C.: Lancet *2* :560, 1967.
23. Blackard, C., *et al.:* Cancer *26* :249–256, 1970.
24. Royal College of General Practitioners: J.R. Coll, Gen. Pract. *13* :267–279, 1967.
25. Inman, W.H.W., *et al.:* Br. Med. J. *2* :193–199, 1968.
26. Vessey, M.P., *et al.:* Br. Med. J. *2* :651–657, 1969.
27. Sartwell, P.E., *et al.:* Am. J. Epidemiol, *90* :365–380, 1969.
28. Collaborative Group for the Study of Stroke in Young Women: N. Engl. J. Med. *288* :871–878, 1973.
29. Collaborative Group for the Study of Stroke in Young Women: J.A.M.A. *231* :718–722, 1975.
30. Mann, J.I., *et al.:* Br. Med. J. *2* :245–248, 1975.
31. Mann, J.I., *et al.:* Br. Med. J. *2* :241–245, 1975.
32. Inman, W.H.W., *et al.:* Br. Med. J. *2* :203–209, 1970.
33. Stolley, P.D., *et al.:* Am. J. Epidemiol, *102* :197–208, 1975.
34. Vessey, M.P., *et al.:* Br. Med. J. *3* :123–126, 1970.
35. Greene, G.R., *et al.:* Am. J. Public Health *62* :680–685, 1972.
36. Rosenberg, L., *et al.:* N. Engl. J. Med. *294* :1256–1259, 1976.
37. Coronary Drug Project Research Group: J.A.M.A. *214* : 1303–1313, 1970.
38. Baum, J., *et al.:* Lancet *2* :926–928, 1973.
39. Mays, E.T., *et al.:* J.A.M.A. *235* :730–732, 1976.
40. Edmondson, H.A., *et al.:* N. Engl. J. Med. *294* :470–472, 1976.
41. Pfeffer, R.I., *et al.:* Am. J. Epidemiol, *103* :445–456, 1976.

INFORMATION FOR THE PATIENT:

WHAT YOU SHOULD KNOW ABOUT ESTROGENS: Estrogens are female hormones produced by the ovaries. The ovaries make several different kinds of estrogens. In addition, scientists have been able to make a variety of synthetic estrogens. As far as we know, all these estrogens have similar properties and therefore much the same usefulness, side effects, and risks. This leaflet is intended to help you understand what estrogens are used for, the risks involved in their use, and how to use them as safely as possible.

This leaflet includes the most important information about estrogens, but not all the information. If you want to know more, you can ask your doctor or pharmacist to let you read the package insert prepared for the doctor.

USES OF ESTROGEN:

Estrogens are prescribed by doctors for a number of purposes, including:

1. To provide estrogen during a period of adjustment when a woman's ovaries no longer produce it, in order to prevent certain uncomfortable symptoms of estrogen deficiency. (All women normally stop producing estrogens, generally between the ages of 45 and 55; this is called the menopause).

2. To prevent symptoms of estrogen deficiency when a woman's ovaries have been removed surgically before the natural menopause.

3. To prevent pregnancy. (Estrogens are given along with a progestogen, another female hormone; these combinations are called oral contraceptives or birth controll pills. Patient labeling is available to women taking oral contraceptives and they will not be discussed in this leaflet).

4. To treat certain cancers in women and men.

THERE IS NO PROPER USE OF ESTROGENS IN A PREGNANT WOMAN.

ESTROGENS IN THE MENOPAUSE: In the natural course of their lives, all women eventually experience a decrease in estrogen production. This usually occurs between ages 45 and 55 but may occur earlier or later. Sometimes the ovaries may need to be removed before natural menopause by an operation, producing a "surgical menopause."

When the amount of estrogen in the blood begins to decrease, many women may develop typical symptoms: Feelings of warmth in the face, neck, and chest or sudden intense episodes of heat and sweating throughout the body (called "hot flashes" or "hot flushes"). These symptoms are sometimes very uncomfortable. A few women eventually develop changes in the vagina (called "atrophic vaginitis") which cause discomfort, especially during and after intercourse.

Estrogens can be prescribed to treat these symptoms of the menopause. It is estimated that considerably more than half of all women undergoing the menopause have only mild symptoms or no symptoms at all and therefore do not need estrogens. Other women may need estrogens for a few months, while their bodies adjust to lower estrogen levels. Sometimes the need will be for periods longer than six months. In an attempt to avoid overstimulation of the

uterus (womb), estrogens are usually given cyclically during each month of use, that is three weeks of pills followed by one week without pills.

Sometimes women experience nervous symptoms or depression during menopause. There is no evidence that estrogens are effective for such symptoms and they should not be used to treat them, although other treatment may be needed.

You may have heard that taking estrogens for long periods (years) after the menopause will keep your skin soft and supple and keep you feeling young. There is no evidence that this is so, however, and such long-term treatment carries important risks.

THE DANGERS OF ESTROGENS:

1. **Cancer of the uterus.** If estrogens are used in the post-menopausal period for more than a year, there is an increased risk of **endometrial cancer** (cancer of the uterus). Women taking estrogens have roughly 5 to 10 times as great a chance of getting this cancer as women who take no estrogens. To put this another way, while a postmenopausal woman not taking estrogens has 1 chance in 1,000 each year of getting cancer of the uterus, a woman taking estrogens has 5 to 10 chances in 1,000 each year. For this reason **it is important to take estrogens only when you really need them.**

   The risk of this cancer is greater the longer estrogens are used and also seems to be greater when larger doses are taken. For this reason, **It is important to take the lowest dose of estrogen that will control symptoms and to take it only as long as it is needed.** If estrogens are needed for longer periods of time, your doctor will want to reevaluate your need for estrogens at least every six months.

   Women using estrogens should report any irregular vaginal bleeding to their doctors; such bleeding may be of no importance, but it can be an early warning of cancer of the uterus. If you have undiagnosed vaginal bleeding, you should not use estrogens until a diagnosis is made and you are certain there is no cancer of the uterus.

2. **Other possible cancers.** Estrogens can cause development of other tumors in animals, such as tumors of the breast, cervix, vagina, or liver, when given for a long time. At present there is no good evidence that women using estrogen in the menopause have an increased risk of such tumors, but there is no way yet to be sure they do not; and one study raises the possibility that use of estrogens in the menopause may increase the risk of breast cancer many years later. This is a further reason to use estrogens only when clearly needed. While you are taking estrogens, it is important that you go to your doctor at least once a year for a physical examination. Also, if members of your family have had breast cancer or if you have had breast nodules or abnormal mammograms (breast x-rays), your doctor may wish to carry out more frequent examinations of your breasts.

3. **Gallbladder disease.** Women who use estrogens after menopause are more likely to develop gallbladder disease needing surgery as women who do not use estrogens. Birth control pills have a similar effect.

4. **Abnormal blood clotting.** Oral contraceptives increase the risk of blood clotting in various parts of the body. This can result in a stroke (if the clot is in the brain), a heart attack (clot in a blood vessel of the heart), or pulmonary embolus (a clot which forms in the legs or pelvis, then breaks off and travels to the lungs). Any of these can be fatal. At this time use of estrogens in the menopause is not known to cause such blood clotting, but this has not been fully studied and there could still prove to be such a risk. It is recommended that if you have had clotting in the legs or lungs or a heart attack or stroke while you were using estrogens or birth control pills, you should not use estrogens (unless they are being used to treat cancer of the breast or prostate). If you have had a stroke or heart attack or if you have angina pectoris, estrogens should be used with great caution and only if clearly needed (for example, if you have severe symptoms of the menopause).

   The larger doses of estrogen used to prevent swelling of the breasts after pregnancy have been reported to cause clotting in the legs and lungs.

SPECIAL WARNING ABOUT PREGNANCY: You should not receive estrogen if you are pregnant. If this should occur, there is a greater than usual chance that the developing child will be born with a birth defect, although the possibility remains fairly small. A female child may have an increased risk of developing cancer of the vagina or cervix later in life (in the teens or twenties). Every possible effort should be made to avoid exposure to estrogens during pregnancy. If exposure occurs, see your doctor.

OTHER EFFECTS OF ESTROGENS: In addition to the serious known risks of estrogens described above, estrogens have the following side effects and potential risks:

1. **Nausea and vomiting.** The most common side effect of estrogen therapy is nausea. Vomiting is less common.

2. **Effects on breasts.** Estrogens may cause breast tenderness or enlargement and may cause the breasts to secrete a liquid. These effects are not dangerous.

3. **Effects on the uterus.** Estrogens may cause benign fibroid tumors of the uterus to get larger.

   Some women will have menstrual bleeding when estrogens are stopped. But if the bleeding occurs on days you are still taking estrogens you should report this to your doctor.

4. **Effect on liver.** Women taking oral contraceptives develop on rare occasions a benign tumor of the liver which can rupture and bleed into the abdomen. So far, these tumors have not been reported in women using estrogens in the menopause, but you should report any swelling or unusual pain or tenderness in the abdomen to your doctor immediately.

   Women with a past history of jaundice (yellowing of the skin and white parts of the eyes) may get jaundice again during estrogen use. If this occurs, stop taking estrogens and see your doctor.

5. **Other effects.** Estrogens may cause excess fluid to be retained in the body. This may make some conditions worse, such as epilepsy, migraine, heart disease, or kidney disease.

SUMMARY: Estrogens have important uses, but they have serious risks as well. You must decide, with your doctor, whether the risks are acceptable to you in view of the benefits of treatment. Except where your doctor has prescribed estrogens for use in special cases of cancer of the breast or prostate, you should not use estrogens if you have cancer of the breast or uterus, are pregnant, have undiagnosed abnormal vaginal bleeding, or have had a stroke, heart attack or angina, or clotting in the legs or lungs in the past while you were taking estrogens.

You can use estrogens as safely as possible by understanding that your doctor will require regular physical examinations while you are taking them and will try to discontinue the drug as soon as possible and use the smallest dose possible. Be alert for signs of trouble including:

1. Abnormal bleeding from the vagina.
2. Pains in the calves or chest or sudden shortness of breath, or coughing blood (indicating possible clots in the legs, heart, or lungs).
3. Severe headaches, dizziness, faintness, or changes in vision (indicating possible developing clots in the brain or eye).
4. Breast lumps (you should ask your doctor how to examine your own breasts).
5. Jaundice (yellowing of the skin).
6. Mental depression.

Based on his or her assessment of your medical needs, your doctor has prescribed this drug for you. Do not give the drug to anyone else.

HOW SUPPLIED

ESTRATEST® H.S. a combination of Esterified Estrogens and Methyltestosterone. Each capsule-shaped Light Green sugar coated Tablet contains: 0.625 mg of Esterified Estrogens, USP and 1.25 mg of Methyltestosterone, USP.

ESTRATEST® a combination of Esterified Estrogens and Methyltestosterone. Each capsule-shaped Dark Green Sugar Coated Tablet contains: 1.25 mg of Esterified Estrogens, USP and 2.5 mg of Methyltestosterone, USP.

SOLVAY PHARMACEUTICALS, INC.

Marietta, GA 30062   4E 0978 Rev 7/94

Shown in Product Identification Guide, page 340

LITHOBID®   ℞
(Lithium Carbonate, USP)
Slow-Release Tablets
300 mg

WARNING

Lithium toxicity is closely related to serum lithium levels, and can occur at doses close to therapeutic levels. Facilities for prompt and accurate serum lithium determinations should be available before initiating therapy (see DOSAGE AND ADMINISTRATION).

DESCRIPTION

LITHOBID® Tablets contain lithium carbonate, a white, odorless alkaline powder with molecular formula Li_2CO_3 and molecular weight 73.89. Lithium is an element of the alkali-metal group with atomic number 3, atomic weight 6.94 and an emission line at 671 nm on the flame photometer.

Each peach-colored, film-coated, slow-release tablet contains 300 mg of lithium carbonate. This slowly dissolving, film-coated tablet is designed to give lower serum lithium peak concentrations than obtained with conventional oral lithium dosage forms. Inactive ingredients consist of calcium stearate, carnauba wax, cellulose compounds, FD&C Blue No. 2 Aluminum Lake, FD&C Red No. 40 Aluminum Lake, FD&C Yellow No. 6 Aluminum Lake, povidone, propylene glycol, sodium chloride, sodium lauryl sulfate, sodium starch glycolate, sorbitol and titanium dioxide.

ACTIONS

Preclinical studies have shown that lithium alters sodium transport in nerve and muscle cells and effects a shift toward intraneuronal metabolism of catecholamines, but the specific biochemical mechanism of lithium action in mania is unknown.

INDICATIONS

Lithium is indicated in the treatment of manic episodes of manic-depressive illness. Maintenance therapy prevents or diminishes the intensity of subsequent episodes in those manic-depressive patients with a history of mania.

Typical symptoms: of mania include pressure of speech, motor hyperactivity, reduced need for sleep, flight of ideas, grandiosity, elation, poor judgment, aggressiveness, and possibly hostility. When given to a patient experiencing a manic episode, lithium may produce a normalization of symptomatology within 1 to 3 weeks.

WARNINGS

Lithium should generally not be given to patients with significant renal or cardiovascular disease, severe debilitation, dehydration, sodium depletion, and to patients receiving diuretics, or angiotensin converting enzyme (ACE) inhibitors, since the risk of lithium toxicity is very high in such patients. If the psychiatric indication is life threatening, and if such a patient fails to respond to other measures, lithium treatment may be undertaken with extreme caution, including daily serum lithium determinations and adjustment to the usually low doses ordinarily tolerated by these individuals. In such instances, hospitalization is a necessity.

Chronic lithium therapy may be associated with diminution of renal concentrating ability, occasionally presenting as nephrogenic diabetes insipidus, with polyuria and polydipsia. Such patients should be carefully managed to avoid dehydration with resulting lithium retention and toxicity. This condition is usually reversible when lithium is discontinued. Morphologic changes with glomerular and interstitial fibrosis and nephron atrophy have been reported in patients on chronic lithium therapy. Morphologic changes have also been seen in manic-depressive patients never exposed to lithium. The relationship between renal function and morphologic changes and their association with lithium therapy have not been established.

Kidney function should be assessed prior to and during lithium therapy. Routine urinalysis and other tests may be used to evaluate tubular function (e.g., urine specific gravity or osmolality following a period of water deprivation, or 24-hour urine volume) and glomerular function (e.g., serum creatinine or creatinine clearance). During lithium therapy, progressive or sudden changes in renal function, even within the normal range, indicate the need for reevaluation of treatment.

An encephalopathic syndrome (characterized by weakness, lethargy, fever, tremulousness and confusion, extrapyramidal symptoms, leukocytosis, elevated serum enzymes, BUN and FBS) has occurred in a few patients treated with lithium plus a neuroleptic, most notably haloperidol. In some instances, the syndrome was followed by irreversible brain damage. Because of possible causal relationship between these events and the concomitant administration of lithium and neuroleptic drugs, patients receiving such combined therapy or patients with organic brain syndrome or other CNS impairment should be monitored closely for early evidence of neurologic toxicity and treatment discontinued promptly if such signs appear. This encephalopathic syndrome may be similar to or the same as Neuroleptic Malignant Syndrome (NMS).

Lithium toxicity is closely related to serum lithium concentrations and can occur at doses close to the therapeutic concentrations (see DOSAGE AND ADMINISTRATION).

Outpatients and their families should be warned that the patient must discontinue lithium therapy and contact his physician if such clinical signs of lithium toxicity as diarrhea, vomiting, tremor, mild ataxia, drowsiness, or muscular weakness occur.

Lithium may prolong the effects of neuromuscular blocking agents. Therefore, neuromuscular blocking agents should be given with caution to patients receiving lithium.

Usage in Pregnancy Adverse effects on nidation in rats, embryo viability in mice, and metabolism in vitro of rat testis and human spermatozoa have been attributed to lithium, as have teratogenicity in submammalian species and cleft palate in mice.

In humans, lithium may cause fetal harm when administered to a pregnant woman. Data from lithium birth registries suggest an increase in cardiac and other anomalies especially Ebstein's anomaly. If this drug is used in women of childbearing potential, or during pregnancy, or if a patient becomes pregnant while taking this drug, the patient should be apprised by their physician of the potential hazard to the fetus.

Usage in Nursing Mothers Lithium is excreted in human milk. Nursing should not be undertaken during lithium

Continued on next page

Lithobid—Cont.

therapy except in rare and unusual circumstances where, in the view of the physician, the potential benefits to the mother outweigh possible hazard to the infant or neonate. Signs and symptoms of lithium toxicity such as hypertonia, hypothermia, cyanosis and ECG changes have been reported in some infants and neonates.

Pediatric Use Safety and effectiveness in pediatric patients under 12 years of age have not been determined; its use in these patients is not recommended.

There has been a report of transient syndrome of acute dystonia and hyperreflexia occurring in a 15 kg pediatric patient who ingested 300 mg of lithium carbonate.

PRECAUTIONS

The ability to tolerate lithium is greater during the acute manic phase and decreases when manic symptoms subside (see DOSAGE AND ADMINISTRATION.)

The distribution space of lithium approximates that of total body water. Lithium is primarily excreted in urine with insignificant excretion in feces. Renal excretion of lithium is proportional to its plasma concentration. The elimination half-life of lithium is approximately 24 hours. Lithium decreases sodium reabsorption by the renal tubules which could lead to sodium depletion. Therefore, it is essential for the patient to maintain a normal diet, including salt, and an adequate fluid intake (2500–3500 mL) at least during the initial stabilization period. Decreased tolerance to lithium has been reported to ensue from protracted sweating or diarrhea and, if such occur, supplemental fluid and salt should be administered under careful medical supervision and lithium intake reduced or suspended until the condition is resolved.

In addition to sweating and diarrhea, concomitant infection with elevated temperatures may also necessitate a temporary reduction or cessation of medication.

Previously existing underlying thyroid disorders do not necessarily constitute a contraindication to lithium treatment. Where hypothyroidism preexists, careful monitoring of thyroid function during lithium stabilization and maintenance allows for correction of changing thyroid parameters and/or adjustment of lithium doses, if any. If hypothyroidism occurs during lithium stabilization and maintenance, supplemental thyroid treatment may be used.

In general, the concomitant use of diuretics or angiotensin converting enzyme (ACE) inhibitors with lithium carbonate should be avoided. In those cases where concomitant use is necessary extreme caution is advised since sodium loss from these drugs may reduce the renal clearance of lithium resulting in increased serum lithium concentrations with the risk of lithium toxicity. When such combinations are used, the lithium dosage may need to be decreased, and more frequent monitoring of lithium serum concentrations is recommended. See WARNINGS for additional caution information.

Concomitant administration of carbamazepine and lithium may increase the risk of neurotoxic side effects.

The following drugs can lower serum lithium concentrations by increasing urinary lithium excretion: acetazolamide, urea, xanthine preparations and alkalinizing agents such as sodium bicarbonate.

Concomitant extended use of iodide preparations, especially potassium iodide, with lithium may produce hypothyroidism. Indomethacin and piroxicam have been reported to significantly increase steady state serum lithium concentrations. In some cases lithium toxicity has resulted from such interactions. There is also some evidence that other nonsteroidal, anti-inflammatory agents may have a similar effect. When such combinations are used, increased serum lithium concentrations monitoring is recommended.

Concurrent use of calcium channel blocking agents with lithium may increase the risk of neurotoxicity in the form of ataxia, tremors, nausea, vomiting, diarrhea and/or tinnitus. Concurrent use of metronidazole with lithium may provoke lithium toxicity due to reduced renal clearance. Patients receiving such combined therapy should be monitored closely. Concurrent use of fluoxetine with lithium has resulted in both increased and decreased serum lithium concentrations. Patients receiving such combined therapy should be monitored closely.

Lithium may impair mental and/or physical abilities. Patients should be cautioned about activities requiring alertness (e.g., operating vehicles or machinery).

Usage in Pregnancy

Pregnancy Category D. (see WARNINGS).

Usage in Nursing Mothers Because of the potential for serious adverse reactions in nursing infants and neonates from lithium, a decision should be made whether to discontinue nursing or to discontinue the drug, taking into account the importance of the drug to the mother (see WARNINGS).

Pediatric Use Safety and effectiveness in pediatric patients below the age of 12 have not been established (see WARNINGS).

Usage in the Elderly

Elderly patients often require lower lithium dosages to achieve therapeutic serum concentrations. They may also exhibit adverse reactions at serum concentrations ordinarily tolerated by younger patients. Additionally, patients with renal impairment may also require lower lithium doses (see WARNINGS).

ADVERSE REACTIONS

The occurrence and severity of adverse reactions are generally directly related to serum lithium concentrations and to individual patient sensitivity to lithium. They generally occur more frequently and with greater severity at higher concentrations.

Adverse reactions may be encountered at serum lithium concentrations below 1.5 mEq/L. Mild to moderate adverse reactions may occur at concentrations from 1.5–2.5 mEq/L, and moderate to severe reactions may be seen at concentrations from 2.0 mEq/L and above.

Fine hand tremor, polyuria and mild thirst may occur during initial therapy for the acute manic phase, and may persist throughout treatment. Transient and mild nausea and general discomfort may also appear during the first few days of lithium administration.

These side effects usually subside with continued treatment or with a temporary reduction or cessation of dosage. If persistent, a cessation of lithium therapy may be required. Diarrhea, vomiting, drowsiness, muscular weakness and lack of coordination may be early signs of lithium intoxication, and can occur at lithium concentrations below 2.0 mEq/L. At higher concentrations giddiness, ataxia, blurred vision, tinnitus and a large output of dilute urine may be seen. Serum lithium concentrations above 3.0 mEq/L may produce a complex clinical picture involving multiple organs and organ systems. Serum lithium concentrations should not be permitted to exceed 2.0 mEq/L during the acute treatment phase.

The following reactions have been reported and appear to be related to serum lithium concentrations, including concentrations within the therapeutic range:

Central Nervous System: tremor, muscle hyperirritability (fasiculations, twitching, clonic movements of whole limbs), hypertonicity, ataxia, choreoathetotic movements, hyperactive deep tendon reflex, extrapyramidal symptoms including acute dystonia, cogwheel rigidity, blackout spells, epileptiform seizures, slurred speech, dizziness, vertigo, downbeat nystagmus, incontinence of urine or feces, somnolence, psychomotor retardation, restlessness, confusion, stupor, coma, tongue movements, tics, tinnitus, hallucinations, poor memory, slowed intellectual functioning, startled response, worsening of organic brain syndromes. Cases of Pseudotumor Cerebri (increased intracranial pressure and papilledema) have been reported with lithium use. If undetected, this condition may result in enlargement of the blind spot, constriction of visual fields and eventual blindness due to optic atrophy. Lithium should be discontinued, if clinically possible, if this syndrome occurs. **Cardiovascular:** cardiac arrhythmia, hypotension, peripheral circulatory collapse, bradycardia, sinus node dysfunction with severe bradycardia (which may result in syncope); **Gastrointestinal:** anorexia, nausea, vomiting, diarrhea, gastritis, salivary gland swelling, abdominal pain, excessive salivation, flatulence, indigestion; **Genitourinary:** glycosuria, decreased creatinine clearance, albuminuria, oliguria, and symptoms of nephrogenic diabetes insipidus including polyuria, thirst and polydipsia; **Dermatologic:** drying and thinning of hair, alopecia, anesthesia of skin, acne, chronic folliculitis, xerosis cutis, psoriasis or its exacerbation, generalized pruritus with or without rash, cutaneous ulcers, angioedema; **Autonomic Nervous System:** blurred vision, dry mouth, impotence/sexual dysfunction; **Thyroid Abnormalities:** euthyroid goiter and/or hypothyroidism (including myxedema) accompanied by lower T_3 and T_4. ^{131}Iodine uptake may be elevated (see PRECAUTIONS). Paradoxically, rare cases of hyperthyroidism have been reported.

EEG Changes: diffuse slowing, widening of frequency spectrum, potentiation and disorganization of background rhythm. **EKG Changes:** reversible flattening, isoelectricity or inversion of T-waves. **Miscellaneous:** fatigue, lethargy, transient scotomata, exophthalmos, dehydration, weight loss, leucocytosis, headache, transient hyperglycemia, hypercalcemia, hyperparathyroidism, albuminuria, excessive weight gain, edematous swelling of ankles or wrists, metallic taste, dysgeusia/taste distortion, salty taste, thirst, swollen lips, tightness in chest, swollen and/or painful joints, fever, polyarthralgia, and dental caries.

Some reports of nephrogenic diabetes insipidus, hyperparathyroidism and hypothyroidism which persist after lithium discontinuation have been received.

A few reports have been received of the development of painful discoloration of fingers and toes and coldness of the extremities within one day of starting lithium treatment. The mechanism through which these symptoms (resembling Raynaud's Syndrome) developed is not known. Recovery followed discontinuance.

DOSAGE AND ADMINISTRATION

Acute Mania Optimal patient response can usually be established with 1800 mg/day in the following dosages:

ACUTE MANIA

	Morning	Afternoon	Nighttime
LITHOBID® Slow-Release Tablets[1]	3 tabs (900 mg)		3 tabs (900 mg)

[1]Can also be administered on 600mg t.i.d. recommended dosing interval.

Such doses will normally produce an effective serum lithium concentration ranging between 1.0 and 1.5 mEq/L. Dosage must be individualized according to serum concentrations and clinical response. Regular monitoring of the patient's clinical state and of serum lithium concentrations is necessary. Serum concentrations should be determined twice per week during the acute phase, and until the serum concentrations and clinical condition of the patient have been stabilized.

Long-Term Control Desirable serum lithium concentrations are 0.6 to 1.2 mEq/L which can usually be achieved with 900–1200 mg/day. Dosage will vary from one individual to another, but generally the following dosages will maintain this concentration.

LONG TERM

	Morning	Afternoon	Nighttime
LITHOBID® Slow-Release Tablets[1]	2 tabs (600 mg)		2 tabs (600 mg)

[1]Can be administered on t.i.d. recommended dosing interval up to 1200mg/day

Serum lithium concentrations in uncomplicated cases receiving maintenance therapy during remission should be monitored at least every two months. Patients abnormally sensitive to lithium may exhibit toxic signs at serum concentrations of 1.0 to 1.5 mEq/L. Elderly patients often respond to reduced dosage, and may exhibit signs of toxicity at serum concentrations ordinarily tolerated by other patients.

N.B.: Blood samples for serum lithium determinations should be drawn immediately prior to the next dose when lithium concentrations are relatively stable (i.e., 8–12 hours after previous dose). Total reliance must not be placed on serum concentrations alone. Accurate patient evaluation requires both clinical and laboratory analysis. LITHOBID® Slow-Release Tablets must be swallowed whole and never chewed or crushed.

OVERDOSAGE

The toxic concentrations for lithium (≥ 1.5 mEq/L) are close to the therapeutic concentrations (0.6–1.2 mEq/L). It is therefore important that patients and their families be cautioned to watch for early toxic symptoms and to discontinue the drug and inform the physician should they occur.(Toxic symptoms are listed in detail under ADVERSE REACTIONS.)

Treatment No specific antidote for lithium poisoning is known. Treatment is supportive. Early symptoms of lithium toxicity can usually be treated by reduction or cessation of dosage of the drug and resumption of the treatment at a lower dose after 24 to 48 hours. In severe cases of lithium poisoning, the first and foremost goal of treatment consists of elimination of this ion from the patient.

Treatment is essentially the same as that used in barbiturate poisoning: 1) gastric lavage, 2) correction of fluid and electrolyte imbalance and 3) regulation of kidney functioning. Urea, mannitol, and aminophylline all produce significant increases in lithium excretion. Hemodialysis is an effective and rapid means of removing the ion from the severely toxic patient. However, patient recovery may be slow. Infection prophylaxis, regular chest X-rays, and preservation of adequate respiration are essential.

HOW SUPPLIED

LITHOBID® (Lithium Carbonate, USP) Slow-Release Tablets, 300 mg, peach-colored imprinted "LITHOBID"

Bottles of 100
NDC 0032-4492-01
Bottles of 1000
NDC 0032-4492-10

Store between 59°–86°F (15°–30°C). Protect from moisture. Dispense in tight, child-resistant container (USP).

Caution: Federal law prohibits dispensing without prescription.

Solvay Pharmaceuticals
Marietta, GA 30062

1E0990 Rev 8/97
©1997 Solvay Pharmaceuticals, Inc.
Shown in Product Identification Guide, page 340

LUVOX® ℞
(Fluvoxamine Maleate) Tablets
25 mg, 50 mg and 100 mg

DESCRIPTION

Fluvoxamine maleate is a selective serotonin (5-HT) reuptake inhibitor (SSRI) belonging to a new chemical series, the 2-aminoethyl oxime ethers of aralkylketones. It is chemically unrelated to other SSRIs and clomipramine. It is chemically designated as 5-methoxy-4′-(trifluoromethyl) valerophenone-(E)-O-(2-aminoethyl)oxime maleate (1:1) and has the empirical formula $C_{15}H_{21}O_2N_2F_3 \cdot C_4H_4O_4$. Its molecular weight is 434.4.
The structural formula is:

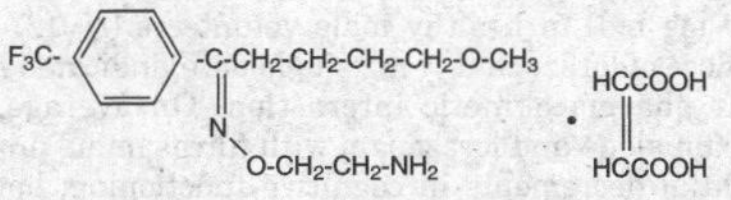

Fluvoxamine maleate is a white or off white, odorless, crystalline powder which is sparingly soluble in water, freely soluble in ethanol and chloroform and practically insoluble in diethyl ether.

LUVOX® (fluvoxamine maleate) Tablets are available in 25 mg, 50 mg and 100 mg strengths for oral administration. In addition to the active ingredient, fluvoxamine maleate, each tablet contains the following inactive ingredients: carnauba wax, hydroxypropyl methylcellulose, mannitol, polyethylene glycol, polysorbate 80, pregelatinized starch (potato), silicon dioxide, sodium stearyl fumarate, starch (corn), and titanium dioxide. The 50 mg and 100 mg tablets also contain synthetic iron oxides.

CLINICAL PHARMACOLOGY

Pharmacodynamics

The mechanism of action of fluvoxamine maleate in Obsessive Compulsive Disorder is presumed to be linked to its specific serotonin reuptake inhibition in brain neurons. In preclinical studies, it was found that fluvoxamine inhibited neuronal uptake of serotonin.

In *in vitro* studies fluvoxamine maleate had no significant affinity for histaminergic, alpha or beta adrenergic, muscarinic, or dopaminergic receptors. Antagonism of some of these receptors is thought to be associated with various sedative, cardiovascular, anticholinergic, and extrapyramidal effects of some psychotropic drugs.

Pharmacokinetics

Bioavailability: The absolute bioavailability of fluvoxamine maleate is 53%. Oral bioavailability is not significantly affected by food.

In a dose proportionality study involving fluvoxamine maleate at 100, 200 and 300 mg/day for 10 consecutive days in 30 normal volunteers, steady state was achieved after about a week of dosing. Maximum plasma concentrations at steady state occurred within 3–8 hours of dosing and reached concentrations averaging 88, 283 and 546 ng/mL, respectively. Thus, fluvoxamine had nonlinear pharmacokinetics over this dose range, i.e., higher doses of fluvoxamine maleate produced disproportionately higher concentrations than predicted from the lower dose.

Distribution/Protein Binding: The mean apparent volume of distribution for fluvoxamine is approximately 25 L/kg, suggesting extensive tissue distribution.

Approximately 80% of fluvoxamine is bound to plasma protein, mostly albumin, over a concentration range of 20 to 2000 ng/mL.

Metabolism: Fluvoxamine maleate is extensively metabolized by the liver; the main metabolic routes are oxidative demethylation and deamination. Nine metabolites were identified following a 5 mg radiolabelled dose of fluvoxamine maleate, constituting approximately 85% of the urinary excretion products of fluvoxamine. The main human metabolite was fluvoxamine acid which, together with its N-acetylated analog, accounted for about 60% of the urinary excretion products. A third metabolite, fluvoxethanol, formed by oxidative deamination, accounted for about 10%. Fluvoxamine acid and fluvoxethanol were tested in an *in vitro* assay of serotonin and norepinephrine reuptake inhibition in rats; they were inactive except for a weak effect of the former metabolite on inhibition of serotonin uptake (1–2 orders of magnitude less potent than the parent compound). Approximately 2% of fluvoxamine was excreted in urine unchanged. (See PRECAUTIONS - Drug Interactions)

Elimination: Following a ^{14}C-labelled oral dose of fluvoxamine maleate (5 mg), an average of 94% of drug-related products was recovered in the urine within 71 hours.

The mean plasma half-life of fluvoxamine at steady state after multiple oral doses of 100 mg/day in healthy, young volunteers was 15.6 hours.

Elderly Subjects: In a study of LUVOX Tablets at 50 and 100 mg comparing elderly (ages 66–73) and young subjects (ages 19–35), mean maximum plasma concentrations in the elderly were 40% higher. The multiple dose elimination half-life of fluvoxamine was 17.4 and 25.9 hours in the elderly compared to 13.6 and 15.6 hours in the young subjects at steady state for 50 and 100 mg doses, respectively.

In elderly patients, the clearance of fluvoxamine was reduced by about 50% and, therefore, LUVOX Tablets should be slowly titrated during initiation of therapy.

Hepatic and Renal Disease: A cross study comparison (healthy subjects vs. patients with hepatic dysfunction) suggested a 30% decrease in fluvoxamine clearance in association with hepatic dysfunction. The mean minimum plasma concentrations in renally impaired patients (creatinine clearance of 5 to 45 mL/min) after 4 and 6 weeks of treatment (50 mg bid, N=13) were comparable to each other, suggesting no accumulation of fluvoxamine in these patients. (See PRECAUTIONS - *Use in Patients with Concomitant Illness*)

Clinical Trials

Adult OCD Studies: The effectiveness of LUVOX Tablets for the treatment of Obsessive Compulsive Disorder (OCD) was demonstrated in two 10-week multicenter, parallel group studies of adult outpatients. Patients in these trials were titrated to a total daily fluvoxamine maleate dose of 150 mg/day over the first two weeks of the trial, following which the dose was adjusted within a range of 100–300 mg/day (on a bid schedule), on the basis of response and tolerance. Patients in these studies had moderate to severe OCD (DSM-III-R), with mean baseline ratings on the Yale-Brown Obsessive Compulsive Scale (Y-BOCS), total score of 23. Patients receiving fluvoxamine maleate experienced mean reductions of approximately 4 to 5 units on the Y-BOCS total score, compared to a 2 unit reduction for placebo patients.

The following table provides the outcome classification by treatment group on the Global Improvement item of the Clinical Global Impressions (CGI) scale for both studies combined.

OUTCOME CLASSIFICATION (%) ON CGI-GLOBAL IMPROVEMENT ITEM FOR COMPLETERS IN POOL OF TWO ADULT OCD STUDIES

Outcome Classification	Fluvoxamine (N = 120)	Placebo (N = 134)
Very Much Improved	13%	2%
Much Improved	30%	10%
Minimally Improved	22%	32%
No Change	31%	51%
Worse	4%	6%

Exploratory analyses for age and gender effects on outcomes did not suggest any differential responsiveness on the basis of age or sex.

Pediatric OCD Study: The effectiveness of LUVOX Tablets for the treatment of OCD was also demonstrated in a 10-week multicenter, parallel group study in a pediatric outpatient population (children and adolescents, ages 8–17). Patients in this study were titrated to a total daily fluvoxamine dose of approximately 100 mg/day over the first two weeks of the trial, following which the dose was adjusted within a range of 50–200 mg/day (on a bid schedule) on the basis of response and tolerance. Patients in these studies had moderate to severe OCD (DSM-III-R) with mean baseline ratings on the Children's Yale-Brown Obsessive Compulsive Scale (CY-BOCS), total score of 24. Patients receiving fluvoxamine maleate experienced mean reductions of approximately 6 units on the CY-BOCS total score, compared to a 3 unit reduction for placebo patients.

The following table provides the outcome classification by treatment group on the Global Improvement item of the Clinical Global Impression (CGI) scale for the pediatric study.

OUTCOME CLASSIFICATION (%) ON CGI-GLOBAL IMPROVEMENT ITEM FOR COMPLETERS IN PEDIATRIC STUDY

Outcome Classification	Fluvoxamine (N = 38)	Placebo (N = 36)
Very Much Improved	21%	11%
Much Improved	18%	17%
Minimally Improved	37%	22%
No Change	16%	44%
Worse	8%	6%

Post hoc exploratory analyses for gender effects on outcomes did not suggest any differential responsiveness on the basis of gender. Further exploratory analyses revealed a prominent treatment effect in the 8–11 age group and essentially no effect in the 12–17 age group. The significance of these results is not known at this time.

INDICATIONS AND USAGE

LUVOX Tablets are indicated for the treatment of obsessions and compulsions in patients with Obsessive Compulsive Disorder (OCD), as defined in the DSM-III-R. The obsessions or compulsions cause marked distress, are time-consuming, or significantly interfere with social or occupational functioning.

The efficacy of LUVOX Tablets was established in three 10-week trials with obsessive compulsive outpatients with the diagnosis of Obsessive Compulsive Disorder as defined in DSM-III-R. (See Clinical Trials under CLINICAL PHARMACOLOGY.)

Obsessive Compulsive Disorder is characterized by recurrent and persistent ideas, thoughts, impulses or images (obsessions) that are ego-dystonic and/or repetitive, purposeful, and intentional behaviors (compulsions) that are recognized by the person as excessive or unreasonable.

The effectiveness of LUVOX Tablets for long-term use, i.e., for more than 10 weeks, has not been systematically evaluated in placebo-controlled trials. Therefore, the physician who elects to use LUVOX Tablets for extended periods should periodically re-evaluate the long-term usefulness of the drug for the individual patient. (See DOSAGE AND ADMINISTRATION)

CONTRAINDICATIONS

Co-administration of terfenadine, astemizole, or cisapride with LUVOX Tablets is contraindicated (see WARNINGS and PRECAUTIONS).

LUVOX Tablets are contraindicated in patients with a history of hypersensitivity to fluvoxamine maleate.

WARNINGS

Potential for Interaction with Monoamine Oxidase Inhibitors

In patients receiving another serotonin reuptake inhibitor drug in combination with monoamine oxidase inhibitors (MAOI), there have been reports of serious, sometimes fatal, reactions including hyperthermia, rigidity, myoclonus, autonomic instability with possible rapid fluctuations of vital signs, and mental status changes that include extreme agitation progressing to delirium and coma. These reactions have also been reported in patients who have discontinued that drug and have been started on a MAOI. Some cases presented with features resembling neuroleptic malignant syndrome. Therefore, it is recommended that LUVOX Tablets not be used in combination with a MAOI, or within 14 days of discontinuing treatment with a MAOI. After stopping LUVOX Tablets, at least 2 weeks should be allowed before starting a MAOI.

Potential Terfenadine, Astemizole, and Cisapride Interactions

Terfenadine, astemizole, and cisapride are all metabolized by the cytochrome P450IIIA4 isozyme, and it has been demonstrated that ketoconazole, a potent inhibitor of IIIA4, blocks the metabolism of these drugs, resulting in increased plasma concentrations of parent drug. Increased plasma concentrations of terfenadine, astemizole, and cisapride cause QT prolongation and have been associated with torsades de pointes-type ventricular tachycardia, sometimes fatal. As noted below, a substantial pharmacokinetic interaction has been observed for fluvoxamine in combination with alprazolam, a drug that is known to be metabolized by the IIIA4 isozyme. Although it has not been definitively demonstrated that fluvoxamine is a potent IIIA4 inhibitor, it is likely to be, given the substantial interaction of fluvoxamine with alprazolam. Consequently, it is recommended that fluvoxamine not be used in combination with either terfenadine, astemizole, or cisapride (see CONTRAINDICATIONS and PRECAUTIONS).

Other Potentially Important Drug Interactions

(Also see PRECAUTIONS - Drug Interactions)

Benzodiazepines: Benzodiazepines metabolized by hepatic oxidation (e.g., alprazolam, midazolam, triazolam, etc.) should be used with caution because the clearance of these drugs is likely to be reduced by fluvoxamine. The clearance of benzodiazepines metabolized by glucuronidation (e.g., lorazepam, oxazepam, temazepam) is unlikely to be affected by fluvoxamine.

Alprazolam - When fluvoxamine maleate (100 mg qd) and alprazolam (1 mg qid) were co-administered to steady state,

Continued on next page

Luvox—Cont.

plasma concentrations and other pharmacokinetic parameters (AUC, C_{max}, $T_{1/2}$) of alprazolam were approximately twice those observed when alprazolam was administered alone; oral clearance was reduced by about 50%. The elevated plasma alprazolam concentrations resulted in decreased psychomotor performance and memory. This interaction, which has not been investigated using higher doses of fluvoxamine, may be more pronounced if a 300 mg daily dose is co-administered, particularly since fluvoxamine exhibits non-linear pharmacokinetics over the dosage range 100–300 mg. If alprazolam is co-administered with LUVOX Tablets, the initial alprazolam dosage should be at least halved and titration to the lowest effective dose is recommended. No dosage adjustment is required for LUVOX Tablets.

Diazepam - The co-administration of LUVOX Tablets and diazepam is generally not advisable. Because fluvoxamine reduces the clearance of both diazepam and its active metabolite, N-desmethyldiazepam, there is a strong likelihood of substantial accumulation of both species during chronic co-administration.

Evidence supporting the conclusion that it is inadvisable to co-administer fluvoxamine and diazepam is derived from a study in which healthy volunteers taking 150 mg/day of fluvoxamine were administered a single oral dose of 10 mg of diazepam. In these subjects (N=8), the clearance of diazepam was reduced by 65% and that of N-desmethyldiazepam to a level that was too low to measure over the course of the 2 week long study.

It is likely that this experience significantly underestimates the degree of accumulation that might occur with repeated diazepam administration. Moreover, as noted with alprazolam, the effect of fluvoxamine may even be more pronounced when it is administered at higher doses.

Accordingly, diazepam and fluvoxamine should not ordinarily be co-administered.

Theophylline: The effect of steady-state fluvoxamine (50 mg bid) on the pharmacokinetics of a single dose of theophylline (375 mg as 442 mg aminophylline) was evaluated in 12 healthy non-smoking, male volunteers. The clearance of theophylline was decreased approximately 3-fold. Therefore, if theophylline is co-administered with fluvoxamine maleate, its dose should be reduced to one third of the usual daily maintenance dose and plasma concentrations of theophylline should be monitored. No dosage adjustment is required for LUVOX Tablets.

Warfarin: When fluvoxamine maleate (50 mg tid) was administered concomitantly with warfarin for two weeks, warfarin plasma concentrations increased by 98% and prothrombin times were prolonged. Thus patients receiving oral anticoagulants and LUVOX Tablets should have their prothrombin time monitored and their anticoagulant dose adjusted accordingly. No dosage adjustment is required for LUVOX Tablets.

PRECAUTIONS
General

Activation of Mania/Hypomania: During premarketing studies involving primarily depressed patients, hypomania or mania occurred in approximately 1% of patients treated with fluvoxamine. In a ten week pediatric OCD study, 2 out of 57 patients (4%) treated with fluvoxamine experienced manic reactions, compared to none of 63 placebo patients. Activation of mania/hypomania has also been reported in a small proportion of patients with major affective disorder who were treated with other marketed antidepressants. As with all antidepressants, LUVOX Tablets should be used cautiously in patients with a history of mania.

Seizures: During premarketing studies, seizures were reported in 0.2% of fluvoxamine-treated patients. LUVOX Tablets should be used cautiously in patients with a history of seizures. It should be discontinued in any patient who develops seizures.

Suicide: The possibility of a suicide attempt is inherent in patients with depressive symptoms, whether these occur in primary depression or in association with another primary disorder such as OCD. Close supervision of high risk patients should accompany initial drug therapy. Prescriptions for LUVOX Tablets should be written for the smallest quantity of tablets consistent with good patient management in order to reduce the risk of overdose.

Use in Patients with Concomitant Illness: Closely monitored clinical experience with LUVOX Tablets in patients with concomitant systemic illness is limited. Caution is advised in administering LUVOX Tablets to patients with diseases or conditions that could affect hemodynamic responses or metabolism.

LUVOX Tablets have not been evaluated or used to any appreciable extent in patients with a recent history of myocardial infarction or unstable heart disease. Patients with these diagnoses were systematically excluded from many clinical studies during the product's premarketing testing. Evaluation of the electrocardiograms for patients with de-

pression or OCD who participated in premarketing studies revealed no differences between fluvoxamine and placebo in the emergence of clinically important ECG changes.

In patients with liver dysfunction, fluvoxamine clearance was decreased by approximately 30%. LUVOX Tablets should be slowly titrated in patients with liver dysfunction during the initiation of treatment.

Information for Patients
Physicians are advised to discuss the following issues with patients for whom they prescribe LUVOX Tablets:

Interference with Cognitive or Motor Performance: Since any psychoactive drug may impair judgement, thinking, or motor skills, patients should be cautioned about operating hazardous machinery, including automobiles, until they are certain that LUVOX Tablets therapy does not adversely affect their ability to engage in such activities.

Pregnancy: Patients should be advised to notify their physicians if they become pregnant or intend to become pregnant during therapy with LUVOX Tablets.

Nursing: Patients receiving LUVOX Tablets should be advised to notify their physicians if they are breast feeding an infant. (See PRECAUTIONS - Nursing Mothers)

Concomitant Medication: Patients should be advised to notify their physicians if they are taking, or plan to take, any prescription or over-the-counter drugs, since there is a potential for clinically important interactions with LUVOX Tablets.

Alcohol: As with other psychotropic medications, patients should be advised to avoid alcohol while taking LUVOX Tablets.

Allergic Reactions: Patients should be advised to notify their physicians if they develop a rash, hives, or a related allergic phenomenon during therapy with LUVOX Tablets.

Laboratory Tests
There are no specific laboratory tests recommended.

Drug Interactions

Potential Interactions with Drugs that Inhibit or are Metabolized by Cytochrome P450 Isozymes: Multiple hepatic cytochrome P450 (CYP450) enzymes are involved in the oxidative biotransformation of a large number of structurally different drugs and endogenous compounds. The available knowledge concerning the relationship of fluvoxamine and the CYP450 enzyme system has been obtained mostly from pharmacokinetic interaction studies conducted in healthy volunteers, but some preliminary in vitro data are also available. Based on a finding of substantial interactions of fluvoxamine with certain of these drugs (see later parts of this section and also WARNINGS for details) and limited in vitro data for the IIIA4 isozyme, it appears that fluvoxamine inhibits the following isozymes that are known to be involved in the metabolism of the listed drugs:

IA2	IIC9	IIIA4
Warfarin	Warfarin	Alprazolam
Theophylline		
Propranolol		

In vitro data suggest that fluvoxamine is a relatively weak inhibitor of the IID6 isozyme.

Approximately 7% of the normal population has a genetic defect that leads to reduced levels of activity of cytochrome P450IID6 isozyme. Such individuals have been referred to as "poor metabolizers" (PM) of drugs such as debrisoquin, dextromethorphan, and tricyclic antidepressants. While none of the drugs studied for drug interactions significantly affected the pharmacokinetics of fluvoxamine, an in vivo study of fluvoxamine single-dose pharmacokinetics in 13 PM subjects demonstrated altered pharmacokinetic properties compared to 16 "extensive metabolizers" (EM): mean Cmax, AUC, and half-life were increased by 52%, 200%, and 62%, respectively, in the PM compared to the EM group. This suggests that fluvoxamine is metabolized, at least in part, by IID6 isozyme. Caution is indicated in patients known to have reduced levels of P450IID6 activity and those receiving concomitant drugs known to inhibit this isozyme (e.g. quinidine).

The metabolism of fluvoxamine has not been fully characterized and the effects of potent P450 isozyme inhibition, such as the ketoconazole inhibition of IIIA4, on fluvoxamine metabolism have not been studied.

A clinically significant fluvoxamine interaction is possible with drugs having a narrow therapeutic ratio such as terfenadine, astemizole, or cisapride, warfarin, theophylline, certain benzodiazepines and phenytoin. If LUVOX Tablets are to be administered together with a drug that is eliminated via oxidative metabolism and has a narrow therapeutic window, plasma levels and/or pharmacodynamic effects of the latter drug should be monitored closely, at least until steady-state conditions are reached (See CONTRAINDICATIONS and WARNINGS).

CNS Active Drugs:
Monoamine Oxidase Inhibitors: See WARNINGS

Alprazolam: See WARNINGS
Diazepam: See WARNINGS
Alcohol: Studies involving single 40 g doses of ethanol (oral administration in one study and intravenous in the other) and multiple dosing with fluvoxamine maleate (50 mg bid) revealed no effect of either drug on the pharmacokinetics or pharmacodynamics of the other.
Carbamazepine: Elevated carbamazepine levels and symptoms of toxicity have been reported with the co-administration of fluvoxamine maleate and carbamazepine.
Clozapine: Elevated serum levels of clozapine have been reported in patients taking fluvoxamine maleate and clozapine. Since clozapine related seizures and orthostatic hypotension appear to be dose related, the risk of these adverse events may be higher when fluvoxamine and clozapine are co-administered. Patients should be closely monitored when fluvoxamine maleate and clozapine are used concurrently.
Lithium: As with other serotonergic drugs, lithium may enhance the serotonergic effects of fluvoxamine and, therefore, the combination should be used with caution. Seizures have been reported with the co-administration of fluvoxamine maleate and lithium.
Lorazepam: A study of multiple doses of fluvoxamine maleate (50 mg bid) in healthy male volunteers (N=12) and a single dose of lorazepam (4 mg single dose) indicated no significant pharmacokinetic interaction. On average, both lorazepam alone and lorazepam with fluvoxamine produced substantial decrements in cognitive functioning; however, the co-administration of fluvoxamine and lorazepam did not produce larger mean decrements compared to lorazepam alone.
Methadone: Significantly increased methadone (plasma level:dose) ratios have been reported when fluvoxamine maleate was administered to patients receiving maintenance methadone treatment, with symptoms of opioid intoxication in one patient. Opioid withdrawal symptoms were reported following fluvoxamine maleate discontinuation in another patient.
Sumatriptan: There have been rare postmarketing reports describing patients with weakness, hyperreflexia, and incoordination following the use of a selective serotonin reuptake inhibitor (SSRI) and sumatriptan. If concomitant treatment with sumatriptan and an SSRI (e.g., fluoxetine, fluvoxamine, paroxetine, sertraline) is clinically warranted, appropriate observation of the patient is advised.
Tacrine: In a study of 13 healthy, male volunteers, a single 40 mg dose of tacrine added to fluvoxamine 100 mg/day administered at steady-state was associated with five- and eight-fold increases in tacrine Cmax and AUC, respectively, compared to the administration of tacrine alone. Five subjects experienced nausea, vomiting, sweating, and diarrhea following co-administration, consistent with the cholinergic effects of tacrine.
Tricyclic Antidepressants (TCAs): Significantly increased plasma TCA levels have been reported with the co-administration of fluvoxamine maleate and amitriptyline, clomipramine or imipramine. Caution is indicated with the co-administration of LUVOX Tablets and TCAs; plasma TCA concentrations may need to be monitored, and the dose of TCA may need to be reduced.
Tryptophan: Tryptophan may enhance the serotonergic effects of fluvoxamine, and the combination should, therefore, be used with caution. Severe vomiting has been reported with the co-administration of fluvoxamine maleate and tryptophan.
Other Drugs:
Theophylline: See WARNINGS
Warfarin: See WARNINGS
Digoxin: Administration of fluvoxamine maleate 100 mg daily for 18 days (N=8) did not significantly affect the pharmacokinetics of a 1.25 mg single intravenous dose of digoxin.
Diltiazem: Bradycardia has been reported with the co-administration of fluvoxamine maleate and diltiazem.
Propranolol and Other Beta-Blockers: Co-administration of fluvoxamine maleate 100 mg per day and propranolol 160 mg per day in normal volunteers resulted in a mean five-fold increase (range 2 to 17) in minimum propranolol plasma concentrations. In this study, there was a slight potentiation of the propranolol-induced reduction in heart rate and reduction in the exercise diastolic pressure.
One case of bradycardia and hypotension and a second case of orthostatic hypotension have been reported with the co-administration of fluvoxamine maleate and metoprolol.
If propranolol or metoprolol is co-administered with LUVOX Tablets, a reduction in the initial beta-blocker dose and more cautious dose titration is recommended. No dosage adjustment is required for LUVOX Tablets.
Co-administration of fluvoxamine maleate 100 mg per day with atenolol 100 mg per day (N=6) did not affect the plasma concentrations of atenolol. Unlike propranolol and metoprolol which undergo hepatic metabolism, atenolol is eliminated primarily by renal excretion.
Effects of Smoking on Fluvoxamine Metabolism: Smokers had a 25% increase in the metabolism of fluvoxamine compared to nonsmokers.

Electroconvulsive Therapy (ECT): There are no clinical studies establishing the benefits or risks of combined use of ECT and fluvoxamine maleate.

Carcinogenesis, Mutagenesis, Impairment of Fertility

Carcinogenesis: There is no evidence of carcinogenicity, mutagenicity or impairment of fertility with fluvoxamine maleate.

There was no evidence of carcinogenicity in rats treated orally with fluvoxamine maleate for 30 months or hamsters treated orally with fluvoxamine maleate for 20 (females) or 26 (males) months. The daily doses in the high dose groups in these studies were increased over the course of the study from a minimum of 160 mg/kg to a maximum of 240 mg/kg in rats, and from a minimum of 135 mg/kg to a maximum of 240 mg/kg in hamsters. The maximum dose of 240 mg/kg is approximately 6 times the maximum human daily dose on a mg/m^2 basis.

Mutagenesis: No evidence of mutagenic potential was observed in a mouse micronucleus test, an *in vitro* chromosome aberration test, or the Ames microbial mutagen test with or without metabolic activation.

Impairment of Fertility: In fertility studies of male and female rats, up to 80 mg/kg/day orally of fluvoxamine maleate, (approximately 2 times the maximum human daily dose on a mg/m^2 basis) had no effect on mating performance, duration of gestation, or pregnancy rate.

Pregnancy

Teratogenic Effects - Pregnancy Category C: In teratology studies in rats and rabbits, daily oral doses of fluvoxamine maleate of up to 80 and 40 mg/kg, respectively (approximately 2 times the maximum human daily dose on a mg/m^2 basis) caused no fetal malformations. However, in other reproduction studies in which pregnant rats were dosed through weaning there was (1) an increase in pup mortality at birth (seen at 80 mg/kg and above but not at 20 mg/kg), and (2) decreases in postnatal pup weights (seen at 160 but not at 80 mg/kg) and survival (seen at all doses; lowest dose tested = 5 mg/kg). (Doses of 5, 20, 80, and 160 mg/kg are approximately 0.1, 0.5, 2, and 4 times the maximum human daily dose on a mg/m^2 basis.) While the results of a cross-fostering study implied that at least some of these results likely occurred secondarily to maternal toxicity, the role of a direct drug effect on the fetuses or pups could not be ruled out. There are no adequate and well-controlled studies in pregnant women. Fluvoxamine maleate should be used during pregnancy only if the potential benefit justifies the potential risk to the fetus.

Labor and Delivery

The effect of fluvoxamine on labor and delivery in humans is unknown.

Nursing Mothers

As for many other drugs, fluvoxamine is secreted in human breast milk. The decision of whether to discontinue nursing or to discontinue the drug should take into account the potential for serious adverse effects from exposure to fluvoxamine in the nursing infant as well as the potential benefits of LUVOX® (fluvoxamine maleate) Tablets therapy to the mother.

Pediatric Use

The efficacy of fluvoxamine maleate for the treatment of Obsessive Compulsive Disorder was demonstrated in a 10-week multicenter placebo controlled study with 120 outpatients ages 8–17. The adverse event profile observed in that study was generally similar to that observed in adult studies with fluvoxamine (see ADVERSE REACTIONS and DOSAGE AND ADMINISTRATION).

Decreased appetite and weight loss have been observed in association with the use of fluvoxamine as well as other SSRIs. Consequently, regular monitoring of weight and growth is recommended if treatment of a child with an SSRI is to be continued long term.

The risks, if any, that may be associated with fluvoxamine's extended use in children and adolescents with OCD have not been systematically assessed. The prescriber should be mindful that the evidence relied upon to conclude that fluvoxamine is safe for use in children and adolescents derived from relatively short term clinical studies and from extrapolation of experience gained with adult patients. In particular, there are no studies that directly evaluate the effects of long term fluvoxamine use on the growth, development, and maturation of children and adolescents. Although there is no affirmative finding to suggest that fluvoxamine possesses a capacity to adversely affect growth, development or maturation, the absence of such findings is not compelling evidence of the absence of the potential of fluvoxamine to have adverse effects in chronic use.

Geriatric Use

Approximately 230 patients participating in controlled premarketing studies with LUVOX Tablets were 65 years of age or over. No overall differences in safety were observed between these patients and younger patients. Other reported clinical experience has not identified differences in response between the elderly and younger patients. However, the clearance of fluvoxamine is decreased by about 50% in elderly compared to younger patients (see Pharmacokinetics under CLINICAL PHARMACOLOGY), and

greater sensitivity of some older individuals also cannot be ruled out. Consequently, LUVOX Tablets should be slowly titrated during initiation of therapy.

ADVERSE REACTIONS

Associated with Discontinuation of Treatment

Of the 1087 OCD and depressed patients treated with fluvoxamine maleate in controlled clinical trials conducted in North America, 22% discontinued treatment due to an adverse event. The most common events (≥1%) associated with discontinuation and considered to be drug related (i.e., those events associated with dropout at a rate at least twice that of placebo) included:

Table 1
ADVERSE EVENTS ASSOCIATED WITH DISCONTINUATION OF TREATMENT IN OCD AND DEPRESSION POPULATIONS

BODY SYSTEM/ ADVERSE EVENT	PERCENTAGE OF PATIENTS FLUVOXAMINE	PLACEBO
BODY AS A WHOLE		
Headache	3%	1%
Asthenia	2%	<1%
Abdominal Pain	1%	0%
DIGESTIVE		
Nausea	9%	1%
Diarrhea	1%	<1%
Vomiting	2%	<1%
Anorexia	1%	<1%
Dyspepsia	1%	<1%
NERVOUS SYSTEM		
Insomnia	4%	1%
Somnolence	4%	<1%
Nervousness	2%	<1%
Agitation	2%	<1%
Dizziness	2%	<1%
Anxiety	1%	<1%
Dry Mouth	1%	<1%

Incidence in Controlled Trials

Commonly Observed Adverse Events in Controlled Clinical Trials:

LUVOX Tablets have been studied in controlled trials of OCD (N=320) and depression (N=1350). In general, adverse event rates were similar in the two data sets as well as in the pediatric OCD study. The most commonly observed adverse events associated with the use of LUVOX Tablets and likely to be drug-related (incidence of 5% or greater and at least twice that for placebo) derived from Table 2 were: *somnolence, insomnia, nervousness, tremor, nausea, dyspepsia, anorexia, vomiting, abnormal ejaculation, asthenia, and sweating.* In a pool of two studies involving only patients with OCD, the following additional events were identified using the above rule: *dry mouth, decreased libido, urinary frequency, anorgasmia, rhinitis and taste perversion.* In a study of pediatric patients with OCD, the following additional events were identified using the above rule: *agitation, depression, dysmenorrhea, flatulence, hyperkinesia, and rash.*

Adverse Events Occurring at an Incidence of 1%: Table 2 enumerates adverse events that occurred in adults at a frequency of 1% or more, and were more frequent than in the placebo group, among patients treated with LUVOX Tablets in two short-term placebo controlled OCD trials (10 week) and depression trials (6 week) in which patients were dosed in a range of generally 100 to 300 mg/day. This table shows the percentage of patients in each group who had at least one occurrence of an event at some time during their treatment. Reported adverse events were classified using a standard COSTART-based Dictionary terminology.

The prescriber should be aware that these figures cannot be used to predict the incidence of side effects in the course of usual medical practice where patient characteristics and other factors may differ from those that prevailed in the clinical trials. Similarly, the cited frequencies cannot be compared with figures obtained from other clinical investigations involving different treatments, uses, and investigators. The cited figures, however, do provide the prescribing physician with some basis for estimating the relative contribution of drug and non-drug factors to the side-effect incidence rate in the population studied.

Table 2
TREATMENT-EMERGENT ADVERSE EVENT INCIDENCE RATES BY BODY SYSTEM IN ADULT OCD AND DEPRESSION POPULATIONS COMBINED[1]

BODY SYSTEM/ ADVERSE EVENT	Percentage of Patients Reporting Event FLUVOXAMINE N=892	PLACEBO N=778
BODY AS WHOLE		
Headache	22	20
Asthenia	14	6
Flu Syndrome	3	2
Chills	2	1
CARDIOVASCULAR		
Palpitations	3	2
DIGESTIVE SYSTEM		
Nausea	40	14
Diarrhea	11	7
Constipation	10	8
Dyspepsia	10	5
Anorexia	6	2
Vomiting	5	2
Flatulence	4	3
Tooth Disorder[2]	3	1
Dysphagia	2	1
NERVOUS SYSTEM		
Somnolence	22	8
Insomnia	21	10
Dry Mouth	14	10
Nervousness	12	5
Dizziness	11	6
Tremor	5	1
Anxiety	5	3
Vasodilation[3]	3	1
Hypertonia	2	1
Agitation	2	1
Decreased Libido	2	1
Depression	2	1
CNS Stimulation	2	1
RESPIRATORY SYSTEM		
Upper Respiratory Infection	9	5
Dyspnea	2	1
Yawn	2	0
SKIN		
Sweating	7	3
SPECIAL SENSES		
Taste Perversion	3	1
Amblyopia[4]	3	2
UROGENITAL		
Abnormal Ejaculation[5,6]	8	1
Urinary Frequency	3	2
Impotence[6]	2	1
Anorgasmia	2	0
Urinary Retention	1	0

[1] Events for which fluvoxamine maleate incidence was equal or less than placebo are not listed in the table above, but include the following: abdominal pain, abnormal dreams, appetite increase, back pain, chest pain, confusion, dysmenorrhea, fever, infection, leg cramps, migraine, myalgia, pain, paresthesia, pharyngitis, postural hypotension, pruritus, rash, rhinitis, thirst and tinnitus.

[2] Includes "toothache", "tooth extraction and abscess," and "caries."

[3] Mostly feeling warm, hot, or flushed.

[4] Mostly "blurred vision."

[5] Mostly "delayed ejaculation."

[6] Incidence based on number of male patients.

Adverse Events in OCD Placebo Controlled Studies Which are Markedly Different (defined as at least a two-fold difference) in Rate from the Pooled Event Rates in OCD and Depression Placebo Controlled Studies: The events in OCD studies with a two-fold decrease in rate compared to event rates in OCD and depression studies were dysphagia and amblyopia (mostly blurred vision). Additionally, there was an approximate 25% decrease in nausea.

The events in OCD studies with a two-fold increase in rate compared to event rates in OCD and depression studies were: *asthenia, abnormal ejaculation (mostly delayed ejaculation), anxiety, infection, rhinitis, anorgasmia (in males), depression, libido decreased, pharyngitis, agitation, impotence, myoclonus/twitch, thirst, weight loss, leg cramps, myalgia and urinary retention.* These events are listed in order of decreasing rates in the OCD trials.

Other Adverse Events in OCD Pediatric Population

In pediatric patients (N=57) treated with LUVOX Tablets, the overall profile of adverse events was generally similar to that seen in adult studies, as shown in Table 2. However, the following adverse events, not appearing in Table 2, were reported in two or more of the pediatric patients and were more frequent with LUVOX Tablets than with placebo: abnormal thinking, cough increase, dysmenorrhea, ecchymosis, emotional lability, epistaxis, hyperkinesia, infection, manic reaction, rash, sinusitis, and weight decrease.

Vital Sign Changes

Comparisons of fluvoxamine maleate and placebo groups in separate pools of short-term OCD and depression trials on (1) median change from baseline on various vital signs variables and on (2) incidence of patients meeting criteria for potentially important changes from baseline on various vital signs variables revealed no important differences between fluvoxamine maleate and placebo.

Continued on next page

Luvox—Cont.

Laboratory Changes

Comparisons of fluvoxamine maleate and placebo groups in separate pools of short-term OCD and depression trials on (1) median change from baseline on various serum chemistry, hematology, and urinalysis variables and on (2) incidence of patients meeting criteria for potentially important changes from baseline on various serum chemistry, hematology, and urinalysis variables revealed no important differences between fluvoxamine maleate and placebo.

ECG Changes

Comparisons of fluvoxamine maleate and placebo groups in separate pools of short-term OCD and depression trials on (1) mean change from baseline on various ECG variables and on (2) incidence of patients meeting criteria for potentially important changes from baseline on various ECG variables revealed no important differences between fluvoxamine maleate and placebo.

Other Events Observed During the Premarketing Evaluation of LUVOX Tablets

During premarketing clinical trials conducted in North America and Europe, multiple doses of fluvoxamine maleate were administered for a combined total of 2737 patient exposures in patients suffering OCD or Major Depressive Disorder. Untoward events associated with this exposure were recorded by clinical investigators using descriptive terminology of their own choosing. Consequently, it is not possible to provide a meaningful estimate of the proportion of individuals experiencing adverse events without first grouping similar types of untoward events into a limited (i.e., reduced) number of standard event categories.

In the tabulations which follow, a standard COSTART-based Dictionary terminology has been used to classify reported adverse events. If the COSTART term for an event was so general as to be uninformative, it was replaced with a more informative term. The frequencies presented, therefore, represent the proportion of the 2737 patient exposures to multiple doses of fluvoxamine maleate who experienced an event of the type cited on at least one occasion while receiving fluvoxamine maleate. All reported events are included in the list below, with the following exceptions: 1) those events already listed in Table 2, which tabulates incidence rates of common adverse experiences in placebo-controlled OCD and depression clinical trials, are excluded; 2) those events for which a drug cause was considered remote (i.e., neoplasia, gastrointestinal carcinoma, herpes simplex, herpes zoster, application site reaction, and unintended pregnancy) are omitted; and 3) events which were reported in only one patient and judged to not be potentially serious are not included. It is important to emphasize that, although the events reported did occur during treatment with fluvoxamine maleate, a causal relationship to fluvoxamine maleate has not been established.

Events are further classified within body system categories and enumerated in order of decreasing frequency using the following definitions: frequent adverse events are defined as those occurring on one or more occasions in at least 1/100 patients; infrequent adverse events are those occurring between 1/100 and 1/1000 patients; and rare adverse events are those occurring in less than 1/1000 patients.

Body as a Whole: *Frequent:* accidental injury, malaise; *Infrequent:* allergic reaction, neck pain, neck rigidity, overdose, photosensitivity reaction, suicide attempt; *Rare:* cyst, pelvic pain, sudden death.

Cardiovascular System: *Frequent:* hypertension, hypotension, syncope, tachycardia; *Infrequent:* angina pectoris, bradycardia, cardiomyopathy, cardiovascular disease, cold extremities, conduction delay, heart failure, myocardial infarction, pallor, pulse irregular, ST segment changes; *Rare:* AV block, cerebrovascular accident, coronary artery disease, embolus, pericarditis, phlebitis, pulmonary infarction, supraventricular extrasystoles.

Digestive System: *Frequent:* elevated liver transaminases; *Infrequent:* colitis, eructation, esophagitis, gastritis, gastroenteritis, gastrointestinal hemorrhage, gastrointestinal ulcer, gingivitis, glossitis, hemorrhoids, melena, rectal hemorrhage, stomatitis; *Rare:* biliary pain, cholecystitis, cholelithiasis, fecal incontinence, hematemesis, intestinal obstruction, jaundice.

Endocrine System: *Infrequent:* hypothyroidism; *Rare:* goiter.

Hemic and Lymphatic Systems: *Infrequent:* anemia, ecchymosis, leukocytosis, lymphadenopathy, thrombocytopenia; *Rare:* leukopenia, purpura.

Metabolic and Nutritional Systems: *Frequent:* edema, weight gain, weight loss; *Infrequent:* dehydration, hypercholesterolemia; *Rare:* diabetes mellitus, hyperglycemia, hyperlipidemia, hypoglycemia, hypokalemia, lactate dehydrogenase increased.

Musculoskeletal System: *Infrequent:* arthralgia, arthritis, bursitis, generalized muscle spasm, myasthenia, tendinous contracture, tenosynovitis; *Rare:* arthrosis, myopathy, pathological fracture.

Nervous System: *Frequent:* amnesia, apathy, hyperkinesia, hypokinesia, manic reaction, myoclonus, psychotic reaction; *Infrequent:* agoraphobia, akathisia, ataxia, CNS depression, convulsion, delirium, delusion, depersonalization, drug dependence, dyskinesia, dystonia, emotional lability, euphoria, extrapyramidal syndrome, gait unsteady, hallucinations, hemiplegia, hostility, hypersomnia, hypochondriasis, hypotonia, hysteria, incoordination, increased salivation, increased libido, neuralgia, paralysis, paranoid reaction, phobia, psychosis, sleep disorder, stupor, twitching, vertigo; *Rare:* akinesia, coma, fibrillations, mutism, obsessions, reflexes decreased, slurred speech, tardive dyskinesia, torticollis, trismus, withdrawal syndrome.

Respiratory System: *Frequent:* cough increased, sinusitis; *Infrequent:* asthma, bronchitis, epistaxis, hoarseness, hyperventilation; *Rare:* apnea, congestion of upper airway, hemoptysis, hiccups, laryngismus, obstructive pulmonary disease, pneumonia.

Skin: *Infrequent:* acne, alopecia, dry skin, eczema, exfoliative dermatitis, furunculosis, seborrhea, skin discoloration, urticaria.

Special Senses: *Infrequent:* accommodation abnormal, conjunctivitis, deafness, diplopia, dry eyes, ear pain, eye pain, mydriasis, otitis media, parosmia, photophobia, taste loss, visual field defect; *Rare:* corneal ulcer, retinal detachment.

Urogenital System: *Infrequent:* anuria, breast pain, cystitis, delayed menstruation[1], dysuria, female lactation[1], hematuria, menopause[1], menorrhagia[1], metrorrhagia[1], nocturia, polyuria, premenstrual syndrome[1], urinary incontinence, urinary tract infection, urinary urgency, urination impaired, vaginal hemorrhage[1], vaginitis[1]; *Rare:* kidney calculus, hematospermia[2], oliguria.

[1] Based on the number of females.

[2] Based on the number of males.

Non-US Postmarketing Reports

Voluntary reports of adverse events in patients taking LUVOX Tablets that have been received since market introduction and are of unknown causal relationship to LUVOX Tablets use include: toxic epidermal necrolysis, Stevens-Johnson syndrome, Henoch-Schoenlein purpura, bullous eruption, priapism, agranulocytosis, neuropathy, aplastic anemia, anaphylactic reaction, hyponatremia, acute renal failure, hepatitis, and severe akinesia with fever when fluvoxamine was co-administered with antipsychotic medication.

DRUG ABUSE AND DEPENDENCE

Controlled Substance Class

LUVOX Tablets are not controlled substances.

Physical and Psychological Dependence

The potential for abuse, tolerance and physical dependence with fluvoxamine maleate has been studied in a nonhuman primate model. No evidence of dependency phenomena was found. The discontinuation effects of LUVOX Tablets were not systematically evaluated in controlled clinical trials. LUVOX Tablets were not systematically studied in clinical trials for potential for abuse, but there was no indication of drug-seeking behavior in clinical trials. It should be noted, however, that patients at risk for drug dependency were systematically excluded from investigational studies of fluvoxamine maleate. Generally, it is not possible to predict on the basis of preclinical or premarketing clinical experience the extent to which a CNS active drug will be misused, diverted, and/or abused once marketed. Consequently, physicians should carefully evaluate patients for a history of drug abuse and follow such patients closely, observing them for signs of fluvoxamine maleate misuse or abuse (i.e., development of tolerance, incrementation of dose, drug -seeking behavior).

OVERDOSAGE

Human Experience

Worldwide exposure to fluvoxamine maleate includes over 37,000 patients treated in clinical trials and an estimated exposure of 4,500,000 patients treated during foreign marketing experience (circa 1992). Of the 354 cases of deliberate or accidental overdose involving fluvoxamine maleate reported from this population, there were 19 deaths. Of the 19 deaths, 2 were in patients taking fluvoxamine maleate alone and the remaining 17 were in patients taking fluvoxamine maleate along with other drugs. In the remaining 335 patients, 309 had complete recovery after gastric lavage or symptomatic treatment. One patient had persistent mydriasis after the event, and a second patient had a bowel infarction requiring a hemicolectomy. In the remaining 24 patients the outcome was unknown. The highest reported overdose of fluvoxamine maleate involved a non-lethal ingestion of 10,000 mg (equivalent of 1–3 months' dosage). The patient fully recovered with no sequelae.

Commonly observed adverse events associated with fluvoxamine maleate overdose included drowsiness, vomiting, diarrhea, and dizziness. Other notable signs and symptoms seen with fluvoxamine maleate overdose (single or mixed drugs) included coma, tachycardia, bradycardia, hypotension, ECG abnormalities, liver function abnormalities, convulsions, and symptoms such as aspiration pneumonitis, respiratory difficulties or hypokalemia that may occur secondary to loss of consciousness or vomiting.

Management of Overdose

1. An unobstructed airway should be established with maintenance of respiration as required. Vital signs and ECG should be monitored.
2. Administration of activated charcoal may be as effective as emesis or lavage and should be considered in treating overdose. Since absorption with overdose may be delayed, measures to minimize absorption may be necessary for up to 24 hours post-ingestion.
3. Maintain close observation as clinically indicated.
4. There are no specific antidotes for LUVOX Tablets.
5. In managing overdosage, consider the possibility of multiple drug involvement. The physician should consider contacting a poison control center for additional information on the treatment of any overdosage.
6. Dialysis is not believed to be beneficial.

DOSAGE AND ADMINISTRATION

Dosage for Adults

The recommended starting dose for LUVOX Tablets in adult patients is 50 mg, administered as a single daily dose at bedtime. In the controlled clinical trials establishing the effectiveness of LUVOX Tablets in OCD, patients were titrated within a dose range of 100 to 300 mg/day. Consequently, the dose should be increased in 50 mg increments every 4 to 7 days, as tolerated, until maximum therapeutic benefit is achieved, not to exceed 300 mg per day. It is advisable that a total daily dose of more than 100 mg should be given in two divided doses. If the doses are not equal, the larger dose should be given at bedtime.

Dosage for Pediatric Population (children and adolescents)

The recommended starting dose for LUVOX Tablets in pediatric populations (ages 8–17 years) is 25 mg, administered as a single daily dose at bedtime. In a controlled clinical trial establishing the effectiveness of LUVOX Tablets in OCD, pediatric patients (ages 8–17) were titrated within a dose range of 50 to 200 mg/day. The dose should be increased in 25 mg increments every 4 to 7 days, as tolerated, until maximum therapeutic benefit is achieved, not to exceed 200 mg per day. It is advisable that a total daily dose of more than 50 mg should be given in two divided doses. If the two divided doses are not equal, the larger dose should be given at bedtime.

Dosage for Elderly or Hepatically Impaired Patients

Elderly patients and those with hepatic impairment have been observed to have a decreased clearance of fluvoxamine maleate. Consequently, it may be appropriate to modify the initial dose and the subsequent dose titration for these patient groups.

Maintenance/Continuation Extended Treatment

Although the efficacy of LUVOX Tablets beyond 10 weeks of dosing for OCD has not been documented in controlled trials, OCD is a chronic condition, and it is reasonable to consider continuation for a responding patient. Dosage adjustments should be made to maintain the patient on the lowest effective dosage, and patients should be periodically reassessed to determine the need for continued treatment.

HOW SUPPLIED

Tablets 25 mg: unscored, white, elliptical, film-coated (debossed "SOLVAY" and "4202" on one side)

Bottles of 100 .... NDC 0032-4202-01
Unit dose pack of 100 .... NDC 0032-4202-11

Tablets 50 mg: scored, yellow, elliptical, film-coated (debossed "SOLVAY" and "4205" on one side and scored on the other)

Bottles of 100 .... NDC 0032-4205-01
Bottles of 1000 .... NDC 0032-4205-10
Unit dose pack of 100 .... NDC 0032-4205-11

Tablets 100 mg: scored, beige, elliptical, film-coated (debossed "SOLVAY" and "4210" on one side and scored on the other)

Bottles of 100 .... NDC 0032-4210-01
Bottles of 1000 .... NDC 0032-4210-10
Unit dose pack of 100 .... NDC 0032-4210-11

LUVOX Tablets should be protected from high humidity and stored at controlled room temperature, 15°–30° C (59°–86° F).

Dispense in tight containers.

Rx only

Solvay
Pharmaceuticals
Marietta, GA 30062
1252
11E Rev 3/98
© 1998 Solvay Pharmaceuticals, Inc.

Shown in Product Identification Guide, page 340

PROMETRIUM   ℞

[prō mē' trium]
(progesterone, USP)
Capsules 100 mg

DESCRIPTION

Each PROMETRIUM® (progesterone, USP) Capsule contains 100 mg micronized progesterone for oral administra-

tion. Progesterone has a molecular weight of 314.47 and an empirical formula of $C_{21}H_{30}O_2$. Progesterone, (pregn-4-ene-3,20-dione) is a white or creamy white, odorless, crystalline powder, practically insoluble in water, soluble in alcohol, acetone, and dioxane, and sparingly soluble in vegetable oils, stable in air, melting between 126° and 131°C. The structural formula is:

Each peach-colored, opaque, soft-gelatin capsule contains 100 mg micronized progesterone as the active ingredient. The inactive ingredients are peanut oil NF, gelatin NF, glycerin USP, lecithin NF, titanium dioxide USP, D&C Yellow No. 10, and FD&C Red No. 40.

CLINICAL PHARMACOLOGY

PROMETRIUM Capsules are an oral dosage form of micronized progesterone which is chemically identical to progesterone of ovarian origin. The oral bioavailability of progesterone is increased through micronization.

Pharmacokinetics

Absorption

After oral administration of progesterone as a micronized soft gelatin capsule formulation, maximum serum concentrations were attained within 3 hours. The absolute bioavailability of micronized progesterone is not known. Table 1 summarizes the mean pharmacokinetic parameters in postmenopausal women after five oral daily doses of PROMETRIUM Capsules as a micronized soft-gelatin capsule formulation:

Table 1

Parameter	PROMETRIUM Capsules Dose QD		
	100 mg	200 mg	300 mg
Cmax (ng/mL)	17.3±21.9[a]	38.1±37.8	60.6±72.5
Tmax (hr)	1.5±0.8	2.3±1.4	1.7±0.6
AUC (0–10) (ng•hr/mL)	43.3±30.8	101.2±66.0	175.7±170.3

[a]Mean ± S.D.

Serum progesterone concentrations appeared linear and dose proportional following multiple dose administration of PROMETRIUM Capsules over the dose range 100 mg/day to 300 mg/day in postmenopausal women. Although doses greater than 300 mg/day were not studied in females, serum concentrations from a study in male volunteers appeared linear and dose proportional between 100 mg/day and 400 mg/day. The pharmacokinetic parameters in male volunteers were generally consistent with those seen in postmenopausal women.

Distribution

Progesterone is approximately 96%–99% bound to serum proteins, primarily to serum albumin (50%–54%) and transcortin (43%–48%).

Metabolism

Progesterone is metabolized primarily by the liver, largely to pregnanediols and pregnanolones. Pregnanediols and pregnanolones are conjugated in the liver to glucuronide and sulfate metabolites. Progesterone metabolites which are excreted in the bile may be deconjugated and may be further metabolized in the gut via reduction, dehydroxylation, and epimerization.

Excretion

The glucuronide and sulfate conjugates of pregnanediol and pregnanolone are excreted in the bile and urine. Progesterone metabolites which are excreted in the bile may undergo enterohepatic recycling or may be excreted in the feces.

Special Populations

The pharmacokinetics of this formulation have not been assessed in low body weight or obese patients.

Race:

There is insufficient information available from trials conducted with PROMETRIUM Capsules to compare progesterone pharmacokinetics in different racial groups.

Drug-Drug Interaction:

The metabolism of progesterone by human liver microsomes was inhibited by ketoconazole (IC_{50} <0.1 µM). Ketoconazole is a known inhibitor of cytochrome P450 3A4, hence these data suggest that other known inhibitors of this enzyme may increase the bioavailability of progesterone. The clinical relevance of the *in vitro* findings are unknown.

Food-Drug Interaction:

Concomitant food ingestion increased the bioavailability of PROMETRIUM Capsules relative to a fasting state when

administered to postmenopausal women at a dose of 200 mg. This effect was further characterized at a single dose of 300 mg in healthy male volunteers. Mean Cmax was slightly increased (9%) when PROMETRIUM Capsules were administered with or 2 hours after a high-fat breakfast relative to the fasting state. In contrast, when the PROMETRIUM Capsules dose was administered 4 hours after the high-fat breakfast, there was a significant increase in Cmax (193%). The corresponding increases in AUC were 47%, 50%, and 102% following administration with breakfast, 2 hours and 4 hours after breakfast, respectively. There was no effect on the time to maximum serum concentrations (Tmax). High intra- and intersubject variability was observed.

Hepatic Insufficiency:

No formal studies have evaluated the effect of hepatic disease on the disposition of progesterone. However, since progesterone is metabolized by the liver, use in patients with severe liver dysfunction or disease is contraindicated (see **CONTRAINDICATIONS**). If treatment with progesterone is indicated in patients with mild to moderate hepatic dysfunction, these patients should be monitored carefully.

Renal Insufficiency:

No formal studies have evaluated the effect of renal disease on the disposition of progesterone. Since progesterone metabolites are eliminated mainly by the kidneys, PROMETRIUM Capsules should be used with caution and only with careful monitoring in patients with renal dysfunction. (See **PRECAUTIONS**.)

Clinical Studies

In a single-center, randomized, double-blind clinical study that included premenopausal women with secondary amenorrhea for at least 90 days, administration of 10 days of micronized progesterone therapy resulted in 80% experiencing withdrawal bleeding within 7 days of the last dose of PROMETRIUM Capsules, 300 mg/day (n=20), compared to 10% of women experiencing withdrawal bleeding in the placebo group (n=21).

The rate of secretory transformation was evaluated in a multicenter, randomized, double-blind clinical study in estrogen-primed postmenopausal women. Micronized progesterone administered orally for 10 days at 400 mg/day (n=22) induced complete secretory changes in the endometrium in 45% of women compared to 0% in the placebo group (n=23).

INDICATIONS AND USAGE

Secondary amenorrhea.

CONTRAINDICATIONS

1. **Known sensitivity to PROMETRIUM Capsules or its ingredients. PROMETRIUM Capsules contain peanut oil and should never be used by patients allergic to peanuts.**
2. Known or suspected pregnancy.
3. Thrombophlebitis, thromboembolic disorders, cerebral apoplexy, or patients with a past history of these conditions.
4. Severe liver dysfunction or disease.
5. Known or suspected malignancy of breast or genital organs.
6. Undiagnosed vaginal bleeding.
7. Missed abortion.
8. As a diagnostic test for pregnancy.

WARNINGS

1. The physician should be alert to the earliest manifestations of thrombotic disorders (thrombophlebitis, cerebrovascular disorders, pulmonary embolism, and retinal thrombosis). Should any of these occur or be suspected, the drug should be discontinued immediately.
2. Discontinue medication pending examination if there is sudden partial or complete loss of vision, or if there is a sudden onset of proptosis, diplopia, or migraine. If examination reveals papilledema or retinal vascular lesions, medication should be withdrawn.
3. The administration of any drug to nursing mothers should be done only when clearly necessary since many drugs are excreted in human milk. Detectable amounts of progestin have been identified in the milk of mothers receiving progestins. The effect of this on the nursing infant has not been determined.
4. Usage in pregnancy is not recommended. A case of cleft palate has been observed in the child of a woman who was using PROMETRIUM Capsules during early pregnancy. Rare instances of fetal death have been reported in pregnant women prescribed PROMETRIUM Capsules for unapproved indications. Definitive causality has not been established.
5. Retrospective studies of morbidity and mortality in Great Britain and studies of morbidity in the United States have shown a statistically significant association between thrombophlebitis, pulmonary embolism, cerebral thrombosis and embolism, and the use of oral contraceptives. The estimate of the relative risk of thromboembolism in the study by Vessey and Doll was about seven fold, while Sartwell and associates in the United States found a relative risk of 4.4, meaning that the users are several times as likely to undergo thromboembolic disease without evident cause as nonusers. The American study also indicated that the risk did not persist after discontinuation of administration, and that it was not enhanced by long-continued administration. The American study was not designed to evaluate a difference between products.

PRECAUTIONS

General

1. The pretreatment physical examination should include special reference to breast and pelvic organs, as well as Papanicolaou smear.
2. Because progesterone may cause some degree of fluid retention, conditions which might be influenced by this factor, such as epilepsy, migraine, asthma, cardiac or renal dysfunction, require careful observation.
3. In cases of breakthrough bleeding, as in any cases of irregular bleeding per vaginum, nonfunctional causes should be borne in mind. In cases of undiagnosed vaginal bleeding, adequate diagnostic measures are indicated.

Table 2

Adverse Experiences (≥5%) Reported in Patients Using 400 mg/day in a Placebo-Controlled Trial in Estrogen-Primed Postmenopausal Women

Adverse Experience	PROMETRIUM Capsules 400 mg N=25	Placebo N=24
	Percentage (%) of Patients	
Fatigue	8	4
Headache	16	8
Dizziness	24	4
Abdominal Distension (Bloating)	8	8
Abdominal Pain (Cramping)	20	13
Diarrhea	8	4
Nausea	8	0
Back Pain	8	8
Musculoskeletal Pain	12	4
Irritability	8	4
Breast Pain	16	8
Infection Viral	12	0
Coughing	8	0

Continued on next page

Prometrium—Cont.

4. Patients who have a history of psychic depression should be carefully observed and the drug discontinued if the depression recurs to a serious degree.
5. Any possible influence of prolonged progestin therapy on pituitary, ovarian, adrenal, hepatic, or uterine functions awaits further study.
6. Diabetic patients should be carefully observed while receiving progestin therapy.
7. The pathologist should be advised of progestin therapy when relevant specimens are submitted.
8. Because of the occurrence of thrombotic disorders (thrombophlebitis, pulmonary embolism, retinal thrombosis, and cerebrovascular disorders) in patients taking estrogen-progestin combinations, the physician should be alert to the earliest manifestation of these disorders, although the mechanism is obscure.
9. Transient dizziness may occur in some patients. Use caution when driving a motor vehicle or operating machinery.

Information for the Patient

See accompanying Patient Insert.

Drug Lab Test Interactions

The following laboratory results may be altered by the use of estrogen-progestin combination drugs:

Increased sulfobromophthalein retention and other hepatic function tests.

Coagulation tests: increase in prothrombin factors VII, VIII, IX and X.

Metyrapone test.

Pregnanediol determination.

Thyroid function: increase in PBI, and butanol extractable protein bound iodine and decrease in T3 uptake values.

In a 3-year study of micronized progesterone 200 mg/day administered for 12 days per 28-day cycle in combination with conjugated estrogens 0.625 mg/day, the concomitant use of conjugated estrogens and micronized progesterone increased HDL-C and triglycerides and decreased LDL-C compared to placebo, and did not impair glucose tolerance.

Carcinogenesis, Mutagenesis, Impairment of Fertility

Progesterone has not been tested for carcinogenicity in animals by the oral route of administration. Other progestational drugs administered to experimental animals by various routes of administration, including orally, have produced tumors in several tissues after exposure to high dosages.

Progesterone did not show evidence of genotoxicity in *in vitro* studies for point mutations or for chromosome damage. *In vivo* animal studies for chromosome damage have yielded positive results in mice at oral doses of 1000 mg/kg and 2000 mg/kg (*Med Sci Res.* 1987;15:703–704).

Exogenously administered progesterone has been shown to inhibit ovulation in a number of species and it is expected that high doses given for an extended duration would impair fertility until the cessation of treatment.

Pregnancy Category X

Progesterone, including PROMETRIUM Capsules, should not be used during pregnancy.

Nursing Mothers

The administration of any drug to nursing mothers should be done only when clearly necessary since many drugs are excreted in human milk. Detectable amounts of progestin have been identified in the milk of nursing mothers receiving progestins. The effect of this on the nursing infant has not been determined.

Pediatric Use

The safety and effectiveness of PROMETRIUM Capsules in pediatric patients have not been established.

ADVERSE REACTIONS

Table 2 lists adverse experiences which were reported in ≥5% of patients receiving PROMETRIUM Capsules, 400 mg/day, in a multicenter, randomized, double-blind, placebo-controlled clinical trial in estrogen-primed (6 weeks) postmenopausal women receiving conjugated equine estrogens 0.625 mg/day and cyclic (10 days per calendar month cycle) PROMETRIUM Capsules at a dose of 400 mg/day for three cycles.

[See table 2 at top of previous page]

The most common adverse experiences reported in ≥5% of patients in all PROMETRIUM Capsules dosage groups studied in this trial (100 mg/day to 400 mg/day) were: dizziness (16%), breast pain (11%), headache (10%), abdominal pain (10%), fatigue (9%), viral infection (7%), abdominal distension (6%), musculoskeletal pain (6%), emotional lability (6%), irritability (5%), and upper respiratory tract infection (5%).

Other adverse events reported in <5% of patients taking PROMETRIUM Capsules include:

Autonomic Nervous System Disorders: dry mouth
Body As A Whole: accidental injury, chest pain, fever
Cardiovascular System Disorders: hypertension
Central and Peripheral Nervous System Disorders: confusion, somnolence, speech disorder
Gastrointestinal System Disorders: constipation, dyspepsia, gastroenteritis, hemorrhagic rectum, hiatus hernia, vomiting
Hearing and Vestibular Disorders: earache
Heart Rate and Rhythm Disorders: palpitation
Metabolic and Nutritional Disorders: edema, edema peripheral
Musculoskeletal System Disorders: arthritis, leg cramps, hypertonia, muscle disorder, myalgia
Myo/Endo/Pericardial and Valve Disorders: angina pectoris
Psychiatric Disorders: anxiety, depression, impaired concentration, insomnia, personality disorder
Reproductive System Disorders: leukorrhea, uterine fibroid, vaginal dryness, fungal vaginitis, vaginitis
Resistance Mechanism Disorders: abscess, herpes simplex
Respiratory System Disorders: bronchitis, nasal congestion, pharyngitis, pneumonitis, sinusitis
Skin and Appendages Disorders: acne, verruca, wound debridement
Urinary System Disorders: urinary tract infection
Vision Disorders: abnormal vision
White Cell and Resistance Disorders: lymphadenopathy

The following adverse experiences have been reported with PROMETRIUM Capsules in other U.S. clinical trials: increased sweating, asthenia, tooth disorder, anorexia, increased appetite, nervousness, and breast enlargement.

The following spontaneous adverse events have been reported during the foreign marketing of PROMETRIUM Capsules: reversible cases of hepatitis and elevated transaminases. These events occurred mainly in patients receiving high doses of up to 1200 mg.

The following additional adverse experiences have been observed in women taking progestins in general: breakthrough bleeding, spotting, change in menstrual flow, amenorrhea, changes in weight (increase or decrease), changes in the cervical squamo-columnar junction and cervical secretions, cholestatic jaundice, anaphylactoid reactions and anaphylaxis, rash (allergic) with and without pruritus, melasma or chloasma, pyrexia, and insomnia.

OVERDOSAGE

No studies on overdosage have been conducted in humans. In the case of overdosage, PROMETRIUM Capsules should be discontinued, and the patient should be treated symptomatically.

DOSAGE AND ADMINISTRATION

PROMETRIUM Capsules may be given as a single daily dose of 400 mg in the evening for 10 days.

HOW SUPPLIED

PROMETRIUM® (progesterone, USP) Capsules 100 mg are round, peach-colored capsules branded with black imprint "SV", available in bottles of 100 capsules (NDC 0032-1708-01).

Store at controlled room temperature at 25°C (77°F).

Dispense in tight, light-resistant container as defined in USP/NF, accompanied by a Patient Insert.

Rx only

Manufactured by:
R. P. Scherer North America
St. Petersburg, FL 33716
Marketed by:
Solvay
Pharmaceuticals, Inc.
Marietta, GA 30062

Copyright ©1998, Solvay Pharmaceuticals, Inc.
All rights reserved.

9536
1E-4 Rev 5/98

Shown in Product Identification Guide, page 340

ROWASA® ℞

[*rō-ā′să*]

(Mesalamine)
Rectal Suspension Enema
4.0 grams/unit (60 mL)
Rectal Suppositories 500 mg

DESCRIPTION

The active ingredient in ROWASA®, is mesalamine, also known as 5-aminosalicylic acid (5-ASA). Chemically, mesalamine is 5-amino-2-hydroxybenzoic acid, and is classified as an anti-inflammatory drug.

The empirical formula is $C_7H_7NO_3$, representing a molecular weight of 153.14. The structural formula is:

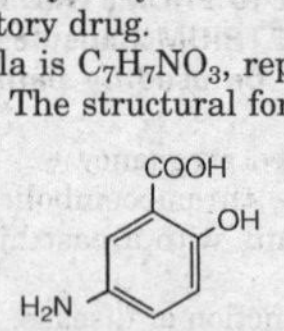

Each rectal suspension enema unit contains 4 grams of mesalamine. In addition to mesalamine the preparation contains the inactive ingredients carbomer 934P, edetate disodium, potassium acetate, potassium metabisulfite, purified water and xanthan gum. Sodium benzoate is added as a preservative. The disposable unit consists of an applicator tip protected by a polyethylene cover and lubricated with USP white petrolatum. The unit has a one-way valve to prevent back flow of the dispensed product.

Each ROWASA® Suppository contains 500 mg of mesalamine in a base of hard Fat NF. Each suppository is individually wrapped in foil.

CLINICAL PHARMACOLOGY

Sulfasalazine is split by bacterial action in the colon into sulfapyridine (SP) and mesalamine (5-ASA). It is thought that the mesalamine component is therapeutically active in ulcerative colitis [A.K. Azad Khan *et al*, **Lancet** 2:892-895 (1977)]. The usual oral dose of sulfasalazine for active ulcerative colitis in adults is two to four grams per day in divided doses. Four grams of sulfasalazine provide 1.6 g of free mesalamine to the colon. Each ROWASA® suspension enema delivers up to 4 g of mesalamine to the left side of the colon. Each ROWASA® suppository delivers 500 mg of mesalamine to the rectum.

The mechanism of action of mesalamine (and sulfasalazine) is unknown, but appears to be topical rather than systemic. Mucosal production of arachidonic acid (AA) metabolites, both through the cyclooxygenase pathways, i.e., prostanoids, and through the lipoxygenase pathways, i.e., leukotrienes (LTs) and hydroxyeicosatetraenoic acids (HETEs) is increased in patients with chronic inflammatory bowel disease, and it is possible that mesalamine diminishes inflammation by blocking cyclooxygenase and inhibiting prostaglandin (PG) production in the colon.

Preclinical Toxicology

Preclinical studies have shown the kidney to be the major target organ for mesalamine toxicity. Adverse renal function changes were observed in rats after a single 600 mg/kg oral dose, but not after a 200 mg/kg dose. Gross kidney lesions, including papillary necrosis, were observed after a single oral >900 mg/kg dose, and after i.v. doses of >214 mg/kg. Mice responded similarly. In a 13-week oral (gavage) dose study in rats, the high dose of 640 mg/kg/day mesalamine caused deaths, probably due to renal failure, and dose-related renal lesions (papillary necrosis and/or multifocal tubular injury) were seen in most rats given the high dose (males and females) as well as in males receiving lower doses 160 mg/kg/day. Renal lesions were not observed in the 160 mg/kg/day female rats. Minimal tubular epithelial damage was seen in the 40 mg/kg/day males and was reversible. In a six-month oral study in dogs, the no-observable dose level of mesalamine was 40 mg/kg/day and doses of 80 mg/kg/day and higher caused renal pathology similar to that described for the rat. In a combined 52-week toxicity and 127-week carcinogenicity study in rats, degeneration in kidneys was observed at doses of 100 mg/kg/day and above admixed with diet for 52 weeks, and at 127 weeks increased incidence of kidney degeneration and hyalinization of basement membranes and Bowman's capsule were seen at 100 mg/kg/day and above. In the 12 month eye toxicity study in dogs, Keratoconjunctivitis Sicca (KCS) occurred at oral doses of 40 mg/kg/day and above. The oral preclinical studies were done with a highly bioavailable suspension where absorption throughout the gastrointestinal tract occurred. The human dose of 4 grams represents approximately 80 mg/kg but when mesalamine is given rectally as a suspension, absorption is poor and limited to the distal colon (see **Pharmacokinetics**). Overt renal toxicity has not been observed (see **ADVERSE REACTIONS** and **PRECAUTIONS**), but the potential must be considered.

Pharmacokinetics

Mesalamine administered rectally as ROWASA® Rectal Suspension Enema is poorly absorbed from the colon and is excreted principally in the feces during subsequent bowel movements. The extent of absorption is dependent upon the retention time of the drug product, and there is considerable individual variation. At steady state, approximately 10 to 30% of the daily 4-gram dose can be recovered in cumulative 24-hour urine collections. Other than the kidney, the organ distribution and other bioavailability characteristics of absorbed mesalamine in man are not known. It is known that the compound undergoes acetylation but whether this process takes place at colonic or systemic sites has not been elucidated.

Whatever the metabolic site, most of the absorbed mesalamine is excreted in the urine as the N-acetyl-5-ASA metabolite. The poor colonic absorption of rectally administered mesalamine is substantiated by the low serum concentration of 5-ASA and N-acetyl-5-ASA seen in ulcerative colitis patients after dosage with mesalamine. Under clinical conditions patients demonstrated plasma levels 10 to 12 hours post mesalamine administration of 2 µg/mL, about two-thirds of which was the N-acetyl metabolite. While the elimination half-life of mesalamine is short (0.5 to 1.5 h), the acetylated metabolite exhibits a half-life of 5 to 10 hours [U. Klotz, **Clin. Pharmacokin.** 10:285-302 (1985)]. In addition, steady state plasma levels demonstrated a lack of accumulation of either free or metabolized drug during repeated daily administrations.

For ROWASA® Suppositories: Following single doses of ROWASA® 500 mg Suppository in normal volunteers, 24-hr urines contained (only) N-acetyl-mesalamine equivalent to 15 to 38% (avg. 24%) of the administered dose. This is commensurate with the finding of 3 to 36% (avg. 10%) in urine in a study of ROWASA® 4 g Rectal Suspension in normals. In that study, 40 to 107% (avg. 75%) of the administered dose was recovered in feces. At steady state in ulcerative colitis patients (N=38) being treated with ROWASA® Rectal Suspension, 24-hr urines contained 0 to 41% (avg. 8%) of the 4 g daily dose and plasma levels 10 to 12-hr post administration ranged from 0 to 2.1 mcg/mL (avg. 0.37 mcg/mL) of mesalamine equivalent (84% as N-acetyl metabolite). Multiple dose pharmacokinetic studies have not been conducted with ROWASA® Suppository nor have plasma levels been reported from single dose studies.

Efficacy

ROWASA® Rectal Suspension Enema: In a placebo-controlled, international, multicenter trial of 153 patients with active distal ulcerative colitis, proctosigmoiditis or proctitis, ROWASA® Rectal Suspension Enema reduced the overall disease activity index (DAI) and individual components as follows:

[See table above]

Differences between ROWASA® and placebo were also statistically different in subgroups of patients on concurrent sulfasalazine and in those having an upper disease boundary between 5 and 20 or 20 and 40 cm. Significant differences between ROWASA® and placebo were not achieved in those subgroups of patients on concurrent prednisone or with an upper disease boundary between 40 and 50 cm.

ROWASA® Suppositories: Two double-blind placebo-controlled multicenter studies were conducted in North America in patients with active ulcerative proctitis. The primary measures of efficacy were the same in both trials. The main difference between the two studies was the dosage regimen: 500 mg three times daily (1.5 g/d) in Study 1 and 500 mg twice daily (1.0 a/d) in Study 2. A total of 173 patients were studies (Study 1, N=79; Study 2, N=94). Patients were evaluated clinically and sigmoidoscopically after three and six weeks of suppository treatment.

Compared to placebo, ROWASA® (mesalamine) Suppository treatment was statistically (p <.01) superior in both trials with respect to stool frequency, rectal bleeding, mucosal appearance, disease severity and overall disease activity after both three and six weeks of treatment. Daily diary records indicated significant improvement in rectal bleeding in the first week of therapy while tenesmus and diarrhea improved significantly within two weeks. Investigators rated patients much improved in 84% and 79% with mesalamine in Studies 1 and 2, respectively compared to 41% and 26% with placebo (p <0.001, p <.001).

Normalization of rectal mucosa was achieved by 62% and 60% of mesalamine treated patients in Studies 1 and 2 compared to 25% and 10% of placebo-treated patients (p <0.001, p <.001). The effectiveness of ROWASA® Suppositories was statistically significant irrespective of sex, extent of proctitis, duration of current episode or duration of disease. Overall the efficacy demonstrated with the twice daily regimen (Study 2) was comparable to that observed with three times daily dosing (Study 1).

INDICATIONS AND USAGE

ROWASA® Rectal Suspension Enema is indicated for the treatment of active mild to moderate distal ulcerative colitis, proctosigmoiditis or proctitis.

ROWASA® Suppositories are indicated for the treatment of active ulcerative proctitis.

CONTRAINDICATIONS

ROWASA® Rectal Suspension Enema is contraindicated for patients known to have hypersensitivity to the drug or any component of this medication.

ROWASA® Suppositories are contraindicated for patients known to have hypersensitivity to mesalamine (5-aminosalicylic acid) or to the suppository vehicle [saturated vegetable fatty acid esters (Hard Fat, NF)].

WARNINGS

ROWASA® Rectal Suspension Enema contains potassium metabisulfite, a sulfite that may cause allergic-type reactions including anaphylactic symptoms and life-threatening or less severe asthmatic episodes in certain susceptible people. The overall prevalence of sulfite sensitivity in the general population is unknown but probably low. Sulfite sensitivity is seen more frequently in asthmatic or in atopic nonasthmatic persons. Epinephrine is the preferred treatment for serious allergic or emergency situations even though epinephrine injection contains sodium or potassium metabisulfite with the above-mentioned potential liabilities. The alternatives to using epinephrine in a life-threatening situation may not be satisfactory. The presence of a sulfite(s) in epinephrine injection should not deter the administration of the drug for treatment of serious allergic or other emergency situations.

EFFECT OF TREATMENT ON SEVERITY OF DISEASE
DATA FROM U.S.-CANADA TRIAL
COMBINED RESULTS OF EIGHT CENTERS
Activity Indices, mean

		N	Baseline	Day 22	End-Point	Change Baseline to End-Point†
Overall DAI	ROWASA®	76	7.42	4.05**	3.37***	-55.07%***
	Placebo	77	7.40	6.03	5.83	-21.58%
Stool Frequency	ROWASA®		1.58	1.11*	1.01**	-0.57*
	Placebo		1.92	1.47	1.50	-0.41
Rectal Bleeding	ROWASA®		1.82	0.59***	0.51***	-1.30***
	Placebo		1.73	1.21	1.11	-0.61
Mucosal Inflammation	ROWASA®		2.17	1.22**	0.96***	-1.21**
	Placebo		2.18	1.74	1.61	-0.56
Physician's Assessment of Disease Severity	ROWASA®		1.86	1.13***	0.88***	-0.97***
	Placebo		1.87	1.62	1.55	-0.30

Each parameter has a 4-point scale with a numerical rating:
0=normal, 1=mild, 2=moderate, 3=severe. The four parameters are added together to produce a maximum overall DAI of 12.
† Percent change for overall DAI only (calculated by taking the average of the change for each individual patient).
* Significant ROWASA®/placebo difference. p<0.05
** Significant ROWASA®/placebo difference. p<0.01
*** Significant ROWASA®/placebo difference. p<0.001

PRECAUTIONS

Mesalamine has been implicated in the production of an acute intolerance syndrome characterized by cramping, acute abdominal pain and bloody diarrhea, sometimes fever, headache and a rash; in such cases prompt withdrawal is required. The patient's history of sulfasalazine intolerance, if any, should be re-evaluated. If a rechallenge is performed later in order to validate the hypersensitivity it should be carried out under close supervision and only if clearly needed, giving consideration to reduced dosage. In the literature one patient previously sensitive to sulfasalazine was rechallenged with 400 mg oral mesalamine; within eight hours she experienced headache, fever, intensive abdominal colic, profuse diarrhea and was readmitted as an emergency. She responded poorly to steroid therapy and two weeks later a pancolectomy was required.

Although renal abnormalities were not noted in the clinical trials with ROWASA® Rectal Suspension Enema, the possibility of increased absorption of mesalamine and concomitant renal tubular damage as noted in the preclinical studies must be kept in mind. Patients on ROWASA®, especially those on concurrent oral products which liberate mesalamine and those with preexisting renal disease, should be carefully monitored with urinalysis, BUN and creatinine studies.

In a clinical trial most patients who were hypersensitive to sulfasalazine were able to take mesalamine enemas without evidence of any allergic reaction. Nevertheless, caution should be exercised when mesalamine is initially used in patients known to be allergic to sulfasalazine. These patients should be instructed to discontinue therapy if signs of rash or fever become apparent.

While using ROWASA® some patients have developed pancolitis. However, extension of upper disease boundary and/or flare-ups occurred less often in the ROWASA® treated group than in the placebo-treated group.

Rare instances of pericarditis have been reported with mesalamine containing products including sulfasalazine. Cases of pericarditis have also been reported as manifestations of inflammatory bowel disease. In the cases reported with ROWASA® there have been positive rechallenges with mesalamine or mesalamine containing products. In one of these cases, however, a second rechallenge with sulfasalazine was negative throughout a 2 month follow-up. Chest pain or dyspnea in patients treated with ROWASA® should be investigated with this information in mind. Discontinuation of ROWASA® may be warranted in some cases, but rechallenge with mesalamine can be performed under careful clinical observation should the continued therapeutic need for mesalamine be present.

Carcinogenesis, Mutagenesis, Impairment of Fertility

Mesalamine caused no increase in the incidence of neoplastic lesions over controls in a two-year study of Wistar rats fed up to 320 mg/kg/day of mesalamine admixed with diet. Mesalamine is not mutagenic to Salmonella typhimurium tester strains TA98, TA100, TA1535, TA1537, TA1538. There were no reverse mutations in an assay using E. coli strain WP2UVRA. There were no effects in an *in vivo* mouse micronucleus assay at 600 mg/kg and in an *in vivo* sister chromatid exchange at doses up to 610 mg/kg. No effects on fertility were observed in rats receiving up to 320 mg/kg/day. The oligospermia and infertility in men associated with sulfasalazine have not been reported with mesalamine.

Pregnancy (Category B)

Teratologic studies have been performed in rats and rabbits at oral doses up to five and eight times respectively, the maximum recommended human dose, and have revealed no evidence of harm to the embryo or the fetus. There are, however, no adequate and well controlled studies in pregnant women for either sulfasalazine or 5-ASA. Because animal reproduction studies are not always predictive of human response, 5-ASA should be used during pregnancy only if clearly needed.

Nursing Mothers

It is not known whether mesalamine or its metabolite(s) are excreted in human milk. As a general rule, nursing should not be undertaken while a patient is on a drug since many drugs are excreted in human milk.

Pediatric Use

Safety and effectiveness in pediatric patients have not been established.

ADVERSE REACTIONS

Clinical Adverse Experience

ROWASA® Rectal Suspension Enema is usually well tolerated. Most adverse effects have been mild and transient.

[See table at top of next page]

ADVERSE REACTIONS OCCURRING IN MORE THAN 1% OF ROWASA® SUPPOSITORY TREATED PATIENTS (COMPARISON TO PLACEBO)

	ROWASA® (N=168)		ROWASA® (N=84)	
SYMPTOM	N	%	N	%
Headache	11	6.5	10	11.9
Flatulence	6	3.6	6	7.1
Abdominal Pain	5	3.0	7	8.3
Diarrhea	5	3.0	5	6.0
Dizziness	5	3.0	2	2.4
Rectal Pain	3	1.8	0	0.0
Upper Resp. Infection	3	1.8	2	2.4
Acne	2	1.2	0	0.0
Asthenia	2	1.2	4	4.8
Colitis	2	1.2	0	0.0
Fever	2	1.2	0	0.0
Generalized Edema	2	1.2	1	1.2
Nausea	2	1.2	6	7.1
Rash	2	1.2	0	0.0

In addition, the following adverse events have been associated with ROWASA® and other mesalamine containing products: nephrotoxicity, pancreatitis, fibrosing alveolitis and elevated liver enzymes. Cases of pancreatitis and fibrosing alveolitis have been reported as manifestations of inflammatory bowel disease as well.

Hair Loss

Mild hair loss characterized by "more hair in the comb" but no withdrawal from clinical trials has been observed in seven of 815 mesalamine patients but none of the placebo-treated patients. In the literature there are at least six additional patients with mild hair loss who received either mesalamine or sulfasalazine. Retreatment is not always associated with repeated hair loss.

Continued on next page

Rowasa—Cont.

OVERDOSAGE

There have been no documented reports of serious toxicity in man resulting from massive overdosing with mesalamine. Under ordinary circumstances, mesalamine absorption from the colon is limited.

DOSAGE AND ADMINISTRATION

ROWASA® Rectal Suspension Enema: The usual dosage of ROWASA® (mesalamine) Rectal Suspension Enema in 60 mL units is one rectal instillation (4 grams) once a day, preferably at bedtime, and retained for approximately eight hours. While the effect of ROWASA® (mesalamine) may be seen within three to twenty-one days, the usual course of therapy would be from three to six weeks depending on symptoms and sigmoidoscopic findings. Studies available to date have not assessed if ROWASA® Rectal Suspension Enema will modify relapse rates after the 6-week short-term treatment.

Patients should be instructed to shake the bottle well to make sure the suspension is homogeneous. The patient should remove the protective sheath from the applicator tip. Holding the bottle at the neck will not cause any of the medication to be discharged. The position most often used is obtained by lying on the left side (to facilitate migration into the sigmoid colon); with the lower leg extended and the upper right leg flexed forward for balance. An alternative is the knee-chest position. The applicator tip should be gently inserted in the rectum pointing toward the umbilicus. A steady squeezing of the bottle will discharge most of the preparation. The preparation should be taken at bedtime with the objective of retaining it all night. Patient instructions are included with every seven units.

ROWASA® Suppositories: The usual dosage of ROWASA® (mesalamine) Suppositories 500 mg is one rectal suppository 2 times daily. The suppository should be retained for one to three hours or longer, if possible, to achieve the maximum benefit. While the effect of ROWASA® Suppositories may be seen within three to twenty-one days, the usual course of therapy would be from three to six weeks depending on symptoms and sigmoidoscopic findings. Studies available to date have not assessed if ROWASA® Suppositories will modify relapse rates after the six-week short-term treatment.

Rx only
Patient Instructions:
NOTE: ROWASA® Suppositories will cause staining of direct contact surfaces, including but not limited to fabrics, flooring, painted surfaces, marble, granite, vinyl, and enamel. Take care in choosing a suitable location for administration of this product.

1. Detach one suppository from strip of suppositories.
2. Hold suppository upright and carefully remove the foil wrapper.
3. Avoid excessive handling of suppository, which is designed to melt at body temperature.
4. Insert suppository completely into rectum with gentle pressure, pointed end first.

HOW SUPPLIED

ROWASA® Rectal Suspension Enema: ROWASA® suspension for rectal administration is an off-white to tan colored suspension. Each disposable enema bottle contains 4.0 grams of mesalamine in 60 mL aqueous suspension. Enema bottles are supplied in boxed, foil-wrapped trays of seven (NDC 0032-1924-82). ROWASA® enemas are for rectal use only.

Patient instructions are included.

Store at controlled room temperature 15° to 30°C (59° to 86°F). Once the foil-wrapped unit of seven bottles is opened, all enemas should be used promptly as directed by your physician. **Contents of enemas removed from the foil pouch may darken with time. Slight darkening will not affect potency, however, enemas with dark brown contents should be discarded.**

ROWASA® Suppositories: ROWASA® Suppositories for rectal administration are available as bullet shaped, light tan suppositories containing 50 mg mesalamine supplied in boxes of 12 or 24 individually foil wrapped suppositories.

Boxes of 12, NDC 0032-1928-46
Boxes of 24, NDC 0032-1928-24

Patient instructions are on back of boxes.
Store at 19° to 26°C (66°–79° F).

NOTE: ROWASA® will cause staining of direct contact surfaces, including but not limited to fabrics, flooring, painted surfaces, marble, granite, vinyl, and enamel. Take care in choosing a suitable location for administration of this product.

Rx only
ROWASA® Rectal Suspension Enema
Manufactured and Marketed By:
Solvay Pharmaceuticals, Inc.
Marietta, GA 30062

ADVERSE REACTIONS OCCURRING IN MORE THAN 0.1% OF ROWASA® RECTAL SUSPENSION ENEMA TREATED PATIENTS (COMPARISON TO PLACEBO)

SYMPTOM	ROWASA® N=815		PLACEBO N=128	
	N	%	N	%
Abdominal Pain/Cramps/Discomfort	66	8.10	10	7.81
Headache	53	6.50	16	12.50
Gas/Flatulence	50	6.13	5	3.91
Nausea	47	5.77	12	9.38
Flu	43	5.28	1	0.78
Tired/Weak/Malaise/Fatigue	28	3.44	8	6.25
Fever	26	3.19	0	0.00
Rash/Spots	23	2.82	4	3.12
Cold/Sore Throat	19	2.33	9	7.03
Diarrhea	17	2.09	5	3.91
Leg/Joint Pain	17	2.09	1	0.78
Dizziness	15	1.84	3	2.34
Bloating	12	1.47	2	1.56
Back Pain	11	1.35	1	0.78
Pain on Insertion of Enema Tip	11	1.35	1	0.78
Hemorrhoids	11	1.35	0	0.00
Itching	10	1.23	1	0.78
Rectal Pain	10	1.23	0	0.00
Constipation	8	0.98	4	3.12
Hair Loss	7	0.86	0	0.00
Peripheral Edema	5	0.61	11	8.59
UTI/Urinary Burning	5	0.61	4	3.12
Rectal Pain/Soreness/Burning	5	0.61	3	2.34
Asthenia	1	0.12	4	3.12
Insomnia	1	0.12	3	2.34

ROWASA® Suppository
Manufactured By:
G & W Laboratories Inc.
South Plainfield, NJ 07080
Marketed By:
Solvay Pharmaceuticals, Inc.
Marietta, GA 30062   Rev. 6/98
Shown in Product Identification Guide, page 340

Advanced Formula ZENATE® ℞
[ze' nãt]
Prenatal Multivitamin/Mineral Supplement Tablets

> **WARNING: Accidental overdose of iron-containing products is a leading cause of fatal poisoning in children under six. Keep this product out of the reach of children. In case of accidental overdose, call a doctor or poison control center immediately.**

DESCRIPTION

Each film-coated tablet contains:

Vitamins:
A*	3,000 I.U.
D (as cholecalciferol)	400 I.U.
E (as dl-alpha tocopheryl acetate)	10 I.U.
C (ascorbic acid)	70 mg
Folic Acid	1 mg
B_1 (as thiamine mononitrate)	1.5 mg
B_2 (riboflavin)	1.6 mg
Niacin (as niacinamide)	17 mg
B_6 (as pyridoxine hydrochloride)	2.2 mg
B_{12} (cyanocobalamin)	2.2 mcg

Minerals:
Calcium (from calcium carbonate)	200 mg
Iodine (from potassium iodide)	175 mcg
Iron (from ferrous fumarate)	65 mg
Magnesium (from magnesium oxide)	100 mg
Zinc (from zinc oxide)	15 mg

* Input as retinyl palmitate and beta-carotene.

Inactive Ingredients: Amorphous Precipitated Silica, Aqueous Shellac, Croscarmellose Sodium, Crospovidone, Hydrogenated Soybean Oil, Hydrogenated Castor Oil, Hydroxypropyl Cellulose, Hydroxypropyl Methylcellulose, Magnesium Stearate, Polyethylene Glycol, Polysorbate 80, Powdered Cellulose, Pregelatinized Starch, and Titanium Dioxide.

INDICATIONS AND USAGE

As a dietary adjunct in nutritional stress associated with periconception, pregnancy and lactation.

CONTRAINDICATIONS

This product is contraindicated in patients with a known hypersensitivity to any of the ingredients.

WARNINGS

See boxed WARNING.

PRECAUTIONS

Folic Acid may obscure pernicious anemia, in that hematologic remission can occur while neurologic manifestations remain progressive.
Information for patients: Do not remove tablets from original unit-dose, child-resistant packaging until use.

ADVERSE REACTIONS

Allergic sensitization has been reported following both oral and parenteral administration of folic acid.

DOSAGE AND ADMINISTRATION

One tablet daily or as directed by physician.

HOW SUPPLIED

Advanced Formula ZENATE® Tablets are white, film-coated, scored, capsule-shaped tablets debossed SOLVAY on one side and 1472 on the other and supplied in child-resistant unit dose foil pouches.
Unit dose pack of 30 tablets (1 x 30) . NDC 0032-1472-26.
Advanced Formula ZENATE® Tablets are supplied in child-resistant unit dose packaging. Do not repackage.
Store at controlled room temperature, 15°-30°C (59°-86°F).
CAUTION: Federal law prohibits dispensing without prescription.
Manufactured by:
Leiner Health Products, Inc.
Garden Grove, CA 92641

Marketed by:
SOLVAY PHARMACEUTICALS, INC.
MARIETTA, GA 30062

3E1030 Rev 3/97

©1997 SOLVAY PHARMACEUTICALS, INC.
Shown in Product Identification Guide, page 340

Somerset Pharmaceuticals, Inc.
**5215 W. LAUREL STREET
SUITE 200
TAMPA, FLORIDA 33607**

For Medical Information Contact:
Generally:
Professional Services Department
(813) 288-0040
FAX: (813) 282-0287
In Emergencies:
(800) 892-8889
FAX: (813) 282-0287

ELDEPRYL® ℞
(SELEGILINE HYDROCHLORIDE) CAPSULES

DESCRIPTION

ELDEPRYL (selegiline hydrochloride) is a levorotatory acetylenic derivative of phenethylamine. It is commonly referred to in the clinical and pharmacological literature as l-deprenyl.

The chemical name is: (R)-(-)-*N*,2-dimethyl-*N*-2-propynylphenethylamine hydrochloride. It is a white to near white crystalline powder, freely soluble in water, chloroform, and methanol, and has a molecular weight of 223.75. The structural formula is as follows:

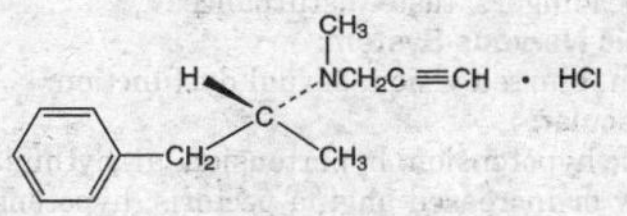

Each aqua blue capsule is band imprinted with the Somerset logo on the cap and "Eldepryl 5 mg" on the body. Each capsule contains 5 mg selegiline hydrochloride. Inactive ingredients are citric acid, lactose, magnesium stearate, and microcrystalline cellulose.

CLINICAL PHARMACOLOGY

The mechanisms accounting for selegiline's beneficial adjunctive action in the treatment of Parkinson's disease are not fully understood. Inhibition of monoamine oxidase, type B, activity is generally considered to be of primary importance; in addition, there is evidence that selegiline may act through other mechanisms to increase dopaminergic activity.

Selegiline is best known as an irreversible inhibitor of monoamine oxidase (MAO), an intracellular enzyme associated with the outer membrane of mitochondria. Selegiline inhibits MAO by acting as a 'suicide' substrate for the enzyme; that is, it is converted by MAO to an active moiety which combines irreversibly with the active site and/or the enzyme's essential FAD cofactor. Because selegiline has greater affinity for type B rather than for type A active sites, it can serve as a selective inhibitor of MAO type B if it is administered at the recommended dose.

MAOs are widely distributed throughout the body; their concentration is especially high in liver, kidney, stomach, intestinal wall, and brain. MAOs are currently subclassified into two types, A and B, which differ in their substrate specificity and tissue distribution. In humans, intestinal MAO is predominantly type A, while most of that in brain is type B.

In CNS neurons, MAO plays an important role in the catabolism of catecholamines (dopamine, norepinephrine and epinephrine) and serotonin. MAOs are also important in the catabolism of various exogenous amines found in a variety of foods and drugs. MAO in the GI tract and liver (primarily type A), for example, is thought to provide vital protection from exogenous amines (e.g., tyramine) that have the capacity, if absorbed intact, to cause a 'hypertensive crisis,' the so-called 'cheese reaction.' (If large amounts of certain exogenous amines gain access to the systemic circulation - e.g., from fermented cheese, red wine, herring, over-the-counter cough/cold medications, etc. - they are taken up by adrenergic neurons and displace norepinephrine from storage sites within membrane bound vesicles. Subsequent release of the displaced norepinephrine causes the rise in systemic blood pressure, etc.)

In theory, since MAO A of the gut is not inhibited, patients treated with selegiline at a dose of 10 mg a day should be able to take medications containing pharmacologically active amines and consume tyramine-containing foods without risk of uncontrolled hypertension. Although rare, a few reports of hypertensive reactions have occurred in patients receiving Eldepryl at the recommended dose, with tyramine-containing foods. In addition, one case of hypertensive crisis has been reported in a patient taking the recommended dose of selegiline and a sympathomimetic medication, ephedrine. The pathophysiology of the 'cheese reaction' is complicated and, in addition to its ability to inhibit MAO B selectively, selegiline's relative freedom from this reaction has been attributed to an ability to prevent tyramine and other indirect acting sympathomimetics from displacing norepinephrine from adrenergic neurons. However, until the pathophysiology of the cheese reaction is more completely understood, it seems prudent to assume that selegiline can ordinarily only be used safely without dietary restrictions at doses where it presumably selectively inhibits MAO B (e.g., 10 mg/day).

In short, attention to the dose dependent nature of selegiline's selectivity is critical if it is to be used without elaborate restrictions being placed on diet and concomitant drug use although, as noted above, a few cases of hypertensive reactions have been reported at the recommended dose. (See WARNINGS and PRECAUTIONS.)

It is important to be aware that selegiline may have pharmacological effects unrelated to MAO B inhibition. As noted above, there is some evidence that it may increase dopaminergic activity by other mechanisms, including interfering with dopamine re-uptake at the synapse. Effects resulting from selegiline administration may also be mediated through its metabolites. Two of its three principal metabolites, amphetamine and methamphetamine, have pharmacological actions of their own; they interfere with neuronal uptake and enhance release of several neurotransmitters (e.g., norepinephrine, dopamine, serotonin). However, the extent to which these metabolites contribute to the effects of selegiline are unknown.

Rationale for the Use of a Selective Monoamine Oxidase Type B Inhibitor in Parkinson's Disease: Many of the prominent symptoms of Parkinson's disease are due to a deficiency of striatal dopamine that is the consequence of a progressive degeneration and loss of a population of dopaminergic neurons which originate in the substantia nigra of the midbrain and project to the basal ganglia or striatum. Early in the course of Parkinson's Disease, the deficit in the capacity of these neurons to synthesize dopamine can be overcome by administration of exogenous levodopa, usually given in combination with a peripheral decarboxylase inhibitor (carbidopa).

With the passage of time, due to the progression of the disease and/or the effect of sustained treatment, the efficacy and quality of the therapeutic response to levodopa diminishes. Thus, after several years of levodopa treatment, the response, for a given dose of levodopa, is shorter, has less predictable onset and offset (i.e., there is 'wearing off'), and is often accompanied by side effects (e.g., dyskinesia, akinesias, on-off phenomena, freezing, etc.).

This deteriorating response is currently interpreted as a manifestation of the inability of the ever decreasing population of intact nigrostriatal neurons to synthesize and release adequate amounts of dopamine.

MAO B inhibition may be useful in this setting because, by blocking the catabolism of dopamine, it would increase the net amount of dopamine available (i.e., it would increase the pool of dopamine). Whether or not this mechanism or an alternative one actually accounts for the observed beneficial effects of adjunctive selegiline is unknown.

Selegiline's benefit in Parkinson's disease has only been documented as an adjunct to levodopa/carbidopa. Whether or not it might be effective as a sole treatment is unknown, but past attempts to treat Parkinson's disease with non-selective MAOI monotherapy are reported to have been unsuccessful. It is important to note that attempts to treat Parkinsonian patients with combinations of levodopa and currently marketed non-selective MAO inhibitors were abandoned because of multiple side effects including hypertension, increase in involuntary movement, and toxic delirium.

Pharmacokinetic Information (Absorption, Distribution, Metabolism and Elimination—ADME):

The absolute bioavailability of selegiline following oral dosing is not known; however, selegiline undergoes extensive metabolism (presumably attributable to presystemic clearance in gut and liver). The major plasma metabolites are N-desmethylselegiline, L-amphetamine and L-methamphetamine. Only N-desmethylselegiline has MAO-B inhibiting activity. The peak plasma levels of these metabolites following a single oral dose of 10 mg are from 4 to almost 20 times greater than that of the maximum plasma concentration of selegiline [1 ng/mL]. The maximum concentrations of amphetamine and methamphetamine, however, are far below those ordinarily expected to produce clinically important effects.

Single oral dose studies do not predict multiple dose kinetics, however. At steady state the peak plasma level of selegiline is 4 fold that obtained following a single dose. Metabolite concentrations increase to a lesser extent, averaging 2 fold that seen after a single dose.

The bioavailability of selegiline is increased 3 to 4 fold when it is taken with food.

The extent of systemic exposure to selegiline at a given dose varies considerably among individuals. Estimates of systemic clearance of selegiline are not available. Following a single oral dose, the mean elimination half-life of selegiline is two hours. Under steady state conditions the elimination half-life increases to ten hours.

Because selegiline's inhibition of MAO-B is irreversible, it is impossible to predict the extent of MAO-B inhibition from steady state plasma levels. For the same reason, it is not possible to predict the rate of recovery of MAO-B activity as a function of plasma levels. The recovery of MAO-B activity is a function of de novo protein synthesis; however, information about the rate of de novo protein synthesis is not yet available. Although platelet MAO-B activity returns to the normal range within 5 to 7 days of selegiline discontinuation, the linkage between platelet and brain MAO-B inhibition is not fully understood nor is the relationship of MAO-B inhibition to the clinical effect established (see Clinical Pharmacology).

Special Populations:

Renal Impairment:

No pharmacokinetic information is available on selegiline or its metabolites in renally impaired subjects.

Hepatic Impairment:

No pharmacokinetic information is available on selegiline or its metabolites in hepatically impaired subjects.

Age:

Although a general conclusion about the effects of age on the pharmacokinetics of selegiline is not warranted because of the size of the sample evaluated (12 subjects greater than 60 years of age, 12 subjects between the ages of 18 to 30), systemic exposure was about twice as great in older as compared to a younger population given a single oral dose of 10 mg.

Gender:

No information is available on the effects of gender on the pharmacokinetics of selegiline.

INDICATIONS AND USAGE

ELDEPRYL is indicated as an adjunct in the management of Parkinsonian patients being treated with levodopa/carbidopa who exhibit deterioration in the quality of their response to this therapy. There is no evidence from controlled studies that selegiline has any beneficial effect in the absence of concurrent levodopa therapy.

Evidence supporting this claim was obtained in randomized controlled clinical investigations that compared the effects of added selegiline or placebo in patients receiving levodopa/carbidopa. Selegiline was significantly superior to placebo on all three principal outcome measures employed: change from baseline in daily levodopa/carbidopa dose, the amount of 'off' time, and patient self-rating of treatment success. Beneficial effects were also observed on other measures of treatment success (e.g., measures of reduced end of dose akinesia, decreased tremor and sialorrhea, improved speech and dressing ability and improved overall disability as assessed by walking and comparison to previous state).

CONTRAINDICATIONS

ELDEPRYL is contraindicated in patients with a known hypersensitivity to this drug.

ELDEPRYL is contraindicated for use with meperidine (DEMEROL & other trade names). This contraindication is often extended to other opioids. (See Drug Interactions.)

WARNINGS

Selegiline should not be used at daily doses exceeding those recommended (10 mg/day) because of the risks associated with nonselective inhibition of MAO. (See CLINICAL PHARMACOLOGY.)

The selectivity of selegiline for MAO B may not be absolute even at the recommended daily dose of 10 mg a day. Rare cases of hypertensive reactions associated with ingestion of tyramine-containing foods have been reported in patients taking the recommended daily dose of selegiline. The selectivity is further diminished with increasing daily doses. The precise dose at which selegiline becomes a non-selective inhibitor of all MAO is unknown, but may be in the range of 30 to 40 mg a day.

Severe CNS toxicity associated with hyperpyrexia and death have been reported with the combination of tricyclic antidepressants and nonselective MAOIs (NARDIL, PARNATE). A similar reaction has been reported for a patient on amitriptyline and ELDEPRYL. Another patient receiving protriptyline and ELDEPRYL developed tremors, agitation, and restlessness followed by unresponsiveness and death two weeks after ELDEPRYL was added. Related adverse events including hypertension, syncope, asystole, diaphoresis, seizures, changes in behavioral and mental status, and muscular rigidity have also been reported in some patients receiving ELDEPRYL and various tricyclic antidepressants.

Serious, sometimes fatal, reactions with signs and symptoms that may include hyperthermia, rigidity, myoclonus, autonomic instability with rapid fluctuations of the vital signs, and mental status changes that include extreme agitation progressing to delirium and coma have been reported with patients receiving a combination of fluoxetine hydrochloride (PROZAC) and non-selective MAOIs. Similar signs have been reported in some patients on the combination of ELDEPRYL (10 mg a day) and selective serotonin reuptake inhibitors including fluoxetine, sertraline and paroxetine.

Since the mechanisms of these reactions are not fully understood, it seems prudent, in general, to avoid this combination of ELDEPRYL and tricyclic antidepressants as well as ELDEPRYL and selective serotonin reuptake inhibitors. At least 14 days should elapse between discontinuation of ELDEPRYL and initiation of treatment with a tricyclic antidepressant or selective serotonin reuptake inhibitors. Because of the long half-lives of fluoxetine and its active metabolite, at least five weeks (perhaps longer, especially if fluoxetine has been prescribed chronically and/or at higher doses) should elapse between discontinuation of fluoxetine and initiation of treatment with ELDEPRYL.

PRECAUTIONS

General:

Some patients given selegiline may experience an exacerbation of levodopa associated side effects, presumably due to the increased amounts of dopamine reaction with super sensitive, post-synaptic receptors. These effects may often be mitigated by reducing the dose of levodopa/carbidopa by approximately 10 to 30%.

Continued on next page

Eldepryl—Cont.

The decision to prescribe selegiline should take into consideration that the MAO system of enzymes is complex and incompletely understood and there is only a limited amount of carefully documented clinical experience with selegiline. Consequently, the full spectrum of possible responses to selegiline may not have been observed in pre-marketing evaluation of the drug. It is advisable, therefore, to observe patients closely for atypical responses.

Information for Patients:

Patients should be advised of the possible need to reduce levodopa dosage after the initiation of ELDEPRYL therapy.

Patients (or their families if the patient is incompetent) should be advised not to exceed the daily recommended dose of 10 mg. The risk of using higher daily doses of selegiline should be explained, and a brief description of the 'cheese reaction' provided. Rare hypertensive reactions with selegiline at recommended doses associated with dietary influences have been reported.

Consequently, it may be useful to inform patients (or their families) about the signs and symptoms associated with MAOI induced hypertensive reactions. In particular, patients should be urged to report, immediately, any severe headache or other atypical or unusual symptoms not previously experienced.

Laboratory Tests:

No specific laboratory tests are deemed essential for the management of patients on ELDEPRYL. Periodic routine evaluation of all patients, however, is appropriate.

Drug Interactions:

The occurrence of stupor, muscular rigidity, severe agitation, and elevated temperature has been reported in some patients receiving the combination of selegiline and meperidine. Symptoms usually resolve over days when the combination is discontinued. This is typical of the interaction of meperidine and MAOIs. Other serious reactions (including severe agitation, hallucinations, and death) have been reported in patients receiving this combination (see **CONTRAINDICATIONS**). Severe toxicity has also been reported in patients receiving the combination of tricyclic antidepressants and ELDEPRYL and selective serotonin reuptake inhibitors and ELDEPRYL. (See **WARNINGS** for details.) One case of hypertensive crisis has been reported in a patient taking the recommended doses of selegiline and a sympathomimetic medication (ephedrine).

Carcinogenesis, Mutagenesis, and Impairment of Fertility:

Assessment of the carcinogenic potential of selegiline in mice and rats is ongoing.

Selegiline did not induce mutations or chromosomal damage when tested in the bacterial mutation assay in Salmonella typhimurium and in an *in vivo* chromosomal aberration assay. While these studies provide some reassurance that selegiline is not mutagenic or clastogenic, they are not definitive because of methodological limitations. No definitive *in vitro* chromosomal aberration or *in vitro* mammalian gene mutation assays have been performed.

The effect of selegiline on fertility has not been adequately assessed.

Pregnancy:

Pregnancy Category C: No teratogenic effects were observed in a study of embryo-fetal development in Sprague-Dawley rats at oral doses of 4, 12, and 36 mg/kg or 4, 12 and 35 times the human therapeutic dose on a mg/m^2 basis. No teratogenic effects were observed in a study of embryo-fetal development in New Zealand White rabbits at oral doses of 5, 25, and 50 mg/kg or 10, 48, and 95 times the human therapeutic dose on a mg/m^2 basis; however, in this study, the number of litters produced at the two higher doses was less than recommended for assessing teratogenic potential. In the rat study, there was a decrease in fetal body weight at the highest dose tested. In the rabbit study, increases in total resorptions and % post-implantation loss, and a decrease in the number of live fetuses per dam occurred at the highest dose tested. In a peri- and postnatal development study in Sprague-Dawley rats (oral doses of 4, 16, and 64 mg/kg or 4, 15, and 62 times the human therapeutic dose on a mg/m^2 basis), an increase in the number of stillbirths and decreases in the number of pups per dam, pup survival, and pup body weight (at birth and throughout the lactation period) were observed at the two highest doses. At the highest dose tested, no pups born alive survived to Day 4 postpartum. Postnatal development at the highest dose tested in dams could not be evaluated because of the lack of surviving pups. The reproductive performance of the untreated offspring was not assessed.

There are no adequate and well-controlled studies in pregnant women. Selegiline should be used during pregnancy only if the potential benefit justifies the potential risk to the fetus.

Nursing Mothers:

It is not known whether selegiline hydrochloride is excreted in human milk. Because many drugs are excreted in human milk, consideration should be given to discontinuing the use of all but absolutely essential drug treatments in nursing women.

Pediatric Use:

The effects of selegiline hydrochloride in children have not been evaluated.

ADVERSE REACTIONS

Introduction:

The number of patients who received selegiline in prospectively monitored pre-marketing studies is limited. While other sources of information about the use of selegiline are available (e.g., literature reports, foreign post-marketing reports, etc.) they do not provide the kind of information necessary to estimate the incidence of adverse events. Thus, overall incidence figures for adverse reactions associated with the use of selegiline cannot be provided. Many of the adverse reactions seen have also been reported as symptoms of dopamine excess.

Moreover, the importance and severity of various reactions reported often cannot be ascertained. One index of relative importance, however, is whether or not a reaction caused treatment discontinuation. In prospective pre-marketing studies, the following events led, in decreasing order of frequency, to discontinuation of treatment with selegiline: nausea, hallucinations, confusion, depression, loss of balance, insomnia, orthostatic hypotension, increased akinetic involuntary movements, agitation, arrhythmia, bradykinesia, chorea, delusions, hypertension, new or increased angina pectoris, and syncope. Events reported only once as a cause of discontinuation are ankle edema, anxiety, burning lips/mouth, constipation, drowsiness/lethargy, dystonia, excess perspiration, increased freezing, gastrointestinal bleeding, hair loss, increased tremor, nervousness, weakness, and weight loss.

Experience with ELDEPRYL obtained in parallel, placebo controlled, randomized studies provides only a limited basis for estimates of adverse reaction rates. The following reactions that occurred with greater frequency among the 49 patients assigned to selegiline as compared to the 50 patients assigned to placebo in the only parallel, placebo controlled trial performed in patients with Parkinson's disease are shown in the following Table. None of these adverse reactions led to a discontinuation of treatment.

INCIDENCE OF TREATMENT-EMERGENT ADVERSE EXPERIENCES IN THE PLACEBO-CONTROLLED CLINICAL TRIAL

Adverse Event	Number of Patients Reporting Events	
	selegiline hydrochloride N=49	placebo N=50
Nausea	10	3
Dizziness/Lightheaded/Fainting	7	1
Abdominal Pain	4	2
Confusion	3	0
Hallucinations	3	1
Dry mouth	3	1
Vivid Dreams	2	0
Dyskinesias	2	5
Headache	2	1

The following events were reported once in either or both groups:

Ache, generalized	1	0
Anxiety/Tension	1	1
Anemia	0	1
Diarrhea	1	0
Hair Loss	0	1
Insomnia	1	1
Lethargy	1	0
Leg pain	1	0
Low back pain	1	0
Malaise	0	1
Palpitations	1	0
Urinary Retention	1	0
Weight Loss	1	0

In all prospectively monitored clinical investigations, enrolling approximately 920 patients, the following adverse events, classified by body system, were reported.

Central Nervous System:

Motor/Coordination/Extrapyramidal:

increased tremor, chorea, loss of balance, restlessness, blepharospasm, increased bradykinesia, facial grimace, falling down, heavy leg, muscle twitch*, myoclonic jerks*, stiff neck, tardive dyskinesia, dystonic symptoms, dyskinesia, involuntary movements, freezing, festination, increased apraxia, muscle cramps.

Mental Status/Behavioral/Psychiatric:

hallucinations, dizziness, confusion, anxiety, depression, drowsiness, behavior/mood change, dreams/nightmares, tiredness, delusions, disorientation, lightheadedness, impaired memory*, increased energy*, transient high*, hollow feeling, lethargy/malaise, apathy, overstimulation, vertigo, personality change, sleep disturbance, restlessness, weakness, transient irritability.

Pain/Altered Sensation:

headache, back pain, leg pain, tinnitus, migraine, supraorbital pain, throat burning, generalized ache, chills, numbness of toes/fingers, taste disturbance.

Autonomic Nervous System:

dry mouth, blurred vision, sexual dysfunction.

Cardiovascular:

orthostatic hypotension, hypertension, arrhythmia, palpitations, new or increased angina pectoris, hypotension, tachycardia, peripheral edema, sinus bradycardia, syncope.

Gastrointestinal:

nausea/vomiting, constipation, weight loss, anorexia, poor appetite, dysphagia, diarrhea, heartburn, rectal bleeding, bruxism*, gastrointestinal bleeding (exacerbation of preexisting ulcer disease).

Genitourinary/Gynecologic/Endocrine:

slow urination, transient anorgasmia*, nocturia, prostatic hypertrophy, urinary hesitancy, urinary retention, decreased penile sensation*, urinary frequency.

Skin and Appendages:

increased sweating, diaphoresis, facial hair, hair loss, hematoma, rash, photosensitivity.

Miscellaneous:

asthma, diplopia, shortness of breath, speech affected.

Postmarketing Reports:

The following experiences were described in spontaneous post-marketing reports. These reports do not provide sufficient information to establish a clear causal relationship with the use of ELDEPRYL.

CNS:

Seizure in dialyzed chronic renal failure patient on concomitant medications.

*indicates events reported only at doses greater than 10 mg/day.

OVERDOSAGE

Selegiline:

No specific information is available about clinically significant overdoses with ELDEPRYL. However, experience gained during selegiline's development reveals that some individuals exposed to doses of 600 mg of d,l-selegiline suffered severe hypotension and psychomotor agitation.

Since the selective inhibition of MAO B by selegiline hydrochloride is achieved only at doses in the range recommended for the treatment of Parkinson's disease (e.g., 10 mg/day), overdoses are likely to cause significant inhibition of both MAO A and MAO B. Consequently, the signs and symptoms of overdose may resemble those observed with marketed non-selective MAO inhibitors [e.g., tranylcypromine (PARNATE), isocarboxazide (MARPLAN), and phenelzine (NARDIL)].

Overdose with Non-Selective MAO Inhibition:

NOTE:

This section is provided for reference; it does not describe events that have actually been observed with selegiline in overdose.

Characteristically, signs and symptoms of non-selective MAOI overdose may not appear immediately. Delays of up to 12 hours between ingestion of drug and the appearance of signs may occur. Importantly, the peak intensity of the syndrome may not be reached for upwards of a day following the overdose. Death has been reported following overdosage. Therefore, immediate hospitalization, with continuous patient observation and monitoring for a period of at least two days following the ingestion of such drugs in overdose, is strongly recommended.

The clinical picture of MAOI overdose varies considerably; its severity may be a function of the amount of drug consumed. The central nervous and cardiovascular systems are prominently involved.

Signs and symptoms of overdosage may include, alone or in combination, any of the following: drowsiness, dizziness, faintness, irritability, hyperactivity, agitation, severe headache, hallucinations, trismus, opisthotonos, convulsions, and coma; rapid and irregular pulse, hypertension, hypotension and vascular collapse; precordial pain, respiratory depression and failure, hyperpyrexia, diaphoresis, and cool, clammy skin.

Treatment Suggestions For Overdose:

NOTE:

Because there is no recorded experience with selegiline overdose, the following suggestions are offered based upon the assumption that selegiline overdose may be modeled by non-selective MAOI poisoning. In any case, up-to-date information about the treatment of overdose can often be obtained from a certified Regional Poison Control Center. Telephone numbers of certified Poison Control Centers are listed in the Physicians' Desk Reference (PDR).

Treatment of overdose with non-selective MAOIs is symptomatic and supportive. Induction of emesis or gastric lavage with instillation of charcoal slurry may be helpful in

early poisoning, provided the airway has been protected against aspiration. Signs and symptoms of central nervous system stimulation, including convulsions, should be treated with diazepam, given slowly intravenously. Phenothiazine derivatives and central nervous system stimulants should be avoided. Hypotension and vascular collapse should be treated with intravenous fluids and, if necessary, blood pressure titration with an intravenous infusion of a dilute pressor agent. It should be noted that adrenergic agents may produce a markedly increased pressor response.

Respiration should be supported by appropriate measures, including management of the airway, use of supplemental oxygen, and mechanical ventilatory assistance, as required.

Body temperature should be monitored closely. Intensive management of hyperpyrexia may be required. Maintenance of fluid and electrolyte balance is essential.

DOSAGE AND ADMINISTRATION

ELDEPRYL is intended for administration to Parkinsonian patients receiving levodopa/carbidopa therapy who demonstrate a deteriorating response to this treatment. The recommended regimen for the administration of ELDEPRYL is 10 mg per day administered as divided doses of 5 mg each taken at breakfast and lunch. There is no evidence that additional benefit will be obtained from the administration of higher doses. Moreover, higher doses should ordinarily be avoided because of the increased risk of side effects.

After two to three days of selegiline treatment, an attempt may be made to reduce the dose of levodopa/carbidopa. A reduction of 10 to 30% was achieved with the typical participant in the domestic placebo controlled trials who was assigned to selegiline treatment. Further reductions of levodopa/carbidopa may be possible during continued selegiline therapy.

HOW SUPPLIED

ELDEPRYL capsules are available containing 5 mg of selegiline hydrochloride. Each aqua blue capsule is band imprinted with the Somerset logo on the cap and "Eldepryl 5 mg" on the body.
They are available as:
  NDC 39506-022-60 bottles of 60 capsules.
  NDC 39506-022-30 bottles of 300 capsules.
Store at controlled room temperature, 59° to 86°F (15° to 30°C).
CAUTION—Federal (USA) law prohibits dispensing without prescription.
SOMERSET
PHARMACEUTICALS, INC.
Tampa, FL 33607
Literature issued February 1997
ELD:R13
  Shown in Product Identification Guide, page 340

Speywood Pharmaceuticals, Inc.
27 MAPLE STREET
MILFORD, MA 01757-3650

Direct Inquiries to:
Customer Service:
(800) 456-7322
Educational Information:
(508) 478-8900
For Medical Information Contact:
In Emergencies:
(800) 456-7322
Sales and Ordering:
(800) 456-7322
Reimbursement Services:
(800) 334-1142

HYATE:C®
Antihemophilic Factor (Porcine)

DESCRIPTION
Antihemophilic Factor (Porcine)—HYATE:C® is a highly purified sterile freeze-dried concentrate of porcine antihemophilic factor (Factor VIII:C) in the form of a white lyophilized powder for reconstitution.

HOW SUPPLIED
Antihemophilic Factor (Porcine)—HYATE:C® is supplied in vials containing between 400-700 porcine units of Factor VIII:C, to be reconstituted with 20mL Sterile Water for Injection U.S.P. (not supplied).
1 Vial   NDC 55688-106-02
Manufactured by:
Speywood Biopharm Ltd.
Ash Road, Wrexham Industrial Estate
Wrexham, Clwyd LL13 9UF

United Kingdom
Tel. 978 661181
US License #1014
Distributed by:
Speywood Pharmaceuticals, Inc.
27 Maple Street
Milford, MA 01757-3650
Tel: (508) 478-8900
FAX (508) 478-1883
For customer service or medical emergency contact: (800) 456-7322
For HYATE: C Reimbursement Services contact (800) 334-1142

EDUCATIONAL MATERIAL

Educational Information concerning Factor VIII Inhibitors or Acquired Hemophilia is available free of charge. Please call or write Speywood Pharmaceuticals, Inc.

Star Pharmaceuticals, Inc.
1990 N.W. 44TH STREET
POMPANO BEACH, FL 33064-8712

Direct Inquiries to:
Scott L. Davidson, President
(954) 971-9704
For Medical Information Contact:
Scott L. Davidson
(800) 845-7827
Sales and Ordering:
(800) 845-7827
FAX: (954) 971-7718
http://www.starpharmaceuticals.com

APHRODYNE®   ℞
[af"ro-din ']
brand of yohimbine hydrochloride

Each scored aqua caplet contains 5.4 mg yohimbine hydrochloride.

HOW SUPPLIED
Bottles of 100 and 1000.
NDC 0076-0401-03 and 04

PROSED®/DS   ℞
Tablets/Double Strength

Each dark blue, round sugar-coated tablet contains:
Methenamine .... 81.6 mg.
Phenyl Salicylate .... 36.2 mg.
Methylene Blue .... 10.8 mg.
Benzoic Acid .... 9.0 mg.
Atropine Sulfate .... 0.06 mg.
Hyoscyamine Sulfate .... 0.06 mg.

HOW SUPPLIED
Bottles of 100
NDC 0076-0108-03

URO–KP–NEUTRAL®   ℞
[ū 'ro-kp-nū 'tral]
Phosphorus Supplement

Each peach capsule-shaped, film coated tablet contains:
Phosphorus .... 258 mg.
Potassium .... 49.4 mg.
Sodium .... 262.4 mg.
Derived from Sodium Phosphate Monobasic Anhydrous, Dipotassium Phosphate Anhydrous, and Disodium Phosphate Anhydrous.

HOW SUPPLIED
Bottles of 100.
NDC 0076-0109-03

UROLENE BLUE®   ℞
[ū 'ro-lene blue]
Methylene Blue Tablets

Each blue coated tablet contains   Methylene blue USP 65 mg.

HOW SUPPLIED
Bottles of 100 and 1000.
NDC 0076-0501-03 & 04

VIRILON®   ℞
[vir 'i-lon]
Methyltestosterone Macro-Beads Capsules
Oral Androgen Macro-Beads

Each capsule contains Methyltestosterone ..... USP 10 mg. In a special base. Look for the grey and white seeds in the black and transparent capsule, available only from Star Pharmaceuticals.

HOW SUPPLIED
Bottles of 100 and 1000.
NDC 0076-0301-03 & 04

VIRILON® IM   ℞
brand of testosterone cypionate
injection sterile solution
200 mg/ml
For Intramuscular Use Only

HOW SUPPLIED
Multiple dose vials of 10 ml containing 200 mg/ml.
NDC 0076-0302-10

Write for complete prescribing information for all Star products.

Stiefel Laboratories, Inc.
255 ALHAMBRA CIRCLE
CORAL GABLES, FL 33134

Direct Inquiries to:
Professional Services Department
(305) 443-3800

BREVOXYL®-4   ℞
[brĕv-ăhx-il]
(benzoyl peroxide 4%)
BREVOXYL®-8   ℞
(benzoyl peroxide 8%)

DESCRIPTION
Brevoxyl-4 and Brevoxyl-8 are topical preparations containing benzoyl peroxide 4% and 8%, respectively, as the active ingredient in a gel vehicle containing purified water, cetyl alcohol, dimethyl isosorbide, fragrance, simethicone, stearyl alcohol and ceteareth-20. The structural formula of benzoyl peroxide is:

CLINICAL PHARMACOLOGY
The exact method of action of benzoyl peroxide in acne vulgaris is not known. Benzoyl peroxide is an antibacterial agent with demonstrated activity against *Propionibacterium acnes*. This action, combined with the mild keratolytic effect of benzoyl peroxide is believed to be responsible for its usefulness in acne.
Benzoyl peroxide is absorbed by the skin where it is metabolized to benzoic acid and excreted as benzoate in the urine.

INDICATIONS AND USAGE
Brevoxyl-4 and Brevoxyl-8 are indicated for use in the topical treatment of mild to moderate acne vulgaris. Brevoxyl may be used as an adjunct in acne treatment regimens including antibiotics, retinoic acid products, and sulfur/salicylic acid containing preparations.

CONTRAINDICATIONS
Brevoxyl-4 and Brevoxyl-8 should not be used in patients who have shown hypersensitivity to benzoyl peroxide or to any of the other ingredients in the product.

PRECAUTIONS
General—For external use only. Avoid contact with eyes and mucous membranes. **AVOID CONTACT WITH HAIR, FABRICS OR CARPETING AS BENZOYL PEROXIDE WILL CAUSE BLEACHING.**

Continued on next page

Brevoxyl-4/Brevoxyl-8—Cont.

Carcinogenesis, Mutagenesis, Impairment of Fertility—Based upon all available evidence, benzoyl peroxide is not considered to be a carcinogen. However, data from a study using mice known to be highly susceptible to cancer suggest that benzoyl peroxide acts as a tumor promoter. The clinical significance of the findings is not known.
Pregnancy: Category C—Animal reproduction studies have not been conducted with benzoyl peroxide. It is also not known whether benzoyl peroxide can cause fetal harm when administered to a pregnant woman or can affect reproduction capacity. Benzoyl peroxide should be used by a pregnant woman only if clearly needed.
Nursing Mothers—It is not known whether this drug is excreted in human milk. Because many drugs are excreted in human milk, caution should be exercised when benzoyl peroxide is administered to a nursing woman.
Pediatric Use—Safety and effectiveness in children below the age of 12 have not been established.

ADVERSE REACTIONS

Contact sensitization reactions are associated with the use of topical benzoyl peroxide products and may be expected to occur in 10 to 25 of 1000 patients. The most frequent adverse reactions associated with benzoyl peroxide use are excessive erythema and peeling which may be expected to occur in 5 of 100 patients. Excessive erythema and peeling most frequently appear during the initial phase of drug use and may normally be controlled by reducing frequency of use.

DOSAGE AND ADMINISTRATION

Therapy may be initiated with either Brevoxyl-4 or Brevoxyl-8. The medication should be applied once or twice daily to affected areas. Frequency of use should be adjusted to obtain the desired clinical response. Gentle cleansing of the affected areas prior to application of Brevoxyl-4 or Brevoxyl-8 may be beneficial. Clinically visible improvement will normally occur by the third week of therapy. Maximum lesion reduction may be expected after approximately eight to twelve weeks of drug use. Continuing use of the drug is normally required to maintain a satisfactory clinical response.

HOW SUPPLIED

Brevoxyl-4 and Brevoxyl-8 are supplied in 42.5 g (1.5 oz) and 90 g (3.1 oz) tubes.
Brevoxyl-4
42.5 g tube NDC 0145-2374-06
90 g tube NDC 0145-2374-08
Brevoxyl-8
42.5 g tube NDC 0145-2384-06
90 g tube NDC 0145-2384-08
Store at controlled room temperature 15°–30°C (59°–86°F).
U.S. Patent No. 4,923,900

BREVOXYL®-4 Cleansing Lotion ℞
[*brev-ăhx-il*]
(benzoyl peroxide 4%)
BREVOXYL-8 Cleansing Lotion ℞
(benzoyl peroxide 8%)

DESCRIPTION

Brevoxyl-4 and Brevoxyl-8 Cleansing Lotions are topical preparations containing benzoyl peroxide as the active ingredient.
Brevoxyl-4 and Brevoxyl-8 Cleansing Lotions contain benzoyl peroxide 4% and 8%, respectively, in a lathering vehicle containing purified water, cetyl alcohol, citric acid, dimethyl isosorbide, docusate sodium, hydroxypropyl methylcellulose, laureth-12, magnesium aluminum silicate, propylene glycol, sodium hydroxide, sodium lauryl sulfoacetate, and sodium octoxynol-2 ethane sulfonate.
The structural formula of benzoyl peroxide is:

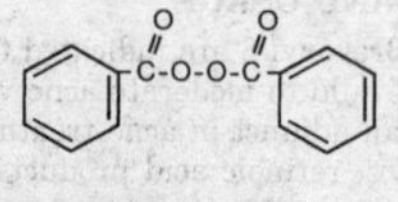

CLINICAL PHARMACOLOGY

The exact method of action of benzoyl peroxide in acne vulgaris is not known. Benzoyl peroxide is an antibacterial agent with demonstrated activity against *Propionibacterium acnes.* This action, combined with the mild keratolytic effect of benzoyl peroxide is believed to be responsible for its usefulness in acne.
Benzoyl peroxide is absorbed by the skin where it is metabolized to benzoic acid and excreted as benzoate in the urine.

INDICATIONS AND USAGE

Brevoxyl-4 and Brevoxyl-8 Cleansing Lotions are indicated for use in the topical treatment of mild to moderate acne vulgaris. Brevoxyl-4 or Brevoxyl-8 Cleansing Lotion may be used as an adjunct in acne treatment regimens including antibiotics, retinoic acid products, and sulfur/salicylic acid containing preparations.

CONTRAINDICATIONS

Brevoxyl-4 and Brevoxyl-8 Cleansing Lotions should not be used in patients who have shown hypersensitivity to benzoyl peroxide or to any of the other ingredients in the product.

PRECAUTIONS

General—For external use only. Avoid contact with eyes and mucous membranes. **AVOID CONTACT WITH HAIR, FABRICS OR CARPETING AS BENZOYL PEROXIDE WILL CAUSE BLEACHING.**
Carcinogenesis, Mutagenesis, Impairment of Fertility—Based upon all available evidence, benzoyl peroxide is not considered to be a carcinogen. However, data from a study using mice known to be highly susceptible to cancer suggest that benzoyl peroxide acts as a tumor promoter. The clinical significance of the findings is not known.
Pregnancy: Category C—Animal reproduction studies have not been conducted with benzoyl peroxide. It is also not known whether benzoyl peroxide can cause fetal harm when administered to a pregnant woman or can affect reproduction capacity. Benzoyl peroxide should be used by a pregnant woman only if clearly needed.
Nursing Mothers—It is not known whether this drug is excreted in human milk. Because many drugs are excreted in human milk, caution should be exercised when benzoyl peroxide is administered to a nursing woman.
Pediatric Use—Safety and effectiveness in children below the age of 12 have not been established.

ADVERSE REACTIONS

Contact sensitization reactions are associated with the use of topical benzoyl peroxide products and may be expected to occur in 10 to 25 of 1000 patients. The most frequent adverse reactions associated with benzoyl peroxide use are excessive erythema and peeling which may be expected to occur in 5 of 100 patients. Excessive erythema and peeling most frequently appear during the initial phase of drug use and may normally be controlled by reducing frequency of use.

DOSAGE AND ADMINISTRATION

Shake well before using. Wash the affected areas once a day during the first week, and twice a day thereafter as tolerated. Wet skin areas to be treated; apply Brevoxyl-4 or Brevoxyl-8 Cleansing Lotion, work to a full lather, rinse thoroughly and pat dry. Frequency of use should be adjusted to obtain the desired clinical response. Clinically visible improvement will normally occur by the third week of therapy. Maximum lesion reduction may be expected after approximately eight to twelve weeks of drug use. Continuing use of the drug is normally required to maintain a satisfactory clinical response.

HOW SUPPLIED

Brevoxyl-4 Cleansing Lotion is supplied in 297 g (10.5 oz) plastic bottles NDC 0145-2310-05.
Brevoxyl-8 Cleansing Lotion is supplied in 297 g (10.5 oz) plastic bottles NDC 0145-2410-05.
Store at controlled room temperature 15°–30°C (59°–86°F).

CLINDETS® ℞
[*klĭn-dĕtz'*]
(Clindamycin Phosphate Pledgets)
1%*
***equivalent to 1% clindamycin**
(10 mg/mL)
FOR EXTERNAL USE ONLY

DESCRIPTION

Clindets® (Clindamycin Phosphate Pledgets) contain clindamycin phosphate, USP at a concentration equivalent to 10 mg clindamycin per milliliter in a vehicle of isopropyl alcohol 52% v/v, propylene glycol and water. Each Clindets® pledget applicator contains approximately 1 mL of Clindamycin Phosphate Topical Solution. Clindamycin Phosphate Topical Solution has a pH range between 4.0 and 7.0.
Clindamycin phosphate is a water soluble ester of the semi-synthetic antibiotic produced by a 7(S)-chloro-substitution of the 7(R)-hydroxyl group of the parent antibiotic lincomycin. It occurs as a white to off-white, hygroscopic, crystalline powder. It is freely soluble in water, slightly soluble in dehydrated alcohol, very slightly soluble in acetone and practically insoluble in chloroform, benzene, and ether. Clindamycin phosphate is odorless or practically odorless, and has a bitter taste.
Chemically, clindamycin phosphate is $C_{18}H_{34}ClN_2O_8PS$. It has the following structural formula:
[See chemical structure at top of next column]

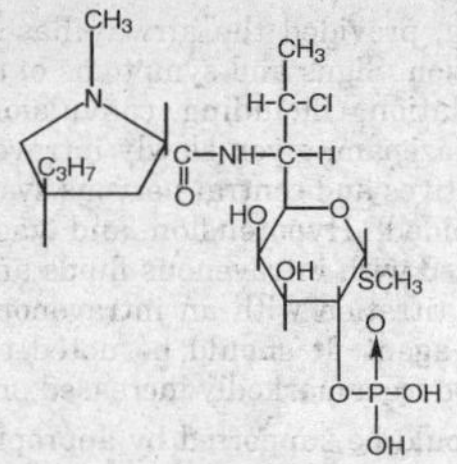

The chemical name for clindamycin phosphate is Methyl 7-chloro-6,7,8-trideoxy-6-(1-methyl-*trans*-4-propyl-L-2-pyrrolidinecarboxamido)-1-thio-L-*threo*-α-D-*galacto*-octopyranoside 2-(dihydrogen phosphate). (MW=504.97)

CLINICAL PHARMACOLOGY

Although clindamycin phosphate is inactive *in vitro*, rapid *in vivo* hydrolysis converts this compound to the antibacterially active clindamycin.
Cross resistance has been demonstrated between clindamycin and lincomycin.
Antagonism has been demonstrated between clindamycin and erythromycin.
Following multiple topical applications of clindamycin phosphate at a concentration equivalent to 10 mg clindamycin per mL in an isopropyl alcohol and water solution, very low levels of clindamycin are present in the serum (0-3 ng/mL) and less than 0.2% of the dose is recovered in urine as clindamycin.
Clindamycin activity has been demonstrated in comedones from acne patients. The mean concentration of antibiotic activity in extracted comedones after application of a Clindamycin Phosphate Pledget for 4 weeks was 597 mcg/g of comedonal material (range 0-1490). Clindamycin *in vitro* inhibits all *Propionibacterium acnes* cultures tested (MICs 0.4 mcg/mL). Free fatty acids on the skin surface have been decreased from approximately 14% to 2% following application of clindamycin.

INDICATIONS AND USAGE

Clindets are indicated in the treatment of acne vulgaris. In view of the potential for diarrhea, bloody diarrhea and pseudomembranous colitis, the physician should consider whether other agents are more appropriate. (See CONTRAINDICATIONS, WARNINGS, and ADVERSE REACTIONS.)

CONTRAINDICATIONS

Clindets are contraindicated in individuals with a history of hypersensitivity to preparations containing clindamycin or lincomycin, a history of regional enteritis or ulcerative colitis, or a history of antibiotic-associated colitis.

WARNINGS

Orally and parenterally administered clindamycin has been associated with severe colitis which may result in patient death. Use of the topical formulation of clindamycin results in absorption of the antibiotic from the skin surface. Diarrhea, bloody diarrhea, and colitis (including pseudomembranous colitis) have been reported with the use of topical and systemic clindamycin.
Studies indicate a toxin(s) produced by *clostridia* is one primary cause of antibiotic-associated colitis. The colitis is usually characterized by severe persistent diarrhea and severe abdominal cramps and may be associated with the passage of blood and mucus. Endoscopic examination may reveal pseudomembranous colitis. Stool culture for *Clostridium difficile* and stool assay for *C. difficile* toxin may be helpful diagnostically.
When significant diarrhea occurs, the drug should be discontinued. Large bowel endoscopy should be considered to establish a definitive diagnosis in cases of severe diarrhea.
Antiperistaltic agents such as opiates and diphenoxylate with atropine may prolong and/or worsen the condition. Vancomycin has been found to be effective in the treatment of antibiotic-associated pseudomembranous colitis produced by *Clostridium difficile*. The usual adult dosage is 500 milligrams to 2 grams of vancomycin orally per day in three to four divided doses administered for 7 to 10 days. Cholestyramine or colestipol resins bind to vancomycin *in vitro*. If both a resin and vancomycin are to be administered concurrently, it may be advisable to separate the time of administration of each drug.
Diarrhea, colitis, and pseudomembranous colitis have been observed to begin up to several weeks following cessation of oral and parenteral therapy with clindamycin.

PRECAUTIONS

General
Clindets contain an alcohol base which will cause burning and irritation of the eyes. In the event of accidental contact with sensitive surfaces (eye, abraded skin, mucous membranes), bathe with copious amounts of cool tap water. The solution has an unpleasant taste and caution should be exercised when applying medication around the mouth.

Treatment Emergent Adverse Event	Number of patients reporting events		
	Solution n=553 (%)	Gel n=148 (%)	Lotion n=160 (%)
Burning	62 (11)	15 (10)	17 (11)
Itching	36 (7)	15 (10)	17 (11)
Burning/Itching	60 (11)	# (-)	# (-)
Dryness	105 (19)	34 (23)	29 (18)
Erythema	86 (16)	10 (7)	22 (14)
Oiliness/Oily Skin	8 (1)	26 (18)	12* (10)
Peeling	61 (11)	# (-)	11 (7)

not recorded   * of 126 subjects

Clindets should be prescribed with caution in atopic individuals.

Drug Interactions
Clindamycin has been shown to have neuromuscular blocking properties that may enhance the action of other neuromuscular blocking agents. Therefore, it should be used with caution in patients receiving such agents.

Pregnancy: Teratogenic effects-Pregnancy Category B
Reproduction studies have been performed in rats and mice using subcutaneous and oral doses of clindamycin ranging from 100 to 600 mg/kg/day and have revealed no evidence of impaired fertility or harm to the fetus due to clindamycin. There are, however, no adequate and well-controlled studies in pregnant women. Because animal reproduction studies are not always predictive of human response, this drug should be used during pregnancy only if clearly needed.

Nursing Mothers
It is not known whether clindamycin is excreted in human milk following use of Clindets. However, orally and parenterally administered clindamycin has been reported to appear in breast milk. Because of the potential for serious adverse reactions in nursing infants, a decision should be made whether to discontinue nursing or to discontinue the drug, taking into account the importance of the drug to the mother.

Pediatric Use
Safety and effectiveness in the pediatric population under the age of 12 has not been established.

ADVERSE REACTIONS
In 18 clinical studies of various topical formulations of clindamycin phosphate using placebo vehicle and/or active comparator drugs as controls, patients experienced a number of treatment emergent adverse dermatological events (see table below).
[See table above]

OVERDOSAGE
Topically applied Clindamycin Phosphate formulations can be absorbed in sufficient amounts to produce systemic effects. (See WARNINGS.)

DOSAGE AND ADMINISTRATION
Apply a thin film using a Clindets applicator for the application of Clindamycin Phosphate Topical Solution twice daily to affected area. More than one pledget may be used. Each pledget should be used only once and then discarded. Remove pledget from foil just before use. Do not use if the seal is broken.
Discard after single use.

HOW SUPPLIED
Clindets® (Clindamycin Phosphate Pledgets) 1%** equivalent to 1% clindamycin (10 mg/mL) is available in the following size:
60 pledget container — NDC 0145-2472-60
Store at controlled room temperature, 15°–30°C (59°–86°F).

LACTICARE®–HC Lotion 1%, 2¹/₂%   ℞
[lăk 'tĭ-kār']
(hydrocortisone lotion, USP)

CONTAINS
Each mL of LactiCare-HC Lotion 1% and 2¹/₂% (hydrocortisone lotion, USP) contains 10 mg and 25 mg respectively of hydrocortisone in a vehicle consisting of carbomer 940, sodium PCA, lactic acid, sodium hydroxide, stearyl alcohol (and) ceteareth-20, glyceryl stearate (and) PEG-100 stearate, cetyl alcohol, isopropyl palmitate, light mineral oil, myristyl lactate, DMDM hydantoin, dehydroacetic acid, fragrance and purified water.

HOW SUPPLIED
Lacticare®-HC Lotion 1% (hydrocortisone lotion, USP) is available in the following size:
118 mL (4 fl oz) bottle NDC 0145-2537-04
Lacticare®-HC Lotion 2¹/₂% (hydrocortisone lotion, USP) is available in the following sizes:
59 mL (2 fl oz) bottle NDC 0145-2538-02
118 mL (4 fl oz) bottle NDC 0145-2538-04

PANOXYL® 5   ℞
[pan 'ăhx-il]
(benzoyl peroxide 5%)
PANOXYL® 10   ℞
(benzoyl peroxide 10%)

HOW SUPPLIED
PanOxyl 5 and PanOxyl 10 are supplied in 56.7 gram and 113.4 gram tubes.
PanOxyl 5
56.7 g (2.0 oz) tube NDC 0145-2372-06
113.4 g (4.0 oz) tube NDC 0145-2372-08
PanOxyl 10
56.7 g (2.0 oz) tube NDC 0145-2373-06
113.4 g (4.0 oz) tube NDC 0145-2373-08
U.S. Patent 4056611

PANOXYL® AQ 2¹/₂   ℞
[pan 'ăhx-il]
(benzoyl peroxide 2¹/₂%)
PANOXYL® AQ 5   ℞
(benzoyl peroxide 5%)
PANOXYL® AQ 10   ℞
(benzoyl peroxide 10%)

HOW SUPPLIED
PanOxyl AQ 2¹/₂, PanOxyl AQ 5, and PanOxyl AQ 10 are supplied in 56.7 gram and 113.4 gram tubes.
PanOxyl AQ 2¹/₂
56.7 g (2.0 oz) tube NDC 0145-2375-06
113.4 g (4.0 oz) tube NDC 0145-2375-08
PanOxyl AQ 5
56.7 g (2.0 oz) tube NDC 0145-2376-06
113.4 g (4.0 oz) tube NDC 0145-2376-08
PanOxyl AQ 10
56.7 g (2.0 oz) tube NDC 0145-2377-06
113.4 g (4.0 oz) tube NDC 0145-2377-08

SULFOXYL® Lotion Regular   ℞
SULFOXYL® Lotion Strong   ℞
[sul 'fox-ul]

HOW SUPPLIED
Sulfoxyl Lotion Regular and Sulfoxyl Lotion Strong are supplied in 59 milliliter (2 fluid ounce) plastic bottles.
Sulfoxyl Lotion Regular   **Sulfoxyl Lotion Strong**
NDC 0145-3518-07   NDC 0145-3519-07

Supergen, Inc.
TWO ANNABEL LANE SUITE 220
SAN RAMON, CA 94583

For Customer Service and Placing Orders Contact:
800-905-5474
FAX: 800-903-5474
For Medical or Drug Information Contact:
Generally:
Professional Services Department:
888-43-SUPER
888-437-8737
FAX: 925-327-7347
In Emergencies:
415-487-8441

MITOMYCIN   ℞
FOR INJECTION, USP

DESCRIPTION
Mitomycin (also known as mitomycin-C) is an antibiotic isolated from the broth of *Streptomyces caespitosus* which has been shown to have antitumor activity. The compound is heat stable, has a high melting point, and is freely soluble in organic solvents.

Mitomycin for Injection is a sterile dry mixture of mitomycin and mannitol, which when reconstituted with Sterile Water for Injection provides a solution for intravenous administration. Mitomycin for Injection is supplied in vials containing 5 mg and 20 mg of mitomycin. Each 5 mg vial of Mitomycin for Injection contains mitomycin 5 mg and mannitol 10 mg. Each 20 mg vial of Mitomycin for Injection contains mitomycin 20 mg and mannitol 40 mg.

Mitomycin is a blue-violet crystalline powder with the molecular formula of $C_{15}H_{18}N_4O_5$ and a molecular weight of 334.33. Its chemical name is 7-amino-9α-methoxymitosane.

HOW SUPPLIED
Mitomycin for Injection, USP
NDC 62701-010-01—5 mg mitomycin in an amber vial, individually packaged in single cartons.
NDC 62701-011-01—20 mg mitomycin in an amber vial, individually packaged in single cartons.

Storage: Store dry powder at controlled room temperatures 15° to 30°C (59° to 86°F), protected from light. Protect reconstituted solution from light. Store solution under refrigeration 2° to 8°C (36° to 46°F), discard after 14 days. If unrefrigerated, discard after 7 days.

Rx Only

NIPENT®   ℞
(pentostatin for injection)

> **WARNING**
>
> NIPENT should be administered under the supervision of a physician qualified and experienced in the use of cancer chemotherapeutic agents. The use of higher doses than those specified (see DOSAGE AND ADMINISTRATION) is not recommended. Dose-limiting severe renal, liver, pulmonary, and CNS toxicities occurred in Phase 1 studies that used NIPENT at higher doses (20–50 mg/m^2 in divided doses over 5 days) than recommended.
>
> In a clinical investigation in patients with refractory chronic lymphocytic leukemia using NIPENT at the recommended dose in combination with fludarabine phosphate, 4 of 6 patients entered in the study had severe or fatal pulmonary toxicity. The use of NIPENT in combination with fludarabine phosphate is not recommended.

DESCRIPTION
NIPENT® (pentostatin for injection) is supplied as a sterile, apyrogenic, lyophilized powder in single-dose vials for intravenous administration. Each vial contains 10 mg of pentostain and 50 mg of Mannitol, USP. The pH of the final product is maintained between 7.0 and 8.5 by addition of sodium hydroxide or hydrochloric acid.

Pentostatin, also known as 2'-deoxycoformycin (DCF), is a potent inhibitor of the enzyme adenosine deaminase and is isolated from fermentation cultures of *Streptomyces antibioticus*. Pentostatin is known chemically as (R)-3-(2–deoxy-β-D-*erythro* -pentofuranosyl)-3,6,7,8-tetrahydroimidazo[4,5-d] [1,3]diazepin-8-ol with a molecular formula of $C_{11}H_{16}N_4O_4$ and a molecular weight of 268.27.

Pentostain is a white to off-white solid, freely soluble in distilled water.

The molecular structure of pentostatin is:

CLINICAL PHARMACOLOGY

Mechanism of Action
Pentostatin is a potent transition state inhibitor of the enzyme adenosine deaminase (ADA). The greatest activity of ADA is found in cells of the lymphoid system with T-cells

Continued on next page

Nipent—Cont.

having higher activity than B-cells and T-cell malignancies higher ADA activity than B-cell malignancies. Pentostatin inhibition of ADA, particularly in the presence of adenosine or deoxyadenosine, leads to cytotoxicity, and this is believed to be due to elevated intracellular levels of dATP which can block DNA synthesis through inhibition of ribonucleotide reductase. Pentostatin can also inhibit RNA synthesis as well as cause increased DNA damage. In addition to elevated dATP, these mechanisms may also contribute to the overall cytotoxic effect of pentostatin. The precise mechanism of pentostain's antitumor effect, however, in hairy cell leukemia is not known.

Pharmacokinetics/Drug Metabolism

A tissue distribution and whole-body autoradiography study in the rat revealed that radioactivity concentrations were highest in the kidneys with very little central nervous system penetration.

In man, following a single dose of 4 mg/m^2 of pentostain infused over 5 minutes, the distribution half-life was 11 minutes, the mean terminal half-life was 5.7 hours, the mean plasma clearance was 68 mL/min/m^2, and approximately 90% of the dose was excreted in the urine as unchanged pentostatin and/or metabolites as measured by adenosine deaminase inhibitory activity. The plasma protein binding of pentostain is low, approximately 4%.

A positive correlation was observed between pentostatin clearance and creatinine clearance (CrCl) in patients with creatinine clearance values ranging from 60 mL/min to 130 mL/min.[1] Pentostatin half-life in patients with renal impairment (CrCl <50 mL/min, n=2) was 18 hours, which was much longer than that observed in patients with normal renal function (CrCl >60 mL/min, n=14), about 6 hours.

CLINICAL STUDIES

The following table provides efficacy results for 4 groups (columns) of patients with hairy cell leukemia: patients who initially received NIPENT, patients who initially received alpha-interferon (IFN), and 2 different groups of patients who received NIPENT after proving to be refractory to, or intolerant of IFN therapy. The first 2 groups represent treatment results from the SWOG 8691 study, a large multicenter study comparing NIPENT and IFN in untreated (frontline) patients with confirmed hairy cell leukemia. The third group represents evaluable patients from the SWOG study who crossed over to NIPENT after initially receiving IFN. The fourth group, labeled NCI Phase 2 studies, displays pooled results of 2 noncomparative studies (MD Anderson and CALGB), in which NIPENT was used to treat patients with confirmed IFN-refractory disease.

In the SWOG 8691 study, NIPENT was administered at a dose of 4 mg/m^2 every 2 weeks. After 6 months of treatment, patients were evaluated for response. If a complete response was achieved, 2 additional doses of NIPENT were administered and then discontinued. If a partial response was achieved. NIPENT was continued for up to an additional 6 months. NIPENT was discontinued for stable disease after 6 months or progressive disease after 2 months of therapy. IFN was administered 3 million units subcutaneously 3 times per week. Patients who achieved a complete or partial response after 6 months of treatment continued on IFN for another 6 months. IFN was discontinued if patients did not achieve a complete or partial response after 6 months of initial treatment or progressed after 2 months. This study allowed crossover of patients intolerant of, or refractory to, initial treatment.

Interferon-refractory patients enrolled into the MD Anderson study received NIPENT at a dose of 4 mg/m^2 every other week for 3 months and responding patients received 3 additional months. CALGB patients received 4 mg/m^2 of NIPENT every other week for 3 months and responding patients were treated monthly for up to 9 additional months. Almost all patients had a PS of 0 to 2 in the Phase 2 and 3 studies.

For each study, a complete response (CR) required clearing of the peripheral blood and bone marrow of all hairy cells, normalization of organomegaly and lymphadenopathy by physical examination, and recovery of hemoglobin to at least 12 g/dL, platelet count to at least 100,000/mm^3, and granulocyte count to at least 1500/mm^3. A partial response (PR) required that the percentage of hairy cells in the blood and bone marrow decrease by more than 50%, enlarged organs and lymph nodes decrease by more than 50% by physical examination, and hematologic parameters had to meet the same criteria as for complete response. The table below reports the response rate for 2 groups of patients: (1) Evaluable, ie, patients who could be evaluated for response and (2) Intent-to-Treat, ie, patients diagnosed with hairy cell leukemia.

[See table below]

The results show that frontline patients treated with NIPENT achieved a significantly higher rate of response than those treated with IFN. The time to recovery of neutrophil and platelet counts was shorter with NIPENT treatment and the estimated duration of response was longer. The response rate in IFN-refractory patients treated with NIPENT was similar to that in NIPENT-treated frontline patients. At a median follow-up duration of 46 months, there was no statistically significant difference in survival between hairy cell leukemia patients initially treated with NIPENT and those initially treated with IFN. However, no definite conclusions regarding survival can be made from these results because they are complicated by the fact that the majority of IFN patients crossed over to NIPENT treatment.

In the Phase 3 SWOG study, 25 patients with hairy cell leukemia died during treatment or follow-up: 18 patients had last received NIPENT (3 of whom had crossed over from IFN), and 7 patients had last received IFN (1 of whom crossed over from NIPENT). Eleven of the 25 deaths occurred within 60 days of the last dose of treatment. Of these, hairy cell leukemia was cited by the investigators as a contributory cause for 1 death in the NIPENT group and 3 deaths in the IFN group. Additionally, infection contributed to the deaths of 3 patients in the NIPENT group and 2 patients in the IFN group. Approximately 4% of hairy cell leukemia patients, in each arm, died more than 60 days after the last dose of either treatment and there was no outstanding cause of death among these patients.

INDICATIONS AND USAGE

NIPENT is indicated as single-agent treatment for both untreated and alpha-interferon-refractory hairy cell leukemia patients with active disease as defined by clinically significant anemia, neutropenia, thrombocytopenia, or disease-related symptoms.

		FRONTLINE		IFN-REFRACTORY[a]	
Parameter		Evaluable NIPENT N=138	Evaluable IFN N=130	SWOG 8691[b] Crossover N=79	NCI Phase 2 Studies N=44
Response Rates (%)					
Evaluable	CR	84	18	85	58
	PR	6	24	4	28
Intent-to-Treat		*N=170*	*N=170*		
	CR	*68*	*14*		
	PR	*5*	*18*		
Median Time to Response (months)					
	CR	6.6	11.5	6.0	4.2
	PR	4.0	6.2	5.8	—
Median Duration of Response (months)					
	CR	NR	8.3	NR	>7.7[c] (CALGB) >15.2[c] (MDA)
	PR	NR	15.2	NR	—
% Estimated to be in Response After 24 Months					
	CR	76	16	85	—
	PR	50	21	—	—
Median Time to Recovery (days)					
ANC (1500/mm^3)		70	106	—	—
Platelets (100,000/mm^3)		22	36	—	—

NR = Not reached by Kaplan-Meier method; ANC = Absolute neutrophil count.
[a]Evaluable patients
[b]Patients either refractory to, or intolerant of, IFN
[c]Kaplan-Meier estimate

CONTRAINDICATIONS

NIPENT is contraindicated in patients who have demonstrated hypersensitivity to NIPENT.

WARNINGS

See Boxed Warning.

Patients with hairy cell leukemia may experience myelosuppression primarily during the first few courses of treatment. Patients with infections prior to NIPENT treatment have in some cases developed worsening of their condition leading to death, whereas others have achieved complete response. Patients with infection should be treated only when the potential benefit of treatment justifies the potential risk to the patient. Efforts should be made to control the infection before treatment is initiated or resumed.

In patients with progressive hairy cell leukemia, the initial courses of NIPENT treatment were associated with worsening of neutropenia. Therefore, frequent monitoring of complete blood counts during this time is necessary. If severe neutropenia continues beyond the initial cycles, patients should be evaluated for disease status, including a bone marrow examination.

Elevations in liver function tests occurred during treatment with NIPENT and were generally reversible.

Renal toxicity was observed at higher doses in early studies; however, in patients treated at the recommended dose, elevations in serum creatinine were usually minor and reversible. There were some patients who began treatment with normal renal function who had evidence of mild to moderate toxicity at a final assessment. (See **DOSAGE AND ADMINISTRATION**.)

Rashes, occasionally severe, were commonly reported and may worsen with continued treatment. Withholding of treatment may be required (See **DOSAGE AND ADMINISTRATION**.)

Acute pulmonary edema and hypotension, leading to death, have been reported in the literature in patients treated with pentostatin in combination with carmustine, etoposide and high dose cyclophosphamide as part of the ablative regimen for bone marrow transplant.

Pregnancy Category D

Pentostatin can cause fetal harm when administered to a pregnant woman. Pentostatin was administered intravenously at doses of 0, 0.01, 0.1, or 0.75 mg/kg/day (0, 0.06, 0.6, and 4.5 mg/m^2) to pregnant rats on days 6 through 15 of gestation. Drug-related maternal toxicity occurred at doses of 0.1 and 0.75 mg/kg/day (0.6 and 4.5 mg/m^2). Teratogenic effects were observed at 0.75 mg/kg/day (4.5 mg/m^2) manifested by increased incidence of various skeletal malformations. In a dose range-finding study, pentostatin was administered intravenously to rats at doses of 0, 0.05, 0.1, 0.5, 0.75, or 1 mg/kg/day (0, 0.3, 0.6, 3, 4.5, 6 mg/m^2) on days 6 through 15 of gestation. Fetal malformations that were observed were an omphalocele at 0.05 mg/kg (0.3 mg/m^2), gastroschisis at 0.75 mg/kg and 1 mg/kg (4.5 and 6 mg/m^2), and a flexure defect of the hindlimbs at 0.75 mg/kg (4.5 mg/m^2). Pentostatin was also shown to be teratogenic in mice when administered as a single 2 mg/kg (6 mg/m^2) intraperitoneal injection on day 7 of gestation. Pentostatin was not teratogenic in rabbits when administered intravenously on days 6 through 18 of gestation at doses of 0, 0.005, 0.01, or 0.02 mg/kg/day (0, 0.015, 0.03, or 0.06 mg/m^2); however, maternal toxicity, abortions, early deliveries, and deaths occurred in all drug-treated groups. There are no adequate and well-controlled studies in pregnant women. If NIPENT is used during pregnancy, or if the patient becomes pregnant while taking (receiving) this drug, the patient should be apprised of the potential hazard to the fetus. Women of childbearing potential receiving NIPENT should be advised to avoid becoming pregnant.

PRECAUTIONS

General

Therapy with NIPENT requires regular patient observation and monitoring of hematologic parameters and blood chemistry values. If severe adverse reactions occur, the drug should be withheld (see **DOSAGE AND ADMINISTRATION**), and appropriate corrective measures should be taken according to the clinical judgment of the physician.

NIPENT treatment should be withheld or discontinued in patients showing evidence of nervous system toxicity.

Information for Patients

Patients should be advised of the signs and symptoms of adverse events associated with NIPENT therapy. (See **ADVERSE REACTIONS**.)

Laboratory Tests

Prior to initiating therapy witn NIPENT, renal function should be assessed with a serum creatinine and/or a creatinine clearance assay. (See **CLINICAL PHARMACOLOGY** and **DOSAGE AND ADMINISTRATION**.) Complete blood counts and serum creatinine should be performed before each dose of NIPENT and at other appropriate periods during therapy (see **DOSAGE AND ADMINISTRATION**). Severe neutropenia has been observed following the early courses of treatment with NIPENT and therefore frequent monitoring of complete blood counts is recommended during this time. If hematologic parameters do not improve with

subsequent courses, patients should be evaluated for disease status, including a bone marrow examination. Periodic monitoring of the peripheral blood for hairy cells should be performed to assess the response to treatment.

In addition, bone marrow aspirates and biopsies may be required at 2 to 3 month intervals to assess the response to treatment.

Drug Interactions

Allopurinol and NIPENT are both associated with skin rashes. Based on clinical studies in 25 refractory patients who received both NIPENT and allopurinol, the combined use of NIPENT and allopurinol did not appear to produce a higher incidence of skin rashes than observed with NIPENT alone. There has been a report of one patient who received both drugs and experienced a hypersensitivity vasculitis that resulted in death. It was unclear whether this adverse event and subsequent death resulted from the drug combination.

Biochemical studies have demonstrated that pentostatin enhances the effects of vidarabine, a purine nucleoside with antiviral activity. The combined use of vidarabine and NIPENT may result in an increase in adverse reactions associated with each drug. The therapeutic benefit of the drug combination has not been established.

The combined use of NIPENT and fludarabine phosphate is not recommended because it may be associated with an increased risk of fatal pulmonary toxicity (see **WARNINGS**). Acute pulmonary edema and hypotension, leading to death, have been reported in the literature in patients treated with pentostatin in combination with carmustine, etoposide and high dose cyclophosphamide as part of the ablative regimen for bone marrow transplant.

Carcinogenesis, Mutagenesis, Impairment of Fertility

Carcinogenesis: No animal carcinogenicity studies have been conducted with pentostatin.

Mutagenesis: Pentostatin was nonmutagenic when tested in *Salmonella typhimurium* strains TA-98, TA-1535, TA-1537, and TA-1538. When tested with strain TA-100, a repeatable statistically significant response trend was observed with and without metabolic activation. The response was 2.1 to 2.2 fold higher than the background at 10 mg/plate, the maximum possible drug concentration. Formulated pentostatin was clastogenic in the *in vivo* mouse bone marrow micronucleus assay at 20, 120, and 240 mg/kg. Pentostatin was not mutagenic to V79 Chinese hamster lung cells at the HGPRT locus exposed 3 hours to concentrations of 1 to 3 mg/mL, with or without metabolic activation. Pentostatin did not significantly increase chromosomal aberrations in V79 Chinese hamster lung cells exposed 3 hours to 1 to 3 mg/mL in the presence or absence of metabolic activation.

Impairment of Fertility: No fertility studies have been conducted in animals; however, in a 5-day intravenous toxicity study in dogs, mild seminiferous tubular degeneration was observed with doses of 1 and 4 mg/kg. The possible adverse effects on fertility in humans have not been determined.

Pregnancy

Pregnancy Category D: (See **WARNINGS**)

Nursing Mothers

It is not known whether NIPENT is excreted in human milk. Because many drugs are excreted in human milk, and because of the potential for serious adverse reactions in nursing infants from pentostatin, a decision should be made whether to discontinue nursing or discontinue the drug, taking into account the importance of NIPENT to the mother.

Pediatric Use

Safety and effectiveness in children or adolescents have not been established.

ADVERSE REACTIONS

Most patients treated for hairy cell leukemia in the five NCI-sponsored Phase 2 and the Phase 3 SWOG study experienced an adverse event. The following table lists the most frequently occurring adverse events in patients treated with NIPENT (both frontline and IFN-refractory patients) compared with IFN (frontline only), regardless of drug association. The drug association of some adverse events is uncertain as they may be associated with the disease itself (eg, infection, hematologic suppression), but other events, such as the gastrointestinal symptoms, rashes, and abnormal liver function tests, can in many cases be attributed to the drug. Most adverse events that were assessed for severity were either mild or moderate, and diminished in frequency with continued therapy.

	Percent of Patients		
All Adverse Events [a]	Frontline, Treated With NIPENT N=180	Frontline, Treated With IFN N=176	IFN-Refractory Treated With NIPENT N=197
Nausea and/or Vomiting	63	22	53 [b]
Fever	46	59	42
Rash	43	30	26
Fatigue	42	55	29
Leukopenia	22	15	60
Pruritus	21	6	10
Coughing/Increased Cough	20	15	17
Myalgia	19	36	11
Chills	19	34	11
Headache	17	29	13
Diarrhea	17	17	15
Abdominal Pain	16	15	4
Anorexia	13	10	16
Upper Respiratory Infection	13	8	16
Asthenia	12	13	10
Stomatitis	12	7	5
Rhinitis	11	15	10
Dyspnea	11	13	8
Anemia	8	5	35
Pain	8	19	20
Pharyngitis	8	11	10
Sweating Increased/ Sweating	8	21	10
Viral Infection	8	17	NR
Infection	7 [c]	2 [c]	36
Arthralgia	6	14	3
Thrombocytopenia	6	6	32
Skin Disorder	4	5	17
Allergic Reaction	2	1	11
Hepatic Disorder/ Elevated Liver Function Tests [d]	2	2	19
Neurologic Disorder, CNS/CNS Toxicity	1	NR	11
Lung Disorder/ Disease	NR	1	12
Nausea	NR	NR	22
Genitourinary Disorder	NR	NR	15

NR = Not Reported
[a] Occurring in more than 10% of patients, in any group, regardless of drug association
[b] Includes only nausea with vomiting
[c] These figures represent only unspecified infections. Refer to infection table.
[d] Elevated liver enzymes and liver disorder for SWOG

The total incidence for all types of infections is considerably higher for both treatment groups in the SWOG 8691 study than is listed in the table above. An intent-to-treat analysis of infections found that 38% of patients treated with NIPENT and 34% of patients treated with IFN averaged 2.4 and 1.9 documented infections during treatment, respectively. The following table lists the different types of infections that were reported as adverse events during the initial phase of the SWOG study. There were no apparent differences in the types of infection between the 2 treatment groups, with the possible exception of herpes zoster which was reported more frequently for NIPENT (8%) than for IFN (1%).

	Percent of Patients	
Type of Infection	Frontline, Treated With NIPENT N=180	Frontline, Treated With IFN N=176
Upper Respiratory Infection	13	8
Rhinitis	11	15
Herpes Zoster	8	1
Pharyngitis	8	11
Viral Infection	8	17
Infection (Unspecified)	7	2
Sinusitis	6	4
Cellulitis	6	3
Bacterial Infection	5	4
Pneumonia	5	7
Conjunctivitis	4	2
Furunculosis	4	<1
Herpes Simplex	4	1
Bronchitis	3	2
Sepsis	3	2
Urinary Tract Infection	3	3
Abscess, Skin	2	4
Moniliasis, Oral	2	<1
Mycotic Infection, Skin	<1	3
Osteomyelitis	1	0

The drug relatedness of the adverse events listed below cannot be excluded. The following adverse events occurred in 3% to 10% of NIPENT-treated patients in the initial phase of the SWOG study:

Body as a Whole—Chest Pain, Death, Face Edema, Peripheral Edema

Cardiovascular System—Hemorrhage, Hypotension

Digestive System—Dental Abnormalities, Dyspepsia, Flatulence, Gingivitis

Hemic and Lymphatic System—Agranulocytosis

Laboratory Deviations—Elevated Creatinine

Musculoskeletal System—Arthralgia

Nervous System—Confusion, Dizziness, Insomnia, Paresthesia, Somnolence

Psychobiologic Function—Anxiety, Depression, Nervousness

Respiratory System—Asthma

Skin & Appendages—Skin Dry, Urticaria

The remaining adverse events which occurred in less than 3% of NIPENT-treated patients during the initial phase of the SWOG study:

Body as a Whole—Flu-like Symptoms, Hangover Effect, Neoplasm

Cardiovascular System—Angina Pectoris, Arrhythmia, A-V Block, Bradycardia, Extrasystoles Ventricular, Heart Arrest, Heart Failure, Hypertension, Pericardial Effusion, Phlebitis, Pulmonary Embolus, Sinus Arrest, Tachycardia, Thrombophlebitis Deep, Vasculitis

Digestive System—Constipation, Dysphagia, Glossitis, Ileus

Hemic and Lymphatic System—Acute Leukemia, Anemia-Hemolytic, Aplastic Anemia

Laboratory Deviations—Hypercalcemia, Hyponatremia

Musculoskeletal System—Arthritis, Gout

Nervous System—Amnesia, Ataxia, Convulsions, Dreaming Abnormal, Dysarthria, Encephalitis, Hyperkinesia, Meningism, Neuralgia, Neuritis, Neuropathy, Paralysis, Syncope, Twitching, Vertigo

Psychobiologic Function—Decrease/Loss Libido, Emotional Liability, Hallucination, Hostility, Neurosis, Thinking Abnormal

Respiratory System—Bronchospasm, Larynx Edema

Skin and Appendages—Acne, Alopecia, Eczema, Petechial Rash, Photosensitivity Reaction

Special Senses—Amblyopia, Deafness, Earache, Eyes Dry, Labyrinthitis, Lacrimation Disorder, Nonreactive Eye, Photophobia, Retinopathy, Tinnitus, Unusual Taste, Vision Abnormal, Watery Eyes

Urogenital System—Amenorrhea, Breast Lump, Impotence, Kidney Function Abnormal, Nephropathy, Renal Failure, Renal Insufficiency, Renal Stone

One patient with hairy cell leukemia treated with NIPENT during another clinical study developed unilateral uveitis with vision loss.

Nineteen (5%) patients withdrew from the Phase 3 SWOG 8691 study because of adverse events; 9 during initial NIPENT treatment, 4 during NIPENT crossover, 5 during initial IFN treatment, and 1 during both initial IFN treatment and NIPENT crossover. In the Phase 2 studies in IFN-refractory hairy cell leukemia, 11% of patients withdrew from treatment with NIPENT due to an adverse event.

OVERDOSAGE

No specific antidote for NIPENT overdose is known. NIPENT administered at higher doses (20 to 50 mg/m^2 in divided doses over 5 days) than recommended was associated with deaths due to severe renal, hepatic, pulmonary, and CNS toxicity. In case of overdose, management would include general supportive measures through any period of toxicity that occurs.

DOSAGE AND ADMINISTRATION

It is recommended that patients receive hydration with 500 to 1,000 mL of 5% Dextrose in 0.5 Normal Saline or equivalent before NIPENT administration. An additional 500 mL of 5% Dextrose or equivalent should be administered after NIPENT is given.

The recommended dosage of NIPENT for the treatment of hairy cell leukemia is 4 mg/m^2 every other week. NIPENT may be administered intravenously by bolus injection or diluted in a larger volume and given over 20 to 30 minutes. (See **Preparation of Intravenous Solution**.)

Higher doses are not recommended.

No extravasation injuries were reported in clinical studies.

The optimal duration of treatment has not been determined. In the absence of major toxicity and with observed continuing improvement, the patient should be treated until a complete response has been achieved. Although not established as required, the administration of two additional doses has been recommended following the achievement of a complete response.

Continued on next page

Nipent—Cont.

All patients receiving NIPENT at 6 months should be assessed for response to treatment. If the patient has not achieved a complete or partial response, treatment with NIPENT should be discontinued.
If the patient has achieved a partial response, NIPENT treatment should be continued in an effort to achieve a complete response. At any time thereafter that a complete response is achieved, two additional doses of NIPENT are recommended. NIPENT treatment should then be stopped. If the best response to treatment at the end of 12 months is a partial response, it is recommended that treatment with NIPENT be stopped.
Withholding or discontinuation of individual doses may be needed when severe adverse reactions occur. Drug treatment should be withheld in patients with severe rash, and withheld or discontinued in patients showing evidence of nervous system toxicity.
NIPENT treatment should be withheld in patients with active infection occurring during the treatment but may be resumed when the infection is controlled.
Patients who have elevated serum creatinine should have their dose withheld and a creatinine clearance determined. There are insufficient data to recommend a starting or a subsequent dose for patients with impaired renal function (creatinine clearance <60 mL/min).
Patients with impaired renal function should be treated only when the potential benefit justifies the potential risk. Two patients with impaired renal function (creatinine clearances 50 to 60 mL/min) achieved complete response without unusual adverse events when treated with 2 mg/m^2.
No dosage reduction is recommended at the start of therapy with NIPENT in patients with anemia, neutropenia, or thrombocytopenia. In addition, dosage reductions are not recommended during treatment in patients with anemia and thrombocytopenia if patients can be otherwise supported hematologically. NIPENT should be temporarily withheld if the absolute neutrophil count falls during treatment below 200 cells/mm^3 in a patient who had an initial neutrophil count greater than 500 cells/mm^3 and may be resumed when the count returns to predose levels.

Preparation of Intravenous Solution

1. Procedures for proper handling and disposal of anticancer drugs should be followed. Several guidelines on this subject have been published.[2–7] There is no general agreement that all of the procedures recommended in the guidelines are necessary or appropriate. Spills and wastes should be treated with a 5% sodium hypochlorite solution prior to disposal.
2. Protective clothing including polyethylene gloves must be worn.
3. Transfer 5 mL of Sterile Water for Injection, USP to the vial containing NIPENT and mix thoroughly to obtain complete dissolution of a solution yielding 2 mg/mL. Parenteral drug products should be inspected visually for particulate matter and discoloration prior to administration.
4. NIPENT may be given intravenously by bolus injection or diluted in a larger volume (25 to 50 mL) with 5% Dextrose Injection, USP or 0.9% Sodium Chloride Injection, USP. Dilution of the entire contents of a reconstituted vial with 25 mL or 50 mL provides a pentostatin concentration of 0.33 mg/mL or 0.18 mg/mL, respectively, for the diluted solutions.
5. NIPENT solution when diluted for infusion with 5% Dextrose Injection, USP or 0.9% Sodium Chloride Injection, USP does not interact with PVC infusion containers or administration sets at concentrations of 0.18 mg/mL to 0.33 mg/mL.

Stability

NIPENT vials are stable at refrigerated storage temperature 2° to 8°C (36° to 46°F) for the period stated on the package. Vials reconstituted or reconstituted and further diluted as directed may be stored at room temperature and ambient light but should be used within 8 hours because NIPENT contains no preservatives.

HOW SUPPLIED

NIPENT (pentostatin for injection) is supplied as a sterile lyophilized white to off-white powder in single-dose vials containing 10 mg of pentostatin. The vials are packed in individual cartons. **NDC 62701-800-01**

Storage: Store NIPENT vials under refrigerated storage conditions 2° to 8°C (36° to 46°F).

Rx Only

REFERENCES

1. Malspeis L, et al. Clinical Pharmacokinetics of 2'-Deoxycoformycin. Cancer Treatment Symposia 2:7–15, 1984.
2. Recommendations for the safe handling of parenteral antineoplastic drugs. NIH publication 83-2621. For sale by the Superintendent of Documents, US Government Printing Office, Washington, NC 20402.
3. AMA council report. Guidelines for handling parenteral antineoplastics. JAMA 253:1590–2, 1985.
4. National Study Commission on Cytotoxic Exposure–Recommendations for handling cytotoxic agents. Available from Louis P. Jeffery, Sc.D., Chairman, National Study Commission on Cytotoxic Exposure, Massachusetts College of Pharmacy and Allied Health Sciences, 179 Longwood Ave, Boston, Massachusetts 02115.
5. Clinical Oncology Society of Australia: Guidelines and recommendations for safe handling of antineoplastic agents. Med J Australia 1:426–8, 1983.
6. Jones RB, et al. Safe handling of chemotherapeutic agents: A report from the Mount Sinai Medical Center. CA: A Cancer Journal for Clinicians 33:258–63, 1983.
7. American Society of Hospital Pharmacists technical assistance bulletin on handling cytotoxic and hazardous drugs. Am J Hosp Pharm 47:1033–49, 1990.

800P2 Rev. April, 1998

TAP Pharmaceuticals Inc.

DEERFIELD, IL 60015

For Medical Information Contact:
Generally:
Medical Department
(800) 622-2011 (LUPRON)
(800) 478-9526 (PREVACID)
In Emergencies:
Medical Department
(800) 622-2011 (LUPRON)
(800) 478-9526 (PREVACID)

LUPRON® ℞

(leuprolide acetate) Injection

DESCRIPTION

LUPRON (leuprolide acetate) Injection is a synthetic nonapeptide analog of naturally occurring gonadotropin releasing hormone (GnRH or LH-RH). The analog possesses greater potency than the natural hormone. The chemical name is 5-Oxo-L-prolyl-L-histidyl-L-tryptophyl-L-seryl-L-tyrosyl-D-leucyl-L-leucyl-L-arginyl-N-ethyl-L-prolinamide acetate (salt) with the following structural formula:
[See chemical structure below]
LUPRON is a sterile, aqueous solution intended for subcutaneous injection. It is available in a 2.8 mL multiple-dose vial containing 5 mg/mL of leuprolide acetate, sodium chloride for tonicity adjustment, 9 mg/mL of benzyl alcohol as a preservative and water for injection. The pH may have been adjusted with sodium hydroxide and/or acetic acid.

CLINICAL PHARMACOLOGY

Leuprolide acetate, an LH-RH agonist, acts as a potent inhibitor of gonadotropin secretion when given continuously and in therapeutic doses. Animal and human studies indicate that following an initial stimulation, chronic administration of leuprolide acetate results in suppression of ovarian and testicular steroidogenesis. This effect is reversible upon discontinuation of drug therapy. Administration of leuprolide acetate has resulted in inhibition of the growth of certain hormone dependent tumors (prostatic tumors in Noble and Dunning male rats and DMBA-induced mammary tumors in female rats) as well as atrophy of the reproductive organs.
In humans, subcutaneous administration of single daily doses of leuprolide acetate results in an initial increase in circulation levels of luteinizing hormone (LH) and follicle stimulating hormone (FSH), leading to a transient increase in levels of the gonadal steroids (testosterone and dihydrotestosterone in males, and estrone and estradiol in premenopausal females). However, continuous daily administration of leuprolide acetate results in decreased levels of LH and FSH in all patients. In males, testosterone is reduced to castrate levels. In pre-menopausal females, estrogens are reduced to post-menopausal levels. These decreases occur within two to four weeks after initiation of treatment, and castrate levels of testosterone in prostatic cancer patients have been demonstrated for periods of up to five years.
Leuprolide acetate is not active when given orally. Bioavailability by subcutaneous administration is comparable to that by intravenous administration. Leuprolide acetate has a plasma half-life of approximately three hours. The metabolism, distribution and excretion of leuprolide acetate in man have not been determined.

INDICATIONS AND USAGE

LUPRON (leuprolide acetate) Injection is indicated in the palliative treatment of advanced prostatic cancer. It offers an alternative treatment of prostatic cancer when orchiectomy or estrogen administration are either not indicated or unacceptable to the patient. In a controlled study comparing LUPRON 1 mg/day given subcutaneously to DES (diethylstilbestrol), 3 mg/day, the survival rate for the two groups was comparable after two years treatment. The objective response to treatment was also similar for the two groups.

CONTRAINDICATIONS

A report of an anaphylactic reaction to synthetic GnRH (Factrel) has been reported in the medical literature.[1]
LUPRON is contraindicated in women who are or may become pregnant while receiving the drug. When administered on day 6 of pregnancy at test dosages of 0.00024, 0.0024, and 0.024 mg/kg (1/600 to 1/6 the human dose) to rabbits, LUPRON produced a dose-related increase in major fetal abnormalities. Similar studies in rats failed to demonstrate an increase in fetal malformations. There was increased fetal mortality and decreased fetal weights with the two higher doses of LUPRON in rabbits and with the highest dose in rats. The effects on fetal mortality are logical consequences of the alterations in hormonal levels brought about by this drug. Therefore, the possibility exists that spontaneous abortion may occur if the drug is administered during pregnancy.

WARNINGS

Isolated cases of worsening of signs and symptoms during the first weeks of treatment have been reported. Worsening of symptoms may contribute to paralysis with or without fatal complications.

PRECAUTIONS

Patients with metastatic vertebral lesions and/or with urinary tract obstruction should be closely observed during the first few weeks of therapy (see "ADVERSE REACTIONS" section).
Patients with known allergies to benzyl alcohol, an ingredient of the drug's vehicle, may present symptoms of hypersensitivity, usually local, in the form of erythema and induration at the injection site.
Information for Patients: See Information for Patients which appears after the "HOW SUPPLIED" section.
Laboratory Tests: Response to leuprolide acetate should be monitored by measuring serum levels of testosterone and acid phosphatase. In the majority of patients, testosterone levels increased above baseline during the first week, declining thereafter to baseline levels or below by the end of the second week of treatment. Castrate levels were reached within two to four weeks and once attained were maintained for as long as drug administration continued. Transient increases in acid phosphatase levels occurred sometimes early in treatment. However, by the fourth week, the elevated levels usually decreased to values at or near baseline.
Drug Interactions: None have been reported.
Carcinogenesis, Mutagenesis, Impairment of Fertility: Two-year carcinogenicity studies were conducted in rats and mice. In rats, a dose-related increase of benign pituitary hyperplasia and benign pituitary adenomas was noted at 24 months when the drug was administered subcutaneously at high daily doses (0.6 to 4 mg/kg). In mice no pituitary abnormalities were observed at a dose as high as 60 mg/kg for two years. Patients have been treated with leuprolide acetate for up to three years with doses as high as 10 mg/day and for two years with doses as high as 20 mg/day without demonstrable pituitary abnormalities.
Mutagenicity studies have been performed with leuprolide acetate using bacterial and mammalian systems. These studies provided no evidence of a mutagenic potential.
Clinical and pharmacologic studies with leuprolide acetate and similar analogs have shown full reversibility of fertility suppression when the drug is discontinued after continuous

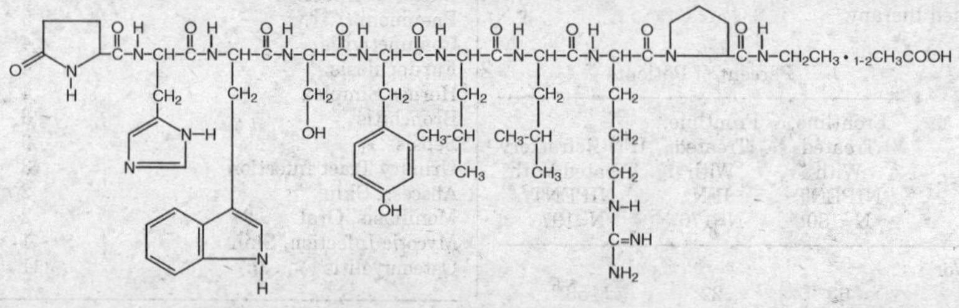

administration for periods of up to 24 weeks. However, no clinical studies have been conducted with leuprolide acetate to assess the reversibility of fertility suppression.

Pregnancy Category X. See "CONTRAINDICATIONS" section.

ADVERSE REACTIONS

In the majority of patients testosterone levels increased above baseline during the first week, declining thereafter to baseline levels or below by the end of the second week of treatment. This transient increase was occasionally associated with a temporary worsening of signs and symptoms, usually manifested by an increase in bone pain (See "WARNINGS" section). In a few cases a temporary worsening of existing hematuria and urinary tract obstruction occurred during the first week. Temporary weakness and paresthesia of the lower limbs have been reported in a few cases.

Potential exacerbations of signs and symptoms during the first few weeks of treatment is a concern in patients with vertebral metastases and/or urinary obstruction which, if aggravated, may lead to neurological problems or increase the obstruction.

In a comparative trial of LUPRON (leuprolide acetate) Injection versus DES, in 5% or more of the patients receiving either drug, the following adverse reactions were reported to have a possible or probable relationship to drug as ascribed by the treating physician. Often, causality is difficult to assess in patients with metastatic prostate cancer. Reactions considered not drug related are excluded.

	LUPRON (N=98)	DES (N=101)
	Number of Reports	
Cardiovascular System		
Congestive heart failure	1	5
ECG changes/ischemia	19	22
High blood pressure	8	5
Murmur	3	8
Peripheral edema	12	30
Phlebitis/thrombosis	2	10
Gastrointestinal System		
Anorexia	6	5
Constipation	7	9
Nausea/vomiting	5	17
Endocrine System		
* Decreased testicular size	7	11
* Gynecomastia/breast tenderness or pain	7	63
* Hot flashes	55	12
* Impotence	4	12
Hemic and Lymphatic System		
Anemia	5	5
Musculoskeletal System		
Bone pain	5	2
Myalgia	3	9
Central/Peripheral Nervous System		
Dizziness/lightheadedness	5	7
General pain	13	13
Headache	7	4
Insomnia/sleep disorders	7	5
Respiratory System		
Dyspnea	2	8
Sinus congestion	5	6
Integumentary System		
Dermatitis	5	8
Urogenital System		
Frequency/urgency	6	8
Hematuria	6	4
Urinary tract infection	3	7
Miscellaneous		
Asthenia	10	10

*Physiologic effect of decreased testosterone.

In this same study, the following adverse reactions were reported in less than 5% of the patients on LUPRON.

Cardiovascular System- Angina, Cardiac arrhythmias, Myocardial infarction, Pulmonary emboli; *Gastrointestinal System* - Diarrhea, Dysphagia, Gastrointestinal bleeding, Gastrointestinal disturbance, Peptic ulcer, Rectal polyps; *Endocrine System* - Libido decrease, Thyroid enlargement; *Musculoskeletal System* - Joint pain; *Central/Peripheral Nervous System* - Anxiety, Blurred vision, Lethargy, Memory disorder, Mood swings, Nervousness, Numbness, Paresthesia, Peripheral neuropathy, Syncope/blackouts, Taste disorders; *Respiratory System* - Cough, Pleural rub, Pneumonia, Pulmonary fibrosis; *Integumentary System* - Carcinoma of skin/ear, Dry skin, Ecchymosis, Hair loss, Itching, Local skin reactions, Pigmentation, Skin lesions; *Urogenital System* - Bladder spasms, Dysuria, Incontinence, Testicular pain, Urinary obstruction; *Miscellaneous* - Depression, Diabetes, Fatigue, Fever/chills, Hypoglycemia, Increased BUN,

Increased calcium, Increased creatinine, Infection/inflammation, Ophthalmologic disorders, Swelling (temporal bone).

The following additional adverse reactions have been reported with LUPRON or LUPRON DEPOT (leuprolide acetate for depot suspension) during other clinical trials and/or during postmarketing surveillance. Reactions considered as nondrug related by the treating physician are excluded.

Cardiovascular System - Hypotension, Transient ischemic attack/stroke; *Gastrointestinal System* - Hepatic dysfunction; *Endocrine System*- Libido increase; *Hemic and Lymphatic System*- Decreased WBC, Hemoptysis; *Musculoskeletal System*- Ankylosing spondylosis, Pelvic fibrosis; *Central/Peripheral Nervous System* - Hearing disorder, Peripheral neuropathy, Spinal fracture/paralysis; *Respiratory System* - Pulmonary infiltrate, Respiratory disorders; *Integumentary System* - Hair growth; *Urogenital System* - Penile swelling, Prostate pain; *Miscellaneous* - Hypoproteinemia, Hard nodule in throat, Weight gain, Increased uric acid.

OVERDOSAGE

In rats subcutaneous administration of 250 to 500 times the recommended human dose, expressed on a per body weight basis, resulted in dyspnea, decreased activity, and local irritation at the injection site. There is no evidence at present that there is a clinical counterpart of this phenomenon. In early clinical trials with leuprolide acetate doses as high as 20 mg/day for up to two years caused no adverse effects differing from those observed with the 1 mg/day dose.

DOSAGE AND ADMINISTRATION

The recommended dose is 1 mg (0.2 mL) administered as a single daily subcutaneous injection. As with other drugs administered chronically by subcutaneous injection, the injection site should be varied periodically.

NOTE: As with all parenteral products, inspect container's solution for discoloration and particulate matter before each use.

HOW SUPPLIED

LUPRON (leuprolide acetate) Injection is a sterile solution supplied in a 2.8 mL multiple-dose vial, **NDC** 0300-3626-28. Store below 77°F (25°C). Do not freeze. Protect from light—store vial in carton until use.

Each 0.2 mL contains 1 mg of leuprolide acetate, sodium chloride for tonicity adjustment, 1.8 mg of benzyl alcohol as preservative and water for injection. The pH may have been adjusted with sodium hydroxide and/or acetic acid.

Caution: Federal (U.S.A.) law prohibits dispensing without a prescription.

U.S. Patent Nos. 4,005,063 and 4,005,194.

REFERENCE

1. MacLeod TL, Eisen A, Sussman GL, et al: Anaphylactic reaction to synthetic luteinizing hormone-releasing hormone. *Fertil Steril* 1987 Sept;48(3):500-502.

INFORMATION FOR PATIENTS

NOTE: Be sure to consult your physician with any questions you may have or for information about LUPRON (leuprolide acetate) Injection and its use.

WHAT IS LUPRON?

LUPRON (leuprolide acetate) Injection is chemically similar to gonadotropin releasing hormone (GnRH or LH-RH) a hormone which occurs naturally in your body.

Normally, your body releases small amounts of LH-RH and this leads to events which stimulate the production of sex hormones.

However, when you inject LUPRON (leuprolide acetate) Injection, the normal events that lead to sex hormone production are interrupted and testosterone is no longer produced by the testes.

LUPRON must be injected because, like insulin which is injected by diabetics, LUPRON is inactive when taken by mouth.

If you were to discontinue the drug for any reason, your body would begin making testosterone again.

DIRECTIONS FOR USING LUPRON

1. Wash hands thoroughly with soap and water.
2. If using a new bottle for the first time, flip off the plastic cover to expose the gray rubber stopper. Wipe metal ring and rubber stopper with an alcohol wipe each time you use LUPRON. Check the liquid in the container. If it is not clear or has particles in it, DO NOT USE IT. Exchange it at your pharmacy for another container.
3. Remove outer wrapping from one syringe. Pull plunger back until the tip of the plunger is at the .2 or 20 unit mark.
4. Take cover off needle. Push the needle through the center of the rubber stopper on the LUPRON bottle.
5. Push the plunger all the way in to inject air into the bottle.
6. Keep the needle in the bottle and turn the bottle upside down. Check to make sure the tip of the needle is in the liquid. Slowly pull back on the plunger, until the syringe fills to the .2 or 20 unit mark.

7. Toward the end of a two-week period, the amount of LUPRON left in the bottle will be small. Take special care to hold the bottle straight and to keep the needle tip in liquid while pulling back on the plunger.
8. Keeping the needle in the bottle and the bottle upside down, check for air bubbles in the syringe. If you see any, push the plunger *slowly* in to push the air bubble back into the bottle. Keep the tip of the needle in the liquid and pull the plunger back again to fill to the .2 or 20 unit mark.
9. Do this again if necessary to eliminate air bubbles. Remove needle from bottle and lay syringe down. DO NOT TOUCH THE NEEDLE OR ALLOW THE NEEDLE TO TOUCH ANY SURFACE.
10. To protect your skin, inject each daily dose at a different body spot.
11. Choose an injection spot. Cleanse the injection spot with another alcohol wipe.
12. Hold the syringe in one hand. Hold the skin taut, or pull up a little flesh with the other hand, as you were instructed.
13. Holding the syringe as you would a pencil, thrust the needle all the way into the skin at a 90° angle.
14. Hold an alcohol wipe down on your skin where the needle is inserted and withdraw the needle at the same angle it was inserted.
15. Use the disposable syringe only once and dispose of it properly as you were instructed. Needles thrown into a garbage bag could accidentally stick someone. NEVER LEAVE SYRINGES, NEEDLES OR DRUGS WHERE CHILDREN CAN REACH THEM.

SOME SPECIAL ADVICE

- You may experience hot flashes when using LUPRON (leuprolide acetate) Injection. During the first few weeks of treatment you may experience increased bone pain, increased difficulty in urinating, and less commonly but most importantly, you may experience the onset or aggravation of nerve symptoms. In any of these events, discuss the symptoms with your doctor.
- You may experience some irritation at the injection site, such as burning, itching or swelling. These reactions are usually mild and go away. If they do not, tell your doctor.
- Do not stop taking your injections because you feel better. You need an injection every day to make sure LUPRON keeps working for you.
- If you need to use an alternate to the syringe supplied with LUPRON, insulin syringes should be utilized.
- When the drug level gets low, take special care to hold the bottle straight up and down and to keep the needle tip in liquid while pulling back on the plunger.
- Do not try to get every last drop out of the bottle. This will increase the possibility of drawing air into the syringe and getting an incomplete dose. Some extra drug has been provided so that you can withdraw the recommended number of doses.
- Tell your pharmacist when you will need LUPRON so it will be at the pharmacy when you need it.
- Store below 77°F (25°C). Do not store near a radiator or other very warm place. Do not freeze. Protect from light - store vial in carton until use.
- Do not leave your drug or hypodermic syringes where anyone can pick them up.
- Keep this and all other medications out of reach of children.

TAP Pharmaceuticals Inc.
Deerfield, IL 60015, U.S.A.
Lupron Injection
manufactured by
Abbott Laboratories,
North Chicago, IL 60064
® – Registered
03-4676-R7
Revised: April, 1996

For Pediatric Use
LUPRON®   ℞
(leuprolide acetate) Injection

DESCRIPTION

Leuprolide acetate is a synthetic nonapeptide analog of naturally occurring gonadotropin releasing hormone (GnRH or LH-RH). The analog possesses greater potency than the natural hormone. The chemical name is 5-Oxo-L-prolyl-L-histidyl -L-tryptophyl-L-seryl -L- tyrosyl-D-leucyl-L-leucyl-L-arginyl-N-ethyl-L-prolinamide acetate (salt) with the following structural formula:
[See chemical structure at top of next page]
LUPRON Injection is a sterile, aqueous solution intended for daily subcutaneous injection.

- A 2.8 mL multiple dose vial contains leuprolide acetate (5 mg/mL), sodium chloride (6.3 mg/mL) for to-

Continued on next page

Lupron for Pediatric Use—Cont.

nicity adjustment, benzyl alcohol as a preservative (9 mg/mL), and water for injection. The pH may have been adjusted with sodium hydroxide and/or acetic acid.

CLINICAL PHARMACOLOGY

Leuprolide acetate, a GnRH agonist, acts as a potent inhibitor of gonadotropin secretion when given continuously and in therapeutic doses. Human studies indicate that following an initial stimulation of gonadotropins, chronic stimulation with leuprolide acetate results in suppression or "downregulation" of these hormones and consequent suppression of ovarian and testicular steroidogenesis. These effects are reversible on discontinuation of drug therapy.

Leuprolide acetate is not active when given orally. In adults, bioavailability by subcutaneous administration is comparable to that by intravenous administration; and leuprolide acetate has a plasma half-life of approximately three hours. The metabolism, distribution and excretion of leuprolide acetate in humans have not been determined. A pharmacokinetic study of leuprolide acetate in children has not been performed.

In children with central precocious puberty (CPP), stimulated and basal gonadotropins are reduced to prepubertal levels. Testosterone and estradiol are reduced to prepubertal levels in males and females respectively. Reduction of gonadotropins will allow for normal physical and psychological growth and development. Natural maturation occurs when gonadotropins return to pubertal levels following discontinuation of leuprolide acetate.

The following physiologic effects have been noted with the chronic administration of leuprolide acetate in this patient population.

1. **Skeletal Growth.** A measurable increase in body length can be noted since the epiphyseal plates will not close prematurely.
2. **Organ growth.** Reproductive organs will return to a prepubertal state.
3. **Menses.** Menses, if present, will cease.

INDICATIONS AND USAGE

LUPRON Injection is indicated in the treatment of children with central precocious puberty. Children should be selected using the following criteria:

1. Clinical diagnosis of CPP (idiopathic or neurogenic) with onset of secondary sexual characteristics earlier than 8 years in females and 9 years in males.
2. Clinical diagnosis should be confirmed prior to initiation of therapy:
   - Confirmation of diagnosis by a pubertal response to a GnRH stimulation test. The sensitivity and methodology of this assay must be understood.
   - Bone age advanced one year beyond the chronological age.
3. Baseline evaluation should also include:
   - Height and weight measurements.
   - Sex steroid levels.
   - Adrenal steroid level to exclude congenital adrenal hyperplasia.
   - Beta human chorionic gonadotropin level to rule out a chorionic gonadotropin secreting tumor.
   - Pelvic/adrenal/testicular ultrasound to rule out a steroid secreting tumor.
   - Computerized tomography of the head to rule out intracranial tumor.

CONTRAINDICATIONS

LUPRON Injection is contraindicated in women who are or may become pregnant while receiving the drug. When administered on day 6 of pregnancy at test dosages of 0.00024, 0.0024, and 0.024 mg/kg (1/1200 to 1/12 the human pediatric dose) to rabbits, LUPRON produced a dose-related increase in major fetal abnormalities. Similar studies in rats failed to demonstrate an increase in fetal malformations. There was increased fetal mortality and decreased fetal weights with the two higher doses of LUPRON in rabbits and with the highest dose in rats. The effects on fetal mortality are logical consequences of the alterations in hormonal levels brought about by this drug. Therefore, the possibility exists that spontaneous abortion may occur if the drug is administered during pregnancy.

Leuprolide acetate is contraindicated in children demonstrating hypersensitivity to GnRH, GnRH agonist analogs, or any of the excipients.

A report of an anaphylactic reaction to synthetic GnRH (Factrel) has been reported in the medical literature.[1]

WARNINGS

During the early phase of therapy, gonadotropins and sex steroids rise above baseline because of the natural stimulatory effect of the drug. Therefore, an increase in clinical signs and symptoms may be observed (see "Clinical Pharmacology" section).

Noncompliance with drug regimen or inadequate dosing may result in inadequate control of the pubertal process. The consequences of poor control include the return of

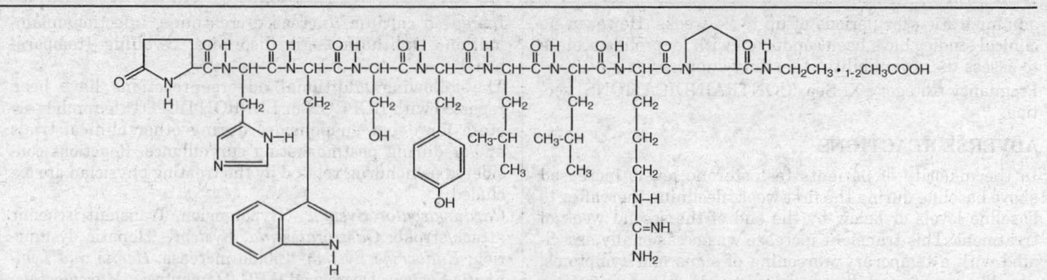

pubertal signs such as menses, breast development, and testicular growth. The long-term consequences of inadequate control of gonadal steroid secretion are unknown, but may include a further compromise of adult stature.

PRECAUTIONS

Patients with known allergies to benzyl alcohol, an ingredient of the vehicle of Lupron Injection, may present symptoms of hypersensitivity, usually local, in the form of erythema and induration at the injection site.

Laboratory Tests: Response to leuprolide acetate should be monitored 1-2 months after the start of therapy with a GnRH stimulation test and sex steroid levels. Measurement of bone age for advancement should be done every 6-12 months.

Sex steroids may increase or rise above prepubertal levels if the dose is inadequate (see "WARNINGS" section). Once a therapeutic dose has been established, gonadotropin and sex steroid levels will decline to prepubertal levels.

Drug Interactions: No pharmacokinetic-based drug-drug interaction studies have been conducted. However, because leuprolide acetate is a peptide that is primarily degraded by peptidase and not by cytochrome P-450 enzymes as noted in specific studies, and the drug is only about 46% bound to plasma proteins, drug interactions would not be expected to occur.

Drug/Laboratory Test Interactions: Administration of leuprolide acetate in therapeutic doses results in suppression of the pituitary-gonadal system. Normal function is usually restored within 4 to 12 weeks after treatment is discontinued.

Information for Parents: Prior to starting therapy with LUPRON Injection, the parent or guardian must be aware of the importance of continuous therapy. Adherence to daily drug administration schedules must be accepted if therapy is to be successful.

- During the first 2 months of therapy, a female may experience menses or spotting. If bleeding continues beyond the second month, notify the physician.
- Any irritation at the injection site should be reported to the physician immediately.
- Report any unusual signs or symptoms to the physician.

Carcinogenesis, Mutagenesis, Impairment of Fertility: A two-year carcinogenicity study was conducted in rats and mice. In rats, a dose-related increase of benign pituitary hyperplasia and benign pituitary adenomas was noted at 24 months when the drug was administered subcutaneously at high daily doses (0.6 to 4 mg/kg). There was a significant but not dose-related increase of pancreatic islet-cell adenomas in females and of testes interstitial cell adenomas in males (highest incidence in the low dose group). In mice, no leuprolide acetate-induced tumors or pituitary abnormalities were observed at a dose as high as 60 mg/kg for two years. Adult patients have been treated with leuprolide acetate for up to three years with doses as high as 10 mg/day and for two years with doses as high as 20 mg/day without demonstrable pituitary abnormalities.

Although no clinical studies have been completed in children to assess the full reversibility of fertility suppression, animal studies (prepubertal and adult rats and monkeys) with leuprolide acetate and other GnRH analogs have shown functional recovery. However, following a study with leuprolide acetate, immature male rats demonstrated tubular degeneration in the testes even after a recovery period. In spite of the failure to recover histologically, the treated males proved to be as fertile as the controls. Also, no histologic changes were observed in the female rats following the same protocol. In both sexes, the offspring of the treated animals appeared normal. The effect of the treatment of the parents on the reproductive performance of the F1 generation was not tested. The clinical significance of these findings is unknown.

Pregnancy Category X. See **"CONTRAINDICATIONS"** section.

Nursing Mothers: It is not known whether leuprolide acetate is excreted in human milk. LUPRON should not be used by nursing mothers.

ADVERSE REACTIONS

Potential exacerbation of signs and symptoms during the first few weeks of treatment (See "PRECAUTIONS" section) is a concern in patients with rapidly advancing central precocious puberty.

In two studies of children with central precocious puberty, in 2% or more of the patients receiving the drug, the following adverse reactions were reported to have a possible or probable relationship to drug as ascribed by the treating physician. Reactions considered not drug related are excluded.

	Number of Patients N = 395	(Percent)
Body as a Whole		
General Pain	7	(2)
Integumentary System		
Acne/Seborrhea	7	(2)
Injection Site Reactions Including Abscess	21	(5)
Rash Including Erythema Multiforme	8	(2)
Urogenital System		
Vaginitis/Bleeding/ Discharge	7	(2)

In those same studies, the following adverse reactions were reported in less than 2% of the patients.

Body as a Whole - Body Odor, Fever, Headache, Infection; *Cardiovascular System* - Syncope, Vasodilation; *Digestive System* - Dysphagia, Gingivitis, Nausea/Vomiting; *Endocrine System* - Accelerated Sexual Maturity; *Metabolic and Nutritional Disorders* - Peripheral Edema, Weight Gain; *Nervous System* - Nervousness, Personality Disorder, Somnolence, Emotional Lability; *Respiratory System* - Epistaxis; *Integumentary System*- Alopecia, Skin Striae; *Urogenital System* - Cervix Disorder, Gynecomastia/Breast Disorders, Urinary Incontinence.

See other package inserts for adverse events reported in other patient populations.

OVERDOSAGE

In rats, subcutaneous administration of 125 to 250 times the recommended human pediatric dose, expressed on a per body weight basis, resulted in dyspnea, decreased activity, and local irritation at the injection site. There is no evidence at present that there is a clinical counterpart of this phenomenon. In early clinical trials using leuprolide acetate in adult patients, doses as high as 20 mg/day for up to two years caused no adverse effects differing from those observed with the 1 mg/day dose.

DOSAGE AND ADMINISTRATION

LUPRON INJECTION can be administered by a patient/parent or health care professional.

The dose of LUPRON Injection must be individualized for each child. The dose is based on a mg/kg ratio of drug to body weight. Younger children require higher doses on a mg/kg ratio.

For either dosage form, after 1-2 months of initiating therapy or changing doses, the child must be monitored with a GnRH stimulation test, sex steroids, and Tanner staging to confirm downregulation. Measurements of bone age for advancement should be monitored every 6-12 months. The dose should be titrated upward until no progression of the condition is noted either clinically and/or by laboratory parameters.

The first dose found to result in adequate downregulation can probably be maintained for the duration of therapy in most children. However, there are insufficient data to guide dosage adjustment as patients move into higher weight categories after beginning therapy at very young ages and low dosages. It is recommended that adequate downregulation be verified in such patients whose weight has increased significantly while on therapy.

As with other drugs administered by injection, the injection site should be varied periodically.

Discontinuation of LUPRON Injection should be considered before age 11 for females and age 12 for males.

The recommended starting dose is 50 mcg/kg/day administered as a single subcutaneous injection. If total downregulation is not achieved, the dose should be titrated upward by 10 mcg/kg/day. This dose will be considered the maintenance dose.

NOTE: As with other parenteral products, inspect container's solution for discoloration and particulate matter before each use.

HOW SUPPLIED

LUPRON (leuprolide acetate) Injection is a sterile solution.

- A 2.8 mL multiple dose vial (NDC 0300-3626-28) contains leuprolide acetate (5 mg/mL), sodium chloride (6.3 mg/mL) for tonicity adjustment, benzyl alcohol as a preservative (9 mg/mL), and water for injection. The pH may have been adjusted with sodium hydroxide and/or acetic acid.
- Store below 77°F (25°C). Do not freeze. Protect from light - store vial in carton until use.
- Use the syringes supplied with LUPRON Injection. Insulin syringes may be substituted for use with Lupron Injection. The volume of drug for the dose will vary depending on the syringe used and the concentration of drug.

Caution: Federal (U.S.A.) law prohibits dispensing without a prescription.

U.S. Patent Nos. 4,005,063; 4,005,194.

REFERENCE

1. MacLeod TL, et al. Anaphylactic reaction to synthetic luteinizing hormone-releasing hormone. *Fertil Steril* 1987 Sept;48(3):500-502.

TAP Pharmaceuticals Inc.
Deerfield, IL 60015, U.S.A.
Lupron Injection
manufactured by
Abbott Laboratories,
North Chicago, IL 60064
® – Registered
03-4676-R7
Revised: April, 1996

This is combined labeling. Examples of different fonts appear below.

- General information
- Information on endometriosis
- **Information on uterine fibroids**

LUPRON DEPOT® 3.75 mg ℞
(leuprolide acetate for depot suspension)

DESCRIPTION

Leuprolide acetate is a synthetic nonapeptide analog of naturally occurring gonadotropin-releasing hormone (GnRH or LH-RH). The analog possesses greater potency than the natural hormone. The chemical name is 5-oxo-L-prolyl-L-histidyl-L-tryptophyl-L-seryl-L-tyrosyl-D-leucyl-L-leucyl-L-arginyl-N-ethyl-L-prolinamide acetate (salt) with the following structural formula:

[See chemical structure above]

LUPRON DEPOT is available in a vial and also in a prefilled dual-chamber syringe. Both contain sterile lyophilized microspheres, which when mixed with diluent, become a suspension which is intended as a monthly intramuscular injection.

The single-dose vial of LUPRON DEPOT contains leuprolide acetate (3.75 mg), purified gelatin (0.65 mg), DL-lactic and glycolic acids copolymer (33.1 mg), and D-mannitol (6.6 mg). The accompanying ampule of diluent contains carboxymethylcellulose sodium (10 mg), D-mannitol (100 mg), polysorbate 80 (2 mg), water for injection, USP, and glacial acetic acid, USP to control pH.

The front chamber of LUPRON DEPOT 3.75 mg prefilled dual-chamber syringe contains leuprolide acetate (3.75 mg), purified gelatin (0.65 mg), DL-lactic and glycolic acids copolymer (33.1 mg), and D-mannitol (6.6 mg). The second chamber of diluent contains carboxymethylcellulose sodium (5 mg), D-mannitol (50 mg), polysorbate 80 (1 mg), water for injection, USP, and glacial acetic acid, USP to control pH.

During the manufacture of LUPRON DEPOT 3.75 mg, acetic acid is lost, leaving the peptide.

CLINICAL PHARMACOLOGY

Leuprolide acetate is a long-acting GnRH analog. A single monthly injection of LUPRON DEPOT 3.75 mg results in an initial stimulation followed by a prolonged suppression of pituitary gonadotropins. Repeated dosing at monthly intervals results in decreased secretion of gonadal steroids; consequently, tissues and functions that depend on gonadal steroids for their maintenance become quiescent. This effect is reversible on discontinuation of drug therapy.

Leuprolide acetate is not active when given orally. Intramuscular injection of the depot formulation provides plasma concentrations of leuprolide over a period of one month.

PHARMACOKINETICS

Absorption: A single dose of LUPRON DEPOT 3.75 mg was administered by intramuscular injection to healthy female volunteers. The absorption of leuprolide was characterized by an initial increase in plasma concentration, with peak concentration ranging from 4.6 to 10.2 ng/mL at four hours postdosing. However, intact leuprolide and an inactive metabolite could not be distinguished by the assay used in the study. Following the initial rise, leuprolide concentrations started to plateau within two days after dosing and remained relatively stable for about four to five weeks with plasma concentrations of about 0.30 ng/mL.

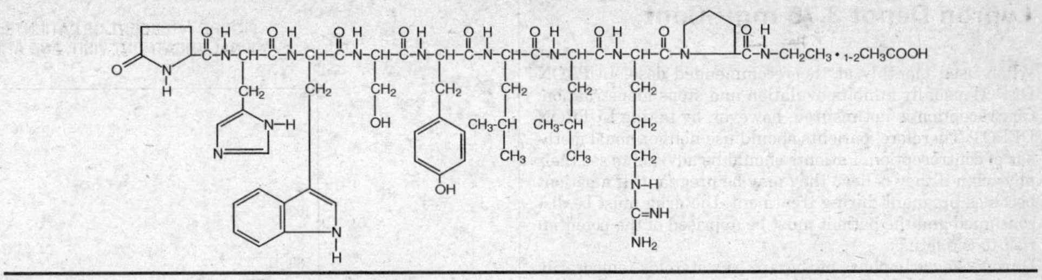

Distribution: The mean steady-state volume of distribution of leuprolide following intravenous bolus administration to healthy male volunteers was 27 L. In vitro binding to human plasma proteins ranged from 43% to 49%.

Metabolism: In healthy male volunteers, a 1 mg bolus of leuprolide administered intravenously revealed that the mean systemic clearance was 7.6 L/h, with a terminal elimination half-life of approximately 3 hours based on a two compartment model.

In rats and dogs, administration of ^{14}C-labeled leuprolide was shown to be metabolized to smaller inactive peptides, a pentapeptide (Metabolite I), tripeptides (Metabolites II and III) and a dipeptide (Metabolite IV). These fragments may be further catabolized.

The major metabolite (M-I) plasma concentrations measured in 5 prostate cancer patients reached maximum concentration 2 to 6 hours after dosing and were approximately 6% of the peak parent drug concentration. One week after dosing, mean plasma M-I concentrations were approximately 20% of mean leuprolide concentrations.

Excretion: Following administration of LUPRON DEPOT 3.75 mg to 3 patients, less than 5% of the dose was recovered as parent and M-I metabolite in the urine.

Special Populations: The pharmacokinetics of the drug in hepatically and renally impaired patients have not been determined.

CLINICAL STUDIES

Endometriosis: In controlled clinical studies, LUPRON DEPOT 3.75 mg monthly for six months was shown to be comparable to danazol 800 mg/day in relieving the clinical sign/symptoms of endometriosis (pelvic pain, dysmenorrhea, dyspareunia, pelvic tenderness, and induration) and in reducing the size of endometrial implants as evidenced by laparoscopy. The clinical significance of a decrease in endometriotic lesions is not known at this time, and in addition laparoscopic staging of endometriosis does not necessarily correlate with the severity of symptoms.

LUPRON DEPOT 3.75 mg monthly induced amenorrhea in 74% and 98% of the patients after the first and second treatment months respectively. Most of the remaining patients reported episodes of only light bleeding or spotting. In the first, second and third post-treatment months, normal menstrual cycles resumed in 7%, 71% and 95% respectively, of those patients who did not become pregnant.

Figure 1 illustrates the percent of patients with symptoms at baseline, final treatment visit and sustained relief at six and 12 months following discontinuation of treatment for the various symptoms evaluated during the study. This included all patients at end of treatment and those who elected to participate at the follow-up periods. This might provide a slight bias in the results at follow-up as 75% of the original patients entered the follow-up study, and 36% were evaluated at six months and 26% at 12 months respectively.

[See figure 1 at top of next page]

Hormonal replacement therapy: Clinical studies suggest that the addition of hormonal replacement therapy (estrogen and/or progestin) to LUPRON is effective in reducing loss of bone mineral density which occurs with LUPRON, without compromising the efficacy of LUPRON in relieving symptoms of endometriosis. The optimal drug/dose is not established.

Uterine Leiomyomata (Fibroids): In controlled clinical trials, administration of LUPRON DEPOT 3.75 mg for a period of three or six months was shown to decrease uterine and fibroid volume, thus allowing for relief of clinical symptoms (abdominal bloating, pelvic pain, and pressure). Excessive vaginal bleeding (menorrhagia and menometrorrhagia) decreased, resulting in improvement in hematologic parameters.

In three clinical trials, enrollment was not based on hematologic status. Mean uterine volume decreased by 41% and myoma volume decreased by 37% at final visit as evidenced by ultrasound or MRI. These patients also experienced a decrease in symptoms including excessive vaginal bleeding and pelvic discomfort. Benefit occurred by three months of therapy, but additional gain was observed with an additional three months of LUPRON DEPOT 3.75 mg. Ninety-five percent of these patients became amenorrheic with 61%, 25%, and 4% experiencing amenorrhea during the first, second, and third treatment months respectively.

Post-treatment follow-up was carried out for a small percentage of LUPRON DEPOT 3.75 mg patients among the 77% who demonstrated a ≥ 25% decrease in uterine volume while on therapy. Menses usually returned within two months of cessation of therapy. Mean time to return to pretreatment uterine size was 8.3 months. Regrowth did not appear to be related to pretreatment uterine volume.

In another controlled clinical study, enrollment was based on hematocrit ≤ 30% and/or hemoglobin ≤ 10.2 g/dL. Administration of LUPRON DEPOT 3.75 mg, concomitantly with iron, produced an increase of ≥ 6% hematocrit and ≥ 2 g/dL hemoglobin in 77% of patients at three months of therapy. The mean change in hematocrit was 10.1% and the mean change in hemoglobin was 4.2 g/dL. Clinical response was judged to be a hematocrit of ≥ 36% and hemoglobin of ≥ 12 g/dL, thus allowing for autologous blood donation prior to surgery. At three months, 75% of patients met this criterion.

At three months, 80% of patients experienced relief from either menorrhagia or menometrorrhagia. As with the previous studies, episodes of spotting and menstrual-like bleeding were noted in some patients.

In this same study, a decrease of ≥ 25% was seen in uterine and myoma volumes in 60% and 54% of patients respectively. LUPRON DEPOT 3.75 mg was found to relieve symptoms of bloating, pelvic pain, and pressure.

There is no evidence that pregnancy rates are enhanced or adversely affected by the use of LUPRON DEPOT 3.75 mg.

INDICATIONS AND USAGE

Endometriosis:

LUPRON DEPOT 3.75 mg is indicated for management of endometriosis, including pain relief and reduction of endometriotic lesions. Experience with LUPRON DEPOT 3.75 mg in females has been limited to women 18 years of age and older treated for 6 months.

Uterine Leiomyomata (Fibroids):

LUPRON DEPOT 3.75 mg concomitantly with iron therapy is indicated for the preoperative hematologic improvement of patients with anemia caused by uterine leiomyomata. The clinician may wish to consider a one-month trial period on iron alone inasmuch as some of the patients will respond to iron alone (see clinical trial results below). LUPRON may be added if the response to iron alone is considered inadequate. Recommended duration of therapy with LUPRON DEPOT 3.75 mg is **up to** three months.

Experience with LUPRON DEPOT in females has been limited to women 18 years of age and older.

PERCENT OF PATIENTS ACHIEVING HEMOGLOBIN ≥ 12 GM/DL

Treatment Group	Week 4	Week 8	Week 12
LUPRON DEPOT 3.75 mg with Iron	41*	71**	79*
Iron Alone	17	40	56

* P-Value < 0.01
** P-Value < 0.001

CONTRAINDICATIONS

1. Hypersensitivity to GnRH, GnRH agonist analogs or any of the excipients in LUPRON DEPOT.
2. Undiagnosed abnormal vaginal bleeding.
3. LUPRON DEPOT is contraindicated in women who are or may become pregnant while receiving the drug. LUPRON DEPOT may cause fetal harm when administered to a pregnant woman. Major fetal abnormalities were observed in rabbits but not in rats after administration of LUPRON DEPOT throughout gestation. There was increased fetal mortality and decreased fetal weights in rats and rabbits (see *Pregnancy* section). The effects on fetal mortality are expected consequences of the alterations in hormonal levels brought about by the drug. If this drug is used during pregnancy or if the patient becomes pregnant while taking this drug, she should be apprised of the potential hazard to the fetus.
4. Use in women who are breast feeding (see *Nursing Mothers* section).
5. A report of an anaphylactic reaction to synthetic GnRH (Factrel) has been reported in the medical literature.[1]

WARNINGS

Safe use of leuprolide acetate in pregnancy has not been established clinically. Before starting treatment with LUPRON DEPOT, pregnancy must be excluded.

Continued on next page

Lupron Depot 3.75 mg—Cont.

When used monthly at the recommended dose, LUPRON DEPOT usually inhibits ovulation and stops menstruation. Contraception is not insured, however, by taking LUPRON DEPOT. Therefore, patients should use nonhormonal methods of contraception. Patients should be advised to see their physician if they believe they may be pregnant. If a patient becomes pregnant during treatment, the drug must be discontinued and the patient must be apprised of the potential risk to the fetus.

During the early phase of therapy, sex steroids temporarily rise above baseline because of the physiologic effect of the drug. Therefore, an increase in clinical signs and symptoms may be observed during the initial days of therapy, but these will dissipate with continued therapy.

PRECAUTIONS

Information for Patients: An information pamphlet for patients is included with the product. Patients should be aware of the following information:

1. Since menstruation should stop with effective doses of LUPRON DEPOT, the patient should notify her physician if regular menstruation persists. Patients missing successive doses of LUPRON DEPOT may experience breakthrough bleeding.

2. Patients should not use LUPRON DEPOT if they are pregnant, breast feeding, have undiagnosed abnormal vaginal bleeding, or are allergic to any of the ingredients in LUPRON DEPOT.

3. Safe use of the drug in pregnancy has not been established clinically. Therefore, nonhormonal method of contraception should be used during treatment. Patients should be advised that if they miss successive doses of LUPRON DEPOT, breakthrough bleeding or ovulation may occur with the potential for conception. If a patient becomes pregnant during treatment, she should discontinue treatment and consult her physician.

4. Adverse events occurring in clinical studies with LUPRON DEPOT that are associated with hypoestrogenism include: hot flashes, headaches, emotional lability, decreased libido, acne, myalgia, reduction in breast size, and vaginal dryness. Estrogen levels returned to normal after treatment was discontinued.

5. The induced hypoestrogenic state **also** results in a small loss in bone density over the course of treatment, some of which may not be reversible. For a period up to six months, this bone loss should not be important. In patients with major risk factors for decreased bone mineral content such as chronic alcohol and/or tobacco use, strong family history of osteoporosis, or chronic use of drugs that can reduce bone mass such as anticonvulsants or corticosteroids, LUPRON DEPOT therapy may pose an additional risk. In these patients, the risks and benefits must be weighed carefully before therapy with LUPRON DEPOT is instituted. Repeated courses of therapy with gonadotropin-releasing hormone analogs beyond six months are not advisable in patients with major risk factors for loss of bone mineral content. Clinical studies sug-

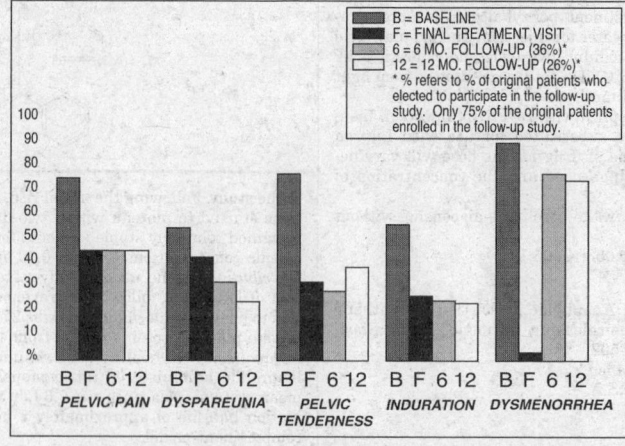

FIGURE 1-PERCENT OF PATIENTS WITH SIGNS/SYMPTOMS AT BASELINE, FINAL TREATMENT VISIT, AND AFTER 6 AND 12 MONTHS OF FOLLOW-UP

B = BASELINE
F = FINAL TREATMENT VISIT
6 = 6 MO. FOLLOW-UP (36%)*
12 = 12 MO. FOLLOW-UP (26%)*
* % refers to % of original patients who elected to participate in the follow-up study. Only 75% of the original patients enrolled in the follow-up study.

gest that the addition of hormonal replacement therapy (estrogen and/or progestin) to LUPRON is effective in reducing loss of bone mineral density which occurs with LUPRON, without compromising the efficacy of LUPRON in relieving symptoms of endometriosis. The optimal drug/dose is not established.

6. Retreatment cannot be recommended since safety data beyond six months are not available.

Drug Interactions: No pharmacokinetic-based drug-drug interaction studies have been conducted with LUPRON DEPOT. However, because leuprolide acetate is a peptide that is primarily degraded by peptidase and not by cytochrome P-450 enzymes as noted in specific studies, and the drug is only about 46% bound to plasma proteins, drug interactions would not be expected to occur.

Drug/Laboratory Test Interactions: Administration of LUPRON DEPOT in therapeutic doses results in suppression of the pituitary-gonadal system. Normal function is usually restored within three months after treatment is discontinued. Therefore, diagnostic tests of pituitary gonadotropic and gonadal functions conducted during treatment and for up to three months after discontinuation of LUPRON DEPOT may be misleading.

Carcinogenesis, Mutagenesis, Impairment of Fertility: A two-year carcinogenicity study was conducted in rats and mice. In rats, a dose-related increase of benign pituitary hyperplasia and benign pituitary adenomas was noted at 24 months when the drug was administered subcutaneously at high daily doses (0.6 to 4 mg/kg). There was a significant but not dose-related increase of pancreatic islet-cell adenomas in females and of testicular interstitial cell adenomas in males (highest incidence in the low dose group).

In mice, no leuprolide acetate-induced tumors or pituitary abnormalities were observed at a dose as high as 60 mg/kg for two years. Patients have been treated with leuprolide acetate for up to three years with doses as high as 10 mg/day and for two years with doses as high as 20 mg/day without demonstrable pituitary abnormalities.

Mutagenicity studies have been performed with leuprolide acetate using bacterial and mammalian systems. These studies provided no evidence of a mutagenic potential.

Clinical and pharmacologic studies in adults (>18 years) with leuprolide acetate and similar analogs have shown reversibility of fertility suppression when the drug is discontinued after continuous administration for periods of up to 24 weeks. Although no clinical studies have been completed in children to assess the full reversibility of fertility suppression, animal studies (prepubertal and adult rats and monkeys) with leuprolide acetate and other GnRH analogs have shown functional recovery.

Pregnancy, Teratogenic Effects: Pregnancy Category X. (See **CONTRAINDICATIONS** section.) When administered on day 6 of pregnancy at test dosages of 0.00024, 0.0024, and 0.024 mg/kg (1/300 to 1/3 the human dose) to rabbits, LUPRON DEPOT produced a dose-related increase in major fetal abnormalities. Similar studies in rats failed to demonstrate an increase in fetal malformations. There was increased fetal mortality and decreased fetal weights with the two higher doses of LUPRON DEPOT in rabbits and with the highest dose (0.024 mg/kg) in rats.

Nursing Mothers: It is not known whether LUPRON DEPOT is excreted in human milk. Because many drugs are excreted in human milk, and because the effects of LUPRON DEPOT on lactation and/or the breast-fed child have not been determined, LUPRON DEPOT should not be used by nursing mothers.

Pediatric Use: See LUPRON DEPOT-PED® (leuprolide acetate for depot suspension) labeling for the safety and effectiveness in children with central precocious puberty.

ADVERSE REACTIONS

Estradiol levels may increase during the first weeks following the initial injection, but then decline to menopausal levels. This transient increase in estradiol can be associated with a temporary worsening of signs and symptoms (see **WARNINGS** section).

As would be expected with a drug that lowers serum estradiol levels, the most frequently reported adverse reactions were those related to hypoestrogenism.

Endometriosis: In controlled studies comparing LUPRON DEPOT 3.75 mg monthly and danazol (800 mg/day) or placebo, adverse reactions most frequently reported and thought to be possibly or probably drug-related are shown in Figure 2.
[See figure 2 at left]

Cardiovascular System - Palpitations, Syncope, Tachycardia; *Gastrointestinal System* - Dry mouth, Thirst, Appetite changes; *Central/Peripheral Nervous System* - Anxiety,* Personality disorder, Memory disorder, Delusions; *Integumentary System* - Ecchymosis, Alopecia, Hair disorder; *Urogenital System* - Dysuria,* Lactation; *Miscellaneous* - Ophthalmologic disorders,* Lymphadenopathy.

Uterine Leiomyomata (Fibroids): In controlled clinical trials comparing LUPRON DEPOT 3.75 mg and placebo, adverse events reported in >5% of patients and thought to be potentially related to drug are noted in the following table.

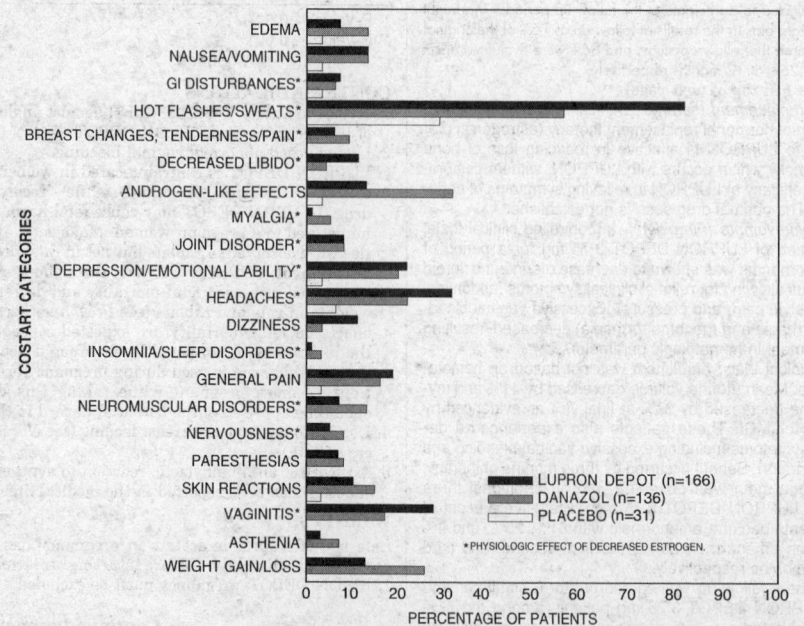

FIGURE 2–ADVERSE EVENTS REPORTED DURING 6 MONTHS OF TREATMENT WITH LUPRON DEPOT 3.75 MG

COSTART CATEGORIES

EDEMA
NAUSEA/VOMITING
GI DISTURBANCES*
HOT FLASHES/SWEATS*
BREAST CHANGES, TENDERNESS/PAIN*
DECREASED LIBIDO*
ANDROGEN-LIKE EFFECTS
MYALGIA*
JOINT DISORDER*
DEPRESSION/EMOTIONAL LABILITY*
HEADACHES*
DIZZINESS
INSOMNIA/SLEEP DISORDERS*
GENERAL PAIN
NEUROMUSCULAR DISORDERS*
NERVOUSNESS*
PARESTHESIAS
SKIN REACTIONS
VAGINITIS*
ASTHENIA
WEIGHT GAIN/LOSS

LUPRON DEPOT (n=166)
DANAZOL (n=136)
PLACEBO (n=31)

* PHYSIOLOGIC EFFECT OF DECREASED ESTROGEN.

PERCENTAGE OF PATIENTS

	Lupron Depot 3.75 mg N=166 (%)	Placebo N=163 (%)
Body as a Whole		
Asthenia	14 (8.4)	8 (4.9)
General pain	14 (8.4)	10 (6.1)

Headache*	43 (25.9)	29 (17.8)
Cardiovascular System		
Hot flashes/sweats*	121 (72.9)	29 (17.8)
Metabolic and Nutritional Disorders		
Edema	9 (5.4)	2 (1.2)
Musculoskeletal System		
Joint disorder*	13 (7.8)	5 (3.1)
Nervous System		
Depression/emotional lability*	18 (10.8)	7 (4.3)
Urogenital System		
Vaginitis*	19 (11.4)	3 (1.8)

Symptoms reported in < 5% of patients included: *Body as Whole* - Body odor, Flu syndrome, Injection site reactions; *Cardiovascular System* - Tachycardia; *Digestive System* - Appetite changes, Dry mouth, GI disturbances, Nausea/vomiting; *Metabolic and Nutritional Disorders* - Weight changes; *Musculoskeletal System* - Myalgia; *Nervous System* - Anxiety, Decreased libido,* Dizziness, Insomnia, Nervousness,* Neuromuscular disorders,* Paresthesias; *Respiratory System* - Rhinitis; *Integumentary System* - Androgen-like effects, Nail disorder, Skin reactions; *Special Senses* - Conjunctivitis, Taste perversion; *Urogenital System* - Breast changes,* Menstrual disorders.
* = Physiologic effect of the drug.

In one controlled clinical trial, patients received a higher dose (7.5 mg) of LUPRON DEPOT. Events seen with this dose that were thought to be potentially related to drug and were not seen at the lower dose included palpitations, syncope, glossitis, ecchymosis, hypesthesia, confusion, lactation, pyelonephritis, and urinary disorders. Generally, a higher incidence of hypoestrogenic effects was observed at the higher dose.

Postmarketing
During postmarketing surveillance, the following adverse events were reported. Like other drugs in this class, mood swings, including depression, have been reported as a physiologic effect of decreased sex steroids. There have been very rare reports of suicidal ideation and attempt. Many, but not all, of these patients had a history of depression or other psychiatric illness. Patients should be counseled on the possibility of worsening of depression.
Symptoms consistent with an anaphylactoid or asthmatic process have been rarely reported. Rash, urticaria, and photosensitivity reactions have also been reported.
Localized reactions including induration and abscess have been reported at the site of injection.
Cardiovascular System - Hypotension; *Hemic and Lymphatic System* - Decreased WBC; *Central/Peripheral Nervous System* - Peripheral neuropathy, Spinal fracture/paralysis; *Musculoskeletal System* - Tenosynovitis-like symptoms; *Urogenital System* - Prostate pain.
See other LUPRON DEPOT and LUPRON Injection package inserts for other events reported in different patient populations.

Changes in Bone Density:
A controlled study in endometriosis patients showed that vertebral bone density as measured by dual energy x-ray absorptiometry (DEXA) decreased by an average of 3.2% at six months compared with the pretreatment value. In this same study, LUPRON DEPOT 3.75 mg alone and LUPRON DEPOT 3.75 mg plus three different hormonal add-back regimens were compared for one year. All add-back groups demonstrated mean changes in bone mineral density of ≤1% from baseline and showed statistically significantly (P-value <0.001) less loss of bone density than the group treated with LUPRON DEPOT 3.75 mg alone, at all time points. Clinical studies suggest that the addition of hormonal replacement therapy (estrogen and/or progestin) to LUPRON is effective in reducing loss of bone mineral density which occurs with LUPRON, without compromising the efficacy of LUPRON in relieving symptoms of endometriosis. The optimal drug/dose is not established.
When LUPRON DEPOT 3.75 mg was administered for three months in uterine fibroid patients, vertebral trabecular bone mineral density as assessed by quantitative digital radiography (QDR) revealed a mean decrease of 2.7% compared with baseline. Six months after discontinuation of therapy, a trend toward recovery was observed. Use of LUPRON DEPOT for longer than three months (uterine fibroids) or six months (endometriosis) or in the presence of other known risk factors for decreased bone mineral content may cause additional bone loss and **is not recommended.**

Changes in Laboratory Values During Treatment:
Plasma Enzymes
Endometriosis: During clinical trials with LUPRON DEPOT 3.75 mg, regular laboratory monitoring revealed that AST levels were more than twice the upper limit of normal in only one patient. There was no clinical or other laboratory evidence of abnormal liver function.
Uterine Leiomyomata (Fibroids): In clinical trials with LUPRON DEPOT 3.75 mg, five (3%) patients had a post-treatment transaminase value that was at least twice the baseline value and above the upper limit of the normal range. None of the laboratory increases were associated with clinical symptoms.

Lipids
Endometriosis: At enrollment, 4% of the LUPRON DEPOT 3.75 mg patients and 1% of the danazol patients had total cholesterol values above the normal range. These patients also had cholesterol values above the normal range at the end of treatment.
Of those patients whose pretreatment cholesterol values were in the normal range, 7% of the LUPRON DEPOT 3.75 mg patients and 9% of the danazol patients had post-treatment values above the normal range.
The mean (±SEM) pretreatment values for total cholesterol from all patients were 178.8 (2.9) mg/dL in the LUPRON DEPOT 3.75 mg groups and 175.3 (3.0) mg/dL in the danazol group. At the end of treatment, the mean values for total cholesterol from all patients were 193.3 mg/dL in the LUPRON DEPOT 3.75 mg group and 194.4 mg/dL in the danazol group. These increases from the pretreatment values were statistically significant (p<0.03) in both groups.
Triglycerides were increased above the upper limit of normal in 12% of the patients who received LUPRON DEPOT 3.75 mg and in 6% of the patients who received danazol.
At the end of treatment, HDL cholesterol fractions decreased below the lower limit of the normal range in 2% of the LUPRON DEPOT 3.75 mg patients compared with 54% of those receiving danazol. LDL cholesterol fractions increased above the upper limit of the normal range in 6% of the patients receiving LUPRON DEPOT 3.75 mg compared with 23% of those receiving danazol. There was no increase in the LDL/HDL ratio in patients receiving LUPRON DEPOT 3.75 mg but there was approximately a two-fold increase in the LDL/HDL ratio in patients receiving danazol.
Uterine Leiomyomata (Fibroids): In patients receiving LUPRON DEPOT 3.75 mg, mean changes in cholesterol (+11 mg/dL to +29 mg/dL), LDL cholesterol (+8 mg/dL to +22 mg/dL), HDL cholesterol (0 to +6 mg/dL), and the LDL/HDL ratio (-0.1 to +0.5) were observed across studies. In the one study in which triglycerides were determined, the mean increase from baseline was 32 mg/dL.
Other Changes
Endometriosis: In comparative studies, the following changes were seen in approximately 5% to 8% of patients. LUPRON DEPOT 3.75 mg was associated with elevations of LDH and phosphorus, and decreases in WBC counts. Danazol therapy was associated with increases in hematocrit, platelet count, and LDH.
Uterine Leiomyomata (Fibroids):
Hematology: (See Clinical Studies section.) In LUPRON DEPOT 3.75 mg treated patients, although there were statistically significant mean decreases in platelet counts from baseline to final visit, the last mean platelet counts were within the normal range. Decreases in total WBC count and neutrophils were observed, but were not clinically significant.
Chemistry: Slight to moderate mean increases were noted for glucose, uric acid, BUN, creatinine, total protein, albumin, bilirubin, alkaline phosphatase, LDH, calcium, and phosphorus. None of these increases were clinically significant.

OVERDOSAGE

In rats subcutaneous administration of 250 to 500 times the recommended human dose, expressed on a per body weight basis, resulted in dyspnea, decreased activity, and local irritation at the injection site. There is no evidence that there is a clinical counterpart of this phenomenon. In early clinical trials using daily subcutaneous leuprolide acetate in patients with prostate cancer, doses as high as 20 mg/day for up to two years caused no adverse effects differing from those observed with the 1 mg/day dose.

DOSAGE AND ADMINISTRATION

LUPRON DEPOT Must Be Administered Under The Supervision Of A Physician.
The recommended dose of LUPRON DEPOT is 3.75 mg, incorporated in a depot formulation. The lyophilized microspheres are to be reconstituted and administered monthly as a single intramuscular injection, in accord with the following directions:
Vial and ampule:
1. Using a syringe with a 22 gauge needle, withdraw 1 mL of diluent from the ampule, and inject it into the vial. (Extra diluent is provided; any remaining should be discarded.)
2. Shake well to thoroughly disperse particles to obtain a uniform suspension. The suspension will appear milky.
3. Withdraw the entire contents of the vial into the syringe and inject it at the time of reconstitution.
Although the potency of the reconstituted suspension has been shown to be stable for 24 hours, since the product does not contain a preservative, the suspension should be discarded if not used immediately.
Prefilled dual-chamber syringe:
1. To prepare for injection, screw the white plunger into the end stopper until the stopper begins to turn.
2. Remove and discard the tab around the base of the needle.
3. Holding the syringe upright, release the diluent by SLOWLY PUSHING the plunger until the first stopper is at the blue line in the middle of the barrel.
4. Gently shake the syringe to thoroughly mix the particles to form a uniform suspension. The suspension will appear milky.

5. If the microspheres (particles) adhere to the stopper, tap the syringe against your finger.
6. Then remove the needle guard and advance the plunger to expel the air from the syringe.
7. Inject the entire contents of the syringe intramuscularly as you would for a normal injection.
Although the potency of the reconstituted suspension has been shown to be stable for 24 hours, since the product does not contain a preservative, the suspension should be discarded if not used immediately.

Endometriosis: The recommended duration of administration is six months. Retreatment cannot be recommended since safety data for retreatment are not available. If the symptoms of endometriosis recur after a course of therapy, and further treatment with LUPRON DEPOT 3.75 mg is contemplated, it is recommended that bone density be assessed before retreatment begins to ensure that values are within normal limits.

Uterine Leiomyomata (Fibroids): Recommended duration of therapy with LUPRON DEPOT 3.75 mg is **up to** 3 months. The symptoms associated with uterine leiomyomata will recur following discontinuation of therapy. If additional treatment with LUPRON DEPOT 3.75 mg is contemplated, bone density should be assessed prior to initiation of therapy to ensure that values are within normal limits.
As with other drugs administered by injection, the injection site should be varied periodically.
The vial of LUPRON DEPOT, the ampule, as well as the prefilled dual-chamber syringe, of diluent may be stored at room temperature.

HOW SUPPLIED

LUPRON DEPOT 3.75 mg is packaged in the following forms:
Kit with vial and ampule   (NDC 0300-3639-01)
Multi-pack with six vials and six ampules   (NDC 0300-3639-06)
Kit with prefilled dual-chamber syringe   (NDC 0300-3641-01)
Each vial and syringe contains sterile lyophilized microspheres which is leuprolide incorporated in a biodegradable copolymer of lactic and glycolic acids. When mixed with diluent, LUPRON DEPOT 3.75 mg is administered as a single monthly IM injection.
No refrigeration necessary. Protect from freezing.
Rx only.

REFERENCE

1. MacLeod TL, et al. Anaphylactic reaction to synthetic luteinizing hormone-releasing hormone. *Fertil Steril* 1987 Sept;48(3):500-502.

U.S. Patent Nos. 4,652,441; 4,677,191; 4,728,721; 4,849,228; 4,917,893; 4,954,298; 5,330,767; 5,476,663; 5,575,987; 5,631,020; 5,631,021; and 5,716,640.
TAP Pharmaceuticals Inc.
Deerfield, Illinois 60015-1595, U.S.A.
LUPRON DEPOT 3.75 mg manufactured by
Takeda Chemical Industries, Ltd.
Osaka, JAPAN 541
for TAP Pharmaceuticals Inc.
®-Registered Trademark
Revised: May, 1998
03-4865-R10 (No. 3639, 3641)
Shown in Product Identification Guide, page 341

LUPRON DEPOT® 7.5 mg ℞
(leuprolide acetate for depot suspension)

DESCRIPTION

Leuprolide acetate is a synthetic nonapeptide analog of naturally occurring gonadotropin-releasing hormone (GnRH or LH-RH). The analog possesses greater potency than the natural hormone. The chemical name is 5-oxo-L-prolyl-L-histidyl-L-tryptophyl-L-seryl-L-tyrosyl-D-leucyl-L-leucyl-L-arginyl-N-ethyl-L-prolinamide acetate (salt) with the following structural formula:
[See chemical structure at top of next page]
LUPRON DEPOT is available in a vial containing sterile lyophilized microspheres, which when mixed with diluent, become a suspension which is intended as a monthly intramuscular injection.
The single-dose vial of LUPRON DEPOT 7.5 mg contains leuprolide acetate (7.5 mg), purified gelatin (1.3 mg), DL-lactic and glycolic acids copolymer (66.2 mg), and D-mannitol (13.2 mg). The accompanying ampule of diluent contains carboxymethylcellulose sodium (10 mg), D-mannitol (100 mg), polysorbate 80 (2 mg), water for injection, USP, and glacial acetic acid, USP to control pH.
During the manufacture of LUPRON DEPOT 7.5 mg, acetic acid is lost, leaving the peptide.

Continued on next page

Lupron Depot 7.5 mg—Cont.

CLINICAL PHARMACOLOGY

Leuprolide acetate, an LH-RH agonist, acts as a potent inhibitor of gonadotropin secretion when given continuously and in therapeutic doses. Animal and human studies indicate that following an initial stimulation, chronic administration of leuprolide acetate results in suppression of ovarian and testicular steroidogenesis. This effect is reversible upon discontinuation of drug therapy. Administration of leuprolide acetate has resulted in inhibition of the growth of certain hormone dependent tumors (prostatic tumors in Noble and Dunning male rats and DMBA-induced mammary tumors in female rats) as well as atrophy of the reproductive organs.

In humans, administration of leuprolide acetate results in an initial increase in circulating levels of luteinizing hormone (LH) and follicle stimulating hormone (FSH), leading to a transient increase in levels of the gonadal steroids (testosterone and dihydrotestosterone in males, and estrone and estradiol in premenopausal females). However, continuous administration of leuprolide acetate results in decreased levels of LH and FSH. In males, testosterone is reduced to castrate levels. In premenopausal females, estrogens are reduced to postmenopausal levels. These decreases occur within two to four weeks after initiation of treatment, and castrate levels of testosterone in prostate cancer patients have been demonstrated for more than five years. Leuprolide acetate is not active when given orally.

PHARMACOKINETICS

Absorption: Following a single LUPRON DEPOT 7.5 mg injection to patients, mean peak leuprolide plasma concentration was almost 20 ng/mL at 4 hours and 0.36 ng/mL at 4 weeks. However, intact leuprolide and an inactive major metabolite could not be distinguished by the assay which was employed in the study. Nondetectable leuprolide plasma concentrations have been observed during chronic LUPRON DEPOT 7.5 mg administration, but testosterone levels appear to be maintained at castrate levels.

Distribution: The mean steady-state volume of distribution of leuprolide following intravenous bolus administration to healthy male volunteers was 27 L. In vitro binding to human plasma proteins ranged from 43% to 49%.

Metabolism: In healthy male volunteers, a 1 mg bolus of leuprolide administered intravenously revealed that the mean systemic clearance was 7.6 L/h, with a terminal elimination half-life of approximately 3 hours based on a two compartment model.

In rats and dogs, administration of ^{14}C-labeled leuprolide was shown to be metabolized to smaller inactive peptides, a pentapeptide (Metabolite I), tripeptides (Metabolites II and III) and a dipeptide (Metabolite IV). These fragments may be further catabolized.

The major metabolite (M-I) plasma concentrations measured in 5 prostate cancer patients reached maximum concentration 2 to 6 hours after dosing and were approximately 6% of the peak parent drug concentration. One week after dosing, mean plasma M-I concentrations were approximately 20% of mean leuprolide concentrations.

Excretion: Following administration of LUPRON DEPOT 3.75 mg to 3 patients, less than 5% of the dose was recovered as parent and M-I metabolite in the urine.

Special Populations: The pharmacokinetics of the drug in hepatically and renally impaired patients have not been determined.

INDICATIONS AND USAGE

LUPRON DEPOT 7.5 mg is indicated in the palliative treatment of advanced prostatic cancer. It offers an alternative treatment of prostatic cancer when orchiectomy or estrogen administration are either not indicated or unacceptable to the patient. In clinical trials, the safety and efficacy of LUPRON DEPOT 7.5 mg does not differ from that of the original daily subcutaneous injection.

CONTRAINDICATIONS

A report of an anaphylactic reaction to synthetic GnRH (Factrel) has been reported in the medical literature.[1]

LUPRON DEPOT is contraindicated in women who are or may become pregnant while receiving the drug. When administered on day 6 of pregnancy at test dosages of 0.00024, 0.0024, and 0.024 mg/kg (1/600 to 1/6 the human dose) to rabbits, LUPRON DEPOT produced a dose-related increase in major fetal abnormalities. Similar studies in rats failed to demonstrate an increase in fetal malformations. There was increased fetal mortality and decreased fetal weights with the two higher doses of LUPRON DEPOT in rabbits and with the highest dose in rats. The effects on fetal mortality are logical consequences of the alterations in hormonal levels brought about by this drug. Therefore, the possibility exists that spontaneous abortion may occur if the drug is administered during pregnancy.

WARNINGS

Isolated cases of worsening of signs and symptoms during the first weeks of treatment have been reported with

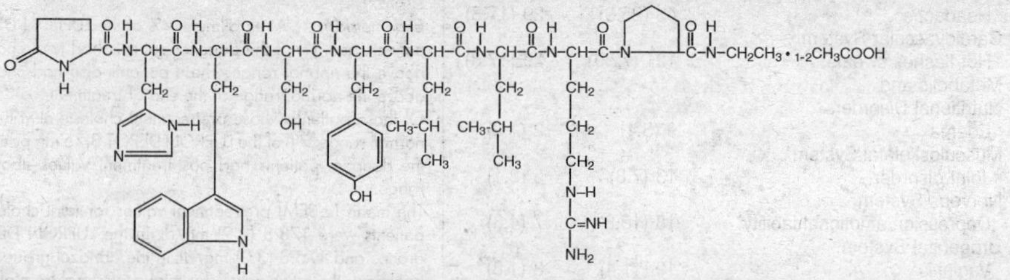

LH-RH analogs. Worsening of symptoms may contribute to paralysis with or without fatal complications. For patients at risk, the physician may consider initiating therapy with daily LUPRON® (leuprolide acetate) Injection for the first two weeks to facilitate withdrawal of treatment if that is considered necessary.

PRECAUTIONS

Patients with metastatic vertebral lesions and/or with urinary tract obstruction should be closely observed during the first few weeks of therapy (see **WARNINGS** section).

Laboratory Tests: Response to LUPRON DEPOT 7.5 mg should be monitored by measuring serum levels of testosterone, as well as prostate-specific antigen and prostatic acid phosphatase. In the majority of patients, testosterone levels increased above baseline during the first week, declining thereafter to baseline levels or below by the end of the second week. Castrate levels were reached within two to four weeks and once achieved were maintained for as long as the patients received their injections. Transient increases in prostatic acid phosphatase levels may occur sometime early in treatment. However, by the fourth week, the elevated levels can be expected to decrease to values at or near baseline.

Drug Interactions: No pharmacokinetic-based drug-drug interaction studies have been conducted with LUPRON DEPOT. However, because leuprolide acetate is a peptide that is primarily degraded by peptidase and not by cytochrome P-450 enzymes as noted in specific studies, and the drug is only about 46% bound to plasma proteins, drug interactions would not be expected to occur.

Drug/Laboratory Test Interactions: Administration of LUPRON DEPOT 3.75 mg in women results in suppression of the pituitary-gonadal system. Normal function is usually restored within three months after treatment is discontinued. Therefore, diagnostic tests of pituitary gonadotropic and gonadal functions conducted during treatment and up to three months after discontinuation of LUPRON DEPOT may be misleading.

Carcinogenesis, Mutagenesis, Impairment of Fertility: Two-year carcinogenicity studies were conducted in rats and mice. In rats, a dose-related increase of benign pituitary hyperplasia and benign pituitary adenomas was noted at 24 months when the drug was administered subcutaneously at high daily doses (0.6 to 4 mg/kg). There was a significant but not dose-related increase of pancreatic islet-cell adenomas in females and of testicular interstitial cell adenomas in males (highest incidence in the low dose group). In mice, no leuprolide acetate-induced tumors or pituitary abnormalities were observed at a dose as high as 60 mg/kg for two years. Patients have been treated with leuprolide acetate for up to three years with doses as high as 10 mg/day and for two years with doses as high as 20 mg/day without demonstrable pituitary abnormalities.

Mutagenicity studies have been performed with leuprolide acetate using bacterial and mammalian systems. These studies provided no evidence of a mutagenic potential.

Clinical and pharmacologic studies in adults (≥18 years) with leuprolide acetate and similar analogs have shown reversibility of fertility suppression when the drug is discontinued after continuous administration for periods of up to 24 weeks.

Pregnancy Category X. (See **CONTRAINDICATIONS** section.)

Pediatric Use: See LUPRON DEPOT-PED® (leuprolide acetate for depot suspension) labeling for the safety and effectiveness of the monthly formulation in children with central precocious puberty.

ADVERSE REACTIONS

In the majority of patients testosterone levels increased above baseline during the first week, declining thereafter to baseline levels or below by the end of the second week of treatment.

Potential exacerbations of signs and symptoms during the first few weeks of treatment is a concern in patients with vertebral metastases and/or urinary obstruction or hematuria which, if aggravated, may lead to neurological problems such as temporary weakness and/or paresthesia of the lower limbs or worsening of urinary symptoms (see **WARNINGS** section).

In a clinical trial of LUPRON DEPOT 7.5 mg, the following adverse reactions were reported to have a possible or probable relationship to drug as ascribed by the treating physician in 5% or more of the patients receiving the drug. **Often, causality is difficult to assess in patients with metastatic prostate cancer.** Reactions considered not drug-related are excluded.

	LUPRON DEPOT 7.5 mg N=56	(Percent)
Cardiovascular System		
Edema	7	(12.5%)
Gastrointestinal System		
Nausea/vomiting	3	(5.4%)
Endocrine System		
*Decreased testicular size	3	(5.4%)
*Hot flashes/sweats	33	(58.9%)
*Impotence	3	(5.4%)
Central/Peripheral Nervous System		
General pain	4	(7.1%)
Respiratory System		
Dyspnea	3	(5.4%)
Miscellaneous		
Asthenia	3	(5.4%)

*Physiologic effect of decreased testosterone.

Laboratory: Elevations of certain parameters were observed, but it is difficult to assess these abnormalities in this population.

SGOT (>2N)	4	(7.1%)
LDH (>2N)	11	(19.6%)
Alkaline phos (>1.5N)	4	(7.1%)

In this same study, the following adverse reactions were reported in less than 5% of the patients on LUPRON DEPOT 7.5 mg.

Cardiovascular System—Angina, Cardiac arrhythmia; *Gastrointestinal System*—Anorexia, Diarrhea; *Endocrine System*—Gynecomastia, Libido decrease; *Musculoskeletal System*—Bone pain, Myalgia; *Central/Peripheral Nervous System*—Paresthesia, Insomnia; *Respiratory System*—Hemoptysis; *Integumentary System*—Dermatitis, Local skin reactions, Hair growth; *Urogenital System*—Dysuria, Frequency/urgency, Hematuria, Testicular pain; *Miscellaneous*—Diabetes, Fever/chills, Hard nodule in throat, Increased calcium, Weight gain, Increased uric acid.

Postmarketing

During postmarketing surveillance, which includes other dosage forms, the following adverse events were reported.

Symptoms consistent with an anaphylactoid or asthmatic process have been rarely reported with GnRH analogs. Rash, urticaria, and photosensitivity reactions have also been reported.

Localized reactions including induration and abscess have been reported at the site of injection.

Cardiovascular System—Hypotension; *Hemic and Lymphatic System*— Decreased WBC; *Central/Peripheral Nervous System*—Peripheral neuropathy, Spinal fracture/paralysis; *Musculoskeletal System*—Tenosynovitis-like symptoms; *Urogenital System*—Prostate pain.

See other LUPRON DEPOT and LUPRON Injection package inserts for other events reported in different patient populations.

OVERDOSAGE

In rats subcutaneous administration of 250 to 500 times the recommended human dose, expressed on a per body weight basis, resulted in dyspnea, decreased activity, and local irritation at the injection site. There is no evidence that there is a clinical counterpart of this phenomenon. In early clinical trials with daily subcutaneous leuprolide acetate, doses as high as 20 mg/day for up to two years caused no adverse effects differing from those observed with the 1 mg/day dose.

DOSAGE AND ADMINISTRATION

LUPRON DEPOT Must Be Administered Under The Supervision Of A Physician.

The recommended dose of LUPRON DEPOT is 7.5 mg, incorporated in a depot formulation. The lyophilized microspheres are to be reconstituted and administered monthly as a single intramuscular injection, in accord with the following directions:

1. Using a syringe with a 22 gauge needle, withdraw 1 mL of diluent from the ampule, and inject it into the vial.

(Extra diluent is provided; any remaining should be discarded.)
2. Shake well to thoroughly disperse particles to obtain a uniform suspension. The suspension will appear milky.
3. Withdraw the entire contents of the vial into the syringe and inject it at the time of reconstitution.

Although the potency of the reconstituted suspension has been shown to be stable for 24 hours, since the product does not contain a preservative, the suspension should be discarded if not used immediately.
As with other drugs administered by injection, the injection site should be varied periodically.
The vial of LUPRON DEPOT 7.5 mg and the ampule of diluent may be stored at room temperature.

HOW SUPPLIED

LUPRON DEPOT 7.5 mg is available in a single use kit (NDC 0300-3629-01) and in a six pack of drug only (NDC 0300-3629-06). Each vial contains sterile lyophilized microspheres which is leuprolide incorporated in a biodegradable copolymer of lactic and glycolic acids. When mixed with 1 mL of diluent, LUPRON DEPOT 7.5 mg is administered as a single monthly IM injection.
An information pamphlet for patients is included with the kit.
No refrigeration necessary. Protect from freezing.
Caution: Federal (U.S.A.) law prohibits dispensing without a prescription.

REFERENCE

1. MacLeod TL, et al. Anaphylactic reaction to synthetic luteinizing hormone-releasing hormone. Fertil Steril 1987 Sept; 48(3):500–502.

U.S. Patent Nos. 4,652,441; 4,677,191; 4,728,721; 4,849,228; 4,917,893; 4,954,298; 5,330,767; and 5,476,663.
TAP Pharmaceuticals Inc.
Deerfield, Illinois 60015-1595, U.S.A.
LUPRON DEPOT 7.5 mg manufactured by
Takeda Chemical Industries, Ltd.
Osaka, JAPAN 541
®—Registered Trademark
(No. 3629)
03-4808-R8–Rev. June, 1997

Shown in Product Identification Guide, page 340

This is combined labeling. Examples of different fonts appear below.
- General information
- Information on endometrosis
- **Information on uterine fibroids**

LUPRON DEPOT®–3 Month 11.25 mg ℞
(leuprolide acetate for depot suspension)

3-MONTH FORMULATION

DESCRIPTION

Leuprolide acetate is a synthetic nonapeptide analog of naturally occurring gonadotropin-releasing hormone (GnRH or LH-RH). The analog possesses greater potency than the natural hormone. The chemical name is 5-oxo-L-prolyl-L-histidyl-L-tryptophyl-L-seryl-L-tyrosyl-D-leucyl-L-leucyl-L-arginyl-N-ethyl-L-prolinamide acetate (salt) with the following structural formula:
[See chemical structure above]

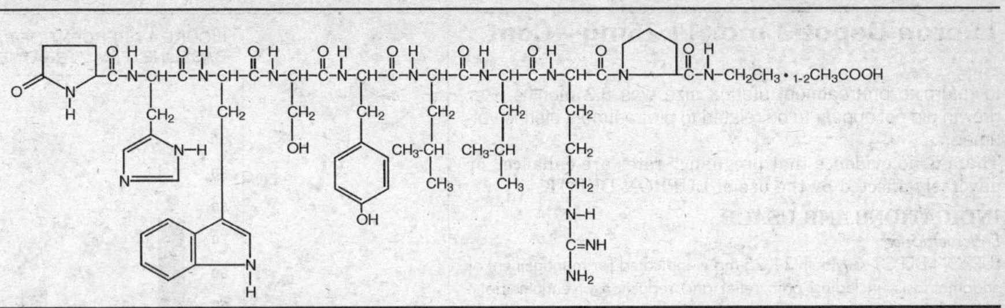

LUPRON DEPOT–3 Month 11.25 mg is available in a vial containing sterile lyophilized microspheres, which when mixed with diluent, become a suspension which is intended as an intramuscular injection.
LUPRON DEPOT–3 Month 11.25 mg is to be given **ONCE EVERY THREE MONTHS.** The single-dose vial contains leuprolide acetate (11.25 mg), polylactic acid (99.3 mg), and D-mannitol (19.45 mg). The accompanying ampule of diluent contains carboxymethylcellulose sodium (10 mg), D-mannitol (100 mg), polysorbate 80 (2 mg), water for injection, USP, and glacial acetic acid, USP to control pH.
During the manufacture of LUPRON DEPOT-3 Month 11.25 mg, acetic acid is lost, leaving the peptide.

CLINICAL PHARMACOLOGY

Leuprolide acetate is a long-acting GnRH analog. A single injection of LUPRON DEPOT–3 Month 11.25 mg will result in an initial stimulation followed by a prolonged suppression of pituitary gonadotropins. Repeated dosing at quarterly (LUPRON DEPOT–3 Month 11.25 mg) intervals results in decreased secretion of gonadal steroids; consequently, tissues and functions that depend on gonadal steroids for their maintenance become quiescent. This effect is reversible on discontinuation of drug therapy.
Leuprolide acetate is not active when given orally.

PHARMACOKINETICS

Absorption: Following a single injection of the three month formulation of LUPRON DEPOT–3 Month 11.25 mg in female subjects, a mean plasma leuprolide concentration of 36.3 ng/mL was observed at 4 hours. Leuprolide appeared to be released at a constant rate following the onset of steady-state levels during the third week after dosing and mean levels then declined gradually to near the lower limit of detection by 12 weeks. The mean (± standard deviation) leuprolide concentration from 3 to 12 weeks was 0.23 ± 0.09 ng/mL. However, intact leuprolide and an inactive major metabolite could not be distinguished by the assay which was employed in the study. The initial burst, followed by the rapid decline to a steady-state level, was similar to the release pattern seen with the monthly formulation.
Distribution: The mean steady-state volume of distribution of leuprolide following intravenous bolus administration to healthy male volunteers was 27 L. In vitro binding to human plasma proteins ranged from 43% to 49%.
Metabolism: In healthy male volunteers, a 1 mg bolus of leuprolide administered intravenously revealed that the mean systemic clearance was 7.6 L/h, with a terminal elimination half-life of approximately 3 hours based on a two compartment model.
In rats and dogs, administration of ^{14}C-labeled leuprolide was shown to be metabolized to smaller inactive peptides, a pentapeptide (Metabolite I), tripeptides (Metabolites II and III) and a dipeptide (Metabolite IV). These fragments may be further catabolized.
The major metabolite (M-I) plasma concentrations measured in 5 prostate cancer patients reached maximum concentration 2 to 6 hours after dosing and were approximately 6% of the peak parent drug concentration. One week after dosing, mean plasma M-I concentrations were approximately 20% of mean leuprolide concentrations.
Excretion: Following administration of LUPRON DEPOT 3.75 mg to 3 patients, less than 5% of the dose was recovered as parent and M-I metabolite in the urine.
Special Populations: The pharmacokinetics of the drug in hepatically and renally impaired patients have not been determined.
Drug Interactions: No pharmacokinetic-based drug-drug interaction studies have been conducted with LUPRON DEPOT. However, because leuprolide acetate is a peptide that is primarily degraded by peptidase and not by cytochrome P-450 enzymes as noted in specific studies, and the drug is only about 46% bound to plasma proteins, drug interactions would not be expected to occur.

CLINICAL STUDIES

In a pharmacokinetic/pharmacodynamic study of healthy female subjects (N=20), the onset of estradiol suppression was observed for individual subjects between day 4 and week 4 after dosing. By the third week following the injection, the mean estradiol concentration (8 pg/mL) was in the menopausal range. Throughout the remainder of the dosing period, mean serum estradiol levels ranged from the menopausal to the early follicular range.
Serum estradiol was suppressed to ≤20 pg/mL in all subjects within four weeks and remained suppressed (≤40 pg/mL) in 80% of subjects until the end of the 12-week dosing interval, at which time two of these subjects had a value between 40 and 50 pg/mL. Four additional subjects had at least two consecutive elevations of estradiol (range 43–240 pg/mL) levels during the 12-week dosing interval, but there was no indication of luteal function for any of the subjects during this period.
LUPRON DEPOT–3 Month 11.25 mg induced amenorrhea in 85% (N=17) of subjects during the initial month and 100% during the second month following the injection. All subjects remained amenorrheic through the remainder of the 12-week dosing interval. Episodes of light bleeding and spotting were reported by a majority of subjects during the first month after the injection and in a few subjects at later time-points. Menses resumed on average 12 weeks (range 2.9 to 20.4 weeks) following the end of the 12-week dosing interval.
LUPRON DEPOT–3 Month 11.25 mg produced similar pharmacodynamic effects in terms of hormonal and menstrual suppression to those achieved with monthly injections of LUPRON DEPOT 3.75 mg during the controlled clinical trials for the management of endometriosis and the anemia caused by uterine fibroids.
Endometriosis: In controlled clinical studies, LUPRON DEPOT 3.75 mg monthly for six months was shown to be comparable to danazol 800 mg/day in relieving the clinical sign/symptoms of endometriosis (pelvic pain, dysmenorrhea, dyspareunia, pelvic tenderness, and induration) and in reducing the size of endometrial implants as evidenced by laparoscopy. The clinical significance of a decrease in endometriotic lesions is not known at this time, and in addition laparoscopic staging of endometriosis does not necessarily correlate with the severity of symptoms.
LUPRON DEPOT 3.75 mg monthly induced amenorrhea in 74% and 98% of the patients after the first and second treatment months respectively. Most of the remaining patients reported episodes of only light bleeding or spotting. In the first, second and third post-treatment months, normal menstrual cycles resumed in 7%, 71% and 95% respectively, of those patients who did not become pregnant.
Figure 1 illustrates the percent of patients with symptoms at baseline, final treatment visit and sustained relief at six and 12 months following discontinuation of treatment for the various symptoms evaluated during the two controlled clinical studies. A total of 166 patients received LUPRON DEPOT 3.75 mg. Seventy-five percent (n=125) of these elected to participate in the follow-up periods. Of these patients, 36% and 24% are included in the six month and 12 month follow-up analysis, respectively. All the patients who had a pain evaluation at baseline and at a minimum of one treatment visit, are included in the Baseline (B) and final treatment visit (F) analysis.
[See figure 1 at top of next page]
Hormonal replacement therapy: Clinical studies suggest that the addition of hormonal replacement therapy (estrogen and/or progestin) to LUPRON is effective in reducing loss of bone mineral density which occurs with LUPRON, without compromising the efficacy of LUPRON in relieving symptoms of endometriosis. The optimal drug/dose is not established.
Uterine Leiomyomata (Fibroids): LUPRON DEPOT 3.75 mg for a period of three to six months was studied in four controlled clinical trials.
In one of these clinical studies, enrollment was based on hematocrit ≤30% and/or hemoglobin ≤10.2 g/dL. Administration of LUPRON DEPOT 3.75 mg, concomitantly with iron, produced an increase of ≥ 6% hematocrit and ≥ 2 g/dL hemoglobin in 77% of patients at three months of therapy. The mean change in hematocrit was 10.1% and the mean change in hemoglobin was 4.2 g/dL. Clinical response was judged to be a hematocrit of ≥ 36% and hemoglobin of ≥ 12 g/dL, thus allowing for autologous blood donation prior to surgery. At two and three months respectively, 71% and 75% of patients met this criterion (Table 1). These data suggest however, that some patients may benefit from iron alone or 1 to 2 months of LUPRON DEPOT 3.75 mg.

Table 1:
PERCENT OF PATIENTS ACHIEVING HEMATOCRIT ≥ 36% AND HEMOGLOBIN ≥ 12 GM/DL

Treatment Group	Week 4	Week 8	Week 12
LUPRON DEPOT 3.75 mg			
with Iron (N=104)	40*	71**	75*
Iron Alone (N=98)	17	39	49

* P-Value <0.01
** P-Value <0.001

Excessive vaginal bleeding (menorrhagia or menometrorrhagia) decreased in 80% of patients at three months. Episodes of spotting and menstrual-like bleeding were noted in 16% of patients at final visit.
In this same study, a decrease of ≥ 25% was seen in uterine and myoma volumes in 60% and 54% of patients respectively. LUPRON DEPOT 3.75 mg was found to relieve symptoms of bloating, pelvic pain, and pressure.
In three other controlled clinical trials, enrollment was not based on hematologic status. Mean uterine volume decreased by 41% and myoma volume decreased by 37% at final visit as evidenced by ultrasound or MRI. These patients also experienced a decrease in symptoms including excessive vaginal bleeding and pelvic discomfort. Ninety-five percent of these patients became amenorrheic with 61%, 25%, and 4% experiencing amenorrhea during the first, second, and third treatment months respectively.
In addition, posttreatment follow-up was carried out in one clinical trial for a small percentage of LUPRON DEPOT 3.75 mg patients (N=46) among the 77% who demonstrated a ≥ 25% decrease in uterine volume while on therapy. Menses usually returned within two months of cessation of therapy. Mean time

Continued on next page

Lupron Depot-3 mo. 11.25mg—Cont.

to return to pretreatment uterine size was 8.3 months. Regrowth did not appear to be related to pretreatment uterine volume.

There is no evidence that pregnancy rates are enhanced or adversely affected by the use of LUPRON DEPOT.

INDICATIONS AND USAGE

Endometriosis:
LUPRON DEPOT–3 Month 11.25 mg is indicated for management of endometriosis, including pain relief and reduction of endometriotic lesions.

Experience with LUPRON DEPOT in females has been limited to women 18 years of age and older treated for no more than 6 months.

Uterine Leiomyomata (Fibroids):
LUPRON DEPOT–3 Month 11.25 mg concomitantly with iron therapy is indicated for the preoperative hematologic improvement of patients with anemia caused by uterine leiomyomata. The clinician may wish to consider a one-month trial period on iron alone inasmuch as some of the patients will respond to iron alone (see Table 1, **CLINICAL STUDIES** section). LUPRON may be added if the response to iron alone is considered inadequate. Recommended therapy is a single injection of LUPRON DEPOT–3 Month 11.25 mg. This dosage form is indicated only for women for whom three months of hormonal suppression is deemed necessary.

Experience with LUPRON DEPOT in females has been limited to women 18 years of age and older treated for no more than 6 months.

CONTRAINDICATIONS

1. Hypersensitivity to GnRH, GnRH agonist analogs or any of the excipients in LUPRON DEPOT. A report of an anaphylactic reaction to synthetic GnRH (Factrel) has been reported in the medical literature.[1]
2. LUPRON DEPOT is contraindicated in women who are or may become pregnant while receiving the drug. LUPRON DEPOT may cause fetal harm when administered to a pregnant woman. Major fetal abnormalities were observed in rabbits but not in rats after administration of LUPRON DEPOT throughout gestation. There was increased fetal mortality and decreased fetal weights in rats and rabbits (see *Pregnancy* section). The effects on fetal mortality are expected consequences of the alterations in hormonal levels brought about by the drug. If this drug is used during pregnancy or if the patient becomes pregnant while taking this drug, she should be apprised of the potential hazard to the fetus.
3. Use in women who are breast feeding (see *Nursing Mothers* section).
4. Undiagnosed abnormal vaginal bleeding.

WARNINGS

1. As the effects of LUPRON DEPOT–3 Month 11.25 mg are present throughout the course of therapy, the drug should only be used in patients who require hormonal suppression for at least three months.
2. Experience with LUPRON DEPOT in females has been limited to six months; therefore, exposure should be limited to six months of therapy.
3. When used at the recommended dose and dosing interval, LUPRON DEPOT usually inhibits ovulation and stops menstruation. Contraception is not insured, however, by taking LUPRON DEPOT. Therefore, patients should use nonhormonal methods of contraception. Patients should be advised to see their physician if they believe they may be pregnant. If a patient becomes pregnant during treatment, the drug must be discontinued and the patient must be apprised of the potential risk to the fetus (see **CONTRAINDICATIONS** section).
4. During the early phase of therapy, sex steroids temporarily rise above baseline because of the physiologic effect of the drug. Therefore, an increase in clinical signs and symptoms may be observed during the initial days of therapy, but these will dissipate with continued therapy.

PRECAUTIONS

Information for Patients: An information pamphlet for patients is included with the product. Patients should be aware of the following information:
1. Since menstruation should stop with effective doses of LUPRON DEPOT, the patient should notify her physician if regular menstruation persists. Patients missing successive doses of LUPRON DEPOT may experience breakthrough bleeding.
2. Patients should not use LUPRON DEPOT if they are pregnant, breast feeding, have undiagnosed abnormal vaginal bleeding, or are allergic to any of the ingredients in LUPRON DEPOT.
3. LUPRON DEPOT is contraindicated for use during pregnancy. Therefore, a nonhormonal method of contraception should be used during treatment. Patients should be advised that if they miss successive doses of LUPRON DEPOT, breakthrough bleeding or ovulation may occur with the potential for conception. If a patient becomes pregnant during treatment, she should discontinue treatment and consult her physician.

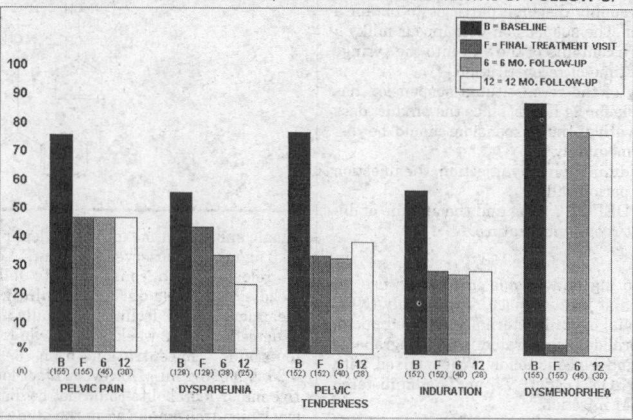

FIGURE 1 - PERCENT OF PATIENTS WITH SIGN/SYMPTOMS OF ENDOMETRIOSIS AT BASELINE, FINAL TREATMENT VISIT, AND AFTER 6 AND 12 MONTHS OF FOLLOW-UP

4. Adverse events occurring in clinical studies with LUPRON DEPOT that are associated with hypoestrogenism include: hot flashes, headaches, emotional lability, decreased libido, acne, myalgia, reduction in breast size, and vaginal dryness. Estrogen levels returned to normal after treatment was discontinued.
5. The induced hypoestrogenic state **also** results in a small loss in bone density over the course of treatment, which may not be fully reversible. In patients with major risk factors for decreased bone mineral content such as chronic alcohol and/or tobacco use, strong family history of osteoporosis, or chronic use of drugs that can reduce bone mass such as anticonvulsants or corticosteroids, LUPRON DEPOT therapy may pose an additional risk. In these patients, the risks and benefits must be weighed carefully before therapy with LUPRON DEPOT is instituted. Clinical studies suggest that the addition of hormonal replacement therapy (estrogen and/or progestin) to LUPRON is effective in reducing loss of bone mineral density which occurs with LUPRON, without compromising the efficacy of LUPRON in relieving symptoms of endometriosis. The optimal drug/dose is not established.
6. Retreatment for more than six months cannot be recommended since safety data beyond six months are not available.

Drug/Laboratory Test Interactions: Administration of LUPRON DEPOT in therapeutic doses results in suppression of the pituitary-gonadal system. Normal function is usually restored within three months after treatment is discontinued. Due to the suppression of the pituitary-gonadal system by LUPRON DEPOT, diagnostic tests of pituitary gonadotropic and gonadal functions conducted during treatment and for up to three months after discontinuation of LUPRON DEPOT may be affected.

Carcinogenesis, Mutagenesis, Impairment of Fertility: A two-year carcinogenicity study was conducted in rats and mice. In rats, a dose-related increase of benign pituitary hyperplasia and benign pituitary adenomas was noted at 24 months when the drug was administered subcutaneously at high daily doses (0.6 to 4 mg/kg). There was a significant but not dose-related increase of pancreatic islet-cell adenomas in females and of testicular interstitial cell adenomas in males (highest incidence in the low dose group). In mice, no leuprolide acetate-induced tumors or pituitary abnormalities were observed at a dose as high as 60 mg/kg for two years. Patients have been treated with leuprolide acetate for up to three years with doses as high as 10 mg/day and for two years with doses as high as 20 mg/day without demonstrable pituitary abnormalities.

Mutagenicity studies have been performed with leuprolide acetate using bacterial and mammalian systems. These studies provided no evidence of a mutagenic potential.

Clinical and pharmacologic studies in adults (> 18 years) with leuprolide acetate and similar analogs have shown reversibility of fertility suppression when the drug is discontinued after continuous administration for periods of up to 24 weeks.

Pregnancy, Teratogenic Effects: Pregnancy Category X. (See **CONTRAINDICATIONS** section.) When administered on day 6 of pregnancy at test dosages of 0.00024, 0.0024, and 0.024 mg/kg (1/300 to 1/3 the human dose) to rabbits, LUPRON DEPOT produced a dose-related increase in major fetal abnormalities. Similar studies in rats failed to demonstrate an increase in fetal malformations. There was increased fetal mortality and decreased fetal weights with the two higher doses of LUPRON DEPOT in rabbits and with the highest dose (0.024 mg/kg) in rats.

Nursing Mothers: It is not known whether LUPRON DEPOT is excreted in human milk. Because many drugs are excreted in human milk, and because the effects of LUPRON DEPOT on lactation and/or the breast-fed child

have not been determined, LUPRON DEPOT should not be used by nursing mothers.

Pediatric Use: Safety and effectiveness of LUPRON DEPOT–3 Month 11.25 mg have not been established in pediatric patients. See LUPRON DEPOT-PED® (leuprolide acetate for depot suspension) labeling for the safety and effectiveness in children with central precocious puberty.

ADVERSE REACTIONS

The **monthly formulation of LUPRON DEPOT 3.75 mg** was utilized in controlled clinical trials that studied the drug in 166 endometriosis and 166 uterine fibroids patients. Adverse events reported in ≥ 5% of patients in either of these populations and thought to be potentially related to drug are noted in the following table.

[See table 2 at bottom of next page]

In these same studies, symptoms reported in < 5% of patients included: *Body as a Whole* - Body odor, Flu syndrome, Injection site reactions; *Cardiovascular System* - Palpitations, Syncope, Tachycardia; *Digestive System* - Appetite changes, Dry mouth, Thirst; *Endocrine System* - Androgen-like effects; *Hemic and Lymphatic Systems*- Ecchymosis, Lymphadenopathy; *Nervous System*- Anxiety,* Insomnia/Sleep disorders,* Delusions, Memory disorder, Personality disorder; *Respiratory System* - Rhinitis; *Skin and Appendages* - Alopecia, Hair disorder, Nail disorder; *Special Senses* - Conjunctivitis, Ophthalmologic disorders,* Taste perversion; *Urogenital System*- Dysuria,* Lactation, Menstrual disorders.

* = Physiologic effect of the drug.

In one controlled clinical trial utilizing the monthly formulation of LUPRON DEPOT, patients diagnosed with uterine fibroids received a higher dose (7.5 mg) of LUPRON DEPOT. Events seen with this dose that were thought to be potentially related to drug and were not seen at the lower dose included glossitis, hypesthesia, lactation, pyelonephritis, and urinary disorders. Generally, a higher incidence of hypoestrogenic effects was observed at the higher dose.

In a pharmacokinetic trial involving 20 healthy female subjects receiving LUPRON DEPOT–3 Month 11.25 mg, a few adverse events were reported with this formulation that were not reported previously. These included face edema, agitation, laryngitis, and ear pain.

Changes in Bone Density:
In controlled clinical studies, patients with endometriosis (six months of therapy) or uterine fibroids (three months of therapy) were treated with LUPRON DEPOT 3.75 mg. In endometriosis patients, vertebral bone density as measured by dual energy x-ray absorptiometry (DEXA) decreased by an average of 3.2% at six months compared with the pretreatment value. In this same study, LUPRON DEPOT 3.75 mg alone and LUPRON DEPOT 3.75 mg plus three different hormonal add-back regimens were compared for one year. All add-back groups demonstrated mean changes in bone mineral density of ≤1% from baseline and showed statistically significantly (P-value <0.001) less loss of bone density than the group treated with LUPRON DEPOT 3.75 mg alone, at all time points. Clinical studies suggest that the addition of hormonal replacement therapy (estrogen and/or progestin) to LUPRON is effective in reducing loss of bone mineral density which occurs with LUPRON, without compromising the efficacy of LUPRON in relieving symptoms of endometriosis. The optimal drug/dose is not established.

When LUPRON DEPOT 3.75 mg was administered for three months in uterine fibroid patients, vertebral trabecular bone mineral density as assessed by quantitative digital radiography (QDR) revealed a mean decrease of 2.7% compared with baseline. Six months after discontinuation of therapy, a trend toward recovery was observed. Use of LUPRON DEPOT for longer than three months (uterine fibroids) or six months (endometriosis) or in the presence of

other known risk factors for decreased bone mineral content may cause additional bone loss **and is not recommended.**

Changes in Laboratory Values During Treatment
Liver Enzymes
Three percent of uterine fibroid patients treated with LUPRON DEPOT 3.75 mg, manifested posttreatment transaminase values that were at least twice the baseline value and above the upper limit of the normal range. None of the laboratory increases were associated with clinical symptoms.
Lipids
Triglycerides were increased above the upper limit of normal in 12% of the endometriosis patients who received LUPRON DEPOT 3.75 mg and in 32% of the subjects receiving LUPRON DEPOT-3 Month 11.25 mg.
Of those endometriosis and uterine fibroid patients whose pretreatment cholesterol values were in the normal range, mean change following therapy was +16 mg/dL to +17 mg/dL in endometriosis patients and +11 mg/dL to +29 mg/dL in uterine fibroid patients. In the endometriosis treated patients, increases from the pretreatment values were statistically significant (p<0.03). There was essentially no increase in the LDL/HDL ratio in patients from either population receiving LUPRON DEPOT 3.75 mg.

Postmarketing
During postmarketing surveillance with other dosage forms and in the same and/or different populations, the following adverse events were reported. Like other drugs in this class, mood swings, including depression, have been reported as a physiologic effect of decreased sex steroids. There have been very rare reports of suicidal ideation and attempt. Many, but not all, of these patients had a history of depression or other psychiatric illness. Patients should be counseled on the possibility of worsening of depression.
Symptoms consistent with an anaphylactoid or asthmatic process have been reported. Rash, urticaria, and photosensitivity reactions have also been reported.
Localized reactions including induration and abscess have been reported at the site of injection.
Symptoms consistent with fibromyalgia (eg: joint and muscle pain, headaches, sleep disorders, gastrointestinal distress, and shortness of breath) have been reported individually and collectively.
Cardiovascular System - Hypotension, Pulmonary embolism; *Hemic and Lymphatic System* - Decreased WBC; *Central/Peripheral Nervous System* - Peripheral neuropathy, Spinal fracture/paralysis; *Musculoskeletal System* - Tenosynovitis-like symptoms; *Urogenital System* - Prostate pain.
See other LUPRON DEPOT and LUPRON Injection package inserts for other events reported in the same and different patient populations.

OVERDOSAGE
In clinical trials using daily subcutaneous leuprolide acetate in patients with prostate cancer, doses as high as 20 mg/day for up to two years caused no adverse effects differing from those observed with the 1 mg/day dose.

DOSAGE AND ADMINISTRATION
LUPRON DEPOT Must Be Administered Under the Supervision of a Physician.
Endometriosis: The recommended dose of LUPRON DEPOT-3 Month 11.25 mg is one injection every three months, for a maximum recommended duration of six months. Retreatment cannot be recommended since safety data for retreatment are not available. If the symptoms of endometriosis recur after a course of therapy, and further treatment with LUPRON DEPOT-3 Month 11.25 mg is contemplated, it is recommended that bone density be assessed before retreatment begins to ensure that values are within normal limits.
Uterine Leiomyomata (Fibroids): The recommended dose of LUPRON DEPOT-3 Month 11.25 mg is one injection. The symptoms associated with uterine leiomyomata will recur following discontinuation of therapy. If additional treatment with LUPRON DEPOT-3 Month 11.25 mg is contemplated, bone density should be assessed prior to initiation of therapy to ensure that values are within normal limits.
Due to different release characteristics, a fractional dose of the 3-month depot formulation is not equivalent to the same dose of the monthly formulation and should not be given.
Incorporated in a depot formulation, the lyophilized microspheres are to be reconstituted and administered as a single intramuscular injection, in accord with the following directions:
1. Using a syringe with a 22 gauge needle, withdraw 1.5 mL of diluent from the ampule, and inject it into the vial. (Extra diluent is provided; any remaining should be discarded.)
2. Shake well to thoroughly disperse particles to obtain a uniform suspension. The suspension will appear milky.
3. Withdraw the entire contents of the vial into the syringe and inject it at the time of reconstitution.
The suspension settles very quickly following reconstitution; therefore, it is preferable that LUPRON DEPOT-3 Month 11.25 mg be mixed and used immediately. Reshake suspension if settling occurs.
Although the potency of the reconstituted suspension has been shown to be stable for 24 hours, since the product does not contain a preservative, the suspension should be discarded if not used immediately.
As with other drugs administered by injection, the injection site should be varied periodically.
The vial of LUPRON DEPOT and the ampule of diluent may be stored at room temperature.

HOW SUPPLIED
LUPRON DEPOT-3 Month 11.25 mg (NDC 0300-3343-01) is available in a single use kit. Each kit contains a vial of sterile lyophilized microspheres which is leuprolide incorporated in a biodegradable polymer of polylactic acid. When mixed with 1.5 mL of accompanying diluent, LUPRON DEPOT-3 Month 11.25 mg is administered as a single IM injection **EVERY THREE MONTHS.**
No refrigeration necessary. Protect from freezing.

Rx only

REFERENCE
1. MacLeod TL, et al. Anaphylactic reaction to synthetic luteinizing hormone-releasing hormone. *Fertil Steril* 1987 Sept;48(3):500-502.

U.S. Patent Nos. 4,652,441; 4,728,721; 4,849,228; 4,917,893; 4,954,298; 5,330,767; 5,476,663; 5,480,656; 5,575,987; 5,631,020; 5,631,021; 5,643,607; and 5,716,640.

TAP Pharmaceuticals Inc.
Deerfield, Illinois 60015-1595, U.S.A.

LUPRON DEPOT-3 Month 11.25 mg
manufactured by
Takeda Chemical Industries, Ltd.
Osaka, JAPAN 541
for TAP Pharmaceuticals Inc.

® - Registered Trademark
Revised: May, 1998
03-4864-R3 (No. 3343)
Shown in Product Identification Guide, page 340

LUPRON DEPOT®-3 Month 22.5 mg ℞
(leuprolide acetate for depot suspension)

3-MONTH FORMULATION

DESCRIPTION
Leuprolide acetate is a synthetic nonapeptide analog of naturally occurring gonadotropin-releasing hormone (GnRH or LH-RH). The analog possesses greater potency than the natural hormone. The chemical name is 5-oxo-L-prolyl-L-histidyl-L-tryptophyl -L- seryl-L-tyrosyl-D-leucyl-L- leucyl-L-arginyl-N-ethyl-L-prolinamide acetate (salt) with the following structural formula:
[See chemical structure at top of next page]
LUPRON DEPOT-3 Month 22.5 mg is available in a vial containing sterile lyophilized microspheres, which when mixed with diluent, become a suspension which is intended as an intramuscular injection to be given **ONCE EVERY THREE MONTHS (84 days).**
The single-dose vial of LUPRON DEPOT-3 Month 22.5 mg contains leuprolide acetate (22.5 mg), polylactic acid (198.6 mg), and D-mannitol (38.9 mg). The accompanying ampule of diluent contains carboxymethylcellulose sodium (10 mg), D-mannitol (100 mg), polysorbate 80 (2 mg), water for injection, USP, and glacial acetic acid, USP to control pH.
During the manufacture of LUPRON DEPOT-3 Month 22.5 mg, acetic acid is lost, leaving the peptide.

CLINICAL PHARMACOLOGY
Leuprolide acetate, an LH-RH agonist, acts as a potent inhibitor of gonadotropin secretion when given continuously and in therapeutic doses. Animal and human studies indicate that following an initial stimulation, chronic administration of leuprolide acetate results in suppression of ovarian and testicular steroidogenesis. This effect is reversible upon discontinuation of drug therapy. Administration of leuprolide acetate has resulted in inhibition of the growth of certain hormone dependent tumors (prostatic tumors in Noble and Dunning male rats and DMBA-induced mammary tumors in female rats) as well as atrophy of the reproductive organs.
In humans, administration of leuprolide acetate results in an initial increase in circulating levels of luteinizing hormone (LH) and follicle stimulating hormone (FSH), leading to a transient increase in levels of the gonadal steroids (testosterone and dihydrotestosterone in males, and estrone and estradiol in premenopausal females). However, continuous administration of leuprolide acetate results in decreased levels of LH and FSH. In males, testosterone is reduced to castrate levels. In premenopausal females, estrogens are reduced to postmenopausal levels. These decreases occur within two to four weeks after initiation of treatment, and castrate levels of testosterone in prostatic cancer patients have been demonstrated for more than five years. Leuprolide acetate is not active when given orally.

PHARMACOKINETICS
Absorption: Following a single injection of the three month formulation of LUPRON DEPOT-3 Month 22.5 mg in patients, mean peak plasma leuprolide concentration of 48.9 ng/mL was observed at 4 hours and then declined to 0.67 ng/mL at 12 weeks. Leuprolide appeared to be released at a constant rate following the onset of steady-state levels during the third week after dosing, providing steady plasma concentrations through the 12-week dosing interval. However, intact leuprolide and an inactive major metabolite could not be distinguished by the assay which was employed in the study. Detectable levels of leuprolide were present at all measurement points in all patients. The initial burst, fol-

---

Table 2:
Adverse Events Reported to be Causally Related to Drug in ≥ 5% of Patients

	Endometriosis (2 Studies)			Uterine Fibroids (4 Studies)	
	LUPRON DEPOT 3.75 mg N=166 N (%)	Danazol N=136 N (%)	Placebo N=31 N (%)	LUPRON DEPOT 3.75 mg N=166 N (%)	Placebo N=163 N (%)
Body as a Whole					
Asthenia	5 (3)	9 (7)	0 (0)	14 (8.4)	8 (4.9)
General pain	31 (19)	22 (16)	1 (3)	14 (8.4)	10 (6.1)
Headache*	53 (32)	30 (22)	2 (6)	43 (25.9)	29 (17.8)
Cardiovascular System					
Hot flashes/sweats*	139 (84)	77 (57)	9 (29)	121 (72.9)	29 (17.8)
Gastrointestinal System					
Nausea/vomiting	21 (13)	17 (13)	1 (3)	8 (4.8)	6 (3.7)
GI disturbances*	11 (7)	8 (6)	1 (3)	5 (3.0)	2 (1.2)
Metabolic and Nutritional Disorders					
Edema	12 (7)	17 (13)	1 (3)	9 (5.4)	2 (1.2)
Weight gain/loss	22 (13)	36 (26)	0 (0)	5 (3.0)	2 (1.2)
Endocrine system					
Acne	17 (10)	27 (20)	0 (0)	0 (0)	0 (0)
Hirsutism	2 (1)	9 (7)	1 (3)	1 (0.6)	0 (0)
Musculoskeletal System					
Joint disorder*	14 (8)	11 (8)	0 (0)	13 (7.8)	5 (3.1)
Myalgia*	1 (1)	7 (5)	0 (0)	1 (0.6)	0 (0)
Nervous System					
Decreased libido*	19 (11)	6 (4)	0 (0)	3 (1.8)	0 (0)
Depression/emotional lability*	36 (22)	27 (20)	1 (3)	18 (10.8)	7 (4.3)
Dizziness*	19 (11)	4 (3)	0 (0)	3 (1.8)	6 (3.7)
Nervousness*	8 (5)	11 (8)	0 (0)	8 (4.8)	1 (0.6)
Neuromuscular disorders*	11 (7)	17 (13)	0 (0)	3 (1.8)	0 (0)
Paresthesias	12 (7)	11 (8)	0 (0)	2 (1.2)	1 (0.6)
Skin and Appendages					
Skin reactions	17 (10)	20 (15)	1 (3)	5 (3.0)	2 (1.2)
Urogenital System					
Breast changes/tenderness/pain*	10 (6)	12 (9)	0 (0)	3 (1.8)	7 (4.3)
Vaginitis*	46 (28)	23 (17)	0 (0)	19 (11.4)	3 (1.8)

Continued on next page

Lupron Depot-3 mo. 22.5mg—Cont.

lowed by the rapid decline to a steady-state level, was similar to the release pattern seen with the monthly formulation.

Distribution: The mean steady-state volume of distribution of leuprolide following intravenous bolus administration to healthy male volunteers was 27 L. In vitro binding to human plasma proteins ranged from 43% to 49%.

Metabolism: In healthy male volunteers, a 1 mg bolus of leuprolide administered intravenously revealed that the mean systemic clearance was 7.6 L/h, with a terminal elimination half-life of approximately 3 hours based on a two compartment model.

In rats and dogs, administration of ^{14}C-labeled leuprolide was shown to be metabolized to smaller inactive peptides, a pentapeptide (Metabolite I), tripeptides (Metabolites II and III) and a dipeptide (Metabolite IV). These fragments may be further catabolized.

The major metabolite (M-I) plasma concentrations measured in 5 prostate cancer patients reached maximum concentration 2 to 6 hours after dosing and were approximately 6% of the peak parent drug concentration. One week after dosing, mean plasma M-I concentrations were approximately 20% of mean leuprolide concentrations.

Excretion: Following administration of LUPRON DEPOT 3.75 mg to 3 patients, less than 5% of the dose was recovered as parent and M-I metabolite in the urine.

Special Populations: The pharmacokinetics of the drug in hepatically and renally impaired patients have not been determined.

CLINICAL STUDIES

In clinical studies, serum testosterone was suppressed to castrate within 30 days in 87 of 92 (95%) patients and within an additional two weeks in three patients. Two patients did not suppress for 15 and 28 weeks, respectively. Suppression was maintained in all of these patients with the exception of transient minimal testosterone elevations in one of them, and in another an increase in serum testosterone to above the castrate range was recorded during the 12 hour observation period after a subsequent injection. This represents stimulation of gonadotropin secretion.

An 85% rate of "no progression" was achieved during the initial 24 weeks of treatment. A decrease from baseline in serum PSA of ≥90% was reported in 71% of the patients and a change to within the normal range (≤3.99 ng/mL) in 63% of the patients.

Periodic monitoring of serum testosterone and PSA levels is recommended, especially if the anticipated clinical or biochemical response to treatment has not been achieved. It should be noted that results of testosterone determinations are dependent on assay methodology. It is advisable to be aware of the type and precision of the assay methodology to make appropriate clinical and therapeutic decisions.

INDICATIONS AND USAGE

LUPRON DEPOT-3 Month 22.5 mg is indicated in the palliative treatment of advanced prostatic cancer. It offers an alternative treatment of prostatic cancer when orchiectomy or estrogen administration are either not indicated or unacceptable to the patient. In clinical trials, the safety and efficacy of LUPRON DEPOT-3 Month 22.5 mg were similar to that of the original daily subcutaneous injection and the monthly depot formulation.

CONTRAINDICATIONS

A report of an anaphylactic reaction to synthetic GnRH (Factrel) has been reported in the medical literature.[1]

LUPRON DEPOT is contraindicated in women who are or may become pregnant while receiving the drug. When administered on day 6 of pregnancy at test dosages of 0.00024, 0.0024, and 0.024 mg/kg (1/600 to 1/6 the human dose) to rabbits, the monthly formulation of LUPRON DEPOT produced a dose-related increase in major fetal abnormalities. Similar studies in rats failed to demonstrate an increase in fetal malformations. There was increased fetal mortality and decreased fetal weights with the two higher doses of the monthly formulation of LUPRON DEPOT in rabbits and with the highest dose in rats. The effects on fetal mortality are logical consequences of the alterations in hormonal levels brought about by this drug. Therefore, the possibility exists that spontaneous abortion may occur if the drug is administered during pregnancy.

WARNINGS

Isolated cases of worsening of signs and symptoms during the first weeks of treatment have been reported with LH-RH analogs. Worsening of symptoms may contribute to paralysis with or without fatal complications. For patients at risk, the physician may consider initiating therapy with daily LUPRON® (leuprolide acetate) Injection for the first two weeks to facilitate withdrawal of treatment if that is considered necessary.

PRECAUTIONS

Patients with metastatic vertebral lesions and/or with urinary tract obstruction should be closely observed during the first few weeks of therapy (see **WARNINGS** section).

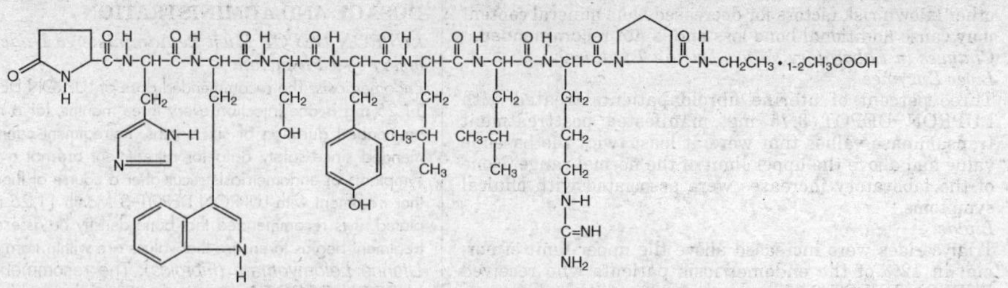

Laboratory Tests: Response to LUPRON DEPOT-3 Month 22.5 mg should be monitored by measuring serum levels of testosterone, as well as prostate-specific antigen and prostatic acid phosphatase. In the majority of patients, testosterone levels increased above baseline during the first week, declining thereafter to baseline levels or below by the end of the second week. Castrate levels were reached within two to four weeks and once achieved were maintained for as long as the patients received their injections.

Drug Interactions: No pharmacokinetic-based drug-drug interaction studies have been conducted with LUPRON DEPOT. However, because leuprolide acetate is a peptide that is primarily degraded by peptidase and not by cytochrome P-450 enzymes as noted in specific studies, and the drug is only about 46% bound to plasma proteins, drug interactions would not be expected to occur.

Drug/Laboratory Test Interactions: Administration of LUPRON DEPOT 3.75 mg in women results in suppression of the pituitary-gonadal system. Normal function is usually restored within one to three months after treatment is discontinued. Therefore, diagnostic tests of pituitary gonadotropic and gonadal functions conducted during treatment and up to three months after discontinuation of LUPRON DEPOT 3.75 mg therapy may be misleading.

Carcinogenesis, Mutagenesis, Impairment of Fertility: Two-year carcinogenicity studies were conducted in rats and mice. In rats, a dose-related increase of benign pituitary hyperplasia and benign pituitary adenomas was noted at 24 months when the drug was administered subcutaneously at high daily doses (0.6 to 4 mg/kg). There was a significant but not dose-related increase of pancreatic islet-cell adenomas in females and of testicular interstitial cell adenomas in males (highest incidence in the low dose group). In mice no pituitary abnormalities were observed at a dose as high as 60 mg/kg for two years. Patients have been treated with leuprolide acetate for up to three years with doses as high as 10 mg/day and for two years with doses as high as 20 mg/day without demonstrable pituitary abnormalities.

Mutagenicity studies have been performed with leuprolide acetate using bacterial and mammalian systems. These studies provided no evidence of a mutagenic potential.

Clinical and pharmacologic studies in adults (≥18 years) with leuprolide acetate and similar analogs have shown reversibility of fertility suppression when the drug is discontinued after continuous administration for periods of up to 24 weeks.

Pregnancy Category X. (See **CONTRAINDICATIONS** section.)

Pediatric Use: See LUPRON DEPOT-PED® (leuprolide acetate for depot suspension) labeling for the safety and effectiveness of the monthly formulation in children with central precocious puberty.

ADVERSE REACTIONS

In the majority of patients testosterone levels increased above baseline during the first week, declining thereafter to baseline levels or below by the end of the second week of treatment.

Potential exacerbations of signs and symptoms during the first few weeks of treatment is a concern in patients with vertebral metastases and/or urinary obstruction or hematuria which, if aggravated, may lead to neurological problems such as temporary weakness and/or paresthesia of the lower limbs or worsening of urinary symptoms (see **WARNINGS** section).

In two clinical trials of LUPRON DEPOT-3 Month 22.5 mg, the following adverse reactions were reported to have a possible or probable relationship to drug as ascribed by the treating physician in 5% or more of the patients receiving the drug. **Often, causality is difficult to assess in patients with metastatic prostate cancer.** Reactions considered not drug-related are excluded.

	LUPRON DEPOT-3 Month 22.5 mg N=94	(Percent)
Body As A Whole		
Asthenia	7	(7.4%)
General Pain	25	(26.6%)
Headache	6	(6.4%)
Injection Site Reaction	13	(13.8%)
Cardiovascular System		
Hot flashes/Sweats*	55	(58.5%)
Digestive System		
GI Disorders	15	(16.0%)
Musculoskeletal System		
Joint Disorders	11	(11.7%)
Central/Peripheral Nervous System		
Dizziness/Vertigo	6	(6.4%)
Insomnia/Sleep Disorders	8	(8.5%)
Neuromuscular Disorders	9	(9.6%)
Respiratory System		
Respiratory Disorders	6	(6.4%)
Skin and Appendages		
Skin Reaction	8	(8.5%)
Urogenital System		
Testicular Atrophy*	19	(20.2%)
Urinary Disorders	14	(14.9%)

In these same studies, the following adverse reactions were reported in less than 5% of the patients on LUPRON DEPOT-3 Month 22.5 mg.

Body As A Whole— Enlarged abdomen, Fever; *Cardiovascular System*—Arrhythmia, Bradycardia, Heart failure, Hypertension, Hypotension, Varicose vein; *Digestive System*— Anorexia, Duodenal ulcer, Increased appetite, Thirst/dry mouth; *Hemic and Lymphatic System*— Anemia, Lymphedema; *Metabolic and Nutritional Disorders*— Dehydration, Edema; *Central / Peripheral Nervous System*— Anxiety, Delusions, Depression, Hypesthesia, Libido decreased*, Nervousness, Paresthesia; *Respiratory System*— Epistaxis, Pharyngitis, Pleural effusion, Pneumonia; *Special Senses*— Abnormal vision, Amblyopia, Dry eyes, Tinnitus; *Urogenital System*— Gynecomastia, Impotence*, Penis disorders, Testis disorders.

Laboratory: Abnormalities of certain parameters were observed, but are difficult to assess in this population. The following were recorded in ≥5% of patients: Increased BUN, Hyperglycemia, Hyperlipidemia (total cholesterol, LDL-cholesterol, triglycerides), Hyperphosphatemia, Abnormal liver function tests, Increased PT, Increased PTT. Additional laboratory abnormalities reported were: Decreased platelets, Decreased potassium and Increased WBC.

* Physiologic effect of decreased testosterone.

Postmarketing

During postmarketing surveillance, which includes other dosage forms, the following adverse events were reported. Symptoms consistent with an anaphylactoid or asthmatic process have been rarely reported. Rash, urticaria, and photosensitivity reactions have also been reported.

Localized reactions including induration and abscess have been reported at the site of injection.

Hemic and Lymphatic System—Decreased WBC; *Central / Peripheral Nervous System*—Peripheral neuropathy, Spinal fracture/paralysis; *Musculoskeletal System*—Tenosynovitis-like symptoms; *Urogenital System*—Prostate pain.

See other LUPRON DEPOT and LUPRON Injection package inserts for other events reported in different patient populations.

OVERDOSAGE

In rats subcutaneous administration of 250 to 500 times the recommended human dose, expressed on a per body weight basis, resulted in dyspnea, decreased activity, and local irritation at the injection site. There is no evidence at present that there is a clinical counterpart of this phenomenon. In early clinical trials with daily subcutaneous leuprolide acetate, doses as high as 20 mg/day for up to two years caused no adverse effects differing from those observed with the 1 mg/day dose.

DOSAGE AND ADMINISTRATION

LUPRON DEPOT Must Be Administered Under The Supervision Of A Physician.

The recommended dose of LUPRON DEPOT-3 Month 22.5 mg to be administered is one injection every three months **(84 days)**. Due to different release characteristics, a fractional dose of this 3-month depot formulation is not equivalent to the same dose of the monthly formulation and should not be given.

Incorporated in a depot formulation, the lyophilized microspheres are to be reconstituted and administered every three months as a single intramuscular injection, in accord with the following directions:

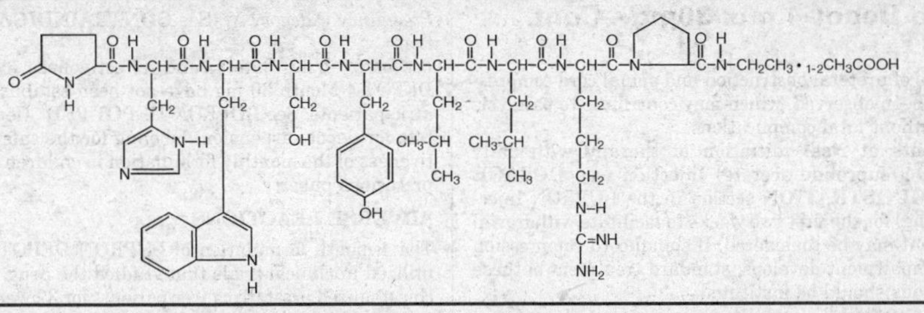

1. Withdraw 1.5 mL of diluent from the ampule, and inject it into the vial. (Extra diluent is provided; any remaining should be discarded.)
2. Shake well to thoroughly disperse particles to obtain a uniform suspension. The suspension will appear milky.
3. Withdraw the entire contents of the vial into the syringe with a 23 gauge or larger needle and inject it at the time of reconstitution. As the suspension settles very quickly following reconstitution, **it is strongly recommended that LUPRON DEPOT-3 Month 22.5 mg be administered immediately**. Reshake suspension if settling occurs.

Although the potency of the reconstituted suspension has been shown to be stable for 24 hours, since the product does not contain a preservative, the suspension should be discarded if not used immediately.

As with other drugs administered by injection, the injection site should be varied periodically.

The vial of LUPRON DEPOT-3 Month 22.5 mg and the ampule of diluent may be stored at room temperature.

HOW SUPPLIED

LUPRON DEPOT — 3 Month 22.5 mg (NDC 0300-3336-01) is available in a single use kit. Each kit contains a vial of sterile lyophilized microspheres which is leuprolide incorporated in a biodegradable polymer of polylactic acid. When mixed with 1.5 mL of accompanying diluent, LUPRON DEPOT-3 Month 22.5 mg is administered as a single IM injection **EVERY THREE MONTHS (84 days).**

An information pamphlet for patients is included with the kit.

No refrigeration necessary. Protect from freezing.

Caution: Federal (U.S.A.) law prohibits dispensing without a prescription.

REFERENCE

1. MacLeod TL, et al. Anaphylactic reaction to synthetic luteinizing hormone-releasing hormone. *Fertil Steril* 1987 Sept; 48(3):500-502.

U.S. Patent Nos. 4,652,441; 4,677,191; 4,728,721; 4,849,228; 4,917,893; 4,954,298; 5,330,767; and 5,476,663.

TAP Pharmaceuticals Inc.
Deerfield, Illinois 60015-1595, U.S.A.
LUPRON DEPOT-3 Month 22.5 mg
manufactured by
Takeda Chemical Industries, Ltd.
Osaka, JAPAN 541
®—Registered trademark
(No. 3336)
03-4771-R3-Revised: March, 1997

Shown in Product Identification Guide, page 340

LUPRON DEPOT®-4 Month 30 mg ℞
(leuprolide acetate for depot suspension)

4-MONTH FORMULATION

DESCRIPTION

Leuprolide acetate is a synthetic nonapeptide analog of naturally occurring gonadotropin-releasing hormone (GnRH or LH-RH). The analog possesses greater potency than the natural hormone. The chemical name is 5-oxo-L-prolyl-L-histidyl-L-tryptophyl-L-seryl-L-tyrosyl-D-leucyl-L-leucyl-L-arginyl-N-ethyl-L-prolinamide acetate (salt) with the following structural formula:

[See chemical structure above]

LUPRON DEPOT-4 Month 30 mg is available in a vial containing sterile lyophilized microspheres, which when mixed with diluent, become a suspension which is intended as an intramuscular injection to be given **ONCE EVERY FOUR MONTHS (16 weeks).**

The single-dose vial of LUPRON DEPOT - 4 Month 30 mg contains leuprolide acetate (30 mg), polylactic acid (264.8 mg), and D-mannitol (51.9 mg). The accompanying ampule of diluent contains carboxymethylcellulose sodium (10 mg), D-mannitol (100 mg), polysorbate 80 (2 mg), water for injection, USP, and glacial acetic acid, USP to control pH.

During the manufacture of LUPRON DEPOT-4 Month 30 mg, acetic acid is lost, leaving the peptide.

CLINICAL PHARMACOLOGY

Leuprolide acetate, an LH-RH agonist, acts as a potent inhibitor of gonadotropin secretion when given continuously and in therapeutic doses. Animal and human studies indicate that following an initial stimulation, chronic administration of leuprolide acetate results in suppression of ovarian and testicular steroidogenesis. This effect is reversible upon discontinuation of drug therapy. Administration of leuprolide acetate has resulted in inhibition of the growth of certain hormone dependent tumors (prostatic tumors in Noble and Dunning male rats and DMBA-induced mammary tumors in female rats) as well as atrophy of the reproductive organs.

In humans, administration of leuprolide acetate results in an initial increase in circulating levels of luteinizing hormone (LH) and follicle stimulating hormone (FSH), leading to a transient increase in levels of the gonadal steroids (testosterone and dihydrotestosterone in males, and estrone and estradiol in premenopausal females). However, continuous administration of leuprolide acetate results in decreased levels of LH and FSH. In males, testosterone is reduced to castrate levels. In premenopausal females, estrogens are reduced to postmenopausal levels. These decreases occur within two to four weeks after initiation of treatment. Castrate levels of testosterone in prostatic cancer patients have been demonstrated for more than five years.

Leuprolide acetate is not active when given orally.

PHARMACOKINETICS

Absorption: Following a single injection of LUPRON DEPOT-4 Month 30 mg in sixteen orchiectomized prostate cancer patients, mean plasma leuprolide concentration of 59.3 ng/mL was observed at 4 hours and the mean concentration then declined to 0.30 ng/mL at 16 weeks. The mean plasma concentration of leuprolide from weeks 3.5 to 16 was 0.44 ± 0.20 ng/mL (range: 0.20–1.06). Leuprolide appeared to be released at a constant rate following the onset of steady-state levels during the fourth week after dosing, providing steady plasma concentrations throughout the 16-week dosing interval. However, intact leuprolide and an inactive major metabolite could not be distinguished by the assay which was employed in the study. The initial burst, followed by the rapid decline to a steady-state level, was similar to the release pattern seen with the other depot formulations.

Distribution: The mean steady-state volume of distribution of leuprolide following intravenous bolus administration to healthy male volunteers was 27 L. In vitro binding to human plasma proteins ranged from 43% to 49%.

Metabolism: In healthy male volunteers, a 1 mg bolus of leuprolide administered intravenously revealed that the mean systemic clearance was 7.6 L/h, with a terminal elimination half-life of approximately 3 hours based on a two compartment model.

In rats and dogs, administration of ^{14}C-labeled leuprolide was shown to be metabolized to smaller inactive peptides, a pentapeptide (Metabolite I), tripeptides (Metabolites II and III) and a dipeptide (Metabolite IV). These fragments may be further catabolized.

The major metabolite (M-I) plasma concentrations measured in 5 prostate cancer patients reached maximum concentration 2 to 6 hours after dosing and were approximately 6% of the peak parent drug concentration. One week after dosing, mean plasma M-I concentrations were approximately 20% of mean leuprolide concentrations.

Excretion: Following administration of LUPRON DEPOT 3.75 mg to 3 patients, less than 5% of the dose was recovered as parent and M-I metabolite in the urine.

Special Populations: The pharmacokinetics of the drug in hepatically and renally impaired patients have not been determined.

Drug Interactions: No pharmacokinetic-based drug-drug interaction studies have been conducted with LUPRON DEPOT. However, because leuprolide acetate is a peptide that is primarily degraded by peptidase and the drug is only about 46% bound to plasma proteins, drug interactions would not be expected to occur.

CLINICAL STUDIES

In an open-label, noncomparative, multicenter clinical study of LUPRON DEPOT-4 Month 30 mg, 49 patients with stage D2 prostatic adenocarcinoma (with no prior treatment) were enrolled. The objectives were to determine whether a 30 mg depot formulation of leuprolide injected once every 16 weeks would reduce and maintain serum testosterone levels at castrate levels (≤ 50 ng/dL), and to assess the safety of the formulation. The study was divided into an initial 32-week treatment phase and a long term treatment phase. Serum testosterone levels were determined biweekly or weekly during the first 32 weeks of treatment. Once the patient completed the initial 32-week treatment period, treatment continued at the investigator's discretion with serum testosterone levels being done every 4 months prior to the injection.

In the majority of patients, testosterone levels increased 50% or more above the baseline during the first week of treatment. Mean serum testosterone subsequently suppressed to castrate levels within 30 days of the first injection in 94% of patients and within 43 days in all 49 patients during the initial 32-week treatment period. The median dosing interval between injections was 112 days. One escape from suppression (two consecutive testosterone values > 50 ng/dL after castrate levels achieved) was noted at Week 16. In this patient, serum testosterone increased to above the castrate range following the second depot injection (Week 16) but returned to the castrate level by Week 18. No adverse events were associated with this rise in serum testosterone. A second patient had a rise in testosterone at Week 17, then returned to the castrate level by Week 18 and remained there through Week 32. In the long term treatment phase two patients experienced testosterone elevations, both at Week 48. Testosterone for one patient returned to the castrate range at Week 52, and one patient discontinued the study at Week 48 due to disease progression.

Secondary efficacy endpoints evaluated in the study were the objective tumor response as assessed by clinical evaluations of tumor burden (complete response, partial response, objectively stable and progression) and evaluations of changes in prostatic involvement and prostate-specific antigen (PSA). These evaluations were performed at Weeks 16 and 32 of the treatment phase. The long term treatment phase monitored PSA at each visit (every 16 weeks). The objective tumor response analysis showed "no progression" (i.e. complete or partial response, or stable disease) in 86% (37/43) of patients at Week 16, and in 77% (37/48) of patients at Week 32. Local disease improved or remained stable in all patients evaluated at Week 16 and/or 32. For patients with elevated baseline PSA, 50% (23/46) had a normal PSA (< 4.0 ng/mL) at Week 16, and 51% (19/37) had a normal PSA at Week 32.

Periodic monitoring of serum testosterone and PSA levels is recommended, especially if the anticipated clinical or biochemical response to treatment has not been achieved. It should be noted that results of testosterone determinations are dependent on assay methodology. It is advisable to be aware of the type and precision of the assay methodology to make appropriate clinical and therapeutic decisions.

Using historical comparisons, the safety and efficacy of LUPRON DEPOT-4 Month 30 mg appear similar to the other LUPRON DEPOT formulations.

INDICATIONS AND USAGE

LUPRON DEPOT-4 Month 30 mg is indicated in the palliative treatment of advanced prostatic cancer.

CONTRAINDICATIONS

1. Hypersensitivity to GnRH, GnRH agonist analogs or any of the excipients in LUPRON DEPOT. Reports of anaphylactic reactions to synthetic GnRH (Factrel) or GnRH agonist analogs have been reported in the medical literature.
2. This formulation is not indicated for use in women (see LUPRON DEPOT 3.75 mg and LUPRON DEPOT-3 Month 11.25 mg package inserts).
3. All formulations of LUPRON DEPOT are contraindicated in women who are or may become pregnant while receiving the drug. LUPRON DEPOT may cause fetal harm when administered to a pregnant woman. Major fetal abnormalities were observed in rabbits but not in rats after administration of LUPRON DEPOT throughout gestation. There was increased fetal mortality and decreased fetal weights in rats and rabbits. The effects on fetal mortality are expected consequences of the alterations in hormonal levels brought about by this drug. Therefore, the possibility exists that spontaneous abortion may occur. If the drug is administered during pregnancy or if the patient becomes pregnant while taking any formulation of LUPRON DEPOT, she should be apprised of the potential hazard to the fetus.

WARNINGS

Initially, LUPRON DEPOT, like other LH-RH agonists, causes increases in serum levels of testosterone to approximately 50% above baseline during the first week of treatment. Transient worsening of symptoms, or the occurrence of additional signs and symptoms of prostate cancer, may occasionally develop during the first few weeks of LUPRON DEPOT treatment. A small number of patients may experience a temporary increase in bone pain, which can be managed symptomatically. As with other LH-RH agonists, iso-

Continued on next page

Lupron Depot-4 mo. 30mg—Cont.

lated cases of ureteral obstruction and spinal cord compression have been observed, which may contribute to paralysis with or without fatal complications.

For patients at risk, initiation of therapy with daily LUPRON® (leuprolide acetate) Injection (see **DOSAGE AND ADMINISTRATION** section in the LUPRON Injection labeling) for the first two weeks to facilitate withdrawal of treatment may be considered. If spinal cord compression or renal impairment develops, standard treatment of these complications should be instituted.

PRECAUTIONS

Information for Patients: An information pamphlet for patients is included with the product.

General: Patients with metastatic vertebral lesions and/or with urinary tract obstruction should be closely observed during the first few weeks of therapy (see **WARNINGS** section).

Laboratory Tests: Response to LUPRON DEPOT-4 Month 30 mg should be monitored by measuring serum levels of testosterone, as well as prostate-specific antigen. In the majority of patients, testosterone levels increased above baseline during the first week, declining thereafter to baseline levels or below by the end of the second week. Castrate levels were reached within two to four weeks and once achieved were maintained in most (45/49) patients for as long as the patients received their injections (see **CLINICAL PHARMACOLOGY, Clinical Studies** section).

Drug Interactions: See **CLINICAL PHARMACOLOGY**.

Drug/Laboratory Test Interactions: Administration of LUPRON DEPOT in therapeutic doses results in suppression of the pituitary-gonadal system. Normal function is usually restored within three months after treatment is discontinued. Due to the suppression of the pituitary-gonadal system by LUPRON DEPOT, diagnostic tests of pituitary gonadotropic and gonadal functions conducted during treatment and for up to three months after discontinuation of LUPRON DEPOT may be affected.

Carcinogenesis, Mutagenesis, Impairment of Fertility: Two-year carcinogenicity studies were conducted in rats and mice. In rats, a dose-related increase of benign pituitary hyperplasia and benign pituitary adenomas was noted at 24 months when the drug was administered subcutaneously at high daily doses (0.6 to 4 mg/kg). There was a significant but not dose-related increase of pancreatic islet-cell adenomas in females and of testicular interstitial cell adenomas in males (highest incidence in the low dose group). In mice no pituitary abnormalities were observed at a dose as high as 60 mg/kg for two years. Patients have been treated with leuprolide acetate for up to three years with doses as high as 10 mg/day and for two years with doses as high as 20 mg/day without demonstrable pituitary abnormalities.

Mutagenicity studies have been performed with leuprolide acetate using bacterial and mammalian systems. These studies provided no evidence of a mutagenic potential.

Clinical and pharmacologic studies in adults (≥ 18 years) with leuprolide acetate and similar analogs have shown reversibility of fertility suppression when the drug is discontinued after continuous administration for periods of up to 24 weeks.

Pregnancy Category X. (See **CONTRAINDICATIONS** section.)

Pediatric Use: Safety and effectiveness of LUPRON DEPOT-4 Month 30 mg have not been established in pediatric patients. See LUPRON DEPOT-PED® (leuprolide acetate for depot suspension) labeling for the safety and effectiveness of the monthly formulation in children with central precocious puberty.

ADVERSE REACTIONS

The 4-month formulation of LUPRON DEPOT 30 mg was utilized in clinical trials that studied the drug in 49 nonorchiectomized prostate cancer patients for 32 weeks or longer and in 24 orchiectomized prostate cancer patients for 20 weeks.

In the majority of nonorchiectomized patients, testosterone levels increased 50% or more above baseline during the first week of treatment with LUPRON DEPOT, declining thereafter to baseline levels or below by the end of the second week of treatment. Therefore, potential exacerbations of signs and symptoms during the first few weeks of treatment are of concern in patients with vertebral metastases and/or urinary obstruction or hematuria which, if aggravated, may lead to neurological problems such as temporary weakness and/or paresthesia of the lower limbs or worsening of urinary symptoms (see **WARNINGS** section).

In the above described clinical trials, the following adverse reactions were reported in ≥ 5% of the patients during the treatment period regardless of causality.

[See table below]

In these same studies, the following adverse reactions were reported in less than 5% of the patients on LUPRON DEPOT - 4 Month 30 mg.

Body As a Whole - Abscess, Accidental injury, Allergic reaction, Cyst, Fever, Generalized edema, Hernia, Neck pain, Neoplasm; *Cardiovascular System* - Atrial fibrillation, Deep thrombophlebitis, Hypertension; *Digestive System* - Anorexia, Eructation, Gastrointestinal hemorrhage, Gingivitis, Gum hemorrhage, Hepatomegaly, Increased appetite, Intestinal obstruction, Peridontal abscess; *Hemic and Lymphatic System* - Lymphadenopathy; *Metabolic and Nutritional Disorders* - Healing abnormal, hypoxia, Weight loss; *Musculoskeletal System* - Leg cramps, Pathological fracture, Ptosis; *Nervous System* - Abnormal thinking, Amnesia, Confusion, Convulsion, Dementia, Depression, Insomnia/sleep disorders, Libido decreased*, Neuropathy, Paralysis; *Respiratory System* - Asthma, Bronchitis, Hiccup, Lung disorder, Sinusitis, Voice alteration; *Skin and Appendages* - Herpes zoster, Melanosis; *Urogenital System* - Bladder carcinoma, epididymitis, Impotence*, Prostate disorder, Testicular atrophy*, Urinary incontinence, Urinary tract infection.

*Due to the expected physiologic effects of decreased testosterone levels.

Laboratory: Abnormalities of certain parameters were observed, but their relationship to drug treatment are difficult to assess in this population. The following were recorded in ≥ 5% of patients: Decreased bicarbonate, Decreased hemoglobin/hematocrit/RBC, Hyperlipidemia (total cholesterol, LDL-cholesterol, triglycerides), Decreased HDL-cholesterol, Eosinophilia, Increased glucose, Increased liver function tests (ALT, AST, GGTP, LDH), Increased phosphorus. Additional laboratory abnormalities were reported: Increased BUN and PT, Leukopenia, Thrombocytopenia, Uricaciduria.

Postmarketing

During postmarketing surveillance, which includes other dosage forms and other patient populations, the following adverse events were reported. Symptoms consistent with an anaphylactoid or asthmatic process have been reported. Rash, urticaria, and photosensitivity reactions have also been reported. Localized reactions including induration and abscess have been reported at the site of injection.

Cardiovascular System - Hypotension; *Hemic and Lymphatic System* - Decreased WBC; *Central/Peripheral Nervous System* - Peripheral neuropathy, Spinal fracture/paralysis; *Musculoskeletal System* - Tenosynovitis-like symptoms; *Urogenital System* - Prostate pain.

Changes in Bone Density: Decreased bone density has been reported in the medical literature in men who have had orchiectomy or who have been treated with an LH-RH agonist analog. In a clinical trial, 25 men with prostate cancer, 12 of whom had been treated previously with leuprolide acetate for at least six months, underwent bone density studies as a result of pain. The leuprolide-treated group had lower bone density scores than the nontreated control group. It can be anticipated that long periods of medical castration in men will have effects on bone density.

See other LUPRON DEPOT and LUPRON Injection package inserts for other events reported in women and pediatric populations.

Adverse Events Reported in ≥5% of Patients Regardless of Causality

LUPRON DEPOT-4 Month 30 mg

	Nonorchiectomized, N=49 Study 013		Orchiectomized, N=24 Study 012	
	N	(%)	N	(%)
Body As a Whole				
Asthenia	6	(12.2)	1	(4.2)
Flu Syndrome	6	(12.2)	0	(0.0)
General Pain	16	(32.7)	1	(4.2)
Headache	5	(10.2)	1	(4.2)
Injection Site Reaction	4	(8.2)	9	(37.5)
Cardiovascular System				
Hot flashes/Sweats*	23	(46.9)	2	(8.3)
Digestive System				
GI Disorders	5	(10.2)	3	(12.5)
Metabolic and Nutritional Disorders				
Dehydration	4	(8.2)	0	(0.0)
Edema	4	(8.2)	5	(20.8)
Musculoskeletal System				
Joint Disorder	8	(16.3)	1	(4.2)
Myalgia	4	(8.2)	0	(0.0)
Nervous System				
Dizziness/Vertigo	3	(6.1)	2	(8.3)
Neuromuscular Disorders	3	(6.1)	1	(4.2)
Paresthesia	4	(8.2)	1	(4.2)
Respiratory System				
Respiratory Disorder	4	(8.2)	1	(4.2)
Skin and Appendages				
Skin Reaction	6	(12.2)	0	(0.0)
Urogenital System				
Urinary Disorders	5	(10.2)	4	(16.7)

OVERDOSAGE

In clinical trials using daily subcutaneous leuprolide acetate in patients with prostate cancer, doses as high as 20 mg/day for up to two years caused no adverse effects differing from those observed with the 1 mg/day dose.

DOSAGE AND ADMINISTRATION

LUPRON DEPOT Must Be Administered Under The Supervision Of A Physician.

The recommended dose of LUPRON DEPOT-4 Month 30 mg to be administered is one injection **EVERY FOUR MONTHS (16 weeks).** Due to different release characteristics, a fractional dose of this 4-month depot formulation is not equivalent to the same dose of the monthly formulation and should not be given.

Incorporated in a depot formulation, the lyophilized microspheres are to be reconstituted and administered **EVERY FOUR MONTHS (16 weeks)** as a single intramuscular injection, in accord with the following directions:

1. Withdraw 1.5 mL of diluent from the ampule, and inject it into the vial. (Extra diluent is provided; any remaining should be discarded.)
2. Shake well to thoroughly disperse particles to obtain a uniform suspension. The suspension will appear milky.
3. Withdraw the entire contents of the vial into the syringe with a 22 gauge or larger needle and inject it at the time of reconstitution. As the suspension settles very quickly following reconstitution, **it is strongly recommended that LUPRON DEPOT-4 Month 30 mg be administered immediately.** Reshake suspension if settling occurs.

Since the product does not contain a preservative, the suspension should be discarded if not used immediately.

As with other drugs administered by injection, the injection site should be varied periodically.

The vial of LUPRON DEPOT-4 Month 30 mg and the ampule of diluent may be stored at room temperature.

HOW SUPPLIED

LUPRON DEPOT-4 Month 30 mg (**NDC** 0300-3673-01) is available in a single use kit. Each kit contains a vial of sterile lyophilized microspheres which is leuprolide incorporated in a biodegradable polymer of polylactic acid, and an ampule of sterile diluent. When mixed with 1.5 mL of the diluent, LUPRON DEPOT-4 Month 30 mg is administered as a single IM injection **EVERY FOUR MONTHS (16 weeks).**

No refrigeration necessary. Protect from freezing.

Caution: Federal (U.S.A.) law prohibits dispensing without a prescription.

U.S. Patent Nos. 4,652,441; 4,677,191; 4,728,721; 4,849,228; 4,917,893; 4,954,298; 5,330,767; 5,476,663; 5,480,656; and 5,575,987.

TAP Pharmaceuticals Inc.
Deerfield, Illinois 60015-1595, U.S.A.
LUPRON DEPOT - 4 Month 30 mg
manufactured by
Takeda Chemical Industries, Ltd.
Osaka, JAPAN 541
®-Registered trademark
Revised: June, 1997
03-4799-R1 (No. 3673)

Shown in Product Identification Guide, page 340

LUPRON DEPOT-PED® ℞

(leuprolide acetate for depot suspension)
7.5 mg, 11.25 mg and 15 mg

DESCRIPTION

Leuprolide acetate is a synthetic nonapeptide analog of naturally occurring gonadotropin-releasing hormone (GnRH or

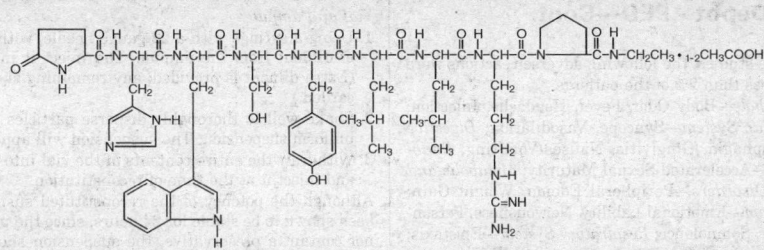

LH-RH). The analog possesses greater potency than the natural hormone. The chemical name is 5-oxo-L-prolyl-L-histidyl -L- tryptophyl-L-seryl-L-tyrosyl-D-leucyl-L-leucyl-L-arginyl-N-ethyl-L-prolinamide acetate (salt) with the following structural formula:

[See chemical structure at right]

LUPRON DEPOT-PED is available in a vial and also in a prefilled dual-chamber syringe. Both contain sterile lyophilized microspheres, which when mixed with diluent, become a suspension which is intended as a single intramuscular injection.

The single-dose vial of LUPRON DEPOT-PED 7.5 mg, 11.25 mg, and 15 mg contains, respectively for each dosage strength, leuprolide acetate (7.5/11.25/15 mg), purified gelatin (1.3/1.95/2.6 mg), DL-lactic and glycolic acids copolymer (66.2/99.3/132.4 mg), and D-mannitol (13.2/19.8/26.4 mg). The accompanying ampule of diluent contains carboxymethylcellulose sodium (10 mg), D-mannitol (100 mg), polysorbate 80 (2 mg), water for injection, USP, and glacial acetic acid, USP to control pH.

The front chamber of LUPRON DEPOT-PED 7.5 mg, 11.25 mg, and 15 mg prefilled dual-chamber syringe contains leuprolide acetate (7.5/11.25/15 mg), purified gelatin (1.3/1.95/2.6 mg), DL-lactic and glycolic acids copolymer (66.2/99.3/132.4 mg), and D-mannitol (13.2/19.8/26.4 mg). The second chamber of diluent contains carboxymethylcellulose sodium (5 mg), D-mannitol (50 mg), polysorbate 80 (1mg), water for injection, USP, and glacial acetic acid, USP to control pH. During the manufacture of LUPRON DEPOT-PED, acetic acid is lost, leaving the peptide.

CLINICAL PHARMACOLOGY

Leuprolide acetate, a GnRH agonist, acts as a potent inhibitor of gonadotropin secretion when given continuously and in therapeutic doses. Human studies indicate that following an initial stimulation of gonadotropins, chronic stimulation with leuprolide acetate results in suppression or "downregulation" of these hormones and consequent suppression of ovarian and testicular steroidogenesis. These effects are reversible on discontinuation of drug therapy.

Leuprolide acetate is not active when given orally.

PHARMACOKINETICS

Absorption: Following a single LUPRON DEPOT 7.5 mg injection to adult patients, mean peak leuprolide plasma concentration was almost 20 ng/mL at 4 hours and then declined to 0.36 ng/mL at 4 weeks. However, intact leuprolide and an inactive major metabolite could not be distinguished by the assay which was employed in the study. Nondetectable leuprolide plasma concentrations have been observed during chronic LUPRON DEPOT 7.5 mg administration, but testosterone levels appear to be maintained at castrate levels.

Distribution: The mean steady-state volume of distribution of leuprolide following intravenous bolus administration to healthy male volunteers was 27 L. In vitro binding to human plasma proteins ranged from 43% to 49%.

Metabolism: In healthy male volunteers, a 1 mg bolus of leuprolide administered intravenously revealed that the mean systemic clearance was 7.6 L/h, with a terminal elimination half-life of approximately 3 hours based on a two compartment model.

In rats and dogs, administration of ^{14}C-labeled leuprolide was shown to be metabolized to smaller inactive peptides, a pentapeptide (Metabolite I), tripeptides (Metabolites II and III) and a dipeptide (Metabolite IV). These fragments may be further catabolized.

The major metabolite (M-I) plasma concentrations measured in 5 prostate cancer patients reached maximum concentration 2 to 6 hours after dosing and were approximately 6% of the peak parent drug concentration. One week after dosing, mean plasma M-I concentrations were approximately 20% of mean leuprolide concentrations.

Excretion: Following administration of LUPRON DEPOT 3.75 mg to 3 patients, less than 5% of the dose was recovered as parent and M-I metabolite in the urine.

Special Populations: The pharmacokinetics of the drug in hepatically and renally impaired patients have not been determined.

CLINICAL STUDIES

In children with central precocious puberty (CPP), stimulated and basal gonadotropins are reduced to prepubertal levels. Testosterone and estradiol are reduced to prepubertal levels in males and females respectively. Reduction of gonadotropins will allow for normal physical and psychological growth and development. Natural maturation occurs when gonadotropins return to pubertal levels following discontinuation of leuprolide acetate.

The following physiologic effects have been noted with the chronic administration of leuprolide acetate in this patient population.

1. **Skeletal Growth.** A measurable increase in body length can be noted since the epiphyseal plates will not close prematurely.
2. **Organ Growth.** Reproductive organs will return to a prepubertal state.
3. **Menses.** Menses, if present, will cease.

In a study of 22 children with central precocious puberty, doses of LUPRON DEPOT were given every 4 weeks and plasma levels were determined according to weight categories as summarized below:

[See table at bottom of next page]

INDICATIONS AND USAGE

LUPRON DEPOT-PED is indicated in the treatment of children with central precocious puberty. Children should be selected using the following criteria:

1. Clinical diagnosis of CPP (idiopathic or neurogenic) with onset of secondary sexual characteristics earlier than 8 years in females and 9 years in males.
2. Clinical diagnosis should be confirmed prior to initiation of therapy:
   • Confirmation of diagnosis by a pubertal response to a GnRH stimulation test. The sensitivity and methodology of this assay must be understood.
   • Bone age advanced one year beyond the chronological age.
3. Baseline evaluation should also include:
   • Height and weight measurements.
   • Sex steroid levels.
   • Adrenal steroid level to exclude congenital adrenal hyperplasia.
   • Beta human chorionic gonadotropin level to rule out a chorionic gonadotropin secreting tumor.
   • Pelvic/adrenal/testicular ultrasound to rule out a steroid secreting tumor.
   • Computerized tomography of the head to rule out intracranial tumor.

CONTRAINDICATIONS

LUPRON DEPOT-PED is contraindicated in women who are or may become pregnant while receiving the drug. When administered on day 6 of pregnancy at test dosages of 0.00024, 0.0024, and 0.024 mg/kg (1/1200 to 1/12 the human pediatric dose) to rabbits, LUPRON DEPOT produced a dose-related increase in major fetal abnormalities. Similar studies in rats failed to demonstrate an increase in fetal malformations. There was increased fetal mortality and decreased fetal weights with the two higher doses of LUPRON DEPOT in rabbits and with the highest dose in rats. The effects on fetal mortality are logical consequences of the alterations in hormonal levels brought about by this drug. Therefore, the possibility exists that spontaneous abortion may occur if the drug is administered during pregnancy.

Leuprolide acetate is contraindicated in children demonstrating hypersensitivity to GnRH, GnRH agonist analogs, or any of the excipients.

A report of an anaphylactic reaction to synthetic GnRH (Factrel) has been reported in the medical literature.[1]

WARNINGS

During the early phase of therapy, gonadotropins and sex steroids rise above baseline because of the natural stimulatory effect of the drug. Therefore, an increase in clinical signs and symptoms may be observed (see **CLINICAL PHARMACOLOGY** section).

Noncompliance with drug regimen or inadequate dosing may result in inadequate control of the pubertal process. The consequences of poor control include the return of pubertal signs such as menses, breast development, and testicular growth. The long-term consequences of inadequate control of gonadal steroid secretion are unknown, but may include a further compromise of adult stature.

PRECAUTIONS

Laboratory Tests: Response to LUPRON DEPOT-PED should be monitored 1–2 months after the start of therapy with a GnRH stimulation test and sex steroid levels. Measurement of bone age for advancement should be done every 6–12 months.

Sex steroids may increase or rise above prepubertal levels if the dose is inadequate (see **WARNINGS** section). Once a therapeutic dose has been established, gonadotropin and sex steroid levels will decline to prepubertal levels.

Drug Interactions: No pharmacokinetic-based drug-drug interaction studies have been conducted. However, because leuprolide acetate is a peptide that is primarily degraded by peptidase and not by cytochrome P-450 enzymes as noted in specific studies, and the drug is only about 46% bound to plasma proteins, drug interactions would not be expected to occur.

Drug/Laboratory Test Interactions: Administration of LUPRON DEPOT 3.75 mg in women results in suppression of the pituitary-gonadal system. Normal function is usually restored within three months after treatment is discontinued. Therefore, diagnostic tests of pituitary gonadotropic and gonadal functions conducted during treatment and for up to three months after discontinuation of LUPRON DEPOT therapy may be misleading.

Information for Parents: Prior to starting therapy with LUPRON DEPOT-PED, the parent or guardian must be aware of the importance of continuous therapy. Adherence to 4 week drug administration schedules must be accepted if therapy is to be successful.

• During the first 2 months of therapy, a female may experience menses or spotting. If bleeding continues beyond the second month, notify the physician.
• Any irritation at the injection site should be reported to the physician immediately.
• Report any unusual signs or symptoms to the physician.

Carcinogenesis, Mutagenesis, Impairment of Fertility: A two-year carcinogenicity study was conducted in rats and mice. In rats, a dose-related increase of benign pituitary hyperplasia and benign pituitary adenomas was noted at 24 months when the drug was administered subcutaneously at high daily doses (0.6 to 4 mg/kg). There was a significant but not dose-related increase of pancreatic islet-cell adenomas in females and of testicular interstitial cell adenomas in males (highest incidence in the low dose group). In mice, no leuprolide acetate-induced tumors or pituitary abnormalities were observed at a dose as high as 60 mg/kg for two years. Adult patients have been treated with leuprolide acetate for up to three years with doses as high as 10 mg/day and for two years with doses as high as 20 mg/day without demonstrable pituitary abnormalities. Although no clinical studies have been completed in children to assess the full reversibility of fertility suppression, animal studies (prepubertal and adult rats and monkeys) with leuprolide acetate and other GnRH analogs have shown functional recovery. However, following a study with leuprolide acetate, immature male rats demonstrated tubular degeneration in the testes even after a recovery period. In spite of the failure to recover histologically, the treated males proved to be as fertile as the controls. Also, no histologic changes were observed in the female rats following the same protocol. In both sexes, the offspring of the treated animals appeared normal. The effect of the treatment of the parents on the reproductive performance of the F1 generation was not tested. The clinical significance of these findings is unknown.

Pregnancy Category X. See **CONTRAINDICATIONS** section.

Nursing Mothers: It is not known whether leuprolide acetate is excreted in human milk. LUPRON should not be used by nursing mothers.

ADVERSE REACTIONS

Potential exacerbation of signs and symptoms during the first few weeks of treatment (See **PRECAUTIONS** section) is a concern in patients with rapidly advancing central precocious puberty.

In two studies of children with central precocious puberty, in 2% or more of the patients receiving the drug, the following adverse reactions were reported to have a possible or probable relationship to drug as ascribed by the treating physician. Reactions considered not drug related are excluded.

	Number of Patients N=395	(Percent)
Body as a Whole		
General Pain	7	(2)
Integumentary System		
Acne/Seborrhea	7	(2)
Injection Site Reactions		
Including Abscess	21	(5)
Rash Including		
Erythema Multiforme	8	(2)
Urogenital System		
Vaginitis/Bleeding/		
Discharge	7	(2)

Continued on next page

Lupron Depot - PED—Cont.

In those same studies, the following adverse reactions were reported in less than 2% of the patients.

Body as a Whole—Body Odor, Fever, Headache, Infection; *Cardiovascular System*—Syncope, Vasodilation; *Digestive System*—Dysphagia, Gingivitis, Nausea/Vomiting; *Endocrine System*—Accelerated Sexual Maturity; *Metabolic and Nutritional Disorders*—Peripheral Edema, Weight Gain; *Nervous System*—Emotional Lability, Nervousness, Personality Disorder, Somnolence; *Respiratory System*—Epistaxis; *Integumentary System*—Alopecia, Skin Striae; *Urogenital System*—Cervix Disorder, Gynecomastia/Breast Disorders, Urinary Incontinence.

Postmarketing

During postmarketing surveillance, which includes other dosage forms, the following adverse events were reported. Symptoms consistent with an anaphylactoid or asthmatic process have been rarely reported. Rash, urticaria, and photosensitivity reactions have also been reported.

Localized reactions including induration and abscess have been reported at the site of injection.

Cardiovascular System—Hypotension; *Hemic and Lymphatic System*—Decreased WBC; *Central/Peripheral Nervous System*—Peripheral neuropathy, Spinal fracture/paralysis; *Musculoskeletal System*—Tenosynovitis-like symptoms; *Urogenital System*—Prostate pain.

See other LUPRON DEPOT and LUPRON Injection package inserts for other events reported in different patient populations.

OVERDOSAGE

In rats, subcutaneous administration of 125 to 250 times the recommended human pediatric dose, expressed on a per body weight basis, resulted in dyspnea, decreased activity, and local irritation at the injection site. There is no evidence at present that there is a clinical counterpart of this phenomenon. In early clinical trials using leuprolide acetate in adult patients, doses as high as 20 mg/day for up to two years caused no adverse effects differing from those observed with the 1 mg/day dose.

DOSAGE AND ADMINISTRATION

LUPRON DEPOT-PED must be administered under the supervision of a physician.

The dose of LUPRON DEPOT-PED must be individualized for each child. The dose is based on a mg/kg ratio of drug to body weight. Younger children require higher doses on a mg/kg ratio.

For each dosage form, after 1-2 months of initiating therapy or changing doses, the child must be monitored with a GnRH stimulation test, sex steroids, and Tanner staging to confirm downregulation. Measurements of bone age for advancement should be monitored every 6-12 months. The dose should be titrated upward until no progression of the condition is noted either clinically and/or by laboratory parameters.

The first dose found to result in adequate downregulation can probably be maintained for the duration of therapy in most children. However, there are insufficient data to guide dosage adjustment as patients move into higher weight categories after beginning therapy at very young ages and low dosages. It is recommended that adequate downregulation be verified in such patients whose weight has increased significantly while on therapy.

Discontinuation of LUPRON DEPOT-PED should be considered before age 11 for females and age 12 for males.

The recommended starting dose is 0.3 mg/kg/4 weeks (minimum 7.5 mg) administered as a single intramuscular injection. The starting dose will be dictated by the child's weight.

≤ 25 kg	7.5 mg
> 25–37.5 kg	11.25 mg
> 37.5 kg	15 mg

If total downregulation is not achieved, the dose should be titrated upward in increments of 3.75 mg every 4 weeks. This dose will be considered the maintenance dose.

The lyophilized microspheres are to be reconstituted and administered as a single intramuscular injection, in accord with the following directions:

Vial and ampule:

1. Using a syringe with a 22 gauge needle, withdraw 1 mL of diluent from the ampule, and inject it into the vial. (Extra diluent is provided; any remaining should be discarded.)
2. Shake well to thoroughly disperse particles to obtain a uniform suspension. The suspension will appear milky.
3. Withdraw the entire contents of the vial into the syringe and inject it at the time of reconstitution.

Although the potency of the reconstituted suspension has been shown to be stable for 24 hours, since the product does not contain a preservative, the suspension should be discarded if not used immediately.

Prefilled dual-chamber syringe:

1. To prepare for injection, screw the white plunger into the end stopper until the stopper begins to turn.
2. Remove and discard the tab around the base of the needle.
3. Holding the syringe upright, release the diluent by SLOWLY PUSHING the plunger until the first stopper is at the blue line in the middle of the barrel.
4. Gently shake the syringe to thoroughly mix the particles to form a uniform suspension. The suspension will appear milky.
5. If the microspheres (particles) adhere to the stopper, tap the syringe against your finger.
6. Then remove the needle guard and advance the plunger to expel the air from the syringe.
7. Inject the entire contents of the syringe intramuscularly as you would for a normal injection.

Although the potency of the reconstituted suspension has been shown to be stable for 24 hours, since the product does not contain a preservative, the suspension should be discarded if not used immediately.

As with other drugs administered by injection, the injection site should be varied periodically.

The vial of LUPRON DEPOT-PED, the ampule of diluent, as well as the prefilled dual-chamber syringe may be stored at room temperature.

HOW SUPPLIED

LUPRON DEPOT-PED (7.5/11.25/15 mg) is packaged in the following forms:

Kit with vial and ampule (7.5 mg)	(NDC 0300-2106-01)
Kit with vial and ampule (11.25 mg)	(NDC 0300-2270-01)
Kit with vial and ampule (15 mg)	(NDC 0300-2437-01)
Kit with prefilled dual-chamber syringe (7.5 mg)	(NDC 0300-2108-01)
Kit with prefilled dual-chamber syringe (11.25 mg)	(NDC 0300-2282-01)
Kit with prefilled dual-chamber syringe (15 mg)	(NDC 0300-2440-01)

Each vial and syringe contains sterile lyophilized microspheres which is leuprolide incorporated in a biodegradable copolymer of lactic and glycolic acids. When mixed with diluent, LUPRON DEPOT-PED is administered as a single IM injection.

An information pamphlet for parents is included with the kit.

No refrigeration necessary. Protect from freezing.

Caution: Federal (U.S.A.) law prohibits dispensing without a prescription.

REFERENCE

1. MacLeod TL, et al. Anaphylactic reaction to synthetic luteinizing hormone-releasing hormone. *Fertil Steril* 1987 Sept;48(3):500–502.

U.S. Patent Nos. 4,652,441; 4,677,191; 4,728,721; 4,849,228; 4,917,893; 4,954,298; 5,330,767; and 5,476,663.

TAP Pharmaceuticals Inc.

Deerfield, IL 60015, U.S.A.

LUPRON DEPOT-PED manufactured by

Takeda Chemical Industries, Ltd.

Osaka, JAPAN 541

®—Registered Trademark

(Nos. 2106, 2270, 2437)

03-4755-R7-Revised: March, 1997

PREVACID®   ℞

[prĕ '-va-sĭd]

(lansoprazole)

Delayed-Release Capsules

DESCRIPTION

The active ingredient in PREVACID (lansoprazole) Delayed-Release Capsules is a substituted benzimidazole, 2-[[[3-methyl -4- (2,2,2-trifluroethoxy) -2- pyridyl]methyl]sulfinyl] benzimidazole, a compound that inhibits gastric acid secretion. Its empirical formula is $C_{16}H_{14}F_3N_3O_2S$ with a molecular weight of 369.37. The structural formula is:

Lansoprazole is a white to brownish-white odorless crystalline powder which melts with decomposition at approximately 166°C. Lansoprazole is freely soluble in dimethylformamide; soluble in methanol; sparingly soluble in ethanol; slightly soluble in ethyl acetate, dichloromethane and acetonitrile; very slightly soluble in ether; and practically insoluble in hexane and water.

Lansoprazole is stable when exposed to light for up to two months. The compound degrades in aqueous solution, the rate of degradation increasing with decreasing pH. At 25°C the $t_{1/2}$ is approximately 0.5 hour at pH 5.0 and approximately 18 hours at pH 7.0.

PREVACID is supplied in delayed-release capsules for oral administration. The delayed-release capsules contain the active ingredient, lansoprazole, in the form of enteric-coated granules and are available in two dosage strengths: 15 mg and 30 mg of lansoprazole per capsule. Each delayed-release capsule contains enteric-coated granules consisting of lansoprazole, hydroxypropyl cellulose, low substituted hydroxypropyl cellulose, colloidal silicon dioxide, magnesium carbonate, methacrylic acid copolymer, starch, talc, sugar sphere, sucrose, polyethylene glycol, polysorbate 80, and titanium dioxide. Components of the gelatin capsule include gelatin, titanium dioxide, D&C Red No. 28, FD&C Blue No. 1, FD&C Green No. 3*, and FD&C Red No. 40.

* PREVACID 15-mg capsules only.

CLINICAL PHARMACOLOGY

Pharmacokinetics and Metabolism

PREVACID Delayed-Release Capsules contain an enteric-coated granule formulation of lansoprazole. Absorption of lansoprazole begins only after the granules leave the stomach. Absorption is rapid, with mean peak plasma levels of lansoprazole occurring after approximately 1.7 hours. Peak plasma concentrations of lansoprazole (C_{max}) and the area under the plasma concentration curve (AUC) of lansoprazole are approximately proportional in doses from 15 mg to 60 mg after single-oral administration. Lansoprazole does not accumulate and its pharmacokinetics are unaltered by multiple dosing.

Absorption

The absorption of lansoprazole is rapid, with mean C_{max} occurring approximately 1.7 hours after oral dosing, and relatively complete with absolute bioavailability over 80%. In healthy subjects, the mean (± SD) plasma half-life was 1.5 (± 1.0) hours. Both C_{max} and AUC are diminished by about 50% if the drug is given 30 minutes after food as opposed to the fasting condition. There is no significant food effect if the drug is given before meals.

Distribution

Lansoprazole is 97% bound to plasma proteins. Plasma protein binding is constant over the concentration range of 0.05 to 5.0 μg/mL.

Metabolism

Lansoprazole is extensively metabolized in the liver. Two metabolites have been identified in measurable quantities in plasma (the hydroxylated sulfinyl and sulfone derivatives of lansoprazole). These metabolites have very little or no antisecretory activity. Lansoprazole is thought to be transformed into two active species which inhibit acid secretion by (H⁺, K⁺)-ATPase within the parietal cell canaliculus, but are not present in the systemic circulation. The plasma elimination half-life of lansoprazole does not reflect its duration of suppression of gastric acid secretion. Thus, the plasma elimination half-life is less than two hours, while the acid inhibitory effect lasts more than 24 hours.

Elimination

Following single-dose oral administration of lansoprazole, virtually no unchanged lansoprazole was excreted in the urine. In one study, after a single oral dose of ^{14}C-lansoprazole, approximately one-third of the administered radiation

Patient Weight Range (kg)	Group Weight Average (kg)	Dose (mg)	Trough Plasma Leuprolide Level Mean ± SD (ng/mL)*
20.2–27.0	22.7	7.5	0.77±0.033
28.4–36.8	32.5	11.25	1.25±1.06
39.3–57.5	44.2	15.0	1.59±0.65

* Group average values determined at Week 4 immediately prior to leuprolide injection. Drug levels at 12 and 24 weeks were similar to respective 4 week levels.

was excreted in the urine and two-thirds was recovered in the feces. This implies a significant biliary excretion of the metabolites of lansoprazole.

Special Populations
Geriatric
The clearance of lansoprazole is decreased in the elderly, with elimination half-life increased approximately 50% to 100%. Because the mean half-life in the elderly remains between 1.9 to 2.9 hours, repeated once daily dosing does not result in accumulation of lansoprazole. Peak plasma levels were not increased in the elderly.

Pediatric
The pharmacokinetics of lansoprazole has not been investigated in patients <18 years of age.

Gender
In a study comparing 12 male and six female human subjects, no gender differences were found in pharmacokinetics and intragastric pH results. (Also see Use in Women.)

Renal Insufficiency
In patients with severe renal insufficiency, plasma protein binding decreased by 1.0%–1.5% after administration of 60 mg of lansoprazole. Patients with renal insufficiency had a shortened elimination half-life and decreased total AUC (free and bound). AUC for free lansoprazole in plasma, however, was not related to the degree of renal impairment, and C_{max} and T_{max} were not different from subjects with healthy kidneys.

Hepatic Insufficiency
In patients with various degrees of chronic hepatic disease, the mean plasma half-life of the drug was prolonged from 1.5 hours to 3.2–7.2 hours. An increase in mean AUC of up to 500% was observed at steady state in hepatically-impaired patients compared to healthy subjects. Dose reduction in patients with severe hepatic disease should be considered.

Race
The pooled mean pharmacokinetic parameters of lansoprazole from twelve U.S. Phase 1 studies (N=513) were compared to the mean pharmacokinetic parameters from two Asian studies (N=20). The mean AUCs of lansoprazole in Asian subjects were approximately twice those seen in pooled U.S. data; however, the inter-individual variability was high. The C_{max} values were comparable.

PHARMACODYNAMICS
Mechanism of action
Lansoprazole belongs to a class of antisecretory compounds, the substituted benzimidazoles, that do not exhibit anticholinergic or histamine H_2-receptor antagonist properties, but that suppress gastric acid secretion by specific inhibition of the (H^+, K^+)-ATPase enzyme system at the secretory surface of the gastric parietal cell. Because this enzyme system is regarded as the acid (proton) pump within the parietal cell, lansoprazole has been characterized as a gastric acid-pump inhibitor, in that it blocks the final step of acid production. This effect is dose-related and leads to inhibition of both basal and stimulated gastric acid secretion irrespective of the stimulus.

Antisecretory activity
After oral administration, lansoprazole was shown to significantly decrease the basal acid output and significantly increase the mean gastric pH and percent of time the gastric pH was >3 and >4. Lansoprazole also significantly reduced meal-stimulated gastric acid output and secretion volume, as well as pentagastrin-stimulated acid output. In patients with hypersecretion of acid, lansoprazole significantly reduced basal and pentagastrin-stimulated gastric acid secretion. Lansoprazole inhibited the normal increases in secretion volume, acidity and acid output induced by insulin.

In a crossover study comparing lansoprazole 15 and 30 mg with omeprazole 20 mg for five days, the following effects on intragastric pH were noted:
[See table below]

After the initial dose in this study, increased gastric pH was seen within 1–2 hours with lansoprazole 30 mg, 2–3 hours with lansoprazole 15 mg, and 3–4 hours with omeprazole 20 mg. After multiple daily dosing, increased gastric pH was seen within the first hour postdosing with lansoprazole 30 mg and within 1–2 hours postdosing with lansoprazole 15 mg and omeprazole 20 mg.

Clarithromycin Susceptibility Test Results and Clinical/Bacteriological Outcomes[a]

Clarithromycin Pretreatment Results	Clarithromycin Post-treatment Results			
	H. pylori negative-eradicated	*H. pylori* positive-not eradicated		
		Post-treatment susceptibility results		
		S[b]　　I[b]	R[b]	No MIC

Triple Therapy 14-Day (lansoprazole 30 mg b.i.d./amoxicillin 1 gm b.i.d./clarithromycin 500 mg b.i.d.) (M95-399, M93-131, M95-392)

Susceptible[b]　112	105			7
Intermediate[b]　3	3			
Resistant[b]　17	6		7	4

Triple Therapy 10-Day (lansoprazole 30 mg b.i.d./amoxicillin 1 gm b.i.d./clarithromycin 500 mg b.i.d.) (M95-399)

Suceptible[b]　42	40	1		1
Intermediate[b]				
Resistant[b]　4	1		3	

[a] Includes only patients with pretreatment clarithromycin susceptibility test results
[b] Susceptible (S) MIC ≤ 0.25 µg/mL, Intermediate (I) MIC 0.5 - 1.0 µg/mL, Resistant (R) MIC ≥ 2 µg/mL.

Acid suppression may enhance the effect of antimicrobials in eradicating *Helicobacter pylori (H. pylori)*. The percentage of time gastric pH was elevated above 5 and 6 was evaluated in a crossover study of PREVACID given q.d., b.i.d. and t.i.d.

Mean Antisecretory Effects After 5 Days of b.i.d. and t.i.d. Dosing

Parameter	PREVACID			
	30 mg q.d.	15 mg b.i.d.	30 mg b.i.d.	30 mg t.i.d.
% Time Gastric pH>5	43	47	59[+]	77[*]
% Time Gastric pH>6	20	23	28	45[*]

[+] (p<0.05) versus PREVACID 30 mg q.d.
[*] (p<0.05) versus PREVACID 30 mg q.d., 15 mg b.i.d. and 30 mg b.i.d.

The inhibition of gastric acid secretion as measured by intragastric pH returns gradually to normal over two to four days after multiple doses. There is no indication of rebound gastric acidity.

Enterochromaffin-like (ECL) cell effects
During lifetime exposure of rats with up to 150 mg/kg/day of lansoprazole dosed seven days per week, marked hypergastrinemia was observed followed by ECL cell proliferation and formation of carcinoid tumors, especially in female rats. (See PRECAUTIONS, Carcinogenesis, Mutagenesis, Impairment of Fertility.)

Gastric biopsy specimens from the body of the stomach from approximately 150 patients treated continuously with lansoprazole for at least one year did not show evidence of ECL cell effects similar to those seen in rat studies. Longer term data are needed to rule out the possibility of an increased risk of the development of gastric tumors in patients receiving long-term therapy with lansoprazole.

Other gastric effects in humans
Lansoprazole did not significantly affect mucosal blood flow in the fundus of the stomach. Due to the normal physiologic effect caused by the inhibition of gastric acid secretion, a decrease of about 17% in blood flow in the antrum, pylorus, and duodenal bulb was seen. Lansoprazole significantly slowed the gastric emptying of digestible solids. Lansoprazole increased serum pepsinogen levels and decreased pepsin activity under basal conditions and in response to meal stimulation or insulin injection. As with other agents that

---

elevate intragastric pH, increases in gastric pH were associated with increases in nitrate-reducing bacteria and elevation of nitrite concentration in gastric juice in patients with gastric ulcer. No significant increase in nitrosamine concentrations was observed.

Serum gastrin effects
In over 2100 patients, median fasting serum gastrin levels increased 50% to 100% from baseline but remained within normal range after treatment with lansoprazole given orally in doses of 15 mg to 60 mg. These elevations reached a plateau within two months of therapy and returned to pretreatment levels within four weeks after discontinuation of therapy.

Endocrine effects
Human studies for up to one year have not detected any clinically significant effects on the endocrine system. Hormones studied include testosterone, luteinizing hormone (LH), follicle stimulating hormone (FSH), sex hormone binding globulin (SHBG), dehydroepiandrosterone sulfate (DHEA-S), prolactin, cortisol, estradiol, insulin, aldosterone, parathormone, glucagon, thyroid stimulating hormone (TSH), triiodothyronine (T_3), thyroxine (T_4), and somatotropic hormone (STH). Lansoprazole in oral doses of 15 to 60 mg for up to one year had no clinically significant effect on sexual function. In addition, lansoprazole in oral doses of 15 to 60 mg for two to eight weeks had no clinically significant effect on thyroid function.

In 24-month carcinogenicity studies in Sprague-Dawley rats with daily dosages up to 150 mg/kg, proliferative changes in the Leydig cells of the testes, including benign neoplasm, were increased compared to control rates.

Other effects
No systemic effects of lansoprazole on the central nervous system, lymphoid, hematopoietic, renal, hepatic, cardiovascular or respiratory systems have been found in humans. No visual toxicity was observed among 56 patients who had extensive baseline eye evaluations, were treated with up to 180 mg/day of lansoprazole and were observed for up to 58 months. Other rat-specific findings after lifetime exposure included focal pancreatic atrophy, diffuse lymphoid hyperplasia in the thymus, and spontaneous retinal atrophy.

CLINICAL PHARMACOLOGY

MICROBIOLOGY
Lansoprazole, clarithromycin and/or amoxicillin have been shown to be active against most strains of *Helicobacter pylori in vitro* and in clinical infections as described in the **INDICATIONS AND USAGE** section.

Helicobacter
Helicobacter pylori
Pretreatment Resistance
Clarithromycin pretreatment resistance (≥ 2.0 µg/mL) was 9.5% (91/960) by E-test and 11.3% (12/106) by agar dilution in the dual and triple therapy clinical trials (M93-125, M93-130, M93-131, M95-392, and M95-399).

Amoxicillin pretreatment susceptible isolates (≤ 0.25 µg/mL) occurred in 97.8% (936/957) and 98.0% (98/100) of the patients in the dual and triple therapy clinical trials by E-test and agar dilution, respectively. Twenty-one of 957 patients (2.2%) by E-test and 2 of 100 patients (2.0%) by agar dilution had amoxicillin pretreatment MICs of > 0.25 µg/mL. One patient on the 14 day triple therapy regimen had

---

Mean Antisecretory Effects after Single and Multiple Daily Dosing

Parameter	Baseline Value	PREVACID				Omeprazole	
		15 mg		30 mg		20 mg	
		Day 1	Day 5	Day 1	Day 5	Day 1	Day 5
Mean 24-Hour pH	2.1	2.7[+]	4.0[+]	3.6[*]	4.9[*]	2.5	4.2[+]
Mean Nighttime pH	1.9	2.4	3.0[+]	2.6	3.8[*]	2.2	3.0[+]
% Time Gastric pH>3	18	33[+]	59[+]	51[*]	72[*]	30[+]	61[+]
% Time Gastric pH>4	12	22[+]	49[+]	41[*]	66[*]	19	51[+]

NOTE: An intragastric pH of >4 reflects a reduction in gastric acid by 99%.
[*] (p<0.05) versus baseline, lansoprazole 15 mg and omeprazole 20 mg.
[+] (p<0.05) versus baseline only.

Continued on next page

Prevacid—Cont.

an unconfirmed pretreatment amoxicillin minimum inhibitory concentration (MIC) of > 256 µg/mL by E-test and the patient was eradicated of *H. pylori*.

[See table at top of previous page]

Patients not eradicated of *H. pylori* following lansoprazole/amoxicillin/clarithromycin triple therapy will likely have clarithromycin resistant *H. pylori*. Therefore, for those patients who fail therapy, clarithromycin susceptibility testing should be done when possible. Patients with clarithromycin resistant *H. pylori* should not be treated with lansoprazole/amoxicillin/clarithromycin triple therapy or with regimens which include clarithromycin as the sole antimicrobial agent.

Amoxicillin Susceptibility Test Results and Clinical/Bacteriological Outcomes

In the dual and triple therapy clinical trials, 82.6% (195/236) of the patients that had pre-treatment amoxicillin susceptible MICs (≤ 0.25 µg/mL) were eradicated of *H. pylori*. Of those with pretreatment amoxicillin MICs of > 0.25 µg/mL, three of six had the *H. pylori* eradicated. A total of 30% (21/70) of the patients failed lansoprazole 30 mg t.i.d./amoxicillin 1 gm t.i.d. dual therapy and a total of 12.8% (22/172) of the patients failed the 10-and-14 day triple therapy regimens. Post-treatment susceptibility results were not obtained on 11 of the patients who failed therapy. Nine of the 11 patients with amoxicillin post-treatment MICs that failed the triple therapy regimen also had clarithromycin resistant *H. pylori* isolates.

Susceptibility Test for *Helicobacter pylori*

The reference methodology for susceptibility testing of *H. pylori* is agar dilution MICs.[1] One to three microliters of an inoculum equivalent to a No. 2 McFarland standard (1 × 10^7 − 1 × 10^8 CFU/mL for *H. pylori*) are inoculated directly onto freshly prepared antimicrobial containing Mueller-Hinton agar plates with 5% aged defibrinated sheep blood (≥ 2 weeks old). The agar dilution plates are incubated at 35°C in a microaerobic environment produced by a gas generating system suitable for campylobacters. After 3 days of incubation, the MICs are recorded as the lowest concentration of antimicrobial agent required to inhibit growth of the organism. The clarithromycin and amoxicillin MIC values should be interpreted according to the following criteria:

Clarithromycin MIC (µg/mL)[a]	Interpretation
≤0.25	Susceptible (S)
0.5-1.0	Intermediate (I)
≥2.0	Resistant (R)

Amoxicillin MIC (µg/mL)[b]	Interpretation
≤0.25	Susceptible (S)

[a] These are tentative breakpoints for the agar dilution methodology and they should not be used to interpret results obtained using alternative methods.
[b] There were not enough organisms with MICs > 0.25 µg/mL to determine a resistance breakpoint.

Standardized susceptibility test procedures require the use of laboratory control microorganisms to control the technical aspects of the laboratory procedures. Standard clarithromycin and amoxicillin powders should provide the following MIC values:

Microorganism	Antimicrobial Agent	MIC (µg/mL)[a]
H. pylori ATCC 43504	Clarithromycin	0.015-0.12 mcg/mL
H. pylori ATCC 43504	Amoxicillin	0.015-0.12 mcg/mL

[a] These are quality control ranges for the agar dilution methodology and they should not be used to control test results obtained using alternative methods.

Reference

1. National Commitee for Clinical Laboratory Standards. Summary Minutes, Subcommittee on Antimicrobial Susceptibility Testing, Tampa, FL, January 11–13, 1998.

CLINICAL STUDIES

Duodenal Ulcer

In a U.S. multicenter, double-blind, placebo-controlled, dose-response (15, 30, and 60 mg of PREVACID once daily) study of 284 patients with endoscopically documented duodenal ulcer, the percentage of patients healed after two and four weeks was significantly higher with all doses of PREVACID than with placebo. There was no evidence of a greater or earlier response with the two higher doses compared with PREVACID 15 mg. Based on this study and the second study described below, the recommended dose of PREVACID in duodenal ulcer is 15 mg per day.

Duodenal Ulcer Healing Rates

Week	PREVACID 15 mg q.d. (N=68)	PREVACID 30 mg q.d. (N=74)	PREVACID 60 mg q.d. (N=70)	Placebo (N=72)
2	42.4%*	35.6%*	39.1%*	11.3%
4	89.4%*	91.7%*	89.9%*	46.1%

*(p≤0.001) versus placebo.

PREVACID 15 mg was significantly more effective than placebo in relieving day and nighttime abdominal pain and in decreasing the amount of antacid taken per day.

In a second U.S. multicenter study, also double-blind, placebo-controlled, dose-comparison (15 and 30 mg of PREVACID once daily), and including a comparison with ranitidine, in 280 patients with endoscopically documented duodenal ulcer, the percentage of patients healed after four weeks was significantly higher with both doses of PREVACID than with placebo. There was no evidence of a greater or earlier response with the higher dose of PREVACID. Although the 15-mg dose of PREVACID was superior to ranitidine at 4 weeks, the lack of significant difference at 2 weeks and the absence of a difference between 30 mg of PREVACID and ranitidine leaves the comparative effectiveness of the two agents undetermined.

Duodenal Ulcer Healing Rates

Week	PREVACID 15 mg q.d. (N=80)	PREVACID 30 mg q.d. (N=77)	Ranitidine 300 mg h.s. (N=82)	Placebo (N=41)
2	35.0%	44.2%	30.5%	34.2%
4	92.3%**	80.3%*	70.5%*	47.5%

* (p≤0.05) versus placebo.
** (p≤0.05) versus placebo and ranitidine.

H. pylori Eradication to Reduce the Risk of Duodenal Ulcer Recurrence

Randomized, double-blind clinical studies performed in the U.S. in patients with *H. pylori* and duodenal ulcer disease (defined as an active ulcer or history of an ulcer within one year) evaluated the efficacy of PREVACID in combination with amoxicillin capsules and clarithromycin tablets as triple 14-day therapy or in combination with amoxicillin capsules as dual 14-day therapy for the eradication of *H. pylori*. Based on the results of these studies, the safety and efficacy of two different eradication regimens were established:

Triple therapy: PREVACID 30 mg b.i.d./amoxicillin 1 gm b.i.d./clarithromycin 500 mg b.i.d.
Dual therapy: PREVACID 30 mg t.i.d./amoxicillin 1 gm t.i.d.

All treatments were for 14 days. *H. pylori* eradication was defined at two negative tests (culture and histology) at 4–6 weeks following the end of treatment.

Triple therapy was shown to be more effective than all possible dual therapy combinations. Dual therapy was shown to be more effective than both monotherapies. Eradication of *H. pylori* has been shown to reduce the risk of duodenal ulcer recurrence.

A randomized, double-blind clinical study performed in the U.S. in patients with *H. pylori* and duodenal ulcer disease (defined as an active ulcer or history of an ulcer within one year) compared the efficacy of PREVACID triple therapy for 10 and 14 days. This study established that the 10-day triple therapy was equivalent to the 14-day triple therapy in eradicating *H. pylori*.

H. pylori Eradication Rates - Triple Therapy
(PREVACID/amoxicillin/clarithromycin)
Percent of Patients Cured
[95% Confidence Interval]
(Number of patients)

Study	Duration	Triple Therapy Evaluable Analysis*	Triple Therapy Intent-to-Treat Analysis#
M93-131	14 days	92[†] [80.0-97.7] (N=48)	86[†] [73.3-93.5] (N=55)
M95-392	14 days	86[‡] [75.7-93.6] (N=66)	83[‡] [72.0-90.8] (N=70)
M95-399[+]	14 days	85 [77.0-91.0] (N=113)	82 [73.9-88.1] (N=126)
	10 days	84 [76.0-89.8] (N=123)	81 [73.9-87.6] (N=135)

* Based on evaluable patients with confirmed duodenal ulcer (active or within one year) and *H. pylori* infection at baseline defined as at least two of three positive endoscopic tests from CLOtest® (Delta West Ltd., Bentley, Australia); histology and/or culture. Patients were included in the analysis if they completed the study. Additionally, if patients dropped out of the study due to an adverse event related to the study drug, they were included in the evaluable analysis as failures of therapy.
# Patients were included in the analysis if they had documented *H. pylori* infection at baseline as defined above and had a confirmed duodenal ulcer (active or within one year). All dropouts were included as failures of therapy.
† (p<0.05) versus PREVACID/amoxicillin and PREVACID/clarithromycin dual therapy
‡ (p<0.05) versus clarithromycin/amoxicillin dual therapy
+ The 95% confidence interval for the difference in eradication rates, 10-day minus 14-day is (-10.5, 8.1) in the evaluable analysis and (-9.7, 9.1) in the intent-to-treat analysis.

H. pylori Eradication Rates - 14-Day Dual Therapy
(PREVACID/amoxicillin)
Percent of Patients Cured
[95% Confidence Interval]
(Number of patients)

Study	Dual Therapy Evaluable Analysis*	Dual Therapy Intent-to-Treat Analysis#
M93-131	77[†] [62.5-87.2] (N=51)	70[†] [56.8-81.2] (N=60)
M95-125	66[‡] [51.9-77.5] (N=58)	61[‡] [48.5-72.9] (N=67)

* Based on evaluable patients with confirmed duodenal ulcer (active or within one year) and *H. pylori* infection at baseline defined as at least two of three positive endoscopic tests from CLOtest®, histology and/or culture. Patients were included in the analysis if they completed the study. Additionally, if patients dropped out of the study due to an adverse event related to the study drug, they were included in the analysis as failures of therapy.
# Patients were included in the analysis if they had documented *H. pylori* infection at baseline as defined above and had a confirmed duodenal ulcer (active or within one year). All dropouts were included as failures of therapy.
† (p<0.05) versus PREVACID alone.
‡ (p<0.05) versus PREVACID alone or amoxicillin alone.

Long-Term Maintenance Treatment of Duodenal Ulcers

PREVACID has been shown to prevent the recurrence of duodenal ulcers. Two independent, double-blind, multicenter, controlled trials were conducted in patients with endoscopically confirmed healed duodenal ulcers. Patients remained healed significantly longer and the number of recurrences of duodenal ulcers was significantly less in patients treated with PREVACID than in patients treated with placebo over a 12-month period.

[See first table at top of next page]

In trial #2, no significant difference was noted between PREVACID 15 mg and 30 mg in maintaining remission.

Gastric Ulcer

In a U.S. multicenter, double-blind, placebo-controlled study of 253 patients with endoscopically documented gastric ulcer, the percentage of patients healed at four and eight weeks was significantly higher with PREVACID 15 mg and 30 mg once a day than with placebo.

Gastric Ulcer Healing Rates

Week	PREVACID 15 mg q.d. (N=65)	PREVACID 30 mg q.d. (N=63)	PREVACID 60 mg q.d. (N=61)	Placebo (N=64)
4	64.6%*	58.1%*	53.3%*	37.5%
8	92.2%*	96.8%*	93.2%*	76.7%

*(p≤0.05) versus placebo.

Patients treated with any PREVACID dose reported significantly less day and night abdominal pain along with fewer days of antacid use and fewer antacid tablets used per day than the placebo group.

Independent substantiation of the effectiveness of PREVACID 30 mg was provided by a meta-analysis of published and unpublished data.

Gastroesophageal Reflux Disease (GERD)

Symptomatic GERD

In a U.S. multicenter, double-blind, placebo-controlled study of 214 patients with frequent GERD symptoms, but no esophageal erosions by endoscopy, significantly greater relief of heartburn associated with GERD was observed with the administration of lansoprazole 15 mg once daily up to 8 weeks than with placebo. No significant additional benefit from lansoprazole 30 mg once daily was observed.

The intent-to-treat analyses demonstrated significant reduction in frequency and severity of day and night heartburn. Data for frequency and severity for the 8-week treatment period were as follows:

[See second table at right]

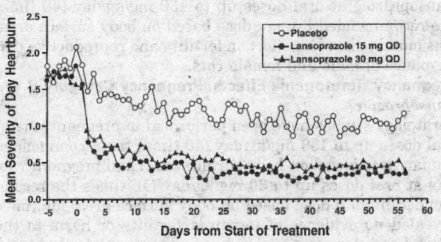

Mean Severity of Day Heartburn By Study Day For Evaluable Patients
(3=Severe, 2=Moderate, 1=Mild, 0=None)

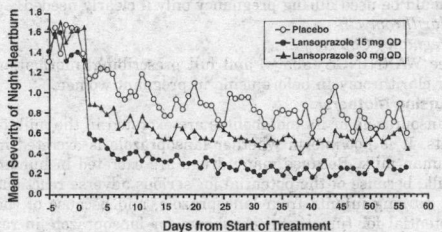

Mean Severity of Night Heartburn By Study Day For Evaluable Patients
(3=Severe, 2=Moderate, 1=Mild, 0=None)

Erosive Esophagitis

In a U.S. multicenter, double-blind, placebo-controlled study of 269 patients entering with an endoscopic diagnosis of esophagitis with mucosal grading of 2 or more and grades 3 and 4 signifying erosive disease, the percentages of patients with healing were as follows:

Erosive Esophagitis Healing Rates

Week	PREVACID 15 mg q.d. (N=69)	PREVACID 30 mg q.d. (N=65)	PREVACID 60 mg q.d. (N=72)	Placebo (N=63)
4	67.6%*	81.3%**	80.6%**	32.8%
6	87.7%*	95.4%*	94.3%*	52.5%
8	90.9%*	95.4%*	94.4%*	52.5%

* (p≤0.001) versus placebo.
** (p≤0.05) versus PREVACID 15 mg and placebo.

In this study, all PREVACID groups reported significantly greater relief of heartburn and less day and night abdominal pain along with fewer days of antacid use and fewer antacid tablets taken per day than the placebo group.

Although all doses were effective, the earlier healing in the higher two doses suggests 30 mg q.d. as the recommended dose.

PREVACID was also compared in a U.S. multicenter, double-blind study to a low dose of ranitidine in 242 patients with erosive reflux esophagitis. PREVACID at a dose of 30 mg was significantly more effective than ranitidine 150 mg b.i.d. as shown below.

Erosive Esophagitis Healing Rates

Week	PREVACID 30 mg q.d. (N=115)	Ranitidine 150 mg b.i.d. (N=127)
2	66.7%*	38.7%
4	82.5%*	52.0%
6	93.0%*	67.8%
8	92.1%*	69.9%

* (p≤0.001) versus ranitidine.

Endoscopic Remission Rates

| Trial | Drug | No. of Pts. | Percent in Endoscopic Remission | | |
			0–3 mo.	0–6 mo.	0–12 mo.
#1	PREVACID 15 mg q.d.	86	90%*	87%*	84%*
	Placebo	83	49%	41%	39%
#2	PREVACID 30 mg q.d.	18	94%*	94%*	85%*
	PREVACID 15 mg q.d.	15	87%*	79%*	70%*
	Placebo	15	33%	0%	0%

%=Life Table Estimate
*(p≤0.001) versus placebo.

Frequency of Heartburn

| Variable | Placebo (n=43) | PREVACID 15 mg (n=80) | PREVACID 30 mg (n=86) |
		Median	
% of Days without Heartburn			
Week 1	0%	71%*	46%*
Week 4	11%	81%*	76%*
Week 8	13%	84%*	82%*
% of Nights without Heartburn			
Week 1	17%	86%*	57%*
Week 4	25%	89%*	73%*
Week 8	36%	92%*	80%*

*(p<0.01) versus placebo.

In addition, patients treated with PREVACID reported less day and nighttime heartburn and took less antacid tablets for fewer days than patients taking ranitidine 150 mg b.i.d. Although this study demonstrates effectiveness of PREVACID in healing erosive esophagitis, it does not represent an adequate comparison with ranitidine because the recommended ranitidine dose for esophagitis is 150 mg q.i.d., twice the dose used in this study.

In the two trials described and in several smaller studies involving patients with moderate to severe erosive esophagitis, PREVACID produced healing rates similar to those shown above.

In a U.S. multicenter, double-blind, active-controlled study, 30 mg of PREVACID was compared with ranitidine 150 mg b.i.d. in 151 patients with erosive reflux esophagitis that was poorly responsive to a minimum of 12 weeks of treatment with at least one H_2-receptor antagonist given at the dose indicated for symptom relief or greater, namely, cimetidine 800 mg/day, ranitidine 300 mg/day, famotidine 40 mg/day or nizatidine 300 mg/day. PREVACID 30 mg was more effective than ranitidine 150 mg b.i.d. in healing reflux esophagitis, and the percentage of patients with healing were as follows. This study does not constitute a comparison of the effectiveness of histamine H_2-receptor antagonists with PREVACID, as all patients had demonstrated unresponsiveness to the histamine H_2-receptor antagonist mode of treatment. It does indicate, however, that PREVACID may be useful in patients failing on a histamine H_2-receptor antagonist.

Reflux Esophagitis Healing Rates in Patients Poorly Responsive to Histamine H_2-Receptor Antagonist Therapy

Week	PREVACID 30 mg q.d. (N=100)	Ranitidine 150 mg b.i.d. (N=51)
4	74.7%*	42.6%
8	83.7%*	32.0%

* (p≤0.001) versus ranitidine.

Long-Term Maintenance Treatment of Erosive Esophagitis

Two independent, double-blind, multicenter, controlled trials were conducted in patients with endoscopically confirmed healed esophagitis. Patients remained in remission significantly longer and the number of recurrences of erosive esophagitis was significantly less in patients treated with PREVACID than in patients treated with placebo over a 12-month period.

[See table at top of next page]

Regardless of initial grade of erosive esophagitis, PREVACID 15 mg and 30 mg were similar in maintaining remission.

Pathological Hypersecretory Conditions Including Zollinger-Ellison Syndrome

In open studies of 57 patients with pathological hypersecretory conditions, such as Zollinger-Ellison (ZE) syndrome with or without multiple endocrine adenomas, PREVACID significantly inhibited gastric acid secretion and controlled associated symptoms of diarrhea, anorexia and pain. Doses ranging from 15 mg every other day to 180 mg per day maintained basal acid secretion below 10 mEq/hr in patients without prior gastric surgery and below 5 mEq/hr in patients with prior gastric surgery.

Initial doses were titrated to the individual patient need, and adjustments were necessary with time in some patients. (See DOSAGE AND ADMINISTRATION.) PREVACID was well tolerated at these high dose levels for prolonged periods (greater than four years in some patients). In most ZE patients, serum gastrin levels were not modified by PREVACID. However, in some patients, serum gastrin increased to levels greater than those present prior to initiation of lansoprazole therapy.

INDICATIONS AND USAGE

Short-Term Treatment of Active Duodenal Ulcer

PREVACID Delayed-Release Capsules are indicated for short-term treatment (up to 4 weeks) for healing and symptom relief of active duodenal ulcer.

H. pylori Eradication to Reduce the Risk of Duodenal Ulcer Recurrence

Triple Therapy (PREVACID/amoxicillin/clarithromycin)

PREVACID Delayed-Release Capsules, in combination with amoxicillin plus clarithromycin as triple therapy, are indicated for the treatment of patients with H. pylori infection and duodenal ulcer disease (active or one-year history of a duodenal ulcer) to eradicate H. pylori. Eradication of H. pylori has been shown to reduce the risk of duodenal ulcer recurrence. (See CLINICAL STUDIES and DOSAGE AND ADMINISTRATION.)

Dual Therapy (PREVACID/amoxicillin)

PREVACID Delayed-Release Capsules, in combination with amoxicillin as dual therapy, are indicated for the treatment of patients with H. pylori infection and duodenal ulcer disease (active or one-year history of a duodenal ulcer) **who are either allergic or intolerant to clarithromycin or in whom resistance to clarithromycin is known or suspected.** (See the clarithromycin package insert, MICROBIOLOGY section.) Eradication of H. pylori has been shown to reduce the risk of duodenal ulcer recurrence. (See CLINICAL STUDIES and DOSAGE AND ADMINISTRATION.)

Maintenance of Healed Duodenal Ulcers

PREVACID Delayed-Release Capsules are indicated to maintain healing of duodenal ulcers. Controlled studies do not extend beyond 12 months.

Short-Term Treatment of Active Benign Gastric Ulcer

PREVACID Delayed-Release Capsules are indicated for short-term treatment (up to 8 weeks) for healing and symptom relief of active benign gastric ulcer.

Gastroesophageal Reflux Disease (GERD)

Short-Term Treatment of Symptomatic GERD

PREVACID Delayed-Release Capsules are indicated for the treatment of heartburn and other symptoms associated with GERD.

Short-Term Treatment of Erosive Esophagitis

PREVACID Delayed-Release Capsules are indicated for short-term treatment (up to 8 weeks) for healing and symptom relief of all grades of erosive esophagitis.

Continued on next page

Prevacid—Cont.

For patients who do not heal with PREVACID for 8 weeks (5–10%), it may be helpful to give an additional 8 weeks of treatment.
If there is a recurrence of erosive esophagitis an additional 8-week course of PREVACID may be considered.

Maintenance of Healing of Erosive Esophagitis
PREVACID Delayed-Release Capsules are indicated to maintain healing of erosive esophagitis. Controlled studies did not extend beyond 12 months.

Pathological Hypersecretory Conditions Including Zollinger-Ellison Syndrome
PREVACID Delayed-Release Capsules are indicated for the long-term treatment of pathological hypersecretory conditions, including Zollinger-Ellison syndrome.

Endoscopic Remission Rates

Trial	Drug	No. of Pts.	Percent in Endoscopic Remission 0–3 mo.	0–6 mo.	0–12 mo.
#1	PREVACID 15 mg q.d.	59	83%*	81%*	79%*
	PREVACID 30 mg q.d.	56	93%*	93%*	90%*
	Placebo	55	31%	27%	24%
#2	PREVACID 15 mg q.d.	50	74%*	72%*	67%*
	PREVACID 30 mg q.d.	49	75%*	72%*	55%*
	Placebo	47	16%	13%	13%

%=Life Table Estimate
*(p≤0.001) versus placebo.

CONTRAINDICATIONS

PREVACID Delayed-Release Capsules are contraindicated in patients with known hypersensitivity to any component of the formulation.
Amoxicillin is contraindicated in patients with a known hypersensitivity to any penicillin. (Please refer to full prescribing information for amoxicillin before prescribing.)
Clarithromycin is contraindicated in patients with a known hypersensitivity to any macrolide antibiotic, and in patients receiving terfenadine therapy who have preexisting cardiac abnormalities or electrolyte disturbances. (Please refer to full prescribing information for clarithromycin before prescribing.)

WARNINGS

CLARITHROMYCIN SHOULD NOT BE USED IN PREGNANT WOMEN EXCEPT IN CLINICAL CIRCUMSTANCES WHERE NO ALTERNATIVE THERAPY IS APPROPRIATE. IF PREGNANCY OCCURS WHILE TAKING CLARITHROMYCIN, THE PATIENT SHOULD BE APPRISED OF THE POTENTIAL HAZARD TO THE FETUS. (SEE WARNINGS IN PRESCRIBING INFORMATION FOR CLARITHROMYCIN.)

Pseudomembranous colitis has been reported with nearly all antibacterial agents, including clarithromycin and amoxicillin, and may range in severity from mild to life threatening. Therefore, it is important to consider this diagnosis in patients who present with diarrhea subsequent to the administration of antibacterial agents.

Treatment with antibacterial agents alters the normal flora of the colon and may permit overgrowth of clostridia. Studies indicate that a toxin produced by *Clostridium difficile* is a primary cause of "antibiotic-associated colitis".
After the diagnosis of pseudomembranous colitis has been established, therapeutic measures should be initiated. Mild cases of pseudomembranous colitis usually respond to discontinuation of the drug alone. In moderate to severe cases, consideration should be given to management with fluids and electrolytes, protein supplementation, and treatment with an antibacterial drug clinically effective against *Clostridium difficile* colitis.
Serious and occasionally fatal hypersensitivity (anaphylactic) reactions have been reported in patients on penicillin therapy. These reactions are more apt to occur in individuals with a history of penicillin hypersensitivity and/or a history of sensitivity to multiple allergens.
There have been well documented reports of individuals with a history of penicillin hypersensitivity reactions who have experienced severe hypersensitivity reactions when treated with a cephalosporin. Before initiating therapy with any penicillin, careful inquiry should be made concerning previous hypersensitivity reactions to penicillins, cephalosporins, and other allergens. If an allergic reaction occurs, amoxicillin should be discontinued and the appropriate therapy instituted.
SERIOUS ANAPHYLACTIC REACTIONS REQUIRE IMMEDIATE EMERGENCY TREATMENT WITH EPINEPHRINE. OXYGEN, INTRAVENOUS STEROIDS, AND AIRWAY MANAGEMENT, INCLUDING INTUBATION, SHOULD ALSO BE ADMINISTERED AS INDICATED.

PRECAUTIONS

General
Symptomatic response to therapy with lansoprazole does not preclude the presence of gastric malignancy.

Information for Patients
PREVACID Delayed-Release Capsules should be taken before eating.
For patients who have difficulty swallowing capsules, PREVACID Delayed-Release Capsules can be opened, and the intact granules contained within can be sprinkled on one tablespoon of applesauce and swallowed immediately. The granules should not be chewed or crushed. The granules have also been shown *in vitro* to remain intact when exposed to apple, cranberry, grape, orange, pineapple, prune, tomato, and V-8® vegetable juice and stored for up to 30 minutes.
For patients who have a nasogastric tube in place, PREVACID Delayed-Release Capsules can be opened and the intact granules mixed in 40 mL of apple juice and injected through the nasogastric tube into the stomach. After administering the granules, the nasogastric tube should be flushed with additional apple juice to clear the tube.

Drug Interactions
Lansoprazole is metabolized through the cytochrome P_{450} system, specifically through the CYP3A and CYP2C19 isozymes. Studies have shown that lansoprazole does not have clinically significant interactions with other drugs metabolized by the cytochrome P_{450} system, such as warfarin, antipyrine, indomethacin, ibuprofen, phenytoin, propranolol, prednisone, diazepam, clarithromycin, or terfenadine in healthy subjects. These compounds are metabolized through various cytochrome P_{450} isozymes including CYP1A2, CYP2C9, CYP2C19, CYP2D6, and CYP3A. When lansoprazole was administered concomitantly with theophylline (CYP1A2, CYP3A), a minor increase (10%) in the clearance of theophylline was seen. Because of the small magnitude and the direction of the effect on theophylline clearance, this interaction is unlikely to be of clinical concern. Nonetheless, individual patients may require additional titration of their theophylline dosage when lansoprazole is started or stopped to ensure clinically effective blood levels.
Lansoprazole has also been shown to have no clinically significant interaction with amoxicillin.
In a single-dose crossover study examining lansoprazole 30 mg and omeprazole 20 mg each administered alone and concomitantly with sucralfate 1 gram, absorption of the proton pump inhibitors was delayed and their bioavailability was reduced by 17% and 16%, respectively, when administered concomitantly with sucralfate. Therefore, proton pump inhibitors should be taken at least 30 minutes prior to sucralfate. In clinical trials, antacids were administered concomitantly with PREVACID Delayed-Release Capsules; this did not interfere with its effect.
Lansoprazole causes a profound and long-lasting inhibition of gastric acid secretion; therefore, it is theoretically possible that lansoprazole may interfere with the absorption of drugs where gastric pH is an important determinant of bioavailability (eg, ketoconazole, ampicillin esters, iron salts, digoxin).

Carcinogenesis, Mutagenesis, Impairment of Fertility
In two 24-month carcinogenicity studies, Sprague-Dawley rats were treated orally with doses of 5 to 150 mg/kg/day, about 1 to 40 times the exposure on a body surface (mg/m^2) basis, of a 50-kg person of average height (1.46 m^2 body surface area) given the recommended human dose of 30 mg/day (22.2 mg/m^2). Lansoprazole produced dose-related gastric enterochromaffin-like (ECL) cell hyperplasia and ECL cell carcinoids in both male and female rats. It also increased the incidence of intestinal metaplasia of the gastric epithelium in both sexes. In male rats, lansoprazole produced a dose-related increase of testicular interstitial cell adenomas. The incidence of these adenomas in rats receiving doses of 15 to 150 mg/kg/day (4 to 40 times the recommended human dose based on body surface area) exceeded the low background incidence (range = 1.4 to 10%) for this strain of rat. Testicular interstitial cell adenoma also occurred in 1 of 30 rats treated with 50 mg/kg/day (13 times the recommended human dose based on body surface area) in a 1-year toxicity study.
In a 24-month carcinogenicity study, CD-1 mice were treated orally with doses of 15 to 600 mg/kg/day, 2 to 80 times the recommended human dose based on body surface area. Lansoprazole produced a dose-related increased incidence of gastric ECL cell hyperplasia. It also produced an increased incidence of liver tumors (hepatocellular adenoma plus carcinoma). The tumor incidences in male mice treated with 300 and 600 mg/kg/day (40 to 80 times the recommended human dose based on body surface area) and female mice treated with 150 to 600 mg/kg/day (20 to 80 times the recommended human dose based on body surface area) exceeded the ranges of background incidences in historical controls for this strain of mice. Lansoprazole treatment produced adenoma of rete testis in male mice receiving 75 to 600 mg/kg/day (10 to 80 times the recommended human dose based on body surface area).
Lansoprazole was not genotoxic in the Ames test, the *ex vivo* rat hepatocyte unscheduled DNA synthesis (UDS) test, the *in vivo* mouse micronucleus test or the rat bone marrow cell chromosomal aberration test. It was positive in *in vitro* human lymphocyte chromosomal aberration assays.
Lansoprazole at oral doses up to 150 mg/kg/day (40 times the recommended human dose based on body surface area) was found to have no effect on fertility and reproductive performance of male and female rats.

Pregnancy: Teratogenic Effects. Pregnancy Category B
Lansoprazole
Teratology studies have been performed in pregnant rats at oral doses up to 150 mg/kg/day (40 times the recommended human dose based on body surface area) and pregnant rabbits at oral doses up to 30 mg/kg/day (16 times the recommended human dose based on body surface area) and have revealed no evidence of impaired fertility or harm to the fetus due to lansoprazole.
There are, however, no adequate or well-controlled studies in pregnant women. Because animal reproduction studies are not always predictive of human response, this drug should be used during pregnancy only if clearly needed.
Clarithromycin
Pregnancy Category C
See WARNINGS (above) and full prescribing information for clarithromycin before using in pregnant women.

Nursing Mothers
Lansoprazole or its metabolites are excreted in the milk of rats. It is not known whether lansoprazole is excreted in human milk. Because many drugs are excreted in human milk, because of the potential for serious adverse reactions in nursing infants from lansoprazole, and because of the potential for tumorigenicity shown for lansoprazole in rat carcinogenicity studies, a decision should be made whether to discontinue nursing or to discontinue the drug, taking into account the importance of the drug to the mother.

Pediatric Use
Safety and effectiveness in pediatric patients have not been established.

Use in Women
Over 800 women were treated with lansoprazole. Ulcer healing rates in females were similar to those in males. The incidence rates of adverse events were also similar to those seen in males.

Use in Geriatric Patients
Ulcer healing rates in elderly patients are similar to those in a younger age group. The incidence rates of adverse events and laboratory test abnormalities are also similar to those seen in younger patients. For elderly patients, dosage and administration of lansoprazole need not be altered for a particular indication.

ADVERSE REACTIONS

Worldwide, over 6100 patients have been treated with lansoprazole in Phase 2–3 clinical trials involving various dosages and durations of treatment. In general, lansoprazole treatment has been well tolerated in both short-term and long-term trials.
The following adverse events were reported by the treating physician to have a possible or probable relationship to drug in 1% or more of PREVACID-treated patients and occurred at a greater rate in PREVACID-treated patients than placebo-treated patients:

Incidence of Possibly or Probably Treatment-Related Adverse Events in Short-term, Placebo-Controlled Studies

Body System/Adverse Event	PREVACID (N=1457) %	Placebo (N=467) %
Body as a Whole		
Abdominal Pain	1.8	1.3
Digestive System		
Diarrhea	3.6	2.6
Nausea	1.4	1.3

Headache was also seen at greater than 1% incidence but was more common on placebo. The incidence of diarrhea was similar between patients who received placebo and pa-

tients who received lansoprazole 15 mg and 30 mg, but higher in the patients who received lansoprazole 60 mg (2.9%, 1.4%, 4.2%, and 7.4%, respectively).

The most commonly reported possibly or probably treatment-related adverse event during maintenance therapy was diarrhea.

Additional adverse experiences occurring in <1% of patients or subjects in domestic and/or international trials, or occurring since the drug was marketed, are shown below within each body system.

Body as a Whole — anaphylactoid-like reaction, asthenia, candidiasis, chest pain (not otherwise specified), edema, fever, flu syndrome, halitosis, infection (not otherwise specified), malaise; *Cardiovascular System* — angina, cerebrovascular accident, hypertension/hypotension, myocardial infarction, palpitations, shock (circulatory failure), vasodilation; *Digestive System* — melena, anorexia, bezoar, cardiospasm, cholelithiasis, constipation, dry mouth/thirst, dyspepsia, dysphagia, eructation, esophageal stenosis, esophageal ulcer, esophagitis, fecal discoloration, flatulence, gastric nodules/fundic gland polyps, gastroenteritis, gastrointestinal hemorrhage, hematemesis, increased appetite, increased salivation, rectal hemorrhage, stomatitis, tenesmus, ulcerative colitis, vomiting; *Endocrine System* — diabetes mellitus, goiter, hyperglycemia/hypoglycemia; *Hematologic and Lymphatis System** — agranulocytosis, anemia, aplastic anemia, hemolysis, hemolytic anemia, leukopenia, neutropenia, pancytopenia, thrombocytopenia, and thrombotic thrombocytopenic purpura; *Metabolic and Nutritional Disorders* — gout, weight gain/loss; *Musculoskeletal System* — arthritis/arthralgia, musculoskeletal pain, myalgia; *Nervous System* — agitation, amnesia, anxiety, apathy, confusion, depression, dizziness/syncope, hallucinations, hemiplegia, hostility aggravated, libido decreased, nervousness, paresthesia, thinking abnormality; *Respiratory System* — asthma, bronchitis, cough increased, dyspnea, epistaxis, hemoptysis, hiccup, pneumonia, upper respiratory inflammation/infection; *Skin and Appendages* — acne, alopecia, pruritis, rash, urticaria; *Special Senses* — blurred vision, deafness, eye pain, visual field defect, otitis media, speech disorder, taste perversion, tinnitus; *Urogenital System* — abnormal menses, albuminuria, breast enlargement/gynecomastia, breast tenderness, glycosuria, hematuria, impotence, kidney calculus, urinary retention.

*The majority of hematologic cases received were foreign-sourced and their relationship to lansoprazole was unclear.

Combination Therapy with Amoxicillin and Clarithromycin

In clinical trials using combination therapy with PREVACID plus amoxicillin and clarithromycin, and PREVACID plus amoxicillin, no adverse reactions peculiar to these drug combinations were observed. Adverse reactions that have occurred have been limited to those that had been previously reported with PREVACID, amoxicillin, or clarithromycin.

Triple Therapy: PREVACID/amoxicillin/clarithromycin

The most frequently reported adverse events for patients who received triple therapy for 14 days were diarrhea (7%), headache (6%), and taste perversion (5%). There were no statistically significant differences in the frequency of reported adverse events between the 10- and 14-day triple therapy regimens. No treatment-emergent adverse events were observed at significantly higher rates with triple therapy than with any dual therapy regimen.

Dual Therapy: PREVACID/amoxicillin

The most frequently reported adverse events for patients who received PREVACID t.i.d. plus amoxicillin t.i.d. dual therapy were diarrhea (8%) and headache (7%). No treatment-emergent adverse events were observed at significantly higher rates with PREVACID t.i.d. plus amoxicillin t.i.d. dual therapy than with PREVACID alone.

For more information on adverse reactions with amoxicillin or clarithromycin, refer to their package inserts, ADVERSE REACTIONS sections.

Laboratory Values

The following changes in laboratory parameters for lansoprazole were reported as adverse events:

Abnormal liver function tests, increased SGOT (AST), increased SGPT (ALT), increased creatinine, increased alkaline phosphatase, increased globulins, increased GGTP, increased/decreased/abnormal WBC, abnormal AG ratio, abnormal RBC, bilirubinemia, eosinophilia, hyperlipemia, increased/decreased electrolytes, increased/decreased cholesterol, increased glucocorticoids, increased LDH, increased/decreased/abnormal platelets, and increased gastrin levels. Additional isolated laboratory abnormalities were reported.

In the placebo controlled studies, when SGOT (AST) and SGPT (ALT) were evaluated, 0.4% (1/250) placebo patients and 0.3% (2/795) lansoprazole patients had enzyme elevations greater than three times the upper limit of normal range at the final treatment visit. None of these patients reported jaundice at any time during the study.

In clinical trials using combination therapy with PREVACID plus amoxicillin and clarithromycin, and PREVACID plus amoxicillin, no increased laboratory abnormalities particular to these drug combinations were observed.

For more information on laboratory value changes with amoxicillin or clarithromycin, refer to their package inserts, ADVERSE REACTIONS section.

OVERDOSAGE

Oral doses up to 5000 mg/kg in rats (approximately 1300 times the recommended human dose based on body surface area) and mice (about 675.7 times the recommended human dose based on body surface area) did not produce deaths or any clinical signs.

Lansoprazole is not removed from the circulation by hemodialysis. In one reported case of overdose, the patient consumed 600 mg of lansoprazole with no adverse reaction.

DOSAGE AND ADMINISTRATION

Short-Term Treatment of Duodenal Ulcer

The recommended adult oral dose is 15 mg once daily for 4 weeks. (See INDICATIONS AND USAGE.)

***H. pylori* Eradication to Reduce the Risk of Duodenal Ulcer Recurrence**

Triple Therapy: PREVACID/amoxicillin/clarithromycin

The recommended adult oral dose is 30 mg PREVACID, 1 gram amoxicillin, and 500 mg clarithromycin, all given twice daily (q 12h) for 10 or 14 days. (See INDICATIONS AND USAGE.)

Dual Therapy: PREVACID/amoxicillin

The recommended adult oral dose is 30 mg PREVACID and 1 gram amoxicillin, each given three times daily (q 8h) for 14 days. (See INDICATIONS AND USAGE.)

Please refer to amoxicillin and clarithromycin full prescribing information for CONTRAINDICATIONS and WARNINGS, and for information regarding dosing in elderly and renally-impaired patients.

Maintenance of Healed Duodenal Ulcers

The recommended adult oral dose is 15 mg once daily. (See CLINICAL STUDIES.)

Short-Term Treatment of Gastric Ulcer

The recommended adult oral dose is 30 mg once daily for up to eight weeks. (See CLINICAL STUDIES.)

Gastroesophageal Reflux Disease (GERD)

Short-Term Treatment of Symptomatic GERD

The recommended adult oral dose is 15 mg once daily for up to 8 weeks.

Short-Term Treatment of Erosive Esophagitis

The recommended adult oral dose is 30 mg once daily for up to 8 weeks. For patients who do not heal with PREVACID for 8 weeks (5-10%), it may be helpful to give an additional 8 weeks of treatment. (See INDICATIONS AND USAGE.)

If there is a recurrence of erosive esophagitis, an additional 8-week course of PREVACID may be considered.

Maintenance of Healing of Erosive Esophagitis

The recommended adult oral dose is 15 mg once daily. (See CLINICAL STUDIES.)

Pathological Hypersecretory Conditions Including Zollinger-Ellison Syndrome

The dosage of PREVACID in patients with pathologic hypersecretory conditions varies with the individual patient. The recommended adult oral starting dose is 60 mg once a day. Doses should be adjusted to individual patient needs and should continue for as long as clinically indicated. Dosages up to 90 mg b.i.d. have been administered. Daily dosages of greater than 120 mg should be administered in divided doses. Some patients with Zollinger-Ellison syndrome have been treated continuously with PREVACID for more than four years.

No dosage adjustment is necessary in patients with renal insufficiency or the elderly. For patients with severe liver disease, dosage adjustment should be considered.

PREVACID Delayed-Release Capsules should be taken before eating. In the clinical trials, antacids were used concomitantly with PREVACID. For patients who have difficulty swallowing capsules, PREVACID Delayed-Release Capsules can be opened, and the intact granules contained within can be sprinkled on one tablespoon of applesauce and swallowed immediately. The granules should not be chewed or crushed. The granules have also been shown *in vitro* to remain intact when exposed to apple, cranberry, grape, orange, pineapple, prune, tomato, and V-8® vegetable juice and stored for up to 30 minutes.

For patients who have a nasogastric tube in place, PREVACID Delayed-Release Capsules can be opened and the intact granules mixed in 40 mL of apple juice and injected through the nasogastric tube into the stomach. After administering the granules, the nasogastric tube should be flushed with additional apple juice to clear the tube.

HOW SUPPLIED

PREVACID Delayed-Release Capsules, 15 mg, are opaque, hard gelatin, colored pink and green with the TAP logo and "PREVACID 15" imprinted on the capsules. The 30 mg are opaque, hard gelatin, colored pink and black with the TAP logo and "PREVACID 30" imprinted on the capsules. They are available as follows:

NDC 0300-1541-30
Unit of use bottles of 30: 15-mg capsules
NDC 0300-1541-13
Bottles of 100: 15-mg capsules
NDC 0300-1541-19
Bottles of 1000: 15-mg capsules
NDC 0300-1541-11
Unit dose package of 100: 15-mg capsules
NDC 0300-3046-13
Bottles of 100: 30-mg capsules
NDC 0300-3046-19
Bottles of 1000: 30-mg capsules
NDC 0300-3046-11
Unit dose package of 100: 30-mg capsules

Storage: PREVACID capsules should be stored in a tight container protected from moisture.

Store between 15°C and 30°C (59°F and 86°F).

℞ only

U.S. Patent Nos. 4,628,098; 4,689,333; 5,013,743; 5,026,560 and 5,045,321.

Manufactured for
TAP Pharmaceuticals Inc.
Deerfield, Illinois 60015-1595, U.S.A.
by Takeda Chemical Industries Limited,
Osaka, Japan 541
®—Registered Trademark
03-4891-R11-Rev. June, 1998

Shown in Product Identification Guide, page 341

PREVPAC™ ℞

(lansoprazole 30-mg capsules, amoxicillin 500-mg capsules, USP, and clarithromycin 500-mg tablets)

THESE PRODUCTS ARE INTENDED ONLY FOR USE AS DESCRIBED. The individual products contained in this package should not be used alone or in combination for other purposes. The information described in this labeling concerns only the use of these products as indicated in this daily administration pack. For information on use of the individual components when dispensed as individual medications outside this combined use for treating *Helicobacter pylori (H. pylori)*, please see the package inserts for each individual product.

DESCRIPTION

PREVPAC consists of a daily administration pack containing two PREVACID 30-mg capsules, four amoxicillin 500-mg capsules, USP, and two clarithromycin 500-mg tablets, for oral administration.

PREVACID® (lansoprazole) Delayed-Release Capsules

The active ingredient in PREVACID capsules is a substituted benzimidazole, 2-[[[3-methyl-4-(2,2,2-trifluoroethoxy)-2-pyridyl] methyl]sulfinyl] benzimidazole, a compound that inhibits gastric acid secretion. Its empirical formula is $C_{16}H_{14}F_3N_3O_2S$ with a molecular weight of 369.37. The structural formula is:

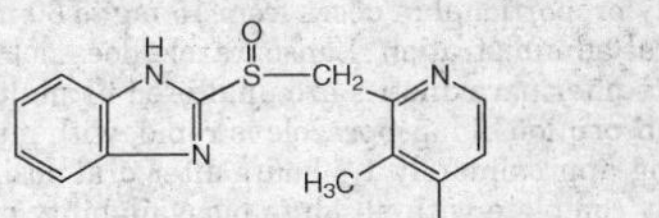

Lansoprazole is a white to brownish-white odorless crystalline powder which melts with decomposition at approximately 166°C. Lansoprazole is freely soluble in dimethylformamide; soluble in methanol; sparingly soluble in ethanol; slightly soluble in ethyl acetate, dichloromethane and acetonitrile; very slightly soluble in ether; and practically insoluble in hexane and water.

Each delayed-release capsule contains enteric-coated granules consisting of lansoprazole (30 mg), hydroxypropyl cellulose, low substituted hydroxypropyl cellulose, colloidal silicon dioxide, magnesium carbonate, methacrylic acid copolymer, starch, talc, sugar sphere, sucrose, polyethylene glycol, polysorbate 80, and titanium dioxide. Components of the gelatin capsule include gelatin, titanium dioxide, D&C Red No. 28, FD&C Blue No. 1, and FD&C Red No. 40.

TRIMOX® (amoxicillin, USP)

Amoxicillin, USP, (2*S*,5*R*,6*R*)-6-[(*R*)-(−)-2-Amino-2-(*p*-hydroxyphenyl) acetamido]-3,3-dimethyl-7-oxo-4-thia-1-azabicyclo[3.2.0]heptane-2-carboxylic acid trihydrate, is a semisynthetic penicillin, an analogue of ampicillin. It has the following chemical structure:

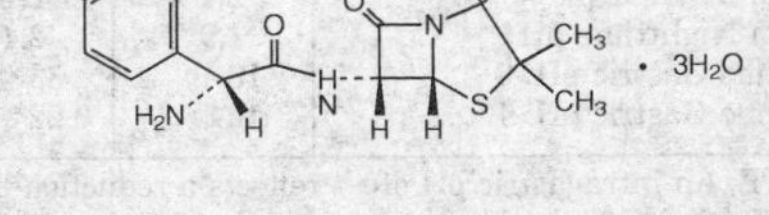

Continued on next page

Prevpac—Cont.

The empirical formula is $C_{16}H_{18}N_3O_5S \bullet 3H_2O$, and the molecular weight is 419.45.
The maroon and light-pink capsules contain amoxicillin trihydrate equivalent to 500 mg of amoxicillin. The inactive ingredient in the capsules is magnesium stearate.
BIAXIN® Filmtab® (clarithromycin tablets)
Clarithromycin is a semi-synthetic macrolide antibiotic. Chemically, it is 6-*0*-methylerythromycin. The molecular formula is $C_{38}H_{69}NO_{13}$, and the molecular weight is 747.96. The structural formula is:

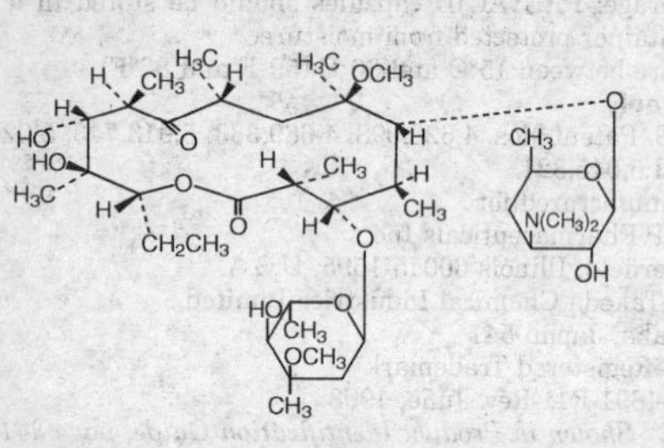

Clarithromycin is a white to off-white crystalline powder. It is soluble in acetone, slightly soluble in methanol, ethanol, and acetonitrile, and practically insoluble in water.
Each yellow oval film-coated tablet contains 500 mg of clarithromycin and the following inactive ingredients: cellulosic polymers, croscarmellose sodium, D&C Yellow No. 10, FD&C Blue No. 1, magnesium stearate, povidone, propylene glycol, silicon dioxide, sorbic acid, sorbitan monooleate, stearic acid, talc, titanium dioxide, and vanillin.

CLINICAL PHARMACOLOGY

Pharmacokinetics

Pharmacokinetics when all three of the PREVPAC components (PREVACID capsules, amoxicillin capsules, clarithromycin tablets) were coadministered has not been studied. Studies have shown no clinically significant interactions of PREVACID and amoxicillin or PREVACID and clarithromycin when administered together. There is no information about the gastric mucosal concentrations of PREVACID, amoxicillin and clarithromycin after administration of these agents concomitantly. The systemic pharmacokinetic information presented below is based on studies in which each product was administered alone.
PREVACID:
PREVACID capsules contain an enteric-coated granule formulation of lansoprazole. Absorption of lansoprazole begins only after the granules leave the stomach. Absorption is rapid, with mean peak plasma levels of lansoprazole occurring after approximately 1.7 hours. Peak plasma concentrations of lansoprazole (C_{max}) and the area under the plasma concentration curve (AUC) of lansoprazole are approximately proportional in doses from 15 mg to 60 mg after single-oral administration. Lansoprazole does not accumulate and its pharmacokinetics are unaltered by multiple dosing.
The absorption of lansoprazole is rapid, with mean C_{max} occurring approximately 1.7 hours after oral dosing, and relatively complete with absolute bioavailability over 80%. In healthy subjects, the mean (± SD) plasma half-life was 1.5 (± 1.0) hours. Both C_{max} and AUC are diminished by about 50% if the drug is given 30 minutes after food as opposed to the fasting condition. There is no significant food effect if the drug is given before meals.
Lansoprazole is 97% bound to plasma proteins. Plasma protein binding is consistent over the concentration range of 0.05 to 5.0 mcg/mL.
Lansoprazole is extensively metabolized in the liver. Two metabolites have been identified in measurable quantities in plasma (the hydroxylated sulfinyl and sulfone derivatives of lansoprazole). These metabolites have very little or no antisecretory activity. Lansoprazole is thought to be transformed into two active species which inhibit acid secretion by (H^+,K^+)-ATPase within the parietal cell canaliculus, but are not present in the systemic circulation. The plasma elimination half-life of lansoprazole does not reflect its duration of suppression of gastric acid secretion. Thus, the plasma elimination half-life is less than two hours while the acid inhibitory effect lasts more than 24 hours.
Following single-dose oral administration of PREVACID, virtually no unchanged lansoprazole was excreted in the urine. In one study, after a single oral dose of ^{14}C-lansoprazole, approximately one-third of the administered radiation was excreted in the urine and two-thirds was recovered in the feces. This implies a significant biliary excretion of the metabolites of lansoprazole.
The clearance of lansoprazole is decreased in the elderly, with elimination half-life increased approximately 50% to 100%. Because the mean half-life in the elderly remains between 1.9 to 2.9 hours, repeated once daily dosing does not result in accumulation of lansoprazole. Peak plasma levels were not increased in the elderly.
In patients with severe renal insufficiency, plasma protein binding decreased by 1.0%–1.5% after administration of 60 mg of lansoprazole. Patients with renal insufficiency had a shortened elimination half-life and decreased total AUC (free and bound). AUC for free lansoprazole in plasma, however, was not related to the degree of renal impairment, and C_{max} and T_{max} were not different from subjects with healthy kidneys.
In patients with various degrees of chronic hepatic disease, the mean plasma half-life of the drug was prolonged from 1.5 hours to 3.2–7.2 hours. An increase in mean AUC of up to 500% was observed at steady state in hepatically-impaired patients compared to healthy subjects. Dose reduction in patients with severe hepatic disease should be considered.
The pooled pharmacokinetic parameters of PREVACID from twelve U.S. Phase I studies (N=513) were compared to the mean pharmacokinetic parameters from two Asian studies (N=20). The mean AUCs of PREVACID in Asian subjects are approximately twice that seen in pooled U.S. data; however, the inter-individual variability is high. The C_{max} values are comparable.
Amoxicillin:
Amoxicillin is stable in the presence of gastric acid and is well absorbed from the gastrointestinal tract and may be given with no regard to food. It diffuses readily into most body tissues and fluids, with the exception of brain and spinal fluid, except when meninges are inflamed. The half-life of amoxicillin is 61.3 minutes. Most of the amoxicillin is excreted unchanged in the urine; its excretion can be delayed by concurrent administration of probenecid. Amoxicillin is not highly protein-bound. In blood serum, amoxicillin is approximately 20% protein-bound as compared to 60% for penicillin G.
Orally administered doses of 500-mg amoxicillin capsules result in average peak blood levels 1 to 2 hours after administration in the range of 5.5 to 7.5 μg/mL.
Detectable serum levels are observed up to eight hours after an orally administered dose of amoxicillin. Approximately 60% of an orally administered dose of amoxicillin is excreted in the urine within 6 to 8 hours.
Clarithromycin:
Clarithromycin is rapidly absorbed from the gastrointestinal tract after oral administration. The absolute bioavailability of 250 mg clarithromycin tablets was approximately 50%. Food slightly delays both the onset of clarithromycin absorption and the formation of the antimicrobially active metabolite, 14-OH clarithromycin, but does not affect the extent of bioavailability. Therefore, clarithromycin tablets may be given without regard to food.
In fasting healthy human subjects, peak serum concentrations were attained within two hours after oral dosing. Steady-state peak serum clarithromycin concentrations were attained in two to three days and were approximately 2 to 3 μg/mL with a 500-mg dose administered every 12 hours. The elimination half-life of clarithromycin was 5 to 7 hours with 500 mg administered every 8 to 12 hours. The nonlinearity of clarithromycin pharmacokinetics is slight at the recommended dose of 500 mg administered every 12 hours. With a 500-mg dose every 8 to 12 hours, the peak steady-state concentration of 14-OH clarithromycin, the principal metabolite, is up to 1 μg/mL and its elimination half-life is about 7 to 9 hours. The steady-state concentration of this metabolite is generally attained within 2 to 3 days.
After a 500-mg tablet every 12 hours, the urinary excretion of clarithromycin is approximately 30%. The renal clearance of clarithromycin approximates the normal glomerular filtration rate. The major metabolite found in urine is 14-OH clarithromycin, which accounts for an additional 10% to 15% of the dose with a 500-mg tablet administered every 12 hours.
The steady-state concentrations of clarithromycin in subjects with impaired hepatic function did not differ from those in normal subjects; however, the 14-OH clarithromycin concentrations were lower in the hepatically impaired subjects. The decreased formation of 14-OH clarithromycin was at least partially offset by an increase in renal clearance of clarithromycin in the subjects with impaired hepatic function when compared to healthy subjects.
The pharmacokinetics of clarithromycin was also altered in subjects with impaired renal function. (See **PRECAUTIONS and DOSAGE AND ADMINISTRATION.**)

Pharmacodynamics

Microbiology

Susceptibility Testing for Helicobacter pylori
In vitro susceptibility testing methods and diagnostic products currently available for determining minimum inhibitory concentrations (MICs) and zone sizes have not been standardized, validated, or approved for testing *H. pylori* microorganisms.
Culture and susceptibility testing should be obtained in patients who fail triple therapy. If resistance to amoxicillin or clarithromycin is demonstrated or susceptibility testing is not possible, alternative antimicrobial therapy is recommended.

Antisecretory activity

After oral administration, lansoprazole was shown to significantly decrease the basal acid output and significantly increase the mean gastric pH and percent of time the gastric pH was >3 and >4. Lansoprazole also significantly reduced meal-stimulated gastric acid output and secretion volume, as well as pentagastrin-stimulated acid output. In patients with hypersecretion of acid, lansoprazole significantly reduced basal and pentagastrin-stimulated gastric acid secretion. Lansoprazole inhibited the normal increases in secretion volume, acidity and acid output induced by insulin.
In a crossover study comparing lansoprazole 15 and 30 mg with omeprazole 20 mg for five days, the following effects on intragastric pH were noted:
[See table below]
After the initial dose in this study, increased gastric pH was seen within 1–2 hours with lansoprazole 30 mg, 2–3 hours with lansoprazole 15 mg, and 3–4 hours with omeprazole 20 mg. After multiple daily dosing, increased gastric pH was seen within the first hour postdosing with lansoprazole 30 mg and within 1–2 hours postdosing with lansoprazole 15 mg and omeprazole 20 mg.
The percentage of time gastric pH was elevated above 5 and 6 was evaluated in a crossover study of PREVACID given q.d., b.i.d. and t.i.d.
[See table at bottom of next page]
The inhibition of gastric acid secretion as measured by intragastric pH returns gradually to normal over two to four days after multiple doses. There is no indication of rebound gastric acidity.

CLINICAL STUDIES

***H. pylori* Eradication to Reduce the Risk of Duodenal Ulcer Recurrence**

Randomized, double-blind clinical studies performed in the U.S. in patients with *H. pylori* and duodenal ulcer disease (defined as an active ulcer or history of an ulcer within one year) evaluated the efficacy of PREVPAC as triple 14-day therapy for the eradication of *H. pylori.* The triple therapy regimen (PREVACID 30 mg BID plus amoxicillin 1 gm BID plus clarithromycin 500 mg BID) produced statistically significantly higher eradication rates than PREVACID plus amoxicillin, PREVACID plus clarithromycin, and amoxicillin plus clarithromycin dual therapies.
H. pylori eradication was defined as two negative tests (culture and histology) at 4 to 6 weeks following the end of treatment.
Triple therapy was shown to be more effective than all possible dual therapy combinations. The combination of PREVACID plus amoxicillin and clarithromycin as triple therapy was effective in eradicating *H. pylori.* Eradication of *H. pylori* has been shown to reduce the risk of duodenal ulcer recurrence.

***H. pylori* Eradication Rates - Triple Therapy**
(PREVACID/amoxicillin/clarithromycin)
Percent of Patients Cured
[95% Confidence Interval]
(Number of Patients)

Study	Triple Therapy Evaluable Analysis*	Triple Therapy Intent-to-Treat Analysis#
M93-131	92† [80.0-97.7] (N=48)	86† [73.3-93.5] (N=55)

Mean Antisecretory Effects after Single and Multiple Daily Dosing

Parameter	Baseline Value	PREVACID 15 mg Day 1	PREVACID 15 mg Day 5	PREVACID 30 mg Day 1	PREVACID 30 mg Day 5	Omeprazole 20 mg Day 1	Omeprazole 20 mg Day 5
Mean 24-Hour pH	2.1	2.7⁺	4.0⁺	3.6*	4.9*	2.5	4.2⁺
Mean Nighttime pH	1.9	2.4	3.0⁺	2.6	3.8*	2.2	3.0⁺
% Time Gastric pH>3	18	33⁺	59⁺	51*	72*	30⁺	61⁺
% Time Gastric pH>4	12	22⁺	49⁺	41*	66*	19	51⁺

NOTE: An intragastric pH of >4 reflects a reduction in gastric acid by 99%.
*(p<0.05) versus baseline, lansoprazole 15 mg and omeprazole 20 mg.
⁺(p<0.05) versus baseline only.

M95-392	86‡ [75.7-93.6] (N=66)	83‡ [72.0-90.8] (N=70)

* Based on evaluable patients with confirmed duodenal ulcer (active or within one year) and *H. pylori* infection at baseline defined as at least two of three positive endoscopic tests from CLOtest® (Delta West Ltd., Bentley, Australia), histology and/or culture. Patients were included in the analysis if they completed the study. Additionally, if patients dropped out of the study due to an adverse event related to the study drug, they were included in the analysis as failures of therapy.

\# Patients were included in the analysis if they had documented *H. pylori* infection at baseline as defined above and had a confirmed duodenal ulcer (active or within one year). All dropouts were included as failures of therapy.

† ($p<0.05$) versus PREVACID/amoxicillin and PREVACID/clarithromycin dual therapy

‡ ($p<0.05$) versus clarithromycin/amoxicillin dual therapy

INDICATIONS AND USAGE

H. pylori Eradication to Reduce the Risk of Duodenal Ulcer Recurrence

The components in PREVPAC (PREVACID, amoxicillin, and clarithromycin) are indicated for the treatment of patients with *H. pylori* infection and duodenal ulcer disease (active or one-year history of a duodenal ulcer) to eradicate *H. pylori*. Eradication of *H. pylori* has been shown to reduce the risk of duodenal ulcer recurrence (See **CLINICAL STUDIES** and **DOSAGE AND ADMINISTRATION**).

CONTRAINDICATIONS

PREVPAC is contraindicated in patients with known hypersensitivity to any component of the formulation of PREVACID, any macrolide antibiotic, or any penicillin.

Concomitant administration of PREVPAC with cisapride, pimozide, or terfenadine is contraindicated. There have been postmarketing reports of drug interactions when clarithromycin and/or erythromycin are co-administered with cisapride, pimozide, or terfenadine resulting in cardiac arrhythmias (QT prolongation, ventricular tachycardia, ventricular fibrillation, and torsades de pointes) most likely due to inhibition of hepatic metabolism of these drugs by erythromycin and clarithromycin. Fatalities have been reported.

WARNINGS

Amoxicillin:

Serious and occasionally fatal hypersensitivity (anaphylactoid) reactions have been reported in patients on penicillin therapy. Although anaphylaxis is more frequent following parenteral therapy, it has occurred in patients on oral penicillins. These reactions are more apt to occur in individuals with a history of penicillin hypersensitivity and/or a history of sensitivity to multiple allergens.

There have been well documented reports of individuals with a history of penicillin hypersensitivity reactions who have experienced severe hypersensitivity reactions when treated with a cephalosporin. Before initiating therapy with any penicillin, careful inquiry should be made concerning previous hypersensitivity reactions to penicillins, cephalosporins, and other allergens. If an allergic reaction occurs, amoxicillin should be discontinued and the appropriate therapy instituted.

SERIOUS ANAPHYLACTOID REACTIONS REQUIRE IMMEDIATE EMERGENCY TREATMENT WITH EPINEPHRINE. OXYGEN, INTRAVENOUS STEROIDS, AND AIRWAY MANAGEMENT, INCLUDING INTUBATION, SHOULD ALSO BE ADMINISTERED AS INDICATED.

Clarithromycin:

CLARITHROMYCIN SHOULD NOT BE USED IN PREGNANT WOMEN EXCEPT IN CLINICAL CIRCUMSTANCES WHERE NO ALTERNATIVE THERAPY IS APPROPRIATE. IF PREGNANCY OCCURS WHILE TAKING CLARITHROMYCIN, THE PATIENT SHOULD BE APPRISED OF THE POTENTIAL HAZARD TO THE FETUS. CLARITHROMYCIN HAS DEMONSTRATED ADVERSE EFFECTS OF PREGNANCY OUTCOME AND/OR EMBRYO-FETAL DEVELOPMENT IN MONKEYS, RATS, MICE, AND RABBITS AT DOSES THAT PRODUCED PLASMA LEVELS 2 TO 17 TIMES THE SERUM LEVELS ACHIEVED IN HUMANS TREATED AT THE MAXIMUM RECOMMENDED HUMAN DOSES. (See PRECAUTIONS - *Pregnancy*).

Pseudomembranous colitis has been reported with nearly all antibacterial agents, including clarithromycin, and may range in severity from mild to life threatening. Therefore, it is important to consider this diagnosis in patients who present with diarrhea subsequent to the administration of antibacterial agents.

Treatment with antibacterial agents alters the normal flora of the colon and may permit overgrowth of clostridia. Studies indicate that a toxin produced by *Clostridium difficile* is a primary cause of "antibiotic-associated colitis."

After the diagnosis of pseudomembranous colitis has been established, therapeutic measures should be initiated. Mild cases of pseudomembranous colitis usually respond to discontinuation of the drug alone. In moderate to severe cases, consideration should be given to management with fluids and electrolytes, protein supplementation, and treatment with an antibacterial drug clinically effective against *Clostridium difficile* colitis.

PRECAUTIONS

Clarithromycin is principally excreted via the liver and kidney. Clarithromycin may be administered without dosage adjustment to patients with hepatic impairment and normal renal function. However, in the presence of severe renal impairment with or without coexisting hepatic impairment, decreased dosage or prolonged dosing intervals may be appropriate.

The possibility of superinfections with mycotic organisms or bacterial pathogens should be kept in mind during therapy. In such cases, discontinue PREVPAC and substitute appropriate treatment.

Symptomatic response to therapy with PREVACID does not preclude the presence of gastric malignancy.

Information for Patients: Each dose of PREVPAC contains four pills: one pink and black capsule (PREVACID), two maroon and light-pink capsules (amoxicillin) and one yellow tablet (clarithromycin). Each dose should be taken twice per day before eating. Patients should be instructed to swallow each pill whole.

Drug Interactions

PREVACID:

PREVACID is metabolized through the cytochrome P_{450} system, specifically through the CYP3A and CYP2C19 isozymes. Studies have shown that PREVACID does not have clinically significant interactions with other drugs metabolized by the cytochrome P_{450} system, such as warfarin, antipyrine, indomethacin, ibuprofen, phenytoin, propranolol, prednisone, diazepam, clarithromycin, or terfenadine in healthy subjects. These compounds are metabolized through various cytochrome P_{450} isozymes including CYP1A2, CYP2C9, CYP2C19, CYP2D6, and CYP3A. When PREVACID was administered concomitantly with theophylline (CYP1A2, CYP3A), a minor increase (10%) in the clearance of theophylline was seen. Because of the small magnitude and the direction of the effect on theophylline clearance, this interaction is unlikely to be of clinical concern. Nonetheless, individual patients may require additional titration of their theophylline dosage when PREVACID is started or stopped to ensure clinically effective blood levels.

PREVACID has also been shown to have no clinically significant interaction with amoxicillin.

In a single-dose crossover study examining PREVACID 30 mg and omeprazole 20 mg each administered alone and concomitantly with sucralfate 1 gram, absorption of the proton pump inhibitors was delayed and their bioavailability was reduced by 17% and 16%, respectively, when administered concomitantly with sucralfate. Therefore, proton pump inhibitors should be taken at least 30 minutes prior to sucralfate. In clinical trials, antacids were administered concomitantly with PREVACID Delayed-Release Capsules; this did not interfere with its effect.

PREVACID causes a profound and long-lasting inhibition of gastric acid secretion; therefore, it is theoretically possible that PREVACID may interfere with the absorption of drugs where gastric pH is an important determinant of bioavailability (eg, ketoconazole, ampicillin esters, iron salts, digoxin).

Clarithromycin:

Clarithromycin use in patients who are receiving theophylline may be associated with an increase of serum theophylline concentrations. Monitoring of serum theophylline concentrations should be considered for patients receiving high doses of theophylline or with baseline concentrations in the upper therapeutic range. In two studies in which theophylline was administered with clarithromycin (a theophylline sustained-release formulation was dosed at either 6.5 mg/kg or 12 mg/kg together with 250 or 500 mg q12h clarithromycin), the steady-state levels of C_{max}, C_{min}, and the area under the serum concentration time curve (AUC) of theophylline increased about 20%.

Concomitant administration of single doses of clarithromycin and carbamazepine has been shown to result in increased plasma concentrations of carbamazepine. Blood level monitoring of carbamazepine may be considered.

When clarithromycin and terfenadine were coadministered, plasma concentrations of the active acid metabolite of terfenadine were threefold higher, on average, than the values observed when terfenadine was administered alone. The pharmacokinetics of clarithromycin and the 14-hydroxy-clarithromycin were not significantly affected by coadministration of terfenadine once clarithromycin reached steady-state conditions. Concomitant administration of clarithromycin with terfenadine is contraindicated. (See **CONTRAINDICATIONS**.)

Spontaneous reports in the postmarketing period suggest that concomitant administration of clarithromycin and oral anticoagulants may potentiate the effects of the oral anticoagulants. Prothrombin times should be carefully monitored while patients are receiving clarithromycin and oral anticoagulants simultaneously.

Elevated digoxin serum concentrations in patients receiving clarithromycin and digoxin concomitantly have also been reported in postmarketing surveillance. Some patients have shown clinical signs consistent with digoxin toxicity, including arrhythmias. Serum digoxin levels should be carefully monitored while patients are receiving digoxin and clarithromycin simultaneously.

For information on interactions between clarithromycin in combination with other drugs which may be administered to HIV-infected patients, see the BIAXIN package insert, Drug Interactions, under the **PRECAUTIONS** section.

The following drug interactions, other than increased serum concentrations of carbamazepine and active acid metabolite of terfenadine, have not been reported in clinical trials with clarithromycin; however, they have been observed with erythromycin products and/or with clarithromycin in postmarketing experience.

Concurrent use of erythromycin or clarithromycin and ergotamine or dihydroergotamine has been associated in some patients with acute ergot toxicity characterized by severe peripheral vasospasm and dysesthesia.

Erythromycin has been reported to decrease the clearance of triazolam and, thus, may increase the pharmacologic effect of triazolam. There have been postmarketing reports of drug interactions and CNS effects (e.g., somnolence and confusion) with the concomitant use of clarithromycin and triazolam.

There have been reports of an interaction between erythromycin and astemizole resulting in QT prolongation and torsades de pointes. Concomitant administration of erythromycin and astemizole is contraindicated. Because clarithromycin is also metabolized by cytochrome P_{450}, concomitant administration of clarithromycin with astemizole is not recommended.

The use of erythromycin and clarithromycin in patients concurrently taking drugs metabolized by the cytochrome P_{450} system may be associated with elevations in serum levels of these other drugs. There have been reports of interactions of erythromycin and/or clarithromycin with carbamazepine, cyclosporine, tacrolimus, hexobarbital, phenytoin, alfentanil, disopyramide, lovastatin, bromocriptine, valproate, terfenadine, cisapride, pimozide, and astemizole. Serum concentrations of drugs metabolized by the cytochrome P_{450} system should be monitored closely in patients concurrently receiving these drugs.

Carcinogenesis, Mutagenesis, Impairment of Fertility

PREVACID:

In two 24-month carcinogenicity studies, Sprague-Dawley rats were treated orally with doses of 5 to 150 mg/kg/day, about 1 to 40 times the exposure on a body surface (mg/m^2) basis, of a 50-kg person of average height (1.46 m^2 body surface area) given the recommended human dose of 30 mg/day (22.2 mg/m^2). Lansoprazole produced dose-related gastric enterochromaffin-like (ECL) cell hyperplasia and ECL cell carcinoids in both male and female rats. It also increased the incidence of intestinal metaplasia of the gastric epithelium in both sexes. In male rats, lansoprazole produced a dose-related increase of testicular interstitial cell adenomas. The incidence of these adenomas in rats receiving doses of 15 to 150 mg/kg/day (4 to 40 times the recommended human dose based on body surface area) exceeded the low background incidence (range = 1.4 to 10%) for this strain of rat. Testicular interstitial cell adenoma also occurred in 1 of 30 rats treated with 50 mg/kg/day (13 times the recommended human dose based on body surface area) in a 1-year toxicity study.

Mean Antisecretory Effects After 5 Days of b.i.d. and t.i.d. Dosing

	PREVACID			
Parameter	30 mg q.d.	15 mg b.i.d.	30 mg b.i.d.	30 mg t.i.d.
% Time Gastric pH>5	43	47	59⁺	77*
% Time Gastric pH>6	20	23	28	45*

⁺($p<0.05$) versus PREVACID 30 mg q.d.

*($p<0.05$) versus PREVACID 30 mg q.d., 15 mg b.i.d. and 30 mg b.i.d.

Continued on next page

Prevpac—Cont.

In a 24-month carcinogenicity study, CD-1 mice were treated orally with doses of 15 to 600 mg/kg/day, 2 to 80 times the recommended human dose based on body surface area. Lansoprazole produced a dose-related increased incidence of gastric ECL cell hyperplasia. It also produced an increased incidence of liver tumors (hepatocellular adenoma plus carcinoma). The tumor incidences in male mice treated with 300 and 600 mg/kg/day (40 to 80 times the recommended human dose based on body surface area) and female mice treated with 150 to 600 mg/kg/day (20 to 80 times the recommended human dose based on body surface area) exceeded the ranges of background incidences in historical controls for this strain of mice. Lansoprazole treatment produced adenoma of rete testis in male mice receiving 75 to 600 mg/kg/day (10 to 80 times the recommended human dose based on body surface area).

Lansoprazole was not genotoxic in the Ames test, the *ex vivo* rat hepatocyte unscheduled DNA synthesis (UDS) test, the *in vivo* mouse micronucleus test or the rat bone marrow cell chromosomal aberration test. It was positive in *in vitro* human lymphocyte chromosomal aberration assays.

Lansoprazole at oral doses up to 150 mg/kg/day (40 times the recommended human dose based on body surface area) was found to have no effect on fertility and reproductive performance of male and female rats.

Amoxicillin:
Long-term studies in animals have not been performed with amoxicillin.

Clarithromycin:
The following *in vitro* mutagenicity tests have been conducted with clarithromycin:

> *Salmonella*/Mammalian Microsomes Test
> Bacterial Induced Mutation Frequency Test
> *In Vitro* Chromosome Aberration Test
> Rat Hepatocyte DNA Synthesis Assay
> Mouse Lymphoma Assay
> Mouse Dominant Lethal Study
> Mouse Micronucleus Test

All tests had negative results except the *In Vitro* Chromosome Aberration Test which was weakly positive in one test and negative in another.

In addition, a Bacterial Reverse-Mutation Test (Ames Test) has been performed on clarithromycin metabolites with negative results.

Fertility and reproduction studies have shown that daily doses of up to 160 mg/kg/day (1.3 times the recommended maximum human dose based on mg/m²) to male and female rats caused no adverse effects on the estrous cycle, fertility, parturition, or number and viability of offspring. Plasma levels in rats after 150 mg/kg/day were 2 times the human serum levels.

In the 150 mg/kg/day monkey studies, plasma levels were 3 times the human serum levels. When given orally at 150 mg/kg/day (2.4 times the recommended maximum human dose based on mg/m²), clarithromycin was shown to produce embryonic loss in monkeys. This effect has been attributed to marked maternal toxicity of the drug at this high dose.

In rabbits, *in utero* fetal loss occurred at an intravenous dose of 33 mg/m², which is 17 times less than the maximum proposed human oral daily dose of 618 mg/m².

Long-term studies in animals have not been performed to evaluate the carcinogenic potential of clarithromycin.

Pregnancy
Teratogenic Effects. Pregnancy Category C
Category C is based on the pregnancy category for clarithromycin.

Four teratogenicity studies in rats (three with oral doses and one with intravenous doses up to 160 mg/kg/day administered during the period of major organogenesis) and two in rabbits at oral doses up to 125 mg/kg/day (approximately 2 times the recommended maximum human dose based on mg/m²) or intravenous doses of 30 mg/kg/day administered during gestation days 6 to 18 failed to demonstrate any teratogenicity from clarithromycin. Two additional oral studies in a different rat strain at similar doses and similar conditions demonstrated a low incidence of cardiovascular anomalies at doses of 150 mg/kg/day administered during gestation days 6 to 15. Plasma levels after 150 mg/kg/day were 2 times the human serum levels. Four studies in mice revealed a variable incidence of cleft palate following oral doses of 1000 mg/kg/day (2 and 4 times the recommended maximum human dose based on mg/m², respectively) during gestation days 6 to 15. Cleft palate was also seen at 500 mg/kg/day. The 1000 mg/kg/day exposure resulted in plasma levels 17 times the human serum levels. In monkeys, an oral dose of 70 mg/kg/day (an approximate equidose of the recommended maximum human dose based on mg/m²) produced fetal growth retardation at plasma levels that were 2 times the human serum levels.

There are no adequate and well-controlled studies of PREVPAC in pregnant women. PREVPAC should be used during pregnancy only if the potential benefit justifies the potential risk to the fetus. (See **WARNINGS**.)

Labor and Delivery
Oral ampicillin-class antibiotics are poorly absorbed during labor. Studies in guinea pigs showed that intravenous administration of ampicillin slightly decreased the uterine tone and frequency of contractions, but moderately increased the height and duration of contractions. However, it is not known whether use of these drugs in humans during labor or delivery has immediate or delayed adverse effects on the fetus, prolongs the duration of labor, or increases the likelihood that forceps delivery or other obstetrical intervention or resuscitation of the newborn will be necessary.

Nursing Mothers
Amoxicillin is excreted in human milk in very small amounts. Because of the potential for serious adverse reactions in nursing infants from PREVPAC, a decision should be made whether to discontinue nursing or to discontinue the drug therapy, taking into account the importance of the therapy to the mother.

Pediatric Use
Safety and effectiveness of PREVPAC in pediatric patients infected with *H. pylori* have not been established (See **CONTRAINDICATIONS** and **WARNINGS**.)

Geriatric Use
Elderly patients may suffer from asymptomatic renal and hepatic dysfunction. Care should be taken when administering PREVPAC to this patient population.

ADVERSE REACTIONS

The most common adverse reaction (≥ 3%) reported in clinical trials when all three components of this therapy were given concomitantly are listed in the table below.

Adverse Reactions Most Frequently Reported in Clinical Trials (≥3%)

Adverse Reaction	Triple Therapy n=138 (%)
Diarrhea	7.0
Headache	6.0
Taste Perversion	5.0

The additional adverse reactions which were reported as possibly or probably related to treatment (< 3%) in clinical trials when all three components of this therapy were given concomitantly are listed below and divided by body system: *Body as a Whole* - abdominal pain; *Digestive System* - dark stools, dry mouth/thirst, glossitis, rectal itching, nausea, oral moniliasis, stomatitis, tongue discoloration, tongue disorder, vomiting; *Musculoskeletal System* - myalgia; *Nervous System* - confusion, dizziness; *Respiratory System* - respiratory disorders; *Skin and Appendages* - skin reactions; *Urogenital System* - vaginitis, vaginal moniliasis.

PREVACID:
The following adverse reactions from the labeling for lansoprazole are provided for information.

Worldwide, over 6100 patients have been treated with lansoprazole in Phase II-III clinical trials involving various dosages and duration of treatment. In general, lansoprazole treatment has been well tolerated in both short-term and long-term trials.

Incidence in Clinical Trials
The following adverse events were reported by the treating physician to have a possible or probable relationship to drug in 1% or more of patients treated with PREVACID capsules and occurred at a greater rate in patients treated with PREVACID capsules than placebo-treated patients:

Incidence of Possibly or Probably Treatment-Related Adverse Events in Short-term, Placebo-Controlled Studies

Body System/Adverse Event	PREVACID (N=1457) %	Placebo (N=467) %
Body as a Whole		
Abdominal Pain	1.8	1.3
Digestive System		
Diarrhea	3.6	2.6
Nausea	1.4	1.3

Headache was also seen at greater than 1% incidence but was more common on placebo. The incidence of diarrhea is similar between placebo and lansoprazole 15 mg and 30 mg patients, but higher in the lansoprazole 60 mg patients (2.9%, 1.4%, 4.2%, and 7.4%, respectively).

The most commonly reported possibly or probably treatment-related adverse event during maintenance therapy was diarrhea.

Additional adverse experiences occurring in <1% of patients or subjects in domestic and/or international trials, or occurring since the drug was marketed, are shown below within each body system.

In short-term and long-term studies, the following adverse events were reported in <1% of the lansoprazole-treated patients:

Body as a Whole - asthenia, candidiasis, chest pain (not otherwise specified), edema, fever, flu syndrome, halitosis, infection (not otherwise specified), malaise; *Cardiovascular System* - angina, cerebrovascular accident, hypertension/hypotension, myocardial infarction, palpitations, shock (circulatory failure), vasodilation; *Digestive System* - melena, anorexia, bezoar, cardiospasm, cholelithiasis, constipation, dry mouth/thirst, dyspepsia, dysphagia, eructation, esophageal stenosis, esophageal ulcer, esophagitis, fecal discoloration, flatulence, gastric nodules/fundic gland polyps, gastroenteritis, gastrointestinal hemorrhage, hematemesis, increased appetite, increased salivation, rectal hemorrhage, stomatitis, tenesmus, ulcerative colitis, vomiting; *Endocrine System* - diabetes mellitus, goiter, hyperglycemia/hypoglycemia; *Hematologic and Lymphatic System** - agranulocytosis, anemia, aplastic anemia, hemolysis, hemolytic anemia, leukopenia, neutropenia, pancytopenia, thrombocytopenia, and thrombotic thrombocytopenic purpura; *Metabolic and Nutritional Disorders* - gout, weight gain/loss; *Musculoskeletal System* - arthritis/arthralgia, musculoskeletal pain, myalgia; *Nervous System* - agitation, amnesia, anxiety, apathy, confusion, depression, dizziness/syncope, hallucinations, hemiplegia, hostility aggravated, libido decreased, nervousness, paresthesia, thinking abnormality; *Respiratory System* - asthma, bronchitis, cough increased, dyspnea, epistaxis, hemoptysis, hiccup, pneumonia, upper respiratory inflammation/infection; *Skin and Appendages* - acne, alopecia, pruritus, rash, urticaria; *Special Senses* - amblyopia, deafness, eye pain, visual field defect, otitis media, taste perversion, tinnitus; *Urogenital System* - abnormal menses, albuminuria, breast enlargement/gynecomastia, breast tenderness, glycosuria, hematuria, impotence, kidney calculus.

* The majority of hematologic cases received were foreign-sourced and their relationship to lansoprazole was unclear.

Laboratory Values
The following changes in laboratory parameters were reported as adverse events.

Abnormal liver function tests, increased SGOT (AST), increased SGPT (ALT), increased creatinine, increased alkaline phosphatase, increased globulins, increased GGTP, increased/decreased/abnormal WBC, abnormal AG ratio, abnormal RBC, bilirubinemia, eosinophilia, hyperlipemia, increased/decreased electrolytes, increased/decreased cholesterol, increased glucocorticoids, increased LDH, increased/decreased/abnormal platelets, and increased gastrin levels. Additional isolated laboratory abnormalities were reported.

In the placebo-controlled studies, when SGOT (AST) and SGPT (ALT) were evaluated, 0.4% (1/250) placebo patients and 0.3% (2/795) lansoprazole patients had enzyme elevations greater than three times the upper limit of normal range at the final treatment visit. None of these patients reported jaundice at any time during the study.

Amoxicillin:
The following adverse reactions from the labeling for amoxicillin are provided for information.

As with other penicillins, it may be expected that untoward reactions will be essentially limited to sensitivity phenomena. They are more likely to occur in individuals who have previously demonstrated hypersensitivity to penicillins and in those with a history of allergy, asthma, hay fever, or urticaria. Glossitis, stomatitis, black "hairy" tongue, nausea, vomiting, and diarrhea have been reported as associated with the use of penicillin. (These reactions are usually associated with oral dosage forms.)

Hypersensitivity Reactions - Skin rashes and urticaria have been reported frequently. A few cases of exfoliative dermatitis and erythema multiforme have been reported. Anaphylaxis is the most serious reaction experienced and has usually been associated with the parenteral dosage form. Urticaria, other skin rashes, and serum sickness-like reactions may be controlled with antihistamines and, if necessary, systemic corticosteroids. Whenever such reactions occur, penicillin should be discontinued unless, in the opinion of the physician, the condition being treated is life threatening and amenable only to penicillin therapy. Serious anaphylactic reactions require the immediate use of epinephrine, oxygen, and intravenous steroids.

Liver - A moderate rise in serum glutamic oxaloacetic transaminase (SGOT) has been noted, particularly in infants, but the significance of this finding is unknown.

Hemic and Lymphatic Systems - Anemia, thrombocytopenia, thrombocytopenic purpura, eosinophilia, leukopenia, and agranulocytosis have been reported during therapy with the penicillins. These reactions are usually reversible on discontinuation of therapy and are believed to be hypersensitivity phenomena.

Clarithromycin:
The following adverse reactions from the labeling for clarithromycin are provided for information.

The majority of side effects observed in clinical trials were of a mild and transient nature. Fewer than 3% of adult patients without mycobacterial infections discontinued therapy because of drug-related side effects.

The most frequently reported events in adults were diarrhea (3%), nausea (3%), abnormal taste (3%), dyspepsia (2%), abdominal pain/discomfort (2%), and headache (2%). Most of these events were described as mild or moderate in severity. Of the reported adverse events, only 1% was described as severe.

Postmarketing Experience:
Allergic reactions ranging from urticaria and mild skin eruptions to rare cases of anaphylaxis and Stevens-Johnson syndrome have occurred. Other spontaneously reported adverse events include glossitis, stomatitis, oral moniliasis, vomiting, tongue discoloration, and dizziness. There have been reports of tooth discoloration in patients treated with clarithromycin. Tooth discoloration is usually reversible with professional dental cleaning. There have been isolated reports of hearing loss, which is usually reversible, occurring chiefly in elderly women. Reports of alterations of the sense of smell, usually in conjunction with taste perversion have also been reported.

Transient CNS events including anxiety, behavioral changes, confusional states, depersonalization, disorientation, hallucinations, insomnia, nightmares, psychosis, tinnitus, and vertigo have been reported during postmarketing surveillance. Events usually resolve with discontinuation of the drug.

Hepatic dysfunction, including increased liver enzymes and hepatocellular and/or cholestatic hepatitis, with or without jaundice, has been infrequently reported with clarithromycin. This hepatic dysfunction may be severe and is usually reversible. In very rare instances, hepatic failure with fatal outcome has been reported and generally has been associated with serious underlying diseases and/or concomitant medications.

Rarely, erythromycin and clarithromycin have been associated with ventricular arrhythmias, including ventricular tachycardia and torsades de pointes in individuals with prolonged QT_C intervals.

Changes in Laboratory Values: Changes in laboratory values with possible clinical significance were as follows: *Hepatic* - elevated SGPT (ALT) <1%, SGOT (AST) <1%, GGT <1%, alkaline phosphatase <1%, total bilirubin <1%; *Hematologic* - decreased WBC <1%, elevated prothrombin time 1%; *Renal* - elevated BUN 4%, elevated serum creatinine <1%. GGT, alkaline phosphatase, and prothrombin time are from adult studies only.

OVERDOSAGE

In case of an overdose, patients should contact a physician, poison control center, or emergency room. There is neither a pharmacologic basis nor data suggesting an increased toxicity of the combination compared to individual components.
Lansoprazole:
Oral doses up to 5000 mg/kg in rats (approximately 1300 times the 30 mg human dose based on body surface area) and mice (about 675.7 times the 30 mg human dose based on body surface area) did not produce deaths or any clinical signs.
Lansoprazole is not removed from the circulation by hemodialysis. In one reported case of overdose, the patient consumed 600 mg of lansoprazole with no adverse reaction.
Amoxicillin:
In case of overdosage, discontinue medication, treat symptomatically and institute supportive measures as required. Amoxicillin can be removed from circulation by hemodialysis.

DOSAGE AND ADMINISTRATION

H. pylori Eradication to Reduce the Risk of Duodenal Ulcer Recurrence
The recommended adult oral dose is 30 mg PREVACID, 1 g amoxicillin, and 500 mg clarithromycin administered together twice daily (morning and evening) for 14 days. (See **INDICATIONS AND USAGE.**)
PREVPAC is not recommended in patients with creatinine clearance less than 30 mL/min.

HOW SUPPLIED

PREVPAC is supplied as an individual daily administration pack, each containing:
PREVACID:
– two opaque, hard gelatin, black and pink PREVACID 30-mg capsules, with the TAP logo and "PREVACID 30" imprinted on the capsules.
TRIMOX:
– four maroon and light-pink amoxicillin 500-mg capsules, USP, with "BRISTOL 7279" imprinted on the capsules.
BIAXIN Filmtab:
– two yellow oval film-coated clarithromycin 500-mg tablets with the Abbott logo and "KL" imprinted in blue on one side of the tablets.
NDC 0300-3702-01 Daily administration pack
Storage: Protect from light and moisture.
Store at a controlled room temperature between 59° F and 86° F (15° C and 30° C).
Caution: Federal (USA) law prohibits dispensing without a prescription.
U.S. Patent No. 5,013,743

Revised: December, 1997
PREVPAC is distributed by TAP Pharmaceuticals Inc.
PREVACID® (lansoprazole) Delayed-Release Capsules Manufactured for
TAP Pharmaceuticals Inc.
Deerfield, Illinois 60015-1595, U.S.A.
by Takeda Chemical Industries, Limited,
Osaka, Japan 541
Distributed by TAP Pharmaceuticals Inc.
TRIMOX® (amoxicillin, USP)
Manufactured by
APOTHECON®
A Bristol-Myers Squibb Company
Princeton, NJ 08540, U.S.A.
BIAXIN® Filmtab® (clarithromycin tablets)
Manufactured by
Abbott Laboratories
North Chicago, IL 60064, U.S.A.
Shown in Product Identification Guide, page 341

Taylor Pharmaceuticals
An Akorn Company
CORPORATE/CUSTOMER SERVICE:
942 CALLE NEGOCIO
SUITE 150
SAN CLEMENTE, CA 92673
SALES:
150 S. WYCKLES ROAD
DECATUR, IL 62525

Direct Inquiries to:
Corporate/customer service:
800-223-9851
Sales:
217-428-1100

ALFENTA® ⓒ℞
[ăl-fĕn 'tä]
(alfentanil hydrochloride)
Injection

DESCRIPTION

ALFENTA (alfentanil hydrochloride) Injection is an opioid analgesic chemically designated as N-[1-[2-(4-ethyl-4, 5-dihydro-5-oxo-1H-tetrazol-1-yl) ethyl]-4-(methoxymethyl)-4-piperidinyl]-N-phenylpropanamide monohydrochloride (1:1) with a molecular weight of 452.98 and an n-octanol: water partition coefficient of 128:1 at pH 7.4.
ALFENTA is a sterile, non-pyrogenic, preservative free aqueous solution containing alfentanil hydrochloride equivalent to 500 μg per mL of alfentanil base for intravenous injection. The solution, which contains sodium chloride for isotonicity, has a pH range of 4–6.

HOW SUPPLIED

Each mL of ALFENTA (alfentanil hydrochloride) Injection for intravenous use contains alfentanil hydrochloride equivalent to 500 μg of alfentanil base. ALFENTA Injection is available as:
NDC 11098-060-02, 2 mL ampoules in packages of 10
NDC 11098-060-05, 5 mL ampoules in packages of 10
NDC 11098-060-10, 10 mL ampoules in packages of 5
NDC 11098-060-20, 20 mL ampoules in packages of 5
U.S. Patent No. 4,167,574
May 1995, November, 1995
Taylor Pharmaceuticals
An Akorn Company

SUFENTA® ⓒ℞
[su-fĕn 'ta]
(sufentanil citrate)
Injection

DESCRIPTION

SUFENTA® (sufentanil citrate) is a potent opioid analgesic chemically designated as N-[-4-(methyoxymethyl) -1- [2- (2-thienyl) ethyl] -4- piperidinyl]-N-phenylpropanamide: 2-hydroxy-1,2,3-propanetricarboxylate (1:1) with a molecular weight of 578.68.
SUFENTA is a sterile, preservative free, aqueous solution containing sufentanil citrate equivalent to 50 μg per mL of sufentanil base for intravenous and epidural injection. The solution has a pH range of 3.5–6.0.

HOW SUPPLIED

SUFENTA (sufentanil citrate) Injection is supplied as a sterile aqueous preservative-free solution for intravenous and epidural use as:
NDC 11098-050-01 50 μg/mL sufentanil base, 1 mL ampoules in packages of 10

NDC 11098-050-02 50 μg/mL sufentanil base, 2 mL ampoules in packages of 10
NDC 11098-050-05 50 μg/mL sufentanil base, 5 mL ampoules in packages of 10
Protect from light. Store at controlled room temperature (59°–77°F/15°–25°C).
U.S. Patent No. 3,998,834
May 1995, September 1995
Taylor Pharmaceuticals
An Akorn Company

UCB Pharma, Inc.
1950 LAKE PARK DRIVE
SMYRNA, GA 30080

Direct Inquiries to:
UCB Pharma, Inc.
1950 Lake Park Drive
Smyrna, GA 30080
(800) 477–7877

For Medical Information Contact:
Suzan E. Leake
Manager, Med. Affairs
770-437-5558
In Emergencies:
Medical Affairs
(800) 477–7877

DURATUSS™ Tablets ℞
120 mg pseudoephedrine hydrochloride and 600 mg guaifenesin

DESCRIPTION

Each long-acting, film-coated, dye-free Duratuss Tablet contains:
Pseudoephedrine Hydrochloride .... 120 mg
Guaifenesin .... 600 mg
Also contains colloidal silicon dioxide, magnesium stearate, microcrystalline cellulose, stearic acid and other ingredients. Film coating composed of hydroxypropyl methylcellulose and polyethylene glycol.
Pseudoephedrine hydrochloride is a nasal decongestant. Chemically it is [S-(R*,R*)]-α-[1-(methylamino)ethyl] benzenemethanol hydrochloride with the following structure:

Guaifenesin is an expectorant. Chemically it is 3-(2-methoxyphenoxy)-1,2 propanediol with the following structure:

CLINICAL PHARMACOLOGY

Pseudoephedrine hydrochloride is an orally effective nasal decongestant that acts on alpha-adrenergic receptors in the mucosa of the respiratory tract producing vasoconstriction. Pseudoephedrine shrinks swollen nasal mucous membranes, reduces tissue hyperemia, edema and nasal congestion and increases nasal airway patency. Drainage of sinus secretions is increased and obstructed Eustachian ostia may be opened. Pseudoephedrine produces little, if any, rebound congestion.
Guaifenesin is an expectorant which enhances the flow of respiratory tract secretions. The enhanced flow of less viscid secretions lubricates irritated respiratory tract membranes, promotes ciliary action and facilitates the removal of inspissated mucus. As a result, sinus and bronchial drainage is improved and nonproductive coughs become more productive and less frequent.

INDICATIONS

Duratuss Tablets are indicated for the relief of nasal congestion due to the common cold, hay fever or other upper respiratory allergies and nasal congestion associated with sinusitis. To promote nasal or sinus drainage; for the relief of Eustachian tube congestion; for adjunctive therapy in serous otitis media; for the symptomatic relief of respiratory

Continued on next page

Duratuss—Cont.

conditions characterized by dry, nonproductive cough and in the presence of tenacious mucus and/or mucus plugs in the respiratory tract.

CONTRAINDICATIONS

Duratuss Tablets are contraindicated in individuals with known hypersensitivity to sympathomimetics, severe hypertension or in patients receiving MAO inhibitors.

PRECAUTIONS

DO NOT CRUSH OR CHEW DURATUSS TABLETS BEFORE INGESTION TO PRESERVE THE LONG-ACTING EFFECT.

Information for Patients: As with other sympathomimetic drugs, Duratuss should be used with caution in the presence of hypertension, hyperthyroidism, diabetes, heart disease, peripheral vascular disease, glaucoma and prostatic hypertrophy.

Laboratory Test Interactions: Guaifenesin interferes with the colorimetric determination of 5-hydroxyindoleacetic acid (5-HIAA) and vanillylmandelic acid (VMA).

Pregnancy Category C.: Animal reproduction studies have not been conducted with pseudoephedrine or guaifenesin. It is also not known whether pseudoephedrine or guaifenesin can cause fetal harm when administered to a pregnant woman or can affect reproduction capacity. Pseudoephedrine and guaifenesin may be given to a pregnant woman only if clearly needed.

Nursing Mothers: Because of potential serious adverse reactions in nursing infants from sympathomimetic amines, pseudoephedrine is contraindicated in nursing mothers.

ADVERSE REACTIONS

Possible adverse reactions include nervousness, insomnia, restlessness or headache. These reactions seldom, if ever, require discontinuation of therapy. Urinary retention may occur in patients with prostatic hypertrophy.

OVERDOSAGE

Since the effects of Duratuss Tablets may last up to 12 hours, treatment of overdosage directed towards supporting the patient and reversing the effects of the drug should be continued for at least that length of time.

Saline cathartics may be useful in hastening the evacuation of unreleased medication.

DOSAGE AND ADMINISTRATION

Adults: 1 tablet every 12 hours. Children 6—12 years of age: one half ($^1/_2$) tablet every 12 hours. Tablet may be broken in half without affecting release of medication but not crushed or chewed.

HOW SUPPLIED

Duratuss™ Tablets (120 mg pseudoephedrine hydrochloride and 600 mg guaifenesin) are supplied as white, film-coated, dye-free, oval-shaped tablets debossed "ucb" on one side and scored and debossed "612" on the other side in bottles of 100 (NDC 50474-612-01), and 500 tablets (NCD 50474-612-50). Store at controlled room temperature, 15°C-30°C (59°F-86°F).

Dispense in a tight, light-resistant container with a child-resistant closure. Protect from light and moisture.

Rx only.

Manufactured for
UCB Pharma, Inc.,
Smyrna, GA 30080
by Mikart, Inc.,
Atlanta, GA 30318

Rev. 5/98

Shown in Product Identification Guide, page 341

DURATUSS™ G TABLETS
guaifenesin 1200 mg
℞

DESCRIPTION

Each long-acting, film coated, dye-free Duratuss G Tablet contains:

Guaifenesin .... 1200 mg

Also contains: microcrystalline cellulose, magnesium stearate and other ingredients. Film coating composed of hydroxypropyl methylcellulose and polyethylene glycol.

Guaifenesin is an expectorant. Chemically, it is 3-(2-methoxyphenoxy)-1,2 propanediol with the following structural formula:

CLINICAL PHARMACOLOGY

Guaifenesin is an expectorant. Expectorants promote and facilitate the removal of respiratory tract secretions by in-

creasing sputum volume and making sputum less viscous. Guaifenesin is readily absorbed from the gastrointestinal tract and is rapidly metabolized and excreted in the urine. Guaifenesin has a plasma half-life of one hour. The major urinary metabolite is beta-(2-methoxyphenoxy) lactic acid.

INDICATIONS AND USAGE

Duratuss G Tablets help loosen phlegm (mucus) and thin bronchial secretions. The result is enhanced flow of less viscid secretions to lubricate irritated mucous membranes and increase the efficiency of the mucociliary mechanism in removing accumulated secretions from the upper and lower airway. As a result, sinus and bronchial drainage is improved and nonproductive coughs become more productive. Duratuss G Tablets are indicated for the temporary relief of symptoms associated with respiratory tract infections and related conditions such as sinusitis, pharyngitis, bronchitis, and allergies, when these conditions are complicated by tenacious mucus and/or mucus plugs and excess secretions.

CONTRAINDICATIONS

Duratuss G Tablets are contraindicated in patients hypersensitive to any of the ingredients.

PRECAUTIONS

TO PRESERVE THE LONG-ACTING EFFECT, DO NOT CRUSH OR CHEW DURATUSS G TABLETS BEFORE INGESTION.

Carcinogenesis, Mutagenesis, Impairment of Fertility: No data are available on the long term potential of guaifenesin for carcinogenesis, mutagenesis, or impairment of fertility in animals or humans.

Teratogenic Effects: Pregnancy Category C: Animal reproduction studies have not been conducted with guaifenesin. Safe use in pregnancy has not been established relative to possible adverse effects on fetal development. Therefore, this product should not be used in pregnant patients, unless in the judgement of the physician, the potential benefits outweigh possible hazards.

Nursing Mothers: It is not known whether guaifenesin is excreted in human milk. Because many drugs are excreted in human milk, caution should be exercised when these products are administered to a nursing mother and a decision should be made whether to discontinue nursing or to discontinue the drug, taking into account the importance of the drug to the mother.

Laboratory Test Interactions: Guaifenesin interferes with the calorimetric determination of 5-HIAA (5-hydroxyindoleacetic acid) and VMA (vanillylmandelic acid).

ADVERSE REACTIONS

Guaifenesin is well tolerated and has a wide margin of safety. Side effects are generally mild and infrequent. Nausea and vomiting are the most frequently occurring side effects. Dizziness, headache and rash (including urticaria) have been reported rarely.

OVERDOSAGE

Overdosage with guaifenesin is unlikely to produce serious toxic effects due to its wide margin of safety.

When laboratory animals were administered guaifenesin in doses up to 5 grams/kg by stomach tube, no toxicity resulted. In severe cases of overdosage, the stomach should be emptied (emesis or gastric lavage) and further absorption prevented. Treatment should be directed toward supporting the patient and reversing the effects of the drug.

DOSAGE AND ADMINISTRATION

Adults and children over 12 years of age: One tablet every 12 hours not to exceed 2 tablets (2400 mg) in 24 hours. Children 6–12 years: One-half ($^1/_2$) tablet every 12 hours not to exceed 1 tablet (1200 mg) in 24 hours. Tablets may be broken in half (but not crushed or chewed) without affecting the release of the medication.

HOW SUPPLIED

Duratuss™ G Tablets (guaifenesin 1200 mg) are supplied as white (dye-free), film-coated, capsule-shaped tablets scored and debossed 'ucb/620' on one side, in bottles of 100 tablets (NDC 50474–620–01), 500 tablets (NDC 50474-620-50) and 1000 tablets (NDC 50474-620-70).

Store at controlled room temperature, 15°-30°C (59°-86°F). Dispense in a tight, light-resistant container with a child-resistant closure. Protect from light and moisture.

Rx only.

Manufactured for
UCB Pharma, Inc.
Smyrna, GA 30080
by Mikart, Inc.
Atlanta, GA 30318

Rev. 5/98

Shown in Product Identification Guide, page 341

DURATUSS™ DM Elixir
20 mg dextromethorphan hydrobromide and 200 mg guaifenesin per 5 mL
℞

DESCRIPTION

Each 5 mL (one teaspoonful) of Duratuss DM Elixir contains:

Dextromethorphan hydrobromide .... 20 mg
Guaifenesin .... 200 mg
Alcohol 5%

Also contains citric acid, high fructose corn syrup, propylene glycol, purified water, saccharin sodium, sodium benzoate, FD&C Red No. 40, FD&C Red No. 3, FD&C Blue No. 1, and artificial flavoring.

Dextromethorphan hydrobromide, a synthetic, nonopioid antitussive, is a salt of the methyl ether of the dextrorotatory isomer of levorphanol, an opioid analgesic. The chemical name is 3-methoxy-17-methyl-9α, 13α, 14α-morphinan hydrobromide monohydrate. It has the following structural formula:

$C_{18}H_{25}NO \cdot HBr \cdot H_2O$ MW = 370.33

Guaifenesin is an expectorant. The chemical name is 3-(2-methoxyphenoxy)-1,2 propanediol. It has the following structural formula:

$C_{10}H_{14}O_4$ MW = 198.22

CLINICAL PHARMACOLOGY

Duratuss DM Elixir combines the cough suppressant dextromethorphan hydrobromide and the expectorant guaifenesin.

Dextromethorphan hydrobromide is a nonopioid antitussive agent. Dextromethorphan temporarily controls and suppresses the cough reflex by a direct action on the cough center. It has no significant analgesic or sedative properties, does not depress respiration or predispose to addiction with usual doses. In therapeutic dosage, dextromethorphan does not inhibit cilliary activity.

Dextromethorphan is rapidly absorbed from the gastrointestinal tract and exerts its effect 15–30 minutes after oral administration. The duration of action is approximately 3–6 hours. Dextromethorphan is rapidly and extensively metabolized by the liver. It is primarily renally excreted as unchanged dextromethorphan and demethylated metabolites including dextrorphan, an active metabolite.

Guaifenesin is an expectorant. Expectorants promote and facilitate the removal of respiratory tract secretions. By increasing respiratory tract fluid, guaifenesin reduces the viscosity of secretions, and facilitates expectoration of retained secretions. Guaifenesin is readily absorbed from the gastrointestinal tract and is rapidly metabolized and renally excreted. Guaifenesin has a plasma half-life of one hour. The major urinary metabolite is beta-(2-methoxyphenoxy) lactic acid.

INDICATIONS AND USAGE

Duratuss DM Elixir temporarily relieves coughs due to minor throat and bronchial irritation as may occur with upper respiratory tract infections or inhaled irritants, when complicated by viscous mucus. Dextromethorphan hydrobromide suppresses the cough control center and relieves coughing. Guaifenesin helps loosen phlegm (mucus) and thin bronchial secretions to rid the bronchial passageways of bothersome mucus, drain bronchial tubes, and make coughs more productive.

CONTRAINDICATIONS

Duratuss DM Elixir is contraindicated in patients hypersensitive to any of the ingredients and in patients receiving monoamine oxidase inhibitor (MAO) therapy, including 14 days after stopping MAOI therapy (see PRECAUTIONS: *Drug Interactions*).

WARNINGS

A persistent cough may be a sign of a serious condition. If cough persists for more than one week or tends to recur, or is accompanied by fever, rash, or persistent headache, patient reevaluation should be considered.

PRECAUTIONS

General: Before prescribing any medication to suppress or modify cough, it is important that the underlying cause of cough is identified, that modification of cough does not increase the risk of clinical or physiological complications, and that appropriate therapy for the primary disease is instituted.

Information for Patients: Patients should be warned not to use this product if they are now taking a prescription monoamine oxidase inhibitor [MAOI] (certain drugs for depres-

sion, psychiatric or emotional conditions, or Parkinson's disease), including 14 days after stopping the MAOI drug. If patients are uncertain whether a prescription drug contains an MAOI, they should be instructed to consult a health professional before taking this product.

Drug Interactions: Serious toxicity (serotonin syndrome) has been reported in patients receiving dextromethorphan hydrobromide and monoamine oxidase inhibitors [MAOIs] concomitantly. Dextromethorphan preparations should not be used in patients receiving MAOIs, including 14 days after stopping the MAOI drug. The use of dextromethorphan hydrobromide may result in additive CNS depressant effects when coadministered with alcohol, antihistamines, psychotropics or other drugs which produce CNS depression.

Laboratory Test Interactions: Guaifenesin interferes with the colorimetric determination of 5-HIAA (5-hydroxyindoleacetic acid) and VMA (vanillylmandelic acid).

Carcinogenesis, Mutagenesis, Impairment of Fertility: No data are available on the long term potential of dextromethorphan hydrobromide or of guaifenesin for carcinogenesis, mutagenesis, or impairment of fertility in animals or humans.

Pregnancy: Teratogenic Effects: Pregnancy Category C: Animal reproduction studies have not been conducted with dextromethorphan hydrobromide or guaifenesin. It is also not known whether dextromethorphan hydrobromide or guaifenesin can cause fetal harm when administered to a pregnant woman or can affect reproduction capacity. Duratuss DM Elixir should be given to a pregnant woman only if clearly needed.

Nursing Mothers: It is not known whether dextromethorphan hydrobromide or guaifenesin is excreted in human milk. Because many drugs are excreted in human milk, caution should be exercised when dextromethorphan hydrobromide or guaifenesin are administered to a nursing woman.

Pediatric Use: The safety and effectiveness of dextromethorphan hydrobromide and guaifenesin in pediatric patients have been established in the age groups 2 years to over 12 years. Safety and effectiveness in pediatric patients below the age of 2 years have not been established. (see DOSAGE AND ADMINISTRATION).

Administration of dextromethorphan may be associated with histamine release and should be used with caution in atopic children.

ADVERSE REACTIONS

Adverse effects associated with dextromethorphan hydrobromide are rare, but nausea and/or other gastrointestinal disturbances, slight dizziness and drowsiness sometimes occur (see also *Drug Interactions*). Guaifenesin is well tolerated and has a wide margin of safety. Adverse effects associated with guaifenesin usually result from doses larger than those required for expectoration. Reported adverse reactions include nausea and vomiting, dizziness, headache and rash (including urticaria).

OVERDOSAGE

Overdosage with dextromethorphan hydrobromide may produce central excitement and mental confusion. Very high doses may produce respiratory depression. Overdosage with guaifenesin is unlikely to produce toxic effects since its toxicity is low. When laboratory animals were administered guaifenesin in doses up to 5 g/kg by stomach tube, no toxicity resulted.

In severe cases of overdosage, the stomach should be emptied (emesis or gastric lavage) and further absorption prevented. Treatment should be directed toward supporting the patient and reversing the effects of the drug.

DOSAGE AND ADMINISTRATION

Adults and children over 12 years of age: One teaspoonful (5 mL) every 4 hours, not to exceed 6 teaspoonfuls in 24 hours. Children 6–12 years: One-half (1/2) teaspoonful (2.5 mL) every 4 hours, not to exceed 3 teaspoonfuls in 24 hours. Children 2–6 years: One-fourth (1/4) teaspoonful (1.25 mL) every 4 hours, not to exceed 1 1/2 teaspoonfuls in 24 hours. It is recommended that caregivers obtain and use a calibrated measuring device for administering this product to a child. Use extreme care in measuring the dosage. Do not exceed the recommended daily dosage except under the advice and supervision of the prescribing physician.

HOW SUPPLIED

Duratuss™ DM Elixir is a purple-colored, fruit-flavored liquid containing 20 mg dextromethorphan hydrobromide and 200 mg guaifenesin per 5 mL with 5% alcohol. It is supplied in containers of 1 pint (473 mL), NDC 50474-630-16 and 1 gallon (3785 mL), NDC 50474-630-28.

Store at controlled room temperature, 15°-30°C (59°-86°F). Dispense in a tight, light-resistant container with a child-resistant closure.

Rx only.

Manufactured for
UCB Pharma, Inc.
Smyrna, GA 30080
by **Vintage Pharmaceuticals, Inc.**
Huntsville, AL 35811

Rev. 5/98

Shown in Product Identification Guide, page 341

DURATUSS™ HD Elixir Ⓒ III

2.5 mg hydrocodone bitartrate
30 mg pseudoephedrine hydrochloride, and
100 mg guaifenesin per 5 mL

DESCRIPTION

Each 5 mL (one teaspoonful) of Duratuss HD Elixir contains:

Hydrocodon Bitartrate	2.5 mg
Pseudoephedrine Hydrochloride	30 mg
Guaifenesin	100 mg
Alcohol	5%

Also contains citric acid anhydrous, glucose liquid, methylparaben, propylene glycol, propylparaben, purified water, saccharin sodium, sorbitol solution, sucrose, FD&C Red #40, natural and artificial flavoring.

WARNING: May be habit forming (see DRUG ABUSE AND DEPENDENCE).

Hydrocodone bitartrate is an antitussive. Chemically it is 4,5α-epoxy-3-methoxy-17-methylmorphinan-6-one-tartrate (1:1) hydrate (2:5) with the following structure:

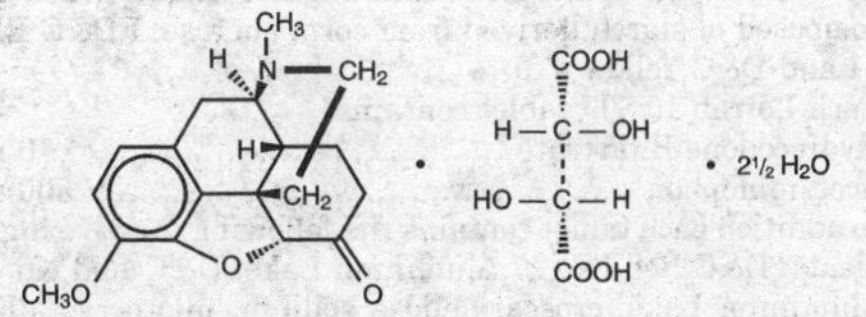

Pseudoephedrine hydrochloride is a nasal decongestant. Chemically it is [S-(R*,R*)]-α-[1-(methylamino)ethyl] benzenemethanol hydrochloride with the following structure:

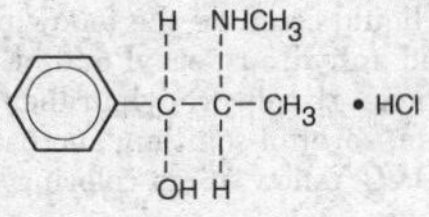

Guaifenesin is an expectorant. Chemically it is 3-(2-methoxyphenoxy)-1,2 propanediol with the following structure:

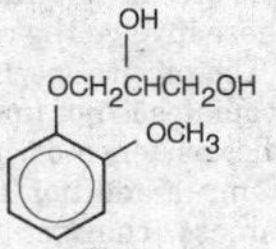

CLINICAL PHARMACOLOGY

Hydrocodone is a semisynthetic narcotic analgesic and antitussive with multiple actions qualitatively similar to those of codeine. Most of these involve the central nervous system and smooth muscle. Hydrocodone suppresses the cough reflex by depressing the medullary cough center. The precise mechanism of action of hydrocodone and other opiates is not known, although it is believed to relate to the existence of opiate receptors in the central nervous system.

Pseudoephedrine hydrochloride is an orally effective nasal decongestant that acts on alpha-adrenergic receptors in the mucosa of the respiratory tract producing vasoconstriction. Pseudoephedrine shrinks swollen nasal mucous membranes, reduces tissue hyperemia, edema and nasal congestion and increases nasal airway patency. Drainage of sinus secretions is increased and obstructed Eustachian ostia may be opened. Pseudoephedrine produces little if any rebound congestion.

Guaifenesin is an expectorant which enhances the flow of respiratory tract secretions. The enhanced flow of less viscid secretions lubricates irritated respiratory tract membranes, promotes cilliary action and facilitates the removal of inspissated mucus. As as result, sinus and bronchial drainage is improved and nonproductive coughs become more productive and less frequent.

INDICATIONS AND USAGE

For exhausting, nonproductive cough accompanying respiratory tract congestion associated with the common cold, influenza, sinusitis, and bronchitis.

CONTRAINDICATIONS

Duratuss HD Elixir is contraindicated in patients with severe hypertension, severe coronary artery disease, and in patients on MAO inhibitor therapy.

Hypersensitivity: Contraindicated in patients with hypersensitivity or idiosyncracy to sympathomimetic amines, phenanthrene derivatives, or to any other formula ingredients.

Nursing Mothers: Contraindicated because of the higher than usual risk for infants for sympathomimetic amines.

WARNINGS

Hydrocodone should be prescribed and administered with the same degree of caution as all oral medications containing a narcotic analgesic. Extreme caution should be exercised in the use of hydrocodone in patients with severe respiratory impairment or patients with impaired respiratory drive.

If sympathomimetic amines are used in patients with hypertension, diabetes mellitus, ischemic heart disease, hyperthyroidism, increased intraocular pressure or prostatic hypertrophy, judicious caution should be exercised (see CONTRAINDICATIONS).

Use in Elderly: The elderly (60 years and older) are more likely to have adverse reactions to sympathomimetics. Overdosage of sympathomimetics in this age group may cause hallucinations, convulsions, CNS depression and death.

PRECAUTIONS

General: Caution should be exercised if used in patients with diabetes, hypertension, cardiovascular diseases, hyperreactivity to ephedrine or decreased respiratory drive (see CONTRAINDICATIONS).

Information for Patients: Hydrocodone may produce drowsiness. Persons who perform hazardous tasks requiring mental alertness or physical coordination should be cautioned accordingly. Concomitant use of hydrocodone with tranquilizers, alcohol or other depressants may produce additive depressant effects. Do not exceed the prescribed dosage.

Drug Interactions: Hydrocodone may potentiate the effects of other narcotics, general anesthetics, tranquilizers, sedatives and hypnotics, tricyclic antidepressants, MAO inhibitors, alcohol, and other CNS depressants. Beta-adrenergic blockers and MAO inhibitors potentiate the sympathomimetic effects of pseudoephedrine. Sympathomimetics may reduce the antihypertensive effects of methyldopa, mecamylamine, reserpine and veratrum alkaloids.

Laboratory Test Interactions: Guaifenesin interferes with the colorimetric determination of 5-hydroxyindoleacetic acid (5-HIAA) and vanillylmandelic acid (VMA).

Pregnancy Category C: Animal reproduction studies have not been conducted with pseudoephedrine, guaifenesin, or hydrocodone. It is also not known whether pseudoephedrine, guaifenesin or hydrocodone can cause fetal harm when administered to a pregnant woman or can affect reproduction capacity. Pseudoephedrine, guaifenesin or hydrocodone may be given to a pregnant woman only if clearly needed.

Nursing Mothers: Because of the potential for serious adverse reactions in nursing infants from sympathomimetic amines, pseudoephedrine is contraindicated in nursing mothers.

ADVERSE REACTIONS

Gastrointestinal upset, nausea, drowsiness and constipation. A slight elevation in serum transaminase levels has been noted.

Individuals hyperreactive to pseudoephedrine may display ephedrine-like reactions such as tachycardia, palpitations, headache, dizziness or nausea. Sympathomimetic drugs have been associated with certain untoward reactions including fear, anxiety, tenseness, restlessness, tremor, weakness, pallor, respiratory difficulty, dysuria, insomnia, hallucinations, convulsions, CNS depression, arrhythmias, and cardiovascular collapse with hypotension. Patient idiosyncrasy to adrenergic agents may be manifested by insomnia, dizziness, weakness, tremor or arrhythmias.

DRUG ABUSE AND DEPENDENCE

Controlled Substance: Hydrocodone in Duratuss HD Elixir is controlled by the Drug Enforcement Administration. Duratuss HD Elixir is a Schedule III controlled substance.

Abuse: Hydrocodone is a narcotic drug related to codeine with similar abuse potential.

Dependence: Hydrocodone can produce drug dependence of the morphine type. Psychic dependence, physical dependence and tolerance may develop if dosage recommendations are greatly exceeded over a prolonged period of time.

OVERDOSAGE

Acute overdosage with Duratuss HD Elixir may produce variable clinical signs as hydrocodone produces CNS depression and cardiovascular depression while pseudoephedrine produces CNS stimulation and variable cardiovascular effects. Hydrocodone is likely to be responsible for most of the severe reactions from overdosage. Pressor amines should be used with great caution when taking pseudoephedrine. Patients with signs of stimulation should be

Continued on next page

Duratuss HD—Cont.

treated conservatively and depressant medications should be avoided if possible because of potential drug interaction with hydrocodone.

DOSAGE AND ADMINISTRATION

Adults: 2 teaspoonfuls (10 mL) every 4–6 hours. Children 6–12 years of age: 1 teaspoonful (5 mL) every 4–6 hours. May be given four times a day as needed. May be taken with meals.

HOW SUPPLIED

Duratuss™ HD Elixir is a red-colored, fruit punch-flavored liquid containing 2.5 mg hydrocodone bitartrate, 30 mg pseudoephedrine hydrochloride, and 100 mg guaifenesin per 5 mL, with 5% alcohol. It is supplied in containers of 1 pint (473 mL), NDC 50474-610-16, and 1 gallon (3785 mL), NDC 50474-610-28.
Store at controlled room temperature, 15°C–30° (59°F–86°F).
Dispense in a tight, light-resistant container with a child-resistant closure.
Rx only.

Manufactured for
UCB Pharma, Inc.,
Smyrna, GA 30080
by **Mikart, Inc.,**
Atlanta, GA 30318

Rev. 5/98

Shown in Product Identification Guide, page 341

Fe50™ Caplets OTC
Extended release iron caplet

Each off-white caplet debossed with the symbol ⊗ contains:
Elemental Iron (ferrous sulfate) .... 50 mg

HOW SUPPLIED

Child-resistant, unit-dose packages of 100 [10×10] caplets; NDC 58436-072-02

LORTAB® 2.5/500 Tablets Ⓒ III
Hydrocodone Bitartrate and Acetaminophen Tablets, USP
2.5 mg/500 mg

LORTAB® 5/500 Tablets Ⓒ III
Hydrocodone Bitartrate and Acetaminophen Tablets, USP
5 mg/500 mg

LORTAB® 7.5/500 Tablets Ⓒ III
Hydrocodone Bitartrate and Acetaminophen Tablets, USP
7.5 mg/500 mg

LORTAB® 10/500 Tablets Ⓒ III
Hydrocodone Bitartrate and Acetaminophen Tablets, USP
10 mg/500 mg

LORTAB® Elixir Ⓒ III
Hydrocodone Bitartrate and Acetaminophen Elixir, 7.5 mg/500 mg per 15 mL

DESCRIPTION

Hydrocodone bitartrate and acetaminophen is supplied in tablet and liquid forms for oral administration.
WARNING: May be habit forming (see PRECAUTIONS, Information for Patients, and DRUG ABUSE AND DEPENDENCE).
Hydrocodone bitartrate is an opioid analgesic and antitussive and occurs as fine, white crystals or as a crystalline powder. It is affected by light. The chemical name is 4,5α-epoxy-3-methoxy-17-methylmorphinan-6-one tartrate (1:1) hydrate (2:5). It has the following structural formula:

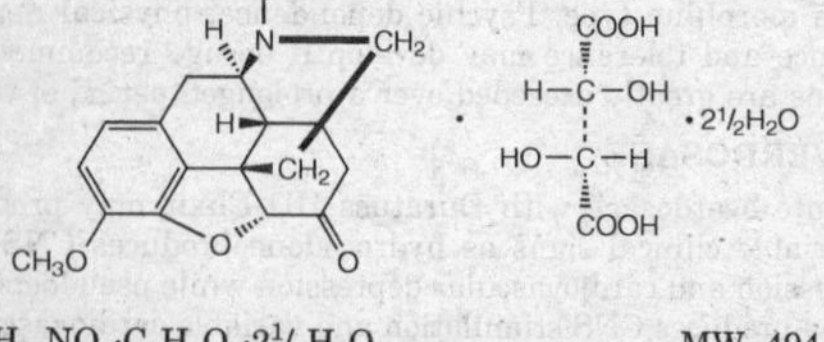

$C_{18}H_{21}NO_3 \cdot C_4H_6O_6 \cdot 2^1/_2H_2O$ MW=494.50

Acetaminophen, 4'-hydroxyacetanilide, a slightly bitter, white, odorless, crystalline powder, is a non-opiate, non-salicylate analgesic and antipyretic. It has the following structural formula:
[See chemical structure at top of next column]

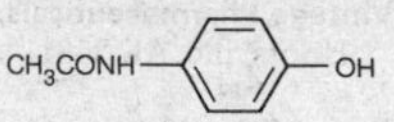

$C_8H_9NO_2$ MW=151.17

Each Lortab 2.5/500 contains:
Hydrocodone Bitartrate .... 2.5 mg
Acetaminophen .... 500 mg
In addition each tablet contains the following inactive ingredients: colloidal silicon dioxide, croscarmellose sodium, crospovidone, microcrystalline cellulose, povidone, pregelatinized starch, stearic acid and sugar spheres which are composed of starch derived from corn, sucrose, FD&C Red #3.
Each Lortab 5/500 contains:
Hydrocodone Bitartrate .... 5 mg
Acetaminophen .... 500 mg
In addition each tablet contains the following inactive ingredients: corn starch, FD&C Blue #1 lake, gelatin, magnesium stearate, microcrystalline cellulose, sugar spheres, povidone, pregelatinized starch, sodium starch glycolate.
Each Lortab 7.5/500 contains:
Hydrocodone Bitartrate .... 7.5 mg
Acetaminophen .... 500 mg
In addition each tablet contains the following inactive ingredients: colloidal silicon dioxide, croscarmellose sodium, crospovidone, microcrystalline cellulose, povidone, pregelatinized starch, stearic acid, and sugar spheres which are composed of starch derived from corn, sucrose, FD&C Blue #1 and D&C Yellow #10.
Each Lortab 10/500 tablet contains:
Hydrocodone Bitartrate .... 10 mg
Acetaminophen .... 500 mg
In addition each tablet contains the following inactive ingredients: D&C Red No. 27 Aluminum Lake, D&C Red No. 30 Aluminum Lake, croscarmellose sodium, microcrystalline cellulose, colloidal silicon dioxide, starch (corn), stearic acid, pregelatinized starch, povidone, and crospovidone.

Lortab Elixir contains:	Per 5 mL	Per 15 mL
Hydrocodone Bitartrate	2.5 mg	7.5 mg
Acetaminophen	167 mg	500 mg
Alcohol	7%	7%

In addition the liquid contains the following inactive ingredients: citric acid anhydrous, ethyl maltol, glycerin, methyl paraben, propylene glycol, propylparaben, purified water, saccharin sodium, sorbitol solution, sucrose, with D&C Yellow #10 and FD&C Yellow #6 as coloring and natural and artificial flavoring.

CLINICAL PHARMACOLOGY

Hydrocodone is a semisynthetic narcotic analgesic and antitussive with multiple actions qualitatively similar to those of codeine. Most of these involve the central nervous system and smooth muscle. The precise mechanism of action of hydrocodone and other opiates is not known, although it is believed to relate to the existence of opiate receptors in the central nervous system. In addition to analgesia, narcotics may produce drowsiness, changes in mood and mental clouding.
The analgesic action of acetaminophen involves peripheral influences, but the specific mechanism is as yet undetermined. Antipyretic activity is mediated through hypothalamic heat regulating centers. Acetaminophen inhibits prostaglandin synthetase. Therapeutic doses of acetaminophen have negligible effects on the cardiovascular or respiratory systems; however, toxic doses may cause circulatory failure and rapid, shallow breathing.
Pharmacokinetics: The behavior of the individual components is described below.
Hydrocodone: Following a 10 mg oral dose of hydrocodone administered to five adult male subjects, the mean peak concentration was 23.6 ± 5.2 ng/mL. Maximum serum levels were achieved at 1.3 ± 0.3 hours and the half-life was determined to be 3.8 ± 0.3 hours. Hydrocodone exhibits a complex pattern of metabolism including O-demethylation, N-demethylation and 6-keto reduction to the corresponding 6-α- and 6-β- hydroxymetabolites.
See OVERDOSAGE for toxicity information.
Acetaminophen: Acetaminophen is rapidly absorbed from the gastrointestinal tract and is distributed throughout most body tissues. The plasma half-life is 1.25 to 3 hours, but may be increased by liver damage and following overdosage. Elimination of acetaminophen is principally by liver metabolism (conjugation) and subsequent renal excretion of metabolites. Approximately 85% of an oral dose appears in the urine within 24 hours of administration, most as the glucuronide conjugate, with small amounts of other conjugates and unchanged drug.
See OVERDOSAGE for toxicity information.

INDICATIONS AND USAGE

Lortab Tablets & Elixir are indicated for the relief of moderate to moderately severe pain.

CONTRAINDICATIONS

This product should not be administered to patients who have previously exhibited hypersensitivity to hydrocodone or acetaminophen.

WARNINGS

Respiratory Depression: At high doses or in sensitive patients, hydrocodone may produce dose-related respiratory depression by acting directly on the brain stem respiratory center. Hydrocodone also affects the center that controls respiratory rhythm, and may produce irregular and periodic breathing.
Head Injury and Increased Intracranial Pressure: The respiratory depressant effects of narcotics and their capacity to elevate cerebrospinal fluid pressure may be markedly exaggerated in the presence of head injury, other intracranial lesions or a preexisting increase in intracranial pressure. Furthermore, narcotics produce adverse reactions which may obscure the clinical course of patients with head injuries.
Acute Abdominal Conditions: The administration of narcotics may obscure the diagnosis or clinical course of patients with acute abdominal conditions.

PRECAUTIONS

General: Special Risk Patients: As with any narcotic analgesic agent, Lortab Tablets & Elixir should be used with caution in elderly or debilitated patients, and those with severe impairment of hepatic or renal function, hypothyroidism, Addison's disease, prostatic hypertrophy or urethral stricture. The usual precautions should be observed and the possibility of respiratory depression should be kept in mind.
Cough Reflex: Hydrocodone suppresses the cough reflex; as with all narcotics, caution should be exercised when Lortab Tablets or Elixir are used postoperatively and in patients with pulmonary disease.
Information for Patients: Hydrocodone, like all narcotics, may impair the mental and/or physical abilities required for the performance of potentially hazardous tasks such as driving a car or operating machinery; patients should be cautioned accordingly.
Alcohol and other CNS depressants may produce an additive CNS depression, when taken with this combination product, and should be avoided.
Hydrocodone may be habit-forming. Patients should take the drug only for as long as it is prescribed, in the amounts prescribed, and no more frequently than prescribed.
Laboratory Tests: In patients with severe hepatic or renal disease, effects of therapy should be monitored with serial liver and/or renal function tests.
Drug Interactions: Patients receiving narcotics, antihistamines, antipsychotics, antianxiety agents, or other CNS depressants (including alcohol) concomitantly with hydrocodone bitartrate and acetaminophen tablets or elixir may exhibit an additive CNS depression. When combined therapy is contemplated, the dose of one or both agents should be reduced.
The use of MAO inhibitors or tricyclic antidepressants with hydrocodone preparations may increase the effect of either the antidepressant or hydrocodone.
Drug/Laboratory Test Interactions: Acetaminophen may produce false-positive test results for urinary 5-hydroxyindoleacetic acid.
Carcinogenesis, Mutagenesis, Impairment of Fertility: No adequate studies have been conducted in animals to determine whether hydrocodone or acetaminophen have a potential for carcinogenesis, mutagenesis, or impairment of fertility.
Pregnancy:
Teratogenic Effects: Pregnancy Category C: There are no adequate and well-controlled studies in pregnant women. Lortab Tablets or Elixir should be used during pregnancy only if the potential benefit justifies the potential risk to the fetus.
Nonteratogenic Effects: Babies born to mothers who have been taking opioids regularly prior to delivery will be physically dependent. The withdrawal signs include irritability and excessive crying, tremors, hyperactive reflexes, increased respiratory rate, increased stools, sneezing, yawning, vomiting, and fever. The intensity of the syndrome does not always correlate with the duration of maternal opioid use or dose. There is no consensus on the best method of managing withdrawal.
Labor and Delivery: As with all narcotics, administration of this product to the mother shortly before delivery may result in some degree of respiratory depression in the newborn, especially if higher doses are used.
Nursing Mothers: Acetaminophen is excreted in breast milk in small amounts, but the significance of its effects on nursing infants is not known. It is not known whether hydrocodone is excreted in human milk. Because many drugs are excreted in human milk and because of the potential for serious adverse reactions in nursing infants from hydrocodone and acetaminophen, a decision should be made whether to discontinue nursing or to discontinue the drug, taking into account the importance of the drug to the mother.

Pediatric Use: Safety and effectiveness in the pediatric population have not been established.

ADVERSE REACTIONS

The most frequently reported adverse reactions are lightheadedness, dizziness, sedation, nausea and vomiting. These effects seem to be more prominent in ambulatory than in non-ambulatory patients, and some of these adverse reactions may be alleviated if the patient lies down.

Other adverse reactions include:

Central Nervous System: Drowsiness, mental clouding, lethargy, impairment of mental and physical performance, anxiety, fear, dysphoria, psychic dependence, mood changes.

Gastrointestinal System: Prolonged administration of Lortab Tablets or Elixir may produce constipation.

Genitourinary System: Ureteral spasm, spasm of vesical sphincters and urinary retention have been reported with opiates.

Respiratory Depression: Hydrocodone bitartrate may produce dose-related respiratory depression by acting directly on brain stem respiratory centers (see OVERDOSAGE).

Dermatological: Skin rash, pruritus.

The following adverse drug events may be borne in mind as potential effects of acetaminophen: allergic reactions, rash, thrombocytopenia, agranulocytosis.

Potential effects of high dosage are listed in the OVERDOSAGE section.

Controlled Substance: Lortab Tablets & Elixir are classified as Schedule III controlled substances.

Abuse and Dependence: Psychic dependence, physical dependence, and tolerance may develop upon repeated administration of narcotics; therefore, this product should be prescribed and administered with caution. However, psychic dependence is unlikely to develop when hydrocodone bitartrate and acetaminophen tablets or elixir are used for a short time for the treatment of pain.

Physical dependence, the condition in which continued administration of the drug is required to prevent the appearance of a withdrawal syndrome, assumes clinically significant proportions only after several weeks of continued narcotic use, although some mild degree of physical dependence may develop after a few days of narcotic therapy. Tolerance, in which increasingly large doses are required in order to produce the same degree of analgesia, is manifested initially by a shortened duration of analgesic effect, and subsequently by decreases in the intensity of analgesia. The rate of development of tolerance varies among patients.

OVERDOSAGE

Following an acute overdosage, toxicity may result from hydrocodone or acetaminophen.

Signs and Symptoms:

Hydrocodone: Serious overdose with hydrocodone is characterized by respiratory depression (a decrease in respiratory rate and/or tidal volume, Cheyne-Stokes respiration, cyanosis), extreme somnolence progressing to stupor or coma, skeletal muscle flaccidity, cold and clammy skin, and sometimes bradycardia and hypotension. In severe overdosage, apnea, circulatory collapse, cardiac arrest and death may occur.

Acetaminophen: In acetaminophen overdosage: dose-dependent, potentially fatal hepatic necrosis is the most serious adverse effect. Renal tubular necrosis, hypoglycemic coma, and thrombocytopenia may also occur.

Early symptoms following a potentially hepatotoxic overdose may include: nausea, vomiting, diaphoresis and general malaise. Clinical and laboratory evidence of hepatic toxicity may not be apparent until 48 to 72 hours post-ingestion.

In adults, hepatic toxicity has rarely been reported with acute overdoses of less than 10 grams or fatalities with less than 15 grams.

Treatment: A single or multiple overdose with hydrocodone and acetaminophen is a potentially lethal polydrug overdose, and consultation with a regional poison control center is recommended.

Immediate treatment includes support of cardiorespiratory function and measures to reduce drug absorption. Vomiting should be induced mechanically, or with syrup of ipecac, if the patient is alert (adequate pharyngeal and laryngeal reflexes). Oral activated charcoal (1 g/kg) should follow gastric emptying. The first dose should be accompanied by an appropriate cathartic. If repeated doses are used, the cathartic might be included with alternate doses as required. Hypotension is usually hypovolemic and should respond to fluids. Vasopressors and other supportive measures should be employed as indicated. A cuffed endo-tracheal tube should be inserted before gastric lavage of the unconscious patient and, when necessary, to provide assisted respiration.

Meticulous attention should be given to maintaining adequate pulmonary ventilation. In severe cases of intoxication, peritoneal dialysis, or preferably hemodialysis may be considered. If hypoprothrombinemia occurs due to acetaminophen overdose, vitamin K should be administered intravenously.

Naloxone, a narcotic antagonist, can reverse respiratory depression and coma associated with opioid overdose. Naloxone hydrochloride 0.4 mg to 2 mg is given parenterally. Since the duration of action of hydrocodone may exceed that of the naloxone, the patient should be kept under continuous surveillance and repeated doses of the antagonist should be administered as needed to maintain adequate respiration. A narcotic antagonist should not be administered in the absence of clinically significant respiratory or cardiovascular depression.

If the dose of acetaminophen may have exceeded 140 mg/kg, acetylcysteine should be administered as early as possible. Serum acetaminophen levels should be obtained, since levels four or more hours following ingestion help predict acetaminophen toxicity. Do not await acetaminophen assay results before initiating treatment. Hepatic enzymes should be obtained initially, and repeated at 24-hour intervals.

Methemoglobinemia over 30% should be treated with methylene blue by slow intravenous administration.

The toxic dose for adults for acetaminophen is 10 g.

DOSAGE AND ADMINISTRATION

Dosage should be adjusted according to severity of pain and response of the patient. However, it should be kept in mind that tolerance to hydrocodone can develop with continued use and that the incidence of untoward effects is dose related.

The usual adult dosage for LORTAB® 2.5/500 tablets is one or two tablets every four to six hours as needed for pain. The total daily dosage should not exceed 8 tablets.

The usual adult dosage for LORTAB® 5/500 tablets is one or two tablets every four to six hours as needed for pain. The total daily dosage should not exceed 8 tablets.

The usual adult dosage for LORTAB® 7.5/500 tablets is one tablet every four to six hours as needed for pain. The total daily dosage should not exceed 6 tablets.

The usual adult dosage for LORTAB® 10/500 tablets is one tablet every four to six hours as needed for pain. The total daily dosage should not exceed 6 tablets.

The usual adult dosage for LORTAB® ELIXIR is one tablespoonful (15 mL) every four to six hours as needed for pain. The total daily dosage should not exceed 6 tablespoonfuls.

HOW SUPPLIED

LORTAB® 2.5/500 (Hydrocodone Bitartrate and Acetaminophen Tablets, USP) contain hydrocodone bitartrate 2.5 mg and acetaminophen 500 mg. They are supplied as white with pink specks, capsule-shaped, bisected tablets, debossed "ucb/901" in containers of 100 tablets NDC 50474-925-01.

LORTAB® 5/500 (Hydrocodone Bitartrate and Acetaminophen Tablets, USP) contain hydrocodone bitartrate 5 mg and acetaminophen 500 mg. They are supplied as white with blue specks, capsule-shaped, bisected tablets, debossed "ucb/902," in containers of 100 tablets NDC 50474-902-01, in containers of 500 tablets NDC 50474-902-50, and in hospital unit-dose packages of 100 tablets [4×25] NDC 50474-902-60.

LORTAB® 7.5/500 (Hydrocodone Bitartrate and Acetaminophen Tablets, USP) contain hydrocodone bitartrate 7.5 mg and acetaminophen 500 mg. They are supplied as white with green specks, capsule-shaped, bisected tablets, debossed "ucb/903," in containers of 100 tablets NDC 50474-907-01, in containers of 500 tablets NDC 50474-907-50, and in hospital unit-dose packages of 100 tablets [4×25] NDC 50474-907-60.

Lortab® 10/500 (Hydrocodone Bitartrate and Acetaminophen Tablets, USP) contain hydrocodone bitartrate 10 mg and acetaminophen 500 mg. They are supplied as pink, capsule-shaped, bisected tablets debossed "ucb/910," in containers of 100 tablets NDC 50474–910–01, 500 tablets NDC 50474–910–50, and in hospital unit-dose packages of 100 tablets [4×25] NDC 50474–910–60.

LORTAB® Elixir (Hydrocodone Bitartrate and Acetaminophen Elixir, 7.5mg/500 mg per 15 mL) is a yellow-colored, tropical fruit punch flavored liquid containing 7.5 mg hydrocodone bitartrate and 500 mg acetaminophen per 15 mL, with 7% alcohol. It is supplied in containers of 1 pint (473 mL) NDC 50474-909-16.

Storage: Store at controlled room temperature, 15°–30°C (59°–86°F).

Dispense in a tight, light-resistant container with a child-resistant closure.

Rx only.

A Schedule CIII Narcotic

Manufactured for:
UCB PHARMA, INC.
Smyrna, GA 30080
Lortab® 2.5/500, Lortab® 7.5/500, Lortab® Elixir
Manufactured by:
Mikart, Inc.
Atlanta, GA 30318
Lortab® 5/500, Lortab® 10/500
Manufactured by:
Mallinckrodt Inc
Hobart, NY 13788

Rev. 5/98

Shown in Product Identification Guide, page 341

LORTAB® ASA (CIII)

Hydrocodone Bitartrate and Aspirin Tablets 5 mg/500 mg

Each tablet contains:

Hydrocodone bitartrate	5 mg
Aspirin	500 mg

HOW SUPPLIED

Bottles of 100; NDC 50474-500-01

Shown in Product Identification Guide, page 341

PRECARE® ℞

PRENATAL MULTI-VITAMIN/MINERAL FILM COATED CAPLET

DESCRIPTION

Each peach film-coated caplet contains:

Vitamin C (ascorbic acid)	50 mg
Calcium (as calcium carbonate)	250 mg
Iron (as ferrous fumarate)	40 mg
Vitmain D (cholecalciferol)	6 mcg
Vitamin E (dl-α-tocopherol acetate)	3.5 mg
Vitamin B_6 (pyridoxine hydrochloride)	2 mg
Folic Acid (folate)	1 mg
Magnesium (as magnesium oxide)	50 mg
Zinc (as zinc sulfate)	15 mg
Copper (as cupric sulfate)	2 mg

INACTIVE INGREDIENTS

Castor Oil, Corn Starch, Ethyl Cellulose, FD&C Yellow #6 Lake, Gelatin, Hydroxypropyl Cellulose, Hydroxypropyl Methylcellulose, Magnesium Stearate, Pharmaceutical Glaze, Polyethylene Glycol, Povidone, Propylene Glycol, Silicon Dioxide, Sodium Benzoate, Sodium Lauryl Sulfate, Sodium Starch Glycolate, Sorbic Acid, Titanium Dioxide.

INDICATIONS

Precare is indicated to provide vitamin and mineral supplementation throughout pregnancy and during the postnatal period—for both lactating and non-lactating mothers. It is also useful for improving nutritional status prior to conception.

CONTRAINDICATIONS

This product is contraindicated in patients with a known hypersensitivity to any of the ingredients.

WARNINGS

Folic acid alone is improper therapy in the treatment of pernicious anemia and other megaloblastic anemias where Vitamin B_{12} is deficient.

WARNING: Accidental overdose of iron-containing products is a leading cause of fatal poisoning in children under 6. Keep this product out of reach of children. In case of accidental overdose, call a doctor or poison control center immediately.

PRECAUTIONS

Folic acid, in doses above 0.1 mg daily may obscure pernicious anemia, in that hematologic remission can occur while neurological manifestations remain progressive.

ADVERSE REACTIONS

Allergic sensitization has been reported following both oral and parenteral administration of folic acid.

DOSAGE AND ADMINISTRATION

One caplet daily between meals or at bedtime, or as prescribed by a physician.

HOW SUPPLIED

Precare caplets for oral administration are supplied as peach film-coated caplets, debossed "nmi" on one side and scored on the other side in child-resistant, unit-dose packages of 30 caplets [3 × 10] (NDC 58436-071-03) and 100 caplets [10 × 10] (NDC 58436-071-02).

STORE AT CONTROLLED ROOM TEMPERATURE, 15°–30°C (59°–86°F).

Rx only.

Manufactured for:
UCB Pharma, Inc. (d/b/a) nmi
Smyrna, GA 30080
Manufactured by:
Schwarz Pharma Manufacturing, Inc.
Seymour, IN 47274

Rev. 5/98

Continued on next page

THEO-24®
℞

(theophylline anhydrous)

Extended-release capsules 100, 200, 300, & 400 mg

DESCRIPTION

Theophylline

Theophylline is structurally classified as a methylxanthine. It occurs as a white, odorless, crystalline powder with a bitter taste. Anhydrous theophylline has the chemical name 1H-Purine-2,6-dione,3,7-dihydro-1,3-dimethyl-, and is represented by the following structural formula:

The molecular formula of anhydrous theophylline is $C_7H_8N_4O_2$ with a molecular weight of 180.17.

Theo-24 is available as capsules intended for oral administration, containing 100 mg, 200 mg, 300 mg, or 400 mg of anhydrous theophylline per capsule, in an extended-release formulation which allows a 24-hour dosing interval for appropriate patients.

Inactive ingredients are edible ink (which contains synthetic black iron oxide, FD&C Blue No. 1, FD&C Blue No. 2, FD&C Yellow No. 6, D&C Yellow No. 10, FD&C Red No. 40), ethylcellulose, gelatin, pharmaceutical glaze, colloidal silicon dioxide, starch, sucrose, talc, titanium dioxide, and coloring agents: 100 mg—includes FD&C Yellow No. 6; 200 mg—FD&C Red No. 3 and D&C Yellow No. 10; 300 mg—FD&C Blue No.1 and FD&C Red No. 40; 400 mg—FD&C Red No. 40 and D&C Red No. 28.

Theo-24® Extended-release capsules meet Drug Release Test 6 as published in the USP 23 monograph for Theophylline Extended-release Capsules.

CLINICAL PHARMACOLOGY

Mechanism of Action;

Theophylline has two distinct actions in the airways of patients with reversible obstruction: smooth muscle relaxation (i.e., bronchodilation) and suppression of the response of the airways to stimuli (i.e., non-bronchodilator prophylactic effects). While the mechanisms of action of theophylline are not known with certainty, studies in animals suggest that bronchodilation is mediated by the inhibition of two isozymes of phosphodiesterase (PDE III and, to a lesser extent, PDE IV) while non-bronchodilator prophylactic actions are probably mediated through one or more different molecular mechanisms that do not involve inhibition of PDE III or antagonism of adenosine receptors. Some of the adverse effects associated with theophylline appear to be mediated by inhibition of PDE III (e.g., hypotension, tachycardia, headache, and emesis) and adenosine receptor antagonism (e.g., alterations in cerebral blood flow).

Theophylline increases the force of contraction of diaphragmatic muscles. This action appears to be due to enhancement of calcium uptake through an adenosine-mediated channel.

Serum Concentration-Effect Relationship:

Bronchodilation occurs over the serum theophylline concentration range of 5–20 mcg/mL. Clinically important improvement in symptom control has been found in most studies to require peak serum theophylline concentrations >10 mcg/mL, but patients with mild disease may benefit from lower concentrations. At serum theophylline concentrations >20 mcg/mL, both the frequency and severity of adverse reactions increase. In general, maintaining peak serum theophylline concentrations between 10 and 15 mcg/mL will achieve most of the drug's potential therapeutic benefit while minimizing the risk of serious adverse events.

Pharmacokinetics:

Overview Theophylline is rapidly and completely absorbed after oral administration in solution or immediate-release solid oral dose form. Theophylline does not undergo any appreciable pre-systemic elimination, distributes freely into fat-free tissues and is extensively metabolized in the liver. The pharmacokinetics of theophylline vary widely among similar patients and cannot be predicted by age, sex, body weight or other demographic characteristics. In addition, certain concurrent illnesses and alterations in normal physiology (see Table I) and co-administration of other drugs (see Table II) can significantly alter the pharmacokinetic characteristics of theophylline. Within-subject variability in metabolism has also been reported in some studies, especially in acutely ill patients. It is, therefore, recommended that serum theophylline concentrations be measured frequently in acutely ill patients (e.g., at 24-hr intervals) and periodically in patients receiving long-term therapy, e.g., at 6–12 month intervals. More frequent measurements should be made in the presence of any condition that may significantly alter theophylline clearance (see PRECAUTIONS, Laboratory Tests).

[See table below]

Absorption Theophylline is rapidly and completely absorbed after oral administration in solution or immediate-release solid oral dosage form. After a single immediate-release dose of 5 mg/kg in adults, a mean peak serum concentration of about 10 mcg/mL (range 5–15 mcg/mL) can be expected 1–2 hr after dose. Co-administration of theophylline with food or antacids does not cause clinically significant changes in the absorption of theophylline from immediate-release dosage forms.

Theo-24 capsules contain hundreds of coated beads of theophylline. Each bead is an individual extended-release delivery system. After dissolution of the capsules these beads are released and distributed in the gastrointestinal tract, thus minimizing the probability of high local concentrations of theophylline at any particular site.

In a 6–day multiple-dose study involving 18 subjects (with theophylline clearance rates between 0.57 and 1.02 mL/kg/min) who had fasted overnight and 2 hours after morning dosing, Theo-24 given once daily in a dose of 1500 mg produced serum theophylline levels that ranged between 5.7 mcg/mL and 22 mcg/mL. The mean minimum and maximum values were 11.6 mcg/mL and 18.1 mcg/mL, respectively, with an average peak-trough difference of 6.5 mcg/mL. The mean percent fluctuation $[(C_{max}-C_{min}/C_{min})\times100]$ equals 80%. A 24-hour single-dose study demonstrated an approximately proportional increase in serum levels as the dose was increased from 600 to 1500 mg.

Taking Theo-24 with a high-fat-content meal may result in a significant increase in the peak serum level and in the extent of absorption of theophylline as compared to administration in the fasted state (see Precautions, Drug/Food Interactions).

Following the single-dose administration (8 mg/kg) of Theo-24 to 20 normal subjects who had fasted overnight and 2 hours after morning dosing, peak serum theophylline concentrations of 4.8 ± 1.5 (SD) mcg/mL were obtained at 13.3 ± 4.7 (SD) hours. The amount of the dose absorbed was approximately 13% at 3 hours, 31% at 6 hours, 55% at 12 hours, 70% at 16 hours, and 88% at 24 hours. The extent of theophylline bioavailability from Theo-24 was comparable to the most widely used 12-hour extended-release product when both products were administered every 12 hours.

Distribution Once theophylline enters the systemic circulation, about 40% is bound to plasma protein, primarily albumin. Unbound theophylline distributes throughout body water, but distributes poorly into body fat. The apparent volume of distribution of theophylline is approximately 0.45 L/kg (range 0.3–0.7 L/kg) based on ideal body weight. Theophylline passes freely across the placenta, into breast milk and into the cerebrospinal fluid (CSF). Saliva theophylline concentrations approximate unbound serum concentrations, but are not reliable for routine or therapeutic monitoring unless special techniques are used. An increase in the volume of distribution of theophylline, primarily due to reduction in plasma protein binding, occurs in premature neonates, patients with hepatic cirrhosis, uncorrected acidemia, the elderly and in women during the third trimester of pregnancy. In such cases, the patient may show signs of toxicity at total (bound + unbound) serum concentrations of theophylline in the therapeutic range (10–20 mcg/mL) due to elevated concentrations of the pharmacologically active unbound drug. Similarly, a patient with decreased theophylline binding may have a sub-therapeutic total drug concentration while the pharmacologically active unbound concentration is in the therapeutic range. If only total serum theophylline concentration is measured, this may lead to an unnecessary and potentially dangerous dose increase. In patients with reduced protein binding, measurement of unbound serum theophylline concentration provides a more reliable means of dosage adjustment than measurement of total serum theophylline concentration. Generally, concentrations of unbound theophylline should be maintained in the range of 6–12 mcg/mL.

Metabolism Following oral dosing, theophylline does not undergo any measurable first-pass elimination. In adults and children beyond one year of age, approximately 90% of the dose is metabolized in the liver. Biotransformation takes place through demethylation to 1-methylxanthine and 3-methylxanthine and hydroxylation to 1,3-dimethyluric acid. 1-methylxanthine is further hydroxylated, by xanthine

Table I. Mean and range of total body clearance and half-life of theophylline related to age and altered physiological states.¶

Population characteristics		Total body clearance* mean (range)†† (mL/kg/min)	Half-life mean (range)††, (hr)
Age			
Premature neonates			
postnatal age 3–15 days		0.29 (0.09–0.49)	30 (17–43)
postnatal age 25–57 days		0.64 (0.04–1.2)	20 (9.4–30.6)
Term infants			
postnatal age 1–2 days		NR†	25.7 (25–26.5)
postnatal age 3–30 weeks		NR†	11 (6–29)
Children			
1–4 years		1.7 (0.5–2.9)	3.4 (1.2–5.6)
4–12 years		1.6 (0.8–2.4)	NR†
13–15 years		0.9 (0.48–1.3)	NR†
6–17 years		1.4 (0.2–2.6)	3.7 (1.5–5.9)
Adults (16–60 years)			
otherwise healthy			
non-smoking asthmatics		0.65 (0.27–1.03)	8.7 (6.1–12.8)
Elderly (>60 years)			
non-smokers with normal cardiac,			
liver, and renal function		0.41 (0.21–0.61)	9.8 (1.6–18)
Concurrent illness or altered physiological state			
Acute pulmonary edema		0.33** (0.07–2.45)	19** (3.1–82)
COPD>60 years, stable			
non-smoker >1 year		0.54 (0.44–0.64)	11 (9.4–12.6)
COPD with cor-pulmonale		0.48 (0.08–0.88)	NR†
Cystic fibrosis (14–28 years)		1.25 (0.31–2.2)	6.0 (1.8–10.2)
Fever associated with			
acute viral respiratory illness			
(children 9–15 years)		NR†	7.0 (1.0–13)
Liver disease -	cirrhosis	0.31** (0.1–0.7)	32** (10–56)
	acute hepatitis	0.35 (0.25–0.45)	19.2 (16.6–21.8)
	cholestasis	0.65 (0.25–1.45)	14.4 (5.7–31.8)
Pregnancy -	1st trimester	NR†	8.5 (3.1–13.9)
	2nd trimester	NR†	8.8 (3.8–13.8)
	3rd trimester	NR†	13.0 (8.4–17.6)
Sepsis with multi-organ failure		0.47 (0.19–1.9)	18.8 (6.3–24.1)
Thyroid disease -	hypothyroid	0.38 (0.13–0.57)	11.6 (8.2–25)
	hyperthyroid	0.8 (0.68–0.97)	4.5 (3.7–5.6)

¶   For various North American patient populations from literature reports. Different rates of elimination and consequent dosage requirements have been observed among other peoples.

*   Clearance represents the volume of blood completely cleared of theophylline by the liver in one minute. Values listed were generally determined at serum theophylline concentrations <20 mcg/mL; clearance may decrease and half-life may increase at higher serum concentrations due to non-linear pharmacokinetics.

†† Reported range or estimated range (mean ± 2 SD) where actual range not reported.

†   NR = not reported or not reported in a comparable format.

** Median

Note: In addition to the factors listed above, theophylline clearance is increased and half-life decreased by low carbohydrate/high protein diets, parenteral nutrition, and daily consumption of charcoal-broiled beef. A high carbohydrate/low protein diet can decrease the clearance and prolong the half-life of theophylline.

oxidase, to 1-methyluric acid. About 6% of a theophylline dose is N-methylated to caffeine. Theophylline demethylation to 3-methylxanthine is catalyzed by cytochrome P-450 1A2, while cytochromes P-450 2E1 and P-450 3A3 catalyze the hydroxylation to 1,3-dimethyluric acid. Demethylation to 1-methylxanthine appears to be catalyzed either by cytochrome P-450 1A2 or a closely related cytochrome. In neonates, the N-demethylation pathway is absent while the function of the hydroxylation pathway is markedly deficient. The activity of these pathways slowly increases to maximal levels by one year of age.

Caffeine and 3-methylxanthine are the only theophylline metabolites with pharmacologic activity. 3–methylxanthine has approximately one tenth the pharmacologic activity of theophylline and serum concentrations in adults with normal renal function are <1 mcg/mL. In patients with end-stage renal disease, 3-methylxanthine may accumulate to concentrations that approximate the unmetabolized theophylline concentration. Caffeine concentrations are usually undetectable in adults regardless of renal function. In neonates, caffeine may accumulate to concentrations that approximate the unmetabolized theophylline concentration and thus, exert a pharmacologic effect.

Both the N-demethylation and hydroxylation pathways of theophylline biotransformation are capacity-limited. Due to the wide intersubject variability of the rate of theophylline metabolism, non-linearity of elimination may begin in some patients at serum theophylline concentrations <10 mcg/mL. Since this non-linearity results in more than proportional changes in serum theophylline concentrations with changes in dose, it is advisable to make increases or decreases in dose in small increments in order to achieve desired changes in serum theophylline concentrations (see DOSAGE AND ADMINISTRATION, Table VI). Accurate prediction of dose-dependency of theophylline metabolism in patients *a priori* is not possible, but patients with very high initial clearance rates (i.e., low steady state serum theophylline concentrations at above average doses) have the greatest likelihood of experiencing large changes in serum theophylline concentration in response to dosage changes.

Excretion In neonates, approximately 50% of the theophylline dose is excreted unchanged in the urine. Beyond the first three months of life, approximately 10% of the theophylline dose is excreted unchanged in the urine. The remainder is excreted in the urine mainly as 1,3-dimethyluric acid (35-40%), 1-methyluric acid (20-25%) and 3-methylxanthine (15-20%). Since little theophylline is excreted unchanged in the urine and since active metabolites of theophylline (i.e., caffeine, 3-methylxanthine) do not accumulate to clinically significant levels even in the face of end-stage renal disease, no dosage adjustment for renal insufficiency is necessary in adults and children >3 months of age. In contrast, the large fraction of the theophylline dose excreted in the urine as unchanged theophylline and caffeine in neonates requires careful attention to dose reduction and frequent monitoring of serum theophylline concentrations in neonates with reduced renal function (See WARNINGS).

Serum concentrations at Steady State After multiple doses of theophylline, steady state is reached in 30–65 hours (average 40 hours) in adults. At steady state, on a dosage regimen with 6-hour intervals, the expected mean trough concentration is approximately 60% of the mean peak concentration, assuming a mean theophylline half-life of 8 hours. The difference between peak and trough concentrations is larger in patients with more rapid theophylline clearance. In patients with high theophylline clearance and half-lives of about 4–5 hours, such as children age 1 to 9 years, the trough serum theophylline concentration may be only 30% of peak with a 6-hour dosing interval. In these patients a slow release formulation would allow a longer dosing interval (8–12 hours) with a smaller peak/trough difference.

Special Populations (See Table I for mean clearance and half-life values)

Geriatric The clearance of theophylline is decreased by an average of 30% in healthy elderly adults (>60 years) compared to healthy young adults. Careful attention to dose reduction and frequent monitoring of serum theophylline concentrations are required in elderly patients (see WARNINGS).

Pediatrics The clearance of theophylline is very low in neonates (see WARNINGS). Theophylline clearance reaches maximal values by one year of age, remains relatively constant until about 9 years of age and then slowly decreases by approximately 50% to adult values at about age 16. Renal excretion of unchanged theophylline in neonates amounts to about 50% of the dose, compared to about 10% in children older than three months and in adults. Careful attention to dosage selection and monitoring of serum theophylline concentrations are required in pediatric patients (see WARNINGS and DOSAGE AND ADMINISTRATION).

Gender Gender differences in theophylline clearance are relatively small and unlikely to be of clinical significance. Significant reduction in theophylline clearance, however, has been reported in women on the 20th day of the menstrual cycle and during the third trimester of pregnancy.

Race Pharmacokinetic differences in theophylline clearance due to race have not been studied.

Renal Insufficiency Only a small fraction, e.g., about 10% of the administered theophylline dose is excreted unchanged in the urine of children greater than three months of age and adults. Since little theophylline is excreted unchanged in the urine and since active metabolites of theophylline (i.e., caffeine, 3-methylxanthine) do not accumulate to clinically significant levels even in the face of end-stage renal disease, no dosage adjustment for renal insufficiency is necessary in adults and children >3 months of age. In contrast, approximately 50% of the administered theophylline dose is excreted unchanged in the urine in neonates. Careful attention to dose reduction and frequent monitoring of serum theophylline concentrations are required in neonates with decreased renal function (see WARNINGS).

Hepatic Insufficiency Theophylline clearance is decreased by 50% or more in patients with hepatic insufficiency (e.g., cirrhosis, acute hepatitis, cholestasis). Careful attention to dose reduction and frequent monitoring of serum theophylline concentrations are required in patients with reduced hepatic function (see WARNINGS).

Congestive Heart Failure (CHF) Theophylline clearance is decreased by 50% or more in patients with CHF. The extent of reduction in theophylline clearance in patients with CHF appears to be directly correlated to the severity of the cardiac disease. Since theophylline clearance is independent of liver blood flow, the reduction in clearance appears to be due to impaired hepatocyte function rather than reduced perfusion. Careful attention to dose reduction and frequent monitoring of serum theophylline concentrations are required in patients with CHF (see WARNINGS).

Smokers Tobacco and marijuana smoking appears to increase the clearance of theophylline by induction of metabolic pathways. Theophylline clearance has been shown to increase by approximately 50% in young adult tobacco smokers and by approximately 80% in elderly tobacco smokers compared to non-smoking subjects. Passive smoke exposure has also been shown to increase theophylline clearance by up to 50%. Abstinence from tobacco smoking for one week causes a reduction of approximately 40% in theophylline clearance. Careful attention to dose reduction and frequent monitoring of serum theophylline concentrations are required in patients who stop smoking (see WARNINGS). Use of nicotine gum has been shown to have no effect on theophylline clearance.

Fever Fever, regardless of its underlying cause, can decrease the clearance of theophylline. The magnitude and duration of the fever appear to be directly correlated to the degree of decrease of theophylline clearance. Precise data are lacking, but a temperature of 39°C (102°F) for at least 24 hours is probably required to produce a clinically significant increase in serum theophylline concentrations. Children with rapid rates of theophylline clearance (i.e., those who require a dose that is substantially larger than average [e.g., >22 mg/kg/day] to achieve a therapeutic peak serum theophylline concentration when afebrile) may be at greater risk of toxic effects from decreased clearance during sustained fever. Careful attention to dose reduction and frequent monitoring of serum theophylline concentrations are required in patients with sustained fever (see WARNINGS).

Miscellaneous

Other factors associated with decreased theophylline clearance include the third trimester of pregnancy, sepsis with multiple organ failure, and hypothyroidism. Careful attention to dose reduction and frequent monitoring of serum theophylline concentrations are required in patients with any of these conditions (see WARNINGS). Other factors associated with increased theophylline clearance include hyperthyroidism and cystic fibrosis.

Clinical Studies:

In patients with chronic asthma, including patients with severe asthma requiring inhaled corticosteroids or alternate-day oral corticosteroids, many clinical studies have shown that theophylline decreases the frequency and severity of symptoms, including nocturnal exacerbations, and decreases the "as needed" use of inhaled $beta_2$ agonists. Theophylline has also been shown to reduce the need for short courses of daily oral prednisone to relieve exacerbations of airway obstruction that are unresponsive to bronchodilators in asthmatics.

In patients with chronic obstructive pulmonary disease (COPD), clinical studies have shown that theophylline decreases dyspnea, air trapping, the work of breathing, and improves contractility of diaphragmatic muscles with little or no improvement in pulmonary function measurements.

INDICATIONS AND USAGE

Theophylline is indicated for the treatment of the symptoms and reversible airflow obstruction associated with chronic asthma and other chronic lung diseases, e.g., emphysema and chronic bronchitis.

CONTRAINDICATIONS

Theo-24 is contraindicated in patients with a history of hypersensitivity to theophylline or other components in the product.

WARNINGS

Concurrent Illness:

Theophylline should be used with extreme caution in patients with the following clinical conditions due to the increased risk of exacerbation of the concurrent condition:

Active peptic ulcer disease
Seizure disorders
Cardiac arrhythmias (not including bradyarrhythmias)

Conditions That Reduce Theophylline Clearance:

There are several readily indentifiable causes of reduced theophylline clearance. ***If the total daily dose is not appropriately reduced in the presence of these risk factors, severe and potentially fatal theophylline toxicity can occur.*** Careful consideration must be given to the benefits and risks of theophylline use and the need for more intensive monitoring of serum theophylline concentrations in patients with the following risk factors:

Age
- Neonates (term and premature)
- Children <1 year
- Elderly (>60 years)

Concurrent Diseases
- Acute pulmonary edema
- Congestive heart failure
- Cor-pulmonale
- Fever; ≥102°F for 24 hours or more; or lesser temperature elevations for longer periods
- Hypothyroidism
- Liver disease; cirrhosis, acute hepatitis
- Reduced renal function in infants <3 months of age
- Sepsis with multi-organ failure
- Shock

Cessation of Smoking

Drug Interactions Adding a drug that inhibits theophylline metabolism (e.g., cimetidine, erythromycin, tacrine) or stopping a concurrently administered drug that enhances theophylline metabolism (e.g., carbamazepine, rifampin). (see PRECAUTIONS, Drug Interactions, Table II).

When Signs or Symptoms of Theophylline Toxicity Are Present:

Whenever a patient receiving theophylline develops nausea or vomiting, particularly repetitive vomiting, or other signs or symptoms consistent with theophylline toxicity (even if another cause may be suspected), additional doses of theophylline should be withheld and a serum theophylline concentration measured immediately. Patients should be instructed not to continue any dosage that causes adverse effects and to withhold subsequent doses until the symptoms have resolved, at which time the clinician may instruct the patient to resume the drug at a lower dosage (see DOSAGE AND ADMINISTRATION, Dosing Guidelines, Table VI).

Dosage Increases:

Increases in the dose of theophylline should not be made in response to an acute exacerbation of symptoms of chronic lung disease since theophylline provides little added benefit to inhaled $beta_2$-selective agonists and systemically administered corticosteroids in this circumstance and increases the risk of adverse effects. A peak steady-state serum theophylline concentration should be measured before increasing the dose in response to persistent chronic symptoms to ascertain whether an increase in dose is safe. Before increasing the theophylline dose on the basis of a low serum concentration, the clinician should consider whether the blood sample was obtained at an appropriate time in relationship to the dose and whether the patient has adhered to the prescribed regimen (see PRECAUTIONS, Laboratory Tests).

As the rate of theophylline clearance may be dose-dependent (i.e., steady-state serum concentrations may increase disproportionately to the increase in dose), an increase in dose based upon a sub-therapeutic serum concentration measurement should be conservative. In general, limiting dose increases to about 25% of the previous total daily dose will reduce the risk of unintended excessive increases in serum theophylline concentration (see DOSAGE AND ADMINISTRATION, Table VI).

PRECAUTIONS

General:

Careful consideration of the various interacting drugs and physiologic conditions that can alter theophylline clearance and require dosage adjustment should occur prior to initiation of theophylline therapy, prior to increases in theophylline dose, and during follow up (see WARNINGS). The dose of theophylline selected for initiation of therapy should be low and, ***if tolerated***, increased slowly over a period of a week or longer with the final dose guided by monitoring serum theophylline concentrations and the patient's clinical response (see DOSAGE AND ADMINISTRATION, Table V).

Continued on next page

Theo-24—Cont.

Monitoring Serum Theophylline Concentrations:

Serum theophylline concentration measurements are readily available and should be used to determine whether the dosage is appropriate. Specifically, the serum theophylline concentration should be measured as follows:

1. When initiating therapy to guide final dosage adjustment after titration.
2. Before making a dose increase to determine whether the serum concentration is sub-therapeutic in a patient who continues to be symptomatic.
3. Whenever signs or symptoms of theophylline toxicity are present.
4. Whenever there is a new illness, worsening of a chronic illness or a change in the patient's treatment regimen that may alter theophylline clearance (e.g., fever >102°F sustained for ≥24 hours, hepatitis, or drugs listed in Table II are added or discontinued).

To guide a dose increase, the blood sample should be obtained at the time of the expected peak serum theophylline concentration; 12 hours after a dose at steady-state (expected peak serum theophylline concentration range is between 5–15 mcg/mL). For most patients, steady-state will be reached after 3 days of dosing when no doses have been missed, no extra doses have been added, and none of the doses have been taken at unequal intervals. A trough concentration (i.e., at the end of the dosing interval) provides no additional useful information and may lead to an inappropriate dose increase since the peak serum theophylline concentration can be two or more times greater than the trough concentration with an extended-release formulation. If the serum sample is drawn more or less than twelve (12) hours after the dose, the results must be interpreted with caution since the concentration may not be reflective of the peak concentration. In contrast, when signs or symptoms of theophylline toxicity are present, the serum sample should be obtained as soon as possible, analyzed immediately, and the result reported to the clinician without delay. In patients in whom decreased serum protein binding is suspected (e.g., cirrhosis, women during the third trimester of pregnancy), the concentration of unbound theophylline should be measured and the dosage adjusted to achieve an unbound concentration of 6-12 mcg/mL.

Saliva concentrations of theophylline cannot be used reliably to adjust dosage without special techniques.

Effects on Laboratory Tests:

As a result of its pharmacological effects, theophylline at serum concentrations within the 10–20 mcg/mL range modestly increases plasma glucose (from a mean of 88 mg% to 98 mg%), uric acid (from a mean of 4 mg/dL to 6 mg/dL), free fatty acids (from a mean of 451 μEq/L to 800 μEq/L, total cholesterol (from a mean of 140 vs 160 mg/dL), HDL (from a mean of 36 to 50 mg/dL), HDL/LDL ratio (from a mean of 0.5 to 0.7), and urinary free cortisol excretion (from a mean of 44 to 63 mcg/24 hr). Theophylline at serum concentrations within the 10–20 mcg/mL range may also transiently decrease serum concentrations of triiodothyronine (144 before, 131 after one week and 142 ng/dL after 4 weeks of theophylline). The clinical importance of these changes should be weighed against the potential therapeutic benefit of theophylline in individual patients.

Information for Patients:

The patient (or parent/care giver) should be instructed to seek medical advice whenever nausea, vomiting, persistent headache, insomnia or rapid heart beat occurs during treatment with theophylline, even if another cause is suspected. The patient should be instructed to contact their clinician if they develop a new illness, especially if accompanied by a persistent fever, if they experience worsening of a chronic illness, if they start or stop smoking cigarettes or marijuana, or if another clinician adds a new medication or discontinues a previously prescribed medication. Patients should be instructed to inform all clinicians involved in their care that they are taking theophylline, especially when a medication is being added or deleted from their treatment. Patients should be instructed to not alter the dose, timing of the dose, or frequency of administration without first consulting their clinician. If a dose is missed, the patient should be instructed to take the next dose at the usually scheduled time and to not attempt to make up for the missed dose.

Patients should be instructed to take this medication each morning at approximately the same time and not to exceed the prescribed dose.

Patients who require a relatively high dose of theophylline should be informed of important considerations relating to time of drug administration and meal content (see PRECAUTIONS, Drug/Food Interactions, and DOSAGE AND ADMINISTRATION).

Drug Interactions:

Drug/Drug Interactions Theophylline interacts with a wide variety of drugs. The interaction may be pharmacodynamic, i.e., alterations in the therapeutic response to theophylline or another drug or occurrence of adverse effects without a change in serum theophylline concentration. More frequently, however, the interaction is pharmacokinetic, i.e., the rate of theophylline clearance is altered by another drug resulting in increased or decreased serum theophylline concentrations. Theophylline only rarely alters the pharmacokinetics of other drugs.

The drugs listed in Table II have the potential to produce clinically significant pharmacodynamic or pharmacokinetic interactions with theophylline. The information in the "Effect" column of Table II assumes that the interacting drug is being added to a steady-state theophylline regimen. If theophylline is being initiated in a patient who is already taking a drug that inhibits theophylline clearance (e.g., cimetidine, erythromycin), the dose of theophylline required to achieve a therapeutic serum theophylline concentration will be smaller. Conversely, if theophylline is being initiated in a patient who is already taking a drug that enhances theophylline clearance (e.g., rifampin), the dose of theophylline required to achieve a therapeutic serum theophylline concentration will be larger. Discontinuation of a concomitant drug that increases theophylline clearance will result in accumulation of theophylline to potentially toxic levels, unless the theophylline dose is appropriately reduced. Discontinuation of a concomitant drug that inhibits theophylline clearance will result in decreased serum theophylline concentrations, unless the theophylline dose is appropriately increased.

The drugs listed in Table III have either been documented not to interact with theophylline or do not produce a clinically significant interaction (i.e., <15% change in theophylline clearance).

The listing of drugs in Tables II and III are current as of January 2, 1996. New interactions are continuously being reported for theophylline, especially with new chemical entities. **The clinician should not assume that a drug does not interact with theophylline if it is not listed in Table II.** Before addition of a newly available drug in a patient receiving theophylline, the package insert of the new drug and/or the medical literature should be consulted to determine if an interaction between the new drug and theophylline has been reported.

[See table II at left and on next page]

Table III. Drugs that have been documented not to interact with theophylline or drugs that produce no clinically significant interaction with theophylline.*

albuterol,	lomefloxacin
systemic and inhaled	mebendazole
amoxicillin	medroxyprogesterone
ampicillin,	methylprednisolone
with or without sulbactam	metronidazole
atenolol	metoprolol
azithromycin	nadolol
caffeine,	nifedipine
dietary ingestion	nizatidine
cefaclor	norfloxacin
co-trimoxazole	ofloxacin
(trimethoprim and	omeprazole
sulfamethoxazole)	prednisone, prednisolone
diltiazem	ranitidine
dirithomycin	rifabutin
enflurane	roxithromycin
famotidine	sorbitol
felodipine	(purgative doses do not
finasteride	inhibit theophylline
hydrocortisone	absorption)
isoflurane	sucralfate
isoniazid	terbutaline, systemic
isradipine	terfenadine
influenza vaccine	tetracycline
ketoconazole	tocainide

* Refer to PRECAUTIONS, Drug Interactions for information regarding table.

Drug/Food Interactions Taking Theo-24 less than one hour before a high-fat-content meal, such as 8 oz whole

Table II. Clinically significant drug interactions with theophylline*.

Drug	Type of Interaction	Effect**
Adenosine	Theophylline blocks adenosine receptors.	Higher doses of adenosine may be required to achieve desired effect.
Alcohol	A single large dose of alcohol (3 mL/kg of whiskey) decreases theophylline clearance for up to 24 hours.	30% increase
Allopurinol	Decreases theophylline clearance at allopurinol doses ≥600 mg/day.	25% increase
Aminoglutethimide	Increases theophylline clearance by induction of microsomal enzyme activity.	25% decrease
Carbamazepine	Similar to aminoglutethimide.	30% decrease
Cimetidine	Decreases theophylline clearance by inhibiting cytochrome P450 1A2.	70% increase
Ciprofloxacin	Similar to cimetidine.	40% increase
Clarithomycin	Similar to erythromycin.	25% increase
Diazepam	Benzodiazepines increase CNS concentrations of adenosine, a potent CNS depressant, while theophylline blocks adenosine receptors.	Larger diazepam doses may be required to produce desired level of sedation. Discontinuation of theophylline without reduction of diazepam dose may result in respiratory depression.
Disulfiram	Decreases theophylline clearance by inhibiting hydroxylation and demethylation.	50% increase
Enoxacin	Similar to cimetidine.	300% increase
Ephedrine	Synergistic CNS effects	Increased frequency of nausea, nervousness, and insomnia.
Erythromycin	Erythromycin metabolite decreases theophylline clearance by inhibiting cytochrome P450 3A3.	35% increase. Erythromycin steady-state serum concentrations decrease by a similar amount.
Estrogen	Estrogen containing oral contraceptives decrease theophylline clearance in a dose-dependent fashion. The effect of progesterone on theophylline clearance is unknown.	30% increase
Flurazepam	Similar to diazepam.	Similar to diazepam.
Fluvoxamine	Similar to cimetidine	Similar to cimetidine
Halothane	Halothane sensitizes the myocardium to catecholamines, theophylline increases release of endogenous catecholamines.	Increased risk of ventricular arrhythmias.
Interferon, human recombinant alpha-A	Decreases theophylline clearance.	100% increase
Isoproterenol (IV)	Increases theophylline clearance.	20% decrease

continued

milk, 2 fried eggs, 2 bacon strips, 2 oz hashed brown potatoes, and 2 slices of buttered toast (about 985 calories, including approximately 71g of fat) may result in a significant increase in peak serum level and in the extent of absorption of theophylline as compared to administration in the fasted state. In some cases (especially with doses of 900 mg or more taken less than one hour before a high-fat-content meal) serum theophylline levels may exceed the 20 mcg/mL level, above which theophylline toxicity is more likely to occur.

The Effect of Other Drugs on Theophylline Serum Concentration Measurements:

Most serum theophylline assays in clinical use are immunoassays which are specific for theophylline. Other xanthines such as caffeine, dyphylline, and pentoxifylline are not detected by these assays. Some drugs (e.g., cefazolin, cephalothin), however, may interfere with certain HPLC techniques. Caffeine and xanthine metabolites in neonates or patients with renal dysfunction may cause the reading from some dry reagent office methods to be higher than the actual serum theophylline concentration.

Carcinogenesis, Mutagenesis, and Impairment of Fertility:

Long term carcinogenicity studies have been carried out in mice (oral doses 30–150 mg/kg) and rats (oral doses 5–75 mg/kg). Results are pending.

Theophylline has been studied in Ames salmonella, *in vivo* and *in vitro* cytogenetics, micronucleus and Chinese hamster ovary test systems and has not been shown to be genotoxic.

In a 14 week continuous breeding study, theophylline, administered to mating pairs of B6C3F$_1$ mice at oral doses of 120, 270 and 500 mg/kg (approximately 1.0–3.0 times the human dose on a mg/m^2 basis) impaired fertility, as evidenced by decreases in the number of live pups per litter, decreases in the mean number of litters per fertile pair, and increases in the gestation period at the high dose as well as decreases in the proportion of pups born alive at the mid and high dose. In 13 week toxicity studies, theophylline was administered to F344 rats and B6C3F$_1$ mice at oral doses of 40–300 mg/kg (approximately 2.0 times the human dose on a mg/m^2 basis). At the high dose, systemic toxicity was observed in both species including decreases in testicular weight.

Pregnancy:

CATEGORY C: There are no adequate and well controlled studies in pregnant women. Additionally, there are no teratogenicity studies in non-rodents (e.g., rabbits). Theophylline was not shown to be teratogenic in CD-1 mice at oral doses up to 400 mg/kg, approximately 2.0 times the human dose on a mg/m^2 basis or in CD-1 rats at oral doses up to 260 mg/kg, approximately 3.0 times the recommended human dose on a mg/m^2 basis. At a dose of 220 mg/kg, embryotoxicity was observed in rats in the absence of maternal toxicity.

Nursing Mothers:

Theophylline is excreted into breast milk and may cause irritability or other signs of mild toxicity in nursing human infants. The concentration of theophylline in breast milk is about equivalent to the maternal serum concentration. An infant ingesting a liter of breast milk containing 10–20 mcg/mL of theophylline day is likely to receive 10–20 mg of theophylline per day. Serious adverse effects in the infant are unlikely unless the mother has toxic serum theophylline concentrations.

Pediatric Use:

Theophylline is safe and effective for the approved indications in pediatric patients (See, INDICATIONS AND USAGE). The maintenance dose of theophylline must be selected with caution in pediatric patients since the rate of theophylline clearance is highly variable across the age range of neonates to adolescents (see CLINICAL PHARMACOLOGY, Table I, WARNINGS, and DOSAGE AND ADMINISTRATION, Table V). Due to the immaturity of theophylline metabolic pathways in infants under the age of one year, particular attention to dosage selection and frequent monitoring of serum theophylline concentrations are required when theophylline is prescribed to pediatric patients in this group.

Geriatric Use:

Elderly patients are at significantly greater risk of experiencing serious toxicity from theophylline than younger patients due to pharmacokinetic and pharmacodynamic changes associated with aging. Theophylline clearance is reduced in patients greater than 60 years of age, resulting in increased serum theophylline concentrations in response to a given theophylline dose. Protein binding may be decreased in the elderly resulting in a larger proportion of the total serum theophylline concentration in the pharmacologically active unbound form. Elderly patients also appear to be more sensitive to the toxic effects of theophylline after chronic overdosage than younger patients. For these reasons, the maximum daily dose of theophylline in patients greater than 60 years of age ordinarily should not exceed 400 mg/day unless the patient continues to be symptomatic and the peak steady state serum theophylline concentration is <10 mcg/mL (see DOSAGE AND ADMINISTRATION). Theophylline doses greater than 400 mg/day should be prescribed with caution in elderly patients.

ADVERSE REACTIONS

Adverse reactions associated with theophylline are generally mild when peak serum theophylline concentrations are <20 mcg/mL and mainly consist of transient caffeine-like adverse effects such as nausea, vomiting, headache, and insomnia. When peak serum theophylline concentrations exceed 20 mcg/mL, however, theophylline produces a wide range of adverse reactions including persistent vomiting, cardiac arrhythmias, and intractable seizures which can be lethal (see OVERDOSE). The transient caffeine-like adverse reactions occur in about 50% of patients when theophylline therapy is initiated at doses higher than recommended initial doses (e.g., >300 mg/day in adults and >12 mg/kg/day in children beyond 1 year of age). During the initiation of theophylline therapy, caffeine-like adverse effects may transiently alter patient behavior, especially in school age children, but this response rarely persists. Initiation of theophylline therapy at a low dose with subsequent slow titration to a predetermined age-related maximum dose will significantly reduce the frequency of these transient adverse effects (see DOSAGE AND ADMINISTRATION, Table V). In a small percentage of patients (<3% of children and <10% of adults) the caffeine-like adverse effects persist during maintenance therapy, even at peak serum theophylline concentrations within the therapeutic range (i.e., 10–20 mcg/mL). Dosage reduction may alleviate the caffeine-like adverse effects in these patients, however, persistent adverse effects should result in a reevaluation of the need for continued theophylline therapy and the potential therapeutic benefit of alternative treatment.

Other adverse reactions that have been reported at serum theophylline concentrations <20 mcg/mL include diarrhea, irritability, restlessness, fine skeletal muscle tremors, and transient diuresis. In patients with hypoxia secondary to COPD, multifocal atrial tachycardia and flutter have been reported at serum theophylline concentrations ≥15 mcg/mL. There have been a few isolated reports of seizures at serum theophylline concentrations <20 mcg/mL in patients with an underlying neurological disease or in elderly patients. The occurrence of seizures in elderly patients with serum theophylline concentrations <20 mcg/mL may be secondary to decreased protein binding resulting in a larger proportion of the total serum theophylline concentration in the pharmacologically active unbound form. The clinical characteristics of the seizures reported in patients with serum theophylline concentrations <20 mcg/mL have generally been milder than seizures associated with excessive serum theophylline concentrations resulting from an overdose (i.e., they have generally been transient, often stopped without anticonvulsant therapy, and did not result in neurological residua).

Table II. Clinically significant drug interactions with theophylline*. (Continued)

Drug	Type of Interaction	Effect**
Ketamine	Pharmacologic	May lower theophylline seizure threshold.
Lithium	Theophylline increases renal lithium clearance.	Lithium dose required to achieve a therapeutic serum concentration increased an average of 60%.
Lorazepam	Similar to diazepam.	Similar to diazepam.
Methotrexate (MTX)	Decreases theophylline clearance.	20% increase after low dose MTX, higher dose MTX may have a greater effect.
Mexiletine	Similar to disulfiram.	80% increase
Midazolam	Similar to diazepam.	Similar to diazepam.
Moricizine	Increases theophylline clearance.	25% decrease
Pancuronium	Theophylline may antagonize non-depolarizing neuromuscular blocking effects, possibly due to phosphodiesterase inhibition.	Larger dose of pancuronium may be required to achieve neuromuscular blockade.
Pentoxifylline	Decreases theophylline clearance.	30% increase
Phenobarbital (PB)	Similar to aminoglutethimide.	25% decrease after two weeks of concurrent PB.
Phenytoin	Phenytoin increases theophylline clearance by increasing microsomal enzyme activity. Theophylline decreases phenytoin absorption.	Serum theophylline and phenytoin concentrations decrease about 40%.
Propafenone	Decreases theophylline clearance and pharmacologic interaction.	40% increase. Beta$_2$ blocking effect may decrease efficacy of theophylline.
Propranolol	Similar to cimetidine and pharmacologic interaction.	100% increase. Beta$_2$ blocking effect may decrease efficacy of theophylline.
Rifampin	Increases theophylline clearance by increasing cytochrome P450 1A2 and 3A3 activity.	20–40% decrease
Sulfinpyrazone	Increases theophylline clearance by increasing demethylation and hydroxylation. Decreases renal clearance of theophylline.	20% decrease
Tacrine	Similar to cimetidine, also increases renal clearance of theophylline.	90% increase
Thiabendazole	Decreases theophylline clearance.	190% increase
Ticlopidine	Decreases theophylline clearance.	60% increase
Troleandomycin	Similar to erythromycin.	33–100% increase depending on troleandomycin dose.
Verapamil	Similar to disulfiram.	20% increase

Table IV. Manifestations of theophylline toxicity.*

	Percentage of patients reported with sign or symptom			
	Acute Overdose (Large Single Ingestion)		Chronic Overdosage (Multiple Excessive Doses)	
Sign/Symptom	Study 1 (n=157)	Study 2 (n=14)	Study 1 (n=92)	Study 2 (n=102)
Asymptomatic	NR**	0	NR**	6
Gastrointestinal				
Vomiting	73	93	30	61
Abdominal Pain	NR**	21	NR**	12
Diarrhea	NR**	0	NR**	14
Hematemesis	NR**	0	NR**	2
Metabolic/Other				
Hypokalemia	85	79	44	43
Hyperglycemia	98	NR**	18	NR**
Acid/base disturbance	34	21	9	5
Rhabdomyolysis	NR**	7	NR**	0

* Refer to PRECAUTIONS, Drug Interactions for further information regarding table.
** Average effect on steady-state theophylline concentration or other clinical effect for pharmacologic interactions. Individual patients may experience larger changes in serum theophylline concentration than the value listed.

Continued on next page

Theo-24—Cont.

Cardiovascular				
Sinus tachycardia	100	86	100	62
Other supraventricular tachycardias	2	21	12	14
Ventricular premature beats	3	21	10	19
Atrial fibrillation or flutter	1	NR**	12	NR**
Multifocal atrial tachycardia	0	NR**	2	NR**
Ventricular arrythmias with hemodynamic instability	7	14	40	0
Hypotension/shock	NR**	21	NR**	8
Neurologic				
Nervousness	NR**	64	NR**	21
Tremors	38	29	16	14
Disorientation	NR**	7	NR**	11
Seizures	5	14	14	5
Death	3	21	10	4

* These data are derived from two studies in patients with serum theophylline concentrations >30 mcg/mL. In the first study (Study #1—Shanon, Ann Intern Med 1993; 119:1161–67), data were prospectively collected from 249 consecutive cases of theophylline toxicity referred to a regional poison center for consultation. In the second study (Study #2—Sessler, Am J Med 1990;88:567–76), data were retrospectively collected from 116 cases with serum theophylline concentrations >30 mcg/mL among 6000 blood samples obtained for measurement of serum theophylline concentrations in three emergency departments. Differences in the incidence of manifestations of theophylline toxicity between the two studies may reflect sample selection as a result of study design (e.g., in Study #1, 48% of the patients had acute intoxications versus only 10% in Study #2) and different methods of reporting results.

**NR = Not reported in a comparable manner.

OVERDOSAGE

General:

The chronicity and pattern of theophylline overdosage significantly influences clinical manifestations of toxicity, management and outcome. There are two common presentations: (1) acute overdose, i.e., ingestion of a single large excessive dose (>10 mg/kg) as occurs in the context of an attempted suicide or isolated medication error, and (2) chronic overdosage, i.e., ingestion of repeated doses that are excessive for the patient's rate of theophylline clearance. The most common causes of chronic theophylline overdosage include patient or care giver error in dosing, clinician prescribing of an excessive dose or a normal dose in the presence of factors known to decrease the rate of theophylline clearance, and increasing the dose in response to an exacerbation of symptoms without first measuring the serum theophylline concentration to determine whether a dose increase is safe.

Severe toxicity from theophylline overdose is a relatively rare event. In one health maintenance organization, the frequency of hospital admissions for chronic overdosage of theophylline was about 1 per 1000 person-years exposure. In another study, among 6000 blood samples obtained for measurement of serum theophylline concentration, for any reason, from patients treated in an emergency department, 7% were in the 20-30 mcg/mL range and 3% were >30 mcg/mL. Approximately two-thirds of the patients with serum theophylline concentrations in the 20-30 mcg/mL range had one or more manifestations of toxicity while >90% of patients with serum theophylline concentrations >30 mcg/mL were clinically intoxicated. Similarly, in other reports, serious toxicity from theophylline is seen principally at serum concentrations >30 mcg/mL.

Several studies have described the clinical manifestations of theophylline overdose and attempted to determine the factors that predict life-threatening toxicity. In general, patients who experience an acute overdose are less likely to experience seizures than patients who have experienced a chronic overdosage, unless the peak serum theophylline concentration is >100 mcg/mL. After a chronic overdosage, generalized seizures, life-threatening cardiac arrhythmias, and death may occur at serum theophylline concentrations >30 mcg/mL. The severity of toxicity after chronic overdosage is more strongly correlated with the patient's age than the peak serum theophylline concentration; patients >60 years are at the greatest risk for severe toxicity and mortality after a chronic overdosage. Pre-existing or concurrent disease may also significantly increase the susceptibility of a patient to a particular toxic manifestation, e.g., patients

with neurologic disorders have an increased risk of seizures and patients with cardiac disease have an increased risk of cardiac arrhythmias for a given serum theophylline concentration compared to patients without the underlying disease.

The frequency of various reported manifestations of theophylline overdose according to the mode of overdose are listed in Table IV.

Other manifestations of theophylline toxicity include increases in serum calcium, creatine kinase, myoglobin and leukocyte count, decreases in serum phosphate and magnesium, acute myocardial infarction, and urinary retention in men with obstructive uropathy.

Seizures associated with serum theophylline concentrations >30 mcg/mL are often resistant to anticonvulsant therapy and may result in irreversible brain injury if not rapidly controlled. Death from theophylline toxicity is most often secondary to cardiorespiratory arrest and/or hypoxic encephalopathy following prolonged generalized seizures or intractable cardiac arrhythmias causing hemodynamic compromise.

Overdose Management:

General Recommendations for Patients with Symptoms of Theophylline Overdose or Serum Theophylline Concentrations >30 mcg/mL (Note: Serum theophylline concentrations may continue to increase after presentation of the patient for medical care.

1. While simultaneously instituting treatment, contact a regional poison center to obtain updated information and advice on individualizing the recommendations that follow.

2. Institute supportive care, including establishment of intravenous access, maintenance of the airway, and electrocardiographic monitoring.

3. Treatment of seizures Because of the high morbidity and mortality associated with theophylline-induced seizures, treatment should be rapid and aggressive. Anticonvulsant therapy should be initiated with an intravenous benzodiazepine, e.g., diazepam, in increments of 0.1-0.2 mg/kg every 1-3 minutes until seizures are terminated. Repetitive seizures should be treated with a loading dose of phenobarbital (20 mg/kg infused over 30-60 minutes). Case reports of theophylline overdose in humans and animal studies suggest that phenytoin is ineffective in terminating theophylline-induced seizures. The doses of benzodiazepines and phenobarbital required to terminate theophylline-induced seizures are close to the doses that may cause severe respiratory depression or respiratory arrest; the clinician should therefore be prepared to provide assisted ventilation. Elderly patients and patients with COPD may be more susceptible to the respiratory depressant effects of anticonvulsants. Barbiturate-induced coma or administration of general anesthesia may be required to terminate repetitive seizures or status epilepticus. General anesthesia should be used with caution in patients with theophylline overdose because fluorinated volatile anesthetics may sensitize the myocardium to endogenous catecholamines released by theophylline. Enflurane appears less likely to be associated with this effect than halothane and may, therefore, be safer. Neuromuscular blocking agents alone should not be used to terminate seizures since they abolish the musculoskeletal manifestations without terminating seizure activity in the brain.

4. Anticipate need for anticonvulsants In patients with theophylline overdose who are at a high risk for theophylline-induced seizures, e.g., patients with acute overdoses and serum theophylline concentrations >100 mcg/mL or chronic overdosage in patients >60 years of age with serum theophylline concentrations >30 mcg/mL, the need for anticonvulsant therapy should be anticipated. A benzodiazepine such as diazepam should be drawn into a syringe and kept at the patient's bedside and medical personnel qualified to treat seizures should be immediately available. In selected patients at high risk for theophylline-induced seizures, consideration should be given to the administration of prophylactic anticonvulsant therapy. Situations where prophylactic anticonvulsant therapy should be considered in high risk patients include anticipated delays in instituting methods for extracorporeal removal of theophylline (e.g., transfer of a high risk patient from one health care facility to another for extracorporeal removal) and clinical circumstances that significantly interfere with efforts to enhance theophylline clearance (e.g., a neonate where dialysis may not be technically feasible or a patient with vomiting unresponsive to antiemetics who is unable to tolerate multiple-dose oral activated charcoal). In animal studies, prophylactic administration of phenobarbital, but not phenytoin, has been shown to delay the onset of theophylline-induced generalized seizures and to increase the dose of theophylline required to induce seizures (i.e., markedly increases the LD_{50}). Although there are no controlled studies in humans, a loading dose of intravenous phenobarbital (20 mg/kg infused over 60 minutes) may delay or prevent life-threatening seizures in high risk patients while efforts to

enhance theophylline clearance are continued. Phenobarbital may cause respiratory depression, particularly in elderly patients and patients with COPD.

5. Treatment of cardiac arrhythmias Sinus tachycardia and simple ventricular premature beats are not harbingers of life-threatening arrhythmias, they do not require treatment in the absence of hemodynamic compromise, and they resolve with declining serum theophylline concentrations. Other arrhythmias, especially those associated with hemodynamic compromise, should be treated with antiarrhythmic therapy appropriate for the type of arrhythmia.

6. Gastrointestinal decontamination Oral activated charcoal (0.5 g/kg up to 20 g and repeat at least once 1-2 hours after the first dose) is extremely effective in blocking the absorption of theophylline throughout the gastrointestinal tract, even when administered several hours after ingestion. If the patient is vomiting, the charcoal should be administered through a nasogastric tube or after administration of an antiemetic. Phenothiazine antiemetics such as prochlorperazine or perphenazine should be avoided since they can lower the seizure threshold and frequently cause dystonic reactions. A single dose of sorbitol may be used to promote stooling to facilitate removal of theophylline bound to charcoal from the gastrointestinal tract. Sorbitol, however, should be dosed with caution since it is a potent purgative which can cause profound fluid and electrolyte abnormalities, particularly after multiple doses. Commercially available fixed combinations of liquid charcoal and sorbitol should be avoided in young children and after the first dose in adolescents and adults since they do not allow for individualization of charcoal and sorbitol dosing. Ipecac syrup should be avoided in theophylline overdoses. Although ipecac induces emesis, it does not reduce the absorption of theophylline unless administered within 5 minutes of ingestion and even then is less effective than oral activated charcoal. Moreover, ipecac-induced emesis may persist for several hours after a single dose and significantly decrease the retention and the effectiveness of oral activated charcoal.

7. Serum theophylline concentration monitoring The serum theophylline concentration should be measured immediately upon presentation, 2-4 hours later, and then at sufficient intervals, e.g., every 4 hours, to guide treatment decisions and to assess the effectiveness of therapy. Serum theophylline concentrations may continue to increase after presentation of the patient for medical care as a result of continued absorption of theophylline from the gastrointestinal tract. Serial monitoring of serum theophylline concentrations should be continued until it is clear that the concentration is no longer rising and has returned to non-toxic levels.

8. General monitoring procedures Electrocardiographic monitoring should be initiated on presentation and continued until the serum theophylline level has returned to a non-toxic level. Serum electrolytes and glucose should be measured on presentation and at appropriate intervals indicated by clinical circumstances. Fluid and electrolyte abnormalities should be promptly corrected. **Monitoring and treatment should be continued until the serum concentration decreases below 20 mcg/mL.**

9. Enhance clearance of theophylline Multiple-dose oral activated charcoal (e.g., 0.5 g/kg up to 20 g, every two hours) increases the clearance of theophylline at least twofold by adsorption of theophylline secreted into gastrointestinal fluids. Charcoal must be retained in, and pass through, the gastrointestinal tract to be effective; emesis should therefore be controlled by administration of appropriate antiemetics. Alternatively, the charcoal can be administered continuously through a nasogastric tube in conjunction with appropriate antiemetics. A single dose of sorbitol may be administered with the activated charcoal to promote stooling to facilitate clearance of the adsorbed theophylline from the gastrointestinal tract. Sorbitol alone does not enhance clearance of theophylline and should be dosed with caution to prevent excessive stooling which can result in severe fluid and electrolyte imbalances. Commercially available fixed combinations of liquid charcoal and sorbitol should be avoided in young children and after the first dose in adolescents and adults since they do not allow for individualization of charcoal and sorbitol dosing. In patients with intractable vomiting, extracorporeal methods of theophylline removal should be instituted (see OVERDOSAGE, Extracorporeal Removal).

Specific Recommendations:

Acute Overdose

A. Serum Concentration >20 <30 mcg/mL
   1. Administer a single dose of oral activated charcoal.
   2. Monitor the patient and obtain a serum theophylline concentration in 2-4 hours to insure that the concentration is not increasing.

B. Serum Concentration >30 <100 mcg/mL
   1. Administer multiple dose oral activated charcoal and measures to control emesis.

2. Monitor the patient and obtain serial theophylline concentrations every 2-4 hours to gauge the effectiveness of therapy and to guide further treatment decisions.

3. Institute extracorporeal removal if emesis, seizures, or cardiac arrhythmias cannot be adequately controlled (see OVERDOSAGE,Extracorporeal Removal).

C. Serum Concentration >100 mcg/mL

1. Consider prophylactic anticonvulsant therapy.

2. Administer multiple-dose oral activated charcoal and measures to control emesis.

3. Consider extracorporeal removal, even if the patient has not experienced a seizure (see OVERDOSAGE, Extracorporeal Removal).

4. Monitor the patient and obtain serial theophylline concentrations every 2-4 hours to gauge the effectiveness of therapy and to guide further treatment decisions.

Chronic Overdosage

A. Serum Concentration >20<30 mcg/mL (with manifestations of theophylline toxicity)

1. Administer a single dose of oral activated charcoal.

2. Monitor the patient and obtain a serum theophylline concentration in 2–4 hours to insure that the concentration is not increasing.

B. Serum Concentration >30 mcg/mL in patients <60 years of age

1. Administer multiple-dose oral activated charcoal and measures to control emesis.

2. Monitor the patient and obtain serial theophylline concentrations every 2–4 hours to gauge the effectiveness of therapy and to guide further treatment decisions.

3. Institute extracorporeal removal if emesis, seizures, or cardiac arrhythmias cannot be adequately controlled (see OVERDOSAGE, Extracorporeal Removal).

C. Serum Concentration >30 mcg/mL in patients ≥60 years of age.

1. Consider prophylactic anticonvulsant therapy.

2. Administer multiple-dose oral activated charcoal and measures to control emesis.

3. Consider extracorporeal removal even if the patient has not experienced a seizure (see OVERDOSAGE, Extracorporeal Removal).

4. Monitor the patient and obtain serial theophylline concentrations every 2–4 hours to gauge the effectiveness of therapy and to guide further treatment decisions.

Extracorporeal Removal:

Increasing the rate of theophylline clearance by extracorporeal methods may rapidly decrease serum concentrations, but the risks of the procedure must be weighed against the potential benefit. Charcoal hemoperfusion is the most effective method of extracorporeal removal, increasing theophylline clearance up to six fold, but serious complications, including hypotension, hypocalcemia, platelet consumption and bleeding diatheses may occur. Hemodialysis is about as efficient as multiple-dose oral activated charcoal and has a lower risk of serious complications than charcoal hemoperfusion. Hemodialysis should be considered as an alternative when charcoal hemoperfusion is not feasible and multiple-dose oral charcoal is ineffective because of intractable emesis. Serum theophylline concentrations may rebound 5–10 mcg/mL after discontinuation of charcoal hemoperfusion or hemodialysis due to redistribution of theophylline from the tissue compartment. Peritoneal dialysis is ineffective for theophylline removal; exchange transfusions in neonates have been minimally effective.

DOSAGE AND ADMINISTRATION

General Considerations:

Theo-24, like other extended-release theophylline products, is intended for patients with relatively continuous or recurring symptoms who have a need to maintain therapeutic serum levels of theophylline. It is not intended for patients experiencing an acute episode of bronchospasm (associated with asthma, chronic bronchitis, or emphysema). Such patients require rapid relief of symptoms and should be treated with an immediate-release or intravenous theophylline preparation (or other bronchodilators) and not with extended-release products.

Patients who metabolize theophylline at a normal or slow rate are reasonable candidates for once-daily dosing with Theo-24. Patients who metabolize theophylline rapidly (e.g, the young, smokers, and some nonsmoking adults) and who have symptoms repeatedly at the end of a dosing interval, will require either increased doses given once a day or preferably, are likely to be better controlled by a schedule of twice-daily dosing. Those patients who require increased daily doses are more likely to experience relatively wide peak-trough differences and may be candidates for twice-a-day dosing with Theo-24.

Patients should be instructed to take this medication each morning at approximately the same time and not to exceed the prescribed dose.

Recent studies suggest that dosing of extended-release theophylline products at night (after the evening meal) results in serum concentrations of theophylline which are not identical to those recorded during waking hours and may be characterized by early trough and delayed peak levels. This appears to occur whether the drug is given as an immediate-release, extended-release, or intravenous product. To avoid this phenomenon when two doses per day are prescribed, it is recommended that the second dose be given 10 to 12 hours after the morning dose and before the evening meal.

Food and posture, along with changes associated with circadian rhythm, may influence the rate of absorption and/or clearance rates of theophylline from extended-release dosage forms administered at night. The exact relationship of these and other factors to nighttime serum concentrations and the clinical significance of such findings require additional study. Therefore, it is not recommended that Theo-24 (when used as a once-a-day product) be administered at night.

Patients who require a relatively high dose of theophylline (i.e., a dose equal to or greater than 900 mg or 13 mg/kg, whichever is less) should not take Theo-24 less than 1 hour before a high-fat-content meal since this may result in a significant increase in peak serum level and in the extent of absorption of theophylline as compared to administration in the fasted state (see PRECAUTIONS, Drug/Food Interactions).

The steady-state peak serum theophylline concentration is a function of the dose, the dosing interval, and the rate of theophylline absorption and clearance in the individual patient. Because of marked individual differences in the rate of theophylline clearance the dose required to achieve a peak serum theophylline concentration in the 10–20 mcg/mL range varies fourfold among otherwise similar patients in the absence of factors known to alter theophylline clearance (e.g., 400–1600 mg/day in adults <60 years old and 10–36 mg/kg/day in children 1–9 years old). For a given population there is no single theophylline dose that will provide both safe and effective serum concentrations for all patients. Administration of the median theophylline dose required to achieve a therapeutic serum theophylline concentration in a given population may result in either subtherapeutic or potentially toxic serum theophylline concentrations in individual patients. For example, at a dose of 900 mg/day in adults <60 years or 22 mg/kg/day in children 1–9 years, the steady-state peak serum theophylline concentration will be <10 mcg/mL in about 30% of patients, 10–20 mcg/mL in about 50% and 20–30 mcg/mL in about 20% of patients. **The dose of theophylline must be individualized on the basis of peak serum theophylline concentration measurements in order to achieve a dose that will provide maximum potential benefit with minimal risk of adverse effects.**

Transient caffeine-like adverse effects and excessive serum concentrations in slow metabolizers can be avoided in most patients by starting with a sufficiently low dose and slowly increasing the dose, if judged to be clinically indicated, in small increments (See Table V). Dose increases should only be made if the previous dosage is well tolerated and at intervals of no less than 3 days to allow serum theophylline concentrations to reach the new steady state. Dosage adjustment should be guided by serum theophylline concentration measurement (see PRECAUTIONS, Laboratory Tests and DOSAGE AND ADMINISTRATION, Table VI). Health care providers should instruct patients and care givers to discontinue any dosage that causes adverse effects, to withhold the medication until these symptoms are gone and to then resume therapy at a lower, previously tolerated dosage (see WARNINGS).

If the patient's symptoms are well controlled, there are no apparent adverse effects, and no intervening factors that might alter dosage requirements (see WARNINGS and PRECAUTIONS), serum theophylline concentrations should be monitored at 6 month intervals for rapidly growing children and at yearly intervals for all others. In acutely ill patients, serum theophylline concentrations should be monitored at frequent intervals, e.g., every 24 hours.

Theophylline distributes poorly into body fat, therefore, mg/kg dose should be calculated on the basis of ideal body weight.

Table V contains theophylline dosing titration schema recommended for patients in various age groups and clinical circumstances. Table VI contains recommendations for theophylline dosage adjustment based upon serum theophylline concentrations. **Application of these general dosing recommendations to individual patients must take into account the unique clinical characteristics of each patient. In general, these recommendations should serve as the upper limit for dosage adjustments in order to decrease the risk of potentially serious adverse events associated with unexpected large increases in serum theophylline concentration.**

Table V. Dosing initiation and titration (as anhydrous theophylline).*

A. Children (12–15 years) and adults (16–60 years) without risk factors for impaired clearance.

Titration Step	*Children <45 kg*	*Children >45 kg and adults*
1. Starting Dosage	12–14 mg/kg/day up to a maximum of 300 mg/day divided Q 24 hrs*	300–400 mg/day[1] divided Q 24 hrs*
2. After 3 days, *if tolerated*, increase dose to:	16 mg/kg/day up to a maximum of 400 mg/day divided Q 24 hrs*	400–600 mg/day[1] Q 24 hrs *
3. After 3 more days, *if tolerated* and *if needed*, increase dose to:	20 mg/kg/day up to a maximum of 600 mg/day divided Q 24 hrs*	As with all theophylline products, doses greater than 600 mg should be titrated according to blood level (see Table VI)

1 If caffeine-like effects occur, then consideration should be given to a lower dose and titrating the dose more slowly (see ADVERSE REACTIONS).

B. Patients with risk factors for impaired clearance, the elderly (>60 years), and those in whom it is not feasible to monitor serum theophylline concentrations: In children 1–15 years of age, the final theophylline dose should not exceed 16 mg/kg/day up to a maximum of 400 mg/day in the presence of risk factors for reduced theophylline clearance (see WARNINGS) or if it is not feasible to monitor serum theophylline concentrations. In adolescents ≥16 years and adults, including the elderly, the final theophylline dose should not exceed 400 mg/day in the presence of risk factors for reduced theophylline clearance (see WARNINGS) or if it is not feasible to monitor serum theophylline concentrations.

* Patients with more rapid metabolism, clinically identified by higher than average dose requirements, should receive a smaller dose more frequently to prevent breakthrough symptoms resulting from low trough concentrations before the next dose. A reliably absorbed slow-release formulation will decrease fluctuations and permit longer dosing intervals.

Table VI. Dosage adjustment guided by serum theophylline concentration.

Peak Serum Concentration	**Dosage Adjustment**
<9.9 mcg/mL	If symptoms are not controlled and current dosage is tolerated, increase dose about 25%. Recheck serum concentration after three days for further dosage adjustment.
10–14.9 mcg/mL	If symptoms are controlled and current dosage is tolerated, maintain dose and recheck serum concentration at 6–12 month intervals.¶ If symptoms are not controlled and current dosage is tolerated consider adding additional medication(s) to treatment regimen.
15–19.9 mcg/mL	Consider 10% decrease in dose to provide greater margin of safety even if current dosage is tolerated.¶
20–24.9 mcg/mL	Decrease dose by 25% even if no adverse effects are present. Recheck serum concentration after 3 days to guide further dosage adjustment.
25–30 mcg/mL	Skip next dose and decrease subsequent doses at least 25% even if no adverse effects are present. Recheck serum concentration after 3 days to guide further dosage adjustment. If symptomatic, consider whether overdose treatment is indicated (see recommendations for chronic overdosage).
>30 mcg/mL	Treat overdose as indicated (see recommendations for chronic overdosage). If theophylline is subsequently resumed, decrease dose by at least 50% and recheck serum concentration after 3 days to guide further dosage adjustment.

Continued on next page

Theo-24—Cont.

¶ Dose reduction and/or serum theophylline concentration measurement is indicated whenever adverse effects are present, physiologic abnormalities that can reduce theophylline clearance occur (e.g., sustained fever), or a drug that interacts with theophylline is added or discontinued (see WARNINGS).

HOW SUPPLIED

Theo-24® (theophylline anhydrous) is supplied in extended-release capsules containing 100, 200, 300 or 400 mg of anhydrous theophylline.

Theo-24 100 mg capsules are yellow-orange and clear, with markings Theo-24, 100 mg, ucb, and 2832, supplied as:

NDC Number	Size
50474-100-01	bottle of 100

Theo-24 200 mg capsules are red-orange and clear, with markings Theo-24, 200 mg, ucb, and 2842, supplied as:

NDC Number	Size
50474-200-01	bottle of 100
50474-200-50	bottle of 500
50474-200-60	carton of 100 unit dose

Theo-24 300 mg capsules are red and clear, with markings Theo-24, 300 mg, ucb, and 2852, supplied as:

NDC Number	Size
50474-300-01	bottle of 100
50474-300-50	bottle of 500
50474-300-60	carton of 100 unit dose

Theo-24 400 mg capsules are pink and clear, with markings Theo-24, 400 mg, ucb, and 2902, supplied as:

NDC Number	Size
50474-400-01	bottle of 100
50474-400-50	bottle of 500

Store below 77°F (25°C).

Rx only.

Manufactured for: Revised: 5/98

UCB Pharma, Inc.
Smyrna, GA 30080
by: **G. D. Searle & Co.,**
Chicago, IL 60680

Shown in Product Identification Guide, page 341

TRINSICON® ℞

[tren 'sa-kon]
Hematinic Concentrate
With Intrinsic Factor
A Highly Potent Oral Antianemia Preparation

DESCRIPTION

Each TRINSICON capsule contains:

Special liver-stomach concentrate (containing intrinsic factor)	240 mg
Vitamin B_{12} (activity equivalent)	15 mcg
Iron, elemental (as ferrous fumarate)	110 mg
Ascorbic acid (vitamin C)	75 mg
Folic acid	0.5 mg

with other factors of vitamin B complex present in the liver-stomach concentrate.

Each capsule also contains FD&C Blue No. 1, D&C Red No. 28, FD&C Red No. 40, D&C Yellow No. 10, gelatin, silicon dioxide, corn starch, edible ink, silicon fluid, sodium lauryl sulfate and titanium dioxide.

CLINICAL PHARMACOLOGY

Vitamin B_{12} with Intrinsic Factor: When secretion of intrinsic factor in gastric juice is inadequate or absent (eg, in Addisonian pernicious anemia or after gastrectomy), vitamin B_{12} in physiologic doses is absorbed poorly, if at all. The resulting deficiency of vitamin B_{12} leads to the clinical manifestations of pernicious anemia. Similar megaloblastic anemias may develop in fish tapeworm *(Diphyllobothrium latum)* infection or after a surgically created small-bowel blind loop; in these situations, treatment requires freeing the host of the parasites or bacteria that appear to compete for the available vitamin B_{12}. Strict vegetarianism and malabsorption syndromes may also lead to vitamin B_{12} deficiency. In the latter case, parenteral therapy, or oral therapy with so-called massive doses of vitamin B_{12} may be necessary for adequate treatment of the patient.

Potency of intrinsic factor concentrates is determined physiologically, ie, by their use in patients with pernicious anemia. The liver-stomach concentrate with intrinsic factor and the vitamin B_{12} contained in two TRINSICON capsules provide $1^1/_2$ times the minimum amount of therapeutic agent that, when given daily in an uncomplicated case of pernicious anemia, will produce a satisfactory reticulocyte response and relief of anemia and symptoms.

Concentrates of intrinsic factor derived from hog gastric, pyloric, and duodenal mucosa have been used successfully in patients who lack intrinsic factor. For example, Fouts et al maintained patients with pernicious anemia in clinical remission with oral therapy (liver extracts or intrinsic factor concentrate with vitamin B_{12}) for as long as 29 years.

After total gastrectomy, Ficarra found multifactor preparations taken orally to be "just as effective in maintaining blood levels as any medication that has to be administered parenterally." His study was based on 24 patients who had survived for five years after total gastrectomy for cancer and who had been taking two TRINSICON capsules daily.

Folic Acid: Folic acid deficiency is the immediate cause of most, if not all, cases of nutritional megaloblastic anemia and of the megaloblastic anemias of pregnancy and infancy; usually, it is also at least partially responsible for the megaloblastic anemias of malabsorption syndromes, eg, tropical and nontropical sprue.

It is apparent that in vitamin B_{12} deficiency (eg, pernicious anemia), lack of this vitamin results in impaired utilization of folic acid. There are other evidences of the close folic acid-vitamin B_{12} interrelationship: (1) B_{12} influences the storage, absorption, and utilization of folic acid, and (2) as a deficiency of B_{12} progresses, the requirement for folic acid increases. However, folic acid does not change the requirement for vitamin B_{12}.

Iron: A very common anemia is that due to iron deficiency. In most cases, the response to iron salts is prompt, safe, and predictable. Within limits, the response is quicker and more certain to large doses of iron than to small doses.

Each TRINSICON (hematinic concentrate with intrinsic factor) capsule furnishes 110 mg of elemental iron (as ferrous fumarate) to provide a maximum response.

Ascorbic Acid: Vitamin C plays a role in anemia therapy. It augments the conversion of folic acid to its active form, folinic acid. In addition, ascorbic acid promotes the reduction of ferric iron in food to the more readily absorbed ferrous form. Severe and prolonged vitamin C deficiency is associated with an anemia that is usually hypochromic but occasionally megaloblastic in type.

INDICATIONS AND USAGE

TRINSICON is a multifactor preparation effective in the treatment of anemias that respond to oral hematinics, including pernicious anemia and other megaloblastic anemias and also iron-deficiency anemia. Therapeutic quantities of hematopoietic factors that are known to be important are present in the recommended daily dose.

CONTRAINDICATIONS

Hemochromatosis and hemosiderosis are contraindications to iron therapy.

WARNINGS:

> WARNING: Accidental overdose of iron-containing products is a leading cause of fatal poisoning in children under 6. Keep this product out of reach of children. In case of accidental overdose, call a doctor or poison control center immediately.

PRECAUTIONS

General: Anemia is a manifestation that requires appropriate investigation to determine its cause or causes.

Folic acid *alone* is unwarranted in the treatment of pure vitamin B_{12} deficiency states, such as pernicious anemia. Folic acid may obscure pernicious anemia in that the blood picture may revert to normal while neurolological manifestations remain progressive.

As with all preparations containing intrinsic factor, resistance may develop in some cases of pernicious anemia to the potentiation of absorption of physiologic doses of vitamin B_{12}. If resistance occurs, parenteral therapy or oral therapy with so-called massive doses of vitamin B_{12} may be necessary for adequate treatment of the patient. No single regimen fits all cases, and the status of the patient observed in follow-up is the final criterion for adequacy of therapy. Periodic clinical and laboratory studies are considered essential and are recommended.

Pregnancy:

Teratogenic Effects: *Pregnancy Category C:* Animal reproduction studies have not been conducted with TRINSICON. It is also not known whether TRINSICON can cause fetal harm when administered to a pregnant woman or can affect reproduction capacity. TRINSICON should be given to a pregnant woman only if clearly needed.

Nursing Mothers: It is not known whether this drug is excreted in human milk. Because many drugs are excreted in human milk, caution should be exercised when TRINSICON is administered to a nursing woman.

Pediatric Use: Safety and effectiveness in children below the age of 10 have not been established.

ADVERSE REACTIONS

Rarely, iron in therapeutic doses produces gastrointestinal reactions, such as diarrhea or constipation. Reducing the dose and administering it with meals will minimize these effects in the iron-sensitive patient.

In extremely rare instances, skin rash suggesting allergy has been noted following the oral administration of liver-stomach material. Allergic sensitization has been reported following both oral and parenteral administration of folic acid.

OVERDOSAGE

Symptoms: Those of iron intoxication, which may include pallor and cyanosis, vomiting, hematemesis, diarrhea, melena, shock, drowsiness, and coma.

Treatment: For specific therapy, exchange transfusion and chelating agents. For general management, gastric and rectal lavage with sodium bicarbonate solution or milk, administration of intravenous fluids and electrolytes, and use of oxygen.

DOSAGE AND ADMINISTRATION

One capsule twice a day. (Two capsules daily produce a standard response in the average uncomplicated case of pernicious anemia.)

HOW SUPPLIED

Dark pink and dark red capsules imprinted "ucb/364" in child-resistant, unit dose packages of 60 capsules [6 × 10] (NDC 50474-364-23), and of 100 capsules [10 × 10] (NDC 50474-364-28).

Rx only.

Manufactured for
UCB Pharma, Inc.
Smyrna, GA 30080
By **Mallinckrodt Inc**
Hobart, NY 13788

Revised 5/98

Shown in Product Identification Guide, page 341

VICON FORTE® Capsules ℞

[vī 'kon for 'tā]
(Therapeutic Vitamins-Minerals)

DESCRIPTION

Each black and orange VICON FORTE capsule for oral administration contains:

Vitamin A	8,000 IU
Vitamin E	50 IU
Ascorbic acid	150 mg
Zinc sulfate, USP*	80 mg
Magnesium sulfate, USP†	70 mg
Niacinamide	25 mg
Thiamine mononitrate	10 mg
d-Calcium pantothenate	10 mg
Manganese chloride	4 mg
Riboflavin	5 mg
Pyridoxine hydrochloride	2 mg
Folic acid	1 mg
Vitamin B_{12} (Cyanocobalamin)	10 mcg

* As 50 mg dried zinc sulfate.
† As 50 mg dried magnesium sulfate.

Each capsule also contains edible ink, FD&C Blue No. 1, FD&C Red No. 40, FD&C Yellow No. 6, gelatin, lactose, magnesium stearate, silicon dioxide, sodium lauryl sulfate, and titanium dioxide.

INDICATIONS AND USAGE

VICON FORTE is indicated for the treatment and/or prevention of vitamin and mineral deficiencies associated with restricted diets, improper food intake, alcoholism, and decreased absorption. VICON FORTE is also indicated in patients with increased requirements for vitamins and minerals due to chronic disease, infection, and burns and in persons using alcohol to excess. Preoperative and postoperative use of VICON FORTE can provide the increased amounts of vitamins and minerals necessary for optimal recovery from the stress of surgery.

CONTRAINDICATIONS

None known.

PRECAUTIONS

General: Folic acid in doses above 0.1 mg daily may obscure pernicious anemia in that hematologic remission can occur while neurological manifestations remain progressive.

DOSAGE AND ADMINISTRATION

One capsule daily or as directed by physician.

HOW SUPPLIED

Orange and black capsules imprinted with "ucb/316" in bottles of 60 (NDC 50474-316-22) and 500 (NDC 50474-316-24) and unit dose packs of 100 (NDC 50474-316-27).

Dispense in tight, light-resistant container with a child resistant closure.

Rx only.

Manufactured for
UCB Pharma, Inc.,
Smyrna, GA 30080
by Mallinckrodt Inc.
Hobart, NY 13788

Revised 5/98

Shown in Product Identification Guide, page 341

U.S. Bioscience, Inc.
ONE TOWER BRIDGE
100 FRONT STREET
WEST CONSHOHOCKEN, PA 19428

Direct Inquiries to:
US Bioscience
(610) 832-0570

For Medical Information or Emergencies Contact:
1-800-872-4672

Ethyol® (amifostine), see Listing under ALZA Pharmaceuticals

HEXALEN®
[hex 'a-len]
(ALTRETAMINE)
CAPSULES
50 mg

Ŗ

WARNINGS
1. HEXALEN® should only be given under the supervision of a physician experienced in the use of antineoplastic agents.
2. Peripheral blood counts should be monitored at least monthly, prior to the initiation of each course of HEXALEN, and as clinically indicated (see Adverse Reactions).
3. Because of the possibility of HEXALEN-related neurotoxicity, neurologic examination should be performed regularly during HEXALEN administration (see Adverse Reactions).

DESCRIPTION
HEXALEN (altretamine), is a synthetic cytotoxic antineoplastic s-triazine derivative. HEXALEN capsules contain 50 mg of altretamine for oral administration. Inert ingredients include lactose, anhydrous and calcium stearate. Altretamine, known chemically as N,N,N',N',N'',N''-hexamethyl-1,3,5-triazine-2,4,6-triamine, has the following structural formula:

Its empirical formula is $C_9H_{18}N_6$ with a molecular weight of 210.28. Altretamine is a white crystalline powder, melting at $172° \pm 1°C$. Altretamine is practically insoluble in water but is increasingly soluble at pH 3 and below.

CLINICAL PHARMACOLOGY
The precise mechanism by which HEXALEN exerts its cytotoxic effect is unknown, although a number of theoretical possibilities have been studied. Structurally, HEXALEN resembles the alkylating agent triethylenemelamine, yet *in vitro* tests for alkylating activity of HEXALEN and its metabolites have been negative. HEXALEN has been demonstrated to be efficacious for certain ovarian tumors resistant to classical alkylating agents. Metabolism of altretamine is a requirement for cytotoxicity. Synthetic monohydroxymethylmelamines, and products of altretamine metabolism, *in vitro* and *in vivo*, can form covalent adducts with tissue macromolecules including DNA, but the relevance of these reactions to antitumor activity is unknown.
HEXALEN is well-absorbed following oral administration in humans, but undergoes rapid and extensive demethylation in the liver, producing variation in altretamine plasma levels. The principal metabolites are pentamethylmelamine and tetramethylmelamine.
Pharmacokinetic studies were performed in a limited number of patients and should be considered preliminary. After oral administration of HEXALEN to 11 patients with advanced ovarian cancer in doses of 120–300 mg/m², peak plasma levels (as measured by gas-chromatographic assay) were reached between 0.5 and 3 hours, varying from 0.2 to 20.8 mg/l. Half-life of the β-phase of elimination ranged from 4.7 to 10.2 hours. Altretamine and metabolites show binding to plasma proteins. The free fractions of altretamine, pentamethylmelamine and tetramethylmelamine are 6%, 25% and 50%, respectively.
Following oral administration of ¹⁴C-ring-labeled altretamine (4 mg/kg), urinary recovery of radioactivity was 61% at 24 hours and 90% at 72 hours. Human urinary metabolites were N-demethylated homologues of altretamine with <1% unmetabolized altretamine excreted at 24 hours.

After intraperitoneal administration of ¹⁴C-ring-labeled altretamine to mice, tissue distribution was rapid in all organs, reaching a maximum at 30 minutes. The excretory organs (liver and kidney) and the small intestine showed high concentrations of radioactivity, whereas relatively low concentrations were found in other organs, including the brain. There have been no formal pharmacokinetic studies in patients with compromised hepatic and/or renal function, though HEXALEN has been administered both concurrently and following nephrotoxic drugs such as cisplatin.
HEXALEN has been administered in 4 divided doses, with meals and at bedtime, though there is no pharmacokinetic data on this schedule nor information from formal interaction studies about the effect of food on its bioavailability or pharmacokinetics.
In two studies in patients with persistent or recurrent ovarian cancer following first-line treatment with cisplatin and/or alkylating agent-based combinations, HEXALEN was administered as a single agent for 14 or 21 days of a 28 day cycle. In the 51 patients with measurable or evaluable disease, there were 6 clinical complete responses, 1 pathologic complete response, and 2 partial responses for an overall response rate of 18%. The duration of these responses ranged from 2 months in a patient with a palpable pelvic mass to 36 months in a patient who achieved a pathologic complete response. In some patients, tumor regression was associated with improvement in symptoms and performance status.

INDICATIONS AND USAGE
HEXALEN (altretamine) is indicated for use as a single agent in the palliative treatment of patients with persistent or recurrent ovarian cancer following first-line therapy with a cisplatin and/or alkylating agent-based combination.

CONTRAINDICATIONS
HEXALEN is contraindicated in patients who have shown hypersensitivity to it. HEXALEN should not be employed in patients with preexisting severe bone marrow depression or severe neurologic toxicity. HEXALEN has been administered safely, however, to patients heavily pretreated with cisplatin and/or alkylating agents, including patients with preexisting cisplatin neuropathies. Careful monitoring of neurologic function in these patients is essential.

WARNINGS
See boxed Warnings.
Concurrent administration of HEXALEN and antidepressants of the monoamine oxidase (MAO) inhibitor class may cause severe orthostatic hypotension. Four patients, all over 60 years of age, were reported to have experienced symptomatic hypotension after 4 to 7 days of concomitant therapy with HEXALEN and MAO inhibitors.
HEXALEN causes mild to moderate myelosuppression and neurotoxicity. Blood counts and a neurologic examination should be performed prior to the initiation of each course of therapy and the dose of HEXALEN adjusted as clinically indicated (see Dosage and Administration).

Pregnancy: Category D
HEXALEN has been shown to be embryotoxic and teratogenic in rats and rabbits when given at doses 2 and 10 times the human dose. HEXALEN may cause fetal damage when administered to a pregnant woman. If HEXALEN is used during pregnancy, or if the patient becomes pregnant while taking the drug, the patient should be appraised of the potential hazard to the fetus. Women of childbearing potential should be advised to avoid becoming pregnant.

PRECAUTIONS
General
Neurologic examination should be performed regularly (see Adverse Reactions).
Laboratory Tests
Peripheral blood counts should be monitored at least monthly, prior to the initiation of each course of HEXALEN, and as clinically indicated (see Adverse Reactions).
Drug Interactions
Concurrent administration of HEXALEN and antidepressants of the MAO inhibitor class may cause severe orthostatic hypotension (see Warnings section). Cimetidine, an inhibitor of microsomal drug metabolism, increased altretamine's half-life and toxicity in a rat model.
Data from a randomized trial of HEXALEN and cisplatin plus or minus pyridoxine in ovarian cancer indicated that pyridoxine significantly reduced neurotoxicity; however, it adversely affected response duration suggesting that pyridoxine should not be administered with HEXALEN and/or cisplatin (1).
Carcinogenesis, Mutagenesis and Impairment of Fertility
The carcinogenic potential of HEXALEN has not been studied in animals, but drugs with similar mechanisms of action have been shown to be carcinogenic. HEXALEN was weakly mutagenic when tested in strain TA100 of *Salmonella typhimurium*. HEXALEN administered to female rats 14 days prior to breeding through the gestation period had no adverse effect on fertility, but decreased post-natal survival at 120 mg/m²/day and was embryocidal at 240 mg/m²/day. Administration of 120 mg/m²/day HEXALEN to male rats for 60 days prior to mating resulted in testicular atrophy, re-

duced fertility and a possible dominant lethal mutagenic effect. Male rats treated with HEXALEN at 450 mg/m²/day for 10 days had decreased spermatogenesis, atrophy of testes, seminal vesicles and ventral prostate.
Pregnancy
Pregnancy Category D: see Warnings section.
Nursing Mothers
It is not known whether altretamine is excreted in human milk. Because there is a possibility of toxicity in nursing infants secondary to HEXALEN treatment of the mother, it is recommended that breast feeding be discontinued if the mother is treated with HEXALEN.
Pediatric Use
The safety and effectiveness of HEXALEN in children have not been established.

ADVERSE REACTIONS
Gastrointestinal
With continuous high-dose daily HEXALEN, nausea and vomiting of gradual onset occur frequently. Although in most instances these symptoms are controllable with antiemetics, at times the severity requires HEXALEN dose reduction or, rarely, discontinuation of HEXALEN therapy. In some instances, a tolerance of these symptoms develops after several weeks of therapy. The incidence and severity of nausea and vomiting are reduced with moderate-dose administration of HEXALEN. In 2 clinical studies of single-agent HEXALEN utilizing a moderate, intermittent dose and schedule, only 1 patient (1%) discontinued HEXALEN due to severe nausea and vomiting.
Neurotoxicity
Peripheral neuropathy and central nervous system symptoms (mood disorders, disorders of consciousness, ataxia, dizziness, vertigo) have been reported. They are more likely to occur in patients receiving continuous high-dose daily HEXALEN than moderate-dose HEXALEN administered on an intermittent schedule. Neurologic toxicity has been reported to be reversible when therapy is discontinued. Data from a randomized trial of HEXALEN and cisplatin plus or minus pyridoxine in ovarian cancer indicated that pyridoxine significantly reduced neurotoxicity; however, it adversely affected response duration suggesting that pyridoxine should not be administered with HEXALEN and/or cisplatin (1).
Hematologic
HEXALEN (altretamine) causes mild to moderate dose-related myelosuppression. Leukopenia below 3000 WBC/mm³ occurred in <15% of patients on a variety of intermittent or continuous dose regimens. Less than 1% had leukopenia below 1000 WBC/mm³. Thrombocytopenia below 50,000 platelets/mm³ was seen in <10% of patients. When given in doses of 8–12 mg/kg/day over a 21 day course, nadirs of leukocyte and platelet counts were reached by 3–4 weeks, and normal counts were regained by 6 weeks. With continuous administration at doses of 6–8 mg/kg/day, nadirs are reached in 6–8 weeks (median).
Data in the following table are based on the experience of 76 patients with ovarian cancer previously treated with a cisplatin-based combination regimen who received single-agent HEXALEN. In one study, HEXALEN, 260 mg/m²/day, was administered for 14 days of a 28 day cycle. In another study, HEXALEN, 6–8 mg/kg/day, was administered for 21 days of a 28 day cycle.

ADVERSE EXPERIENCES IN 76 PREVIOUSLY TREATED OVARIAN CANCER PATIENTS RECEIVING SINGLE-AGENT HEXALEN

Adverse Experiences	% Patients
Gastrointestinal	
Nausea and Vomiting	33
Mild to Moderate	32
Severe	1
Increased Alkaline Phosphatase	9
Neurologic	
Peripheral Sensory Neuropathy	31
Mild	22
Moderate to Severe	9
Anorexia and Fatigue	1
Seizures	1
Hematologic	
Leukopenia	5
WBC 2000–2999/mm³	4
WBC <2000/mm³	1
Thrombocytopenia	9
Platelets 75,000–99,000/mm³	6
Platelets <75,000/mm³	3
Anemia	33
Mild	20
Moderate to Severe	13

Continued on next page

Hexalen—Cont.

Renal	
Serum Creatinine 1.6–3.75 mg/dl	7
BUN	9
25–40 mg%	5
41–60 mg%	3
>60 mg%	1

Additional adverse reaction information is available from 13 single-agent altretamine studies (total of 1014 patients) conducted under the auspices of the National Cancer Institute. The treated patients had a variety of tumors and many were heavily pretreated with other chemotherapies; most of these trials utilized high, continuous daily doses of altretamine (6–12 mg/kg/day). In general, adverse reaction experiences were similar in the two trials described above. Additional toxicities, not reported in the above table, included hepatic toxicity, skin rash, pruritus and alopecia, each occurring in <1% of patients.

OVERDOSAGE

No case of acute overdosage in humans has been described. The oral LD50 dose in rats was 1050 mg/kg and 437 mg/kg in mice.

DOSAGE AND ADMINISTRATION

HEXALEN is administered orally. Doses are calculated on the basis of body surface area.

HEXALEN may be administered either for 14 or 21 consecutive days in a 28 day cycle at a dose of 260 mg/m^2/day. The total daily dose should be given as 4 divided oral doses after meals and at bedtime. There is no pharmacokinetic information supporting this dosing regimen and the effect of food on HEXALEN bioavailability or pharmacokinetics has not been evaluated.

HEXALEN should be temporarily discontinued (for 14 days or longer) and subsequently restarted at 200 mg/m^2/day for any of the following situations:

1) Gastrointestinal intolerance unresponsive to symptomatic measures;
2) White blood count <2000/mm^3 or granulocyte count <1000/mm^3;
3) Platelet count <75,000/mm^3;
4) Progressive neurotoxicity.

If neurologic symptoms fail to stabilize on the reduced dose schedule, HEXALEN should be discontinued indefinitely.

Procedures for proper handling and disposal of anticancer drugs should be considered. Several guidelines on this subject have been published (2–8). There is no general agreement that all of the procedures recommended in the guidelines are necessary or appropriate.

HOW SUPPLIED

HEXALEN (altretamine) is available in 50 mg clear, hard gelatin capsules in bottles of 100 (**NDC** 58178-001-70). The capsules are imprinted with the following inscription: USB001. Store at controlled room temperature 15°–30°C (59°–86°F).

REFERENCES

1. Wiernik PH, et al. Hexamethylmelamine and Low or Moderate Dose Cisplatin With or Without Pyridoxine for Treatment of Advanced Ovarian Carcinoma: A Study of the Eastern Cooperative Oncology Group. *Cancer Investigation* 10(1): 1–9, 1992.
2. Recommendations for the Safe Handling of Parenteral Antineoplastic Drugs. NIH Publication No. 83-2621. For sale by the Superintendent of Documents, U.S. Government Printing Office, Washington, D.C. 20402.
3. AMA Council Report. Guidelines for Handling Parenteral Antineoplastics. *Journal of the American Medical Association* March 15, 1985.
4. National Study Commission on Cytotoxic Exposure—Recommendation for Handling Cytotoxic Agents. Available from Louis P. Jeffrey, Sc.D., Director of Pharmacy Services, Rhode Island Hospital, 593 Eddy Street, Providence, Rhode Island 02902.
5. Clinical Oncological Society of Australia: Guidelines and Recommendations for Safe Handling of Antineoplastic Agents. *Medical Journal of Australia* 1:426–428, 1983.
6. Jones, RB, et al. Safe Handling of Chemotherapeutic Agents: A Report from the Mount Sinai Medical Center. *CA —A Cancer Journal for Clinicians* Sept/Oct, 258–263, 1983.
7. American Society of Hospital Pharmacists Technical Assistance Bulletin on Handling Cytotoxic Drugs in Hospitals. *American Journal of Hospital Pharmacy* 42:131–137, 1985.
8. OSHA Work Practice Guidelines for Personnel Dealing with Cytotoxic (Antineoplastic) Drugs. *American Journal of Hospital Pharmacy* 43:1193–1204, 1986.

Manufactured by:
Applied Analytical Industries, Inc.
Wilmington, NC 28405
or
Heumann Pharma GmbH
90478 Nürnberg
Germany
Distributed By: **U.S. Bioscience**
West Conshohocken, PA 19428
1-800-USBIOSC
(1-800-872-4672)
Revision Date 7/98 **PE**

Shown in Product Identification Guide, page 341

NEUTREXIN® ℞

[n(y)ü-trex 'in]

(trimetrexate glucuronate for injection)

WARNINGS

NEUTREXIN (TRIMETREXATE GLUCURONATE FOR INJECTION) MUST BE USED WITH CONCURRENT LEUCOVORIN (LEUCOVORIN PROTECTION) TO AVOID POTENTIALLY SERIOUS OR LIFE-THREATENING TOXICITIES (SEE PRECAUTIONSAND DOSAGE AND ADMINISTRATION).

DESCRIPTION

Neutrexin is the brand name for trimetrexate glucuronate. Trimetrexate, a 2,4-diaminoquinazoline, non-classical folate antagonist, is a synthetic inhibitor of the enzyme dihydrofolate reductase (DHFR). Neutrexin is available as a sterile lyophilized powder in multi-dose vials, containing trimetrexate glucuronate equivalent to either 200 mg or 25 mg of trimetrexate without any preservatives or excipients. The powder is reconstituted prior to intravenous infusion (see **DOSAGE AND ADMINISTRATION, RECONSTITUTION AND DILUTION**).

Trimetrexate glucuronate is chemically known as 2,4-diamino-5-methyl-6-[(3,4,5-trimethoxyanilino)methyl] quinazoline mono-D-glucuronate, and has the following structure:

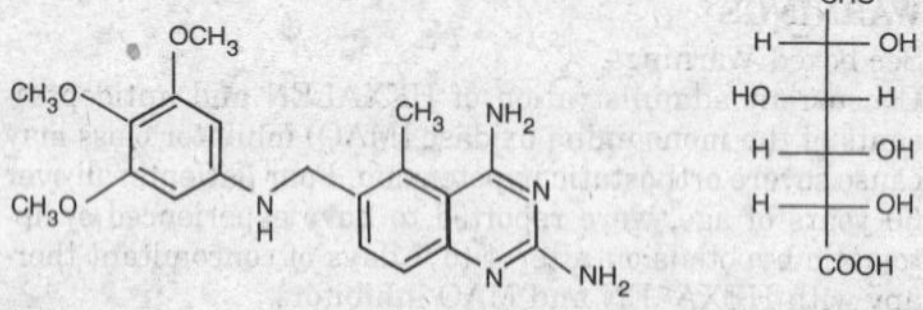

The empirical formula for trimetrexate glucuronate is $C_{19}H_{23}N_5O_3 \cdot C_6H_{10}O_7$ with a molecular weight of 563.56. The active ingredient, trimetrexate free base, has an empirical formula of $C_{19}H_{23}N_5O_3$ with a molecular weight of 369.42. Trimetrexate glucuronate for injection is a pale greenish-yellow powder or cake. Trimetrexate glucuronate is soluble in water (>50 mg/mL), whereas trimetrexate free base is practically insoluble in water (<0.1 mg/mL). The pKa of trimetrexate free base in 50% methanol/water is 8.0. The logarithm$_{10}$ of the partition coefficient of trimetrexate free base between octanol and water is 1.63.

CLINICAL PHARMACOLOGY

Mechanism of Action

In vitro studies have shown that trimetrexate is a competitive inhibitor of dihydrofolate reductase (DHFR) from bacterial, protozoan, and mammalian sources. DHFR catalyzes the reduction of intracellular dihydrofolate to the active coenzyme tetrahydrofolate. Inhibition of DHFR results in the depletion of this coenzyme, leading directly to interference with thymidylate biosynthesis, as well as inhibition of folate-dependent formyltransferases, and indirectly to inhibition of purine biosynthesis. The end result is disruption of DNA, RNA, and protein synthesis, with consequent cell death.

Leucovorin (folinic acid) is readily transported into mammalian cells by an active, carrier-mediated process and can be assimilated into cellular folate pools following its metabolism. *In vitro* studies have shown that leucovorin provides a source of reduced folates necessary for normal cellular biosynthetic processes. Because the *Pneumocystis carinii* organism lacks the reduced folate carrier-mediated transport system, leucovorin is prevented from entering the organism. Therefore, at concentrations achieved with therapeutic doses of trimetrexate plus leucovorin, the selective transport of trimetrexate, but not leucovorin, into the *Pneumocystis carinii* organism allows the concurrent administration of leucovorin to protect normal host cells from the cytotoxicity of trimetrexate without inhibiting the antifolate's inhibition of *Pneumocystis carinii.* It is not known if considerably higher doses of leucovorin would affect trimetrexate's effect on *Pneumocystis carinii.*

Microbiology

Trimetrexate inhibits, in a dose-related manner, *in vitro* growth of the trophozoite stage of rat *Pneumocystis carinii* cultured on human embryonic lung fibroblast cells. Trimetrexate concentrations between 3 and 54.1 µM were shown to inhibit the growth of trophozoites. Leucovorin alone at a concentration of 10 µM did not alter either the growth of the trophozoites or the anti-pneumocystis activity of trimetrexate. Resistance to trimetrexate's antimicrobial activity against *Pneumocystis carinii* has not been studied.

Pharmacokinetics

Trimetrexate pharmacokinetics were assessed in six patients with acquired immunodeficiency syndrome (AIDS) who had *Pneumocystis carinii* pneumonia (4 patients) or toxoplasmosis (2 patients). Trimetrexate was administered intravenously as a bolus injection at a dose of 30 mg/m^2/day along with leucovorin 20 mg/m^2 every 6 hours for 21 days. Trimetrexate clearance (mean ± SD) was 38 ± 15 mL/min/m^2 and volume of distribution at steady state (Vd_{ss}) was 20 ± 8 L/m^2. The plasma concentration time profile declined in a biphasic manner over 24 hours with a terminal half-life of 11 ± 4 hours.

The pharmacokinetics of trimetrexate without the concomitant administration of leucovorin have been evaluated in cancer patients with advanced solid tumors using various dosage regimens. The decline in plasma concentrations over time has been described by either biexponential or triexponential equations. Following the single-dose administration of 10 to 130 mg/m^2 to 37 patients, plasma concentrations were obtained for 72 hours. Nine plasma concentration time profiles were described as biexponential. The alpha phase half-life was 57 ± 28 minutes, followed by a terminal phase with a half-life of 16 ± 3 hours. The plasma concentrations in the remaining patients exhibited a triphasic decline with half-lives of 8.6 ± 6.5 minutes, 2.4 ± 1.3 hours, and 17.8 ± 8.2 hours.

Trimetrexate clearance in cancer patients has been reported as 53 ± 41 mL/min (14 patients) and 32 ± 18 mL/min/m^2 (23 patients) following single-dose administration. After a five-day infusion of trimetrexate to 16 patients, plasma clearance was 30 ± 8 mL/min/m^2.

Renal clearance of trimetrexate in cancer patients has varied from about 4 ± 2 mL/min/m^2 to 10 ± 6 mL/min/m^2. Ten to 30% of the administered dose is excreted unchanged in the urine. Considering the free fraction of trimetrexate, active tubular secretion may possibly contribute to the renal clearance of trimetrexate. Renal clearance has been associated with urine flow, suggesting the possibility of tubular reabsorption as well.

The Vd_{ss} of trimetrexate in cancer patients after single-dose administration and for whom plasma concentrations were obtained for 72 hours was 36.9 ± 17.6 L/m^2 (n=23) and 0.62 ± 0.24 L/kg (n=14). Following a constant infusion of trimetrexate for five days, Vd_{ss} was 32.8 ± 16.6 L/m^2. The volume of the central compartment has been estimated as 0.17 ± 0.08 L/kg and 4.0 ± 2.9 L/m^2.

There have been inconsistencies in the reporting of trimetrexate protein binding. The *in vitro* plasma protein binding of trimetrexate using ultrafiltration is approximately 95% over the concentration range of 18.75 to 1000 ng/mL. There is a suggestion of capacity limited binding (saturable binding) at concentrations greater than about 1000 ng/mL, with free fraction progressively increasing to about 9.3% as concentration is increased to 15 µg/mL. Other reports have declared trimetrexate to be greater than 98% bound at concentrations of 0.1 to 10 µg/mL; however, specific free fractions were not stated. The free fraction of trimetrexate also has been reported to be about 15 to 16% at a concentration of 60 ng/mL, increasing to about 20% at a trimetrexate concentration of 6 µg/mL.

Trimetrexate metabolism in man has not been characterized. Preclinical data strongly suggest that the major metabolic pathway is oxidative O-demethylation, followed by conjugation to either glucuronide or the sulfate. N-demethylation and oxidation is a related minor pathway. Preliminary findings in humans indicate the presence of a glucuronide conjugate with DHFR inhibition and a demethylated metabolite in urine.

The presence of metabolite(s) in human plasma following the administration of trimetrexate is suggested by the differences seen in trimetrexate plasma concentrations when measured by HPLC and a nonspecific DHFR inhibition assay. The profiles are similar initially, but diverge with time; concentrations determined by DHFR being higher than those determined by HPLC. This suggests the presence of one or more metabolites with DHFR inhibition activity. After intravenous administration of trimetrexate to humans, urinary recovery averaged about 40%, using a DHFR assay, in comparison to 10% urinary recovery as determined by HPLC, suggesting the presence of one or more metabolites that retain inhibitory activity against DHFR. Fecal recovery of trimetrexate over 48 hours after intravenous administration ranged from 0.09 to 7.6% of the dose as determined by DHFR inhibition and 0.02 to 5.2% of the dose as determined by HPLC.

The pharmacokinetics of trimetrexate have not been determined in patients with renal insufficiency or hepatic dysfunction.

INDICATIONS AND USAGE

Neutrexin (trimetrexate glucuronate for injection) with concurrent leucovorin administration (leucovorin protection) is indicated as an alternative therapy for the treatment of moderate-to-severe *Pneumocystis carinii* pneumonia (PCP) in immunocompromised patients, including patients with the acquired immunodeficiency syndrome (AIDS), who are intolerant of, or are refractory to, trimethoprim-sulfamethoxazole therapy or for whom trimethoprim-sulfamethoxazole is contraindicated.

This indication is based on the results of a randomized, controlled double-blind trial comparing Neutrexin with concurrent leucovorin protection (TMTX/LV) to trimethoprim-sulfamethoxazole (TMP/SMX) in patients with moderate-to-severe *Pneumocystis carinii* pneumonia, as well as results of a Treatment IND. These studies are summarized below:

Neutrexin Comparative Study with TMP/SMX: This double-blind, randomized trial initiated by the AIDS Clinical Trials Group (ACTG) in 1988 was designed to compare the safety and efficacy of TMTX/LV to that of TMP/SMX for the treatment of histologically confirmed, moderate-to-severe PCP, defined as (A-a) baseline gradient >30 mmHg, in patients with AIDS.

Of the 220 patients with histologically confirmed PCP, 109 were randomized to receive TMTX/LV and 111 to TMP/SMX. Study patients randomized to TMTX/LV treatment were to receive 45 mg/m^2 of TMTX daily for 21 days plus 20 mg/m^2 of LV every 6 hours for 24 days. Those randomized to TMP/SMX were to receive 5 mg/kg TMP plus 25 mg/kg SMX four times daily for 21 days.

Response to therapy, defined as alive and off ventilatory support at completion of therapy, with no change in antipneumocystis therapy, or addition of supraphysiologic doses of steroids, occurred in fifty percent of patients in each treatment group.

The observed mortality in the TMTX/LV treatment group was approximately twice that in the TMP/SMX treatment group (95% CI: 0.99–4.11). Thirty of 109 (27%) patients treated with TMTX/LV and 18 of 111 (16%) patients receiving TMP/SMX died during the 21-day treatment course or 4-week follow-up period. Twenty-seven of 30 deaths in the TMTX/LV arm were attributed to PCP; all 18 deaths in the TMP/SMX arm were attributed to PCP.

A significantly smaller proportion of patients who received TMTX/LV compared to TMP/SMX failed therapy due to toxicity (10% vs. 25%), and a significantly greater proportion of patients failed due to lack of efficacy (40% vs. 24%). Six patients (12%) who responded to TMTX/LV relapsed during the one-month follow-up period; no patient responding to TMP/SMX relapsed during this period. Information is not available as to whether these patients received prophylaxis therapy for PCP.

Treatment IND: The FDA granted a Treatment IND for Neutrexin with leucovorin protection in February 1988 to make Neutrexin therapy available to HIV-infected patients with histologically confirmed PCP who had disease refractory to or who are intolerant of TMP/SMX and/or intravenous pentamidine.

Over 500 physicians in the United States participated in the Treatment IND. Of the first 753 patients enrolled, 577 were evaluable for efficacy. Of these, 227 patients were intolerant of both TMP/SMX and pentamidine (IST—patients intolerant of both standard therapies), 146 were intolerant of one therapy and refractory to the other (RIST-patients refractory to one therapy and intolerant of the other) and 204 were refractory to both therapies (RST-refractory to both standard therapies). This was a very ill patient population; 38% required ventilatory support at entry (Table 1). These studies did not have concurrent control groups.

[See table 1 above]

The overall survival rate one month after completion of TMTX/LV as salvage therapy was 48%. Patients who had not responded to treatment with both TMP/SMX and pentamidine, of whom 63% required mechanical ventilation at entry, achieved a survival rate of 25% following treatment with TMTX/LV. Survival was 67% in patients who were intolerant to both TMP/SMX and pentamidine (Table 2).

[See table 2 above]

In the Treatment IND, 12% of the patients discontinued Neutrexin therapy (with leucovorin protection) for toxicity.

CONTRAINDICATIONS

Neutrexin (trimetrexate glucuronate for injection) is contraindicated in patients with clinically significant sensitivity to trimetrexate, leucovorin, or methotrexate.

WARNINGS

Neutrexin (trimetrexate glucuronate for injection) must be used with concurrent leucovorin to avoid potentially serious or life-threatening complications including bone marrow suppression, oral and gastrointestinal mucosal ulceration, and renal and hepatic dysfunction. Leucovorin therapy must extend for 72 hours past the last dose of Neutrexin.

Patients should be informed that failure to take the recommended dose and duration of leucovorin can lead to fatal toxicity. Patients should be closely monitored for the development of serious hematologic adverse reactions (see **PRECAUTIONS** and **DOSAGE AND ADMINISTRATION**).

Neutrexin can cause fetal harm when administered to a pregnant woman. Trimetrexate has been shown to be fetotoxic and teratogenic in rats and rabbits. Rats administered 1.5 and 2.5 mg/kg/day intravenously on gestational days 6–15 showed substantial postimplantation loss and severe inhibition of maternal weight gain. Trimetrexate administered intravenously to rats at 0.5 and 1.0 mg/kg/day on gestational days 6–15 retarded normal fetal development and was teratogenic. Rabbits administered trimetrexate intravenously at daily doses of 2.5 and 5.0 mg/kg/day on gestational days 6–18 resulted in significant maternal and fetal toxicity. In rabbits, trimetrexate at 0.1 mg/kg/day was teratogenic in the absence of significant maternal toxicity. These effects were observed using doses 1/20 to 1/2 the equivalent human therapeutic dose based on a mg/m^2 basis. Teratogenic effects included skeletal, visceral, ocular, and cardiovascular abnormalities. If Neutrexin is used during pregnancy, or if the patient becomes pregnant while taking this drug, the patient should be apprised of the potential hazard to the fetus. Women of childbearing potential should be advised to avoid becoming pregnant.

PRECAUTIONS
General

Patients receiving Neutrexin (trimetrexate glucuronate for injection) may experience severe hematologic, hepatic, renal, and gastrointestinal toxicities. Caution should be used in treating patients with impaired hematologic, renal, or hepatic function. Patients who require concomitant therapy with nephrotoxic, myelosuppressive, or hepatotoxic drugs should be treated with Neutrexin at the discretion of the physician and monitored carefully. To allow for full therapeutic doses of Neutrexin, treatment with zidovudine should be discontinued during Neutrexin therapy.

Neutrexin-associated myelosuppression, stomatitis, and gastrointestinal toxicities generally can be ameliorated by adjusting the dose of leucovorin. Mild elevations in transaminases and alkaline phosphatase have been observed with Neutrexin administration and are usually not cause for modification of Neutrexin therapy (see **DOSAGE AND ADMINISTRATION**). Seizures have been reported rarely (<1%) in AIDS patients receiving Neutrexin; however, a causal relationship has not been established. Trimetrexate is a known inhibitor of histamine metabolism. Hypersensitivity/allergic type reactions including but not limited to rash, chills/rigors, fever, diaphoresis and dyspnea, have occurred with trimetrexate primarily when it is administered as a bolus infusion or at doses higher than those recom-

Continued on next page

TABLE 1
TREATMENT IND
Baseline Characteristics

	IST (n = 227)	RIST (n = 146)	RST (n = 204)	TOTAL (n = 577)
Ventilatory Support Required n (%)	39(17)	50(34)	129(63)	218(38)
Median Days on Standard Therapy	10	12	16	14
First Episode of PCP n (%)	104(46)	103(71)	190(93)	397(69)

TABLE 2
TREATMENT IND
Survival Rate One Month After Completion of Neutrexin Therapy

	IST		RIST		RST	
All Patients	153/227	(67%)	73/146	(50%)	50/204	(25%)
Baseline Ventilatory Support	9/39	(23%)	15/50	(30%)	18/129	(14%)
No Baseline Ventilatory Support	144/188	(77%)	58/96	(60%)	32/75	(43%)

TABLE 3
NEUTREXIN COMPARATIVE TRIAL
Comparison of Adverse Events Reported for ≥1% of Patients

Adverse Events	Number and Percent (%) of Patients with Adverse Events			
	TMTX/LV (n = 109)		TMP/SMX (n = 111)	
Non-Laboratory Adverse Events:				
Fever	9	(8.3)	14	(12.6)
Rash/Pruritus	6	(5.5)	14	(12.6)
Nausea/Vomiting	5	(4.6)[a]	15	(13.5)[a]
Confusion	3	(2.8)	3	(2.7)
Fatigue	2	(1.8)	0	(0.0)
Hematologic Toxicity:				
Neutropenia (≤1000/mm^3)	33	(30.3)	37	(33.3)
Thrombocytopenia (≤75,000/mm^3)	11	(10.1)	17	(15.3)
Anemia (Hgb <8 g/dL)	8	(7.3)	10	(9.0)
Hepatotoxicity:				
Increased AST (>5 × ULN[b])	15	(13.8)	10	(9.0)
Increased ALT (>5 × ULN)	12	(11.0)	13	(11.7)
Increased Alkaline Phosphatase (>5 × ULN)	5	(4.6)	3	(2.7)
Increased Bilirubin (2.5 × ULN)	2	(1.8)	1	(0.9)
Renal:				
Increased Serum Creatinine (>3 × ULN)	1	(0.9)	2	(1.8)
Electrolyte Imbalance:				
Hyponatremia	5	(4.6)	10	(9.0)
Hypocalcemia	2	(1.8)	0	(0.0)
No. of Patients With at least one Adverse Event[c]	58	(53.2)	60	(54.1)

a Statistically significant difference between treatment groups (Chi-square: p = 0.022)
b ULN = Upper limit of normal range
c Patients could have reported more than one adverse event; therefore, the sum of adverse events exceeds the number of patients

Neutrexin—Cont.

mended for PCP, and most frequently in combination with 5FU and leucovorin. In rare cases, anaphylactoid reactions, including acute hypotension and loss of consciousness have occurred.

Neutrexin has not been evaluated clinically for the treatment of concurrent pulmonary conditions such as bacterial, viral, or fungal pneumonia or mycobacterial diseases. *In vitro* activity has been observed against *Toxoplasma gondii*, *Mycobacterium avium* complex, gram positive cocci, and gram negative rods. If clinical deterioration is observed in patients, they should be carefully evaluated for other possible causes of pulmonary disease and treated with additional agents as appropriate.

Laboratory Tests

Patients receiving Neutrexin and leucovorin protection should be seen frequently by a physician. Blood tests to assess the following parameters should be performed at least twice a week during therapy: hematology (absolute neutrophil counts [ANC], platelets), renal function (serum creatinine, BUN), and hepatic function (AST, ALT, alkaline phosphatase).

Drug Interactions

Since trimetrexate is metabolized by a P450 enzyme system, drugs that induce or inhibit this drug metabolizing enzyme system may elicit important drug-drug interactions that may alter trimetrexate plasma concentrations. Agents that might be coadministered with trimetrexate in AIDS patients for other indications that could elicit this activity include erythromycin, rifampin, rifabutin, ketoconazole, and fluconazole. *In vitro* perfusion of isolated rat liver has shown that cimetidine caused a significant reduction in trimetrexate metabolism and that acetaminophen altered the relative concentration of trimetrexate metabolites possibly by competing for sulfate metabolites. Based on an *in vitro* rat liver model, nitrogen substituted imidazole drugs (clotrimazole, ketoconazole, miconazole) were potent, non-competitive inhibitors of trimetrexate metabolism. Patients medicated with these drugs and trimetrexate should be carefully monitored.

Carcinogenesis, Mutagenesis, Impairment of Fertility

Carcinogenesis: Long term studies in animals to evaluate the carcinogenic potential of trimetrexate have not been performed.

Mutagenesis: Trimetrexate was not mutagenic when tested using the standard Ames *Salmonella* mutagenicity assay with and without metabolic activation. Trimetrexate did not induce mutations in Chinese hamster lung cells or sister-chromatid exchange in Chinese hamster ovary cells. Trimetrexate did induce an increase in the chromosomal aberration frequency of cultured Chinese hamster lung cells; however, trimetrexate showed no clastogenic activity in a mouse micronucleus assay.

Impairment of fertility: No studies have been conducted to evaluate the potential of trimetrexate to impair fertility. However, during standard toxicity studies conducted in mice and rats, degeneration of the testes and spermatocytes including the arrest of spermatogenesis was observed.

Pregnancy, Teratogenic Effects- See WARNINGS.

Pregnancy Category D

Nursing Mothers

It is not known if trimetrexate is excreted in human milk. Because many drugs are excreted in human milk and because of the potential for serious adverse reactions in nursing infants from trimetrexate, it is recommended that breast feeding be discontinued if the mother is treated with Neutrexin.

Pediatric Use

The safety and effectiveness of Neutrexin for the treatment of histologically confirmed PCP has not been established for patients under 18 years of age. Two children, ages 15 months and 9 months, were treated with trimetrexate and leucovorin using a dose of 45 mg/m² of trimetrexate per day for 21 days and 20 mg/m² of leucovorin every 6 hours for 24 days. There were no serious or unexpected adverse effects.

ADVERSE REACTIONS

Because many patients who participated in clinical trials of Neutrexin (trimetrexate glucuronate for injection) had complications of advanced HIV disease, it is difficult to distinguish adverse events caused by Neutrexin from those resulting from underlying medical conditions.

Table 3 lists the adverse events that occurred in ≥1% of the patients who participated in the Comparative Study of Neutrexin plus leucovorin versus TMP/SMX.

[See table 3 on previous page]

Laboratory toxicities were generally manageable with dose modification of trimetrexate/leucovorin (see DOSAGE AND ADMINISTRATION).

Table 4 lists the adverse events resulting in discontinuation of study therapy in the Neutrexin Comparative Study with TMP/SMX. Twenty-nine percent of the patients on the TMP/SMX arm discontinued therapy due to adverse events compared to 10% of the patients treated with TMTX/LV (p <0.001).

TABLE 4
NEUTREXIN COMPARATIVE TRIAL
Adverse Events Resulting in Discontinuation of Therapy

Adverse Events	Number and Percent (%) of Patients Discontinued for Adverse Events[b]	
	TMTX/LV (n = 109)	TMP/SMX (n = 111)
Non-Laboratory Adverse Events:		
Rash/Pruritus	3 (2.8)	5 (4.5)
Fever	2 (1.8)	4 (3.6)
Nausea/Vomiting	1 (0.9)	8 (7.2)
Neurologic Toxicity	1 (0.9)[c]	2 (1.8)
Hematologic Toxicity:		
Neutropenia (≤1000/mm³)	4 (3.7)	6 (5.4)
Thrombocytopenia (≤75,000/mm³)	0 (0.0)	4 (3.6)
Anemia (Hgb <8 g/dL)	0 (0.0)	4 (3.6)
Hepatotoxicity:		
Increased AST (>5 × ULN[a])	3 (2.8)	9 (8.1)
Increased ALT (>5 × ULN)	1 (0.9)	4 (3.6)
Increased Alkaline Phosphatase (>5 × ULN)	0 (0.0)	1 (0.9)
Electrolyte Imbalance:		
Hyponatremia	0 (0.0)	3 (2.7)
No. of Patients Discontinuing Therapy Due to an Adverse Event [b]	11 (10.1)[d]	32 (28.8)[d]

a ULN = Upper limit of normal range
b Patients could discontinue therapy due to more than one toxicity; therefore the sum exceeds number of patients who discontinued due to toxicity
c Patient discontinued TMTX/LV due to seizure, though causal relationship could not be established
d Statistically significant difference between treatment groups (Chi-square: p < 0.001)

TABLE 5
DOSE MODIFICATIONS FOR HEMATOLOGIC TOXICITY

Toxicity Grade	Neutrophils (Polys and Bands)	Platelets	Recommended Dosages of	
			Neutrexin	Leucovorin
1	>1000/mm³	>75,000/mm³	45 mg/m² once daily	20 mg/m² every 6 hours
2	750–1000/mm³	50,000–75,000/mm³	45 mg/m² once daily	40 mg/m² every 6 hours
3	500–749/mm³	25,000–49,999/mm³	22 mg/m² once daily	40 mg/m² every 6 hours
4	<500/mm³	<25,000/mm³	Day 1–9 Discontinue Day 10–21 Interrupt up to 96 hours[a]	40 mg/m² every 6 hours

a If Grade 4 hematologic toxicity occurs prior to Day 10, Neutrexin should be discontinued. Leucovorin (40 mg/m², q6h) should be administered for an additional 72 hours. If Grade 4 hematologic toxicity occurs at Day 10 or later, Neutrexin may be held up to 96 hours to allow counts to recover. If counts recover to Grade 3 within 96 hours, Neutrexin should be administered at a dose of 22 mg/m² and leucovorin maintained at 40 mg/m², q6h. When counts recover to Grade 2 toxicity, Neutrexin dose may be increased to 45 mg/m², but the leucovorin dose should be maintained at 40 mg/m² for the duration of treatment. If counts do not improve to ≤ Grade 3 toxicity within 96 hours, Neutrexin should be discontinued. Leucovorin at a dose of 40 mg/m², q6h should be administered for 72 hours following the last dose of Neutrexin.

[See table 4 above]
Hematologic toxicity was the principal dose-limiting side effect.

OVERDOSAGE

Neutrexin (trimetrexate glucuronate for injection) administered without concurrent leucovorin can cause lethal complications. There has been no extensive experience in humans receiving single intravenous doses of trimetrexate greater than 90 mg/m²/day with concurrent leucovorin. The toxicities seen at this dose were primarily hematologic. In the event of overdose, Neutrexin should be stopped and leucovorin should be administered at a dose of 40 mg/m² every 6 hours for 3 days. The LD$_{50}$ of intravenous trimetrexate in mice is 62 mg/kg (186 mg/m²).

DOSAGE AND ADMINISTRATION

Caution: Neutrexin (trimetrexate glucuronate for injection) must be administered with concurrent leucovorin (leucovorin protection) to avoid potentially serious or life-threatening toxicities. Leucovorin therapy must extend for 72 hours past the last dose of Neutrexin.

Neutrexin (trimetrexate glucuronate for injection) is administered at a dose of 45 mg/m² once daily by intravenous infusion over 60 minutes. Leucovorin must be administered daily during treatment with Neutrexin and for 72 hours past the last dose of Neutrexin. Leucovorin may be administered intravenously at a dose of 20 mg/m² over 5 to 10 minutes every 6 hours for a total daily dose of 80 mg/m², or orally as 4 doses of 20 mg/m² spaced equally throughout the day. The oral dose should be rounded up to the next higher 25 mg increment. The recommended course of therapy is 21 days of Neutrexin and 24 days of leucovorin.

Neutrexin and leucovorin may alternatively be dosed on a mg/kg basis, depending on the patients body weight, using the conversion factors shown in the table below:

Body Weight (kg)	Neutrexin Dose (mg/kg/day)	Leucovorin Dose (mg/kg/qid)
<50	1.5	0.6
50-80	1.2	0.5
>80	1.0	0.5

Dosage Modifications

Hematologic toxicity: Neutrexin (trimetrexate glucuronate for injection) and leucovorin doses should be modified based on the worst hematologic toxicity according to the following table. If leucovorin is given orally, doses should be rounded up to the next higher 25 mg increment.
[See table 5 above]

Hepatic toxicity: Transient elevation of transaminases and alkaline phosphatase have been observed in patients treated with Neutrexin. Interruption of treatment is advisable if transaminase level or alkaline phosphatase levels increase to >5 times the upper limit of normal range.

Renal toxicity: Interruption of Neutrexin is advisable if serum creatinine levels increase to >2.5 mg/dL and the elevation is considered to be secondary to Neutrexin.

Other toxicities: Interruption of treatment is advisable in patients who experience severe mucosal toxicity that interferes with oral intake. Treatment should be discontinued for fever (oral temperature ≥ 105°F/40.5°C) that cannot be controlled with antipyretics.

Leucovorin therapy must extend for 72 hours past the last dose of Neutrexin.

RECONSTITUTION AND DILUTION

Each vial of Neutrexin (trimetrexate glucuronate for injection) should be reconstituted in accordance with labeled instructions with either 5% Dextrose Injection, USP, or Sterile Water for Injection, USP, to yield a concentration of 12.5 mg of trimetrexate per mL (complete dissolution should occur within 30 seconds). The reconstituted product will appear as a pale greenish-yellow solution and must be inspected visually prior to dilution. **Do not use if cloudiness or precipitate is observed.** Neutrexin should not be reconstituted with solutions containing either chloride ion or leucovorin, since precipitation occurs instantly.

After reconstitution, the solution is stable for 2 days at room temperature, 5 days at refrigeration (2–8°C) or 8 days frozen (−10 to −20°C).

Reconstituted solution should be further diluted with 5% Dextrose Injection, USP, to yield a final concentration of 0.25 to 2 mg of trimetrexate per mL. The diluted solution should be administered by intravenous infusion over 60 minutes. Neutrexin should not be mixed with solutions containing either chloride ion or leucovorin, since precipitation occurs instantly. It is stable under refrigeration or at room temperature for up to 24 hours. Do not freeze. Discard any unused portion after 24 hours. The intravenous line must be flushed thoroughly with at least 10 mL of 5% Dextrose Injection, USP, before and after administering Neutrexin. Leucovorin protection may be administered prior to or following Neutrexin. In either case, the intravenous line must be flushed thoroughly with at least 10 mL of 5% Dextrose Injection, USP. Leucovorin calcium for injection should be diluted according to the instructions in the leucovorin package insert, and administered over 5 to 10 minutes every 6 hours.

Caution: Parenteral products should be inspected visually for particulate matter and discoloration prior to administration, whenever solution and container permit. Neutrexin forms a precipitate instantly upon contact with chloride ion or leucovorin, therefore it should not be added to solutions containing sodium chloride or other anions. Neutrexin and leucovorin solutions must be administered separately. Intravenous lines should be flushed with at least 10 mL of 5% Dextrose Injection, USP, between Neutrexin and leucovorin infusions.

HANDLING AND DISPOSAL

If Neutrexin (trimetrexate glucuronate for injection) contacts the skin or mucosa, immediately wash thoroughly with soap and water. Procedures for proper disposal of cytotoxic drugs should be considered. Several guidelines on this subject have been published (1–5).

HOW SUPPLIED

Neutrexin (trimetrexate glucuronate for injection) is supplied as a sterile lyophilized powder in either 5 mL or 30 mL multi-dose vials. Each 5 mL vial contains trimetrexate glucuronate equivalent to 25 mg of trimetrexate. Each 30 mL vial contains trimetrexate glucuronate equivalent to 200 mg trimetrexate. The 5 mL vials are packaged and available in two market presentations as listed below:

10 Pack—10 vials in a white chip-board carton (NDC 58178-020-10)

50 Pack—2 trays of 25 vials per shrink-wrapped tray (NDC 58178-020-50)

The 30 mL vials are packaged and available as listed below:

Single Pack—1 vial (NDC 58178-021-01)

Store at controlled room temperature 15° to 30°C (59° to 86°F). **Protect from exposure to light.**

U.S. Patents 4,376,858; 4,694,007

REFERENCES

1. AMA Council Report. Guidelines for Handling Parenteral Antineoplastics. *Journal of the American Medical Association* March 15, 1985.
2. Clinical Oncological Society of Australia: Guidelines and Recommendations for Safe Handling of Antineoplastic Agents. *Medical Journal of Australia* 1:426–428, 1983.
3. Jones RB, et al. Safe Handling of Chemotherapeutic Agents: A Report from the Mount Sinai Medical Center. *CA–A Cancer Journal for Clinicians* Sept/Oct, 258–263, 1983.
4. American Society of Hospital Pharmacists Technical Assistance Bulletin on Handling Cytotoxic Drugs in Hospitals. *American Journal of Hospital Pharmacy* 42: 131–137, 1985.
5. OSHA Work Practice Guidelines for Personnel Dealing with Cytotoxic (Antineoplastic) Drugs. *American Journal of Hospital Pharmacy* 43: 1193–1204, 1986.

Distributed by:
U.S. Bioscience, Inc.
West Conshohocken, PA 19428

© 1998 U.S. Bioscience, Inc.   1-800-USBIOSC
Revision Date 8/98   (1-800-872-4672)
Shown in Product Identification Guide, page 341

U.S. Pharmaceutical Corporation
2401-C MELLON COURT
DECATUR, GA 30035

Direct Inquiries to:
Peter J. Krebs, Ph.D.
CEO Management Unit
(800) 330-3040,
or
Raymond F. Meyer, R.Ph.,
Marketing Director, (SE)
(800) 330-3040
or
Clayton W. Bishop
Director of Sales Development (SW)
(512) 847-3357

HEMOCYTE™ Tablets   OTC
(ferrous fumarate 324 mg.)

HOW SUPPLIED

Boxes of 100 child-proof tablets NDC 52747-307-70
Boxes of 30 child-proof tablets NDC 52747-307-30

HEMOCYTE PLUS™ Tabules   ℞
Iron-Vitamin-Mineral Complex

DESCRIPTION

Each tabule contains:

Ferrous Fumarate (anhydrous)	324 mg.
[Equivalent to about 106 mg. of Elemental Iron]	
Sodium Ascorbate (Vit. C)	200 mg.
Vit. B-1—Thiamine Mononitrate	10 mg.
Vit. B-2—Riboflavin	6 mg.
Vit. B-6—Pyridoxine HCl	5 mg.
Vit. B-12—Cyanocobalamin Concentrate	5mcg.
Folic Acid	1 mg.
Niacinamide	30 mg.
Calcium Pantothenate	10 mg.
Zinc (as Zinc Sulfate)	18.2 mg.
Magnesium (as Magnesium Sulfate)	6.9 mg.
Manganese (as Manganese Sulfate)	1.3 mg.
Copper (as Copper Sulfate)	0.8 mg.

HOW SUPPLIED

Boxes of 100 child-proof tablets NDC 52747-308-70
Boxes of 30 child-proof tablets NDC 52747-308-30

HEMOCYTE-F ELIXIR   ℞
Iron, Folic Acid, and Vitamin B12 Complex

DESCRIPTION

Each Teaspoon Contains:

Elemental Iron	100 mg
(As a polysaccharide-iron complex)	
Folic Acid	1 mg
Vitamin B12	25 mcg
Alcohol	10%
(Sugar Free)	

HOW SUPPLIED

Bottles of 16 oz.

HEMOCYTE–F TABLETS   ℞

DESCRIPTION

Each tablet contains:

Ferrous Fumarate (anhydrous)	324 mg.
Folic Acid	1 mg.

HOW SUPPLIED

Boxes of 100 child proof tablets NDC 52747-306-70
Boxes of 30 child proof tablets NDC 52747-306-30

MAGSAL™ TABLETS   ℞

DESCRIPTION

Each tablet contains:

Magnesium Salicylate	600 mg.
Phenyltoloxamine Dihydrogen Citrate	25 mg.

HOW SUPPLIED

Bottles of 100 NDC 52747-321-60

MEDIGESIC® Capsules   ℞

DESCRIPTION

Each capsule or tablet contains:

Butalbital*	50 mg
*WARNING: May be habit forming.	
Acetaminophen	325 mg
Caffeine	40 mg

HOW SUPPLIED

Capsules: Bottles of 100 NDC 52747-600-60

MEDIPLEX ULTRA   OTC
(Vitamin-Mineral Complex)

DESCRIPTION

Each tabule contains:

Vitamin E - dl-alpha Tocopheryl Acetate	100 I.U.
Vitamin C-Ascorbic Acid	300 mg.
Vitamin B12 - Cyanocabalmin Concentrate	25 mcg
Vitamin B1 - Thiamine	25 mg.
Niacinamide	100 mg.
Folic Acid	0.4 mg.
Vitamin B6 - Pyridoxine	10 mg.
Vitamin B2 - Riboflavin	10 mg.
Calcium Pantothenate	25 mg.
Zinc (as Zinc Sulfate)	18 mg.
Magnesium (as Magnesium Sulfate)	7 mg.
Manganese (as Manganese Sulfate)	1.3 mg.
Copper (as Cupric Sulfate)	0.8 mg.

HOW SUPPLIED

Bottles of 100 NDC 52747-305-70

NOREL PLUS   ℞
Decongestant–Analgesic–Antihistaminic

DESCRIPTION

Each yellow and white capsule for oral administration contains:

Acetaminophen	325 mg
Phenyltoloxamine Dihydrogen Citrate	25 mg
Phenylpropanolamine Hydrochloride	25 mg
Chlorpheniramine Maleate	4 mg

HOW SUPPLIED

Bottles of 100 NDC 52747-128-60

Unimed Pharmaceuticals, Inc.
2150 E. LAKE COOK ROAD
BUFFALO GROVE, IL 60089-1862

Direct Inquiries to:
(847) 541-2525

ANADROL®-50   Ⅲ ℞
[ană-drŏl]
(oxymetholone)
50 mg Tablets

DESCRIPTION

ANADROL (oxymetholone) tablets for oral administration each contain 50 mg of the steroid oxymetholone, a potent anabolic and androgenic drug.

The chemical name for oxymetholone is 17β-hydroxy-2-(hydroxymethylene)-17-methyl-5α-androstan-3-one. The structural formula is:

Inactive Ingredients—   lactose
                               magnesium stearate
                               povidone
                               starch

CLINICAL PHARMACOLOGY

Anabolic steroids are synthetic derivatives of testosterone. Nitrogen balance is improved with anabolic agents but only

Continued on next page

Anadrol-50—Cont.

when there is sufficient intake of calories and protein. Whether this positive nitrogen balance is of primary benefit in the utilization of protein-building dietary substances has not been established. Oxymetholone enhances the production and urinary excretion of erythropoietin in patients with anemias due to bone marrow failure and often stimulates erythropoiesis in anemias due to deficient red cell production.

Certain clinical effects and adverse reactions demonstrate the androgenic properties of this class of drugs. Complete dissociation of anabolic and androgenic effects has not been achieved. The actions of anabolic steroids are therefore similar to those of male sex hormones with the possibility of causing serious disturbances of growth and sexual development if given to young children. They suppress the gonadotropic functions of the pituitary and may exert a direct effect upon the testes.

INDICATIONS AND USAGE

ANADROL-50 is indicated in the treatment of anemias caused by deficient red cell production. Acquired aplastic anemia, congenital aplastic anemia, myelofibrosis and the hypoplastic anemias due to the administration of myelotoxic drugs often respond. ANADROL-50 should not replace other supportive measures such as transfusion, correction of iron, folic acid, vitamin B_{12} or pyridoxine deficiency, antibacterial therapy and the appropriate use of corticosteroids.

CONTRAINDICATIONS

1. Carcinoma of the prostate or breast in male patients.
2. Carcinoma of the breast in females with hypercalcemia; androgenic anabolic steroids may stimulate osteolytic resorption of bones.
3. Oxymetholone can cause fetal harm when administered to pregnant women. It is contraindicated in women who are or may become pregnant. If the patient becomes pregnant while taking the drug, she should be apprised of the potential hazard to the fetus.
4. Nephrosis or the nephrotic phase of nephritis.
5. Hypersensitivity to the drug.
6. Severe hepatic dysfunction.

WARNINGS

The following conditions have been reported in patients receiving androgenic anabolic steroids as a general class of drugs:

Peliosis hepatis, a condition in which liver and sometimes splenic tissue is replaced with blood-filled cysts, has been reported in patients receiving androgenic anabolic steroid therapy. These cysts are sometimes present with minimal hepatic dysfunction, but at other times they have been associated with liver failure. They are often not recognized until life-threatening liver failure or intra-abdominal hemorrhage develops. Withdrawal of drug usually results in complete disappearance of lesions.

Liver cell tumors are also reported. Most often these tumors are benign and androgen-dependent, but fatal malignant tumors have been reported. Withdrawal of drug often results in regression or cessation of progression of the tumor. However, hepatic tumors associated with androgens or anabolic steroids are much more vascular than other hepatic tumors and may be silent until life-threatening intra-abdominal hemorrhage develops.

Blood lipid changes that are known to be associated with increased risk of atherosclerosis are seen in patients treated with androgens and anabolic steroids. These changes include decreased high density lipoprotein and sometimes increased low density lipoprotein. The changes may be very marked and could have a serious impact on the risk of atherosclerosis and coronary artery disease.

Cholestatic hepatitis and jaundice occur with 17-alpha-alkylated androgens at relatively low doses. Clinical jaundice may be painless, with or without pruritus. It may also be associated with acute hepatic enlargement and right upper-quadrant pain, which has been mistaken for acute (surgical) obstruction of the bile duct. Drug-induced jaundice is usually reversible when the medication is discontinued. Continued therapy has been associated with hepatic coma and death. Because of the hepatoxicity associated with oxymetholone administration, periodic liver function tests are recommended.

In patients with breast cancer, anabolic steroid therapy may cause hypercalcemia by stimulating osteolysis. In this case, the drug should be discontinued.

Edema with or without congestive heart failure may be a serious complication in patients with pre-existing cardiac, renal or hepatic disease. Concomitant administration with adrenal steroids or ACTH may add to the edema. This is generally controllable with appropriate diuretic and/or digitalis therapy.

Geriatric male patients treated with androgenic anabolic steroids may be at an increased risk for the development of prostate hypertrophy and prostatic carcinoma.

Anabolic steroids have not been shown to enhance athletic ability.

PRECAUTIONS

General:

Women should be observed for signs of virilization (deepening of the voice, hirsutism, acne and clitoromegaly). To prevent irreversible change, drug therapy must be discontinued when mild virilism is first detected. Such virilization is usual following androgenic anabolic steroid use at high doses. Some virilizing changes in women are irreversible even after prompt discontinuance of therapy and are not prevented by concomitant use of estrogens. Menstrual irregularities, including amenorrhea, may also occur.

The insulin or oral hypoglycemic dosage may need adjustment in diabetic patients who receive anabolic steroids.

Anabolic steroids may cause suppression of clotting factors II, V, VII and X, and an increase in prothrombin time.

Information for the patient:

The physician should instruct patients to report any of the following side effects of androgens.

Adult or Adolescent Males: Too frequent or persistent erections of the penis, appearance or aggravation of acne.

Women: Hoarseness, acne, changes in menstrual periods or more hair on the face.

All Patients: Any nausea, vomiting, changes in skin color or ankle swelling.

Laboratory Tests:

Women with disseminated breast carcinoma should have frequent determination of urine and serum calcium levels during the course of androgenic anabolic steroid therapy (see WARNINGS).

Because of the hepatoxicity associated with the use of 17-alpha-alkylated androgens, liver function tests should be obtained periodically.

Periodic (every 6 months) x-ray examinations of bone age should be made during treatment of prepubertal patients to determine the rate of bone maturation and the effects of androgenic anabolic steroid therapy on the epiphyseal centers.

Anabolic steroids have been reported to lower the level of high-density lipoproteins and raise the level of low-density lipoproteins. These changes usually revert to normal on discontinuation of treatment. Increased low-density lipoproteins and decreased high-density lipoproteins are considered cardiovascular risk factors. Serum lipids and high-density lipoprotein cholesterol should be determined periodically.

Hemoglobin and hematocrit should be checked periodically for polycythemia in patients who are receiving high doses of anabolics.

Because iron deficiency anemia has been observed in some patients treated with oxymetholone, periodic determination of the serum iron and iron binding capacity is recommended. If iron deficiency is detected, it should be appropriately treated with supplementary iron.

Oxymetholone has been shown to decrease 17-ketosteroid excretion.

Drug Interaction:

Anabolic steroids may increase sensitivity to anticoagulants; therefore, dosage of an anticoagulant may have to be decreased in order to maintain the prothrombin time at the desired therapeutic level.

Drug/Laboratory Test Interferences:

Therapy with androgenic anabolic steroids may decrease levels of thyroxine-binding globulin resulting in decreased total T_4 serum levels and increased resin uptake of T_3 and T_4. Free thyroid hormone levels remain unchanged and there is no clinical evidence of thyroid dysfunction. Altered tests usually persist for 2 to 3 weeks after stopping anabolic therapy.

Anabolic steroids may cause an increase in prothrombin time.

Anabolic steroids have been shown to alter fasting blood sugar and glucose tolerance tests.

Carcinogenesis, Mutagenesis, Impairment of Fertility:

Animal data: Testosterone has been tested by subcutaneous injection and implantation in mice and rats. The implant induced cervical-uterine tumors in mice, which metastasized in some cases. There is suggestive evidence that injection of testosterone into some strains of female mice increases their susceptibility to hepatoma. Testosterone is also known to increase the number of tumors and decrease the degree of differentiation of chemically induced carcinomas of the liver in rats.

Human data: There are rare reports of hepatocellular carcinoma in patients receiving long-term therapy with androgens in high doses. Withdrawal of the drugs did not lead to regression of the tumors in all cases.

Geriatric patients treated with androgens may be at an increased risk of developing prostatic hypertrophy and prostatic carcinoma although conclusive evidence to support this concept is lacking.

This compound has not been tested for mutagenic potential. However, as noted above, carcinogenic effects have been attributed to treatment with androgenic hormones. The potential carcinogenic effects likely occur through a hormonal mechanism rather than by a direct chemical interaction mechanism.

Impairment of fertility was not tested directly in animal species. However, as noted below under ADVERSE REACTIONS, oligospermia in males and amenorrhea in females are potential adverse effects of treatment with ANADROL® Tablets. Therefore, impairment of fertility is a possible outcome of treatment with ANADROL.

Pregnancy:

Pregnancy category X. See CONTRAINDICATIONS.

Nursing Mothers:

It is not known whether anabolics are excreted in human milk. Because of the potential for serious adverse reactions in nursed infants from anabolics, women who take oxymetholone should not nurse.

Pediatric Use:

Anabolic/androgenic steroids should be used very cautiously in children and only by specialists who are aware of their effects on bone maturation.

Anabolic agents may accelerate epiphyseal maturation more rapidly than linear growth in children, and the effect may continue for 6 months after the drug has been stopped. Therefore, therapy should be monitored by x-ray studies at 6-month intervals in order to avoid the risk of compromising the adult height.

ADVERSE REACTIONS

Hepatic:

Cholestatic jaundice with, rarely, hepatic necrosis and death. Hepatocellular neoplasms and peliosis hepatis have been reported in association with long-term androgenic anabolic steroid therapy (see WARNINGS).

Genitourinary System:

In Men:

Prepubertal: Phallic enlargement and increased frequency of erections.

Postpubertal: Inhibition of testicular function, testicular atrophy and oligospermia, impotence, chronic priapism, epididymitis, bladder irritability and decrease in seminal volume.

In Women:

Clitoral enlargement, menstrual irregularities.

In Both Sexes:

Increased or decreased libido.

CNS: Excitation, insomnia.

Gastrointestinal: Nausea, vomiting, diarrhea.

Hematologic: Bleeding in patients on concomitant anticoagulant therapy, iron-deficiency anemia.

Leukemia has been observed in patients with aplastic anemia treated with oxymetholone. The role, if any, of oxymetholone is unclear because malignant transformation has been seen in blood dyscrasias and leukemia has been reported in patients with aplastic anemia who have not been treated with oxymetholone.

Breast: Gynecomastia.

Larynx: Deepening of the voice in women.

Hair: Hirsutism and male-pattern baldness in women, male-pattern of hair loss in postpubertal males.

Skin: Acne (especially in women and prepubertal boys).

Skeletal: Premature closure of epiphyses in children (see PRECAUTIONS, Pediatric Use), muscle cramps.

Body as a Whole: Chills.

Fluid and Electrolytes: Edema, retention of serum electrolytes (sodium, chloride, potassium, phosphate, calcium).

Metabolic/Endocrine: Decreased glucose tolerance (see PRECAUTIONS), increased serum levels of low-density lipoproteins and decreased levels of high-density lipoproteins (see PRECAUTIONS, Laboratory Tests), increased creatine and creatinine excretion, increased serum levels of creatinine phosphokinase (CPK). Reversible changes in liver function tests also occur, including increased bromsulphalein (BSP) retention and increases in serum bilirubin, glutamic oxaloacetic transaminase (SGOT), and alkaline phosphatase.

DRUG ABUSE AND DEPENDENCE

Controlled Substance:

ANADROL-50 is considered to be a controlled substance and is listed in Schedule III.

OVERDOSAGE

There have been no reports of acute overdosage with anabolics.

DOSAGE AND ADMINISTRATION

The recommended daily dose in children and adults is 1–5 mg/kg body weight per day. The usual effective dose is 1–2 mg/kg/day but higher doses may be required, and the dose should be individualized. Response is not often immediate, and a minimum trial of three to six months should be given. Following remission, some patients may be maintained without the drug; others may be maintained on an estab-

lished lower daily dosage. A continued maintenance dose is usually necessary in patients with congenital aplastic anemia.

HOW SUPPLIED

ANADROL-50 (oxymetholone) is supplied in bottles of 100 white scored tablets imprinted with 8633 and UNIMED (NDC 0051-8633-33).

Store at 15° to 30°C (59° to 86°F).

CAUTION: Federal law prohibits dispensing without prescription.

6/17/97

Manufactured for
Unimed Pharmaceuticals, Inc.
Buffalo Grove IL 60089
by Oread, Inc.
Palo Alto, CA 94304
Shown in Product Identification Guide, page 341

MARINOL®   ℂ ℞
(dronabinol)
Capsules

Dronabinol is a cannabinoid designated chemically as (6a*R*-*trans*)-6a,7,8,10a-tetrahydro-6,6,9-trimethyl-3-pentyl-6*H*-dibenzol[*b,d*]pyran-1-ol. Dronabinol has the following empirical and structural formula:

$C_{21}H_{30}O_2$ (molecular weight = 314.47)

Dronabinol, delta-9-tetrahydrocannabinol (delta-9-THC), is naturally-occurring and has been extracted from *Cannabis sativa* L. (marijuana).

Dronabinol is also chemically synthesized and is a light-yellow resinous oil that is sticky at room temperature and hardens upon refrigeration. Dronabinol is insoluble in water and is formulated in sesame oil. It has a pK_a of 10.6 and an octanol-water partition coefficient: 6,000:1 at pH 7.

Capsules for oral administration: Marinol is supplied as round, soft gelatin capsules containing either 2.5 mg, 5 mg, or 10 mg dronabinol. Each Marinol capsule is formulated with the following inactive ingredients: sesame oil, gelatin, glycerin, methylparaben, propylparaben, FD&C Yellow No. 6 (5 mg and 10 mg), and titanium dioxide.

HOW SUPPLIED

MARINOL® CAPSULES (dronabinol solution in sesame oil in soft gelatin capsules)

2.5 mg white capsules (identified RL).
NDC 0054-2601-11: Bottles of 25 capsules.
NDC 0054-2601-21: Bottles of 60 capsules.
NDC 0054-2601-25: Bottles of 100 capsules.

5 mg dark brown capsules (identified RL).
NDC 0054-2602-11: Bottles of 25 capsules.
NDC 0054-2602-25: Bottles of 100 capsules.

10 mg orange capsules (identified RL).
NDC 0054-2603-11: Bottles of 25 capsules.
NDC 0054-2603-21: Bottles of 60 capsules.

MARINOL® is a registered trademark of Unimed Pharmaceuticals, Inc. and is marketed by Roxane Laboratories, Inc. under license from Unimed Pharmaceuticals, Inc. Manufactured by Banner Pharmacaps, Inc. Chatsworth CA 91311

DEA ORDER FORM REQUIRED
Rx only

4056050   **Revised June 1998**
068   © RLI, 1998
Roxane
Laboratories, Inc.
Columbus, Ohio 43216
Shown in Product Identification Guide, page 341

MAXAQUIN®   ℞
[*măx 'ah-kwĭn*]
(lomefloxacin hydrochloride)
Film-coated Tablets

DESCRIPTION

Maxaquin (lomefloxacin HCl) is a synthetic broad-spectrum antimicrobial agent for oral administration. Lomefloxacin

HCl, a difluoroquinolone, is the monohydrochloride salt of (±)-1-ethyl-6,8-difluoro-1,4-dihydro-7-(3-methyl-1-piperazinyl)-4-oxo-3-quinolinecarboxylic acid. Its empirical formula is $C_{17}H_{19}F_2N_3O_3 \cdot HCl$, and its structural formula is:

Lomefloxacin HCl is a white to pale yellow powder with a molecular weight of 387.8. It is slightly soluble in water and practically insoluble in alcohol. Lomefloxacin HCl is stable to heat and moisture but is sensitive to light in dilute aqueous solution.

Maxaquin is available as a film-coated tablet formulation containing 400 mg of lomefloxacin base, present as the hydrochloride salt. The base content of the hydrochloride salt is 90.6%. The inactive ingredients are carboxymethylcellulose calcium, hydroxypropyl cellulose, hydroxypropyl methylcellulose, lactose, magnesium stearate, polyethylene glycol, polyoxyl 40 stearate, and titanium dioxide.

CLINICAL PHARMACOLOGY

Pharmacokinetics in healthy volunteers: In 6 fasting healthy male volunteers, approximately 95% to 98% of a single oral dose of lomefloxacin was absorbed. Absorption was rapid following single doses of 200 and 400 mg (T_{max} 0.8 to 1.4 hours). Mean plasma concentration increased proportionally between 100 and 400 mg as shown below:

Dose (mg)	Mean Peak Plasma Concentration (µg/mL)	Area Under Curve (AUC) (µg/mL)
100	0.8	5.6
200	1.4	10.9
400	3.2	26.1

In 6 healthy male volunteers administered 400 mg of lomefloxacin on an empty stomach qd for 7 days, the following mean pharmacokinetic parameter values were obtained:

C_{max}	2.8 µg/mL
C_{min}	0.27 µg/mL
$AUC_{0-24 h}$	25.9 µg·h/mL
T_{max}	1.5 h
$t_{1/2}$	7.75 h

The elimination half-life in 8 subjects with normal renal function was approximately 8 hours. At 24 hours postdose, subjects with normal renal function receiving single doses of 200 or 400 mg had mean plasma lomefloxacin concentrations of 0.10 and 0.24 µg/mL, respectively. Steady-state concentrations were achieved within 48 hours of initiating therapy with one-a-day dosing. There was no drug accumulation with single-daily dosing in patients with normal renal function.

Approximately 65% of an orally administered dose was excreted in the urine as unchanged drug in patients with normal renal function. Following a 400-mg dose of lomefloxacin administered qd for 7 days, the mean urine concentration 4 hours postdose was in excess of 300 µg/mL. The mean urine concentration exceeded 35 µg/mL for at least 24 hours after dosing.

Following a single 400-mg dose, the solubility of lomefloxacin in urine usually exceeded its peak urinary concentration 2- to 6-fold. In this study, urine pH affected the solubility of lomefloxacin with solubilities ranging from 7.8 mg/mL at pH 5.2, to 2.4 mg/mL at pH 6.5, and 3.03 mg/mL at pH 8.12. The urinary excretion of lomefloxacin was virtually complete within 72 hours after cessation of dosing, with approximately 65% of the dose being recovered as parent drug and 9% as its glucuronide metabolite. The mean renal clearance was 145 mL/min in subjects with normal renal function (GFR = 120 mL/min). This may indicate tubular secretion.

Food effect: When lomefloxacin and food were administered concomitantly, the rate of drug absorption was delayed (T_{max} increased to 2 hours [delayed by 41%], C_{max} decreased by 18%), and the extent of absorption (AUC) was decreased by 12%.

Pharmacokinetics in the geriatric population: In 16 healthy elderly volunteers (61 to 76 years of age) with normal renal function for their age, the half-life of lomefloxacin (mean of 8 hours) and its peak plasma concentration (mean of 4.2 µg/mL) following a single 400-mg dose were similar to those in 8 younger subjects dosed with a single 400-mg dose. Thus, drug absorption appears unaffected in the elderly. Plasma clearance was, however, reduced in this elderly population by approximately 25%, and the AUC was increased by approximately 33%. This slower elimination most likely reflects the decreased renal function normally observed in the geriatric population.

Pharmacokinetics in renally impaired patients: In 8 patients with creatinine clearance (Cl_{Cr}) between 10 and 40 mL/min/1.73 m^2, the mean AUC after a single 400-mg dose of lomefloxacin increased 335% over the AUC demonstrated in patients with a $Cl_{Cr} > 80$ mL/min/1.73 m^2. Also, in these patients, the mean $t_{1/2}$ increased to 21 hours. In 8 patients with $Cl_{Cr} < 10$ mL/min/1.73 m^2, the mean AUC after a single 400-mg dose of lomefloxacin increased 700% over the AUC demonstrated in patients with a $Cl_{Cr} > 80$ mL/min/1.73 m^2. In these patients with $Cl_{Cr} < 10$ mL/min/1.73 m^2, the mean $t_{1/2}$ increased to 45 hours. The plasma clearance of lomefloxacin was closely correlated with creatinine clearance, ranging from 31 mL/min/1.73 m^2 when creatinine clearance was zero to 271 mL.min/1.73 m^2 at a normal creatinine clearance of 110 mL/min/1.73 m^2. Peak lomefloxacin concentrations were not affected by the degree of renal function when single doses of lomefloxacin were administered. Adjustment of dosage schedules for patients with such decreases in renal function is warranted. (See **Dosage and Administration**.)

Pharmacokinetics in patients with cirrhosis: In 12 patients with histologically confirmed cirrhosis, no significant changes in rate or extent of lomefloxacin exposure (C_{max}, T_{max}, $t_{1/2}$, or AUC) were observed when they were administered 400 mg of lomefloxacin as a single dose. No data are available in cirrhotic patients treated with multiple doses of lomefloxacin. Cirrhosis does not appear to reduce the nonrenal clearance of lomefloxacin. There does not appear to be a need for a dosage reduction in cirrhotic patients, provided adequate renal function is present.

Metabolism and pharmacodynamics of lomefloxacin: Lomefloxacin is minimally metabolized although 5 metabolites have been identified in human urine. The glucuronide metabolite is found in the highest concentration and accounts for approximately 9% of the administered dose. The other 4 metabolites together account for < 0.5% of the dose.

Approximately 10% of an oral dose was recovered as unchanged drug in the feces.

Serum protein binding of lomefloxacin is approximately 10%.

The following are mean tissue- or fluid-to-plasma ratios of lomefloxacin following oral administration. Studies have not been conducted to assess the penetration of lomefloxacin into human cerebrospinal fluid.

Tissue or Body Fluid	Mean Tissue- or Fluid-to-Plasma Ratio
Bronchial mucosa	2.1
Bronchial secretions	0.6
Prostatic tissue	2.0
Sputum	1.3
Urine	140.0

In two studies including 74 healthy volunteers, the minimal dose of UVA light needed to cause erythema (MED-UVA) was inversely proportional to plasma lomefloxacin concentration. The MED-UVA values (16 hours and 12 hours postdose) were significantly higher than the MED-UVA values 2 hours postdose at steady state. Increasing the interval between lomefloxacin dosing and exposure to UVA light increased the amount of light energy needed for photoreaction. In a study of to 27 healthy volunteers, the steady state AUC values and C_{min} values were equivalent whether the drug was administered in the morning or in the evening.

Microbiology: Lomefloxacin is a bactericidal agent with in vitro activity against a wide range of gram-negative and gram-positive organisms. The bactericidal action of lomefloxacin results from interference with the activity of the bacterial enzyme DNA gyrase, which is needed for the transcription and replication of bacterial DNA. The minimum bactericidal concentration (MBC) generally does not exceed the minimum inhibitory concentration (MIC) by more than a factor of 2, except for staphylococci, which usually have MBCs 2 to 4 times the MIC.

Lomefloxacin has been shown to be active against most strains of the following organisms both in vitro and in clinical infections: (See **Indications and Usage**.)

Gram-positive aerobes
Staphylococcus saprophyticus

Gram-negative aerobes
Citrobacter diversus
Enterobacter cloacae
Escherichia coli
Haemophilus influenzae
Klebsiella pneumoniae
Moraxella catarrhalis
Proteus mirabilis
Pseudomonas aeruginosa (urinary tract only—See **Indications and Usage** and **Warnings**)

The following in vitro data are available; however, their clinical significance is unknown.

Lomefloxacin exhibits in vitro MICs of 2 µg/mL or less against most strains of the following organisms; however,

Continued on next page

Maxaquin—Cont.

the safety and effectiveness of lomefloxacin in treating clinical infections due to these organisms have not been established in adequate and well-controlled trials:

Gram-positive aerobes
Staphylococcus aureus (including methicillin-resistant strains)
Staphylococcus epidermidis (including methicillin-resistant strains)
Gram-negative aerobes
Aeromonas hydrophila
Citrobacter freundii
Enterobacter aerogenes
Enterobacter agglomerans
Haemophilus parainfluenzae
Hafnia alvei
Klebsiella oxytoca
Klebsiella ozaenae
Morganella morganii
Proteus vulgaris
Providencia alcalifaciens
Providencia rettgeri
Serratia liquefaciens
Serratia marcescens
Other organisms:
Legionella pneumophila
Beta-lactamase production should have no effect on the in vitro activity of lomefloxacin.
Most group A, B, D, and G streptococci, *Streptococcus pneumoniae, Pseudomonas cepacia, Ureaplasma urealyticum, Mycoplasma hominis,* and anaerobic bacteria are resistant to lomefloxacin.
Lomefloxacin appears slightly less active in vitro when tested at acidic pH. An increase in inoculum size has little effect on the in vitro activity of lomefloxacin. In vitro resistance to lomefloxacin develops slowly (multiple-step mutation). Rapid one-step development of resistance occurs only rarely ($<10^{-9}$) in vitro.
Cross-resistance between lomefloxacin and other quinolone-class antimicrobial agents has been reported; however, cross-resistance between lomefloxacin and members of other classes of antimicrobial agents, such as aminoglycosides, penicillins, tetracyclines, cephalosporins, or sulfonamides has not yet been reported. Lomefloxacin is active in vitro against some strains of cephalosporin- and aminoglycoside-resistant gram-negative bacteria.

Susceptibility tests
Diffusion techniques: Quantitative methods that require measurement of zone diameters give the most precise estimate of the susceptibility of bacteria to antimicrobial agents. One such standardized procedure[1] that has been recommended for use with disks to test the susceptibility of organisms to lomefloxacin uses the 10-µg lomefloxacin disk. Interpretation involves correlation of the diameter obtained in the disk test with the MIC for lomefloxacin.
Reports from the laboratory giving results of the standard single-disk susceptibility test with a 10-µg lomefloxacin disk should be interpreted according to the following criteria:

Zone Diameter (mm)	Interpretation
≥22	Susceptible (S)
19–21	Intermediate (I)
≤18	Resistant (R)

A report of "susceptible" indicates that the pathogen is likely to be inhibited by generally achievable drug concentrations. A report of "intermediate" indicates that the result should be considered equivocal, and, if the organism is not fully susceptible to alternative clinically feasible drugs, the test should be repeated. This category provides a buffer zone that prevents small uncontrolled technical factors from causing major discrepancies in interpretation. A report of "resistant" indicates that achievable drug concentrations are unlikely to be inhibitory, and other therapy should be selected.
Standardized susceptibility test procedures require the use of laboratory control organisms. The 10-µg lomefloxacin disk should give the following zone diameters:

Organism	Zone Diameter (mm)
S aureus (ATCC 25923)	23–29
E coli (ATCC 25922)	27–33
P aeruginosa (ATCC 27853)	22–28

Dilution techniques: Use a standardized dilution method[2] (broth, agar, or microdilution) or equivalent with lomefloxacin powder. The MIC values obtained should be interpreted according to the following criteria:

MIC (µg/mL)	Interpretation
≤2	Susceptible (S)
4	Intermediate (I)
≥8	Resistant (R)

As with standard diffusion techniques, dilution methods require the use of laboratory control organisms. Standard lomefloxacin powder should provide the following MIC values:

Organism	MIC (µg/mL)
S aureus (ATCC 29213)	0.25–2.0
E coli (ATCC 25922)	0.03–0.12
P aeruginosa (ATCC 27853)	1.0–4.0

INDICATIONS AND USAGE

Treatment:
Maxaquin (lomefloxacin HCl) film-coated tablets are indicated for the treatment of adults with mild to moderate infections caused by susceptible strains of the designated microorganisms in the conditions listed below: (See **Dosage and Administration** for specific dosing recommendations.)
LOWER RESPIRATORY TRACT
Acute Bacterial Exacerbation of Chronic Bronchitis caused by *Haemophilus influenzae* or *Moraxella catarrhalis.**
NOTE: MAXAQUIN IS NOT INDICATED FOR THE EMPIRIC TREATMENT OF ACUTE BACTERIAL EXACERBATION OF CHRONIC BRONCHITIS WHEN IT IS PROBABLE THAT *S PNEUMONIAE* IS A CAUSATIVE PATHOGEN. *S PNEUMONIAE* EXHIBITS IN VITRO RESISTANCE TO LOMEFLOXACIN, AND THE SAFETY AND EFFICACY OF LOMEFLOXACIN IN THE TREATMENT OF PATIENTS WITH ACUTE BACTERIAL EXACERBATION OF CHRONIC BRONCHITIS CAUSED BY *S PNEUMONIAE* HAVE NOT BEEN DEMONSTRATED. IF LOMEFLOXACIN IS TO BE PRESCRIBED FOR GRAM-STAIN-GUIDED EMPIRIC THERPY OF ACUTE BACTERIAL EXACERBATION OF CHRONIC BRONCHITIS, IT SHOULD BE USED ONLY IF SPUTUM GRAM STAIN DEMONSTRATES AN ADEQUATE QUALITY OF SPECIMEN (>25 PMNs/LPF) AND THERE IS BOTH A PREDOMINANCE OF GRAM-NEGATIVE MICROORGANISMS AND NOT A PREDOMINANCE OF GRAM-POSITIVE MICROORGANISMS.
URINARY TRACT
Uncomplicated Urinary Tract Infections (cystitis) caused by *Escherichia coli, Klebsiella pneumoniae, Proteus mirabilis,* or *Staphylococcus saprophyticus.* (See **DOSAGE AND ADMINISTRATION** and **CLINICAL STUDIES—UNCOMPLICATED CYSTITIS.**)
Complicated Urinary Tract Infections caused by *Escherichia coli, Klebsiella pneumoniae, Proteus mirabilis, Pseudomonas aeruginosa, Citrobacter diversus,** or *Enterobacter cloacae.**
NOTE: In clinical trials with patients experiencing complicated urinary tract infections (UTIs) due to *P aeruginosa,* 12 of 16 patients had the microorganism eradicated from the urine after therapy with lomefloxacin. None of the patients had concomitant bacteremia. Serum levels of lomefloxacin do not reliably exceed the MIC of *Pseudomonas* isolates. THE SAFETY AND EFFICACY OF LOMEFLOXACIN IN TREATING PATIENTS WITH *PSEUDOMONAS* BACTEREMIA HAVE NOT BEEN ESTABLISHED.
*Although treatment of infections due to this microorganism in this organ system demonstrated a clinically acceptable overall outcome, efficacy was studied in fewer than 10 infections.
Appropriate culture and susceptibility tests should be performed before antimicrobial treatment in order to isolate and identify microorganisms causing infection and to determine their susceptibility to lomefloxacin. In patients with UTIs, therapy with Maxaquin film-coated tablets may be initiated before results of these tests are known; once these results become available, appropriate therapy should be continued. In patients with an acute bacterial exacerbation of chronic bronchitis, therapy should not be started empirically with lomefloxacin when there is a probability the causative pathogen is *S pneumoniae.*
Beta-lactamase production should have no effect on lomefloxacin activity.

Prevention/prophylaxis:
Maxaquin is indicated preoperatively for the prevention of infection in the following situations:
- Transrectal prostate biopsy: to reduce the incidence of urinary tract infection, in the early and late postoperative periods (3–5 days and 3–4 weeks postsurgery).
- Transurethral surgical procedures: to reduce the incidence of urinary tract infection in the early postoperative period (3–5 days postsurgery).

Efficacy in decreasing the incidence of infections other than urinary tract infection has not been established. Maxaquin, like all drugs for prophylaxis of transurethral surgical procedures, usually should not be used in minor urologic procedures for which prophylaxis is not indicated (eg, simple cystoscopy or retrograde pyelography). (See **Dosage and Administration.**)

CONTRAINDICATIONS

Maxaquin (lomefloxacin HCl) is contraindicated in persons with a history of hypersensitivity to lomefloxacin or any member of the quinolone group of antimicrobial agents.

WARNINGS

MODERATE TO SEVERE PHOTOTOXIC REACTIONS HAVE OCCURRED IN PATIENTS EXPOSED TO DIRECT OR INDIRECT SUNLIGHT OR TO ARTIFICAL ULTRAVIOLET LIGHT (eg, sunlamps) DURING OR FOLLOWING TREATMENT WITH LOMEFLOXACIN. THESE REACTIONS HAVE ALSO OCCURRED IN PATIENTS EXPOSED TO SHADED OR DIFFUSE LIGHT, INCLUDING EXPOSURE THROUGH GLASS. PATIENTS SHOULD BE ADVISED TO DISCONTINUE LOMEFLOXACIN THERAPY AT THE FIRST SIGNS OR SYMPTOMS OF A PHOTOTOXICITY REACTION SUCH AS A SENSATION OF SKIN BURNING, REDNESS, SWELLING, BLISTERS, RASH, ITCHING, OR DERMATITIS.
These phototoxic reactions have occurred with and without the use of sunscreens or sunblocks. Single doses of lomefloxacin have been associated with these types of reactions. In a few cases, recovery was prolonged for several weeks. As with some other types of phototoxicity, there is the potential for exacerbation of the reaction on re-exposure to sunlight or artificial ultraviolet light prior to complete recovery from the reaction. In rare cases, reactions have recurred up to several weeks after stopping lomefloxacin therapy.
EXPOSURE TO DIRECT OR INDIRECT SUNLIGHT (EVEN WHEN USING SUNSCREENS OR SUNBLOCKS) SHOULD BE AVOIDED WHILE TAKING LOMEFLOXACIN AND FOR SEVERAL DAYS FOLLOWING THERAPY. LOMEFLOXACIN THERAPY SHOULD BE DISCONTINUED IMMEDIATELY AT THE FIRST SIGNS OR SYMPTOMS OF PHOTOTOXICITY.
THE SAFETY AND EFFICACY OF LOMEFLOXACIN IN PEDIATRIC PATIENTS, ADOLESCENTS (UNDER THE AGE OF 18 YEARS), PREGNANT WOMEN, AND LACTATING WOMEN HAVE NOT BEEN ESTABLISHED. (See **PRECAUTIONS—*Pregnancy; Nursing Mothers;*** and ***Pediatric Use.***) The oral administration of multiple doses of lomefloxacin to juvenile dogs at 0.3 times and to rats at 5.4 times the recommended adult human dose based on mg/m^2 (0.6 and 34 times the recommended adult human dose based on mg/kg, respectively) caused arthropathy and lameness. Histopathologic examination of the weight-bearing joints of these animals revealed permanent lesions of the cartilage. Other quinolones also produce erosions of cartilage of weight-bearing joints and other signs of arthropathy in juvenile animals of various species. (See **Animal Pharmacology.**)
The safety and efficacy of lomefloxacin in the treatment of acute bacterial exacerbation of chronic bronchitis due to *S pneumoniae* have not been demonstrated. This product should not be used empirically in the treatment of acute bacterial exacerbation of chronic bronchitis when it is probable that *S pneumoniae* is a causative pathogen.
In clinical trials of complicated UTIs due to *P aeruginosa,* 12 of 16 patients had the microorganism eradicated from the urine after therapy with lomefloxacin. No patients had concomitant bacteremia. Serum levels of lomefloxacin do not reliably exceed the MIC of *Pseudomonas* isolates. THE SAFETY AND EFFICACY OF LOMEFLOXACIN IN TREATING PATIENTS WITH *PSEUDOMONAS* BACTEREMIA HAVE NOT BEEN ESTABLISHED.
Convulsions have been reported in patients receiving lomefloxacin. Whether the convulsions were directly related to lomefloxacin administration has not yet been established. However, convulsions, increased intracranial pressure, and toxic psychoses have been reported in patients receiving other quinolones. Quinolones may also cause central nervous system (CNS) stimulation, which may lead to tremors, restlessness, lightheadedness, confusion, and hallucinations. If any of these reactions occurs in patients receiving lomefloxacin, the drug should be discontinued and appropriate measures instituted. No evidence of an effect of lomefloxacin on the electrical activity of the brain has been demonstrated. Lomefloxacin does not alter cerebral blood flow or cerebral glucose uptake in the CNS based on positron emission tomography. However, until more information becomes available, lomefloxacin, like all other quinolones, should be used with caution in patients with known or suspected CNS disorders, such as severe cerebral arteriosclerosis, epilepsy, or other factors that predispose to seizures. (See **Adverse Reactions.**)
Serious and occasionally fatal hypersensitivity (anaphylactoid or anaphylactic) reactions, some following the first dose, have been reported in patients receiving quinolone therapy. Some reactions were accompanied by cardiovascular collapse, loss of consciousness, tingling, pharyngeal or facial edema, dyspnea, urticaria, or itching. Only a few of these patients had a history of previous hypersensitivity reactions. Serious hypersensitivity reactions have also been reported following treatment with lomefloxacin. If an allergic reaction to lomefloxacin occurs, discontinue the drug. Serious acute hypersensitivity reactions may require immediate emergency treatment with epinephrine. Oxygen, intra-

venous fluids, antihistamines, corticosteroids, pressor amines, and airway management, including intubation, should be administered as indicated.

Pseudomembranous colitis has been reported with nearly all antibacterial agents, including lomefloxacin, and may range from mild to life-threatening in severity. Therefore, it is important to consider this diagnosis in patients who present with diarrhea subsequent to the administration of antibacterial agents. Treatment with antimicrobial agents alters the normal flora of the colon and may permit overgrowth of clostridia. Studies indicate that a toxin produced by *Clostridium difficile* is a primary cause of "antibiotic-associated colitis." After the diagnosis of pseudomembranous colitis has been established, therapeutic measures should be initiated. Mild cases of pseudomembranous colitis usually respond to discontinuation of drug alone. In moderate to severe cases, consideration should be given to management with fluids and electrolytes, protein supplementation, and treatment with an antibacterial drug clinically effective against *C difficile* colitis.

Ruptures of the shoulder, hand, and Achilles tendons that required surgical repair or resulted in prolonged disability have been reported with lomefloxacin. Lomefloxacin should be discontinued if the patient experiences pain, inflammation, or rupture of a tendon. Patients should rest and refrain from exercise until the diagnosis of tendinitis or tendon rupture has been confidently excluded. Tendon rupture can occur at any time during or after therapy with lomefloxacin.

Infection	Unit Dose	Frequency	Duration	Daily Dose
Acute bacterial exacerbation of chronic bronchitis	400 mg	qd	10 days	400 mg
Uncomplicated cystitis in females caused by *E. coli*	400 mg	qd	3 days	400 mg
(see **CLINICAL STUDIES—UNCOMPLICATED CYSTITIS.**)				
Uncomplicated cystitis caused by *K pneumoniae, P mirabilis,* or *S saprophyticus*	400 mg	qd	10 days	400 mg
Complicated UTI	400 mg	qd	14 days	400 mg

PRECAUTIONS

General:

Alteration of the dosage regimen is recommended for patients with impairment of renal function (Cl_{Cr} < 40 mL/min/1.73 m^2). (See **Dosage and Administration.**)

Information for patients:

Patients should be advised

- to avoid to the maximum extent possible direct or indirect sunlight (including exposure through glass and exposure through sunscreens and sunblocks) and artificial ultraviolet light (eg, sunlamps) during treatment with lomefloxacin and for several days after therapy;
- that they may reduce the risk of developing phototoxicity from sunlight by taking the daily dose of lomefloxacin at least 12 hours before exposure to the sun (eg, in the evening);
- to discontinue lomefloxacin therapy at the first signs or symptoms of phototoxicity reaction such as a sensation of skin burning, redness, swelling, blisters, rash, itching, or dermatitis;
- that a patient who has experienced a phototoxic reaction should avoid re-exposure to sunlight and artificial ultraviolet light until he has completely recovered from the reaction. In rare cases, reactions have recurred up to several weeks after stopping lomefloxacin therapy.
- to drink fluid liberally;
- that lomefloxacin can be taken without regard to meals;
- that mineral supplements or vitamins with iron or minerals should not be taken within the 2-hour period before or after taking lomefloxacin (see **Drug Interactions**);
- that sucralfate or antacids containing magnesium or aluminum should not be taken within 4 hours before or 2 hours after taking lomefloxacin (see **Drug Interactions**);
- that lomefloxacin can cause dizziness and lightheadedness and, therefore, patients should know how they react to lomefloxacin before they operate an automobile or machinery or engage in activities requiring mental alertness and coordination;
- to discontinue treatment and inform their physician if they experience pain, inflammation, or rupture of a tendon, and to rest and refrain from exercise until the diagnosis of tendinitis or tendon rupture has been confidently excluded;
- that lomefloxacin may be associated with hypersensitivity reactions, even following the first dose, and to discontinue the drug at the first sign of a skin rash or other allergic reaction.

Drug Interactions:

Theophylline: In three pharmacokinetic studies including 46 normal, healthy subjects, theophylline clearance and concentration were not significantly altered by the addition of lomefloxacin. In clinical studies where patients were on chronic theophylline therapy, lomefloxacin had no measurable effect on the mean distribution of theophylline concentrations or the mean estimates of theophylline clearance. Though individual theophylline levels fluctuated, there were no clinically significant symptoms of drug interaction.

Antacids and sucralfate: Sucralfate and antacids containing magnesium or aluminum form chelation complexes with lomefloxacin and interfere with its bioavailability. Sucralfate administered 2 hours before lomefloxacin resulted in a slower rate of absorption (mean C_{max} decreased by 30% and mean T_{max} increased by 1 hour) and a lesser extent of absorption (mean AUC decreased by approximately 25%). Magnesium- and aluminum-containing antacids, administered concomitantly with lomefloxacin, significantly decreased the bioavailability (48%) of lomefloxacin. Separating the doses of antacid and lomefloxacin minimizes this decrease in bioavailability; therefore, administration of these agents should precede lomefloxacin dosing by 4 hours or follow lomefloxacin dosing by at least 2 hours.

Caffeine: Two hundred mg of caffeine (equivalent to 1 to 3 cups of American coffee) was administered to 16 normal, healthy volunteers who had achieved steady-state blood concentrations of lomefloxacin after being dosed at 400 mg qd. This did not result in any statistically or clinically relevant changes in the pharmacokinetic parameters of either caffeine or its major metabolite, paraxanthine. No data are available on potential interactions in individuals who consume greater than 200 mg of caffeine per day or in those, such as the geriatric population, who are generally believed to be more susceptible to the development of drug-induced CNS-related adverse effects. Other quinolones have demonstrated moderate to marked interference with the metabolism of caffeine, resulting in a reduced clearance, a prolongation of plasma half-life, and an increase in symptoms that accompany high levels of caffeine.

Cimetidine: Cimetidine has been demonstrated to interfere with the elimination of other quinolones. This interference has resulted in significant increases in half-life and AUC. The interaction between lomefloxacin and cimetidine has not been studied.

Cyclosporine: Elevated serum levels of cyclosporine have been reported with concomitant use of cyclosporine with other members of the quinolone class. Interaction between lomefloxacin and cyclosporine has not been studied.

Omeprazole: No clinically significant changes in lomefloxacin pharmacokinetics (AUC, C_{max}, or T_{max}) were observed when a single dose of lomefloxacin 400 mg was given after multiple doses of omeprazole (20 mg qd) in 13 healthy volunteers. Changes in omeprazole pharmacokinetics were not studied.

Phenytoin: No significant differences were observed in mean phenytoin AUC. C_{max}, C_{min} or T_{max} (although C_{max} increased by 11%) when extended phenytoin sodium capsules (100 mg tid) were coadministered with lomefloxacin (400 mg qd) for five days in 15 healthy males. Lomefloxacin is unlikely to have a significant effect on phenytoin metabolism.

Probenecid: Probenecid slows the renal elimination of lomefloxacin. An increase of 63% in the mean AUC and increases of 50% and 4%, respectively, in the mean T_{max} and mean C_{max} were noted in 1 study of 6 individuals.

Terfenadine: No clinically significant changes occurred in heart rate or corrected QT intervals, or in terfenadine metabolite or lomefloxacin pharmacokinetics, during concurrent administration of lomefloxacin and terfenadine at steady-state in 28 healthy males.

Warfarin: Quinolones may enhance the effects of the oral anticoagulant, warfarin, or its derivatives. When these products are administered concomitantly, prothrombin or other suitable coagulation tests should be monitored closely. However, no clinically or statistically significant differences in prothrombin time ratio or warfarin enantiomer pharmacokinetics were observed in a small study of 7 healthy males who received both warfarin and lomefloxacin under steady-state conditions.

Carcinogenesis, mutagenesis, impairment of fertility:

Carcinogenesis: Hairless (Skh-1) mice were exposed to UVA light for 3.5 hours five times every two weeks for up to 52 weeks while concurrently being administered lomefloxacin. The lomefloxacin doses used in this study caused a phototoxic response. In mice treated with both UVA and lomefloxacin concomitantly, the time to development of skin tumors was 16 weeks. In mice treated concomitantly in this model with both UVA and other quinolones, the times to development of skin tumors ranged from 28 to 52 weeks.

Ninety-two percent (92%) of the mice treated concomitantly with both UVA and lomefloxacin developed well-differentiated squamous cell carcinomas of the skin. These squamous cell carcinomas were nonmetastatic and were endophytic in character. Two-thirds of these squamous cell carcinomas contained large central keratinous inclusion masses and were thought to arise from the vestigial hair follicles in these hairless animals.

In this model, mice treated with lomefloxacin alone did not develop skin or systemic tumors.

There are no data from similar models using pigmented mice and/or fully haired mice.

The clinical significance of these findings to humans is unknown.

Mutagenesis: One in vitro mutagenicity test (CHO/HGPRT assay) was weakly positive at lomefloxacin concentrations ≥226 μg/mL and negative at concentrations <226 μg/mL. Two other in vitro mutagenicity tests (chromosomal aberrations in Chinese hamster ovary cells, chromosomal aberrations in human lymphocytes) and two in vivo mouse micronucleus mutagenicity tests were all negative.

Impairment of fertility: Lomefloxacin did not affect the fertility of male and female rats at oral doses up to 8 times the recommended human dose based on mg/m^2 (34 times the recommended human dose based on mg/kg).

Pregnancy: Teratogenic effects. Pregnancy Category C.

Reproductive function studies have been performed in rats at doses up to 8 times the recommended human dose based on mg/m^2 (34 times the recommended human dose based mg/kg), and no impaired fertility or harm to the fetus was reported due to lomefloxacin. Increased incidence of fetal loss in monkeys has been observed at approximately 3 to 6 times the recommended human dose based on mg/m^2 (6 to 12 times the recommended human dose based on mg/kg). No teratogenicity has been observed in rats and monkeys at up to 16 times the recommended human dose exposure. In the rabbit, maternal toxicity and associated fetotoxicity, decreased placental weight, and variations of the coccygeal vertebrae occurred at doses 2 times the recommended human exposure based on mg/m^2. There are, however, no adequate and well-controlled studies in pregnant women. Lomefloxacin should be used during pregnancy only if the potential benefit justifies the potential risk to the fetus.

Nursing mothers:

It is not known whether lomefloxacin is excreted in human milk. However, it is known that other drugs of this class are excreted in human milk and that lomefloxacin is excreted in the milk of lactating rats. Because of the potential for serious adverse reactions from lomefloxacin in nursing infants, a decision should be made whether to discontinue nursing or to discontinue the drug, taking into account the importance of the drug to the mother.

Pediatric use:

The safety and effectiveness of lomefloxacin in pediatric patients and adolescents less than 18 years of age have not been established. Lomefloxacin causes arthropathy in juvenile animals of several species. (See **Warnings** and **Animal Pharmacology**.)

Geriatric use:

Of the total number of patients in clinical trials of lomefloxacin, 25% were ≥65 years of age. No overall differences in effectiveness or safety were observed between these patients and younger patients. (See **Clinical Pharmacology**—*Pharmacokinetics in the geriatric population.*)

ADVERSE REACTIONS

In clincial trials, most of the adverse events reported were mild to moderate in severity and transient in nature. During these clinical investigations, 5,623 patients received Maxaquin. In 2.2% of the patients, lomefloxacin was discontinued because of adverse events, primarily involving the gastrointestinal system (0.7%), skin (0.7%), or CNS (0.5%).

Adverse clinical events:

The events with the highest incidence (≥1%) in patients, regardless of relationship to drug, were headache (3.6%), nausea (3.5%), photosensitivity (2.3%) [see **Warnings**], dizziness (2.1%), diarrhea (1.4%), and abdominal pain (1.2%).

Additional clinical events reported in <1% of patients treated with Maxaquin, regardless of relationship to drug, are listed below:

Autonomic: increased sweating, dry mouth, flushing, syncope.

Continued on next page

Maxaquin—Cont.

Body as a whole: fatigue, back pain, malaise, asthenia, chest pain, face edema, hot flashes, influenza-like symptoms, edema, chills, allergic reaction, anaphylactoid reaction, decreased heat tolerance.

Cardiovascular: tachycardia, hypertension, hypotension, myocardial infarction, angina pectoris, cardiac failure, bradycardia, arrhythmia, phlebitis, pulmonary embolism, extrasystoles, cerebrovascular disorder, cyanosis, cardiomyopathy.

Central and peripheral nervous system: tremor, vertigo, paresthesias, twitching, hypertonia, convulsions, hyperkinesia, coma.

Gastrointestinal: dyspepsia, vomiting, flatulence, constipation, gastrointestinal bleeding, dysphagia, stomatitis, tongue discoloration, gastrointestinal inflammation.

Hearing: earache, tinnitus.

Hematologic: purpura, lymphadenopathy, thrombocythemia, anemia, thrombocytopenia, increased fibrinolysis.

Hepatic: abnormal liver function.

Metabolic: thirst, hyperglycemia, hypoglycemia, gout.

Musculoskeletal: arthralgia, myalgia, leg cramps.

Ophthalmologic: abnormal vision, conjunctivitis, photophobia, eye pain, abnormal lacrimation.

Psychiatric: insomnia, nervousness, somnolence, anorexia, depression, confusion, agitation, increased appetite, depersonalization, paranoid reaction, anxiety, paroniria, abnormal thinking, concentration impairment.

Reproductive system: Female: vaginal moniliasis, vaginitis, leukorrhea, menstrual disorder, perineal pain, intermenstrual bleeding. Male: epididymitis, orchitis.

Resistance mechanism: viral infection, moniliasis, fungal infection.

Respiratory: respiratory infection, rhinitis, pharyngitis, dyspnea, cough, epistaxis, bronchospasm, respiratory disorder, increased sputum, stridor, respiratory depression.

Skin/Allergic: pruritus, rash, urticaria, skin exfoliation, bullous eruption, eczema, skin disorder, acne, skin discoloration, skin ulceration, angiodema. (See also *Body as a whole.*)

Special senses: taste perversion.

Urinary: hematuria, micturition disorder, dysuria, strangury, anuria.

Adverse laboratory events:

Changes in laboratory parameters, listed as adverse events, without regard to drug relationship include:

Hematologic: monocytosis (0.2%), eosinophilia (0.1%), leukopenia (0.1%), leukocytosis (0.1%).

Renal: elevated BUN (0.1%), decreased potassium (0.1%), increased creatinine (0.1%).

Hepatic: elevations of ALT (SGPT) (0.4%), AST (SGOT) (0.3%), bilirubin (0.1%), alkaline phosphatase (0.1%).

Additional laboratory changes occurring in <0.1% in the clinical studies included: elevation of serum gamma glutamyl transferase, decrease in total protein or albumin, prolongation of prothrombin time, anemia, decrease in hemoglobin, thrombocythemia, thrombocytopenia, abnormalities of urine specific gravity or serum electrolytes, increased albumin, elevated ESR, albuminuria, macrocytosis.

Quinolone-class adverse events:

Post-marketing adverse events: Adverse events reported from worldwide marketing experience with lomefloxacin are: anaphylaxis, cardiopulmonary arrest, laryngeal or pulmonary edema, ataxia, cerebral thrombosis, hallucinations, painful oral mucosa, pseudomembranous colitis, hemolytic anemia, hepatitis, tendinitis, diplopia, photophobia, phobia, exfoliative dermatitis, hyperpigmentation, Stevens-Johnson syndrome, toxic epidermal necrolysis, dysgeusia, interstitial nephritis, polyuria, renal failure, urinary retention, and vasculitis.

Quinolone-class adverse events: Additional quinolone-class adverse events include: erythema nodosum, hepatic necrosis, possible exacerbation of myasthenia gravis, dysphasia, nystagmus, intestinal perforation, manic reaction, renal calculi, acidosis and hiccough.

Laboratory adverse events include: agranulocytosis, elevation of serum triglycerides, elevation of serum cholesterol, elevation of blood glucose, elevation of serum potassium, albuminuria, candiduria, and crystalluria.

OVERDOSAGE

Information on overdosage in humans is limited. In the event of acute overdosage, the stomach should be emptied by inducing vomiting or by gastric lavage, and the patient should be carefully observed and given supportive treatment. Adequate hydration must be maintained. Hemodialysis or peritoneal dialysis is unlikely to aid in the removal of lomefloxacin as < 3% is removed by these modalities.

Clinical signs of acute toxicity in rodents progressed from salivation to tremors, decreased activity, dyspnea, and clonic convulsions prior to death. These signs were noted in rats and mice as lomefloxacin doses were increased.

STUDIES 1, 2, AND 3

U.S. AND CANADIAN STUDIES				
	Lomefloxacin 3-Day Treatment	Norfloxacin 3-Day Treatment	Ofloxacin 3-Day Treatment	Trimethoprim/ sulfamethoxazole 10-Day Treatment
E coli	133/135 (99%)	36/39 (92%)	65/67 (97%)	33/34 (97%)
K pneumoniae	7/7 (100%)	2/2 (100%)	4/4 (100%)	2/2 (100%)
P mirabilis	8/8 (100%)	1/1 (100%)	2/2 (100%)	1/1 (100%)
S saprophyticus	11/11 (100%)	3/3 (100%)	1/1 (100%)	0/0

SWEDISH STUDY			
	Lomefloxacin 3-Day Treatment	Lomefloxacin 7-Day Treatment	Norfloxacin 7-Day Treatment
E coli	101/109 (93%)	102/104 (98%)	108/110 (98%)
K pneumoniae	2/2 (100%)	5/5 (100%)	1/1 (100%)
P mirabilis	0/0	6/6 (100%)	4/4 (100%)
S saprophyticus	11/17 (65%)	23/23 (100%)	16/16 (100%)

DOSAGE AND ADMINISTRATION

Maxaquin (lomefloxacin HCl) may be taken without regard to meals. Risk of reaction to solar UVA light may be reduced by taking Maxaquin at least 12 hours before exposure to the sun (eg, in the evening). (See **Clinical Pharmacology**.) See **Indications and Usage** for information on appropriate pathogens and patient populations.

Treatment:

Patients with normal renal function: The recommended daily dose of Maxaquin is described in the following chart: [See table at top of previous page]

Elderly patients: No dosage adjustment is needed for elderly patients with normal renal function ($Cl_{Cr} \geq 40$ mL/min/1.73 m^2).

Patients with impaired renal function: Lomefloxacin is primarily eliminated by renal excretion. (See **Clinical Pharmacology**.) Modification of dosage is recommended in patients with renal dysfunction. In patients with a creatinine clearance > 10 mL/min/1.73 m^2 but < 40 mL/min/1.73 m^2, the recommended dosage is an initial loading dose of 400 mg followed by daily maintenance doses of 200 mg (1/2 tablet) once daily for the duration of treatment. It is suggested that serial determinations of lomefloxacin levels be performed to determine any necessary alteration in the appropriate next dosing interval.

If only the serum creatinine is known, the following formula may be used to estimate creatinine clearance.

Men: $$\frac{(\text{weight in kg}) \times (140 - \text{age})}{(72) \times \text{serum creatinine (mg/dL)}}$$

Women: $(0.85) \times$ (calculated value for men)

Dialysis patients: Hemodialysis removes only a negligible amount of lomefloxacin (3% in 4 hours). Hemodialysis patients should receive an initial loading dose of 400 mg followed by daily maintenance doses of 200 mg (1/2 tablet) once daily for the duration of treatment.

Patients with cirrhosis: Cirrhosis does not reduce the non-renal clearance of lomefloxacin. The need for a dosage reduction in this population should be based on the degree of renal function of the patient and on the plasma concentrations. (See **Clinical Pharmacology** and **Dosage and Administration–***Patients with impaired renal function.*)

Prevention/prophylaxis:

The recommended dose of Maxaquin is described in the following chart:

Procedure	Dose	Oral Administration
Transrectal prostate biopsy	400 mg single dose	1–6 hours prior to procedure
Transurethral surgical procedures*	400 mg single dose	2–6 hours prior to procedure

* When preoperative prophylaxis is considered appropriate.

HOW SUPPLIED

Maxaquin (lomefloxacin HCl) is supplied as a scored, film-coated tablet containing the equivalent of 400 mg of lomefloxacin base present as the hydrochloride. The tablet is oval, white, and film-coated with "MAXAQUIN 400" debossed on one side and scored on the other side and is supplied in:

NDC Number	Size
0051-1651-02	bottle of 20
0051-1651-32	carton of 100 unit dose

Store at 59° to 77°F (15° to 25°C).

Caution: Federal law prohibits dispensing without prescription.

CLINICAL STUDIES—UNCOMPLICATED CYSTITIS

In three controlled clinical studies of uncomplicated cystitis in females, two performed in the United States and one in Canada, lomefloxacin was compared to other oral antimicrobial agents. In these studies, using very strict evaluability criteria and microbiological criteria at 5–9 days post-therapy follow-up, the following bacterial eradication outcomes were obtained:

[See first table above]

STUDY 4

In a controlled clinical study of uncomplicated cystitis performed in Sweden, lomefloxacin 3-day treatment was compared with lomefloxacin 7-day treatment and norfloxacin 7-day treatment. In this study, using very strict evaluability criteria and microbiological criteria at 5–9 days post-therapy follow-up, the following bacterial eradication outcomes were obtained:

[See second table above]

ANIMAL PHARMACOLOGY

Lomefloxacin and other quinolones have been shown to cause arthropathy in juvenile animals. Arthropathy, involving multiple diarthrodial joints, was observed in juvenile dogs administered lomefloxacin at doses as low as 4.5 mg/kg for 7 to 8 days (0.3 times the recommended human dose based on mg/m^2 or 0.6 times the recommended human dose based on mg/kg). In juvenile rats, no changes were observed in the joints with doses up to 91 mg/kg for 7 days (2 times the recommended human dose based on mg/m^2 or 11 times the recommended human dose based on mg/kg). (See **Warnings**.)

In a 13-week oral rat study, gamma globulin decreased when lomefloxacin was administered at less than the recommended human exposure. Beta globulin decreased when lomefloxacin was administered at 0.6 to 2 times the recommended human dose based on mg/m^2. The A/G ratio increased when lomefloxacin was administered at 6 to 20 times the human dose. Following a 4-week recovery period, beta globulins in the females and A/G ratios in the females returned to control values. Gamma globulin values in the females and beta and gamma globulins and A/G ratios in the males were still statistically significantly different from control values. No effects on globulins were seen in oral studies in dogs or monkeys in the limited number of specimens collected.

Twenty-seven NSAIDs, administered concomitantly with lomefloxacin, were tested for seizure induction in mice at approximately 2 times the recommended human dose based on mg/m^2. At a dose of lomefloxacin equivalent to the recommended human exposure based on mg/m^2 (10 times the human dose based on mg/kg), only fenbufen, when coadministered, produced an increase in seizures.

Crystalluria and ocular toxicity, seen with some related quinolones, were not observed in any lomefloxacin-treated animals, either in studies designed to look for these effects specifically or in subchronic and chronic toxicity studies in rats, dogs, and monkeys.

Long-term, high-dose systemic use of other quinolones in experimental animals has caused lenticular opacities; however, this finding was not observed with lomefloxacin.

REFERENCES

1. National Committee for Clinical Laboratory Standards, *Performance Standards for Antimicrobial Disk Susceptibility Tests*–4th ed. Approved Standard NCCLS Document M2–A4, vol 10, No. 7, NCCLS, Villanova, Pa, 1990. **2.** National Committee for Clinical Laboratory Standards. *Methods for Dilution Antimicrobial Susceptibility Tests for Bacteria that Grow Aerobically*–2nd ed. Approved Standard NCCLS Document M7–A2, vol 10, No. 8 NCCLS, Villanova, PA, 1990.

8/7/97 · A05229-1

Manufactured for
Unimed Pharmaceuticals, Inc.
Buffalo Grove IL 60089
by Searle & Co.
San Juan PR 00936
Maxaquin is a registered trademark of G.D. Searle & Co.
Shown in Product Identification Guide, page 341

Upsher-Smith Laboratories, Inc.

14905 23RD AVE. NORTH
MINNEAPOLIS, MN 55447

For Medical Information Contact:
Write: Professional Services Department
or call: (800) 654-2299
(during business hours-8:00 am to 5:00 pm CST)

AMLACTIN™ 12% OTC
[ăm'-lăk-tĭn]
Cosmetic Lotion and Cream

DESCRIPTION

AMLACTIN™ Lotion and Cream are a special formulation of 12% lactic acid, neutralized with ammonium hydroxide to form ammonium lactate, that provides a lotion pH of 4.5-5.5. Lactic acid, an alpha-hydroxy acid, has been reported as an effective, naturally occurring humectant in the skin. It has beneficial effects on dry, scaly skin and itching associated with this condition.

HOW SUPPLIED

225g (8oz) plastic bottle: List No. 0245-0023-22
400g (14 oz) plastic bottle: List No. 0245-0023-40
140g (4.9 oz) tube: List No. 0245-0024-14

KLOR–CON® POWDER Rx
[klōr 'kon]
Potassium Chloride for Oral Solution, USP
20 mEq (1.5 g) per packet

DESCRIPTION

Each packet contains 1.5 g potassium chloride providing potassium 20 mEq and chloride 20 mEq. Fruit-flavored with artificial color and sweetener (saccharin) added.

HOW SUPPLIED

KLOR-CON® Powder 20 mEq: Cartons of 30 and 100 packets.
30's NDC 0245-0035-30, 100's NDC 0245-0035-01

KLOR-CON®/25 POWDER Rx
[klōr 'kon]
Potassium Chloride for Oral Solution, USP
25 mEq (1.875 g) per packet

DESCRIPTION

Each packet contains 1.875 g potassium chloride providing potassium 25 mEq and chloride 25 mEq. Fruit-flavored with artificial color and sweetener (saccharin) added.

HOW SUPPLIED

KLOR-CON®/25 Powder 25 mEq:
Cartons of 30, 100 and 250 packets.
30's NDC 0245-0037-30, 100's NDC 0245-0037-01
250's NDC 0245-0037-25 .

KLOR–CON® 8/KLOR–CON® 10 Rx
[klōr 'kon]
Potassium Chloride
Extended–release Tablets, USP
8 mEq and 10 mEq

DESCRIPTION

KLOR-CON® Extended-release Tablets, USP are a solid oral dosage form of potassium chloride. Each contains 600 mg or 750 mg of potassium chloride equivalent to 8 mEq or 10 mEq of potassium in a wax matrix tablet. This formulation is intended to slow the release of potassium so that the likelihood of a high localized concentration of potassium chloride within the gastrointestinal tract is reduced.

HOW SUPPLIED

Film coated, Klor-Con 8 (blue), Klor-Con 10 (yellow), imprinted round tablets containing:
600 mg potassium chloride (equivalent to 8 mEq) in bottles of 100 (NDC 0245-0040-11), bottles of 500 (NDC 0245-0040-15), unit-dose packages of 100 (NDC 0245-0040-01), bulk packs of 5,000 for repack only (NDC 0245-0040-55), and bulk packs of 10,000 for repack only (NDC 0245-0040-00);
750 mg potassium chloride (equivalent to 10 mEq) in bottles of 100 (NDC 0245-0041-11), bottles of 500 (NDC 0245-0041-15), unit-dose packages of 100 (NDC 0245-0041-01), bulk packs of 5,000 for repack only (NDC 0245-0041-55), and bulk packs of 10,000 for repack only (NDC 0245-0041-00).
Shown in Product Identification Guide, page 341

KLOR-CON®/EF 25mEq Rx
[klōr 'kon]
Potassium Bicarbonate Effervescent Tablets for Oral Solution, USP

DESCRIPTION

Each effervescent tablet in solution provides 25 mEq (978 mg) potassium as bicarbonate and citrate. Fruit-flavored with artificial color and sweetener (saccharin) added.

HOW SUPPLIED

KLOR-CON®/EF 25 mEq effervescent tablets in cartons of 30 and 100 individually wrapped tablets.
30's NDC 0245-0039-30, 100's NDC 0245-0039-01

NIACOR® Rx
[nī 'ă-kōr]
NIACIN TABLETS, USP
500 mg

DESCRIPTION

Niacin or nicotinic acid, a water-soluble B complex vitamin and antihyperlipidemic agent, is 3-pyridinecarboxylic acid. Each NIACOR® tablet, for oral administration, contains 500 mg of nicotinic acid.

HOW SUPPLIED

NIACOR® is available in bottles of 100 tablets (NDC 0245-0067-11).

OMS® Concentrate Ⓒ Rx
Morphine Sulfate (Immediate-release) Concentrated Oral Solution, 20 mg per ml

DESCRIPTION

Each ml of OMS® Concentrate contains:
Morphine Sulfate .... 20 mg
(WARNING: May be habit forming)

HOW SUPPLIED

NDC 0245–0167–31: Bottle of 30 ml with calibrated dropper.
NDC 0245–0167–04: Bottle of 120 ml with calibrated dropper.
DEA ORDER FORM REQUIRED

PACERONE® Rx
[pă-sĕ-rōn]
(Amiodarone HCl)
Tablets, 200 mg

DESCRIPTION

Pacerone® (Amiodarone HCl) is a member of a new class of antiarrhythmic drugs with predominantly Class III (Vaughan Williams' classification) effects, available for oral administration as pink, scored tablets containing 200 mg of amiodarone hydrochloride. The inactive ingredients present are lactose monohydrate, magnesium stearate, povidone, pregelatinized corn starch, sodium starch glycolate, stearic acid, FD&C Red 40 and FD&C Yellow 6.

Amiodarone hydrochloride, the active ingredient in Pacerone®, is a benzofuran derivative: 2-butyl-3-benzofuranyl 4-[2-(diethylamino)-ethoxy]-3,5-diiodophenyl ketone, hydrochloride. It is not chemically related to any other available antiarrhythmic drug.
The structural formula is as follows:

$C_{25}H_{29}I_2NO_3 \cdot HCl$ Molecular Weight: 681.8

Amiodarone HCl is a white to cream-colored crystalline powder. It is slightly soluble in water, soluble in alcohol, and freely soluble in chloroform. It contains 37.3% iodine by weight.

CLINICAL PHARMACOLOGY

ELECTROPHYSIOLOGY/MECHANISMS OF ACTION
In animals, amiodarone HCl is effective in the prevention or suppression of experimentally induced arrhythmias. The antiarrhythmic effect of amiodarone may be due to at least two major properties: 1) a prolongation of the myocardial cell-action potential duration and refractory period and 2) noncompetitive alpha- and beta-adrenergic inhibition.
Amiodarone prolongs the duration of the action potential of all cardiac fibers while causing minimal reduction of dV/dt (maximal upstroke velocity of the action potential). The refractory period is prolonged in all cardiac tissues. Amiodarone increases the cardiac refractory period without influencing resting membrane potential, except in automatic cells where the slope of the prepotential is reduced, generally reducing automaticity. These electrophysiologic effects are reflected in a decreased sinus rate of 15 to 20%, increased PR and QT intervals of about 10%, the development of U-waves, and changes in T-wave contour. These changes should not require discontinuation of Pacerone® as they are evidence of its pharmacological action, although amiodarone can cause marked sinus bradycardia or sinus arrest and heart block. On rare occasions, QT prolongation has been associated with worsening of arrhythmia (see "**WARNINGS**").
HEMODYNAMICS
In animal studies and after intravenous administration in man, amiodarone relaxes vascular smooth muscle, reduces peripheral vascular resistance (afterload), and slightly increases cardiac index. After oral dosing, however, amiodarone produces no significant change in left ventricular ejection fraction (LVEF), even in patients with depressed LVEF. After acute intravenous dosing in man, amiodarone may have a mild negative inotropic effect.
PHARMACOKINETICS
Following oral administration in man, amiodarone is slowly and variably absorbed. The bioavailability of amiodarone is approximately 50%, but has varied between 35 and 65% in various studies. Maximum plasma concentrations are attained 3 to 7 hours after a single dose. Despite this, the onset of action may occur in 2 to 3 days, but more commonly takes 1 to 3 weeks, even with loading doses. Plasma concentrations with chronic dosing at 100 to 600 mg/day are approximately dose proportional, with a mean 0.5 mg/L increase for each 100 mg/day. These means, however, include considerable individual variability.
Amiodarone has a very large but variable volume of distribution, averaging about 60 L/kg, because of extensive accumulation in various sites, especially adipose tissue and highly perfused organs, such as the liver, lung, and spleen. One major metabolite of amiodarone, desethylamiodarone, has been identified in man; it accumulates to an even greater extent in almost all tissues. The pharmacological activity of this metabolite, however, is not known. During chronic treatment, the plasma ratio of metabolite to parent compound is approximately one.
The main route of elimination is via hepatic excretion into bile, and some enterohepatic recirculation may occur. However, its kinetics in patients with hepatic insufficiency have not been elucidated. Amiodarone has a very low plasma clearance with negligible renal excretion, so that it does not appear necessary to modify the dose in patients with renal failure. In patients with renal impairment, the plasma concentration of amiodarone is not elevated. Neither amiodarone nor its metabolite is dialyzable.
In patients, following discontinuation of chronic oral therapy, amiodarone has been shown to have a biphasic elimination with an initial one-half reduction of plasma levels after 2.5 to 10 days. A much slower terminal plasma-elimination phase shows a half-life of the parent compound ranging from 26 to 107 days, with a mean of approximately 53 days and most patients in the 40- to 55-day range. In the absence of a loading-dose period, steady-state plasma concentrations, at constant oral dosing, would therefore be reached beween 130 and 535 days, with an average of 265 days. For the metabolite, the mean plasma-elimination half-life was approximately 61 days. These data probably reflect an initial elimination of drug from well-perfused tissue (the 2.5- to 10-day half-life phase), followed by a terminal phase representing extremely slow elimination from poorly perfused tissue compartments such as fat.
The considerable intersubject variation in both phases of elimination, as well as uncertainty as to what compartment is critical to drug effect, requires attention to individual responses once arrhythmia control is achieved with loading doses because the correct maintenance dose is determined, in part, by the elimination rates. Daily maintenance doses of Pacerone® should be based on individual patient requirements (see "**DOSAGE AND ADMINISTRATION**").
Amiodarone and its metabolite have a limited transplacental transfer of approximately 10 to 50%. The parent drug and its metabolite have been detected in breast milk.
Amiodarone is highly protein-bound (approximately 96%).

Continued on next page

Pacerone—Cont.

Although electrophysiologic effects, such as prolongation of QTc, can be seen within hours after a parenteral dose of amiodarone, effects on abnormal rhythms are not seen before 2 to 3 days and usually require 1 to 3 weeks, even when a loading dose is used. There may be a continued increase in effect for longer periods still. There is evidence that the time to effect is shorter when a loading-dose regimen is used. Consistent with the slow rate of elimination, antiarrhythmic effects persist for weeks or months after Pacerone® is discontinued, but the time of recurrence is variable and unpredictable. In general, when the drug is resumed after recurrence of the arrhythmia, control is established relatively rapidly compared to the initial response, presumably because tissue stores were not wholly depleted at the time of recurrence.

PHARMACODYNAMICS

There is no well-established relationship of plasma concentration to effectiveness, but it does appear that concentrations much below 1 mg/L are often ineffective and that levels above 2.5 mg/L are generally not needed. Within individuals, dose reductions and ensuing decreased plasma concentrations can result in loss of arrhythmia control. Plasma-concentration measurements can be used to identify patients whose levels are unusually low, and who might benefit from a dose increase, or unusually high, and who might have dosage reduction in the hope of minimizing side effects. Some observations have suggested a plasma concentration, dose, or dose/duration relationship for side effects such as pulmonary fibrosis, liver-enzyme elevations, corneal deposits and facial pigmentation, peripheral neuropathy, gastrointestinal and central nervous system effects.

MONITORING EFFECTIVENESS

Predicting the effectiveness of any antiarrhythmic agent in long-term prevention of recurrent ventricular tachycardia and ventricular fibrillation is difficult and controversial, with highly qualified investigators recommending use of ambulatory monitoring, programmed electrical stimulation with various stimulation regimens, or a combination of these, to assess response. There is no present consensus on many aspects of how best to assess effectiveness, but there is a reasonable consensus of some aspects:
1. If a patient with a history of cardiac arrest does not manifest a hemodynamically unstable arrhythmia during electrocardiographic monitoring prior to treatment, assessment of the effectiveness of amiodarone requires some provocative approach, either exercise or programmed electrical stimulation (PES).
2. Whether provocation is also needed in patients who do manifest their life-threatening arrhythmia spontaneously is not settled, but there are reasons to consider PES or other provocation in such patients. In the fraction of patients whose PES-inducible arrhythmia can be made noninducible by amiodarone (a fraction that has varied widely in various series from less than 10% to almost 40%, perhaps due to different stimulation criteria), the prognosis has been almost uniformly excellent, with very low recurrence (ventricular tachycardia or sudden death) rates. More controversial is the meaning of continued inducibility. There has been an impression that continued inducibility in amiodarone patients may not foretell a poor prognosis but, in fact, many observers have found greater recurrence rates in patients who remain inducible than in those who do not. A number of criteria have been proposed, however, for identifying patients who remain inducible but who seem likely nonetheless to do well on Pacerone®. These criteria include increased difficulty of induction (more stimuli or more rapid stimuli), which has been reported to predict a lower rate of recurrence, and ability to tolerate the induced ventricular tachycardia without severe symptoms, a finding that has been reported to correlate with better survival but not with lower recurrence rates. While these criteria require confirmation and further study in general, *easier* inducibility or *poorer* tolerance of the induced arrhythmia should suggest consideration of a need to revise treatment.

Several predictors of success not based on PES have also been suggested, including complete elimination of all non-sustained ventricular tachycardia on ambulatory monitoring and very low premature ventricular-beat rates (less than 1 VPB/1,000 normal beats).

While these issues remain unsettled for amiodarone, as for other agents, the prescriber of Pacerone® should have access to (direct or through referral), and familiarity with, the full range of evaluatory procedures used in the care of patients with life-threatening arrhythmias.

It is difficult to describe the effectiveness rates of Pacerone®, as these depend on the specific arrhythmia treated, the success criteria used, the underlying cardiac disease of the patient, the number of drugs tried before resorting to Pacerone®, the duration of follow-up, the dose of amiodarone HCl, the use of additional antiarrhythmic agents, and many other factors. As amiodarone has been studied principally in patients with refractory life-threatening ventricular arrhythmias, in whom drug therapy must be selected on the basis of response and cannot be assigned arbitrarily, randomized comparisons with other agents or placebo have not been possible. Reports of series of treated patients with a history of cardiac arrest and mean follow-up of one year or more have given mortality (due to arrhythmia) rates that were highly variable, ranging from less than 5% to over 30%, with most series in the range of 10 to 15%. Overall arrhythmia-recurrence rates (fatal and nonfatal) also were highly variable (and, as noted above, depended on response to PES and other measures), and depend on whether patients who do not seem to respond initially are included. In most cases, considering only patients who seemed to respond well enough to be placed on long-term treatment, recurrence rates have ranged from 20 to 40% in series with a mean follow-up of a year or more.

INDICATIONS AND USAGE

Because of the life-threatening side effects and the substantial management difficulties associated with amiodarone use (see "WARNINGS" below), Pacerone® (Amiodarone HCl) is indicated only for the treatment of the following documented, life-threatening recurrent ventricular arrhythmias when these have not responded to documented adequate doses of other available antiarrhythmics or when alternative agents could not be tolerated.
1. Recurrent ventricular fibrillation.
2. Recurrent hemodynamically unstable ventricular tachycardia.

As is the case for other antiarrhythmic agents, there is no evidence from controlled trials that the use of amiodarone HCl favorably affects survival.

Pacerone® (Amiodarone HCl) should be used only by physicians familiar with and with access to (directly or through referral) the use of all available modalities for treating recurrent life-threatening ventricular arrhythmias, and who have access to appropriate monitoring facilities, including in-hospital and ambulatory continuous electrocardiographic monitoring and electrophysiologic techniques.

Because of the life-threatening nature of the arrhythmias treated, potential interactions with prior therapy, and potential exacerbation of the arrhythmia, initiation of therapy with Pacerone® should be carried out in the hospital.

CONTRAINDICATIONS

Pacerone® is contraindicated in severe sinus-node dysfunction, causing marked sinus bradycardia; second- and third-degree atrioventricular block; and when episodes of bradycardia have caused syncope (except when used in conjunction with a pacemaker).

Pacerone® is contraindicated in patients with a known hypersensitivity to the drug.

WARNINGS

> Pacerone® is intended for use only in patients with the indicated life-threatening arrhythmias because its use is accompanied by substantial toxicity.
>
> Amiodarone has several potentially fatal toxicities, the most important of which is pulmonary toxicity (hypersensitivity pneumonitis or interstitial/alveolar pneumonitis) that has resulted in clinically manifest disease at rates as high as 10 to 17% in some series of patients with ventricular arrhythmias given doses around 400 mg/day, and as abnormal diffusion capacity without symptoms in a much higher percentage of patients. Pulmonary toxicity has been fatal about 10% of the time. Liver injury is common with amiodarone, but is usually mild and evidenced only by abnormal liver enzymes. Overt liver disease can occur, however, and has been fatal in a few cases. Like other antiarrhythmics, amiodarone can exacerbate the arrhythmia, e.g., by making the arrhythmia less well tolerated or more difficult to reverse. This has occurred in 2 to 5% of patients in various series, and significant heart block or sinus bradycardia has been seen in 2 to 5%. All of these events should be manageable in the proper clinical setting in most cases. Although the frequency of such proarrhythmic events does not appear greater with amiodarone than with many other agents used in this population, the affects are prolonged when they occur. Even in patients at high risk of arrhythmic death, in whom the toxicity of amiodarone is an acceptable risk, Pacerone® poses major management problems that could be life-threatening in a population at risk of sudden death, so that every effort should be made to utilize alternative agents first.
>
> The difficulty of using Pacerone® effectively and safely itself poses a significant risk to patients. Patients with the indicated arrhythmias must be hospitalized while the loading dose of Pacerone® is given, and a response generally requires at least one week, usually two or more. Because absorption and elimination are variable, maintenance-dose selection is difficult, and it is not unusual to require dosage decrease or discontinuation of treatment. In a retrospective survey of 192 patients with ventricular tachyarrhythmias, 84 required dose reduction and 18 required at least temporary discontinu-

ation because of adverse effects, and several series have reported 15 to 20% overall frequencies of discontinuation due to adverse reactions. The time at which a previously controlled life-threatening arrhythmia will recur after discontinuation or dose adjustment is unpredictable, ranging from weeks to months. The patient is obviously at great risk during this time and may need prolonged hospitalization. Attempts to substitute other antiarrhythmic agents when Pacerone® must be stopped will be made difficult by the gradually, but unpredictably, changing amiodarone body burden. A similar problem exists when amiodarone is not effective; it still poses the risk of an interaction with whatever subsequent treatment is tried.

MORTALITY

In the National Heart, Lung and Blood Institute's Cardiac Arrhythmia Suppression Trial (CAST), a long-term, multi-centered, randomized, double-blind study in patients with asymptomatic non-life-threatening ventricular arrhythmias who had had myocardial infarctions more than six days but less than two years previously, an excessive mortality or non-fatal cardiac arrest rate was seen in patients treated with encainide or flecainide (56/730) compared with that seen in patients assigned to matched placebo-treated groups (22/725). The average duration of treatment with encainide or flecainide in this study was ten months.

The applicability of these results to other populations (e.g., those without recent myocardial infarctions) or to amiodarone-treated patients is uncertain. While definitive controlled trials with amiodarone are in progress, pooled analysis of small controlled studies in patients with structural heart disease (including post-myocardial infarction) have not shown excess mortality in the amiodarone-treated population.

PULMONARY TOXICITY

Amiodarone may cause a clinical syndrome of cough and progressive dyspnea accompanied by functional, radiographic, gallium-scan, and pathological data consistent with pulmonary toxicity, the frequency of which varies from 2 to 7% in most published reports, but is as high as 10 to 17% in some reports. Therefore, when Pacerone® therapy is initiated, a baseline chest X-ray and pulmonary-function tests, including diffusion capacity, should be performed. The patient should return for a history, physical exam, and chest X-ray every 3 to 6 months.

Preexisting pulmonary disease does not appear to increase the risk of developing pulmonary toxicity; however, these patients have a poorer prognosis if pulmonary toxicity does develop.

Pulmonary toxicity secondary to amiodarone seems to result from either indirect or direct toxicity as represented by hypersensitivity pneumonitis or interstitial/alveolar pneumonitis, respectively.

Hypersensitivity pneumonitis usually appears earlier in the course of therapy, and rechallenging these patients with Pacerone® results in a more rapid recurrence of greater severity. Bronchoalveolar lavage is the procedure of choice to confirm this diagnosis, which can be made when a T suppressor/cytotoxic (CD8-positive) lymphocytosis is noted. Steroid therapy should be instituted and Pacerone® therapy discontinued in these patients.

Interstitial/alveolar pneumonitis may result from the release of oxygen radicals and/or phospholipidosis and is characterized by findings of diffuse alveolar damage, interstitial pneumonitis or fibrosis in lung biopsy specimens. Phospholipidosis (foamy cells, foamy macrophages), due to inhibition of phospholipase, will be present in most cases of amiodarone-induced pulmonary toxicity; however, these changes also are present in approximately 50% of all patients on amiodarone therapy. These cells should be used as markers of therapy, but not as evidence of toxicity. A diagnosis of amiodarone-induced interstitial/alveolar pneumonitis should lead, at a minimum, to dose reduction or, preferably, to withdrawal of the Pacerone® to establish reversibility, especially if other acceptable antiarrhythmic therapies are available. Where these measures have been instituted, a reduction in symptoms of amiodarone-induced pulmonary toxicity was usually noted within the first week, and a clinical improvement was greatest in the first two to three weeks. Chest X-ray changes usually resolve within two to four months. According to some experts, steroids may prove beneficial.

Prednisone in doses of 40 to 60 mg/day or equivalent doses of other steroids have been given and tapered over the course of several weeks depending upon the condition of the patient. In some cases rechallenge with amiodarone at a lower dose has not resulted in return of toxicity. Recent reports suggest that the use of lower loading and maintenance doses of amiodarone are associated with a decreased incidence of amiodarone-induced pulmonary toxicity.

In a patient receiving Pacerone®, any new respiratory symptoms should suggest the possibility of pulmonary toxicity, and the history, physical exam, chest X-ray, and pulmonary-function tests (with diffusion capacity) should be repeated and evaluated. A 15% decrease in diffusion capacity

has a high sensitivity but only a moderate specificity for pulmonary toxicity; as the decrease in diffusion capacity approaches 30%, the sensitivity decreases but the specificity increases. A gallium scan also may be performed as part of the diagnostic workup.

Fatalities, secondary to pulmonary toxicity, have occurred in approximately 10% of cases. However, in patients with life-threatening arrhythmias, discontinuation of Pacerone® therapy due to suspected drug-induced pulmonary toxicity should be undertaken with caution, as the most common cause of death in these patients is sudden cardiac death. Therefore, every effort should be made to rule out other causes of respiratory impairment (i.e., congestive heart failure with Swan-Ganz catheterization if necessary, respiratory infection, pulmonary embolism, malignancy, etc.) before discontinuing Pacerone® in these patients. In addition, bronchoalveolar lavage, trans-bronchial lung biopsy and/or open lung biopsy may be necessary to confirm the diagnosis, especially in those cases where no acceptable alternative therapy is available.

If a diagnosis of amiodarone-induced hypersensitivity pneumonitis is made, Pacerone® should be discontinued, and treatment with steroids should be instituted. If a diagnosis of amiodarone-induced interstitial/alveolar pneumonitis is made, steroid therapy should be instituted and, preferably, Pacerone® discontinued or, at a minimum, reduced in dosage. Some cases of amiodarone-induced interstitial/alveolar pneumonitis may resolve following a reduction in Pacerone® dosage in conjunction with the administration of steroids. In some patients, rechallenge at a lower dose has not resulted in return of interstitial/alveolar pneumonitis; however, in some patients (perhaps because of severe alveolar damage) the pulmonary lesions have not been reversible.

WORSENED ARRHYTHMIA

Amiodarone, like other antiarrhythmics, can cause serious exacerbation of the presenting arrhythmia, a risk that may be enhanced by the presence of concomitant antiarrhythmics. Exacerbation has been reported in about 2 to 5% in most series, and has included new ventricular fibrillation, incessant ventricular tachycardia, increased resistance to cardioversion, and polymorphic ventricular tachycardia associated with QT prolongation (Torsade de Pointes). In addition, amiodarone has caused symptomatic bradycardia or sinus arrest with suppression of escape foci in 2 to 4% of patients.

LIVER INJURY

Elevations of hepatic enzyme levels are seen frequently in patients exposed to amiodarone and in most cases are asymptomatic. If the increase exceeds three times normal, or doubles in a patient with an elevated baseline, discontinuation of Pacerone® or dosage reduction should be considered. In a few cases in which biopsy has been done, the histology has resembled that of alcoholic hepatitis or cirrhosis. Hepatic failure has been a rare cause of death in patients treated with amiodarone.

PREGNANCY: PREGNANCY CATEGORY D

Amiodarone has been shown to be embryotoxic (increased fetal resorption and growth retardation) in the rat when given orally at a dose of 200 mg/kg/day (18 times the maximum recommended maintenance dose). Similar findings have been noted in one strain of mice at a dose of 5 mg/kg/day (approximately 1/2 the maximum recommended maintenance dose) and higher, but not in a second strain nor in the rabbit at doses up to 100 mg/kg/day (9 times the maximum recommended maintenance dose).

Neonatal hypo- or hyperthyroidism

Amiodarone can cause fetal harm when administered to a pregnant woman. Although amiodarone use during pregnancy is uncommon, there have been a small number of published reports of congenital goiter/hypothyroidism and hyperthyroidism. If Pacerone® (Amiodarone HCl) is used during pregnancy, or if the patient becomes pregnant while taking Pacerone®, the patient should be apprised of the potential hazard to the fetus.

In general, Pacerone® should be used during pregnancy only if the potential benefit to the mother justifies the unknown risk to the fetus.

PRECAUTIONS

CORNEAL MICRODEPOSITS; IMPAIRMENT OF VISION

Corneal microdeposits appear in the majority of adults treated with amiodarone. They are usually discernible only by slit-lamp examination, but give rise to symptoms such as visual halos or blurred vision in as many as 10% of patients. Corneal microdeposits are reversible upon reduction of dose or termination of treatment. Asymptomatic microdeposits are not a reason to reduce dose or discontinue treatment.

PHOTOSENSITIVITY

Amiodarone has induced photosensitization in about 10% of patients; some protection may be afforded by the use of sunbarrier creams or protective clothing. During long-term treatment, a blue-gray discoloration of the exposed skin may occur. The risk may be increased in patients of fair complexion or those with excessive sun exposure, and may be related to cumulative dose and duration of therapy.

THYROID ABNORMALITIES

Amiodarone inhibits peripheral conversion of thyroxine (T_4) to triiodothyronine (T_3) and may cause increased thyroxine levels, decreased T_3 levels, and increased levels of inactive reverse T_3 (rT_3) in clinically euthyroid patients. It is also a potential source of large amounts of inorganic iodine. Because of its release of inorganic iodine, or perhaps for other reasons, amiodarone can cause either hypothyroidism or hyperthyroidism. Thyroid function should be monitored prior to treatment and periodically thereafter, particularly in elderly patients, and in any patient with a history of thyroid nodules, goiter, or other thyroid dysfunction. Because of the slow elimination of amiodarone and its metabolites, high plasma iodide levels, altered thyroid function, and abnormal thyroid-function tests may persist for several weeks or even months following Pacerone® withdrawal.

Hypothyroidism has been reported in 2 to 4% of patients in most series, but in 8 to 10% in some series. This condition may be identified by relevant clinical symptoms and particularly by elevated serum TSH levels. In some clinically hypothyroid amiodarone-treated patients, free thyroxine index values may be normal. Hypothyroidism is best managed by Pacerone® dose reduction and/or thyroid hormone supplement. However, therapy must be individualized, and it may be necessary to discontinue Pacerone® in some patients.

Hyperthyroidism occurs in about 2% of patients receiving amiodarone, but the incidence may be higher among patients with prior inadequate dietary iodine intake. Amiodarone-induced hyperthyroidism usually poses a greater hazard to the patient than hypothyroidism because of the possibility of arrhythmia breakthrough or aggravation. In fact, IF ANY NEW SIGNS OF ARRHYTHMIA APPEAR, THE POSSIBILITY OF HYPERTHYROIDISM SHOULD BE CONSIDERED. Hyperthyroidism is best identified by relevant clinical symptoms and signs, accompanied usually by abnormally elevated levels of serum T_3 RIA, and further elevations of serum T_4, and a subnormal serum TSH level (using a sufficiently sensitive TSH assay). The finding of a flat TSH response to TRH is confirmatory of hyperthyroidism and may be sought in equivocal cases. Since arrhythmia breakthroughs may accompany amiodarone-induced hyperthyroidism, aggressive medical treatment is indicated, including, if possible, dose reduction or withdrawal of Pacerone®. The institution of antithyroid drugs, beta-adrenergic blockers and/or temporary corticosteroid therapy may be necessary. The action of antithyroid drugs may be especially delayed in amiodarone-induced thyrotoxicosis because of substantial quantities of preformed thyroid hormones stored in the gland. Radioactive iodine therapy is contraindicated because of the low radioiodine uptake associated with amiodarone-induced hyperthyroidism. Experience with thyroid surgery in this setting is extremely limited, and this form of therapy runs the theoretical risk of inducing thyroid storm. Amiodarone-induced hyperthyroidism may be followed by a transient period of hypothyroidism.

SURGERY

Hypotension Postbypass: Rare occurrences of hypotension upon discontinuation of cardiopulmonary bypass during open-heart surgery in patients receiving amiodarone have been reported. The relationship of this event to Pacerone® therapy is unknown.

Adult Respiratory Distress Syndrome (ARDS): Postoperatively, rare occurrences of ARDS have been reported in patients receiving amiodarone therapy who have undergone either cardiac or noncardiac surgery. Although patients usually responded well to vigorous respiratory therapy, in rare instances the outcome has been fatal. Until further studies have been performed, it is recommended that FiO_2 and the determinants of oxygen delivery to the tissues (e.g., SaO_2, PaO_2) be closely monitored in patients on amiodarone.

LABORATORY TESTS

Elevations in liver enzymes (SGOT and SGPT) can occur. Liver enzymes in patients on relatively high maintenance doses should be monitored on a regular basis. Persistent significant elevations in the liver enzymes or hepatomegaly should alert the physician to consider reducing the maintenance dose of Pacerone® or discontinuing therapy.

Amiodarone alters the results of thyroid-function tests, causing an increase in serum T_4 and serum reverse T_3, and a decline in serum T_3 levels. Despite these biochemical changes, most patients remain clinically euthyroid.

DRUG INTERACTIONS

Although only a small number of drug-drug interactions with amiodarone have been explored formally, most of these have shown such an interaction. The potential for other interactions should be anticipated, particularly for drugs with potentially serious toxicity, such as other antiarrhythmics. If such drugs are needed, their dose should be reassessed and, where appropriate, plasma concentration measured.

In view of the long and variable half-life of amiodarone, potential for drug interactions exists not only with concomitant medication but also with drugs administered after discontinuation of Pacerone®.

Cyclosporine

Concomitant use of amiodarone and cyclosporine has been reported to produce persistently elevated plasma concentrations of cyclosporine resulting in elevated creatinine, despite reduction in dose of cyclosporine.

Digitalis

Administration of amiodarone to patients receiving digoxin therapy regularly results in an increase in the serum digoxin concentration that may reach toxic levels with resultant clinical toxicity. **On initiation of Pacerone®, the need for digitalis therapy should be reviewed and the dose reduced by approximately 50% or discontinued.** If digitalis treatment is continued, serum levels should be closely monitored and patients observed for clinical evidence of toxicity. These precautions probably should apply to digitoxin administration as well.

Anticoagulants

Potentiation of warfarin-type anticoagulant response is almost always seen in patients receiving amiodarone and can result in serious or fatal bleeding. **The dose of the anticoagulant should be reduced by one-third to one-half, and prothrombin times should be monitored closely.**

Antiarrhythmic Agents

Other antiarrhythmic drugs, such as quinidine, procainamide, disopyramide, and phenytoin, have been used concurrently with amiodarone.

There have been case reports of increased steady-state levels of quinidine, procainamide, and phenytoin during concomitant therapy with amiodarone. In general, any added antiarrhythmic drug should be initiated at a lower than usual dose with careful monitoring.

In general, combination of Pacerone® with other antiarrhythmic therapy should be reserved for patients with life-threatening ventricular arrhythmias who are incompletely responsive to a single agent or incompletely responsive to amiodarone. During transfer to Pacerone®, the dose levels of previously administered agents should be reduced by 30 to 50% several days after the addition of Pacerone®, when arrhythmia suppression should be beginning. The continued need for the other antiarrhythmic agent should be reviewed after the effects of amiodarone have been established, and discontinuation ordinarily should be attempted. If the treatment is continued, these patients should be particularly carefully monitored for adverse effects, especially conduction disturbances and exacerbation of tachyarrhythmias, as Pacerone® is continued. In Pacerone® treated patients who require additional antiarrhythmic therapy, the initial dose of such agents should be approximately half of the usual recommended dose.

Pacerone® should be used with caution in patients receiving beta-blocking agents or calcium antagonists because of the possible potentiation of bradycardia, sinus arrest, and AV block; if necessary, Pacerone® can continue to be used after insertion of a pacemaker in patients with severe bradycardia or sinus arrest.

[See table at top of next page]

ELECTROLYTE DISTURBANCES

Since antiarrhythmic drugs may be ineffective or may be arrhythmogenic in patients with hypokalemia, any potassium or magnesium deficiency should be corrected before instituting Pacerone® therapy.

CARCINOGENESIS, MUTAGENESIS, IMPAIRMENT OF FERTILITY

Amiodarone HCl reduced fertility of male and female rats at a dose level of 90 mg/kg/day (8 times highest recommended human maintenance dose).

Amiodarone caused a statistically significant, dose-related increase in the incidence of thyroid tumors (follicular adenoma and/or carcinoma) in rats. The incidence of thyroid tumors was greater than control even at the lowest dose level of amiodarone HCl tested, i.e., 5 mg/kg/day or approximately equal to 1/2 the highest recommended human maintenance dose. Mutagenicity studies (Ames, micronucleus, and lysogenic tests) with amiodarone were negative.

PREGNANCY: PREGNANCY CATEGORY D

See "WARNINGS".

LABOR AND DELIVERY

It is not known whether the use of Pacerone® during labor or delivery has any immediate or delayed adverse effects. Preclinical studies in rodents have not shown any effect of amiodarone on the duration of gestation or on parturition.

NURSING MOTHERS

Amiodarone is excreted in human milk, suggesting that breast-feeding could expose the nursing infant to a significant dose of the drug. Nursing offspring of lactating rats administered amiodarone have been shown to be less viable and have reduced body-weight gains. Therefore, when Pacerone® therapy is indicated, the mother should be advised to discontinue nursing.

PEDIATRIC USE

The safety and effectiveness of Pacerone® in pediatric patients have not been established.

ADVERSE REACTIONS

Adverse reactions have been very common in virtually all series of patients treated with amiodarone HCl for ventricular arrhythmias with relatively large doses of drug (400 mg/day and above), occurring in about three-fourths of all patients and causing discontinuation in 7 to 18%. The most

Continued on next page

Pacerone—Cont.

serious reactions are pulmonary toxicity, exacerbation of arrhythmia, and rare serious liver injury (see "**WARNINGS**"), but other adverse effects constitute important problems. They are often reversible with dose reduction and virtually always reversible with cessation of amiodarone treatment. Most of the adverse effects appear to become more frequent with continued treatment beyond six months, although rates appear to remain relatively constant beyond one year. The time and dose relationships of adverse effects are under continued study.

Neurologic problems are extremely common, occurring in 20 to 40% of patients and including malaise and fatigue, tremor and involuntary movements, poor coordination and gait, and peripheral neuropathy; they are rarely a reason to stop therapy and may respond to dose reductions.

Gastrointestinal complaints, most commonly nausea, vomiting, constipation, and anorexia, occur in about 25% of patients but rarely require discontinuation of drug. These commonly occur during high-dose administration (i.e., loading dose) and usually respond to dose reduction or divided doses.

Asymptomatic corneal microdeposits are present in virtually all adult patients who have been on drug for more than 6 months. Some patients develop eye symptoms of halos, photophobia, and dry eyes. Vision is rarely affected and drug discontinuation is rarely needed.

Dermatological adverse reactions occur in about 15% of patients, with photosensitivity being most common (about 10%). Sunscreen and protection from sun exposure may be helpful, and drug discontinuation is not usually necessary. Prolonged exposure to amiodarone occasionally results in a blue-gray pigmentation. This is slowly and occasionally incompletely reversible on discontinuation of drug but is of cosmetic importance only.

Cardiovascular adverse reactions, other than exacerbation of the arrhythmias, include the uncommon occurrence of congestive heart failure (3%) and bradycardia. Bradycardia usually responds to dosage reduction but may require a pacemaker for control. CHF rarely requires drug discontinuation. Cardiac conduction abnormalities occur infrequently and are reversible on discontinuation of drug.

The following side-effect rates are based on a retrospective study of 241 patients treated for 2 to 1,515 days (mean 441.3 days).

The following side effects were each reported in 10 to 33% of patients:
Gastrointestinal: Nausea and vomiting.

The following side effects were each reported in 4 to 9% of patients:
Dermatologic: Solar dermatitis/photosensitivity.
Neurologic: Malaise and fatigue, tremor/abnormal involuntary movements, lack of coordination, abnormal gait/ataxia, dizziness, paresthesias.
Gastrointestinal: Constipation, anorexia.
Ophthalmologic: Visual disturbances.
Hepatic: Abnormal liver-function tests.
Respiratory: Pulmonary inflammation or fibrosis.

The following side effects were each reported in 1 to 3% of patients:
Thyroid: Hypothyroidism, hyperthyroidism.
Neurologic: Decreased libido, insomnia, headache, sleep disturbances.
Cardiovascular: Congestive heart failure, cardiac arrhythmias, SA node dysfunction.
Gastrointestinal: Abdominal pain.
Hepatic: Nonspecific hepatic disorders.
Other: Flushing, abnormal taste and smell, edema, abnormal salivation, coagulation abnormalities.

The following side effects were each reported in less than 1% of patients:
Blue skin discoloration, rash, spontaneous ecchymosis, alopecia, hypotension, and cardiac conduction abnormalities.

Rare occurrences of hepatitis, cholestatic hepatitis, cirrhosis, optic neuritis, epididymitis, vasculitis, pseudotumor cerebri, and thrombocytopenia have been reported in patients receiving amiodarone.

In surveys of almost 5,000 patients treated in open U.S. studies and in published reports of treatment with amiodarone HCl, the adverse reactions most frequently requiring discontinuation of drug included pulmonary infiltrates of fibrosis, paroxysmal ventricular tachycardia, congestive heart failure, and elevation of liver enzymes. Other symptoms causing discontinuations less often included visual disturbances, solar dermatitis, blue skin discoloration, hyperthyroidism, and hypothyroidism.

SUMMARY OF DRUG INTERACTIONS WITH Pacerone®

Concomitant Drug	Onset (days)	Magnitude	Recommended Dose Reduction of Concomitant Drug
Warfarin	3 to 4	Increases prothrombin time by 100%	↓ 1/3 to 1/2
Digoxin	1	Increases serum concentration by 70%	↓ 1/2
Quinidine	2	Increases serum concentration by 33%	↓ 1/3 to 1/2 (or discontinue)
Procainamide	<7	Increases plasma concentration by 55%; NAPA* concentration by 33%	↓ 1/3 (or discontinue)

*NAPA = n-acetyl procainamide.

OVERDOSAGE

There have been a few reported cases of amiodarone HCl overdose in which 3 to 8 grams were taken. There were no deaths or permanent sequelae. Animal studies indicate that amiodarone HCl has a high oral LD_{50} (>3,000 mg/kg).

In addition to general supportive measures, the patient's cardiac rhythm and blood pressure should be monitored and if bradycardia ensues, a β-adrenergic agonist or a pacemaker may be used. Hypotension with inadequate tissue perfusion should be treated with positive inotropic and/or vasopressor agents. Neither amiodarone nor its metabolite is dialyzable.

DOSAGE AND ADMINISTRATION

BECAUSE OF THE UNIQUE PHARMACOKINETIC PROPERTIES, DIFFICULT DOSING SCHEDULE, AND SEVERITY OF THE SIDE EFFECTS IF PATIENTS ARE IMPROPERLY MONITORED, PACERONE® SHOULD BE ADMINISTERED ONLY BY PHYSICIANS WHO ARE EXPERIENCED IN THE TREATMENT OF LIFE-THREATENING ARRHYTHMIAS WHO ARE THOROUGHLY FAMILIAR WITH THE RISKS AND BENEFITS OF AMIODARONE THERAPY, AND WHO HAVE ACCESS TO LABORATORY FACILITIES CAPABLE OF ADEQUATELY MONITORING THE EFFECTIVENESS AND SIDE EFFECTS OF TREATMENT.

In order to insure that an antiarrhythmic effect will be observed without waiting several months, loading doses are required. A uniform, optimal dosage schedule for administration of Pacerone® has not been determined. Individual patient titration is suggested according to the following guidelines.

For life-threatening ventricular arrhythmias, such as ventricular fibrillation or hemodynamically unstable ventricular tachycardia: Close monitoring of the patients is indicated during the loading phase, particularly until risk of recurrent ventricular tachycardia or fibrillation has abated. Because of the serious nature of the arrhythmia and the lack of predictable time course of effect, loading should be performed in a hospital setting. Loading doses of 800 to 1,600 mg/day are required for 1 to 3 weeks (occasionally longer) until initial therapeutic response occurs. (Administration of Pacerone® in divided doses with meals is suggested for total daily doses of 1,000 mg or higher, or when gastrointestinal intolerance occurs.) If side effects become excessive, the dose should be reduced.

Elimination of recurrence of ventricular fibrillation and tachycardia usually occurs within 1 to 3 weeks, along with reduction in complex and total ventricular ectopic beats.

Upon starting Pacerone® therapy, an attempt should be made to gradually discontinue prior antiarrhythmic drugs (see "**PRECAUTIONS, DRUG INTERACTIONS**"). When adequate arrhythmia control is achieved, or if side effects become prominent, Pacerone® dose should be reduced to 600 to 800 mg/day for one month and then to the maintenance dose, usually 400 mg/day (see "**CLINICAL PHARMACOLOGY**, MONITORING EFFECTIVENESS"). Some patients may require larger maintenance doses, up to 600 mg/day, and some can be controlled on lower doses. Pacerone® may be administered as a single daily dose, or in patients with severe gastrointestinal intolerance, as a b.i.d. dose. In each patient, the chronic maintenance dose should be determined according to antiarrhythmic effect as assessed by symptoms, Holter recordings, and/or programmed electrical stimulation and by patient tolerance. Plasma concentrations may be helpful in evaluating nonresponsiveness or unexpectedly severe toxicity (see "**CLINICAL PHARMACOLOGY**").

The lowest effective dose should be used to prevent the occurrence of side effects. In all instances, the physician must be guided by the severity of the individual patient's arrhythmia and response to therapy.

When dosage adjustments are necessary, the patient should be closely monitored for an extended period of time because of the long and variable half-life of amiodarone and the difficulty in predicting the time required to attain a new steady-state level of drug. Dosage suggestions are summarized below:
[See table below]

HOW SUPPLIED

Pacerone® (Amiodarone HCl) Tablets, 200 mg, are available in bottles of 60 tablets (NDC 0245-0147-60), bottles of 500 tablets (NDC 0245-0147-15), and in unit dose cartons of 100 tablets (10 cards containing 10 tablets each) (NDC 0245-0147-01).

Pacerone® Tablets are pink, round, flat-faced, scored, uncoated tablets, debossed with "P₂₀₀" on the unscored side, and "U-S" above and "0147" below the score on the reverse side.

STORAGE

Store at room temperature, approximately 25°C (77°F). Protect from light and moisture.

Dispense in a tight, light-resistant container with a child-resistant closure.

Rx only.

Manufactured by: UPSHER-SMITH LABORATORIES, INC., Minneapolis, MN 55447

Certain manufacturing operations have been performed by other firms.

Rev. 0398

Shown in Product Identification Guide, page 341

PREVALITE® ℞
[prĕ 'vă līt]
(Cholestyramine for Oral Suspension, USP)

DESCRIPTION

Prevalite® (Cholestyramine for Oral Suspension, USP), the chloride salt of a basic anion exchange resin, a cholesterol-lowering agent, is intended for oral administration.

HOW SUPPLIED

Available in cartons of forty-two and sixty single-dose packets and in cans containing 231 grams. 5.5 grams of Prevalite® contain 4 grams of anhydrous cholestyramine resin.
NDC 0245-0036-42 Cartons of 42, 5.5 g packets
NDC 0245-0036-60 Cartons of 60, 5.5 g packets
NDC 0245-0036-23 Cans, 231 g (42 doses)
Please refer to the *PDR for Generics* for full prescribing information.

RMS® Suppositories ℃ ℞
(Rectal Morphine Sulfate)

DESCRIPTION

Suppositories contain 5, 10, 20, or 30 mg of morphine sulfate. Morphine sulfate suppositories are prepared from a hydrogenated vegetable oil base and other ingredients (contains BHA and BHT as preservatives), and are suitable for rectal administration.

HOW SUPPLIED

RMS® Suppositories are individually sealed in color-coded wrappers to aid in identification. 5 mg suppositories (white

	Loading Dose (Daily)		Adjustment and Maintenance Dose (Daily)		
Ventricular Arrhythmias	1 to 3 weeks		~1 month		usual maintenance
	800 to 1,600 mg		600 to 800 mg		400 mg

wrapper/blue print), NDC 0245-0160-12, 12 per carton. 10 mg suppositories (white wrapper/green print), NDC 0245-0161-12, 12 per carton. 20 mg suppositories (white wrapper/red print), NDC 0245-0162-12, 12 per carton. 30 mg suppositories (white wrapper/gold print), NDC 0245-0163-12, 12 per carton.

DEA ORDER FORM REQUIRED

SSKI®   Rx
Potassium Iodide Oral Solution, USP
(Saturated) 1 g/ml

DESCRIPTION

SSKI® (Potassium Iodide Oral Solution, USP) is a saturated solution of potassium iodide containing 1 g of potassium iodide per ml.

HOW SUPPLIED

SSKI® (Potassium Iodide Oral Solution, USP) is supplied in 1 fluid ounce (30 ml) bottles (NDC 0245-0003-31) with a calibrated dropper marked to deliver 0.3 ml (300 mg) and 0.6 ml (600 mg); and 8 fluid ounce (237 ml) bottles (NDC 0245-0003-08).

Notice: When exposed to cold temperatures, crystallization may occur, but on warming and shaking, the crystals will redissolve. If the solution turns brownish yellow in color, it should be discarded.

SLO–NIACIN® Tablets   OTC
(polygel® controlled-release niacin)
Dietary Supplement

DESCRIPTION

Slo-Niacin® Tablets are manufactured utilizing a unique, patented polygel® controlled-release delivery system. This exclusive technology assures the gradual and measured release of niacin (nicotinic acid) and is designed to reduce the incidence of flushing and itching commonly associated with niacin use. Slo-Niacin® Tablets are available in 250 mg, 500 mg, and 750 mg strengths.

HOW SUPPLIED

250 mg tablets in bottles of 100: List No. 0245–0062–11
500 mg tablets in bottles of 100: List No. 0245–0063–11
750 mg tablets in bottles of 100: List No. 0245–0064–11
U.S. Patent No. 5,126,145 and 5,268,181
Shown in Product Identification Guide, page 341

USANA, Incorporated
3838 WEST PARKWAY BOULEVARD
SALT LAKE CITY, UTAH 84120-6336

Direct Inquiries to:
Ph: (801) 954 7860
Fax: (801) 954 7658

CALMAG PLUS
[kaél maēg plus]

COMPOSITION

Each CalMag Plus tablet contains the following minerals:

Calcium (as citrate)	135 mg
Magnesium (as aminoate*)	90 mg
Silicon (as aminoate*)	2.25 mg
Boron (as aminoate*)	330 mcg
Vitamin D	40 IU

*Amino acid chelate from rice protein

ADVANTAGES

Each table contains a balanced blend of calcium, magnesium, vitamin D, boron and silicon; five nutrients required for bone development, bone remodeling and skeletal health. This non-prescription product meets USP guidelines for potency (as applicable), uniformity and disintegration, and is manufactured according to pharmaceutical cGMP standards.

RECOMMENDED USE

Take 4–8 tablets by mouth daily.

SUPPLIED

Capsule-shaped tablet, mottled greenish-white color, with clear film coating, and with USANA imprint. In bottle of 240 tablets.
Shown in Product Identification Guide, page 341

CHELATED MINERAL
[chē'-latĕd mineral]

COMPOSITION

Each Chelated Mineral contains the following minerals:

Calcium (as citrate)	90 mg
Magnesium (as aminoate*)	100 mg
Zinc (as citrate)	6.7 mg
Manganese (as aminoate*)	1.7 mg
Boron (as aminoate*)	1 mg
Copper (as aminoate*)	1 mg
Chromium (as picolinate)	100 mcg
Iodine (as potassium iodide)	75 mcg
Selenium (as aminoate*)	66.7 mcg
Molybdenum (as aminoate*)	16 mcg
Trace minerals	33 mg

*amino acid chelate from rice protein.

ADVANTAGES

Each tablet contains a complete and balanced blend of essential minerals in bioavailable forms. The Chelated Mineral is designed to be taken with USANA's Mega Antioxidant to provide the full complement of essential nutrients required for health. This non-prescription product meets USP guidelines for potency (as applicable), uniformity and disintegration, and is manufactured according to pharmaceutical cGMP standards.

RECOMMENDED USE

Take 3 tablets by mouth daily, one in the morning and two in the evening.

SUPPLIED

Oblong shaped tablet, off-white color, with clear film coating and with USANA imprint. In bottle of 90 tablets.
Shown in Product Identification Guide, page 341

COQUINONE™
[cokwinōun]

COMPOSITION

Each CoQuinone™ contains the following:

Coenzyme Q10	10 mg
Alpha Lipoic Acid	12.5 mg

ADVANTAGES

CoQuinone™ contains a hydrosoluble form of Coenzyme Q10 (CoQ10) that is 2.5 times more bioavailable than material supplied in dry tablet/capsule formulas. The higher blood levels of CoQ10 supplied enhance mitochondrial production of ATP. CoQ10 is a rate-limiting factor in the electron transport chain involved in mitochondrial production of ATP. It is also involved in neutralizing free radicals generated during ATP production. As such, CoQ10 helps the body maintain healthy skeletal and cardiac muscle. Alpha lipoic acid is included in the formula as a lipid-soluble antioxidant to recycle CoQ10 from the prooxidant form to the antioxidant form. This non-prescription product meets USP guidelines for uniformity and disintegration and is manufactured according to cGMP standards.

RECOMMENDED USE

Take 2 or 3 capsules by mouth daily.

SUPPLIED

Oval shaped, soft gelatin capsule, orange-colored, opaque, imprinted with USANA in white edible ink. Capsules contain an orange colored liquid. In bottle of 60 soft-gel capsules.
Shown in Product Identification Guide, page 341

MEGA ANTIOXIDANT
[mēga aenti-óksid'nt]

COMPOSITION

Each Mega Antioxidant contains the following vitamins and antioxidants:

Beta carotene	5,670 IU
Vitamin C (as Poly C, a blend of calcium, zinc, potassium and magnesium ascorbates)	433 mg
Vitamin D	67 IU
Vitamin E	150 IU
Vitamin K	20 mcg
Vitamin B1 (Thiamine HCl)	9 mg
Vitamin B2 (Riboflavin)	9 mg
Niacin and Niacinamide	13.3 mg
Vitamin B6 (Pyridoxine HCl)	9 mg
Folate	333 mcg
Vitamin B12 (Cyanocobalamin)	20 mcg
Biotin	16.7 mcg
Pantothenic Acid	30 mg
Bioflavonoid Complex (Rutin, Quercetin, Hesperidin, Green Tea Extract, Bilberry Extract)	69.4 mg
Inositol	50 mg
Choline Bitartrate	33.3 mg
Cruciferrous Extract	33.3 mg
N-Acetyl-L-Cysteine	21.7 mg
Para-Aminobenzoic Acid	16.7 mg
Bromelain	16.7 mg
Alpha-Lipoic Acid	5 mg
Coenzyme Q10	4 mg
Reduced Glutathione	3.3 mg
Broccoli Concentrate	3.3 mg
Mixed Carotenoids (Lutein and Zeaxanthin)	67 mcg

ADVANTAGES

A comprehensive and balanced formula containing the essential vitamins and antioxidants at levels substantially higher than RDA amounts. In addition to the traditionally recognized essential nutrients, the formula contains a unique blend of dietary antioxidants including mixed carotenoids, a bioflavonoid complex, cruciferous extracts and a glutathione complex to provide full-spectrum antioxidant protection. This formula is designed to be taken with USANA's Chelated Mineral to provide the full compliment of essential nutrients required for health. This non-prescription product meets USP guidelines for potency (as applicable), uniformity and disintegration, and is manufactured according to pharmaceutical cGMP standards.

RECOMMENDED USE

Three tablets by mouth daily, spread throughout the day, at or near mealtimes.

SUPPLIED

Oblong shaped tablets, mottled orange-brown color, with clear film coating and with USANA imprint. In bottle of 90 tablets.
Shown in Product Identification Guide, page 341

PROFLAVANOL®
[prou fléivanol]

COMPOSITION

Each Proflavanol contains the following:

Vitamin C (Poly C)	100 mg
Grape seed extract	30 mg
Ascorbyl palmitate	12 mg

ADVANTAGES

A potent antioxidant formula combining the proanthocyanidins (bioflavonoids) from standardized grape seed extract with vitamin C in the form of ascorbate salts and ascorbyl palmitate. Proflavanol is designed to be taken as a stand-alone antioxidant, or preferably in combination with USANA's Mega Antioxidant and Chelated Mineral to provide additional antioxidant protection. This non-prescription product meets USP guidelines for uniformity and disintegration and is manufactured according to pharmaceutical cGMP standards.

RECOMMENDED USE

Take 2–4 tablets by mouth daily.

SUPPLIED

Round, buff colored tablet, with clear film coating, without imprint or distinguishing marks. In bottle of 90 tablets.
Shown in Product Identification Guide, page 341

IDENTIFICATION PROBLEM?
Turn to the **Product Identification Guide,**
where you'll find more than
1600 products pictured in actual
size and full color.

Vitaline Corporation

**385 WILLIAMSON WAY
ASHLAND, OR 97520**

Direct Inquiries to:
Jed D. Meese, Technical Director
(800) 648-4755
(541) 482-9231
FAX: (541) 482-9112
E-Mail: jmeese@vitaline.com

L–CARNITINE USP   OTC
250mg Tablets, 500mg Scored Caplets and 500mg Chewable Wafers

L–CARNITINE
500mg Capsules (from 736mg L-Carnitine Tartrate)

DESCRIPTION
Carnitine is a naturally occurring substance, and is essential for fatty acid oxidation and energy production. Without it, long-chain fatty acids cannot cross from cellular cytoplasm into the mitochondria and out again, resulting in loss of energy and toxic accumulations of free fatty acids. Ninety-five percent of the body's carnitine is found in cardiac and skeletal tissue; these muscles rely upon fatty acid oxidation for most of their energy.

INDICATIONS
Dietary supplementation of L-Carnitine for individuals who may benefit from supplementation of this essential nutrient. Renal dialysis patients and individuals with immune system deficiencies may benefit from L-Carnitine supplementation.

WARNINGS
None reported.

SUGGESTED USE
As a dietary supplement: Adults, one gram daily or as directed by physician, registered dietitian or nutritionist. Children, as directed by physician.

HOW SUPPLIED
250mg tablets in bottles of 90 NDC 54022-2100-1
500mg scored caplets in bottles of 30 NDC 54022-2120-1
500mg chewable wafers in bottles of 30 NDC 54022-2700-1
500mg capsules in bottles of 30 NDC 54022-2800-1

REFERENCES
1. Effect of Oral L-Carnitine on Serum Myoglobin in Hemodialysis Patients. *Renal Failure. 18(1):91-96, 1996*
2. Effects of L-Carnitine on Erythrocyte Acyl-CoA, Free CoA, and Glycerophospholipid Acyltransferase in Uremia. Delosreyes B, et al. *American Journal of Clinical Nutrition. 67(3):386–390, March 1998*
3. Carnitine and its Derivatives in Cardiovascular Disease. Arsenian MA, *Progress in Cardiovascular Diseases, 40(3): 265–286, Nov.-Dec. 1997*

COENZYME Q$_{10}$ OTC
(Ubiquinone)
200mg, 100mg & 60mg Chewable Wafers, and 200mg, 60mg & 25mg Tablets

DESCRIPTION
Coenzyme Q$_{10}$ (CoQ$_{10}$) is an essential nutrient that is a co-factor in the mitochondrial electron transport chain, the biochemical pathway in cellular respiration from which ATP and metabolic energy are derived. Since nearly all cellular functions are dependent on energy, CoQ$_{10}$ is essential for the health of all human tissues and organs. The involvement of CoQ$_{10}$ as a redox carrier of the respiratory chain is well established on the basis of both reconstitution studies and kinetic evidence.

In addition to CoQ$_{10}$'s vital role in cellular energy production, it also functions as a powerful, highly effective antioxidant. These functions of CoQ$_{10}$ support normal heart function. Studies show that CoQ$_{10}$ also enhances vitamin E's ability to destroy free radicals.

SUGGESTED USE
As a dietary supplement: Adults, 60mg–200mg daily or as directed by physician or registered dietitian. Children, as directed by physician.

ADVERSE REACTIONS
None reported.

HOW SUPPLIED
Bottles of 30, 60, 500 and 1000.
200mg with 400 I.U. Vitamin E chewable wafers, NDC 54022-2091, 100mg with 300 I.U. Vitamin E chewable wafers, NDC 54022-2090, 60mg chewable wafers, NDC 54022-2085, 200mg tablets, NDC 54022-8002, 60mg tablets, NDC 54022-2081, 25mg tablets, NDC 54022-2055

REFERENCES
1) Introduction to Coenzyme Q$_{10}$. *Langsjoen, Peter H., M.D., F.A.C.C., Tyler, TX 75701, 1996*
2) Coenzyme Q10 Attenuates the 1-methyl-4-phenyl-1-1, 2, 3, 6-tetrahydropyridine (MPTP) Induced Loss of Striatal Dopamine and Dopaminergic Axons in Aged Mice. Beale MF, et al. *Brain Research 783:109–114, 1998*
3) Absorption, Tolerability, and Effects on Mitochondrial Activity of Oral Coenzyme Q10 in Parkinsonian Patients. Shultz C.W., et al. *Neurology, 50:793–795, March 1998*
4) Heart Muscle and Plasma Vitamin Q with Heart Transplantation. *Karlsson J., Semb B., Can J Carol, 13(2):147, February 1997*
5) Neuroprotective Strategies for Treatment of Lesions Produced by Mitochondrial Toxins: Implications for Neurodegenerative Diseases. Beal M.F., et al. *Neuroscience, 71(4): 1043-1048, 1996*

VIVUS, Inc.

**605 EAST FAIRCHILD DRIVE
MOUNTAIN VIEW, CA 94043**

Direct Inquiries to:
(888) 345-6873

For Medical Information or Emergencies Contact:
Medical Services Department @ VIVUS:
(650) 934-5200
(650) 934-5209
FAX: (415) 325-2173

ACTIS®   ℞
[ac-tis]
VENOUS FLOW CONTROLLER

DESCRIPTION
The ACTIS® device is designed to enhance erections by slowing venous outflow from the penis, which aids the normal erection process. The ACTIS device consists of an adjustable elastomeric loop, placed around the base of the penis which allows for a wide range of compression pressures. An O ring and ball-locking unit allow for easy adjustment of tension.

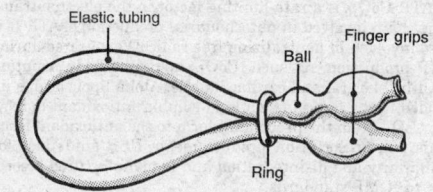

Elastic tubing — Ball — Finger grips — Ring

The ACTIS Device

INDICATIONS AND USAGE
The ACTIS device is indicated for the treatment of erectile dysfunction and is designed to maintain penile rigidity by restricting penile venous outflow.

Blood flows into the penis through arteries deep in the tissues and flows out through the veins near the surface of the penis. The ACTIS device works by closing the veins while allowing blood to flow into the penis, producing an erection.

CONTRAINDICATIONS
- Known hypersensitivity to natural (latex) or synthetic rubber
- Abnormally formed penis
- Men for whom sexual activity is inadvisable
- Conditions that may result in bleeding or long-lasting erections, such as: sickle cell anemia or trait, leukemia, tumor of the bone marrow (multiple myeloma) or conditions that either increase or decrease blood clotting

PRECAUTIONS
- Patients should consult their physician if any complications occur. Discontinue use if such conditions persist.
- Do not fall asleep wearing the ACTIS device. Tension should not be maintained for more than 30 minutes. Prolonged tension may damage the penis.
- Use the least constrictive tension that will maintain an erection. Excessive tension may lead to discomfort and could cause damage to the penis.
- Frequent use or excessive tension of the ACTIS device may result in ecchymosis (i.e. bruising) at the penoscrotal junction.
- Allow 60 minutes between uses.
- Do not use while under the influence of alcohol or drugs.
- The ACTIS device is not a contraceptive (birth control method).

Caution: This Product Contains Natural Rubber Latex Which May Cause Allergic Reactions.

Information for Patients:
Patients should be instructed how to use the ACTIS device. A patient package insert must be given to each patient prior to using the device.

ADVERSE REACTIONS
- Pain or redness of the penis
- Prolonged erection (Please note: If your erection is rigid for more than 4 hours, call your doctor promptly)

TO USE THE ACTIS DEVICE

To stretch the ACTIS device: Grasp the loop of the ACTIS device wih the left hand. Note that the end of the tubing with the ball is on top **(Figure 1)**.

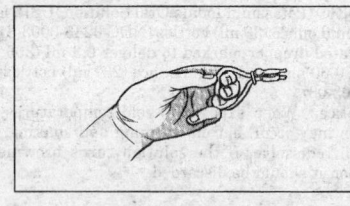

Figure 1

With the right hand, grasp the loop next to the O ring and stretch the ACTIS device **(Figure 2)**.

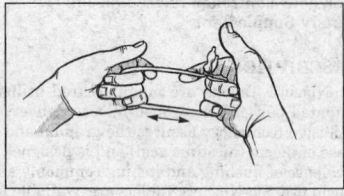

Figure 2

To place around the shaft of the penis: Place the end of the penis through the stretched loop and slide the ACTIS device over the shaft of the penis **(Figure 3)** until it is positioned around the base **(see Figure 5)**.

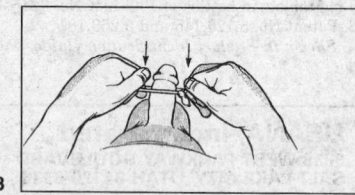

Figure 3

To position the ACTIS device: The ACTIS device should be placed so that the loop encircles the base of the penis. The portion of the tubing with the ball should be on the top side of the penis. Grasp the fingergrip end (lower end) of the tubing without the ball. Pull horizontally away from the penis until the ACTIS device is gently snug around the base of the penis **(Figure 4)**.

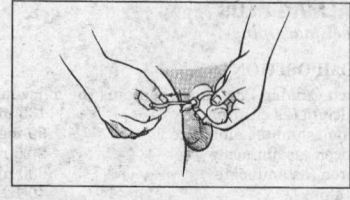

Figure 4

When the ACTIS device is initially positioned, the ends of the tubing should be located on the side of the shaft of the penis with the ball on top.

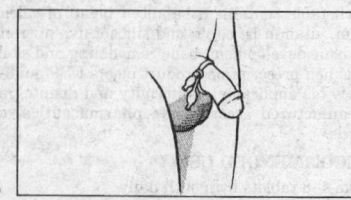

Figure 5

To achieve proper tension: Grasp the fingergrip on the end of the tubing without the ball and pull down **(Figure 6)**. The ACTIS device should be tight enough to keep the blood from leaving the penis. Excessive tension may lead to discomfort and could cause damage to the penis.

If the erection is not rigid enough, massage the area behind the scrotum as this may push more blood into the penis. As the penis becomes erect, the ACTIS device may be tightened or loosened to achieve the desired erection while maintaining maximum comfort.

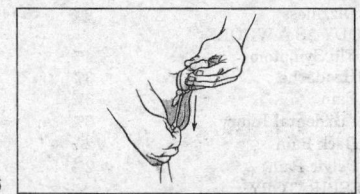

Figure 6

To loosen the tension: After intercourse or if the erection is uncomfortably rigid, the ACTIS device may be loosened by pulling up on the end of the tubing with the ball **(Figure 7)**. Once fully loosened, the ACTIS device can be easily removed by sliding the loop over the end of the penis.

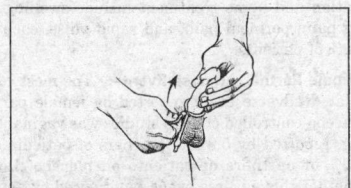

Figure 7

CARE AND REPLACEMENT OF THE ACTIS DEVICE
Care of the ACTIS device: The ACTIS device is designed for multiple use and should be cleaned after use with warm water and ordinary hand soap. Oil-based lubricants may alter the elasticity and should not be used.
Replacement: Repeated use of the ACTIS device may result in deterioration of the tubing. It is recommended that the ACTIS device be replaced after 6 months of use.
Medical information line at VIVUS 1–888–345–6873.
ACTIS is manufactured for VIVUS, Inc., Mountain View, CA 94043
Caution: Federal law restricts this device to sale by or on the order of a physician.
ACTIS® IS A REGISTERED TRADEMARK OF VIVUS, INC. IN THE U.S. AND OTHER COUNTRIES.
VIVUS, Inc.
Mountain View, CA 94043
Shown in Product Identification Guide, page 341

MUSE®   ℞
(alprostadil)
urethral suppository

DESCRIPTION
MUSE® (alprostadil) is a single-use, medicated transurethral system for the delivery of alprostadil to the male urethra. Alprostadil is suspended in polyethylene glycol 1450 (as excipient) and is formed into a medicated pellet (microsuppository) measuring 1.4 mm in diameter by 3 mm or 6 mm in length) that resides in the tip of a translucent hollow applicator. MUSE is administered by inserting the applicator stem into the urethra after urination. The pellet containing alprostadil is delivered by depressing the applicator button (see Figure 1). The components of the delivery system are constructed of medical grade polypropylene. Each MUSE system is packaged in an individual foil pouch.

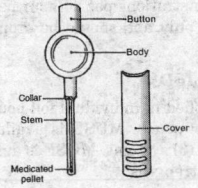

Figure 1: Diagram of the MUSE Transurethral System

Figure 1: Diagram of the MUSE Transurethral System
The active ingredient in MUSE is alprostadil, which is chemically identical to the naturally occurring eicosanoid, prostaglandin E_1 (PGE_1). The chemical name for alprostadil is prost-13-en-1-oic acid, 11,15-dihydroxy-9-oxo-(11α, 13E, 15S)-(1R,2R,3R)-3-hydroxy-2-[(E)-(3S)-3-hydroxy-1-octenyl]-5-oxo-cyclopentane heptanoic acid, and the molecular weight is 354.49. The empirical formula is $C_{20}H_{34}O_5$. The structural formula of alprostadil is represented below:
[See chemical structure at top of next column]

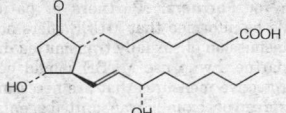

Alprostadil is a white to off-white crystalline powder with a melting point between 115° and 116°C. Its solubility at 35°C is 8000 mcg per 100 mL double-distilled water. The inactive ingredient in MUSE is polyethylene glycol 1450, USP. There are no other active agents or excipients in MUSE.
MUSE is available in 4 dosage strengths: 125 mcg, 250 mcg, 500 mcg, and 1000 mcg.

CLINICAL PHARMACOLOGY
Mechanism of Action: Prostaglandin E_1 is a naturally occurring acidic lipid that is synthesized from fatty acid precursors by most mammalian tissues and has a variety of pharmacologic effects. Human seminal fluid is a rich source of prostaglandins, including PGE_1 and PGE_2, and the total concentration of prostaglandins in ejaculate has been estimated to be approximately 100–200 mcg/mL. In vitro, alprostadil (PGE_1) has been shown to cause dose-dependent smooth muscle relaxation in isolated corpus cavernosum and corpus spongiosum preparations. Additionally, vasodilation has been demonstrated in isolated cavernosal artery segments that were pre-contracted with either norepinephrine or prostaglandin $F_{2\alpha}$. When alprostadil was injected into the corpus cavernosum of pigtail monkeys in vivo, dose-dependent increases in cavernosal artery blood flow were observed.
In human studies using Doppler duplex ultrasonography, intraurethral administration of 500 mcg of MUSE resulted in an increase in cavernosal artery diameter and a 5- to 10-fold increase in peak systolic flow velocities. These results suggest that intraurethral alprostadil is absorbed from the urethra, transported throughout the erectile bodies by communicating vessels between the corpus spongiosum and corpora cavernosa, and able to induce vasodilation of the targeted vascular beds.
The vasodilatory effects of alprostadil on the cavernosal arteries and the trabecular smooth muscle of the corpora cavernosa result in rapid arterial inflow and expansion of the lacunar spaces within the corpora. As the expanded corporal sinusoids are compressed against the tunica albuginea, venous outflow through subtunical vessels is impeded and penile rigidity develops. This process is referred to as the corporal veno-occlusive mechanism.
The most notable systemic effects of alprostadil are vasodilation, inhibition of platelet aggregation, and stimulation of intestinal and uterine smooth muscle. Intravenous doses of 1 to 10 micrograms per kilogram of body weight lower blood pressure in mammals by decreasing peripheral resistance. Reflex increases in cardiac output and heart rate may accompany these effects.
Pharmacokinetics: About 80% of alprostadil administered by MUSE is absorbed within 10 minutes and is rapidly cleared from the systemic circulation by the lungs, leaving barely detectable systemic blood levels.
Absorption: MUSE is designed to deliver alprostadil directly to the urethral lining for transfer via the corpus spongiosum to the corpora cavernosa. Intraurethral administration of MUSE is preceded by urination, and the residual urine disperses the medicated pellet, permitting alprostadil to be absorbed by the urethral mucosa. The transurethral absorption of alprostadil after MUSE administration is biphasic. Initial absorption is rapid, with approximately 80% of an administered dose absorbed within 10 minutes. The mean time to the maximum plasma PGE_1 concentration after a 1000 mcg intraurethral dose of MUSE is approximately 16 minutes.
In 10 normal human volunteers, endogenous PGE_1 levels in the ejaculate averaged 31 mcg (range 0–161 mcg). In these same volunteers, an average of 123 mcg of additional PGE_1 (range 30–369 mcg) was present in the ejaculate obtained 10 minutes after the highest dose (1000 mcg) of MUSE. The mean total endogenous PGE content (PGE_1, PGE_2, 19-OH-PGE_1, and 19-OH-PGE_2) of the ejaculate in these subjects was 444 mcg (range 0–1423 mcg).
Distribution: Following MUSE administration, alprostadil is absorbed from the urethral mucosa into the corpus spongiosum. A portion of the administered dose is transported to the corpora cavernosa through collateral vessels, while the remainder passes into the pelvic venous circulation through veins draining the corpus spongiosum. The half-life of alprostadil in humans is short, varying between 30 seconds and 10 minutes, depending on the body compartment in which it is measured and the physiological status of the subject. Nearly all of the alprostadil entering the central venous circulation is removed in a single pass through the lungs; thus peripheral venous plasma levels of PGE_1 are low or undetectable (<2 picograms/mL) after MUSE administration. The mean maximum plasma PGE_1 concentration following intraurethral administration of the highest dose of MUSE (1000 mcg) was barely detectable (11.4 picograms/

mL). In a study of 14 subjects, the plasma PGE_1 level was shown to be undetectable within 60 minutes of MUSE administration in most subjects.
Metabolism: Alprostadil is rapidly metabolized locally by enzymatic oxidation of the 15-hydroxyl group to 15-keto-PGE_1. The enzyme catalyzing this process has been isolated from many tissues in the lower genitourinary tract including the urethra, prostate, and corpus cavernosum. 15-keto-PGE_1 retains little (1–2%) of the biological activity of PGE_1. 15-keto-PGE_1 is rapidly reduced at the C_{13}–C_{14} position to form the most abundant metabolite in plasma, 13, 14-dihydro, 15-keto PGE_1 (DHK-PGE_1), which is biologically inactive. The majority of DHK-PGE_1 is further metabolized to smaller prostaglandin remnants that are cleared primarily by the kidney and liver. Between 60% and 90% of PGE_1 has been shown to be metabolized after 1 pass through the pulmonary capillary beds.
Excretion: After intravenous administration of tritium-labeled alprostadil in man, labeled drug disappears rapidly from the blood in the first 10 minutes, and by 1 hour radioactivity in the blood reaches a low level. The metabolites of alprostadil are excreted primarily by the kidney, with approximately 90% of an administered intravenous dose excreted in the urine within 24 hours of dosing. The remainder is excreted in the feces. There is no evidence of tissue retention of alprostadil or its metabolites following intravenous administration.
Pharmacokinetics in Special Populations:
Pulmonary Disease: The near-complete pulmonary first-pass metabolism of PGE_1 is the primary factor influencing the systemic pharmacokinetics of MUSE and is a reason that peripheral venous plasma levels of PGE_1 are low or undetectable (<2 picograms/mL) following MUSE administration. Patients with pulmonary disease therefore may have a reduced capacity to clear the drug. In patients with the adult respiratory distress syndrome (ARDS), pulmonary extraction of intravascularly administered alprostadil was reduced by approximately 15% compared to a control group of patients with normal respiratory function (66±3.2% vs. 78±2.4%).
Geriatrics: The effects of age on the pharmacokinetics of alprostadil have not been evaluated.

CLINICAL TRIALS
The MUSE system was evaluated in 7 placebo-controlled trials of various design in over 2500 patients with a history of erectile dysfunction of various etiologies. These trials assessed erectile function in the clinic and sexual intercourse in outpatient settings. In studies of sexual performance, patients were screened in the clinic, generally using doses of 125 mcg to 1000 mcg, for a satisfactory erectile response, then sent home with the selected dose or placebo for evaluation of sexual performance. Not all patients beginning titration had a successful dose and some patients could not tolerate MUSE, principally because of penile pain, so that the success rates in the studies described below must be understood to represent response rates only in patients who were successfully titrated.
In 2 identical multicenter, double-blind, placebo-controlled, parallel-group studies, 1511 monogamous and heterosexual patients with a mean 4-year history of erectile dysfunction and at least a 3-month history of no erections adequate for sexual intercourse without medical assistance, were enrolled and began dose titration in the clinic with doses between 125 mcg and 1000 mcg. 996 patients (66%) completed dose titration, achieved an erection sufficient for intercourse, and were randomized equally to placebo or active treatment and followed during at-home treatment for up to 3 months. 874 patients and partners completed 3 months of follow-up. About 10%, 20%, 30%, and 40% of patients were titrated to 125 mcg, 250 mcg, 500 mcg, and 1000 mcg, respectively. Couples on active therapy were more likely to have at least 1 successful sexual intercourse (65% vs. 19%) than were couples on placebo. Among patients who reported successful intercourse at least once with active treatment, approximately 7 of 10 MUSE systems resulted in successful sexual intercourse. Results were similar in patients with erectile dysfunction stemming from surgery or trauma, diabetes, vascular disease, or other etiologies, and were similar in Caucasians and non-Caucasians. In administrations resulting in sexual intercourse, the duration of erections sufficient for penetration was 6 minutes on placebo and 16 minutes on active drug. Successful therapy with MUSE was associated with improvement in the quality of life measures of "emotional well-being" for patients and "relationship with partner" for both patients and their female partners.

INDICATIONS AND USAGE
MUSE is indicated for the treatment of erectile dysfunction. Studies that established benefit demonstrated improvements in success rates for sexual intercourse compared with similarly administered placebo.

CONTRAINDICATIONS
MUSE is contraindicated in men with any of the following:
1. Known hypersensitivity to alprostadil.

Continued on next page

MUSE—Cont.

2. Abnormal penile anatomy: MUSE is contraindicated in patients with urethral stricture, balanitis (inflammation/infection of the glans of the penis), severe hypospadias and curvature, and in patients with acute or chronic urethritis.
3. Sickle cell anemia or trait, thrombocythemia, polycythemia, multiple myeloma: MUSE is contraindicated in patients who are prone to venous thrombosis or who have a hyperviscosity syndrome and are therefore at increased risk of priapism (rigid erection lasting 6 or more hours).
4. MUSE should not be used in men for whom sexual activity is inadvisable (see General Precautions).
5. MUSE should not be used for sexual intercourse with a pregnant woman unless the couple uses a condom barrier.

WARNINGS

Because of the potential for symptomatic hypotension and syncope, which occurred in 3% and 0.4%, respectively, of patients during in-clinic dosing, MUSE titration should be carried out under medical supervision. During post-marketing surveillance syncope occurring within one hour of administration has been reported. Patients should be cautioned to avoid activities, such as driving or hazardous tasks, where injury could result if hypotension or syncope were to occur after MUSE administration.

PRECAUTIONS

General Precautions:

1. A complete medical history and physical examination should be undertaken to exclude reversible causes of erectile dysfunction prior to the initiation of MUSE therapy. In addition, underlying disorders that might preclude the use of MUSE (see CONTRAINDICATIONS) should be sought.
2. *Cardiovascular effects:* During in-clinic dosing, patients should be monitored for symptoms of hypotension, and the lowest effective dose of MUSE should be prescribed.
3. *Hematologic effects:* Patients administering MUSE improperly may be at risk of urethral abrasion resulting in minor bleeding or spotting. Patients on anticoagulant therapy or with bleeding disorders may be at higher risk of bleeding. Patients on anticoagulant therapy have been safely treated with MUSE; however, the risk/benefit ratio in these patients should be considered prior to prescribing MUSE.
4. *Resumption of sexual activity:* Sexual intercourse is considered a vigorous physical activity, and it increases heart rate as well as cardiac work. Physicians may want to examine the cardiac fitness of patients prior to treating erectile dysfunction.
5. *Priapism and prolonged erection:* In clinical trials of MUSE, priapism (rigid erection lasting ≥6 hours) and prolonged erection (rigid erection lasting 4 hours and <6 hours) were reported infrequently (<0.1% and 0.3% of patients, respectively). Nevertheless, these events are a potential risk of pharmacologic therapy and can cause penile injury. Physicians should lower the dose or consider discontinuing MUSE treatment in any patient who develops priapism or prolonged erection.
6. *Drug-Drug Interactions:* Because there are low or undetectable (<2 picograms/mL) amounts of alprostadil found in the peripheral venous circulation following MUSE administration, systemic drug-drug interactions with MUSE are unlikely. Although formal studies have not been conducted, the concomitant use of MUSE and antihypertensive medications may increase the risk of hypotension. It is therefore advised that caution be used in the administration of MUSE to individuals on anti-hypertensive medications. In addition, the presence of medications in the circulation that attenuate erectile function may influence the response to MUSE.
7. *Drug-Device Interactions:* Use of MUSE in patients with penile implants has not been studied.
8. *Sexual Preference:* There is no experience in homosexual men and no experience with other than vaginal intercourse.

Information for Patients: Patients should be informed that MUSE offers no protection from the transmission of sexually transmitted diseases. Patients and partners who use MUSE need to be counseled about the protective measures that are necessary to guard against the spread of sexually transmitted agents, including the human immunodeficiency virus (HIV).

Although unreported in clinical trials, there is the possibility that an overdosage of MUSE can cause priapism, a painful erection of the penis sustained for hours and unrelieved by sexual intercourse or masturbation. This condition is serious and, if untreated, it can lead to permanent inability to have an erection. Patients who experience a prolonged erection should seek prompt medical attention.

Patients should be instructed how to administer MUSE. A patient package insert must be given to each patient at the initiation of MUSE therapy.

Information for Partners: Partners of patients using MUSE should be informed that MUSE offers no protection from the transmission of sexually transmitted diseases. Patients and partners who use MUSE should be counseled about the protective measures that are necessary to guard against the spread of sexually transmitted agents, including the human immunodeficiency virus (HIV). Human semen contains PGE_1, but additional amounts may be present from MUSE administration (see CLINICAL PHARMACOLOGY). Partners who have experienced an extended period of sexual abstinence should be encouraged to seek advice from a health care professional prior to resuming sexual intercourse. The use of a water-based lubricant may facilitate vaginal penetration.

It is recommended that couples using MUSE employ adequate contraception if the female partner is of childbearing potential. There is no information on the effects on early pregnancy of PGE_1 at the levels received by female partners. MUSE has no contraceptive properties. MUSE should not be used if the female partner is pregnant, unless the couple uses a condom barrier.

Carcinogenesis, Mutagenesis, Impairment of Fertility: Long-term carcinogenicity studies of alprostadil have not been conducted. Alprostadil showed no evidence of mutagenicity in vitro in the Ames bacterial reverse mutation test, the unscheduled DNA synthesis assay in rat hepatocytes, or the Chinese hamster ovary forward gene mutation assay; nor was there evidence of mutagenicity in vivo in the mouse micronucleus assay. Alprostadil concentrations increased chromosomal aberrations above control incidence in the in vitro Chinese hamster ovary chromosomal aberration assay. In dogs, sperm concentration, morphology, and motility were unaffected by daily intraurethral administration of up to 3000 mcg MUSE (alprostadil) for 13 weeks (200 mcg/kg/day or about 3.5 times the maximum recommended daily dose adjusted for body surface area). Alprostadil concentrations of 400 mcg/mL had no effect on human sperm motility or viability in vitro.

Pregnancy: Pregnancy Category C: Alprostadil has been shown to be embryotoxic (decreased fetal weight) when administered as a subcutaneous bolus to pregnant rats at doses as low as 500 mcg/kg/day. Doses of 2000 mcg/kg/day resulted in increased resorptions, reduced numbers of live fetuses, increased incidences of visceral and skeletal variations (primarily left umbilical artery and generalized reduction in ossification of the entire skeleton) and gross visceral and skeletal malformations (primarily edema, hydrocephaly, anophthalmia/microphthalmia, and skeletal anomalies). The latter dose produced maternal toxicity (ataxia, lethargy, diarrhea, and retarded body weight gain). When administered by continuous intravenous infusion, evidence of embryotoxicity (decreased fetal weight gain and increased incidence of hydroureter) was observed at 2000 mcg/kg/day, a dose that was also associated with a decrease in maternal weight gain. Intravaginal administration of up to 4000 mcg/day of MUSE (alprostadil) to pregnant rabbits (1100 mcg/kg/day or about 12.5 times the maximum recommended daily dose adjusted for body surface area) resulted in no evidence of harm to the fetus. MUSE should not be used for sexual intercourse with a pregnant woman unless the couple uses a condom barrier.

Nursing Mothers and Pediatric Use: MUSE is not indicated for use in newborns, children, or women.

ADVERSE REACTIONS

In-Clinic Titration: In the 2 largest double-blind, parallel, placebo-controlled trials, 1511 patients received MUSE at least 1 time in the clinic setting. The most frequently reported drug-related side effects during in-clinic titration included pain in the penis (36%), urethra (13%), or testes (5%). These discomforts were most commonly reported as mild and transient, but about 7% of patients withdrew at this stage because of adverse events. Urethral bleeding/spotting and other minor abrasions to the urethra were reported in approximately 3% of patients. Symptomatic lowering of blood pressure (hypotension) occurred in 3% of patients; in addition, some lowering of blood pressure may occur without symptoms. Dizziness was reported in 4% of patients. Syncope (fainting) was reported by 0.4% of patients. (See **WARNINGS**).

Home Treatment: 996 patients (66% of those who began titration) were studied during the home treatment portion of 2 Phase III placebo-controlled studies. Fewer than 2% of patients discontinued from these studies primarily because of adverse events. The following table summarizes the frequency of adverse events reported by patients using MUSE or placebo.

Adverse Events Reported by ≥2% of Patients Treated with MUSE and More Common than on Placebo At Home in Phase III Placebo-Controlled Clinical Studies for up to 3 Months

Event	MUSE n = 486	Placebo n = 511
UROGENITAL SYSTEM		
Penile Pain	32%	3%
Urethral Burning	12%	4%
Minor Urethral Bleeding/Spotting	5%	1%
Testicular Pain	5%	1%
NERVOUS SYSTEM		
Dizziness	2%	<1%
BODY AS A WHOLE		
Flu Symptoms	4%	2%
Headache	3%	2%
Pain	3%	1%
Accidental Injury	3%	2%
Back Pain	2%	1%
Pelvic Pain	2%	<1%
RESPIRATORY		
Rhinitis	2%	<1%
Infection	3%	2%

Other drug-related side effects observed during in-clinic titration and home treatment include swelling of leg veins, leg pain, perineal pain, and rapid pulse, each occurring in <2% of patients.

Female Partner Adverse Events: The most common drug-related adverse event reported by female partners during placebo-controlled clinical studies was vaginal burning/itching, reported by 5.8% of partners of patients on active vs. 0.8% of partners of patients on placebo. It is unknown whether this adverse event experienced by female partners was a result of the medication or a result of resuming sexual intercourse, which occurred much more frequently in partners of patients on active medication.

OVERDOSAGE

Overdosage has not been reported with MUSE. Overdosage with MUSE may result in hypotension, persistent penile pain, and possibly priapism (rigid erection lasting ≥6h). Priapism can result in permanent worsening of erectile function. Patients suspected of overdosage who develop these symptoms should be kept under medical supervision until systemic or local symptoms have resolved.

DOSAGE AND ADMINISTRATION

MUSE is a transurethral delivery system available in 4 dosage strengths: 125 mcg, 250 mcg, 500 mcg, and 1000 mcg. MUSE should be administered as needed to achieve an erection. The onset of effect is within 5–10 minutes after administration. The duration of effect is approximately 30–60 minutes. However, the actual duration will vary from patient to patient. Each patient should be instructed by a medical professional on proper technique for administering MUSE prior to self-administration. The maximum frequency of use is no more than 2 systems per 24-hour period.

Initiation of Therapy: Dose titration should be administered under the supervision of a physician to test a patient's responsiveness to MUSE, to demonstrate proper administration technique (see detailed instructions for MUSE administration in patient package insert), and to monitor for evidence of hypotension (see **WARNINGS**). Patients should be individually titrated to the lowest dose that is sufficient for sexual intercourse. The lower doses of MUSE (125 mcg or 250 mcg) are recommended for initial dosing. If necessary, the dose should be increased (or decreased) on separate occasions in a stepwise manner until the patient achieves an erection that is sufficient for sexual intercourse.

Home Treatment Regimen: MUSE should be used as needed to achieve an erection. The maximum frequency of use is 2 administrations per 24-hour period. Each MUSE is for single use only and should be properly discarded after use.

HOW SUPPLIED

MUSE is supplied in individual foil pouches containing one (1) system per pouch. MUSE is available in unit cartons containing six (6) systems. MUSE is available in the following 4 dosage strengths:

Dosage Strength	NDC Numbers		Identifying Package Color
	Carton	Pouch	
125 mcg	62541-110-06	62541-110-01	Tan
250 mcg	62541-120-06	62541-120-01	Green
500 mcg	62541-130-06	62541-130-01	Blue
1000 mcg	62541-140-06	62541-140-01	Burgundy

STORAGE AND HANDLING

Store unopened foil pouches in a refrigerator at 2°–8°C (36°–46°F). Do not expose MUSE to temperatures above

30°C (86°F). MUSE may be kept by the patient at room temperature (below 30°C or 86°F) for up to 14 days prior to use. Caution: Federal law prohibits dispensing without prescription.

Medical information line at VIVUS 1-888-345-MUSE (1-888-345-6873).

MUSE® IS A REGISTERED TRADEMARK OF VIVUS, INC. IN THE U.S. AND OTHER COUNTRIES.

Revised February 1998

PATIENT INFORMATION

Please read this pamphlet before using MUSE® (alprostadil). This pamphlet is a quick reference source on important information about MUSE for you and your partner. **Before administering MUSE, please review the patient video and education booklet. These materials provide visual instruction and more detailed information as well as practical tips on how to use MUSE.**

WHAT IS MUSE?

MUSE represents a unique approach for the treatment of erectile dysfunction, commonly called impotence. It is based on the discovery that the urethra (the normal pathway for urine) can absorb certain medications into the surrounding erectile tissues thereby creating an erection. There are 4 dose strengths available: 125, 250, 500, and 1000 micrograms. The MUSE applicator (Fig. 1) contained in each foil pouch is intended for 1 administration only. Your dose of MUSE will be determined by you and your physician. After administration, the erection process will begin within 5–10 minutes, and may last 30–60 minutes. However, the actual duration will vary from patient to patient.

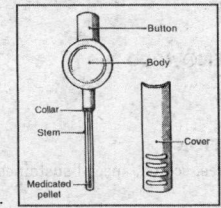

Figure 1.

WHAT IS MUSE USED FOR?

MUSE is indicated for the treatment of erectile dysfunction. Erectile dysfunction is the inability to attain or maintain an erection sufficient for sexual intercourse.

WHO SHOULD NOT USE MUSE?

You should not use MUSE if you have any of the following:
- Known hypersensitivity to alprostadil (the active medication in MUSE)
- An abnormally formed penis
- Have been advised not to undertake sexual activity
- Conditions that might result in long-lasting erections, such as sickle cell anemia or trait, leukemia, or tumor of the bone marrow (multiple myeloma)
- MUSE should not be used for sexual intercourse with a pregnant woman unless the couple uses a condom barrier.

WHAT ARE THE POSSIBLE SIDE EFFECTS OF MUSE?

The most common side effects that have been observed using MUSE follow:
- Aching in the penis, testicles, legs, and in the perineum (area between the penis and rectum)
- Warmth or burning sensation in the urethra
- Redness of the penis due to increased blood flow
- Minor urethral bleeding or spotting due to improper administration.

Side effects reported less frequently:
- Prolonged erection— PLEASE NOTE: IF YOUR ERECTION IS RIGID FOR MORE THAN 4 HOURS, CALL YOUR DOCTOR PROMPTLY.
- Swelling of leg veins
- Light-headedness/Dizziness
- Fainting— PLEASE NOTE: AFTER USING MUSE, YOU SHOULD AVOID ACTIVITIES, SUCH AS DRIVING OR HAZARDOUS TASKS, WHERE INJURY COULD RESULT IF DIZZINESS OR FAINTING WERE TO OCCUR. IN PATIENTS EXPERIENCING THESE SYMPTOMS, THE SYMPTOMS HAVE USUALLY OCCURRED DURING INITIATION OF THERAPY AND WITHIN ONE HOUR OF MUSE ADMINISTRATION.
- Rapid pulse.

If you have a history of fainting be sure to discuss this with your doctor prior to using MUSE. If you do experience dizziness or feel faint, this may be due to the lowering of your blood pressure. Lie down immediately and raise your legs. If symptoms persist, call your doctor promptly. Because of the potential for these side effects, MUSE titration should be carried out under medical supervision.

Changing Your Dosage

It is assumed that you and your doctor have determined the proper dose of MUSE. If you suspect that your dose needs to be increased or decreased to achieve the response that works best for you, please call your doctor to determine if your dose needs to be reevaluated. Do not use MUSE more than twice in a 24-hour period.

WHAT ARE THE POSSIBLE SIDE EFFECTS OF MUSE FOR YOUR PARTNER?

The most common reported side effects observed in women whose partners use MUSE are mild vaginal itching or burning. Using a water-based lubricant can help to make vaginal penetration easier. Your partner may want to consult her health care provider if she has not had sexual intercourse for an extended period of time.

IMPORTANT INFORMATION FOR YOU AND YOUR PARTNER

Pregnancy

MUSE has no contraceptive properties.

Because MUSE has not been tested during human pregnancy, it is recommended that couples use adequate contraception if the female partner is of childbearing potential. MUSE should not be used for sexual intercourse with a pregnant woman unless the couple uses a condom barrier.

Sexually Transmitted Diseases

MUSE will not protect you or your partner from sexually transmitted diseases like chlamydia, gonorrhea, herpes simplex virus, viral hepatitis, human immunodeficiency virus (HIV—the virus that causes AIDS), human papilloma virus (genital warts), and syphilis. Latex condoms can protect against these sexually transmitted diseases.

HOW SHOULD I STORE MUSE?

It is recommended that MUSE be stored in a refrigerator. MUSE may be kept at room temperature (less than 30°C/86°F) for up to 14 days prior to use. It is very important that MUSE not be exposed to temperatures above 30°C/86°F since this will make MUSE ineffective. MUSE should not be exposed to high temperatures or placed in direct sunlight.

Storage when traveling

When traveling, store MUSE in a portable ice pack or cooler. Do not store in the trunk of a car or in baggage storage areas where MUSE may be exposed to extremes in temperature.

HOW TO ADMINISTER MUSE:

1. Immediately prior to administration, urinate and gently shake the penis several times to remove excess urine. A moist urethra makes administration of MUSE easier. The medicated pellet has been specially developed to dissolve in the small quantity of urine that remains in the urethra after urination.

2. Open the foil pouch by tearing fully across the notched edge (Fig. 2). Let the MUSE slide out of the pouch. Save the pouch for discarding the MUSE applicator later.

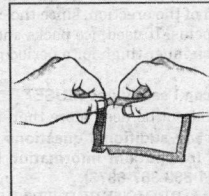

Figure 2.

3. To remove the protective cover from the applicator stem (Fig. 3), hold the body of the applicator with your thumb and forefinger. Twist the body and pull out the applicator from the cover, being careful not to push in or pull out the applicator button. Avoid touching the applicator stem and tip. Save the cover for discarding the MUSE applicator later.

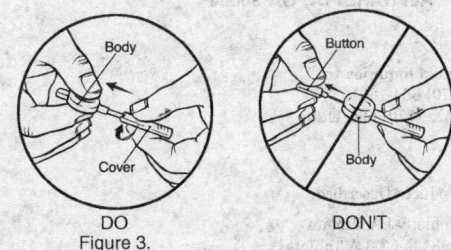

DO
Figure 3.

DON'T

4. Visually inspect the MUSE. The MUSE system is see-through, and you will be able to see the medicated pellet at the end of the stem. Make sure that the pellet is present before insertion (Fig. 4).
[See figure at top of next column]

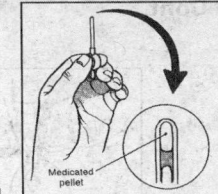

Medicated pellet

Figure 4.

5. Hold the applicator in a way which is the most comfortable for you (Fig. 5A and 5B).

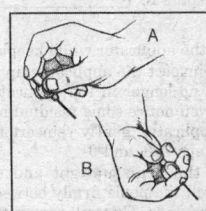

Figure 5.

6. Please review Figure 6A, the anatomy of the penis.

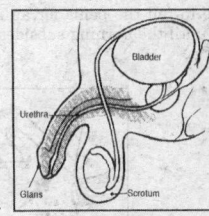

Bladder

Urethra

Glans   Scrotum

Figure 6A.

While sitting or standing, whichever is more comfortable for you, take several seconds to gently and slowly stretch the penis upward to its full length, with gentle compression from top to bottom of the glans (Fig. 6B). This straightens and opens the urethra. Slowly insert the MUSE stem into the urethra up to the collar (Fig. 6C). If you feel any discomfort or a pulling sensation, withdraw the applicator slightly and then gently reinsert.

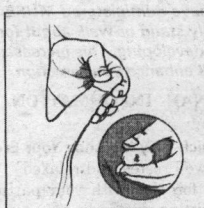

Figure 6B.

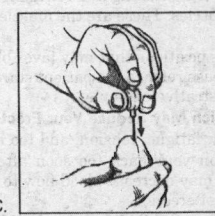

Figure 6C.

7. Gently and completely push down (Fig. 7) the button at the top of the applicator until it stops. It is important to do this to ensure that the medicated pellet is completely released. Hold the applicator in this position for 5 seconds.

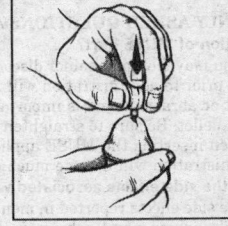

Figure 7.

8. Gently rock the applicator from side to side. This will separate the medicated pellet from the applicator tip (Fig. 8). If you apply too much pressure you may scratch the lining of the urethra causing it to bleed.
[See figure at top of next page]

Continued on next page

MUSE—Cont.

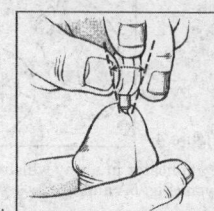

Figure 8.

9. Remove the applicator while keeping the penis upright.
10. Visually inspect the applicator tip to see that the medication is no longer in the applicator. Do not touch the stem. If you notice some residual medication in the end of the applicator, gently reinsert into the urethra and repeat steps 7, 8, and 9.
11. Holding the penis upright and stretched to its full length, roll the penis firmly between your hands for at least 10 seconds. This will ensure that the medication is adequately distributed along the walls of the urethra (Fig. 9). If you feel a burning sensation, it may help to continue to roll the penis for an additional 30–60 seconds or until the burning subsides.

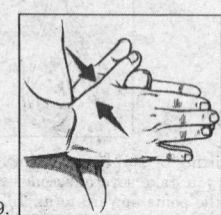

Figure 9.

12. Remember, each MUSE is good for a single administration only. Replace the cover on the MUSE applicator, place in the opened foil pouch, fold, and discard as normal household waste.

After you have administered MUSE, it is important to sit, or preferably stand or walk about for 10 minutes while the erection is developing. This increases blood flow to the penis and will enhance your erection.

ADDITIONAL INFORMATION AND PRACTICAL TIPS

Factors Which May Enhance Your Erection:
• Being well rested and relaxed
• Sexual foreplay with your partner or self-stimulation while sitting or standing
• Pelvic exercises (for example, Kegel exercises)—these consist of tightening and releasing your pelvic and buttock muscles. These are the muscles you use to stop urination
• Various positions that may favor blood flow into the penis. Please refer to the patient starter booklet and video for illustrative examples.

Factors Which May Reduce Your Erection:
• Anxiety, fatigue, tension, and too much alcohol
• Lying on your back too soon after administration of MUSE may decrease blood flow to the penis and result in loss of erection
• Urination or dribbling immediately following administration may result in loss of medication from the urethra
• Using medications that contain decongestants, such as over-the-counter cold remedies, allergy, sinus medications, and appetite suppressants, may block the effect of MUSE.

COMMONLY ASKED QUESTIONS ABOUT MUSE
Will insertion of MUSE hurt?
At first, you may feel some minor discomfort from insertion. Urinating prior to administration will reduce the chance of discomfort or abrasions and is important for dissolving the medicated pellet. Be sure to straighten your penis to its full length when inserting the MUSE applicator. With repeated use, administration will become much easier.

What are the side effects associated with MUSE?
Most of the side effects reported in men are relatively minor and include burning and aching in the penis and groin. Rarely noted are prolonged erection, light-headedness, dizziness, fainting, rapid pulse, and swelling of the leg veins. If you feel dizzy, light-headed, faint, or experience rapid pulse, lie down immediately and raise your legs. If symptoms persist, call your doctor promptly. Because of the potential for these side effects, MUSE titration should be carried out under medical supervision.

(See also: "WHAT ARE THE POSSIBLE SIDE EFFECTS OF MUSE?")
In women, mild vaginal itching and burning have been observed.

After I administer MUSE, can we immediately lie down and begin sexual activity?
You can begin sexual activity, but having the man lie down, especially on his back shortly after administration, is not recommended. This will reduce blood flow to the penis and may reduce the erection. It is important to sit, stand or walk about for 10 minutes after administration. Many couples have used this time to incorporate various types of foreplay. After this initial period, you can assume different positions leading to sexual intercourse. Some couples have noticed that the erection is better maintained in positions that favor blood flow into the penis during intercourse.
Please review the video and patient starter booklet available from your doctor which illustrates various positions that will enhance your erection.

How long will the effect of MUSE last?
An erection should begin within 5–10 minutes after administering MUSE. The duration of effect is approximately 30–60 minutes. However, the actual duration will vary from patient to patient.

What will the erection be like? How will it compare to the erections I had when I was younger?
An effective dose of MUSE should produce an erection sufficient for sexual intercourse. MUSE may not create an erection such as those you experienced when you were younger. Some patients may experience some mild pain and aching in the penis or groin area. Also, your erection may continue after orgasm.

How do I know if I have the correct dose of MUSE?
You and your physician will determine the appropriate dose of MUSE. If your erection cannot be maintained for the time needed to have foreplay and sexual intercourse, you may need to have your dose increased. Similarly, an erection that lasts longer than desired may require a dose decrease. Call your doctor if you suspect you may require a dosing adjustment.

After my erection is over, will my penis feel sensitive?
Your penis may feel full, warm, and somewhat sensitive to the touch. These effects are normal and may last a few hours.

Can I reuse MUSE?
No. MUSE is intended for single-dose application only.

How do I dispose of the MUSE applicator?
After you have administered MUSE, replace the cap on the applicator, place in the opened foil pouch, fold, and discard as normal household waste.

If my erection lasts longer than desired, what should I do?
Note: Call your doctor promptly if you have a rigid erection that lasts more than 4 hours.
An application of ice packs to the inner thigh may shorten the duration of the erection, since the cold will restrict blood flow to the penis. If used, ice packs should be applied alternately to each inner thigh for a period not exceeding 10 minutes.

How often can I safely use MUSE?
MUSE should not be used more than twice per day.

If you have any additional questions about MUSE, please call the toll free patient information line at VIVUS 1-888-367-MUSE (1-888-367-6873).
MUSE® IS A REGISTERED TRADEMARK OF VIVUS, INC. IN THE U.S. AND OTHER COUNTRIES.
VIVUS, Inc.
Mountain View, CA 94043   February 1998
Shown in Product Identification Guide, page 341

Wakefield Pharmaceuticals, Inc.
310 MAXWELL ROAD, SUITE 100
ALPHARETTA, GA 30004

Direct Inquiries to:
(770) 664-1661
FAX: (770) 664-1126

Products Described:
Biohist®-LA Tablets
Muco-Fen®-LA Tablets
Muco-Fen® 800 Tablets
Muco-Fen® 1200 Tablets
Muco-Fen® DM Tablets
Profen II® Tablets
Profen II DM® Tablets
Profen LA® Tablets

BIOHIST®-LA Tablets ℞
Antihistamine, Decongestant

DESCRIPTION
Each dye-free, scored, special sustained release tablet contains:
Carbinoxamine Maleate .... 8 mg
Pseudoephedrine HCl .... 120 mg

DOSAGE
12 yrs. and older, 1 Tablet b.i.d.

HOW SUPPLIED
Bottles of 100 (NDC 59310-101-10)

MUCO-FEN® 800 Tablets ℞
[mū-co-fin]
Guaifenesin

DESCRIPTION
Each dye-free, scored, special sustained release tablet contains:
Guaifenesin .... 800 mg

DOSAGE
12 yrs. and older, 1 Tablet b.i.d., not to exceed 2400 mg/day. Children 6 to 12, 1/2 Tablet b.i.d., not to exceed 1200 mg/day.

HOW SUPPLIED
Bottles of 100 (NDC 59310-109-10)

MUCO-FEN® 1200 ℞
[mū-co-fin]
Guaifenesin

DESCRIPTION
Each dye-free, scored, special sustained release tablet contains:
Guaifenesin .... 1200 mg.

DOSAGE
12 years and older, 1 tablet b.i.d., not to exceed 2400 mg./day. Children 6 to 12, one half tablet every 12 hours, not to exceed 1200 mg. per day.

HOW SUPPLIED
Bottles of 100 (NDC 59310-0120-10)

MUCO-FEN® DM Tablets ℞
[mū-co-fin]
Dextromethorphan Hydrobromide/Guaifenesin

DESCRIPTION
Each dye free, scored, special sustained release tablet contains:
Dextromethorphan Hydrobromide .... 30 mg
Guaifenesin .... 600 mg

DOSAGE
12 yrs. and older, 1 or 2 Tablets b.i.d.
Children 6 to 12, 1 Tablet b.i.d.

HOW SUPPLIED
Bottles of 100 (NDC 59310-108-10)

MUCO-FEN® LA Tablets ℞
[mū-co-fin]
Guaifenesin

DESCRIPTION
Each dye-free, scored, special sustained release tablet contains:
Guaifenesin .... 600 mg

DOSAGE
12 yrs. and older, 1 or 2 Tablets b.i.d.
Children 6 to 12, 1 Tablet b.i.d.

HOW SUPPLIED
Bottles of 100 (NDC 59310-102-10)

PROFEN-LA® Tablets ℞
[Pró-fin]
Phenylpropanolamine HCl/Guaifenesin

DESCRIPTION
Each dye-free, scored, special sustained release tablet contains:

Phenylpropanolamine HCl .... 75 mg
Guaifenesin .... 600 mg

DOSAGE

12 yrs. and older, 1 Tablet b.i.d.
Children 6 to 12, 1/2 Tablet b.i.d.

HOW SUPPLIED

Bottle of 100 (NDC 59310-104-10)

PROFEN II® Tablets ℞

[*Pro' -fin*]
Phenylpropanolamine HCl/Guaifenesin

DESCRIPTION

Each dye-free, scored, special sustained release tablet contains:
Phenylpropanolamine HCl .... 37.5 mg
Guaifenesin .... 600 mg

DOSAGE

12 yrs. and older, 1 or 2 Tablets b.i.d.
Children 6 to 12, 1 Tablet b.i.d.

HOW SUPPLIED

Bottles of 100 (NDC 59310-107-10)

PROFEN II DM® TABLETS ℞

[*pro '-fin*]
**Phenylpropanolamine HCl/Guaifenesin/
Dextromethorphan Hydrobromide**

DESCRIPTION

Each dye-free, scored, special sustained release tablet contains:
Phenylpropanolamine HCl .... 37.5 mg.
Guaifenesin .... 600 mg.
Dextromethorphan HBr .... 30 mg.

DOSAGE

12 yrs. and older, 1 or 2 tablets b.i.d. children 6 to 12, 1 tablet b.i.d.

HOW SUPPLIED

Bottles of 100 (NDC 59310-110-10)

Wallace Laboratories

**P.O. BOX 1001
CRANBURY, NJ 08512**

For Medical Information, Contact:
Generally:
Professional Services
800-526-3840
After Hours and Weekend Emergencies:
(609) 655-6474

Wallace Laboratories
Sales and Ordering:
Div. of Carter-Wallace, Inc
P.O. Box 1001
Cranbury, NJ 08512

AQUATENSEN® ℞

**(methyclothiazide tablets, USP, 5 mg)
Tablets**

ASTELIN® ℞

**(azelastine hydrochloride)
Nasal Spray, 137 mcg
For Intranasal Use Only**

DESCRIPTION

Astelin® (azelastine hydrochloride) Nasal Spray, 137 micrograms (mcg), is an antihistamine formulated as a metered-spray solution for intranasal administration. Azelastine hydrochloride occurs as a white, almost odorless, crystalline powder with a bitter taste. It has a molecular weight of 418.37. It is sparingly soluble in water, methanol, and propylene glycol and slightly soluble in ethanol, octanol, and glycerine. It has a melting point of about 225°C and the pH of a saturated solution is between 5.0 and 5.4. Its chemical name is (±)-1-(2H)-phthalazinone,4-[(4-chlorophenyl) methyl]-2-(hexahydro-1-methyl-1H-azepin-4-yl)-, monohydro-

chloride. Its molecular formula is $C_{22}H_{24}ClN_3O \cdot HCl$ with the following chemical structure:

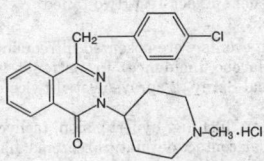

Astelin® Nasal Spray contains 0.1% azelastine hydrochloride in an aqueous solution at pH 6.8 ± 0.3. It also contains benzalkonium chloride (125 mcg/mL), edetate disodium, hydroxypropyl methyl cellulose, citric acid, dibasic sodium phosphate, sodium chloride, and purified water.
After priming, each metered spray delivers a 0.137 mL mean volume containing 137 mcg of azelastine hydrochloride (equivalent to 125 mcg of azelastine base). Each bottle can deliver 100 metered sprays.

CLINICAL PHARMACOLOGY

Azelastine hydrochloride, a phthalazinone derivative, exhibits histamine H_1-receptor antagonist activity in isolated tissues, animal models, and humans. Astelin® Nasal Spray is administered as a racemic mixture with no difference in pharmacologic activity noted between the enantiomers in *in vitro* studies. The major metabolite, desmethylazelastine, also possesses H_1-receptor antagonist activity.

Pharmacokinetics and Metabolism

After intranasal administration, the systemic bioavailability of azelastine hydrochloride is approximately 40%. Maximum plasma concentrations (Cmax) are achieved in 2–3 hours. Based on intravenous and oral administration, the elimination half-life, steady-state volume of distribution, and plasma clearance are 22 hours, 14.5 L/kg and 0.5 L/h/kg, respectively. Approximately 75% of an oral dose of radiolabeled azelastine hydrochloride was excreted in the feces with less than 10% as unchanged azelastine. Azelastine is oxidatively metabolized to the principal active metabolite, desmethylazelastine, by the cytochrome P450 enzyme system. The specific P450 isoforms responsible for the biotransformation of azelastine have not been identified; however, clinical interaction studies with the known CYP3A4 inhibitor erythromycin failed to demonstrate a pharmacokinetic interaction. In a multiple-dose, steady-state drug interaction study in normal volunteers, cimetidine (400 mg twice daily), a nonspecific P450 inhibitor, raised orally administered mean azelastine (4 mg twice daily) concentrations by approximately 65%.
The major active metabolite, desmethylazelastine, was not measurable (below assay limits) after single-dose intranasal administration of azelastine hydrochloride. After intranasal dosing of azelastine hydrochloride to steady-state, plasma concentrations of desmethylazelastine range from 20–50% of azelastine concentrations. When azelastine hydrochloride is administered orally, desmethylazelastine has an elimination half-life of 54 hours. Limited data indicate that the metabolite profile is similar when azelastine hydrochloride is administered via the intranasal or oral route.
In vitro studies with human plasma indicate that the plasma protein binding of azelastine and desmethylazelastine are approximately 88% and 97%, respectively.
Azelastine hydrochloride administered intranasally at doses above two sprays per nostril twice daily for 29 days resulted in greater than proportional increases in Cmax and area under the curve (AUC) for azelastine.
Studies in healthy subjects administered oral doses of azelastine hydrochloride demonstrated linear responses in Cmax and AUC.

Special Populations
Following oral administration, pharmacokinetic parameters were not influenced by age, gender, or hepatic impairment. Based on oral, single-dose studies, renal insufficiency (creatine clearance <50 mL/min) resulted in a 70–75% higher Cmax and AUC compared to normal subjects. Time to maximum concentration was unchanged.
Oral azelastine has been safely administered to over 1400 asthmatic subjects, supporting the safety of administering Astelin® Nasal Spray to allergic rhinitis patients with asthma.

Pharmacodynamics
In a placebo-controlled study (95 subjects with allergic rhinitis), there was no evidence of an effect of Astelin® Nasal Spray (2 sprays per nostril twice daily for 56 days) on cardiac repolarization as represented by the corrected QT interval (QTc) of the electrocardiogram. At higher oral exposures (≥ 4 mg twice daily), a nonclinically significant mean change in the QTc (3–7 millisecond increase) was observed. Interaction studies investigating the cardiac repolarization effects of concomitantly administered oral azelastine hydro-

chloride and erythromycin or ketoconazole were conducted. Oral erythromycin had no effect on azelastine pharmacokinetics or QTc based on analysis of serial electrocardiograms. Ketoconazole interfered with the measurement of azelastine plasma levels; however, no effects on QTc were observed (see PRECAUTIONS, Drug Interactions).

Clinical Trials
U.S. placebo-controlled clinical trials of Astelin® Nasal Spray included 322 patients with seasonal allergic rhinitis who received two sprays per nostril twice a day for up to 4 weeks. These trials included 55 pediatric patients ages 12 to 16 years. Astelin® Nasal Spray significantly improved a complex of symptoms, which included rhinorrhea, sneezing, and nasal pruritis.
In dose-ranging trials, Astelin® Nasal Spray administration resulted in a decrease in symptoms, which reached statistical significance from saline placebo within 3 hours after initial dosing and persisted over the 12-hour dosing interval. There were no findings on nasal examination in an 8-week study that suggested any adverse effect of azelastine on the nasal mucosa.

INDICATIONS AND USAGE

Astelin® Nasal Spray is indicated for the treatment of the symptoms of seasonal allergic rhinitis such as rhinorrhea, sneezing, and nasal pruritis in adults and children 12 years and older.

CONTRAINDICATIONS

Astelin® Nasal Spray is contraindicated in patients with a known hypersensitivity to azelastine hydrochloride or any of its components.

PRECAUTIONS

Activities Requiring Mental Alertness: In clinical trials, the occurrence of somnolence has been reported in some patients taking Astelin® Nasal Spray; due caution should therefore be exercised when driving a car or operating potentially dangerous machinery. Concurrent use of Astelin® Nasal Spray with alcohol or other CNS depressants should be avoided because additional reductions in alertness and additional impairment of CNS performance may occur.
Information for Patients: Patients should be instructed to use Astelin® Nasal Spray only as prescribed. For the proper use of the nasal spray and to attain maximum improvement, the patient should read and follow carefully the accompanying patient instructions. Patients should be instructed to prime the delivery system before initial use and after storage for 3 or more days (see PATIENT INSTRUCTIONS FOR USE). Patients should also be instructed to store the bottle upright at room temperature with the pump tightly closed and out of the reach of children. In case of accidental ingestion by a young child, seek professional assistance or contact a poison control center immediately.
Patients should be advised against the concurrent use of Astelin® Nasal Spray with other antihistamines without consulting a physician. Patients who are, or may become, pregnant should be told that this product should be used in pregnancy or during lactation only if the potential benefit justifies the potential risks to the fetus or nursing infant. Patients should be advised to assess their individual responses to Astelin® Nasal Spray before engaging in any activity requiring mental alertness, such as driving a car or operating machinery. Patients should be advised that the concurrent use of Astelin® Nasal Spray with alcohol or other CNS depressants may lead to additional reductions in alertness and impairment of CNS performance and should be avoided (see Drug Interactions).
Drug Interactions: Concurrent use of Astelin® Nasal Spray with alcohol or other CNS depressants should be avoided because additional reductions in alertness and additional impairment of CNS performance may occur.
Cimetidine (400 mg twice daily) increased the mean Cmax and AUD of orally administered azelastine hydrochloride (4 mg twice daily) by approximately 65%. Ranitidine hydrochloride (150 mg twice daily) had no effect on azelastine pharmacokinetics.
Interaction studies investigating the cardiac effects, as measured by the corrected QT interval (QTc), of concomitantly administered oral azelastine hydrochloride and erythromycin or ketoconazole were conducted. Oral erythromycin (500 mg three times daily for seven days) had no effect on azelastine pharmacokinetics or QTc based on analyses of serial electrocardiograms. Ketoconazole (200 mg twice daily for seven days) interfered with the measurement of azelastine plasma concentrations; however, no effects on QTc were observed.
No significant pharmacokinetic interaction was observed with the coadministration of an oral 4 mg dose of azelastine hydrochloride twice daily and theophylline 300 mg or 400 mg twice daily.
Geriatric Use: U.S. placebo-controlled clinical trials included 11 patients above the age of 60 years who were treated with Astelin® Nasal Spray. While this number is very small and no substantial conclusions can be drawn, the

Continued on next page

Astelin—Cont.

adverse events in this group were similar to patients under age 60 years.

Carcinogenesis, Mutagenesis, Impairment of Fertility: Carcinogenicity studies in rats and mice with oral azelastine hydrochloride for 24 months at doses up to 30 mg/kg/day and 25 mg/kg/day, respectively (240 and 100 times the maximum recommended human daily intranasal dose on a mg/m^2 basis), revealed no evidence of carcinogenicity. Azelastine hydrochloride showed no genotoxic effects in the Ames test, DNA repair test, mouse lymphoma forward mutation assay, mouse micronucleus test, or chromosomal aberration test in rat bone marrow.

Reproduction and fertility studies in rats showed no effects on male or female fertility at oral doses of up to 30 mg/kg/day (240 times the maximum recommended human daily intranasal dose on a mg/m^2 basis). At 68.6 mg/kg/day (550 times the maximum recommended human daily intranasal dose on a mg/m^2 basis), the duration of estrous cycles was prolonged and copulatory activity and the number of pregnancies were decreased. The numbers of corpora lutea and implantations were decreased; however, the implantation ratio was not affected.

Pregnancy Category C: Azelastine hydrochloride has been shown to be embryotoxic, fetotoxic, and teratogenic (external and skeletal abnormalities) in mice at an oral dose of 68.6 mg/kg/day (280 times the maximum recommended human daily intranasal dose on a mg/m^2 basis).

At an oral dose of 30 mg/kg/day (240 times the maximum recommended human daily intranasal dose on a mg/m^2 basis), delayed ossification (undeveloped metacarpus), and the incidence of 14th rib were increased in rats. At 68.6 mg/kg/day (550 times the maximum recommended human daily intranasal dose on a mg/m^2 basis) azelastine hydrochloride caused abortion and fetotoxic effects in rats.

The relevance to humans of these skeletal findings noted at only high drug exposure levels is unknown.

There are no adequate and well-controlled clinical studies in pregnant women. Astelin® Nasal Spray should be used during pregnancy only if the potential benefit justifies the potential risk to the fetus.

Nursing Mothers: It is not known whether azelastine hydrochloride is excreted in human milk. Because many drugs are excreted in human milk, caution should be used when Astelin® Nasal Spray is administered to a nursing woman.

Pediatric Use: Safety and efficacy of Astelin® Nasal Spray in pediatric patients below the age of 12 years have not been established.

ADVERSE REACTIONS

Adverse experience information for Astelin® Nasal Spray is derived from six well-controlled, 2-day to 8-week clinical studies which included 391 patients who received Astelin® Nasal Spray at a dose of 2 sprays per nostril twice daily. In placebo-controlled efficacy trials, the incidence of discontinuation due to adverse reactions in patients receiving Astelin® Nasal Spray was not significantly different from vehicle placebo (2.2% vs 2.8%, respectively).

In these clinical studies, adverse events that occurred statistically significantly more often in patients treated with Astelin® Nasal Spray versus vehicle placebo included bitter taste (19.7% vs 0.6%), somnolence (11.5% vs 5.4%), weight increase (2.0% vs 0%), and myalgia (1.5% vs 0%).

The following adverse events were reported with frequencies ≥2% in the Astelin® Nasal Spray treatment group and more frequently than placebo in short-term (≤2 days) and long-term (2–8 weeks) clinical trials.

ADVERSE EVENT	Astelin® Nasal Spray n=391	Vehicle Placebo n=353
Bitter Taste*	19.7	0.6
Headache	14.8	12.7
Somnolence*	11.5	5.4
Nasal Burning	4.1	1.7
Pharyngitis	3.8	2.8
Dry Mouth	2.8	1.7
Paroxysmal Sneezing	3.1	1.1
Nausea	2.8	1.1
Rhinitis	2.3	1.4
Fatigue	2.3	1.4
Dizziness	2.0	1.4
Epistaxis	2.0	1.4
Weight Increase*	2.0	0.0

*P<0.05, Fisher's Exact Test (two-tailed)

The following events were observed infrequently (<2% and exceeding placebo incidence) in patients who received Astelin® Nasal Spray (2 sprays/nostril twice daily) in U.S. clinical trials.

Cardiovascular: flushing, hypertension, tachycardia.

Dermatological: contact dermatitis, eczema, hair and follicle infection, furunculosis.

Digestive: constipation, gastroenteritis, glossitis, ulcerative stomatitis, vomiting, increased SGPT, aphthous stomatitis.

Metabolic and Nutritional: increased appetite.

Musculoskeletal: myalgia, temporomandibular dislocation.

Neurological: hyperkinesia, hypoesthesia, vertigo.

Psychological: anxiety, depersonalization, depression, nervousness, sleep disorder, thinking abnormal.

Respiratory: bronchospasm, coughing, throat burning, laryngitis.

Special Senses: conjunctivitis, eye abnormality, eye pain, watery eyes, taste loss.

Urogenital: albuminuria, amenorrhea, breast pain, hematuria, increased urinary frequency.

Whole Body: allergic reaction, back pain, herpes simplex, viral infection, malaise, pain in extremities, abdominal pain.

In controlled trials involving nasal and oral azelastine hydrochloride formulations, there were infrequent occurrences of hepatic transaminase elevations. The clinical relevance of these reports has not been established.

OVERDOSAGE

There have been no reported overdosages with Astelin® Nasal Spray. Acute overdosage by adults with this dosage form is unlikely to result in clinically significant adverse events, other than increased somnolence, since one bottle of Astelin® Nasal Spray contains 17 mg of azelastine hydrochloride. Clinical studies in adults with single doses of the oral formulation of azelastine hydrochloride (up to 16 mg) have not resulted in increased incidence of serious adverse events. General supportive measures should be employed if overdosage occurs. There is no known antidote to Astelin® Nasal Spray. Oral ingestion of antihistamines has the potential to cause serious adverse effects in young children. Accordingly, Astelin® Nasal Spray should be kept out of the reach of children. Oral doses greater than 120 mg/kg (480 times the maximum recommended human daily intranasal dose on a mg/m^2 basis) produced significant mortality in mice. Responses seen prior to mortality were tremor, convulsions, decreased muscle tone, and salivation. Single doses as high as 10 mg/kg (270 times the maximum recommended human daily intranasal dose on a mg/m^2 basis) were well tolerated in dogs, but single doses of 20 mg/kg were lethal.

DOSAGE AND ADMINISTRATION

The recommended dose of Astelin® Nasal Spray in adults and children 12 years and older is two sprays per nostril twice daily. Before initial use, the screw cap on the bottle should be replaced with the pump unit and the delivery system should be primed with 4 sprays or until a fine mist appears. When 3 or more days have elapsed since the last use, the pump should be reprimed with 2 sprays or until a fine mist appears.

CAUTION: Avoid spraying in the eyes.

Directions for Use: Illustrated patient instructions for proper use accompany each package of Astelin® Nasal Spray.

HOW SUPPLIED

Astelin® (azelastine hydrochloride) Nasal Spray, 137 mcg, (NDC 0037-0241-10) is supplied as a package containing a total of 200 metered sprays in two high-density polyethylene (HDPE) bottles fitted with screw caps. A separate metered-dose spray pump unit and a leaflet of patient instructions are also provided. The spray pump unit is packaged in a polyethylene wrapper and consists of a nasal spray pump fitted with a blue safety clip and a blue plastic dust cover. Each Astelin® (azelastine hydrochloride) Nasal Spray, 137 mcg, bottle contains 17 mg (1 mg/mL) of azelastine hydrochloride to be used with the supplied metered-dose spray pump unit. Each bottle can deliver 100 metered sprays. Each spray delivers a mean of 0.137 mL solution containing 137 mcg of azelastine hydrochloride.

ATTENTION: The imprinted expiration date applies to the product in the bottles with screw caps. After the spray pump is inserted into the first bottle of the dispensing package, both bottles of product should be discarded after 3 months, not to exceed the expiration date imprinted on the label.

Storage: Store at controlled room temperature 20°–25°C (68°–77°F). Protect from freezing.

CAUTION: Federal law prohibits dispensing without a prescription.

Manufactured under license from
ASTA Medica AG, Germany
by **WALLACE LABORATORIES**
Division of Carter-Wallace, Inc.
Cranbury, New Jersey 08512-0181
©1991, 1997 Carter-Wallace, Inc.
IN-023S3-05A   Rev. 8/97
Shown in Product Identification Guide, page 341

DEPEN® ℞
(penicillamine tablets, USP)
Titratable Tablets

> Physicians planning to use penicillamine should thoroughly familiarize themselves with its toxicity, special dosage considerations, and therapeutic benefits. Penicillamine should never be used casually. Each patient should remain constantly under the close supervision of the physician. Patients should be warned to report promptly any symptoms suggesting toxicity.

DESCRIPTION

Penicillamine is 3-mercapto-D-valine, a disease modifying antirheumatic drug. It is a white or practically white, crystalline powder, freely soluble in water, slightly soluble in alcohol, and insoluble in ether, acetone, benzene, and carbon tetrachloride. Although its configuration is D, it is levorotatory as usually measured:

$$[\alpha] \begin{smallmatrix} \\ 25° \\ D \end{smallmatrix} = -62.5° \pm 2.0° (C = 1, 1N NaOH)$$

The empirical formula is $C_5H_{11}NO_2S$, giving it a molecular weight of 149.21. The structural formula is:

$$\begin{array}{c} CH_3\ H \\ |\quad | \\ HS-C\cdots C\cdots COOH \\ |\quad | \\ CH_3\ NH_2 \end{array}$$

It reacts readily with formaldehyde or acetone to form a thiazolidine-carboxylic acid.

Depen® (penicillamine tablets, USP) Titratable Tablets for oral administration contain 250 mg of penicillamine.

Other ingredients (inactive): edetate disodium, hydroxypropyl methylcellulose, lactose, magnesium stearate, magnesium trisilicate, polyethylene glycol, povidone, simethicone emulsion, starch, and stearic acid.

CLINICAL PHARMACOLOGY

Penicillamine is a chelating agent recommended for the removal of excess copper in patients with Wilson's disease. From *in vitro* studies which indicate that one atom of copper combines with two molecules of penicillamine, it would appear that one gram of penicillamine should be followed by the excretion of about 200 milligrams of copper; however, the actual amount excreted is about one percent of this.

Penicillamine also reduces excess cystine excretion in cystinuria. This is done, at least in part, by disulfide interchange between penicillamine and cystine, resulting in formation of penicillamine-cysteine disulfide, a substance that is much more soluble than cystine and is excreted readily.

Penicillamine interferes with the formation of cross-links between tropocollagen molecules and cleaves them when newly formed.

The mechanism of action of penicillamine in rheumatoid arthritis is unknown, although it appears to suppress disease activity. Unlike cytotoxic immunosuppressants, penicillamine markedly lowers IgM rheumatoid factor but produces no significant depression in absolute levels of serum immunoglobulins. Also unlike cytotoxic immunosuppressants, which act on both, penicillamine *in vitro* depresses T-cell activity but not B-cell activity.

In vitro, penicillamine dissociates macroglobulins (rheumatoid factor) although the relationship of the activity to its effect in rheumatoid arthritis is not known.

In rheumatoid arthritis, the onset of therapeutic response to DEPEN may not be seen for two or three months. In those patients who respond, however, the first evidence of suppression of symptoms such as pain, tenderness, and swelling usually is generally apparent within three months. The optimum duration of therapy has not been determined. If remissions occur, they may last from months to years but usually require continued treatment (see DOSAGE AND ADMINISTRATION).

In all patients receiving penicillamine, it is important that DEPEN be given on an empty stomach, at least one hour before meals or two hours after meals, and at least one hour apart from any other drug, food or milk. This permits maximum absorption and reduces the likelihood of inactivation by metal binding in the gastrointestinal tract.

Methodology for determining the bioavailability of penicillamine is not available; however, penicillamine is known to be a very soluble substance.

INDICATIONS

DEPEN is indicated in the treatment of Wilson's disease, cystinuria, and in patients with severe, active rheumatoid arthritis who have failed to respond to an adequate trial of conventional therapy. Available evidence suggests that DEPEN is not of value in alkylosing spondylitis.

Wilson's Disease—Wilson's disease (hepatolenticular degeneration) results from the interaction of an inherited defect and an abnormality in copper metabolism. The metabolic defect, which is the consequence of the autosomal inheritance of one abnormal gene from each parent, manifests itself in a greater positive copper balance than normal. As a result, copper is deposited in several organs and appears eventually to produce pathologic effects most prominently seen in the brain, where degeneration is widespread; in the liver, where fatty infiltration, inflammation, and hepatocellular damage progress to postnecrotic cirrhosis; in the kidney, where tubular and glomerular dysfunction results; and in the eye, where characteristic corneal copper deposits are known as Kayser-Fleischer rings.

Two types of patients require treatment for Wilson's disease: (1) the symptomatic, and (2) the asymptomatic in whom it can be assumed the disease will develop in the future if the patient is not treated.

Diagnosis, suspected on the basis of family or individual history, physical examination, or a low serum concentration of ceruloplasmin*, is confirmed by the demonstration of Kayser-Fleischer rings or, particularly in the asymtpomatic patient, by the quantitative demonstration in a liver biopsy specimen of a concentration of copper in excess of 250 mcg/g dry weight.

* For quantitative test for serum ceruloplasmin see: Morell, A.G.; Windsor, J.; Sternlieb, I; Scheinberg, I.H.: Measurement of the concentration of ceruloplasmin in serum by determination of its oxidase activity, in "Laboratory Diagnosis of Liver Disease," F.W. Sunderman; F.W. Sunderman, Jr., (eds.), St. Louis, Warren H. Green, Inc., 1968, pp. 193–195.

Treatment has two objectives:

(1) to minimize dietary intake and absorption of copper.

(2) to promote excretion of copper deposited in tissues.

The first objective is attained by a daily diet that contains no more than one or two milligrams of copper. Such a diet should exclude, most importantly, chocolate, nuts, shellfish, mushrooms, liver, molasses, broccoli, and cereals enriched with copper, and be composed to as great an extent as possible of foods with a low copper content. Distilled or demineralized water should be used if the patient's drinking water contains more than 0.1 mg of copper per liter.

For the second objective, a copper chelating agent is used. In symptomatic patients, this treatment usually produces marked neurologic improvement, fading of Kayser-Fleischer rings, and gradual amelioration of hepatic dysfunction and psychic disturbances.

Clinical experience to date suggests that life is prolonged with the above regimen.

Noticeable improvement may not occur for one to three months. Occasionally, neurologic symptoms become worse during initiation of therapy with DEPEN. Despite this, the drug should not be discontinued permanently. Although temporary interruption may result in clinical improvement of the neurological symptoms, it carries an increased risk of developing a sensitivity reaction upon resumption of therapy (See WARNINGS).

Treatment of asymptomatic patients has been carried out for over ten years. Symptoms and signs of the disease appear to be prevented indefinitely if daily treatment with DEPEN can be continued.

Cystinuria—Cystinuria is characterized by excessive urinary excretion of the dibasic amino acids, arginine, lysine, ornithine, and cystine, and the mixed disulfide of cysteine and homocysteine. The metabolic defect that leads to cystinuria is inherited as an autosomal, recessive trait. Metabolism of the affected amino acids is influenced by at least two abnormal factors: (1) defective gastrointestinal absorption and (2) renal tubular dysfunction.

Arginine, lysine, ornithine, and cysteine are soluble substances, readily excreted. There is no apparent pathology connected with their excretion in excessive quantities.

Cystine, however, is so slightly soluble at the usual range of urinary pH that it is not excreted readily, and so crystallizes and forms stones in the urinary tract. Stone formation is the only known pathology in cystinuria. Normal daily output of cystine is 40 to 80 mg. In cystinuria, output is greatly increased and may exceed 1 g/day. At 500 to 600 mg/day, stone formation is almost certain. When it is more than 300 mg/day, treatment is indicated.

Conventional treatment is directed at keeping urinary cystine diluted enough to prevent stone formation, keeping the urine alkaline enough to dissolve as much cystine as possible, and minimizing cystine production by a diet low in methionine (the major dietary precursor of cystine). Patients must drink enough fluid to keep urine specific gravity below 1.010, take enough alkali to keep urinary pH at 7.5 to 8, and maintain a diet low in methionine. This diet is not recommended in growing children and probably is contraindicated in pregnancy because of its low protein content (see PRECAUTIONS).

When these measures are inadequate to control recurrent stone formation, DEPEN may be used as additional therapy. When patients refuse to adhere to conventional treatment, DEPEN may be a useful substitute. It is capable of keeping cystine excretion to near normal values, thereby hindering stone formation and the serious consequences of pyelonephritis and impaired renal function that develop in some patients.

Bartter and colleagues depict the process by which penicillamine interacts with cystine to form penicillamine-cysteine mixed disulfide as:

$$CSSC + PS' \rightleftarrows CS' + CSSP$$

$$PSSP + CS' \rightleftarrows PS' + CSSP$$

$$CSSC + PSSP \rightleftarrows 2\ CSSP$$

CSSC = cystine
CS′ = deprotonated cysteine
PSSP = penicillamine
PS′ = deprotonated penicillamine sulfhydryl
CSSP = penicillamine-cysteine mixed disulfide

In this process, it is assumed that the deprotonated form of penicillamine, PS′, is the active factor in bringing about the disulfide interchange.

Rheumatoid Arthritis—Because DEPEN can cause severe adverse reactions, its use in rheumatoid arthritis should be restricted to patients who have severe, active disease and who have failed to respond to an adequate trial of conventional therapy. Even then, benefit-to-risk ratio should be carefully considered. Other measures, such as rest, physiotherapy, salicylates, and corticosteroids should be used, when indicated, in conjunction with DEPEN (see PRECAUTIONS).

CONTRAINDICATIONS

Except for treatment of Wilson's disease or certain cases of cystinuria, use of penicillamine during pregnancy is contraindicated (see WARNINGS).

Although breast milk studies have not been reported in animals or humans, mothers on therapy with penicillamine should not nurse their infants.

Patients with a history of penicillamine-related aplastic anemia or agranulocytosis should not be restarted on penicillamine (see WARNINGS and ADVERSE REACTIONS).

Because of its potential for causing renal damage, penicillamine should not be administered for rheumatoid arthritis patients with a history or other evidence of renal insufficiency.

WARNINGS

The use of penicillamine has been associated with fatalities due to certain diseases, such as aplastic anemia, agranulocytosis, thrombocytopenia, Goodpasture's syndrome, and myasthenia gravis.

Because of the potential for serious hematological and renal adverse reactions to occur at any time, routine urinalysis, white and differential blood cell count, hemoglobin determination, and direct platelet count must be done every two weeks for at least the first six months of penicillamine therapy and monthly thereafter. Patients should be instructed to report promptly the development of signs and symptoms of granulocytopenia and/or thrombocytopenia such as fever, sore throat, chills, bruising, or bleeding. The above laboratory studies should then be promptly repeated.

Leukopenia and thrombocytopenia have been reported to occur in up to five percent of patients during penicillamine therapy. Leukopenia is of the granulocytic series and may or may not be associated with an increase in eosinophils. A confirmed reduction in WBC below 3500 per cubic mL mandates discontinuance of penicillamine therapy. Thrombocytopenia may be on an idiosyncratic basis with decreased or absent megakaryocytes in the marrow, when it is part of an aplastic anemia. In other cases the thrombocytopenia is presumably on an immune basis since the number of megakaryocytes in the marrow has been reported to be normal or sometimes increased. The development of a platelet count below 100,000 per cubic mL, even in the absence of clinical bleeding, requires at least temporary cessation of penicillamine therapy. A progressive fall in either platelet count or WBC in three successive determinations, even though values are still within the normal range, likewise requires at least temporary cessation.

Proteinuria and/or hematuria may develop during therapy and may be warning signs of membranous glomerulopathy which can progress to a nephrotic syndrome. Close observation of these patients is essential. In some patients the proteinuria disappears with continued therapy; in others penicillamine must be discontinued. When a patent develops proteinuria or hematuria the physician must ascertain whether it is a sign of drug-induced glomerulopathy or is unrelated to penicillamine.

Rheumatoid arthritis patients who develop moderate degrees of proteinuria may be continued cautiously on penicillamine therapy, provided that quantitative 24-hour urinary protein determinations are obtained at intervals of one to two weeks. Penicillamine dosage should not be increased under these circumstances. Proteinuria which exceeds 1 g/24 hours, or proteinuria which is progressively increasing requires either discontinuance of the drug or a reduction in the dosage. In some patients, proteinuria has been reported to clear following reduction in dosage.

In rheumatoid arthritis patients, penicillamine should be discontinued if unexplained gross hematuria or persistent microscopic hematuria develops.

In patients with Wilson's disease or cystinuria the risks of continued penicillamine therapy in patients manifesting potentially serious urinary abnormalities must be weighed against the expected therapeutic benefits.

When penicillamine is used in cystinuria, an annual x-ray for renal stones is advised. Cystine stones form rapidly, sometimes in six months.

Up to one year or more may be required for any urinary abnormalities to disappear after penicillamine has been discontinued.

Because of rare reports of intrahepatic cholestasis and toxic hepatitis, liver function tests are recommended every six months for the duration of therapy.

Goodpasture's syndrome has occurred rarely. The development of abnormal urinary findings associated with hemoptysis and pulmonary infiltrates on x-ray requires immediate cessation of penicillamine.

Obliterative bronchiolitis has been reported rarely. The patient should be cautioned to report immediately pulmonary symptoms such as exertional dyspnea, unexplained cough, or wheezing. Pulmonary function studies should be considered at that time.

Myasthenic syndrome sometimes progressing to myasthenia gravis has been reported. Ptosis and diplopia, with weakness of the extraocular mucles, are often early signs of myasthenia. In the majority of cases, symptoms of myasthenia have receded after withdrawal of penicillamine.

Most of the various forms of pemphigus have occurred during treatment with penicillamine. Pemphigus vulgaris and pemphigus foliaceus are reported most frequently, usually as a late complication of therapy. The seborrhea-like characteristics of pemphigus foliaceus may obscure an early diagnosis. When pemphigus is suspected, DEPEN should be discontinued. Treatment has consisted of high doses of corticosteroids alone or, in some cases, concomitantly with an immunosuppressant. Treatment may be required for only a few weeks or months, but may need to be continued for more than a year.

Once instituted for Wilson's disease or cystinuria, treatment with penicillamine should, as a rule, be continued on a daily basis. Interruptions for even a few days have been followed by sensitivity reactions after reinstitution of therapy.

Use in Pregnancy—Penicillamine has been shown to be teratogenic in rats when given in doses 6 times higher than the highest dose recommended for human use (based on a standard weight of 50 kg). Skeletal defects, cleft palates, and fetal toxicity (resorptions) have been reported.

There are no controlled studies on the use of penicillamine in pregnant women. Although normal outcomes have been reported, characteristic congenital cutis laxa and associated birth defects have been reported in infants born of mothers who received therapy with penicillamine during pregnancy. Penicillamine should be used in women of childbearing potential only when the expected benefits outweigh the possible hazards. Women on therapy with penicillamine who are of childbearing potential should be apprised of this risk, advised to report promptly any missed menstrual periods or other indications of possible pregnancy, and followed closely for early recognition of pregnancy.

Wilson's Disease—Reported experience* shows that continued treatment with penicillamine throughout pregnancy protects the mother against relapse of the Wilson's disease, and that discontinuation of penicillamine has deleterious effects on the mother.

* Scheinberg, I.H., Sternlieb, I.: *N Engl J Med 293:* 1300–1302, December 18, 1975.

If penicillamine is administered during pregnancy to patients with Wilson's disease, it is recommended that the daily dosage be limited to 1 g. If cesarean section is planned, the daily dosage should be limited to 250 mg during the last six weeks of pregnancy and postoperatively until wound healing is complete.

Cystinuria—If possible, penicillamine should not be given during pregnancy to women with cystinuria (see CONTRAINDICATIONS). There are reports of women with cystinuria on therapy with penicillamine who gave birth to infants with generalized connective tissue defects who died following abdominal surgery. If stones continue to form in these patients, the benefits of therapy to the mother must be evaluated against the risk to the fetus.

Continued on next page

Depen—Cont.

Rheumatoid Arthritis—Penicillamine should not be administered to rheumatoid arthritis patients who are pregnant (see CONTRAINDICATIONS) and should be discontinued promptly in patients in whom pregnancy is suspected or diagnosed.
There is a report that a woman with rheumatoid arthritis treated with less than one gram a day of penicillamine during pregnancy gave birth (cesarean delivery) to an infant with growth retardation, flattened face with broad nasal bridge, low set ears, short neck with loose skin folds, and unusually lax body skin.

PRECAUTIONS

Some patients may experience drug fever, a marked febrile response to penicillamine, usually in the second or third week following initiation of therapy. Drug fever may sometimes be accompanied by a macular cutaneous eruption.
In the case of drug fever in patients with Wilson's disease or cystinuria, penicillamine should be temporarily discontinued until the reaction subsides. Then penicillamine should be reinstituted with a small dose that is gradually increased until the desired dosage is attained. Systemic steroid therapy may be necessary, and is usually helpful, in such patients in whom toxic reactions develop a second or third time.
In the case of drug fever in rheumatoid arthritis patients, because other treatments are available, penicillamine should be discontinued and another therapeutic alternative tried, since experience indicates that the febrile reaction will recur in a very high percentage of patients upon readministration of penicillamine.
The skin and mucous membranes should be observed for allergic reactions. Early and late rashes have occurred. Early rash occurs during the first few months of treatment and is more common. It is usually a generalized pruritic, erythematous, maculopapular, or morbilliform rash and resembles the allergic rash seen with other drugs. Early rash usually disappears within days after stopping penicillamine and seldom recurs when the drug is restarted at a lower dosage. Pruritus and early rash may often be controlled by the concomitant administration of antihistamines. Less commonly, a late rash may be seen, usually after six months or more of treatment, and requires discontinuation of penicillamine. It is usually on the trunk, is accompanied by intense pruritus, and is usually unresponsive to topical corticosteroid therapy. Late rash may take weeks to disappear after penicillamine is stopped and usually recurs if the drug is restarted.
The appearance of a drug eruption accompanied by fever, arthralgia, lymphadenopathy, or other allergic manifestations usually requires discontinuation of penicillamine. Certain patients will develop a positive antinuclear antibody (ANA) test and some of these may show a lupus erythematosus-like syndrome similar to drug-induced lupus associated with other drugs. The lupus erythemastosus-like syndrome is not associated with hypocomplementemia and may be present without nephropathy. The development of a positive ANA test does not mandate discontinuance of the drug; however, the physician should be alerted to the possibility that a lupus erythematosus-like syndrome may develop in the future.
Some patients may develop oral ulcerations which in some cases have the appearance of aphthous stomatitis. The stomatitis usually recurs on rechallenge but often clears on a lower dosage. Although rare, cheilosis, glossitis, and gingivostomatitis have also been reported. These oral lesions are frequently dose-related and may preclude further increase in penicillamine dosage or require discontinuation of the drug.
Hypogeusia (a blunting or diminution in taste perception) has occurred in some patients. This may last two to three months or more and may develop into a total loss of taste; however, it is usually self-limited, despite continued penicillamine treatment. Such taste impairment is rare in patients with Wilson's disease.
Penicillamine should not be used in patients who are receiving concurrently gold therapy, antimalarial or cytotoxic drugs, oxyphenbutazone, or phenylbutazone because these drugs are also associated with similar serious hematologic and renal adverse reactions. Patients who have had gold salt therapy discontinued due to a major toxic reaction may be at greater risk of serious adverse reactions with penicillamine, but not necessarily of the same type.
Patients who are allergic to penicillin may theoretically have cross-sensitivity to penicillamine. The possibility of reactions from contamination of penicillamine by trace amounts of penicillin has been eliminated now that penicillamine is being produced synthetically rather than as a degradation product of penicillin.
Because of their dietary restrictions, patients with Wilson's disease and cystinuria should be given 25 mg/day of pyridoxine during therapy, since penicillamine increases the requirement for this vitamin. Patients also may receive benefit from a multivitamin preparation, although there is no evidence that deficiency of any vitmain other than pyridoxine is associated with penicillamine. In Wilson's disease, multivitamin preparations must be copper-free.
Rheumatoid arthritis patients whose nutrition is impaired should also be given a daily supplement of pyridoxine. Mineral supplements should not be given, since they may block the response to penicillamine.
Iron deficiency may develop, especially in children and in menstruating women. In Wilson's disease, this may be a result of adding the effects of the low copper diet, which is probably also low in iron, and the penicillamine to the effects of blood loss or growth. In cystinuria, a low methionine diet may contribute to iron deficiency, since it is necessarily low in protein. If necessary, iron may be given in short courses, but a period of two hours should elapse between administration of penicillamine and iron, since orally administered iron has been shown to reduce the effects of penicillamine.
Penicillamine causes an increase in the amount of soluble collagen. In the rat this results in inhibition of normal healing and also a decrease in tensile strength of intact skin. In man this may be the cause of increased skin friability at sites especially subject to pressure or trauma, such as shoulders, elbows, knees, toes, and buttocks. Extravasations of blood may occur and may appear as purpuric areas, with external bleeding if the skin is broken, or as vesicles containing dark blood. Neither type is progressive. There is no apparent association with bleeding elsewhere in the body and no associated coagulation defect has been found. Therapy with penicillamine may be continued in the presence of these lesions. They may not recur if dosage is reduced. Other reported effects probably due to the action of penicillamine on collagen are excessive wrinkling of the skin and development of small, white papules at venipuncture and surgical sites.
The effects of penicillamine on collagen and elastin make it advisable to consider a reduction in dosage to 250 mg/day when surgery is contemplated. Reinstitution of full therapy should be delayed until wound healing is complete.
Carcinogenesis—Long-term animal carcinogenicity studies have not been done with penicillamine. There is a report that five of ten autoimmune disease-prone NZB hybrid mice developed lymphocytic leukemia after 6 months' intraperitoneal treatment with a dose of 400 mg/kg penicillamine 5 days per week.
Nursing Mothers—See CONTRAINDICATIONS.
Pediatric Use—The efficacy of DEPEN in pediatric patients with juvenile rheumatoid arthritis has not been established.

ADVERSE REACTIONS

Penicillamine is a drug with a high incidence of untoward reactions, some of which are potentially fatal. Therefore, it is mandatory that patients receiving penicillamine therapy remain under close medical supervision throughout the period of drug administration (see WARNINGS and PRECAUTIONS).
Reported incidences (%) for the most commonly occurring adverse reactions in rheumatoid arthritis patients are noted, based on 17 representative clinical trials reported in the literature (1270 patients).
Allergic—Generalized pruritus, early and late rashes (5%), pemphigus (see WARNINGS), and drug eruptions which may be accompanied by fever, arthralgia, or lymphadenopathy have occurred (see WARNINGS and PRECAUTIONS). Some patients may show lupus erythematosus-like syndrome similar to drug-induced lupus produced by other pharmacological agents (see PRECAUTIONS).
Urticaria and exfoliative dermatitis have occurred.
Thyroiditis has been reported; hypoglycemia in association with anti-insulin antibodies has been reported. These reactions are extremely rare.
Some patients may develop a migratory polyarthralgia, often with objective synovitis (see DOSAGE AND ADMINISTRATION).
Gastrointestinal—Anorexia, epigastric pain, nausea, vomiting, or occasional diarrhea may occur (17%).
Isolated cases of reactivated peptic ulcer have occurred, as have hepatic dysfunction and pancreatitis. Intrahepatic cholestasis and toxic hepatitis have been reported rarely. There have been a few reports of increased serum alkaline phosphatase, lactic dehydrogenase, and positive cephalin flocculation and thymol turbidity tests.
Some patients may report a blunting, diminution, or total loss of taste perception (12%); or may develop oral ulcerations. Although rare, cheilosis, glossitis, and gingivostomatitis have been reported (see PRECAUTIONS).
Gastrointestinal side effects are usually reversible following cessation of therapy.
Hematological—Penicillamine can cause bone marrow depression (see WARNINGS). Leukopenia (2%) and thrombocytopenia (4%) have occurred. Fatalities have been reported as a result of thrombocytopenia, agranulocytosis, aplastic anemia, and sideroblastic anemia.
Thrombotic thrombocytopenic purpura, hemolytic anemia, red cell aplasia, monocytosis, leukocytosis, eosinophilia, and thrombocytosis have also been reported.
Renal—Patients on penicillamine therapy may develop proteinuria (6%) and/or hematuria which, in some, may progress to the development of the nephrotic syndrome as a result of an immune complex membranous glomerulopathy (see WARNINGS).
Central Nervous System—Tinnitus, optic neuritis, and peripheral sensory and motor neuropathies (including polyradiculoneuropathy, i.e., Guillain-Barre Syndrome) have been reported. Muscular weakness may or may not occur with the peripheral neuropathies.
Neuromuscular—Myasthenia gravis (see WARNINGS).
Other—Adverse reactions that have been reported rarely include thrombophlebitis; hyperpyrexia (see PRECAUTIONS); falling hair or alopecia; lichen planus; polymyositis; dermatomyositis; mammary hyperplasia; elastosis perforans serpiginosa; toxic epidermal necrolysis; anetoderma (cutaneous macular atrophy); and Goodpasture's syndrome, a severe and ultimately fatal glomerulonephritis associated with intra-alveloar hemorrhage (see WARNINGS). Fatal renal vasculitis has also been reported. Allergic alveolitis, obliterative bronchiolitis, interstitial pneumonitis, and pulmonary fibrosis have been reported in patients with severe rheumatoid arthritis, some of whom were receiving penicillamine. Bronchial asthma also has been reported.
Increased skin friability, excessive wrinkling of skin, and development of small, white papules at venipuncture and surgical sites have been reported (see PRECAUTIONS).
The chelating action of the drug may cause increased excretion of other heavy metals such as zinc, mercury, and lead.
There have been reports associating penicillamine with leukemia. However, circumstances involving these reports are such that a cause and effect relationship to the drug has not been established.

DOSAGE AND ADMINISTRATION

In all patients receiving penicillamine, it is important that DEPEN be given on an empty stomach, at least one hour before meals or two hours after meals, and at least one hour apart from any other drug, food, or milk. Because penicillamine increases the requirement for pyridoxine, patients may require a daily supplement of pyridoxine (see PRECAUTIONS).
Wilson's Disease—Optimal dosage can be determined by measurement of urinary copper excretion and the determination of free copper in the serum. The urine must be collected in copper-free glassware and should be quantitatively analyzed for copper before and soon after initiation of therapy with DEPEN.
Determination of 24-hour urinary copper excretions is of greatest value in the first week of therapy with penicillamine. In the absence of any drug reaction, a dose between 0.75 and 1.5 g that results in an initial 24-hour cupriuresis of over 2 mg should be continued for about three months, by which time the most reliable method of monitoring maintenance treatment is the determination of free copper in the serum. This equals the difference between quantitatively determined total copper and ceruloplasmin-copper. Adequately treated patients will usually have less than 10 mcg free copper/dL of serum. It is seldom necessary to exceed a dosage of 2 g/day. If the patient is intolerant to therapy with DEPEN, alternative treatment is trientine hydrochloride.
In patients who cannot tolerate as much as 1 g/day initially, initiating dosage with 250 mg/day, and increasing gradually to the requisite amount, gives closer control of the effects of the drug and may help to reduce the incidence of adverse reactions.
Cystinuria—It is recommended that DEPEN be used along with conventional therapy. By reducing urinary cystine, it decreases crystalluria and stone formation. In some instances, it has been reported to decease the size of, and even to dissolve, stones already formed.
The usual dosage of DEPEN in the treatment of cystinuria is 2 g/day for adults, with a range of 1 to 4 g/day. For pediatric patients, dosage can be based on 30 mg/kg/day. The total daily amount should be divided into four doses. If four equal doses are not feasible, give the larger portion at bedtime. If adverse reactions necessitate a reduction in dosage, it is important to retain the bedtime dose
Initiating dosage with 250 mg/day, and increasing gradually to the requisite amount, gives closer control of the effects of the drug and may help to reduce the incidence of adverse reactions.
In addition to taking DEPEN, patients should drink copiously. It is especially important to drink about a pint of fluid at bedtime and another pint once during the night when urine is more concentrated and more acid than during the day. The greater the fluid intake, the lower the required dosage of DEPEN.
Dosage must be individualized to an amount that limits cystine excretion to 100–200 mg/day in those with no history of stones, and below 100 mg/day in those who have had stone formation and/or pain. Thus, in determining dosage, the inherent tubular defect, the patient's size, age, and rate of growth, and his diet and water intake all must be taken into consideration.

The standard nitroprusside cyanide test has been reported useful as a qualitative measure of the effective dose*: Add 2 mL of freshly prepared 5 percent sodium cyanide to 5 mL of a 24-hour aliquot of protein-free urine and let stand ten minutes. Add 5 drops of freshly prepared 5 percent sodium nitroprusside and mix. Cystine will turn the mixture magenta. If the result is negative, it can be assumed that cystine excretion is less than 100 mg/g creatinine.

* Lotz, M., Potts, J.T. and Bartter, F.C.: *BritMed J 2*: 521, August 28, 1965 (in Medical Memoranda).

Although penicillamine is rarely excreted unchanged, it also will turn the mixture magenta. If there is any question as to which substance is causing the reaction, a ferric chloride test can be done to eliminate doubt: Add 3 percent ferric chloride dropwise to the urine. Penicillamine will turn the urine an immediate and quickly fading blue. Cystine will not produce any change in appearance.

Rheumatoid Arthritis—The principal rule of treatment with DEPEN in rheumatoid arthritis is patience. The onset of therapeutic response is typically delayed. Two or three months may be required before the first evidence of a clinical response is noted (see CLINICAL PHARMACOLOGY). When treatment with DEPEN has been interrupted because of adverse reactions or other reasons, the drug should be reintroduced cautiously by starting with a lower dosage and increasing slowly.

Initial Therapy—The currently recommended dosage regimen in rheumatoid arthritis begins with a single daily dose of 125 mg or 250 mg which is thereafter increased at one to three month intervals, by 125 mg or 250 mg/day, as patient response and tolerance indicate. If a satisfactory remission of symptoms is achieved, the dose associated with the remission should be continued (see Maintenance Therapy). If there is no improvement and there are no signs of potentially serious toxicity after two to three months of treatment with doses of 500–750 mg/day, increases of 250 mg/day at two to three month intervals may be continued until a satisfactory remission occurs (see Maintenance Therapy) or signs of toxicity develop (see WARNINGS and PRECAUTIONS). If there is no discernible improvement after three to four months of treatment with 1000 to 1500 mg of penicillamine/day, it may be assumed the patient will not respond and DEPEN should be discontinued.

Maintenance Therapy—The maintenance dosage of DEPEN must be individualized, and may require adjustment during the course of treatment. Many patients respond satisfactorily to a dosage within the 500–750 mg/day range. Some need less.

Changes in maintenance dosage levels may not be reflected clinically or in the erythrocyte sedimentation rate for two to three months after each dosage adjustment.

Some patients will subsequently require an increase in the maintenance dosage to achieve maximal disease suppression. In those patients who do respond, but who evidence incomplete suppression of their disease after the first six to nine months of treatment, the daily dosage of DEPEN may be increased by 125 mg or 250 mg/day at three-month intervals. It is unusual in current practice to employ a dosage in excess of 1 g/day, but up to 1.5 g/day has sometimes been required.

Management of Exacerbations—During the course of treatment some patients may experience an exacerbation of disease activity following an initial good response. These may be self-limited and can subside within twelve weeks. They are usually controlled by the addition of nonsteroidal anti-inflammatory drugs, and only if the patient has demonstrated a true "escape" phenomenon (as evidenced by failure of the flare to subside within this time period) should an increase in the maintenance dose ordinarily be considered. In the rheumatoid patient, migratory polyarthralgia due to penicillamine is extremely difficult to differentiate from an exacerbation of the rheumatoid arthritis. Discontinuance or a substantial reduction in the dosage of DEPEN for up to several weeks will usually determine which of these processes is responsible for the arthralgia.

Duration of Therapy—The optimum duration of DEPEN therapy in rheumatoid arthritis has not been determined. If the patient has been in remission for six months or more, a gradual, stepwise dosage reduction in decrements of 125 mg or 250 mg/day at approximately three month intervals may be attempted.

Concomitant Drug Therapy—DEPEN should not be used in patients who are receiving gold therapy, antimalarial or cytotoxic drugs, oxyphenbutazone, or phenylbutazone (see PRECAUTIONS). Other measures, such as salicylates, other nonsteroidal anti-inflammatory drugs or systemic corticosteroids may be continued when DEPEN is initiated. After improvement commences, analgesic and anti-inflammatory drugs may be slowly discontinued as symptoms permit. Steroid withdrawal must be done gradually, and many months of DEPEN treatment may be required before steroids can be completely eliminated.

Dosage Frequency—Based on clinical experience, dosages up to 500 mg/day can be given as a single daily dose. Dosages in excess of 500 mg/day should be administered in divided doses.

HOW SUPPLIED

Depen® (penicillamine tablets, USP) Titratable Tablets: 250 mg scored, oval, white tablets coded with 37-4401 and Wallace; available in bottles of 100 (NDC 0037-4401-01). Storage: Store at controlled room temperature 20°–25°C (68°–77°F). Protect from moisture. Dispense in a tight container.

WALLACE LABORATORIES
Division of Carter-Wallace, Inc.
Cranbury, New Jersey 08512
Manufactured under license from ASTA Medica AG, Frankfurt, Federal Republic of Germany

IN-030F2-10   Rev. 12/96

DIUTENSEN®–R   ℞
(methyclothiazide and reserpine)
Tablets

FELBATOL®   ℞
(felbamate)
Tablets 400 mg and 600 mg,
Oral Suspension 600 mg/5 mL

Before Prescribing Felbatol® (felbamate), the physician should be thoroughly familiar with the details of this prescribing information.
FELBATOL® SHOULD NOT BE USED BY PATIENTS UNTIL THERE HAS BEEN A COMPLETE DISCUSSION OF THE RISKS AND THE PATIENT, PARENT, OR GUARDIAN HAS PROVIDED WRITTEN INFORMED CONSENT (SEE PATIENT INFORMATION/CONSENT SECTION).

WARNING
1. APLASTIC ANEMIA
THE USE OF FELBATOL® (felbamate) IS ASSOCIATED WITH A MARKED INCREASE IN THE INCIDENCE OF APLASTIC ANEMIA. ACCORDINGLY, FELBATOL® SHOULD ONLY BE USED IN PATIENTS WHOSE EPILEPSY IS SO SEVERE THAT THE RISK OF APLASTIC ANEMIA IS DEEMED ACCEPTABLE IN LIGHT OF THE BENEFITS CONFERRED BY ITS USE (SEE **INDICATIONS**). ORDINARILY, A PATIENT SHOULD NOT BE PLACED ON AND/OR CONTINUED ON FELBATOL® WITHOUT CONSIDERATION OF APPROPRIATE EXPERT HEMATOLOGIC CONSULTATION.
AMONG FELBATOL® TREATED PATIENTS, APLASTIC ANEMIA (PANCYTOPENIA IN THE PRESENCE OF A BONE MARROW LARGELY DEPLETED OF HEMATOPOIETIC PRECURSORS) OCCURS AT AN INCIDENCE THAT MAY BE MORE THAN A 100 FOLD GREATER THAN THAT SEEN IN THE UNTREATED POPULATION (I.E., 2 TO 5 PER MILLION PERSONS PER YEAR). THE RISK OF DEATH IN PATIENTS WITH APLASTIC ANEMIA GENERALLY VARIES AS A FUNCTION OF ITS SEVERITY AND ETIOLOGY; CURRENT ESTIMATES OF THE OVERALL CASE FATALITY RATE ARE IN THE RANGE OF 20 TO 30%, BUT RATES AS HIGH AS 70% HAVE BEEN REPORTED IN THE PAST.
THERE ARE TOO FEW FELBATOL® ASSOCIATED CASES, AND TOO LITTLE KNOWN ABOUT THEM TO PROVIDE A RELIABLE ESTIMATE OF THE SYNDROME'S INCIDENCE OR ITS CASE FATALITY RATE OR TO IDENTIFY THE FACTORS, IF ANY, THAT MIGHT CONCEIVABLY BE USED TO PREDICT WHO IS AT GREATER OR LESSER RISK.
IN MANAGING PATIENTS ON FELBATOL®, IT SHOULD BE BORNE IN MIND THAT THE CLINICAL MANIFESTATION OF APLASTIC ANEMIA MAY NOT BE SEEN UNTIL AFTER A PATIENT HAS BEEN ON FELBATOL® FOR SEVERAL MONTHS (E.G., ONSET OF APLASTIC ANEMIA AMONG FELBATOL® EXPOSED PATIENTS FOR WHOM DATA ARE AVAILABLE HAS RANGED FROM 5 TO 30 WEEKS). HOWEVER, THE INJURY TO BONE MARROW STEM CELLS THAT IS HELD TO BE ULTIMATELY RESPONSIBLE FOR THE ANEMIA MAY OCCUR WEEKS TO MONTHS EARLIER. ACCORDINGLY, PATIENTS WHO ARE DISCONTINUED FROM FELBATOL® REMAIN AT RISK FOR DEVELOPING ANEMIA FOR A VARIABLE, AND UNKNOWN, PERIOD AFTERWARDS.
IT IS NOT KNOWN WHETHER OR NOT THE RISK OF DEVELOPING APLASTIC ANEMIA CHANGES WITH DURATION OF EXPOSURE. CONSEQUENTLY, IT IS NOT SAFE TO ASSUME THAT A PATIENT WHO HAS BEEN ON FELBATOL® WITHOUT SIGNS OF HEMATOLOGIC ABNORMALITY FOR LONG PERIODS OF TIME IS WITHOUT RISK.
IT IS NOT KNOWN WHETHER OR NOT THE DOSE OF FELBATOL® AFFECTS THE INCIDENCE OF APLASTIC ANEMIA.
IT IS NOT KNOWN WHETHER OR NOT CONCOMITANT USE OF ANTIEPILEPTIC DRUGS AND/OR OTHER DRUGS AFFECTS THE INCIDENCE OF APLASTIC ANEMIA.
APLASTIC ANEMIA TYPICALLY DEVELOPS WITHOUT PREMONITORY CLINICAL OR LABORATORY SIGNS, THE FULL BLOWN SYNDROME PRESENTING WITH SIGNS OF INFECTION, BLEEDING, OR ANEMIA. ACCORDINGLY, ROUTINE BLOOD TESTING CANNOT BE RELIABLY USED TO REDUCE THE INCIDENCE OF APLASTIC ANEMIA, BUT, IT WILL, IN SOME CASES, ALLOW THE DETECTION OF THE HEMATOLOGIC CHANGES BEFORE THE SYNDROME DECLARES ITSELF CLINICALLY. FELBATOL® SHOULD BE DISCONTINUED IF ANY EVIDENCE OF BONE MARROW DEPRESSION OCCURS.
2. HEPATIC FAILURE
HEPATIC FAILURE RESULTING IN FATALITIES HAS BEEN REPORTED WITH A MARKED INCREASE IN THE FREQUENCY IN PATIENTS RECEIVING FELBATOL® (felbamate). ACCORDINGLY, FELBATOL® SHOULD ONLY BE USED IN PATIENTS WHOSE EPILEPSY IS SO SEVERE THAT THE RISK OF LIVER FAILURE IS OUTWEIGHED BY THE POTENTIAL BENEFITS OF SEIZURE CONTROL.
ALTHOUGH FULL INFORMATION IS NOT YET AVAILABLE, THE NUMBER OF CASES REPORTED GREATLY EXCEEDS THE NUMBER THAT IS EXPECTED BASED ON THE ANNUAL INCIDENCE OF ACUTE LIVER FAILURE IN THE UNITED STATES (I.E., ABOUT 2,000 CASES PER YEAR).
THERE ARE TOO FEW FELBATOL® ASSOCIATED CASES OF HEPATIC FAILURE AND TOO LITTLE KNOWN ABOUT THEM TO PROVIDE EITHER A RELIABLE ESTIMATE OF ITS INCIDENCE OR TO IDENTIFY THE FACTORS, IF ANY, THAT MIGHT BE USED TO PREDICT WHICH PATIENT IS AT GREATER OR LESSER RISK.
IT IS NOT KNOWN WHETHER OR NOT THE RISK OF DEVELOPING HEPATIC FAILURE CHANGES WITH DURATION OF EXPOSURE.
IT IS NOT KNOWN WHETHER OR NOT THE DOSAGE OF FELBATOL® AFFECTS THE INCIDENCE OF HEPATIC FAILURE.
IT IS NOT KNOWN WHETHER CONCOMITANT USE OF OTHER ANTIEPILEPTIC DRUGS AND/OR OTHER DRUGS AFFECTS THE INCIDENCE OF HEPATIC FAILURE.
FELBATOL® SHOULD NOT BE PRESCRIBED FOR ANYONE WITH A HISTORY OF HEPATIC DYSFUNCTION.
PATIENTS PRESCRIBED FELBATOL® SHOULD HAVE LIVER FUNCTION TESTS (AST, ALT, BILIRUBIN) PERFORMED BEFORE INITIATING FELBATOL® AND AT 1- TO 2-WEEK INTERVALS WHILE TREATMENT CONTINUES. A PATIENT WHO DEVELOPS ABNORMAL LIVER FUNCTION TESTS SHOULD BE IMMEDIATELY WITHDRAWN FROM FELBATOL® TREATMENT.

DESCRIPTION

Felbatol® (felbamate) is an antiepileptic available as 400 mg and 600 mg tablets and as a 600 mg/5 mL suspension for oral administration. Its chemical name is 2-phenyl-1,3-propanediol dicarbamate.

Felbamate is a white to off-white crystalline powder with a characteristic odor. It is very slightly soluble in water, slightly soluble in ethanol, sparingly soluble in methanol, and freely soluble in dimethyl sulfoxide. The molecular weight is 238.24; felbamate's molecular formula is $C_{11}H_{14}N_2O_4$; its structural formula is:

The inactive ingredients for Felbatol® (felbamate) tablets 400 mg and 600 mg are starch, microcrystalline cellulose, croscarmellose sodium, lactose, magnesium stearate, FD&C Yellow No. 6, D&C Yellow No. 10, and FD&C Red No. 40

Continued on next page

Felbatol—Cont.

(600 mg tablets only). The inactive ingredients for Felbatol® (felbamate) suspension 600 mg/5 mL are sorbitol, glycerin, microcrystalline cellulose, carboxymethylcellulose sodium, simethicone, polysorbate 80, methylparaben, saccharin sodium, propylparaben, FD&C Yellow No. 6, FD&C Red No. 40, flavorings, and purified water.

CLINICAL PHARMACOLOGY

Mechanism of Action:

The mechanism by which felbamate exerts its anticonvulsant activity is unknown, but in animal test systems designed to detect anticonvulsant activity, felbamate has properties in common with other marketed anticonvulsants. Felbamate is effective in mice and rats in the maximal electroshock test, the subcutaneous pentylenetetrazol seizure test, and the subcutaneous picrotoxin seizure test. Felbamate also exhibits anticonvulsant activity against seizures induced by intracerebroventricular administration of glutamate in rats and N-methyl-D,L-aspartic acid in mice. Protection against maximal electroshock-induced seizures suggests that felbamate may reduce seizure spread, an effect possibly predictive of efficacy in generalized tonic-clonic or partial seizures. Protection against pentylenetetrazol-induced seizures suggests that felbamate may increase seizure threshold, an effect considered to be predictive of potential efficacy in absence seizures.

Receptor-binding studies *in vitro* indicate that felbamate has weak inhibitory effects on GABA-receptor binding, benzodiazepine receptor binding, and is devoid of activity at the MK-801 receptor binding site of the NMDA receptor-ionophore complex. However, felbamate does interact as an antagonist at the strychnine-insensitive glycine recognition site of the NMDA receptor-ionophore complex. Felbamate is not effective in protecting chick embryo retina tissue against the neurotoxic effects of the excitatory amino acid agonists NMDA, kainate, or quisqualate *in vitro*.

The monocarbamate, p-hydroxy, and 2-hydroxy metabolites were inactive in the maximal electroshock-induced seizure test in mice. The monocarbamate and p-hydroxy metabolites had only weak (0.2 to 0.6) activity compared with felbamate in the subcutaneous pentylenetetrazol seizure test. These metabolites did not contribute significantly to the anticonvulsant action of felbamate.

Pharmacokinetics:

The numbers in the pharmacokinetic section are mean ± standard deviation.

Felbamate is well-absorbed after oral administration. Over 90% of the radioactivity after a dose of 1000 mg ^{14}C felbamate was found in the urine. Absolute bioavailability (oral vs. parenteral) has not been measured. The tablet and suspension were each shown to be bioequivalent to the capsule used in clinical trials, and pharmacokinetic parameters of the tablet and suspension are similar. There was no effect of food on absorption of the tablet; the effect of food on absorption of the suspension has not been evaluated.

Following oral administration, felbamate is the predominant plasma species (about 90% of plasma radioactivity). About 40–50% of absorbed dose appears unchanged in urine, and an additional 40% is present as unidentified metabolites and conjugates. About 15% is present as parahydroxyfelbamate, 2-hydroxyfelbamate, and felbamate monocarbamate, none of which have significant anticonvulsant activity.

Binding of felbamate to human plasma protein was independent of felbamate concentrations between 10 and 310 micrograms/mL. Binding ranged from 22% to 25%, mostly to albumin, and was dependent on the albumin concentration.

Felbamate is excreted with a terminal half-life of 20–23 hours, which is unaltered after multiple doses. Clearance after a single 1200 mg dose is 26±3 mL/hr/kg, and after multiple daily doses of 3600 mg is 30±8 mL/hr/kg. The apparent volume of distribution was 756±82 mL/kg after a 1200 mg dose. Felbamate Cmax and AUC are proportionate to dose after single and multiple doses over a range of 100–800 mg single doses and 1200–3600 mg daily doses. Cmin (trough) blood levels are also dose proportional. Multiple daily doses of 1200, 2400, and 3600 mg gave Cmin values of 30±5, 55±8, and 83±21 micrograms/mL (N=10 patients). Linear and dose proportional pharmacokinetics were also observed at doses above 3600 mg/day up to the maximum dose studied of 6000 mg/day. Felbamate gave dose proportional steady-state peak plasma concentrations in children age 4–12 over a range of 15, 30, and 45 mg/kg/day with peak concentrations of 17, 32, and 49 micrograms/mL.

The effects of race and gender on felbamate pharmacokinetics have not been systematically evaluated, but plasma concentrations in males (N=5) and females (N=4) given felbamate have been similar. The effects of felbamate kinetics on hepatic functional impairment have not been evaluated.

Renal Impairment: Felbamate's single dose monotherapy pharmacokinetic parameters were evaluated in 12 otherwise healthy individuals with renal impairment. Reduced felbamate clearance and a longer half-life were associated with diminishing renal function.

Pharmacodynamics:

Typical Physiologic Responses:

1. Cardiovascular:

In adults, there is no effect of felbamate on blood pressure. Small but statistically significant mean increases in heart rate were seen during adjunctive therapy and monotherapy; however, these mean increases of up to 5 bpm were not clinically significant. In children, no clinically relevant changes in blood pressure or heart rate were seen during adjunctive therapy or monotherapy with felbamate.

2. Other Physiologic Effects:

The only other change in vital signs was a mean decrease of approximately 1 respiration per minute in respiratory rate during adjunctive therapy in children. In adults, statistically significant mean reductions in body weight were observed during felbamate monotherapy and adjunctive therapy. In children, there were mean decreases in body weight during adjunctive therapy and monotherapy; however, these mean changes were not statistically significant. These mean reductions in adults and children were approximately 5% of the mean weights at baseline.

CLINICAL STUDIES

The results of controlled clinical trials established the efficacy of Felbatol® (felbamate) as monotherapy and adjunctive therapy in adults with partial-onset seizures with or without secondary generalization and in partial and generalized seizures associated with Lennox-Gastaut syndrome in children.

Felbatol® Monotherapy Trials in Adults

Felbatol® (3600 mg/day given QID) and low-dose valproate (15 mg/kg/day) were compared as monotherapy during a 112-day treatment period in a multicenter and a single-center double-blind efficacy trial. Both trials were conducted according to an identical study design. During a 56-day baseline period, all patients had at least four partial-onset seizures per 28 days and were receiving one antiepileptic drug at a therapeutic level, the most common being carbamazepine. In the multicenter trial, baseline seizure frequencies were 12.4 per 28 days in the Felbatol® group and 21.3 per 28 days in the low-dose valproate group. In the single-center trial, baseline seizure frequencies were 18.1 per 28 days in the Felbatol® group and 15.9 per 28 days in the low-dose valproate group. Patients were converted to monotherapy with Felbatol® or low-dose valproic acid during the first 28 days of the 112-day treatment period. Study endpoints were completion of 112 study days or fulfilling an escape criterion. Criteria for escape relative to baseline were: (1) twofold increase in monthly seizure frequency, (2) twofold increase in highest 2-day seizure frequency, (3) single generalized tonic-clonic seizure (GTC) if none occurred during baseline, or (4) significant prolongation of GTCs. The primary efficacy variable was the number of patients in each treatment group who met escape criteria.

In the multicenter trial, the percentage of patients who met escape criteria was 40% (18/45) in the Felbatol® group and 78% (39/50) in the low-dose valproate group. In the single-center trial, the percentage of patients who met escape criteria was 14% (3/21) in the Felbatol® group and 90% (19/21) in the low-dose valproate group. In both trials, the difference in the percentage of patients meeting escape criteria was statistically significant (P<.001) in favor of Felbatol®. These two studies by design were intended to demonstrate the effectiveness of Felbatol® monotherapy. The studies were not designed or intended to demonstrate comparative efficacy of the two drugs. For example, valproate was not used at the maximally effective dose.

Felbatol® Adjunctive Therapy Trials in Adults

A double-blind, placebo-controlled crossover trial consisted of two 10-week outpatient treatment periods. Patients with refractory partial-onset seizures who were receiving phenytoin and carbamazepine at therapeutic levels were administered Felbatol® (felbamate) as add-on therapy at a starting dosage of 1400 mg/day in three divided doses, which was increased to 2600 mg/day in three divided doses. Among the 56 patients who completed the study, the baseline seizure frequency was 20 per month. Patients treated with Felbatol® had fewer seizures than patients treated with placebo for each treatment sequence. There was a 23% (P=.018) difference in percentage seizure frequency reduction in favor of Felbatol®.

Felbatol® 3600 mg/day given QID and placebo were compared in a 28-day double-blind add-on trial in patients who had their standard antiepileptic drugs reduced while undergoing evaluations for surgery of intractable epilepsy. All patients had confirmed partial-onset seizures with or without generalization, seizure frequency during surgical evaluation not exceeding an average of four partial seizures per day or more than one generalized seizure per day, and a minimum average of one partial or generalized tonic-clonic seizure per day for the last 3 days of the surgical evaluation. The primary efficacy variable was time to fourth seizure after randomization to treatment with Felbatol® or placebo. Thirteen (46%) of 28 patients in the Felbatol® group versus 29 (88%) of 33 patients in the placebo group experienced a fourth seizure. The median times to fourth seizure were greater than 28 days in the Felbatol® group and 5 days in the placebo group. The difference between Felbatol® and placebo in time to fourth seizure was statistically significant (P=.002) in favor of Felbatol®.

Felbatol® Adjunctive Therapy Trial in Children with Lennox-Gastaut Syndrome

In a 70-day double-blind, placebo-controlled add-on trial in the Lennox-Gastaut syndrome, Felbatol® 45 mg/kg/day given QID was superior to placebo in controlling the multiple seizure types associated with this condition. Patients had at least 90 atonic and/or atypical absence seizures per month while receiving therapeutic dosages of one or two other antiepileptic drugs. Patients had a past history of using an average of eight antiepileptic drugs. The most commonly used antiepileptic drug during the baseline period was valproic acid. The frequency of all types of seizures during the baseline period was 1617 per month in the Felbatol® group and 716 per month in the placebo group. Statistically significant differences in the effect on seizure frequency favored Felbatol® over placebo for total seizures (26% reduction vs 5% increase, P<.001), atonic seizures (44% reduction vs 7% reduction, P=.002), and generalized tonic-clonic seizures (40% reduction vs 12% increase, P=.017). Parent/guardian global evaluations based on impressions of quality of life with respect to alertness, verbal responsiveness, general well-being, and seizure control significantly (P<.001) favored Felbatol® over placebo.

When efficacy was analyzed by gender in four well-controlled trials of felbamate as adjunctive and monotherapy for partial-onset seizures and Lennox-Gastaut syndrome, a similar response was seen in 122 males and 142 females.

INDICATIONS AND USAGE

Felbatol® is not indicated as a first line antiepileptic treatment (see **Warnings**). Felbatol® is recommended for use only in those patients who respond inadequately to alternative treatments and whose epilepsy is so severe that a substantial risk of aplastic anemia and/or liver failure is deemed acceptable in light of the benefits conferred by its use.

If these criteria are met and the patient has been fully advised of the risk and has provided written, informed consent, Felbatol® can be considered for either monotherapy or adjunctive therapy in the treatment of partial seizures, with and without generalization, in adults with epilepsy and as adjunctive therapy in the treatment of partial and generalized seizures associated with Lennox-Gastaut syndrome in children.

CONTRAINDICATIONS

Felbatol® is contraindicated in patients with known hypersensitivity to Felbatol®, its ingredients, or known sensitivity to other carbamates. It should not be used in patients with a history of any blood dyscrasia or hepatic dysfunction.

WARNINGS

See Boxed Warning regarding aplastic anemia and hepatic failure.

Antiepileptic drugs should not be suddenly discontinued because of the possibility of increasing seizure frequency.

PRECAUTIONS

A study in otherwise healthy individuals with renal dysfunction indicated that prolonged half-life and reduced clearance of felbamate are associated with diminishing renal function. Felbamate should be used with caution in patients with renal dysfunction (**see DOSAGE AND ADMINISTRATION**).

Information for Patients: Patients should be informed that the use of Felbatol® is associated with aplastic anemia and hepatic failure, potentially fatal conditions acutely or over a long term.

The physician should obtain written, informed consent prior to initiation of Felbatol® therapy (see **PATIENT INFORMATION/CONSENT** section).

Aplastic anemia in the general population is relatively rare. The absolute risk for the individual patient is not known with any degree of reliability, but patients on Felbatol® may be at more than a 100 fold greater risk for developing the syndrome than the general population.

The long term outlook for patients with aplastic anemia is variable. Although many patients are apparently cured, others require repeated transfusions and other treatments for relapses, and some, although surviving or years, ultimately develop serious complications that sometimes prove fatal (e.g., leukemia).

At present there is no way to predict who is likely to get aplastic anemia, nor is there a documented effective means to monitor the patient so as to avoid and/or reduce the risk. Patients with a history of any blood dyscrasia should not receive Felbatol®.

Patients should be advised to be alert for signs of infection, bleeding, easy bruising, or signs of anemia (fatigue, weakness, lassitude, etc.) and should be advised to report to the physician immediately if any such signs or symptoms appear.

Hepatic failure in the general population is relatively rare. The absolute risk for an individual patient is not known with any degree of reliability but patients on Felbatol® are at a greater risk for developing hepatic failure than the general population.

At present, there is no way to predict who is likely to develop hepatic failure, however, patients with a history of hepatic dysfunction should not be started on Felbatol®.

Patients should be advised to follow their physician's directives for liver function testing both before starting Felbatol® (felbamate) and at frequent intervals while taking Felbatol®.

Laboratory Tests: Full hematologic evaluations should be performed before Felbatol® therapy, frequently during therapy, and for a significant period of time after discontinuation of Felbatol® therapy. While it might appear prudent to perform frequent CBCs in patients continuing on Felbatol®, there is no evidence that such monitoring will allow early detection of marrow suppression before aplastic anemia occurs. (See **Boxed Warnings**.) Complete pretreatment blood counts, including platelets and reticulocytes should be obtained as a baseline. If any hematologic abnormalities are detected during the course of treatment, immediate consultation with a hematologist is advised. Felbatol® should be discontinued if any evidence of bone marrow depression occurs.

Liver function testing (AST, ALT, bilirubin) should be done before Felbatol® is started and at 1- to 2-week intervals while the patient is taking Felbatol®. If any liver abnormalities are detected during the course of treatment, Felbatol® should be discontinued immediately. (see **PATIENT INFORMATION/CONSENT**).

Drug Interactions:

The drug interaction data described in this section were obtained from controlled clinical trials and studies involving otherwise healthy adults with epilepsy.

Use in Conjunction with Other Antiepileptic Drugs (See DOSAGE AND ADMINISTRATION):

The addition of Felbatol® to antiepileptic drugs (AEDs) affects the steady-state plasma concentrations of AEDs. The net effect of these interactions is summarized in the following table:

AED Coadministered	AED Concentration	Felbatol® Concentration
Phenytoin	↑	↓
Valproate	↑	↔**
Carbamazepine (CBZ) *CBZ epoxide	↓ ↑	↓
Phenobarbital	↑	↓

*Not administered, but an active metabolite of carbamazepine.

**No significant effect.

Specific Effects of Felbatol® on Other Antiepileptic Drugs:

Phenytoin: Felbatol® causes an increase in steady-state phenytoin plasma concentrations. In 10 otherwise healthy subjects with epilepsy ingesting phenytoin, the steady-state trough (Cmin) phenytoin plasma concentration was 17±5 micrograms/mL. The steady-state Cmin increased to 21±5 micrograms/mL when 1200 mg/day of felbamate was coadministered. Increasing the felbamate dose to 1800 mg/day in six of these subjects increased the steady-state phenytoin Cmin to 25±7 micrograms/mL. In order to maintain phenytoin levels, limit adverse experiences, and achieve the felbamate dose of 3600 mg/day, a phenytoin dose reduction of approximately 40% was necessary for eight of these 10 subjects.

In a controlled clinical trial, a 20% reduction of the phenytoin dose at the initiation of Felbatol® therapy resulted in phenytoin levels comparable to those prior to Felbatol® administration.

Carbamazepine: Felbatol® causes a decrease in the steady-state carbamazepine plasma concentrations and an increase in the steady-state carbamazepine epoxide plasma concentration. In nine otherwise healthy subjects with epilepsy ingesting carbamazepine, the steady-state trough (Cmin) carbamazepine concentration was 8±2 micrograms/mL. The carbamazepine steady-state Cmin decreased 31% to 5±1 micrograms/mL when felbamate (3000 mg/day, divided into three doses) was coadministered. Carbamazepine epoxide steady-state Cmin concentrations increased 57% from 1.0±0.3 to 1.6±0.4 micrograms/mL with the addition of felbamate.

In clinical trials, similar changes in carbamazepine and carbamazepine epoxide were seen.

Valproate: Felbatol® causes an increase in steady-state valproate concentrations. In four subjects with epilepsy ingesting valproate, the steady-state trough (Cmin) valproate plasma concentration was 63±16 micrograms/mL. The steady-state Cmin increased to 78±14 micrograms/mL when 1200 mg/day of felbamate was coadministered. Increasing the felbamate dose to 2400 mg/day increased the steady-state valproate Cmin to 96±25 micrograms/mL. Corresponding values for free valproate Cmin concentrations were 7±3, 9±4, and 11±6 micrograms/mL for 0, 1200, and 2400 mg/day Felbatol®, respectively. The ratios of the AUCs of unbound valproate to the AUCs of the total valproate were 11.1%, 13.0%, and 11.5%, with coadministration of 0, 1200, and 2400 mg/day of Felbatol®, respectively. This indicates that the protein binding of valproate did not change appreciably with increasing doses of Felbatol®.

Phenobarbital: Coadministration of felbamate with phenobarbital causes an increase in phenobarbital plasma concentrations. In 12 otherwise healthy male volunteers ingesting phenobarbital, the steady-state trough (Cmin) phenobarbital concentration was 14.2 micrograms/mL. The steady-state Cmin concentration increased to 17.8 micrograms/mL when 2400 mg/day of felbamate was coadministered for one week.

Effects of Other Antiepileptic Drugs on Felbatol®:

Phenytoin: Phenytoin causes an approximate doubling of the clearance of Felbatol® (felbamate) at steady state and, therefore, the addition of phenytoin causes an approximate 45% decrease in the steady-state trough concentrations of Felbatol® as compared to the same dose of Felbatol® given as monotherapy.

Carbamazepine: Carbamazepine causes an approximate 50% increase in the clearance of Felbatol® at steady state and, therefore, the addition of carbamazepine results in an approximate 40% decrease in the steady-state trough concentrations of Felbatol® as compared to the same dose of Felbatol® given as monotherapy.

Valproate: Available data suggest that there is no significant effect of valproate on the clearance of Felbatol® at steady state. Therefore, the addition of valproate is not expected to cause a clinically important effect on Felbatol® (felbamate) plasma concentrations.

Phenobarbital: It appears that phenobarbital may reduce plasma felbamate concentrations. Steady-state plasma felbamate concentrations were found to be 29% lower than the mean concentrations of a group of newly diagnosed subjects with epilepsy also receiving 2400 mg of felbamate a day.

Effects of Antacids on Felbatol®:

The rate and extent of absorption of a 2400 mg dose of Felbatol® as monotherapy given as tablets was not affected when coadministered with antacids.

Effects of Erythromycin on Felbatol®:

The coadministration of erythromycin (1000 mg/day) for 10 days did not alter the pharmacokinetic parameters of Cmax, Cmin, AUC, Cl/kg or tmax at felbamate daily doses of 3000 or 3600 mg/day in 10 otherwise healthy subjects with epilepsy.

Effects of Felbatol® on Low-Dose Combination Oral Contraceptives:

A group of 24 nonsmoking, healthy white female volunteers established on an oral contraceptive regimen containing 30 µg ethinyl estradiol and 75 µg gestodene for at least 3 months received 2400 mg/day of felbamate from midcycle (day 15) to midcycle (day 14) of two consecutive oral contraceptive cycles. Felbamate treatment resulted in a 42% decrease in the gestodene AUC 0–24, but no clinically relevant effect was observed on the pharmacokinetic parameters of ethinyl estradiol. No volunteer showed hormonal evidence of ovulation, but one volunteer reported intermenstrual bleeding during felbamate treatment.

Drug/Laboratory Test Interactions: There are no known interactions of Felbatol® with commonly used laboratory tests.

Carcinogenesis, Mutagenesis, Impairment of Fertility: Carcinogenicity studies were conducted in mice and rats. Mice received felbamate as a feed admixture for 92 weeks at doses of 300, 600, and 1200 mg/kg and rats were also dosed by feed admixture for 104 weeks at doses of 30, 100, and 300 (males) or 10, 30, and 100 (females) mg/kg. The maximum doses in these studies produced steady-state plasma concentrations that were equal to or less than the steady-state plasma concentrations in epileptic patients receiving 3600 mg/day. There was a statistically significant increase in hepatic cell adenomas in high-dose male and female mice and in high-dose female rats. Hepatic hypertrophy was significantly increased in a dose-related manner in mice, primarily males, but also in females. Hepatic hypertrophy was not found in female rats. The relationship between the occurrence of benign hepatocellular adenomas and the finding of liver hypertrophy resulting from liver enzyme induction has not been examined. There was a statistically significant increase in benign interstitial cell tumors of the testes in high-dose male rats receiving felbamate. The relevance of these findings to humans is unknown.

As a result of the synthesis process, felbamate could contain small amounts of two known animal carcinogens, the genotoxic compound ethyl carbamate (urethane) and the nongenotoxic compound methyl carbamate. It is theoretically possible that a 50 kg patient receiving 3600 mg of felbamate could be exposed to up to 0.72 micrograms of urethane and 1800 micrograms of methyl carbamate. These daily doses are approximately 1/35,000 (urethane) and 1/5,500 (methyl carbamate) on a mg/kg basis, and 1/10,000 (urethane) and 1/1,600 (methyl carbamate) on a mg/m^2 basis, of the dose levels shown to be carcinogenic in rodents. Any presence of these two compounds in felbamate used in the lifetime carcinogenicity studies was inadequate to cause tumors.

Microbial and mammalian cell assays revealed no evidence of mutagenesis in the Ames *Salmonella*/microsome plate test, CHO/HGPRT mammalian cell forward gene mutation assay, sister chromatid exchange assay in CHO cells, and bone marrow cytogenetics assay.

Reproduction and fertility studies in rats showed no effects on male or female fertility at oral doses of up to 13.9 times the human total daily dose of 3600 mg on a mg/kg basis, or up to 3 times the human total daily dose on a mg/m^2 basis.

Pregnancy: Pregnancy Category C. The incidence of malformations was not increased compared to control in offspring of rats or rabbits given doses up to 13.9 times (rat) and 4.2 times (rabbit) the human daily dose on a mg/kg basis, or 3 times (rat) and less than 2 times (rabbit) the human daily dose on a mg/m^2 basis. However, in rats, there was a decrease in pup weight and an increase in pup deaths during lactation. The cause for these deaths is not known. The no effect dose for rat pup mortality was 6.9 times the human dose on a mg/kg basis or 1.5 times the human dose on a mg/m^2 basis.

Placental transfer of felbamate occurs in rat pups. There are, however, no studies in pregnant women. Because animal reproduction studies are not always predictive of human response, this drug should be used during pregnancy only if clearly needed.

Labor and Delivery: The effect of felbamate on labor and delivery in humans is unknown.

Nursing Mothers: Felbamate has been detected in human milk. The effect on the nursing infant is unknown (see **Pregnancy** section).

Pediatric Use: The safety and effectiveness of Felbatol® in children other than those with Lennox-Gastaut syndrome has not been established.

Geriatric Use: No systematic studies in geriatric patients have been conducted. Clinical studies of Felbatol® did not include sufficient numbers of patients aged 65 and over to determine whether they respond differently from younger patients. Other reported clinical experience has not identified differences in responses between the elderly and younger patients. In general, dosage selection for an elderly patient should be cautious, usually starting at the low end of the dosing range, reflecting the greater frequency of decreased hepatic, renal, or cardiac function, and of concomitant disease or other drug therapy.

ADVERSE REACTIONS

The most common adverse reactions seen in association with Felbatol® (felbamate) in adults during monotherapy are anorexia, vomiting, insomnia, nausea, and headache. The most common adverse reactions seen in association with Felbatol® in adults during adjunctive therapy are anorexia, vomiting, insomnia, nausea, dizziness, somnolence, and headache.

The most common adverse reactions seen in association with Felbatol® in children during adjunctive therapy are anorexia, vomiting, insomnia, headache, and somnolence.

The dropout rate because of adverse experiences or intercurrent illnesses among adult felbamate patients was 12 percent (120/977). The dropout rate because of adverse experiences or intercurrent illnesses among pediatric felbamate patients was six percent (22/357). In adults, the body systems associated with causing these withdrawals in order of frequency were: digestive (4.3%), psychological (2.2%), whole body (1.7%), neurological (1.5%), and dermatological (1.5%). In children, the body systems associated with causing these withdrawals in order of frequency were: digestive (1.7%), neurological (1.4%), dermatological (1.4%), psychological (1.1%), and whole body (1.0%). In adults, specific events with an incidence of 1% or greater associated with causing these withdrawals, in order of frequency were: anorexia (1.6%), nausea (1.4%), rash (1.2%), and weight decrease (1.1%). In children, specific events with an incidence of 1% or greater associated with causing these withdrawals, in order of frequency was rash (1.1%).

Incidence in Clinical Trials:

The prescriber should be aware that the figures cited in the following table cannot be used to predict the incidence of side effects in the course of usual medical practice where patient characteristics and other factors differ from those which prevailed in the clinical trials. Similarly, the cited frequencies cannot be compared with figures obtained from other clinical investigations involving different investigators, treatments, and uses including the use of Felbatol® (felbamate) as adjunctive therapy where the incidence of adverse events may be higher due to drug interactions. The cited figures, however, do provide the prescribing physician

Continued on next page

Felbatol—Cont.

with some basis for estimating the relative contribution of drug and nondrug factors to the side effect incidence rate in the population studied.

Adults
Incidence in Controlled Clinical Trials—Monotherapy Studies in Adults:
The table that follows enumerates adverse events that occurred at an incidence of 2% or more among 58 adult patients who received Felbatol® monotherapy at dosages of 3600 mg/day in double-blind controlled trials. Reported adverse events were classified using standard WHO-based dictionary terminology.

Adults
Treatment-Emergent Adverse Event
Incidence in Controlled Monotherapy Trials

Body System/Event	Felbatol®* (N=58) %	Low Dose Valproate** (N=50) %
Body as a Whole		
Fatigue	6.9	4.0
Weight Decrease	3.4	0
Face Edema	3.4	0
Central Nervous System		
Insomnia	8.6	4.0
Headache	6.9	18.0
Anxiety	5.2	2.0
Dermatological		
Acne	3.4	0
Rash	3.4	0
Digestive		
Dyspepsia	8.6	2.0
Vomiting	8.6	2.0
Constipation	6.9	2.0
Diarrhea	5.2	0
SGPT Increased	5.2	2.0
Metabolic/Nutritional		
Hypophosphatemia	3.4	0
Respiratory		
Upper Respiratory Tract Infection	8.6	4.0
Rhinitis	6.9	0
Special Senses		
Diplopia	3.4	4.0
Otitis Media	3.4	0
Urogenital		
Intramenstrual Bleeding	3.4	0
Urinary Tract Infection	3.4	2.0

*3600 mg/day;
**15 mg/kg/day

Incidence in Controlled Add-On Clinical Studies in Adults:
The table that follows enumerates adverse events that occurred at an incidence of 2% or more among 114 adult patients who received Felbatol® adjunctive therapy in add-on controlled trials at dosages up to 3600 mg/day. Reported adverse events were classified using standard WHO-based dictionary terminology.
Many adverse experiences that occurred during adjunctive therapy may be a result of drug interactions. Adverse experiences during adjunctive therapy typically resolved with conversion to monotherapy, or with adjustment of the dosage of other antiepileptic drugs.

Adults
Treatment-Emergent Adverse Event
Incidence in Controlled Add-On Trials

Body System/Event	Felbatol® (N=114) %	Placebo (N=43) %
Body as a Whole		
Fatigue	16.8	7.0
Fever	2.6	4.7
Chest Pain	2.6	0
Central Nervous System		
Headache	36.8	9.3
Somnolence	19.3	7.0
Dizziness	18.4	14.0
Insomnia	17.5	7.0
Nervousness	7.0	2.3
Tremor	6.1	2.3
Anxiety	5.3	4.7
Gait Abnormal	5.3	0
Depression	5.3	0
Paraesthesia	3.5	2.3
Ataxia	3.5	0
Mouth Dry	2.6	0
Stupor	2.6	0

Body System/Event	Felbatol® %	Placebo %
Dermatological		
Rash	3.5	4.7
Digestive		
Nausea	34.2	2.3
Anorexia	19.3	2.3
Vomiting	16.7	4.7
Dyspepsia	12.3	7.0
Constipation	11.4	2.3
Diarrhea	5.3	2.3
Abdominal Pain	5.3	0
SGPT Increased	3.5	0
Musculoskeletal		
Myalgia	2.6	0
Respiratory		
Upper Respiratory Tract Infection	5.3	7.0
Sinusitis	3.5	0
Pharyngitis	2.6	0
Special Senses		
Diplopia	6.1	0
Taste Perversion	6.1	0
Vision Abnormal	5.3	2.3

Children
Incidence in a Controlled Add-On Trial in Children with Lennox-Gastaut Syndrome:
The table that follows enumerates adverse events that occurred more than once among 31 pediatric patients who received Felbatol® up to 45 mg/kg/day or a maximum of 3600 mg/day. Reported adverse events were classified using standard WHO-based dictionary terminology.

Children
Treatment-Emergent Adverse Event
Incidence in a Controlled Add-On Lennox-Gastaut Trial

Body System/Event	Felbatol® (N=31) %	Placebo (N=27) %
Body as a Whole		
Fever	22.6	11.1
Fatigue	9.7	3.7
Weight Decrease	6.5	0
Pain	6.5	0
Central Nervous System		
Somnolence	48.4	11.1
Insomnia	16.1	14.8
Nervousness	16.1	18.5
Gait Abnormal	9.7	0
Headache	6.5	18.5
Thinking Abnormal	6.5	3.7
Ataxia	6.5	3.7
Urinary Incontinence	6.5	7.4
Emotional Lability	6.5	0
Miosis	6.5	0
Dermatological		
Rash	9.7	7.4
Digestive		
Anorexia	54.8	14.8
Vomiting	38.7	14.8
Constipation	12.9	0
Hiccup	9.7	3.7
Nausea	6.5	0
Dyspepsia	6.5	3.7
Hematologic		
Purpura	12.9	7.4
Leukopenia	6.5	0
Respiratory		
Upper Respiratory Tract Infection	45.2	25.9
Pharyngitis	9.7	3.7
Coughing	6.5	0
Special Senses		
Otitis Media	9.7	0

Other Events Observed in Association with the Administration of Felbatol® (felbamate):
In the paragraphs that follow, the adverse clinical events, other than those in the preceding tables, that occurred in a total of 977 adults and 357 children exposed to Felbatol® (felbamate) and that are reasonably associated with its use are presented. They are listed in order of decreasing frequency. Because the reports cite events observed in open-label and uncontrolled studies, the role of Felbatol® in their causation cannot be reliably determined.
Events are classified within body system categories and enumerated in order of decreasing frequency using the following definitions: frequent adverse events are defined as those occurring on one or more occasions in at least 1/100 patients; infrequent adverse events are those occurring in 1/100–1/1000 patients; and rare events are those occurring in fewer than 1/1000 patients.

Event frequencies are calculated as the number of patients reporting an event divided by the total number of patients (N=1334) exposed to Felbatol®.
Body as a Whole: *Frequent:* Weight increase, asthenia, malaise, influenza-like symptoms; *Rare:* anaphylactoid reaction, chest pain substernal.
Cardiovascular: *Frequent:* Palpitation, tachycardia; *Rare:* supraventricular tachycardia.
Central Nervous System: *Frequent:* Agitation, psychological disturbance, aggressive reaction; *Infrequent:* hallucination, euphoria, suicide attempt, migraine.
Digestive: *Frequent:* SGOT increased; *Infrequent:* esophagitis, appetite increased; *Rare:* GGT elevated.
Hematologic: *Infrequent:* Lymphadenopathy, leukopenia, leukocytosis, thrombocytopenia, granulocytopenia; *Rare:* antinuclear factor test positive, qualitative platelet disorder, agranulocytosis.
Metabolic/Nutritional: *Infrequent:* Hypokalemia, hyponatremia, LDH increased, alkaline phosphatase increased, hypophosphatemia; *Rare:* creatinine phosphokinase increased.
Musculoskeletal: *Infrequent:* Dystonia.
Dermatological: *Frequent:* Pruritus; *Infrequent:* urticaria, bullous eruption; *Rare:* buccal mucous membrane swelling, Stevens-Johnson Syndrome.
Special Senses: *Rare:* Photosensitivity allergic reaction.
Postmarketing Adverse Event Reports:
Voluntary reports of adverse events in patients taking Felbatol® (usually in conjunction with other drugs) have been received since market introduction and may have no causal relationship with the drug(s). These include the following by body system:
Body as a Whole: neoplasm, sepsis, L.E. syndrome, SIDS, sudden death, edema, hypothermia, rigors, hyperpyrexia.
Cardiovascular: atrial fibrillation, atrial arrhythmia, cardiac arrest, torsade de pointes, cardiac failure, hypotension, hypertension, flushing, thrombophlebitis, ischemic necrosis, gangrene, peripheral ischemia, bradycardia, Henoch-Schönlein purpura (vasculitis).
Central & Peripheral Nervous System: delusion, paralysis, mononeuritis, cerebrovascular disorder, cerebral edema, coma, manic reaction, encephalopathy, paranoid reaction, nystagmus, choreoathetosis, extrapyramidal disorder, confusion, psychosis, status epilepticus, dyskinesia, dysarthria, respiratory depression, apathy, concentration impaired.
Dermatological: abnormal body odor, sweating, lichen planus, livedo reticularis, alopecia, toxic epidermal necrolysis.
Digestive: (Refer to **WARNINGS**) hepatitis, hepatic failure, G.I. hemorrhage, hyperammonemia, pancreatitis, hematemesis, gastritis, rectal hemorrhage, flatulence, gingival bleeding, acquired megacolon, ileus, intestinal obstruction, enteritis, ulcerative stomatitis, glossitis, dysphagia, jaundice, gastric ulcer, gastric dilatation, gastroesophageal reflux.
Fetal Disorders: fetal death, microcephaly, genital malformation, anencephaly, encephalocele.
Hematologic: (Refer to **WARNINGS**) increased and decreased prothrombin time, anemia, hypochromic anemia, aplastic anemia, pancytopenia, hemolytic uremic syndrome, increased mean corpuscular volume (mcv) with and without anemia, coagulation disorder, embolism-limb, disseminated intravascular coagulation, eosinophilia, hemolytic anemia.
Metabolic/Nutritional: hypernatremia, hypoglycemia, SIADH, hypomagnesemia, dehydration, hyperglycemia, hypocalcemia.
Musculoskeletal: arthralgia, muscle weakness, involuntary muscle contraction, rhabdomyolysis.
Respiratory: dyspnea, pneumonia, pneumonitis, hypoxia, epistaxis, pleural effusion, respiratory insufficiency, pulmonary hemorrhage, asthma.
Special Senses: hemianopsia, decreased hearing, conjunctivitis.
Urogenital: menstrual disorder, acute renal failure, hepatorenal syndrome, hematuria, urinary retention, nephrosis, vaginal hemorrhage, abnormal renal function, dysuria, placental disorder.

DRUG ABUSE AND DEPENDENCE

Abuse: Abuse potential was not evaluated in human studies.
Dependence: Rats administered felbamate orally at doses 8.3 times the recommended human dose 6 days each week for 5 consecutive weeks demonstrated no signs of physical dependence as measured by weight loss following drug withdrawal on day 7 of each week.

OVERDOSAGE

Four subjects inadvertently received Felbatol® (felbamate) as adjunctive therapy in dosages ranging from 5400 to 7200 mg/day for durations between 6 and 51 days. One subject who received 5400 mg/day as monotherapy for 1 week reported no adverse experiences. Another subject attempted suicide by ingesting 12,000 mg of Felbatol® in a 12-hour period. The only adverse experiences reported were mild gastric distress and a resting heart rate of 100 bpm. No serious adverse reactions have been reported.
General supportive measures should be employed if overdosage occurs. It is not known if felbamate is dialyzable.

Dosage Table (adults)

	WEEK 1	WEEK 2	WEEK 3
Dosage reduction of concomitant AEDs	REDUCE original dose by 20–33%*	REDUCE original dose by up to an additional 1/3*	REDUCE as clinically indicated
Felbatol® Dosage	1200 mg/day Initial dose	2400 mg/day Therapeutic dosage range	3600 mg/day Therapeutic dosage range

* See **Adjunctive** and **Conversion to Monotherapy** sections.

DOSAGE AND ADMINISTRATION

Felbatol® (felbamate) has been studied as monotherapy and adjunctive therapy in adults and as adjunctive therapy in children with seizures associated with Lennox-Gastaut syndrome. As Felbatol® is added to or substituted for existing AEDs, it is strongly recommended to reduce the dosage of those AEDs in the range of 20–33% to minimize side effects (see **Drug Interactions** subsection).

Felbamate should be used with caution in patients with renal dysfunction. Adjunctive therapy with medications which affect felbamate plasma concentrations, especially AEDS, may warrant further reductions in felbamate daily doses in patients with renal dysfunction.

Adults (14 years of age and over)

The majority of patients received 3600 mg/day in clinical trials evaluating its use as both monotherapy and adjunctive therapy.

Monotherapy: (Initial therapy) Felbatol® (felbamate) has not been systematically evaluated as initial monotherapy. Initiate Felbatol® at 1200 mg/day in divided doses three or four times daily. The prescriber is advised to titrate previously untreated patients under close clinical supervision, increasing the dose in 600-mg increments every 2 weeks to 2400 mg/day based on clinical response and thereafter to 3600 mg/day if clinically indicated.

Conversion to Monotherapy: Initiate Felbatol® at 1200 mg/day in divided doses three or four times daily. Reduce the dosage of concomitant AEDs by one-third at initiation of Felbatol® therapy. At week 2, increase the Felbatol® dosage to 2400 mg/day while reducing the dosage of other AEDs up to an additional one-third of their original dosage. At week 3, increase the Felbatol® dosage up to 3600 mg/day and continue to reduce the dosage of other AEDs as clinically indicated.

Adjunctive Therapy: Felbatol® should be added at 1200 mg/day in divided doses three or four times daily while reducing present AEDs by 20% in order to control plasma concentrations of concurrent phenytoin, valproic acid, phenobarbital, and carbamazepine and its metabolites. Further reductions of the concomitant AEDs dosage may be necessary to minimize side effects due to drug interactions. Increase the dosage of Felbatol® by 1200 mg/day increments at weekly intervals to 3600 mg/day. Most side effects seen during Felbatol® adjunctive therapy resolve as the dosage of concomitant AEDs is decreased.

[See table above]

While the above Felbatol® conversion guidelines may result in a Felbatol® 3600 mg/day dose within 3 weeks, in some patients titration to a 3600 mg/day Felbatol® dose has been achieved in as little as 3 days with appropriate adjustment of other AEDs.

Children with Lennox-Gastaut Syndrome (Ages 2–14 years)

Adjunctive Therapy: Felbatol® should be added at 15 mg/kg/day in divided doses three or four times daily while reducing present AEDs by 20% in order to control plasma levels of concurrent phenytoin, valproic acid, phenobarbital, and carbamazepine and its metabolites. Further reductions of the concomitant AEDs dosage may be necessary to minimize side effects due to drug interactions. Increase the dosage of Felbatol® by 15 mg/kg/day increments at weekly intervals to 45 mg/kg/day. Most side effects seen during Felbatol® adjunctive therapy resolve as the dosage of concomitant AEDs is decreased.

HOW SUPPLIED

Felbatol® (felbamate) Tablets, 400 mg, are yellow, scored, capsule-shaped tablets, debossed "0430" on one side and "WALLACE" on the other; available in Bottles of 100 (NDC 0037-0430-01) and Unit Dose 100's (NDC 0037-0430-11). Felbatol® (felbamate) Tablets, 600 mg, are peach-colored, scored, capsule-shaped tablets, debossed "0431" on one side and "WALLACE" on the other; available in Bottles of 100 (NDC 0037-0431-01) and Unit Dose 100's (NDC 0037-0431-11). Felbatol® (felbamate) Oral Suspension, 600 mg/5 mL, is peach-colored; available in 8 oz bottles (NDC 0037-0442-67) and 32 oz bottles (NDC 0037-0442-17).

Shake suspension well before using. Store at controlled room temperature 20°–25°C (68°–77°F). Dispense in tight container.

WALLACE LABORATORIES,
Division of Carter-Wallace, Inc.
Cranbury, NJ 08512

PATIENT INFORMATION/CONSENT

FELBATOL® (felbamate) SHOULD NOT BE USED BY PATIENTS UNTIL THERE HAS BEEN A COMPLETE DISCUSSION OF THE RISKS AND WRITTEN INFORMED CONSENT HAS BEEN OBTAINED.

IMPORTANT INFORMATION AND WARNING:
Felbatol®, taken by itself or with other prescription and/or non-prescription drugs, can result in severe, potentially fatal blood abnormality ("aplastic anemia") and/or severe, potentially fatal liver damage.

PATIENT CONSENT:
My [My son, daughter, ward, _____'s] treatment with Felbatol® has been personally explained to me by Dr. _____

The following points of information, among others, have been specifically discussed and made clear and I have had the opportunity to ask any questions concerning this information:

1. I, _____ (Patient's Name), understanding that Felbatol® is used to treat certain types of seizures and my physician has told me that I have this type(s) of seizures;
INITIALS: _____

2. I understand that Felbatol® is being used since my seizures have not been satisfactorily treated with other antiepileptic drugs;
INITIALS: _____

3. I understand that there is a serious risk that I could develop aplastic anemia and/or liver failure, both of which are potentially fatal, by using Felbatol®;
INITIALS: _____

4. I understand that there are no laboratory tests which will predict if I am at an increased risk for one of the potentially fatal conditions;
INITIALS: _____

5. I understand that I should have the recommended blood work before my treatment with Felbatol® is begun or continued and then every 1–2 weeks while taking Felbatol®. I understand that although this blood work may help detect if I develop one of these conditions, it may do so only after significant, irreversible and potentially fatal damage has already occurred;
INITIALS: _____

6. If I am currently taking another antiepileptic drug, I understand that the manufacturer of Felbatol® recommends that the dosage of these other drugs be decreased by a certain amount when Felbatol® is started; if my physician determines that this should not be done in my case, he/she has explained the reason(s) for this decision;
INITIALS: _____

7. I understand that I must immediately report any unusual symptoms to Dr._____ and be especially aware of any rashes, easy bruising, bleeding, sore throats, fever, and/or dark urine;
INITIALS: _____

I now authorize Dr. _____
to begin my treatment with Felbatol®; OR, if my treatment has already begun with Felbatol®, to continue such treatment.

Patient, Parent, or Guardian

Address

Telephone

PHYSICIAN STATEMENT:
I have fully explained to the patient, _____ the nature and purpose of the treatment with Felbatol® (felbamate) and the potential risks associated with that treatment. I have asked the patient if he/she has any questions regarding this treatment or the risks and have answered those questions to the best of my ability. I also acknowledge that I have read and understand the prescribing information listed above.

Physician _____ **Date** _____

NOTE TO PHYSICIAN: It is strongly recommended that you retain a signed copy of the informed consent with the patient's medical records.

SUPPLY OF PATIENT INFORMATION/CONSENT FORMS:
A supply of "Patient Information/Consent" forms as printed above is available, free of charge, from your local Wallace representative, or may be obtained by calling 609-655-6147. Permission to use the above Patient Information/Consent by photocopy reproduction is also hereby granted by Carter-Wallace, Inc.

IN-00431-09 PP Rev. 3/98
Shown in Product Identification Guide, page 341

LUFYLLIN®
(dyphylline)
Elixir
℞

LUFYLLIN® Tablets
(dyphylline tablets, USP, 200 mg)
℞

LUFYLLIN®–400 Tablets
(dyphylline tablets, USP, 400 mg)
℞

DESCRIPTION

LUFYLLIN (dyphylline), a xanthine derivative, is a bronchodilator available for oral administration as tablets containing 200 mg and 400 mg of dyphylline. Other ingredients: magnesium stearate, microcrystalline cellulose.

Chemically, dyphylline is 7-(2,3-dihydroxypropyl)-theophylline, a white, extremely bitter, amorphous powder that is freely soluble in water and soluble in alcohol to the extent of 2 g/100 mL. Dyphylline forms a neutral solution that is stable in gastrointestinal fluids over a wide range of pH.

The molecular formula for dyphylline is $C_{10}H_{14}N_4O_4$ with a molecular weight of 254.25. Its structural formula is:

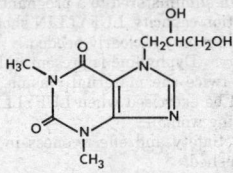

CLINICAL PHARMACOLOGY

Dyphylline is a xanthine derivative with pharmacologic actions similar to theophylline and other members of this class of drugs. Its primary action is that of bronchodilation, but it also exhibits peripheral vasodilatory and other smooth muscle relaxant activity to a lesser degree. The bronchodilatory action of dyphylline, as with other xanthines, is thought to be mediated through competitive inhibition of phosphodiesterase with a resulting increase in cyclic AMP producing relaxation of bronchial smooth muscle. LUFYLLIN is well tolerated and produces less nausea than aminophylline and other alkaline theophylline compounds when administered orally. Unlike the hydrolyzable salts of theophylline, dyphylline is not converted to free theophylline *in vivo*. It is absorbed rapidly in therapeutically active form and in healthy volunteers reaches a mean peak plasma concentration of 17.1 mcg/mL in approximately 45 minutes following a single oral dose of 1000 mg. of LUFYLLIN.

Dyphylline exerts its bronchodilatory effects directly and, unlike theophylline, is excreted unchanged by the kidneys without being metabolized by the liver. Because of this, dyphylline pharmacokinetics and plasma levels are not influenced by various factors that affect liver function and hepatic enzyme activity, such as smoking, age, congestive heart failure, or concomitant use of drugs which affect liver function.

The elimination half-life of dyphylline is approximately two hours (1.8–2.1 hr) and approximately 88% of a single oral dose can be recovered from the urine unchanged. The renal clearance would be correspondingly reduced in patients with impaired renal function. In anuric patients, the half-life may be increased 3 to 4 times normal.

Dyphylline plasma levels are dose-related and generally predictable. The range of plasma levels within which dyphylline can be expected to produce effective brohchodilation has not been determined.

Continued on next page

Lufyllin Tablets—Cont.

Dyphylline plasma concentrations can be accurately determined using high pressure liquid chromatography (HPLC)* or gas-liquid chromatography (GLC).

---

*See Valia, et al., J. Chromatogr. 221: 170 (1980). Small quantities of pure dyphylline powder may be obtained from Wallace Laboratories, Cranbury, N.J. The internal standard, β-hydroxyethyl-theophylline, may be obtained from companies supplying analytical chemicals.

INDICATIONS AND USAGE

For relief of acute bronchial asthma and for reversible bronchospasm associated with chronic bronchitis and emphysema.

CONTRAINDICATIONS

Hypersensitivity to dyphylline or related xanthine compounds.

WARNINGS

LUFYLLIN is not indicated in the management of status asthmaticus, which is a serious medical emergency.

Although the relationship between plasma levels of dyphylline and appearance of toxicity is unknown, excessive doses may be expected to be associated with an increased risk of adverse effects.

PRECAUTIONS

General: Use LUFYLLIN with caution in patients with severe cardiac disease, hypertension, hyperthyroidism, acute myocardial injury, or peptic ulcer.

Drug interactions: Synergism between xanthine bronchodilators (e.g., theophylline), ephedrine, and other sympathomimetic bronchodilators has been reported. This should be considered whenever these agents are prescribed concomitantly.

Concurrent administration of dyphylline and probenecid, which competes for tubular secretion, has been shown to increase the plasma half-life of dyphylline (see Clinical Pharmacology).

Carcinogenesis, mutagenesis, impairment of fertility: No long-term animal studies have been performed with LUFYLLIN.

Pregnancy: Teratogenic effects—Pregnancy Category C. Animal reproduction studies have not been conducted with LUFYLLIN. It is also not known if LUFYLLIN can cause fetal harm when administered to a pregnant woman or can affect reproduction capacity. LUFYLLIN should be given to a pregnant woman only if clearly needed.

Nursing mothers: Dyphylline is present in human milk at approximately twice the maternal plasma concentration. Caution should be exercised when LUFYLLIN is administered to a nursing woman.

Pediatric use: Safety and effectiveness in children have not been established.

ADVERSE REACTIONS

Adverse reactions with the use of LUFYLLIN have been infrequent, relatively mild, and rarely required reduction in dosage or withdrawal of therapy.

The following adverse reactions which have been reported with other xanthine bronchodilators, and which have most often been related to excessive drug plasma levels, should be considered as potential adverse effects when dyphylline is administered:

Gastrointestinal: nausea, vomiting, epigastric pain, hematemesis, diarrhea.

Central nervous system: headache, irritability, restlessness, insomnia, hyperexcitability, agitation, muscle twitching, generalized clonic and tonic convulsions.

Cardiovascular: palpitation, tachycardia, extrasystoles, flushing, hypotension, circulatory failure, ventricular arrhythmias.

Respiratory: tachypnea.

Renal: albuminuria, gross and microscopic hematuria, diuresis.

Other: hyperglycemia, inappropriate ADH syndrome.

OVERDOSAGE

There have been no reports, in the literature, of overdosage with LUFYLLIN. However, the following information based on reports of theophylline overdosage are considered typical of the xanthine class of drugs and should be kept in mind.

Signs and symptoms: Restlessness, anorexia, nausea, vomiting, diarrhea, insomnia, irritability, and headache. Marked overdosage with resulting severe toxicity has produced agitation, severe vomiting, dehydration, excessive thirst, tinnitus, cardiac arrhythmias, hyperthermia, diaphoresis, and generalized clonic and tonic convulsions. Cardiovascular collapse has also occurred, with some fatalities. Seizures have occurred in some cases associated with very high theophylline plasma concentrations, without any premonitory symptoms of toxicity.

Treatment: There is no specific antidote for overdosage with drugs of the xanthine class. Symptomatic treatment and general supportive measures should be instituted with careful monitoring and maintenance of vital signs, fluids, and electrolytes. The stomach should be emptied by inducing emesis if the patient is conscious and responsive, or by gastric lavage, taking care to protect against aspiration, especially in stuporous or comatose patients. Maintenance of an adequate airway is essential in case oxygen or assisted respiration is needed. Sympathomimetic agents should be avoided but sedatives such as short-acting barbiturates may be useful.

Dyphylline is dialyzable and, although not recommended as a routine procedure in overdosage cases, hemodialysis may be of some benefit when severe intoxication is present or when the patient has not responded to general supportive and symptomatic treatment.

DOSAGE AND ADMINISTRATION

Dosage should be individually titrated according to the severity of the condition and the response of the patient.

Usual adult dosage: Up to 15 mg/kg every six hours.

Appropriate dosage adjustments should be made in patients with impaired renal function (see Clinical Pharmacology).

HOW SUPPLIED

LUFYLLIN Tablets contain 200 mg dyphylline and are white, rectangular, scored on one side and imprinted WALLACE 521 on the other side.

The tablets are available in bottles of 100 (NDC 0037-0521-92), 1000 (NDC 0037-0521-97), and 5000 (NDC 0037-0521-98).

LUFYLLIN-400 Tablets contain 400 mg dyphylline and are white, capsule-shaped, scored on one side and imprinted WALLACE 731 on the other side. The tablets are available in bottles of 100 (NDC 0037-0731-92), 1000 (NDC 0037-0731-97), and 2500 (NDC 0037-0731-99).

Storage: Store at controlled room temperature 15°–30°C (59°–86°F).

Dispense in a tight container.

CAUTION: Federal law prohibits dispensing without prescription.

WALLACE LABORATORIES

Division of CARTER-WALLACE, INC.
Cranbury, New Jersey 08512
IN-0521-06   Rev. 8/97

LUFYLLIN®-GG   ℞
(dyphylline and guaifenesin
tablets and elixir, USP)
Tablets and Elixir

DESCRIPTION

LUFYLLIN®-GG is a bronchodilator/expectorant combination available for oral administration as *Tablets* and *Elixir.*

Each Tablet contains:

Dyphylline	200 mg
Guaifenesin	200 mg

Other ingredients: corn starch, D&C Yellow No. 10, magnesium aluminium silicate, magnesium stearate, microcrystalline cellulose.

Each 15 mL (one tablespoonful) of Elixir contains:

Dyphylline	100 mg
Guaifenesin	100 mg
Alcohol (by volume)	17%

Other ingredients: citric acid, FD&C Yellow No. 6, flavor (artificial), purified water, saccharin sodium, sodium citrate, sucrose.

Dyphylline is 7-(2,3-dihydroxypropyl)-theophylline, a white, extremely bitter, amorphous powder that is fully soluble in water and soluble in alcohol to the extent of 2 g/100 mL. Dyphylline forms a neutral solution that is stable in gastrointestinal fluids over a wide range of pH.

CLINICAL PHARMACOLOGY

Dyphylline is a xanthine derivative with pharmacologic actions similar to theophylline and other members of this class of drugs. Its primary action is that of bronchodilation, but it also exhibits peripheral vasodilatory and other smooth muscle relaxant activity to a lesser degree. The bronchodilatory action of dyphylline, as with as other xanthines, is thought to be mediated through competitive inhibition of phosphodiesterase with a resulting increase in cyclic AMP producing relaxation of bronchial smooth muscle. Dyphylline in LUFYLLIN-GG is well tolerated and produces less nausea than aminophylline and other alkaline theophylline compounds when administered orally. Unlike the hydrolyzable salts of theophylline, dyphylline is not converted to free theophylline *in vivo.* It is absorbed rapidly in therapeutically active form and in healthy volunteers reaches a mean peak plasma concentration of 17.1 mcg/mL in approximately 45 minutes following a single oral dose of 1000 mg of dyphylline.

Dyphylline exerts its bronchodilatory effects directly and, unlike theophylline, is excreted unchanged by the kidneys without being metabolized by the liver. Because of this, dyphylline pharmacokinetics and plasma levels are not influenced by various factors that affect liver function and hepatic enzyme activity, such as smoking, age, or concomitant use of drugs which affect liver function.

The elimination half-life of dyphylline is approximately two hours (1.8–2.1 hr) and approximately 88% of a single oral dose can be recovered from the urine unchanged. The renal clearance would be correspondingly reduced in patients with impaired renal function. In anuric patients, the half-life may be increased 3 to 4 times normal.

Dyphylline plasma levels are dose-related and generally predictable. The therapeutic range of plasma levels within which dyphylline can be expected to produce effective bronchodilation has not been determined.

Dyphylline plasma concentrations can be accurately determined using high pressure liquid chromatography (HPLC)* or gas-liquid chromatography (GLC).

Guaifenesin is an expectorant whose action helps increase the output of thin respiratory tract fluid to facilitate mucociliary clearance and removal of inspissated mucus.

---

*See Valia, et al, J Chromatogr. 221: 170 (1980). Small quantities of pure dyphylline powder may be obtained from Wallace Laboratories, Cranbury, N.J. The internal standard, β-hydroxyethyl-theophylline, may be obtained from companies supplying analytical chemicals.

INDICATIONS AND USAGE

For relief of acute bronchial asthma and for reversible bronchospasm associated with chronic bronchitis and emphysema.

CONTRAINDICATIONS

Hypersensitivity to any of the ingredients or related compounds.

WARNINGS

LUFYLLIN-GG is not indicated in the management of status asthmaticus, which is a serious medical emergency.

Although the relationship between plasma levels of dyphylline and appearance of toxicity is unknown, excessive doses may be expected to be associated with an increased risk of adverse effects.

PRECAUTIONS

General: Use LUFYLLIN-GG with caution in patients with severe cardiac disease, hypertension, hyperthyroidism, acute myocardial injury or peptic ulcer.

Drug interactions: Synergism between xanthine bronchodilators (e.g., theophylline), ephedrine and other sympathomimetic bronchodilators has been reported. This should be considered whenever these agents are prescribed concomitantly.

Concurrent administration of dyphylline and probenecid, which competes for tubular secretion, has been shown to increase plasma half-life of dyphylline (see Clinical Pharmacology).

Carcinogenesis, mutagenesis, impairment of fertility: No long-term animal studies have been performed with LUFYLLIN-GG.

Pregnancy: Teratogenic effects—Pregnancy Category C. Animal reproduction studies have not been conducted with LUFYLLIN-GG. It is also not known whether the product can cause fetal harm when administered to a pregnant woman or can affect reproduction capacity. LUFYLLIN-GG should be given to a pregnant woman only if clearly needed.

Nursing mothers: Dyphylline is present in human milk at approximately twice the maternal plasma concentration. Caution should be exercised when LUFYLLIN-GG is administered to a nursing woman.

Pediatric use: Safety and effectiveness in children below the age of six have not been established. Use caution when administering to children six years of age or older.

ADVERSE REACTIONS

LUFYLLIN-GG may cause nausea, headache, cardiac palpitation and CNS stimulation. Postprandial administration may help avoid gastric discomfort.

The following adverse reactions which have been reported with other xanthine bronchodilators, and which have most often been related to excessive drug plasma levels, should be considered as potential adverse effects when dyphylline is administered:

Gastrointestinal: nausea, vomiting, epigastric pain, hematemesis, diarrhea.

Central nervous system: headache, irritability, restlessness, insomnia, hyperexcitability, agitation, muscle twitching, generalized clonic and tonic convulsions.

Cardiovascular: palpitation, tachycardia, extrasystoles, flushing, hypotension, circulatory failure, ventricular arrhythmias.

Respiratory: tachypnea.

Renal: albuminuria, gross and microscopic hematuria, diuresis.

Other: hyperglycemia, inappropriate ADH syndrome.

OVERDOSAGE

There have been no reports, in the literature, of overdosage with LUFYLLIN-GG. However, the following information based on reports of theophylline overdosage are considered typical of the xanthine class of drugs and should be kept in mind.

Signs & symptoms: Restlessness, anorexia, nausea, vomiting, diarrhea, insomnia, irritability, and headache. Marked overdosage with resulting severe toxicity has produced agitation, severe vomiting, dehydration, excessive thirst, tinnitus, cardiac arrhythmias, hyperthermia, diaphoresis, and generalized clonic and tonic convulsions. Cardiovascular collapse has also occurred, with some fatalities. Seizures have occurred in some cases associated with very high theophylline plasma concentrations, without any premonitory symptoms of toxicity.

Treatment: There is no specific antidote for overdosage with drugs of the xanthine class. Symptomatic treatment and general supportive measures should be instituted with careful monitoring and maintenance of vital signs, fluids and electrolytes. The stomach should be emptied by inducing emesis if the patient is conscious and responsive, or by gastric lavage, taking care to protect against aspiration, especially in stuporous or comatose patients. Maintenance of an adequate airway is essential in case oxygen or assisted respiration is needed. Sympathomimetic agents should be avoided but sedatives such as short-acting barbiturates may be useful.

Dyphylline is dialyzable and, although not recommended as a routine procedure in overdosage cases, hemodialysis may be of some benefit when severe intoxication is present or when the patient has not responded to general supportive and symptomatic treatment.

DOSAGE AND ADMINISTRATION

Dosage should be individually titrated according to the severity of the condition and the response of the patient.

Usual adult dosage:

One tablet or 30 mL (two tablespoonfuls) elixir, four times daily.

Children above age six:

One-half to one tablet or 15 to 30 mL (one to two tablespoonfuls) elixir, three or four times daily.

Not recommended for use in children below age six: (see Precautions).

HOW SUPPLIED

LUFYLLIN-GG Tablets (dyphylline 200 mg and guaifenesin 200 mg) are round, convex, light yellow, scored on one side and imprinted on the other side with WALLACE 541. The tablets are available in bottles of 100 (NDC 0037-0541-92), 1000 (NDC 0037-0541-97), and 3000 (NDC 0037-0541-96), and in boxes of 100 unit-dose (NDC 0037-0541-85).

LUFYLLIN-GG Elixir (dyphylline 100 mg, quaifenesin 100 mg and alcohol 17% by volume per 15 mL) is a clear, light yellow-orange liquid with a mild wine-like odor and taste. The elixir is available in bottles of one pint (NDC 0037-0545-68) and one gallon (NDC 0037-0545-69).

Storage:

Tablets and Elixir—Store at controlled room temperature 15°–30°C (59°–86°F).

Dispense in a tight container.

CAUTION: Federal law prohibits dispensing without prescription.

WALLACE LABORATORIES
Division of CARTER-WALLACE, INC.
Cranbury, New Jersey 08512
IN-0541-06 Rev. 2/95

MALTSUPEX® OTC

(malt soup extract)
Powder, Liquid, Tablets

(See PDR For Nonprescription Drugs.)

MILTOWN® CIV ℞

(meprobamate tablets, USP)

DESCRIPTION

Meprobamate is a white powder with a *characteristic odor* and a bitter taste. It is slightly soluble in water, freely soluble in acetone and alcohol, and sparingly soluble in ether. The structural formula of meprobamate is:

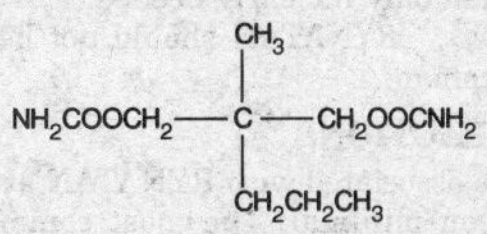

'Miltown'-200 contains 200 mg meprobamate per tablet. Other ingredients: acacia, carnauba wax, corn starch, gelatin, magnesium carbonate, magnesium stearate, methylcellulose, shellac, sugar, talc, titanium dioxide, white wax and other ingredients.

'Miltown'-400 contains 400 mg meprobamate per tablet. Other ingredients: corn starch, magnesium stearate, methylcellulose.

ACTIONS

Meprobamate is a carbamate derivative which has been shown in animal studies to have effects at multiple sites in the central nervous system, including the thalamus and limbic system.

INDICATIONS

'Miltown' (meprobamate) is indicated for the management of anxiety disorders or for the short-term relief of the symptoms of anxiety. Anxiety or tension associated with the stress of everyday life usually do not require treatment with an anxiolytic.

The effectiveness of 'Miltown' in long-term use, that is, more than 4 months, has not been assessed by systematic clinical studies. The physician should periodically reassess the usefulness of the drug for the individual patient.

CONTRAINDICATIONS

Acute intermittent porphyria as well as allergic or idiosyncratic reactions to meprobamate or related compounds such as carisoprodol, mebutamate, tybamate or carbromal.

WARNINGS

Drug Dependence

Physical dependence, psychological dependence, and abuse have occurred. When chronic intoxication from prolonged use occurs, it usually involves ingestion of greater than recommended doses and is manifested by ataxia, slurred speech, and vertigo. Therefore, careful supervision of dose and amounts prescribed is advised, as well as avoidance of prolonged administration, especially for alcoholics and other patients with a known propensity for taking excessive quantities of drugs.

Sudden withdrawal of the drug after prolonged and excessive use may precipitate recurrence of pre-existing symptoms, such as anxiety, anorexia, or insomnia, or withdrawal reactions, such as vomiting, ataxia, tremors, muscle twitching, confusional states, hallucinosis, and, rarely, convulsive seizures. Such seizures are more likely to occur in persons with central nervous system damage or pre-existent or latent convulsive disorders. Onset of withdrawal symptoms occurs usually within 12 to 48 hours after discontinuation of meprobamate; symptoms usually cease within the next 12 to 48 hours.

When excessive dosage has continued for weeks or months, dosage should be reduced gradually over a period of one or two weeks rather than abruptly stopped. Alternatively, a short-acting barbiturate may be substituted, then gradually withdrawn.

Potentially Hazardous Tasks

Patients should be warned that this drug may impair the mental and/or physical abilities required for the performance of potentially hazardous tasks such as driving a motor vehicle or operating machinery.

Additive Effects

Since the effects of meprobamate and alcohol or meprobamate and other CNS depressants or psychotropic drugs may be additive, appropriate caution should be exercised with patients who take more than one of these agents simultaneously.

Usage in Pregnancy and Lactation

An increased risk of congenital malformations associated with the use of minor tranquilizers (meprobamate, chlordiazepoxide, and diazepam) during the first trimester of pregnancy has been suggested in several studies. Because use of these drugs is rarely a matter of urgency, their use during this period should almost always be avoided. The possibility that a woman of childbearing potential may be pregnant at the time of institution of therapy should be considered. Patients should be advised that if they become pregnant during therapy or intend to become pregnant they should communicate with their physician about the desirability of discontinuing the drug.

Meprobamate passes the placental barrier. It is present both in umbilical cord blood at or near maternal plasma levels and in breast milk of lactating mothers at concentrations two to four times that of maternal plasma. When use of meprobamate is contemplated in breast-feeding patients, the drug's higher concentration in breast milk as compared to maternal plasma levels should be considered.

Usage in Children

'Miltown'-200 and 'Miltown'-400 should not be administered to children under age six, since there is a lack of documented evidence for safety and effectiveness in this age group.

PRECAUTIONS

The lowest effective dose should be administered, particularly to elderly and/or debilitated patients, in order to preclude oversedation.

The possibility of suicide attempts should be considered and the least amount of drug feasible should be dispensed at any one time.

Meprobamate is metabolized in the liver and excreted by the kidney; to avoid its excess accumulation, caution should be exercised in administration to patients with compromised liver or kidney function.

Meprobamate occasionally may precipitate seizures in epileptic patients.

ADVERSE REACTIONS

Central Nervous System

Drowsiness, ataxia, dizziness, slurred speech, headache, vertigo, weakness, paresthesias, impairment of visual accommodation, euphoria, overstimulation, paradoxical excitement, fast EEG activity.

Gastrointestinal

Nausea, vomiting, diarrhea.

Cardiovascular

Palpitations, tachycardia, various forms of arrhythmia, transient ECG changes, syncope; also, hypotensive crises (including one fatal case).

Allergic or Idiosyncratic

Allergic or idiosyncratic reactions are usually seen within the period of the first to fourth dose in patients having had no previous contact with the drug. Milder reactions are characterized by an itchy, urticarial, or erythematous maculopapular rash which may be generalized or confined to the groin. Other reactions have included leukopenia, acute nonthrombocytopenic purpura, petechiae, ecchymoses, eosinophilia, peripheral edema, adenopathy, fever, fixed drug eruption with cross reaction to carisoprodol, and cross sensitivity between meprobamate/mebutamate and meprobamate/carbromal.

More severe hypersensitivity reactions, rarely reported, include hyperpyrexia, chills, angioneurotic edema, bronchospasm, oliguria, and anuria. Also, anaphylaxis, erythema multiforme, exfoliative dermatitis, stomatitis, proctitis, Stevens-Johnson syndrome, and bullous dermatitis, including one fatal case of the latter following administration of meprobamate in combination with prednisolone.

In case of allergic or idiosyncratic reactions to meprobamate, discontinue the drug and initiate appropriate symptomatic therapy, which may include epinephrine, antihistamines, and in severe cases corticosteroids. In evaluating possible allergic reactions, also consider allergy to excipients.

Hematologic

(See also **Allergic or Idiosyncratic.**) Agranulocytosis and aplastic anemia have been reported. These cases rarely were fatal. Rare cases of thrombocytopenic purpura have been reported.

Other

Exacerbation of porphyric symptoms.

DOSAGE AND ADMINISTRATION

'Miltown'-200 and 400:

The usual adult daily dosage is 1200 mg to 1600 mg, in three or four divided doses; a daily dosage above 2400 mg is not recommended. The usual daily dosage for children ages six to twelve is 200 mg to 600 mg, in two or three divided doses.

Not recommended for children under age 6 (see **Usage in Children**).

OVERDOSAGE

Suicidal attempts with meprobamate have resulted in drowsiness, lethargy, stupor, ataxia, coma, shock, vasomotor and respiratory collapse. Some suicidal attempts have been fatal.

The following data on meprobamate tablets have been reported in the literature and from other sources. These data are not expected to correlate with each case (considering factors such as individual susceptibility and length of time from ingestion to treatment), but represent the **usual ranges** reported.

Acute simple overdose (meprobamate alone): Death has been reported with ingestion of as little as 12 g meprobamate and survival with as much as 40 g.

Blood Levels:

0.5 – 2.0 mg% represents the usual blood level range of meprobamate after therapeutic doses. The level may occasionally be as high as 3.0 mg%.

3 – 10 mg% usually corresponds to findings of mild to moderate symptoms of overdosage, such as stupor or light coma.

10 – 20 mg% usually corresponds to deeper coma, requiring more intensive treatment. Some fatalities occur.

At levels greater than 20%, more fatalities than survivals can be expected.

Acute combined overdose (meprobamate with alcohol or other CNS depressants or psychotropic drugs): Since effects can be additive, a history of ingestion of a low dose of meprobamate plus any of these compounds (or of a relative low

Continued on next page

Miltown—Cont.

blood or tissue level) cannot be used as a prognostic indicator.

In cases where excessive doses have been taken, sleep ensues rapidly and blood pressure, pulse, and repiratory rates are reduced to basal levels. Any drug remaining in the stomach should be removed and symptomatic therapy given. Should respiration or blood pressure become compromised, respiratory assistance, central nervous system stimulants, and pressor agents should be administered cautiously as indicated. Meprobamate is metabolized in the liver and excreted by the kidney. Diuresis, osmotic (mannitol) diuresis, peritoneal dialysis, and hemodialysis have been used successfully. Careful monitoring of urinary output is necessary and caution should be taken to avoid overhydration. Relapse and death, after initial recovery, have been attributed to incomplete gastric emptying and delayed absorption. Meprobamate can be measured in biologic fluids by two methods: colorimetric (Hoffman, A.J. and Ludwig, B.J.: *J Amer Pharm Assn 48:* 740, 1959) and gas chromatographic (Douglas, J.F. et al.: *Anal Chem 39:* 956, 1967).

HOW SUPPLIED

'Miltown'-200: 200 mg white, sugar-coated tablets coded 37-1101 and Wallace; available in bottles of 100 (NDC 0037-1101-01).

'Miltown'-400: 400 mg white, scored tablets coded 37-1001 and Wallace; available in bottles of 100 (NDC 0037-1001-01), 500 (NDC 0037-1001-03), and 1000 (NDC 0037-1001-02).

Storage: Store at controlled room temperature 15°–30°C (59°–86°F). Dispense in a tight container.

CAUTION: Federal law prohibits dispensing without prescription.

WALLACE LABORATORIES

Division of Carter-Wallace, Inc.
Cranbury, New Jersey 08512

IN-070J2-08   Rev. 7/97

ORGANIDIN® NR*
(*Newly Reformulated)
(guaifenesin)
Tablets and Liquid   ℞

Professional Labeling Information and Directions for Use
This product labeled for sale on prescription only.

DESCRIPTION

ORGANIDIN® NR* (*Newly Reformulated) (guaifenesin) is an expectorant available for oral administration as tablets and liquid.

Each tablet contains 200 mg guaifenesin, USP.

Other ingredients: Microcrystalline cellulose, corn starch, croscarmellose sodium, magnesium stearate, FD&C Red No. 40.

Each teaspoonful (5 mL) of liquid contains 100 mg guaifenesin, USP.

Other ingredients: Citric acid, caramel, glycerin, sorbitol solution, propylene glycol, saccharin sodium, sodium benzoate, flavor compound (raspberry), purified water.

Guaifenesin (glycerol guaiacolate) has the chemical name 3-(2-methoxyphenoxy)-1,2-propanediol. Its molecular formula is $C_{10}H_{14}O_4$, with a molecular weight of 198.21. It is a white, colorless crystalline substance with a slightly bitter aromatic taste. One gram dissolves in 20 mL water at 25°C; freely soluble in ethanol. Guaifenesin is readily absorbed from the GI tract and is rapidly metabolized and excreted in the urine. Guaifenesin has a plasma half-life of one hour. The major urinary metabolite is beta-(2-methoxyphenoxy) lactic acid.

CLINICAL PHARMACOLOGY

Guaifenesin is an expectorant the action of which promotes or facilitates the removal of secretions from the respiratory tract. By increasing sputum volume and making sputum less viscous, guaifenesin facilitates expectoration of retained secretions.

INDICATIONS AND USAGE

Helps loosen phlegm (mucus) and thin bronchial secretions to rid the bronchial passageways of bothersome mucus, drain bronchial tubes, and make coughs more productive. Helps loosen phlegm and thin bronchial secretions in patients with stable chronic bronchitis.

CONTRAINDICATIONS

ORGANIDIN® NR* (*Newly Reformulated) is contraindicated in patients hypersensitive to any of the ingredients.

PRECAUTIONS

Carcinogenesis, Mutagenesis, Impairment of Fertility. Animal studies to assess the long-term carcinogenic and mu-

tagenic potential or the effect of fertility in animals or humans have not been performed.

Pregnancy

Teratogenic Effects—Pregnancy Category C: Animal reproduction studies have not been conducted. Safe use in pregnancy has not been established relative to possible adverse effects on fetal development. Therefore, this product should not be used in pregnant patients, unless in the judgment of the physician, the potential benefits outweigh possible hazards.

Nursing Mothers: It is not known whether guaifenesin is excreted in human milk. Because many drugs are excreted in human milk, caution should be exercised when these products are administered to a nursing woman and a decision should be made whether to discontinue nursing or to discontinue the drug, taking into account the importance of the drug to the mother.

Laboratory Test Interactions: Guaifenesin or its metabolites may cause color interference with the VMA (vanillylmandelic acid) test for catechols. It may also falsely elevate the level of urinary 5-HIAA (5-hydroxyindoleacetic acid) in certain serotonin metabolite chemical tests because of color interference.

ADVERSE REACTIONS

Guaifenesin is well tolerated and has a wide margin of safety. Side effects have been generally mild and infrequent. Nausea and vomiting are the side effects that occur most commonly. Dizziness, headache, and rash (including urticaria) have been reported rarely.

OVERDOSAGE

The acute toxicity of guaifenesin is low and overdosage is unlikely to produce serious toxic effects. In laboratory animals no toxicity resulted when guaifenesin was administered by stomach tube in doses up to 5 grams/kg.

In massive overdosage the stomach should be emptied (emesis and/or gastric lavage) and further absorption prevented. Treatment is symptomatic and supportive.

DOSAGE AND ADMINISTRATION

Tablets—Adults and children 12 years of age and older: One to 2 tablets (200 mg to 400 mg) every four hours, not to exceed 2400 mg (12 tablets) in 24 hours.

Liquid—Adults and children 12 years of age and older: Two to four teaspoonfuls (200 mg to 400 mg) every four hours, not to exceed 2400 mg (24 teaspoonfuls) in 24 hours. *Children 6 years to under 12 years of age:* One to two teaspoonfuls (100 mg to 200 mg) every four hours, not to exceed 1200 mg (12 teaspoonfuls) in 24 hours.

Children 2 years to under 6 years of age: $^1/_2$ to 1 teaspoonful (50 mg to 100 mg) every four hours, not to exceed 600 mg (6 teaspoonfuls) in 24 hours.

Children 6 mo. to under 2 years of age: A common dosage is $^1/_4$ to $^1/_2$ teaspoonful (25 to 50 mg) every four hours, not to exceed 300 mg (3 teaspoonfuls) in 24 hours. Individualized dosage should be determined by evaluation of patient.

HOW SUPPLIED

Tablet—Each round scored rose-colored tablet contains 200 mg guaifenesin USP—available in bottles of 100 (NDC 0037-4312-01).

Liquid—Each teaspoonful (5 mL) contains 100 mg guaifenesin—available as a clear amber liquid in bottles of 1 pint (NDC 0037-4214-10) and 1 gallon (NDC 0037-4214-20)

Storage—Store at controlled room temperature—15°–30°C (59°–86°F). Protect from light. Keep bottle tightly closed.

ORGANIDIN® NR* (*Newly Reformulated) (guaifenesin) Tablets are Manufactured and Distributed by:

WALLACE LABORATORIES

Division of CARTER-WALLACE, Inc.
Cranbury, NJ 08512

ORGANIDIN® NR* (*Newly Reformulated) (guaifenesin) Liquid is distributed by:

WALLACE LABORATORIES

Division of CARTER-WALLACE, Inc.
Cranbury, NJ 08512

Manufactured by:
Denver Chemical (Puerto Rico) Inc.
Subsidiary of Carter-Wallace, Inc.
Humacao, Puerto Rico 00791
IN-046F8-01   Rev. 7/94

Shown in Product Identification Guide, page 342

RYNA®
(Liquid)
RYNA–C®
(Liquid)   ℭ
RYNA–CX®
(Liquid)   ℭ

(See PDR For Nonprescription Drugs.)

RYNATAN®
Tablets
Pediatric Suspension
RYNATAN®-S*
Pediatric Suspension   ℞

DESCRIPTION

RYNATAN® is an antihistamine/nasal decongestant combination available for oral administration as *Tablets* and as *Pediatric Suspension.* Each tablet contains:

Phenylephrine Tannate	25 mg
Chlorpheniramine Tannate	8 mg
Pyrilamine Tannate	25 mg

Other ingredients: corn starch, dibasic calcium phosphate, magnesium stearate, methylcellulose, polygalacturonic acid, talc.

Each 5 mL (one teaspoonful) of the Pediatric Suspension contains:

Phenylephrine Tannate	5 mg
Chlorpheniramine Tannate	2 mg
Pyrilamine Tannate	12.5 mg

Other ingredients: benzoic acid, FD&C Red No. 3, flavors (natural and artificial), glycerin, kaolin, magnesium aluminum silicate, methylparaben, pectin, purified water, saccharin sodium, sucrose.

CLINICAL PHARMACOLOGY

RYNATAN combines the sympathomimetic decongestant effect of phenylephrine with the antihistaminic actions of chlorpheniramine and pyrilamine.

INDICATIONS AND USAGE

RYNATAN is indicated for symptomatic relief of the coryza and nasal congestion associated with the common cold, sinusitis, allergic rhinitis and other upper respiratory tract conditions. Appropriate therapy should be provided for the primary disease.

CONTRAINDICATIONS

RYNATAN is contraindicated for newborns, nursing mothers and patients sensitive to any of the ingredients or related compounds.

WARNINGS

Use with caution in patients with hypertension, cardiovascular disease, hyperthyroidism, diabetes, narrow angle glaucoma or prostatic hypertrophy. Use with caution or avoid use in patients taking monoamine oxidase (MAO) inhibitors, or within 14 days of stopping such treatment. This product contains antihistamines which may cause drowsiness and may have additive central nervous system (CNS) effects with alcohol or other CNS depressants (e.g., hypnotics, sedatives, tranquilizers).

PRECAUTIONS

General: Antihistamines are more likely to cause dizziness, sedation and hypotension in elderly patients. Antihistamines may cause excitation, particularly in children, but their combination with sympathomimetics may cause either mild stimulation or mild sedation.

Information for patients: Caution patients against drinking alcoholic beverages or engaging in potentially hazardous activities requiring alertness, such as driving a car or operating machinery while using this product. Patients should be warned not to use this product if they are now taking a prescription monoamine oxidase inhibitor (MAOI) (certain drugs for depression, psychiatric or emotional conditions, or Parkinson's disease), or for 2 weeks after stopping the MAOI drug. If patients are uncertain whether a prescription drug contains an MAOI, they should be instructed to consult a health professional before taking such a product.

Drug Interactions: MAO inhibitors may prolong and intensify the anticholinergic effects of antihistamines and the overall effects of sympathomimetic agents.

Carcinogenesis, mutagenesis, impairment of fertility: No long term animal studies have been performed with RYNATAN®.

Pregnancy: Teratogenic effects: Pregnancy Category C. Animal reproduction studies have not been conducted with RYNATAN. It is also not known whether RYNATAN can cause fetal harm when administered to a pregnant woman or can affect reproduction capacity. RYNATAN should be given to a pregnant woman only if clearly needed.

Nursing mothers: RYNATAN should not be administered to a nursing woman.

ADVERSE REACTIONS

Adverse effects associated with RYNATAN at recommended doses have been minimal. The most common have been drowsiness, sedation, dryness of mucous membranes, and gastrointestinal effects. Serious side effects with oral antihistamines or sympathomimetics have been rare.

OVERDOSAGE

Signs & Symptoms: May vary from CNS depression to stimulation (restlessness to convulsions). Antihistamine overdosage in young children may lead to convulsions and death. Atropine-like signs and symptoms may be prominent.

Treatment: Induce vomiting if it has not occurred spontaneously. Precautions must be taken against aspiration especially in infants, children and comatose patients. If gastric lavage is indicated, isotonic or half-isotonic saline solution is preferred. Stimulants should not be used. If hypotension is a problem, vasopressor agents may be considered.

DOSAGE AND ADMINISTRATION

Administer the recommended dose every 12 hours.
RYNATAN Tablets: Adults—1 or 2 tablets.
RYNATAN Pediatric Suspension: Children over six years of age —5 to 10 mL (1 to 2 teaspoonfuls); Children two to six years of age —2.5 to 5 mL (1/2 to 1 teaspoonful); *Children under two years of age*—Titrate dose individually.

HOW SUPPLIED

RYNATAN® Tablets (phenylephrine tannate 25 mg, chlorpheniramine tannate 8 mg, and pyrilamine tannate 25 mg): buff-colored, capsule-shaped, scored on one side and imprinted WALLACE 713 on the other side. The tablets are available in bottles of 100 (NDC 0037-0713-92), 500 (NDC 0037-0713-96), and 2000 (NDC 0037-0713-95).
RYNATAN® Pediatric Suspension (phenylephrine tannate 5 mg, chlorpheniramine tannate 2 mg, and pyrilamine tannate 12.5 mg per 5 mL): pink with strawberry-currant flavor in 4 fl oz **unit of use** container with a 10 mL graduated oral syringe and fitment (NDC 0037-0715-67, labeled RYNATAN®-S*) and in pint bottles (NDC 0037-0715-68).
Storage: RYNATAN Tablets—Store at controlled room temperature 15°–30°C (59°–86°F).
RYNATAN Pediatric Suspension—Store at controlled room temperature 15°–30°C (59°–86°F).
Dispense in a tight container.
CAUTION: Federal law prohibits dispensing without prescription.
*RYNATAN®-S is RYNATAN Pediatric Suspension either in a 4 fl oz **unit of use** container with a 10 mL graduated oral syringe and fitment or in a 15 mL sample container.

WALLACE LABORATORIES
Division of CARTER-WALLACE, INC.
Cranbury, New Jersey 08512
IN-0713-08 Rev. 4/95
Shown in Product Identification Guide, page 342

RYNATUSS® ℞
Tablets
Pediatric Suspension

DESCRIPTION

RYNATUSS® is an antitussive/antihistamine/nasal decongestant/bronchodilator combination available for oral administration as *Tablets* and as *Pediatric Suspension*
Each tablet contains:

Carbetapentane Tannate	60 mg
Chlorpheniramine Tannate	5 mg
Ephedrine Tannate	10 mg
Phenylephrine Tannate	10 mg

Other ingredients: corn starch, dibasic calcium phosphate, FD&C Blue No. 1, FD&C Red No. 40, magnesium stearate, methylcellulose, polygalacturonic acid, povidone, talc.
Each 5 mL (one teaspoonful) of the Pediatric Suspension contains:

Carbetapentane Tannate	30 mg
Chlorpheniramine Tannate	4 mg
Ephedrine Tannate	5 mg
Phenylephrine Tannate	5 mg

Other ingredients: benzoic acid, FD&C Blue No. 1, FD&C Red No. 3, FD&C Red No. 40, FD&C Yellow No. 5 (see Precautions), flavors (natural and artificial), glycerin, Kaolin, magnesium aluminum silicate, methylparaben, pectin, purified water, saccharin sodium, sucrose.

CLINICAL PHARMACOLOGY

RYNATUSS combines the antitussive action of carbetapentane, the sympathomimetic decongestant effect of phenylephrine, the antihistaminic action of chlorpheniramine, and the bronchodilator action of ephedrine.

INDICATIONS AND USAGE

RYNATUSS is indicated for the symptomatic relief of cough associated with respiratory tract conditions such as the common cold, bronchial asthma, acute and chronic bronchitis. Appropriate therapy should be provided for the primary disease.

CONTRAINDICATIONS

RYNATUSS is contraindicated for newborns, nursing mothers, and patients who are sensitive to any of the ingredients or related compounds.

WARNINGS

Use with caution in patients with hypertension, cardiovascular disease, hyperthyroidism, diabetes, narrow angle glaucoma, or prostatic, hypertrophy. Do not use in patients taking monoamine oxidase (MAO) inhibitors, or for 14 days after stopping treatment with an MAOI.
This product contains antihistamines which may cause drowsiness and may have additive central nervous system (CNS) effects with alcohol or other CNS depressants (e.g., hypnotics, sedatives, tranquilizers).

PRECAUTIONS

For RYNATUSS Pediatric Suspension only: This product contains FD&C Yellow No. 5 (tartrazine) which may cause allergic-type reactions (including bronchial asthma) in certain susceptible individuals. Although the overall incidence of FD&C Yellow No. 5 (tartrazine) sensitivity in the general population is low, it is frequently seen in patients who also have aspirin hypersensitivity.
General: Antihistamines are more likely to cause dizziness, sedation, and hypotension in elderly patients. Antihistamines may cause excitation, particularly in children, but their combination with sympathomimetics may cause either mild stimulation or mild sedation.
Information for patients: Caution patients against drinking alcoholic beverages or engaging in potentially hazardous activities requiring alertness, such as driving a car or operating machinery, while using this product. Patients should be warned not to use this product if they are now taking a prescription monoamine oxidase inhibitor (MAOI) (certain drugs for depression, psychiatric or emotional conditions, or Parkinson's disease), or for 2 weeks after stopping the MAOI drug. If patients are uncertain whether a prescription drug contains an MAOI, they should be instructed to consult a health professional before taking such a product.
Drug Interactions: MAO inhibitors may prolong and intensify the anticholinergic effects of antihistamines and the overall effects of sympathomimetic agents.
Carcinogenesis, mutagenesis, impairment of fertility: No long term animal studies have been performed with RYNATUSS.
Pregnancy: Teratogenic effects: Pregnancy Category C. Animal reproduction studies have not been conducted with RYNATUSS. It is also not known whether RYNATUSS can cause fetal harm when administered to a pregnant woman or can affect reproduction capacity. RYNATUSS should be given to a pregnant woman only if clearly needed.
Nursing mothers: RYNATUSS should not be administered to a nursing woman.

ADVERSE REACTIONS

Adverse effects associated with RYNATUSS at recommended doses have been minimal. The most common have been drowsiness, sedation, dryness of mucous membranes, and gastrointestinal effects. Serious side effects with oral antihistamines or sympathomimetics have been rare.

OVERDOSAGE

Signs and symptoms: May vary from CNS depression to stimulation (restlessness to convulsions). Antihistamine overdosage in young children may lead to convulsions and death. Atropine-like signs and symptoms may be prominent.
Treatment: Induce vomiting if it has not occurred spontaneously. Precautions must be taken against aspiration especially in infants, children, and comatose patients. If gastric lavage is indicated, isotonic or half-isotonic saline solution is preferred. Stimulants should not be used. If hypotension is a problem, vasopressor agents may be considered.

DOSAGE AND ADMINISTRATION

Administer the recommended dose every 12 hours.
RYNATUSS Tablets: Adults – 1 to 2 tablets.
RYNATUSS Pediatric Suspension: *Children over six years of age*– 5 to 10 mL (1 to 2 teaspoonfuls); *Children two to six years of age*– 2.5 to 5 mL (1/2 to 1 teaspoonful); *Children under two years of age*– Titrate dose individually.

HOW SUPPLIED

RYNATUSS® Tablets are mauve, capsule-shaped, scored on one side and imprinted WALLACE 717 on the other side, containing in each tablet: carbetapentane tannate 60 mg, chlorpheniramine tannate 5 mg, ephedrine tannate 10 mg, phenylephrine tannate 10 mg, available in bottles of 100 (NDC 0037-0717-92), 500 (NDC 0037-0717-96), and 2000 (NDC 0037-0717-95).
RYNATUSS® Pediatric Suspension is pink with strawberry-currant flavor, containing in each 5 mL (one teaspoonful): carbetapentane tannate 30 mg, chlorpheniramine tannate 4 mg, ephedrine tannate 5 mg, phenylephrine tannate 5 mg, available in bottles of 8 fl oz (NDC 0037-0718-67) and one pint (NDC 0037-0718-68).
Storage: RYNATUSS Tablets and RYNATUSS Pediatric Suspension: Store at controlled room temperature 15°–30°C (59°–86°F).
Dispense in a tight container.

WALLACE LABORATORIES
Division of CARTER-WALLACE, INC.
Cranbury, New Jersey 08512
IN-0717-05 Rev: 1/95
Shown in Product Identification Guide, page 342

SOMA® ℞
(carisoprodol)
Tablets, USP

DESCRIPTION

'SOMA' (carisoprodol) Tablets, USP is available as 350 mg round, white tablets. Chemically, carisoprodol is N-isopropyl-2-methyl-2-propyl-1,3-propanediol dicarbamate. Carisoprodol is a white, crystalline powder, having a mild, characteristic odor and a bitter taste. It is very slightly soluble in water; freely soluble in alcohol, in chloroform, and in acetone; its solubility is practically independent of pH. Carisoprodol is present as a racemic mixture. The molecular formula is $C_{12}H_{24}N_2O_4$, with a molecular weight of 260.33. The structural formula is:

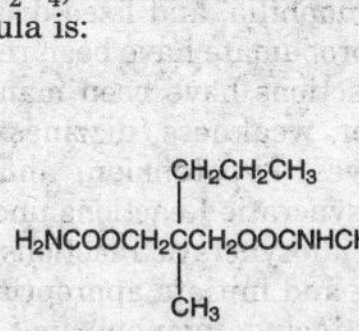
CH₂CH₂CH₃
H₂NCOOCH₂CCH₂OOCNHCH(CH₃)₂
CH₃

Other ingredients: alginic acid, magnesium stearate, potassium sorbate, starch, tribasic calcium phosphate.

ACTIONS

Carisoprodol produces muscle relaxation in animals by blocking interneuronal activity in the descending reticular formation and spinal cord. The onset of action is rapid and effects last four to six hours.

INDICATIONS

Carisoprodol is indicated as an adjunct to rest, physical therapy, and other measures for the relief of discomfort associated with acute, painful musculoskeletal conditions. The mode of action of this drug has not been clearly identified, but may be related to its sedative properties. Carisoprodol does not directly relax tense skeletal muscles in man.

CONTRAINDICATIONS

Acute intermittent porphyria as well as allergic or idiosyncratic reactions to carisoprodol or related compounds.

WARNINGS

Idiosyncratic Reactions—On very rare occasions, the first dose of carisoprodol has been followed by idiosyncratic symptoms appearing within minutes or hours. Symptoms reported include: extreme weakness, transient quadriplegia, dizziness, ataxia, temporary loss of vision, diplopia, mydriasis, dysarthria, agitation, euphoria, confusion, and disorientation. Symptoms usually subside over the course of the next several hours. Supportive and symptomatic therapy, including hospitalization, may be necessary.
Usage in Pregnancy and Lactation—Safe usage of this drug in pregnancy or lactation has not been established. Therefore, use of this drug in pregnancy, in nursing mothers, or in women of childbearing potential requires that the potential benefits of the drug be weighed against the potential hazards to mother and child. Carisoprodol is present in breast milk of lactating mothers at concentrations two to four times that of maternal plasma. This factor should be taken into account when use of the drug is contemplated in breast-feeding patients.
Usage in Children—Because of limited clinical experience, 'SOMA' is not recommended for use in patients under 12 years of age.
Potentially Hazardous Tasks—Patients should be warned that this drug may impair the mental and/or physical abilities required for the performance of potentially hazardous tasks such as driving a motor vehicle or operating machinery.
Additive Effects—Since the effects of carisoprodol and alcohol or carisoprodol and other CNS depressants or psychotropic drugs may be additive, appropriate caution should be exercised with patients who take more than one of these agents simultaneously.
Drug Dependence—In dogs, no withdrawal symptoms occurred after abrupt cessation of carisoprodol from dosages as high as 1 gm/kg/day. In a study in man, abrupt cessation of 100 mg/kg/day (about five times the recommended daily adult dosage) was followed in some subjects by mild withdrawal symptoms such as abdominal cramps, insomnia, chilliness, headache, and nausea. Delirium and convulsions did not occur. In clinical use, psychological dependence and

Continued on next page

Soma—Cont.

abuse have been rare, and there have been no reports of significant abstinence signs. Nevertheless, the drug should be used with caution in addiction-prone individuals.

PRECAUTIONS

Carisoprodol is metabolized in the liver and excreted by the kidney; to avoid its excess accumulation, caution should be exercised in administration to patients with compromised liver or kidney function.

ADVERSE REACTIONS

Central Nervous System —Drowsiness and other CNS effects may require dosage reduction. Also observed: dizziness, vertigo, ataxia, tremor, agitation, irritability, headache, depressive reactions, syncope, and insomnia. (See also Idiosyncratic Reactions under "Warnings.")

Allergic or Idiosyncratic —Allergic or idiosyncratic reactions occasionally develop. They are usually seen within the period of the first to fourth dose in patients having had no previous contact with the drug. Skin rash, erythema multiforme, pruritus, eosinophilia, and fixed drug eruption with cross reaction to meprobamate have been reported with carisoprodol. Severe reactions have been manifested by asthmatic episodes, fever, weakness, dizziness, angioneurotic edema, smarting eyes, hypotension, and anaphylactoid shock. (See also Idiosyncratic Reactions under "Warnings.") In case of allergic or idiosyncratic reactions to carisoprodol, discontinue the drug and initiate appropriate symptomatic therapy, which may include epinephrine, antihistamines, and in severe cases corticosteroids. In evaluating possible allergic reactions, also consider allergy to excipients (information on excipients is available to physicians on request).

Cardiovascular —Tachycardia, postural hypotension, and facial flushing.

Gastrointestinal —Nausea, vomiting, hiccup, and epigastric distress.

Hematologic —Leukopenia, in which other drugs or viral infection may have been responsible, and pancytopenia, attributed to phenylbutazone, have been reported. No serious blood dyscrasias have been attributed to carisoprodol.

DOSAGE AND ADMINISTRATION

The usual adult dosage of 'SOMA' (carisoprodol) Tablets, USP is one 350 mg tablet, three times daily and at bedtime. Usage in patients under age 12 is not recommended.

OVERDOSAGE

Overdosage of carisoprodol has produced stupor, coma, shock, respiratory depression, and, very rarely, death. The effects of an overdosage of carisoprodol and alcohol or other CNS depressants or psychotropic agents can be additive even when one of the drugs has been taken in the usual recommended dosage. Any drug remaining in the stomach should be removed and symptomatic therapy given. Should respiration or blood pressure become compromised, respiratory assistance, central nervous system stimulants, and pressor agents should be administered cautiously as indicated. Carisoprodol is metabolized in the liver and excreted by the kidney. Although carisoprodol overdosage experience is limited, the following types of treatment have been used successfully with the related drug meprobamate: diuresis, osmotic (mannitol) diuresis, peritoneal dialysis, and hemodialysis (carisoprodol is dialyzable). Careful monitoring of urinary output is necessary and caution should be taken to avoid overhydration. Observe for possible relapse due to incomplete gastric emptying and delayed absorption. Carisoprodol can be measured in biological fluids by gas chromatography (Douglas, J. F. et al.: *J Pharm Sci 58:* 145, 1969).

HOW SUPPLIED

'SOMA' (carisoprodol) Tablets, USP 350 mg: Round, convex, white tablets, inscribed with 'SOMA' on one side and 37-WALLACE 2001 on the other side, are available in bottles of 100 (NDC 0037-2001-01) and 500 (NDC 0037-2001-03), and unit-dose packages of 100 (NDC 0037-2001-85).

Storage: Store at controlled room temperature 15°–30°C (59°–86°F).

Dispense in a tight container.

WALLACE LABORATORIES
Division of CARTER-WALLACE, INC.
Cranbury, New Jersey 08512
IN-090H2-10   Rev. 9/94
Shown in Product Identification Guide, page 342

SOMA® COMPOUND   ℞
(carisoprodol and aspirin tablets, USP)
carisoprodol 200 mg + aspirin 325 mg
TABLETS

DESCRIPTION

SOMA Compound is a combination product containing carisoprodol, a centrally-acting muscle relaxant, plus aspirin, an analgesic with antipyretic and anti-inflammatory prop-

erties. It is available as a two-layered, white and orange, round tablet for oral administration. Each tablet contains carisoprodol, USP 200 mg and aspirin 325 mg. Chemically, carisoprodol is N-isopropyl-2-methyl-2-propyl-1,3-propanediol dicarbamate. Its empirical formula is $C_{12}H_{24}N_2O_4$, with a molecular weight of 260.33. The structural formula is:

$$CH_2CH_2CH_3$$
$$|$$
$$H_2NCOOCH_2CCH_2OOCNHCH(CH_3)_2$$
$$|$$
$$CH_3$$

Other ingredients: croscarmellose sodium, FD&C Red #40, FD&C Yellow #6, hydroxypropyl methylcellulose, magnesium stearate, microcrystalline cellulose, povidone, starch, stearic acid.

CLINICAL PHARMACOLOGY

Carisoprodol: Carisoprodol is a centrally-acting muscle relaxant that does not directly relax tense skeletal muscles in man. The mode of action of carisoprodol in relieving acute muscle spasm of local origin has not been clearly identified, but may be related to its sedative properties. In animals, carisoprodol has been shown to produce muscle relaxation by blocking interneuronal activity and depressing transmission of polysynaptic neurons in the spinal cord and in the descending reticular formation of the brain. The onset of action is rapid and lasts four to six hours.

Carisoprodol is metabolized in the liver and is excreted by the kidneys. It is dialyzable by peritoneal and hemodialysis.

Aspirin: Aspirin is a nonnarcotic analgesic with anti-inflammatory and antipyretic activity. Inhibition of prostaglandin biosynthesis appears to account for most of its anti-inflammatory and for at least part of its analgesic and antipyretic properties.

Aspirin is rapidly absorbed and almost totally hydrolyzed to salicylic acid following oral administration. Although aspirin has a half-life of only about 15 minutes, the apparent biologic half-life of salicylic acid in the therapeutic plasma concentration range is between 6 and 12 hours. Salicylic acid is eliminated by renal excretion and by biotransformation to inactive metabolites. Clearance of salicylic acid in the high-dose range is sensitive to urinary pH (see *Drug Interactions*) and is reduced by renal dysfunction.

INDICATIONS AND USAGE

SOMA Compound is indicated as an adjunct to rest, physical therapy, and other measures for the relief of pain, muscle spasm, and limited mobility associated with acute, painful musculoskeletal conditions.

CONTRAINDICATIONS

Acute intermittent porphyria; bleeding disorders; allergic or idiosyncratic reactions to carisoprodol, aspirin or related compounds.

WARNINGS

On very rare occasions, the first dose of carisoprodol has been followed by an idiosyncratic reaction with symptoms appearing within minutes or hours. These may include extreme weakness, transient quadriplegia, dizziness, ataxia, temporary loss of vision, diplopia, mydriasis, dysarthia, agitation, euphoria, confusion, and disorientation. Although symptoms usually subside over the course of the next several hours, discontinue SOMA Compound and initiate appropriate supportive and symptomatic therapy, which may include epinephrine and/or antihistamines. In severe cases, corticosteroids may be necessary. Severe reactions have been manifested by asthmatic episodes, fever, weakness, dizziness, angioneurotic edema, smarting eyes, hypotension, and anaphylactoid shock.

The effects of carisoprodol with agents such as alcohol, other CNS depressants, or psychotropic drugs may be additive. Appropriate caution should be exercised with patients who may take one or more of these agents simultaneously with SOMA Compound.

PRECAUTIONS

General: To avoid excessive accumulation of carisoprodol, aspirin, or their metabolites, use SOMA Compound with caution in patients with compromised liver or kidney function, or in elderly or debilitated patients (see CLINICAL PHARMACOLOGY).

Use with caution in patients with history of gastritis or peptic ulcer, in patients on anticoagulant therapy, and in addiction-prone individuals.

Information for Patients: Caution patients that this drug may impair the mental and/or physical abilities required for the performance of potentially hazardous tasks such as driving a motor vehicle or operating machinery.

Caution patients with a predisposition for gastrointestinal bleeding that concomitant use of aspirin and alcohol may have an additive effect in this regard.

Caution patients that dosage of medications used for gout, arthritis, or diabetes may have to be adjusted when aspirin is administered or discontinued (see *Drug Interactions*).

Drug Interactions: Clinically important interactions may occur when certain drugs are administered concomitantly with aspirin or aspirin-containing preparations.

1. *Oral Anticoagulants*—By interfering with platelet function or decreasing plasma prothrombin concentration, aspirin enhances the potential for bleeding in patients on anticoagulants.

2. *Methotrexate*—aspirin enhances the toxic effects of this drug.

3. *Probenecid and Sulfinpyrazone*—large doses of aspirin reduce the uricosuric effect of both drugs. Renal excretion of salicylate may also be reduced.

4. *Oral Antidiabetic Drugs*—enhancement of hypoglycemia may occur.

5. *Antacids*—to the extent that they raise urinary pH, antacids may substantially decrease plasma salicylate concentrations; conversely, their withdrawal can result in a substantial increase.

6. *Ammonium Chloride*—this and other drugs that acidify a relatively alkaline urine can elevate plasma salicylate concentrations.

7. *Ethyl Alcohol*—enhanced aspirin-induced fecal blood loss has been reported.

8. *Corticosteroids*—salicylate plasma levels may be decreased when adrenal corticosteroids are given, and may be increased substantially when they are discontinued.

Carcinogenesis, Mutagenesis, Impairment of Fertility: No long-term studies have been done with SOMA Compound.

Pregnancy—Teratogenic Effects: Pregnancy Category C. Adequate animal reproduction studies have not been conducted with SOMA Compound. It is also not known whether SOMA Compound can cause fetal harm when administered to a pregnant woman or can affect reproduction capacity. SOMA Compound should be given to a pregnant woman only if clearly needed.

Studies in rodents have shown salicylates to be teratogenic when given in early gestation, and embryocidal when given in later gestation in doses considerably greater than usual therapeutic doses in humans. Studies in women who took aspirin during pregnancy have not demonstrated an increased incidence of congenital abnormalities in the offspring.

Labor and Delivery: Ingestion of aspirin near term or prior to delivery may prolong delivery or lead to bleeding in mother, fetus, or neonate.

Nursing Mothers: Carisoprodol is excreted in human milk in concentrations two-to-four times that in maternal plasma. Aspirin is excreted in human milk in moderate amounts and can produce a bleeding tendency in nursing infants. Because of the potential for serious adverse reactions in nursing infants, a decision should be made whether to discontinue nursing or the drug, taking into account the importance of the drug to the mother.

Pediatric Use: Safety and effectiveness in children below the age of twelve have not been established.

ADVERSE REACTIONS

If severe reactions occur, discontinue SOMA Compound and initiate appropriate symptomatic and supportive therapy.

The following side effects which have occurred with the administration of the individual ingredients alone may also occur with the combination.

Carisoprodol: Central Nervous System—Drowsiness is the most frequent complaint and along with other CNS effects may require dosage reduction. Observed less frequently are dizziness, vertigo and ataxia. Tremor, agitation, irritability, headache, depressive reactions, syncope, and insomnia have been infrequent or rare.

Idiosyncratic—Idiosyncratic reactions are very rare. They are usually seen within the period of the first to fourth dose in patients having had no previous contact with the drug (see WARNINGS).

Allergic—Skin rash, erythema multiforme, pruritus, eosinophilia, and fixed drug eruptions with cross-reaction to meprobamate have been reported. If allergic reactions occur, discontinue SOMA Compound and treat symptomatically. In evaluating possible allergic reactions, also consider allergy to excipients (information on excipients is available to physicians on request).

Cardiovascular—Tachycardia, postural hypotension, and facial flushing.

Gastrointestinal—Nausea, vomiting, epigastric distress, and hiccup.

Hematologic—No serious blood dyscrasias have been attributed to carisoprodol alone. Leukopenia and pancytopenia have been reported, very rarely, in situations in which other drugs or viral infections may have been responsible.

Aspirin: The most common adverse reactions associated with the use of aspirin have been gastrointestinal, including nausea, vomiting, gastritis, occult bleeding, constipation, and diarrhea. Gastric erosion, angioedema, asthma, rash,

pruritus and urticaria have been reported less commonly. Tinnitus is a sign of high serum salicylate levels (see OVERDOSAGE).

Aspirin Intolerance—Allergic type reactions in aspirin-sensitive individuals may involve the respiratory tract or the skin. Symptoms of the former range from rhinorrhea and shortness of breath to severe asthma, and the latter may consist of urticaria, edema, rash, or angioedema (giant hives). These may occur independently or in combination.

DRUG ABUSE AND DEPENDENCE

Abuse: In clinical use, abuse has been rare.
Dependence: In clinical use, dependence with SOMA Compound has been rare, and there have been no reports of significant abstinence signs. Nevertheless, the following information on the individual ingredients should be kept in mind.
Carisoprodol—In dogs, no withdrawal symptoms occurred after abrupt cessation of carisoprodol from dosages as high as 1 gm/kg/day. In a study in man, abrupt cessation of 100 mg/kg/day (about five times the recommended daily adult dosage) was followed in some subjects by mild withdrawal symptoms such as abdominal cramps, insomnia, chills, headache, and nausea. Delirium and convulsions did not occur (see PRECAUTIONS).

OVERDOSAGE

Signs and Symptoms: Any of the following which have been reported with the individual ingredients may occur and may be modified to a varying degree by the effects of the other ingredients present in SOMA Compound.
Carisoprodol—Stupor, coma, shock, respiratory depression, and, very rarely, death. Overdosage with carisoprodol in combination with alcohol, other CNS depressants, or psychotropic agents can have additive effects, even when one of the agents has been taken in the usually recommended dosage.
Aspirin—Headache, tinnitus, hearing difficulty, dim vision, dizziness, lassitude, hyperpnea, rapid breathing, thirst, nausea, vomiting, sweating and occasionally diarrhea are characteristic of mild to moderate salicylate poisoning. Salicylate poisoning should be considered in children with symptoms of vomiting, hyperpnea, and hyperthermia.
Hyperpnea is an early sign of salicylate poisoning, but dyspnea supervenes at plasma levels above 50 mg/dL. These respiratory changes eventually lead to serious acid-base disturbances. Metabolic acidosis is a constant finding in infants but occurs in older children only with severe poisoning; adults usually exhibit respiratory alkalosis initially and acidosis terminally.
Other symptoms of severe salicylate poisoning include hyperthermia, dehydration, delirium, and mental disturbances. Skin eruptions, GI hemorrhage, or pulmonary edema are less common. Early CNS stimulation is replaced by increasing depression, stupor, and coma. Death is usually due to respiratory failure or cardiovascular collapse.
Treatment: *General:* Provide symptomatic and supportive treatment, as indicated. Any drug remaining in the stomach should be removed using appropriate procedures and caution to protect the airway and prevent aspiration, especially in the stuporous or comatose patient. Incomplete gastric emptying with delayed absorption of carisoprodol has been reported as a cause for relapse. Should respiration or blood pressure become compromised, respiratory assistance, central nervous system stimulants, and pressor agents should be administered cautiously, as indicated.
Carisoprodol: The following have been used successfully in overdosage with the related drug meprobamate: diuretics, osmotic (mannitol) diuresis, peritoneal dialysis, and hemodialysis (see CLINICAL PHARMACOLOGY). Careful monitoring of urinary output is necessary and caution should be taken to avoid overhydration. Carisoprodol can be measured in biological fluid by gas chromatography (Douglas, J. F., et al: *J Pharm Sci 58:* 145, 1969).
Aspirin—Since there are no specific antidotes for salicylate poisoning, the aim of treatment is to enhance elimination of salicylate and prevent or reduce further absorption; to correct any fluid, electrolyte or metabolic imbalance; and to provide general and cardiorespiratory support. If acidosis is present, intravenous sodium bicarbonate must be given, along with adequate hydration, until salicylate levels decrease to within the therapeutic range. To enhance elimination, forced diuresis and alkalinization of the urine may be beneficial. The need for hemoperfusion or hemodialysis is rare and should be used only when other measures have failed.

DOSAGE AND ADMINISTRATION

Usual Adult Dosage: 1 or 2 tablets, four times daily.
Not recommended for use in children under age twelve (see PRECAUTIONS).

HOW SUPPLIED

SOMA Compound Tablets (carisoprodol, USP 200 mg and aspirin 325 mg) are round, convex, two-layered and inscribed on the white layer with SOMA C and on the light orange layer with WALLACE 2103. The tablets are available in bottles of 100 (NDC 0037-2103-01) and 500 (NDC 0037-2103-03) and unit-dose packages of 100 (NDC 0037-2103-85).
Storage: Store at controlled room temperature 15°–30°C (59°–86°F). Protect from moisture.
Dispense in a tight container.

WALLACE LABORATORIES
Division of CARTER-WALLACE, INC.
Cranbury, New Jersey 08512
IN-094E2-12   Rev. 9/93
Patent No. 4534973
Shown in Product Identification Guide, page 342

SOMA® COMPOUND with CODEINE   ⓒ ℞
(carisoprodol, aspirin and codeine phosphate tablets, USP)
carisoprodol 200 mg + aspirin 325 mg + codeine phosphate 16 mg—Warning: May be habit-forming TABLETS

DESCRIPTION

'Soma' Compound with Codeine is a combination product containing carisoprodol, a centrally-acting muscle relaxant, plus aspirin, an analgesic with antipyretic and anti-inflammatory properties and codeine phosphate, a centrally-acting narcotic analgesic. It is available as a two-layered, white and yellow, oval-shaped tablet for oral administration. Each tablet contains carisoprodol 200 mg, aspirin 325 mg, and codeine phosphate 16 mg. Chemically, carisoprodol is N-isopropyl-2-methyl-2-propyl-1,3-propanediol dicarbamate. Its empirical formula is $C_{12}H_{24}N_2O_4$, with a molecular weight of 260.33. The structural formula is:

$$CH_2CH_2CH_3$$
$$|$$
$$H_2NCOOCH_2CCH_2OOCNHCH(CH_3)_2$$
$$|$$
$$CH_3$$

Other ingredients: croscarmellose sodium, D&C Yellow #10, hydroxypropyl methylcellulose, magnesium stearate, microcrystalline cellulose, povidone, sodium metabisulfite, starch, stearic acid.

CLINICAL PHARMACOLOGY

Carisoprodol: Carisoprodol is a centrally-acting muscle relaxant that does not directly relax tense skeletal muscles in man. The mode of action of carisoprodol in relieving acute muscle spasm of local origin has not been clearly identified, but may be related to its sedative properties. In animals, carisoprodol has been shown to produce muscle relaxation by blocking interneuronal activity and depressing transmission of polysynaptic neurons in the spinal cord and in the descending reticular formation of the brain. The onset of action is rapid and lasts four to six hours.
Carisoprodol is metabolized in the liver and is excreted by the kidneys. It is dialyzable by peritoneal and hemodialysis.
Aspirin: Aspirin is a non-narcotic analgesic with anti-inflammatory and antipyretic activity. Inhibition of prostaglandin biosynthesis appears to account for most of its anti-inflammatory and for at least part of its analgesic and antipyretic properties.
Aspirin is rapidly absorbed and almost totally hydrolyzed to salicylic acid following oral administration. Although aspirin has a half-life of only about 15 minutes, the apparent biologic half-life of salicylic acid in the therapeutic plasma concentration range is between 6 and 12 hours. Salicylic acid is eliminated by renal excretion and by biotransformation to inactive metabolites. Clearance of salicylic acid in the high-dose range is sensitive to urinary pH (see *Drug Interactions*) and is reduced by renal dysfunction.
Codeine Phosphate: Codeine phosphate is a centrally-acting narcotic-analgesic. Its actions are qualitatively similar to morphine, but its potency is substantially less.
Clinical studies have shown that combining aspirin and codeine produces a significant additive effect in analgesic efficacy.

INDICATIONS AND USAGE

'Soma' Compound with Codeine is indicated as an adjunct to rest, physical therapy, and other measures for the relief of pain, muscle spasm, and limited mobility associated with acute, painful musculoskeletal conditions when the additional action of codeine is desired.

CONTRAINDICATIONS

Acute intermittent porphyria; bleeding disorders; allergic or idiosyncratic reactions to carisoprodol, aspirin, codeine, or related compounds.

WARNINGS

On very rare occasions, the first dose of carisoprodol has been followed by idiosyncratic reactions, with symptoms appearing within minutes or hours. These may include extreme weakness, transient quadriplegia, dizziness, ataxia, temporary loss of vision, diplopia, mydriasis, dysarthria, agitation, euphoria, confusion, and disorientation. Although symptoms usually subside over the course of the next several hours, discontinue 'Soma' Compound with Codeine and initiate appropriate supportive and symptomatic therapy, which may include epinephrine and/or antihistamines. In severe cases, corticosteroids may be necessary. Severe reactions have been manifested by asthmatic episodes, fever, weakness, dizziness, angioneurotic edema, smarting eyes, hypotension, and anaphylactoid shock.
The effects of carisoprodol with agents such as alcohol, other CNS depressants, or psychotropic drugs may be additive. Appropriate caution should be exercised with patients who take one or more of these agents simultaneously with Soma Compound with Codeine.
Contains sodium metabisulfite, a sulfite that may cause allergic-type reactions including anaphylactic symptoms and life-threatening or less severe asthmatic episodes in certain susceptible people. The overall prevalence of sulfite sensitivity in the general population is unknown and probably low. Sulfite sensitivity is seen more frequently in asthmatic than in nonasthmatic people.

PRECAUTIONS

General: To avoid excessive accumulation of carisoprodol, aspirin, or their metabolites, use 'Soma' Compound with Codeine with caution in patients with compromised liver or kidney function, or in elderly or debilitated patients (see CLINICAL PHARMACOLOGY).
Use with caution in patients with history of gastritis or peptic ulcer, in patients on anticoagulant therapy, and in addiction-prone individuals.
Information for Patients: Caution patients that this drug may impair the mental and/or physical abilities required for the performance of potentially hazardous tasks such as driving a motor vehicle or operating machinery.
Caution patients with a predisposition for gastrointestinal bleeding that concomitant use of aspirin and alcohol may have an additive effect in this regard.
Caution patients that dosage of medications used for gout, arthritis, or diabetes may have to be adjusted when aspirin is administered or discontinued (see *Drug Interactions*).
Drug Interactions: Clinically important interactions may occur when certain drugs are administered concomitantly with aspirin or aspirin-containing drugs.
1. *Oral Anticoagulants*—By interfering with platelet function or decreasing plasma prothrombin concentration, aspirin enhances the potential for bleeding in patients on anticoagulants.
2. *Methotrexate*—aspirin enhances the toxic effects of this drug.
3. *Probenecid and Sulfinpyrazone*—large doses of aspirin reduce the uricosuric effect of both drugs. Renal excretion of salicylate may also be reduced.
4. *Oral Antidiabetic Drugs*—enhancement of hypoglycemia may occur.
5. *Antacids*—to the extent that they raise urinary pH, antacids may substantially decrease plasma salicylate concentrations; conversely, their withdrawal can result in a substantial increase.
6. *Ammonium Chloride*—this and other drugs that acidify a relatively alkaline urine can elevate plasma salicylate concentrations.
7. *Ethyl Alcohol*—enhanced aspirin-induced fecal blood loss has been reported.
8. *Corticosteroids*—salicylate plasma levels may be decreased when adrenal corticosteroids are given, and may be increased substantially when they are discontinued.
Carcinogenesis, Mutagenesis, Impairment of Fertility: No long-term studies have been done with 'Soma' Compound with Codeine.
Pregnancy—Teratogenic Effects: Pregnancy Category C. Adequate animal reproduction studies have not been conducted with 'Soma' Compound with Codeine. It is also not known whether 'Soma' Compound with Codeine can cause fetal harm when administered to a pregnant woman or can affect reproduction capacity. 'Soma' Compound with Codeine should be given to a pregnant woman only if clearly needed. Studies in rodents have shown salicylates to be teratogenic when given in early gestation, and embryocidal when given in later gestation in doses considerably greater than usual therapeutic doses in humans. Studies in women who took aspirin during pregnancy have not demonstrated an increased incidence of congenital abnormalities in the offspring.
Labor and Delivery: Ingestion of aspirin near term or prior to delivery may prolong delivery or lead to bleeding in mother, fetus, or neonate.
Nursing Mothers: Carisoprodol is excreted in human milk in concentrations two-to-four times that in maternal plasma. Aspirin is excreted in human milk in moderate amounts and can produce a bleeding tendency in nursing

Continued on next page

Soma Compound w/Codeine—Cont.

infants. Because of the potential for serious adverse reactions in nursing infants, a decision should be made whether to discontinue nursing or the drug, taking into account the importance of the drug to the mother.

Pediatric Use: Safety and effectiveness in children below the age of twelve have not been established.

ADVERSE REACTIONS

If severe reactions occur, discontinue 'Soma' Compound with Codeine and initiate appropriate symptomatic and supportive therapy.

The following side effects which have occurred with the administration of the individual ingredients alone may also occur with the combination.

Carisoprodol: *Central Nervous System*—Drowsiness is the most frequent complaint and along with other CNS effects may require dosage reduction. Observed less frequently are dizziness, vertigo and ataxia. Tremor, agitation, irritability, headache, depressive reactions, syncope, and insomnia have been infrequent or rare.

Idiosyncratic—Idiosyncratic reactions are very rare. They are usually seen within the period of the first to fourth dose in patients having had no previous contact with the drug (see WARNINGS).

Allergic—Skin rash, erythema multiforme, pruritus, eosinophilia, and fixed drug eruptions with cross-reaction to meprobamate have been reported. If allergic reactions occur, discontinue 'Soma' Compound with Codeine and treat symptomatically. In evaluating possible allergic reactions, also consider allergy to excipients (information on excipients is available to physicians on request).

Cardiovascular—Tachycardia, postural hypotension, and facial flushing.

Gastrointestinal—Nausea, vomiting, epigastric distress and hiccup.

Hematologic—No serious blood dyscrasias have been attributed to carisoprodol alone. Leukopenia and pancytopenia have been reported, very rarely, in situations in which other drugs or viral infections may have been responsible.

Aspirin: The most common adverse reactions associated with the use of aspirin have been gastrointestinal, including nausea, vomiting, gastritis, occult bleeding, constipation and diarrhea. Gastric erosion, angioedema, asthma, rash, pruritus and urticaria have been reported less commonly. Tinnitus is a sign of high serum salicylate levels (see OVERDOSAGE).

Aspirin Intolerance—Allergic type reactions in aspirin-sensitive individuals may involve the respiratory tract or the skin. Symptoms of the former range from rhinorrhea and shortness of breath to severe asthma, and the latter may consist of urticaria, edema, rash, or angioedema (giant hives). These may occur independently or in combination.

Codeine Phosphate: Nausea, vomiting, constipation, miosis, sedation, and dizziness have been reported.

DRUG ABUSE AND DEPENDENCE

Controlled Substance: Schedule C-III (see PRECAUTIONS).

Abuse: In clinical use, abuse has been rare.

Dependence: In clinical use, dependence with 'Soma' Compound with Codeine has been rare and there have been no reports of significant abstinence signs. Nevertheless, the following information on the individual ingredients should be kept in mind.

Carisoprodol—In dogs, no withdrawal symptoms occurred after abrupt cessation of carisoprodol from dosages as high as 1 gm/kg/day. In a study in man, abrupt cessation of 100 mg/kg/day (about five times the recommended daily adult dosage) was followed in some subjects by mild withdrawal symptoms such as abdominal cramps, insomnia, chills, headache, and nausea. Delirium and convulsions did not occur (see PRECAUTIONS).

Codeine Phosphate—Drug dependence of the morphine type may result.

OVERDOSAGE

Signs and Symptoms: Any of the following which have been reported with the individual ingredients may occur and may be modified to a varying degree by the effects of the other ingredients present in 'Soma' Compound with Codeine.

Carisoprodol—Stupor, coma, shock, respiratory depression and, very rarely, death. Overdosage with carisoprodol in combination with alcohol, other CNS depressants, or psychotropic agents can have additive effects, even when one of the agents has been taken in the usually recommended dosage.

Aspirin—Headache, tinnitus, hearing difficulty, dim vision, dizziness, lassitude, hyperpnea, rapid breathing, thirst, nausea, vomiting, sweating and occasionally diarrhea are characteristic of mild to moderate salicylate poisoning. Salicylate poisoning should be considered in children with symptoms of vomiting, hyperpnea, and hyperthermia.

Hyperpnea is an early sign of salicylate poisoning, but dyspnea supervenes at plasma levels above 50 mg/dl. These respiratory changes eventually lead to serious acid-base disturbances. Metabolic acidosis is a constant finding in infants but occurs in older children only with severe poisoning; adults usually exhibit respiratory alkalosis initially and acidosis terminally.

Other symptoms of severe salicylate poisoning include hyperthermia, dehydration, delirium, and mental disturbances. Skin eruptions, GI hemorrhage, or pulmonary edema are less common. Early CNS stimulation is replaced by increasing depression, stupor, and coma. Death is usually due to respiratory failure or cardiovascular collapse.

Codeine Phosphate—pinpoint pupils, CNS depression, coma, respiratory depression, and shock.

Treatment: *General*—Provide symptomatic and supportive treatment, as indicated. Any drug remaining in the stomach should be removed using appropriate procedures and caution to protect the airway and prevent aspiration, especially in the stuporous or comatose patient. Incomplete gastric emptying with delayed absorption of carisoprodol has been reported as a cause for relapse. Should respiration or blood pressure become compromised, respiratory assistance, central nervous system stimulants, and pressor agents should be administered cautiously, as indicated.

Carisoprodol—The following have been used successfully in overdosage with the related drug meprobamate: diuretics, osmotic (mannitol) diuresis, peritoneal dialysis, and hemodialysis (see CLINICAL PHARMACOLOGY). Careful monitoring of urinary output is necessary and caution should be taken to avoid overhydration. Carisoprodol can be measured in biological fluid by gas chromatography (Douglas, J. F., et al: *J Pharm Sci* 58: 145, 1969).

Aspirin—Since there are no specific antidotes for salicylate poisoning, the aim of treatment is to enhance elimination of salicylate and prevent or reduce further absorption; to correct any fluid, electrolyte or metabolic imbalance; and to provide general and cardiorespiratory support. If acidosis is present, intravenous sodium bicarbonate must be given, along with adequate hydration, until salicylate levels decrease to within the therapeutic range. To enhance elimination, forced diuresis and alkalinization of the urine may be beneficial. The need for hemoperfusion or hemodialysis is rare and should be used only when other measures have failed.

Codeine Phosphate—Narcotic antagonists, such as nalorphine and levallorphan, may be indicated.

DOSAGE AND ADMINISTRATION

Usual Adult Dosage: 1 or 2 tablets, four times daily. Not recommended for use in children under age twelve.

HOW SUPPLIED

'Soma' Compound with Codeine Tablets (carisoprodol, USP 200 mg, aspirin 325 mg, and codeine phosphate, USP 16 mg) are oval, convex, two-layered and inscribed on the white layer with SOMA CC and on the yellow layer with WALLACE 2403. The tablets are available in bottles of 100 (NDC 0037-2403-01).

Storage: Store at controlled room temperature 15°–30°C (59°–86°F). Protect from moisture.

Dispense in a tight container.

WALLACE LABORATORIES
Division of CARTER-WALLACE, INC.
Cranbury, New Jersey 08512
IN-095E2–12   Rev. 9/93
                                      Patent No. 4534974
Shown in Product Identification Guide, page 342

TUSSI-ORGANIDIN® DM NR*   ℞
(*Newly Reformulated) Liquid

TUSSI-ORGANIDIN® DM-S† NR*
(*Newly Reformulated) Liquid
(guaifenesin, dextromethorphan hydrobromide)

**Professional Labeling Information and Directions for Use
This product labeled for sale on prescription only.**

DESCRIPTION

TUSSI-ORGANIDIN® DM NR* (*Newly Reformulated) Liquid is a clear yellow liquid with a raspberry flavor.
Each 5 mL (1 teaspoon) contains:
Guaifenesin, USP .... 100 mg
Dextromethorphan Hydrobromide, USP .... 10 mg
Other ingredients: Citric acid, D&C Yellow No. 10, FD&C Red No. 40, flavor (artificial), glycerin, propylene glycol, purified water, saccharin sodium, sodium benzoate, sorbitol.
Guaifenesin (glyceryl guaiacolate) has the chemical name 3-(2-methoxyphenoxy)-1,2-propanediol. Its molecular formula is $C_{10}H_{14}O_4$, with a molecular weight of 198.21. It is a white, colorless crystalline substance with a slightly bitter aromatic taste. One gram dissolves in 20 mL water at 25°C; freely soluble in ethanol. Guaifenesin is readily absorbed from the GI tract and is rapidly metabolized and excreted in

the urine. Guaifenesin has a plasma half-life of one hour. The major urinary metabolite is beta-(2-methoxyphenoxy) lactic acid.

CLINICAL PHARMACOLOGY

TUSSI-ORGANIDIN® DM NR* (*Newly Reformulated) combines the expectorant, guaifenesin and the cough suppressant, dextromethorphan hydrobromide. Guaifenesin is an expectorant the action of which promotes or facilitates the removal of secretions from the respiratory tract. By increasing sputum volume and making sputum less viscous, guaifenesin facilitates expectoration of retained secretions. Dextromethorphan is a synthetic nonopioid cough suppressant, the dextro isomer of the codeine analogue of levorphanol. Dextromethorphan acts centrally to elevate the threshold for coughing, but does not have addictive, analgesic or sedative actions and does not produce respiratory depression with usual doses.

INDICATIONS AND USAGE

Temporarily relieves cough due to minor throat and bronchial irritation as may occur with the common cold or inhaled irritants. Calms the cough control center and relieves coughing. Helps loosen phlegm (mucus) and thin bronchial secretions to rid the bronchial passageways of bothersome mucus, drain bronchial tubes, and make coughs more productive.

CONTRAINDICATIONS

Hypersensitivity to any of the ingredients. The use of dextromethorphan-containing products is contraindicated in patients receiving monoamine oxidase inhibitors (MAOIs).

PRECAUTIONS

Carcinogenesis, Mutagenesis, Impairment of Fertility: Animal studies to assess the long-term carcinogenic and mutagenic potential or the effect on fertility in animals or humans of TUSSI-ORGANIDIN DM NR* (*Newly Reformulated) Liquid have not been performed.

Pregnancy.

Teratogenic Effects—Pregnancy Category C: Animal reproduction studies have not been conducted. Safe use in pregnancy has not been established relative to possible adverse effects on fetal development. Therefore, this product should not be used in pregnant patients, unless in the judgment of the physician, the potential benefits outweigh possible hazards.

Nursing Mothers: It is not known whether guaifenesin or dextromethorphan is excreted in human milk. Because many drugs are excreted in human milk, caution should be exercised when these products are administered to a nursing woman and a decision should be made whether to discontinue nursing or to discontinue the drug, taking into account the importance of the drug to the mother.

Laboratory Test Interactions: Guaifenesin or its metabolites may cause color interference with the VMA (vanillylmandelic acid) test for catechols. It may also falsely elevate the level of urinary 5-HIAA (5-hydroxyindoleacetic acid) in certain serotonin metabolite chemical tests because of color interference.

Drug Interactions: Serious toxicity may result if dextromethorphan is coadministered with monoamine oxidase inhibitors (MAOIs). The use of dextromethorphan hydrobromide may result in additive CNS depressant effects when coadministered with alcohol, antihistamines, psychotropics or other drugs which produce CNS depression.

Information for Patients: Patients should be warned not to use this product if they are now taking a prescription monoamine oxidase inhibitor (MAOI) (certain drugs for depression, psychiatric or emotional conditions, or Parkinson's disease), or for 2 weeks after stopping the MAOI drug. If patients are uncertain whether a prescription drug contains an MAOI, they should be instructed to consult a health professional before taking such a product.

ADVERSE REACTIONS

Guaifenesin is well tolerated and has a wide margin of safety. Nausea and vomiting are the side effecs that occur most commonly. Other reported adverse reactions have included dizziness, headache and rash (including urticaria). Rare drowsiness or mild gastrointestinal disturbances are the only side effects associated with dextromethorphan in clinical use. (see also Drug Interactions)

OVERDOSAGE

Overdosage with guaifenesin is unlikely to produce toxic effects since its toxicity is low. Guaifenesin, when administered by stomach tube to test animals in doses up to 5 grams/kg, produced no signs of toxicity. In severe cases of overdosage, treatment should be aimed at reducing further absorption of the drug. Gastric emptying (emesis and/or gastric lavage) is recommended as soon as possible after ingestion.

Overdosage with dextromethorphan may produce excitement and mental confusion. Very high doses may produce respiratory depression. One case of toxic psychosis (hyper-

activity, marked visual and auditory hallucinations) after ingestion of a single 300 mg dose of dextromethorphan has been reported.

DOSAGE AND ADMINISTRATION

Adults and children 12 years of age and older: 2 teaspoonfuls (10 mL) every four hours not to exceed 12 teaspoonfuls (60 mL) in 24 hours.

Children 6 years to under 12 years of age: 1 teaspoonful (5 mL) every four hours not to exceed 6 teaspoonfuls (30 mL) in 24 hours.

Children 2 to under 6 years of age: 1/2 teaspoonful (2.5 mL) every four hours not to exceed 3 teaspoonfuls (15 mL) in 24 hours.

Children 6 mo. to under 2 years of age: A common dosage is 1/8 teaspoonful to 1/4 teaspoonful (0.6 mL to 1.25 mL) every 4 hours or 1/2 teaspoonful (2.5 mL) every 6–8 hours, not to exceed 1.5 teaspoonfuls (7.5 mL) in 24 hours. Individualized dosage should be determined by evaluation of patient.

HOW SUPPLIED

Guaifenesin 100 mg and dextromethorphan hydrobromide 10 mg per 5 mL of clear yellow liquid in bottles of one pint (NDC 0037-4714-10) and one gallon (NDC 0037-4714-20), and 4 fl oz (NDC 0037-4714-01) labeled TUSSI-ORGANIDIN® DM-S† NR.*

Storage—Store at controlled room temperature—15°–30°C (59°–86°F). Protect from light. Keep bottle tightly closed.

†TUSSI-ORGANIDIN® DM-S NR* is TUSSI-ORGANIDIN® DM NR* Liquid either in a 4 fl oz unit of use container with a 10 mL graduated oral syringe and fitment or in a 30 mL sample container.

TUSSI-ORGANIDIN® DM NR* (*Newly Reformulated) Liquid is distributed by:

WALLACE LABORATORIES
Division of CARTER-WALLACE, Inc.
Cranbury, NJ 08512

Manufactured by:
Denver Chemical (Puerto Rico) Inc.
Subsidiary of Carter-Wallace, Inc.
Humacao, Puerto Rico 00791
IN-053J8-01   Rev. 7/94
Shown in Product Identification Guide, page 342

TUSSI-ORGANIDIN® NR*   Ⓒ
(*Newly Reformulated) Liquid

TUSSI-ORGANIDIN®-S NR*   Ⓒ
(*Newly Reformulated) Liquid
(guaifenesin, codeine phosphate.

Warning: May be habit-forming)

Professional Labeling Information and Directions for Use
This product labeled for sale on prescription only.
DESCRIPTION
TUSSI-ORGANIDIN® NR* (*Newly Reformulated) Liquid Ⓒ is a clear red liquid with a raspberry flavor for oral administration.

Each 5 mL (1 teaspoonful) contains:

Guaifenesin, USP .... 100 mg
Codeine Phosphate, USP .... 10 mg
(Warning: May be habit-forming)

Other ingredients: Citric acid, FD&C Red No. 40, flavor (artificial), glycerin, propylene glycol, purified water, saccharin sodium, sodium benzoate, sorbitol.

Guaifenesin (glyceryl guaiacolate) has the chemical name 3-(2-methoxyphenoxy)-1,2-propanediol. Its molecular formula is $C_{10}H_{14}O_4$, with a molecular weight of 198.21. It is a white, colorless crystalline substance with a slightly bitter aromatic taste. One gram dissolves in 20 mL water at 25°C; freely soluble in ethanol. Guaifenesin is readily absorbed from the GI tract and is rapidly metabolized and excreted in the urine. Guaifenesin has a plasma half-life of one hour. The major urinary metabolite is beta-(2-methoxyphenoxy) lactic acid.

CLINICAL PHARMACOLOGY

TUSSI-ORGANIDIN® NR* (*Newly Reformulated) combines the expectorant, guaifenesin and the cough suppressant, codeine. Guaifenesin is an expectorant the action of which promotes or facilitates the removal of secretions from the respiratory tract. By increasing sputum volume and making sputum less viscous, guaifenesin facilitates expectoration of retained secretions. Codeine is a centrally acting antitussive agent.

INDICATIONS AND USAGE

Temporarily relieves cough due to minor throat and bronchial irritation as may occur with the common cold or inhaled irritants. Calms the cough control center and relieves coughing. Helps loosen phlegm (mucus) and thin bronchial secretions to rid the bronchial passageways of bothersome mucus, drain bronchial tubes, and make cough more productive.

CONTRAINDICATIONS
Hypersensitivity to any of the ingredients.
PRECAUTIONS
Information for Patients: Patients should be warned about engaging in activities requiring mental alertness, such as driving a car or operating dangerous machinery.

Drug Interactions: The use of codeine may result in additive CNS depressant effects when coadministered with alcohol, antihistamines, psychotropics or other drugs which produce CNS depression.

Carcinogenesis, Mutgenesis, Impairment of Fertility: Animal studies of TUSSI-ORGANIDIN® NR* (*Newly Reformulated) Liquid to assess the long-term carcinogenic and mutagenic potential or the effect on fertility in animals or humans have not been performed.

Pregnancy.

Teratogenic Effects—Pregnancy Category C: Animal reproduction studies have not been conducted. Safe use in pregnancy has not been established relative to possible adverse effects on fetal development. Therefore, this product should not be used in pregnant patients, unless in the judgment of a physician, the potential benefits outweigh possible hazards.

Nursing Mothers: Because the hepatic enzyme system which acts to conjugate codeine to an inactive glucuronide (an important inactivation pathway) is not fully developed in infants less than 6 months of age, the use of codeine is contraindicated in nursing mothers.

Laboratory Test Interactions: Guaifenesin or its metabolites may cause color interference with the vanillylmandelic acid (VMA) test for catechols. It may also falsely elevate the level of urinary 5-hydroxyindoleacetic acid (5-HIAA) in certain serotonin metabolite chemical tests because of color interference.

ADVERSE REACTIONS

Guaifenesin is well tolerated and has a wide margin of safety. Nausea and vomiting are the side effects that occur most commonly. Other reported adverse reactions have included dizziness, headache and rash (including urticaria).

Codeine: Nausea, vomiting, constipation, drowsiness and miosis have been reported. Higher doses may induce euphoria, light-headedness, dizziness, drowsiness and depression of respiration. Pruritus and skin rashes have been rare.

DRUG ABUSE AND DEPENDENCE

Controlled Substance—Schedule V.
Dependence—Codeine may be habit forming.

OVERDOSAGE

If overdosage occurs, treat symptomatically. Gastric emptying (emesis and/or gastric lavage) is recommended.

Severe intoxication with codeine may result in dyspnea, vertigo, double vision, delusions, hallucinations, speech disturbances, excitement, restlessness, delirium, constricted pupils, respiratory depression (slow and shallow breathing), Cheyne-Stokes respiration, circulatory collapse, stupor or coma.

Treatment of overdosage consists primarily of support of vital functions, especially maintenance of codeine-induced respiratory depression. The narcotic antagonist naloxone is a specific antidote for respiratory depression which may result from overdose or unusual sensitivity from narcotics.

DOSAGE AND ADMINISTRATION

Adults and children 12 years of age and older: 2 teaspoonfuls every four hours, not to exceed 12 teaspoonfuls in 24 hours.

Children 6 years to under 12 years of age: 1 teaspoonful every four hours, not to exceed 6 teaspoonfuls in a 24 hour period.

Children 2 to under 6 years of age: Oral dosage is based on 1 mg/kg/day of codeine administered in four equal divided doses.

The average body weight for each age group may also be used to determine codeine dosage as follows:

For children 2 years of age (average body weight 12 kg) the oral dosage is 1.5 mL (3 mg codeine + 30 mg guaifenesin) TUSSI-ORGANIDIN® NR* (*Newly Reformulated) Liquid every 4–6 hr, not to exceed 6 mL (12 mg codeine + 120 mg guaifenesin) in a 24 hr period.

For children 3 years of age (average 14 kg): 1.75 mL (3.5 mg codeine + 35 mg guaifenesin) every 4–6 hours, not to exceed 7 mL (14 mg codeine + 140 mg guaifenesin) in 24 hours.

For children 4 years of age (average 16 kg): 2 mL (4.0 mg codeine + 40 mg guaifenesin) every 4–6 hours, not to exceed 8 mL (16 mg codeine + 160 mg guaifenesin) in 24 hours.

For children 5 years of age (average 18 kg): 2.25 mL (4.5 mg codeine + 45 mg guaifenesin) every 4–6 hours, not to exceed 9 mL (18 mg codeine + 180 mg guaifenesin) in 24 hours.

Patients should be instructed to obtain and use a dispensing device (such as a dropper calibrated for age and weight) to

administer the drug to a child, to use extreme care in measuring dosage, and not to exceed the recommended daily dosage.

CODEINE IS NOT RECOMMENDED FOR USE IN CHILDREN UNDER 2 YEARS OF AGE.

Children under 2 years of age may be more susceptible to the respiratory depressant effects of codeine, including respiratory arrest, coma and death.

PATIENTS SHOULD BE ADVISED TO KEEP THIS AND ALL DRUGS OUT OF THE REACH OF CHILDREN AND TO SEEK PROFESSIONAL ASSISTANCE OR CONTACT A POISON CONTROL CENTER IMMEDIATELY IN CASE OF ACCIDENTAL OVERDOSE.

HOW SUPPLIED

Guaifenesin 100 mg and codeine phosphate 10 mg per 5 mL of clear red liquid in bottles of one pint (NDC 0037-4814-10), one gallon (NDC 0037-4814-20), and 4 fl oz (NDC 0037-4814-01) labeled TUSSI-ORGANIDIN®-S† NR*

Storage—Store at controlled room temperature—15°–30°C (59°–86°F). Protect from light. Keep bottle tightly closed.

†TUSSI-ORGANIDIN®-S NR* is TUSSI-ORGANIDIN® NR* Liquid either in a 4 fl oz unit of use container with a 10 mL graduated oral syringe and fitment or in a 30 mL sample container.

TUSSI-ORGANIDIN® NR* (*Newly Reformulated) Liquid Ⓒ is distributed by:
WALLACE LABORATORIES
Division of CARTER-WALLACE, Inc.
Cranbury, NJ 08512

Manufactured by:
Denver Chemical (Puerto Rico) Inc.
Subsidiary of Carter-Wallace, Inc.
Humacao, Puerto Rico 00791
IN-052J8-01   Rev. 7/94
Shown in Product Identification Guide, page 342

VASCOR®   ℞
brand of bepridil hydrochloride
Tablets

Marketed jointly by McNeil Pharmaceutical and Wallace Laboratories. See McNeil Pharmaceutical for product information.

VōSoL®   ℞
OTIC SOLUTION
(acetic acid otic solution, USP)
VōSoL® HC   ℞
OTIC SOLUTION
(hydrocortisone and acetic acid otic solution, USP)

DESCRIPTION

VōSoL (acetic acid otic solution, USP) is a solution of acetic acid (2%), in a propylene glycol vehicle containing propylene glycol diacetate (3%), benzethonium chloride (0.02%), and sodium acetate (0.015%). The empirical formula for acetic acid is CH_3COOH, with a molecular weight of 60.05. The structural formula is:

$$\begin{array}{c} H \quad O \\ | \quad || \\ H-C-C-OH \\ | \\ H \end{array}$$

VōSoL is available as a nonaqueous otic solution buffered at pH 3 for use in the external ear canal.

VōSoL HC (hydrocortisone and acetic acid otic solution, USP) is a solution containing hydrocortisone (1%) and acetic acid (2%), in a propylene glycol vehicle containing propylene glycol diacetate (3%), benzethonium chloride (0.02%), sodium acetate (0.015%) and citric acid (0.05%). The empirical formulas for acetic acid and hydrocortisone are CH_3COOH and $C_{21}H_{30}O_5$, with a molecular weight of 60.05 and 362.46, respectively. The structural formulas are:

$$\begin{array}{c} H \quad O \\ | \quad || \\ H-C-C-OH \\ | \\ H \end{array}$$

Acetic Acid

Continued on next page

VoSol—Cont.

Chemically, hydrocortisone is:
Pregn-4-ene-3,20-dione,
11,17,21-trihydroxy-(11β)-.

VōSoL HC is available as a nonaqueous otic solution buffered at pH 3 for use in the external ear canal.

CLINICAL PHARMACOLOGY

VōSoL—Acetic acid is antibacterial and antifungal; propylene glycol is hydrophilic and provides a low surface tension; benzethonium chloride is a surface active agent that promotes contact of the solution with tissues.

VōSoL HC—Acetic acid is antibacterial and antifungal; hydrocortisone is antiinflammatory, antiallergic and antipruritic; propylene glycol is hydrophilic and provides a low surface tension; benzethonium chloride is a surface active agent that promotes contact of the solution with tissues.

INDICATIONS AND USAGE

VōSoL—For the treatment of superficial infections of the external auditory canal caused by organisms susceptible to the action of the antimicrobial.

VōSoL HC—For the treatment of superficial infections of the external auditory canal caused by organisms susceptible to the action of the antimicrobial, complicated by inflammation.

CONTRAINDICATIONS

VōSoL—Hypersensitivity to VōSoL or any of the ingredients. Perforated-tympanic membrane is considered a contraindication to the use of any medication in the external ear canal.

VōSoL HC—Hypersensitivity to VōSoL HC or any of the ingredients; herpes simplex, vaccinia and varicella. Perforated tympanic membrane is considered a contraindication to the use of any medication in the external ear canal.

WARNINGS

VōSoL—Discontinue promptly if sensitization or irritation occurs.

VōSoL HC—Discontinue promptly if sensitization or irritation occurs.

PRECAUTIONS

VōSoL—Transient stinging or burning may be noted occasionally when the solution is first instilled into the acutely inflamed ear.

VōSoL HC—Transient stinging or burning may be noted occasionally when the solution is first instilled into the acutely inflamed ear.

PEDIATRIC USE

VōSoL—Safety and effectiveness in pediatric patients below the age of 3 years have not been established.

VōSoL HC—Safety and effectiveness in pediatric patients below the age of 3 years have not been established.

ADVERSE REACTIONS

VōSoL—Stinging or burning may be noted occasionally; local irritation has occurred very rarely.

VōSoL HC—Stinging or burning may be noted occasionally; local irritation has occurred very rarely.

DOSAGE AND ADMINISTRATION

VōSoL—Carefully remove all cerumen and debris to allow VōSoL to contact infected surfaces directly. To promote continuous contact, insert a wick of cotton saturated with VōSoL into the ear canal; the wick may also be saturated after insertion. Instruct the patient to keep the wick in for at least 24 hours and to keep it moist by adding 3 to 5 drops of VōSoL every 4 to 6 hours. The wick may be removed after 24 hours but the patient should continue to instill 5 drops of VōSoL 3 or 4 times daily thereafter, for as long as indicated. In pediatric patients, 3 to 4 drops may be sufficient due to the smaller capacity of the ear canal.

VōSoL HC—Carefully remove all cerumen and debris to allow VōSoL HC to contact infected surfaces directly. To promote continuous contact, insert a wick of cotton saturated with VōSoL HC into the ear canal; the wick may also be saturated after insertion. Instruct the patient to keep the wick in for at least 24 hours and to keep it moist by adding 3 to 5 drops of VōSoL HC every 4 to 6 hours. The wick may be removed after 24 hours but the patient should continue to instill 5 drops of VōSoL HC 3 or 4 times daily thereafter for as long as indicated. In pediatric patients, 3 or 4 drops may be sufficient due to the smaller capacity of the ear canal.

HOW SUPPLIED

VōSoL (acetic acid otic solution, USP), containing 2% acetic acid, is available in 15 mL (NDC 0037-3611-10) measured-drop, safety-tip plastic bottles.

VōSoL HC (Hydrocortisone and acetic acid otic solution, USP), containing hydrocortisone (1%) and acetic acid (2%), is available in 10 mL, measured-drop, safety-tip plastic bottles (NDC 0037-3811-12).

STORAGE

VōSoL—Store at room temperature, 20°–25°C (68°–77°F). Keep container tightly closed.

VōSoL HC—Store at room temperature, 20°–25°C (68°–77°F). Keep container tightly closed.

WALLACE LABORATORIES

Division of CARTER-WALLACE, INC.
Cranbury, New Jersey 08512

VōSoL—IN-056S3–04D   Rev. 8/97
VōSoL HC—IN-056H9–04D

Warner Chilcott Laboratories

PROFESSIONAL PRODUCTS DIVISION
ROCKAWAY 80 CORPORATE CENTER
100 ENTERPRISE DRIVE
SUITE 280
ROCKAWAY, NJ 07866

Direct Inquiries to:
(800) 521-8813
Product/Medical Information:
(800) 521-8813
(973) 442-3236
Medical Emergency Contact:
After hours and weekend
(303) 739-1110

Following is the list of products belonging to our **PROFESSIONAL PRODUCTS DIVISION**

CHOLEDYL SA®   ℞
[Ko '-le-dil]
Oxtriphylline Extended-release Tablets, USP
400mg, 600mg

DORYX®   ℞
[Dor '-ix]
Coated Doxycycline Hyclate Pellets
100mg

ERYC®   ℞
[Er 'ik]
Erythromycin delayed-release Capsules, USP
250mg

MANDELAMINE®   ℞
[Man-del '-a-meen]
Methenamine Mandelate Tablets, USP
.5gm, 1gr

PYRIDIUM®   ℞
[Per-i '-deum]
Phenazopyridine Hydrochloride Tablets, USP
100mg, 200mg

PYRIDIUM® PLUS   ℞

LoCHOLEST™ POWDER   ℞
(CHOLESTYRAMINE FOR
ORAL SUSPENSION, USP)

DESCRIPTION

LoCHOLEST™ Powder (Cholestyramine for Oral Suspension, USP) the chloride salt of a basic anion exchange resin, a cholesterol lowering agent, is intended for oral administration. Cholestyramine resin is quite hydrophilic, but insoluble in water. Cholestyramine resin is not absorbed from the digestive tract. Nine grams of LoCHOLEST™ Powder (Cholestyramine for Oral Suspension, USP) contain 4 grams of cholestyramine resin. It is represented by the following structural formula:
[See chemical structure at top of next column]
Inactive ingredients: citric acid anhydrous, fructose, mono ammonium glycrrhizinate, pectin, propylene glycol alginate, sorbitol, sucrose, xanthan gum, artificial strawberry flavor, D&C Red No. 30 aluminum lake.

CLINICAL PHARMACOLOGY

Cholesterol is probably the sole precursor of bile acids. During normal digestion, bile acids are secreted into the intestines. A major portion of the bile acids is absorbed from the

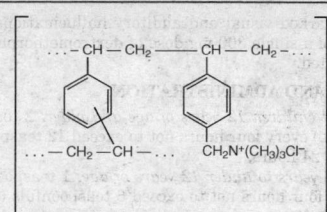

Representation of structure of main polymeric groups

intestinal tract and returned to the liver via the enterohepatic circulation. Only very small amounts of bile acids are found in normal serum.

Cholestyramine resin adsorbs and combines with the bile acids in the intestine to form an insoluble complex which is excreted in the feces. This results in a partial removal of bile acids from the enterohepatic circulation by preventing their absorption.

The increased fecal loss of bile acids due to cholestyramine resin administration leads to an increased oxidation of cholesterol to bile acids, a decrease in beta lipoprotein or low density lipoprotein plasma levels and a decrease in serum cholesterol levels. Although in man, cholestyramine resin produces an increase in hepatic synthesis of cholesterol, plasma cholesterol levels fall.

In patients with partial biliary obstruction, the reduction of serum bile acid levels by cholestyramine resin reduces excess bile acids deposited in the dermal tissue with resultant decrease in pruritus.

Clinical Studies

In a large, placebo-controlled, multi-clinic study, LRC-CPPT[1], hypercholesterolemic subjects treated with cholestyramine resin had mean reduction in total and low-density lipoprotein cholesterol (LDL-C) which exceeded those for diet and placebo treatment by 7.2% and 10.4%, respectively. Over the seven-year study period the cholestyramine resin group experienced a 19% reduction (relative to the incidence in the placebo group) in the combined rate of coronary heart disease death plus non-fatal myocardial infarction (cumulative incidence of 7% cholestyramine resin and 8.6% placebo). The subjects included in the study were men aged 35 to 59 with serum cholesterol levels above 265 mg/dL and no previous history of heart disease. It is not clear to what extent these findings can be extrapolated to females and other segments of the hypercholesterolemic population. (See also PRECAUTIONS: Carcinogenesis, Mutagenesis, Impairment of Fertility.)

Two controlled clinical trials have examined the effects of cholestyramine monotherapy upon coronary atherosclerotic lesions using coronary arteriography. In the NHLBI Type II coronary intervention trial[2], 116 patients (80% male) with coronary artery disease (CAD) documented by arteriography were randomized to cholestyramine resin or placebo for five years of treatment. Final study arteriography revealed progression of coronary artery disease in 49% of placebo patients compared to 32% of the cholestyramine resin group (p<0.05).

In the St. Thomas Atherosclerosis Regression Study (STARS)[3], 90 hypercholesterolemic men with CAD were randomized to three blinded treatments: usual care, lipid-lowering diet, and lipid-lowering diet plus cholestyramine resin. After 36 months, follow-up coronary arteriography revealed progression of disease in 46% of usual care patients, 15% of patients on lipid-lowering diet and 12% of those receiving diet plus cholestyramine resin (p<0.02). The mean absolute width of coronary segments decreased in the usual care group, increased slightly (0.003 mm) in the diet group and increased by 0.103 mm in the diet plus cholestyramine group (p<0.05). Thus in these randomized controlled clinical trials using coronary arteriography, cholestyramine resin monotherapy has been demonstrated to slow progression[2,3] and promote regression[3] of atherosclerotic lesions in the coronary arteries of patients with coronary artery disease.

The effect of intensive lipid-lowering therapy on coronary atherosclerosis has been assessed by arteriography in hyperlipidemic patients. In these randomized, controlled clinical trials, patients were treated for two to four years by either conventional methods (diet, placebo, or in some cases low dose resin), or intensive combination therapy using diet plus colestipol (an anion exchange resin with a mechanism of action and an effect on serum lipids similar to that of Lo-CHOLEST™ Powder plus either nicotinic acid or lovastatin. When compared to conventional measures, intensive lipid-lowering combination therapy significantly reduced the frequency of progression and increased the frequency of regression of coronary atherosclerotic lesions in patients with or at risk for coronary artery disease.

INDICATIONS AND USAGE

1) LoCHOLEST™ Powder is indicated as adjunctive therapy to diet for the reduction of elevated serum cholesterol in patients with primary hypercholesterolemia (elevated low

density lipoprotein [LDL] cholesterol) who do not respond adequately to diet. LoCHOLEST™ Powder may be useful to lower LDL cholesterol in patients who also have hypertriglyceridemia, but it is not indicated where hypertriglyceridemia is the abnormality of most concern.

Therapy with lipid-altering agents should be a component of multiple risk factor intervention in those individuals at significantly increased risk for atherosclerotic vascular disease due to hypercholesterolemia. Treatment should begin and continue with dietary therapy specific for the type of hyperlipoproteinemia determined prior to initiation of drug therapy. Excess body weight may be an important factor and caloric restriction for weight normalization should be addressed prior to drug therapy in the overweight.

Prior to initiating therapy with cholestyramine resin, secondary causes of hypercholesterolemia (e.g., poorly controlled diabetes mellitus, hypothyroidism, nephrotic syndrome, dysproteinemias, obstructive liver disease, other drug therapy, alcoholism), should be excluded, and a lipid profile performed to assess Total cholesterol, HDL-C, and triglycerides (TG). For individuals with TG less than 400 mg/dL (<4.5 mmol/L), LDL-C can be estimated using the following equation:

$$\text{LDL-C} = \text{Total cholesterol} - [(\text{TG}/5) + \text{HDL-C}]$$

For TG levels > 400 mg/dL, this equation is less accurate and LDL-C concentrations should be determined by ultracentrifugation. In hypertriglyceridemia patients, LDL-C may be low or normal despite elevated Total-C. In such cases cholestyramine resin may not be indicated.

Serum cholesterol and triglyceride levels should be determined periodically based on NCEP guidelines to confirm initial and adequate long-term response. A favorable trend in cholesterol reduction should occur during the first month of cholestyramine resin therapy. The therapy should be continued to sustain cholesterol reduction. If adequate cholesterol reduction is not attained, increasing the dosage of cholestyramine resin or adding other lipid-lowering agents in combination with cholestyramine resin should be considered.

Since the goal of treatment is to lower LDL-C the NCEP[4] recommends that LDL-C levels be used to initiate and assess treatment response. If LDL-C levels are not available then Total-C alone may be used to monitor long-term therapy. A lipoprotein analysis (including LDL-C determination) should be carried out once a year. The NCEP treatment guidelines are summarized below.

		LDL-Cholesterol mg/dL (mmol/L)	
Definite Atherosclerotic Disease*	Two or More Other Risk Factors**	Initiation Level	Goal
NO	NO	≥190 (≥4.9)	<160 (<4.1)
NO	YES	≥160 (≥4.1)	<130 (<3.4)
YES	YES or NO	≥130 (≥3.4)	≤100 (≤2.6)

* Coronary heart disease or peripheral vascular disease (including symptomatic carotid artery disease).

** Other risk factors for coronary heart disease (CHD) include: age (males ≥45 years; females: ≥55 years or premature menopause without estrogen replacement therapy); family history of premature CHD; current cigarette smoking; hypertension, confirmed HDL-C <35 mg/dL (<0.91 mmol/L); and diabetes mellitus. Subtract one risk factor if HDL-C is ≥ 60 mg/dL (≥1.6 mmol/L).

Cholestyramine resin monotherapy has been demonstrated to retard the rate of progression[2,3] and increase the rate of regression[3] of coronary atherosclerosis.

2) LoCHOLEST™ Powder is indicated for the relief of pruritus associated with partial biliary obstruction. Cholestyramine resin has been shown to have a variable effect on serum cholesterol in these patients. Patients with primary biliary cirrhosis may exhibit an elevated cholesterol as part of their disease.

CONTRAINDICATIONS

LoCHOLEST™ Powder is contraindicated in patients with complete biliary obstruction where bile is not secreted into the intestine and in those individuals who have shown hypersensitivity to any of its components.

PRECAUTION

General: Chronic use of cholestyramine resin may be associated with increased bleeding tendency due to hypoprothrombinemia associated with Vitamin K deficiency. This will usually respond promptly to parenteral Vitamin K_1 and recurrences can be prevented by oral administration of vitimin K_1. Reduction of serum or red cell folate has been reported over long term administration of cholestyramine resin. Supplementation with folic acid should be considered in these cases.

There is a possibility that prolonged use of cholestyramine resin, since it is a chloride form of anion exchange resin, may produce hyperchloremic acidosis. This would especially be true in younger and smaller patients where the relative dosage may be higher. Caution should also be exercised in patients with renal insufficiency or volume depletion, and in patients receiving concomitant spironolactone.

Cholestyramine resin may produce or worsen preexisting constipation. The dosage should be increased gradually in patients to minimize the risk of developing fecal impaction. In patients with pre-existing constipation, the starting dose should be 1 pouch or 1 scoop once daily for 5 to 7 days, increasing to twice daily with monitoring of constipation and of serum lipoproteins, at least twice, 4 to 6 weeks apart. Increased fluid intake and fiber intake should be encouraged to alleviate constipation and a stool softener may occasionally be indicated. If the initial dose is well tolerated, the dose may be increased as needed by one dose/day (at monthly intervals) with periodic monitoring of serum lipoproteins. If constipation worsens or the desired therapeutic response is not achieved at one to six doses/day, combination therapy or alternate therapy should be considered. Particular effort should be made to avoid constipation in patients with symptomatic coronary artery disease. Constipation associated with cholestyramine resin may aggravate hemorrhoids.

Information for Patients: Inform your physician if you are pregnant or plan to become pregnant or are breast-feeding. Drink plenty of fluids and mix each 9 gram dose of LoCHOLEST™ Powder (Cholestyramine for Oral Suspension, USP) in at least 2 to 6 ounces of fluid before taking. Sipping or holding the resin suspension in the mouth for prolonged periods may lead to changes in the surface of the teeth resulting in discoloration, erosion of enamel or decay, good oral hygiene should be maintained.

Laboratory Tests: Serum cholesterol levels should be determined frequently during the first few months of therapy and periodically thereafter. Serum triglyceride levels should be measured periodically to detect whether significant changes have occurred.

The LRC-CPPT showed a dose-related increase in serum triglycerides of 10.7% to 17.1% in the cholestyramine-treated group, compared with an increase of 7.9% to 11.7% in the placebo group. Based on the mean values and adjusted for the placebo group, the cholestyramine-treated group showed an increase of 5% over pre-entry levels the first year of the study and an increase of 4.3% the seventh year.

Drug Interactions:

Cholestyramine resin may delay or reduce the absorption of concomitant oral medication such as phenylbutazone, warfarin, thiazide diuretics (acidic) or propranolol (basic), as well as tetracycline, penicillin G, phenobarbital, thyroid and thyroxine preparations, estrogens and progestins, and digitalis. Interference with the absorption of oral phosphate supplements has been observed with another positively-charged bile acid sequestrant. Cholestyramine resin may interfere with the pharmacokinetics of drugs that undergo enterohepatic circulation. The discontinuance of cholestyramine resin could pose a hazard to health if a potentially toxic drug such as digitalis has been titrated to a maintenance level while the patient was taking cholestyramine resin.

Because cholestyramine binds bile acids, cholestyramine resin may interfere with normal fat digestion and absorption and thus may prevent absorption of fat soluble vitamins such as A, D, E, and K. When cholestyramine resin is given for long periods of time, concomitant supplementation with water-miscible (or parenteral) forms of fat-soluble vitamins should be considered.

SINCE CHOLESTYRAMINE RESIN MAY BIND OTHER DRUGS GIVEN CONCURRENTLY, IT IS RECOMMENDED THAT PATIENTS TAKE OTHER DRUGS AT LEAST 1 HOUR BEFORE OR 4 TO 6 HOURS AFTER CHOLESTYRAMINE RESIN (OR AT AS GREAT AN INTERVAL AS POSSIBLE) TO AVOID IMPEDING THEIR ABSORPTION.

Carcinogenesis, Mutagenesis, Impairment of Fertility: In studies conducted in rats in which cholestyramine resin was used as a tool to investigate the role of various intestinal factors, such as fat, bile salts and microbial flora, in the development of intestinal tumors induced by potent carcinogens, the incidence of such tumors was observed to be greater in cholestyramine resin-treated rats than in control rats.

The relevance of this laboratory observation from studies in rats to the clinical use of cholestyramine resin is not known. In the LRC-CPPT study referred to above, the total incidence of fatal and nonfatal neoplasms was similar in both treatment groups. When the many different categories of tumors are examined, various alimentary system cancers were somewhat more prevalent in the cholestyramine group. The small numbers and the multiple categories prevent conclusions from being drawn. However, in view of the fact that cholestyramine resin is confined to the GI tract and not absorbed, and in light of the animal experiments referred to above, a six-year post-trial follow-up of the LRC-CPPT[5] patient population has been completed (a total of 13.4 years of in-trial plus post-trial follow-up) and revealed no significant difference in the incidence of cause-specific mortality or cancer morbidity between cholestyramine and placebo treated patients.

Pregnancy: Pregnancy Category C. There are no adequate and well controlled studies in pregnant women. The use of cholestyramine in pregnancy or lactation or by women of childbearing age requires that the potential benefits of drug therapy be weighted against the possible hazards to the mother and child. Cholestyramine is not absorbed systemically, however, it is known to interfere with absorption of fat-soluble vitamins; accordingly, regular prenatal supplementation may not be adequate (see PRECAUTIONS: Drug Interactions).

Nursing Mothers: Caution should be exercised when cholestyramine resin is administered to a nursing mother. The possible lack of proper vitamin absorption described in the "Pregnancy" section may have an effect on nursing infants.

Pediatric Use: Although an optimal dosage schedule has not been established, standard texts ([6–7]) list a usual pediatric dose of 240 mg/kg/day of anhydrous cholestyramine resin in two to three divided doses, normally not to exceed 8 g/day with dose titration based on response and tolerance. In calculating pediatric dosages, 44.4 mg of anhydrous cholestyramine resin are contained in 100 mg of LoCHOLEST™.

The effects of long-term drug administration, as well as its effect in maintaining lowered cholesterol levels in pediatric patients, are unknown. Also see "ADVERSE REACTIONS".

ADVERSE REACTIONS

The most common adverse reaction is constipation. When used as a cholesterol-lowering agent predisposing factors for most complaints of constipation are high dose and increased age (more than 60 years old). Most instances of constipation are mild, transient, and controlled with conventional therapy. Some patients require a temporary decrease in dosage or discontinuation of therapy.

Less Frequent Adverse Reactions- Abdominal discomfort and/or pain, flatulence, nausea, vomiting, diarrhea, eructation, anorexia, steatorrhea, bleeding tendencies due to hypoprothrombinemia (Vitamin K deficiency) as well as Vitamin A (one case of night blindness reported) and D deficiencies, hyperchloremic acidosis in children, osteoporosis, rash and irritation of the skin, tongue and perianal area. Rare reports of intestinal obstruction, including two deaths, have been reported in pediatric patients.

Occasional calcified material has been observed in the biliary tree, including calcification of the gallbladder, in patients to whom cholestyramine resin has been given. However, this may be a manifestation of the liver disease and not drug related.

One patient experienced biliary colic on each of three occasions on which he took a cholestyramine for oral suspension product. One patient diagnosed as acute abdominal symptom complex was found to have a "pasty mass" in the transverse colon on x-ray.

Other events (not necessarily drug related) reported in patients taking cholestyramine resin include:

Gastrointestinal – GI-rectal bleeding, black stools, hemorrhoidal bleeding, bleeding from known duodenal ulcer, dysphagia, hiccups, ulcer attack, sour taste, pancreatitis, rectal pain, diverticulitis.

Laboratory test changes - Liver function abnormalities.

Hematologic - Prolonged prothrombin time, ecchymosis, anemia.

Hypersensitivity - Urticaria, asthma, wheezing, shortness of breath.

Musculoskeletal - Backache, muscle and joint pains, arthritis.

Neurologic - Headache, anxiety, vertigo, dizziness, fatigue, tinnitus, syncope, drowsiness, femoral nerve pain, paresthesia.

Eye - Uveitis.

Renal - Hematuria, dysuria, burnt odor to urine, diuresis.

Miscellaneous - Weight loss, weight gain, increased libido, swollen glands, edema, dental bleeding, dental caries, erosion of tooth enamel, tooth discoloration.

OVERDOSAGE

Overdosage of cholestyramine resin has been reported in a patient taking 150% of the maximum recommended daily dosage for a period of several weeks. No ill effects were reported. Should an overdosage occur, the chief potential harm would be obstruction of the gastrointestinal tract. The location of such potential obstruction, the degree of obstruction, and the presence or absence of normal gut motility would determine treatment.

DOSAGE AND ADMINISTRATION

The recommended starting adult dose for LoCHOLEST™ Powder is 1 pouch or 1 level scoopful (9 grams of LoC-

Continued on next page

LoCholest—Cont.

HOLEST™ Powder contains 4 grams of anhydrous cholestyramine resin) once or twice a day. The recommended maintenance dose for LoCHOLEST™ Powder is 2 to 4 pouches or scoopfuls daily (8 to 16 grams anhydrous cholestyramine resin) divided into two doses. It is recommended that increases in dose be gradual with periodic assessment of lipid/lipoprotein levels at intervals of not less than 4 weeks. The maximum recommended daily dose is 6 pouches or scoopfuls of LoCHOLEST™ Powder (24 grams of anhydrous cholestyramine resin). The suggested time of administration is at mealtime but may be modified to avoid interference with absorption of other medication. Although the recommended dosing schedule is twice daily, LoCHOLEST™ Powder may be administered in 1 to 6 doses per day.

LoCHOLEST™ Powder should not be taken in its dry form. Always mix the dry powder with water or other fluids before ingesting. See Preparation Instructions.

Concomitant Therapy

Preliminary evidence suggests that the lipid-lowering effects of cholestyramine on total and LDL-cholesterol are enhanced when combined with a HMG-CoA reductase inhibitor, e.g., pravastatin, lovastatin, simvastatin, and fluvastatin. Additive effects on LDL-cholesterol are also seen with combined nicotinic acid/cholestyramine therapy. See the Drug Interactions subsection of the PRECAUTIONS section for recommendations on administering concomitant therapy

Preparation

The color of LoCHOLEST™ Powder may vary somewhat from batch to batch but this variation does not affect the performance of the product. Place the contents of one single-dose pouch or one level scoopful of LoCHOLEST™ Powder in a glass or cup. Add at least 2 to 6 ounces of water or the beverage of your choice. Stir to a uniform consistency.

LoCHOLEST™ Powder may also be mixed with highly fluid soups or pulpy fruits with a high moisture content such as applesauce or crushed pineapple.

HOW SUPPLIED

LoCHOLEST™ Powder strawberry flavor is available in cartons of sixty 9 gram pouches and in cans containing 378 grams. Nine grams of LoCHOLEST™ Powder contain 4 grams of anhydrous cholestyramine resin.

NDC 0047-2008-20 Carton of 60 pouches

NDC 0047-2008-22 Can, 378 g (containing a scoop that is not interchangeable with scoops from other products)

Storage:

Store at controlled room temperature 15°–30°C (59°–86°F).

Rx only

REFERENCES

1. The Lipid Research Clinics Coronary Primary Prevention Trial Results: (I) Reduction in Incidence of Coronary Heart Disease: (II) The Relationship of Reduction in Incidence of Coronary Heart Disease to Cholesterol Lowering. *JAMA*. 1984;251:351–374.
2. Brensike JF, Levy RI, Kelsey SF, et al. Effects of therapy with cholestyramine in progression of coronary arteriosclerosis, results of the NHLBI type II coronary intervention study. Circulation 1984;69:313–24.
3. Watts GF, Lewis B, Brunt JNH, Lewis ES, et al. Effects on coronary artery disease of lipid-lowering diet, or diet plus cholestyramine, in the St. Thomas Atherosclerosis Regression Study (STARS). Lancet 1992;339:563–69.
4. National Cholesterol Education Program. Second Report of the Exper5t Panel on Detection, Evaluation, and Treatment of High Blood Cholesterol in Adults (Adult Treatment Panel II).Circulation 1994 Mar;89 (3): 1333–445.
5. The Lipid Research Clinics Investigators. The Lipid Research Clinics Coronary Primary Prevention Trial Results of 6 Years of Post-Trial Follow-up. Arch Interm Med 1992; 152:1399–1410.
6. Behrman RE et al (eds): *Nelson, Textbook of Pediatrics*, ed 15. Philadelphia, PA, WB Saunders Company, 1996.
7. Takemoto CK et al (eds): *Pediatric Dosage Handbook*, ed 3. Cleveland/Akron, OH, Lexi-Comp, Inc., 1996/1997.

Manufactured for:
Warner Chilcott Laboratories
100 Enterprise Dr.
Rockaway, NJ 07866
Manufactured by:
Eon Labs Manufacturing, Inc.

Rev. 03/98
MF0938REV0398
Flat #11469
2008-G012

Shown in Product Identification Guide, page 342

LoCHOLEST™ Light Powder ℞
(CHOLESTYRAMINE FOR ORAL SUSPENSION, USP LIGHT)

DESCRIPTION

LoCHOLEST™ Light Powder (Cholestyramine for Oral Suspension, USP Light), the chloride salt of a basic anion exchange resin, a cholesterol-lowering agent, is intended for oral administration. Cholestyramine resin is quite hydrophilic, but insoluble in water. Cholestyramine resin is not absorbed from the digestive tract. Each 5.7 grams of LoCHOLEST™ Light Powder (Cholestyramine for Oral Suspension, USP Light) contain 4 grams of cholestyramine resin. It is represented by the following structural formula:

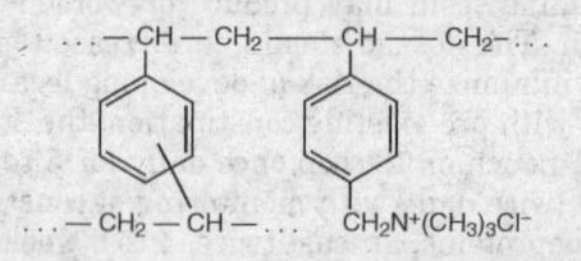

Representation of structure of main polymeric groups

Inactive Ingredients: aspartame, citric acid anhydrous, colloidal silicon dioxide, fructose, mannitol, mono ammonium glycrrhizinate, pectin, propylene glycol alginate, sorbitol, xanthan gum, artificial strawberry flavor, D&C Red No. 30 aluminum lake.

CLINICAL PHARMACOLOGY

Cholesterol is probably the sole precursor of bile acids. During normal digestion, bile acids are secreted into the intestines. A major portion of the bile acids is absorbed from the intestinal tract and returned to the liver via the enterohepatic circulation. Only very small amounts of bile acids are found in normal serum.

Cholestyramine resin adsorbs and combines with the bile acids in the intestine to form an insoluble complex which is excreted in the feces. This results in a partial removal of bile acids from the enterohepatic circulation by preventing their absorption.

The increased fecal loss of bile acids due to cholestyramine resin administration leads to an increased oxidation of cholesterol to bile acids, a decrease in beta lipoprotein or low density lipoprotein plasma levels and a decrease in serum cholesterol levels. Although in man, cholestyramine resin produces an increase in hepatic synthesis of cholesterol, plasma cholesterol levels fall.

In patients with partial biliary obstruction, the reduction of serum bile acid levels by cholestyramine resin reduces excess bile acids deposited in the dermal tissue with resultant decrease in pruritus.

Clinical Studies

In a large, placebo-controlled, multi-clinic study, LRC-CPPT[1], hypercholesterolemic subjects treated with cholestyramine resin had mean reductions in total and low-density lipoprotein cholesterol (LDL-C) which exceeded those for diet and placebo treatment by 7.2% and 10.4%, respectively. Over the seven-year study period the cholestyramine resin group experienced a 19% reduction (relative to the incidence in the placebo group) in the combined rate of coronary heart disease death plus non-fatal myocardial infarction (cumulative incidences of 7% cholestyramine resin and 8.6% placebo). The subjects included in the study were men aged 35 to 59 with serum cholesterol levels above 265 mg/dL and no previous history of heart disease. It is not clear to what extent these findings can be extrapolated to females and other segments of the hypercholesterolemic population. (See also PRECAUTIONS: Carcinogenesis, Mutagenesis, Impairment of Fertility.)

Two controlled clinical trials have examined the effects of cholestyramine monotherapy upon coronary atherosclerotic lesions using coronary arteriography. In the NHLBI Type II Coronary Intervention Trial[2], 116 patients (80% male) with coronary artery disease (CAD) documented by arteriography were randomized to cholestyramine resin or placebo for five years of treatment. Final study arteriography revealed progression of coronary artery disease in 49% of placebo patients compared to 32% of the cholestyramine resin group ($p<0.05$).

In the St. Thomas Atherosclerosis Regression Study (STARS)[3], 90 hypercholesterolemic men with CAD were randomized to three blinded treatments: usual care, lipid-lowering diet, and lipid-lowering diet plus cholestyramine resin. After 36 months, follow-up coronary arteriography revealed progression of disease in 46% of usual care patients, 15% of patients on lipid-lowering diet and 12% of those receiving diet plus cholestyramine resin ($p<0.02$). The mean absolute width of coronary segments decreased in the usual care group, increased slightly (0.003 mm) in the diet group and increased by 0.103 mm in the diet plus cholestyramine group ($p<0.05$). Thus in these randomized controlled clinical trials using coronary arteriography, cholestyramine resin monotherapy has been demonstrated to slow progression[2,3] and promote regression[3] of atherosclerotic lesions in the coronary arteries of patients with coronary artery disease.

The effect of intensive lipid-lowering therapy on coronary atherosclerosis has been assessed by arteriography in hyperlipidemic patients. In these randomized, controlled clinical trials, patients were treated for two to four years by either conventional measures (diet, placebo, or in some cases low dose resin), or intensive combination therapy using diet plus colestipol (an anion exchange resin with a mechanism of action and an effect similar on serum lipids to that of LoCHOLEST™ Light Powder plus either nicotinic acid or lovastatin. When compared to conventional measures, intensive lipid-lowering combination therapy significantly reduced the frequency of progression and increased the frequency of regression of coronary atherosclerotic lesions in patients with or at risk for coronary artery disease.

INDICATIONS AND USAGE

1) LoCHOLEST™ Light Powder is indicated as adjunctive therapy to diet for the reduction of elevated serum cholesterol in patients with primary hypercholesterolemia (elevated low density lipoprotein [LDL] cholesterol) who do not respond adequately to diet. LoCHOLEST™ Light Powder may be useful to lower LDL cholesterol in patients who also have hypertriglyceridemia, but it is not indicated where hypertriglyceridemia is the abnormality of most concern.

Therapy with lipid-altering agents should be a component of multiple risk factor intervention in those individuals at significantly increased risk for atherosclerotic vascular disease due to hypercholesterolemia. Treatment should begin and continue with dietary therapy specific for the type of hyperlipoproteinemia determined prior to initiation of drug therapy. Excess body weight may be an important factor and caloric restriction for weight normalization should be addressed prior to drug therapy in the overweight.

Prior to initiating therapy with cholestyramine resin, secondary causes of hypercholesterolemia (e.g., poorly controlled diabetes mellitus, hypothyroidism, nephrotic syndrome, dysproteinemias, obstructive liver disease, other drug therapy, alcoholism), should be excluded, and a lipid profile performed to assess Total cholesterol, HDL-C, and triglycerides (TG). For individuals with TG less than 400 mg/dL (<4.5 mmol/L), LDL-C can be estimated using the following equation:

$$\text{LDL-C} = \text{Total cholesterol} - [(\text{TG}/5) + \text{HDL-C}]$$

For TG levels > 400 mg/dL, this equation is less accurate and LDL-C concentrations should be determined by ultracentrifugation. In hypertriglyceridemic patients, LDL-C may be low or normal despite elevated Total-C. In such cases cholestyramine resin may not be indicated.

Serum cholesterol and triglyceride levels should be determined periodically based on NCEP guidelines to confirm initial and adequate long-term response. A favorable trend in cholesterol reduction should occur during the first month of cholestyramine resin therapy. The therapy should be continued to sustain cholesterol reduction. If adequate cholesterol reduction is not attained, increasing the dosage of cholestyramine resin or adding other lipid-lowering agents in combination with cholestyramine resin should be considered.

Since the goal of treatment is to lower LDL-C, the NCEP[4] recommends that LDL-C levels be used to initiate and assess treatment response. If LDL-C levels are not available then Total-C alone may be used to monitor long-term therapy. A lipoprotein analysis (including LDL-C determination) should be carried out once a year. The NCEP treatment guidelines are summarized below.

		LDL-Cholesterol mg/dL (mmol/L)	
Definite Atherosclerotic Disease*	Two or More Other Risk Factors**	Initiation Level	Goal
NO	NO	≥190 (≥4.9)	<160 (<4.1)
NO	YES	≥160 (≥4.1)	<130 (<3.4)
YES	YES or NO	≥130 (≥3.4)	≤100 (≤2.6)

*Coronary heart disease or peripheral vascular disease (including symptomatic carotid artery disease).

**Other risk factors for coronary heart disease (CHD) include: age (males ≥45 years; females: ≥55 years or premature menopause without estrogen replacement therapy); family history of premature CHD; current cigarette smoking; hypertension; confirmed HDL-C <35 mg/dL (<0.91 mmol/L); and diabetes mellitus. Subtract one risk factor if HDL-C is ≥60 mg/dL (≥1.6 mmol/L).

Cholestyramine resin monotherapy has been demonstrated to retard the rate of progression[2,3] and increase the rate of regression[3] of coronary atherosclerosis.

2) LoCHOLEST™ Light Powder is indicated for the relief of pruritus associated with partial biliary obstruction. Cholestyramine resin has been shown to have a variable effect on serum cholesterol in these patients. Patients with primary biliary cirrhosis may exhibit an elevated cholesterol as part of their disease.

CONTRAINDICATIONS

LoCHOLEST™ Light Powder is contraindicated in patients with complete biliary obstruction where bile is not secreted into the intestine and in those individuals who have shown hypersensitivity to any of its components.

WARNING

PHENYLKETONURICS: LoCHOLEST™ LIGHT POWDER CONTAINS 22.4 MG PHENYLALANINE PER 5.7 GRAM DOSE.

PRECAUTIONS

General

Chronic use of cholestyramine resin may be associated with increased bleeding tendency due to hypoprothrombinemia associated with Vitamin K deficiency. This will usually respond promptly to parenteral Vitamin K_1 and recurrences can be prevented by oral administration of Vitamin K_1. Reduction of serum or red cell folate has been reported over long term administration of cholestyramine resin. Supplementation with folic acid should be considered in these cases.

There is possibility that prolonged use of cholestyramine resin, since it is a chloride form of anion exchange resin, may produce hyperchloremic acidosis. This would especially be true in younger and smaller patients where the relative dosage may be higher. Caution should be exercised in patients with renal insufficiency or volume depletion, and in patients receiving concomitant spironolactone.

Cholestyramine resin may produce or worsen preexisting constipation. The dosage should be increased gradually in patients to minimize the risk of developing fecal impaction. In patients with preexisting constipation, the starting dose should be 1 pouch or 1 scoop once daily for 5 to 7 days, increasing to twice daily with monitoring of constipation and of serum lipoproteins, at least twice, 4 to 6 weeks apart. Increased fluid intake and fiber intake should be encouraged to alleviate constipation and a stool softener may occasionally be indicated. If the initial dose is well tolerated, the dose may be increased as needed by one dose/day (at monthly intervals) with periodic monitoring of serum lipoproteins. If constipation worsens or the desired therapeutic response is not achieved at one to six doses/day, combination therapy or alternate therapy should be considered. Particular effort should be made to avoid constipation in patients with symptomatic coronary artery disease. Constipation associated with cholestyramine resin may aggravate hemorrhoids.

Information for Patients: Inform your physician if you are pregnant or plan to become pregnant or are breast-feeding. Drink plenty of fluids and mix each 5.7 gram dose of LoCHOLEST™ Light Powder (Cholestyramine for Oral Suspension, USP Light) in at least 2 to 3 ounces of fluid before taking. Sipping or holding the resin suspension in the mouth for prolonged periods may lead to changes in the surface of the teeth resulting in discoloration, erosion of enamel or decay; good oral hygiene should be maintained.

Laboratory Tests: Serum cholesterol levels should be determined frequently during the first few months of therapy and periodically thereafter. Serum triglyceride levels should be measured periodically to detect whether significant changes have occurred.

The LRC-CPPT showed a dose-related increase in serum triglycerides of 10.7% to 17.1% in the cholestyramine-treated group, compared with an increase of 7.9% to 11.7% in the placebo group. Based on the mean values and adjusting for the placebo group, the cholestyramine-treated group showed an increase of 5% over pre-entry levels the first year of the study and an increase of 4.3% the seventh year.

Drug Interactions: Cholestyramine resin may delay or reduce the absorption of concomitant oral medication such as phenylbutazone, warfarin, thiazide diuretics (acidic) or propranolol (basic), as well as tetracycline, penicillin G, phenobarbital, thyroid and thyroxine preparations, estrogens and progestins, and digitalis. Interference with the absorption of oral phosphate supplements has been observed with another positively-charged bile acid sequestrant. Cholestyramine resin may interfere with the pharmacokinetics of drugs that undergo enterohepatic circulation. The discontinuance of cholestyramine resin could pose a hazard to health if a potentially toxic drug such as digitalis has been titrated to a maintenance level while the patient was taking cholestyramine resin.

Because cholestyramine binds bile acids, cholestyramine resin may interfere with normal fat digestion and absorption and thus may prevent absorption of fat-soluble vitamins such as A, D, E and K. When cholestyramine resin is given for long periods of time, concomitant supplementation with water-miscible (or parenteral) forms of fat soluble vitamins should be considered.

SINCE CHOLESTYRAMINE RESIN MAY BIND OTHER DRUGS GIVEN CONCURRENTLY, IT IS RECOMMENDED THAT PATIENTS TAKE OTHER DRUGS AT LEAST 1 HOUR BEFORE OR 4 TO 6 HOURS AFTER CHOLESTYRAMINE RESIN (OR AT AS GREAT AN INTERVAL AS POSSIBLE) TO AVOID IMPEDING THEIR ABSORPTION.

Carcinogenesis, Mutagenesis, Impairment of Fertility:

In studies conducted in rats in which cholestyramine resin was used as a tool to investigate the role of various intestinal factors, such as fat, bile salts and microbial flora, in the development of intestinal tumors induced by potent carcinogens, the incidence of such tumors was observed to be greater in cholestyramine resin-treated rats than in control rats.

The relevance of this laboratory observation from studies in rats to the clinical use of cholestyramine resin is not known. In the LRC-CPPT study referred to above, the total incidence of fatal and nonfatal neoplasms was similar in both treatment groups. When the many different categories of tumors are examined, various alimentary system cancers were somewhat more prevalent in the cholestyramine group. The small numbers and the multiple categories prevent conclusions from being drawn. However, in view of the fact that cholestyramine resin is confined to the GI tract and not absorbed, and in light of the animal experiments referred to above, a six-year post-trial follow-up of the LRC-CPPT[5] patient population has been completed (a total of 13.4 years of in-trial plus post-trial follow-up) and revealed no significant difference in the incidence of cause-specific mortality or cancer morbidity between cholestyramine and placebo treated patients.

Pregnancy: Pregnancy Category C. There are no adequate and well controlled studies in pregnant women. The use of cholestyramine in pregnancy or lactation or by women of childbearing age requires that the potential benefits of drug therapy be weighted against the possible hazards to the mother and child. Cholestyramine is not absorbed systemically, however, it is known to interfere with absorption of fat-soluble vitamins; accordingly, regular prenatal supplementation may not be adequate (see PRECAUTIONS, Drug Interactions).

Nursing Mothers: Caution should be exercised when cholestyramine resin is administered to a nursing mother. The possible lack of proper vitamin absorption described in the "Pregnancy" section may have an effect on nursing infants.

Pediatric Use: Although an optimal dosage schedule has not been established, standard texts [6-7] list a usual pediatric dose of 240 mg/kg/day of anhydrous cholestyramine resin in two to three divided doses, normally not to exceed 8 g/day with dose titration based on response and tolerance. In calculating pediatric dosages, 70.2 mg of anhydrous cholestyramine resin are contained in 100 mg of LoCHOLEST™ Light.

The effects of long-term drug administration, as well as its effect in maintaining lowered cholesterol levels in pediatric patients, are unknown. Also see "ADVERSE REACTIONS".

ADVERSE REACTIONS

The most common adverse reaction is constipation. When used as a cholesterol-lowering agent predisposing factors for most complaints of constipation are high dose and increased age (more than 60 years old). Most instances of constipation are mild, transient, and controlled with conventional therapy. Some patients require a temporary decrease in dosage or discontinuation of therapy.

Less Frequent Adverse Reactions—Abdominal discomfort and/or pain, flatulence, nausea, vomiting, diarrhea, eructation, anorexia, steatorrhea, bleeding tendencies due to hypoprothrombinemia (Vitamin K deficiency) as well as Vitamin A (one case of night blindness reported) and D deficiencies, hyperchloremic acidosis in children, osteoporosis, rash and irritation of the skin, tongue and perianal area. Rare reports of intestinal obstruction, including two deaths, have been reported in pediatric patients.

Occasional calcified material has been observed in the biliary tree, including calcification of the gallbladder, in patients to whom cholestyramine resin has been given. However, this may be a manifestation of the liver disease and not drug related.

One patient experienced biliary colic on each of three occasions on which he took a cholestyramine for oral suspension product. One patient diagnosed as acute abdominal symptom complex was found to have a "pasty mass" in the transverse colon on x-ray.

Other events (not necessarily drug related) reported in patients taking cholestyramine resin include:

Gastrointestinal—GI-rectal bleeding, black stools, hemorrhoidal bleeding, bleeding from known duodenal ulcer, dysphagia, hiccups, ulcer attack, sour taste, pancreatitis, rectal pain, diverticulitis.

Laboratory test changes—Liver function abnormalities.

Hematologic—Prolonged prothrombin time, ecchymosis, anemia.

Hypersensitivity—Urticaria, asthma, wheezing, shortness of breath.

Musculoskeletal—Backache, muscle and joint pains, arthritis.

Neurologic—Headache, anxiety, vertigo, dizziness, fatigue, tinnitus, syncope, drowsiness, femoral nerve pain, paresthesia.

Eye—Uveitis.

Renal—Hematuria, dysuria, burnt odor to urine, diuresis.

Miscellaneous—Weight loss, weight gain, increased libido, swollen glands, edema, dental bleeding, dental caries, erosion of tooth enamel, tooth discoloration.

OVERDOSAGE

Overdosage of cholestyramine resin has been reported in a patient taking 150% of the maximum recommended daily dosage for a period of several weeks. No ill effects were reported. Should an overdosage occur, the chief potential harm would be obstruction of the gastrointestinal tract. The location of such potential obstruction, the degree of obstruction, and the presence or absence of normal gut motility would determine treatment.

DOSAGE AND ADMINISTRATION

The recommended starting adult dose for LoCHOLEST™ Light Powder is one pouch or one level scoopful (5.7 grams of LoCHOLEST™ Light Powder contains 4 grams of anhydrous cholestyramine resin) once or twice a day. The recommended maintenance dose for LoCHOLEST™ Light Powder is 2 to 4 pouches or scoopfuls daily (8 to 16 grams anhydrous cholestyramine resin) divided into two doses. It is recommended that increases in dose be gradual with periodic assessment of lipid/lipoprotein levels at intervals of not less than 4 weeks. The maximum recommended daily dose is 6 pouches or scoopfuls of LoCHOLEST™ Light Powder (24 grams of anhydrous cholestyramine resin). The suggested time of administration is at mealtime but may be modified to avoid interference with absorption of other medications. Although the recommended dosing schedule is twice daily, LoCHOLEST™ Light Powder may be administered in 1 to 6 doses per day.

LoCHOLEST™ Light Powder should not be taken in its dry form. Always mix the dry powder with water or other fluids before ingesting. See Preparation Instructions.

Concomitant Therapy

Preliminary evidence suggests that the lipid-lowering effects of cholestyramine on total and LDL-cholesterol are enhanced when combined with a HMG-CoA reductase inhibitor, e.g., pravastatin, lovastatin, simvastatin, and fluvastatin. Additive effects on LDL-cholesterol are also seen with combined nicotinic acid/cholestyramine therapy. See the Drug Interactions subsection of the PRECAUTIONS section for recommendations on administering concomitant therapy.

Preparation

The color of LoCHOLEST™ Light Powder may vary somewhat from batch to batch but this variation does not affect the performance of the product. Place the contents of one single-dose pouch or one level scoopful of LoCHOLEST™ Light Powder in a glass or cup. Add at least 2 to 3 ounces of water or the beverage of your choice. Stir to a uniform consistency.

LoCHOLEST™ Light Powder may also be mixed with highly fluid soups or pulpy fruits with a high moisture content such as applesauce or crushed pineapple.

HOW SUPPLIED

LoCHOLEST™ Light Powder strawberry flavor is available in cartons of sixty 5.7 gram pouches and in cans containing 239.4 grams. Each 5.7 gram dose of LoCHOLEST™ Light Powder contains 4 grams of anhydrous cholestyramine resin.

NDC 0047-2009-20 Carton of 60 pouches

NDC 0047-2009-22 Can, 239.4 g (containing a scoop that is not interchangeable with scoops from other products)

Storage: Store at controlled room temperature 15°–30°C (59°-86°F).

Rx only

REFERENCES

1. The Lipid Research Clinics Coronary Primary Prevention Trial Results: (I) Reduction in Incidence of Coronary Heart Disease; (II) The Relationship of Reduction in Incidence of Coronary Heart Disease to Cholesterol Lowering. *JAMA.* 1984; 251:351–374.
2. Brensike JF, Levy RI, Kelsey SF, et al. Effects of therapy with cholestyramine on progression of coronary arteriosclerosis: results of the NHLBI type II coronary intervention study. *Circulation* 1984; 69:313–24.
3. Watte, GF, Lewis B, Brunt JNH, Lewis ES, et al. Effects on coronary artery disease of lipid-lowering diet, or diet plus cholestyramine, in the St. Thomas Atherosclerosis Regression Study (STARS). *Lancet* 1992; 339:563–69.
4. National Cholesterol Education Program. Second Report of the Expert panel on Detection, Evaluation, and Treatment of High Blood Cholesterol in Adults (Adult Treatment Panel II). *Circulation* 1994 Mar, 89 (3):1333–445.
5. The Lipid Research Clinics Investigators. The Lipid Research Clinics Coronary Primary Prevention Trial Results of 6 Years of Post-Trial Follow-up. *Arch Intern Med* 1992; 152:1399–1410.
6. Behrman RE et al (eds): *Nelson, Textbook of Pediatrics,* ed 15. Philadelphia, PA, WB Saunders Company, 1996.
7. Takemoto CK et al (eds): *Pediatric Dosage Handbook,* ed 3. Cleveland/Akron, OH, Lexi-Comp, Inc., 1996/1997.

Manufactured for:
Warner Chilcott Laboratories
100 Enterprise Dr.
Rockaway, NJ 07866

Continued on next page

LoCholest Light—Cont.

Manufactured by:
Eon Labs Manufacturing, Inc.
Rev. 03/98
MF0937REV0398
Flat #11470
2009—G012
Shown in Product Identification Guide, page 342

NATAFORT®   Ŗ
PRENATAL MULTIVITAMIN TABLET WITH IRON

FOR USE BEFORE, DURING, AND AFTER PREGNANCY

Caution—Federal law prohibits dispensing without prescription.

Each white, film-coated tablet contains:
VITAMINS

Vitamin A (as vitamin A acetate and beta-carotene)	1000 IU
Vitamin D₃ (cholecalciferol)	400 IU
Vitamin E (dl-alpha tocopheryl acetate)	11 IU
Vitamin C (ascorbic acid)	120 mg
Folic Acid	1 mg
Thiamine Mononitrate (vitamin B₁)	2 mg
Riboflavin (vitamin B₂)	3 mg
Niacinamide	20 mg
Vitamin B₆ (pyridoxine HCl)	10 mg
Vitamin B₁₂ (cyanocobalamin)	12 mcg

MINERAL

Iron (as carbonyl iron)	60 mg

Each tablet also contains lactose monohydrate, magnesium stearate, microcrystalline cellulose, pregelatinized starch, sodium starch glycolate, stearic acid, and other ingredients.

INDICATIONS:

To provide vitamin and mineral supplementation throughout pregnancy and during the postnatal period, for both the lactating and non-lactating mother. It is also useful for improving nutritional status prior to conception.

DOSAGE:

One tablet daily, or as directed by a physician.

> **WARNING**
> Accidental overdose of iron-containing products is a leading cause of fatal poisoning in children under 6. Keep this product out of the reach of children. In case of accidental overdose, call a doctor or poison control center immediately.

CAUTION:

Folic acid may partially correct the hematological damage due to Vitamin B₁₂ deficiency of pernicious anemia, while the associated neurological damage progresses. In rare instances, allergic hypersensitivity has been reported following administration of folic acid.

DISPENSE: In a tight, light-resistant container as defined by the USP.

STORAGE: Store at controlled room temperature 15°–30°C (59°–86°F).

KEEP THIS AND ALL MEDICATIONS OUT OF THE REACH OF CHILDREN.

Manufactured by: Amide Pharmaceutical, Inc.
Little Falls, NJ 07424
Manufactured for: Warner Chilcott, Inc.
100 Enterprise Drive, Rockaway, NJ 07866 USA
7922-00
0226G010
Lot No.
Exp. Date
Shown in Product Identification Guide, page 342

VECTRIN®   Ŗ
(minocycline hydrochloride capsules, USP)

DESCRIPTION

Minocycline hydrochloride, a semisynthetic derivative of tetracycline is [4 S-(4α,4aα,5aα,12aα)]-4,7-Bis(dimethylamino)-1,4,4a,5,5a,6,11,12a-octahydro-3, 10, 12, 12a-tetrahydroxy-1,11-dioxo-2-naphthacene-carboxamide monohydrochloride. Its structural formula is:
[See chemical structure at top of next column]

$C_{23}H_{27}N_3O_7 \cdot HCl$ M.W. 493.94

Each Vectrin capsule, for oral administration, contains minocycline hydrochloride equivalent to 50 or 100 mg minocycline. In addition, each capsule contains the following inactive ingredients: magnesium stearate, NF and pregelatinized starch, NF (corn). The capsule shell contains gelatin, NF; silicon dioxide, NF; sodium lauryl sulfate, NF; and titanium dioxide. The 50-mg capsule shell also contains D&C yellow #10, and FD&C red #40. The 100-mg capsule shell also contains FD&C blue #1.

CLINICAL PHARMACOLOGY

Following oral administration of minocycline hydrochloride capsules, absorption from the gastrointestinal tract is rapid. Following a single dose of minocycline hydrochloride administered to normal fasting adult volunteers, maximum serum concentrations were attained in 1 to 4 hours. The serum half-life in normal volunteers ranged from approximately 11 hours to 22 hours.

When minocycline hydrochloride capsules were given concomitantly with a meal which included dairy products, the extent of absorption was not noticeably influenced. The peak plasma concentrations were slightly decreased and delayed by one hour when administered with food, compared to dosing under fasting conditions.

In previous studies with minocycline hydrochloride, the minocycline serum half-life ranged from 11 to 16 hours in 7 patients with hepatic dysfunction, and from 18 to 69 hours in 5 patients with renal dysfunction. The urinary and fecal recovery of minocycline when administered to 12 normal volunteers is one-half to one-third that of other tetracyclines.

Microbiology—The tetracyclines are primarily bacteriostatic and are thought to exert their antimicrobial effect by the inhibition of protein synthesis. The tetracyclines, including minocycline, have similar antimicrobial spectra of activity against a wide range of gram-positive and gram-negative organisms. Cross-resistance of these organisms to tetracyclines is common.

While *in vitro* studies have demonstrated the susceptibility of most strains of the following microorganisms, clinical efficacy for infections other than those included in the INDICATIONS AND USAGE section has not been documented.

GRAM-NEGATIVE BACTERIA:
Bartonella bacilliformis
Brucella species
Campylobacter fetus
Francisella tularensis
Haemophilus ducreyi
Haemophilus influenzae
Listeria monocytogenes
Neisseria gonorrhoeae
Vibrio cholerae
Yersinia pestis

Because many strains of the following groups of gram-negative microorganisms have been shown to be resistant to tetracyclines, culture and susceptibility tests are especially recommended:

Acinetobacter species
Bacteroides species
Enterobacter aerogenes
Escherichia coli
Klebsiella species
Shigella species

GRAM-POSITIVE BACTERIA:
Because many strains of the following groups of gram-positive microorganisms have been shown to be resistant to tetracyclines, culture and susceptibility testing are especially recommended. Up to 44 percent of *Streptococcus pyogenes* strains have been found to be resistant to tetracycline drugs. Therefore, tetracyclines should not be used for streptococcal disease unless the organism has been demonstrated to be susceptible.

Alpha hemolytic streptococci (viridans group)
Streptococcus pneumoniae
Streptococcus pyogenes

OTHER MICROORGANISMS:
Actinomyces species
Bacillus anthracis
Balantidium coli
Borrelia recurrentis
Chlamydia psittaci
Chlamydia trachomatis
Clostridium species
Entamoeba species
Fusobacterium fusiforme
Propionibacterium acnes
Treponema pallidum
Treponema pertenue
Ureaplasma urealyticum

Susceptibility Tests

Diffusion Techniques—The use of antibiotic disk susceptibility test methods which measure zone diameter gives an accurate estimation of susceptibility of microorganisms to minocycline HCl. One such standard procedure[1] has been recommended for use with disks for testing antimicrobials.

Either the 30 mcg tetracycline-class disk or the 30 mcg minocycline disk should be used for the determination of the susceptibility of microorganisms to minocycline.

With this type of procedure a report of "susceptible" from the laboratory indicates that the infecting organism is likely to respond to therapy. A report of "intermediate susceptibility" suggests that the organism would be susceptible if a high dosage is used or if the infection is confined to tissues and fluids (eg, urine) in which high antibiotic levels are attained. A report of "resistant" indicates that the infecting organism is not likely to respond to therapy. With either the tetracycline-class disk or the minocycline disk, zone sizes of 19 mm or greater indicate susceptibility, zone sizes of 14 mm or less indicate resistance, and zone sizes of 15 to 18 mm indicate intermediate susceptibility.

Standardized procedures require the use of laboratory control organisms. The 30 mcg tetracycline disk should give zone diameters between 19 and 28 mm for *Staphylococcus aureus* ATCC 25923 and between 18 and 25 mm for *Escherichia coli* ATCC 25922. The 30 mcg minocycline disk should give zone diameters between 25 and 30 mm for *S. aureus* ATCC 25923 and between 19 and 25 mm for *E. coli* ATCC 25922.

Dilution Techniques—When using the NCCLS agar dilution or broth dilution (including microdilution) method[2] or equivalent, a bacterial isolate may be considered susceptible if the MIC (minimal inhibitory concentration) of minocycline is 4 mcg/mL or less. Organisms are considered resistant if the MIC is 16 mcg/mL or greater. Organisms with an MIC value of less than 16 mcg/mL but greater than 4 mcg/mL are expected to be susceptible if a high dosage is used or if the infection is confined to tissues and fluids (eg, urine) in which high antibiotic levels are attained.

As with standard diffusion methods, dilution procedures require the use of laboratory control organisms. Standard tetracycline or minocycline powder should give MIC values of 0.25 mcg/mL to 1.0 mcg/mL for *S. aureus* ATCC 25923, and 1.0 mcg/mL to 4.0 mcg/mL for *E. coli* ATCC 25922.

INDICATIONS AND USAGE

Vectrin capsules are indicated in the treatment of the following infections due to susceptible strains of the designated microorganisms:

Rocky Mountain spotted fever, typhus fever and the typhus group, Q fever, rickettsialpox and tick fevers caused by Rickettsiae

Respiratory tract infections caused by *Mycoplasma pneumoniae.*

Lymphogranuloma venereum caused by *Chlamydia trachomatis.*

Psittacosis (ornithosis) due to *Chlamydia psittaci.*

Trachoma caused by *Chlamydia trachomatis*, although the infectious agent is not always eliminated, as judged by immunofluorescence

Inclusion conjunctivitis caused by *Chlamydia trachomatis.*

Nongonococcal urethritis in adults caused by *Ureaplasma urealyticum* or *Chlamydia trachomatis.*

Relapsing fever due to *Borrelia recurrentis.*

Chancroid caused by *Haemophilus ducreyi*

Plague due to *Yersinia pestis.*

Tularemia due to *Francisella tularensis.*

Cholera caused by *Vibrio cholerae.*

Campylobacter fetus infections caused by *Campylobacter fetus.*

Brucellosis due to *Brucella species* (in conjunction with streptomycin).

Bartonellosis due to *Bartonella bacilliformis.*

Granuloma inguinale caused by *Calymmatobacterium granulomatis*

Minocycline is indicated for treatment of infections caused by the following gram-negative microorganisms when bacteriologic testing indicates appropriate susceptibility to the drug:

Escherichia coli.
Enterobacter aerogenes.
Shigella species.
Acinetobacter species

Respiratory tract infections caused by *Haemophilus influenzae.*

Respiratory tract and urinary tract infections caused by *Klebsiella* species.

Vectrin capsules are indicated for the treatment of infections caused by the following gram-positive microorganisms when bacteriologic testing indicates appropriate susceptibility to the drug:

Upper respiratory tract infections caused by *Streptococcus pneumoniae.*

Skin and skin structure infections caused by *Staphylococcus aureus*. (Note: Minocycline is not the drug of choice in the treatment of any type of staphylococcal infection.)

Uncomplicated urethritis in men due to *Neisseria gonorrhoeae* and for the treatment of other gonococcal infections when penicillin is contraindicated.

When penicillin is contraindicated, minocycline is an alternative drug in the treatment of the following infections:

PRODUCT INFORMATION WARNER CHILCOTT/3213

Infections in women caused by *Neisseria gonorrhoeae.*
Syphilis caused by *Treponema pallidum.*
Yaws caused by *Treponema pertenue.*
Listeriosis due to *Listeria monocytogenes.*
Anthrax due to *Bacillus anthracis.*
Vincent's infection caused by *Fusobacterium fusiforme.*
Actinomycosis caused by *Actinomyces israelii.*
Infections caused by *Clostridium* species.

In *acute intestinal amebiasis,* minocycline may be a useful adjunct to amebicides.

In severe *acne*, Vectrin may be useful adjunctive therapy.

Oral minocycline is indicated in the treatment of asymptomatic carriers of *Neisseria meningitidis* to eliminate meningococci from the nasopharynx. In order to preserve the usefulness of minocycline in the treatment of asymptomatic meningococcal carrier, diagnostic laboratory procedures, including serotyping and susceptibility testing, should be performed to establish the carrier state and the correct treatment. It is recommended that the prophylactic use of minocycline be reserved for situations in which the risk of meningococcal meningitis is high.

Oral minocycline is not indicated for the treatment of meningococcal infection.

Although no controlled clinical efficacy studies have been conducted, limited clinical data show that oral minocycline hydrochloride has been used successfully in the treatment of infections caused by *Mycobacterium marinum.*

CONTRAINDICATIONS

This drug is contraindicated in persons who have shown hypersensitivity to any of the tetracyclines.

WARNINGS

VECTRIN CAPSULES, LIKE OTHER TETRACYCLINE-CLASS ANTIBIOTICS, CAN CAUSE FETAL HARM WHEN ADMINISTERED TO A PREGNANT WOMAN. IF ANY TETRACYCLINE IS USED DURING PREGNANCY, OR IF THE PATIENT BECOMES PREGNANT WHILE TAKING THESE DRUGS, THE PATIENT SHOULD BE APPRISED OF THE POTENTIAL HAZARD TO THE FETUS. THE USE OF DRUGS OF THE TETRACYCLINE CLASS DURING TOOTH DEVELOPMENT (LAST HALF OF PREGNANCY, INFANCY, AND CHILDHOOD TO THE AGE OF 8 YEARS) MAY CAUSE PERMANENT DISCOLORATION OF THE TEETH (YELLOW-GRAY-BROWN).

This adverse reaction is more common during long-term use of the drug but has been observed following repeated short-term courses. Enamel hypoplasia has also been reported. TETRACYCLINE DRUGS, THEREFORE, SHOULD NOT BE USED DURING TOOTH DEVELOPMENT UNLESS OTHER DRUGS ARE NOT LIKELY TO BE EFFECTIVE OR ARE CONTRAINDICATED.

All tetracyclines form a stable calcium complex in any bone-forming tissue. A decrease in fibula growth rate has been observed in young animals (rats and rabbits) given oral tetracycline in doses of 25 mg/kg every six hours. This reaction was shown to be reversible when the drug was discontinued.

Results of animal studies indicate that tetracyclines cross the placenta, are found in fetal tissues, and can have toxic effects on the developing fetus (often related to retardation of skeletal development). Evidence of embryotoxicity has been noted in animals treated early in pregnancy.

The antianabolic action of the tetracyclines may cause an increase in BUN. While this is not a problem in those with normal renal function, in patients with significantly impaired function, higher serum levels of tetracycline may lead to azotemia, hyperphosphatemia, and acidosis. If renal impairment exists, even usual oral or parenteral doses may lead to excessive systemic accumulations of the drug and possible liver toxicity. Under such conditions, lower than usual total doses are indicated, and if therapy is prolonged, serum level determinations of the drug may be advisable.

Photosensitivity manifested by an exaggerated sunburn reaction has been observed in some individuals taking tetracyclines. This has been reported rarely with minocycline.

Central nervous system side effects including lightheadedness, dizziness, or vertigo have been reported with minocycline therapy. Patients who experience these symptoms should be cautioned about driving vehicles or using hazardous machinery while on minocycline therapy. These symptoms may disappear during therapy and usually disappear rapidly when the drug is discontinued.

PRECAUTIONS

General

As with other antibiotic preparations, use of this drug may result in overgrowth of nonsusceptible organisms, including fungi. If superinfection occurs, the antibiotic should be discontinued and appropriate therapy instituted.

Pseudotumor cerebri (benign intracranial hypertension) in adults has been associated with the use of tetracyclines. The usual clinical manifestations are headache and blurred vision. Bulging fontanels have been associated with the use of tetracyclines in infants. While both of these conditions and related symptoms usually resolve after discontinuation of the tetracycline, the possibility for permanent sequelae exists.

Incision and drainage or other surgical procedures should be performed in conjunction with antibiotic therapy when indicated.

Information for Patients

Photosensitivity manifested by an exaggerated sunburn reaction has been observed in some individuals taking tetracyclines. Patients apt to be exposed to direct sunlight or ultraviolet light should be advised that this reaction can occur with tetracycline drugs, and treatment should be discontinued at the first evidence of skin erythema. This reaction has been reported rarely with use of minocycline.

Patients who experience central nervous system symptoms (see WARNINGS) should be cautioned about driving vehicles or using hazardous machinery while on minocycline therapy.

Concurrent use of tetracycline may render oral contraceptives less effective (see Drug Interactions).

Laboratory Tests

In venereal disease when coexistent syphilis is suspected, a dark-field examination should be done before treatment is started and the blood serology repeated monthly for at least four months.

In long-term therapy, periodic laboratory evaluations of organ systems, including hematopoietic, renal, and hepatic studies should be performed.

Drug Interactions

Because tetracyclines have been shown to depress plasma prothrombin activity, patients who are on anticoagulant therapy may require downward adjustment of their anticoagulant dosage.

Since bacteriostatic drugs may interfere with the bactericidal action of penicillin, it is advisable to avoid giving tetracycline-class drugs in conjunction with penicillin.

Absorption of tetracyclines is impaired by antacids containing aluminum, calcium or magnesium and iron-containing preparations.

The concurrent use of tetracycline and methoxyflurane has been reported to result in fatal renal toxicity.

Concurrent use of tetracyclines may render oral contraceptives less effective.

Drug/Laboratory Test Interactions

False elevations of urinary catecholamine levels may occur due to interference with the fluorescence test.

Carcinogenesis, Mutagenesis, Impairment of Fertility

Dietary administration of minocycline in long-term tumorigenicity studies in rats resulted in evidence of thyroid tumor production. Minocycline has also been found to produce thyroid hyperplasia in rats and dogs. In addition, there has been evidence of oncogenic activity in rats in studies with related antibiotic, oxytetracycline (ie., adrenal and pituitary tumors). Likewise, although mutagenicity studies of minocycline have not been conducted, positive results in *in vitro* mammalian cell assays (ie, mouse lymphoma and Chinese hamster lung cells) have been reported for related antibiotics (tetracycline hydrochloride and oxytetracycline). Segment I (fertility and general reproduction) studies have provided evidence that minocycline impairs fertility in male rats.

Teratogenic Effects *Pregnancy*: Pregnancy Category D (see WARNINGS).

Labor and Delivery

The effect of tetracyclines on labor and delivery is unknown.

Nursing Mothers

Tetracyclines are excreted in human milk.

Because of the potential for serious adverse reactions in nursing infants from the tetracyclines, a decision should be made whether to discontinue nursing or discontinue the drug, taking into account the importance of the drug to the mother (see WARNINGS).

Pediatric Use: see WARNINGS.

ADVERSE REACTIONS

Due to oral minocycline's virtually complete absorption, side effects to the lower bowel, particularly diarrhea, have been infrequent. The following adverse reactions have been observed in patients receiving tetracyclines.

Gastrointestinal: Anorexia, nausea, vomiting, diarrhea, glossitis, dysphagia, enterocolitis, pancreatitis, inflammatory lesions (with monilial overgrowth) in the anogenital region, and increases in liver enzymes. Rarely, hepatitis and liver failure have been reported. Rare instances of esophagitis and esophageal ulcerations have been reported in patients taking the tetracycline-class antibiotics in capsule and tablet form. Most of these patients took the medication immediately before going to bed (see DOSAGE AND ADMINISTRATION).

Skin: Maculopapular and erythematous rashes. Exfoliative dermatitis has been reported but is uncommon. Fixed drug eruptions, including balanitis, have been rarely reported. Erythema multiforme and rarely Stevens-Johnson syndrome have been reported. Photosensitivity is discussed above (see WARNINGS). Pigmentation of the skin and mucous membranes has been reported.

Renal toxicity: Elevations in BUN have been reported and are apparently dose related (see WARNINGS).

Hypersensitivity reactions: Urticaria, angioneurotic edema, polyarthralgia, anaphylaxis, anaphylactoid purpura, pericarditis, exacerbation of systemic lupus erythematosus and rarely pulmonary infiltrates with eosinophilia have been reported. A transient lupus-like syndrome has also been reported.

Blood: Hemolytic anemia, thrombocytopenia, neutropenia, and eosinophilia have been reported.

Central nervous system: Bulging fontanels in infants and benign intracranial hypertension (pseudotumor cerebri) in adults (see PRECAUTIONS—General) have been reported.

Other: When given over prolonged periods, tetracyclines have been reported to produce brown-black microscopic discoloration of the thyroid glands. Very rare cases of abnormal thyroid function have been reported.

Tooth discoloration in pediatric patients less than 8 years of age (see WARNINGS) and also rarely, in adults have been reported. Decreased hearing has been rarely reported in patients on minocycline hydrochloride.

OVERDOSAGE

In case of overdosage, discontinue medication, treat symptomatically and institute supportive measures.

DOSAGE AND ADMINISTRATION

THE USUAL DOSAGE AND FREQUENCY OF ADMINISTRATION OF MINOCYCLINE DIFFERS FROM THAT OF THE OTHER TETRACYCLINES. EXCEEDING THE RECOMMENDED DOSAGE MAY RESULT IN AN INCREASED INCIDENCE OF SIDE EFFECTS.

Minocycline hydrochloride capsules may be taken with or without food.

ADULTS: The usual dosage of Vectrin (minocycline hydrochloride capsules) is 200 mg initially followed by 100 mg every 12 hours. Alternatively, if more frequent doses are preferred, two or four 50 mg capsules may be given initially followed by one 50 mg capsule four times daily.

FOR PEDIATRIC POPULATION ABOVE 8 YEARS OF AGE: The usual dosage of Vectrin (minocycline hydrochloride capsules) is 4 mg/kg initially followed by 2 mg/kg every 12 hours.

Uncomplicated gonococcal infections other than urethritis and anorectal infections in men: 200 mg initially, followed by 100 mg every 12 hours for a minimum of four days, with post-therapy cultures within 2 to 3 days.

In the treatment of uncomplicated gonococcal urethritis in men, 100 mg every 12 hours for five days is recommended.

For the treatment of syphilis, the usual dosage of Vectrin (minocycline hydrochloride capsules) should be administered over a period of 10 to 15 days. Close follow-up, including laboratory tests, is recommended.

In the treatment of meningococcal carrier state, the recommended dosage is 100 mg every 12 hours for five days.

Mycobacterium marinum infections: Although optimal doses have not been established, 100 mg every 12 hours for 6 to 8 weeks have been used successfully in a limited number of cases.

Uncomplicated nongonococcal urethral infection in adults caused by *Chlamydia trachomatis* or *Ureaplasma urealyticum*: 100 mg orally, every 12 hours for at least seven days.

Ingestion of adequate amounts of fluids along with capsule and tablet forms of drugs in the tetracycline-class is recommended to reduce the risk of esophageal irritation and ulceration.

In patients with renal impairment (see WARNINGS) the total dosage should be decreased by either reducing the recommended individual doses and/or by extending the time intervals between doses.

HOW SUPPLIED

Vectrin (minocycline hydrochloride capsules USP), equivalent to 50 mg or 100 mg minocycline, are supplied as:

50 mg orange opaque, size #3, capsules imprinted Vectrin 50 mg:

Bottles of 100	N 0047-0687-24
Bottles of 1000	N 0047-0687-32

100 mg blue opaque, size #2, capsules imprinted Vectrin 100 mg:

Bottles of 50	N 0047-0688-19
Bottles of 1000	N 0047-0688-32

Storage Conditions: Store at controlled room temperature 15°–30° C (59°–86° F). Protect from light.

Caution—Federal law prohibits dispensing without prescription.

ANIMAL PHARMACOLOGY AND TOXICOLOGY

Minocycline HCl has been observed to cause a dark discoloration of the thyroid in experimental animals (rats, minipigs, dogs, and monkeys). In the rat, chronic treatment with minocycline hydrochloride has resulted in goiter accompanied by elevated radioactive iodine uptake and evidence of thyroid tumor production. Minocycline hydrochloride has also been found to produce thyroid hyperplasia in rats and dogs.

Continued on next page

Vectrin—Cont.

REFERENCES

1. National Committee for Clinical Laboratory Standards, Approved Standard: *Performance Standards for Antimicrobial Disk Susceptibility Tests*, 3rd Edition, Vol. 4(16): M2-A3, Villanova, PA. December 1984.
2. National Committee for Clinical Laboratory Standards, Approved Standard: *Methods for Dilution Antimicrobial Susceptibility Tests for Bacteria that Grow Aerobically*, 2nd Edition, Vol. 5(22): M7-A, Villanova, PA. December 1985.
0687G021
Issued November 1996
Manufactured for:
WARNER CHILCOTT, INC.
100 Enterprise Drive
Rockaway, NJ 07866 USA
By: Warner-Lambert Company
Morris Plains, NJ 07950 USA
Shown in Product Identification Guide, page 342

Warner Chilcott Laboratories
ROCKAWAY 80 CORPORATE CENTER
100 ENTERPRISE DRIVE
SUITE 280
ROCKAWAY, NJ 07866

Direct Inquiries to:
800-521-8813
Product/Medical Information
800-521-8813
973-442–3236
After Hours and Weekend Medical Emergencies:
303-739-1110

PRODUCT

Albuterol Inhalation Aerosol, 90 mcg	Rx
Amoxicillin Tablets, USP (Chewable) 250 mg	Rx
Amoxicillin Capsules, USP 250 mg	Rx
Amoxicillin Capsules, USP 500 mg	Rx
Amoxicillin for Oral Suspension, USP 125 mg/5 mL	Rx
Amoxicillin for Oral Suspension, USP 250 mg/5 mL	Rx
Ampicillin Capsules, USP 250 mg	Rx
Ampicillin Capsules, USP 500 mg	Rx
Ampicillin for Oral Suspension, USP 125 mg/5 mL	Rx
Ampicillin for Oral Suspension, USP 250 mg/5 mL	Rx
Benzonatate Capsules USP 100 mg	
Desipramine HCl Tablets, USP 25 mg	Rx
Desipramine HCl Tablets, USP 50 mg	Rx
Desipramine HCl Tablets, USP 75 mg	Rx
Doxycycline Hyclate Capsules, USP 50 mg	Rx
Doxycycline Hyclate Capsules, USP 100 mg	Rx
Gemfibrozil Tablets USP 600 mg	Rx
Glipizide Tablets USP 5 mg	Rx
Glipizide Tablets USP 10 mg	Rx
Guanabenz Acetate USP Tablets USP 4 mg	Rx
Guanabenz Acetate USP Tablets USP 8 mg	Rx
Guanfacine HCl Tablets 1 mg	Rx
Guanfacine HCl Tablets 2 mg	Rx
Hydrocodone and acetaminophen Tablets 5/500 mg	©/Rx
Hydrocodone Bitartrate and Acetaminophen Tablets 2.5 mg/500 mg	©/Rx
Hydrocodone Bitartrate and Acetaminophen Tablets, USP 7.5 mg/650 mg	©/Rx
Hydrocodone Bitartrate and Acetaminophen Tablets, USP 10 mg/650 mg	©/Rx
Hydrocodone Bitartrate and acetaminophen Tablets 7.5/500 mg	©/Rx
Hydrocodone Bitartrate and acetaminophen Tablets 7.5/750 mg	©/Rx
Ibuprofen Tablets, USP 400 mg	Rx
Ibuprofen Tablets, USP 600 mg	Rx
Ibuprofen Tablets, USP 800 mg	Rx
Indomethacin Extended-Release Capsules, 75 mg	Rx
Loxapine Succinate Capsules 5 mg Base	Rx
Loxapine Succinate Capsules 10 mg Base	Rx
Loxapine Succinate Capsules 25 mg Base	Rx
Loxapine Succinate Capsules 50 mg Base	Rx

Nelova™ 1/35E (norethindrone 1 mg and ethinyl estradiol 35 mcg)	Rx
Nelova™ 0.5/35E (norethindrone 0.5 mg and ethinyl estradiol 35 mcg)	Rx
Nelova™ 10/11 (norethindrone 0.5 mg and ethinyl estradiol 35 mcg)	Rx
Nelova™ 1/50M (norethindrone 1 mg and mestranol 50 mcg)	Rx
Penicillin V Potassium Tablets, USP 250 mg	Rx
Penicillin V Potassium Tablets, USP 500 mg	Rx
Penicillin VPotassium for Oral Solution, USP 125 mg/5 mL	Rx
Penicillin VPotassium for Oral Solution, USP 250 mg/5 mL	Rx
Potassium Chloride Extended-Release Tablets, USP 8 mEq (600 mg)	Rx
Potassium Chloride Extended Release Tablets, USP 10 mEq (750 mg)	Rx
Propranolol HCl Tablets, USP 10 mg	Rx
Propranolol HCl Tablets, USP 20 mg	Rx
Propranolol HCl Tablets, USP 40 mg	Rx
Propranolol HCl Tablets, USP 60 mg	Rx
Propranolol HCl Tablets, USP 80 mg	Rx
Theophylline Extended-Release Tablets 100 mg	Rx
Theophylline Extended-Release Tablets 200 mg	Rx
Theophylline Extended-Release Tablets 300 mg	Rx
Theophylline Extended–Release Tablets 450 mg	
Transdermal-NTG (Nitroglycerin Transdermal System) 0.2 mg/hour	Rx
Transdermal-NTG (Nitroglycerin Transdermal System) 0.4 mg/hour	Rx
Transdermal-NTG (Nitroglycerin Transdermal System) 0.6 mg/hour	Rx
Trazodone HCl Tablets USP 50 mg	Rx
Trazodone HCl Tablets USP 100 mg	Rx
Trazodone HCl Tablets USP 150 mg	Rx
Verapamil HCl Tablets 80 mg	Rx
Verapamil HCl Tablets 120 mg	Rx
Verapamil Sustained Release Tablets 180 mg	Rx
Verapamil Sustained Release Tablets 240 mg	Rx

Warner-Lambert
Consumer Healthcare
201 TABOR ROAD
MORRIS PLAINS, NJ 07950

Direct Inquiries and For Medical Information Contact:
Consumer Affairs
1-(800) 223-0182
(See PDR For Nonprescription Drugs)

ACTIFED® COLD & ALLERGY Tablets   OTC
[ăk '-tĭ-fĕd]

Pseudoephedrine HCl (60 mg)
Triprolidine HCl (2.5 mg)
Nasal Decongestant/Antihistamine

ACTIFED® COLD & SINUS   OTC
Caplets and Tablets
[ăk 'tĭ-fĕd]

Acetaminophen (500 mg)
Pseudoephedrine HCl (30 mg)
Triprolidine HCl (1.25 mg)
Pain Reliever-Fever Reducer/
Nasal Decongestant/Antihistamine

ANUSOL® HC-1 Ointment   OTC
[an '-ū-sōl]

Hydrocortisone Acetate (equivalent to 1% Hydrocortisone)
Hydrocortisone Anti-Itch Ointment

ANUSOL® Hemorrhoidal Ointment   OTC
[an '-ū-sōl]

Pramoxine HCl (1%)
Zinc Oxide (12.5%)
Mineral Oil
Protectant/External Analgesic

ANUSOL® Hemorrhoidal Suppositories   OTC
[an' -ū -sōl]

Topical Starch (51%)
Protectant

BENADRYL® ALLERGY CHEWABLES   OTC
[bě '-nă-drĭl]

Diphenhydramine HCl (12.5 mg)
Antihistamine

BENADRYL® ALLERGY/COLD Tablets   OTC
[bě '-nă-drĭl]

Acetaminophen (500 mg)
Diphenhydramine HCl (12.5 mg)
Pseudoephedrine HCl (30 mg)
Pain Reliever-Fever Reducer/
Antihistamine/Nasal Decongestant

BENADRYL®ALLERGY/CONGESTION   OTC
Tablets
[bě '-nă-drĭl]

Diphenhydramine HCl (25 mg)
Pseudoephedrine HCl (60 mg)
Antihistamine/Nasal Decongestant

BENADRYL® ALLERGY/CONGESTION   OTC
Liquid
[bě '-nă-drĭl]

Diphenhydramine HCl (12.5 mg)
Pseudoephedrine HCl (30 mg)
Antihistamine/Nasal Decongestant

BENADRYL® ALLERGY Kapseal Capsules   OTC
[bě '-nă-drĭl]

Diphenhydramine HCl (25 mg)
Antihistamine

BENADRYL® ALLERGY Liquid   OTC
[bě '-nă-drĭl]

Diphenhydramine HCl (12.5 mg)
Antihistamine

BENADRYL® ALLERGY Ultratab Tablets   OTC
[bě '-nă-drĭl]

Diphenhydramine HCl (25 mg)
Antihistamine

BENADRYL® ALLERGY/SINUS Headache   OTC
Caplets & Gelcaps
[bě '-nă-drĭl]

Acetaminophen (500 mg)
Diphenhydramine HCl (12.5 mg)
Pseudoephedrine HCl (30 mg)
Pain Reliever/Antihistamine/Nasal Decongestant

BENADRYL® DYE-FREE ALLERGY Liqui-gels®   OTC
[bě '-nă-drĭl]

Diphenhydramine HCl (25 mg)
Antihistamine

BENADRYL® DYE-FREE ALLERGY Liquid   OTC
[bě '-nă-drĭl]

Diphenhydramine HCl (12.5 mg)
Antihistamine

BENADRYL® Itch Relief Stick OTC
Extra Strength
[bĕ '-nă-drĭl]

Diphenhydramine HCl (2%)
Zinc Acetate (0.1%)
Topical Analgesic/Skin Protectant

BENADRYL® Itch Stopping Cream OTC
[bĕ '-nă-drĭl]
Original Strength
Diphenhydramine HCl (1%)
Zinc Acetate (0.1%)
Topical Analgesic/Skin Protectant
Extra Strength
Diphenhydramine HCl (2%)
Zinc Acetate (0.1%)
Topical Analgesic/Skin Protectant

BENADRYL® Itch Stopping Gel OTC
[bĕ '-nă-drĭl]
Original Strength
Diphenhydramine HCl (1%)
Topical Analgesic
Extra Strength
Diphenhydramine HCl (2%)
Topical Analgesic

BENADRYL® Itch Stopping Spray OTC
[bĕ '-nă-drĭl]
Original Strength
Diphenhydramine HCl (1%)
Zinc Acetate (0.1%)
Topical Analgesic/Skin Protectant
Extra Strength
Diphenyhydramine HCl (2%)
Zinc Acetate (0.1%)
Topical Analgesic/Skin Protectant

BENYLIN® ADULT Formula OTC
[bĕ '-nă-lĭn]

Dextromethorphan HBr (15 mg)
Cough Suppressant

BENYLIN® EXPECTORANT OTC
[bĕ '-nă-lĭn]

Dextromethorphan HBr (5 mg)
Guaifenesin (100 mg)
Cough Suppressant/Expectorant

BENYLIN® MULTI-SYMPTOM OTC
[bĕ '-nă-lĭn]

Dextromethorphan HBr (5 mg)
Guaifenesin (100 mg)
Pseudoephedrine HCl (15 mg)
Cough Suppressant/Expectorant/Nasal Decongestant

BENYLIN® PEDIATRIC OTC
[bĕ '-nă-lĭn]

Dextromethorphan HBr (7.5 mg)
Cough Suppressant

CALADRYL® CLEAR Lotion OTC
[kăl '-ă-drĭl]

Pramoxine HCl (1%)
Zinc Acetate (0.1%)
Skin Protectant/External Analgesic

CALADRYL® Cream for Kids OTC
[kăl '-ă-drĭl]

Calamine (8%)
Pramoxine HCl (1%)
External Analgesic/Skin Protectant

CALADRYL® Lotion OTC
[kăl '-ă-drĭl]

Calamine (8%)
Pramoxine HCl (1%)
External Analgesic/Skin Protectant

COOL MINT LISTERINE® OTC
[lĭs 'tər ēn]

Eucalyptol (0.092%)
Menthol (0.042%)
Methyl Salicylate (0.060%)
Thymol (0.064%)
Antiseptic

FRESHBURSH LISTERINE® OTC
[lĭs 'tər ēn]

Eucalyptol (0.092%)
Menthol (0.042%)
Methyl Salicylate (0.060%)
Thymol (0.064%)
Antiseptic

LISTERINE® Antiseptic OTC
[lĭs 'tər ēn]

Eucalyptol (0.092%)
Menthol (0.042%)
Methyl Salicylate (0.060%)
Thymol (0.064%)
Antiseptic

LISTERMINT® OTC
Alcohol-Free Mouthwash
[lĭs 'tər mĭnt]

LUBRIDERM® Daily UV Lotion OTC
with Sunscreen
[lū brĭ dĕrm]

Octyl Methoxycinnamate (7.5%)
Octyl Salicylate (4%)
Oxybenzone (3%)
Moisturizer/Sun Protection

NEOSPORIN® ORIGINAL Ointment OTC
[nē "ō-spōr 'in]

Bacitracin Zinc (400 units)
Neomycin (3.5 mg)
Polymyxin B Sulfate (5000 units)
First Aid Antibiotic

NEOSPORIN® + PAIN RELIEF OTC
Maximum Strength Cream
[nē "ō-spor 'in]

Neomycin (3.5 mg)
Polymyxin B Sulfate (10,000 units)
Pramoxine HCl (10 mg)
First Aid Antibiotic/Pain Relieving Cream

NEOSPORIN® + PAIN RELIEF OTC
Maximum Strength Ointment
[nē "ō-spor 'in]

Bacitracin Zinc (500 units)
Neomycin (3.5 mg)
Polymyxin B Sulfate (10,000 units)
Pramoxine HCl (10 mg)
First Aid Antibiotic/Pain Relieving Ointment

NIX® Creme Rinse OTC
[nĭks]

Permethrin (280 mg)
Lice Treatment

POLYSPORIN® Ointment OTC
[pah "lē-spor 'in]

Bacitracin Zinc (500 Units in a special
White Petrolatum Base)
Polymyxin B Sulfate (10,000 Units)
First Aid Antibiotic

POLYSPORIN® Powder OTC
[pah "lē-spor 'in]

Bacitracin Zinc (500 units in a Lactose Base)
Polymyxin B Sulfate (10,000 units)
First Aid Antibiotic

SINUTAB® Non-Drying Liquid Caps OTC
[sîn 'ū tăb]

Guaifenesin (200 mg)
Pseudoephedrine HCl (30 mg)
Expectorant/Nasal Decongestant

SINUTAB® SINUS ALLERGY OTC
Maximum Strength
Caplets & Tablets
[sîn 'ū tăb]

Acetaminophen (500 mg)
Chlorpheniramine Maleate (2 mg)
Pseudoephedrine HCl (30 mg)
Pain Reliever/Antihistamine/Nasal Decongestant

SINUTAB® SINUS Maximum Strength OTC
Without Drowsiness Caplets & Tablets
[sîn 'ū tăb]

Acetaminophen (500 mg)
Pseudoephedrine HCl (30 mg)
Pain Reliever/Nasal Decongestant

SUDAFED® 12 Hour Tablets OTC
[sū 'dah-fĕd "]

Pseudoephedrine HCl (120 mg)
Long Acting Nasal Decongestant

SUDAFED® 24 Hour Tablets OTC
[sū 'dah-fĕd]

Pseudoephedrine HCl (240 mg)
Long-Acting Nasal Decongestant

SUDAFED® COLD & ALLERGY Tablets OTC
[sū 'dah-fĕd "]

Chlorpheniramine Maleate (4 mg)
Pseudoephedrine HCl (60 mg)
Antihistamine/Nasal Decongestant

SUDAFED® COLD & COUGH Liquid Caps OTC
[sū 'dah-fĕd "]

Acetaminophen (250 mg)
Dextromethorphan HBr (10 mg)
Guaifenesin (100 mg)
Pseudoephedrine HCl (30 mg)
Pain Reliever-Fever Reducer/Cough
Suppressant/Expectorant/Nasal Decongestant

SUDAFED® Cold & Sinus Liquid Caps OTC
[sū 'dah-fĕd "]

Acetaminophen (325 mg)
Pseudoephedrine HCl (30 mg)
Pain Reliever-Fever Reducer/
Nasal Decongestant

SUDAFED® Severe Cold Formula OTC
Maximum Strength
Caplets & Tablets
[sū 'dah-fĕd "]

Acetaminophen (500 mg)
Dextromethorphan Hydrobromide (15 mg)
Pseudoephedrine HCl (30 mg)
Pain Reliever-Fever Reducer/
Cough Suppressant/Nasal Decongestant

Continued on next page

Consult 1999 PDR® supplements and future editions for revisions

SUDAFED® NASAL DECONGESTANT 30 mg
Tablets OTC
[sū 'dah-fĕd "]

Pseudoephedrine HCl (30 mg)
Nasal Decongestant

SUDAFED® NON-DRYING SINUS
Liquid Caps OTC
[sū 'dah-fĕd "]

Guaifenesin (200 mg)
Pseudoephedrine HCl (30 mg)
Expectorant/Nasal Decongestant

SUDAFED® SINUS
OTC
Maximum Strength
Caplets and Tablets
[sū 'dah-fĕd "]

Acetaminophen (500 mg)
Pseudoephedrine HCl (30 mg)
Pain Reliever/Nasal Decongestant

CHILDREN'S SUDAFED® COLD & COUGH OTC
Liquid
[sū 'dah-fĕd "]

Dextromethorphan HBr (5 mg)
Pseudoephedrine HCl (15 mg)
Cough Suppressant/Nasal Decongestant

CHILDREN'S SUDAFED® NASAL
DECONGESTANT Chewables OTC
[sū 'dah-fĕd "]

Pseudoephedrine HCl (15 mg)
Nasal Decongestant

CHILDREN'S SUDAFED® NASAL
DECONGESTANT Liquid OTC
[sū 'dah-fĕd]

Pseudoephedrine HCl (15 mg)
Nasal Decongestant

TUCKS® Medicated Pads OTC
[tŭks]

Witch Hazel (50%)
Astringent

TUCKS® Take Alongs Towelettes OTC
[tŭks]

Witch Hazel (50%)
Astringent

ZANTAC® 75 OTC
[zan ' tak]

Ranitidine Hydrochloride (84 mg)
(equivalent to 75 mg ranitidine)
Acid Reducer

NOTICE
Before prescribing or administering
any product described in
PHYSICIANS' DESK REFERENCE
check the **PDR Supplements**
for revised information.

Watson Laboratories, Inc.
311 BONNIE CIRCLE
CORONA, CA 91720

Address Inquiries to:
Customer Service Department
Telephone: 800/272-5525
FAX: 909/735-2871

The following list of Watson Laboratories products is provided to facilitate identification. It includes the color(s) and identification codes for all tablets and capsules.

PRODUCT	IDENTIFICATION CODE
GENERIC NAME	(Front/Back*)
Description	
Color(s), Shape	
ACEBUTOLOL	
HYDROCHLORIDE	WATSON 437/200 mg
Capsules, 200 mg ℞	
Red/Gray	
ACEBUTOLOL	
HYDROCHLORIDE	WATSON 438/400 mg
Capsules, 400 mg ℞	
Maroon/Green	
ALBUTEROL SULFATE	
Syrup, 2 mg/5 ml ℞	
Clear, orange-yellow	
ALPRAZOLAM	WATSON 682/0.25
Tablets, USP, 0.25 mg Ⓝ ℞	BiConvex, Scored
White, Oval	
ALPRAZOLAM	WATSON 683/0.5
Tablets, USP, 0.5 mg Ⓝ ℞	BiConvex, Scored
Peach, Oval	
ALPRAZOLAM	WATSON 684/1.0
Tablets, USP, 1 mg Ⓝ ℞	BiConvex, Scored
Blue, Oval,	
AMILORIDE HCl & HCTZ	WATSON 685/5-50
Tablets, USP, 5mg/50 mg ℞	Scored
Peach, Round	
AMOXAPINE	WATSON 379/Bisected
Tablets, USP, 25 mg ℞	
White, Round	
AMOXAPINE	WATSON 380/Bisected
Tablets, USP, 50 mg ℞	
Salmon, Round	
AMOXAPINE	WATSON 381/Bisected
Tablets, USP, 100 mg ℞	
Blue, Round	
AMOXAPINE	WATSON 382/Bisected
Tablets, USP, 150 mg ℞	
Peach, Round	
BACLOFEN	WATSON 686/10
Tablets, USP, 10 mg ℞	Scored
White, Oval	
BACLOFEN	WATSON 687/20
Tablets, USP, 20 mg ℞	Scored
White, Round	
BUTALBITAL, ASPIRIN, CAFFEINE,	
and CODEINE PHOSPHATE	WATSON/425
Capsules, USP 50 mg/325 mg/40 mg/30 mg Ⓒ ℞	
Blue/Yellow	
CAPTOPRIL	WATSON 688/12.5
Tablets, USP, 12.5 mg ℞	Scored
White, Capsule-shaped	
CAPTOPRIL	WATSON 689/25
Tablets, USP, 25 mg ℞	Quadrisect Scored
White, Round	
CAPTOPRIL	WATSON 690/50
Tablets, USP, 50 mg ℞	Scored
White, Football shaped	
CAPTOPRIL	WATSON 691/100
Tablets, USP, 100 mg ℞	Scored
White, Football shaped	
CARISOPRODOL	WATSON/784
Tablets, ℞	
white round	
CHLORDIAZEPOXIDE HCL	WATSON/785 cap
Capsules, 5 mg ℞	5 mg body
green op/yellow op	
10 mg ℞	WATSON/786 cap
black op/green op	10 mg body
25 mg ℞	WATSON/787 cap
green op/white op	25 mg body
CHLORDIAZEPOXIDE HCL	WATSON/788 body
Capsules, ℞	5–2.5 mg cap
white op/white op	
CHLORZOXAZONE	WATSON 693/500
Tablets, USP, 500 mg ℞	Partial-Scored
Green, Capsule-shaped	

PRODUCT	IDENTIFICATION CODE
CLOMIPHENE CITRATE	WATSON/781
Tablets, 50 mg ℞	
off white round	
CLOMIPRAMINE HYDROCHLORIDE	WATSON
Capsules, 25 mg ℞	594/25 mg
Opaque Blue/Opaque Blue	
CLOMIPRAMINE HYDROCHLORIDE	WATSON
Capsules, 50 mg ℞	595/50 mg
Opaque Yellow/Opaque Yellow	
CLOMIPRAMINE HYDROCHLORIDE	WATSON
Capsules, 75 mg ℞	596/75 mg
Opaque Green/Opaque Green	
CLONAZEPAM	WATSON 746
Tablets, USP, 0.5 mg Ⓒ ℞	Biconvex, Scored
yellow/round	
CLONAZEPAM	WATSON 747
Tablets, USP, 1 mg Ⓒ ℞	Biconvex, Scored
aqua/round	
CLONAZEPAM	WATSON 748
Tablets, USP, 2 mg Ⓒ ℞	Biconvex, Scored
white/round	
CLORAZEPATE DIPOTASSIUM	WATSON 363/3.75
Tablets, 3.75 mg Ⓒ ℞	Scored
Light Blue, Round	
CLORAZEPATE DIPOTASSIUM	WATSON 364/7.5
Tablets, 7.5 mg Ⓒ ℞	Scored
Light beige, Round	
CLORAZEPATE DIPOTASSIUM	WATSON 365/15
Tablets, 15 mg Ⓒ ℞	Scored
Pink, Round	
CYCLOBENZAPRINE HYDRO-	
CHLORIDE ℞	WATSON/418
Tablets, USP, 10 mg	Scored
Dark Yellow, Round	
DESIPRAMINE HCL	
Tablets, 25 mg ℞	WATSON/808
yellow round	
50 mg ℞	WATSON/809
green round	
75 mg ℞	WATSON/544
orange round	
100 mg ℞	WATSON/545
peach round	
DICYCLOMINE HCL	
Capsules, 10 mg ℞	WATSON/794 cap
dk blue/dk blue	10 mg body
Tablets 20 mg ℞	WATSON/795
blue round	
DIETHYLPROPION HCL	
Tablets, 25 mg ℞	WATSON/783
white round	
DIETHYLPROPION HCL	
Extended Release Tablets, 75 mg ℞	WATSON/802
white capsule shaped	
DILTIAZEM	120/WATSON/662
Extended release	
Capsules, 120 mg	
DILTIAZEM	180/WATSON/663
Extended release	
Capsules, 180 mg	
DILTIAZEM	240/WATSON/664
Extended release	
Capsule, 240 mg	
DILTIAZEM HCL	
Tablets, 30 mg ℞	WATSON/775
blue round	
60 mg ℞	WATSON/776
white round	
90 mg ℞	WATSON/777
blue oblong	
120 mg ℞	WATSON/778
white oblong	
DOXEPIN HYDROCHLORIDE	WATSON 695/10 mg
Capsules, USP, 10 mg ℞	
Scarlet/Pink Opaque	
DOXEPIN HYDROCHLORIDE	WATSON 696/25 mg
Capsules, USP, 25 mg ℞	
Blue/Pink Opaque	
DOXEPIN HYDROCHLORIDE	WATSON 697/50 mg
Capsules, USP, 50 mg ℞	
Pink/Flesh Opaque	
ESTAZOLAM	WATSON 744/1
Tablets, 1 mg Ⓒ ℞	
White, diamond shaped	
ESTAZOLAM	WATSON 745/2
Tablets, 2 mg Ⓒ ℞	
Dark Pink, diamond shaped	
ESTRADIOL	WATSON 528/Scored
Tablets, USP, 0.5 mg ℞	
White, Round	
ESTRADIOL	WATSON 487/Scored
Tablets, USP, 1 mg ℞	
Gray, Round	
ESTRADIOL	WATSON 488/Scored
Tablets, USP, 2 mg ℞	
Light Green, Round	

ESTROPIPATE · WATSON 414/Scored
Tablets, USP, 0.75 mg ℞
(calculated as sodium
estrone sulfate 0.625 mg)
Yellow, Round
ESTROPIPATE · WATSON 415/Scored
Tablets, USP, 1.5 mg ℞
(calculated as sodium
estrone sulfate 1.25 mg)
Peach, Round
ESTROPIPATE · WATSON 416/Scored
Tablets, USP, 3 mg ℞
(calculated as sodium
estrone sulfate 2.5 mg)
Blue, Round
ETODOLAC · WATSON 735/200 mg
Capsules, 200 mg ℞
Gray/Brown opaque
ETODOLAC · WATSON 736/300
Capsules, 300 mg ℞
Gray/Red
ETODOLAC · WATSON 667/400
Tablets, 400 mg ℞
Yellow Capsule Shaped, Film Coated, Biconvex
FUROSEMIDE · WATSON 300/Blank
Tablets, USP, 20 mg ℞
White, Round
FUROSEMIDE · WATSON/311
Tablets, USP, 20 mg ℞
White, Oval
FUROSEMIDE · WATSON 301/Scored
Tablets, USP, 40 mg ℞
White, Round
FUROSEMIDE · WATSON 302/Scored
Tablets, USP, 80 mg ℞
White, Round
GEMFIBROZIL · WATSON 454/Bisected
Tablets, USP, 600 mg ℞
White, Film-coated Oval
GLIPIZIDE · WATSON 460/Scored
Tablets, USP, 5 mg ℞
White, Round
GLIPIZIDE · WATSON 461/Scored
Tablets, USP, 10 mg ℞
White, Round
GUANABENZ ACETATE · WATSON 451/Blank
Tablets, USP, 4 mg ℞
Orange, Round
GUANABENZ ACETATE · WATSON 452/Blank
Tablets, USP, 8 mg ℞
Grey, Round
GUANFACINE HYDROCHLORIDE · WATSON 444/Blank
Tablets, 1 mg ℞ USP
Pink, Round, Biconvex
GUANFACINE HYDROCHLORIDE · WATSON 453/Blank
Tablets, 2 mg ℞ USP
Peach, Round, Biconvex
HYDROCODONE BITARTRATE and APAP · WATSON
Tablets, USP, 2.5 mg/500 mg ℂ ℞ · 388/Bisected
White, Oblong
HYDROCODONE BITARTRATE and APAP · WATSON
Tablets, USP, 5 mg/500 mg ℂ ℞ · 349/Bisected
White, Capsule-shaped
HYDROCODONE BITARTRATE and APAP · WATSON
Tablets, USP, 7.5 mg/500 mg ℂ ℞ · 385/Bisected
White, Capsule-shaped
HYDROCODONE BITARTRATE and APAP · WATSON
Tablets, USP, 7.5 mg/650 mg ℂ ℞ · 502/Bisected
Pink, Capsule-shaped
HYDROCODONE BITARTRATE and APAP · WATSON
Tablets, USP, 7.5 mg/750 mg ℂ ℞ · 387/Bisected
White, Oblong
HYDROCODONE BITARTRATE and APAP · WATSON
Tablets, USP, 10 mg/500 mg ℂ ℞ · 540/Bisected
Blue, Capsule-Shaped
HYDROCODONE BITARTRATE and APAP · WATSON
Tablets, USP, 10 mg/650mg ℂ ℞ · 503/Bisected
Light Green, Capsule-Shaped
HYDROXYCHLOROQUINE
SULFATE · WATSON 698/200
Tablets, USP, 200 mg ℞
White/Off-White, Oval, Film-coated
HYDROXYZINE
HYDROCHLORIDE · WATSON 699/10
Tablets, USP, 10 mg ℞
Orange, Round, Film-coated
HYDROXYZINE
HYDROCHLORIDE · WATSON 700/25
Tablets, USP, 25 mg ℞
Green, Round, Film-coated
HYDROXYZINE · WATSON 704/50
HYDROCHLORIDE
Tablets, USP, 50 mg ℞
Yellow, Round, Film-coated
HYDROXYZINE PAMOATE
Capsules, 25 mg ℞ · WATSON/800
dk green op/lt green

50 mg ℞ · WATSON/801
green op/white op
INDAPAMIDE · WATSON 527/Blank
Tablets, USP, 1.25 mg ℞
Orange, Film Coated, Round
INDAPAMIDE · WATSON 504/Blank
Tablets, USP, 2.5 mg ℞
White, Film Coated, Round
LORAZEPAM · ROYCE/240 Scored 0.5
Tablets, USP, 0.5 mg ℂᵥ ℞
White, Round
LORAZEPAM · ROYCE/241 Scored 1.0
Tablets, USP, 1 mg ℂᵥ ℞
White, Round
LORAZEPAM · ROYCE/242 Scored 2.0
Tablets, USP, 2 mg ℂᵥ ℞
White, Round
LOXAPINE · WATSON 369/5 mg
Capsules, USP, 5 mg ℞
White/white
LOXAPINE · WATSON 370/10 mg
Capsules, USP, 10 mg ℞
Yellow/white
LOXAPINE · WATSON 371/25 mg
Capsules, USP, 25 mg ℞
Green/white
LOXAPINE · WATSON 372/50 mg
Capsules, USP, 50 mg ℞
Blue/white
MAPROTILINE HYDROCHLORIDE · WATSON/373
Tablets, USP, 25 mg ℞ · (Partial Bisect)
Peach, Film Coated, Oval
MAPROTILINE HYDROCHLORIDE · WATSON
Tablets, USP, 50 mg ℞ · 374/Scored
Peach, Film Coated, Round
MAPROTILINE HYDROCHLORIDE · WATSON/375
Tablets, USP, 75 mg ℞ · (Partial Bisect)
White, Film Coated, Oval
MECLIZINE HCL
Tablets, 12.5 mg ℞ · WATSON/802
blue/white oval
25 mg ℞ · WATSON/803
yellow/white oval
MEPERIDINE HYDROCHLORIDE
Tablets, 50 mg USP ℞ ℂ · WATSON/726/50
white, round, biconvex
Tablets, 100 mg USP ℞ ℂ · WATSON/727/100
white, round, biconvex
MEPROBAMATE
Tablets, 200 mg ℞ · WATSON/804
white round scored
400 mg ℞ · WATSON/805
white round convex
METHOCARBAMOL
Tablets, 500 mg ℞ · WATSON/806
white round scored
750 mg ℞ · WATSON/807
white capsule shaped
METHYLPREDNISOLONE
Tablets, 4 mg ℞ · WATSON/790
white oval quadrisect
METOCLOPRAMIDE HYDROCHLORIDE · WATSON
Tablets, 10 mg ℞ · 312/Scored
White, Round
METOPROLOL TARTRATE · WATSON 462/Scored
Tablets, USP, 50 mg ℞
Pink, Film Coated, Round
METOPROLOL TARTRATE · WATSON 463/Scored
Tablets, USP, 100 mg ℞
Light Blue, Film Coated, Round
MEXILETINE HYDROCHLORIDE · WATSON 491/150 mg
Capsules, USP, 150 mg ℞
Brown/Light Brown
MEXILETINE HYDROCHLORIDE · WATSON 492/200 mg
Capsules, USP, 200 mg ℞
Brown/Brown
MEXILETINE HYDROCHLORIDE · WATSON 493/250 mg
Capsules, USP, 250 mg ℞
Brown/Light Green
NAPROXEN
Tablets, 250 mg ℞ · WATSON/821
white round
375 mg ℞ · WATSON/822
gray capsule shaped
500 mg ℞ · WATSON/791
white capsule shaped
NAPROXEN SODIUM
Tablets, 275 mg ℞ · WATSON/792
white oval
550 mg ℞ · WATSON/793
green oval
OXYBUTYNIN CHLORIDE
Tablets, 5 mg ℞ · WATSON/779
pale blue round

OXYCODONE and
ACETAMINOPHEN · WATSON 737/5–500 mg
Capsules, USP 5 mg/500 mg ℂ
Opaque White and Opaque Red
OXYCODONE and ACETAMINOPHEN · WATSON 749
Tablets, USP 5 mg/325 mg ℂ
White, Round, Bisected
OXYCODONE HYDROCHLORIDE
Tablets, 5 mg USP ℂ · WATSON/774
white, round
OXYCODONE and ASPIRIN
Tablets 4.5 mg/0.38 mg/325 mg USP ℂ ℞
PENTAZOCINE &
NALOXONE HCl · WATSON 395/50/0.5
Tablets, USP, 50 mg/0.5 ℂᵥ ℞ · *Scored*
Light Green, Capsule Shaped
PERPHENAZINE/AMITRIPTYLINE
HYDROCHLORIDE · WATSON 706/2–10
Tablets, USP, 2 mg/10 mg ℞ · *Biconvex*
Blue, Round,
PERPHENAZINE/AMITRIPTYLINE
HYDROCHLORIDE · WATSON 707/2–25
Tablets, USP, 2 mg/25 mg ℞ · *Biconvex*
Light Orange, Round
PERPHENAZINE/AMITRIPTYLINE
HYDROCHLORIDE · WATSON 708/4–10
Tablets, USP, 4 mg/10 mg ℞ · *Biconvex*
Beige, Round
PERPHENAZINE/AMITRIPTYLINE
HYDROCHLORIDE · WATSON 709/4–25
Tablets, USP, 4 mg/25 mg ℞ · *Biconvex*
Yellow, Round
PINDOLOL · WATSON 710/5
Tablets, USP, 5 mg ℞ · *Scored*
White, Round
PINDOLOL · WATSON 711/10
Tablets, USP, 10 mg ℞ · *Scored*
White, Round
PIROXICAM · WATSON 712/10 mg
Capsules, USP, 10 mg ℞
Light Blue/White
PIROXICAM · WATSON 713/20 mg
Capsules, USP, 20 mg ℞
Light Blue/Light Blue
PREDNISONE
Tablets, 5 mg ℞ · WATSON/830
white round
10 mg ℞ · WATSON/831
white round
20 mg ℞ · WATSON/832
peach round
50 mg ℞ · WATSON/797
white round
PROPOXYPHENE HYDROCHLORIDE
& ACETAMINOPHEN · WATSON 714/65–650
Tablets USP 65/650 mg ℂ
Orange, Oblong
PROPRANOLOL HYDROCHLORIDE · WATSON 305/
Tablets, USP, 10 mg ℞ · *Scored*
Orange, Round
PROPRANOLOL HYDROCHLORIDE · WATSON 306/
Tablets, USP, 20 mg ℞ · *Scored*
Blue, Round
PROPRANOLOL HYDROCHLORIDE · WATSON 307/
Tablets, USP, 40 mg ℞ · *Scored*
Green, Round
PROPRANOLOL HYDROCHLORIDE · WATSON 352/
Tablets, USP, 60 mg ℞ · *Scored*
Pink, Round
PROPRANOLOL HYDROCHLORIDE · WATSON 308/
Tablets, USP, 80 mg ℞ · *Scored*
Yellow, Round
QUININE SULFATE · WATSON 716/325 mg
Capsules, USP, 325 mg ℞
Opaque White/Opaque White
QUININE SULFATE · WATSON 715/260 mg
Tablets, USP, 260 mg ℞
White, Round
RANITIDINE
Tablets, 150 mg ℞ · WATSON/760
beige round
300 mg ℞ · WATSON/761
beige capsule shaped
SILVER SULFADIAZINE
Cream, 1% ℞
white
SUCRALFATE
Tablets, 1 gm ℞ · WATSON/780
lt blue oblong
SULFASALAZINE
Tablets, 500 mg ℞ · WATSON/796
mustard round bisect
TRIAMTERENE and
HYDROCHLOROTHIAZIDE · WATSON 424/Scored
Tablets, USP, 37.5 mg/25 mg ℞
Light green, Round

Continued on next page

Product Listing—Cont.

TRIAMTERENE and HYDROCHLOROTHIAZIDE Tablets, USP, 75 mg/50 mg ℞ *Yellow, Round*	WATSON 348/Scored
VERAPAMIL HYDROCHLORIDE Tablets, USP, 40 mg ℞ *Light Peach, Film Coated, Round*	WATSON 404/Blank
VERAPAMIL HYDROCHLORIDE Tablets, USP, 80 mg ℞ *White, Film Coated, Round*	WATSON 343/Scored
VERAPAMIL HYDROCHLORIDE Tablets, USP, 80 mg ℞ *Light peach, Film Coated, Round*	WATSON 344/Scored
VERAPAMIL HYDROCHLORIDE Tablets, USP, 120 mg ℞ *White, Film Coated, Round*	WATSON 345/Scored
VERAPAMIL HYDROCHLORIDE Tablets, USP, 120 mg ℞ *Peach, Film Coated, Round*	WATSON 346/Scored
YOHIMBINE HYDROCHLORIDE Tablets, 5.4 mg ℞ *White, Round*	WATSON 717/5.4 *Biconvex, Scored*

ORAL CONTRACEPTIVE PRODUCTS:
(available in 21 day and 28 day packs)

NORETHINDRONE AND ETHINYL ESTRADIOL TABLETS USP: ℞

NECON® 0.5/35 (0.5 mg norethindrone and 35 mcg ethinyl estradiol)	WATSON/507
NECON® 1/35 (1 mg norethindrone and 35 mcg ethinyl estradiol)	WATSON/508
NECON® 10/11 (10 tablets—each contains 0.5 mg norethindrone and 35 mcg ethinyl estradiol; 11 tablets—each contains 1 mg norethindrone and 35 mcg ethinyl estradiol.)	10 tablets of WATSON/507 and 11 tablets of WATSON/508

NORETHINDRONE AND MESTRANOL TABLETS USP: ℞

NECON® 1/50 (1 mg norethindrone and 50 mcg mestranol)	WATSON/510

ETHYNODIOL DIACETATE AND ETHINYL ESTRADIOL TABLETS USP: ℞

ZOVIA® 1/35E (1 mg ethynodiol diacetate and 35 mcg ethinyl estradiol)	WATSON 383/Blank
ZOVIA® 1/50E (1 mg ethynodiol diacetate and 50 mcg ethinyl estradiol)	WATSON 384/Blank

DILACOR XR® ℞
[dĭl 'a-kor]
(diltiazem HCl)
Extended-release Capsules

PRODUCT OVERVIEW

KEY FACTS

Dilacor XR capsules contain multiple units of diltiazem HCl Extended-release 60 mg, resulting in 120 mg, 180 mg or 240 mg dosage strengths.

Dilacor XR capsules contain a degradable controlled-release tablet formulation designed to release diltiazem over a 24-hour period. Geomatrix™, a registered trademark of Jago Research AG, Zollikon, Switzerland, is a patented controlled-release system incorporated in the tablets.

MAJOR USES

Dilacor XR is indicated for the treatment of hypertension. Diltiazem hydrochloride may be used alone or in combination with other antihypertensive medications, such as diuretics.

Dilacor XR is indicated for the management of chronic stable angina.

Dosage: Hypertension. Dosages must be adjusted to each patient's needs, starting with 180 or 240 mg once-daily. Based on the antihypertensive effect, the dose may be adjusted as needed. Individual patients, particularly ≥ 60 years of age, may respond to a lower dose of 120 mg. The usual dosage range studied in clinical trials was 180 to 480 mg once daily. Current clinical experience with the 540 mg dose is limited, the dose may be increased to 540 mg with little or no increased risk of adverse reactions. Doses should not exceed 540 mg once-daily.

Dosage: Angina. Dosages for the treatment of angina should be adjusted to each patient's needs, starting with a dose of 120 mg once daily, which may be titrated to doses of up to 480 mg once daily. When necessary, titration may be carried out over a 7 to 14 day period.

SAFETY INFORMATION

Diltiazem hydrochloride is contraindicated in: (1) patients with sick sinus syndrome except in the presence of a functioning ventricular pacemaker; (2) patients with second or third degree AV block except in the presence of a functioning ventricular pacemaker; (3) patients with hypotension (less than 90 mmHg systolic); (4) patients who have demonstrated hypersensitivity to the drug; and (5) patients with acute myocardial infarction and pulmonary congestion as documented by X-ray on admission.

PRESCRIBING INFORMATION

DILACOR XR® ℞
(diltiazem HCl)
Extended-release Capsules

DESCRIPTION

Dilacor XR® (diltiazem hydrochloride) is a calcium ion influx inhibitor (slow channel blocker or calcium antagonist). Chemically, diltiazem hydrochloride is 1,5-Benzothiazepin-4(5H)one,3- (acetyloxy) -5- [2-(dimethylamino) ethyl]-2,3-dihydro-2-(4-methoxyphenyl)-, monohydrochloride, (+)-cis-. Its molecular formula is $C_{22}H_{26}N_2O_4S$ HCl and its molecular weight is 450.98. Its structural formula is as follows:

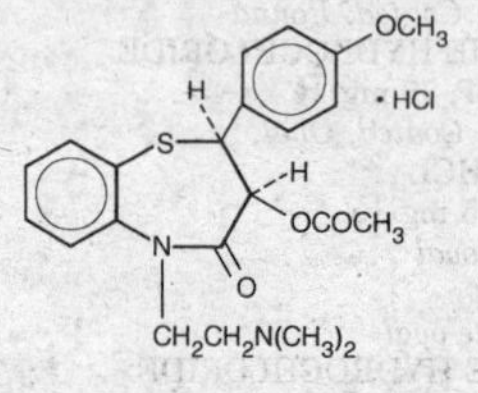

Diltiazem hydrochloride is a white to off-white crystalline powder with a bitter taste. It is soluble in water, methanol and chloroform. Dilacor XR complies with USP Drug Release Test #2.

Dilacor XR capsules contain multiple units of diltiazem HCl Extended-release 60 mg, resulting in 120 mg, 180 mg or 240 mg dosage strengths allowing for the controlled release of diltiazem HCl over a 24-hour period.

Inactive Ingredients: Dilacor XR capsules also contain mannitol, ethyl cellulose, hydroxypropyl methylcellulose, hydrogenated castor oil, ferric oxides, silicon dioxide, magnesium stearate, gelatin, D&C Yellow No. 10, FD&C Red No. 40, D&C Red No. 28, and titanium dioxide. The 120 mg dosage form contains pregelatinized starch.

For oral administration.

CLINICAL PHARMACOLOGY

The therapeutic benefits of diltiazem hydrochloride are believed to be related to its ability to inhibit the influx of calcium ions during membrane depolarization of cardiac and vascular smooth muscle.

Mechanisms of Action. *Hypertension:* Dilacor XR produces its antihypertensive effect primarily by relaxation of vascular smooth muscle with a resultant decrease in peripheral vascular resistance. The magnitude of blood pressure reduction is related to the degree of hypertension; thus hypertensive individuals experience an antihypertensive effect, whereas there is only a modest fall in blood pressure in normotensives.

Angina: Diltiazem HCl has been shown to produce increases in exercise tolerance, probably due to its ability to reduce myocardial oxygen demand. This is accomplished via reductions in heart rate and systemic blood pressure at submaximal and maximal work loads.

Diltiazem has been shown to be a potent dilator of coronary arteries, both epicardial and subendocardial. Spontaneous and ergonovine-induced coronary artery spasm are inhibited by diltiazem.

In animal models, diltiazem interferes with the slow inward (depolarizing) current in excitable tissue. It causes excitation-contraction uncoupling in various myocardial tissues without changes in the configuration of the action potential. Diltiazem produces relaxation of coronary vascular smooth muscle and dilation of both large and small coronary arteries at drug levels which cause little or no negative inotropic effect. The resultant increases in coronary blood flow (epicardial and subendocardial) occur in ischemic and nonischemic models and are accompanied by dose-dependent decreases in systemic blood pressure and decreases in peripheral resistance.

Hemodynamic and Electrophysiologic Effects: Like other calcium antagonists, diltiazem decreases sinoatrial and atrioventricular conduction in isolated tissues and has a negative inotropic effect in isolated preparations. In the intact animal, prolongation of the AH interval can be seen at higher doses.

In man, diltiazem prevents spontaneous and ergonovine-provoked coronary artery spasm. It causes a decrease in peripheral vascular resistance and a modest fall in blood pressure in normotensive individuals. In exercise tolerance studies in patients with ischemic heart disease, diltiazem reduces the double product (HR × SBP) for any given work load. Studies to date, primarily in patients with good ventricular function, have not revealed evidence of a negative inotropic effect. Cardiac output, ejection fraction and left ventricular end diastolic pressure have not been affected. Such data have no predictive value with respect to effects in patients with poor ventricular function. Increased heart failure has, however, been reported in occasional patients with pre-existing impairment of ventricular function. There are as yet few data on the interaction of diltiazem and beta-blockers in patients with poor ventricular function. Resting heart rate is usually slightly reduced by diltiazem.

Dilacor XR produces antihypertensive effects both in the supine and standing positions. Postural hypotension is infrequently noted upon suddenly assuming an upright position. Diltiazem decreases vascular resistance, increases cardiac output (by increasing stroke volume), and produces a slight decrease or no change in heart rate. No reflex tachycardia is associated with the chronic antihypertensive effects.

During dynamic exercise, increases in diastolic pressure are inhibited while maximum achievable systolic pressure is usually reduced. Heart rate at maximum exercise does not change or is slightly reduced.

Diltiazem antagonizes the renal and peripheral effects of angiotensin II. No increased activity of the renin-angiotensin-aldosterone axis has been observed. Chronic therapy with diltiazem produces no change or an increase in plasma catecholamines. Hypertensive animal models respond to diltiazem with reductions in blood pressure and increased urinary output and natriuresis without a change in the urinary sodium/potassium ratio. In man, transient natriuresis and kaliuresis have been reported, but only in high intravenous doses of 0.5 mg/kg of body weight.

Diltiazem-associated prolongation of the AH interval is not more pronounced in patients with first-degree heart block. In patients with sick sinus syndrome, diltiazem significantly prolongs sinus cycle length (up to 50% in some cases). Intravenous diltiazem in doses of 20 mg prolongs AH conduction time and AV node functional and effective refractory periods approximately 20%.

In two short-term, double-blind, placebo-controlled studies, 303 hypertensive patients were treated with once-daily Dilacor XR in doses of up to 540 mg. There were no instances of greater than first-degree atrioventricular block, and the maximum increase in the PR interval was .08 seconds. No patients were prematurely discontinued from the medication due to symptoms related to prolongation of the PR interval.

Pharmacodynamics: In one short-term, double-blind, placebo-controlled study, Dilacor XR 120, 240, 360 and 480 mg/day demonstrated a dose-related antihypertensive response among patients with mild to moderate hypertension. Statistically significant decreases in trough mean supine diastolic blood pressure were seen through four weeks of treatment: 120 mg/day (−5.1 mmHg); 240 mg/day (−6.9 mmHg); 360 mg/day (−6.9 mmHg); and 480 mg/day (−10.6 mmHg). Statistically significant decreases in trough mean supine systolic blood pressure were also seen through four weeks of treatment: 120 mg/day (−2.6 mmHg); 240 mg/day (−6.5 mmHg); 360 mg/day (−4.8 mmHg); and 480 mg/day (−10.6 mmHg). The proportion of evaluable patients exhibiting a therapeutic response (supine diastolic blood pressure <90 mmHg or decrease >10 mmHg) was greater as the dose increased: 31%, 42%, 48% and 69% with the 120, 240, 360 and 480 mg/day diltiazem groups, respectively. Similar findings were observed for standing systolic and diastolic blood pressures. The trough (24 hours after a dose) antihypertensive effect of Dilacor XR retained more than one-half of the response seen at peak (3–6 hours after administration).

Significant reductions of mean supine blood pressure (at trough) in patients with mild to moderate hypertension were also seen in a short-term, double-blind, dose-escalation, placebo-controlled study after 2 weeks of once-daily Dilacor XR 180 mg/day (diastolic: −6.1 mmHg; systolic: −4.7 mmHg) and again, 2 weeks after escalation to 360 mg/day (diastolic: −9.3 mmHg; systolic: −7.2 mmHg). However, a further increase in dose to 540 mg/day for 2 weeks provided only a minimal further increase in the antihypertensive effect (diastolic: −10.2 mmHg; systolic: −6.7 mmHg).

Dilacor XR, given at 120 mg, 240 mg, and 480 mg/day, in a randomized, multicenter, double-blind, placebo-controlled, parallel group, dose-ranging study, in 189 patients with chronic angina, demonstrated a dose-related increase in exercise time by Exercise Tolerance Test (ETT) and a reduction in rates of anginal attacks (based on individual patients diaries). The improvement in total exercise time (using the Bruce protocol), measured at trough exercise periods, for placebo, 120 mg, 240 mg, and 480 mg, was 20, 37, 49, and 56 seconds, respectively.

Pharmacokinetics and Metabolism: Diltiazem is well-absorbed from the gastrointestinal tract, and is subject to an extensive first-pass effect. When given as an immediate release oral formulation, the absolute bioavailability (com-

pared to intravenous administration) of diltiazem is approximately 40%. Diltiazem undergoes extensive hepatic metabolism in which 2% to 4% of the unchanged drug appears in the urine. Total radioactivity measurement following short IV administration in healthy volunteers suggests the presence of other unidentified metabolites which attain higher concentrations than those of diltiazem and are more slowly eliminated; half-life of total radioactivity is about 20 hours compared to 2 to 5 hours for diltiazem. *In-vitro* binding studies show diltiazem HCl is 70% to 80% bound to plasma proteins. Competitive *in-vitro* ligand binding studies have also shown diltiazem HCl binding is not altered by therapeutic concentrations of digoxin, HCTZ, phenylbutazone, propranolol, salicylic acid, or warfarin. The plasma elimination half-life of diltiazem is approximately 3.0 to 4.5 hours. Desacetyldiltiazem, the major metabolite of diltiazem, which is also present in the plasma at concentrations of 10% to 20% of the parent drug, is approximately 25% to 50% as potent a coronary vasodilator as diltiazem. Therapeutic blood levels of diltiazem hydrochloride appear to be in the range of 40-200 ng/mL. There is a departure from linearity when dose strengths are increased; the half-life is slightly increased with dose.

A study that compared patients with normal hepatic function to patients with cirrhosis found an increase in half-life and a 69% increase in bioavailability in the hepatically impaired patients. Patients with severely impaired renal function showed no difference in the pharmacokinetic profile of diltiazem compared to patients with normal renal function. Dilacor XR capsules contain a degradable controlled-release tablet formulation designed to release diltiazem over a 24-hour period. Geomatrix™, a registered trademark of Jago Research AG, Zollikon, Switzerland, is a patented controlled-release system incorporated in the tablets. Controlled absorption of diltiazem begins within 1 hour, with maximum plasma concentrations being achieved 4 to 6 hours after administration. The apparent steady-state half-life of diltiazem following once-daily administration of Dilacor XR capsules ranges from 5 to 10 hours. This prolongation of half-life is attributed to continued absorption of diltiazem rather than to alterations in its elimination.

The absolute bioavailability of diltiazem from a single dose of dilacor XR (compared to intravenous administration) is 41% (±14). This value was shown to be similar to the 40% systemic availability reported following administration of an immediate release diltiazem HCl formulation.

As the dose of Dilacor XR capsules is increased from a daily dose of 120 mg to 240 mg, there is an increase in the AUC of 2.3 fold. When the dose is increased from 240 mg to 360 mg, AUC increases 1.6 fold and when increased from 240 mg to 480 mg, AUC increases 2.4 fold.

In-vivo release of diltiazem occurs throughout the gastrointestinal tract, with controlled release still occurring for up to 24 hours after administration, as determined by radiolabelled methods. As the once-daily dose of Dilacor XR was increased, departures from linearity were noted. There were disproportionate increases in area under the curve for doses from 120 mg to 480 mg.

The presence of food did not affect the ability of Dilacor XR to maintain a controlled release of the drug and did not impact its sustained release properties over 24 hours after administration. However, simultaneous administration of Dilacor XR with a high-fat breakfast resulted in increases in AUC of 13% and 19%, and in C$_{max}$ by 37% and 51%, respectively.

INDICATIONS AND USAGE

Dilacor XR is indicated for the treatment of hypertension. Diltiazem hydrochloride may be used alone or in combination with other antihypertensive medications, such as diuretics.

Dilacor XR is indicated for the management of chronic stable angina.

CONTRAINDICATIONS

Diltiazem hydrochloride is contraindicated in: (1) patients with sick sinus syndrome except in the presence of a functioning ventricular pacemaker; (2) patients with second or third degree AV block except in the presence of a functioning ventricular pacemaker; (3) patients with hypotension (less than 90 mmHg systolic); (4) patients who have demonstrated hypersensitivity to the drug; and (5) patients with acute myocardial infarction and pulmonary congestion as documented by X-ray on admission.

WARNINGS

Cardiac Conduction: Diltiazem hydrochloride prolongs AV node refractory periods without significantly prolonging sinus node recovery time, except in patients with sick sinus syndrome. This effect may rarely result in abnormally slow heart rates (particularly in patients with sick sinus syndrome) or second, or third degree AV block (22 of 10,119 patients, or 0.2%); 41% of these 22 patients were receiving concomitant β-adrenoceptor antagonists versus 17% of the total group. Concomitant use of diltiazem with beta-blockers or digitalis may result in additive effects on cardiac conduc-

tion. A patient with Prinzmetal's angina developed periods of asystole (2 to 5 seconds) after a single 60 mg dose of diltiazem.

Congestive Heart Failure: Although diltiazem has a negative inotropic effect in isolated animal tissue preparations, hemodynamic studies in humans with normal ventricular function have not shown a reduction in cardiac index nor consistent negative effects on contractility (dp/dt). An acute study of oral diltiazem in patients with impaired ventricular function (ejection fraction of 24% ± 6%) showed improvement in indices of ventricular function without significant decrease in contractile function (dp/dt). Worsening of congestive heart failure has been reported in patients with preexisting impairment of ventricular function. Experience with the use of diltiazem hydrochloride in combination with beta-blockers in patients with impaired ventricular function is limited. Caution should be exercised when using this combination.

Hypotension: Decreases in blood pressure associated with diltiazem hydrochloride therapy may occasionally result in symptomatic hypotension.

Acute Hepatic Injury: Mild elevations of serum transaminases with and without concomitant elevation in alkaline phosphatase and bilirubin have been observed in clinical studies. Such elevations were usually transient and frequently resolved even with continued diltiazem treatment. In rare instances, significant elevations in alkaline phosphatase, LDH, SGOT, SGPT, and other phenomena consistent with acute hepatic injury have been noted. These reactions tended to occur early after therapy initiation (1 to 6 weeks) and have been reversible upon discontinuation of drug therapy. The relationship to diltiazem is uncertain in some cases, but probable in some others (see **PRECAUTIONS**).

PRECAUTIONS

General: Diltiazem hydrochloride is extensively metabolized by the liver and is excreted by the kidneys and in bile. As with any drug given over prolonged periods, laboratory parameters should be monitored at regular intervals. The drug should be used with caution in patients with impaired renal or hepatic function. In subacute and chronic dog and rat studies designed to produce toxicity, high doses of diltiazem were associated with hepatic damage. In special subacute hepatic studies, oral doses of 125 mg/kg and higher in rats were associated with histological changes in the liver which were reversible when the drug was discontinued. In dogs, doses of 20 mg/kg were also associated with hepatic changes; however, these changes were reversible with continued dosing.

Dermatological events (see **ADVERSE REACTIONS**) may be transient and may disappear despite continued use of diltiazem hydrochloride. However, skin eruptions progressing to erythema multiforme and/or exfoliative dermatitis have also been infrequently reported. Should a dermatologic reaction persist, the drug should be discontinued.

Although Dilacor XR utilizes a slowly disintegrating matrix, caution should still be used in patients with preexisting severe gastrointestinal narrowing (pathologic or iatrogenic). There have been no reports of obstructive symptoms in patients with known strictures in association with the ingestion of Dilacor XR.

Information for Patients: Dilacor XR capsules should be taken on an empty stomach. Patients should be cautioned that the Dilacor XR capsules should not be opened, chewed or crushed, and should be swallowed whole.

Drug Interaction: Due to the potential for additive effects, caution and careful titration are warranted in patients receiving diltiazem hydrochloride concomitantly with any agents known to affect cardiac contractility and/or conduction. (See **WARNINGS**.) Pharmacologic studies indicate that there may be additive effects in prolonging AV conduction when using beta-blockers or digitalis concomitantly with diltiazem hydrochloride. (See **WARNINGS**.) As with all drugs, care should be exercised when treating patients with multiple medications. Diltiazem hydrochloride undergoes biotransformation by cytochrome P-450 mixed function oxidase. Co-administration of diltiazem hydrochloride with other agents which follow the same route of biotransformation may result in the competitive inhibition of metabolism. Especially in patients with renal and/or hepatic impairment, dosages of similarly metabolized drugs, particularly those of low therapeutic ratio such as cyclosporin, may require adjustment when starting or stopping concomitantly administered diltiazem hydrochloride to maintain optimum therapeutic blood levels. Concomitant administration of diltiazem with carbamazepine has been reported to result in elevated plasma levels of carbamazepine, resulting in toxicity in some cases.

Beta-Blockers: Controlled and uncontrolled domestic studies suggest that concomitant use of diltiazem hydrochloride and beta-blockers is usually well-tolerated, but available data are not sufficient to predict the effects of concomitant treatment in patients with left ventricular dysfunction or cardiac conduction abnormalities. Administration of diltiazem hydrochloride concomitantly with propranolol in five

normal volunteers resulted in increased propranolol levels in all subjects and the bioavailability of propranolol was increased approximately 50%. If combination therapy is initiated or withdrawn in conjunction with propranolol, an adjustment in the propranolol dose may be warranted. (See **WARNINGS.**)

Cimetidine: A study in six healthy volunteers has shown a significant increase in peak diltiazem plasma levels (58%) and area-under-the-curve (53%) after a 1-week course of cimetidine at 1,200 mg per day and diltiazem 60 mg per day. Ranitidine produced smaller, nonsignificant increases. The effect may be mediated by cimetidine's known inhibition of hepatic cytochrome P-450, the enzyme system responsible for the first-pass metabolism of diltiazem. Patients currently receiving diltiazem therapy should be carefully monitored for a change in pharmacological effect when initiating and discontinuing therapy with cimetidine. An adjustment in the diltiazem dose may be warranted.

Digitalis: Administration of diltiazem hydrochloride with digoxin in 24 healthy male subjects increased plasma digoxin concentrations approximately 20%. Another investigator found no increase in digoxin levels in 12 patients with coronary artery disease. Since there have been conflicting results regarding the effect of digoxin levels, it is recommended that digoxin levels be monitored when initiating, adjusting, and discontinuing diltiazem hydrochloride therapy to avoid possible over- or under-digitalization. (See **WARNINGS.**)

Anesthetics: The depression of cardiac contractility, conductivity, and automaticity as well as the vascular dilation associated with anesthetics may be potentiated by calcium channel blockers. When used concomitantly, anesthetics and calcium channel blockers should be titrated carefully.

Carcinogenesis, Mutagenesis, Impairment of Fertility: A 24-month study in rats and an 18-month study in mice showed no evidence of carcinogenicity. There was also no mutagenic response *in vitro* or *in vivo* in mammalian cell assays or *in vitro* in bacteria. No evidence of impaired fertility was observed in male or female rats at oral doses of up to 100 mg/kg/day.

Pregnancy: *(Category C.)* Reproduction studies have been conducted in mice, rats and rabbits. Administration of doses ranging from 4 to 6 times (depending on species) the upper limit of the optimum dosage range in clinical trials (480 mg q.d. or 8 mg/kg q.d. for a 60 kg patient) has resulted in embryo and fetal lethality. These studies have revealed, in one species or another, a propensity to cause abnormalities of the skeleton, heart, retina and tongue. Also observed were reductions in early individual pup weights and pup survival, prolonged delivery and increased incidence of stillbirths.

There are no well-controlled studies in pregnant women; therefore, use diltiazem hydrochloride in pregnant women only if the potential benefit justifies the potential risk to the fetus.

Nursing Mothers: Diltiazem is excreted in human milk. One report suggests that concentrations in breast milk may approximate serum levels. If use of diltiazem hydrochloride is deemed essential, an alternative method of infant feeding should be instituted.

Pediatric Use: Safety and effectiveness in pediatric patients have not been established.

ADVERSE REACTIONS

Serious adverse reactions to diltiazem hydrochloride have been rare in studies with other formulations, as well as with Dilacor XR®. It should be recognized, however, that patients with impaired ventricular function and cardiac conduction abnormalities have usually been excluded from these studies.

Hypertension: The most common adverse events (frequency ≥1%) in placebo-controlled, clinical hypertension studies with Dilacor XR using daily doses up to 540 mg, are listed in the table below with placebo-treated patients included for comparison.

MOST COMMON ADVERSE EVENTS IN
DOUBLE-BLIND, PLACEBO-CONTROLLED
HYPERTENSION TRIALS

Adverse Events (COSTART Term)	Dilacor XR®* n=303 # pts (%)	Placebo n=87 # pts (%)
rhinitis	29 (9.6)	7 (8.0)
headache	27 (8.9)	12 (13.8)
pharyngitis	17 (5.6)	4 (4.6)
constipation	11 (3.6)	2 (2.3)
cough increase	9 (3.0)	2 (2.3)
flu syndrome	7 (2.3)	1 (1.1)
edema, peripheral	7 (2.3)	0 (0.0)
myalgia	7 (2.3)	0 (0.0)
diarrhea	6 (2.0)	0 (0.0)
vomiting	6 (2.0)	0 (0.0)
sinusitis	6 (2.0)	1 (1.1)
asthenia	5 (1.7)	0 (0.0)

Continued on next page

Dilacor XR—Cont.

pain, back	5 (1.7)	2 (2.3)
nausea	5 (1.7)	1 (1.1)
dyspepsia	4 (1.3)	0 (0.0)
vasodilatation	4 (1.3)	0 (0.0)
injury, accident	4 (1.3)	0 (0.0)
pain, abdominal	3 (1.0)	0 (0.0)
arthrosis	3 (1.0)	0 (0.0)
insomnia	3 (1.0)	0 (0.0)
dyspnea	3 (1.0)	0 (0.0)
rash	3 (1.0)	1 (1.1)
tinnitus	3 (1.0)	0 (0.0)

*Adverse events occurring in 1% or more of patients receiving Dilacor XR.

Angina: The most common adverse events (frequency ≥1%) in a placebo-controlled, short-term (2 week) clinical angina study with Dilacor XR are listed in the table below with placebo-treated patients included for comparison. In this trial, following a placebo phase, patients were randomly assigned to once-daily doses of either 120, 240 or 480 mg of Dilacor XR.

MOST COMMON ADVERSE EVENTS IN A DOUBLE-BLIND, PLACEBO-CONTROLLED SHORT-TERM, ANGINA TRIAL

Adverse Events (COSTART Term)	Dilacor XR®* n=139 # pts (%)	Placebo n=50 # pts (%)
asthenia	5 (3.6)	2 (4.0)
headache	4 (2.9)	3 (6.0)
pain, back	4 (2.9)	1 (2.0)
rhinitis	4 (2.9)	1 (2.0)
constipation	3 (2.2)	1 (2.0)
nausea	3 (2.2)	0 (0.0)
edema, peripheral	3 (2.2)	1 (2.0)
dizziness	3 (2.2)	0 (0.0)
cough, increased	3 (2.2)	0 (0.0)
bradycardia	2 (1.4)	0 (0.0)
fibrillation, atrial	2 (1.4)	0 (0.0)
arthralgia	2 (1.4)	0 (0.0)
dream, abnormal	2 (1.4)	0 (0.0)
dyspnea	2 (1.4)	0 (0.0)
pharyngitis	2 (1.4)	1 (2.0)

* Adverse events occurring in 1% or more of patients receiving Dilacor XR.

Infrequent Adverse Events: The following additional events (COSTART Terms), listed by body system, were reported infrequently (less than 1%) in all subjects, hypertensive (n=425) or angina (n=318) patients who received Dilacor XR, or with other formulations of diltiazem.

Hypertension: *Cardiovascular:* First-degree AV block, arrhythmia, postural hypotension, tachycardia, pallor, palpitations, phlebitis, ECG abnormality, ST elevation.

Nervous System: Vertigo, hypertonia, paresthesia, dizziness, somnolence.

Digestive System: Dry mouth, anorexia, tooth disorder, eructation.

Skin and Appendages: Sweating, urticaria, skin hypertrophy (nevus).

Respiratory System: Epistaxis, bronchitis, respiratory disorder.

Urogenital System: Cystitis, kidney calculus, impotence, dysmenorrhea, vaginitis, prostate disease.

Metabolic and Nutritional Disorders: Gout, edema.

Musculoskeletal System: Arthralgia, bursitis, bone pain.

Hemic and Lymphatic System: Lymphadenopathy.

Body as a Whole: Pain, unevaluable reaction, neck pain, neck rigidity, fever, chest pain, malaise.

Special Senses: Amblyopia (blurred vision), ear pain.

Angina: *Cardiovascular:* Palpitations, AV block, sinus bradycardia, bigeminal extrasystole, angina pectoris, hypertension, hypotension, myocardial infarct, myocardial ischemia, syncope, vasodilatation, ventricular extrasystole.

Nervous System: Abnormal thinking, neuropathy, paresthesia.

Digestive System: Diarrhea, dyspepsia, vomiting, colitis, flatulence, GI hemorrhage, stomach ulcers.

Skin and Appendages: Contact dermatitis, pruritus, sweating.

Respiratory System: Respiratory distress.

Urogenital System: Kidney failure, pyelonephritis, urinary tract infection.

Metabolic and Nutritional Disorders: Weight increase.

Musculoskeletal System: Myalgia.

Body as a Whole: Chest pain, accidental injury, infection.

Special Senses: Eye hemorrhage, ophthalmitis, otitis media, taste perversion, tinnitus.

There have been post-marketing reports of Stevens-Johnson syndrome and toxic epidermal necrolysis associated with the use of diltiazem hydrochloride.

OVERDOSAGE OR EXAGGERATED RESPONSE

Overdosage experience with oral diltiazem hydrochloride has been limited. The administration of ipecac to induce vomiting and activated charcoal to reduce drug absorption have been advocated as initial means of intervention. In addition to gastric lavage, the following measures should also be considered:

Bradycardia: Administer atropine (0.60 mg to 1.0 mg). If there is no response to vagal blockade, administer isoproterenol cautiously.

High-Degree AV Block: Treat as for bradycardia above. Fixed high-degree AV block should be treated with cardiac pacing.

Cardiac Failure: Administer inotropic agents (dopamine or dobutamine) and diuretics.

Hypotension: Vasopressors (*e.g.* dopamine, or levarterenol bitartrate).

Actual treatment and dosage should depend on the severity of the clinical situation as well as the judgment and experience of the treating physician.

Due to extensive metabolism, plasma concentrations after a standard dose of diltiazem can vary over tenfold, which significantly limits their value in evaluating cases of overdosage.

Charcoal hemoperfusion has been used successfully as an adjunct therapy to hasten drug elimination. Overdoses with as much as 10.8 gm of oral diltiazem have been successfully treated using appropriate supportive care.

DOSAGE AND ADMINISTRATION

Hypertensive or anginal patients who are treated with other formulations of diltiazem can safely be switched to Dilacor XR capsules at the nearest equivalent total daily dose. Subsequent titration to higher or lower doses may, however, be necessary and should be initiated as clinically indicated. Studies have shown a slight increase in the rate of absorption of Dilacor XR, when ingested with a high-fat breakfast; therefore, administration in the morning on an empty stomach is recommended.

Patients should be cautioned that the Dilacor XR capsules should not be opened, chewed or crushed and should be swallowed whole.

Dosage: *Hypertension:* Dosages must be adjusted to each patient's needs, starting with 180 mg or 240 mg once-daily. Based on the antihypertensive effect, the dose may be adjusted as needed. Individual patients, particularly ≥ 60 years of age, may respond to a lower dose of 120 mg. The usual dosage range studied in clinical trials was 180 mg to 480 mg once daily. Current clinical experience with the 540 mg dose is limited; the dose may be increased to 540 mg with little or no increased risk of adverse reactions. Doses should not exceed 540 mg once-daily.

While a dose of Dilacor XR given once-daily may produce an antihypertensive effect similar to the same total daily dose given in divided doses, individual dose adjustment may be needed.

Dosage: *Angina:* Dosages for the treatment of angina should be adjusted to each patient's needs, starting with a dose of 120 mg once-daily, which may be titrated to doses of up to 480 mg once-daily. When necessary, titration may be carried out over a 7 to 14 day period.

Concomitant Use with Other Cardiovascular Agents.

1. *Sublingual Nitroglycerin* may be taken as required to abort acute anginal attacks during diltiazem hydrochloride therapy.
2. *Prophylactic Nitrate Therapy*—Diltiazem hydrochloride may be safely co-administered with short- and long-acting nitrates.
3. *Beta-blockers.* (See **WARNINGS** and **PRECAUTIONS**.)
4. *Antihypertensives*—Diltiazem hydrochloride has an additive antihypertensive effect when used with other antihypertensive agents. Therefore, the dosage of diltiazem hydrochloride or the concomitant antihypertensives may need to be adjusted when adding one to the other.

HOW SUPPLIED

[See table at bottom of page]

National Stock Number

Strength	Size	NSN
120 mg	Bottles of 100	6505-01-365-8942
	Bottles of 1000	6505-01-393-7440
180 mg	Bottles of 100	6505-01-355-3602
	Bottles of 1000	6505-01-393-7319
240 mg	Bottles of 100	6505-01-355-3601
	Bottles of 1000	6505-01-393-7437

STORE AT CONTROLLED ROOM TEMPERATURE, 20 to 25°C (68 to 77°F). [See USP].

Keep out of the reach of children.

Caution: Federal law prohibits dispensing without prescription.

U.S. Patent Nos. 4,839,177 and 5,422,123
Manufactured for: WATSON PHARMA
A Division of Watson Laboratories, Inc.
Corona, CA 91720
by Centeon LLC, Kankakee, IL 60901
Rev. 12/97   14100   IN-1005N
WATSON LABORATORIES, INC
CORONA, CA 91720
Shown in Product Identification Guide, page 342

Strength	Size	NDC 52544-	Color		Markings
120 mg	Bottles of 30	732-30	gold cap		Dilacor XR 120 mg
	Bottles of 100	732-01	white body		
	Bottles of 1000	732-10			
180 mg	Bottles of 30	733-30	orange cap		Dilacor XR 180 mg
	Bottles of 100	733-01	white body		
	Unit Dose 100	733-44			
	Bottles of 1000	733-10			
240 mg	Bottles of 30	734-30	brown cap		Dilacor XR 240 mg
	Bottles of 100	734-01	white body		
	Unit Dose 100	734-44			
	Bottles of 1000	734-10			

LEVORA® 0.15/30-21 Tablets   ℞
[lĕ-vŏra]
(levonorgestrel and ethinyl estradiol tablets, USP)

LEVORA® 0.15/30-28 Tablets
[lĕ-vŏra]
(levonorgestrel and ethinyl estradiol tablets, USP)

Patients should be counseled that this product does not protect against HIV infection (AIDS) and other sexually transmitted diseases.
ORAL CONTRACEPTIVE AGENTS

DESCRIPTION

Levora® 0.15/30-21 Tablets provide an oral contraceptive regimen consisting of 21 white tablets containing levonorgestrel 0.15 mg and ethinyl estradiol 0.03 mg.

Levora® 0.15/30-28 Tablets provide an oral contraceptive regimen consisting of 21 white tablets containing levonorgestrel 0.15 mg and ethinyl estradiol 0.03 mg followed by 7 peach tablets containing inert ingredients.

Levonorgestrel is a totally synthetic progestogen with the chemical name (-)-13-Ethyl-17-hydroxy-18,19-dinor-17α-pregn-4-en-20-yn-3-one. Ethinyl estradiol is an estrogen with the chemical name 19-Nor-17α-pregna-1,3,5(10)-trien-20-yne-3,17-diol. Their structural formula follow:
[See chemical structures at top of next column]
The white Levora® 0.15/30 tablets contain the following inactive ingredients: croscarmellose sodium, lactose, magnesium stearate, microcrystalline cellulose, and povidone.

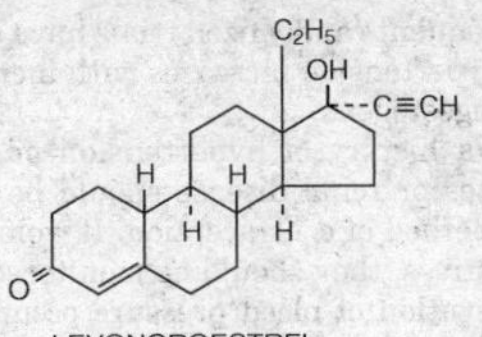
LEVONORGESTREL

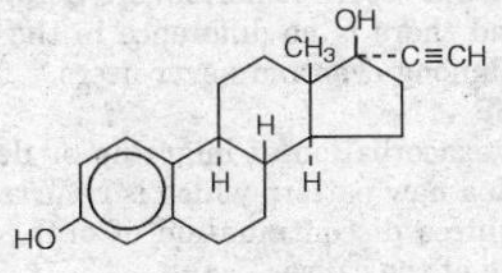
ETHINYL ESTRADIOL

The inactive peach tablets in the 28-day regimen of Levora® 0.15/30 contain the following inactive ingredients: FD&C Yellow No. 6, lactose, magnesium stearate, povidone, and starch (corn).

CLINICAL PHARMACOLOGY

Combination oral contraceptives act by suppression of gonadotrophins. Although the primary mechanism of this action is inhibition of ovulation, other alterations include changes in the cervical mucus (which increase the difficulty of sperm entry into the uterus) and the endometrium (which may reduce the likelihood of implantation).

INDICATIONS AND USAGE

Oral contraceptives are indicated for the prevention of pregnancy in women who elect to use this product as a method of contraception

Oral contraceptives are highly effective. Table I lists the typical accidental pregnancy rates for users of combination oral contraceptives and other methods of contraception.[1] The efficacy of these contraceptive methods, except sterilization, depends upon the reliability with which they are used. Correct and consistent use of methods can result in lower failure rates.

TABLE I: PERCENTAGE OF WOMEN EXPERIENCING A CONTRACEPTIVE FAILURE DURING THE FIRST YEAR OF PERFECT USE AND FIRST YEAR OF TYPICAL USE

	% of Women Experiencing an Accidental Pregnancy within the First Year of Use	
Method	Typical Use[a]	Percent Use[b]
Chance	85	85
Spermicides	21	6
Periodic abstinence	20	1-9
Withdrawal	19	4
Cap		
Parous	36	26
Nulliparous	18	9
Sponge		
Parous	36	20
Nulliparous	18	9
Diaphragm	18	6
Condom		
Female	21	5
Male	12	3
Pill	3	
Progestin only		0.5
Combined		0.1
IUD		
Progesterone	2	1.5
Copper T 380A	0.8	0.6
Injection (Depo-Provera)	0.3	0.3
Implants (Norplant)	0.09	0.09
Female sterilization	0.4	0.4
Male sterilization	0.15	0.10

Adapted with permission.[1]

[a] Among *typical* couples who initiate use of a method (not necessarily for the first time), the percentage who experience an accidental pregnancy during the first year if they do not stop use for any other reason.

[b] Among couples who initiate use of a method (not necessarily for the first time) and who use it *perfectly* (both consistently and correctly), the percentage who experience an accidental pregnancy during the first year if they do not stop use for any other reason.

CONTRAINDICATIONS

Oral contraceptives should not be used in women who have the following conditions:

- Thrombophlebitis or thromboembolic disorders
- A past history of deep vein thrombophlebitis or thromboembolic disorders
- Cerebral vascular or coronary artery disease
- Known or suspected carcinoma of the breast
- Carcinoma of the endometrium or other known or suspected estrogen-dependent neoplasia
- Undiagnosed abnormal genital bleeding
- Cholestatic jaundice of pregnancy or jaundice with prior pill use
- Hepatic adenomas, carcinomas or benign liver tumors
- Known or suspected pregnancy

WARNINGS

Cigarette smoking increases the risk of serious cardiovascular side effects from oral contraceptive use. This risk increases with age and with heavy smoking (15 or more cigarettes per day) and is quite marked in women over 35 years of age. Women who use oral contraceptives should be strongly advised not to smoke.

The use of oral contraceptives is associated with increased risks of several serious conditions including myocardial infraction, thromboembolism, stroke, hepatic neoplasia, and gallbladder disease, although the risk of serious morbidity or mortality is very small in healthy women without underlying risk factors. The risk of morbidity and mortality increases significantly in the presence of other underlying risk factors such as hypertension, hyperlipidemias, hypercholesterolemia, obesity and diabetes.[2-5]

Practitioners prescribing oral contraceptives should be familiar with the following information relating to these risks.

The information contained in this package insert is principally based on studies carried out in patients who used oral contraceptives with higher formulations of both estrogens and progestogens than those in common use today. The effect of long-term use of the oral contraceptives with lower formulations of both estrogens and progestogens remains to be determined.

Throughout this labeling, epidemiological studies reported are of two types: retrospective or case control studies and prospective or cohort studies.[6-11] Case control studies provide a measure of the relative risk of a disease. Relative risk, the *ratio* of the incidence of a disease among oral contraceptive users to that among non-users, cannot be assessed directly from case control studies, but the odds ratio obtained is a measure of relative risk. The relative risk does not provide information on the actual clinical occurrence of a disease. Cohort studies provide not only a measure of the relative risk but of a measure of attributable risk, which is the *difference* in the incidence of disease between oral contraceptive users and non-users. The attributable risk does provide information about the actual occurrence of a disease in the population. (Adapted from ref. 12 and 13 with the author's permission.) For further information, the reader is referred to a text on epidemiological methods.

1. THROMBOEMBOLIC DISORDERS AND OTHER VASCULAR PROBLEMS

a. Myocardial infarction

An increased risk of myocardial infarction has been attributed to oral contractive use. This risk is primarily in smokers or women with other underlying risk factors for coronary artery disease such as hypertension, hypercholesterolemia, morbid obesity and diabetes.[2-5, 13] The relative risk of heart attack for current oral contraceptive users has been estimated to be 2 to 6.[2, 14-19] The risk is very low under the age of 30. However, there is the possibility of a risk of cardiovascular disease even in very young women who take oral contraceptives.

Smoking in combination with oral contraceptive use has been shown to contribute substantially to the incidence of myocardial infractions in women in their mid-thirties or older, with smoking accounting for the majority of excess cases.[20]

Mortality rates associated with circulatory disease have been shown to increase substantially in smokers over the age of 35 and non-smokers over the age of 40 among women who use oral contraceptives (see Table II).[16]

TABLE II: CIRCULATORY DISEASE MORTALITY RATES PER 100, 000 WOMAN YEARS BY AGE, SMOKING STATUS AND ORAL CONTRACEPTIVE USE

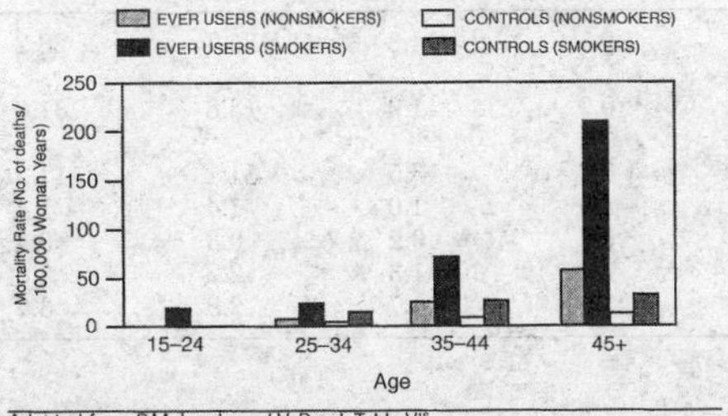
EVER USERS (NONSMOKERS)
CONTROLS (NONSMOKERS)
EVER USERS (SMOKERS)
CONTROLS (SMOKERS)
Mortality Rate (No. of deaths/ 100,000 Woman Years)
250
200
150
100
50
0
15–24
25–34
35–44
45+
Age

Adapted from P.M. Layde and V. Beral, Table V[16]

Oral contraceptives may compound the effects of well-known risk factors such as hypertension, diabetes, hyperlipidemias, hypercholesterolemia age and obesity.[3, 13, 21] In particular, some progestogens are known to decrease HDL cholesterol and cause glucose intolerance, while estrogens may create a state of hyperinsulinism.[21-25] Oral contraceptives have been shown to increase blood pressure among users (see **WARNINGS**, section 9). Similar effects on risk factors have been associated with an increased risk of heart disease. Oral contraceptives must be used with caution in women with cardiovascular disease risk factors.

b. Thromboembolism

An increased risk of thromboembolic and thrombotic disease associated with the use of oral contraceptives is well established. Case control studies have found the relative risk of users compared to non-users to be 3 for the first episode of superficial venous thrombosis, 4 to 11 for deep vein thrombosis or pulmonary embolism, and 1.5 to 6 for women with predisposing conditions for venous thromboembolic disease.[12, 13, 26-31] Cohort studies have shown the relative risk to be somewhat lower, about 3 for new cases and about 4.5 for new cases requiring hospitalization.[32] The risk of thromboembolic disease due to oral contraceptives is not related to length of use and disappears after pill use is stopped.[12]

A 2- to 6-fold increase in relative risk of post-operative thromboembolic complications has been reported with the use of oral contraceptives. The relative risk of venous thrombosis in women who have predisposing conditions is twice that of women without such medical conditions.[83] If feasible, oral contraceptives should be discontinued at least 4 weeks prior to and for 2 weeks after elective surgery and during and following prolonged immobilization. Since the immediate postpartum period also is associated with an increased risk of thromboembolism, oral contraceptives should be started no earlier than 4 to 6 weeks after delivery in women who elect not to breast feed.[33]

c. Cerebrovascular diseases

An increase in both the relative and attributable risks of cerebrovascular events (thrombotic and hemorrhagic strokes) has been shown in users of oral contraceptives. In general, the risk is greatest among older (>35 years), hypertensive women who also smoke. Hypertension was found to be a risk factor for both users and non-users for both types of strokes while smoking interacted to increase the risk for hemorrhagic strokes.[34]

In a large study, the relative risk of thrombotic strokes has been shown to range from 3 for normotensive users to 14 for users with severe hypertension.[35] The relative risk of hemorrhagic stroke is reported to be 1.2 for non-smokers who used oral contraceptives, 2.6 for smokers who did not use oral contraceptives, 7.6 for smokers who used oral contraceptives, 1.8 for normotensive users and 25.7 for users with severe hypertension.[35] The attributable risk also is greater in women in their mid-thirties or older and among smokers.[13]

d. Dose-related risk of vascular disease with oral contraceptives

A positive association has been observed between the amount of estrogen and progestogen in oral contraceptives and the risk of vascular disease.[36-38] A decline in serum high-density lipoproteins (HDL) has been reported with many progestational agents.[22-24] A decline in serum high-density lipoproteins has been associated with an increased incidence of ischemic heart disease.[39] Because estrogens increase HDL cholesterol, the net effect of an oral contraceptive depends on a balance achieved between doses of estrogen and progestogen and the nature and absolute amount of progestogens used in the contraceptives. The amount of both hormones should be considered in the choice of an oral contraceptive.[37]

Minimizing exposure to estrogen and progestogen is in keeping with good principles of therapeutics. For any particular estrogen/progestogen combination, the dosage regimen prescribed should be one which contains the least amount of estrogen and progestogen that is compatible with a low failure rate and the needs of the individual patient. New acceptors of oral contraceptive agents should be started on preparations containing the lowest estrogen content that produces satisfactory results for the individual.

e. Persistence of risk of vascular disease

There are three studies which have shown persistence of risk of vascular disease for ever-users of oral contraceptives.[17, 34, 40] In a study in the United States, the risk of developing myocardial infarction after discontinuing oral contraceptives persists for at least 9 years for women 40-49 years who had used oral contraceptives for 5 or more years, but this increased risk was not demonstrated in other age groups.[17] In another study in Great Britain, the risk of developing cerebrovascular disease persisted for at least 6 years after discontinuation of oral contraceptives, although excess risk was very small.[40] There is a significantly increased relative risk of subarachnoid hemorrhage after ter-

Continued on next page

Levora—Cont.

mination of use of oral contraceptives.[34] However, these studies were performed with oral contraceptive formulations containing 50 mcg or higher of estrogen.

2. ESTIMATES OF MORTALITY FROM CONTRACEPTIVE USE

One study gathered data from a variety of sources which have estimated the mortality rates associated with different methods of contraception at different ages (see Table III).[41] These estimates include the combined risk of death associated with contraceptive methods plus the risk attributable to pregnancy in the event of method failure. Each method of contraception has its specific benefits and risks. The study concluded that with the exception of oral contraceptive users 35 and older who smoke and 40 and older who do not smoke, mortality associated with all methods of birth control is low and below that associated with childbirth. The observation of a possible increase in risk of mortality with age for oral contraceptive users is based on data gathered in the 1970's–but not reported in the U.S. until 1983.[16, 41] However, current clinical practice involves the use of lower estrogen dose formulations combined with careful restriction of oral contraceptive use to women who do not have the various risk factors listed in this labeling.

Because of these changes in practice and, also, because of some limited new data which suggest that the risk of cardiovascular disease with the use of oral contraceptives may now be less than previously observed,[78, 79] the Fertility and Maternal Health Drugs Advisory Committee was asked to review the topic in 1989. The Committee concluded that although cardiovascular disease risks may be increased with oral contraceptive use after age 40 in healthy non-smoking women (even with the newer low-dose formulations), there are greater potential health risks associated with pregnancy in older women and with the alternative surgical and medical procedures which may be necessary if such women do not have access to effective and acceptable means of contraception.

Therefore, the Committee recommended that the benefits of oral contraceptive use by healthy non-smoking women over 40 may outweigh the possible risks. Of course, older women, as all women who take oral contraceptives, should take the lowest possible dose formulation that is effective.[80]

[See table III below]

3. CARCINOMA OF THE BREAST AND REPRODUCTIVE ORGANS

Numerous epidemiological studies have been performed on the incidence of breast, endometrial, ovarian and cervical cancer in women using oral contraceptives. The overwhelming evidence in the literature suggests that use of oral contraceptives is not associated with an increase in the risk of developing breast cancer, regardless of the age and parity of first use or with most of the marketed brands and doses.[42-44] The Cancer and Steroid Hormone (CASH) study also showed no latent effect on the risk of breast cancer for at least a decade following long-term use.[43] A few studies have shown a slightly increased relative risk of developing breast cancer,[44-47] although the methodology of these studies, which included differences in examination of users and non-users and differences in age at start of use, has been questioned.[47-49] Some studies have reported an increased relative risk of developing breast cancer, particularly at a younger age. This increased relative risk appears to be related to duration of use.[81-82]

Some studies suggest that oral contraceptive use has been associated with an increase in the risk of cervical intraepithelial neoplasia in some populations of women.[50-53] However, there continues to be controversy about the extent to which such findings may be due to differences in sexual behavior and other factors.

In spite of many studies of the relationship between oral contraceptive use and breast or cervical cancers, a cause and effect relationship has not been established.

4. HEPATIC NEOPLASIA

Benign hepatic adenomas are associated with oral contraceptive use although the incidence of benign tumors is rare in the United States. Indirect calculations have estimated the attributable risk to be in the range of 3.3 cases per 100,000 for users, a risk that increases after 4 or more years of use.[54] Rupture of rare, benign, hepatic adenomas may cause death through intra-abdominal hemorrhage.[55-56]

Studies in the United States and Britain have shown an increased risk of developing hepatocellular carcinoma in long-term (>8 years) oral contraceptive users,[57-59] However, these cancers are extremely rare in the United States and the attributable risk (the excess incidence) of liver cancers in oral contraceptive users approaches less than 1 per 1,000,000 users.

5. OCULAR LESIONS

There have been clinical case reports of retinal thrombosis associated with the use of oral contraceptives. Oral contraceptives should be discontinued if there is unexplained partial or complete loss of vision; onset of proptosis or diplopia; papilledema; or retinal vascular lesions. Appropriate diagnostic and therapeutic measures should be undertaken immediately.

6. ORAL CONTRACEPTIVE USE BEFORE OR DURING EARLY PREGNANCY

Extensive epidemiological studies have revealed no increased risk of birth defects in women who have used oral contraceptives prior to pregnancy.[60-62] Studies also do not suggest a teratogenic effect, particularly insofar as cardiac anomalies and limb reduction defects are concerned, when taken inadvertently during early pregnancy.[60,61,63,64]

The administration of oral contraceptives to induce withdrawal bleeding should not be used as a test for pregnancy. Oral contraceptives should not be used during pregnancy to treat threatened or habitual abortion.

It is recommended that for any patient who has missed 2 consecutive periods, pregnancy should be ruled out before continuing oral contraceptives use. If the patient has not adhered to the prescribed schedule, the possibility of pregnancy should be considered at the first missed period. Oral contraceptive use should be discontinued if pregnancy is confirmed.

7. GALLBLADDER DISEASE

Earlier studies have reported an increased lifetime relative risk of gallbladder surgery in users of oral contraceptives and estrogens.[65-66] More recent studies, however, have shown that the relative risk of developing gallbladder disease among oral contraceptive users may be minimal.[67] The recent findings of minimal risk may be related to the use of oral contraceptive formulations containing lower hormonal doses of estrogens and progestogens.[68]

8. CARBOHYDRATE AND LIPID METABOLIC EFFECTS

Oral contraceptives have been shown to cause glucose intolerance in a significant percentage of users.[25] Oral contraceptives containing greater than 75 mcg of estrogen cause hyperinsulinism, while lower doses of estrogen cause less glucose intolerance.[70] Progestogens increase insulin secretion and create insulin resistance, this effect varying with different progestational agents.[25, 71] However, in the non-diabetic woman, oral contraceptives appear to have no effect on fasting blood glucose.[69] Because of these demonstrated effects, prediabetic and diabetic women should be carefully observed while taking oral contraceptives.

Some women may develop persistent hypertriglyceridemia while on the pill.[72] As discussed earlier (see **WARNINGS**, sections 1a. and 1d.), changes in serum triglycerides and lipoprotein levels have been reported in oral contraceptive users.[23]

9. ELEVATED BLOOD PRESSURE

An increase in blood pressure have been reported in women taking oral contraceptives and this increase is more likely in older oral contraceptive users and with continued use.[73, 84] Data from the Royal College of General Practitioners and subsequent randomized trials have shown that the incidence of hypertension increases with increasing concentrations of progestogens.

Women with a history of hypertension or hypertension-related diseases or renal disease should be encouraged to use another method of contraception. If women elect to use oral contraceptives, they should be monitored closely and if significant elevation of blood pressure occurs, oral contraceptives should be discontinued. For most women, elevated blood pressure will return to normal after stopping oral contraceptives and there is no difference in the occurrence of hypertension among ever-and never-users.[73-75]

10. HEADACHE

The onset or exacerbation of migraine or development of headache with a new pattern which is recurrent, persistent or severe requires discontinuation of oral contraceptives and evaluation of the cause.

11. BLEEDING IRREGULARITIES

Breakthrough bleeding and spotting are sometimes encountered in patients on oral contraceptives, especially during the first 3 months of use. Non-hormonal causes should be considered and adequate diagnostic measures taken to rule out malignancy or pregnancy in the event of breakthrough bleeding, as in the case of any abnormal vaginal bleeding. If pathology has been excluded, time or a change to another formulation may solve the problem. In the event of amenorrhea, pregnancy should be ruled out.

Some woman may encounter post-pill amenorrhea or oligomenorrhea, especially when such a condition was pre-existent.

PRECAUTIONS

GENERAL

Patients should be counseled that this product does not protect against HIV infection (AIDS) and other sexually transmitted diseases.

1. PHYSICAL EXAMINATION AND FOLLOW-UP

It is good medical practice for all women to have annual history and physical examinations, including women using oral contraceptives. The physical examination, however, may be deferred until after initiation of oral contraceptives if requested by the woman and judged appropriate by the clinician. The physical examination should include special reference to blood pressure, breasts, abdomen and pelvic organs, including cervical cytology, and relevant laboratory tests. In case of undiagnosed, persistent or recurrent abnormal vaginal bleeding, appropriate measures should be conducted to rule out malignancy. Women with a strong family history of breast cancer or who have breast nodules should be monitored with particular care.

2. LIPID DISORDERS

Women who are being treated for hyperlipidemias should be followed closely if they elect to use oral contraceptives. Some progestogens may elevate LDL levels and may render the control of hyperlipidemias more difficult.

3. LIVER FUNCTION

If jaundice develops in any woman receiving oral contraceptives the medication should be discontinued. Steroid hormones may be poorly metabolized in patients with impaired liver function.

4. FLUID RETENTION

Oral contraceptives may cause some degree of fluid retention. They should be prescribed with caution, and only with careful monitoring, in patients with conditions which might be aggravated by fluid retention.

5. EMOTIONAL DISORDERS

Women with a history of depression should be carefully observed and the drug discontinued if depression recurs to a serious degree.

6. CONTACT LENSES

Contact lens wearers who develop visual changes or changes in lens tolerance should be assessed by an ophthalmologist.

7. DRUG INTERACTIONS

Reduced efficacy and increased incidence of breakthrough bleeding and menstrual irregularities have been associated with concomitant use of rifampin. A similar association, though less marked, has been suggested with barbiturates, phenylbutazone, phenytoin sodium, and possibly with griseofulvin, ampicillin and tetracyclines.[76]

8. INTERACTIONS WITH LABORATORY TESTS

Certain endocrine and liver function tests and blood components may be affected by oral contraceptives:

a. Increased prothrombin and factors VII, VIII, IX and X; decreased antithrombin 3; increased norepinephrine-induced platelet aggregability.

b. Increased thyroid binding globulin (TBG) leading to increased circulating total thyroid hormone, as measured by protein-bound iodine (PBI), T4 by column or by radioimmunoassay. Free T3 resin uptake is decreased, reflecting the elevated TBG. Free T4 concentration is unaltered.

c. Other binding proteins may be elevated in the serum.

d. Sex steroid binding globulins are increased and result in elevated levels of total circulating sex steroids and corticoids; however, free or biologically active levels remain unchanged.

TABLE III: ESTIMATED ANNUAL NUMBER OF BIRTH-RELATED OR METHOD-RELATED DEATHS ASSOCIATED WITH CONTROL OF FERTILITY PER 100,000 NONSTERILE WOMEN, BY FERTILITY CONTROL METHOD ACCORDING TO AGE

Method of control and outcome	15–19	20–24	25–29	30–34	35–39	40–44
No fertility control methods*	7.0	7.4	9.1	14.8	25.7	28.2
Oral contraceptives non-smoker**	0.3	0.5	0.9	1.9	13.8	31.6
Oral contraceptives smoker**	2.2	3.4	6.6	13.5	51.1	117.2
IUD**	0.8	0.8	1.0	1.0	1.4	1.4
Condom*	1.1	1.6	0.7	0.2	0.3	0.4
Diaphragm/Spermicide*	1.9	1.2	1.2	1.3	2.2	2.8
Periodic abstinence*	2.5	1.6	1.6	1.7	2.9	3.6

*Deaths are birth-related

**Deaths are method-related

Estimates adapted from H.W. Ory, Table 3[41]

e. Triglycerides may be increased.
f. Glucose tolerance may be decreased.
g Serum folate levels may be depressed by oral contraceptive therapy. This may be of clinical significance if a woman becomes pregnant shortly after discontinuing oral contraceptives.

9. CARCINOGENESIS
See **WARNINGS** section.

10. PREGNANCY
Pregnancy Category X. See **CONTRAINDICATIONS** and **WARNINGS** sections.

11. NURSING MOTHERS
Small amounts of oral contraceptive steroids have been identified in the milk of nursing mothers and a few adverse effects on the child have been reported, including jaundice and breast enlargement. In addition, oral contraceptives given in the postpartum period may interfere with lactation by decreasing the quantity and quality of breast milk. If possible, the nursing mother should be advised not to use oral contraceptives but to use other forms of contraception until she has completely weaned her child.

INFORMATION FOR THE PATIENT
See **PATIENT LABELING** printed below.

ADVERSE REACTIONS

An increased risk of the following serious adverse reactions has been associated with the use of oral contraceptives (see **WARNINGS** section):

- Thrombophlebitis
- Arterial thromboembolism
- Pulmonary embolism
- Myocardial infarction
- Cerebral hemorrhage
- Cerebral thrombosis
- Hypertension
- Gallbladder disease
- Hepatic adenomas, carcinomas or benign liver tumors

There is evidence of an association between the following conditions and the use of oral contraceptives, although additional confirmatory studies are needed:

- Mesenteric thrombosis
- Retinal thrombosis

The following adverse reactions have been reported in patients receiving oral contraceptives and are believed to be drug-related:

- Nausea
- Vomiting
- Gastrointestinal symptoms (such as abdominal cramps and bloating)
- Breakthrough bleeding
- Spotting
- Change in menstrual flow
- Amenorrhea
- Temporary infertility after discontinuation of treatment
- Edema
- Melasma which may persist
- Breast changes: tenderness, enlargement, secretion
- Change in weight (increase or decrease)
- Change in cervical erosion and secretion
- Diminution in lactation when given immediately postpartum
- Cholestatic jaundice
- Migraine
- Rash (allergic)
- Mental depression
- Reduced tolerance to carbohydrates
- Vaginal candidiasis
- Change in corneal curvature (steepening)
- Intolerance to contact lenses

The following adverse reactions have been reported in users of oral contraceptives and the association has been neither confirmed nor refuted:

- Pre-menstrual syndrome
- Cataracts
- Changes in appetite
- Cystitis-like syndrome
- Headache
- Nervousness
- Dizziness
- Hirsutism
- Loss of scalp hair
- Erythema multiforme
- Erythema nodosum
- Hemorrhagic eruption
- Vaginitis
- Porphyria
- Impaired renal function
- Hemolytic uremic syndrome
- Budd-Chiari syndrome
- Acne
- Changes in libido
- Colitis

OVERDOSAGE

Serious ill effects have not been reported following acute ingestion of large doses of oral contraceptives by young children. Overdosage may cause nausea, and withdrawal bleeding may occur in females.

NON-CONTRACEPTIVE HEALTH BENEFITS
The following non-contraceptive health benefits related to the use of oral contraceptives are supported by epidemiological studies which largely utilized oral contraceptive formulations containing estrogen doses exceeding 0.035 mg of ethinyl estradiol or 0.05 mg of mestranol.[6-11]

Effects on menses:

- Increased menstrual cycle regularity
- Decreased blood loss and decreased incidence of iron deficiency anemia
- Decreased incidence of dysmenorrhea

Effects related to inhibition of ovulation:

- Decreased incidence of functional ovarian cysts
- Decreased incidence of ectopic pregnancies

Effects from long-term use:

- Decreased incidence of fibroadenomas and fibrocystic disease of the breast
- Decreased incidence of acute pelvic inflammatory disease
- Decreased incidence of endometrial cancer
- Decreased incidence of ovarian cancer

DOSAGE AND ADMINISTRATION

To achieve maximum contraceptive effectiveness, oral contraceptives must be taken exactly as directed and at intervals not exceeding 24 hours.

21-Day Schedule: For a DAY 1 START, count the first day of menstrual flow as Day 1 and the first tablet (white) is then taken on Day 1. For a SUNDAY START when menstrual flow begins on or before Sunday, the first tablet (white) is taken on that day. With either a DAY 1 START or SUNDAY START, 1 tablet is taken each day at the same time for 21 days. No tablets are taken for 7 days, then, whether bleeding has stopped or not, a new course is started of 1 tablet a day for 21 days. This institutes a 3 weeks on, 1 week off dosage regimen.

28-Day Schedule: For a DAY 1 START, count the first day of menstrual flow as Day 1 and the first tablet (white) is then taken on Day 1. For a SUNDAY START when menstrual flow begins on or before Sunday, the first tablet (white) is taken on that day. With either a DAY 1 START or SUNDAY START, 1 tablet (white) is taken each day at the same time for 21 days. Then the peach tablets are taken for 7 days, whether bleeding has stopped or not. After all 28 tablets have been taken, whether bleeding has stopped or not, the same dosage schedule is repeated beginning on the following day.

INSTRUCTIONS TO PATIENTS

- To achieve maximum contraceptive effectiveness, the oral contraceptive pill must be taken exactly as directed and at intervals not exceeding 24 hours.
- Important: Women should be instructed to use an additional method of protection until after the first 7 days of administration *in the initial cycle.*
- Due to the normally increased risk of thromboembolism occurring postpartum, women should be instructed not to initiate treatment with oral contraceptives earlier than 4 weeks after a full-term delivery. If pregnancy is terminated in the first 12 weeks, the patient should be instructed to start oral contraceptives immediately or within 7 days. If pregnancy is terminated after 12 weeks, the patient should be instructed to start oral contraceptives after 2 weeks.[33, 77]
- If spotting or breakthrough bleeding should occur, the patient should continue the medication according to the schedule. Should spotting or breakthrough bleeding persist, the patient should notify her physician.
- If the patient misses 1 pill, she should be instructed to take it as soon as she remembers and then take the next pill at the regular time. The patient should be advised that missing a pill can cause spotting or light bleeding and that she may be a little sick to her stomach on the days she takes the missed pill with her regularly scheduled pill. If the patient has missed more than one pill, see DETAILED PATIENT LABELING: HOW TO TAKE THE PILL, WHAT TO DO IF YOU MISS PILLS.
- Use of oral contraceptives in the event of a missed menstrual period:
  1. If the patient has not adhered to the prescribed dosage regimen, the possibility of pregnancy should be considered after the first missed period and oral contraceptives should be withheld until pregnancy has been ruled out.
  2. If the patient has adhered to the prescribed regimen and misses 2 consecutive periods, pregnancy should be ruled out before continuing the contraceptive regimen.

HOW SUPPLIED

Levora® 0.15/30-21 Tablets (levonorgestrel and ethinyl estradiol tablets, USP): Each white tablet is unscored, round in shape, with "15/30" debossed on one side and "WATSON" on the other side, and contains 0.15 mg levonorgestrel and 0.03 mg ethinyl estradiol. Levora® 0.15/30-21 is packaged in cartons of six tablet dispensers. Each dispenser contains 21 white (active) tablets.

Levora® 0.15/30-28 Tablets (levonorgestrel and ethinyl estradiol tablets, USP): Each white tablet is unscored, round in shape, with "15/30" debosssed on one side and "WATSON" on the other side, and contains 0.15 mg levonorgestrel and 0.03 mg ethinyl estradiol. Levora® 0.15/30-28 is packaged in cartons of six tablet dispensers. Each tablet dispenser contains 21 white (active) tablets and 7 peach (inert) tablets. Inert tablets are unscored, round in shape with "WATSON" debossed on one side and PI on the other side.

Rx only
Store at controlled room temperature 15°-25°C (59°-77°F).

REFERENCES

1. Hatcher, R.A., Trussell, J., Stewart, F., et al.: *Contraceptive Technology: Sixteenth Revised Edition*, New York, NY, 1994. **2.** Mann, J., et al.: *Br Med J* 2(5956)241-245, 1975. **3.** Knopp, R.H.: *J Reprod Med* 31(9):913-921, 1986. **4.** Mann, J.I., et al.: *Br Med J* 2:445-447, 1976. **5.** Ory, H.: *JAMA* 237: 2619-2622, 1977. **6.** The Cancer and Steroid Hormone Study of the Centers for Disease Control: *JAMA* 249(2): 1596-1599, 1983. **7.** The Cancer and Steroid Hormone Study of the Centers for Disease Control: *JAMA* 257(6):796-800, 1987. **8.** Ory, H.W.: *JAMA* 228(1):68-69, 1974. **9.** Ory, H.W., et al.: *N Eng J Med* 294:419-422, 1976. **10.** Ory, H.W.: *Fam Plann Perspect* 14:182-184, 1982. **11.** Ory, H.W., et al.: *Making Choices*, New York, The Alan Guttmacher Institute, 1983. **12.** Stadel, B.: *N Eng J Med* 305(11):612-618, 1981. **13.** Stadel, B.: *N Eng J Med* 305(12):672-677, 1981. **14.** Adam, S., et al.: *Br J Obstet Gynaecol* 88:838-845, 1981. **15.** Mann, J., et al.: *Br Med J* 2(5965):245-248, 1975. **16.** Royal College of General Practitioners' Oral Contraceptive Study: *Lancet* 1:541-546, 1981. **17.** Slone, D., et al.: *N Eng J Med* 305(8):420-424, 1981. **18.** Vessey, M.P.: *Br J Fam Plann* 6(supplement):1-12, 1980. **19.** Russell-Briefel, R., et al.: *Prev Med* 15:352-362, 1986. **20.** Goldbaum, G., et al.: *JAMA* 258(10):1339-1342, 1987. **21.** LaRosa, J.C.: *J Reprod Med* 31(9):906-912, 1986. **22.** Krauss, R.M., et al.: *Am J Obstet Gynecol* 145:446-452, 1983. **23.** Wahl, P., et al.: *N Eng J Med* 308(15):862-867, 1983. **24.** Wynn, V., et al.: *Am J Obstet Gynecol* 142(6):766-771, 1982. **25.** Wynn, V., et al.: *J Reprod Med* 31(9):892-897, 1986. **26.** Inman, W.H., et al.: *Br Med J* 2(5599):193-199, 1968. **27.** Maguire, M.G., et al.: *Am J Epidemiol* 110 (2):188-195, 1979. **28.** Petitti, D., et al.: *JAMA* 242(11):1150-1154, 1979. **29.** Vessey, M.P., et al.: *Br Med J* 2(5599):199-205, 1968. **30.** Vessey, M.P., et al.: *Br Med J* 2(5658):651-657, 1969. **31.** Porter, J.B., et al.: *Obstet Gynecol* 59(3):299-302, 1982. **32.** Vessey, M.P., et al.: *J Biosoc Sci* 8:373-427, 1976. **33.** Mishell, D.R., et al.: *Reproductive Endocrinology*, Philadelphia, F.A. Davis Co., 1979. **34.** Pettiti, D.B., et al.: *Lancet* 2:234-236, 1978. **35.** Collaborative Group for the Study of Stroke in Young Women: *JAMA* 231(7):718-722, 1975. **36.** Inman, W.H., et al.: *Br Med J* 2:203-209, 1970. **37.** Meade, T.W., et al.: *Br Med J* 280(6224):1157-1161, 1980. **38.** Kay, C.R., *Am J Obstet Gynecol* 142(6):762-765, 1982. **39.** Gordon, T., et al.: *Am J Med* 62:707-714, 1977. **40.** Royal College of General Practitioners' Oral Contraception Study: *J Coll Gen Pract* 33:75-82, 1983. **41.** Ory, H.W.: *Fam Plann Perspect* 15(2):57-63, 1983. **42.** Paul, C., et al.: *Br Med J* 293:723-725, 1986. **43.** The Cancer and Steroid Hormone Study of the Centers for Disease Control: *N Eng J Med* 315(7):405-411, 1986. **44.** Pike, M.C., et al.: *Lancet* 2:926-929, 1983. **45.** Miller, D.R., et al.: *Obstet Gynecol* 68:863-868, 1986. **46.** Olsson, H., et al.: *Lancet* 2:748-749, 1985. **47.** McPherson, K., et al.: *Br J Cancer* 56:653-660, 1987. **48.** Huggins, G.R., et al.: *Fetil Steril* 47(5):733-761, 1987. **49.** McPherson, K., et al.: *Br Med J* 293:709-710, 1986. **50.** Ory, H., et al.: *Am J Obstet Gynecol* 124(6):573-577, 1976. **51.** Vessey, M.P., et al.: *Lancet* 2:930, 1983. **52.** Brinton, L.A., et al.: *Int J Cancer* 38: 339-344, 1986. **53.** WHO Collaborative Study of Neoplasia and Steroid Contraceptives: *Br Med J* 290:961-965, 1985. **54.** Rooks, J.B., et al.: *JAMA* 242(7):644-648, 1979.**55.** Bein, N.N., et al.: *Br J Surg* 64: 433-435, 1977. **56.** Klatskin, G.: *Gastroenterology* 73:386-394, 1977. **57.** Henderson, B.E., et al.: *Br J Cancer* 48:437-440, 1983. **58.** Neuberger, J., et al.: *Br Med J* 292:1355-1357, 1986. **59.** Forman, D., et al.: *Br Med J* 292:1357-1361, 1986. **60.** Harlap, S., et al.: *Obstet Gynecol* 55(4):447-452, 1980. **61.** Savolainen, E., et al.: *Am J Obstet Gynecol* 140(5):521-524, 1981. **62.** Janerich, D.T., et al.: *Am J Epidemiol* 112(1):73-79, 1980. **63.** Ferencz, C., et al.: *Teratology* 21:225-259, 1980. **64.** Rothman, K.J., et al.: *Am J Epidemiol*, 109(4):433-439, 1979. **65.** Boston Collaborative Drug Surveillance Program: *Lancet* 1:1399-1404, 1973. **66.** Royal College of General Practioners: *Oral contraceptives and health*. New York, Pittman, 1974. **67.** Rome Group for the Epidemiology and Prevention of Cholelithiasis: *Am J Epidemiol* 119(5):796-805, 1984. **68.** Strom, B.L., et al.: *Clin Pharmacol Ther* 39(3):335-341, 1986. **69.** Perlman, J.A., et al.: *J Chronic Dis* 38(10):857-864, 1985. **70.** Wynn, V., et al.: *Lancet* 1:1045-1049, 1979. **71.** Wynn, V.: *Progesterone and Progestin*, New York, Raven Press, 1983. **72.** Wynn, V., et al.: *Lancet* 2:720-723, 1966. **73.** Fisch, I.R., et al.: *JAMA* 237(23):2499-2503, 1977. **74.** Laragh, J.H.: *Am J Obstet Gynecol* 126(1):141-147, 1976. **75.** Ramcharan, S., et al.: *Pharmacology of Steroid Contraceptive Drugs*,

Continued on next page

Levora—Cont.

New York, Raven Press, 1977. **76.** Stockley, I.; *Pharm J* 216: 140-143, 1976. **77.** Dickey, R.P.: *Managing Contraceptive Pill Patients*, Oklahoma, Creative Informatics Inc., 1984. **78.** Porter, J.B., Hunter, J., Jick, H., et al.: *Obstet Gynecol* 1985;66:1-4. **79.** Porter, J.B., Hershel, J., Walker, A.M.: *Obstet Gynecol* 1987;70:29-32. **80.** Fertility and Maternal Health Drugs Advisory Committee, F.D.A., October, 1989. **81.** Schlesselman, J., Stadel, B.V., Murray, P., Lai, S.: *Breast cancer in relation to early use of oral contraceptives. JAMA* 1988;259:1828-1833. **82.** Hennekens, C.H., Speizer, F.E., Lipnick, R.J., Rosner, B., Bain, C., Belanger, C., Stampfer, M.J., Willett, W., Peto, R.: *A case—control study of oral contraceptive use and breast cancer*. JNCI 1984;72:39-42. **83.** Royal College of General Practitioners: *Oral contraceptives, venous thrombosis, and varicose veins. J Coll Gen Pract* 28:393-399, 1978. **84.** Royal College of General Practitioners' Oral Contraception Study: *Effect on hypertension and benign breast disease of progestogen component in combined oral contraceptives, Lancet* 1:624, 1977.

Manufactured for
WATSON PHARMA
A Division of
Watson Laboratories, Inc.
Corona, CA 91720
By Patheon Inc.
Mississauga, ON L5N 7K9 CANADA

Address medical inquiries to:
WATSON PHARMA
Medical Information
PO Box 1900
Corona, CA 91718
WATSON PHARMA

Printed in USA

Shown in Product Identification Guide, page 342

LOXITANE® ℞
LOXAPINE SUCCINATE
Capsules

LOXITANE® C ℞
LOXAPINE HYDROCHLORIDE
Oral Concentrate
For Oral Use

LOXITANE® IM ℞
LOXAPINE HYDROCHLORIDE
For Intramuscular Use Only

DESCRIPTION

LOXITANE loxapine, a dibenzoxazepine compound, represents a subclass of tricyclic antipsychotic agents, chemically distinct from the thioxanthenes, butyrophenones, and phenothiazines. Chemically, it is 2-Chloro-11-(4-methyl-1-piperazinyl)-dibenz[*b,f*] [1,4]oxazepine. It is present in capsules as the succinate salt, and in the concentrate and parenteral primarily as the hydrochloride salt.

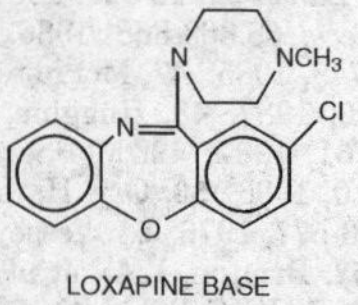

LOXAPINE BASE

CAPSULES — Each capsule contains loxapine succinate equivalent to 5, 10, 25, or 50 mg of loxapine base and the following inactive ingredients: Blue 1, Gelatin, Lactose, Magnesium Stearate, Titanium Dioxide, and Yellow 10. Additionally, the 5 mg capsule contains Red 33, the 10 mg capsule contains Red 28 and Red 33, and the 25 mg capsule contains FD&C Yellow No. 6.

ORAL CONCENTRATE — Each mL contains loxapine hydrochloride equivalent to 25 mg of loxapine base and propylene glycol as an inactive ingredient.

Hydrochloric acid and, if necessary, sodium hydroxide are used to adjust pH to approximately 5.8 during manufacture.

INTRAMUSCULAR — (Sterile) - Not for Intravenous Use - Each mL contains loxapine hydrochloride equivalent to 50 mg of loxapine base. Inactive Ingredients: Polysorbate 80 NF 5% w/v, Propylene Glycol 70% v/v, and Water for Injection qs ad 100% v.

Hydrochloric acid and, if necessary, sodium hydroxide are used to adjust pH to approximately 5.5 during manufacture.

CLINICAL PHARMACOLOGY

Pharmacodynamics

Pharmacologically, loxapine is a tranquilizer for which the exact mode of action has not been established. However, changes in the level of excitability of subcortical inhibitory areas have been observed in several animal species in association with such manifestations of tranquilization as calming effects and suppression of aggressive behavior.

In normal human volunteers, signs of sedation were seen within 20 to 30 minutes after administration, were most pronounced within 1 1/2 to three hours, and lasted through 12 hours. Similar timing of primary pharmacologic effects was seen in animals.

Absorption, Distribution, Metabolism, and Excretion

After administration of LOXITANE as an oral solution, systemic bioavailability of the parent drug was only about one third that after an equivalent intramuscular dose (25 mg base) in male volunteers. C_{max} for the parent drug was similar for the IM and oral administrations, whereas T_{max} was significantly longer for the IM administration than the oral administration (approximately 5 vs 1 hour). The lower systemic availability of the parent drug after oral administration as compared to the IM administration may be due to first pass metabolism of the oral form.

This is supported by the finding that two metabolites found in serum (8-hydroxyloxapine and 8-hydroxydesmethylloxapine) were formed to a lesser extent after IM administration of loxapine as compared to oral administration.

The apparent half-life of loxapine after oral and IM administration is approximately four hours (range, 1 to 14 hours) and 12 hours (range, 8 to 23 hours), respectively. The extended half-life for the IM administration as compared to the oral administration may be explained by prolonged absorption of loxapine from the muscle during the concurrent elimination process.

Loxapine is extensively metabolized, and urinary recovery over 48 hours resulted in recoveries of approximately 30% and 40% of an IM and orally administered loxapine dose as five metabolites.

INDICATIONS AND USAGE

LOXITANE is indicated for the management of the manifesta-tions of psychotic disorders. The antipsychotic efficacy of LOXITANE was established in clinical studies which enrolled newly hospitalized and chronically hospitalized acutely ill schizophrenic patients as subjects.

CONTRAINDICATIONS

LOXITANE is contraindicated in comatose or severe drug-induced depressed states (alcohol, barbiturates, narcotics, etc.).

LOXITANE is contraindicated in individuals with known hypersensitivity to dibenzoxazepines.

WARNINGS

Tardive Dyskinesia

Tardive dyskinesia, a syndrome consisting of potentially irreversible, involuntary, dyskinetic movements may develop in patients treated with neuroleptic (antipsychotic) drugs. Although the prevalence of the syndrome appears to be highest among the elderly, especially elderly women, it is impossible to rely upon prevalence estimates to predict, at the inception of neuroleptic treatment, which patients are likely to develop the syndrome. Whether neuroleptic drug products differ in their potential to cause tardive dyskinesia is unknown.

Both the risk of developing the syndrome and the likelihood that it will become irreversible are believed to increase as the duration of treatment and the total cumulative dose of neuroleptic drugs administered to the patient increase. However, the syndrome can develop, although much less commonly, after relatively brief treatment periods at low doses.

There is no known treatment for established cases of tardive dyskinesia, although the syndrome may remit, partially or completely, if neuroleptic treatment is withdrawn. Neuroleptic treatment itself, however, may suppress (or partially suppress) the signs and symptoms of the syndrome and thereby may possibly mask the underlying disease process. The effect that symptomatic suppression has upon the long-term course of the syndrome is unknown.

Given these considerations, neuroleptics should be prescribed in a manner that is most likely to minimize the occurrence of tardive dyskinesia. Chronic neuroleptic treatment should generally be reserved for patients who suffer from a chronic illness that, (1) is known to respond to neuroleptic drugs, and (2) for whom alternative, equally effective, but potentially less harmful treatments are *not* available or appropriate. In patients who do require chronic treatment, the smallest dose and the shortest duration of treatment producing a satisfactory clinical response should be sought. The need for continued treatment should be reassessed periodically.

If signs and symptoms of tardive dyskinesia appear in a patient on neuroleptics, drug discontinuation should be considered. However, some patients may require treatment despite the presence of the syndrome. (See **ADVERSE REACTIONS** and **Information for Patients** sections.)

Neuroleptic Malignant Syndrome (NMS)

A potentially fatal symptom complex sometimes referred to as Neuroleptic Malignant Syndrome (NMS) has been reported in association with antipsychotic drugs. Clinical manifestations of NMS are hyperpyrexia, muscle rigidity, altered mental status, and evidence of autonomic instability (irregular pulse or blood pressure, tachycardia, diaphoresis, and cardiac dysrhythmias).

The diagnostic evaluation of patients with this syndrome is complicated. In arriving at a diagnosis, it is important to identify cases where the clinical presentation includes both serious medical illness (e.g., pneumonia, systemic infection, etc.) and untreated or inadequately treated extrapyramidal signs and symptoms (EPS). Other important considerations in the differential diagnosis include central anticholinergic toxicity, heat stroke, drug fever, and primary central nervous system (CNS) pathology.

The management of NMS should include: (1) immediate discontinuation of antipsychotic drugs and other drugs not essential to concurrent therapy, (2) intensive symptomatic treatment and medical monitoring, and (3) treatment of any concomitant serious medical problems for which specific treatments are available. There is no general agreement about specific pharmacological treatment regimens for uncomplicated NMS.

If a patient requires antipsychotic drug treatment after recovery from NMS, the potential reintroduction of drug therapy should be carefully considered. The patient should be carefully monitored, since recurrences of NMS have been reported.

LOXITANE, like other tranquilizers, may impair mental and/or physical abilities, especially during the first few days of therapy. Therefore, ambulatory patients should be warned about activities requiring alertness (e.g., operating vehicles or machinery) and about concomitant use of alcohol and other CNS depressants.

LOXITANE has not been evaluated for the management of behavioral complications in patients with mental retardation, and therefore, it cannot be recommended.

PRECAUTIONS

General

LOXITANE should be used with extreme caution in patients with a history of convulsive disorders since it lowers the convulsive threshold. Seizures have been reported in patients receiving LOXITANE at antipsychotic dose levels, and may occur in epileptic patients even with maintenance of routine anticonvulsant drug therapy.

LOXITANE has an antiemetic effect in animals. Since this effect may also occur in man, LOXITANE may mask signs of overdosage of toxic drugs and may obscure conditions such as intestinal obstruction and brain tumor.

LOXITANE should be used with caution in patients with cardiovascular disease. Increased pulse rates have been reported in the majority of patients receiving antipsychotic doses; transient hypotension has been reported. In the presence of severe hypotension requiring vasopressor therapy, the preferred drugs may be norepinephrine or angiotensin. Usual doses of epinephrine may be ineffective because of inhibition of its vasopressor effect by LOXITANE.

The possibility of ocular toxicity from loxapine cannot be excluded at this time. Therefore, careful observation should be made for pigmentary retinopathy and lenticular pigmentation since these have been observed in some patients receiving certain other antipsychotic drugs for prolonged periods.

Because of possible anticholinergic action, the drug should be used cautiously in patients with glaucoma or a tendency to urinary retention, particularly with concomitant administration of anticholinergic-type antiparkinson medication.

Experience to date indicates the possibility of a slightly higher incidence of extrapyramidal effects following intramuscular administration than normally anticipated with oral formulations. The increase may be attributable to higher plasma levels following intramuscular injection.

Neuroleptic drugs elevate prolactin levels; the elevation persists during chronic administration. Tissue culture experiments indicate that approximately one third of human breast cancers are prolactin dependent *in vitro*, a factor of potential importance if the prescription of these drugs is contemplated in a patient with a previously detected breast cancer. Although disturbances such as galactorrhea, amenorrhea, gynecomastia, and impotence have been reported, the clinical significance of elevated serum prolactin levels is unknown for most patients. An increase in mammary neoplasms has been found in rodents after chronic administration of neuroleptic drugs. Neither clinical studies nor epidemiologic studies conducted to date, however, have shown an association between chronic administration of these drugs and mammary tumorigenesis; the available evidence is considered too limited to be conclusive at this time.

Information for Patients

Given the likelihood that some patients exposed chronically to neuroleptics will develop tardive dyskinesia, it is advised that all patients in whom chronic use is contemplated be given, if possible, full information about this risk. The decision to inform patients and/or their guardians must obviously take into account the clinical circumstances and the competency of the patient to understand the information provided.

Drug Interactions

There have been rare reports of significant respiratory depression, stupor and/or hypotension with the concomitant use of loxapine and lorazepam.

The risk of using loxapine in combination with CNS-active drugs has not been systematically evaluated. Therefore, caution is advised if the concomitant administration of loxapine and CNS-active drugs is required.

Usage in Pregnancy

Safe use of LOXITANE during pregnancy or lactation has not been established; therefore, its use in pregnancy, in nursing mothers, or in women of childbearing potential requires that the benefits of treatment be weighed against the possible risks to mother and child. No embryotoxicity or teratogenicity was observed in studies in rats, rabbits or dogs although, with the exception of one rabbit study, the highest dosage was only two times the maximum recommended human dose and in some studies it was below this dose. Perinatal studies have shown renal papillary abnormalities in offspring of rats treated from midpregnancy with doses of 0.6 and 1.8 mg/kg, doses which approximate the usual human dose but which are considerably below the maximum recommended human dose.

Nursing Mothers

The extent of the excretion of LOXITANE or its metabolites in human milk is not known. However, LOXITANE and its metabolites have been shown to be transported into the milk of lactating dogs. LOXITANE administration to nursing women should be avoided if clinically possible.

Pediatric Use

Safety and effectiveness of LOXITANE in pediatric patients have not been established.

ADVERSE REACTIONS

CNS Effects: Manifestations of adverse effects on the central nervous system, other than extrapyramidal effects, have been seen infrequently. Drowsiness, usually mild, may occur at the beginning of therapy or when dosage is increased. It usually subsides with continued LOXITANE® therapy. The incidence of sedation has been less than that of certain aliphatic phenothiazines and slightly more than the piperazine phenothiazines. Dizziness, faintness, staggering gait, shuffling gait, muscle twitching, weakness, insomnia, agitation, tension, seizures, akinesia, slurred speech, numbness, and confusional states have been reported. Neuroleptic malignant syndrome (NMS) has been reported (see **WARNINGS**).

Extrapyramidal Reactions - Neuromuscular (extrapyramidal) reactions during the administration of LOXITANE have been reported frequently, often during the first few days of treatment. In most patients, these reactions involved parkinsonian-like symptoms such as tremor, rigidity, excessive salivation, and masked facies. Akathisia (motor restlessness) also has been reported relatively frequently. These symptoms are usually not severe and can be controlled by reduction of LOXITANE dosage or by administration of antiparkinson drugs in usual dosage. Dystonic and dyskinetic reactions have occurred less frequently, but may be more severe. Dystonias include spasms of muscles of the neck and face, tongue protrusion, and oculogyric movement. Dyskinetic reactions have been described in the form of choreoathetoid movements. These reactions sometimes require reduction or temporary withdrawal of loxapine dosage in addition to appropriate counteractive drugs.

Persistent Tardive Dyskinesia - As with all antipsychotic agents, tardive dyskinesia may appear in some patients on long-term therapy or may appear after drug therapy has been discontinued. The risk appears to be greater in elderly patients on high-dose therapy, especially females. The symptoms are persistent and in some patients appear to be irreversible. The syndrome is characterized by rhythmical involuntary movement of the tongue, face, mouth, or jaw (e.g., protrusion of tongue, puffing of cheeks, puckering of mouth, chewing movements). Sometimes these may be accompanied by involuntary movements of extremities.

There is no known effective treatment for tardive dyskinesia; antiparkinson agents usually do not alleviate the symptoms of this syndrome. It is suggested that all antipsychotic agents be discontinued if these symptoms appear. Should it be necessary to reinstitute treatment, or increase the dosage of the agent, or switch to a different antipsychotic agent, the syndrome may be masked. It has been suggested that fine vermicular movements of the tongue may be an early sign of the syndrome, and if the medication is stopped at that time the syndrome may not develop.

Cardiovascular Effects: Tachycardia, hypotension, hypertension, orthostatic hypotension, light-headedness, and syncope have been reported.

A few cases of ECG changes similar to those seen with phenothiazines have been reported. It is not known whether these were related to LOXITANE administration.

Hematologic: Rarely, agranulocytosis, thrombocytopenia, leukopenia.

Skin: Dermatitis, edema (puffiness of face), pruritus, rash, alopecia, and seborrhea have been reported with loxapine.

Anticholinergic Effects: Dry mouth, nasal congestion, constipation, blurred vision, urinary retention, and paralytic ileus have occurred.

Gastrointestinal: Nausea and vomiting have been reported in some patients. Hepatocellular injury (i.e., SGOT/SGPT elevation) has been reported in association with loxapine administration and rarely, jaundice and/or hepatitis questionably related to LOXITANE treatment.

Other Adverse Reactions: Weight gain, weight loss, dyspnea, ptosis, hyperpyrexia, flushed facies, headache, paresthesia, and polydipsia have been reported in some patients. Rarely, galactorrhea, amenorrhea, gynecomastia, and menstrual irregularity of uncertain etiology have been reported.

OVERDOSAGE

Signs and symptoms of overdosage will depend on the amount ingested and individual patient tolerance. As would be expected from the pharmacologic actions of the drug, the clinical findings may range from mild depression of the CNS and cardiovascular systems to profound hypotension, respiratory depression, and unconsciousness. The possibility of occurrence of extrapyramidal symptoms and/or convulsive seizures should be kept in mind. Renal failure following loxapine overdosage has also been reported.

The treatment of overdosage is essentially symptomatic and supportive. Early gastric lavage and extended dialysis might be expected to be beneficial. Centrally-acting emetics may have little effect because of the antiemetic action of loxapine. In addition, emesis should be avoided because of the possibility of aspiration of vomitus. Avoid analeptics, such as pentylenetetrazol, which may cause convulsions. Severe hypotension might be expected to respond to the administration of levarterenol or phenylephrine. EPINEPHRINE SHOULD NOT BE USED SINCE ITS USE IN A PATIENT WITH PARTIAL ADRENERGIC BLOCKADE MAY FURTHER LOWER THE BLOOD PRESSURE. Severe extrapyramidal reactions should be treated with anticholinergic antiparkinson agents or diphenhydramine hydrochloride, and anticonvulsant therapy should be initiated as indicated. Additional measures include oxygen and intravenous fluids.

DOSAGE AND ADMINISTRATION

LOXITANE is administered, usually in divided doses, two to four times a day. Daily dosage (in terms of base equivalents) should be adjusted to the individual patient's needs as assessed by the severity of symptoms and previous history of response to antipsychotic drugs.

Oral Administration

Initial dosage of 10 mg twice daily is recommended, although in severely disturbed patients initial dosage up to a total of 50 mg daily may be desirable. Dosage should then be increased fairly rapidly over the first seven to ten days until there is effective control of psychotic symptoms. The usual therapeutic and maintenance range is 60 to 100 mg daily. However, as with other antipsychotic drugs, some patients respond to lower dosage and others require higher dosage for optimal benefit. Daily dosage higher than 250 mg is not recommended.

LOXITANE C Oral Concentrate should be mixed with orange or grapefruit juice shortly before administration. Use only the enclosed calibrated (10 mg, 15 mg, 25 mg, 50 mg) dropper for dosage.

Maintenance Therapy

For maintenance therapy, dosage should be reduced to the lowest level compatible with symptom control; many patients have been maintained satisfactorily at dosages in the range of 20 to 60 mg daily.

Intramuscular Administration

LOXITANE IM is utilized for prompt symptomatic control in the acutely agitated patient and in patients whose symptoms render oral medication temporarily impractical. During clinical trial there were only rare reports of significant local tissue reaction.

LOXITANE IM is administered by intramuscular (not intravenous) injection in doses of 12.5 mg (1/4 mL) to 50 mg (1 mL) at intervals of four to six hours or longer, both dose and interval depending on patient response. Many patients have responded satisfactorily to twice-daily dosage. As described above for oral administration, attention is directed to the necessity for dosage adjustment on an individual basis over the early days of loxapine administration.

Once the desired symptomatic control is achieved and the patient is able to take medication orally, loxapine should be administered in capsule or oral concentrate form. Usually this should occur within five days.

HOW SUPPLIED

LOXITANE®, loxapine succinate, Capsules are available in the following base equivalent strengths:

5 mg - Hard shell, opaque, dark-green capsules printed with "" over "WATSON" on one half and "LOXITANE" over "5 mg" on the other, are supplied as follows: NDC 52544-811-01 - Bottle of 100s

10 mg - Hard shell, opaque, with yellow body and a dark-green cap, printed with " " over "WATSON" on one half and "LOXITANE" over "10 mg" on the other, are supplied as follows:
NDC 52544-812-01 - Bottle of 100s
NDC 52544-812-10 - Bottle of 1000s

25 mg - Hard shell, opaque, with a light-green body and a dark-green cap, printed with "" over "WATSON" on one half and "LOXITANE" over "25 mg" on the other, are supplied as follows:
NDC 52544-813-01 - Bottle of 100s
NDC 52544-813-10 - Bottle of 1000s

50 mg - Hard shell, opaque, with a blue body and a dark-green cap, printed with "" over "WATSON" on one half and "LOXITANE" over "50 mg" on the other, are supplied as follows:
NDC 52544-814-01 - Bottle of 100s
NDC 52544-814-10 - Bottle of 1000s

Store at controlled room temperature 15°–30°C (59°–86°F).

LOXITANE® C, loxapine hydrochloride, Oral Concentrate is supplied as follows:

NDC 52544-815-34 - 4 fl oz (120 mL) with calibrated dropper.

Each mL contains loxapine HCl equivalent to 25 mg of loxapine base.

Store at controlled room temperature 20°–25°C (68°–77°F).

DO NOT FREEZE.

mfd for: WATSON PHARMA
A Division of Watson Laboratories, Inc.
Corona, CA 91720
by: LEDERLE PHARMACEUTICAL DIVISION
of American Cyanamid Company
Pearl River, NY 10965

LOXITANE® IM, loxapine hydrochloride, for intramuscular use only is supplied as follows:

NDC 52544-816-79 - 10 mL multi-dose vial

Each mL contains loxapine HCl equivalent to 50 mg of loxapine base.

Keep package closed to protect from light. Intensification of the straw color to a light amber will not alter potency or therapeutic efficacy; if noticeably discolored, ampul or vial should not be used.

Store at controlled room temperature 15°–30°C (59°–86°F).

DO NOT FREEZE.

Rx only

mfd for: WATSON PHARMA
A Division of Watson Laboratories, Inc.
Corona, CA 91720
by: LEDERLE PARENTERALS, INC.
Carolina, Puerto Rico 00987

CI 5062-1 Issued May 4, 1998

Shown in Product Identification Guide, page 342

MICROZIDE™ Capsules ℞

(Hydrochlorothiazide 12.5 mg)

DESCRIPTION

Microzide™ (hydrochlorothiazide 12.5 mg) is the 3,4-dihydro derivative of chlorothiazide. Its chemical name is 6-chloro-3,4-dihydro-2*H*-1,2,4-benzothiadiazine-7-sulfonamide 1,1-dioxide. Its empirical formula is $C_7H_8ClN_3O_4S_2$; its molecular weight is 297.72; and its structural formula is:

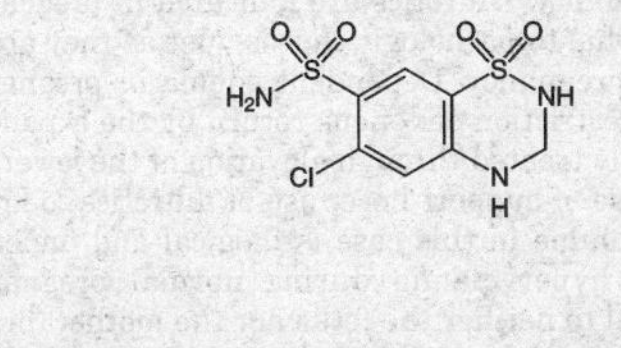

It is a white, or practically white, crystalline powder which is slightly soluble in water, but freely soluble in sodium hydroxide solution.

MICROZIDE is supplied as 12.5 mg capsules for oral use. Each capsule contains the following inactive ingredients: colloidal silicon dioxide, corn starch, D&C Red #28, D&C Yellow #10, FD&C Blue #1, gelatin, lactose monohydrate, magnesium stearate, titanium dioxide and other ingredients.

CLINICAL PHARMACOLOGY

Hydrochlorothiazide blocks the reabsorption of sodium and chloride ions, and it thereby increases the quantity of sodium traversing the distal tubule and the volume of water excreted. A portion of the additional sodium presented to the distal tubule is exchanged there for potassium and hydrogen ions. With continued use of hydrochlorothiazide and depletion of sodium, compensatory mechanisms tend to increase this exchange and may produce excessive loss of potassium, hydrogen and chloride ions. Hydrochlorothiazide also decreases the excretion of calcium and uric acid, may increase the excretion of iodide and may reduce glomerular filtration rate. Metabolic toxicities associated with excessive electrolyte changes caused by hydrochlorothiazide have been shown to be dose-related.

Continued on next page

Microzide—Cont.

Pharmacokinetics and Metabolism: Hydrochlorothiazide is well absorbed (65% to 75%) following oral administration. Absorption of hydrochlorothiazide is reduced in patients with congestive heart failure.

Peak plasma concentrations are observed within 1 to 5 hours of dosing, and range from 70 to 490 ng/mL following oral doses of 12.5 to 100 mg. Plasma concentrations are linearly related to the administered dose. Concentrations of hydrochlorothiazide are 1.6 to 1.8 times higher in whole blood than in plasma. Binding to serum proteins has been reported to be approximately 40% to 68%. The plasma elimination half-life has been reported to be 6 to 15 hours. Hydrochlorothiazide is eliminated primarily by renal pathways. Following oral doses of 12.5 to 100 mg, 55% to 77% of the administered dose appears in urine and greater than 95% of the absorbed dose is excreted in urine as unchanged drug. In patients with renal disease, plasma concentrations of hydrochlorothiazide are increased and the elimination half-life is prolonged.

When MICROZIDE is administered with food, its bioavailability is reduced by 10%, the maximum plasma concentration is reduced by 20%, and the time to maximum concentration increases from 1.6 to 2.9 hours.

Pharmacodynamics: Acute antihypertensive effects of thiazides are thought to result from a reduction in blood volume and cardiac output, secondary to a natriuretic effect, although a direct vasodilatory mechanism has also been proposed. With chronic administration, plasma volume returns toward normal, but peripheral vascular resistance is decreased. The exact mechanism of the antihypertensive effect of hydrochlorothiazide is not known.

Thiazides do not affect normal blood pressure. Onset of action occurs within 2 hours of dosing, peak effect is observed at about 4 hours, and activity persists for up to 24 hours.

Clinical Studies: In an 87 patient 4-week double-blind, placebo controlled, parallel group trial, patients who received MICROZIDE had reductions in seated systolic and diastolic blood pressure that were significantly greater than those seen in patients who received placebo. In published placebo-controlled trials comparing 12.5 mg of hydrochlorothiazide to 25 mg, the 12.5 mg dose preserved most of the placebo-corrected blood pressure reduction seen with 25 mg.

INDICATIONS AND USAGE

MICROZIDE is indicated in the management of hypertension either as the sole therapeutic agent, or in combination with other antihypertensives. Unlike potassium sparing combination diuretic products, MICROZIDE may be used in those patients in whom the development of hyperkalemia cannot be risked, including patients taking ACE inhibitors.

Usage in Pregnancy: The routine use of diuretics in an otherwise healthy woman is inappropriate and exposes mother and fetus to unnecessary hazard. Diuretics do not prevent development of toxemia of pregnancy, and there is no satisfactory evidence that they are useful in the treatment of developed toxemia.

Edema during pregnancy may arise from pathological causes or from the physiologic and mechanical consequences of pregnancy. Diuretics are indicated in pregnancy when edema is due to pathologic causes, just as they are in the absence of pregnancy. Dependent edema in pregnancy resulting from restriction of venous return by the expanded uterus is properly treated through elevation of the lower extremities and use of support hose; use of diuretics to lower intravascular volume in this case is illogical and unnecessary. There is hypervolemia during normal pregnancy which is harmful to neither the fetus nor the mother (in the absence of cardiovascular disease), but which is associated with edema, including generalized edema in the majority of pregnant women. If this edema produces discomfort, increased recumbency will often provide relief. In rare instances this edema may cause extreme discomfort which is not relieved by rest. In these cases a short course of diuretics may provide relief and may be appropriate.

CONTRAINDICATIONS

Hydrochlorothiazide is contraindicated in patients with anuria. Hypersensitivity to this product or other sulfonamide derived drugs is also contraindicated.

WARNINGS

Diabetes and Hypoglycemia: Latent diabetes mellitus may become manifest and diabetic patients given thiazides may require adjustment of their insulin dose.

Renal Disease: Cumulative effects of the thiazides may develop in patients with impaired renal function. In such patients, thiazides may precipitate azotemia.

PRECAUTIONS

Electrolyte and Fluid Balance Status: In published studies, clinically significant hypokalemia has been consistently less common in patients who received 12.5 mg of hydrochlorothiazide than in patients who received higher doses. Nevertheless, periodic determination of serum electrolytes should be performed in patients who may be at risk for the development of hypokalemia. Patients should be observed for signs of fluid or electrolyte disturbances, i.e. hyponatremia, hypochloremic alkalosis, and hypokalemia and hypomagnesemia.

Warning signs or symptoms of fluid and electrolyte imbalance include dryness of mouth, thirst, weakness, lethargy, drowsiness, restlessness, muscle pains or cramps, muscular fatigue, hypotension, oliguria tachycardia, and gastrointestinal disturbances such as nausea and vomiting.

Hypokalemia may develop, especially with brisk diuresis when severe cirrhosis is present, during concomitant use of corticosteroid or adrenocorticotropic hormone (ACTH) or after prolonged therapy. Interference with adequate oral electrolyte intake will also contribute to hypokalemia. Hypokalemia and hypomagnesemia can provoke ventricular arrhythmias or sensitize or exaggerate the response of the heart to the toxic effects of digitalis. Hypokalemia may be avoided or treated by potassium supplementation or increased intake of potassium rich foods.

Dilutional hyponatremia is life-threatening and may occur in edematous patients in hot weather; appropriate therapy is water restriction rather than salt administration, except in rare instances when the hyponatremia is life-threatening. In actual salt depletion, appropriate replacement is the therapy of choice.

Hyperuricemia: Hyperuricemia or acute gout may be precipitated in certain patients receiving thiazide diuretics.

Impaired Hepatic Function: Thiazides should be used with caution in patients with impaired hepatic function. They can precipitate hepatic coma in patients with severe liver disease.

Parathyroid Disease: Calcium excretion is decreased by thiazides, and pathologic changes in the parathyroid glands, with hypercalcemia and hypophosphatemia, have been observed in a few patients on prolonged thiazide therapy.

Drug Interactions: When given concurrently the following drugs may interact with thiazide diuretics:

Alcohol, barbiturates, or narcotics—potentiation of orthostatic hypotension may occur.

Antidiabetic drugs—(oral agents and insulin) dosage adjustment of the antidiabetic drug may be required.

Other antihypertensive drugs—additive effect or potentiation.

Cholestyramine and colestipol resins—Cholestyramine and colestipol resins bind the hydrochlorothiazide and reduce its absorption from the gastrointestinal tract by up to 85 and 43 percent, respectively.

Corticosteroid, ACTH—intensified electrolyte depletion, particularly hypokalemia.

Pressor amines (e.g., norepinephrine)—possible decreased response to pressor amines but not sufficient to preclude their use.

Skeletal muscle relaxants, nondepolarizing (e.g., tubocurarine)—possible increased responsiveness to the muscle relaxant

Lithium—generally should not be given with diuretics. Diuretic agents reduce the renal clearance of lithium and greatly increase the risk of lithium toxicity. Refer to the package insert for lithium preparations before use of such preparations with MICROZIDE.

Non-steroidal anti-inflammatory drugs—In some patients, the administration of a non-steroidal anti-inflammatory agent can reduce the diuretic, natriuretic, and antihypertensive effects of loop, potassium-sparing and thiazide diuretics. When MICROZIDE and non-steroidal anti-inflammatory agents are used concomitantly, the patients should be observed closely to determine if the desired effect of the diuretic is obtained.

Drug/Laboratory Test Interactions: Thiazides should be discontinued before carrying out tests for parathyroid function (see PRECAUTIONS, *General*).

Carcinogenesis, Mutagenesis, Impairment of Fertility: Two-year feeding studies in mice and rats conducted under the auspices of the National Toxicology Program (NTP) uncovered no evidence of a carcinogenic potential of hydrochlorothiazide in female mice (at doses of up to approximately 600 mg/kg/day) or in male and female rats (at doses of approximately 100 mg/kg/day). The NTP, however, found equivocal evidence for hepatocarcinogenicity in male mice. Hydrochlorothiazide was not genotoxic *in vitro* in the Ames mutagenicity assay of *Salmonella typhimurium* strains TA 98, TA 100, TA 1535, TA 1537, and TA 1538 and in the Chinese Hamster Ovary (CHO) test for chromosomal aberrations, or *in vivo* in assays using mouse germinal cell chromosomes, Chinese hamster bone marrow chromosomes, and the *Drosophila* sex-linked recessive lethal trait gene. Positive test results were obtained only in the *in vitro* CHO Sister Chromatid Exchange (clastogenicity) and in the Mouse Lymphoma Cell (mutagenicity) assays, using concentrations of hydrochlorothiazide from 43 to 1300 µg/mL, and in the *Aspergillus nidulans* non-disjunction assay at an unspecified concentration.

Hydrochlorothiazide had no adverse effects on the fertility of mice and rats of either sex in studies wherein these species were exposed, via their diet, to doses of up to 100 and 4 mg/kg, respectively, prior to conception and throughout gestation.

Pregnancy:

Teratogenic Effects —Pregnancy Category B: Studies in which hydrochlorothiazide was orally administered to pregnant mice and rats during their respective periods of major organogenesis at doses up to 3000 and 1000 mg hydrochlorothiazide/kg, respectively, provided no evidence of harm to the fetus.

There are, however, no adequate and well-controlled studies in pregnant women. Because animal reproduction studies are not always predictive of human response, this drug should be used during pregnancy only if clearly needed.

Nonteratogenic Effects: Thiazides cross the placental barrier and appear in cord blood. There is a risk of fetal or neonatal jaundice, thrombocytopenia, and possibly other adverse reactions that have occurred in adults.

Nursing Mothers: Thiazides are excreted in breast milk. Because of the potential for serious adverse reactions in nursing infants, a decision should be made whether to discontinue nursing or to discontinue hydrochlorothiazide, taking into account the importance of the drug to the mother.

Pediatric Use: Safety and effectiveness in pediatric patients have not been established.

Elderly Use: A greater blood pressure reduction and an increase in side effects may be observed in the elderly (i.e. >65 years) with hydrochlorothiazide. Starting treatment when the lowest available dose of hydrochlorothiazide (12.5 mg) is therefore recommended. If further titration is required, 12.5 mg increments should be utilized.

ADVERSE REACTIONS

The adverse reactions associated with hydrochlorothiazide have been shown to be dose related. In controlled clinical trials, the adverse events reported with doses of 12.5 mg hydrochlorothiazide once daily were comparable to placebo. The following adverse reactions have been reported for doses of hydrochlorothiazide 25 mg and greater and, within each category, are listed in the order of decreasing severity.

Body as a whole: Weakness.

Cardiovascular: Hypotension including orthostatic hypotension (may be aggravated by alcohol, barbiturates, narcotics or antihypertensive drugs).

Digestive: Pancreatitis, jaundice (intrahepatic cholestatic jaundice), diarrhea, vomiting, sialadenitis, cramping, constipation, gastric irritation, nausea, anorexia.

Hematologic: Aplastic anemia, agranulocytosis, leukopenia, hemolytic anemia, thrombocytopenia.

Hypersensitivity: Anaphylactic reactions, necrotizing angiitis (vasculitis and cutaneous vasculitis), respiratory distress including pneumonitis and pulmonary edema, photosensitivity, fever, urticaria, rash, purpura.

Metabolic: Electrolyte imbalance (see **PRECAUTIONS**), hyperglycemia, glycosuria, hyperuricemia.

Musculoskeletal: Muscle spasm.

Nervous System/Psychiatric: Vertigo, paresthesia, dizziness, headache, restlessness.

Renal: Renal failure, renal dysfunction, interstitial nephritis (See **WARNINGS**).

Skin: Erythema multiforme including Stevens-Johnson syndrome, exfoliative dermatitis including toxic epidermal necrolysis, alopecia.

Special Senses: Transient blurred vision, xanthopsia.

Urogenital: Impotence.

Whenever adverse reactions are moderate or severe, thiazide dosage should be reduced or therapy withdrawn.

OVERDOSAGE

The most common signs and symptoms observed are those caused by electrolyte depletion (hypokalemia, hypochloremia, hyponatremia) and dehydration resulting from excessive diuresis. If digitalis has also been administered, hypokalemia may accentuate cardiac arrhythmias.

In the event of overdosage, symptomatic and supportive measures should be employed. Emesis should be induced or gastric lavage performed. Correct dehydration, electrolyte imbalance, hepatic coma and hypotension by established procedures. If required, give oxygen or artificial respiration for respiratory impairment. The degree to which hydrochlorothiazide is removed by hemodialysis has not been established.

The oral LD_{50} of hydrochlorothiazide is greater than 10 g/kg in the mouse and rat.

DOSAGE AND ADMINISTRATION

For Control of Hypertension: The adult initial dose of MICROZIDE is one capsule given once daily whether given alone or in combination with other antihypertensives. Total daily doses greater than 50 mg are not recommended.

HOW SUPPLIED

MICROZIDE capsules are #4 Teal Opaque/Teal Opaque two piece hard gelatin capsules imprinted with MICROZIDE and 12.5 mg in black ink. They are supplied in bottles of 100 with child resistant closures (NDC 52544-622-01).

Storage: Keep container tightly closed. Protect from light, moisture, freezing, −20°C (−4°F) and store at room temperature, 15–30°C (59–86°F).

Caution: Federal law prohibits dispensing without prescription.

Manufactured by
Watson Laboratories, Inc.
Copiague, NY 11726
13304
R2 1/97

Shown in Product Identification Guide, page 342

NECON® ℞

[*nē-con*]
**(norethindrone and
ethinyl estradiol tablets, USP)**

12621
Necon 1/35-21
Necon 1/35-28
(norethindrone and ethinyl estradiol tablets, USP)
Necon 10/11-21
Necon 10/11-28
(norethindrone and ethinyl estradiol tablets, USP)
Necon 0.5/35-21
Necon 0.5/35-28
(norethindrone and ethinyl estradiol tablets, USP)
Necon 1/50-21
Necon 1/50-28
(norethindrone and mestranol tablets, USP)

Patients should be counseled that this product does not protect against HIV infection (AIDS) and other sexually transmitted diseases.

DESCRIPTION

Necon 1/35-21 and *Necon 1/35-28 (Norethindrone and Ethinyl Estradiol Tablets, USP).* Each dark yellow tablet contains 1 mg of norethindrone and 35 mcg of ethinyl estradiol, and the inactive ingredients include microcrystalline cellulose, lactose (anhydrous), magnesium stearate, polacrilin potassium and povidone. In addition, the coloring agent is D&C Yellow No. 10. Each white tablet in the Necon 1/35-28 package is a placebo containing no active ingredients and the inactive ingredients include microcrystalline cellulose, lactose (anhydrous), and magnesium stearate.

Necon 0.5/35-21 and *Necon 0.5/35-28 (Norethindrone and Ethinyl Estradiol Tablets, USP).* Each light yellow tablet contains 0.5 mg of norethindrone and 35 mcg of ethinyl estradiol, and the inactive ingredients include microcrystalline cellulose, lactose (anhydrous), magnesium stearate, polacrilin potassium and povidone. In addition, the coloring agent is D&C Yellow No. 10. Each white tablet in the Necon 0.5/35-28 package is a placebo containing no active ingredients and the inactive ingredients include microcrystalline cellulose, lactose (anhydrous), and magnesium stearate.

Necon 10/11-21 and *Necon 10/11-28 (Norethindrone and Ethinyl Estradiol Tablets, USP).* Each light yellow tablet (10) contains 0.5 mg of norethindrone and 35 mcg of ethinyl estradiol. Each dark yellow tablet (11) contains 1 mg of norethindrone and 35 mcg of ethinyl estradiol. The inactive ingredients include microcrystalline cellulose, lactose (anhydrous), magnesium stearate, polacrilin potassium and povidone. In addition, the coloring agent is D&C Yellow No. 10. Each white tablet in the Necon 10/11-28 package is a placebo containing no active ingredients and the inactive ingredients include microcrystalline cellulose, lactose (anhydrous), and magnesium stearate.

Necon 1/50-21 and *Necon 1/50-28 (Norethindrone and Mestranol Tablets, USP).* Each light blue tablet contains 1 mg of norethindrone and 50 mcg of mestranol, and the inactive ingredients include microcrystalline cellulose, lactose (anhydrous), magnesium stearate, polacrilin potassium and povidone. In addition, the coloring agent is FD&C Blue No. 1 Aluminum Lake. Each white tablet in the Necon 1/50-28 package is a placebo containing no active ingredients and the inactive ingredients include microcrystalline cellulose, lactose (anhydrous), and magnesium stearate.

The chemical name for norethindrone is 17-hydroxy-19-*nor*-17α-pregn-4-en-20-yn-3-one. The chemical name of ethinyl estradiol is 19-nor-17α-pregna-1, 3, 5(10)-trien-20-yne-3, 17-diol. The chemical name for mestranol is 3-methoxy-19-nor-17α-pregna-1, 3, 5(10)-trien-20-yn-17-ol. The structural formulas are as follows:

NORETHINDRONE
M.W. = 298.42

ETHINYL ESTRADIOL
M.W. = 296.41

MESTRANOL
M.W. = 310.44

Therapeutic class: Oral contraceptive

CLINICAL PHARMACOLOGY

Combination oral contraceptives act primarily by suppression of gonadotropins. Although the primary mechanism of this action is inhibition of ovulation, other alterations in the genital tract, including changes in the cervical mucus (which increase the difficulty of sperm entry into the uterus) and the endometrium (which may reduce the likelihood of implantation) may also contribute to contraceptive effectiveness.

INDICATIONS AND USAGE

Necon 1/35, Necon 0.5/35, Necon 10/11 and Necon 1/50 are indicated for the prevention of pregnancy in women who elect to use oral contraceptives as a method of contraception.

Oral contraceptives are highly effective. Table 1 lists the typical accidental pregnancy rates for users of combination oral contraceptives and other methods of contraception. The efficacy of these contraceptive methods, except sterilization, depends upon the reliability with which they are used. Correct and consistent use of methods can result in lower failure rates.

[See table 1 at top of next page]

CONTRAINDICATIONS

Oral contraceptives should not be used in women who have the following conditions:

• Thrombophlebitis or thromboembolic disorders
• A past history of deep vein thrombophlebitis or thromboembolic disorders
• Cerebral vascular disease, myocardial infarction or coronary artery disease, or a past history of these conditions
• Known or suspected carcinoma of the breast, or a history of this condition
• Known or suspected carcinoma of the female reproductive organs or suspected estrogen-dependent neoplasia, or a history of these conditions
• Undiagnosed abnormal genital bleeding
• History of cholestatic jaundice of pregnancy or jaundice with prior oral contraceptive use
• Past or present, benign or malignant liver tumors
• Known or suspected pregnancy

WARNINGS

> **Cigarette smoking increases the risk of serious adverse effects on the heart and blood vessels from oral contraceptive use. This risk increases with age and with heavy smoking (15 or more cigarettes per day) and is quite marked in women over 35 years of age. Women who use oral contraceptives are strongly advised not to smoke.**

The use of oral contraceptives is associated with increased risk of several serious conditions including venous and arterial thromboembolism, thrombotic and hemorrhagic stroke, myocardial infarction, liver tumors or other liver lesions, and gallbladder disease. The risk of morbidity and mortality increases significantly in the presence of other risk factors such as hypertension, hyperlipidemia, obesity, and diabetes mellitus.

Practitioners prescribing oral contraceptives should be familiar with the following information relating to these and other risks. The information contained herein is principally based on studies carried out in patients who use oral contraceptives with formulations containing higher amounts of estrogens and progestogens than those in common use today. The effect of long-term use of the oral contraceptives with lesser amounts of both estrogens and progestogens remains to be determined.

Throughout this labeling, epidemiological studies reported are of two types: retrospective case-control studies and prospective cohort studies. Case-control studies provide an es-

timate of the relative risk of a disease, which is defined as the *ratio* of the incidence of a disease among oral contraceptive users to that among nonusers. The relative risk (or odds ratio) does not provide information about the actual clinical occurrence of a disease. Cohort studies provide a measure of both the relative risk and the attributable risk. The latter is the *difference* in the incidence of disease between oral contraceptive users and nonusers. The attributable risk does provide information about the actual occurrence or incidence of a disease in the subject population. For further information, the reader is referred to a text on epidemiological methods.

1. Thromboembolic disorders and other vascular problems
a. Myocardial infarction

An increased risk of myocardial infarction has been associated with oral contraceptive use.[2–21] This increased risk is primarily in smokers or in women with other underlying risk factors for coronary artery disease such as hypertension, obesity, diabetes, and hypercholesterolemia. The relative risk for myocardial infarction in current oral contraceptive users has been estimated to be 2 to 6. The risk is very low under the age of 30. However, there is the possibility of a risk of cardiovascular disease even in very young women who take oral contraceptives.

Smoking in combination with oral contraceptive use has been reported to contribute substantially to the risk of myocardial infarction in women in the mid-thirties or older, with smoking accounting for the majority of excess cases.[22] Mortality rates associated with circulatory disease have been shown to increase substantially in smokers, especially in those 35 years of age and older among women who use oral contraceptives (see Figure 1, Table 2).

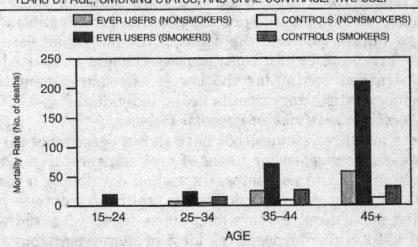

FIGURE 1. CIRCULATORY DISEASE MORTALITY RATES PER 100,000 WOMEN—YEARS BY AGE, SMOKING STATUS, AND ORAL CONTRACEPTIVE USE.[14]

Adapted from Layde and Beral.[14]

Oral contraceptives may compound the effects of well-known cardiovascular risk factors such as hypertension, diabetes, hyperlipidemias, hypercholesterolemia, age, cigarette smoking, and obesity. In particular, some progestogens decrease HDL cholesterol[23–31] and cause glucose intolerance, while estrogens may create a state of hyperinsulinism.[32] Oral contraceptives have been shown to increase blood pressure among some users (see **WARNING** No. 9). Similar effects on risk factors have been associated with an increased risk of heart disease.

b. Thromboembolism

An increased risk of thromboembolic and thrombotic disease associated with the use of oral contraceptives is well established.[17, 33–51] Case-control studies have estimated the relative risk to be 3 for the first episode of superficial venous thrombosis, 4 to 11 for deep vein thrombosis or pulmonary embolism, and 1.5 to 6 for women with predisposing conditions for venous thromboembolic disease.[34–37, 45, 46] Cohort studies have shown the relative risk to be somewhat lower, about 3 for new cases (subjects with no past history of venous thrombosis or varicose veins) and about 4.5 for new cases requiring hospitalization.[42, 47, 48] The risk of venous thromboembolic disease associated with oral contraceptives is not related to duration of use.

A two- to seven-fold increase in relative risk of postoperative thromboembolic complications has been reported with the use of oral contraceptives.[38, 39] The relative risk of venous thrombosis in women who have predisposing conditions is about twice that of women without such medical conditions.[43] If feasible, oral contraceptives should be discontinued at least 4 weeks prior to and for 2 weeks after elective surgery of a type associated with an increased risk of thromboembolism, and also during and following prolonged immobilization. Since the immediate postpartum period is also associated with an increased risk of thromboembolism, oral contraceptives should be started no earlier than 4 to 6 weeks after delivery in women who elect not to breast feed.

c. Cerebrovascular disease

Both the relative and attributable risks of cerebrovascular events (thrombotic and hemorrhagic strokes) have been reported to be increased with oral contraceptive use,[14, 17, 18, 34, 42, 46, 52–59] although, in general, the risk was greatest among older (over 35 years) hypertensive women who also smoked. Hypertension was reported to be a risk factor for both users

Continued on next page

Necon—Cont.

and nonusers for both types of strokes, while smoking increased the risk factor for both users and nonusers for both types of strokes, while smoking increased the risk for hemorrhagic strokes.

In one large study,[52] the relative risk for thrombotic stroke was reported as 9.5 times greater in users than in nonusers. It ranged from 3 for normotensive users to 14 for users with severe hypertension.[54] The relative risk for hemorrhagic stroke was reported to be 1.2 for nonsmokers who used oral contraceptives, 1.9 to 2.6 for smokers who did not use oral contraceptives, 6.1 to 7.6 for smokers who used oral contraceptives, 1.8 for normotensive users, and 25.7 for users with severe hypertension. The risk is also greater in older women and among smokers.

d. Dose-related risk of vascular disease with oral contraceptives

A positive association has been reported between the amount of estrogen and progestogen in oral contraceptives and the risk of vascular disease.[41, 43, 53, 59–64] A decline in serum high density lipoproteins (HDL) has been reported with many progestogens.[23–31] A decline in serum high density lipoproteins has been associated with an increased incidence of ischemic heart disease.[65] Because estrogens increase HDL-cholesterol, the net effect of an oral contraceptive depends on the balance achieved between doses of estrogen and progestogen and the nature and absolute amount of progestogens used in the contraceptives. The amount of both steroids should be considered in the choice of an oral contraceptive.

Minimizing exposure to estrogen and progestogen is in keeping with good principles of therapeutics. For any particular estrogen-progestogen combination, the dosage regimen prescribed should be one that contains the least amount of estrogen and progestogen that is compatible with a low failure rate and the needs of the individual patient. New acceptors of oral contraceptives should be started on preparations containing the lowest estrogen content that produces satisfactory results in the individual.

e. Persistence of risk of vascular disease

There are three studies that have shown persistence of risk of vascular disease for users of oral contraceptives. In a study in the United States, the risk of developing myocardial infarction after discontinuing oral contraceptives persisted for at least 9 years for women 40–49 years old who had used oral contraceptives for 5 or more years, but this increased risk was not demonstrated in other age groups.[16] Another American study reported former use of oral contraceptives was significantly associated with increased risk of subarachnoid hemorrhage.[57] In another study, in Great Britain, the risk of developing non-rheumatic heart disease plus hypertension, subanoid hemorrhage, cerebral thrombosis, and transient ischemic attacks persisted for at least 6 years after discontinuation of oral contraceptives, although the excess risk was small.[14, 18, 66] It should be noted that these studies were performed with oral contraceptive formulations containing 50 mcg or more of estrogens.

2. Estimates of mortality from contraceptive use

One study[67] gathered data from a variety of sources that have estimated the mortality rates associated with different methods of contraception at different ages. (Table 2). These estimates include the combined risk of death associated with contraceptive methods plus the risk attributable to pregnancy in the event of method failure. Each method of contraception has its specific benefits and risks. The study concluded that, with the exception of oral contraceptive users 35 and older who smoke and 40 and older who do not smoke, mortality associated with all methods of birth control is low and below that associated with childbirth. The observation of a possible increase in risk of mortality with age of oral contraceptive users is based on data gathered in the 1970's, but not reported until 1983.[67] However, current clinical practice involves the use of lower estrogen dose formulations combined with careful restriction of oral contraceptive use to women who do not have various risk factors listed in this labeling.

Because of these changes in practice and, also, because of some limited new data that suggest that the risk of cardiovascular disease with the use of oral contraceptives may now be less than previously observed,[48, 152] the Fertility and Maternal Health Drugs Advisory Committee was asked to review the topic in 1989. The Committee concluded that, although cardiovascular disease risks may be increased with oral contraceptive use after age 40 in healthy, nonsmoking women (even with the newer low-dose formulations), there are greater potential health risks associated with pregnancy in older women and with the alternative surgical and medical procedures that may be necessary if such women do not have access to effective and acceptable means of contraception.

Therefore, the Committee recommended that the benefits of oral contraceptive use by healthy nonsmoking women over 40 may outweigh the possible risks. Of course, older women, as all women who take oral contraceptives, should take the lowest possible dose formulation that is effective.

[See table below]

Adapted from Ory.[67]

3. Carcinoma of the breast and reproductive organs

Numerous epidemiological studies have been performed on the incidence of breast, endometrial, ovarian, and cervical cancer in women using oral contraceptives. While there are conflicting reports, most studies suggest that the use of oral contraceptives is not associated with an overall increase in the risk of developing breast cancer.[17, 40, 68–78] Some studies have reported an increased relative risk of developing breast cancer, particularly at a young age.[79–102, 51] This increased relative risk appears to be related to duration of use.

Some studies suggested that oral contraceptive use was associated with an increase in the risk of cervical intrepithelial neoplasia, dysplasia, erosion, carcinoma, or microglandular dysplasia in some populations of women.[17, 50, 103–115] However, there continues to be controversy about the extent to which such findings may be due to differences in sexual behavior and other factors.

In spite of many studies of the relationship between oral contraceptive use and breast and cervical cancers, a cause and effect relationship has not been established.

4. Hepatic neoplasia

Benign hepatic adenomas and other hepatic lesions have been associated with oral contraceptive use,[116–121] although the incidence of such benign tumors is rare in the United States. Indirect calculations have estimated the attributable risk to be in the range of 3.3 cases per 100,000 for users, a risk that increases after 4 or more years of use.[120] Rupture of benign, hepatic adenomas or other lesions may cause death through intraabdominal hemorrhage. Therefore, such lesions should be considered in women presenting with abdominal pain and tenderness, abdominal mass, or shock. About one quarter of the cases presented because of abdominal masses, up to one half had signs and symptoms of acute intraperitoneal hemorrhage.[121] Diagnosis may prove difficult.

Studies from the U.S.,[122–150] Great Britain,[123–124] and Italy[125] have shown an increased risk of hepatocellular carcinoma in long-term (>8 years; relative risk of 7–20) oral contraceptive users. However, these cancers are rare in the United States, and the attributable risk (the excess incidence) of liver cancers in oral contraceptive users approaches less than 1 per 1,000,000 users.

5. Ocular Lesions

There have been reports of retinal thrombosis and other ocular lesions associated with the use of oral contraceptives. Oral contraceptives should be discontinued if there is unexplained, gradual or sudden, partial or complete loss of vision, onset of proptosis or diplopia, papilledema, or any evidence of retinal vascular lesions. Appropriate diagnostic and therapeutic measures should be undertaken immediately.

6. Oral contraceptive use before or during pregnancy

Extensive epidemiological studies have revealed no increased risk of birth defects in women who have used oral contraceptives prior to pregnancy.[126, 129] The majority of recent studies also do not suggest a teratogenic effect, particularly insofar as cardiac anomalies and limb reduction defects are concerned,[126, 129] when the pill is taken inadvertently during early pregnancy.

The administration of oral contraceptives to induce withdrawal bleeding should not be used as a test for pregnancy. Oral contraceptives should not be used during pregnancy to treat threatened or habitual abortion. It is recommended that for any patient who has missed two consecutive periods, pregnancy should be ruled out before continuing oral contraceptive use. If the patient has not adhered to the prescribed schedule, the possibility of pregnancy should be considered at the time of the first missed period and further use of oral contraceptives should be withheld until pregnancy has been ruled out. Oral contraceptive use should be discontinued if pregnancy is confirmed.

7. Gallbladder disease

Earlier studies reported an increased lifetime relative risk of gallbladder surgery in users of oral contraceptives and estrogens.[40, 42, 53, 70] More recent studies, however, have shown that the relative risk of developing gallbladder disease among oral contraceptive users may be minimal.[130–132] The recent findings of minimal risk may be related to the use of oral contraceptive formulations containing lower doses of estrogens and progestogens.

TABLE 1. LOWEST EXPECTED AND TYPICAL FAILURE RATES
DURING THE FIRST YEAR OF CONTINUOUS USE OF A METHOD.
PERCENT OF WOMEN EXPERIENCING AN ACCIDENTAL PREGNANCY
IN THE FIRST YEAR OF CONTINUOUS USE.[1]

Method	Lowest Expected*	Typical**
No contraception	85	85
Oral contraceptives		
Combined	0.1	N/A***
Progestogen only	0.5	N/A***
Diaphragm with spermicidal cream or jelly	6	18
Spermicides alone (foam, creams, jellies and vaginal suppositories)	3	21
Vaginal sponge		
Nulliparous	6	18
Parous	9	28
IUD (medicated)		
Progesterone	2	N/A***
Copper T 380A	0.8	N/A***
Condom without spermicides	2	12
Periodic abstinence (all methods)	1–9	20
Female sterilization	0.2	0.4
Male sterilization	0.1	0.15

Adapted from Trussel et al.[1]

  * The authors' best guess of the percentage of women expected to experience an accidental pregnancy among couples who initiate a method (not necessarily for the first time) and who use it consistently and correctly during the first year if they do not stop for any other reason.

  ** This term represents "typical" couples who initiate use of a method (not necessarily for the first time), who experience an accidental pregnancy during the first year if they do not stop for any reason.

  *** N/A—Data not available

TABLE 2. ANNUAL NUMBER OF BIRTH-RELATED OR METHOD-RELATED DEATHS
ASSOCIATED WITH CONTROL OF FERTILITY
PER 100,000 NONSTERILE WOMEN, BY FERTILITY CONTROL METHOD ACCORDING TO AGE.[67]

Method of control	15–19	20–24	25–29	30–34	35–39	40–44
No fertility control methods*	7.0	7.4	9.1	14.8	25.7	28.2
Oral contraceptives						
nonsmoker**	0.3	0.5	0.9	1.9	13.8	31.6
smoker**	2.2	3.4	6.6	13.5	51.1	117.2
IUD**	0.8	0.8	1.0	1.0	1.4	1.4
Condom*	1.1	1.6	0.7	0.2	0.3	0.4
Diaphragm/spermicide*	1.9	1.2	1.2	1.3	2.2	2.8
Periodic abstinence*	2.5	1.6	1.6	1.7	2.9	3.6

  * Deaths are birth-related
  ** Deaths are method-related

8. Carbohydrate and lipid metabolic effects

Oral contraceptives have been shown to cause a decrease in glucose tolerance in a significant percentage of users.[32] This effect has been shown to be directly related to estrogen dose.[133] Progestogens increase insulin secretion and create insulin resistance, the effect varying with different progestational agents.[32, 134] However, in the nondiabetic woman, oral contraceptives appear to have no effect on fasting blood glucose. Because of these demonstrated effects, prediabetic and diabetic women should be carefully observed while taking oral contraceptives.

Some women may have persistent hypertriglyceridemia while on the pill. As discussed earlier (see **WARNINGS** 1a and 1d), changes in serum triglycerides and lipoprotein levels have been reported in oral contraceptive users.[23-31, 135, 136]

9. Elevated blood pressure

An increase in blood pressure has been reported in women taking oral contraceptives[50, 53, 137-139] and this increase is more likely in older oral contraceptive users[137] and with extended duration of use.[53] Data from the Royal College of General Practitioners[138] and subsequent randomized trials have shown that the incidence of hypertension increases with increasing concentrations of progestogens.

Women with a history of hypertension or hypertension-related disease, or renal disease[139] should be encouraged to use another method of contraception. If such women elect to use oral contraceptives, they should be monitored closely and if significant elevation of blood pressure occurs, oral contraceptives should be discontinued. For most women, elevated blood pressure will return to normal after stopping oral contraceptives,[137] and there is no difference in the occurrence of hypertension among ever- and never-users.[140]

10. Headache

The onset or exacerbation of migraine or the development of headache of a new pattern that is recurrent, persistent, or severe requires discontinuation of oral contraceptives and evaluation of the cause.

11. Bleeding Irregularities

Breakthrough bleeding and spotting are sometimes encountered in patients on oral contraceptives, especially during the first three months of use. Nonhormonal causes should be considered and adequate diagnostic measures taken to rule out malignancy or pregnancy in the event of breakthrough bleeding, as in the case of any abnormal vaginal bleeding. If a pathologic basis has been excluded, time alone or a change to another formulation may solve the problem. In the event of amenorrhea, pregnancy should be ruled out.

PRECAUTIONS

1. Physical examination and follow-up

A complete medical history and physical examination should be completed prior to the initiation or reinstitution of oral contraceptives and at least annually during the use of oral contraceptives. These physical examinations should include special reference to blood pressure, breasts, abdomen, and pelvic organs, including cervical cytology, and relevant laboratory tests. In case of undiagnosed, persistent, or recurrent abnormal vaginal bleeding, appropriate diagnostic measures should be conducted to rule out malignancy. Women with a strong family history of breast cancer or who have breast nodules should be monitored with particular care.

2. Lipid disorders

Women who are being treated for hyperlipidemias should be followed closely if they elect to use oral contraceptives. Some progestogens may elevate LDL levels and may render the control of hyperlipidemias more difficult.

3. Liver function

If jaundice develops in any woman receiving oral contraceptives, they should be discontinued. Steroids may be poorly metabolized in patients with impaired liver function and should be administered with caution in such patients. Cholestatic jaundice has been reported after combined treatment with oral contraceptives and troleandomycin. Hepatotoxicity following a combination of oral contraceptives and cyclosporine has also been reported.

4. Fluid retention

Oral contraceptives may cause some degree of fluid retention. They should be prescribed with caution, and only with careful monitoring, in patients with conditions that might be aggravated by fluid retention, such as convulsive disorders, migraine syndrome, asthma, or cardiac, hepatic, or renal dysfunction.

5. Emotional disorders

Women with a history of depression should be carefully observed and the drug discontinued if depression recurs to a serious degree.

6. Contact lenses

Contact lens wearers who develop visual changes or changes in lens tolerance should be assessed by an ophthalmologist.

7. Drug interactions

Reduced efficacy and increased incidence of breakthrough bleeding and menstrual irregularities have been associated with concomitant use of rifampin. A similar association, though less marked, has been suggested for barbiturates, phenylbutazone, phenytoin sodium, and possibly with griseofulvin, ampicillin, and tetracyclines.

8. Laboratory test interactions

Certain endocrine and liver function tests and blood components may be affected by oral contraceptives:

a. Increased prothrombin and factors VII, VIII, IX and X; decreased antithrombin III; increased platelet aggregability.
b. Increased thyroid binding globulin (TBG), leading to increased circulating total thyroid hormone as measured by protein-bound iodine (PBI), T_4 by column or by radioimmunoassay. Free T_3 resin uptake is decreased, reflecting the elevated TBG; free T_4 concentration is unaltered.
c. Other binding proteins may be elevated in the serum.
d. Sex-steroid binding globulins are increased and result in elevated levels of total circulating sex steroids and corticoids; however, free or biologically active levels remain unchanged.
e. Triglycerides and phospholipids may be increased.
f. Glucose tolerance may be decreased.
g. Serum folate levels may be depressed. This may be of clinical significance if a woman becomes pregnant shortly after discontinuing oral contraceptives.
h. Increased sulfobromophthalein and other abnormalities in liver function tests may occur.
i. Plasma levels of trace minerals may be altered.
j. Response to the metyrapone test may be reduced.

9. CARCINOGENESIS

See **WARNINGS**.

10. PREGNANCY

Pregnancy Category X. See **CONTRAINDICATIONS** and **WARNINGS**.

11. Nursing mothers

Small amounts of oral contraceptive steroids have been identified in the milk of nursing mothers[141-143] and a few adverse effects on the child have been reported, including jaundice and breast enlargement. In addition, oral contraceptives given in the postpartum period may interfere with lactation by decreasing the quantity and quality of breast milk. If possible, the nursing mother should be advised not to use oral contraceptives, but to use other forms of contraception until she has completely weaned her child.

12. Venereal diseases

Oral contraceptives are of no value in the prevention or treatment of venereal disease. The prevalence of cervical *Chlamydia trachomatis* and *Neisseria gonorrhoeae* in oral contraceptive users is increased several-fold.[144, 145] It should not be assumed that oral contraceptives afford protection against pelvic inflammatory disease from chlamydia.[144]

13. General

a. The pathologist should be advised of oral contraceptive therapy when relevant specimens are submitted.
b. Treatment with oral contraceptives may mask the onset of the climacteric. (See **WARNINGS** regarding risks in this age group.)

Patients should be counseled that this product does not protect against HIV infection (AIDS) and other sexually transmitted diseases.

14. Information for the patient

See patient labeling, in package insert.

ADVERSE REACTIONS

An increased risk of the following serious adverse reactions has been associated with the use of oral contraceptives (See **WARNINGS**):

- Thrombophlebitis and thrombosis
- Arterial thromboembolism
- Pulmonary embolism
- Myocardial infarction and coronary thrombosis
- Cerebral hemorrhage
- Cerebral thrombosis
- Hypertension
- Gallbladder disease
- Benign and malignant liver tumors, and other hepatic lesions

There is evidence of an association between the following conditions and the use of oral contraceptives, although additional confirmatory studies are needed:

- Mesenteric thrombosis
- Neuro-ocular lesions (eg, retinal thrombosis and optic neuritis)

The following adverse reactions have been reported in patients receiving oral contraceptives and are believed to be drug-related:

- Nausea
- Vomiting
- Gastrointestinal symptoms (such as abdominal cramps and bloating)
- Breakthrough bleeding
- Spotting
- Change in menstrual flow
- Amenorrhea during or after use
- Temporary infertility after discontinuation of use
- Edema
- Chloasma or melasma, which may persist

- Breast changes: tenderness, enlargement, secretion
- Change in weight (increase or decrease)
- Change in cervical erosion or secretion
- Diminution in lactation when given immediately postpartum
- Cholestatic jaundice
- Migraine
- Rash (allergic)
- Mental depression
- Reduced tolerance to carbohydrates
- Vaginal candidiasis
- Change in corneal curvature (steepening)
- Intolerance to contact lenses

The following adverse reactions or conditions have been reported in users of oral contraceptives and the association has been neither confirmed nor refuted:

- Premenstrual syndrome
- Cataracts
- Changes in appetite
- Cystitis-like syndrome
- Headache
- Nervousness
- Dizziness
- Hirsutism
- Loss of scalp hair
- Erythema multiforme
- Erythema nodosum
- Hemorrhagic eruption
- Vaginitis
- Porphyria
- Impaired renal function
- Hemolytic uremic syndrome
- Acne
- Changes in libido
- Colitis
- Budd-Chiari syndrome
- Endocervical hyperplasia or ectropion

OVERDOSAGE

Serious ill effects have not been reported following acute ingestion of large doses of oral contraceptives by young children.[180, 181] Overdosage may cause nausea, and withdrawal bleeding may occur in females.

NON-CONTRACEPTIVE HEALTH BENEFITS

The following non-contraceptive health benefits related to the use of oral contraceptives are supported by epidemiological studies that largely utilized oral contraceptive formulations containing estrogen doses exceeding 35 mcg of ethinyl estradiol or 50 mcg of mestranol.[148, 149]

Effects on menses:
- Increased menstrual cycle regularity
- Decreased blood loss and decreased risk of iron-deficiency anemia
- Decreased frequency of dysmenorrhea

Effects related to inhibition of ovulation:
- Decreased risk of functional ovarian cysts
- Decreased risk of ectopic pregnancies

Effects from long-term use:
- Decreased risk of fibroadenomas and fibrocystic disease of the breast
- Decreased risk of acute pelvic inflammatory disease
- Decreased risk of endometrial cancer
- Decreased risk of ovarian cancer
- Decreased risk of uterine fibroids

DOSAGE AND ADMINISTRATION

To achieve maximum contraceptive effectiveness, oral contraceptives must be taken exactly as directed and at intervals of 24 hours.

IMPORTANT: The patient should be instructed to use an additional method of protection until after the first week of administration *in the initial cycle.*

The possibility of ovulation and conception prior to initiation of use should be considered.

Necon 1/35-21, Necon 1/35-28, Necon 0.5/35-21, Necon 0.5/35-28, Necon 10/11-21, Necon 10/11-28, Necon 1/50-21 and Necon 1/50-28 Dosage Schedules

The Necon 1/35-21, Necon 0.5/35-21, Necon 10/11-21, and Necon 1/50-21 tablet dispenser contain 21 tablets arranged in three numbered rows of 7 tablets each.

The Necon 1/35-28, Necon 0.5/35-28, Necon 10/11-28, and Necon 1/50-28 tablet dispenser contain 21 colored active tablets arranged in three numbered rows of 7 tablets each, followed by a fourth row of 7 white placebo tablets.

Days of the week are printed above the tablets, starting with Sunday on the left.

Two dosage schedules are described, one of which may be more convenient or suitable than the other for an individual patient.

Schedule #1: Sunday start. The patient begins taking Necon 1/35-21, Necon 1/35-28, Necon 0.5/35-21, Necon 0.5/35-28, Necon 10/11-21, Necon 10/11-28, Necon 1/50-21 or Necon 1/50-28 from the first row of her package, one tablet daily, starting on the first Sunday after the onset of menstruation.

Continued on next page

Necon—Cont.

If the patient's period begins on Sunday she takes her first tablet the very same day. The 21st tablet or the 28th tablet, depending on whether the patient is taking the 21- or 28-tablet course, will then be taken on a Saturday.

Subsequent cycles:

21-tablet course—The patient begins a new 21-tablet course on the eighth day, Sunday, after taking her last tablet. All subsequent cycles will also begin on Sunday, one tablet being taken each day for 3 weeks followed by a week of no-pill-taking.

28-tablet course—The patient begins a new 28-tablet course on the next day, Sunday, and all subsequent cycles will also begin on Sunday, one tablet being taken each and every day. With a Sunday-start schedule, a woman whose period begins on the day of or 1 to 4 days before taking the first tablet should expect a diminution of flow and fewer menstrual days. The initial cycle will likely be shortened by from 1 to 5 days. Thereafter, cycles should be about 28 days in length.

Schedule #2: Day 5 start. The patient begins taking Necon 1/35-21, Necon 0.5/35-21, or Necon 1/50-21 from the first row of her package, one tablet daily, starting with the pill day which corresponds to day 5 of her menstrual cycle; the first day of menstruation is counted as day 1. After the last (Saturday) tablet in row #3 has been taken, if any remain in the first row, the patient completes her 21-tablet schedule starting with Sunday in row #1.

Subsequent cycles: The patient begins a new 21-tablet course on the eighth day after taking her last tablet, again starting the same day of the week on which she began her first course. All subsequent cycles will also begin on that same day, one tablet being taken each day for 3 weeks followed by a week of no-pill taking.

Special notes

Spotting or breakthrough bleeding. If spotting (bleeding insufficient to require a pad) or breakthrough bleeding (heavier bleeding similar to a menstrual flow) occurs when these products are used for contraception, the patient should continue taking her tablets as directed. The incidence of spotting or breakthrough bleeding is minimal, most frequently occurring in the first cycle. Ordinarily spotting or breakthrough bleeding will stop within a week. Usually the patient will begin to cycle regularly within two to three courses of tablet-taking. In the event of spotting or breakthrough bleeding organic causes should be borne in mind. (See **WARNING** No. 11)

Missed menstrual periods. Withdrawal flow will normally occur 2 or 3 days after the last active tablet is taken. Failure of withdrawal bleeding ordinarily does not mean that the patient is pregnant, providing the dosage schedule has been correctly followed. (See **WARNING** No. 6)

If the patient has *not* adhered to the prescribed dosage regimen, the possibility of pregnancy should be considered after the first missed period, and oral contraceptives should be withheld until pregnancy has been ruled out.

If the patient has adhered to the prescribed regimen and misses two consecutive periods, pregnancy should be ruled out before continuing the contraceptive regimen.

The first intermenstrual interval after discontinuing the tablets is usually prolonged; consequently, a patient for whom a 28-day cycle is usual might not begin to menstruate for 35 days or longer. Ovulation in such prolonged cycles will occur correspondingly later in the cycle. Posttreatment cycles after the first one however, are usually typical for the individual woman prior to taking tablets. (See **WARNING** No. 11)

Missed tablets. If a woman misses taking one active tablet, the missed tablet should be taken as soon as it is remembered. In addition, the next tablet should be taken at the usual time. If two consecutive active tablets are missed the dosage should be doubled for the next 2 days. The regular schedule should then be resumed, but an additional method of protection is recommended for the remainder of the cycle. While there is little likelihood of ovulation if only one active tablet is missed, the possibility of spotting or breakthrough bleeding is increased and should be expected if two or more successive active tablets are missed. However, the possibility of ovulation increases with each successive day that scheduled active tablets are missed.

If one or more placebo tablets of Necon 1/35-28, Necon 0.5/35-28, Necon 10/11-28, or Necon 1/50-28 are missed, the Necon 1/35-28, Necon 0.5/35-28, Necon 10/11-28, or Necon 1/50-28 schedule should be resumed on the following Sunday (the eighth day after the last white tablet was taken). Omission of placebo tablets in the 28-tablet courses does not increase the possibility of conception provided that this schedule is followed.

HOW SUPPLIED

Necon 1/35: (Norethindrone and Ethinyl Estradiol Tablets, USP) Each dark yellow Necon 1/35 tablet is round in shape, with a debossed WATSON on one side and 508 on the other side, and contains 1 mg of norethindrone and 35 mcg of ethinyl estradiol.

Necon 1/35-21 (NDC 52544-508-21) is packaged in cartons of six tablet dispensers of 21 tablets each.

Necon 1/35-28 (NDC 52544-552-28) is packaged in cartons of six tablet dispensers. Each dispenser contains 21 dark yellow tablets and 7 white placebo tablets. (Placebo tablets have a debossed WATSON on one side and P on the other side.)

Necon 0.5/35: (Norethindrone and Ethinyl Estradiol Tablets, USP) Each light yellow Necon 0.5/35 tablet is round in shape, with a debossed WATSON on one side and 507 on the other side, and contains 0.5 mg of norethindrone and 35 mcg of ethinyl estradiol.

Necon 0.5/35-21 (NDC 52544-507-21) is packaged in cartons of six tablet dispensers of 21 tablets each.

Necon 0.5/35-28 (NDC 52544-550-28) is packaged in cartons of six tablet dispensers. Each dispenser contains 21 light yellow tablets and 7 white placebo tablets. (Placebo tablets have a debossed WATSON on one side and P on the other side.)

Necon 10/11: (Norethindrone and Ethinyl Estradiol Tablets, USP) Each light yellow Necon 10/11 tablet is round in shape, with a debossed WATSON on one side and 507 on the other side, and contains 0.5 mg of norethindrone and 35 mcg of ethinyl estradiol. Each dark yellow Necon 10/11 tablet is round in shape, with a debossed WATSON on one side and 508 on the other side, and contains 1 mg of norethindrone and 35 mcg of ethinyl estradiol.

Necon 10/11-21 (NDC 52544-553-21) is packaged in cartons of six tablet dispensers. Each dispenser contains 10 light yellow tablets and 11 dark yellow tablets.

Necon 10/11-28 (NDC 52544-553-28) is packaged in cartons of six tablet dispensers. Each dispenser contains 10 light yellow tablets and 11 dark yellow tablets and 7 white placebo tablets (Placebo tablets have a debossed WATSON on one side and P on the other side).

Necon 1/50: (Norethindrone and Mestranol Tablets, USP) Each light blue Necon 1/50 tablet is round in shape, with a debossed WATSON on one side and 510 on the other side, and contains 1 mg of norethindrone and 50 mcg of mestranol.

Necon 1/50-21 (NDC 52544-510-21) is packaged in cartons of six tablet dispensers of 21 tablets each.

Necon 1/50-28 (NDC 52544-556-28) is packaged in cartons of six tablet dispensers. Each dispenser contains 21 light blue tablets and 7 white placebo tablets. (Placebo tablets have a debossed WATSON on one side and P on the other side).

Store at controlled room temperature 15°–30°C (59°–86°F).

CAUTION: Federal Law prohibits dispensing without prescription.

REFERENCES

1. Trussel J, et al. *Stud Fam Plann.* 1987;18(Sept-Oct);237; and 1990;21(Jan-Feb):51. **2.** Mann JI, et al. *Br Med J.* 1975;2(May 3):241. **3.** Mann JI, et al. *Br Med J.* 1975;3(Sept 13):631. **4.** Mann JI, et al. *Br Med J.* 1975;2(May 3):245. **5.** Mann JI, et al. *Br Med J.* 1976;2(Aug 21):445. **6.** Arthes FG, et al. *Chest.* 1976;70(Nov):574. **7.** Jain AK. *Am J Obstet Gynecol.* 1976;301(Oct 1):126 and *Stud Fam Plann.* 1977;8(March):50. **8.** Ory HW. *JAMA.* 1977;237(June 13): 2619. **9.** Jick H, et al. *JAMA.* 1978;240(Dec 1):2548. **10.** Jick H, et al. *JAMA.* 1978;240(Dec 1):2548. **11.** Shapiro S, et al. *Lancet.* 1979;1(April 7):743. **12.** Rosenberg L, et al. *Am J Epidemiol.* 1980;111(Jan):59. **13.** Krueger DE, et al. *Am J Epidemiol.* 1980;111(June):655. **14.** Layde P, et al. *Lancet.* 1981;1(March 7):541. **15.** Adam SA, et al. *Br J Obstet Gynaecol.* 1981;88(Aug):838. **16.** Slone D, et al. *N Engl J Med.* 1981;305(Aug 20):420. **17.** Ramcharan S, et al. *The Walnut Creek Contraceptive Drug Study.* Vol 3. US Govt Ptg Off. 1981; and *J Reprod Med.* 1980;25(Dec):346. **18.** Layde PM, et al. *J R Coll Gen Pract.* 1983;33(Feb):75. **19.** Rosenberg L, et al. *JAMA.* 1985;253(May 24/31):2965. **20.** Mant D, et al. *J Epidemiol Community Health.* 1987;41(Sept):215. **21.** Croft P, et al. *Br Med J.* 1989;2998(Jan 21):165. **22.** Goldbaum GM, et al. *JAMA.* 1987;258(Sept 11):1339. **23.** Bradley DD, et al. *N Engl J Med.* 1978;299(July 6):17. **24.** Tikkanen MJ. *J Reprod Med.* 1986;31(Sept suppl):898. **25.** Lipson A, et al. *Contraception.* 1986;34(Aug):121. **26.** Burkman RT, et al. *Obstet Gynecol.* 1988;71(Jan):33. **27.** Knopp RH. *J Reprod Med.* 1986;31(Sept Suppl):913. **28.** Krauss RM, et al. *Am J Obstet Gynecol.* 1983;145(Feb 15):446. **29.** Wahl P, et al. *N Engl J Med.* 1983;308(April 14):862. **30.** Wynn V, et al. *Am J Obstet Gynecol.* 1982;142(March 15):766. **31.** LaRosa JC. *J Reprod Med.* 1986;31(Sept Suppl):906. **32.** Wynn V, et al. *J Reprod Med.* 1986;31(Sept Suppl):892. **33.** Royal College of General Practitioners. *JR Coll Gen Pract.* 1967;13(May): 267. **34.** Inman WHW, et al. *Br Med J.* 1968(April 27);193. **35.** Vessey MP, et al. *Br Med J.* 1968;2(April 27):199. **36.** Vessey MP, et al. *Br Med J.* 1969;2(June 14):651. **37.** Sartwell PE, et al. *Am J Epidemiol.* 1969;90(Nov):365. **38.** Vessey MP, et al. *Br Med J.* 1970;3(July 18):123. **39.** Greene GR, et al. *Am J Public Health.* 1972;62(May):680. **40.** Boston Collaborative Drug Surveillance Programme. *Lancet.* 1973;1(June 23):1399. **41.** Stolley PD, et al. *Am J Epidemiol.* 1975;102(Sept):197. **42.** Vessey MP, et al. *J Biosoc Sci.* 1976;8(Oct):373. **43.** Kay CR, *JR Coll Gen Pract.* 1978;28(July):393. **44.** Petitti DB, et al. *Am J Epidemiol.* 1978;108(Dec):480. **45.** Maquire MG, et al. *Am J Epidemiol.* 1979;110(Aug):188. **46.** Petitti DB, et al. *JAMA.* 1979;242(Sept 14):1150. **47.** Porter JB, et al. *Obstet Gynecol.* 1982;59(March):299. **48.** Porter JB, et al. *Obstet Gynecol.* 1985;66(July):1. **49.** Vessey MP, et al. *Br Med J.* 1986;292(Feb 22):526. **50.** Hoover R, et al. *Am J Public Health.* 1978;68(April):335. **51.** Vessey MP, *Br J Fam Plann.* 1980;6(Oct suppl):1. **52.** Collaborative Group for the Study of Stroke in Young Women. *N Engl J Med.* 1973;288(April 26):871. **53.** Royal College of General Practitioners. *Oral Contraceptives and Health.* New York, NY: Pitman Publ Corp; May 1974. **54.** Collaborative Group for the Study of Stroke in Young Women. *JAMA.* 1975;231(Feb 17):718. **55.** Beral V. *Lancet* . 1976;2(Nov 13):1047. **56.** Vessey MP, et al. *Lancet.* 1977;2(Oct 8);731; and 1981;1(March 7):549. **57.** Petitti DB, et al. *Lancet.* 1978;2(July 29):234. **58.** Inman WHW. *Br Med J.* 1979;2(Dec 8):1468. **59.** Vessey MP, et al. *Br Med J.* 1984;289(Sept 1):530. **60.** Inman WHW, et al. *Br Med J.* 1970;2(April 25):203. **61.** Meade TW, et al. *Br Med J.* 1980;280(May 10):1157. **62.** Bottiger LE, et al. *Lancet.* 1980;1(May 24):1097. **63.** Kay CR. *Am J Obstet Gynecol.* 1982;142(March 15):762. **64.** Vessey MP, et al. *Br Med J.* 1986;292(Feb 22):526. **65.** Gordon T, et al. *Am J Med.* 1977;62(May):707. **66.** Beral V, et al. *Lancet.* 1977;2(Oct 8): 727. **67.** Ory H. *Fam Plann Perspect.* 1983;15(March-April): 57. **68.** Arthes FG, et al. *Cancer.* 1971;28(Dec):1391. **69.** Vessey MP, et al. *Br Med J.* 1972;3(Sept 23):719. **70.** Boston Collaborative Drug Surveillance Program. *N Engl J Med.* 1974;290(Jan 3):15. **71.** Vessey MP, et al. *Lancet.* 1975;1(April 26):941. **72.** Casagrande J, et al. *J Natl Cancer Inst.* 1976;56(April):839. **73.** Kelsey JL, et al. *Am M Epidemiol.* 1978;107(March):236. **74.** Kay CR. *Br Med J.* 1981;282(June 27):2089. **75.** Vessey MP, et al. *Br Med J.* 1981;282(June 27):2093. **76.** The Cancer and Steroid Hormone Study of the Centers for Disease Control and the National Institute of Child Health and Human Development. Oral contraceptive use and the risk of breast cancer. *N Engl J Med.* 1986;315(Aug 14):405. **77.** Paul C, et al. *Br Med J.* 1986;293(Sept 20):723. **78.** Miller DR, et al. *Obstet Gynecol.* 1986;68(Dec):863. **79.** Pike MC, et al. *Lancet.* 1983;2(Oct 22):926. **80.** McPherson K, et al. *Br J Cancer.* 1987;56(Nov): 653. **81.** Hoover R, et al. *N Engl J Med.* 1976;295(Aug 19): 401. **82.** Lees AW, et al. *Int J Cancer.* 1978;22(Dec):700. **83.** Brinton LA, et al. *J Natl Cancer Inst.* 1979;62(Jan):37. **84.** Black MM. *Pathol Res Pract.* 1980;166:491; and *Cancer.* 1980;46(Dec):2747; and *Cancer.* 1983;51(June):2147. **85.** Clavel F, et al. *Bull Cancer* (Paris). 1981;68(Dec):449. **86.** Brinton LA, et al. *Int J Epidemiol.* 1982;11(Dec):316. **87.** Harris NV, et al. *Am J Epidemiol.* 1982;116(Oct):643. **88.** Jick H, et al. *Am J Epidemiol.* 1980;112(Nov):577. **89.** McPherson K, et al. *Lancet.* 1983;2(Dec 17):1414. **90.** Hoover R, et al. *J Natl Cancer Inst.* 1981;67(Oct):815. **91.** Jick H, et al. *Am J Epidemiol.* 1980;112(Nov):586. **92.** Meirik O, et al. *Lancet.* 1986;2(Sept 20):650. **93.** Fasal E, et al. *J Natl Cancer Inst.* 1975;55(Oct):767. **94.** Paffenbarger RS, et al. *Cancer.* 1977;39(April suppl):1887. **95.** Stadel BV, et al. *Contraception.* 1988;38(Sept):287. **96.** Miller DR, et al. *Am J Epidemiol.* 1989;129(Feb):269. **97.** Kay CR, et al. *Br J Cancer.* 1988;58(Nov):675. **98.** Miller DR, et al. *Obstet Gynecol.* 1986;68(Dec):863. **99.** Olsson H, et al. *Lancet.* 1985;1(March 30):748. **100.** Chilvers C, et al. *Lancet.* 1989;1(May 6):973. **101.** Huggins GR, et al. *Fertil Steril.* 1987;47(May):733. **102.** Pike MC, et al. *Br J Cancer.* 1981;43(Jan):72. **103.** Ory H, et al. *Am J Obstet Gynecol.* 1976;124(March 15):573. **104.** Stern E, et al. *Science.* 1977;196(June 24):1460. **105.** Pertiz E, et al. *Am J Epidemiol.* 1977;106(Dec):462. **106.** Ory HW, et al. In: Garattini S, Berendes H, eds. *Pharmacology of Steroid Contraceptive Drugs.* New York, NY:Raven Press;1977: 211-224. **107.** Meisels A, et al. *Cancer.* 1977;40(Dec):3076. **108.** Goldacre MJ, et al. *Br Med J.* 1978;1(March 25):748. **109.** Swan SH, et al. *Am J Obstet Gynecol.* 1981;139(Jan 1): 52. **110.** Vessey MP, et al. *Lancet.* 1983;2(Oct 22):930. **111.** Dallenbach-Hellweg G. *Pathol Res Pract.* 1984;179;38. **112.** Thomas DB, et al. *Br Med J.* 1985;290(March 30):961. **113.** Brinton LA, et al. *Int J Cancer.* 1986;38(Sept):339. **114.** Ebeling K, et al. *Int J Cancer.* 1987;39(April):427. **115.** Beral V, et al. *Lancet.* 1988;2(Dec 10):1331.**116.** Baum JK, et al. *Lancet.* 1973;2(Oct 27):926.**117.** Edmondson HA, et al. *N Engl J Med.* 1976;294(Feb 26):470. **118.** Bein NN, et al. *Br J Surg.* 1977;64(June):433. **119.** Klatskin G. *Gastroenterology.* 1977;73(Aug):386. **120.** Rooks JB, et al. *JAMA.* 1979;242(Aug 17):644. **121.** Sturtevant FM. In: Moghissi K, ed. *Controversies in Contraception.* Baltimore, MD; Wil-

liams & Wilkins; 1979:93–150. **122.** Henderson BE, et al. *Br J Cancer.* 1983;48(July):437. **123.** Neuberger J, et al. *Br Med J.* 1986;292(May 24):1355. **124.** Forman D, et al. *Br Med J.* 1986;292(May 24):1357. **125.** La Vecchia C, et al. *Br J Cancer.* 1989;59(March):460. **126.** Savolainen E, et al. *Am J Obstet Gynecol.* 1981;140(July 1):521. **127.** Ferencz C, et al. *Teratology.* 1980;21(April):225. **128.** Rothman KJ, et al. *Am J Epidemiol.* 1979;109(April):433. **129.** Harlap S, et al. *Obstet Gynecol.* 1980;55(April)447. **130.** Layde PM, et al. *J Epidemiol Community Health.* 1982;36(Dec):274. **131.** Rome Group for the Epidemiology and Prevention of Cholelithiasis (GREPCO). *Am J Epidemiol.* 1984;119(May):796. **132.** Strom BL, et al. *Clin Pharmacol Ther.* 1986;39(March):335. **133.** Wynn V. In: Bardin CE, et al. eds. *Progesterone and Progestins.* New York, NY:Raven Press;1983:395-410. **134.** Perlman JA, et al. *J Chron Dis.* 1985;38(Oct):857. **135.** Powell MG, et al. *Obstet Gynecol.* 1984;63(June):764. **136.** Wynn V, et al. *Lancet.* 1966;2(Oct 1):720. **137.** Firsch IR, et al. *JAMA.* 1977;237(June 6):2499. **138.** Kay CR. *Lancet.* 1977;1(March 19):624. **139.** Laragh JH. *Am J Obstet Gynecol.* 1976;126(Sept 1):141. **140.** Ramcharan S. In: Garattini S, Gerendes HW, eds. *Pharmacology of Steroid Contraceptive Drugs.* New York, NY:Raven Press;1977:277-288. **141.** Laumas KR, et al. *Am J Obstet Gynecol.* 1967;98(June 1):411. **142.** Saxena BN, et al. *Contraception.* 1977;16(Dec):605. **143.** Nilsson S, et al. *Contraception.* 1978;17(Feb):131. **144.** Washington AE, et al. *JAMA.* 1985;253(April 19):2246. **145.** Louv WC, et al. *Am J Obstet Gynecol.* 1989;160(Feb):396. **146.** Francis WG, et al. *Can Med Assoc J.* 1965;92(Jan 23):191. **147.** Verhulst HL, et al. *J Clin Pharmacol.* 1967;7(Jan-Feb):9. **148.** Ory HW. *Fam Plann Perspect.* 1982;14(July-Aug):182. **149.** Ory HW, et al. *Making Choices Evaluating the Health Risks and Benefits of Birth Control Methods.* New York, NY: The Alan Guttmacher Institute. 1983. **150.** Palmer JR, et al. *Am J Epidemiol.* 1989;130(Nov):878. **151.** Romeiu I, et al. *J Natl Cancer Inst.* 1989;81(Sept):1313. **152.** Porter JB, et al. *Obstet Gynecol.* 1987;70(July):29.

Manufactured by
WATSON LABORATORIES, INC.
Corona, CA 91720 Revised August 17, 1993

Necon 1/35-21
Necon 1/35-28
Necon 0.5/35-21
Necon 0.5/35-28
Necon 10/11-21
Necon 10/11-28
(norethindrone and ethinyl estradiol tablets, USP)
Necon 1/50-21
Necon 1/50-28
(norethindrone and mestranol tablets USP)

Shown in Product Identification Guide, page 342

NOR-QD® Tablets ℞
(norethindrone 0.35 mg)

PHYSICIAN LABELING

Patients should be counseled that this product does not protect against HIV infection (AIDS) and other sexually transmitted diseases.

DESCRIPTION

Each yellow NOR-QD® tablet provides a continuous oral contraceptive regimen of 0.35 mg norethindrone daily, and the inactive ingredients include D&C Yellow No. 10, FD&C Yellow No. 6, lactose, magnesium stearate, povidone, and starch.
The chemical name for norethindrone is 17-Hydroxy-19-Nor-17α-pregn-4-en-20-yn-3-one. The structural formula follows:

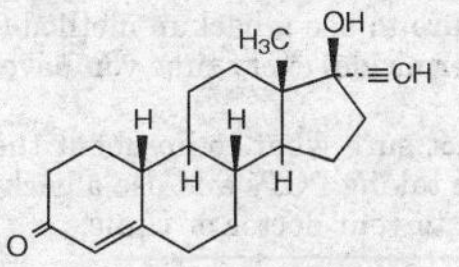

norethindrone

Therapeutic class = oral contraceptive.

CLINICAL PHARMACOLOGY

1. Mode of Action. NOR-QD® progestin-only oral contraceptives prevent conception by suppressing ovulation in approximately half of users, thickening the cervical mucus to inhibit sperm penetration, lowering the midcycle LH and FSH peaks, slowing the movement of the ovum through the fallopian tubes, and altering the endometrium.
2. Pharmacokinetics. Serum progestin levels peak about two hours after oral administration, followed by rapid distribution and elimination. By 24 hours after drug ingestion, serum levels are near baseline, making efficacy dependent upon rigid adherence to the dosing schedule. There are large variations in serum levels among individual users. Progestin-only administration results in lower steady-state serum progestin levels and a shorter elimination half-life than concomitant administration with estrogens.

INDICATIONS AND USAGE

1. Indications. Progestin-only oral contraceptives are indicated for the prevention of pregnancy.
2. Efficacy. If used perfectly, the first-year failure rate for progestin-only oral contraceptives is 0.5%. However, the typical failure rate is estimated to be closer to 5%, due to late or omitted pills. The following table lists the pregnancy rates for users of all major methods of contraception.

Table 1.
Comparison of reversible contraceptive methods:
Percent of women experiencing a contraceptive failure (pregnancy) during the first year of use.

Method	Percent of women experiencing a pregnancy within the first year of use: Average Use	Perfect Use
No contraception	85	85
Spermicides	21	6
Periodic abstinence	20	1–9[1]
Withdrawal	19	4
Cervical caps		
Given birth	36	26
Never given birth	18	9
Diaphragms	18	6
Condoms		
Female	21	5
Male	12	3
Pills	3	
Progestin-only		0.5
Combined		0.1
IUDs		
Progesterone	2	1.5
Copper T 380A	0.8	0.6
Injectables	0.3	0.3
Implant	0.09	0.09

Adapted with permission.[2]

1. Depending on method (calendar, ovulation, symptom-thermal, post-ovulation)
2. Hatcher RA, Trussel J, Stewart F, Stewart GK, Kowal D, Guest F, Cates W, Pollcar M. Contraceptive Technology 1994-1996, New York, NY: Irvington Publishers, 1994.

CONTRAINDICATIONS

Progestin-only oral contraceptives should not be used by women who currently have the following conditions:
- Known or suspected pregnancy
- Known or suspected carcinoma of the breast
- Undiagnosed abnormal genital bleeding
- Hypersensitivity to any component of this product
- Benign or malignant liver tumors
- Acute liver disease

WARNINGS

Cigarette smoking greatly increases the possibility of suffering heart attacks and strokes. Women who use oral contraceptives are strongly advised not to smoke.
Nor-QD does not contain estrogen and, therefore, this insert does not discuss the serious health risks that have been associated with the estrogen component of combined oral contraceptives. The health care provider is referred to the prescribing information of combined oral contraceptives for a discussion of those risks, including, but not limited to, an increased risk of serious cardiovascular disease in women who smoke, carcinoma of the breast and reproductive organs, hepatic neoplasia, and changes in carbohydrates and lipid metabolism. The relationship between progestin-only oral contraceptives and these risks have not been established and there are no studies definitely linking progestin-only pill (POP) use to an increased risk of heart attack or stroke.
The physician should remain alert to the earliest manifestation of symptoms of any serious disease and discontinue oral contraceptive therapy when appropriate.
1. Ectopic pregnancy. The incidence of ectopic pregnancies for progestin-only oral contraceptive users is 5 per 1000 woman-years. Up to 10% of pregnancies reported in clinical studies of progestin-only oral contraceptive users are extrauterine. Although symptoms of ectopic pregnancy should be watched for, a history of ectopic pregnancy need not be considered a contraindication to use of this contraceptive method. Health providers should be alert to the possibility of an ectopic pregnancy in women who become pregnant or complain of lower abdominal pain while on progestin-only oral contraceptives.
2. Delayed follicular atresia/Ovarian cysts. If follicular development occurs, atresia of the follicle is sometimes delayed, and the follicle may continue to grow beyond the size it would attain in a normal cycle. Generally these enlarged follicles disappear spontaneously. Often they are asymptomatic; in some cases they are associated with mild abdominal pain. Rarely they may twist or rupture, requiring surgical intervention.
3. Irregular genital bleeding. Irregular menstrual patterns are common among women using progestin-only oral contraceptives. If genital bleeding is suggestive of infection, malignancy or other abnormal conditions, such nonpharmacologic causes should be ruled out. If prolonged amenorrhea occurs, the possibility of pregnancy should be evaluated.
4. Carcinoma of the breast and reproductive organs. Some epidemiologic studies of oral contraceptive users have reported an increased relative risk of developing breast cancer, particularly at a younger age and apparently related to duration of use. These studies have predominantly involved combined oral contraceptives and there is insufficient data to determine whether the use of POPs similarly increases the risk. Women with breast cancer should not use oral contraceptives because the role of female hormones in breast cancer has not been fully determined.
Some studies suggest that oral contraceptive use has been associated with an increase in the risk of cervical intraepithelial neoplasia in some populations of women. However, there continues to be controversy about the extent to which such findings may be due to differences in sexual behavior and other factors. There is insufficient data to determine whether the use of POPs increases the risk of developing cervical intraepithelial neoplasia.
5. Hepatic neoplasia. Benign hepatic adenomas are associated with combined oral contraceptive use, although the incidence of benign tumors is rare in the United States. Rupture of benign, hepatic adenomas may cause death through intraabdominal hemorrhage.
Studies from Britain and the U.S. have shown an increased risk of developing hepatocellular carcinoma in combined oral contraceptive users. However, these cancers are rare. There is insufficient data to determine whether POPs increase the risk of developing hepatic neoplasia.

PRECAUTIONS

1. General. Patients should be counseled that this product does not protect against HIV infection (AIDS) and other sexually transmitted diseases.
2. Physical examination and followup. It is considered good medical practice for sexually active women using oral contraceptives to have annual history and physical examinations. The physical examination may be deferred until after initiation of oral contraceptives if requested by the women and judged appropriate by the clinician.
3. Carbohydrates and lipid metabolism. Some users may experience slight deterioration in glucose tolerance, with increases in plasma insulin but women with diabetes mellitus who use progestin-only oral contraceptives do not generally experience changes in their insulin requirements. Nonetheless, prediabetic and diabetic women in particular should be carefully monitored while taking POPs.
Lipid metabolism is occasionally affected in that HDL, HDL_2, and apolipoprotein A-I and A-II may be decreased; hepatic lipase may be increased. There is no effect on total cholesterol, HDL_3, LDL, or VLDL.
4. Drug interactions. The effectiveness of progestin-only pills is reduced by hepatic enzyme-inducing drugs such as the anticonvulsants phenytoin, carbamazepine, and barbiturates, and the antituberculosis drug rifampin. No significant interaction has been found with broad-spectrum antibiotics.
5. Interactions with laboratory tests. The following endocrine tests may be affected by progestin-only oral contraceptive use:
- Sex hormone-binding globulin (SHBG) concentrations may be decreased.
- Thyroxine concentrations may be decreased, due to a decrease in thyroid binding globulin (TBG).

6. Carcinogenesis. See **WARNINGS** section.
7. Pregnancy. Many studies have found no effects on fetal development associated with long-term use of contraceptive doses of oral progestins. The few studies of infant growth and development that have been conducted have not demonstrated significant adverse effects. It is nonetheless prudent to rule out suspected pregnancy before initiating any hormonal contraceptive use.
8. Nursing mothers. No adverse effects have been found on breastfeeding performance or on the health, growth or development of the infant. Small amounts of progestin pass into the breast milk, resulting in steroid levels in infant plasma of 1–6% of the levels of maternal plasma.

Continued on next page

Nor-QD—Cont.

9. Fertility following discontinuation: The limited available data indicate a rapid return of normal ovulation and fertility following discontinuation of progestin-only oral contraceptives.

10. Headache. The onset or exacerbation of migraine or the development of severe headache with focal neurological symptoms which is recurrent or persistent requires discontinuation of progestin-only contraceptives and evaluation of the cause.

11. Pediatric use. Safety and efficacy of Nor-QD have been established in women of reproductive age. Safety and efficacy are expected to be the same for postpubertal adolescents under the age of 16 and for users 16 years and older. Use of this product before menarche is not indicated.

INFORMATION FOR THE PATIENT

1. See **PATIENT LABELING** for detailed information.

2. Counseling issues. The following points should be discussed with prospective users before prescribing progestin-only oral contraceptives.

- The necessity of taking pills at the same time every day, including throughout all bleeding episodes.
- The need to use a backup method such as condoms and spermicides for the next 48 hours whenever a progestin-only contraceptive is taken 3 or more hours late.
- The potential side effects of progestin-only oral contraceptives, particularly menstrual irregularities.
- The need to inform the clinician of prolonged episodes of bleeding, amenorrhea or severe abdominal pain.
- The importance of using a barrier method in addition to progestin-only oral contraceptives if a woman is at risk of contracting or transmitting STDs/HIV.

ADVERSE REACTIONS

- Menstrual irregularity is the most frequently reported side effect.
- Frequent and irregular bleeding are common, while long duration of bleeding episodes and amenorrhea are less likely.
- Headache, breast tenderness, nausea, and dizziness are increased among progestin-only oral contraceptive users in some studies.
- Androgenic side effects such as acne, hirsutism, and weight gain occur rarely.

OVERDOSAGE

There have been no reports of serious ill effects from overdosage, including ingestion by children.

DOSAGE AND ADMINISTRATION

To achieve maximum contraceptive effectiveness, NOR-QD® must be taken exactly as directed. One tablet is taken every day, at the same time. Administration is continuous, with no interruption between pill packs. See **PATIENT LABELING** for detailed instructions.

HOW SUPPLIED

NOR-QD® (norethindrone) tablets are available in 42-tablet dispensers.
Rx only
STORAGE
Store at controlled room temperature 15°–25°C (59°–77°F).

REFERENCE

McCann M, and Potter L. Progestin-Only Oral Contraceptives: A Comprehensive Review. Contraception, 50:60 (Suppl. 1), December 1994.

DETAILED INFORMATION FOR THE PATIENT

This product (like all oral contraceptives) is used to prevent pregnancy. It does not protect against HIV infection (AIDS) and other sexually transmitted diseases.

INTRODUCTION

This leaflet is about birth control pills that contain one hormone, a progestin. Please read this leaflet before you begin to take your pills. It is meant to be used along with talking with your doctor or clinic.

Progestin-only pills are often called "POPs" or "the minipill." POPs have less progestin than the combined birth control pill (or "the pill") which contains both an estrogen and a progestin.

HOW EFFECTIVE ARE POPS?

About 1 in 200 POPs users will get pregnant in the first year if they all take POPs perfectly (that is, on time, every day). About 1 in 20 "typical" POPs users (including women who are late taking pills or miss pills) gets pregnant in the first year of use. The following table will help you compare the efficacy of different methods.

Table 1.
Comparison of reversible contraceptive methods: Percent of women who become pregnant during the first year of use.

Method	Percent of women experiencing a pregnancy within the first year of use	
	Average Use	Perfect Use
No contraception	85	85
Spermicides	21	6
Periodic abstinence	20	1–9[1]
Withdrawal	19	4
Cervical caps		
Given birth	36	26
Never given birth	18	9
Diaphragms	18	6
Condoms		
Female	21	5
Male	12	3
Pills	3	
POPs		0.5
Combined pills		0.1
IUDs		
Progesterone	2	1.5
Copper T 380A	0.8	0.6
Injectables	0.3	0.3
Implant	0.09	0.09

Adapted with permission.[2]

1. Depending on method (calendar, ovulation, symptom-thermal, post-ovulation)
2. Hatcher RA, Trussel J, Stewart F, Stewart GK, Kowal D, Guest F, Cates W, Pollcar M. Contraceptive Technology 1994-1996. New York, NY: Irvington Publishers, 1994.

HOW DO POPS WORK?

- They make the cervical mucus at the entrance to the womb (the uterus) too thick for the sperm to get through to the egg.
- They prevent ovulation (release of the egg from the ovary) in about half the time.
- They also affect other hormones, the fallopian tubes and the lining of the uterus.

YOU SHOULD NOT TAKE POPS

- If there is any chance you may be pregnant.
- If you have breast cancer.
- If you have bleeding between your periods which has not been diagnosed.
- If you are taking certain drugs for epilepsy (seizures) or for TB. (See **USING POPS WITH OTHER MEDICINES** below.)
- If you are hypersensitive or allergic to any component of this product.
- If you have liver tumors, either benign or cancerous.
- If you have acute liver disease.

RISKS OF TAKING POPS

WARNING: If you have sudden or severe pain in your lower abdomen or stomach area, you may have an ectopic pregnancy or an ovarian cyst. If this happens, you should contact your doctor or clinic immediately.

1. Ectopic pregnancy. An ectopic pregnancy is a pregnancy outside the womb. Because POPs protect against pregnancy, the chance of having a pregnancy outside the womb is very low. If you do get pregnant while taking POPs, you have a slightly higher chance that the pregnancy will be ectopic than do users of some other birth control methods.

2. Ovarian cysts. These cysts are small sacs of fluid in the ovary. They are more common among POP users than among users of most other birth control methods. They usually disappear without treatment and rarely cause problems.

3. Cancer of the reproductive organs and breasts. Some studies in women who use combined oral contraceptives that contain both estrogen and a progestin have reported an increase in the risk of developing breast cancer, particularly at a younger age and apparently related to duration of use. There is insufficient data to determine whether the use of POPs similarly increases this risk.

Some studies have found an increase in the incidence of cancer of the cervix in women who use oral contraceptives. However, this finding may be related to factors other than the use of oral contraceptives and there is insufficient data to determine whether the use of POPs increases the risk of developing cancer of the cervix.

4. Liver tumors. In rare cases, combined oral contraceptives can cause benign but dangerous liver tumors. These benign liver tumors can rupture and cause fatal internal bleeding. In addition, a possible but not definite association has been found with combined oral contraceptives and liver cancers in studies in which a few women who developed these very rare cancers were found to have used combined oral contraceptives for long periods of time. There is insuf-ficient data to determine whether POPs increase the risk of liver tumors.

SEXUALLY-TRANSMITTED DISEASES (STDS)

WARNING: POPs do not protect against getting or giving someone HIV (AIDS) or any other STD, such as chlamydia, gonorrhea, genital warts or herpes.

SIDE EFFECTS

1. Irregular bleeding. The most common side effect of POPs is a change in menstrual bleeding. Your periods may be either early or late, and you may have some spotting between periods. Taking pills late or missing pills can also result in some spotting or bleeding.

2. Other side effects. Less common side effects include headaches, tender breasts, nausea and dizziness. Weight gain, acne and extra hair on your face and body have been reported, but are rare.

If you are concerned about any of these side effects, check with your doctor or clinic.

USING POPS WITH OTHER MEDICINES

Before taking a POP, inform your health care provider of any other medication, including over-the-counter medicine, that you may be taking.

If you are taking medicines for seizures (epilepsy) or tuberculosis (TB), tell your doctor or clinic. These medicines can make POPs less effective:

Medicines for seizures:
- Phenytoin (Dilantin®)
- Carbamazepine (Tegretol®)
- Phenobarbital

Medicine for TB:
- Rifampin (Rifampicin)

Before you begin taking any new medicines be sure your doctor or clinic knows you are taking birth control pills that contain a progestin.

HOW TO TAKE POPS

IMPORTANT POINTS TO REMEMBER

- POPs must be taken at the same time every day, so choose a time and then take the pill at that same time every day. Every time you take a pill late, and especially if you miss a pill, you are more likely to get pregnant.
- Start the next pack the day after the last pack is finished. There is no break between packs. Always have your next pack of pills ready.
- You may have some menstrual spotting between periods. Do not stop taking your pills if this happens.
- If you vomit soon after taking a pill, use a backup method (such as condom and/or spermicide) for 48 hours.
- If you want to stop taking POPs, you can do so at any time, but, if you remain sexually active and don't wish to become pregnant, be certain to use another birth control method.
- If you are not sure about how to take POPs, ask your doctor or clinic.

STARTING POPS

- It's best to take your first POP on the first day of your menstrual period.
- If you decide to take your first POP on another day, use a backup method (such as condom and/or spermicide) every time you have sex during the next 48 hours.
- If you have had a miscarriage or an abortion, you can start POPs the next day.

IF YOU ARE LATE OR MISS TAKING YOUR POPS

- If you are more than 3 hours late or you miss one or more POPs:
  1. TAKE a missed pill as soon as you remember that you missed it,
  2. THEN go back to taking POPs at your regular time,
  3. BUT be sure to use a backup method (such as condom and/or spermicide) every time you have sex for the next 48 hours.
- If you are not sure what to do about the pills you have missed, keep taking POPs and use a backup method until you can talk to your doctor or clinic.

IF YOU ARE BREASTFEEDING

- If you are fully breastfeeding (not giving your baby any food or formula), you may start your pills 6 weeks after delivery.
- If you are partially breastfeeding (giving your baby some food or formula), you should start taking pills by 3 weeks after delivery.

IF YOU ARE SWITCHING PILLS

- If you are switching from the combined pills to POPs, take the first POP the day after you finish the last active combined pill. Do not take any of the 7 inactive pills from the

combined pill pack. You should know that many women have irregular periods after switching to POPs, but this is normal and to be expected.

- If you are switching from POPs to the combined pills, take the first active combined pill on the first day of your period, even if your POPs pack is not finished.
- If you switch to another brand of POPs, start the new brand anytime.
- If you are breastfeeding, you can switch to another method of birth control at any time, except do not switch to the combined pills until you stop breastfeeding or at least until 6 months after delivery.

PREGNANCY WHILE ON THE PILL

If you become pregnant, or think you might be, stop taking POPs and contact your physician. Even though research has shown that POPs do not cause harm to the unborn baby, it is always best not to take any drugs or medicines that you don't need when you are pregnant.

You should get a pregnancy test:
- If your period is late and you took one or more pills late or missed taking them and had sex without a backup method.
- Anytime you miss 2 periods in a row.

WILL POPS AFFECT YOUR ABILITY TO GET PREGNANT LATER?

If you want to become pregnant, simply stop taking POPs. POPs will not delay your ability to get pregnant.

BREASTFEEDING

If you are breastfeeding, POPs will not affect the quality or amount of your breastmilk or the health of your nursing baby.

OVERDOSE

No serious problems have been reported when many pills were taken by accident, even by a small child, so there is usually no reason to treat an overdose.

OTHER QUESTIONS OR CONCERNS

Cigarette smoking greatly increases the possibility of suffering heart attacks and strokes. Women who use oral contraceptives are strongly advised not to smoke.

Diabetic women taking POPs do not generally require changes in the amount of insulin they are taking. However, your physician may monitor you more closely under these conditions.

If you have any questions or concerns, check with your doctor or clinic. You can also ask for the more detailed "professional package labeling" written for doctors and other health care providers.

HOW TO STORE YOUR POPs

Store your POPs at room temperature 15°–25°C (59°–77°F).

Be certain to read new revisions of this leaflet. You may check the date of the most recent revision by phoning the manufacturer toll-free at 1-800-272-5525 or by writing to the address below:

Revised: Feb. 26, 1998

Address medical inquiries to:
Medical Information Department
Watson Laboratories, Inc.
311 Bonnie Circle
Corona, CA 91720
Manufactured for:
WATSON PHARMA
A Division of Watson Laboratories, Inc.
Corona, CA 91720
by Syntex Inc.
Humacao, PR 00791
Shown in Product Identification Guide, page 342

NORCO™ TABLETS　　　　　　　　　　CⅢ Rx

DESCRIPTION

NORCO™ (Hydrocodone bitartrate and acetaminophen) is supplied in tablet form for oral administration.

Hydrocodone bitartrate is an opioid analgesic and antitussive and occurs as fine, white crystals or as a crystalline powder. It is affected by light. The chemical name is 4,5α-epoxy-3-methoxy-17-methylmorphinan-6-one tartrate (1:1) hydrate (2:5). It has the following structural formula:
[See first chemical structure at top of next column]

Acetaminophen, 4¹-hydroxyacetanilide, a slightly bitter, white, odorless, crystalline powder, is a non-opiate, non-salicylate analgesic and antipyretic. It has the following structural formula:
[See second chemical structure at top of next column]

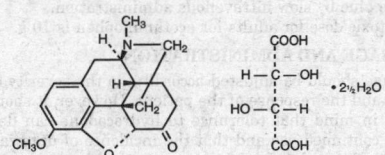

$C_{18}H_{21}NO_3 \cdot C_4H_6O_6 \cdot 2\frac{1}{2}H_2O$　　　　　　　MW=494.50

$C_8H_9NO_2$　　　　　　　　　　　　MW=151.17

Each NORCO™ tablet contains:

Hydrocodone Bitartrate	10 mg
(**WARNING:** May be habit forming)	
Acetaminophen	325 mg

In addition, each tablet contains the following inactive ingredients: croscarmellose sodium, crospovidone, D&C yellow #10 aluminum lake, magnesium stearate, microcrystalline cellulose, pregelatinized starch, povidone and stearic acid.

CLINICAL PHARMACOLOGY

Hydrocodone is a semisynthetic narcotic analgesic and antitussive with multiple actions qualitatively similar to those of codeine. Most of these involve the central nervous system and smooth muscle. The precise mechanism of action of hydrocodone and other opiates is not known, although it is believed to relate to the existence of opiate receptors in the central nervous system. In addition to analgesia, narcotics may produce drowsiness, changes in mood and mental clouding.

The analgesic action of acetaminophen involves peripheral influences, but the specific mechanism is as yet undetermined. Antipyretic activity is mediated through hypothalamic heat regulating centers. Acetaminophen inhibits prostaglandin synthetase. Therapeutic doses of acetaminophen have negligible effects on the cardiovascular or respiratory systems; however, toxic doses may cause circulatory failure and rapid, shallow breathing.

Pharmacokinetics: The behavior of the individual components is described below.

Hydrocodone: Following a 10 mg oral dose of hydrocodone administered to five adult male subjects, the mean peak concentration was 23.6 ± 5.2 ng/mL. Maximum serum levels were achieved at 1.3 ± 0.3 hours and the half-life was determined to be 3.8 ± 0.3 hours. Hydrocodone exhibits a complex pattern of metabolism including O-demethylation, N-demethylation and 6-keto reduction to the corresponding 6-α- and 6-β-hydroxymetabolites.

See **OVERDOSAGE** for toxicity information.

Acetaminophen: Acetaminophen is rapidly absorbed from the gastrointestinal tract and is distributed throughout most body tissues. The plasma half-life is 1.25 to 3 hours, but may be increased by liver damage and following overdosage. Elimination of acetaminophen is principally by liver metabolism (conjugation) and subsequent renal excretion of metabolites. Approximately 85% of an oral dose appears in the urine within 24 hours of administration, most as the glucuronide conjugate, with small amounts of other conjugates and unchanged drug.

See **OVERDOSAGE** for toxicity information.

INDICATIONS AND USAGE

NORCO™ Tablets are indicated for the relief of moderate to moderately severe pain.

CONTRAINDICATIONS

NORCO™ Tablets should not be administered to patients who have previously exhibited hypersensitivity to hydrocodone or acetaminophen.

WARNINGS

Respiratory Depression: At high doses or in sensitive patients, hydrocodone may produce dose-related respiratory depression by acting directly on the brain stem respiratory center. Hydrocodone also affects the center that controls respiratory rhythm, and may produce irregular and periodic breathing.

Head Injury and Increased Intracranial Pressure: The respiratory depressant effects of narcotics and their capacity to elevate cerebrospinal fluid pressure may be markedly exaggerated in the presence of head injury, other intracranial lesions or a pre-existing increase in intracranial pressure.

Furthermore, narcotics produce adverse reactions which may obscure the clinical course of patients with head injuries.

Acute Abdominal Conditions: The administration of narcotics may obscure the diagnosis or clinical course of patients with acute abdominal conditions.

PRECAUTIONS

General: Special Risk Patients: As with any narcotic analgesic agent, NORCO™ Tablets should be used with caution in elderly or debilitated patients, and those with severe impairment of hepatic or renal function, hypothyroidism, Addison's disease, prostatic hypertrophy or urethral stricture. The usual precautions should be observed and the possibility of respiratory depression should be kept in mind.

Cough reflex: Hydrocodone suppresses the cough reflex; as with all narcotics, caution should be exercised when NORCO™ Tablets are used postoperatively and in patients with pulmonary disease.

Information for Patients: NORCO™ Tablets, like all narcotics, may impair mental and/or physical abilities required for the performance of potentially hazardous tasks such as driving a car or operating machinery; patients should be cautioned accordingly.

Alcohol and other CNS depressants may produce an additive CNS depression, when taken with this combination product, and should be avoided.

Hydrocodone may be habit-forming. Patients should take the drug only for as long as it is prescribed, in the amounts prescribed, and no more frequently than prescribed.

Laboratory Tests: In patients with severe hepatic or renal disease, effects of therapy should be monitored with serial liver and/or renal function tests.

Drug Interactions: Patients receiving narcotics, antihistamines, antipsychotics, antianxiety agents, or other CNS depressants (including alcohol) concomitantly with NORCO™ Tablets may exhibit an additive CNS depression. When combined therapy is contemplated, the dose of one or both agents should be reduced.

The use of MAO inhibitors or tricyclic antidepressants with hydrocodone preparations may increase the effect of either the antidepressant or hydrocodone.

Drug/Laboratory Test Interactions: Acetaminophen may produce false-positive test results for urinary 5-hydroxyindoleacetic acid.

Carcinogenesis, Mutagenesis, Impairment of Fertility: No adequate studies have been conducted in animals to determine whether hydrocodone or acetaminophen have a potential for carcinogenesis, mutagenesis, or impairment of fertility.

Pregnancy:

Teratogenic Effects: Pregnancy Category C: There are no adequate and well-controlled studies in pregnant women. NORCO™ Tablets should be used during pregnancy only if the potential benefit justifies the potential risk to the fetus.

Nonteratogenic Effects: Babies born to mothers who have been taking opioids regularly prior to delivery will be physically dependent. The withdrawal signs include irritability and excessive crying, tremors, hyperactive reflexes, increased respiratory rate, increased stools, sneezing, yawning, vomiting and fever. The intensity of the syndrome does not always correlate with the duration of maternal opioid use or dose. There is no consensus on the best method of managing withdrawal.

Labor and Delivery: As with all narcotics, administration of NORCO™ Tablets to the mother shortly before delivery may result in some degree of respiratory depression in the newborn, especially if higher doses are used.

Nursing Mothers: Acetaminophen is excreted in breast milk in small amounts, but the significance of its effects on nursing infants is not known. It is not known whether hydrocodone is excreted in human milk. Because many drugs are excreted in human milk and because of the potential for serious adverse reactions in nursing infants from NORCO™ Tablets, a decision should be made whether to discontinue nursing or to discontinue the drug, taking into account the importance of the drug to the mother.

Pediatric Use: Safety and effectiveness in pediatric patients have not been established.

ADVERSE REACTIONS

The most frequently reported adverse reactions are lightheadedness, dizziness, sedation, nausea and vomiting. These effects seem to be more prominent in ambulatory than in nonambulatory patients, and some of these adverse reactions may be alleviated if the patient lies down.

Other adverse reactions include:

Central Nervous System: Drowsiness, mental clouding, lethargy, impairment of mental and physical performance, anxiety, fear, dysphoria, psychic dependence, mood changes.

Gastrointestinal System: Prolonged administration of NORCO™ Tablets may produce constipation.

Genitourinary System: Ureteral spasm, spasm of vesical sphincters and urinary retention have been reported with opiates.

Continued on next page

Norco—Cont.

Respiratory Depression: Hydrocodone bitartrate may produce dose-related respiratory depression by acting directly on brain stem respiratory centers (see **OVERDOSAGE**).

Dermatological: Skin rash, pruritus.

The following adverse drug events may be borne in mind as potential effects of acetaminophen: allergic reactions, rash, thrombocytopenia, agranulocytosis.

Potential effects of high dosage are listed in the **OVERDOSAGE** section.

DRUG ABUSE AND DEPENDENCE

Controlled Substance: NORCO™ Tablets are classified as a Schedule III controlled substance.

Abuse and Dependence: Psychic dependence, physical dependence, and tolerance may develop upon repeated administration of narcotics; therefore, NORCO™ Tablets should be prescribed and administered with caution. However, psychic dependence is unlikely to develop when NORCO™ Tablets are used for a short time for the treatment of pain.

Physical dependence, the condition in which continued administration of the drug is required to prevent the appearance of a withdrawal syndrome, assumes clinically significant proportions only after several weeks, of continued narcotic use, although some mild degree of physical dependence may develop after a few days of narcotic therapy. Tolerance, in which increasingly large doses are required in order to produce the same degree of analgesia, is manifested initially by a shortened duration of analgesic effect, and subsequently by decreases in the intensity of analgesia. The rate of development of tolerance varies among patients.

OVERDOSAGE

Following an acute overdosage, toxicity may result from hydrocodone or acetaminophen.

Signs and Symptoms

Hydrocodone: Serious overdose with hydrocodone is characterized by respiratory depression (a decrease in respiratory rate and/or tidal volume, Cheyne-Stokes respiration, cyanosis), extreme somnolence progressing to stupor or coma, skeletal muscle flaccidity, cold and clammy skin, and sometimes bradycardia and hypotension. In severe overdosage, apnea, circulatory collapse, cardiac arrest and death may occur.

Acetaminophen: In acetaminophen overdosage: dose-dependent, potentially fatal hepatic necrosis is the most serious adverse effect. Renal tubular necrosis, hypoglycemic coma and thrombocytopenia may also occur.

Early symptoms following a potentially hepatotoxic overdose may include: nausea, vomiting, diaphoresis and general malaise. Clinical and laboratory evidence of hepatic toxicity may not be apparent until 48 to 72 hours post-ingestion.

In adults, hepatic toxicity has rarely been reported with acute overdoses of less than 10 grams, or fatalities with less than 15 grams.

Treatment: A single or multiple overdose with hydrocodone and acetaminophen is a potentially lethal polydrug overdose, and consultation with a regional poison control center is recommended.

Immediate treatment includes support of cardiorespiratory function and measures to reduce drug absorption. Vomiting should be induced mechanically, or with syrup of ipecac, if the patient is alert (adequate pharyngeal and laryngeal reflexes). Oral activated charcoal (1 g/kg) should follow gastric emptying. The first dose should be accompanied by an appropriate cathartic. If repeated doses are used, the cathartic might be required with alternate doses as required. Hypotension is usually hypovolemic and should respond to fluids. Vasopressors and other supportive measures should be employed as indicated. A cuffed endo-tracheal tube should be inserted before gastric lavage of the unconscious patient and, when necessary, to provide assisted respiration.

Meticulous attention should be given to maintaining adequate pulmonary ventilation. In severe cases of intoxication, peritoneal dialysis, or preferably hemodialysis may be considered. If hypoprothrombinemia occurs due to acetaminophen overdose, vitamin K should be administered intravenously.

Naloxone, a narcotic antagonist, can reverse respiratory depression and coma associated with opioid overdose. Naloxone hydrochloride 0.4 mg to 2 mg is given parenterally. Since the duration of action of hydrocodone may exceed that of the naloxone, the patient should be kept under continuous surveillance and repeated doses of the antagonist should be administered as needed to maintain adequate respiration. A narcotic antagonist should not be administered in the absence of clinically significant respiratory or cardiovascular depression.

If the dose of acetaminophen may have exceeded 140 mg/kg, acetylcysteine should be administered as early as possible. Serum acetaminophen levels should be obtained, since levels four or more hours following ingestion help predict acet-

aminophen toxicity. Do not await acetaminophen assay results before initiating treatment. Hepatic enzymes should be obtained initially, and repeated at 24-hour intervals. Methemoglobinemia over 30% should be treated with methylene blue by slow intravenous administration.

The toxic dose for adults for acetaminophen is 10 g.

DOSAGE AND ADMINISTRATION

Dosage should be adjusted according to the severity of the pain and the response of the patient. However, it should be kept in mind that tolerance to hydrocodone can develop with continued use and that the incidence of untoward effects is dose related.

The usual adult dosage is one tablet every four to six hours as needed for pain. The total daily dosage should not exceed 6 tablets.

HOW SUPPLIED

NORCO™ is supplied as a yellow, capsule-shaped tablet containing 10 mg hydrocodone bitartrate and 325 mg acetaminophen, bisected on one side and debossed with "NORCO 539" on the other side.

Bottles of 100   NDC 52544-539-01
Bottles of 500   NDC 52544-539-05

Store at controlled room temperature, 15° - 30°C (59°-86°F).

Dispense in a tight, light-resistant container with a child-resistant closure.

WATSON PHARMA
A division of
Watson Laboratories   Revised May 15, 1998
Corona, CA 91720   13095

Shown in Product Identification Guide, page 342

TRIVORA® –21 Tablets
–28 Tablets   ℞
**(levonorgestrel and
ethinyl estradiol tablets, USP)–triphasic regimen**

Patients should be counseled that this product does not protect against HIV infection (AIDS) and other sexually transmitted diseases.

ORAL CONTRACEPTIVE AGENTS

DESCRIPTION

Trivora-21 Tablets provide an oral contraceptive regimen of 6 blue tablets followed by 5 white tablets and 10 pink tablets. Each blue tablet contains levonorgestrel 0.05 mg and ethinyl estradiol 0.03 mg, each white tablet contains levonorgestrel 0.075 mg and ethinyl estradiol 0.04 mg and each pink tablet contains levonorgestrel 0.125 mg and ethinyl estradiol 0.03 mg.

Trivora-28 tablets provide a continuous oral contraceptive regimen of 6 blue tablets, 5 white tablets, 10 pink tablets and then 7 peach tablets. Each blue tablet contains

levonorgestrel 0.05 mg and ethinyl estradiol 0.03 mg, each white tablet contains levonorgestrel 0.075 mg and ethinyl estradiol 0.04 mg, each pink tablet contains levonorgestrel 0.125 mg and ethinyl estradiol 0.03 mg and each peach tablet contains inert ingredients.

Levonorgestrel is a totally synthetic progestogen with the chemical name (−)-13-Ethyl-17-hydroxy-18, 19-dinor-17α-pregn-4-en-20-yn-3-one. Ethinyl estradiol is an estrogen with the chemical name 19-Nor-17α-pregna-1,3,5(10)-trien-20-yne-3,17-diol. Their structural formulae follow:

LEVONORGESTREL
$C_{21}H_{28}O_2$
M.W. = 312.45

ETHINYL ESTRADIOL
$C_{20}H_{24}O_2$
M.W. = 296.41

The inactive ingredients present in all the tablets are lactose monohydrate, magnesium stearate, povidone, starch (corn) plus the following dyes:

Blue tablet: FD&C Blue #1
Pink tablet: FD&C Red #40
Peach tablet: FD&C Yellow #6

CLINICAL PHARMACOLOGY

Combination oral contraceptives act by suppression of gonadotrophins. Although the primary mechanism of this action is inhibition of ovulation, other alterations include changes in the cervical mucus (which increase the difficulty of sperm entry into the uterus) and the endometrium (which may reduce the likelihood of implantation).

INDICATIONS AND USAGE

Oral contraceptives are indicated for the prevention of pregnancy in women who elect to use this product as a method of contraception.

Oral contraceptives are highly effective. Table I lists the typical accidental pregnancy rates for users of combination oral contraceptives and other methods of oral contracep-

TABLE I: PERCENTAGE OF WOMEN EXPERIENCING A CONTRACEPTIVE FAILURE DURING THE FIRST YEAR OF PERFECT USE AND FIRST YEAR OF TYPICAL USE
% of Women Experiencing an Accidental Pregnancy within the First Year of Use

Method	Typical Use[a]	Perfect Use[b]
Chance	85	85
Spermicides	21	6
Periodic abstinence	20	1-9
Withdrawal	19	4
Cap		
Parous	36	26
Nulliparous	18	9
Sponge		
Parous	36	20
Nulliparous	18	9
Diaphragm	18	6
Condom		
Female	21	5
Male	12	3
Pill	3	
Progestin only		0.5
Combined		0.1
IUD		
Progesterone	2	1.5
Copper T 380A	0.8	0.6
Injection (Depo-Provera)	0.3	0.3
Implants (Norplant)	0.09	0.09
Female Sterilization	0.4	0.4
Male Sterilization	0.15	0.10

Adapted with permission[1].

---

[a]Among *typical* couples who initiate use of a method (not necessarily for the first time), the percentage who experience an accidental pregnancy during the first year if they do not stop use for any other reason.

[b]Among couples who initiate use of a method (not necessarily for the first time) and who use it *perfectly* (both consistently and correctly), the percentage who experience an accidental pregnancy during the first year if they do not stop use for any other reason.

tion.[1] The efficacy of these contraceptive methods, except sterilization, depends upon the reliability with which they are used. Correct and consistent use of methods can result in lower failure rates.
[See table 1 at bottom of previous page]

CONTRAINDICATIONS

Oral contraceptives should not be used in women who have the following conditions:
• Thrombophlebitis or thromboembolic disorders
• A past history of deep vein thrombophlebitis or thromboembolic disorders
• Cerebral vascular or coronary artery disease
• Known or suspected carcinoma of the breast
• Carcinoma of the endometrium or other known or suspected estrogen-dependent neoplasia
• Undiagnosed abnormal genital bleeding
• Cholestatic jaundice of pregnancy or jaundice with prior pill use
• Hepatic adenomas, carcinomas or benign liver tumors
• Known or suspected pregnancy

WARNINGS

> **Cigarette smoking increases the risk of serious cardiovascular side effects from oral contraceptive use. This risk increases with age and with heavy smoking (15 or more cigarettes per day) and is quite marked in women over 35 years of age. Women who use oral contraceptives should be strongly advised not to smoke.**

The use of oral contraceptives is associated with increased risks of several serious conditions, including myocardial infarction, thromboembolism, stroke, hepatic neoplasia, and gallbladder disease, although the risk of serious morbidity or mortality is very small in healthy women without underlying risk factors. The risk of morbidity and mortality increases significantly in the presence of other underlying risk factors such as hypertension, hyperlipidemias, hypercholesterolemia, obesity and diabetes.[2–5]

Practitioners prescribing oral contraceptives should be familiar with the following information relating to these risks. The information contained in this package insert is principally based on studies carried out in patients who used oral contraceptives with higher formulations of both estrogens and progestogens than those in common use today. The effect of long-term use of the oral contraceptives with lower formulations of both estrogens and progestogens remains to be determined.

Throughout this labeling, epidemiological studies reported are of two types: retrospective or case control studies and prospective or cohort studies. Case control studies provide a measure of the relative risk of a disease. Relative risk, the *ratio* of the incidence of a disease among oral contraceptive users to that among non-users, cannot be assessed directly from case control studies, but the odds ratio obtained is a measure of relative risk. The relative risk does not provide information on the actual clinical occurrence of a disease. Cohort studies provide not only a measure of the relative risk but a measure of attributable risk, which is the *difference* in the incidence of disease between oral contraceptive users and non-users. The attributable risk does not provide information about the actual occurrence of a disease in the population. (Adapted from ref. 12 and 13 with the author's permission.) For further information, the reader is referred to a text on epidemiological methods.

1. THROMBOEMBOLIC DISORDERS AND OTHER VASCULAR PROBLEMS

a. Myocardial Infarction

An increased risk of myocardial infarction has been attributed to oral contraceptive use. This risk is primarily in smokers or women with other underlying risk factors for coronary artery disease such as hypertension, hypercholesterolemia, morbid obesity and diabetes.[2–5, 13] The relative risk of heart attack for current oral contraceptive users has been estimated to be 2 to 6.[2, 14–19] The risk is very low under the age of 30. However, there is the possibility of a risk of cardiovascular disease even in very young women who take oral contraceptives.

Smoking in combination with oral contraceptive use has been shown to contribute substantially to the incidence of myocardial infarctions in women in their mid-thirties or older, with smoking accounting for the majority of excess cases.[20]

Mortality rates associated with circulatory disease have been shown to increase substantially in smokers over the age of 35 and non-smokers over the age of 40 among women who use oral contraceptives (see Table II).[16]

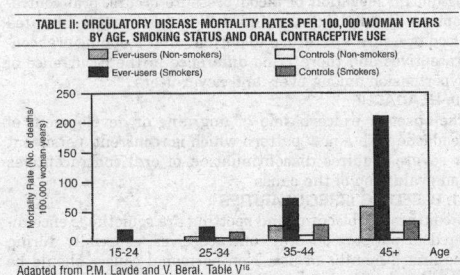

TABLE II: CIRCULATORY DISEASE MORTALITY RATES PER 100,000 WOMAN YEARS BY AGE, SMOKING STATUS AND ORAL CONTRACEPTIVE USE

Ever-users (Non-smokers)   Controls (Non-smokers)
Ever-users (Smokers)   Controls (Smokers)

Adapted from P.M. Layde and V. Beral. Table V[16]

Oral contraceptives may compound the effects of well-known risk factors such as hypertension, diabetes, hyperlipidemias, hypercholesterolemia, age and obesity.[3, 13, 21] In particular, some progestogens are known to decrease HDL cholesterol and cause glucose intolerance, while estrogens may create a state of hyperinsulinism.[21–25] Oral contraceptives have been shown to increase blood pressure among users (see **WARNINGS**, section 9). Similar effects on risk factors have been associated with an increased risk of heart disease. Oral contraceptives must be used with caution in women with cardiovascular disease risk factors.

b. Thromboembolism

An increased risk of thromboembolic and thrombotic disease associated with the use of oral contraceptives is well established. Case control studies have found the relative risk of users compared to nonusers to be 3 for the first episode of superficial venous thrombosis, 4 to 11 for deep vein thrombosis or pulmonary embolism, and 1.5 to 6 for women with predisposing conditions for venous thromboembolic disease.[12, 13, 26–31] Cohort studies have shown the relative risk to be somewhat lower, about 3 for new cases and about 4.5 for new cases requiring hospitalization.[32] The risk of thromboembolic disease due to oral contraceptives is not related to length of use and disappears after pill use is stopped.[12]

A 2- to 6-fold increase in relative risk of post-operative thromboembolic complications has been reported with the use of oral contraceptives. The relative risk of venous thrombosis in women who have predisposing conditions is twice that of women without such medical conditions.[83] If feasible, oral contraceptives should be discontinued at least 4 weeks prior to and for 2 weeks after elective surgery and during and following prolonged immobilization. Since the immediate postpartum period also is associated with an increased risk of thromboembolism, oral contraceptives should be started no earlier than 4 to 6 weeks after delivery in women who elect not to breast feed.[33]

c. Cerebrovascular diseases

An increase in both the relative and attributable risks of cerebrovascular events (thrombotic and hemorrhagic strokes) has been shown in users of oral contraceptives. In general, the risk is greatest among older (>35 years), hypertensive women who also smoke. Hypertension was found to be a risk factor for both users and non-users for both types of strokes while smoking interacted to increase the risk for hemorrhagic strokes.[34]

In a large study, the relative risk of thrombotic strokes has been shown to range from 3 for normotensive users to 14 for users with severe hypertension.[35] The relative risk of hemorrhagic stroke is reported to be 1.2 for non-smokers who used oral contraceptives, 2.6 for smokers who did not use oral contraceptives, 7.6 for smokers who used oral contraceptives, 1.8 for normotensive users and 25.7 for users with severe hypertension.[35] The attributable risk also is greater in women in their mid-thirties or older and among smokers.[13]

d. Dose-related risk of vascular disease from oral contraceptives

A positive association has been observed between the amount of estrogen and progestogen in oral contraceptives and the risk of vascular disease.[36–38] A decline in serum high-density lipoproteins (HDL) has been reported with many progestational agents.[22–24] A decline in serum high-density lipoproteins has been associated with an increased incidence of ischemic heart disease.[39] Because estrogens increase HDL cholesterol, the net effect of an oral contraceptive depends on a balance achieved between doses of estrogen and progestogen and the nature and absolute amount of progestogens used in the contraceptives. The amount of both hormones should be considered in the choice of an oral contraceptive.[37]

Minimizing exposure to estrogen and progestogen is in keeping with good principles of therapeutics. For any particular estrogen/progestogen combination, the dosage regimen prescribed should be one which contains the least amount of estrogen and progestogen that is compatible with a low failure rate and the needs of the individual patient. New acceptors of oral contraceptive agents should be started on preparations containing the lowest estrogen content that produces satisfactory results for the individual.

e. Persistence of risk of vascular disease

There are three studies which have shown persistence of risk of vascular disease for ever-users of oral contraceptives.[17, 34, 40] In a study in the United States, the risk of developing myocardial infarction after discontinuing oral contraceptives persists for at least 9 years for women 40–49 years who had used oral contraceptives for 5 or more years, but this increased risk was not demonstrated in other age groups.[17] In another study in Great Britain, the risk of developing cerebrovascular disease persisted for at least 6 years after discontinuation of oral contraceptives, although excess risk was very small.[40] There is a significantly increased relative risk of subarachnoid hemorrhage after termination of use of oral contraceptives.[34] However, these studies were performed with oral contraceptive formulations containing 50 μg or higher of estrogen.

2. ESTIMATES OF MORTALITY FROM CONTRACEPTIVE USE

One study gathered data from a variety of sources which have estimated the mortality rates associated with different methods of contraception at different ages (see Table III).[41] These estimates include the combined risk of death associated with contraceptive methods plus the risk attributable to pregnancy in the event of method failure. Each method of contraception has its specific benefits and risks. The study concluded that with the exception of oral contraceptive users 35 and older who smoke and 40 and older who do not smoke, mortality associated with all methods of birth control is low and below that associated with childbirth. The observation of a possible increase in risk of mortality with age for oral contraceptive users is based on data gathered in the 1970s – but not reported in the U.S. until 1983.[16, 41] However, current clinical practice involves the use of lower estrogen dose formulations combined with careful restriction of oral contraceptive use to women who do not have the various risk factors listed in this labeling.

Because of these changes in practice and, also, because of some limited new data which suggest that the risk of cardiovascular disease with the use of oral contraceptives may now be less than previously observed,[78, 79] the Fertility and Maternal Health Drugs Advisory Committee was asked to review the topic in 1989. The Committee concluded that although cardiovascular disease risks may be increased with oral contraceptive use after age 40 in healthy non-smoking women (even with the newer low-dose formulations), there are greater potential health risks associated with pregnancy in older women and with the alternative surgical and medical procedures which may be necessary if such women do not have access to effective and acceptable means of contraception.

Therefore, the Committee recommended that the benefits of oral contraceptive use by healthy non-smoking women over 40 may outweigh the possible risks. Of course, older women, as all women who take oral contraceptives, should take the lowest possible dose formulation that is effective.[80]
[See table III at left]

TABLE III: ESTIMATED ANNUAL NUMBER OF BIRTH-RELATED OR METHOD-RELATED DEATHS ASSOCIATED WITH CONTROL OF FERTILITY PER 100,000 NONSTERILE WOMEN, BY FERTILITY CONTROL METHOD ACCORDING TO AGE

Method of control and outcome	15-19	20-24	25-29	30-34	35-39	40-44
No fertility control methods*	7.0	7.4	9.1	14.8	25.7	28.2
Oral contraceptives non-smoker**	0.3	0.5	0.9	1.9	13.8	31.6
Oral contraceptives smoker	2.2	3.4	6.6	13.5	51.1	117.2
IUD**	0.8	0.8	1.0	1.0	1.4	1.4
Condom*	1.1	1.6	0.7	0.2	0.3	0.4
Diaphragm/Spermicide*	1.9	1.2	1.2	1.3	2.2	2.8
Periodic abstinence*	2.5	1.6	1.6	1.7	2.7	3.6

*Deaths are birth-related
**Deaths are method-related

Estimates adapted from H.W. Ory, Table 3[41]

Continued on next page

Trivora—Cont.

3. CARCINOMA OF THE REPRODUCTIVE ORGANS AND BREASTS

Numerous epidemiological studies have been performed on the incidence of breast, endometrial, ovarian and cervical cancer in women using oral contraceptives. The overwhelming evidence in the literature suggests that use of oral contraceptives is not associated with an increase in the risk of developing breast cancer, regardless of the age and parity of first use or with most of the marketed brands and doses.[42–44] The Cancer and Steroid Hormone (CASH) study also showed no latent effect on the risk of breast cancer for at least a decade following long-term use.[43] A few studies have shown increased relative risk of developing breast cancer,[44–47] although the methodology of these studies, which included differences in examination of users and non-users and differences in age at start of use, has been questioned.[47–49] Some studies have reported an increased relative risk of developing breast cancer, particularly at a younger age. This increased relative risk appears to be related to duration of use.[81, 82]

Some studies suggest that oral contraceptive use has been associated with an increase in the risk of cervical intraepithelial neoplasia in some populations of women.[50–53] However, there continues to be controversy about the extent to which such findings may be due to differences in sexual behavior and other factors.

In spite of many studies of the relationship between oral contraceptive use and breast or cervical cancer, a cause and effect relationship has not been established.

4. HEPATIC NEOPLASIA

Benign hepatic adenomas are associated with oral contraceptive use although the incidence of benign tumors is rare in the United States. Indirect calculations have estimated the attributable risk to be in the range of 3.3 cases per 100,000 for users, a risk that increases after 4 or more years of use.[54] Rupture of rare, benign, hepatic adenomas may cause death through intra-abdominal hemorrhage.[55–56]

Studies in the United States and Britain have shown an increased risk of developing hepatocellular carcinoma in the long-term (>8 years) oral contraceptive users.[57–59] However, these cancers are extremely rare in the United States and the attributable risk (the excess incidence) of liver cancers in oral contraceptive users approaches less than 1 per 1,000,000 users.

5. OCULAR LESIONS

There have been clinical case reports of retinal thrombosis associated with the use of oral contraceptives. Oral contraceptives should be discontinued if there is unexplained partial or complete loss of vision; onset of proptosis or diplopia; papilledema; or retinal vascular lesions. Appropriate diagnostic and therapeutic measures should be undertaken immediately.

6. ORAL CONTRACEPTIVE USE BEFORE OR DURING EARLY PREGNANCY

Extensive epidemiological studies have revealed no increased risk of birth defects in women who have used oral contraceptives prior to pregnancy.[60–62] Studies also do not suggest a teratogenic effect, particularly insofar as cardiac anomalies and limb reduction defects are concerned, when taken inadvertently during early pregnancy.[60, 61, 63, 64]

The administration of oral contraceptives to induce withdrawal bleeding should not be used as a test for pregnancy. Oral contraceptives should not be used during pregnancy to treat threatened or habitual abortion.

It is recommended that for any patient who has missed 2 consecutive periods, pregnancy should be ruled out before continuing oral contraceptive use. If the patient has not adhered to the prescribed schedule, the possibility of pregnancy should be considered at the first missed period. Oral contraceptive use should be discontinued if pregnancy is confirmed.

7. GALLBLADDER DISEASE

Earlier studies have reported an increased lifetime relative risk of gallbladder surgery in users of oral contraceptives and estrogens.[65–66] More recent studies, however, have shown that the relative risk of developing gallbladder disease among oral contraceptive users may be minimal.[67] The recent findings of minimal risk may be related to the use of oral contraceptive formulations containing lower hormonal doses of estrogens and progestogens.[68]

8. CARBOHYDRATE AND LIPID METABOLIC EFFECTS

Oral contraceptives have been shown to cause glucose intolerance in a significant percentage of users.[25] Oral contraceptives containing greater than 75 µg of estrogen cause hyperinsulinism, while lower doses of estrogen cause less glucose intolerance.[70] Progestogens increase insulin secretion and create insulin resistance, this effect varying with different progestational agents.[25, 71] However, in the non-diabetic woman, oral contraceptives appear to have no effect on fasting blood glucose.[69] Because of these demonstrated effects, prediabetic and diabetic women should be carefully observed while taking oral contraceptives.

Some women may develop persistent hypertriglyceridemia while on the pill.[72] As discussed earlier (see **WARNINGS**, sections 1a. and 1d.), changes in serum triglycerides and lipoprotein levels have been reported in oral contraceptive users.[23]

9. ELEVATED BLOOD PRESSURE

An increase in blood pressure has been reported in women taking oral contraceptives and this increase is more likely in older oral contraceptive users and with continued use.[73,84] Data from the Royal College of General Practitioners and subsequent randomized trials have shown that the incidence of hypertension increases with increasing concentrations of progestogens.

Women with a history of hypertension or hypertension-related diseases or renal disease should be encouraged to use another method of contraception. If women elect to use oral contraceptives, they should be monitored closely and if significant elevation of blood pressure occurs, oral contraceptives should be discontinued. For most women, elevated blood pressure will return to normal after stopping oral contraceptives and there is no difference in the occurrence of hypertension among ever- and never-users.[73–75]

10. HEADACHE

The onset or exacerbation of migraine or development of headache with a new pattern which is recurrent, persistent or severe requires discontinuation of oral contraceptives and evaluation of the cause.

11. BLEEDING IRREGULARITIES

Breakthrough bleeding and spotting are sometimes encountered in patients on oral contraceptives, especially during the first 3 months of use. Non-hormonal causes should be considered and adequate diagnostic measures taken to rule out malignancy or pregnancy in the event of breakthrough bleeding, as in the case of any abnormal vaginal bleeding. If pathology has been excluded, time or a change to another formulation may solve the problem. In the event of amenorrhea, pregnancy should be ruled out.

Some women may encounter post-pill amenorrhea or oligomenorrhea, especially when such a condition was pre-existent.

PRECAUTIONS

GENERAL

Patients should be counseled that this product does not protect against HIV infection (AIDS) and other sexually transmitted diseases.

1. PHYSICAL EXAMINATION AND FOLLOW-UP

It is good medical practice for all women to have annual history and physical examinations, including women using oral contraceptives. The physical examination, however, may be deferred until after initiation of oral contraceptives if requested by the woman and judged appropriate by the clinician. The physical examination should include special reference to blood pressure, breasts, abdomen and pelvic organs, including cervical cytology, and relevant laboratory tests. In case of undiagnosed, persistent or recurrent abnormal vaginal bleeding, appropriate measures should be conducted to rule out malignancy. Women with a strong family history of breast cancer or who have breast nodules should be monitored with particular care.

2. LIPID DISORDERS

Women who are being treated for hyperlipidemias should be followed closely if they elect to use oral contraceptives. Some progestogens may elevate LDL levels and may render the control of hyperlipidemias more difficult.

3. LIVER FUNCTION

If jaundice develops in any woman receiving oral contraceptives the medication should be discontinued. Steroid hormones may be poorly metabolized in patients with impaired liver function.

4. FLUID RETENTION

Oral contraceptives may cause some degree of fluid retention. They should be prescribed with caution, and only with careful monitoring, in patients with conditions which might be aggravated by fluid retention.

5. EMOTIONAL DISORDERS

Women with a history of depression should be carefully observed and the drug discontinued if depression recurs to a serious degree.

6. CONTACT LENSES

Contact lens wearers who develop visual changes or changes in lens tolerance should be assessed by an ophthalmologist.

7. DRUG INTERACTIONS

Reduced efficacy and increased incidence of breakthrough bleeding and menstrual irregularities have been associated with concomitant use of rifampin. A similar association though less marked, has been suggested with barbiturates, phenylbutazone, phenytoin sodium, and possibly with griseofulvin, ampicillin and tetracyclines.[76]

8. INTERACTIONS WITH LABORATORY TESTS

Certain endocrine and liver function tests and blood components may be affected by oral contraceptives:

a. Increased prothrombin and factors VII, VIII, IX, and X; decreased antithrombin 3; increased norepinephrine-induced platelet aggregability.

b. Increased thyroid binding globulin (TBG) leading to increased circulating total thyroid hormone, as measured by protein-bound iodine (PBI), T4 by column or by radioimmunoassay. Free T3 resin uptake is decreased, reflecting the elevated TBG. Free T4 concentration is unaltered.

c. Other binding proteins may be elevated in serum.

d. Sex steroid binding globulins are increased and result in elevated levels of total circulating sex steroids and corticoids; however, free or biologically active levels remain unchanged.

e. Triglycerides may be increased.

f. Glucose tolerance may be decreased.

g. Serum folate levels may be depressed by oral contraceptive therapy. This may be of clinical significance if a woman becomes pregnant shortly after discontinuing oral contraceptives.

9. CARCINOGENESIS

See **WARNINGS** section.

10. PREGNANCY

Pregnancy Category X. See **CONTRAINDICATIONS** and **WARNINGS** sections.

11. NURSING MOTHERS

Small amounts of oral contraceptive steroids have been identified in the milk of nursing mothers and a few adverse effects on the child have been reported, including jaundice and breast enlargement. In addition, oral contraceptives given in the postpartum period may interfere with lactation by decreasing the quantity and quality of breast milk. If possible, the nursing mother should be advised not to use oral contraceptives while breast feeding. She should use another method of contraception since breast feeding provides only partial protection from becoming pregnant and this partial protection decreases significantly as she breast feeds for longer periods of time. The nursing mother should consider starting oral contraceptives only after she has weaned her child completely.

INFORMATION FOR THE PATIENT

See **PATIENT LABELING** printed below.

ADVERSE REACTIONS

An increased risk of the following serious adverse reactions has been associated with the use of oral contraceptives (see **WARNINGS** section):

- Thrombophlebitis
- Arterial thromboembolism
- Pulmonary embolism
- Myocardial infarction
- Cerebral hemorrhage
- Cerebral thrombosis
- Hypertension
- Gallbladder disease
- Hepatic adenomas, carcinomas or benign liver tumors

There is evidence of an association between the following conditions and the use of oral contraceptives, although additional confirmatory studies are needed:

- Mesenteric thrombosis
- Retinal thrombosis

The following adverse reactions have been reported in patients receiving oral contraceptives and are believed to be drug-related:

- Nausea
- Vomiting
- Gastrointestinal symptoms (such as abdominal cramps and bloating)
- Breakthrough bleeding
- Spotting
- Changes in menstrual flow
- Amenorrhea
- Temporary infertility after discontinuation of treatment
- Edema
- Melasma which may persist
- Breast changes; tenderness, enlargement, secretion
- Change in weight (increase or decrease)
- Change in cervical erosion and secretion
- Diminution in lactation when given immediately postpartum
- Cholestatic jaundice
- Migraine
- Rash (allergic)
- Mental depression
- Reduced tolerance to carbohydrates
- Vaginal candidiasis
- Change in corneal curvature (steepening)
- Intolerance to contact lenses

The following adverse reactions have been reported in users of oral contraceptives and the association has been neither confirmed nor refuted:

- Pre-menstrual syndrome
- Cataracts
- Changes in appetite
- Cystitis-like syndrome
- Headache
- Nervousness
- Dizziness
- Hirsutism

- Loss of scalp hair
- Erythema multiforme
- Erythema nodosum
- Hemorrhagic eruption
- Vaginitis
- Porphyria
- Impaired renal function
- Hemolytic uremic syndrome
- Budd-Chiari syndrome
- Acne
- Changes in libido
- Colitis

OVERDOSAGE

Serious ill effects have not been reported following acute ingestion of large doses of oral contraceptives by young children. Overdosage may cause nausea, and withdrawal bleeding may occur in females.

HEALTH BENEFITS FROM ORAL CONTRACEPTIVES

The following health benefits related to the use of oral contraceptives are supported by epidemiological studies which largely utilized oral contraceptive formulations containing estrogen doses exceeding 0.035 mg of ethinyl estradiol or 0.05 mg of mestranol.[6–11]

Effects on menses:
- Increased menstrual cycle regularity
- Decreased blood loss and decreased incidence of iron deficiency anemia
- Decreased incidence of dysmenorrhea

Effects related to inhibition of ovulation:
- Decreased incidence of functional ovarian cysts
- Decreased incidence of ectopic pregnancies

Effects from long-term use:
- Decreased incidence of fibroadenomas and fibrocystic disease of the breast
- Decreased incidence of acute pelvic inflammatory disease
- Decreased incidence of endometrial cancer
- Decreased incidence of ovarian cancer.

DOSAGE AND ADMINISTRATION

To achieve maximum contraceptive effectiveness, oral contraceptives must be taken exactly as directed and at intervals exceeding 24 hours.

21-Day Schedule: For a DAY 1 START, count the first day of menstrual flow as Day 1 and first blue tablet is then taken on Day 1. For a SUNDAY START, when menstrual flow begins on or before Sunday, the first blue tablet is taken on that day. With either a DAY 1 START or SUNDAY START, 1 blue tablet is taken for 6 days, then 1 white tablet for 5 days, then 1 pink tablet for 10 days. With either a DAY 1 START or SUNDAY START, 1 tablet is taken each day at the same time for 21 days. No tablets are taken for 7 days, then, whether bleeding has stopped or not, a new course is started of 1 tablet a day for 21 days. This institutes 3 weeks on, 1 week off dosage regimen.

28-Day Schedule: For a DAY 1 START, count the first day of menstrual flow as Day 1 and the first blue tablet is then taken on Day 1. For a SUNDAY START when menstrual flow begins on or before Sunday, the first blue tablet is taken on that day. With either a DAY 1 START or SUNDAY START, 1 blue tablet is taken for 6 days, then 1 white tablet for 5 days, then 1 pink tablet for 10 days, then 1 peach (inert) tablet for 7 days. With either a DAY 1 START or SUNDAY START, 1 tablet is taken each day at the same time for 28 days. After all 28 tablets are taken, whether bleeding has stopped or not, the same dosage schedule is repeated beginning on the following day.

INSTRUCTIONS TO PATIENTS

- To achieve maximum contraceptive effectiveness, the oral contraceptive pill must be taken exactly as directed and at intervals not exceeding 24 hours.
- Important: Women should be instructed to use an additional method of protection until after the first 7 days of administration *in the initial cycle.*
- Due to the normally increased risk of thromboembolism occurring postpartum, women should be instructed not to initiate treatment with oral contraceptives earlier than 4 weeks after a full-term delivery. If pregnancy is terminated in the first 12 weeks, the patient should be instructed to start oral contraceptives immediately or within 7 days. If pregnancy is terminated after 12 weeks, the patient should be instructed to start oral contraceptives after 2 weeks.[33, 77]
- If spotting or breakthrough bleeding should occur, the patient should continue the medication according to the schedule. Should spotting or breakthrough bleeding persist, the patient should notify her physician.
- If the patient misses 1 pill, she should be instructed to take it as soon as she remembers and then take the next pill at the regular time. The patient should be advised that missing a pill can cause spotting or light bleeding and that she may be a little sick to her stomach on the days she takes the missed pill with her regularly scheduled pill. If the patient has missed more than one pill, see DETAILED PATIENT LABELING: HOW TO TAKE THE PILL, WHAT TO DO IF YOU MISS PILLS.
- Use of oral contraceptives in the event of a missed menstrual period:

1. If the patient has not adhered to the prescribed dosage regimen, the possibility of pregnancy should be considered after the first missed period and oral contraceptives should be withheld until pregnancy has been ruled out.
2. If the patient has adhered to the prescribed regimen and misses 2 consecutive periods, pregnancy should be ruled out before continuing the contraceptive regimen.

HOW SUPPLIED

Trivora®-21 Tablets are available in 21-tablet blister cards. Six blister cards are packaged in a carton. All the tablets are unscored, round in shape. The blue tablets are debossed with "WATSON" on one side and "50/30" on the other side. The white tablets are debossed with "WATSON" on one side and "75/40" on the other side. The pink tablets are debossed with "WATSON" on one side and "125/30" on the other side. Trivora®-28 Tablets are available in 28-tablet blister cards. Six blister cards are packaged in a carton. Trivora®-28 Tablets contain the same 21 active tablets as Trivora®-21 Tablets with 7 additional inert tablets. The peach inert tablets are unscored, round in shape with "WATSON" on one side and "P1" on the other side.

Rx only

Store at controlled room temperature 15°–30°C (59°–86°F).

REFERENCES

1. Hatcher, R.A. Trussell, J., Stewart, F., et al.: *Contraceptive Technology: Sixteenth Revised Edition,* New York, NY 1994.
2. Mann, J., et al.: *Br Med J* 2(5956):241–245, 1975.
3. Knopp, R.H.: *J Reprod Med* 31(9):913–921, 1986.
4. Mann, J.I., et al.: *Br Med J* 2:445–447, 1976.
5. Ory, H.: *JAMA* 237:2619–2622, 1977.
6. The Cancer and Steroid Hormone Study of the Centers for Disease Control: *JAMA* 249(2):1596–1599, 1983.
7. The Cancer and Steroid Hormone Study of the Centers for Disease Control: *JAMA* 257(6):796–800. 1987.
8. Ory, H.W.: *JAMA* 228(1):68–69, 1974.
9. Ory, H.W., et al.: *N Engl J Med* 294:419–422, 1976.
10. Ory, H.W.: *Fam Plann Perspect* 14:182–184, 1982.
11. Ory, H.W. et al.: *Making Choices,* New York, The Alan Guttmacher Institute, 1983.
12. Stadel, B.: *N Engl J Med* 305(11):612–618, 1981.
13. Stadel, B.: *N Engl J Med* 305(12):672–677, 1981.
14. Adam, S., et al.: *Br J Obstet Gynaecol* 88:838–845, 1981.
15. Mann, J., et al.: *Br Med J* 2(5965):245–248, 1975.
16. Royal College of General Practitioners' Oral Contraceptive Study: *Lancet* 1:541–546, 1981.
17. Slone, D., et al.: *N Engl J Med* 305(8):420–424, 1981.
18. Vessey, M.P.: *Br J Fam Plann* 6 (supplement):1–12, 1980.
19. Russell-Briefel, R., et al.: *Prev Med* 15:352–362, 1986.
20. Goldbaum, G., et al.: *JAMA* 258(10):1339–1342, 1987.
21. LaRosa, J.C.: *J Reprod Med* 31 (9):906–912, 1986.
22. Krauss, R.M., et al.: *Am J Obstet Gynecol* 145:446–452, 1983.
23. Wahl, P., et al.: *N Engl J Med* 308(15)862–867, 1983.
24. Wynn, V., et al.: *Am J Obstet Gynecol* 142(6):766–771, 1982.
25. Wynn, V., et al.: *J Reprod Med* 31(9):892–897, 1986.
26. Inman, W.H., et al.: *Br Med J* 2(5599):193–199, 1968.
27. Maguire, M.G., et al.: *Am J Epidemiol* 110(2):188–195, 1979.
28. Petitti, D., et al.: *JAMA* 242(11):1150–1154, 1979.
29. Vessey, M.P., et al.: *Br Med J* 2(5599):199–205, 1968.
30. Vessey, M.P., et al.: *Br Med J* 2(5658):651–657, 1969.
31. Porter, J.B., et al.: *Obstet Gynecol* 59(3):299–302, 1982.
32. Vessey, M.P., et al.: *J Biosoc Sci* 8:373–427, 1976.
33. Mishell, D.R., et al.: *Reproductive Endocrinology,* Philadelphia, F.A. Davis Co., 1979.
34. Petitti, D.B., et al.: *Lancet* 2:234–236, 1978.
35. Collaborative Group for the Study of Stroke in Young Women: *JAMA* 231(7):718–722, 1975.
36. Inman, W.H., et al.: *Br Med J* 2:203–209, 1970.
37. Meade, T.W., et al.: *Br Med J* 280(6224):1157–1161, 1980.
38. Kay, C.R.: *Am J Obstet Gynecol* 142(6):762–765, 1982.
39. Gordon, T., et al.: *Am J Med* 62:707–714, 1977.
40. Royal College of General Practitioners' Oral Contraception Study: *J Coll Gen Pract* 33:75–82, 1983.
41. Ory, H.W.: *Fam Plann Perspect* 15(2):57–63, 1983.
42. Paul, C., et al.: *Br Med J* 293:723–725, 1986.
43. The Cancer and Steroid Hormone Study of the Centers for Disease Control: *N Engl J Med* 315(7):405–411, 1986.
44. Pike, M.C., et al.: *Lancet* 2:926–929, 1983.
45. Miller, D.R., et al.: *Obstet Gynecol* 68:863–868, 1986.
46. Olsson, H., et al.: *Lancet* 2:748–749, 1985.
47. McPherson, K., et al.: *Br J Cancer* 56:653–660, 1987.
48. Huggins, G.R., et al.: *Fertil Steril* 47(5):733–761, 1987.
49. McPherson, K., et al.: *Br Med J* 293:709–710, 1986.
50. Ory, H., et al.: *Am J Obstet Gynecol* 124(6):573–577, 1976.
51. Vessey, M.P., et al.: *Lancet* 2:930, 1983.
52. Brinton, L.A., et al.: *Int J Cancer* 38:339–344, 1986.
53. WHO Collaborative Study of Neoplasia and Steroid Contraceptives: *Br Med J* 290:961–965, 1985.
54. Rooks, J.B., et al.: *JAMA* 242(7):644–648, 1979.
55. Bein, N.N., et al.: *Br J Surg* 64:433–435, 1977.
56. Klatskin, G., *Gastroenterology* 73:386–394, 1977.
57. Henderson, B.E., et al.: *Br J Cancer* 48:437–440, 1983.
58. Neuberger, J., et al.: *Br Med J* 292:1355–1357, 1986.
59. Forman, D., et al.: *Br Med J* 292:1357–1361, 1986.
60. Harlap, S., et al.: *Obstet Gynecol* 55(4):447–452, 1980.
61. Savolainen, E., et al.: *Am J Obstet Gynecol* 140(5):521–524, 1981.
62. Janerich, D.T., et al.: *Am J Epidemiol* 112(1):73–79, 1980.
63. Ferencz, C., et al., *Teratology* 21:225–239, 1980.
64. Rothman, K.J., et al.: *Am J Epidemiol* 109(4):433–439, 1979.
65. Boston Collaborative Drug Surveillance Program: *Lancet* 1:1399–1404, 1973.
66. Royal College of General Practitioners: *Oral contraceptives and health,* New York, Pittman, 1974.
67. Rome Group for the Epidemiology and Prevention of Cholelithiasis: *Am J Epidemiol* 119(5):796–805, 1984.
68. Strom, B.L., et al.: *Clin Pharmacol Ther* 39(3):335–341, 1986.
69. Perlman, J.A., et al.: *J Chronic Dis* 38(10):857–864, 1985.
70. Wynn, V., et al.: *Lancet* 1:1045–1049, 1979.
71. Wynn, V.: *Progesterone and Progestin,* New York, Raven Press, 1983.
72. Wynn, V., et al.: *Lancet* 2:720–723, 1966.
73. Fisch, I.R., et al.: *JAMA* 237(23):2499–2503, 1977.
74. Laragh, J.H.: *Am J Obstet Gynecol* 126(1):141–147, 1976.
75. Ramcharan, S., et al.: *Pharmacology of Steroid Contraceptive Drugs,* New York, Raven Press, 1977.
76. Stockley, I.: *Pharm J* 216:140–143, 1976.
77. Dickey, R.P.: *Managing Contraceptive Pill Patients,* Oklahoma, Creative Informatics Inc., 1984.
78. Porter, J.B., Hunter, J., Jick, H., et al.: *Obstet Gynecol* 1985:66:1–4.
79. Porter, J.B., Hershel, J., Walker, A.M.: *Obstet Gynecol* 1987:70:29–32.
80. Fertility and Maternal Health Drugs Advisory Committee, F.D.A., October, 1989.
81. Schlesselman, J., Stadel, B.V., Murray, P., Lai, S.: *Breast cancer in relation to early use of oral contraceptives.* JAMA 1988:259:1828–1833.
82. Hennekens, C.H., Speizer, F.E., Lipnick, R.J., Rosner, B., Bain, C., Belanger, C., Stampfer, M.J., Willett, W., Peto, R.: *A case-control study of oral contraceptive use and breast cancer.* JNCI 1984; 72:39–42.
83. Royal College of General Practitioners: *Oral contraceptives, venous thrombosis, and varicose veins. J Coll Gen Pract* 28:393–399, 1978.
84. Royal College of General Practitioners' Oral Contraception Study: *Effect on hypertension and benign breast disease of progestogen component in combined oral contraceptives. Lancet* 1:624, 1977.

Manufactured for WATSON PHARMA a division of Watson Laboratories, Inc.
Corona, CA 91720 (USA)
By Syntex (FP) Inc.
Humacao, PR 00791
Revised: Feb. 26, 1998

Trivora®-21 Tablets
Trivora®-28 Tablets

(levonorgestrel and ethinyl estradiol tablets, USP)–triphasic regimen

Shown in Product Identification Guide, page 343

ZOVIA ℞

[*zō vĭa*]

(ethynodiol diacetate and ethinyl estradiol tablets, USP)

Zovia 1/35E-21
Zovia 1/35E-28
Zovia 1/50E-21
Zovia 1/50E-28

(Ethynodiol Diacetate and Ethinyl Estradiol Tablets, USP)

Patients should be counseled that this product does not protect against HIV infection (AIDS) and other sexually transmitted diseases.

DESCRIPTION

Zovia 1/35E-21 and Zovia 1/35E-28. Each light pink tablet contains 1 mg of ethynodiol diacetate and 35 mcg of ethinyl estradiol, and the inactive ingredients include microcrystalline cellulose, lactose (anhydrous), magnesium stearate, polacrilin potassium and povidone. In addition, the coloring agents are D&C Yellow No. 10 and D&C Red No. 30. Each white tablet in the Zovia 1/35E-28 package is a placebo con-

Continued on next page

Zovia—Cont.

taining no active ingredients and the inactive ingredients include microcrystalline cellulose, lactose (anhydrous) and magnesium stearate.

Zovia 1/50E-21 and Zovia 1/50E-28. Each pink tablet contains 1 mg of ethynodiol diacetate and 50 mcg of ethinyl estradiol, and the inactive ingredients iinclude microcrystalline cellulose, lactose (anhydrous), magnesium stearate, polacrilin piotassium and povidone. In addition, the coloring agents are D&C Yellow No. 10 and D&C Red No. 30. Each white tablet in the Zovia 1/50E-28 package is a placebo containing no active ingredients, and the inactive ingredients include microcrystalline cellulose, lactose (anhydrous) and magnesium stearate.

The chemical name for ethynodiol diacetate is 19-nor-17α-pregn-4-en-20-yne-3β, 17-diol diacetate, and for ethinyl estradiol it is 19-nor-17α-pregn-1, 3, 5 (10)-trien-20-yne-3, 17-diol. The structural formulas are as follows:
Therapeutic class: Oral contraceptive

ethynodiol diacetate
M.W. = 384.51

ethinyl estradiol
M.W. = 296.41

CLINICAL PHARMACOLOGY

Combination oral contraceptives act primarily by suppression of gonadotropins. Although the primary mechanism of this action is inhibition of ovulation, other alterations in the genital tract, including changes in the cervical mucus (which increase the difficulty of sperm entry into the uterus) and the endometrium (which may reduce the likelihood of implantation) may also contribute to contraceptive effectiveness.

INDICATIONS AND USAGE

Zovia 1/35E and Zovia 1/50E are indicated for the prevention of pregnancy in women who elect to use oral contraceptives as a method of contraception.
Oral contraceptives are highly effective. Table 1 lists the typical accidental pregnancy rates for users of combination oral contraceptives and other methods of contraception. The efficacy of these contraceptive methods, except sterilization and progestogen implants and injections, depends upon the reliability with which they are used. Correct and consistent use of methods can result in lower failure rates.

Table 1. Lowest expected and typical failure rates during the first year of continuous use of a method. Percent of women experiencing an accidental pregnancy in the first year of continuous use.[1, 1a]

Method	Lowest Expected*	Typical**
No contraception	85	85
Oral contraceptives		
Combined	0.1	N/A***
Progestogen only	0.5	N/A***
Diaphragm with spermicidal		
cream or jelly	6	18
Spermicides alone		
(foam, creams, jellies		
and vaginal suppositories	3	21
Vaginal sponge		
Nulliparous	6	18
Parous	9	28
IUD (medicated)		
Progesterone	2	N/A***
Copper T 380A	0.8	N/A***
Condom without spermicides	2	12
Periodic abstinence		
(all methods)	1-9	20
Progestogen injections	0.3	0.3
Progestogen implants	0.2	0.2
Female sterilization	0.2	0.4
Male sterilization	0.1	0.15

Adapted from Trussel et al[1]

* The authors' best guess of the percentage of women expected to experience an accidental pregnancy among couples who initiate a method (not necessarily for the first time) and who use it consistently and correctly during the first year if they do not stop for any other reason.

** This term represents "typical" couples who initiate use of a method (not necessarily for the first time), who experience an accidental pregnancy during the first year if they do not stop for any other reason.

*** N/A—Data not available

CONTRAINDICATIONS

Oral contraceptives should not be used in women who have the following conditions:

- Thrombophlebitis or thromboembolic disorders
- A past history of deep vein thrombophlebitis or thromboembolic disorders
- Cerebral vascular disease, myocardial infarction, or coronary artery disease, or a past history of these conditions
- Known or suspected carcinoma of the breast, or a history of this condition
- Known or suspected carcinoma of the female reproductive organs or suspected estrogen-dependent neoplasia, or a history of these conditions
- Undiagnosed abnormal genital bleeding
- History of cholestatic jaundice of pregnancy or jaundice with prior oral contraceptive use
- Past or present, benign or malignant liver tumors
- Known or suspected pregnancy

WARNINGS

> Cigarette smoking increases the risk of serious cardiovascular side effects from oral contraceptive use. This risk increases with age and with heavy smoking (15 or more cigarettes per day) and is quite marked in women over 35 years of age. Women who use oral contraceptives should be strongly advised not to smoke.

The use of oral contraceptives is associated with increased risk of several serious conditions including venous and arterial thromboembolism, thrombotic and hemorrhagic stroke, myocardial infarction, liver tumors or other liver lesions, and gallbladder disease. The risk of morbidity and mortality increases signficantly in the presence of other risk factors such as hypertension, hyperlipidemia, obesity, and diabetes mellitus.

Practitioners prescribing oral contraceptives should be familiar with the following information relating to these and other risks.

The information contained herein is principally based on studies carried out in patients who use oral contraceptives with formulations containing higher amounts of estrogens and progestogens than those in common use today. The effect of long-term use of the oral contraceptives with lesser amounts of both estrogens and progestogens remains to be determined.

Throughout this labeling, epidemiological studies reported are of two types: retrospective case-control studies and prospective cohort studies. Case-control studies provide an estimate of the relative risk of a disease, which is defined as the *ratio* of the incidence of a disease among oral contraceptive users to that among nonusers. The relative risk (or odds ratio) does not provide information about the actual clinical occurrence of a disease. Cohort studies provide a measure of both the relative risk and the attributable risk. the latter is the *difference* in the incidence of disease between oral contraceptive users and nonusers. The attributable risk does provide information about the actual occurrence or incidence of a disease in the subject population. For further information, the reader is referred to a text on epidemiological methods.

1. Thromboembolic disorders and other vascular problems.
a. Myocardial infarction. An increased risk of myocardial infarction has been associated with oral contraceptive use.[2-21] This increased risk is primarily in smokers or in women with other underlying risk factors for coronary artery disease such as hypertension, obesity, diabetes, and hypercholesterolemia. The relative risk for myocardial infarction in current oral contraceptive users has been estimated to be 2 to 6. The risk is very low under the age of 30. However, there is the possibility of a risk of cardiovascular disease even in very young women who take oral contraceptives. Smoking in combination with oral contraceptive use has been reported to contribute substantially to the risk of myocardial infarction in women in their mid-thirties or older, with smoking accounting for the majority of excess cases.[22] Mortality rates associated with circulatory disease have been shown to increase substantially in smokers, especially in those 35 years of age and older among women who use oral contraceptives (see Figure 1, Table 2).

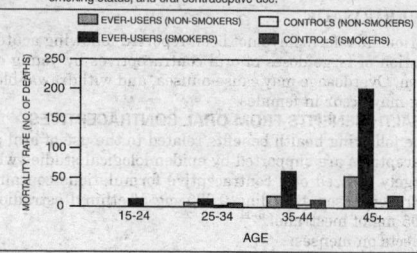

Figure 1. Circulatory disease mortality rates per 100,000 women—years by age, smoking status, and oral contraceptive use.[14]

Adapted from Layde and Beral.[14]

Oral contraceptives may compound the effects of well-known cardiovascular risk factors such as hypertension, diabetes, hyperlipidemias, hypercholesterolemia, age, cigarette smoking, and obesity. In particular, some progestogens decrease HDL cholesterol[23-31] and cause glucose intolerance, while estrogens may create a state of hyperinsulinism.[32] Oral contraceptives have been shown to increase blood pressure among some users (see **WARNING** No. 9). Similar effects on risk factors have been associated with an increased risk of heart disease.

b. Thromboembolism. An increased risk of thromboembolic and thrombolic disease associated with the use of oral contraceptives is well established.[17, 33-51] Case-control studies have estimated the relative risk to be 3 for the first episode of superficial venous thrombosis, 4 to 11 for deep vein thrombosis or pulmonary embolism, and 1.5 to 6 for women with predisposing conditions for venous thromboembolic disease.[34-37, 45, 46] Cohort studies have shown the relative risk to be somewhat lower, about 3 for new cases (subjects with no past history of venous thrombosis or varicose veins) and about 4.5 for new cases requiring hospitalization.[42, 47, 48] The risk of venous thromboemblic disease associated with oral contraceptives is not related to duration of use.

A two- to seven-fold increase in relative risk of postoperative thromboembolic complications have been reported with the use of oral contraceptives.[38, 39] The relative risk of venous thrombosis in women who have predisposing conditions is about twice that of women without such medical conditions.[43] If feasible, oral contraceptives should be discontinued at least 4 weeks prior to and for 2 weeks after elective surgery of a type associated with an increased risk of thromboembolism, and also during and following prolonged immobilization. Since the immediate postpartum period is also associated with an increased risk of thromboembolism, oral contraceptives should be started no earlier than 4 to 6 weeks after delivery in women who elect not to breast feed.

c. Cerebrovascular diseases. Both the relative and attributable risks of cerebrovascular events (thrombotic and hemorrhagic strokes) have been reported to be increased with oral contraceptive use,[14, 17, 18, 34, 42, 46, 52-59] although, in general, the risk was greatest among older (over 35 years) hypertensive women who also smoked. Hypertension was reported to be a risk factor for both users and nonusers, for both types of strokes, while smoking increased the risk for hemorrhagic strokes.

In one large study,[52] the relative risk for thrombotic stroke was reported as 9.5 times greater in users than in nonusers. It ranged from 3 for normotensive users to 14 for users with severe hypertension.[54] The relative risk for hemorrhagic stroke was reported to be 1.2 for nonsmokers who used oral contraceptives, 1.9 to 2.6 for smokers who did not use oral contraceptives, 6.1 to 7.6 for smokers who used oral contraceptives, 1.8 for normotensive users, and 25.7 for users with severe hypertension. The risk is also greater in older women and among smokers.

d. Dose-related risk of vascular disease with oral contraceptives. A positive association has been reported between the amount of estrogen and progestogen in oral contraceptives and the risk of vascular disease.[41, 43, 53, 59-64] A decline in serum high density lipoproteins (HDL) has been reported with many progestogens.[23-31] A decline in serum high density lipoproteins has been associated with an increased incidence of ischemic heart disease.[65] Because estrogens increase HDL-cholesterol, the net effect of an oral contraceptive depends on the balance achieved between doses of estrogen and progestogen and the nature and absolute amount of progestogens used in the contraceptives. The amount of both steroids should be considered in the choice of an oral contraceptive.

Minimizing exposure to estrogen and progestogen is in keeping with good principles of therapeutics. For any particular estrogen-progestogen combination, the dosage regimen prescribed should be one that contains the least amount of estrogen and progestogen that is compatible with a low failure rate and the needs of the individual patient. New acceptors of oral contraceptives should be started on preparations containing the lowest estrogen content that produces satisfactory results in the individual.

e. Persistance of risk of vascular disease. There are three studies that have shown persistence of risk of vascular disease for users of oral contraceptives. In a study in the United States, the risk of developing myocardial infarction after discontinuing oral contraceptives persisted for at least 9 years for women 40–49 years old who had used oral contraceptives for 5 or more years, but this increased risk was not demonstrated in other age groups.[16] Another American study reported former use of oral contraceptives was significantly associated with increased risk of subaracnoid hemorrhage.[57] In another study, in Great Britain, the risk of developing nonrheumatic heart disease plus hypertension, subarachnoid hemorrhage, cerebral thrombosis, and transient ischemic attacks persisted for at least 6 years after discontinuation of oral contraceptives, although the excess risk was small.[14, 18, 66] It should be noted that these studies were performed with oral contraceptive formulations containing 50 mcg or more of estrogens.

2. Estimates of mortality from contraceptive use. One study[67] gathered data from a variety of sources that have estimated the mortality rates associated with different methods of contraception at different ages. (Table 2). These estimates include the combined risk of death associated with contraceptive methods plus the risk attributable to pregnancy in the event of method failure. Each method of contraception has its specific benefits and risks. The study concluded that, with the exception of oral contraceptive users 35 and older who smoke and 40 or older who do not smoke, mortality associated with all methods of birth control is low and below that associated with childbirth. The observation of a possible increase in risk of mortality with age of oral contraceptive users is based on data gathered in the 1970's, but not reported until 1983.[67] However, current clinical practice involves the use of lower estrogen dose formulations combined with careful restriction of oral contraceptive use to women who do not have the various risk fators listed in this labeling.

Because of these changes in practice and, also, because of some limited new data that suggest that the risk of cardiovascular disease with the use of oral contraceptives may now be less than previously observed,[48, 152] the Fertility and Maternal Health Drugs Advisory Committee was asked to review the topic in 1989. The Committee concluded that, although cardiovascular disease risks may be increased with oral contraceptive use after age 40 in healthy nonsmoking women (even with the newer low-dose formulations), there are greater potential health risks associated with pregnancy in older women and with the alternative surgical and medical procedures that may be necessary if such women do not have access to effective and acceptable means of contraception.

Therefore, the Committee recommended that the benefits of oral contraceptive use by healthy nonsmoking women over 40 may outweigh the possible risks. Of course, older women, as all women who take oral contraceptives, should take the lowest possible dose formulation that is effective.

[See table 2 above]

3. Carcinoma of the breast and reproductive organs. Numerous epidemiological studies have been performed on the incidence of breast, endometrial, ovarian, and cervical cancer in women using oral contraceptives. While there are conflicting reports, most studies suggest that the use of oral contraceptives is not associated with an overall increase in the risk of developing breast cancer.[17, 40, 68–78] Some studies have reported an increased relative risk of developing breast cancer, particularly at a young age.[79–102, 51] This increased relative risk appears to be related to duration of use.

Some studies suggested that oral contraceptive use was associated with an increase in the risk of cervical intraepithelial neoplasia, dysplasia, erosion, carcinoma, or microglandular dysplasia in some populations of women.[17, 50, 103–115] However, there continues to be controversy about the extent to which such findings may be due to differences in sexual behavior and other factors.

In spite of many studies of the relationship between oral contraceptive use and breast and cervical cancers, a cause and effect relationship has not been established.

4. Hepatic neoplasia. Benign hepatic adenomas and other hepatic lesions have been associated with oral contraceptive use,[116–121] although the incidence of such benign tumors is rare in the United States. Indirect calculations have estimated the attributable risk to be in the range of 3.3 cases per 100,000 for users, a risk that increases after 4 or more years of use.[120] Rupture of benign, hepatic adenomas or other lesions may case death through intraabdominal hemorrhage. Therefore, such lesions should be considered in

TABLE 2. Annual number of birth-related or method-related deaths associated with control of fertility per 100,000 nonsterile women, by fertility control method according to age.[67]

Method of control	15–19	20–24	25–29	30–34	35–39	40–44
No fertility control methods*	7.0	7.4	9.1	14.8	25.7	28.2
Oral contraceptives nonsmoker**	0.3	0.5	0.9	1.9	13.8	31.6
smoker**	2.2	3.4	6.6	13.5	51.1	117.2
IUD**	0.8	0.8	1.0	1.0	1.4	1.4
Condom*	1.1	1.6	0.7	0.2	0.3	0.4
Diaphragm/Spermicide*	1.9	1.2	1.2	1.3	2.2	2.8
Periodic abstinence*	2.5	1.6	1.6	1.7	2.9	3.6

Adapted from Ory.[67]

* Deaths are birth-related
** Deaths are method-related

women presenting with abdominal pain and tenderness, abdominal mass, or shock. About one quarter of the cases presented because of abdominal masses, up to one half had signs and symptoms of acute intraperitoneal hemorrhage.[121] Diagnosis may prove difficult.

Studies from the U.S.,[122, 150] Great Britain,[123, 124] and Italy[125] have shown an increased risk of hepatocellular carcinoma in long-term (>8 years; relative risk of 7–20) oral contraceptive users. However, these cancers are rare in the United States, and the attributable risk (the excess incidence) of liver cancers in oral contraceptive users approaches less than 1 per 1,000,000 users.

5. Ocular lesions. There have been reports of retinal thrombosis and other ocular lesions associated with the use of oral contraceptives. Oral contraceptives should be discontinued if there is unexplained, gradual or sudden, partial or complete loss of vision; onset of proptosis or diplopia; papilledema; or any evidence of retinal vascular lesions. Appropriate diagnostic and therapeutic measures should be undertaken immediately.

6. Oral contraceptive use before or during pregnancy. Extensive epidemiological studies have revealed no increased risk of birth defects in women who have used oral contracepties prior to pregnancy.[126, 129] The majority of recent studies also do not suggest a teratogenic effect, particularly insofar as cardiac anomalies and limb reduction defects are concerned,[126, 129] when the pill is taken inadvertently during early pregnancy.

The administration of oral contraceptives to induce withdrawal bleeding should not be used as a test for pregnancy. Oral contraceptives should not be used during pregnancy to treat threatened or habitual abortion. It is recommended that for any patient who has missed two consecutive periods, pregnancy should be ruled out before continuing oral contraceptive use. If the patient has not adhered to the prescribed schedule, the possibility of pregnancy should be considered at the time of the first missed period and further use of oral contraceptives should be withheld until pregnancy has been ruled out. Oral contraceptive use should be discontinued if pregnancy is confirmed.

7. Gallbladder disease. Earlier studies reported an increased lifetime relative risk of gallbladder surgery in users of oral contraceptives and estrogens.[40, 42, 53, 70] More recent studies, however, have shown that the relative risk of developing gallbladder disease among oral contraceptive users may be minimal.[130–132] The recent findings of minimal risk may be related to the use of oral contraceptive formulations containing lower doses of estrogens and progestogens.

8. Carbohydrate and lipid metabolic effects. Oral contraceptives have been shown to cause a decrease in glucose tolerance in a signficant percentage of users.[32] This effect has been shown to be directly related to estrogen dose.[133] Progestogens increase insulin secretion and create insulin resistance, the effect varying with different progestational agents.[32, 134] However, in the nondiabetic woman, oral contraceptives appear to have no effect on fasting blood glucose. Because of these demonstrated effects, prediabetic and diabetic women should be carefully observed while taking oral contraceptives.

Some women may have persistent hypertriglyceridemia while on the pill. As discussed earlier (see **WARNINGS** 1a and 1d), changes in serum triglycerides and lipoprotein levels have been reported in oral contraceptive users.[23–31, 135, 136]

9. Elevated blood pressure. An increase in blood pressure has been reported in women taking oral contraceptives[50, 53, 137–139] and this increase is more likely in older oral contraceptive users[137] and with extended duration of use.[53] Data from the Royal College of General Practitioners[138] and subsequent randomized trials have shown that the incidence of hypertension increases with increasing concentration of progestogens.

Women with a history of hypertension or hypertension-related disease, or renal disease[139] should be encouraged to use another method of contraception. If such women elect to use oral contraceptives, they should be monitored closely and if significant elevation of blood pressure occurs, oral contraceptives should be discontinued. For most women, elevated blood pressure will return to normal after stopping oral contraceptives,[137] and there is no difference in the occurrence of hypertension among ever- and never-users.[140]

10. Headache. The onset or exacerbation of migraine or the development of headache of a new pattern that is recurrent, persistent, or severe requires discontinuation of oral contraceptives and evaluation of the cause.

11. Bleeding irregularities. Breakthrough bleeding and spotting are sometimes encountered in patients on oral contraceptives, especially during the first three months of use. Nonhormonal causes should be considered and adequate diagnostic measures taken to rule out malignancy or pregnancy in the event of breakthrough bleeding, as in the case of any abnormal vaginal bleeding. If a pathologic basis has been excluded, time alone or a change to another formulation may solve the problem. In the event of amenorrhea, pregnancy should be ruled out.

PRECAUTIONS

1. Physical examination and follow-up. It is good medical practice for all women to have annual history and physical examinations, including women using oral contraceptives. The physical examination, however, may be deferred until after initiation of oral contraceptives if requested by the woman and judged appropriate by the clinician. The physical examination should include special reference to blood pressure, breasts, abdomen, and pelvic organs, including cervical cytology, and relevant laboratory tests. In case of undiagnosed, persistent, or recurrent abnormal vaginal bleeding, appropriate diagnostic measures should be conducted to rule out malignancy. women with a strong family history of breast cancer or who have breast nodules should be monitored with particular care.

2. Lipid disorders. Women who are being treated for hyperlipidemias should be folowed closely if they elect to use oral contraceptives. Some preogestogens may elevate LDL levels and may render the control of hyperlipidemias more difficult.

3. Liver function. If jaundice develops in any woman receiving oral contraceptives, they should be discontinued. Steroids may be poorly metabolized in patients with impaired liver function and should be administered with caution in such patients. Cholestatic jaundice has been reported after combined treatment with oral contraceptives and troleandomycin. Hepatotoxicity following a combination of oral contraceptives and and cyclosporine has also been reported.

4. Fluid retention. Oral contraceptives may cause some degree of fluid retention. They should be prescribed with caution, and only with careful monitoring, in patients with conditions that might be aggravated by fluid retention, such as convulsive disorders, migraine syndrome, asthma, or cardiac, hepatic, or renal dysfunction.

5. Emotional disorders. Women with a history of depression should be carefully observed and the drug discontinued if depression recurs to a serious degree.

6. Contact lenses. Contact lens wearers who develop visual changes or changes in lens tolerance should be assessed by an ophthalmologist.

Continued on next page

Zovia—Cont.

7. Drug Interactions. Reduced efficacy and increased incidence of breakthrough bleeding and menstrual irregularities have been associated with concomitant use of rifampin. A similar association, though less marked, has been suggested for barbiturates, phenylbutazone, phenytoin sodium, and possibly with griseofulvin, ampicillin, and tetracyclines.
8. Laboratory test interactions. Certain endocrine and liver function tests and blood components may be affected by oral contraceptives:
a. Increased prothrombin and factors VII, VIII, IX and X; decreased antithrombin III; increased platelet aggregability.
b. Increased thyroid binding globulin (TBG), leading to increased circulating total thyroid hormone as measured by protein-bound iodine (PBI), T_4 by column or by radioimmunoassay. Free T_3 resin uptake is decreased, reflecting the elevated TBG; free T_4 concentration is unaltered.
c. Other binding proteins may be elevated in the serum.
d. Sex-steroid binding globulins are increased and result in elevated levels of total circulating sex steroids and corticoids; however, free or biologically active levels remain unchanged.
e. Triglycerides and phospholipids may be increased.
f. Glucose tolerance may be decreased.
g. Serum folate levels may be depressed. This may be of clinical signficance if a woman becomes pregnant shortly after discontinuing oral contraceptives.
h. Increased sulfobromophthalein and other abnormalities in liver function tests may occur.
i. Plasma levels of trace minerals may be altered.
j. Response to the metyrapone test may be reduced.
9. Carcinogenesis. See **WARNINGS.**
10. Pregnancy. Pregnancy Category X. See **CONTRAINDICATIONS** and **WARNINGS.**
11. Nursing mother. Small amounts of oral contraceptive steroids have been identified in the milk of nursing mothers[141–143] and a few adverse effects on the child have been reported, including jaundice and breast enlargement. In addition, oral contraceptives give in the postpartum period may interfere with lactation by decreasing the quantity and quality of breast milk. If possible, the nursing mother should be advised not to use oral contraceptives, but to use other forms of contraception until she has completely weaned her child.
12. Venereal diseases. Oral contraceptives are of no value in the prevention or treatment of venereal disease. The prevalence of cervical *Chlamydia trachomatis* and *Neisseria gonorrhoeae* in oral contraceptive users is increased severalfold.[144, 145] It should not be assumed that oral contraceptives afford protection against pelvic inflammatory disease from chlamydia.[144] Patients should be counseled that this product does not protect against HIV infection (AIDS) and other sexually transmitted diseases.
13. General.
a. The pathologist should be advised of oral contraceptive therapy when relevant specimens are submitted.
b. Treatment with oral contraceptives may mask the onset of the climacteric. (See **WARNINGS** regarding risks in this age group.)

INFORMATION FOR THE PATIENT
See patient labeling printed below.

ADVERSE REACTIONS
An increased risk of the following serious adverse reactions has been associated with the use of oral contraceptives (see **WARNINGS**):
- Thrombophlebitis and thrombosis
- Arterial thromboembolism
- Pulmonary embolism
- Myocardial infarction and coronary thrombosis
- Cerebral hemorrhage
- Cerebral thrombosis
- Hypertension
- Gallbladder disease
- Benign and malignant liver tumors, and other hepatic lesions

There is evidence of an association between the following conditions and the use of oral contraceptives, although additional confirmatory studies are needed:
- Mesenteric thrombosis
- Neuro-ocular lesions (e.g., retinal thrombosis and optic neuritis)

The following adverse reactions have been reported in patients receiving oral contraceptives and are believed to be drug-related:
- Nausea
- Vomiting
- Gastrointestinal symptoms (such as abdominal cramps and bloating)
- Breakthrough bleeding
- Spotting
- Change in menstrual flow
- Amenorrhea during or after use
- Temporary infertility after discontinuation of use
- Edema
- Chloasma or melasma, which may persist
- Breast changes: tenderness, enlargement, secretion
- Change in weight (increase or decrease)
- Change in cervical erosion or secretion
- Diminution in lactation when given immediately postpartum
- Cholestatic jaundice
- Migraine
- Rash (allergic)
- Mental depression
- Reduced tolerance to carbohydrates
- Vaginal candidiasis
- Change in corneal curvature (steepening)
- Intolerance to contact lenses

The following adverse reactions or conditions have been reported in users of oral contraceptives and the association has been neither confirmed nor refuted:
- Premenstrual syndrome
- Cataracts
- Changes in appetite
- Cystitis-like syndrome
- Headache
- Nervousness
- Dizziness
- Hirsutism
- Loss of scalp hair
- Erythema multiforme
- Erythema nodosum
- Hemorrhagic eruption
- Vaginitis
- Porphyria
- Impaired renal function
- Hemolytic uremic syndrome
- Acne
- Changes in libido
- Colitis
- Budd-Chiari syndrome
- Endocervical hyperplasia or ectropion

OVERDOSAGE
Serious ill effects have not been reported following acute ingestion of large doses of oral contraceptives by young children.[180, 181] Overdosage may cause nausea, and withdrawal bleeding may occur in females.

NON-CONTRACEPTIVE HEALTH BENEFITS
The following non-contraceptive health benefits related to the use of oral contraceptives are supported by epidemiological studies that largely utilized oral contraceptive formulations containing estrogen doses exceeding 35 mcg of ethinyl estradiol or 50 mcg of mestranol.[148, 149]
Effects on menses:
- Increased menstrual cycle regularity
- Decreased blood loss and decreased risk of iron-deficiency anemia
- Decreased frequency of dysmenorrhea

Effects related to inhibition of ovulation:
- Decreased risk of functional ovarian cysts
- Decreasd risk of ectopic pregnancies

Effects from long-term use:
- Decreased risk of fibroadenomas and fibrocystic disease of the breast
- Decreased risk of acute pelvic inflammatory disease
- Decreased risk of endometrial cancer
- Decreased risk of ovarian cancer
- Decreased risk of uterine fibroids

DOSAGE AND ADMINISTRATION
To achieve maximum contraceptive effectiveness, oral contraceptives must be taken exactly as directed and at intervals of 24 hours.
IMPORTANT: If the Sunday start schedule is selected, the patient should be instructed to use an additional method of protection until after the first week of administration *in the initial cycle.*
The possibility of ovulation and conception prior to initiation of use should be considered.

Zovia 1/35E-21 and Zovia 1/35E-28
Zovia 1/50E-21 and Zovia 1/50E-28
Dosage Schedules
The Zovia 1/35E-21 and Zovia 1/50E-21 tablet dispensers contain 21 tablets arranged in three numbered rows of 7 tablets each.
The Zovia 1/35E-28 and Zovia 1/50E-28 tablet dispensers contain 21 colored active tablets arranged in three numbered rows of 7 tablets each, followed by a fourth row of 7 white placebo tablets.
Days of the week are printed above the tablets, starting with Sunday on the left.
Two dosage schedules are described, one of which may be more convenient or suitable than the other for an individual patient.
Schedule #1: Sunday start. The patient begins taking Zovia 1/35E-21, Zovia 1/35E-28, Zovia 1/50E-21, or Zovia 1/50E-28 from the first row of her package, one tablet daily, starting on the first Sunday after the onset of menstruation. If the patient's period begins on a Sunday she takes her first tablet that very same day. The 21st tablet or the 28th tablet, depending on whether the patient is taking the 21- or 28-tablet course, will be taken on a Saturday.
Subsequent cycles:
21-tablet course—The patient begins a new 21-tablet course on the eighth day. Sunday, after taking her last tablet. All subsequent cycles will also begin on Sunday, one tablet being taken each day for 3 weeks followed by a week of no pill-taking.
28-tablet course—The patient begins a new 28-tablet course on the next day, Sunday, and all subsequent cycles will also begin on Sunday, one tablet being taken each and every day.
With a Sunday-start schedule, a woman whose period begins on the day of or 1 to 4 days before taking the first tablet should expect a diminution of flow and fewer menstrual days. The initial cycle will likely be shortened by from 1 to 5 days. Thereafter, cycles should be about 28 days in length.
Schedule #2: Day 1 start. The patient begins taking Zovia 1/35E-21 or Zovia 1/50E-21 from the first row of her package, one tablet daily, starting with the pill day which corresponds to day 1 of her menstrual cycle; the first day of menstruation is counted as day 1. After the last (Saturday) tablet in row #3 has been taken, if any remain in the first row, the patient completes her 21-tablet schedule starting with Sunday in row #1.
Subsequent cycles: The patient begins a new 21-tablet course on the eighth day after taking her last tablet, again starting the same day of the week on which she began her first course. All subsequent cycles will also begin on that same day, one tablet being taken each day for 3 weeks followed by a week of no pill-taking.

Special notes
Spotting, breakthrough bleeding, or nausea. If spotting (bleeding insufficient to require a pad), breakthrough bleeding (heavier bleeding similar to a menstrual flow), or nausea occurs the patient should continue taking her tablets as directed. The incidence of spotting, breakthrough bleeding or nausea is minimal, most frequently occurring in the first cycle. Ordinarily spotting or breakthrough bleeding will stop within a week. Usually the patient will begin to cycle regularly within two to three courses of tablet-taking. In the event of spotting or breakthrough bleeding organic causes should be borne in mind. (see **WARNING** No. 11)
Missed menstrual periods. Withdrawal flow will normally occur 2 or 3 days after the last active tablet is taken. Failure of withdrawal bleeding ordinarily does not mean that the patient is pregnant, providing the dosage schedule has been correctly followed. (See **WARNING** No. 6)
If the patient has *not* adhered to the prescribed dosage regimen, the possibility of pregnancy should be considered after the first missed period, and oral contraceptives should be withheld until pregnancy has been ruled out.
If the patient has adhered to the prescribed regimen and misses two consecutive periods, pregnancy should be ruled out before continuing the contraceptive regimen.
The first intermenstrual interval after discontinuing the tablets is usually prolonged; consequently, a patient for whom a 28-day cycle is usual might not begin to menstruate for 35 days or longer. Ovulation in such prolonged cycles will occur correspondingly later in the cycle. Posttreatment cycles after the first one, however, are usually typical for the individual woman prior to taking tablets. (See **WARNING** No. 11)
Missed tablets. If a woman misses taking one active tablet, the missed tablet should be taken as soon as it is remembered. In addition, the next tablet should be taken at the usual time. If two consecutive active tablets are missed in week 1 or week 2 of the dispenser, the dosage should be doubled for the next 2 days. The regular schedule should then be resumed, but an additional method of protection must be used as backup for the next 7 days if she has sex during that time or she may become pregnant.
If two consecutive active tablets are missed in week 3 of the dispenser or three consecutive active tablets are missed during any of the first 3 weeks of the dispenser, direct the patient to do one of the following: Day 1 Starters should discard the rest of the dispenser and begin a new dispenser that same day; Sunday Starters should continue to take 1 tablet daily until Sunday, discard the rest of the dispenser and begin a new dispenser that same day. The patient may not have a period this month; however, if she has missed two consecutive periods, pregnancy should be ruled out. An additional method of protection must be used as a backup for the next 7 days after the tablets are missed if she has sex during that time or she may become pregnant.
While there is little likelihood of ovulation if only one active tablet is missed, the possibility of spotting or breakthrough bleeding is increased and should be expected if two or more successive active tablets are missed. However, the possibility of ovulation increases with each successive day that scheduled active tablets are missed.
If one or more placebo tablets of Zovia 1/35E-28 or Zovia 1/50E-28 are missed, the Zovia 1/35E-28 or Zovia 1/50E-28 schedule should be resumed on the following Sunday (the eighth day after the last colored tablet was taken). Omis-

sion of placebo tablets in the 28-tablet courses does not increase the possibility of conception provided that this schedule is followed.

HOW SUPPLIED

Zovia 1/35E: Each light pink Zovia 1/35E tablet is round in shape, unscored, debossed with WATSON 383 and contains 1 mg of ethynodiol diacetate and 35 mcg of ethinyl estradiol.
Zovia 1/35E-21 (NDC 52544-532-21) is packaged in cartons of six tablet dispensers of 21 tablets each.
Zovia 1/35E-28 (NDC 52544-383-28) is packaged in cartons of six tablet dispensers. Each dispenser contains 21 light pink tablet and 7 white placebo tablets. (Placebo tablets have a debossed WATSON on one side and P on the other side.)

Zovia 1/50E: Each pink Zovia 1/50E tablet is round in shape, unscored, debossed with WATSON 384 and contains 1 mg of ethynodiol diacetate and 50 mcg of ethinyl estradiol.
Zovia 1/50E-21 (NDC 52544-533-21) is packaged in cartons of six tablet dispensers of 21 tablets each.
Zovia 1/50E-28 (NDC 52544-384-28) is packaged in cartons of six tablet dispensers. Each dispenser contains 21 pink tablets and 7 white placebo tablets. (Placebo tablets have a debosssed WATSON on one side and P on the other side).
Store at controlled room temperature 15°–30°C (59°–86°F).

CAUTION: Federal law prohibits dispensing without prescription.

REFERENCES

1. Trussel J, et al. *Stud Fam Plann.* 1987;18(Sept-Oct); and 1990;21(Jan-Feb):51. **1a.** *Physicians' Desk Reference* 47th ed. Orudell, NJ: Medical Economics Co Inc; 1993;2598–2601. **2.** Mann JI, et al. *Br Med J.* 1975;2(May 3):241. **3.** Mann JI, et al. *Br Med J.* 1975;3(Sept13):631. **4.** Mann JI, et al. *Br Med J.* 1975;2(May 3):245. **5.** Mann JI, et al. Br Med J. 1976;2(Aug 21):445. **6.** Arthes FG, et al. *Chest.* 1976;70(Nov):574. **7.** Jain AK, *Am J Obstet Gynecol.* 1976;301(Oct 1):126 and *Stud Fam Plann.* 1977;8(March): 50. **8.** Ory HW. *JAMA.* 1977;237(June 13);2619. **9.** Jick H, et al. *JAMA.* 1978;239(April 3):1403, 1407. **10.** Jick H, et al. *JAMA.* 1978;240(Dec 1):2548. **11.** Shapiro S, et al. *Lancet.* 1979;1(April 7):743. **12.** Rosenberg L, et al. *Am J Epidemiol.* 1980;111(Jan):59. **13.** Krueger DE, et al. *Am J Epidemiol.* 1980;111(June):655. **14.** Layde P, et al. *Lancet.* 1981;1(March 7):541. **15.** Adam SA, et al. *Br J Obstet Gynaecol.* 1981;88(Aug):838. **16.** Slone D, et al. *N Engl J Med* 1981;305(Aug 20):420. **17.** Ramcharan S, et al. *The Walnut Creek Contraceptive Drug Study. Vol 3.* US Govt Ptg Off. 1981; and *J Reprod Med.* 1980;25(Dec):346. **18.** Layde PM, et al. *J R Coll Gen Pract.* 1983;33(Feb):75. **19.** Rosenberg L, et al. *JAMA.* 1985;253(May 24/31):2965. **20.** Mant D, et al. *J Epidemiol Community Health.* 1987;41(Sept):215. **21.** Croft P, et al. *Br Med J.* 1989;298(Jan 21):165. **22.** Goldbaum GM, et al. *JAMA.* 1987;258(Sept 11):1339. **23.** Bradley DD, et al. *N Engl J Med.* 1978;299(July 6):17. **24.** Tikkanen MJ. *J Reprod Med.* 1986;31(Sept suppl):898. **25.** Lipson A, et al. *Contraception.* 1986;34(Aug):121. **26.** Burkman RT, et al. *Obstet Gynecol.* 1988; 71(Jan):33. **27.** Knopp RH, *J Reprod Med.* 1986;31(Sept suppl):913. **28.** Krauss RM, et al. *Am J Obstet Gynecol.* 1983;145(Feb 15):446. **29.** Wahl P, et al. *N Engl J Med.* 1983;308(April 14):862. **30.** Wynn V, et al. *Am J Obstet Gynecol.* 1982;142(March 15):766. **31.** LaRosa JC. *J Reprod Med.* 1986;31(Sept suppl):906. **32.** Wynn V, et al. *J Reprod Med.* 1986;31(Sept suppl):892. **33.** Royal College of General Practitioners. *JR Coll Gen Pract.* 1967;13(May):267. **34.** Inman WHW, et al. *Br Med J.* 1968;(April 27):193. **35.** Vessey MP, et al. *Br Med J.* 1968;2(April 27):199. **36.** Vessey MP, et al. *Br Med J.* 1969;2(June14):651. **37.** Sartwell PE, et al. *Am J Epidemiol.* 1969;90(Nov):365. **38.** Vessey MP, et al. *Br Med J.* 1970;3(July 18):123. **39.** Greene GR, et al. *Am J Public Health.* 1972;62(May):680. **40.** Boston Collaborative Drug Surveillance Programme. *Lancet.* 1973;1(June 23):1399. **41.** Stolley PD, et al. *Am J Epidemiol.* 1975;102(Sept):197. **42.** Vessey MP, et al. *J Biosoc Sci.* 1976;8(Oct):373. **43.** Kay CR, *Jr Coll Gen Pract.* 1978;28(July):393. **44.** Petitti DB, et al. *Am J Epidemiol.* 1978;108(Dec):480. **45.** Maguire MG, et al. *Am J Epidemiol.* 1979;110(Aug):188. **46.** Petitti DB, et al. *JAMA.* 1979;242(Sept 14):1150. **47.** Porter JB, et al. *Obstet Gynecol.* 1982;59(March):299. **48.** Porter JB, et al. *Obstet Gynecol.* 1985;66(July):1. **49.** Vessey MP, et al. *Br Med J.* 1986;292(Feb 22):526. **50.** Hoover R, et al. *Am J Public Health.* 1978;68(April):335. **51.** Vessey MP, *Br J Fam Plann.* 1980;6(Oct suppl):1. **52.** Collaborative Group for the Study of Stroke in Young Women. *N Engl J Med.* 1973;288(April 26):871. **53.** Royal College of General Practitioners. *Oral Contraceptives and Health.* New York, NY: Pitman Publ Corp; May 1974. **54.** Collaborative Group for the Study of Stroke in Young Women. *JAMA.* 1975;231(Feb 17):718. **55.** Beral V. *Lancet.* 1976;2(Nov 13):1047. **56.** Vessey MP, et al. *Lancet.* 1977;2(Oct 8):731; and 1981;1(March 7):549. **57.** Petitti DB, et al. *Lancet.* 1978;2(July 29):234. **58.** Inman WHW. *Br Med J.* 1979;2(Dec 8):1468. **59.** Vessy MP, et al. *Br Med J.* 1984;289(Sept 1):530. **60.** Inman WHW, et al. *Br Med J.* 1970;2(April 25):203. **61.** Meade TW, et al. *Br Med J.* 1980;280(May 10):1157. **62.** Bottiger LE, et al. *Lancet.* 1980;1(May 24):1097. **63.** Kay CR, *Am J Obstet Gynecol.* 1982;142(March 15):762. **64.** Vessey MP, et al. *Br Med J.* 1986;292(Feb 22):526. **65.** Gordon T, et al. *Am J Med.* 1977;62(May):707. **66.** Beral V, et al. *Lancet.* 1977;2 (Oct 8): 727. **67.** Ory H. *Fam Plann Perspect.* 1983;15(March-April): 57. **68.** Arthes FG, et al. *Cancer.* 1971;28(Dec):1391. **69.** Vessey MP, et al. *Br Med J.* 1972;3(Sept 23):719. **70.** Boston Collaborative Drug Surveilance Program. *N Engl J Med.* 1974;290(Jan3):15. **71.** Vessey MP, et al. *Lancet.* 1975;1(April 26):941. **72.** Casagrande J, et al. *J Natl Cancer Inst.* 1976;56(April):839. **73.** Kelsey, JL, et al. *Am J Epidemiol.* 1978;107(March):236. **74.** Kay CR, *Br Med J.* 1981;282(June 27):2089. **75.** Vessey MP, et al. *Br Med J.* 1981;282(June 27):2093. **76.** The Cancer and Steroid Hormone Study of the Center for Disease Control and the National Institute of Child Health and Human Development. Oral contraceptive use and the risk of breast cancer. *N Engl J Med.* 1986;315(Aug 14):405. **77.** Paul C, et al. *Br Med J.* 1986; 293(Sept 20):723. **78.** Miller DR, et al. *Obstet Gynecol.* 1986;68(Dec):863. **79.** Pike MC, et al. *Lancet.* 1983;2(Oct 22):926. **80.** McPherson K, et al. *Br J Cancer.* 1987;56(Nov): 653. **81.** Hoover R, et al. *N Engl J Med.* 1976;295(Aug 19): 401. **82.** Lees AW, et al. *Int J Cancer.* 1978;22(Dec):700. **83.** Brinton LA, et al. *J Natl Cancer Inst.* 1979;62(Jan):37. **84.** Black MM, *Pathol Res Pract.* 1980;166:491; and *Cancer.* 1980;46(Dec):2747; and *Cancer.* 1983;51 June):2147. **85.** Clavel F, et al. *Bull Cancer* (Paris). 1981;68(Dec):449. **86.** Brinton LA, et al. *Int J Epidemiol.* 1982;11(Dec):316. **87.** Harris NV, et al. *Am J Epidemiol.* 1982;116(Oct):643. **88.** Jick H, et al. *Am J Epidemiol.* 1980;112(Nov):577. **89.** McPherson K, et al. *Lancet.* 1983;2(Dec 17):1414. **90.** Hoover R, et al. *J Natl Cancer Inst.* 1981;67(Oct):815. **91.** Jick H, et al. *Am J Epidemiol.* 1980;112(Nov):586. **92.** Meirik O, et al. *Lancet.* 1986;2(Sept 20):650. **93.** Fasal E, et al. *J Natl Cancer Inst.* 1975;55(Oct):767. **94.** Paffenbarger RS, et al. *Cancer.* 1977;39(April suppl):1887. **95.** Stadel BV, et al. *Contraception.* 1988;38(Sept): 287. **96.** Miller DR, et al. *Am J Epidemiol.* 1989;129(Feb):269. **97.** Kay CR, et al. *Br J Cancer.* 1988;58(Nov):675. **98.** Miller DR, et al. *Obstet Gynecol.* 1986;68(Dec):863. **99.** Olsson H, et al. *Lancet.* 1985;1(March 30):748. **100.** Chilvers C, et al. *Lancet.* 1989;1(May 6):973. **101.** Huggins GR, et al. *Fertil Steril.* 1987;47(May):733. **102.** Pike MC, et al. *Br J Cancer.* 1981;43(Jan):72. **103.** Ory H, et al. *Am J Obstet Gynecol.* 1976;124(March 15):573. **104.** Stern E, et al. *Science.* 1977;196(June 24):1460. **105.** Pertiz E, et al. *Am J Epidemiol.* 1977;106(Dec):462. **106.** Ory HW, et al. In: Garattini S, Berendes H, eds. *Pharmacology of Steroid Contraceptive Drugs.* New York, NY: Raven Press; 1977;211-224. **107.** Meisels A, et al. *Cancer.* 1977;40(Dec): 3076. **108.** Goldacre MJ, et al. *Br Med J.* 1978;1(March 25): 748. **109.** Swan SH, et al. *Am J Obstet Gynecol.* 1981;139(Jan 1):52. **110.** Vessey MP, et al. *Lancet.* 1983;2(Oct 22):930. **111.** Dallenbach-Hellweg G. *Pathol Res Pract.* 1984:179:38. **112.** Thomas DB, et al. *Br Med J.* 1985;290(March 30):961. **113.** Brinton LA, et al. *Int J Cancer.* 1986;38 (Sept):339. **114.** Ebeling K, et al. *Int J Cancer.* 1987;39(April):427. **115.** Beral V, et al. *Lancet.* 1988;2(Dec 10):1331. **116.** Baum JK, et al. *Lancet.* 1973;2(Oct 27):926. **117.** Edmondson HA, et al. *N Engl J Med.* 1976;294(Feb 26): 470. **118.** Bein NN, et al. *Br J Surg.* 1977;64(June):433. **119.** Klatskin G. *Gastroenterology.* 1977;73 (Aug):386. **120.** Rooks JB, et al. *JAMA.* 1979;242(Aug 17):644. **121.** Sturtevant FM. In: Moghissi K, ed. *Controversies in Contraception..* Baltimore, MD: Williams & Wilkins; 1979:93-150. **122.** Henderson BE, et al. *Br J Cancer.* 1983;48(July):437. **123.** Neuberger J, et al. *Br Med J.* 1986;292(May 24):1355. **124.** Forman D, et al. *Br Med J.* 1986;292(May 24):1357. **125.** La Vecchia C, et al. *Br J Cancer.* 1989;59(March):460. **126.** Savolainen E, et al. *Am J Obstet Gynecol.* 1981;140(July 1): 521. **127.** Ferencz C, et al. *Teratology.* 1980;21(April):225. **128.** Rothman KJ, et al. *Am J Epidemiol.* 1979;109(April): 433. **129.** Harlap S, et al. *Obstet Gynecol.* 1980;55(April): 447. **130.** Layde PM, et al. *J Epidemiol Community Health.* 1982;36(Dec):274. **131.** Rome Group for the Epidemiology and Prevention of Cholelithiasis (GREPCO). *Am J Epidemiol.* 1984;119(May):796. **132.** Strom BL, et al. *Clin Pharmacol Ther.* 1986;39(March):335. **133.** Wynn V. In: Bardin CE, et al. eds. *Progesterone and Progestins.* New York, NY: Raven Press;1983:395-410. **134.** Perlman JA, et al. *J Chron Dis.* 1985;38(Oct)857. **135.** Powell MG, et al. *Obstet Gynecol.* 1984;63(June):764. **136.** Wynn V, et al. *Lancet.* 1966;2(Oct 1):720. **137.** Firsch IR, et al. *JAMA.* 1977;237(June 6):2499. **138.** Kay CR. *Lancet.* 1977;1(March 19):624. **139.** Laragh JH, *Am J Obstet Gynecol.* 1976;126(Sept 1):141. **140.** Ramcharan S. In: Garattini S, Berendes HW, eds. *Pharmacology of Steroid Contraceptive Drugs.* New York, NY: Raven Press; 1977:277-288. **141.** Laumas KR, et al. *Am J Obstet Gynecol.* 1967;98(June 1):411. **142.** Saxena BN, et al. *Contraception.* 1977;16(Dec):605. **143.** Nilsson S. et al. *Contraception.* 1978;17(Feb):131. **144.** Washington AE, et al. *JAMA.* 1985;253(April 19):2246. **145.** Louv WC, et al. *Am J Obstet Gynecol.* 1989;160(Feb):396. **146.** Francis WG, et al. *Can Med Assoc J.* 1965;92(Jan 23):191. **147.** Verhulst HL, et al. *J Clin Pharmacol.* 1967;7(Jan-Feb):9. **148.** Ory HW, *Fam Plann Perspect.* 1982;14(July-Aug):182.**149.** Ory HW, et al. *Making Choices Evaluating the Health Risks and Benefits of Birth Control Methods.* New York, NY: The Alan Guttmacher Institute; 1983. **150.** Palmer JR, et al. *Am J Epidemiol.* 1989;130(Nov):878. **151.** Romieu I, et al. *J Natl Cancer Inst.* 1989;81(Sept):1313. **152.** Porter JB, et al. *Obstet Gynecol.* 1987;70(July):29.

Manufactured by
Watson Laboratories, Inc.,
Corona, CA 91720 12178-2

Revised, December 8, 1995

Zovia 1/35E-21
Zovia 1/35E-28
Zovia 1/50E-21
Zovia 1/50E-28
(Ethynodiol Diacetate and Ethinyl Estradiol Tablets, USP)
Shown in Product Identification Guide, page 343

WE Pharmaceuticals, Inc.

P.O. BOX 1142
RAMONA, CA, 92065

Direct Inquiries to:
(760) 788-9155
For Medical Emergencies Contact:
(760) 788-9155

AH-CHEW® Chewable Tablets ℞

Each tablet contains chlorpheniramine maleate 2mg. phenylephrine HCl 10mg. methscopolamine nitrate 1.25mg.

DOSAGE

12 yrs. & Older 1 or 2 Tabs (Q.I.D.), 6–12 yrs. 1 Tab (Q.I.D.).

HOW SUPPLIED

Bottles of 100, NDC# 59196-003-01

AH-CHEW®D Chewable Tablets ℞

Each tablet contains phenylephrine HCl 10mg.

DOSAGE

12 yrs. & Older 1 or 2 Tabs (Q.I.D.), 6–12 yrs. 1 Tab (Q.I.D.)

HOW SUPPLIED

Bottles of 100, NDC# 59196-007-01

D-FEDA® II Tablets ℞

Each tablet contains pseudoephedrine HCl 60 mg, guaifenesin 600 mg.

DOSAGE

12 yrs. & Older 1 or 2 Tabs (B.I.D.), 6–12 yrs. 1 Tab (B.I.D.), 2–6 Yrs. $^1/_2$ Tab (B.I.D.).

HOW SUPPLIED

Bottles of 100, NDC #59196-005-01

E-Z SPACER® ℞

Portable Drug Delivery System for use with metered dose inhalers.

HOW SUPPLIED

One Unit plus Instructions for Single Patient Use.
NDC #59196-009-01

E-Z SPACER® MASK (SMALL) ℞

For use with E-Z Spacer Drug Delivery System (contains no Latex)

HOW SUPPLIED

One mask plus instructions for Single Patient Use.
NDC #59196-020-01

HUMAVENT® L.A. Tablets ℞

600 mg Guaifenesin

HOW SUPPLIED

NDC # 59196-008-01 Bottles of 100
59196-008-05 Bottles of 500

OMNIHIST® L.A. Tablets ℞

Each tablet contains chlorpheniramine maleate 8 mg, phenylephrine HCl 20 mg, methscopolamine nitrate 2.5 mg.

DOSAGE

12 yrs. & Older 1 Tab (B.I.D.), 6–12 yrs. $^1/_2$ Tab (B.I.D.)

Continued on next page

Omnihist L.A.—Cont.

HOW SUPPLIED

Bottles of 100, NDC #59196-002-01

PREDNISOLONE SYRUP, USP   ℞ Only

DESCRIPTION

Contains Prednisolone 15 mg per 5 mL.

HOW SUPPLIED

Prednisolone Syrup, USP, is a cherry flavored red liquid containing 15 mg of Prednisolone in each 5 mL (teaspoonful) and is supplied in 240 mL bottles (NDC 59196-0010-24) and 480 mL bottles (NDC 59196-0010-48).

SINUVENT® Tablets   ℞

Each tablet contains phenylpropanolamine HCl 75mg, guaifenesin 600mg.

DOSAGE

12 yrs. & Older 1 Tab (B.I.D.), 6–12 yrs. $^1/_2$ Tab (B.I.D.)

HOW SUPPLIED

Bottles of 100, NDC# 59196-001-01

ULTRABROM® Capsules   ℞

Each capsule contains brompheniramine maleate 12mg, pseudoephedrine HCl 120mg.

DOSAGE

12 yrs. and Older 1 Cap (B.I.D.)

HOW SUPPLIED

Bottles of 100, NDC# 59196-006-01

ULTRABROM® PD Capsules   ℞

Each capsule contains brompheniramine maleate 6mg, pseudoephedrine HCl 60mg.

DOSAGE

12 yrs. & Older 1 or 2 Caps B.I.D., 6–12 yrs. 1 Cap B.I.D.

HOW SUPPLIED

Bottles of 100, NDC# 59196-004-01

Westlake Laboratories, Inc.
24700 CENTER RIDGE ROAD
CLEVELAND, OH 44145

Direct Inquiries to:
Customer Service
 (888) WSTLAKE (978–5253)
Fax (216) 835–2177
Internet: www.westlake-labs.com

BEVITAMEL   OTC
[bē-vīt ´ə-měl]
Melatonin-B-Vitamin Supplement

DESCRIPTION

Each tablet contains:

	Amount	% U.S.RDA*
Melatonin	3 mg	***
Vitamin B12	1000 µg	16667
Folic Acid	400 µg	100

* U.S. Recommended Daily Amount (RDA) established by the U.S. Food and Drug Administration (FDA).

*** The U.S.RDA has not been established by the U.S. FDA.

INDICATIONS

Bevitamel can be used to enhance the natural sleep process. Vitamin B12 and Folic Acid can be used to assist the metabolism of blood homocysteine.

CONTRAINDICATIONS

Product NOT intended for the treatment of Pernicious anemia

WARNINGS

Keep out of reach of children and store in a cool dry place. Tamper-resistant package, do not use if outer seal is missing or broken.

PRECAUTIONS

The dose size and timing may need to be adjusted by the physician to provide maximum effect for individual patients.

Individuals taking other medications, or with autoimmune, seizure or endocrine disorders and pregnant or lactating women, should consult a physician prior to use.

ADVERSE REACTIONS

None known.

DOSAGE AND ADMINISTRATION

One tablet sub-lingual approximately 30 minutes before bedtime as directed by a physician. Fractional tablets may be taken when indicated.

OVERDOSAGE

None known.

HOW SUPPLIED

BEVITAMEL is supplied as a pink bisected sub-lingual tablet (60 per bottle).

Westwood-Squibb
Pharmaceuticals, Inc.
100 FOREST AVENUE
BUFFALO, NY 14213

For Medical Information Contact:
Generally:
Consumer Affairs Department:
1-800-333-0950
Adverse Drug Experiences
and Product Defects Reporting call during business hours only:
1-800-333-0950

CAPITROL®   ℞
(chloroxine 2%)
Shampoo

Rx only.

DESCRIPTION

CAPITROL is an antibacterial shampoo containing 2% (w/w) chloroxine (each gram contains 20 mg chloroxine) suspended in a base of sodium octoxynol-2 ethane sulfonate, water, PEG-6 lauramide, dextrin, sodium lauryl sulfoacetate, sodium dioctyl sulfosuccinate, 1% benzyl alcohol, PEG-14M, magnesium aluminum silicate, fragrance, EDTA, and color. May contain citric acid to adjust pH.

Chloroxine is a synthetic antibacterial compound that is effective in the treatment of dandruff and seborrheic dermatitis when incorporated in a shampoo.

The chemical name of chloroxine is 5,7-dichloro-8-hydroxyquinoline. The chemical structure of chloroxine is:

CLINICAL PHARMACOLOGY

Well controlled studies demonstrate Capitrol effectively reduces the excess scaling in patients with dandruff or seborrheic dermatitis. Though the cause of dandruff is not known, it is thought to be the result of accelerated mitotic activity in the epidermis. The presumed mechanism of action to reduce scaling would be to slow down the mitotic activity.

The role of microbes in seborrheic dermatitis is not known; however, *Staphylococcus aureus* and *Pityrosporon* species are often present in increased numbers during the course of the disease. Chloroxine is antibacterial, inhibiting the growth of Gram-positive as well as some Gram-negative organisms. Antifungal activity against some dermatophytes and yeasts also has been shown.

The absorption, metabolism and pharmacokinetics of Capitrol in humans have not been studied.

INDICATIONS AND USAGE

Capitrol is indicated in the treatment of dandruff and mild-to-moderately severe seborrheic dermatitis of the scalp. Clinical studies indicate that improvement may be observed after 14 days of therapy.

CONTRAINDICATIONS

Capitrol is contraindicated in those patients with a history of hypersensitivity to any of the listed ingredients.

WARNINGS

Capitrol should not be used on acutely inflamed (exudative) lesions of the scalp.

PRECAUTIONS

Information for patients: Exercise care to prevent Capitrol from entering the eyes. If contact occurs, the patient should flush eyes with cool water. Discoloration of light-colored hair (e.g. blond, gray or bleached) may follow use of this preparation.

Irritation and a burning sensation on the scalp and adjacent areas have been reported.

Drug/Laboratory Test Interactions: There is no known interference of Capitrol with laboratory tests.

Carcinogenesis, Mutagenesis: No long term studies in animals have been performed to evaluate the carcinogenic potential of Capitrol.

Results of the *in vitro* Ames Salmonella/Microsome Plate test show that Capitrol does not demonstrate genetic activity and is considered non-mutagenic.

Pregnancy Category C: Animal reproduction studies have not been conducted with Capitrol. It is also not known whether Capitrol can cause fetal harm when administered to a pregnant woman or can affect reproduction capacity. Capitrol should be given to a pregnant woman only if clearly needed.

Nursing Mothers: It is not known whether this drug is excreted in human milk. Because many drugs are excreted in human milk, caution should be exercised when Capitrol is administered to a nursing woman.

Pediatric Use: Specific studies to demonstrate the safety and effectiveness for use of Capitrol in children have not been conducted.

ADVERSE REACTION

One patient out of 225 in clinical studies was reported to have contact dermatitis.

OVERDOSAGE

The acute oral LD_{50} in mice was found to be 200 mg/kg and in rats 450 mg/kg. On the basis of these animal studies, Capitrol may be considered practically non-toxic.

DOSAGE AND ADMINISTRATION

Shake well. Capitrol should be massaged thoroughly onto the wet scalp, avoiding contact with the eyes. Lather should remain on the scalp for approximately three minutes, then rinsed. The application should be repeated and the scalp rinsed thoroughly. Two treatments per week are usually sufficient.

HOW SUPPLIED

Capitrol shampoo contains 2% (w/w) chloroxine (20 mg chloroxine per gram) and is supplied in 110g plastic bottles (NDC 0072-6850-04).

Store at room temperature.

WATER BASE **DESQUAM-E™ 2.5 Emollient Gel** (2.5% benzoyl peroxide)	℞
WATER BASE **DESQUAM-E™ 5 Emollient Gel** (5% benzoyl peroxide)	℞
WATER BASE **DESQUAM-E™ 10 Emollient Gel** (10% benzoyl peroxide)	℞
WATER BASE **DESQUAM-X® 5 Gel** (5% Benzoyl Peroxide)	℞
WATER BASE **DESQUAM-X® 10 Gel** (10% Benzoyl Peroxide)	℞
WATER BASE **DESQUAM-X® 5 Wash** (5% benzoyl peroxide)	℞
WATER BASE **DESQUAM-X 10 ® Wash** (10% benzoyl peroxide)	℞
DESQUAM-X® 10 Bar (10% benzoyl peroxide)	℞

Rx only.

DESCRIPTION

DESQUAM-E 2.5, DESQUAM-E 5 and DESQUAM-E 10 brand topical anti-acne gels contain benzoyl peroxide (2.5, 5 and 10%) in a water-base vehicle of carbomer 940, diisopropanolamine, disodium edetate, docusate sodium, methyl gluceth-20 and polyquaternium-7.

DESQUAM-X 5 and DESQUAM-X 10 brand topical anti-acne gels contain benzoyl peroxide (5 and 10%), in a water-base vehicle of carbomer 940, disodium edetate and laureth-4. May contain diisopropanolamine or triethanolamine to adjust pH.

DESQUAM-X[5] and DESQUAM-X[10] brand topical therapeutic anti-acne cleansers contain benzoyl peroxide (5% and 10%) in a lathering water base of sodium octoxynol-3 sulfonate, dioctyl sodium sulfosuccinate, magnesium aluminum silicate, methylcellulose and EDTA.

DESQUAM-X 10 brand therapeutic anti-acne BAR contains 10% benzoyl peroxide, boric acid, cellulose gum, dextrin (may contain wheat starch), disodium EDTA, docusate sodium, lactic acid, PEG-14M, sodium lauryl sulfoacetate (or sodium dodecyl benzene sulfonate and trisodium sulfosuccinate), sorbitol, urea and water.

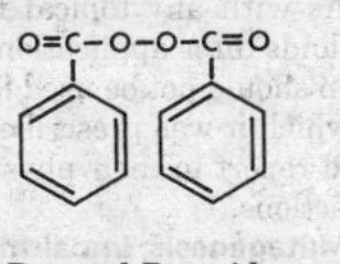

Benzoyl Peroxide

CLINICAL PHARMACOLOGY

The effectiveness of benzoyl peroxide in the treatment of acne vulgaris is primarily attributable to its antibacterial activity, especially with respect to *Propionibacterium acnes,* the predominant organism in sebaceous follicles and comedones. The antibacterial activity of this compound is presumably due to the release of active or free-radical oxygen capable of oxidizing bacterial proteins. In acne patients treated topically with benzoyl peroxide, resolution of the acne usually coincides with reduction in the level of *P. acnes* and free fatty acids (FFA). Mild desquamation is another observed action of topically applied benzoyl peroxide and may also play a role in the drug's effectiveness in acne. Studies also indicate that topical benzoyl peroxide may exert a sebostatic effect with a resultant reduction of skin surface lipids.

Benzoyl peroxide has been shown to be absorbed by the skin, where it is metabolized to benzoic acid and then excreted as benzoate in the urine.

INDICATIONS AND USAGE

DESQUAM-E (5 or 10) EMOLLIENT GEL is indicated for the topical treatment of mild to moderate acne vulgaris and as an adjunct in therapeutic regimens including antibiotics, retinoic acid products and sulfur or salicylic acid-containing preparations. DESQUAM-E EMOLLIENT GEL has been shown effective in the treatment of the following acne lesion types: papules, pustules, open and closed comedones. Clinical studies have demonstrated therapeutic response after two to three weeks.

DESQUAM-X (5 or 10) GEL is indicated for the topical treatment of mild to moderate acne vulgaris and as an adjunct in therapeutic regimens including antibiotics, retinoic acid products and sulfur or salicylic acid-containing preparations. DESQUAM-X GEL has been shown effective in the treatment of the following acne lesion types: papules, pustules, open and closed comedones. Clinical studies have demonstrated therapeutic response after two to three weeks. DESQUAM-X GEL may also be used as adjunctive treatment for nodulo-cystic acne (acne conglobata), although its effectiveness for this condition has not been proven.

DESQUAM-X (5 or 10) WASH is indicated for the topical treatment of mild to moderate acne. In more severe cases, it may be used as an adjunct in therapeutic regimens including benzoyl peroxide gels, antibiotics, retinoic acid products and sulfur/salicylic acid-containing preparations. The improvement of the treated condition is dependent on the degree and type of acne, the frequency of use of DESQUAM-X WASH and the nature of other therapies employed.

DESQUAM-X 10 BAR is indicated for the topical treatment of acne. It may be used as an adjunct in therapeutic regimens including benzoyl peroxide gels, antibiotics, retinoic acid products and sulfur/salicylic acid-containing preparations. The improvement of the treated condition is dependent on the degree and type of acne, the frequency of use of DESQUAM-X 10 BAR and the nature of other therapies employed.

CONTRAINDICATIONS

This product should not be used in patients known to be sensitive to benzoyl peroxide or any of the other listed ingredients.

PRECAUTIONS

General: Avoid contact with eyes and other mucous membranes. For external use only. In patients known to be sensitive to the following substances, there is a possibility of cross-sensitization: benzoic acid derivatives (including certain topical anesthetics) and cinnamon.

Information for Patients: This product may bleach colored fabric or hair. Concurrent use with PABA-containing sunscreens may result in transient discoloration of the skin.

Carcinogenesis, Mutagenesis, Impairment of Fertility: Based upon considerable evidence, benzoyl peroxide is not considered to be a carcinogen. However, in one study, using mice known to be highly susceptible to cancer, there was evidence for benzoyl peroxide as a tumor promoter. Benzoyl peroxide has been found to be inactive as a mutagen in the *Ames Salmonella* and other assays, including the mouse dominant lethal assay. This assay is frequently used to assess the effect of substances on spermatogenesis.

Pregnancy (Category C): Animal reproduction studies have not been conducted with benzoyl peroxide. It is also not known whether benzoyl peroxide can cause fetal harm when administered to a pregnant woman or can affect reproductive capacity. Benzoyl peroxide should be given to a pregnant woman only if clearly needed.

Nursing Mothers: It is not known whether this drug is excreted in human milk. Caution should be exercised when benzoyl peroxide is administered to a nursing woman.

Pediatric Use: Safety and effectiveness in children below the age of 12 have not been established.

ADVERSE REACTIONS

Adverse reactions which may be encountered with topical benzoyl peroxide include excessive drying (manifested by marked peeling, erythema and possible edema), and allergic contact sensitization.

Excessive dryness would appear to occur in approximately 2 patients in 50.

Pertinent literature indicates that allergic sensitization to benzoyl peroxide may occur in 10 to 25 patients in 1,000. There is one reference that reports an occurrence of sensitization in 5 of 100 patients.

OVERDOSAGE

In the event that excessive scaling, erythema or edema occur, the use of this preparation should be discontinued. If the reaction is judged to be due to excessive use and not allergenicity, after symptoms and signs subside, a reduced dosage schedule may be cautiously tried.

To hasten resolution of the adverse effects, emollients, cool compresses and/or topical corticosteroid preparations may be used.

DOSAGE AND ADMINISTRATION

DESQUAM-E EMOLLIENT GEL should be gently rubbed into all affected areas once or twice daily. Suitable cleansing of the affected area should precede application. In fair-skinned individuals or under excessively drying conditions, it is suggested that therapy be initiated with one application daily. The degree of drying or peeling may be controlled by modification of dose frequency or drug concentration. The use of DESQUAM-E EMOLLIENT GEL may be continued as long as deemed necessary.

DESQUAM-X GEL should be gently rubbed into all affected areas once or twice daily. Suitable cleansing of the affected area should precede application. In fair-skinned individuals or under excessively drying conditions, it is suggested that therapy be initiated with one application daily. The degree of drying or peeling may be controlled by modification of dose frequency or drug concentration. The use of DESQUAM-X GEL may be continued as long as deemed necessary.

DESQUAM-X (5 or 10) WASH—

Shake well before use. Wash affected areas once or twice daily, avoiding contact with eyes or mucous membranes. Wet skin areas to be treated prior to administration; apply DESQUAM-X WASH, work to a full lather, rinse thoroughly and pat dry. The amount of drying or peeling may be controlled by modification of dose frequency or drug concentration.

DESQUAM-X 10 BAR—

Wash entire area gently with fingertips for 1 to 2 minutes 2 or 3 times daily or as physician directs. Rinse well. The desired degree of dryness and peeling may be obtained by regulating frequency of use.

HOW SUPPLIED

DESQUAM-E 2.5 EMOLLIENT GEL

1.5 oz. (42.5g)	Plastic Tubes	NDC 0072-6003-45

DESQUAM-E 5 EMOLLIENT GEL

1.5 oz. (42.5g)	Plastic Tubes	NDC 0072-6103-45

DESQUAM-E 10 EMOLLIENT GEL

1.5 oz. (42.5g)	Plastic Tubes	NDC 0072-6203-45

Store at controlled room temperature (59°–86°F).

DESQUAM-X 5 GEL

1.5 oz. (42.5 g)	Plastic Tubes	NDC 0072-6621-01
3 oz. (85 g)	Plastic Tubes	NDC 0072-6621-03

DESQUAM-X 10 GEL

1.5 oz. (42.5 g)	Plastic Tubes	NDC 0072-6721-01
3 oz. (85 g)	Plastic Tubes	NDC 0072-6721-03

Store at controlled room temperature (59°–86° F).

DESQUAM-X WASH (5%)

5 oz.	Plastic Bottle	NDC 0072-6905-05

DESQUAM-X WASH (10%)

5 oz.	Plastic Bottle	NDC 0072-7000-05

Store at controlled room temperature (59°–86°F; 15°–30°C).

DESQUAM-X BAR (10%):
3.75 oz.
carton
NDC 0072-2000-04
Store at controlled room temperature (59°–86°F).

DOVONEX® ℞

[dōvă-nex]
(calcipotriene cream)
Cream, 0.005%
FOR TOPICAL DERMATOLOGIC USE ONLY.
Not for ophthalmic, oral or intravaginal use.

DESCRIPTION

DOVONEX (calcipotriene cream) Cream contains calcipotriene monohydrate, a synthetic vitamin D_3 derivative, for topical dermatological use.

Chemically, calcipotriene monohydrate is (5Z,7E,22E,24S)-24-cyclopropyl-9, 10-secochola-5,7,10(19), 22-tetraene-1α,3β,24-triol monohydrate, with empirical formula $C_{27}H_{40}O_3 \cdot H_2O$, a molecular weight of 430.6, and the following structural formula:

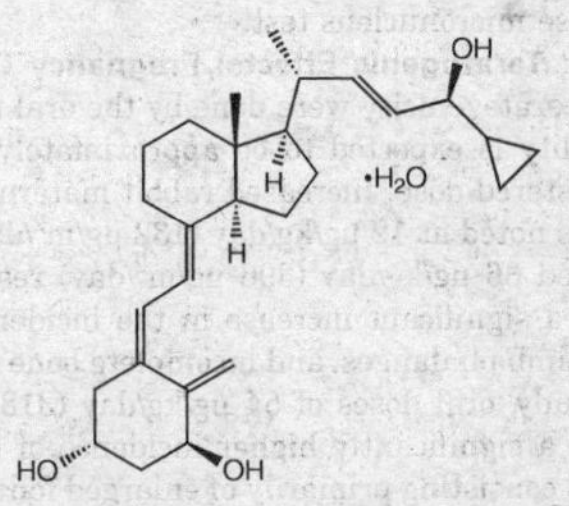

Calcipotriene monohydrate is a white or off-white crystalline substance. DOVONEX Cream contains calcipotriene monohydrate equivalent to 50 μg/g anhydrous calcipotriene in a cream base of cetearyl alcohol, ceteth-20, diazolidinyl urea, dichlorobenzyl alcohol, dibasic sodium phosphate, edetate disodium, glycerin, mineral oil, petrolatum, and water.

CLINICAL PHARMACOLOGY

In humans, the natural supply of vitamin D depends mainly on exposure to the ultraviolet rays of the sun for conversion of 7-dehydrocholesterol to vitamin D_3 (cholecalciferol) in the skin. Calcipotriene is a synthetic analog of vitamin D_3.

Clinical studies with radiolabelled calcipotriene ointment indicate that approximately 6% (±3%, SD) of the applied dose of calcipotriene is absorbed systemically when the ointment is applied topically to psoriasis plaques or 5% (±2.6%, SD) when applied to normal skin, and much of the absorbed active is converted to inactive metabolites within 24 hours of application. Systemic absorption of the cream has not been studied.

Vitamin D and its metabolites are transported in the blood, bound to specific plasma proteins. The active form of the vitamin, 1,25-dihydroxy vitamin D_3 (calcitriol) is known to be recycled via the liver and excreted in the bile. Calcipotriene metabolism following systemic uptake is rapid and occurs via a similar pathway to the natural hormone.

CLINICAL STUDIES

Adequate and well-controlled trials of patients treated with DOVONEX Cream have demonstrated improvement usually beginning after 2 weeks of therapy. This improvement continued with approximately 50% of patients showing at least marked improvement in the signs and symptoms of psoriasis after 8 weeks of therapy, but only approximately 4% showed complete clearing.

INDICATIONS AND USAGE

DOVONEX (calcipotriene cream) Cream, 0.005%, is indicated for the treatment of plaque psoriasis. The safety and effectiveness of topical calcipotriene in dermatoses other than psoriasis have not been established.

CONTRAINDICATIONS

DOVONEX Cream is contraindicated in those patients with a history of hypersensitivity to any of the components of the preparation. It should not be used by patients with demonstrated hypercalcemia or evidence of vitamin D toxicity. DOVONEX Cream should not be used on the face.

PRECAUTIONS

General: Use of DOVONEX Cream may cause transient irritation of both lesions and surrounding uninvolved skin. If irritation develops, DOVONEX Cream should be discontinued.

Reversible elevation of serum calcium has occurred with use of topical calcipotriene. If elevation in serum calcium outside the normal range should occur, discontinue treatment until normal calcium levels are restored.

Continued on next page

Dovonex Cream—Cont.

Information for Patients: Patients using DOVONEX Cream should receive the following information and instructions:

1. This medication is to be used only as directed by the physician. It is for external use only. Avoid contact with the face or eyes. As with any topical medication, patients should wash their hands after application.
2. This medication should not be used for any disorder other than that for which it was prescribed.
3. Patients should report to their physician any signs of adverse reactions.

Carcinogenesis, Mutagenesis, Impairment of Fertility: Animal studies have not been conducted to evaluate the carcinogenic potential of calcipotriene. Studies in rats at doses up to 54 µg/kg/day (318 µg/m^2/day) of calcipotriene indicated no impairment of fertility or general reproductive performance.

Calcipotriene did not elicit any mutagenic effects in the Ames mutagenicity assay, the mouse lymphoma TK locus assay, the human lymphocyte chromosome aberration test, or the mouse micronucleus test.

Pregnancy: Teratogenic Effects: Pregnancy Category C. Studies of teratogenicity were done by the oral route where bioavailability is expected to be approximately 40–60% of the administered dose. Increased rabbit maternal and fetal toxicity was noted at 12 µg/kg/day (132 µg/m^2/day). Rabbits administered 36 µg/kg/day (396 µg/m^2/day) resulted in fetuses with a significant increase in the incidence of pubic bones, forelimb phalanges, and incomplete bone ossification. In a rat study, oral doses of 54 µg/kg/day (318 µg/m^2/day) resulted in a significantly higher incidence of skeletal abnormalities consisting primarily of enlarged fontanelles and extra ribs. The enlarged fontanelles are most likely due to calcipotriene's effect upon calcium metabolism. The maternal and fetal calculated no-effect exposures in the rat (43.2 µg/m^2/day) and rabbit (17.6 µg/m^2/day) studies are approximately equal to the expected human systemic exposure level (18.5 µg/m^2/day) from dermal applicatioin. There are no adequate and well-controlled studies in pregnant women. Therefore, DOVONEX Cream should be used during pregnancy only if the potential benefit justifies the potential risk to the fetus.

Nursing Mothers: There is evidence that maternal 1,25-dihydroxy vitamin D_3 (calcitriol) may enter the fetal circulation, but it is not known whether it is excreted in human milk. The systemic disposition of calcipotriene is expected to be similar to that of the naturally occurring vitamin. Because many drugs are excreted in human milk, caution should be exercised when DOVONEX Cream is administered to a nursing woman.

Pediatric Use: Safety and effectiveness of DOVONEX Cream in pediatric patients have not been established. Because of a higher ratio of skin surface area to body mass, pediatric patients are at greater risk than adults of systemic adverse effects when they are treated with topical medication.

ADVERSE REACTIONS

In controlled clinical trials, the most frequent adverse experiences reported for DOVONEX Cream were cases of skin irritation which occurred in approximately 10–15% of patients. Rash, pruritus, dermatitis, and worsening of psoriasis were reported in 1 to 10% of patients.

OVERDOSAGE

Topically applied calcipotriene can be absorbed in sufficient amounts to produce systemic effects. Elevated serum calcium has been observed with excessive use of topical calcipotriene. If elevation in serum calcium should occur, discontinue treatment until normal calcium levels are restored (See PRECAUTIONS).

DOSAGE AND ADMINISTRATION

Apply a thin layer of DOVONEX Cream to the affected skin twice daily and rub in gently and completely. The safety and efficacy of DOVONEX Cream have been demonstrated in patients treated for eight weeks.

HOW SUPPLIED

DOVONEX Cream is available in 30 g, 60 g, and 100 g aluminum tubes. Store at controlled room temperature 15°–25°C (59°–77°F). Do not freeze.

Rx only

Manufactured by
Leo Laboratories Ltd.,
Dublin, Ireland
©1994 Distributed by
Westwood-Squibb Pharmaceuticals Inc.,
Buffalo, NY, USA 14213
A Bristol-Myers Squibb Company
1996 03-6012-0

DOVONEX® ℞

[*dō vă-nex*]

(calcipotriene ointment), 0.005%

For topical dermatologic use only. Not for ophthalmic, oral or intravaginal use.

DESCRIPTION

DOVONEX (calcipotriene ointment) contains the compound calcipotriene, a synthetic vitamin D_3 derivative for topical dermatological use.

Chemically, calcipotriene is (5Z, 7E, 22E, 24S)-24-cyclopropyl-9,10-secochola-5,7,10(19),22-tetraene-1α, 3β, 24-triol-, with the empirical formula $C_{27}H_{40}O_3$, a molecular weight of 412.6, and the following structural formula:

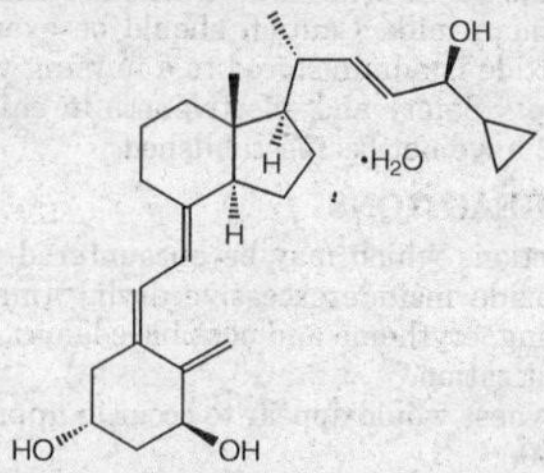

Calcipotriene is a white or off-white crystalline substance. DOVONEX contains calcipotriene 50 µg/g in an ointment base of dibasic sodium phosphate, edetate disodium, mineral oil, petrolatum, propylene glycol, tocopherol, steareth-2 and water.

CLINICAL PHARMACOLOGY

In humans, the natural supply of vitamin D depends mainly on exposure to the ultraviolet rays of the sun for conversion of 7-dehydrocholesterol to vitamin D_3 (cholecalciferol) in the skin. Calcipotriene is a synthetic analog of vitamin D_3.

Clinical studies with radiolabelled ointment indicate that approximately 6% (±3%, SD) of the applied dose of calcipotriene is absorbed systemically when the ointment is applied topically to psoriasis plaques or 5% (±2.6%, SD) when applied to normal skin, and much of the absorbed active is converted to inactive metabolites within 24 hours of application.

Vitamin D and its metabolites are transported in the blood, bound to specific plasma proteins. The active form of the vitamin, 1,25-dihydroxy vitamin D_3 (calcitriol), is known to be recycled via the liver and excreted in the bile. Calcipotriene metabolism following systemic uptake is rapid, and occurs via a similar pathway to the natural hormone. The primary metabolites are much less potent than the parent compound.

There is evidence that maternal 1,25-dihydroxy vitamin D_3 (calcitriol) may enter the fetal circulation, but it is not known whether it is excreted in human milk. The systemic disposition of calcipotriene is expected to be similar to that of the naturally occurring vitamin.

CLINICAL STUDIES: Adequate and well-controlled trials of patients treated with DOVONEX have demonstrated improvement usually beginning after two weeks of therapy. This improvement continued in patients using Dovonex once daily and twice daily. After 8 weeks of once daily Dovonex, 56.7% of patients showed at least marked improvements (6.4% showed complete clearing). After 8 weeks of twice daily Dovonex, 70.0% of patients showed at least marked improvement (11.3% showed complete clearing).

Subtracting percentages of patients using placebo (vehicle only) from percentages of patients using Dovonex who had at least marked improvements after 8 weeks yields 39.9% for once daily and 49.6% for twice daily. This adjustment for placebo effect indicates that what might appear to be differences between once and twice daily use may reflect differences in the studies independent from the frequency of dosing. Although there was a numerical difference in comparison across studies, twice daily dosing has not been shown to be superior in efficacy to once daily dosing.

Over 400 patients have been treated in open label clinical studies of DOVONEX for periods of up to one year. In half of these studies, patients who previously had not responded well to DOVONEX were excluded. The adverse events in these extended studies included skin irritation in approximately 25% of patients and worsening of psoriasis in approximately 10% of patients. In one of these open label studies, half of the patients no longer required DOVONEX by 16 weeks of treatment, because of satisfactory therapeutic results.

INDICATIONS AND USAGE

DOVONEX (calcipotriene ointment), 0.005%, is indicated for the treatment of moderate plaque psoriasis in adults. The safety and effectiveness of topical calcipotriene in dermatoses other than psoriasis have not been established.

CONTRAINDICATIONS

DOVONEX is contraindicated in those patients with a history of hypersensitivity to any of the components of the preparation. It should not be used by patients with demonstrated hypercalcemia or evidence of vitamin D toxicity. DOVONEX should not be used on the face.

PRECAUTIONS

General

Use of DOVONEX may cause irritation of lesions and surrounding uninvolved skin. If irritation develops, DOVONEX should be discontinued.

Transient, rapidly reversible elevation of serum calcium has occurred with use of DOVONEX. If elevation in serum calcium outside the normal range should occur, discontinue treatment until normal calcium levels are restored.

Information for patients: Patients using DOVONEX should receive the following information and instructions:

1. This medication is to be used as directed by the physician. It is for external use only. Avoid contact with the face or eyes. As with any topical medication, patients should wash hands after application.
2. This medication should not be used for any disorder other than that for which it was prescribed.
3. Patients should report to their physician any signs of local adverse reactions.

Carcinogenesis, Mutagenesis, Impairment of fertility: Long-term animal studies have not been conducted to evaluate the carcinogenic potential of calcipotriene. Studies in rats at doses up to 54 µg/kg/day (318 µg/m^2/day) of calcipotriene indicated no impairment of fertility or general reproductive performance.

Calcipotriene did not elicit any mutagenic effects in the Ames mutagenicity assay, the mouse lymphoma TK locus assay, the human lymphocyte chromosome aberration test or the mouse micronucleus test.

Pregnancy; Teratogenic Effects; Pregnancy Category C. Studies of teratogenicity were done by the oral route where bioavailability is expected to be approximately 40–60% of the administered dose. In rabbits, increased maternal and fetal toxicity were noted at a dosage of 12 µg/kg/day (132 µg/m^2/day); a dosage of 36 µg/kg/day (396 µg/m^2/day) resulted in a significant increase in the incidence of incomplete ossification of the pubic bones and forelimb phalanges of fetuses. In a rat study, a dosage of 54 µg/kg/day (318 µg/m^2/day) resulted in a significantly increased incidence of skeletal abnormalities (enlarged fontanelles and extra ribs). The enlarged fontanelles are most likely due to calcipotriene's effect upon calcium metabolism. The estimated maternal and fetal no-effect exposure levels in the rat (43.2 µg/m^2/day) and rabbit (17.6 µg/m^2/day) studies are approximately equal to the expected human systemic exposure level (18.5 µg/m^2/day) from dermal application. There are no adequate and well-controlled studies in pregnant women. Therefore, DOVONEX Ointment should be used during pregnancy only if the potential benefit justifies the potential risk to the fetus.

Nursing mothers: It is not known whether calcipotriene is excreted in human milk. Because many drugs are excreted in human milk, caution should be exercised when DOVONEX is administered to a nursing woman.

Pediatric Use: Safety and effectiveness of DOVONEX in children have not been established. Because of a higher ratio of skin surface area to body mass, children are at greater risk than adults of systemic adverse effects when they are treated with topical medication.

Geriatric Use: Of the total number of patients in clinical studies of calcipotriene ointment, approximately 12 % were 65 or older, while approximately 4% were 75 and over. The results of an analysis of severity of skin-related adverse events showed a statistically significant difference for subjects over 65 years (more severe) compared to those under 65 years (less severe).

ADVERSE REACTIONS

In controlled clinical trials, the most frequent adverse reactions reported for DOVONEX were burning, itching, and skin irritation, which occurred in approximately 10–15% of patients. Erythema, dry skin, peeling, rash, dermatitis, worsening of psoriasis including development of facial/scalp psoriasis were reported in 1 to 10% of patients. Other experiences reported in less than 1% of patients included skin atrophy, hyperpigmentation, hypercalcemia, and folliculitis. Once daily dosing has not been shown to be superior in safety to twice daily dosing.

OVERDOSAGE

Topically applied DOVONEX can be absorbed in sufficient amounts to produce systemic effects. Elevated serum calcium has been observed with excessive use of DOVONEX.

DOSAGE AND ADMINISTRATION

Apply a thin layer of DOVONEX to the affected skin once or twice daily, and rub in gently and completely.

HOW SUPPLIED

DOVONEX Ointment is available in 30 g, 60 g, and 100 g aluminum tubes. Store at controlled room temperature 15°–25°C (59°–77°F). Do not freeze.

Rx only.

Manufactured by Leo Laboratories Ltd.,
Dublin, Ireland   5/97
©1997 Distributed by Westwood-Squibb Pharmaceuticals
Inc., Buffalo, N.Y., U.S.A. 14213
A Bristol-Myers Squibb Company

DOVONEX®
(calcipotriene solution)
Scalp Solution, 0.005%

℞

FOR TOPICAL DERMATOLOGIC USE ONLY.
Not for ophthalmic, oral or intravaginal use.

DESCRIPTION

DOVONEX (calcipotriene solution) Scalp Solution 0.005%,
is a colorless topical solution containing 0.005% calcipotriene in a vehicle of isopropanol (51% v/v) propylene glycol,
hydroxypropyl cellulose, sodium citrate, menthol and water.
The chemical name of calcipotriene is (5Z, 7E, 22E, 24S)-24-
cyclopropyl-9,10-secochola-5,7,10(19), 22-tetraene-1α,3β,
24-triol, with the empirical formula $C_{27}H_{40}O_3$, a molecular
weight of 412.6, and the following structural formula:

CLINICAL PHARMACOLOGY

In humans, the natural supply of vitamin D depends mainly
on exposure to the ultraviolet rays of the sun for conversion
of 7-dehydrocholesterol to vitamin D_3 (cholecalciferol) in the
skin. Calcipotriene is a synthetic analog of vitamin D_3.
Although the precise mechanism of calcipotriene's antipsoriatic action is not fully understood, *in vitro* evidence suggests that calcipotriene is roughly equipotent to the natural
vitamin in its effects on proliferation and differentiation of a
variety of cell types. Calcipotriene has also been shown, in
animal studies, to be 100–200 times less potent in its effects
on calcium utilization than the natural hormone.
Clinical studies with radiolabelled calcipotriene solution indicate that less than 1% of the applied dose of calcipotriene
is absorbed through the scalp when the solution (2.0 mL) is
applied topically to normal skin or psoriasis plaques
(160 cm²) for 12 hours, and that much of the absorbed calcipotriene is converted to inactive metabolites within 24
hours of application.
Vitamin D and its metabolites are transported in the blood,
bound to specific plasma proteins. The active form of the vitamin, 1,25-dihydroxy vitamin D_3 (calcitriol), is known to be
recycled via the liver and excreted in the bile. Calcipotriene
metabolism following systemic uptake is rapid, and occurs
via a similar pathway to the natural hormone. The primary
metabolites are much less potent than the parent compound.
There is evidence that maternal 1,25-dihydroxy vitamin D_3
(calcitriol) may enter the fetal circulation, but it is not
known whether it is excreted in human milk. The systemic
disposition of calcipotriene is expected to be similar to that
of the naturally occurring vitamin.

CLINICAL STUDIES

Adequate and well-controlled trials of patients treated with
DOVONEX Scalp Solution, 0.005%, have demonstrated improvement usually beginning after 2 weeks of therapy. This
improvement continued with approximately 31% of patients
appearing either cleared (14%) or almost cleared (17%) after
8 weeks of therapy.

INDICATIONS AND USAGE

DOVONEX (calcipotriene solution) Scalp Solution, 0.005%,
is indicated for the topical treatment of chronic, moderately
severe psoriasis of the scalp. The safety and effectiveness of
topical calcipotriene in dermatoses other than psoriasis
have not been established.

CONTRAINDICATIONS

DOVONEX Scalp Solution, 0.005%, is contraindicated in
those patients with acute psoriatic eruptions or a history of
hypersensitivity to any of the components of the preparation. It should not be used by patients with demonstrated
hypercalcemia or evidence of vitamin D toxicity.

WARNINGS

Avoid contact with the eyes or mucous membranes. Discontinue use if a sensitivity reaction occurs or if excessive irritation develops on uninvolved skin areas.
Drug product is flammable. Keep away from open flame.

PRECAUTIONS

General: Use of DOVONEX Scalp Solution, 0.005%, may
cause transient irritation of both lesions and surrounding
uninvolved skin. If irritation develops, DOVONEX Scalp Solution, 0.005% should be discontinued.
For external use only. Keep out of the reach of children. Always wash hands thoroughly after use.
Reversible elevation of serum calcium has occurred with use
of topical calcipotriene. If elevation in serum calcium outside the normal range should occur, discontinue treatment
until normal calcium levels are restored.
Information for Patients: Patients using DOVONEX Scalp
Solution, 0.005% should receive the following information
and instructions:
1. This medication is to be used only as directed by the physician. It is for external use only. Avoid contact with the
   face or eyes. As with any topical medication, patients
   should wash their hands after application.
2. This medication should not be used for any disorder other
   than that for which it was prescribed.
3. Patients should report to their physician any signs of adverse reactions.
Carcinogenesis, Mutagenesis, Impairment of Fertility: Animal studies have not been conducted to evaluate the carcinogenic potential of calcipotriene. Studies in rats at doses
up to 54 µg/kg/day (318 µg/m²/day) of calcipotriene indicated
no impairment of fertility or general reproductive performance.
Calcipotriene did not elicit any mutagenic effects in the
Ames mutagenicity assay, the mouse lymphoma TK locus
assay, the human lymphocyte chromosome aberration test
or the mouse micronucleus test.
Pregnancy: Teratogenic Effects: Pregnancy Category C:
Studies of teratogenicity were done by the oral route where
bioavailability is expected to be approximately 40–60% of
the administered dose. Increased rabbit maternal and fetal
toxicity was noted at 12 µg/kg/day (132 µg/m²/day). Rabbits
administered 36 µg/kg/day (396 µg/m²/day) resulted in fetuses with a significant increase in the incidences of pubic
bones, forelimb phalanges, and incomplete bone ossification.
In a rat study, oral doses of 54 µg/kg/day (318 µg/m²/day)
resulted in a significantly higher incidence of skeletal abnormalities consisting primarily of enlarged fontanelles and
extra ribs. The enlarged fontanelles are most likely due to
calcipotriene's effect upon calcium metabolism. The maternal and fetal calculated no-effect exposures in the rat (43.2
µg/m²/day) the rabbit (17 µg/m²/day) studies are greater
than the expected human systemic exposure level (0.13 µg/
m²/day) from dermal application. There are no adequate
and well-controlled studies in pregnant women. Therefore,
DOVONEX Scalp Solution, 0.005%, should be used during
pregnancy only if the potential benefit justifies the potential
risk to the fetus.
Nursing Mothers: There is evidence that maternal 1,25-
dihydroxy vitamin D_3 (calcitriol) may enter the fetal circulation, but it is not known whether it is excreted in human
milk. The systemic disposition of calcipotriene is expected to
be similar to that of the naturally occurring vitamin. Because many drugs are excreted in human milk, caution
should be exercised when DOVONEX Scalp Solution,
0.005%, is administered to a nursing woman.
Pediatric Use: Safety and effectiveness of DOVONEX Scalp
Solution, 0.005%, in pediatric patients have not been specifically established. Because of a higher ratio of skin surface
area to body mass, pediatric patients are at greater risk
than adults of systemic adverse effects when they are
treated with topical medication.

ADVERSE REACTIONS

In controlled clinical trials, the most frequent adverse reactions reported to be related to DOVONEX Scalp Solution,
0.005%, use were transient burning, stinging and tingling,
which occurred in approximately 23% of patients. Rash was
reported in about 11% of patients. Dry skin, irritation and
worsening of psoriasis was reported in 1–5% of patients.
Skin atrophy, hyperpigmentation, hypercalcemia, and folliculitis were not observed in these studies, but cannot be excluded.

OVERDOSAGE

Topically applied calcipotriene can be absorbed in sufficient
amounts to produce systemic effects. Elevated serum calcium has been observed with excessive use of topical calcipotriene. If elevation in serum calcium should occur, discontinue treatment until normal calcium levels are restored.
(See PRECAUTIONS.)

DOSAGE AND ADMINISTRATION

Comb the hair to remove scaly debris and after suitably
parting, apply DOVONEX Scalp Solution, 0.005%, twice
daily, only to the lesions, and rub in gently and completely,
taking care to prevent the solution spreading onto the forehead. The safety and efficacy of DOVONEX Scalp Solution,
0.005%, have been demonstrated in patients treated for
eight weeks.

Keep DOVONEX Scalp Solution, 0.005%, well away from
the eyes. Avoid application of the solution to uninvolved
scalp margins. **Always wash hands thoroughly after use.**

HOW SUPPLIED

DOVONEX Scalp Solution, 0.005%, is available in 60 mL
plastic bottles. Store at controlled room temperature 15°–
25°C (59°–77°F). Avoid sunlight. Do not freeze.
Rx only.
Manufactured by
Leo Pharmaceutical Products, Ltd.
Ballerup, Denmark
©1995 Distributed by
Westwood-Squibb Pharmaceuticals Inc.
Buffalo, N.Y., U.S.A. 14213
A Bristol-Myers Squibb Company
revised 2/97   011785-00

EURAX®
(crotamiton USP)
Lotion/Cream
Scabicide/Antipruritic

℞

For topical use only. Not for opthalmic use.
Rx only.

DESCRIPTION

EURAX, crotamiton USP, is a scabicidal and antipruritic
agent available as a cream or lotion for topical use only. EU-
RAX provides 10% (w/w) of the synthetic, crotamiton USP,
in a vanishing-cream or emollient-lotion base containing:
water, petrolatum, propylene glycol, steareth-2, cetyl alcohol, dimethicone, laureth-23, fragrance, magnesium aluminum silicate, carbomer-934, sodium hydroxide, diazolidinyl
urea, methylchloroisothiazolinone, methylisothiazolinone
and magnesium nitrate. In addition, the cream contains
glyceryl stearate. Crotamiton is N-ethyl-N-(o-methylphe-
nyl)-2-butenamide and its structural formula is:

Crotamiton USP is a colorless to slightly yellowish oil, having a faint amine-like odor. It is miscible with alcohol and
with methanol. Crotamiton is a mixture of the *cis* and *trans*
isomers. Its molecular weight is 203.28.

CLINICAL PHARMACOLOGY

EURAX has scabicidal and antipruritic actions. The mechanisms of these actions are not known.

INDICATIONS AND USAGE

For eradication of scabies (*Sarcoptes scabiei*) and for symptomatic treatment of pruritic skin.

CONTRAINDICATIONS

EURAX should not be applied topically to patients who develop a sensitivity or are allergic to it or who manifest a
primary irritation response to topical medications.

WARNINGS

If severe irritation or sensitization develops, treatment with
this product should be discontinued and appropriate therapy instituted.

PRECAUTIONS

General: EURAX should not be applied in the eyes or
mouth because it may cause irritation. It should not be applied to acutely inflamed skin or raw or weeping surfaces
until the acute inflammation has subsided.
Information for Patients: See "Directions for patients with
scabies."
Drug Interactions: None known.
Carcinogenesis, Mutagenesis, Impairment of Fertility:
Long-term carcinogenicity studies in animals have not been
conducted.
Pregnancy (Category C): Animal reproduction studies
have not been conducted with EURAX. It is also not known
whether EURAX can cause fetal harm when applied topically to a pregnant woman or can affect reproduction capacity. EURAX should be given to a pregnant woman only if
clearly needed.
Pediatric Use: Safety and effectiveness in children have
not been established.

ADVERSE REACTIONS

Allergic sensitivity or primary irritation reactions may occur in some patients.

OVERDOSAGE

There is no specific information on the effect of overtreatment with repeated topical applications in humans. Acute

Continued on next page

Eurax—Cont.

toxicity (after accidental oral administration in children): Highest known doses ingested: Cream: children—2g (age 1½ years); Lotion: 1 ounce (age 2 years). A death was reported but cause was not confirmed.

Oral LD$_{50}$ in animals (mg/kg): rats, 2212; mice, 2011.

Signs and symptoms (of oral ingestion): Burning sensation in the mouth, irritation of the buccal, esophageal and gastric mucosa, nausea, vomiting, abdominal pain.

Treatment: There is no specific antidote if taken orally. General measures to eliminate the drug and reduce its absorption, combined with symptomatic treatment, are recommended.

DOSAGE AND ADMINISTRATION

LOTION: Shake well before using—*In Scabies:* Thoroughly massage into the skin of the whole body from the chin down, paying particular attention to all folds and creases. A second application is advisable 24 hours later. Clothing and bed linen should be changed the next morning. A cleansing bath should be taken 48 hours after the last application. *In Pruritus:* Massage gently into affected areas until medication is completely absorbed. Repeat as needed.

DIRECTIONS FOR PATIENTS WITH SCABIES

1. Take a routine bath or shower. Thoroughly massage EURAX cream or lotion into the skin from the chin to the toes including folds and creases.
2. A second application is advisable 24 hours later.
3. This 60 gram tube or bottle is sufficient for two applications.
4. Clothing and bed linen should be changed the next day. Contaminated clothing and bed linen may be dry-cleaned, or washed in the hot cycle of the washing machine.
5. A cleansing bath should be taken 48 hours after the last application.

HOW SUPPLIED

Cream: 60g tubes (NDC 0072-2103-60; NSN 6505-00-116-0200).

Lotion: 60g (2 oz.) bottles (NDC 0072-2203-60, NSN 6505-01-153-4423). 454g (16 oz.) bottles (NDC 0072-2203-16). Store at room temperature.

EXELDERM®
(sulconazole nitrate)
Cream, 1.0%
For topical use only. Not for ophthalmic use.

Rx only.

DESCRIPTION

EXELDERM (sulconazole nitrate) CREAM, 1.0% is a broad-spectrum antifungal agent intended for topical application. Sulconazole nitrate, the active ingredient in EXELDERM CREAM, is an imidazole derivative with in vitro antifungal and antiyeast activity. Its chemical name is (±)-1-[2.4-dichloro-β-[(p-chlorobenzyl)-thio]-phenethyl] imidazole mononitrate and it has the following chemical structure:

Sulconazole nitrate is a white to off-white crystalline powder with a molecular weight of 460.77. It is freely soluble in pyridine; slightly soluble in ethanol, acetone, and chloroform: and very slightly soluble in water. It has a melting point of about 130°C.

EXELDERM CREAM contains sulconazole nitrate 10 mg/g in an emollient cream base consisting of propylene glycol, stearyl alcohol, isopropyl myristate, cetyl alcohol, polysorbate 60, sorbitan monostearate, glyceryl stearate (and) PEG-100 stearate, ascorbyl palmitate, and purified water, with sodium hydroxide and/or nitric acid added to adjust the pH.

CLINICAL PHARMACOLOGY

Sulconazole nitrate is an imidazole derivative with broad-spectrum antifungal activity that inhibits the growth in vitro of the common pathogenic dermatophytes including *Trichophyton rubrum, Trichophyton mentagrophytes, Epidermophyton floccosum* and *Microsporum canis*. It also inhibits (*in vitro*) the organism responsible for tinea versicolor, *Malassezia furfur*. Sulconazole nitrate has been shown to be active *in vitro* against the following microorganisms, although clinical efficacy has not been established: *Candida albicans* and certain gram positive bacteria.

A modified Draize test showed no allergic contact dermatitis and a phototoxicity study showed no phototoxic or photoallergic reaction to sulconazole nitrate cream. Maximization tests with sulconazole nitrate cream showed no evidence of contact sensitization or irritation.

INDICATIONS AND USAGE

EXELDERM (sulconazole nitrate) CREAM, 1.0% is an antifungal agent indicated for the treatment of tinea pedis (athlete's foot), tinea cruris, and tinea corporis caused by *Trichophyton rubrum, Trichophyton mentagrophytes, Epidermophyton floccosum,* and *Microsporum canis,** and for the treatment of tinea versicolor.

*Efficacy for this organism in the organ system was studied in fewer than ten infections.

CONTRAINDICATIONS

EXELDERM (sulconazole nitrate) CREAM, 1.0% is contraindicated in patients who have a history of hypersensitivity to any of its ingredients.

PRECAUTIONS

General: EXELDERM (sulconazole nitrate) CREAM, 1.0% is for external use only. Avoid contact with the eyes. If irritation develops, the cream should be discontinued and appropriate therapy instituted.

Information for Patients: Patients should be told to use EXELDERM CREAM as directed by the physician, to use it externally only, and to avoid contact with the eyes.

Carcinogenesis, Mutagenesis, Impairment of Fertility: Long-term animal studies to determine carcinogenic potential have not been performed. In vitro studies have shown no mutagenic activity.

Pregnancy (Category C): There are no adequate and well controlled studies in pregnant women. Sulconazole nitrate should be used during pregnancy only if clearly needed. Sulconazole nitrate has been shown to be embryotoxic in rats when given in doses of 125 times the adult human dose (in mg/kg). The drug was not teratogenic in rats or rabbits at oral doses of 50 mg/kg/day.

Sulconazole nitrate given orally to rats at a dose 125 times the human dose resulted in prolonged gestation and dystocia. Several females died during the prenatal period, most likely due to labor complications.

Nursing Mothers: It is not known whether sulconazole nitrate is excreted in human milk. Caution should be exercised when sulconazole nitrate is administered to a nursing woman.

Pediatric Use: Safety and effectiveness in children have not been established.

ADVERSE REACTIONS

There were no systemic effects and only infrequent cutaneous adverse reactions in 1185 patients treated with sulconazole nitrate cream in controlled clinical trials. Approximately 3% of these patients reported itching, 3% burning or stinging, and 1% redness. These complaints did not usually interfere with treatment.

CLINICAL STUDIES

In a vehicle-controlled study for the treatment of tinea pedis (moccasin type) due to *T. rubrum*, after 4–6 weeks of treatment 69% of patients on the active drug and 19% of patients on the drug vehicle had become KOH and culture negative. In addition, 68% of patients on the active drug and 20% of patients on the drug vehicle showed a good or excellent clinical response.

DOSAGE AND ADMINISTRATION

A small amount of cream should be gently massaged into the affected and surrounding skin areas once or twice daily, except in tinea pedis, where administration should be twice daily.

Early relief of symptoms is experienced by the majority of patients and clinical improvement may be seen fairly soon after treatment is begun; however, tinea corporis/cruris and tinea versicolor should be treated for 3 weeks and tinea pedis for 4 weeks to reduce the possibility of recurrence.

If significant clinical improvement is not seen after 4 to 6 weeks of treatment, an alternate diagnosis should be considered.

HOW SUPPLIED

EXELDERM (sulconazole nitrate) CREAM, 1.0%:

15 g tube—NDC 0072-8200-15
30 g tube—NDC 0072-8200-30
60 g tube—NDC 0072-8200-60
Avoid excessive heat, above 40°C (104°F).

EXELDERM®
(sulconazole nitrate)
Solution, 1.0%
For topical use only. Not for ophthalmic use.

Rx only.

DESCRIPTION

EXELDERM (sulconazole nitrate) SOLUTION, 1.0% is a broad-spectrum antifungal agent intended for topical application. Sulconazole nitrate, the active ingredient in EXELDERM SOLUTION, is an imidazole derivative with antifungal and antiyeast activity. Its chemical name is (±)-1-[2.4-dichloro-β-[(p-chlorobenzyl)-thio]-phenethyl] imidazole mononitrate and it has the following chemical structure:

Sulconazole nitrate is a white to off-white crystalline powder with a molecular weight of 460.77. It is freely soluble in pyridine; slightly soluble in ethanol, acetone, and chloroform; and very slightly soluble in water. It has a melting point of about 130°C.

EXELDERM SOLUTION contains sulconazole nitrate 10 mg/mL in a solution of propylene glycol, poloxamer 407, polysorbate 20, butylated hydroxyanisole, and purified water, with sodium hydroxide and, if necessary, nitric acid added to adjust the pH.

CLINICAL PHARMACOLOGY

Sulconazole nitrate is an imidazole derivative that inhibits the growth of the common pathogenic dermatophytes including *Trichophyton rubrum, Trichophyton mentagrophytes, Epidermophyton floccosum,* and *Microsporum canis*. It also inhibits the organism responsible for tinea versicolor, *Malassezia furfur*, and certain gram positive bacteria.

A maximization test with sulconazole nitrate solution showed no evidence of irritation or contact sensitization.

INDICATIONS AND USAGE

EXELDERM (sulconazole nitrate) SOLUTION, 1.0% is a broad-spectrum antifungal agent indicated for the treatment of tinea cruris and tinea corporis caused by *Trichophyton rubrum, Trichophyton mentagrophytes, Epidermophyton floccosum,* and *Microsporum canis;* and for treatment of tinea versicolor. Effectiveness has not been proven in tinea pedis (athlete's foot).

Symptomatic relief usually occurs within a few days after starting EXELDERM SOLUTION and clinical improvement usually occurs within one week.

CONTRAINDICATIONS

EXELDERM (sulconazole nitrate) SOLUTION, 1.0% is contraindicated in patients who have a history of hypersensitivity to any of the ingredients.

PRECAUTIONS

General: EXELDERM (sulconazole nitrate) SOLUTION, 1.0% is for external use only. Avoid contact with the eyes. If irritation develops, the solution should be discontinued and appropriate therapy instituted.

Information for Patients: Patients should be told to use EXELDERM SOLUTION as directed by the physician, to use it externally only, and to avoid contact with the eyes.

Carcinogenesis, Mutagenesis, Impairment of Fertility: Long-term animal studies to determine carcinogenic potential have not been performed. In vitro studies have shown no mutagenic activity.

Pregnancy: Pregnancy Category C: Sulconazole nitrate has been shown to be embryotoxic in rats when given in doses 125 times the human dose (in mg/kg). The drug at this dose given orally to rats also resulted in prolonged gestation and dystocia. Several females died during the perinatal period, most likely due to labor complications. Sulconazole nitrate was not teratogenic in rats or rabbits at oral doses of 50 mg/kg/day.

There are no adequate and well-controlled studies in pregnant women. Sulconazole nitrate should be used during pregnancy only if the potential benefit justifies the potential risk to the fetus.

Nursing Mothers: It is not known whether this drug is excreted in human milk. Because many drugs are excreted in human milk, caution should be exercised when sulconazole nitrate is administered to a nursing woman.

Pediatric Use: Safety and effectiveness in children have not been established.

ADVERSE REACTIONS

There were no systemic effects and only infrequent cutaneous adverse reactions in 370 patients treated with sulconazole nitrate solution in controlled clinical trials. Approximately 1% of these patients reported itching and 1% burning or stinging. These complaints did not usually interfere with treatment.

DOSAGE AND ADMINISTRATION

A small amount of the solution should be gently massaged into the affected and surrounding skin areas once or twice daily.

Symptomatic relief usually occurs within a few days after starting EXELDERM (sulconazole nitrate) SOLUTION, 1.0%, and clinical improvement usually occurs within one week. To reduce the possibility of recurrence, tinea cruris, tinea corporis, and tinea versicolor should be treated for 3 weeks.
If significant clinical improvement is not seen after 4 weeks of treatment, an alternate diagnosis should be considered.

HOW SUPPLIED
EXELDERM SOLUTION, 1.0%
30 mL Plastic Bottle NDC 0072-8400-30
Avoid excessive heat, above 40°C (104°F), and protect from light.

HALOG Cream ℞
Halcinonide Cream USP 0.1%
HALOG Ointment ℞
Halcinonide Ointment USP 0.1%
HALOG Solution ℞
Halcinonide Topical Solution USP 0.1%
HALOG-E Cream ℞
Halcinonide Cream USP 0.1%
For dermatologic use only.
Not for ophthalmic use.

Rx Only.

DESCRIPTION
The topical corticosteroids constitute a class of primarily synthetic steroids used as anti-inflammatory and antipruritic agents. The steroids in this class include halcinonide. Halcinonide is designated chemically as 21-Chloro-9-fluoro-11β, 16α, 17-trihydroxypregn-4-ene-3,20-dione cyclic 16,17-acetal with acetone.

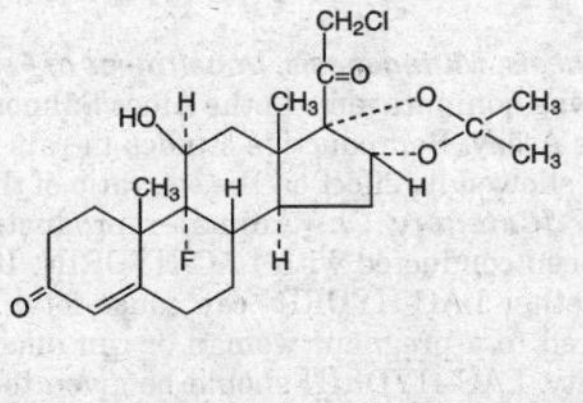

$C_{24}H_{32}ClFO_5$, MW 454.96, CAS-3093-35-4

Each gram of 0.1% HALOG Cream (Halcinonide Cream) contains 1 mg halcinonide in a specially formulated cream base consisting of glyceryl monostearate NF XII, cetyl alcohol, isopropyl palmitate, dimethicone 350, polysorbate 60, titanium dioxide, propylene glycol, and purified water.
Each gram of 0.1% **HALOG Ointment (Halcinonide Ointment)** contains 1 mg halcinonide in Plastibase® (Plasticized Hydrocarbon Gel), a polyethylene and mineral oil gel base with polyethylene glycol 400, polyethylene glycol 6000 distearate, polyethylene glycol 300, polyethylene glycol 1450, and butylated hydroxytoluene as an antioxidant.
Each mL of 0.1% **HALOG Solution (Halcinonide Topical Solution)** contains 1 mg halcinonide with edetate disodium, polyethylene glycol 300, purified water, and butylated hydroxytoluene as an antioxidant.
Each gram of 0.1% **HALOG-E Cream (Halcinonide Cream)** contains 1 mg halcinonide in a hydrophilic vanishing cream base consisting of propylene glycol, dimethicone 350, castor oil, cetearyl alcohol (and) ceteareth-20, propylene glycol stearate, white petrolatum, and purified water. This formulation is water-washable, greaseless, and nonstaining, with moisturizing and emollient properties.

CLINICAL PHARMACOLOGY
Topical corticosteroids share anti-inflammatory, antipruritic and vasoconstrictive actions.
The mechanism of anti-inflammatory activity of the topical corticosteroids is unclear. Various laboratory methods, including vasoconstrictor assays, are used to compare and predict potencies and/or clinical efficacies of the topical corticosteroids. There is some evidence to suggest that a recognizable correlation exists between vasoconstrictor potency and therapeutic efficacy in man.

PHARMACOKINETICS
The extent of percutaneous absorption of topical corticosteroids is determined by many factors including the vehicle, the integrity of the epidermal barrier, and the use of occlusive dressings.
Topical corticosteroids can be absorbed from normal intact skin. Inflammation and/or other disease processes in the skin increase percutaneous absorption. Occlusive dressings substantially increase the percutaneous absorption of topical corticosteroids. Thus, occlusive dressings may be a valuable therapeutic adjunct for treatment of resistant dermatoses (see DOSAGE AND ADMINISTRATION).
Once absorbed through the skin, topical corticosteroids are handled through pharmacokinetic pathways similar to systemically administered corticosteroids. Corticosteroids are bound to plasma proteins in varying degrees. Corticosteroids are metabolized primarily in the liver and are then excreted by the kidneys. Some of the topical corticosteroids and their metabolites are also excreted into the bile.

INDICATIONS AND USAGE
HALOG (Halcinonide) preparations are indicated for the relief of the inflammatory and pruritic manifestations of corticosteroid-responsive dermatoses.

CONTRAINDICATIONS
Topical corticosteroids are contraindicated in those patients with a history of hypersensitivity to any of the components of the preparations.

PRECAUTIONS
General
Systemic absorption of topical corticosteroids has produced reversible hypothalamic-pituitary-adrenal (HPA) axis suppression, manifestations of Cushing's syndrome, hyperglycemia, and glucosuria in some patients.
Conditions which augment systemic absorption include the application of the more potent steroids, use over large surface areas, prolonged use, and the addition of occlusive dressings.
Therefore, patients receiving a large dose of any potent topical steroid applied to a large surface area or under an occlusive dressing should be evaluated periodically for evidence of HPA axis suppression by using the urinary free cortisol and ACTH stimulation tests, and for impairment of thermal homeostasis. If HPA axis suppression or elevation of the body temperature occurs, an attempt should be made to withdraw the drug, to reduce the frequency of application, substitute a less potent steroid, or use a sequential approach when utilizing the occlusive technique.
Recovery of HPA axis function and thermal homeostasis are generally prompt and complete upon discontinuation of the drug. Infrequently, signs and symptoms of steroid withdrawal may occur, requiring supplemental systemic corticosteroids. Occasionally, a patient may develop a sensitivity reaction to a particular occlusive dressing material or adhesive and a substitute material may be necessary.
Children may absorb proportionally larger amounts of topical corticosteroids and thus be more susceptible to systemic toxicity (see PRECAUTIONS, Pediatric Use).
If irritation develops, topical corticosteroids should be discontinued and appropriate therapy instituted.
In the presence of dermatological infections, the use of an appropriate antifungal or antibacterial agent should be instituted. If a favorable response does not occur promptly, the corticosteroid should be discontinued until the infection has been adequately controlled.
These preparations are not for ophthalmic use.
Information for the Patient
Patients using topical corticosteroids should receive the following information and instructions:
1. These medications are to be used as directed by the physician. They are for dermatologic use only. Avoid contact with the eyes.
2. Patients should be advised not to use these medications for any disorder other than for which it was prescribed.
3. The treated skin area should not be bandaged or otherwise covered or wrapped as to be occlusive unless directed by the physician.
4. Patients should report any signs of local adverse reactions especially under occlusive dressing.
5. Parents of pediatric patients should be advised not to use tight-fitting diapers or plastic pants on a child being treated in the diaper area, as these garments may constitute occlusive dressings.

Laboratory Tests
A urinary free cortisol test and ACTH stimulation test may be helpful in evaluating HPA axis suppression.
Carcinogenesis, Mutagenesis, and Impairment of Fertility
Long-term animal studies have not been performed to evaluate the carcinogenic potential or the effect on fertility of topical corticosteroids. Studies to determine mutagenicity with prednisolone and hydrocortisone showed negative results.
Pregnancy: Teratogenic Effects
Category C. Corticosteroids are generally teratogenic in laboratory animals when administered systemically at relatively low dosage levels. The more potent corticosteroids have been shown to be teratogenic after dermal application in laboratory animals. There are no adequate and well-controlled studies in pregnant women on teratogenic effects from topically applied corticosteroids. Therefore, topical corticosteroids should be used during pregnancy only if the potential benefit justifies the potential risk to the fetus. Drugs of this class should not be used extensively on pregnant patients, in large amounts, or for prolonged periods of time.
Nursing Mothers
It is not known whether topical administration of corticosteroids could result in sufficient systemic absorption to produce detectable quantities in breast milk. Systemically administered corticosteroids are secreted into breast milk in quantities **not** likely to have a deleterious effect on the infant. Nevertheless, caution should be exercised when topical corticosteroids are administered to a nursing woman.
Pediatric Use
Pediatric patients may demonstrate greater susceptibility to topical corticosteroid-induced HPA axis suppression and Cushing's syndrome than mature patients because of a larger skin surface area to body weight ratio.
HPA axis suppression, Cushing's syndrome, and intracranial hypertension have been reported in children receiving topical corticosteroids. Manifestations of adrenal suppression in children include linear growth retardation, delayed weight gain, low plasma cortisol levels, and absence of response to ACTH stimulation. Manifestations of intracranial hypertension include bulging fontanelles, headaches, and bilateral papilledema.
Administration of topical corticosteroids to children should be limited to the least amount compatible with an effective therapeutic regimen. Chronic corticosteroid therapy may interfere with the growth and development of children.

ADVERSE REACTIONS
The following local adverse reactions are reported infrequently with topical corticosteroids, but may occur more frequently with the use of occlusive dressings (reactions are listed in an approximate decreasing order of occurrence): burning, itching, irritation, dryness, folliculitis, hypertrichosis, acneiform eruptions, hypopigmentation, perioral dermatitis, allergic contact dermatitis, maceration of the skin, secondary infection, skin atrophy, striae, and miliaria.

OVERDOSAGE
Topically applied corticosteroids can be absorbed in sufficient amounts to produce systemic effects (see PRECAUTIONS, General).

DOSAGE AND ADMINISTRATION
HALOG Creams (Halcinonide Cream): Apply the 0.1% HALOG Cream (Halcinonide Cream) to the affected area two to three times daily. Rub in gently.
HALOG Ointment (Halcinonide Ointment): Apply a thin film of 0.1% HALOG Ointment (Halcinonide Ointment) to the affected area two to three times daily.
HALOG Solution (Halcinonide Topical Solution): Apply HALOG Solution (Halcinonide Topical Solution) 0.1% to the affected area two to three times daily.
HALOG-E Cream (Halcinonide Cream): Apply HALOG-E Cream (Halcinonide Cream) 0.1% to the affected area one to three times daily. Rub in gently.
Occlusive Dressing Technique
Occlusive dressings may be used for the management of psoriasis or other recalcitrant conditions.
HALOG Cream (Halcinonide Cream) 0.1% and HALOG-E Cream (Halcinonide Cream) 0.1%: Gently rub a small amount of the cream into the lesion until it disappears. Reapply the preparation leaving a thin coating on the lesion, cover with a pliable nonporous film, and seal the edges. If needed, additional moisture may be provided by covering the lesion with a dampened clean cotton cloth before the nonporous film is applied or by briefly wetting the affected area with water immediately prior to applying the medication. The frequency of changing dressings is best determined on an individual basis. It may be convenient to apply HALOG/ HALOG-E Cream under an occlusive dressing in the evening and to remove the dressing in the morning (i.e., 12-hour occlusion). When utilizing the 12-hour occlusion regimen, additional cream should be applied, without occlusion, during the day. Reapplication is essential at each dressing change.
If an infection develops, the use of occlusive dressings should be discontinued and appropriate antimicrobial therapy instituted.
HALOG Ointment (Halcinonide Ointment) 0.1%: Apply a thin film of the ointment to the lesion, cover with a pliable nonporous film, and seal the edges. If needed, additional moisture may be provided by covering the lesion with a dampened clean cotton cloth before the nonporous film is applied or by briefly wetting the affected area with water immediately prior to applying the medication. The frequency of changing dressings is best determined on an individual basis. It may be convenient to apply HALOG Ointment under an occlusive dressing in the evening and to remove the dressing in the morning (i.e., 12-hour occlusion). When utilizing the 12-hour occlusion regimen, additional ointment should be applied, without occlusion, during the day. Reapplication is essential at each dressing change.
If an infection develops, the use of occlusive dressings should be discontinued and appropriate antimicrobial therapy instituted.

Continued on next page

Halog—Cont.

HALOG Solution (Halcinonide Topical Solution) 0.1%: Apply the solution to the lesion, cover with a pliable nonporous film, and seal the edges. If needed, additional moisture may be provided by covering the lesion with a dampened clean cotton cloth before the nonporous film is applied or by briefly wetting the affected area with water immediately prior to applying the medication. The frequency of changing dressings is best determined on an individual basis. It may be convenient to apply HALOG solution under an occlusive dressing in the evening and to remove the dressing in the morning (i.e., 12-hour occlusion). When utilizing the 12-hour occlusion regimen, additional solution should be applied, without occlusion, during the day. Reapplication is essential at each dressing change.

If an infection develops, the use of occlusive dressings should be discontinued and appropriate antimicrobial therapy instituted.

HOW SUPPLIED

HALOG Cream (Halcinonide Cream USP)
0.1%: tubes containing 15 g (NDC 0003-1482-15), 30 g (NDC 0003-1482-20), 60 g (NDC 0003-1482-30); and jars containing 240 g (NDC 0003-1482-40) of cream.

HALOG Ointment (Halcinonide Ointment USP)
0.1%: tubes containing 15 g (NDC 0003-0248-15), 30 g (NDC 0003-0248-20), and 60 g (NDC 0003-0248-30); and jars containing 240 g (NDC 0003-0248-40) of ointment.

HALOG Solution (Halcinonide Topical Solution USP)
0.1%: plastic squeeze bottles containing 20 mL (NDC 0003-0249-15) and 60 mL (NDC 0003-0249-20) of solution.

HALOG-E Cream (Halcinonide Cream USP)
0.1%: 30 g (NDC 0003-1494-21), and 60 g (NDC 0003-1494-31) of cream.

Storage

HALOG Cream (Halcinonide Cream USP)
Store at room temperature; avoid excessive heat (104°F).

HALOG Ointment (Halcinonide Ointment USP)
Store at room temperature; avoid excessive heat (104°F).

HALOG Solution (Halcinonide Topical Solution USP)
Store at room temperature; avoid freezing and temperatures above 104°F.

HALOG-E Cream (Halcinonide Cream USP)
Store at room temperature; avoid freezing and refrigeration.

LAC-HYDRIN® 12%*   ℞
(ammonium lactate cream) Cream
For Dermatologic use only. Not for ophthalmic, oral or intravaginal use.

Rx only

DESCRIPTION

*Lac-Hydrin is a formulation of 12% lactic acid neutralized with ammonium hydroxide, as ammonium lactate, with a pH of 4.4-5.4. Lac-Hydrin Cream also contains water, light mineral oil, glyceryl stearate, polyoxyl 100 stearate, propylene glycol, polyoxyl 40 stearate, glycerin, cetyl alcohol, magnesium aluminum silicate, laureth-4, methyl and propyl parabens, methylcellulose, and quaternium-15. Lactic acid is a racemic mixture of 2-hydroxypropanoic acid and has the following structural formula:

$$\begin{array}{c} COOH \\ | \\ CHOH \\ | \\ CH_3 \end{array}$$

CLINICAL PHARMACOLOGY

Lactic acid is an alpha-hydroxy acid. It is a normal constituent of tissues and blood. The alpha-hydroxy acids (and their salts) are felt to act as humectants when applied to the skin. This property may influence hydration of the stratum corneum. In addition, lactic acid, when applied to the skin, may act to decrease corneocyte cohesion. The mechanism(s) by which this is accomplished is not yet known.

An *in vitro* study of percutaneous absorption of Lac-Hydrin Cream using human cadaver skin indicates that approximately 6.1% of the material was absorbed after 68 hours.

INDICATIONS AND USAGE

Lac-Hydrin Cream is indicated for the treatment of ichthyosis vulgaris and xerosis.

CONTRAINDICATIONS

None known.

WARNING

Use of this product should be discontinued if hypersensitivity to any of the ingredients is noted. Sun exposure (natural or artificial sunlight) to areas of the skin treated with Lac-Hydrin Cream should be minimized or avoided (see Precautions section).

PRECAUTIONS

General: For external use only. Stinging or burning may occur when applied to skin with fissures, erosions, or that is

otherwise abraded (for example, after shaving the legs). Caution is advised when used on the face because of the potential for irritation. The potential for post-inflammatory hypo- or hyperpigmentation has not been studied.

Information for patients: Patients using Lac-Hydrin Cream should receive the following information and instructions:

1. This medication is to be used as directed by the physician, and should not be used for any disorder other than for which it was prescribed. Caution is advised when used on the face because of the potential for irritation. It is for external use only. Avoid contact with eyes, lips, or mucous membranes.
2. Patients should minimize or avoid use of this product on areas of the skin that may be exposed to natural or artificial sunlight, including the face. If sun exposure is unavoidable, clothing should be worn to protect the skin.
3. This medication may cause stinging or burning when applied to skin with fissures, erosions, or abrasions (for example, after shaving the legs).
4. If the skin condition worsens with treatment, the medication should be promptly discontinued.

Carcinogenesis, Mutagenesis, Impairment of Fertility: Carcinogenesis: A long-term photocarcinogenicity study in hairless albino mice suggested that topically applied 12% ammonium lactate cream enhanced the rate of ultraviolet light-induced skin tumor formation. Although the biologic significance of these results to humans is not clear, patients should minimize or avoid use of this product on areas of the skin that may be exposed to natural or artificial sunlight, including the face. Long-term dermal carcinogenicity studies in animals have not been conducted to evaluate the carcinogenic potential of ammonium lactate.

Pregnancy: Teratogenic effects: Pregnancy Category C. Animal reproduction studies have not been conducted with Lac-Hydrin Cream. It is also not known whether Lac-Hydrin Cream can cause fetal harm when administered to a pregnant woman or can affect reproduction capacity. Lac-Hydrin Cream should be given to a pregnant woman only if clearly needed.

Nursing Mothers: Although lactic acid is a normal constituent of blood and tissues, it is not known to what extent this drug affects normal lactic acid levels in human milk. Because many drugs are excreted in human milk, caution should be exercised when Lac-Hydrin Cream is administered to a nursing woman.

Pediatric Use: The safety and effectiveness of Lac-Hydrin Cream have not been established in pediatric patients less than 12 years old. Potential systemic toxicity from percutaneous absorption has not been studied. Because of the increased surface area to body weight ratio in pediatric patients, the systemic burden of lactic acid may be increased.

ADVERSE REACTIONS

In controlled clinical trials of patients with ichthyosis vulgaris, the most frequent adverse reactions in patients treated with Lac-Hydrin Cream were rash (including erythema and irritation) and burning/stinging. Each was reported in approximately 10-15% of patients. In addition, itching was reported in approximately 5% of patients.

In controlled clinical trials of patients with xerosis, the most frequent adverse reactions in patients treated with Lac-Hydrin Cream were transient burning, in about 3% of patients, stinging, dry skin and rash, each reported in approximately 2% of patients.

DOSAGE AND ADMINISTRATION

Apply to the affected areas and rub in thoroughly. Use twice daily or as directed by a physician.

HOW SUPPLIED

Lac-Hydrin Cream is available in cartons of 280 g (2-140 g plastic tubes). Store at controlled room temperature, 15-30°C (59-86°F).

©1994 WESTWOOD-SQUIBB PHARMACEUTICALS, INC.
Buffalo, N.Y., U.S.A. 14213   03-5982-1
A Bristol-Myers Squibb Company Revised August 20, 1996

LAC–HYDRIN® 12%*   ℞
(ammonium lactate)
Lotion
For topical use only. Not for ophthalmic use.

RX only.

DESCRIPTION

*LAC-HYDRIN, specially formulates 12% lactic acid neutralized with ammonium hydroxide, as ammonium lactate to provide a lotion pH of 4.5–5.5. LAC-HYDRIN also contains light mineral oil, glyceryl stearate, PEG-100 stearate, propylene glycol, polyoxyl 40 stearate, glycerin, magnesium aluminum silicate, laureth-4, cetyl alcohol, methyl and propylparabens, methylcellulose, fragrance, and water. Lactic acid is a racemic mixture of 2-hydroxypropanoic acid and has the following structural formula:
[See chemical structure at top of next column]

$$\begin{array}{c} COOH \\ | \\ CHOH \\ | \\ CH_3 \end{array}$$

CLINICAL PHARMACOLOGY

It is generally accepted that the water content of the stratum corneum is a controlling factor in maintaining skin flexibility. When the stratum corneum contains more than 10% water it remains soft and pliable; however, when the water content drops below 10% the stratum corneum becomes less flexible and rough, and may exhibit scaling and cracking and the underlying skin may become irritated. Symptomatic relief of dry skin is provided by skin protectants containing hygroscopic substances (humectants) which increase skin moisture. Lactic acid, an α-hydroxy acid, is reported to be one of the most effective naturally occurring humectants in the skin. The α-hydroxy acids (and their salts), in addition to having beneficial effects on dry skin, have also been shown to reduce excessive epidermal keratinization in patients with hyperkeratotic conditions (e.g., ichthyosis).

Pharmacokinetics: The mechanism of action of topically applied neutralized lactic acid is not yet known.

INDICATIONS AND USAGE

LAC-HYDRIN is indicated for the treatment of dry, scaly skin (xerosis) and ichthyosis vulgaris and for temporary relief of itching associated with these conditions.

CONTRAINDICATIONS

Known hypersensitivity to any of the label ingredients.

PRECAUTIONS

General: For external use only. Avoid contact with eyes, lips or mucous membranes. Caution is advised when used on the face of fair-skinned individuals since irritation may occur. A mild, transient stinging may occur on application to abraded or inflamed areas or in individuals with sensitive skin.

Carcinogenesis, Mutagenesis, Impairment of Fertility: LAC-HYDRIN was nonmutagenic in the Ames/Salmonella/Microsome Plate Assay. Reproductive studies in rats given lactic acid orally showed no effect on the sex ratio of the offspring.

Pregnancy (Category C): Animal reproduction studies have not been conducted with LAC-HYDRIN. It is also not known whether LAC-HYDRIN can cause fetal harm when administered to a pregnant woman or can affect reproduction capacity. LAC-HYDRIN should be given to a pregnant woman only if clearly needed.

Nursing Mothers: Although lactic acid is a normal constituent of blood and tissues, it is not known to what extent this drug affects normal lactic acid levels in human milk. Because many drugs are excreted in human milk, caution should be exercised when LAC-HYDRIN is administered to a nursing woman.

Pediatric Use: Safety and effectiveness of LAC-HYDRIN have been demonstrated in infants and children. No unusual toxic effects were reported.

ADVERSE REACTIONS

The most frequent adverse experiences in patients with xerosis are transient stinging (1 in 30 patients), burning (1 in 30 patients), erythema (1 in 50 patients) and peeling (1 in 60 patients). Other adverse reactions which occur less frequently are irritation, eczema, petechiae, dryness and hyperpigmentation.

Due to the more severe initial skin conditions associated with ichthyosis, there was a higher incidence of transient stinging, burning and erythema (each occurring in 1 in 10 patients).

OVERDOSAGE

The oral administration of LAC-HYDRIN to rats and mice showed this drug to be practically non-toxic (LD$_{50}$>15 ml/kg).

DOSAGE AND ADMINISTRATION

Shake well. Apply to the affected areas and rub in thoroughly. Use twice daily or as directed by a physician.

HOW SUPPLIED

225g (NDC 0072-5712-08; NSN 6505-01-216-6274) plastic bottle and 400g (NDC 0072-5712-14) plastic bottle.
Store at controlled room temperature (15°–30°C; 59°–86°F).

MOISTUREL® CREAM   OTC
Fragrance Free Skin Protectant—Moisturizer

COMPOSITION

Active Ingredients: Dimethicone 1%, petrolatum 30%. Also contains: Water, glycerin, PG dioctanoate, cetyl alcohol, steareth-2, PVP/hexadecene copolymer, laureth-23, magnesium aluminum silicate, diazolidinyl urea, carbomer-934, sodium hydroxide, methylchloroisothiazolinone and methylisothiazolinone.

ACTIONS AND USES

A highly effective, concentrated formula clinically proven to relieve dry skin and designed not to cause acne or blemishes. Ideal for sensitive skin. Free of lanolins, fragrances, and parabens that can sensitize or irritate skin.

Helps prevent and temporarily protects chafed, chapped, cracked or windburned skin. For temporary protection of minor cuts, scrapes, burns and sunburn. Helps treat and prevent minor skin irritation due to diaper rash and helps seal out wetness.

WARNINGS

For external use only. Avoid contact with the eyes. Not to be applied over puncture wounds or infections.

ADMINISTRATION AND DOSAGE

Apply liberally as often as needed. If used for diaper rash, change wet diapers promptly, cleanse the diaper area and allow to dry. Apply cream liberally with each changing.

HOW SUPPLIED

4 oz. (113g) (NDC 0072-9500-04) and 16 oz. (453g) (NDC 0072-9500-16) plastic jars.

MOISTUREL® LOTION   OTC
Skin Protectant—Moisturizer

COMPOSITION

Active Ingredient: Dimethicone 3%. Also contains: Water, petrolatum, glycerin, stearreth-2, cetyl alcohol, benzyl alcohol, laureth-23, magnesium aluminum silicate, carbomer-934, sodium hydroxide, potassium sorbate.

ACTION AND USES

Quick absorbing, long lasting formula that leaves the skin feeling smooth and soft. Clinically proven to relieve dry skin and designed not to cause acne. Free of lanolins and parabens that can irritate sensitive skin. Generalized dry skin. Helps prevent and temporarily protects chafed, chapped, cracked or windburned skin. Helps treat and prevent minor skin irritation due to diaper rash and helps seal out wetness.

WARNINGS

For external use only. Avoid contact with the eyes. Not to be applied over puncture wounds or infections.

ADMINISTRATION AND DOSAGE

Apply liberally as often as needed to soothe and soften sensitive skin. If used for diaper rash, change wet diapers promptly, cleanse the diaper area and allow to dry. Apply lotion liberally with each changing.

HOW SUPPLIED

8 oz. (226g) (NDC 0072-9100-08) and 14 oz. (397g) (NDC 0072-9100-14) plastic bottles.

MYCOSTATIN® CREAM   ℞
[mīk 'o-stat "in]
Nystatin Cream USP
MYCOSTATIN® TOPICAL POWDER
Nystatin Topical Powder USP
FOR TOPICAL USE ONLY • NOT FOR OPHTHALMIC USE

DESCRIPTION

Nystatin is a polyene antifungal antibiotic obtained from *Streptomyces nursei*.
Structural formula:

Mycostatin® Cream (Nystatin Cream) and Mycostatin® Topical Powder (Nystatin Topical Powder) are for dermatologic use.

MYCOSTATIN® (Nystatin) **Cream** for topical use, contains 100,000 USP nystatin units per gram. Inactive ingredients: aluminum hydroxide concentrated wet gel, titanium dioxide, propylene glycol, cetearyl alcohol (and) ceteareth-20, white petrolatum, sorbitol solution, glyceryl monostearate, polyethylene glycol monostearate, sorbic acid and simethicone.

MYCOSTATIN® (Nystatin) **Topical Powder** contains 100,000 USP nystatin units per gram dispersed in talc.

CLINICAL PHARMACOLOGY
Pharmacokinetics
Nystatin is not absorbed from intact skin or mucous membrane.

Microbiology

Nystatin is an antibiotic which is both fungistatic and fungicidal *in vitro* against a wide variety of yeasts and yeast-like fungi, including *Candida albicans, C. parapsilosis, C. tropicalis, C. guilliermondi, C. pseudotropicalis, C. krusei, Torulopsis glabrata, Tricophyton rubrum, T. mentagrophytes*.

Nystatin acts by binding to sterols in the cell membrane of susceptible species resulting in a change in membrane permeability and the subsequent leakage of intracellular components. On repeated subculturing with increasing levels of nystatin, *Candida albicans* does not develop resistance to nystatin. Generally, resistance to nystatin does not develop during therapy. However, other species of *Candida (C. tropicalis, C. guilliemondi, C. krusei*, and *C. stellatoides)* become quite resistant on treatment with nystatin and simultaneously become cross resistant to amphotericin as well. This resistance is lost when the antibiotic is removed.

Nystatin exhibits no appreciable activity against bacteria, protozoa, or viruses.

INDICATIONS AND USAGE

Nystatin topical preparations are indicated in the treatment of cutaneous or mucocutaneous mycotic infections caused by *Candida albicans* and other susceptible *Candida* species.

These preparations are not indicated for systemic, oral, intravaginal or ophthalmic use.

CONTRAINDICATIONS

Nystatin topical preparations are contraindicated in patients with a history of hypersensitivity to **any** of their components.

PRECAUTIONS
General
Nystatin, topical preparations should not be used for the treatment of systemic, oral, intravaginal or ophthalmic infections.
If irritation or sensitization develops, treatment should be discontinued and appropriate measures taken as indicated. It is recommended that KOH smears, cultures, or other diagnostic methods be used to confirm the diagnosis of cutaneous or mucocutaneous candidiasis and to rule out infection caused by other pathogens.
INFORMATION FOR THE PATIENT
Patients using these medications should receive the following information and instructions:
1. The patient should be instructed to use these medications as directed (including the replacement of missed doses). These medications are not for any disorder other than that for which they are prescribed.
2. Even if symptomatic relief occurs within the first few days of treatment, the patient should be advised not to interrupt or discontinue therapy until the prescribed course of treatment is completed.
3. If symptoms of irritation develop, the patient should be advised to notify the physician promptly.
Laboratory Tests
If there is a lack of therapeutic response, KOH smears, cultures, or other diagnostic methods should be repeated.
Carcinogenesis, Mutagenesis, Impairment of Fertility
No long-term animal studies have been performed to evaluate the carcinogenic potential of nystatin. No studies have been performed to determine the mutagenicity of nystatin or its effects on male or female fertility.
Pregnancy: Teratogenic Effects
Category C. Animal reproduction studies have not been conducted with any nystatin topical preparation. It also is not known whether these preparations can cause fetal harm when used by a pregnant woman or can affect reproductive capacity. Nystatin topical preparations should be prescribed for a pregnant woman only if the potential benefit to the mother outweighs the potential risk to the fetus.
Nursing Mothers
It is not known whether nystatin is excreted in human milk. Caution should be exercised when nystatin is prescribed for a nursing woman.
Pediatric Use
Safety and effectiveness have been established in the pediatric population from birth to 16 years.
(See **DOSAGE AND ADMINISTRATION**.)

ADVERSE REACTIONS

The frequency of adverse events reported in patients using Mycostatin® preparations is less than 0.1%. The more common events that were reported include allergic reactions, burning, itching, rash, eczema, and pain on application.
(See **PRECAUTIONS: General**.)

DOSAGE AND ADMINISTRATION

Very moist lesions are best treated with the topical dusting powder.
MYCOSTATIN® Cream
Adults and Pediatric Patients (Neonates and Older):
Apply liberally to affected areas twice daily or as indicated until healing is complete.

MYCOSTATIN® Topical Powder
Adults and Pediatric Patients (Neonates and Older):
Apply to candidal lesions two or three times daily until healing is complete. For fungal infection of the feet caused by *Candida* species, the powder should be dusted on the feet, as well as, in all foot wear.

HOW SUPPLIED

MYCOSTATIN® Cream: 100,000 units nystatin per gram in an aqueous, perfumed vanishing cream base, in 30 g (NDC 0003-0579-31) tubes.
MYCOSTATIN® Topical Powder: 100,000 units nystatin per gram in 15 g (NDC 0003-0593-20) plastic squeeze bottles.
ALSO AVAILABLE
MYCOSTATIN® (Nystatin) is also available as vaginal tablets and in oral formulations (pastilles, suspension, tablets). See package inserts for complete prescribing information.
STORAGE
MYCOSTATIN® Cream: Store at room temperature, avoid freezing.
MYCOSTATIN® Topical Powder: Store at room temperature, avoid excessive heat (40° C/104° F). Keep tightly closed.
Rx only.
© 1997 Westwood-Squibb Pharmaceuticals Inc.
Buffalo, N.Y., U.S.A. 14213
A Bristol-Myers Squibb Company
J3-327G   51-007275-00   Printed in USA
Revised April 1997   51-007275-00   J3-327G

T-STAT®   ℞
(erythromycin) 2.0% Topical Solution and Pads
For topical use only. Not for ophthalmic use.

Rx only.

DESCRIPTION

Erythromycin is an antibiotic produced from a strain of Streptomyces erythraeus. It is basic and readily forms salts with acids. Each ml of T-STAT (erythromycin). 2.0% Topical Solution contains 20 mg of erythromycin base in a vehicle consisting of alcohol (71.2%), propylene glycol and fragrance. It may contain citric acid to adjust pH.

ACTIONS

Although the mechanism by which T-STAT Solution acts in reducing inflammatory lesions of acne vulgaris is unknown, it is presumably due to its antibiotic action.

INDICATIONS

T-STAT Solution is indicated for the topical control of acne vulgaris.

CONTRAINDICATIONS

T-STAT Solution is contraindicated in persons who have shown hypersensitivity to any of its ingredients.

WARNING

The safe use of T-STAT (erythromycin) 2.0% Solution during pregnancy or lactation has not been established.

PRECAUTIONS

General—The use of antibiotic agents may be associated with the overgrowth of antibiotic-resistant organisms. If this occurs, administration of this drug should be discontinued and appropriate measures taken.
Information for Patients—T-STAT Solution is for external use only and should be kept away from the eyes, nose, mouth, and other mucous membranes. Concomitant topical acne therapy should be used with caution because a cumulative irritant effect may occur, especially with the use of peeling, desquamating, or abrasive agents.
Carcinogensis, Mutagenesis, Impairment of Fertility— Long-term animal studies to evaluate carcinogenic potential, mutagenicity, or the effect on fertility of erythromycin have not been performed.
Pregnancy: Pregnancy Category C.—Animal reproduction studies have not been conducted with erythromycin. It is also not known whether erythromycin can cause fetal harm when administered to a pregnant woman or can affect reproduction capacity. Erythromycin should be given to a pregnant woman only if clearly needed.
Nursing Mothers—Erythromycin is excreted in breast milk. Caution should be exercised when erythromycin is administered to a nursing woman.

ADVERSE REACTIONS

Adverse conditions reported include dryness, tenderness, pruritus, desquamation, erythema, oiliness, and burning sensation. Irritation of the eyes has also been reported. A case of generalized urticarial reaction, possibly related to the drug, which required the use of systemic steroid therapy has been reported.

Continued on next page

T-Stat—Cont.

DOSAGE AND ADMINISTRATION

T-STAT Solution or Pads should be applied over the affected area twice a day after the skin is thoroughly washed with warm water and soap and patted dry. Acne lesions on the face, neck, shoulder, chest, and back may be treated in this manner. Additional pads may be used, if needed.
This medication should be applied with applicator top or the disposable applicator pads. If fingertips or pads are used, wash hands after application. Drying and peeling may be controlled by reducing the frequency of applications.

HOW SUPPLIED

T-STAT Solution, 60 ml plastic bottle with optional applicator, NDC 0072-8300-60. T-STAT Pads, 60 disposable premoistened applicator pads in a plastic jar. NDC 0072-8303-60. Store in a dry place at temperatures between 15°C and 25°C (59°F and 77°F).

ULTRAVATE® ℞

(halobetasol propionate cream)
Cream, 0.05%
For Dermatological Use Only. Not for Ophthalmic Use.

Rx only.

DESCRIPTION

ULTRAVATE (halobetasol propionate cream) Cream contains halobetasol propionate, a synthetic corticosteroid for topical dermatological use. The corticosteroids constitute a class of primarily synthetic steroids used topically as an anti-inflammatory and antipruritic agent.
Chemically halobetasol propionate is 21-chloro-6α, 9-difluoro-11β, 17-dihydroxy-16β-methylpregna-1, 4-diene-3-20-dione, 17 propionate, $C_{25}H_{31}ClF_2O_5$. It has the following structural formula:

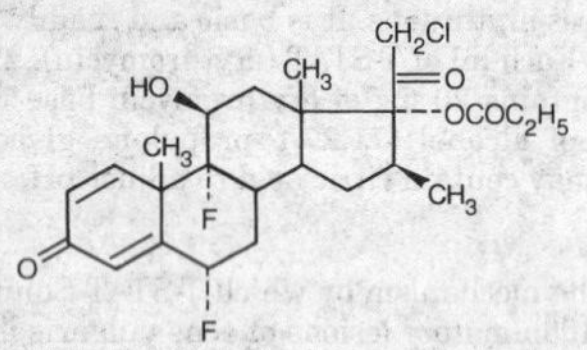

Halobetasol propionate has the molecular weight of 485. It is a white crystalline powder insoluble in water.
Each gram of ULTRAVATE Cream contains 0.5 mg/g of halobetasol propionate in a cream base of cetyl alcohol, glycerin, isopropyl isostearate, isopropyl palmitate, steareth-21, diazolidinyl urea, methylchloroisothiazolinone, methylisothiazolinone and water.

CLINICAL PHARMACOLOGY

Like other topical corticosteroids, halobetasol propionate has anti-inflammatory, antipruritic and vasoconstrictive actions. The mechanism of the anti-inflammatory activity of the topical corticosteroids, in general, is unclear. However, corticosteroids are thought to act by the induction of phospholipase A_2 inhibitory proteins, collectively called lipocortins. It is postulated that these proteins control the biosynthesis of potent mediators of inflammation such as prostaglandins and leukotrienes by inhibiting the release of their common precursor arachidonic acid. Arachidonic acid is released from membrane phospholipids by phospholipase A_2.
Pharmacokinetics—The extent of percutaneous absorption of topical corticosteroids is determined by many factors including the vehicle and the integrity of the epidermal barrier. Occlusive dressings with hydrocortisone for up to 24 hours have not been demonstrated to increase penetration; however, occlusion of hydrocortisone for 96 hours markedly enhances penetration. Topical corticosteroids can be absorbed from normal intact skin. Inflammation and/or other disease processes in the skin may increase percutaneous absorption.
Human and animal studies indicate that less than 6% of the applied dose of halobetasol propionate enters the circulation with 96 hours following topical administration of the cream. Studies performed with ULTRAVATE (halobetasol propionate cream) Cream indicate that it is in the super-high range of potency as compared with other topical corticosteroids.

INDICATIONS AND USAGE

ULTRAVATE (halobetasol propionate cream) Cream 0.05% is a super-high potency corticosteroid indicated for the relief of the inflammatory and pruritic manifestations of corticosteroid-responsive dermatoses. Treatment beyond two consecutive weeks is not recommended, and the total dosage should not exceed 50 g/week because of the potential for the drug to suppress the hypothalamic-pituitary-adrenal (HPA) axis.

CONTRAINDICATIONS

ULTRAVATE (halobetasol propionate cream) Cream is contraindicated in those patients with a history of hypersensitivity to any of the components of the preparation.

PRECAUTIONS

General: Systemic absorption of topical corticosteroids can produce reversible hypothalamic-pituitary-adrenal (HPA) axis suppression with the potential for glucocorticosteroid insufficiency after withdrawal of treatment. Manifestations of Cushing's syndrome, hyperglycemia, and glucosuria can also be produced in some patients by systemic absorption of topical corticosteroids while on treatment.
Patients applying a topical steroid to a large surface area or to areas under occlusion should be evaluated periodically for evidence of HPA axis suppression. This may be done by using the ACTH stimulation, A.M. plasma cortisol, and urinary free-cortisol tests. Patients receiving super potent corticosteroids should not be treated for more than 2 weeks at a time and only small areas should be treated at any one time due to increased risk of HPA suppression.
ULTRAVATE (halobetasol propionate cream) Cream produced HPA axis suppression when used in divided doses at 7 grams per day for one week in patients with psoriasis. These effects were reversible upon discontinuation of treatment.
If HPA axis suppression is noted, an attempt should be made to withdraw the drug, to reduce the frequency of application, or to substitute a less potent corticosteroid. Recovery of HPA axis function is generally prompt upon discontinuation of topical corticosteroids. Infrequently, signs and symptoms of glucocorticosteroids insufficiency may occur requiring supplemental systemic corticosteroids. For information on systemic supplementation, see prescribing information for those products.
Pediatric patients may be more susceptible to systemic toxicity from equivalent doses due to their larger skin surface to body mass ratios (See PRECAUTIONS: Pediatric Use).
If irritation develops, ULTRAVATE (halobetasol propionate cream) Cream should be discontinued and appropriate therapy instituted. Allergic contact dermatitis with corticosteroids is usually diagnosed by observing failure to heal rather than noting a clinical exacerbation as with most topical products not containing corticosteroids. Such an observation should be corroborated with appropriate diagnostic patch testing.
If concomitant skin infections are present or develop, an appropriate antifungal or antibacterial agent should be used. If a favorable response does not occur promptly, use of ULTRAVATE (halobetasol propionate cream) Cream should be discontinued until the infection has been adequately controlled.
ULTRAVATE (halobetasol propionate cream) Cream should not be used in the treatment of rosacea or perioral dermatitis, and it should not be used on the face, groin, or in the axillae.
Information for Patients: Patients using topical corticosteroids should receive the following information and instructions:
1. The medication is to be used as directed by the physician. It is for external use only. Avoid contact with the eyes.
2. The medication should not be used for any disorder other than that for which it was prescribed.
3. The treated skin area should not be bandaged, otherwise covered or wrapped, so as to be occlusive unless directed by the physician.
4. Patients should report to the their physician any signs of local adverse reactions.
5. Parents of pediatric patients should be advised not to use tight-fitting diapers or plastic pants on a child being treated in the diaper area, as these garments may constitute occlusive dressing.

Laboratory Tests: The following tests may be helpful in evaluating patients for HPA axis suppression: ACTH-stimulation test; A.M. plasma cortisol test; Urinary free-cortisol test.
Carcinogenesis, mutagenesis, and Impairment of fertility: Long-term animal studies have not been performed to evaluate the carcinogenic potential of halobetasol propionate.
Positive mutagenicity effects were observed in two genotoxicity assays. Halobetasol propionate was positive in a Chinese hamster micronucleus test, and in a mouse lymphoma gene mutation assay *in vitro*.
Studies in the rat following oral administration at dose levels up to 50 µg/kg/day indicated no impairment of fertility or general reproductive performance.
In other genotoxicity testing, halobetasol propionate was not found to be genotoxic in the Ames/Salmonella assay, in the sister chromatid exchange test in somatic cells of the Chinese hamster, in chromosome aberration studies of germinal and somatic cells of rodents, and in a mammalian spot test to determine point mutations.
Pregnancy: *Teratogenic effects: Pregnancy Category C:* Corticosteroids have been shown to be teratogenic in laboratory animals when administered systemically at relatively low dosage levels. Some corticosteroids have been shown to be teratogenic after dermal application in laboratory animals. Halobetasol propionate has been shown to be teratogenic in SPF rats and chinchilla-type rabbits when given systemically during gestation at doses of 0.04 to 0.1 mg/kg in rats and 0.01 mg/kg in rabbits. These doses are approximately 13.33 and 3 times, respectively, the human topical dose of ULTRAVATE (halobetasol propionate cream) Cream. Halobetasol propionate was embryotoxic in rabbits but not in rats.
Cleft palate was observed in both rats and rabbits. Omphalocele was seen in rats, but not in rabbits.
There are no adequate and well-controlled studies of the teratogenic potential of halobetasol propionate in pregnant women. ULTRAVATE (halobetasol propionate cream) Cream should be used during pregnancy only if the potential benefit justifies the potential risk to the fetus.
Nursing Mothers: Systemically administered corticosteroids appear in human milk and could suppress growth, interfere with endogenous corticosteroid production, or cause other untoward effects. It is not known whether topical administration of corticosteroids could result in sufficient systemic absorption to produce detectable quantities in human milk. Because many drugs are excreted in human milk, caution should be exercised when ULTRAVATE (halobetasol propionate cream) Cream is administered to a nursing woman.
Pediatric Use: Safety and effectiveness of ULTRAVATE (halobetasol propionate cream) Cream in pediatric patients have not been established and use in pediatric patients under 12 is not recommended. Because of a higher ratio of skin surface area to body mass, pediatric patients are at a greater risk than adults of HPA axis suppression and Cushing's syndrome when they are treated with topical corticosteroids. They are therefore also at greater risk of adrenal insufficiency during or after withdrawal of treatment. Adverse effects including striae have been reported with inappropriate use of topical corticosteroids in infants and children.
HPA axis suppression, Cushing's syndrome, linear growth retardation, delayed weight gain and intracranial hypertension have been reported in children receiving topical corticosteroids. Manifestations of adrenal suppression in children include low plasma cortisol levels and an absence of response to ACTH stimulation. Manifestations of intracranial hypertension include bulging fontanelles, headaches, and bilateral papilledema.

ADVERSE REACTIONS

In controlled clinical trials, the most frequent adverse events reported for ULTRAVATE (halobetasol propionate cream) Cream included stinging, burning or itching in 4.4% of the patients. Less frequently reported adverse reactions were dry skin, erythema, skin atrophy, leukoderma, vesicles and rash.
The following additional local adverse reactions are reported infrequently with topical corticosteroids, and they may occur more frequently with high potency corticosteroids, such as ULTRAVATE (halobetasol propionate cream) Cream. These reactions are listed in an approximate decreasing order of occurrence: folliculitis, hypertrichosis, acneiform eruptions, hypopigmentation, perioral dermatitis, allergic contact dermatitis, secondary infection, striae and miliaria.

OVERDOSAGE

Topically applied ULTRAVATE (halobetasol propionate cream) Cream can be absorbed in sufficient amounts to produce systemic effects (see PRECAUTIONS).

DOSAGE AND ADMINISTRATION

Apply a thin layer of ULTRAVATE (halobetasol propionate cream) Cream to the affected skin once or twice daily, as directed by your physician, and rub in gently and completely.
ULTRAVATE (halobetasol propionate cream) Cream is a high potency topical corticosteroids; therefore, treatment should be limited to two weeks, and amounts greater than 50 g/wk should not be used. As with other corticosteroids, therapy should be discontinued when control is achieved. If no improvement is seen within 2 weeks, reassessment of diagnosis may be necessary.
ULTRAVATE (halobetasol propionate cream) Cream should not be used with occlusive dressings.

HOW SUPPLIED

ULTRAVATE CREAM, 0.05% is supplied in the following tube sizes:
15 g (NDC 0072-1400-15)
50 g (NDC 0072-1400-50)
Store between 15° and 30°C (59° and 86°F).
WESTWOOD
SQUIBB™

A Bristol-Myers Squibb Company
Buffalo, New York U.S.A. 14213 03-5994-0

ULTRAVATE® ℞
(halobetasol propionate ointment)
Ointment, 0.05%
For Dermatological Use Only. Not for Ophthalmic Use.

Rx only.

DESCRIPTION

ULTRAVATE (halobetasol propionate ointment) Ointment contains halobetasol propionate, a synthetic corticosteroid for topical dermatological use. The corticosteroids constitute a class of primarily synthetic steroids used topically as an anti-inflammatory and antipruritic agent.

Chemically halobetasol propionate is 21-chloro-6α, 9-difluoro-11β, 17-dihydroxy-16β-methylpregna-1, 4-diene-3-20-dione, 17-propionate, $C_{25}H_{31}ClF_2O_5$. It has the following structural formula:

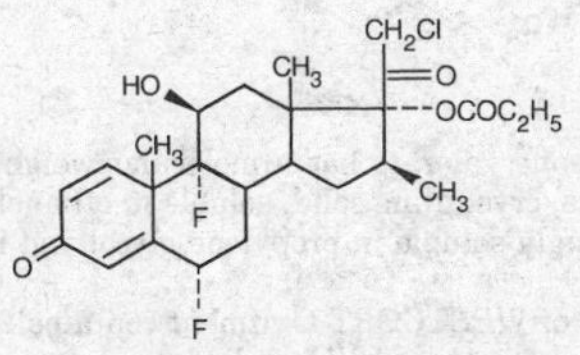

Halobetasol propionate has the molecular weight of 485. It is a white crystalline powder insoluble in water.

Each gram of ULTRAVATE Ointment contains 0.5 mg/g of halobetasol propionate in a base of aluminum stearate, beeswax, pentaerythritol cocoate, petrolatum, propylene glycol, sorbitan sesquioleate, and stearyl citrate.

CLINICAL PHARMACOLOGY

Like other topical corticosteroids, halobetasol propionate has anti-inflammatory, antipruritic and vasoconstrictive actions. The mechanism of the anti-inflammatory activity of the topical corticosteroids, in general, is unclear. However, corticosteroids are thought to act by the induction of phospholipase A_2 inhibitory proteins, collectively called lipocortins. It is postulated that these proteins control the biosynthesis of potent mediators of inflammation such as prostaglandins and leukotrienes by inhibiting the release of their common precursor arachidonic acid. Arachidonic acid is released from membrane phospholipids by phospholipase A_2.

Pharmacokinetics

The extent of percutaneous absorption of topical corticosteroids is determined by many factors including the vehicle and the integrity of the epidermal barrier. Occlusive dressings with hydrocortisone for up to 24 hours have not been demonstrated to increase penetration; however, occlusion of hydrocortisone for 96 hours markedly enhances penetration. Topical corticosteroids can be absorbed from normal intact skin. Inflammation and/or other disease processes in the skin may increase percutaneous absorption.

Human and animal studies indicate that less than 6% of the applied dose of halobetasol propionate enters the circulation within 96 hours following topical administration of the ointment.

Studies performed with ULTRAVATE (halobetasol propionate ointment) Ointment indicate that it is in the super-high range of potency as compared with other topical corticosteroids.

INDICATIONS AND USAGE

ULTRAVATE (halobetasol propionate ointment) Ointment 0.05% is a super-high potency corticosteroid indicated for the relief of the inflammatory and pruritic manifestations of corticosteroid-responsive dermatoses. Treatment beyond two consecutive weeks is not recommended, and the total dosage should not exceed 50 g/week because of the potential for the drug to suppress the hypothalamic-pituitary-adrenal (HPA) axis.

CONTRAINDICATIONS

ULTRAVATE (halobetasol propionate ointment) Ointment is contraindicated in those patients with a history of hypersensitivity to any of the components of the preparation.

PRECAUTIONS

General: Systemic absorption of topical corticosteroids can produce reversible hypothalamic-pituitary-adrenal (HPA) axis suppression with the potential for glucocorticosteroid insufficiency after withdrawal of treatment. Manifestations of Cushing's syndrome, hyperglycemia, and glucosuria can also be produced in some patients by systemic absorption of topical corticosteroids while on treatment.

Patients applying a topical steroid to a large surface area or to areas under occlusion should be evaluated periodically for evidence of HPA axis suppression. This may be done by using the ACTH stimulation, A.M. plasma cortisol, and urinary free-cortisol tests. Patients receiving super potent corticosteroids should not be treated for more than 2 weeks at a time and only small areas should be treated at any one time due to the increased risk of HPA suppression.

ULTRAVATE (halobetasol propionate ointment) Ointment produced HPA axis suppression when used in divided doses at 7 grams per day for one week in patients with psoriasis. These effects were reversible upon discontinuation of treatment.

If HPA axis suppression is noted, an attempt should be made to withdraw the drug, to reduce the frequency of application, or to substitute a less potent corticosteroid. Recovery of HPA axis function is generally prompt upon discontinuation of topical corticosteroids. Infrequently, signs and symptoms of glucocorticosteroid insufficiency may occur requiring supplemental systemic corticosteroids. For information on systemic supplementation, see prescribing information for those products.

Pediatric patients may be more susceptible to systemic toxicity from equivalent doses due to their larger skin surface to body mass ratios (See PRECAUTIONS: Pediatric Use).

If irritation develops, ULTRAVATE (halobetasol propionate ointment) Ointment should be discontinued and appropriate therapy instituted. Allergic contact dermatitis with corticosteroids is usually diagnosed by observing failure to heal rather than noting a clinical exacerbation as with most topical products not containing corticosteroids. Such an observation should be corroborated with appropriate diagnostic patch testing.

If concomitant skin infections are present or develop, an appropriate antifungal or antibacterial agent should be used. If a favorable response does not occur promptly, use of ULTRAVATE (halobetasol propionate ointment) Ointment should be discontinued until the infection has been adequately controlled.

ULTRAVATE (halobetasol propionate ointment) Ointment should not be used in the treatment of rosacea or perioral dermatitis, and it should not be used on the face, groin, or in the axillae.

Information for Patients

Patients using topical corticosteroids should receive the following information and instructions:

1. The medication is to be used as directed by the physician. It is for external use only. Avoid contact with the eyes.
2. The medication should not be used for any disorder other than that for which it was prescribed.
3. The treated skin area should not be bandaged, otherwise covered or wrapped, so as to be occlusive unless directed by the physician.
4. Patients should report to their physician any signs of local adverse reactions.
5. Parents of pediatric patients should be advised not to use tight-fitting diapers or plastic pants on a child being treated in the diaper area, as these garments may constitute occlusive dressing.

Laboratory Tests

The following tests may be helpful in evaluating patients for HPA axis suppression: ACTH-stimulation test; A.M. plasma cortisol test; Urinary free-cortisol test.

Carcinogenesis, mutagenesis, and Impairment of fertility

Long-term animal studies have not been performed to evaluate the carcinogenic potential of halobetasol propionate. Positive mutagenicity effects were observed in two genotoxicity assays. Halobetasol propionate was positive in a Chinese hamster micronucleus test, and in a mouse lymphoma gene mutation assay *in vitro*.

Studies in the rat following oral administration at dose levels up to 50 µg/kg/day indicated no impairment of fertility or general reproductive performance.

In other genotoxicity testing, halobetasol propionate was not found to be genotoxic in the Ames/Salmonella assay, in the sister chromatid exchange test in somatic cells of the Chinese hamster, in chromosome aberration studies of germinal and somatic cells of rodents, and in a mammalian spot test to determine point mutations.

Pregnancy

Teratogenic effects: Pregnancy Category C: Corticosteroids have been shown to be teratogenic in laboratory animals when administered systemically at relatively low dosage levels. Some corticosteroids have been shown to be teratogenic after dermal application in laboratory animals.

Halobetasol propionate has been shown to be teratogenic in SPF rats and chinchilla-type rabbits when given systematically during gestation at doses of 0.04 to 0.1 mg/kg in rats and 0.01 mg/kg in rabbits. These doses are approximately 13, 33 and 3 times, respectively, the human topical dose of ULTRAVATE (halobetasol propionate ointment) Ointment. Halobetasol propionate was embryotoxic in rabbits but not in rats.

Cleft palate was observed in both rats and rabbits. Omphalocele was seen in rats, but not in rabbits.

There are no adequate and well-controlled studies of the teratogenic potential of halobetasol propionate in pregnant women. ULTRAVATE (halobetasol propionate ointment) Ointment should be used during pregnancy only if the potential benefit justifies the potential risk to the fetus.

Nursing Mothers

Systematically administered corticosteroids appear in human milk and could suppress growth, interfere with endogenous corticosteroid production, or cause other untoward effects. It is not known whether topical administration of corticosteroids could result in sufficient systemic absorption to produce detectable quantities in human milk. Because many drugs are excreted in human milk, caution should be exercised when ULTRAVATE (halobetasol propionate ointment) Ointment is administered to a nursing woman.

Pediatric Use

Safety and effectiveness of ULTRAVATE (halobetasol propionate ointment) Ointment in pediatric patients have not been established and use in pediatric patients under 12 is not recommended. Because of a higher ratio of skin surface area to body mass, pediatric patients are at a greater risk than adults of HPA axis suppression and Cushing's syndrome when they are treated with topical corticosteroids. They are therefore also at greater risk of adrenal insufficiency during or after withdrawal of treatment. Adverse effects including striae have been reported with inappropriate use of topical corticosteroids in infants and children.

HPA axis suppression, Cushing's syndrome, linear growth retardation, delayed weight gain and intracranial hypertension have been reported in children receiving topical corticosteroids. Manifestations of adrenal suppression in children include low plasma cortisol levels and an absence of response to ACTH stimulation. Manifestations of intracranial hypertension include bulging fontanelles, headaches, and bilateral papilledema.

ADVERSE REACTIONS

In controlled clinical trials, the most frequent adverse events reported for ULTRAVATE (halobetasol propionate ointment) Ointment included stinging or burning in 1.6% of the patients. Less frequently reported adverse reactions were pustulation, erythema, skin atrophy, leukoderma, acne, itching, secondary infection, telangiectasia, urticaria, dry skin, miliaria, paresthesia, and rash.

The following additional local adverse reactions are reported infrequently with topical corticosteroids, and they may occur more frequently with high potency corticosteroids, such as ULTRAVATE (halobetasol propionate ointment) Ointment. These reactions are listed in an approximate decreasing order of occurrence: folliculitis, hypertrichosis, acneiform eruptions, hypopigmentation, perioral dermatitis, allergic contact dermatitis, secondary infection, striae and miliaria.

OVERDOSAGE

Topically applied ULTRAVATE (halobetasol propionate ointment) Ointment can be absorbed in sufficient amounts to produce systemic effects (see **PRECAUTIONS**).

DOSAGE AND ADMINISTRATION

Apply a thin layer of ULTRAVATE (halobetasol propionate ointment) Ointment to the affected skin once or twice daily, as directed by your physician, and rub in gently and completely.

ULTRAVATE (halobetasol propionate ointment) Ointment is a high potency topical corticosteroid; therefore, treatment should be limited to two weeks, and amounts greater than 50 g/wk should not be used. As with other corticosteroids, therapy should be discontinued when control is achieved. If no improvement is seen within 2 weeks, reassessment of diagnosis may be necessary.

ULTRAVATE (halobetasol propionate ointment) Ointment should not be used with occlusive dressings.

HOW SUPPLIED

ULTRAVATE OINTMENT, 0.05% is supplied in the following tube sizes:
15 g (NDC 0072-1450-15)
50 g (NDC 0072-1450-50)
Store between 15° and 30°C (59° and 86°F).

WESTWOOD SQUIBB™
©1995 Westwood-Squibb Pharmaceuticals Inc.
A Bristol-Myers Squibb Company
Buffalo, New York U.S.A. 14213   03-5995-1

WESTCORT® ℞
(hydrocortisone valerate)
Cream, 0.2%

For topical use only. Not for use in eyes.

Rx only.

DESCRIPTION

WESTCORT CREAM is a topical formulation containing hydrocortisone valerate, a non-fluorinated steroid. It has the chemical name Pregn-4-ene-3,20-dione. 11, 21-dihydroxy-17-[(1-oxopentyl) oxy]-, (11β)-; the empirical formula is: $C_{26}H_{38}O_6$; the molecular weight is 446.58, and the CAS registry number is: 57524-89-7. The structural formula is:
[See chemical structure at top of next column]

Each gram of Westcort Cream contains 2.0 mg hydrocortisone valerate in a hydrophilic base composed of white pet-

Continued on next page

Westcort Cream—Cont.

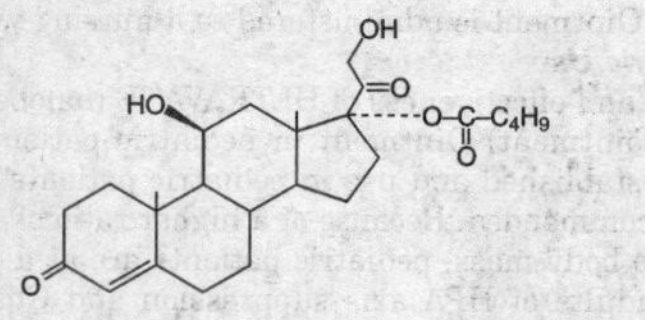

rolatum, stearyl alcohol, propylene glycol, amphoteric-9, carbomer 940, dried sodium phosphate, sodium lauryl sulfate, sorbic acid and water.

CLINICAL PHARMACOLOGY

Topical corticosteroids share anti-inflammatory, anti-pruritic and vasoconstrictive actions.

The mechanism of anti-inflammatory activity of the topical corticosteroids is unclear.[1] Various laboratory methods, including vasoconstrictor assays, are used to compare and predict potencies and/or clinical efficacies of the topical corticosteroids.[2] There is some evidence to suggest that a recognizable correlation exists between vasoconstrictor potency and therapeutic efficacy in man.[3]

Pharmacokinetics—The extent of percutaneous absorption of topical corticosteroids is determined by many factors including the vehicle, the integrity of the epidermal barrier, and the use of occlusive dressings.[4,5,6]

Topical corticosteroids can be absorbed from normal intact skin.[5,6,7] Inflammation and/or other disease processes in the skin increase percutaneous absorption.[8] Occlusive dressings substantially increase the percutaneous absorption of topical corticosteroids.[4,7] Thus, occlusive dressings may be valuable therapeutic adjunct for treatment of resistant dermatoses (see DOSAGE AND ADMINISTRATION).

Once absorbed through the skin, topical corticosteroids are handled through pharmacokinetic pathways similar to systemically administered corticosteroids. Corticosteroids are bound to plasma proteins in varying degrees. Corticosteroids are metabolized primarily in the liver and are then excreted by the kidneys. Some of the topical corticosteroids and their metabolites are also excreted into the bile.

INDICATIONS AND USAGE

Westcort Cream is indicated for the relief of the inflammatory and pruritic manifestations of the corticosteroid-responsive dermatoses.

CONTRAINDICATIONS

Topical corticosteroids are contraindicated in those patients with a history of hypersensitivity to any of the components of the preparation.

PRECAUTIONS

General—Systemic absorption of topical corticosteroids has produced reversible hypothalamic-pituitary-adrenal (HPA) axis suppression, manifestations of Cushing's syndrome, hyperglycemia, and glucosuria in some patients.[9]

Conditions which augment systemic absorption include the application of the more potent steroids, use over large surface areas, prolonged use, and the addition of occlusive dressings.[10]

Therefore, patients receiving a large dose of a potent topical steroid applied to a large surface area or under an occlusive dressing should be evaluated periodically for evidence of HPA axis suppression by using the urinary free cortisol and ACTH stimulation tests. If HPA axis suppression is noted, an attempt should be made to withdraw the drug, to reduce the frequency of application, or to substitute a less potent steroid.

Recovery of HPA axis function is generally prompt and complete upon discontinuation of the drug.[10] Infrequently, signs and symptoms of steroid withdrawal may occur, requiring supplemental systemic corticosteroids.[11,12]

Children may absorb proportionally larger amounts of topical corticosteroids and thus be more susceptible to systemic toxicity.[13,14] (see PRECAUTIONS—*Pediatric Use*).

If irritation develops, topical corticosteroids should be discontinued and appropriate therapy instituted.

In the presence of dermatological infections, the use of an appropriate antifungal or antibacterial agent should be instituted. If a favorable response does not occur promptly, the corticosteroid should be discontinued until the infection has been adequately controlled.

Information for the Patient—Patients using topical corticosteroids should receive the following information and instructions:

1. This medication is to be used as directed by the physician. It is for external use only. Avoid contact with the eyes.
2. Patients should be advised not to use this medication for any disorder other than for which it was prescribed.
3. The treated skin area should not be bandaged or otherwise covered or wrapped as to be occlusive unless directed by the physician.
4. Patients should report any signs of local adverse reactions especially under occlusive dressing.
5. Parents of pediatric patients should be advised not to use tight-fitting diapers or plastic pants on a child being treated in the diaper area, as these garments may constitute occlusive dressing.

Laboratory Tests—The following tests may be helpful in evaluating the HPA axis suppression:

Urinary free cortisol test
ACTH stimulation test

Carcinogenesis, Mutagenesis, and Impairment of Fertility—Long-term animal studies have not been performed to evaluate the carcinogenic potential or the effect on fertility of topical corticosteroids.

Studies to determine mutagenicity with prednisolone and hydrocortisone have revealed negative results.[15,16]

Pregnancy (Category C)—Corticosteroids are generally teratogenic in laboratory animals when administered systemically at relatively low dosage levels. The more potent corticosteroids have been shown to be teratogenic after dermal application in laboratory animals. There are no adequate and well-controlled studies in pregnant women on teratogenic effects from topically applied corticosteroids. Therefore, topical corticosteroids should be used during pregnancy only if the potential benefit justifies the potential risk to the fetus. Drugs of this class should not be used extensively on pregnant patients, in large amounts, or for prolonged periods of time.

Nursing Mothers—It is not known whether topical administration of corticosteroids could result in sufficient systemic absorption to produce detectable quantities in breast milk. Systemically administered corticosteroids are secreted into breast milk in quantities *not* likely to have a deleterious effect on the infant.[17,18] Nevertheless, caution should be exercised when topical corticosteroids are administered to a nursing woman.

Pediatric Use—*Pediatric patients may demonstrate greater susceptibility to topical corticosteroid-induced HPA axis suppression and Cushing's syndrome than mature patients because of a larger skin surface area to body weight ratio.*

Hypothalamic-pituitary-adrenal (HPA) axis suppression, Cushing's syndrome, and intracranial hypertension have been reported in children receiving topical corticosteroids. Manifestations of adrenal suppression in children include linear growth retardation, delayed weight gain, low plasma cortisol levels, and absence of response to ACTH stimulation. Manifestations of intracranial hypertension include bulging fontanelles, headaches, and bilateral papilledema.

Administration of topical corticosteroids to children should be limited to the least amount compatible with an effective therapeutic regimen. Chronic corticosteroid therapy may interfere with the growth and development of children.

ADVERSE REACTIONS

The following local adverse reactions are reported infrequently with topical corticosteroids, but may occur more frequently with the use of occlusive dressings. These reactions are listed in an approximate decreasing order of occurrence: burning, itching, irritation, dryness, folliculitis, hypertrichosis, acneiform eruptions, hypopigmentation, perioral dermatitis, allergic contact dermatitis, maceration of the skin, secondary infection, skin atrophy, striae, miliaria.

OVERDOSAGE

Topically applied corticosteroids can be absorbed in sufficient amounts to produce systemic effects (see PRECAUTIONS).

DOSAGE AND ADMINISTRATION

Westcort Cream should be applied to the affected area as a thin film two or three times daily depending on the severity of the condition.

Occlusive dressings may be used for the management of psoriasis or recalcitrant conditions.

If an infection develops, the use of occlusive dressings should be discontinued and appropriate antimicrobial therapy instituted.

HOW SUPPLIED

WESTCORT CREAM, 0.2% is supplied in the following tube sizes:

15 g NDC 0072-8100-15; NSN 6505-01-093-9901
45 g NDC 0072-8100-45; NSN 6505-01-083-9901
60 g NDC 0072-8100-60
Store below 78°F (26°C).

©1982, 1990 WESTWOOD-SQUIBB PHARMACEUTICALS, INC.

Buffalo, N.Y., U.S.A. 14213 03-5971-0
A Bristol-Myers Squibb Company

WESTCORT® ℞

(hydrocortisone valerate ointment)
Ointment, 0.2%
For Dermatologic Use Only. Not for Ophthalmic Use.
Rx only.

DESCRIPTION

Ointment contains hydrocortisone valerate, 11, 21-dihydroxy-17-[(1-oxopentyl)oxy]-,(11β)-pregn-4-ene-3, 20-dione, a synthetic corticosteroid for topical dermatologic use. The corticosteroids constitute a class of primarily synthetic steroids used topically as anti-inflammatory and antipruritic agents.

Chemically, hydrocortisone valerate is $C_{26}H_{38}O_6$. It has the following structural formula:

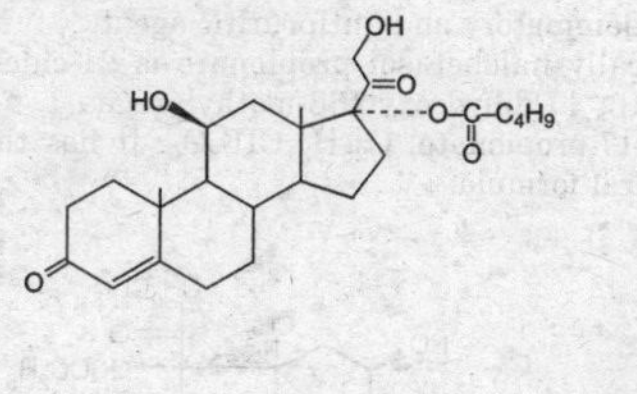

Hydrocortisone valerate has a molecular weight of 446.58. It is a white, crystalline solid, soluble in ethanol and methanol, sparingly soluble in propylene glycol and insoluble in water.

Each gram of WESTCORT Ointment contains 2 mg hydrocortisone valerate in a hydrophilic base composed of white petrolatum, stearyl alcohol, propylene glycol, sorbic acid, sodium lauryl sulfate, carbomer 934, dried sodium phosphate, mineral oil, steareth-2, steareth-100, and water.

CLINICAL PHARMACOLOGY

Like other topical corticosteroids, hydrocortisone valerate has anti-inflammatory, anti-pruritic and vasoconstrictive properties. The mechanism of the anti-inflammatory activity of the topical steroids, in general, is unclear. However, corticosteroids are thought to act by the induction of phospholipase A_2 inhibitory proteins, collectively called lipocortins. It is postulated that these proteins control the biosynthesis of potent mediators of inflammation such as prostaglandins and leukotrienes by inhibiting the release of their common precursor arachidonic acid. Arachidonic acid is released from membrane phospholipids by phospholipase A_2.

Pharmacokinetics: The extent of percutaneous absorption of topical corticosteroids is determined by many factors including the vehicle and the integrity of the epidermal barrier. Occlusive dressings with hydrocortisone for up to 24 hours have not been demonstrated to increase penetration; however, occlusion of hydrocortisone for 96 hours markedly enhances penetration. Topical corticosteroids can be absorbed from normal intact skin. Inflammation and/or other disease processes in the skin may increase percutaneous absorption.

Studies performed with WESTCORT Ointment indicate that it is in the medium range of potency as compared with other topical corticosteroids.

INDICATIONS AND USAGE

WESTCORT Ointment is a medium potency corticosteroid indicated for the relief of the inflammatory and pruritic manifestations of corticosteroid responsive dermatoses.

CONTRAINDICATIONS

WESTCORT Ointment is contraindicated in those patients with a history of hypersensitivity to any of the components of the preparation.

PRECAUTIONS

General: Systemic absorption of topical corticosteroids can produce reversible hypothalamic-pituitary-adrenal (HPA) axis suppression with the potential for glucocorticosteroid insufficiency after withdrawal of treatment. Manifestations of Cushing's syndrome, hyperglycemia, and glucosuria can also be produced in some patients by systemic absorption of topical corticosteroids while on treatment.

Patients applying a topical steroid to a large surface area or to areas under occlusion should be evaluated periodically for evidence of HPA axis suppression. This may be done by using the ACTH stimulation, A.M. plasma cortisol, and urinary free cortisol tests.

WESTCORT Ointment has produced mild, reversible adrenal suppression when used under occlusion for 5 days or on extensive areas of psoriasis for 3–4 weeks.

If HPA axis suppression is noted, an attempt should be made to withdraw the drug, to reduce the frequency of application, or to substitute a less potent corticosteroid. Recovery of HPA axis function is generally prompt upon discontinuation of topical corticosteroids. Infrequently, signs and symptoms of glucocorticosteroid insufficiency may occur, requiring supplemental systemic corticosteroids. For information on systemic supplementation, see prescribing information for these products.

Pediatric patients may be more susceptible to systemic toxicity from equivalent doses due to their larger skin surface to body mass ratios. (See PRECAUTIONS—Pediatric Use)

If irritation develops, WESTCORT Ointment should be discontinued and appropriate therapy instituted. Allergic con-

tact dermatitis with corticosteroids is usually diagnosed by observing a failure to heal rather than noting a clinical exacerbation, as with most topical products not containing corticosteroids. Such an observation should be corroborated with appropriate diagnostic patch testing.
If concomitant skin infections are present or develop, an appropriate antifungal or antibacterial agent should be used. If a favorable response does not occur promptly, use of WESTCORT Ointment should be discontinued until the infection has been adequately controlled.
Information for Patients: Patients using topical corticosteroids should receive the following information and instructions:
1. This medication is to be used as directed by the physician. It is for external use only. Avoid contact with the eyes.
2. This medication should not be used for any disorder other than that for which it was prescribed.
3. The treated skin area should not be bandaged, otherwise covered or wrapped, so as to be occlusive unless directed by the physician.
4. Patients should report to their physician any signs of local adverse reactions.
5. This medication should not be used on the face, underarms, or groin areas unless directed by the physician.
6. As with other corticosteroids, therapy should be discontinued when control is achieved. If no improvement is seen within 2 weeks, contact the physician.

Laboratory Tests: The following tests may be helpful in evaluating patients for HPA axis suppression:
ACTH stimulation test
A.M. plasma cortisol test
Urinary free cortisol test
Carcinogenesis, mutagenesis, and impairment of fertility: Long-term animal studies have not been performed to evaluate the carcinogenic potential of hydrocortisone valerate. WESTCORT Ointment was shown to be non-mutagenic in the Ames-Salmonella/Microsome Plate Test.
There are no studies which assess the effects of hydrocortisone valerate on fertility and general reproductive performance.
Pregnancy: *Teratogenic Effects: Pregnancy Category C:* Corticosteroids have been shown to be teratogenic in laboratory animals when administered systematically at relatively low dosage levels. Some corticosteroids have been shown to be teratogenic after dermal application in laboratory animals.
Hydrocortisone valerate was found to be teratogenic in rabbits treated topically with a daily dose 5 times the estimated average human dose. However, there was no evidence of teratogenicity in rats treated topically with 22 times the estimated average human dose.
There are no adequate and well-controlled studies in pregnant women. WESTCORT Ointment should be used during pregnancy only if the potential benefit justifies the potential risk to the fetus.
Nursing Mothers: Systematically administered corticosteroids appear in human milk and could suppress growth, interfere with endogenous corticosteroid production, or cause other untoward effects. It is not known whether topical administration of corticosteroids could result in sufficient systemic absorption to produce detectable quantities in human milk. Because many drugs are excreted in human milk, caution should be exercised when WESTCORT Ointment is administered to a nursing woman.
Pediatric Use: Safety and effectiveness in pediatric patients have not been established. Because of a higher ratio of skin surface area to body mass, pediatric patients are at a greater risk than adults of HPA axis suppression and Cushing's syndrome when they are treated with topical corticosteroids. They are therefore also at a greater risk of adrenal insufficiency during and/or after withdrawal of treatment. Adverse effects including striae have been reported with inappropriate use of topical corticosteroids in infants and children. (See PRECAUTIONS)
HPA axis suppression, Cushing's syndrome, linear growth retardation, delayed weight gain, and intracranial hypertension have been reported in children receiving topical corticosteroids. Manifestations of adrenal suppression in children include low plasma cortisol levels, and an absence of response to ACTH stimulation. Manifestations of intracranial hypertension include bulging fontanelles, headaches, and bilateral papilledema.

ADVERSE REACTIONS
In controlled clinical trials, the total incidence of adverse reactions associated with the use of WESTCORT Ointment was approximately 12%. These include worsening of condition (2%), transient itching (2%), irritation (1%) and redness (1%).
The following additional local adverse reactions have been reported with topical corticosteroids, and they may occur more frequently with the use of occlusive dressings. These reactions are listed in an approximate decreasing order of occurrence: burning, dryness, folliculitis, acneiform eruptions, hypopigmentation, perioral dermatitis, allergic contact dermatitis, secondary infection, skin atrophy, striae, and miliaria.

OVERDOSAGE
Topically applied WESTCORT Ointment can be absorbed in sufficient amounts to produce systemic effects (see PRECAUTIONS).

DOSAGE AND ADMINISTRATION
WESTCORT Ointment should be applied to the affected area as a thin film two or three times daily depending on the severity of the condition.
As with other corticosteroids, therapy should be discontinued when control is achieved. If no improvement is seen within 2 weeks, reassessment of the diagnosis may be necessary.
WESTCORT Ointment should not be used with occlusive dressings unless directed by a physician. WESTCORT Ointment should not be applied in the diaper area if the patient requires diapers or plastic pants as these garments may constitute occlusive dressing.

HOW SUPPLIED
WESTCORT OINTMENT, 0.2% is supplied in the following tube sizes:
15 g NDC 0072-7800-15
45 g NDC 0072-7800-45
60 g NDC 0072-7800-60
Store between 59°–78°F (15°–26°C)
WESTWOOD SQUIBB™
©1995 Westwood-Squibb Pharmaceuticals Inc., Buffalo, NY, USA 14213 03-5996-0
A Bristol-Myers Squibb Company

Whitby Pharmaceuticals, Inc.

The following products previously marketed by Whitby Pharmaceuticals are now marketed by UCB Pharma, Inc. Please see UCB Pharma, Inc.

Duratuss™ ℞
Duratuss™ HD Elixir ⒸIII, ℞
Lortab® Tablets ⒸIII, ℞
Lortab® Elixir ⒸIII, ℞
Lortab® ASA ⒸIII, ℞
Theo-24® ℞
Trinsicon® ℞
Vicon®Forte ℞

Women First HealthCare, Inc.

12220 EL CAMINO REAL
SUITE 400
SAN DIEGO, CA 92130

Direct Inquiries to:
Ph: (888) 950-2246
Fax: (888) 950-2248

ORTHO-EST® ℞
(estropipate tablets, USP)

WARNINGS:
1. ESTROGENS HAVE BEEN REPORTED TO INCREASE THE RISK OF ENDOMETRIAL CARCINOMA IN POSTMENOPAUSAL WOMEN.
Close clinical surveillance of all women taking estrogens is important. Adequate diagnostic measures, including endometrial sampling when indicated, should be undertaken to rule out malignancy in all cases of undiagnosed persistent or recurring abnormal vaginal bleeding. There is no evidence that "natural" estrogens are more or less hazardous than "synthetic" estrogens at equi-estrogenic doses.
2. ESTROGENS SHOULD NOT BE USED DURING PREGNANCY.
There is no indication for estrogen therapy during pregnancy or during the immediate postpartum period. Estrogens are ineffective for the prevention or treatment of threatened, or habitual abortion. Estrogens are not indicated for the prevention of postpartum breast engorgement.
Estrogen therapy during pregnancy is associated with an increased risk of congenital defects in the reproductive organs of the fetus, and possibly other birth defects. Studies of women who received diethylstilbestrol (DES) during pregnancy have shown that female offspring have an increased risk of vaginal adenosis, squamous cell dysplasia of the uterine cervix, and clear cell vaginal cancer later in life; male offspring have an increased risk of urogenital abnormalities and possibly testicular cancer later in life. The 1985 DES Task Force concluded that use of DES during pregnancy is associated with a subsequent increased risk of breast cancer in the mothers, although a causal relationship remains unproven and the observed level of excess risk is similar to that for a number of other breast cancer risk factors.

DESCRIPTION ORTHO-EST (estropipate tablets USP), (formerly piperazine estrone sulfate), is a natural estrogenic substance prepared from purified crystalline estrone, solubilized as the sulfate and stabilized with piperazine. It is appreciably soluble in water and has almost no odor or taste—properties which are ideally suited for oral administration. The amount of piperazine in ORTHO-EST is not sufficient to exert a pharmacological action. Its addition ensures solubility, stability and uniform potency of the estrone sulfate. Chemically, estropipate, molecular weight: 436.56, is represented by estra-1,3,5(10)-trien-17-one, 3-(sulfooxy)-, compound with piperazine (1:1). The structural formula may be represented as follows:

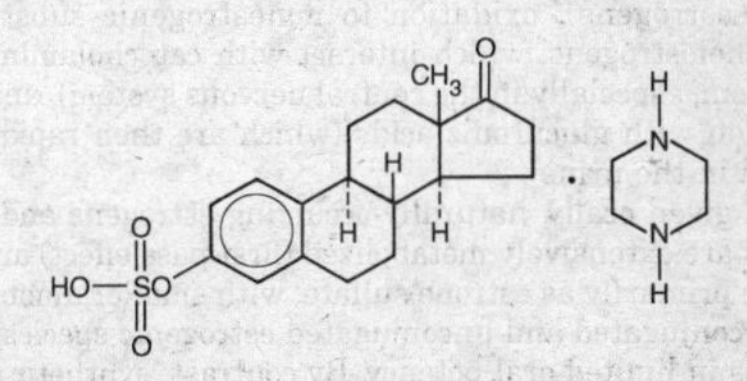

ORTHO-EST is available as tablets for oral administration containing either 0.75 mg (ORTHO-EST .625) or 1.5 mg (ORTHO-EST 1.25) estropipate. (Calculated as sodium estrone sulfate .625 mg and 1.25 mg respectively).
Inactive Ingredients:
Each tablet contains: Lactose, magnesium stearate and pregelatinized starch. ORTHO-EST 1.25 also contains: D&C Red No. 7 Calcium Lake, FD&C Blue No. 2 Aluminium Lake.

CLINICAL PHARMACOLOGY
Estrogen drug products act by regulating the transcription of a limited number of genes. Estrogens diffuse through cell membranes, distribute themselves throughout the cell, and bind to and activate the nuclear estrogen receptor, a DNA-binding protein which is found in estrogen-responsive tissues. The activated estrogen receptor binds to specific DNA sequences, or hormone-response elements, which enhance the transcription of adjacent genes and in turn lead to the observed effects. Estrogen receptors have been identified in tissues of the reproductive tract, breast, pituitary, hypothalamus, liver, and bone of women.
Estrogens are important in the development and maintenance of the female reproductive system and secondary sex characteristics. By a direct action, they cause growth and development of the uterus, Fallopian tubes, and vagina. With other hormones, such as pituitary hormones and progestrone, they cause enlargement of the breasts through promotion of ductal growth, stromal development, and the accretion of fat. Estrogens are intricately involved with other hormones, especially progestrone, in the processes of the ovulatory menstrual cycle and pregnancy, and affect the release of pituitary gonadotropins. They also contribute to the shaping of the skeleton, maintenance of tone and elasticity of urogenital structures, changes in the epiphyses of the long bones that allow for the pubertal growth spurt and its termination, and pigmentation of the nipples and genitals.
Estrogens occur naturally in several forms. The primary source of estrogen in normally cycling adult women is the ovarian follicle, which secretes 70 to 500 micrograms of estradiol daily, depending on the phase of the menstrual cycle. This is converted primarily to estrone, which circulates in roughly equal proportion to estradiol, and to small amounts of estriol. After menopause, most endogenous estrogen is produced by conversion of androstenedione, secreted by the adrenal cortex, to estrone by peripheral tissues. Thus, estrone-especially in its sulfate ester form—is the most abundant circulating estrogen in postmenopausal women. Although circulating estrogens exist in a dynamic equilibrium of metabolic interconversions, estradiol is the principal intracellular human estrogen and is substantially more potent than estrone or estriol at the receptor.
Estrogens used in therapy are well absorbed through the skin, mucous membranes, and gastrointestinal tract. When applied for a local action, absorption is usually sufficient to

Continued on next page

Ortho-Est—Cont.

cause systemic effects. When conjugated with aryl and alkyl groups for parenteral administration, the rate of absorption of oily preparations is slowed with a prolonged duration of action, such that a single intramuscular injection of estradiol valerate or estradiol cypionate is absorbed over several weeks.

Administered estrogens and their esters are handled within the body essentially the same as the endogenous hormones. Metabolic conversion of estrogens occurs primarily in the liver (first pass effect), but also at local target tissue sites. Complex metabolic processes result in a dynamic equilibrium of circulating conjugated and unconjugated estrogenic forms which are continually interconverted, especially between estrone and estradiol and between esterified and unesterified forms. Although naturally-occurring estrogens circulate in the blood largely bound to sex hormone-binding globulin and albumin, only unbound estrogens enter target tissue cells. A significant proportion of the circulating estrogen exists as sulfate conjugates, especially estrone sulfate, which serves as a circulating reservoir for the formation of more active estrogenic species. A certain proportion of the estrogen is excreted into the bile and then reabsorbed from the intestine. During this enterohepatic recirculation, estrogens are desulfated and resulfated and undergo degradation through conversion to less active estrogens (estriol and other estrogens), oxidation to nonestrogenic substances (catecholestrogens, which interact with catecholamine metabolism, especially in the central nervous system), and conjugation with glucuronic acids (which are then rapidly excreted in the urine).

When given orally, naturally-occurring estrogens and their esters are extensively metabolized (first pass effect) and circulate primarily as estrone sulfate, with smaller amounts of other conjugated and unconjugated estrogenic species. This results in limited oral potency. By contrast, synthetic estrogens, such as ethinyl estradiol and the nonsteroidal estrogens, are degraded very slowly in the liver and other tissues, which results in their high intrinsic potency. Estrogen drug products administered by non-oral routes are not subject to first-pass metabolism, but also undergo significant hepatic uptake, metabolism, and enterohepatic recycling.

INDICATIONS AND USAGE

Estrogen drug products are indicated in the:

1. Treatment of moderate to severe vasomotor symptoms associated with the menopause. There is no adequate evidence that estrogens are effective for nervous symptoms or depression which might occur during menopause and they should not be used to treat these conditions.
2. Treatment of vulval and vaginal atrophy.
3. Treatment of hypoestrogenism due to hypogonadism, castration or primary ovarian failure.
4. Prevention of osteoporosis.

Since estrogen administration is associated with risk, selection of patients should ideally be based on prospective identification of risk factors for developing osteoporosis. Unfortunately, there is no certain way to identify those women who will develop osteoporotic fractures. Most prospective studies of efficacy for this indication have been carried out in white menopausal women, without stratification by other risk factors, and tend to show a universally salutary effect on bone. Thus, patient selection must be individualized based on the balance of risks and benefits. A more favorable risk/benefit ratio exists in a hysterectomized woman because she has no risk of endometrial cancer (see BOXED WARNINGS).

Estrogen replacement therapy reduces bone resorption and retards or halts postmenopausal bone loss. Case-control studies have shown an approximately 60 percent reduction in hip and wrist fractures in women whose extrogen replacement was begun within a few years of menopause. Studies also suggest that estrogen reduces the rate of vertebral fractures. Even when started as late as 6 years after menopause, estrogen prevents further loss of bone mass for as long as the treatment is continued. The results of a double-blind, placebo-controlled two-year study have shown that treatment with one tablet of estropipate .75 daily for 25 days (of a 31-day cycle per month) prevents vertebral bone mass loss in postmenopausal women. When estrogen therapy is discontinued, bone mass declines at a rate comparable to the immediate postmenopausal period. There is no evidence that estrogen replacement therapy restores bone mass to premenopausal levels.

At skeletal maturity there are sex and race differences in both the total amount of bone present and its density, in favor of men and blacks. Thus, women are at higher risk than men because they start with less bone mass and, for several years following natural or induced menopause, the rate of bone mass decline is accelerated. White and Asian women are at higher risk than black women.

Early menopause is one of the strongest predictors for the development of osteoporosis. In addition, other factors affecting the skeleton which are associated with osteoporosis include genetic factors (small build, family history), endocrine factors (nulliparity, thyrotoxicosis, hyperparathyroidism, Cushing's syndrome, hyperprolactinemia, Type I diabetes), lifestyle (cigarette smoking, alcohol abuse, sedentary exercise habits) and nutrition (below average body weight, dietary calcium intake).

The mainstays of prevention and management of osteoporosis are estrogen, an adequate lifetime calcium intake, and exercise. Postmenopausal women absorb dietary calcium less efficiently than premenopausal women and require an average of 1500 mg/day of elemental calcium to remain in neutral calcium balance. By comparison, premenopausal women require about 1000 mg/day and the average calcium intake in the USA is 400-600 mg/day. Therefore, when not contraindicated, calcium supplementation may be helpful.

Weight-bearing exercise and nutrition may be important adjuncts to the prevention and management of osteoporosis. Immobilization and prolonged bed rest produce rapid bone loss, while weight-bearing exercise has been shown both to reduce bone loss and to increase bone mass. The optimal type and amount of physical activity that would prevent osteoporosis have not been established, however in two studies an hour of walking and running exercises twice or three times weekly significantly increased lumbar spine bone mass.

CONTRAINDICATIONS

Estrogens should not be used in individuals with any of the following conditions:

1. Known or suspected pregnancy (see BOXED WARNINGS). Estrogens may cause fetal harm when administered to a pregnant woman.
2. Undiagnosed abnormal genital bleeding.
3. Known or suspected cancer of the breast except in appropriately selected patients being treated for metastatic disease.
4. Known or suspected estrogen-dependent neoplasia.
5. Active thrombophlebitis or thromboembolic disorders.

WARNINGS

1. ***Induction of malignant neoplasms.***

Endometrial cancer. The reported endometrial cancer risk among unopposed estrogen users is about 2- to 12-fold greater than in nonusers, and appears dependent on duration of treatment and on estrogen dose. Most studies show no significant increased risk associated with use of estrogens for less than one year. The greatest risk appears associated with prolonged use—with increased risks of 15-to 24-fold for five to ten years or more. In three studies, persistence of risk was demonstrated for 8 to over 15 years after cessation of estrogen treatment. In one study a significant decrease in the incidence of endometrial cancer occurred six months after estrogen withdrawal. Concurrent progestin therapy may offset this risk but the overall health impact in postmenopausal women is not known (see PRECAUTIONS).

Breast cancer. While the majority of studies have not shown an increased risk of breast cancer in women who have ever used estrogen replacement therapy, some have reported a moderately increased risk (relative risks of 1.3- 2.0) in those taking higher doses or those taking lower doses for prolonged periods of time, especially in excess of 10 years. Other studies have not shown this relationship.

Congenital lesions with malignant potential. Estrogen therapy during pregnancy is associated with an increased risk of fetal congenital reproductive tract disorders, and possibly other birth defects. Studies of women who received DES during pregnancy have shown that female offspring have an increased risk of vaginal adenosis, squamous cell dysplasia of the uterine cervix, and clear cell vaginal cancer later in life; male offspring have an increased risk of urogenital abnormalities and possibly testicular cancer later in life. Although some of these changes are benign, others are precursors of malignancy.

2. ***Gallbladder disease.*** Two studies have reported a 2- to 4-fold increase in the risk of gallbladder disease requiring surgery in women receiving postmenopausal estrogens.

3. ***Cardiovascular disease.*** Large doses of estrogen (5 mg conjugated estrogens per day), comparable to those used to treat cancer of the prostate and breast, have been shown in a large prospective clinical trial in men to increase the risks of nonfatal myocardial infarction, pulmonary embolism, and thrombophlebitis. These risks cannot necessarily be extrapolated from men to women. However, to avoid the theoretical cardiovascular risk to women caused by high estrogen doses, the dose for estrogen replacement therapy should not exceed the lowest effective dose.

4. ***Elevated blood pressure.*** Occasional blood pressure increases during estrogen replacement therapy have been attributed to idiosyncratic reactions to estrogens. More often, blood pressure has remained the same or has dropped. One study showed that postmenopausal estrogen users have higher blood pressure than nonusers. Two other studies showed slightly lower blood pressure among estrogen users compared to nonusers. Postmenopausal estrogen use does not increase the risk of stroke. Nonetheless, blood pressure should be monitored at regular intervals with estrogen use.

5. ***Hypercalcemia.*** Administration of estrogens may lead to severe hypercalcemia in patients wtih breast cancer and bone metastases. If this occurs, the drug should be stopped and appropriate measures taken to reduce the serum calcium level.

PRECAUTIONS

A. *General*

1. **Addition of a progestin.** Studies of the addition of a progestin for seven or more days of a cycle of estrogen administration have reported a lowered incidence of endometrial hyperplasia which would otherwise be induced by estrogen treatment. Morphological and biochemical studies of endometrium suggest that 10 to 14 days of progestin are needed to provide maximal maturation of the endometrium and to eliminate any hyperplastic changes. There are possible additional risks which may be associated with the inclusion of progestins in estrogen replacement regimens. These include: (1) adverse effects on lipoprotein metabloism (lowering HDL and raising LDL) which may diminish the possible cardioprotective effect of estrogen therapy (see PRECAUTIONS, D.4., below); (2) impairment of glucose tolerance; and (3) possible enhancement of mitotic activity in breast epithelial tissue (although few epidemiological data are available to address this point). The choice of progestin, its dose, and its regimen may be important in minimizing these adverse effects, but these issues remain to be clarified.

2. **Physical examination.** A complete medical and family history should be taken prior to the initiation of any estrogen therapy. The pretreatment and periodic physical examinations should include special reference to blood pressure, breasts, abdomen, and pelvic organs, and should include a Papanicolaou smear. As a general rule, estrogen should not be prescribed for longer than one year without reexamining the patient.

3. **Hypercoagulability.** Some studies have shown that women taking estrogen replacement therapy have hypercoagulability, primarily related to decreased antithrombin activity. This effect appears dose- and duration-dependent and is less pronounced than that associated with oral contraceptive use. Also, postmenopausal women tend to have increased coagulation parameters at baseline compared to premenopausal women. There is some suggestion that low dose postmenopausal mestranol may increase the risk of thromboembolism, although the majority of studies (of primarily conjugated estrogens users) report no such increase. There is insufficient information on hypercoagulability in women who have had previous thromboembolic disease.

4. **Familial hyperlipoproteinemia.** Estrogen therapy may be associated with massive elevations of plasma triglycerides leading to pancreatitis and other complications in patients with familial defects of lipoprotein metabolism.

5. **Fluid retention.** Because estrogens may cause some degree of fluid retention, conditions which might be exacerbated by this factor, such as asthma, epilepsy, migraine, and cardiac or renal dysfunction, require careful observation.

6. **Uterine bleeding and mastodynia.** Certain patients may develop undesirable manifestations of estrogenic stimulation, such as abnormal uterine bleeding and mastodynia.

7. **Impaired liver function.** Estrogen may be poorly metabolized in patients with impaired liver function and should be administered with caution.

B. *Information for the Patient.* See text of Patient Package Insert below.

C. *Laboratory Tests.* Estrogen administration should generally be guided by clinical response at the smallest dose, rather than laboratory monitoring, for relief of symptoms for those indications in which symptoms are observable.

D. *Drug/Laboratory Test Interactions.*

Accelerated prothrombin time, partial thromboplastin time, and platelet aggregation time; increased platelet count; increased factors II, VII antigen, VIII antigen, VIII coagulant activity, IX, X, XII, VII—X complex, II—VII—X complex, and beta-thromboglobulin; decreased levels of anti-factor Xa and antithrombin III, decreased antithrombin III activity; increased levels of fibrinogen and fibrinogen activity; increased plasminogen antigen and activity.

Increased thyroid-binding globulin (TBG) leading to increased circulating total thyroid hormone, as measured by protein-bound iodine (PBI), T4 levels (by column or by radioimmunoassay) or T3 levels by radioimmunoassay. T3 resin uptake is decreased, reflecting the elevated TBG. Free T4 and free T3 concentrations are unaltered.

Other binding proteins may be elevated in serum, i.e., corticosteroid binding globulin (CBG), sex hormone-binding globulin (SHBG), leading to increased circulating corticosteroids and sex steroids respectively. Free or biologically active hormone concentrations are unchanged. Other plasma proteins may be increased (angiotensinogen/renin substrate, alpha-I-antitrypsin, ceruloplasmin).

Increased plasma HDL and HDL-2 subfraction concentrations, reduced LDL cholesterol concentration, increased triglycerides levels.

Impaired glucose tolerance.

Reduced response to metyrapone test.

Reduced serum folate concentration.

E. *Carcinogenesis, Mutagenesis, and Impairment of Fertility.* Long-term continuous administration of natural and synthetic estrogens in certain animal species increases the frequency of carcinomas of the breast, uterus, cervix, vagina, testis, and liver. See "CONTRAINDICATIONS" and "WARNINGS" sections.

F. *Pregnancy Category X.* Estrogens should not be used during pregnancy. See "CONTRAINDICATIONS" and BOXED WARNING.

G. *Nursing Mothers.* As a general principle, the administration of any drug to nursing mothers should be done only when clearly necessary since many drugs are excreted in human milk. In addition, estrogen administration to nursing mothers has been shown to decrease the quantity and quality of the milk.

ADVERSE REACTIONS

The following additional adverse reactions have been reported with estrogen therapy (see WARNINGS regarding induction of neoplasia, adverse effects on the fetus, increased incidence of gallbladder disease, cardiovascular disease, elevated blood pressure, and hypercalcemia).

1. *Genitourinary system.*
Changes in vaginal bleeding pattern and abnormal withdrawal bleeding or flow; breakthrough bleeding, spotting.
Increase in size of uterine leiomyomata.
Vaginal candidiasis.
Change in amount of cervical secretion.
2. *Breast.*
Tenderness, enlargement.
3. *Gastrointestinal.*
Nausea, vomiting.
Abdominal cramps, bloating.
Cholestatic jaundice.
Increased incidence of gallbladder disease.
4. *Skin.*
Chloasma or melasma that may persist when drug is discontinued.
Erythema multiforme.
Erythema nodosum.
Hemorrhagic eruption.
Loss of scalp hair.
Hirsuitism.
5. *Eyes.*
Steepening of corneal curvature.
Intolerance to contact lenses.
6. *Central Nervous System.*
Headache, migraine, dizziness.
Mental depression.
Chorea.
7. *Miscellaneous.*
Increase or decrease in weight.
Reduced carbohydrate tolerance.
Aggravation of porphyria.
Edema.
Changes in libido.

OVERDOSAGE

Serious ill effects have not been reported following acute ingestion of large doses of estrogen-containing oral contraceptives by young children. Overdosage of estrogen may cause nausea and vomiting, and withdrawal bleeding may occur in females.

DOSAGE AND ADMINISTRATION

1. For treatment of moderate to severe vasomotor symptoms, vulval and vaginal atrophy associated with the menopause, the lowest dose and regimen that will control symptoms should be chosen and medication should be discontinued as promptly as possible.
Attempts to discontinue or taper medication should be made at 3-month to 6-month intervals.
Usual dosage ranges:
Vasomotor symptoms—0.75 mg to 6 mg estropipate per day. The lowest dose that will control symptoms should be chosen. If the patient has not menstruated within the last two months or more, cyclic administration is started arbitrarily. If the patient is menstruating, cyclic administration is started on day 5 of bleeding.
Vulval and vaginal atrophy—0.75 mg to 6 mg estropipate daily, depending upon the tissue response of the individual patient. The lowest dose that will control symptoms should be chosen. Administer cyclically.
2. For treatment of female hypoestrogenism due to hypogonadism, castration, or primary ovarian failure.
Usual dosage ranges:
Female hypogonadism—A daily dose of 1.5 mg to 9 mg estropipate may be given for the first three weeks of a theoretical cycle, followed by a rest period of eight to ten days. The lowest dose that will control symptoms should be chosen. If bleeding does not occur by the end of this period, the same dosage schedule is repeated. The number of courses of estrogen therapy necessary to produce bleeding may vary depending on the responsiveness of the endometrium. If satisfactory withdrawal bleeding does not occur, an oral progestogen may be given in addition to estrogen during the third week of the cycle.

Female castration or primary ovarian failure—A daily dose of 1.5 mg to 9 mg estropipate may be given for the first three weeks of a theoretical cycle, followed by a rest period of eight to ten days. Adjust dosage upward or downward according to the severity of symptoms and response of the patient. For maintenance, adjust dosage to lowest level that will provide effective control.
Treated patients with an intact uterus should be monitored closely for signs of endometrial cancer and appropriate diagnostic measures should be taken to rule out malignancy in the event of persistent or recurring abnormal vaginal bleeding.
3. For prevention of osteoporosis. A daily dose of one ORTHO-EST .625 (0.75 mg estropipate) tablet for 25 days of a 31-day cycle per month.

HOW SUPPLIED

ORTHO-EST (estropipate tablets, USP) is supplied as ORTHO-EST .625 (0.75 mg estropipate; calculated as sodium estrone sulfate 0.625 mg), white, diamond-shaped tablets, scored on one side and imprinted with WFHC 101 on the other, NDC 64248-101-01; and ORTHO-EST 1.25 (1.5 mg estropipate; calculated as sodium estrone sulfate 1.25 mg), lavender, diamond-shaped tablets, scored on one side and imprinted with WFHC 102 on the other, NDC 64248-102-01. Both tablet sizes are available in bottles of 100.
Tablets are standardized to provide uniform estrone activity and are scored to provide dosage flexibility.
Dispense in tight, light-resistant containers as defined in the USP.
Store below 30°C (86°F).

PATIENT INFORMATION

WHAT YOU SHOULD KNOW ABOUT ESTROGENS

ORTHO-EST
(estropipate tablets, USP)

INTRODUCTION

This leaflet describes when and how to use estrogens, and the risks and benefits of estrogen treatment.
Estrogens have important benefits but also some risks. You must decide, with your doctor, whether the risks to you of estrogen use are acceptable because of their benefits. If you use estrogens, check with your doctor to be sure you are using the lowest possible dose that works, and that you do not use them longer than necessary. How long you need to use estrogens will depend on the reason for use.

WARNINGS

ESTROGENS INCREASE THE RISK OF CANCER OF THE UTERUS IN WOMEN WHO HAVE HAD THEIR MENOPAUSE ("CHANGE OF LIFE").
If you use any estrogen-containing drug, it is important to visit your doctor regularly and report any unusual vaginal bleeding right away. Vaginal bleeding after menopause may be a warning sign of uterine cancer. Your doctor should evaluate any unusual vaginal bleeding to find out the cause.
ESTROGENS SHOULD NOT BE USED DURING PREGNANCY.
Estrogens do not prevent miscarriage (spontaneous abortion) and are not needed in the days following childbirth. If you take estrogens during pregnancy, your unborn child has a greater than usual chance of having birth defects. The risk of developing these defects is small, but clearly larger than the risk in children whose mothers did not take estrogens during pregnancy. These birth defects may affect the baby's urinary system and sex organs. Daughters born to mothers who took DES (an estrogen drug) have a higher than usual chance of developing cancer of the vagina or cervix when they become teenagers or young adults. Sons may have a higher than usual chance of developing cancer of the testicles when they become teenagers or young adults.

USES OF ESTROGEN

(Not every estrogen drug is approved for every use listed in this section. If you want to know which of these possible uses are approved for the medicine prescribed for you, ask your doctor or pharmacist to show you the professional labeling. You can also look up the specific estrogen product in a book called the "Physicians' Desk Reference", which is available in many book stores and public libraries. Generic drugs carry virtually the same labeling information as their brand name versions.)

• **To reduce moderate or severe menopausal symptoms.**
Estrogens are hormones made by the ovaries of normal women. Between ages 45 and 55, the ovaries normally stop making estrogens. This leads to a drop in body estrogen levels which causes the "change of life" or menopause (the end of monthly menstrual periods). If both ovaries are removed during an operation before natural menopause takes place, the sudden drop in estrogen levels causes "surgical menopause".
When the estrogen levels begin dropping, some women develop very uncomfortable symptoms, such as feelings of

warmth in the face, neck, and chest, or sudden intense episodes of heat and sweating ("hot flashes" or "hot flushes"). Using estrogen drugs can help the body adjust to lower estrogen levels and reduce these symptoms. Most women have only mild menopausal symptoms or none at all and do not need to use estrogen drugs for these symptoms. Others may need to take estrogens for a few months while their bodies adjust to lower estrogen levels. The majority of women do not need estrogen replacement for longer than six months for these symptoms.

• **To treat vulval and vaginal atrophy** (itching, burning, dryness in or around the vagina, difficulty or burning on urination) associated with menopause.
• **To treat certain conditions in which a young women's ovaries do not produce enough estrogen naturally.**
• **To treat certain types of abnormal vaginal bleeding due to hormonal imbalance when your doctor has found no serious cause of the bleeding.**
• **To treat certain cancers in special situations, in men and women.**
• **To prevent thinning of bones.**

Osteoporosis is a thinning of the bones that makes them weaker and allows them to break more easily. The bones of the spine, wrists and hips break more often in osteoporosis. Both men and women start to lose bone mass after about age 40, but women lose bone mass faster after the menopause. Using estrogens after the menopause slows down bone thinning and may prevent bones from breaking. Lifelong adequate calcium intake, either in the diet (such as dairy products) or by calcium supplements (to reach a total daily intake of 1000 milligrams per day before menopause or 1500 milligrams per day after menopause), may help to prevent osteoporosis. Regular weight-bearing exercise (like walking and running for an hour, two or three times a week) may also help to prevent osteoporosis. Before you change your calcium intake or exercise habits, it is important to discuss these lifestyle changes with your doctor to find out if they are safe for you.

Since estrogen use has some risks, only women who are likely to develop osteoporosis should use estrogens for prevention. Women who are likely to develop osteoporosis often have the following characteristics: white or Asian race, slim, cigarette smokers, and a family history of osteoporosis in a mother, sister, or aunt. Women who have relatively early menopause, often because their ovaries were removed during an operation ("surgical menopause"), are more likely to develop osteoporosis than women whose menopause happens at the average age.

WHO SHOULD NOT USE ESTROGENS

Estrogens should not be used:
• **During pregnancy (see BOXED WARNING).**
If you think you may be pregnant, do not use any form of estrogen-containing drug. Using estrogens while you are pregnant may cause your unborn child to have birth defects. Estrogens do not prevent miscarriage.
• **If you have unusual vaginal bleeding which has not been evaluated by your doctor (see BOXED WARNING).**
• Unusual vaginal bleeding can be a warning sign of cancer of the uterus, especially if it happens after menopause. Your doctor must find out the cause of the bleeding so that he or she can recommend the proper treatment. Taking estrogens without visiting your doctor can cause you serious harm if your vaginal bleeding is caused by cancer of the uterus.
• **If you have had cancer.**
Since estrogens increase the risk of certain types of cancer, you should not use estrogens if you have ever had cancer of the breast or uterus, unless your doctor recommends that the drug may help in the cancer treatment. (For certain patients with breast or prostate cancer, estrogens may help.)
• **If you have any circulation problems.**
Estrogen drugs should not be used except in unusually special situations in which your doctor judges that you need estrogen therapy so much that the risks are acceptable. Men and women with abnormal blood clotting conditions should avoid estrogen use (see DANGERS OF ESTROGENS, below).
• **When they do not work.**
During menopause, some women develop nervous symptoms or depression. Estrogens do not relieve these symptoms. You may have heard that taking estrogens for years after menopause will keep your skin soft and supple and keep you feeling young. There is no evidence for these claims and such long-term estrogen use may have serious risks.
• **After childbirth or when breastfeeding a baby.**
Estrogens should not be used to try to stop the breasts from filling with milk after a baby is born. Such treatment may increase the risk of developing blood clots (see DANGERS OF ESTROGENS, below).
If you are breastfeeding, you should avoid using any drugs because many drugs pass through to the baby in the milk. While nursing a baby, you should take drugs only on the advice of your health care provider.

Continued on next page

Ortho-Est—Cont.

DANGERS OF ESTROGENS

- **Cancer of the uterus.**

Your risk of developing cancer of the uterus gets higher the longer you use estrogens and the larger doses you use. One study showed that after women stop taking estrogens, this higher cancer risk quickly returns to the usual level of risk (as if you had never used estogen therapy). Three other studies showed that the cancer risk stayed high for 8 to more than 15 years after stopping estrogen treatment. **Because of this risk, IT IS IMPORTANT TO TAKE THE LOWEST DOSE THAT WORKS AND TO TAKE IT ONLY AS LONG AS YOU NEED IT.**

Using progestin therapy together with estrogen therapy may reduce the higher risk of uterine cancer related to estrogen use (but see OTHER INFORMATION, below).

If you have had your uterus removed (total hysterectomy), there is no danger of developing cancer of the uterus.

- **Cancer of the breast.**

Most studies have not shown a higher risk of breast cancer in women who have ever used estrogens. However, some studies have reported that breast cancer developed more often (up to twice the usual rate) in women who used estrogens for long periods of time (especially more than 10 years), or who used higher doses for shorter time periods.

Regular breast examinations by a health professional and monthly self-examination are recommended for all women.

- **Gallbladder disease.**

Women who use estrogens after menopause are more likely to develop gallbladder disease needing surgery than women who do not use estrogens.

- **Abnormal blood clotting.**

Taking estrogens may cause changes in your blood clotting system. These changes allow the blood to clot more easily, possibly allowing clots to form in your bloodstream. If blood clots do form in your bloodstream, they can cut off the blood supply to vital organs, causing serious problems. These problems may include a stroke (by cutting off blood to the brain), a heart attack (by cutting off blood to the heart), a pulmonary embolus (by cutting off blood to the lungs), or other problems. Any of these conditions may cause death or serious long-term disability. However, most studies of low dose estrogen usage by women do not show an increased risk of these complications.

SIDE EFFECTS

In addition to the risks listed above, the following side effects have been reported with estrogen use:

Nausea and vomiting

Breast tenderness or enlargement.

Enlargement of benign tumors ("fibroids") of the uterus.

Retention of excess fluid. This may make some conditions worsen, such as asthma, epilepsy, migraine, heart disease, or kidney disease.

A spotty darkening of the skin, particularly on the face.

REDUCING RISK OF ESTROGEN USE

If you use estrogens, you can reduce your risks by doing these things:

- **See your doctor regularly.** While you are using estrogens, it is important to visit your doctor at least once a year for a check up. If you develop vaginal bleeding while taking estrogens, you may need further evaluation. If members of your family have had breast cancer or if you have ever had breast lumps or an abnormal mammogram (breast X ray), you may need to have more frequent breast examinations.
- **Reassess your need for estrogens.** You and your doctor should reevaluate whether or not you still need estrogens at least every six months.
- **Be alert for signs of trouble.** If any of these warning signals (or any other unusual symptoms) happen while you are using estrogens, call your doctor immediately:

Abnormal bleeding from the vagina (possible uterine cancer).

Pains in the calves or chest, sudden shortness of breath, or coughing blood (possible clot in the legs, heart, or lungs).

Severe headache or vomiting, dizziness, faintness, changes in vision or speech, weakness or numbness of an arm or leg (possible clot in the brain or eye).

Breast lumps (possible breast cancer, ask your doctor or health professional to show you how to examine your breasts monthly).

Yellowing of the skin or eyes (possible liver problem).

Pain, swelling, or tenderness in the abdomen (possible gallbladder problem).

OTHER INFORMATION

Some doctors may choose to prescribe a progestin, a different hormonal drug, for you to take together with your estrogen treatment. Progestins lower your risk of developing endometrial hyperplasia (a possible pre-cancerous condition of the uterus) while using estrogens. Taking estrogens and progestins together may also protect you from the higher risk of uterine cancer, but this has not been clearly established. Combined use of progestin and estrogen treatment may have additional risks, however. The possible risks include unhealthy effects on blood fats (especially a lowering of HDL cholesterol, the "good" blood fat which protects against heart disease risk), unhealthy effects on blood sugar (which might worsen a diabetic condition), and a possible further increase in the breast cancer risk which may be associated with long-term estrogen use. The type of progestin drug used and its dosage schedule may be important in minimizing these effects.

Your doctor has prescribed this drug for you and you alone. Do not give the drug to anyone else.

If you will be taking calcium supplements as part of the treatment to help prevent osteoporosis, check with your doctor about how much to take.

Keep this and all drugs out of the reach of children. In case of overdose, call your doctor, hospital or poison control center immediately.

This leaflet provides a summary of the most important information about estrogens. If you want more information, ask your doctor or pharmacist to show you the professional labeling. The professional labeling is also published in a book called the "Physicians' Desk Reference," which is available in book stores and public libraries. Generic drugs carry virtually the same labeling information as their brand name versions.

HOW SUPPLIED

ORTHO-EST .625 (estropipate tablets USP, 0.75 mg) is a white, diamond-shaped tablet.

ORTHO-EST 1.25 (estropipate tablets USP, 1.5 mg) is a lavender, diamond-shaped tablet.

Distributed by:
Women First HealthCare, Inc.
San Diego, CA 92130
Manufactured by:
OMJ Pharmaceuticals, Inc.
Manati, Puerto Rico 00674
© OMJ 1998
634-20-181-1

Shown in Product Identification Guide, page 343

Wyeth-Ayerst Laboratories

Division of American Home Products Corporation
P.O. BOX 8299
PHILADELPHIA, PA 19101

Direct General Inquiries to:
(610) 688-4400

For Medical Information Contact:
Medical Affairs
Day: (800) 934-5556
8:30 AM to 4:30 PM (Eastern Standard Time),
Weekdays only
In Emergencies:
Day: (800) 934-5556
Night: (610) 688-4400
(Emergencies only;
non-emergencies should wait until the next day)

For prescribing information for products of Elkins-Sinn Incorporated, see page 963 of the 1999 PDR; ESI Lederle Inc. see page 992; Lederle Laboratories, see page 1510; and page 2634 for products of A.H. Robins Company. Information for these products can also be obtained by writing to Professional Service, Wyeth-Ayerst Laboratories, P.O. Box 8299, Philadelphia, PA 19101, or by contacting your local Wyeth-Ayerst representative.

Product Identification Codes

The following is a numerical list of National Drug Code (NDC) numbers with their corresponding product names for all oral solid dosage forms listed under Wyeth-Ayerst Laboratories.

Numerical Listing

PRODUCTS MANUFACTURED BY WYETH LABORATORIES INC.

Product Ident. Code	Product
1	Equanil® (meprobamate) Tablet 400 mg. CIV
2	Equanil® (meprobamate) Tablet 200 mg. CIV
6	Serax® (oxazepam) Capsule 15 mg. CIV
13	Amphojel® [dried aluminum hydroxide gel (hydrated alumina)] Tablet 0.6 Gm. (10 gr.)
19	Phenergan® (promethazine HCl) Tablet 12.5 mg.
27	Phenergan® (promethazine HCl) Tablet 25 mg.
51	Serax® (oxazepam) Capsule 10 mg. CIV
52	Serax® (oxazepam) Capsule 30 mg. CIV
56	Ovral® (each tablet contains 0.5 mg. norgestrel with 0.05 mg. ethinyl estradiol) Tablet, white
62	Ovrette® (norgestrel) Tablet
64	Ativan® (lorazepam) Tablet 1 mg. CIV
65	Ativan® (lorazepam) Tablet 2 mg. CIV
73	Wytensin® (guanabenz acetate) Tablet 4 mg.
74	Wytensin® (guanabenz acetate) Tablet 8 mg.
75	Nordette®-21 (each tablet contains 0.15 mg. levonorgestrel with 0.03 mg. ethinyl estradiol) Tablet
78	Lo/Ovral® (each tablet contains 0.3 mg. norgestrel with 0.03 mg. ethinyl estradiol) Tablet, white
81	Ativan® (lorazepam) Tablet 0.5 mg. CIV
85	Wygesic® (each tablet contains 65 mg. propoxyphene HCl, U.S.P., and 650 mg. acetaminophen, U.S.P.) Tablet CIV
91	Equagesic® (meprobamate with aspirin) Tablet
119	Amphojel® [dried aluminum hydroxide gel (hydrated alumina)] Tablet 0.3 Gm. (5 gr.)
227	Phenergan® (promethazine HCl) Tablet 50 mg.
261	Mepergan® Fortis (meperidine HCl and promethazine HCl) Capsule CII
308	Meperidine HCl Tablet USP 50 mg. CII
317	Serax® (oxazepam) Tablet 15 mg. CIV
445	Ovral®-28 pink inert tablet
486	Nordette®-28, Lo/Ovral®-28 pink inert tablet
559	Wymox® (amoxicillin) Capsule 250 mg.
560	Wymox® (amoxicillin) Capsule 500 mg.
650	Alesse™-28 green inert tablet
690	Oruvail® (ketoprofen extended-release capsules) 200 mg.
701	Effexor® (venlafaxine HCl) Tablet 25 mg.
703	Effexor® (venlafaxine HCl) Tablet 50 mg.
704	Effexor® (venlafaxine HCl) Tablet 75 mg.
705	Effexor® (venlafaxine HCl) Tablet 100 mg.
771	Ismo® (isosorbide dinitrate) Tablet 20 mg.
781	Effexor® (venlafaxine HCl) Tablet 37.5 mg.
821	Oruvail® (ketoprofen extended-release capsules) 100 mg.
822	Oruvail® (ketoprofen extended-release capsules) 150 mg.
833	Effexor® XR (venlafaxine HCl) Extended-Release Capsules, 75 mg.
836	Effexor® XR (venlafaxine HCl) Extended-Release Capsules, 150 mg.
837	Effexor® XR (venlafaxine HCl) Extended-Release Capsules, 37.5 mg.
901	Naprelan® (naproxen sodium controlled-release tablet) 375 mg.
902	Naprelan® (naproxen sodium controlled-release tablet) 500 mg.
912	Alesse™ (each tablet contains 0.10 mg levonorgestrel and 0.02 mg ethinyl estradiol), pink
2511	Ovral®-28 Pilpak® (21 white tablets each containing 0.5 mg. norgestrel with 0.05 mg. ethinyl estradiol and 7 pink inert tablets)
2514	Lo/Ovral®-28 Pilpak® (21 white tablets each containing 0.3 mg. norgestrel with 0.03 mg. ethinyl estradiol and 7 pink inert tablets)
2533	Nordette®-28 Pilpak® (21 light-orange tablets each containing 0.15 mg. levonorgestrel with 0.03 mg ethinyl estradiol and 7 pink inert tablets)
2535	Triphasil®-21 Tablets (levonorgestrel and ethinyl estradiol tablets—triphasic regimen)
2536	Triphasil®-28 Tablets (levonorgestrel and ethinyl estradiol tablets—triphasic regimen)
4126	Isordil® Sublingual Tablet 5 mg
4130	Trecator®-SC (ethionamide) Tablet 250 mg
4132	Surmontil® (trimipramine maleate) Capsule 25 mg
4133	Surmontil® (trimipramine maleate) Capsule 50 mg
4139	Isordil® (isosorbide dinitrate) Sublingual Tablet 2.5 mg
4148	Cyclospasmol® (cyclandelate) Capsule 400 mg
4152	Isordil® (isosorbide dinitrate) 5 Titradose Tablet 5 mg
4153	Isordil® (isosorbide dinitrate) 10 Titradose Tablet 10 mg
4154	Isordil® (isosorbide dinitrate) 20 Titradose Tablet 20 mg
4158	Surmontil® (trimipramine) Capsule 100 mg
4159	Isordil® (isosorbide dinitrate) 30 Titradose Tablet 30 mg
4161	Isordil® (isosorbide dinitrate) Sublingual Tablet 10 mg
4177	Sectral® (acebutolol HCl) Capsule 200 mg
4179	Sectral® (acebutolol HCl) Capsule 400 mg
4181	Orudis® (ketoprofen capsule) 50 mg
4186	Orudis® (ketoprofen capsule) 25 mg
4187	Orudis® (ketoprofen capsule) 75 mg
4188	Cordarone® (amiodarone) Tablet 200 mg

4191 Synalgos®-DC (each capsule contains 16 mg. dihydrocodeine bitartrate, 356.4 mg. aspirin, and 30 mg. caffeine) Capsule

4192 Isordil® (isosorbide dinitrate) 40 Titradose Tablet 40 mg

PRODUCTS MANUFACTURED BY AYERST LABORATORIES INC.

243 Atromid-S® (clofibrate) Capsule 500 mg.
421 Inderal® (propranolol HCl) Tablet 10 mg.
422 Inderal® (propranolol HCl) Tablet 20 mg.
424 Inderal® (propranolol HCl) Tablet 40 mg.
426 Inderal® (propranolol HCl) Tablet 60 mg.
428 Inderal® (propranolol HCl) Tablet 80 mg.
435 Grisactin® Ultra (griseofulvin ultramicrosize) Tablet 250 mg.
437 Grisactin® Ultra (griseofulvin ultramicrosize) Tablet 330 mg.
443 Grisactin® 250 (griseofulvin, microsize) Capsule 250 mg.
444 Grisactin® 500 (griseofulvin, microsize) Tablet 500 mg.
455 Inderide® LA (each capsule contains 80 mg. Inderal® LA [propranolol HCl] and 50 mg. hydrochlorothiazide) Capsule
457 Inderide® LA (each capsule contains 120 mg. Inderal® LA [propranolol HCl] and 50 mg. hydrochlorothiazide) Capsule
459 Inderide® LA (each capsule contains 160 mg. Inderal® LA [propranolol HCl] and 50 mg. hydrochlorothiazide) Capsule
470 Inderal® LA (propranolol HCl) Capsule 60 mg.
471 Inderal® LA (propranolol HCl) Capsule 80 mg.
473 Inderal® LA (propranolol HCl) Capsule 120 mg.
479 Inderal® LA (propranolol HCl) Capsule 160 mg.
484 Inderide® (each tablet contains 40 mg. Inderal® [propranolol HCl] and 25 mg. hydrochlorothiazide) Tablet
488 Inderide® (each tablet contains 80 mg. Inderal® [propranolol HCl] and 25 mg. hydrochlorothiazide) Tablet
702 Diucardin® (hydroflumethiazide) Tablet 50 mg.
738 Lodine® (etodolac capsule) 200 mg.
739 Lodine® (etodolac capsule) 300 mg.
761 Lodine® (etodolac tablet) 400 mg.
787 Lodine® (etodolac tablet) 500 mg.
809 Antabuse® (disulfiram) Tablet 250 mg.
810 Antabuse® (disulfiram) Tablet 500 mg.
829 Lodine® XL (etodolac extended-release tablet) 400 mg.
831 Lodine® XL (etodolac extended-release tablet) 600 mg.
839 Lodine® XL (etodolac extended-release tablet) 500 mg.
864 Premarin® (conjugated estrogens tablets, USP) Tablet 0.9 mg.
865 Premarin® (conjugated estrogens tablets, USP) Tablet 2.5 mg.
866 Premarin® (conjugated estrogens tablets, USP) Tablet 1.25 mg.
867 Premarin® (conjugated estrogens tablets, USP) Tablet 0.625 mg.
868 Premarin® (conjugated estrogens tablets, USP) Tablet 0.3 mg.
875 Prempro™ (conjugated estrogens/medroxyprogesterone acetate 0.625 mg./2.5 mg. [continuous regimen] Tablets)
975 Prempro (conjugated estrogens/medroxyprogesterone acetate 0.625 mg./5 mg [continuous regimen] Tablets)
2573 Premphase® (conjugated estrogens/medroxyprogesterone acetate 0.625 mg./5 mg. [sequential regimen] Tablets)

ALESSE™-21 Tablets ℞
[ă 'lĕs]

levonorgestrel and ethinyl estradiol tablets

Patients should be counseled that this product does not protect against HIV infection (AIDS) and other sexually transmitted diseases.

DESCRIPTION
21 pink active tablets each containing 0.10 mg of levonorgestrel, d(-)-13β-ethyl-17α-ethinyl-17β-hydroxygon-4-en-3-one, a totally synthetic progestogen, and 0.02 mg of ethinyl estradiol, 17α-ethinyl-1,3,5(10)-estratriene-3, 17β-diol. The inactive ingredients present are cellulose, hydroxypropyl methylcellulose, iron oxide, lactose, magnesium stearate, polacrilin potassium, polyethylene glycol, titanium dioxide, and wax E.
[See chemical structures in next column]

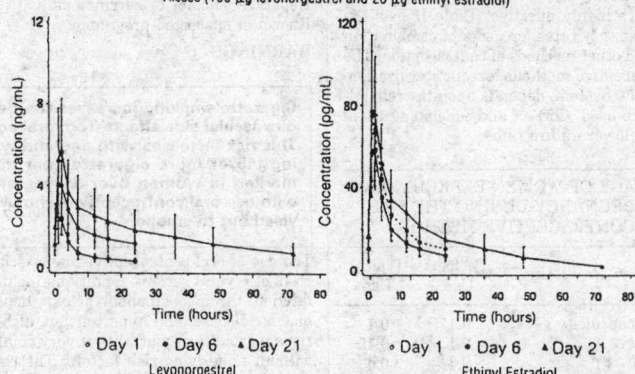

Levonorgestrel

Ethinyl Estradiol

CLINICAL PHARMACOLOGY
Combination oral contraceptives act by suppression of gonadotropins. Although the primary mechanism of this action is inhibition of ovulation, other alterations include changes in the cervical mucus (which increase the difficulty of sperm entry into the uterus) and the endometrium (which reduce the likelihood of implantation).

PHARMACOKINETICS
Absorption
No specific investigation of the absolute bioavailability of Alesse in humans has been conducted. However, literature indicates that levonorgestrel is rapidly and completely absorbed after oral administration (bioavailability about 100%) and is not subject to first-pass metabolism. Ethinyl estradiol is rapidly and almost completely absorbed from the gastrointestinal tract but, due to first-pass metabolism in gut mucosa and liver, the bioavailability of ethinyl estradiol is between 38% and 48%.

After a single dose of Alesse to 22 women under fasting conditions, maximum serum concentrations of levonorgestrel are 2.8 ± 0.9 ng/mL (mean ± SD) at 1.6 ± 0.9 hours. At steady state, attained from day 19 onwards, maximum levonorgestrel concentrations of 6.0 ± 2.7 ng/mL are reached at 1.5 ± 0.5 hours after the daily dose. The minimum serum levels of levonorgestrel at steady state are 1.9 ± 1.0 ng/mL. Observed levonorgestrel concentrations increased from day 1 (single dose) to days 6 and 21 (multiple doses) by 34% and 96%, respectively (Figure 1). Unbound levonorgestrel concentrations increased from day 1 to days 6 and 21 by 25% and 83%, respectively. The kinetics of total levonorgestrel are non-linear due to an increase in binding of levonorgestrel to sex hormone binding globulin (SHBG), which is attributed to increased SHBG levels that are induced by the daily administration of ethinyl estradiol.
Following a single dose, maximum serum concentrations of ethinyl estradiol of 62 ± 21 pg/mL are reached at 1.5 ± 0.5 hours. At steady state, attained from at least day 6 onwards, maximum concentrations of ethinyl estradiol were 77 ± 30 pg/mL and were reached at 1.3 ± 0.7 hours after the daily dose. The minimum serum levels of ethinyl estradiol at steady state are 10.5 ± 5.1 pg/mL. Ethinyl estradiol concentrations did not increase from days 1 to 6, but did increase by 19% from days 1 to 21 (Figure 1).
[See Figure 1 above]
Table I provides a summary of levonorgestrel and ethinyl estradiol pharmacokinetic parameters.
[See table 1 at bottom of next page]
Distribution
Levonorgestrel in serum is primarily bound to SHBG. Ethinyl estradiol is about 97% bound to plasma albumin. Ethinyl estradiol does not bind to SHBG, but induces SHBG synthesis.
Metabolism
Levonorgestrel: The most important metabolic pathway occurs in the reduction of the Δ4-3-oxo group and hydroxylation at positions 2α, 1β, and 16β, followed by conjugation. Most of the metabolites that circulate in the blood are sulfates of 3α,5β-tetrahydro-levonorgestrel, while excretion occurs predominantly in the form of glucuronides. Some of the parent levonorgestrel also circulates as 17β-sulfate. Metabolic clearance rates may differ among individuals by several-fold, and this may account in part for the wide variation observed in levonorgestrel concentrations among users.
Ethinyl estradiol: Cytochrom P450 enzymes (CYP3A4) in the liver are responsible for the 2-hydroxylation that is the major oxidative reaction. The 2-hydroxy metabolite is further transformed by methylation and glucuronidation prior to urinary and fecal excretion. Levels of Cytochrome P450 (CYP3A) vary widely among individuals and can explain the variation in rates of ethinyl estradiol 2-hydroxylation. Ethinyl estradiol is excreted in the urine and feces as glucuronide and sulfate conjugates, and undergoes enterohepatic circulation.
Excretion
The elimination half-life for levonorgestrel is approximately 36 ± 13 hours at steady state. Levonorgestrel and its metabolites are primarily excreted in the urine (40% to 68%) and about 16% to 48% are excreted in feces. The elimination half-life of ethinyl estradiol is 18 ± 4.7 hours at steady state.

SPECIAL POPULATIONS
Race
Based on the pharmacokinetic study with Alesse, there are no apparent differences in pharmacokinetic parameters among women of different races.
Hepatic Insufficiency
No formal studies have evaluated the effect of hepatic disease on the disposition of Alesse. However, steroid hormones may be poorly metabolized in patients with impaired liver function.
Renal Insufficiency
No formal studies have evaluated the effect of renal disease on the disposition of Alesse.
Drug-Drug Interactions
Interactions between ethinyl estradiol and other drugs have been reported in the literature.
- *Interactions with Absorption:* Diarrhea may increase gastrointestinal motility and reduce hormone absorption. Similarly, any drug which reduces gut transit time may reduce hormone concentrations in the blood.
- *Interactions with Metabolism:*
  Gastrointestinal wall: Sulfation of ethinyl estradiol has been shown to occur in the gastrointestinal (GI) wall. Therefore, drugs which act as competitive inhibitors for sulfation in the GI wall may increase ethinyl estradiol bioavailability (e.g., ascorbic acid).
  Hepatic metabolism: Interactions can occur with drugs that induce microsomal enzymes which can decrease ethinyl estradiol concentrations (e.g., rifampin, barbiturates, phenylbutazone, phenytoin, griseofulvin).
- *Interference with Enterohepatic Circulation:* Some clinical reports suggest that enterohepatic circulation of estrogens may decrease when certain antibiotic agents are given, which may reduce ethinyl estradiol concentrations (e.g., ampicillin, tetracycline).
- *Interference in the Metabolism of Other Drugs:* Ethinyl estradiol may interfere with the metabolism of other drugs by inhibiting hepatic microsomal enzymes or by inducing hepatic drug conjugation, particularly glucuronidation. Accordingly, plasma and tissue concentrations may either be increased or decreased, respectively (e.g., cyclosporine, theophylline).

INDICATIONS AND USAGE
Oral contraceptives are indicated for the prevention of pregnancy in women who elect to use this product as a method of contraception.

Continued on next page

FIGURE 1
Mean (SE) levonorgestrel and ethinyl estradiol serum concentrations in 22 subjects receiving Alesse (100 μg levonorgestrel and 20 μg ethinyl estradiol)

• Day 1 • Day 6 ▲ Day 21
Levonorgestrel

• Day 1 • Day 6 ▲ Day 21
Ethinyl Estradiol

Alesse-21—Cont.

Oral contraceptives are highly effective. Table II lists the typical accidental pregnancy rates for users of combination oral contraceptives and other methods of contraception. The efficacy of these contraceptive methods, except sterilization, the IUD, and Norplant® System, depends upon the reliability with which they are used. Correct and consistent use of methods can result in lower failure rates.

TABLE II: PERCENTAGE OF WOMEN EXPERIENCING AN UNINTENDED PREGNANCY DURING THE FIRST YEAR OF USE OF A CONTRACEPTIVE METHOD

Method	Perfect Use	Typical Use
Norplant® System (6 capsules)	0.1	0.1
Male sterilization	0.1	0.15
Female sterilization	0.4	0.4
Depo-Provera® (injectable progestogen)	0.3	0.3
Oral contraceptives		
Combined	0.1	NA
Progestin only	0.5	NA
IUD		
Progesterone	1.5	2.0
Copper T 380A	0.6	0.8
Condom (male) without spermicide	3	12
(female) without spermicide	5	21
Cervical cap		
Nulliparous women	9	18
Parous women	26	36
Diaphragm with spermicidal		
cream or jelly	6	18
Spermicides alone		
(foam, creams, jellies, and vaginal		
suppositories)	6	21
Periodic abstinence (all methods)	1-9*	20
Withdrawal	4	19
No contraception (planned pregnancy)	85	85

NA - not available

*Depending on method (calendar, ovulation, symptothermal, post-ovulation)

Adapted from Hatcher RA et al., *Contraceptive Technology*, 16th Revised Edition. New York, NY: Irvington Publishers, 1994.

In a clinical trial with Alesse, 1,477 subjects had 7,720 cycles of use and a total of 5 pregnancies were reported. This represents an overall pregnancy rate of 0.84 per 100 woman-years. This rate includes patients who did not take the drug correctly. One or more pills were missed during 1,479 (18.8%) of the 7,870 cycles; thus all tablets were taken during 6,391 (81.2%) of the 7,870 cycles. Of the total 7,870 cycles, a total of 150 cycles were excluded from the calculation of the Pearl index due to the use of backup contraception and/or missing 3 or more consecutive pills.

CONTRAINDICATIONS

Oral contraceptives should not be used in women with any of the following conditions:

Thrombophlebitis or thromboembolic disorders

A past history of deep-vein thrombophlebitis or thromboembolic disorders

Cerebrovascular or coronary artery disease

Known or suspected carcinoma of the breast

Carcinoma of the endometrium or other known or suspected estrogen-dependent neoplasia

Undiagnosed abnormal genital bleeding

Cholestatic jaundice of pregnancy or jaundice with prior pill use

Hepatic adenomas or carcinomas

Known or suspected pregnancy

WARNINGS

> Cigarette smoking increases the risk of serious cardiovascular side effects from oral-contraceptive use. This risk increases with age and with heavy smoking (15 or more cigarettes per day) and is quite marked in women over 35 years of age. Women who use oral contraceptives should be strongly advised not to smoke.

The use of oral contraceptives is associated with increased risks of several serious conditions including myocardial infarction, thromboembolism, stroke, hepatic neoplasia, gallbladder disease, and hypertension, although the risk of serious morbidity or mortality is very small in healthy women without underlying risk factors. The risk of morbidity and mortality increases significantly in the presence of other underlying risk factors such as hypertension, hyperlipidemias, obesity and diabetes.

Practitioners prescribing oral contraceptives should be familiar with the following information relating to these risks. The information contained in this package insert is principally based on studies carried out in patients who used oral contraceptives with higher formulations of estrogens and progestogens than those in common use today. The effect of long-term use of the oral contraceptives with lower doses of both estrogens and progestogens remains to be determined. Throughout this labeling, epidemiological studies reported are of two types: retrospective or case control studies and prospective or cohort studies. Case control studies provide a measure of the relative risk of disease, namely, a ratio of the incidence of a disease among oral-contraceptive users to that among nonusers. The relative risk does not provide information on the actual clinical occurrence of a disease. Cohort studies provide a measure of attributable risk, which is the difference in the incidence of disease between oral-contraceptive users and nonusers. The attributable risk does provide information about the actual occurrence of a disease in the population. For further information, the reader is referred to a text on epidemiological methods.

1. THROMBOEMBOLIC DISORDERS AND OTHER VASCULAR PROBLEMS

a. Myocardial Infarction

An increased risk of myocardial infarction has been attributed to oral-contraceptive use. This risk is primarily in smokers or women with other underlying risk factors for coronary-artery disease such as hypertension, hypercholesterolemia, morbid obesity, and diabetes. The relative risk of heart attack for current oral-contraceptive users has been estimated to be two to six. The risk is very low under the age of 30.

Smoking in combination with oral-contraceptive use has been shown to contribute substantially to the incidence of myocardial infarction in women in their mid-thirties or older with smoking accounting for the majority of excess cases. Mortality rates associated with circulatory disease have been shown to increase substantially in smokers over the age of 35 and nonsmokers over the age of 40 (Table III) among women who use oral contraceptives.

[See figure at top of next column]

Oral contraceptives may compound the effects of well-known risk factors, such as hypertension, diabetes, hyperlipidemias, age and obesity. In particular, some progestogens are known to decrease HDL cholesterol and cause glucose intolerance, while estrogens may create a state of hyperinsulinism. Oral contraceptives have been shown to

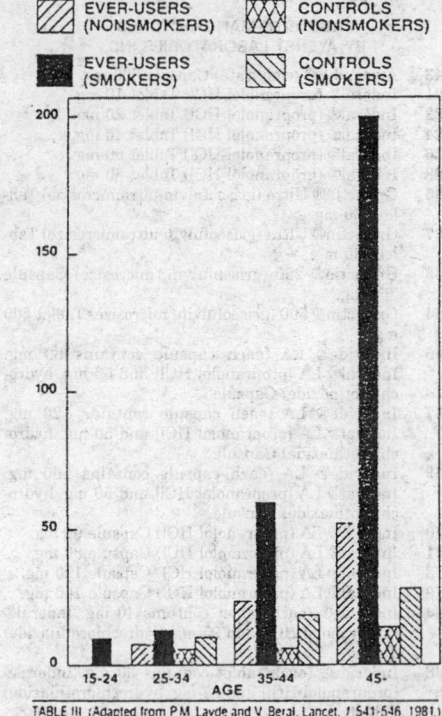

CIRCULATORY DISEASE MORTALITY RATES PER 100,000 WOMAN YEARS BY AGE, SMOKING STATUS AND ORAL-CONTRACEPTIVE USE

TABLE III ; Adapted from P.M. Layde and V. Beral. Lancet. *1* 541-546, 1981.)

increase blood pressure among users (see section 9 in "Warnings"). Similar effects on risk factors have been associated with an increased risk of heart disease. Oral contraceptives must be used with caution in women with cardiovascular disease risk factors.

b. Thromboembolism

An increased risk of thromboembolic and thrombotic disease associated with the use of oral contraceptives is well established. Case control studies have found the relative risk of users compared to non-users to be 3 for the first episode of superficial venous thrombosis, 4 to 11 for deep-vein thrombosis or pulmonary embolism, and 1.5 to 6 for women with predisposing conditions for venous thromboembolic disease. Cohort studies have shown the relative risk to be somewhat lower, about 3 for new cases and about 4.5 for new cases requiring hospitalization. The risk of thromboembolic disease due to oral contraceptives is not related to length of use and disappears after pill use is stopped.

A two- to four-fold increase in relative risk of postoperative thromboembolic complications has been reported with the use of oral contraceptives. The relative risk of venous thrombosis in women who have predisposing conditions is twice that of women without such medical conditions. If feasible, oral contraceptives should be discontinued at least four weeks prior to and for two weeks after elective surgery of a type associated with an increase in risk of thromboembolism and during and following prolonged immobilization. Since the immediate postpartum period is also associated with an increased risk of thromboembolism, oral contraceptives should be started no earlier than four to six weeks after delivery in women who elect not to breast-feed, or a midtrimester pregnancy termination.

c. Cerebrovascular diseases

Oral contraceptives have been shown to increase both the relative and attributable risks of cerebrovascular events (thrombotic and hemorrhagic strokes), although, in general, the risk is greatest among older (>35 years), hypertensive women who also smoke. Hypertension was found to be a risk factor for both users and nonusers, for both types of strokes, while smoking interacted to increase the risk for hemorrhagic strokes.

In a large study, the relative risk of thrombotic strokes has been shown to range from 3 for normotensive users to 14 for users with severe hypertension. The relative risk of hemorrhagic stroke is reported to be 1.2 for nonsmokers who used oral contraceptives, 2.6 for smokers who did not use oral contraceptives, 7.6 for smokers who used oral contraceptives, 1.8 for normotensive users and 25.7 for users with severe hypertension. The attributable risk is also greater in older women.

d. Dose-related risk of vascular disease from oral contraceptives

A positive association has been observed between the amount of estrogen and progestogen in oral contraceptives

TABLE 1: MEAN (SD) PHARMACOKINETIC PARAMETERS OF ALESSE OVER A 21-DAY DOSING PERIOD

Day	C_{max} ng/mL	T_{max} h	AUC ng·h/mL	CL/F mL/h/kg	Vλz/F L/kg	SHBG nmol/L
Levonorgestrel						
1	2.75 (0.88)	1.6 (0.9)	35.2 (12.8)	53.7 (20.8)	2.66 (1.09)	57 (18)
6	4.52 (1.79)	1.5 (0.7)	46.0 (18.8)	40.8 (14.5)	2.05 (0.86)	81 (25)
21	6.00 (2.65)	1.5 (0.5)	68.3 (32.5)	28.4 (10.3)	1.43 (0.62)	93 (40)

Day	pg/mL	h	pg·h/mL	L/h/kg	L/kg	fu %
Unbound Levonorgestrel						
1	51.2 (12.9)	1.6 (0.9)	654 (201)	2.79 (0.97)	135.9 (41.8)	1.92 (0.30)
6	77.9 (22.0)	1.5 (0.7)	794 (240)	2.24 (0.59)	112.4 (40.5)	1.80 (0.24)
21	103.6 (36.9)	1.5 (0.5)	1177 (452)	1.57 (0.49)	78.6 (29.7)	1.78 (0.19)

Day	pg/mL	h	pg·h/mL	mL/h/kg	L/kg	
Ethinyl Estradiol						
1	62.0 (20.5)	1.5 (0.5)	653 (227)	567 (204)	14.3 (3.7)	
6	76.7 (29.9)	1.3 (0.7)	604 (231)	610 (196)	15.5 (4.0)	
21	82.3 (33.2)	1.4 (0.6)	776 (308)	486 (179)	12.4 (4.1)	

and the risk of vascular disease. A decline in serum high-density lipoproteins (HDL) has been reported with many progestational agents. A decline in serum high-density lipoproteins has been associated with an increased incidence of ischemic heart disease. Because estrogens increase HDL cholesterol, the net effect of an oral contraceptive depends on a balance achieved between doses of estrogen and progestogen and the nature and absolute amount of progestogen used in the contraceptive. The amount of both hormones should be considered in the choice of an oral contraceptive.

Minimizing exposure to estrogen and progestogen is in keeping with good principles of therapeutics. For any particular estrogen/progestogen combination, the dosage regimen prescribed should be one which contains the least amount of estrogen and progestogen that is compatible with a low failure rate and the needs of the individual patient. New acceptors of oral-contraceptive agents should be started on preparations containing less than 50 mcg of estrogen.

e. *Persistence of risk of vascular disease*

There are two studies which have shown persistence of risk of vascular disease for ever-users of oral contraceptives. In a study in the United States, the risk of developing myocardial infarction after discontinuing oral contraceptives persists for at least 9 years for women 40–49 years who had used oral contraceptives for five or more years, but this increased risk was not demonstrated in other age groups. In another study in Great Britain, the risk of developing cerebrovascular disease persisted for at least 6 years after discontinuation of oral contraceptives, although excess risk was very small. However, both studies were performed with oral contraceptive formulations containing 50 micrograms or higher of estrogens.

2. ESTIMATES OF MORTALITY FROM CONTRACEPTIVE USE

One study gathered data from a variety of sources which have estimated the mortality rate associated with different methods of contraception at different ages (Table IV). These estimates include the combined risk of death associated with contraceptive methods plus the risk attributable to pregnancy in the event of method failure. Each method of contraception has its specific benefits and risks. The study concluded that with the exception of oral-contraceptive users 35 and older who smoke and 40 and older who do not smoke, mortality associated with all methods of birth control is less than that associated with childbirth. The observation of a possible increase in risk of mortality with age for oral-contraceptive users is based on data gathered in the 1970's—but not reported until 1983. However, current clinical practice involves the use of lower estrogen dose formulations combined with careful restriction of oral-contraceptive use to women who do not have the various risk factors listed in this labeling.

Because of these changes in practice and, also, because of some limited new data which suggest that the risk of cardiovascular disease with the use of oral contraceptives may now be less than previously observed, the Fertility and Maternal Health Drugs Advisory Committee was asked to review the topic in 1989. The Committee concluded that although cardiovascular disease risks may be increased with oral-contraceptive use after age 40 in healthy nonsmoking women (even with the newer low-dose formulations), there are greater potential health risks associated with pregnancy in older women and with the alternative surgical and medical procedures which may be necessary if such women do not have assess to effective and acceptable means of contraception.

Therefore, the Committee recommended that the benefits of oral-contraceptive use by healthy nonsmoking women over 40 may outweigh the possible risks. Of course, older women, as all women who take oral contraceptives, should take the lowest possible dose formulation that is effective.

TABLE IV: ANNUAL NUMBER OF BIRTH-RELATED OR METHOD-RELATED DEATHS ASSOCIATED WITH CONTROL OF FERTILITY PER 100,000 NONSTERILE WOMEN, BY FERTILITY-CONTROL METHOD AND ACCORDING TO AGE

Method of control and outcome	15-19	20-24	25-29	30-34	35-39	40-44
No fertility-control methods*	7.0	7.4	9.1	14.8	25.7	28.2
Oral contraceptives nonsmoker**	0.3	0.5	0.9	1.9	13.8	31.6
Oral contraceptives smoker**	2.2	3.4	6.6	13.5	51.1	117.2
IUD**	0.8	0.8	1.0	1.0	1.4	1.4
Condom*	1.1	1.6	0.7	0.2	0.3	0.4
Diaphragm/ spermicide*	1.9	1.2	1.2	1.3	2.2	2.8
Periodic abstinence*	2.5	1.6	1.6	1.7	2.9	3.6

* Deaths are birth related
**Deaths are method related
Adapted from H.W. Ory, Family Planning Perspectives, *15:* 57-63, 1983.

3. CARCINOMA OF THE REPRODUCTIVE ORGANS

Numerous epidemiological studies have been performed on the incidence of breast, endometrial, ovarian and cervical cancer in women using oral contraceptives. The overwhelming evidence in the literature suggests that use of oral contraceptives is not associated with an increase in the risk of developing breast cancer, regardless of the age and parity of first use or with most of the marketed brands and doses. The Cancer and Steroid Hormone (CASH) study also showed no latent effect on the risk of breast cancer for at least a decade following long-term use. A few studies have shown a slightly increased relative risk of developing breast cancer, although the methodology of these studies, which included differences in examination of users and nonusers and differences in age at start of use, has been questioned. Some studies suggest that oral-contraceptive use has been associated with an increase in the risk of cervical intraepithelial neoplasia in some populations of women. However, there continues to be controversy about the extent to which such findings may be due to differences in sexual behavior and other factors.

In spite of many studies of the relationship between oral-contraceptive use and breast and cervical cancers, a cause-and-effect relationship has not been established.

4. HEPATIC NEOPLASIA

Benign hepatic adenomas are associated with oral-contraceptive use, although the incidence of these benign tumors is rare in the United States. Indirect calculations have estimated the attributable risk to be in the range of 3.3 cases/100,000 for users, a risk that increases after four or more years of use. Rupture of rare, benign, hepatic adenomas may cause death through intra-abdominal hemorrhage.

Studies from Britain have shown an increased risk of developing hepatocellular carcinoma in long-term (>8 years) oral-contraceptive users. However, these cancers are extremely rare in the U.S. and the attributable risk (the excess incidence) of liver cancers in oral-contraceptive users approaches less than one per million users.

5. OCULAR LESIONS

There have been clinical case reports of retinal thrombosis associated with the use of oral contraceptives. Oral contraceptives should be discontinued if there is unexplained partial or complete loss of vision; onset of proptosis or diplopia; papilledema; or retinal vascular lesions. Appropriate diagnostic and therapeutic measures should be undertaken immediately.

6. ORAL-CONTRACEPTIVE USE BEFORE OR DURING EARLY PREGNANCY

Extensive epidemiological studies have revealed no increased risk of birth defects in women who have used oral contraceptives prior to pregnancy. Studies also do not suggest a teratogenic effect, particularly in so far as cardiac anomalies and limb-reduction defects are concerned, when taken inadvertently during early pregnancy.

The administration of oral contraceptives to induce withdrawal bleeding should not be used as a test for pregnancy. Oral contraceptives should not be used during pregnancy to treat threatened or habitual abortion.

It is recommended that for any patient who has missed two consecutive periods, pregnancy should be ruled out before continuing oral-contraceptive use. If the patient has not adhered to the prescribed schedule, the possibility of pregnancy should be considered at the time of the first missed period. Oral-contraceptive use should be discontinued if pregnancy is confirmed.

7. GALLBLADDER DISEASE

Earlier studies have reported an increased lifetime relative risk of gallbladder surgery in users of oral contraceptives and estrogens. More recent studies, however, have shown that the relative risk of developing gallbladder disease among oral-contraceptive users may be minimal. The recent findings of minimal risk may be related to the use of oral-contraceptive formulations containing lower hormonal doses of estrogens and progestogens.

8. CARBOHYDRATE AND LIPID METABOLIC EFFECTS

Oral contraceptives have been shown to cause glucose intolerance in a significant percentage of users. Oral contraceptives containing greater than 75 micrograms of estrogens cause hyperinsulinism, while lower doses of estrogen cause less glucose intolerance. Progestogens increase insulin secretion and create insulin resistance, this effect varying with different progestational agents. However, in the nondiabetic woman, oral contraceptives appear to have no effect on fasting blood glucose. Because of these demonstrated effects, prediabetic and diabetic women should be carefully observed while taking oral contraceptives.

A small proportion of women will have persistent hypertriglyceridemia while on the pill. As discussed earlier (see "**Warnings**" 1a. and 1d.), changes in serum triglycerides and lipoprotein levels have been reported in oral-contraceptive users.

9. ELEVATED BLOOD PRESSURE

An increase in blood pressure has been reported in women taking oral contraceptives and this increase is more likely in older oral-contraceptive users and with continued use. Data from the Royal College of General Practitioners and subsequent randomized trials have shown that the incidence of hypertension increases with increasing quantities of progestogens.

Women with a history of hypertension or hypertension-related diseases, or renal disease should be encouraged to use another method of contraception. If women with hypertension elect to use oral contraceptives, they should be monitored closely and if significant elevation of blood pressure occurs, oral contraceptives should be discontinued. For most women, elevated blood pressure will return to normal after stopping oral contraceptives, and there is no difference in the occurrence of hypertension among ever- and never-users.

10. HEADACHE

The onset or exacerbation of migraine or development of headache with a new pattern that is recurrent, persistent or severe requires discontinuation of oral contraceptives and evaluation of the cause.

11. BLEEDING IRREGULARITIES

Breakthrough bleeding and spotting are sometimes encountered in patients on oral contraceptives, especially during the first three months of use. The type and dose of progestogen may be important. Nonhormonal causes should be considered and adequate diagnostic measures taken to rule out malignancy or pregnancy in the event of breakthrough bleeding, as in the case of any abnormal vaginal bleeding. If pathology has been excluded, time or a change to another formulation may solve the problem. In the event of amenorrhea, pregnancy should be ruled out.

Some women may encounter post-pill amenorrhea or oligomenorrhea, especially when such a condition was preexistent.

PRECAUTIONS

Patients should be counseled that this product does not protect against HIV infection (AIDS) and other sexually transmitted diseases.

1. PHYSICAL EXAMINATION AND FOLLOW-UP

A periodic history and physical examination is appropriate for all women, including women using oral contraceptives. The physical examination, however, may be deferred until after initiation of oral contraceptives if requested by the woman and judged appropriate by the clinician. The physical examination should include special reference to blood pressure, breasts, abdomen and pelvic organs, including cervical cytology, and relevant laboratory tests. In case of undiagnosed, persistent or recurrent abnormal vaginal bleeding, appropriate diagnostic measures should be conducted to rule out malignancy. Women with a strong family history of breast cancer or who have breast nodules should be monitored with particular care.

2. LIPID DISORDERS

Women who are being treated for hyperlipidemias should be followed closely if they elect to use oral contraceptives. Some progestogens may elevate LDL levels and may render the control of hyperlipidemias more difficult. (See "**Warnings**," 1d.)

3. LIVER FUNCTION

If jaundice develops in any woman receiving such drugs, the medication should be discontinued. Steroid hormones may be poorly metabolized in patients with impaired liver function.

4. FLUID RETENTION

Oral contraceptives may cause some degree of fluid retention. They should be prescribed with caution, and only with careful monitoring, in patients with conditions which might be aggravated by fluid retention.

5. EMOTIONAL DISORDERS

Patients becoming significantly depressed while taking oral contraceptives should stop the medication and use an alternative method of contraception in an attempt to determine whether the symptom is drug related. Women with a history of depression should be carefully observed and the drug discontinued if depression recurs to a serious degree.

6. CONTACT LENSES

Contact-lens wearers who develop visual changes or changes in lens tolerance should be assessed by an ophthalmologist.

7. DRUG INTERACTIONS

Reduced efficacy and increased incidence of breakthrough bleeding and menstrual irregularities have been associated with concomitant use of rifampin. A similar association, though less marked, has been suggested with barbiturates, phenylbutazone, phenytoin, and possibly with griseofulvin, ampicillin, and tetracyclines.

Continued on next page

Alesse-21—Cont.

8. INTERACTIONS WITH LABORATORY TESTS
Certain endocrine- and liver-function tests and blood components may be affected by oral contraceptives:
a. Increased prothrombin and factors VII, VIII, IX, and X; decreased antithrombin 3; increased norepinephrine-induced platelet aggregability.
b. Increased thyroid-binding globulin (TBG) leading to increased circulating total thyroid hormone, as measured by protein-bound iodine (PBI), T4 by column or by radioimmunoassay. Free T3 resin uptake is decreased, reflecting the elevated TBG; free T4 concentration is unaltered.
c. Other binding proteins may be elevated in serum.
d. Sex-hormone binding globulins are increased and result in elevated levels of total circulating sex steroids; however, free or biologically active levels remain unchanged.
e. Triglycerides may be increased.
f. Glucose tolerance may be decreased.
g. Serum folate levels may be depressed by oral-contraceptive therapy. This may be of clinical significance if a woman becomes pregnant shortly after discontinuing oral contraceptives.
9. CARCINOGENESIS
See "**Warnings**" section.
10. PREGNANCY
Pregnancy Category X. See "**Contraindications**" and "**Warnings**" sections.
11. NURSING MOTHERS
Small amounts of oral-contraceptive steroids have been identified in the milk of nursing mothers, and a few adverse effects on the child have been reported, including jaundice and breast enlargement. In addition, oral contraceptives given in the postpartum period may interfere with lactation by decreasing the quantity and quality of breast milk. If possible, the nursing mother should be advised not to use oral contraceptives but to use other forms of contraception until she has completely weaned her child.
INFORMATION FOR THE PATIENT
See Patient Labeling Printed Below.

ADVERSE REACTIONS

An increased risk of the following serious adverse reactions has been associated with the use of oral contraceptives (see "**Warnings**" section):
Thrombophlebitis
Arterial thromboembolism
Pulmonary embolism
Myocardial infarction
Cerebral hemorrhage
Cerebral thrombosis
Hypertension
Gallbladder disease
Hepatic adenomas or benign liver tumors
There is evidence of an association between the following conditions and the use of oral contraceptives, although additional confirmatory studies are needed:
Mesenteric thrombosis
Retinal thrombosis
The following adverse reactions have been reported in patients receiving oral contraceptives and are believed to be drug related:
Nausea
Vomiting
Gastrointestinal symptoms (such as abdominal cramps and bloating)
Breakthrough bleeding
Spotting
Change in menstrual flow
Amenorrhea
Temporary infertility after discontinuation of treatment
Edema
Melasma which may persist
Breast changes: tenderness, enlargement, secretion
Change in weight (increase or decrease)
Change in cervical erosion and secretion
Diminution in lactation when given immediately postpartum
Cholestatic jaundice
Migraine
Rash (allergic)
Mental depression
Reduced tolerance to carbohydrates
Vaginal candidiasis
Change in corneal curvature (steepening)
Intolerance to contact lenses
The following adverse reactions have been reported in users of oral contraceptives and the association has been neither confirmed nor refuted:
Premenstrual syndrome
Cataracts
Optic neuritis
Changes in appetite
Cystitis-like syndrome
Headache
Nervousness
Dizziness
Hirsutism
Loss of scalp hair
Erythema multiforme
Erythema nodosum
Hemorrhagic eruption
Vaginitis
Porphyria
Impaired renal function
Hemolytic uremic syndrome
Budd-Chiari syndrome
Acne
Changes in libido
Colitis

OVERDOSAGE

Serious ill effects have not been reported following acute ingestion of large doses of oral contraceptives by young children. Overdosage may cause nausea, and withdrawal bleeding may occur in females.

Noncontraceptive Health Benefits
The following noncontraceptive health benefits related to the use of oral contraceptives are supported by epidemiological studies which largely utilized oral-contraceptive formulations containing doses exceeding 0.035 mg of ethinyl estradiol or 0.05 mg of mestranol.
Effects on menses:
Increased menstrual cycle regularity
Decreased blood loss and decreased incidence of iron-deficiency anemia
Decreased incidence of dysmenorrhea
Effects related to inhibition of ovulation:
Decreased incidence of functional ovarian cysts
Decreased incidence of ectopic pregnancies
Effects from long-term use:
Decreased incidence of fibroadenomas and fibrocystic disease of the breast
Decreased incidence of acute pelvic inflammatory disease
Decreased incidence of endometrial cancer
Decreased incidence of ovarian cancer

DOSAGE AND ADMINISTRATION

To achieve maximum contraceptive effectiveness, Alesse™ must be taken exactly as directed and at intervals not exceeding 24 hours. The dispenser should be kept in the wallet supplied to avoid possible fading of the pills. If the pills fade, patients should continue to take them as directed.
The dosage of Alesse-21 is one pink tablet daily for 21 consecutive days, followed by 7 days when no tablets are taken. It is recommended that Alesse-21 tablets be taken at the same time each day.
Sunday start:
During the first cycle of medication, the patient is instructed to begin taking Alesse-21 on the first Sunday after the onset of menstruation. If menstruation begins on a Sunday, the first tablet (pink) is taken that day. One pink tablet should be taken daily for 21 consecutive days, followed by seven days when no tablet is taken. Withdrawal bleeding should usually occur within three days following discontinuation of pink tablets. During the first cycle, contraceptive reliance should not be placed on Alesse-21 until a pink tablet has been taken daily for 7 consecutive days. The possibility of ovulation and conception prior to initiation of medication should be considered.
The patient begins her next and all subsequent 21-day courses of tablets on the same day of the week (Sunday) on which she began her first course, following the same schedule: 21 days on pink tablets—7 days when no tablets are taken. If in any cycle the patient starts tablets later than the proper day, she should protect herself against pregnancy by using another method of birth control until she has taken a pink tablet daily for 7 consecutive days.
Day 1 start:
During the first cycle of medication, the patient is instructed to begin taking Alesse-21 during the first 24 hours of her period (day one of her menstrual cycle). One pink tablet should be taken daily for 21 consecutive days. Withdrawal bleeding should usually occur within three days following discontinuation of pink tablets. If medication is begun on day one of the menstrual cycle, no back-up contraception is necessary. If Alesse-21 tablets are started later than day one of the first menstrual cycle or postpartum, contraceptive reliance should not be placed on Alesse-21 tablets until after the first 7 consecutive days of administration. The possibility of ovulation and conception prior to initiation of medication should be considered.
When the patient is switching from a 21-day regimen of tablets, she should wait 7 days after her last tablet before she starts Alesse. She will probably experience withdrawal bleeding during that week. She should be sure that no more than 7 days pass after her previous 21-day regimen. When the patient is switching from a 28-day regimen of tablets, she should start her first pack of Alesse on the day after her last tablet. She should not wait any days between packs.
If spotting or breakthrough bleeding occur, the patient is instructed to continue on the same regimen. This type of bleeding is usually transient and without significance; however, if the bleeding is persistent or prolonged, the patient is advised to consult her physician. While there is little likelihood of ovulation occurring if only one or two pink tablets are missed, the possibility of ovulation increases with each successive day that scheduled pink tablets are missed. Although the occurrence of pregnancy is unlikely if Alesse is taken according to directions, if withdrawal bleeding does not occur, the possibility of pregnancy must be considered. If the patient has not adhered to the prescribed schedule (missed one or more tablets or started taking them on a day later than she should have), the probability of pregnancy should be considered at the time of the first missed period and appropriate diagnostic measures taken before the medication is resumed. If the patient has adhered to the prescribed regimen and misses two consecutive periods, pregnancy should be ruled out before continuing the contraceptive regimen.
The risk of pregnancy increases with each active (pink) tablet missed. For additional patient instructions regarding missed tablets, see the "WHAT TO DO IF YOU MISS PILLS" section in the **DETAILED PATIENT LABELING** below.
In the nonlactating mother, Alesse may be initiated postpartum, for contraception. When the tablets are administered in the postpartum period, the increased risk of thromboembolic disease associated with the postpartum period must be considered (See "**Contraindications**", "**Warnings**", and "**Precautions**" concerning thromboembolic disease).

HOW SUPPLIED

Alesse™-21 tablets (0.10 mg levonorgestrel and 0.02 mg ethinyl estradiol) are available in packages of 3 MINI-PACK™ dispensers of 21 tablets each, NDC 0008-0912-02, as follows:
21 active tablets. NDC 0008-0912, pink, round tablet marked "W" and "912".
Store at controlled room temperature 20°-25° C (68°-77° F).
References available upon request.

Brief Summary Patient Package Insert

This product (like all oral contraceptives) is intended to prevent pregnancy. It does not protect against HIV infection (AIDS) and other sexually transmitted diseases.
Oral contraceptives, also known as "birth-control pills" or "the pill", are taken to prevent pregnancy, and when taken correctly, have a failure rate of less than 1.0% per year when used without missing any pills. The typical failure rate of large numbers of pill users is less than 3.0% per year when women who miss pills are included. For most women oral contraceptives are also free of serious or unpleasant side effects. However, forgetting to take pills considerably increases the chances of pregnancy.
For the majority of women, oral contraceptives can be taken safely. But there are some women who are at high risk of developing certain serious diseases that can be life-threatening or may cause temporary or permanent disability or death. The risks associated with taking oral contraceptives increase significantly if you:
- smoke.
- have high blood pressure, diabetes, high cholesterol.
- have or have had clotting disorders, heart attack, stroke, angina pectoris, cancer of the breast or sex organs, jaundice, or malignant or benign liver tumors.

You should not take the pill if you suspect you are pregnant or have unexplained vaginal bleeding.

Cigarette smoking increases the risk of serious adverse effects on the heart and blood vessels from oral-contraceptive use. This risk increases with age and with heavy smoking (15 or more cigarettes per day) and is quite marked in women over 35 years of age. Women who use oral contraceptives should not smoke.

Most side effects of the pill are not serious. The most common such effects are nausea, vomiting, bleeding between menstrual periods, weight gain, breast tenderness, and difficulty wearing contact lenses. These side effects, especially nausea and vomiting, may subside within the first three months of use.
The serious side effects of the pill occur very infrequently, especially if you are in good health and do not smoke. However, you should know that the following medical conditions have been associated with or made worse by the pill:
1. Blood clots in the legs (thrombophlebitis), lungs (pulmonary embolism), stoppage or rupture of a blood vessel in the brain (stroke), blockage of blood vessels in the heart (heart attack and angina pectoris) or other organs of the body. As mentioned above, smoking increases the risk of heart attacks and strokes and subsequent serious medical consequences.
2. Liver tumors, which may rupture and cause severe bleeding. A possible but not definite association has been found with the pill and liver cancer. However, liver cancers are extremely rare. The chance of developing liver cancer from using the pill is thus even rarer.

3. High blood pressure, although blood pressure usually returns to normal when the pill is stopped.

The symptoms associated with these serious side effects are discussed in the detailed leaflet given to you with your supply of pills. Notify your doctor or health-care provider if you notice any unusual physical disturbances while taking the pill. In addition, drugs such as rifampin, as well as some anticonvulsants and some antibiotics, may decrease oral-contraceptive effectiveness.

Studies to date of women taking the pill have not shown an increase in the incidence of cancer of the breast or cervix. There is, however, insufficient evidence to rule out the possibility that pills may cause such cancers.

Taking the pill provides some important noncontraceptive benefits. These include less painful menstruation, less menstrual blood loss and anemia, fewer pelvic infections, and fewer cancers of the ovary and the lining of the uterus.

Be sure to discuss any medical condition you may have with your health-care provider. Your health-care provider will take a medical and family history before prescribing oral contraceptives and will examine you. The physical examination may be delayed to another time if you request it and the health-care provider believes that it is appropriate to postpone it. You should be reexamined at least once a year while taking oral contraceptives. The detailed patient information leaflet gives you further information which you should read and discuss with your health-care provider.

This product (like all oral contraceptives) is intended to prevent pregnancy. It does not protect against transmission of HIV (AIDS) and other sexually transmitted diseases such as chlamydia, genital herpes, genital warts, gonorrhea, hepatitis B, and syphilis.

DETAILED PATIENT LABELING

This product (like all oral contraceptives) is intended to prevent pregnancy. It does not protect against HIV infection (AIDS) and other sexually transmitted diseases.

INTRODUCTION

Any woman who considers using oral contraceptives (the birth-control pill or the pill) should understand the benefits and risks of using this form of birth control. This leaflet will give you much of the information you will need to make this decision and will also help you determine if you are at risk of developing any of the serious side effects of the pill. It will tell you how to use the pill properly so that it will be as effective as possible.

However, this leaflet is not a replacement for a careful discussion between you and your health-care provider. You should discuss the information provided in this leaflet with him or her, both when you first start taking the pill and during your revisits. You should also follow your health-care provider's advice with regard to regular check-ups while you are on the pill.

EFFECTIVENESS OF ORAL CONTRACEPTIVES

Oral contraceptives or "birth-control pills" or "the pill" are used to prevent pregnancy and are more effective than other nonsurgical methods of birth control. When they are taken correctly, the chance of becoming pregnant is less than 1.0% per year when used perfectly, without missing any pills. Typical failure rates are less than 3.0% per year. The chance of becoming pregnant increases with each missed pill during the menstrual cycle.

In comparison, typical failure rates for other methods of birth control during the first year of use are as follows:
IUD: 3%
DEPO-PROVERA® (injectable progestogen): 0.3%
NORPLANT® SYSTEM (implants): 0.1%
Diaphragm with spermicides: 18%
Spermicides alone: 21%
Male condom alone: 12%
Female condom alone: 21%
Cervical cap
  Nulliparous women: 18%
  Parous women: 36%
Periodic abstinence: 20%
No methods: 85%

WHO SHOULD NOT TAKE ORAL CONTRACEPTIVES

> **Cigarette smoking increases the risk of serious adverse effects on the heart and blood vessels from oral-contraceptive use. This risk increases with age and with heavy smoking (15 or more cigarettes per day) and is quite marked in women over 35 years of age. Women who use oral contraceptives should not smoke.**

Some women should not use the pill. For example, you should not take the pill if you are pregnant or think you may be pregnant. You should also not use the pill if you have had any of the following conditions:
• Heart attack or stroke.
• Blood clots in the legs (thrombophlebitis), lungs (pulmonary embolism), or eyes.
• Blood clots in the deep veins of your legs.
• Known or suspected breast cancer or cancer of the lining of the uterus, cervix or vagina.
• Liver tumor (benign or cancerous).

Or, if you have any of the following:
• Chest pain (angina pectoris).
• Unexplained vaginal bleeding (until a diagnosis is reached by your doctor).
• Yellowing of the whites of the eyes or of the skin (jaundice) during pregnancy or during previous use of the pill.
• Known or suspected pregnancy.

Tell your health-care provider if you have ever had any of these conditions. Your health-care provider can recommend another method of birth control.

OTHER CONSIDERATIONS BEFORE TAKING ORAL CONTRACEPTIVES

Tell your health-care provider if you or any family member has ever had:
• Breast nodules, fibrocystic disease of the breast, an abnormal breast X ray or mammogram.
• Diabetes.
• Elevated cholesterol or triglycerides.
• High blood pressure.
• Migraine or other headaches or epilepsy.
• Mental depression.
• Gallbladder, heart or kidney disease.
• History of scanty or irregular menstrual periods.

Women with any of these conditions should be checked often by their health-care provider if they choose to use oral contraceptives. Also, be sure to inform your doctor or health-care provider if you smoke or are on any medications.

RISKS OF TAKING ORAL CONTRACEPTIVES

1. Risk of developing blood clots

Blood clots and blockage of blood vessels are the most serious side effects of taking oral contraceptives and can be fatal. In particular, a clot in the legs can cause thrombophlebitis and a clot that travels to the lungs can cause a sudden blocking of the vessel carrying blood to the lungs. Rarely, clots occur in the blood vessels of the eye and may cause blindness, double vision, or impaired vision.

If you take oral contraceptives and need elective surgery, need to stay in bed for a prolonged illness, or have recently delivered a baby, you may be at risk of developing blood clots. You should consult your doctor about stopping oral contraceptives three to four weeks before surgery and not taking oral contraceptives for two weeks after surgery or during bed rest. You should also not take oral contraceptives soon after delivery of a baby or a midtrimester pregnancy termination. It is advisable to wait for at least four weeks after delivery if you are not breast-feeding. If you are breast-feeding, you should wait until you have weaned your child before using the pill (See also the section on breast-feeding in "GENERAL PRECAUTIONS.")

2. Heart attacks and strokes

Oral contraceptives may increase the tendency to develop strokes (stoppage or rupture of blood vessels in the brain) and angina pectoris and heart attacks (blockage of blood vessels in the heart). Any of these conditions can cause death or serious disability.

Smoking greatly increases the possibility of suffering heart attacks and strokes. Furthermore, smoking and the use of oral contraceptives greatly increase the chances of developing and dying of heart disease.

3. Gallbladder disease

Oral-contraceptive users probably have a greater risk than nonusers of having gallbladder disease, although this risk may be related to pills containing high doses of estrogens.

4. Liver tumors

In rare cases, oral contraceptives can cause benign but dangerous liver tumors. These benign liver tumors can rupture and cause fatal internal bleeding. In addition, a possible but not definite association has been found with the pill and liver cancers in two studies in which a few women who developed these very rare cancers were found to have used oral contraceptives for long periods. However, liver cancers are extremely rare. The chance of developing liver cancer from using the pill is thus even rarer.

5. Cancer of the reproductive organs

There is, at present, no confirmed evidence that oral contraceptives increase the risk of cancer of the reproductive organs in human studies. Several studies have found no overall increase in the risk of developing breast cancer. However, women who use oral contraceptives and have a strong family history of breast cancer or who have breast nodules or abnormal mammograms should be closely followed by their doctors.

Some studies have found an increase in the incidence of cancer of the cervix in women who use oral contraceptives. However, this finding may be related to factors other than the use of oral contraceptives.

ESTIMATED RISK OF DEATH FROM A BIRTH CONTROL METHOD OR PREGNANCY

All methods of birth control and pregnancy are associated with a risk of developing certain diseases which may lead to disability or death. An estimate of the number of deaths associated with different methods of birth control and pregnancy has been calculated and is shown in the following table.

ANNUAL NUMBER OF BIRTH-RELATED OR METHOD-RELATED DEATHS ASSOCIATED WITH CONTROL OF FERTILITY PER 100,000 NONSTERILE WOMEN, BY FERTILITY-CONTROL METHOD AND ACCORDING TO AGE

Method of control and outcome	15-19	20-24	25-29	30-34	35-39	40-44
No fertility-control methods*	7.0	7.4	9.1	14.8	25.7	28.2
Oral contraceptives nonsmoker**	0.3	0.5	0.9	1.9	13.8	31.6
Oral contraceptives smoker**	2.2	3.4	6.6	13.5	51.1	117.2
IUD**	0.8	0.8	1.0	1.0	1.4	1.4
Condom*	1.1	1.6	0.7	0.2	0.3	0.4
Diaphragm/ spermicide*	1.9	1.2	1.2	1.3	2.2	2.8
Periodic abstinence*	2.5	1.6	1.6	1.7	2.9	3.6

* Deaths are birth related
** Deaths are method related

In the above table, the risk of death from any birth-control method is less than the risk of childbirth, except for oral-contraceptive users over the age of 35 who smoke and pill users over the age of 40 even if they do not smoke. It can be seen in the table that for women aged 15 to 39, the risk of death was highest with pregnancy (7 to 26 deaths per 100,000 women, depending on age). Among pill users who do not smoke, the risk of death was always lower than that associated with pregnancy for any age group, except for those women over the age of 40, when the risk increases to 32 deaths per 100,000 women, compared to 28 associated with pregnancy at that age. However, for pill users who smoke and are over the age of 35, the estimated number of deaths exceeds those for other methods of birth control. If a woman is over the age of 40 and smokes, her estimated risk of death is four times higher (117/100,000 women) than the estimated risk associated with pregnancy (28/100,000 women) in that age group.

The suggestion that women over 40 who don't smoke should not take oral contraceptives is based on information from older high-dose pills and on less-selective use of pills than is practiced today. An Advisory Committee of the FDA discussed this issue in 1989 and recommended that the benefits of oral-contraceptive use by healthy, nonsmoking women over 40 years of age may outweigh the possible risks. However, all women, especially older women, are cautioned to use the lowest-dose pill that is effective.

WARNING SIGNALS

If any of these adverse effects occur while you are taking oral contraceptives, call your doctor immediately:
• Sharp chest pain, coughing of blood, or sudden shortness of breath (indicating a possible clot in the lung).
• Pain in the calf (indicating a possible clot in the leg).
• Crushing chest pain or heaviness in the chest (indicating a possible heart attack).
• Sudden severe headache or vomiting, dizziness or fainting, disturbances of vision or speech, weakness, or numbness in an arm or leg (indicating a possible stroke).
• Sudden partial or complete loss of vision (indicating a possible clot in the eye).
• Breast lumps (indicating possible breast cancer or fibrocystic disease of the breast; ask your doctor or health-care provider to show you how to examine your breasts).
• Severe pain or tenderness in the stomach area (indicating a possibly ruptured liver tumor).
• Difficulty in sleeping, weakness, lack of energy, fatigue, or change in mood (possibly indicating severe depression).
• Jaundice or a yellowing of the skin or eyeballs, accompanied frequently by fever, fatigue, loss of appetite, dark-colored urine, or light-colored bowel movements (indicating possible liver problems).

SIDE EFFECTS OF ORAL CONTRACEPTIVES

1. Vaginal bleeding

Irregular vaginal bleeding or spotting may occur while you are taking the pills. Irregular bleeding may vary from slight staining between menstrual periods to breakthrough bleeding which is a flow much like a regular period. Irregular bleeding occurs most often during the first few months of oral-contraceptive use, but may also occur after you have been taking the pill for some time. Such bleeding may be temporary and usually does not indicate any serious problems. It is important to continue taking your pills on schedule. If the bleeding occurs in more than one cycle or lasts for more than a few days, talk to your doctor or health-care provider.

Continued on next page

Alesse-21—Cont.

2. *Contact lenses*
If you wear contact lenses and notice a change in vision or an inability to wear your lenses, contact your doctor or health-care provider.
3. *Fluid retention*
Oral contraceptives may cause edema (fluid retention) with swelling of the fingers or ankles and may raise your blood pressure. If you experience fluid retention, contact your doctor or health-care provider.
4. *Melasma*
A spotty darkening of the skin is possible, particularly of the face.
5. *Other side effects*
Other side effects may include change in appetite, headache, nervousness, depression, dizziness, loss of scalp hair, rash, and vaginal infections.
If any of these side effects bother you, call your doctor or health-care provider.

GENERAL PRECAUTIONS

1. *Missed periods and use of oral contraceptives before or during early pregnancy.*
There may be times when you may not menstruate regularly after you have completed taking a cycle of pills. If you have taken your pills regularly and miss one menstrual period, continue taking your pills for the next cycle but be sure to inform your health-care provider before doing so. If you have not taken the pills daily as instructed and missed a menstrual period, or if you missed two consecutive menstrual periods, you may be pregnant. Check with your health-care provider immediately to determine whether you are pregnant. Do not continue to take oral contraceptives until you are sure you are not pregnant, but continue to use another method of contraception.
There is no conclusive evidence that oral-contraceptive use is associated with an increase in birth defects, when taken inadvertently during early pregnancy. Previously, a few studies had reported that oral contraceptives might be associated with birth defects, but these studies have not been confirmed. Nevertheless, oral contraceptives or any other drugs should not be used during pregnancy unless clearly necessary and prescribed by your doctor. You should check with your doctor about risks to your unborn child of any medication taken during pregnancy.
2. *While breast-feeding*
If you are breast-feeding, consult your doctor before starting oral contraceptives. Some of the drug will be passed on to the child in the milk. A few adverse effects on the child have been reported, including yellowing of the skin (jaundice) and breast enlargement. In addition, oral contraceptives may decrease the amount and quality of your milk. If possible, do not use oral contraceptives while breast-feeding. You should use another method of contraception since breast-feeding provides only partial protection from becoming pregnant and this partial protection decreases significantly as you breast-feed for longer periods of time. You should consider starting oral contraceptives only after you have weaned your child completely.
3. *Laboratory tests*
If you are scheduled for any laboratory tests, tell your doctor you are taking birth-control pills. Certain blood tests may be affected by birth-control pills.
4. *Drug interactions*
Certain drugs may interact with birth-control pills to make them less effective in preventing pregnancy or cause an increase in breakthrough bleeding. Such drugs include rifampin, drugs used for epilepsy such as barbiturates (for example, phenobarbital) and phenytoin (Dilantin is one brand of this drug), phenylbutazone (Butazolidin is one brand) and possibly certain antibiotics. You may need to use an additional method of contraception during any cycle in which you take drugs that can make oral contraceptives less effective.

HOW TO TAKE THE PILL

This product (like all oral contraceptives) is intended to prevent pregnancy. It does not protect against transmission of HIV (AIDS) and other sexually transmitted diseases such as chlamydia, genital herpes, genital warts, gonorrhea, hepatitis B, and syphilis.

IMPORTANT POINTS TO REMEMBER

BEFORE YOU START TAKING YOUR PILLS:
1. BE SURE TO READ THESE DIRECTIONS:
Before you start taking your pills.
And
Anytime you are not sure what to do.
2. THE RIGHT WAY TO TAKE THE PILL IS TO TAKE ONE PILL EVERY DAY AT THE SAME TIME.
If you miss pills you could get pregnant. This includes starting the pack late. The more pills you miss, the more likely you are to get pregnant.
3. MANY WOMEN HAVE SPOTTING OR LIGHT BLEEDING, OR MAY FEEL SICK TO THEIR STOMACH DURING THE FIRST 1–3 PACKS OF PILLS.
If you feel sick to your stomach, do not stop taking the pill. The problem will usually go away. If it doesn't go away, check with your doctor or clinic.
4. MISSING PILLS CAN ALSO CAUSE SPOTTING OR LIGHT BLEEDING, even when you make up these missed pills. On the days you take 2 pills to make up for missed pills, you could also feel a little sick to your stomach.
5. IF YOU HAVE VOMITING OR DIARRHEA, for any reason, or IF YOU TAKE SOME MEDICINES, including some antibiotics, your pills may not work as well.
Use a back-up method (such as condoms or foam) until you check with your doctor or clinic.
6. IF YOU HAVE TROUBLE REMEMBERING TO TAKE THE PILL, talk to your doctor or clinic about how to make pill-taking easier or about using another method of birth control.
7. IF YOU HAVE ANY QUESTIONS OR ARE UNSURE ABOUT THE INFORMATION IN THIS LEAFLET, call your doctor or clinic.

***BEFORE* YOU START TAKING YOUR PILLS**

1. DECIDE WHAT TIME OF DAY YOU WANT TO TAKE YOUR PILL. It is important to take it at about the same time every day.
2. LOOK AT YOUR PILL PACK TO SEE IF IT HAS 21 OR 28 PILLS.
The *21-pill pack* has 21 "active" pink pills (with hormones) to take for 3 weeks, followed by 1 week without pills.
The *28-pill pack* has 21 "active" pink pills (with hormones) to take for 3 weeks, followed by 1 week of reminder light-green pills (without hormones).
3. ALSO FIND:
1) where on the pack to start taking pills, and
2) in what order to take the pills (follow the arrow).
4. BE SURE YOU HAVE READY AT ALL TIMES:
ANOTHER KIND OF BIRTH CONTROL (such as condoms or foam) to use as a back-up in case you miss pills.

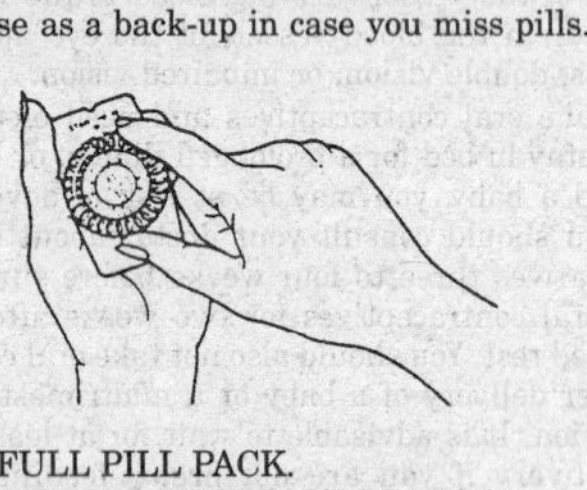

AN EXTRA, FULL PILL PACK.

WHEN TO START THE *FIRST* PACK OF PILLS:

You have a choice of which day to start taking your first pack of pills.
Decide with your doctor or clinic which is the best day for you. Pick a time of day which will be easy to remember.

DAY 1 START:

1. Take the first "active" pink pill of the first pack during the *first 24 hours of your period.*
2. You will not need to use a back-up method of birth control, since you are starting the pill at the beginning of your period.

SUNDAY START:

1. Take the first "active" pink pill of the first pack on the *Sunday after your period starts*, even if you are still bleeding. If your period begins on Sunday, start the pack that same day.
2. *Use another method of birth control* as a back-up method if you have sex anytime from the Sunday you start your first pack until the next Sunday (7 days). Condoms or foam are good back-up methods of birth control.

WHAT TO DO DURING THE MONTH

1. TAKE ONE PILL AT THE SAME TIME EVERY DAY UNTIL THE PACK IS EMPTY.
Do not skip pills even if you are spotting or bleeding between monthly periods or feel sick to your stomach (nausea).
Do not skip pills even if you do not have sex very often.

2. WHEN YOU FINISH A PACK OR SWITCH YOUR BRAND OF PILLS:
21 pills: Wait 7 days to start the next pack. You will probably have your period during that week. Be sure that no more than 7 days pass between 21-day packs.
28 pills: Start the next pack on the day after your last "reminder" pill. Do not wait any days between packs.

WHAT TO DO IF YOU MISS PILLS

If you **MISS 1** pink "active" pill:
1. Take it as soon as you remember. Take the next pill at your regular time. This means you take 2 pills in 1 day.
2. You do not need to use a back-up birth-control method if you have sex.

If you **MISS 2** pink "active" pills in a row in **WEEK 1 OR WEEK 2** of your pack:
1. Take 2 pills on the day you remember and 2 pills the next day.
2. Then take 1 pill a day until you finish the pack.
3. You MAY BECOME PREGNANT if you have sex in the 7 *days* after you miss pills. You MUST use another birth-control method (such as condoms or foam) as a back-up for those 7 days.

If you **MISS 2** pink "active" pills in a row in **THE 3rd WEEK:**
1. ***If you are a Day 1 Starter:***
THROW OUT the rest of the pill pack and start a new pack that same day.
If you are a Sunday Starter:
Keep taking 1 pill every day until Sunday.
On Sunday, THROW OUT the rest of the pack and start a new pack of pills that same day.
2. You may not have your period this month but this is expected.
However, if you miss your period 2 months in a row, call your doctor or clinic because you might be pregnant.
3. You MAY BECOME PREGNANT if you have sex in the 7 *days* after you miss pills. You MUST use another birth-control method (such as condoms or foam) as a back-up for those 7 days.

If you **MISS 3 OR MORE** pink "active" pills in a row (during the first 3 weeks):
1. ***If you are a Day 1 Starter:***
THROW OUT the rest of the pill pack and start a new pack that same day.
If you are a Sunday Starter:
Keep taking 1 pill every day until Sunday.
On Sunday, THROW OUT the rest of the pack and start a new pack of pills that same day.
2. You may not have your period this month but this is expected.
However, if you miss your period 2 months in a row, call your doctor or clinic because you might be pregnant.
3. You MAY BECOME PREGNANT if you have sex in the 7 *days* after you miss pills. You MUST use another birth-control method (such as condoms or foam) as a back-up for those 7 days.

A REMINDER FOR THOSE ON 28-DAY PACKS:

If you forget any of the 7 light-green "reminder" pills in Week 4:
THROW AWAY the pills you missed.
Keep taking 1 pill each day until the pack is empty.
You do not need a back-up method if you start your next pack on time.

FINALLY, IF YOU ARE STILL NOT SURE WHAT TO DO ABOUT THE PILLS YOU HAVE MISSED:

Use a BACK-UP METHOD anytime you have sex.
KEEP TAKING ONE PILL EACH DAY until you can reach your doctor or clinic.

Pregnancy due to pill failure
The incidence of pill failure resulting in pregnancy is approximately less than 1.0% if taken every day as directed, but more typical failure rates are less than 3.0%. If failure does occur, the risk to the fetus is minimal.

RISKS TO THE FETUS

If you do become pregnant while using oral contraceptives, the risk to the fetus is small, on the order of no more than one per thousand. You should, however, discuss the risks to the developing child with your doctor.

Pregnancy after stopping the pill
There may be some delay in becoming pregnant after you stop using oral contraceptives, especially if you had irregular menstrual cycles before you used oral contraceptives. It may be advisable to postpone conception until you begin menstruating regularly once you have stopped taking the pill and desire pregnancy.
There does not appear to be any increase in birth defects in newborn babies when pregnancy occurs soon after stopping the pill.

Overdosage
Serious ill effects have not been reported following ingestion of large doses of oral contraceptives by young children. Overdosage may cause nausea and withdrawal bleeding in females. In case of overdosage, contact your health-care provider or pharmacist.

Other information
Your health-care provider will take a medical and family history before prescribing oral contraceptives and will examine you. The physical examination may be delayed to another time if you request it and the health-care provider believes that it is appropriate to postpone it. You should be reexamined at least once a year. Be sure to inform your health-care provider if there is a family history of any of the conditions listed previously in this leaflet. Be sure to keep all appointments with your health-care provider, because this is a time to determine if there are early signs of side effects of oral-contraceptive use.
Do not use the drug for any condition other than the one for which it was prescribed. This drug has been prescribed specifically for you; do not give it to others who may want birth-control pills.

HEALTH BENEFITS FROM ORAL CONTRACEPTIVES

In addition to preventing pregnancy, use of oral contraceptives may provide certain benefits. They are:

- Menstrual cycles may become more regular.
- Blood flow during menstruation may be lighter, and less iron may be lost. Therefore, anemia due to iron deficiency is less likely to occur.
- Pain or other symptoms during menstruation may be encountered less frequently.
- Ovarian cysts may occur less frequently.
- Ectopic (tubal) pregnancy may occur less frequently.
- Noncancerous cysts or lumps in the breast may occur less frequently.
- Acute pelvic inflammatory disease may occur less frequently.
- Oral-contraceptive use may provide some protection against developing two forms of cancer: cancer of the ovaries and cancer of the lining of the uterus.

If you want more information about birth-control pills, ask your doctor or pharmacist. They have a more technical leaflet called the Professional Labeling which you may wish to read.

Manufactured by:
Wyeth Laboratories Inc.
A Wyeth-Ayerst Company
Philadelphia, PA 19101

Shown in Product Identification Guide, page 343

ALESSE™-28   ℞
[ă 'lĕs]
levonorgestrel and ethinyl estradiol tablets

Patients should be counseled that this product does not protect against HIV infection (AIDS) and other sexually transmitted diseases.

DESCRIPTION

21 pink active tablets each containing 0.10 mg of levonorgestrel, d(-)-13β-ethyl-17α-ethinyl-17β-hydroxygon-4-en-3-one, a totally synthetic progestogen, and 0.02 mg of ethinyl estradiol, 17α-ethinyl-1,3,5(10)-estratriene-3, 17β-diol. The inactive ingredients present are cellulose, hydroxypropyl methylcellulose, iron oxide, lactose, magnesium stearate, polacrilin potassium, polyethylene glycol, titanium dioxide, and wax E.
7 light-green inert tablets, each containing cellulose, FD&C blue no. 1, hydroxypropyl methylcellulose, iron oxide, lactose, magnesium stearate, polacrilin potassium, polyethylene glycol, titanium dioxide, and wax E.

Levonorgestrel

Ethinyl Estradiol

CLINICAL PHARMACOLOGY
See ALESSE™-21.

INDICATIONS AND USAGE
See ALESSE-21.

CONTRAINDICATIONS
See ALESSE-21.

WARNINGS
See ALESSE-21.

PRECAUTIONS
See ALESSE-21.
Drug Interactions: See ALESSE-21.
Carcinogenesis: See ALESSE-21.
Pregnancy: See ALESSE-21.
Nursing Mothers: See ALESSE-21.
Information for the Patient: See Alesse-21.

ADVERSE REACTIONS
See Alesse-21.

OVERDOSAGE
See Alesse-21.

NONCONTRACEPTIVE HEALTH BENEFITS
See Alesse-21.

DOSAGE AND ADMINISTRATION
To achieve maximum contraceptive effectiveness, Alesse™ must be taken exactly as directed and at intervals not ex-

ceeding 24 hours. The dispenser should be kept in the wallet supplied to avoid possible fading of the pills. If the pills fade, patients should continue to take them as directed.
The dosage of Alesse-28 is one pink tablet daily for 21 consecutive days, followed by one light-green inert tablet daily for 7 consecutive days, according to the prescribed schedule. It is recommended that Alesse-28 tablets be taken at the same time each day.
Sunday start:
During the first cycle of medication, the patient is instructed to begin taking Alesse-28 on the first Sunday after the onset of menstruation. If menstruation begins on a Sunday, the first tablet (pink) is taken that day. One pink tablet should be taken daily for 21 consecutive days, followed by one light-green inert tablet daily for seven consecutive days. Withdrawal bleeding should usually occur within three days following discontinuation of pink tablets. During the first cycle, contraceptive reliance should not be placed on Alesse-28 until a pink tablet has been taken daily for 7 consecutive days. The possibility of ovulation and conception prior to initiation of medication should be considered.
The patient begins her next and all subsequent 28-day courses of tablets on the same day of the week (Sunday) on which she began her first course, following the same schedule: 21 days on pink tablets—7 days on light-green inert tablets. If in any cycle the patient starts tablets later than the proper day, she should protect herself against pregnancy by using another method of birth control until she has taken a pink tablet daily for 7 consecutive days.
Day 1 start:
During the first cycle of medication, the patient is instructed to begin taking Alesse-28 during the first 24 hours of her period (day one of her menstrual cycle). One pink tablet should be taken daily for 21 consecutive days, followed by one light-green inert tablet daily for seven consecutive days. Withdrawal bleeding should usually occur within three days following discontinuation of pink tablets. If medication is begun on day one of the menstrual cycle, no back-up contraception is necessary. If Alesse-28 tablets are started later than day one of the first menstrual cycle or postpartum, contraceptive reliance should not be placed on Alesse-28 tablets until after the first 7 consecutive days of administration. The possibility of ovulation and conception prior to initiation of medication should be considered.
When the patient is switching from a 21-day regimen of tablets, she should wait 7 days after her last tablet before she starts Alesse. She will probably experience withdrawal bleeding during that week. She should be sure that no more than 7 days pass after her previous 21-day regimen. When the patient is switching from a 28-day regimen of tablets, she should start her first pack of Alesse on the day after her last tablet. She should not wait any days between packs.
If spotting or breakthrough bleeding occur, the patient is instructed to continue on the same regimen. This type of bleeding is usually transient and without significance; however, if the bleeding is persistent or prolonged, the patient is advised to consult her physician. While there is little likelihood of ovulation occurring if only one or two pink tablets are missed, the possibility of ovulation increases with each successive day that scheduled pink tablets are missed. Although the occurrence of pregnancy is unlikely if Alesse is taken according to directions, if withdrawal bleeding does not occur, the possibility of pregnancy must be considered. If the patient has not adhered to the prescribed schedule (missed one or more tablets or started taking them on a day later than she should have), the probability of pregnancy should be considered at the time of the first missed period and appropriate diagnostic measures taken before the medication is resumed. If the patient has adhered to the prescribed regimen and misses two consecutive periods, pregnancy should be ruled out before continuing the contraceptive regimen.
The risk of pregnancy increases with each active (pink) tablet missed. For additional patient instructions regarding missed tablets, see the "WHAT TO DO IF YOU MISS PILLS" section in the **DETAILED PATIENT LABELING** below. In the nonlactating mother, Alesse may be initiated postpartum, for contraception. When the tablets are administered in the postpartum period, the increased risk of thromboembolic disease associated with the postpartum period must be considered (See "**Contraindications**", "**Warnings**", and "**Precautions**" concerning thromboembolic disease).

HOW SUPPLIED
Alesse™-28 tablets (0.10 mg levonorgestrel and 0.02 mg ethinyl estradiol) are available in packages of 3 MINI-PACK™ dispensers of 28 tablets each, NDC 0008-2576-02, as follows:
21 active tablets, NDC 0008-0912, pink, round tablet marked "w" and "912".
7 inert tablets, NDC 0008-0650, light-green, round tablet marked "w" and "650".
Store at controlled room temperature 20°–25° C (68°–77° F).
References available upon request.

BRIEF SUMMARY PATIENT PACKAGE INSERT
See Alesse-21.

DETAILED PATIENT LABELING
See Alesse-21.
Manufactured by:
Wyeth Laboratories Inc.
A Wyeth-Ayerst Company
Philadelphia, PA 19101
Shown in Product Identification Guide, page 343

AMPHOJEL®   OTC
[am 'fo-jel]
(aluminum hydroxide gel)
ORAL SUSPENSION • TABLETS

COMPOSITION

Suspension—Peppermint flavored—Each teaspoonful (5 ml) contains 320 mg of aluminum hydroxide [Al(OH)₃] as a gel, and not more than 0.10 mEq of sodium. The inactive ingredients present are calcium benzoate, glycerin, hydroxypropyl methylcellulose, menthol, peppermint oil, potassium butylparaben, potassium propylparaben, saccharin, simethicone, sorbitol solution, and water.
Suspension—Without flavor—Each teaspoonful (5 ml) contains 320 mg of aluminum hydroxide [Al (OH)₃] as a gel. The inactive ingredients present are butylparaben, calcium benzoate, glycerin, hydroxypropyl methylcellulose, methylparaben, propylparaben, saccharin, simethicone, sorbitol solution, and water.
Tablets available in 0.3 g and 0.6 g strengths. Each contains, respectively, the equivalent of 300 mg and 600 mg aluminum hydroxide as a dried gel. The inactive ingredients present are artificial and natural flavors, cellulose, hydrogenated vegetable oil, magnesium stearate, polacrilin potassium, saccharin, starch, and talc. The 0.3 g (5 grain) strength is equivalent to about 1 teaspoonful of the suspension and the 0.6 g (10 grain) strength is equivalent to about 2 teaspoonfuls. Each 0.3 g tablet contains 0.08 mEq of sodium and each 0.6 g tablet contains 0.13 mEq of sodium.

INDICATIONS

For the symptomatic relief of hyperacidity associated with the diagnosis of peptic ulcer, gastritis, peptic esophagitis, gastric hyperacidity, and hiatal hernia.

DOSAGE

Suspension—two teaspoonfuls followed by a sip of water if desired, five or six times daily, between meals and on retiring. Two teaspoonfuls have the capacity to neutralize 20 mEq of acid. *Tablets*—Two tablets of the 0.3 g strength, or one tablet of the 0.6 g strength, five or six times daily between meals and on retiring. Two tablets have the capacity to neutralize 16 mEq of acid.
It is unnecessary to chew the 0.3 g tablet before swallowing with water. After chewing the 0.6 g tablet, one-half glass of water should be sipped.

WARNINGS

Patients are advised not to take more than 12 teaspoonfuls (60 ml) or twelve (12) 0.3 g tablets or six (6) 0.6 g tablets in a 24-hour period or use this maximum dosage for more than two weeks except under the advice and supervision of a physician. Prolonged use of aluminum-containing antacids in patients with renal failure may result in or worsen dialysis osteomalacia. Elevated tissue aluminum levels contribute to the development of dialysis encephalopathy and osteomalacia syndromes. Also, a number of cases of dialysis encephalopathy have been associated with elevated aluminum levels in the dialysate water. Small amounts of aluminum are absorbed from the gastrointestinal tract and renal excretion of aluminum is impaired in renal failure. Prolonged use of aluminum-containing antacids in such patients may contribute to increased plasma levels of aluminum. Aluminum is not well removed by dialysis because it is bound to albumin and transferrin, which do not cross dialysis membranes. As a result, aluminum is deposited in bone, and dialysis osteomalacia may develop when large amounts of aluminum are ingested orally by patients with impaired renal function. Pregnant women and nursing mothers are advised to seek the advice of a health professional before using this product.

PRECAUTION

May cause constipation.

DRUG INTERACTION PRECAUTIONS

Antacids may interact with certain prescription drugs.
This product must not be taken if the patient is presently taking a prescription antibiotic drug containing any form of tetracycline.
If patients are presently taking a prescription drug, they are advised to check with their physicians before taking this product.

Continued on next page

Amphojel—Cont.

Keep tightly closed and store at room temperature, Approx. 77°F (25°C). Suspension should be shaken well before use. Avoid freezing. Keep this and all drugs out of the reach of children.

HOW SUPPLIED

Suspension—Peppermint flavored; without flavor—bottles of 12 fluidounces. *Tablets*—a convenient auxiliary dosage form—0.3 g (5 gr.), bottles of 100; 0.6 g (10 gr.), boxes of 100.
Manufactured by:
Wyeth Laboratories Inc.
A Wyeth-Ayerst Company
Philadelphia, PA 19101

ANTABUSE® ℞

[*an 'tah-būse*]
(disulfiram)
IN ALCOHOLISM

Caution: Federal law prohibits dispensing without prescription.

> **WARNING**
>
> Antabuse should *never* be administered to a patient when he is in a state of alcohol intoxication, or without his full knowledge.
> The physician should instruct relatives accordingly.

DESCRIPTION

CHEMICAL NAME: bis(diethylthiocarbamoyl) disulfide
STRUCTURAL FORMULA:

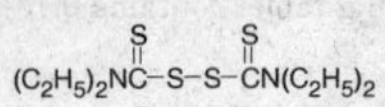

Antabuse occurs as a white to off-white, odorless, and almost tasteless powder, soluble in water to the extent of about 20 mg in 100 mL, and in alcohol to the extent of about 3.8 g in 100 mL.
Antabuse contains these inactive ingredients: magnesium aluminum silicate; magnesium stearate, NF; povidone, USP; starch, NF.

ACTION

Antabuse produces a sensitivity to alcohol which results in a highly unpleasant reaction when the patient under treatment ingests even small amounts of alcohol.
Antabuse blocks the oxidation of alcohol at the acetaldehyde stage. During alcohol metabolism following Antabuse intake, the concentration of acetaldehyde occurring in the blood may be 5- to 10-times higher than that found during metabolism of the same amount of alcohol alone.
Accumulation of acetaldehyde in the blood produces a complex of highly unpleasant symptoms referred to hereinafter as the Antabase-alcohol reaction. This reaction, which is proportional to the dosage of both Antabuse and alcohol, will persist as long as alcohol is being metabolized. Antabuse does not appear to influence the rate of alcohol elimination from the body.
Antabuse is absorbed slowly from the gastrointestinal tract and eliminated slowly from the body. One (or even two) weeks after a patient has taken his last dose of Antabuse, ingestion of alcohol may produce unpleasant symptoms.
Prolonged administration of Antabuse does not produce tolerance; the longer a patient remains on therapy, the more exquisitely sensitive he becomes to alcohol.

INDICATION

Antabuse is an aid in the management of selected chronic alcoholic patients who *want* to remain in a state of enforced sobriety so that supportive and psychotherapeutic treatment may be applied to best advantage.
Antabuse is not a cure for alcoholism. When used alone, without proper motivation and supportive therapy, it is unlikely that it will have any substantive effect on the drinking pattern of the chronic alcoholic.

CONTRAINDICATIONS

Patients who are receiving or have recently received metronidazole, paraldehyde, alcohol, or alcohol-containing preparations, e.g., cough syrups, tonics and the like, should not be given Antabuse.
Antabuse is contraindicated in the presence of severe myocardial disease or coronary occlusion, psychoses, and hypersensitivity to disulfiram or to other thiuram derivatives used in pesticides and rubber vulcanization.

WARNINGS

> Antabuse should *never* be administered to a patient when he is in a state of alcohol intoxication, or without his full knowledge.
> The physician should instruct relatives accordingly.

The patient must be fully informed of the Antabuse-alcohol reaction. He must be strongly cautioned against surreptitious drinking while taking the drug, and he must be fully aware of possible consequences. He should be warned to avoid alcohol in disguised form, i.e., in sauces, vinegars, cough mixtures, and even aftershave lotions and back rubs. He should also be warned that reactions may occur with alcohol up to 14 days after ingesting Antabuse.
THE ANTABUSE-ALCOHOL REACTION:
Antabuse plus alcohol, even small amounts, produces flushing, throbbing in head and neck, throbbing headache, respiratory difficulty, nausea, copious vomiting, sweating, thirst, chest pain, palpitation, dyspnea, hyperventilation, tachycardia, hypotension, syncope, marked uneasiness, weakness, vertigo, blurred vision, and confusion. In severe reactions there may be respiratory depression, cardiovascular collapse, arrhythmias, myocardial infarction, acute congestive heart failure, unconsciousness, convulsions, and death.
The intensity of the reaction varies with each individual but is generally proportional to the amounts of Antabuse and alcohol ingested. Mild reactions may occur in the sensitive individual when the blood alcohol concentration is increased to as little as 5 to 10 mg per 100 mL. Symptoms are fully developed at 50 mg per 100 mL, and unconsciousness usually results when the blood alcohol level reaches 125 to 150 mg.

The duration of the reaction varies from 30 to 60 minutes, to several hours in the more severe cases, or as long as there is alcohol in the blood.

DRUG INTERACTIONS
Disulfiram appears to decrease the rate at which certain drugs are metabolized and therefore may increase the blood levels and the possibility of clinical toxicity of drugs given concomitantly.

DISULFIRAM SHOULD BE USED WITH CAUTION IN THOSE PATIENTS RECEIVING PHENYTOIN AND ITS CONGENERS, SINCE THE CONCOMITANT ADMINISTRATION OF THESE TWO DRUGS CAN LEAD TO PHENYTOIN INTOXICATION. PRIOR TO ADMINISTERING DISULFIRAM TO A PATIENT ON PHENYTOIN THERAPY, A BASELINE PHENYTOIN SERUM LEVEL SHOULD BE OBTAINED. SUBSEQUENT TO INITIATION OF DISULFIRAM THERAPY, SERUM LEVELS OF PHENYTOIN SHOULD BE DETERMINED ON DIFFERENT DAYS FOR EVIDENCE OF AN INCREASE OR FOR A CONTINUING RISE IN LEVELS. INCREASED PHENYTOIN LEVELS SHOULD BE TREATED WITH APPROPRIATE DOSAGE ADJUSTMENT.
It may be necessary to adjust the dosage of oral anticoagulants upon beginning or stopping disulfiram, since disulfiram may prolong prothrombin time.
Patients taking isoniazid when disulfiram is given should be observed for the appearance of unsteady gait or marked changes in mental status; the disulfiram should be discontinued if such signs appear.
In rats, simultaneous ingestion of disulfiram and nitrite in the diet for 78 weeks has been reported to cause tumors, and it has been suggested that disulfiram may react with nitrites in the rat stomach to form a nitrosamine, which is tumorigenic. Disulfiram alone in the rats' diet did not lead to such tumors. The relevance of this finding to humans is not known at this time.
CONCOMITANT CONDITIONS
Because of the possibility of an accidental Antabuse-alcohol reaction, Antabuse should be used with extreme caution in patients with any of the following conditions: diabetes mellitus, hypothyroidism, epilepsy, cerebral damage, chronic and acute nephritis, hepatic cirrhosis or insufficiency.
USAGE IN PREGNANCY
The safe use of this drug in pregnancy has not been established. Therefore, Antabuse should be used during pregnancy only when, in the judgment of the physician, the probable benefits outweigh the possible risks.

PRECAUTIONS

Patients with a history of rubber contact dermatitis should be evaluated for hypersensitivity to thiuram derivatives before receiving Antabuse (see "Contraindications").
It is suggested that every patient under treatment carry an *Identification Card*, stating that he is receiving Antabuse and describing the symptoms most likely to occur as a result of the Antabuse-alcohol reaction. In addition, this card should indicate the physician or institution to be contacted in an emergency. (Cards may be obtained from Wyeth-Ayerst Laboratories upon request.)
Alcoholism may accompany or be followed by dependence on narcotics or sedatives. Barbiturates and Antabuse have been administered concurrently without untoward effects; the possibility of initiating a new abuse should be considered.
Baseline and follow-up transaminase tests (10 to 14 days) are suggested to detect any hepatic dysfunction that may result with Antabuse therapy. In addition, a complete blood count and a sequential multiple analysis-12 (SMA-12) test should be made every six months.
Patients taking Antabuse Tablets should not be exposed to ethylene dibromide or its vapors. This precaution is based on preliminary results of animal research currently in progress that suggest a toxic interaction between inhaled ethylene dibromide and ingested disulfiram resulting in a higher incidence of tumors and mortality in rats. A correlation between this finding and humans, however, has not been demonstrated.

ADVERSE REACTIONS

(See "Contraindications," "Warnings," and "Precautions.")
OPTIC NEURITIS, PERIPHERAL NEURITIS, POLYNEURITIS, AND PERIPHERAL NEUROPATHY MAY OCCUR FOLLOWING ADMINISTRATION OF ANTABUSE.
Multiple cases of hepatitis, including both cholestatic and fulminant hepatitis, have been reported to be associated with administration of Antabuse.
Occasional skin eruptions are, as a rule, readily controlled by concomitant administration of an antihistaminic drug.
In a small number of patients, a transient mild drowsiness, fatigability, impotence, headache, acneform eruptions, allergic dermatitis, or a metallic or garlic-like aftertaste may be experienced during the first two weeks of therapy. These complaints usually disappear spontaneously with the continuation of therapy, or with reduced dosage.
Psychotic reactions have been noted, attributable in most cases to high dosage, combined toxicity (with metronidazole or isoniazid), or to the unmasking of underlying psychoses in patients stressed by the withdrawal of alcohol.

DOSAGE AND ADMINISTRATION

Antabuse should never be administered until the patient has abstained from alcohol for at least 12 hours.
INITIAL DOSAGE SCHEDULE
In the first phase of treatment, a *maximum* of 500 mg daily is given in a single dose for one to two weeks. Although usually taken in the morning, Antabuse may be taken on retiring by patients who experience a sedative effect. Alternatively, to minimize, or eliminate, the sedative effect, dosage may be adjusted downward.
MAINTENANCE REGIMEN
The average maintenance dose is 250 mg daily (range, 125 to 500 mg); it should not exceed 500 mg daily.

Note: Occasionally patients, while seemingly on adequate maintenance doses of Antabuse, report that they are able to drink alcoholic beverages with impunity and without any symptomatology. All appearances to the contrary, such patients must be presumed to be disposing of their tablets in some manner without actually taking them. Until such patients have been observed reliably taking their daily Antabuse Tablets (preferably crushed and well mixed with liquid), it cannot be concluded that Antabuse is ineffective.
DURATION OF THERAPY
The daily, uninterrupted administration of Antabuse must be continued until the patient is fully recovered socially and a basis for permanent self-control is established. Depending on the individual patient, maintenance therapy may be required for months, or even years.
TRIAL WITH ALCOHOL
During early experience with Antabuse, it was thought advisable for each patient to have at least one supervised alcohol-drug reaction. More recently, the test reaction has been largely abandoned. Furthermore, such a test reaction should never be administered to a patient over 50 years of age. A clear, detailed, and convincing description of the reaction is felt to be sufficient in most cases.
However, where a test reaction is deemed necessary, the suggested procedure is as follows:

After the first one to two weeks' therapy with 500 mg daily, a drink of 15 mL ($^1/_2$ oz) of 100 proof whiskey, or equivalent, is taken slowly. This test dose of alcoholic beverage may be repeated once only, so that the total dose does not exceed 30 mL (1 oz) of whiskey. Once a reaction develops, no more alcohol should be consumed. Such tests should be carried out only when the patient is hospitalized, or comparable supervision and facilities, including oxygen, are available.
MANAGEMENT OF ANTABUSE-ALCOHOL REACTION:
In severe reactions, whether caused by an excessive test dose or by the patient's unsupervised ingestion of alcohol, supportive measures to restore blood pressure and treat shock should be instituted. Other recommendations include: oxygen, carbogen (95% oxygen and 5% carbon dioxide), vitamin C intravenously in massive doses (1 g), and ephedrine sulfate. Antihistamines have also been used intravenously. Potassium levels should be monitored, particularly in patients on digitalis, since hypokalemia has been reported.

HOW SUPPLIED

Antabuse® (disulfiram) Tablets are available in the following dosage strengths:
250 mg, NDC 0046-0809-81, white-to-off-white, octagonal-shaped, scored, compressed tablet, embossed with a stylized "A" on one side and imprinted with "ANTABUSE" and "250" on the scored reverse side, in bottles of 100 tablets.
500 mg, NDC 0046-0810-50, white-to-off-white, octagonal-shaped, scored compressed tablet, embossed with a stylized "A" on one side and imprinted with "ANTABUSE" and "500" on the scored reverse side, in bottles of 50 tablets.
Store at room temperature, approximately 25°C.
Dispense in a tight, light-resistant container as defined in the USP
Manufactured by:
Ayerst Laboratories Inc.
A Wyeth-Ayerst Company
Philadelphia, PA 19101
Shown in Product Identification Guide, page 343

ANTIVENIN ℞
(CROTALIDAE)
[an "te ven 'in]
POLYVALENT
(equine origin)

IMPORTANT

Pit viper bites may cause severe tissue damage or fatal envenomation, or both. The physician responsible for treatment of an envenomated patient should be familiar with the contents of this brochure and the pertinent medical literature concerning current concepts of first-aid and general supportive therapy as presented in the references listed at the end of this pamphlet.

COMPOSITION

Antivenin (Crotalidae) Polyvalent, Wyeth, is a refined and concentrated preparation of serum globulins obtained by fractionating blood from healthy horses immunized with the following venoms: *Crotalus adamanteus* (Eastern diamond rattlesnake), *C. atrox* (Western diamond rattlesnake), *C. durissus terrificus* (tropical rattlesnake, Cascabel), and *Bothrops atrox* ("Fer-de-lance"). Phenol, 0.25%, and thimerosal, 0.005%, are added as preservatives. The product is standardized by its ability to neutralize the lethal action of standard venoms by intravenous injection in mice.[1] Dried from the frozen state, the lyophilized serum has a moisture content of less than 1% and is soluble on addition of the diluent contained in each package (Bacteriostatic Water for Injection, USP, with preservative: 0.001% phenylmercuric nitrate).
Antivenin (Crotalidae) Polyvalent, Wyeth (hereinafter referred to as Antivenin) contains protective substances capable of neutralizing the toxic effects of venoms of crotalids (pit vipers) native to North, Central, and South America, including rattlesnakes *(Crotalus, Sistrurus)*; copperhead and cottonmouth moccasins *(Agkistrodon)*, including *A. halys* of Korea and Japan; the Fer-de-lance and other species of *Bothrops*; the tropical rattler (*Crotalus durissus* and similar species); the Cantil (*A. bilineatus*); and bushmaster *(Lachesis mutus)* of South and Central America.

INDICATION

Antivenin is indicated only for the treatment of envenomation caused by bites of those crotalids (pit vipers) specified in the immediately preceding paragraph.

PIT VIPER BITES AND ENVENOMATION

The symptoms, signs, and severity of snake-venom poisoning resulting from pit viper bites depend on many factors, including, but not limited to, the following variables: species, age, and size of the biting snake; the number and location of bite(s); the depth of venom deposit by the snake's fangs; the condition of the snake's fangs and venom glands; the length of time the snake "hangs on"; the age, general health, and size of the victim; the type and efficacy of any first-aid treatment rendered in an attempt to remove venom and how soon such treatment was applied. In any venomous snake bite, the actual amount of venom introduced into the victim is always an unknown. Even the type of clothing or leg-footwear through which the snake's fangs pass may affect the amount of venom delivered by the bite. Although most North American pit vipers tend to bite and introduce venom superficially, their fangs may get hung-up in the subcutaneous tissues during the biting act and can penetrate deeper tissues during the attempt to release the bitten part. In some bites the fangs may penetrate into muscle. In such cases, the usual local superficial manifestations of envenomation may not appear early in the course of poisoning. In bites by some species, systemic evidence of envenomation may be present in the absence of significant local manifestations. It may be difficult to determine the severity of envenomation during the first several hours after a pit viper bite and estimates of severity may need to be revised as poisoning progresses. It must be remembered, too, that not all pit viper bites result in envenomation. In approximately 20% of rattlesnake bites, the snake may not inject any venom. The local and systemic symptoms and signs of envenomation include the following:
LOCAL:
Fang puncture(s).
Swelling—edema is usually seen around the site of bite within five minutes. It may progress rapidly and involve the entire extremity within an hour. More than 95% of all snakebites are inflicted on extremities.[2] Generally, however, edema spreads more slowly, usually over a period of 8 or more hours. Swelling is usually most severe following envenomation by the Eastern diamondback; less severe after bites by the Western diamondback, prairie, timber, red, Pacific, Mojave, and blacktailed rattlers, the sidewinder and cottonmouth moccasins; least severe after bites by copperheads, massasaugas, and pygmy rattlers.
Ecchymosis and discoloration of the skin—often appear in the area of the bite within a few hours. Vesicules may form within a few hours and are usually present at 24 hours. Hemorrhagic blebs and petechiae are common. Necrosis may develop, necessitating amputation of an extremity or a portion thereof.
Pain—frequently a complaint of the victim beginning shortly after the bite by most pit vipers. Pain may be absent after bites by Mojave rattlers.
SYSTEMIC:
Weakness; faintness; nausea; sweating; numbness or tingling around the mouth, tongue, scalp, fingers, toes, site of bite; muscle fasciculations; hypotension; prolongation of bleeding and clotting times; hemoconcentration, early followed by a decrease in erythrocytes; thrombocytopenia; hematuria; proteinuria; vomiting, including hematemesis; melena; hemoptysis; epistaxis. In fatal poisoning, a frequent cause of death is associated with destruction of erythrocytes and changes in capillary permeability, especially of the pulmonary vascular system, leading to pulmonary edema; hemoconcentration usually occurs early, probably as a result of plasma loss secondary to vascular permeability; the hemoglobin may fall, and bleeding may occur throughout the body as early as 6 hours after the bite. Renal involvement is not uncommon. Mojave rattler venom may cause neuromuscular changes leading to respiratory failure.
An estimate of the severity of envenomation should be made as soon as possible and before any Antivenin is administered. The amount (volume) of the first dose of Antivenin is determined on this estimate of severity. Every symptom, sign, laboratory-test result, and any other pertinent information should be considered in estimating severity—local manifestations; systemic manifestations, including abnormal laboratory findings; species and size of the biting snake, if known; number and location of bite(s); size and health of the patient; type of first-aid treatment rendered; and interval between bite and arrival for treatment. Russell et al,[3] and Wingert and Wainschel[4] grade severity as follows:
No envenomation—no local or systemic manifestations.
Minimal envenomation—local swelling and other local changes; no systemic manifestations; normal laboratory findings.
Moderate envenomation—swelling progressing beyond the site of bite and one or more systemic manifestations; abnormal laboratory findings, for example, a fall in hematocrit or platelets.
Severe envenomation—marked local response, severe systemic manifestations and significant alteration in laboratory findings.
Parrish and Hayes,[5] McCollough and Gennaro,[6] and Watt and Gennaro[7] have used a Grade 0 (no envenomation) through Grade IV (very severe) classification of severity which was developed for the most part in treatment of envenomation by the Eastern diamondback and timber rattlers. This classification is more dependent on local manifestations, or the absence thereof, as the venoms of these species seem to be more consistent in inducing local tissue damage.
Any suspected envenomation should be treated as a medical emergency, and until careful observation provides clear evidence that envenomation has not occurred or is minimal, the following procedures are recommended:
Monitor vital signs at frequent intervals: Blood pressure, pulse, respiration.
Draw sufficient blood as soon as possible for baseline laboratory studies, including type and cross-match, CBC, hematocrit, platelet count, prothrombin time, clot retraction, bleeding and coagulation times, BUN, electrolytes, bilirubin. Some of these studies may need to be repeated at daily intervals, or less, depending on the severity of envenomation and the response to treatment. During the first 4 or 5 days of severe envenomations, hemoglobin, hematocrit, and platelet counts should be carried out several times a day.
Obtain urine samples at frequent intervals for analysis, with special attention to microscopic examination for presence of erythrocytes.
Chart fluid intake and urine output.
Measure and record the circumference of the bitten extremity just proximal to the bite and at one or more additional points each several inches closer to the trunk. Repeat measurements every 15-30 minutes to obtain information about progression of edema.
Have available and ready for immediate use: oxygen, resuscitation equipment including airway, tourniquet, epinephrine, injectable antihistaminic agents and corticosteroids.
Start an intravenous infusion in one or two extremities: one line to be used for supportive therapy, if needed, such as whole blood, plasma, packed red cells, specific clotting factors, platelet transfusion, plasma expanders; the other line to be used for administration of Antivenin and electrolytes.
Carry out and interpret a skin test for horse-serum sensitivity. (See "Precautions" section below.)

DOSAGE AND ADMINISTRATION

Before administration, read "Precautions" and "Systemic Reactions" sections below. Since the possibility of a severe immediate reaction (anaphylaxis) exists whenever a horse-serum-containing product is administered, appropriate therapeutic agents, including a tourniquet, airway, oxygen, epinephrine, an injectable pressor amine, and corticosteroid, must be available and ready for immediate use. Constant attendance and observation of the patient for untoward reactions are mandatory when Antivenin is administered. Should any systemic reaction occur, administration should be discontinued immediately and appropriate treatment initiated.
The intravenous route of administration is preferred, and probably should always be used for moderate or severe envenomation. Intravenous administration is mandatory if venom-induced shock is present. To be most effective, Antivenin should be administered within 4 hours of the bite; it is less effective when given after 8 hours and may be of questionable value after 12 hours. However, it is recommended that Antivenin therapy be given in severe poisonings, even if 24 hours have elapsed since the time of the bite. It should be kept in mind that maximum blood levels of Antivenin may not be obtained for 8 or more hours after intramuscular administration.
For intravenous-drip use, prepare a 1:1 to 1:10 dilution of reconstituted Antivenin in Sodium Chloride Injection, USP, or 5% Dextrose Injection, USP. To avoid foaming, mix by gently swirling rather than shaking. Allow the initial 5 to 10 mL to infuse over a 3- to 5-minute period, with careful observation of the patient for evidence of untoward reaction. If no symptoms or signs of an immediate systemic reaction appear, continue the infusion with delivery at the maximum safe rate for intravenous fluid administration. The dilution of Antivenin to be used, the type of electrolyte solution used for dilution, and the rate of intravenous delivery of the diluted Antivenin must take into consideration the age, weight, and cardiac status of the patient; the severity of envenomation; the total amount and type of parenteral fluids it is anticipated will be given or are needed; and the interval between bite and initiation of specific therapy.
It is important to give as soon as possible the entire initial dose of Antivenin as based on the best estimate of the severity of envenomation at the time treatment is begun. The following initial doses are recommended:[3,4,8]
no envenomation—none
minimal envenomation—20-40 mL (contents of 2 to 4 vials)
moderate envenomation—50-90 mL (contents of 5 to 9 vials)
severe envenomation—100-150 mL or more (contents of 10 to 15 or more vials)
These recommended initial-dosage volumes are in general accord with those of others.[5-7,9]
The need for additional Antivenin must be based on the clinical response to the initial dose and continuing assessment of the severity of poisoning. If swelling continues to progress or if systemic symptoms or signs of envenomation increase in severity or if new manifestations appear, for example, fall in hematocrit or hypotension, administer an additional 10 to 50 mL (contents of 1 to 5 vials) intravenously.
Envenomation by large snakes in children or small adults requires larger doses of Antivenin. The amount administered to a child is not based on weight.
If Antivenin is given intramuscularly, it should be given into a large muscle mass, preferably the gluteal area, with care to avoid nerve trunks. Antivenin should never be injected into a finger or toe.
The effectiveness of corticosteroids in treatment of envenomation per se or venom shock is not resolved. Russell[3] and others[9,10] believe corticosteroids may mask the seriousness of hypovolemia in moderate or severe poisoning and have little, if any, effect on the local-tissue response to rattler venoms. Corticosteroids should not be given simultaneously with Antivenin on a routine basis or during the acute state of envenomation; however, their use may be necessary to treat immediate allergic reactions to Antivenin, and corticosteroids are the agents of choice for treating serious delayed reactions to Antivenin.

Continued on next page

Antivenin-Crotalidae—Cont.

Snakes' mouths do not harbor *Clostridium tetani*. However, appropriate tetanus prophylaxis is indicated, since tetanus spores may be carried into the fang puncture wounds by dirt present on skin at time of bite or by nonsterile first-aid procedures.

A broad-spectrum antibiotic in adequate dosage is indicated if local tissue damage is evident.

Shock following envenomation is treated like shock resulting from hypovolemia from any cause, including administration of whole blood, plasma, albumin, or other plasma expanders, as indicated.

Aspirin or codeine is usually adequate for relieving pain. Sedation with phenobarbital or mild tranquilizers may be used if indicated, but not in the presence of respiratory failure.

The bitten extremity should not be packed in ice, and so-called "cryotherapy" is contraindicated.

Compartment syndromes may complicate pit viper envenomations, especially those caused by bites on the lower extremities. Prompt surgical consultation is indicated whenever a closed-compartment syndrome is suspected.[3,12]

Defibrination and disseminated intravascular coagulation (DIC) syndromes have been associated with envenomation caused by some pit vipers native to the United States, and appropriate therapy may be indicated.[3,9,10,13–17]

TECHNIC FOR RECONSTITUTING THE DRIED ANTIVENIN

Pry off the small metal disc in the cap over the diaphragms of the vials of Antivenin and diluent. Swab the exposed surface of the rubber diaphragms of both vials with an appropriate germicide. With a sterile 10 mL syringe and needle, withdraw the diluent (Bacteriostatic Water for Injection, USP, containing phenylmercuric nitrate 1:100,000) from the vial of diluent and inject it into the vial of Antivenin. Gentle agitation will hasten complete dissolution of the lyophilized Antivenin.

PRECAUTIONS

Before administration of any product prepared from horse serum, appropriate measures must be taken in an effort to detect the presence of dangerous sensitivity: (1) A careful review of the patient's history, including any report of (a) asthma, hay fever, urticaria, or other allergic manifestations; (b) allergic reactions upon exposure to horses; and (c) prior injections of horse serum. (2) A suitable test for detection of sensitivity. A skin test should be performed in every patient prior to administration, regardless of clinical history.

Skin test—Inject intracutaneously 0.02 to 0.03 mL of a 1:10 dilution of Normal Horse Serum or Antivenin. A control test on the opposite extremity, using Sodium Chloride Injection, USP, facilitates interpretation. Use of larger amounts for the skin-test dose increases the likelihood of false-positive reactions, and in the exquisitely sensitive patient, increases the risk of a systemic reaction from the skin-test dose. A 1:100 or greater dilution should be used for preliminary skin testing if the history suggests sensitivity. A positive reaction to a skin test occurs within five to thirty minutes and is manifested by a wheal with or without pseudopodia and surrounding erythema. In general, the shorter the interval between injection and the beginning of the skin reaction, the greater the sensitivity.

If the history is negative for allergy and the result of a skin test is negative, proceed with administration of Antivenin as outlined above. If the history is positive and a skin test is strongly positive, administration may be dangerous, especially if the positive sensitivity test is accompanied by systemic allergic manifestations. In such instances, the risk of administering Antivenin must be weighed against the risk of withholding it, keeping in mind that severe envenomation can be fatal. (See last paragraph of this section.)

A negative allergic history and absence of reaction to a properly applied skin test do not rule out the possibility of an immediate reaction. Also, a negative skin test has no bearing on whether or not delayed serum reactions (serum sickness) will occur after administration of the full dose.

If the history is negative, and the skin test is mildly or questionably positive, administer as follows to reduce the risk of a severe immediate systemic reaction: (a) Prepare, in separate sterile vials or syringes, 1:100 and 1:10 dilutions of Antivenin. (b) Allow at least 15 minutes between injections and proceed with the next dose if no reaction follows the previous dose. (c) Inject subcutaneously, using a tuberculin-type syringe, 0.1, 0.2, and 0.5 mL of the 1:100 dilution at 15-minute intervals; repeat with the 1:10 dilution, and finally undiluted Antivenin. (d) If a systemic reaction occurs after any injection, place a tourniquet proximal to the site of injections and administer an appropriate dose of epinephrine, 1:1000, proximal to the tourniquet or into another extremity. Wait at least 30 minutes before injecting another dose. The amount of the next dose should be the same as the last that did not evoke a reaction. (e) If no reaction occurs after 0.5 mL of undiluted Antivenin has been administered,

switch to the intramuscular route and continue doubling the dose at 15-minute intervals until the entire dose has been injected intramuscularly or proceed to the intravenous route as described above under "Dosage and Administration."

Obviously, if the just-described schedule is used, 3 to 5 or more hours would be required to administer the initial dose suggested for a moderate or severe envenomation, and time is an important factor in neutralization of venom in a critically ill patient. Wingert and Wainschel[4] have described a procedure based on the experience of their group which they have used in some severely envenomated patients who have positive sensitivity tests: 50 to 100 mg of diphenhydramine hydrochloride is given intravenously, followed by slow intravenous infusion of diluted Antivenin for 15 to 20 minutes while carefully observing the patient for symptoms and signs of anaphylaxis; if anaphylaxis does not occur, Antivenin is continued, maintaining close observation of the patient. Patients who require Antivenin but develop signs of impending anaphylaxis in spite of this or the procedure described earlier present a difficult problem, and consultation should be sought.

SYSTEMIC REACTIONS

A. The immediate reaction (shock, anaphylaxis) usually occurs within 30 minutes. Symptoms and signs may develop before the needle is withdrawn and may include apprehension, flushing, itching, urticaria; edema of the face, tongue, and throat; cough, dyspnea, cyanosis, vomiting, and collapse.

B. Serum sickness usually occurs 5 to 24 days after administration. The incubation period may be less than 5 days, especially in those who have received horse-serum-containing preparations in the past. The usual symptoms and signs are malaise, fever, urticaria, lymphadenopathy, edema, arthralgia, nausea, and vomiting. Occasionally, neurological manifestations develop, such as meningismus or peripheral neuritis. Peripheral neuritis usually involves the shoulders and arms. Pain and muscle weakness are frequently present, and permanent atrophy may develop.

REFERENCES

1. GINGRICH, W. & HOHENADEL, J.: Standardization of polyvalent antivenin. "Venoms", edited by E. Buckley and N. Porges. Publication No. 44, Amer. Assoc. for the Advancement of Science, Washington, D.C., 1956, Pages 337–80.
2. PARRISH, H.: Incidence of treated snakebite in the United States. Pub. Hlth. Rep. *81* :269, 1966.
3. RUSSELL, F., et al.: Snake venom poisoning in the United States. Experiences with 550 cases. JAMA *233* :341, 1975. RUSSELL, F.: Venomous bites and stings: Poisonous snakes. In The Merck Manual of Diagnosis and Therapy, pp. 2450–2456, 14th Ed., 1982.
4. WINGERT, W. and WAINSCHEL, J.: Diagnosis and management of envenomation by poisonous snakes. South. Med. J. *68* :1015, 1975.
5. PARRISH, H. & HAYES, R.: Hospital management of pit viper venenations. Clinical Toxicol. *3* :501, 1970.
6. McCOLLOUGH, N. & GENNARO, J.: Diagnosis, symptoms, treatment and sequelae of envenomation by *Crotalus adamanteus* and Genus *Agkistrodon*. J. Florida Med. Assoc. *55* :327, 1968.
7. WATT, C. & GENNARO, J.: Pit viper bites in South Georgia and North Florida. Tr. South. Surg. Assoc. *77* :378, 1966.
8. MINTON, S.: Venom Diseases: Snakebite. In Textbook of Medicine, P. Beeson and W. McDermott (Eds.), pp. 88–92, Saunders, Philadelphia, 1975.
9. VAN MIEROP, L.: Snakebite symposium. J. Florida Med. Assoc. *63* :101, 1976.
10. ARNOLD, R.: Treatment of snakebite. JAMA *236* : 1843, 1976; Controversies and hazards in the treatment of pit viper bites. South Med. J. *72* :902, 1979.
11. Poisonous Snakes of the World. U.S. Government Printing Office, Washington, D.C., NAVMED, 1965.
12. GARFIN, S. et al.: Rattlesnake bites: Current concepts. Clin. Orthop. *140* :50, 1979; Role of surgical decompression in treatment of rattlesnake bites. Surg. Forum *30* :502, 1979.
13. VAN MIEROP, L. & KITCHENS, C.: Defibrination syndrome following bites by the Eastern diamondback rattlesnake. J. Florida Med. Assoc. *67* :21, 1980.
14. HASIBA, U. et al.: DIC-like syndrome after envenomation by the snake, *Crotalus horridus horridus*. New Eng. J. Med. *292* :505, 1975.
15. WEISS, H. et al.: Afibrinogenemia in man following the bite of a rattlesnake (*Crotalus adamanteus*). Am. J. Med. *47* :625, 1969.
16. SIVAPRASAD, R. & CANTINI, E.: Western diamondback rattlesnake (*Crotalus atrox*) poisoning. Postgrad. Med. *71* :223, 1982.
17. SABBACK, M. et al.: A study of the treatment of pit viper envenomization in 45 patients. J. Trauma *17* :569, 1977.

HOW SUPPLIED

Each combination package contains one vacuum vial to yield 10 mL of serum—to be used immediately after reconstitution or within 48 hr of reconstitution if stored at 2–8°C.—(with preservatives: phenol 0.25% and thimerosal [mercury derivative] 0.005%). One vial containing 10 mL of Bacteriostatic Water for Injection, USP (with preservative: phenylmercuric nitrate 0.001%). One 1 mL vial of normal horse serum (diluted 1:10) as sensitivity testing material with preservatives: thimerosal (mercury derivative) 0.005% and phenol 0.35%. Not returnable.

Manufactured by: Wyeth Laboratories Inc., A Wyeth-Ayerst Company, Marietta, PA 17547.

ANTIVENIN ℞
(Micrurus fulvius)
[an "te ven 'in]
(equine origin)
North American Coral Snake Antivenin

COMPOSITION

Each combination package contains one vial of lyophilized Antivenin (Micrurus fulvius) with 0.25% phenol and 0.005% thimerosal (mercury derivative) as preservatives (before lyophilization); one vial of diluent containing 10 mL of Bacteriostatic Water for Injection, U.S.P., with phenylmercuric nitrate (0.001%) as preservative.

HOW SUPPLIED

Combination packages as described (not returnable).
Manufactured by Wyeth Laboratories Inc., A Wyeth-Ayerst Company, Marietta, PA 17547.
For prescribing information write to Professional Service, Wyeth-Ayerst Laboratories, P.O. Box 8299, Philadelphia, PA 19101, or contact your local Wyeth-Ayerst representative.

A.P.L.® ℞
(chorionic gonadotropin for injection, USP)
For Intramuscular Injection Only

Rx only

DESCRIPTION

Human chorionic gonadotropin (HCG), a polypeptide hormone produced by the human placenta, is composed of an alpha and a beta subunit. The alpha subunit is essentially identical to the alpha subunits of the human pituitary gonadotropins, luteinizing hormone (LH) and follicle-stimulating hormone (FSH), as well as to the alpha subunit of human thyroid stimulating hormone (TSH). The beta subunits of these hormones differ in amino acid sequence.

A.P.L. (chorionic gonadotropin, USP) is a gonad-stimulating principle obtained from the urine of pregnant women. It is a sterile, amorphous powder prepared by cryodesiccation, and is freely soluble in water.

When reconstituted with the accompanying 10 mL of sterile diluent water, each SECULE® vial contains:

5,000 USP units of chorionic gonadotropin, 2.0% benzyl alcohol, 0.9% lactose, and not more than 0.2% phenol;
10,000 USP units of chorionic gonadotropin, 2.0% benzyl alcohol, 1.8% lactose, and not more than 0.2% phenol;
20,000 USP units of chorionic gonadotropin, 2.0% benzyl alcohol, 3.6% lactose, and not more than 0.2% phenol.

The pH is adjusted with sodium hydroxide or hydrochloric acid.

After reconstitution, store refrigerated and use within 30 days.

THIS PRODUCT IS FOR INTRAMUSCULAR INJECTION ONLY.

HOW SUPPLIED

A.P.L.® (chorionic gonadotropin for injection, USP)
NDC 0046-0970-10 — Each package provides:
(1) One vial containing 5,000 USP units chorionic gonadotropin in dry form, and
(2) One 10 mL ampul sterile diluent.
NDC 0046-0971-10 — Each package provides:
(1) One vial containing 10,000 USP units chorionic gonadotropin in dry form, and
(2) One 10 mL ampul sterile diluent.
NDC 0046-0972-10 — Each package provides:
(1) One vial containing 20,000 USP units chorionic gonadotropin in dry form, and
(2) One 10 mL ampul sterile diluent.
The product is assayed in accord with USP method; USP potency units are defined in terms of the USP Chorionic Gonadotropin Reference Standard.

When reconstituted with 10 mL of accompanying sterile diluent, the resulting solutions also contain 2.0% benzyl alcohol, not more than 0.2% phenol, and the following concentrations of lactose: No. 970, 0.9%; No. 971, 1.8%; No. 972, 3.6%. The pH is adjusted with sodium hydroxide or hydrochloric acid.

Directions for Reconstitution
Withdraw sterile air from lyophilized vial. Remove 10 mL from diluent ampule and add to lyophilized vial; agitate gently until powder is completely dissolved.
MAY BE STORED FOR 30 DAYS IN A REFRIGERATOR AFTER RECONSTITUTION.
Manufactured by:
Ayerst Laboratories Inc.
A Wyeth-Ayerst Company
Philadelphia, PA 19101
For prescribing information write to Professional Service, Wyeth-Ayerst Laboratories, P.O. Box 8299, Philadelphia, PA 19101, or contact your local Wyeth-Ayerst representative.

ATIVAN® Ⓒ℞
[*ăt ĭ-văn*]
(lorazepam)
Injection

DESCRIPTION

Lorazepam, a benzodiazepine with antianxiety, sedative, and anticonvulsant effects, is intended for intramuscular or intravenous routes of administration. It has the chemical formula: 7-chloro-5-(2-chlorophenyl)-1,3-dihydro-3-hydroxy-2*H*-1,4-benzodiazepin-2-one. The molecular weight is 321.16, and the C.A.S. No. is [846-49-1].
Lorazepam is a nearly white powder almost insoluble in water. Each mL of sterile injection contains either 2.0 or 4.0 mg of lorazepam, 0.18 mL polyethylene glycol 400 in propylene glycol with 2.0% benzyl alcohol as preservative.

CLINICAL PHARMACOLOGY

Lorazepam interacts with the γ-aminobutyric acid (GABA)-benzodiazepine receptor complex, which is widespread in the brain of humans as well as other species. This interaction is presumed to be responsible for lorazepam's mechanism of action. Lorazepam exhibits relatively high and specific affinity for its recognition site but does not displace GABA. Attachment to the specific binding site enhances the affinity of GABA for its receptor site on the same receptor complex. The pharmacodynamic consequences of benzodiazepine agonist actions include antianxiety effects, sedation, and reduction of seizure activity. The intensity of action is directly related to the degree of benzodiazepine receptor occupancy.

Effects in Pre-Operative Patients
Intravenous or intramuscular administration of the recommended dose of 2 mg to 4 mg of Ativan Injection to adult patients is followed by dose-related effects of sedation (sleepiness or drowsiness), relief of preoperative anxiety, and lack of recall of events related to the day of surgery in the majority of patients. The clinical sedation (sleepiness or drowsiness) thus noted is such that the majority of patients are able to respond to simple instructions whether they give the appearance of being awake or asleep. The lack of recall is relative rather than absolute, as determined under conditions of careful patient questioning and testing, using props designed to enhance recall. The majority of patients under these reinforced conditions had difficulty recalling perioperative events or recognizing props from before surgery. The lack of recall and recognition was optimum within 2 hours following intramuscular administration and 15 to 20 minutes after intravenous injection.
The intended effects of the recommended adult dose of Ativan Injection usually last 6 to 8 hours. In rare instances, and where patients received greater than the recommended dose, excessive sleepiness and prolonged lack of recall were noted. As with other benzodiazepines, unsteadiness, enhanced sensitivity to CNS-depressant effects of ethyl alcohol and other drugs were noted in isolated and rare cases for greater than 24 hours.

Physiologic Effects in Healthy Adults
Studies in healthy adult volunteers reveal that intravenous lorazepam in doses up to 3.5 mg/70 kg does not alter sensitivity to the respiratory stimulating effect of carbon dioxide and does not enhance the respiratory-depressant effects of doses of meperidine up to 100 mg/70 kg (also determined by carbon dioxide challenge) as long as patients remain sufficiently awake to undergo testing. Upper airway obstruction has been observed in rare instances where the patient received greater than the recommended dose and was excessively sleepy and difficult to arouse (see **WARNINGS** and **ADVERSE REACTIONS**.)
Clinically employed doses of Ativan Injection do not greatly affect the circulatory system in the supine position or employing a 70-degree tilt test. Doses of 8 mg to 10 mg of intravenous lorazepam (2 to $2^1/_2$ times the maximum recommended dosage) will produce loss of lid reflexes within 15 minutes.
Studies in 6 healthy young adults who received lorazepam injection and no other drugs revealed that visual tracking (the ability to keep a moving line centered) was impaired for a mean of 8 hours following administration of 4 mg of intramuscular lorazepam and 4 hours following administration of 2 mg intramuscularly with considerable subject variation. Similar findings were noted with pentobarbital, 150 and 75 mg. Although this study showed that both lorazepam and pentobarbital interfered with eye-hand coordination, the data are insufficient to predict when it would be safe to operate a motor vehicle or engage in a hazardous occupation or sport.

Pharmacokinetics and Metabolism
Absorption
Intravenous
A 4-mg dose provides an initial concentration of 70 ng/mL.
Intramuscular
Following intramuscular administration, lorazepam is completely and rapidly absorbed reaching peak concentrations within 3 hours. A 4-mg dose provides a C_{max} of approximately 48 ng/mL. Following administration of 1.5 to 5.0 mg of lorazepam IM, the amount of lorazepam delivered to the circulation is proportional to the dose administered.
Distribution / Metabolism / Elimination
At clinically relevant concentrations, lorazepam is 91±2% bound to plasma proteins; its volume of distribution is approximately 1.3 L/kg. Unbound lorazepam penetrates the blood/brain barrier freely by passive diffusion, a fact confirmed by CSF sampling. Following parenteral administration, the terminal half-life and total clearance averaged 14.5±5 hours and 1.1±0.4 mL/min/kg, respectively.
Lorazepam is extensively conjugated to the 3-O-phenolic glucuronide in the liver and is known to undergo enterohepatic recirculation. Lorazepam glucuronide is an inactive metabolite and is eliminated mainly by the kidneys.
Following a single 2-mg oral dose of ^{14}C-lorazepam to 8 healthy subjects, 88±4% of the administered dose was recovered in urine and 7±2% was recovered in feces. The percent of administered dose recovered in urine as lorazepam glucuronide was 74±4%. Only 0.3% of the dose was recovered as unchanged lorazepam, and the remainder of the radioactivity represented minor metabolites.

Special Populations
Effect of Age
Pediatrics
NEONATES (BIRTH TO 1 MONTH)
Following a single 0.05 mg/kg (n=4) or 0.1 mg/kg (n=6) intravenous dose of lorazepam, *mean total clearance normalized to body weight was reduced by 80% compared to normal adults*, terminal half-life was prolonged 3-fold, and volume of distribution was decreased by 40% in neonates with asphyxia neonatorum compared to normal adults. All neonates were of ≥ 37 weeks of gestational age.
INFANTS (1 MONTH UP TO 2 YEARS)
There is no information on the pharmacokinetic profile of lorazepam in infants in the age range of 1 month to 2 years.
CHILDREN (2 YEARS TO 12 YEARS)
Total (bound and unbound) lorazepam had a 50% higher mean volume of distribution (normalized to body-weight) and a 30% longer mean half-life in children with acute lymphocytic leukemia in complete remission (2 to 12 years, n=37) compared to normal adults (n=10). *Unbound* lorazepam clearance normalized to body-weight was comparable in children and adults.
ADOLESCENTS (12 YEARS TO 18 YEARS)
Total (bound and unbound) lorazepam had a 50% higher mean volume of distribution (normalized to body-weight) and a mean half-life that has two fold greater in adolescents with acute lymphocytic leukemia in complete remission (12 to 18 years, n=13) compared to normal adults (n=10). *Unbound* lorazepam clearance normalized to body-weight was comparable in adolescents and adults.
Elderly
Following single intravenous doses of 1.5 to 3 mg of Ativan Injection, mean total body clearance of lorazepam decreased by 20% in 15 elderly subjects of 60 to 84 years of age compared to that in 15 younger subjects of 19 to 38 years of age. Consequently, no dosage adjustment appears to be necessary in elderly subjects based solely on their age.
Effect of Gender
Gender has no effect on the pharmacokinetics of lorazepam.
Effect of Race
Young Americans (n=15) and Japanese subjects (n=7) had very comparable mean total clearance value of 1.0 mL/min/kg. However, elderly Japanese subjects had a 20% lower mean total clearance than elderly Americans, 0.59 mL/min/kg vs. 0.77 mL/min/kg, respectively.
Patients with Renal Insufficiency
Because the kidney is the primary route of elimination of lorazepam glucuronide, renal impairment would be expected to compromise its clearance. This should have no direct effect on the glucuronidation (and inactivation) of lorazepam. There is a possibility that the enterohepatic circulation of lorazepam glucuronide leads to a reduced efficiency of the net clearance of lorazepam in this population. Six normal subjects, six patients with renal impairment (Cl_{cr} of 22±9 mL/min), and four patients on chronic maintenance hemodialysis were given single 1.5 to 3.0 mg intravenous doses of lorazepam. Mean volume of distribution and terminal half-life values of lorazepam were 40% and 25% higher, respectively, in renally impaired patients than in normal subjects. Both parameters were 75% higher in patients undergoing hemodialysis than in normal subjects. Overall, though, in this group of subjects the mean total clearance of lorazepam did not change. About 8% of the administered intravenous dose was removed as intact lorazepam during the 6-hour dialysis session.
The kinetics of lorazepam glucuronide were markedly affected by renal dysfunction. The mean terminal half-life was prolonged by 55% and 125% in renally impaired patients and patients under hemodialysis, respectively, as compared to normal subjects. The mean metabolic clearance decreased by 75% and 90% in renally impaired patients and patients under hemodialysis, respectively, as compared with normal subjects. About 40% of the administered lorazepam intravenous dose was removed as glucuronide conjugate during the 6-hour dialysis session.
Hepatic Disease
Because cytochrome oxidation is not involved with the metabolism of lorazepam, liver disease would not be expected to have an effect on metabolic clearance. This prediction is supported by the observation that following a single 2 mg intravenous dose of lorazepam, cirrhotic male patients (n=13) and normal male subjects (n=11) exhibited no substantive difference in their ability to clear lorazepam.
Effect of Smoking
Administration of a single 2 mg intravenous dose of lorazepam showed that there was no difference in any of the pharmacokinetic parameters of lorazepam between cigarette smokers (n=10, mean=31 cigarettes per day) and nonsmoking subjects (n=10) who were matched for age, weight and gender.

Clinical Studies
The effectiveness of Ativan Injection in status epilepticus was established in two multi-center controlled trials in 177 patients. With rare exceptions, patients were between 18 and 65 years of age. More than half the patients in each study had tonic-clonic status epilepticus; patients with simple partial and complex partial status epilepticus comprised the rest of the population studied, along with a smaller number of patients who had the absence status.
One study (n=58) was a double-blind active-control trial comparing Ativan Injection and diazepam. Patients were randomized to receive Ativan 2 mg IV (with an additional 2 mg IV if needed) or diazepam 5 mg IV (with an additional 5 mg IV if needed). The primary outcome measure was a comparison of the proportion of responders in each treatment group, where a responder was defined as a patient whose seizures stopped within 10 minutes after treatment and who continued seizure-free for at least an additional 30 minutes. Twenty-four of the 30 (80%) patients were deemed responders to Ativan and 16/28 (57%) patients were deemed responders to diazepam (p=0.04). Of the 24 Ativan responders, 23 received both 2 mg infusions.
Non-responders to Ativan 4 mg were given an additional 2 to 4 mg Ativan; non-responders to diazepam 10 mg were given an additional 5 to 10 mg diazepam. After this additional dose administration, 28/30 (93%) of patients randomized to Ativan and 24/28 (86%) of patients randomized to diazepam were deemed responders, a difference that was not statistically significant.
Although this study provides support for the efficacy of Ativan as the treatment for status epilepticus, it cannot speak reliably or meaningfully to the comparative performance of either diazepam (Valium) or lorazepam (Ativan Injection) under the conditions of actual use.
A second study (n=119) was a double-blind dose-comparison trial with 3 doses of Ativan Injection: 1 mg, 2 mg, and 4 mg. Patients were randomized to receive one of the three doses of Ativan. The primary outcome and definition of responder were as in the first study. Twenty-five of 41 patients (61%) responded to 1 mg Ativan; 21/37 patients (57%) responded to 2 mg Ativan; and 31/41 (76%) responded to 4 mg Ativan. The p-value for a statistical test of the difference between the Ativan 4-mg dose group and the Ativan 1-mg dose group was 0.08 (two-sided). Data from all randomized patients were used in this test.
Although analyses failed to detect an effect of age, sex, or race on the effectiveness of Ativan in status epilepticus, the numbers of patients evaluated were too few to allow a definitive conclusion about the role these factors may play.

INDICATIONS AND USAGE

Status Epilepticus
Ativan Injection is indicated for the treatment of status epilepticus.

Preanesthetic
Ativan Injection is indicated in adult patients for preanesthetic medication, producing sedation (sleepiness or drowsiness), relief of anxiety, and a decreased ability to recall events related to the day of surgery. It is most useful in those patients who are anxious about their surgical proce-

Continued on next page

Ativan Injection—Cont.

dure and who would prefer to have diminished recall of the events of the day of surgery (see **PRECAUTIONS**, **Information for Patients**).

CONTRAINDICATIONS

Ativan Injection is contraindicated in patients with a known sensitivity to benzodiazepines or its vehicle (polyethylene glycol, propylene glycol and benzyl alcohol), in patients with acute narrow-angle glaucoma, or in patients with sleep apnea syndrome. It is also contraindicated in patients with severe respiratory insufficiency, except in those patients requiring relief of anxiety and/or diminished recall of events while being mechanically ventilated. The use of Ativan Injection intra-arterially is contraindicated because, as with other injectable benzodiazepines, inadvertent intra-arterial injection may produce arteriospasm resulting in gangrene which may require amputation (see **WARNINGS**).

WARNINGS

Use in Status Epilepticus
Management of Status Epilepticus
Status epilepticus is a potentially life-threatening condition associated with a high risk of permanent neurological impairment, if inadequately treated. The treatment of status, however, requires far more than the administration of an anticonvulsant agent. It involves observation and management of all parameters critical to maintaining vital function and the capacity to provide support of those functions as required. Ventilatory support must be readily available. The use of benzodiazepines, like Ativan Injection, is ordinarily only one step of a complex and sustained intervention which may require additional interventions (e.g., concomitant intravenous administration of phenytoin). Because status epilepticus may result from a correctable acute cause such as hypoglycemia, hyponatremia, or other metabolic or toxic derangement, such an abnormality must be immediately sought and corrected. Furthermore, patients who are susceptible to further seizure episodes should receive adequate maintenance antiepileptic therapy.
Any health care professional who intends to treat a patient with status epilepticus should be familiar with this package insert and the pertinent medical literature concerning current concepts for the treatment of status epilepticus. A comprehensive review of the considerations critical to the informed and prudent management of status epilepticus cannot be provided in drug product labeling. The archival medical literature contains many informative references on the management of status epilepticus, among them the report of the working group on status epilepticus of the Epilepsy Foundation of America "Treatment of Convulsive Status Epilepticus" (JAMA 1993; 270:854–859). As noted in the report just cited, it may be useful to consult with a neurologist if a patient fails to respond (e.g., fails to regain consciousness).
For the treatment of status epilepticus, the usual recommended dose of Ativan Injection is 4 mg given slowly (2 mg/min) for patients 18 years and older. If seizures cease, no additional Ativan Injection is required. If seizures continue or recur after a 10- to 15- minute observation period, an additional 4 mg intravenous dose may be slowly administered. *Experience with further doses of Ativan is very limited.* The usual precautions in treating status epilepticus should be employed. An intravenous infusion should be started, vital signs should be monitored, an unobstructed airway should be maintained, and artificial ventilation equipment should be available.
Respiratory Depression
The most important risk associated with the use of Ativan Injection in status epilepticus is respiratory depression. Accordingly, airway patency must be assured and respiration monitored closely. Ventilatory support should be given as required.
Excessive Sedation
Because of its prolonge duration of action, the prescriber should be alert to the possibility, especially when multiple doses have been given, that the sedative effects of lorazepam may add to the impairment of consciousness seen in the post-ictal state.
Preanesthetic Use
AIRWAY OBSTRUCTION MAY OCCUR IN HEAVILY SEDATED PATIENTS. INTRAVENOUS LORAZEPAM AT ANY DOSE, WHEN GIVEN EITHER ALONE OR IN COMBINATION WITH OTHER DRUGS ADMINISTERED DURING ANESTHESIA, MAY PRODUCE HEAVY SEDATION; THEREFORE, EQUIPMENT NECESSARY TO MAINTAIN A PATENT AIRWAY AND TO SUPPORT RESPIRATION/VENTILATION SHOULD BE AVAILABLE.
As is true of similar CNS-acting drugs, the decision as to when patients who have received injectable lorazepam, particularly on an outpatient basis, may again operate machinery, drive a motor vehicle, or engage in hazardous or other activities requiring attention and coordination must be individualized. It is recommended that no patient engage in such activities for a period of 24 to 48 hours or until the

effects of the drug, such as drowsiness, have subsided, whichever is longer. Impairment of performance may persist for greater intervals because of extremes of age, concomitant use of other drugs, stress of surgery, or the general condition of the patient.
Clinical trials have shown that patients over the age of 50 years may have a more profound and prolonged sedation with intravenous lorazepam (see also **DOSAGE AND ADMINISTRATION, Preanesthetic**).
As with all central-nervous-system-depressant drugs, care should be exercised in patients given injectable lorazepam as premature ambulation may result in injury from falling. There is no added beneficial effect from the addition of scopolamine to injectable lorazepam, and their combined effect may result in an increased incidence of sedation, hallucination and irrational behavior.
General (All Uses)
PRIOR TO INTRAVENOUS USE, ATIVAN INJECTION MUST BE DILUTED WITH AN EQUAL AMOUNT OF COMPATIBLE DILUENT (see **DOSAGE AND ADMINISTRATION**). INTRAVENOUS INJECTION SHOULD BE MADE SLOWLY AND WITH REPEATED ASPIRATION. CARE SHOULD BE TAKEN TO DETERMINE THAT ANY INJECTION WILL NOT BE INTRA-ARTERIAL AND THAT PERIVASCULAR EXTRAVASATION WILL NOT TAKE PLACE. IN THE EVENT THAT A PATIENT COMPLAINS OF PAIN DURING INTENDED INTRAVENOUS INJECTION OF ATIVAN INJECTION, THE INJECTION SHOULD BE STOPPED IMMEDIATELY TO DETERMINE IF INTRA-ARTERIAL INJECTION OR PERIVASCULAR EXTRAVASATION HAS TAKEN PLACE.
Since the liver is the most likely site of conjugation of lorazepam and since excretion of conjugated lorazepam (glucuronide) is a renal function, this drug is not recommended for use in patients with hepatic and/or renal *failure*. Ativan should be used with caution in patients with mild-to-moderate hepatic or renal disease (see **DOSAGE AND ADMINISTRATION**).
Pregnancy
ATIVAN MAY CAUSE FETAL DAMAGE WHEN ADMINISTERED TO PREGNANT WOMEN. Ordinarily, Ativan Injection should not be used during pregnancy except in serious or life-threatening conditions where safer drugs cannot be used or are ineffective. Status epilepticus may represent such a serioius life-threatening condition.
An increased risk of congenital malformations associated with the use of minor tranquilizers (chlordiazepoxide, diazepam and meprobamate) during the first trimester of pregnancy has been suggested in several studies. In humans, blood levels obtained from umbilical cord blood indicate placental transfer of lorazepam and lorazepam glucuronide.
Reproductive studies in animals were performed in mice, rats, and two strains of rabbits. Occasional anomalies (reduction of tarsals, tibia, metatarsals, malrotated limbs, gastroschisis, malformed skull, and microphthalmia) were seen in drug-treated rabbits without relationship to dosage. Although all of these anomalies were not present in the concurrent control group, they have been reported to occur randomly in historical controls. At doses of 40 mg/kg orally or 4 mg/kg intravenously and higher, there was evidence of fetal resorption and increased fetal loss in rabbits which was not seen at lower doses.
The possibility that a woman of childbearing potential may be pregnant at the time of therapy should be considered.
There are insufficient data regarding obstetrical safety of parenteral lorazepam, including use in cesarean section. Such use, therefore, is not recommended.
Endoscopic Procedures
There are insufficient data to support the use of Ativan Injection for outpatient endoscopic procedures. Inpatient endoscopic procedures require adequate recovery room observation time.
When Ativan Injection is used for peroral endoscopic procedures, adequate topical or regional anesthesia is recommended to minimize reflex activity associated with such procedures.

PRECAUTIONS

General
The additive central-nervous-system effects of other drugs such as phenothiazines, narcotic analgesics, barbiturates, antidepressants, scopolamine, and monoamine-oxidase inhibitors, should be borne in mind when these other drugs are used concomitantly with or during the period of recovery from Ativan Injection (see **CLINICAL PHARMACOLOGY** and **WARNINGS**).
Extreme caution must be used when administering Ativan Injection to elderly patients, very ill patients, or to patients with limited pulmonary reserve because of the possibility that hypoventilation and/or hypoxic cardiac arrest may occur. Resuscitative equipment for ventilatory support should be readily available. (See **WARNINGS** and **DOSAGE AND ADMINISTRATION**.)
When lorazepam injection is used IV as the premedicant prior to regional or local anesthesia, the possibility of excessive sleepiness or drowsiness may interfere with patient co-

operation in determining levels of anesthesia. This is most likely to occur when greater than 0.05 mg/kg is given and when narcotic analgesics are used concomitantly with the recommended dose (see **ADVERSE REACTIONS**).
As with all benzodiazepines, paradoxical reactions may occur in rare instances and in an unpredictable fashion (see **ADVERSE REACTIONS**). In these instances, further use of the drug in these patients should be considered with caution.
There have been reports of possible propylene glycol toxicity (e.g., lactic acidosis, hyperosmolality, hypotension) and possible polyethylene glycol toxicity (e.g., acute tubular necrosis) during administration of Ativan Injection at higher than recommended doses. Symptoms may be more likely to develop in patients with renal impairment.
Information for Patients
Patients should be informed of the pharmacological effects of the drug, including sedation, relief of anxiety, and lack of recall, the duration of these effects (about 8 hours), and be apprised of the risks as well as the benefits to be derived from its use.
Patients who receive Ativan Injection as a premedicant should be cautioned that driving a motor vehicle, operating machinery, or engaging in hazardous or other activities requiring attention and coordination, should be delayed for 24 to 48 hours following the injection or until the effects of the drug, such as drowsiness, have subsided, whichever is longer. Sedatives, tranquilizers and narcotic analgesics may produce a more prolonged and profound effect when administered along with injectable Ativan. This effect may take the form of excessive sleepiness or drowsiness and, on rare occasions, interfere with recall and recognition of events of the day of surgery and the day after.
Patients should be advised that getting out of bed unassisted may result in falling and injury if undertaken within 8 hours of receiving lorazepam injection. Since tolerance for CNS depressants will be diminished in the presence of Ativan Injection, these substances should either be avoided or taken in reduced dosage. Alcoholic beverages should not be consumed for at least 24 to 48 hours after receiving lorazepam injectable due to the additive effects on central-nervous-system depression seen with benzodiazepines in general. Elderly patients should be told that Ativan Injection may make them very sleepy for a period longer than 6 to 8 hours following surgery.
Laboratory Tests
In clinical trials, no laboratory test abnormalities were identified with either single or multiple doses of Ativan Injection. These tests included: CBC, urinalysis, SGOT, SGPT, bilirubin, alkaline phosphatase, LDH, cholesterol, uric acid, BUN, glucose, calcium, phosphorus, and total proteins.
Drug Interactions
Ativan Injection, like other injectable benzodiazepines, produces additive depression of the central nervous system when administered with other CNS depressants such as ethyl alcohol, phenothiazines, barbiturates, MAO inhibitors, and other antidepressants.
When scopolamine is used concomitantly with injectable lorazepam, an increased incidence of sedation, hallucinations and irrational behavior has been observed.
There have been rare reports of significant respiratory depression, stupor and/or hypotension with the concomitant use of loxapine and lorazepam.
Marked sedation, excessive salivation, ataxia, and, rarely, death have been reported with the concomitant use of clozapine and lorazepam.
Apnea, coma, bradycardia, arrhythmia, heart arrest, and death have been reported with the concomitant use of haloperidol and lorazepam.
The risk of using lorazepam in combination with scopolamine, loxapine, clozapine, haloperidol, or other CNS-depressant drugs has not been systematically evaluated. Therefore, caution is advised if the concomitant administration of lorazepam and these drugs is required.
Concurrent administration of any of the following drugs with lorazepam had no effect on the pharmacokinetics of lorazepam; metoprolol, cimetidine, ranitidine, disulfiram, propranolol, metronidazole, and propoxyphene. No change in Ativan dosage is necessary when concomitantly given with any of these drugs.
Lorazepam-Valproate Interaction
Concurrent administration of lorazepam (2 mg intravenously) with valproate (250 mg twice daily orally for 3 days) to 6 healthy male subjects resulted in decreased total clearance of lorazepam by 40% and decreased formation rate of lorazepam glucuronide by 55%, as compared with lorazepam administered alone. Accordingly, lorazepam plasma concentrations were about two-fold higher for at least 12 hours post-dose administration during valproate treatment. Lorazepam dosage should be reduced to 50% of the normal adult dose when this drug combination is prescribed in patients (see also **DOSAGE AND ADMINISTRATION**).
Lorazepam-Oral Contraceptive Steroids Interaction
Coadministration of lorazepam (2 mg intravenously) with oral contraceptive steroids (norethindrone acetate, 1 mg,

and ethinyl estradiol, 50 µg, for at least 6 months) to healthy females (n=7) was associated with a 55% decrease in half-life, a 50% increase in the volume of distribution, thereby resulting in an almost 3.7-fold increase in total clearance of lorazepam as compared with control healthy females (n=8). It may be necessary to increase the dose of Ativan in female patients who are concomitantly taking oral contraceptives (see also **DOSAGE AND ADMINISTRATION**).

Lorazepam-Probenecid Interaction

Concurrent administration of lorazepam (2 mg intravenously) with probenecid (500 mg orally every 6 hours) to 9 healthy volunteers resulted in a prolongation of lorazepam half-life by 130% and a decrease in its total clearance by 45%. No change in volume of distribution was noted during probenecid co-treatment. Ativan dosage needs to be reduced by 50% when coadministered with probenecid (see also **DOSAGE AND ADMINISTRATION**).

Drug/Laboratory Test Interactions

No laboratory test abnormalities were identified when lorazepam was given alone or concomitantly with another drug, such as narcotic analgesics, inhalation anesthetics, scopolamine, atropine, and a variety of tranquilizing agents.

Carcinogenesis, Mutagenesis, Impairment of Fertility

No evidence of carcinogenic potential emerged in rats and mice during an 18-month study with oral lorazepam. No studies regarding mutagenesis have been performed. The results of pre-implantation study in rats, in which the oral lorazepam dose was 20 mg/kg dose, showed no impairment of fertility.

Pregnancy

Teratogenic Effects—Pregnancy Category D (See **WARNINGS**.)

Labor and Delivery

There are insufficient data to support the use of Ativan Injection during labor and delivery, including cesarean section; therefore, its use in this clinical circumstance is not recommended.

Nursing Mothers

Lorazepam has been detected in human breast milk, Therefore, lorazepam should not be administered to nursing mothers because, like other benzodiazepines, the possibility exists that lorazepam may sedate or otherwise adversely affect the infant.

Pediatric Use

Status Epilepticus

The safety of Ativan in pediatric patients with status epilepticus has not been systematically evaluated.

Open-label studies described in the medical literature included 273 pediatric/adolescent patients; the age range was from a few hours old to 18 years of age. Paradoxical excitation was observed in 10% to 30% of the pediatric patients under 8 years of age and was characterized by tremors, agitation, euphoria, logorrhea, and brief episodes of visual hallucinations. Parodoxical excitation in pediatric patients also has also been reported with other benzodiazepines when used for status epilepticus, as an anesthesia, or for pre-chemotherapy treatment.

Pediatric patients (as well as adults) with atypical petit mal status epilepticus have developed brief tonic-clonic seizures shortly after Ativan was given. This "paradoxical" effect was also reported for diazepam and clonazepam. Nevertheless, the development of seizures after treatment with benzodiazepines is probably rare, based on the incidence in the uncontrolled treatment series reported (i.e., seizures were not observed for 112 pediatric patients and 18 adults or during approximately 400 doses.).

Preanesthetic

There are insufficient data to support the efficacy of injectable lorazepam as a preanesthetic agent in patients less than 18 years of age.

General

Seizure activity and myoclonus have been reported to occur following administration of Ativan Injection, especially in very low birth weight neonates.

Pediatric patients may exhibit a sensitivity to benzyl alcohol, polyethelene glycol and propylene glycol, components of Ativan Injection (see also **CONTRAINDICATIONS**). The "gasping syndrome," characterized by central nervous system depression, metabolic acidosis, gasping respirations, and high levels of benzyl alcohol and its metabolites found in the blood and urine, has been associated with benzyl alcohol dosages >99 mg/kg/day in neonates and low-birth-weight neonates. Additional symptoms may include gradual neurological deterioration, seizures, intracranial hemorrhage, hematologic abnormalities, skin breakdown, hepatic and renal failure, hypotension, bradycardia, and cardiovascular collapse. Central nervous system toxicity, including seizures and intraventricular hemorrhage, as well as unresponsiveness, tachypnea, tachycardia, and diaphoresis have been associated with propylene glycol toxicity. Although normal therapeutic doses of Ativan Injection contain very small amounts of these compounds, premature and low-birth-weight infants as well as pediatric patients receiving high dosages may be more susceptible to their effects.

Geriatric Use

Status Epilepticus

Age over 65 years may be associated with a greater incidence of central nervous system depression and more respiratory depression.

ADVERSE REACTIONS

Status Epilepticus

The most important adverse clinical event caused by the use of Ativan Injection is repiratory depression (see **WARNINGS**).

The adverse clinical events most commonly observed with the use of Ativan Injection in clinical trials evaluating its use in status epilepticus were hypotension, somnolence, and respiratory failure.

Incidence in Controlled Clinical Trials

All adverse events were recorded during the trials by the clinical investigators using terminology of their own choosing. Similar types of events were grouped into standardized categories using modified COSTART dictionary terminology. These categories are used in the table and listings below with the frequencies representing the proportion of individuals exposed to Ativan Injection or to comparative therapy.

The prescriber should be aware that these figures cannot be used to predict the frequency of adverse events in the course of usual medical practice where patient characteristics and other factors may differ from those prevailing during clinical studies. Similarly, the cited frequencies cannot be directly compared with figures obtained from other clinical investigators involving different treatment, uses, or investigators. An inspection of these frequencies, however, does provide the prescribing physician with one basis to estimate the relative contribution of drug and nondrug factors to the adverse event incidences in the population studied.

Commonly Observed Adverse Events in a Controlled Dose-Comparison Clinical Trial

Table 1 lists the treatment-emergent adverse events that occurred in the patients treated with Ativan Injection in a dose-comparison trial of Ativan 1 mg, 2 mg, and 4 mg.

TABLE 1. NUMBER (%) OF STUDY EVENTS IN A DOSE COMPARISON CLINICAL TRIAL

Body System Event	Ativen Injection (n=130)[a]
Any Study Event (1 or more)[b]	16 (12.3%)
Body as a whole	
Infection	1 (<1%)
Cardiovascular system	
Hypotension	2 (1.5%)
Digestive system	
Liver function tests abnormal	1 (<1%)
Nausea	1 (<1%)
Vomiting	1 (<1%)
Metabolic and Nutritional	
Acidosis	1 (<1%)
Nervous system	
Brain edema	1 (<1%)
Coma	1 (<1%)
Convulsion	1 (<1%)
Somnolence	2 (1.5%)
Thinking abnormal	1 (<1%)
Respiratory system	
Hyperventilation	1 (<1%)
Hypoventilation	1 (<1%)
Respiratory failure	2 (1.5%)
Terms not classifiable	
Injection site reaction	1 (<1%)
Urogenital system	
Cystitis	1 (<1%)

a: One hundred and thirty (130) patients received Ativan Injection.

b: Totals are not necessarily the sum of the individual study events because a patient may report two or more different study events in the same body system.

Commonly Observed Adverse Events in Active-Controlled Clinical Trials

In two studies, patients who completed the course of treatment for status epilepticus were permitted to be reenrolled and to receive treatment for a second status episode, given that there was a sufficient interval between the two episodes. Safety was determined from all treatment episodes for all intent-to-treat patients, i.e., from all "patient-episodes." Table 2 lists the treatment emergent adverse events that occurred in at least 1% of the patient-episodes in which Ativan Injection or diazepam was given. The table represents the pooling of results from the two controlled trials.

[See table 2 at bottom of next page]

These trials were not designed or intended to demonstrate the comparative safety of the two treatments.

The overall adverse experience profile for Ativan was similar between women and men. There are insufficient data to support a statement regarding the distribution of adverse events by race. Generally, age greater than 65 years may be associated with a greater incidence of central-nervous-system depression and more respiratory depression.

Other Events Observed During the Pre-marketing Evaluation of Ativan Injection for the Treatment of Status Epilepticus

Ativan Injection, active comparators, and Ativan Injection in combination with a comparator were administered to 488 individuals during controlled and open-label clinical trials. Because of reenrollments, these 488 patients participated in a total of 521 patient-episodes. Ativan Injection alone was given in 69% of these patient-episodes (n=360). The safety information below is based on data available from 326 of these patient-episodes in which Ativan Injection was given alone.

All adverse events that were seen once are listed, except those already included in previous listings (Table 1 and Table 2).

Study events were classified by body system in descending frequency by using the following definitions: frequent adverse events were those that occurred in at least 1/100 individuals; infrequent study events were those that occurred in 1/100 to 1/1000 individuals.

Frequent and Infrequent Study Events

BODY AS A WHOLE-	Infrequent: asthenia, chills, headache, infection.
DIGESTIVE SYSTEM-	Infrequent: abnormal liver function test, increased salivation, nausea, vomiting.
METABOLIC AND NUTRITIONAL-	Infrequent: acidosis, alkaline phosphatase increased.
NERVOUS SYSTEM-	Infrequent: agitation, ataxia, brain edema, coma, confusion, hallucinations, myoclonus, stupor, thinking abnormal, tremor.
RESPIRATORY SYSTEM-	Frequent: apnea; Infrequent: hyperventilation, hypoventilation, respiratory disorder.
TERMS NOT CLASSIFIABLE-	Infrequent: injection site reaction.
UROGENTIAL SYSTEM-	Infrequent cystitis.

Preanesthetic

Central Nervous System

The most frequent adverse drug event reported with injectable lorazepam is a central-nervous-system depression. The incidence varied from one study to another, depending on the dosage, route of administration, use of other central-nervous-system depressants, and the investigator's opinion concerning the degree and duration of desired sedation. Excessive sleepiness and drowsiness were the most common consequence of CNS depression. This interfered with patient cooperation in approximately 6% (25/446) of patients undergoing regional anesthesia, causing difficulty in assessing levels of anesthesia. Patients over 50 years of age had a higher incidence of excessive sleepiness or drowsiness when compared with those under 50 (21/106 versus 24/245) when lorazepam was given intravenously (see **DOSAGE AND ADMINISTRATION**). On rare occasion (3/1580) the patient was unable to give personal identification in the operating room on arrival, and one patient fell when attempting premature ambulation in the postoperative period.

Symptoms such as restlessness, confusion, depression, crying, sobbing, and delirium occurred in about 1.3% (20/1580). One patient injured himself by picking at his incision during the immediate postoperative period.

Hallucinations were present in about 1% (14/1580) of patients and were visual and self-limiting.

An occasional patient complained of dizziness, diplopia and/or blurred vision. Depressed hearing was infrequently reported during the peak-effect period.

An occasional patient had a prolonged recovery room stay, either because of excessive sleepiness or because of some form of inappropriate behavior. The latter was seen most commonly when scopolamine was given concomitantly as a premedicant.

Limited information derived from patients who were discharged the day after receiving injectable lorazepam showed one patient complained of some unsteadiness of gait and a reduced ability to perform complex mental functions. Enhanced sensitivity to alcoholic beverages has been reported more than 24 hours after receiving injectable lorazepam, similar to experience with other benzodiazepines.

Continued on next page

Ativan Injection—Cont.

Local Effects

Intramuscular injection of lorazepam has resulted in pain at the injection site, a sensation of burning, or observed redness in the same area in a very variable incidence from one study to another. The overall incidence of pain and burning was about 17% (146/859) in the immediate postinjection period and about 1.4% (12/859) at the 24-hour observation time. Reactions at the injection site (redness) occurred in approximately 2% (17/859) in the immediate postinjection period and were present 24 hours later in about 0.8% (7/859).

Intravenous administration of lorazepam resulted in painful responses in 13/771 patients or approximately 1.6% in the immediate postinjection period, and 24 hours later 4/771 patients or about 0.5% still complained of pain. Redness did not occur immediately following intravenous injection but was noted in 19/771 patients at the 24-hour observation period. This incidence is similar to that observed with an intravenous infusion before lorazepam is given. Intra-arterial injection may produce arteriospasm resulting in gangrene which may require amputation (see CONTRAINDICATIONS).

Cardiovascular System

Hypertension (0.1%) and hypotension (0.1%) have occasionally been observed after patients have received injectable lorazepam.

Respiratory System

Five patients (5/446) who underwent regional anesthesia were observed to have airway obstruction. This was believed due to excessive sleepiness at the time of the procedure and resulted in temporary hypoventilation. In this instance, appropriate airway management may become necessary (see also CLINICAL PHARMACOLOGY, WARNINGS and PRECAUTIONS).

Other Adverse Experiences

Skin rash, nausea and vomiting have occasionally been noted in patients who have received injectable lorazepam combined with other drugs during anesthesia and surgery.

Paradoxical Reactions

As with all benzodiazepines, parodoxical reactions such as stimulation, mania, irritability, restlessness, agitation, aggression, psychosis, hostility, rage, or hallucinations may occur in rare instances and in an unpredictable fashion. In these instances, further use of the drug in these patients should be considered with caution (see PRECAUTIONS, General).

Postmarketing Reports

Voluntary reports of other adverse events temporally associated with the use of Ativan Injection that have been received since market introduction and that may have no causal relationship with the use of Ativan Injection include the following: acute brain syndrome, aggravation of pheochromocytoma, amnesia, apnea/respiratory arrest, arrhythmia, bradycardia, brain edema, coagulation disorder, coma, convulsion, gastrointestinal hemorrhage, heart arrest/failure, heart block, liver damage, lung edema, lung hemorrhage, nervousness, neuroleptic malignant syndrome, paralysis, pericardial effusion, pneumothorax, pulmonary hypertension, tachycardia, thrombocytopenia, urinary incontinence, ventricular arrhythmia.

Fatalities also have been reported, usually in patients on concomitant medications (e.g., respiratory depressants) and/or with other medical conditions (e.g., obstructive sleep apnea).

DRUG ABUSE AND DEPENDENCE

Controlled Substance Class

Lorazepam is a controlled substance in Schedule IV.

Abuse and Physical and Psychological Dependence

As with other benzodiazepines, Ativan Injection has a potential for abuse and may lead to dependence. Physicians should be aware that repeated doses over a prolonged period of time may result in physical and psychological dependence and withdrawal symptoms, following abrupt discontinuance, similar in character to those noted with barbiturates and alcohol.

OVERDOSAGE

Symptoms

Overdosage of benzodiazepines is usually manifested by varying degrees of central-nervous-system depression, ranging from drowsiness to coma. In mild cases symptoms include drowsiness, mental confusion and lethargy. In more serious examples, symptoms may include ataxia, hypotonia, hypotension, hypnosis, stages one (1) to three (3) coma, and, very rarely, death.

Treatment

Treatment of overdosage is mainly supportive until the drug is eliminated from the body. Vital signs and fluid balance should be carefully monitored in conjunction with close observation of the patient. An adequate airway should be maintained and assisted respiration used as needed. With normally functioning kidneys, forced diuresis with intravenous fluids and electrolytes may accelerate elimination of benzodiazepines from the body. In addition, osmotic diuretics, such as mannitol, may be effective as adjunctive measures. In more critical situations, renal dialysis and exchange blood transfusions may be indicated. Lorazepam does not appear to be removed in significant quantities by dialysis, although lorazepam glucuronide may be highly dialyzable. The value of dialysis has not been adequately determined for lorazepam.

The benzodiazepine antagonist flumazenil may be used in hospitalized patients as an adjunct to, not as a substitute for, proper management of benzodiazepine overdose. **The prescriber should be aware of a risk of seizure in association with flumazenil treatment, particularly in long-term benzodiazepine users and in cyclic antidepressant overdose.** The complete flumazenil package insert including CONTRAINDICATIONS, WARNINGS and PRECAUTIONS should be consulted prior to use.

DOSAGE AND ADMINISTRATION

Ativan must never be used without individualization of dosage particularly when used with other medications capable of producing central-nervous-system depression.

EQUIPMENT NECESSARY TO MAINTAIN A PATENT AIRWAY SHOULD BE IMMEDIATELY AVAILABLE PRIOR TO INTRAVENOUS ADMINISTRATION OF LORAZEPAM (see WARNINGS).

Status Epilepticus

General Advice

Status epilepticus is a potentially life-threatening condition associated with a high risk of permanent neurological impairment, if inadequately treated. The treatment of status, however, requires far more than the administration of an anticonvulsant agent. It involves observation and management of all parameters critical to maintaining vital function and the capacity to provide support of those functions as required. Ventilatory support must be readily available. The use of benzodiazepines, like Ativan Injection, is ordinarily only an initial step of a complex and sustained intervention which may require additional interventions, (e.g., concomitant intravenous administration of phenytoin). Because status epilepticus may result from a correctable acute cause such as hypoglycemia, hyponatremia, or other metabolic or toxic derangement, such an abnormality must be immediately sought and corrected. Furthermore, patients who are susceptible to further seizure episodes should receive adequate maintenance antiepileptic therapy.

Any health care professional who intends to treat a patient with status epilepticus should be familiar with this package insert and the pertinent medical literature concerning current concepts for the treatment of status epilepticus. A comprehensive review of the considerations critical to the informed and prudent management of status epilepticus cannot be provided in drug product labeling. The archival medical literature contains many informative references on the management of status epilepticus, among them the report of the working group on status epilepticus of the Epilepsy Foundation of America "Treatment of Convulsive Status Epilepticus" (JAMA 1993; 270:854–859). As noted in the report just cited, it may be useful to consult with a neurologist if a patient fails to respond (e.g., fails to regain consciousness).

Intravenous Injection

For the treatment of status epilepticus, the usual recommended dose of Ativan Injection is 4 mg given slowly (2 mg/min) for patients 18 years and older. If seizures cease, no additional Ativan Injection is required. If seizures continue or recur after a 10- to 15-minute observation period, an additional 4 mg intravenous dose may be slowly administered. *Experience with further doses of Ativan is very limited.* The usual precautions in treating status epilepticus should be employed. An intravenous infusion should be started, vital signs should be monitored, an unobstructed airway should be maintained, and artificial ventilation equipment should be available.

Intramuscular Injection

IM Ativan is not preferred in the treatment of status epilepticus because therapeutic lorazepam levels may not be reached as quickly as with IV administration. However, when an intravenous port is not available, the IM route may prove useful (see CLINICAL PHARMACOLOGY, Pharmacokinetics and Metabolism).

Pediatric

The safety of Ativan in pediatric patients has not been established.

Preanesthetic

Intramuscular Injection

For the designated indications as a premedicant, the usual recommended dose of lorazepam for intramuscular injection is 0.05 mg/kg up to a maximum of 4 mg. As with all premedicant drugs, the dose should be individualized (see also CLINICAL PHARMACOLOGY, WARNINGS, PRECAUTIONS, and ADVERSE REACTIONS). Doses of other central-nervous-system depressant drugs should be reduced (see PRECAUTIONS). *For optimum effect, measured as lack of recall, intramuscular lorazepam should be administered at least 2 hours before the anticipated operative procedure.* Narcotic analgesics should be administered at their usual preoperative time.

There are insufficient data to support efficacy or make dosage recommendations for intramuscular lorazepam in patients less than 18 years of age; therefore, such use is not recommended.

Intravenous Injection

For the primary purpose of sedation and relief of anxiety, the usual recommended initial dose of lorazepam for intravenous injection is 2 mg total, or 0.02 mg/lb (0.044 mg/kg), whichever is smaller. This dose will suffice for sedating most adult patients and ordinarily should not be exceeded in patients over 50 years of age. In those patients in whom a greater likelihood of lack of recall for perioperative events would be beneficial, larger doses as high as 0.05 mg/kg up to a total of 4 mg may be administered (see CLINICAL PHARMACOLOGY, WARNINGS, PRECAUTIONS, and ADVERSE REACTIONS). Doses of other injectable central-nervous-system-depressant drugs ordinarily should be reduced (see PRECAUTIONS). *For optimum effect, mea-*

TABLE 2. NUMBER (%) OF STUDY EVENTS IN ACTIVE CONTROLLED CLINICAL TRIALS

Body System Event	Ativan Injection (n=85)[a]	Diazepam (n=80)[a]
Any Study Event (1 or more)[b]	14 (16.5%)	11 (13.8%)
Body as a whole		
Headache	1 (1.2%)	1 (1.3%)
Cardiovascular system		
Hypotension	2 (2.4%)	0
Hemic and lymphatic system		
Hypochromic anemia	0	1 (1.3%)
Leukocytosis	0	1 (1.3%)
Thrombocythemia	0	1 (1.3%)
Nervous system		
Coma	1 (1.2%)	1 (1.3%)
Somnolence	3 (3.5%)	3 (3.8%)
Stupor	1 (1.2%)	0
Respiratory system		
Hypoventilation	1 (1.2%)	2 (2.5%)
Apnea	1 (1.2%)	1 (1.3%)
Respiratory failure	2 (2.4%)	1 (1.3%)
Respiratory disorder	1 (1.2%)	0

a: The number indicates the number of "patient-episodes." Patient-episodes were used rather than "patients" because a total of 7 patients were reenrolled for the treatment of a second episode of status: 5 patients received Ativan Injection on two occasions that were far enough apart to establish the diagnosis of status epilepticus for each episode, and, using the same time criterion, 2 patients received diazepam on two occasions.

b: Totals are not necessarily the sum of the individual study events because a patient may report two or more different study events in the same body system.

sured as lack of recall, intravenous lorazepam should be administered 15 to 20 minutes before the anticipated operative procedure.

There are insufficient data to support efficacy or make dosage recommendations for intravenous lorazepam in patients less than 18 years of age; therefore, such use is not recommended.

Dose Administration in Special Populations

Elderly Patients and Patients with Hepatic Disease

No dosage adjustments are needed in elderly patients and in patients with hepatic disease.

Patients with Renal Disease

For acute dose administration, adjustment is not needed for patients with renal disease. However, in patients with renal disease, caution should be exercised if frequent doses are given over relatively short periods of time (see also **CLINICAL PHARMACOLOGY**).

Dose Adjustment Due to Drug Interactions

The dose of Ativan should be reduced by 50% when coadministered with probenecid or valproate (see **PRECAUTIONS, Drug Interactions**).

It may be necessary to increase the dose of Ativan in female patients who are concomitantly taking oral contraceptives.

Administration

The **TUBEX® BLUNT POINTE**™ Sterile Cartridge Unit is suitable for substances to be administered intravenously. It is intended for use with injection sets specifically manufactured as "needle-less" injection systems. As of the date of this circular, **TUBEX BLUNT POINTE** is compatible with LifeShield® Prepierced Reseal injection site, InterLink® Injection Site, SafeLine® Injection Site, User-Gard® Intermittent Injection Cap, and SafSite® reflux valve.

The **TUBEX** Sterile Cartridge-Needle Unit is suitable for substances to be administered intravenously or intramuscularly.

When given intramuscularly, Ativan Injection, undiluted, should be injected deep in the muscle mass.

Injectable Ativan can be used with atropine sulfate, narcotic analgesics, other parenterally used analgesics, commonly used anesthetics, and muscle relaxants.

Immediately prior to intravenous use, Ativan Injection must be diluted with an equal volume of compatible solution. Contents should be mixed thoroughly by gently inverting the container repeatedly until a homogenous solution results. Do not shake vigorously, as this will result in air entrapment. When properly diluted, the drug may be injected directly into a vein or into the tubing of an existing intravenous infusion (see above for tubing products compatible with the **BLUNT POINTE** Sterile Cartridge Unit). The rate of injection should not exceed 2.0 mg per minute.

Parenteral drug products should be inspected visually for particulate matter and discoloration prior to administration, whenever solution and container permit. Do not use if solution is discolored or contains a precipitate.

Ativan Injection is compatible for dilution purposes with the following solutions: Sterile Water for Injection, USP; Sodium Chloride Injection, USP; 5% Dextrose Injection, USP.

HOW SUPPLIED

Ativan® (lorazepam) Injection is available in **TUBEX® BLUNT POINTE**™ Sterile Cartridge Units and Sterile Cartridge-Needle Units (22 gauge × 1¼ inch needle), in boxes of 10 **TUBEX®** as follows:

1 mg per 0.5 mL, NDC 0008-0581-50, 0.5 mL fill in 1 mL size **BLUNT POINTE**™

1 mg per 0.5 mL, NDC 0008-0581-07, 0.5 mL fill in 1 mL size

2 mg per mL, NDC 0008-0581-52, 1 mL fill in 2 mL size **BLUNT POINTE**™

2 mg per mL, NDC 0008-0581-02, 1 mL fill in 2 mL size

4 mg per mL, NDC 0008-0570-50, 1 mL fill in 2 mL size **BLUNT POINTE**™

4 mg per mL, NDC 0008-0570-02, 1 mL fill in 2 mL size

For IM or IV injection.

Protect from light.

Store in a refrigerator.

Use carton to protect contents from light.

ALSO AVAILABLE

TUBEX® BLUNT POINTE™ Sterile Cartridge Units and Sterile Cartridge-Needle Units (22 gauge × 1¼ inch needle), packaged in boxes of 10 **TUBEX®** in TAMP-R-TEL® tamper-resistant packages as follows:

1 mg per 0.5 mL, NDC 0008-0581-51, 0.5 mL fill in 1 mL size **BLUNT POINTE**™

1 mg per 0.5 mL, NDC 0008-0581-05, 0.5 mL fill in 1 mL size

2 mg per mL, NDC 0008-0581-53, 1 mL fill in 2 mL size **BLUNT POINTE**™

2 mg per mL, NDC 0008-0581-06, 1 mL fill in 2 mL size

4 mg per mL, NDC 0008-0570-51, 1 mL fill in 2 mL size **BLUNT POINTE**™

4 mg per mL, NDC 0008-0570-05, 1 mL fill in 2 mL size

Single-dose and multiple-dose vials are available as follows:

2 mg per mL, NDC 0008-0581-15, 1 mL vial and NDC 0008-0581-13, 10 mL vial

4 mg per mL, NDC 0008-0570-15, 1 mL vial and NDC 0008-0570-13, 10 mL vial

TUBEX is a registered trademark of Wyeth-Ayerst Laboratories. **BLUNT POINTE** is a trademark of Wyeth-Ayerst Laboratories.

InterLink is a registered trademark of Baxter International, Inc.

LifeSheild is a registered trademark of Abbott Laboratories.

SafeLine is a registered trademark of McGaw, Inc.

SafSite is a registered trademark of B. Braun Medical, Inc.

User-Gard is a registered trademark of Arrow International, Inc.

Manufactured by:
Wyeth Laboratories Inc.
A Wyeth-Ayerst Company
Philadelphia, PA 19101

ATIVAN® Ⓒ℞
[at 'i-van]
(lorazepam)
Tablets

DESCRIPTION

Ativan (lorazepam), an antianxiety agent, has the chemical formula, 7-chloro-5-(*o*-chlorophenyl)-1,3-dihydro-3-hydroxy-2*H*-1,4-benzodiazepin-2-one.

It is a nearly white powder almost insoluble in water. Each Ativan (lorazepam) tablet, to be taken orally, contains 0.5 mg, 1 mg, or 2 mg of lorazepam. The inactive ingredients present are lactose and other ingredients.

CLINICAL PHARMACOLOGY

Studies in healthy volunteers show that in single high doses Ativan (lorazepam) has a tranquilizing action on the central nervous system with no appreciable effect on the respiratory or cardiovascular systems.

Ativan (lorazepam) is readily absorbed with an absolute bioavailability of 90 percent. Peak concentrations in plasma occur approximately 2 hours following administration. The peak plasma level of lorazepam from a 2 mg dose is approximately 20 ng/mL.

The mean half-life of unconjugated lorazepam in human plasma is about 12 hours and for its major metabolite, lorazepam glucuronide, about 18 hours. At clinically relevant concentrations, lorazepam is approximately 85% bound to plasma proteins. Ativan (lorazepam) is rapidly conjugated at its 3-hydroxy group into lorazepam glucuronide which is then excreted in the urine. Lorazepam glucuronide has no demonstrable CNS activity in animals.

The plasma levels of lorazepam are proportional to the dose given. There is no evidence of accumulation of lorazepam on administration up to six months.

Studies comparing young and elderly subjects have shown that the pharmacokinetics of lorazepam remain unaltered with advancing age.

INDICATIONS AND USAGE

Ativan (lorazepam) is indicated for the management of anxiety disorders or for the short-term relief of the symptoms of anxiety or anxiety associated with depressive symptoms. Anxiety or tension associated with the stress of everyday life usually does not require treatment with an anxiolytic.

The effectiveness of Ativan (lorazepam) in long-term use, that is, more than 4 months, has not been assessed by systematic clinical studies. The physician should periodically reassess the usefulness of the drug for the individual patient.

CONTRAINDICATIONS

Ativan (lorazepam) is contraindicated in patients with known sensitivity to the benzodiazepines or with acute narrow-angle glaucoma.

WARNINGS

Ativan (lorazepam) is not recommended for use in patients with a primary depressive disorder or psychosis. As with all patients on CNS-acting drugs, patients receiving lorazepam should be warned not to operate dangerous machinery or motor vehicles and that their tolerance for alcohol and other CNS depressants will be diminished.

PHYSICAL AND PSYCHOLOGICAL DEPENDENCE

Withdrawal symptoms, similar in character to those noted with barbiturates and alcohol (convulsions, tremor, abdominal and muscle cramps, vomiting, and sweating), have occurred following abrupt discontinuance of lorazepam. The more severe withdrawal symptoms have usually been limited to those patients who received excessive doses over an extended period of time. Generally milder withdrawal symptoms (e.g., dysphoria and insomnia) have been reported following abrupt discontinuance of benzodiazepines taken continuously at therapeutic levels for several months. Consequently, after extended therapy, abrupt discontinuation should generally be avoided and a gradual dosage-tapering schedule followed. Addiction-prone individuals (such as drug addicts or alcoholics) should be under careful surveillance when receiving lorazepam or other psychotropic agents because of the predisposition of such patients to habituation and dependence.

PRECAUTIONS

In patients with depression accompanying anxiety, a possibility for suicide should be borne in mind.

For elderly or debilitated patients, the initial daily dosage should not exceed 2 mg in order to avoid oversedation.

The usual precautions for treating patients with impaired renal or hepatic function should be observed.

In patients where gastrointestinal or cardiovascular disorders coexist with anxiety, it should be noted that lorazepam has not been shown to be of significant benefit in treating the gastrointestinal or cardiovascular component.

Esophageal dilation occurred in rats treated with lorazepam for more than one year at 6 mg/kg/day. The no-effect dose was 1.25 mg/kg/day (approximately 6 times the maximum human therapeutic dose of 10 mg per day). The effect was reversible only when the treatment was withdrawn within two months of first observation of the phenomenon. The clinical significance of this is unknown. However, use of lorazepam for prolonged periods and in geriatric patients requires caution, and there should be frequent monitoring for symptoms of upper G.I. disease.

Safety and effectiveness of Ativan (lorazepam) in children of less than 12 years have not been established.

INFORMATION FOR PATIENTS

To assure the safe and effective use of Ativan (lorazepam), patients should be informed that, since benzodiazepines may produce psychological and physical dependence, it is advisable that they consult with their physician before either increasing the dose or abruptly discontinuing this drug.

ESSENTIAL LABORATORY TESTS

Some patients on Ativan (lorazepam) have developed leukopenia, and some have had elevations of LDH. As with other benzodiazepines, periodic blood counts and liver-function tests are recommended for patients on long-term therapy.

CLINICALLY SIGNIFICANT DRUG INTERACTIONS

The benzodiazepines, including Ativan (lorazepam), produce CNS-depressant effects when administered with such medications as barbiturates or alcohol.

CARCINOGENESIS AND MUTAGENESIS

No evidence of carcinogenic potential emerged in rats during an 18-month study with Ativan (lorazepam). No studies regarding mutagenesis have been performed.

PREGNANCY

Reproductive studies in animals were performed in mice, rats, and two strains of rabbits. Occasional anomalies (reduction of tarsals, tibia, metatarsals, malrotated limbs, gastroschisis, malformed skull, and microphthalmia) were seen in drug-treated rabbits without relationship to dosage. Although all of these anomalies were not present in the concurrent control group, they have been reported to occur randomly in historical controls. At doses of 40 mg/kg and higher, there was evidence of fetal resorption and increased fetal loss in rabbits which was not seen at lower doses.

The clinical significance of the above findings is not known. However, an increased risk of congenital malformations associated with the use of minor tranquilizers (chlordiazepoxide, diazepam, and meprobamate) during the first trimester of pregnancy has been suggested in several studies. Because the use of these drugs is rarely a matter of urgency, the use of lorazepam during this period should almost always be avoided. The possibility that a woman of childbearing potential may be pregnant at the time of institution of therapy should be considered. Patients should be advised that if they become pregnant, they should communicate with their physician about the desirability of discontinuing the drug.

In humans, blood levels obtained from umbilical cord blood indicate placental transfer of lorazepam and lorazepam glucuronide.

NURSING MOTHERS

It is not known whether oral lorazepam is excreted in human milk like the other benzodiazepine tranquilizers. As a general rule, nursing should not be undertaken while a patient is on a drug, since many drugs are excreted in human milk.

ADVERSE REACTIONS

Adverse reactions, if they occur, are usually observed at the beginning of therapy and generally disappear on continued medication or upon decreasing the dose. In a sample of about 3,500 anxious patients, the most frequent adverse reaction to Ativan (lorazepam) is sedation (15.9%), followed by dizziness (6.9%), weakness (4.2%), and unsteadiness (3.4%). Less frequent adverse reactions are disorientation, depression, nausea, change in appetite, headache, sleep disturbance, agitation, dermatological symptoms, eye-function disturbance, together with various gastrointestinal symptoms and autonomic manifestations. The incidence of sedation and unsteadiness increased with age.

Continued on next page

Ativan Tablets—Cont.

Small decreases in blood pressure have been noted but are not clinally significant, probably being related to the relief of anxiety produced by Ativan (lorazepam).
Transient amnesia or memory impairment has been reported in association with the use of benzodiazepines.

OVERDOSAGE

In the management of overdosage with any drug, it should be borne in mind that multiple agents may have been taken.
SYMPTOMS
Overdosage of benzodiazepines is usually manifested by varing degrees of central nervous system depression ranging from drowsiness to coma. In mild cases, symptoms include drowsiness, mental confusion and lethary. In more serious cases, and especially when other drugs or alcohol were ingested, symptoms may include ataxia, hypotonia, hypotension, hypnotic state, stage one (1) to three (3) coma, and very rarely, death.
MANAGEMENT
Induced vomiting and/or gastric lavage should be undertaken, followed by general supportive care, monitoring of vital signs, and close observation of the patient.
Hypotension, though unlikely, usually may be controlled with norepinephrine bitartrate injection. The value of dialysis has not been adequately determined for lorazepam. The benzodiazepine antagonist flumazenil may be used in hospitalized patients as an adjunct to, not as a substitute for, proper management of benzodiazepine overdose.
The prescriber should be aware of a risk of seizure in association with flumazenil treatment, particularly in long-term benzodiazepine users and in cyclic antidepressant overdose. The complete flumazenil package insert including "**Contraindications**," "**Warnings**," and "**Precautions**" should be consulted prior to use.

DOSAGE AND ADMINISTRATION

Ativan (lorazepam) is administered orally. For optimal results, dose, frequency of administration, and duration of therapy should be individualized according to patient response. To facilitate this, 0.5 mg, 1 mg, and 2 mg tablets are available.
The usual range is 2 to 6 mg/day given in divided doses, the largest dose being taken before bedtime, but the daily dosage may vary from 1 to 10 mg/day.
For anxiety, most patients require an initial dose of 2 to 3 mg/day given b.i.d. or t.i.d.
For insomnia due to anxiety or transient situational stress, a single daily dose of 2 to 4 mg may be given, usually at bedtime.
For elderly or debilitated patients, an initial dosage of 1 to 2 mg/day in divided doses is recommended, to be adjusted as needed and tolerated.
The dosage of Ativan (lorazepam) should be increased gradually when needed to help avoid adverse effects. When higher dosage is indicated, the evening dose should be increased before the daytime doses.

HOW SUPPLIED

Ativan® (lorazepam) Tablets are available in the following dosage strengths:
0.5 mg, NDC 0008-0081, white, five-sided tablet with a raised "A" on one side and "WYETH" and "81" on reverse side, in bottles of 100 and 500 tablets.
1 mg, NDC 0008-0064, white, five-sided tablet with a raised "A" on one side and "WYETH" and "64" on scored reverse side, in bottles of 100, 500, and 1000 tablets.
2 mg, NDC 0008-0065, white, five-sided tablet with a raised "A" on one side and "WYETH" and "65" on scored reverse side, in bottles of 100, 500, and 1000 tablets.
BOTTLES:
Keep tightly closed.
Store at controlled room temperature.
Dispense in tight container.
The appearance of ATIVAN tablets is a registered trademark of Wyeth-Ayerst Laboratories.
Manufactured by:
Wyeth Laboratories Inc.
A Wyeth-Ayerst Company
Philadelphia, PA 19101
Shown in Product Identification Guide, page 343

ATROMID-S® ℞

[ă 'trō-mid s]
Capsules
(clofibrate capsules)
Antilipidemic agent for reduction of elevated serum lipids

Caution: Federal law prohibits dispensing without prescription.

DESCRIPTION

Atromid-S Capsules (clofibrate capsules) is ethyl 2-(p-chlorophenoxy)-2-methyl-propionate, an antilipidemic agent.
structural formula

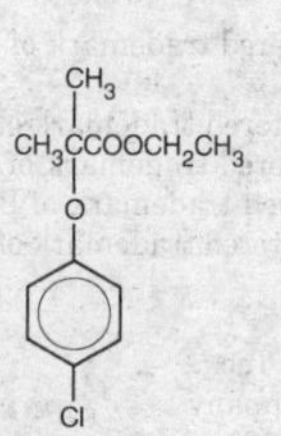
CH3
CH3CCOOCH2CH3
O
Cl

Its molecular formula is $C_{12}H_{15}O_3Cl$, molecular weight 242.7, and boiling point 148–150°C at 25 mm Hg. It is a stable, colorless to pale-yellow liquid with a faint odor and characteristic taste, soluble in common solvents but not in water. Each Atromid-S Capsule contains 500 mg clofibrate for oral administration.
Atromid-S Capsules contain the following inactive ingredients: D&C Red No. 28, D&C Red No. 30, D&C Yellow No. 10, FD&C Blue No. 1, FD&C Red No. 28, FD&C Red No. 40, FD&C Yellow No. 6, gelatin.

CLINICAL PHARMACOLOGY

Atromid-S is an antilipidemic agent. It acts to lower elevated serum lipids by reducing the very low-density lipoprotein fraction (S_f 20–400) rich in triglycerides. Serum cholesterol may be decreased, particularly in those patients whose cholesterol elevation is due to the presence of IDL as a result of Type III hyperlipoproteinemia.
The mechanism of action has not been established definitively. Clofibrate may inhibit the hepatic release of lipoproteins (particularly VLDL), potentiate the action of lipoprotein lipase, and increase the fecal excretion of neutral sterols.
Between 95% and 99% of an oral dose of clofibrate is excreted in the urine as free and conjugated clofibric acid; thus, the absorption of clofibrate is virtually complete. The half-life of clofibric acid in normal volunteers averages 18 to 22 hours (range 14 to 35 hours) but can vary by up to 7 hours in the same subject at different times. Clofibric acid is highly protein-bound (95% to 97%). In subjects undergoing continuous clofibrate treatment, 1 g q12h, plasma concentrations of clofibric acid range from 120 to 125 mcg/mL to an approximate peak of 200 mcg/mL.
Several investigators have observed in their studies that clofibrate may produce a decrease in cholesterol linoleate but an increase in palmitoleate and oleate, the latter being considered atherogenic in experimental animals. The significance of this finding is unknown at this time.
Reduction of triglycerides in some patients treated with clofibrate or certain of its chemically and clinically similar analogs may be associated with an increase in LDL cholesterol. Increase in LDL cholesterol has been observed in patients whose cholesterol is initially normal.
Animal studies suggest that clofibrate interrupts cholesterol biosynthesis prior to mevalonate formation.

INDICATIONS AND USAGE

The initial treatment of choice for hyperlipidemia is dietary therapy specific for the type of hyperlipidemia.[1]
Excess body weight and alcoholic intake may be important factors in hypertriglyceridemia and should be addressed prior to any drug therapy. Physical exercise can be an important ancillary measure. Estrogen therapy, some beta-blockers, and thiazide diuretics may also be associated with increases in plasma triglycerides. Discontinuation of such products may obviate the need for specific antilipidemic therapy. Contributory diseases such as hypothyroidism or diabetes mellitus should be looked for and adequately treated. The use of drugs should be considered only when reasonable attempts have been made to obtain satisfactory results with nondrug methods. If the decision ultimately is to use drugs, the patient should be instructed that this does not reduce the importance of adhering to diet.
Because Atromid-S is associated with certain serious adverse findings reported in two large clinical trials (see "**WARNINGS**"), agents other than clofibrate may be more suitable for a particular patient.
Atromid-S is indicated for Primary Dysbetalipoproteinemia (Type III hyperlipidemia) that does not respond adequately to diet.
Atromid-S may be considered for the treatment of adult patients with very high serum-triglyceride levels (Type IV and V hyperlipidemia) who present a risk of abdominal pain and pancreatitis and who do not respond adequately to a determined dietary effort to control them. Patients who present such risk typically have serum triglycerides over 2000 mg/dl and have elevations of VLDL-cholesterol as well as fasting chylomicrons (Type V hyperlipidemia). Subjects who consistently have total serum or plasma triglycerides below 1000 mg/dl are unlikely to present a risk of pancreatitis. Atromid-S therapy may be considered for those subjects with triglyceride elevations between 1000 and 2000 mg/dl who have a history of pancreatitis or of recurrent abdominal pain typical of pancreatitis. It is recognized that some Type IV patients with triglycerides under 1000 mg/dl may, through dietary or alcoholic indiscretion, convert to a Type V pattern with massive triglyceride elevations accompanying fasting chylomicronemia, but the influence of Atromid-S therapy on the risk of pancreatitis in such situations has not been adequately studied.
Atromid-S is not useful for the hypertriglyceridemia of Type I hyperlipidemia, where elevations of chylomicrons and plasma triglycerides are accompanied by normal levels of very low-density lipoprotein (VLDL). Inspection of plasma refrigerated for 12 to 14 hours is helpful in distinguishing Types I, IV, and V hyperlipoproteinemia.[2]
Atromid-S has not been shown to be effective for prevention of coronary heart disease.
The biochemical response to Atromid-S is variable, and it is not always possible to predict from the lipoprotein type or other factors which patients will obtain favorable results. LDL cholesterol, as well as triglycerides, should be rechecked during the first several months of therapy in order to detect rises in LDL cholesterol that often accompany fibric-acid-type drug-induced reductions in elevated triglycerides. It is essential that lipid levels be reassessed periodically and that the drug be discontinued in any patient in whom lipids do not show significant improvement.

CONTRAINDICATIONS

Clofibrate is contraindicated in pregnant women. While teratogenic studies have not demonstrated any effect attributable to clofibrate, it is known that serum of the rabbit fetus accumulates a higher concentration of clofibrate than that found in maternal serum, and it is possible that the fetus may not have developed the enzyme system required for the excretion of clofibrate.
It is contraindicated in patients with clinically significant hepatic or renal dysfunction. Rhabdomyolysis and severe hyperkalemia have been reported in association with preexisting renal insufficiency.
It is contraindicated in patients with primary biliary cirrhosis, since it may raise the already elevated cholesterol in these cases.
It is contraindicated in patients with a known hypersensitivity to clofibrate.
It is contraindicated in nursing women (see "**PRECAUTIONS**").

WARNINGS

In a large study involving 5,000 patients in a clofibrate-treated group and 5,000 in a placebo-treated group followed for an average of five years on drug or placebo and one year beyond (the WHO study), there was a statistically significant 44% higher age-adjusted total mortality in the clofibrate-treated group than in a comparable placebo group. The excess deaths were due to noncardiovascular causes; half of this difference was due to malignancy; other causes of death included postcholecystectomy complications and pancreatitis.[3] In another prospective study involving 1,000 clofibrate- and 3,000 placebo-treated patients followed for an average of six years on drug or placebo (the Coronary Drug Project study), the noncardiovascular mortality rate, including that of malignancy, was not significantly different in the clofibrate- and placebo-treated groups.[4] This should not be interpreted to mean that clofibrate is not associated with an increased risk of noncardiovascular death, because the patients in the Coronary Drug Project were much older than those in the WHO study and they all had had a previous myocardial infarction, so that the deaths in the Coronary Drug Project were overwhelmingly due to cardiovascular causes, and it would have been very difficult to discern a clofibrate-associated risk of death due to noncardiovascular causes if it existed. Both studies demonstrated that clofibrate users have twice the risk of developing cholelithiasis and cholecystitis requiring surgery as do nonusers.

A potential benefit of clofibrate was, however, reported in the WHO study which involved patients with hypercholesterolemia and no history of myocardial infarction or angina pectoris. In this study, there was a statistically significant 25% decrease in subsequent nonfatal myocardial infarctions in the clofibrate-treated group when compared with the placebo group. There was no difference in incidence of fatal myocardial infarction in the two groups. In the Coronary Drug Project study, which involved patients with or without hypercholesterolemia and/or hypertriglyceridemia and with a history of previous myocardial infarction, there was no significant difference in incidence of either nonfatal or fatal myocardial infarction between the clofibrate- and placebo-treated groups.[3]

As a result of these and other studies, the following can be stated:

1. Clofibrate, in general, causes a relatively modest reduction of serum cholesterol and a somewhat greater reduction of serum triglycerides. In Type III hyperlipidemia, however, substantial reductions of both cholesterol and triglycerides can occur with clofibrate use.

2. No study to date has shown a convincing reduction in incidence of *fatal* myocardial infarction.

3. A significantly increased incidence of cholelithiasis has been demonstrated consistently in clofibrate-treated groups, and an increase in morbidity from this complication and mortality from cholecystectomy must be anticipated during clofibrate treatment.

4. Several types of other undesirable events have been associated in a statistically significant way with clofibrate administration in the WHO and the Coronary Drug Project studies. There was an increase in incidence of noncardiovascular deaths reported in the WHO study. There was an increase in cardiac arrhythmias, intermittent claudication, and definite or suspected thromboembolic events, and angina reported in the Coronary Drug Project, which was not, however, reported in the WHO study.

5. Administration of clofibrate to mice and rats in long-term studies at 1 to 2 times the maximum recommended human dose (based on surface area, mg/m²), resulted in a higher incidence of benign and malignant liver tumors than in controls.

There was an increase in benign Leydig cell tumors in male rats treated at 400 mg/kg/day or 2 times the maximum recommended human dose in one study. A comparative carcinogenicity study was also done in rats comparing three drugs in this class: fenofibrate (10 and 60 mg/kg; 0.3 and 1.6 times the human dose), clofibrate (400 mg/kg; 1.6 times the human dose), and gemfibrozil (250 mg/kg; 1.7 times the human dose). Pancreatic acinar adenomas were increased in males and females on fenofibrate; hepatocellular carcinoma and pancreatic acinar adenomas were increased in males and hepatic neoplastic nodules in females treated with clofibrate; hepatic neoplastic nodules were increased in males and females treated with gemfibrozil while testicular interstitial cell tumors were increased in males on all three drugs.

6. Administration of clofibrate to male monkeys at dosages of 1 to 2 times the maximum recommended human dose resulted in increases in mortality of 2- to 5-fold. As in the case of men in the WHO study, no single cause of death was identified.

BECAUSE OF THE TUMORIGENICITY OF CLOFIBRATE IN RODENTS AND THE POSSIBLE INCREASED RISK OF MALIGNANCY ASSOCIATED WITH CLOFIBRATE IN THE HUMAN, AS WELL AS THE INCREASED RISK OF CHOLELITHIASIS, AND BECAUSE THERE IS NOT, TO DATE, SUBSTANTIAL EVIDENCE OF A BENEFICIAL EFFECT ON CARDIOVASCULAR MORTALITY FROM CLOFIBRATE, THIS DRUG SHOULD BE UTILIZED ONLY FOR THOSE PATIENTS DESCRIBED IN THE "INDICATIONS AND USAGE" SECTION, AND SHOULD BE DISCONTINUED IF SIGNIFICANT LIPID RESPONSE IS NOT OBTAINED.

Concomitant Anticoagulants
CAUTION SHOULD BE EXERCISED WHEN ANTICOAGULANTS ARE GIVEN IN CONJUNCTION WITH ATROMID-S®. THE DOSAGE OF THE ANTICOAGULANT SHOULD BE REDUCED USUALLY BY ONE-HALF (DEPENDING ON THE INDIVIDUAL CASE) TO MAINTAIN THE PROTHROMBIN TIME AT THE DESIRED LEVEL TO PREVENT BLEEDING COMPLICATIONS. FREQUENT PROTHROMBIN DETERMINATIONS ARE ADVISABLE UNTIL IT HAS BEEN DEFINITELY DETERMINED THAT THE PROTHROMBIN LEVEL HAS BEEN STABILIZED.

Skeletal Muscle
Myalgia, myositis, myopathy, and rhabdomyolysis with or without elevation of CPK have been associated with Atromid-S therapy. Consideration should be given to withholding or discontinuing drug therapy in any patient with a risk factor predisposing to the development of renal failure secondary to rhabdomyolysis, including: severe acute infection; hypotension; major surgery; trauma; severe metabolic, endocrine, or electrolyte disorders; and uncontrolled seizures. Atromid-S therapy should be discontinued if markedly elevated CPK levels occur or myositis is diagnosed.

Avoidance of Pregnancy
Strict birth-control procedures must be exercised by women of child-bearing potential. In patients who plan to become pregnant, clofibrate should be withdrawn several months before conception. Because of the possibility of pregnancy occurring despite birth-control precautions in patients taking clofibrate, the possible benefits of the drug to the patient must be weighed against possible hazards to the fetus. (See "Pregnancy" section.)

PRECAUTIONS
General
Before instituting therapy with clofibrate, attempts should be made to control serum lipids with appropriate dietary regimens, weight loss in obese patients, control of diabetes mellitus, etc.

Because of the long-term administration of a drug of this nature, adequate baseline studies should be performed to determine that the patient has significantly elevated serum lipid levels. Frequent determinations of serum lipids should be obtained during the first few months of Atromid-S administration, and periodic determinations made thereafter. The drug should be withdrawn after three months if response is inadequate. However, in the case of xanthoma tuberosum, the drug should be employed for longer periods (even up to one year) provided that there is a reduction in the size and/or number of the xanthomata.

Since cholelithiasis is a possible side effect of clofibrate therapy, appropriate diagnostic procedures should be performed if signs and symptoms related to disease of the biliary system should occur.

Clofibrate may produce "flu-like" symptoms (muscular aching, soreness, cramping) associated with increased creatine kinase levels indicative of drug-induced myopathy. The physician should differentiate this from actual viral and/or bacterial disease.

Use with caution in patients with peptic ulcer, since reactivation has been reported. Whether this is drug related is unknown.

Various cardiac arrhythmias have been reported with the use of clofibrate.

Laboratory Tests
Subsequent serum lipid determinations should be done to detect a paradoxical rise in serum cholesterol or triglyceride levels. Clofibrate will not alter the seasonal variations of serum cholesterol: peak elevations in midwinter and late summer and decreases in fall and spring. If the drug is discontinued, the patient should be continued on an appropriate hypolipidemic diet, and serum lipids should be monitored until stabilized, as a rise in these values to or above the original baseline may occur.

During clofibrate therapy, frequent serum-transaminase determinations and other liver-function tests should be performed, since the drug may produce abnormalities in these parameters. These effects are usually reversible when the drug is discontinued. Hepatic biopsies are usually within normal limits. If the hepatic-function tests steadily rise or show excessive abnormalities, the drug should be withdrawn. Therefore, use with caution in those patients with a past history of jaundice or hepatic disease.

Complete blood counts should be done periodically since anemia, and more frequently, leukopenia have been reported in patients who have been taking clofibrate.

Drug Interactions
Caution should be exercised when anticoagulants are given in conjunction with Atromid-S. Usually, the dosage of the anticoagulant should be reduced by one-half (depending on the individual case) to maintain the prothrombin time at the desired level to prevent bleeding complications. Frequent prothrombin determinations are advisable until it has been determined definitely that the prothrombin level has been stabilized.

Atromid-S may displace acidic drugs such as phenytoin or tolbutamide from their binding sites. Caution should be exercised when treating patients with either of these drugs or other highly protein-bound drugs and Atromid-S. The hypoglycemic effect of tolbutamide has been reported to increase when Atromid-S is given concurrently.

Fulminant rhabdomyolysis has been seen as early as three weeks after initiation of combined therapy with another fibrate and lovastatin but may be seen after several months. For these reasons, it is felt that, in most subjects who have had an unsatisfactory lipid response to either drug alone, the possible benefits of combined therapy with lovastatin and a fibrate do not outweigh the risks of severe myopathy, rhabdomyolysis, and acute renal failure. While it is not known whether this interaction occurs with fibrates other than gemfibrozil, myopathy and rhabdomyolysis have occasionally been associated with the use of fibrates alone, including clofibrate. Therefore, the combined use of lovastatin with fibrates should generally be avoided.

Carcinogenesis, Mutagenesis, Impairment of Fertility
See "WARNINGS" section for information on carcinogenesis and mutagenesis.

Arrest of spermatogenesis has been seen in both dogs and monkeys at doses approximately 2 times the maximum recommended human dose (based on surface area).

Electron microscopy studies have demonstrated peroxisomal proliferation following clofibrate administration to the rat. Changes in peroxisome morphology and numbers have been observed in humans after treatment with several members of the fibrate class, including clofibrate, when liver biopsies were compared before and after treatment in the same individual.

Pregnancy
Teratogenic effects

Pregnancy Category C. Animal reproduction studies have not been conducted with Atromid-S. It is also not known whether Atromid-S can cause fetal harm when administered to a pregnant woman or can affect reproductive capacity. However, animal reproduction studies with clofibrate plus androsterone showed increases in neonatal deaths and pup mortality during lactation.

Nursing Mothers
Atromid-S is contraindicated in lactating women, since an active metabolite (CPIB) has been measured in breast milk.

Pediatric Use
Safety and efficacy in pediatric patients have not been established.

ADVERSE REACTIONS
The most common is nausea. Less frequently encountered gastrointestinal reactions are vomiting, loose stools, dyspepsia, flatulence, and abdominal distress. Reactions reported less often than gastrointestinal ones are headache, dizziness, and fatigue; muscle cramping, aching, and weakness; skin rash, urticaria, and pruritus; dry brittle hair, and alopecia.

The following reported adverse reactions are listed alphabetically by systems:

Cardiovascular
Increased or decreased angina.
Cardiac arrhythmias.
Both swelling and phlebitis at site of xanthomas.

Dermatologic
Allergic reactions including urticaria.
Skin rash.
Pruritus.
Dry skin and dry, brittle hair.
Alopecia.
Toxic epidermal necrolysis.
Erythema multiforme.
Stevens-Johnson syndrome.

Gastrointestinal
Gallstones.
Nausea.
Vomiting.
Diarrhea.
Gastrointestinal upset (bloating, flatulence, abdominal distress).
Hepatomegaly (not associated with hepatotoxicity).
Stomatitis and gastritis.

Genitourinary
Findings consistent with renal dysfunction as evidenced by dysuria, hematuria, proteinuria, decreased urine output. One patient's renal biopsy suggested "allergic reaction."
Impotence and decreased libido.

Hematologic
Leukopenia.
Potentiation of anticoagulant effect.
Anemia.
Eosinophilia.
Agranulocytosis.

Musculoskeletal
Myalgia (muscle cramping, aching, weakness).
"Flu-like" symptoms.
Myositis.
Myopathy.
Rhabdomyolysis in the setting of preexisting renal insufficiency.
Arthralgia.

Neurologic
Fatigue, weakness, drowsiness.
Dizziness.
Headache.

Miscellaneous
Weight gain.
Polyphagia.

Laboratory Findings
Abnormal liver-function tests as evidenced by increased transaminase (SGOT and SGPT), BSP retention, and increased thymol turbidity.
Proteinuria.
Increased creatine phosphokinase.
Hyperkalemia in association with renal insufficiency and continuous ambulatory peritoneal dialysis treatment.

Reported adverse reactions whose direct relationship with the drug has not been established: peptic ulcer, gastrointestinal hemorrhage, rheumatoid arthritis, tremors, increased perspiration, systemic lupus erythematosus, blurred vision, gynecomastia, thrombocytopenic purpura.

Continued on next page

Atromid-S—Cont.

OVERDOSAGE

While there has been no reported case of overdosage, should it occur, symptomatic supportive measures should be taken.

DOSAGE AND ADMINISTRATION

Initial: The recommended dosage for adults is 2 g daily in divided doses. Some patients may respond to a lower dosage.

Maintenance: Same as for initial dosage.

HOW SUPPLIED

Atromid-S Capsules (clofibrate capsules)—Each orange, oblong, soft-gelatin capsule contains 500 mg clofibrate, in bottles of 100 (NDC 0046-0243-81).

The appearance of these orange, oblong, soft-gelatin capsules is a trademark of Wyeth-Ayerst Laboratories.

Store at room temperature, approximately 25° C (77° F).

Dispense in a well-closed, light-resistant container as defined in the USP.

Avoid freezing and excessive heat.

REFERENCES

1. Coronary Risk Handbook (1973). American Heart Association.
2. Nikkila, EA: Familial lipoprotein lipase deficiency and related disorders of chylomicron metabolism. In Stanbury JB et al (eds): The Metabolic Basis of Inherited Disease, 5th ed., McGraw-Hill, 1983, Chap. 30. p.622–642.
3. Report from the Committee of Principal Investigators: A cooperative trial in the primary prevention of ischaemic heart disease using clofibrate. Br Heart J *40* :1069, 1978.
4. The Coronary Drug Project Research Group: Clofibrate and niacin in coronary heart disease. JAMA *231* :360, 1975.

Manufactured for
Ayerst Laboratories Inc.
A Wyeth-Ayerst Company
Philadelphia, PA 19101

Shown in Product Identification Guide, page 343

AURALGAN® ℞

[*aw-răl 'găn*]

Otic Solution

Caution: Federal law prohibits dispensing without prescription.

DESCRIPTION

Each mL contains:

Antipyrine	54.0 mg
Benzocaine	14.0 mg
Glycerin dehydrated q.s. to	1.0 mL

(contains not more than 0.6% moisture)
(also contains oxyquinoline sulfate)

TOPICAL DECONGESTANT AND ANALGESIC

Auralgan is an otic solution containing antipyrine, benzocaine, and dehydrated glycerin. The solution congeals at 0° C (32° F), but returns to normal consistency, unchanged, at room temperature.

The structures of the components are:

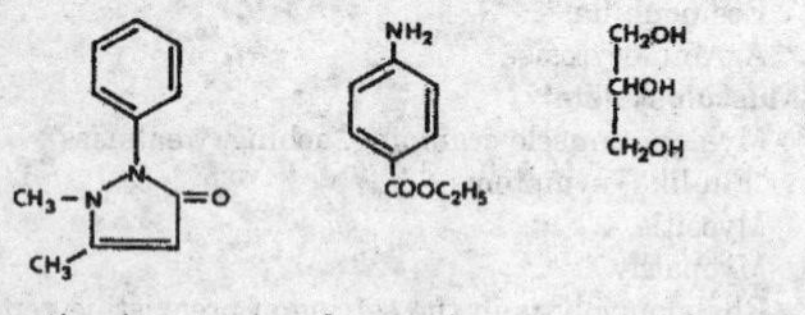

antipyrine benzocaine glycerin

CLINICAL PHARMACOLOGY

Auralgan combines the hygroscopic property of dehydrated glycerin with the analgesic action of antipyrine and benzocaine to relieve pressure, reduce inflammation and congestion, and alleviate pain and discomfort in acute otitis media. Auralgan does not blanch the tympanic membrane or mask the landmarks and, therefore, does not distort the otoscopic picture.

INDICATIONS AND USAGE

ACUTE OTITIS MEDIA OF VARIOUS ETIOLOGIES

— prompt relief of pain and reduction of inflammation in the congestive and serous stages

— adjuvant therapy during systemic antibiotic administration for resolution of the infection

Because of the close anatomical relationship of the eustachian tube to the nasal cavity, otitis media is a frequent problem, especially in children in whom the tube is shorter, wider, and more horizontal than in adults.

REMOVAL OF CERUMEN

—facilitates the removal of excessive or impacted cerumen

CONTRAINDICATIONS

Hypersensitivity to any of the components or substances related to them.

Perforated tympanic membrane is considered a contraindication to the use of any medication in the external ear canal.

WARNINGS

Discontinue promptly if sensitization or irritation occurs.

PRECAUTIONS

CARCINOGENESIS, MUTAGENESIS, IMPAIRMENT OF FERTILITY

No long-term studies in animals or humans have been conducted

PREGNANCY CATEGORY C

Animal reproduction studies have not been conducted with Auralgan. It is also not known whether Auralgan can cause fetal harm when administered to a pregnant woman, or can affect reproduction capacity. Auralgan should be given to a pregnant woman only if clearly needed.

NURSING MOTHERS

It is not known whether this drug is excreted in human milk. Because many drugs are excreted in human milk, caution should be exercised when Auralgan is administered to a nursing woman.

DOSAGE AND ADMINISTRATION

ACUTE OTITIS MEDIA

Instill Auralgan permitting the solution to run along the wall of the canal until it is filled. Avoid touching the ear with dropper. Then moisten a cotton pledget with Auralgan and insert into meatus. Repeat every one to two hours until pain and congestion are relieved.

REMOVAL OF CERUMEN

Before: Instill Auralgan three times daily for two or three days to help detach cerumen from wall of canal and facilitate removal.

After: Auralgan is useful for drying out the canal or relieving discomfort.

Before and after removal of cerumen, a cotton pledget moistened with Auralgan should be inserted into the meatus following instillation.

Note: Do not rinse dropper after use.

Replace dropper in bottle after each use. Hold dropper assembly by screw cap and, without compressing the rubber bulb, insert into drug container and screw down tightly.

Protect the solution from light and heat, and do not use if it is brown or contains a precipitate.

DISCARD THIS PRODUCT SIX MONTHS AFTER DROPPER IS FIRST PLACED IN THE DRUG SOLUTION.

HOW SUPPLIED

Auralgan® Otic Solution, in package containing 10 mL bottle with separate dropper-screw cap attachment (NDC 0046-1000-10).

Store at room temperature (approximately 25° C).

Manufactured by:
Ayerst Laboratories Inc.
A Wyeth-Ayerst Company
Philadelphia, PA 19101

BICILLIN® C-R ℞

[*bī-sil 'in*]

(penicillin G benzathine and penicillin G procaine suspension)

INJECTION
FOR DEEP INTRAMUSCULAR INJECTION ONLY

DESCRIPTION

Bicillin C-R (penicillin G benzathine and penicillin G procaine suspension), contains equal amounts of the benzathine and procaine salts of penicillin G. It is available for deep intramuscular injection.

Penicillin G benzathine is prepared by the reaction of dibenzylethylene diamine with two molecules of penicillin G. It is chemically designated as (2*S*, 5*R*, 6*R*)-3,3-Dimethyl-7-oxo-6-(2-phenylacetamido)-4-thia-1-azabicyclo [3.2.0] heptane-2-carboxylic acid compound with *N,N'*-dibenzylethylenediamine (2:1), tetrahydrate. It occurs as a white, crystalline powder and is very slightly soluble in water and sparingly soluble in alcohol.

Penicillin G procaine, (2*S*, 5*R*, 6*R*)-3,3-Dimethyl-7-oxo-6-(2-phenylacetamido)-4-thia-1-azabicyclo [3.2.0] heptane-2-carboxylic acid compound with 2-(diethylamino)ethyl p-aminobenzoate (1:1) monohydrate, is an equimolar salt of procaine and penicillin G. It occurs as white crystals or a white, microcrystalline powder and is slightly soluble in water.

Bicillin C-R (penicillin G benzathine and penicillin G procaine suspension) contains in each mL the equivalent of 150,000 units of penicillin G as the benzathine salt and 150,000 units of penicillin G as the procaine salt in a stabilized aqueous suspension with sodium citrate buffer; and as w/v, approximately 0.5% lecithin, 0.55% carboxymethylcellulose, 0.55% povidone, 0.1% methylparaben, and 0.01% propylparaben.

Each disposable syringe (4 mL size) contains the equivalent of 2,400,000 units of penicillin G comprising: the equivalent of 1,200,000 units of penicillin G as the benzathine salt and the equivalent of 1,200,000 units of penicillin G as the procaine salt in a stabilized aqueous suspension with sodium citrate buffer; and as w/v, approximately 0.5% lecithin, 0.55% carboxymethylcellulose, 0.55% povidone, 0.1% methylparaben, and 0.01% propylparaben.

Each **TUBEX** cartridge (1 mL size) contains the equivalent of 600,000 units of penicillin G comprising: the equivalent of 300,000 units penicillin G as the benzathine salt and the equivalent of 300,000 units penicillin G as the procaine salt in a stabilized aqueous suspension with sodium citrate buffer; and as w/v, approximately 0.5% lecithin, 0.55% carboxymethylcellulose, 0.55% povidone, 0.1% methylparaben, and 0.01% propylparaben.

Each **TUBEX** cartridge (2 mL size) contains the equivalent of 1,200,000 units of penicillin G comprising: the equivalent of 600,000 units of penicillin G as the benzathine salt and the equivalent of 600,000 units of penicillin G as the procaine salt in a stabilized aqueous suspension with sodium citrate buffer; and as w/v, approximately 0.5% lecithin, 0.55% carboxymethylcellulose, 0.55% povidone, 0.1% methylparaben, and 0.01% propylparaben.

Bicillin C-R suspension in the multiple-dose-vial formulation, disposable-syringe formulation, and the **TUBEX** formulation is viscous and opaque. Read **CONTRAINDICATIONS, WARNINGS, PRECAUTIONS,** and **DOSAGE AND ADMINISTRATION** sections prior to use.

CLINICAL PHARMACOLOGY

General

Penicillin G benzathine and penicillin G procaine have a low solubility and, thus, the drugs are slowly released from intramuscular injection sites. The drugs are hydrolyzed to penicillin G. This combination of hydrolysis and slow absorption results in blood serum levels much lower but more prolonged than other parenteral penicillins.

Intramuscular administration of 600,000 units of Bicillin C-R in adults usually produces peak blood levels of 1.0 to 1.3 units per mL within 3 hours; this level falls to an average concentration of 0.32 units per mL at 12 hours, 0.19 units per mL at 24 hours, and 0.03 units per mL at seven days.

Intramuscular administration of 1,200,000 units of Bicillin C-R in adults usually produces peak blood levels of 2.1 to 2.6 units per mL within 3 hours; this level falls to an average concentration of 0.75 units per mL at 12 hours, 0.28 units per mL at 24 hours, and 0.04 units per mL at seven days.

Approximately 60% of penicillin G is bound to serum protein. The drug is distributed throughout the body tissues in widely varying amounts. Highest levels are found in the kidneys with lesser amounts in the liver, skin, and intestines. Penicillin G penetrates into all other tissues and the spinal fluid to a lesser degree. With normal kidney function, the drug is excreted rapidly by tubular excretion. In neonates and young infants and in individuals with impaired kidney function, excretion is considerably delayed.

Microbiology

Penicillin G exerts a bactericidal action against penicillin-susceptible microorganisms during the stage of active multiplication. It acts through the inhibition of biosynthesis of cell-wall mucopeptide. It is not active against the penicillinase-producing bacteria, which include many strains of staphylococci.

The following *in vitro* data are available, but their clinical significance is unknown. Penicillin G exerts high *in vitro* activity against staphylococci (except penicillinase-producing strains), streptococci (Groups A, C, G, H, L, and M), and pneumococci. Other organisms susceptible to penicillin G are *Neisseria gonorrhoeae, Corynebacterium diphtheriae, Bacillus anthracis,* Clostridia species, *Actinomyces bovis, Streptobacillus moniliformis, Listeria monocytogenes,* and Leptospira species. *Treponema pallidum* is extremely susceptible to the bactericidal action of penicillin G.

Susceptibility Test: If the Kirby-Bauer method of disc susceptibility is used, a 10-unit penicillin disc should give a zone greater than 28 mm when tested against a penicillin-sensitive bacterial strain.

INDICATIONS AND USAGE

This drug is indicated in the treatment of moderately severe infections due to penicillin-G-susceptible microorganisms that are susceptible to serum levels common to this particular dosage form. Therapy should be guided by bacteriological studies (including susceptibility testing) and by clinical response.

Bicillin C-R is indicated in the treatment of the following in adults and pediatric patients:

Moderately severe to severe infections of the upper-respiratory tract, scarlet fever, erysipelas, and skin and soft-tissue infections due to susceptible streptococci.

NOTE: Streptococci in Groups A, C, G, H, L, and M are very sensitive to penicillin G. Other groups, including Group D (enterococci), are resistant. Penicillin G sodium or potassium is recommended for streptococcal infections with bacteremia.

Moderately severe pneumonia and otitis media due to susceptible pneumococci.

NOTE: Severe pneumonia, empyema, bacteremia, pericarditis, meningitis, peritonitis, and arthritis of pneumococcal etiology are better treated with penicillin G sodium or potassium during the acute stage.

When high, sustained serum levels are required, penicillin G sodium or potassium, either IM or IV, should be used. This drug should not be used in the treatment of venereal diseases, including syphilis, gonorrhea, yaws, bejel, and pinta.

CONTRAINDICATIONS

A previous hypersensitivity reaction to any penicillin or to procaine is a contraindication.

Do not inject into or near an artery or nerve.

WARNINGS

The combination of penicillin G benzathine and penicillin G procaine should only be prescribed for the indications listed in this insert.

SERIOUS AND OCCASIONALLY FATAL HYPERSENSITIVITY (ANAPHYLACTIC) REACTIONS HAVE BEEN REPORTED IN PATIENTS ON PENICILLIN THERAPY. THESE REACTIONS ARE MORE LIKELY TO OCCUR IN INDIVIDUALS WITH A HISTORY OF PENICILLIN HYPERSENSITIVITY AND/OR A HISTORY OF SENSITIVITY TO MULTIPLE ALLERGENS. THERE HAVE BEEN REPORTS OF INDIVIDUALS WITH A HISTORY OF PENICILLIN HYPERSENSITIVITY WHO HAVE EXPERIENCED SEVERE REACTIONS WHEN TREATED WITH CEPHALOSPORINS. BEFORE INITIATING THERAPY WITH BICILLIN C-R, CAREFUL INQUIRY SHOULD BE MADE CONCERNING PREVIOUS HYPERSENSITIVITY REACTIONS TO PENICILLINS, CEPHALOSPORINS AND OTHER ALLERGENS. IF AN ALLERGIC REACTION OCCURS, BICILLIN C-R SHOULD BE DISCONTINUED AND APPROPRIATE THERAPY INSTITUTED. SERIOUS ANAPHYLACTIC REACTIONS REQUIRE IMMEDIATE EMERGENCY TREATMENT WITH EPINEPHRINE, OXYGEN, INTRAVENOUS STEROIDS AND AIRWAY MANAGEMENT, INCLUDING INTUBATION, SHOULD ALSO BE ADMINISTERED AS INDICATED.

Pseudomembranous colitis has been reported with nearly all antibacterial agents, including penicillin, and may range in severity from mild to life-threatening. Therefore, it is important to consider this diagnosis in patients who present with diarrhea subsequent to the administration of any antibacterial agent.

Treatment with antibacterial agents alters the normal flora of the colon and may permit overgrowth of clostridia. Studies indicate that a toxin produced by *Clostridium difficile* is one primary cause of "antibiotic-associated colitis".

After the diagnosis of pseudomembranous colitis has been established, appropriate therapeutic measures should be initiated. Mild cases of pseudomembranous colitis usually respond to drug discontinuation alone. In moderate to severe cases, consideration should be given to management with fluids and electrolytes, protein supplementation, and treatment with an antibacterial drug clinically effective against *C. difficile* colitis.

Inadvertent intravascular administration, including inadvertent direct intra-arterial injection or injection immediately adjacent to arteries, of Bicillin C-R and other penicillin preparations has resulted in severe neurovascular damage, including transverse myelitis with permanent paralysis, gangrene requiring amputation of digits and more proximal portions of extremities, and necrosis and sloughing at and surrounding the injection site. Such severe effects have been reported following injections into the buttock, thigh, and deltoid areas. Other serious complications of suspected intravascular administration which have been reported include immediate pallor, mottling or cyanosis of the extremity both distal and proximal to the injection site followed by bleb formation; severe edema requiring anterior and/or posterior compartment fasciotomy in the lower extremity. The above-described severe effects and complications have most often occurred in infants and small children. Prompt consultation with an appropriate specialist is indicated if any evidence of compromise of the blood supply occurs at, proximal to, or distal to the site of injection.[1-9] See **CONTRAINDICATIONS**, **PRECAUTIONS**, and **DOSAGE AND ADMINISTRATION** sections.

Quadriceps femoris fibrosis and atrophy have been reported following repeated intramuscular injections of penicillin preparations into the anterolateral thigh.

Injection into or near a nerve may result in permanent neurological damage.

PRECAUTIONS

General

Penicillin should be used with caution in individuals with histories of significant allergies and/or asthma.

Care should be taken to avoid intravenous or intra-arterial administration, or injection into or near major peripheral nerves or blood vessels, since such injections may produce neurovascular damage. See **CONTRAINDICATIONS**, **WARNINGS**, and **DOSAGE AND ADMINISTRATION** sections.

A small percentage of patients are sensitive to procaine. If there is a history of sensitivity, make the usual test: Inject intradermally 0.1 mL of a 1 to 2 percent procaine solution. Development of an erythema, wheal, flare, or eruption indicates procaine sensitivity. Sensitivity should be treated by the usual methods, including barbiturates, and procaine penicillin preparations should not be used. Antihistaminics appear beneficial in treatment of procaine reactions.

The use of antibiotics may result in overgrowth of nonsusceptible organisms. Constant observation of the patient is essential. If new infections due to bacteria or fungi appear during therapy, the drug should be discontinued and appropriate measures taken.

Whenever allergic reactions occur, penicillin should be withdrawn unless, in the opinion of the physician, the condition being treated is life-threatening and amenable only to penicillin therapy.

In prolonged therapy with penicillin, and particularly with high-dosage schedules, periodic evaluation of the renal and hematopoietic systems is recommended.

Laboratory Tests

In streptococcal infections, therapy must be sufficient to eliminate the organism; otherwise, the sequelae of streptococcal disease may occur. Cultures should be taken following completion of treatment to determine whether streptococci have been eradicated.

Drug Interactions

Tetracycline, a bacteriostatic antibiotic, may antagonize the bactericidal effect of penicillin, and concurrent use of these drugs should be avoided.

Concurrent administration of penicillin and probenecid increases and prolongs serum penicillin levels by decreasing the apparent volume of distribution and slowing the rate of excretion by competitively inhibiting renal tubular secretion of penicillin.

Pregnancy Category B

Reproduction studies performed in the mouse, rat, and rabbit have revealed no evidence of impaired fertility or harm to the fetus due to penicillin G. Human experience with the penicillins during pregnancy has not shown any positive evidence of adverse effects on the fetus. There are, however, no adequate and well-controlled studies in pregnant women showing conclusively that harmful effects of these drugs on the fetus can be excluded. Because animal reproduction studies are not always predictive of human response, this drug should be used during pregnancy only if clearly needed.

Nursing Mothers

Soluble penicillin G is excreted in breast milk. Caution should be exercised when penicillin G benzathine and penicillin G procaine are administered to a nursing woman.

Carcinogenesis, Mutagenesis, Impairment of Fertility

No long-term animal studies have been conducted with these drugs.

Pediatric Use

See **INDICATIONS AND USAGE** and **DOSAGE AND ADMINISTRATION**.

ADVERSE REACTIONS

As with other penicillins, untoward reactions of the sensitivity phenomena are likely to occur, particularly in individuals who have previously demonstrated hypersensitivity to penicillins or in those with a history of allergy, asthma, hay fever, or urticaria.

The following have been reported with parenteral penicillin G:

General: Hypersensitivity reactions including the following: skin eruptions (maculopapular to exfoliative dermatitis), urticaria, laryngeal edema, fever, eosinophilia; other serum-sickness-like reactions (including chills, fever, edema, arthralgia, and prostration); anaphylaxis including shock and death. Note: Urticaria, other skin rashes, and serum-sickness-like reactions may be controlled with antihistamines and, if necessary, systemic corticosteriods. Whenever such reactions occur, penicillin G should be discontinued unless, in the opinion of the physician, the condition being treated is life-threatening and amenable only to therapy with penicillin G. Serious anaphylactic reactions require immediate emergency treatment with epinephrine. Oxygen, intravenous steroids, and airway management, including intubation, should also be administered as indicated.

Gastrointestinal: Pseudomembranous colitis. Onset of pseudomembranous colitis symptoms may occur during or after antibacterial treatment. (See **WARNINGS**).

Hematologic: Hemolytic anemia, leukopenia, thrombocytopenia.

Neurologic: Neuropathy.

Urogenital: Nephropathy.

The following adverse events have been temporally associated with parenteral administration of the penicillin G benzathine:

Body as a Whole: Hypersensitivity reactions including allergic vasculitis, pruritus, fatigue, asthenia, and pain; aggravation of existing disorder; headache.

Cardiovascular: Cardiac arrest; hypotension; tachycardia; palpitations; pulmonary hypertension; pulmonary embolism; vasodilatation; vasovagal reaction; cerebrovascular accident; syncope.

Gastrointestinal: Nausea, vomiting, blood in stool; intestinal necrosis.

Hemic and Lymphatic: Lymphadenopathy.

Injection Site: Injection site reactions including pain, inflammation, lump, abscess, necrosis, edema, hemorrhage, cellulitis, hypersensitivity, atrophy, ecchymosis, and skin ulcer. Neurovascular reactions including warmth, vasospasm, pallor, mottling, gangrene, numbness of the extremities, cyanosis of the extremities, and neurovascular damage.

Metabolic: Elevated BUN, creatinine, and SGOT.

Musculoskeletal: Joint disorder, periostitis, exacerbation of arthritis; myoglobinuria; rhabdomyolysis.

Nervous System: Nervousness; tremors; dizziness; somnolence; confusion; anxiety; euphoria; transverse myelitis; seizures; coma. A syndrome manifested by a variety of CNS symptoms such as severe agitation with confusion, visual and auditory hallucinations, and a fear of impending death (Hoigne's syndrome), has been reported after administration of penicillin G procaine and, less commonly, after injection of the combination of penicillin G benzathine and penicillin G procaine. Other symptoms associated with this syndrome, such as psychosis, seizures, dizziness, tinnitus, cyanosis, palpitations, tachycardia, and/or other abnormal perception in taste, also may occur.

Respiratory: Hypoxia; apnea; dyspnea.

Skin: Diaphoresis.

Special Senses: Blurred vision; blindness.

Urogenital: Neurogenic bladder, hematuria; proteinuria; renal failure; impotence; priapism.

OVERDOSAGE

Penicillin in overdosage has the potential to cause neuromuscular hyperirritability or convulsive seizures.

DOSAGE AND ADMINISTRATION

Administer by DEEP, INTRAMUSCULAR INJECTION in the upper, outer quadrant of the buttock. In neonates, infants and small children, the midlateral aspect of the thigh may be preferable. When doses are repeated, vary the injection site.

When using the multiple-dose vial:

Shake multiple-dose vial vigorously before withdrawing the desired dose.

Due to the viscous nature of this medication, a 23 gauge or larger bore needle should be used to withdraw medication from the vial and for patient administration. A smaller bore needle, such as a 24 or 25 gauge, is not recommended.

After selection of the proper site and insertion of the needle into the selected muscle, aspirate by pulling back on the plunger. While maintaining negative pressure for 2 to 3 seconds, carefully observe the neck of the syringe immediately proximal to the needle hub for appearance of blood or any discoloration. Blood or "typical blood color" may *not* be seen if a blood vessel has been entered—only a mixture of blood and Bicillin C-R. The appearance of any discoloration is reason to withdraw the needle and discard the syringe. If it is elected to inject at another site, a new syringe and needle should be used. If no blood or discoloration appears, inject the contents of the syringe slowly. Discontinue delivery of the dose if the subject complains of severe immediate pain at the injection site or if in infants and young children symptoms or signs occur suggesting onset of severe pain.

When using the **TUBEX** cartridge:

The Wyeth-Ayerst **TUBEX**® cartridge for this product incorporates several features that are designed to facilitate the visualization of blood on aspiration if a blood vessel is inadvertently entered.

[See figure at top of next column]

The design of this cartridge is such that blood which enters its needle will be quickly visualized as a red or dark-colored "spot." This "spot" will appear on the barrel of the glass cartridge immediately proximal to the blue hub. The **TUBEX** is designed with two orientation marks, in order to determine where the "spot" can be seen. First insert and secure the cartridge in the **TUBEX** injector in the usual fashion. Locate the yellow rectangle at the base of the blue hub. This yellow rectangle is aligned with the blood visualization "spot." An imaginary straight line, drawn from this yellow rectangle to the shoulder of the glass cartridge, will point to the area on the cartridge where the "spot" can be visualized. When the needle cover is removed, a second yellow rectangle will be visible. The second yellow rectangle is also aligned with the blood visualization "spot" to assist the operator in locating this "spot." If the 2 mL metal or plastic syringe is used, the glass cartridge should be rotated by turning the plunger of the syringe clockwise until the yellow rectangle is visualized. If the 1 mL metal syringe is used, it will not be possible to continue to rotate the glass cartridge clockwise once it is properly engaged and fully threaded; it can, however, then be rotated counterclockwise as far as necessary to properly

Continued on next page

Bicillin C-R—Cont.

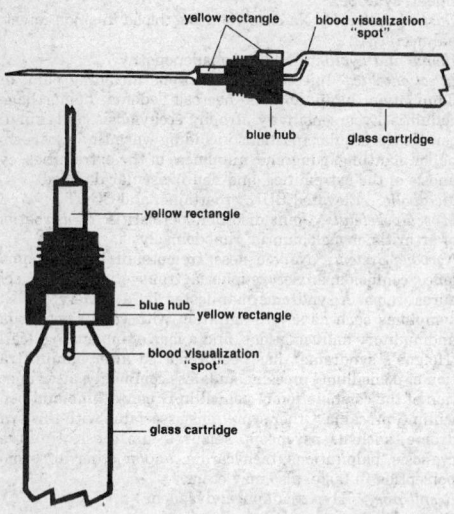

yellow rectangle

blood visualization "spot"

blue hub

glass cartridge

yellow rectangle

blue hub — yellow rectangle

blood visualization "spot"

glass cartridge

orient the yellow rectangles and locate the observation area. (In this same area in some cartridges, a dark spot may sometimes be visualized prior to injection. This is the proximal end of the needle and does not represent a foreign body in, or other abnormality of, the suspension.)

Thus, before the needle is inserted into the selected muscle, it is important for the operator to orient the yellow rectangle so that any blood which may enter after needle insertion and during aspiration can be visualized in the area on the cartridge where it will appear and not be obscured by any obstructions.

After selection of the proper site and insertion of the needle into the selected muscle, aspirate by pulling back on the plunger. While maintaining negative pressure for 2 to 3 seconds, carefully observe the neck of the glass **TUBEX** cartridge immediately proximal to the blue plastic needle hub for appearance of blood or any discoloration. Blood or "typical blood color" may *not* be seen if a blood vessel has been entered—only a mixture of blood and Bicillin C-R. The appearance of any discoloration is reason to withdraw the needle and discard the **TUBEX**. If it is elected to inject at another site, a new **TUBEX** cartridge should be used. If no blood or discoloration appears, inject the contents of the **TUBEX** slowly. Discontinue delivery of the dose if the subject complains of severe immediate pain at the injection site or if, especially in neonates, infants and young children, symptoms or signs occur suggesting onset of severe pain.

Some **TUBEX** cartridges may contain a small air bubble which may be disregarded since it does not affect administration of the product. DO NOT clear any air bubbles from the cartridge or needle as this may interfere with the visualization of any blood or discoloration during aspiration.

Because of the high concentration of suspended material in this product, the needle may be blocked if the injection is not made at a slow, steady rate.

When using the disposable syringe:

The Wyeth-Ayerst disposable syringe for this product incorporates several new features that are designed to facilitate its use.

A single small indentation, or "dot," has been punched into the metal ring that surrounds the neck of the syringe near the base of the needle. It is important that this "dot" be placed in a position so that it can be easily visualized by the operator following the intramuscular insertion of the syringe needle.

After selection of the proper site and insertion of the needle into the selected muscle, aspirate by pulling back on the plunger. While maintaining negative pressure for 2 to 3 seconds, carefully observe the barrel of the syringe immediately proximal to the location of the "dot" for appearance of blood or any discoloration. Blood or "typical blood color" may *not* be seen if a blood vessel has been entered—only a mixture of blood and Bicillin C-R. The appearance of any discoloration is reason to withdraw the needle and discard the syringe. If it is elected to inject at another site, a new syringe should be used. If no blood or discoloration appears, inject the contents of the syringe slowly. Discontinue delivery of the dose if the subject complains of severe immediate pain at the injection site or if in infants and young children symptoms or signs occur suggesting onset of severe pain.

Some disposable syringes may contain a small air bubble which may be disregarded, since it does not affect administration of the product.

Because of the high concentration of suspended material in this product, the needle may be blocked if the injection is not made at a slow, steady rate.

Streptococcal Infections Group A —Infections of the upper-respiratory tract, skin and soft-tissue infections, scarlet fever, and erysipelas.

The following doses are recommended:

Adults and pediatric patients over 60 lbs. in weight: 2,4000,000 units

Pediatric patients from 30 to 60 lbs.: 900,000 units to 1,200,000 units

Pediatric patients under 30 lbs.: 600,000 units

NOTE: Treatment with the recommended dosage is usually given at a single session using multiple IM sites when indicated. An alternative dosage schedule may be used, giving one-half ($\frac{1}{2}$) the total dose on day 1 and one-half ($\frac{1}{2}$) on day 3. This will also insure the penicillinemia required over a 10-day period; however, this alternate schedule should be used only when the physician can be assured of the patient's cooperation.

Pneumococcal Infections (Except Pneumococcal Meningitis)

600,000 units in pediatric patients and 1,200,000 units in adults, repeated every 2 or 3 days until the temperature is normal for 48 hours. Other forms of penicillin may be necessary for severe cases.

Parenteral drug products should be inspected visually for particulate matter and discoloration prior to administration whenever solution and container permit.

HOW SUPPLIED

Bicillin® C-R (penicillin G benzathine and penicillin G procaine suspension) is supplied in packages of 10 **TUBEX®** Sterile Cartridge-Needle Units as follows:

1 mL size, containing 600,000 units per **TUBEX®** (21 gauge, thin-wall 1 inch needle for pediatric use), NDC 0008-0026-37.

2 mL size, containing 1,200,000 units per **TUBEX®** (21 gauge, thin-wall 1 inch needle for pediatric use), NDC 0008-0026-36.

2 mL size, containing 1,200,000 units per **TUBEX®** (21 gauge, thin-wall 1-1/4 inch needle), NDC 0008-0026-35

Store in a refrigerator.

Keep from freezing.

Also Available

Bicillin C-R (penicillin G benzathine and penicillin G procaine suspension) is also available in packages of 10 disposable syringes as follows:

4 mL size, 2,400,000 units per syringe (18 gauge × 2 inch needle), NDC 0008-0026-22.

Bicillin C-R (penicillin G benzathine and penicillin G procaine suspension) is also available in packages of single multiple-dose vials as follows:

10 mL size, 300,000 units per mL, NDC 0008-0176-01.

Store in a refrigerator.

Keep from freezing.

Shake multiple-dose vials well before using.

REFERENCES

1. SHAW, E.: Transverse myelitis from injection of penicillin. *Am. J. Dis. Child., 111* :548, 1966.
2. KNOWLES, J.: Accidental intra-arterial injection of penicillin. *Am. J. Dis. Child., 111* :552, 1966.
3. DARBY, C., et al: Ischemia following an intragluteal injection of benzathine-procaine penicillin G mixture in a one-year-old boy. *Clin. Pediatrics, 12* :485, 1973.
4. BROWN, L. & NELSON, A.: Postinfectious intravascular thrombosis with gangrene. *Arch. Surg., 94* :652, 1967.
5. BORENSTINE, J.: Transverse myelitis and penicillin (Correspondence). *Am. J. Dis. Child., 112* :166, 1966.
6. ATKINSON, J.: Transverse myelopathy secondary to penicillin injection. *J. Pediatrics, 75* :867, 1969.
7. TALBERT, J, et al: Gangrene of the foot following intramuscular injection in the lateral thigh: A case report with recommendations for prevention. *J. Pediatrics, 70* :110, 1967.
8. FISHER, T.: Medicolegal affairs. *Canad. Med. Assoc. J., 112* :395, 1975.
9. SCHANZER, H. et al: Accidental intraarterial injection of penicillin G. *JAMA, 242* :1289, 1979.

Manufactured by:

Wyeth Laboratories Inc.

A Wyeth-Ayerst Company

Philadelphia, PA 19101

BICILLIN® C-R 900/300   ℞

[bī-sĭl ′ĭn]

(penicillin G benzathine and penicillin G procaine suspension)

INJECTION

FOR DEEP INTRAMUSCULAR INJECTION ONLY

DESCRIPTION

Bicillin C-R 900/300 (penicillin G benzathine and penicillin G procaine suspension) contains the equivalent of 900,000

units of penicillin G as the benzathine and 300,000 units of penicillin G as the procaine salts. It is available for deep intramuscular injection.

Penicillin G benzathine is prepared by the reaction of dibenzylethylene diamine with two molecules of penicillin G. It is chemically designated as (2S, 5R, 6R)-3,3-Dimethyl-7-oxo-6-(2-phenylacetamido)-4-thia-1-azabicyclo[3.2.0]heptane-2-carboxylic acid compound with N,N'-dibenzylethylenediamine (2:1), tetrahydrate. It occurs as a white, crystalline powder and is very slightly soluble in water and sparingly soluble in alcohol.

Penicillin G procaine, (2S, 5R, 6R)-3,3-Dimethyl-7-oxo-6-(2-phenylacetamido)-4-thia-1-azabicyclo[3.2.0] heptane-2- carboxylic acid compound with 2-(diethylamino)ethyl p-aminobenzoate compound (1:1) monohydrate, is an equimolar salt of procaine and penicillin G. It occurs as white crystals or a white, microcrystalline powder and is slightly soluble in water.

Each **TUBEX®** cartridge (2 mL size) contains the equivalent to 1,200,000 units of penicillin G as follows: penicillin G benzathine equivalent to 900,000 units of penicillin G and penicillin G procaine equivalent to 300,000 units of penicillin G in a stabilized aqueous suspension with sodium citrate buffer; and as w/v, approximately 0.5% lecithin, 0.55% carboxymethylcellulose, 0.55% povidone, 0.1% methylparaben, and 0.01% propylparaben.

Bicillin C-R 900/300 suspension in **TUBEX** formulation is viscous and opaque. Read **CONTRAINDICATIONS, WARNINGS, PRECAUTIONS,** and **DOSAGE AND ADMINISTRATION** sections prior to use.

CLINICAL PHARMACOLOGY

General

Penicillin G benzathine and penicillin G procaine have a low solubility and, thus, the drugs are slowly released from intramuscular injection sites. The drugs are hydrolyzed to penicillin G. This combination of hydrolysis and slow absorption results in blood serum levels much lower but more prolonged than other parenteral penicillins. Intramuscular administration of 1,200,000 units of Bicillin C-R 900/300 in patients weighing 100 to 140 lbs. usually produces average blood levels of 0.24 units/mL at 24 hours, 0.039 units/mL at 7 days, and 0.024 units/mL at 10 days.

Approximately 60% of penicillin G is bound to serum protein. The drug is distributed throughout the body tissues in widely varying amounts. Highest levels are found in the kidneys with lesser amounts in the liver, skin, and intestines. Penicillin G penetrates into all other tissues and the spinal fluid to a lesser degree. With normal kidney function, the drug is excreted rapidly by tubular excretion. In neonates and young infants and in individuals with impaired kidney function, excretion is considerably delayed.

Microbiology

Penicillin G exerts a bactericidal action against penicillin-susceptible microorganisms during the stage of active multiplication. It acts through the inhibition of biosynthesis of cell-wall mucopeptide. It is not active against the penicillinase-producing bacteria, which include many strains of staphylococci.

The following *in vitro* data are available, but their clinical significance is unknown. Penicillin G exerts high *in vitro* activity against staphylococci (except penicillinase-producing strains), streptococci (Groups A, C, G, H, L, and M), and pneumococci. Other organisms susceptible to penicillin G are *Neisseria gonorrhoeae, Corynebacterium diphtheriae, Bacillus anthracis,* Clostridia species, *Actinomyces bovis, Streptobacillus moniliformis, Listeria monocytogenes,* and Leptospira species. *Treponema pallidum* is extremely susceptible to the bactericidal action of penicillin G.

Susceptibility Test: If the Kirby-Bauer method of disc susceptibility is used, a 10-unit penicillin disc should give a zone greater than 28 mm when tested against a penicillin-susceptible bacterial strain.

INDICATIONS AND USAGE

Bicillin C-R 900/300 is indicated in the treatment of infections as described below that are susceptible to serum levels characteristic of this particular dosage form. Therapy should be guided by bacteriological studies (including susceptibility testing) and by clinical response.

Bicillin C-R 900/300 is indicated in the treatment of the following in pediatric patients:

Moderately severe to severe infections of the upper-respiratory tract, scarlet fever, erysipelas, and skin and soft-tissue infections due to susceptible streptococci.

NOTE: Streptococci in Groups A, C, G, H, L, and M are very susceptible to penicillin G. Other groups, including Group D (enterococci), are resistant. Penicillin G sodium or potassium is recommended for streptococcal infections with bacteremia.

Moderately severe pneumonia and otitis media due to susceptible pneumococci.

NOTE: Severe pneumonia, empyema, bacteremia, pericarditis, meningitis, peritonitis, and arthritis of pneumococcal etiology are better treated with penicillin G sodium or potassium during the acute stage.

When high, sustained serum levels are required, penicillin G sodium or potassium, either IM or IV, should be used. This drug should not be used in the treatment of venereal diseases, including syphilis, gonorrhea, yaws, bejel, and pinta.

CONTRAINDICATIONS

A previous hypersensitivity reaction to any penicillin or to procaine is a contraindication.

Do not inject into or near an artery or nerve.

WARNINGS

The combination of penicillin G benzathine and penicillin G procaine should only be prescribed for the indications listed in this insert.

SERIOUS AND OCCASIONALLY FATAL HYPERSENSITIVITY (ANAPHYLACTIC) REACTIONS HAVE BEEN REPORTED IN PATIENTS ON PENICILLIN THERAPY. THESE REACTIONS ARE MORE LIKELY TO OCCUR IN INDIVIDUALS WITH A HISTORY OF PENICILLIN HYPERSENSITIVITY AND/OR A HISTORY OF SENSITIVITY TO MULTIPLE ALLERGENS. THERE HAVE BEEN REPORTS OF INDIVIDUALS WITH A HISTORY OF PENICILLIN HYPERSENSITIVITY WHO HAVE EXPERIENCED SEVERE REACTIONS WHEN TREATED WITH CEPHALOSPORINS. BEFORE INITIATING THERAPY WITH BICILLIN C-R 900/300, CAREFUL INQUIRY SHOULD BE MADE CONCERNING PREVIOUS HYPERSENSITIVITY REACTIONS TO PENICILLINS, CEPHALOSPORINS AND OTHER ALLERGENS, IF AN ALLERGIC REACTION OCCURS, BICILLIN C-R 900/300 SHOULD BE DISCONTINUED AND APPROPRIATE THERAPY INSTITUTED. **SERIOUS ANAPHYLACTIC REACTIONS REQUIRE IMMEDIATE EMERGENCY TREATMENT WITH EPINEPHRINE. OXYGEN, INTRAVENOUS STEROIDS AND AIRWAY MANAGEMENT, INCLUDING INTUBATION, SHOULD ALSO BE ADMINISTERED AS INDICATED.**

Pseudomembranous colitis has been reported with nearly all antibacterial agents, including penicillin, and may range in severity from mild to life-threatening. Therefore, it is important to consider this diagnosis in patients who present with diarrhea subsequent to the administration of any antibacterial agent.

Treatment with antibacterial agents alters the normal flora of the colon and may permit overgrowth of clostridia. Studies indicate that a toxin produced by *Clostridium difficile* is one primary cause of "antibiotic colitis".

After the diagnosis of pseudomembranous colitis has been established, appropriate therapeutic measures should be initiated. Mild cases of pseudomembranous colitis usually respond to drug discontinuation alone. In moderate to severe cases, consideration should be given to management with fluids and electrolytes, protein supplementation, and treatment with an antibacterial drug clinically effective against *C. difficile* colitis.

Inadvertent intravascular administration, including inadvertent direct intra-arterial injection or injection immediately adjacent to arteries, of Bicillin C-R 900/300 and other penicillin preparations has resulted in severe neurovascular damage, including transverse myelitis with permanent paralysis, gangrene requiring amputation of digits and more proximal portions of extremities, and necrosis and sloughing at and surrounding the injection site. Such severe effects have been reported following injections into the buttock, thigh, and deltoid areas. Other serious complications of suspected intravascular administration which have been reported include immediate pallor, mottling, or cyanosis of the extremity both distal and proximal to the injection site, followed by bleb formation; severe edema requiring anterior and/or posterior compartment fasciotomy in the lower extremity. The above-described severe effects and complications have most often occurred in infants and small children. Prompt consultation with an appropriate specialist is indicated if any evidence of compromise of the blood supply occurs at, proximal to, or distal to the site of injection.[1–9] See **CONTRAINDICATIONS**, **PRECAUTIONS**, and **DOSAGE AND ADMINISTRATION** sections.

Quadriceps femoris fibrosis and atrophy have been reported following repeated intramuscular injections of penicillin preparations into the anterolateral thigh.

Injection into or near a nerve may result in permanent neurological damage.

PRECAUTIONS

General

Penicillin should be used with caution in individuals with histories of significant allergies and/or asthma.

Care should be taken to avoid intravenous or intra-arterial administration, or injection into or near major peripheral nerves or blood vessels, since such injections may produce neurovascular damage. See **CONTRAINDICATIONS, WARNINGS**, and **DOSAGE AND ADMINISTRATION** sections.

A small percentage of patients are sensitive to procaine. If there is a history of sensitivity, make the usual test: Inject intradermally 0.1 mL of a 1 to 2 percent procaine solution. Development of an erythema, wheal, flare, or eruption indicates procaine sensitivity. Sensitivity should be treated by the usual methods, including barbiturates, and procaine penicillin preparations should not be used. Antihistaminics appear beneficial in treatment of procaine reactions.

The use of antibiotics may result in overgrowth of nonsusceptible organisms. Constant observation of the patient is essential. If new infections due to bacteria or fungi appear during therapy, the drug should be discontinued and appropriate measures taken.

Whenever allergic reactions occur, penicillin should be withdrawn unless, in the opinion of the physician, the condition being treated is life-threatening and amenable only to penicillin therapy.

In prolonged therapy with penicillin, and particularly with high-dosage schedules, periodic evaluation of the renal and hematopoietic systems is recommended.

Laboratory Tests

In streptococcal infections, therapy must be sufficient to eliminate the organism; otherwise, the sequelae of streptococcal disease may occur. Cultures should be taken following completion of treatment to determine whether streptococci have been eradicated.

Drug Interactions

Tetracycline, a bacteriostatic antibiotic, may antagonize the bactericidal effect of penicillin, and concurrent use of these drugs should be avoided.

Concurrent administration of penicillin and probenecid increases and prolongs serum penicillin levels by decreasing the apparent volume of distribution and slowing the rate of excretion by competitively inhibiting renal tubular secretion of penicillin.

Pregnancy Category B

Reproduction studies performed in the mouse, rat, and rabbit have revealed no evidence of impaired fertility or harm to the fetus due to penicillin G. Human experience with the penicillins during pregnancy has not shown any positive evidence of adverse effects on the fetus. There are, however, no adequate and well-controlled studies in pregnant women showing conclusively that harmful effects of these drugs on the fetus can be excluded. Because animal reproduction studies are not always predictive of human response, this drug should be used during pregnancy only if clearly needed.

Nursing Mothers

Soluble penicillin G is excreted in breast milk. Caution should be exercised when penicillin G benzathine and penicillin G procaine are administered to a nursing woman.

Carcinogeneses, Mutagenesis, Impairment of Fertility

No long-term animal studies have been conducted with these drugs.

Pediatric Use

See **INDICATIONS AND USAGE** and **DOSAGE AND ADMINISTRATION**.

ADVERSE REACTIONS

As with other penicillins, untoward reactions of the sensitivity phenomena are likely to occur, particularly in individuals who have previously demonstrated hypersensitivity to penicillins or in those with a history of allergy, asthma, hay fever, or urticaria.

The following have been reported with parenteral penicillin G:

General: Hypersensitivity reactions including the following; skin eruptions (maculopapular to exfoliative dermatitis), urticaria, laryngeal edema, fever, eosinophilia; other serum-sickness-like reactions (including chills, fever, edema, arthralgia, and prostration); anaphylaxis including shock and death. NOTE: Urticaria, other skin rashes, and serum sickness-like reactions may be controlled with antihistamines and, if necessary, systemic corticosteroids.

Whenever such reactions occur, penicillin G should be discontinued unless, in the opinion of the physician, the condition being treated is life-threatening and amenable only to therapy with penicillin G. Serious anaphylactic reactions require immediate emergency treatment with epinephrine. Oxygen, intravenous steroids, and airway management, including intubation, should also be administered as indicated.

Gastrointestinal: Pseudomembranous colitis. Onset of pseudomembranous colitis symptoms may occur during or after antibacterial treatment. (See **WARNINGS**.)

Hematologic: Hemolytic anemia, leukopenia, thrombocytopenia.

Neurologic: Neuropathy.

Urogenital: Nephropathy.

The following adverse events have been temporally associated with parenteral administration of penicillin G benzathine:

Body as a Whole: Hypersensitivity reactions including allergic vasculitis, pruritus, fatigue, asthenia, and pain; aggravation of existing disorder; headache.

Cardiovascular: Cardiac arrest; hypotension; tachycardia; palpitations; pulmonary hypertension; pulmonary embolism; vasodilatation; vasovagal reaction; cerebrovascular accident; syncope.

Gastrointestinal: Nausea, vomiting; blood in stool; intestinal necrosis.

Hemic and Lymphatic: Lymphadenopathy.

Injection Site: Injection site reactions including pain, inflammation, lump, abscess, necrosis, edema, hemorrhage, cellulitis, hypersensitivity, atrophy, ecchymosis, and skin ulcer. Neurovascular reactions including warmth, vasospasm, pallor, mottling, gangrene, numbness of the extremities, cyanosis of the extremities, and neurovascular damage.

Metabolic: Elevated BUN, creatinine, and SGOT.

Musculoskeletal: Joint disorder; periostitis; exacerbation of arthritis; myoglobinuria; rhabdomyolysis.

Nervous System: Nervousness; tremors; dizziness; somnolence; confusion; anxiety; euphoria; transverse myelitis; seizures; coma. A syndrome manifested by a variety of CNS symptoms such as severe agitation with confusion, visual and auditory hallucinations, and a fear of impending death (Hoigne's syndrome), has been reported after administration of penicillin G procaine and, less commonly, after injection of the combination of penicillin G benzathine and penicillin G procaine. Other symptoms associated with this syndrome, such as psychosis, seizures, dizziness, tinnitus, cyanosis, palpitations, tachycardia, and/or abnormal perception in taste, also may occur.

Respiratory: Hypoxia; apnea; dyspnea.

Skin: Diaphoresis.

Special Senses: Blurred vision; blindness.

Urogenital: Neurogenic bladder; hematuria; proteinuria; renal failure; impotence; priapism.

OVERDOSAGE

Penicillin in overdosage has the potential to cause neuromuscular hyperirritability or convulsive seizures.

DOSAGE AND ADMINISTRATION

Administer by DEEP, INTRAMUSCULAR INJECTION in the upper, outer quadrant of the buttock. In neonates, infants and small children, the midlateral aspect of the thigh may be preferable. When doses are repeated, vary the injection site.

The Wyeth-Ayerst **TUBEX** cartridge for this product incorporates several features that are designed to facilitate the visualization of blood on aspiration if a blood vessel is inadvertently entered.

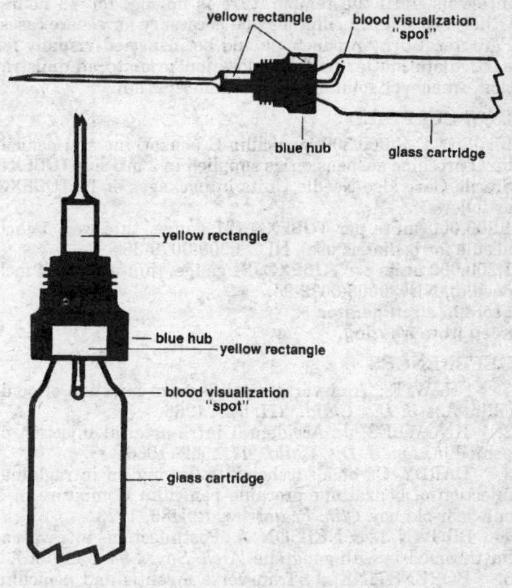

The design of this cartridge is such that blood which enters its needle will be quickly visualized as a red or dark-colored "spot." This "spot" will appear on the barrel of the glass cartridge immediately proximal to the blue hub. The **TUBEX** is designed with two orientation marks, in order to determine where the "spot" can be seen. First insert and secure the cartridge in the **TUBEX** injector in the usual fashion. Locate the yellow rectangle at the base of the blue hub. This yellow rectangle is aligned with the blood visualization "spot." An imaginary straight line, drawn from this yellow rectangle to the shoulder of the glass cartridge, will point to the area on the cartridge where the "spot" can be visualized. When the needle cover is removed, a second yellow rectangle will be visible. The second yellow rectangle is also aligned with the blood visualization "spot" to assist the operator in locating the "spot." If the 2 mL metal or plastic syringe is used, the glass cartridge should be rotated by turning the plunger of the syringe clockwise until the yellow rectangle is visualized. If the 1 mL metal syringe is used, it will not be possible to continue to rotate the glass cartridge clockwise once it is properly engaged and fully threaded; it can, however, then be rotated counterclockwise as far as necessary to properly orient the yellow rectangles and locate the observation area. (In this same area in some cartridges, a dark spot may

Continued on next page

Bicillin C-R 900/300—Cont.

sometimes be visualized prior to injection. This is the proximal end of the needle and does not represent a foreign body in, or other abnormality of, the suspension.)

Thus, before the needle is inserted into the selected muscle, it is important for the operator to orient the yellow rectangle so that any blood which may enter after needle insertion and during aspiration can be visualized in the area on the cartridge where it will appear and not be obscured by any obstructions.

After selection of the proper site and insertion of the needle into the selected muscle, aspirate by pulling back on the plunger. While maintaining negative pressure for 2 to 3 seconds, carefully observe the neck of the glass **TUBEX** cartridge immediately proximal to the blue plastic needle hub for appearance of blood or any discoloration.

Blood or "typical blood color" may *not* be seen if a blood vessel has been entered—only a mixture of blood and Bicillin C-R 900/300. The appearance of any discoloration is reason to withdraw the needle and discard the **TUBEX**. If it is elected to inject at another site, a new **TUBEX** cartridge should be used. If no blood or discoloration appears, inject the contents of the **TUBEX** slowly. Discontinue delivery of the dose if the subject complains of severe immediate pain at the injection site or if, especially in neonates, infants and young children, symptoms or signs occur suggesting onset of severe pain.

Some **TUBEX** cartridges may contain a small air bubble which may be disregarded, since it does not affect administration of the product. DO NOT clear any air bubbles from the cartridge or needle as this may interfere with the visualization of any blood or discoloration during aspiration.

Because of the high concentration of suspended material in this product, the needle may be blocked if the injection is not made at a slow, steady rate.

Streptococcal Infections

Group A Infections of the upper-respiratory tract, skin and soft-tissue infections, scarlet fever, and erysipelas: A single injection of Bicillin C-R 900/300 is usually sufficient for the treatment of Group A streptococcal infections in pediatric patients.

Pneumococcal Infections (except pneumococcal meningitis)

One TUBEX Bicillin C-R 900/300 repeated at 2- or 3-day intervals until the temperature is normal for 48 hours. Other forms of penicillin may be necessary for severe cases.

Parenteral drug products should be inspected visually for particulate matter and discoloration prior to administration, whenever solution and container permit.

HOW SUPPLIED

Bicillin® C-R 900/300 (penicillin G benzathine and penicillin G procaine suspension) is supplied in 2 mL size **TUBEX®** Sterile Cartridge-Needle Units in packages of 10 **TUBEX®** as follows:

1,200,000 units per **TUBEX®** (21 gauge, thin-wall 1 inch needle for pediatric use), NDC 0008-0079-36.

1,200,000 units per **TUBEX®** (21 gauge, thin-wall 1-1/4 inch needle), NDC 0008-0079-35.

Store in a refrigerator.
Keep from freezing.

REFERENCES

1. SHAW, E.: Transverse myelitis from injection of penicillin. *Am. J. Dis. Child., 111:* 548, 1966.
2. KNOWLES, J.: Accidental intra-arterial injection of penicillin. *Am. J. Dis. Child., 111:* 552, 1966.
3. DARBY, C., et al: Ischemia following an intragluteal injection of benzathine-procaine penicillin G mixture in a one-year-old boy. *Clin. Pediatrics, 12:* 485, 1973.
4. BROWN, L. & NELSON, A.: Postinfectious intravascular thrombosis with gangrene. *Arch. Surg., 94:* 652, 1967.
5. BORENSTINE, J.: Transverse myelitis and penicillin (Correspondence). *Am. J. Dis. Child., 112:* 166, 1966.
6. ATKINSON, J.: Transverse myelopathy secondary to penicillin injection. *J. Pediatrics, 75:* 867, 1969.
7. TALBERT, J. et al: Gangrene of the foot following intramuscular injection in the lateral thigh: A case report with recommendations for prevention. *J. Pediatrics, 70:* 110, 1967.
8. FISHER, T.: Medicolegal affairs. *Canad. Med. Assoc. J., 112:* 395, 1975.
9. SCHANZER, H. et al: Accidental intra-arterial injection of penicillin G. *JAMA, 242:* 1289, 1979.

Manufactured by:
Wyeth Laboratories Inc.
A Wyeth-Ayerst Company
Philadelphia, PA 19101

BICILLIN® L-A ℞

[bī-sil 'in]

(penicillin G benzathine suspension)
INJECTION
FOR DEEP INTRAMUSCULAR INJECTION ONLY

DESCRIPTION

Bicillin L-A (penicillin G benzathine suspension) is prepared by the reaction of dibenzylethylene diamine with two molecules of penicillin G. It is chemically designated as (2*S*, 5*R*, 6*R*) 3,3-Dimethyl-7-oxo -6- (2-phenylacetamido) -4-thia-1-azabicyclo[3.2.0]heptane-2-carboxylic acid compound with *N,N* '-dibenzylethylenediamine (2:1), tetrahydrate.

It is available for deep intramuscular injection. It contains penicillin G benzathine in aqueous suspension with sodium citrate buffer and, as w/v, approximately 0.5% lecithin, 0.6% carboxymethylcellulose, 0.6% povidone, 0.1% methylparaben, and 0.01% propylparaben. It occurs as a white, crystalline powder and is very slightly soluble in water and sparingly soluble in alcohol.

Bicillin L-A suspension in the multiple-dose vial formulation, disposable syringe formulation and **TUBEX** formulation is viscous and opaque. The multiple-dose vial formulation contains the equivalent of 300,000 units per mL of penicillin G as the benzathine salt. The disposable syringe formulation is available in a 4 mL size containing the equivalent of 2,400,000 units of penicillin G as the benzathine salt. The **TUBEX** formulation is available in 1 mL and 2 mL **TUBEX** Sterile Cartridge-Needle Units containing the equivalent of 600,000 units and 1,200,000 units respectively of penicillin G as the benzathine salt. Read **CONTRAINDICATIONS, WARNINGS, PRECAUTIONS,** and **DOSAGE AND ADMINISTRATION** sections prior to use.

CLINICAL PHARMACOLOGY

General

Penicillin G benzathine has an extremely low solubility and, thus, the drug is slowly released from intramuscular injection sites. The drug is hydrolyzed to penicillin G. This combination of hydrolysis and slow absorption results in blood serum levels much lower but much more prolonged than other parenteral penicillins.

Intramuscular administration of 300,000 units of penicillin G benzathine in adults results in blood levels of 0.03 to 0.05 units per mL, which are maintained for 4 to 5 days. Similar blood levels may persist for 10 days following administration of 600,000 units and for 14 days following administration of 1,200,000 units. Blood concentrations of 0.003 units per mL may still be detectable 4 weeks following administration of 1,200,000 units.

Approximately 60% of penicillin G is bound to serum protein. The drug is distributed throughout the body tissues in widely varying amounts. Highest levels are found in the kidneys with lesser amounts in the liver, skin, and intestines. Penicillin G penetrates into all other tissues and the spinal fluid to a lesser degree. With normal kidney function, the drug is excreted rapidly by tubular excretion. In neonates and young infants and in individuals with impaired kidney function, excretion is considerably delayed.

Microbiology

Penicillin G exerts a bactericidal action against penicillin-susceptible microorganisms during the stage of active multiplication. It acts through the inhibition of biosynthesis of cell-wall mucopeptide. It is not active against the penicillinase-producing bacteria, which include many strains of staphylococci.

The following *in vitro* data are available, but their clinical significance is unknown. Penicillin G exerts high *in vitro* activity against staphylococci (except penicillinase-producing strains), streptococci (Groups A, C, G, H, L, and M), and pneumococci. Other organisms susceptible to penicillin G are *Neisseria gonorrhoeae, Corynebacterium diphtheriae, Bacillus anthracis,* Clostridia species, *Actinomyces bovis, Streptobacillus moniliformis, Listeria monocytogenes,* and Leptospira species. *Treponema pallidum* is extremely susceptible to the bactericidal action of penicillin G.

Susceptibility Test: If the Kirby-Bauer method of disc susceptibility is used, a 20-unit penicillin disc should give a zone greater than 28 mm when tested against a penicillin-susceptible bacterial strain.

INDICATIONS AND USAGE

Intramuscular penicillin G benzathine is indicated in the treatment of infections due to penicillin-G-sensitive microorganisms that are susceptible to the low and very prolonged serum levels common to this particular dosage form. Therapy should be guided by bacteriological studies (including sensitivity tests) and by clinical response.

The following infections will usually respond to adequate dosage of intramuscular penicillin G benzathine:

Mild-to-moderate infections of the upper respiratory tract due to susceptible streptococci.

Venereal infections —Syphilis, yaws, bejel, and pinta.

Medical Conditions in which Penicillin G Benzathine Therapy is Indicated as Prophylaxis:

Rheumatic fever and/or chorea—Prophylaxis with penicillin G benzathine has proven effective in preventing recurrence of these conditions. It has also been used as follow-up prophylactic therapy for rheumatic heart disease and acute glomerulonephritis.

CONTRAINDICATIONS

A history of a previous hypersensitivity reaction to any of the penicillins is a contraindication.

Do not inject into or near an artery or nerve.

WARNINGS

Penicillin G benzathine should only be prescribed for the indications listed in this insert.

SERIOUS AND OCCASIONALLY FATAL HYPERSENSITIVITY (ANAPHYLACTIC) REACTIONS HAVE BEEN REPORTED IN PATIENTS ON PENICILLIN THERAPY. THESE REACTIONS ARE MORE LIKELY TO OCCUR IN INDIVIDUALS WITH A HISTORY OF PENICILLIN HYPERSENSITIVITY AND/OR A HISTORY OF SENSITIVITY TO MULTIPLE ALLERGENS. THERE HAVE BEEN REPORTS OF INDIVIDUALS WITH A HISTORY OF PENICILLIN HYPERSENSITIVITY WHO HAVE EXPERIENCED SEVERE REACTIONS WHEN TRATED WITH CEPHALOSPORINS. BEFORE INITIATING THERAPY WITH BICILLIN L-A, CAREFUL INQUIRY SHOULD BE MADE CONCERNING PREVIOUS HYPERSENSITIVITY REACTIONS TO PENICILLINS, CEPHALOSPORINS AND OTHER ALLERGENS. IF AN ALLERGIC REACTION OCCURS, BICILLIN L-A SHOULD BE DISCONTINUED AND APPROPRIATE THERAPY INSTITUTED. **SERIOUS ANAPHYLACTIC REACTIONS REQUIRE IMMEDIATE EMERGENCY TREATMENT WITH EPINEPHRINE, OXYGEN, INTRAVENOUS STEROIDS AND AIRWAY MANAGEMENT, INCLUDING INTUBATION, SHOULD ALSO BE ADMINISTERED AS INDICATED.**

Pseudomembranous colitis has been reported with nearly all antibacterial agents, including penicillin, and may range in severity from mild to life-threatening. Therefore, it is important to consider this diagnosis in patients who present with diarrhea subsequent to the administration of any antibacterial agent.

Treatment with antibacterial agents alter the normal flora of the colon and may permit overgrowth of clostridia. Studies indicate that a toxin produced by *Clostridium difficile* is one primary cause of "antibiotic-associated colitis".

After the diagnosis of pseudomembranous colitis has been established, appropriate therapeutic measures should be initiated. Mild cases of pseudomembranous colitis usually respond to drug discontinuation alone. In moderate to severe cases, consideration should be given to management with fluids and electrolytes, protein supplementation, and treatment with an antibacterial drug clinically effective against *C. difficile* colitis.

Inadvertent intravascular administration, including inadvertent direct intra-arterial injection or injection immediately adjacent to arteries, of Bicillin L-A and other penicillin preparations has resulted in severe neurovascular damage, including transverse myelitis with permanent paralysis, gangrene requiring amputation of digits and more proximal portions of extremities, and necrosis and sloughing at and surrounding the injection site. Such severe effects have been reported following injections into the buttock, thigh, and deltoid areas. Other serious complications of suspected intravascular administration which have been reported include immediate pallor, mottling, or cyanosis of the extremity both distal and proximal to the injection site, followed by bleb formation; severe edema requiring anterior and/or posterior compartment fasciotomy in the lower extremity. The above-described severe effects and complications have most often occurred in infants and small children. Prompt consultation with an appropriate specialist is indicated if any evidence of compromise of the blood supply occurs at, proximal to, or distal to the site of injection.[1-9] See **CONTRAINDICATIONS, PRECAUTIONS,** and **DOSAGE AND ADMINISTRATION** sections.

Quadriceps femoris fibrosis and atrophy have been reported following repeated intramuscular injections of penicillin preparations into the anterolateral thigh.

Injection into or near a nerve may result in permanent neurological damage.

PRECAUTIONS

General

Penicillin should be used with caution in individuals with histories of significant allergies and/or asthma.

Care should be taken to avoid intravenous or intra-arterial administration, or injection into or near major peripheral nerves or blood vessels, since such injection may produce neurovascular damage. See **CONTRAINDICATIONS, WARNINGS,** and **DOSAGE AND ADMINISTRATION** sections.

Prolonged use of antibiotics may promote the overgrowth of nonsusceptible organisms, including fungi. Should superinfection occur, appropriate measures should be taken.

Laboratory Tests

In streptococcal infections, therapy must be sufficient to eliminate the organism; otherwise, the sequelae of streptococcal disease may occur. Cultures should be taken following completion of treatment to determine whether streptococci have been eradicated.

Drug Interactions

Tetracycline, a bacteriostatic antibiotic, may antagonize the bactericidal effect of penicillin, and concurrent use of these drugs should be avoided.

Concurrent administration of penicillin and probenecid increases and prolongs serum penicillin levels by decreasing

the apparent volume of distribution and slowing the rate of excretion by competitively inhibiting renal tubular secretion of penicillin.

Pregnancy Category B

Reproduction studies performed in the mouse, rat, and rabbit have revealed no evidence of impaired fertility or harm to the fetus due to penicillin G. Human experience with the penicillins during pregnancy has not shown any positive evidence of adverse effects on the fetus. There are, however, no adequate and well-controlled studies in pregnant women showing conclusively that harmful effects of these drugs on the fetus can be excluded. Because animal reproduction studies are not always predictive of human response, this drug should be used during pregnancy only if clearly needed.

Nursing Mothers

Soluble penicillin G is excreted in breast milk. Caution should be exercised when penicillin G benzathine is administered to a nursing woman.

Carcinogenesis, Mutagenesis, Impairment Of Fertility

No long-term animal studies have been conducted with this drug.

Pediatric Use

See **INDICATIONS AND USAGE** and **DOSAGE AND ADMINISTRATION**.

ADVERSE REACTIONS

As with other penicillins, untoward reactions of the sensitivity phenomena are likely to occur, particularly in individuals who have previously demonstrated hypersensitivity to penicillins or in those with a history of allergy, asthma, hay fever, or urticaria.

As with other treatments for syphilis, the Jarisch-Herxheimer reaction has been reported.

The following have been reported with parenteral penicillin G:

General: Hypersensitivity reactions including the following: skin eruptions (maculopapular to exfoliative dermatitis), urticaria, laryngeal edema, fever, eosinophilia; other serum sickness-like reactions (including chills, fever, edema, arthralgia, and prostration); and anaphylaxis including shock and death. Note: Urticaria, other skin rashes, and serum sickness-like reactions may be controlled with antihistamines and, if necessary, systemic corticosteroids. Whenever such reactions occur, penicillin G should be discontinued unless, in the opinion of the physician, the condition being treated is life-threatening and amenable only to therapy with penicillin G. Serious anaphylactic reactions require immediate emergency treatment with epinephrine. Oxygen, intravenous steroids, and airway management, including intubation, should also be administered as indicated.

Gastrointestinal: Pseudomembranous colitis. Onset of pseudomembranous colitis symptoms may occur during or after antibacterial treatment. See **WARNINGS**.

Hematologic: Hemolytic anemia, leukopenia, thrombocytopenia.

Neurologic: Neuropathy.

Urogenital: Nephropathy.

The following adverse events have been temporally associated with parenteral administration of penicillin G benzathine, although a causal relationship has not necessarily been established:

Body as a Whole: Hypersensitivity reactions including allergic vasculitis, pruritus, fatigue, asthenia, and pain; aggravation of existing disorder; headache.

Cardiovascular: Cardiac arrest; hypotension; tachycardia; palpitations; pulmonary hypertension; pulmonary embolism; vasodilatation; vasovagal reaction; cerebrovascular accident; syncope.

Gastrointestinal: Nausea, vomiting; blood in stool; intestinal necrosis.

Hemic and Lymphatic: Lymphadenopathy.

Injection Site: Injection site reactions including pain, inflammation, lump, abscess, necrosis, edema, hemorrhage, cellulitis, hypersensitivity, atrophy, ecchymosis, and skin ulcer. Neurovascular reactions including warmth, vasospasm, pallor, mottling, gangrene, numbness of the extremities, and neurovascular damage.

Metabolic: Elevated BUN, creatinine, and SGOT.

Musculoskeletal: Joint disorder; periostitis; exacerbation of arthritis; myoglobinura; rhabdomyolysis.

Nervous System: Nervousness; tremors; dizziness; somnolence; confusion; anxiety; euphoria; transverse myelitis; seizures; coma. A syndrome manifested by a variety of CNS symptoms such as severe agitation with confusion, visual and auditory hallucinations, and a fear of impending death (Hoigne's syndrome), has been reported after administration of penicillin G procaine and, less commonly, after injection of the combination of penicillin G benzathine and penicillin G procaine. Other symptoms associated with this syndrome, such as psychosis, seizures, dizziness, tinnitus, cyanosis, palpitations, tachycardia, and/or abnormal perception in taste, also may occur.

Respiratory: Hypoxia; apnea; dyspnea.

Skin: Diaphoresis.

Special Senses: Blurred vision; blindness.

Urogenital: Neurogenic bladder; hematuria; proteinuria; renal failure; impotence; priapism.

OVERDOSAGE

Penicillin in overdosage has the potential to cause neuromuscular hyperirritability or convulsive seizures.

DOSAGE AND ADMINISTRATION

Due to the viscous nature of this medication, a 23 gauge or larger bore needle should be used to withdraw medication from the vial and for patient administration. A smaller bore needle, such as a 24 or 25 gauge, is not recommended.

Streptococcal (Group A) Upper-respiratory infections (for example, pharyngitis)

Adults—a single injection of 1,200,000 units; older pediatric patients—a single injection of 900,000 units; infants and pediatric patients under 60 lbs.—300,000 to 600,000 units.

Syphilis

Primary, secondary, and latent—2,400,000 units (1 dose). Late (tertiary and neurosyphilis)—2,400,000 units at 7-day intervals for three doses.

Congenital—under 2 years of age: 50,000 units/kg/body weight; ages 2 to 12 years: adjust dosage based on adult dosage schedule.

Yaws, Bejel, and Pinta—1,200,000 units (1 injection).

Prophylaxis—for rheumatic fever and glomerulonephritis. Following an acute attack, penicillin G benzathine (parenteral) may be given in doses of 1,200,000 units once a month or 600,000 units every 2 weeks.

Administer by DEEP INTRAMUSCULAR INJECTION in the upper, outer quadrant of the buttock. In neonates, infants and small children, the midlateral aspect of the thigh may be preferable. When doses are repeated, vary the injection site.

When using the multiple-dose vial:

After selection of the proper site and insertion of the needle into the selected muscle, aspirate by pulling back on the plunger. While maintaining negative pressure for 2 to 3 seconds, carefully observe the barrel of the syringe immediately proximal to the needle hub for appearance of blood or any discoloration. Blood or "typical blood color" may *not* be seen if a blood vessel has been entered—only a mixture of blood and Bicillin L-A. The appearance of any discoloration is reason to withdraw the needle and discard the syringe. If it is elected to inject at another site, a new syringe and needle should be used. If no blood or discoloration appears, inject the contents of the syringe slowly. Discontinue delivery of the dose if the subject complains of severe immediate pain at the injection site or if in infants and young children symptoms or signs occur suggesting onset of severe pain.

Because of the high concentration of suspended material in this product, the needle may be blocked if the injection is not made at a slow, steady rate.

When using the **TUBEX** cartridge:

The Wyeth-Ayerst **TUBEX®** cartridge for this product incorporates several features that are designed to facilitate the visualization of blood on aspiration if a blood vessel is inadvertently entered.

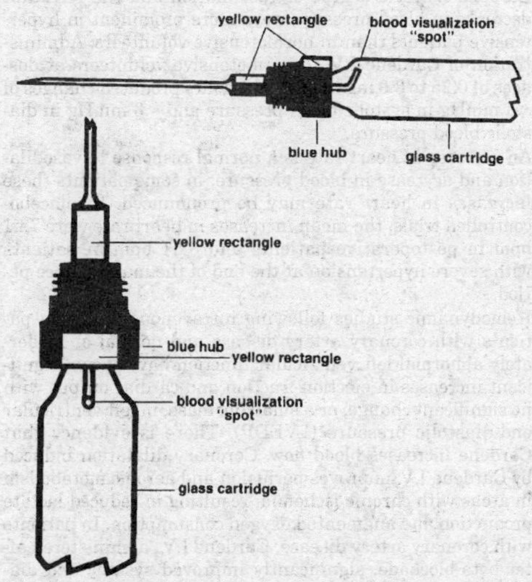

The design of this cartridge is such that blood which enters its needle will be quickly visualized as a red or dark-colored "spot." This "spot" will appear on the barrel of the glass cartridge immediately proximal to the blue hub. The **TUBEX** is designed with two orientation marks, in order to determine where the "spot" can be seen. First insert and secure the cartridge in the **TUBEX** injector in the usual fashion. Locate the yellow rectangle at the base of the blue hub. This yellow rectangle is aligned with the blood visualization "spot." An imaginary straight line, drawn from this yellow rectangle to the shoulder of the glass cartridge, will point to the area on the cartridge where the "spot" can be visualized. When the needle cover is removed, a second yellow rectangle will be visible. The second yellow rectangle is also aligned with the blood visualization "spot" to assist the operator in locating this "spot." If the 2 mL metal or plastic syringe is used, the glass cartridge should be rotated by turning the plunger of the syringe clockwise until the yellow rectangle is visualized. If the 1 mL metal syringe is used, it will not be possible to continue to rotate the glass cartridge clockwise once it is properly engaged and fully threaded; it can, however, then be rotated counterclockwise as far as necessary to properly orient the yellow rectangles and locate the observation area. (In this same area in some cartridges, a dark spot may sometimes be visualized prior to injection. This is the proximal end of the needle and does not represent a foreign body in, or other abnormality of, the suspension.)

Thus, before the needle is inserted into the selected muscle, it is important for the operator to orient the yellow rectangle so that any blood which may enter after needle insertion and during aspiration can be visualized in the area on the cartridge where it will appear and not be obscured by any obstructions.

After selection of the proper site and insertion of the needle into the selected muscle, aspirate by pulling back on the plunger. While maintaining negative pressure for 2 to 3 seconds, carefully observe the barrel of the cartridge in the area previously identified (see above) for the appearance of a red or dark-colored "spot."

Blood or "typical blood color" may not be seen if a blood vessel has been entered—only a mixture of blood and Bicillin L-A. The appearance of any discoloration is reason to withdraw the needle and discard the glass **TUBEX** cartridge. If it is elected to inject at another site, a new cartridge should be used. If no blood or discoloration appears, inject the contents of the cartridge slowly. Discontinue delivery of the dose if the subject complains of severe immediate pain at the injection site or if, especially in infants and young children, symptoms or signs occur suggesting onset of severe pain.

Some **TUBEX** cartridges may contain a small air bubble which may be disregarded, since it does not affect administration of the product.

DO NOT clear any air bubbles from the cartridge or needle as this may interfere with the visualization of any blood or discoloration during aspiration.

Because of the high concentration of suspended material in this product, the needle may be blocked if the injection is not made at a slow, steady rate.

When using the disposable syringe:

The Wyeth-Ayerst disposable syringe for this product incorporates several new features that are designed to facilitate its use.

A single small indentation, or "dot," has been punched into the metal ring that surrounds the neck of the syringe near the base of the needle. It is important that this "dot" be placed in a position so that it can be easily visualized by the operator following the intramuscular insertion of the syringe needle.

After selection of the proper site and insertion of the needle into the selected muscle, aspirate by pulling back on the plunger. While maintaining negative pressure for 2 to 3 seconds, carefully observe the barrel of the syringe immediately proximal to the location of the "dot" for appearance of blood or any discoloration. Blood or "typical blood color" may *not* be seen if a blood vessel has been entered—only a mixture of blood and Bicillin L-A. The appearance of any discoloration is reason to withdraw the needle and discard the syringe. If it is elected to inject at another site, a new syringe should be used. If no blood or discoloration appears, inject the contents of the syringe slowly. Discontinue delivery of the dose if the subject complains of severe immediate pain at the injection site or if in infants and young children symptoms or signs occur suggesting onset of severe pain.

Some disposable syringes may contain a small air bubble which may be disregarded, since it does not affect administration of the product.

Because of the high concentration of suspended material in this product, the needle may be blocked if the injection is not made at a slow, steady rate.

Parenteral drug products should be inspected visually for particulate matter and discoloration prior to administration whenever solution and container permit.

HOW SUPPLIED

Bicillin® L-A (penicillin G benzathine suspension) is supplied in packages of 10 **TUBEX®** Sterile Cartridge-Needle Units as follows:

1 mL size, containing 600,000 units per **TUBEX®** (21 gauge, thin-wall 1 inch needle for pediatric use), NDC 0008-0021-37.

2 mL size, containing 1,200,000 units per **TUBEX®** (21 gauge, thin-wall 1–1/4 inch needle), NDC 0008-0021-35.

Continued on next page

Bicillin L-A—Cont.

Store in a refrigerator.
Keep from freezing.

ALSO AVAILABLE

Bicillin L-A (penicillin G benzathine suspension) is also available in packages of 10 disposable syringes as follows: 4 mL size, containing 2,400,000 units per syringe (18 gauge × 2 inch needle), NDC 0008-0021-12

Bicillin L-A (penicillin G benzathine suspension) is also available in packages of single multiple-dose vials as follows:

10 mL size, 300,000 units per mL, NDC 0008-0163-01.

Store in a refrigerator.
Keep from freezing.
Shake multiple-dose vials well before using.

REFERENCES

1. SHAW, E.: Transverse myelitis from injection of penicillin. *Am. J. Dis. Child., 111:* 548, 1966.
2. KNOWLES, J.: Accidental intra-arterial injection of penicillin. *Am. J. Dis. Child., 111:* 552, 1966.
3. DARBY, C., et al: Ischemia following an intragluteal injection of benzathine-procaine penicillin G mixture in a one-year-old boy. *Clin. Pediatrics, 12:* 485, 1973.
4. BROWN, L. & NELSON, A.: Postinfectious intravascular thrombosis with gangrene. *Arch. Surg., 94:* 652, 1967.
5. BORENSTINE, J.: Transverse myelitis and penicillin (Correspondence). *Am. J. Dis. Child., 112:* 166, 1966.
6. ATKINSON, J.: Transverse myelopathy secondary to penicillin injection. *J. Pediatrics, 75:* 867, 1969.
7. TALBERT, J. et al: Gangrene of the foot following intramuscular injection in the lateral thigh: A case report with recommendations for prevention. *J. Pediatrics, 70:* 110, 1967.
8. FISHER, T.: Medicolegal affairs. *Canad. Med. Assoc. J., 112:* 395, 1975.
9. SCHANZER, H. et al: Accidental intra-arterial injection of penicillin G. *JAMA, 242:* 1289, 1979.

Manufactured by:
Wyeth Laboratories Inc.
A Wyeth-Ayerst Company
Philadelphia, PA 19101

BIOLOGICALS

Each of the biological products distributed by Wyeth-Ayerst Laboratories is listed separately in alphabetical order under the Product Information Sections either herein, for those manufactured by Wyeth Laboratories Inc., or under the Lederle listing for those manufactured by Lederle Laboratories Division, American Cyanamid Company.

For prescribing information on the products listed—and for which information is not provided—write to Professional Service, Wyeth-Ayerst Laboratories, P.O. Box 8299, Philadelphia, PA 19101, or contact your local Wyeth-Ayerst representative.

CARDENE® I.V. ℞

[*kăr 'deen*]
(nicardipine hydrochloride)

DESCRIPTION

Cardene (nicardipine HCl) is a calcium ion influx inhibitor (slow channel blocker or calcium channel blocker). Cardene I.V. for intravenous administration contains 2.5 mg/mL of nicardipine hydrochloride.

Nicardipine hydrochloride is a dihydropyridine derivative with IUPAC (International Union of Pure and Applied Chemistry) chemical name (±)-2-(benzyl-methyl amino) ethyl methyl 1,4-dihydro-2,6-dimethyl-4-(*m*-nitrophenyl)-3,5-pyridinedicarboxylate monohydrochloride and has the following structure:

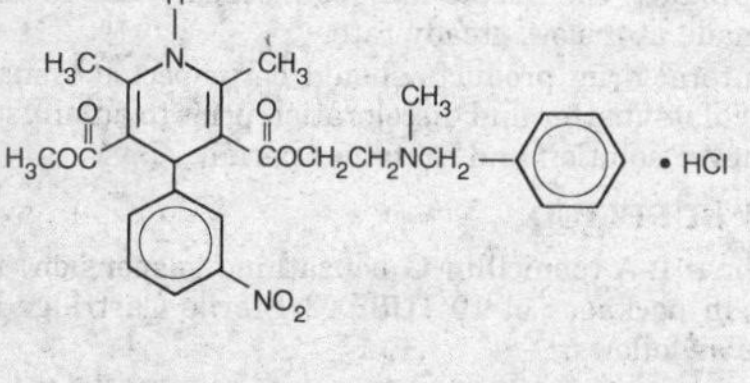

$C_{26}H_{29}N_3O_6 \cdot HCl$

Nicardipine hydrochloride is a greenish-yellow, odorless, crystalline powder that melts at about 169°C. It is freely soluble in chloroform, methanol, and glacial acetic acid, sparingly soluble in anhydrous ethanol, slightly soluble in n-butanol, water, 0.01 M potassium dihydrogen phosphate, acetone, and dioxane, very slightly soluble in ethyl acetate, and practically insoluble in benzene, ether, and hexane. It has a molecular weight of 515.99.

Cardene I.V. is available as a sterile, non-pyrogenic, clear, yellow solution in 10 mL ampuls for intravenous infusion after dilution. Each mL contains 2.5 mg nicardipine hydrochloride in Water for Injection, USP, with 48.00 mg Sorbitol, NF, buffered to pH 3.5 with 0.525 mg citric acid monohydrate, USP, and 0.09 mg sodium hydroxide, NF. Additional citric acid and/or sodium hydroxide may have been added to adjust pH.

CLINICAL PHARMACOLOGY

MECHANISM OF ACTION

Nicardipine inhibits the transmembrane influx of calcium ions into cardiac muscle and smooth muscle without changing serum calcium concentrations. The contractile processes of cardiac muscle and vascular smooth muscle are dependent upon the movement of extracellular calcium ions into these cells through specific ion channels. The effects of nicardipine are more selective to vascular smooth muscle than cardiac muscle. In animal models, nicardipine produced relaxation of coronary vascular smooth muscle at drug levels which cause little or no negative inotropic effect.

PHARMACOKINETICS AND METABOLISM

Following infusion, nicardipine plasma concentrations decline tri-exponentially, with a rapid early distribution phase (α-half-life of 2.7 minutes), an intermediate phase (β-half-life of 44.8 minutes), and a slow terminal phase (γ-half-life of 14.4 hours) that can only be detected after long-term infusions. Total plasma clearance (Cl) is 0.4 L/hr·kg, and the apparent volume of distribution (V_d) using a non-compartment model is 8.3 L/kg. The pharmacokinetics of Cardene I.V. are linear over the dosage range of 0.5 to 40.0 mg/hr.

Rapid dose-related increases in nicardipine plasma concentrations are seen during the first two hours after the start of an infusion of Cardene I.V. Plasma concentrations increase at a much slower rate after the first few hours, and approach steady state at 24 to 48 hours. On termination of the infusion, nicardipine concentrations decrease rapidly, with at least a 50% decrease during the first two hours post-infusion. The effects of nicardipine on blood pressure significantly correlate with plasma concentrations.

Nicardipine is highly protein bound (>95%) in human plasma over a wide concentration range.

Cardene I.V. has been shown to be rapidly and extensively metabolized by the liver. After coadministration of a radioactive intravenous dose of Cardene I.V. with an oral 30 mg dose given every 8 hours, 49% of the radioactivity was recovered in the urine and 43% in the feces within 96 hours. None of the dose was recovered as unchanged nicardipine. Nicardipine does not induce or inhibit its own metabolism and does not induce or inhibit hepatic microsomal enzymes.

The steady-state pharmacokinetics of nicardipine are similar in elderly hypertensive patients (>65 years) and young healthy adults.

HEMODYNAMICS

Cardene I.V. produces significant decreases in systemic vascular resistance. In a study of intra-arterially administered Cardene I.V., the degree of vasodilation and the resultant decrease in blood pressure were more prominent in hypertensive patients than in normotensive volunteers. Administration of Cardene I.V. to normotensive volunteers at dosages of 0.25 to 3.0 mg/hr for eight hours produced changes of <5 mmHg in systolic blood pressure and <3 mmHg in diastolic blood pressure.

An increase in heart rate is a normal response to vasodilation and decrease in blood pressure; in some patients these increases in heart rate may be pronounced. In placebo-controlled trials, the mean increases in heart rate were 7±1 bpm in postoperative patients and 8±1 bpm in patients with severe hypertension at the end of the maintenance period.

Hemodynamic studies following intravenous dosing in patients with coronary artery disease and normal or moderately abnormal left ventricular function have shown significant increases in ejection fraction and cardiac output with no significant change, or a small decrease, in left ventricular end-diastolic pressure (LVEDP). There is evidence that Cardene increases blood flow. Coronary dilatation induced by Cardene I.V. improves perfusion and aerobic metabolism in areas with chronic ischemia, resulting in reduced lactate production and augmented oxygen consumption. In patients with coronary artery disease, Cardene I.V., administered after beta-blockade, significantly improved systolic and diastolic left ventricular function. In congestive heart failure patients with impaired left ventricular function, Cardene I.V. increased cardiac output both at rest and during exercise. Decreases in left ventricular end-diastolic pressure were also observed. However, in some patients with severe left ventricular dysfunction, it may have a negative inotropic effect and could lead to worsened failure.

"Coronary steal" has not been observed during treatment with Cardene I.V. (Coronary steal is the detrimental redistribution of coronary blood flow in patients with coronary artery disease from underperfused areas toward better perfused areas.) Cardene I.V. has been shown to improve systolic shortening in both normal and hypokinetic segments of myocardial muscle. Radionuclide angiography has confirmed that wall motion remained improved during increased oxygen demand. (Occasional patients have developed increased angina upon receiving Cardene capsules. Whether this represents coronary steal in these patients, or is the result of increased heart rate and decreased diastolic pressure, is not clear.)

In patients with coronary artery disease, Cardene I.V. improves left ventricular diastolic distensibility during the early filling phase, probably due to a faster rate of myocardial relaxation in previously underperfused areas. There is little or no effect on normal myocardium, suggesting the improvement is mainly by indirect mechanisms such as afterload reduction and reduced ischemia. Cardene I.V. has no negative effect on myocardial relaxation at therapeutic doses. The clinical benefits of these properties have not yet been demonstrated.

ELECTROPHYSIOLOGIC EFFECTS

In general, no detrimental effects on the cardiac conduction system have been seen with Cardene I.V. During acute electrophysiologic studies, it increased heart rate and prolonged the corrected QT interval to a minor degree. It did not affect sinus node recovery or SA conduction times. The PA, AH, and HV intervals* or the functional and effective refractory periods of the atrium were not prolonged. The relative and effective refractory periods of the His-Purkinje system were slightly shortened.

---

*PA=conduction time from high to low right atrium; AH=conduction time from low right atrium to His bundle deflection, or AV nodal conduction time; HV=conduction time through the His bundle and the bundle branch-Purkinje system.

HEPATIC FUNCTION

Because nicardipine is extensively metabolized by the liver, plasma concentrations are influenced by changes in hepatic function. In a clincial study with Cardene capsules in patients with severe liver disease, plasma concentrations were elevated and the half-life was prolonged (see "**Precautions**"). Similar results were obtained in patients with hepatic disease when Cardene I.V. (nicardipine hydrochloride) was administered for 24 hours at 0.6 mg/hr.

RENAL FUNCTION

When Cardene I.V. was given to mild to moderate hypertensive patients with moderate degrees of renal impairment, significant reduction in glomerular filtration rate (GFR) and effective renal plasma flow (RPF) was observed. No significant differences in liver blood flow were observed in these patients. A significantly lower systemic clearance and higher area under the curve (AUC) were observed.

When Cardene capsules (20 mg or 30 mg TID) were given to hypertensive patients with impaired renal function, mean plasma concentrations, AUC, and C_{max} were approximately two-fold higher than in healthy controls. There is a transient increase in electrolyte excretion, including sodium (see "**Precautions**").

Acute bolus administration of Cardene I.V. (2.5 mg) in healthy volunteers decreased mean arterial pressure and renal vascular resistance; glomerular filtration rate (GFR), renal plasma flow (RPF), and the filtration fraction were unchanged. In healthy patients undergoing abdominal surgery, Cardene I.V. (10 mg over 20 minutes) increased GFR with no change in RPF when compared with placebo. In hypertensive Type II diabetic patients with nephropathy, Cardene capsules (20 mg TID) did not change RPF and GFR, but reduced renal vascular resistance.

PULMONARY FUNCTION

In two well-controlled studies of patients with obstructive airway disease treated with Cardene capsules, no evidence of increased bronchospasm was seen. In one of the studies, Cardene capsules improved forced expiratory volume 1 second (FEV 1) and forced vital capacity (FVC) in comparison with metoprolol. Adverse experiences reported in a limited number of patients with asthma, reactive airway disease, or obstructive airway disease are similar to all patients treated with Cardene capsules.

EFFECTS IN HYPERTENSION

In patients with mild to moderate chronic stable essential hypertension, Cardene I.V. (0.5. to 4.0 mg/hr) produced dose-dependent decreases in blood pressure, although only the decreases at 4.0 mg/hr were statistically different from placebo. At the end of a 48-hour infusion at 4.0 mg/hr, the decreases were 26.0 mmHg (17%) in systolic blood pressure and 20.7 mmHg (20%) in diastolic blood pressure.

In other settings (e.g., patients with severe or postoperative hypertension), Cardene I.V. (5 to 15 mg/hr) produced dose-dependent decreases in blood pressure. Higher infusion rates produced therapeutic responses more rapidly. The mean time to therapeutic response for severe hypertension, defined as diastolic blood pressure ≤95 mmHg or ≥25 mmHg decrease and systolic blood pressure ≤160 mmHg, was 77 ±5.2 minutes. The average maintenance dose was 8.0 mg/hr. The mean time to therapeutic response for post-

operative hypertension, defined as ≥15% reduction in diastolic or systolic blood pressure, was 11.5 ±0.8 minutes. The average maintenance dose was 3.0 mg/hr.

INDICATION AND USAGE
Cardene I.V. is indicated for the short-term treatment of hypertension when oral therapy is not feasible or not desirable.

For prolonged control of blood pressure, patients should be transferred to oral medication as soon as their clinical condition permits (see "Dosage and Administration").

CONTRAINDICATIONS
Cardene I.V. is contraindicated in patients with known hypersensitivity to the drug.

Cardene I.V. is also contraindicated in patients with advanced aortic stenosis because part of the effect of Cardene I.V. is secondary to reduced afterload.

Reduction of diastolic pressure in these patients may worsen rather than improve myocardial oxygen balance.

WARNINGS
BETA-BLOCKER WITHDRAWAL
Nicardipine is not a beta-blocker and therefore gives no protection against the dangers of abrupt beta-blocker withdrawal; any such withdrawal should be by gradual reduction of dose of beta-blocker.

RAPID DECREASES IN BLOOD PRESSURE
No clinical events have been reported suggestive of a too rapid decrease in blood pressure with Cardene I.V. However, as with any antihypertensive agent, blood pressure lowering should be accomplished over as long a time as is compatible with the patient's clinical status.

USE IN PATIENTS WITH ANGINA
Increases in frequency, duration, or severity of angina have been seen in chronic oral therapy with Cardene capsules. Induction or exacerbation of angina has been seen in less than 1% of coronary artery disease patients treated with Cardene I.V. The mechanism of this effect has not been established.

USE IN PATIENTS WITH CONGESTIVE HEART FAILURE
Cardene I.V. reduced afterload without impairing myocardial contractility in preliminary hemodynamic studies of CHF patients. However, in vitro and in some patients, a negative inotropic effect has been observed. Therefore, caution should be exercised when using Cardene I.V., particularly in combination with a beta-blocker, in patients with CHF or significant left ventricular dysfunction.

USE IN PATIENTS WITH PHEOCHROMOCYTOMA
Only limited clinical experience exists in use of Cardene I.V. for patients with hypertension associated with pheochromocytoma. Caution should therefore be exercised when using the drug in these patients.

PERIPHERAL VEIN INFUSION SITE
To minimize the risk of peripheral venous irritation, it is recommended that the site of infusion of Cardene I.V. be changed every 12 hours.

PRECAUTIONS
GENERAL
Blood Pressure: Because Cardene I.V. decreases peripheral resistance, monitoring of blood pressure during administration is required. Cardene I.V., like other calcium channel blockers, may occasionally produce symptomatic hypotension. Caution is advised to avoid systemic hypotension when administering the drug to patients who have sustained an acute cerebral infarction or hemorrhage.

Use in Patients with Impaired Hepatic Function: Since nicardipine is metabolized in the liver, the drug should be used with caution in patients with impaired liver function or reduced hepatic blood flow. The use of lower dosages should be considered.

Nicardipine administered intravenously has been reported to increase hepatic venous pressure gradient by 4 mmHg in cirrhotic patients at high doses (5 mg/20 min). Cardene I.V. should therefore be used with caution in patients with portal hypertension.

Use in Patients with Impaired Renal Function: When Cardene I.V. was given to mild to moderate hypertensive patients with moderate renal impairment, a significantly lower systemic clearance and higher AUC was observed. These results are consistent with those seen after oral administration of nicardipine. Careful dose titration is advised when treating renal impaired patients.

DRUG INTERACTIONS
Since Cardene I.V. may be administered to patients already being treated with other medications, including other antihypertensive agents, careful monitoring of these patients is necessary to detect and promptly treat any undesired effects from concomitant administration.

BETA-BLOCKERS
In most patients, Cardene I.V. can safely be used concomitantly with beta-blockers. However, caution should be exercised when using Cardene I.V. in combination with a beta-blocker in congestive heart failure patients (see "Warnings").

CIMETIDINE
Cimetidine has been shown to increase nicardipine plasma concentrations with Cardene capsule administration. Patients receiving the two drugs concomitantly should be carefully monitored. Data with other histamine-2 antagonists are not available.

DIGOXIN
Studies have shown that Cardene capsules usually do not alter digoxin plasma concentrations. However, as a precaution, digoxin levels should be evaluated when concomitant therapy with Cardene I.V. is initiated.

FENTANYL ANESTHESIA
Hypotension has been reported during fentanyl anesthesia with concomitant use of a beta-blocker and a calcium channel blocker. Even though such interactions were not seen during clinical studies with Cardene I.V. (nicardipine hydrochloride), an increased volume of circulating fluids might be required if such an interaction were to occur.

CYCLOSPORINE
Concomitant administration of Cardene capsules and cyclosporine results in elevated plasma cyclosporine levels. Plasma concentrations of cyclosporine should therefore be closely monitored during Cardene I.V. administration, and the dose of cyclosporine reduced accordingly.

IN VITRO INTERACTION
The plasma protein binding of nicardipine was not altered when therapeutic concentrations of furosemide, propranolol, dipyridamole, warfarin, quinidine, or naproxen were added to human plasma *in vitro*.

CARCINOGENESIS, MUTAGENESIS, IMPAIRMENT OF FERTILITY
Rats treated with nicardipine in the diet (at concentrations calculated to provide daily dosage levels of 5, 15, or 45 mg/kg/day) for two years showed a dose-dependent increase in thyroid hyperplasia and neoplasia (follicular adenoma/carcinoma). One- and three-month studies in the rat have suggested that these results are linked to a nicardipine-induced reduction in plasma thyroxine (T4) levels with a consequent increase in plasma levels of thyroid stimulating hormone (TSH). Chronic elevation of TSH is known to cause hyperstimulation of the thyroid. In rats on an iodine deficient diet, nicardipine administration for one month was associated with thyroid hyperplasia that was prevented by T4 supplementation. Mice treated with nicardipine in the diet (at concentrations calculated to provide daily dosage levels of up to 100 mg/kg/day) for up to 18 months showed no evidence of neoplasia of any tissue and no evidence of thyroid changes. There was no evidence of thyroid pathology in dogs treated with up to 25 mg nicardipine/kg/day for one year and no evidence of effects of nicardipine on thyroid function (plasma T4 and TSH) in man. There was no evidence of a mutagenic potential of nicardipine in a battery of genotoxicity tests conducted on microbial indicator organisms, in micronucleus tests in mice and hamsters, or in a sister chromatid exchange study in hamsters. No impairment of fertility was seen in male or female rats administered nicardipine at oral doses as high as 100 mg/kg/day (50 times the 40 mg TID maximum recommended dose in man, assuming a patient weight of 60 kg).

Pregnancy Category C: Cardene® I.V. at doses up to 5 mg/kg/day to pregnant rats and up to 0.5 mg/kg/day to pregnant rabbits produced no embryotoxicity or teratogenicity. Embryotoxicity was seen at 10 mg/kg/day in rats and at 1 mg/kg/day in rabbits, but no teratogenicity was observed at these doses.

Nicardipine was embryocidal when administered orally to pregnant Japanese White rabbits, during organogenesis, at 150 mg/kg/day (a dose associated with marked body weight gain suppression in the treated doe), but not at 50 mg/kg/day (25 times the maximum recommended dose in man). No adverse effects on the fetus were observed when New Zealand albino rabbits were treated, during organogenesis, with up to 100 mg nicardipine/kg/day (a dose associated with significant mortality in the treated doe). In pregnant rats administered nicardipine orally at up to 100 mg/kg/day (50 times the maximum recommended human dose) there was no evidence of embryolethality or teratogenicity. However, dystocia, reduced birth weights, reduced neonatal survival, and reduced neonatal weight gain were noted. There are no adequate and well-controlled studies in pregnant women. Cardene should be used during pregnancy only if the potential benefit justifies the potential risk to the fetus.

NURSING MOTHERS
Studies in rats have shown significant concentrations of nicardipine in maternal milk. For this reason, it is recommended that women who wish to breastfeed should not be given this drug.

PEDIATRIC USE
Safety and efficacy in patients under the age of 18 have not been established.

USE IN THE ELDERLY
No significant difference has been observed in the antihypertensive effect of Cardene I.V. in elderly patients (≥65 years) compared with other adult patients in clinical studies.

ADVERSE EXPERIENCES
Two hundred forty-four patients participated in two multicenter, double-blind, placebo controlled trials of Cardene I.V. Adverse experiences were generally not serious and most were expected consequences of vasodilation. Adverse experiences occasionally required dosage adjustment. Therapy was discontinued in approximately 12% of patients, mainly due to hypotension, headache, and tachycardia. [See table above]

Percent of Patients with Adverse Experiences During the Double-Blind Portion of Controlled Trials		
Adverse Experience	Cardene (n=144)	Placebo (n=100)
Body as a Whole		
Headache	14.6	2.0
Asthenia	0.7	0.0
Abdominal pain	0.7	0.0
Chest pain	0.7	0.0
Cardiovascular		
Hypotension	5.6	1.0
Tachycardia	3.5	0.0
ECG abnormality	1.4	0.0
Postural hypotension	1.4	0.0
Ventricular extrasystoles	1.4	0.0
Extrasystoles	0.7	0.0
Hemopericardium	0.7	0.0
Hypertension	0.7	0.0
Supraventricular tachycardia	0.7	0.0
Syncope	0.7	0.0
Vasodilation	0.7	0.0
Ventricular tachycardia	0.7	0.0
Digestive		
Nausea/vomiting	4.9	1.0
Injection Site		
Injection site reaction	1.4	0.0
Injection site pain	0.7	0.0
Metabolic and Nutritional		
Hypokalemia	0.7	0.0
Nervous		
Dizziness	1.4	0.0
Hypesthesia	0.7	0.0
Intracranial hemorrhage	0.7	0.0
Paresthesia	0.7	0.0
Respiratory		
Dyspnea	0.7	0.0
Skin and Appendages		
Sweating	1.4	0.0
Urogenital		
Polyuria	1.4	0.0
Hematuria	0.7	0.0

Continued on next page

Cardene I.V.—Cont.

RARE EVENTS
The following rare events have been reported in clinical trials or in the literature in association with the use of intravenously administered nicardipine.
Body as a Whole: fever, neck pain
Cardiovascular: angina pectoris, atrioventricular block, ST segment depression, inverted T wave, deep-vein thrombophlebitis
Digestive: dyspepsia
Hemic and Lymphatic: thrombocytopenia
Metabolic and Nutritional: hypophosphatemia, peripheral edema
Nervous: confusion, hypertonia
Respiratory: respiratory disorder
Special Senses: conjunctivitis, ear disorder, tinnitus
Urogenital: urinary frequency
Sinus node dysfunction and myocardial infarction, which may be due to disease progression, have been seen in patients on chronic therapy with orally administered nicardipine.

OVERDOSAGE
Several overdosages with orally administered nicardipine have been reported. One adult patient allegedly ingested 600 mg of nicardipine [standard (immediate release) capsules], and another patient, 2160 mg of the sustained release formulation of nicardipine. Symptoms included marked hypotension, bradycardia, palpitations, flushing, drowsiness, confusion and slurred speech. All symptoms resolved without sequelae. An overdosage occurred in a one year old child who ingested half of the powder in a 30 mg nicardipine standard capsule. The child remained asymptomatic. Based on results obtained in laboratory animals, lethal overdose may cause systemic hypotension, bradycardia (following initial tachycardia) and progressive atrioventricular conduction block. Reversible hepatic function abnormalities and sporadic focal hepatic necrosis were noted in some animal species receiving very large doses of nicardipine.
For treatment of overdosage, standard measures including monitoring of cardiac and respiratory functions should be implemented. The patient should be positioned so as to avoid cerebral anoxia. Frequent blood pressure determinations are essential. Vasopressors are clinically indicated for patients exhibiting profound hypotension. Intravenous calcium gluconate may help reverse the effects of calcium entry blockade.

DOSAGE AND ADMINISTRATION
Cardene I.V. (nicardipine hydrochloride) is intended for intravenous use. DOSAGE MUST BE INDIVIDUALIZED depending upon the severity of hypertension and the response of the patient during dosing.
Blood pressure should be monitored both during and after the infusion; too rapid or excessive reduction in either systolic or diastolic blood pressure during parenteral treatment should be avoided.
PREPARATION
WARNING: AMPULS MUST BE DILUTED BEFORE INFUSION
Dilution: Cardene I.V. is administered by slow continuous infusion at a CONCENTRATION OF 0.1 MG/ML. Each ampul (25 mg) should be diluted with 240 mL of compatible intravenous fluid (see below), resulting in 250 mL of solution at a concentration of 0.1 mg/mL.
Cardene I.V. has been found to be compatible and stable in glass or polyvinyl chloride containers for 24 hours at controlled room temperature with:
Dextrose (5%) Injection, USP
Dextrose (5%) and Sodium Chloride (0.45%) Injection, USP
Dextrose (5%) and Sodium Chloride (0.9%) Injection, USP
Dextrose (5%) with 40 mEq Potassium, USP
Sodium Chloride (0.45%) Injection, USP
Sodium Chloride (0.9%) Injection, USP
Cardene I.V. is NOT compatible with Sodium Bicarbonate (5%) Injection, USP, or Lactated Ringer's Injection, USP.
THE DILUTED SOLUTION IS STABLE FOR 24 HOURS AT ROOM TEMPERATURE.
Inspection: As with all parenteral drugs, Cardene I.V. should be inspected visually for particulate matter and discoloration prior to administration, whenever solution and container permit. Cardene I.V. is normally light yellow in color.

DOSAGE
As a Substitute for Oral Nicardipine Therapy
The intravenous infusion rate required to produce an average plasma concentration equivalent to a given oral dose at steady state is shown in the following table:

Oral Cardene Dose	Equivalent I.V. Infusion Rate
20 mg q8h	0.5 mg/hr
30 mg q8h	1.2 mg/hr
40 mg q8h	2.2 mg/hr

For Initiation of Therapy in a Drug Free Patient
The time course of blood pressure decrease is dependent on the initial rate of infusion and the frequency of dosage adjustment.
Cardene I.V. is administered by slow continuous infusion at a CONCENTRATION OF 0.1 MG/ML. With constant infusion, blood pressure begins to fall within minutes. It reaches about 50% of its ultimate decrease in about 45 minutes and does not reach final steady state for about 50 hours.
When treating acute hypertensive episodes in patients with chronic hypertension, discontinuation of infusion is followed by a 50% offset of action in 30±7 minutes but plasma levels of drug and gradually decreasing antihypertensive effects exist for about 50 hours.
Titration: For gradual reduction in blood pressure, initiate therapy at 50 mL/hr (5.0 mg/hr). If desired blood pressure reduction is not achieved at this dose, the infusion rate may be increased by 25 mL/hr (2.5 mg/hr) every 15 minutes up to a maximum of 150 mL/hr (15.0 mg/hr), until desired blood pressure reduction is achieved. For more rapid blood pressure reduction, initiate therapy at 50 mL/hr (5.0 mg/hr). If desired blood pressure reduction is not achieved at this dose, the infusion rate may be increased by 25 mL/hr (2.5 mg/hr) every 5 minutes up to a maximum of 150 mL/hr (15.0 mg/hr), until desired blood pressure reduction is achieved. Following achievement of the blood pressure goal, the infusion rate should be decreased to 30 mL/hr (3 mg/hr).
Maintenance: The rate of infusion should be adjusted as needed to maintain desired response.
CONDITIONS REQUIRING INFUSION ADJUSTMENT
Hypotension or Tachycardia: If there is concern of impending hypotension or tachycardia, the infusion should be discontinued. When blood pressure has stabilized, infusion of Cardene I.V. may be restarted at low doses such as 30–50 mL/hr (3.0–5.0 mg/hr) and adjusted to maintain desired blood pressure.
Infusion Site Changes: Cardene I.V. should be continued as long as blood pressure control is needed. The infusion site should be changed every 12 hours if administered via peripheral vein.
Impaired Cardiac, Hepatic, or Renal Function: Caution is advised when titrating Cardene I.V. in patients with congestive heart failure or impaired hepatic or renal function (see "Precautions").
TRANSFER TO ORAL ANTIHYPERTENSIVE AGENTS
If treatment includes transfer to an oral antihypertensive agent other than Cardene capsules, therapy should generally be initiated upon discontinuation of Cardene I.V. If Cardene capsules are to be used, the first dose of a TID regimen should be administered 1 hour prior to discontinuation of the infusion.

HOW SUPPLIED
Cardene I.V. (nicardipine hydrochloride) is available in packages of 10 ampuls of 10 mL as follows:
25 mg (2.5 mg/mL), NDC 0008-0812-02.
Store at controlled room temperature, 20°–25° C (68°–77° F).
Freezing does not adversely affect the product, but exposure to elevated temperatures should be avoided.
Protect from light. Store ampuls in carton until used.
Caution: Federal law prohibits dispensing without prescription.
U.S. Patent Nos. 3,985,758; 4,880,823; and 5,164,405
Cardene® is a registered trademark of Syntex (U.S.A.) Inc.
Manufactured under license
from Syntex (U.S.A.) Inc. by
Wyeth Laboratories Inc.
A Wyeth-Ayerst Company
Philadelphia, PA 19101

CEROSE®–DM   OTC
[se-rōs ' DM]

(See PDR For Nonprescription Drugs.)

CHOLERA VACCINE   ℞
USP

DESCRIPTION
Cholera Vaccine, USP is a sterile suspension of equal parts of Ogawa and Inaba serotypes of killed *Vibrio cholerae (V. comma)* in buffered sodium chloride injection. The Inaba and Ogawa strains of *V. cholerae* are grown on trypticase soy agar medium, removed from the medium with buffered sodium chloride injection and killed by the addition of 0.5 percent phenol. Phenol in a concentration of 0.5 percent is also used as the preservative in the finished vaccine. The vaccine contains 8 units of each serotype antigen (Ogawa and Inaba) per milliliter.

Cholera vaccine may be injected intracutaneously (intradermally), subcutaneously or intramuscularly.

CLINICAL PHARMACOLOGY
Cholera vaccine is used for active immunization against cholera. Field studies carried out in endemic cholera areas have shown cholera vaccines to be approximately 50% effective in reducing incidence of disease and for only 3 to 6 months. Use of cholera vaccine does not prevent transmission of infection.

INDICATION AND USAGE
Active immunization against cholera is indicated only for individuals traveling to or residing in countries where cholera is endemic or epidemic.

CONTRAINDICATIONS
Use of cholera vaccine should be postponed in the presence of any acute illness.
A history of severe systemic reaction or allergic response following a prior dose of cholera vaccine is a contraindication to further use.

WARNINGS
DO NOT INJECT INTRAVENOUSLY.
Cholera vaccine should not be administered intramuscularly to persons with thrombocytopenia or any coagulation disorder that would contraindicate intramuscular injection.

PRECAUTIONS
GENERAL
A separate, sterilized syringe and needle should be used for each patient to prevent transmission of hepatitis B virus and other infectious agents from one person to another.
Before delivering the dose intramuscularly or subcutaneously, aspirate to help avoid inadvertent injection into a blood vessel.
Before the injection of any biological, the physician should take all precautions known for prevention of allergic or other side reactions. This should include: a review of the patient's history regarding possible sensitivity; and a knowledge of the recent literature pertaining to the use of the biological concerned.
Epinephrine (1:1000) should be available for immediate use when this product is injected.
DRUG INTERACTIONS
Some data suggest that administration of cholera and yellow fever vaccines within three weeks of each other may result in decreased levels of antibody response to both vaccines as compared with administration at longer intervals. However, there is no evidence that protection to either disease is diminished following simultaneous administration.[1] It is currently recommended that, when feasible, cholera and yellow fever vaccines should be administered at a minimal interval of three weeks, unless time constraints preclude this. If the vaccines cannot be administered at least three weeks apart, they should be given simultaneously.[2]

PREGNANCY
Pregnancy Category C
Animal reproduction studies have not been conducted with cholera vaccine. It is also not known whether cholera vaccine can cause fetal harm when administered to a pregnant woman or can affect reproductive capacity. However, as with other inactivated bacterial vaccines, its use is not contraindicated during pregnancy unless the intended recipient has manifested significant systemic or allergic reaction following administration of prior doses. Use of cholera vaccine during pregnancy should be individualized to reflect actual need.[1,3]

ADVERSE REACTIONS
Local reactions manifested by erythema, induration, pain, and tenderness at the site of injection occur in most recipients, and such local reactions may persist for a few days. Recipients frequently develop malaise, headache, and mild-to-moderate temperature elevations which may persist for 1 to 2 days.[1,4]

DOSAGE AND ADMINISTRATION
Shake vial vigorously before withdrawing each dose.
Parenteral drug products should be inspected visually for presence of particulate matter and discoloration prior to use.
The primary immunizing course consists of two doses administered one week to one month or more apart. The table below summarizes the recommended doses for both primary and booster immunizations by age, volume (mL), and route of administration.[3,5] The intracutaneous (intradermal) route is satisfactory for persons 5 years of age and older, but higher levels of antibody may be achieved in children less than 5 years old by the subcutaneous or intramuscular routes.

Dose number	Route & Age			
	Intra-dermal	Subcutaneous or Intramuscular		
	5 years and over	6 mos-4 years	5–10 years	Over 10 years
1 & 2	0.2 mL	0.2 mL	0.3 mL	0.5 mL
Boosters	0.2 mL	0.2 mL	0.3 mL	0.5 mL

In areas where cholera is epidemic or endemic, booster doses should be given every six months.
The primary immunizing series need never be repeated for booster doses to be effective.
Before injection, the rubber diaphragm of the vial and the skin over the site to be injected should be cleansed and prepared with a suitable germicide.

HOW SUPPLIED

Cholera Vaccine, USP, is supplied as 1.5 and 20 mL vials.

STORAGE

Keep between 2° and 8°C (35° and 46°F).
Keep from freezing.

REFERENCES

1. Recommendation of the Immunization Practices Advisory Committee (ACIP). General recommendations on immunization. MMWR 32(1):1, 1983.
2. Recommendations of the Immunization Practices Advisory Committee (ACIP). Yellow fever vaccine. MMWR 32(52):679, 1984.
3. Recommendation of the Public Health Service Advisory Committee on Immunization Practices—Cholera Vaccine. MMWR 27(20):173, 1978.
4. GANGAROSA, E. and FAICH, G.: Cholera: The risk to American travelers. Ann. Int. Med. 74:412, 1971.
5. Report of the Committee on Infectious Diseases, American Academy of Pediatrics, 1982 (Red Book).

U S Gov't License No. 3
Manufactured by:
Wyeth Laboratories Inc.
A Wyeth-Ayerst Company
Marietta, PA 17547

CORDARONE® ℞

[kŏr 'dă-rōn]
(amiodarone HCl)
Tablets

DESCRIPTION

Cordarone is a member of a new class of antiarrhythmic drugs with predominantly Class III (Vaughan Williams' classification) effects, available for oral administration as pink, scored tablets containing 200 mg of amiodarone hydrochloride. The inactive ingredients present are colloidal silicon dioxide, lactose, magnesium stearate, povidone, starch, and FD&C Red 40. Cordarone is a benzofuran derivative: 2-butyl -3-benzofuranyl 4-[2-(diethylamino)-ethoxy]-3,5-diiodophenyl ketone hydrochloride. It is not chemically related to any other available antiarrhythmic drug.
The structural formula is as follows:

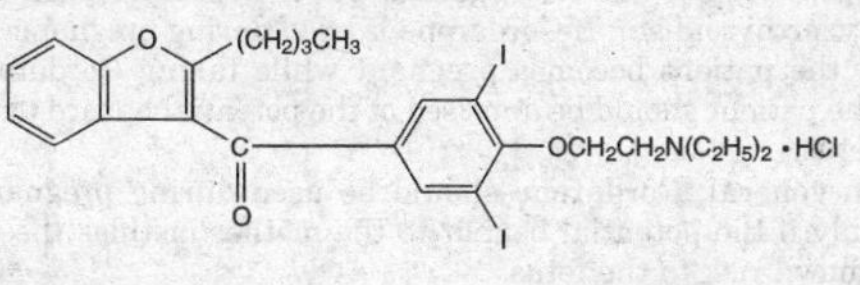

$C_{25}H_{29}I_2NO_3 \cdot HCl$ Molecular Weight: 681.8

Amiodarone HCl is a white to cream-colored crystalline powder. It is slightly soluble in water, soluble in alcohol, and freely soluble in chloroform. It contains 37.3% iodine by weight.

CLINICAL PHARMACOLOGY

Electrophysiology/Mechanisms of Action

In animals, Cordarone is effective in the prevention or suppression of experimentally induced arrhythmias. The antiarrhythmic effect of Cordarone may be due to at least two major properties: 1) a prolongation of the myocardial cell-action potential duration and refractory period and 2) noncompetitive α- and β-adrenergic inhibition.
Cordarone prolongs the duration of the action potential of all cardiac fibers while causing minimal reduction of dV/dt (maximal upstroke velocity of the action potential). The refractory period is prolonged in all cardiac tissues. Cordarone increases the cardiac refractory period without influencing resting membrane potential, except in automatic cells where the slope of the prepotential is reduced, generally reducing automaticity. These electrophysiologic effects are reflected in a decreased sinus rate of 15 to 20%, increased PR and QT intervals of about 10%, the development of U-waves, and changes in T-wave contour. These changes should not require discontinuation of Cordarone as they are evidence of its pharmacological action, although Cordarone can cause marked sinus bradycardia or sinus arrest and heart block. On rare occasions, QT prolongation has been associated with worsening of arrhythmia (see "**WARNINGS**").

Hemodynamics

In animal studies and after intravenous administration in man, Cordarone relaxes vascular smooth muscle, reduces peripheral vascular resistance (afterload), and slightly increases cardiac index. After oral dosing, however, Cordarone produces no significant change in left ventricular ejection fraction (LVEF), even in patients with depressed LVEF. After acute intravenous dosing in man, Cordarone may have a mild negative inotropic effect.

Pharmacokinetics

Following oral administration in man, Cordarone is slowly and variably absorbed. The bioavailability of Cordarone is approximately 50%, but has varied between 35 and 65% in various studies. Maximum plasma concentrations are attained 3 to 7 hours after a single dose. Despite this, the onset of action may occur in 2 to 3 days, but more commonly takes 1 to 3 weeks, even with loading doses. Plasma concentrations with chronic dosing at 100 to 600 mg/day are approximately dose proportional, with a mean 0.5 mg/L increase for each 100 mg/day. These means, however, include considerable individual variability.
Cordarone has a very large but variable volume of distribution, averaging about 60 L/kg, because of extensive accumulation in various sites, especially adipose tissue and highly perfused organs, such as the liver, lung, and spleen. One major metabolite of Cordarone, desethylamiodarone, has been identified in man; it accumulates to an even greater extent in almost all tissues. The pharmacological activity of this metabolite, however, is not known. During chronic treatment, the plasma ratio of metabolite to parent compound is approximately one.
The main route of elimination is via hepatic excretion into bile, and some enterohepatic recirculation may occur. However, its kinetics in patients with hepatic insufficiency have not been elucidated. Cordarone has a very low plasma clearance with negligible renal excretion, so that it does not appear necessary to modify the dose in patients with renal failure. In patients with renal impairment, the plasma concentration of Cordarone is not elevated. Neither Cordarone nor its metabolite is dialyzable.
In patients, following discontinuation of chronic oral therapy, Cordarone has been shown to have a biphasic elimination with an initial one-half reduction of plasma levels after 2.5 to 10 days. A much slower terminal plasma-elimination phase shows a half-life of the parent compound ranging from 26 to 107 days, with a mean of approximately 53 days and most patients in the 40- to 55-day range. In the absence of a loading-dose period, steady-state plasma concentrations, at constant oral dosing, would therefore be reached between 130 and 535 days, with an average of 265 days. For the metabolite, the mean plasma-elimination half-life was approximately 61 days. These data probably reflect an initial elimination of the drug from well-perfused tissue (the 2.5- to 10-day half-life phase), followed by a terminal phase representing extremely slow elimination from poorly perfused tissue compartments such as fat.
The considerable intersubject variation in both phases of elimination, as well as uncertainty as to what compartment is critical to drug effect, requires attention to individual responses once arrhythmia control is achieved with loading doses because the correct maintenance dose is determined, in part, by the elimination rates. Daily maintenance doses of Cordarone should be based on individual patient requirements (see "**DOSAGE AND ADMINISTRATION**").
Cordarone and its metabolite have a limited transplacental transfer of approximately 10 to 50%. The parent drug and its metabolite have been detected in breast milk.
Cordarone is highly protein-bound (approximately 96%).
Although electrophysiologic effects, such as prolongation of QTc, can be seen within hours after a parenteral dose of Cordarone, effects on abnormal rhythms are not seen before 2 to 3 days and usually require 1 to 3 weeks, even when a loading dose is used. There may be a continued increase in effect for longer periods still. There is evidence that the time to effect is shorter when a loading-dose regimen is used.
Consistent with the slow rate of elimination, antiarrhythmic effects persist for weeks or months after Cordarone is discontinued, but the time of recurrence is variable and unpredictable. In general, when the drug is resumed after recurrence of the arrhythmia, control is established relatively rapidly compared to the initial response, presumably because tissue stores were not wholly depleted at the time of recurrence.

Pharmacodynamics

There is no well-established relationship of plasma concentration to effectiveness, but it does appear that concentrations much below 1 mg/L are often ineffective and that levels above 2.5 mg/L are generally not needed. Within individuals dose reductions and ensuing decreased plasma concentrations can result in loss of arrhythmia control. Plasma-concentration measurements can be used to identify patients whose levels are unusually low, and who might benefit from a dose increase, or unusually high, and who might have dosage reduction in the hope of minimizing side effects. Some observations have suggested a plasma concentration, dose, or dose/duration relationship for side effects such as pulmonary fibrosis, liver-enzyme elevations, corneal deposits and facial pigmentation, peripheral neuropathy, gastrointestinal and central nervous system effects.

Monitoring Effectiveness

Predicting the effectiveness of any antiarrhythmic agent in long-term prevention of recurrent ventricular tachycardia and ventricular fibrillation is difficult and controversial, with highly qualified investigators recommending use of ambulatory monitoring, programmed electrical stimulation with various stimulation regimens, or a combination of these, to assess response. There is no present consensus on many aspects of how best to assess effectiveness, but there is a reasonable consensus on some aspects:

1. If a patient with a history of cardiac arrest does not manifest a hemodynamically unstable arrhythmia during electrocardiographic monitoring prior to treatment, assessment of the effectiveness of Cordarone requires some provocative approach, either exercise or programmed electrical stimulation (PES).
2. Whether provocation is also needed in patients who do manifest their life-threatening arrhythmia spontaneously is not settled, but there are reasons to consider PES or other provocation in such patients. In the fraction of patients whose PES-inducible arrhythmia can be made noninducible by Cordarone (a fraction that has varied widely in various series from less than 10% to almost 40%, perhaps due to different stimulation criteria), the prognosis has been almost uniformly excellent, with very low recurrence (ventricular tachycardia or sudden death) rates. More controversial is the meaning of continued inducibility. There has been an impression that continued inducibility in Cordarone patients may not foretell a poor prognosis but, in fact, many observers have found greater recurrence rates in patients who remain inducible than in those who do not. A number of criteria have been proposed, however, for identifying patients who remain inducible but who seem likely nonetheless to do well on Cordarone. These criteria include increased difficulty of Induction (more stimuli or more rapid stimuli), which has been reported to predict a lower rate of recurrence, and ability to tolerate the induced ventricular tachycardia without severe symptoms, a finding that has been reported to correlate with better survival but not with lower recurrence rates. While these criteria require confirmation and further study in general, *easier* inducibility or *poorer* tolerance of the induced arrhythmia should suggest consideration of a need to revise treatment.

Several predictors of success not based on PES have also been suggested, including complete elimination of all nonsustained ventricular tachycardia on ambulatory monitoring and very low premature ventricular-beat rates (less than 1 VPB/1,000 normal beats).
While these issues remain unsettled for Cordarone, as for other agents, the prescriber of Cordarone should have access to (direct or through referral), and familiarity with, the full range of evaluatory procedures used in the care of patients with life-threatening arrhythmias.
It is difficult to describe the effectiveness rates of Cordarone, as these depend on the specific arrhythmia treated, the success criteria used, the underlying cardiac disease of the patient, the number of drugs tried before resorting to Cordarone, the duration of follow-up, the dose of Cordarone, the use of additional antiarrhythmic agents, and many other factors. As Cordarone has been studied principally in patients with refractory life-threatening ventricular arrhythmias, in whom drug therapy must be selected on the basis of response and cannot be assigned arbitrarily, randomized comparisons with other agents or placebo have not been possible. Reports of series of treated patients with a history of cardiac arrest and mean follow-up of one year or more have given mortality (due to arrhythmia) rates that were highly variable, ranging from less than 5% to over 30%, with most series in the range of 10 to 15%. Overall arrhythmia-recurrence rates (fatal and nonfatal) also were highly variable (and, as noted above, depended on response to PES and other measures), and depend on whether patients who do not seem to respond initially are included. In most cases, considering only patients who seemed to respond well enough to be placed on long-term treatment, recurrence rates have ranged from 20 to 40% in series with a mean follow-up of a year or more.

INDICATIONS AND USAGE

Because of its life-threatening side effects and the substantial management difficulties associated with its use (see "**WARNINGS**" below), Cordarone is indicated only for the treatment of the following documented, life-threatening re-

Continued on next page

Cordarone Tablets—Cont.

current ventricular arrhythmias when these have not responded to documented adequate doses of other available antiarrhythmics or when alternative agents could not be tolerated.
1. Recurrent ventricular fibrillation.
2. Recurrent hemodynamically unstable ventricular tachycardia.

As is the case for other antiarrhythmic agents, there is no evidence from controlled trials that the use of Cordarone favorably affects survival.

Cordarone should be used only by physicians familiar with and with access to (directly or through referral) the use of all available modalities for treating recurrent life-threatening ventricular arrhythmias, and who have access to appropriate monitoring facilities, including in-hospital and ambulatory continuous electrocardiographic monitoring and electrophysiologic techniques. Because of the life-threatening nature of the arrhythmias treated, potential interactions with prior therapy, and potential exacerbation of the arrhythmia, initiation of therapy with Cordarone should be carried out in the hospital.

CONTRAINDICATIONS

Cordarone is contraindicated in severe sinus-node dysfunction, causing marked sinus bradycardia; second- and third-degree atrioventricular block; and when episodes of bradycardia have caused syncope (except when used in conjunction with a pacemaker).

Cordarone is contraindicated in patients with a known hypersensitivity to the drug.

WARNINGS

Cordarone is intended for use only in patients with the indicated life-threatening arrhythmias because its use is accompanied by substantial toxicity.

Cordarone has several potentially fatal toxicities, the most important of which is pulmonary toxicity (hypersensitivity pneumonitis or interstitial/alveolar pneumonitis) that has resulted in clinically manifest disease at rates as high as 10 to 17% in some series of patients with ventricular arrhythmias given doses around 400 mg/day, and as abnormal diffusion capacity without symptoms in a much higher percentage of patients. Pulmonary toxicity has been fatal about 10% of the time. Liver injury is common with Cordarone, but is usually mild and evidenced only by abnormal liver enzymes. Overt liver disease can occur, however, and has been fatal in a few cases. Like other antiarrhythmics, Cordarone can exacerbate the arrhythmia, e.g., by making the arrhythmia less well tolerated or more difficult to reverse. This has occurred in 2 to 5% of patients in various series, and significant heart block or sinus bradycardia has been seen in 2 to 5%. All of these events should be manageable in the proper clinical setting in most cases. Although the frequency of such proarrhythmic events does not appear greater with Cordarone than with many other agents used in this population, the effects are prolonged when they occur.

Even in patients at high risk of arrhythmic death, in whom the toxicity of Cordarone is an acceptable risk, Cordarone poses major management problems that could be life-threatening in a population at risk of sudden death, so that every effort should be made to utilize alternative agents first.

The difficulty of using Cordarone effectively and safely itself poses a significant risk to patients. Patients with the indicated arrhythmias must be hospitalized while the loading dose of Cordarone is given, and a response generally requires at least one week, usually two or more. Because absorption and elimination are variable, maintenance-dose selection is difficult, and it is not unusual to require dosage decrease or discontinuation of treatment. In a retrospective survey of 192 patients with ventricular tachyarrhythmias, 84 required dose reduction and 18 required at least temporary discontinuation because of adverse effects, and several series have reported 15 to 20% overall frequencies of discontinuation due to adverse reactions. The time at which a previously controlled life-threatening arrhythmia will recur after discontinuation or dose adjustment is unpredictable, ranging from weeks to months. The patient is obviously at great risk during this time and may need prolonged hospitalization. Attempts to substitute other antiarrhythmic agents when Cordarone must be stopped will be made difficult by the gradually, but unpredictably, changing amiodarone body burden. A similar problem exists when Cordarone is not effective; it still poses the risk of an interaction with whatever subsequent treatment is tried.

Mortality

In the National Heart, Lung and Blood Institute's Cardiac Arrhythmia Suppression Trial (CAST), a long-term, multi-centered, randomized, double-blind study in patients with asymptomatic non-life-threatening ventricular arrhythmias who had had myocardial infarctions more than six days but less than two years previously, an excessive mortality or non-fatal cardiac arrest rate was seen in patients treated with encainide or flecainide (56/730) compared with that seen in patients assigned to matched placebo-treated groups (22/725). The average duration of treatment with encainide or flecainide in this study was ten months.

The applicability of these results to other populations (e.g., those without recent myocardial infarctions) or to Cordarone-treated patients is uncertain. While definitive controlled trials with Cordarone are in progress, pooled analysis of small controlled studies in patients with structural heart disease (including post-myocardial infarction) have not shown excess mortality in the Cordarone-treated population.

Pulmonary Toxicity

Cordarone may cause a clinical syndrome of cough and progressive dyspnea accompanied by functional, radiographic, gallium-scan, and pathological data consistent with pulmonary toxicity, the frequency of which varies from 2 to 7% in most published reports, but is as high as 10 to 17% in some reports. Therefore, when Cordarone therapy is initiated, a baseline chest X ray and pulmonary-function tests, including diffusion capacity, should be performed. The patient should return for a history, physical exam, and chest X ray every 3 to 6 months.

Preexisting pulmonary disease does not appear to increase the risk of developing pulmonary toxicity; however, these patients have a poorer prognosis if pulmonary toxicity does develop.

Pulmonary toxicity secondary to Cordarone seems to result from either indirect or direct toxicity as represented by hypersensitivity pneumonitis or interstitial/alveolar pneumonitis, respectively.

Hypersensitivity pneumonitis usually appears earlier in the course of therapy, and rechallenging these patients with Cordarone results in a more rapid recurrence of greater severity. Bronchoalveolar lavage is the procedure of choice to confirm this diagnosis, which can be made when a T suppressor/cytotoxic (CD8-positive) lymphocytosis is noted. Steroid therapy should be instituted and Cordarone therapy discontinued in these patients.

Interstitial/alveolar pneumonitis may result from the release of oxygen radicals and/or phospholipidosis and is characterized by findings of diffuse alveolar damage, interstitial pneumonitis or fibrosis in lung biopsy specimens. Phospholipidosis (foamy cells, foamy macrophages), due to inhibition of phospholipase, will be present in most cases of Cordarone-induced pulmonary toxicity; however, these changes also are present in approximately 50% of all patients on Cordarone therapy. These cells should be used as markers of therapy, but not as evidence of toxicity. A diagnosis of Cordarone-induced interstitial/alveolar pneumonitis should lead, at a minimum, to dose reduction or, preferably, to withdrawal of the Cordarone to establish reversibility, especially if other acceptable antiarrhythmic therapies are available. Where these measures have been instituted, a reduction in symptoms of amiodarone-induced pulmonary toxicity was usually noted within the first week, and a clinical improvement was greatest in the first two to three weeks. Chest X ray changes usually resolve within two to four months. According to some experts, steroids may prove beneficial. Prednisone in doses of 40 to 60 mg/day or equivalent doses of other steroids have been given and tapered over the course of several weeks depending upon the condition of the patient. In some cases rechallenge with Cordarone at a lower dose has not resulted in return of toxicity. Recent reports suggest that the use of lower loading and maintenance doses of Cordarone are associated with a decreased incidence of Cordarone-induced pulmonary toxicity.

In a patient receiving Cordarone, any new respiratory symptoms should suggest the possibility of pulmonary toxicity, and the history, physical exam, chest X ray, and pulmonary-function tests (with diffusion capacity) should be repeated and evaluated. A 15% decrease in diffusion capacity has a high sensitivity but only a moderate specificity for pulmonary toxicity; as the decrease in diffusion capacity approaches 30%, the sensitivity decreases but the specificity increases. A gallium scan also may be performed as part of the diagnostic workup.

Fatalities, secondary to pulmonary toxicity, have occurred in approximately 10% of cases. However, in patients with life-threatening arrhythmias, discontinuation of Cordarone therapy due to suspected drug-induced pulmonary toxicity should be undertaken with caution, as the most common cause of death in these patients is sudden cardiac death. Therefore, every effort should be made to rule out other causes of respiratory impairment (i.e., congestive heart failure with Swan-Ganz catheterization if necessary, respiratory infection, pulmonary embolism, malignancy, etc.) before discontinuing Cordarone in these patients. In addition, bronchoalveolar lavage, transbronchial lung biopsy and/or open lung biopsy may be necessary to confirm the diagnosis, especially in those cases where no acceptable alternative therapy is available.

If a diagnosis of Cordarone-induced hypersensitivity pneumonitis is made, Cordarone should be discontinued, and treatment with steroids should be instituted. If a diagnosis of Cordarone-induced interstitial/alveolar pneumonitis is made, steroid therapy should be instituted and, preferably, Cordarone discontinued or, at a minimum, reduced in dosage. Some cases of Cordarone-induced interstitial/alveolar pneumonitis may resolve following a reduction in Cordarone dosage in conjunction with the administration of steroids. In some patients, rechallenge at a lower dose has not resulted in return of interstitial/alveolar pneumonitis; however, in some patients (perhaps because of severe alveolar damage) the pulmonary lesions have not been reversible.

Worsened Arrhythmia

Cordarone, like other antiarrhythmics, can cause serious exacerbation of the presenting arrhythmia, a risk that may be enhanced by the presence of concomitant antiarrhythmics. Exacerbation has been reported in about 2 to 5% in most series, and has included new ventricular fibrillation, incessant ventricular tachycardia, increased resistance to cardioversion, and polymorphic ventricular tachycardia associated with QT prolongation (Torsade de Pointes). In addition, Cordarone has caused symptomatic bradycardia or sinus arrest with suppression of escape foci in 2 to 4% of patients.

Liver Injury

Elevations of hepatic enzyme levels are seen frequently in patients exposed to Cordarone and in most cases are asymptomatic. If the increase exceeds three times normal, or doubles in a patient with an elevated baseline, discontinuation of Cordarone or dosage reduction should be considered. In a few cases in which biopsy has been done, the histology has resembled that of alcoholic hepatitis or cirrhosis. Hepatic failure has been a rare cause of death in patients treated with Cordarone.

Loss Of Vision

Cases of optic neuropathy and/or optic neuritis, usually resulting in visual impairment, have been reported in patients treated with amiodarone. In some cases, visual impairment has progressed to permanent blindness. Optic neuropathy and/or neuritis may occur at any time following initiation of therapy. A causal relationship to the drug has not been clearly established. If symptoms of visual impairment appear, such as changes in visual acuity and decreases in peripheral vision, prompt ophthalmic examination is recommended. Appearance of optic neuropathy and/or neuritis calls for re-evaluation of Cordarone therapy. The risks and complications of antiarrhythmic therapy with Cordarone must be weighed against its benefits in patients whose lives are threatened by cardiac arrhythmias. Regular ophthalmic examination, including fundoscopy and slit-lamp examination, is recommended during administration of Cordarone. (See "**ADVERSE REACTIONS.**")

Pregnancy: Pregnancy Category D

Cordarone has been shown to be embryotoxic (increased fetal resorption and growth retardation) in the rat when given orally at a dose of 200 mg/kg/day (18 times the maximum recommended maintenance dose). Similar findings have been noted in one strain of mice at a dose of 5 mg/kg/day (approximately $^1/_2$ the maximum recommended maintenance dose) and higher, but not in a second strain nor in the rabbit at doses up to 100 mg/kg/day (9 times the maximum recommended maintenance dose).

Neonatal hypo- or hyperthyroidism

Cordarone can cause fetal harm when administered to a pregnant woman. Although Cordarone use during pregnancy is uncommon, there have been a small number of published reports of congenital goiter/hypothyroidism and hyperthyroidism. If Cordarone is used during pregnancy, or if the patient becomes pregnant while taking Cordarone, the patient should be apprised of the potential hazard to the fetus.

In general, Cordarone should be used during pregnancy only if the potential benefit to the mother justifies the unknown risk to the fetus.

PRECAUTIONS

Impairment of Vision

Optic Neuropathy and/or Neuritis

Cases of optic neuropathy and optic neuritis have been reported (see "**WARNINGS**").

Corneal Microdeposits

Corneal microdeposits appear in the majority of adults treated with Cordarone. They are usually discernible only by slit-lamp examination, but give rise to symptoms such as visual halos or blurred vision in as many as 10% of patients. Corneal microdeposits are reversible upon reduction of dose or termination of treatment. Asymptomatic microdeposits alone are not a reason to reduce dose or discontinue treatment (see "**ADVERSE REACTIONS**").

Neurologic

Chronic administration of oral amiodarone in rare instances may lead to the development of peripheral neuropathy that may resolve when amiodarone is discontinued, but this resolution has been slow and incomplete.

Photosensitivity

Cordarone has induced photosensitization in about 10% of patients; some protection may be afforded by the use of sunbarrier creams or protective clothing. During long-term treatment, a blue-gray discoloration of the exposed skin may occur. The risk may be increased in patients of fair complexion or those with excessive sun exposure, and may be related to cumulative dose and duration of therapy.

Thyroid Abnormalities

Cordarone inhibits peripheral conversion of thyroxine (T_4) to triiodothyronine (T_3) and may cause increased thyroxine levels, decreased T_3 levels, and increased levels of inactive reverse T_3 (rT_3) in clinically euthyroid patients. It is also a potential source of large amounts of inorganic iodine. Because of its release of inorganic iodine, or perhaps for other reasons, Cordarone can cause either hypothyroidism or hyperthyroidism. Thyroid function should be monitored prior to treatment and periodically thereafter, particularly in elderly patients, and in any patient with a history of thyroid nodules, goiter, or other thyroid dysfunction. Because of the slow elimination of Cordarone and its metabolites, high plasma iodide levels, altered thyroid function, and abnormal thyroid-function tests may persist for several weeks or even months following Cordarone withdrawal.

Hypothyroidism has been reported in 2 to 4% of patients in most series, but in 8 to 10% in some series. This condition may be identified by relevant clinical symptoms and particularly by elevated serum TSH levels. In some clinically hypothyroid amiodarone-treated patients, free thyroxine index values may be normal. Hypothyroidism is best managed by Cordarone dose reduction and/or thyroid hormone supplement. However, therapy must be individualized, and it may be necessary to discontinue Cordarone in some patients.

Hyperthyroidism occurs in about 2% of patients receiving Cordarone, but the incidence may be higher among patients with prior inadequate dietary iodine intake. Cordarone-induced hyperthyroidism usually poses a greater hazard to the patient than hypothyroidism because of the possibility of arrhythmia breakthrough or aggravation. In fact, IF ANY NEW SIGNS OF ARRHYTHMIA APPEAR, THE POSSIBILITY OF HYPERTHYROIDISM SHOULD BE CONSIDERED. Hyperthyroidism is best identified by relevant clinical symptoms and signs, accompanied usually by abnormally elevated levels of serum T_3 RIA, and further elevations of serum T_4, and a subnormal serum TSH level (using a sufficiently sensitive TSH assay). The finding of a flat TSH response to TRH is confirmatory of hyperthyroidism and may be sought in equivocal cases. Since arrhythmia breakthroughs may accompany Cordarone-induced hyperthyrodism, aggressive medical treatment is indicated, including, if possible, dose reduction or withdrawal of Cordarone. The institution of antithyroid drugs, β-adrenergic blockers and/or temporary corticosteroid therapy may be necessary. The action of antithyroid drugs may be especially delayed in amiodarone-induced thyrotoxicosis because of substantial quantities of preformed thyroid hormones stored in the gland. Radioactive iodine therapy is contraindicated because of the low radioiodine uptake associated with amiodarone-induced hyperthyroidism. Experience with thyroid surgery in this setting is extremely limited, and this form of therapy runs the theoretical risk of inducing thyroid storm. Cordarone-induced hyperthyroidism may be followed by a transient period of hypothyroidism.

Surgery

Hypotension Postbypass: Rare occurrences of hypotension upon discontinuation of cardiopulmonary bypass during open-heart surgery in patients receiving Cordarone have been reported. The relationship of this event to Cordarone therapy is unknown.

Adult Respiratory Distress Syndrome (ARDS): Postoperatively, rare occurrences of ARDS have been reported in patients receiving Cordarone therapy who have undergone either cardiac or noncardiac surgery. Although patients usually respond well to vigorous respiratory therapy, in rare instances the outcome has been fatal. Until further studies have been performed, it is recommended that FiO_2 and the determinants of oxygen delivery to the tissues (e.g., SaO_2, PaO_2) be closely monitored in patients on Cordarone.

Laboratory Tests

Elevations in liver enzymes (SGOT and SGPT) can occur. Liver enzymes in patients on relatively high maintenance doses should be monitored on a regular basis. Persistent significant elevations in the liver enzymes or hepatomegaly should alert the physician to consider reducing the maintenance dose of Cordarone or discontinuing therapy.

Cordarone alters the results of thyroid-function tests, causing an increase in serum T_4 and serum reverse T_3, and a decline in serum T_3 levels. Despite these biochemical changes, most patients remain clinically euthyroid.

Drug Interactions

Although only a small number of drug-drug interactions with Cordarone have been explored formally, most of these have shown such an interaction. The potential for other interactions should be anticipated, particularly for drugs with potentially serious toxicity, such as other antiarrhythmics.

SUMMARY OF DRUG INTERACTIONS WITH CORDARONE

Concomitant Drug	Interaction — Onset (days)	Interaction — Magnitude	Recommended Dose Reduction of Concomitant Drug
Warfarin	3 to 4	Increases prothrombin time by 100%	↓ $^1/_3$ to $^1/_2$
Digoxin	1	Increases serum concentration by 70%	↓ $^1/_2$
Quinidine	2	Increases serum concentration by 33%	↓ $^1/_3$ to $^1/_2$ (or discontinue)
Procainamide	<7	Increases plasma concentration by 55%; NAPA* concentration by 33%	↓ $^1/_3$ (or discontinue)

*NAPA = n-acetyl procainamide.

	Loading Dose (Daily)	Adjustment and Maintenance Dose (Daily)	
Ventricular Arrhythmias	1 to 3 weeks	~1 month	usual maintenance
	800 to 1,600 mg	600 to 800 mg	400 mg

If such drugs are needed, their dose should be reassessed and, where appropriate, plasma concentration measured.

In view of the long and variable half-life of Cordarone, potential for drug interactions exists not only with concomitant medication but also with drugs administered after discontinuation of Cordarone.

Cyclosporine
Concomitant use of amiodarone and cyclosporine has been reported to produce persistently elevated plasma concentrations of cyclosporine resulting in elevated creatinine, despite reduction in dose of cyclosporine.

Digitalis
Administration of Cordarone to patients receiving digoxin therapy regularly results in an increase in the serum digoxin concentration that may reach toxic levels with resultant clinical toxicity. On initiation of Cordarone, the need for digitalis therapy should be reviewed and the dose reduced by approximately 50% or discontinued. If digitalis treatment is continued, serum levels should be closely monitored and patients observed for clinical evidence of toxicity. These precautions probably should apply to digitoxin administration as well.

Anticoagulants
Potentiation of warfarin-type anticoagulant response is almost always seen in patients receiving Cordarone and can result in serious or fatal bleeding. The dose of the anticoagulant should be reduced by one-third to one-half, and prothrombin times should be monitored closely.

Antiarrhythmic Agents
Other antiarrhythmic drugs, such as quinidine, procainamide, disopyramide, and phenytoin, have been used concurrently with Cordarone.

There have been case reports of increased steady-state levels of quinidine, procainamide, and phenytoin during concomitant therapy with Cordarone. In general, any added antiarrhythmic drug should be initiated at a lower than usual dose with careful monitoring.

In general, combination of Cordarone with other antiarrhythmic therapy should be reserved for patients with life-threatening ventricular arrhythmias who are incompletely responsive to a single agent or incompletely responsive to Cordarone. During transfer to Cordarone the dose levels of previously administered agents should be reduced by 30 to 50% several days after the addition of Cordarone, when arrhythmia suppression should be beginning. The continued need for the other antiarrhythmic agent should be reviewed after the effects of Cordarone have been established, and discontinuation ordinarily should be attempted. If the treatment is continued, these patients should be particularly carefully monitored for adverse effects, especially conduction disturbances and exacerbation of tachyarrhythmias, as Cordarone is continued. In Cordarone-treated patients who require additional antiarrhythmic therapy, the initial dose of such agents should be approximately half of the usual recommended dose.

Cordarone should be used with caution in patients receiving β-blocking agents or calcium antagonists because of the possible potentiation of bradycardia, sinus arrest, and AV block; if necessary, Cordarone can continue to be used after insertion of a pacemaker in patients with severe bradycardia or sinus arrest.

[See first table above]

Electrolyte Disturbances

Since antiarrhythmic drugs may be ineffective or may be arrhythmogenic in patients with hypokalemia, any potassium or magnesium deficiency should be corrected before instituting Cordarone therapy.

Carcinogenesis, Mutagenesis, Impairment of Fertility

Cordarone reduced fertility of male and female rats at a dose level of 90 mg/kg/day (8 × highest recommended human maintenance dose).

Cordarone caused a statistically significant, dose-related increase in the incidence of thyroid tumors (follicular adenoma and/or carcinoma) in rats. The incidence of thyroid tumors was greater than control even at the lowest dose level of Cordarone tested, i.e., 5 mg/kg/day or approximately equal to $^1/_2$ the highest recommended human maintenance dose. Mutagenicity studies (Ames, micronucleus, and lysogenic tests) with Cordarone were negative.

Pregnancy: Pregnancy Category D
See "WARNINGS."

Labor and Delivery
It is not known whether the use of Cordarone during labor or delivery has any immediate or delayed adverse effects. Preclinical studies in rodents have not shown any effect of Cordarone on the duration of gestation or on parturition.

Nursing Mothers
Cordarone is excreted in human milk, suggesting that breast-feeding could expose the nursing infant to a significant dose of the drug. Nursing offspring of lactating rats administered Cordarone have been shown to be less viable and have reduced body-weight gains. Therefore, when Cordarone therapy is indicated, the mother should be advised to discontinue nursing.

Pediatric Use
The safety and effectiveness of Cordarone in pediatric patients have not been established.

ADVERSE REACTIONS

Adverse reactions have been very common in virtually all series of patients treated with Cordarone for ventricular arrhythmias with relatively large doses of drug (400 mg/day and above), occurring in about three-fourths of all patients and causing discontinuation in 7 to 18%. The most serious reactions are pulmonary toxicity, exacerbation of arrhythmia, and rare serious liver injury (see "WARNINGS"), but other adverse effects constitute important problems. They are often reversible with dose reduction or cessation of Cordarone treatment. Most of the adverse effects appear to become more frequent with continued treatment beyond six months, although rates appear to remain relatively constant beyond one year. The time and dose relationships of adverse effects are under continued study.

Neurologic problems are extremely common, occurring in 20 to 40% of patients and including malaise and fatigue, tremor and involuntary movements, poor coordination and gait, and peripheral neuropathy; they are rarely a reason to stop therapy and may respond to dose reductions or discontinuation (see "PRECAUTIONS").

Gastrointestinal complaints, most commonly nausea, vomiting, constipation, and anorexia, occur in about 25% of patients but rarely require discontinuation of drug. These commonly occur during high-dose administration (i.e., loading dose) and usually respond to dose reduction or divided doses.

Ophthalmic abnormalities including optic neuropathy and/or optic neuritis, in some cases progressing to permanent blindness, papilledema, corneal degeneration, photosensitivity, eye discomfort, scotoma, lens opacities, and macular degeneration have been reported. (See "WARNINGS.") Asymptomatic corneal microdeposits are present in virtually all adult patients who have been on drug for more than 6 months. Some patients develop eye symptoms of halos, photophobia, and dry eyes. Vision is rarely affected and drug discontinuation is rarely needed.

Dermatological adverse reactions occur in about 15% of patients, with photosensitivity being most common (about 10%). Sunscreen and protection from sun exposure may be helpful, and drug discontinuation is not usually necessary. Prolonged exposure to Cordarone occasionally results in a blue-gray pigmentation. This is slowly and occasionally incompletely reversible on discontinuation of drug but is of cosmetic importance only.

Cardiovascular adverse reactions, other than exacerbation of the arrhythmias, include the uncommon occurrence of congestive heart failure (3%) and bradycardia. Bradycardia

Continued on next page

Cordarone Tablets—Cont.

usually responds to dosage reduction but may require a pacemaker for control. CHF rarely requires drug discontinuation. Cardiac conduction abnormalities occur infrequently and are reversible on discontinuation of drug.

Hepatitis, cholestatic hepatitis, cirrhosis, epididymitis, vasculitis, pseudotumor cerebri, thrombocytopenia, angioedema, bronchiolitis obliterans organizing pneumonia (possibly fatal), pleuritis, pancreatitis, toxic epidermal necrolysis, pancytopenia, and neutropenia also have been reported in patients receiving Cordarone.

The following side-effect rates are based on a retrospective study of 241 patients treated for 2 to 1,515 days (mean 441.3 days).

The following side effects were reported in 10 to 33% of patients:

Gastrointestinal: Nausea and vomiting.

The following side effects were each reported in 4 to 9% of patients:

Dermatologic: Solar dermatitis/photosensitivity.

Neurologic: Malaise and fatigue, tremor/abnormal involuntary movements, lack of coordination, abnormal gait/ataxia, dizziness, paresthesias.

Gastrointestinal: Constipation, anorexia.

Ophthalmologic: Visual disturbances.

Hepatic: Abnormal liver-function tests.

Respiratory: Pulmonary inflammation or fibrosis.

The following side effects were each reported in 1 to 3% of patients:

Thyroid: Hypothyroidism, hyperthyroidism.

Neurologic: Decreased libido, insomnia, headache, sleep disturbances.

Cardiovascular: Congestive heart failure, cardiac arrhythmias, SA node dysfunction.

Gastrointestinal: Abdominal pain.

Hepatic: Nonspecific hepatic disorders.

Other: Flushing, abnormal taste and smell, edema, abnormal salivation, coagulation abnormalities.

The following side effects were each reported in less than 1% of patients:

Blue skin discoloration, rash, spontaneous ecchymosis, alopecia, hypotension, and cardiac conduction abnormalities.

In surveys of almost 5,000 patients treated in open U.S. studies and in published reports of treatment with Cordarone, the adverse reactions most frequently requiring discontinuation of Cordarone included pulmonary infiltrates or fibrosis, paroxysmal ventricular tachycardia, congestive heart failure, and elevation of liver enzymes. Other symptoms causing discontinuations less often included visual disturbances, solar dermatitis, blue skin discoloration, hyperthyroidism and hypothyroidism.

OVERDOSAGE

There have been a few reported cases of Cordarone overdose in which 3 to 8 grams were taken. There were no deaths or permanent sequelae. Animal studies indicate that Cordarone has a high oral LD_{50} (>3,000 mg/kg).

In addition to general supportive measures, the patient's cardiac rhythm and blood pressure should be monitored, and if bradycardia ensues, a β-adrenergic agonist or a pacemaker may be used. Hypotension with inadequate tissue perfusion should be treated with positive inotropic and/or vasopressor agents. Neither Cordarone nor its metabolite is dialyzable.

DOSAGE AND ADMINISTRATION

BECAUSE OF THE UNIQUE PHARMACOKINETIC PROPERTIES, DIFFICULT DOSING SCHEDULE, AND SEVERITY OF THE SIDE EFFECTS IF PATIENTS ARE IMPROPERLY MONITORED, CORDARONE SHOULD BE ADMINISTERED ONLY BY PHYSICIANS WHO ARE EXPERIENCED IN THE TREATMENT OF LIFE-THREATENING ARRHYTHMIAS WHO ARE THOROUGHLY FAMILIAR WITH THE RISKS AND BENEFITS OF CORDARONE THERAPY, AND WHO HAVE ACCESS TO LABORATORY FACILITIES CAPABLE OF ADEQUATELY MONITORING THE EFFECTIVENESS AND SIDE EFFECTS OF TREATMENT.

In order to insure that an antiarrhythmic effect will be observed without waiting several months, loading doses are required. A uniform, optimal dosage schedule for administration of Cordarone has not been determined. Individual patient titration is suggested according to the following guidelines.

For life-threatening ventricular arrhythmias, such as ventricular fibrillation or hemodynamically unstable ventricular tachycardia: Close monitoring of the patients is indicated during the loading phase, particularly until risk of recurrent ventricular tachycardia or fibrillation has abated. Because of the serious nature of the arrhythmia and the lack of predictable time course of effect, loading should be performed in a hospital setting. Loading doses of 800 to 1,600 mg/day are required for 1 to 3 weeks (occasionally longer) until initial therapeutic response occurs. (Administration of Cordarone in divided doses with meals is suggested for total daily doses of 1,000 mg or higher, or when gastrointestinal intolerance occurs.) If side effects become excessive, the dose should be reduced. Elimination of recurrence of ventricular fibrillation and tachycardia usually occurs within 1 to 3 weeks, along with reduction in complex and total ventricular ectopic beats.

Upon starting Cordarone therapy, an attempt should be made to gradually discontinue prior antiarrhythmic drugs (see section on "**Drug Interactions**"). When adequate arrhythmia control is achieved, or if side effects become prominent, Cordarone dose should be reduced to 600 to 800 mg/day for one month and then to the maintenance dose, usually 400 mg/day (see "**CLINICAL PHARMACOLOGY—Monitoring Effectiveness**"). Some patients may require larger maintenance doses, up to 600 mg/day, and some can be controlled on lower doses. Cordarone may be administered as a single daily dose, or in patients with severe gastrointestinal intolerance, as a b.i.d. dose. In each patient, the chronic maintenance dose should be determined according to antiarrhythmic effect as assessed by symptoms, Holter recordings, and/or programmed electrical stimulation and by patient tolerance. Plasma concentrations may be helpful in evaluating nonresponsiveness or unexpectedly severe toxicity (see "**CLINICAL PHARMACOLOGY**").

The lowest effective dose should be used to prevent the occurrence of side effects. In all instances, the physician must be guided by the severity of the individual patient's arrhythmia and response to therapy.

When dosage adjustments are necessary, the patient should be closely monitored for an extended period of time because of the long and variable half-life of Cordarone and the difficulty in predicting the time required to attain a new steady-state level of drug. Dosage suggestions are summarized below:

[See second table at top of previous page]

HOW SUPPLIED

Cordarone® (amiodarone HCl) Tablets are available in bottles of 60 tablets and in Redipak® cartons containing 100 tablets (10 blister strips of 10) as follows:

200 mg, NDC 0008-4188, round, convex-faced, pink tablets with a raised "C" and marked "200" on one side, with reverse side scored and marked "Wyeth" and "4188."

Keep tightly closed.

Store at room temperature, approximately 25° C (77° F).

Protect from light.

Dispense in a light-resistant, tight container.

Use carton to protect contents from light.

Caution: Federal law prohibits dispensing without prescription.

Manufactured for
Wyeth Laboratories Inc.
A Wyeth-Ayerst Company
Philadelphia, PA 19101
by Sanofi Winthrop Industrie
1, rue de la Vierge
33440 Ambares, France

Shown in Product Identification Guide, page 343

CORDARONE® INTRAVENOUS ℞
(amiodarone hydrochloride)

DESCRIPTION

Cordarone Intravenous (Cordarone I.V.) contains amiodarone HCl ($C_{25}H_{29}I_2NO_3 \cdot HCl$), a class III antiarrhythmic drug. Amiodarone HCl is (2-butyl-3-benzofuranyl)[4-[2-(diethylamino)ethoxy]-3,5-diiodophenyl]methanone hydrochloride. Amiodarone HCl has the following structural formula:

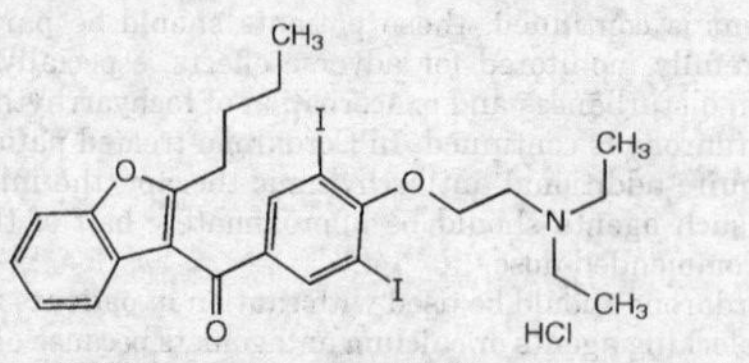

Amiodarone HCl is a white to slightly yellow crystalline powder, and is very slightly soluble in water. It has a molecular weight of 681.78 and contains 37.3% iodine by weight. Cordarone I.V. is a sterile clear, pale-yellow solution visually free from particulates. Each milliliter of the Cordarone I.V. formulation contains 50 mg of amiodarone HCl, 20.2 mg of benzyl alcohol, 100 mg of polysorbate 80, and water for injection.

CLINICAL PHARMACOLOGY

MECHANISMS OF ACTION

Amiodarone is generally considered a class III antiarrhythmic drug, but it possesses electrophysiologic characteristics of all four Vaughan Williams classes. Like class I drugs, amiodarone blocks sodium channels at rapid pacing frequencies, and like class II drugs, it exerts a noncompetitive antisympathetic action. One of its main effects, with prolonged administration, is to lengthen the cardiac action potential, a class III effect. The negative chronotropic effect of amiodarone in nodal tissues is similar to the effect of class IV drugs. In addition to blocking sodium channels, amiodarone blocks myocardial potassium channels, which contributes to slowing of conduction and prolongation of refractoriness. The antisympathetic action and the block of calcium and potassium channels are responsible for the negative dromotropic effects on the sinus node and for the slowing of conduction and prolongation of refractoriness in the atrioventricular (AV) node. Its vasodilatory action can decrease cardiac workload and consequently myocardial oxygen consumption.

Cordarone I.V. administration prolongs intranodal conduction (Atrial-His, AH) and refractoriness of the atrioventricular node (ERP AVN), but has little or no effect on sinus cycle length (SCL), refractoriness of the right atrium and right ventricle (ERP RA and ERP RV), repolarization (QTc), intraventricular conduction (QRS), and infranodal conduction (His-ventricular, HV). A comparison of the electrophysiologic effects of Cordarone I.V. and oral Cordarone is shown in the table below.

EFFECTS OF INTRAVENOUS AND ORAL CORDARONE ON ELECTROPHYSIOLOGIC PARAMETERS

Formulation	SCL	QRS	QTc	AH	HV	ERP RA	ERP RV	ERP AVN
I.V.	↔	↔	↔	↑	↔	↔	↔	↑
Oral	↑	↔	↑	↑	↔	↑	↑	↑

↔No change

At higher doses (>10 mg/kg) of Cordarone I.V., prolongation of the ERP RV and modest prolongation of the QRS have been seen. These differences between oral and intravenous administration suggest that the initial acute effects of Cordarone I.V. may be predominantly focused on the AV node, causing an intranodal conduction delay and increased nodal refractoriness due to slow channel blockade (class IV activity) and noncompetitive adrenergic antagonism (class II activity).

PHARMACOKINETICS AND METABOLISM

Amiodarone exhibits complex disposition characteristics after intravenous administration. Peak serum concentrations after single 5 mg/kg 15-minute intravenous infusions in healthy subjects range between 5 and 41 mg/L. Peak concentrations after 10-minute infusions of 150 mg Cordarone I.V. in patients with ventricular fibrillation (VF) or hemodynamically unstable ventricular tachycardia (VT) range between 7 and 26 mg/L. Due to rapid distribution, serum concentrations decline to 10% of peak values within 30 to 45 minutes after the end of the infusion. In clinical trials, after 48 hours of continued infusions (125, 500, or 1000 mg/day) plus supplemental (150 mg) infusions (for recurrent arrhythmias), amiodarone mean serum concentrations between 0.7 to 1.4 mg/L were observed (n=260).

N-desethylamiodarone (DEA) is the major active metabolite of amiodarone in humans. DEA serum concentrations above 0.05 mg/L are not usually seen until after several days of continuous infusion but with prolonged therapy reach approximately the same concentration as amiodarone. The enzymes responsible for the N-deethylation are believed to be the cytochrome P-450 3A (CYP3A) subfamily, principally CYP3A4. This isozyme is present in both the liver and intestines. The highly variable systemic availability of oral amiodarone may be attributed potentially to large interindividual variability in CYP3A4 activity.

Amiodarone is eliminated primarily by hepatic metabolism and biliary excretion and there is negligible excretion of amiodarone or DEA in urine. Neither amiodarone nor DEA is dialyzable. Amiodarone and DEA cross the placenta and both appear in breast milk.

No data are available on the activity of DEA in humans, but in animals, it has significant electrophysiologic and antiarrhythmic effects generally similar to amiodarone itself. DEA's precise role and contribution to the antiarrhythmic activity of oral amiodarone are not certain. The development of maximal ventricular class III effects after oral Cordarone administration in humans correlates more closely with DEA accumulation over time than with amiodarone accumulation. On the other hand (see CLINICAL TRIALS), after Cordarone I.V. administration, there is evidence of activity well before significant concentrations of DEA are attained.

The following table summarizes the mean ranges of pharmacokinetic parameters of amiodarone reported in single dose i.v. (5 mg/kg over 15 min) studies of healthy subjects.

PHARMACOKINETIC PROFILE AFTER I.V. AMIODARONE ADMINISTRATION

Drug	Clearance (mL/h/kg)	V_c (L/kg)	V_{ss} (L/kg)	$t_{1/2}$ (days)
Amiodarone	90–158	0.2	40–84	20–47
Desethylamiodarone	197–290	—	68–168	≥AMI $t_{1/2}$

Notes: V_c and V_{ss} denote the central and steady-state volumes of distribution from i.v. studies.
"—" denotes not available.

Desethylamiodarone clearance and volume involve an unknown biotransformation factor.

The systemic availability of ***oral*** amiodarone in healthy subjects ranges between 33% and 65%.

From *in vitro* studies, the protein binding of amiodarone is >96%.

In clinical studies of 2 to 7 days, clearance of amiodarone after intravenous administration in patients with VT and VF ranged between 220 and 440 mL/h/kg. Age, sex, renal disease, and hepatic disease (cirrhosis) do not have marked effects on the disposition of amiodarone or DEA. Renal impairment does not influence the pharmacokinetics of amiodarone. After a single dose of Cordarone I.V. in cirrhotic patients, significantly lower C_{max} and average concentration values are seen for DEA, but mean amiodarone levels are unchanged. Normal subjects over 65 years of age show lower clearances (about 100 mL/hr/kg) than younger subjects (about 150 mL/hr/kg) and an increase in $t_{1/2}$ from about 20 to 47 days. In patients with severe left ventricular dysfunction, the pharmacokinetics of amiodarone are not significantly altered but the terminal disposition $t_{1/2}$ of DEA is prolonged. Although no dosage adjustment for patients with renal, hepatic, or cardiac abnormalities has been defined during chronic treatment with ***oral*** Cordarone, close clinical monitoring is prudent for elderly patients and those with severe left ventricular dysfunction.

There is no established relationship between drug concentration and therapeutic response for short-term intravenous use. Steady-state amiodarone concentrations of 1 to 2.5 mg/L have been associated with antiarrhythmic effects and acceptable toxicity following chronic ***oral*** Cordarone therapy.

PHARMACODYNAMICS

Cordarone I.V. has been reported to produce negative inotropic and vasodilatory effects in animals and humans. In clinical studies of patients with refractory VF or hemodynamically unstable VT, treatment-emergent, drug-related hypotension occurred in 288 of 1836 patients (16%) treated with Cordarone I.V. No correlations were seen between the baseline ejection fraction and the occurrence of clinically significant hypotension during infusion of Cordarone I.V.

CLINICAL TRIALS

Apart from studies in patients with VT or VF, described below, there are two other studies of amiodarone showing an antiarrhythmic effect before significant levels of DEA could have accumulated. A placebo-controlled study of i.v. amiodarone (300 mg over 2 hours followed by 1200 mg/day) in post-coronary artery bypass graft patients with supraventricular and 2- to 3-consecutive-beat ventricular arrhythmias showed a reduction in arrhythmias from 12 hours on. A baseline-controlled study using a similar i.v. regimen in patients with recurrent, refractory VT/VF also showed rapid onset of antiarrhythmic activity; amiodarone therapy reduced episodes of VT by 85% compared to baseline.

The acute effectiveness of Cordarone I.V. in suppressing recurrent VF or hemodynamically unstable VT is supported by two randomized, parallel, dose-response studies of approximately 300 patients each. In these studies, patients with at least two episodes of VF or hemodynamically unstable VT in the preceding 24 hours were randomly assigned to receive doses of approximately 125 or 1000 mg over the first 24 hours, an 8-fold difference. In one study, a middle dose of approximately 500 mg was evaluated. The dose regimen consisted of an initial rapid loading infusion, followed by a slower 6-hour loading infusion, and then an 18-hour maintenance infusion. The maintenance infusion was continued up to hour 48. Additional 10-minute infusions of 150 mg Cordarone I.V. were given for "breakthrough" VT/VF more frequently to the 125-mg dose group, thereby considerably reducing the planned 8-fold differences in total dose to 1.8- and 2.6- fold, respectively, in the two studies.

The prospectively defined primary efficacy end point was the rate of VT/VF episodes per hour. For both studies, the median rate was 0.02 episodes per hour in patients receiving the high dose and 0.07 episodes per hour in patients receiving the low dose, or approximately 0.5 versus 1.7 episodes per day (p=0.07, 2-sided, in both studies). In one study, the time to first episode of VT/VF was significantly prolonged (approximately 10 hours in patients receiving the low dose and 14 hours in patients receiving the high dose). In both studies, significantly fewer supplemental infusions were given to patients in the high-dose group. Mortality was not affected in these studies; at the end of double-blind therapy or after 48 hours, all patients were given open access to whatever treatment (including Cordarone I.V.) was deemed necessary.

INDICATIONS AND USAGE

Cordarone I.V. is indicated for initiation of treatment and prophylaxis of frequently recurring ventricular fibrillation and hemodynamically unstable ventricular tachycardia in patients refractory to other therapy. Cordarone I.V. also can be used to treat patients with VT/VF for whom oral Cordarone is indicated, but who are unable to take oral medication. During or after treatment with Cordarone I.V., patients may be transferred to oral Cordarone theray (see **DOSAGE AND ADMINISTRATION**).

Cordarone I.V. should be used for acute treatment until the patient's ventricular arrhythmias are stabilized. Most patients will require this therapy for 48 to 96 hours, but Cordarone I.V. may be safely administered for longer periods if necessary.

CONTRAINDICATIONS

Cordarone I.V. is contraindicated in patients with known hypersensitivity to any of the components of Cordarone I.V., or in patients with cardiogenic shock, marked sinus bradycardia, and second- or third-degree AV block unless a functioning pacemaker is available.

WARNINGS

HYPOTENSION

Hypotension is the most common adverse effect seen with Cordarone I.V. In clinical trials, treatment-emergent, drug-related hypotension was reported as an adverse effect in 288 (16%) of 1836 patients treated with Cordarone I.V. Clinically significant hypotension during infusions was seen most often in the first several hours of treatment and was not dose related, but appeared to be related to the rate of infusion. Hypotension necessitating alterations in Cordarone I.V. therapy was reported in 3% of patients, with permanent discontinuation required in less than 2% of patients. Hypotension should be treated initially by slowing the infusion; additional standard therapy may be needed, including the following: vasopressor drugs, positive inotropic agents, and volume expansion. ***The initial rate of infusion should be monitored closely and should not exceed that prescribed in*** **DOSAGE AND ADMINISTRATION**.

BRADYCARDIA AND AV BLOCK

Drug-related bradycardia occurred in 90 (4.9%) of 1836 patients in clinical trials while they were receiving Cordarone I.V. for life-threatening VT/VF; it was not dose-related. Bradycardia should be treated by slowing the infusion rate or discontinuing Cordarone I.V. In some patients, inserting a pacemaker is required. Despite such measures, bradycardia was progressive and terminal in 1 patient during the controlled trials. Patients with a known predisposition to bradycardia or AV block should be treated with Cordarone I.V. in a setting where a temporary pacemaker is available.

LONG-TERM USE

See labeling for oral Cordarone. There has been limited experience in patients receiving Cordarone I.V. for longer than 3 weeks.

NEONATAL HYPO- OR HYPERTHYROIDISM

Although ***oral*** Cordarone use during pregnancy is uncommon, there have been a small number of published reports of congenital goiter/hypothyroidism and hyperthyroidism. If Cordarone I.V. is administered during pregnancy, the patient should be apprised of the potential hazard to the fetus.

PRECAUTIONS

Cordarone I.V. should be administered only by physicians who are experienced in the treatment of life-threatening arrhythmias, who are thoroughly familiar with the risks and benefits of Cordarone therapy, and who have access to facilities adequate for monitoring the effectiveness and side effects of treatment.

LIVER ENZYME ELEVATIONS

Elevations of blood hepatic enzyme values—alanine aminotransferase (ALT), aspartate aminotransferase (AST), and gamma-glutamyl transferase (GGT)—are seen commonly in patients with immediately life-threatening VT/VF. Interpreting elevated AST activity can be difficult because the values may be elevated in patients who have had recent myocardial infarction, congestive heart failure, or multiple electrical defibrillations. Approximately 54% of patients receiving Cordarone I.V. in clinical studies had baseline liver enzyme elevations, and 13% had clinically significant elevations. In 81% of patients with both baseline and on-therapy data available, the liver enzyme elevations either improved during therapy or remained at baseline levels. Baseline abnormalities in hepatic enzymes are not a contraindication to treatment.

Two (2) cases of fatal hepatocellular necrosis after treatment with Cordarone I.V. have been reported. The patients, one 28 years of age and the other 60 years of age, were treated for atrial arrhythmias with an initial infusion of 1500 mg over 5 hours, a rate much higher than recommended. Both patients developed hepatic and renal failure within 24 hours after the start of Cordarone I.V. treatment and died on day 14 and day 4, respectively. Because these episodes of hepatic necrosis may have been due to the rapid rate of infusion with possible rate-related hypotension, ***the initial rate of infusion should be monitored closely and should not exceed that prescribed in*** **DOSAGE AND ADMINISTRATION**.

In patients with life-threatening arrhythmias, the potential risk of hepatic injury should be weighed against the potential benefit of Cordarone I.V. therapy, but patients receiving Cordarone I.V. should be monitored carefully for evidence of progressive hepatic injury. Consideration should be given to reducing the rate of administration or withdrawing Cordarone I.V. in such cases.

PROARRHYTHMIA

Like all antiarrhythmic agents, Cordarone I.V. may cause a worsening of existing arrhythmias or precipitate a new arrhythmia. Proarrhythmia, primarily torsades de pointes, has been associated with prolongation by Cordarone I.V. of the QTc interval to 500 ms or greater. Although QTc prolongation occurred frequently in patients receiving Cordarone I.V., torsades de pointes or new-onset VF occurred infrequently (less than 2%). Patients should be monitored for QTc prolongation during infusion with Cordarone I.V.

PULMONARY DISORDERS

ARDS

Two percent (2%) of patients were reported to have adult respiratory distress syndrome (ARDS) during clinical studies. ARDS is a disorder characterized by bilateral, diffuse pulmonary infiltrates with pulmonary edema and varying degrees of respiratory insufficiency. The clinical and radiographic picture can arise after a variety of lung injuries, such as those resulting from trauma, shock, prolonged cardiopulmonary resuscitation, and aspiration pneumonia, conditions present in many of the patients enrolled in the clinical studies. It is not possible to determine what role, if any, Cordarone I.V. played in causing or exacerbating the pulmonary disorder in those patients.

Pulmonary fibrosis

Only 1 of more than 1000 patients treated with Cordarone I.V. in clinical studies developed pulmonary fibrosis. In that patient, the condition was diagnosed 3 months after treatment with Cordarone I.V., during which time she received ***oral*** Cordarone. Pulmonary toxicity is a well-recognized complication of long-term Cordarone use (see labeling for oral Cordarone).

SURGERY

Close perioperative monitoring is recommended in patients undergoing general anesthesia who are on amiodarone therapy as they may be more sensitive to the myocardial depressant and conduction effects of halogenated inhalational anesthetics.

DRUG INTERACTIONS

Amiodarone can inhibit metabolism mediated by cytochrome P-450 enzymes, probably accounting for the significant effects of oral Cordarone (and presumably Cordarone I.V.) on the pharmacokinetics of various therapeutic agents including digoxin, quinidine, procainamide, warfarin (CYP2C9), dextromethorphan (CYP2D6), and cyclosporine (CYP3A4). Hemodynamic and electrophysiologic interactions have also been observed after concomitant administration with propranolol, diltiazem, and verapamil. Conversely, agents producing a significant effect on amiodarone pharmacokinetics include phenytoin, cimetidine, and cholestyramine. Because of the long half-life of amiodarone, drug interactions may persist long after discontinuation of drug administration. Few data are available on drug interactions with Cordarone I.V. Except as noted, the following tables summarize the important interactions between ***oral*** Cordarone and other therapeutic agents.

SUMMARY OF DRUG INTERACTIONS WITH CORDARONE
Drugs Whose Effects May Be Increased by Cordarone

Concomitant Drug	Interaction
Warfarin	Increases prothrombin time.
Digoxin	Increases serum concentration.
Quinidine	Increases serum concentration.
Procainamide	Increases serum concentration, NAPA concentration.
Disopyramide	Increases QT prolongation which could cause arrhythmia.
Fentanyl	May cause hypotension, bradycardia, decreased cardiac output.
Flecainide	Reduces the dose of flecainide needed to maintain therapeutic plasma concentrations.
Lidocaine	**Oral:** Sinus bradycardia was observed in a patient receiving oral Cordarone who was given lidocaine for local anesthesia. **I.V.:** Seizure associated with increased lidocaine concentrations was observed in one patient.
Cyclosporine	Produces persistently elevated plasma concentrations of cyclosporine resulting in elevated creatinine, despite reduction in dose of cyclosporine.

Continued on next page

Cordarone Intravenous—Cont.

Study Event	Controlled Studies (n=814)		Open-Label Studies (n=1022)		Total (n=1836)	
Body as a Whole						
Fever	24	(2.9%)	13	(1.2%)	37	(2.0%)
Cardiovascular System						
Bradycardia	49	(6.0%)	41	(4.0%)	90	(4.9%)
Congestive heart failure	18	(2.2%)	21	(2.0%)	39	(2.1%)
Heart arrest	29	(3.5%)	26	(2.5%)	55	(2.9%)
Hypotension	165	(20.2%)	123	(12.0%)	288	(15.6%)
Ventricular tachycardia	15	(1.8%)	30	(2.9%)	45	(2.4%)
Digestive System						
Liver function test abnormal	35	(4.2%)	29	(2.8%)	64	(3.4%)
Nausea	29	(3.5%)	43	(4.2%)	72	(3.9%)

SUMMARY OF DRUG INTERACTIONS WITH CORDARONE
Drugs that May Interfere with the Actions of Cordarone

Concomitant Drug	Interaction
Cholestyramine	Increases enterohepatic elimination of amiodarone and may reduce serum levels and $t_{1/2}$.
Cimetidine	Increases serum amiodarone levels.
Phenytoin	Decreases serum amiodarone levels.

Potential drug class interactions with Cordarone
Beta Blockers: Since Cordarone has weak beta blocking activity, use with beta blocking agents could increase risk of hypotension and bradycardia.
Calcium Channel Blockers: Cordarone inhibits atrioventricular conduction and decreases myocardial contractility, increasing the risk of AV block with verapamil or diltiazem or of hypotension with any calcium channel blocker.
Volatile Anesthetic Agents: (see **Precautions**—SURGERY).
In addition to the interactions noted above, chronic (>2 weeks) *oral* Cordarone administration impairs metabolism of phenytoin, dextromethorphan, and methotrexate.

ELECTROLYTE DISTURBANCES
Patients with hypokalemia or hypomagnesemia should have the condition corrected whenever possible before being treated with Cordarone I.V., as these disorders can exaggerate the degree of QTc prolongation and increase the potential for torsades de pointes. Special attention should be given to electrolyte and acid-base balance in patients experiencing severe or prolonged diarrhea or in patients receiving concomitant diuretics.

CARCINOGENESIS, MUTAGENESIS, IMPAIRMENT OF FERTILITY
No carcinogenicity studies were conducted with Cordarone I.V. However, *oral* Cordarone caused a statistically significant, dose-related increase in the incidence of thyroid adenomas in rats. The incidence of thyroid adenomas in rats was greater than the incidence in controls even at the lowest tested dose of 5 mg/kg/day (about 0.1 times the maximum recommended oral human maintenance dose in mg/m²).
Mutagenicity studies conducted with amiodarone HCl (Ames, micronucleus, and lysogenic induction tests) were negative.
No fertility studies were conducted with Cordarone I.V. However, *oral* Cordarone administration resulted in reduced fertility of rats at a dose of 90 mg/kg/day (about 1.3 times the maximum recommended oral human maintenance dose in mg/m²). No significant effects on fertility occurred at 30 mg/kg/day.

PREGNANCY
Category D. See **WARNINGS** and NEONATAL HYPO- OR HYPERTHYROIDISM.
In addition to causing infrequent congenital goiter/hypothyroidism and hyperthyroidism, amiodarone has caused a variety of adverse effects in animals.
In a reproductive study in which amiodarone was given intravenously to rabbits at dosages of 5, 10, or 25 mg/kg per day (about 0.1, 0.3, and 0.7 times the maximum recommended human dose [MRHD] on a body surface area basis), maternal deaths occurred in all groups, including controls. Embryotoxicity (as manifested by fewer full-term fetuses and increased resorptions with concomitantly lower litter weights) occurred at dosages of 10 mg/kg and above. No evidence of embryotoxicity was observed at 5 mg/kg and no teratogenicity was observed at any dosages.
In a teratology study in which amiodarone was administered by continuous i.v. infusion to rats at dosages of 25, 50, or 100 mg/kg per day (about 0.4, 0.7, and 1.4 times the MRHD when compared on a body surface area basis), maternal toxicity (as evidenced by reduced weight gain and food consumption) and embryotoxicity (as evidenced by increased resorptions, decreased live litter size, reduced body weights, and retarded sternum and metacarpal ossification) were observed in the 100 mg/kg group.
Cordarone I.V. should be used during pregnancy only if the potential benefit to the mother justifies the risk to the fetus.

NURSING MOTHERS
Amiodarone is excreted in human milk, suggesting that breast-feeding could expose the nursing infant to a significant dose of the drug. Nursing offspring of lactating rats administered amiodarone have demonstrated reduced viability and reduced body weight gains. The risk of exposing the infant to amiodarone should be weighed against the potential benefit of arrhythmia suppression in the mother. The mother should be advised to discontinue nursing.

LABOR AND DELIVERY
It is not known whether the use of Cordarone during labor or delivery has any immediate or delayed adverse effects. Preclinical studies in rodents have not shown any effect on the duration of gestation or on parturition.

PEDIATRIC USAGE
The safety and efficacy of Cordarone in the pediatric population have not been established; therefore, its use in pediatric patients is not recommended.

ADVERSE REACTIONS
In a total of 1836 patients in controlled and uncontrolled clinical trials, 14% of patients received Cordarone I.V. for at least 1 week, 5% received it for at least 2 weeks, 2% received it for at least 3 weeks, and 1% received it for more than 3 weeks, without an increased incidence of severe adverse reactions. The mean duration of therapy in these studies was 5.6 days; median exposure was 3.7 days.
The most important treatment-emergent adverse effects were hypotension, asystole/cardiac arrest/electromechanical dissociation (EMD), cardiogenic shock, congestive heart failure, bradycardia, liver function test abnormalities, VT, and AV block. Overall, treatment was discontinued for about 9% of the patients because of adverse effects. The most common adverse effects leading to discontinuation of Cordarone I.V. therapy were hypotension (1.6%), asystole/cardiac arrest/EMD (1.2%), VT (1.1%), and cardiogenic shock (1%).
The following table lists the most common (incidence ≥2%) treatment-emergent adverse events during Cordarone I.V. therapy considered at least possibly drug-related. These data were collected from the Wyeth-Ayerst clinical trials involving 1836 patients with life-threatening VT/VF. Data from all assigned treatment groups are pooled because none of the adverse events appeared to be dose-related.
[See table at top right of page]
Other treatment-emergent possibly drug-related adverse events reported in less than 2% of patients receiving Cordarone I.V. in Wyeth-Ayerst controlled and uncontrolled studies included the following: abnormal kidney function, atrial fibrillation, diarrhea, increased ALT, increased AST, lung edema, nodal arrhythmia, prolonged QT interval, respiratory disorder, shock, sinus bradycardia, Stevens-Johnson syndrome, thrombocytopenia, VF, and vomiting.
In postmarketing surveillance, toxic epidermal necrolysis also has been reported with amiodarone therapy.

OVERDOSAGE
The most likely effects of an inadvertent overdose of Cordarone I.V. are hypotension, cardiogenic shock, bradycardia, AV block, and hepatotoxicity. Hypotension and cardiogenic shock should be treated by slowing the infusion rate or with standard therapy: vasopressor drugs, positive inotropic agents, and volume expansion. Bradycardia and AV block may require temporary pacing. Hepatic enzyme concentrations should be monitored closely.

Amiodarone is not dialyzable.

DOSAGE AND ADMINISTRATION
Amiodarone shows considerable interindividual variation in response. Thus, although a starting dose adequate to suppress life-threatening arrhythmias is needed, close monitoring with adjustment of dose as needed is essential. The recommended starting dose of Cordarone I.V. is about 1000 mg over the first 24 hours of therapy, delivered by the following infusion regimen:

CORDARONE I.V. DOSE RECOMMENDATIONS — FIRST 24 HOURS —

Loading infusions

First Rapid:	**150 mg over the FIRST 10 minutes (15 mg/min).** Add 3 mL of Cordarone I.V. (150 mg) to 100 mL D₅W (concentration = 1.5 mg/mL). Infuse 100 mL over 10 minutes.
Followed by Slow:	**360 mg over the NEXT 6 hours (1 mg/min).** Add 18 mL of Cordarone I.V. (900 mg) to 500 mL D₅W (concentration = 1.8 mg/mL).
Maintenance infusion	**540 mg over the REMAINING 18 hours (0.5 mg/min).** Decrease the rate of the slow loading infusion to 0.5 mg/min.

After the first 24 hours, the maintenance infusion rate of 0.5 mg/min (720 mg/24 hours) should be continued utilizing a concentration of 1 to 6 mg/mL (Cordarone I.V. concentrations greater than 2 mg/mL should be administered via a central venous catheter). In the event of breakthrough episodes of VF or hemodynamically unstable VT, 150-mg supplemental infusions of Cordarone I.V. mixed in 100 mL of D₅W may be administered. Such infusions should be administered over 10 minutes to minimize the potential for hypotension. The rate of the maintenance infusion may be increased to achieve effective arrhythmia suppression.
The first 24-hour dose may be individualized for each patient; however, in controlled clinical trials, mean daily doses above 2100 mg were associated with an increased risk of hypotension. The initial infusion rate should not exceed 30 mg/min.
Based on the experience from clinical studies of Cordarone I.V., a maintenance infusion of up to 0.5 mg/min can be cautiously continued for 2 to 3 weeks regardless of the patient's age, renal function, or left ventricular function. There has been limited experience in patients receiving Cordarone I.V. for longer than 3 weeks.

AMIODARONE HCl SOLUTION STABILITY

Solution	Concentration (mg/mL)	Container	Comments
5% Dextrose in Water (D₅W)	1.0–6.0	PVC	Physically compatible, with amiodarone loss <10% at 2 hours.
5% Dextrose in Water (D₅W)	1.0–6.0	Polyolefin, Glass	Physically compatible, with no amiodarone loss at 24 hours.

Y-SITE INJECTION INCOMPATIBILITY

Drug	Vehicle	Amiodarone Concentration	Comments
Aminophylline	D₅W	4 mg/mL	Precipitate
Cefamandole Nafate	D₅W	4 mg/mL	Precipitate
Cefazolin Sodium	D₅W	4 mg/mL	Precipitate
Mezlocillin Sodium	D₅W	4 mg/mL	Precipitate
Heparin Sodium	D₅W	—	Precipitate
Sodium Bicarbonate	D₅W	3 mg/mL	Precipitate

The surface properties of solutions containing injectable amiodarone are altered such that the drop size may be reduced. This reduction may lead to underdosage of the patient by up to 30% if drop counter infusion sets are used. Cordarone I.V. must be delivered by a volumetric infusion pump.

Cordarone I.V. should, whenever possible, be administered through a central venous catheter dedicated to that purpose. An in-line filter should be used during administration. Cordarone I.V. concentrations greater than 3 mg/mL in D_5W have been associated with a high incidence of peripheral vein phlebitis; however, concentrations of 2.5 mg/mL or less appear to be less irritating. Therefore, for infusions longer than 1 hour, Cordarone I.V. concentrations should not exceed 2 mg/mL unless a central venous catheter is used.

Cordarone I.V. infusions exceeding 2 hours must be administered in glass or polyolefin bottles containing D_5W. Use of evacuated glass containers for admixing Cordarone I.V. is not recommended as incompatibility with a buffer in the container may cause precipitation.

It is well known that amiodarone adsorbs to polyvinyl chloride (PVC) tubing and the clinical trial dose administration schedule was designed to account for this adsorption. All of the clinical trials were conducted using PVC tubing and its use is therefore recommended. The concentrations and rates of infusion provided in **DOSAGE AND ADMINISTRATION** reflect doses identified in these studies. It is important that the recommended infusion regimen be followed closely.

Cordarone I.V. does not need to be protected from light during administration.

[See first table at bottom of previous page]

ADMIXTURE INCOMPATIBILITY

Cordarone I.V. in D_5W is incompatible with the drugs shown below.

[See second table at bottom of previous page]

INTRAVENOUS TO ORAL TRANSITION

Patients whose arrhythmias have been suppressed by Cordarone I.V. may be switched to oral Cordarone. The optimal dose for changing from intravenous to oral administration of Cordarone I.V. will depend on the dose of Cordarone I.V. already administered, as well as the bioavailability of oral Cordarone. When changing to oral Cordarone therapy, clinical monitoring is recommended, particularly for elderly patients.

The following table provides suggested doses of oral Cordarone to be initiated after varying durations of Cordarone I.V. administration. These recommendations are made on the basis of a comparable total body amount of amiodarone delivered by the intravenous and oral routes, based on 50% bioavailability of oral amiodarone.

RECOMMENDATIONS FOR ORAL DOSAGE AFTER I.V. INFUSION

Duration of Cordarone I.V. Infusion#	Initial Daily Dose of Oral Cordarone
<1 week	800–1600 mg
1—3 weeks	600–800 mg
>3 weeks*	400 mg

\# Assuming a 720 mg/day infusion (0.5 mg/min).

* Cordarone I.V is not intended for maintenance treatment.

HOW SUPPLIED

Cordarone® I.V. (amiodarone HCl) is available in packages of 10 ampuls (2 cartons each containing 5 ampuls, 3 mL each, as follows:
50 mg per mL, NDC 0008-0814-01.
Store at room temperature, 15° to 25°C (59° to 77°F).
Protect from light and excessive heat.
Use carton to protect contents from light until used.
Manufactured by:
Wyeth Laboratories Inc.
A Wyeth-Ayerst Company
Philadelphia, PA 19101
by arrangement with Sanofi S.A.

CRINONE™ 4%
CRINONE™ 8%

R

[crĭ ′nōn]
(progesterone gel)

DESCRIPTION

CRINONE™ (progesterone gel) is a bioadhesive vaginal gel containing micronized progesterone in an emulsion system, which is contained in single use, one piece polyethylene vaginal applicators. The carrier vehicle is an oil in water emulsion containing the water swellable, but insoluble polymer, polycarbophil. The progesterone is partially soluble in both the oil and water phase of the vehicle, with the majority of

the progesterone existing as a suspension. Physically, CRINONE has the appearance of a soft, white to off-white gel.

The active ingredient, progesterone, is present in either a 4% or an 8% concentration (w/w). The chemical name for progesterone is pregn-4-ene-3,20-dione. It has an empirical formula of $C_{21}H_{30}O_2$ and a molecular weight of 314.5. The structural formula is:

Progesterone exists in two polymorphic forms. Form 1, which is the form used in CRINONE, exists as white orthorhombic prisms with a melting point of 127–131°C.

Each applicator delivers 1.125 grams of CRINONE gel containing either 45 mg (4% gel) or 90 mg (8% gel) of progesterone in a base containing glycerin, mineral oil, polycarbophil, carbomer 934P, hydrogenated palm oil glyceride, sorbic acid, sodium hydroxide and purified water.

CLINICAL PHARMACOLOGY

Progesterone is a naturally occurring steroid that is secreted by the ovary, placenta, and adrenal gland. In the presence of adequate estrogen, progesterone transforms a proliferative endometrium into a secretory endometrium. Progesterone is essential for the development of decidual tissue, and the effect of progesterone on the differentiation of glandular epithelia and stroma has been extensively studied. Progesterone is necessary to increase endometrial receptivity for implantation of an embryo. Once an embryo is implanted, progesterone acts to maintain the pregnancy. Normal or near-normal endometrial responses to oral estradiol and intramuscular progesterone have been noted in functionally agonadal women through the sixth decade of life. Progesterone administration decreases the circulatory levels of gonadotropins.

Pharmacokinetics

Absorption

Due to sustained release properties of CRINONE, progesterone absorption is prolonged with an absorption half-life of approximately 25–50 hours, and an elimination half-life of 5–20 minutes. Therefore, the pharmacokinetics of CRINONE are rate-limited by absorption rather than by elimination.

The bioavailability of progesterone in CRINONE was determined relative to progesterone administered intramuscularly. In a single dose cross-over study, 20 healthy, estrogenized postmenopausal women received 45 mg or 90 mg progesterone vaginally in CRINONE 4% or CRINONE 8%, or 45 mg or 90 mg progesterone intramuscularly. The pharmacokinetic parameters (mean ± standard deviation) are shown in Table 1.

[See table 1 below]

The multiple dose pharmacokinetics of CRINONE 4% and CRINONE 8% administered every other day and CRINONE 8% administered daily or twice daily for 12 days were studied in 10 healthy, estrogenized postmenopausal women in two separate studies. Steady state was achieved within the first 24 hours after initiation of treatment. The pharmacokinetic parameters (mean ± standard deviation) after the last administration of CRINONE 4% or 8% derived from these studies are shown in Table 2.

[See table 2 at bottom of next page]

Distribution

Progesterone is extensively bound to serum proteins (≈ 96–99%), primarily to serum albumin and corticosteroid binding globulin.

Metabolism

The major urinary metabolite of oral progesterone is 5β-pregnan-3α, 20α-diol glucuronide which is present in plasma in the conjugated form only. Plasma metabolites also include 5β-pregnan-3α-ol-20-one (5β-pregnanolone) and 5α-pregnan-3α-ol-20-one (5α-pregnanolone).

Excretion

Progesterone undergoes both biliary and renal elimination. Following an injection of labeled progesterone, 50–60% of the excretion of progesterone metabolites occurs via the kidney; approximately 10% occurs via the bile and feces, the second major excretory pathway. Overall recovery of labeled material accounts for 70% of an administered dose, with the remainder of the dose not characterized with respect to elimination. Only a small portion of unchanged progesterone is excreted in the bile.

Clinical Studies

Assisted Reproductive Technology

In a single-center, open-label study (COL 1620-007US), 99 women (aged 28–47 years) with either partial (n=84) or premature ovarian failure (n=15) who were candidates to receive a donor oocyte transfer as an Assisted Reproductive Technology ("ART") procedure were randomized to receive either CRINONE 8% twice daily (n=68) or intramuscular progesterone 100 mg daily (n=31). The study was divided into three phases (Pilot, Donor Egg and Treatment). The first phase of the study consisted of a test Pilot Cycle to ensure that the administration of transdermal estradiol and progesterone would adequately prime the endometrium to receive the donor egg. The second phase was the Donor Egg Cycle during which a fertilized oocyte was implanted. CRINONE 8% was administered beginning the evening of Day 14 of the Pilot and Donor Egg cycles. Subjects with partial ovarian function also underwent a Pre-Pilot Cycle and a Pre-Donor Egg Cycle during which time they were administered only leuprolide acetate to suppress remaining ovarian function. The Pre-Pilot Cycle, Pilot Cycle, Pre-Donor Egg Cycle, and Donor Egg Cycle each lasted approximately 34 days. The third phase of the study consisted of a 10-week treatment period to maintain a pregnancy until placental autonomy was achieved.

Sixty-one women received CRINONE 8% as part of the Pilot Cycle to determine their endometrial response. Of the 55 evaluable endometrial biopsies in the CRINONE 8% group performed on Day 25–27, all were histologically "in-phase", consistent with luteal phase biopsy specimens of menstruating women at comparable time intervals. Fifty-four women who received CRINONE 8% and had a histologically "in-phase" biopsy received a donor oocyte transfer. Among these 54 CRINONE-treated women, clinical pregnancies (assessed about week 10 after transfer by clinical examination, ultrasound and/or β-hCG levels) occurred in 26 women (48%). In these 54 women, 17 women (31%) delivered a total of 25 newborns, seven women (13%) had a spontaneous abortion and two women (4%) had an elective abortion.

In a second study (COL1620-F01), CRINONE 8% was used in luteal phase support of women with tubal or idiopathic infertility due to endometriosis and normal ovulatory cycles, undergoing *in vitro* fertilization ("IVF") procedures. All women received a GnRH analog to suppress endogenous

Continued on next page

TABLE 1
Single Dose Relative Bioavailability

	CRINONE 4%	45 mg Intramuscular Progesterone	CRINONE 8%	90 mg Intramuscular Progesterone
C_{max} (ng/mL)	13.15 ± 6.49	39.06 ± 13.68	14.87 ± 6.32	53.76 ± 14.9
$C_{avg\ 0\text{-}24}$ (ng/mL)	6.94 ± 4.24	22.41 ± 4.92	6.98 ± 3.21	28.98 ± 8.75
$AUC_{0\text{-}96}$ (ng•hr/mL)	288.63 ± 273.72	806.26 ± 102.75	296.78 ± 129.90	1378.91 ± 176.39
T_{max} (hr)	5.6 ± 1.84	8.2 ± 6.43	6.8 ± 3.3	9.2 ± 2.7
$t_{1/2}$ (hr)	55.13 ± 28.04	28.05 ± 16.87	34.8 ± 11.3	19.6 ± 6.0
F (%)	27.6		19.8	

C_{max} – maximum progesterone serum concentration
$C_{avg\ 0\text{-}24}$ – average progesterone serum concentration over 24 hours
$AUC_{0\text{-}96}$ – area under the drug concentration versus time curve from 0-96 hours post dose
T_{max} – time to maximum progesterone concentration
$t_{1/2}$ – elimination half-life
F – relative bioavailability

Crinone—Cont.

progesterone, human menopausal gonadotropins, and human chorionic gonadotropin. In this multi-center, open-label study, 139 women (aged 22–38 years) received CRINONE 8% once daily beginning within 24 hours of embryo transfer and continuing through Day 30 post-transfer. Clinical pregnancies assessed at Day 90 post-transfer were seen in 36 (26%) of women. Thirty-two women (23%) delivered newborns and four women (3%) had a spontaneous abortion. (See **PRECAUTIONS**, subsection **Pregnancy**)

Secondary Amenorrhea

In three parallel, open-label studies (COL1620-004US, COL1620-005US, COL1620-009US), 127 women (aged 18–44) with hypothalamic amenorrhea or premature ovarian failure were randomized to receive either CRINONE 4% (n=62) or CRINONE 8% (n=65). All women were treated with either conjugated estrogens 0.625 mg daily (n=100) or transdermal estradiol (delivering 50 mcg/day) twice weekly (n=27).

Estrogen therapy was continuous for the entire three 28-day cycle studies. At Day 15 of the second cycle (six weeks after initiating estrogen replacement), women who demonstrated adequate response to estrogen therapy (by ultrasound) and who continued to be amenorrheic received CRINONE every other day for six doses (Day 15 through Day 25 of the cycle).

In cycle 2, CRINONE 4% induced bleeding in 79% of women and CRINONE 8% induced bleeding in 77% of women. In the third cycle, estrogen was continued and CRINONE was administered every other day beginning on Day 15 for six doses. On Day 24 an endometrial biopsy was performed. In 53 women who received CRINONE 4%, biopsy results were as follows: 7% proliferative, 40% late secretory, 19% mid secretory, 13% early secretory, 7% atrophic, 6% menstrual endometrium, 6% inactive endometrium and 2% negative endometrium. In 54 women who received CRINONE 8%, biopsy results were as follows: 44% late secretory, 19% mid secretory, 11% early secretory, 19% atrophic, 5% menstrual endometrium and 2% "oral contraceptive like" endometrium.

INDICATIONS AND USAGE

Assisted Reproductive Technology

CRINONE 8% is indicated for progesterone supplementation or replacement as part of an Assisted Reproductive Technology ("ART") treatment for infertile women with progesterone deficiency.

Secondary Amenorrhea

CRINONE 4% is indicated for the treatment of secondary amenorrhea.

CRINONE 8% is indicated for use in women who have failed to respond to treatment with CRINONE 4%.

CONTRAINDICATIONS

CRINONE should not be used in individuals with any of the following conditions:

1. Known sensitivity to CRINONE (progesterone or any of the other ingredients)
2. Undiagnosed vaginal bleeding
3. Liver dysfunction or disease
4. Known or suspected malignancy of the breast or genital organs
5. Missed abortion
6. Active thrombophlebitis or thromboembolic disorders, or a history of hormone-associated thrombophlebitis or thromboembolic disorders.

WARNINGS

The physician should be alert to the earliest manifestations of thrombotic disorders (thrombophlebitis, cerebrovascular disorders, pulmonary embolism, and retinal thrombosis). Should any of these occur or be suspected, the drug should be discontinued immediately.

Progesterone and progestins have been used to prevent miscarriage in women with a history of recurrent spontaneous pregnancy losses. No adequate evidence is available to show that they are effective for this purpose.

PRECAUTIONS
General

1. The pretreatment physical examination should include special reference to breast and pelvic organs, as well as Papanicolaou smear.
2. In cases of breakthrough bleeding, as in all cases of irregular vaginal bleeding, nonfunctional causes should be considered. In cases of undiagnosed vaginal bleeding, adequate diagnostic measures should be undertaken.
3. Because progestogens may cause some degree of fluid retention, conditions which might be influenced by this factor (e.g., epilepsy, migraine, asthma, cardiac or renal dysfunction) require careful observation.
4. The pathologist should be advised of progesterone therapy when relevant specimens are submitted.
5. Patients who have a history of psychic depression should be carefully observed and the drug discontinued if the depression recurs to a serious degree.
6. A decrease in glucose tolerance has been observed in a small percentage of patients on estrogen-progestin combination drugs. The mechanism of this decrease is not known. For this reason, diabetic patients should be carefully observed while receiving progestin therapy.

Information for Patients

The product should not be used concurrently with other local intravaginal therapy. If other local intravaginal therapy is to be used concurrently, there should be at least a 6-hour period before or after CRINONE™ administration.

Drug Interactions

No drug interactions have been assessed with CRINONE.

Carcinogenesis, Mutagenesis, Impairment of Fertility

Nonclinical toxicity studies to determine the potential of CRINONE to cause carcinogenicity or mutagenicity have not been performed. The effect of CRINONE on fertility has not been evaluated in animals.

Pregnancy (See **CLINICAL PHARMACOLOGY**, subsection **Clinical Studies**)

CRINONE 8% has been used to support embryo implantation and maintain pregnancies through its use as part of ART treatment regimens in two clinical studies (studies COL1620–007US and COL1620-F01). In the first study (COL1620-007US), 54 CRINONE-treated women had donor oocyte transfer procedures, and clinical pregnancies occurred in 26 women (48%). The outcomes of these 26 pregnancies were as follows: one woman had an elective termination of pregnancy at 19 weeks due to congenital malformations (omphalocele) associated with a chromosomal abnormality; one woman pregnant with triplets had an elective termination of her pregnancy; seven women spontaneously aborted their pregnancy; and 17 women delivered 25 apparently normal newborns.

In the second study (COL1620-F01), CRINONE 8% was used in the luteal phase support of women undergoing *in vitro* fertilization ("IVF") procedures. In this multi-center, open-label study, 139 women received CRINONE 8% once daily beginning within 24 hours of embryo transfer and continuing through Day 30 post-transfer.

Clinical pregnancies assessed at Day 90 post-transfer were seen in 36 (26%) of women. Thirty-two women (23%) delivered newborns and four women (3%) had a spontaneous abortion. Of the 47 newborns delivered, one had a teratoma associated with a cleft palate; one had respiratory distress syndrome; 44 were apparently normal and one was lost to follow-up.

Pediatric Use

Safety and effectiveness in pediatric patients have not been established.

Nursing Mothers

Detectable amounts of progestins have been identified in the milk of mothers receiving them. The effect of this on the nursing infant has not been determined.

ADVERSE REACTIONS
Assisted Reproductive Technology

In a study of 61 women with ovarian failure undergoing a donor oocyte transfer procedure receiving CRINONE 8% twice daily, treatment-emergent adverse events occurring in 5% or more of the women are shown in Table 3.

TABLE 3
Treatment-Emergent Adverse Events
in ≥5% of Women Receiving CRINONE 8%
Twice Daily
Study COL1620-007US (n=61)

Body as a Whole	
Bloating	7%
Cramps NOS	15%
Pain	8%
Central and Peripheral Nervous System	
Dizziness	5%
Headache	13%
Gastro-Intestinal System	
Nausea	7%
Reproductive, Female	
Breast Pain	13%
Moniliasis Genital	5%
Vaginal Discharge	7%
Skin and Appendages	
Pruritus Genital	5%

In a second clinical study of 139 women using CRINONE 8% once daily for luteal phase support while undergoing an *in vitro* fertilization procedure, treatment-emergent adverse events reported in ≥5% of the women are shown in Table 4.

TABLE 4
Treatment-Emergent Adverse Events
in ≥5% of Women Receiving CRINONE 8%
Once Daily
Study COL1620-F01 (n=139)

Body as a Whole	
Abdominal Pain	12%
Perineal Pain Female	17%
Central and Periphal Nervous System	
Headache	17%
Gastro-Intestinal System	
Constipation	27%
Diarrhea	8%
Nausea	22%
Vomiting	5%
Musculo-Skeletal System	
Arthralgia	8%
Psychiatric	
Depression	11%
Libido Decreased	10%
Nervousness	16%
Somnolence	27%
Reproductive, Female	
Breast Enlargement	40%

TABLE 2
Multiple Dose Pharmacokinetics

	Assisted Reproductive Technology		Secondary Amenorrhea	
	Daily Dosing 8%	Twice Daily Dosing 8%	Every Other Day Dosing 4%	Every Other Day Dosing 8%
C_{max} (ng/mL)	15.97 ± 5.05	14.57 ± 4.49	13.21 ± 9.46	13.67 ± 3.58
C_{avg} (ng/mL)	8.99 ± 3.53	11.6 ± 3.47	4.05 ± 2.85	6.75 ± 2.83
T_{max} (hr)	5.40 ± 0.97	3.55 ± 2.48	6.67 ± 3.16	7.00 ± 2.88
$AUC_{0-\tau}$ (ng•hr/mL)	391.98 ± 153.28	138.72 ± 41.58	242.15 ± 167.88	438.36 ± 223.36
$t_{1/2}$ (hr)	45.00 ± 34.70	25.91 ± 6.15	49.87 ± 31.20	39.08 ± 12.88

Dyspareunia	6%
Urinary System	
Nocturia	13%

Secondary Amenorrhea

In three studies, 127 women with secondary amenorrhea received estrogen replacement therapy and CRINONE 4% or 8% every other day for six doses. Treatment emergent adverse events during estrogen and CRINONE treatment that occurred in 5% or more of women are shown in Table 5.

TABLE 5
Treatment Emergent Adverse Events in ≥5% of Women
Receiving Estrogen Treatment and CRINONE Every
Other Day
Studies COL1620-004US, COL1620-005US,
COL1620-009US

	Estrogen +CRINONE 4% n = 62	Estrogen +CRINONE 8% n = 65
Body as a Whole		
Abdominal Pain	3 (5%)	6 (9%)
Appetite Increased	3 (5%)	5 (8%)
Bloating	8 (13%)	8 (12%)
Cramps NOS	12 (19%)	17 (26%)
Fatigue	13 (21%)	14 (22%)
Central and Peripheral Nervous System		
Headache	12 (19%)	10 (15%)
Gastro-Intestinal System		
Nausea	5 (8%)	4 (6%)
Musculo-Skeletal System		
Back Pain	5 (8%)	2 (3%)
Myalgia	5 (8%)	0 (0%)
Psychiatric		
Depression	12 (19%)	10 (15%)
Emotional Lability	14 (23%)	14 (22%)
Sleep Disorder	11 (18%)	12 (18%)
Reproductive, Female		
Vaginal Discharge	7 (11%)	2 (3%)
Resistance Mechanism		
Upper Respiratory Tract Infection	3 (5%)	5 (8%)
Skin and Appendages		
Pruritis genital	1 (2%)	4 (6%)

Additional adverse events reported in women at a frequency <5% in the CRINONE ART and secondary amenorrhea studies and not listed in the tables above include:
Autonomic Nervous System—mouth dry, sweating increased
Body as a Whole—abnormal crying, allergic reaction, allergy, appetite decreased, asthenia, edema, face edema, fever, hot flushes, influenza-like symptoms, water retention, xerophthalmia
Cardiovascular, General—syncope
Central and Peripheral Nervous System—migraine, tremor
Gastro-Intestinal—dyspepsia, eructation, flatulence, gastritis, toothache
Metabolic and Nutritional—thirst
Musculo-Skeletal System—cramps legs, leg pain, skeletal pain
Neoplasm—benign cyst
Platelet, Bleeding & Clotting—purpura
Psychiatric—aggressive reactions, forgetfulness, insomnia
Red Blood Cell—anemia
Reproductive, Female—dysmenorrhea, premenstrual tension, vaginal dryness
Resistance Mechanism—infection, pharyngitis, sinusitis, urinary tract infection
Respiratory System—asthma, dyspnea, hyperventilation, rhinitis

Skin and Appendages—acne, pruritus, rash, seborrhea, skin discoloration, skin disorder, urticaria
Urinary System—cystitis, dysuria, micturition frequency
Vision Disorders—conjunctivitis

OVERDOSAGE

There have been no reports of overdosage with CRINONE. In the case of overdosage, however, discontinue CRINONE, treat the patient symptomatically, and institute supportive measures.
As with all prescription drugs, this medicine should be kept out of the reach of children.

DOSAGE AND ADMINISTRATION

Assisted Reproductive Technology—CRINONE 8% is administered vaginally at a dose of 90 mg once daily in women who require progesterone supplementation. CRINONE 8% is administered vaginally at a dose of 90 mg twice daily in women with partial or complete ovarian failure who require progesterone replacement. If pregnancy occurs, treatment may be continued until placental autonomy is achieved, up to 10–12 weeks.
Secondary Amenorrhea—CRINONE 4% is administered vaginally every other day up to a total of six doses. For women who fail to respond, a trial of CRINONE 8% every other day up to a total of six doses may be instituted. It is important to note that a dosage increase from the 4% gel can only be accomplished by using the 8% gel. Increasing the volume of gel administered does not increase the amount of progesterone absorbed.
SEE CRINONE PATIENT INFORMATION SHEET—HOW TO USE CRINONE

HOW SUPPLIED

CRINONE™ is available in the following strengths:
4% gel (45 mg) in a single use, one piece, disposable, white polyethylene vaginal applicator with a twist-off top. Each applicator contains 2.6 g of gel and delivers 1.125 g of gel.
    NDC – 0008-0907-02 – 6 Single-use prefilled applicators.
8% gel (90 mg) in a single use, one piece, disposable, white polyethylene vaginal applicator with a twist-off top. Each applicator contains 2.6 g of gel and delivers 1.125 g of gel.
    NDC – 0008-0908-02 – 6 Single-use prefilled applicators.
    NDC – 0008-0908-03 – 18 Single-use prefilled applicators (3 boxes of 6).
Each applicator is wrapped and sealed in a foil overwrap.
Store at controlled room temperature below 25°C (77°F).
Caution: Federal law prohibits dispensing without prescription.
U.S. Patent Numbers 4,615,697 and 5,543,150.

Distributed by
Wyeth Laboratories Inc.
A Wyeth-Ayerst Company
Philadelphia, PA 19101

PATIENT INFORMATION

CRINONE™ 8%
(progesterone gel)
For Vaginal Use Only

FOR PROGESTERONE SUPPLEMENTATION OR REPLACEMENT AS PART OF AN ASSISTED REPRODUCTIVE TECHNOLOGY ("ART") TREATMENT FOR INFERTILE WOMEN WITH PROGESTERONE DEFICIENCY
Please read this information carefully before you start to use CRINONE and each time your prescription is renewed, in case anything has changed. This leaflet does not take the place of discussions with your doctor. If you still have any questions, ask your doctor or health-care provider.

About CRINONE
CRINONE is a specially formulated vaginal gel which contains the natural female hormone called progesterone. CRINONE is indicated for the treatment of infertility associated with progesterone deficiency.

Understanding the role of CRINONE in your infertility treatment
Progesterone is one of the hormones essential for maintaining a pregnancy. If you are undergoing ART treatment and your doctor has determined your body does not produce enough progesterone on its own, CRINONE may be prescribed to provide the progesterone you need.
The progesterone in CRINONE will help prepare the lining of your uterus so that it is ready to receive and nourish a fertilized egg. If pregnancy occurs, CRINONE may be supplemented for 10–12 weeks until production of progesterone by the placenta is adequate.

When you should not use CRINONE
• *If you are allergic to progesterone, progesterone-like drugs, or any of the inactive ingredients in the gel.*
• *If you have unusual vaginal bleeding which has not been evaluated by your doctor.*
• *If you have liver disease.*
• *If you have known or suspected cancer of the breast or genital organs.*
• *If you have a miscarriage and your physician suspects some tissue is still in the uterus.*
• *If you have or have had blood clots in the legs, lungs, eyes, or elsewhere.*

Risks of CRINONE
• *Risk to the fetus.* Birth defects have been reported in the offspring of women who were using CRINONE during early pregnancy. These included an abdominal wall defect and a cleft palate. A causal association has been neither confirmed nor refuted. You should check with your doctor about the risks to your unborn child of any medication taken during pregnancy.
• *Abnormal blood clotting.* Blood clots have been reported with the use of estrogens and progestational drugs (alone or in combination). If blood clots do form in your bloodstream, they can cut off the blood supply to vital organs, causing serious problems. These problems may include a stroke (by cutting off blood to part of the brain), a heart attack (by cutting off blood to part of the heart), a pulmonary embolus (by cutting off blood to part of the lungs), or other problems. Any of these conditions may cause death or serious long-term disability. Call your doctor immediately if you suspect you have any of these conditions. He or she may advise you to stop using this drug.

Possible side effects of CRINONE
In addition to the risks listed above, the following side effects have been reported with CRINONE used either for progesterone supplementation or for replacement as part of an ART treatment for infertile women with progesterone deficiency. Consult your doctor if you experience any of the side effects mentioned below, or other side effects.

SIDE EFFECTS REPORTED AT A FREQUENCY OF 5% OR GREATER
• abdominal pain; perineal pain
• headache
• constipation; diarrhea; nausea
• joint pain
• depression; decreased libido; nervousness; sleepiness*
• breast enlargement
• excessive urination at night

SIDE EFFECTS REPORTED AT A FREQUENCY RANGING FROM 1% to 5%
• allergy; bloating; cramps; fatigue; pain
• dizziness*
• vomiting
• mood swings
• breast pain
• difficult or painful intercourse; genital itching; genital yeast infection; vaginal discharge
• urinary tract infection

SIDE EFFECTS REPORTED AT A FREQUENCY OF LESS THAN 1%
• fever; flu-like syndrome
• water retention†
• gastrointestinal discomfort; gas; abdominal distention
• back pain; leg pain
• insomnia
• sinusitis; upper respiratory tract infection
• asthma
• acne; itching
• painful or difficult urination; frequent urination

*If you experience dizziness or sleepiness, do not drive or operate machinery.
†This may worsen some conditions such as asthma, epilepsy, migraine, heart disease, or kidney disease.

PRECAUTIONS

Be alert for unusual signs and symptoms. If any of these warning signals (or any other unusual symptoms) happen while you are using CRINONE, call your doctor immediately:
• Abnormal bleeding from the vagina.
• Pains in the calves or chest, a sudden shortness of breath or coughing blood indicating possible clots in the legs, heart, or lungs.
• Severe headache or vomiting, dizziness, faintness, or changes in vision or speech, weakness or numbness of an arm or leg indicating possible clots in the brain or eye.
• Breast lumps, which could be associated with fibrocystic disorders, fibroadenoma, or breast cancer. (Ask your doctor or health-care provider to show you how to examine your breasts monthly.)
• Yellowing of the skin and/or white of the eyes indicating possible liver problems.

How CRINONE works
CRINONE has been formulated to be administered through the vagina. The moisturizing gel in CRINONE forms a coating on the walls of the vagina which allows for absorption of progesterone through the vaginal tissue.
Small, white globules may appear as a discharge, even several days after usage. CRINONE contains no irritating perfumes or dyes.

Other information
1. Your doctor has prescribed this drug for you and you alone. Do not give this drug to anyone else.
2. This medication was prescribed for your particular medical condition. Do not use it for another condition.
3. Keep this and all drugs out of the reach of children.

Continued on next page

Crinone—Cont.

How to use CRINONE

The dosage is one application of the 8% gel (90 mg of progesterone) vaginally, daily or twice daily as directed by your doctor. If you become pregnant, your doctor may decide to continue treatment for up to 10 to 12 weeks.

CRINONE is to be applied directly from the specially designed sealed applicator into the vagina. The applicator is designed to deliver a premeasured dose of CRINONE. A small amount of gel will be left in the tube after usage. Do not be concerned because you will still be receiving the appropriate dosage. Remove the applicator from the sealed wrapper. DO NOT remove the twist-off tab at this time.

1. Hold the applicator by the thick end. Shake down several times like a thermometer to ensure that the contents are at the thin end.

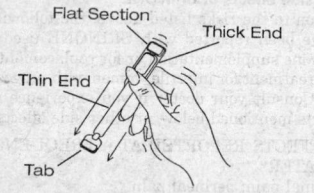

2. Hold the applicator by the flat section of the thick end. Twist off and discard the tab at the other end. To avoid a partial release of the gel before insertion, DO NOT squeeze the thick end while twisting off the tab.

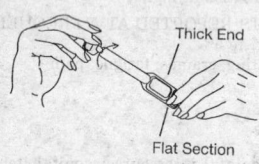

3. The applicator may be inserted into the vagina while you are in a sitting position or when lying on your back with your knees bent. Gently insert the thin end well into the vagina.

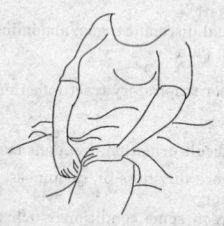

4. Squeeze the thick end of the applicator to deposit the gel. Remove the applicator and discard it into a waste container. Do not be concerned if a small amount of gel is left in the applicator. You will still be receiving the appropriate dosage.

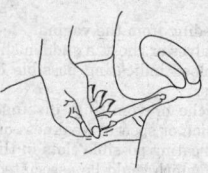

5. CRINONE coats the vaginal mucosa to provide long-lasting release of progesterone. Small, white globules may appear as a discharge, even several days after usage. It is not unusual, but if you are concerned, discuss this with your doctor.

If you forget a dose of CRINONE, use it as soon as you remember, but do not use more than the recommended daily dose.

CRINONE should not be used at the same time that you are using other vaginal therapy.

This leaflet provides the most important information about CRINONE. If you want to read more, ask your doctor or pharmacist to let you read the professional leaflet. You may need their help to understand some of the information.

How Supplied

CRINONE is available as 8% gel (90 mg of progesterone). Each box of the 8% gel contains eighteen single use, disposable vaginal applicators with a twist-off tab.

Each applicator is wrapped and sealed in a foil overwrap.

CRINONE should be stored at controlled room temperature below 25°C (77°F).

Do not use CRINONE after the expiration date which is printed on the box.

PATIENT INFORMATION

CRINONE™ 4% and CRINONE™ 8%
(progesterone gel)
For Vaginal Use Only

FOR THE TREATMENT OF SECONDARY AMENORRHEA (ABSENCE OF MENSES IN WOMEN WHO HAVE PREVIOUSLY HAD A MENSTRUAL PERIOD)

Please read this information carefully before you start to use CRINONE and each time your prescription is renewed, in case anything has changed. This leaflet does not take the place of discussions with your doctor. If you still have any questions, ask your doctor or health-care provider.

About CRINONE

CRINONE is a specially formulated vaginal gel which contains the natural female hormone called progesterone. CRINONE is indicated for the treatment of secondary amenorrhea due to progesterone deficiency.

Understanding the role of CRINONE in the treatment of your menstrual irregularities

Progesterone is one of the hormones essential for regular menstrual periods. If your doctor has determined your body does not produce enough progesterone on its own, CRINONE may be prescribed to provide the progesterone you need.

When you do not produce enough progesterone, menstrual irregularities can occur. CRINONE can provide you with the progesterone needed during a normal menstrual cycle.

When you should not use CRINONE: See PATIENT INFORMATION for CRINONE 8% above.

Risks of CRINONE: See PATIENT INFORMATION for CRINONE 8% above.

Possible side effects of CRINONE

In addition to the risks listed above, the following side effects have been reported in studies with CRINONE used for the treatment of menstrual irregularities due to progesterone deficiency. In these studies, women were treated with estrogen prior to and during CRINONE therapy. All side effects reported at a frequency of 5% or greater after CRINONE was added to estrogen therapy also were reported with estrogen therapy alone. Consult your doctor if you experience any of the side effects mentioned below, or other side effects.

SIDE EFFECTS REPORTED AT A FREQUENCY OF 5% OR GREATER

- abdominal pain; increased appetite; bloating; cramps; fatigue
- headache
- nausea
- back pain
- depression; mood swings; sleep disorder
- vaginal discharge
- upper respiratory tract infection

SIDE EFFECTS REPORTED AT A FREQUENCY RANGING FROM 1% to 5%

- increased sweating
- allergy; flu-like symptoms; hot flushes; pain
- dizziness*
- migraine; tremor
- gas; gastrointestinal discomfort
- thirst
- leg pain; muscle pain
- insomnia; nervousness; sleepiness*
- breast pain; painful menstruation
- infection; genital yeast infection
- acne; genital itching; rash; skin disorder
- frequent urination

SIDE EFFECTS REPORTED AT A FREQUENCY OF LESS THAN 1%

- dry mouth
- abnormal crying; allergic reaction; decreased appetite; dry eyes; edema; face edema; perineal pain; water retention†; weakness
- fainting
- abdominal distention; gastritis; toothache
- joint pain; leg cramps; skeletal pain
- benign cyst
- bruising
- aggressive reaction; forgetfulness
- anemia
- premenstrual tension; vaginal dryness
- sore throat
- hyperventilation; shortness of breath; rhinitis
- hives; itching; seborrhea; skin discoloration
- cystitis; painful or difficult urination
- conjunctivitis

*If you experience dizziness or sleepiness, do not drive or operate machinery.

†This may worsen some conditions such as asthma, epilepsy, migraine, heart disease, or kidney disease.

PRECAUTIONS: See PATIENT INFORMATION for CRINONE 8% above.

How CRINONE works: See PATIENT INFORMATION for CRINONE 8% above.

Other information: See PATIENT INFORMATION for CRINONE 8% above.

How to use CRINONE

The dosage is one application of the 4% gel (45 mg of progesterone) vaginally, every other day as directed by your doctor, for a total of six doses. In some cases, your doctor may prescribe the 8% gel (90 mg of progesterone) every other day, for a total of six doses.

It is important to note that a dosage increase from the 4% gel can only be accomplished by using the 8% gel. Increasing the volume of gel administered does not increase the amount of progesterone absorbed.

CRINONE is to be applied directly from the specially designed sealed applicator into the vagina. The applicator is designed to deliver a premeasured dose of CRINONE. A small amount of gel will be left in the tube after usage. Do not be concerned because you will still be receiving the appropriate dosage. Remove the applicator from the sealed wrapper. DO NOT remove the twist-off tab at this time.

Steps for How to use CRINONE: See PATIENT INFORMATION for CRINONE 8% above.

HOW SUPPLIED

CRINONE is available in two strengths: 4% gel (45 mg of progesterone) and 8% gel (90 mg of progesterone).

Each box of the 4% gel contains six single use, disposable vaginal applicators with a twist-off tab. Each box of the 8% gel contains eighteen single use, disposable vaginal applicators with a twist-off tab. Each applicator is wrapped and sealed in a foil overwrap.

CRINONE should be stored at controlled room temperature below 25°C (77°F).

Do not use CRINONE after the expiration date which is printed on the box.

Distributed by
Wyeth Laboratories Inc.
A Wyeth-Ayerst Company
Philadelphia, PA 19101
Shown in Product Identification Guide, page 343

DIUCARDIN® ℞
[dī"ū-car'din]
(hydroflumethiazide tablets, USP)

DESCRIPTION

Diucardin (hydroflumethiazide) is an oral thiazide (benzothiadiazine) diuretic-antihypertensive agent.

Diucardin is available as 50 mg tablets for oral administration.

Chemical name: 3,4-Dihydro-6-(trifluoromethyl)-2H-1,2,4-benzothiadiazine-7-sulfonamide 1,1-dioxide.

Structural formula:

Hydroflumethiazide is an odorless white to cream-colored, finely divided, crystalline powder. It has a melting point between 270° and 275° C. Hydroflumethiazide is freely soluble in acetone, soluble in alcohol, and very slightly soluble in water.

The inactive ingredients contained in Diucardin tablets are: lactose, magnesium stearate, microcrystalline cellulose, povidone, and starch.

CLINICAL PHARMACOLOGY

Hydroflumethiazide is incompletely but fairly rapidly absorbed from the gastrointestinal tract. It appears to have a biphasic biological half-life with an estimated alpha-phase of about 2 hours and an estimated beta-phase of about 17 hours; it has a metabolite with a longer half-life, which is extensively bound to the red blood cells. Hydroflumethiazide is excreted in the urine; its metabolite has also been detected in the urine.

The mechanism of action results in an interference with the renal tubular mechanism of electrolyte reabsorption. At maximal therapeutic dosage, all thiazides are approximately equal in their diuretic potency. The mechanism whereby thiazides function in the control of hypertension is unknown.

INDICATIONS AND USAGE

Diucardin is indicated as adjunctive therapy in edema associated with congestive heart failure, hepatic cirrhosis, and corticosteroid and estrogen therapy.

Diucardin has also been found useful in edema due to various forms of renal dysfunction such as: nephrotic syndrome; acute glomerulonephritis; and chronic renal failure.

Diucardin is indicated in the management of hypertension either as the sole therapeutic agent or to enhance the effect of other antihypertensive drugs in the more severe forms of hypertension.

USAGE IN PREGNANCY

The routine use of diuretics in an otherwise healthy woman is inappropriate and exposes mother and fetus to unnecessary hazard. Diuretics do not prevent development of toxemia of pregnancy, and there is no satisfactory evidence that they are useful in the treatment of developed toxemia.

Edema during pregnancy may arise from pathological causes or from the physiologic and mechanical consequences of pregnancy. Thiazides are indicated in pregnancy when edema is due to pathologic causes just as they are in the absence of pregnancy (however, see "Precautions—PREGNANCY" below).

Dependent edema in pregnancy, resulting from restriction of venous return by the expanded uterus, is properly treated through elevation of the lower extremities and use of support hose. Use of diuretics to lower intravascular volume in this case is illogical and unnecessary. There is hypervolemia during normal pregnancy which is harmful to neither the fetus nor the mother (in absence of cardiovascular disease), but which is associated with edema, including generalized edema, in the majority of pregnant women. If this edema produces discomfort, increased recumbency will often provide relief. In rare instances, this edema may cause extreme discomfort which is not relieved by rest. In these cases, a short course of diuretics may provide relief and may be appropriate.

CONTRAINDICATIONS

Anuria.

Hypersensitivity to this or other sulfonamide-derived drugs.

WARNINGS

Diucardin should be used with caution in severe renal disease. In patients with renal disease, thiazides may precipitate azotemia. Cumulative effects of the drug may develop in patients with impaired renal function.

Thiazides should be used with caution in patients with impaired hepatic function or progressive liver disease, since minor alterations of fluid and electrolyte balance may precipitate hepatic coma.

Thiazides may add to or potentiate the action of other antihypertensive drugs. Potentiation occurs with ganglionic or peripheral adrenergic blocking drugs.

Sensitivity reactions may occur in patients with a history of allergy or bronchial asthma.

The possibility of exacerbation or activation of systemic lupus erythematosus has been reported.

PRECAUTIONS

GENERAL

All patients receiving thiazide therapy should be observed for clinical signs of fluid or electrolyte imbalance: namely, hyponatremia, hypochloremic alkalosis, and hypokalemia. Serum and urine electrolyte determinations are particularly important when the patient is vomiting excessively or receiving parenteral fluids. Medication such as digitalis may also influence serum electrolytes. Warning signs, irrespective of cause, are: dryness of mouth, thirst, weakness, lethargy, drowsiness, restlessness, muscle pains or cramps, muscular fatigue, hypotension, oliguria, tachycardia, and gastrointestinal disturbances such as nausea and vomiting.

Hypokalemia may develop with thiazides as with any other potent diuretic, especially with brisk diuresis, when severe cirrhosis is present, or during concomitant use of corticosteroids or ACTH.

Interference with adequate oral electrolyte intake will also contribute to hypokalemia. Digitalis therapy may exaggerate metabolic effects of hypokalemia, especially with reference to myocardial activity.

Any chloride deficit is generally mild and usually does not require specific treatment except under extraordinary circumstances (as in liver disease or renal disease). Dilutional hyponatremia may occur in edematous patients in hot weather; appropriate therapy is water restriction, rather than administration of salt, except in rare instances when the hyponatremia is life-threatening. In actual salt depletion, appropriate replacement is the therapy of choice.

Hyperuricemia may occur or frank gout may be precipitated in certain patients receiving thiazide therapy.

Insulin requirements in diabetic patients may be increased, decreased, or unchanged. Latent diabetes mellitus may become manifested during thiazide administration.

The antihypertensive effects of the drug may be enhanced in the post-sympathectomy patient.

If progressive renal impairment becomes evident, as indicated by a rising creatinine or blood urea nitrogen, a careful reappraisal of therapy is necessary with consideration given to withholding or discontinuing diuretic therapy.

Thiazides may decrease serum PBI levels without signs of thyroid disturbance.

Lithium generally should not be given with diuretics because they reduce its renal clearance and increase the risk of lithium toxicity. Read circulars for lithium preparations before use of such concomitant therapy with Diucardin.

Thiazides have been shown to increase the urinary excretion of magnesium; this may result in hypomagnesemia.

Calcium excretion is decreased by thiazides. Pathological changes in the parathyroid gland with hypercalcemia and hypophosphatemia have been observed in a few patients on prolonged thiazide therapy. The common complications of hyperparathyroidism, such as renal lithiasis, bone resorption, and peptic ulceration, have not been seen.

LABORATORY TESTS

Periodic determination of serum electrolytes to detect possible electrolyte imbalance should be performed at appropriate intervals.

DRUG INTERACTIONS

Anticoagulants, oral

(Effects may be decreased when used concurrently with thiazide diuretics; dosage adjustments may be necessary.)

Antigout medications

(Thiazide diuretics may raise the level of blood uric acid; dosage adjustment of antigout medications may be necessary to control hyperuricemia and gout.)

Antihypertensive medications, other, especially diazoxide, or preanesthetic and anesthetic agents used in surgery or skeletal-muscle relaxants, nondepolarizing, used in surgery

(Effects may be potentiated when used concurrently with thiazide diuretics; dosage adjustments may be necessary.)

Amphotericin B or Corticosteroids or Corticotropin (ACTH)

(Concurrent use with thiazide diuretics may intensify electrolyte imbalance, particularly hypokalemia.)

Cardiac glycosides

(Concurrent use with thiazide diuretics may enhance the possibility of digitalis toxicity associated with hypokalemia.)

Colestipol

(May inhibit gastrointestinal absorption of the thiazide diuretics; administration 1 hour before or 4 hours after colestipol is recommended.)

Hypoglycemics

(Thiazide diuretics may raise blood glucose levels; for adult-onset diabetics, dosage adjustment of hypoglycemic medications may be necessary during and after thiazide diuretic therapy; insulin requirements may be increased, decreased, or unchanged.)

Lithium salts

(Concurrent use with thiazide diuretics is not recommended, as they may provoke lithium toxicity because of reduced renal clearance.)

Methenamine

(Effectiveness may be decreased when used concurrently with thiazide diuretics because of alkalinization of the urine.)

Nonsteroidal anti-inflammatory agents

(In some patients, the steroidal anti-inflammatory agent can reduce the diuretic, natriuretic, and antihypertensive effects of loop, potassium sparing, and thiazide diuretics. Therefore, when hydroflumethiazide and nonsteroidal anti-inflammatory agents are used concomitantly, the patient should be observed closely to determine if the desired effect of the diuretic is obtained.)

Norepinephrine

(Thiazides may decrease arterial responsiveness to norepinephrine. This diminution is not sufficient to preclude effectiveness of the pressor agent for therapeutic use.)

Tubocurarine

(Thiazide drugs may increase the responsiveness to tubocurarine.)

DIAGNOSTIC INTERFERENCE—With expected physiologic effects:

Blood and urine glucose levels (usually only in patients with a predisposition for glucose intolerance) and

Serum bilirubin levels (by displacement from albumin binding) and

Serum calcium levels (thiazide diuretics should be discontinued before parathyroid-function tests are carried out) and

Serum uric acid levels (may be increased)

Serum magnesium, potassium, and sodium levels (may be decreased; serum magnesium levels may increase in uremic patients)

Serum protein-bound iodine (PBI) levels (may be decreased)

Thiazides should be discontinued before carrying out tests for parathyroid function (see "Precautions—GENERAL, Calcium excretion").

CARCINOGENESIS, MUTAGENESIS, IMPAIRMENT OF FERTILITY

No studies have been performed to evaluate carcinogenic or mutagenic potential of Diucardin or the potential of Diucardin to impair fertility.

PREGNANCY

Teratogenic Effects—Pregnancy Category C

Animal reproduction studies have not been conducted with Diucardin. It is also not known whether Diucardin can

cause fetal harm when administered to a pregnant woman or can affect reproduction capacity. Diucardin should be given to a pregnant woman only if clearly needed.

Nonteratogenic Effects

Fetal or neonatal jaundice, thrombocytopenia, and possibly other adverse reactions which have occurred in the adult.

NURSING MOTHERS

Thiazides appear in breast milk. If use of the drug is deemed essential, the patient may consider stopping nursing.

PEDIATRIC USE

Safety and effectiveness in children have not been established.

ADVERSE REACTIONS

The following adverse reactions have been observed, but there is not enough systematic collection of data to support an estimate of their frequency.

GASTROINTESTINAL SYSTEMS

Anorexia, gastric irritation, nausea, vomiting, cramping, diarrhea, constipation, jaundice (intrahepatic cholestatic jaundice), pancreatitis, sialadenitis.

CENTRAL NERVOUS SYSTEM

Dizziness, vertigo, paresthesias, headache, xanthopsia.

HEMATOLOGIC

Leukopenia, agranulocytosis, thrombocytopenia, aplastic anemia, hemolytic anemia.

CARDIOVASCULAR

Orthostatic hypotension (may be aggravated by alcohol, barbiturates, or narcotics).

DERMATOLOGIC—HYPERSENSITIVITY

Purpura, photosensitivity, rash, urticaria, necrotizing angiitis (vasculitis, cutaneous vasculitis), fever, respiratory distress including pneumonitis, anaphylactic reactions.

OTHER

Hyperglycemia, glycosuria, hyperuricemia, muscle spasm, weakness, restlessness, transient blurred vision.

Whenever adverse reactions are moderate or severe, thiazide dosage should be reduced or therapy withdrawn.

OVERDOSAGE

SIGNS AND SYMPTOMS

Diuresis, lethargy progressing to coma, with minimal cardiorespiratory depression and with or without significant serum electrolyte changes or dehydration; GI irritation; hypermotility; transient elevation in BUN level.

TREATMENT

Empty stomach by gastric lavage, taking care to avoid aspiration. Monitor serum electrolyte levels and renal function, and institute supportive measures, as required to maintain hydration, electrolyte balance, respiration, and cardiovascular and renal function. Treat GI effects symptomatically.

DOSAGE AND ADMINISTRATION

The average adult diuretic dose is 25 to 200 mg per day. The average adult antihypertensive dose is 50 to 100 mg per day. Therapy should be individualized according to patient response. This therapy should be titrated to gain maximal response as well as the minimal dose possible to maintain that therapeutic response.

HOW SUPPLIED

Diucardin®—Each scored, white oval compressed tablet, inscribed "DIUCARDIN 50," contains 50 mg hydroflumethiazide, in bottles of 100 (NDC 0046-0702-81).

Store at room temperature (approximately 25° C)

Dispense in a well-closed container as defined in the USP

Caution: Federal law prohibits dispensing without prescription.

Manufactured by:

Ayerst Laboratories Inc.

A Wyeth-Ayerst Company

Philadelphia, PA 19101

Shown in Product Identification Guide, page 343

EFFEXOR®
(venlafaxine hydrochloride)
Tablets

℞

DESCRIPTION

Effexor (venlafaxine hydrochloride) is a structurally novel antidepressant for oral administration. It is chemically unrelated to tricyclic, tetracyclic, or other available antidepressant agents. It is designated (R/S)-1-[2-(dimethylamino)-1-(4-methoxyphenyl)ethyl] cyclohexanol hydrochloride or (±)-1-[α-[(dimethylamino)methyl]-p-methoxybenzyl] cyclohexanol hydrochloride and has the empirical formula of $C_{17}H_{27}NO_2$ HCl. Its molecular weight is 313.87. The structural formula is shown below.

[See chemical structure at top of next column]

Continued on next page

Effexor—Cont.

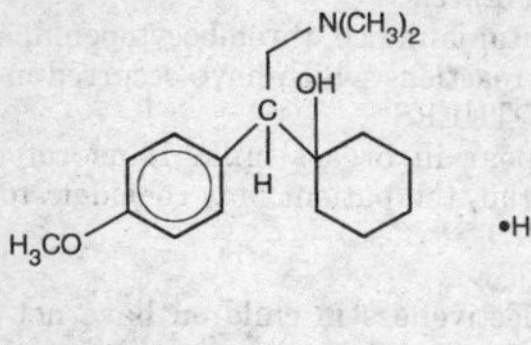

venlafaxine hydrochloride

Venlafaxine hydrochloride is a white to off-white crystalline solid with a solubility of 572 mg/mL in water (adjusted to ionic strength of 0.2 M with sodium chloride). Its octanol: water (0.2 M sodium chloride) partition coefficient is 0.43. Compressed tablets contain venlafaxine hydrochloride equivalent to 25 mg, 37.5 mg, 50 mg, 75 mg, or 100 mg venlafaxine. Inactive ingredients consist of cellulose, iron oxides, lactose, magnesium stearate, and sodium starch glycolate.

CLINICAL PHARMACOLOGY

Pharmacodynamics

The mechanism of the antidepressant action of venlafaxine in humans is believed to be associated with its potentiation of neurotransmitter activity in the CNS. Preclinical studies have shown that venlafaxine and its active metabolite, O-desmethylvenlafaxine (ODV), are potent inhibitors of neuronal serotonin and norepinephrine reuptake and weak inhibitors of dopamine reuptake. Venlafaxine and ODV have no significant affinity for muscarinic, histaminergic, or α-1 adrenergic receptors *in vitro*. Pharmacologic activity at these receptors is hypothesized to be associated with the various anticholinergic, sedative, and cardiovascular effects seen with other psychotropic drugs. Venlafaxine and ODV do not possess monoamine oxidase (MAO) inhibitory activity.

Pharmacokinetics

Venlafaxine is well absorbed and extensively metabolized in the liver. O-desmethylvenlafaxine (ODV) is the only major active metabolite. On the basis of mass balance studies, at least 92% of a single dose of venlafaxine is absorbed. Approximately 87% of a venlafaxine dose is recovered in the urine within 48 hours as either unchanged venlafaxine (5%), unconjugated ODV (29%), conjugated ODV (26%), or other minor inactive metabolites (27%). Renal elimination of venlafaxine and its metabolites is the primary route of excretion. The relative bioavailability of venlafaxine from a tablet was 100% when compared to an oral solution. Food has no significant effect on the absorption of venlafaxine or on the formation of ODV.

The degree of binding of venlafaxine to human plasma is 27%±2% at concentrations ranging from 2.5 to 2215 ng/mL. The degree of ODV binding to human plasma is 30%±12% at concentrations ranging from 100 to 500 ng/mL. Protein-binding-induced drug interactions with venlafaxine are not expected.

Steady-state concentrations of both venlafaxine and ODV in plasma were attained within 3 days of multiple-dose therapy. Venlafaxine and ODV exhibited linear kinetics over the dose range of 75 to 450 mg total dose per day (administered on a q8h schedule). Plasma clearance, elimination half-life and steady-state volume of distribution were unaltered for both venlafaxine and ODV after multiple-dosing. Mean±SD steady-state plasma clearance of venlafaxine and ODV is 1.3±0.6 and 0.4±0.2 L/h/kg, respectively; elimination half-life is 5±2 and 11±2 hours, respectively; and steady-state volume of distribution is 7.5±3.7 L/kg and 5.7±1.8 L/kg, respectively. When equal daily doses of venlafaxine were administered as either b.i.d. or t.i.d. regimens, the drug exposure (AUC) and fluctuation in plasma levels of venlafaxine and ODV were comparable following both regimens.

Age and Gender

A pharmacokinetic analysis of 404 venlafaxine-treated patients from two studies involving both b.i.d. and t.i.d. regimens showed that dose-normalized trough plasma levels of either venlafaxine or ODV were unaltered due to age or gender differences. Dosage adjustment based upon the age or gender of a patient is generally not necessary (see **"DOSAGE AND ADMINISTRATION"**).

Liver Disease

In 9 patients with hepatic cirrhosis, the pharmacokinetic disposition of both venlafaxine and ODV was significantly altered after oral administration of venlafaxine. Venlafaxine elimination half-life was prolonged by about 30%, and clearance decreased by about 50% in cirrhotic patients compared to normal subjects. ODV elimination half-life was prolonged by about 60% and clearance decreased by about 30% in cirrhotic patients compared to normal subjects. A large degree of intersubject variability was noted. Three patients with more severe cirrhosis had a more substantial decrease in venlafaxine clearance (about 90%) compared to normal subjects.

Dosage adjustment is necessary in these patients (see **"DOSAGE AND ADMINISTRATION"**).

Renal Disease

In a renal impairment study, venlafaxine elimination half-life after oral administration was prolonged by about 50% and clearance was reduced by about 24% in renally impaired patients (GFR =10-70 mL/min), compared to normal subjects. In dialysis patients, venlafaxine elimination half-life was prolonged by about 180% and clearance was reduced by about 57% compared to normal subjects. Similarly, ODV elimination half-life was prolonged by about 40% although clearance was unchanged in patients with renal impairment (GFR =10-70 mL/min) compared to normal subjects. In dialysis patients, ODV elimination half-life was prolonged by about 142% and clearance was reduced by about 56%, compared to normal subjects. A large degree of intersubject variability was noted.

Dosage adjustment is necessary in these patients (see **"DOSAGE AND ADMINISTRATION"**).

CLINICAL TRIALS

The efficacy of Effexor (venlafaxine hydrochloride) as a treatment for depression was established in 5 placebo-controlled, short-term trials. Four of these were 6-week trials in outpatients meeting DSM-III or DSM-III-R criteria for major depression: two involving dose titration with Effexor in a range of 75 to 225 mg/day (t.i.d. schedule), the third involving fixed Effexor doses of 75, 225, and 375 mg/day (t.i.d. schedule), and the fourth involving doses of 25, 75, and 200 mg/day (b.i.d. schedule). The fifth was a 4-week study of inpatients meeting DSM-III-R criteria for major depression with melancholia whose Effexor doses were titrated in a range of 150 to 375 mg/day (t.i.d schedule). In these 5 studies, Effexor was shown to be significantly superior to placebo on at least 2 of the following 3 measures: Hamilton Depression Rating Scale (total score), Hamilton depressed mood item, and Clinical Global Impression—Severity of Illness rating. Doses from 75 to 225 mg/day were superior to placebo in outpatient studies and a mean dose of about 350 mg/day was effective in inpatients. Data from the 2 fixed-dose outpatient studies were suggestive of a dose-response relationship in the range of 75 to 225 mg/day. There was no suggestion of increased response with doses greater than 225 mg/day.

While there were no efficacy studies focusing specifically on an elderly population, elderly patients were included among the patients studied. Overall, approximately $^{2}/_{3}$ of all patients in these trials were women. Exploratory analyses for age and gender effects on outcome did not suggest any differential responsiveness on the basis of age or sex.

INDICATIONS AND USAGE

Effexor (venlafaxine hydrochloride) is indicated for the treatment of depression.

The efficacy of Effexor in the treatment of depression was established in 6-week controlled trials of outpatients whose diagnoses corresponded most closely to the DSM-III or DSM-III-R category of major depressive disorder and in a 4-week controlled trial of inpatients meeting diagnostic criteria for major depressive disorder with melancholia (see **"CLINICAL PHARMACOLOGY"**).

A major depressive episode implies a prominent and relatively persistent depressed or dysphoric mood that usually interferes with daily functioning (nearly every day for at least 2 weeks); it should include at least 4 of the following 8 symptoms: change in appetite, change in sleep, psychomotor agitation or retardation, loss of interest in usual activities or decrease in sexual drive, increased fatigue, feelings of guilt or worthlessness, slowed thinking or impaired concentration, and a suicide attempt or suicidal ideation.

The effectiveness of Effexor in long-term use, that is, for more than 4 to 6 weeks, has not been systematically evaluated in controlled trials. Therefore, the physician who elects to use Effexor for extended periods should periodically re-evaluate the long-term usefulness of the drug for the individual patient.

CONTRAINDICATIONS

Effexor (venlafaxine hydrochloride) is contraindicated in patients known to be hypersensitive to it.

Concomitant use in patients taking monoamine oxidase inhibitors (MAOIs) is contraindicated (see **"WARNINGS"**).

WARNINGS

Potential for Interaction with Monoamine Oxidase Inhibitors

Adverse reactions, some of which were serious, have been reported in patients who have recently been discontinued from a monoamine oxidase inhibitor (MAOI) and started on Effexor, or who have recently had Effexor therapy discontinued prior to initiation of an MAOI. These reactions have included tremor, myoclonus, diaphoresis, nausea, vomiting, flushing, dizziness, hyperthermia with features resembling neuroleptic malignant syndrome, seizures, and death. In patients receiving antidepressants with pharmacological properties similar to venlafaxine in combination with a monoamine oxidase inhibitor, there have also been reports of serious, sometimes fatal, reactions. For a selective serotonin reuptake inhibitor, these reactions have included hyperthermia, rigidity, myoclonus, autonomic instability with possible rapid fluctuations of vital signs, and mental status changes that include extreme agitation progressing to delirium and coma. Some cases presented with features resembling neuroleptic malignant syndrome. Severe hyperthermia and seizures, sometimes fatal, have been reported in association with the combined use of tricyclic antidepressants and MAOIs. These reactions have also been reported in patients who have recently discontinued these drugs and have been started on an MAOI. Therefore, it is recommended that Effexor not be used in combination with an MAOI, or within at least 14 days of discontinuing treatment with an MAOI. Based on the half-life of Effexor, at least 7 days should be allowed after stopping Effexor before starting an MAOI.

Sustained Hypertension

Venlafaxine treatment is associated with sustained increases in blood pressure. (1) In a premarketing study comparing three fixed doses of venlafaxine (75, 225, and 375 mg/day) and placebo, a mean increase in supine diastolic blood pressure (SDBP) of 7.2 mm Hg was seen in the 375 mg/day group at week 6 compared to essentially no changes in the 75 and 225 mg/day groups and a mean decrease in SDBP of 2.2 mm Hg in the placebo group. (2) An analysis for patients meeting criteria for sustained hypertension (defined as treatment-emergent SDBP ≥ 90 mm Hg *and* ≥ 10 mm Hg above baseline for 3 consecutive visits) revealed a dose-dependent increase in the incidence of sustained hypertension for venlafaxine:

Probability of Sustained Elevation in SDBP (Pool of Premarketing Venlafaxine Studies)

Treatment Group	Incidence of Sustained Elevation in SDBP
Venlafaxine	
<100 mg/day	3%
101–200 mg/day	5%
201–300 mg/day	7%
>300 mg/day	13%
Placebo	2%

An analysis of the patients with sustained hypertension and the 19 venlafaxine patients who were discontinued from treatment because of hypertension (<1% of total venlafaxine-treated group) revealed that most of the blood pressure increases were in a modest range (10–15 mm Hg, SDBP). Nevertheless, sustained increases of this magnitude could have adverse consequences. Therefore, it is recommended that patients receiving venlafaxine have regular monitoring of blood pressure. For patients who experience a sustained increase in blood pressure while receiving venlafaxine, either dose reduction or discontinuation should be considered.

PRECAUTIONS

General

Anxiety and Insomnia

Treatment-emergent anxiety, nervousness, and insomnia were more commonly reported for venlafaxine-treated patients compared to placebo-treated patients in a pooled analysis of short-term, double-blind, placebo-controlled depression studies:

Symptom	Venlafaxine n = 1033	Placebo n = 609
Anxiety	6%	3%
Nervousness	13%	6%
Insomnia	18%	10%

Anxiety, nervousness, and insomnia led to drug discontinuation in 2%, 2%, and 3%, respectively, of the patients treated with venlafaxine in the phase 2–3 depression studies.

Changes in Appetite and Weight

Treatment-emergent anorexia was more commonly reported for venlafaxine-treated (11%) than placebo-treated patients (2%) in the pool of short-term, double-blind, placebo-controlled depression studies. A dose-dependent weight loss was often noted in patients treated with venlafaxine for several weeks. Significant weight loss, especially in underweight depressed patients, may be an undesirable result of venlafaxine treatment. A loss of 5% or more of body weight

occurred in 6% of patients treated with venlafaxine compared with 1% of patients treated with placebo and 3% of patients treated with another antidepressant. However, discontinuation for weight loss associated with venlafaxine was uncommon (0.1% of venlafaxine-treated patients in the phase 2–3 depression trials).

Activation of Mania/Hypomania

During phase 2–3 trials, hypomania or mania occurred in 0.5% of patients treated with venlafaxine. Activation of mania/hypomania has also been reported in a small proportion of patients with major affective disorder who were treated with other marketed antidepressants. As with all antidepressants, Effexor (venlafaxine hydrochloride) should be used cautiously in patients with a history of mania.

Seizures

During premarketing testing, seizures were reported in 0.26% (8/3082) of venlafaxine-treated patients. Most seizures (5 of 8) occurred in patients receiving doses of 150 mg/day or less. Effexor should be used cautiously in patients with a history of seizures. It should be discontinued in any patient who develops seizures.

Suicide

The possibility of a suicide attempt is inherent in depression and may persist until significant remission occurs. Close supervision of high-risk patients should accompany initial drug therapy. Prescriptions for Effexor should be written for the smallest quantity of tablets consistent with good patient management in order to reduce the risk of overdose.

Use in Patients with Concomitant Illness

Clinical experience with Effexor in patients with concomitant systemic illness is limited. Caution is advised in administering Effexor to patients with diseases or conditions that could affect hemodynamic responses or metabolism.

Effexor has not been evaluated or used to any appreciable extent in patients with a recent history of myocardial infarction or unstable heart disease. Patients with these diagnoses were sytematically excluded from many clinical studies during the product's premarketing testing. Evaluation of the electrocardiograms for 769 patients who received Effexor in 4- to 6-week double-blind placebo-controlled trials, however, showed that the incidence of trial-emergent conduction abnormalities did not differ from that with placebo. The mean heart rate in Effexor-treated patients was increased relative to baseline by about 4 beats per minute.

In patients with renal impairment (GFR=10-70 mL/min) or cirrhosis of the liver, the clearances of venlafaxine and its active metabolite were decreased, thus prolonging the elimination half-lives of these substances. A lower dose may be necessary (see "**DOSAGE AND ADMINISTRATION**"). Effexor (venlafaxine hydrochloride), like all antidepressants, should be used with caution in such patients.

Information for Patients

Physicians are advised to discuss the following issues with patients for whom they prescribe Effexor:

Interference with Cognitive and Motor Performance

Clinical studies were performed to examine the effects of venlafaxine on behavioral performance of healthy individuals. The results revealed no clinically significant impairment of psychomotor, cognitive, or complex behavior performance. However, since any psychoactive drug may impair judgment, thinking, or motor skills, patients should be cautioned about operating hazardous machinery, including automobiles, until they are reasonably certain that Effexor therapy does not adversely affect their ability to engage in such activities.

Pregnancy

Patients should be advised to notify their physician if they become pregnant or intend to become pregnant during therapy.

Nursing

Patients should be advised to notify their physician if they are breast-feeding an infant.

Concomitant Medication

Patients should be advised to inform their physicians if they are taking, or plan to take, any prescription or over-the-counter drugs, since there is a potential for interactions.

Alcohol

Although Effexor has not been shown to increase the impairment of mental and motor skills caused by alcohol, patients should be advised to avoid alcohol while taking Effexor.

Allergic Reactions

Patients should be advised to notify their physician if they develop a rash, hives, or a related allergic phenomenon.

Laboratory Tests

There are no specific laboratory tests recommended.

Drug Interactions

As with all drugs, the potential for interaction by a variety of mechanisms is a possibility.

Drugs Highly Bound to Plasma Protein

Venlafaxine is not highly bound to plasma proteins; therefore, administration of Effexor to a patient taking another drug that is highly protein bound should not cause increased free concentrations of the other drug.

Lithium

The steady-state pharmacokinetics of venlafaxine administered as 50 mg every 8 hours were not affected when a single 600 mg oral dose of lithium was administered to 12 healthy male subjects. O-desmethylvenlafaxine (ODV) was also unaffected. Venlafaxine had no effect on the pharmacokinetics of lithium.

Diazepam

Under steady-state conditions for venlafaxine administered as 50 mg every 8 hours, a single 10 mg dose of diazepam did not appear to affect the pharmacokinetics of either venlafaxine or ODV in 18 healthy male subjects. Venlafaxine also did not have any effect on the pharmacokinetics of diazepam or its active metabolite, desmethyldiazepam.

Administration of Effexor did not affect the psychomotor and psychometric effects induced by diazepam.

Cimetidine

Concomitant administration of cimetidine and Effexor in a steady-state study for both drugs resulted in inhibition of first-pass metabolism of venlafaxine in 18 healthy subjects. The oral clearance of venlafaxine was reduced by about 43%, and the exposure (AUC) and maximum concentration (C_{max}) of the drug were increased by about 60%. However, co-administration of cimetidine had no apparent effect on the pharmacokinetics of ODV, which is present in much greater quantity in the circulation than is venlafaxine. Consequently, the overall pharmacological activity of venlafaxine plus ODV is expected to increase only slightly, and no dosage adjustment should be necessary for most normal adults. However, for patients with pre-existing hypertension, and for elderly patients or patients with hepatic dysfunction, the interaction associated with the concomitant use of Effexor (venlafaxine hydrochloride) and cimetidine is not known and potentially could be more pronounced. Therefore, caution is advised with such patients.

Alcohol

A single dose of ethanol (0.5 g/kg) had no effect on the pharmacokinetics of venlafaxine or ODV when venlafaxine was administered as a 50 mg dose every 8 hours in 15 healthy male subjects. The administration of Effexor in a stable regimen did not exaggerate the psychomotor and psychometric effects induced by ethanol in these same subjects when they were not receiving Effexor.

Haloperidol

Venlafaxine administered under steady-state conditions at 75 mg every 12 hours in 24 healthy subjects decreased total oral-dose clearance (Cl/F) of a single 2 mg dose of haloperidol by 42%, which resulted in a 70% increase in haloperidol AUC. In addition, the haloperidol C_{max} increased 88% when coadministered with venlafaxine, but the haloperidol elimination half-life ($t_{1/2}$) was unchanged. The mechanism explaining this finding is unknown.

Drugs that Inhibit Cytochrome P450 Isoenzymes

CYP2D6 Inhibitors: *In vitro* and *in vivo* studies indicate that venlafaxine is metabolized to its active metabolite, ODV, by CYP2D6, the isoenzyme that is responsible for the genetic polymorphism seen in the metabolism of many antidepressants. Therefore, the potential exists for a drug interaction between drugs that inhibit CYP2D6-mediated metabolism and venlafaxine. However, although imipramine partially inhibited the CYP2D6-mediated metabolism of venlafaxine, resulting in higher plasma concentrations of venlafaxine and lower plasma concentrations of ODV, the total concentration of active compounds (venlafaxine plus ODV) was not affected. Additionally, in a clinical study involving CYP2D6-poor and -extensive metabolizers, the total concentration of active compounds (venlafaxine plus ODV), was similar in the two metabolizer groups. Therefore, no dosage adjustment is required when venlafaxine is coadministered with a CYP2D6 inhibitor.

CYP3A4 Inhibitors: *In vitro* studies indicate that venlafaxine is likely metabolized to a minor, less active metabolite, N-desmethylvenlafaxine, by CYP3A4. Because CYP3A4 is typically a minor pathway relative to CYP2D6 in the metabolism of venlafaxine, the potential for a clinically significant drug interaction between drugs that inhibit CYP3A4-mediated metabolism and venlafaxine is small.

The concomitant use of venlafaxine with a drug treatment(s) that potently inhibits both CYP2D6 and CYP3A4, the primary metabolizing enzymes for venlafaxine, has not been studied. Therefore, caution is advised should a patient's therapy include venlafaxine and any agent(s) that produce potent simultaneous inhibition of these two enzyme systems.

Drugs Metabolized by Cytochrome P450 Isoenzymes

CYP2D6: *In vitro* studies indicate that venlafaxine is a relatively weak inhibitor of CYP2D6. These findings have been confirmed in a clinical drug interaction study comparing the effect of venlafaxine to that of fluoxetine on the CYP2D6-mediated metabolism of dextromethorphan to dextrorphan.

Imipramine–Venlafaxine did not inhibit the CYP2D6-mediated metabolism of imipramine or its active metabolite, desipramine. However, the renal clearance of 2-hydroxydesipramine was reduced with coadministration of venlafaxine.

Risperidone–Venlafaxine administered under steady-state conditions at 75 mg every 12 hours slightly inhibited the CYP2D6-mediated metabolism of risperidone (administered as a single 1 mg oral dose) to its active metabolite, 9-hydroxyrisperidone, resulting in an approximate 32% increase in risperidone AUC. However, venlafaxine coadministration did not significantly alter the pharmacokinetic profile of the total active moiety (risperidone plus 9-hydroxyrisperidone).

CYP3A4: Venlafaxine did not inhibit CYP3A4 *in vitro*. This finding was confirmed *in vivo* by clinical drug interaction studies in which venlafaxine did not inhibit the metabolism of several CYP3A4 substrates, including alprazolam, diazepam, and terfenadine.

CYP1A2: Venlafaxine did not inhibit CYP1A2 *in vitro*. This finding was confirmed *in vivo* by a clinical drug interaction study in which venlafaxine did not inhibit the metabolism of caffeine, a CYP1A2 substrate.

CYP2C9: Venlafaxine did not inhibit CYP2C9 *in vitro*. The clinical significance of this finding is unknown.

CYP2C19: Venlafaxine did not inhibit the metabolism of diazepam which is partially metabolized by CYP2C19 (see *"Diazepam"* above).

Monoamine Oxidase Inhibitors

See **"CONTRAINDICATIONS"** and **"WARNINGS."**

CNS-Active Drugs

The risk of using venlafaxine in combination with other CNS-active drugs has not been systematically evaluated (except in the case of those CNS-active drugs noted above). Consequently, caution is advised if the concomitant administration of venlafaxine and such drugs is required.

Electroconvulsive Therapy

There are no clinical data establishing the benefit of electroconvulsive therapy combined with Effexor treatment.

Postmarketing Spontaneous Drug Interaction Reports

See "**ADVERSE REACTIONS**, **Postmarketing Reports**."

Carcinogenesis, Mutagenesis, Impairment of Fertility

Carcinogenesis

Venlafaxine was given by oral gavage to mice for 18 months at doses up to 120 mg/kg per day, which was 16 times, on a mg/kg basis, and 1.7 times on a mg/m^2 basis, the maximum recommended human dose. Venlafaxine was also given to rats by oral gavage for 24 months at doses up to 120 mg/kg per day. In rats receiving the 120 mg/kg dose, plasma levels of venlafaxine were 1 times (male rats) and 6 times (female rats) the plasma levels of patients receiving the maximum recommended human dose. Plasma levels of the O-desmethyl metabolite were lower in rats than in patients receiving the maximum recommended dose. Tumors were not increased by venlafaxine treatment in mice or rats.

Mutagenicity

Venlafaxine and the major human metabolite, O-desmethylvenlafaxine (ODV), were not mutagenic in the Ames reverse mutation assay in Salmonella bacteria or the CHO/HGPRT mammalian cell forward gene mutation assay. Venlafaxine was also not mutagenic in the *in vitro* BALB/c-3T3 mouse cell transformation assay, the sister chromatid exchange assay in cultured CHO cells, or the *in vivo* chromosomal aberration assay in rat bone marrow. ODV was not mutagenic in the *in vitro* CHO cell chromosomal aberration assay. There was a clastogenic response in the *in vivo* chromosomal aberration assay in rat bone marrow in male rats receiving 200 times, on a mg/kg basis, or 50 times, on a mg/m^2 basis, the maximum human daily dose. The no effect dose was 67 times (mg/kg) or 17 times (mg/m^2) the human dose.

Impairment of Fertility

Reproduction and fertility studies in rats showed no effects on male or female fertility at oral doses of up to 8 times the maximum recommended human daily dose on a mg/kg basis, or up to 2 times on a mg/m^2 basis.

Pregnancy

Teratogenic Effects—Pregnancy Category C

Venlafaxine did not cause malformations in offspring of rats or rabbits given doses up to 11 times (rat) or 12 times (rabbit) the maximum recommended human daily dose on a mg/kg basis, or 2.5 times (rat) and 4 times (rabbit) the human daily dose on a mg/m^2 basis. However, in rats, there was a decrease in pup weight, an increase in stillborn pups, and an increase in pup deaths during the first 5 days of lactation, when dosing began during pregnancy and continued until weaning. The cause of these deaths is not known. These effects occurred at 10 times (mg/kg) or 2.5 times (mg/m^2) the maximum human daily dose. The no effect dose for rat pup mortality was 1.4 times the human dose on a mg/kg basis or 0.25 times the human dose on a mg/m^2 basis. There are no adequate and well-controlled studies in pregnant

Continued on next page

Effexor—Cont.

women. Because animal reproduction studies are not always predictive of human response, this drug should be used during pregnancy only if clearly needed.

Labor and Delivery
The effect of Effexor® (venlafaxine hydrochloride) on labor and delivery in humans is unknown.

Nursing Mothers
It is not known whether venlafaxine hydrochloride or its metabolites are excreted in human milk. Because many drugs are excreted in human milk, caution should be exercised when Effexor is administered to a nursing woman.

Usage in Children
Safety and effectiveness in individuals below 18 years of age have not been established.

Geriatric Use
Of the 2,897 patients in phase 2–3 depression studies with Effexor, 12% (357) were 65 years of age or over. No overall differences in effectiveness or safety were observed between these patients and younger patients, and other reported clinical experience has not identified differences in response between the elderly and younger patients. However, greater sensitivity of some older individuals cannot be ruled out.

ADVERSE REACTIONS

Associated with Discontinuation of Treatment
Nineteen percent (537/2897) of venlafaxine patients in phase 2–3 depression studies discontinued treatment due to an adverse event. The more common events ($\geq 1\%$) associated with discontinuation and considered to be drug-related (i.e., those events associated with dropout at a rate approximately twice or greater for venlafaxine compared to placebo) included:

CNS	Venlafaxine	Placebo
Somnolence	3%	1%
Insomnia	3%	1%
Dizziness	3%	—
Nervousness	2%	—
Dry mouth	2%	—
Anxiety	2%	1%
Gastrointestinal		
Nausea	6%	1%
Urogenital		
Abnormal ejaculation*	3%	—
Other		
Headache	3%	1%
Asthenia	2%	—
Sweating	2%	—

* Percentages based on the number of males.
— Less than 1%

Incidence in Controlled Trials
Commonly Observed Adverse Events in Controlled Clinical Trials
The most commonly observed adverse events associated with the use of Effexor® (incidence of 5% or greater) and not seen at an equivalent incidence among placebo-treated patients (i.e., incidence for Effexor at least twice that for placebo), derived from the 1% incidence table below, were asthenia, sweating, nausea, constipation, anorexia, vomiting, somnolence, dry mouth, dizziness, nervousness, anxiety, tremor, and blurred vision as well as abnormal ejaculation/orgasm and impotence in men.

Adverse Events Occurring at an Incidence of 1% or More Among Effexor-Treated Patients
The table that follows enumerates adverse events that occurred at an incidence of 1% or more, and were more frequent than in the placebo group, among Effexor-treated patients who participated in short-term (4- to 8-week) placebo-controlled trials in which patients were administered doses in a range of 75 to 375 mg/day. This table shows the percentage of patients in each group who had at least one episode of an event at some time during their treatment. Reported adverse events were classified using a standard COSTART-based Dictionary terminology.

The prescriber should be aware that these figures cannot be used to predict the incidence of side effects in the course of usual medical practice where patient characteristics and other factors differ from those which prevailed in the clinical trials. Similarly, the cited frequencies cannot be compared with figures obtained from other clinical investigations involving different treatments, uses and investigators. The cited figures, however, do provide the prescribing physician with some basis for estimating the relative contribution of drug and nondrug factors to the side effect incidence rate in the population studied.

[See table 1 at right]

Dose Dependency of Adverse Events
A comparison of adverse event rates in a fixed-dose study comparing Effexor (venlafaxine hydrochloride) 75, 225, and 375 mg/day with placebo revealed a dose dependency for some of the more common adverse events associated with Effexor use, as shown in the table that follows. The rule for including events was to enumerate those that occurred at an incidence of 5% or more for at least one of the venlafaxine groups and for which the incidence was at least twice the placebo incidence for at least one Effexor group. Tests for potential dose relationships for these events (Cochran-Armitage Test, with a criterion of exact 2-sided p-value ≤ 0.05) suggested a dose-dependency for several adverse events in this list, including chills, hypertension, anorexia, nausea, agitation, dizziness, somnolence, tremor, yawning, sweating, and abnormal ejaculation.

[See table 2 at bottom of next page]

Adaptation to Certain Adverse Events
Over a 6-week period, there was evidence of adaptation to some adverse events with continued therapy (e.g., dizziness and nausea), but less to other effects (e.g., abnormal ejaculation and dry mouth).

Vital Sign Changes
Effexor (venlafaxine hydrochloride) treatment (averaged over all dose groups) in clinical trials was associated with a mean increase in pulse rate of approximately 3 beats per minute, compared to no change for placebo. It was associated with mean increases in diastolic blood pressure ranging from 0.7 to 2.5 mm Hg averaged over all dose groups, compared to mean decreases ranging from 0.9 to 3.8 mm Hg for placebo. However, there is a dose dependency for blood pressure increase (see "WARNINGS").

Laboratory Changes
Of the serum chemistry and hematology parameters monitored during clinical trials with Effexor, a statistically significant difference with placebo was seen only for serum cholesterol, i.e., patients treated with Effexor had mean increases from baseline of 3 mg/dL, a change of unknown clinical significance.

ECG Changes
In an analysis of ECGs obtained in 769 patients treated with Effexor and 450 patients treated with placebo in controlled clinical trials, the only statistically significant difference observed was for heart rate, i.e., a mean increase from baseline of 4 beats per minute for Effexor.

Other Events Observed During the Premarketing Evaluation of Venlafaxine
During its premarketing assessment, multiple doses of Effexor were administered to 2181 patients in phase 2 and 3 studies. The conditions and duration of exposure to Effexor varied greatly, and included (in overlapping categories) open and double-blind studies, uncontrolled and controlled studies, inpatient and outpatient studies, fixed-dose and titration studies. Untoward events associated with this exposure were recorded by clinical investigators using terminology of their own choosing. Consequently, it is not possible to

---

TABLE 1
Treatment-Emergent Adverse Experience Incidence in
4- to 8-Week Placebo-Controlled Clinical Trials[1]

Body System	Preferred Term	Effexor (n=1033)	Placebo (n=609)
Body as a Whole	Headache	25%	24%
	Asthenia	12%	6%
	Infection	6%	5%
	Chills	3%	—
	Chest pain	2%	1%
	Trauma	2%	1%
Cardiovascular	Vasodilatation	4%	3%
	Increased blood pressure/hypertension	2%	—
	Tachycardia	2%	—
	Postural hypotension	1%	—
Dermatological	Sweating	12%	3%
	Rash	3%	2%
	Pruritus	1%	—
Gastrointestinal	Nausea	37%	11%
	Constipation	15%	7%
	Anorexia	11%	2%
	Diarrhea	8%	7%
	Vomiting	6%	2%
	Dyspepsia	5%	4%
	Flatulence	3%	2%
Metabolic	Weight loss	1%	—
Nervous System	Somnolence	23%	9%
	Dry mouth	22%	11%
	Dizziness	19%	7%
	Insomnia	18%	10%
	Nervousness	13%	6%
	Anxiety	6%	3%
	Tremor	5%	1%
	Abnormal dreams	4%	3%
	Hypertonia	3%	2%
	Paresthesia	3%	2%
	Libido decreased	2%	—
	Agitation	2%	—
	Confusion	2%	1%
	Thinking abnormal	2%	1%
	Depersonalization	1%	—
	Depression	1%	—
	Urinary retention	1%	—
	Twitching	1%	—
Respiration	Yawn	3%	—
Special Senses	Blurred vision	6%	2%
	Taste perversion	2%	—
	Tinnitus	2%	—
	Mydriasis	2%	—
Urogenital System	Abnormal ejaculation/orgasm	12%[2]	—[2]
	Impotence	6%[2]	—[2]
	Urinary frequency	3%	2%
	Urination impaired	2%	—
	Orgasm disturbance	2%[3]	—[3]
	Menstrual disorder	1%[3]	—[3]

[1] Events reported by at least 1% of patients treated with Effexor (venlafaxine hydrochloride) are included, and are rounded to the nearest %. Events for which the Effexor incidence was equal to or less than placebo are not listed in the table, but included the following: abdominal pain, pain, back pain, flu syndrome, fever, palpitation, increased appetite, myalgia, arthralgia, amnesia, hypesthesia, rhinitis, pharyngitis, sinusitis, cough increased, urinary tract infection, and dysmenorrhea[3]
—Incidence less than 1%.
[2] Incidence based on number of male patients.
[3] Incidence based on number of female patients.

provide a meaningful estimate of the proportion of individuals experiencing adverse events without first grouping similar types of untoward events into a smaller number of standardized event categories.

In the tabulations that follow, reported adverse events were classified using a standard COSTART-based Dictionary terminology. The frequencies presented, therefore, represent the proportion of the 2181 patients exposed to multiple doses of Effexor who experienced an event of the type cited on at least one occasion while receiving Effexor. All reported events are included except those already listed in Table 1 and those events for which a drug cause was remote. If the COSTART term for an event was so general as to be uninformative, it was replaced with a more informative term. It is important to emphasize that, although the events reported occurred during treatment with Effexor, they were not necessarily caused by it.

Events are further categorized by body system and listed in order of decreasing frequency according to the following definitions: frequent adverse events are those occurring on one or more occasions in at least 1/100 patients (only those not already listed in the tabulated results from placebo-controlled trials appear in this listing); infrequent adverse events are those occurring in 1/100 to 1/1000 patients; rare events are those occurring in fewer than 1/1000 patients.

Body as a whole—Frequent: accidental injury, malaise, neck pain; Infrequent: abdomen enlarged, allergic reaction, cyst, face edema, generalized edema, hangover effect, hernia, intentional injury, moniliasis, neck rigidity, overdose, chest pain substernal, pelvic pain, photosensitivity reaction, suicide attempt; Rare: appendicitis, body odor, carcinoma, cellulitis, halitosis, ulcer, withdrawal syndrome.

Cardiovascular system—Infrequent: migraine; Infrequent: angina pectoris, extrasystoles, hypotension, peripheral vascular disorder (mainly cold feet and/or cold hands), syncope, thrombophlebitis; Rare: arrhythmia, first-degree atrioventricular block, bradycardia, bundle branch block, mitral valve disorder, mucocutaneous hemorrhage, sinus bradycardia, varicose vein.

Digestive system—Frequent: dysphagia, eructation; Infrequent: colitis, tongue edema, esophagitis, gastritis, gastroenteritis, gingivitis, glossitis, rectal hemorrhage, hemorrhoids, melena, stomatitis, stomach ulcer, mouth ulceration; Rare: cheilitis, cholecystitis, cholelithiasis, hematemesis, gum hemorrhage, hepatitis, ileitis, jaundice, oral moniliasis, intestinal obstruction, proctitis, increased salivation, soft stools, tongue discoloration, esophageal ulcer, peptic ulcer syndrome.

Endocrine system—Rare: goiter, hyperthyroidism, hypothyroidism.

Hemic and lymphatic system—Frequent: ecchymosis; Infrequent: anemia, leukocytosis, leukopenia, lymphadenopathy, lymphocytosis, thrombocythemia, thrombocytopenia, WBC abnormal; Rare: basophilia, cyanosis, eosinophilia, erythrocytes abnormal.

Metabolic and nutritional—Frequent: peripheral edema, weight gain; Infrequent: alkaline phosphatase increased, creatinine increased, diabetes mellitus, edema, glycosuria, hypercholesteremia, hyperglycemia, hyperlipemia, hyperuricemia, hypoglycemia, hypokalemia, SGOT increased, thirst; Rare: alcohol intolerance, bilirubinemia, BUN increased, gout, hemochromatosis, hyperkalemia, hyperphosphatemia, hypoglycemic reaction, hyponatremia, hypophosphatemia, hypoproteinemia, SGPT increased, uremia.

Musculoskeletal system—Infrequent: arthritis, arthrosis, bone pain, bone spurs, bursitis, joint disorder, myasthenia, tenosynovitis; Rare: osteoporosis.

Nervous system—Frequent: emotional lability, trismus, vertigo; Infrequent: apathy, ataxia, circumoral paresthesia, CNS stimulation, euphoria, hallucinations, hostility, hyperesthesia, hyperkinesia, hypertonia, hypotonia, incoordination, libido increased, manic reaction, myoclonus, neuralgia, neuropathy, paranoid reaction, psychosis, psychotic depression, sleep disturbance, abnormal speech, stupor, torticollis; Rare: akathisia, akinesia, alcohol abuse, aphasia, bradykinesia, cerebrovascular accident, loss of consciousness, delusions, dementia, dystonia, hypokinesia, neuritis, nystagmus, reflexes increased, seizures.

Respiratory system—Frequent: bronchitis, dyspnea; Infrequent: asthma, chest congestion, epistaxis, hyperventilation, laryngismus, laryngitis, pneumonia, voice alteration; Rare: atelectasis, hemoptysis, hypoxia, pleurisy, pulmonary embolus, sleep apnea, sputum increased.

Skin and appendages—Infrequent: acne, alopecia, brittle nails, contact dermatitis, dry skin, herpes simplex, herpes zoster, maculopapular rash, urticaria; Rare: skin atrophy, exfoliative dermatitis, fungal dermatitis, lichenoid dermatitis, hair discoloration, eczema, furunculosis, hirsutism, skin hypertrophy, leukoderma, psoriasis, pustular rash, vesiculobullous rash.

Special senses—Frequent: abnormal vision, ear pain; Infrequent: cataract, conjunctivitis, corneal lesion, diplopia, dry eyes, exophthalmos, eye pain, otitis media, parosmia, photophobia, subconjunctival hemorrhage, taste loss, visual field defect; Rare: blepharitis, chromatopsia, conjunctival edema, deafness, glaucoma, hyperacusis, keratitis, labyrinthitis, miosis, papilledema, decreased pupillary reflex, scleritis.

Urogenital system—Frequent: anorgasmia, dysuria, hematuria, metrorrhagia*, urination impaired, vaginitis*; Infrequent: albuminuria, amenorrhea*, kidney calculus, cystitis, leukorrhea, menorrhagia*, nocturia, bladder pain, breast pain, kidney pain, polyuria, prostatitis*, pyelonephritis, pyuria, urinary incontinence, urinary urgency, uterine fibroids enlarged*, uterine hemorrhage*, vaginal hemorrhage*, vaginal moniliasis*; Rare: abortion*, breast engorgement, breast enlargement, calcium crystalluria, female lactation*, hypomenorrhea*, menopause*, prolonged erection*, uterine spasm*.

---

* Based on the number of male or female patients as appropriate.

Postmarketing Reports

Voluntary reports of other adverse events temporally associated with the use of EFFEXOR that have been received since market introduction and that may have no causal relationship with the use of EFFEXOR include the following: abnormal gait, agranulocytosis, anaphylaxis, aplastic anemia, bruxism, catatonia, congenital anomalies, congestive heart failure, CPK increased, deep vein thrombophlebitis, dehydration, delirium, EKG abnormalities (such as atrial fibrillation, bigeminy, supraventricular tachycardia, ventricular extrasystole, ventricular tachycardia), epidermal necrosis/Stevens-Johnson Syndrome, extrapyramidal symptoms (including tardive dyskinesia), heart arrest, hemorrhage (including eye and gastrointestinal bleeding), hepatic events (including GGT elevation; abnormalities of unspecified liver function tests; liver damage, necrosis, or failure; and fatty liver), involuntary movements, LDH increased, myocardial infarction, neuroleptic malignant syndrome-like events (including a case of a 10-year-old who may have been taking methylphenidate, was treated and recovered), pancreatitis, panic, prolactin increased, renal failure, serotonin syndrome, shock-like electrical sensations (in some cases, subsequent to the discontinuation of Effexor or tapering of dose), and syndrome of inappropriate antidiuretic hormone secretion.

There have been reports of elevated clozapine levels that were temporally associated with adverse events, including seizures, following the addition of venlafaxine. There have been reports of increases in prothrombin time, partial thromboplastin time, or INR when venlafaxine was given to patients receiving warfarin therapy.

DRUG ABUSE AND DEPENDENCE

Controlled Substance Class

Effexor (venlafaxine hydrochloride) is not a controlled substance.

Physical and Psychological Dependence

In vitro studies revealed that venlafaxine has virtually no affinity for opiate, benzodiazepine, phencyclidine (PCP), or N-methyl-D-aspartic acid (NMDA) receptors.

Venlafaxine was not found to have any significant CNS stimulant activity in rodents. In primate drug discrimination studies, venlafaxine showed no significant stimulant or depressant abuse liability.

While the discontinuation effects of Effexor have not been systematically evaluated in controlled clinical trials, a retrospective survey of new events occurring during taper or following discontinuation revealed the following six events that occurred at an incidence of at least 5% and for which the incidence for Effexor was at least twice the placebo incidence: asthenia, dizziness, headache, insomnia, nausea, and nervousness. Therefore, it is recommended that the dosage be tapered gradually and the patient monitored (see "DOSAGE AND ADMINISTRATION").

While Effexor has not been systematically studied in clinical trials for its potential for abuse, there was no indication of drug-seeking behavior in the clinical trials. However, it is not possible to predict on the basis of premarketing experience the extent to which a CNS active drug will be misused, diverted, and/or abused once marketed. Consequently, physicians should carefully evaluate patients for history of drug abuse and follow such patients closely, observing them for signs of misuse or abuse of Effexor (e.g., development of tolerance, incrementation of dose, drug-seeking behavior).

OVERDOSAGE

Human Experience

There were 14 reports of acute overdose with Effexor (venlafaxine hydrochloride), either alone or in combination with other drugs and/or alcohol, among the patients included in the premarketing evaluation. The majority of the reports involved ingestions in which the total dose of Effexor taken was estimated to be no more than several-fold higher than the usual therapeutic dose. The 3 patients who took the highest doses were estimated to have ingested approximately 6.75 g, 2.75 g, and 2.5 g. The resultant peak plasma levels of venlafaxine for the latter 2 patients were 6.24 and 2.35 µg/mL, respectively, and the peak plasma levels of O-desmethylvenlafaxine were 3.37 and 1.30 µg/mL, respectively. Plasma venlafaxine levels were not obtained for the

TABLE 2
Treatment-Emergent Adverse Experience Incidence in a Dose Comparison Trial

Body System/ Preferred Term	Placebo (n=92)	Effexor (mg/day)		
		75 (n=89)	225 (n=89)	375 (n=88)
Body as a Whole				
Abdominal pain	3.3%	3.4%	2.2%	8.0%
Asthenia	3.3%	16.9%	14.6%	14.8%
Chills	1.1%	2.2%	5.6%	6.8%
Infection	2.2%	2.2%	5.6%	2.3%
Cardiovascular System				
Hypertension	1.1%	1.1%	2.2%	4.5%
Vasodilatation	0.0%	4.5%	5.6%	2.3%
Digestive System				
Anorexia	2.2%	14.6%	13.5%	17.0%
Dyspepsia	2.2%	6.7%	6.7%	4.5%
Nausea	14.1%	32.6%	38.2%	58.0%
Vomiting	1.1%	7.9%	3.4%	6.8%
Nervous System				
Agitation	0.0%	1.1%	2.2%	4.5%
Anxiety	4.3%	11.2%	4.5%	2.3%
Dizziness	4.3%	19.1%	22.5%	23.9%
Insomnia	9.8%	22.5%	20.2%	13.6%
Libido decreased	1.1%	2.2%	1.1%	5.7%
Nervousness	4.3%	21.3%	13.5%	12.5%
Somnolence	4.3%	16.9%	18.0%	26.1%
Tremor	0.0%	1.1%	2.2%	10.2%
Respiratory System				
Yawn	0.0%	4.5%	5.6%	8.0%
Skin and Appendages				
Sweating	5.4%	6.7%	12.4%	19.3%
Special Senses				
Abnormality of accommodation	0.0%	9.1%	7.9%	5.6%
Urogenital System				
Abnormal ejaculation/orgasm	0.0%	4.5%	2.2%	12.5%
Impotence	0.0%	5.8%	2.1%	3.6%
(Number of men)	(n=63)	(n=52)	(n=48)	(n=56)

Continued on next page

Effexor—Cont.

patient who ingested 6.75 g of venlafaxine. All 14 patients recovered without sequelae. Most patients reported no symptoms. Among the remaining patients, somnolence was the most commonly reported symptom. The patient who ingested 2.75 g of venlafaxine was observed to have 2 generalized convulsions and a prolongation of QTc to 500 msec, compared with 405 msec at baseline. Mild sinus tachycardia was reported in 2 of the other patients.

In postmarketing experience, there have been reports of fatalities in patients taking overdoses of venlafaxine, predominantly in combination with alcohol and/or other drugs.

Overdosage Management

Treatment should consist of those general measures employed in the management of overdosage with any antidepressant. Ensure an adequate airway, oxygenation, and ventilation. Monitoring of cardiac rhythm and vital signs is recommended. General supportive and symptomatic measures are also recommended. Use of activated charcoal, induction of emesis, or gastric lavage should be considered. Due to the large volume of distribution of venlafaxine hydrochloride, forced diuresis, dialysis, hemoperfusion and exchange transfusion are unlikely to be of benefit. No specific antidotes for Effexor are known.

In managing overdosage, consider the possibility of multiple drug involvement. The physician should consider contacting a poison control center on the treatment of any overdose.

DOSAGE AND ADMINISTRATION

Initial Treatment

The recommended starting dose for Effexor is 75 mg/day, administered in two or three divided doses, taken with food. Depending on tolerability and the need for further clinical effect, the dose may be increased to 150 mg/day. If needed, the dose should be further increased up to 225 mg/day. When increasing the dose, increments of up to 75 mg/day should be made at intervals of no less than 4 days. In outpatient settings there was no evidence of usefulness of doses greater than 225 mg/day for moderately depressed patients, but more severely depressed inpatients responded to a mean dose of 350 mg/day. Certain patients, including more severely depressed patients, may therefore respond more to higher doses, up to a maximum of 375 mg/day, generally in three divided doses.

Dosage for Patients with Hepatic Impairment

Given the decrease in clearance and increase in elimination half-life for both venlafaxine and ODV that is observed in patients with hepatic cirrhosis compared to normal subjects (see **"CLINICAL PHARMACOLOGY"**), it is recommended that the total daily dose be reduced by 50% in patients with moderate hepatic impairment. Since there was much individual variability in clearance between patients with cirrhosis, it may be necessary to reduce the dose even more than 50%, and individualization of dosing may be desirable in some patients.

Dosage for Patients with Renal Impairment

Given the decrease in clearance for venlafaxine and the increase in elimination half-life for both venlafaxine and ODV that is observed in patients with renal impairment (GFR = 10-70 mL/min) compared to normals (see **"CLINICAL PHARMACOLOGY"**), it is recommended that the total daily dose be reduced by 25% in patients with mild to moderate renal impairment. It is recommended that the total daily dose be reduced by 50% and the dose be withheld until the dialysis treatment is completed (4 hrs) in patients undergoing hemodialysis. Since there was much individual variability in clearance between patients with renal impairment, individualization of dosing may be desirable in some patients.

Dosage for Elderly Patients

No dose adjustment is recommended for elderly patients on the basis of age. As with any antidepressant, however, caution should be exercised in treating the elderly. When individualizing the dosage, extra care should be taken when increasing the dose.

Maintenance/Continuation/Extended Treatment

There is no body of evidence available to answer the question of how long a patient should continue to be treated with Effexor. It is generally agreed that acute episodes of major depression require several months or longer of sustained pharmacologic therapy. Whether the dose of antidepressant needed to induce remission is identical to the dose needed to maintain and/or sustain euthymia is unknown.

Discontinuing Effexor (venlafaxine hydrochloride)

When discontinuing Effexor after more than 1 week of therapy, it is generally recommended that the dose be tapered to minimize the risk of discontinuation symptoms. Patients who have received Effexor for 6 weeks or more should have their dose tapered gradually over a 2-week period.

SWITCHING PATIENTS TO OR FROM A MONOAMINE OXIDASE INHIBITOR

At least 14 days should elapse between discontinuation of an MAOI and initiation of therapy with Effexor. In addition, at least 7 days should be allowed after stopping Effexor before starting an MAOI (see **"CONTRAINDICATIONS"** and **"WARNINGS"**).

HOW SUPPLIED

Effexor® (venlafaxine HCl tablets) is available in bottles of 100 tablets and in Redipak® cartons of 100 tablets (10 blister strips of 10) in the following dosage strengths (expressed in equivalent amounts of venlafaxine):

25 mg, NDC 0008-0701-02, peach, shield-shaped tablet with "25" and a "W" on one side and "701" on scored reverse side.

37.5 mg, NDC 0008-0781-02, peach, shield-shaped tablet with "37.5" and a "W" on one side and "781" on scored reverse side.

50 mg, NDC 0008-0703-02, peach, shield-shaped tablet with "50" and a "W" on one side and "703" on scored reverse side.

75 mg, NDC 0008-0704-02, peach, shield-shaped tablet with "75" and a "W" on one side and "704" on scored reverse side.

100 mg, NDC 0008-0705-02, peach, shield-shaped tablet with "100" and a "W" on one side and "705" on scored reverse side.

The appearance of these tablets is a trademark of Wyeth-Ayerst Laboratories.

Store at controlled room temperature, 20°C to 25°C (68°F to 77°F), in a dry place.

Dispense in a well-closed container as defined in the USP.

Manufactured by:
Wyeth Laboratories Inc.
A Wyeth-Ayerst Company
Philadelphia, PA 19101

Shown in Product Identification Guide, page 343

EFFEXOR® XR ℞

[ĕf-fĕks'ŏr XR]

(venlafaxine hydrochloride)
Extended Release Capsules

DESCRIPTION

Effexor XR is an extended release capsule for oral administration that contains venlafaxine hydrochloride, a structurally novel antidepressant. Venlafaxine hydrochloride is chemically unrelated to tricyclic, tetracyclic, or other available antidepressant agents. It is designated (R/S)-1-[2-(dimethylamino)-1-(4-methoxyphenyl) ethyl] cyclohexanol hydrochloride or (±)-1-[α-[(dimethylamino)methyl]-p-methoxybenzyl] cyclohexanol hydrochloride and has the empirical formula of $C_{17}H_{27}NO_2$ hydrochloride. Its molecular weight is 313.87. The structural formula is shown below.

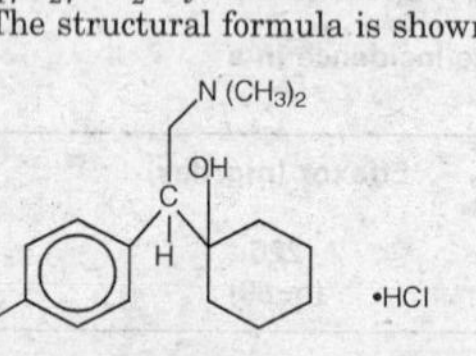

venlafaxine hydrochloride

Venlafaxine hydrochloride is a white to off-white crystalline solid with a solubility of 572 mg/mL in water (adjusted to ionic strength of 0.2 M with sodium chloride). Its octanol: water (0.2 M sodium chloride) partition coefficient is 0.43.

Effexor XR is formulated as an extended release capsule for once-a-day oral administration. Drug release is controlled by diffusion through the coating membrane on the spheroids and is not pH dependent. Capsules contain venlafaxine hydrochloride equivalent to 37.5 mg, 75 mg, or 150 mg venlafaxine. Inactive ingredients consist of cellulose, ethylcellulose, gelatin, hydroxypropyl methylcellulose, iron oxide, and titanium dioxide.

CLINICAL PHARMACOLOGY

Pharmacodynamics

The mechanism of the antidepressant action of venlafaxine in humans is believed to be associated with its potentiation of neurotransmitter activity in the CNS. Preclinical studies have shown that venlafaxine and its active metabolite, O-desmethylvenlafaxine (ODV), are potent inhibitors of neuronal serotonin and norepinephrine reuptake and weak inhibitors of dopamine reuptake. Venlafaxine and ODV have no significant affinity for muscarinic cholinergic, H_1-histaminergic, or α_1-adrenergic receptors *in vitro*. Pharmacologic activity at these receptors is hypothesized to be associated with the various anticholinergic, sedative, and cardiovascular effects seen with other psychotropic drugs. Venlafaxine and ODV do not possess monoamine oxidase (MAO) inhibitory activity.

Pharmacokinetics

Steady-state concentrations of venlafaxine and ODV in plasma are attained within 3 days of oral multiple dose therapy. Venlafaxine and ODV exhibited linear kinetics over the dose range of 75 to 450 mg/day. Mean±SD steady-state plasma clearance of venlafaxine and ODV is 1.3±0.6 and 0.4±0.2 L/h/kg, respectively; apparent elimination half-life is 5±2 and 11±2 hours, respectively; and apparent (steady-state) volume of distribution is 7.5±3.7 and 5.7±1.8 L/kg, respectively. Venlafaxine and ODV are minimally bound at therapeutic concentrations to plasma proteins (27 and 30%, respectively).

Absorption

Venlafaxine is well absorbed and extensively metabolized in the liver. O-desmethylvenlafaxine (ODV) is the only major active metabolite. On the basis of mass balance studies, at least 92% of a single dose of venlafaxine is absorbed. The absolute bioavailability of venlafaxine is about 45%.

Administration of Effexor XR (150 mg q24 hours) generally resulted in lower C_{max} (150 ng/mL for venlafaxine and 260 ng/mL for ODV) and later T_{max} (5.5 hours for venlafaxine and 9 hours for ODV) than for immediate release venlafaxine tablets (C_{max}'s for immediate release 75 mg q12 hours were 225 ng/mL for venlafaxine and 290 ng/mL for ODV; T_{max}'s were 2 hours for venlafaxine and 3 hours for ODV). When equal daily doses of venlafaxine were administered as either an immediate release tablet or the extended release capsule, the exposure to both venlafaxine and ODV was similar for the two treatments, and the fluctuation in plasma concentrations was slightly lower with the Effexor XR capsule. Effexor XR, therefore, provides a slower rate of absorption but the same extent of absorption compared with the immediate release tablet.

Food did not affect the bioavailability of venlafaxine or its active metabolite, ODV. Time of administration (AM vs PM) did not affect the pharmacokinetics of venlafaxine and ODV from the 75 mg Effexor XR capsule.

Metabolism and Excretion

Following absorption, venlafaxine undergoes extensive presystemic metabolism in the liver, primarily to ODV, but also to N-desmethylvenlafaxine, N,O-didesmethylvenlafaxine, and other minor metabolites. *In vitro* studies indicate that the formation of ODV is catalyzed by CYP2D6; this has been confirmed in a clinical study showing that patients with low CYP2D6 levels ("poor metabolizers") had increased levels of venlafaxine and reduced levels of ODV compared to people with normal CYP2D6 ("extensive metabolizers"). The differences between the CYP2D6 poor and extensive metabolizers, however, is not expected to be clinically important because the sum of venlafaxine and ODV is similar in the two groups and venlafaxine and ODV are pharmacologically approximately equiactive and equipotent.

Approximately 87% of a venlafaxine dose is recovered in the urine within 48 hours as unchanged venlafaxine (5%), unconjugated ODV (29%), conjugated ODV (26%), or other minor inactive metabolites (27%). Renal elimination of venlafaxine and its metabolites is thus the primary route of excretion.

Special Populations

Age and Gender: A population pharmacokinetic analysis of 404 venlafaxine-treated patients from two studies involving both b.i.d. and t.i.d. regimens showed that dose-normalized trough plasma levels of either venlafaxine or ODV were unaltered by age or gender differences. Dosage adjustment based on the age or gender of a patient is generally not necessary (see **"DOSAGE AND ADMINISTRATION"**).

Extensive/Poor Metabolizers: Plasma concentrations of venlafaxine were higher in CYP2D6 poor metabolizers than extensive metabolizers. Because the total exposure (AUC) of venlafaxine and ODV was similar in poor and extensive metabolizer groups, however, there is no need for different venlafaxine dosing regimens for these two groups.

Liver Disease: In 9 patients with hepatic cirrhosis, the pharmacokinetic disposition of both venlafaxine and ODV was significantly altered after oral administration of venlafaxine. Venlafaxine elimination half-life was prolonged by about 30%, and clearance decreased by about 50% in cirrhotic patients compared to normal subjects. ODV elimination half-life was prolonged by about 60% and clearance decreased by about 30% in cirrhotic patients compared to normal subjects. A large degree of intersubject variability was noted. Three patients with more severe cirrhosis had a more substantial decrease in venlafaxine clearance (about 90%) compared to normal subjects. Dosage adjustment is necessary in these patients (see **"DOSAGE AND ADMINISTRATION"**).

Renal Disease: In a renal impairment study, venlafaxine elimination half-life after oral administration was prolonged by about 50% and clearance was reduced by about 24% in renally impaired patients (GFR=10–70 mL/min), compared to normal subjects. In dialysis patients, venlafaxine elimination half-life was prolonged by about 180% and clearance was reduced by about 57% compared to normal subjects. Similarly, ODV elimination half-life was prolonged by about 40% although clearance was unchanged in patients with renal impairment (GFR=10–70 mL/min) compared to normal subjects. In dialysis patients, ODV elimination half-life was prolonged by about 142% and clearance was reduced by about 56% compared to normal subjects. A large degree of intersubject variability was noted. Dosage adjustment is necessary in these patients (see **"DOSAGE AND ADMINISTRATION"**).

Clinical Trials

The efficacy of Effexor XR (venlafaxine hydrochloride) extended release capsules as a treatment for depression was

established in two placebo-controlled, short-term, flexible-dose studies in adult outpatients meeting DSM-III-R or DSM-IV criteria for major depression.

A 12-week study utilizing Effexor XR doses in a range 75–150 mg/day (mean dose for completers was 136 mg/day) and an 8-week study utilizing Effexor XR doses in a range 75–225 mg/day (mean dose for completers was 177 mg/day) both demonstrated superiority of Effexor XR over placebo on the HAM-D total score, HAM-D Depressed Mood Item, the MADRS total score, the CGI Severity of Illness scale, and the CGI Global Improvement scale. In both studies, Effexor XR was also significantly better than placebo for certain factors of the HAM-D, including the anxiety/somatization factor, the cognitive disturbance factor, and the retardation factor, as well as for the psychic anxiety score.

A 4-week study of inpatients meeting DSM-III-R criteria for major depression with melancholia utilizing Effexor (the immediate release form of venlafaxine) in a range of 150 to 375 mg/day (t.i.d. schedule) demonstrated superiority of Effexor over placebo. The mean dose in completers was 350 mg/day. Examination of gender subsets of the population studied did not reveal any differential responsiveness on the basis of gender.

INDICATIONS AND USAGE

Effexor XR (venlafaxine hydrochloride) extended release capsules is indicated for the treatment of depression.

The efficacy of Effexor XR in the treatment of depression was established in 8- and 12-week controlled trials of outpatients whose diagnoses corresponded most closely to the DSM-III-R or DSM-IV category of major depressive disorder (see "Clinical Trials").

A major depressive episode (DSM-IV) implies a prominent and relatively persistent (nearly every day for at least 2 weeks) depressed mood or the loss of interest or pleasure in nearly all activities, representing a change from previous functioning, and includes the presence of at least five of the following nine symptoms during the same two-week period: depressed mood, markedly diminished interest or pleasure in usual activities, significant change in weight and/or appetite, insomnia or hypersomnia, psychomotor agitation or retardation, increased fatigue, feelings of guilt or worthlessness, slowed thinking or impaired concentration, a suicide attempt or suicidal ideation.

The efficacy of Effexor (the immediate release form of venlafaxine) in the treatment of depression in inpatients meeting diagnostic criteria for major depressive disorder with melancholia was established in a 4-week controlled trial (see "Clinical Trials"). The safety and efficacy of Effexor XR in hospitalized depressed patients has not been adequately studied.

The effectiveness of Effexor XR in long-term use, that is, for more than 12 weeks, has not been systematically evaluated in controlled trials. The physician who elects to use Effexor XR for extended periods should periodically re-evaluate the long-term usefulness of the drug for the individual patient (See "DOSAGE AND ADMINISTRATION").

CONTRAINDICATIONS

Effexor XR (venlafaxine hydrochloride) extended release capsules is contraindicated in patients known to be hypersensitive to venlafaxine hydrochloride.

Concomitant use in patients taking monoamine oxidase inhibitors (MAOIs) is contraindicated (see "WARNINGS").

WARNINGS

Potential For Interaction With Monoamine Oxidase Inhibitors

Adverse reactions, some of which were serious, have been reported in patients who have recently been discontinued from a monoamine oxidase inhibitor (MAOI) and started on venlafaxine, or who have recently had venlafaxine therapy discontinued prior to initiation of an MAOI. These reactions have included tremor, myoclonus, diaphoresis, nausea, vomiting, flushing, dizziness, hyperthermia with features resembling neuroleptic malignant syndrome, seizures, and death. In patients receiving antidepressants with pharmacological properties similar to venlafaxine in combination with an MAOI, there have also been reports of serious, sometimes fatal, reactions. For a selective serotonin reuptake inhibitor, these reactions have included hyperthermia, rigidity, myoclonus, autonomic instability with possible rapid fluctuations of vital signs, and mental status changes that include extreme agitation progressing to delirium and coma. Some cases presented with features resembling neuroleptic malignant syndrome. Severe hyperthermia and seizures, sometimes fatal, have been reported in association with the combined use of tricyclic antidepressants and MAOIs. These reactions have also been reported in patients who have recently discontinued these drugs and have been started on an MAOI. The effects of combined use of venlafaxine and MAOIs have not been evaluated in humans or animals. Therefore, because venlafaxine is an inhibitor of both norepinephrine and serotonin reuptake, it is recommended that Effexor XR (venlafaxine hydrochloride) extended release capsules not be used in combination with an MAOI, or within at least 14 days of

discontinuing treatment with an MAOI. Based on the half-life of venlafaxine, at least 7 days should be allowed after stopping venlafaxine before starting an MAOI.

Sustained Hypertension

Venlafaxine is associated with sustained increases in blood pressure in some patients. Among patients treated with 75–375 mg per day of Effexor XR in premarketing studies, 3% (19/705) experienced sustained hypertension [defined as treatment-emergent supine diastolic blood pressure (SDBP) ≥90 mm Hg and ≥10 mm Hg above baseline for 3 consecutive on-therapy visits]. Experience with the immediate release venlafaxine showed that sustained hypertension was dose related, increasing from 3–7% at 100–300 mg per day to 13% at doses above 300 mg per day. An insufficient number of patients received mean doses of Effexor XR > 300 mg/day to fully evaluate the incidence of sustained blood pressure at these higher doses.

In placebo-controlled premarketing depression studies with Effexor XR 75–225 mg/day, a final on-drug mean increase in supine diastolic blood pressure (SDBP) of 1.2 mm Hg was observed for Effexor XR-treated patients compared with a mean decrease of 0.2 mm Hg for placebo-treated patients.

In premarketing depression studies, 0.7% (5/705) of the Effexor XR-treated patients discontinued treatment because of elevated blood pressure. Among these patients, most of the blood pressure increases were in a modest range (12–16 mm Hg, SDBP).

Sustained increases of SDBP could have adverse consequences. Therefore, it is recommended that patients receiving Effexor XR have regular monitoring of blood pressure. For patients who experience a sustained increase in blood pressure while receiving venlafaxine, either dose reduction or discontinuation should be considered.

PRECAUTIONS

General

Insomnia and Nervousness

Treatment-emergent insomnia and nervousness were more commonly reported for patients treated with Effexor XR (venlafaxine hydrochloride) extended release capsules than with placebo in a pooled analysis of short-term depression studies, as shown in Table 1.

TABLE 1
Incidence of Insomnia and Nervousness in Placebo-Controlled Trials

Symptom	Effexor XR (n = 357)	Placebo (n = 285)
Insomnia	17%	11%
Nervousness	10%	5%

Insomnia and nervousness each led to drug discontinuation in 0.9% of the patients treated with Effexor XR in Phase 3 studies.

Changes in Appetite and Weight

Treatment-emergent anorexia was more commonly reported for Effexor XR-treated (8%) than placebo-treated patients (4%) in the pool of short-term depression studies. Significant weight loss, especially in underweight depressed patients, may be an undesirable result of Effexor XR treatment. A loss of 5% or more of body weight occurred in 7% of Effexor XR-treated and 2% of placebo-treated patients in placebo-controlled trials. Discontinuation rates for anorexia and weight loss associated with Effexor XR were low (1.0% and 0.1%, respectively, of Effexor XR-treated patients in Phase 3 studies).

Activation of Mania/Hypomania

During premarketing experience, mania or hypomania occurred in 0.3% of Effexor XR-treated patients compared with 0% of placebo patients. In all premarketing depression trials with Effexor, mania or hypomania occurred in 0.5% of venlafaxine-treated patients compared with 0% of placebo patients. Mania/hypomania has also been reported in a small proportion of patients with mood disorders who were treated with other marketed antidepressants. As with all antidepressants, Effexor XR should be used cautiously in patients with a history of mania.

Seizures

During premarketing experience, no seizures occurred among 705 Effexor XR-treated patients. In all premarketing depression trials with Effexor, seizures were reported at various doses in 0.3% (8/3082) of venlafaxine-treated patients. Effexor XR, like other antidepressants, should be used cautiously in patients with a history of seizures and should be discontinued in any patient who develops seizures.

Suicide

The possibility of a suicide attempt is inherent in depression and may persist until significant remission occurs. Close supervision of high-risk patients should accompany initial drug therapy. Prescriptions for Effexor XR should be written for the smallest quantity of capsules consistent with good patient management in order to reduce the risk of overdose.

Use in Patients With Concomitant Illness

Premarketing experience with venlafaxine in patients with concomitant systemic illness is limited. Caution is advised in administering Effexor XR to patients with diseases or conditions that could affect hemodynamic responses or metabolism.

Venlafaxine has not been evaluated or used to any appreciable extent in patients with a recent history of myocardial infarction or unstable heart disease. Patients with these diagnoses were systematically excluded from many clinical studies during venlafaxine's premarketing testing. The electrocardiograms for 357 patients who received Effexor XR and 285 patients who received placebo in 8- to 12-week double-blind, placebo-controlled trials were analyzed. The mean change from baseline in corrected QT interval (QT$_c$) for Effexor XR-treated patients was increased relative to that for placebo-treated patients (increase of 4.7 msec for Effexor XR and decrease of 1.9 msec for placebo). In these same trials, the mean change from baseline in heart rate for Effexor XR-treated patients was significantly higher than that for placebo (a mean increase of 4 beats per minute for Effexor XR and 1 beat per minute for placebo). The clinical significance of these changes is unknown. Evaluation of the electrocardiograms for 769 patients who received immediate release Effexor in 4- to 6-week double-blind, placebo-controlled trials showed that the incidence of trial-emergent conduction abnormalities did not differ from that with placebo.

In patients with renal impairment (GFR = 10–70 mL/min) or cirrhosis of the liver, the clearances of venlafaxine and its active metabolites were decreased, thus prolonging the elimination half-lives of these substances. A lower dose may be necessary (see "DOSAGE AND ADMINISTRATION"). Effexor XR, like all antidepressants, should be used with caution in such patients.

Information for Patients

Physicians are advised to discuss the following issues with patients for whom they prescribe Effexor XR (venlafaxine hydrochloride) extended release capsules:

Interference With Cognitive and Motor Performance

Clinical studies were performed to examine the effects of venlafaxine on behavioral performance of healthy individuals. The results revealed no clinically significant impairment of psychomotor, cognitive, or complex behavior performance. However, since any psychoactive drug may impair judgment, thinking, or motor skills, patients should be cautioned about operating hazardous machinery, including automobiles, until they are reasonably certain that venlafaxine therapy does not adversely affect their ability to engage in such activities.

Concomitant Medication

Patients should be advised to inform their physicians if they are taking, or plan to take, any prescription or over-the-counter drugs, since there is a potential for interactions.

Alcohol

Although venlafaxine has been shown not to increase the impairment of mental and motor skills caused by alcohol, patients should be advised to avoid alcohol while taking venlafaxine.

Allergic Reactions

Patients should be advised to notify their physician if they develop a rash, hives, or a related allergic phenomenon.

Pregnancy

Patients should be advised to notify their physician if they become pregnant or intend to become pregnant during therapy.

Nursing

Patients should be advised to notify their physician if they are breast-feeding an infant.

Laboratory Tests

There are no specific laboratory tests recommended.

Drug Interactions

As with all drugs, the potential for interaction by a variety of mechanisms is a possibility.

Alcohol

A single dose of ethanol (0.5 g/kg) had no effect on the pharmacokinetics of venlafaxine or O-desmethylvenlafaxine (ODV) when venlafaxine was administered at 150 mg/day in 15 healthy male subjects. Additionally, administration of venlafaxine in a stable regimen did not exaggerate the psychomotor and psychometric effects induced by ethanol in these same subjects when they were not receiving venlafaxine.

Cimetidine

Concomitant administration of cimetidine and venlafaxine in a steady-state study for both drugs resulted in inhibition of first-pass metabolism of venlafaxine in 18 healthy subjects. The oral clearance of venlafaxine was reduced by about 43%, and the exposure (AUC) and maximum concentration (C$_{max}$) of the drug were increased by about 60%. However, coadministration of cimetidine had no apparent effect on the pharmacokinetics of ODV, which is present in much greater quantity in the circulation than venlafaxine. The overall pharmacological activity of venlafaxine plus

Continued on next page

Effexor-XR—Cont.

ODV is expected to increase only slightly, and no dosage adjustment should be necessary for most normal adults. However, for patients with pre-existing hypertension, and for elderly patients or patients with hepatic dysfunction, the interaction associated with the concomitant use of venlafaxine and cimetidine is not known and potentially could be more pronounced. Therefore, caution is advised with such patients.

Diazepam

Under steady-state conditions for venlafaxine administered at 150 mg/day, a single 10 mg dose of diazepam did not appear to affect the pharmacokinetics of either venlafaxine or ODV in 18 healthy male subjects. Venlafaxine also did not have any effect on the pharmacokinetics of diazepam or its active metabolite, desmethyldiazepam, or affect the psychomotor and psychometric effects induced by diazepam.

Haloperidol

Venlafaxine administered under steady-state conditions at 150 mg/day in 24 healthy subjects decreased total oral-dose clearance (Cl/F) of a single 2 mg dose of haloperidol by 42%, which resulted in a 70% increase in haloperidol AUC. In addition, the haloperidol C_{max} increased 88% when coadministered with venlafaxine, but the haloperidol elimination half-life ($t_{1/2}$) was unchanged. The mechanism explaining this finding is unknown.

Lithium

The steady-state pharmacokinetics of venlafaxine administered at 150 mg/day were not affected when a single 600 mg oral dose of lithium was administered to 12 healthy male subjects. ODV also was unaffected. Venlafaxine had no effect on the pharmacokinetics of lithium.

Drugs Highly Bound to Plasma Proteins

Venlafaxine is not highly bound to plasma proteins; therefore, administration of Effexor XR to a patient taking another drug that is highly protein bound should not cause increased free concentrations of the other drug.

Drugs that Inhibit Cytochrome P450 Isoenzymes

CYP2D6 Inhibitors: *In vitro* and *in vivo* studies indicate that venlafaxine is metabolized to its active metabolite, ODV, by CYP2D6, the isoenzyme that is responsible for the genetic polymorphism seen in the metabolism of many antidepressants. Therefore, the potential exists for a drug interaction between drugs that inhibit CYP2D6-mediated metabolism of venlafaxine, reducing the metabolism of venlafaxine to ODV, resulting in increased plasma concentrations of venlafaxine and decreased concentrations of the active metabolite. CYP2D6 inhibitors such as quinidine would be expected to do this, but the effect would be similar to what is seen in patients who are genetically CYP2D6 poor metabolizers (See "*Metabolism and Excretion*" under "**CLINICAL PHARMACOLOGY**"). Therefore, no dosage adjustment is required when venlafaxine is coadministered with a CYP2D6 inhibitor.

The concomitant use of venlafaxine with a drug treatment(s) that potently inhibits both CYP2D6 and CYP3A4, the primary metabolizing enzymes for venlafaxine, has not been studied. Therefore, caution is advised should a patient's therapy include venlafaxine and any agent(s) that produce simultaneous inhibition of these two enzyme systems.

Drugs Metabolized by Cytochrome P450 Isoenzymes

CYP2D6: *In vitro* studies indicate that venlafaxine is a relatively weak inhibitor of CYP2D6. These findings have been confirmed in a clinical drug interaction study comparing the effect of venlafaxine with that of fluoxetine on the CYP2D6-mediated metabolism of dextromethorphan to dextrorphan.

Imipramine—Venlafaxine did not affect the pharmacokinetics of imipramine and 2-OH-imipramine. However, desipramine AUC, C_{max}, and C_{min} increased by about 35% in the presence of venlafaxine. The 2-OH-desipramine AUC's increased by at least 2.5 fold (with venlafaxine 37.5 mg q12h) and by 4.5 fold (with venlafaxine 75 mg q12h). Imipramine did not affect the pharmacokinetics of venlafaxine and ODV. The clinical significance of elevated 2-OH-desipramine levels is unknown.

Risperidone—Venlafaxine administered under steady-state conditions at 150 mg/day slightly inhibited the CYP2D6-mediated metabolism of risperidone (administered as a single 1 mg oral dose) to its active metabolite, 9-hydroxyrisperidone, resulting in an approximate 32% increase in risperidone AUC. However, venlafaxine coadministration did not significantly alter the pharmacokinetic profile of the total active moiety (risperidone plus 9-hydroxyrisperidone).

CYP3A4: Venlafaxine did not inhibit CYP3A4 *in vitro*. This finding was confirmed *in vivo* by clinical drug interaction studies in which venlafaxine did not inhibit the metabolism of several CYP3A4 substrates, including alprazolam, diazepam, and terfenadine.

CYP1A2: Venlafaxine did not inhibit CYP1A2 *in vitro*. This finding was confirmed *in vivo* by a clinical drug interaction study in which venlafaxine did not inhibit the metabolism of caffeine, a CYP1A2 substrate.

CYP2C9: Venlafaxine did not inhibit CYP2C9 *in vitro*. The clinical significance of this finding is unknown.

CYP2C19: Venlafaxine did not inhibit the metabolism of diazepam, which is partially metabolized by CYP2C19 (see "*Diazepam*" above).

Monoamine Oxidase Inhibitors

See "**CONTRAINDICATIONS**" and "**WARNINGS**."

CNS-Active Drugs

The risk of using venlafaxine in combination with other CNS-active drugs has not been systematically evaluated (except in the case of those CNS-active drugs noted above). Consequently, caution is advised if the concomitant administration of venlafaxine and such drugs is required.

Electroconvulsive Therapy

There are no clinical data establishing the benefit of electroconvulsive therapy combined with Effexor XR (venlafaxine hydrochloride) extended release capsules treatment.

Carcinogenesis, Mutagenesis, Impairment of Fertility

Carcinogenesis

Venlafaxine was given by oral gavage to mice for 18 months at doses up to 120 mg/kg per day, which was 1.7 times the maximum recommended human dose on a mg/m^2 basis. Venlafaxine was also given to rats by oral gavage for 24 months at doses up to 120 mg/kg per day. In rats receiving the 120 mg/kg dose, plasma concentrations of venlafaxine at necropsy were 1 times (male rats) and 6 times (female rats) the plasma concentrations of patients receiving the maximum recommended human dose. Plasma concentrations of the O-desmethyl metabolite were lower in rats than in patients receiving the maximum recommended dose. Tumors were not increased by venlafaxine treatment in mice or rats.

Mutagenesis

Venlafaxine and the major human metabolite, O-desmethylvenlafaxine (ODV), were not mutagenic in the Ames reverse mutation assay in Salmonella bacteria or the Chinese hamster ovary/HGPRT mammalian cell forward gene mutation assay. Venlafaxine was also not mutagenic or clastogenic in the *in vitro* BALB/c-3T3 mouse cell transformation assay, the sister chromatid exchange assay in cultured Chinese hamster ovary cells, or in the *in vivo* chromosomal aberration assay in rat bone marrow. ODV was not clastogenic in the *in vitro* Chinese hamster ovary cell chromosomal aberration assay, but elicited a clastogenic response in the *in vivo* chromosomal aberration assay in rat bone marrow.

Impairment of Fertility

Reproduction and fertility studies in rats showed no effects on male or female fertility at oral doses of up to 2 times the maximum recommended human dose on a mg/m^2 basis.

Pregnancy

Teratogenic Effects—Pregnancy Category C

Venlafaxine did not cause malformations in offspring of rats or rabbits given doses up to 2.5 times (rat) or 4 times (rabbit) the maximum recommended human daily dose on a mg/m^2 basis. However, in rats, there was a decrease in pup weight, an increase in stillborn pups, and an increase in pup deaths during the first 5 days of lactation, when dosing began during pregnancy and continued until weaning. The cause of these deaths is not known. These effects occurred at 2.5 times (mg/m^2) the maximum human daily dose. The no effect dose for rat pup mortality was 0.25 times the human dose on a mg/m^2 basis. There are no adequate and well-controlled studies in pregnant women. Because animal reproduction studies are not always predictive of human response, this drug should be used during pregnancy only if clearly needed.

Labor and Delivery

The effect of venlafaxine on labor and delivery in humans is unknown.

Nursing Mothers

It is not known whether venlafaxine or its metabolites are excreted in human milk. Because many drugs are excreted in human milk, caution should be exercised when venlafaxine is administered to a nursing woman.

Pediatric Use

Safety and effectiveness in pediatric patients have not been established.

Geriatric Use

Approximately 4% of Effexor® XR-treated patients in placebo-controlled premarketing trials were 65 years of age or over. Of 2,897 Effexor-treated patients in premarketing phase depression studies, 12% (357) were 65 years of age or over. No overall differences in effectiveness or safety were observed between geriatric patients and younger patients, and other reported clinical experience has not identified differences in response between the elderly and younger patients. However, greater sensitivity of some older individuals cannot be ruled out.

ADVERSE REACTIONS

The information included in the Adverse Findings Observed in Short-Term, Placebo-Controlled Studies with Effexor XR subsection is based on data from a pool of three 8- and 12-week controlled clinical trials (includes two U.S. trials and one European trial) with Effexor XR. Information on additional adverse events associated with Effexor XR in the entire development program for the formulation and with Effexor (the immediate release formulation of venlafaxine) is included in the "**Other Adverse Events Observed During the Premarketing Evaluation of Effexor and Effexor XR**" subsection (See also "**WARNINGS**" and "**PRECAUTIONS**").

Adverse Findings Observed in Short-Term, Placebo-Controlled Studies With Effexor XR

Adverse Events Associated with Discontinuation of Treatment

Approximately 11% of the 357 patients who received Effexor XR (venlafaxine hydrochloride) extended release capsules in placebo-controlled clinical trials discontinued treatment due to an adverse experience, compared to 6% of the 285 placebo-treated patients in those studies. The most common events leading to discontinuation and considered drug related (i.e., leading to discontinuation in at least 1% of the Effexor XR-treated patients at a rate at least twice that of placebo) are shown in Table 2.

TABLE 2
Common Adverse Events Leading to Discontinuation of Treatment in Placebo-Controlled Trials[1]

	Percentage of Patients Discontinuing Due to Adverse Event	
	Effexor XR (n=357)	Placebo (n=285)
Digestive		
Nausea	4%	<1%
Anorexia	1%	<1%
Dry Mouth	1%	0%
Nervous		
Dizziness	2%	1%
Insomnia	1%	<1%
Somnolence	2%	<1%

[1] In U.S. placebo-controlled trials, the following were also common events leading to discontinuation and were considered to be drug-related for Effexor XR-treated patients (% Effexor XR [n=192], % Placebo [n=202]); hypertension (1%, <1%); diarrhea (1%, 0%); paresthesia (1%, 0%); tremor (1%, 0%); abnormal vision, mostly blurred vision (1%, 0%); and abnormal, mostly delayed, ejaculation (1%, 0%).

Adverse Events Occurring at an Incidence of 2% or More Among Effexor XR-Treated Patients

Table 3 enumerates the incidence, rounded to the nearest percent, of treatment-emergent adverse events that occurred during acute therapy (up to 12 weeks) of depression in 2% or more of patients treated with Effexor XR (dose range of 75 to 225 mg/day) where the incidence in patients treated with Effexor XR was greater than the incidence in placebo-treated patients. The table shows the percentage of patients in each group who had at least one episode of an event at some time during their treatment. Reported adverse events were classified using a standard COSTART-based Dictionary terminology.

The prescriber should be aware that these figures cannot be used to predict the incidence of side effects in the course of usual medical practice where patient characteristics and other factors differ from those which prevailed in the clinical trials. Similarly, the cited frequencies cannot be compared with figures obtained from other clinical investigations involving different treatments, uses and investigators. The cited figures, however, do provide the prescribing physician with some basis for estimating the relative contribution of drug and nondrug factors to side effect incidence in the population studied.

Commonly Observed Adverse Events from Table 3: Note in particular the following adverse events that occurred in at least 5% of Effexor XR patients and at a rate at least twice that of the placebo group for all placebo-controlled trials: Abnormal ejaculation, gastrointestinal complaints (nausea, dry mouth, and anorexia), CNS complaints (dizziness, somnolence, and abnormal dreams), and sweating. In the two U.S. placebo-controlled trials, the following additional events occurred in at least 5% of Effexor XR-treated patients (n=192) and at a rate at least twice that of the placebo group: Abnormalities of sexual function (impotence in men, anorgasmia in women, and libido decreased), gastrointestinal complaints (constipation and flatulence), CNS complaints (insomnia, nervousness, and tremor), problems of special senses (abnormal vision), cardiovascular effects (hypertension and vasodilatation), and yawning.

TABLE 3
Treatment-Emergent Adverse Event Incidence in Short-Term Placebo-Controlled Effexor XR Clinical Trials in Depressed Patients[1,2]

Body System Preferred Term	% Reporting Event	
	Effexor XR (n=357)	Placebo (n=285)
Body as a Whole		
Asthenia	8%	7%
Cardiovascular System		
Vasodilatation[3]	4%	2%
Hypertension	4%	1%
Digestive System		
Nausea	31%	12%
Constipation	8%	5%
Anorexia	8%	4%
Vomiting	4%	2%
Flatulence	4%	3%
Metabolic/Nutritional		
Weight Loss	3%	0%
Nervous System		
Dizziness	20%	9%
Somnolence	17%	8%
Insomnia	17%	11%
Dry Mouth	12%	6%
Nervousness	10%	5%
Abnormal Dreams[4]	7%	2%
Tremor	5%	2%
Depression	3%	<1%
Paresthesia	3%	1%
Libido Decreased	3%	<1%
Agitation	3%	1%
Respiratory System		
Pharyngitis	7%	6%
Yawn	3%	0%
Skin		
Sweating	14%	3%
Special Senses		
Abnormal Vision[5]	4%	<1%
Urogenital System		
Abnormal Ejaculation[6,7]	16%	<1%
Impotence[7]	4%	<1%
Anorgasmia (female)[8,9]	3%	<1%

[1] Incidence, rounded to the nearest %, for events reported by at least 2% of patients treated with Effexor XR, except the following events which had an incidence equal to or less than placebo: abdominal pain, accidental injury, anxiety, back pain, bronchitis, diarrhea, dysmenorrhea, dyspepsia, flu syndrome, headache, infection, pain, palpitation, rhinitis, and sinusitis.
[2] <1% indicates an incidence greater than zero but less than 1%.
[3] Mostly "hot flashes."
[4] Mostly "vivid dreams," "nightmares," and "increased dreaming."
[5] Mostly "blurred vision" and "difficulty focusing eyes."
[6] Mostly "delayed ejaculation."
[7] Incidence is based on the number of male patients.
[8] Mostly "delayed orgasm" or "anorgasmia."
[9] Incidence is based on the number of female patients.

Vital Sign Changes

Effexor XR (venlafaxine hydrochloride) extended release capsules treatment for up to 12 weeks in premarketing placebo-controlled depression trials was associated with a mean final on-therapy increase in pulse rate of approximately 2 beats per minute, compared with 1 beat per minute for placebo. (See the **"Sustained Hypertension"** section of **"WARNINGS"** for effects on blood pressure.)

Laboratory Changes

Effexor XR (venlafaxine hydrochloride) extended release capsules treatment for up to 12 weeks in premarketing placebo-controlled depression trials was associated with a mean final on-therapy increase in serum cholesterol concentration of approximately 1.5 mg/dL. This change is of unknown clinical significance.

ECG Changes

(See the *"Use in Patients with Concomitant Illnesses"* section of **"PRECAUTIONS"**).

Other Adverse Events Observed During the Premarketing Evaluation of Effexor and Effexor XR

During its premarketing assessment, multiple doses of Effexor XR were administered to 705 patients in phase 3 depression studies and Effexor was administered to 96 patients. In addition, in the premarketing assessment of Effexor, multiple doses were administered to 2897 patients in phase 2–3 depression studies. The conditions and duration of exposure to venlafaxine in both development programs varied greatly, and included (in overlapping categories) open and double-blind studies, uncontrolled and controlled studies, inpatient (Effexor only) and outpatient studies, fixed-dose, and titration studies. Untoward events associated with this exposure were recorded by clinical in-

vestigators using terminology of their own choosing. Consequently, it is not possible to provide a meaningful estimate of the proportion of individuals experiencing adverse events without first grouping similar types of untoward events into a smaller number of standardized event categories.

In the tabulations that follow, reported adverse events were classified using a standard COSTART-based Dictionary terminology. The frequencies presented, therefore, represent the proportion of the 3698 patients exposed to multiple doses of either formulation of venlafaxine who experienced an event of the type cited on at least one occasion while receiving venlafaxine. All reported events are included except those already listed in Table 3 and those events for which a drug cause was remote. If the COSTART term for an event was so general as to be uninformative, it was replaced with a more informative term. It is important to emphasize that, although the events reported occurred during treatment with venlafaxine, they were not necessarily caused by it.

Events are further categorized by body system and listed in order of decreasing frequency according to the following definitions: **frequent** adverse events are those occurring on one or more occasions in at least 1/100 patients (only those not already listed in the tabulated results from placebo-controlled trials appear in this listing); **infrequent** adverse events are those occurring in 1/100 to 1/1000 patients; **rare** events are those occurring in fewer than 1/1000 patients. Events not observed with Effexor XR are shown in *italics*.

Body as a whole - **Frequent**: chest pain substernal, chills, fever; **Infrequent**: *face edema, intentional injury*, malaise, moniliasis, neck rigidity, *pelvic pain*, photosensitivity reaction, suicide attempt; **Rare**: *appendicitis, carcinoma, cellulitis, withdrawal syndrome.*

Cardiovascular system - **Frequent**: migraine, postural hypotension, tachycardia; **Infrequent**: angina pectoris, arrhythmia, bundle branch block, congestive heart failure, extrasystoles, hypotension, myocardial infarct, *peripheral vascular disorder (mainly cold feet and/or cold hands),* syncope, *thrombophlebitis;* **Rare**: *arteritis, first-degree atrioventricular block,* bigeminy, *bradycardia, cerebral ischemia,* coronary artery disease, *heart arrest, mitral valve disorder, mucocutaneous hemorrhage, pallor.*

Digestive system - **Frequent**: eructation, increased appetite; **Infrequent**: bruxism, colitis, dysphagia, *tongue edema, esophagitis,* gastritis, gastroenteritis, gastrointestinal ulcer, gingivitis, glossitis, hemorrhoids, rectal hemorrhage, *melena,* oral moniliasis, stomatitis, mouth ulceration; **Rare**: *cheilitis, cholecystitis, cholelithiasis,* hematemesis, *gastrointestinal hemorrhage,* gum hemorrhage, *hepatitis, ileitis, jaundice, intestinal obstruction, proctitis,* increased salivation, *soft stools, tongue discoloration.*

Endocrine system - **Rare**: goiter, hyperthyroidism, hypothyroidism, thyroid nodule, thyroiditis.

Hemic and lymphatic system - **Frequent**: ecchymosis; **Infrequent**: anemia, *leukocytosis, leukopenia, lymphadenopathy, lymphocytosis, thrombocythemia, thrombocytopenia;* **Rare**: *basophilia, cyanosis, eosinophilia.*

Metabolic and nutritional - **Frequent**: edema, weight gain; **Infrequent**: *alkaline phosphatase increased, creatinine increased, diabetes mellitus, glycosuria, hypercholesteremia, hyperglycemia,* hyperlipemia, *hyperuricemia, hypoglycemia, hypokalemia,* SGOT increased, thirst; **Rare**: *alcohol intolerance, bilirubinemia, BUN increased, dehydration, gout, hemochromatosis, hypercalcinuria, hyperkalemia, hyperphosphatemia, hyponatremia, hypophosphatemia, hypoproteinemia, SGPT increased, uremia.*

Musculoskeletal system - **Frequent**: arthralgia, myalgia; **Infrequent**: arthritis, *arthrosis,* bone pain, *bone spurs,* bursitis, leg cramps, myasthenia, tenosynovitis; **Rare**: *myopathy, osteoporosis, osteosclerosis, pathological fracture, rheumatoid arthritis, tendon rupture.*

Nervous system - **Frequent**: amnesia, confusion, depersonalization, emotional lability, hypertonia, hypesthesia, trismus, vertigo; **Infrequent**: apathy, ataxia, *circumoral paresthesia,* CNS stimulation, euphoria, *hallucinations,* hostility, hyperesthesia, hyperkinesia, hypotonia, incoordination, *libido increased,* manic reaction, myoclonus, neuralgia, neuropathy, *paranoid reaction, psychosis,* psychotic depression, seizure, *abnormal speech,* stupor, *torticollis,* twitching; **Rare**: *akathisia, akinesia, alcohol abuse,* aphasia, *bradykinesia, buccoglossal syndrome, cerebrovascular accident,* loss of consciousness, *delusions, dementia, dystonia,* facial paralysis, abnormal gait, *Guillain-Barré syndrome,* hypokinesia, *neuritis, nystagmus,* reflexes decreased, *reflexes increased,* suicidal ideation.

Respiratory system - **Frequent**: cough increased, dyspnea; **Infrequent**: asthma, chest congestion, epistaxis, hyperventilation, *laryngismus,* laryngitis, pneumonia, voice alteration; **Rare**: *atelectasis, hemoptysis, hypoventilation,* hypoxia, pleurisy, *pulmonary embolus, sleep apnea.*

Skin and appendages - **Frequent**: pruritus, rash; **Infrequent**: acne, alopecia, brittle nails, contact dermatitis, dry skin, eczema, skin hypertrophy, maculopapular rash, psoriasis, urticaria; **Rare**: erythema nodosum, *skin atrophy,* exfoliative dermatitis, lichenoid dermatitis, *hair discoloration,* skin discoloration, *furunculosis, hirsutism, leukoderma, pustular rash, vesiculobullous rash, seborrhea.*

Special senses- **Frequent**: abnormality of accommodation, mydriasis, taste perversion, tinnitus; **Infrequent**: *cataract,* conjunctivitis, *corneal lesion,* diplopia, dry eyes, *exophthalmos, eye pain,* hyperacusis, otitis media, parosmia, *photophobia,* taste loss, visual field defect; **Rare**: *blepharitis, chromatopsia, conjunctival edema, deafness, glaucoma, retinal hemorrhage, subconjunctival hemorrhage, keratitis,* labyrinthitis, miosis, *papilledema, decreased pupillary reflex,* otitis externa, scleritis, uveitis.

Urogenital system- **Frequent**: anorgasmia (male),* metrorrhagia,* prostatitis,* urinary frequency, urinary retention, urination impaired, vaginitis*; **Infrequent**: abnormal orgasm (female),* albuminuria, amenorrhea,* cystitis, dysuria, hematuria, *kidney calculus, female lactation,* leukorrhea,* menorrhagia,* nocturia, bladder pain, *breast pain,* polyuria, pyelonephritis, pyuria, urinary incontinence, urinary urgency, vaginal hemorrhage*; **Rare**: *abortion,* anuria, breast engorgement, breast enlargement, fibrocystic breast, calcium crystalluria, cervicitis,* gynecomastia (male),* ovarian cyst,* prolonged erection,* hypomenorrhea,* kidney function abnormal, mastitis, menopause,* kidney pain, salpingitis,* urolithiasis, uterine hemorrhage,* uterine spasm.*

*Based on the number of men and women as appropriate.

DRUG ABUSE AND DEPENDENCE

Controlled Substance Class

Effexor XR (venlafaxine hydrochloride) extended release capsules is not a controlled substance.

Physical and Psychological Dependence

In vitro studies revealed that venlafaxine has virtually no affinity for opiate, benzodiazepine, phencyclidine (PCP), or N-methyl-D-aspartic acid (NMDA) receptors.

Venlafaxine was not found to have any significant CNS stimulant activity in rodents. In primate drug discrimination studies, venlafaxine showed no significant stimulant or depressant abuse liability.

The discontinuation effects of Effexor XR have not been systematically evaluated in controlled clinical trials (See "DOSAGE AND ADMINISTRATION").

While venlafaxine has not been systematically studied in clinical trials for its potential for abuse, there was no indication of drug-seeking behavior in the clinical trials. However, it is not possible to predict on the basis of premarketing experience the extent to which a CNS active drug will be misused, diverted, and/or abused once marketed. Consequently, physicians should carefully evaluate patients for history of drug abuse and follow such patients closely, observing them for signs of misuse or abuse of venlafaxine (e.g., development of tolerance, incrementation of dose, drug-seeking behavior).

OVERDOSAGE

Human Experience

Among the patients included in the premarketing evaluation of Effexor XR, there were 2 reports of acute overdosage with Effexor XR, either alone or in combination with other drugs. One patient took a combination of 6 g of Effexor XR and 2.5 mg of lorazepam. This patient was hospitalized, treated symptomatically, and recovered without any untoward effects. The other patient took 2.85 g of Effexor XR. This patient reported paresthesia of all four limbs but recovered without sequelae.

Among the patients included in the premarketing evaluation with Effexor, there were 14 reports of acute overdose with venlafaxine, either alone or in combination with other drugs and/or alcohol. The majority of the reports involved ingestions in which the total dose of venlafaxine taken was estimated to be no more than several-fold higher than the usual therapeutic dose. The 3 patients who took the highest doses were estimated to have ingested approximately 6.75 g, 2.75 g, and 2.5 g. The resultant peak plasma levels of venlafaxine for the latter 2 patients were 6.24 and 2.35 μg/mL, respectively, and the peak plasma levels of O-desmethylvenlafaxine were 3.37 and 1.30 μg/mL, respectively. Plasma venlafaxine levels were not obtained for the patient who ingested 6.75 g of venlafaxine. All 14 patients recovered without sequelae. Most patients reported no symptoms. Among the remaining patients, somnolence was the most commonly reported symptom. The patient who ingested 2.75 g of venlafaxine was observed to have 2 generalized convulsions and a prolongation of QTc to 500 msec compared with 405 msec at baseline. Mild sinus tachycardia was reported in 2 of the other patients.

In postmarketing experience, there have been reports of fatalities in patients taking overdoses of venlafaxine, predominantly in combination with alcohol and/or other drugs.

Management of Overdosage

Treatment should consist of those general measures employed in the management of overdosage with any antidepressant. Ensure an adequate airway, oxygenation, and ventilation. Monitoring of cardiac rhythm and vital signs is recommended. General supportive and symptomatic measures are also recommended. Use of activated charcoal, induction of emesis, or gastric lavage should be considered.

Continued on next page

Effexor-XR—Cont.

Due to the large volume of distribution of venlafaxine, forced diuresis, dialysis, hemoperfusion and exchange transfusion are unlikely to be of benefit. No specific antidotes for venlafaxine are known.

In managing overdosage, consider the possibility of multiple drug involvement. The physician should consider contacting a poison control center on the treatment of any overdose.

DOSAGE AND ADMINISTRATION

Initial Treatment

For most patients, the recommended starting dose for Effexor XR is 75 mg/day, administered in a single dose. In the clinical trials establishing the efficacy of Effexor XR in moderately depressed outpatients, the initial dose of venlafaxine was 75 mg/day. For some patients, it may be desirable to start at 37.5 mg/day for 4 to 7 days, to allow new patients to adjust to the medication before increasing to 75 mg/day. While the relationship between dose and antidepressant response for Effexor XR has not been adequately explored, patients not responding to the initial 75 mg/day dose may benefit from dose increases to a maximum of approximately 225 mg/day. Dose increases should be in increments of up to 75 mg/day, as needed, and should be made at intervals of not less than 4 days, since steady state plasma levels of venlafaxine and its major metabolite are achieved in most patients by 4 days. In the clinical trials establishing efficacy, upward titration was permitted at intervals of 2 weeks or more; the average doses were about 140–180 mg/day (see "**Clinical Trials**" under "**CLINICAL PHARMACOLOGY**").

It should be noted that, while the maximum recommended dose for moderately depressed outpatients is also 225 mg/day for Effexor (the immediate release form of venlafaxine), more severely depressed inpatients in one study of the development program for that product responded to a mean dose of 350 mg/day (range of 150 to 375 mg/day). Whether or not higher doses of Effexor XR are needed for more severely depressed patients is unknown; however, the experience with Effexor XR doses higher than 225 mg/day is very limited.

Effexor XR should be administered in a single daily dose with food, either in the morning or in the evening, at approximately the same time each day. Each capsule should be swallowed whole with fluid and not divided, crushed, chewed, or placed in water.

Switching Patients From Effexor Tablets

Depressed patients who are currently being treated at a therapeutic dose with Effexor may be switched to Effexor XR at the nearest equivalent dose (mg/day), e.g., 37.5 mg venlafaxine two-times-a-day to 75 mg Effexor XR once daily. However, individual dosage adjustments may be necessary.

Patients With Hepatic Impairment

Given the decrease in clearance and increase in elimination half-life for both venlafaxine and ODV that is observed in patients with hepatic cirrhosis compared with normal subjects (see "**CLINICAL PHARMACOLOGY**"), it is recommended that the starting dose be reduced by 50% in patients with moderate hepatic impairment. Because there was much individual variability in clearance between patients with cirrhosis, individualization of dosage may be desirable in some patients.

Patients With Renal Impairment

Given the decrease in clearance for venlafaxine and the increase in elimination half-life for both venlafaxine and ODV that is observed in patients with renal impairment (GFR = 10–70 mL/min) compared with normal subjects (see "**CLINICAL PHARMACOLOGY**"), it is recommended that the total daily dose be reduced by 25%–50%. In patients undergoing hemodialysis, it is recommended that the total daily dose be reduced by 50% and that the dose be withheld until the dialysis treatment is completed (4 hrs). Because there was much individual variability in clearance between patients with renal impairment, individualization of dosage may be desirable in some patients.

Elderly Patients

No dose adjustment is recommended for elderly patients on the basis of age. As with any antidepressant, however, caution should be exercised in treating the elderly. When individualizing the dosage, extra care should be taken when increasing the dose.

Maintenance/Extended Treatment

There is no body of evidence available from controlled trials to indicate how long the depressed patient should be treated with Effexor XR. It is generally agreed, however, that pharmacological treatment for acute episodes of depression should continue for up to six months or longer. Whether the dose of antidepressant needed to induce remission is identical to the dose needed to maintain euthymia is unknown.

Discontinuing Effexor XR

When discontinuing Effexor XR after more than 1 week of therapy, it is generally recommended that the dose be tapered to minimize the risk of discontinuation symptoms. In clinical trials with Effexor XR, tapering was achieved by reducing the daily dose by 75 mg at 1 week intervals. Individualization of tapering may be necessary. While the discontinuation effects of Effexor XR have not been systematically evaluated in controlled clinical trials, a retrospective survey of new events occurring during taper or following discontinuation revealed the following six events that occurred at an incidence of at least 3% and for which the incidence for Effexor XR was at least twice the placebo incidence: dizziness, dry mouth, insomnia, nausea, nervousness, and sweating.

Switching Patients To or From a Monoamine Oxidase Inhibitor

At least 14 days should elapse between discontinuation of an MAOI and initiation of therapy with Effexor XR. In addition, at least 7 days should be allowed after stopping Effexor XR before starting an MAOI (see "**CONTRAINDICATIONS**" and "**WARNINGS**").

HOW SUPPLIED

Effexor® XR (venlafaxine hydrochloride) extended release capsules are available in bottles of 100 capsules and in Redipak® cartons of 100 capsules (10 blister strips of 10) in the following dosage strengths:

37.5 mg, NDC 0008-0837, gray cap/peach body with "W" and Effexor XR" on the cap and "37.5" on the body.

75 mg, NDC 0008-0833, peach cap and body with "W" and Effexor XR" on the cap and "75" on the body.

150 mg, NDC 0008-0836, dark orange cap and body with "W" and Effexor XR" on the cap and "150" on the body.

The appearance of these capsules is a trademark of Wyeth-Ayerst Laboratories.

Store at controlled room temperature, 20°C to 25°C (68°F to 77°F).

Manufactured by:
Wyeth Laboratories Inc.
A Wyeth-Ayerst Company
Philadelphia, PA 19101

Shown in Product Identification Guide, page 343

EQUAGESIC® ℂ ℞

[*ek ″wa-je ′zik*]
(meprobamate with aspirin)

DESCRIPTION

Each tablet of Equagesic contains 200 mg meprobamate and 325 mg aspirin. The inactive ingredients present are cellulose, D&C Yellow 10, FD&C Red 3, FD&C Yellow 6, hydrogenated vegetable oil, magnesium stearate, polacrilin potassium, and starch.

HOW SUPPLIED

Equagesic® (meprobamate with aspirin) Tablets, 200 mg meprobamate and 325 mg aspirin, are available as follows: NDC 0008-0091, pink and yellow, double-layer, round, scored tablet marked "WYETH" and "91", in bottles of 100 tablets.

Store at room temperature, approx. 25°C (77°F).
Keep tightly closed.
Protect from light.
Dispense in light-resistant, tight container.

The appearance of EQUAGESIC tablets is a registered trademark of Wyeth-Ayerst Laboratories.

Manufactured by:
Wyeth Laboratories Inc.
A Wyeth-Ayerst Company
Philadelphia, PA 19101

For full prescribing information write to Professional Service, Wyeth-Ayerst Laboratories, P.O. Box 8299, Philadelphia, PA 19101, or contact your local Wyeth-Ayerst representative.

EQUANIL® ℂ ℞

[*ek ′wah-nil*]
(meprobamate)
Tablets

DESCRIPTION

Meprobamate is a white powder with a characteristic odor and a bitter taste. It is slightly soluble in water, freely soluble in acetone and alcohol, and sparingly soluble in ether. Equanil tablets contain 200 mg or 400 mg meprobamate. The inactive ingredients present are lactose, methylcellulose, polacrilin potassium, and stearic acid.

HOW SUPPLIED

Equanil® (meprobamate) Tablets are available in the following dosage strengths:

200 mg, NDC 0008-0002, white, five-sided tablet marked "WYETH" and "2", in bottles of 100 tablets.

400 mg, NDC 0008-0001, white, round, scored tablet marked "WYETH" and "1", in bottles of 100 and 500 tablets.

Keep tightly closed.
Dispense in tight container.
Store at room temperature, approximately 25°C (77°F).

Manufactured by:
Wyeth Laboratories Inc.
A Wyeth-Ayerst Company
Philadelphia, PA 19101

For prescribing information write to Professional Service, Wyeth-Ayerst Laboratories, P.O. Box 8299, Philadelphia, PA 19101, or contact your local Wyeth-Ayerst representative.

FACTREL® ℞

[*făc-trĕl* ′]
(gonadorelin hydrochloride)
Synthetic Luteinizing Hormone Releasing Hormone (LH-RH)
DIAGNOSTIC USE ONLY

HOW SUPPLIED

LYOPHILIZED POWDER

in single-dose Secule® vials containing 100 mcg (NDC 0046-0507-05) and 500 mcg (NDC 0046-0509-05) gonadorelin as the hydrochloride with 100 mg lactose, USP. Each Secule® vial is accompanied by one ampul containing 2 mL sterile diluent of 2% benzyl alcohol in sterile water.

Secule® —Registered trademark to designate a vial containing an injectable preparation in dry form.

For full prescribing information turn to the Diagnostic Product Information section of this edition of the PDR.

FLUOTHANE® ℞

[*flū ′o-thăn*]
(halothane, USP)
Inhalation

Caution: Federal law prohibits dispensing without prescription.

DESCRIPTION

Fluothane (halothane, USP) is supplied as a liquid and is vaporized for use as an inhalation anesthetic. It is 2-bromo-2-chloro-1, 1, 1-trifluoro-ethane and has the following structural formula:

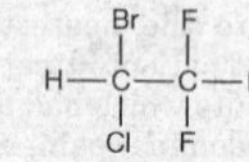

$C_2HBrClF_3$

The molecular weight is 197.38. The drug substance halothane molecule has an asymmetric carbon atom; the commercial product is a racemic mixture. Resolution of the mixture has not been reported.*

*Klaus Florey, editor, Analytical Profiles of Drug Substances, Vol. 1, page 127, (1972).

Halothane is miscible with alcohol, chloroform, ether, and other fat solvents.

The specific gravity is 1.872–1.877 at 20°C, and the boiling point (range) is 49°C–51°C at 760 mm Hg. The vapor pressure is 243 mm Hg at 20°C. The blood/gas coefficient is 2.5 at 37°C, and the olive oil/water coefficient is 220 at 37°C. Vapor concentrations within anesthetic range are nonirritating and have a pleasant odor.

Fluothane is nonflammable, and its vapors mixed with oxygen in proportions from 0.5 to 50% (v/v) are not explosive. Fluothane does not decompose in contact with warm soda lime. When moisture is present, the vapor attacks aluminum, brass, and lead, but not copper. Rubber, some plastics, and similar materials are soluble in Fluothane; such materials will deteriorate rapidly in contact with Fluothane vapor or liquid. Stability of Fluothane is maintained by the addition of 0.01% thymol (w/w), up to 0.00025% ammonia (w/w).

CLINICAL PHARMACOLOGY

Fluothane is an inhalation anesthetic. Induction and recovery are rapid, and depth of anesthesia can be rapidly altered. Fluothane progressively depresses respiration. There may be tachypnea with reduced tidal volume and alveolar ventilation. Fluothane is not an irritant to the respiratory tract, and no increase in salivary or bronchial secretions ordinarily occurs. Pharyngeal and laryngeal reflexes are rapidly obtunded. It causes bronchodilation. Hypoxia, acidosis, or apnea may develop during deep anesthesia.

Fluothane reduces the blood pressure and frequently decreases the pulse rate. The greater the concentration of the drug, the more evident these changes become. Atropine may reverse the bradycardia. Fluothane does not cause the release of catecholamines from adrenergic stores. Fluothane also causes dilation of the vessels of the skin and skeletal muscles.

Cardiac arrhythmias may occur during Fluothane anesthesia. These include nodal rhythm, AV dissociation, ventricu-

lar extrasystoles, and asystole. Fluothane sensitizes the myocardial conduction system to the action of epinephrine and norepinephrine, and the combination may cause serious cardiac arrhythmias. Fluothane increases cerebrospinal-fluid pressure. Fluothane produces moderate muscular relaxation. Muscle relaxants are used as adjuncts in order to maintain lighter levels of anesthesia. Fluothane augments the action of nondepolarizing relaxants and ganglionic-blocking agents. Fluothane is a potent uterine relaxant.

The mechanism(s) whereby Fluothane and other substances induce general anesthesia is unknown. Fluothane is a very potent anesthetic in humans, with a minimum alveolar concentration (MAC) determined to be 0.64%. The MAC has been found to decrease with age (see MAC table in "Dosage and Administration").

INDICATIONS AND USAGE

Fluothane (halothane, USP) is indicated for the induction and maintenance of general anesthesia.

CONTRAINDICATIONS

Fluothane is not recommended for obstetrical anesthesia except when uterine relaxation is required.

WARNINGS

When previous exposure to Fluothane was followed by unexplained hepatic dysfunction and/or jaundice, consideration should be given to the use of other agents.

PRECAUTIONS

GENERAL

Fluothane should be used in vaporizers that permit a reasonable approximation of output, and preferably of the calibrated type. The vaporizer should be placed out of circuit in closed-circuit rebreathing systems; otherwise, overdosage is difficult to avoid. The patient should be closely observed for signs of overdosage, i.e., depression of blood pressure, pulse rate, and ventilation, particularly during assisted or controlled ventilation.

Fluothane increases cerebrospinal-fluid pressure. Therefore, in patients with markedly raised intracranial pressure, if Fluothane is indicated, administration should be preceded by measures ordinarily used to reduce cerebrospinal-fluid pressure. Ventilation should be carefully assessed, and it may be necessary to assist or control ventilation to ensure adequate oxygenation and carbon dioxide removal. In susceptible individuals, halothane anesthesia may trigger a skeletal-muscle hypermetabolic state leading to a high oxygen demand and the clinical syndrome known as malignant hyperthermia. The syndrome includes nonspecific features such as muscle rigidity, tachycardia, tachypnea, cyanosis, arrhythmias, and unstable blood pressure. (It should also be noted that many of these nonspecific signs may appear with light anesthesia, acute hypoxia, etc.) An increase in overall metabolism may be reflected in an elevated temperature (which may rise rapidly, early or late in the case, but usually is not the first sign of augmented metabolism) and an increased usage of the CO_2 absorption system (hot canister). PaO_2 and pH may decrease, and hyperkalemia and a base deficit may appear. Treatment includes discontinuance of triggering agents (e.g., halothane), administration of intravenous dantrolene, and application of supportive therapy. Such therapy includes vigorous efforts to restore body temperature to normal, respiratory and circulatory support as indicated, and management of electrolyte-fluid-acid-base derangements. Renal failure may appear later, and urine flow should be sustained if possible. It should be noted that the syndrome of malignant hyperthermia secondary to halothane appears to be rare.

INFORMATION FOR PATIENTS

When appropriate, as in some cases where discharge is anticipated soon after general anesthesia, patients should be cautioned not to drive automobiles, operate hazardous machinery, or engage in hazardous sports for 24 hours or more (depending on the total dose of Fluothane, condition of the patient, and consideration given to other drugs administered after anesthesia).

DRUG INTERACTIONS

Epinephrine or norepinephrine should be employed cautiously, if at all, during Fluothane (halothane, USP) anesthesia, since their simultaneous use may induce ventricular tachycardia or fibrillation.

Nondepolarizing relaxants and ganglionic-blocking agents should be administered cautiously, since their actions are augmented by Fluothane (halothane, USP).

Clinical experience and animal experiments suggest that pancuronium should be given with caution to patients receiving chronic tricyclic antidepressant therapy who are anesthetized with halothane, because severe ventricular arrhythmias may result from such usage.

CARCINOGENESIS, MUTAGENESIS, IMPAIRMENT OF FERTILITY

An 18-month inhalational carcinogenicity study of halothane at 0.05% in the mouse revealed no evidence of anesthetic-related carcinogenicity. This concentration is equivalent to 24 hours of 1% halothane.

Mutagenesis testing of halothane revealed both positive and negative results. In the rat, one-year exposure to trace concentrations of halothane (1 and 10 ppm) and nitrous oxide produced chromosomal damage to spermatogonia cells and bone marrow cells. Negative mutagenesis tests included: Ames bacterial assay, Chinese hamster lung fibroblast assay, sister chromatid exchange in Chinese hamster ovary cells, and human leukocyte culture assay.

Reproduction studies of halothane (10 ppm) and nitrous oxide in the rat caused decreased fertility. This trace concentration corresponds to 1/1000 the human maintenance dose.

PREGNANCY

Teratogenic Effects: Pregnancy Category C. Some studies have shown Fluothane to be teratogenic, embryotoxic, and fetotoxic in the mouse, rat, hamster, and rabbit at subanesthetic and/or anesthetic concentrations. There are no adequate and well-controlled studies in pregnant women. Fluothane should be used during pregnancy only if the potential benefit justifies the potential risk to the fetus.

LABOR AND DELIVERY

The uterine relaxation obtained with Fluothane, unless carefully controlled, may fail to respond to ergot derivatives and oxytocic posterior pituitary extract.

NURSING MOTHERS

It is not known whether this drug is excreted in human milk. Because many drugs are excreted in human milk, caution should be exercised when Fluothane is administered to a nursing woman.

PEDIATRIC USE

Extensive clinical experience reveals that maintenance concentrations of halothane are generally higher in infants and children, and that maintenance requirements decrease with age. See MAC table, based upon age, in "Dosage and Administration."

ADVERSE REACTIONS

The following adverse reactions have been reported: mild, moderate, and severe hepatic dysfunction (including hepatic necrosis); cardiac arrest; hypotension; respiratory arrest; cardiac arrhythmias; hyperpyrexia; shivering; nausea; and emesis.

OVERDOSAGE

In the event of overdosage, or what may appear to be overdosage, drug administration should be stopped, and assisted or controlled ventilation with pure oxygen initiated.

DOSAGE AND ADMINISTRATION

Fluothane may be administered by the nonrebreathing technique, partial rebreathing, or closed technique. The induction dose varies from patient to patient but is usually within the range of 0.5% to 3%. The maintenance dose varies from 0.5% to 1.5%.

Fluothane may be administered with either oxygen or a mixture of oxygen and nitrous oxide.

Fluothane should not be kept indefinitely in vaporizer bottles not specifically designed for its use. Thymol does not volatilize along with Fluothane and, therefore, accumulates in the vaporizer and may, in time, impart a yellow color to the remaining liquid or to wicks in vaporizers. The development of such discoloration may be used as an indicator that the vaporizer should be drained and cleaned, and the discolored Fluothane (halothane, USP) discarded. Accumulation of thymol may be removed by washing with diethyl ether. After cleaning a wick or vaporizer, make certain all the diethyl ether has been removed before reusing the equipment to avoid introducing ether into the system.

Because of the more rapid uptake of Fluothane and the increased blood concentration required for anesthesia in younger patients, the minimum alveolar concentration (MAC)[1] values will decrease with age as follows:

Age	MAC %
Infants	1.08
3 yrs.	0.91
10 yrs.	0.87
15 yrs.	0.92
24 yrs.	0.84
42 yrs.	0.76
81 yrs.	0.64

HOW SUPPLIED

Fluothane® (halothane, USP) is available in unit packages of 125 mL (NDC 0046-3125-81) and 250 mL (NDC 0046-3125-82) of halothane, USP, stabilized with 0.01% thymol (w/w) and up to 0.00025% ammonia (w/w).

HANDLING AND STORAGE

Store at room temperature (approximately 25°C) in a tight, closed container.
Protect from light.
Use carton to protect contents from light.

PHYSICIAN REFERENCE

1. Gregory, GA et al: *Anesthesiology* 1969; *30*(5):488–491.
Manufactured for:
Ayerst Laboratories Inc.
A Wyeth-Ayerst Company
Philadelphia, PA 19101
By ICI Chemicals and Polymers Ltd.
Runcorn, Cheshire, U.K.

GRISACTIN® ℞
[grĭz-ăc 'tĭn]
(griseofulvin) microsize

Caution: Federal law prohibits dispensing without prescription.

DESCRIPTION

Griseofulvin is an oral fungistatic antibiotic for the treatment of superficial mycoses. It is derived from a species of *Penicillium*.

Grisactin is produced by a special process that fractures griseofulvin particles into minute crystals of irregular shape offering a greater and more effective surface area for increased gastrointestinal absorption.

Grisactin Capsules and Tablets contain the following inactive ingredients:

- 250 mg capsules: black iron oxide, D&C Yellow No. 10, FD&C Blue No. 2, FD&C Red No. 40, FD&C Yellow No. 6, gelatin, lactose, magnesium stearate, titanium dioxide, water.
- 500 mg tablets: calcium carboxymethylcellulose, D&C Red No. 36, gelatin, magnesium stearate, starch.

HOW SUPPLIED

GRISACTIN (griseofulvin) microsize—
GRISACTIN 250, each capsule contains 250 mg, in bottles of 100 (NDC 0046-0443-81) and 500 (NDC 0046-0443-85).
GRISACTIN 500, each tablet (scored) contains 500 mg, in bottles of 60 (NDC 0046-0444-60).
Store at room temperature (approximately 25°C)
Dispense in a well-closed container as defined in the USP
Manufactured by:
Ayerst Laboratories Inc.
A Wyeth-Ayerst Company
Philadelphia, PA 19101
For prescribing information write to Professional Service, Wyeth-Ayerst Laboratories, P.O. Box 8299, Philadelphia, PA 19101, or contact your local Wyeth-Ayerst representative.
Shown in Product Identification Guide, page 343

GRISACTIN® Ultra ℞
[grĭz-ăc 'tĭn ŭl' trä]
(griseofulvin ultramicrosize)

Caution: Federal law prohibits dispensing without prescription.

DESCRIPTION

Griseofulvin is an oral fungistatic antibiotic for the treatment of superficial mycoses. It is derived from a species of *Penicillium*.

Grisactin Ultra tablets contain griseofulvin ultramicrosize in 250 mg and 330 mg dosage strengths.

Grisactin Ultra tablets contain the following inactive ingredients: lactose, magnesium stearate, microcrystalline cellulose, sodium starch glycolate.

HOW SUPPLIED

Grisactin® Ultra tablets, 250 mg: white, square shaped, compressed tablets impressed with the trade name and dosage strength, in bottles of 100 (NDC 0046-0435-81).
Grisactin® Ultra tablets, 330 mg: white, wide-oval shaped, compressed tablets impressed with the trade name and dosage strength, in bottles of 100 (NDC 0046-0437-81).
Store at room temperature (approximately 25° C)
Dispense in a well-closed container as defined in the USP
Manufactured by:
Ayerst Laboratories Inc.
A Wyeth-Ayerst Company
Philadelphia, PA 19101
For prescribing information write to Professional Service, Wyeth-Ayerst Laboratories, P.O. Box 8299, Philadelphia, PA 19101, or contact your local Wyeth-Ayerst representative.
Shown in Product Identification Guide, page 343

HEPARIN ℞
[hep 'ăh-rĭn]

Lock Flush Solution, USP

Caution: Federal law prohibits dispensing without prescription.

Heparin Lock Flush Solution is intended for maintenance of patency of intravenous injection devices only and is not to be used for anticoagulant therapy.

DESCRIPTION

TUBEX® Heparin Lock Flush Solution, USP is a sterile solution. Each mL contains either 10 or 100 USP units heparin sodium derived from porcine intestinal mucosa (stan-

Continued on next page

Heparin Lock Flush—Cont.

dardized for use as an anticoagulant) in normal saline solution, and not more than 10 mg benzyl alcohol as a preservative. The pH range is 5.0 to 7.5.

The potency is determined by biological assay using a USP reference standard based upon units of heparin activity per milligram.

Heparin is a heterogenous group of straight-chain anionic mucopolysaccharides, called glycosaminoglycans, having anticoagulant properties. Although others may be present, the main sugars occurring in heparin are: (1) α-L-iduronic acid 2-sulfate, (2) 2-deoxy-2-sulfamino-α-D-glucose 6-sulfate, (3) β-D-glucuronic acid, (4) 2-acetamido-2-deoxy-α-D-glucose, and (5) α-L-iduronic acid. These sugars are present in decreasing amounts, usually in the order (2) > (1) > (4) > (3) > (5), and are joined by glycosidic linkages forming polymers of varying sizes. Heparin is strongly acidic because of its content of covalently linked sulfate and carboxylic acid groups. In heparin sodium, the acidic protons of the sulfate units are partially replaced by sodium ions.

STRUCTURE OF HEPARIN SODIUM (representative subunits):

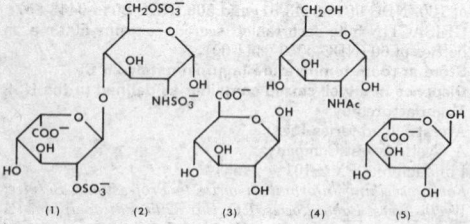

(1) (2) (3) (4) (5)

CLINICAL PHARMACOLOGY

Heparin inhibits reactions that lead to the clotting of blood and the formation of fibrin clots both *in vitro* and *in vivo*. Heparin acts at multiple sites in the normal coagulation systems. Small amounts of heparin in combination with antithrombin III (heparin cofactor) can inhibit thrombosis by inactivating activated Factor X and inhibiting the conversion of prothrombin to thrombin. Once active thrombosis has developed, larger amounts of heparin can inhibit further coagulation by inactivating thrombin and preventing the conversion of fibrinogen to fibrin. Heparin also prevents the formation of a stable fibrin clot by inhibiting the activation of the fibrin stabilizing factor.

Bleeding time is usually unaffected by heparin. Clotting time is prolonged by full therapeutic doses of heparin; in most cases, it is not measurably affected by low doses of heparin.

Loglinear plots of heparin plasma concentrations with time, for a wide range of dose levels, are linear which suggests the absence of zero order processes. Liver and the reticuloendothelial system are the sites of biotransformation. The biphasic elimination curve, a rapidly declining alpha phase ($t_{1/2}$ = 10 min.), and after the age of 40 a slower beta phase, indicates uptake in organs. The absence of a relationship between anticoagulant half-life and concentration half-life may reflect factors such as protein binding of heparin.

Heparin does not have fibrinolytic activity; therefore, it will not lyse existing clots.

INDICATIONS AND USAGE

Heparin Lock Flush Solution, USP is intended to maintain patency of an indwelling venipuncture device designed for intermittent injection or infusion therapy or blood sampling. Heparin Lock Flush Solution, USP may be used following initial placement of the device in the vein, after each injection of a medication or after withdrawal of blood for laboratory tests. (See "**Dosage and Administration**, MAINTENANCE OF PATENCY OF INTRAVENOUS DEVICES," for direction for use.)

Heparin Lock Flush Solution, USP is not to be used for anticoagulant therapy.

CONTRAINDICATIONS

Heparin sodium should not be used in patients with the following conditions:

severe thrombocytopenia; an uncontrollable active bleeding state (see "**Warnings**"), except when this is due to disseminated intravascular coagulation.

WARNINGS

This product contains benzyl alcohol as a preservative. Benzyl alcohol has been reported to be associated with a fatal "Gasping Syndrome" in premature neonates.

Neonatologists do not advise the use of 100 units/mL concentration because of the risk of bleeding, especially in low birth weight neonates.

Heparin is not intended for intramuscular use.

HYPERSENSITIVITY

Patients with documented hypersensitivity to heparin should be given the drug only in clearly life-threatening situations. (See "**Adverse Reactions**, HYPERSENSITIVITY.")

HEMORRHAGE

Hemorrhage can occur at virtually any site in patients receiving heparin. An unexplained fall in hematocrit, fall in blood pressure or any other unexplained symptom should lead to serious consideration of a hemorrhagic event.

Heparin sodium should be used with extreme caution in infants and in patients with disease states in which there is increased danger of hemorrhage. Some of the conditions in which increased danger of hemorrhage exists are:

Cardiovascular—subacute bacterial endocarditis, severe hypertension.

Surgical—during and immediately following (a) spinal tap or spinal anesthesia or (b) major surgery, especially involving the brain, spinal cord, or eye.

Hematologic—conditions associated with increased bleeding tendencies, such as hemophilia, thrombocytopenia and some vascular purpuras.

Gastrointestinal—ulcerative lesions and continuous tube drainage of the stomach or small intestine.

Other—menstruation, liver disease with impaired hemostasis.

THROMBOCYTOPENIA

Thrombocytopenia has been reported to occur in patients receiving heparin with a reported incidence of 0 to 30%. Mild thrombocytopenia (count greater than $100,000/mm^3$) may remain stable or reverse even if heparin is continued. However, thrombocytopenia of any degree should be monitored closely. If the count falls below $100,000/mm^3$ or if recurrent thrombosis develops (see **Precautions**, GENERAL, *White-clot Syndrome*), the heparin product should be discontinued. If continued heparin therapy is essential, administration of heparin from a different organ source can be reinstituted with caution.

PRECAUTIONS

GENERAL

In infants, the cumulative amounts of heparin and benzyl alcohol received from the frequent administration of Heparin Lock Flush Solution, USP during a 24–hour period should be considered.

Precautions must be exercised when drugs which are incompatible with heparin are administered through an indwelling intravenous catheter containing Heparin Lock Flush Solution, USP. (See "**Dosage and Administration**, MAINTENANCE OF PATENCY OF INTRAVENOUS DEVICES.")

White-clot Syndrome

It has been reported that patients on heparin may develop new thrombus formation in association with thrombocytopenia, resulting from irreversible aggregation of platelets induced by heparin, the so-called "white-clot syndrome." The process may lead to severe thromboembolic complications like skin necrosis, gangrene of the extremities that may lead to amputation, myocardial infarction, pulmonary embolism, stroke, and possibly death. Therefore, heparin administration should be promptly discontinued if a patient develops new thrombosis in association with thrombocytopenia.

Increased Risk in Older Women

A higher incidence of bleeding has been reported in women over 60 years of age.

LABORATORY TESTS

Periodic platelet counts, hematocrits and tests for occult blood in stool are recommended during the entire course of heparin use (see "**Dosage and Administration**").

DRUG INTERACTIONS

Platelet Inhibitors

Drugs such as acetylsalicylic acid, dextran, phenylbutazone, ibuprofen, indomethacin, dipyridamole, hydroxychloroquine, and others that interfere with platelet-aggregation reactions (the main hemostatic defense of heparinized patients) may induce bleeding and should be used with caution in patients receiving heparin sodium.

Other Interactions

Digitalis, tetracyclines, nicotine, or antihistamines may partially counteract the anticoagulant action of heparin sodium.

CARCINOGENESIS, MUTAGENESIS, IMPAIRMENT OF FERTILITY

No long-term studies in animals have been performed to evaluate carcinogenic potential of heparin sodium. Also, no reproduction studies in animals have been performed concerning mutagenesis or impairment of fertility.

PREGNANCY

Teratogenic Effects —Pregnancy Category C

Animal reproduction studies have not been conducted with heparin sodium. It is also not known whether heparin sodium can cause fetal harm when administered to a pregnant woman or can affect reproduction capacity. Heparin sodium should be given to a pregnant woman only if clearly needed.

Nonteratogenic Effects

Heparin does not cross the placental barrier.

NURSING MOTHERS

Heparin is not excreted in human milk.

PEDIATRIC USE

Heparin Lock Flush Solution, USP is not recommended for use in the neonate (see "**Warnings**").

ADVERSE REACTIONS

HEMORRHAGE

Hemorrhage is the chief complication that may result from heparin use (see "**Warnings**, HEMORRHAGE"). An overly prolonged clotting time or minor bleeding during therapy can usually be controlled by withdrawing the drug (see "**Overdosage**").

LOCAL IRRITATION

Local irritation and erythema have been reported with the use of Heparin Lock Flush Solution, USP.

HYPERSENSITIVITY

Generalized hypersensitivity reactions have been reported, with chills, fever, and urticaria as the most usual manifestations, and asthma, rhinitis, lacrimation, headache, nausea and vomiting, and anaphylactoid reactions, including shock, occurring more rarely. Itching and burning, especially on the plantar side of the feet, may occur.

Thrombocytopenia has been reported to occur in patients receiving heparin with a reported incidence of 0 to 30%. While often mild and of no obvious clinical significance, such thrombocytopenia can be accompanied by severe thromboembolic complications, such as skin necrosis, gangrene of the extremities that may lead to amputation, myocardial infarction, pulmonary embolism, stroke, and possibly death. (See "**Warnings**" and "**Precautions**.")

Certain episodes of painful, ischemic and cyanosed limbs have been attributed, in the past, to allergic vasospastic reactions. Whether these are, in fact, identical to the thrombocytopenia-associated complications remains to be determined.

OVERDOSAGE

SYMPTOMS

Bleeding is the chief sign of heparin overdosage. Nosebleeds, blood in urine, or tarry stools may be noted as the first sign of bleeding. Easy bruising or petechial formations may precede frank bleeding.

TREATMENT—Neutralization of Heparin Effect

When clinical circumstances (bleeding) require reversal of heparinization, protamine sulfate (1% solution) by slow infusion will neutralize heparin sodium. No more than 50 mg should be administered, very slowly, in any 10-minute period. Each mg of protamine sulfate neutralizes approximately 100 USP heparin units. The amount of protamine required decreases over time as heparin is metabolized. Although the metabolism of heparin is complex, it may, for the purpose of choosing a protamine dose, be assumed to have a half-life of about $1/2$ hour after intravenous injection.

Administration of protamine sulfate can cause severe hypotensive and anaphylactoid reactions. Because fatal reactions, often resembling anaphylaxis, have been reported, the drug should be given only when resuscitation techniques and treatment of anaphylactoid shock are readily available.

For additional information consult the labeling of Protamine Sulfate Injection, USP products.

DOSAGE AND ADMINISTRATION

Parenteral drug products should be inspected visually for particulate matter and discoloration prior to administration, whenever solution and container permit. Slight discoloration does not alter potency.

Heparin Lock Flush Solution, USP is **not recommended for use in the neonate** (see "**Warnings**").

MAINTENANCE OF PATENCY OF INTRAVENOUS DEVICES

To prevent clot formation in a heparin lock set or central venous catheter following its proper insertion, Heparin Lock Flush Solution, USP is injected via the injection hub in a quantity sufficient to fill the entire device. This solution should be replaced each time the device is used. Aspirate before administering any solution via the device in order to confirm patency and location of needle or catheter tip. If the drug to be administered is incompatible with heparin, the entire device should be flushed with normal saline before and after the medication is administered; following the second saline flush, Heparin Lock Flush Solution, USP may be reinstilled into the device. The device manufacturer's instructions should be consulted for specifics concerning its use. Usually this dilute heparin solution will maintain anticoagulation within the device for up to 4 hours.

Note: Since repeated injections of small doses of heparin can alter tests for activated partial thromboplastin time (APTT), a baseline value for APTT should be obtained prior to insertion of an intravenous device.

WITHDRAWAL OF BLOOD SAMPLES

Heparin Lock Flush Solution, USP may also be used after each withdrawal of blood for laboratory tests. When heparin would interfere with or alter the results of blood tests, the

heparin solution should be cleared from the device by aspirating and discarding it before withdrawing the blood sample.

The **TUBEX® BLUNT POINTE™** Sterile Cartridge Unit is suitable for substances to be administered intravenously. It is intended for use with injection sets specifically manufactured as "needle-less" injection systems. As of the date of this circular, **TUBEX BLUNT POINTE** is compatible with LifeShield® Prepierced Reseal injection site, Interlink® Injection Site, and SafeLine® Injection Site, User-Gard® Intermittent Injection Cap, and Safesite® reflux valve.

HOW SUPPLIED

Heparin Lock Flush Solution, USP is available in **TUBEX® BLUNT POINTE™** Sterile Cartridge Units and in **TUBEX®** Sterile Cartridge-Needle Units.

Each 1 mL size **TUBEX®** contains one of the following concentrations of heparin sodium, in packages of 50 **TUBEX®**:
10 USP Units per mL:
NDC 0008-0523-50, **BLUNT POINTE™**.
NDC 0008-0523-01, (25 gauge × $^5/_8$ inch needle).
100 USP Units per mL:
NDC 0008-0487-50, **BLUNT POINTE™**.
NDC 0008-0487-01, (25 gauge × $^5/_8$ inch needle).

Each 2.5 mL size **TUBEX®** contains one of the following concentrations of heparin sodium in packages of 50 **TUBEX®**:
25 USP Units per **TUBEX®** (10 USP Units per mL):
NDC 0008-0523-51, **BLUNT POINTE™**.
NDC 0008-0523-02, (25 gauge × $^5/_8$ inch needle).
250 USP Units per **TUBEX®** (100 USP Units per mL):
NDC 0008-0487-51, **BLUNT POINTE™**.
NDC 0008-0487-03, (25 gauge × $^5/_8$ inch needle).

Do not use if solution is discolored or contains a precipitate
Store at controlled room temperature, 20° to 25°C (68° to 77°F) [see USP].
Do not freeze
Single use only. Discard any unused solution after initial use.

TUBEX is a registered trademark of Wyeth-Ayerst Laboratories.
BLUNT POINTE is a trademark of Wyeth-Ayerst Laboratories.
InterLink is a registered trademark of Baxter International, Inc.
LifeShield is a registered trademark of Abbott Laboratories.
SafeLine is a registered trademark of McGaw, Inc.
SafSite is a registered trademark of B. Braun Medical, Inc.
User-Gard is a registered trademark of Arrow International, Inc.

Manufactured by:
Wyeth Laboratories Inc.
A Wyeth-Ayerst Company
Philadelphia, PA 19101

HEPARIN ℞
[*hĕp 'ăh-rĭn*]
Sodium Injection, USP

Caution: Federal law prohibits dispensing without prescription.

DESCRIPTION

TUBEX® Heparin Sodium Injection, USP, is a sterile solution. Each mL contains 1,000, 2,500, 5,000, 7,500, 10,000, 15,000, or 20,000 USP units heparin sodium, derived from porcine intestinal mucosa (standardized for use as an anticoagulant), in water for injection, and not more than 10 mg benzyl alcohol as a preservative.

The potency is determined by biological assay, using a USP reference standard based upon units of heparin activity per milligram.

The pH range is 5.0 to 7.5.

Heparin is a heterogenous group of straight-chain anionic mucopolysaccharides, called glycosaminoglycans, having anticoagulant properties. Although others may be present, the main sugars occurring in heparin are: (1) α-L-iduronic acid 2-sulfate, (2) 2-deoxy-2-sulfamino-α-D-glucose 6-sulfate, (3) β-D-glucuronic acid, (4) 2-acetamido-2-deoxy-α-D-glucose, and (5) α-L-iduronic acid. These sugars are present in decreasing amounts, usually in the order (2) > (1) > (4) > (3) > (5), and are joined by glycosidic linkages, forming polymers of varying sizes. Heparin is strongly acidic because of its content of covalently linked sulfate and carboxylic acid groups. In heparin sodium, the acidic protons of the sulfate units are partially replaced by sodium ions.

STRUCTURE OF HEPARIN SODIUM (representative subunits):
[See chemical structure at top of next column]

CLINICAL PHARMACOLOGY

Heparin inhibits reactions that lead to the clotting of blood and the formation of fibrin clots both *in vitro* and *in vivo.* Heparin acts at multiple sites in the normal coagulation system. Small amounts of heparin in combination with anti-

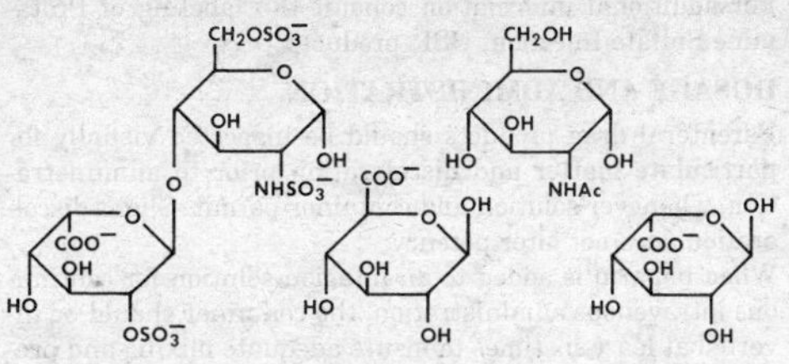

(1) (2) (3) (4) (5)

thrombin III (heparin cofactor) can inhibit thrombosis by inactivating activated Factor X and inhibiting the conversion of prothrombin to thrombin. Once active thrombosis has developed, larger amounts of heparin can inhibit further coagulation by inactivating thrombin and preventing the conversion of fibrinogen to fibrin. Heparin also prevents the formation of a stable fibrin clot by inhibiting the activation of the fibrin-stabilizing factor.

Bleeding time is usually unaffected by heparin. Clotting time is prolonged by full therapeutic doses of heparin; in most cases, it is not measurably affected by low doses of heparin.

Peak plasma levels of heparin are achieved 2 to 4 hours following subcutaneous administration, although there are considerable individual variations. Loglinear plots of heparin plasma concentrations with time, for a wide range of dose levels, are linear which suggests the absence of zero order processes. Liver and the reticulo-endothelial system are the sites of biotransformation. The biphasic elimination curve, a rapidly declining alpha phase ($t_{1/2}$ = 10 min.), and after the age of 40 a slower beta phase, indicates uptake in organs. The absence of a relationship between anticoagulant half-life and concentration half-life may reflect factors such as protein binding of heparin.

Heparin does not have fibrinolytic activity; therefore, it will not lyse existing clots.

INDICATIONS AND USAGE

Heparin sodium injection is indicated for anticoagulant therapy in prophylaxis and treatment of venous thrombosis and its extension, in low-dose regimen for prevention of postoperative deep venous thrombosis and pulmonary embolism in patients undergoing major abdominothoracic surgery who are at risk of developing thromboembolic disease (see "**Dosage and Administration**"); for prophylaxis and treatment of pulmonary embolism, in atrial fibrillation with embolization, for diagnosis and treatment of acute and chronic consumptive coagulopathies (disseminated intravascular coagulation), for prevention of clotting in arterial and cardiac surgery, and for prophylaxis and treatment of peripheral arterial embolism.

Heparin may also be employed as an anticoagulant in blood transfusions, extracorporeal circulation, dialysis procedures, and in blood samples for laboratory purposes.

CONTRAINDICATIONS

Heparin sodium should not be used in patients:
with severe thrombocytopenia;
in whom suitable blood-coagulation tests—e.g., the whole-blood clotting time, partial thromboplastin time, etc.—cannot be performed at appropriate intervals (this contraindication refers to full-dose heparin; there is usually no need to monitor coagulation parameters in patients receiving low-dose heparin);
with an uncontrollable active bleeding state (see "**Warnings**"), except when this is due to disseminated intravascular coagulation.

WARNINGS

Heparin is not intended for intramuscular use.

HYPERSENSITIVITY

Patients with documented hypersensitivity to heparin should be given the drug only in clearly life-threatening situations.

HEMORRHAGE

Hemorrhage can occur at virtually any site in patients receiving heparin. An unexplained fall in hematocrit, fall in blood pressure or any other unexplained symptom should lead to serious consideration of a hemorrhagic event.

Heparin sodium should be used with extreme caution in disease states in which there is increased danger of hemorrhage. Some of the conditions in which increased danger of hemorrhage exists are:

Cardiovascular —subacute bacterial endocarditis, severe hypertension.

Surgical —during and immediately following (a) spinal tap or spinal anesthesia or (b) major surgery, especially involving the brain, spinal cord or eye.

Hematologic —conditions associated with increased bleeding tendencies, such as hemophilia, thrombocytopenia and some vascular purpuras.

Gastrointestinal —ulcerative lesions and continuous tube drainage of the stomach or small intestine.

Other —Menstruation, liver disease with impaired hemostasis.

COAGULATION TESTING

When heparin sodium is administered in therapeutic amounts, its dosage should be regulated by frequent blood-coagulation tests. If the coagulation test is unduly prolonged or if hemorrhage occurs, heparin sodium should be discontinued promptly (see "**Overdosage**").

THROMBOCYTOPENIA

Thrombocytopenia has been reported to occur in patients receiving heparin with a reported incidence of 0 to 30%. Mild thrombocytopenia (count greater than 100,000/mm^3) may remain stable or reverse even if heparin is continued. However, thrombocytopenia of any degree should be monitored closely. If the count falls below 100,000/mm^3 or if recurrent thrombosis develops (see "**PRECAUTIONS**, GENERAL *White-clot Syndrome,*"), the heparin product should be discontinued. If continued heparin therapy is essential, administration of heparin from a different organ source can be reinstituted with caution.

MISCELLANEOUS

This product contains benzyl alcohol as preservative. Benzyl alcohol has been reported to be associated with a fatal "Gasping Syndrome" in premature neonates.

PRECAUTIONS

GENERAL

White-clot Syndrome

It has been reported that patients on heparin may develop new thrombus formation in association with thrombocytopenia, resulting from irreversible aggregation of platelets induced by heparin, the so-called "white-clot syndrome." The process may lead to severe thromboembolic complications like skin necrosis, gangrene of the extremities that may lead to amputation, myocardial infarction, pulmonary embolism, stroke, and possibly death. Therefore, heparin administration should be promptly discontinued if a patient develops new thrombosis in association with thrombocytopenia.

Heparin Resistance

Increased resistance to heparin is frequently encountered in fever, thrombosis, thrombophlebitis, infections with thrombosing tendencies, myocardial infarction, cancer, and in postsurgical patients.

Increased Risk in Older Women

A higher incidence of bleeding has been reported in women over 60 years of age.

LABORATORY TESTS

Periodic platelet counts, hematocrits and tests for occult blood in stool are recommended during the entire course of heparin therapy, regardless of the route of administration (see "**Dosage and Administration**").

DRUG INTERACTIONS

Oral Anticoagulants

Heparin sodium may prolong the one-stage prothrombin time. Therefore, when heparin sodium is given with dicumarol or warfarin sodium, a period of at least 5 hours after the last intravenous dose or 24 hours after the last subcutaneous dose should elapse before blood is drawn if a valid prothrombin time is to be obtained.

Platelet Inhibitors

Drugs such as acetylsalicylic acid, dextran, phenylbutazone, ibuprofen, indomethacin, dipyridamole, hydroxychloroquine, and others that interfere with platelet-aggregation reactions (the main hemostatic defense of heparinized patients) may induce bleeding and should be used with caution in patients receiving heparin sodium.

Other Interactions

Digitalis, tetracyclines, nicotine, or antihistamines may partially counteract the anticoagulant action of heparin sodium.

DRUG/LABORATORY TEST INTERACTIONS

Hyperaminotransferasemia

Significant elevations of aminotransferase (SGOT [S-AST] and SGPT [S-ALT]) levels have occurred in a high percentage of patients (and healthy subjects) who have received heparin. Since aminotransferase determinations are important in the differential diagnosis of myocardial infarction, liver disease and pulmonary emboli, increases that might be caused by drugs (like heparin) should be interpreted with caution.

CARCINOGENESIS, MUTAGENESIS, IMPAIRMENT OF FERTILITY

No long-term studies in animals have been performed to evaluate carcinogenic potential of heparin. Also, no reproduction studies in animals have been performed concerning mutagenesis or impairment of fertility.

PREGNANCY

Teratogenic Effects—Pregnancy Category C

Animal reproduction studies have not been conducted with heparin sodium. It is also not known whether heparin sodium can cause fetal harm when administered to a preg-

Continued on next page

Heparin Injection—Cont.

nant woman or can affect reproduction capacity. Heparin sodium should be given to a pregnant woman only if clearly needed.

Nonteratogenic Effects

Heparin does not cross the placental barrier.

NURSING MOTHERS

Heparin is not excreted in human milk.

PEDIATRIC USE

See "**Dosage and Administration.**"

ADVERSE REACTIONS

HEMORRHAGE

Hemorrhage is the chief complication that may result from heparin therapy (see "**Warnings**").

An overly prolonged clotting time or minor bleeding during therapy can usually be controlled by withdrawing the drug (see "**Overdosage**"). It should be appreciated that gastrointestinal- or urinary-tract bleeding during anticoagulant therapy may indicate the presence of an underlying occult lesion. Bleeding can occur at any site but certain specific hemorrhagic complications may be difficult to detect:

a. Adrenal hemorrhage, with resultant acute adrenal insufficiency, has occurred during anticoagulant therapy. Therefore, such treatment should be discontinued in patients who develop signs and symptoms of acute adrenal hemorrhage and insufficiency. Initiation of corrective therapy should not depend on laboratory confirmation of the diagnosis, since any delay in an acute situation may result in the patient's death.

b. Ovarian (corpus luteum) hemorrhage developed in a number of women of reproductive age receiving short- or long-term anticoagulant therapy. This complication, if unrecognized, may be fatal.

c. Retroperitoneal hemorrhage.

LOCAL IRRITATION

Local irritation, erythema, mild pain, hematoma, or ulceration may follow deep, subcutaneous (intrafat) injection of heparin sodium. These complications are much more common after intramuscular use, and such use is not recommended.

HYPERSENSITIVITY

Generalized hypersensitivity reactions have been reported, with chills, fever, and urticaria as the most usual manifestations, and asthma, rhinitis, lacrimation, headache, nausea and vomiting, and anaphylactoid reactions, including shock, occurring more rarely. Itching and burning, especially on the plantar side of the feet, may occur.

Thrombocytopenia has been reported to occur in patients receiving heparin with a reported incidence of 0 to 30%. While often mild and of no obvious clinical significance, such thrombocytopenia can be accompanied by severe thromboembolic complications such as skin necrosis, gangrene of the extremities that may lead to amputation, myocardial infarction, pulmonary embolism, stroke, and possibly death. (See "**Warnings**," and "**Precautions**.")

Certain episodes of painful, ischemic and cyanosed limbs have been attributed, in the past, to allergic vasospastic reactions. Whether these are, in fact, identical to the thrombocytopenia-associated complications remains to be determined.

MISCELLANEOUS

Osteoporosis following long-term administration of high doses of heparin, cutaneous necrosis after systemic administration, suppression of aldosterone synthesis, delayed transient alopecia, priapism, and rebound hyperlipemia on discontinuation of heparin sodium have also been reported. Significant elevations of aminotransferase (SGOT [S-AST] and SGPT [S-ALT]) levels have occurred in a high percentage of patients (and healthy subjects) who have received heparin.

OVERDOSAGE

SYMPTOMS

Bleeding is the chief sign of heparin overdosage. Nosebleeds, blood in urine, or tarry stools may be noted as the first sign of bleeding. Easy bruising or petechial formations may precede frank bleeding.

TREATMENT—Neutralization of Heparin Effect

When clinical circumstances (bleeding) require reversal of heparinization, protamine sulfate (1% solution) by slow infusion will neutralize heparin sodium. No more than 50 mg should be administered, very slowly, in any 10-minute period. Each mg of protamine sulfate neutralizes approximately 100 USP heparin units. The amount of protamine required decreases over time as heparin is metabolized. Although the metabolism of heparin is complex, it may, for the purpose of choosing a protamine dose, be assumed to have a half-life of about $1/_2$ hour after intravenous injection.

Administration of protamine sulfate can cause severe hypotensive and anaphylactoid reactions. Because fatal reactions, often resembling anaphylaxis, have been reported, the drug should be given only when resuscitation techniques and treatment of anaphylactoid shock are readily available.

For additional information consult the labeling of Protamine Sulfate Injection, USP, products.

DOSAGE AND ADMINISTRATION

Parenteral drug products should be inspected visually for particulate matter and discoloration prior to administration, whenever solution and container permit. Slight discoloration does not alter potency.

When heparin is added to an infusion solution for continuous intravenous administration, the container should be inverted at least six times to insure adequate mixing and prevent pooling of the heparin in the solution.

Heparin sodium is not effective by oral administration and should be given by intermittent intravenous injection, intravenous infusion, or deep subcutaneous (intrafat, i.e., above the iliac crest or abdominal fat layer) injection. *The intramuscular route of administration should be avoided because of the frequent occurrence of hematoma at the injection site.*

The **TUBEX® BLUNT POINTE**™ Sterile Cartridge Unit is suitable for substances to be administered intravenously. It is intended for use with injection sets specifically manufactured as "needle-less" injection systems. As of the date of this circular, **TUBEX BLUNT POINTE** is compatible with LifeShield® Prepierced Reseal injection site, InterLink® Injection Site, and SafeLine® Injection Site, User-Gard® Intermittent Injection Cap, and SafSite® reflux valve.

The dosage of heparin sodium should be adjusted according to the patient's coagulation-test results. When heparin is given by continuous intravenous infusion, the coagulation time should be determined approximately every 4 hours in the early stages of treatment. When the drug is administered intermittently by intravenous injection, coagulation tests should be performed before each injection during the early stages of treatment and at appropriate intervals thereafter. Dosage is considered adequate when the activated partial thromboplastin time (APTT) is 1.5 to 2 times normal or when the whole-blood clotting time is elevated approximately 2.5 to 3 times the control value. After deep subcutaneous (intrafat) injections, tests for adequacy of dosage are best performed on samples drawn 4 to 6 hours after the injections.

Periodic platelet counts, hematocrits and tests for occult blood in stool are recommended during the entire course of heparin therapy, regardless of the route of administration.

CONVERTING TO ORAL ANTICOAGULANT

When an oral anticoagulant of the coumarin or similar type is to be begun in patients already receiving heparin sodium, baseline and subsequent tests of prothrombin activity must be determined at a time when heparin activity is too low to affect the prothrombin time. This is about 5 hours after the last IV bolus and 24 hours after the last subcutaneous dose. If continuous IV heparin infusion is used, prothrombin time can usually be measured at any time.

In converting from heparin to an oral anticoagulant, the dose of the oral anticoagulant should be the usual initial amount, and thereafter prothrombin time should be determined at the usual intervals. To ensure continuous anticoagulation, it is advisable to continue full heparin therapy for several days after the prothrombin time has reached the therapeutic range. Heparin therapy may then be discontinued without tapering.

THERAPEUTIC ANTICOAGULANT EFFECT WITH FULL-DOSE HEPARIN

Although dosage must be adjusted for the individual patient according to the results of suitable laboratory tests, the following dosage schedules may be used as guidelines:

[See table below]

PEDIATRIC USE

Follow recommendations of appropriate pediatric reference texts. In general, the following dosage schedule may be used as a guideline.

Initial Dose: 50 units/kg (IV, drip).

Maintenance Dose: 100 units/kg (IV, drip) every four hours, or 20,000 units/M²/24 hours continuously.

SURGERY OF THE HEART AND BLOOD VESSELS

Patients undergoing total body perfusion for open-heart surgery should receive an initial dose of not less than 150 units of heparin sodium per kilogram of body weight. Frequently, a dose of 300 units of heparin sodium per kilogram of body weight is used for procedures estimated to last less than 60 minutes or 400 units per kilogram for those estimated to last longer than 60 minutes.

LOW-DOSE PROPHYLAXIS OF POSTOPERATIVE THROMBOEMBOLISM

A number of well-controlled clinical trials have demonstrated that low-dose heparin prophylaxis, given just prior to and after surgery, will reduce the incidence of postoperative deep-vein thrombosis in the legs, as measured by the I-125 fibrinogen technique and venography, and of clinical pulmonary embolism. The most widely used dosage has been 5,000 units 2 hours before surgery and 5,000 units every 8 to 12 hours thereafter for 7 days or until the patient is fully ambulatory, whichever is longer. The heparin is given by deep subcutaneous injection in the arm or abdomen with a fine needle (25 to 26 gauge) to minimize tissue trauma. A concentrated solution of heparin sodium is recommended. Such prophylaxis should be reserved for patients over 40 undergoing major surgery. Patients with bleeding disorders, those having neurosurgery, spinal anesthesia, eye surgery, or potentially sanguineous operations should be excluded, as well as patients receiving oral anticoagulants or platelet-active drugs (see "**Warnings**"). The value of such prophylaxis in hip surgery has not been established. The possibility of increased bleeding during surgery or postoperatively should be borne in mind. If such bleeding occurs, discontinuance of heparin and neutralization with protamine sulfate is advisable. If clinical evidence of thromboembolism develops despite low-dose prophylaxis, full therapeutic doses of anticoagulants should be given unless contraindicated. All patients should be screened prior to heparinization to rule out bleeding disorders, and monitoring should be performed with appropriate coagulation tests just prior to surgery. Coagulation-test values should be normal or only slightly elevated. There is usually no need for daily monitoring of the effect of low-dose heparin in patients with normal coagulation parameters.

EXTRACORPOREAL DIALYSIS USE

Follow equipment manufacturer's operating directions carefully.

BLOOD TRANSFUSION

Addition of 400 to 600 USP units per 100 mL of whole blood. Usually, 7,500 USP units of heparin sodium are added to 100 mL of Sterile Sodium Chloride Injection (or 75,000 USP units per 1,000 mL of Sterile Sodium Chloride Injection) and mixed, and from this sterile solution, 6 to 8 mL is added per 100 mL of whole blood.

LABORATORY SAMPLES

Addition of 70 to 150 units of heparin sodium per 10 to 20 mL sample of whole blood is usually employed to prevent coagulation of the sample. Leukocyte counts should be performed on heparinized blood within two hours after addition of the heparin. Heparinized blood should not be used for isoagglutinin, complement, erythrocyte fragility tests, or platelet counts.

HOW SUPPLIED

Heparin Sodium Injection, USP, is available in **TUBEX®** Sterile Cartridge-Needle Units.

Method of Administration	Frequency	Recommended Dose [based on 150 lb (68 kg) patient]
Deep, Subcutaneous (Intrafat Injection)	Initial Dose	5,000 units by IV injection followed by 10,000–20,000 units of a concentrated solution, subcutaneously
A different site should be used for each injection to prevent the development of massive hematoma.	Every 8 hours	8,000–10,000 units of a concentrated solution
	(or) Every 12 hours	15,000–20,000 units of a concentrated solution
Intermittent Intravenous Injection	Initial Dose	10,000 units, either undiluted or in 50–100 mL isotonic sodium chloride injection
	Every 4 to 6 hours	5,000–10,000 units, either undiluted or in 50–100 mL isotonic sodium chloride injection
Intravenous Infusion	Initial Dose	5,000 units by IV injection
	Continuous	20,000–40,000 units in 1,000 mL of isotonic sodium chloride solution for infusion/day

Each 1 mL size **TUBEX** contains one of the following concentrations of heparin sodium:
1,000 USP Units per mL
NDC 0008–0275–01, (22 gauge × $1^1/_4$ inch needle), in packages of 10 **TUBEX**.
2,500 USP Units per mL
NDC 0008–0482–01, (25 gauge × $^5/_8$ inch needle), in packages of 10 **TUBEX**.
5,000 USP Units per 0.5 mL (10,000 USP Units per mL)
NDC 0008–0277–02, (25 gauge ×$^5/_8$ inch needle), in packages of 10 **TUBEX**.
NDC 0008–0277–03, (25 gauge × $^5/_8$ inch needle), in packages of 50 **TUBEX**.
5,000 USP Units per mL
NDC 0008–0278–02, (25 gauge × $^5/_8$ inch needle), in packages of 10 **TUBEX**.
7,500 USP Units per mL
NDC 0008–0293–01, (25 gauge × $^5/_8$ inch needle), in packages of 10 **TUBEX**.
10,000 USP Units per mL
NDC 0008–0277–01, (25 gauge × $^5/_8$ inch needle), in packages of 10 **TUBEX**.
20,000 USP Units per mL
NDC 0008–0276–01, (25 gauge × $^5/_8$ inch needle), in packages of 10 **TUBEX**.
Heparin Sodium Injection, USP, 1,000 USP Units per mL, is also available in packages of 10 **TUBEX® BLUNT POINTE™** Sterile Cartridge Units, NDC 0008–0275–50.
Store at controlled room temperature, 20°–25°C (68°–77°F) [see USP].
Do not freeze.
Do not use if solution is discolored or contains a precipitate.
Manufactured by:
Wyeth Laboratories Inc.
A Wyeth-Ayerst Company
Philadelphia, PA 19101

INDERAL® ℞
[*ĭn 'der-al*]
(propranolol hydrochloride)

Caution: Federal law prohibits dispensing without prescription.

DESCRIPTION

Inderal (propranolol hydrochloride) is a synthetic beta-adrenergic receptor blocking agent chemically described as 1-(Isopropylamino)-3-(1-naphthyloxy)-2-propanol hydrochloride. Its structural formula is

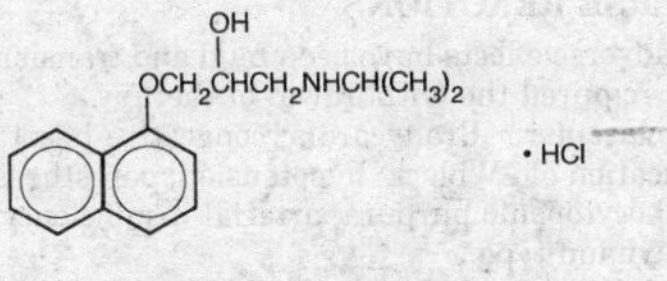

Propranolol hydrochloride is a stable, white, crystalline solid which is readily soluble in water and ethanol. Its molecular weight is 295.81.
Inderal is available as 10 mg, 20 mg, 40 mg, 60 mg, and 80 mg tablets for oral administration and as a 1 mg/mL sterile injectable solution for intravenous administration.
The inactive ingredients contained in Inderal Tablets are: lactose, magnesium stearate, microcrystalline cellulose, and stearic acid. In addition, Inderal 10 mg and 80 mg Tablets contain FD&C Yellow No. 6 and D&C Yellow No. 10; Inderal 20 mg Tablets contain FD&C Blue No. 1; Inderal 40 mg Tablets contain FD&C Blue No. 1, FD&C Yellow No. 6, and D&C Yellow No. 10; Inderal 60 mg Tablets contain D&C Red No. 30.

CLINICAL PHARMACOLOGY

Inderal is a nonselective beta-adrenergic receptor blocking agent possessing no other autonomic nervous system activity. It specifically competes with beta-adrenergic receptor stimulating agents for available receptor sites. When access to beta-receptor sites is blocked by Inderal, the chronotropic, inotropic, and vasodilator responses to beta-adrenergic stimulation are decreased proportionately.
Propranolol is almost completely absorbed from the gastrointestinal tract, but a portion is immediately bound by the liver. Peak effect occurs in one to one- and one-half hours. The biologic half-life is approximately four hours.
There is no simple correlation between dose or plasma level and therapeutic effect, and the dose-sensitivity range as observed in clinical practice is wide. The principal reason for this is that sympathetic tone varies widely between individuals. Since there is no reliable test to estimate sympathetic tone or to determine whether total beta blockade has been achieved, proper dosage requires titration.
The mechanism of the antihypertensive effect of Inderal has not been established. Among the factors that may be involved in contributing to the antihypertensive action are (1) decreased cardiac output, (2) inhibition of renin release by the kidneys, and (3) diminution of tonic sympathetic nerve outflow from vasomotor centers in the brain. Although total peripheral resistance may increase initially, it readjusts to or below the pretreatment level with chronic use. Effects on plasma volume appear to be minor and somewhat variable. Inderal has been shown to cause a small increase in serum potassium concentration when used in the treatment of hypertensive patients.
In angina pectoris, propranolol generally reduces the oxygen requirement of the heart at any given level of effort by blocking the catecholamine-induced increases in the heart rate, systolic blood pressure, and the velocity and extent of myocardial contraction. Propranolol may increase oxygen requirements by increasing left ventricular fiber length, end diastolic pressure, and systolic ejection period. The net physiologic effect of beta-adrenergic blockade is usually advantageous and is manifested during exercise by delayed onset of pain and increased work capacity. Propranolol exerts its antiarrhythmic effects in concentrations associated with beta-adrenergic blockade, and this appears to be its principal antiarrhythmic mechanism of action. In dosages greater than required for beta blockade, Inderal also exerts a quinidine-like or anesthetic-like membrane action, which affects the cardiac action potential. The significance of the membrane action in the treatment of arrhythmias is uncertain.
The mechanism of the antimigraine effect of propranolol has not been established. Beta-adrenergic receptors have been demonstrated in the pial vessels of the brain.
The specific mechanism of Inderal's antitremor effects has not been established, but beta-2 (noncardiac) receptors may be involved. A central effect is also possible. Clinical studies have demonstrated that Inderal is of benefit in exaggerated physiological and essential (familial) tremor.
Beta-receptor blockade can be useful in conditions in which, because of pathologic or functional changes, sympathetic activity is detrimental to the patient. But there are also situations in which sympathetic stimulation is vital. For example, in patients with severely damaged hearts, adequate ventricular function is maintained by virtue of sympathetic drive, which should be preserved. In the presence of AV block greater than first degree, beta blockade may prevent the necessary facilitating effect of sympathetic activity on conduction. Beta blockade results in bronchial constriction by interfering with adrenergic bronchodilator activity, which should be preserved in patients subject to bronchospasm.
Propranolol is not significantly dialyzable.
The Beta-Blocker Heart Attack Trial (BHAT) was a National Heart, Lung and Blood Institute-sponsored multicenter, randomized, double-blind, placebo-controlled trial conducted in 31 U.S. centers (plus one in Canada) in 3,837 persons without history of severe congestive heart failure or presence of recent heart failure; certain conduction defects; angina since infarction, who had survived the acute phase of myocardial infarction. Propranolol was administered at either 60 or 80 mg t.i.d. based on blood levels achieved during an initial trial of 40 mg t.i.d. Therapy with Inderal, begun 5 to 21 days following infarction, was shown to reduce overall mortality up to 39 months, the longest period of follow-up. This was primarily attributable to a reduction in cardiovascular mortality. The protective effect of Inderal was consistent regardless of age, sex, or site of infarction. Compared with placebo, total mortality was reduced 39% at 12 months and 26% over an average follow-up period of 25 months. The Norwegian Multicenter Trial in which propranolol was administered at 40 mg q.i.d. gave overall results which support the findings in the BHAT.
Although the clinical trials used either t.i.d. or q.i.d. dosing, clinical, pharmacologic, and pharmacokinetic data provide a reasonable basis for concluding that b.i.d. dosing with propranolol should be adequate in the treatment of postinfarction patients.

Clinical
In the BHAT, patients on Inderal were prescribed either 180 mg/day (82% of patients) or 240 mg/day (18% of patients). Patients were instructed to take the medication 3 times a day at mealtimes. This dosing schedule would result in an overnight dosing interval of 12 to 14 hours which is similar to the dosing interval for a b.i.d regimen. In addition, blood samples were drawn at various times and analyzed for propranolol. When the patients were grouped into tertiles based on the blood levels observed and the mortality in the upper and lower tertiles was compared, there was no evidence that blood levels affected mortality.

Pharmacologic
Studies in normal volunteers have shown that a 90 mg b.i.d. regimen maintains beta blockade at, or above, the minimum for 60 mg t.i.d. dosing for 24 hours even though differences occurred at two time intervals. At 10 to 12 hours after the first dose of the day, t.i.d. dosing gave more beta blockade than b.i.d. dosing; at 20 to 24 hours the trend of the relationship was reversed. These relationships were similar in direction to those observed for plasma propranolol levels. (See "**Pharmacokinetic.**")

Pharmacokinetic
A bioavailability study in normal volunteers showed that the blood levels produced by 180 mg/day given b.i.d. are below those provided by the same daily dosage given t.i.d. at 10 to 12 hours after the first dose of the day, but above those of a t.i.d. regimen at 20 to 24 hours. However, the blood levels produced by b.i.d. dosing were always equivalent to or above the minimum for t.i.d. dosing throughout the 24 hours. In addition, the mean AUC on the fourth day for the b.i.d. regimen was about 17% greater than for the t.i.d. regimen (1,194 *vs.* 1,024 ng/mL·hr).

INDICATIONS AND USAGE

Hypertension
Inderal is indicated in the management of hypertension. It may be used alone or used in combination with other antihypertensive agents, particularly a thiazide diuretic. Inderal is not indicated in the management of hypertensive emergencies.

Angina Pectoris Due to Coronary Atherosclerosis
Inderal is indicated for the long-term management of patients with angina pectoris.

Cardiac Arrhythmias
1) Supraventricular arrhythmias
   a) Paroxysmal atrial tachycardias, particularly those arrhythmias induced by catecholamines or digitalis or associated with the Wolff-Parkinson-White syndrome. (See W-P-W under "**WARNINGS.**")
   b) Persistent sinus tachycardia which is noncompensatory and impairs the well-being of the patient.
   c) Tachycardias and arrhythmias due to thyrotoxicosis when causing distress or increased hazard and when immediate effect is necessary as adjunctive, short-term (2 to 4 weeks) therapy. May be used with, but not in place of, specific therapy. (See "**Thyrotoxicosis**" under "**WARNINGS.**")
   d) Persistent atrial extrasystoles which impair the well-being of the patient and do not respond to conventional measures.
   e) Atrial flutter and fibrillation when ventricular rate cannot be controlled by digitalis alone, or when digitalis is contraindicated.
2) Ventricular tachycardias.
   Ventricular arrhythmias do not respond to propranolol as predictably as do the supraventricular arrhythmias.
   a) Ventricular tachycardias
   With the exception of those induced by catecholamines or digitalis, Inderal is not the drug of first choice. In critical situations when cardioversion techniques or other drugs are not indicated or are not effective, Inderal may be considered. If, after consideration of the risks involved, Inderal is used, it should be given intravenously in low dosage and very slowly. (See "**DOSAGE AND ADMINISTRATION.**") *Care in the administration of* Inderal *with constant electrocardiographic monitoring is essential as the failing heart requires some sympathetic drive for maintenance of myocardial tone.*
   b) Persistent premature ventricular extrasystoles which do not respond to conventional measures and impair the well-being of the patient.
3) Tachyarrhythmias of digitalis intoxication
   If digitalis-induced tachyarrhythmias persist following discontinuance of digitalis and correction of electrolyte abnormalities, they are usually reversible with *oral* Inderal. Severe bradycardia may occur. (See "**Overdosage.**")
   Intravenous propranolol hydrochloride is reserved for life-threatening arrhythmias. Temporary maintenance with oral therapy may be indicated. (See "**DOSAGE AND ADMINISTRATION.**")
4) Resistant tachyarrhythmias due to excessive catecholamine action during anesthesia
   Tachyarrhythmias due to excessive catecholamine action during anesthesia may sometimes arise because of release of endogenous catecholamines or administration of catecholamines. When usual measures fail in such arrhythmias, Inderal may be given intravenously to abolish them. All general inhalation anesthetics produce some degree of myocardial depression. Therefore, when Inderal is used to treat arrhythmias during anesthesia, it should be used with extreme caution and constant ECG and central venous pressure monitoring. (See "**WARNINGS.**")

Myocardial Infarction
Inderal is indicated to reduce cardiovascular mortality in patients who have survived the acute phase of myocardial infarction and are clinically stable.

Migraine
Inderal is indicated for the prophylaxis of common migraine headache. The efficacy of propranolol in the treatment of a migraine attack that has started has not been established, and propranolol is not indicated for such use.

Continued on next page

Inderal—Cont.

Essential Tremor
Inderal is indicated in the management of familial or hereditary essential tremor. Familial or essential tremor consists of involuntary, rhythmic, oscillatory movements, usually limited to the upper limbs. It is absent at rest but occurs when the limb is held in a fixed posture or position against gravity and during active movement. Inderal causes a reduction in the tremor amplitude but not in the tremor frequency. Inderal is not indicated for the treatment of tremor associated with Parkinsonism.

Hypertrophic Subaortic Stenosis
Inderal is useful in the management of hypertrophic subaortic stenosis, especially for treatment of exertional or other stress-induced angina, palpitations, and syncope. Inderal also improves exercise performance. The effectiveness of propranolol hydrochloride in this disease appears to be due to a reduction of the elevated outflow pressure gradient, which is exacerbated by beta-receptor stimulation. Clinical improvement may be temporary.

Pheochromocytoma
After primary treatment with an alpha-adrenergic blocking agent has been instituted, Inderal may be useful as *adjunctive* therapy if the control of tachycardia becomes necessary before or during surgery. It is hazardous to use Inderal unless alpha-adrenergic blocking drugs are already in use, since this would predispose to serious blood pressure elevation. Blocking only the peripheral dilator (beta) action of epinephrine leaves its constrictor (alpha) action unopposed. In the event of hemorrhage or shock, there is a disadvantage in having both beta and alpha blockade since the combination prevents the increase in heart rate and peripheral vasoconstriction needed to maintain blood pressure.

With inoperable or metastatic pheochromocytoma, Inderal may be useful as an adjunct to the management of symptoms due to excessive beta-receptor stimulation.

CONTRAINDICATIONS
Inderal is contraindicated in 1) cardiogenic shock, 2) sinus bradycardia and greater than first degree block, 3) bronchial asthma, 4) congestive heart failure (see "**WARNINGS**") unless the failure is secondary to a tachyarrhythmia treatable with Inderal.

WARNINGS

Cardiac Failure
Sympathetic stimulation may be a vital component supporting circulatory function in patients with congestive heart failure, and its inhibition by beta blockade may precipitate more severe failure. Although beta blockers should be avoided in overt congestive heart failure, if necessary, they can be used with close follow-up in patients with a history of failure who are well compensated and are receiving digitalis and diuretics. Beta-adrenergic blocking agents do not abolish the inotropic action of digitalis on heart muscle.

In Patients Without a History of Heart Failure,
continued use of beta blockers can, in some cases, lead to cardiac failure. Therefore, at the first sign or symptom of heart failure, the patient should be digitalized and/or treated with diuretics, and the response observed closely, or Inderal should be discontinued (gradually, if possible).

In Patients with Angina Pectoris, there have been reports of exacerbation of angina and, in some cases, myocardial infarction, following *abrupt* discontinuance of Inderal therapy. Therefore, when discontinuance of Inderal is planned, the dosage should be gradually reduced over at least a few weeks and the patient should be cautioned against interruption or cessation of therapy without the physician's advice. If Inderal therapy is interrupted and exacerbation of angina occurs, it usually is advisable to reinstitute Inderal therapy and take other measures appropriate for the management of unstable angina pectoris. Since coronary artery disease may be unrecognized, it may be prudent to follow the above advice in patients considered at risk of having occult atherosclerotic heart disease who are given propranolol for other indications.

NONALLERGIC BRONCHOSPASM (E.G., CHRONIC BRONCHITIS, EMPHYSEMA)
PATIENTS WITH BRONCHOSPASTIC DISEASES SHOULD IN GENERAL NOT RECEIVE BETA BLOCKERS. Inderal should be administered with caution since it may block bronchodilation produced by endogenous and exogenous catecholamine stimulation of beta receptors.

Major Surgery
The necessity or desirability of withdrawal of beta-blocking therapy prior to major surgery is controversial. It should be noted, however, that the impaired ability of the heart to respond to reflex adrenergic stimuli may augment the risks of general anesthesia and surgical procedures.

Inderal, like other beta blockers, is a competitive inhibitor of beta-receptor agonists and its effects can be reversed by administration of such agents, e.g., dobutamine or isoproterenol. However, such patients may be subject to protracted severe hypotension. Difficulty in starting and maintaining the heartbeat has also been reported with beta blockers.

Diabetes and Hypoglycemia
Beta-adrenergic blockade may prevent the appearance of certain premonitory signs and symptoms (pulse rate and pressure changes) of acute hypoglycemia in labile insulin-dependent diabetes. In these patients, it may be more difficult to adjust the dosage of insulin. Hypoglycemic attacks may be accompanied by a precipitous elevation of blood pressure. Propranolol therapy, particularly in infants and children, diabetic or not, has been associated with hypoglycemia especially during fasting as in preparation for surgery. Hypoglycemia also has been found after this type of drug therapy and prolonged physical exertion and has occurred in renal insufficiency, both during dialysis and sporadically, in subjects on propranolol.

Thyrotoxicosis
Beta blockade may mask certain clinical signs of hyperthyroidism. Therefore, abrupt withdrawal of propranolol may be followed by an exacerbation of symptoms of hyperthyroidism, including thyroid storm. Propranolol may change thyroid-function tests, increasing T_4 and reverse T_3 and decreasing T_3.

In Patients With Wolff-Parkinson-White Syndrome, several
cases have been reported in which, after propranolol, the tachycardia was replaced by a severe bradycardia requiring a demand pacemaker. In one case this resulted after an initial dose of 5 mg propranolol.

PRECAUTIONS

General
Propranolol should be used with caution in patients with impaired hepatic or renal function. Inderal is not indicated for the treatment of hypertensive emergencies.

Beta-adrenoreceptor blockade can cause reduction of intraocular pressure. Patients should be told that Inderal may interfere with the glaucoma screening test. Withdrawal may lead to a return of increased intraocular pressure.

Risk of anaphylactic reaction. While taking beta blockers, patients with a history of severe anaphylactic reaction to a variety of allergens may be more reactive to repeated challenge, either accidental, diagnostic, or therapeutic. Such patients may be unresponsive to the usual doses of epinephrine used to treat allergic reaction.

Clinical Laboratory Tests
Elevated blood urea levels in patients with severe heart disease, elevated serum transaminase, alkaline phosphatase, lactate dehydrogenase.

Drug Interactions
Patients receiving catecholamine-depleting drugs such as reserpine should be closely observed if Inderal is administered. The added catecholamine-blocking action may produce an excessive reduction of resting sympathetic nervous activity, which may result in hypotension, marked bradycardia, vertigo, syncopal attacks, or orthostatic hypotension.

Caution should be exercised when patients receiving a beta blocker are administered a calcium-channel blocking drug, especially intravenous verapamil, for both agents may depress myocardial contractility or atrioventricular conduction. On rare occasions, the concomitant intravenous use of a beta blocker and verapamil has resulted in serious adverse reactions, especially in patients with severe cardiomyopathy, congestive heart failure or recent myocardial infarction.

Blunting of the antihypertensive effect of beta-adrenoceptor blocking agents by nonsteroidal anti-inflammatory drugs has been reported.

Hypotension and cardiac arrest have been reported with the concomitant use of propranolol and haloperidol.

Aluminum hydroxide gel greatly reduces intestinal absorption of propranolol.

Ethanol slows the rate of absorption of propranolol.

Phenytoin, phenobarbitone, and *rifampin* accelerate propranolol clearance.

Chlorpromazine, when used concomitantly with propranolol, results in increased plasma levels of both drugs.

Antipyrine and *lidocaine* have reduced clearance when used concomitantly with propranolol.

Thyroxine may result in a lower than expected T_3 concentration when used concomitantly with propranolol.

Cimetidine decreases the hepatic metabolism of propranolol, delaying elimination and increasing blood levels.

Theophylline clearance is reduced when used concomitantly with propranolol.

Carcinogenesis, Mutagenesis, Impairment of Fertility
In dietary administration studies in which mice and rats were treated with propranolol for up to 18 months at doses of up to 150 mg/kg/day, there was no evidence of drug-related tumorigenesis. In a study in which both male and female rats were exposed to propranolol in their diets at concentrations of up to 0.05%, from 60 days prior to mating and throughout pregnancy and lactation for two generations, there were no effects on fertility. Based on differing results from Ames Tests performed by different laboratories, there is equivocal evidence for a genotoxic effect of propranolol in bacteria (*S. typhimurium* strain TA 1538).

Pregnancy: Pregnancy Category C
In a series of reproductive and developmental toxicology studies, propranolol was given to rats by gavage or in the diet throughout pregnancy and lactation. At doses of 150 mg/kg/day (> 10 times the maximum recommended human daily dose of propranolol on a body weight basis), but not at doses of 80 mg/kg/day, treatment was associated with embryotoxicity (reduced litter size and increased resorption sites) as well as neonatal toxicity (deaths). Propranolol also was administered (in the feed) to rabbits (throughout pregnancy and lactation) at doses as high as 150 mg/kg/day (> 15 times the maximum recommended daily human dose). No evidence of embryo or neonatal toxicity was noted.

There are no adequate and well-controlled studies in pregnant women. Intrauterine growth retardation has been reported in neonates whose mothers received propranolol during pregnancy. Neonates whose mothers are receiving propranolol at parturition have exhibited bradycardia, hypoglycemia and respiratory depression. Adequate facilities for monitoring these infants at birth should be available. Inderal should be used during pregnancy only if the potential benefit justifies the potential risk to the fetus.

Nursing Mothers
Inderal is excreted in human milk. Caution should be exercised when Inderal is administered to a nursing woman.

Pediatric Use
High serum propranolol levels have been noted in patients with Down's syndrome (trisomy 21), suggesting that the bioavailability of propranolol may be increased in patients with this condition.

Evaluation of the effects of propranolol in pediatric patients, relative to the drug's efficacy and safety, has not been as systematically performed as in adults. Information is available in the medical literature to allow fair estimates, and specific dosing information has been reasonably studied.

Cardiovascular diseases that are common to adults and children are generally as responsive to propranolol intervention in children as they are in adults.

Adverse reactions are also similar: for example, bronchospasm and congestive heart failure related to propranolol therapy have been reported in pediatric patients and occur through the same mechanisms as previously described in adults.

The normal echocardiogram evolves through a series of changes as the heart matures during growth and development in pediatric patients. Should echocardiography be used to monitor propranolol therapy in pediatric patients, the age-related changes in the echocardiogram need to be borne in mind.

ADVERSE REACTIONS
Most adverse effects have been mild and transient and have rarely required the withdrawal of therapy.

Cardiovascular: Bradycardia; congestive heart failure; intensification of AV block; hypotension; paresthesia of hands; thrombocytopenic purpura; arterial insufficiency, usually of the Raynaud type.

Central Nervous System: Light-headedness; mental depression manifested by insomnia, lassitude, weakness, fatigue; reversible mental depression progressing to catatonia; visual disturbances; hallucinations, vivid dreams, an acute reversible syndrome characterized by disorientation for time and place, short-term memory loss, emotional lability, slightly clouded sensorium, and decreased performance on neuropsychometrics. Total daily doses above 160 mg (when administered as divided doses of greater than 80 mg each) may be associated with an increased incidence of fatigue, lethargy, and vivid dreams.

Gastrointestinal: Nausea, vomiting, epigastric distress, abdominal cramping, diarrhea, constipation, mesenteric arterial thrombosis, ischemic colitis.

Allergic: Pharyngitis and agranulocytosis, erythematous rash, fever combined with aching and sore throat, laryngospasm, and respiratory distress.

Respiratory: Bronchospasm.

Hematologic: Agranulocytosis, nonthrombocytopenic purpura, thrombocytopenic purpura.

Autoimmune: In extremely rare instances, systemic lupus erythematosus has been reported.

Miscellaneous: Alopecia, LE-like reactions, psoriasiform rashes, dry eyes, male impotence, and Peyronie's disease have been reported rarely. Oculomucocutaneous reactions involving the skin, serous membranes and conjunctivae reported for a beta blocker (practolol) have not been associated with propranolol.

DOSAGE AND ADMINISTRATION
The dosage range for Inderal is different for each indication.

Oral

Hypertension—*Dosage must be individualized.*
The usual initial dosage is 40 mg Inderal twice daily, whether used alone or added to a diuretic. Dosage may be increased gradually until adequate blood pressure control is

achieved. The usual maintenance dosage is 120 mg to 240 mg per day. In some instances a dosage of 640 mg a day may be required. The time needed for full antihypertensive response to a given dosage is variable and may range from a few days to several weeks.

While twice-daily dosing is effective and can maintain a reduction in blood pressure throughout the day, some patients, especially when lower doses are used, may experience a modest rise in blood pressure toward the end of the 12-hour dosing interval. This can be evaluated by measuring blood pressure near the end of the dosing interval to determine whether satisfactory control is being maintained throughout the day. If control is not adequate, a larger dose, or 3-times-daily therapy may achieve better control.

Angina Pectoris—*Dosage must be individualized.*

Total daily doses of 80 mg to 320 mg, when administered orally, twice a day, three times a day, or four times a day, have been shown to increase exercise tolerance and to reduce ischemic changes in the ECG. If treatment is to be discontinued, reduce dosage gradually over a period of several weeks. (See "**WARNINGS**.")

Arrhythmias—10 mg to 30 mg three or four times daily, before meals and at bedtime.

Myocardial Infarction—The recommended daily dosage is 180 mg to 240 mg per day in divided doses. Although a t.i.d. regimen was used in the Beta-Blocker Heart Attack Trial and a q.i.d. regimen in the Norwegian Multicenter Trial, there is a reasonable basis for the use of either a t.i.d. or b.i.d. regimen (see "**CLINICAL PHARMACOLOGY**"). The effectiveness and safety of daily dosages greater than 240 mg for prevention of cardiac mortality have not been established. However, higher dosages may be needed to effectively treat coexisting diseases such as angina or hypertension (see above).

Migraine—*Dosage must be individualized.*

The initial oral dose is 80 mg Inderal daily in divided doses. The usual effective dose range is 160 mg to 240 mg per day. The dosage may be increased gradually to achieve optimum migraine prophylaxis. If a satisfactory response is not obtained within four to six weeks after reaching the maximum dose, Inderal therapy should be discontinued. It may be advisable to withdraw the drug gradually over a period of several weeks.

Essential Tremor—*Dosage must be individualized.*

The initial dosage is 40 mg Inderal twice daily. Optimum reduction of essential tremor is usually achieved with a dose of 120 mg per day. Occasionally, it may be necessary to administer 240 mg to 320 mg per day.

Hypertrophic Subaortic Stenosis—20 mg to 40 mg three or four times daily, before meals and at bedtime.

Pheochromocytoma—*Preoperatively*—60 mg daily in divided doses for three days prior to surgery, concomitantly with an alpha-adrenergic blocking agent.

—*Management of inoperable tumor* —30 mg daily in divided doses.

Use in Pediatric Patients: Intravenous administration of Inderal is not recommended in pediatric patients. Oral dosage for treating hypertension requires individual titration, beginning with a 1.0 mg per kg (body weight) per day dosage regimen (i.e., 0.5 mg per kg b.i.d.).

The usual pediatric dosage range is 2 mg to 4 mg per kg per day in two equally divided doses (i.e., 1.0 mg per kg b.i.d. to 2.0 mg per kg b.i.d.). Pediatric dosage calculated by weight (recommended) generally produces propranolol plasma levels in a therapeutic range similar to that in adults. On the other hand, pediatric doses calculated on the basis of body surface area (*not* recommended) usually result in plasma levels above the mean adult therapeutic range. Doses above 16 mg per kg per day should not be used in pediatric patients. If treatment with Inderal is to be discontinued, a gradually decreasing dose titration over a 7- to 14-day period is necessary.

Intravenous

Parenteral drug products should be inspected visually for particulate matter and discoloration prior to administration, whenever solution and container permit.

Intravenous administration is reserved for life-threatening arrhythmias or those occurring under anesthesia. The usual dose is from 1 mg to 3 mg administered under careful monitoring, e.g., electrocardiographic, central venous pressure. The rate of administration should not exceed 1 mg (1 mL) per minute to diminish the possibility of lowering blood pressure and causing cardiac standstill. Sufficient time should be allowed for the drug to reach the site of action even when a slow circulation is present. If necessary, a second dose may be given after two minutes. Thereafter, additional drug should not be given in less than four hours. Additional Inderal should not be given when the desired alteration in rate and/or rhythm is achieved.

Transference to oral therapy should be made as soon as possible.

The intravenous administration of Inderal has not been evaluated adequately in the management of hypertensive emergencies.

Overdosage

Inderal is not significantly dialyzable. In the event of overdosage or exaggerated response, the following measures should be employed:

General—If ingestion is or may have been recent, evacuate gastric contents, taking care to prevent pulmonary aspiration.

Bradycardia—ADMINISTER ATROPINE (0.25 mg to 1.0 mg); IF THERE IS NO RESPONSE TO VAGAL BLOCKADE, ADMINISTER ISOPROTERENOL CAUTIOUSLY.

Cardiac Failure—DIGITALIZATION AND DIURETICS.

Hypotension — VASOPRESSORS, *e.g.*, LEVARTERENOL OR EPINEPHRINE (THERE IS EVIDENCE THAT EPINEPHRINE IS THE DRUG OF CHOICE).

Bronchospasm — ADMINISTER ISOPROTERENOL AND AMINOPHYLLINE.

HOW SUPPLIED

Inderal®
(propranolol hydrochloride)

Tablets

INDERAL 10—Each hexagonal-shaped, orange, scored tablet, embossed with an "I" and imprinted with "INDERAL 10", contains 10 mg propranolol hydrochloride, in bottles of 100 (NDC 0046-0421-81); 1,000 (NDC 0046-0421-91); and 5,000 (NDC 0046-0421-95). Also in Unit Dose packages of 100 (NDC 0046-0421-99).

Store at room temperature (approximately 25° C).

Dispense in a well-closed container as defined in the USP.

INDERAL 20—Each hexagonal-shaped, blue, scored tablet, embossed with an "I" and imprinted with "INDERAL 20", contains 20 mg propranolol hydrochloride, in bottles of 100 (NDC 0046-0422-81); 1,000 (NDC 0046-0422-91); and 5,000 (NDC 0046-0422-95). Also in Unit Dose packages of 100 (NDC 0046-0422-99).

Store at room temperature (approximately 25° C).

Dispense in a well-closed, light-resistant container as defined in the USP.

Protect from light.

Use carton to protect contents from light.

INDERAL 40—Each hexagonal-shaped, green, scored tablet, embossed with an "I" and imprinted with "INDERAL 40", contains 40 mg propranolol hydrochloride, in bottles of 100 (NDC 0046-0424-81); 1,000 (NDC 0046-0424-91); and 5,000 (NDC 0046-0424-95). Also in Unit Dose packages of 100 (NDC 0046-0424-99).

Store at room temperature (approximately 25° C).

Dispense in a well-closed, light-resistant container as defined in the USP.

Protect from light.

Use carton to protect contents from light.

INDERAL 60—Each hexagonal-shaped, pink, scored tablet, embossed with an "I" and imprinted with "INDERAL 60", contains 60 mg propranolol hydrochloride, in bottles of 100 (NDC 0046-0426-81); and 1,000 (NDC 0046-0426-91).

Store at room temperature (approximately 25° C).

Dispense in a well-closed container as defined in the USP.

INDERAL 80—Each hexagonal-shaped, yellow, scored tablet, embossed with an "I" and imprinted with "INDERAL 80", contains 80 mg propranolol hydrochloride, in bottles of 100 (NDC 0046-0428-81); 1,000 (NDC 0046-0428-91); and 5,000 (NDC 0046-0428-95).

Store at room temperature (approximately 25° C).

Dispense in a well-closed container as defined in the USP.

The appearance of these tablets is a registered trademark of Wyeth-Ayerst Laboratories.

Injectable

—Each mL contains 1 mg of propranolol hydrochloride in Water for Injection. The pH is adjusted with citric acid. Supplied as: 1 mL ampuls in boxes of 10 (NDC 0046-3265-10).

Store at room temperature (approximately 25°C).

Protect from freezing or excessive heat.

Manufactured by:
Ayerst Laboratories Inc.
A Wyeth-Ayerst Company
Philadelphia, PA 19101

Shown in Product Identification Guide, page 343

INDERAL® LA ℞

[ĭn 'der-al]

(propranolol hydrochloride)

Long-Acting Capsules

Caution: Federal law prohibits dispensing without prescription.

DESCRIPTION

Inderal (propranolol hydrochloride) is a synthetic beta-adrenergic receptor-blocking agent chemically described as 1-(Isopropylamino)-3-(1-naphthyloxy)-2-propanol hydrochloride. Its structural formula is

[See chemical structure at top of next column]

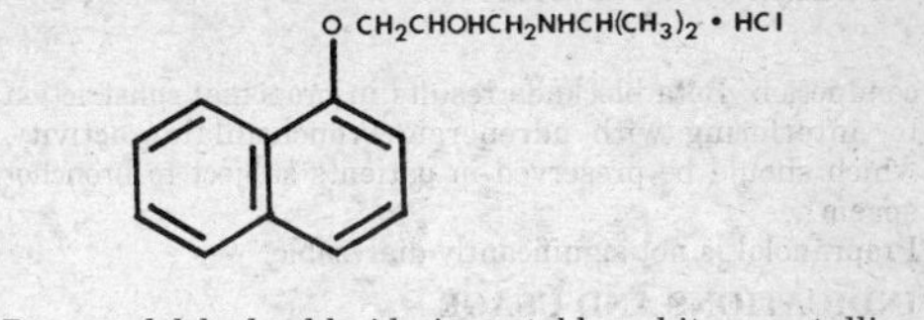
O CH₂CHOHCH₂NHCH(CH₃)₂ • HCl

Propranolol hydrochloride is a stable, white, crystalline solid which is readily soluble in water and ethanol. Its molecular weight is 295.81.

Inderal LA is formulated to provide a sustained release of propranolol hydrochloride. Inderal LA is available as 60 mg, 80 mg, 120 mg, and 160 mg capsules.

Inderal LA capsules contain the following inactive ingredients: cellulose, ethylcellulose, gelatin capsules, hydroxypropyl methylcellulose, and titanium dioxide. In addition, Inderal LA 60 mg, 80 mg, and 120 mg capsules contain D&C Red No. 28 and FD&C Blue No. 1; Inderal LA 160 mg capsules contain FD&C Blue No. 1.

These capsules comply with USP Drug Release Test 1.

CLINICAL PHARMACOLOGY

Inderal is a nonselective, beta-adrenergic receptor-blocking agent possessing no other autonomic nervous system activity. It specifically competes with beta-adrenergic receptor-stimulating agents for available receptor sites. When access to beta-receptor sites is blocked by Inderal, the chronotropic, inotropic, and vasodilator responses to beta-adrenergic stimulation are decreased proportionately.

Inderal LA Capsules (60, 80, 120, and 160 mg) release propranolol HCl at a controlled and predictable rate. Peak blood levels following dosing with Inderal LA occur at about 6 hours, and the apparent plasma half-life is about 10 hours. When measured at steady state over a 24-hour period the areas under the propranolol plasma concentration-time curve (AUCs) for the capsules are approximately 60% to 65% of the AUCs for a comparable divided daily dose of Inderal Tablets. The lower AUCs for the capsules are due to greater hepatic metabolism of propranolol, resulting from the slower rate of absorption of propranolol. Over a twenty-four (24) hour period, blood levels are fairly constant for about twelve (12) hours, then decline exponentially.

Inderal LA should not be considered a simple mg-for-mg substitute for conventional propranolol and the blood levels achieved do not match (are lower than) those of two to four times daily dosing with the same dose. When changing to Inderal LA from conventional propranolol, a possible need for retitration upwards should be considered, especially to maintain effectiveness at the end of the dosing interval. In most clinical settings, however, such as hypertension or angina where there is little correlation between plasma levels and clinical effect, Inderal LA has been therapeutically equivalent to the same mg dose of conventional Inderal as assessed by 24-hour effects on blood pressure and on 24-hour exercise responses of heart rate, systolic pressure, and rate pressure product. Inderal LA can provide effective beta blockade for a 24-hour period.

The mechanism of the antihypertensive effect of Inderal has not been established. Among the factors that may be involved in contributing to the antihypertensive action are: (1) decreased cardiac output, (2) inhibition of renin release by the kidneys, and (3) diminution of tonic sympathetic nerve outflow from vasomotor centers in the brain. Although total peripheral resistance may increase initially, it readjusts to or below the pretreatment level with chronic use. Effects on plasma volume appear to be minor and somewhat variable. Inderal has been shown to cause a small increase in serum potassium concentration when used in the treatment of hypertensive patients.

In angina pectoris, propranolol generally reduces the oxygen requirement of the heart at any given level of effort by blocking the catecholamine-induced increases in the heart rate, systolic blood pressure, and the velocity and extent of myocardial contraction. Propranolol may increase oxygen requirements by increasing left ventricular fiber length, end diastolic pressure, and systolic ejection period. The net physiologic effect of beta-adrenergic blockade is usually advantageous and is manifested during exercise by delayed onset of pain and increased work capacity.

In dosages greater than required for beta blockade, Inderal also exerts a quinidine-like or anesthetic-like membrane action which affects the cardiac action potential. The significance of the membrane action in the treatment of arrhythmias is uncertain.

The mechanism of the antimigraine effect of propranolol has not been established. Beta-adrenergic receptors have been demonstrated in the pial vessels of the brain.

Beta-receptor blockade can be useful in conditions in which, because of pathologic or functional changes, sympathetic activity is detrimental to the patient. But there are also situations in which sympathetic stimulation is vital. For example, in patients with severely damaged hearts, adequate ventricular function is maintained by virtue of sympathetic drive, which should be preserved. In the presence of AV block, greater than first degree, beta blockade may prevent the necessary facilitating effect of sympathetic activity on

Continued on next page

Inderal LA—Cont.

conduction. Beta blockade results in bronchial constriction by interfering with adrenergic bronchodilator activity, which should be preserved in patients subject to bronchospasm.

Propranolol is not significantly dialyzable.

INDICATIONS AND USAGE

Hypertension

Inderal LA is indicated in the management of hypertension; it may be used alone or used in combination with other antihypertensive agents, particularly a thiazide diuretic. Inderal LA is not indicated in the management of hypertensive emergencies.

Angina Pectoris Due to Coronary Atherosclerosis

Inderal LA is indicated for the long-term management of patients with angina pectoris.

Migraine

Inderal LA is indicated for the prophylaxis of common migraine headache. The efficacy of propranolol in the treatment of a migraine attack that has started has not been established, and propranolol is not indicated for such use.

Hypertrophic Subaortic Stenosis

Inderal LA is useful in the management of hypertrophic subaortic stenosis, especially for treatment of exertional or other stress-induced angina, palpitations, and syncope. Inderal LA also improves exercise performance. The effectiveness of propranolol hydrochloride in this disease appears to be due to a reduction of the elevated outflow pressure gradient which is exacerbated by beta-receptor stimulation. Clinical improvement may be temporary.

CONTRAINDICATIONS

Inderal is contraindicated in 1) cardiogenic shock; 2) sinus bradycardia and greater than first-degree block; 3) bronchial asthma; 4) congestive heart failure (see "**WARNINGS**"), unless the failure is secondary to a tachyarrhythmia treatable with Inderal.

WARNINGS

Cardiac Failure: Sympathetic stimulation may be a vital component supporting circulatory function in patients with congestive heart failure, and its inhibition by beta blockade may precipitate more severe failure. Although beta blockers should be avoided in overt congestive heart failure, if necessary, they can be used with close follow-up in patients with a history of failure who are well compensated and are receiving digitalis and diuretics. Beta-adrenergic blocking agents do not abolish the inotropic action of digitalis on heart muscle.

In Patients Without a History of Heart Failure, continued use of beta blockers can, in some cases, lead to cardiac failure. Therefore, at the first sign or symptom of heart failure, the patient should be digitalized and/or treated with diuretics, and the response observed closely, or Inderal should be discontinued (gradually, if possible).

In Patients With Angina Pectoris, there have been reports of exacerbation of angina and, in some cases, myocardial infarction, following *abrupt* discontinuance of Inderal therapy. Therefore, when discontinuance of Inderal is planned, the dosage should be gradually reduced over at least a few weeks, and the patient should be cautioned against interruption or cessation of therapy without the physician's advice. If Inderal therapy is interrupted and exacerbation of angina occurs, it usually is advisable to reinstitute Inderal therapy and take other measures appropriate for the management of unstable angina pectoris. Since coronary artery disease may be unrecognized, it may be prudent to follow the above advice in patients considered at risk of having occult atherosclerotic heart disease who are given propranolol for other indications.

Nonallergic Bronchospasm (e.g., Chronic Bronchitis, Emphysema)—PATIENTS WITH BRONCHOSPASTIC DISEASES SHOULD IN GENERAL NOT RECEIVE BETA BLOCKERS. Inderal should be administered with caution since it may block bronchodilation produced by endogenous and exogenous catecholamine stimulation of beta receptors.

Major Surgery: The necessity or desirability of withdrawal of beta-blocking therapy prior to major surgery is controversial. It should be noted, however, that the impaired ability of the heart to respond to reflex adrenergic stimuli may augment the risks of general anesthesia and surgical procedures.

Inderal, like other beta blockers, is a competitive inhibitor of beta-receptor agonists and its effects can be reversed by administration of such agents, e.g., dobutamine or isoproterenol. However, such patients may be subject to protracted severe hypotension. Difficulty in starting and maintaining the heartbeat has also been reported with beta blockers.

Diabetes and Hypoglycemia: Beta-adrenergic blockade may prevent the appearance of certain premonitory signs and symptoms (pulse rate and pressure changes) of acute hypoglycemia in labile insulin-dependent diabetes. In these patients, it may be more difficult to adjust the dosage of insulin. Hypoglycemic attacks may be accompanied by a precipitous elevation of blood pressure.

Propranolol therapy, particularly in infants and children, diabetic or not, has been associated with hypoglycemia especially during fasting as in preparation for surgery. Hypoglycemia also has been found after this type of drug therapy and prolonged physical exertion and has occurred in renal insufficiency, both during dialysis and sporadically, in subjects on propranolol.

Thyrotoxicosis: Beta blockade may mask certain clinical signs of hyperthyroidism. Therefore, abrupt withdrawal of propranolol may be followed by an exacerbation of symptoms of hyperthyroidism, including thyroid storm. Propranolol may change thyroid-function tests, increasing T_4 and reverse T_3, and decreasing T_3.

In Patients With Wolff-Parkinson-White Syndrome, several cases have been reported in which, after propranolol, the tachycardia was replaced by a severe bradycardia requiring a demand pacemaker. In one case this resulted after an initial dose of 5 mg propranolol.

PRECAUTIONS

General

Propranolol should be used with caution in patients with impaired hepatic or renal function. Inderal is not indicated for the treatment of hypertensive emergencies.

Beta-adrenoreceptor blockade can cause reduction of intraocular pressure. Patients should be told that Inderal may interfere with the glaucoma screening test. Withdrawal may lead to a return of increased intraocular pressure.

Risk of anaphylactic reaction. While taking beta blockers, patients with a history of severe anaphylactic reaction to a variety of allergens may be more reactive to repeated challenge, either accidental, diagnostic, or therapeutic. Such patients may be unresponsive to the usual doses of epinephrine used to treat allergic reaction.

Clinical Laboratory Tests

Elevated blood urea levels in patients with severe heart disease, elevated serum transaminase, alkaline phosphatase, lactate dehydrogenase.

Drug Interactions

Patients receiving catecholamine-depleting drugs such as reserpine should be closely observed if Inderal is administered. The added catecholamine-blocking action may produce an excessive reduction of resting sympathetic nervous activity which may result in hypotension, marked bradycardia, vertigo, syncopal attacks, or orthostatic hypotension.

Caution should be exercised when patients receiving a beta blocker are administered a calcium-channel-blocking drug, especially intravenous verapamil, for both agents may depress myocardial contractility or atrioventricular conduction. On rare occasions, the concomitant intravenous use of a beta blocker and verapamil has resulted in serious adverse reactions, especially in patients with severe cardiomyopathy, congestive heart failure or recent myocardial infarction.

Blunting of the antihypertensive effect of beta-adrenoceptor blocking agents by nonsteroidal anti-inflammatory drugs has been reported.

Hypotension and cardiac arrest have been reported with the concomitant use of propranolol and haloperidol.

Aluminum hydroxide gel greatly reduces intestinal absorption of propranolol.

Ethanol slows the rate of absorption of propranolol.

Phenytoin, phenobarbitone, and *rifampin* accelerate propranolol clearance.

Chlorpromazine, when used concomitantly with propranolol, results in increased plasma levels of both drugs.

Antipyrine and *lidocaine* have reduced clearance when used concomitantly with propranolol.

Thyroxine may result in a lower than expected T_3 concentration when used concomitantly with propranolol.

Cimetidine decreases the hepatic metabolism of propranolol, delaying elimination and increasing blood levels.

Theophylline clearance is reduced when used concomitantly with propranolol.

Carcinogenesis, Mutagenesis, Impairment of Fertility

In dietary administration studies in which mice and rats were treated with propranolol for up to 18 months at doses of up to 150 mg/kg/day, there was no evidence of drug-related tumorigenesis. In a study in which both male and female rats were exposed to propranolol in their diets at concentrations of up to 0.05%, from 60 days prior to mating and throughout pregnancy and lactation for two generations, there were no effects on fertility. Based on differing results from Ames Tests performed by different laboratories, there is equivocal evidence for a genotoxic effect of propranolol in bacteria (*S. typhimurium* strain TA 1538).

Pregnancy: Pregnancy Category C

In a series of reproductive and developmental toxicology studies, propranolol was given to rats by gavage or in the diet throughout pregnancy and lactation. At doses of 150 mg/kg/day (> 10 times the maximum recommended human daily dose of propranolol on a body weight basis), but not at doses of 80 mg/kg/day, treatment was associated with embryotoxicity (reduced litter size and increased resorption sites) as well as neonatal toxicity (deaths). Propranolol also was administered (in the feed) to rabbits (throughout pregnancy and lactation) at doses as high as 150 mg/kg/day (> 15 times the maximum recommended daily human dose). No evidence of embryo or neonatal toxicity was noted. There are no adequate and well-controlled studies in pregnant women. Intrauterine growth retardation has been reported in neonates whose mothers received propranolol during pregnancy. Neonates whose mothers are receiving propranolol at parturition have exhibited bradycardia, hypoglycemia and respiratory depression. Adequate facilities for monitoring these infants at birth should be available. Inderal should be used during pregnancy only if the potential benefit justifies the potential risk to the fetus.

Nursing Mothers

Inderal is excreted in human milk. Caution should be exercised when Inderal is administered to a nursing woman.

Pediatric Use

Safety and effectiveness in pediatric patients have not been established.

ADVERSE REACTIONS

Most adverse effects have been mild and transient and have rarely required the withdrawal of therapy.

Cardiovascular: Bradycardia; congestive heart failure; intensification of AV block; hypotension; paresthesia of hands; thrombocytopenic purpura; arterial insufficiency, usually of the Raynaud type.

Central Nervous System: Light-headedness, mental depression manifested by insomnia, lassitude, weakness, fatigue; reversible mental depression progressing to catatonia; visual disturbances; hallucinations; vivid dreams; an acute reversible syndrome characterized by disorientation for time and place, short-term memory loss, emotional lability, slightly clouded sensorium, and decreased performance on neuropsychometrics. For immediate formulations, fatigue, lethargy, and vivid dreams appear dose related.

Gastrointestinal: Nausea, vomiting, epigastric distress, abdominal cramping, diarrhea, constipation, mesenteric arterial thrombosis, ischemic colitis.

Allergic: Pharyngitis and agranulocytosis; erythematous rash, fever combined with aching and sore throat; laryngospasm, and respiratory distress.

Respiratory: Bronchospasm.

Hematologic: Agranulocytosis, nonthrombocytopenic purpura, thrombocytopenic purpura.

Autoimmune: In extremely rare instances, systemic lupus erythematosus has been reported.

Miscellaneous: Alopecia, LE-like reactions, psoriasiform rashes, dry eyes, male impotence, and Peyronie's disease have been reported rarely. Oculomucocutaneous reactions involving the skin, serous membranes and conjunctivae reported for a beta blocker (practolol) have not been associated with propranolol.

DOSAGE AND ADMINISTRATION

Inderal LA provides propranolol hydrochloride in a sustained-release capsule for administration once daily. If patients are switched from Inderal Tablets to Inderal LA Capsules, care should be taken to assure that the desired therapeutic effect is maintained. Inderal LA should not be considered a simple mg-for-mg substitute for Inderal. Inderal LA has different kinetics and produces lower blood levels. Retitration may be necessary, especially to maintain effectiveness at the end of the 24-hour dosing interval.

Hypertension

Dosage must be individualized. The usual initial dosage is 80 mg Inderal LA once daily, whether used alone or added to a diuretic. The dosage may be increased to 120 mg once daily or higher until adequate blood pressure control is achieved. The usual maintenance dosage is 120 to 160 mg once daily. In some instances a dosage of 640 mg may be required. The time needed for full hypertensive response to a given dosage is variable and may range from a few days to several weeks.

Angina Pectoris

Dosage must be individualized. Starting with 80 mg Inderal LA once daily, dosage should be gradually increased at three- to seven-day intervals until optimal response is obtained. Although individual patients may respond at any dosage level, the average optimal dosage appears to be 160 mg once daily. In angina pectoris, the value and safety of dosage exceeding 320 mg per day have not been established. If treatment is to be discontinued, reduce dosage gradually over a period of a few weeks (see "**WARNINGS**").

Migraine

Dosage must be individualized. The initial oral dose is 80 mg Inderal LA once daily. The usual effective dose range is 160 to 240 mg once daily. The dosage may be increased gradually to achieve optimal migraine prophylaxis. If a satisfactory response is not obtained within four to six weeks after reaching the maximal dose, Inderal LA therapy should be discontinued. It may be advisable to withdraw the drug gradually over a period of several weeks.

Hypertrophic Subaortic Stenosis
80 to 160 mg Inderal LA once daily.

Pediatric Dosage
At this time the data on the use of the drug in this age group are too limited to permit adequate directions for use.

OVERDOSAGE

Inderal is not significantly dialyzable. In the event of overdosage or exaggerated response, the following measures should be employed:

General
If ingestion is, or may have been, recent, evacuate gastric contents, taking care to prevent pulmonary aspiration.

Bradycardia
ADMINISTER ATROPINE (0.25 to 1.0 mg); IF THERE IS NO RESPONSE TO VAGAL BLOCKADE, ADMINISTER ISOPROTERENOL CAUTIOUSLY.

Cardiac Failure
DIGITALIZATION AND DIURETICS.

Hypotension
VASOPRESSORS, e.g., LEVARTERENOL OR EPINEPHRINE (THERE IS EVIDENCE THAT EPINEPHRINE IS THE DRUG OF CHOICE).

Bronchospasm
ADMINISTER ISOPROTERENOL AND AMINOPHYLLINE.

HOW SUPPLIED

Inderal® LA Capsules (propranolol hydrochloride)
Each white/light-blue capsule, identified by 3 narrow bands, 1 wide band, and "INDERAL LA 60," contains 60 mg of propranolol hydrochloride in bottles of 100 (NDC 0046-0470-81) and in bottles of 1,000 (NDC 0046-0470-91).
Each light-blue capsule, identified by 3 narrow bands, 1 wide band, and "INDERAL LA 80," contains 80 mg of propranolol hydrochloride in bottles of 100 (NDC 0046-0471-81) and in bottles of 1,000 (NDC 0046-0471-91). Also available in a Unit Dose package of 100 (NDC 0046-0471-99).
Each light-blue/dark-blue capsule, identified by 3 narrow bands, 1 wide band, and "INDERAL LA 120," contains 120 mg of propranolol hydrochloride in bottles of 100 (NDC 0046-0473-81) and in bottles of 1,000 (NDC 0046-0473-91). Also available in a Unit Dose package of 100 (NDC 0046-0473-99).
Each dark-blue capsule, identified by 3 narrow bands, 1 wide band, and "INDERAL LA 160," contains 160 mg of propranolol hydrochloride in bottles of 100 (NDC 0046-0479-81) and in bottles of 1,000 (NDC 0046-0479-91). Also available in a Unit Dose package of 100 (NDC 0046-0479-99).
The appearance of these capsules is a registered trademark of Wyeth-Ayerst Laboratories.
Store at room temperature (approximately 25° C).
Protect from light, moisture, freezing, and excessive heat.
Dispense in a tight, light-resistant container as defined in the USP.
Use carton to protect contents from light.
Manufactured by:
Ayerst Laboratories Inc.
A Wyeth-Ayerst Company
Philadelphia, PA 19101
Shown in Product Identification Guide, page 343

INDERIDE® ℞

[*ĭn 'de-rīde*]
(propranolol hydrochloride
[INDERAL®] and hydrochlorothiazide)

Caution: Federal law prohibits dispensing without prescription.

DESCRIPTION

Inderide Tablets for oral administration combine two antihypertensive agents: Inderal (propranolol hydrochloride), a beta-adrenergic blocking agent, and hydrochlorothiazide, a thiazide diuretic-antihypertensive. Inderide 40/25 Tablets contain 40 mg propranolol hydrochloride and 25 mg hydrochlorothiazide; Inderide 80/25 Tablets contain 80 mg propranolol hydrochloride and 25 mg hydrochlorothiazide.
Inderal (propranolol hydrochloride) is a synthetic beta-adrenergic receptor-blocking agent chemically described as 1-(Isopropylamino)-3-(1-naphthyloxy)-2-propanol hydrochloride. Its structural formula is:

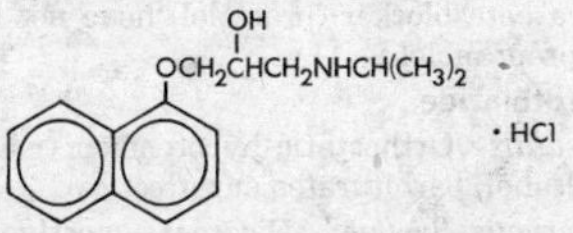

Propranolol hydrochloride is a stable, white, crystalline solid which is readily soluble in water and ethanol. Its molecular weight is 295.81.

Hydrochlorothiazide is a white, or practically white, practically odorless, crystalline powder. It is slightly soluble in water; freely soluble in sodium hydroxide solution; sparingly soluble in methanol; insoluble in ether, chloroform, benzene, and dilute mineral acids. Its chemical name is: 6-Chloro-3,4-dihydro-2H-1,2,4-benzothiadiazine-7-sulfonamide1,1-dioxide. Its structural formula is:

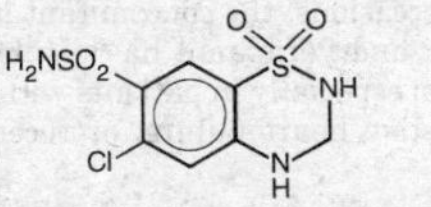

The inactive ingredients contained in Inderide Tablets are lactose, magnesium stearate, microcrystalline cellulose, stearic acid, and yellow ferric oxide.

CLINICAL PHARMACOLOGY

Propranolol hydrochloride (Inderal®)
Propranolol hydrochloride is a nonselective beta-adrenergic receptor blocking agent possessing no other autonomic nervous system activity. It specifically competes with beta-adrenergic receptor stimulating agents for available receptor sites. When access to beta-receptor sites is blocked by propranolol, the chronotropic, inotropic, and vasodilator responses to beta-adrenergic stimulation are decreased proportionately.
Propranolol is almost completely absorbed from the gastrointestinal tract, but a portion is immediately metabolized by the liver on its first pass through the portal circulation.
Peak effect occurs in one to one-and-one-half hours. The biologic half-life is approximately four hours. Propranolol is not significantly dialyzable. There is no simple correlation between dose or plasma level and therapeutic effect, and the dose-sensitivity range, as observed in clinical practice, is wide. The principal reason for this is that sympathetic tone varies widely between individuals. Since there is no reliable test to estimate sympathetic tone or to determine whether total beta blockade has been achieved, proper dosage requires titration.
The mechanism of the antihypertensive effects of propranolol has not been established. Among the factors that may be involved in contributing to the antihypertensive action are (1) decreased cardiac output, (2) inhibition of renin release by the kidneys, and (3) diminution of tonic sympathetic nerve outflow from vasomotor centers in the brain. Although total peripheral resistance may increase initially, it readjusts to, or below, the pretreatment level with chronic use. Effects on plasma volume appear to be minor and somewhat variable. Propranolol has been shown to cause a small increase in serum potassium concentration when used in the treatment of hypertensive patients. Propranolol hydrochloride decreases heart rate, cardiac output, and blood pressure.
Beta-receptor blockade can be useful in conditions in which, because of pathologic or functional changes, sympathetic activity is detrimental to the patient. But there are also situations in which sympathetic stimulation is vital. For example, in patients with severely damaged hearts, adequate ventricular function is maintained by virtue of sympathetic drive, which should be preserved. In the presence of AV block greater than first degree, beta blockade may prevent the necessary facilitating effect of sympathetic activity on conduction. Beta blockade results in bronchial constriction by interfering with adrenergic bronchodilator activity, which should be preserved in patients subject to bronchospasm.
The proper objective of beta-blockade therapy is to decrease adverse sympathetic stimulation, but not to the degree that may impair necessary sympathetic support.

Hydrochlorothiazide
Hydrochlorothiazide is a benzothiadiazine (thiazide) diuretic closely related to chlorothiazide. The mechanism of the antihypertensive effect of the thiazides is unknown. Thiazides do not affect normal blood pressure.
Thiazides affect the renal tubular mechanism of electrolyte reabsorption. At maximal therapeutic dosage, all thiazides are approximately equal in their diuretic potency.
Thiazides increase excretion of sodium and chloride in approximately equivalent amounts. Natriuresis causes a secondary loss of potassium and bicarbonate. Onset of diuretic action of hydrochlorothiazide occurs in two hours, and the peak effect in about four hours. Its action persists for approximately six to 12 hours. Thiazides are eliminated rapidly by the kidney.

INDICATIONS AND USAGE

Inderide is indicated in the management of hypertension.
This fixed combination is not indicated for initial therapy of hypertension. Hypertension requires therapy titrated to the individual patient. If the fixed combination represents the dosage so determined, its use may be more convenient in patient management.

CONTRAINDICATIONS

Propranolol hydrochloride (Inderal®)
Propranolol is contraindicated in: 1) cardiogenic shock; 2) sinus bradycardia and greater than first-degree block; 3) bronchial asthma; 4) congestive heart failure (see **WARNINGS**) unless the failure is secondary to a tachyarrhythmia treatable with propranolol.

Hydrochlorothiazide
Hydrochlorothiazide is contraindicated in patients with anuria or hypersensitivity to this or other sulfonamide-derived drugs.

WARNINGS

Propranolol hydrochloride (Inderal®)
Cardiac Failure: Sympathetic stimulation is a vital component supporting circulatory function in congestive heart failure, and inhibition with beta blockade always carries the potential hazard of further depressing myocardial contractility and precipitating cardiac failure. Propranolol acts selectively without abolishing the inotropic action of digitalis on the heart muscle (i.e., that of supporting the strength of myocardial contractions). In patients already receiving digitalis, the positive inotropic action of digitalis may be reduced by propranolol's negative inotropic effect. The effects of propranolol and digitalis are additive in depressing AV conduction.
Patients Without a History of Heart Failure: Continued depression of the myocardium over a period of time can, in some cases, lead to cardiac failure. In rare instances, this has been observed during propranolol therapy. Therefore, at the first sign or symptom of impending cardiac failure, patients should be fully digitalized and/or given additional diuretic, and the response observed closely: a) if cardiac failure continues, despite adequate digitalization and diuretic therapy, propranolol therapy should be withdrawn (gradually, if possible); b) if tachyarrhythmia is being controlled, patients should be maintained on combined therapy and the patient closely followed until threat of cardiac failure is over.

Angina Pectoris: There have been reports of exacerbation of angina and, in some cases, myocardial infarction following *abrupt* discontinuation of propranolol therapy. Therefore, when discontinuance of propranolol is planned, the dosage should be gradually reduced and the patient should be carefully monitored. In addition, when propranolol is prescribed for angina pectoris, the patient should be cautioned against interruption or cessation of therapy without the physician's advice. If propranolol therapy is interrupted and exacerbation of angina occurs, it usually is advisable to reinstitute propranolol therapy and take other measures appropriate for the management of unstable angina pectoris. Since coronary artery disease may be unrecognized, it may be prudent to follow the above advice in patients considered at risk of having occult atherosclerotic heart disease, who are given propranolol for other indications.

Nonallergic Bronchospasm (e.g., chronic bronchitis, emphysema): PATIENTS WITH BRONCHOSPASTIC DISEASES SHOULD, IN GENERAL, NOT RECEIVE BETA BLOCKERS. Propranolol should be administered with caution since it may block bronchodilation produced by endogenous and exogenous catecholamine stimulation of beta receptors.
Major Surgery: The necessity or desirability of withdrawal of beta-blocking therapy prior to major surgery is controversial. It should be noted, however, that the impaired ability of the heart to respond to reflex adrenergic stimuli may augment the risks of general anesthesia and surgical procedures.
Propranolol, like other beta blockers, is a competitive inhibitor of beta-receptor agonists, and its effects can be reversed by administration of such agents, e.g., dobutamine or isoproterenol. However, such patients may be subject to protracted severe hypotension. Difficulty in starting and maintaining the heartbeat has also been reported with beta blockers.
Diabetes and Hypoglycemia: Beta-adrenergic blockade may prevent the appearance of certain premonitory signs and symptoms (pulse rate and pressure changes) of acute hypoglycemia in labile insulin-dependent diabetes. In these patients, it may be more difficult to adjust the dosage of insulin. Hypoglycemic attack may be accompanied by a precipitous elevation of blood pressure.
Propranolol therapy, particularly in infants and children, diabetic or not, has been associated with hypoglycemia especially during fasting as in preparation for surgery. Hypoglycemia also has been found after this type of drug therapy and prolonged physical exertion and has occurred in renal insufficiency, both during dialysis and sporadically, in subjects on propranolol.
Thyrotoxicosis: Beta blockade may mask certain clinical signs of hyperthyroidism. Therefore, abrupt withdrawal of propranolol may be followed by an exacerbation of symptoms of hyperthyroidism, including thyroid storm. Propranolol may change thyroid-function tests, increasing T_4 and reverse T_3, and decreasing T_3.

Continued on next page

Inderide—Cont.

Wolff-Parkinson-White Syndrome: Several cases have been reported in which, after propranolol, the tachycardia was replaced by a severe bradycardia requiring a demand pacemaker. In one case this resulted after an initial dose of 5 mg propranolol.

Hydrochlorothiazide

Thiazides should be used with caution in severe renal disease. In patients with renal disease, thiazides may precipitate azotemia. In patients with impaired renal function, cumulative effects of the drug may develop.

Thiazides should also be used with caution in patients with impaired hepatic function or progressive liver disease, since minor alterations of fluid and electrolyte balance may precipitate hepatic coma.

Thiazides may add to or potentiate the action of other antihypertensive drugs. Potentiation occurs with ganglionic or peripheral adrenergic-blocking drugs.

Sensitivity reactions may occur in patients with a history of allergy or bronchial asthma. The possibility of exacerbation or activation of systemic lupus erythematosus has been reported.

PRECAUTIONS

General

Propranolol hydrochloride (Inderal®)

Propranolol should be used with caution in patients with impaired hepatic or renal function. Inderide is not indicated for the treatment of hypertensive emergencies.

Risk of anaphylactic reaction: While taking beta blockers, patients with a history of severe anaphylactic reaction to a variety of allergens may be more reactive to repeated challenge, either accidental, diagnostic, or therapeutic. Such patients may be unresponsive to the usual doses of epinephrine used to treat allergic reaction.

Hydrochlorothiazide

All patients receiving thiazide therapy should be observed for clinical signs of fluid or electrolyte imbalance, namely hyponatremia, hypochloremic alkalosis, and hypokalemia. Serum and urine electrolyte determinations are particularly important when the patient is vomiting excessively or receiving parenteral fluids. Medication such as digitalis may also influence serum electrolytes. Warning signs, irrespective of cause, are: dryness of mouth, thirst, weakness, lethargy, drowsiness, restlessness, muscle pains or cramps, muscular fatigue, hypotension, oliguria, tachycardia, and gastrointestinal disturbances such as nausea and vomiting.

Hypokalemia may develop, especially with brisk diuresis or when severe cirrhosis is present.

Interference with adequate oral electrolyte intake will also contribute to hypokalemia. Hypokalemia can sensitize or exaggerate the response of the heart to the toxic effects of digitalis (e.g., increased ventricular irritability).

Hypokalemia may be avoided or treated by use of potassium supplements or foods with a high potassium content.

Any chloride deficit is generally mild, and usually does not require specific treatment except under extraordinary circumstances (as in liver or renal disease). Dilutional hyponatremia may occur in edematous patients in hot weather; appropriate therapy is water restriction rather than administration of salt, except in rare instances when the hyponatremia is life-threatening. In actual salt depletion, appropriate replacement is the therapy of choice.

Hyperuricemia may occur or frank gout may be precipitated in certain patients receiving thiazide therapy.

Diabetes mellitus which has been latent may become manifest during thiazide administration.

The antihypertensive effects of the drug may be enhanced in the postsympathectomy patient.

If progressive renal impairment becomes evident, consider withholding or discontinuing diuretic therapy.

Calcium excretion is decreased by thiazides. Pathologic changes in the parathyroid gland with hypercalcemia and hypophosphatemia have been observed in a few patients on prolonged thiazide therapy. The common complications of hyperparathyroidism, such as renal lithiasis, bone resorption, and peptic ulceration, have not been seen.

Information for Patients

Beta-adrenoreceptor blockade can cause reduction of intraocular pressure. Patients should be told that Inderide may interfere with the glaucoma screening test. Withdrawal may lead to a return of increased intraocular pressure.

Laboratory Tests

Propranolol hydrochloride (Inderal®)

Elevated blood urea levels in patients with severe heart disease, elevated serum transaminase, alkaline phosphatase, lactate dehydrogenase.

Hydrochlorothiazide

Periodic determination of serum electrolytes to detect possible electrolyte imbalance should be performed at appropriate intervals.

Drug/Drug Interactions

Propranolol hydrochloride (Inderal®)

Patients receiving catecholamine-depleting drugs such as reserpine should be closely observed if Inderide is administered. The added catecholamine-blocking action may produce an excessive reduction of resting sympathetic nervous activity, which may result in hypotension, marked bradycardia, vertigo, syncopal attacks, or orthostatic hypotension.

Caution should be exercised when patients receiving a beta blocker are administered a calcium-channel blocking drug, especially intravenous verapamil, for both agents may depress myocardial contractility or atrioventricular conduction. On rare occasions, the concomitant intravenous use of a beta blocker and verapamil has resulted in serious adverse reactions, especially in patients with severe cardiomyopathy, congestive heart failure, or recent myocardial infarction.

Blunting of the antihypertensive effect of beta-adrenoceptor blocking agents by nonsteroidal anti-inflammatory drugs has been reported.

Hypotension and cardiac arrest have been reported with the concomitant use of propranolol and haloperidol.

Aluminum hydroxide gel greatly reduces intestinal absorption of propranolol.

Ethanol slows the rate of absorption of propranolol.

Phenytoin, phenobarbitone, and rifampin accelerate propranolol clearance.

Chlorpromazine, when used concomitantly with propranolol, results in increased plasma levels of both drugs.

Antipyrine and *lidocaine* have reduced clearance when used concomitantly with propranolol.

Thyroxine may result in a lower than expected T_3 concentration when used concomitantly with propranolol.

Cimetidine decreases the hepatic metabolism of propranolol, delaying elimination and increasing blood levels.

Theophylline clearance is reduced when used concomitantly with propranolol.

Hydrochlorothiazide

Thiazide drugs may increase the responsiveness to tubocurarine.

Thiazides may decrease arterial responsiveness to norepinephrine. This diminution is not sufficient to preclude effectiveness of the pressor agent for therapeutic use.

Insulin requirements in diabetic patients may be increased, decreased, or unchanged.

Hypokalemia may develop during concomitant use of corticosteroids or ACTH.

Drug/Laboratory Test Interactions

Hydrochlorothiazide

Thiazides may decrease serum PBI levels without signs of thyroid disturbance.

Thiazides should be discontinued before carrying out tests for parathyroid function (see **"PRECAUTIONS—General"**).

Carcinogenesis, Mutagenesis, Impairment of Fertility

Combinations of propranolol and hydrochlorothiazide have not been evaluated for carcinogenic or mutagenic potential or for potential to adversely affect fertility.

Propranolol hydrochloride (Inderal®)

In dietary administration studies in which mice and rats were treated with propranolol for up to 18 months at doses of up to 150 mg/kg/day, there was no evidence of drug-related tumorigenesis. In a study in which both male and female rats were exposed to propranolol in their diets at concentrations of up to 0.05%, from 60 days prior to mating and throughout pregnancy and lactation for two generations, there were no effects on fertility. Based on differing results from Ames Tests performed by different laboratories, there is equivocal evidence for a genotoxic effect of propranolol in bacteria (*S. typhimurium* strain TA 1538).

Hydrochlorothiazide

Two-year feeding studies in mice and rats conducted under the auspices of the National Toxicology Program (NTP) uncovered no evidence of a carcinogenic potential of hydrochlorothiazide in female mice (at doses of up to approximately 600 mg/kg/day) or in male and female rats (at doses of up to approximately 100 mg/kg/day). The NTP, however, found equivocal evidence for hepatocarcinogenicity in male mice.

Hydrochlorothiazide was not genotoxic *in vitro* in the Ames bacterial mutagen assay (*S. typhimurium* strains TA 98, TA 100, TA 1535, TA 1537 and TA 1538) or in the Chinese Hamster Ovary (CHO) test for chromosomal aberrations. Nor was it genotoxic *in vivo* in assays using mouse germinal cell chromosomes, Chinese hamster bone marrow chromosomes, and the *Drosophila* sex-linked recessive lethal trait gene. Positive test results were obtained in the *in vitro* CHO Sister Chromatid Exchange (clastogenicity), Mouse Lymphoma Cell (mutagenicity) and *Aspergillus nidulans* non-disjunction assays.

Hydrochlorothiazide had no adverse effects on the fertility of mice and rats of either sex in studies wherein these species were exposed, via their diet, to doses of up to 100 mg/kg and 4 mg/kg, respectively, prior to mating and throughout gestation.

Pregnancy: Pregnancy Category C

Combinations of propranolol and hydrochlorothiazide have not been evaluated for effects on pregnancy in animals. Nor are there adequate and well-controlled studies of propranolol, hydrochlorothiazide, or Inderide in pregnant women. Inderide should be used during pregnancy only if the potential benefit justifies the potential risk to the fetus.

Propranolol hydrochloride (Inderal®)

In a series of reproduction and developmental toxicology studies, propranolol was given to rats by gavage or in the diet throughout pregnancy and lactation. At doses of 150 mg/kg/day (>30 times the dose of propranolol contained in the maximum recommended human daily dose of Inderide), but not at doses of 80 mg/kg/day, treatment was associated with embryotoxicity (reduced liter size and increased resorption sites) as well as neonatal toxicity (deaths). Propranolol also was administered (in the feed) to rabbits (throughout pregnancy and lactation) at doses as high as 150 mg/kg/day (>45 times the dose of propranolol contained in the maximum recommended daily human dose of Inderide). No evidence of embryo or neonatal toxicity was noted.

Intrauterine growth retardation has been reported in human neonates whose mothers received propranolol during pregnancy. Neonates whose mothers received propranolol at parturition have exhibited bradycardia, hypoglycemia and respiratory depression. Adequate facilities for monitoring these infants at birth should be available.

Hydrochlorothiazide

Studies in which hydrochlorothiazide was orally administered to pregnant mice and rats at doses of up to 3000 and 1000 mg/kg/day, respectively, provided no evidence of harm to the fetus.

Thiazides cross the placental barrier and appear in cord blood. The use of thiazides in pregnant women requires that the anticipated benefit be weighed against possible hazards to the fetus. These hazards include fetal or neonatal jaundice, thrombocytopenia, and possibly other adverse reactions that have occurred in the adult.

Nursing Mothers

Propranolol hydrochloride (Inderal®)

Propranolol is excreted in human milk. Caution should be exercised when Inderide is administered to a nursing woman.

Hydrochlorothiazide

Thiazides appear in breast milk. If the use of drug is deemed essential, the patient should stop nursing.

Pediatric Use

Safety and effectiveness in pediatric patients have not been established.

ADVERSE REACTIONS

The following adverse reactions have been observed, but there is not enough systematic collection of data to support an estimate of their frequency. Within each category, adverse reactions are listed in decreasing order of severity. Although many side effects are mild and transient, some require discontinuation of therapy.

Propranolol hydrochloride (Inderal®)

Cardiovascular: Congestive heart failure; hypotension; intensification of AV block; bradycardia; thrombocytopenic purpura; arterial insufficiency, usually of the Raynaud type; paresthesia of hands.

Central Nervous System: Reversible mental depression progressing to catatonia; mental depression manifested by insomnia, lassitude, weakness, fatigue; an acute reversible syndrome characterized by disorientation for time and place, short-term memory loss, emotional lability, slightly clouded sensorium, decreased performance on neuropsychometrics; hallucinations; visual disturbances; vivid dreams; light-headedness. Total daily doses above 160 mg (when administered as divided doses of greater than 80 mg each) may be associated with an increased incidence of fatigue, lethargy, and vivid dreams.

Gastrointestinal: Mesenteric arterial thrombosis; ischemic colitis; nausea, vomiting, epigastric distress, abdominal cramping, diarrhea, constipation.

Allergic: Laryngospasm and respiratory distress; pharyngitis and agranulocytosis; fever combined with aching and sore throat; erythematous rash.

Respiratory: Bronchospasm.

Hematologic: Agranulocytosis; nonthrombocytopenic purpura; thrombocytopenic purpura.

Autoimmune: In extremely rare instances, systemic lupus erythematosus has been reported.

Miscellaneous: Male impotence. Alopecia, LE-like reactions, psoriasiform rashes, dry eyes, and Peyronie's disease have been reported rarely. Oculomucocutaneous reactions involving the skin, serous membranes, and conjunctivae reported for a beta blocker (practolol) have not been associated with propranolol.

Hydrochlorothiazide

Cardiovascular: Orthostatic hypotension (may be aggravated by alcohol, barbiturates or narcotics).

Central Nervous System: Dizziness, vertigo, headache, xanthopsia, paresthesias.

Gastrointestinal: Pancreatitis; jaundice (intrahepatic cholestatic jaundice); sialadenitis; anorexia, nausea, vomiting, gastric irritation, cramping, diarrhea, constipation.

Hypersensitivity: Anaphylactic reactions; necrotizing angiitis (vasculitis, cutaneous vasculitis); respiratory distress including pneumonitis; fever; urticaria, rash, purpura, photosensitivity.
Hematologic: Aplastic anemia, agranulocytosis, leukopenia, thrombocytopenia.
Miscellaneous: Hyperglycemia, glycosuria; hyperuricemia; muscle spasm; weakness; restlessness; transient blurred vision.
Whenever adverse reactions are moderate or severe, thiazide dosage should be reduced or therapy withdrawn.

OVERDOSAGE

The propranolol hydrochloride component may cause bradycardia, cardiac failure, hypotension, or bronchospasm. Propranolol is not significantly dialyzable.
The hydrochlorothiazide component can be expected to cause diuresis. Lethargy of varying degree may appear and may progress to coma within a few hours, with minimal depression of respiration and cardiovascular function, and in the absence of significant serum electrolyte changes or dehydration. The mechanism of central nervous system depression with thiazide overdosage is unknown. Gastrointestinal irritation and hypermotility can occur, temporary elevation of BUN has been reported, and serum electrolyte changes could occur, especially in patients with impairment of renal function.
The oral LD_{50} dosages in rats and mice for propranolol, hydrochlorothiazide, and combined propranolol/hydrochlorothiazide (40/25, 80/25) are 364 to 533 mg/kg, greater than 2,750 to 5,000 mg/kg, and 538 to 845 mg/kg, respectively.

Treatment

The following measures should be employed:
General—If ingestion is, or may have been, recent, evacuate gastric contents, taking care to prevent pulmonary aspiration.
Bradycardia—Administer atropine (0.25 to 1.0 mg). If there is no response to vagal blockade, administer isoproterenol cautiously.
Cardiac Failure—Digitalization and diuretics.
Hypotension—Vasopressors, e.g., levarterenol or epinephrine.
Bronchospasm—Administer isoproterenol and aminophylline.
Stupor or Coma—Administer supportive therapy as clinically warranted.
Gastrointestinal Effects—Though usually of short duration, these may require symptomatic treatment.
Abnormalities in BUN and/or Serum Electrolytes—Monitor serum electrolyte levels and renal function; institute supportive measures as required individually to maintain hydration, electrolyte balance, respiration, and cardiovascular-renal function.

DOSAGE AND ADMINISTRATION

The dosage must be determined by individual titration.
Hydrochlorothiazide can be given at doses of 12.5 to 50 mg per day when used alone. The initial dose of propranolol is 80 mg daily, and it may be increased gradually until optimal blood pressure control is achieved. The usual effective dose when used alone is 160 to 480 mg per day.
One Inderide Tablet twice daily can be used to administer up to 160 mg of propranolol and 50 mg of hydrochlorothiazide. For doses of propranolol greater than 160 mg the combination products are not appropriate, because their use would lead to an excessive dose of the thiazide component.
When necessary, another antihypertensive agent may be added gradually beginning with 50 percent of the usual recommended starting dose to avoid an excessive fall in blood pressure.

HOW SUPPLIED

Inderide 40/25
Each hexagonal-shaped, off-white, scored tablet, embossed with an "I" and imprinted with "INDERIDE 40/25," contains 40 mg propranolol hydrochloride (Inderal®) and 25 mg hydrochlorothiazide, in bottles of 100 (NDC 0046-0484-81) and 1,000 (NDC 0046-0484-91).
Inderide 80/25
Each hexagonal-shaped, off-white, scored tablet, embossed with an "I" and imprinted with "INDERIDE 80/25," contains 80 mg propranolol hydrochloride (Inderal®) and 25 mg hydrochlorothiazide, in bottles of 100 (NDC 0046-0488-81).

Store at room temperature (approximately 25° C).

Protect from moisture, freezing, and excessive heat.

Dispense in a well-closed container as defined in the USP.

The appearance of these tablets is a registered trademark of Wyeth-Ayerst Laboratories.
Manufactured by:
Ayerst Laboratories Inc.
A Wyeth-Ayerst Company
Philadelphia, PA 19101

Shown in Product Identification Guide, page 343

INDERIDE® LA ℞

[*in 'de-rīde*]
(propranolol hydrochloride and hydrochlorothiazide)
Long-Acting Capsules

No. 455—Each Inderide® LA 80/50 Capsule contains:
Propranolol hydrochloride
(Inderal® LA) .... 80 mg
Hydrochlorothiazide .... 50 mg
No. 457—Each Inderide® LA 120/50 Capsule contains:
Propranolol hydrochloride
(Inderal® LA) .... 120 mg
Hydrochlorothiazide .... 50 mg
No. 459—Each Inderide® LA 160/50 Capsule contains:
Propranolol hydrochloride
(Inderal® LA) .... 160 mg
Hydrochlorothiazide .... 50 mg
Caution: Federal law prohibits dispensing without prescription.

DESCRIPTION

Inderide LA is indicated in the once-daily management of hypertension.
Inderide LA combines two antihypertensive agents: Inderal (propranolol hydrochloride), a beta-adrenergic receptor-blocking agent, and hydrochlorothiazide, a thiazide diuretic-antihypertensive. Inderide LA is formulated to provide a sustained release of propranolol hydrochloride. Hydrochlorothiazide in Inderide LA exists in a conventional (not sustained-release) formulation.
Inderal (propranolol hydrochloride) is a synthetic beta-adrenergic receptor-blocking agent chemically described as 1-(Isopropylamino)-3-(1-naphthyloxy)-2-propanol hydrochloride. Its structural formula is:

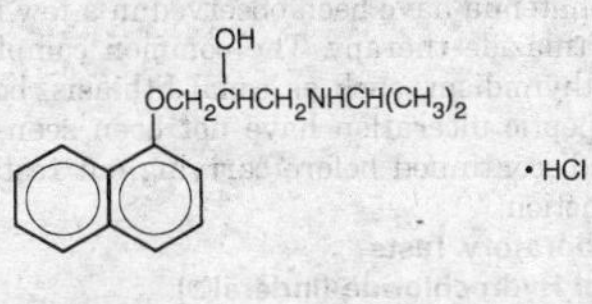

Propranolol hydrochloride is a stable, white, crystalline solid which is readily soluble in water and ethanol. Its molecular weight is 295.81.
Hydrochlorothiazide is a white, or practically white, practically odorless, crystalline powder. It is slightly soluble in water; freely soluble in sodium hydroxide solution; sparingly soluble in methanol; insoluble in ether, chloroform, benzene, and dilute mineral acids. Its chemical name is 6-Chloro-3,4-dihydro-2H-1,2,4-benzothiadiazine-7-sulfonamide 1,1-dioxide. Its structural formula is:

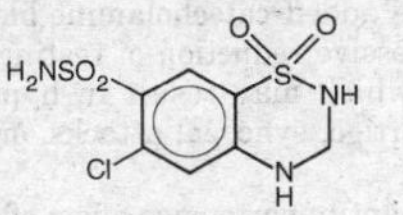

Inderide LA contains the following inactive ingredients: calcium carbonate, ethylcellulose, gelatin capsules, hydroxypropyl methylcellulose, lactose, magnesium stearate, microcrystalline cellulose, sodium lauryl sulfate, sodium starch glycolate, titanium dioxide, and D&C Yellow No. 10. In addition, Inderide LA 80/50 mg and 120/50 mg Capsules contain D&C Red No. 33; Inderide LA 120/50 mg and 160/50 mg Capsules contain FD&C Blue No. 1 and FD&C Red No. 40.

CLINICAL PHARMACOLOGY

Propranolol Hydrochloride (Inderal®)

Inderal is a nonselective, beta-adrenergic receptor-blocking agent possessing no other autonomic nervous system activity. It specifically competes with beta-adrenergic receptor-stimulating agents for available receptor sites. When access to beta-receptor sites is blocked by Inderal, the chronotropic, inotropic, and vasodilator responses to beta-adrenergic stimulation are decreased proportionately.
Inderide LA Capsules (80/50, 120/50, and 160/50 mg) release propranolol hydrochloride at a controlled and predictable rate. Peak propranolol blood levels following dosing with Inderide LA occur at about 6 hours, and the apparent plasma half-life is about 10 hours. Over a 24-hour period, propranolol blood levels are fairly constant for about 12 hours, then decline exponentially. When measured at steady state over a 24-hour period, the areas under the propranolol plasma concentration-time curve (AUCs) for the capsules are approximately 60% to 65% of the AUCs for a comparable divided daily dose of Inderal Tablets. The lower AUCs for the capsules are due to greater hepatic metabolism of propranolol resulting from the slower rate of absorption of propranolol.
Inderide LA should not be considered a simple mg-for-mg substitute for conventional Inderide Tablets, and the propranolol blood levels achieved do not match (are lower than) those of twice-daily dosing of Inderide Tablets with the same dose. When changing to Inderide LA from conventional Inderide Tablets, a possible need for retitration upwards should be considered.
The mechanism of the antihypertensive effect of propranolol has not been established. Among the factors that may be involved in contributing to the antihypertensive action are: (1) decreased cardiac output, (2) inhibition of renin release by the kidneys, and (3) diminution of tonic sympathetic nerve outflow from vasomotor centers in the brain.
Propranolol hydrochloride decreases heart rate, cardiac output, and blood pressure. Although total peripheral vascular resistance may increase initially, it readjusts to or below the pretreatment level with chronic usage. Effects on plasma volume appear to be minor and somewhat variable. Inderal has been shown to cause a small increase in serum potassium concentration when used in the treatment of hypertensive patients.
Beta-receptor blockade is useful in conditions in which, because of pathologic or functional changes, sympathetic activity is excessive or inappropriate, and detrimental to the patient. But there are also situations in which sympathetic stimulation is vital. For example, in patients with severely damaged hearts, adequate ventricular function is maintained by virtue of sympathetic drive, which should be preserved. In the presence of AV block, beta blockade may prevent the necessary facilitating effect of sympathetic activity on conduction. Beta blockade results in bronchial constriction by interfering with adrenergic bronchodilator activity, which should be preserved in patients subject to bronchospasm.
The proper objective of beta-blockade therapy is to decrease adverse sympathetic stimulation, but not to the degree that may impair necessary sympathetic support.

Hydrochlorothiazide

Hydrochlorothiazide is a benzothiadiazine (thiazide) diuretic closely related to chlorothiazide. The mechanism of the antihypertensive effect of the thiazides is unknown. Thiazides usually do not affect normal blood pressure.
Thiazides affect the renal tubular mechanism of electrolyte reabsorption. At maximal therapeutic dosage, all thiazides are approximately equal in their diuretic efficacy.
Thiazides increase excretion of sodium and chloride in approximately equivalent amounts. Natriuresis causes a secondary loss of potassium and bicarbonate.
Onset of diuretic action of thiazides occurs in 2 hours, and the peak effect in about 4 hours. Its action persists for approximately 6 to 12 hours. Thiazides are eliminated rapidly by the kidney. The hydrochlorothiazide in Inderide LA is a conventional (not sustained-release) formulation.

INDICATIONS AND USAGE

Inderide LA is indicated in the management of hypertension.
This fixed-combination drug is not indicated for initial therapy of hypertension. Hypertension requires therapy titrated to the individual patient. If the fixed combination represents the dosage so determined, its use may be more convenient in patient management. The treatment of hypertension is not static, but must be reevaluated as conditions in each patient warrant.

CONTRAINDICATIONS

Propranolol Hydrochloride (Inderal®)

Propranolol is contraindicated in: 1) cardiogenic shock; 2) sinus bradycardia and greater than first-degree block; 3) bronchial asthma; 4) congestive heart failure (see **WARNINGS**), unless the failure is secondary to a tachyarrhythmia treatable with propranolol.

Hydrochlorothiazide

Hydrochlorothiazide is contraindicated in patients with anuria or hypersensitivity to this or other sulfonamide-derived drugs.

WARNINGS

Propranolol Hydrochloride (Inderal®)

Cardiac Failure: Sympathetic stimulation may be a vital component supporting circulatory function in patients with congestive heart failure, and its inhibition by beta blockade may precipitate more severe failure. Although beta blockers should be avoided in overt congestive heart failure, if necessary, they can be used with close follow-up in patients with a history of failure who are well compensated and are receiving digitalis and diuretics. Beta-adrenergic blocking agents do not abolish the inotropic action of digitalis on heart muscle.
In Patients Without a History of Heart Failure, continued use of beta blockers can, in some cases, lead to cardiac failure. Therefore, at the first sign or symptom of heart failure, the patient should be digitalized and/or treated with diuretics, and the response observed closely, or propranolol should be discontinued (gradually, if possible).

Continued on next page

Inderide LA—Cont.

In Patients with Angina Pectoris, there have been reports of exacerbation of angina and, in some cases, myocardial infarction, following *abrupt* discontinuance of propranolol therapy. Therefore, when discontinuance of propranolol is planned, the dosage should be gradually reduced and the patient carefully monitored. In addition, when propranolol is prescribed for angina pectoris, the patient should be cautioned against interruption or cessation of therapy without the physician's advice. If propranolol therapy is interrupted and exacerbation of angina occurs, it usually is advisable to reinstitute propranolol therapy and take other measures appropriate for the management of unstable angina pectoris. Since coronary artery disease may be unrecognized, it may be prudent to follow the above advice in patients considered at risk of having occult atherosclerotic heart disease who are given propranolol for other indications.

Thyrotoxicosis: Beta blockade may mask certain clinical signs of hyperthyroidism. Therefore, abrupt withdrawal of propranolol may be followed by an exacerbation of symptoms of hyperthyroidism, including thyroid storm. Propranolol does not distort thyroid function tests.

In Patients With Wolff-Parkinson-White Syndrome, several cases have been reported in which, after propranolol, the tachycardia was replaced by a severe bradycardia requiring a demand pacemaker. In one case this resulted after an initial dose of 5 mg propranolol.

Major Surgery: The necessity or desirability of withdrawal of beta-blocking therapy prior to major surgery is controversial. It should be noted, however, that the impaired ability of the heart to respond to reflex adrenergic stimuli may augment the risks of general anesthesia and surgical procedures.

Nonallergic Bronchospasm (e.g., *chronic bronchitis, emphysema*): PATIENTS WITH BRONCHOSPASTIC DISEASES SHOULD, IN GENERAL, NOT RECEIVE BETA BLOCKERS. Inderal should be administered with caution since it may block bronchodilation produced by endogenous and exogenous catecholamine stimulation of beta receptors.

Diabetes and Hypoglycemia: Beta-adrenergic blockade may prevent the appearance of certain premonitory signs and symptoms (pulse rate and pressure changes) of acute hypoglycemia in labile insulin-dependent diabetes. In these patients, it may be more difficult to adjust the dosage of insulin. Hypoglycemic attacks may be accompanied by a precipitous elevation of blood pressure.

Propranolol therapy, particularly in infants and children, diabetic or not, has been associated with hypoglycemia especially during fasting as in preparation for surgery. Hypoglycemia also has been found after this type of drug therapy and prolonged physical exertion and has occurred in renal insufficiency, both during dialysis and sporadically, in subjects on propranolol.

Hydrochlorothiazide

Thiazides should be used with caution in severe renal disease. In patients with renal disease, thiazides may precipitate azotemia. In patients with impaired renal function, cumulative effects of the drug may develop.

Thiazides should also be used with caution in patients with impaired hepatic function or progressive liver disease, since minor alterations of fluid and electrolyte balance may precipitate hepatic coma.

Thiazides may add to or potentiate the action of other antihypertensive drugs. Potentiation occurs with ganglionic or peripheral adrenergic-blocking drugs.

Sensitivity reactions may occur in patients with a history of allergy or bronchial asthma. The possibility of exacerbation or activation of systemic lupus erythematosus has been reported.

PRECAUTIONS

General

Propranolol Hydrochloride (Inderal®)

Propranolol should be used with caution in patients with impaired hepatic or renal function. Propranolol is not indicated for the treatment of hypertensive emergencies.

Beta-adrenoreceptor blockade can cause reduction of intraocular pressure. Patients should be told that propranolol may interfere with the glaucoma screening test. Withdrawal may lead to a return of increased intraocular pressure.

Risk of anaphylactic reaction: While taking beta blockers, patients with a history of severe anaphylactic reaction to a variety of allergens may be more reactive to repeated challenge, either accidental, diagnostic, or therapeutic. Such patients may be unresponsive to the usual doses of epinephrine used to treat allergic reaction.

Hydrochlorothiazide

All patients receiving thiazide therapy should be observed for clinical signs of fluid or electrolyte imbalance, namely: Hyponatremia, hypochloremic alkalosis, and hypokalemia. Serum and urine electrolyte determinations are particu-

larly important when the patient is vomiting excessively or receiving parenteral fluids. Medication such as digitalis may also influence serum electrolytes. Warning signs irrespective of cause are: Dryness of mouth, thirst, weakness, lethargy, drowsiness, restlessness, muscle pains or cramps, muscular fatigue, hypotension, oliguria, tachycardia, and gastrointestinal disturbances such as nausea and vomiting. Hypokalemia may develop, especially with brisk diuresis, when severe cirrhosis is present or during concomitant use of corticosteroids or ACTH.

Interference with adequate oral electrolyte intake will also contribute to hypokalemia. Hypokalemia can sensitize or exaggerate the response of the heart to the toxic effect of digitalis (e.g., increased ventricular irritability).

Hypokalemia may be avoided or treated by use of potassium supplements, such as foods with a high potassium content. Any chloride deficit is generally mild and usually does not require specific treatment, except under extraordinary circumstances (as in liver or renal disease). Dilutional hyponatremia may occur in edematous patients in hot weather; appropriate therapy is water restriction, rather than administration of salt, except in rare instances when the hyponatremia is life-threatening. In actual salt depletion, appropriate replacement is the therapy of choice.

Hyperuricemia may occur or frank gout may be precipitated in certain patients receiving thiazide therapy.

Insulin requirements in diabetic patients may be increased, decreased, or unchanged. Diabetes mellitus which has been latent may become manifest during thiazide administration.

If progressive renal impairment becomes evident, consider withholding or discontinuing diuretic therapy.

Thiazides may decrease serum PBI levels without signs of thyroid disturbance.

Calcium excretion is decreased by thiazides. Pathologic changes in the parathyroid gland with hypercalcemia and hypophosphatemia have been observed in a few patients on prolonged thiazide therapy. The common complications of hyperparathyroidism, such as renal lithiasis, bone resorption, and peptic ulceration have not been seen. Thiazides should be discontinued before carrying out tests for parathyroid function.

Clinical Laboratory Tests

Propranolol Hydrochloride (Inderal®)

Elevated blood urea levels in patients with severe heart disease, elevated serum transaminase, alkaline phosphatase, lactate dehydrogenase.

Hydrochlorothiazide

Periodic determination of serum electrolytes to detect possible electrolyte imbalance should be performed at appropriate intervals.

Drug Interactions

Propranolol Hydrochloride (Inderal®)

Patients receiving catecholamine-depleting drugs, such as reserpine, should be closely observed if propranolol is administered. The added catecholamine-blocking action may produce an excessive reduction of resting sympathetic nervous activity, which may result in hypotension, marked bradycardia, vertigo, syncopal attacks, or orthostatic hypotension.

Blunting of the antihypertensive effect of beta-adrenoceptor blocking agents by nonsteroidal anti-inflammatory drugs has been reported.

Hypotension and cardiac arrest have been reported with the concomitant use of propranolol and haloperidol.

Hydrochlorothiazide

Thiazide drugs may increase the responsiveness to tubocurarine.

The antihypertensive effects of thiazides may be enhanced in the postsympathectomy patient. Thiazides may decrease arterial responsiveness to norepinephrine. This diminution is not sufficient to preclude effectiveness of the pressor agent for therapeutic use.

Carcinogenesis, Mutagenesis, Impairment of Fertility

Combinations of propranolol and hydrochlorothiazide have not been evaluated for carcinogenic or mutagenic potential or for potential to adversely affect fertility.

Propranolol Hydrochloride (Inderal®)

In dietary administration studies in which mice and rats were treated with propranolol for up to 18 months at doses of up to 150 mg/kg/day, there was no evidence of drug-related tumorigenesis. In a study in which both male and female rats were exposed to propranolol in their diets at concentrations of up to 0.05%, from 60 days prior to mating and throughout pregnancy and lactation for two generations, there were no effects on fertility. Based on differing results from Ames Tests performed by different laboratories, there is equivocal evidence for a genotoxic effect of propranolol in bacteria (*S. typhimurium* strain TA 1538).

Hydrochlorothiazide

Two-year feeding studies in mice and rats conducted under the auspices of the National Toxicology Program (NTP) uncovered no evidence of a carcinogenic potential of hydrochlorothiazide in female mice (at doses of up to approximately 600 mg/kg/day) or in male and female rats (at doses of up to

approximately 100 mg/kg/day). The NTP, however, found equivocal evidence for hepatocarcinogenicity in male mice. Hydrochlorothiazide was not genotoxic *in vitro* in the Ames bacterial mutagen assay (*S. typhimurium* strains TA 98, TA 100, TA 1535, TA 1537 and TA 1538) or in the Chinese Hamster Ovary (CHO) test for chromosomal aberrations. Nor was it genotoxic *in vivo* in assays using mouse germinal cell chromosomes, Chinese hamster bone marrow chromosomes, and the *Drosophila* sex-linked recessive lethal trait gene. Positive test results were obtained in the *in vitro* CHO Sister Chromatid Exchange (clastogenicity), Mouse Lymphoma Cell (mutagenicity) and *Aspergillus nidulans* non-disjunction assays.

Hydrochlorothiazide had no adverse effects on the fertility of mice and rats of either sex in studies wherein these species were exposed, via their diets, to doses of up to 100 mg/kg and 4 mg/kg, respectively, prior to mating and throughout gestation.

Pregnancy: Pregnancy Category C

Combinations of propranolol and hydrochlorothiazide have not been evaluated for effects on pregnancy in animals. Nor are there adequate and well-controlled studies of propranolol, hydrochlorothiazide, or Inderide in pregnant women. Inderide should be used during pregnancy only if the potential benefit justifies the potential risk to the fetus.

Propranolol Hydrochloride (Inderal®)

In a series of reproductive and developmental toxicology studies, propranolol was given to rats by gavage or in the diet throughout pregnancy and lactation. At doses of 150 mg/kg/day (>30 times the dose of propranolol contained in the maximum recommended human daily dose of Inderide), but not at doses of 80 mg/kg/day, treatment was associated with embryotoxicity (reduced litter size and increased resorption sites) as well as neonatal toxicity (deaths). Propranolol also was administered (in the feed) to rabbits (throughout pregnancy and lactation) at doses as high as 150 mg/kg/day (>45 times the dose of propranolol contained in the maximum recommended daily human dose of Inderide). No evidence of embryo or neonatal toxicity was noted. Intrauterine growth retardation has been reported in human neonates whose mothers received propranolol during pregnancy. Neonates whose mothers received propranolol at parturition have exhibited bradycardia, hypoglycemia and respiratory depression. Adequate facilities for monitoring these infants at birth should be available.

Hydrochlorothiazide

Studies in which hydrochlorothiazide was orally administered to pregnant mice and rats at doses of up to 3000 and 1000 mg/kg/day, respectively, provided no evidence of harm to the fetus.

Thiazides cross the placental barrier and appear in cord blood. The use of thiazides in pregnant women requires that the anticipated benefit be weighed against possible hazards to the fetus. These hazards include fetal or neonatal jaundice, thrombocytopenia, and possibly other adverse reactions that have occurred in the adult.

Nursing Mothers

Propranolol and thiazides are excreted in human milk. Caution should be exercised when Inderide LA is administered to a nursing woman.

Pediatric Use

Safety and effectiveness in pediatric patients have not been established.

ADVERSE REACTIONS

Propranolol Hydrochloride (Inderal®)

Most adverse effects have been mild and transient and have rarely required the withdrawal of therapy.

Cardiovascular: Bradycardia; congestive heart failure; intensification of AV block; hypotension; paresthesia of hands; thrombocytopenic purpura; arterial insufficiency, usually of the Raynaud type.

Central Nervous System: Light-headedness; mental depression manifested by insomnia, lassitude, weakness, fatigue; reversible mental depression progressing to catatonia; visual disturbances; hallucinations; an acute reversible syndrome characterized by disorientation for time and place, short-term memory loss, emotional lability, slightly clouded sensorium, and decreased performance on neuropsychometrics.

Gastrointestinal: Nausea, vomiting, epigastric distress, abdominal cramping, diarrhea, constipation, mesenteric arterial thrombosis, ischemic colitis.

Allergic: Pharyngitis and agranulocytosis; erythematous rash; fever combined with aching and sore throat; laryngospasm and respiratory distress.

Respiratory: Bronchospasm.

Hematologic: Agranulocytosis; nonthrombocytopenic purpura, thrombocytopenic purpura.

Autoimmune: In extremely rare instances, systemic lupus erythematosus has been reported.

Miscellaneous: Alopecia, LE-like reactions; psoriasiform rashes; dry eyes; male impotence; and Peyronie's disease have been reported rarely. Oculomucocutaneous reactions

involving the skin, serous membrances, and conjunctivae reported for a beta blocker (practolol) have not been associated with propranolol.

Hydrochlorothiazide

Gastrointestinal: Anorexia, gastric irritation, nausea, vomiting, cramping; diarrhea; constipation; jaundice (intrahepatic cholestatic jaundice); pancreatitis; sialadenitis.

Central Nervous System: Dizziness, vertigo; paresthesias; headache; xanthopsia.

Hematologic: Leukopenia; agranulocytosis; thrombocytopenia; aplastic anemia.

Cardiovascular: Orthostatic hypotension (may be aggravated by alcohol, barbiturates, or narcotics).

Hypersensitivity: Purpura; photosensitivity; rash; urticaria; necrotizing angiitis (vasculitis, cutaneous vasculitis); fever; respiratory distress, including pneumonitis; anaphylactic reactions.

Other: Hyperglycemia; glycosuria; hyperuricemia; muscle spasm; weakness; restlessness; transient blurred vision.

Whenever adverse reactions are moderate or severe, thiazide dosage should be reduced or therapy withdrawn.

OVERDOSAGE OR EXAGGERATED RESPONSE

The propranolol hydrochloride (Inderal) component may cause bradycardia, cardiac failure, hypotension, or bronchospasm.

The hydrochlorothiazide component can be expected to cause diuresis. Lethargy of varying degree may appear and may progress to coma within a few hours, with minimal depression of respiration and cardiovascular function, and in the absence of significant serum electrolyte changes or dehydration. The mechanism of central nervous system depression with thiazide overdosage is unknown. Gastrointestinal irritation and hypermotility can occur; temporary elevation of BUN has been reported and serum electrolyte changes could occur, especially in patients with impairment of renal function.

Treatment

The following measures should be employed:

General: If ingestion is, or may have been, recent, evacuate gastric contents, taking care to prevent pulmonary aspiration.

Bradycardia: Administer atropine (0.25 to 1.0 mg). If there is no response to vagal blockade, administer isoproterenol cautiously.

Cardiac Failure: Digitalization and diuretics.

Hypotension: Vasopressors, e.g., levarterenol or epinephrine.

Bronchospasm: Administer isoproterenol and aminophylline.

Stupor or Coma: Administer supportive therapy as clinically warranted.

Gastrointestinal Effects: Though usually of short duration, these may require symptomatic treatment.

Abnormalities in BUN and/or Serum Electrolytes: Monitor serum electrolyte levels and renal function; institute supportive measures, as required individually, to maintain hydration, electrolyte balance, respiration, and cardiovascular function.

DOSAGE AND ADMINISTRATION

The dosage must be determined by individual titration.

Hydrochlorothiazide can be given at doses of 12.5 to 50 mg per day when used alone. The initial dose of propranolol is 80 mg daily, and it may be increased gradually until optimal blood pressure control is achieved. The usual effective dose, when used alone, is 160 to 480 mg per day.

One Inderide LA Capsule once a day can be used to administer up to 160 mg of propranolol and 50 mg of hydrochlorothiazide. For doses of propranolol greater than 160 mg, the combination products are not appropriate because their use would lead to an excessive dose of the thiazide component.

Inderide LA provides propranolol hydrochloride in a sustained-release form and hydrochlorothiazide in conventional formulation, for once-daily administration. If patients are switched from Inderide Tablets (or Inderal plus hydrochlorothiazide) to Inderide LA, care should be taken to ensure that the desired therapeutic effect is maintained. Inderide LA should not be considered a mg-for-mg substitute for Inderide or Inderal plus hydrochlorothiazide. Inderide LA has different kinetics and produces lower blood levels. Retitration may be necessary, especially to maintain effectiveness at the end of the 24-hour dosing interval.

When necessary, another antihypertensive agent may be added gradually, beginning with 50% of the usual recommended starting dose, to avoid an excessive fall in blood pressure.

HOW SUPPLIED

Each beige capsule, identified by one wide band and 3 narrow bands, all in gold, and "Inderide LA 80/50", contains 80 mg of propranolol hydrochloride (Inderal® LA) and 50 mg of hydrochlorothiazide, in bottles of 100 (NDC 0046- 0455-81).

Each beige/brown capsule, identified by one wide band and 3 narrow bands, all in gold, and "Inderide LA 120/50", contains 120 mg of propranolol hydrochloride (Inderal® LA) and 50 mg of hydrochlorothiazide, in bottles of 100 (NDC 0046-0457-81).

Each brown capsule, identified by one wide band and 3 narrow bands, all in gold, and "Inderide LA 160/50", contains 160 mg of propranolol hydrochloride (Inderal® LA) and 50 mg of hydrochlorothiazide, in bottles of 100 (NDC 0046-0459-81).

Store at room temperature (approximately 25° C).

Protect from light, moisture, freezing, and excessive heat. Dispense in a tight, light-resistant container as defined in the USP.

The appearance of these capsules is a registered trademark of Wyeth-Ayerst Laboratories.

Manufactured by:
Ayerst Laboratories
A Wyeth-Ayerst Company
Philadelphia, PA 19101

Shown in Product Identification Guide, page 343

INFLUENZA VIRUS VACCINE, ℞
TRIVALENT, TYPES A AND B
(chromatograph- and filter-purified subvirion antigen)
FluShield®
[flū' sheeld]
1998-99 formula
DO NOT INJECT INTRAVENOUSLY

Rx only

DESCRIPTION

FluShield® (Influenza Virus Vaccine, Trivalent, Types A and B [Purified Subvirion]) is a sterile injectable for administration intramuscularly.

FluShield is prepared from the allantoic fluids of chick embryos inoculated with a specific type of influenza virus. During processing, not more than 5 µg of gentamicin sulfate per mL is added. The harvested virus is concentrated, purified, then inactivated with formaldehyde.

FluShield, Trivalent (chromatograph- and filter-purified subvirion antigen), is concentrated and refined by a column-chromatographic procedure. At the same time, addition of tri(n)butylphosphate and Polysorbate 80, USP to the column-eluting fluids effects inactivation and disruption of a significant proportion of the virus to smaller subunit particles. The recovered subvirion (split-virus) suspension is freed of substantial portions of the disrupting agents by dialysis and of other undesirable materials by selective filtration through membranes of controlled pore size.

The viral antigen content has been standardized by immunodiffusion tests, according to current U.S. Public Health Service requirements. Each dose (0.5 mL) contains the proportions and not less than the microgram amounts of hemagglutinin antigens (µg HA) representative of the specific components recommended for the 1998-99 season: 15 µg HA of A/Beijing/262/95 (H1N1), 15 µg HA of A/Sydney/5/97 (H3N2), and 15 µg HA of B/Harbin/7/94 (B/Beijing/184/93-like).

The vaccine contains 1:10,000 thimerosal (mercury derivative) as a preservative. Gentamicin sulfate is used during manufacturing but is not detectable in the final product by current assay procedures.

CLINICAL PHARMACOLOGY

The administration of inactivated influenza vaccine to high-risk persons each year before the influenza season is the single most important influenza-control measure.[1]

The injection of antigens prepared from inactivated influenza virus stimulates the production of specific antibodies. Any protection afforded is only against those strains of virus from which the vaccine is prepared or closely related strains. With the passing of time, there may be major antigenic changes in the prevalent strains, or there may be continuous and progressive antigenic variation within a given virus subtype over time (antigenic drift), so that infection or immunization with one strain may not induce immunity to distantly related strains. Field studies of influenza vaccines conducted on many occasions since the 1940's have shown marked variation in efficacy, as measured by protection from disease, ranging from undemonstrable to 70-80%. The PHS regularly reviews the antigenic characteristics of circulating strains in order to select those to be included in the contemporary vaccine.

Based upon the epidemiological data available through the early months of 1998 the Federal Government determined, after consultation with advisory groups, that the influenza vaccines to be distributed in 1998-99 will be trivalent, including 15 µg HA each of strains that are antigenically similar to A/Beijing/262/95, A/Sydney/5/97, and B/Beijing/184/93.

INDICATIONS AND USAGE

As with any vaccine, FluShield may not protect 100% of individuals receiving the vaccine. FluShield is recommended for 1) high-risk persons 6 months of age or older and for their medical-care providers or household contacts and 2) for other persons who wish to reduce their chances of acquiring influenza. FluShield should only be administered if it is prescribed by a health-care provider whose license includes the prescribing of biologicals.

Guidelines for the use of vaccine among different groups are given below.

Target Groups for Vaccination

Groups at increased risk for influenza-related complications:

1. Persons 65 years of age or older.
2. Residents of nursing homes and other chronic-care facilities housing patients of any age with chronic medical conditions.
3. Adults and children with chronic disorders of the pulmonary or cardiovascular systems, including children with asthma.
4. Adults and children who have required regular medical follow-up or hospitalization during the preceding year because of chronic metabolic diseases (including diabetes mellitus), renal dysfunction, hemoglobinopathies, or immunosuppression (including immunosuppression caused by medications).
5. Children and teenagers (aged 6 months to 18 years) who are receiving long-term aspirin therapy and, therefore, may be at risk of developing Reye's syndrome after influenza infection.
6. Women who will be in the second or third trimester of pregnancy during the influenza season.[1]

Although animal reproductive studies have not been conducted, the prescribing health-care provider should be aware of the recommendations of the Advisory Committee on Immunization Practices (ACIP), which are incorporated below. Influenza-associated excess mortality among pregnant women has not been documented, except during the pandemics of 1918–19 and 1957–58. However, because death-certificate data often do not indicate whether a woman was pregnant at the time of death, studies conducted during interpandemic periods may underestimate the impact of influenza in this population. Case reports and limited studies suggest that pregnancy may increase the risk for serious medical complications of influenza as a result of increases in heart rate, stroke volume and oxygen consumption, decreases in lung capacity, and changes in immunologic function. A recent study of the impact of influenza during 17 interpandemic influenza seasons documented that the relative risk of hospitalization for selected cardiorespiratory conditions among pregnant women increased from 1.4 during weeks 14–20 of gestation to 4.7 during weeks 37–42 compared with rates among women who were 1–6 months postpartum. Women in their third trimester of pregnancy were hospitalized at a rate comparable to that of nonpregnant women who have high-risk medical conditions for whom influenza vaccine has traditionally been recommended. Using data from this study, it was estimated that an average of 1 to 2 hospitalizations among pregnant women could be prevented for every 1,000 pregnant women immunized.[1]

On the basis of these and other data that suggest that influenza infection may cause increased morbidity in women during the second and third trimesters of pregnancy, the ACIP recommends that women who will be beyond the first trimester of pregnancy (14 weeks' gestation) during the influenza season be vaccinated. Pregnant women who have medical conditions that increase their risk for complications from influenza should be vaccinated before the influenza season, regardless of the stage of pregnancy. Studies of influenza immunization of more than 2,000 pregnant women have demonstrated no adverse fetal effects associated with influenza vaccine; however, more data are needed (see **"PRECAUTIONS—Pregnancy"**).[1]

Elderly persons and persons with certain chronic diseases may develop lower postvaccination antibody titers than healthy young adults and thus may remain susceptible to influenza-related upper-respiratory-tract infections. However, even if such persons develop influenza illness despite vaccination, the vaccine has been shown to be effective in helping to prevent lower-respiratory-tract involvement or other secondary complications, thereby reducing the risk of hospitalization and death.[1]

Groups that can transmit influenza to persons at high risk:

Persons who are clinically or subclinically infected can transmit influenza virus to persons at high risk whom they care for or with whom they live. Some persons at high-risk, e.g., the elderly, transplant recipients, and persons with acquired immunodeficiency syndrome (AIDS), can have a low antibody response to influenza vaccine. Efforts to help protect these members of high-risk groups against influenza might be improved by reducing the likelihood of influenza exposure from their caregivers. Therefore, the following groups should be vaccinated:

1. Physicians, nurses, and other personnel in both hospital and outpatient settings.
2. Employees of nursing homes and chronic-care facilities who have contact with patients or residents.

Continued on next page

FluShield—Cont.

3. Providers of home care to high-risk persons (e.g., visiting nurses, volunteer workers).
4. Household members (including children) of persons in high-risk groups.[1]

Vaccination of Other Groups

General population:
Physicians should administer influenza vaccine to any person who wishes to reduce the likelihood of becoming ill with influenza caused by the strains incorporated into this year's vaccine. Persons who provide essential community services should be considered for vaccination to minimize disruption of essential activities during influenza outbreaks. Students or other healthy individuals in institutional settings (e.g., those who reside in dormitories) should be encouraged to receive vaccine to minimize the disruption of routine activities during epidemics.[1]

Persons infected with human immunodeficiency virus (HIV):
Limited information exists regarding the frequency and severity of influenza illness among HIV-infected persons, but reports suggest that symptoms might be prolonged and the risk of complications increased for some HIV-infected persons. Influenza vaccine has produced protective antibody titers against influenza in vaccinated HIV-infected persons who have minimal AIDS-related symptoms and high CD4+ T-lymphocyte cell counts. In patients who have advanced HIV disease and low CD4+ T-lymphocyte cell counts, however, influenza vaccine may not induce protective antibody titers; a second dose of vaccine does not improve the immune response for these persons.

Recent studies have examined the effect on influenza vaccination on replication of HIV type 1 (HIV-1). Although some studies have demonstrated a transient (i.e., 2- to 4-week) increase in replication of HIV-1 in the plasma or peripheral blood mononuclear cells of HIV-infected persons after vaccine administration, other studies using similar laboratory techniques have not indicated any substantial increase in replication. Deterioration of CD4+ T-lymphocyte cell counts and progression of clinical HIV disease have not been demonstrated among HIV-infected persons who receive vaccine. Because influenza can result in serious illness and complications and because influenza vaccination may result in protective antibody titers, vaccination will benefit many HIV-infected patients.[1]

Nursing mothers:
Influenza vaccine does not affect the safety of breastfeeding for mothers or infants. Breastfeeding does not adversely affect immune response and is not a contraindication for vaccination.[1]

Persons traveling to foreign countries:
The risk of exposure to influenza during foreign travel varies, depending on season and destination. Influenza can occur throughout the year in the tropics; the season of greatest influenza activity in the Southern Hemisphere is April through September. Because of the short incubation period for influenza, exposure to the virus during travel can result in clinical illness that begins during travel, an inconvenience or potential danger, especially for persons at increased risk for complications. Persons preparing to travel to the tropics at any time of year or to the Southern Hemisphere from April through September should review their vaccination histories. If they were not vaccinated the previous fall or winter, they should consider influenza vaccination prior to travel. Persons in the high-risk categories especially should be encouraged to receive the most current vaccine. Persons at high risk who received the previous season's vaccine prior to travel should be revaccinated in the fall or winter with the current vaccine.[1]

Immunization programs:
If this product is to be used in an immunization program sponsored by an organization WHERE A TRADITIONAL PHYSICIAN/PATIENT RELATIONSHIP DOES NOT EXIST, each participant (or legal guardian) should be made aware of the possible risks and adverse events that have been associated with the use of influenza virus vaccines, including the possible risk of a form of paralysis sometimes known as Guillain-Barré syndrome. Information about possible side effects and adverse events is presented below, and informed consent, preferably written, should be obtained from the intended recipient (or legal guardian) before vaccine administration. FluShield is a prescription product and shall only be administered upon prescription by a health-care provider who is licensed to prescribe biologicals. The prescribing health-care provider should be familiar with the text of this insert, including the "**CONTRAINDICATIONS**," "**PRECAUTIONS**," and "**ADVERSE REACTIONS**" sections.

Simultaneous Administration of Pneumococcal or Pediatric Vaccines

The target groups for influenza and pneumococcal vaccination overlap considerably. For persons at high risk who have not previously been vaccinated with pneumococcal vaccine, health-care providers should strongly consider administering pneumococcal and influenza vaccine concurrently. These vaccines can be administered at the same time at different sites without increasing side effects.[1] However, influenza vaccine is given annually, whereas pneumococcal vaccine is not.[2]

Children at high risk for influenza-related complications can receive influenza vaccine with routine pediatric vaccines, including pertussis vaccine (DTaP or DTP), with administration at different sites recommended. Because influenza vaccine can cause fever when administered to young children, DTaP (which is less frequently associated with fever and other adverse events) is preferable to DTP.

CONTRAINDICATIONS

FLUSHIELD SHOULD NOT BE ADMINISTERED TO INDIVIDUALS WITH A HISTORY OF HYPERSENSITIVITY (ALLERGY) TO CHICKEN EGG OR TO ANY COMPONENT(S) OF INFLUENZA VIRUS VACCINE, INCLUDING THIMEROSAL, WITHOUT FIRST CONSULTING A PHYSICIAN (see "**ADVERSE REACTIONS**"). Before being vaccinated, persons known to be hypersensitive to egg protein or other components should be given a skin test or other allergy-evaluating test, using the influenza virus vaccine as the antigen. Persons with adverse reactions to such testing should not be vaccinated. Chemoprophylaxis may be indicated for prevention of influenza A in such persons. However, persons with a history of anaphylactic hypersensitivity to vaccine components but who are also at highest risk for complications of influenza infections may benefit from vaccine after appropriate evaluation and desensitization.[1]

Persons with a past history of Guillain-Barré syndrome (GBS) should not be given influenza virus vaccine (see "**ADVERSE REACTIONS**").

Persons with acute febrile illnesses usually should not be vaccinated until their symptoms have abated. However, minor illnesses with or without fever should not contraindicate the use of influenza virus vaccine, particularly in children with a mild upper-respiratory-tract infection or allergic rhinitis.[1,3]

WARNINGS

Patients with impaired immune responsiveness, whether due to the use of immunosuppressive therapy (including irradiation, large amounts of corticosteroids, antimetabolites, alkylating agents, and cytotoxic agents), a genetic defect, HIV infection, leukemia, lymphoma, generalized malignancy, or other causes, may have a reduced antibody response to active immunization procedures. Short-term (less than 2 weeks) oral corticosteroid therapy or administration via topical (skin or eyes) or inhalation routes, or intra-articular, bursal, or tendon injections should not be immunosuppressive.[4] Inactivated vaccines are not a risk to immunocompromised individuals, although their efficacy may be substantially reduced. Because patients with immunodeficiencies may not have an adequate response to immunizing agents, they may remain susceptible despite having received an appropriate vaccine. If feasible, specific serum antibody titers or other immunologic responses may be determined after immunization to assess immunity.[3] Chemoprophylaxis may be indicated for high-risk persons who are expected to have a poor antibody response to influenza vaccine.[1]

Product contains latex rubber closure.

PRECAUTIONS

General

Influenza virus is remarkably capricious antigenically, and significant changes may occur from time to time. *It is known definitely that FluShield, as now constituted, is not effective against all possible strains of influenza virus. Any protection afforded is only against those strains of virus from which the vaccine is prepared or against closely related strains.*

Influenza vaccine often contains one or more antigens used in previous years. However, immunity declines during the year following immunization. Therefore, revaccination on a yearly basis is necessary to provide optimal protection for the current season. REMAINING 1997-1998 VACCINE SHOULD NOT BE USED.

Epinephrine injection (1:1000) must be immediately available should an acute anaphylactoid reaction occur due to any component of the vaccine.

A separate sterile syringe and needle should be used for each patient to prevent transmission of hepatitis B or other infectious agents from one person to another. Reusable glass syringes and needles should be heat-sterilized.

Vaccine sterility and stability cannot be assured if unit doses are withdrawn form the multidose vial and allowed to remain in syringes for longer than a few minutes prior to injection into patients.

Do not inject into or near a blood vessel or nerve.

Health-care professionals should administer FluShield with caution to patients with a possible history of latex sensitivity, since its packaging contains dry natural rubber.

Drug Interactions

There have been conflicting reports[5–15] on the effects of influenza virus vaccine on the elimination of some drugs metabolized by the hepatic cytochrome P-450 system. Hypoprothrombinemia in patients receiving warfarin and elevated theophylline serum concentrations have occurred. Most studies have failed to show any adverse effects of influenza vaccine in patients receiving these drugs. Nevertheless, monitoring for possible enhanced drug effect or toxicity is indicated for those persons taking theophylline preparations or warfarin sodium.

Individuals receiving therapy with immunosuppressive agents (large amounts of corticosteroids, antimetabolites, alkylating agents, cytotoxic agents) may not respond optimally to active immunization procedures (see "**WARNINGS**").

Pregnancy

Pregnancy Category C:
Animal reproduction studies have not been conducted with influenza virus vaccine. It is also not known whether influenza virus vaccine can cause fetal harm when administered to a pregnant woman or can affect reproduction capacity. Influenza virus vaccine should be given to a pregnant woman only if clearly needed.

The benefits of preventing influenza-related complications versus the theoretical risk of fetal harm should be considered, and discussed with the patient before administering influenza vaccine to a pregnant woman. The ACIP states that, if used during pregnancy, administration of influenza virus vaccine after 14 weeks of gestation may be preferable to avoid coincidental association of the vaccine with early pregnancy loss[1] (see "**INDICATIONS AND USAGE, Target Groups for Vaccination**").

Geriatric Use

The effectiveness of influenza vaccine in preventing or attenuating illness varies, depending primarily on the age and immunocompetence of the vaccine recipient and the degree of similarity between the virus strains included in the vaccine and those that circulate during the influenza season. When a good match exists between vaccine and circulating viruses, influenza vaccine has been shown to prevent illness in approximately 70%–90% of healthy persons aged <65 years. In these circumstances, studies also have indicated that the effectiveness of influenza vaccine in preventing hospitalization for pneumonia and influenza among elderly persons living in settings other than nursing homes or similar chronic-care facilities ranges from 30% to 70%.[1]

Among elderly persons residing in nursing homes, influenza vaccine is most effective in preventing severe illness, secondary complications, and death. Studies of this population have indicated that the vaccine can be 50–60% effective in preventing hospitalization and pneumonia and 80% effective in preventing death, even though efficacy in preventing influenza may often be in the range of 30%–40% among the frail elderly. Achieving a high rate of vaccination among nursing home residents can reduce the spread of infection in a facility, thus preventing disease through herd immunity. Vaccination of health-care workers in nursing homes also has been effective in reducing the impact of influenza among residents.[1]

Pediatric Use

The safety and effectiveness of influenza virus vaccine in pediatric patients under 6 months of age have not been established. However, the ACIP recommends influenza vaccination in certain circumstances for persons 6 months of age or older (see "**INDICATIONS AND USAGE, Target Groups for Vaccination**" and "**DOSAGE AND ADMINISTRATION**").[1]

ADVERSE REACTIONS

Side effects of influenza vaccination are generally inconsequential in adults and occur at low frequency, but at younger ages side effects may be more common.

BECAUSE INFLUENZA VACCINE CONTAINS ONLY NONINFECTIOUS VIRUSES, IT CANNOT CAUSE INFLUENZA. Occasional cases of respiratory disease following vaccination represent coincidental illnesses unrelated to influenza vaccination.[1]

The most frequent side effect of vaccination is soreness at the vaccination site for up to 2 days. These local reactions generally are mild and rarely interfere with the ability to conduct usual daily activities.[1] With vaccines in general, it is not uncommon for patients to note at or around the injection site the following minor reactions: swelling or edema; pain or tenderness; redness, erythema, inflammation, or skin discoloration; induration or mass; or hypersensitivity reaction.

In addition, the following types of systemic reactions have occurred:

Fever, malaise, myalgia, and other systemic symptoms can occur following vaccination and most often affect persons who have had no exposure to the influenza virus antigens in the vaccine (e.g., young children). These reactions begin 6 to 12 hours after vaccination and can persist for 1 or 2 days.[1]

Other systemic events that have been reported include: arthralgia, asthenia, chills, dizziness, headache, lymphadenopathy, pruritus, rash, vomiting, diarrhea, and pharyngitis. Recent placebo-controlled trials suggest that in elderly persons and healthy young adults, split-virus influenza vac-

cine is not associated with higher rates of systemic symptoms (e.g., fever, malaise, myalgia, and headache) when compared with placebo injections.[1]

Immediate, presumably allergic, reactions such as hives, angioedema, allergic asthma, or systemic anaphylaxis occur rarely after influenza vaccination. These reactions probably result from hypersensitivity to some vaccine component—the majority of reactions are most likely related to residual egg protein. Although current influenza vaccines contain only a small quantity of egg protein, this protein can induce immediate hypersensitivity reactions among persons who have severe egg allergy. Persons who have developed hives, have had swelling of the lips or tongue, or experienced acute respiratory distress or collapse after eating eggs should consult a physician for appropriate evaluation to help determine if vaccine should be administered. Persons who have documented immunoglobulin E (IgE)-mediated hypersensitivity to eggs, including those who have had occupational asthma or other allergic responses due to exposure to egg protein, might also be at increased risk for reactions from influenza vaccine and similar consultation should be considered. The protocol for influenza vaccination developed by Murphy and Strunk may be considered for patients who have egg allergies and medical conditions that place them at increased risk for influenza-associated complications.[16]

Hypersensitivity reactions to any vaccine component can occur. Although exposure to vaccines containing thimerosal can lead to induction of hypersensitivity, most patients do not develop reactions to thimerosal when administered as a component of vaccines even when patch or intradermal tests for thimerosal indicate hypersensitivity. When reported, hypersensitivity to thimerosal has usually consisted of local, delayed-type hypersensitivity reactions.[1]

There have been rare reports of Guillain-Barré syndrome (GBS) following receipt of influenza virus vaccine. GBS is an uncommon illness characterized by ascending paralysis which is usually self-limited and reversible. Though most persons with GBS recover without residual weakness, approximately 5% of cases are fatal. Before 1976, no association of GBS with influenza vaccine use was recognized.

Information from the Centers for Disease Control and Prevention, and ACIP recommendations regarding GBS are incorporated below. Although the 1976 swine influenza vaccine was associated with an increased frequency of GBS, evidence for a causal relationship of GBS with subsequent vaccines prepared from other virus strains is less clear. However, obtaining strong evidence for a possible small increase in risk is difficult for a rare condition such as GBS, which has an annual background incidence of only 1 to 2 cases per 100,000 adults. During three of four influenza seasons studied from 1977 through 1991, the point estimates of the overall relative risk for GBS after influenza vaccination were slightly elevated but were not statistically significant in any of these studies. However, in a recent study of the 1992-1993 and 1993-1994 seasons, investigators found an elevation in the overall relative risk for GBS of 1.83 (95% confidence interval=1.12-3.00) during the 6 weeks following vaccination, representing an excess of an estimated 0.1 to 0.2 cases of GBS per 100,000 persons vaccinated; the combined number of GBS cases peaked 2 weeks after vaccination. The increase in the relative risk and the increased number of cases in the second week after vaccination may be the result of vaccination but also could be due to other factors (e.g., confounding or diagnostic bias) rather than a true vaccine-related risk.[1]

Among persons who received the swine influenza vaccine in 1976, the rate of GBS that exceeded the background rate was slightly less than one case per 100,000 vaccinations. The estimated risk for GBS in subsequent years was much lower than 1:100,000 and substantially less than that for severe influenza, which could be prevented by vaccination, especially for persons aged ≥ 65 years and those who have medical indications for influenza vaccination.[1] During different epidemics occurring from 1972 through 1981, estimated rates of influenza-associated hospitalization have ranged from approximately 200 to 300 hospitalizations per million population for previously healthy persons aged 5–44 years and from 2,000 to >10,000 hospitalizations per million population for persons aged ≥65 years. During epidemics from 1972–73 through 1994–95, estimated rates of influenza-associated death have ranged from approximately 300 to >1,500 per million persons aged ≥65 years, who account for more than 90% of all influenza-associated deaths.

The average case-fatality ratio of GBS is 6% and increases with age. However, no evidence indicates that the case-fatality ratio for GBS differs among vaccinated and non-vaccinated persons.

Whereas the incidence of GBS in the general population is very low, persons with a history of GBS have a substantially greater likelihood of subsequently developing GBS than persons without such a history. Thus, the likelihood of coincidentally developing GBS after influenza vaccination is expected to be greater among persons with a history of GBS than among persons with no history of this syndrome. Whether influenza vaccination might be causally associated with this risk for recurrence is not known.[1] Avoiding subsequent influenza vaccination of persons known to have developed GBS within 6 weeks of a previous influenza vaccination seems prudent. Candidates for influenza virus vaccine should be made aware of the possible risks, including GBS, and the benefits of administration.

Other neurologic disorders not defined as GBS, including encephalopathies, facial paralysis, unspecified neuritis, encephalitis, peripheral nerve disease, brachial neuritis, optic neuritis, demyelinating disease, labyrinthitis and meningitis have been temporally associated with influenza vaccination.[17] Rarely, transverse myelitis has been reported.[18]

ADVERSE EVENT REPORTING

The manufacturer and lot number of the vaccine administered should be recorded in the vaccine recipient's permanent medical record, along with the date of administration of the vaccine and the name, address, and title of the person administering the vaccine. Any adverse events following immunizations should be reported by the health-care professional to the U.S. Department of Health and Human Services (DHHS). The U.S. DHHS has established the Vaccine Adverse Event Reporting System (VAERS) to accept all reports of suspected adverse events after administration of any vaccine. The toll-free number for VAERS forms and information is 800-822-7967.

DOSAGE AND ADMINISTRATION

Although influenza virus vaccine often contains one or more antigens used in previous years, immunity declines during the year following vaccination. Therefore, a history of vaccination in any previous year with a vaccine containing one or more antigens included in the current vaccine does NOT preclude the need for revaccination for the 1998–1999 influenza season to help provide optimal protection. REMAINING 1997–1998 VACCINE SHOULD NOT BE USED.

Influenza vaccine may be offered to high-risk persons presenting for routine care or hospitalization beginning in September, but not until new vaccine is available (see "INDICATIONS AND USAGE, Vaccination of Other Groups, *Persons traveling to foreign countries*" for foreign travel-related exceptions). Opportunities to vaccinate persons at high risk for complications of influenza should not be missed. In the United States, influenza activity generally peaks between late December and early March, and high levels of influenza activity infrequently occur in the contiguous 48 states before December. Therefore, the optimal time for vaccination for high-risk persons usually is the period from October through mid-November. In facilities such as nursing homes it is particularly important to avoid administering vaccine too far in advance of the influenza season because antibody levels may begin to decline within a few months of vaccination. Vaccination may be undertaken as soon as current vaccine is available (e.g., September) if regional influenza activity is expected to begin earlier than December.[1]

Children less than 9 years of age who have not been vaccinated previously should receive two doses with at least 1 month between doses to maximize the chance of a satisfactory antibody response to all three vaccine antigens. The second dose should be given before December, if possible. Vaccine should continue to be offered to both children and adults up to and even after influenza virus activity is documented in a community.[1]

Parenteral drug products should be inspected visually for particulate matter and discoloration prior to administration, whenever solution and container permit.

DO NOT INJECT INTRAVENOUSLY. Injections of FluShield are recommended to be given intramuscularly. The recommended site is the deltoid muscle for adults and older children. The preferred site for infants and young children is the anterolateral aspect of the thigh musculature. Because of lack of adequate evaluation of other routes in high-risk persons, the preferred route of vaccination is intramuscularly whenever possible. Before injection, the skin over the site to be injected should be cleansed with a suitable germicide. After insertion of the needle, aspirate to help avoid inadvertent injection into a blood vessel.

AGE GROUP	DOSAGE SCHEDULE
9 years and older	0.5 mL (one dose)
3 to 8 years	0.5 mL (1 or 2 doses)*
6 to 35 months	0.25 mL (1 or 2 doses)*

For those under 13 years, only split-virus (subvirion) vaccine is recommended.

*Two doses are recommended for children under 9 years who are receiving influenza virus vaccine for the first time. With the 2-dose regimen, allow 4 weeks or more between doses. Both doses are recommended for maximum protection.

Immunogenicity and reactogenicity of split- and whole-virus vaccines are similar in adults when used according to the recommended dosage.[1]

HOW SUPPLIED

Influenza Virus Vaccine, Trivalent, Types A and B, (Purified Subvirion), FluShield®, is available in vials of 5 mL as follows:

NDC 0008-0981-01
NDC 0008-0981-35 (Non-returnable)
ALSO AVAILABLE
TUBEX® Sterile Cartridge-Needle Units, 0.5 mL fill in 1 mL size (25 gauge × 5/8 inch needle), in packages of 10 **TUBEX** as follows:
NDC 0008-0981-02
NDC 0008-0981-45 (Non-returnable)
STORAGE
Store between 2°–8°C (35°–46°F). Potency is destroyed by freezing; do not use FluShield that has been frozen.

REFERENCES

1. Prevention and control of influenza: Recommendations of the Advisory Committee on Immunization Practices (ACIP). MMWR-May 1, 1998; 47 (No. RR-6).
2. Prevention of Pneumococcal Disease: Recommendations of the Advisory Committee on Immunization Practices (ACIP). MMWR-April 4, 1997; 46 (No. RR-8).
3. American Academy of Pediatrics: Report of the Committee on Infectious Diseases. 24th ed. Elk Grove Village, IL, American Academy of Pediatrics, 1997.
4. Recommendations of the Advisory Committee on Immunization Practices (ACIP): Use of vaccines and immune globulins in persons with altered immunocompetence. MMWR-April 9, 1993; 42 (No. RR-4).
5. KRAMER, P., and McCLAIN, C.: Depression of aminopyrine metabolism by influenza vaccination. NEJM 1981; 305: 1262.
6. RENTON, K. et al: Decreased elimination of theophylline after influenza vaccination. Can Med Assoc J 1980; 123: 288.
7. GOLDSTEIN, R.S. et al: Decreased elimination of theophylline after influenza vaccination. Can Med Assoc J 1982; 126: 470.
8. BRITTON, L. and RUBEN, F.L.: Serum and theophylline levels after influenza vaccination. Can Med Assoc J 1982; 126: 1375.
9. FISCHER, R.G. et al: Influence of trivalent influenza vaccine on serum theophylline levels. Can Med Assoc J 1982; 126: 1312–13.
10. SAN JOAQUIN, V.H., REYES, S., AND MARKS, M.I.: Influenza vaccination in asthmatic children on maintenance theophylline therapy. Clin Pediatrics 1982; 21: 724–6.
11. STULTS, B. AND HASISAKI, P.: Influenza vaccination and theophylline pharmacokinetics in patients with chronic obstructive lung disease. West J Med 1983; 139: 651–4.
12. PATRIARCA, P.A. et al: Influenza vaccination and warfarin or theophylline toxicity in nursing-home residents. NEJM 1983; 308: 1601.
13. MEREDITH, C.G. et al: Effects of influenza virus vaccine on hepatic drug metabolism. Clin Pharm Ther 1985; 37: 396–401.
14. LIPSKY, B.A. et al: Influenza vaccination and warfarin anticoagulation. Ann Int Med 1984; 100: 835–7.
15. KRAMER, P. et al: Effect of influenza vaccine on warfarin anticoagulation. Clin Pharmacol Ther 1984; 35: 416.
16. MURPHY, K.R. and STRUNK, R.L.: Safe administration of influenza vaccine in asthmatic children hypersensitive to egg proteins. J Pediatr 1985; 106: 931–3.
17. RETAILLIAU, H. et al: Illness after influenza vaccination reported through a nation-wide surveillance system, 1976–1977. Am J Epidemiol 1980; 111: 170.
18. BAKSHI, R. AND MAZZIOTTA, J.C.: Acute transverse myelitis after influenza vaccination: Magnetic resonance imaging findings. J Neuroimaging 1996; 6: 248–250.

U.S. Gov't. License No. 3
Manufactured by:
Wyeth Laboratories Inc.
A Wyeth-Ayerst Company
Marietta, PA 17547

ISMO® ℞
[ĭs 'mō]
(isosorbide mononitrate)
20 mg tablets

DESCRIPTION

Isosorbide mononitrate is 1,4:3,6-dianhydro-D-glucitol,5-nitrate, an organic nitrate whose structural formula is:

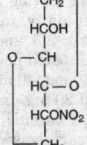

and whose molecular weight is 191.14. The organic nitrates are vasodilators, active on both arteries and veins.

Continued on next page

Ismo—Cont.

Each Ismo® tablet contains 20 mg of isosorbide mononitrate. The inactive ingredients in each tablet are D&C Yellow 10 Aluminum Lake, FD&C Yellow 6 Aluminum Lake, hydroxypropyl methylcellulose, lactose, magnesium stearate, microcrystalline cellulose, polyethylene glycol, polysorbate 20, povidone, silicon dioxide, sodium starch glycolate, titanium dioxide and hydroxypropyl cellulose.

CLINICAL PHARMACOLOGY

Isosorbide mononitrate is the major active metabolite of isosorbide dinitrate (ISDN), and most of the clinical activity of the dinitrate is attributable to the mononitrate.

The principal pharmacological action of isosorbide mononitrate, due to its nitric oxide metabolite, is direct relaxation of vascular smooth muscle. The result is dilatation of peripheral arteries and veins, especially the latter. Dilation of the veins promotes peripheral pooling of blood and decreases venous return to the heart, thereby reducing left ventricular end-diastolic pressure and pulmonary capillary wedge pressure (preload). Arteriolar relaxation reduces systemic vascular resistance, systolic arterial pressure, and mean arterial pressure (afterload). Dilatation of the coronary arteries also occurs. The relative importance of preload reduction, afterload reduction, and coronary dilatation remains undefined.

PHARMACODYNAMICS

Dosing regimens for most chronically used drugs are designed to provide plasma concentrations that are continuously greater than a minimally effective concentration. This strategy is inappropriate for organic nitrates. Several well-controlled clinical trials have used exercise testing to assess the antianginal efficacy of continuously delivered nitrates. In the large majority of these trials, active agents were indistinguishable from placebo after 24 hours (or less) of continuous therapy. Attempts to overcome tolerance by dose escalation, even to doses far in excess of those used acutely, have consistently failed. Only after nitrates have been absent from the body for several hours has their antianginal efficacy been restored.

The drug-free interval sufficient to avoid tolerance to isosorbide mononitrate has not been completely defined. In the only regimen of twice-daily isosorbide mononitrate that has been shown to avoid development of tolerance, the two doses of Ismo tablets are given 7 hours apart, so there is a gap of 17 hours between the second dose of each day and the first dose of the next day. Taking account of the relatively long half-life of isosorbide mononitrate this result is consistent with those obtained for other organic nitrates.

The same twice-daily regimen of Ismo tablets successfully avoided significant rebound/withdrawal effects. The incidence and magnitude of such phenomena have appeared, in studies of other nitrates, to be highly dependent upon the schedule of nitrate administration.

PHARMACOKINETICS

In humans, isosorbide mononitrate is not subject to first pass metabolism in the liver. The absolute bioavailability of isosorbide mononitrate from Ismo tablets is nearly 100%. Maximum serum concentrations of isosorbide mononitrate are achieved 30 to 60 minutes after ingestion of Ismo.

The volume of distribution of isosorbide mononitrate is approximately 0.6 L/kg, and less than 4% is bound to plasma proteins. It is cleared from the serum by denitration to isosorbide; glucuronidation to the mononitrate glucuronide; and denitration/hydration to sorbitol. None of these metabolites is vasoactive. Less than 1% of administered isosorbide mononitrate is eliminated in the urine.

The overall elimination half-life of isosorbide mononitrate is about 5 hours; the rate of clearance is the same in healthy young adults, in patients with various degrees of renal, hepatic, or cardiac dysfunction, and in the elderly. In a single-dose study, the pharmacokinetics of isosorbide mononitrate were dose-proportional up to at least 60 mg.

CLINICAL TRIALS

Controlled trials of single doses of Ismo tablets have demonstrated that antianginal activity is present about 1 hour after dosing, with peak effect seen from 1–4 hours after dosing.

In placebo-controlled trials lasting 2–3 weeks, Ismo tablets were administered twice daily, in asymmetric regimens (with interdosing intervals of 7 and 17 hours) designed to avoid tolerance. One trial tested doses of 10 mg and 20 mg; one trial tested doses of 20 mg, 40 mg, and 60 mg; and three trials tested only doses of 20 mg. In each trial, the subjects were persons with known chronic stable angina, and the primary measure of efficacy was exercise tolerance on a standardized treadmill test. After initial dosing and for at least 3 weeks, exercise tolerance in patients treated with Ismo 20 mg tablets was significantly greater than that seen in patients treated with placebo, although there was some attenuation of effect with time. Treatment with Ismo tablets was superior to placebo for at least 12 hours after the first

dose (i.e., 5 hours after the second dose) of each day. Significant tolerance and rebound phenomena were not observed. The 10-mg dose was not unequivocally superior to placebo, while the effect of the 40-mg dose was similar to that of the 20-mg dose. The 60-mg dose appeared to be less effective, and it was associated with a rebound phenomenon (early-morning worsening).

INDICATIONS AND USAGE

Ismo tablets are indicated for the prevention of angina pectoris due to coronary artery disease. The onset of action of oral isosorbide mononitrate is not sufficiently rapid for this product to be useful in aborting an acute anginal episode.

CONTRAINDICATIONS

Allergic reactions to organic nitrates are extremely rare, but they do occur. Isosorbide mononitrate is contraindicated in patients who are allergic to it.

WARNINGS

The benefits of isosorbide mononitrate in patients with acute myocardial infarction or congestive heart failure have not been established. Because the effects of isosorbide mononitrate are difficult to terminate rapidly, this drug is not recommended in these settings.

If isosorbide mononitrate is used in these conditions, careful clinical or hemodynamic monitoring must be used to avoid the hazards of hypotension and tachycardia.

PRECAUTIONS

GENERAL

Severe hypotension, particularly with upright posture, may occur with even small doses of isosorbide mononitrate. This drug should therefore be used with caution in patients who may be volume depleted or who, for whatever reason, are already hypotensive. Hypotension induced by isosorbide mononitrate may be accompanied by paradoxical bradycardia and increased angina pectoris.

Nitrate therapy may aggravate the angina caused by hypertrophic cardiomyopathy.

In industrial workers who have had long-term exposure to unknown (presumably high) doses of organic nitrates, tolerance clearly occurs. Chest pain, acute myocardial infarction, and even sudden death have occurred during temporary withdrawal of nitrates from these workers, demonstrating the existence of true physical dependence. The importance of these observations to the routine, clinical use of oral isosorbide mononitrate is not known.

INFORMATION FOR PATIENTS

Patients should be told that the antianginal efficacy of Ismo tablets can be maintained by carefully following the prescribed schedule of dosing (two doses taken 7 hours apart). For most patients, this can be accomplished by taking the first dose on awakening and the second dose 7 hours later. As with other nitrates, daily headaches sometimes accompany treatment with isosorbide mononitrate. In patients who get these headaches, the headaches are a marker of the activity of the drug. Patients should resist the temptation to avoid headaches by altering the schedule of their treatment with isosorbide mononitrate, since loss of headache may be associated with simultaneous loss of antianginal efficacy. Aspirin and/or acetaminophen, on the other hand, often successfully relieve isosorbide mononitrate-induced headaches with no deleterious effect on isosorbide mononitrate's antianginal efficacy.

Treatment with isosorbide mononitrate may be associated with light-headedness on standing, especially just after rising from a recumbent or seated position. This effect may be more frequent in patients who have also consumed alcohol.

DRUG INTERACTIONS

The vasodilating effects of isosorbide mononitrate may be additive with those of other vasodilators. Alcohol, in particular, has been found to exhibit additive effects of this variety.

Marked symptomatic orthostatic hypotension has been reported when calcium channel blockers and organic nitrates were used in combination. Dose adjustments of either class of agents may be necessary.

CARCINOGENESIS, MUTAGENESIS, AND IMPAIRMENT OF FERTILITY

No carcinogenic effects were observed in mice exposed to oral isosorbide mononitrate for 104 weeks at doses of up to 900 mg/kg/day (102 × the human exposure comparing body surface area). Rats treated with 900 mg/kg/day for 26 weeks (225 × the human exposure comparing body surface area) and 500 mg/kg/day for the remaining 95 to 111 weeks (males and females, respectively) showed no evidence of tumors.

No mutagenic activity was seen in a variety of *in vitro* and *in vivo* assays.

No adverse effects on fertility were observed when isosorbide mononitrate was administered to male and female rats at doses up to 500 mg/kg/day (125 × the human exposure comparing body surface area).

PREGNANCY CATEGORY C

Isosorbide mononitrate has been shown to be associated with stillbirths and neonatal death in rats receiving 500 mg/kg/day of isosorbide mononitrate (125 × the human expo-

sure comparing body surface area). At 250 mg/kg/day, no adverse effects on reproduction and development were reported.

In rats and rabbits receiving isosorbide mononitrate at up to 250 mg/kg/day, no developmental abnormalities, fetal abnormalities, or other effects upon reproductive performance were detected; these doses are larger than the maximum recommended human dose by factors between 70 (body-surface-area basis in rabbits) and 310 (body-weight basis, either species). In rats receiving 500 mg/kg/day, there were small but statistically significant increases in the rates of prolonged gestation, prolonged parturition, stillbirth, and neonatal death; and there were small but statistically significant decreases in birth weight, live litter size, and pup survival.

There are no adequate and well-controlled studies in pregnant women. Isosorbide mononitrate should be used during pregnancy only if the potential benefit justifies the potential risk to the fetus.

NURSING MOTHERS

It is not known whether isosorbide mononitrate is excreted in human milk. Because many drugs are excreted in human milk, caution should be exercised when isosorbide mononitrate is administered to a nursing woman.

PEDIATRIC USE

Safety and effectiveness of isosorbide mononitrate in pediatric patients have not been established.

ADVERSE REACTIONS

The table below shows the frequencies of the adverse reactions observed in more than 1% of the subjects (a) in 6 placebo-controlled domestic studies in which patients in the active-treatment arm received 20 mg of isosorbide mononitrate twice daily, and (b) in all studies in which patients received isosorbide mononitrate in a variety of regimens. In parentheses, the same table shows the frequencies with which these adverse reactions led to discontinuation of treatment. Overall, 11% of the patients who received isosorbide mononitrate in the six controlled U.S. studies discontinued treatment because of adverse reactions. Most of these discontinued because of headache. "Dizziness" and nausea were also frequently associated with withdrawal from these studies.

Frequency of Adverse Reactions (Discontinuations)*					
	6 Controlled Studies			92 Clinical Studies	
Dose	Placebo		20 mg		(varied)
Patients	204		219		3344
Headache	9%	(0%)	38%	(9%)	19% (4.3%)
Dizziness	1%	(0%)	5%	(1%)	3% (0.2%)
Nausea, Vomiting	<1%	(0%)	4%	(3%)	2% (0.2%)

* Some individuals discontinued for multiple reasons.

Other adverse reactions, each reported by fewer than 1% of exposed patients, and in many cases of uncertain relation to drug treatment, were:

Cardiovascular: angina pectoris, arrhythmias, atrial fibrillation, hypotension, palpitations, postural hypotension, premature ventricular contractions, supraventricular tachycardia, syncope.

Dermatologic: pruritus, rash.

Gastrointestinal: abdominal pain, diarrhea, dyspepsia, tenesmus, tooth disorder, vomiting.

Genitourinary: dysuria, impotence, urinary frequency.

Miscellaneous: asthenia, blurred vision, cold sweat, diplopia, edema, malaise, neck stiffness, rigors.

Musculoskeletal: arthralgia.

Neurologic: agitation, anxiety, confusion, dyscoordination, hypoesthesia, hypokinesia, increased appetite, insomnia, nervousness, nightmares.

Respiratory: bronchitis, pneumonia, upper-respiratory tract infection.

Extremely rarely, ordinary doses of organic nitrates have caused methemoglobinemia in normal-seeming patients; for further discussion of its diagnosis and treatment see under OVERDOSAGE.

OVERDOSAGE

HEMODYNAMIC EFFECTS

The ill effects of isosorbide mononitrate overdose are generally the results of isosorbide mononitrate's capacity to induce vasodilatation, venous pooling, reduced cardiac output, and hypotension. These hemodynamic changes may have protean manifestations, including increased intracranial pressure, with any or all of persistent throbbing headache, confusion, and moderate fever; vertigo; palpitations; visual disturbances; nausea and vomiting (possibly with colic and even bloody diarrhea); syncope (especially in the upright

posture); air hunger and dyspnea, later followed by reduced ventilatory effort; diaphoresis, with the skin either flushed or cold and clammy; heart block and bradycardia; paralysis; coma; seizures and death.

Laboratory determinations of serum levels of isosorbide mononitrate and its metabolites are not widely available, and such determinations have, in any event, no established role in the management of isosorbide mononitrate overdose.

There are no data suggesting what dose of isosorbide mononitrate is likely to be life-threatening in humans. In rats and mice, there is significant lethality at doses of 2000 mg/kg and 3000 mg/kg, respectively.

No data are available to suggest physiological maneuvers (e.g., maneuvers to change the pH of the urine) that might accelerate elimination of isosorbide mononitrate. In particular, dialysis is known to be ineffective in removing isosorbide mononitrate from the body.

No specific antagonist to the vasodilator effects of isosorbide mononitrate is known, and no intervention has been subject to controlled study as a therapy of isosorbide mononitrate overdose. Because the hypotension associated with isosorbide mononitrate overdose is the result of venodilatation and arterial hypovolemia, prudent therapy in this situation should be directed toward an increase in central fluid volume. Passive elevation of the patient's legs may be sufficient, but intravenous infusion of normal saline or similar fluid may also be necessary.

The use of epinephrine or other arterial vasoconstrictors in this setting is likely to do more harm than good.

In patients with renal disease or congestive heart failure, therapy resulting in central volume expansion is not without hazard. Treatment of isosorbide mononitrate overdose in these patients may be subtle and difficult, and invasive monitoring may be required.

METHEMOGLOBINEMIA

Methemoglobinemia has been reported in patients receiving other organic nitrates, and it probably could also occur as a side effect of isosorbide mononitrate. Certainly nitrate ions liberated during metabolism of isosorbide mononitrate can oxidize hemoglobin into methemoglobin. Even in patients totally without cytochrome b_5 reductase activity, however, and even assuming that the nitrate moiety of isosorbide mononitrate is quantitatively applied to oxidation of hemoglobin, about 2 mg/kg of isosorbide mononitrate should be required before any of these patients manifests clinically significant ($\geq$ 10%) methemoglobinemia. In patients with normal reductase function, significant production of methemoglobin should require even larger doses of isosorbide mononitrate. In one study in which 36 patients received 2 to 4 weeks of continuous nitroglycerin therapy at 3.1 to 4.4 mg/hr (equivalent, in total administered dose of nitrate ions, to 7.8 to 11.1 mg of isosorbide mononitrate per hour), the average methemoglobin level measured was 0.2%; this was comparable to that observed in parallel patients who received placebo.

Notwithstanding these observations, there are case reports of significant methemoglobinemia in association with moderate overdoses of organic nitrates. None of the affected patients had been thought to be unusually susceptible.

Methemoglobin levels are available from most clinical laboratories. The diagnosis should be suspected in patients who exhibit signs of impaired oxygen delivery despite adequate cardiac output and adequate arterial pO_2. Classically, methemoglobinemic blood is described as chocolate brown, without color change on exposure to air.

When methemoglobinemia is diagnosed, the treatment of choice is methylene blue, 1 to 2 mg/kg intravenously.

DOSAGE AND ADMINISTRATION

The recommended regimen of Ismo tablets is 20 mg (one tablet) twice daily, with the two doses given 7 hours apart. For most patients, this can be accomplished by taking the first dose on awakening and the second dose 7 hours later. Dosage adjustments are not necessary for elderly patients or patients with altered renal or hepatic function.

As noted above (**CLINICAL PHARMACOLOGY**), multiple studies of organic nitrates have shown that maintenance of continuous 24-hour plasma levels results in refractory tolerance. The dosing regimen for Ismo tablets provides a daily nitrate-free interval to avoid the development of this tolerance.

As also noted under **CLINICAL PHARMACOLOGY,** well-controlled studies have shown that tolerance to Ismo tablets is avoided when using the twice-daily regimen in which the two doses are given 7 hours apart. This regimen has been shown to have antianginal efficacy beginning 1 hour after the first dose and lasting at least 5 hours after the second dose. The duration (if any) of antianginal activity beyond 12 hours has not been studied; large controlled studies with other nitrates suggest that no dosing regimen should be expected to provide more than about 12 hours of continuous antianginal efficacy per day.

In clinical trials, Ismo tablets have been administered in a variety of regimens. Single doses less than 20 mg have not been adequately studied, while single doses greater than 20 mg have demonstrated no greater efficacy than doses of 20 mg.

HOW SUPPLIED

Ismo® (isosorbide mononitrate) tablets, 20 mg, are available in bottles of 100 (NDC 0008-0771-01) and in unit dose packages of 10 blister strips of 10 tablets (NDC 0008-0771-02). Each orange, round, film-coated tablet is engraved "ISMO 20" on one side and scored on the reverse side.

Store at controlled room temperature between 20°C and 25°C (68°F and 77°F).

Dispense in tight container.

Manufactured by:
Wyeth Laboratories Inc.
A Wyeth-Ayerst Company
Philadelphia, PA 19101
Distributed jointly with:
Boehringer Mannheim Pharmaceuticals Corp.
Rockville, MD 20850

Shown in Product Identification Guide, page 343

ISORDIL® ℞

(isosorbide dinitrate)
Sublingual Tablets

DESCRIPTION

Isosorbide dinitrate (ISDN) is 1,4:3,6-dianhydro-D-glucitol 2,5-dinitrate, an organic nitrate whose structural formula is and whose molecular weight is 236.14. The organic nitrates are vasodilators, active on both arteries and veins.

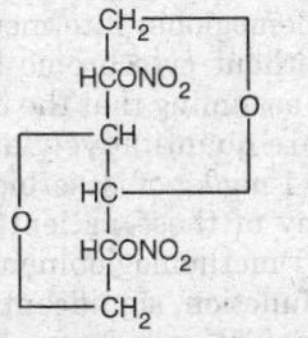

Isosorbide dinitrate is a white, crystalline, odorless compound which is stable in air and in solution, has a melting point of 70°C and has an optical rotation of +134° (c=1.0, alcohol, 20°C). Isosorbide dinitrate is freely soluble in organic solvents such as acetone, alcohol, and ether, but is only sparingly soluble in water.

Each Isordil® Sublingual tablet contains 2.5, 5, or 10 mg of isosorbide dinitrate. The inactive ingredients in each tablet are cellulose, lactose, magnesium stearate, and starch. The 2.5 mg dosage strength also contains D&C Yellow 10 and FD&C Yellow 6, and the 5 mg dosage strength also contains FD&C Red 40.

CLINICAL PHARMACOLOGY

The principal pharmacological action of isosorbide dinitrate is relaxation of vascular smooth muscle and consequent dilatation of peripheral arteries and veins, especially the latter. Dilatation of the veins promotes peripheral pooling of blood and decreases venous return to the heart, thereby reducing left ventricular end-diastolic pressure and pulmonary capillary wedge pressure (preload). Arteriolar relaxation reduces systemic vascular resistance, systolic arterial pressure, and mean arterial pressure (afterload). Dilatation of the coronary arteries also occurs. The relative importance of preload reduction, afterload reduction, and coronary dilatation remains undefined.

Dosing regimens for most chronically used drugs are designed to provide plasma concentrations that are continuously greater than a minimally effective concentration. This strategy is inappropriate for organic nitrates. Several well-controlled clinical trials have used exercise testing to assess the anti-anginal efficacy of continuously-delivered nitrates. In the large majority of these trials, active agents were no more effective than placebo after 24 hours (or less) of continuous therapy. Attempts to overcome nitrate tolerance by dose escalation, even to doses far in excess of those used acutely, have consistently failed. Only after nitrates have been absent from the body for several hours has their anti-anginal efficacy been restored.

PHARMACOKINETICS

Bioavailability of ISDN after single sublingual doses is 40 to 50%. Multiple-dose studies of sublingual ISDN pharmacokinetics have not been reported; multiple-dose studies of ingested ISDN have observed progressive increases in bioavailability during chronic therapy. Serum levels of ISDN reach their maxima 10 to 15 minutes after sublingual dosing.

Once absorbed, the volume of distribution of isosorbide dinitrate is 2 to 4 L/kg, and this volume is cleared at the rate of 2 to 4 L/min, so ISDN's half-life in serum is about an hour. Since the clearance exceeds hepatic blood flow, considerable extrahepatic metabolism must also occur. Clearance is affected primarily by denitration to the 2-mononitrate (15 to 25%) and the 5-mononitrate (75 to 85%).

Both metabolites have biological activity, especially the 5-mononitrate. With an overall half-life of about 5 hours, the 5-mononitrate is cleared from the serum by denitration to isosorbide, glucuronidation to the 5-mononitrate glucuronide, and denitration/hydration to sorbitol. The 2-mononitrate has been less well studied, but it appears to participate in the same metabolic pathways, with a half-life of about 2 hours.

The daily dose-free interval sufficient to avoid tolerance to organic nitrates has not been well defined. Studies of nitroglycerin (an organic nitrate with a very short half-life) have shown that daily dose-free intervals of 10 to 12 hours are usually sufficient to minimize tolerance. Daily dose-free intervals that have succeeded in avoiding tolerance during trials of moderate doses (*e.g.,* 30 mg) of immediate-release ISDN have generally been somewhat longer (at least 14 hours), but this is consistent with the longer half-lives of ISDN and its active metabolites.

Few well-controlled clinical trials of organic nitrates have been designed to detect rebound or withdrawal effects. In one such trial, however, subjects receiving nitroglycerin had *less* exercise tolerance at the end of the daily dose-free interval than the parallel group receiving placebo. The incidence, magnitude, and clinical significance of similar phenomena in patients receiving ISDN have not been studied.

CLINICAL TRIALS

In a controlled trial in which 0.4 mg of sublingual nitroglycerin took 1.9 minutes to begin to produce an anti-anginal effect, 5 mg of sublingual ISDN took 3.4 minutes to begin to produce a similar effect. In the same trial, the anti-anginal effect of the sublingual nitroglycerin was evident for about an hour, while that of the sublingual ISDN lasted about 2 hours.

In other controlled trials, the anti-anginal efficacy of sublingual ISDN has persisted for periods ranging from 30 minutes up to 4 hours.

Multiple-dose trials of sublingual ISDN have not been reported. Multiple-dose trials of ingested formulations of ISDN have shown that ISDN's anti-anginal efficacy is substantially attenuated by tolerance unless the daily regimen includes a dose-free interval of at least 14 hours. The daily dose-free interval necessary in any chronic regimen using sublingual ISDN is not known.

From large, well-controlled studies of other nitrates, it is reasonable to believe that the maximal achievable daily duration of anti-anginal effect from isosorbide dinitrate is about 12 hours. No dosing regimen for isosorbide dinitrate has, however, ever actually been shown to achieve this duration of effect. In the absence of data from multiple-dose trials, and considering the capacity of organic nitrates to induce tolerance, it is not reasonable to assume that multiple sublingual ISDN tablets taken during the course of a day will all have similar effects.

INDICATIONS AND USAGE

Isordil Sublingual tablets are indicated for the prevention and treatment of angina pectoris due to coronary artery disease. However, because the onset of action of sublingual ISDN is significantly slower than that of sublingual nitroglycerin, sublingual ISDN is not the drug of first choice for abortion of an acute anginal episode.

CONTRAINDICATIONS

Allergic reactions to organic nitrates are extremely rare, but they do occur. Isordil is contraindicated in patients who are allergic to isosorbide dinitrate or any of its other ingredients.

WARNINGS

The benefits of sublingual isosorbide dinitrate in patients with acute myocardial infarction or congestive heart failure have not been established. If one elects to use isosorbide dinitrate in these conditions, careful clinical or hemodynamic monitoring must be used to avoid the hazards of hypotension and tachycardia.

PRECAUTIONS

GENERAL

Severe hypotension, particularly with upright posture, may occur with even small doses of isosorbide dinitrate. This drug should therefore be used with caution in patients who may be volume depleted or who, for whatever reason, are already hypotensive. Hypotension induced by isosorbide dinitrate may be accompanied by paradoxical bradycardia and increased angina pectoris.

Nitrate therapy may aggravate the angina caused by hypertrophic cardiomyopathy.

As tolerance to isosorbide dinitrate develops, the effect of sublingual nitroglycerin on exercise tolerance, although still observable, is somewhat blunted.

Some clinical trials in angina patients have provided nitroglycerin for about 12 continuous hours of every 24-hour day. During the daily dose-free interval in some of these trials, anginal attacks have been more easily provoked than before treatment, and patients have demonstrated hemodynamic

Continued on next page

Isordil Tablets—Cont.

rebound and *decreased* exercise tolerance. The importance of these observations to the routine, clinical use of sublingual isosorbide dinitrate is not known.

In industrial workers who have had long-term exposure to unknown (presumably high) doses of organic nitrates, tolerance clearly occurs. Chest pain, acute myocardial infarction, and even sudden death have occurred during temporary withdrawal of nitrates from these workers, demonstrating the existence of true physical dependence.

INFORMATION FOR PATIENTS

Patients should be told that the anti-anginal efficacy of isosorbide dinitrate is strongly related to its dosing regimen, so the prescribed schedule of dosing should be followed carefully. In particular, daily headaches sometimes accompany treatment with isosorbide dinitrate. In patients who get these headaches, the headaches are a marker of the activity of the drug. Patients should resist the temptation to avoid headaches by altering the schedule of their treatment with isosorbide dinitrate, since loss of headache may be associated with simultaneous loss of anti-anginal efficacy. Aspirin and/or acetaminophen, on the other hand, often successfully relieve isosorbide dinitrate-induced headaches with no deleterious effect on isosorbide dinitrate's anti-anginal efficacy.

Treatment with isosorbide dinitrate may be associated with lightheadedness on standing, especially just after rising from a recumbent or seated position. This effect may be more frequent in patients who have also consumed alcohol.

DRUG INTERACTIONS

The vasodilating effects of isosorbide dinitrate may be additive with those of other vasodilators. Alcohol, in particular, has been found to exhibit additive effects of this variety.

CARCINOGENESIS, MUTAGENESIS, IMPAIRMENT OF FERTILITY

No long-term studies in animals have been performed to evaluate the carcinogenic potential of isosorbide dinitrate. In a modified two-litter reproduction study, there was no remarkable gross pathology and no altered fertility or gestation among rats fed isosorbide dinitrate at 25 or 100 mg/kg/day.

PREGNANCY CATEGORY C

At oral doses 35 and 150 times the maximum recommended human daily dose, isosorbide dinitrate has been shown to cause a dose-related increase in embryotoxicity (increase in mummified pups) in rabbits. There are no adequate, well-controlled studies in pregnant women. Isosorbide dinitrate should be used during pregnancy only if the potential benefit justifies the potential risk to the fetus.

NURSING MOTHERS

It is not known whether isosorbide dinitrate is excreted in human milk. Because many drugs are excreted in human milk, caution should be exercised when isosorbide dinitrate is administered to a nursing woman.

PEDIATRIC USE

Safety and effectiveness in pediatric patients have not been established.

ADVERSE REACTIONS

Adverse reactions to isosorbide dinitrate are generally dose-related, and almost all of these reactions are the result of isosorbide dinitrate's activity as a vasodilator. Headache, which may be severe, is the most commonly reported side effect. Headache may be recurrent with each daily dose, especially at higher doses. Transient episodes of lightheadedness, occasionally related to blood pressure changes, may also occur. Hypotension occurs infrequently, but in some patients it may be severe enough to warrant discontinuation of therapy. Syncope, crescendo angina, and rebound hypertension have been reported but are uncommon.

Extremely rarely, ordinary doses of organic nitrates have caused methemoglobinemia in normal-seeming patients. Methemoglobinemia is so infrequent at these doses that further discussion of its diagnosis and treatment is deferred (see "**Overdosage**").

Data are not available to allow estimation of the frequency of adverse reactions during treatment with Isordil® Sublingual tablets.

OVERDOSAGE

HEMODYNAMIC EFFECTS

The ill effects of isosorbide dinitrate overdose are generally the results of isosorbide dinitrate's capacity to induce vasodilatation, venous pooling, reduced cardiac output, and hypotension. These hemodynamic changes may have protean manifestations, including increased intracranial pressure, with any or all of persistent throbbing headache, confusion, and moderate fever; vertigo; palpitations; visual disturbances; nausea and vomiting (possibly with colic and even bloody diarrhea); syncope (especially in the upright posture); air hunger and dyspnea, later followed by reduced ventilatory effort; diaphoresis, with the skin either flushed or cold and clammy; heart block and bradycardia; paralysis; coma; seizures; and death.

Laboratory determinations of serum levels of isosorbide dinitrate and its metabolites are not widely available, and such determinations have, in any event, no established role in the management of isosorbide dinitrate overdose.

There are no data suggesting what dose of isosorbide dinitrate is likely to be life-threatening in humans. In rats, the median acute lethal dose (LD_{50}) was found to be 1100 mg/kg.

No data are available to suggest physiological maneuvers (*e.g.*, maneuvers to change the pH of the urine) that might accelerate elimination of isosorbide dinitrate and its active metabolites. Similarly, it is not known which, if any, of these substances can usefully be removed from the body by hemodialysis.

No specific antagonist to the vasodilator effects of isosorbide dinitrate is known, and no intervention has been subject to controlled studies as a therapy for isosorbide dinitrate overdose. Because the hypotension associated with isosorbide dinitrate overdose is the result of venodilatation and arterial hypovolemia, prudent therapy in this situation should be directed toward increase in central fluid volume. Passive elevation of the patient's legs may be sufficient, but intravenous infusion of normal saline or similar fluid may also be necessary.

The use of epinephrine or other arterial vasoconstrictors in this setting is likely to do more harm than good.

In patients with renal disease or congestive heart failure, therapy resulting in central volume expansion is not without hazard. Treatment of isosorbide dinitrate overdose in these patients may be subtle and difficult, and invasive monitoring may be required.

METHEMOGLOBINEMIA

Nitrate ions liberated during metabolism of isosorbide dinitrate can oxidize hemoglobin into methemoglobin. Even in patients totally without cytochrome b_5 reductase activity, however, and even assuming that the nitrate moieties of isosorbide dinitrate are quantitatively applied to oxidation of hemoglobin, about 1 mg/kg of isosorbide dinitrate should be required before any of these patients manifests clinically significant ($\geq$10%) methemoglobinemia. In patients with normal reductase function, significant production of methemoglobin should require even larger doses of isosorbide dinitrate. In one study in which 36 patients received 2 to 4 weeks of continuous nitroglycerin therapy at 3.1 to 4.4 mg/hr (equivalent, in total administered dose of nitrate ions, to 4.8 to 6.9 mg of bioavailable isosorbide dinitrate per hour), the average methemoglobin level measured was 0.2%; this was comparable to that observed in parallel patients who received placebo.

Notwithstanding these observations, there are case reports of significant methemoglobinemia in association with moderate overdoses of organic nitrates. None of the affected patients had been thought to be unusually susceptible.

Methemoglobin levels are available from most clinical laboratories. The diagnosis should be suspected in patients who exhibit signs of impaired oxygen delivery despite adequate cardiac output and adequate arterial pO_2. Classically, methemoglobinemic blood is described as chocolate brown, without color change on exposure to air.

When methemoglobinemia is diagnosed, the treatment of choice is methylene blue, 1 to 2 mg/kg intravenously.

DOSAGE AND ADMINISTRATION

As noted under "**Clinical Pharmacology**," multiple-dose studies with ISDN and other nitrates have shown that maintenance of continuous 24-hour plasma levels results in refractory tolerance. Every dosing regimen for ISDN must provide a daily dose-free interval to minimize the development of this tolerance. In the case of sublingual tablets, it is probably true that one of the daily dose-free intervals must be somewhat longer than 14 hours.

As also noted under "**Clinical Pharmacology**," the efficacy of daily doses after the first dose has never been demonstrated.

Large controlled studies with other nitrates suggest that no dosing regimen with Isordil Sublingual tablets should be expected to provide more than about 12 hours of continuous anti-anginal efficacy per day.

A patient anticipating activity likely to cause angina should take one Isordil Sublingual tablet (2.5 to 5 mg) about 15 minutes before the activity is expected to begin. Isordil Sublingual tablets may be used to abort an acute anginal episode, but its use is recommended only in patients who fail to respond to sublingual nitroglycerin.

HOW SUPPLIED

Isordil® (isosorbide dinitrate) Sublingual Tablets are available as follows:

2.5 mg, round, yellow tablets imprinted "2.5" on one side and "W" on reverse side:
NDC 0008-4139-01, bottles of 100.
NDC 0008-4139-03, bottles of 500.
NDC 0008-4139-05, Redipak® cartons of 100 (10 blister strips of 10).

5 mg, round, pink tablets imprinted "5" on one side and "W" on reverse side:
NDC 0008-4126-01, bottles of 100.
NDC 0008-4126-03, bottles of 500.
NDC 0008-4126-07, Redipak cartons of 100 (10 blister strips of 10).

Store at room temperature, approximately 25°C (77°F)
Protect from light
Keep bottles tightly closed
Dispense in a light-resistant, tight container
Use carton to protect blisters from light

10 mg, round, white tablets imprinted "10" on one side and "Wyeth" on reverse side:
NDC 0008-4161-01, bottles of 100.

Store at room temperature, approximately 25°C (77°F)
Keep tightly closed
Dispense in a tight container

ALSO AVAILABLE

Oral Titradose® Tablets in the following dosage strengths:
5 mg, NDC 0008-4152, in bottles of 100, 500 or 1,000 and in Redipak cartons of 100 (10 blister strips of 10).
10 mg, NDC 0008-4153, in bottles of 100, 500 or 1,000 and in Redipak cartons of 100 (10 blister strips of 10).
20 mg, NDC 0008-4154, in bottles of 100 or 500 and in Redipak cartons of 100 (10 blister strips of 10).
30 mg, NDC 0008-4159, in bottles of 100 or 500 and in Redipak cartons of 100 (10 blister strips of 10).
40 mg, NDC 0008-4192, in bottles of 100 and in Redipak cartons of 100 (10 blister strips of 10).
Tembids® Tablets, 40 mg, controlled-release tablets, NDC 0008-4125, in bottles of 100, 500 or 1,000.
Tembids® Capsules, 40 mg, controlled-release capsules, NDC 0008-4140, in bottles of 100 or 500.

Manufactured by:
Wyeth Laboratories Inc.
A Wyeth-Ayerst Company
Philadelphia, PA 19101

Shown in Product Identification Guide, page 344

ISORDIL® TITRADOSE® ℞
(isosorbide dinitrate)
Tablets

DESCRIPTION

Isosorbide dinitrate (ISDN) is 1,4:3,6-dianhydro-D-glucitol 2,5-dinitrate, an organic nitrate whose structural formula is and whose molecular weight is 236.14. The organic nitrates are vasodilators, active on both arteries and veins.

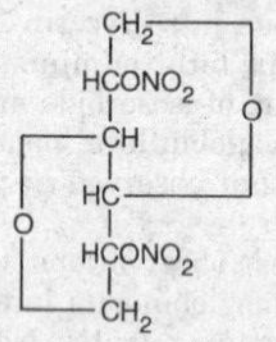

Isosorbide dinitrate is a white, crystalline, odorless compound which is stable in air and in solution, has a melting point of 70°C and has an optical rotation of +134° (c=1.0, alcohol, 20°C). Isosorbide dinitrate is freely soluble in organic solvents such as acetone, alcohol, and ether, but is only sparingly soluble in water.

Each Isordil® Titradose® tablet contains 5, 10, 20, 30, or 40 mg of isosorbide dinitrate. The inactive ingredients in each tablet are lactose, cellulose, and magnesium stearate. The 5 mg, 20 mg, 30 mg, and 40 mg dosage strengths also contain the following: 5 mg—FD&C Red 40; 20 mg and 40 mg—D&C Yellow 10, FD&C Blue 1, and FD&C Yellow 6; 30 mg—FD&C Blue 1.

CLINICAL PHARMACOLOGY

The principal pharmacological action of isosorbide dinitrate is relaxation of vascular smooth muscle and consequent dilatation of peripheral arteries and veins, especially the latter. Dilatation of the veins promotes peripheral pooling of blood and decreases venous return to the heart, thereby reducing left ventricular end-diastolic pressure and pulmonary capillary wedge pressure (preload). Arteriolar relaxation reduces systemic vascular resistance, systolic arterial pressure, and mean arterial pressure (afterload). Dilatation of the coronary arteries also occurs. The relative importance of preload reduction, afterload reduction, and coronary dilatation remains undefined.

Dosing regimens for most chronically used drugs are designed to provide plasma concentrations that are continuously greater than a minimally effective concentration. This strategy is inappropriate for organic nitrates. Several well-controlled clinical trials have used exercise testing to assess the anti-anginal efficacy of continuously-delivered nitrates. In the large majority of these trials, active agents were no more effective than placebo after 24 hours (or less) of continuous therapy. Attempts to overcome nitrate tolerance by dose escalation, even to doses far in excess of those used

acutely, have consistently failed. Only after nitrates have been absent from the body for several hours has their anti-anginal efficacy been restored.

PHARMACOKINETICS

Absorption of isosorbide dinitrate after oral dosing is nearly complete, but bioavailability is highly variable (10% to 90%), with extensive first-pass metabolism in the liver. Serum levels reach their maxima about an hour after ingestion. The average bioavailability of ISDN is about 25%; most studies have observed progressive increases in bioavailability during chronic therapy.

Once absorbed, the volume of distribution of isosorbide dinitrate is 2 to 4 L/kg, and this volume is cleared at the rate of 2 to 4 L/min, so ISDN's half-life in serum is about an hour. Since the clearance exceeds hepatic blood flow, considerable extrahepatic metabolism must also occur. Clearance is affected primarily by denitration to the 2-mononitrate (15 to 25%) and the 5-mononitrate (75 to 85%).

Both metabolites have biological activity, especially the 5-mononitrate. With an overall half-life of about 5 hours, the 5-mononitrate is cleared from the serum by denitration to isosorbide, glucuronidation to the 5-mononitrate glucuronide, and denitration/hydration to sorbitol. The 2-mononitrate has been less well studied, but it appears to participate in the same metabolic pathways, with a half-life of about 2 hours.

The daily dose-free interval sufficient to avoid tolerance to organic nitrates has not been well defined. Studies of nitroglycerin (an organic nitrate with a very short half-life) have shown that daily dose-free intervals of 10 to 12 hours are usually sufficient to minimize tolerance. Daily dose-free intervals that have succeeded in avoiding tolerance during trials of moderate doses (*e.g.,* 30 mg) of immediate-release ISDN have generally been somewhat longer (at least 14 hours), but this is consistent with the longer half-lives of ISDN and its active metabolites.

Few well-controlled clinical trials of organic nitrates have been designed to detect rebound or withdrawal effects. In one such trial, however, subjects receiving nitroglycerin had *less* exercise tolerance at the end of the daily dose-free interval than the parallel group receiving placebo. The incidence, magnitude, and clinical significance of similar phenomena in patients receiving ISDN have not been studied.

CLINICAL TRIALS

In clinical trials, immediate-release oral isosorbide dinitrate has been administered in a variety of regimens, with total daily doses ranging from 30 mg to 480 mg. Controlled trials of single oral doses of isosorbide dinitrate have demonstrated effective reductions in exercise-related angina for up to 8 hours. Anti-anginal activity is present about 1 hour after dosing.

Most controlled trials of multiple-dose oral ISDN taken every 12 hours (or more frequently) for several weeks have shown statistically significant anti-anginal efficacy for only 2 hours after dosing. Once-daily regimens, and regimens with one daily dose-free interval of at least 14 hours (*e.g.,* a regimen providing doses at 0800, 1400, and 1800 hours), have shown efficacy after the first dose of each day that was similar to that shown in the single-dose studies cited above. The effects of the second and later doses have been smaller and shorter-lasting than the effect of the first.

From large, well-controlled studies of other nitrates, it is reasonable to believe that the maximum achievable daily duration of anti-anginal effect from isosorbide dinitrate is about 12 hours. No dosing regimen for isosorbide dinitrate has, however, ever actually been shown to achieve this duration of effect. One study of 8 patients, who were administered a pretitrated dose (average 27.5 mg) of immediate-release ISDN at 0800, 1300, and 1800 hours for 2 weeks, revealed that significant anti-anginal effectiveness was discontinuous and totaled about 6 hours in a 24 hour period.

INDICATIONS AND USAGE

Isordil Titradose tablets are indicated for the prevention of angina pectoris due to coronary artery disease. The onset of action of immediate-release oral isosorbide dinitrate is not sufficiently rapid for this product to be useful in aborting an acute anginal episode.

CONTRAINDICATIONS

Allergic reactions to organic nitrates are extremely rare, but they do occur. Isordil Titradose is contraindicated in patients who are allergic to isosorbide dinitrate or any of its other ingredients.

WARNINGS

The benefits of immediate-release oral isosorbide dinitrate in patients with acute myocardial infarction or congestive heart failure have not been established. If one elects to use isosorbide dinitrate in these conditions, careful clinical or hemodynamic monitoring must be used to avoid the hazards of hypotension and tachycardia. Because the effects of oral isosorbide dinitrate are so difficult to terminate rapidly, this formulation is not recommended in these settings.

PRECAUTIONS

GENERAL

Severe hypotension, particularly with upright posture, may occur with even small doses of isosorbide dinitrate. This drug should therefore be used with caution in patients who may be volume depleted or who, for whatever reason, are already hypotensive. Hypotension induced by isosorbide dinitrate may be accompanied by paradoxical bradycardia and increased angina pectoris.

Nitrate therapy may aggravate the angina caused by hypertrophic cardiomyopathy.

As tolerance to isosorbide dinitrate develops, the effect of sublingual nitroglycerin on exercise tolerance, although still observable, is somewhat blunted.

Some clinical trials in angina patients have provided nitroglycerin for about 12 continuous hours of every 24-hour day. During the daily dose-free interval in some of these trials, anginal attacks have been more easily provoked than before treatment, and patients have demonstrated hemodynamic rebound and *decreased* exercise tolerance. The importance of these observations to the routine, clinical use of immediate-release oral isosorbide dinitrate is not known.

In industrial workers who have had long-term exposure to unknown (presumably high) doses of organic nitrates, tolerance clearly occurs. Chest pain, acute myocardial infarction, and even sudden death have occurred during temporary withdrawal of nitrates from these workers, demonstrating the existence of true physical dependence.

INFORMATION FOR PATIENTS

Patients should be told that the anti-anginal efficacy of isosorbide dinitrate is strongly related to its dosing regimen, so the prescribed schedule of dosing should be followed carefully. In particular, daily headaches sometimes accompany treatment with isosorbide dinitrate. In patients who get these headaches, the headaches are a marker of the activity of the drug. Patients should resist the temptation to avoid headaches by altering the schedule of their treatment with isosorbide dinitrate, since loss of headache may be associated with simultaneous loss of anti-anginal efficacy. Aspirin and/or acetaminophen, on the other hand, often successfully relieve isosorbide dinitrate-induced headaches with no deleterious effect on isosorbide dinitrate's anti-anginal efficacy.

Treatment with isosorbide dinitrate may be associated with lightheadedness on standing, especially just after rising from a recumbent or seated position. This effect may be more frequent in patients who have also consumed alcohol.

DRUG INTERACTIONS

The vasodilating effects of isosorbide dinitrate may be additive with those of other vasodilators. Alcohol, in particular, has been found to exhibit additive effects of this variety.

CARCINOGENESIS, MUTAGENESIS, IMPAIRMENT OF FERTILITY

No long-term studies in animals have been performed to evaluate the carcinogenic potential of isosorbide dinitrate. In a modified two-litter reproduction study, there was no remarkable gross pathology and no altered fertility or gestation among rats fed isosorbide dinitrate at 25 or 100 mg/kg/day.

PREGNANCY CATEGORY C

At oral doses 35 and 150 times the maximum recommended human daily dose, isosorbide dinitrate has been shown to cause a dose-related increase in embryotoxicity (increase in mummified pups) in rabbits. There are no adequate, well-controlled studies in pregnant women. Isosorbide dinitrate should be used during pregnancy only if the potential benefit justifies the potential risk to the fetus.

NURSING MOTHERS

It is not known whether isosorbide dinitrate is excreted in human milk. Because many drugs are excreted in human milk, caution should be exercised when isosorbide dinitate is administered to a nursing woman.

PEDIATRIC USE

Safety and effectiveness in pediatric patients have not been established.

ADVERSE REACTIONS

Adverse reactions to isosorbide dinitrate are generally dose-related, and almost all of these reactions are the result of isosorbide dinitrate's activity as a vasodilator. Headache, which may be severe, is the most commonly reported side effect. Headache may be recurrent with each daily dose, especially at higher doses. Transient episodes of lightheadedness, occasionally related to blood pressure changes, may also occur. Hypotension occurs infrequently, but in some patients it may be severe enough to warrant discontinuation of therapy. Syncope, crescendo angina, and rebound hypertension have been reported but are uncommon.

Extremely rarely, ordinary doses of organic nitrates have caused methemoglobinemia in normal-seeming patient. Methemoglobinemia is so infrequent at these doses that further discussion of its diagnosis and treatment is deferred (see "**Overdosage**").

Data are not available to allow estimation of the frequency of adverse reactions during treatment with Isordil® Titradose® tablets.

OVERDOSAGE

HEMODYNAMIC EFFECTS

The ill effects of isosorbide dinitrate overdose are generally the results of isosorbide dinitrate's capacity to induce vasodilatation, venous pooling, reduced cardiac output, and hypotension. These hemodynamic changes may have protean manifestations, including increased intracranial pressure, with any or all of persistent throbbing headache, confusion, and moderate fever; vertigo; palpitations; visual disturbances; nausea and vomiting (possibly with colic and even bloody diarrhea); syncope (especially in the upright posture); air hunger and dyspnea, later followed by reduced ventilatory effort; diaphoresis, with the skin either flushed or cold and clammy; heart block and bradycardia; paralysis; coma; seizures; and death.

Laboratory determinations of serum levels of isosorbide dinitrate and its metabolites are not widely available, and such determinations have, in any event, no established role in the management of isosorbide dinitrate overdose.

There are no data suggesting what dose of isosorbide dinitrate is likely to be life-threatening in humans. In rats, the median acute lethal dose (LD_{50}) was found to be 1100 mg/kg.

No data are available to suggest physiological maneuvers (*e.g.,* maneuvers to change the pH of the urine) that might accelerate elimination of isosorbide dinitrate and its active metabolites. Similarly, it is not known which, if any, of these substances can usefully be removed from the body by hemodialysis.

No specific antagonist to the vasodilator effects of isosorbide dinitrate is known, and no intervention has been subject to controlled studies as a therapy for isosorbide dinitrate overdose. Because the hypotension associated with isosorbide dinitrate overdose is the result of venodilatation and arterial hypovolemia, prudent therapy in this situation should be directed toward increase in central fluid volume. Passive elevation of the patient's legs may be sufficient, but intravenous infusion of normal saline or similar fluid may also be necessary.

The use of epinephrine or other arterial vasoconstrictors in this setting is likely to do more harm than good.

In patients with renal disease or congestive heart failure, therapy resulting in central volume expansion is not without hazard. Treatment of isosorbide dinitrate overdose in these patients may be subtle and difficult, and invasive monitoring may be required.

METHEMOGLOBINEMIA

Nitrate ions liberated during metabolism of isosorbide dinitrate can oxidize hemoglobin into methemoglobin. Even in patients totally without cytochrome b_5 reductase activity, however, and even assuming that the nitrate moieties of isosorbide dinitrate are quantitatively applied to oxidation of hemoglobin, about 1 mg/kg of isosorbide dinitrate should be required before any of these patients manifests clinically significant (≥10%) methemoglobinemia. In patients with normal reductase function, significant production of methemoglobin should require even larger doses of isosorbide dinitrate. In one study in which 36 patients received 2 to 4 weeks of continuous nitroglycerin therapy at 3.1 to 4.4 mg/hr (equivalent, in total administered dose of nitrate ions, to 4.8 to 6.9 mg of bioavailable isosorbide dinitrate per hour), the average methemoglobin level measured was 0.2%; this was comparable to that observed in parallel patients who received placebo.

Notwithstanding these observations, there are case reports of significant methemoglobinemia in association with moderate overdoses of organic nitrates. None of the affected patients had been thought to be unusually susceptible.

Methemoglobin levels are available from most clinical laboratories. The diagnosis should be suspected in patients who exhibit signs of impaired oxygen delivery despite adequate cardiac output and adequate arterial pO_2. Classically, methemoglobinemic blood is described as chocolate brown, without color change on exposure to air.

When methemoglobinemia is diagnosed, the treatment of choice is methylene blue, 1 to 2 mg/kg intravenously.

DOSAGE AND ADMINISTRATION

As noted under "**Clinical Pharmacology**," multiple-dose studies with ISDN and other nitrates have shown that maintenance of continuous 24-hour plasma levels results in refractory tolerance. Every dosing regimen for Isordil Titradose tablets must provide a daily dose-free interval to minimize the development of this tolerance. With immediate-release ISDN, it appears that one daily dose-free interval must be at least 14 hours long.

As also noted under "**Clinical Pharmacology**," the effects of the second and later doses have been smaller and shorter-lasting than the effects of the first.

Large controlled studies with other nitrates suggest that no dosing regimen with Isordil Titradose tablets should be expected to provide more than about 12 hours of continuous anti-anginal efficacy per day.

As with all titratable drugs, it is important to administer the minimum dose which produces the desired clinical effect. The ususal starting dose of Isordil Titradose is 5 mg to

Continued on next page

Isordil Titradose—Cont.

20 mg, two or three times daily. For maintenance therapy, 10 mg to 40 mg, two or three times daily is recommended. Some patients may require higher doses. A daily dose-free interval of at least 14 hours is advisable to minimize tolerance. The optimal interval will vary with the individual patient, dose and regimen.

HOW SUPPLIED

Isordil® (isosorbide dinitrate) Oral Titradose® Tablets are available as follows:
5 mg, round, pink tablets imprinted "WYETH 4152" on one side and deeply scored on reverse side:
NDC 0008-4152-01, bottles of 100.
NDC 0008-4152-02, bottles of 500.
NDC 0008-4152-03, bottles of 1,000.
NDC 0008-4152-05, Redipak® cartons of 100 (10 blister strips of 10).
Store at room temperature, approximately 25°C (77°F)
Protect from light
Keep bottles tightly closed
Dispense in a light-resistant, tight container
Use carton to protect blisters from light
10 mg, round, white tablets imprinted "WYETH 4153" on one side and deeply scored on reverse side:
NDC 0008-4153-01, bottles of 100.
NDC 0008-4152-02, bottles of 500.
NDC 0008-4153-03, bottles of 1,000.
NDC 0008-4153-05, Redipak cartons of 100 (10 blister strips of 10).
Store at room temperature, approximately 25°C (77°F)
Keep bottles tightly closed
Dispense in a tight container
20 mg, round, green tablets imprinted "WYETH 4154" on one side and deeply scored on reverse side:
NDC 0008-4154-01, bottles of 100.
NDC 0008-4154-02, bottles of 500.
NDC 0008-4154-05, Redipak cartons of 100 (10 blister strips of 10).
30 mg, round, blue tablets imprinted "WYETH 4159" on one side and deeply scored on reverse side:
NDC 0008-4159-01, bottles of 100.
NDC 0008-4159-02, bottles of 500.
NDC 0008-4159-04, Redipak cartons of 100 (10 blister strips of 10).
40 mg, round, light green tablets imprinted "WYETH 4192" on one side and deeply scored on reverse side:
NDC 0008-4192-01, bottles of 100.
NDC 0008-4192-04, Redipak cartons of 100 (10 blister strips of 10).
Store at room temperature, approximately 25°C (77°F)
Protect from light
Keep bottles tightly closed
Dispense in a light-resistant, tight container
Use carton to protect blisters from light
US Pat No. Re. 29077
The appearances of these tablets are trademarks of Wyeth-Ayerst Laboratories.
ALSO AVAILABLE
Sublingual Tablets, 2.5 mg, NDC 0008-4139, in bottles of 100 or 500 and in Redipak cartons of 100 (10 blister strips of 10).
Sublingual Tablets, 5 mg, NDC 0008-4126, in bottles of 100 or 500 and in Redipak cartons of 100 (10 blister strips of 10).
Sublingual Tablets, 10 mg, NDC 0008-4161, in bottles of 100.
Tembids® Tablets, 40 mg, controlled-release tablets, NDC 0008-4125, in bottles of 100, 500 or 1,000.
Tembids® Capsules, 40 mg, controlled-release capsules, NDC 0008-4140, in bottles of 100 or 500.
Manufactured by:
Wyeth Laboratories Inc.
A Wyeth-Ayerst Company
Philadelphia, PA 19101

Shown in Product Identification Guide, page 344

LODINE® ℞

[lō 'deen]
(etodolac capsules and tablets)

DESCRIPTION

Lodine® (etodolac capsules and tablets) is a pyranocarboxylic acid chemically designated as (±) 1,8-diethyl-1,3,4,9-tetrahydropyrano-[3,4-b]indole-1-acetic acid. The structural formula for etodolac is shown below:

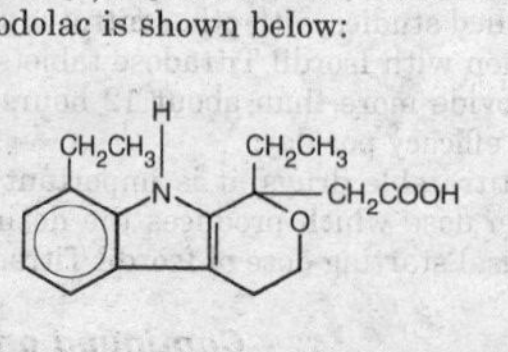

The empirical formula for etodolac is $C_{17}H_{21}NO_3$. The molecular weight of the base is 287.37. It has a pKa of 4.65 and an n-octanol:water partition coefficient of 11.4 at pH 7.4. Etodolac is a white crystalline compound, insoluble in water but soluble in alcohols, chloroform, dimethyl sulfoxide, and aqueous polyethylene glycol.
Inactive ingredients are:
— *in capsules:* cellulose, gelatin, iron oxides, lactose, magnesium stearate, povidone, sodium lauryl sulfate, sodium starch glycolate, and titanium dioxide.
— *in tablets:* cellulose, hydroxypropyl methylcellulose, lactose, magnesium stearate, polyethylene glycol, polysorbate 80, povidone, sodium starch glycolate, and titanium dioxide. The 400 mg tablets contain D&C Yellow #10, FD&C Blue #2, and FD&C Yellow #6 as color additives. The 500 mg tablets contain FD&C Blue #2 only.
Lodine is available in 200 and 300 mg capsules, and 400 and 500 mg tablets, for oral administration.

CLINICAL PHARMACOLOGY

PHARMACOLOGY
Etodolac is a nonsteroidal anti-inflammatory drug (NSAID) that exhibits anti-inflammatory, analgesic, and antipyretic activities in animal models. The mechanism of action of etodolac, like that of other NSAIDs, is not known but is believed to be associated with the inhibition of prostaglandin biosynthesis.
Lodine is a racemic mixture of [-]R- and [+]S-etodolac. As with other NSAIDs, it has been demonstrated in animals that the [+]S-form is biologically active. Both enantiomers are stable and there is no [-]R to [+]S conversion *in vivo*.
PHARMACODYNAMICS
Analgesia was demonstrable $^1/_2$ hour following single doses of 200 to 400 mg Lodine, with the peak effect occurring in 1 to 2 hours. The analgesic effect generally lasted for 4 to 6 hours (see **Clinical Trials**).
PHARMACOKINETICS
The pharmacokinetics of etodolac have been evaluated in 267 normal subjects, 44 elderly patients (>65 years old), 19 patients with renal failure (creatinine clearance 37 to 88 mL/min), 9 patients on hemodialysis, and 10 patients with compensated hepatic cirrhosis.
Etodolac, when administered orally, exhibits kinetics that are well described by a two-compartment model with first-order absorption.
Lodine has no apparent pharmacokinetic interaction when administered with phenytoin, glyburide, furosemide or hydrochlorothiazide.
ABSORPTION
Etodolac is well absorbed and had a relative bioavailability of 100% when 200 mg capsules were compared with a solution of etodolac. Based on mass balance studies, the systemic availability of etodolac from either the tablet or capsule formulation, is at least 80%. Etodolac does not undergo significant first-pass metabolism following oral administration. Mean (± 1 SD) peak plasma concentrations range from approximately 14 ± 4 to 37 ± 9 µg/mL after 200 to 600 mg single doses and are reached in 80 ± 30 minutes (see Table 1 for summary of pharmacokinetic parameters). The dose-proportionality based on AUC (the area under the plasma concentration-time curve) is linear following doses up to 600 mg every 12 hours. Peak concentrations are dose proportional for both total and free etodolac following doses up to 400 mg every 12 hours, but following a 600 mg dose, the peak is about 20% higher than predicted on the basis of lower doses.

Table 1. Etodolac Steady-State Pharmacokinetic Parameters
(N=267)

Kinetic Parameters	Mean ± SD
Extent of oral absorption (bioavailability) [F]	≥80%
Oral-dose clearance [CL/F]	47 ± 16 mL/h/kg
Steady-state volume [V_{ss}/F]	362 ± 129 mL/kg
Distribution half-life [$t_{1/2}$,α]	0.71 ± 0.50 h
Terminal half-life [$t_{1/2}$, β]	7.3 ± 4.0 h

Antacid Effects
The extent of absorption of etodolac is not affected when Lodine is administered with an antacid. Coadministration with an antacid decreases the peak concentration reached by about 15 to 20%, with no measurable effect on time-to-peak.
Food Effects
The extent of absorption of etodolac is not affected when Lodine is administered after a meal. Food intake, however, reduces the peak concentration reached by approximately one half and increases the time-to-peak concentration by 1.4 to 3.8 hours.
Distribution
Etodolac has an apparent steady-state volume of distribution about 0.362 L/kg. Within the therapeutic dose range, etodolac is more than 99% bound to plasma proteins. The free fraction is less than 1% and is independent of etodolac total concentration over the dose range studied.
Metabolism
Etodolac is extensively metabolized in the liver, with renal elimination of etodolac and its metabolites being the primary route of excretion. The intersubject variability of etodolac plasma levels, achieved after recommended doses, is substantial.
Protein Binding
Data from *in vitro* studies, using peak serum concentrations at reported therapeutic doses in humans, show that the etodolac free fraction is not significantly altered by acetaminophen, ibuprofen, indomethacin, naproxen, piroxicam, chlorpropamide, glipizide, glyburide, phenytoin, and probenecid.
Elimination
The mean plasma clearance of etodolac, following oral dosing is 47 (± 16) mL/h/kg, and terminal disposition half-life is 7.3 (± 4.0) hours. Approximately 72% of the administered dose is recovered in the urine as the following, indicated as % of the administered dose:

— etodolac, unchanged	1%
— etodolac glucuronide	13%
— hydroxylated metabolites (6-, 7-, and 8-OH)	5%
— hydroxylated metabolite glucuronides	20%
— unidentified metabolites	33%

Fecal excretion accounted for 16% of the dose.
SPECIAL POPULATIONS
Elderly Patients
In clinical studies, etodolac clearance was reduced by about 15% in older patients (>65 years of age). In these studies, age was shown not to have any effect on etodolac half-life or protein binding, and there was no change in expected drug accumulation. No dosage adjustment is generally necessary in the elderly on the basis of pharmacokinetics. The elderly may need dosage adjustment, however, on the basis of body size (see **Precautions**—GERIATRIC POPULATION), as they may be more sensitive to antiprostaglandin effects than younger patients (see **Precautions**—GERIATRIC POPULATION).
Renal Impairment
Studies in patients with mild-to-moderate renal impairment (creatinine clearance 37 to 88 mL/min) showed no significant differences in the disposition of total and free etodolac. In patients undergoing hemodialysis, there was a 50% greater apparent clearance of total etodolac, due to a 50% greater unbound fraction. Free etodolac clearance was not altered, indicating the importance of protein binding in etodolac's disposition. Nevertheless, etodolac is not dialyzable.
Hepatic Impairment
In patients with compensated hepatic cirrhosis, the disposition of total and free etodolac is not altered. Although no dosage adjustment is generally required in this patient population, etodolac clearance is dependent on hepatic function and could be reduced in patients with severe hepatic failure.

CLINICAL TRIALS

ANALGESIA
Controlled clinical trials in analgesia were single-dose, randomized, double-blind, parallel studies in three pain models, including dental extractions. The analgesic effective dose for Lodine established in these acute pain models was 200 to 400 mg. The onset of analgesia occurred approximately 30 minutes after oral administration. Lodine 200 mg provided efficacy comparable to that obtained with aspirin (650 mg). Lodine 400 mg provided efficacy comparable to that obtained with acetaminophen with codeine (600 mg + 60 mg). The peak analgesic effect was between 1 to 2 hours. Duration of relief averaged 4 to 5 hours for 200 mg of Lodine and 5 to 6 hours for 400 mg of Lodine as measured by when approximately half of the patients required remedication.
OSTEOARTHRITIS
The use of Lodine in managing the signs and symptoms of osteoarthritis of the hip or knee was assessed in double-blind, randomized, controlled clinical trials in 341 patients. In patients with osteoarthritis of the knee, Lodine, in doses of 600 to 1000 mg/day, was better than placebo in two studies. The clinical trials in osteoarthritis used b.i.d. dosage regimens.
RHEUMATOID ARTHRITIS
In a 3-month study with 426 patients, Lodine 300 mg b.i.d. was effective in management of rheumatoid arthritis and comparable in efficacy to piroxicam 20 mg/day. In a long-term study with 1,446 patients in which 60% of patients completed 6 months of therapy and 20% completed 3 years of therapy, Lodine in a dose of 500 mg b.i.d. provided efficacy comparable to that obtained with ibuprofen 600 mg q.i.d. In clinical trials of rheumatoid arthritis patients, Lodine has been used in combination with gold, d-penicillamine, chloroquine, corticosteroids, and methotrexate.

INDICATIONS AND USAGE

Lodine is indicated for acute and long-term use in the management of signs and symptoms of osteoarthritis and rheumatoid arthritis. Lodine is also indicated for the management of pain.

CONTRAINDICATIONS

Lodine is contraindicated in patients with known hypersensitivity to etodolac. Lodine should not be given to patients who have experienced asthma, urticaria, or other allergic-type reactions after taking aspirin or other NSAIDs. Severe, rarely fatal, anaphylactic-like reactions to Lodine have been reported in such patients (see **Warnings**—ANAPHYLACTOID REACTIONS).

WARNINGS

RISK OF GASTROINTESTINAL (GI) ULCERATION, BLEEDING, AND PERFORATION WITH NONSTEROIDAL ANTI-INFLAMMATORY DRUG (NSAID) THERAPY

Serious GI toxicity, such as bleeding, ulceration, and perforation, can occur at any time, with or without warning symptoms, in patients treated chronically with NSAIDs. Although minor upper GI problems, such as dyspepsia, are common, usually developing early in therapy, physicians should remain alert for ulceration and bleeding in patients treated chronically with NSAIDs, even in the absence of previous GI-tract symptoms. In patients observed in clinical trials of such agents for several months' to 2 years' duration, symptomatic upper GI ulcers, gross bleeding, or perforation appears to occur in approximately 1% of patients treated for 3 to 6 months and in about 2% to 4% of patients treated for 1 year. Physicians should inform patients about the signs and/or symptoms of serious GI toxicity and what steps to take if they occur.

Studies to date have not identified any subset of patients not at risk of developing peptic ulceration and bleeding. Except for a prior history of serious GI events and other risk factors known to be associated with peptic ulcer disease, such as alcoholism, smoking, etc., no risk factors (e.g., age, sex) have been associated with increased risk. Elderly or debilitated patients seem to tolerate ulceration or bleeding less well than other individuals, and most spontaneous reports of fatal GI events are in this population. Studies to date are inconclusive concerning the relative risk of various NSAIDs in causing such reactions. High doses of any NSAID probably carry a greater risk of these reactions, although controlled clinical trials showing this do not exist in most cases. In considering the use of relatively large doses (within the recommended dosage range), sufficient benefit should be anticipated to offset the potential increased risk of GI toxicity.

ANAPHYLACTOID REACTIONS

Anaphylactoid reactions may occur in patients without prior exposure to etodolac. Lodine should not be given to patients with the aspirin triad. The triad typically occurs in asthmatic patients who experience rhinitis with or without nasal polyps, or who exhibit severe, potentially fatal bronchospasm after taking aspirin or other nonsteroidal anti-inflammatory drugs. Fatal reactions have been reported in such patients (see **Contraindications** and **Precautions**—*Pre-existing Asthma*). Emergency help should be sought in cases where an anaphylactoid reaction occurs.

ADVANCED RENAL DISEASE

In cases with advanced kidney disease, as with other NSAIDs, treatment with Lodine should only be initiated with close monitoring of the patient's kidney function (see **Precautions**—*Renal Effects*).

PREGNANCY

In late pregnancy, as with other NSAIDs, Lodine should be avoided because it may cause premature closure of the ductus arteriosus (see **Precautions**—*Teratogenic Effects—Pregnancy Category C*).

PRECAUTIONS

GENERAL PRECAUTIONS

Renal Effects

As with other NSAIDs, long-term administration of etodolac to rats has resulted in renal papillary necrosis and other renal medullary changes. Renal pelvic transitional epithelial hyperplasia, a spontaneous change occurring with variable frequency, was observed with increased frequency in treated male rats in a 2-year chronic study.

A second form of renal toxicity encountered with Lodine, as with other NSAIDs, is seen in patients with conditions in which renal prostaglandins have a supportive role in the maintenance of renal perfusion. In these patients, administration of a nonsteroidal anti-inflammatory drug may cause a dose-dependent reduction in prostaglandin formation and, secondarily, in renal blood flow, which may precipitate overt renal decompensation. Patients at greatest risk of this reaction are those with impaired renal function, heart failure, or liver dysfunction; those taking diuretics; and the elderly. Discontinuation of nonsteroidal anti-inflammatory drug therapy is usually followed by recovery to the pretreatment state.

Etodolac metabolites are eliminated primarily by the kidneys. The extent to which the inactive glucuronide metabolites may accumulate in patients with renal failure has not been studied. As with other drugs whose metabolites are excreted by the kidney, the possibility that adverse reactions (not listed in **Adverse Reactions**) may be attributable to these metabolites should be considered.

Hepatic Effects

Borderline elevations of one or more liver tests may occur in up to 15% of patients taking NSAIDs, including Lodine. These abnormalities may disappear, remain essentially unchanged, or progress with continued therapy. Meaningful elevations of ALT or AST (approximately three or more times the upper limit of normal) have been reported in approximately 1% of patients in clinical trials with Lodine. A patient with symptoms and/or signs suggesting liver dysfunction, or in whom an abnormal liver test has occurred, should be evaluated for evidence of the development of a more severe hepatic reaction while on therapy with Lodine. Rare cases of liver necrosis and hepatic failure, some of them with fatal outcomes have been reported. If clinical signs and symptoms consistent with liver disease develop, or if systemic manifestations occur (e.g. eosinophilia, rash, etc.), Lodine should be discontinued.

Hematological Effects

Anemia is sometimes seen in patients receiving NSAIDs including Lodine. This may be due to fluid retention, GI blood loss, or an incompletely described effect upon erythropoiesis. Patients on long-term treatment with NSAIDs, including Lodine, should have their hemoglobin or hematocrit checked if they exhibit any signs or symptoms of anemia.

All drugs which inhibit the biosynthesis of prostaglandins may interfere to some extent with platelet function and vascular responses to bleeding.

Fluid Retention and Edema

Fluid retention and edema have been observed in some patients taking NSAIDs, including Lodine. Therefore, Lodine should be used with caution in patients with fluid retention, hypertension, or heart failure.

Pre-existing Asthma

About 10% of patients with asthma may have aspirin-sensitive asthma. The use of aspirin in patients with aspirin-sensitive asthmas has been associated with severe bronchospasm which can be fatal. Since cross reactivity, including bronchospasm, between aspirin and other nonsteroidal anti-inflammatory drugs has been reported in such aspirin-sensitive patients, etodolac should not be administered to patients with this form of aspirin sensitivity and should be used with caution in all patients with pre-existing asthma.

INFORMATION FOR PATIENTS

Lodine, like other drugs of its class, can cause discomfort and, rarely, more serious side effects, such as gastrointestinal bleeding, which may result in hospitalization and even fatal outcomes.

Physicians may wish to discuss with their patients the potential risks (see **Warnings**, **Precautions**, **Adverse Reactions**) and likely benefits of nonsteroidal anti-inflammatory drug treatment.

Patients on Lodine should report to their physicians signs or symptoms of gastrointestinal ulceration or bleeding, blurred vision or other eye symptoms, skin rash, weight gain, or edema.

Because serious gastrointestinal tract ulcerations and bleeding can occur without warning symptoms, physicians should follow chronically treated patients for the signs and symptoms of ulcerations and bleeding and should inform them of the importance of this follow-up (see **Warnings**—RISK OF GI ULCERATION, BLEEDING AND PERFORATION WITH NONSTEROIDAL ANTI-INFLAMMATORY THERAPY).

Patients should also be instructed to seek medical emergency help in case of an occurrence of anaphylactoid reactions (see **Warnings**).

LABORATORY TESTS

Patients on long-term treatment with Lodine, as with other NSAIDs, should have their hemoglobin or hematocrit checked periodically for signs or symptoms of anemia. Appropriate measures should be taken in case such signs of anemia occur.

If clinical signs and symptoms consistent with liver disease develop or if systemic manifestations occur (e.g., eosinophilia, rash, etc.) and if abnormal liver tests are detected, persist or worsen, Lodine should be discontinued.

DRUG INTERACTIONS

Antacids

The concomitant administration of antacids has no apparent effect on the extent of absorption of Lodine. However, antacids can decrease the peak concentration reached by 15% to 20% but have no detectable effect on the time-to-peak.

Aspirin

When Lodine is administered with aspirin, its protein binding is reduced, although the clearance of free etodolac is not altered. The clinical significance of this interaction is not known; however, as with other NSAIDs, concomitant administration of Lodine and aspirin is not generally recommended because of the potential of increased adverse effects.

Warfarin

Short-term pharmacokinetic studies have demonstrated that concomitant administration of warfarin and Lodine results in reduced protein binding of warfarin, but there was no change in the clearance of free warfarin. There was no significant difference in the pharmacodynamic effect of warfarin administered alone and warfarin administered with Lodine as measured by prothrombin time. Thus, concomitant therapy with warfarin and Lodine should not require dosage adjustment of either drug. However, there have been a few spontaneous reports of prolonged prothrombin times in Lodine-treated patients receiving concomitant warfarin therapy. Caution should be exercised because interactions have been seen with other NSAIDs.

Cyclosporin, Digoxin, Lithium, Methotrexate

Lodine, like other NSAIDs, through effects on renal prostaglandins, may cause changes in the elimination of these drugs leading to elevated serum levels of digoxin, lithium, and methotrexate and increased toxicity. Nephrotoxicity associated with cyclosporine may also be enhanced. Patients receiving these drugs who are given Lodine, or any other NSAID, and particularly those patients with altered renal function, should be observed for the development of the specific toxicities of these drugs.

Phenylbutazone

Phenylbutazone causes increase (by about 80%) in the free fraction of etodolac. Although *in vivo* studies have not been done to see if etodolac clearance is changed by coadministration of phenylbutazone, it is not recommended that they be coadministered.

DRUG/LABORATORY TEST INTERACTIONS

The urine of patients who take Lodine can give a false-positive reaction for urinary bilirubin (urobilin) due to the presence of phenolic metabolites of etodolac. Diagnostic dip-stick methodology, used to detect ketone bodies in urine, has resulted in false-positive findings in some patients treated with Lodine. Generally, this phenomenon has not been associated with other clinically significant events. No dose relationship has been observed.

Lodine treatment is associated with a small decrease in serum uric acid levels. In clinical trials, mean decreases of 1 to 2 mg/dL were observed in arthritic patients receiving etodolac (600 mg to 1000 mg/day) after 4 weeks of therapy. These levels then remained stable for up to 1 year of therapy.

CARCINOGENESIS, MUTAGENESIS, AND IMPAIRMENT OF FERTILITY

No carcinogenic effect of etodolac was observed in mice or rats receiving oral doses of 15 mg/kg/day (45 to 89 mg/m^2, respectively) or less for periods of 2 years or 18 months, respectively. Etodolac was not mutagenic in *in vitro* tests performed with *S. typhimurium* and mouse lymphoma cells as well as in an *in vivo* mouse micronucleus test. However, data from the *in vitro* human peripheral lymphocyte test showed an increase in the number of gaps (3.0 to 5.3% unstained regions in the chromatid without dislocation) among the Lodine-treated cultures (50 to 200 µg/mL) compared to negative controls (2.0%); no other difference was noted between the controls and drug-treated groups. Etodolac showed no impairment of fertility in male and female rats up to oral doses of 16 mg/kg (94 mg/m^2). However, reduced implantation of fertilized eggs occurred in the 8 mg/kg group.

PREGNANCY

Teratogenic Effects—Pregnancy Category C

In teratology studies, isolated occurrences of alterations in limb development were found and included polydactyly, oligodactyly, syndactyly, and unossified phalanges in rats and oligodactyly and synostosis of metatarsals in rabbits. These were observed at dose levels (2 to 14 mg/kg/day) close to human clinical doses. However, the frequency and the dosage group distribution of these findings in initial or repeated studies did not establish a clear drug or dose-response relationship.

There are no adequate or well-controlled studies in pregnant women. Lodine should be used during pregnancy only if the potential benefits justify the potential risk to the fetus. Because of the known effects of NSAIDs on parturition and on the human fetal cardiovascular system with respect to closure of the ductus arteriosus, use during late pregnancy should be avoided.

LABOR AND DELIVERY

In rat studies with etodolac, as with other drugs known to inhibit prostaglandin synthesis, an increased incidence of dystocia, delayed parturition, and decreased pup survival occurred. The effects of Lodine on labor and delivery in pregnant women are unknown.

NURSING MOTHERS

It is not known whether etodolac is excreted in human milk. Because many drugs are excreted in human milk and because of the potential for serious adverse reactions in nursing infants from etodolac, a decision should be made

Continued on next page

Lodine—Cont.

whether to discontinue nursing or to discontinue the drug taking into account the importance of the drug to the mother.

PEDIATRIC USE

Safety and effectiveness in pediatric patients have not been established.

GERIATRIC POPULATION

As with any NSAID, however, caution should be exercised in treating the elderly, and when individualizing their dosage, extra care should be taken when increasing the dose because the elderly seem to tolerate NSAID side effects less well than younger patients. In patients 65 years and older, no substantial differences in the side effect profile of Lodine were seen compared with the general population (see **Clinical Pharmacology—**PHARMACOKINETICS.)

ADVERSE REACTIONS

Adverse-reaction information for Lodine was derived from 2,629 arthritic patients treated with Lodine in double-blind and open-label clinical trials of 4 to 320 weeks in duration and worldwide postmarketing surveillance studies. In clinical trials, most adverse reactions were mild and transient. The discontinuation rate in controlled clinical trials, because of adverse events, was up to 10% for patients treated with Lodine.

New patient complaints (with an incidence greater than or equal to 1%) are listed below by body system. The incidences were determined from clinical trials involving 465 patients with osteoarthritis treated with 300 to 500 mg of Lodine b.i.d. (i.e., 600 to 1000 mg/day).

INCIDENCE GREATER THAN OR EQUAL TO 1%—PROBABLY CAUSALLY RELATED

Body as a whole—Chills and fever.

Digestive system—Dyspepsia (10%), abdominal pain*, diarrhea*, flatulence*, nausea*, constipation, gastritis, melena, vomiting.

Nervous system—Asthenia/malaise*, dizziness*, depression, nervousness.

Skin and appendages—Pruritus, rash.

Special senses—Blurred vision, tinnitus.

Urogenital system—Dysuria, urinary frequency.

*Drug-related patient complaints occurring in 3 to 9% of patients treated with Lodine.

Drug-related patient-complaints occurring in fewer than 3%, but more than 1%, are unmarked.

INCIDENCE LESS THAN 1%—PROBABLY CAUSALLY RELATED

(Adverse reactions reported only in worldwide postmarketing experience, not seen in clinical trials, are considered rarer and are italicized)

Body as a whole—*Allergic reaction, anaphylactoid reaction.*

Cardiovascular system—Hypertension, congestive heart failure, flushing, palpitations, syncope, *vasculitis (including necrotizing and allergic).*

Digestive system—Thirst, dry mouth, ulcerative stomatitis, anorexia, eructation, elevated liver enzymes, *cholestatic hepatitis,* hepatitis, *cholestatic jaundice, duodenitis, jaundice, hepatic failure, liver necrosis,* peptic ulcer with or without bleeding and/or perforation, *intestinal ulceration, pancreatitis.*

Hemic and lymphatic system—Ecchymosis, anemia, thrombocytopenia, bleeding time increased, *agranulocytosis, hemolytic anemia, leukopenia, neutropenia, pancytopenia.*

Metabolic and nutritional—Edema, serum creatinine increase, *hyperglycemia in previously controlled diabetic patients.*

Nervous system—Insomnia, somnolence.

Respiratory system—Asthma.

Skin and appendages—Angioedema, sweating, urticaria, vesiculobullous rash, *cutaneous vasculitis with purpura, Stevens-Johnson Syndrome,* hyperpigmentation, *erythema multiforme.*

Special senses—Photophobia, transient visual disturbances.

Urogenital system—*Elevated BUN, renal failure, renal insufficiency, renal papillary necrosis.*

INCIDENCE LESS THAN 1%—CAUSAL RELATIONSHIP UNKNOWN (Medical events occurring under circumstances where causal relationship to Lodine is uncertain. These reactions are listed as alerting information for physicians)

Body as a whole—Infection, headache.

Cardiovascular system—Arrhythmias, myocardial infarction, cerebrovascular accident.

Digestive system—Esophagitis with or without stricture or cardiospasm, colitis.

Metabolic and nutritional—Change in weight.

Nervous system—Paresthesia, confusion.

Respiratory system—Bronchitis, dyspnea, pharyngitis, rhinitis, sinusitis.

Skin and appendages—Alopecia, maculopapular rash, photosensitivity, skin peeling.

Special senses—Conjunctivitis, deafness, taste perversion.

Urogenital system—Cystitis, hematuria, leukorrhea, renal calculus, interstitial nephritis, uterine bleeding irregularities.

OVERDOSAGE

Symptoms following acute NSAID overdose are usually limited to lethargy, drowsiness, nausea, vomiting, and epigastric pain, which are generally reversible with supportive care. Gastrointestinal bleeding can occur and coma has occurred following massive ibuprofen or mefenamic-acid overdose. Hypertension, acute renal failure, and respiratory depression may occur but are rare. Anaphylactoid reactions have been reported with therapeutic ingestion of NSAIDs, and may occur following overdose.

Patients should be managed by symptomatic and supportive care following an NSAID overdose. There are no specific antidotes. Gut decontamination may be indicated in patients seen within 4 hours of ingestion with symptoms or following a large overdose (5 to 10 times the usual dose). This should be accomplished via emesis and/or activated charcoal (60 to 100 g in adults, 1 to 2 g/kg in children) with an osmotic cathartic. Forced diuresis, alkalinization of the urine, hemodialysis, or hemoperfusion would probably not be useful due to etodolac's high protein binding.

DOSAGE AND ADMINISTRATION

As with other NSAIDs, the lowest dose and longest dosing interval should be sought for each patient. Therefore, after observing the response to initial therapy with Lodine, the dose and frequency should be adjusted to suit an individual patient's needs.

Dosage adjustment of Lodine is generally not required in patients with mild to moderate renal impairment. Etodolac should be used with caution in such patients, because, as with other NSAIDs, it may further decrease renal function in some patients with impaired renal function. (see **Precautions**—GENERAL PRECAUTIONS, *Renal Effects).*

ANALGESIA

The recommended total daily dose of Lodine for acute pain is up to 1000 mg, given as 200–400 mg every 6 to 8 hours. In some patients, if the potential benefits outweigh the risks; the dose may be increased to 1200 mg/day in order to achieve a therapeutic benefit that might not have been achieved with 1000 mg/day. Doses of etodolac greater than 1000 mg/day have not been adequately evaluated in well-controlled clinical trials.

OSTEOARTHRITIS AND RHEUMATOID ARTHRITIS

The recommended starting dose of Lodine for the management of the signs and symptoms of osteoarthritis or rheumatoid arthritis is: 300 mg b.i.d., t.i.d., or 400 mg b.i.d., or 500 mg b.i.d. During long-term administration, the dose of Lodine may be adjusted up or down depending on the clinical response of the patient. A lower dose of 600 mg/day may suffice for long-term administration. In patients who tolerate 1000 mg/day, the dose may be increased to 1200 mg/day when a higher level of therapeutic activity is required. When treating patients with higher doses, the physician should observe sufficient increased clinical benefit to justify the higher dose. Physicians should be aware that doses above 1000 mg/day have not been adequately evaluated in well-controlled clinical trials.

In chronic conditions, a therapeutic response to therapy with Lodine is sometimes seen within one week of therapy, but most often is observed by two weeks. After a satisfactory response has been achieved, the patient's dose should be reviewed and adjusted as required.

HOW SUPPLIED

Lodine (etodolac capsules and tablets) is available as:

Lodine® (etodolac capsules) Capsules

200 mg capsules (light gray with one wide red band with LODINE 200/white with two narrow red bands)

— in bottles of 100, NDC 0046-0738-81

— in unit-dose packages of 100, NDC 0046-0738-99

300 mg capsules (light gray with one red band with LODINE 300/light gray with two narrow red bands)

— in bottles of 100, NDC 0046-0739-81

— in unit-dose packages of 100, NDC 0046-0739-99

Store at controlled room temperature 20°–25°C (68°–77°F), protected from moisture.

Lodine® (etodolac tablets) Tablets

400 mg tablets (yellow-orange, oval, film-coated tablet, debossed LODINE 400 on one side)

— in bottles of 100, NDC 0046-0761-81

— in unit-dose packages of 100, NDC 0046-0761-99

Store at controlled room temperature 20°–25°C (68°–77°F). Store tablets in original container until ready to use. Dispense in light-resistant container.

500 mg tablets (blue, oval, film-coated tablet, branded LODINE 500 on one side)

— in bottles of 100, NDC 0046-0787-81

— in unit-dose packages of 100, NDC 0046-0787-99

Store at controlled room temperature 20°–25°C (68°–77°F). Store tablets in original container until ready to use. Dispense in light-resistant container.

The appearance of these capsules is a registered trademark of Wyeth-Ayerst Laboratories and the appearance of these tablets is a trademark of Wyeth-Ayerst Laboratories.

Caution: Federal law prohibits dispensing without prescription.

Manufactured by:
Ayerst Laboratories
A Wyeth-Ayerst Company
Philadelphia, PA 19101

Shown in Product Identification Guide, page 344

LODINE® XL ℞

[lō 'deen XL]

(etodolac extended-release tablets)

DESCRIPTION

Lodine® XL (etodolac extended-release tablets) contains etodolac in an extended-release formulation. Etodolac is a pyranocarboxylic acid, chemically designated as (±) 1,8-diethyl-1,3,4,9-tetrahydropyrano-[3,4-b]indole-1-acetic acid. The structural formula is shown below:

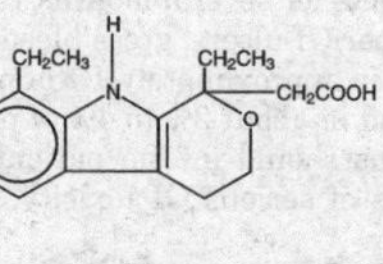

The empirical formula is $C_{17}H_{21}NO_3$. The molecular weight of the base is 287.37. It has a pKa of 4.65 and an n-octanol: water partition coefficient of 11.4 at pH 7.4. Etodolac is a white crystalline compound, insoluble in water, but soluble in alcohols, chloroform, dimethyl sulfoxide, and aqueous polyethylene glycol.

The inactive ingredients are dibasic sodium phosphate, ethylcellulose, hydroxypropyl methylcellulose, lactose, magnesium stearate, polyethylene glycol, and titanium dioxide. In addition, the 400 mg tablets also contain FD&C Red #40, and FD&C Yellow #6 as color additives and polysorbate 80. The 500 mg tablets also contain D&C Yellow #10, FD&C Blue #2, and iron oxide as color additives and polysorbate 80. The 600 mg tablets also contain hydroxypropyl cellulose and iron oxide. Lodine XL is available in 400, 500 and 600 mg tablets, for oral administration.

CLINICAL PHARMACOLOGY

PHARMACOLOGY

Etodolac is a nonsteroidal anti-inflammatory drug (NSAID) that exhibits anti-inflammatory, analgesic, and antipyretic activities in animal models. The mechanism of action of etodolac, like that of other NSAIDs, is not known, but is believed to be associated with the inhibition of prostaglandin biosynthesis.

PHARMACOKINETICS

The activity of Lodine XL is due to the parent drug, etodolac. The free fraction is less than 1% and is independent of concentration over the therapeutic range. Etodolac is not dialyzable. Etodolac is extensively metabolized in the liver, with renal elimination of its metabolites. The terminal half-life ranges between 7.3 and 8.3 hours. Less than 1% of the dose is excreted unchanged in urine.

Absorption

Lodine and Lodine XL both contain etodolac, but differ in their release characteristics. The systemic availability of etodolac from Lodine XL is generally greater than 80%. After administration of 400 mg of Lodine XL, a C_{max} of 8.6 µg/mL was observed 3 to 12 hours post dose. Peak concentrations are dose proportional for both total and free etodolac following Lodine doses up to 400 mg every 12 hours, but following a 600 mg dose, the peak is about 20% higher than predicted on the basis of lower doses. After oral administration of Lodine XL in doses of 800 mg once daily, peak concentrations are dose proportional for both total and free etodolac whereas peak concentrations following 1200 mg Lodine XL once daily were about 20% lower than that predicted by lower doses. Table 1 shows the comparison of pharmacokinetic parameters for etodolac and Lodine XL.

[See table 1 at top of next page]

Antacid Effects

The extent of absorption of etodolac is not affected when etodolac is administered with an antacid. Coadministration with an antacid decreases the peak concentration reached by about 15 to 20%, with no measurable effect on time-to-peak.

Food Effects

Following administration of Lodine XL, etodolac is well absorbed with peak plasma concentrations occurring 3 to 12 hours after dosing. Food produced a much faster rise in plasma levels with time to peak concentrations (T_{max}) rang-

TABLE 1

Kinetic Parameters	Mean ± SD	
	Lodine	Lodine XL
Extent of oral absorption (bioavailability) [F]	≥80%	≥80%
Time to Peak Concentration [t_{max}]	1.7 ± 1.3 h	6.9 ± 3.3 h
Oral-dose clearance [CL/F]	47 ± 16 mL/h/kg	40 ± 19 mL/h/kg
Steady-state volume [V_{ss}/F]	362 ± 129 mL/kg	308 ± 110 mL/kg
Apparent half-life [$t_{1/2}$,β]	7.3 ± 4.0 h	8.3 ± 2.4 h

ing from 1.5 to 6 hours after dosing. The extent of absorption of etodolac after administration of Lodine XL is not affected by a high-fat meal. Although the high-fat meal produced a significantly higher peak concentration (54% increase) following a 600 mg dose of Lodine XL, this is 40% less than that observed following a single 400 mg dose of Lodine (standard release) administered under fasted conditions.

Distribution

Etodolac has an apparent steady-state volume of distribution between 308 and 362 mL/kg. Within the therapeutic dose range, etodolac is more than 99% bound to plasma proteins. The free fraction is less than 1% and is independent of etodolac total concentration over the dose range studied.

Protein Binding

Data from *in vitro* studies, using peak serum concentrations at reported therapeutic doses in humans, show that the etodolac free fraction is not significantly altered by acetaminophen, ibuprofen, indomethacin, naproxen, piroxicam, chlorpropamide, glipizide, glyburide, phenytoin, and probenecid.

Metabolism

Etodolac does not undergo significant first-pass metabolism following oral administration. It is extensively metabolized in the liver, with renal elimination of etodolac and its metabolites being the primary route of excretion. Etodolac has no apparent pharmacokinetic interaction when administered with phenytoin, glyburide, furosemide, hydrochlororthiazide, or methotrexate (see **Precautions**—DRUG INTERACTIONS).

Elimination

The mean plasma clearance of etodolac is in the range of 40 to 47 mL/h/kg. The terminal disposition half-life is approximately 7 to 8 hours. Approximately 72% of the administered dose is recovered in the urine as the following, indicated as % of the administered dose:

—etodolac, unchanged	1%
—etodolac glucuronide	13%
—hydroxylated metabolites (6-, 7-, and 8-OH)	5%
—hydroxylated metabolite glucuronides	20%
—unidentified metabolites	33%

Fecal excretion accounted for 16% of the dose.

SPECIAL POPULATIONS

Elderly Patients

In clinical studies, etodolac clearance was reduced by about 15% in older patients (>65 years of age). In these studies, age was not shown to have any effect on half-life or protein binding, and demonstrated no change in expected drug accumulation. No dosage adjustment is generally necessary in the elderly on the basis of pharmacokinetics. The elderly may need dosage adjustment, however, as they may be more sensitive to antiprostaglandin effects than younger patients (see **Precautions**—GERIATRIC POPULATION).

Renal Impairment

Studies in patients with mild-to-moderate renal impairment (creatinine clearance 37 to 88 mL/min) showed no significant differences in the disposition of total and free etodolac. However, etodolac should be used with caution in such patients because, as with other NSAIDs, it may further decrease renal function in some patients.

In patients undergoing hemodialysis, there was a 50% greater apparent clearance of total etodolac, due to a 50% greater unbound fraction. Free etodolac clearance was not altered, indicating the importance of protein binding in etodolac's disposition. Nevertheless, etodolac is not dialyzable.

Hepatic Impairment

In patients with compensated hepatic cirrhosis, the disposition of total and free etodolac is not altered. Although no dosage adjustment is generally required in this patient population, etodolac clearance is dependent on hepatic function and could be reduced in patients with severe hepatic failure.

CLINICAL TRIALS

The use of Lodine XL in managing the signs and symptoms of osteoarthritis of the knee was assessed in double-blind, randomized, controlled clinical trials in 451 patients. In patients with osteoarthritis of the knee, Lodine XL in doses of 400 mg to 1200 mg, given once daily, provided efficacy comparable to etodolac given 300 mg b.i.d. to 400 mg t.i.d.

INDICATIONS AND USAGE

Lodine XL is indicated for the management of the signs and symptoms of osteoarthritis and rheumatoid arthritis.

CONTRAINDICATIONS

Lodine XL is contraindicated in patients with known hypersensitivity to etodolac. Lodine XL should not be given to patients who have experienced asthma, urticaria, or other allergic-type reactions after taking aspirin or other NSAIDs. Severe, rarely fatal, anaphylactic-like reactions to etodolac have been reported in such patients (see **Warnings**—ANAPHYLACTOID REACTIONS).

WARNINGS

RISK OF GASTROINTESTINAL (GI) ULCERATION, BLEEDING, AND PERFORATION WITH NONSTEROIDAL, ANTI-INFLAMMATORY DRUG (NSAID) THERAPY.

Serious GI toxicity, such as bleeding, ulceration, and perforation, can occur at any time, with or without warning symptoms, in patients treated chronically with NSAIDs. Although minor upper GI problems, such as dyspepsia, are common, usually developing early in therapy, physicians should remain alert for ulceration and bleeding in patients treated chronically with NSAIDs, even in the absence of previous GI-tract symptoms. In patients observed in clinical trials of such agents for several months to 2 years' duration, symptomatic upper GI ulcers, gross bleeding, or perforation appear to occur in approximately 1% of patients treated for 3 to 6 months and in about 2% to 4% of patients treated for 1 year. Physicians should inform patients about the signs and/or symptoms of serious GI toxicity and what steps to take if they occur.

Studies to date have not identified any subset of patients not at risk of developing peptic ulceration and bleeding. Except for a prior history of serious GI events and other risk factors known to be associated with peptic ulcer disease, such as alcoholism, smoking, etc., no risk factors (e.g., age, sex) have been associated with increased risk. Elderly or debilitated patients seem to tolerate ulceration or bleeding less well than other individuals, and most spontaneous reports of fatal GI events are in this population. Studies to date are inconclusive concerning the relative risk of various NSAIDs in causing such reactions. High doses of any NSAID probably carry a greater risk of these reactions, although controlled clinical trials showing this do not exist in most cases. In considering the use of relatively large doses (within the recommended dosage range), sufficient benefit should be anticipated to offset the potential increased risk of GI toxicity.

ANAPHYLACTOID REACTIONS

Anaphylactoid reactions may occur in patients without prior exposure to etodolac. Lodine XL should not be given to patients with the aspirin triad. The triad typically occurs in asthmatic patients who experience rhinitis with or without nasal polyps, or who exhibit severe, potentially fatal bronchospasm after taking aspirin or other NSAIDs. Fatal reactions have been reported in such patients (see **Contraindications** and **Precautions**—*Pre-existing Asthma*). Emergency help should be sought in cases where an anaphylactoid reaction occurs.

ADVANCED RENAL DISEASE

In cases with advanced kidney disease, as with other NSAIDs, treatment with Lodine XL should only be initiated with close monitoring of the patient's kidney function (see **Precautions**—*Renal Effects*).

PREGNANCY

In late pregnancy, as with other NSAIDs, Lodine XL should be avoided because it may cause premature closure of the ductus arteriosus (see **Precautions**—*Teratogenic Effects*).

PRECAUTIONS

GENERAL PRECAUTIONS

Renal Effects

As with other NSAIDs, long-term administration of etodolac to rats has resulted in renal papillary necrosis and other renal medullary changes. Renal pelvic transitional epithelial hyperplasia, a spontaneous change occurring with variable frequency, was observed with increased frequency in treated male rats in a 2-year chronic study.

A second form of renal toxicity encountered with etodolac, as with other NSAIDs, is seen in patients with conditions in which renal prostaglandins have a supportive role in the maintenance of renal perfusion. In these patients, administration of a nonsteroidal anti-inflammatory drug may cause a dose-dependent reduction in prostaglandin formation and, secondarily, in renal blood flow, which may precipitate overt renal decompensation. Patients at greatest risk of this reaction are those with impaired renal function, heart failure, or liver dysfunction; those taking diuretics; and the elderly. Discontinuation of nonsteroidal anti-inflammatory drug therapy is usually followed by recovery to the pretreatment state. Etodolac metabolites are eliminated primarily by the kidneys. The extent to which the inactive glucuronide metabolites may accumulate in patients with renal failure has not been studied. As with other drugs whose metabolites are excreted by the kidney, the possibility that adverse reactions (not listed in **Adverse Reactions**) may be attributable to these metabolites should be considered.

Hepatic Effects

Borderline elevations of one or more liver tests may occur in up to 15% of patients taking NSAIDs, including Lodine XL. These abnormalities may disappear, remain essentially unchanged, or progress with continued therapy. Meaningful elevations of ALT or AST (approximately three or more times the upper limit of normal) have been reported in approximately 1% of patients in clinical trials with etodolac. A patient with symptoms and/or signs suggesting liver dysfunction, or in whom an abnormal liver test has occurred, should be evaluated for evidence of the development of a more severe hepatic reaction while on therapy with Lodine XL. Rare cases of liver necrosis and hepatic failure, some of them with fatal outcomes have been reported. If clinical signs and symptoms consistent with liver disease develop, or if systemic manifestations occur (e.g., eosinophilia, rash, etc.), Lodine XL should be discontinued.

Hematological Effects

Anemia is sometimes seen in patients receiving etodolac or other NSAIDs. This may be due to fluid retention, GI blood loss, or an incompletely described effect upon erythropoiesis. Patients on long-term treatment with NSAIDs, including Lodine XL, should have their hemoglobin or hematocrit checked if they develop signs or symptoms of anemia. All drugs which inhibit the biosynthesis of prostaglandins may interfere to some extent with platelet function and vascular responses to bleeding.

Fluid Rentention and Edema

Fluid rentention and edema have been observed in some patients taking NSAIDs, including Lodine XL. Therefore, Lodine XL should be used with caution in patients with fluid retention, hypertension, or heart failure.

Pre-existing Asthma

About 10% of patients with asthma may have aspirin-sensitive asthma. The use of aspirin in patients with aspirin-sensitive asthma has been associated with severe bronchospasm which can be fatal. Since cross reactivity, including bronchospasm, between aspirin and other nonsteroidal anti-inflammatory drugs has been reported in such aspirin-sensitive patients, etodolac should not be administered to patients with this form of aspirin-sensitivity and should be used with caution in all patients with pre-existing asthma.

INFORMATION FOR PATIENTS

Lodine® XL, like other drugs of its class, can cause discomfort and, rarely, more serious side effects, such as gastrointestinal bleeding, which may result in hospitalization and even fatal outcomes.

Patients on Lodine XL should report to their physicians signs or symptoms of gastrointestinal ulceration or bleeding, blurred vision or other eye symptoms, skin rash, weight gain, or edema.

Because serious gastrointestinal tract ulcerations and bleeding can occur without warning symptoms, physicians should follow chronically treated patients for the signs and symptoms of ulcerations and bleeding and patients should be informed of the importance of this follow-up (see **Warnings**—RISK OF GI ULCERATION, BLEEDING AND PERFORATION WITH NONSTEROIDAL ANTI-INFLAMMATORY THERAPY).

Patients should also be instructed to seek medical emergency help in case of an occurrence of an anaphylactoid reaction (see **Warnings**).

LABORATORY TESTS

Patients on long-term treatment with Lodine XL, as with other NSAIDs, should have their hemoglobin or hematocrit checked periodically for signs or symptoms of anemia. Appropriate measures should be taken in case such signs of anemia occur.

If clinical signs and symptoms consistent with liver disease develop or if systemic manifestations occur (e.g., eosinophilia, rash, etc.) and if abnormal liver tests are detected, persist or worsen, Lodine XL should be discontinued.

DRUG INTERACTIONS

Antacids

The concomitant administration of antacids has no apparent effect on the extent of absorption of etodolac. However, antacids can decrease the peak concentration by 15% to 20%, but have no detectable effect on the time-to-peak concentration.

Aspirin

When etodolac is administered with aspirin, its protein binding is reduced, although the clearance of free etodolac is not altered. The clinical significance of this interaction is

Continued on next page

Lodine XL—Cont.

not known; however, as with other NSAIDs, concomitant administration of Lodine XL and aspirin is not generally recommended because of the potential of increased adverse effects.

Warfarin

Short-term pharmacokinetic studies have demonstrated that concomitant administration of warfarin and etodolac results in reduced protein binding of warfarin, but there was no change in the clearance of free warfarin. There was no significant difference in the pharmacodynamic effect of warfarin administered alone and warfarin administered with etodolac as measured by prothrombin time. Thus, concomitant therapy with warfarin and Lodine XL should not require dosage adjustment of either drug. However, there have been a few spontaneous reports of prolonged prothrombin times in etodolac-treated patients receiving concomitant warfarin therapy. Caution should be exercised because interactions have been seen with other NSAIDs.

Cyclosporine, Digoxin, Lithium

Etodolac, like other NSAIDs, through effects on renal prostaglandins, may cause changes in the elimination of these drugs leading to elevated serum levels of digoxin, lithium and increased toxicity. Nephrotoxicity associated with cyclosporine may also be enhanced. Patients receiving these drugs who are given, Lodine XL or any other NSAID, and particularly those patients with altered renal function, should be observed for the development of the specific toxicities of these drugs.

Phenylbutazone

Phenylbutazone causes an increase (by about 80%) in the free fraction of etodolac. Although *in vivo* studies have not been done to see if etodolac clearance is changed by coadministration of phenylbutazone, it is not recommended that they be coadministered.

DRUG/LABORATORY TEST INTERACTIONS

The urine of patients who take etodolac can give a false-positive reaction for urinary bilirubin (urobilin) due to the presence of phenolic metabolites of etodolac. Diagnostic dipstick methodology, used to detect ketone bodies in urine, has resulted in false-positive findings in some patients treated with etodolac. Generally, this phenomenon has not been associated with other clinically significant events. No dose relationship has been observed.

Etodolac treatment is associated with a small decrease in serum uric acid levels. In clinical trials, mean decreases of 1 to 2 mg/dL were observed in arthritic patients receiving etodolac (600 mg to 1000 mg/day) after 4 weeks of therapy. These levels then remained stable for up to 1 year of therapy.

CARCINOGENESIS, MUTAGENESIS, AND IMPAIRMENT OF FERTILITY

No carcinogenic effect of etodolac was observed in mice or rats receiving oral doses of 15 mg/kg/day (45 to 89 mg/m^2, respectively) or less for periods of 18 months or 2 years, respectively. Etodolac was not mutagenic in *in vitro* tests performed with *S. typhimurium* and mouse lymphoma cells as well as in an *in vivo* mouse micronucleus test. However, data from the *in vitro* human peripheral lymphocyte test showed an increase in the number of gaps (3% to 5% unstained regions in the chromatid without dislocation) among the etodolac-treated cultures (50 to 200 µg/mL) compared to negative controls (2%); no other difference was noted between the controls and drug-treated groups. Etodolac showed no impairment of fertility in male and female rats up to oral doses of 16 mg/kg (94 mg/m^2). However, reduced implantation of fertilized eggs occurred in the 8 mg/kg group.

PREGNANCY

Teratogenic Effects—Pregnancy Category C

In teratology studies, isolated occurrences of alterations in limb development were found and included polydactyly, oligodactyly, syndactyly, and unossified phalanges in rats and oligodactyly and synostosis of metatarsals in rabbits. These were observed at dose levels (2 to 14 mg/kg/day) close to human clinical doses. However, the frequency and the dosage group distribution of these findings in initial or repeated studies did not establish a clear drug or dose-response relationship.

There are no adequate or well-controlled studies in pregnant women. Lodine XL should be used during pregnancy only if the potential benefits justify the potential risk to the fetus. Because of the known effects of NSAIDs on parturition and on the human fetal cardiovascular system with respect to closure of the ductus arteriosus, use during late pregnancy should be avoided.

LABOR AND DELIVERY

In rat studies with etodolac, as with other drugs known to inhibit prostaglandin synthesis, an increased incidence of dystocia, delayed parturition, and decreased pup survival occurred. The effects of Lodine XL on labor and delivery in pregnant women are unknown.

NURSING MOTHERS

It is not known whether this drug is excreted in human milk. Because many drugs are excreted in human milk and because of the potential for serious adverse reactions in nursing infants from etodolac, a decision should be made whether to discontinue nursing or to discontinue the drug, taking into account the importance of the drug to the mother.

PEDIATRIC USE

Safety and effectiveness in pediatric patients have not been established.

GERIATRIC POPULATION

As with any NSAID, caution should be exercised in treating the elderly, and when individualizing their dosage, extra care should be taken when increasing the dose because the elderly seem to tolerate NSAID side effects less well than younger patients. In patients 65 years and older, no substantial differences in the side effect profile of Lodine XL were seen compared with the general population (see **Clinical Pharmacology**—PHARMACOKINETICS).

ADVERSE REACTIONS

In clinical trials most adverse experiences were mild and transient. The discontinuation rate in controlled clinical trials, because of adverse experiences, was up to 10% for patients treated with etodolac.

The following adverse experiences have been reported with the use of etodolac:

INCIDENCE GREATER THAN OR EQUAL TO 1%—PROBABLY CAUSALLY RELATED

Body as a whole—Chills and fever.

Digestive system—Dyspepsia (10%), abdominal pain*, diarrhea*, flatulence*, nausea*, constipation, gastritis, melena, vomiting.

Nervous system—Asthenia/malaise*, dizziness*, depression, nervousness.

Skin and appendages—Pruritus, rash.

Special senses—Blurred vision, tinnitus.

Urogenital system—Dysuria, urinary frequency.

*Drug-related patient complaints occurring in 3 to 9% of patients treated with etodolac.

Drug-related patient-complaints occurring in fewer than 3%, but more than 1%, are unmarked.

INCIDENCE LESS THAN 1%—PROBABLY CAUSALLY RELATED

(Adverse reactions reported only in worldwide postmarketing experience, not seen in clinical trials, are considered rarer and are italicized):

Body as a whole—*Allergic reaction, anaphylactoid reaction.*

Cardiovascular system—Hypertension, congestive heart failure, flushing, palpitations, syncope, *vasculitis (including necrotizing and allergic).*

Digestive system—Thirst, dry mouth, ulcerative stomatitis, anorexia, eructation, elevated liver enzymes, *cholestatic hepatitis,* hepatitis, *cholestatic jaundice, duodenitis, jaundice, hepatic failure, liver necrosis,* peptic ulcer with or without bleeding and/or perforation, *intestinal ulceration, pancreatitis.*

Hemic and lymphatic system—Ecchymosis, anemia, thrombocytopenia, bleeding time increased, *agranulocytosis, hemolytic anemia, leukopenia, neutropenia, pancytopenia.*

Metabolic and nutritional—Edema, serum creatinine increase, *hyperglycemia in previously controlled diabetic patients.*

Nervous system—Insomnia, somnolence.

Respiratory system—Asthma.

Skin and appendages—Angioedema, sweating, urticaria, vesiculobullous rash, *cutaneous vasculitis with purpura, Stevens-Johnson Syndome,* hyperpigmentation, *erythema multiforme.*

Special senses—Photophobia, transient visual disturbances.

Urogenital system—*Elevated BUN, renal failure, renal insufficiency, renal papillary necrosis.*

INCIDENCE LESS THAN 1%—CAUSAL RELATIONSHIP UNKNOWN (Medical events occurring under circumstances where causal relationship to etodolac is uncertain. These reactions are listed as alerting information for physicians):

Body as s whole—Infection, headache.

Cardiovasacular system—Arrhythmias, myocardial infarction, cerebrovascular accident.

Digestive system—Esophagitis with or without stricture or cardiospasm, colitis.

Metabolic and nutritional—Change in weight.

Nervous system—Paresthesia, confusion.

Respiratory system—Bronchitis, dyspnea, pharyngitis, rhinitis, sinusitis.

Skin and appendages—Alopecia, maculopapular rash, photosensitivity, skin peeling.

Special senses—Conjunctivitis, deafness, taste perversion.

Urogenital system—Cystitis, hematuria, leukorrhea, renal calculus, interstitial nephritis, uterine bleeding irregularities.

OVERDOSAGE

Symptoms following acute NSAID overdose are usually limited to lethargy, drowsiness, nausea, vomiting, and epigastric pain, which are generally reversible with supportive care.

Gastrointestinal bleeding can occur and coma has occurred following NSAID overdose. Hypertension, acute renal failure, and respiratory depression may occur but are rare. Anaphylactoid reactions have been reported with therapeutic ingestion of NSAIDs, and may occur following overdose.

Patients should be managed by symptomatic and supportive care following an NSAID overdose. There are no specific antidotes. Gut decontamination may be indicated in patients seen within 4 hours of ingestion with symptoms or following a large overdose (5 to 10 times the usual dose). This should be accomplished via emesis and/or activated charcoal (60 to 100 g in adults, 1 to 2 g/kg in children) with an osmotic cathartic. Forced diuresis, alkalinization of the urine, hemodialysis, or hemoperfusion would probably not be useful due to etodolac's high protein binding.

DOSAGE AND ADMINISTRATION

The recommended dose of Lodine XL is 400 to 1000 mg, given once daily. As with other NSAIDs, the lowest effective dose should be sought for each patient. During long-term administration, the dose of Lodine XL may be adjusted up or down depending on the clinical response up to a maximum dose of 1000 mg/day. In chronic conditions, a therapeutic response to therapy with Lodine XL is sometimes seen within one week of therapy, but most often is observed by two weeks. After a satisfactory response has been achieved, the patient's dose should be reviewed and adjusted as required.

HOW SUPPLIED

Lodine® XL (etodolac extended-release tablets) is available as:

400 mg tablets (orange-red, capsular-oval shaped, biconvex film-coated tablet, branded LODINE XL 400 on one side)
—in bottles of 100, NDC 0046-0829-81

500 mg tablets (grey-green, capsular-oval shaped, biconvex film-coated tablet, branded Lodine XL 500 on one side)
—in bottles of 100, NDC 0046-0839-81

600 mg tablets (light grey, capsular-oval shaped, biconvex film-coated tablet, branded LODINE XL 600 on one side)
—in bottles of 100, NDC 0046-0831-81

Store at controlled room temperature 20°–25°C (68°–77°F). Protect from excessive heat and humidity.

Caution: Federal law prohibits dispensing without prescription.

Manufactured by:
Ayerst Laboratories Inc.
A Wyeth-Ayerst Company
Philadelphia, PA 19101

Shown in Product Identification Guide, page 344

LO/OVRAL® ℞

[*lōh-ōh 'vral*]

Tablets

(norgestrel and ethinyl estradiol tablets)

Patients should be counseled that this product does not protect against HIV infection (AIDS) and other sexually transmitted diseases.

DESCRIPTION

Each LO/OVRAL tablet contains 0.3 mg of norgestrel (*dl*-13-beta-ethyl-17-alpha-ethinyl-17-beta-hydroxygon-4-en-3-one), a totally synthetic progestogen, and 0.03 mg of ethinyl estradiol (19-nor-17α-pregna-1,3,5 (10)-trien-20-yne-3,17-diol). The inactive ingredients present are cellulose, lactose, magnesium stearate, and polacrilin potassium.

CLINICAL PHARMACOLOGY

Combination oral contraceptives act by suppression of gonadotropins. Although the primary mechanism of this action is inhibition of ovulation, other alterations include changes in the cervical mucus (which increase the difficulty of sperm entry into the uterus) and the endometrium (which reduce the likelihood of implantation).

INDICATIONS AND USAGE

Oral contraceptives are indicated for the prevention of pregnancy in women who elect to use this product as a method of contraception.

Oral contraceptives are highly effective. Table I lists the typical accidental pregnancy rates for users of combination oral contraceptives and other methods of contraception. The efficacy of these contraceptive methods, except sterilization and the IUD, depends upon the reliability with which they are used. Correct and consistent use of methods can result in lower failure rates.

TABLE I: LOWEST EXPECTED AND TYPICAL FAILURE RATES DURING THE FIRST YEAR OF CONTINUOUS USE OF A METHOD

% of Women Experiencing an Accidental Pregnancy in the First Year of Continuous Use

Method	Lowest Expected*	Typical**
(No Contraception)	(85)	(85)
Oral contraceptives		3
combined	0.1	N/A***
progestin only	0.5	N/A***
Diaphragm with spermicidal cream or jelly	6	18
Spermicides alone (foams and vaginal suppositories)	3	21
Vaginal Sponge		
nulliparous	6	18
multiparous	9	28
DEPO-PROVERA®		
(injectable progestogen)	0.3	0.3
NORPLANT® SYSTEM		
(implants)	0.2#	0.2#
IUD		3
progesterone	2	N/A***
copper T 380A	0.8	N/A***
Condom without spermicides	2	12
Periodic abstinence		
(all methods)	1–9	20
Female sterilization	0.2	0.4
Male sterilization	0.1	0.15

Adapted from J. Trussell et al., Table 1, Studies in Family Planning, *21*(1): Jan.–Feb. 1990.

* The authors' best guess of the percentage of women expected to experience an accidental pregnancy among couples who initiate a method (not necessarily for the first time) and who use it consistently and correctly during the first year if they do not stop for any other reason.

** This term represents "typical" couples who initiate use of a method (not necessarily for the first time), who experience an accidental pregnancy during the first year if they do not stop use for any other reason.

*** N/A—Data not available.

\# This data is based on NORPLANT® SYSTEM clinical trials.

CONTRAINDICATIONS

Oral contraceptives should not be used in women with any of the following conditions:
Thrombophlebitis or thromboembolic disorders.
A past history of deep-vein thrombophlebitis or thromboembolic disorders.
Cerebral-vascular or coronary-artery disease.
Known or suspected carcinoma of the breast.
Carcinoma of the endometrium or other known or suspected estrogen-dependent neoplasia.
Undiagnosed abnormal genital bleeding.
Cholestatic jaundice of pregnancy or jaundice with prior pill use.
Hepatic adenomas or carcinomas.
Known or suspected pregnancy.

WARNINGS

Cigarette smoking increases the risk of serious cardiovascular side effects from oral-contraceptive use. This risk increases with age and with heavy smoking (15 or more cigarettes per day) and is quite marked in women over 35 years of age. Women who use oral contraceptives should be strongly advised not to smoke.

The use of oral contraceptives is associated with increased risks of several serious conditions including myocardial infarction, thromboembolism, stroke, hepatic neoplasia, gallbladder disease, and hypertension, although the risk of serious morbidity or mortality is very small in healthy women without underlying factors. The risk of morbidity and mortality increases significantly in the presence of other underlying risk factors such as hypertension, hyperlipidemias, obesity, and diabetes.

Practitioners prescribing oral contraceptives should be familiar with the following information relating to these risks. The information contained in this package insert is based principally on studies carried out in patients who used oral contraceptives with higher formulations of estrogens and progestogens than those in common use today. The effect of long-term use of the oral contraceptives with lower formulations of both estrogens and progestogens remains to be determined.

Throughout this labeling, epidemiological studies reported are of two types: retrospective or case control studies and prospective or cohort studies. Case control studies provide a measure of the relative risk of disease, namely, a ratio of the incidence of a disease among oral-contraceptive users to that among nonusers. The relative risk does not provide information on the actual clinical occurrence of a disease. Cohort studies provide a measure of attributable risk, which is the difference in the incidence of disease between oral-contraceptive users and nonusers. The attributable risk does provide information about the actual occurrence of a disease in the population. For further information, the reader is referred to a text on epidemiological methods.

1. THROMBOEMBOLIC DISORDERS AND OTHER VASCULAR PROBLEMS

a. *Myocardial infarction*

An increased risk of myocardial infarction has been attributed to oral-contraceptive use. This risk is primarily in smokers or women with other underlying risk factors for coronary-artery disease such as hypertension, hypercholesterolemia, morbid obesity, and diabetes. The relative risk of heart attack for current oral-contraceptive users has been estimated to be two to six. The risk is very low under the age of 30.

Smoking in combination with oral-contraceptive use has been shown to contribute substantially to the incidence of myocardial infarctions in women in their mid-thirties or older with smoking accounting for the majority of excess cases. Mortality rates associated with circulatory disease have been shown to increase substantially in smokers over the age of 35 and nonsmokers over the age of 40 (Table II) among women who use oral contraceptives.

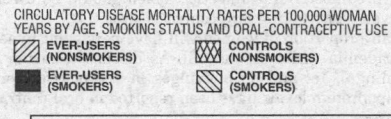

CIRCULATORY DISEASE MORTALITY RATES PER 100,000 WOMAN YEARS BY AGE, SMOKING STATUS AND ORAL-CONTRACEPTIVE USE

EVER-USERS (NONSMOKERS)
EVER-USERS (SMOKERS)
CONTROLS (NONSMOKERS)
CONTROLS (SMOKERS)

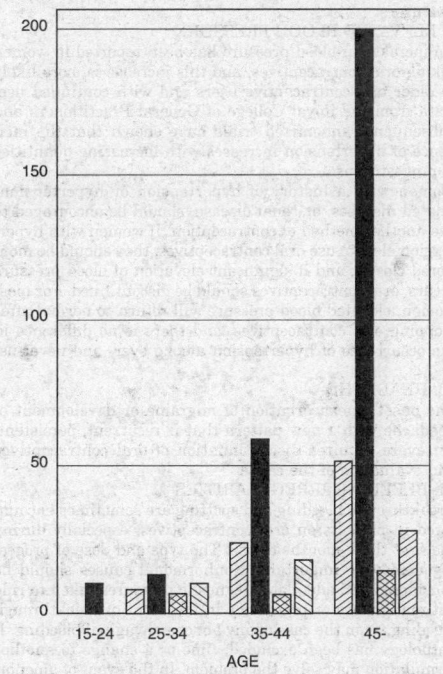

AGE

TABLE II. (Adapted from P.M. Layde and V. Beral, Lancet, *1*:541–546, 1981.)

Oral contraceptives may compound the effects of well-known risk factors, such as hypertension, diabetes, hyperlipidemias, age, and obesity. In particular, some progestogens are known to decrease HDL cholesterol and cause glucose intolerance, while estrogens may create a state of hyperinsulinism. Oral contraceptives have been shown to increase blood pressure among users (see section 9 in "Warnings"). Similar effects on risk factors have been associated with an increased risk of heart disease. Oral contraceptives must be used with caution in women with cardiovascular disease risk factors.

b. *Thromboembolism*

An increased risk of thromboembolic and thrombotic disease associated with the use of oral contraceptives is well established. Case control studies have found the relative risk of users compared to nonusers to be 3 for the first episode of superficial venous thrombosis, 4 to 11 for deep-vein thrombosis or pulmonary embolism, and 1.5 to 6 for women with predisposing conditions for venous thromboembolic

disease. Cohort studies have shown the relative risk to be somewhat lower, about 3 for new cases and about 4.5 for new cases requiring hospitalization. The risk of thromboembolic disease due to oral contraceptives is not related to length of use and disappears after pill use is stopped.

A two- to four-fold increase in relative risk of postoperative thromboembolic complications has been reported with the use of oral contraceptives. The relative risk of venous thrombosis in women who have predisposing conditions is twice that of women without such medical conditions. If feasible, oral contraceptives should be discontinued at least four weeks prior to and for two weeks after elective surgery of a type associated with an increase in risk of thromboembolism and during and following prolonged immobilization. Since the immediate postpartum period is also associated with an increased risk of thromboembolism, oral contraceptives should be started no earlier than four to six weeks after delivery in women who elect not to breast-feed, or a midtrimester pregnancy termination.

c. *Cerebrovascular diseases*

Oral contraceptives have been shown to increase both the relative and attributable risks of cerebrovascular events (thrombotic and hemorrhagic strokes), although, in general, the risk is greatest among older (>35 years), hypertensive women who also smoke. Hypertension was found to be a risk factor for both users and nonusers, for both types of strokes, while smoking interacted to increase the risk for hemorrhagic strokes.

In a large study, the relative risk of thrombotic strokes has been shown to range from 3 for normotensive users to 14 for users with severe hypertension. The relative risk of hemorrhagic stroke is reported to be 1.2 for nonsmokers who used oral contraceptives, 2.6 for smokers who did not use oral contraceptives, 7.6 for smokers who used oral contraceptives, 1.8 for normotensive users, and 25.7 for users with severe hypertension. The attributable risk is also greater in older women.

d. *Dose-related risk of vascular disease from oral contraceptives*

A positive association has been observed between the amount of estrogen and progestogen in oral contraceptives and the risk of vascular disease. A decline in serum high-density lipoproteins (HDL) has been reported with many progestational agents. A decline in serum high-density lipoproteins has been associated with an increased incidence of ischemic heart disease. Because estrogens increase HDL cholesterol, the net effect of an oral contraceptive depends on a balance achieved between doses of estrogen and progestogen and the nature and absolute amount of progestogen used in the contraceptive. The amount of both hormones should be considered in the choice of an oral contraceptive.

Minimizing exposure to estrogen and progestogen is in keeping with good principles of therapeutics. For any particular estrogen/progestogen combination, the dosage regimen prescribed should be one which contains the least amount of estrogen and progestogen that is compatible with a low failure rate and the needs of the individual patient. New acceptors of oral-contraceptive agents should be started on preparations containing less than 50 mcg of estrogen.

e. *Persistence of risk of vascular disease*

There are two studies which have shown persistence of risk of vascular disease for ever-users of oral contraceptives. In a study in the United States, the risk of developing myocardial infarction after discontinuing oral contraceptives persists for at least 9 years for women 40 to 49 years who had used oral contraceptives for five or more years, but this increased risk was not demonstrated in other age groups. In another study in Great Britain, the risk of developing cerebrovascular disease persisted for at least 6 years after discontinuation of oral contraceptives, although excess risk was very small. However, both studies were performed with oral-contraceptive formulations containing 50 micrograms or higher of estrogens.

2. ESTIMATES OF MORTALITY FROM CONTRACEPTIVE USE

One study gathered data from a variety of sources which have estimated the mortality rate associated with different methods of contraception at different ages (Table III). These estimates include the combined risk of death associated with contraceptive methods plus the risk attributable to pregnancy in the event of method failure. Each method of contraception has its specific benefits and risks. The study concluded that with the exception of oral-contraceptive users 35 and older who smoke and 40 and older who do not smoke, mortality associated with all methods of birth control is less than that associated with childbirth. The observation of a possible increase in risk of mortality with age for oral-contraceptive users is based on data gathered in the 1970's—but not reported until 1983. However, current clinical practice involves the use of lower estrogen dose formulations combined with careful restriction of oral-contraceptive use to women who do not have the various risk factors listed in this labeling.

Continued on next page

Lo/Ovral—Cont.

Because of these changes in practice and, also, because of some limited new data which suggest that the risk of cardiovascular disease with the use of oral contraceptives may now be less than previously observed, the Fertility and Maternal Health Drugs Advisory Committee was asked to review the topic in 1989. The Committee concluded that although cardiovascular-disease risks may be increased with oral-contraceptive use after age 40 in healthy nonsmoking women (even with the newer low-dose formulations), there are greater potential health risks associated with pregnancy in older women and with the alternative surgical and medical procedures which may be necessary if such women do not have access to effective and acceptable means of contraception.
Therefore, the Committee recommended that the benefits of oral-contraceptive use by healthy nonsmoking women over 40 may outweigh the possible risks. Of course, older women, as all women who take oral contraceptives, should take the lowest possible dose formulation that is effective.
[See table III below]
3. CARCINOMA OF THE REPRODUCTIVE ORGANS
Numerous epidemiological studies have been performed on the incidence of breast, endometrial, ovarian, and cervical cancer in women using oral contraceptives. The overwhelming evidence in the literature suggests that use of oral contraceptives is not associated with an increase in the risk of developing breast cancer, regardless of the age and parity of first use or with most of the marketed brands and doses. The Cancer and Steroid Hormone (CASH) study also showed no latent effect on the risk of breast cancer for at least a decade following long-term use. A few studies have shown a slightly increased relative risk of developing breast cancer, although the methodology of these studies, which included differences in examination of users and nonusers and differences in age at start of use, has been questioned. Some studies suggest that oral-contraceptive use has been associated with an increase in the risk of cervical intraepithelial neoplasia in some populations of women. However, there continues to be controversy about the extent to which such findings may be due to differences in sexual behavior and other factors.
In spite of many studies of the relationship between oral-contraceptive use and breast and cervical cancers, a cause-and-effect relationship has not been established.
4. HEPATIC NEOPLASIA
Benign hepatic adenomas are associated with oral-contraceptive use, although the incidence of benign tumors is rare in the United States. Indirect calculations have estimated the attributable risk to be in the range of 3.3 cases/100,000 for users, a risk that increases after four or more years of use. Rupture of rare, benign, hepatic adenomas may cause death through intra-abdominal hemorrhage.
Studies from Britain have shown an increased risk of developing hepatocellular carcinoma in long-term (>8 years) oral-contraceptive users. However, these cancers are extremely rare in the U.S., and the attributable risk (the excess incidence) of liver cancers in oral-contraceptive users approaches less than one per million users.
5. OCULAR LESIONS
There have been clincial case reports of retinal thrombosis associated with the use of oral contraceptives. Oral contraceptives should be discontinued if there is unexplained partial or complete loss of vision; onset of proptosis or diplopia; papilledema; or retinal vascular lesions. Appropriate diagnostic and therapeutic measures should be undertaken immediately.
6. ORAL-CONTRACEPTIVE USE BEFORE OR DURING EARLY PREGNANCY
Extensive epidemiological studies have revealed no increased risk of birth defects in women who have used oral contraceptives prior to pregnancy. Studies also do not suggest a teratogenic effect, particularly insofar as cardiac anomalies and limb reduction defects are concerned, when taken inadvertently during early pregnancy.
The administration of oral contraceptives to induce withdrawal bleeding should not be used as a test for pregnancy. Oral contraceptives should not be used during pregnancy to treat threatened or habitual abortion.
It is recommended that for any patient who has missed two consecutive periods, pregnancy should be ruled out before continuing oral-contraceptive use. If the patient has not adhered to the prescribed schedule, the possibility of pregnancy should be considered at the time of the first missed period. Oral-contraceptive use should be discontinued if pregnancy is confirmed.
7. GALLBLADDER DISEASE
Earlier studies have reported an increased lifetime relative risk of gallbladder surgery in users of oral contraceptives and estrogens. More recent studies, however, have shown that the relative risk of developing gallbladder disease among oral-contraceptive users may be minimal. The recent findings of minimal risk may be related to the use of oral-contraceptive formulations containing lower hormonal doses of estrogens and progestogens.
8. CARBOHYDRATE AND LIPID METABOLIC EFFECTS
Oral contraceptives have been shown to cause glucose intolerance in a significant percentage of users. Oral contraceptives containing greater than 75 micrograms of estrogens cause hyperinsulinism, while lower doses of estrogen cause less glucose intolerance. Progestogens increase insulin secretion and create insulin resistance, this effect varying with different progestational agents. However, in the nondiabetic woman, oral contraceptives appear to have no effect on fasting blood glucose. Because of these demonstrated effects, prediabetic and diabetic women should be carefully observed while taking oral contraceptives.
A small proportion of women will have persistent hypertriglyceridemia while on the pill. As discussed earlier (see "Warnings", 1a. and 1d.), changes in serum triglycerides and lipoprotein levels have been reported in oral-contraceptive users.
9. ELEVATED BLOOD PRESSURE
An increase in blood pressure has been reported in women taking oral contraceptives, and this increase is more likely in older oral-contraceptive users and with continued use. Data from the Royal College of General Practitioners and subsequent randomized trials have shown that the incidence of hypertension increases with increasing quantities of progestogens.
Women with a history of hypertension or hypertension-related diseases, or renal disease, should be encouraged to use another method of contraception. If women with hypertension elect to use oral contraceptives, they should be monitored closely, and if significant elevation of blood pressure occurs, oral contraceptives should be discontinued. For most women, elevated blood pressure will return to normal after stopping oral contraceptives, and there is no difference in the occurrence of hypertension among ever- and never-users.
10. HEADACHE
The onset or exacerbation of migraine or development of headache with a new pattern that is recurrent, persistent, or severe requires discontinuation of oral contraceptives and evaluation of the cause.
11. BLEEDING IRREGULARITIES
Breakthrough bleeding and spotting are sometimes encountered in patients on oral contraceptives, especially during the first three months of use. The type and dose of progestogen may be important. Nonhormonal causes should be considered and adequate diagnostic measures taken to rule out malignancy or pregnancy in the event of breakthrough bleeding, as in the case of any abnormal vaginal bleeding. If pathology has been excluded, time or a change to another formulation may solve the problem. In the event of amenorrhea, pregnancy should be ruled out.

TABLE III—ANNUAL NUMBER OF BIRTH-RELATED OR METHOD-RELATED DEATHS ASSOCIATED WITH CONTROL OF FERTILITY PER 100,000 NONSTERILE WOMEN, BY FERTILITY-CONTROL METHOD AND ACCORDING TO AGE

Method of control and outcome	15–19	20–24	25–29	30–34	35–39	40–44
No fertility-control methods*	7.0	7.4	9.1	14.8	25.7	28.2
Oral contraceptives non-smoker**	0.3	0.5	0.9	1.9	13.8	31.6
Oral contraceptives smoker**	2.2	3.4	6.6	13.5	51.1	117.2
IUD**	0.8	0.8	1.0	1.0	1.4	1.4
Condom*	1.1	1.6	0.7	0.2	0.3	0.4
Diaphragm/ spermicide*	1.9	1.2	1.2	1.3	2.2	2.8
Periodic abstinence*	2.5	1.6	1.6	1.7	2.9	3.6

* Deaths are birth related
** Deaths are method related
Adapted from H.W. Ory, Family Planning Perspectives, *15*:57–63, 1983.

Some women may encounter post-pill amenorrhea or oligomenorrhea, especially when such a condition was preexistent.

PRECAUTIONS

Patients should be counseled that this product does not protect against HIV infection (AIDS) and other sexually transmitted diseases.

1. PHYSICAL EXAMINATION AND FOLLOW-UP
A periodic history and physical examination is appropriate for all women, including women using oral contraceptives. The physical examination, however, may be deferred until after initiation of oral contraceptives if requested by the woman and judged appropriate by the clinician. The physical examination should include special reference to blood pressure, breasts, abdomen and pelvic organs, including cervical cytology, and relevant laboratory tests. In case of undiagnosed, persistent or recurrent abnormal vaginal bleeding, appropriate measures should be conducted to rule out malignancy. Women with a strong family history of breast cancer or who have breast nodules should be monitored with particular care.
2. LIPID DISORDERS
Women who are being treated for hyperlipidemias should be followed closely if they elect to use oral contraceptives. Some progestogens may elevate LDL levels and may render the control of hyperlipidemias more difficult. (See "Warnings", 1d.).
3. LIVER FUNCTION
If jaundice develops in any woman receiving such drugs, the medication should be discontinued. Steroid hormones may be poorly metabolized in patients with impaired liver function.
4. FLUID RETENTION
Oral contraceptives may cause some degree of fluid retention. They should be prescribed with caution, and only with careful monitoring, in patients with conditions which might be aggravated by fluid retention.
5. EMOTIONAL DISORDERS
Patients becoming significantly depressed while taking oral contraceptives should stop the medication and use an alternate method of contraception in an attempt to determine whether the symptom is drug related. Women with a history of depression should be carefully observed and the drug discontinued if depression recurs to a serious degree.
6. CONTACT LENSES
Contact-lens wearers who develop visual changes or changes in lens tolerance should be assessed by an ophthalmologist.
7. DRUG INTERACTIONS
Reduced efficacy and increased incidence of breakthrough bleeding and menstrual irregularities have been associated with concomitant use of rifampin. A similar association, though less marked, has been suggested with barbiturates, phenylbutazone, phenytoin sodium, and possibly with griseofulvin, ampicillin, and tetracyclines.
8. INTERACTIONS WITH LABORATORY TESTS
Certain endocrine- and liver-function tests and blood components may be affected by oral contraceptives:
a. Increased prothrombin and factors VII, VIII, IX, and X; decreased antithrombin 3; increased norepinephrine-induced platelet aggregability.
b. Increased thyroid-binding globulin (TBG) leading to increased circulating total thyroid hormone, as measured by protein-bound iodine (PBI), T4 by column or by radioimmunoassay. Free T3 resin uptake is decreased, reflecting the elevated TBG; free T4 concentration is unaltered.
c. Other binding proteins may be elevated in serum.
d. Sex-binding globulins are increased and result in elevated levels of total circulating sex steroids and corticoids; however, free or biologically active levels remain unchanged.
e. Triglycerides may be increased.
f. Glucose tolerance may be decreased.
g. Serum folate levels may be depressed by oral-contraceptive therapy. This may be of clinical significance if a woman becomes pregnant shortly after discontinuing oral contraceptives.
9. CARCINOGENESIS
See "Warnings" section.
10. PREGNANCY
Pregnancy Category X. See "Contraindications" and "Warnings" sections.
11. NURSING MOTHERS
Small amounts of oral-contraceptive steroids have been identified in the milk of nursing mothers, and a few adverse effects on the child have been reported, including jaundice and breast enlargement. In addition, oral contraceptives given in the postpartum period may interfere with lactation by decreasing the quantity and quality of breast milk. If possible, the nursing mother should be advised not to use oral contraceptives but to use other forms of contraception until she has completely weaned her child.

INFORMATION FOR THE PATIENT
See Patient Labeling Printed Below.

ADVERSE REACTIONS

An increased risk of the following serious adverse reactions has been associated with the use of oral contraceptives (see "Warnings" section):
Thrombophlebitis.
Arterial thromboembolism.
Pulmonary embolism.
Myocardial infarction.
Cerebral hemorrhage.
Cerebral thrombosis.
Hypertension.
Gallbladder disease.
Hepatic adenomas or benign liver tumors.
There is evidence of an association between the following conditions and the use of oral contraceptives, although additional confirmatory studies are needed:
Mesenteric thrombosis.
Retinal thrombosis.
The following adverse reactions have been reported in patients receiving oral contraceptives and are believed to be drug related:
Nausea.
Vomiting.
Gastrointestinal symptoms (such as abdominal cramps and bloating).
Breakthrough bleeding.
Spotting.
Change in menstrual flow.
Amenorrhea.
Temporary infertility after discontinuation of treatment.
Edema.
Melasma which may persist.
Breast changes: tenderness, enlargement, secretion.
Change in weight (increase or decrease).
Change in cervical erosion and secretion.
Diminution in lactation when given immediately postpartum.
Cholestatic jaundice.
Migraine.
Rash (allergic).
Mental depression.
Reduced tolerance to carbohydrates.
Vaginal candidiasis.
Change in corneal curvature (steepening).
Intolerance to contact lenses.
The following adverse reactions have been reported in users of oral contraceptives, and the association has been neither confirmed nor refuted:
Congenital anomalies.
Premenstrual syndrome.
Cataracts.
Optic neuritis.
Changes in appetite.
Cystitis-like syndrome.
Headache.
Nervousness.
Dizziness.
Hirsutism.
Loss of scalp hair.
Erythema multiforme.
Erythema nodosum.
Hemorrhagic eruption.
Vaginitis.
Porphyria.
Impaired renal function.
Hemolytic uremic syndrome.
Budd-Chiari syndrome.
Acne.
Changes in libido.
Colitis.
Sickle-cell disease.
Cerebral-vascular disease with mitral valve prolapse.
Lupus-like syndromes.

OVERDOSAGE

Serious ill effects have not been reported following acute ingestion of large doses of oral contraceptives by young children. Overdosage may cause nausea, and withdrawal bleeding may occur in females.

NONCONTRACEPTIVE HEALTH BENEFITS

The following noncontraceptive health benefits related to the use of oral contraceptives are supported by epidemiological studies which largely utilized oral-contraceptive formulations containing doses exceeding 0.035 mg of ethinyl estradiol or 0.05 mg of mestranol.
Effects on menses:
Increased menstrual cycle regularity.
Decreased blood loss and decreased incidence of iron-deficiency anemia.
Decreased incidence of dysmenorrhea.
Effects related to inhibition of ovulation:
Decreased incidence of functional ovarian cysts.
Decreased incidence of ectopic pregnancies.

Effects from long-term use:
Decreased incidence of fibroadenomas and fibrocystic disease of the breast.
Decreased incidence of acute pelvic inflammatory disease.
Decreased incidence of endometrial cancer.
Decreased incidence of ovarian cancer.

DOSAGE AND ADMINISTRATION

To achieve maximum contraceptive effectiveness, LO/OVRAL must be taken exactly as directed and at intervals not exceeding 24 hours.
The dosage of LO/OVRAL is one tablet daily for 21 consecutive days per menstrual cycle according to prescribed schedule. Tablets are then discontinued for 7 days (three weeks on, one week off).
It is recommended that LO/OVRAL tablets be taken at the same time each day, preferably after the evening meal or at bedtime.
During the first cycle of medication, the patient is instructed to take one LO/OVRAL tablet daily for twenty-one consecutive days, beginning on the first day (Day 1 Start) of her menstrual cycle or on the Sunday after her period begins (Sunday Start). (The first day of menstruation is day one.) The tablets are then discontinued for one week (7 days). Withdrawal bleeding should usually occur within 3 days following discontinuation of LO/OVRAL. (For Day 1 Start: If LO/OVRAL is first taken later than the first day of the first menstrual cycle of medication or postpartum, contraceptive reliance should not be placed on LO/OVRAL until after the first seven consecutive days of administration. For Sunday Start: Contraceptive reliance should not be placed on LO/OVRAL until after the first seven consecutive days of administration. The possibility of ovulation and conception prior to initiation of medication should be considered.)
The patient begins her next and all subsequent 21-day courses of LO/OVRAL tablets on the same day of the week that she began her first course, following the same schedule: 21 days on—7 days off. She begins taking her tablets on the 8th day after discontinuance, regardless of whether or not a menstrual period has occurred or is still in progress. Any time a new cycle of LO/OVRAL is started later than the 8th day, the patient should be protected by another means of contraception until she has taken a tablet daily for seven consecutive days.
If spotting or breakthrough bleeding occurs, the patient is instructed to continue on the same regimen. This type of bleeding is usually transient and without significance; however, if the bleeding is persistent or prolonged, the patient is advised to consult her physician. Although the occurrence of pregnancy is highly unlikely if LO/OVRAL is taken according to directions, if withdrawal bleeding does not occur, the possibility of pregnancy must be considered. If the patient has not adhered to the prescribed schedule (missed one or more tablets or started taking them on a day later than she should have), the probability of pregnancy should be considered at the time of the first missed period and appropriate diagnostic measures taken before the medication is resumed. If the patient has adhered to the prescribed regimen and misses two consecutive periods, pregnancy should be ruled out before continuing the contraceptive regimen.
For additional patient instructions regarding missed pills, see the "WHAT TO DO IF YOU MISS PILLS" section in the **DETAILED PATIENT LABELING** below.
Any time the patient misses two or more tablets, she should also use another method of contraception until she has taken a tablet daily for seven consecutive days. If breakthrough bleeding occurs following missed tablets, it will usually be transient and of no consequence. While there is little likelihood of ovulation occurring if only one or two tablets are missed, the possibility of ovulation increases with each successive day that scheduled tablets are missed.
In the nonlactating mother, LO/OVRAL may be initiated postpartum, for contraception. When the tablets are administered in the postpartum period, the increased risk of thromboembolic disease associated with the postpartum period must be considered (see "Contraindications," "Warnings", and "Precautions" concerning thromboembolic disease). It is to be noted that early resumption of ovulation may occur if Parlodel® (bromocriptine mesylate) has been used for the prevention of lactation.

HOW SUPPLIED

LO/OVRAL® Tablets (0.3 mg norgestrel and 0.03 mg ethinyl estradiol) are available in packages of 6 PILPAK® dispensers with 21 tablets each as follows:
NDC 0008-0078, white, round tablet marked "WYETH" and "78".
Store at room temperature, approx. 25°C (77°F).
References available upon request.
Brief Summary Patient Package Insert
This product (like all oral contraceptives) is intended to prevent pregnancy. It does not protect against HIV infection (AIDS) and other sexually transmitted diseases.
Oral contraceptives, also known as "birth-control pills" or "the pill," are taken to prevent pregnancy, and when taken correctly, have a failure rate of less than 1.0% per year when used without missing any pills. The typical failure rate of

large numbers of pill users is less than 3.0% per year when women who miss pills are included. For most women oral contraceptives are also free of serious or unpleasant side effects. However, forgetting to take pills considerably increases the chances of pregnancy.
For the majority of women, oral contraceptives can be taken safely. But there are some women who are at high risk of developing certain serious diseases that can be life-threatening or may cause temporary or permanent disability or death. The risks associated with taking oral contraceptives increase significantly if you:
• smoke
• have high blood pressure, diabetes, high cholesterol
• have or have had clotting disorders, heart attack, stroke, angina pectoris, cancer of the breast or sex organs, jaundice, or malignant or benign liver tumors.
You should not take the pill if you suspect you are pregnant or have unexplained vaginal bleeding.

Cigarette smoking increases the risk of serious adverse effects on the heart and blood vessels from oral-contraceptive use. This risk increases with age and with heavy smoking (15 or more cigarettes per day) and is quite marked in women over 35 years of age. Women who use oral contraceptives should not smoke.

Most side effects of the pill are not serious. The most common such effects are nausea, vomiting, bleeding between menstrual periods, weight gain, breast tenderness, and difficulty wearing contact lenses. These side effects, especially nausea and vomiting, may subside within the first three months of use.
The serious side effects of the pill occur very infrequently, especially if you are in good health and do not smoke. However, you should know that the following medical conditions have been associated with or made worse by the pill:
1. Blood clots in the legs (thrombophlebitis), lungs (pulmonary embolism), stoppage or rupture of a blood vessel in the brain (stroke), blockage of blood vessels in the heart (heart attack or angina pectoris) or other organs of the body. As mentioned above, smoking increases the risk of heart attacks and strokes and subsequent serious medical consequences.
2. Liver tumors, which may rupture and cause severe bleeding. A possible but not definite association has been found with the pill and liver cancer. However, liver cancers are extremely rare. The chance of developing liver cancer from using the pill is thus even rarer.
3. High blood pressure, although blood pressure usually returns to normal when the pill is stopped.
The symptoms associated with these serious side effects are discussed in the detailed leaflet given to you with your supply of pills. Notify your doctor or health-care provider if you notice any unusual physical disturbances while taking the pill. In addition, drugs such as rifampin, as well as some anticonvulsants and some antibiotics, may decrease oral contraceptive effectiveness.
Studies to date of women taking the pill have not shown an increase in the incidence of cancer of the breast or cervix. There is, however, insufficient evidence to rule out the possibility that pills may cause such cancers.
Taking the pill provides some important noncontraceptive benefits. These include less painful menstruation, less menstrual blood loss and anemia, fewer pelvic infections, and fewer cancers of the ovary and the lining of the uterus.
Be sure to discuss any medical condition you may have with your health-care provider. Your health-care provider will take a medical and family history before prescribing oral contraceptives and will examine you. The physical examination may be delayed to another time if you request it and the health-care provider believes that it is appropriate to postpone it. You should be reexamined at least once a year while taking oral contraceptives. The detailed patient information leaflet gives you further information which you should read and discuss with your health-care provider.

DETAILED PATIENT LABELING

This product (like all oral contraceptives) is intended to prevent pregnancy. It does not protect against HIV infection (AIDS) and other sexually transmitted diseases.
INTRODUCTION
Any woman who considers using oral contraceptives (the birth- control pill or the pill) should understand the benefits and risks of using this form of birth control. This leaflet will give you much of the information you will need to make this decision and will also help you determine if you are at risk of developing any of the serious side effects of the pill. It will tell you how to use the pill properly so that it will be as effective as possible. However, this leaflet is not a replacement for a careful discussion between you and your health-care provider. You should discuss the information provided in this leaflet with him or her, both when you first start taking the pill and during your revisits. You should also follow your health-care provider's advice with regard to regular check-ups while you are on the pill.

Continued on next page

Lo/Ovral—Cont.

EFFECTIVENESS OF ORAL CONTRACEPTIVES
Oral contraceptives or "birth-control pills" or "the pill" are used to prevent pregnancy and are more effective than other nonsurgical methods of birth control. When they are taken correctly, the chance of becoming pregnant is less than 1.0% when used perfectly, without missing any pills. Typical failure rates are less than 3.0% per year. The chance of becoming pregnant increases with each missed pill during the menstrual cycle.
In comparison, typical failure rates for other nonsurgical methods of birth control during the first year of use are as follows:
IUD: 3%
DEPO-PROVERA® (injectable progestogen): 0.3%
NORPLANT® SYSTEM (implants): 0.2%
Diaphragm with spermicides: 18%
Spermicides alone: 21%
Male condom alone: 12%
Periodic abstinence: 20%
No methods: 85%

WHO SHOULD NOT TAKE ORAL CONTRACEPTIVES

Cigarette smoking increases the risk of serious adverse effects on the heart and blood vessels from oral-contraceptive use. This risk increases with age and with heavy smoking (15 or more cigarettes per day) and is quite marked in women over 35 years of age. Women who use oral contraceptives should not smoke.

Some women should not use the pill. For example, you should not take the pill if you are pregnant or think you may be pregnant. You should also not use the pill if you have had any of the following conditions:
- Heart attack or stroke.
- Blood clots in the legs (thrombophlebitis), lungs (pulmonary embolism), or eyes.
- Blood clots in the deep veins of your legs.
- Known or suspected breast cancer or cancer of the lining of the uterus, cervix, or vagina.
- Liver tumor (benign or cancerous).

Or, if you have any of the following:
- Chest pain (angina pectoris).
- Unexplained vaginal bleeding (until a diagnosis is reached by your doctor).
- Yellowing of the whites of the eyes or of the skin (jaundice) during pregnancy or during previous use of the pill.
- Known or suspected pregnancy.

Tell your health-care provider if you have ever had any of these conditions. Your health-care provider can recommend another method of birth control.

OTHER CONSIDERATIONS BEFORE TAKING ORAL CONTRACEPTIVES
Tell your health-care provider if you or any family member has ever had:
- Breast nodules, fibrocystic disease of the breast, an abnormal breast X ray or mammogram.
- Diabetes.
- Elevated cholesterol or triglycerides.
- High blood pressure.
- Migraine or other headaches or epilepsy.
- Mental depression.
- Gallbladder, heart, or kidney disease.
- History of scanty or irregular menstrual periods.

Women with any of these conditions should be checked often by their health-care provider if they choose to use oral contraceptives. Also, be sure to inform your doctor or health-care provider if you smoke or are on any medications.

RISKS OF TAKING ORAL CONTRACEPTIVES
1. Risk of developing blood clots
Blood clots and blockage of blood vessels are the most serious side effects of taking oral contraceptives and can be fatal. In particular, a clot in the legs can cause thrombophlebitis and a clot that travels to the lungs can cause a sudden blocking of the vessel carrying blood to the lungs. Rarely, clots occur in the blood vessels of the eye and may cause blindness, double vision, or impaired vision.
If you take oral contraceptives and need elective surgery, need to stay in bed for a prolonged illness, or have recently delivered a baby, you may be at risk of developing blood clots. You should consult your doctor about stopping oral contraceptives three to four weeks before surgery and not taking oral contraceptives for two weeks after surgery or during bed rest. You should also not take oral contraceptives soon after delivery of a baby or a midtrimester pregnancy termination. It is advisable to wait for at least four weeks after delivery if you are not breast-feeding. If you are breast-feeding, you should wait until you have weaned your child before using the pill. (See also the section on breast-feeding in "General Precautions".)
2. Heart attacks and strokes
Oral contraceptives may increase the tendency to develop strokes (stoppage or rupture of blood vessels in the brain) and angina pectoris and heart attacks (blockage of blood vessels in the heart). Any of these conditions can cause death or serious disability.
Smoking greatly increases the possibility of suffering heart attacks and strokes. Furthermore, smoking and the use of oral contraceptives greatly increase the chances of developing and dying of heart disease.
3. Gallbladder disease
Oral-contraceptive users probably have a greater risk than nonusers of having gallbladder disease, although this risk may be related to pills containing high doses of estrogens.
4. Liver tumors
In rare cases, oral contraceptives can cause benign but dangerous liver tumors. These benign liver tumors can rupture and cause fatal internal bleeding. In addition, a possible but not definite association has been found with the pill and liver cancers in two studies in which a few women who developed these very rare cancers were found to have used oral contraceptives for long periods. However, liver cancers are extremely rare. The chance of developing liver cancer from using the pill is thus even rarer.
5. Cancer of the reproductive organs
There is, at present, no confirmed evidence that oral contraceptives increase the risk of cancer of the reproductive organs in human studies. Several studies have found no overall increase in the risk of developing breast cancer. However, women who use oral contraceptives and have a strong family history of breast cancer or who have breast nodules or abnormal mammograms should be closely followed by their doctors.
Some studies have found an increase in the incidence of cancer of the cervix in women who use oral contraceptives. However, this finding may be related to factors other than the use of oral contraceptives.

ESTIMATED RISK OF DEATH FROM A BIRTH-CONTROL METHOD OR PREGNANCY
All methods of birth control and pregnancy are associated with a risk of developing certain diseases which may lead to disability or death. An estimate of the number of deaths associated with different methods of birth control and pregnancy has been calculated and is shown in the following table.
[See table below]
In the above table, the risk of death from any birth-control method is less than the risk of childbirth, except for oral-contraceptive users over the age of 35 who smoke and pill users over the age of 40 even if they do not smoke. It can be seen in the table that for women aged 15 to 39, the risk of death was highest with pregnancy (7 to 26 deaths per 100,000 women, depending on age). Among pill users who do not smoke, the risk of death was always lower than that associated with pregnancy for any age group, except for those women over the age of 40, when the risk increases to 32 deaths per 100,000 women, compared to 28 associated with pregnancy at that age. However, for pill users who smoke and are over the age of 35, the estimated number of deaths exceeds those for other methods of birth control. If a woman is over the age of 40 and smokes, her estimated risk of death is four times higher (117/100,000 women) than the estimated risk associated with pregnancy (28/100,000 women) in that age group.
The suggestion that women over 40 who don't smoke should not take oral contraceptives is based on information from older high-dose pills and on less-selective use of pills than is practiced today. An Advisory Committee of the FDA discussed this issue in 1989 and recommended that the benefits of oral-contraceptive use by healthy, nonsmoking women over 40 years of age may outweigh the possible risks. However, all women, especially older women, are cautioned to use the lowest-dose pill that is effective.

WARNING SIGNALS
If any of these adverse effects occur while you are taking oral contraceptives, call your doctor immediately:
- Sharp chest pain, coughing of blood, or sudden shortness of breath (indicating a possible clot in the lung).
- Pain in the calf (indicating a possible clot in the leg).
- Crushing chest pain or heaviness in the chest (indicating a possible heart attack).
- Sudden severe headache or vomiting, dizziness or fainting, disturbances of vision or speech, weakness, or numbness in an arm or leg (indicating a possible stroke).
- Sudden partial or complete loss of vision (indicating a possible clot in the eye).
- Breast lumps (indicating possible breast cancer or fibrocystic disease of the breast; ask your doctor or health-care provider to show you how to examine your breasts).
- Severe pain or tenderness in the stomach area (indicating a possibly ruptured liver tumor).
- Difficulty in sleeping, weakness, lack of energy, fatigue, or change in mood (possibly indicating severe depression).
- Jaundice or a yellowing of the skin or eyeballs, accompanied frequently by fever, fatigue, loss of appetite, dark-colored urine, or light-colored bowel movements (indicating possible liver problems).

SIDE EFFECTS OF ORAL CONTRACEPTIVES
1. Vaginal bleeding
Irregular vaginal bleeding or spotting may occur while you are taking the pills. Irregular bleeding may vary from slight staining between menstrual periods to breakthrough bleeding which is a flow much like a regular period. Irregular bleeding occurs most often during the first few months of oral-contraceptive use, but may also occur after you have been taking the pill for some time. Such bleeding may be temporary and usually does not indicate any serious problems. It is important to continue taking your pills on schedule. If the bleeding occurs in more than one cycle or lasts for more than a few days, talk to your doctor or health-care provider.
2. Contact lenses
If you wear contact lenses and notice a change in vision or an inability to wear your lenses, contact your doctor or health-care provider.
3. Fluid retention
Oral contraceptives may cause edema (fluid retention) with swelling of the fingers or ankles and may raise your blood pressure. If you experience fluid retention, contact your doctor or health-care provider.
4. Melasma
A spotty darkening of the skin is possible, particularly of the face.
5. Other side effects
Other side effects may include change in appetite, headache, nervousness, depression, dizziness, loss of scalp hair, rash, and vaginal infections.
If any of these side effects bother you, call your doctor or health-care provider.

GENERAL PRECAUTIONS
1. Missed periods and use of oral contraceptives before or during early pregnancy
There may be times when you may not menstruate regularly after you have completed taking a cycle of pills. If you have taken your pills regularly and miss one menstrual period, continue taking your pills for the next cycle but be sure to inform your health-care provider before doing so. If you have not taken the pills daily as instructed and missed a menstrual period, or if you missed two consecutive menstrual periods, you may be pregnant. Check with your health-care provider immediately to determine whether you are pregnant. Do not continue to take oral contraceptives until you are sure you are not pregnant, but continue to use another method of contraception.
There is no conclusive evidence that oral-contraceptive use is associated with an increase in birth defects when taken

ANNUAL NUMBER OF BIRTH-RELATED OR METHOD-RELATED DEATHS ASSOCIATED WITH CONTROL OF FERTILITY PER 100,000 NONSTERILE WOMEN, BY FERTILITY-CONTROL METHOD AND ACCORDING TO AGE

Method of control and outcome	15–19	20–24	25–29	30–34	35–39	40–44
No fertility-control methods*	7.0	7.4	9.1	14.8	25.7	28.2
Oral contraceptives nonsmoker**	0.3	0.5	0.9	1.9	13.8	31.6
Oral contraceptives smoker**	2.2	3.4	6.6	13.5	51.1	117.2
IUD**	0.8	0.8	1.0	1.0	1.4	1.4
Condom*	1.1	1.6	0.7	0.2	0.3	0.4
Diaphragm/ spermicide*	1.9	1.2	1.2	1.3	2.2	2.8
Periodic abstinence*	2.5	1.6	1.6	1.7	2.9	3.6

* Deaths are birth related
** Deaths are method related

inadvertently during early pregnancy. Previously, a few studies had reported that oral contraceptives might be associated with birth defects, but these studies have not been confirmed. Nevertheless, oral contraceptives or any other drugs should not be used during pregnancy unless clearly necessary and prescribed by your doctor. You should check with your doctor about risks to your unborn child of any medication taken during pregnancy.

2. While breast-feeding

If you are breast-feeding, consult your doctor before starting oral contraceptives. Some of the drug will be passed on to the child in the milk. A few adverse effects on the child have been reported, including yellowing of the skin (jaundice) and breast enlargement. In addition, oral contraceptives may decrease the amount and quality of your milk. If possible, do not use oral contraceptives while breast-feeding. You should use another method of contraception since breast-feeding provides only partial protection from becoming pregnant, and this partial protection decreases significantly as you breast-feed for longer periods of time. You should consider starting oral contraceptives only after you have weaned your child completely.

3. Laboratory tests

If you are scheduled for any laboratory tests, tell your doctor you are taking birth-control pills. Certain blood tests may be affected by birth-control pills.

4. Drug interactions

Certain drugs may interact with birth-control pills to make them less effective in preventing pregnancy or cause an increase in breakthrough bleeding. Such drugs include rifampin, drugs used for epilepsy such as barbiturates (for example, phenobarbital) and phenytoin (Dilantin is one brand of this drug), phenylbutazone (Butazolidin is one brand), and possibly certain antibiotics. You may need to use an additional method of contraception during any cycle in which you take drugs that can make oral contraceptives less effective.

HOW TO TAKE THE PILL

This product (like all oral contraceptives) is intended to prevent pregnancy. It does not protect against transmission of HIV (AIDS) and other sexually transmitted diseases such as chlamydia, genital herpes, genital warts, gonorrhea, hepatitis B, and syphilis.

IMPORTANT POINTS TO REMEMBER

BEFORE YOU START TAKING YOUR PILLS:

1. BE SURE TO READ THESE DIRECTIONS:

Before you start taking your pills.

Anytime you are not sure what to do.

2. THE RIGHT WAY TO TAKE THE PILL IS TO TAKE ONE PILL EVERY DAY AT THE SAME TIME.

If you miss pills you could get pregnant. This includes starting the pack late. The more pills you miss, the more likely you are to get pregnant.

3. MANY WOMEN HAVE SPOTTING OR LIGHT BLEEDING, OR MAY FEEL SICK TO THEIR STOMACH DURING THE FIRST 1-3 PACKS OF PILLS.

If you feel sick to your stomach, do not stop taking the pill. The problem will usually go away. If it doesn't go away, check with your doctor or clinic.

4. MISSING PILLS CAN ALSO CAUSE SPOTTING OR LIGHT BLEEDING, even when you make up these missed pills.

On the days you take 2 pills to make up for missed pills, you could also feel a little sick to your stomach.

5. IF YOU HAVE VOMITING OR DIARRHEA, for any reason, or IF YOU TAKE SOME MEDICINES, including some antibiotics, your pills may not work as well. Use a back-up method (such as condoms or foam) until you check with your doctor or clinic.

6. IF YOU HAVE TROUBLE REMEMBERING TO TAKE THE PILL, talk to your doctor or clinic about how to make pill-taking easier or about using another method of birth control.

7. IF YOU HAVE ANY QUESTIONS OR ARE UNSURE ABOUT THE INFORMATION IN THIS LEAFLET, call your doctor or clinic.

NORDETTE®- 21, OVRAL®, LO/OVRAL®, NORDETTE®- 28, OVRAL®-28, AND LO/OVRAL®-28

BEFORE YOU START TAKING YOUR PILLS

1. DECIDE WHAT TIME OF DAY YOU WANT TO TAKE YOUR PILL.

It is important to take it at about the same time every day.

2. LOOK AT YOUR PILL PACK TO SEE IF IT HAS 21 OR 28 PILLS:

The *21-pill pack* has 21 "active" white or light-orange pills (with hormones) to take for 3 weeks, followed by 1 week without pills.

The *28-pill pack* has 21 "active" white or light-orange pills (with hormones) to take for 3 weeks, followed by 1 week of reminder pink pills (without hormones).

3. ALSO FIND:

1) where on the pack to start taking pills, and

2) in what order to take the pills (follow the arrows).

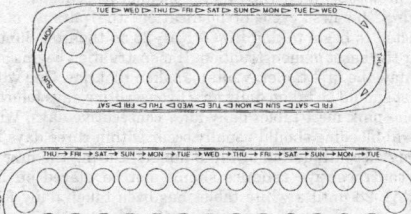

4. BE SURE YOU HAVE READY AT ALL TIMES:

ANOTHER KIND OF BIRTH CONTROL (such as condoms or foam) to use as a back-up in case you miss pills.

AN EXTRA, FULL PILL PACK.

WHEN TO START THE *FIRST* PACK OF PILLS

For the 21-day pill pack you have two choices of which day to start taking your first pack of pills. (See **DAY 1 START** or **SUNDAY START** directions below.) Decide with your doctor or clinic which is the best day for you. The 28-day pill pack accommodates a **SUNDAY START** only. For either pill pack pick a time of day which will be easy to remember.

DAY 1 START:

These instructions are for the 21-day pill pack only. The 28-day pill pack does not accommodate a **DAY 1 START** dosage regimen.

1. Take the first "active" white or light-orange pill of the first pack during the *first 24 hours of your period.*

2. You will not need to use a back-up method of birth control, since you are starting the pill at the beginning of your period.

SUNDAY START:

These instructions are for either the 21-day or the 28-day pill pack.

1. Take the first "active" white or light-orange pill of the first pack on the *Sunday after your period starts,* even if you are still bleeding. If your period begins on Sunday, start the pack that same day.

2. *Use another method of birth control* as a back-up method if you have sex anytime from the Sunday you start your first pack until the next Sunday (7 days). Condoms or foam are good back-up methods of birth control.

WHAT TO DO DURING THE MONTH

1. TAKE ONE PILL AT THE SAME TIME EVERY DAY UNTIL THE PACK IS EMPTY.

Do not skip pills even if you are spotting or bleeding between monthly periods or feel sick to your stomach (nausea).

Do not skip pills even if you do not have sex very often.

2. WHEN YOU FINISH A PACK OR SWITCH YOUR BRAND OF PILLS:

21 pills: Wait 7 days to start the next pack. You will probably have your period during that week. Be sure that no more than 7 days pass between 21-day packs.

28 pills: Start the next pack on the day after your last "reminder" pill. Do not wait any days between packs.

WHAT TO DO IF YOU MISS PILLS

If you **MISS** 1 white or light-orange "active" pill:

1. Take it as soon as you remember. Take the next pill at your regular time. This means you take 2 pills in 1 day.

2. You do not need to use a back-up birth control method if you have sex.

If you **MISS** 2 white or light-orange "active" pills in a row in **WEEK 1 or WEEK 2** of your pack:

1. Take 2 pills on the day you remember and 2 pills the next day.

2. Then take 1 pill a day until you finish the pack.

3. You MAY BECOME PREGNANT if you have sex in the 7 *days* after you miss pills. You MUST use another birth control method (such as condoms or foam) as a back-up for those 7 days.

If you **MISS** 2 white or light-orange "active" pills in a row in **THE 3rd WEEK:**

The *Day 1 Starter* instructions are for the 21-day pill pack only. The 28-day pill pack does not accommodate a **DAY 1 START** dosage regimen. The *Sunday Starter* instructions are for either the 21-day or 28-day pill pack.

1. *If you are a Day 1 Starter:*

THROW OUT the rest of the pill pack and start a new pack that same day.

If you are a Sunday Starter:

Keep taking 1 pill every day until Sunday.

On Sunday, THROW OUT the rest of the pack and start a new pack of pills that same day.

2. You may not have your period this month but this is expected. However, if you miss your period 2 months in a row, call your doctor or clinic because you might be pregnant.

3. You MAY BECOME PREGNANT if you have sex in the 7 *days* after you miss pills. You MUST use another birth control method (such as condoms or foam) as a back-up for those 7 days.

If you **MISS 3 OR MORE** white or light-orange "active" pills in a row (during the first 3 weeks):

The *Day 1 Starter* instructions are for the 21-day pill pack only. The 28-day pill pack does not accommodate a **DAY 1 START** dosage regimen. The *Sunday Starter* instructions are for either the 21-day or 28-day pill pack.

1. *If you are a Day 1 Starter:*

THROW OUT the rest of the pill pack and start a new pack that same day.

If you are a Sunday Starter:

Keep taking 1 pill every day until Sunday.

On Sunday, THROW OUT the rest of the pack and start a new pack of pills that same day.

2. You may not have your period this month but this is expected. However, if you miss your period 2 months in a row, call your doctor or clinic because you might be pregnant.

3. You MAY BECOME PREGNANT if you have sex in the 7 *days* after you miss pills. You MUST use another birth control method (such as condoms or foam) as a back-up for those 7 days.

A REMINDER FOR THOSE ON 28-DAY PACKS:

If you forget any of the 7 pink "reminder" pills in Week 4:

THROW AWAY the pills you missed.

Keep taking 1 pill each day until the pack is empty.

You do not need a back-up method if you start your next pack on time.

FINALLY, IF YOU ARE STILL NOT SURE WHAT TO DO ABOUT THE PILLS YOU HAVE MISSED:

Use a BACK-UP METHOD anytime you have sex.

KEEP TAKING ONE PILL EACH DAY until you can reach your doctor or clinic.

OVRETTE®

Ovrette is administered on a continuous daily dosage schedule, one tablet each day, every day of the year. Take the first tablet on the first day of your menstrual period. Tablets should be taken at the same time every day, without interruption, whether bleeding occurs or not. If bleeding is prolonged (more than 8 days) or unusually heavy, you should contact your doctor.

Forgotten pills

The risk of pregnancy increases with each tablet missed. Therefore, it is very important that you take one tablet daily as directed. If you miss one tablet, take it as soon as you remember and also take your next tablet at the regular time. If you miss two tablets, take one of the missed tablets as soon as you remember, as well as your regular tablet for that day at the proper time. Furthermore, you should use another method of birth control in addition to taking Ovrette until you have taken fourteen days (2 weeks) of medication.

If more than two tablets have been missed, Ovrette should be discontinued immediately and another method of birth control used until the start of your next menstrual period. Then you may resume taking Ovrette.

Pregnancy due to pill failure

The incidence of pill failure resulting in pregnancy is approximately less than 1.0% if taken every day as directed, but more typical failure rates are less than 3.0%. If failure does occur, the risk to the fetus is minimal.

RISKS TO THE FETUS

If you do become pregnant while using oral contraceptives, the risk to the fetus is small, on the order of no more than one per thousand. You should, however, discuss the risks to the developing child with your doctor.

Pregnancy after stopping the pill

There may be some delay in becoming pregnant after you stop using oral contraceptives, especially if you had irregular menstrual cycles before you used oral contraceptives. It may be advisable to postpone conception until you begin menstruating regularly once you have stopped taking the pill and desire pregnancy.

There does not appear to be any increase in birth defects in newborn babies when pregnancy occurs soon after stopping the pill.

Overdosage

Serious ill effects have not been reported following ingestion of large doses of oral contraceptives by young children. Overdosage may cause nausea and withdrawal bleeding in females. In case of overdosage, contact your health-care provider or pharmacist.

Continued on next page

Lo/Ovral—Cont.

Other information

Your health-care provider will take a medical and family history before prescribing oral contraceptives and will examine you. The physical examination may be delayed to another time if you request it and the health-care provider believes that it is appropriate to postpone it. You should be reexamined at least once a year. Be sure to inform your health-care provider if there is a family history of any of the conditions listed previously in this leaflet. Be sure to keep all appointments with your health-care provider, because this is a time to determine if there are early signs of side effects of oral-contraceptive use.

Do not use the drug for any condition other than the one for which it was prescribed. This drug has been prescribed specifically for you; do not give it to others who may want birth-control pills.

HEALTH BENEFITS FROM ORAL CONTRACEPTIVES

In addition to preventing pregnancy, use of oral contraceptives may provide certain benefits. They are:

- Menstrual cycles may become more regular
- Blood flow during menstruation may be lighter, and less iron may be lost. Therefore, anemia due to iron deficiency is less likely to occur.
- Pain or other symptoms during menstruation may be encountered less frequently
- Ovarian cysts may occur less frequently
- Ectopic (tubal) pregnancy may occur less frequently
- Noncancerous cysts or lumps in the breast may occur less frequently
- Acute pelvic inflammatory disease may occur less frequently
- Oral-contraceptive use may provide some protection against developing two forms of cancer: cancer of the ovaries and cancer of the lining of the uterus.

If you want more information about birth-control pills, ask your doctor or pharmacist. They have a more technical leaflet called the Professional Labeling which you may wish to read.

Manufactured by:
Wyeth Laboratories Inc.
A Wyeth-Ayerst Company
Philadelphia, PA 19101

Shown in Product Identification Guide, page 344

LO/OVRAL®-28 ℞
[lōh-ōh ′vrăl-28]
Tablets
(norgestrel and ethinyl estradiol tablets)

Patients should be counseled that this product does not protect against HIV infection (AIDS) and other sexually transmitted diseases.

DESCRIPTION

21 white LO/OVRAL tablets, each containing 0.3 mg of norgestrel (*dl* -13-beta-ethyl-17-alpha-ethinyl-17-beta-hydroxygon-4-en-3-one), a totally synthetic progestogen, and 0.03 mg of ethinyl estradiol (19-nor-17α-pregna-1,3,5(10)-trien-20-yne-3,17-diol), and 7 pink inert tablets. The inactive ingredients present are cellulose, D&C Red 30, lactose, magnesium stearate, and polacrilin potassium.

CLINICAL PHARMACOLOGY

See LO/OVRAL®.

INDICATIONS AND USAGE

See LO/OVRAL.

CONTRAINDICATIONS

See LO/OVRAL.

WARNINGS

See LO/OVRAL.

PRECAUTIONS

See LO/OVRAL.
Drug Interactions: See LO/OVRAL.
Carcinogenesis: See LO/OVRAL.
Pregnancy: See LO/OVRAL.
Nursing Mothers: See LO/OVRAL.
Information for the Patient: See LO/OVRAL.

ADVERSE REACTIONS

See LO/OVRAL.

OVERDOSAGE

See LO/OVRAL.

NONCONTRACEPTIVE HEALTH BENEFITS

See LO/OVRAL.

DOSAGE AND ADMINISTRATION

To achieve maximum contraceptive effectiveness, LO/OVRAL-28 must be taken exactly as directed and at intervals not exceeding 24 hours.

The dosage of LO/OVRAL-28 is one white tablet daily for 21 consecutive days, followed by one pink inert tablet daily for 7 consecutive days, according to prescribed schedule. It is recommended that tablets be taken at the same time each day, preferably after the evening meal or at bedtime.

During the first cycle of medication, the patient is instructed to begin taking LO/OVRAL-28 on the first Sunday after the onset of menstruation. If menstruation begins on a Sunday, the first tablet (white) is taken that day. One white tablet should be taken daily for 21 consecutive days followed by one pink inert tablet daily for 7 consecutive days. Withdrawal bleeding should usually occur within three days following discontinuation of white tablets. During the first cycle, contraceptive reliance should not be placed on LO/OVRAL-28 until a white tablet has been taken daily for 7 consecutive days. The possibility of ovulation and conception prior to initiation of medication should be considered. The patient begins her next and all subsequent 28-day courses of tablets on the same day of the week (Sunday) on which she began her first course, following the same schedule: 21 days on white tablets—7 days on pink inert tablets.

If in any cycle the patient starts tablets later than the proper day, she should protect herself by using another method of birth control until she has taken a white tablet daily for 7 consecutive days.

If spotting or breakthrough bleeding occurs, the patient is instructed to continue on the same regimen. This type of bleeding is usually transient and without significance; however, if the bleeding is persistent or prolonged, the patient is advised to consult her physician. Although the occurrence of pregnancy is highly unlikely if LO/OVRAL-28 is taken according to directions, if withdrawal bleeding does not occur, the possibility of pregnancy must be considered. If the patient has not adhered to the prescribed schedule (missed one or more tablets or started taking them on a day later than she should have), the probability of pregnancy should be considered at the time of the first missed period and appropriate diagnostic measures taken before the medication is resumed. If the patient has adhered to the prescribed regimen and misses two consecutive periods, pregnancy should be ruled out before continuing the contraceptive regimen.

For additional patient instructions regarding missed pills, see the "WHAT TO DO IF YOU MISS PILLS" section in the DETAILED PATIENT LABELING for LO/OVRAL.

Any time the patient misses two or more white tablets, she should also use another method of contraception until she has taken a white tablet daily for seven consecutive days. If the patient misses one or more pink tablets, she is still protected against pregnancy provided she begins taking white tablets again on the proper day.

If breakthrough bleeding occurs following missed white tablets, it will usually be transient and of no consequence. While there is little likelihood of ovulation occurring if only one or two white tablets are missed, the possibility of ovulation increases with each successive day that scheduled white tablets are missed.

In the nonlactating mother, LO/OVRAL-28 may be initiated postpartum, for contraception. When the tablets are administered in the postpartum period, the increased risk of thromboembolic disease associated with the postpartum period must be considered (see "Contraindications," "Warnings," and "Precautions" concerning thromboembolic disease). It is to be noted that early resumption of ovulation may occur if Parlodel® (bromocriptine mesylate) has been used for the prevention of lactation.

HOW SUPPLIED

LO/OVRAL®-28 Tablets (0.3 mg norgestrel and 0.03 mg ethinyl estradiol) are available in packages of 6 PILPAK® dispensers, each containing 28 tablets as follows:

21 active tablets, NDC 0008-0078, white, round tablet marked "WYETH" and "78".

7 inert tablets, NDC 0008-0486, pink, round tablet marked "WYETH" and "486".

ALSO AVAILABLE:

LO/OVRAL®-28 Tablets (0.3 mg norgestrel and 0.03 mg ethinyl estradiol) are available in packages of 12 PILPAK® dispensers for clinic use only, each containing 28 tablets as follows:

21 active tablets, NDC 0008-0078, white, round tablet marked "WYETH" and "78".

7 inert tablets, NDC 0008-0486, pink, round tablet marked "WYETH" and "486".

Store at room temperature, approx. 25°C (77°F).

References available upon request.

Brief Summary Patient Package Insert: See LO/OVRAL.
DETAILED PATIENT LABELING: See LO/OVRAL.

HOW TO TAKE THE PILL

For Lo/Ovral-28 PILPAK® Dispenser, See LO/OVRAL.
For Lo/Ovral-28 Clinic Pilpak®, See below.
HOW TO TAKE THE PILL

This product (like all oral contraceptives) is intended to prevent pregnancy. It does not protect against transmission of

HIV (AIDS) and other sexually transmitted diseases such as chlamydia, genital herpes, genital warts, gonorrhea, hepatitis B, and syphilis.

IMPORTANT POINTS TO REMEMBER

BEFORE YOU START TAKING YOUR PILLS:

1. BE SURE TO READ THESE DIRECTIONS:
Before you start taking your pills.
Anytime you are not sure what to do.

2. THE RIGHT WAY TO TAKE THE PILL IS TO TAKE ONE PILL EVERY DAY AT THE SAME TIME.
If you miss pills you could get pregnant. This includes starting the pack late. The more pills you miss, the more likely you are to get pregnant.

3. MANY WOMEN HAVE SPOTTING OR LIGHT BLEEDING, OR MAY FEEL SICK TO THEIR STOMACH DURING THE FIRST 1–3 PACKS OF PILLS.
If you feel sick to your stomach, do not stop taking the pill. The problem will usually go away. If it doesn't go away, check with your doctor or clinic.

4. MISSING PILLS CAN ALSO CAUSE SPOTTING OR LIGHT BLEEDING, even when you make up these missed pills.
On the days you take 2 pills to make up for missed pills, you could also feel a little sick to your stomach.

5. IF YOU HAVE VOMITING OR DIARRHEA, for any reason, or IF YOU TAKE SOME MEDICINES, including some antibiotics, your pills may not work as well. Use a back-up method (such as condoms or foam) until you check with your doctor or clinic.

6. IF YOU HAVE TROUBLE REMEMBERING TO TAKE THE PILL, talk to your doctor or clinic about how to make pill-taking easier or about using another method of birth control.

7. IF YOU HAVE ANY QUESTIONS OR ARE UNSURE ABOUT THE INFORMATION IN THIS LEAFLET, call your doctor or clinic.

NORDETTE®-21, OVRAL®, LO/OVRAL®, NORDETTE®-28, OVRAL®-28, AND LO/OVRAL®-28

BEFORE YOU START TAKING YOUR PILLS

1. DECIDE WHAT TIME OF DAY YOU WANT TO TAKE YOUR PILL.
It is important to take it at about the same time every day.

2. LOOK AT YOUR PILL PACK TO SEE IF IT HAS 21 OR 28 PILLS:
The *21-pill pack* has 21 "active" white or light-orange pills (with hormones) to take for 3 weeks, followed by 1 week without pills.
The *28-pill pack* has 21 "active" white or light-orange pills (with hormones) to take for 3 weeks, followed by 1 week of reminder pink pills (without hormones).

3. ALSO FIND:
1) where on the pack to start taking pills,
2) in what order to take the pills (follow the arrows), and
3) the week numbers as shown in the picture below.

4. BE SURE YOU HAVE READY AT ALL TIMES:
ANOTHER KIND OF BIRTH CONTROL (such as condoms or foam) to use as a back-up in case you miss pills.
AN EXTRA, FULL PILL PACK.

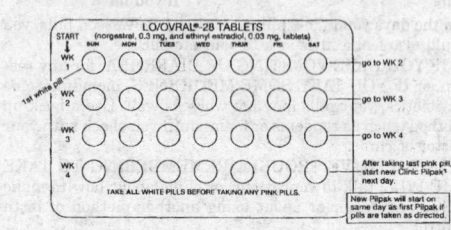

WHEN TO START THE *FIRST* PACK OF PILLS:

For the 21-day pill pack you have two choices of which day to start taking your first pack of pills. (See **DAY 1 START** or **SUNDAY START** directions below.) Decide with your doctor or clinic which is the best day for you. The 28-day pill pack accommodates a **SUNDAY START** only. For either pill pack pick a time of day which will be easy to remember.
DAY 1 START:
These instructions are for the 21-day pill pack only. The 28-day pill pack does not accommodate a **DAY 1 START** dosage regimen.

1. Take the first "active" white or light-orange pill of the first pack during the *first 24 hours of your period*.
2. You will not need to use a back-up method of birth control, since you are starting the pill at the beginning of your period.

SUNDAY START:

These instructions are for either the 21-day or the 28-day pill pack.

1. Take the first "active" white or light-orange pill of the first pack on the *Sunday after your period starts,* even if you are still bleeding. If your period begins on Sunday, start the pack that same day.

2. *Use another method of birth control* as a back-up method if you have sex anytime from the Sunday you start your first pack until the next Sunday (7 days). Condoms or foam are good back-up methods of birth control.

WHAT TO DO DURING THE MONTH:

1. TAKE ONE PILL AT THE SAME TIME EVERY DAY UNTIL THE PACK IS EMPTY.

Do not skip pills even if you are spotting or bleeding between monthly periods or feel sick to your stomach (nausea).

Do not skip pills even if you do not have sex very often.

2. WHEN YOU FINISH A PACK OR SWITCH YOUR BRAND OF PILLS:

21 pills: Wait 7 days to start the next pack. You will probably have your period during that week. Be sure that no more than 7 days pass between 21-day packs.

28 pills: Start the next pack on the day after your last "reminder" pill. Do not wait any days between packs.

WHAT TO DO IF YOU MISS PILLS

If you **MISS 1** white or light-orange "active" pill:

1. Take it as soon as you remember. Take the next pill at your regular time. This means you take 2 pills in 1 day.

2. You do not need to use a back-up birth control method if you have sex.

If you **MISS 2** white or light-orange "active" pills in a row in **WEEK 1 OR WEEK 2** of your pack:

1. Take 2 pills on the day you remember and 2 pills the next day.

2. Then take 1 pill a day until you finish the pack.

3. You MAY BECOME PREGNANT if you have sex in the 7 *days* after you miss pills. You MUST use another birth control method (such as condoms or foam) as a back-up for those 7 days.

If you **MISS 2** white or light-orange "active" pills in a row in **THE 3rd WEEK:**

The *Day 1 Starter* instructions are for the 21-day pill pack only. The 28-day pill pack does not accommodate a **DAY 1 START** dosage regimen. The *Sunday Starter* instructions are for either the 21-day or 28-day pill pack.

1. *If you are a Day 1 Starter:*

THROW OUT the rest of the pill pack and start a new pack that same day.

If you are a Sunday Starter:

Keep taking 1 pill every day until Sunday.

On Sunday, THROW OUT the rest of the pack and start a new pack of pills that same day.

2. You may not have your period this month but this is expected.

However, if you miss your period 2 months in a row, call your doctor or clinic because you might be pregnant.

3. You MAY BECOME PREGNANT if you have sex in the 7 *days* after you miss pills. You MUST use another birth control method (such as condoms or foam) as a back-up for those 7 days.

If you **MISS 3 OR MORE** white or light-orange "active" pills in a row (during the first 3 weeks):

The *Day 1 Starter* instructions are for the 21-day pill pack only. The 28-day pill pack does not accommodate a **DAY 1 START** dosage regimen. The *Sunday Starter* instructions are for either the 21-day or 28-day pill pack.

1. *If you are a Day 1 Starter:*

THROW OUT the rest of the pill pack and start a new pack that same day.

If you are a Sunday Starter:

Keep taking 1 pill every day until Sunday.

On Sunday, THROW OUT the rest of the pack and start a new pack of pills that same day.

2. You may not have your period this month but this is expected.

However, if you miss your period 2 months in a row, call your doctor or clinic because you might be pregnant.

3. You MAY BECOME PREGNANT if you have sex in the 7 *days* after you miss pills. You MUST use another birth control method (such as condoms or foam) as a back-up for those 7 days.

A REMINDER FOR THOSE ON 28-DAY PACKS:

If your forget any of the 7 pink "reminder" pills in Week 4: THROW AWAY the pills you missed.

Keep taking 1 pill each day until the pack is empty.

You do not need a back-up method if you start your next pack on time.

FINALLY, IF YOU ARE STILL NOT SURE WHAT TO DO ABOUT THE PILLS YOU HAVE MISSED:

Use a BACK-UP METHOD anytime you have sex.

KEEP TAKING ONE PILL EACH DAY until you can reach your doctor or clinic.

OVRETTE®

Ovrette is administered on a continuous daily dosage schedule, one tablet each day, every day of the year. Take the first tablet on the first day of your menstrual period. Tablets should be taken at the same time every day without interruption, whether bleeding occurs or not. If bleeding is prolonged (more than 8 days) or unusually heavy, you should contact your doctor.

Forgotten pills

The risk of pregnancy increases with each tablet missed. Therefore, it is very important that you take one tablet daily as directed. If you miss one tablet, take it as soon as you remember and also take your next tablet at the regular time. If you miss two tablets, take one of the missed tablets as soon as you remember, as well as your regular tablet for that day at the proper time. Furthermore, you should use another method of birth control in addition to taking Ovrette until you have taken fourteen days (2 weeks) of medication.

If more than two tablets have been missed, Ovrette should be discontinued immediately and another method of birth control used until the start of your next menstrual period. Then you may resume taking Ovrette.

Pregnancy due to pill failure

The incidence of pill failure resulting in pregnancy is approximately less than 1.0% if taken every day as directed, but more typical failure rates are less than 3.0%. If failure does occur, the risk to the fetus is minimal.

RISKS TO THE FETUS

If you do become pregnant while using oral contraceptives, the risk to the fetus is small, on the order of no more than one per thousand. You should, however, discuss the risks to the developing child with your doctor.

Pregnancy after stopping the pill

There may be some delay in becoming pregnant after you stop using oral contraceptives, especially if you had irregular menstrual cycles before you used oral contraceptives. It may be advisable to postpone conception until you begin menstruating regularly once you have stopped taking the pill and desire pregnancy.

There does not appear to be any increase in birth defects in newborn babies when pregnancy occurs soon after stopping the pill.

Overdosage

Serious ill effects have not been reported following ingestion of large doses of oral contraceptives by young children. Overdosage may cause nausea and withdrawal bleeding in females. In case of overdosage, contact your health-care provider or pharmacist.

Other information

Your health-care provider will take a medical and family history before prescribing oral contraceptives and will examine you. The physical examination may be delayed to another time if you request it and the health-care provider believes that it is appropriate to postpone it. You should be reexamined at least once a year. Be sure to inform your health-care provider if there is a family history of any of the conditions listed previously in this leaflet. Be sure to keep all appointments with your health-care provider, because this is a time to determine if there are early signs of side effects of oral-contraceptive use.

Do not use the drug for any condition other than the one for which it was prescribed. This drug has been prescribed specifically for you; do not give it to others who may want birth-control pills.

HEALTH BENEFITS FROM ORAL CONTRACEPTIVES: See LO/OVRAL.

Manufactured by:

Wyeth Laboratories Inc.

A Wyeth-Ayerst Company

Philadelphia, PA 19101

Shown in Product Identification Guide, page 344

MEPERGAN®   Ⓒ ℞

[mep 'er-gan]

(meperidine HCl and
promethazine HCl)
Injection

DESCRIPTION

This product is available in concentration providing 25 mg each of meperidine hydrochloride and promethazine hydrochloride per mL with 0.1 mg edetate disodium, 0.04 mg cal-

cium chloride, and not more than 0.75 mg sodium formaldehyde sulfoxylate, 0.25 mg sodium metabisulfite, and 5 mg phenol with sodium acetate buffer.

ACTIONS

Meperidine hydrochloride is a narcotic analgesic with multiple actions qualitatively similar to those of morphine. Phenergan®, promethazine HCl, is a phenothiazine derivative that has several different pharmacologic properties including antihistaminic, sedative, and antiemetic actions.

INDICATIONS

As a preanesthetic medication when analgesia and sedation are indicated. As an adjunct to local and general anesthesia.

CONTRAINDICATIONS

Hypersensitivity to meperidine or promethazine.

Under no circumstances should Mepergan be given by intra-arterial injection, due to the likelihood of severe arteriospasm and the possibility of resultant gangrene (see "**Warnings**").

Mepergan should not be given by the subcutaneous route; evidence of chemical irritation has been noted, and necrotic lesions have resulted on rare occasions following subcutaneous injection. The preferred parenteral route of administration is by deep intramuscular injection.

Meperidine is contraindicated in patients who are receiving monoamine oxidase inhibitors (MAOI) or those who have received such agents within 14 days. Therapeutic doses of meperidine have inconsistently precipitated unpredictable, severe, and occasionally fatal reactions in patients who have received such agents within 14 days. The mechanism of these reactions is unclear. Some have been characterized by coma, severe respiratory depression, cyanosis, and hypotension and have resembled the syndrome of acute narcotic overdose. In other reactions the predominant manifestations have been hyperexcitability, convulsions, tachycardia, hyperpyrexia, and hypertension. Although it is not known that other narcotics are free of the risk of such reactions, virtually all of the reported reactions have occurred with meperidine. If a narcotic is needed in such patients, a sensitivity test should be performed in which repeated, small, incremental doses of morphine are administered over the course of several hours while the patient's condition and vital signs are under careful observation.

(Intravenous hydrocortisone or prednisolone have been used to treat severe reactions, with the addition of intravenous chlorpromazine in those cases exhibiting hypertension and hyperpyrexia. The usefulness and safety of narcotic antagonists in the treatment of these reactions is unknown.)

WARNINGS

Mepergan Injection contains sodium metabisulfite, a sulfite that may cause allergic-type reactions, including anaphylactic symptoms and life-threatening or less severe asthmatic episodes, in certain susceptible people. The overall prevalence of sulfite sensitivity in the general population is unknown and probably low. Sulfite sensitivity is seen more frequently in asthmatic than in nonasthmatic people.

Tolerance and Addiction Liability

Warning—may be habit-forming

DRUG DEPENDENCE

Meperidine can produce drug dependence of the morphine type and therefore has the potential for being abused. Psychic dependence, physical dependence, and tolerance may develop upon repeated administration of meperidine, and it should be prescribed and administered with the same degree of caution appropriate to the use of morphine. Like other narcotics, meperidine is subject to the provisions of the Federal narcotic laws.

INTERACTION WITH OTHER CENTRAL NERVOUS SYSTEM DEPRESSANTS

Meperidine should be used with great caution and in reduced dosage in patients who are concurrently receiving other narcotic analgesics, general anesthetics, phenothiazines, other tranquilizers, sedative-hypnotics, tricyclic antidepressants, and other CNS depressants (including alcohol). Respiratory depression, hypotension, and profound sedation or coma may result.

The sedative action of promethazine hydrochloride is additive to the sedative effects of central nervous system depressants; therefore, agents such as alcohol, barbiturates, and narcotic analgesics should either be eliminated or given in reduced dosage in the presence of promethazine hydrochloride. When given concomitantly with promethazine hydrochloride, the dose of barbiturates should be reduced by at least one-half and the dose of analgesic depressants, such as morphine or meperidine, should be reduced by one-quarter to one-half.

HEAD INJURY AND INCREASED INTRACRANIAL PRESSURE

The respiratory-depressant effects of meperidine and its capacity to elevate cerebrospinal-fluid pressure may be markedly exaggerated in the presence of head injury, other intracranial lesions, or a preexisting increase in intracranial

Continued on next page

Mepergan—Cont.

pressure. Furthermore, narcotics produce adverse reactions which may obscure the clinical course of patients with head injuries. In such patients, meperidine must be used with extreme caution and only if its use is deemed essential.

INADVERTENT INTRA-ARTERIAL INJECTION

Due to the close proximity of arteries and veins in the areas most commonly used for intravenous injection, extreme care should be exercised to avoid perivascular extravasation or inadvertent intra-arterial injection of Mepergan. Reports compatible with inadvertent intra-arterial injection suggest that pain, severe chemical irritation, severe spasm of distal vessels, and resultant gangrene requiring amputation is likely under such circumstances. Intravenous injection was intended in all the cases reported, but perivascular extravasation or arterial placement of the needle is now suspect. There is no proven successful management of this condition after it occurs, although sympathetic block and heparinization are commonly employed during the acute management because of the results of animal experiments with other known arteriolar irritants. Aspiration of dark blood does not preclude intra-arterial needle placement, because blood is discolored upon contact with promethazine. Use of syringes with rigid plungers or of small bore needles might obscure typical arterial backflow if this is relied upon alone.

INTRAVENOUS USE

If necessary, meperidine may be given intravenously, but the injection should be given very slowly, preferably in the form of a diluted solution. Rapid intravenous injection of narcotic analgesics, including meperidine, increases the incidence of adverse reactions; severe respiratory depression, apnea, hypotension; peripheral circulatory collapse, and cardiac arrest have occurred. Meperidine should not be administered intravenously unless a narcotic antagonist and the facilities for assisted or controlled respiration are immediately available. When meperidine is given parenterally, especially intravenously, the patient should be lying down. When used intravenously, Mepergan should be given at a rate not to exceed 1 mL (25 mg of each component) per minute. When administering any irritant drug intravenously, it is usually preferable to inject it through the tubing of an intravenous infusion set that is known to be functioning satisfactorily. In the event that a patient complains of pain during intended intravenous injection of Mepergan, the injection should immediately be stopped to provide for evaluation of possible arterial placement or perivascular extravasation.

ASTHMA AND OTHER RESPIRATORY CONDITIONS

Meperidine should be used with extreme caution in patients having an acute asthmatic attack, patients with chronic obstructive pulmonary disease or cor pulmonale, patients having a substantially decreased respiratory reserve, and patients with preexisting respiratory depression, hypoxia, or hypercapnia. In such patients, even usual therapeutic doses of narcotics may decrease respiratory drive while simultaneously increasing airway resistance to the point of apnea.

HYPOTENSIVE EFFECT

The administration of meperidine may result in severe hypotension in an individual whose ability to maintain his blood pressure has already been compromised by a depleted blood volume or concurrent administration of drugs such as the phenothiazines or certain anesthetics.

USAGE IN AMBULATORY PATIENTS

Meperidine may impair the mental and/or physical abilities required for the performance of potentially hazardous tasks, such as driving a car or operating machinery. The patient should be cautioned accordingly.

Meperidine, like other narcotics, may produce orthostatic hypotension in ambulatory patients.

USAGE IN PREGNANCY AND LACTATION

Meperidine should not be used in pregnant women prior to the labor period, unless in the judgment of the physician the potential benefits outweigh the possible hazards, because safe use in pregnancy prior to labor has not been established relative to possible adverse effects on fetal development.

When used as an obstetrical analgesic, meperidine crosses the placental barrier and can produce respiratory depression in the newborn; resuscitation may be required (see "**Overdosage**").

Meperidine appears in the milk of nursing mothers receiving the drug.

PRECAUTIONS

SUPRAVENTRICULAR TACHYCARDIAS

Meperidine should be used with caution in patients with atrial flutter and other supraventricular tachycardias because of a possible vagolytic action which may produce a significant increase in the ventricular response rate.

CONVULSIONS

Meperidine may aggravate preexisting convulsions in patients with convulsive disorders. If dosage is escalated substantially above recommended levels because of tolerance development, convulsions may occur in individuals without a history of convulsive disorders.

ACUTE ABDOMINAL CONDITIONS

The administration of meperidine or other narcotics may obscure the diagnosis or clinical course in patients with acute abdominal conditions.

SPECIAL-RISK PATIENTS

Meperidine should be given with caution, and the initial dose should be reduced in certain patients, such as the elderly or debilitated, and those with severe impairment of hepatic or renal function, hypothyroidism, Addison's disease, and prostatic hypertrophy or urethral stricture.

Antiemetics may mask the symptoms of an unrecognized disease and thereby interfere with diagnosis.

Patients in pain who have received inadequate or no analgesia have been noted to develop "athetoid-like" movements of the upper extremities following the parenteral administration of promethazine. These symptoms usually disappear upon adequate control of the pain.

Ambulatory patients should be cautioned against driving automobiles or operating dangerous machinery until it is known that they do not become drowsy or dizzy from promethazine hydrochloride therapy.

ADVERSE REACTIONS

The major hazards of meperidine, as with other narcotic analgesics, are respiratory depression and, to a lesser degree, circulatory depression; respiratory arrest, shock, and cardiac arrest have occurred.

The most frequently observed adverse reactions include light-headedness, dizziness, sedation, nausea, vomiting, and sweating. These effects seem to be more prominent in ambulatory patients and in those who are not experiencing severe pain. In such individuals, lower doses are advisable. Some adverse reactions in ambulatory patients may be alleviated if the patient lies down.

Other adverse reactions include:

CENTRAL NERVOUS SYSTEM

Euphoria, dysphoria, weakness, headache, agitation, tremor, uncoordinated muscle movements, transient hallucinations and disorientation, visual disturbances and, rarely, extrapyramidal reactions.

GASTROINTESTINAL

Dry mouth, constipation, biliary-tract spasm.

CARDIOVASCULAR

Flushing of the face, tachycardia, bradycardia, palpitation, faintness, syncope.

Cardiovascular effects from promethazine have been rare. Minor increases in blood pressure and occasional mild hypotension have been reported. Venous thrombosis at the injection site has been reported. Intra-arterial injection of Mepergan may result in gangrene of the affected extremity (see "**Warnings**").

GENITOURINARY

Urinary retention.

ALLERGIC

Pruritus, urticaria, other skin rashes, wheal and flare over the vein with IV injection.

Photosensitivity, although extremely rare, has been reported. Occurrence of photosensitivity may be a contraindication to further treatment with promethazine or related drugs.

OTHER

Pain at injection site; local tissue irritation, induration, and possible tissue necrosis, particularly when injection is repeated at same site; antidiuretic effect.

Patients may occasionally complain of autonomic reactions, such as dryness of the mouth, blurring of vision and, rarely, dizziness following the use of promethazine.

Very rare cases have been reported where patients receiving promethazine have developed leukopenia. In one instance agranulocytosis has been reported. In nearly every instance reported, other toxic agents known to have caused these conditions have been associated with the administration of promethazine.

DOSAGE AND ADMINISTRATION

Parenteral drug products should be inspected visually for particulate matter and discoloration prior to administration, whenever solution and container permit.

WARNING—BARBITURATES ARE NOT CHEMICALLY COMPATIBLE IN SOLUTION WITH MEPERGAN (MEPERIDINE HYDROCHLORIDE AND PROMETHAZINE HYDROCHLORIDE) AND SHOULD NOT BE MIXED IN THE SAME SYRINGE.

Mepergan is usually administered intramuscularly. However, in certain specific situations, the intravenous route may be employed. INADVERTENT INTRA-ARTERIAL INJECTION CAN RESULT IN GANGRENE OF THE AFFECTED EXTREMITY (see "**Warnings**"). SUBCUTANEOUS ADMINISTRATION IS CONTRAINDICATED, AS IT MAY RESULT IN TISSUE NECROSIS (see "**Contraindications**"). INJECTION INTO OR NEAR PERIPHERAL NERVES MAY RESULT IN PERMANENT NEUROLOGICAL DEFICIT.

When used intravenously, the rate should not be greater than 1 mL of Mepergan (25 mg of each component) per minute; it is preferable to inject through the tubing of an intravenous infusion set that is known to be functioning satisfactorily.

The TUBEX® BLUNT POINTE™ Sterile Cartridge Unit is suitable for substances to be administered intravenously only. It is intended for use with injection sets specifically manufactured as "needle-less" injection systems. TUBEX® BLUNT POINTE™ is compatible with Abbott's LifeShield® prepierced reseal injection site, Baxter's InterLink® Injection Site, and B. Braun Medical's SafSite® Reflux Valve, Consult manufacturer's recommendations regarding "Directions for Use" of the "needle-less" system. It is also intended for admixture with, and convenient administration of various medicaments when using Drug Vial Adapters for "needle-less" injection systems.

The TUBEX® Sterile Cartridge-Needle Unit is suitable for substances to be administered intravenously or intramuscularly.

The TUBEX® Sterile Cartridge-Needle Unit is designed for single-dose use. VIALS should be used when required doses are fractions of a milliliter, as indicated below.

ADULT DOSE: 1 to 2 mL (25 to 50 mg of each component) per single injection, which can be repeated every 3 to 4 hours.

CHILDREN 12 YEARS OF AGE AND UNDER: 0.5 mg of each component per pound of body weight. The dosage may be repeated every 3 to 4 hours as necessary.

For preanesthetic medication the usual adult dose is 2 mL (50 mg of each component) intramuscularly with or without appropriate atropine-like drug. Atropine sulfate, 0.3 to 0.4 mg, or scopolamine hydrobromide, 0.25 to 0.4 mg, in sterile solution may be mixed in the same syringe with Mepergan. Repeat doses of 50 mg or less of both promethazine and meperidine may be administered by either route at 3- to 4-hour intervals, as necessary. As an adjunct to local or general anesthesia, the usual dose is 2 mL (50 mg each of meperidine and promethazine).

OVERDOSAGE

SYMPTOMS

Serious overdose with meperidine is characterized by respiratory depression (a decrease in respiratory rate and/or tidal volume, Cheyne-Stokes respiration, cyanosis), extreme somnolence progressing to stupor or coma, skeletal muscle flaccidity, cold and clammy skin, and sometimes bradycardia and hypotension. In severe overdosage, particularly by the intravenous route, apnea, circulatory collapse, cardiac arrest, and death may occur.

TREATMENT

Primary attention should be given to the reestablishment of adequate respiratory exchange through provision of a patent airway and institution of assisted or controlled ventilation. The narcotic antagonist, naloxone hydrochloride, is a specific antidote against respiratory depression which may result from overdosage or unusual sensitivity to narcotics, including meperidine. The usual initial adult dose of naloxone is 0.4 to 2.0 mg, administered intravenously. If the desired degree of counteraction and improvement in respiratory functions is not obtained, this dosage can be repeated at two- to three-minute intervals while resuscitation efforts continue. If 10 mg of naloxone have been administered without an improvement in the clinical situation, the diagnosis of Mepergan overdose should be questioned.

An antagonist should not be administered in absence of clinically significant respiratory or cardiovascular depression.

Oxygen, intravenous fluids, vasopressors, and other supportive measures should be employed as indicated.

NOTE: In an individual physically dependent on narcotics, the administration of the usual dose of a narcotic antagonist will precipitate an acute withdrawal syndrome. The severity of this syndrome will depend on the degree of physical dependence and the dose of antagonist administered. The use of narcotic antagonists in such individuals should be avoided if possible. If a narcotic antagonist must be used to treat serious respiratory depression in the physically dependent patient, the antagonist should be administered with extreme care and only one-tenth to one-fifth the usual initial dose administered.

Attempted suicides with promethazine have resulted in deep sedation, coma, rarely convulsions and cardiorespiratory symptoms compatible with the depth of sedation present. Extrapyramidal reactions may be treated with anticholinergic antiparkinson agents, diphenhydramine, or barbiturates.

If severe hypotension occurs, levarterenol or phenylephrine may be indicated. Epinephrine is probably best avoided, since it has been suggested that promethazine overdosage could produce a partial alpha-adrenergic blockade.

A paradoxical reaction, characterized by hyperexcitability and nightmares, has been reported in children receiving large single doses of promethazine.

HOW SUPPLIED

Mepergan® (meperidine HCl and promethazine HCl) Injection is available in TUBEX® BLUNT POINTE™ Sterile

Cartridge Units and Sterile Cartridge-Needle Units, in boxes of 10 TUBEX in TAMP-R-TEL® tamper-resistant packages as follows:

NDC 0008-0235-50, 2 mL size Blunt Pointe™

NDC 0008-0235-01, 2 mL size (22 gauge x 1-1/4 inch needle).

Mepergan (meperidine HCl and promethazine HCl) Injection is also available in vials as follows:

NDC 0008-0234, 10 mL vial.

Do not use if solution is discolored or contains a precipitate.

Protect from light

Use carton to protect contents from light

Store at room temperature, approximately 25° C (77° F)

Manufactured by:

Wyeth Laboratories Inc.

A Wyeth-Ayerst Company

Philadelphia, PA 19101

NAPRELAN®   ℞

[nă′ prĕ-lăn]

(naproxen sodium)

CONTROLLED RELEASE TABLETS

Equivalent to 375 mg and 500 mg naproxen

DESCRIPTION

Naprelan contains naproxen sodium, a member of the arylacetic acid group of nonsteroidal anti-inflammatory drugs (NSAIDs).

Naprelan uses the proprietary IPDAS™ (Intestinal Protective Drug Absorption System) technology. It is a rapidly disintegrating tablet system combining an immediate release component and a sustained release component of microparticles that are widely dispersed, allowing absorption of the active ingredient throughout the gastrointestinal (GI) tract, maintaining blood levels over 24 hours.

The chemical name for naproxen sodium is 2-naphthaleneacetic acid, 6-methoxy-α-methyl-sodium salt, (S)- with the following structural formula:

Naproxen sodium

Molecular Formula: $C_{14}H_{13}NaO_3$

Molecular Weight: 252.24

Naproxen sodium is an odorless crystalline powder, white to creamy in color. It is soluble in methanol and water.

Naprelan contains 412.5 mg or 550 mg of naproxen sodium, equivalent to 375 mg and 500 mg of naproxen and 37.5 mg and 50 mg sodium respectively. Each Naprelan tablet also contains the following inactive ingredients: ammonio methacrylate copolymer Type A, ammonio methacrylate copolymer Type B, citric acid, crospovidone, magnesium stearate, methacrylic acid copolymer Type A, microcrystalline cellulose, povidone, and talc. The tablet coating contains hydroxypropyl methylcellulose, polyethylene glycol, and titanium dioxide.

CLINICAL PHARMACOLOGY

Naproxen is a nonsteroidal anti-inflammatory drug (NSAID), with analgesic and antipyretic properties. As with other NSAIDs, its mode of action is not fully understood; however, its ability to inhibit prostaglandin synthesis may be involved in the anti-inflammatory effect.

PHARMACOKINETICS

Although naproxen itself is well absorbed, the sodium salt form is more rapidly absorbed resulting in higher peak plasma levels for a given dose. Approximately 30% of the total naproxen sodium dose in Naprelan is present in the dosage form as an immediate release component. The remaining naproxen sodium is coated as microparticles to provide sustained release properties. After oral administration, plasma levels of naproxen are detected within 30 minutes of dosing, with peak plasma levels occurring approximately 5 hours after dosing. The observed terminal elimination half-life of naproxen from both immediate release naproxen sodium and Naprelan is approximately 15 hours. Steady state levels of naproxen are achieved in 3 days and the degree of naproxen accumulation in the blood is consistent with this.

[See figure at top of next column]

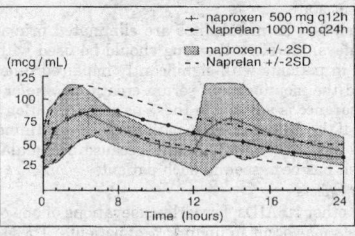

Plasma Naproxen Concentrations
Mean of 24 Subjects (+/-2SD)
(Steady State, Day 5)

— naproxen 500 mg q12h
— Naprelan 1000 mg q24h
naproxen +/-2SD
Naprelan +/-2SD

Pharmacokinetic Parameters at Steady State Day 5 (Mean of 24 Subjects)

Para-meter (units)	naproxen 500 mg Q12h/5 days (1000 mg)			Naprelan 2 x 500 mg tablets (1000 mg) Q24h/5 days		
	Mean	SD	Range	Mean	SD	Range
AUC 0-24 (mcgxh/mL)	1446	168	1167–1858	1448	145	1173–1774
C_{max} (mcg/mL)	95	13	71–117	94	13	74–127
C_{avg} (mcg/mL)	60	7	49–77	60	6	49–74
C_{min} (mcg/mL)	36	9	13–51	33	7	23–48
T_{max} (hrs)	3	1	1–4	5	2	2–10

Absorption

Naproxen itself is rapidly and completely absorbed from the GI tract with an *in vivo* bioavailability of 95%. Based on the pharmacokinetic profile, the absorption phase of Naprelan occurs in the first 4–6 hours after administration. This coincides with disintegration of the tablet in the stomach, transit of the sustained release microparticles through the small intestine and into the proximal large intestine. An *in vivo* imaging study has been performed in healthy volunteers which confirms rapid disintegration of the tablet matrix and dispersion of the microparticles.

The absorption rate from the sustained release particulate component of Naprelan is slower than that for conventional naproxen sodium tablets. It is this prolongation of drug absorption processes which maintains plasma levels and allows for once daily dosing.

Food Effects

No significant food effects were observed when twenty-four subjects were given a single dose of Naprelan 500 mg either after an overnight fast or 30 minutes after a meal. In common with conventional naproxen and naproxen sodium formulations, food causes a slight decrease in the rate of naproxen absorption following Naprelan administration.

Distribution

Naproxen has a volume of distribution of 0.16 L/kg. At therapeutic levels naproxen is greater than 99% albumin-bound. At doses of naproxen greater than 500 mg/day there is a less than proportional increase in plasma levels due to an increase in clearance caused by saturation of plasma protein binding at higher doses. However the concentration of unbound naproxen continues to increase proportionally to dose. Naprelan exhibits similar dose proportional characteristics.

Metabolism

Naproxen is extensively metabolized to 6-0-desmethyl naproxen and both parent and metabolites do not induce metabolizing enzymes.

Elimination

The elimination half-life of Naprelan and conventional naproxen is approximately 15 hours. Steady state conditions are attained after 2–3 doses of Naprelan. Most of the drug is excreted in the urine, primarily as unchanged naproxen (less than 1%), 6-0-desmethyl naproxen (less than 1%) and their glucuronide or other conjugates (66–92%). A small amount (<5%) of the drug is excreted in the feces. The rate of excretion has been found to coincide closely with the rate of clearance from the plasma. In patients with renal failure metabolites may accumulate.

Special Populations

Pediatric Use

No pediatric studies have been performed with Naprelan, thus safety of Naprelan in pediatric populations has not been established.

Renal Insufficiency

Naproxen pharmacokinetics have not been determined in subjects with renal insufficiency. Given that naproxen is me-

tabolized and conjugates are primarily excreted by the kidneys, the potential exists for naproxen metabolites to accumulate in the presence of renal insufficiency.

CLINICAL STUDIES

RHEUMATOID ARTHRITIS

The use of Naprelan for the management of the signs and symptoms of rheumatoid arthritis was assessed in a 12 week double-blind, randomized, placebo and active-controlled study in 348 patients. Two Naprelan 500 mg tablets (1000 mg) once daily and naproxen 500 mg tablets twice daily (1000 mg) were more effective than placebo. Clinical effectiveness was demonstrated at one week and continued for the duration of the study.

OSTEOARTHRITIS

The use of Naprelan for the management of the signs and symptoms of osteoarthritis of the knee was assessed in a 12 week double-blind, placebo and active-controlled study in 347 patients. Two Naprelan 500 mg tablets (1000 mg) once daily and naproxen 500 mg tablets twice daily (1000 mg) were more effective than placebo. Clinical effectiveness was demonstrated at one week and continued for the duration of the study.

ANALGESIA

The onset of the analgesic effect of Naprelan was seen within 30 minutes in a pharmacokinetic/pharmacodynamic study of patients with pain following oral surgery. In controlled clinical trials, naproxen has been used in combination with gold, D-penicillamine, methotrexate and corticosteroids. Its use in combination with salicylate is not recommended because there is evidence that aspirin increases the rate of excretion of naproxen and data are inadequate to demonstrate that naproxen and aspirin produce greater improvement over that achieved with aspirin alone. In addition, as with other NSAIDs the combination may result in higher frequency of adverse events than demonstrated for either product alone.

SPECIAL STUDIES

In a double-blind randomized, parallel group study, 19 subjects received either two Naprelan 500 mg tablets (1000 mg) once daily or naproxen 500 mg tablets (1000 mg) twice daily for 7 days. Mucosal biopsy scores and endoscope scores were lower in the subjects who received Naprelan. In another double-blind, randomized, crossover study, 23 subjects received two Naprelan 500 mg tablets (1000 mg) once daily, naproxen 500 mg tablets (1000 mg) twice daily and aspirin 650 mg four times daily (2600 mg) for 7 days each. There were significantly fewer duodenal erosions seen with Naprelan than with either naproxen or aspirin. There were significantly fewer gastric erosions with both Naprelan and naproxen than with aspirin.

The clinical significance of these findings is unknown.

INDIVIDUALIZATION OF DOSAGE

RHEUMATOID ARTHRITIS, OSTEOARTHRITIS, AND ANKYLOSING SPONDYLITIS

Naprelan like other NSAIDs shows considerable variation in response. The recommended starting dose of Naprelan in adults is two Naprelan 375 mg tablets (750 mg) once daily, or two Naprelan 500 mg tablets (1000 mg) once daily. Patients already taking naproxen 250 mg, 375 mg or 500 mg twice daily (morning and evening) may have their total daily dose replaced with Naprelan as a single daily dose.

During long-term administration, the dose of Naprelan may be adjusted up or down depending on the clinical response of the patient.

In patients who tolerate lower doses of Naprelan well, the dose may be increased to three Naprelan 500 mg tablets (1500 mg) once daily for limited periods when a higher level of anti-inflammatory/analgesic activity is required. When treating patients, especially at the higher dose levels, the physician should observe sufficient increased clinical benefit to offset the potential increased risk. (See **CLINICAL PHARMACOLOGY**). The lowest effective dose should be sought and used in every patient.

Symptomatic improvement in arthritis usually begins within one week; however, treatment for two weeks may be required to achieve a therapeutic benefit. A lower dose should be considered in patients with renal or hepatic impairment or in elderly patients (see **PRECAUTIONS**). Studies indicate that although total plasma concentration of naproxen is unchanged, the unbound plasma fraction of naproxen is increased in the elderly. Caution is advised when high doses are required and some adjustment of dosage may be required in elderly patients. As with other drugs used in the elderly it is prudent to use the lowest effective dose.

ANALGESIA, DYSMENORRHEA, BURSITIS, AND TENDINITIS

The recommended starting dose is two Naprelan 500 mg tablets (1000 mg) once daily. For patients requiring greater analgesic benefit, three Naprelan 500 mg tablets (1500 mg) may be used for a limited period. Thereafter, the total daily dose should not exceed two Naprelan 500 mg tablets (1000 mg).

Continued on next page

Naprelan—Cont.

ACUTE GOUT

The recommended dose on the first day is two or three Naprelan 500 mg tablets (1000–1500 mg) once daily, followed by two Naprelan 500 mg tablets (1000 mg) once daily, until the attack has subsided.

INDICATIONS AND USAGE

Naprelan is indicated for the treatment of rheumatoid arthritis, osteoarthritis, ankylosing spondylitis, tendinitis, bursitis, and acute gout. It is also indicated in the relief of mild to moderate pain and the treatment of primary dysmenorrhea.

CONTRAINDICATIONS

All naproxen products are contraindicated in patients who have had allergic reactions to prescription as well as to over-the-counter products containing naproxen. Anaphylactoid reactions may occur in patients without previous known exposure or hypersensitivity to aspirin, naproxen, or other NSAIDs, or in individuals with a history of angioedema, urticaria, bronchospastic reactivity (e.g., asthma), and nasal polyps. Anaphylactoid reactions, like anaphylaxis, may have a fatal outcome. Therefore, careful questioning of patients for such things as asthma, nasal polyps, urticaria, and hypotension associated with NSAIDs before starting therapy is important. In addition, if such symptoms occur during therapy, treatment with Naprelan should be discontinued.

WARNINGS

RISK OF GI ULCERATION, BLEEDING AND PERFORATION WITH NSAID THERAPY

Serious GI toxicity, such as bleeding, ulceration, and perforation, can occur at any time, with or without warning symptoms, in patients treated chronically with NSAID therapy. Although minor upper GI problems, such as dyspepsia, are common, usually developing early in therapy, physicians should remain alert for ulcerations and bleeding in patients treated chronically with NSAIDs even in the absence of previous GI tract symptoms. In patients observed in clinical trials with naproxen of several months to two years duration, symptomatic upper GI ulcers, gross bleeding or perforation appear to occur in approximately 1% of patients treated for 3–6 months, and in about 2–4% of patients treated for one year. Physicians should inform patients about the signs and/or symptoms of serious GI toxicity and what steps to take if they occur.

Studies to date with all naproxen products have not identified any subset of patients not at risk of developing peptic ulceration and bleeding or any differences between different naproxen products in their propensity to cause peptic ulceration and bleeding. Except for a prior history of serious GI events and other risk factors known to be associated with peptic ulcer disease, such as alcoholism, smoking etc., no risk factors (e.g., age, sex) have been associated with increased risk. Elderly or debilitated patients seem to tolerate ulceration or bleeding less well than other individuals and most spontaneous reports of fatal GI events are in this population. Studies to date are inconclusive concerning the relative risk of various NSAIDs in causing such reactions. High doses of any NSAID probably carry a greater risk of these reactions, although controlled clinical trials showing this do not exist in most cases. In considering the use of relatively large doses (within the recommended dosage range), sufficient benefit should be anticipated to offset the potential increased risk of GI toxicity.

PRECAUTIONS

GENERAL

NAPRELAN SHOULD NOT BE USED CONCOMITANTLY WITH OTHER NAPROXEN PRODUCTS SINCE THEY ALL CIRCULATE IN THE PLASMA AS THE NAPROXEN ANION.
The antipyretic and anti-inflammatory activities of the drug may reduce fever and inflammation, thus diminishing their utility as diagnostic signs.

Because of adverse eye findings in animal studies with drugs of this class, it is recommended that ophthalmic studies be carried out if any change or disturbance in vision occurs.

Renal Effects

As with other NSAIDs, long term administration of naproxen to animals has resulted in renal papillary necrosis and other abnormal renal pathology. In humans, there have been reports of acute interstitial nephritis, hematuria, proteinuria, and occasionally nephrotic syndrome associated with naproxen-containing products and other NSAIDs since they have been marketed.

A second form of renal toxicity has been seen in patients taking naproxen as well as other NSAIDs. In patients with prerenal conditions with reduction in renal blood flow or blood volume, renal prostaglandins have a supportive role in the maintenance of renal perfusion. Administration of a NSAID may cause a dose-dependent reduction in prostaglandin formation and may precipitate overt renal decompensation. Patients at greatest risk of this reaction are those with impaired renal function, heart failure, liver dysfunction, diuretic use, and the elderly. Discontinuation of NSAID therapy is typically followed by recovery to the pretreatment state.

Naproxen and its metabolites are eliminated primarily by the kidneys, therefore the drug should be used with great caution in patients with significantly impaired renal function and the monitoring of serum creatinine and/or creatinine clearance is advised in these patients. Caution should be used if the drug is given to patients with creatinine clearance of less than 20 mL/minute because accumulation of naproxen has been seen in such patients.

Hepatic Effects

As with other NSAIDs, borderline elevations of one or more liver tests may occur in up to 15% of patients. These abnormalities may progress, may remain essentially unchanged, or may resolve with continued therapy. The ALT (SGPT) is probably the most sensitive indicator of liver dysfunction. Meaningful (3 times the upper limit of normal) elevations of ALT (SGPT) or AST (SGOT) occurred in controlled clinical trials in less than 1% of patients. A patient with symptoms and/or signs suggesting liver dysfunction, or in whom an abnormal liver test has occurred, should be evaluated for evidence of the development of more severe hepatic reaction while on therapy with naproxen. Severe hepatic reactions, including jaundice and cases of fatal hepatitis have been reported with naproxen as with other NSAIDs. Although such reactions are rare, if abnormal liver tests persist or worsen, if clinical signs and symptoms consistent with liver disease develop, or if systemic manifestations occur (e.g. eosinophilia, rash, fever, etc.), naproxen should be discontinued. Chronic alcoholic liver disease and probably other diseases with decreased or abnormal plasma proteins (albumin) reduce the total plasma concentration of naproxen, but the plasma concentration of unbound naproxen is increased. Caution is advised when high doses are required and some adjustment of dosage may be required in these patients. It is prudent to use the lowest effective dose.

Fluid Retention and Edema

Peripheral edema has been observed in some patients receiving naproxen. Naprelan (naproxen sodium) tablets contain 37.5 mg or 50 mg of sodium (1.5 mEq or 2.0 mEq respectively). This should be considered in patients whose overall intake of sodium must be severely restricted. For these reasons, Naprelan should be used with caution in patients with fluid retention, hypertension or heart failure.

INFORMATION FOR PATIENTS

Naprelan, like other drugs of its class, is not free of side effects. This formulation of naproxen can cause discomfort and, rarely, there are more serious side effects, such as GI bleeding, which may result in hospitalization and even fatal outcomes. NSAIDs are often essential agents in the management of arthritis and have a major role in the treatment of pain but they also may be commonly employed for conditions which are less serious. Physicians may wish to discuss with their patients the potential risks (see **WARNINGS, PRECAUTIONS,** and **ADVERSE REACTIONS**) and likely benefits of Naprelan treatment. Caution should be exercised by patients whose activities require alertness if they experience drowsiness, dizziness, vertigo or depression during therapy with naproxen.

LABORATORY TESTS

Because serious GI tract ulceration and bleeding can occur without warning symptoms, physicians should follow patients chronically treated with Naprelan for the signs and symptoms of ulceration and bleeding, and should inform them of the importance of this follow-up and what they should do if certain signs and symptoms do appear. Patients with initial hemoglobin values of 10 grams or less who are to receive long-term therapy should have hemoglobin values determined periodically. (See **WARNINGS**—RISK OF GI ULCERATION, BLEEDING AND PERFORATION WITH NSAID THERAPY).

DRUG INTERACTIONS

The use of NSAIDs in patients who are receiving ACE inhibitors may potentiate renal disease states (See **PRECAUTIONS**—*Renal Effects*). *In vitro* studies have shown that naproxen anion, because of its affinity for protein, may displace from their binding site other drugs which are also albumin-bound (see **CLINICAL PHARMACOLOGY**—PHARMACOKINETICS).

Theoretically, the naproxen anion itself could likewise be displaced. Short-term controlled studies failed to show that taking the drug significantly affects prothrombin times when administered to individuals on coumarin-type anticoagulants. Caution is advised nonetheless, since interactions have been seen with other nonsteroidal agents of this class. Similarly, patients receiving the drug and a hydantoin, sulfonamide or sulfonylurea should be observed for signs of toxicity to these drugs.

Concomitant administration of naproxen and aspirin is not recommended because naproxen is displaced from its binding sites during the concomitant administration of aspirin, resulting in lower plasma concentrations and peak plasma levels.

The natriuretic effect of furosemide has been reported to be inhibited by some drugs of this class. Inhibition of renal lithium clearance leading to increases in plasma lithium concentrations has also been reported. Naproxen and other NSAIDs can reduce the antihypertensive effect of propranolol and other beta-blockers.

Probenecid given concurrently increases naproxen anion plasma levels and extends its plasma half-life significantly. Caution should be used if naproxen is administered concomitantly with methotrexate. Naproxen, naproxen sodium and other NSAIDs have been reported to reduce the tubular secretion of methotrexate in an animal model, possibly increasing the toxicity of methotrexate.

DRUG/LABORATORY TEST INTERACTIONS

Naproxen may decrease platelet aggregation and prolong bleeding time. This effect should be kept in mind when bleeding times are determined. The administration of naproxen may result in increased urinary values for 17-ketogenic steroids because of an interaction between the drug and/or its metabolites with m-dinitrobenzene used in this assay. Although 17-hydroxy-corticosteroid measurements (Porter-Silber test) do not appear to be artifactually altered, it is suggested that therapy with naproxen be temporarily discontinued 72 hours before adrenal function tests are performed if the Porter-Silber test is to be used.

Naproxen may interfere with some urinary assays of 5-hydroxyindoleacetic acid (5HIAA).

CARCINOGENESIS

A two year study was performed in rats to evaluate the carcinogenic potential of naproxen at doses of 8 mg/kg/day, 16 mg/kg/day, and 24 mg/kg/day (50 mg/m^2, 100 mg/m^2, and 150 mg/m^2). The maximum dose used was 0.28 times the systemic exposure to humans at the recommended dose. No evidence of tumorigenicity was found.

PREGNANCY

Teratogenic Effects: Pregnancy Category B

Reproduction studies have been performed in rats at 20 mg/kg/day (125 mg/m^2/day, 0.23 times the human systemic exposure) rabbits at 20 mg/kg/day (220 mg/m^2/day, 0.27 times the human systemic exposure) and mice at 170 mg/kg/day (510 mg/m^2/day, 0.28 times the human systemic exposure) with no evidence of impaired fertility or harm to the fetus due to the drug. There are no adequate and well-controlled studies in pregnant women. Because animal reproduction studies are not always predictive of human response, Naprelan should be used during pregnancy only if the potential benefits justify the potential risks to the fetus.

Nonteratogenic Effects

There is some evidence to suggest that when inhibitors of prostaglandin synthesis are used to delay preterm labor there is an increased risk of neonatal complications such as necrotizing enterocolitis, patent ductus arteriosus, and intracranial hemorrhage. Naproxen treatment given in the late pregnancy to delay parturition has been associated with persistent pulmonary hypertension, renal dysfunction, and abnormal prostaglandin E levels in preterm infants. Because of the known effect of drugs of this class on the human fetal cardiovascular system (closure of ductus arteriosus), use during third trimester should be avoided.

NURSING MOTHERS

The naproxen anion has been found in the milk of lactating women at a concentration of approximately 1% of that found in the plasma. Because of the possible adverse effects of prostaglandin-inhibiting drugs on neonates, use in nursing mothers should be avoided.

PEDIATRIC USE

No pediatric studies have been performed with Naprelan, thus safety of Naprelan in pediatric populations has not been established.

ADVERSE REACTIONS

As with all drugs in this class, the frequency and severity of adverse events depends on several factors: the dose of the drug and duration of treatment; the age, the sex, physical condition of the patient; any concurrent medical diagnoses or individual risk factors.

The following adverse reactions are divided into three parts based on frequency and whether or not the possibility exists of a causal relationship between drug usage and these adverse events. In those reactions listed as "Probable Causal Relationship" there is at least one case for each adverse reaction where there is evidence to suggest that there is a causal relationship between drug usage and the reported event. The adverse reactions reported were based on the results from two double-blind controlled clinical trials of three months duration with an additional nine month open-label extension. A total of 542 patients received Naprelan either in the double-blind period or in the nine month open-label extension. Of these 542 patients, 232 received Naprelan, 167 were initially treated with Naprosyn and 143 were initially treated with placebo. Adverse reactions reported by patients who received Naprelan are shown by body system. Those adverse reactions observed with naproxen but not reported in controlled trials with Naprelan are italicized.

The most frequent adverse events from the double-blind and open-label clinical trials were headache (15%), followed

by dyspepsia (14%), and flu syndrome (10%). The incidence of other adverse events occurring in 3%–9% of the patients are marked with an asterisk.

Those reactions occurring in less than 3% of the patients are unmarked.

INCIDENCE GREATER THAN 1% (PROBABLE CAUSAL RELATIONSHIP)

Body as a Whole—Pain (back)*, pain*, infection*, fever, injury (accident), asthenia, pain chest, headache (15%), flu syndrome (10%).

Gastrointestinal—Nausea*, diarrhea*, constipation*, abdominal pain*, flatulence, gastritis, vomiting, dysphagia, dyspepsia (14%), *heartburn*, *stomatitis*.

Hematologic—Anemia, ecchymosis.

Respiratory—Pharyngitis*, rhinitis*, sinusitis*, bronchitis, cough increased.

Renal—Urinary tract infection*, cystitis.

Dermatologic—Skin rash*, *skin eruptions*, *ecchymoses*, *purpura*.

Metabolic and Nutrition—Peripheral edema, hyperglycemia.

Central Nervous System—Dizziness, paresthesia, insomnia, *drowsiness*, *lightheadedness*.

Cardiovascular—Hypertension, *edema*, *dyspnea*, *palpitations*.

Musculoskeletal—Cramps (leg), myalgia, arthralgia, joint disorder, tendon disorder.

Special Senses—*Tinnitus*, *hearing disturbances, visual disturbances*.

General—*Thirst*.

INCIDENCE LESS THAN 1% (PROBABLE CAUSAL RELATIONSHIP)

Body as a Whole—Abscess, monilia, neck rigid, pain neck, abdomen enlarged, carcinoma, cellulitis, edema general, LE syndrome, malaise, mucous membrane disorder, allergic reaction, pain pelvic.

Gastrointestinal—Anorexia, cholecystitis, cholelithiasis, eructation, GI hemorrhage, rectal hemorrhage, stomatitis aphthous, stomatitis ulcer, ulcer mouth, ulcer stomach, periodontal abscess, cardiospasm, colitis, esophagitis, gastroenteritis, GI disorder, rectal disorder, tooth disorder, hepatosplenomegaly, liver function abnormality, melena, ulcer esophagus, *hematemesis, jaundice, pancreatitis, necrosis*.

Renal—Dysmenorrhea, dysuria, kidney function abnormality, nocturia, prostate disorder, pyelonephritis, carcinoma breast, urinary incontinence, kidney calculus, kidney failure, menorrhagia, metrorrhagia, neoplasm breast, nephrosclerosis, hematuria, pain kidney, pyuria, urine abnormal, urinary frequency, urinary retention, uterine spasm, vaginitis, *glomerular nephritis, hyperkalemia, interstitial nephritis, nephrotic syndrome, renal disease, renal failure, renal papillary necrosis*.

Hematologic—Leukopenia, bleeding time increased, eosinophilia, abnormal RBC, abnormal WBC, thrombocytopenia, *agranulocytosis, granulocytopenia*.

Central Nervous System—Depression, anxiety, hypertonia, nervousness, neuralgia, neuritis, vertigo, amnesia, confusion, co-ordination, abnormal diplopia, emotional lability, hematoma subdural, paralysis, *dream abnormalities, inability to concentrate, muscle weakness*.

Dermatologic: Angiodermatitis, herpes simplex, dry skin, sweating, ulcer skin, acne, alopecia, dermatitis contact, eczema, herpes zoster, nail disorder, skin necrosis, subcutaneous nodule, pruritis, urticaria, neoplasm skin, *photosensitive dermatitis, photosensitivity reactions resembling porphyria cutanea tarda, epidermolysis bullosa*.

Special Senses—Amblyopia scleritis, cataract, conjunctivitis, deaf, ear disorder, keratoconjunctivitis, lacrimation disorder, otitis media, pain eye.

Cardiovascular—Angina pectoris, coronary artery disease, myocardial infarction, deep thrombophlebitis, vasodilation, vascular anomaly, arrhythmia, bundle branch block, abnormal ECG, heart failure right, hemorrhage, migraine, aortic stenosis, syncope, tachycardia, *congestive heart failure*.

Respiratory—Asthma, dyspnea, lung edema, laryngitis, lung disorder, epistaxis, pneumonia, respiratory distress, respiratory disorder, *eosinophilic pneumonitis*.

Musculoskeletal—Myasthenia, bone disorder, spontaneous bone fracture, fibrotendinitis, bone pain, ptosis, spasm general, bursitis.

Metabolic and Nutrition—Creatinine increase, glucosuria, hypercholesteremia, albuminuria, alkalosis, BUN increased, dehydration, edema, glucose tolerance decrease, hyperuricemia, hypokalemia, SGOT increase, SGPT increase, weight decrease.

General—*Anaphylactoid reactions, angioneurotic edema, menstrual disorders, hypoglycemia, pyrexia (chills and fevers)*.

INCIDENCE LESS THAN 1% (CAUSAL RELATIONSHIP UNKNOWN)

Other adverse reactions listed in the naproxen package label, but not reported by those who received Naprelan are shown in italics. These observations are being listed as alerting information to the physician.

Hematologic—*Aplastic anemia, hemolytic anemia*.

Central Nervous System: *Aseptic meningitis, cognitive dysfunction*.

Dermatologic—*Epidermal necrolysis, erythema multiforme, Stevens-Johnson syndrome*.

Gastrointestinal—*Non-peptic GI ulceration, ulcerative stomatitis*.

Cardiovascular—*Vasculitis*.

OVERDOSAGE

Significant naproxen overdosage may be characterized by drowsiness, heartburn, indigestion, nausea, or vomiting. Because naproxen sodium may be rapidly absorbed, high and early blood levels should be anticipated. A few patients have experienced seizures, but it is not clear whether or not these were drug-related. It is not known what dose of the drug would be life threatening. The oral LD$_{50}$ of the drug is 500 mg/kg in rats, 1200 mg/kg in mice, 4000 mg/kg in hamsters and greater than 1000 mg/kg in dogs.

Should a patient ingest a large number of tablets, accidentally or purposefully, the stomach may be emptied and usual supportive measures employed. In animals 0.5 g/kg of activated charcoal was effective in reducing plasma levels of naproxen. Hemodialysis does not decrease the plasma concentration of naproxen because of the high degree of its protein binding.

DOSAGE AND ADMINISTRATION

RHEUMATOID ARTHRITIS, OSTEOARTHRITIS, AND ANKYLOSING SPONDYLITIS

The usual daily dose of Naprelan is two Naprelan 375 mg tablets (750 mg) once daily, or two Naprelan 500 mg tablets (1000 mg) once a day. Both larger and smaller doses may be required in individual patients (see **Individualization of Dosage**). Regardless of indication, the dosage should be individualized to achieve effective dose and minimize adverse events, however the maximum daily dose is three Naprelan 500 mg once daily.

MANAGEMENT OF PAIN, PRIMARY DYSMENORRHEA, AND ACUTE TENDINITIS AND BURSITIS

The recommended starting dose is two Naprelan 500 mg tablets (1000 mg) once daily. For patients requiring greater analgesic benefit, three Naprelan 500 mg tablets (1500 mg) may be used for a limited period. Thereafter, the total daily dose should not exceed two Naprelan 500 mg tablets (1000 mg).

ACUTE GOUT

The recommended dose on the first day is two to three Naprelan 500 mg tablets (1000–1500 mg) once daily, followed by two Naprelan 500 mg tablets (1000 mg) once daily, until the attack has subsided.

HOW SUPPLIED

Naprelan® (naproxen sodium) Controlled Release Tablets are available as follows:

Naprelan 375: white, capsule-shaped tablet with "W" on one side and "901" on the reverse; in bottles of 100; NDC 0008-0901-03. Each tablet contains 412.5 mg naproxen sodium equivalent to 375 mg naproxen.

Naprelan 500: white, capsule-shaped tablet with "W" on one side and "902" on the reverse; in bottles of 75; NDC 0008-0902-02. Each tablet contains 550 mg naproxen sodium equivalent to 500 mg naproxen.

Caution: Federal law prohibits dispensing without prescription.

US Patent Pending.

Store at controlled room temperature, 20°–25° C (68°–77° F).

Dispense in a well-closed container.

Manufactured for
Wyeth Laboratories Inc.
A Wyeth-Ayerst Company
Philadelphia, PA 19101
by
élan pharma ltd.
Athlone, Ireland

Shown in Product Identification Guide, page 344

NORDETTE®–21 ℞
[nŏr-dĕt '-21]
TABLETS
(levonorgestrel and ethinyl estradiol tablets)

Patients should be counseled that this product does not protect against HIV infection (AIDS) and other sexually transmitted diseases.

DESCRIPTION

ORAL CONTRACEPTIVE

Each Nordette tablet contains 0.15 mg of levonorgestrel (d(-)13 beta-ethyl-17-alpha-ethinyl-17-beta-hydroxygon-4-en-3-one), a totally synthetic progestogen, and 0.03 mg of ethinyl estradiol (19-nor-17α-pregna-1,3,5 (10)-trien-20-yne-3,17-diol). The inactive ingredients present are cellulose, FD&C Yellow 6, lactose, magnesium stearate, and polacrilin potassium.

CLINICAL PHARMACOLOGY

Combination oral contraceptives act by suppression of gonadotropins. Although the primary mechanism of this action is inhibition of ovulation, other alterations include changes in the cervical mucus (which increase the difficulty of sperm entry into the uterus) and the endometrium (which reduce the likelihood of implantation).

INDICATIONS AND USAGE

Oral contraceptives are indicated for the prevention of pregnancy in women who elect to use this product as a method of contraception.

Oral contraceptives are highly effective. Table I lists the typical accidental pregnancy rates for users of combination oral contraceptives and other methods of contraception. The efficacy of these contraceptive methods, except sterilization and the IUD, depends upon the reliability with which they are used. Correct and consistent use of methods can result in lower failure rates.

TABLE I: LOWEST EXPECTED AND TYPICAL FAILURE RATES DURING THE FIRST YEAR OF CONTINUOUS USE OF A METHOD
% of Women Experiencing an Accidental Pregnancy in the First Year of Continuous Use

Method	Lowest Expected*	Typical**
(No Contraception)	(85)	(85)
Oral contraceptives		3
combined	0.1	N/A***
progestin only	0.5	N/A***
Diaphragm with spermicidal cream or jelly	6	18
Spermicides alone (foams and vaginal suppositories)	3	21
Vaginal Sponge		
nulliparous	6	18
multiparous	9	28
DEPO-PROVERA® (injectable progestogen)	0.3	0.3
NORPLANT® SYSTEM (implants)	0.2#	0.2#
IUD		3
progesterone	2	N/A***
copper T 380A	0.8	N/A***
Condom without spermicides	2	12
Periodic abstinence (all methods)	1–9	20
Female sterilization	0.2	0.4
Male sterilization	0.1	0.15

Adapted from J. Trussell et al., Table 1, Studies in Family Planning, *21(1)*. Jan.–Feb. 1990.

---

* The authors' best guess of the percentage of women expected to experience an accidental pregnancy among couples who initiate a method (not necessarily for the first time) and who use it consistently and correctly during the first year if they do not stop use for any other reason.

** This term represents "typical" couples who initiate use of a method (not necessarily for the first time), who experience an accidental pregnancy during the first year if they do not stop use for any other reason.

*** N/A—Data not available

This data is based on NORPLANT® SYSTEM clinical trials.

CONTRAINDICATIONS

Oral contraceptives should not be used in women with any of the following conditions:

Thrombophlebitis or thromboembolic disorders.
A past history of deep-vein thrombophlebitis or thromboembolic disorders.
Cerebral-vascular or coronary-artery disease.
Known or suspected carcinoma of the breast.
Carcinoma of the endometrium or other known or suspected estrogen-dependent neoplasia.
Undiagnosed abnormal genital bleeding.
Cholestatic jaundice of pregnancy or jaundice with prior pill use.
Hepatic adenomas or carcinomas.
Known or suspected pregnancy.

WARNINGS

Cigarette smoking increases the risk of serious cardiovascular side effects from oral-contraceptive use. This risk increases with age and with heavy smoking (15 or more cigarettes per day) and is quite

Continued on next page

Nordette-21—Cont.

marked in women over 35 years of age. Women who use oral contraceptives should be strongly advised not to smoke.

The use of oral contraceptives is associated with increased risks of several serious conditions including myocardial infarction, thromboembolism, stroke, hepatic neoplasia, gallbladder disease, and hypertension, although the risk of serious morbidity or mortality is very small in healthy women without underlying risk factors. The risk of morbidity and mortality increases significantly in the presence of other underlying risk factors such as hypertension, hyperlipidemias, obesity, and diabetes.

Practitioners prescribing oral contraceptives should be familiar with the following information relating to these risks. The information contained in this package insert is based principally on studies carried out in patients who used oral contraceptives with higher formulations of estrogens and progestogens than those in common use today. The effect of long-term use of the oral contraceptives with lower formulations of both estrogens and progestogens remains to be determined.

Throughout this labeling, epidemiological studies reported are of two types: retrospective or case control studies and prospective or cohort studies. Case control studies provide a measure of the relative risk of disease, namely, a ratio of the incidence of a disease among oral-contraceptive users to that among nonusers. The relative risk does not provide information on the actual clinical occurrence of a disease. Cohort studies provide a measure of attributable risk, which is the difference in the incidence of disease between oral-contraceptive users and nonusers. The attributable risk does provide information about the actual occurrence of a disease in the population. For further information, the reader is referred to a text on epidemiological methods.

1. THROMBOEMBOLIC DISORDERS AND OTHER VASCULAR PROBLEMS

a. Myocardial infarction

An increased risk of myocardial infarction has been attributed to oral-contraceptive use. This risk is primarily in smokers or women with other underlying risk factors for coronary-artery disease such as hypertension, hypercholesterolemia, morbid obesity, and diabetes. The relative risk of heart attack for current oral-contraceptive users has been estimated to be two to six. The risk is very low under the age of 30.

Smoking in combination with oral-contraceptive use has been shown to contribute substantially to the incidence of myocardial infarctions in women in their mid-thirties or older with smoking accounting for the majority of excess cases. Mortality rates associated with circulatory disease have been shown to increase substantially in smokers over the age of 35 and nonsmokers over the age of 40 (Table II) among women who use oral contraceptives.

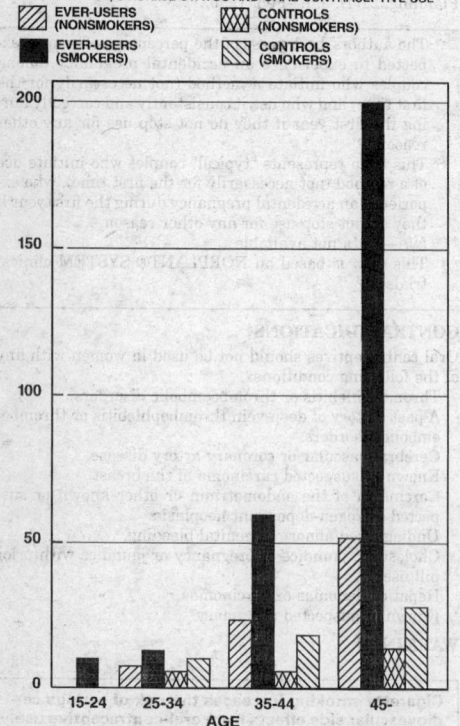

CIRCULATORY DISEASE MORTALITY RATES PER 100,000 WOMAN YEARS BY AGE, SMOKING STATUS AND ORAL-CONTRACEPTIVE USE

- ▨ EVER-USERS (NONSMOKERS)
- ■ EVER-USERS (SMOKERS)
- ▩ CONTROLS (NONSMOKERS)
- ▨ CONTROLS (SMOKERS)

TABLE II. (Adapted from P.M. Layde and V. Beral, Lancet. 1:541–546, 1981.)

Oral contraceptives may compound the effects of well-known risk factors, such as hypertension, diabetes, hyperlipidemias, age, and obesity. In particular, some progestogens are known to decrease HDL cholesterol and cause glucose intolerance, while estrogens may create a state of hyperinsulinism. Oral contraceptives have been shown to increase blood pressure among users (see section 9 in "Warnings"). Similar effects on risk factors have been associated with an increased risk of heart disease. Oral contraceptives must be used with caution in women with cardiovascular disease risk factors.

b. Thromboembolism

An increased risk of thromboembolic and thrombotic disease associated with the use of oral contraceptives is well established. Case control studies have found the relative risk of users compared to nonusers to be 3 for the first episode of superficial venous thrombosis, 4 to 11 for deep-vein thrombosis or pulmonary embolism, and 1.5 to 6 for women with predisposing conditions for venous thromboembolic disease. Cohort studies have shown the relative risk to be somewhat lower, about 3 for new cases and about 4.5 for new cases requiring hospitalization. The risk of thromboembolic disease due to oral contraceptives is not related to length of use and disappears after pill use is stopped.

A two- to four-fold increase in relative risk of postoperative thromboembolic complications has been reported with the use of oral contraceptives. The relative risk of venous thrombosis in women who have predisposing conditions is twice that of women without such medical conditions. If feasible, oral contraceptives should be discontinued at least four weeks prior to and for two weeks after elective surgery of a type associated with an increase in risk of thromboembolism and during and following prolonged immobilization. Since the immediate postpartum period is also associated with an increased risk of thromboembolism, oral contraceptives should be started no earlier than four to six weeks after delivery in women who elect not to breast-feed, or a midtrimester pregnancy termination.

c. Cerebrovascular diseases

Oral contraceptives have been shown to increase both the relative and attributable risks of cerebrovascular events (thrombotic and hemorrhagic strokes), although, in general, the risk is greatest among older (>35 years), hypertensive women who also smoke. Hypertension was found to be a risk factor for both users and nonusers, for both types of strokes, while smoking interacted to increase the risk for hemorrhagic strokes.

In a large study, the relative risk of thrombotic strokes has been shown to range from 3 for normotensive users to 14 for users with severe hypertension. The relative risk of hemorrhagic stroke is reported to be 1.2 for nonsmokers who used oral contraceptives, 2.6 for smokers who did not use oral contraceptives, 7.6 for smokers who used oral contraceptives, 1.8 for normotensive users and 25.7 for users with severe hypertension. The attributable risk is also greater in older women.

d. Dose-related risk of vascular disease from oral contraceptives

A positive association has been observed between the amount of estrogen and progestogen in oral contraceptives and the risk of vascular disease. A decline in serum high-density lipoproteins (HDL) has been reported with many progestational agents. A decline in serum high-density lipoproteins has been associated with an increased incidence of ischemic heart disease. Because estrogens increase HDL cholesterol, the net effect of an oral contraceptive depends on a balance achieved between doses of estrogen and progestogen and the nature and absolute amount of progestogen used in the contraceptive. The amount of both hor-

mones should be considered in the choice of an oral contraceptive.

Minimizing exposure to estrogen and progestogen is in keeping with good principles of therapeutics. For any particular estrogen/progestogen combination, the dosage regimen prescribed should be one which contains the least amount of estrogen and progestogen that is compatible with a low failure rate and the needs of the individual patient. New acceptors of oral-contraceptive agents should be started on preparations containing less than 50 mcg of estrogen.

e. Persistence of risk of vascular disease

There are two studies which have shown persistence of risk of vascular disease for ever-users of oral contraceptives. In a study in the United States, the risk of developing myocardial infarction after discontinuing oral contraceptives persists for at least 9 years for women 40 to 49 years who had used oral contraceptives for five or more years, but this increased risk was not demonstrated in other age groups. In another study in Great Britain, the risk of developing cerebrovascular disease persisted for at least 6 years after discontinuation of oral contraceptives, although excess risk was very small. However, both studies were performed with oral-contraceptive formulations containing 50 micrograms or higher of estrogens.

2. ESTIMATES OF MORTALITY FROM CONTRACEPTIVE USE

One study gathered data from a variety of sources which have estimated the mortality rate associated with different methods of contraception at different ages (Table III). These estimates include the combined risk of death associated with contraceptive methods plus the risk attributable to pregnancy in the event of method failure. Each method of contraception has its specific benefits and risks. The study concluded that with the exception of oral-contraceptive users 35 and older who smoke and 40 and older who do not smoke, mortality associated with all methods of birth control is less than that associated with childbirth. The observation of a possible increase in risk of mortality with age for oral-contraceptive users is based on data gathered in the 1970's—but not reported until 1983. However, current clinical practice involves the use of lower estrogen dose formulations combined with careful restriction of oral-contraceptive use to women who do not have the various risk factors listed in this labeling.

Because of these changes in practice and, also, because of some limited new data which suggest that the risk of cardiovascular disease with the use of oral contraceptives may now be less than previously observed, the Fertility and Maternal Health Drugs Advisory Committee was asked to review the topic in 1989. The Committee concluded that although cardiovascular-disease risks may be increased with oral-contraceptive use after age 40 in healthy nonsmoking women (even with the newer low-dose formulations), there are greater potential health risks associated with pregnancy in older women and with the alternative surgical and medical procedures which may be necessary if such women do not have access to effective and acceptable means of contraception.

Therefore, the Committee recommended that the benefits of oral-contraceptive use by healthy nonsmoking women over 40 may outweigh the possible risks. Of course, older women, as all women who take oral contraceptives, should take the lowest possible dose formulation that is effective.

[See table III below]

3. CARCINOMA OF THE REPRODUCTIVE ORGANS

Numerous epidemiological studies have been performed on the incidence of breast, endometrial, ovarian, and cervical cancer in women using oral contraceptives. The overwhelming evidence in the literature suggests that the use of oral contraceptives is not associated with an increase in the risk

TABLE III—ANNUAL NUMBER OF BIRTH-RELATED OR METHOD-RELATED DEATHS ASSOCIATED WITH CONTROL OF FERTILITY PER 100,000 NONSTERILE WOMEN, BY FERTILITY-CONTROL METHOD ACCORDING TO AGE

Method of control and outcome	15–19	20–24	25–29	30–34	35–39	40–44
No fertility-control methods*	7.0	7.4	9.1	14.8	25.7	28.2
Oral contraceptives nonsmoker**	0.3	0.5	0.9	1.9	13.8	31.6
Oral contraceptives smoker**	2.2	3.4	6.6	13.5	51.1	117.2
IUD**	0.8	0.8	1.0	1.0	1.4	1.4
Condom*	1.1	1.6	0.7	0.2	0.3	0.4
Diaphragm/spermicide*	1.9	1.2	1.2	1.3	2.2	2.8
Periodic abstinence*	2.5	1.6	1.6	1.7	2.9	3.6

* Deaths are birth related
** Deaths are method related

Adapted from H.W. Ory, Family Planning Perspectives, 15:57–63, 1983.

of developing breast cancer, regardless of the age and parity of first use or with most of the marketed brands and doses. The Cancer and Steroid Hormone (CASH) study also showed no latent effect on the risk of breast cancer for at least a decade following long-term use. A few studies have shown a slightly increased relative risk of developing breast cancer, although the methodology of these studies, which included differences in examination of users and nonusers and differences in age at start of use, has been questioned.

Some studies suggest that oral-contraceptive use has been associated with an increase in the risk of cervical intraepithelial neoplasia in some populations of women. However, there continues to be controversy about the extent to which such findings may be due to differences in sexual behavior and other factors.

In spite of many studies of the relationship between oral-contraceptive use and breast and cervical cancers, a cause-and-effect relationship has not been established.

4. HEPATIC NEOPLASIA
Benign hepatic adenomas are associated with oral-contraceptive use, although the incidence of benign tumors is rare in the United States. Indirect calculations have estimated the attributable risk to be in the range of 3.3 cases/100,000 for users, a risk that increases after four or more years of use. Rupture of rare, benign, hepatic adenomas may cause death through intra-abdominal hemorrhage.

Studies from Britain have shown an increased risk of developing hepatocellular carcinoma in long-term (>8 years) oral-contraceptive users. However, these cancers are extremely rare in the U.S. and the attributable risk (the excess incidence) of liver cancers in oral-contraceptive users approaches less than one per million users.

5. OCULAR LESIONS
There have been clincial case reports of retinal thrombosis associated with the use of oral contraceptives. Oral contraceptives should be discontinued if there is unexplained partial or complete loss of vision; onset of proptosis or diplopia; papilledema; or retinal vascular lesions. Appropriate diagnostic and therapeutic measures should be undertaken immediately.

6. ORAL-CONTRACEPTIVE USE BEFORE OR DURING EARLY PREGNANCY
Extensive epidemiological studies have revealed no increased risk of birth defects in women who have used oral contraceptives prior to pregnancy. Studies also do not suggest a teratogenic effect, particularly insofar as cardiac anomalies and limb-reduction defects are concerned, when taken inadvertently during early pregnancy.

The administration of oral contraceptives to induce withdrawal bleeding should not be used as a test for pregnancy. Oral contraceptives should not be used during pregnancy to treat threatened or habitual abortion.

It is recommended that for any patient who has missed two consecutive periods, pregnancy should be ruled out before continuing oral-contraceptive use. If the patient has not adhered to the prescribed schedule, the possibility of pregnancy should be considered at the time of the first missed period. Oral-contraceptive use should be discontinued until pregnancy is confirmed.

7. GALLBLADDER DISEASE
Earlier studies have reported an increased lifetime relative risk of gallbladder surgery in users of oral contraceptives and estrogens. More recent studies, however, have shown that the relative risk of developing gallbladder disease among oral-contraceptive users may be minimal. The recent findings of minimal risk may be related to the use of oral-contraceptive formulations containing lower hormonal doses of estrogens and progestogens.

8. CARBOHYDRATE AND LIPID METABOLIC EFFECTS
Oral contraceptives have been shown to cause glucose intolerance in a significant percentage of users. Oral contraceptives containing greater than 75 micrograms of estrogens cause hyperinsulinism, while lower doses of estrogen cause less glucose intolerance. Progestogens increase insulin secretion and create insulin resistance, this effect varying with different progestational agents. However, in the nondiabetic woman, oral contraceptives appear to have no effect on fasting blood glucose. Because of these demonstrated effects, prediabetic and diabetic women should be carefully observed while taking oral contraceptives.

A small proportion of women will have persistent hypertriglyceridemia while on the pill. As discussed earlier (see "Warnings" 1a and 1d), changes in serum triglycerides and lipoprotein levels have been reported in oral-contraceptive users.

9. ELEVATED BLOOD PRESSURE
An increase in blood pressure has been reported in women taking oral contraceptives, and this increase is more likely in older oral-contraceptive users and with continued use. Data from the Royal College of General Practitioners and subsequent randomized trials have shown that the incidence of hypertension increases with increasing quantities of progestogens.

Women with a history of hypertension or hypertension-related diseases, or renal disease, should be encouraged to use another method of contraception. If women with hyper-

tension elect to use oral contraceptives, they should be monitored closely, and if significant elevation of blood pressure occurs, oral contraceptives should be discontinued. For most women, elevated blood pressure will return to normal after stopping oral contraceptives, and there is no difference in the occurrence of hypertension among ever- and never-users.

10. HEADACHE
The onset or exacerbation of migraine or development of headache with a new pattern that is recurrent, persistent, or severe requires discontinuation of oral contraceptives and evaluation of the cause.

11. BLEEDING IRREGULARITIES
Breakthrough bleeding and spotting are sometimes encountered in patients on oral contraceptives, especially during the first three months of use. The type and dose of progestogen may be important. Non-hormonal causes should be considered and adequate diagnostic measures taken to rule out malignancy or pregnancy in the event of breakthrough bleeding, as in the case of any abnormal vaginal bleeding. If pathology has been excluded, time or a change to another formulation may solve the problem. In the event of amenorrhea, pregnancy should be ruled out.

Some women may encounter post-pill amenorrhea or oligomenorrhea, especially when such a condition was preexistent.

PRECAUTIONS

Patients should be counseled that this product does not protect against HIV infection (AIDS) and other sexually transmitted diseases.

1. PHYSICAL EXAMINATION AND FOLLOW-UP
A periodic history and physical examination is appropriate for all women, including women using oral contraceptives. The physical examination, however, may be deferred until after initiation of oral contraceptives if requested by the woman and judged appropriate by the clinician. The physical examination should include special reference to blood pressure, breasts, abdomen and pelvic organs, including cervical cytology, and relevant laboratory tests. In case of undiagnosed, persistent or recurrent abnormal vaginal bleeding, appropriate diagnostic measures should be conducted to rule out malignancy. Women with a strong family history of breast cancer or who have breast nodules should be monitored with particular care.

2. LIPID DISORDERS
Women who are being treated for hyperlipidemias should be followed closely if they elect to use oral contraceptives. Some progestogens may elevate LDL levels and may render the control of hyperlipidemias more difficult. (See "Warnings," 1d.)

3. LIVER FUNCTION
If jaundice develops in any woman receiving such drugs, the medication should be discontinued. Steroid hormones may be poorly metabolized in patients with impaired liver function.

4. FLUID RETENTION
Oral contraceptives may cause some degree of fluid retention. They should be prescribed with caution, and only with careful monitoring, in patients with conditions which might be aggravated by fluid retention.

5. EMOTIONAL DISORDERS
Patients becoming significantly depressed while taking oral contraceptives should stop the medication and use an alternate method of contraception in an attempt to determine whether the symptom is drug related. Women with a history of depression should be carefully observed and the drug discontinued if depression recurs to a serious degree.

6. CONTACT LENSES
Contact-lens wearers who develop visual changes or changes in lens tolerance should be assessed by an ophthalmologist.

7. DRUG INTERACTIONS
Reduced efficacy and increased incidence of breakthrough bleeding and menstrual irregularities have been associated with concomitant use of rifampin. A similar assocation, though less marked, has been suggested with barbiturates, phenylbutazone, phenytoin sodium, and possibly with griseofulvin, ampicillin and tetracyclines.

8. INTERACTIONS WITH LABORATORY TESTS
Certain endocrine- and liver-function tests and blood components may be affected by oral contraceptives:

a. Increased prothrombin and factors VII, VIII, IX, and X; decreased antithrombin 3; increased norepinephrine-induced platelet aggregability.

b. Increased thyroid-binding globulin (TBG) leading to increased circulating total thyroid hormone, as measured by protein-bound iodine (PBI), T4 by column or by radioimmunoassay. Free T3 resin uptake is decreased, reflecting the elevated TBG; free T4 concentration is unaltered.

c. Other binding proteins may be elevated in serum.

d. Sex-binding globulins are increased and result in elevated levels of total circulating sex steroids and corticoids; however, free or biologically active levels remain unchanged.

e. Triglycerides may be increased.

f. Glucose tolerance may be decreased.

g. Serum folate levels may be depressed by oral-contraceptive therapy. This may be of clinical significance if a woman becomes pregnant shortly after discontinuing oral contraceptives.

9. CARCINOGENESIS
See "Warnings" section.

10. PREGNANCY
Pregnancy Category X. See "Contraindications" and "Warnings" sections.

11. NURSING MOTHERS
Small amounts of oral-contraceptive steroids have been identified in the milk of nursing mothers, and a few adverse effects on the child have been reported, including jaundice and breast enlargement. In addition, oral contraceptives given in the postpartum period may interfere with lactation by decreasing the quantity and quality of breast milk. If possible, the nursing mother should be advised not to use oral contraceptives but to use other forms of contraception until she has completely weaned her child.

INFORMATION FOR THE PATIENT
See LO/OVRAL.

ADVERSE REACTIONS

An increased risk of the following serious adverse reactions has been associated with the use of oral contraceptives (see "Warnings" section):

Thrombophlebitis.
Arterial thromboembolism.
Pulmonary embolism.
Myocardial infarction.
Cerebral hemorrhage.
Cerebral thrombosis.
Hypertension.
Gallbladder disease.
Hepatic adenomas or benign liver tumors.

There is evidence of an association between the following conditions and the use of oral contraceptives, although additional confirmatory studies are needed:

Mesenteric thrombosis.
Retinal thrombosis.

The following adverse reactions have been reported in patients receiving oral contraceptives and are believed to be drug related:

Nausea.
Vomiting.
Gastrointestinal symptoms (such as abdominal cramps and bloating).
Breakthrough bleeding.
Spotting.
Change in menstrual flow.
Amenorrhea.
Temporary infertility after discontinuation of treatment.
Edema.
Melasma which may persist.
Breast changes: tenderness, enlargement, secretion.
Change in weight (increase or decrease).
Change in cervical erosion and secretion.
Diminution in lactation when given immediately postpartum.
Cholestatic jaundice.
Migraine.
Rash (allergic).
Mental depression.
Reduced tolerance to carbohydrates.
Vaginal candidiasis.
Change in corneal curvature (steepening).
Intolerance to contact lenses.

The following adverse reactions have been reported in users of oral contraceptives, and the association has been neither confirmed nor refuted:

Congenital anomalies.
Premenstrual syndrome.
Cataracts.
Optic neuritis.
Changes in appetite.
Cystitis-like syndrome.
Headache.
Nervousness.
Dizziness.
Hirsutism.
Loss of scalp hair.
Erythema multiforme.
Erythema nodosum.
Hemorrhagic eruption.
Vaginitis.
Porphyria.
Impaired renal function.
Hemolytic uremic syndrome.
Budd-Chiari syndrome.
Acne.
Changes in libido.
Colitis.
Sickle-cell disease.
Cerebral-vascular disease with mitral valve prolapse.
Lupus-like syndromes.

Continued on next page

Nordette-21—Cont.

OVERDOSAGE

Serious ill effects have not been reported following acute ingestion of large doses of oral contraceptives by young children. Overdosage may cause nausea, and withdrawal bleeding may occur in females.

NONCONTRACEPTIVE HEALTH BENEFITS

The following noncontraceptive health benefits related to the use of oral contraceptives are supported by epidemiological studies which largely utilized oral-contraceptive formulations containing doses exceeding 0.035 mg of ethinyl estradiol or 0.05 mg of mestranol.
Effects on menses:
Increased menstrual cycle regularity.
Decreased blood loss and decreased incidence of iron-deficiency anemia.
Decreased incidence of dysmenorrhea.
Effects related to inhibition of ovulation:
Decreased incidence of functional ovarian cysts.
Decreased incidence of ectopic pregnancies.
Effects from long-term use:
Decreased incidence of fibroadenomas and fibrocystic disease of the breast.
Decreased incidence of acute pelvic inflammatory disease.
Decreased incidence of endometrial cancer.
Decreased incidence of ovarian cancer.

DOSAGE AND ADMINISTRATION

To achieve maximum contraceptive effectiveness, Nordette-21 must be taken exactly as directed and at intervals not exceeding 24 hours.

The dosage of Nordette-21 is one tablet daily for 21 consecutive days per menstrual cycle according to prescribed schedule. Tablets are then discontinued for 7 days (three weeks on, one week off).

It is recommended that Nordette-21 tablets be taken at the same time each day, preferably after the evening meal or at bedtime.

During the first cycle of medication, the patient is instructed to take one Nordette-21 tablet daily for twenty-one consecutive days, beginning on the first day (Day 1 Start) of her menstrual cycle or on the Sunday after her period begins (Sunday Start). (The first day of menstruation is day one.) The tablets are then discontinued for one week (7 days). Withdrawal bleeding should usually occur within 3 days following discontinuation of Nordette-21. (For Day 1 Start: If Nordette-21 is first taken later than the first day of the first menstrual cycle of medication or postpartum, contraceptive reliance should not be placed on Nordette-21 until after the first seven consecutive days of administration. For Sunday Start: Contraceptive reliance should not be placed on Nordette-21 until after the first seven consecutive days of administration. The possibility of ovulation and conception prior to initiation of medication should be considered.)

The patient begins her next and all subsequent 21-day courses of Nordette-21 tablets on the same day of the week that she began her first course, following the same schedule: 21 days on—7 days off. She begins taking her tablets on the 8th day after discontinuance , regardless of whether or not a menstrual period has occurred or is still in progress. Any time a new cycle of Nordette-21 is started later than the 8th day, the patient should be protected by another means of contraception until she has taken a tablet daily for seven consecutive days.

If spotting or breakthrough bleeding occurs, the patient is instructed to continue on the same regimen. This type of bleeding is usually transient and without significance; however, if the bleeding is persistent or prolonged the patient is advised to consult her physician. Although the occurrence of pregnancy is highly unlikely if Nordette-21 is taken according to directions, if withdrawal bleeding does not occur, the possibility of pregnancy must be considered. If the patient has not adhered to the prescribed schedule (missed one or more tablets or started taking them on a day later than she should have), the probability of pregnancy should be considered at the time of the first missed period and appropriate diagnostic measures taken before the medication is resumed. If the patient has adhered to the prescribed regimen and misses two consecutive periods, pregnancy should be ruled out before continuing the contraceptive regimen.

For additional patient instructions regarding missed pills, see the "WHAT TO DO IF YOU MISS PILLS" section in the **DETAILED PATIENT LABELING** for LO/OVRAL.

Any time the patient misses one or two tablets, she should also use another method of contraception until she has taken a tablet daily for seven consecutive days. If breakthrough bleeding occurs following missed tablets, it will usually be transient and of no consequence. While there is little likelihood of ovulation occurring if only one or two tablets are missed, the possibility of ovulation increases with each successive day that scheduled tablets are missed.

In the nonlactating mother, Nordette-21 may be initiated postpartum, for contraception. When the tablets are administered in the postpartum period, the increased risk of thromboembolic disease associated with the postpartum period must be considered (see "Contraindications," "Warnings," and "Precautions" concerning thromboembolic disease). It is to be noted that early resumption of ovulation may occur if Parlodel® (bromocriptine mesylate) has been used for the prevention of lactation.

HOW SUPPLIED

Nordette®-21 Tablets (0.15 mg levonorgestrel and 0.03 mg ethinyl estradiol) are available in 6 PILPAK® dispensers of 21 tablets each as follows: NDC 0008-0075-01, light-orange, round tablet marked "WYETH" and "75".
Store at room temperature, approx. 25°C (77°F).

References available upon request.

Brief Summary Patient Package Insert: See Lo/Ovral.
DETAILED PATIENT LABELING: See Lo/Ovral.
Manufactured by:
Wyeth Laboratories Inc.
A Wyeth-Ayerst Company
Philadelphia, PA 19101
Shown in Product Identification Guide, page 344

NORDETTE®-28

[nŏr-dĕt '-28]
TABLETS
(levonorgestrel and ethinyl estradiol tablets)

Patients should be counseled that this product does not protect against HIV infection (AIDS) and other sexually transmitted diseases.

DESCRIPTION

21 light-orange Nordette tablets, each containing 0.15 mg of levonorgestrel (d (-)-13 beta-ethyl -17-alpha-ethinyl-17-beta-hydroxygon-4-en-3-one), a totally synthetic progestogen, and 0.03 mg of ethinyl estradiol (19-nor-17α-pregna-1,3,5 (10)-trien-20-yne-3,17-diol), and 7 pink inert tablets. The inactive ingredients present are cellulose, D&C Red 30, FD&C Yellow 6, lactose, magnesium stearate, and polacrilin potassium.

CLINICAL PHARMACOLOGY

See NORDETTE®-21

INDICATIONS AND USAGE

See NORDETTE-21

CONTRAINDICATIONS

See NORDETTE-21

WARNINGS

See NORDETTE-21

PRECAUTIONS

See NORDETTE-21
Drug Interactions: See NORDETTE-21
Carcinogenesis: See NORDETTE-21
Nursing Mothers: See NORDETTE-21
Information for the Patient: See LO/OVRAL.

ADVERSE REACTIONS

See NORDETTE-21

OVERDOSAGE

See NORDETTE-21

NONCONTRACEPTIVE HEALTH BENEFITS

See NORDETTE-21

DOSAGE AND ADMINISTRATION

To achieve maximum contraceptive effectiveness, Nordette-28 must be taken exactly as directed and at intervals not exceeding 24 hours.

The dosage of Nordette-28 is one light-orange tablet daily for 21 consecutive days, followed by one pink inert tablet daily for 7 consecutive days, according to prescribed schedule.

It is recommended that tablets be taken at the same time each day, preferably after the evening meal or at bedtime. During the first cycle of medication, the patient is instructed to begin taking Nordette-28 on the first Sunday after the onset of menstruation. If menstruation begins on a Sunday, the first tablet (light-orange) is taken that day. One light-orange tablet should be taken daily for 21 consecutive days, followed by one pink inert tablet daily for 7 consecutive days. Withdrawal bleeding should usually occur within three days following discontinuation of light-orange tablets. During the first cycle, contraceptive reliance should not be placed on Nordette-28 until a light-orange tablet has been taken daily for 7 consecutive days. The possibility of ovulation and conception prior to initiation of medication should be considered.

The patient begins her next and all subsequent 28-day courses of tablets on the same day of the week (Sunday) on which she began her first course, following the same schedule: 21 days on light-orange tablets—7 days on pink inert tablets. If in any cycle the patient starts tablets later than the proper day, she should protect herself by using another method of birth control until she has taken a light-orange tablet daily for 7 consecutive days.

If spotting or breakthrough bleeding occurs, the patient is instructed to continue on the same regimen. This type of bleeding is usually transient and without significance; however, if the bleeding is persistent or prolonged, the patient is advised to consult her physician. Although the occurrence of pregnancy is highly unlikely if Nordette-28 is taken according to directions, if withdrawal bleeding does not occur, the possibility of pregnancy must be considered. If the patient has not adhered to the prescribed schedule (missed one or more tablets or started taking them on a day later than she should have), the probability of pregnancy should be considered at the time of the first missed period and appropriate diagnostic measures taken before the medication is resumed. If the patient has adhered to the prescribed regimen and misses two consecutive periods, pregnancy should be ruled out before continuing the contraceptive regimen.

For additional patient instructions regarding missed pills, see the "WHAT TO DO IF YOU MISS PILLS" section in the **DETAILED PATIENT LABELING** for LO/OVRAL.

Any time the patient misses two or more light-orange tablets, she should also use another method of contraception until she has taken a light-orange tablet daily for seven consecutive days. If the patient misses one or more pink tablets, she is still protected against pregnancy **provided** she begins taking light-orange tablets again on the proper day. If breakthrough bleeding occurs following missed light-orange tablets, it will usually be transient and of no consequence. While there is little likelihood of ovulation occurring if only one or two light-orange tablets are missed, the possibility of ovulation increases with each successive day that scheduled light-orange tablets are missed.

In the nonlactating mother, Nordette-28 may be initiated postpartum, for contraception. When the tablets are administered in the postpartum period, the increased risk of thromboembolic disease associated with the postpartum period must be considered (see "Contraindications", "Warnings", and "Precautions" concerning thromboembolic disease). It is to be noted that early resumption of ovulation may occur if Parlodel® (bromocriptine mesylate) has been used for the prevention of lactation.

HOW SUPPLIED

Nordette®-28 Tablets (0.15 mg levonorgestrel and 0.03 mg ethinyl estradiol) are available in 6 PILPAK® dispensers, each containing 28 tablets as follows:
21 active tablets, NDC 0008-2533, light-orange, round tablet marked "WYETH" and "75".
7 inert tablets, NDC 0008-0486, pink, round tablet marked "WYETH" and "486".
ALSO AVAILABLE:
Nordette®-28 Tablets (0.15 mg levonorgestrel and 0.03 mg ethinyl estradiol) are available in packages of 12 PILPAK® dispensers for clinic use only, each containing 28 tablets as follows:
21 active tablets, NDC 0008-2533, light-orange, round tablet marked "WYETH" and "75".
7 inert tablets, NDC 0008-0486, pink, round tablet marked "WYETH" and "486".
References available upon request.

Brief Summary Patient Package Insert: See LO/OVRAL.

Store at room temperature, approx. 25°C (77°F).
DETAILED PATIENT LABELING: See LO/OVRAL.
HOW TO TAKE THE PILL
For Nordette-28 PILPAK® Dispenser, See LO/OVRAL.
For Nordette-28 Clinic Pilpak®, See below.
HOW TO TAKE THE PILL
This product (like all oral contraceptives) is intended to prevent pregnancy. It does not protect against transmission of HIV (AIDS) and other sexually transmitted diseases such as chlamydia, genital herpes, genital warts, gonorrhea, hepatitis B, and syphilis.

IMPORTANT POINTS TO REMEMBER

BEFORE YOU START TAKING YOUR PILLS:
1. BE SURE TO READ THESE DIRECTIONS:
Before you start taking your pills.
Anytime you are not sure what to do.
2. THE RIGHT WAY TO TAKE THE PILL IS TO TAKE ONE PILL EVERY DAY AT THE SAME TIME.
If you miss pills you could get pregnant. This includes starting the pack late. The more pills you miss, the more likely you are to get pregnant.
3. MANY WOMEN HAVE SPOTTING OR LIGHT BLEEDING, OR MAY FEEL SICK TO THEIR STOMACH DURING THE FIRST 1–3 PACKS OF PILLS.
If you feel sick to your stomach, do not stop taking the pill. The problem will usually go away. If it doesn't go away, check with your doctor or clinic.

4. MISSING PILLS CAN ALSO CAUSE SPOTTING OR LIGHT BLEEDING, even when you make up these pills. On the days you take 2 pills to make up for missed pills, you could also feel a little sick to your stomach.

5. IF YOU HAVE VOMITING OR DIARRHEA, for any reason, or IF YOU TAKE SOME MEDICINES, including some antibiotics, your pills may not work as well. Use a back-up method (such as condoms or foam) until you check with your doctor or clinic.

6. IF YOU HAVE TROUBLE REMEMBERING TO TAKE THE PILL, talk to your doctor or clinic about how to make pill-taking easier or about using another method of birth control.

7. IF YOU HAVE QUESTIONS OR ARE UNSURE ABOUT THE INFORMATION IN THIS LEAFLET, call your doctor or clinic.

NORDETTE®-21, OVRAL®, LO/OVRAL®, NORDETTE®-28, OVRAL®-28, AND LO/OVRAL®-28.

BEFORE YOU START TAKING YOUR PILLS

1. DECIDE WHAT TIME OF DAY YOU WANT TO TAKE YOUR PILL
It is important to take it at about the same time every day.
2. LOOK AT YOUR PILL PACK TO SEE IF IT HAS 21 OR 28 PILLS:
The *21-pill pack* has 21 "active" white or light-orange pills (with hormones) to take for 3 weeks, followed by 1 week without pills.
The *28-pill pack* has 21 "active" white or light-orange pills (with hormones) to take for 3 weeks, followed by 1 week of reminder pink pills (without hormones).
3. ALSO FIND:
1) where on the pack to start taking the pills,
2) in what order to take the pills (follow the arrows), and
3) the week numbers as shown in the picture below.

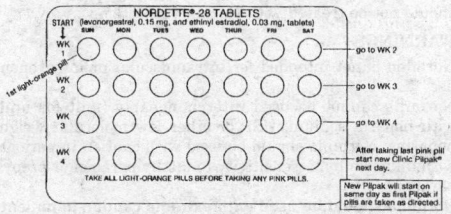

4. BE SURE YOU HAVE READY AT ALL TIMES.
ANOTHER KIND OF BIRTH CONTROL (such as condoms or foam) to use as a back-up in case you miss pills.
AND EXTRA, FULL PILL PACK

WHEN YOU START THE *FIRST* PACK OF PILLS:

For the 21-day pill pack you have two choices of which day to start taking your first pack of pills. (See **DAY 1 START** or **SUNDAY START** directions below.) Decide with your doctor or clinic which is the best day for you. The 28-day pill pack accommodates a **SUNDAY START** only. For either pill pack pick a time of day which will be easy to remember.
DAY 1 START:
These instructions are for the 21-day pill pack only. The 28-day pill pack does not accommodate a **DAY 1 START** dosage regimen.
1. Take the first "active" white or light-orange pill on the first pack during the *first 24 hours of your period.*
2. You will not need to use a back-up method of birth control, since you are starting the pill at the beginning of your period.
SUNDAY START:
These instructions are for either the 21-day or the 28-day pill pack.
1. Take the first "active" white or light-orange pill of the first pack on the *Sunday after your period starts,* even if you are still bleeding. If your period begins on Sunday, start the pack that same day.
2. *Use another method of birth control* as a back-up method if you have sex anytime from the Sunday you start your first pack until the next Sunday (7 days). Condoms or foam are good back-up methods of birth control.

WHAT TO DO DURING THE MONTH:

1. **TAKE ONE PILL AT THE SAME TIME EVERY DAY UNTIL THE PACK IS EMPTY.**
Do not skip pills even if you are spotting or bleeding between monthly periods or feel sick to your stomach (nausea).
Do not skip pills even if you do not have sex very often.
2. **WHEN YOU FINISH A PACK OR SWITCH YOUR BRAND OF PILLS:**
21 pills: Wait 7 days to start the next pack. You will probably have your period during that week. Be sure that no more than 7 days pass between 21-day packs.

28 pills: Start the next pack on the day after your last "reminder" pill.
Do not wait any days between packs.

WHAT TO DO IF YOU MISS PILLS

If you **MISS 1** white or light-orange "active" pill:
1. Take it as soon as you remember. Take the next pill at your regular time. This means you take 2 pills in 1 day.
2. You do not need to use a back-up birth control method if you have sex.
If you **MISS 2** white or light-orange "active" pills in a row in **WEEK 1 OR WEEK 2** of your pack:
1. Take 2 pills on the day you remember and 2 pills the next day.
2. Then take 1 pill a day until you finish the pack.
3. You MAY BECOME PREGNANT if you have sex in the 7 *days* after you miss pills. You MUST use another birth control method (such as condoms or foam) as a back-up for those 7 days.
If you **MISS 2** white or light-orange "active" pills in a row in **THE 3rd WEEK:**
The *Day 1 Starter* instructions are for the 21-day pill pack only. The 28-day pill pack does not accommodate a **DAY 1 START** dosage regimen. The *Sunday Starter* instructions are for either the 21-day or 28-day pill pack.
1. *If you are a Day 1 Starter:*
THROW OUT the rest of the pill pack and start a new pack that same day.
If you are a Sunday Starter:
Keep taking 1 pill every day until Sunday.
On Sunday, THROW OUT the rest of the pack and start a new pack of pills that same day.
2. You may not have your period this month but this is expected. However, if you miss your period 2 months in a row, call your doctor or clinic because you might be pregnant.
3. You MAY BECOME PREGNANT if you have sex in the 7 *days* after you miss pills. You MUST use another method (such as condoms or foam) as a back-up for those 7 days.
If you **MISS 3 OR MORE** white or light-orange "active" pills in a row (during the first 3 weeks):
The *Day 1 Starter* instructions are for the 21-day pill pack only. The 28-day pill pack does not accommodate a **DAY 1 START** dosage regimen. The *Sunday Starter* instructions are for either the 21-day or 28-day pill pack.
1. *If you are a Day 1 Starter*
THROW OUT the rest of the pill pack and start a new pack that same day.
If you are a Sunday Starter
Keep taking 1 pill every day until Sunday.
On Sunday, THROW OUT the rest of the pack and start a new pack of pills that same day.
2. You may not have your period this month but this is expected. However, if you miss your period 2 months in a row, call your doctor or clinic because you might be pregnant.
3. You MAY BECOME PREGNANT if you have sex in the 7 *days* after you miss pills. YOU MUST use another birth control method (such as condoms or foam) as back-up for those 7 days.

A REMINDER FOR THOSE ON 28-DAY PACKS:

If you forget any of the 7 pink "reminder" pills in Week 4:
THROW AWAY the pills you missed.
Keep taking 1 pill each day until the pack is empty.
You do not need a back-up method if you start your next pack on time.

FINALLY, IF YOU ARE STILL NOT SURE WHAT TO DO ABOUT THE PILLS YOU HAVE MISSED:

Use a BACK-UP METHOD anytime you have sex.
KEEP TAKING ONE PILL EACH DAY until you can reach your doctor or clinic.
OVRETTE®
Ovrette is administered on a continuous daily dosage schedule, one tablet daily each day, every day of the year. Take the first tablet on the first day of your menstrual period. Tablets should be taken at the same time every day, without interruption, whether bleeding occurs or not. If bleeding is prolonged (more than 8 days) or unusually heavy, you should contact your doctor.
Forgotten pills
The risk of pregnancy increases with each tablet missed. Therefore, it is very important that you take one tablet daily as directed. If you miss one tablet, take it as soon as you remember and also take your next tablet at the regular time. If you miss two tablets, take one of the missed tablets as soon as you remember, as well as your regular tablet for that day at the proper time. Furthermore, you should use another method of birth control in addition to taking Ovrette until you have taken fourteen days (2 weeks) of medication.
If more than two tablets have been missed, Ovrette should be discontinued immediately and another method of birth control used until the start of your next menstrual period. Then you may resume taking Ovrette.

Pregnancy due to pill failure
The incidence of pill failure resulting in pregnancy is approximately less than 1.0% if taken every day as directed, but more typical failure rates are less than 3.0%. If failure does occur, the risk to the fetus is minimal.
RISKS TO THE FETUS
If you do become pregnant while using oral contraceptives, the risk to the fetus is small, on the order of no more than ten per thousand. You should, however, discuss the risks to the developing child with your doctor.
Pregnancy after stopping the pill
There may be some delay in becoming pregnant after you stop using oral contraceptives, especially if you had irregular menstrual cycles before you used oral contraceptives. It may be advisable to postpone conception until you begin menstruating regularly once you have stopped taking the pill and desire pregnancy.
There does not appear to be any increase in birth defects in newborn babies when pregnancy occurs soon after stopping the pill.
Overdosage
Serious ill effects have not been reported following ingestion of large doses of oral contraceptives by young children. Overdosage may cause nausea and withdrawal bleeding in females. In case of overdosage, contact your health-care provider or pharmacist.
Other information
Your health-care provider will take a medical and family history before prescribing oral contraceptives and will examine you. The physical examination may be delayed to another time if you request it and the health-care provider believes that it is appropriate to postpone it. You should be reexamined at least once a year. Be sure to inform your health-care provider if there is a family history of any of the conditions listed previously in this leaflet. Be sure to keep all appointments with your health-care provider, because this is a time to determine if there are early signs of side effects of oral-contraceptive use.
Do not use the drug for any condition other than the one for which it was prescribed. This drug has been prescribed specifically for you; do not give it to others who may want birth-control pills.
HEALTH BENEFITS FROM ORAL CONTRACEPTIVES: See LO/OVRAL.
Manufactured by:
Wyeth Laboratories Inc.
A Wyeth-Ayerst Company
Philadelphia, PA 19101
Shown in Product Identification Guide, page 344

NORMIFLO® ℞

[*nōr 'mĭ-flō*]
(ardeparin sodium)
Injection

SPINAL/EPIDURAL HEMATOMAS
When neuraxial anesthesia (epidural/spinal anesthesia) or spinal puncture is employed, patients anticoagulated or scheduled to be anticoagulated with low molecular weight heparins or heparinoids for prevention of thromboembolic complications are at risk of developing an epidural or spinal hematoma which can result in long-term or permanent paralysis.
The risk of these events is increased by the use of indwelling epidural catheters for administration of analgesia or by the concomitant use of drugs affecting hemostasis such as non steroidal anti-inflammatory drugs (NSAIDs), platelet inhibitors, or other anticoagulants. The risk also appears to be increased by traumatic or repeated epidural or spinal puncture.
Patients should be frequently monitored for signs and symptoms of neurological impairment. If neurologic compromise is noted, urgent treatment is necessary.
The physician should consider the potential benefit versus risk before neuraxial intervention in patients anticoagulated or to be anticoagulated for thromboprophylaxis (see also WARNINGS, Hemorrhage and PRECAUTIONS, Drug Interactions).

DESCRIPTION

Normiflo® (ardeparin sodium) Injection is a sterile, clear, colorless to light-yellow solution for subcutaneous administration. It is available in concentrations of 5,000 and 10,000 anti-Factor Xa Units/0.5 mL (anti-Xa U/0.5 mL). The anti-Xa to anti-IIa ratio range is from 1.7 to 2.4.
Ardeparin sodium is a low molecular weight heparin. It is a partially depolymerized porcine mucosal heparin that has the same molecular subunits as heparin sodium, USP. Ardeparin sodium has smaller polymer chains consisting of de-

Continued on next page

Normiflo—Cont.

rivatives of D-glucosamine (N-sulfated, N-acetylated, and/or O-sulfated) and hexuronic acid (L-iduronic acid or D-glucuronic acid, including O-sulfated derivatives).

Ardeparin sodium has an average molecular weight range of 6,000 ± 350 daltons. The structure of ardeparin sodium (representative subunits) is:

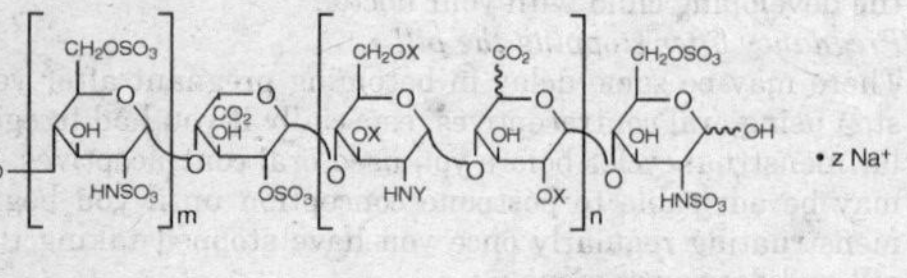

m=0 or 1 n=7–9 X=H or SO_3^- Y=SO_3^-, $COCH_3$

The Na content (z) is variable and dependent on X and Y.

Each **5,000 anti-Xa U/0.5 mL TUBEX® Sterile Cartridge-Needle Unit** contains 5,000 anti-Xa Units of ardeparin sodium with 50 mg glycerin, 0.75 mg methylparaben, 0.5 mg sodium metabisulfite, 0.075 mg propylparaben, 1 N sodium hydroxide solution (to adjust pH), and water for injection.

Each **10,000 anti-Xa U/0.5 mL TUBEX® Sterile Cartridge-Needle Unit** contains 10,000 anti-Xa Units of ardeparin sodium with 50 mg glycerin, 0.65 mg methylparaben, 0.5 mg sodium metabisulfite, 0.065 mg propylparaben, 1 N sodium hydroxide solution (to adjust pH), and water for injection.

The pH of Normiflo Injection is 4.5 to 7.0.

CLINICAL PHARMACOLOGY

Ardeparin inhibits reactions that lead to the clotting of blood and the formation of fibrin clots both *in vitro* and *in vivo*. Ardeparin acts at multiple sites in the normal coagulation system. Ardeparin binds to and accelerates the activity of antithrombin III, thereby inhibiting thrombosis by inactivating Factor Xa and thrombin. Ardeparin also inhibits thrombin by binding to heparin cofactor II.

Ardeparin is a low molecular weight heparin which has antithrombotic properties. In humans, ardeparin is characterized by a higher ratio of anti-Factor Xa to anti-Factor IIa activity (about 2) than unfractionated heparin (about 1 or less).

At the recommended dosages, ardeparin has no effect on prothrombin time (PT) test results. The activated partial thromboplastin time (APTT) may show no effect from ardeparin or may be somewhat prolonged. In three controlled, multicenter trials, 16% of orthopedic surgery patients receiving Normiflo at 50 anti-Xa U/kg every 12h had at least one APTT result ≥ 40 seconds while on therapy, while only 5% had at least one value ≥ 50 seconds on therapy.

Pharmacokinetics/Pharmacodynamics

Plasma concentrations of ardeparin cannot be measured directly. Therefore, changes in plasma serine protease activity that are considered important in hemostasis and that are affected by ardeparin are used to evaluate the pharmacokinetic and pharmacodynamic properties of ardeparin. The pharmacokinetic profiles of ardeparin anti-Xa and anti-IIa activities were studied in healthy young volunteers and in patients with different degrees of renal insufficiency.

When single 60-mg subcutaneous doses of Normiflo (5,400 anti-Xa Units) and heparin sodium, USP (9,600 anti-Xa Units) were given to humans, the peak anti-Xa plasma levels produced by ardeparin were about twice as high as those produced by heparin sodium, USP, and the ardeparin anti-Xa half-life in plasma was longer than that for heparin sodium, USP. The Normiflo dose produced greater activity in a clot-based anti-Xa assay (ie, Heptest®), but similar activity in terms of APTT and anti-IIa activities.

Normiflo, when administered subcutaneously, exhibits characteristics that are well described by a one-compartment pharmacokinetic model with apparent first-order absorption. Mean (± SD) peak plasma anti-Xa activity was 0.09 ± 0.03 to 0.32 ± 0.05 U/mL after 30 to 100 anti-Xa U/kg single doses, and was reached in 2.7 ± 0.6 hours. Similarly, mean plasma anti-IIa activity was barely detectable after 30 anti-Xa U/kg and was 0.07 ± 0.02 U/mL after 100 anti-Xa U/kg single doses, and was reached in 3.0 ± 1.0 hours.

Ardeparin is well absorbed following a single 90 anti-Xa U/kg subcutaneous dose with mean absolute bioavailability of 92 ± 16% based on anti-Xa activity and 63 ± 19% based on anti-IIa activity. The lower bioavailability determined for anti-IIa activity is not unexpected because the anti-IIa activity may be associated with the larger heparin molecules which may be less readily absorbed.

The dose proportionality of ardeparin based on plasma anti-Xa AUC (the area under the plasma concentration versus time curve) is slightly nonlinear following single subcutaneous doses from 30 to 100 anti-Xa U/kg. With each doubling of the dose, the anti-Xa AUC is about 25% higher than would be expected with linear dose proportionality. However, ardeparin anti-IIa activity exhibits linear dose proportionality over the same dose range.

The mean plasma clearances of ardeparin anti-Xa and anti-IIa activities in normal volunteers following a single 90 anti-Xa U/kg intravenous bolus dose are 30 ± 7 and 46 ± 16 mL/h/kg, respectively, and the mean disposition half-lives are 3.3 ± 2.4 and 1.2 ± 0.3 hours, respectively. Similar steady-state volumes of distribution are exhibited for ardeparin anti-Xa (99 ± 37 mL/kg) and anti-IIa (79 ± 12 mL/kg) activity; these volumes are slightly larger than the blood volume.

In early clinical trials, subcutaneous Normiflo was administered as a fixed dose. Analysis of plasma anti-Xa activity 6 and 12 hours after dose administration showed plasma levels to be lower in patients of greater body weight. Subsequently, when Normiflo was administered by actual patient body weight, plasma anti-Xa levels were relatively constant over a great range of body weight. These results, confirmed in large clinical trials (see *Population Pharmacokinetic Profile*), support subcutaneous dosing by actual patient body weight.

Normiflo intravenous bolus doses were administered to 12 patients with impaired renal function (creatinine clearance below 70 mL/min), 13 patients undergoing hemodialysis, and normal volunteers. The mean clearance of ardeparin anti-Xa and anti-IIa activities was reduced in the patients with impaired renal function, compared to the normal volunteers, by about one-fourth to one-half, and the half-life was prolonged by 50 to 100%. Ardeparin clearance was similarly reduced in patients with moderate and severe renal impairment. However, in two large clinical trials in the prophylaxis of venous thromboembolic disease following elective orthopedic surgery, the anti-Xa activity was similar for patients with normal renal function (n = 345) and for patients with partially impaired renal function (creatinine clearance between 17 and 70 mL/min, n = 316). Clotting and bleeding rates did not correlate with creatinine clearance.

Because of the lack of correlation between the degree of renal impairment and clotting and bleeding rates and because ardeparin clearance was not reduced more in patients with end-stage renal impairment than in patients with mild to moderate renal impairment, no dosage adjustment appears necessary for patients with renal disease when treated with dosages recommended for venous thromboembolic disease prophylaxis (see **PRECAUTIONS**).

Based on a study in hemodialysis patients given single 100 anti-Xa U/kg doses of Normiflo during dialysis, ardeparin does not appear to be dialyzable.

Population Pharmacokinetic Profile—In two large-scale clinical trials, 934 patients undergoing hip or knee replacement surgery were administered either 50 anti-Xa U/kg every 12h or 90 anti-Xa U/kg once a day subcutaneously for up to 14 days, and plasma samples were collected before each morning dose and 6 hours later. Population pharmacokinetic methods were used to analyze the plasma anti-Xa activity from the 12,525 plasma samples from these studies. The results indicated that Normiflo was appropriately dosed by patients weight and that age or gender do not need to be considered in dosing Normiflo.

Clinical Trials

Prophylaxis of Deep Vein Thrombosis Which May Lead to Pulmonary Embolism After Knee Replacement Surgery

Normiflo has been shown to prevent deep vein thrombosis (DVT) of the lower extremities which may lead to pulmonary embolism in three controlled clinical trials in patients who underwent elective knee replacement surgery.

The first study in patients undergoing elective knee replacement surgery compared two Normiflo dosing regimens with warfarin. Normiflo treatment was initiated postoperatively on the evening of the day of surgery and was continued for up to 10 days. Normiflo 50 anti-Xa U/kg, administered twice daily (every 12 hours), was found to be more effective in preventing DVT than warfarin administered at the initial dose of 5 mg on the day before surgery and then once a day at a dose adjusted to INR 2.0 – 3.0. Once-daily dosing with Normiflo at 90 anti-Xa U/kg resulted in a DVT rate intermediate between the rates observed with twice daily dosing of Normiflo and with warfarin (see table below).

[See first table below]

The second study in patients undergoing elective knee replacement surgery compared Normiflo at 50 anti-Xa U/kg every 12h, begun postoperatively, combined with graduated compression stockings to placebo combined with graduated compression stockings. Normiflo treatment was initiated on the first postoperative day and was continued for up to 14 days. Normiflo combined with graduated compression stockings was more effective than graduated compression stockings alone in preventing DVT (see table below).

[See second table below]

The third study in patients undergoing elective knee replacement surgery compared Normiflo at 50 anti-Xa U/kg every 12h initiated postoperatively on the evening of the day of surgery and continued for up to 14 days with warfarin administered at the initial dose of 6 mg on the day before surgery, followed by 4 mg on the day of surgery, and then postoperatively once a day at a dose adjusted to INR 2.0 – 3.0. Normiflo was found to be more effective than warfarin. The 27% DVT rate for patients receiving Normiflo 50 anti-Xa U/kg every 12h was significantly lower (p = 0.019) than the 38% DVT rate for patients receiving warfarin.

The results of these trials support the recommended dosing regimen of Normiflo 50 anti-Xa U/kg, administered every 12 hours, initiated postoperatively within the first 24 hours (see **DOSAGE AND ADMINISTRATION**).

INDICATIONS AND USAGE

Normiflo is indicated for the prevention of deep vein thrombosis which may lead to pulmonary embolism following knee replacement surgery.

CONTRAINDICATIONS

Normiflo should not be used in patients with active major bleeding, hypersensitivity to the drug, or thrombocytopenia associated with a positive *in vitro* test for anti-platelet antibodies in the presence of Normiflo. Patients with a known hypersensitivity to ardeparin sodium or to pork products should not be treated with Normiflo Injection.

WARNINGS

Normiflo is not intended for intramuscular or intravenous use.

Normiflo cannot be used interchangeably (unit for unit) with heparin sodium, USP or other low molecular weight heparins. Normiflo should be used with caution in patients with a known hypersensitivity to methylparaben or propylparaben.

Normiflo should be used with extreme caution in patients with a history of heparin-induced thrombocytopenia.

Hypersensitivity

Normiflo contains metabisulfite, a sulfite that may cause allergic-type reactions including anaphylactic symptoms and life-threatening or less severe asthmatic episodes in certain susceptible people. The overall prevalence of sulfite sensitivity in the general population in unknown and probably low. Sulfite sensitivity is seen more frequently in asthmatic than in nonasthmatic people.

Hemorrhage

Bleeding can occur at virtually any site in patients receiving Normiflo. An unexplained fall in hematocrit, fall in blood pressure, or any other unexplained symptom should lead to serious consideration of a bleeding event.

Spinal or epidural hematomas can occur with the associated use of low molecular weight heparins or heparinoids and neuraxial (spinal/epidural) anesthesia or spinal puncture which can result in long-term or permanent paralysis. The risk of these events is higher with the use of post-operative indwelling epidural catheters or concomitant use of additional drugs affecting hemostasis such as NSAIDs (see boxed WARNING.)

Normiflo, like other anticoagulants, should be used with extreme caution in patients with conditions in which there is an increased risk of hemorrhage, such as bacterial endocarditis, congenital or acquired bleeding disorders, active ulcer-

PERCENT DVT IN PATIENTS UNDERGOING KNEE REPLACEMENT SURGERY

Treatment	n	% DVT
Normiflo 50 a-Xa U/kg every 12h	150	26*
Normiflo 90 a-Xa U/kg once a day	149	29**
Warfarin, daily dose adjusted to INR 2.0 –3.0	147	43

*Compared to warfarin p = 0.004.
**Compared to warfarin, p = 0.028.

PERCENT DVT IN PATIENTS UNDERGOING KNEE REPLACEMENT SURGERY

Treatment	n	% DVT
Normiflo 50 a-Xa U/kg every 12h with graduated compression stockings	94	29*
Placebo with graduated compression stockings	99	58

*Compared to placebo, p < 0.001.

ative or angiodysplastic gastrointestinal diseases, severe uncontrolled hypertension, hemorrhagic stroke, or shortly after brain, spinal, or ophthalmologic surgery, or in patients treated concomitantly with platelet inhibitors.

Thrombocytopenia

In controlled clinical trials of patients with knee replacement surgery, there was an equivalent postoperative incidence of thrombocytopenia in patients who received Normiflo and in patients who received either warfarin, aspirin, or placebo. Thrombocytopenia with platelet counts of less than 100,000/mm^3 occurred at a rate of 2% in patients given Normiflo, 2% in patients given warfarin, 1% in patients given aspirin, and 0% in patients given placebo. Thrombocytopenia with platelet counts of less than 50,000/mm^3 occurred at a rate of 0.1% in patients given Normiflo, 0% in patients given warfarin, 0% in patients given aspirin, and 0% in patients given placebo. Immune-type thrombocytopenia has occurred, rarely, in clinical trials. Therefore, patient platelet counts should be monitored.

PRECAUTIONS
General

Normiflo should not be mixed with other injections or infusions.

Normiflo should be used with caution in patients with bleeding diathesis, recent gastrointestinal bleeding, thrombocytopenia or platelet defects, severe liver disease, hypertensive or diabetic retinopathy, or in patients undergoing invasive procedures, particularly if they are receiving other drugs which are known to interfere with hemostasis.

Clinical safety and efficacy trials in patients with severe renal failure have not been performed and no information exists in this population to correlate anti-Xa activity with either clotting or bleeding rates. In the absence of such data, Normiflo should be used with caution in patients with severe renal failure.

Patients should be observed closely for bleeding if Normiflo is administered during or immediately following diagnostic lumbar puncture, epidural anesthesia, or spinal anesthesia.

If thromboembolism develops despite ardeparin prophylaxis, Normiflo should be discontinued and appropriate treatment should be initiated.

Laboratory Tests

It is recommended during therapy with Normiflo to monitor complete blood counts including platelet counts, urinalysis, and occult blood in stools. Routine monitoring of coagulation parameters (APTT) is not required during thromboprophylaxis with Normiflo.

When administered at recommended prophylaxis doses, routine coagulation tests such as Prothrombin Time [PT] and Activated Partial Thromboplastin Time [APTT] are relatively insensitive measures of Normiflo activity and, therefore, unsuitable for monitoring.

Drug Interactions

Patients receiving Normiflo should be observed closely if they are also receiving agents such as anticoagulants or platelet inhibitors, including aspirin and NSAIDs, that can induce or augment bleeding.

Drug/Laboratory Test Interactions
Hyperaminotransferasemia

In controlled clinical trials, asymptomatic increases in aspartate (SGOT/AST) and alanine (SGPT/ALT) aminotransferase levels greater than 3 times the upper limit of normal of the laboratory reference range have been reported in 2 of 16 and 4 of 16 normal subjects, respectively, and in 5.5% and 8.7% of patients, respectively, during treatment with Normiflo. Similar increases in aminotransferase levels have also been observed in patients and normal volunteers treated with heparin and other low molecular weight heparins. Such elevations are fully reversible and are rarely associated with increases in bilirubin. Because aminotransferase determinations are important in the differential diagnosis of myocardial infarction, liver disease and pulmonary embolism, elevations that might be caused by drugs like Normiflo should be interpreted with caution.

Serum triglycerides

Ardeparin sodium, like heparin sodium, USP, is known to increase activity of lipoprotein lipase. However, as with heparin sodium, USP, paradoxical elevations in serum triglyceride levels have been seen in clinical trials with Normiflo.

Carcinogenesis, Mutagenesis, and Impairment of Fertility

No long-term studies in animals have been performed to evaluate the carcinogenic potential of ardeparin sodium. Ardeparin sodium was not genotoxic in the *in vitro* tests including the Ames test, the Chinese Hamster Ovarian Cell (CHO/HGPRT) forward mutation test, and the *in vivo* tests including the mouse micronucleus test or the rat bone marrow cell chromosome aberration test. Ardeparin sodium at subcutaneous doses up to 3,180 anti-Xa U/kg/day (19,080 anti-Xa U/m^2/day, approximately 5 times the recommended human dose based on body surface area) in male rats and 1,590 anti-Xa U/kg/day (9,540 anti-Xa U/m^2/day, approximately 3 times the recommended human dose based on body surface area) in female rats was found to have no effect on fertility and reproductive performance.

HEMORRHAGIC EVENTS OCCURRING IN 2% OR MORE OF PATIENTS TREATED WITH NORMIFLO 50 ANTI-Xa U/kg EVERY 12 HOURS IN CONTROLLED STUDIES: % OF PATIENTS

Adverse Event	Normiflo 50 Anti-Xa U/kg every 12h (n = 877) Attributed by Investigator to Drug	All[a]	Warfarin once a day (n = 682) Attributed by Investigator to Drug	All[a]	Aspirin 650 mg twice a day (n = 90) Attributed by Investigator to Drug	All[a]	Placebo (n = 124) Attributed by Investigator to Drug	All[a]
Hemorrhage[b]	5%	7%	4%	5%	6%	7%	<1%	3%
Injection site hematoma/hemorrhage	7%	7%	7%	7%[c]	NA[d]	NA	0%	0%
Ecchymosis	2%	3%	2%	2%	0%	1%	2%	2%

a: All adverse events regardless of causality.
b: Includes adverse events described as excessive intraoperative bleeding, postoperative surgical site hematoma or hemorrhage, postoperative nonsurgical site hematoma or hemorrhage, bleeding requiring an invasive procedure, and bleeding requiring discontinuation from study.
c: Based on data from 279 warfarin-treated patients who received blinded placebo injections. The other warfarin-treated patients did not receive placebo injections.
d: NA = not applicable. No aspirin-treated patients received blinded placebo injections.

NONHEMORRHAGIC ADVERSE EVENTS OCCURRING IN 5% OR MORE OF PATIENTS TREATED WITH NORMIFLO 50 ANTI-Xa U/kg EVERY 12 HOURS IN CONTROLLED STUDIES: % OF PATIENTS

Adverse Event[a]	Normiflo 50 Anti-Xa U/kg every 12h (n = 877) Attributed by Investigator to Drug	All[b]	Warfarin once a day (n = 682) Attributed by Investigator to Drug	All[b]	Aspirin 650 mg twice a day (n = 90) Attributed by Investigator to Drug	All[b]	Placebo (n = 124) Attributed by Investigator to Drug	All[b]
Fever	3%	17%	1%	16%	3%	10%	<1%	10%
Anemia	8%	16%	3%	9%	32%	37%	11%	17%
Nausea	3%	14%	3%	19%	7%	10%	<1%	7%
Constipation	<1%	8%	1%	7%	0%	4%	0%	<1%
Pruritus/rash[c]	2%	6%	2%	6%	0%	1%	0%	<1%
Vomiting	1%	7%	<1%	9%	2%	2%	0%	4%
Confusion	<1%	5%	<1%	4%	1%	2%	0%	6%

a: Less than 1% of the adverse events listed in this table were described as serious.
b: All adverse events regardless of causality.
c: Includes both local and systemic events.

Pregnancy, Teratogenic Effects: Pregnancy Category C

Teratology studies have been performed in pregnant rats at subcutaneous (the prescribed route of administration) doses up to 1,590 anti-Xa U/kg/day (9,540 anti-Xa U/m^2/day, approximately 3 times the recommended human dose based on body surface area) and in pregnant rabbits at subcutaneous doses up to 3,180 anti-Xa U/kg/day (34,980 anti-Xa U/m^2/day, approximately 10 times the recommended human dose based on body surface area) and have revealed no evidence of impaired fertility or harm to the fetus due to ardeparin sodium.

However, intravenously administered ardeparin sodium has been shown to be teratogenic in rats (scoliosis) at a dose of 4,240 anti-Xa U/kg/day (25,440 anti-Xa U/m^2/day, approximately 7 times the recommended human dose based on body surface area) and in rabbits (interventricular septal defects, stenosis of the aortic arch and pulmonary trunk, and fused sternebrae) at doses of 3,744 anti-Xa U/kg/day and above (41,184 anti-Xa U/m^2/day, approximately 11 times the recommended human dose based on body surface area).

There are no adequate and well-controlled studies in pregnant women. Ardeparin sodium should be used during pregnancy only if the potential benefit justifies the potential risk to the fetus.

Nursing Mothers

It is not known if ardeparin is excreted in human milk. Because many drugs are excreted in human milk, caution should be exercised when ardeparin sodium is administered to a nursing woman.

Pediatric Use

Safety and effectiveness in pediatric patients have not been established.

Geriatric Use

The controlled clinical trials with Normiflo® included subjects aged 18 to 92 years. The mean age was 67 years. Although the rate of clotting in all treatment groups was consistently higher in older patients than in those younger than 65 years, the DVT rates were uniformly lower in patients treated with Normiflo than with comparators. No significant differences in safety were seen in subjects greater than 65 compared to those less than 65 years of age.

ADVERSE REACTIONS

Adverse reaction information for Normiflo was derived from 1,719 patients undergoing elective orthopedic surgery who were treated with subcutaneous Normiflo in controlled and uncontrolled clinical trials of up to 14 days in duration.

In controlled studies, most adverse events reported with Normiflo or other anticoagulants were related to bleeding, as expected.

Hemorrhage

In controlled clinical trials of Normiflo, clinically important bleeding events were defined two ways: as *major bleeding* events (1 trial) or as *clinically significant bleeding* events (3 trials).

In 1 trial, *major bleeding* events were defined as overt bleeding associated with either a decrease in hemoglobin of $\geq$ 2 g/dL or transfusion of $\geq$ 2 units of blood, or bleeding events that were intracranial, intraocular, retroperitoneal, or intra-articular. The results from this trial are shown in the following table.

NUMBER (%) OF PATIENTS WITH MAJOR BLEEDS

Bleeding Event	Normiflo 50 Anti-Xa U/kg every 12h (n = 122)	Placebo (n =124)
Major Bleed	2 (2%)	2 (2%)

In 3 other trials, clinically important bleeding events were defined more broadly as *clinically significant bleeding* events and included moderate bleeding events. *Clinically significant bleeding* events were defined as hemorrhagic events that were considered moderate or severe by the investigator, required discontinuation from the study, or required an invasive diagnostic or therapeutic procedure. In these 3 trials, 7% of patients treated with Normiflo 50 anti-Xa U/kg every 12 hours had *clinically significant bleeding* events. The rates of *clinically significant bleeding* events in these trials for the comparators warfarin and aspirin were 5% and 1%, respectively.

In controlled clinical trials of Normiflo, 17% of patients experienced at least 1 hemorrhagic adverse event, including mild events and injection site hematoma/bruising. The following table shows the hemorrhagic events reported for 2% or more of patients treated with Normiflo 50 anti-Xa U/kg every 12h in controlled clinical trials, regardless of causality. The percentage of drug-related adverse events is also shown for each adverse event listed.

[See first table at top of page]

Continued on next page

Normiflo—Cont.

Additional hemorrhagic events that occurred in less than 2% of Normiflo-treated patients in clinical trials were: epistaxis, gastrointestinal hemorrhage, hematemesis, hematuria, melena, petechiae, rectal hemorrhage, retroperitoneal hemorrhage, and stools abnormal (guaiac- or heme-positive stools).

Thrombocytopenia

During clinical trials, thrombocytopenia, defined as a platelet count of 100,000/mm^3 or less, occurred at a rate of 2% in patients given Normiflo, 2% in patients given warfarin, 1% in patients given aspirin, and 0% in patients given placebo. When thrombocytopenia was defined as a platelet count of 50,000/mm^3 or less, the rate of occurrence was 0.1% in patients given Normiflo and 0% in patients given warfarin, aspirin, or placebo, Immune-type thrombocytopenia has occurred rarely in clinical trials with Normiflo. Cases of postoperative thrombocytosis were also reported.

Other

Nonhemorrhagic adverse events reported in patients treated with Normiflo, warfarin, aspirin, or placebo in controlled clinical trials, and that occurred at a rate of at least 5% in the Normiflo 50 anti-Xa U/kg group, regardless of causality, are shown in the table below. The percentage of drug-related adverse events is also shown for reach adverse event listed.

[See second table at top of previous page]

Other adverse reactions that were reported with the use of Normiflo in clinical trials were allergic reaction (ie, maculopapular rash, vesiculobullous rash, and urticaria), arthralgia, cerebrovascular accident, chest pain, dizziness, dyspnea, headache, injection site reactions (ie, edema hypersensitivity, inflammation, and pain), insomnia, local reaction to procedure, and peripheral edema.

OVERDOSAGE

Bleeding is the expected chief sign of Normiflo overdosage. Bleeding at the surgical site or at venipuncture sites may be noted as the first sign of bleeding. Epistaxis, hematuria, or blood in stools may also be noted. Easy bruising or petechiae may precede frank bleeding.

Most bleeding in patients receiving Normiflo can be controlled by discontinuing Normiflo, applying pressure to the site, if possible, and replacing volume and hemostatic blood elements (eg, fresh frozen plasma, platelets) as required.

In the event that this is ineffective, or a known overdosage of Normiflo has occurred in a bleeding patient, protamine sulfate can be administered. One mg of protamine sulfate neutralizes approximately 100 anti-Xa Units of administered Normiflo. The anti-IIa activity of intravenously administered Normiflo is completely neutralized within ten minutes following an intravenous infusion dose of equal weight protamine sulfate (about 1 mg protamine sulfate for each 100 anti-Xa Units of administered Normiflo). The anti-Xa and Heptest® activities of ardeparin are reduced by about 75% within 10 minutes and are almost completely neutralized within 30 minutes after protamine sulfate administration. If protamine sulfate is given and bleeding persists, approximately two hours later, blood should be drawn and residual anti-Xa levels determined. Additional protamine sulfate can be administered if clinically important bleeding persists or if anti-Xa levels remain higher than desired.

Because protamine sulfate may cause anaphylactoid reactions that can be life threatening, it should be given only when resuscitation techniques and treatment of anaphylactic shock are available (see protamine sulfate labeling for additional information).

At the lowest tested single subcutaneous dose of 13,250 anti-Xa U/kg, ardeparin sodium was lethal to mice and rats (11 to 21 times the recommended human dose based on body surface area). Symptoms of acute toxicity were ataxia, clonic convulsions, bradypnea, dyspnea, and bleeding from the injection site.

DOSAGE AND ADMINISTRATION

Dosage

In patients undergoing elective orthopedic surgery for knee replacement, the recommended subcutaneous dose of Normiflo is 50 anti-Xa U per kg of body weight every 12 hours. Treatment should begin the evening of the day of surgery or the following morning and is continued for up to 14 days or until the patient is fully ambulatory, whichever is shorter.

To calculate the volume (mL) for a 50 anti-Xa U/kg subcutaneous dose:

Using Normiflo 5,000 anti-Xa U/0.5 mL (recommended for patients weighing up to 100 kg [220 lb])

Patient's weight (kg) × 0.005 mL/kg = volume to be administered (mL) subcutaneously

Using Normiflo 10,000 anti-Xa U/0.5 mL (recommended for patients weighing more than 100 kg [220 lb])

Patient's weight (kg) × 0.0025 mL/kg = volume to be administered (mL) subcutaneously

The **volume** of Normiflo to be administered for a range of patient weights is shown in the following table.

[See table below]

Administration

Normiflo is administered by deep (intra-fat) subcutaneous injection. The intramuscular route of administration should not be used in order to avoid the possible occurrence of hematoma at the injection site. Extrude air and excess medication from the **TUBEX®** Sterile Cartridge-Needle Unit before injection.

Subcutaneous injection technique: Patients should be sitting or lying down and Normiflo should be administered by deep subcutaneous injection, Normiflo may be injected in the abdomen (avoiding the navel), the anterior aspect of the thighs, or the outer aspect of the upper arms. The administration site should vary with each injection. A skin fold, held between the thumb and forefinger, must be lifted; the entire length of the needle is inserted into the fold at a 45 to 90-degree angle. Before injecting, draw back on the plunger to ensure that the needle is not in the intravascular space. To minimize bruising, do not rub the injection site after completing the injection.

Normiflo is a clear, colorless to light-yellow solution and as with other parenteral drug products should be inspected visually for particulate matter and discoloration prior to administration.

HOW SUPPLIED

Normiflo® (ardeparin sodium) Injection is supplied in **TUBEX®** Sterile Cartridge-Needle Unit, in concentrations of 5,000 anti-Xa U/0.5 mL and 10,000 anti-Xa U/0.5 mL. The two strengths are available as follows:

- 5,000 anti-Xa U in 0.5 mL:
  (25 gauge × 5/8 inch needle), NDC 0008-0860-01, in packages of 10 **TUBEX®** Sterile Cartridge-Needle Units
- 10,000 anti-Xa U in 0.5 mL:
  (25 gauge × 5/8 inch needle), NDC 0008-0861-01, in packages of 10 **TUBEX®** Sterile Cartridge-Needle Units

Store at room temperature, 15° to 25°C (59° to 77°F).

Caution: Federal law prohibits dispensing without prescription.

Manufactured by:
Wyeth Laboratories Inc.
A Wyeth-Ayerst Company
Philadelphia, PA 19101

NORPLANT® SYSTEM ℞

[nŏr ' plănt]

(levonorgestrel implants)

Patients should be counseled that this product does not protect against HIV infection (AIDS) and other sexually transmitted diseases.

Prescribing Information

DESCRIPTION

The NORPLANT SYSTEM kit contains levonorgestrel implants, a set of six flexible closed capsules made of silicone rubber tubing (Silastic®, dimethylsiloxane/methylvinylsiloxane copolymer), each containing 36 mg of the progestin levonorgestrel contained in an insertion kit to facilitate implantation. The capsules are sealed with Silastic (polydimethylsiloxane) adhesive and sterilized. Each capsule is 2.4 mm in diameter and 34 mm in length. The capsules are inserted in a superficial plane beneath the skin of the upper arm.

Information contained herewith regarding safety and efficacy was derived from studies which used two slightly different Silastic tubing formulations. The formulation being used in the NORPLANT SYSTEM has slightly higher release rates of levonorgestrel and at least comparable efficacy.

Evidence indicates that the dose of levonorgestrel provided by the NORPLANT SYSTEM is initially about 85 mcg/day followed by a decline to about 50 mcg/day by 9 months and to about 35 mcg/day by 18 months with a further decline thereafter to about 30 mcg/day. The NORPLANT SYSTEM is a progestin-only product and does not contain estrogen.

Levonorgestrel, (d(-)-13-beta-ethyl-17-alpha-ethinyl-17-beta-hydroxygon-4-en-3-one), the active ingredient in the NORPLANT SYSTEM, has a molecular weight of 312.46 and the following structural formula:

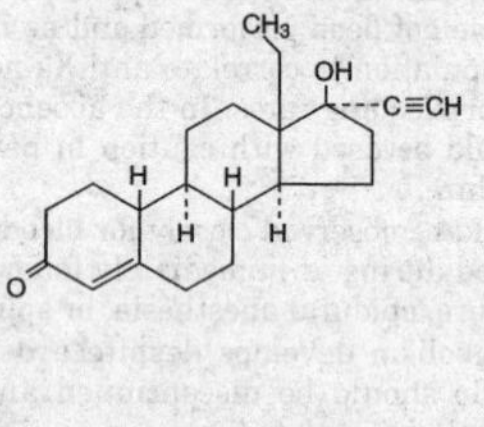

Levonorgestrel

CLINICAL PHARMACOLOGY

Levonorgestrel is a totally synthetic and biologically active progestin which exhibits no significant estrogenic activity and is highly progestational. The absolute configuration conforms to that of D-natural steroids. Levonorgestrel is not subjected to a "first-pass" effect and is virtually 100% bioavailable. Plasma concentrations average approximately 0.30 ng/mL over 5 years but are highly variable as a function of individual metabolism and body weight.

Diffusion of levonorgestrel through the wall of each capsule provides a continuous low dose of the progestin. Resulting blood levels are substantially below those generally observed among users of combination oral contraceptives containing the progestins norgestrel or levonorgestrel. Because of the range of variability in blood levels and variation in individual response, blood levels alone are not predictive of the risk of pregnancy in an individual woman.

At least two mechanisms are active in preventing pregnancy: ovulation inhibition and thickening of the cervical mucus. Other mechanisms may add to these contraceptive effects.

Levonorgestrel concentrations among women show considerable variation depending on individual clearance rates, body weight, and possibly other factors. Levonorgestrel concentrations reach a maximum, or near maximum, within 24 hours after placement with mean values of 1600 ± 1100 pg/mL. They decline rapidly over the first month partially due to a circulating protein, SHBG, that binds levonorgestrel and which is depressed by the presence of levonorgestrel. At 3 months, mean levels decline to values of around 400 pg/mL while concentrations normalized to a 60 kg body weight were 327 ± 119 (SD) pg/mL at 12 months with further decline by 1.4 pg/mL/month to reach 258 ± 95 (SD) pg/mL at 60 months. Concentrations decreased with increasing body weight by a mean of 3.3 pg/mL/kg. After capsule removal, mean concentrations drop to below 100 pg/mL by 96 hours and to below assay sensitivity (50 pg/mL) by 5 to 14 days. Fertility rates return to levels comparable to those seen in the general population of women using no method of contraception. Circulating concentrations can be used to forecast the risk of pregnancy only in a general statistical sense. Mean concentrations associated with pregnancy have been 210 ± 60 (SD) pg/mL. However, in clinical studies, 20 percent of women had one or more values below 200 pg/mL but an average annual gross pregnancy rate of less than 1.0 per 100 women through 5 years.

Although lipoprotein levels were altered in several clinical studies with the NORPLANT SYSTEM, the long-term clinical effects of these changes have not been determined. A decrease in total cholesterol levels has been reported in all lipoprotein studies and reached statistical significance in several. Both increases and decreases in high-density lipoprotein (HDL) levels have been reported in clinical trials. No statistically significant increases have been reported in the ratio of total cholesterol to HDL-cholesterol. Low-den-

VOLUME OF NORMIFLO TO BE ADMINISTERED BY PATIENT WEIGHT

Patient Weight in Pounds	Patient Weight in Kilograms	Volume of Normiflo (mL) 5,000 anti-Xa U/0.5 mL	10,000 anti-Xa U/0.5 mL
45-54	20-24	0.10	
55-76	25-34	0.15	
77-98	35-44	0.20	
99-120	45-54	0.25	
121-142	55-64	0.30	
143-164	65-74	0.35	
165-186	75-84	0.40	
187-208	85-94	0.45	
209-230	95-104	0.50	0.25
231-285	105-129		0.30
286-329	130-149		0.35
330-373	150-169		0.40
374-417	170-189		0.45
418-440	190-200		0.50

TABLE 1
Annual and Five-Year Cumulative Pregnancy Rates
Per 100 Users by Weight Class

Weight class	year 1	year 2	year 3	year 4	year 5	Cumulative
<50 kg (<110 lbs)	0.2	0	0	0	0	0.2
50–59 kg (110–130 lbs)	0.2	0.5	0.4	2.0	0.4	3.4
60–69 kg (131–153 lbs)	0.4	0.5	1.6	1.7	0.8	5.0
≥70 kg (≥154 lbs)	0	1.1	5.1	2.5	0	8.5
All	0.2	0.5	1.2	1.6	0.4	3.9

sity lipoprotein (LDL) levels decreased during NORPLANT SYSTEM use. Triglyceride levels also decreased from pretreatment values.

INDICATIONS AND USAGE

The NORPLANT SYSTEM is indicated for the prevention of pregnancy and is a long-term (up to 5 years) reversible contraceptive system. The capsules should be removed by the end of the 5th year. New capsules may be inserted at that time if continuing contraceptive protection is desired.

In multicenter trials with the NORPLANT SYSTEM, involving 2470 women, the relationship between body weight and efficacy was investigated. Tabulated below is the pregnancy experience as a function of body weight. Because NORPLANT SYSTEM is a long-term method of contraception, this is reported over five years of use.

[See table 1 above]

Typically, pregnancy rates with contraceptive methods are reported for only the first year of use as shown below. The efficacy of these contraceptive methods, except the IUD and sterilization, depends in part on the reliability of use. The efficacy of the NORPLANT SYSTEM does not depend on patient compliance. However, no contraceptive method is 100% effective.

TABLE 2
Lowest Expected and Typical Failure Rates (%)
During the First Year of Use of a Contraceptive Method

Method	Lowest Expected	Typical
NORPLANT SYSTEM (6 capsules)	0.09	0.09
Male Sterilization	0.1	0.15
Female Sterilization	0.4	0.4
DEPO-PROVERA® (injectable progestogen)	0.3	0.3
Oral contraceptives		3
Combined	0.1	NA
Progestin only	0.5	NA
IUD		
Progesterone	1.5	2.0
Copper T 380A	0.6	0.8
Condom (male) without spermicide	3	12
(female) without spermicide	5	21
Cervical Cap		
Nulliparous women	9	18
Parous women	26	36
Diaphragm with spermicidal cream or jelly	6	18
Spermicides alone (foam, creams, jellies, and vaginal suppositories)	6	21
Periodic abstinence (all methods)	1–9*	20
Withdrawal	4	19
No contraception (planned pregnancy)	85	85

NA—not available

* Depending on method (calendar, ovulation, symptothermal, post-ovulation) Adapted from Hatcher, RA et al. *Contraceptive Technology*, 16th Revised Edition. New York, NY: Irvington Publishers, 1994.

NORPLANT SYSTEM gross annual discontinuation and continuation rates are summarized in Table 3.
[See table 3 at top of next page]

CONTRAINDICATIONS

1. Active thrombophlebitis or thromboembolic disorders. There is insufficient information regarding women who have had previous thromboembolic disease.
2. Undiagnosed abnormal genital bleeding.
3. Known or suspected pregnancy.
4. Acute liver disease; benign or malignant liver tumors.
5. Known or suspected carcinoma of the breast.
6. History of idiopathic intracranial hypertension.
7. Hypersensitivity to levonorgestrel or any of the other components of the NORPLANT SYSTEM.

WARNINGS

A. WARNINGS BASED ON EXPERIENCE WITH THE NORPLANT SYSTEM

1. *Bleeding Irregularities*

Most women can expect some variation in menstrual bleeding patterns. Irregular menstrual bleeding, intermenstrual spotting, prolonged episodes of bleeding and spotting, and amenorrhea occur in some women. Irregular bleeding patterns associated with the NORPLANT SYSTEM could mask symptoms of cervical or endometrial cancer. Overall, these irregularities diminish with continuing use. Since some NORPLANT SYSTEM users experience periods of amenorrhea, missed menstrual periods cannot serve as the only means of identifying early pregnancy. Pregnancy tests should be performed whenever a pregnancy is suspected. Six (6) weeks or more of amenorrhea after a pattern of regular menses may signal pregnancy. If pregnancy occurs, the capsules must be removed.

Although bleeding irregularities have occurred in clinical trials, proportionately more women had increases rather than decreases in hemoglobin concentrations, a difference that was highly statistically significant. This finding generally indicates that reduced menstrual blood loss is associated with the use of the NORPLANT SYSTEM. In rare instances, blood loss did result in hemoglobin values consistent with anemia.

2. *Ovarian Cysts   (Delayed Follicular Atresia)*

If follicular development occurs with the NORPLANT SYSTEM, atresia of the follicle is sometimes delayed, and the follicle may continue to grow beyond the size it would attain in a normal cycle. These enlarged follicles cannot be distinguished clinically from ovarian cysts. In the majority of women, enlarged follicles will spontaneously disappear and should not require surgery. Rarely, they may twist or rupture, sometimes causing abdominal pain, and surgical intervention may be required.

3. *Ectopic Pregnancies*

Ectopic pregnancies have occurred among NORPLANT SYSTEM users, although clinical studies have shown no increase in the rate of ectopic pregnancies per year among NORPLANT SYSTEM users as compared with users of no method or of IUDs. The incidence among NORPLANT SYSTEM users was 1.3 per 1000 woman-years, a rate significantly below the rate that has been estimated for noncontraceptive users in the United States (2.7 to 3.0 per 1000 woman-years). The risk of ectopic pregnancy may increase with the duration of NORPLANT SYSTEM use and possibly with increased weight of the user. Physicians should be alert to the possibility of an ectopic pregnancy among women using the NORPLANT SYSTEM who become pregnant or complain of lower-abdominal pain. Any patient who presents with lower-abdominal pain must be evaluated to rule out ectopic pregnancy.

4. *Foreign-body Carcinogenesis*

Rarely, cancers have occurred at the site of foreign-body intrusions or old scars. None has been reported in NORPLANT SYSTEM clinical trials. In rodents, which are highly susceptible to such cancers, the incidence decreases with decreasing size of the foreign body. Because of the resistance of human beings to these cancers and because of the small size of the capsules, the risk to users of the NORPLANT SYSTEM is judged to be minimal.

5. *Thromboembolic Disorders and Other Vascular Problems*

An increased risk of thromboembolic and thrombotic disease (pulmonary embolism, superficial venous thrombosis, and deep-vein thrombosis) has been found to be associated with the use of combination oral contraceptives. The relative risk has been estimated to be 4- to 11-fold higher for users than for nonusers. There have also been post-marketing reports of these events coincident with NORPLANT SYSTEM use. The reports of thrombophlebitis and superficial phlebitis have more commonly occurred in the arm of insertion. Some of these cases have been associated with trauma to that arm.

Cerebrovascular Disorders: Combination oral contraceptives have been shown to increase both the relative and attributable risks of cerebrovascular events (thrombotic and hemorrhagic strokes), although, in general, the risk is greatest among older (>35 years) hypertensive women who also smoke. Hypertension was found to be a risk factor for both users and nonusers for both types of strokes, while smoking interacted to increase the risk for hemorrhagic strokes. There have been post-marketing reports of stroke coincident with NORPLANT SYSTEM use.

Myocardial Infarction: An increased risk of myocardial infarction has been attributed to combination oral-contraceptive use. This is thought to be primarily thrombotic in origin and is related to the estrogen component of combination oral contraceptives. This increased risk occurs primarily in smokers or in women with other underlying risk factors for coronary-artery disease, such as family history of coronary-artery disease, hypertension, hypercholesterolemia, morbid obesity, and diabetes. The current relative risk of heart attack for combination oral-contraceptive users has been estimated as 2 to 6 times the risk for nonusers. The absolute risk is very low for women under 30 years of age.

Studies indicate a significant trend toward higher rates of myocardial infarctions and strokes with increasing doses of progestin in combination oral contraceptives. However, a recent study showed no increased risk of myocardial infarction associated with the past use of levonorgestrel-containing combination oral contraceptives. There have been post-marketing reports of myocardial infarction coincident with NORPLANT SYSTEM use.

Patients who develop active thrombophlebitis or thromboembolic disease should have the NORPLANT SYSTEM capsules removed. Removal should also be considered in women who will be subjected to prolonged immobilization due to surgery or other illnesses.

6. *Use Before or During Early Pregnancy*

Extensive epidemiological studies have revealed no increased risk of birth defects in women who have used oral contraceptives prior to pregnancy. Studies also do not suggest a teratogenic effect, particularly insofar as cardiac anomalies and limb-reduction defects are concerned, when taken inadvertently during early pregnancy. There is no evidence suggesting that the risk associated with NORPLANT SYSTEM use is different.

There have been rare reports of congenital anomalies in offspring of women who were using the NORPLANT SYSTEM inadvertently during early pregnancy. A cause and effect relationship is not believed to exist.

7. *Idiopathic Intracranial Hypertension*

Idiopathic intracranial hypertension (pseudotumor cerebri, benign intracranial hypertension) is a disorder of unknown etiology which is seen most commonly in obese females of reproductive age. There have been reports of idiopathic intracranial hypertension in NORPLANT SYSTEM users. A cardinal sign of idiopathic intracranial hypertension is papilledema; early symptoms may include headache (associated with a change in frequency, pattern, severity, or persistence; of particular importance are those headaches that are unremitting in nature) and visual disturbances. Patients with these symptoms, particularly obese patients or those with recent weight gain, should be screened for papilledema and, if present, the patient should be referred to a neurologist for further diagnosis and care. NORPLANT SYSTEM should be removed from patients experiencing this disorder.

B. WARNINGS BASED ON EXPERIENCE WITH COMBINATION (PROGESTIN PLUS ESTROGEN) ORAL CONTRACEPTIVES

1. *Cigarette Smoking*

Cigarette smoking increases the risk of serious cardiovascular side effects from the use of combination oral contraceptives. This risk increases with age and with heavy smoking (15 or more cigarettes per day) and is quite marked in women over 35 years old. While this is believed to be an estrogen-related effect, it is not known whether a similar risk exists with progestin-only methods such as the NORPLANT SYSTEM; however, women who use the NORPLANT SYSTEM should be advised not to smoke.

2. *Elevated Blood Pressure*

Increased blood pressure has been reported in users of combination oral contraceptives. The prevalence of elevated blood pressure increases with long exposure. Although there were no statistically significant trends among NORPLANT SYSTEM users in clinical trials, physicians should be aware of the possibility of elevated blood pressure with the NORPLANT SYSTEM.

3. *Carcinoma*

Numerous epidemiological studies have been performed to determine the incidence of breast, endometrial, ovarian, and cervical cancer in women using combination oral contraceptives. Recent evidence in the literature suggests that use of combination oral contraceptives is not associated with an increased risk of developing breast cancer in the overall population of users. The Cancer and Steroid Hormone (CASH) study also showed no latent effect on the risk of breast cancer for at least a decade following long-term use. However, some of these same recent studies have shown an increased relative risk of breast cancer in certain subgroups of combination oral-contraceptive users, although no consistent pattern of findings has been identified. This information should be considered when prescribing the NORPLANT SYSTEM.

Continued on next page

Norplant—Cont.

Some studies suggest that combination oral-contraceptive use has been associated with an increase in the risk of cervical intraepithelial neoplasia in some populations of women. However, there continues to be controversy about the extent to which such findings may be due to differences in sexual behavior and other factors. In spite of many studies of the relationship between combination oral-contraceptive use and breast and cervical cancers, a cause-and-effect relationship has not been established.
Evidence indicates that combination oral contraceptives may decrease the risk of ovarian and endometrial cancer. Irregular bleeding patterns associated with the NORPLANT SYSTEM could mask symptoms of cervical or endometrial cancer.

4. *Hepatic Tumors*
Hepatic adenomas have been found to be associated with the use of combination oral contraceptives with an estimated incidence of about 3 occurrences per 100,000 users per year, a risk that increases after 4 or more years of use. Although benign, hepatic adenomas may rupture and cause death through intra-abdominal hemorrhage. The contribution of the progestin component of oral contraceptives to the development of hepatic adenomas is not known.

5. *Ocular Lesions*
There have been clinical case reports of retinal thrombosis associated with the use of oral contraceptives. Although it is believed that this adverse reaction is related to the estrogen component of oral contraceptives, the NORPLANT SYSTEM capsules should be removed if there is unexplained partial or complete loss of vision; onset of proptosis or diplopia; papilledema; or retinal vascular lesions. Appropriate diagnostic and therapeutic measures should be undertaken immediately.

6. *Gallbladder Disease*
Earlier studies have reported an increased lifetime relative risk of gallbladder surgery in users of oral contraceptives and estrogens. More recent studies, however, have shown that the relative risk of developing gallbladder disease among oral-contraceptive users may be minimal. The recent findings of minimal risk may be related to the use of oral-contraceptive formulations containing lower hormonal doses of estrogens and progestins. The association of this risk with use of the NORPLANT SYSTEM progestin-only method is not known.

PRECAUTIONS

GENERAL
Patients should be counseled that this product does not protect against HIV infection (AIDS) and other sexually transmitted diseases.

1. *Physical Examination and Follow-Up*
A complete medical history and physical examination should be taken prior to the implantation or reimplantation of NORPLANT SYSTEM capsules and at least annually during its use. These physical examinations should include special reference to the implant site, blood pressure, breasts, abdomen and pelvic organs, including cervical cytology and relevant laboratory tests. In case of undiagnosed, persistent or recurrent abnormal vaginal bleeding, appropriate diagnostic measures should be conducted to rule out malignancy. Women with a strong family history of breast cancer or who have breast nodules should be monitored with particular care.

2. *Carbohydrate and Lipid Metabolism*
An altered glucose tolerance characterized by decreased insulin sensitivity following glucose loading has been found in some users of combination and progestin-only oral contraceptives. The effects of the NORPLANT SYSTEM on carbohydrate metabolism appear to be minimal. In a study in which pretreatment serum-glucose levels were compared with levels after 1 and 2 years of NORPLANT SYSTEM use, no statistically significant differences in mean serum-glucose levels were evident 2 hours after glucose loading. The clinical significance of these findings is unknown, but diabetic patients should be carefully observed while using the NORPLANT SYSTEM.
Women who are being treated for hyperlipidemias should be followed closely if they elect to use the NORPLANT SYSTEM. Some progestins may elevate LDL levels and may render the control of hyperlipidemias more difficult. (See "Warnings," A.5.)

3. *Liver Function*
If jaundice develops in any women while using the NORPLANT SYSTEM, consideration should be given to removing the capsules. Steroid hormones may be poorly metabolized in patients with impaired liver function.

4. *Fluid Retention*
Steroid contraceptives may cause some degree of fluid retention. They should be prescribed with caution, and only with careful monitoring, in patients with conditions which might be aggravated by fluid retention.

5. *Emotional Disorders*
Consideration should be given to removing NORPLANT SYSTEM capsules in women who become significantly depressed since the symptom may be drug-related. Women with a history of depression should be carefully observed and removal considered if depression recurs to a serious degree.

TABLE 3
Annual and Five-Year Cumulative Rates per 100 Users

	year 1	year 2	year 3	year 4	year 5	Cumulative
Pregnancy	0.2	0.5	1.2	1.6	0.4	3.9
Bleeding Irregularities	9.1	7.9	4.9	3.3	2.9	25.1
Medical (excl. bleeding irreg.)	6.0	5.6	4.1	4.0	5.1	22.4
Personal	4.6	7.7	11.7	10.7	11.7	38.7
Continuation	81.0	77.4	79.2	76.7	77.6	29.5

6. *Contact Lenses*
Contact-lens wearers who develop visual changes or changes in lens tolerance should be assessed by an ophthalmologist.

7. *Autoimmune Disease*
Autoimmune diseases such as scleroderma, systemic lupus erythematosus and rheumatoid arthritis occur in the general population and more frequently among women of childbearing age. There have been rare reports of various autoimmune diseases, including the above, in NORPLANT SYSTEM users; however, the rate of reporting is significantly less than the expected incidence for these diseases. Studies have raised the possibility of developing antibodies against silicone-containing devices; however, the specificity and clinical relevance of these antibodies are unknown. While it is believed that the occurrence of autoimmune disease among NORPLANT SYSTEM users is coincidental, health-care providers should be alert to the earliest manifestations.

8. *Insertion and Removal*
To be sure that the woman is not pregnant at the time of capsule placement and to assure contraceptive effectiveness during the first cycle of use, it is advisable that insertion be done during the first 7 days of the menstrual cycle or immediately following an abortion. However, NORPLANT SYSTEM capsules may be inserted at any time during the cycle provided pregnancy has been excluded and a nonhormonal contraceptive method is used for at least 7 days following insertion. Insertion is not recommended before 6 weeks post-partum in breast-feeding women.
Insertion and removal are not difficult procedures but instructions must be followed closely. It is strongly advised that all health-care professionals who insert and remove NORPLANT SYSTEM capsules be instructed in the procedures before they attempt them. A proper insertion just under the skin will facilitate removals. Proper NORPLANT SYSTEM insertion and removal should result in minimal scarring. If the capsules are placed too deeply, they can be harder to remove. There have been infrequent reports of the use of general anesthesia during the removal procedure; it is generally not required. Before initiating the removal procedure, all NORPLANT SYSTEM capsules should be located via palpation. If all six capsules cannot be palpated, they may be localized via ultrasound (7 MHz), X ray, or compression mammography. If all capsules cannot be removed at the first attempt, removal should be attempted later when the site has healed. Bruising may occur at the implant site during insertion or removal. Other cutaneous reactions that have been reported include blistering, ulcerations and sloughing. There have been reports of arm pain, numbness and tingling following these procedures. In some women, hyperpigmentation occurs over the implantation site but is usually reversible following removal. See detailed Insertion and Removal Instructions below.

9. *Infections*
Infection at the implant site, including cellulitis, has been uncommon. Attention to aseptic technique and proper insertion and removal of the NORPLANT SYSTEM capsules reduces the possibility of infection. If infection occurs, suitable treatment should be instituted. If infection persists, the capsules should be removed.

10. *Capsule Expulsion and Displacement*
Expulsion of capsules was uncommon. It occurred more frequently when placement of the capsules was extremely shallow, too close to the incision, or when infection was present. Replacement of an expelled capsule must be accomplished using a new sterile capsule. If infection is present, it should be treated and cured before replacement. Contraceptive efficacy may be inadequate with fewer than 6 capsules.
There have been reports of capsule displacement (i.e., movement) most of which involve minor changes in the positioning of the capsules. However, infrequent reports of significant displacement (a few to several inches) have been received. Some reports have been associated with pain or discomfort. In the event that capsule movement occurs, the removal technique may need to be modified, such as additional incisions or visits.

11. *Provisions for Removal*
Women should be advised that the capsules will be removed at any time for any reason. The removal should be done on such request or at the end of 5 years of usage by personnel instructed in the removal technique.
Upon removal, NORPLANT SYSTEM capsules should be disposed of in accordance with Center for Disease Control Guidelines for the handling of biohazardous waste.

DRUG INTERACTIONS
Reduced efficacy (pregnancy) has been reported for NORPLANT SYSTEM users taking phenytoin and carbamazepine. These drugs may increase the metabolism of levonorgestrel through induction of microsomal liver enzymes. NORPLANT SYSTEM users should be warned of the possibility of decreased efficacy with the use of the drugs exhibiting enzyme-inducing activity such as those noted above and rifampicin. For women receiving long-term therapy with hepatic enzyme inducers, another method of contraception should be considered.

DRUG/LABORATORY TEST INTERACTIONS
Certain endocrine tests may be affected by NORPLANT SYSTEM use:
1. Sex-hormone-binding globulin concentrations are decreased.
2. Thyroxine concentrations may be slightly decreased and triiodothyronine uptake increased.

CARCINOGENESIS
See "**Warnings**" section.

PREGNANCY
Pregnancy Category X. See "**Warnings**" section.

NURSING MOTHERS
Steroids are not considered the contraceptives of first choice for breast-feeding women. Levonorgestrel has been identified in the breast milk. The health of breast-fed infants whose mothers began using the NORPLANT SYSTEM during the 5th to 7th week postpartum was evaluated: no significant effects were observed on the growth or development of infants who were followed to 12 months of age. No data are available on use in breast-feeding mothers earlier than this after parturition.

INFORMATION FOR THE PATIENT
See Patient Labeling.
Two copies of the Patient Labeling are included to help describe the characteristics of the NORPLANT SYSTEM to the patient. One copy should be provided to the patient. Patients should also be advised that the Prescribing Information is available to them at their request. It is recommended that propective users be fully informed about the risks and benefits associated with use of the NORPLANT SYSTEM, with other forms of contraception, and with no contraception at all. It is also recommended that prospective users be fully informed about the insertion and removal procedures. Health-care providers may wish to obtain informed consent from all patients in light of the techniques involved with insertion and removal.

ADVERSE REACTIONS

The following adverse reactions have been associated with the NORPLANT SYSTEM during the first year of use. They include:

Many bleeding days or prolonged bleeding	27.6%
Spotting	17.1%
Amenorrhea	9.4%
Irregular (onsets of) bleeding	7.6%
Frequent bleeding onsets	7.0%
Scanty bleeding	5.2%
Pain or itching near implant site (usually transient)	3.7%
Infection at implant site	0.7%

In addition, removal difficulties have been reported with a frequency of 6.2%, which is based on 849 removals occurring through 5 years of use.
Clinical studies comparing NORPLANT® SYSTEM users with other contraceptive method users suggest that the following adverse reactions occurring during the first year are probably associated with NORPLANT SYSTEM use. These adverse reactions have also been reported post-marketing:
Headache
Nervousness/Anxiety
Nausea/Vomiting
Dizziness

Adnexal enlargement
Dermatitis/Rash
Acne
Change of appetite
Mastalgia
Weight gain
Hirsutism, hypertrichosis, and scalp-hair loss
In addition, the following adverse reactions have been reported with a frequency of 5% or greater during the first year and are possibly related to NORPLANT SYSTEM use:
Breast discharge
Cervicitis
Musculoskeletal pain
Abdominal discomfort
Leukorrhea
Vaginitis
The following adverse reactions have been reported post-marketing with an incidence of less than 1% and are possibly related to NORPLANT SYSTEM use:
Emotional lability
Idiopathic intracranial hypertension (IIH, pseudotumor cerebri, benign intracranial hypertension)
Dysmenorrhea
Migraine
Arm pain
Numbness
Tingling
Depression
The following adverse reactions have been reported post-marketing with an incidence of less than 1%. These events occurred under circumstances where a causal relationship to the NORPLANT SYSTEM is unknown. These reactions are listed as information for physicians:
Congenital anomalies
Pulmonary embolism
Superficial venous thrombosis
Deep-vein thrombosis
Myocardial infarction
Thrombotic thrombocytopenic purpura (TTP)
Stroke
Pruritus
Urticaria
Asthenia (fatigue/weakness)

OVERDOSAGE

Overdosage can result if more than six capsules of the NORPLANT SYSTEM are in situ. All implanted NORPLANT SYSTEM capsules should be removed before inserting a new set of NORPLANT SYSTEM capsules. Overdosage may cause fluid retention with its associated effects and uterine bleeding irregularities.

DOSAGE AND ADMINISTRATION

The NORPLANT SYSTEM consists of six Silastic® capsules, each containing 36 mg of the progestin, levonorgestrel. The total administered (implanted) dose is 216 mg. Implantation of all six capsules should be performed during the first 7 days of the onset of menses by a health-care professional instructed in the NORPLANT SYSTEM insertion technique. Insertion is subdermal in the midportion of the upper arm about 8 to 10 cm above the elbow crease. Distribution should be in a fanlike pattern, about 15 degrees apart, for a total of 75 degrees. Proper insertion will facilitate later removal. (See section on Insertion/Removal.)

HOW SUPPLIED

The NORPLANT SYSTEM Kit includes the following items:
1 NORPLANT SYSTEM (levonorgestrel implants), a set of six implants (capsules)
1 NORPLANT SYSTEM trocar
1 Scalpel
1 Forceps
1 Syringe
2 Syringe needles
1 Package of skin closures
3 Packages of gauze sponges
1 Stretch bandage
1 Surgical drape (fenestrated)
2 Surgical drapes
Store at room temperature away from excess heat and moisture.
Note: The indented statement below is required by the Federal government's Clean Air Act for all products containing or manufactured with chlorofluorocarbons (CFC's).
  WARNING: Manufactured with dichlorodifluoromethane, a substance which harms public health and environment by destroying ozone in the upper atmosphere.
A notice similar to the above WARNING has been placed in the patient information leaflet of this product under Environmental Protection Agency (EPA) regulations. The patient's warning states that the patient should consult his or her physician if there are questions about alternatives. Dichlorodifluoromethane is a chemical used in the sterilization process of the NORPLANT SYSTEM and is not contained in the product itself.
NDC 0008-2564-01
References available upon request.

INSTRUCTIONS FOR INSERTION AND REMOVAL

The NORPLANT SYSTEM consists of six levonorgestrel-releasing capsules that are inserted subdermally in the medial aspect of the upper arm.
The NORPLANT SYSTEM provides up to 5 years of effective contraceptive protection.
The basis for successful use and subsequent removal of NORPLANT SYSTEM capsules is a correct and carefully performed subdermal insertion of the six capsules. It is recommended that health-care professionals performing insertions or removals of NORPLANT SYSTEM capsules avail themselves of instruction and supervision in the proper technique prior to attempting these procedures. During insertion, special attention should be given to the following:
— asepsis.
— correct subdermal placement of the capsules.
— careful technique to minimize tissue trauma.
This will help to avoid infections and excessive scarring at the insertion area and will help keep the capsules from being inserted too deeply in the tissue. If the capsules are placed too deeply, they will be more difficult to remove than correctly placed subdermal capsules.

INSERTION PROCEDURE

Insertion should be performed within seven days from the onset of menses. However, NORPLANT SYSTEM capsules may be inserted at any time during the cycle provided pregnancy has been excluded and a nonhormonal contraceptive method is used for at least 7 days following insertion. It is recommended that a complete history and physical examination, including a gynecologic examination, be performed before the insertion of NORPLANT SYSTEM capsules. Determine if the subject has any allergies to the antiseptic or anesthetic to be used or contraindications to progestin-only contraception. If none are found, the capsules are inserted using the procedure outlined below.
One NORPLANT SYSTEM set consists of six capsules in a sterile pouch. The insertion is performed under aseptic conditions using a trocar to place the capsules under the skin.

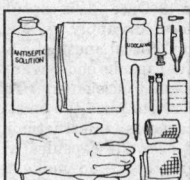

Figure 1: The following equipment is recommended for the insertion:
—an examining table for the patient to lie on.
—sterile surgical drapes, sterile gloves (free of talc), antiseptic solution.
—local anesthetic, needles, and syringe.
—#11 scalpel, #10 trocar, forceps
—skin closure, sterile gauze, and compresses.

The plastic cover and tray are NOT STERILE.

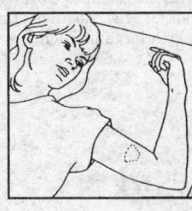

Figure 2: Have the patient lie on her back on the examination table with her left arm (if the patient is left-handed, the right arm) flexed at the elbow and externally rotated so that her hand is lying by her head. The capsules will be inserted subdermally through a small 2-mm incision and positioned in a fanlike manner with the fan opening towards the shoulder.

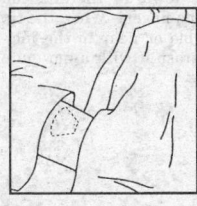

Figure 3: Prep the patient's upper arm with antiseptic solution; cover the arm above and below the insertion area with a sterile cloth. The optimal insertion area is in the inside of the upper arm about 8 to 10 cm above the elbow crease.

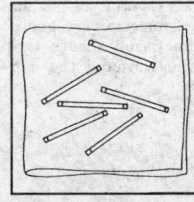

Figure 4: Open the sterile NORPLANT SYSTEM package carefully by pulling apart the sheets of the pouch, allowing the capsules to fall onto a sterile drape. Count the six capsules.

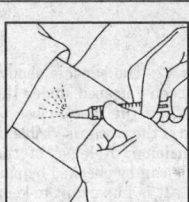

Figure 5: After determining the absence of known allergies to the anesthetic agent or related drugs, fill a 5-mL syringe with the local anesthetic. Since blood loss is minimal with this procedure, use of epinephrine-containing anesthetics is not considered necessary. Anesthetize the insertion area by first inserting the needle under the skin and injecting a small amount of anesthetic. Then anesthetize six areas about 4 to 4.5 cm long, to mimic the fanlike position of the implanted capsules.

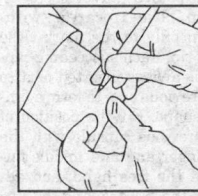

Figure 6: Use the scalpel to make a small incision (about 2 mm) just through the dermis of the skin.
Alternatively, the trocar may be inserted directly through the skin without making an incision with the scalpel. The bevel of the trocar should always face up during the insertion.

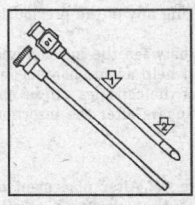

Figure 7: The trocar has two marks on it. The first mark is closer to the hub and indicates how far the trocar should be introduced under the skin before the loading of each capsule. The second mark is close to the tip and indicates how much of the trocar should remain under the skin following the insertion of each implant.

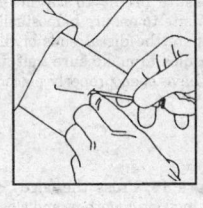

Figure 8: Insert the tip of the trocar through the incision beneath the skin at a shallow angle. Once the trocar is inserted, it should be oriented with the the bevel up toward the skin to keep the capsules in a superficial plane. It is important to keep the trocar subdermal by tenting the skin with the trocar, as failure to do so may result in deep placement of the capsules and could make removal more difficult.

Advance the trocar gently under the skin to the first mark near the hub of the trocar. The tip of the trocar is now at a distance of about 4 to 4.5 cm from the incision.
Do not force the trocar, and if resistance is felt, try another direction.

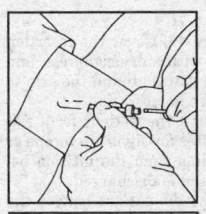

Figure 9: When the trocar has been inserted the appropriate distance, remove the obturator and load the first capsule into the trocar using the thumb and forefinger.

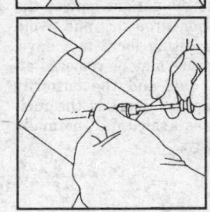

Figure 10: Gently advance the capsule with the obturator towards the tip of the trocar until you feel resistance. Never force the obturator.

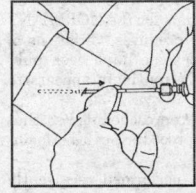

Figure 11: Hold the obturator steady, and bring the trocar back until it touches the handle of the obturator.

Continued on next page

Norplant—Cont.

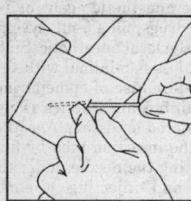

Figure 12: The capsule should have been released under the skin when the mark close to the tip of the trocar is visible in the incision. Release of the capsule can be checked by palpation. It is important to keep the obturator steady and not to push the capsule into the tissue.

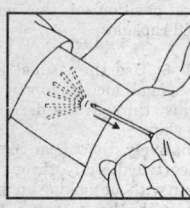

Figure 13: Do not remove the trocar from the incision until all capsules have been inserted. The trocar is withdrawn only to the mark close to its tip. Each succeeding capsule is always inserted next to the previous one, to form a fan-like shape. Fix the position of the previous capsule with the forefinger and and middle finger of the free hand, and advance the trocar along the tips of the fingers. This will ensure a suitable distance of about 15 degrees between capsules and keep the trocar from puncturing any of the previously inserted capsules.

Leave a distance of about 5 mm between the incision and the tips of the capsules. This will help avoid spontaneous expulsions. The correct position of the capsules can be ensured by feeling them with the fingers after the insertion has been completed.

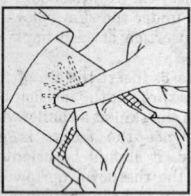

Figure 14: After placement of the sixth capsule, a sterile gauze may be used to apply pressure briefly to the insertion site to ensure hemostasis. Palpate the distal ends of the capsules to make sure that all six have been properly placed.

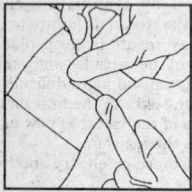

Figure 15: Press the edges of the incision together, and close the incision with a skin closure. Suturing the incision should not be necessary.

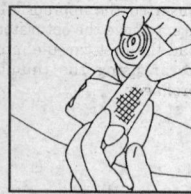

Figure 16: Cover the insertion area with a dry compress, and wrap gauze around the arm to ensure hemostasis.

Observe the patient for a few minutes for signs of syncope or bleeding from the incision before she is discharged.

Advise the patient to keep the insertion area dry and avoid heavy lifting for 2 to 3 days. The gauze may be removed after 1 day, and the butterfly bandage as soon as the incision has healed, i.e., normally in 3 days.

REMOVAL PROCEDURE

Described below is a removal procedure which was developed and used during the clinical trials for the NORPLANT SYSTEM. As with many surgical procedures, variations of the technique have appeared and some have been published. No one particular procedure routinely appears to have any advantage over another.

It is recommended that removals be prescheduled so that preparations for carrying out the procedure can be facilitated.

Removal of the capsules should be performed very gently and will usually take more time than insertion. Capsules are sometimes nicked, cut, or broken during removal. The incidence of overall removal difficulties, including damage to capsules, has been 13.2 percent. Less than half of these removal difficulties have caused inconvenience to the patient. If the removal of some of the capsules proves difficult, have the patient return for another visit. The remaining capsule(s) will be easier to remove after the area is healed. It may be appropriate to seek consultation or provide referral for patients in whom initial attempts at capsule removal prove difficult. If contraception is still desired, a barrier method should be advised until all capsules are removed. The position of the patient and the asepsis are the same as for insertion.

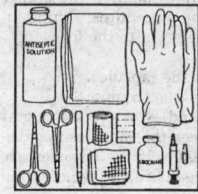

Figure 17: The following equipment is needed for the removal:
—an examining table for the patient to lie on.
—sterile surgical drapes, sterile gloves (free of talc), antiseptic solution.
—local anesthetic, needles, and syringe.
—#11 scalpel, forceps (straight and curved mosquito).
—skin closure, sterile gauze, and compresses.

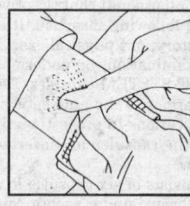

Figure 18: Palpate the capsules to make sure that all six capsules have been located, marking their position with a sterile marker. If all six capsules cannot be palpated, they may be localized via ultrasound (7 MHz), X ray, or compression mammography.

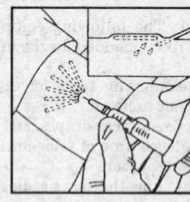

Figure 19: Once all six capsules are located, apply a small amount of local anesthetic *under* the capsule ends nearest the original incision site. This will serve to raise the ends of the capsules. Anesthetic injected over the capsules will obscure them and make removal more difficult. Additional small amounts of the anesthetic can be used for the removal of each of the capsules, if required.

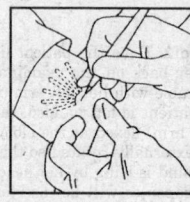

Figure 20: Make a 4-mm incision with the scalpel close to the ends of the capsules. Do not make a large incision.

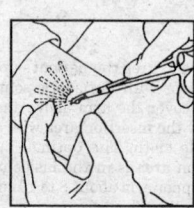

Figure 21: Push each capsule gently towards the incision with the fingers. When the tip is visible or near to the incision, grasp it with a mosquito forceps.

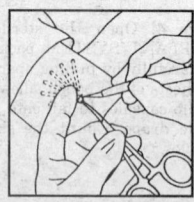

Figure 22: Use the scalpel, forceps, or gauze to very gently open the tissue sheath that has formed around the capsule.

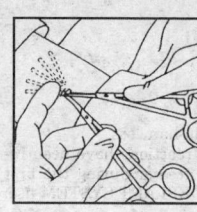

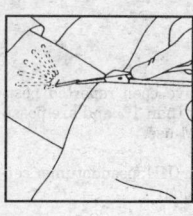

Figures 23 and 24: Remove the capsule from the incision with the second forceps.

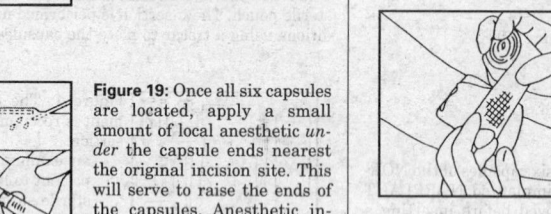

Figures 25 and 26: After the procedure is completed, the incision is closed and bandaged as with insertion. The upper arm should be kept dry for a few days.

Following removal, fertility rates return to levels comparable to those seen in the general population of women using no method of contraception, and a pregnancy may occur at any time. If the patient wishes to continue using the method, a new set of NORPLANT SYSTEM capsules can be inserted through the same incision in the same or opposite direction.

HINTS

Insertion

— Counselling of the patient on the benefits and side effects of the method prior to insertion will greatly increase patient satisfaction.
— Correct subdermal placement of the capsules will facilitate removal.
— Before insertion, apply the anesthetic just beneath the skin so as to raise the dermis above the underlying tissue.
— Never force the trocar.
— To ensure subdermal placement, the trocar with bevel up should be supported by the index finger and should visibly raise the skin at all times during insertion.
— To avoid damaging the previous implanted capsule, stabilize the capsule with your forefinger and middle finger and advance the trocar alongside the finger tips at an angle of 15 degrees.
— After insertion, make a drawing for the patient's file showing the location of the 6 capsules and describe any variations in placement. This will greatly aid removal.

Removal

— Alternate removal techniques have been developed.
— The removal of the implanted capsules will usually take a little more time than the insertion.
— Before initiating removal, all capsules should be located by palpation. If all six capsules cannot be palpated, they may be localized via ultrasound (7 MHz), X ray, or compression mammography.
— Before removal, apply the anesthetic *under* the capsule ends nearest the original incision site.
— If the removal of some of the capsules proves difficult, interrupt the procedure and have the patient return for another visit. The remaining capsule(s) will be easier to remove after the area is healed.
— It may be appropriate to seek consultation or provide referral for patients in whom initial attempts at capsule removal prove difficult.

Distributed by
Wyeth Laboratories Inc.
A Wyeth-Ayerst Company
Philadelphia, PA 19101

Shown in Product Identification Guide, page 344

OMNIPEN®

[om ′nī-pen]
(ampicillin)
for ORAL SUSPENSION

DESCRIPTION

Omnipen (ampicillin) is a semisynthetic penicillin derived from the basic penicillin nucleus, 6-amino-penicillanic acid. Ampicillin is designated chemically as (2S, 5R, 6R)-6-[(R)-2-Amino -2- phenylacetamido] -3,3- dimethyl -7- oxo -4- thia-1-aza-bicyclo [3.2.0]heptane-2-carboxylic acid. The molecular formula for ampicillin is $C_{16}H_{19}N_3O_4S$ with a molecular weight of 349.40.

Omnipen for oral suspension is a powder which when reconstituted as directed yields a suspension of 125 mg or 250 mg ampicillin anhydrous, per 5 mL. The inactive ingredients present are artificial flavors, colloidal silicon dioxide, methylparaben, propylparaben, sodium benzoate, sodium citrate, sucrose, and water. Each dosage strength of suspension also contains the following:

125 mg per 5 mL—carboxymethylcellulose sodium, FD&C Blue 1, FD&C Red 40, FD&C Yellow 6, and natural flavors; 250 mg per 5 mL—D&C Red 28.

CLINICAL PHARMACOLOGY

Ampicillin is bactericidal at low concentrations and is clinically effective not only against the gram-positive organisms usually susceptible to penicillin G, but also against a variety of gram-negative organisms. It is stable in the presence of gastric acid and is well absorbed from the gastrointestinal tract. It diffuses readily into most body tissues and fluids; however, penetration into the cerebrospinal fluid and brain occurs only with meningeal inflammation.

Ampicillin is excreted largely unchanged in the urine; its excretion can be delayed by concurrent administration of probenecid which inhibits the renal tubular secretion of ampicillin. In blood serum, ampicillin is the least bound of all the penicillins; an average of about 20% of the drug is bound to the plasma proteins as compared to 60 to 90% for the other penicillins. Blood serum levels of approximately 2 mcg/mL are attained within 1 to 2 hours following a 250 mg oral dose given to fasting adults. Detectable amounts persist for about 6 hours.

MICROBIOLOGY

While in vitro studies have demonstrated the susceptibility of most strains of the following microorganisms, clinical efficacy for infections other than those included in the "**Indications and Usage**" section has not been documented.

Gram-Positive

Alpha- and beta-hemolytic streptococci, *Streptococcus pneumoniae,* staphylococci (non-penicillinase-producing), *Bacillus anthracis, Clostridium* sp., *Corynebacterium xerose,* and most strains of enterococci.

Gram-Negative

Hemophilus influenzae, Neisseria gonorrhoeae, Neisseria meningitidis, Proteus mirabilis, and many strains of Salmonella (including *S. typhosa*), Shigella, and *Escherichia coli.* NOTE: Ampicillin is inactivated by penicillinase and therefore is ineffective against penicillinase-producing organisms including certain strains of staphylococci, *Pseudomonas aeruginosa, P. vulgaris, Klebsiella pneumoniae, Enterobacter aerogenes,* and some strains of *E. coli.* Ampicillin is not active against Rickettsia, Mycoplasma, and "large viruses" (Miyagawanella).

Testing for Susceptibility

The invading organism should be cultured and its susceptibility demonstrated as a guide to therapy. If the Kirby-Bauer method of disc susceptibility is used, a 10 mcg ampicillin disc should be used to determine the relative in vitro susceptibility.

INDICATIONS AND USAGE

Omnipen (ampicillin) for Oral Suspension is indicated in the treatment of infections caused by susceptible strains of the following microorganisms:

Infections of the genitourinary tract including gonorrhea—E. coli, P. mirabilis, enterococci, *Shigella, S. typhosa* and other *Salmonella,* and non-penicillinase-producing *N. gonorrhoeae.*

*Infections of the respiratory tract—*Non-penicillinase-producing *H. influenzae* and staphylococci, and streptococci including *Streptococcus pneumoniae.*

Infections of the gastrointestinal tract—Shigella, S. typhosa and other *Salmonella, E. coli, P. mirabilis* and enterococci.

Meningitis—N. meningitidis.

Bacteriology studies to determine the causative organisms and their sensitivity to ampicillin should be performed. Therapy may be instituted prior to the results of susceptibility testing.

CONTRAINDICATIONS

The use of this drug is contraindicated in individuals with a history of a previous hypersensitivity reaction to any of the penicillins. Ampicillin is also contraindicated in infections caused by penicillinase-producing organisms.

WARNINGS

Serious and occasionally fatal hypersensitivity (anaphylactic) reactions have been reported in patients on penicillin therapy. Although anaphylaxis is more frequent following parenteral administration, it has occurred in patients on oral penicillins. These reactions are more apt to occur in individuals with a history of penicillin hypersensitivity and/or history of sensitivity to multiple allergens.

There have been well-documented reports of individuals with a history of penicillin hypersensitivity who experienced severe hypersensitivity reactions when treated with cephalosporins. Before initiating therapy with any penicillin, careful inquiry should be made concerning previous hypersensitivity reactions to penicillins, cephalosporins, or other allergens. If an allergic reaction occurs, the drug should be discontinued and appropriate therapy instituted. **Serious anaphylactoid reactions require immediate emergency treatment with epinephrine. Oxygen, intravenous steroids, and airway management, including intubation, should also be administered as indicated.**

PRECAUTIONS

GENERAL

Prolonged use of antibiotics may promote the overgrowth of nonsusceptible organisms, including fungi. Should superinfection occur, appropriate measures should be taken.

Patients with gonorrhea who also have syphilis should be given additional appropriate parenteral penicillin treatment.

Treatment with ampicillin does not preclude the need for surgical procedures, particularly in staphylococcal infections.

INFORMATION FOR THE PATIENT

1. The patient should inform the physician of any history of sensitivity to allergens, including previous hypersensitivity reactions to penicillins and cephalosporins (see "**Warnings**").

2. The patient should discontinue ampicillin and contact the physician immediately if any side effect occurs (see "**Warnings**").

3. Ampicillin should be taken with a full glass (8 oz) of water, one-half hour before or two hours after meals.

4. Diabetic patients should consult with the physician before changing diet or dosage of diabetes medication (see "**Precautions**—DRUG/LABORATORY TEST INTERACTION").

LABORATORY TESTS

In prolonged therapy, and particularly with high dosage regimens, periodic evaluation of the renal, hepatic, and hematopoietic systems is recommended.

In streptococcal infections, therapy must be sufficient to eliminate the organism (10 days minimum); otherwise the sequelae of streptococcal disease may occur. Cultures should be taken following completion of treatment to determine whether streptococci have been eradicated.

Cases of gonococcal infection with a suspected lesion of syphilis should have darkfield examinations ruling out syphilis before receiving ampicillin. Patients who do not have suspected lesions of syphilis and are treated with ampicillin should have a follow-up serologic test for syphilis each month for four months to detect syphilis that may have been masked by treatment for gonorrhea.

DRUG INTERACTIONS

When administered concurrently, the following drugs may interact with ampicillin:

Allopurinol—Increased possibility of skin rash, particularly in hyperuricemic patients, may occur.

Bacteriostatic antibiotics—Chloramphenicol, erythromycins, sulfonamides, or tetracyclines may interfere with the bactericidal effect of penicillins. This has been demonstrated *in vitro;* however, the clinical significance of this interaction is not well-documented.

Oral contraceptives—May be less effective and increased breakthrough bleeding may occur.

Probenecid—May decrease renal tubular secretion of ampicillin resulting in increased blood levels and/or ampicillin toxicity.

DRUG/LABORATORY TEST INTERACTION

After treatment with ampicillin, a false-positive reaction for glucose in the urine may occur with copper sulfate tests (Benedict's solution, Fehling's solution, or Clinitest® tablets) but not with enzyme based tests such as Clinistix® and TesTape®.

CARCINOGENESIS, MUTAGENESIS, IMPAIRMENT OF FERTILITY

Long-term studies in animals have not been performed to evaluate carcinogenesis, mutagenesis, or impairment of fertility in males or females.

PREGNANCY: TERATOGENIC EFFECTS

CATEGORY B

Reproduction studies in animals have revealed no evidence of impaired fertility or harm to the fetus due to penicillin. There are, however, no adequate and well-controlled studies in pregnant women. Because animal reproduction studies are not always predictive of human response, penicillin should be used during pregnancy only if clearly needed.

LABOR AND DELIVERY

Oral ampicillin-class antibiotics are poorly absorbed during labor. Studies in guinea pigs showed that intravenous administration of ampicillin slightly decreased the uterine tone and frequency of contractions, but moderately increased the height and duration of contractions. However, it is not known whether use of these drugs in humans during labor or delivery has immediate or delayed adverse effects on the fetus, prolongs the duration of labor, or increases the likelihood that forceps delivery or other obstetrical intervention or resuscitation of the newborn will be necessary.

NURSING MOTHERS

Ampicillin-class antibiotics are excreted in milk. Ampicillin use by nursing mothers may lead to sensitization of infants; therefore, a decision should be made whether to discontinue nursing or to discontinue ampicillin, taking into account the importance of the drug to the mother.

PEDIATRIC USE

Penicillins are excreted primarily unchanged by the kidney; therefore, the incompletely developed renal function in neonates and young infants will delay the excretion of penicillin. Administration to neonates and young infants should be limited to the lowest dosage compatible with an effective therapeutic regimen (see "**Dosage and Administration**").

ADVERSE REACTIONS

As with other penicillins, it may be expected that untoward reactions will be essentially limited to sensitivity phenomena. They are more likely to occur in individuals who have previously demonstrated hypersensitivity to penicillins and in those with a history of allergy, asthma, hay fever, or urticaria.

The following adverse reactions have been reported as associated with the use of ampicillin:

Gastrointestinal: glossitis, stomatitis, nausea, vomiting, enterocolitis, pseudomembranous colitis, and diarrhea. These reactions are usually associated with oral dosage forms of the drug.

Hypersensitivity Reactions: an erythematous, mildly pruritic, maculopapular skin rash has been reported fairly frequently. The rash, which usually does not develop within the first week of therapy, may cover the entire body, including the soles, palms, and oral mucosa. The eruption usually disappears in three to seven days. Other hypersensitivity reactions that have been reported are: skin rash, pruritis, urticaria, erythema multiforme, and an occasional case of exfoliative dermatitis. Anaphylaxis is the most serious reaction experienced and has usually been associated with the parenteral dosage form of the drug.

NOTE: Urticaria, other skin rashes, and serum sickness-like reactions may be controlled by antihistamines and, if necessary, systemic corticosteroids. Whenever such reactions occur, ampicillin should be discontinued unless, in the opinion of the physician, the condition being treated is life-threatening and amenable only to ampicillin therapy. Serious anaphylactic reactions require emergency measures (see **WARNINGS**).

Liver: A moderate elevation in serum glutamic-oxaloacetic transaminase (SGOT) has been noted, but the significance of this finding is unknown.

Hemic and Lymphatic Systems: Anemia, thrombocytopenia, thrombocytopenic purpura, eosinophilia, leukopenia, and agranulocytosis have been reported during therapy with penicillins. These reactions are usually reversible on discontinuation of therapy and are believed to be hypersensitivity phenomena.

Other adverse reactions that have been reported with the use of ampicillin are laryngeal stridor and high fever. An occasional patient may complain of sore mouth or tongue as with any oral penicillin preparation.

OVERDOSAGE

In case of overdosage, discontinue medication, treat symptomatically and institute supportive measures as required. In patients with renal function impairment, ampicillin-class antibiotics can be removed by hemodialysis but not by peritoneal dialysis.

DOSAGE AND ADMINISTRATION

Adults and children weighing over 20 kg:

For genitourinary- or gastrointestinal-tract infections other than gonorrhea in men and women—the usual dose is 500 mg q.i.d. in equally spaced doses (i.e., 500 mg every 6 hours); larger doses may be required for severe or chronic infections.

For the treatment of gonorrhea in both men and women—a single oral dose of 3.5 grams of ampicillin with 1 gram of probenecid administered simultaneously is recommended. Physicians are cautioned to use no less than the above recommended dosage for the treatment of gonorrhea. Follow-up cultures should be obtained from the original site(s) of infection 7 to 14 days after therapy. In women, it is also desirable to obtain culture test-of-cure from both the

Continued on next page

Omnipen—Cont.

endocervical and anal canals. Prolonged intensive therapy is needed for complications such as prostatitis and epididymitis.

For respiratory-tract infections—the usual dose is 250 mg q.i.d. in equally spaced doses (i.e., 250 mg every 6 hours).

Children weighing 20 kg or less:

For genitourinary- or gastrointestinal-tract infections—the usual dose is 100 mg/kg/day total, administered q.i.d. in equally divided and spaced doses (i.e., every 6 hours).

For respiratory infections—the usual dose is 50 mg/kg/day total, administered in equally divided and spaced doses three to four times daily (i.e., every 8 to every 6 hours).

Doses for children should not exceed doses recommended for adults.

In all patients, irrespective of age and weight: Larger doses may be required for severe or chronic infections. Although ampicillin is resistant to degradation by gastric acid, it should be administered at least one-half hour before or two hours after meals for maximal absorption. Except for the single-dose regimen for gonorrhea referred to above, therapy should be continued for a minimum of 48 to 72 hours after the patient becomes asymptomatic or evidence of bacterial eradication has been obtained. In infections caused by hemolytic strains of streptococci, a minimum of 10 days' treatment is recommended to guard against the risk of rheumatic fever or glomerulonephritis (see "**Precautions—LABORATORY TESTS**").

In the treatment of chronic urinary or gastrointestinal infections, frequent bacteriologic and clinical appraisal is necessary during therapy and may be necessary for several months afterwards. Stubborn infections may require treatment for several weeks. Smaller doses than those indicated above should not be used.

HOW SUPPLIED

Omnipen® (ampicillin) for Oral Suspension is available in the following dosage strengths as a powder, which when reconstituted as directed yields a palatable suspension:

125 mg per 5 mL, NDC 0008-0054, white powder in bottles to make 100 mL, 150 mL, or 200 mL of salmon-colored suspension.

250 mg per 5 mL, NDC 0008-0055, white powder in bottles to make 100 mL, 150 mL, or 200 mL of pink suspension.

Store at room temperature [approximately 25° C (77° F)] before reconstitution.

Shake well before using.

Keep tightly closed.

When stored in refrigerator discard unused portion after 14 days, or when stored at room temperature discard unused portion after 7 days (250 mg per 5 mL).

When stored in refrigerator discard unused portion after 14 days (125 mg per 5 mL).

Manufactured by:
Wyeth Laboratories Inc.
A Wyeth-Ayerst Company
Philadelphia, PA 19101

ORUDIS® ℞
[ō "roo 'dĭs]
(ketoprofen)
Capsules

ORUVAIL® ℞
[or 'ü văl]
(ketoprofen)
Extended-Release
Capsules

DESCRIPTION

Ketoprofen is a nonsteroidal anti-inflammatory drug. The chemical name for ketoprofen is 2-(3-benzoylphenyl)-propionic acid with the following structural formula:

Its empirical formula is $C_{16}H_{14}O_3$, with a molecular weight of 254.29. It has a pKa of 5.94 in methanol:water (3:1) and an n-octanol:water partition coefficient of 0.97 (buffer pH 7.4).

Ketoprofen is a white or off-white, odorless, nonhygroscopic, fine to granular powder, melting at about 95° C. It is freely soluble in ethanol, chloroform, acetone, ether and soluble in benzene and strong alkali, but practically insoluble in water at 20° C.

Orudis capsules contain 25 mg, 50 mg, or 75 mg of ketoprofen for oral administration. The inactive ingredients present are D&C Yellow 10, FD&C Blue 1, FD&C Yellow 6, gelatin,

lactose, magnesium stearate, and titanium dioxide. The 25 mg dosage strength also contains D&C Red 28 and FD&C Red 40.

Each Oruvail 100 mg, 150 mg, or 200 mg capsule contains ketoprofen in the form of hundreds of coated pellets. The dissolution of the pellets is pH dependent with optimum dissolution occurring at pH 6.5–7.5. There is no dissolution at pH 1.

In addition to the active ingredient, each 100 mg, 150 mg, or 200 mg capsule of Oruvail contains the following inactive ingredients: D&C Red 22, D&C Red 28, FD&C Blue 1, ethyl cellulose, gelatin, shellac, silicon dioxide, sodium lauryl sulfate, starch, sucrose, talc, titanium dioxide, and other proprietary ingredients. The 100 and 150 mg capsules also contain D&C Yellow 10 and FD&C Green 3.

CLINICAL PHARMACOLOGY

Ketoprofen is a nonsteroidal anti-inflammatory drug with analgesic and antipyretic properties.

The anti-inflammatory, analgesic, and antipyretic properties of ketoprofen have been demonstrated in classical animal and *in vitro* test systems. In anti-inflammatory models ketoprofen has been shown to have inhibitory effects on prostaglandin and leukotriene synthesis, to have antibradykinin activity, as well as to have lysosomal membrane-stabilizing action. However, its mode of action, like that of other nonsteroidal anti-inflammatory drugs, is not fully understood.

PHARMACODYNAMICS

Ketoprofen is a racemate with only the S enantiomer possessing pharmacological activity. The enantiomers have similar concentration time curves and do not appear to interact with one another.

An analgesic effect-concentration relationship for ketoprofen was established in an oral surgery pain study with Orudis. The effect-site rate constant (k_{e0}) was estimated to be 0.9 hour^{-1} (95% confidence limits: 0 to 2.1), and the concentration (Ce_{50}) of ketoprofen that produced one-half the maximum PID (pain intensity difference) was 0.3 µg/mL (95% confidence limits: 0.1 to 0.5). Thirty-three (33) to 68% of patients had an onset of action (as measured by reporting some pain relief) within 30 minutes following a single oral dose in postoperative pain and dysmenorrhea studies. Pain relief (as measured by remedication) persisted for up to 6 hours in 26 to 72% of patients in these studies.

PHARMACOKINETICS

General

Orudis and Oruvail capsules both contain ketoprofen. They differ only in their release characteristics. Orudis capsules release drug in the stomach whereas the pellets in Oruvail capsules are designed to resist dissolution in the low pH of gastric fluid but release drug at a controlled rate in the higher pH environment of the small intestine (see "**DESCRIPTION**").

Irrespective of the pattern of release, the systemic availability (F_s) when either oral formulation is compared with IV administration is approximately 90% in humans. For 75 to 200 mg single doses, the area under the curve has been shown to be dose proportional. The figure depicts the plasma time curves associated with both products.

Ketoprofen is >99% bound to plasma proteins, mainly to albumin.

Separate sections follow which delineate differences between Orudis and Oruvail capsules.

Absorption

Orudis capsules—Ketoprofen is rapidly and well-absorbed, with peak plasma levels occurring within 0.5 to 2 hours.

Oruvail capsules—Ketoprofen is also well-absorbed from this dosage form, although an observable increase in plasma levels does not occur until approximately 2 to 3 hours after taking the formulation. Peak plasma levels are usually reached 6 to 7 hours after dosing. (See Figure and Table, below).

When ketoprofen is administered with food, its total bioavailability (AUC) is not altered; however, the rate of absorption from either dosage form is slowed.

Orudis capsules—Food intake reduces C_{max} by approximately one-half and increases the mean time to peak concentration (t_{max}) from 1.2 hours for fasting subjects (range, 0.5 to 3 hours) to 2.0 hours for fed subjects (range, 0.75 to 3 hours). The fluctuation of plasma peaks may also be influenced by circadian changes in the absorption process.

Concomitant administration of magnesium hydroxide and aluminum hydroxide does not interfere with absorption of ketoprofen from Orudis capsules.

Oruvail capsules—Administration of Oruvail with a high-fat meal causes a delay of about 2 hours in reaching the C_{max}; neither the total bioavailability (AUC) nor the C_{max} is affected. Circadian changes in the absorption process have not been studied.

The administration of antacids or other drugs which may raise stomach pH would not be expected to change the rate or extent of absorption of ketoprofen from Oruvail capsules.

Multiple Dosing

Steady-state concentrations of ketoprofen are attained within 24 hours after commencing treatment with Orudis or Oruvail capsules. In studies with healthy male volunteers, trough levels at 24 hours following administration of Oruvail 200 mg capsules were 0.4 mg/L compared with 0.07 mg/L at 24 hours following administration of Orudis 50 mg capsules QID (12 hours) or 0.13 mg/L following administration of Orudis 75 mg capsules TID for 12 hours. Thus, relative to the peak plasma concentration, the accumulation of ketoprofen after multiple doses of Oruvail or Orudis capsules is minimal.

The figure below shows a reduction in peak height and area after the second 50 mg dose. This is probably due to a combination of food effects, circadian effects, and plasma sampling times. It is unclear to what extent each factor contributes to the loss of peak height and area.

The shaded area represents ±1 standard deviation (S.D.) around the mean for Orudis or Oruvail.

KETOPROFEN PLASMA CONCENTRATIONS IN SUBJECTS RECEIVING 200 MG OF ORUVAIL ONCE A DAY (QD), OR ORUDIS 50 MG EVERY 4 HOURS FOR 16 HOURS

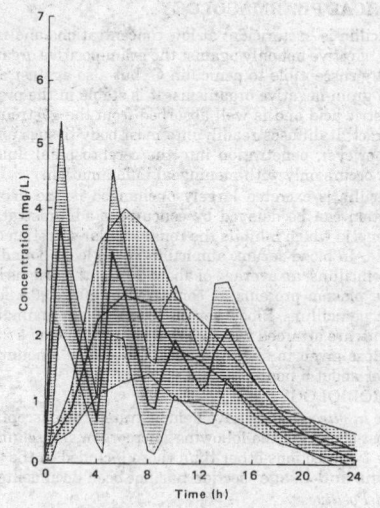

COMPARISON OF PHARMACOKINETIC PARAMETERS# FOR ORUDIS AND ORUVAIL

Kinetic Parameters	Orudis (4×50 mg)	Oruvail (1×200 mg)
Extent of oral absorption (bioavailability) F_s (%)	90	90
Peak plasma levels C_{max} (mg/L)		
Fasted	3.9±1.3	3.1±1.2
Fed	2.4±1.0	3.4±1.3
Time to peak concentration t_{max} (h)		
Fasted	1.2±0.6	6.8±2.1
Fed	2.0±0.8	9.2±2.6
Area under plasma concentration-time curve AUC_{0-24h} (mg·h/L)		
Fasted	32.1±7.2	30.1±7.9
Fed	36.6±8.1	31.3±8.1
Oral-dose clearance CL/F (L/h)	6.9±0.8	6.8±1.8
Half-life $t_{1/2}$ (h) [See footnote 1]	2.1±1.2	5.4±2.2

Values expressed are mean ± standard deviation
[1] In the case of Oruvail, absorption is slowed, intrinsic clearance is unchanged, but because the rate of elimination is dependent on absorption, the half-life is prolonged.

Metabolism

The metabolic fate of ketoprofen is glucuronide conjugation to form an unstable acyl-glucuronide. The glucuronic acid moiety can be converted back to the parent compound. Thus, the metabolite serves as a potential reservoir for parent drug, and this may be important in persons with renal insufficiency, whereby the conjugate may accumulate in the serum and undergo deconjugation back to the parent drug

(see "**Special Populations**: *Renally impaired*").The conjugates are reported to appear only in trace amounts in plasma in healthy adults, but are higher in elderly subjects—presumably because of reduced renal clearance. It has been demonstrated that in elderly subjects following multiple doses (50 mg every 6 h), the ratio of conjugated to parent ketoprofen AUC was 30% and 3%, respectively for the S & R enantiomers.

There are no known active metabolites of ketoprofen. Ketoprofen has been shown not to induce drug-metabolizing enzymes.

Elimination

The plasma clearance of ketoprofen is approximately 0.08 L/kg/h with a V_d of 0.1 L/kg after IV administration. The elimination half-life of ketoprofen has been reported to be 2.05±0.58 h (Mean ± S.D.) following IV administration, from 2 to 4 h following administration of Orudis capsules, and 5.4±2.2 h after administration of Oruvail 200 mg capsules. In cases of slow drug absorption, the elimination rate is dependent on the absorption rate and thus $t_{1/2}$ relative to an IV dose appears prolonged.

After a single 200 mg dose of Oruvail, the plasma levels decline slowly, and average 0.4 mg/L after 24 hours (see Figure above).

In a 24-hour period, approximately 80% of an administered dose of ketoprofen is excreted in the urine, primarily as the glucuronide metabolite.

Enterohepatic recirculation of the drug has been postulated, although biliary levels have never been measured to confirm this.

Special Populations

Elderly: Clearance and unbound fraction

The plasma and renal clearance of ketoprofen is reduced in the elderly (mean age, 73 years) compared to a younger normal population (mean age, 27 years). Hence, ketoprofen peak concentration and AUC increase with increasing age. In addition, there is a corresponding increase in unbound fraction with increasing age. Data from one trial suggest that the increase is greater in women than in men. It has not been determined whether age-related changes in absorption among the elderly contribute to the changes in bioavailability of ketoprofen.

Orudis capsules—In a study conducted with young and elderly men and women, results for subjects older than 75 years of age showed that free drug AUC increased by 40% and C_{max} increased by 60% as compared with estimates of the same parameters in young subjects (those younger than 35 years of age; see "**INDIVIDUALIZATION OF DOSAGE**").

Also in the elderly, the ratio of intrinsic clearance/availability decreased by 35% and plasma half-life was prolonged by 26%. This reduction is thought to be due to a decrease in hepatic extraction associated with aging.

Oruvail capsules—The effects of age and gender on ketoprofen disposition were investigated in 2 small studies in which elderly male and female subjects received Oruvail 200 mg capsules. The results were compared with those from another study conducted in healthy young men.

Compared to the younger subject group, the elimination half-life in the elderly was prolonged by 54% and total drug C_{max} and AUC were 40% and 70% higher, respectively. Plasma concentrations in the elderly after single doses and at steady state were essentially the same. Thus, no drug accumulation occurs.

In comparison to younger subjects taking the immediate-release formulation (Orudis), there was a decrease of 16% and 25% in total drug C_{max} and AUC, respectively, among the elderly. Free drug data are not available for Oruvail.

Renally impaired

Studies of the effects of renal-function impairment have been small. They indicate a decrease in clearance in patients with impaired renal function. In 23 patients with renal impairment, free ketoprofen peak concentration was not significantly elevated, but free ketoprofen clearance was reduced from 15 L/kg/h for normal subjects to 7 L/kg/h in patients with mildly impaired renal function, and to 4 L/kg/h in patients with moderately to severely impaired renal function. The elimination $t_{1/2}$ was prolonged from 1.6 hours in normal subjects to approximately 3 hours in patients with mild renal impairment, and to approximately 5 to 9 hours in patients with moderately to severely impaired renal function.

No studies have been conducted in patients with renal impairment taking Oruvail capsules (see "**INDIVIDUALIZATION OF DOSAGE**").

Hepatically impaired

For patients with alcoholic cirrhosis, no significant changes in the kinetic disposition of Orudis capsules were observed relative to age-matched normal subjects: the plasma clearance of drug was 0.07 L/kg/h in 26 hepatically impaired patients. The elimination half-life was comparable to that observed for normal subjects. However, the unbound (biologically active) fraction was approximately doubled, probably due to hypoalbuminemia and high variability which was observed in the pharmacokinetics for cirrhotic patients. Therefore, these patients should be carefully monitored and daily doses of ketoprofen kept at the minimum providing the desired therapeutic effect.

No studies have been conducted in patients with heptic impairment taking Oruvail capsules (see "**INDIVIDUALIZATION OF DOSAGE**").

CLINICAL TRIALS

Rheumatoid Arthritis and Osteoarthritis

The efficacy of ketoprofen has been demonstrated in patients with rheumatoid arthritis and osteoarthritis. Using standard assessments of therapeutic response, there were no detectable differences in effectiveness or in the incidence of adverse events in crossover comparison of Orudis and Oruvail. In other trials, ketoprofen demonstrated effectiveness comparable to aspirin, ibuprofen, naproxen, piroxicam, diclofenac and indomethacin. In some of these studies there were more dropouts due to gastrointestinal side effects among patients on ketoprofen than among patients on other NSAIDs.

In studies with patients with rheumatoid arthritis, ketoprofen was administered in combination with gold salts, antimalarials, low-dose methotrexate, d-penicillamine, and/or corticosteroids with results comparable to those seen with control nonsteroidal drugs.

Management of Pain

The effectiveness of Orudis as a general-purpose analgesic has been studied in standard pain models which have shown the effectiveness of doses of 25 to 150 mg. Doses of 25 mg were superior to placebo. Doses larger than 25 mg generally could not be shown to be significantly more effective, but there was a tendency toward faster onset and greater duration of action with 50 mg, and, in the case of dysmenorrhea, a significantly greater effect overall with 75 mg. Doses greater than 50 to 75 mg did not have increased analgesic effect. Studies in postoperative pain have shown that Orudis in doses of 25 to 100 mg was comparable to 650 mg of acetaminophen with 60 mg of codeine, or 650 mg of acetaminophen with 10 mg of oxycodone. Ketoprofen tended to be somewhat slower in onset; peak pain relief was about the same and the duration of the effect tended to be 1 to 2 hours longer, particularly with the higher doses of ketoprofen.

The use of Oruvail in patients with acute pain is not recommended, since, in comparison to Orudis, Oruvail would be expected to have a delayed analgesic response due to its extended-release characteristics.

INDIVIDUALIZATION OF DOSAGE

The recommended starting dose of ketoprofen in otherwise healthy patients is Orudis, 75 mg three times or 50 mg four times a day, or Oruvail, 200 mg administered once a day. Smaller doses of Orudis or Oruvail should be utilized initially in small individuals or in debilitated or elderly patients. The recommended maximum daily dose of ketoprofen is 300 mg/day for Orudis or 200 mg/day for Oruvail. Concomitant use of Orudis and Oruvail is not recommended.

If minor side effects appear, they may disappear at a lower dose which may still have an adequate therapeutic effect. If well tolerated but not optimally effective, the dosage may be increased. Individual patients may show a better response to 300 mg of Orudis daily as compared to 200 mg, although in well-controlled clinical trials patients on 300 mg did not show greater mean effectiveness. They did, however, show an increased frequency of upper- and lower-GI distress and headaches. It is of interest that women also had an increased frequency of these adverse effects compared to men. When treating patients with 300 mg/day, the physician should observe sufficient increased clinical benefit to offset potential increased risk.

In patients with mildly impaired renal function, the maximum recommended total daily dose of Orudis or Oruvail is 150 mg. In patients with a more severe renal impairment (GFR less than 25 mL/min/1.73 m^2 or end-stage renal impairment), the maximum total daily dose of Orudis or Oruvail should not exceed 100 mg.

In elderly patients, renal function may be reduced with apparently normal serum creatinine and/or BUN levels. Therefore, it is recommended that the initial dosage of Orudis or Oruvail should be reduced for patients over 75 years of age.

It is recommended that for patients with impaired liver function and serum albumin concentration less than 3.5 g/dL, the maximum initial total daily dose of Orudis or Oruvail should be 100 mg. All patients with metabolic impairment, particularly those with both hypoalbuminemia and reduced renal function, may have increased levels of free (biologically active) ketoprofen and should be closely monitored. The dosage may be increased to the range recommended for the general population, if necessary, only after good individual tolerance has been ascertained.

Because hypoalbuminemia and reduced renal function both increase the fraction of free drug (biologically active form), patients who have both conditions may be at greater risk of adverse effects. Therefore, it is recommended that such patients also be started on lower doses of Orudis or Oruvail and closely monitored.

As with other nonsteroidal anti-inflammatory drugs, the predominant adverse effects of ketoprofen are gastrointestinal. To attempt to minimize these effects, physicians may wish to prescribe that Orudis or Oruvail be taken with antacids, food, or milk. Although food delays the absorption of both formulations (see "**CLINICAL PHARMACOLOGY**"), in most of the clinical trials ketoprofen was taken with food or milk.

Physicians may want to make specific recommendations to patients about when they should take Orudis or Oruvail in relation to food and/or what patients should do if they experience minor GI symptoms associated with either formulation.

INDICATIONS AND USAGE

Orudis or Oruvail are indicated for the management of the signs and symptoms of rheumatoid arthritis and osteoarthritis. Oruvail is not recommended for treatment of acute pain because of its extended-release characteristics (see "**PHARMACOKINETICS**").

Orudis is indicated for the management of pain. Orudis is also indicated for treatment of primary dysmenorrhea.

CONTRAINDICATIONS

Ketoprofen is contraindicated in patients who have shown hypersensitivity to it. Ketoprofen should not be given to patients in whom aspirin or other nonsteroidal anti-inflammatory drugs induce asthma, urticaria, or other allergic-type reactions, because severe, rarely fatal, anaphylactic reactions to ketoprofen have been reported in such patients.

WARNINGS

Risk of GI Ulceration, Bleeding and Perforation with NSAID Therapy

Serious gastrointestinal toxicity, such as bleeding, ulceration, and perforation, can occur at any time with or without warning symptoms, in patients treated chronically with NSAID therapy. Although minor upper-gastrointestinal problems, such as dyspepsia, are common, usually developing early in therapy, physicians should remain alert for ulceration and bleeding in patients treated chronically with NSAIDs even in the absence of previous GI-tract symptoms. In patients observed in clinical trials of several months to two years' duration, symptomatic upper-GI ulcers, gross bleeding, or perforation appear to occur in approximately 1% of patients treated for 3 to 6 months, and in about 2–4% of patients treated for one year. Physicians should inform patients about the signs and/or symptoms of serious GI toxicity and what steps to take if they occur.

Studies to date have not identified any subset of patients not at risk of developing peptic ulceration and bleeding. Except for a prior history of serious GI events and other risk factors known to be associated with peptic ulcer disease, such as alcoholism, smoking, etc., no other risk factors (e.g., age, sex) have been associated with increased risk. Elderly or debilitated patients seem to tolerate ulceration or bleeding less well than other individuals, and most spontaneous reports of fatal GI events are in this population. Studies to date are inconclusive concerning the relative risk of various NSAIDs in causing such reactions. High doses of any NSAID probably carry a greater risk of these reactions, although controlled clinical trials showing this do not exist in most cases. In considering the use of relatively large doses (within the recommended dosage range), sufficient benefit should be anticipated to offset the potential increased risk of GI toxicity.

GENERAL PRECAUTIONS

Ketoprofen and other nonsteroidal anti-inflammatory drugs cause nephritis in mice and rats associated with chronic administration. Rare cases of interstitial nephritis or nephrotic syndrome have been reported in humans with ketoprofen since it has been marketed.

A second form of renal toxicity has been seen in patients with conditions leading to a reduction in renal blood flow or blood volume, where renal prostaglandins have a supportive role in the maintenance of renal blood flow. In these patients, administration of a nonsteroidal anti-inflammatory drug results in a dose-dependent decrease in prostaglandin synthesis and, secondarily, in renal blood flow which may precipitate overt renal failure. Patients at greatest risk of this reaction are those with impaired renal function, heart failure, liver dysfunction, those taking diuretics, and the elderly. Discontinuation of nonsteroidal anti-inflammatory drug therapy is typically followed by recovery to the pretreatment state.

Since ketoprofen is primarily eliminated by the kidneys and its pharmacokinetics are altered by renal failure (see "**CLINICAL PHARMACOLOGY**"), patients with significantly impaired renal function should be closely monitored, and a reduction of dosage should be anticipated to avoid accumulation of ketoprofen and/or its metabolites (see "**INDIVIDUALIZATION OF DOSAGE**").

Continued on next page

Orudis/Oruvail—Cont.

As with other nonsteroidal anti-inflammatory drugs, borderline elevations of one or more liver function tests may occur in up to 15% of patients. These abnormalities may progress, may remain essentially unchanged, or may disappear with continued therapy. The ALT (SGPT) test is probably the most sensitive indicator of liver dysfunction. Meaningful (3 times the upper limit of normal) elevations of ALT or AST (SGOT) occurred in controlled clinical trials in less than 1% of patients. A patient with symptoms and/or signs suggesting liver dysfunction, or in whom an abnormal liver test has occurred, should be evaluated for evidence of the development of a more severe hepatic reaction while on therapy with ketoprofen. Serious hepatic reactions, including jaundice, have been reported from post-marketing experience with ketoprofen as well as with other nonsteroidal anti-inflammatory drugs.

In patients with chronic liver disease with reduced serum albumin levels, ketoprofen's pharmacokinetics are altered (see "**CLINICAL PHARMACOLOGY**"). Such patients should be closely monitored, and a reduction of dosage should be anticipated to avoid high blood levels of ketoprofen and/or its metabolites (see "**INDIVIDUALIZATION OF DOSAGE**").

If steroid dosage is reduced or eliminated during therapy, it should be reduced slowly and the patients observed closely for any evidence of adverse effects, including adrenal insufficiency and exacerbation of symptoms of arthritis.

Anemia is commonly observed in rheumatoid arthritis and is sometimes aggravated by nonsteroidal anti-inflammatory drugs, which may produce fluid retention or significant gastrointestinal blood loss in some patients. Patients on long-term treatment with NSAIDs, including Orudis or Oruvail, should have their hemoglobin or hematocrit checked if they develop signs or symptoms of anemia.

Peripheral edema has been observed in approximately 2% of patients taking ketoprofen. Therefore, as with other nonsteroidal anti-inflammatory drugs, ketoprofen should be used with caution in patients with fluid retention, hypertension, or heart failure.

Information for Patients

Orudis or Oruvail contain ketoprofen. Like other drugs of its class, ketoprofen is not free of side effects. The side effects of these drugs can cause discomfort and, rarely, there are more serious side effects, such as gastrointestinal bleeding, which may result in hospitalization and even fatal outcomes.

NSAIDs are often essential agents in the management of arthritis and have a major role in the treatment of pain, but they also may be commonly employed for conditions which are less serious. Physicians may wish to discuss with their patients the potential risks (see "**WARNINGS**," "**GENERAL PRECAUTIONS**," and "**ADVERSE REACTIONS**" sections) and likely benefits of NSAID treatment, particularly when the drugs are used for less serious conditions where treatment without NSAIDs may represent an acceptable alternative to both the patient and physician.

Because aspirin causes an increase in the level of unbound ketoprofen, patients should be advised not to take aspirin while taking ketoprofen (see "**Drug Interactions**"). It is possible that minor adverse symptoms of gastric intolerance may be prevented by administering Orudis with antacids, food, or milk. Oruvail has not been studied with antacids. Because food and milk do affect the rate but not the extent of absorption (see "**CLINICAL PHARMACOLOGY**"), physicians may want to make specific recommendations to patients about when they should take ketoprofen in relation to food and/or what patients should do if they experience minor GI symptoms associated with ketoprofen therapy.

Laboratory Tests

Because serious GI-tract ulceration and bleeding can occur without warning symptoms, physicians should follow chronically treated patients for the signs and symptoms of ulceration and bleeding and should inform them of the importance of this follow-up (see "**WARNINGS**—Risk of GI Ulceration, Bleeding and Perforation with NSAID Therapy**").

Drug Interactions

The following drug interactions were studied with ketoprofen doses of 200 mg/day. The possibility of increased interaction should be kept in mind when Orudis doses greater than 50 mg as a single dose or 200 mg of ketoprofen per day are used concomitantly with highly bound drugs.

1. Antacids

Concomitant administration of magnesium hydroxide and aluminum hydroxide does not interfere with the rate or extent of the absorption of ketoprofen administered as Orudis.

2. Aspirin

Ketoprofen does not alter aspirin absorption; however, in a study of 12 normal subjects, concurrent administration of aspirin decreased ketoprofen protein binding and increased ketoprofen plasma clearance from 0.07 L/kg/h without aspirin to 0.11 L/kg/h with aspirin. The clinical significance of these changes has not been adequately studied. Therefore, concurrent use of aspirin and ketoprofen is not recommended.

3. Diuretic

Hydrochlorothiazide, given concomitantly with ketoprofen, produces a reduction in urinary potassium and chloride excretion compared to hydrochlorothiazide alone. Patients taking diuretics are at greater risk of developing renal failure secondary to a decrease in renal blood flow caused by prostaglandin inhibition (see "**GENERAL PRECAUTIONS**").

4. Digoxin

In a study in 12 patients with congestive heart failure where ketoprofen and digoxin were concomitantly administered, ketoprofen did not alter the serum levels of digoxin.

5. Warfarin

In a short-term controlled study in 14 normal volunteers, ketoprofen did not significantly interfere with the effect of warfarin on prothrombin time. Bleeding from a number of sites may be a complication of warfarin treatment and GI bleeding a complication of ketoprofen treatment. Because prostaglandins play an important role in hemostasis and ketoprofen has an effect on platelet function as well (see "**DRUG/LABORATORY TEST INTERACTIONS: EFFECT ON BLOOD COAGULATION**"), concurrent therapy with ketoprofen and warfarin requires close monitoring of patients on both drugs.

6. Probenecid

Probenecid increases both free and bound ketoprofen by reducing the plasma clearance of ketoprofen to about one-third, as well as decreasing its protein binding. Therefore, the combination of ketoprofen and probenecid is not recommended.

7. Methotrexate

Ketoprofen, like other NSAIDs, may cause changes in the elimination of methotrexate leading to elevated serum levels of the drug and increased toxicity.

8. Lithium

Nonsteroidal anti-inflammatory agents have been reported to increase steady-state plasma lithium levels. It is recommended that plasma lithium levels be monitored when ketoprofen is co-administered with lithium.

Drug/Laboratory Test Interactions:

Effect on Blood Coagulation

Ketoprofen decreases platelet adhesion and aggregation. Therefore, it can prolong bleeding time by approximately 3 to 4 minutes from baseline values. There is no significant change in platelet count, prothrombin time, partial thromboplastin time, or thrombin time.

Carcinogenesis, Mutagenesis, Impairment of Fertility

Chronic oral toxicity studies in mice (up to 32 mg/kg/day; 96 mg/m^2/day) did not indicate a carcinogenic potential for ketoprofen. The maximum recommended human therapeutic dose is 300 mg/day for a 60 kg patient with a body surface area of 1.6 m^2, which is 5 mg/kg/day or 185 mg/m^2/day. Thus the mice were treated at 0.5 times the maximum human daily dose based on surface area.

A 2-year carcinogenicity study in rats, using doses up to 6.0 mg/kg/day (36 mg/m^2/day), showed no evidence of tumorigenic potential. All groups were treated for 104 weeks except the females receiving 6.0 mg/kg/day (36 mg/m^2/day) where the drug treatment was terminated in week 81 because of low survival; the remaining rats were sacrificed after week 87. Their survival in the groups treated for 104 weeks was within 6% of the control group. An earlier 2-year study with doses up to 12.5 mg/kg/day (75 mg/m^2/day) also showed no evidence of tumorigenicity, but the survival rate was low and the study was therefore judged inconclusive. Ketoprofen did not show mutagenic potential in the Ames Test. Ketoprofen administered to male rats (up to 9 mg/kg/day; or 54 mg/m^2/day) had no significant effect on reproductive performance or fertility. In female rats administered 6 or 9 mg/kg/day (36 or 54 mg/m^2/day), a decrease in the number of implantation sites has been noted. The dosages of 36 mg/m^2/day in rats represent 0.2 times the maximum recommended human dose of 185 mg/m^2/day (see above).

Abnormal spermatogenesis or inhibition of spermatogenesis developed in rats and dogs at high doses, and a decrease in the weight of the testes occurred in dogs and baboons at high doses.

Teratogenic Effects: Pregnancy Category B

In teratology studies ketoprofen administered to mice at doses up to 12 mg/kg/day (36 mg/m^2/day) and rats at doses up to 9 mg/kg/day (54 mg/m^2/day), the approximate equivalent of 0.2 times the maximum recommended therapeutic dose of 185 mg/m^2/day, showed no teratogenic or embryotoxic effects. In separate studies in rabbits, maternally toxic doses were associated with embryotoxicity but not teratogenicity.

There are no adequate and well-controlled studies in pregnant women. Because animal teratology studies are not always predictive of the human response, ketoprofen should be used during pregnancy only if the potential benefit justifies the risk.

Labor and Delivery

The effects of ketoprofen on labor and delivery in pregnant women are unknown. Studies in rats have shown ketoprofen at doses of 6 mg/kg (36 mg/m^2/day, approximately equal to 0.2 times the maximum recommended human dose) pro-

longs pregnancy when given before the onset of labor. Because of the known effects of prostaglandin-inhibiting drugs on the fetal cardiovascular system (closure of ductus arteriosus), use of ketoprofen during late pregnancy should be avoided.

Nursing Mothers

Data on secretion in human milk after ingestion of ketoprofen do not exist. In rats, ketoprofen at doses of 9 mg/kg (54 mg/m^2/day; approximately 0.3 times the maximum human therapeutic dose) did not affect perinatal development. Upon administration to lactating dogs, the milk concentration of ketoprofen was found to be 4 to 5% of the plasma drug level. As with other drugs that are excreted in milk, ketoprofen is not recommended for use in nursing mothers.

Pediatric Use

Ketoprofen is not recommended for use in pediatric patients, because its safety and effectiveness have not been studied in the pediatric population.

ADVERSE REACTIONS

The incidence of common adverse reactions (above 1%) was obtained from a population of 835 Orudis-treated patients in double-blind trials lasting from 4 to 54 weeks and in 622 Oruvail-treated (200 mg/day) patients in trials lasting from 4 to 16 weeks.

Minor gastrointestinal side effects predominated; upper gastrointestinal symptoms were more common than lower gastrointestinal symptoms. In crossover trials in 321 patients with rheumatoid arthritis or osteoarthritis, there was no difference in either upper or lower gastrointestinal symptoms between patients treated with 200 mg of Oruvail once a day or 75 mg of Orudis TID (225 mg/day). Peptic ulcer or GI bleeding occurred in controlled clinical trials in less than 1% of 1,076 patients; however, in open label continuation studies in 1,292 patients the rate was greater than 2%.

The incidence of peptic ulceration in patients on NSAIDs is dependent on many risk factors including age, sex, smoking, alcohol use, diet, stress, concomitant drugs such as aspirin and corticosteroids, as well as the dose and duration of treatment with NSAIDs (see "**WARNINGS**").

Gastrointestinal reactions were followed in frequency by central nervous system side effects, such as headache, dizziness, or drowsiness. The incidence of some adverse reactions appears to be dose-related (see "**DOSAGE AND ADMINISTRATION**"). Rare adverse reactions (incidence less than 1%) were collected from one or more of the following sources: foreign reports to manufacturers and regulatory agencies, publications, and U.S. clinical trials, and/or U.S. postmarketing spontaneous reports.

Reactions are listed below under body system, then by incidence or number of cases in decreasing incidence.

Incidence Greater than 1% (Probable Causal Relationship)

Digestive: Dyspepsia (11%), nausea*, abdominal pain*, diarrhea*, constipation*, flatulence*, anorexia, vomiting, stomatitis.

Nervous System: Headache*, dizziness, CNS inhibition (i.e., pooled reports of somnolence, malaise, depression, etc.) or excitation (i.e., insomnia, nervousness, dreams, etc.)*.

Special Senses: Tinnitus, visual disturbance.

Skin and Appendages: Rash.

Urogenital: Impairment of renal function (edema, increased BUN)*, signs or symptoms of urinary-tract irritation.

* Adverse events occurring in 3 to 9% of patients.

Incidence Less than 1% (Probable Causal Relationship)

Body as a Whole: Chills, facial edema, infection, pain, allergic reaction, anaphylaxis.

Cardiovascular: Hypertension, palpitation, tachycardia, congestive heart failure, peripheral vascular disease, vasodilation.

Digestive: Appetite increased, dry mouth, eructation, gastritis, rectal hemorrhage, melena, fecal occult blood, salivation, peptic ulcer, gastrointestinal perforation, hematemesis, intestinal ulceration, hepatic dysfunction, hepatitis, cholestatic hepatitis, jaundice.

Hemic: Hypocoagulability, agranulocytosis, anemia, hemolysis, purpura, thrombocytopenia.

Metabolic and Nutritional: Thirst, weight gain, weight loss, hyponatremia.

Musculoskeletal: Myalgia.

Nervous System: Amnesia, confusion, impotence, migraine, paresthesia, vertigo.

Respiratory: Dyspnea, hemoptysis, epistaxis, pharyngitis, rhinitis, bronchospasm, laryngeal edema.

Skin and Appendages: Alopecia, eczema, pruritus, purpuric rash, sweating, urticaria, bullous rash, exfoliative dermatitis, photosensitivity, skin discoloration, onycholysis, toxic epidermal necrolysis, erythema multiforme, Stevens-Johnson syndrome.

Special Senses: Conjunctivitis, conjunctivitis sicca, eye pain, hearing impairment, retinal hemorrhage and pigmentation change, taste perversion.

Urogenital: Menometrorrhagia, hematuria, renal failure, interstitial nephritis, nephrotic syndrome.

Incidence Less than 1% (Causal Relationship Unknown)

The following rare adverse reactions, whose causal relationship to ketoprofen is uncertain, are being listed to serve as alerting information to the physician.

Body as a Whole: Septicemia, shock.

Cardiovascular: Arrhythmias, myocardial infarction.

Digestive: Buccal necrosis, ulcerative colitis, microvesicular steatosis, pancreatitis.

Endocrine: Diabetes mellitus (aggravated).

Nervous System: Dysphoria, hallucination, libido disturbance, nightmares, personality disorder, aseptic meningitis.

Urogenital: Acute tubulopathy, gynecomastia.

OVERDOSAGE

Signs and symptoms following acute NSAID overdose are usually limited to lethargy, drowsiness, nausea, vomiting, and epigastric pain, which are generally reversible with supportive care. Respiratory depression, coma, or convulsions have occurred following large ketoprofen overdoses. Gastrointestinal bleeding, hypotension, hypertension, or acute renal failure may occur, but are rare.

Patients should be managed by symptomatic and supportive care following an NSAID overdose. There are no specific antidotes. Gut decontamination may be indicated in patients with symptoms seen within 4 hours (longer for sustained-release products) or following a large overdose (5 to 10 times the usual dose). This should be accomplished via emesis and/or activated charcoal (60 to 100 g in adults, 1 to 2 g/kg in children) with a saline cathartic or sorbitol added to the first dose. Forced diuresis, alkalinization of the urine, hemodialysis or hemoperfusion would probably not be useful due to ketoprofen's high protein binding.

Case reports include twenty-six overdoses: 6 were in children, 16 in adolescents, and 4 in adults. Five of these patients had minor symptoms (vomiting in 4, drowsiness in 1 child). A 12-year-old girl had tonic-clonic convulsions 1–2 hours after ingesting an unknown quantity of ketoprofen and 1 or 2 tablets of acetaminophen with hydrocodone. Her ketoprofen level was 1128 mg/L (56 times the upper therapeutic level of 20 mg/L) 3–4 hours post ingestion. Full recovery ensued 18 hours after ingestion following management with intubation, diazepam, and activated charcoal. A 45-year-old woman ingested twelve 200 mg Oruvail and 375 mL vodka, was treated with emesis and supportive measures 2 hours after ingestion, and recovered completely with her only complaint being mild epigastric pain.

DOSAGE AND ADMINISTRATION

Rheumatoid Arthritis and Osteoarthritis

The recommended starting dose of ketoprofen in otherwise healthy patients is for Orudis 75 mg three times or 50 mg four times a day, or for Oruvail 200 mg administered once a day. Smaller doses of Orudis or Oruvail should be utilized initially in small individuals, in debilitated or elderly patients. The recommended maximum daily dose of ketoprofen is 300 mg/day for Orudis or 200 mg/day for Oruvail (see **"INDIVIDUALIZATION OF DOSAGE"**).

Dosages higher than 300 mg/day of Orudis or 200 mg/day of Oruvail are not recommended because they have not been studied. Concomitant use of Orudis and Oruvail is not recommended. Relatively smaller people may need smaller doses (See **"INDIVIDUALIZATION OF DOSAGE"**).

Management of Pain and Dysmenorrhea

The usual dose of Orudis recommended for mild-to-moderate pain and dysmenorrhea is 25 to 50 mg every 6 to 8 hours as necessary. A smaller dose should be utilized initially in small individuals, in debilitated or elderly patients, or in patients with renal or liver disease (see **"GENERAL PRECAUTIONS"**). A larger dose may be tried if the patient's response to a previous dose was less than satisfactory, but doses above 75 mg have not been shown to give added analgesia. Daily doses above 300 mg are not recommended because they have not been adequately studied. Because of its typical nonsteroidal anti-inflammatory drug-side-effect profile, including as its principal adverse effect GI side effects (see **"WARNINGS"** and **"ADVERSE REACTIONS"**), higher doses of Orudis should be used with caution and patients receiving them observed carefully (see **"INDIVIDUALIZATION OF DOSAGE"**).

Oruvail is not recommended for use in treating acute pain because of its extended-release characteristics.

HOW SUPPLIED

Orudis® (ketoprofen) Capsules are available as follows:

25 mg, NDC 0008-4186, dark-green and red capsule marked "WYETH 4186" on one side and "ORUDIS 25" on the reverse side, in bottles of 100 capsules.

50 mg, NDC 0008-4181, dark-green and light-green capsule marked "WYETH 4181" on one side and "ORUDIS 50" on the reverse side, in bottles of 100 capsules.

75 mg, NDC 0008-4187, dark-green and white capsule marked "WYETH 4187" on one side and "ORUDIS 75" on the reverse side, in bottles of 100 and 500 capsules, and in Redipak® cartons of 100, each containing 10 blister strips of 10 capsules.

Oruvail® (ketoprofen) Extended-Release Capsules are available as follows:

100 mg, NDC 0008-0821, opaque pink and dark-green capsule marked with two radial bands and "ORUVAIL 100" in bottles of 100 capsules.

150 mg, NDC 0008-0822, opaque pink and light-green capsule marked with two radial bands and "ORUVAIL 150" in bottles of 100 capsules.

200 mg, NDC 0008-0690, opaque pink and off-white capsule marked with two radial bands and "ORUVAIL 200" in bottles of 100 capsules and in Redipak® cartons each containing 10 blister strips of 10 capsules.

Keep tightly closed.

Store at room temperature, approximately 25° C (77° F).

Dispense in a tight container.

Oruvail capsules should be protected from direct light and excessive heat and humidity.

The appearance of these capsules is a registered trademark of Wyeth-Ayerst Laboratories.

Caution: Federal law prohibits dispensing without prescription.

By arrangement with Rhone-Poulenc Rorer France.

Orudis Capsules manufactured and distributed by Wyeth Laboratories Inc.

Oruvail Capsules distributed by Wyeth Laboratories Inc.

Wyeth Laboratories Inc.

A Wyeth-Ayerst Company

Philadelphia, PA 19101

Shown in Product Identification Guide, page 344

OVRAL®   ℞

[ōh 'vrăl]

TABLETS

(norgestrel and ethinyl estradiol tablets)

Patients should be counseled that this product does not protect against HIV infection (AIDS) and other sexually transmitted diseases.

DESCRIPTION

Each Ovral tablet contains 0.5 mg of norgestrel (dl -13-beta-ethyl-17-alpha-ethinyl -17- beta-hydroxygon -4- en -3- one), a totally synthetic progestogen, and 0.05 mg of ethinyl estradiol (19-nor-17α-pregna-1,3,5 (10)-trien-20-yne-3,17-diol). The inactive ingredients present are cellulose, lactose, magnesium stearate, and polacrilin potassium.

CLINICAL PHARMACOLOGY

See LO/OVRAL®.

INDICATIONS AND USAGE

Oral contraceptives are indicated for the prevention of pregnancy in women who elect to use this product as a method of contraception.

Oral contraceptive products such as Ovral or Ovral®-28, which contain 50 mcg of estrogen, should not be used unless medically indicated.

Oral contraceptives are highly effective. Table I lists the typical accidental pregnancy rates for users of combination oral contraceptives and other methods of contraception. The efficacy of these contraceptive methods, except sterilization and the IUD, depends upon the reliability with which they are used. Correct and consistent use of methods can result in lower failure rates.

TABLE I: LOWEST EXPECTED AND TYPICAL
FAILURE RATES DURING THE FIRST YEAR OF
CONTINUOUS USE OF A METHOD

% of Women Experiencing an Accidental Pregnancy in the First Year of Continuous Use

Method	Lowest Expected*	Typical**
(No Contraception)	(85)	(85)
Oral contraceptives		3
combined	0.1	N/A***
progestin only	0.5	N/A***
Diaphragm with spermicidal cream or jelly	6	18
Spermicides alone (foams and vaginal suppositories)	3	21
Vaginal Sponge		
nulliparous	6	18
multiparous	9	28
DEPO-PROVERA® (injectable progestogen)	0.3	0.3
NORPLANT® SYSTEM (implants)	0.2#	0.2#
IUD		3
progesterone	2	N/A***
copper T 380A	0.8	N/A***
Condom without spermicides	2	12
Periodic abstinence (all methods)	1–9	20
Female sterilization	0.2	0.4
Male sterilization	0.1	0.15

Adapted from J. Trussell et al., Table 1, Studies in Family Planning, *21(1)*: Jan.–Feb. 1990.

---

* The authors' best guess of the percentage of women expected to experience an accidental pregnancy among couples who initiate a method (not necessarily for the first time) and who use it consistently and correctly during the first year if they do not stop for any other reason.

** This term represents "typical" couples who initiate use of a method (not necessarily for the first time), who experience an accidental pregnancy during the first year if they do not stop use for any other reason.

*** N/A—Data not available

\# This data is based on NORPLANT® SYSTEM clinical trials.

CONTRAINDICATIONS

See LO/OVRAL.

WARNINGS

See LO/OVRAL.

1. THROMBOEMBOLIC DISORDERS AND OTHER VASCULAR PROBLEMS.
   a. *Myocardial infarction:* See LO/OVRAL.
   b. *Thromboembolism:* See LO/OVRAL.
   c. *Cerebrovascular diseases:* See LO/OVRAL.
   d. *Dose-related risk of vascular disease from oral contraceptives*

   A positive association has been observed between the amount of estrogen and progestogen in oral contraceptives and the risk of vascular disease. A decline in serum high-density lipoproteins (HDL) has been reported with many progestational agents. A decline in serum high-density lipoproteins has been associated with an increased incidence of ischemic heart disease. Because estrogens increase HDL cholesterol, the net effect of an oral contraceptive depends on a balance achieved between doses of estrogen and progestogen and the nature and absolute amount of progestogen used in the contraceptive. The amount of both hormones should be considered in the choice of an oral contraceptive.

   Minimizing exposure to estrogen and progestogen is in keeping with good principles of therapeutics. For any particular estrogen/progestogen combination, the dosage regimen prescribed should be one which contains the least amount of estrogen and progestogen that is compatible with a low failure rate and the needs of the individual patient. New acceptors of oral-contraceptive agents should be started on preparations containing less than 50 mcg of estrogen. Products containing 50 mcg of estrogen should be used only when medically indicated.

   e. *Persistence of risk of vascular disease:* See LO/OVRAL.
2. ESTIMATES OF MORTALITY FROM ORAL CONTRACEPTIVES: See LO/OVRAL.
3. CARCINOMA OF THE REPRODUCTIVE ORGANS: See LO/OVRAL.
4. HEPATIC NEOPLASIA: See LO/OVRAL.
5. OCULAR LESIONS: See LO/OVRAL.
6. ORAL-CONTRACEPTIVE USE BEFORE OR DURING EARLY PREGNANCY: See LO/OVRAL.
7. GALLBLADDER DISEASE: See LO/OVRAL.
8. CARBOHYDRATE AND LIPID METABOLIC EFFECTS: See LO/OVRAL.
9. ELEVATED BLOOD PRESSURE: See LO/OVRAL.
10. HEADACHE: See LO/OVRAL.
11. BLEEDING IRREGULARITIES: See LO/OVRAL.

PRECAUTIONS

See LO/OVRAL.

Drug Interactions: See LO/OVRAL.

Carcinogenesis: See LO/OVRAL.

Pregnancy: See LO/OVRAL.

Nursing Mothers: See LO/OVRAL.

Information For the Patient: See LO/OVRAL.

ADVERSE REACTIONS

See LO/OVRAL.

OVERDOSAGE

See LO/OVRAL.

NONCONTRACEPTIVE HEALTH BENEFITS

See LO/OVRAL.

Continued on next page

Ovral—Cont.

DOSAGE AND ADMINISTRATION

To achieve maximum contraceptive effectiveness, Ovral must be taken exactly as directed and at intervals not exceeding 24 hours.

The dosage of Ovral is one tablet daily for 21 consecutive days per menstrual cycle according to prescribed schedule. Tablets are then discontinued for 7 days (three weeks on, one week off).

It is recommended that Ovral tablets be taken at the same time each day, preferably after the evening meal or at bedtime.

During the first cycle of medication, the patient is instructed to take one Ovral tablet daily for twenty-one consecutive days, beginning on the first day (Day 1 Start) of her menstrual cycle or on the Sunday after her period begins (Sunday Start). (The first day of menstruation is day one.) The tablets are then discontinued for one week (7 days). Withdrawal bleeding should usually occur within 3 days following discontinuation of Ovral. (For Day 1 Start: If Ovral is first taken later than the first day of the first menstrual cycle of medication or postpartum, contraceptive reliance should not be placed on Ovral until after the first seven consecutive days of administration. For Sunday Start: Contraceptive reliance should not be placed on Ovral until after the first seven consecutive days of administration. The possibility of ovulation and conception prior to initiation of medication should be considered.) The patient begins her next and all subsequent 21-day courses of Ovral tablets on the same day of the week that she began her first course, following the same schedule: 21 days on—7 days off. She begins taking her tablets on the 8th day after discontinuance, regardless of whether or not a menstrual period has occurred or is still in progress. Any time a new cycle of Ovral is started later than the 8th day, the patient should be protected by another means of contraception until she has taken a tablet daily for seven consecutive days.

If spotting or breakthrough bleeding occurs, the patient is instructed to continue on the same regimen. This type of bleeding is usually transient and without significance; however, if the bleeding is persistent or prolonged, the patient is advised to consult her physician. Although the occurrence of pregnancy is highly unlikely if Ovral is taken according to directions, if withdrawal bleeding does not occur, the possibility of pregnancy must be considered. If the patient has not adhered to the prescribed schedule (missed one or more tablets or started taking them on a day later than she should have), the probability of pregnancy should be considered at the time of the first missed period and appropriate diagnostic measures taken before the medication is resumed. If the patient has adhered to the prescribed regimen and misses two consecutive periods, pregnancy should be ruled out before continuing the contraceptive regimen.

For additional patient instructions regarding missed pills, see the "WHAT TO DO IF YOU MISS PILLS" section in the DETAILED PATIENT LABELING for LO/OVRAL.

Any time the patient misses two or more tablets, she should also use another method of contraception until she has taken a tablet daily for seven consecutive days. If breakthrough bleeding occurs following missed tablets, it will usually be transient and of no consequence. While there is little likelihood of ovulation occurring if only one or two tablets are missed, the possibility of ovulation increases with each successive day that scheduled tablets are missed.

In the nonlactating mother, Ovral may be initiated postpartum, for contraception. When the tablets are administered in the postpartum period, the increased risk of thromboembolic disease associated with the postpartum period must be considered (see "Contraindications," "Warnings," and "Precautions" concerning thromboembolic disease). It is to be noted that early resumption of ovulation may occur if Parlodel® (bromocriptine mesylate) has been used for the prevention of lactation.

HOW SUPPLIED

Ovral® Tablets (0.5 mg norgestrel and 0.05 mg ethinyl estradiol), are available in packages of 6 PILPAK® dispensers with 21 tablets each as follows:
NDC 0008-0056-01, white, round tablet marked "WYETH" and "56".
Store at room temperature, approx. 25° C (77° F).

References available upon request.
Brief Summary Patient Package Insert: See LO/OVRAL.
DETAILED PATIENT LABELING
This product (like all oral contraceptives) is intended to prevent pregnancy. It does not protect against HIV infection (AIDS) and other sexually transmitted diseases.
INTRODUCTION
You should not use Ovral or Ovral-28, which contain higher doses of estrogen than other oral contraceptives, unless specifically recommended by your health-care provider. Any woman who considers using oral contraceptives (the birth-control pill or the pill) should understand the benefits and

risks of using this form of birth control. This leaflet will give you much of the information you will need to make this decision and will also help you determine if you are at risk of developing any of the serious side effects of the pill. It will tell you how to use the pill properly so that it will be as effective as possible. However, this leaflet is not a replacement for a careful discussion between you and your health-care provider. You should discuss the information provided in this leaflet with him or her, both when you first start taking the pill and during your revisits. You should also follow your health-care provider's advice with regard to regular check-ups while you are on the pill.

EFFECTIVENESS OF ORAL CONTRACEPTIVES: See LO/OVRAL.
WHO SHOULD NOT TAKE ORAL CONTRACEPTIVES: See LO/OVRAL.
OTHER CONSIDERATIONS BEFORE TAKING ORAL CONTRACEPTIVES: See LO/OVRAL.
RISKS OF TAKING ORAL CONTRACEPTIVES: See LO/OVRAL.
ESTIMATED RISK OF DEATH FROM A BIRTH-CONTROL METHOD OR PREGNANCY: See LO/OVRAL.
WARNING SIGNALS: See LO/OVRAL.
SIDE EFFECTS OF ORAL CONTRACEPTIVES: See LO/OVRAL.
GENERAL PRECAUTIONS: See LO/OVRAL.
HOW TO TAKE THE PILL: See LO/OVRAL.
RISKS TO THE FETUS: See LO/OVRAL.
HEALTH BENEFITS FROM ORAL CONTRACEPTIVES: See LO/OVRAL.
Manufactured by:
Wyeth Laboratories Inc.
A Wyeth-Ayerst Company
Philadelphia, PA 19101
Shown in Product Identification Guide, page 344

OVRAL®-28

[ōh 'vral-28]
Tablets
(norgestrel and ethinyl estradiol tablets)

℞

Patients should be counseled that this product does not protect against HIV infection (AIDS) and other sexually transmitted diseases.

DESCRIPTION

21 white Ovral tablets, each containing 0.5 mg of norgestrel (*dl* -13-beta-ethyl-17-alpha-ethinyl-17-beta-hydroxygon-4-en-3-one), a totally synthetic progestogen, and 0.05 mg of ethinyl estradiol (19-nor-17α-pregna-1,3,5 (10)-trien-20-yne-3,17-diol), and 7 pink inert tablets. The inactive ingredients present are cellulose, D&C Red 30, lactose, magnesium stearate, and polacrilin potassium.

CLINICAL PHARMACOLOGY
See LO/OVRAL®.

INDICATIONS AND USAGE
See OVRAL®.

CONTRAINDICATIONS
See LO/OVRAL.

WARNINGS
See OVRAL.

PRECAUTIONS
See LO/OVRAL.
Drug Interactions: See LO/OVRAL.
Carcinogenesis: See LO/OVRAL.
Pregnancy: See LO/OVRAL.
Nursing Mothers: See LO/OVRAL.
Information for the Patient: See LO/OVRAL.

ADVERSE REACTIONS
See LO/OVRAL.

OVERDOSAGE
See LO/OVRAL.

NONCONTRACEPTIVE HEALTH BENEFITS
See LO/OVRAL

DOSAGE AND ADMINISTRATION

To achieve maximum contraceptive effectiveness, Ovral-28 must be taken exactly as directed and at intervals not exceeding 24 hours.

The dosage of Ovral-28 is one white tablet daily for 21 consecutive days, followed by one pink inert tablet daily for 7 consecutive days, according to prescribed schedule.

It is recommended that Ovral-28 tablets be taken at the same time each day, preferably after the evening meal or at bedtime.

During the first cycle of medication, the patient is instructed to begin taking Ovral-28 on the first Sunday after the onset of menstruation. If menstruation begins on a Sunday, the first tablet (white) is taken that day. One white tab-

let should be taken daily for 21 consecutive days followed by one pink inert tablet daily for 7 consecutive days. Withdrawal bleeding should usually occur within three days following discontinuation of white tablets. During the first cycle, contraceptive reliance should not be placed on Ovral-28 until a white tablet has been taken daily for 7 consecutive days. The possibility of ovulation and conception prior to initiation of medication should be considered.

The patient begins her next and all subsequent 28-day courses of tablets on the same day of the week (Sunday) on which she began her first course, following the same schedule: 21 days on white tablets—7 days on pink inert tablets. If in any cycle the patient starts tablets later than the proper day, she should protect herself by using another method of birth control until she has taken a white tablet daily for 7 consecutive days.

If spotting or breakthrough bleeding occurs, the patient is instructed to continue on the same regimen. This type of bleeding is usually transient and without significance; however, if the bleeding is persistent or prolonged, the patient is advised to consult her physician. Although the occurrence of pregnancy is highly unlikely if Ovral-28 is taken according to directions, if withdrawal bleeding does not occur, the possibility of pregnancy must be considered. If the patient has not adhered to the prescribed schedule (missed one or more tablets or started taking them on a day later than she should have), the probability of pregnancy should be considered at the time of the first missed period and appropriate diagnostic measures taken before the medication is resumed. If the patient has adhered to the prescribed regimen and misses two consecutive periods, pregnancy should be ruled out before continuing the contraceptive regimen.

For additional patient instructions regarding missed pills, see the "WHAT TO DO IF YOU MISS PILLS" section in the DETAILED PATIENT LABELING for LO/OVRAL.

Any time the patient misses two or more white tablets, she should also use another method of contraception until she has taken a white tablet daily for seven consecutive days. If the patient misses one or more pink tablets, she is still protected against pregnancy **provided** she begins taking white tablets again on the proper day.

If breakthrough bleeding occurs following missed white tablets, it will usually be transient and of no consequence. While there is little likelihood of ovulation occurring if only one or two white tablets are missed, the possibility of ovulation increases with each successive day that scheduled white tablets are missed.

In the nonlactating mother, Ovral-28 may be initiated postpartum, for contraception. When the tablets are administered in the postpartum period, the increased risk of thromboembolic disease associated with the postpartum period must be considered (see "Contraindications", "Warnings", and "Precautions" concerning thromboembolic disease). It is to be noted that early resumption of ovulation may occur if Parlodel® (bromocriptine mesylate) has been used for the prevention of lactation.

HOW SUPPLIED

Ovral®-28 Tablets (0.5 mg norgestrel and 0.05 mg ethinyl estradiol) are available in packages of 6 PILPAK® dispensers, each containing 28 tablets as follows:
21 active tablets, NDC 0008-0056, white, round tablet marked "WYETH" and "56".
7 inert tablets, NDC 0008-0445, pink, round tablet marked "WYETH" and "445".
Store at room temperature, approx. 25°C (77°F).

References available upon request.

Brief Summary Patient Package Insert: See LO/OVRAL.
DETAILED PATIENT LABELING: See OVRAL.
Manufactured by:
Wyeth Laboratories Inc.
A Wyeth-Ayerst Company
Philadelphia, PA 19101.
Shown in Product Identification Guide, page 344

OVRETTE®

[oh-vret ']
Tablets
(norgestrel tablets)

℞

Patients should be counseled that this product does not protect against HIV infection (AIDS) and other sexually transmitted diseases.
Each OVRETTE tablet contains 0.075 mg of norgestrel (*dl* - 13-beta-ethyl-17-alpha-ethinyl-17-beta-hydroxygon-4-en-3-one). The inactive ingredients present are cellulose, FD&C Yellow 5, lactose, magnesium stearate, and polacrilin potassium.

DESCRIPTION
Each OVRETTE tablet contains 0.075 mg of a single active steroid ingredient, norgestrel, a totally synthetic progestogen. The available data suggest that the d (-)enantiomeric form of norgestrel is the biologically active portion. This form amounts to 0.0375 mg per OVRETTE tablet.

CLINICAL PHARMACOLOGY

The primary mechanism through which OVRETTE prevents conception is not known, but progestogen-only contraceptives are known to alter the cervical mucus, exert a progestational effect on the endometrium, interfering with implantation, and, in some patients, suppress ovulation.

INDICATIONS AND USAGE

See LO/OVRAL®.

CONTRAINDICATIONS

See LO/OVRAL.

WARNINGS

See LO/OVRAL.

PRECAUTIONS

See LO/OVRAL.

INFORMATION FOR THE PATIENT

See LO/OVRAL.

DRUG INTERACTIONS

See LO/OVRAL.

CARCINOGENESIS

See LO/OVRAL.

PREGNANCY

See LO/OVRAL.

NURSING MOTHERS

See LO/OVRAL.

ADVERSE REACTIONS

See LO/OVRAL.

OVERDOSAGE

See LO/OVRAL.

DOSAGE AND ADMINISTRATION

To achieve maximum contraceptive effectiveness, OVRETTE must be taken exactly as directed and at intervals not exceeding 24 hours.

OVRETTE is administered on a continuous daily dosage regimen starting on the first day of menstruation, i.e., one tablet each day, every day of the year.

Tablets should be taken at the same time each day and continued daily, without interruption, whether bleeding occurs or not. The patient should be advised that, if prolonged bleeding occurs, she should consult her physician. In the nonlactating mother, OVRETTE may be initiated postpartum, for contraception. When the tablets are administered in the postpartum period, the increased risk of thromboembolic disease associated with the postpartum period must be considered (see "Contraindications," "Warnings," and "Precautions" concerning thromboembolic disease). It is to be noted that early resumption of ovulation may occur if Parlodel® (bromocriptine mesylate) has been used for the prevention of lactation.

The risk of pregnancy increases with each tablet missed. If the patient misses one tablet, she should be instructed to take it as soon as she remembers and to also take her next tablet at the regular time. If she misses two tablets, she should take one of the missed tablets as soon as she remembers, as well as taking her regular tablet for that day at the proper time. Furthermore, she should use a method of nonhormonal contraception in addition to taking OVRETTE until fourteen tablets have been taken. If more than 2 tablets have been missed, OVRETTE should be discontinued immediately and a method of nonhormonal contraception should be used until menses has appeared or pregnancy has been excluded. If menses does not appear within 45 days from the last period, a method of nonhormonal contraception should be substituted until the start of the next menstrual period or an appropriate diagnostic procedure is performed to rule out pregnancy.

HOW SUPPLIED

OVRETTE® Tablets (0.075 mg norgestrel) are available in packages of 6 PILPAK® dispensers with 28 tablets each as follows: NDC 0008-0062-01, yellow, round tablet marked "WYETH" and "62".

Store at room temperature, approx. 25°C (77°F).

REFERENCES

Available upon request.
Brief Summary Patient Package Insert: See LO/OVRAL
DETAILED PATIENT LABELING: See LO/OVRAL.
HOW TO TAKE THE PILL
This product (like all oral contraceptives) is intended to prevent pregnancy. It does not protect against transmission of HIV (AIDS) and other sexually transmitted diseases such as chlamydia, genital herpes, genital warts, gonorrhea, hepatitis B, and syphillis.

1. *General Instructions*
You must take your pill every day according to the instructions. Oral contraceptives are most effective if taken no more than 24 hours apart. Take your pill at the same time

every day so that you are less likely to forget to take it. You will then maintain an effective dose of the oral contraceptive in your body.

If your doctor has scheduled you for surgery, or you need prolonged bed rest, he or she may suggest that you stop taking the pill four weeks before surgery to avoid an increased risk of blood clots. It is also advisable not to start oral contraceptives sooner than four weeks after delivery of a baby or a midtrimester pregnancy termination.

Ovrette is administered on a continuous daily dosage schedule, one tablet each day, every day of the year. Take the first tablet on the first day of your menstrual period. Tablets should be taken at the same time every day, without interruption, whether bleeding occurs or not. If bleeding is prolonged (more than 8 days) or unusually heavy, you should contact your doctor.

SPOTTING OR BREAKTHROUGH BLEEDING
Spotting is slight staining between menstrual periods which may not even require a pad. Breakthrough bleeding is a flow much like a regular period, requiring sanitary protection. Spotting is more common than breakthrough bleeding, and both occur more often in the first few cycles than in later cycles. These types of bleeding are usually temporary and without significance. It is important to continue taking your pills on schedule. If the bleeding persists for more than a few days, consult your doctor.

2. *If you forget to take your pill*
The risk of pregnancy increases with each tablet missed. Therefore, it is very important that you take one tablet daily as directed. If you miss one tablet, take it as soon as you remember and also take your next tablet at the regular time. If you miss two tablets, take one of the missed tablets as soon as you remember, as well as your regular tablet for that day at the proper time. Furthermore, you should use another method of birth control in addition to taking Ovrette until you have taken fourteen days (2 weeks) of medication.

If more than two tablets have been missed, Ovrette should be discontinued immediately and another method of birth control used until the start of your next menstrual period. Then you may resume taking Ovrette.

At times there may be no menstrual period after a cycle of pills. Therefore, if you miss one menstrual period but have taken the pills **exactly as you were supposed to,** continue as usual into the next cycle. If you have not taken the pills correctly and miss a menstrual period, or if it is 45 days or more from the start of your last menstrual period, you may be pregnant and should stop taking oral contraceptives until your doctor determines whether or not you are pregnant. Until you can get to your doctor, use another form of nonhormonal contraception. If two consecutive menstrual periods are missed, you should stop taking pills until it is determined by a physician whether you are pregnant.

3. *Pregnancy due to pill failure*
The incidence of pill failure resulting in pregnancy is approximately less than 1.0% if taken every day as directed, but more typical failure rates are less than 3.0%. If failure does occur, the risk to the fetus is minimal.

4. *Risks to the fetus*
If you do become pregnant while using oral contraceptives, the risk to the fetus is small, on the order of no more than one per thousand. You should, however, discuss the risks to the developing child with your doctor.

5. *Pregnancy after stopping the pill*
There may be some delay in becoming pregnant after you stop using oral contraceptives, especially if you had irregular menstrual cycles before you used oral contraceptives. It may be advisable to postpone conception until you begin menstruating regularly once you have stopped taking the pill and desire pregnancy.

There does not appear to be any increase in birth defects in newborn babies when pregnancy occurs soon after stopping the pill.

6. *Overdosage*
Serious ill effects have not been reported following ingestion of large doses of oral contraceptives by young children. Overdosage may cause nausea and withdrawal bleeding in females. In case of overdosage, contact your health-care provider or pharmacist.

7. *Other information*
Your health-care provider will take a medical and family history before prescribing oral contraceptives and will examine you. The physical examination may be delayed to another time if you request it and the health-care provider believes that it is appropriate to postpone it. You should be reexamined at least once a year. Be sure to inform your health-care provider if there is a family history of any of the conditions listed previously in this leaflet. Be sure to keep all appointments with your health-care provider, because this is a time to determine if there are early signs of side effects of oral-contraceptive use.

Do not use the drug for any condition other than the one for which is was prescribed. This drug has been prescribed specifically for you; do not give it to others who may want birth control pills.

HEALTH BENEFITS FROM ORAL CONTRACEPTIVES

In addition to preventing pregnancy, use of oral contraceptives may provide certain benefits.
They are:
- Menstrual cycles may become more regular.
- Blood flow during menstruation may be lighter, and less iron may be lost. Therefore, anemia due to iron deficiency is less likely to occur.
- Pain or other symptoms during menstruation may be encountered less frequently.
- Ovarian cysts may occur less frequently.
- Ectopic (tubal) pregnancy may occur less frequently.
- Noncancerous cysts or lumps in the breast may occur less frequently.
- Acute pelvic inflammatory disease may occur less frequently.
- Oral-contraceptive use may provide some protection against developing two forms of cancer: cancer of the ovaries and cancer of the lining of the uterus.

If you want more information about birth-control pills, ask you doctor or pharmacist. They have a more technical leaflet called the Professional Labeling which you may wish to read.

Manufactured by:
Wyeth Laboratories Inc.
A Wyeth-Ayerst Company
Philadelphia, PA 19101

PEN • VEE® K   ℞
[*pĕn-vee-kāy*]
(penicillin V potassium)

DESCRIPTION

Penicillin V is the phenoxymethyl analog of penicillin G. Penicillin V potassium is the potassium salt of penicillin V. Pen-Vee K tablets contain penicillin V potassium equivalent to 250 mg (400,000 units) or 500 mg (800,000 units) penicillin V. The inactive ingredients present are carboxymethylcellulose sodium, magnesium stearate, and stearic acid. The 250 mg dosage strength also contains lactose.

Pen-Vee K for oral solution is a powder which when reconstituted as directed yields a solution of penicillin V potassium equivalent to 125 mg (200,000 units) or 250 mg (400,000 units) penicillin V per 5 mL. The inactive ingredients present are artificial and natural flavors, citric acid, FD&C Red 40, saccharin sodium, sodium benzoate, sodium citrate, sodium propionate, sucrose, and water. The 250 mg per 5 mL dosage strength also contains edetate disodium and FD&C Yellow 6.

ACTION AND PHARMACOLOGY

Penicillin V exerts a bactericidal action against penicillin-sensitive microorganisms during the stage of active multiplication. It acts through the inhibition of biosynthesis of cell-wall mucopeptide. It is not active against the penicillinase-producing bacteria, which include many strains of staphylococci. The drug exerts high *in vitro* activity against staphylococci (except penicillinase-producing strains), streptococci (groups A, C, G, H, L, and M), and pneumococci. Other organisms sensitive *in vitro* to penicillin V are *Corynebacterium diphtheriae, Bacillus anthracis,* Clostridia, *Actinomyces bovis, Streptobacillus moniliformis, Listeria monocytogenes,* Leptospira, and *Neisseria gonorrhoeae. Treponema pallidum* is extremely sensitive.

The potassium salt of penicillin V has the distinct advantage over penicillin G in resistance to inactivation by gastric acid. It may be given with meals; however, blood levels are slightly higher when the drug is given on an empty stomach. Average blood levels are two to five times higher than the levels following the same dose of oral penicillin G and also show much less individual variation.

Once absorbed, penicillin V is about 80% bound to serum protein. Tissue levels are highest in the kidneys, with lesser amounts in the liver, skin, and intestines. Small amounts are found in all other body tissues and the cerebrospinal fluid. The drug is excreted as rapidly as it is absorbed in individuals with normal kidney function; however, recovery of the drug from the urine indicates that only about 25% of the dose given is absorbed. In neonates, young infants, and individuals with impaired kidney function, excretion is considerably delayed.

INDICATIONS

Penicillin V potassium is indicated in the treatment of mild to moderately severe infections due to penicillin G-sensitive microorganisms. Therapy should be guided by bacteriological studies (including sensitivity tests) and by clinical response.

Note: Severe pneumonia, empyema, bacteremia, pericarditis, meningitis, and arthritis should not be treated with penicillin V during the acute stage.

Indicated surgical procedures should be performed.

Continued on next page

Pen • Vee K—Cont.

The following infections will usually respond to adequate dosage of penicillin V.

Streptococcal infections (without bacteremia). Mild-to-moderate infections of the upper respiratory tract, scarlet fever, and mild erysipelas.

Note: Streptococci in groups A, C, G, H, L, and M are very sensitive to penicillin. Other groups, including group D (enterococcus), are resistant.

Pneumococcal infections. Mild to moderately severe infections of the respiratory tract.

Staphylococcal infections—penicillin G-sensitive. Mild infections of the skin and soft tissues.

Note: Reports indicate an increasing number of strains of staphylococci resistant to penicillin G, emphasizing the need for culture and sensitivity studies in treating suspected staphylococcal infections.

Fusospirochetosis (Vincent's gingivitis and pharyngitis)—Mild to moderately severe infections of the oropharynx usually respond to therapy with oral penicillin.

Note: Necessary dental care should be accomplished in infections involving the gum tissue.

Medical conditions in which oral penicillin therapy is indicated as prophylaxis:

For the prevention of recurrence following rheumatic fever and/or chorea: Prophylaxis with oral penicillin on a continuing basis has proven effective in preventing recurrence of these conditions.

Although no controlled clinical efficacy studies have been conducted, penicillin V has been suggested by the American Heart Association and the American Dental Association for use as an oral regimen for prophylaxis against bacterial endocarditis in patients who have congenital heart disease or rheumatic or other acquired valvular heart disease when they undergo dental procedures and surgical procedures of the upper respiratory tract.[1] Oral penicillin should not be used in those patients at particularly high risk for endocarditis (e.g., those with prosthetic heart valves or surgically constructed systemic-pulmonary shunts). Penicillin V should not be used as adjunctive prophylaxis for genitourinary instrumentation or surgery, lower-intestinal-tract surgery, sigmoidoscopy, and childbirth. Since it may happen that *alpha* hemolytic streptococci relatively resistant to penicillin may be found when patients are receiving continuous oral penicillin for secondary prevention of rheumatic fever, prophylactic agents other than penicillin may be chosen for these patients and prescribed in addition to their continuous rheumatic fever prophylactic regimen.

Note: When selecting antibiotics for the prevention of bacterial endocarditis, the physician or dentist should read the full joint statement of the American Heart Association and the American Dental Association.[1]

CONTRAINDICATIONS

A previous hypersensitivity reaction to any penicillin is a contraindication.

WARNINGS

Serious and occasionally fatal hypersensitivity (anaphylactoid) reactions have been reported in patients on penicillin therapy. Although anaphylaxis is more frequent following parenteral therapy, it has occurred in patients on oral penicillins. These reactions are more apt to occur in individuals with a history of sensitivity to multiple allergens.

There have been well-documented reports of individuals with a history of penicillin hypersensitivity reactions who have experienced severe hypersensitivity reactions when treated with a cephalosporin. Before therapy with a penicillin, careful inquiry should be made concerning previous hypersensitivity reactions to penicillins, cephalosporins, and other allergens. If an allergic reaction occurs, the drug should be discontinued and the patient treated with the usual agents, e.g., pressor amines, antihistamines, and corticosteroids.

PRECAUTIONS

Penicillin should be used with caution in individuals with histories of significant allergies and/or asthma.

The oral route of administration should not be relied upon in patients with severe illness, or with nausea, vomiting, gastric dilatation, cardiospasm, or intestinal hypermotility. Occasional patients will not absorb therapeutic amounts of orally administered penicillin.

In streptococcal infections, therapy must be sufficient to eliminate the organism (10-day minimum); otherwise the sequelae of streptococcal disease may occur. Cultures should be taken following completion of treatment to determine whether streptococci have been eradicated.

Prolonged use of antibiotics may promote the overgrowth of nonsusceptible organisms, including fungi. Should superinfection occur, appropriate measures should be taken.

ADVERSE REACTIONS

Although the incidence of reactions to oral penicillins has been reported with much less frequency than following parenteral therapy, it should be remembered that all degrees of hypersensitivity, including fatal anaphylaxis, have been reported with oral penicillin.

The most common reactions to oral penicillin are nausea, vomiting, epigastric distress, diarrhea, and black hairy tongue. The hypersensitivity reactions reported are skin eruptions (maculopapular to exfoliative dermatitis), urticaria and other serum-sicknesslike reactions, laryngeal edema, and anaphylaxis. Fever and eosinophilia may frequently be the only reaction observed. Hemolytic anemia, leukopenia, thrombocytopenia, neuropathy, and nephropathy are infrequent reactions and usually associated with high doses of parenteral penicillin.

DOSAGE AND ADMINISTRATION

The dosage of penicillin V should be determined according to the sensitivity of the causative microorganisms and the severity of infection, and adjusted to the clinical response of the patient.

The usual dosage recommendations for adults and children 12 years and over are as follows:

Streptococcal infections—mild to moderately severe—of the upper respiratory tract and including scarlet fever and erysipelas: 125 to 250 mg (200,000 to 400,000 units) every 6 to 8 hours for 10 days.

Pneumococcal infections—mild to moderately severe—of the respiratory tract, including otitis media: 250 to 500 mg (400,000 to 800,000 units) every 6 hours until the patient has been afebrile for at least 2 days.

Staphylococcal infections—mild infections of skin and soft tissue (culture and sensitivity tests should be performed): 250 to 500 mg (400,000 to 800,000 units) every 6 to 8 hours.

Fusospirochetosis (Vincent's infection) of the oropharynx. Mild to moderately severe infections: 250 to 500 mg (400,000 to 800,000 units) every 6 to 8 hours.

For the prevention of recurrence following rheumatic fever and/or chorea: 125 to 250 mg (200,000 to 400,000 units) twice daily on a continuing basis.

For prophylaxis against bacterial endocarditis[1] in patients with congenital heart disease or rheumatic or other acquired valvular heart disease when undergoing dental procedures or surgical procedures of the upper respiratory tract: 2.0 gram of penicillin V (1.0 gram for children under 60 lbs.) 1 hour before the procedure, and then, 1.0 gram (500 mg for children under 60 lbs.) 6 hours later.

HOW SUPPLIED

Pen·Vee® K (penicillin V potassium) Tablets contain penicillin V potassium equivalent to 250 mg (400,000 units) or 500 mg (800,000 units) penicillin V. They are white, round, scored tablets, supplied as follows:

250 mg (400,000 units), NDC 0008-0059, marked "WYETH" and "59", in bottles of 100 or 500 tablets, and in Redipak® cartons of 100 individually wrapped tablets.

500 mg (800,000 units), NDC 0008-0390, marked "WYETH" and "390", in bottles of 100 or 500 tablets, and in Redipak® cartons of 100 individually wrapped tablets.

Keep tightly closed.

Store at room temperature, approximately 25°C (77°F).

Dispense in tight container.

Pen·Vee® K (penicillin V potassium) for Oral Solution is available as a powder which when reconstituted as directed yields a palatable solution of penicillin V potassium equivalent to 125 mg (200,000 units) or 250 mg (400,000 units) penicillin V per 5 mL and is supplied as follows:

125 mg (200,000 units) per 5 mL, NDC 0008-0004, faint pink powder, in bottles to make 100 mL or 200 mL of red solution.

250 mg (400,000 units) per 5 mL, NDC 0008-0036, light peach-colored powder, in bottles to make 100 mL, 150 mL, or 200 mL of light-orange solution.

Keep tightly closed.

Store at room temperature [approximately 25°C (77°F)] before reconstitution.

After reconstitution, solution must be stored in a refrigerator.

Discard any unused portion after 14 days.

REFERENCE

1. American Heart Association. 1984. Prevention of bacterial endocarditis. Circulation *70(6):1123A–1127A*.

Manufactured by:
Wyeth Laboratories Inc.
A Wyeth-Ayerst Company
Philadelphia, PA 19101

PHENERGAN® ℞

[*fĕn 'ĕr-găn*]

(promethazine HCl Injection, USP)
INJECTION

DESCRIPTION

Promethazine HCl (10*H*-Phenothiazine-10-ethanamine, *N,N*,α-trimethyl-, monohydrochloride, (±)-) has the following structural formula:

[See chemical structure at top of next column]

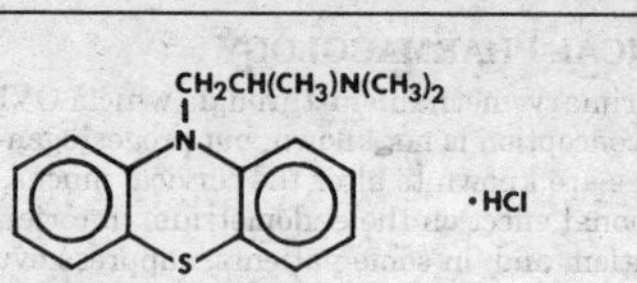

Each mL contains promethazine hydrochloride, either 25 mg or 50 mg, edetate disodium 0.1 mg, calcium chloride 0.04 mg, sodium metabisulfite 0.25 mg and phenol 5 mg in Water for Injection. pH 4.0–5.5; buffered with acetic acid-sodium acetate. Sealed under nitrogen.

Each mL of the **TUBEX®** and **TUBEX® BLUNT POINTE™** Sterile Cartridge Units contains either 25 or 50 mg promethazine hydrochloride with 0.1 mg edetate disodium, 0.04 mg calcium chloride, not more than 5 mg monothioglycerol and 5 mg phenol with sodium acetate-acetic acid buffer. Sealed under nitrogen.

ACTIONS

Promethazine hydrochloride, a phenothiazine derivative, possesses antihistaminic, sedative, antimotion-sickness, antiemetic, and anticholinergic effects. The duration of action is generally from four to six hours. The major side reaction of this drug is sedation. As an antihistamine, it acts by competitive antagonism but does not block the release of histamine. It antagonizes in varying degrees most but not all of the pharmacological effects of histamine.

INDICATIONS AND USAGE

The injectable form of promethazine hydrochloride is indicated for the following conditions:

1. Amelioration of allergic reactions to blood or plasma.
2. In anaphylaxis as an adjunct to epinephrine and other standard measures after the acute symptoms have been controlled.
3. For other uncomplicated allergic conditions of the immediate type when oral therapy is impossible or contraindicated.
4. Active treatment of motion sickness.
5. Preoperative, postoperative, and obstetric (during labor) sedation.
6. Prevention and control of nausea and vomiting associated with certain types of anesthesia and surgery.
7. As an adjunct to analgesics for the control of postoperative pain.
8. For sedation and relief of apprehension and to produce light sleep from which the patient can be easily aroused.
9. Intravenously in special surgical situations, such as repeated bronchoscopy, ophthalmic surgery, and poor-risk patients, with reduced amounts of meperidine or other narcotic analgesic as an adjunct to anesthesia and analgesia.

CONTRAINDICATIONS

Promethazine is contraindicated in comatose states, in patients who have received large amounts of central-nervous-system depressants (alcohol, sedative-hypnotics, including barbiturates, general anesthetics, narcotics, narcotic analgesics, tranquilizers, etc.), and in patients who have demonstrated an idiosyncrasy or hypersensitivity to promethazine.

Under no circumstances should promethazine be given by intra-arterial injection due to the likelihood of severe arteriospasm and the possibility of resultant gangrene (see "**WARNINGS**").

Phenergan Injection should not be given by the subcutaneous route; evidence of chemical irritation has been noted, and necrotic lesions have resulted on rare occasions following subcutaneous injection. The preferred parenteral route of administration is by deep intramuscular injection.

WARNINGS

Promethazine HCl Injection (ampuls only) contains sodium metabisulfite, a sulfite that may cause allergic-type reactions, including anaphylactic symptoms and life-threatening or less severe asthmatic episodes, in certain susceptible people. The overall prevalence of sulfite sensitivity in the general population is unknown and probably low. Sulfite sensitivity is seen more frequently in asthmatic than in nonasthmatic people.

Promethazine may impair the mental and/or physical abilities required for the performance of potentially hazardous tasks, such as driving a vehicle or operating machinery. The concomitant use of alcohol, sedative hypnotics (including barbiturates), general anesthetics, narcotics, narcotic analgesics, tranquilizers or other central-nervous-system depressants may have an additive sedative effect. Patients should be warned accordingly.

USAGE IN PREGNANCY

The safe use of promethazine has not been established with respect to the possible adverse effects upon fetal development. Therefore, the need for the use of this drug during pregnancy should be weighed against the possible but unknown hazards to the developing fetus.

USE IN CHILDREN

Excessively large dosages of antihistamines, including promethazine, in children may cause hallucinations, convul-

sions, and sudden death. In children who are acutely ill associated with dehydration, there is an increased susceptibility to dystonias with the use of promethazine hydrochloride injection.

CAUTION SHOULD BE EXERCISED WHEN ADMINISTERING PHENERGAN TO CHILDREN. ANTIEMETICS ARE NOT RECOMMENDED FOR TREATMENT OF UNCOMPLICATED VOMITING IN CHILDREN, AND THEIR USE SHOULD BE LIMITED TO PROLONGED VOMITING OF KNOWN ETIOLOGY. THE EXTRAPYRAMIDAL SYMPTOMS WHICH CAN OCCUR SECONDARY TO PHENERGAN ADMINISTRATION MAY BE CONFUSED WITH THE CNS SIGNS OF UNDIAGNOSED PRIMARY DISEASE, e.g., ENCEPHALOPATHY OR REYE'S SYNDROME. THE USE OF PHENERGAN SHOULD BE AVOIDED IN CHILDREN WHOSE SIGNS AND SYMPTOMS MAY SUGGEST REYE'S SYNDROME OR OTHER HEPATIC DISEASES.

USE IN THE ELDERLY (APPROXIMATELY 60 YEARS OR OLDER)

Since therapeutic requirements for sedative drugs tend to be less in elderly patients, the dosage of Phenergan should be reduced for these patients.

OTHER CONSIDERATIONS

Drugs having anticholinergic properties should be used with caution in patients with asthmatic attack, narrow-angle glaucoma, prostatic hypertrophy, stenosing peptic ulcer, pyloroduodenal obstruction, and bladder-neck obstruction.

Promethazine should be used with caution in patients with bone-marrow depression. Leukopenia and agranulocytosis have been reported, usually when Phenergan has been used in association with other known toxic agents.

INADVERTENT INTRA-ARTERIAL INJECTION

Due to the close proximity of arteries and veins in the areas most commonly used for intravenous injection, extreme care should be exercised to avoid perivascular extravasation or inadvertent intra-arterial injection. Reports compatible with inadvertent intra-arterial injection of promethazine, usually in conjunction with other drugs intended for intravenous use, suggest that pain, severe chemical irritation, severe spasm of distal vessels, and resultant gangrene requiring amputation are likely under such circumstances. Intravenous injection was intended in all the cases reported, but perivascular extravasation or arterial placement of the needle is now suspect. There is no proven successful management of this condition after it occurs, although sympathetic block and heparinization are commonly employed during the acute management because of the results of animal experiments with other known arteriolar irritants. Aspiration of dark blood does not preclude intra-arterial needle placement, because blood is discolored upon contact with promethazine. Use of syringes with rigid plungers or of small bore needles might obscure typical arterial backflow if this is relied upon alone.

When used intravenously, promethazine hydrochloride should be given in a concentration no greater than 25 mg per mL and at a rate not to exceed 25 mg per minute. When administering any irritant drug intravenously, it is usually preferable to inject it through the tubing of an intravenous infusion set that is known to be functioning satisfactorily. In the event that a patient complains of pain during intended intravenous injection of promethazine, the injection should immediately be stopped to provide for evaluation of possible arterial placement or perivascular extravasation.

PRECAUTIONS

Promethazine may significantly affect the actions of other drugs. It may increase, prolong, or intensify the sedative action of central-nervous-system depressants, such as alcohol, sedative hypnotics (including barbiturates), general anesthetics, narcotics, narcotic analgesics, tranquilizers, etc. When given concomitantly with promethazine hydrochloride, the dose of barbiturates should be reduced by at least one-half, and the dose of narcotics should be reduced by one-quarter to one-half. Dosage must be individualized. Excessive amounts of promethazine relative to a narcotic may lead to restlessness and motor hyperactivity in the patient with pain; these symptoms usually disappear with adequate control of the pain. Promethazine should be used cautiously in persons with cardiovascular disease or impairment of liver function.

Although reversal of the vasopressor effect of epinephrine has not been reported with promethazine, the possibility should be considered in case of promethazine overdose.

ADVERSE REACTIONS

CNS EFFECTS

Drowsiness is the most prominent CNS effect of this drug. Extrapyramidal reactions may occur with high doses; this is almost always responsive to a reduction in dosage. Other reported reactions include dizziness, lassitude, tinnitus, incoordination, fatigue, blurred vision, euphoria, diplopia, nervousness, insomnia, tremors, convulsive seizures, oculogyric crises, excitation, catatonic-like states, and hysteria.

CARDIOVASCULAR EFFECTS

Tachycardia, bradycardia, faintness, dizziness, and increases and decreases in blood pressure have been reported following the use of promethazine hydrochloride injection. Venous thrombosis at the injection site has been reported. INTRA-ARTERIAL INJECTION MAY RESULT IN GANGRENE OF THE AFFECTED EXTREMITY ("see **WARNINGS**").

GASTROINTESTINAL

Nausea and vomiting have been reported, usually in association with surgical procedures and combination drug therapy.

ALLERGIC REACTIONS

These include urticaria, dermatitis, asthma, and photosensitivity. Angioneurotic edema has been reported.

OTHER REPORTED REACTIONS

Leukopenia and agranulocytosis, usually when Phenergan has been used in association with other known toxic agents, have been reported. Thrombocytopenic purpura and jaundice of the obstructive type have been associated with the use of promethazine. The jaundice is usually reversible on discontinuation of the drug. Subcutaneous injection has resulted in tissue necrosis. Nasal stuffiness may occur. Dry mouth has been reported.

LABORATORY TESTS

The following laboratory tests may be affected in patients who are receiving therapy with promethazine hydrochloride:

Pregnancy Tests—Diagnostic pregnancy tests based on immunological reactions between HCG and anti-HCG may result in false-negative or false-positive interpretations.

Glucose Tolerance Test—An increase in glucose tolerance has been reported in patients receiving promethazine hydrochloride.

PARADOXICAL REACTIONS (OVERDOSAGE)

Hyperexcitability and abnormal movements, which have been reported in children following a single administration of promethazine, may be manifestations of relative overdosage, in which case, consideration should be given to the discontinuation of the promethazine and to the use of other drugs. Respiratory depression, nightmares, delirium, and agitated behavior have also been reported in some of these patients.

DRUG INTERACTIONS

NARCOTICS AND BARBITURATES

The CNS-depressant effects of narcotics and barbiturates are additive with promethazine hydrochloride.

MONOAMINE OXIDASE INHIBITORS (MAOI)

Drug interactions, including an increased incidence of extrapyramidal effects, have been reported when some MAOI and phenothiazines are used concomitantly. Although such a reaction has not been reported with promethazine, the possibility should be considered.

DOSAGE AND ADMINISTRATION

The preferred parenteral route of administration for promethazine hydrochloride is by deep intramuscular injection. The proper intravenous administration of this product is well tolerated, but use of this route is not without some hazard.

INADVERTENT INTRA-ARTERIAL INJECTION CAN RESULT IN GANGRENE OF THE AFFECTED EXTREMITY (see "Warnings"). SUBCUTANEOUS INJECTION IS CONTRAINDICATED, AS IT MAY RESULT IN TISSUE NECROSIS (see "Contraindications"). When used intravenously, promethazine hydrochloride should be given in concentration no greater than 25 mg/mL at a rate not to exceed 25 mg per minute; it is preferable to inject through the tubing of an intravenous infusion set that is known to be functioning satisfactorily.

The **TUBEX® BLUNT POINTE™** Sterile Cartridge Unit is suitable for substances to be administered intravenously only. It is intended for use with injection sets specifically manufactured as "needle-less" injection systems. As of the date of this circular, the **TUBEX BLUNT POINTE** is compatible with LifeShield® Prepierced Reseal injection site, InterLink® Injection Site, SafeLine® Injection Site, UserGard® Intermittent Injection Cap, and SafSite® reflux valve*.

The **TUBEX®** Sterile Cartridge-Needle Unit is suitable for substances to be administered intravenously or intramuscularly.

ALLERGIC CONDITIONS

The average adult dose is 25 mg. This dose may be repeated within two hours if necessary, but continued therapy, if indicated, should be via the oral route as soon as existing circumstances permit. After initiation of treatment, dosage should be adjusted to the smallest amount adequate to relieve symptoms. The average adult dose for amelioration of allergic reactions to blood or plasma is 25 mg.

SEDATION

In hospitalized adult patients, nighttime sedation may be achieved by a dose of 25 to 50 mg of promethazine hydrochloride.

PREOPERATIVE AND POSTOPERATIVE USE

As an adjunct to preoperative or postoperative medication, 25 to 50 mg of promethazine hydrochloride in adults may be combined with appropriately reduced doses of analgesics and atropine-like drugs as desired. Dosage of concomitant analgesic or hypnotic medication should be reduced accordingly.

NAUSEA AND VOMITING

For control of nausea and vomiting, the usual adult dose is 12.5 to 25 mg, not to be repeated more frequently than every four hours. When used for control of postoperative nausea and vomiting, the medication may be administered either intramuscularly or intravenously and dosage of analgesics and barbiturates reduced accordingly.

OBSTETRICS

Phenergan in doses of 50 mg will provide sedation and relieve apprehension in the early stages of labor. When labor is definitely established, 25 to 75 mg (average dose, 50 mg) promethazine hydrochloride may be given intramuscularly or intravenously with an appropriately reduced dose of any desired narcotic. Amnesic agents may be administered as necessary. If necessary, Phenergan with a reduced dose of analgesic may be repeated once or twice at four-hour intervals in the course of a normal labor. A maximum total dose of 100 mg of promethazine may be administered during a 24-hour period to patients in labor.

CHILDREN

In children under the age of 12 years, the dosage should not exceed half that of the suggested adult dose. As an adjunct to premedication, the suggested dose is 0.5 mg per lb. of body weight in combination with an equal dose of narcotic or barbiturate and the appropriate dose of an atropine-like drug. Antiemetics should not be used in vomiting of unknown etiology in children.

MANAGEMENT OF OVERDOSAGE

Signs and symptoms of overdosage range from mild depression of the central nervous system and cardiovascular system to profound hypotension, respiratory depression, and unconsciousness. Stimulation may be evident, especially in children and geriatric patients. Atropine-like signs and symptoms—dry mouth, fixed, dilated pupils, flushing, etc., as well as gastrointestinal symptoms, may occur. The treatment of overdosage is essentially symptomatic and supportive. Early gastric lavage may be beneficial if promethazine has been taken orally. Centrally acting emetics are of little use.

Avoid analeptics, which may cause convulsions. Severe hypotension usually responds to the administration of levarterenol or phenylephrine. EPINEPHRINE SHOULD NOT BE USED, since its use in a patient with partial adrenergic blockade may further lower the blood pressure. Extrapyramidal reactions may be treated with anticholinergic antiparkinson agents, diphenhydramine, or barbiturates. Additional measures include oxygen and intravenous fluids. Limited experience with dialysis indicates that it is not helpful.

Parenteral drug products should be inspected visually for particulate matter and discoloration prior to administration, whenever solution and container permit.

HOW SUPPLIED

Phenergan® Injection (Promethazine HCl Injection, USP) is available as follows:

25 mg/mL, 1 mL ampuls packaged in 25s (NDC 0008-0063-01)

50 mg/mL, 1 mL ampuls packaged in 25s (NDC 0008-0746-01).

STORAGE

Protect from light. Keep covered in carton until time of use

Store at controlled room temperature 15°–30°C (59°–86°F). Do not use if soluton has developed color or contains a precipitate.

ALSO AVAILABLE

Phenergan® (promethazine HCl) Injection is available in the following dosage strengths in **TUBEX® BLUNT POINTE™** Sterile Cartridge Units and Sterile Cartridge-Needle Units, packaged in boxes of 10 **TUBEX®** as follows: 25 mg per mL, NDC 0008-0416-50, 1 mL size **BLUNT POINTE™**.

25 mg per mL, NDC 0008-0416-01, 1 mL size (22 gauge × 1–1/4 inch needle).

50 mg per mL, NDC 0008-0417-01, 1 mL size (22 gauge × 1–1/4 inch needle).

Store at room temperature, between 15°-25°C (59°-77°F).

Protect from light.

Use carton to protect contents from light.

Do not use if solution is discolored or contains a precipitate.

Manufactured by:
Wyeth Laboratories Inc.
A Wyeth-Ayerst Company
Philadelphia, PA 19101

Consult 1999 PDR® supplements and future editions for revisions

PHENERGAN® ℞
[*fĕn ′ĕr-găn*]
(promethazine hydrochloride)
Syrup Plain and
PHENERGAN® ℞
(promethazine hydrochloride)
Syrup Fortis

DESCRIPTION

Each teaspoon (5 mL) of Phenergan Syrup Plain contains 6.25 mg promethazine hydrochloride in a flavored syrup base with a pH between 4.7 and 5.2. Alcohol 7%. The inactive ingredients present are artificial and natural flavors, citric acid, D&C Red 33, D&C Yellow 10, FD&C Blue 1, FD&C Yellow 6, glycerin, saccharin sodium, sodium benzoate, sodium citrate, sodium propionate, water, and other ingredients.

Each teaspoon (5 mL) of Phenergan Syrup Fortis contains 25 mg promethazine hydrochloride in a flavored syrup base with a pH between 5.0 and 5.5. Alcohol 1.5%. The inactive ingredients present are artificial and natural flavors, citric acid, saccharin sodium, sodium benzoate, sodium propionate, water, and other ingredients.

Promethazine hydrochloride is a racemic compound; the empirical formula is $C_{17}H_{20}N_2S{\cdot}HCl$ and its molecular weight is 320.88.

Promethazine hydrochloride, a phenothiazine derivative, is designated chemically as 10*H*-Phenothiazine-10-ethanamine, *N,N*,α-trimethyl-, monohydrochloride, (±)- with the following structural formula:

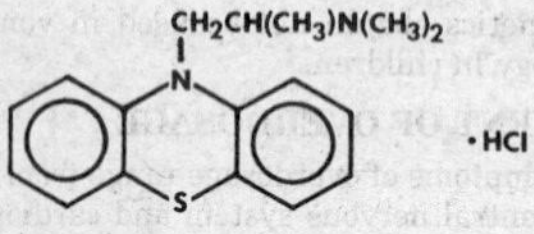

Promethazine hydrochloride occurs as a white to faint yellow, practically odorless, crystalline powder which slowly oxidizes and turns blue on prolonged exposure to air. It is soluble in water and freely soluble in alcohol.

CLINICAL PHARMACOLOGY

Promethazine is a phenothiazine derivative which differs structurally from the antipsychotic phenothiazines by the presence of a branched side chain and no ring substitution. It is thought that this configuration is responsible for its relative lack (1/10 that of chlorpromazine) of dopaminergic (CNS) action.

Promethazine is an H_1 receptor blocking agent. In addition to its antihistaminic action, it provides clinically useful sedative and antiemetic effects. In therapeutic dosage, promethazine produces no significant effects on the cardiovascular system.

Promethazine is well absorbed from the gastrointestinal tract. Clinical effects are apparent within 20 minutes after oral administration and generally last four to six hours, although they may persist as long as 12 hours. Promethazine is metabolized by the liver to a variety of compounds; the sulfoxides of promethazine and N-demethylpromethazine are the predominant metabolites appearing in the urine.

INDICATIONS AND USAGE

Phenergan is useful for:
Perennial and seasonal allergic rhinitis.
Vasomotor rhinitis.
Allergic conjunctivitis due to inhalant allergens and foods.
Mild, uncomplicated allergic skin manifestations of urticaria and angioedema.
Amelioration of allergic reactions to blood or plasma.
Dermographism.
Anaphylactic reactions, as adjunctive therapy to epinephrine and other standard measures, after the acute manifestations have been controlled.
Preoperative, postoperative, or obstetric sedation.
Prevention and control of nausea and vomiting associated with certain types of anesthesia and surgery.
Therapy adjunctive to meperidine or other analgesics for control of postoperative pain.
Sedation in both children and adults, as well as relief of apprehension and production of light sleep from which the patient can be easily aroused.
Active and prophylactic treatment of motion sickness.
Antiemetic therapy in postoperative patients.

CONTRAINDICATIONS

Promethazine is contraindicated in individuals known to be hypersensitive or to have had an idiosyncratic reaction to promethazine or to other phenothiazines.

Antihistamines are contraindicated for use in the treatment of lower respiratory tract symptoms including asthma.

WARNINGS

Promethazine may cause marked drowsiness. Ambulatory patients should be cautioned against such activities as driving or operating dangerous machinery until it is known that they do not become drowsy or dizzy from promethazine therapy.

The sedative action of promethazine hydrochloride is additive to the sedative effects of central nervous system depressants; therefore, agents such as alcohol, narcotic analgesics, sedatives, hypnotics, and tranquilizers should either be eliminated or given in reduced dosage in the presence of promethazine hydrochloride. When given concomitantly with promethazine hydrochloride, the dose of barbiturates should be reduced by at least one-half, and the dose of analgesic depressants, such as morphine or meperidine, should be reduced by one-quarter to one-half.

Promethazine may lower seizure threshold. This should be taken into consideration when administering to persons with known seizure disorders or when giving in combination with narcotics or local anesthetics which may also affect seizure threshold.

Sedative drugs or CNS depressants should be avoided in patients with a history of sleep apnea.

Antihistamines should be used with caution in patients with narrow-angle glaucoma, stenosing peptic ulcer, pyloroduodenal obstruction, and urinary bladder obstruction due to symptomatic prostatic hypertrophy and narrowing of the bladder neck.

Administration of promethazine has been associated with reported cholestatic jaundice.

PRECAUTIONS

GENERAL

Promethazine should be used cautiously in persons with cardiovascular disease or with impairment of liver function.

INFORMATION FOR PATIENTS

Phenergan may cause marked drowsiness or impair the mental and/or physical abilities required for the performance of potentially hazardous tasks, such as driving a vehicle or operating machinery. Ambulatory patients should be told to avoid engaging in such activities until it is known that they do not become drowsy or dizzy from Phenergan therapy. Children should be supervised to avoid potential harm in bike riding or in other hazardous activities.

The concomitant use of alcohol or other central nervous system depressants, including narcotic analgesics, sedatives, hypnotics, and tranquilizers, may have an additive effect and should be avoided or their dosage reduced.

Patients should be advised to report any involuntary muscle movements or unusual sensitivity to sunlight.

DRUG INTERACTIONS

The sedative action of promethazine is additive to the sedative effects of other central nervous system depressants, including alcohol, narcotic analgesics, sedatives, hypnotics, tricyclic antidepressants, and tranquilizers; therefore, these agents should be avoided or administered in reduced dosage to patients receiving promethazine.

DRUG/LABORATORY TEST INTERACTIONS

The following laboratory tests may be affected in patients who are receiving therapy with promethazine hydrochloride:

Pregnancy Tests

Diagnostic pregnancy tests based on immunological reactions between HCG and anti-HCG may result in false-negative or false-positive interpretations.

Glucose Tolerance Test

An increase in blood glucose has been reported in patients receiving promethazine.

CARCINOGENESIS, MUTAGENESIS, IMPAIRMENT OF FERTILITY

Long-term animal studies have not been performed to assess the carcinogenic potential of promethazine, nor are there other animal or human data concerning carcinogenicity, mutagenicity, or impairment of fertility with this drug. Promethazine was nonmutagenic in the *Salmonella* test system of Ames.

PREGNANCY

Teratogenic Effects —Pregnancy Category C

Teratogenic effects have not been demonstrated in rat-feeding studies at doses of 6.25 and 12.5 mg/kg of promethazine. These doses are from approximately 2.1 to 4.2 times the maximum recommended total daily dose of promethazine for a 50-kg subject, depending upon the indication for which the drug is prescribed. Specific studies to test the action of the drug on parturition, lactation, and development of the animal neonate were not done, but a general preliminary study in rats indicated no effect on these parameters. Although antihistamines, including promethazine, have been found to produce fetal mortality in rodents, the pharmacological effects of histamine in the rodent do not parallel those in man. There are no adequate and well-controlled studies of promethazine in pregnant women. Phenergan should be used during pregnancy only if the potential benefit justifies the potential risk to the fetus.

Nonteratogenic Effects

Promethazine taken within two weeks of delivery may inhibit platelet aggregation in the newborn.

LABOR AND DELIVERY

Phenergan, in appropriate dosage form, may be used alone or as an adjunct to narcotic analgesics during labor and delivery. (See "**Indications and Usage**" and "**Dosage and Administration.**")
See also "*Nonteratogenic Effects*."

NURSING MOTHERS

It is not known whether promethazine is excreted in human milk. Caution should be exercised when promethazine is administered to a nursing woman.

PEDIATRIC USE

This product should not be used in children under 2 years of age because safety for such use has not been established.

ADVERSE REACTIONS

Nervous System —Sedation, sleepiness, occasional blurred vision, dryness of mouth, dizziness; rarely confusion, disorientation, and extrapyramidal symptoms such as oculogyric crisis, torticollis, and tongue protrusion (usually in association with parenteral injection or excessive dosage).
Cardiovascular —Increased or decreased blood pressure.
Dermatologic —Rash, rarely photosensitivity.
Hematologic —Rarely leukopenia, thrombocytopenia; agranulocytosis (1 case).
Gastrointestinal —Nausea and vomiting.

OVERDOSAGE

Signs and symptoms of overdosage with promethazine range from mild depression of the central nervous system and cardiovascular system to profound hypotension, respiratory depression, and unconsciousness.

Stimulation may be evident, especially in children and geriatric patients. Convulsions may rarely occur. A paradoxical reaction has been reported in children receiving single doses of 75 mg to 125 mg orally, characterized by hyperexcitability and nightmares.

Atropinelike signs and symptoms—dry mouth, fixed, dilated pupils, flushing, as well as gastrointestinal symptoms, may occur.

TREATMENT

Treatment of overdosage is essentially symptomatic and supportive. Only in cases of extreme overdosage or individual sensitivity do vital signs, including respiration, pulse, blood pressure, temperature, and EKG need to be monitored. Activated charcoal orally or by lavage may be given, or sodium or magnesium sulfate orally as a cathartic. Attention should be given to the reestablishment of adequate respiratory exchange through provision of a patent airway and institution of assisted or controlled ventilation. Diazepam may be used to control convulsions. Acidosis and electrolyte losses should be corrected. Note that any depressant effects of promethazine are not reversed by naloxone. Avoid analeptics which may cause convulsions.

Severe hypotension usually responds to the administration of norepinephrine or phenylephrine. EPINEPHRINE SHOULD NOT BE USED, since its use in patients with partial adrenergic blockade may further lower the blood pressure.

Limited experience with dialysis indicates that it is not helpful.

DOSAGE AND ADMINISTRATION

ALLERGY

The average oral dose is 25 mg taken before retiring; however, 12.5 mg may be taken before meals and on retiring, if necessary. Children tolerate this product well. Single 25-mg doses at bedtime or 6.25 to 12.5 mg taken three times daily will usually suffice. After initiation of treatment in children or adults, dosage should be adjusted to the smallest amount adequate to relieve symptoms.

Phenergan Rectal Suppositories may be used if the oral route is not feasible, but oral therapy should be resumed as soon as possible if continued therapy is indicated.

The administration of promethazine hydrochloride in 25-mg doses will control minor transfusion reactions of an allergic nature.

MOTION SICKNESS

The average adult dose is 25 mg taken twice daily. The initial dose should be taken one-half to one hour before anticipated travel and be repeated 8 to 12 hours later, if necessary. On succeeding days of travel, it is recommended that 25 mg be given on arising and again before the evening meal. For children, Phenergan Tablets, Syrup, or Rectal Suppositories, 12.5 to 25 mg, twice daily, may be administered.

NAUSEA AND VOMITING

The average effective dose of Phenergan for the active therapy of nausea and vomiting in children or adults is 25 mg. When oral medication cannot be tolerated, the dose should be given parenterally (cf. Phenergan Injection) or by rectal suppository. 12.5- to 25-mg doses may be repeated, as necessary, at 4- to 6-hour intervals.

For nausea and vomiting in children, the usual dose is 0.5 mg per pound of body weight, and the dose should be adjusted to the age and weight of the patient and the severity of the condition being treated.

For prophylaxis of nausea and vomiting, as during surgery and the postoperative period, the average dose is 25 mg repeated at 4- to 6-hour intervals, as necessary.
SEDATION
This product relieves apprehension and induces a quiet sleep from which the patient can be easily aroused. Administration of 12.5 to 25 mg Phenergan by the oral route or by rectal suppository at bedtime will provide sedation in children. Adults usually require 25 to 50 mg for nighttime, presurgical, or obstetrical sedation.
PRE- AND POSTOPERATIVE USE
Phenergan in 12.5- to 25-mg doses for children and 50-mg doses for adults the night before surgery relieves apprehension and produces a quiet sleep.
For preoperative medication children require doses of 0.5 mg per pound of body weight in combination with an equal dose of meperidine and the appropriate dose of an atropine-like drug.
Usual adult dosage is 50 mg Phenergan with an equal amount of meperidine and the required amount of a belladonna alkaloid.
Postoperative sedation and adjunctive use with analgesics may be obtained by the administration of 12.5 to 25 mg in children and 25- to 50-mg doses in adults.
Phenergan Syrup Plain and Phenergan Syrup Fortis are not recommended for children under 2 years of age.

HOW SUPPLIED

Phenergan® (Promethazine Hydrochloride) Syrup Plain is a clear, green solution supplied as follows:
NDC 0008-0549-02, case of 24 bottles of 4 fl. oz. (118 mL).
NDC 0008-0549-03, bottle of 1 pint (473 mL).
Phenergan® (Promethazine Hydrochloride) Syrup Fortis is a clear, light straw-colored solution supplied as follows:
NDC 0008-0231-01, bottle of 1 pint (473 mL).
Keep bottles tightly closed.
Store at Room Temperature, between 15° C and 25° C (59° F and 77° F).
Protect from light.
Dispense in light-resistant, glass, tight containers.
Manufactured by:
Wyeth Laboratories Inc.
A Wyeth-Ayerst Company
Philadelphia, PA 19101

PHENERGAN® ℞

[fĕn ′ĕr-găn]
(promethazine HCl)
TABLETS •
SUPPOSITORIES

DESCRIPTION

Each tablet of Phenergan contains 12.5 mg, 25 mg, or 50 mg promethazine hydrochloride. The inactive ingredients present are lactose, magnesium stearate, and methylcellulose. Each dosage strength also contains the following:
12.5 mg—FD&C Yellow 6 and saccharin sodium;
25 mg—saccharin sodium;
50 mg—FD&C Red 40.
Each rectal suppository of Phenergan contains 12.5 mg, 25 mg, or 50 mg promethazine hydrochloride with ascorbyl palmitate, silicon dioxide, white wax, and cocoa butter.
Promethazine hydrochloride is a racemic compound; the empirical formula is $C_{17}H_{20}N_2S{\cdot}HCl$ and its molecular weight is 320.88.
Promethazine hydrochloride, a phenothiazine derivative, is designated chemically as 10*H*-Phenothiazine-10-ethanamine, *N,N*,α-trimethyl-, monohydrochloride, (±)- with the following structural formula:

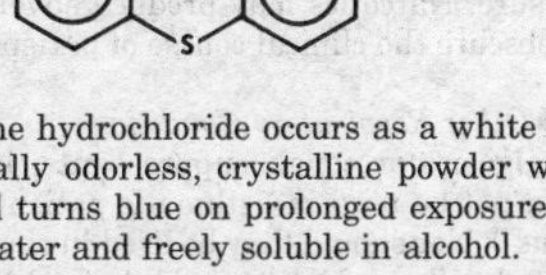

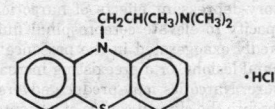

CH2CH(CH3)N(CH3)2
N
S
•HCl

Promethazine hydrochloride occurs as a white to faint yellow, practically odorless, crystalline powder which slowly oxidizes and turns blue on prolonged exposure to air. It is soluble in water and freely soluble in alcohol.

CLINICAL PHARMACOLOGY

Promethazine is a phenothiazine derivative which differs structurally from the antipsychotic phenothiazines by the presence of a branched side chain and no ring substitution. It is thought that this configuration is responsible for its relative lack ($^1/_{10}$ that of chlorpromazine) of dopaminergic (CNS) action.
Promethazine is an H_1 receptor blocking agent. In addition to its antihistaminic action, it provides clinically useful sedative and antiemetic effects. In therapeutic dosage, promethazine produces no significant effects on the cardiovascular system.
Promethazine is well absorbed from the gastrointestinal tract. Clinical effects are apparent within 20 minutes after oral administration and generally last four to six hours, although they may persist as long as 12 hours. Promethazine is metabolized by the liver to a variety of compounds; the sulfoxides of promethazine and N-demethylpromethazine are the predominant metabolites appearing in the urine.

INDICATIONS AND USAGE

Phenergan, either orally or by suppository, is useful for:
Perennial and seasonal allergic rhinitis.
Vasomotor rhinitis.
Allergic conjunctivitis due to inhalant allergens and foods.
Mild, uncomplicated allergic skin manifestations of urticaria and angioedema.
Amelioration of allergic reactions to blood or plasma.
Dermographism.
Anaphylactic reactions, as adjunctive therapy to epinephrine and other standard measures, after the acute manifestations have been controlled.
Preoperative, postoperative, or obstetric sedation.
Prevention and control of nausea and vomiting associated with certain types of anesthesia and surgery.
Therapy adjunctive to meperidine or other analgesics for control of postoperative pain.
Sedation in both children and adults, as well as relief of apprehension and production of light sleep from which the patient can be easily aroused.
Active and prophylactic treatment of motion sickness.
Antiemetic therapy in postoperative patients.

CONTRAINDICATIONS

Promethazine is contraindicated in individuals known to be hypersensitive or to have had an idiosyncratic reaction to promethazine or to other phenothiazines.
Antihistamines are contraindicated for use in the treatment of lower respiratory tract symptoms including asthma.

WARNINGS

Promethazine may cause marked drowsiness. Ambulatory patients should be cautioned against such activities as driving or operating dangerous machinery until it is known that they do not become drowsy or dizzy from promethazine therapy.
The sedative action of promethazine hydrochloride is additive to the sedative effects of central nervous system depressants; therefore, agents such as alcohol, narcotic analgesics, sedatives, hypnotics, and tranquilizers should either be eliminated or given in reduced dosage in the presence of promethazine hydrochloride. When given concomitantly with promethazine hydrochloride, the dose of barbiturates should be reduced by at least one-half, and the dose of analgesic depressants, such as morphine or meperidine, should be reduced by one-quarter to one-half.
Promethazine may lower seizure threshold. This should be taken into consideration when administering to persons with known seizure disorders or when giving in combination with narcotics and local anesthetics which may also affect seizure threshold.
Sedative drugs or CNS depressants should be avoided in patients with a history of sleep apnea.
Antihistamines should be used with caution in patients with narrow-angle glaucoma, stenosing peptic ulcer, pyloroduodenal obstruction, and urinary bladder obstruction due to symptomatic prostatic hypertrophy and narrowing of the bladder neck.
Administration of promethazine has been associated with reported cholestatic jaundice.

PRECAUTIONS

GENERAL
Promethazine should be used cautiously in persons with cardiovascular disease or with impairment of liver function.
INFORMATION FOR PATIENTS
Phenergan may cause marked drowsiness or impair the mental and/or physical abilities required for the performance of potentially hazardous tasks, such as driving a vehicle or operating machinery. Ambulatory patients should be told to avoid engaging in such activities until it is known that they do not become drowsy or dizzy from Phenergan therapy. Children should be supervised to avoid potential harm in bike riding or in other hazardous activities.
The concomitant use of alcohol or other central nervous system depressants, including narcotic analgesics, sedatives, hypnotics, and tranquilizers, may have an additive effect and should be avoided or their dosage reduced.
Patients should be advised to report any involuntary muscle movements or unusual sensitivity to sunlight.
DRUG INTERACTIONS
The sedative action of promethazine is additive to the sedative effects of other central nervous system depressants, including alcohol, narcotic analgesics, sedatives, hypnotics, tricyclic antidepressants, and tranquilizers; therefore, these agents should be avoided or administered in reduced dosage to patients receiving promethazine.
DRUG/LABORATORY TEST INTERACTIONS
The following laboratory tests may be affected in patients who are receiving therapy with promethazine hydrochloride:
Pregnancy Tests
Diagnostic pregnancy tests based on immunological reactions between HCG and anti-HCG may result in false-negative or false-positive interpretations.
Glucose Tolerance Test
An increase in blood glucose has been reported in patients receiving promethazine.
CARCINOGENESIS, MUTAGENESIS, IMPAIRMENT OF FERTILITY
Long-term animal studies have not been performed to assess the carcinogenic potential of promethazine, nor are there other animal or human data concerning carcinogenicity, mutagenicity, or impairment of fertility with this drug. Promethazine was nonmutagenic in the *Salmonella* test system of Ames.
PREGNANCY
Teratogenic Effects —Pregnancy Category C
Teratogenic effects have not been demonstrated in rat-feeding studies at doses of 6.25 and 12.5 mg/kg of promethazine. These doses are from approximately 2.1 to 4.2 times the maximum recommended total daily dose of promethazine for a 50-kg subject, depending upon the indication for which the drug is prescribed. Specific studies to test the action of the drug on parturition, lactation, and development of the animal neonate were not done, but a general preliminary study in rats indicated no effect on these parameters. Although antihistamines, including promethazine, have been found to produce fetal mortality in rodents, the pharmacological effects of histamine in the rodent do not parallel those in man. There are no adequate and well-controlled studies of promethazine in pregnant women. Phenergan should be used during pregnancy only if the potential benefit justifies the potential risk to the fetus.
Nonteratogenic Effects
Promethazine taken within two weeks of delivery may inhibit platelet aggregation in the newborn.
LABOR AND DELIVERY
Phenergan, in appropriate dosage form, may be used alone or as an adjunct to narcotic analgesics during labor and delivery. (See "**Indications and Usage**" and "**Dosage and Administration**.")
See also "*Nonteratogenic Effects*."
NURSING MOTHERS
It is not known whether promethazine is excreted in human milk. Caution should be exercised when promethazine is administered to a nursing woman.
PEDIATRIC USE
This product should not be used in children under 2 years of age because safety for such use has not been established.

ADVERSE REACTIONS

Nervous System —Sedation, sleepiness, occasional blurred vision, dryness of mouth, dizziness; rarely confusion, disorientation, and extrapyramidal symptoms such as oculogyric crisis, torticollis, and tongue protrusion (usually in association with parenteral injection or excessive dosage).
Cardiovascular —Increased or decreased blood pressure.
Dermatologic —Rash, rarely photosensitivity.
Hematologic —Rarely leukopenia, thrombocytopenia; agranulocytosis (1 case).
Gastrointestinal —Nausea and vomiting.

OVERDOSAGE

Signs and symptoms of overdosage with promethazine range from mild depression of the central nervous system and cardiovascular system to profound hypotension, respiratory depression, and unconsciousness.
Stimulation may be evident, especially in children and geriatric patients. Convulsions may rarely occur. A paradoxical reaction has been reported in children receiving single doses of 75 mg to 125 mg orally, characterized by hyperexcitability and nightmares.
Atropine-like signs and symptoms—dry mouth, fixed, dilated pupils, flushing, as well as gastrointestinal symptoms, may occur.
TREATMENT
Treatment of overdosage is essentially symptomatic and supportive. Only in cases of extreme overdosage or individual sensitivity do vital signs, including respiration, pulse, blood pressure, temperature, and EKG, need to be monitored. Activated charcoal orally or by lavage may be given, or sodium or magnesium sulfate orally as a cathartic. Attention should be given to the reestablishment of adequate respiratory exchange through provision of a patent airway and institution of assisted or controlled ventilation. Diazepam may be used to control convulsions. Acidosis and electrolyte losses should be corrected. Note that any depressant effects of promethazine are not reversed by naloxone. Avoid analeptics which may cause convulsions.
Severe hypotension usually responds to the administration of norepinephrine or phenylephrine. EPINEPHRINE

Continued on next page

Phenergan Tabs/Supp.—Cont.

SHOULD NOT BE USED, since its use in patients with partial adrenergic blockade may further lower the blood pressure.
Limited experience with dialysis indicates that it is not helpful.

DOSAGE AND ADMINISTRATION

ALLERGY
The average oral dose is 25 mg taken before retiring; however, 12.5 mg may be taken before meals and on retiring, if necessary. Children tolerate this product well. Single 25-mg doses at bedtime or 6.25 to 12.5 mg taken three times daily will usually suffice. After initiation of treatment in children or adults, dosage should be adjusted to the smallest amount adequate to relieve symptoms. The administration of promethazine hydrochloride in 25-mg doses will control minor transfusion reactions of an allergic nature.

MOTION SICKNESS
The average adult dose is 25 mg taken twice daily. The initial dose should be taken one-half to one hour before anticipated travel and be repeated 8 to 12 hours later, if necessary. On succeeding days of travel, it is recommended that 25 mg be given on arising and again before the evening meal. For children, Phenergan Tablets, Syrup, or Rectal Suppositories, 12.5 to 25 mg, twice daily, may be administered.

NAUSEA AND VOMITING
The average effective dose of Phenergan for the active therapy of nausea and vomiting in children or adults is 25 mg. When oral medication cannot be tolerated, the dose should be given parenterally (cf. Phenergan Injection) or by rectal suppository. 12.5- to 25-mg doses may be repeated, as necessary, at 4- to 6-hour intervals.
For nausea and vomiting in children, the usual dose is 0.5 mg per pound of body weight, and the dose should be adjusted to the age and weight of the patient and the severity of the condition being treated.
For prophylaxis of nausea and vomiting, as during surgery and the postoperative period, the average dose is 25 mg repeated at 4- to 6-hour intervals, as necessary.

SEDATION
This product relieves apprehension and induces a quiet sleep from which the patient can be easily aroused. Administration of 12.5 to 25 mg Phenergan by the oral route or by rectal suppository at bedtime will provide sedation in children. Adults usually require 25 to 50 mg for nighttime, presurgical, or obstetrical sedation.

PRE- AND POSTOPERATIVE USE
Phenergan in 12.5- to 25-mg doses for children and 50-mg doses for adults the night before surgery relieves apprehension and produces a quiet sleep.
For preoperative medication children require doses of 0.5 mg per pound of body weight in combination with an equal dose of meperidine and the appropriate dose of an atropine-like drug.
Usual adult dosage is 50 mg Phenergan with an equal amount of meperidine and the required amount of a belladonna alkaloid.
Postoperative sedation and adjunctive use with analgesics may be obtained by the administration of 12.5 to 25 mg in children and 25- to 50-mg doses in adults.
Phenergan Tablets and Phenergan Rectal Suppositories are not recommended for children under 2 years of age.

HOW SUPPLIED

Phenergan® (promethazine HCl) Tablets are available as follows:
12.5 mg, orange tablet with "WYETH" on one side and "19" on the scored reverse side.
NDC 0008-0019-01, bottle of 100 tablets.
25 mg, white tablet with "WYETH" and "27" on one side and scored on the reverse side.
NDC 0008-0027-02, bottle of 100 tablets.
NDC 0008-0027-07, Redipak® carton of 100 tablets (10 blister strips of 10).
50 mg, pink tablet with "WYETH" on one side and "227" on the other side.
NDC 0008-0227-01, bottle of 100 tablets.
Keep tightly closed.
Store at room temperature, between 15°C and 25°C (59°F and 77°F).
Protect from light.
Dispense in light-resistant, tight container.
Use carton to protect contents from light.
Phenergan® (promethazine HCl) Rectal Suppositories are available in boxes of 12 as follows:
12.5 mg, ivory, torpedo-shaped suppository wrapped in copper-colored foil, NDC 0008-0498-01.
25 mg, ivory, torpedo-shaped suppository wrapped in light-green foil, NDC 0008-0212-01.
50 mg, ivory, torpedo-shaped suppository wrapped in blue foil, NDC 0008-0229-01.
Store refrigerated between 2°–8°C (36°–46°F).
Dispense in well-closed container.
Manufactured by:
Wyeth Laboratories Inc.
A Wyeth-Ayerst Company
Philadelphia, PA 19101
Shown in Product Identification Guide, page 344

PHENERGAN® C-V ℞

[fĕn ′ĕr-găn]
with codeine
(Warning—may be habit-forming)
(Promethazine Hydrochloride and Codeine Phosphate) Syrup

DESCRIPTION

Each teaspoon (5 mL) of Phenergan with codeine contains 10 mg codeine phosphate (Warning—may be habit-forming) and 6.25 mg promethazine hydrochloride in a flavored syrup base with a pH between 4.7 and 5.2. Alcohol 7%. The inactive ingredients present are artificial and natural flavors, citric acid, D&C Red 33, FD&C Blue 1, FD&C Yellow 6, glycerine, saccharin sodium, sodium benzoate, sodium citrate, sodium propionate, water, and other ingredients.
Codeine is one of the naturally occurring phenanthrene alkaloids of opium derived from the opium poppy; it is classified pharmacologically as a narcotic analgesic. Codeine phosphate may be chemically named as (5α,6α)-7,8-didehydro-4, 5-epoxy-3-methoxy-17-methylmorphinan-6-ol phosphate (1:1) (salt) hemihydrate with the following structural formula:

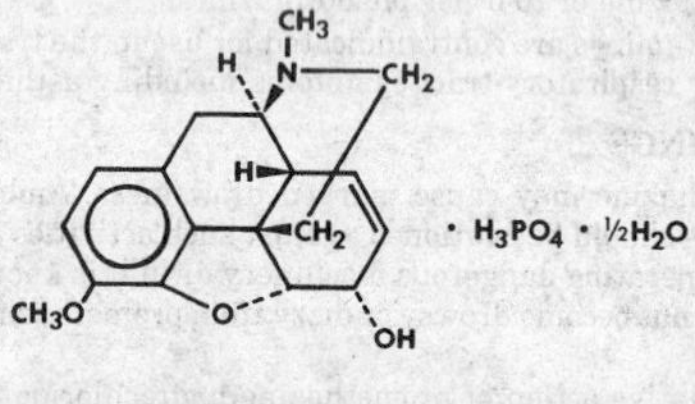

The phosphate salt of codeine occurs as white, needle-shaped crystals or white crystalline powder. Codeine phosphate is freely soluble in water and slightly soluble in alcohol, with a molecular weight of 406.37. The empirical formula is $C_{18}H_{21}NO_3 \cdot H_3PO_4 \cdot {}^1/_2H_2O$, and the stereochemistry is 5α, 6α isomer as indicated in the structure.
Promethazine hydrochloride is a racemic compound; the empirical formula is $C_{17}H_{20}N_2S \cdot HCl$ and its molecular weight is 320.88.
Promethazine hydrochloride, a phenothiazine derivative, is designated chemically as 10*H*-Phenothiazine-10-ethanamine, *N,N*,α-trimethyl-, monohydrochloride, (±)-. with the following structural formula:

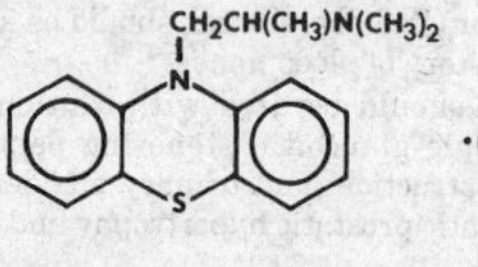

Promethazine hydrochloride occurs as a white to faint yellow, practically odorless, crystalline powder which slowly oxidizes and turns blue on prolonged exposure to air. It is soluble in water and freely soluble in alcohol.

CLINICAL PHARMACOLOGY

CODEINE
Narcotic analgesics, including codeine, exert their primary effects on the central nervous system and gastrointestinal tract. The analgesic effects of codeine are due to its central action; however, the precise sites of action have not been determined, and the mechanisms involved appear to be quite complex. Codeine resembles morphine both structurally and pharmacologically, but its actions at the doses of codeine used therapeutically are milder, with less sedation, respiratory depression, and gastrointestinal, urinary, and pupillary effects. Codeine produces an increase in biliary tract pressure, but less than morphine or meperidine. Codeine is less constipating than morphine.
Codeine has good antitussive activity, although less than that of morphine at equal doses. It is used in preference to morphine, because side effects are infrequent at the usual antitussive dose of codeine.
Codeine in oral therapeutic dosage does not usually exert major effects on the cardiovascular system.
Narcotic analgesics may cause nausea and vomiting by stimulating the chemoreceptor trigger zone (CTZ); however, they also depress the vomiting center, so that subsequent doses are unlikely to produce vomiting. Nausea is minimal after usual oral doses of codeine.
Narcotic analgesics cause histamine release, which appears to be responsible for wheals or urticaria sometimes seen at the site of injection on parenteral administration. Histamine release may also produce dilation of cutaneous blood vessels, with resultant flushing of the face and neck, pruritus, and sweating.
Codeine and its salts are well absorbed following both oral and parenteral administration. Codeine is about 2/3 as effective orally as parenterally. Codeine is metabolized primarily in the liver by enzymes of the endoplasmic reticulum, where it undergoes O-demethylation, N-demethylation, and partial conjugation with glucuronic acid. The drug is excreted primarily in the urine, largely as inactive metabolites and small amounts of free and conjugated morphine. Negligible amounts of codeine and its metabolites are found in the feces.
Following oral or subcutaneous administration of codeine, the onset of analgesia occurs within 15 to 30 minutes and lasts for four to six hours.
The cough-depressing action, in animal studies, was observed to occur 15 minutes after oral administration of codeine, peak action at 45 to 60 minutes after ingestion. The duration of action, which is dose-dependent, usually did not exceed 3 hours.

PROMETHAZINE
Promethazine is a phenothiazine derivative which differs structurally from the antipsychotic phenothiazines by the presence of a branched side chain and no ring substitution. It is thought that this configuration is responsible for its lack (1/10 that of chlorpromazine) of dopaminergic (CNS) action.
Promethazine is an H_1 receptor blocking agent. In addition to its antihistaminic action, it provides clinically useful sedative and antiemetic effects. In therapeutic dosages, promethazine produces no significant effects on the cardiovascular system.
Promethazine is well absorbed from the gastrointestinal tract. Clinical effects are apparent within 20 minutes after oral administration and generally last four to six hours, although they may persist as long as 12 hours. Promethazine is metabolized by the liver to a variety of compounds; the sulfoxides of promethazine and N-demethylpromethazine are the predominant metabolites appearing in the urine.

INDICATIONS AND USAGE

Phenergan with codeine is indicated for the temporary relief of coughs and upper respiratory symptoms associated with allergy or the common cold.

CONTRAINDICATIONS

Codeine is contraindicated in patients with a known hypersensitivity to the drug.
Promethazine is contraindicated in individuals known to be hypersensitive or to have had an idiosyncratic reaction to promethazine or to other phenothiazines.
Antihistamines and codeine are both contraindicated for use in the treatment of lower respiratory tract symptoms, including asthma.

WARNINGS

CODEINE
Dosage of codeine SHOULD NOT BE INCREASED if cough fails to respond; an unresponsive cough should be reevaluated in 5 days or sooner for possible underlying pathology, such as foreign body or lower respiratory tract disease.
Codeine may cause or aggravate constipation.
Respiratory depression leading to arrest, coma, and death has occurred with the use of codeine antitussives in young children, particularly in the under-one-year infants whose ability to deactivate the drug is not fully developed.
Administration of codeine may be accompanied by histamine release and should be used with caution in atopic children.
Head Injury and Increased Intracranial Pressure
The respiratory-depressant effects of narcotic analgesics and their capacity to elevate cerebrospinal fluid pressure may be markedly exaggerated in the presence of head injury, intracranial lesions, or a preexisting increase in intracranial pressure. Narcotics may produce adverse reactions which may obscure the clinical course of patients with head injuries.
Asthma and Other Respiratory Conditions
Narcotic analgesics or cough suppressants, including codeine, should not be used in asthmatic patients (see "Contraindications"). Nor should they be used in acute febrile illness associated with productive cough or in chronic respiratory disease where interference with ability to clear the tracheobronchial tree of secretions would have a deleterious effect on the patient's respiratory function.
Hypotensive Effect
Codeine may produce orthostatic hypotension in ambulatory patients.

PROMETHAZINE
Promethazine may cause marked drowsiness. Ambulatory patients should be cautioned against such activities as driving or operating dangerous machinery until it is known that they do not become drowsy or dizzy from promethazine therapy.

The sedative action of promethazine hydrochloride is additive to the sedative effects of central nervous system depressants; therefore, agents such as alcohol, narcotic analgesics, sedatives, hypnotics, and tranquilizers should either be eliminated or given in reduced dosage in the presence of promethazine hydrochloride. When given concomitantly with promethazine hydrochloride, the dose of barbiturates should be reduced by at least one-half, and the dose of analgesic depressants, such as morphine or meperidine, should be reduced by one-quarter to one-half.

Promethazine may lower seizure threshold. This should be taken into consideration when administering to persons with known seizure disorders or when giving in combination with narcotics or local anesthetics which may also affect seizure threshold.

Sedative drugs or CNS depressants should be avoided in patients with a history of sleep apnea.

Antihistamines should be used with caution in patients with narrow-angle glaucoma, stenosing peptic ulcer, pyloroduodenal obstruction, and urinary bladder obstruction due to symptomatic prostatic hypertrophy and narrowing of the bladder neck.

Administration of promethazine has been associated with reported cholestatic jaundice.

PRECAUTIONS

Animal reproduction studies have not been conducted with the drug combination—promethazine and codeine. It is not known whether this drug combination can cause fetal harm when administered to a pregnant woman or can affect reproduction capacity. Phenergan with codeine should be given to a pregnant woman only if clearly needed.

GENERAL

Narcotic analgesics, including codeine, should be administered with caution and the initial dose reduced in patients with acute abdominal conditions, convulsive disorders, significant hepatic or renal impairment, fever, hypothyroidism, Addison's disease, ulcerative colitis, prostatic hypertrophy, in patients with recent gastrointestinal or urinary tract surgery, and in the very young or elderly or debilitated patients.

Promethazine should be used cautiously in persons with cardiovascular disease or with impairment of liver function.

INFORMATION FOR PATIENTS

Phenergan with codeine may cause marked drowsiness or may impair the mental and/or physical abilities required for the performance of potentially hazardous tasks, such as driving a vehicle or operating machinery. Ambulatory patients should be told to avoid engaging in such activities until it is known that they do not become drowsy or dizzy from Phenergan with codeine therapy. Children should be supervised to avoid potential harm in bike riding or in other hazardous activities.

The concomitant use of alcohol or other central nervous system depressants, including narcotic analgesics, sedatives, hypnotics, and tranquilizers, may have an additive effect and should be avoided or their dosage reduced.

Patients should be advised to report any involuntary muscle movements or unusual sensitivity to sunlight.

Codeine, like other narcotic analgesics, may produce orthostatic hypotension in some ambulatory patients. Patients should be cautioned accordingly.

DRUG INTERACTIONS

CODEINE

In patients receiving MAO inhibitors, an initial small test dose is advisable to allow observation of any excessive narcotic effects or MAOI interaction.

PROMETHAZINE

The sedative action of promethazine is additive to the effects of other central nervous system depressants, including alcohol, narcotic analgesics, sedatives, hypnotics, tricyclic antidepressants, and tranquilizers; therefore, these agents should be avoided or administered in reduced dosage to patients receiving promethazine.

DRUG/LABORATORY TEST INTERACTIONS

Because narcotic analgesics may increase biliary tract pressure, with resultant increases in plasma amylase or lipase levels, determination of these enzyme levels may be unreliable for 24 hours after a narcotic analgesic has been given.

The following laboratory tests may be affected in patients who are receiving therapy with promethazine hydrochloride:

Pregnancy Tests

Diagnostic pregnancy tests based on immunological reactions between HCG and anti-HCG may result in false-negative or false-positive interpretations.

Glucose Tolerance Test

An increase in blood glucose has been reported in patients receiving promethazine.

CARCINOGENESIS, MUTAGENESIS, IMPAIRMENT OF FERTILITY

Long-term animal studies have not been performed to assess the carcinogenic potential of codeine or of promethazine, nor are there other animal or human data concerning carcinogenicity, mutagenicity, or impairment of fertility with these agents. Codeine has been reported to show no evidence of carcinogenicity or mutagenicity in a variety of test systems, including the micronucleus and sperm abnormality assays and the *Salmonella* assay. Promethazine was nonmutagenic in the *Salmonella* test system of Ames.

PHENERGAN WITH CODEINE

Adults	1 teaspoon (5 mL) every 4 to 6 hours, not to exceed 30.0 mL in 24 hours.
Children 6 years to under 12 years	1/2 to 1 teaspoon (2.5 to 5 mL) every 4 to 6 hours, not to exceed 30.0 mL in 24 hours.
Children under 6 years (weight: 18 kg or 40 lbs)	1/4 to 1/2 teaspoon (1.25 to 2.5 mL) every 4 to 6 hours, not to exceed 9.0 mL in 24 hours.
Children under 6 years (weight: 16 kg or 35 lbs)	1/4 to 1/2 teaspoon (1.25 to 2.5 mL) every 4 to 6 hours, not to exceed 8.0 mL in 24 hours.
Children under 6 years (weight: 14 kg or 30 lbs)	1/4 to 1/2 teaspoon (1.25 to 2.5 mL) every 4 to 6 hours, not to exceed 7.0 mL in 24 hours.
Children under 6 years (weight: 12 kg or 25 lbs)	1/4 to 1/2 teaspoon (1.25 to 2.5 mL) every 4 to 6 hours, not to exceed 6.0 mL in 24 hours.

Phenergan with codeine is not recommended for children under 2 years of age.

PREGNANCY

Teratogenic Effects —Pregnancy Category C

CODEINE

A study in rats and rabbits reported no teratogenic effect of codeine administered during the period of organogenesis in doses ranging from 5 to 120 mg/kg. In the rat, doses at the 120-mg/kg level, in the toxic range for the adult animal, were associated with an increase in embryo resorption at the time of implantation. In another study a single 100-mg/kg dose of codeine administered to pregnant mice reportedly resulted in delayed ossification in the offspring.

There are no studies in humans, and the significance of these findings to humans, if any, is not known.

PROMETHAZINE

Teratogenic effects have not been demonstrated in rat-feeding studies at doses of 6.25 and 12.5 mg/kg of promethazine. These doses are 8.3 and 16.7 times the maximum recommended total daily dose of promethazine for a 50-kg subject. Specific studies to test the action of the drug on parturition, lactation, and development of the animal neonate were not done, but a general preliminary study in rats indicated no effect on these parameters. Although antihistamines, including promethazine, have been found to produce fetal mortality in rodents, the pharmacological effects of histamine in the rodent do not parallel those in man. There are no adequate and well-controlled studies of promethazine in pregnant women.

Phenergan with codeine should be used during pregnancy only if the potential benefit justifies the potential risk to the fetus.

Nonteratogenic Effects

Dependence has been reported in newborns whose mothers took opiates regularly during pregnancy. Withdrawal signs include irritability, excessive crying, tremors, hyperreflexia, fever, vomiting, and diarrhea. Signs usually appear during the first few days of life.

Promethazine taken within two weeks of delivery may inhibit platelet aggregation in the newborn.

LABOR AND DELIVERY

Narcotic analgesics cross the placental barrier. The closer to delivery and the larger the dose used, the greater the possibility of respiratory depression in the newborn. Narcotic analgesics should be avoided during labor if delivery of a premature infant is anticipated. If the mother has received narcotic analgesics during labor, newborn infants should be observed closely for signs of respiratory depression. Resuscitation may be required (see "**Overdosage**"). The effect of codeine, if any, on the later growth, development, and functional maturation of the child is unknown.

See also "*Nonteratogenic Effects*."

NURSING MOTHERS

Some studies, but not others, have reported detectable amounts of codeine in breast milk. The levels are probably not clinically significant after usual therapeutic dosage. The possibility of clinically important amounts being excreted in breast milk in individuals abusing codeine should be considered.

It is not known whether promethazine is excreted in human milk.

Caution should be exercised when Phenergan with codeine is administered to a nursing woman.

PEDIATRIC USE

This product should not be used in children under 2 years of age because safety for such use has not been established.

ADVERSE REACTIONS

CODEINE

Nervous System —CNS depression, particularly respiratory depression, and to a lesser extent circulatory depression; light-headedness, dizziness, sedation, euphoria, dysphoria, headache, transient hallucination, disorientation, visual disturbances, and convulsions.

Cardiovascular —Tachycardia, bradycardia, palpitation, faintness, syncope, orthostatic hypotension (common to narcotic analgesics).

Gastrointestinal —Nausea, vomiting, constipation, and biliary tract spasm. Patients with chronic ulcerative colitis may experience increased colonic motility; in patients with acute ulcerative colitis, toxic dilation has been reported.

Genitourinary —Oliguria, urinary retention; antidiuretic effect has been reported (common to narcotic analgesics).

Allergic —Infrequent pruritus, giant urticaria, angioneurotic edema, and laryngeal edema.

Other —Flushing of the face, sweating and pruritus (due to opiate-induced histamine release); weakness.

PROMETHAZINE

Nervous System —Sedation, sleepiness, occasional blurred vision, dryness of mouth, dizziness; rarely confusion, disorientation, and extrapyramidal symptoms such as oculogyric crisis, torticollis, and tongue protrusion (usually in association with parenteral injection or excessive dosage).

Cardiovascular —Increased or decreased blood pressure.

Dermatologic —Rash, rarely photosensitivity.

Hematologic —Rarely leukopenia, thrombocytopenia; agranulocytosis (1 case).

Gastrointestinal —Nausea and vomiting.

DRUG ABUSE AND DEPENDENCE

CONTROLLED SUBSTANCE

Phenergan with codeine is a Schedule V Controlled Substance.

ABUSE

Codeine is known to be subject to abuse; however, the abuse potential of oral codeine appears to be quite low. Even parenteral codeine does not appear to offer the psychic effects sought by addicts to the same degree as heroin or morphine. However, codeine must be administered only under close supervision to patients with a history of drug abuse or dependence.

DEPENDENCE

Psychological dependence, physical dependence, and tolerance are known to occur with codeine.

OVERDOSAGE

CODEINE

Serious overdose with codeine is characterized by respiratory depression (a decrease in respiratory rate and/or tidal volume, Cheyne-Stokes respiration, cyanosis), extreme somnolence progressing to stupor or coma, skeletal muscle flaccidity, cold and clammy skin, and sometimes bradycardia and hypotension. The triad of coma, pinpoint pupils, and respiratory depression is strongly suggestive of opiate poisoning. In severe overdosage, particularly by the intravenous route, apnea, circulatory collapse, cardiac arrest, and death may occur. Promethazine is additive to the depressant effects of codeine.

It is difficult to determine what constitutes a standard toxic or lethal dose. However, the lethal oral dose of codeine in an adult is reported to be in the range of 0.5 to 1.0 gram. Infants and children are believed to be relatively more sensitive to opiates on a body-weight basis. Elderly patients are also comparatively intolerant to opiates.

PROMETHAZINE

Signs and symptoms of overdosage with promethazine range from mild depression of the central nervous system and cardiovascular system to profound hypotension, respiratory depression, and unconsciousness.

Stimulation may be evident, especially in children and geriatric patients. Convulsions may rarely occur. A paradoxical reaction has been reported in children receiving single doses of 75 mg to 125 mg orally, characterized by hyperexcitability and nightmares.

Atropine-like signs and symptoms—dry mouth, fixed, dilated pupils, flushing, as well as gastrointestinal symptoms, may occur.

TREATMENT

The treatment of overdosage with Phenergan with codeine is essentially symptomatic and supportive. Only in cases of extreme overdosage or individual sensitivity do vital signs including respiration, pulse, blood pressure, temperature, and EKG need to be monitored. Activated charcoal orally or by lavage may be given, or sodium or magnesium sulfate orally as a cathartic. Attention should be given to the reestablishment of adequate respiratory exchange through pro-

Continued on next page

Phenergan w/Codeine—Cont.

vision of a patent airway and institution of assisted or controlled ventilation. The narcotic antagonist, naloxone hydrochloride, may be administered when significant respiratory depression occurs with Phenergan with codeine; any depressant effects of promethazine are not reversed with naloxone. Diazepam may be used to control convulsions. Avoid analeptics, which may cause convulsions. Acidosis and electrolyte losses should be corrected. A rise in temperature or pulmonary complications may signal the need for institution of antibiotic therapy.
Severe hypotension usually responds to the administration of norepinephrine or phenylephrine. EPINEPHRINE SHOULD NOT BE USED, since its use in a patient with partial adrenergic blockade may further lower the blood pressure.
Limited experience with dialysis indicates that it is not helpful.

DOSAGE AND ADMINISTRATION

The average effective dose is given in the following table:
[See table at top of previous page]

HOW SUPPLIED

Phenergan® with codeine is a clear, purple solution supplied as follows:
NDC 0008-0550-02, case of 24 bottles of 4 fl. oz. (118 mL).
NDC 0008-0550-03, bottle of 1 pint (473 mL).
Keep tightly closed—Store at room temperature, between 15° C and 25° C (59° F and 77° F).
Protect from light.
Dispense in light-resistant, glass, tight container.
Manufactured by:
Wyeth Laboratories Inc.
A Wyeth-Ayerst Company
Philadelphia, PA 19101

PHENERGAN® ℞

[fĕn 'ĕr-găn]
with dextromethorphan
(Promethazine Hydrochloride and Dextromethorphan Hydrobromide)
Syrup

DESCRIPTION

Each teaspoon (5 mL) of Phenergan with dextromethorphan contains 6.25 mg promethazine hydrochloride and 15 mg dextromethorphan hydrobromide in a flavored syrup base with a pH between 4.7 and 5.2. Alcohol 7%. The inactive ingredients present are artificial and natural flavors, citric acid, D&C Yellow 10, FD&C Yellow 6, glycerin, saccharin sodium, sodium benzoate, sodium citrate, sodium propionate, water, and other ingredients.
Promethazine hydrochloride is a racemic compound; the empirical formula is $C_{17}H_{20}N_2S{\cdot}HCl$ and its molecular weight is 320.88.
Promethazine hydrochloride, a phenothiazine derivative, is designated chemically as 10*H*-Phenothiazine-10-ethanamine, *N,N*,α-trimethyl-, monohydrochloride, (±)-, with the following structural formula:

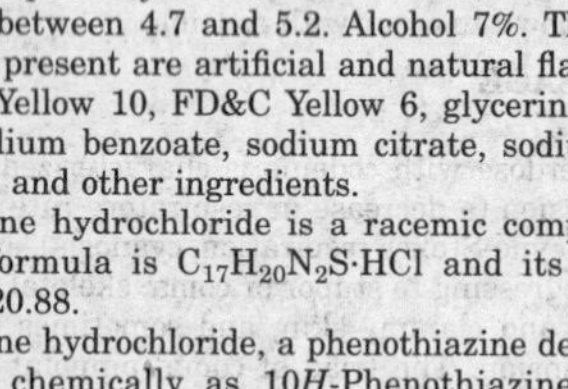

Promethazine hydrochloride occurs as a white to faint yellow, practically odorless, crystalline powder which slowly oxidizes and turns blue on prolonged exposure to air. It is soluble in water and freely soluble in alcohol.
Dextromethorphan hydrobromide is a salt of the methyl ether of the dextrorotatory isomer of levorphanol, a narcotic analgesic. It is chemically named as 3-methoxy-17-methyl-9α, 13α, 14α-morphinan hydrobromide monohydrate with the following structural formula:

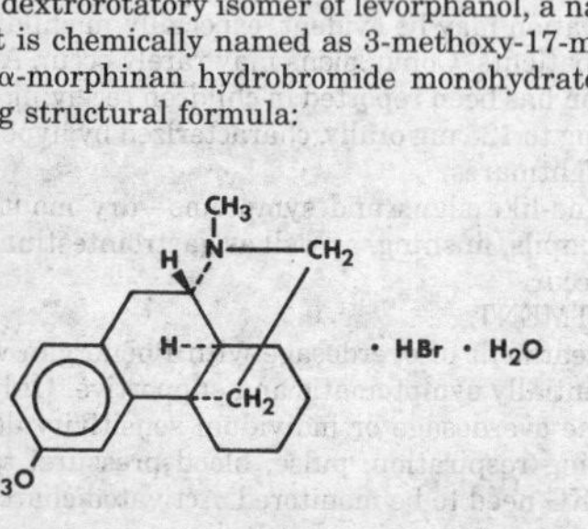

Dextromethorphan hydrobromide monohydrate occurs as white crystals, is sparingly soluble in water, and is freely soluble in alcohol. The empirical formula is $C_{18}H_{25}NO{\cdot}HBr{\cdot}H_2O$, and the molecular weight of the monohydrate is 370.33. Dextromethorphan HBr monohydrate is dextrorotatory with a specific rotation of +27.6 degrees in water (20 degrees C, sodium D-line).

CLINICAL PHARMACOLOGY

PROMETHAZINE
Promethazine is a phenothiazine derivative which differs structurally from the antipsychotic phenothiazines by the presence of a branched side chain and no ring substitution. It is thought that this configuration is responsible for its relative lack (1/10 that of chlorpromazine) of dopaminergic (CNS) action.
Promethazine is an H_1 receptor blocking agent. In addition to its antihistaminic action, it provides clinically useful sedative and antiemetic effects. In therapeutic dosages, promethazine produces no significant effects on the cardiovascular system.
Promethazine is well absorbed from the gastrointestinal tract. Clinical effects are apparent within 20 minutes after oral administration and generally last four to six hours, although they may persist as long as 12 hours. Promethazine is metabolized by the liver to a variety of compounds; the sulfoxides of promethazine and N-demethylpromethazine are the predominant metabolites appearing in the urine.
DEXTROMETHORPHAN
Dextromethorphan is an antitussive agent and, unlike the isomeric levorphanol, it has no analgesic or addictive properties.
The drug acts centrally and elevates the threshold for coughing. It is about equal to codeine in depressing the cough reflex. In therapeutic dosage dextromethorphan does not inhibit ciliary activity.
Dextromethorphan is rapidly absorbed from the gastrointestinal tract and exerts its effect in 15 to 30 minutes. The duration of action after oral administration is approximately three to six hours. Dextromethorphan is metabolized primarily by liver enzymes undergoing O-demethylation, N-demethylation, and partial conjugation with glucuronic acid and sulfate. In humans, (+)-3-hydroxy-N-methylmorphinan, (+)-3-hydroxymorphinan, and traces of unmetabolized drug were found in urine after oral administration.

INDICATIONS AND USAGE

Phenergan with dextromethorphan is indicated for the temporary relief of coughs and upper respiratory symptoms associated with allergy or the common cold.

CONTRAINDICATIONS

Promethazine is contraindicated in individuals known to be hypersensitive or to have had an idiosyncratic reaction to promethazine or to other phenothiazines.
Antihistamines are contraindicated for use in the treatment of lower respiratory tract symptoms, including asthma.
Dextromethorphan should not be used in patients receiving a monoamine oxidase inhibitor (MAOI) (see "PRECAUTIONS—DRUG INTERACTIONS").

WARNINGS

PROMETHAZINE
Promethazine may cause marked drowsiness. Ambulatory patients should be cautioned against such activities as driving or operating dangerous machinery until it is known that they do not become drowsy or dizzy from promethazine therapy.
The sedative action of promethazine hydrochloride is additive to the sedative effects of central nervous system depressants; therefore, agents such as alcohol, narcotic analgesics, sedatives, hypnotics, and tranquilizers should either be eliminated or given in reduced dosage in the presence of promethazine hydrochloride. When given concomitantly with promethazine hydrochloride, the dose of barbiturates should be reduced by at least one-half, and the dose of analgesic depressants, such as morphine or meperidine, should be reduced by one-quarter to one-half.
Promethazine may lower seizure threshold. This should be taken into consideration when administering to persons with known seizure disorders or when giving in combination with narcotics or local anesthetics which may also affect seizure threshold.
Sedative drugs or CNS depressants should be avoided in patients with a history of sleep apnea.
Antihistamines should be used with caution in patients with narrow-angle glaucoma, stenosing peptic ulcer, pyloroduodenal obstruction, and urinary bladder obstruction due to symptomatic prostatic hypertrophy and narrowing of the bladder neck.
Administration of promethazine has been associated with reported cholestatic jaundice.
DEXTROMETHORPHAN
Administration of dextromethorphan may be accompanied by histamine release and should be used with caution in atopic children.

PRECAUTIONS

Animal reproduction studies have not been conducted with the drug combination—promethazine and dextromethorphan. It is not known whether this drug combination can cause fetal harm when administered to a pregnant woman or can affect reproduction capacity. Phenergan with dextromethorphan should be given to a pregnant woman only if clearly needed.
GENERAL
Promethazine should be used cautiously in persons with cardiovascular disease or with impairment of liver function. Dextromethorphan should be used with caution in sedated patients, in the debilitated, and in patients confined to the supine position.
INFORMATION FOR PATIENTS
Phenergan with dextromethorphan may cause marked drowsiness or impair the mental and/or physical abilities required for the performance of potentially hazardous tasks, such as driving a vehicle or operating machinery. Ambulatory patients should be told to avoid engaging in such activities until it is known that they do not become drowsy or dizzy from Phenergan with dextromethorphan therapy. Children should be supervised to avoid potential harm in bike riding or in other hazardous activities.
The concomitant use of alcohol or other central nervous system depressants, including narcotic analgesics, sedatives, hypnotics, and tranquilizers, may have an additive effect and should be avoided or their dosage reduced.
Patients should be advised to report any involuntary muscle movements or unusual sensitivity to sunlight.
DRUG INTERACTIONS
Hyperpyrexia, hypotension, and death have been reported coincident with the coadministration of monoamine oxidase (MAO) inhibitors and products containing dextromethorphan. Thus, concomitant administration of Phenergan with dextromethorphan and MAO inhibitors should be avoided (see "**Contraindications**").
The sedative action of promethazine is additive to the sedative effects of other central nervous system depressants, including alcohol, narcotic analgesics, sedatives, hypnotics, tricyclic antidepressants, and tranquilizers; therefore, these agents should be avoided or administered in reduced dosage to patients receiving promethazine.
DRUG/LABORATORY TEST INTERACTIONS
The following laboratory tests may be affected in patients who are receiving therapy with promethazine hydrochloride:
Pregnancy Tests
Diagnostic pregnancy tests based on immunological reactions between HCG and anti-HCG may result in false-negative or false-positive interpretations.
Glucose Tolerance Test
An increase in blood glucose has been reported in patients receiving promethazine.
CARCINOGENESIS, MUTAGENESIS, IMPAIRMENT OF FERTILITY
Long-term animal studies have not been performed to assess the carcinogenic potential of promethazine or of dextromethorphan. There are no animal or human data concerning the carcinogenicity, mutagenicity, or impairment of fertility with these drugs. Promethazine was nonmutagenic in the *Salmonella* test system of Ames.
PREGNANCY
Teratogenic Effects —Pregnancy Category C
Teratogenic effects have not been demonstrated in rat-feeding studies at doses of 6.25 and 12.5 mg/kg of promethazine. These doses are 8.3 and 16.7 times the maximum recommended total daily dose for a 50-kg subject. Specific studies to test the action of the drug on parturition, lactation, and development of the animal neonate were not done, but a general preliminary study in rats indicated no effect on these parameters. Although antihistamines, including promethazine, have been found to produce fetal mortality in rodents, the pharmacological effects of histamine in the rodent do not parallel those in man. There are no adequate and well-controlled studies of promethazine in pregnant women.
Phenergan with dextromethorphan should be used during pregnancy only if the potential benefit justifies the potential risk to the fetus.
Nonteratogenic Effects
Promethazine taken within two weeks of delivery may inhibit platelet aggregation in the newborn.
LABOR AND DELIVERY
See "*Nonteratogenic Effects.*"
NURSING MOTHERS
It is not known whether promethazine or dextromethorphan is excreted in human milk. Caution should be exercised when Phenergan with dextromethorphan is administered to a nursing woman.
PEDIATRIC USE
This product should not be used in children under 2 years of age because safety for that use has not been established.

ADVERSE REACTIONS

PROMETHAZINE
Nervous System —Sedation, sleepiness, occasional blurred vision, dryness of mouth, dizziness; rarely confusion, disorientation, and extrapyramidal symptoms such as oculogyric crisis, torticollis, and tongue protrusion (usually in association with parenteral injection or excessive dosage).
Cardiovascular —Increased or decreased blood pressure.
Dermatologic —Rash, rarely photosensitivity.

Hematologic —Rarely leukopenia, thrombocytopenia; agranulocytosis (1 case).
Gastrointestinal —Nausea and vomiting.

DEXTROMETHORPHAN

Dextromethorphan hydrobromide occasionally causes slight drowsiness, dizziness, and gastrointestinal disturbances.

DRUG ABUSE AND DEPENDENCE

According to the WHO Expert Committee on Drug Dependence, dextromethorphan could produce very slight psychic dependence but no physical dependence.

OVERDOSAGE

PROMETHAZINE

Signs and symptoms of overdosage with promethazine range from mild depression of the central nervous system and cardiovascular system to profound hypotension, respiratory depression, and unconsciousness.

Stimulation may be evident, especially in children and geriatric patients. Convulsions may rarely occur. A paradoxical reaction has been reported in children receiving single doses of 75 mg to 125 mg orally, characterized by hyperexcitability and nightmares.

Atropine-like signs and symptoms—dry mouth, fixed, dilated pupils, flushing, as well as gastrointestinal symptoms, may occur.

DEXTROMETHORPHAN

Dextromethorphan may produce central excitement and mental confusion. Very high doses may produce respiratory depression. One case of toxic psychosis (hyperactivity, marked visual and auditory hallucinations) after ingestion of a single dose of 20 tablets (300 mg) of dextromethorphan has been reported.

TREATMENT

Treatment of overdosage with Phenergan with dextromethorphan is essentially symptomatic and supportive. Only in cases of extreme overdosage or individual sensitivity do vital signs including respiration, pulse, blood pressure, temperature, and EKG need to be monitored. Activated charcoal orally or by lavage may be given, or sodium or magnesium sulfate orally as a cathartic. Attention should be given to the reestablishment of adequate respiratory exchange through provision of a patent airway and institution of assisted or controlled ventilation. Diazepam may be used to control convulsions. Acidosis and electrolyte losses should be corrected. The antidotal efficacy of narcotic antagonists to dextromethorphan has not been established; note that any of the depressant effects of promethazine are not reversed by naloxone. Avoid analeptics, which may cause convulsions.

Severe hypotension usually responds to the administration of norepinephrine or phenylephrine. EPINEPHRINE SHOULD NOT BE USED, since its use in a patient with partial adrenergic blockade may further lower the blood pressure.

Limited experience with dialysis indicates that it is not helpful.

DOSAGE AND ADMINISTRATION

The average effective dose for adults is one teaspoon (5 mL) every 4 to 6 hours, not to exceed 30.0 mL in 24 hours. For children 6 years to under 12 years of age, the dose is one-half to one teaspoon (2.5 to 5.0 mL) every 4 to 6 hours, not to exceed 20.0 mL in 24 hours. For children 2 years to under 6 years of age, the dose is one-quarter to one-half teaspoon (1.25 to 2.5 mL) every 4 to 6 hours, not to exceed 10.0 mL in 24 hours.

Phenergan with dextromethorphan is not recommended for children under 2 years of age.

HOW SUPPLIED

Phenergan® with dextromethorphan (Promethazine Hydrochloride and Dextromethorphan Hydrobromide) Syrup is a clear, yellow solution supplied as follows:

NDC 0008-0548-02, case of 24 bottles of 4 fl. oz. (118 mL).
NDC 0008-0548-03, bottle of 1 pint (473 mL).

Keep bottles tightly closed and store at room temperature between 15° and 25°C (59° and 77°F).

Protect from light.

Dispense in light-resistant, glass, tight containers.

Manufactured by:
Wyeth Laboratories Inc.
A Wyeth-Ayerst Company
Philadelphia, PA 19101

PHENERGAN® VC ℞

[*fĕn 'ĕr-găn*]

(Promethazine Hydrochloride and Phenylephrine Hydrochloride) Syrup

DESCRIPTION

Each teaspoon (5 mL) of Phenergan VC contains 6.25 mg promethazine hydrochloride and 5 mg phenylephrine hydrochloride in a flavored syrup base with a pH between 4.7 and 5.2. Alcohol 7%. The inactive ingredients present are artificial and natural flavors, citric acid, FD&C Yellow 6, glycerin, saccharin sodium, sodium benzoate, sodium citrate, sodium propionate, water, and other ingredients.

Promethazine hydrochloride is a racemic compound; the empirical formula is $C_{17}H_{20}N_2S{\cdot}HCl$ and its molecular weight is 320.88.

Promethazine hydrochloride, a phenothiazine derivative, is designated chemically as 10*H*-Phenothiazine-10-ethanamine. *N,N*,α-trimethyl-, monohydrochloride, (±)- with the following structural formula:

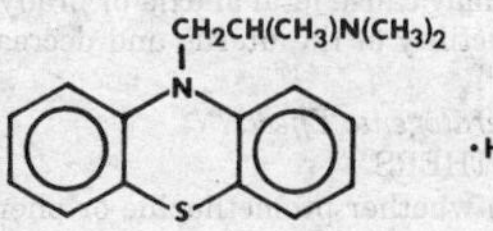

Promethazine hydrochloride occurs as white to faint yellow, practically odorless, crystalline powder which slowly oxidizes and turns blue on prolonged exposure to air. It is soluble in water and freely soluble in alcohol.

Phenylephrine hydrochloride is a sympathomimetic amine salt. It may be chemically named as 3-hydroxy-α-[(methylamino)methyl]-benzenemethanol hydrochloride and has the following chemical formula:

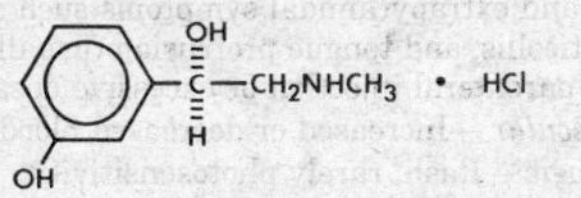

Phenylephrine hydrochloride occurs as white or nearly white crystals, having a bitter taste. It is freely soluble in water and alcohol, with a molecular weight of 203.67. The empirical formula is $C_9H_{13}NO_2{\cdot}HCl$, and the stereochemistry is R-isomer as indicated in the structure; Specific Rotation—between −42° and −47.5°. Phenylephrine hydrochloride is subject to oxidation and must be protected from light and air.

CLINICAL PHARMACOLOGY

PROMETHAZINE

Promethazine is a phenothiazine derivative which differs structurally from the antipsychotic phenothiazines by the presence of a branched side chain and no ring substitution. It is thought that this configuration is responsible for its relative lack (1/10 that of chlorpromazine) of dopaminergic (CNS) action.

Promethazine is an H_1 receptor blocking agent. In addition to its antihistaminic action, it provides clinically useful sedative and antiemetic effects. In therapeutic dosages, promethazine produces no significant effects on the cardiovascular system.

Promethazine is well absorbed from the gastrointestinal tract. Clinical effects are apparent within 20 minutes after oral administration and generally last four to six hours, although they may persist as long as 12 hours. Promethazine is metabolized by the liver to a variety of compounds; the sulfoxides of promethazine and N-demethylpromethazine are the predominant metabolites appearing in the urine.

PHENYLEPHRINE

Phenylephrine is a potent postsynaptic α-receptor agonist with little effect on β receptors of the heart. Phenylephrine has no effect on β-adrenergic receptors of the bronchi or peripheral blood vessels. A direct action at receptors accounts for the greater part of its effects, only a small part being due to its ability to release norepinephrine.

Therapeutic doses of phenylephrine mainly cause vasoconstriction. Phenylephrine increases resistance and, to a lesser extent, decreases capacitance of blood vessels. Total peripheral resistance is increased, resulting in increased systolic and diastolic blood pressure. Pulmonary arterial pressure is usually increased, and renal blood flow is usually decreased. Local vasoconstriction and hemostasis occur following topical application or infiltration of phenylephrine into tissues.

The main effect of phenylephrine on the heart is bradycardia; it produces a positive inotropic effect on the myocardium in doses greater than those usually used therapeutically. Rarely, the drug may increase the irritability of the heart, causing arrhythmias. Cardiac output is decreased slightly. Phenylephrine increases the work of the heart by increasing peripheral arterial resistance.

Phenylephrine has a mild central stimulant effect.

Following oral administration or topical application of phenylephrine to the mucosa, constriction of blood vessels in the nasal mucosa relieves nasal congestion associated with allergy or head colds. Following oral administration, nasal decongestion may occur within 15 or 20 minutes and may persist for up to 4 hours.

Phenylephrine is irregularly absorbed from and readily metabolized in the gastrointestinal tract. Phenylephrine is metabolized in the liver and intestine by monoamine oxidase. The metabolites and their route and rate of excretion have not been identified. The pharmacologic action of phenylephrine is terminated at least partially by uptake of the drug into tissues.

INDICATIONS AND USAGE

Phenergan VC is indicated for the temporary relief of upper respiratory symptoms, including nasal congestion, associated with allergy or the common cold.

CONTRAINDICATIONS

Promethazine is contraindicated in individuals known to be hypersensitive or to have had an idiosyncratic reaction to promethazine or to other phenothiazines.

Antihistamines are contraindicated for use in the treatment of lower respiratory tract symptoms or asthma.

Phenylephrine is contraindicated in patients with hypertension or with peripheral vascular insufficiency (ischemia may result with risk of gangrene or thrombosis of compromised vascular beds). Phenylephrine should not be used in patients known to be hypersensitive to the drug or in those receiving a monoamine oxidase inhibitor (MAOI).

WARNINGS

PROMETHAZINE

Promethazine may cause marked drowsiness. Ambulatory patients should be cautioned against such activities as driving or operating dangerous machinery until it is known that they do not become drowsy or dizzy from promethazine therapy.

The sedative action of promethazine hydrochloride is additive to the sedative effects of central nervous system depressants; therefore, agents such as alcohol, narcotic analgesics, sedatives, hypnotics, and tranquilizers should either be eliminated or given in reduced dosage in the presence of promethazine hydrochloride. When given concomitantly with promethazine hydrochloride, the dose of barbiturates should be reduced by at least one-half, and the dose of analgesic depressants, such as morphine or meperidine, should be reduced by one-quarter to one-half.

Promethazine may lower seizure threshold. This should be taken into consideration when administering to persons with known seizure disorders or when giving in combination with narcotics or local anesthetics which may also affect seizure threshold.

Sedative drugs or CNS depressants should be avoided in patients with a history of sleep apnea.

Antihistamines should be used with caution in patients with narrow-angle glaucoma, stenosing peptic ulcer, pyloroduodenal obstruction, and urinary bladder obstruction due to symptomatic prostatic hypertrophy and narrowing of the bladder neck.

Administration of promethazine has been associated with reported cholestatic jaundice.

PHENYLEPHRINE

Because phenylephrine is an adrenergic agent, it should be given with caution to patients with thyroid diseases, diabetes mellitus, and heart diseases or those receiving tricyclic antidepressants.

Men with symptomatic, benign prostatic hypertrophy can experience urinary retention when given oral nasal decongestants.

Phenylephrine can cause a decrease in cardiac output, and extreme caution should be used when administering the drug, parenterally or orally, to patients with arteriosclerosis, to elderly individuals, and/or to patients with initially poor cerebral or coronary circulation.

Phenylephrine should be used with caution in patients taking diet preparations, such as amphetamines or phenylpropanolamine, because synergistic adrenergic effects could result in serious hypertensive response and possible stroke.

PRECAUTIONS

Animal reproduction studies have not been conducted with the drug combination—promethazine and phenylephrine. It is not known whether this drug combination can cause fetal harm when administered to a pregnant woman or can affect reproduction capacity. Phenergan VC should be given to a pregnant woman only if clearly needed.

GENERAL

Promethazine should be used cautiously in persons with cardiovascular disease or impairment of liver function.

Phenylephrine should be used with caution in patients with cardiovascular disease, particularly hypertension.

INFORMATION FOR PATIENTS

Phenergan VC may cause marked drowsiness or impair the mental and/or physical abilities required for the performance of potentially hazardous tasks, such as driving a vehicle or operating machinery. Ambulatory patients should be told to avoid engaging in such activities until it is known that they do not become drowsy or dizzy from Phenergan VC therapy. Children should be supervised to avoid potential harm in bike riding or other hazardous activities.

Continued on next page

Phenergan VC—Cont.

The concomitant use of alcohol or other central nervous system depressants, including narcotic analgesics, sedatives, hypnotics, and tranquilizers, may have an additive effect and should be avoided or their dosage reduced.

Patients should be advised to report any involuntary muscle movements or unusual sensitivity to sunlight.

DRUG INTERACTIONS
PROMETHAZINE

The sedative action of promethazine is additive to the sedative effects of other central nervous system depressants, including alcohol, narcotic analgesics, sedatives, hypnotics, tricyclic antidepressants, and tranquilizers; therefore, these agents should be avoided or administered in reduced dosage to patients receiving promethazine.

[See table below]

DRUG/LABORATORY TEST INTERACTIONS

The following laboratory tests may be affected in patients who are receiving therapy with promethazine hydrochloride:

Pregnancy Tests

Diagnostic pregnancy tests based on immunological reactions between HCG and anti-HCG may result in false-negative or false-positive interpretations.

Glucose Tolerance Test

An increase in blood glucose has been reported in patients receiving promethazine.

CARCINOGENESIS, MUTAGENESIS, IMPAIRMENT OF FERTILITY
PROMETHAZINE

Long-term animal studies have not been performed to assess the carcinogenic potential of promethazine, nor are there other animal or human data concerning carcinogenicity, mutagenicity, or impairment of fertility with this drug. Promethazine was nonmutagenic in the *Salmonella* test system of Ames.

PHENYLEPHRINE

A study which followed the development of cancer in 143,574 patients over a four-year period indicated that in 11,981 patients who received phenylephrine (systemic or topical), there was no statistically significant association between the drug and cancer at any or all sites.

Long-term animal studies have not been performed to assess the carcinogenic potential of phenylephrine, nor are there other animal or human data concerning mutagenicity.

A study of the effects of adrenergic drugs on ovum transport in rabbits indicated that treatment with phenylephrine did not alter incidence of pregnancy; the number of implantations was significantly reduced when high doses of the drug were used.

PREGNANCY

Teratogenic Effects —Pregnancy Category C

PROMETHAZINE

Teratogenic effects have not been demonstrated in rat-feeding studies at doses of 6.25 and 12.5 mg/kg of promethazine. These doses are 8.3 and 16.7 times the maximum recommended total daily dose of promethazine for a 50-kg subject. Specific studies to test the action of the drug on parturition, lactation, and development of the animal neonate were not done, but a general preliminary study in rats indicated no effect on these parameters. Although antihistamines, including promethazine, have been found to produce fetal mortality in rodents, the pharmacological effects of histamine in the rodent do not parallel those in man. There are no adequate and well-controlled studies of promethazine in pregnant women.

PHENYLEPHRINE

A study in rabbits indicated that continued moderate overexposure to phenylephrine (3 mg/day) during the second half of pregnancy (22nd day of gestation to delivery) may contribute to perinatal wastage, prematurity, premature labor, and possibly fetal anomalies; when phenylephrine (3 mg/day) was given to rabbits during the first half of pregnancy (3rd day after mating for seven days), a significant number gave birth to litters of low birth weight. Another

study showed that phenylephrine was associated with anomalies of aortic arch and with ventricular septal defect in the chick embryo.

Phenergan VC should be used during pregnancy only if the potential benefit justifies the potential risk to the fetus.

Nonteratogenic Effects

Promethazine taken within two weeks of delivery may inhibit platelet aggregation in the newborn.

LABOR AND DELIVERY

Administration of phenylephrine to patients in late pregnancy or labor may cause fetal anoxia or bradycardia by increasing contractility of the uterus and decreasing uterine blood flow.

See also *"Nonteratogenic Effects."*

NURSING MOTHERS

It is not known whether promethazine or phenylephrine is excreted in human milk.

Caution should be exercised when Phenergan VC is administered to a nursing woman.

PEDIATRIC USE

This product should not be used in children under 2 years of age because safety for such use has not been established.

ADVERSE REACTIONS
PROMETHAZINE

Nervous System —Sedation, sleepiness, occasional blurred vision, dryness of mouth, dizziness; rarely confusion, disorientation, and extrapyramidal symptoms such as oculogyric crisis, torticollis, and tongue protrusion (usually in association with parenteral injection or excessive dosage).

Cardiovascular —Increased or decreased blood pressure.

Dermatologic —Rash, rarely photosensitivity.

Hematologic —Rarely leukopenia, thrombocytopenia; agranulocytosis (1 case).

Gastrointestinal —Nausea and vomiting.

PHENYLEPHRINE

Nervous System —Restlessness, anxiety, nervousness, and dizziness.

Cardiovascular —Hypertension (see **"Warnings"**).

Other —Precordial pain, respiratory distress, tremor, and weakness.

Overdosage
PROMETHAZINE

Signs and symptoms of overdosage with promethazine range from mild depression of the central nervous system and cardiovascular system to profound hypotension, respiratory depression, and unconsciousness.

Stimulation may be evident, especially in children and geriatric patients. Convulsions may rarely occur. A paradoxical reaction has been reported in children receiving single doses of 75 mg to 125 mg orally, characterized by hyperexcitability and nightmares.

Atropine-like signs and symptoms—dry mouth, fixed, dilated pupils, flushing, as well as gastrointestinal symptoms, may occur.

PHENYLEPHRINE

Signs and symptoms of overdosage with phenylephrine include hypertension, headache, convulsions, cerebral hemorrhage, and vomiting. Ventricular premature beats and short paroxysms of ventricular tachycardia may also occur. Headache may be a symptom of hypertension. Bradycardia may also be seen early in phenylephrine overdosage through stimulation of baroreceptors.

TREATMENT

Treatment of overdosage with Phenergan VC is essentially symptomatic and supportive. Only in cases of extreme overdosage or individual sensitivity do vital signs including respiration, pulse, blood pressure, temperature, and EKG need to be monitored. Activated charcoal orally or by lavage may be given, or sodium or magnesium sulfate orally as a cathartic. Attention should be given to the reestablishment of adequate respiratory exchange through provision of a patent airway and institution of assisted or controlled ventilation. Diazepam may be used to control convulsions. Acidosis and

electrolyte losses should be corrected. Note that any depressant effects of promethazine are not reversed by naloxone. Avoid analeptics which may cause convulsions.

Severe hypotension usually responds to the administration of norepinephrine or phenylephrine. EPINEPHRINE SHOULD NOT BE USED, since its use in patients with partial adrenergic blockade may further lower the blood pressure.

Limited experience with dialysis indicates that it is not helpful.

DOSAGE AND ADMINISTRATION

The recommended adult dose is one teaspoon (5 mL) every 4 to 6 hours, not to exceed 30.0 mL in 24 hours. For children 6 years to under 12 years of age, the dose is one-half to one teaspoon (2.5 to 5.0 mL) repeated at 4- to 6-hour intervals, not to exceed 30.0 mL in 24 hours. For children 2 years to under 6 years of age, the dose is one-quarter to one-half teaspoon (1.25 to 2.5 mL) every 4 to 6 hours.

Phenergan VC is not recommended for children under 2 years of age.

HOW SUPPLIED

Phenergan® VC (Promethazine Hydrochloride and Phenylephrine Hydrochloride) Syrup, is a clear, orange-yellow solution supplied as follows:

NDC 0008-0551-02, case of 24 bottles of 4 fl. oz. (118 mL).
NDC 0008-0551-03, bottle of 1 pint (473 mL).

Keep bottles tightly closed and store at room temperature between 15° and 25°C (59° and 77°F).
Protect from light.
Dispense in light-resistant, glass, tight containers.
Manufactured by:
Wyeth Laboratories Inc.
A Wyeth-Ayerst Company
Philadelphia, PA 19101

PHENERGAN® VC   C B
[fĕn 'ĕr-gan]
with codeine
(Warning—may be habit-forming)
(Promethazine Hydrochloride,
Phenylephrine Hydrochloride, and
Codeine Phosphate) Syrup

DESCRIPTION

Each teaspoon (5 mL) of Phenergan VC with codeine contains 10 mg codeine phosphate (Warning—may be habit-forming), 6.25 mg promethazine hydrochloride, and 5 mg phenylephrine hydrochloride in a flavored syrup base with a pH between 4.7 and 5.2. Alcohol 7%. The inactive ingredients present are artificial and natural flavors, citric acid, D&C Red 33, FD&C Yellow 6, glycerin, saccharin sodium, sodium benzoate, sodium citrate, sodium propionate, water, and other ingredients.

Codeine is one of the naturally occurring phenanthrene alkaloids derived from the opium poppy; it is classified pharmacologically as a narcotic analgesic. Codeine phosphate may be chemically named as $(5\alpha,6\alpha)$–7,8–didehydro–4,5–epoxy–3–methoxy–17–methylmorphinan–6–ol phosphate (1:1) (salt) hemihydrate with the following structural formula:

The phosphate salt of codeine occurs as white, needle-shaped crystals or white crystalline powder. Codeine phosphate is freely soluble in water and slightly soluble in alcohol, with a molecular weight of 406.37. The empirical formula is $C_{18}H_{21}NO_3 \cdot H_3PO_4 \cdot ^1/_2 H_2O$, and the stereochemistry is $5\alpha, 6\alpha$ isomer as indicated in the structure.

Promethazine hydrochloride is a racemic compound; the empirical formula is $C_{17}H_{20}N_2S \cdot HCl$ and its molecular weight is 320.88.

Promethazine hydrochloride, a phenothiazine derivative, is designated chemically as 10*H*-Phenothiazine-10-ethanamine, *N,N,α*-trimethyl-, monohydrochloride, (±)- with the following structural formula:

[See chemical structure at top of next column]

Promethazine hydrochloride occurs as a white to faint yellow, practically odorless, crystalline powder which slowly oxidizes and turns blue on prolonged exposure to air. It is soluble in water and freely soluble in alcohol.

Phenylephrine hydrochloride is a sympathomimetic amine salt. It may be chemically named as 3-hydroxy-α-[(methyl-

---

PHENERGAN VC

PHENYLEPHRINE

Drug	Effect
Phenylephrine with prior administration of monoamine oxidase inhibitors (MAOI).	Cardiac pressor response potentiated. May cause acute hypertensive crisis.
Phenylephrine with tricyclic antidepressants.	Pressor response increased.
Phenylephrine with ergot alkaloids.	Excessive rise in blood pressure.
Phenylephrine with bronchodilator sympathomimetic agents and with epinephrine or other sympathomimetics.	Tachycardia or other arrhythmias may occur.
Phenylephrine with prior administration of propranolol or other β-adrenergic blockers.	Cardiostimulating effects blocked.
Phenylephrine with atropine sulfate.	Reflex bradycardia blocked; pressor response enhanced.
Phenylephrine with prior administration of phentolamine or other α-adrenergic blockers.	Pressor response decreased.
Phenylephrine with diet preparations, such as amphetamines or phenylpropanolamine.	Synergistic adrenergic response.

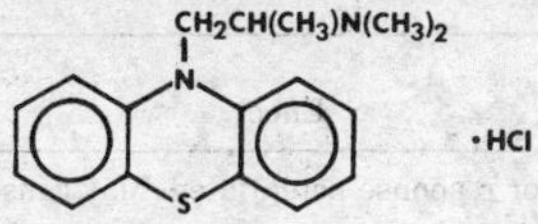

amino)methyl]-benzenemethanol hydrochloride and has the following chemical formula:

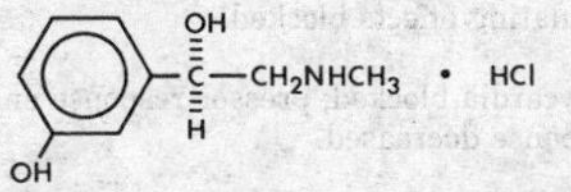

Phenylephrine hydrochloride occurs as white or nearly white crystals, having a bitter taste. It is freely soluble in water and alcohol, with a molecular weight of 203.67. The empirical formula is $C_9H_{13}NO_2 \cdot HCl$, and the stereochemistry is R-isomer as indicated in the structure; Specific Rotation—between −42° and −47.5°. Phenylephrine hydrochloride is subject to oxidation and must be protected from light and air.

CLINICAL PHARMACOLOGY

CODEINE: Narcotic analgesics, including codeine, exert their primary effects on the central nervous system and gastrointestinal tract. The analgesic effects of codeine are due to its central action; however, the precise sites of action have not been determined, and the mechanisms involved appear to be quite complex. Codeine resembles morphine both structurally and pharmacologically, but its actions at the doses of codeine used therapeutically are milder, with less sedation, respiratory depression, and gastrointestinal, urinary, and pupillary effects. Codeine produces an increase in biliary tract pressure, but less than morphine or meperidine. Codeine is less constipating than morphine.

Codeine has good antitussive activity, although less than that of morphine at equal doses. It is used in preference to morphine, because side effects are infrequent at the usual antitussive dose of codeine.

Codeine in oral therapeutic dosage does not usually exert major effects on the cardiovascular system.

Narcotic analgesics may cause nausea and vomiting by stimulating the chemoreceptor trigger zone (CTZ); however, they also depress the vomiting center, so that subsequent doses are unlikely to produce vomiting. Nausea is minimal after usual oral doses of codeine.

Narcotic analgesics cause histamine release, which appears to be responsible for wheals or urticaria sometimes seen at the site of injection on parenteral administration. Histamine release may also produce dilation of cutaneous blood vessels, with resultant flushing of the face and neck, pruritus, and sweating.

Codeine and its salts are well absorbed following both oral and parenteral administration. Codeine is about $^2/_3$ as effective orally as parenterally. Codeine is metabolized primarily in the liver by enzymes of the endoplasmic reticulum, where it undergoes O-demethylation, N-demethylation, and partial conjugation with glucuronic acid. The drug is excreted primarily in the urine, largely as inactive metabolites and small amounts of free and conjugated morphine. Negligible amounts of codeine and its metabolites are found in the feces.

Following oral or subcutaneous administration of codeine, the onset of analgesia occurs within 15 to 30 minutes and lasts for four to six hours.

The cough-depressing action, in animal studies, was observed to occur 15 minutes after oral administration of codeine, peak action at 45 to 60 minutes after ingestion. The duration of action, which is dose-dependent, usually did not exceed 3 hours.

PROMETHAZINE: Promethazine is a phenothiazine derivative which differs structurally from the antipsychotic phenothiazines by the presence of a branched side chain and no ring substitution. It is thought that this configuration is responsible for its relative lack ($^1/_{10}$ that of chlorpromazine) of dopaminergic (CNS) action.

Promethazine is an H_1 receptor blocking agent. In addition to its antihistaminic action, it provides clinically useful sedative and antiemetic effects. In therapeutic dosages, promethazine produces no significant effects on the cardiovascular system.

Promethazine is well absorbed from the gastrointestinal tract. Clinical effects are apparent within 20 minutes after oral administration and generally last four to six hours, although they may persist as long as 12 hours. Promethazine is metabolized by the liver to a variety of compounds; the sulfoxides of promethazine and N-demethylpromethazine are the predominant metabolites appearing in the urine.

PHENYLEPHRINE: Phenylephrine is a potent postsynaptic α-receptor agonist with little effect on β receptors of the heart. Phenylephrine has no effect on β-adrenergic receptors of the bronchi or peripheral blood vessels. A direct action at receptors accounts for the greater part of its effects, only a small part being due to its ability to release norepinephrine.

Therapeutic doses of phenylephrine mainly cause vasoconstriction. Phenylephrine increases resistance and, to a lesser extent, decreases capacitance of blood vessels. Total peripheral resistance is increased, resulting in increased systolic and diastolic blood pressure. Pulmonary arterial pressure is usually increased, and renal blood flow is usually decreased. Local vasoconstriction and hemostasis occur following topical application or infiltration of phenylephrine into tissues.

The main effect of phenylephrine on the heart is bradycardia; it produces a positive inotropic effect on the myocardium in doses greater than those usually used therapeutically. Rarely, the drug may increase the irritability of the heart, causing arrhythmias. Cardiac output is decreased slightly. Phenylephrine increases the work of the heart by increasing peripheral arterial resistance.

Phenylephrine has a mild central stimulant effect.

Following oral administration or topical application of phenylephrine to the mucosa, constriction of blood vessels in the nasal mucosa relieves nasal congestion associated with allergy or head colds. Following oral administration, nasal decongestion may occur within 15 or 20 minutes and may persist for up to 4 hours.

Phenylephrine is irregularly absorbed from and readily metabolized in the gastrointestinal tract. Phenylephrine is metabolized in the liver and intestine by monoamine oxidase. The metabolites and their route and rate of excretion have not been identified. The pharmacologic action of phenylephrine is terminated at least partially by uptake of the drug into tissues.

INDICATIONS AND USAGE

Phenergan VC with codeine is indicated for the temporary relief of coughs and upper respiratory symptoms, including nasal congestion, associated with allergy or the common cold.

CONTRAINDICATIONS

Codeine is contraindicated in patients with a known hypersensitivity to the drug.

Promethazine is contraindicated in individuals known to be hypersensitive or to have had an idiosyncratic reaction to promethazine or to other phenothiazines.

Phenylephrine is contraindicated in patients with hypertension or with peripheral vascular insufficiency (ischemia may result with risk of gangrene or thrombosis of compromised vascular beds). Phenylephrine should not be used in patients known to be hypersensitive to the drug or in those receiving a monoamine oxidase inhibitor (MAOI).

Antihistamines and codeine are both contraindicated for use in the treatment of lower respiratory tract symptoms, including asthma.

WARNINGS

CODEINE: Dosage of codeine SHOULD NOT BE INCREASED if cough fails to respond; an unresponsive cough should be reevaluated in 5 days or sooner for possible underlying pathology, such as foreign body or lower respiratory tract disease.

Codeine may cause or aggravate constipation.

Respiratory depression leading to arrest, coma, and death has occurred with the use of codeine antitussives in young children, particularly in the under-one-year infants whose ability to deactivate the drug is not fully developed.

Administration of codeine may be accompanied by histamine release and should be used with caution in atopic children.

Head Injury and Increased Intracranial Pressure

The respiratory-depressant effects of narcotic analgesics and their capacity to elevate cerebrospinal fluid pressure may be markedly exaggerated in the presence of head injury, intracranial lesions, or a preexisting increase in intracranial pressure. Narcotics may produce adverse reactions which may obscure the clinical course of patients with head injuries.

Asthma and Other Respiratory Conditions

Narcotic analgesics or cough suppressants, including codeine, should not be used in asthmatic patients (see "**Contraindications**"). Nor should they be used in acute febrile illness associated with productive cough or in chronic respiratory disease where interference with ability to clear the tracheobronchial tree of secretions would have a deleterious effect on the patient's respiratory function.

Hypotensive Effect

Codeine may produce orthostatic hypotension in ambulatory patients.

PROMETHAZINE: Promethazine may cause marked drowsiness. Ambulatory patients should be cautioned against such activities as driving or operating dangerous machinery until it is known that they do not become drowsy or dizzy from promethazine therapy.

The sedative action of promethazine hydrochloride is additive to the sedative effects of central nervous system depressants; therefore, agents such as alcohol, narcotic analgesics, sedatives, hypnotics, and tranquilizers should either be eliminated or given in reduced dosage in the presence of promethazine hydrochloride. When given concomitantly with promethazine hydrochloride, the dose of barbiturates should be reduced by at least one-half, and the dose of analgesic depressants, such as morphine or meperidine, should be reduced by one-quarter to one-half.

Promethazine may lower seizure threshold. This should be taken into consideration when administering to persons with known seizure disorders or when giving in combination with narcotics or local anesthetics which may also affect seizure threshold.

Sedative drugs or CNS depressants should be avoided in patients with a history of sleep apnea. Antihistamines should be used with caution in patients with narrow-angle glaucoma, stenosing peptic ulcer, pyloroduodenal obstruction, and urinary bladder obstruction due to symptomatic prostatic hypertrophy and narrowing of the bladder neck.

Administration of promethazine has been associated with reported cholestatic jaundice.

PHENYLEPHRINE: Because phenylephrine is an adrenergic agent, it should be given with caution to patients with thyroid diseases, diabetes mellitus, and heart diseases or those receiving tricyclic antidepressants.

Men with symptomatic, benign prostatic hypertrophy can experience urinary retention when given oral nasal decongestants.

Phenylephrine can cause a decrease in cardiac output, and extreme caution should be used when administering the drug, parenterally or orally, to patients with arteriosclerosis, to elderly individuals, and/or to patients with initially poor cerebral or coronary circulation.

Phenylephrine should be used with caution in patients taking diet preparations, such as amphetamines or phenylpropanolamine, because synergistic adrenergic effects could result in serious hypertensive response and possible stroke.

PRECAUTIONS

Animal reproduction studies have not been conducted with the drug combination—promethazine, phenylephrine, and codeine. It is not known whether this drug combination can cause fetal harm when administered to a pregnant woman or can affect reproduction capacity. Phenergan VC with codeine should be given to a pregnant woman only if clearly needed.

GENERAL

Narcotic analgesics, including codeine, should be administered with caution and the initial dose reduced in patients with acute abdominal conditions, convulsive disorders, significant hepatic or renal impairment, fever, hypothyroidism, Addison's disease, ulcerative colitis, prostatic hypertrophy, in patients with recent gastrointestinal or urinary tract surgery, and in the very young or elderly or debilitated patients.

Promethazine should be used cautiously in persons with cardiovascular disease or with impairment of liver function.

Phenylephrine should be used with caution in patients with cardiovascular disease, particularly hypertension.

INFORMATION FOR PATIENTS

Phenergan VC with codeine may cause marked drowsiness or impair the mental and/or physical abilities required for the performance of potentially hazardous tasks, such as driving a vehicle or operating machinery. Ambulatory patients should be told to avoid engaging in such activities until it is known that they do not become drowsy or dizzy from Phenergan VC with codeine therapy. Children should be supervised to avoid potential harm in bike riding or in other hazardous activities.

The concomitant use of alcohol or other central nervous system depressants, including narcotic analgesics, sedatives, hypnotics, and tranquilizers, may have an additive effect and should be avoided or their dosage reduced.

Patients should be advised to report any involuntary muscle movements or unusual sensitivity to sunlight.

Codeine, like other narcotic analgesics, may produce orthostatic hypotension in some ambulatory patients. Patients should be cautioned accordingly.

DRUG INTERACTIONS

CODEINE: In patients receiving MAO inhibitors, an initial small test dose is advisable to allow observation of any excessive narcotic effects or MAOI interaction.

PROMETHAZINE: The sedative action of promethazine is additive to the effects of other central nervous system depressants, including alcohol, narcotic analgesics, sedatives, hypnotics, tricyclic antidepressants, and tranquilizers; therefore, these agents should be avoided or administered in reduced dosage to patients receiving promethazine.

[See first table at top of next page]

DRUG/LABORATORY TEST INTERACTIONS

Because narcotic analgesics may increase biliary tract pressure, with resultant increases in plasma amylase or lipase levels, determination of these enzyme levels may be unreliable for 24 hours after a narcotic analgesic has been given.

Continued on next page

Phenergan VC w/Codeine—Cont.

The following laboratory tests may be affected in patients who are receiving therapy with promethazine hydrochloride:

Pregnancy Tests

Diagnostic pregnancy tests based on immunological reactions between HCG and anti-HCG may result in false-negative or false-positive interpretations.

Glucose Tolerance Test

An increase in blood glucose has been reported in patients receiving promethazine.

CARCINOGENESIS, MUTAGENESIS, IMPAIRMENT OF FERTILITY

CODEINE AND PROMETHAZINE

Long-term animal studies have not been performed to assess the carcinogenic potential of codeine or of promethazine, nor are there other animal or human data concerning carcinogenicity, mutagenicity, or impairment of fertility with these agents. Codeine has been reported to show no evidence of carcinogenicity or mutagenicity in a variety of test systems, including the micronucleus and sperm abnormality assays and the *Salmonella* assay. Promethazine was nonmutagenic in the *Salmonella* test system of Ames.

PHENYLEPHRINE

A study which followed the development of cancer in 143,574 patients over a four-year period indicated that in 11,981 patients who received phenylephrine (systemic or topical), there was no statistically significant association between the drug and cancer at any or all sites.

Long-term animal studies have not been performed to assess the carcinogenic potential of phenylephrine, nor are there other animal or human data concerning mutagenicity.

A study of the effects of adrenergic drugs on ovum transport in rabbits indicated that treatment with phenylephrine did not alter incidence of pregnancy; the number of implantations was significantly reduced when high doses of the drug were used.

PREGNANCY

Teratogenic Effects —Pregnancy Category C

CODEINE: A study in rats and rabbits reported no teratogenic effect of codeine administered during the period of organogenesis in doses ranging from 5 to 120 mg/kg. In the rat, doses at the 120-mg/kg level, in the toxic range for the adult animal, were associated with an increase in embryo resorption at the time of implantation. In another study a single 100-mg/kg dose of codeine administered to pregnant mice reportedly resulted in delayed ossification in the offspring.

There are no studies in humans, and the significance of these findings to humans, if any, is not known.

PROMETHAZINE: Teratogenic effects have not been demonstrated in rat-feeding studies at doses of 6.25 and 12.5 mg/kg of promethazine. These doses are 8.3 and 16.7 times the maximum recommended total daily dose for a 50-kg subject. Specific studies to test the action of the drug on parturition, lactation, and development of the animal neonate were not done, but a general preliminary study in rats indicated no effect on these parameters. Although antihistamines, including promethazine, have been found to produce fetal mortality in rodents, the pharmacological effects of histamine in the rodent do not parallel those in man. There are no adequate and well-controlled studies of promethazine in pregnant women.

PHENYLEPHRINE: A study in rabbits indicated that continued moderate overexposure to phenylephrine (3 mg/day) during the second half of pregnancy (22nd day of gestation to delivery) may contribute to perinatal wastage, prematurity, premature labor, and possibly fetal anomalies; when phenylephrine (3 mg/day) was given to rabbits during the first half of pregnancy (3rd day after mating for seven days), a significant number gave birth to litters of low birth weight. Another study showed that phenylephrine was associated with anomalies of aortic arch and with ventricular septal defect in the chick embryo.

Phenergan VC with codeine should be used during pregnancy only if the potential benefit justifies the potential risk to the fetus.

Nonteratogenic Effects

Dependence has been reported in newborns whose mothers took opiates regularly during pregnancy. Withdrawal signs include irritability, excessive crying, tremors, hyperreflexia, fever, vomiting, and diarrhea. Signs usually appear during the first few days of life.

Promethazine taken within two weeks of delivery may inhibit platelet aggregation in the newborn.

LABOR AND DELIVERY

Narcotic analgesics cross the placental barrier. The closer to delivery and the larger the dose used, the greater the possibility of respiratory depression in the newborn. Narcotic analgesics should be avoided during labor if delivery of a premature infant is anticipated. If the mother has received narcotic analgesics during labor, newborn infants should be observed closely for signs of respiratory depression. Resuscitation may be required (see "**Overdosage**"). The effect of codeine, if any, on the later growth, development, and functional maturation of the child is unknown.

Administration of phenylephrine to patients in late pregnancy or labor may cause fetal anoxia or bradycardia by increasing contractility of the uterus and decreasing uterine blood flow.

See also "*Nonteratogenic Effects.*"

NURSING MOTHERS

Some studies, but not others, have reported detectable amounts of codeine in breast milk. The levels are probably not clinically significant after usual therapeutic dosage. The possibility of clinically important amounts being excreted in breast milk in individuals abusing codeine should be considered.

It is not known whether either phenylephrine or promethazine is excreted in human milk.

Caution should be exercised when Phenergan VC with codeine is administered to a nursing woman.

PEDIATRIC USE

This product should not be used in children under 2 years of age because safety for such use has not been established.

ADVERSE REACTIONS

CODEINE

Nervous System —CNS depression, particularly respiratory depression, and to a lesser extent circulatory depression; light-headedness, dizziness, sedation, euphoria, dysphoria, headache, transient hallucination, disorientation, visual disturbances, and convulsions.

Cardiovascular —Tachycardia, bradycardia, palpitation, faintness, syncope, orthostatic hypotension (common to narcotic analgesics).

Gastrointestinal —Nausea, vomiting, constipation, and biliary tract spasm. Patients with chronic ulcerative colitis may experience increased colonic motility; in patients with acute ulcerative colitis, toxic dilation has been reported.

Genitourinary —Oliguria, urinary retention; antidiuretic effect has been reported (common to narcotic analgesics).

Allergic —Infrequent pruritus, giant urticaria, angioneurotic edema, and laryngeal edema.

Other —Flushing of the face, sweating and pruritus (due to opiate-induced histamine release); weakness.

PROMETHAZINE

Nervous System —Sedation, sleepiness, occasional blurred vision, dryness of mouth, dizziness; rarely confusion, disorientation, and extrapyramidal symptoms such as oculogyric crisis, torticollis, and tongue protrusion (usually in association with parenteral injection or excessive dosage).

Cardiovascular —Increased or decreased blood pressure.

Dermatologic —Rash, rarely photosensitivity.

Hematologic —Rarely leukopenia, thrombocytopenia; agranulocytosis (1 case).

Gastrointestinal —Nausea and vomiting.

PHENYLEPHRINE

Nervous System —Restlessness, anxiety, nervousness, and dizziness.

Cardiovascular —Hypertension (see "**Warnings**").

Other —Precordial pain, respiratory distress, tremor, and weakness.

PHENERGAN VC WITH CODEINE

PHENYLEPHRINE

Drug	Effect
Phenylephrine with prior administration of monoamine oxidase inhibitors (MAOI).	Cardiac pressor response potentiated. May cause acute hypertensive crisis.
Phenylephrine with tricyclic antidepressants.	Pressor response increased.
Phenylephrine with ergot alkaloids.	Excessive rise in blood pressure.
Phenylephrine with bronchodilator sympathomimetic agents and with epinephrine or other sympathomimetics.	Tachycardia or other arrhythmias may occur.
Phenylephrine with prior administration of propranolol or other β-adrenergic blockers.	Cardiostimulating effects blocked.
Phenylephrine with atropine sulfate.	Reflex bradycardia blocked; pressor response enhanced.
Phenylephrine with prior administration of phentolamine or other α-adrenergic blockers.	Pressor response decreased.
Phenylephrine with diet preparations, such as amphetamines or phenylpropanolamine.	Synergistic adrenergic response.

PHENERGAN VC WITH CODEINE

Adults	1 teaspoon (5 mL) every 4 to 6 hours, not to exceed 30.0 mL in 24 hours.
Children 6 years to under 12 years	1/2 to 1 teaspoon (2.5 to 5 mL) every 4 to 6 hours, not to exceed 30.0 mL in 24 hours.
Children under 6 years (weight: 18 kg or 40 lbs)	1/4 to 1/2 teaspoon (1.25 to 2.5 mL) every 4 to 6 hours, not to exceed 9.0 mL in 24 hours.
Children under 6 years (weight: 16 kg or 35 lbs)	1/4 to 1/2 teaspoon (1.25 to 2.5 mL) every 4 to 6 hours, not to exceed 8.0 mL in 24 hours.
Children under 6 years (weight: 14 kg or 30 lbs)	1/4 to 1/2 teaspoon (1.25 to 2.5 mL) every 4 to 6 hours, not to exceed 7.0 mL in 24 hours.
Children under 6 years (weight: 12 kg or 25 lbs)	1/4 to 1/2 teaspoon (1.25 to 2.5 mL) every 4 to 6 hours, not to exceed 6.0 mL in 24 hours.

Phenergan VC with codeine is not recommended for children under 2 years of age.

DRUG ABUSE AND DEPENDENCE

CONTROLLED SUBSTANCE

Phenergan VC with codeine is a Schedule V Controlled Substance.

ABUSE

Codeine is known to be subject to abuse; however, the abuse potential of oral codeine appears to be quite low. Even parenteral codeine does not appear to offer the psychic effects sought by addicts to the same degree as heroin or morphine. However, codeine must be administered only under close supervision to patients with a history of drug abuse or dependence.

DEPENDENCE

Psychological dependence, physical dependence, and tolerance are known to occur with codeine.

OVERDOSAGE

CODEINE: Serious overdose with codeine is characterized by respiratory depression (a decrease in respiratory rate and/or tidal volume, Cheyne-Stokes respiration, cyanosis), extreme somnolence progressing to stupor or coma, skeletal muscle flaccidity, cold and clammy skin, and sometimes bradycardia and hypotension. The triad of coma, pinpoint pupils, and respiratory depression is strongly suggestive of opiate poisoning. In severe overdosage, particularly by the intravenous route, apnea, circulatory collapse, cardiac arrest, and death may occur. Promethazine is additive to the depressant effects of codeine.

It is difficult to determine what constitutes a standard toxic or lethal dose. However, the lethal oral dose of codeine in an adult is reported to be in the range of 0.5 to 1.0 gram. Infants and children are believed to be relatively more sensitive to opiates on a body-weight basis. Elderly patients are also comparatively intolerant to opiates.

PROMETHAZINE: Signs and symptoms of overdosage with promethazine range from mild depression of the central nervous system and cardiovascular system to profound hypotension, respiratory depression, and unconsciousness. Stimulation may be evident, especially in children and geriatric patients. Convulsions may rarely occur. A paradoxical reaction has been reported in children receiving single doses of 75 mg to 125 mg orally, characterized by hyperexcitability and nightmares.

Atropine-like signs and symptoms—dry mouth, fixed, dilated pupils, flushing, as well as gastrointestinal symptoms, may occur.

PHENYLEPHRINE: Signs and symptoms of overdosage with phenylephrine include hypertension, headache, convulsions, cerebral hemorrhage, and vomiting. Ventricular premature beats and short paroxysms of ventricular tachycardia may also occur. Headache may be a symptom of hypertension. Bradycardia may also be seen early in phenylephrine overdosage through stimulation of baroreceptors.

TREATMENT

Treatment of overdosage with Phenergan VC with codeine is essentially symptomatic and supportive. Only in cases of extreme overdosage or individual sensitivity do vital signs including respiration, pulse, blood pressure, temperature, and EKG need to be monitored. Activated charcoal orally or by lavage may be given, or sodium or magnesium sulfate

orally as a cathartic. Attention should be given to the reestablishment of adequate respiratory exchange through provision of a patent airway and institution of assisted or controlled ventilation. The narcotic antagonist, naloxone hydrochloride, may be administered when significant respiratory depression occurs with Phenergan VC with codeine; any depressant effects of promethazine are not reversed by naloxone. Diazepam may be used to control convulsions. Avoid analeptics, which may cause convulsions. Acidosis and electrolyte losses should be corrected. A rise in temperature or pulmonary complications may signal the need for institution of antibiotic therapy.

Severe hypotension usually responds to the administration of norepinephrine or phenylephrine. EPINEPHRINE SHOULD NOT BE USED, since its use in a patient with partial adrenergic blockade may further lower the blood pressure.

Limited experience with dialysis indicates that it is not helpful.

DOSAGE AND ADMINISTRATION

The average effective dose is given in the following table: [See second table at top of previous page]

HOW SUPPLIED

Phenergan® VC with codeine is a clear, reddish-orange solution supplied as follows:

NDC 0008-0552-02, case of 24 bottles of 4 fl. oz. (118 mL).
NDC 0008-0552-03, bottle of 1 pint (473 mL).
Keep tightly closed—Stored at room temperature, between 15° C and 25° C (59° F and 77° F).
Protect from light.
Dispense in light-resistant, glass, tight container.
Manufactured by:
Wyeth Laboratories Inc.
A Wyeth-Ayerst Company
Philadelphia, PA 19101

PREMARIN® INTRAVENOUS   ℞

[prĕm 'a-rĭn]
(conjugated estrogens, USP)
for Injection
Specially prepared for Intravenous &
Intramuscular use

Rx only

1. ESTROGENS HAVE BEEN REPORTED TO INCREASE THE RISK OF ENDOMETRIAL CARCINOMA.

Three independent, case-controlled studies have reported an increased risk of endometrial cancer in postmenopausal women exposed to exogenous estrogens for more than one year.[1–3] This risk was independent of the other known risk factors for endometrial cancer. These studies are further supported by the finding that incidence rates of endometrial cancer have increased sharply since 1969 in eight different areas of the United States with population-based cancer-reporting systems, an increase which may be related to the rapidly expanding use of estrogens during the last decade.[4]

The three case-controlled studies reported that the risk of endometrial cancer in estrogen users was about 4.5 to 13.9 times greater than in nonusers. The risk appears to depend on both duration of treatment[1] and on estrogen dose.[3] In view of these findings, when estrogens are used for the treatment of menopausal symptoms, the lowest dose that will control symptoms should be utilized and medication should be discontinued as soon as possible. When prolonged treatment is medically indicated, the patient should be reassessed, on at least a semi-annual basis, to determine the need for continued therapy. Although the evidence must be considered preliminary, one study suggests that cyclic administration of low doses of estrogen may carry less risk than continuous administration.[3] It therefore appears prudent to utilize such a regimen.

Close clinical surveillance of all women taking estrogens is important. In all cases of undiagnosed persistent or recurring abnormal vaginal bleeding, adequate diagnostic measures should be undertaken to rule out malignancy.

There is no evidence at present that "natural" estrogens are more or less hazardous than "synthetic" estrogens at equiestrogenic doses.

2. ESTROGENS SHOULD NOT BE USED DURING PREGNANCY.

The use of female sex hormones, both estrogens and progestogens, during early pregnancy may seriously damage the offspring. It has been shown that females exposed *in utero* to diethylstilbestrol, a nonsteroidal estrogen, have an increased risk of developing, in later life, a form of vaginal or cervical cancer that is ordinarily extremely rare.[5,6] This risk has been estimated as not greater than 4 per 1,000 exposures.[7] Furthermore, a

high percentage of such exposed women (from 30% to 90%) have been found to have vaginal adenosis,[8–12] epithelial changes of the vagina and cervix. Although these changes are histologically benign, it is not known whether they are precursors of malignancy. Although similar data are not available with the use of other estrogens, it cannot be presumed they would not induce similar changes.

Several reports suggest an association between intrauterine exposure to female sex hormones and congenital anomalies, including congenital heart defects and limb-reduction defects.[13–16] One case-controlled study[16] estimated a 4.7-fold increased risk of limb-reduction defects in infants exposed *in utero* to sex hormones (oral contraceptives, hormone withdrawal tests for pregnancy, or attempted treatment for threatened abortion). Some of these exposures were very short and involved only a few days of treatment. The data suggest that the risk of limb-reduction defects in exposed fetuses is somewhat less than 1 per 1,000.

In the past, female sex hormones have been used during pregnancy in an attempt to treat threatened or habitual abortion. There is considerable evidence that estrogens are ineffective for these indications, and there is no evidence from well-controlled studies that progestogens are effective for these uses.

If Premarin Intravenous (conjugated estrogens, USP) for injection is used during pregnancy, or if the patient becomes pregnant while taking this drug, she should be apprised of the potential risks to the fetus, and the advisability of pregnancy continuation.

DESCRIPTION

Each Secule® vial contains 25 mg of conjugated estrogens, USP, in a sterile lyophilized cake which also contains lactose 200 mg, sodium citrate 12.2 mg, and simethicone 0.2 mg. The pH is adjusted with sodium hydroxide or hydrochloric acid. A sterile diluent (5 mL) containing 2% benzyl alcohol in sterile water is provided for reconstitution. The reconstituted solution is suitable for intravenous or intramuscular injection.

Premarin (conjugated estrogens, USP) is a mixture of estrogens, obtained exclusively from natural sources, occurring as the sodium salts of water-soluble estrogen sulfates blended to represent the average composition of material derived from pregnant mares' urine. It contains estrone, equilin, and 17 α-dihydroequilin, together with smaller amounts of 17 α-estradiol, equilenin, and 17 α-dihydroequilenin as salts of their sulfate esters.

CLINICAL PHARMACOLOGY

Estrogens are important in the development and maintenance of the female reproductive system and secondary sex characteristics. They promote growth and development of the vagina, uterus, and fallopian tubes, and enlargement of the breasts. Indirectly, they contribute to the shaping of the skeleton, maintenance of tone and elasticity of urogenital structures, changes in the epiphyses of the long bones that allow for the pubertal growth spurt and its termination, growth of axillary and pubic hair, and pigmentation of the nipples and genitals. Decline of estrogenic activity at the end of the menstrual cycle can bring on menstruation, although the cessation of progesterone secretion is the most important factor in the mature ovulatory cycle. However, in the preovulatory or nonovulatory cycle, estrogen is the primary determinant in the onset of menstruation. Estrogens also affect the release of pituitary gonadotropins.

The pharmacologic effects of conjugated estrogens are similar to those of endogenous estrogens. They are soluble in water and may be administered by intravenous or intramuscular injection.

In responsive tissues (female genital organs, breasts, hypothalamus, pituitary) estrogens enter the cell and are transported into the nucleus. As a result of estrogen action, specific RNA and protein synthesis occurs.

Metabolism and inactivation occur primarily in the liver. Some estrogens are excreted into the bile; however, they are reabsorbed from the intestine and returned to the liver through the portal venous system. Water-soluble estrogen conjugates are strongly acidic and, therefore, ionized in body fluids, which favor excretion through the kidneys since tubular reabsorption is minimal.

INDICATION

Premarin Intravenous (conjugated estrogens, USP) for injection is indicated in the treatment of abnormal uterine bleeding due to hormonal imbalance in the absence of organic pathology.

CONTRAINDICATIONS

Estrogens should not be used in women with any of the following conditions:

1. Known or suspected cancer of the breast, except in appropriately selected patients being treated for metastatic disease.
2. Known or suspected estrogen-dependent neoplasia.
3. Known or suspected pregnancy (see Boxed Warning).

4. Undiagnosed abnormal genital bleeding.
5. Active thrombophlebitis or thromboembolic disorders.
6. A past history of thrombophlebitis, thrombosis, or thromboembolic disorders associated with previous estrogen use (except when used in treatment of breast malignancy).

WARNINGS

1. *Induction of malignant neoplasms.* Long-term, continuous administration of natural and synthetic estrogens in certain animal species increases the frequency of carcinomas of the breast, cervix, vagina, and liver. There are now reports that estrogens increase the risk of carcinoma of the endometrium in humans (see Boxed Warning).

At the present time there is no satisfactory evidence that estrogens given to postmenopausal women increase the risk of cancer of the breast,[17] although a recent long-term follow-up of a single physician's practice has raised this possibility.[18] Because of the animal data, there is a need for caution in prescribing estrogens for women with a strong family history of breast cancer, or who have breast nodules, fibrocystic disease, or abnormal mammograms.

2. *Gallbladder disease.* A recent study has reported a 2- to 3-fold increase in the risk of surgically confirmed gallbladder disease in women receiving postmenopausal estrogens,[17] similar to the 2-fold increase previously noted in users of oral contraceptives.[19,24a]

3. *Effects similar to those caused by estrogen-progestogen oral contraceptives.* There are several serious adverse effects of oral contraceptives, some of which have not, up to now, been documented as consequences of postmenopausal estrogen therapy. This may reflect the comparatively low doses of estrogen used in postmenopausal women. It would be expected that the larger doses of estrogen used to treat prostatic or breast cancer are more likely to result in these adverse effects, and, in fact, it has been shown that there is an increased risk of thrombosis in men receiving estrogens for prostatic cancer.[20–23]

a. *Thromboembolic disease.* It is now well established that users of oral contraceptives have an increased risk of various thromboembolic and thrombotic vascular diseases, such as thrombophlebitis, pulmonary embolism, stroke, and myocardial infarction.[24–31] Cases of retinal thrombosis, mesenteric thrombosis, and optic neuritis have been reported in oral-contraceptive users. There is evidence that the risk of several of these adverse reactions is related to the dose of the drug.[32,33] An increased risk of postsurgery thromboembolic complications has also been reported in users of oral contraceptives.[34,35] If feasible, estrogen should be discontinued at least 4 weeks before surgery of the type associated with an increased risk of thromboembolism, or during periods of prolonged immobilization.

Is some studies, women on estrogen replacement therapy, given alone or in combination with a progestin, have been reported to have an increased risk of thrombophlebitis, and/or thromboembolic disease. The physician should be aware of the possibility of thrombotic disorders (thrombophlebitis, retinal thrombosis, cerebral embolism, and pulmonary embolism) during estrogen replacement therapy and be alert to their earliest manifestations. Should any of these occur or be suspected, estrogen replacement therapy should be discontinued immediately. Patients who have risk factors for thrombotic disorders should be kept under careful observation. Subgroups of women who have underlying risk factors, or who are receiving relatively large doses of estrogens, may have increased risk. Therefore estrogens should not be used in persons with active thrombophlebitis or thromboembolic disorders, and they should not be used (except in treatment of malignancy) in persons with a history of such disorders in association with estrogen use. They should be used with caution in patients with cerebral vascular or coronary artery disease and only for those in whom estrogens are clearly needed.

Large doses of estrogen (5 mg conjugated estrogens per day), comparable to those used to treat cancer of the prostate and breast, have been shown in a large prospective clinical trial in men[36] to increase the risk of nonfatal myocardial infarction, pulmonary embolism, and thrombophlebitis. When estrogen doses of this size are used, any of the thromboembolic and thrombotic adverse effects associated with oral contraceptives or estrogen replacement therapy should be considered a clear risk.

b. *Hepatic adenoma.* Benign hepatic adenomas appear to be associated with the use of oral contraceptives.[37–39] Although benign and rare, these may rupture and may cause death through intra-abdominal hemorrhage. Such lesions have not yet been reported in association with other estrogen or progestogen preparations but should be considered in estrogen users having abdominal pain and tenderness, abdominal mass, or hypovolemic shock. Hepatocellular carcinoma has also been reported in women taking estrogen-containing oral contraceptives.[38] The relationship of this malignancy to these drugs is not known at this time.

Continued on next page

Premarin Intravenous—Cont.

c. *Elevated blood pressure.* Women using oral contraceptives sometimes experience increased blood pressure which, in most cases, returns to normal on discontinuing the drug. There is now a report that this may occur with use of estrogens in the menopause[40] and blood pressure should be monitored with estrogen use, especially if high doses are used.

d. *Glucose tolerance.* A worsening of glucose tolerance has been observed in a significant percentage of patients on estrogen-containing oral contraceptives. For this reason, diabetic patients should be carefully observed while receiving estrogen.

4. *Hypercalcemia.* Administration of estrogens may lead to severe hypercalcemia in patients with breast cancer and bone metastases. If this occurs, the drug should be stopped and appropriate measures taken to reduce the serum calcium level.

PRECAUTIONS

A. General Precautions

1. A complete medical and family history should be taken prior to the initiation of any estrogen therapy. The pretreatment and periodic physical examinations should include special reference to blood pressure, breasts, abdomen, and pelvic organs, and should include a Papanicolaou smear. As a general rule, estrogen should not be prescribed for longer than one year without another physical examination being performed.

2. Fluid retention—Because estrogens may cause some degree of fluid retention, conditions which might be influenced by this factor such as asthma, epilepsy, migraine, and cardiac or renal dysfunction, require careful observation.

3. Certain patients may develop undesirable manifestations of excessive estrogenic stimulation, such as abnormal or excessive uterine bleeding, mastodynia, etc.

4. Oral contraceptives appear to be associated with an increased incidence of mental depression.[24a] Although it is not clear whether this is due to the estrogenic or progestogenic component of the contraceptive, patients with a history of depression should be carefully observed.

5. Preexisting uterine leiomyomata may increase in size during estrogen use.

6. The pathologist should be advised of estrogen therapy when relevant specimens are submitted.

7. Patients with a past history of jaundice during pregnancy have an increased risk of recurrence of jaundice while receiving estrogen-containing oral-contraceptive therapy. If jaundice develops in any patient receiving estrogen, the medication should be discontinued while the cause is investigated.

8. Estrogens may be poorly metabolized in patients with impaired liver function and they should be administered with caution in such patients.

9. Because estrogens influence the metabolism of calcium and phosphorus, they should be used with caution in patients with metabolic bone diseases that are associated with hypercalcemia or in patients with renal insufficiency.

10. Because of the effects of estrogens on epiphyseal closure, they should be used judiciously in young patients in whom bone growth is not yet complete.

11. Certain endocrine and liver function tests may be affected by estrogen-containing oral contraceptives. The following similar changes may be expected with larger doses of estrogen:

a. Increased sulfobromophthalein retention.

b. Increased prothrombin and factors VII, VIII, IX, and X; decreased antithrombin 3; increased norepinephrine-induced platelet aggregability.

c. Increased thyroid binding globulin (TBG) leading to increased circulating total thyroid hormone, as measured by PBI, T4 by column, or T4 by radioimmunoassay. Free T3 resin uptake is decreased, reflecting the elevated TBG; free T4 concentration is unaltered.

d. Impaired glucose tolerance.

e. Decreased pregnanediol excretion.

f. Reduced response to metyrapone test.

g. Reduced serum folate concentration.

h. Increased serum triglyceride and phospholipid concentration.

12. Familial hyperlipoproteinemia. Estrogen therapy may be associated with massive elevations of plasma triglycerides leading to pacreatitis and other complications in patients with familial defects of lipoprotein metabolism.

B. Information for the Patient

See text which appears after the "PHYSICIAN REFERENCES."

C. Pregnancy Category X

See **CONTRAINDICATIONS** and Boxed Warning.

D. Nursing Mothers

As a general principle, the administration of any drug to nursing mothers should be done only when clearly necessary, since many drugs are excreted in human milk.

ADVERSE REACTIONS

(See **"WARNINGS"** regarding induction of neoplasia, adverse effects on the fetus, increased incidence of gallbladder disease, and adverse effects similar to those of oral contraceptives, including thromboembolism.) The following additional adverse reactions have been reported with estrogenic therapy, including oral contraceptives:

1. *Genitourinary system:* Breakthrough bleeding, spotting, change in menstrual flow; dysmenorrhea; premenstrual-like syndrome; amenorrhea during and after treatment; increase in size of uterine fibromyomata; vaginal candidiasis; change in cervical erosion and in degree of cervical secretion; cystitis-like syndrome.

2. *Breasts:* Tenderness, enlargement, secretion.

3. *Gastrointestinal:* Nausea, vomiting; abdominal cramps, bloating; cholestatic jaundice; pancreatitis.

4. *Skin:* Chloasma or melasma which may persist when drug is discontinued; erythema multiforme; erythema nodosum; hemorrhagic eruption; loss of scalp hair; hirsutism.

5. *Cardiovascular:* Venous thromboembolism; pulmonary embolism.

6. *Eyes:* Steepening of corneal curvature; intolerance to contact lenses.

7. *CNS:* Headache, migraine, dizziness; mental depression; chorea.

8. *Miscellaneous:* Increase or decrease in weight; reduced carbohydrate tolerance; aggravation of porphyria; edema; changes in libido.

ACUTE OVERDOSAGE

Numerous reports of ingestion of large doses of estrogen-containing oral contraceptives by young children indicate that acute serious ill effects do not occur. Overdosage of estrogen may cause nausea, and withdrawal bleeding may occur in females.

DOSAGE AND ADMINISTRATION

Abnormal uterine bleeding due to hormonal imbalance: One 25 mg injection, intravenously or intramuscularly. Intravenous use is preferred since more rapid response can be expected from this mode of administration.

Repeat in 6 to 12 hours if necessary. The use of Premarin® Intravenous (conjugated estrogens, USP) for injection does not preclude the advisability of other appropriate measures. The usual precautionary measures governing intravenous administration should be adhered to. Injection should be made SLOWLY to obviate the occurrence of flushes.

Infusion of Premarin Intravenous (conjugated estrogens, USP) for injection with other agents is not generally recommended. In emergencies, however, when an infusion has already been started it may be expedient to make the injection into the tubing just distal to the infusion needle. If so used, compatibility of solutions must be considered.

Compatibility of solutions: Premarin Intravenous is compatible with normal saline, dextrose, and invert sugar solutions. IT IS NOT COMPATIBLE WITH PROTEIN HYDROLYSATE, ASCORBIC ACID, OR ANY SOLUTION WITH AN ACID pH.

Treated patients with an intact uterus should be monitored closely for signs of endometrial cancer, and appropriate diagnostic measures should be taken to rule out malignancy in the event of persistent or recurring abnormal vaginal bleeding.

Directions For Storage and Reconstitution

Storage before reconstitution: Store package in refrigerator, 2°–8°C (36°–46°F).

To reconstitute: First withdraw air from Secule® vial so as to facilitate introduction of sterile diluent. Then, flow the sterile diluent slowly against side of Secule® vial and agitate gently. DO NOT SHAKE VIOLENTLY.

Storage after reconstitution: It is common practice to utilize the reconstituted solution within a few hours. If it is necessary to keep the reconstituted solution for more than a few hours, store the reconstituted solution under refrigeration (2°–8°C). Under these conditions, the solution is stable for 60 days, and is suitable for use unless darkening or precipitation occurs.

HOW SUPPLIED

NDC 0046-0749-05—Each package provides: (1) One Secule® vial containing 25 mg of conjugated estrogens, USP, for injection (also lactose 200 mg, sodium citrate 12.2 mg, and simethicone 0.2 mg). The pH is adjusted with sodium hydroxide or hydrochloric acid. (2) One 5 mL ampul sterile diluent with 2% benzyl alcohol in sterile water.

Premarin Intravenous (conjugated estrogens, USP) for injection is prepared by cryodesiccation.

SECULE®—Registered trademark to designate a vial containing an injectable preparation in dry form.

PHYSICIAN REFERENCES

1. Ziel, H. K. *et al.*: N. Engl. J. Med. *293* :1167–1170, 1975.
2. Smith, D. C. *et al.*: N. Engl. J. Med. *293* :1164–1167, 1975.
3. Mack, T. M. *et al.*: N. Engl. J. Med. *294* :1262–1267, 1976.
4. Weiss, N. S. *et al.*: N. Engl. J. Med. *294* :1259–1262, 1976.
5. Herbst, A. L. *et al.*: N. Engl. J. Med. *284* :878–881, 1971.
6. Greenwald, P. *et al.*: N. Engl. J. Med. *285* :390–392, 1971.
7. Lanier, A. *et al.*: Mayo Clin. Proc. *48* :793–799, 1973.
8. Herbst, A. *et al.*: Obstet. Gynecol. *40* :287–298, 1972.
9. Herbst, A. *et al.*: Am. J. Obstet. Gynecol. *118* :607–615, 1974.
10. Herbst, A. *et al.*: N. Engl. J. Med. *292* :334–339, 1975.
11. Stafl, A. *et al.*: Obstet. Gynecol. *43* :118–128, 1974.
12. Sherman, A. I. *et al.*: Obstet. Gynecol. *44* :531–545, 1974.
13. Gal, I. *et al.*: Nature *216* :83, 1967.
14. Levy, E. P. *et al.*: Lancet *1* :611, 1973.
15. Nora, J. *et al.*: Lancet *1* :941–942, 1973.
16. Janerich, D. T. *et al.*: N. Engl. J. Med. *291* :697–700, 1974.
17. Boston Collaborative Drug Surveillance Program: N. Engl. J. Med. *290* :15–19, 1974.
18. Hoover, R. *et al.*: N. Engl. J. Med. *295* :401–405, 1976.
19. Boston Collaborative Drug Surveillance Program: Lancet *1* :1399–1404, 1973.
20. Daniel, D. G. *et al.*: Lancet *2* :287–289, 1967.
21. The Veterans Administration Cooperative Urological Research Group: J. Urol. *98* :516–522, 1967.
22. Bailar, J. C.: Lancet *2* :560, 1967.
23. Blackard, C. *et al.*: Cancer *26* :249–256, 1970.
24. Royal College of General Practitioners: J. R. Coll. Gen. Pract. *13* :267–279, 1967.
24a. Royal College of General Practitioners: Oral Contraceptives and Health, New York, Pitman Corp., 1974.
25. Inman, W. H. W. *et al.*: Br. Med. J. *2* :193–199, 1968.
26. Vessey, M. P. *et al.*: Br. Med. J. *2* :651–657, 1969.
27. Sartwell, P. E. *et al.*: Am. J. Epidemiol. *90* :365–380, 1969.
28. Collaborative Group for the Study of Stroke in Young Women: N. Engl. J. Med. *288* :871–878, 1973.
29. Collaborative Group for the Study of Stroke in Young Women: J.A.M.A. *231* :718–722, 1975.
30. Mann, J. I. *et al.*: Br. Med. J. *2* :245–248, 1975.
31. Mann, J. I. *et al.*: Br. Med. J. *2* :241–245, 1975.
32. Inman, W. H. W. *et al.*: Br. Med. J. *2* :203–209, 1970.
33. Stolley, P. D. *et al.*: Am. J. Epidemiol. *102* :197–208, 1975.
34. Vessey, M. P. *et al.*: Br. Med. J. *3* :123–126, 1970.
35. Greene, G. R., *et al.*: Am. J. Public Health *62* :680–685, 1972.
36. Coronary Drug Project Research Group: J.A.M.A. *214* : 1303–1313, 1970.
37. Baum, J. *et al.*: Lancet *2* :926–928, 1973.
38. Mays, E. T. *et al.*: J.A.M.A. *235* :730–732, 1976.
39. Edmondson, H. A. *et al.*: N. Engl. J. Med. *294* :470–472, 1976.
40. Pfeffer, R. I. *et al.*: Am. J. Epidemiol. *103* :445–456, 1976.

INFORMATION FOR THE PATIENT

What You Should Know About Estrogens

Estrogens are female hormones produced by the ovaries. The ovaries make several different kinds of estrogens. In addition, scientists have been able to make a variety of synthetic estrogens. As far as we know, all these estrogens have similar properties and, therefore, much the same usefulness, side effects, and risks. This leaflet is intended to help you understand what estrogens are used for, the risks involved in their use, and how to use them as safely as possible.

This leaflet includes the most important information about estrogens, but not all the information. If you want to know more, you should ask your doctor for more information, or you can ask your doctor or pharmacist to let you read the package insert prepared for the doctor.

Uses of Estrogen

THERE IS NO PROPER USE OF ESTROGENS IN A PREGNANT WOMAN: Estrogens are prescribed by doctors for a number of purposes, including:

1. To provide estrogen during a period of adjustment when a woman's ovaries stop producing a majority of her estrogens, in order to prevent certain uncomfortable symptoms of estrogen deficiency. (With the menopause, which generally occurs between the ages of 45 and 55, women produce a much smaller amount of estrogens.)

2. To prevent symptoms of estrogen deficiency when a woman's ovaries have been removed surgically before the natural menopause.

3. To prevent pregnancy. (Estrogens are given along with a progestogen, another female hormone; these combinations are called oral contraceptives, or birth-control pills. Patient labeling is available to women taking oral contraceptives and they will not be discussed in this leaflet.)

4. To treat certain cancers in women and men.

Estrogens in the Menopause

In the natural course of their lives, all women eventually experience a decrease in estrogen production. This usually occurs between ages 45 and 55, but may occur earlier or later. Sometimes the ovaries may need to be removed before natural menopause by an operation, producing a "surgical menopause."

When the amount of estrogen in the blood begins to decrease, many women may develop typical symptoms: feelings of warmth in the face, neck, and chest, or sudden intense episodes of heat and sweating throughout the body (called "hot flashes" or "hot flushes"). These symptoms are sometimes very uncomfortable. Some women may also develop changes in the vagina (called "atrophic vaginitis") that cause discomfort, especially during and after intercourse.

Estrogens can be prescribed to treat these symptoms of the menopause. It is estimated that considerably more than half of all women undergoing the menopause have only mild symptoms or no symptoms at all and, therefore, do not need estrogens. Other women may need estrogens for a few months, while their bodies adjust to lower estrogen levels. Sometimes the need will be for periods longer than six months. In an attempt to avoid overstimulation of the uterus (womb), estrogens are usually given cyclically during each month of use, such as three weeks of pills followed by one week without pills.

Sometimes women experience nervous symptoms or depression during menopause. There is no evidence that estrogens are effective for such symptoms without associated vasomotor symptoms. In the absence of vasomotor symptoms, estrogens should not be used to treat nervous symptoms, although other treatment may be needed.

You may have heard that taking estrogens for long periods (years) after the menopause will keep your skin soft and supple and keep you feeling young. There is no evidence that this is so, however, and such long-term treatment carries important risks.

The Dangers of Estrogens

1. *Endometrial cancer.* There are reports that if estrogens are used in the postmenopausal period for more than a year, there is an increased risk of *endometrial cancer* (cancer of the lining of the uterus). Women taking estrogens have roughly 5- to 10-times as great a chance of getting this cancer as women who take no estrogens. To put this another way, while a postmenopausal woman not taking estrogens has 1 chance in 1,000 each year of getting endometrial cancer, a woman taking estrogens has 5 to 10 chances in 1,000 each year. For this reason *it is important to take estrogens only when they are really needed.*

The risk of this cancer is greater the longer estrogens are used and when larger doses are taken. Therefore, you should not take more estrogen than your doctor prescribes. *It is important to take the lowest dose of estrogen that will control symptoms and to take it only as long as it is needed.* If estrogens are needed for longer periods of time, your doctor will want to reevaluate your need for estrogens at least every six months.

Women using estrogens should report any vaginal bleeding to their doctors; such bleeding may be of no importance, but it can be an early warning of endometrial cancer. If you have undiagnosed vaginal bleeding, you should not use estrogens until a diagnosis is made and you are certain there is no endometrial cancer.

Note: If you have had your uterus removed (total hysterectomy), there is no danger of developing endometrial cancer.

2. *Other possible cancers.* Estrogens can cause development of other tumors in animals, such as tumors of the breast, cervix, vagina, or liver, when given for a long time. At present there is no good evidence that women using estrogen in the menopause have an increased risk of such tumors, but there is no way yet to be sure they do not; and one study raises the possibility that use of estrogens in the menopause may increase the risk of breast cancer many years later. This is a further reason to use estrogens only when clearly needed. While you are taking estrogens, it is important that you go to your doctor at least once a year for a physical examination. Also, if members of your family have had breast cancers, or if you have breast nodules, or abnormal mammograms (breast X rays), your doctor may wish to carry out more frequent examinations of your breasts.

3. *Gallbladder disease.* Women who use estrogens after menopause are more likely to develop gallbladder disease needing surgery than women who do not use estrogens. Birth-control pills have a similar effect.

4. *Abnormal blood clotting.* Taking estrogens may increase the risk of blood clotting in various parts of the body. This can result in a stroke (if the clot is in the brain), a heart attack (a clot in a blood vessel of the heart), or a pulmonary embolus (a clot which forms in the legs or pelvis, then breaks off and travels to the lungs). Any of these can be fatal.

It is recommended that if you have had clotting in the legs or lungs, or a heart attack or stroke, while you were using estrogens or birth-control pills, you should not use estrogens

(unless they are being used to treat cancer of the breast or prostate). If you have had a stroke or heart attack, or if you have angina pectoris, estrogens should be used with great caution and only if clearly needed (for example, if you have severe symptoms of the menopause).

5. *Inflammation of the pancreas (Pancreatitis).* Women with high triglyceride levels may have an increased risk of developing inflammation of the pancreas.

Special Warning About Pregnancy

You should not receive estrogen if you are pregnant. If this should occur, there is a greater than usual chance that the developing child will be born with a birth defect, although the possibility remains fairly small. A female child may have an increased risk of developing cancer of the vagina or cervix later in life (in the teens or twenties). Every possible effort should be made to avoid exposure to estrogens during pregnancy. If exposure occurs, see your doctor.

Other Effects of Estrogens

In addition to the serious known risks of estrogens described above, estrogens have the following side effects and potential risks:

1. *Nausea and vomiting.* The most common side effect of estrogen therapy is nausea. Vomiting is less common.

2. *Effects on breasts.* Estrogens may cause breast tenderness or enlargement and may cause the breasts to secrete a liquid. These effects are not dangerous.

3. *Effects on the uterus.* Estrogens may cause benign fibroid tumors of the uterus to get larger.

4. *Effects on liver.* Women taking oral contraceptives develop, on rare occasions, a tumor of the liver which can rupture and bleed into the abdomen and may cause death. So far, these tumors have not been reported in women using estrogens in the menopause, but you should report any swelling or unusual pain or tenderness in the abdomen to your doctor immediately.

Women with a past history of jaundice (yellowing of the skin and white parts of the eyes) may get jaundice again during estrogen use. If this occurs, stop taking estrogens and see your doctor.

5. *Other effects.* Estrogens may cause excess fluid to be retained in the body. This may make some conditions worse, such as asthma, epilepsy, migraine, heart disease, or kidney disease.

Summary

Estrogens have important uses, but they have serious risks as well. You must decide, with your doctor, whether the risks are acceptable to you in view of the benefits of treatment. Except where your doctor has prescribed estrogens for use in special cases of cancer of the breast or prostate, you should not use estrogens if you have cancer of the breast or uterus, are pregnant, have undiagnosed abnormal vaginal bleeding, clotting in the legs or lungs, or have had a stroke, heart attack or angina, or clotting in the legs or lungs in the past while you were taking estrogens.

You can use estrogens as safely as possible by understanding that your doctor will require regular physical examinations while you are taking them, will try to discontinue the drug as soon as possible, and use the smallest dose possible. Be alert for signs of trouble including:

1. Abnormal bleeding from the vagina.

2. Pains in the calves or chest, or sudden shortness of breath, or coughing blood.

3. Severe headache, dizziness, faintness, or changes in vision.

4. Breast lumps (you should ask your doctor how to examine your own breasts).

5. Jaundice (yellowing of the skin).

6. Mental depression.

Your doctor has prescribed this drug for you and you alone. Do not give the drug to anyone else.

HOW SUPPLIED

Premarin® (conjugated estrogens tablets, USP) tablets for oral administration.

Premarin® Vaginal Cream—Premarin® in a nonliquefying base, designed for vaginal use.

Premarin® Intravenous—Premarin® specially prepared for intravenous and intramuscular use.

Manufactured by:
Ayerst Laboratories Inc.
A Wyeth-Ayerst Company
Philadelphia, PA 19101

PREMARIN®
[prĕm 'a-rĭn]
(conjugated estrogens tablets, USP)

Caution: Federal law prohibits dispensing without prescription.

℞

> 1. ESTROGENS HAVE BEEN REPORTED TO INCREASE THE RISK OF ENDOMETRIAL CARCINOMA IN POSTMENOPAUSAL WOMEN.
>
> Close clinical surveillance of all women taking estrogens is important. Adequate diagnostic measures, including endometrial sampling when indicated, should be undertaken to rule out malignancy in all cases of undiagnosed persistent or recurring abnormal vaginal bleeding. There is currently no evidence that "natural" estrogens are more or less hazardous than "synthetic" estrogens at equiestrogenic doses.
>
> 2. ESTROGENS SHOULD NOT BE USED DURING PREGNANCY.
>
> Estrogen therapy during pregnancy is associated with an increased risk of congenital defects in the reproductive organs of the male and female fetus, an increased risk of vaginal adenosis, squamous cell dysplasia of the uterine cervix, and vaginal cancer in the female later in life. The 1985 DES Task Force concluded that women who used DES during their pregnancies may subsequently experience an increased risk of breast cancer. However, a causal relationship is still unproven, and the observed level of risk is similar to that for a number of other breast-cancer risk factors.
>
> There is no indication for estrogen therapy during pregnancy. Estrogens are ineffective for the prevention or treatment of threatened or habitual abortion.

DESCRIPTION

Premarin (conjugated estrogens tablets, USP) for oral administration contains a mixture of estrogens obtained exclusively from natural sources, occurring as the sodium salts of water-soluble estrogen sulfates blended to represent the average composition of material derived from pregnant mares' urine. It contains estrone, equilin, and 17 α-dihydroequilin, together with smaller amounts of 17 α-estradiol, equilenin, and 17 α-dihydroequilenin as salts of their sulfate esters. Tablets for oral administration are available in 0.3 mg, 0.625 mg, 0.9 mg, 1.25 mg, and 2.5 mg strengths of conjugated estrogens.

Premarin Tablets contain the following inactive ingredients: calcium phosphate tribasic, calcium sulfate, carnauba wax, cellulose, glyceryl monooleate, lactose, magnesium stearate, methylcellulose, pharmaceutical glaze, polyethylene glycol, stearic acid, sucrose, titanium dioxide.

— 0.3 mg tablets also contain: D&C Yellow No. 10, FD&C Blue No. 1, FD&C Blue No. 2, FD&C Yellow No. 6; these tablets comply with USP Drug Release Test 1.

— 0.625 mg tablets also contain: FD&C Blue No. 2, D&C Red No. 27, FD&C Red No. 40; these tablets comply with USP Drug Release Test 1.

— 0.9 mg tablets also contain: D&C Red No. 6, D&C Red No. 7; these tablets comply with USP Drug Release Test 2.

— 1.25 mg tablets also contain: black iron oxide, D&C Yellow No. 10, FD&C Yellow No. 6, talc; these tablets comply with USP Drug Release Test 3.

— 2.5 mg tablets also contain: FD&C Blue No. 2, D&C Red No. 7, talc; these tablets comply with USP Drug Release Test 3.

CLINICAL PHARMACOLOGY

Estrogens are important in the development and maintenance of the female reproductive system and secondary sex characteristics. They promote growth and development of the vagina, uterus, and fallopian tubes, and enlargement of the breasts. Indirectly, they contribute to the shaping of the skeleton, maintenance of tone and elasticity of urogenital structures, changes in the epiphyses of the long bones that allow for the pubertal growth spurt and its termination, growth of axillary and pubic hair, and pigmentation of the nipples and genitals. Decline of estrogenic activity at the end of the menstrual cycle can bring on menstruation, although the cessation of progesterone secretion is the most important factor in the mature ovulatory cycle. However, in the preovulatory or nonovulatory cycle, estrogen is the primary determinant in the onset of menstruation. Estrogens also affect the release of pituitary gonadotropins.

The pharmacologic effects of conjugated estrogens are similar to those of endogenous estrogens. They are soluble in water and are well absorbed from the gastrointestinal tract. In responsive tissues (female genital organs, breasts, hypothalamus, pituitary) estrogens enter the cell and are transported into the nucleus. As a result of estrogen action, specific RNA and protein synthesis occurs.

Metabolism and inactivation occur primarily in the liver. Some estrogens are excreted into the bile; however, they are reabsorbed from the intestine and returned to the liver through the portal venous system. Water-soluble estrogen conjugates are strongly acidic and are ionized in body fluids, which favor excretion through the kidneys since tubular reabsorption is minimal.

INDICATIONS AND USAGE

Premarin (conjugated estrogens tablets, USP) is indicated in the treatment of:

Continued on next page

Premarin Tablets—Cont.

1. Moderate to severe vasomotor symptoms associated with the menopause. There is no adequate evidence that estrogens are effective for nervous symptoms or depression which might occur during menopause and they should not be used to treat these conditions.

2. Atrophic vaginitis.

3. Osteoporosis (loss of bone mass). The mainstays of prevention and management of osteoporosis are estrogen and calcium; exercise and nutrition may be important adjuncts. Estrogen replacement therapy is the most effective single modality for the prevention of osteoporosis in women. Estrogen reduces bone resorption and retards or halts postmenopausal bone loss. Case-controlled studies have shown an approximately 60-percent reduction in hip and wrist fractures in women whose estrogen replacement was begun within a few years of menopause. Studies also suggest that estrogen reduces the rate of vertebral fractures. Even when started as late as 6 years after menopause, estrogen prevents further loss of bone mass but does not restore it to premenopausal levels. The lowest effective dose for prevention and treatment of osteoporosis should be utilized. (See "DOSAGE AND ADMINISTRATION.")

Women are at higher risk than men because they have less bone mass, and for several years following natural or induced menopause, the rate of bone mass decline is accelerated. Early menopause is one of the strongest predictors for the development of osteoporosis. White women are at higher risk than black women, and white men are at higher risk than black men. Women who are underweight also have osteoporosis more often than overweight women. Cigarette smoking may be an additional factor in increasing risk. Calcium deficiency has been implicated in the pathogenesis of this disease. Therefore, when not contraindicated, it is recommended that postmenopausal women receive an elemental calcium intake of 1000 to 1500 mg/day.

Immobilization and prolonged bed rest produce rapid bone loss, while weight-bearing exercise has been shown both to reduce bone loss and to increase bone mass. The optimal type and amount of physical activity that would prevent osteoporosis have not been established.

4. Hypoestrogenism due to hypogonadism, castration, or primary ovarian failure.

5. Breast cancer (for palliation only) in appropriately selected women and men with metastatic disease.

6. Advanced androgen-dependent carcinoma of the prostate (for palliation only).

CONTRAINDICATIONS

Estrogens should not be used in women (or men) with any of the following conditions:

1. Known or suspected pregnancy (see Boxed Warning). Estrogen may cause fetal harm when administered to a pregnant woman.

2. Known or suspected cancer of the breast except in appropriately selected patients being treated for metastatic disease.

3. Known or suspected estrogen-dependent neoplasia.

4. Undiagnosed abnormal genital bleeding.

5. Active thrombophlebitis or thromboembolic disorders. However, there is insufficient information regarding women who have had previous thromboembolic disease.

Premarin Tablets should not be used in patients hypersensitive to their ingredients.

WARNINGS

1. *Induction of malignant neoplasms.* Some studies have suggested a possible increased incidence of breast cancer in those women on estrogen therapy taking higher doses for prolonged periods of time. The majority of studies, however, have not shown an association with the usual doses used for estrogen replacement therapy. Women on this therapy should have regular breast examinations and should be instructed in breast self-examination. The reported endometrial cancer risk among estrogen users was about 4-fold or greater than in nonusers and appears dependent on duration of treatment and on estrogen dose. There is no significant increased risk associated with the use of estrogens for less than one year. The greatest risk appears associated with prolonged use—five years or more. In one study, persistence of risk was demonstrated for 10 years after cessation of estrogen treatment. In another study, a significant decrease in the incidence of endometrial cancer occurred six months after estrogen withdrawal.

Estrogen therapy during pregnancy is associated with an increased risk of fetal congenital reproductive-tract disorders. In females there is an increased risk of vaginal adenosis, squamous-cell dysplasia of the cervix, and cancer later in life; in the male, urogenital abnormalities. Although some of these changes are benign, it is not known whether they are precursors of malignancy.

2. *Gallbladder disease.* A study has reported a 2.5-fold increase in the risk of surgically-confirmed gallbladder disease in women receiving postmenopausal estrogens.

3. *Thromboembolic Disorders and Other Vascular Problems.* In some studies, women on estrogen replacement therapy, given alone or in combination with a progestin, have been reported to have an increased risk of thrombophlebitis, and/or thromboembolic disease. Large doses of estrogen (5 mg conjugated estrogens per day), comparable to those used to treat cancer of the prostate and breast, have been shown in a large prospective clinical trial in men to increase the risk of nonfatal myocardial infarction, pulmonary embolism, and thrombophlebitis. The physician should be aware of the possibility of thrombotic disorders (thrombophlebitis, retinal thrombosis, cerebral embolism, and pulmonary embolism) during estrogen replacement therapy and be alert to their earliest manifestations. Should any of these occur or be suspected, estrogen replacement therapy should be discontinued immediately. Patients who have risk factors for thrombotic disorders should be kept under careful observation.

4. *Elevated blood pressure.* There is no evidence that this may occur with use of estrogens in the menopause. However, blood pressure should be monitored with estrogen use, especially if high doses are used.

5. *Hypercalcemia.* Administration of estrogens may lead to severe hypercalcemia in patients with breast cancer and bone metastases. If this occurs, the drug should be stopped and appropriate measures taken to reduce the serum calcium level.

PRECAUTIONS

A. General

1. *Addition of a progestin.* Studies of the addition of a progestin for seven or more days of a cycle of estrogen administration have reported a lowered incidence of endometrial hyperplasia. Morphological and biochemical studies of endometrium suggest that 10 to 13 days of progestin are needed to provide maximal maturation of the endometrium and to eliminate any hyperplastic changes. Whether this will provide protection from endometrial carcinoma has not been clearly established. There are possible additional risks which may be associated with the inclusion of progestin in estrogen replacement regimens. The potential risks include adverse effects on carbohydrate and lipid metabolism. The choice of progestin and dosage may be important in minimizing these adverse effects.

2. *Physical examination.* A complete medical and family history should be taken prior to the initiation of any estrogen therapy. The pretreatment and periodic physical examinations should include special reference to blood pressure, breasts, abdomen, and pelvic organs, and should include a Papanicolaou smear. As a general rule, estrogen should not be prescribed for longer than one year without another physical examination being performed.

3. *Familial hyperlipoproteinemia.* Estrogen therapy may be associated with massive elevations of plasma triglycerides leading to pancreatitis and other complications in patients with familial defects of lipoprotein metabolism.

4. *Fluid retention.* Because estrogens may cause some degree of fluid retention, conditions which might be influenced by this factor, such as asthma, epilepsy, migraine, and cardiac or renal dysfunction, require careful observation.

5. *Uterine bleeding and mastodynia.* Certain patients may develop undesirable manifestations of estrogenic stimulation, such as abnormal uterine bleeding and mastodynia.

6. *Uterine fibroids.* Preexisting uterine leiomyomata may increase in size during prolonged high-dose estrogen use.

7. *Impaired liver function.* Estrogens may be poorly metabolized in patients with impaired liver function and should be administered with caution.

8. *Hypercalcemia and renal insufficiency.* Prolonged use of estrogens can alter the metabolism of calcium and phosphorus. Estrogens should be used with caution in patients with metabolic bone disease.

B. Information for the Patient

See text of Patient Package Insert which appears after the "HOW SUPPLIED" section.

C. Laboratory Tests

Clinical response at the smallest dose should generally be the guide to estrogen administration for relief of symptoms for those indications in which symptoms are observable. However, for prevention and treatment of osteoporosis see "DOSAGE AND ADMINISTRATION" section. Tests used to measure adequacy of estrogen replacement therapy include serum estrone and estradiol levels and suppression of serum gonadotrophin levels.

D. Drug/Laboratory Test Interactions

Some of these drug/laboratory test interactions have been observed only with estrogen-progestin combinations (oral contraceptives):

1. Increased prothrombin and factors VII, VIII, IX and X; decreased antithrombin 3; increased norepinephrine-induced platelet aggregability, decreased fibrinolysis.

2. Increased thyroid-binding globulin (TBG) leading to increased circulating total thyroid hormone, as measured by T4 levels determined either by column or by radioimmunoassay. Free T3 resin uptake is decreased, reflecting the elevated TBG; free T4 concentration is unaltered.

3. Impaired glucose tolerance.

4. Reduced response to metyrapone test.

5. Reduced serum folate concentration.

E. Mutagenesis and Carcinogenesis

Long-term continuous administration of natural and synthetic estrogens in certain animal species increases the frequency of carcinomas of the breast, cervix, vagina, and liver.

F. PREGNANCY CATEGORY X

Estrogens should not be used during pregnancy. (See CONTRAINDICATIONS and Boxed Warning.)

G. NURSING MOTHERS

As a general principle, the administration of any drug to nursing mothers should be done only when clearly necessary since many drugs are excreted in human milk.

ADVERSE REACTIONS

(See "WARNINGS" regarding induction of neoplasia, adverse effects on the fetus, increased incidence of gallbladder disease.) The following additional adverse reactions have been reported with estrogen therapy.

1. *Genitourinary system.* Changes in vaginal bleeding pattern and abnormal withdrawal bleeding or flow. Breakthrough bleeding, spotting. Increase in size of uterine fibromyomata. Vaginal candidiasis. Change in amount of cervical secretion.

2. *Breasts.* Tenderness, enlargement.

3. *Gastrointestinal.* Nausea, vomiting; abdominal cramps, bloating; cholestatic jaundice, pancreatitis.

4. *Skin.* Chloasma or melasma that may persist when drug is discontinued; erythema multiforme; erythema nodosum; hemorrhagic eruption; loss of scalp hair; hirsutism.

5. *Cardiovascular.* Venous thromboembolism; pulmonary embolism.

6. *Eyes.* Steepening of corneal curvature; intolerance of contact lenses.

7. *CNS.* Headache, migraine, dizziness; mental depression; chorea.

8. *Miscellaneous.* Increase or decrease in weight; reduced carbohydrate tolerance; aggravation of porphyria; edema; changes in libido.

ACUTE OVERDOSAGE

Numerous reports of ingestion of large doses of estrogen-containing oral contraceptives by young children indicate that acute serious ill effects do not occur. Overdosage of estrogen may cause nausea and vomiting.

DOSAGE AND ADMINISTRATION

1. For treatment of moderate to severe vasomotor symptoms and atrophic vaginitis associated with the menopause. The lowest dose that will control symptoms should be chosen, and medication should be discontinued as promptly as possible.

Attempts to discontinue or taper medication should be made at 3-month to 6-month intervals.

USUAL DOSAGE RANGES

Vasomotor symptoms—1.25 mg daily. If the patient has not menstruated within the last two months or more, cyclic administration is started arbitrarily. If the patient is menstruating, cyclic (e.g., three weeks on and one week off) administration is started on day 5 of bleeding.

Atrophic vaginitis—0.3 mg to 1.25 mg or more daily, depending upon the tissue response of the individual patient. Administer cyclically.

2. Hypoestrogenism due to:

a. Female hypogonadism—2.5 mg to 7.5 mg daily, in divided doses for 20 days, followed by a rest period of 10 days' duration. If bleeding does not occur by the end of this period, the same dosage schedule is repeated. The number of courses of estrogen therapy necessary to produce bleeding may vary depending on the responsiveness of the endometrium.

If bleeding occurs before the end of the 10-day period, begin a 20-day estrogen-progestin cyclic regimen with Premarin, 2.5 mg to 7.5 mg daily in divided doses, for 20 days. During the last five days of estrogen therapy, give an oral progestin. If bleeding occurs before this regimen is concluded, therapy is discontinued and may be resumed on the fifth day of bleeding.

b. Female castration or primary ovarian failure— 1.25 mg daily, cyclically. Adjust dosage, upward or downward, according to severity of symptoms and response of the patient. For maintenance, adjust dosage to lowest level that will provide effective control.

3. Osteoporosis (loss of bone mass)—0.625 mg daily. Administration should be cyclic (e.g., three weeks on and one week off).

4. Advanced androgen-dependent carcinoma of the prostate, for palliation only—1.25 mg to 2.5 mg three times daily. The effectiveness of therapy can be judged by phosphatase determinations as well as by symptomatic improvement of the patient.

5. Breast cancer (for palliation only) in appropriately selected women and men with metastatic disease. Suggested dosage is 10 mg three times daily for a period of at least three months.

Treated patients with an intact uterus should be monitored closely for signs of endometrial cancer, and appropriate diagnostic measures should be taken to rule out malignancy in the event of persistent or recurring abnormal vaginal bleeding.

HOW SUPPLIED

Premarin® (conjugated estrogens tablets, USP)

— Each oval purple tablet contains 2.5 mg, in bottles of 100 (NDC 0046-0865-81) and 1,000 (NDC 0046-0865-91).

— Each oval yellow tablet contains 1.25 mg, in bottles of 100 (NDC 0046-0866-81); 1,000 (NDC 0046-0866-91); 5,000 (NDC 0046-0866-95); and Unit-Dose packages of 100 (NDC 0046-0866-99).

— Each oval white tablet contains 0.9 mg, in bottles of 100 (NDC 0046-0864-81).

— Each oval maroon tablet contains 0.625 mg, in bottles of 100 (NDC 0046-0867-81); 1,000 (NDC 0046-0867-91); 5,000 (NDC 0046-0867-95); and Unit-Dose packages of 100 (NDC 0046-0867-99).

— Each oval green tablet contains 0.3 mg, in bottles of 100 (NDC 0046-0868-81) and 1,000 (NDC 0046-0868-91).

The appearance of these tablets is a trademark of Wyeth-Ayerst Laboratories.

Store at room temperature (approximately 25° C).
Dispense in a well-closed container as defined in the USP.

INFORMATION FOR THE PATIENT

This leaflet describes when and how to use estrogens and the risks of estrogen treatment.

ESTROGEN DRUGS

Estrogens have several important uses but also some risks. You must decide, with your doctor, whether the risks of estrogens are acceptable in view of their benefits. If you decide to start taking estrogens, check with your doctor to make sure you are using the lowest possible effective dose. The length of treatment with estrogens will depend upon the reason for use. This should also be discussed with your doctor.

USES OF ESTROGEN

To reduce menopausal symptoms. Estrogens are hormones produced by the ovaries. The decrease in the amount of estrogen that occurs in all women, usually between ages 45 and 55, causes the menopause. Sometimes the ovaries are removed by an operation, causing "surgical menopause." When the amount of estrogen begins to decrease, some women develop very uncomfortable symptoms, such as feelings of warmth in the face, neck and chest or sudden intense episodes of heat and sweating ("hot flashes"). The use of drugs containing estrogens can help the body adjust to lower estrogen levels.

Most women have none or only mild menopausal symptoms and do not need estrogens. Other women may need estrogens for a few months while their bodies adjust to lower estrogen levels. The majority of women do not need estrogen replacement for longer than six months for these symptoms.

To prevent brittle bones. After age 40, and especially after menopause, some women develop osteoporosis. This is a thinning of the bones that makes them weaker and more likely to break, often leading to fractures of vertebrae, hip, and wrist bones. Taking estrogens after the menopause slows down bone loss and may prevent bones from breaking. Eating foods that are high in calcium (such as milk products) or taking calcium supplements (1000 to 1500 milligrams per day) and certain types of exercise may also help prevent osteoporosis.

Since estrogen use is associated with some risk, its use in the prevention of osteoporosis should be confined to women who appear to be susceptible to this condition. The following characteristics are often present in women who are likely to develop osteoporosis: white race, thinness, and cigarette smoking.

Women who had their menopause by the surgical removal of their ovaries at a relatively young age are good candidates for estrogen replacement therapy to prevent osteoporosis.

To treat certain types of abnormal uterine bleeding due to hormonal imbalance.

To treat atrophic vaginitis (itching, burning, dryness in or around the vagina).

To treat certain cancers.

WHEN ESTROGENS SHOULD NOT BE USED

Estrogens should not be used:

During pregnancy. Although the possibility is fairly small, there is a greater risk of having a child born with a birth defect if you take estrogens during pregnancy. A male child may have an increased risk of developing abnormalities of the urinary system and sex organs. A female child may have an increased risk of developing cancer of the vagina or cervix in her teens or twenties. Estrogen is not effective in preventing miscarriage (abortion).

If you have had any heart or circulation problems. Estrogen therapy should be used only after consultation with your

physician and only in recommended doses. Patients with a tendency for abnormal blood clotting should avoid estrogen use (see below).

If you have had cancer. Since estrogens increase the risk of certain cancers, you should not take estrogens if you have ever had cancer of the breast or uterus. In certain situations, your doctor may choose to use estrogen in the treatment of breast cancer.

When they are ineffective. Sometimes women experience nervous symptoms or depression during menopause. There is no evidence that estrogens are effective for such symptoms. You may have heard that taking estrogens for long periods (years) after menopause will keep your skin soft and supple and keep you feeling young. There is no evidence that this is so and such long-term treatment may carry serious risks.

DANGERS OF ESTROGENS

Cancer of the uterus. The risk of cancer of the uterus increases the longer estrogens are used and when larger doses are taken. One study showed that when estrogens are discontinued, this increased risk of cancer seems to fall off quickly. In another study, the persistence of risk was demonstrated for 10 years after stopping estrogen treatment. Because of this risk, *it is important to take the lowest dose of estrogen that will control your symptoms and to take it only as long as you need it.* There is a higher risk of cancer of the uterus if you are overweight, diabetic, or have high blood pressure.

If you have had your uterus removed (total hysterectomy), there is no danger of developing cancer of the uterus.

Cancer of the breast. The majority of studies have shown no association with the usual doses used for estrogen replacement therapy and breast cancer. Some studies have suggested a possible increased incidence of breast cancer in those women taking estrogens for prolonged periods of time and especially if higher doses are used.

Regular breast examinations by a health professional and self-examination are recommended for women receiving estrogen therapy, as they are for all women.

Gallbladder disease. Women who use estrogens after menopause are more likely to develop gallbladder disease needing surgery than women who do not use estrogens.

Inflammation of the pancreas. Women with high triglyceride levels may have an increased risk of developing inflammation of the pancreas.

Abnormal blood clotting. Taking estrogens may increase the risk of blood clots. These clots can cause a stroke, heart attack or pulmonary embolus, any of which may be fatal.

SIDE EFFECTS

In addition to the risks listed above, the following side effects have been reported with estrogen use:

• Nausea and vomiting.
• Breast tenderness or enlargement.
• Enlargement of benign tumors of the uterus.
• Retention of excess fluid. This may make some conditions worsen, such as asthma, epilepsy, migraine, heart disease, or kidney disease.
• A spotty darkening of the skin, particularly on the face.

REDUCING RISK OF ESTROGEN USE

If you decide to take estrogens, you can reduce your risks by carefully monitoring your treatment.

See your doctor regularly. While you are taking estrogens, it is important that you visit your doctor at least once a year for a physical examination. If members of your family have had breast cancer or if you have ever had breast nodules or an abnormal mammogram (breast X ray), you may need to have more frequent breast examinations.

Reevaluate your need for estrogens. You and your doctor should reevaluate your need for estrogens at least every six months.

Be alert for signs of trouble. Report these or any other unusual side effects to your doctor immediately:

• Abnormal bleeding from the vagina.
• Pains in the calves or chest, a sudden shortness of breath or coughing blood (indicating possible clots in the legs, heart, or lungs).
• Severe headache, dizziness, faintness, or changes in vision, indicating possible clots in the brain or eye).
• Breast lumps.
• Yellowing of the skin.
• Pain, swelling, or tenderness in the abdomen.

OTHER INFORMATION

Some physicians may choose to prescribe another hormonal drug to be used in association with estrogen treatment. These drugs, progestins, have been reported to lower the frequency of occurrence of a possible precancerous condition of the uterine lining. Whether this will provide protection from uterine cancer has not been clearly established. There are possible additional risks that may be associated with the inclusion of a progestin in estrogen treatment. The possible risks include unfavorable effects on blood fats and sugars. The choice of progestin and its dosage may be important in minimizing these effects.

Your doctor has prescribed this drug for you and you alone. Do not give the drug to anyone else.

If you will be taking calcium supplements as part of the treatment to help prevent osteoporosis, check with your doctor about the amounts recommended.

Keep this and all drugs out of the reach of children. In case of overdose, call your doctor, hospital, or poison control center immediately.

This leaflet provides the most important information about estrogens. If you want to read more, ask your doctor or pharmacist to let you read the professional labeling.

HOW SUPPLIED

Premarin® (conjugated estrogens tablets, USP)—tablets for oral administration.

Each oval purple tablet contains 2.5 mg.
Each oval yellow tablet contains 1.25 mg.
Each oval white tablet contains 0.9 mg.
Each oval maroon tablet contains 0.625 mg.
Each oval green tablet contains 0.3 mg.

The appearance of these tablets is a trademark of Wyeth-Ayerst Laboratories.

Manufactured by:
Ayerst Laboratories Inc.
A Wyeth-Ayerst Company
Philadelphia, PA 19101

Shown in Product Identification Guide, page 344

PREMARIN®   ℞
[prĕm 'a-rin]
(conjugated estrogens)
VAGINAL CREAM
in a nonliquefying base

Rx only

1. ESTROGENS HAVE BEEN REPORTED TO INCREASE THE RISK OF ENDOMETRIAL CARCINOMA.

Three independent, case-controlled studies have reported an increased risk of endometrial cancer in postmenopausal women exposed to exogenous estrogens for more than one year.[1-3] This risk was independent of the other known risk factors for endometrial cancer. These studies are further supported by the finding that incidence rates of endometrial cancer have increased sharply since 1969 in eight different areas of the United States with population-based cancer-reporting systems, an increase which may be related to the rapidly expanding use of estrogens during the last decade.[4]

The three case-controlled studies reported that the risk of endometrial cancer in estrogen users was about 4.5 to 13.9 times greater than in nonusers. The risk appears to depend on both duration of treatment[1] and on estrogen dose.[3] In view of these findings, when estrogens are used for the treatment of menopausal symptoms, the lowest dose that will control symptoms should be utilized and medication should be discontinued as soon as possible. When prolonged treatment is medically indicated, the patient should be reassessed, on at least a semi-annual basis, to determine the need for continued therapy. Although the evidence must be considered preliminary, one study suggests that cyclic administration of low doses of estrogen may carry less risk than continuous administration.[3] It therefore appears prudent to utilize such a regimen.

Close clinical surveillance of all women taking estrogens is important. In all cases of undiagnosed persistent or recurring abnormal vaginal bleeding, adequate diagnostic measures should be undertaken to rule out malignancy.

There is no evidence at present that "natural" estrogens are more or less hazardous than "synthetic" estrogens at equiestrogenic doses.

2. ESTROGENS SHOULD NOT BE USED DURING PREGNANCY.

The use of female sex hormones, both estrogens and progestogens, during early pregnancy may seriously damage the offspring. It has been shown that females exposed *in utero* to diethylstilbestrol, a nonsteroidal estrogen, have an increased risk of developing, in later life, a form of vaginal or cervical cancer that is ordinarily extremely rare.[5,6] This risk has been estimated as not greater than 4 per 1,000 exposures.[7] Furthermore, a high percentage of such exposed women (from 30% to 90%) have been found to have vaginal adenosis,[8-12] epithelial changes of the vagina and cervix. Although these changes are histologically benign, it is not known whether they are precursors of malignancy. Although similar data are not available with the use of other estrogens, it cannot be presumed they would not induce similar changes.

Continued on next page

Premarin Vaginal Cream—Cont.

Several reports suggest an association between intrauterine exposure to female sex hormones and congenital anomalies, including congenital heart defects and limb-reduction defects.[13–16] One case-controlled study[16] estimated a 4.7-fold increased risk of limb-reduction defects in infants exposed *in utero* to sex hormones (oral contraceptives, hormone withdrawal tests for pregnancy, or attempted treatment for threatened abortion). Some of these exposures were very short and involved only a few days of treatment. The data suggest that the risk of limb-reduction defects in exposed fetuses is somewhat less than 1 per 1,000.

In the past, female sex hormones have been used during pregnancy in an attempt to treat threatened or habitual abortion. There is considerable evidence that estrogens are ineffective for these indications, and there is no evidence from well-controlled studies that progestogens are effective for these uses.

If Premarin (conjugated estrogens) Vaginal Cream is used during pregnancy, or if the patient becomes pregnant while taking this drug, she should be apprised of the potential risks to the fetus, and the advisability of pregnancy continuation.

DESCRIPTION

Each gram of Premarin® (conjugated estrogens) Vaginal Cream contains 0.625 mg conjugated estrogens, USP in a nonliquefying base containing cetyl esters wax, cetyl alcohol, white wax, glyceryl monostearate, propylene glycol monostearate, methyl stearate, benzyl alcohol, sodium lauryl sulfate, glycerin, and mineral oil. Premarin Vaginal Cream is applied intravaginally.

Premarin (conjugated estrogens) is a mixture of estrogens obtained exclusively from natural sources, occurring as the sodium salts of water-soluble estrogen sulfates blended to represent the average composition of material derived from pregnant mares' urine. It contains estrone, equilin, and 17 α-dihydroequilin, together with smaller amounts of 17 α-estradiol, equilenin, and 17 α-dihydroequilenin as salts of their sulfate esters.

CLINICAL PHARMACOLOGY

Estrogens are important in the development and maintenance of the female reproductive system and secondary sex characteristics. They promote growth and development of the vagina, uterus, and fallopian tubes, and enlargement of the breasts. Indirectly, they contribute to the shaping of the skeleton, maintenance of tone and elasticity of urogenital structures, changes in the epiphyses of the long bones that allow for the pubertal growth spurt and its termination, growth of axillary and pubic hair, and pigmentation of the nipples and genitals. Decline of estrogenic activity at the end of the menstrual cycle can bring on menstruation, although the cessation of progesterone secretion is the most important factor in the mature ovulatory cycle. However, in the preovulatory or nonovulatory cycle, estrogen is the primary determinant in the onset of menstruation. Estrogens also affect the release of pituitary gonadotropins.

The pharmacologic effects of conjugated estrogens are similar to those of endogenous estrogens. They are soluble in water and may be absorbed from mucosal surfaces after local administration.

In responsive tissues (female genital organs, breasts, hypothalamus, pituitary) estrogens enter the cell and are transported into the nucleus. As a result of estrogen action, specific RNA and protein synthesis occurs.

Metabolism and inactivation occur primarily in the liver. Some estrogens are excreted into the bile; however, they are reabsorbed from the intestine and returned to the liver through the portal venous system. Water-soluble estrogen conjugates are strongly acidic and, therefore, ionized in body fluids, which favor excretion through the kidneys since tubular reabsorption is minimal.

INDICATIONS AND USAGE

Premarin (conjugated estrogens) Vaginal Cream is indicated in the treatment of atrophic vaginitis and kraurosis vulvae.

Premarin Vaginal Cream HAS NOT BEEN SHOWN TO BE EFFECTIVE FOR ANY PURPOSE DURING PREGNANCY AND ITS USE MAY CAUSE SEVERE HARM TO THE FETUS (SEE BOXED WARNING).

CONTRAINDICATIONS

Estrogens should not be used in women with any of the following conditions:

1. Known or suspected cancer of the breast except in appropriately selected patients being treated for metastatic disease.
2. Known or suspected estrogen-dependent neoplasia.
3. Known or suspected pregnancy (see Boxed Warning).
4. Undiagnosed abnormal genital bleeding.
5. Active thrombophlebitis or thromboembolic disorders.

6. A past history of thrombophlebitis, thrombosis, or thromboembolic disorders associated with previous estrogen use (except when used in treatment of breast malignancy). Premarin Vaginal Cream should not be used in patients hypersensitive to its ingredients.

WARNINGS

1. *Induction of malignant neoplasms.* Long-term, continuous administration of natural and synthetic estrogens in certain animal species increases the frequency of carcinomas of the breast, cervix, vagina, and liver. There are now reports that estrogens increase the risk of carcinoma of the endometrium in humans (see Boxed Warning).

At the present time there is no satisfactory evidence that estrogens given to postmenopausal women increase the risk of cancer of the breast,[17] although a recent long-term follow-up of a single physician's practice has raised this possibility.[18] Because of the animal data, there is a need for caution in prescribing estrogens for women with a strong family history of breast cancer or who have breast nodules, fibrocystic disease, or abnormal mammograms.

2. *Gallbladder disease.* A recent study has reported a 2- to 3-fold increase in the risk of surgically confirmed gallbladder disease in women receiving postmenopausal estrogens,[17] similar to the 2-fold increase previously noted in users of oral contraceptives.[19,24a]

3. *Effects similar to those caused by estrogen-progestogen oral contraceptives.* There are several serious adverse effects of oral contraceptives, some of which have not, up to now, been documented as consequences of postmenopausal estrogen therapy. This may reflect the comparatively low doses of estrogen used in postmenopausal women. It would be expected that the larger doses of estrogen used to treat prostatic or breast cancer are more likely to result in these adverse effects, and, in fact, it has been shown that there is an increased risk of thrombosis in men receiving estrogens for prostatic cancer.[20–23]

a. *Thromboembolic disease.* It is now well established that users of oral contraceptives have an increased risk of various thromboembolic and thrombotic vascular diseases, such as thrombophlebitis, pulmonary embolism, stroke, and myocardial infarction.[24–31] Cases of retinal thrombosis, mesenteric thrombosis, and optic neuritis have been reported in oral-contraceptive users. There is evidence that the risk of several of these adverse reactions is related to the dose of the drug.[32,33] An increased risk of postsurgery thromboembolic complications has also been reported in users of oral contraceptives.[34,35] If feasible, estrogen should be discontinued at least 4 weeks before surgery of the type associated with an increased risk of thromboembolism, or during periods of prolonged immobilization.

In some studies, women on estrogen replacement therapy, given alone or in combination with a progestin, have been reported to have an increased risk of thrombophlebitis, and/or thromboembolic disease. The physician should be aware of the possibility of thrombotic disorders (thrombophlebitis, retinal thrombosis, cerebral embolism, and pulmonary embolism) during estrogen replacement therapy and be alert to their earliest manifestations. Should any of these occur or be suspected, estrogen replacement therapy should be discontinued immediately. Patients who have risk factors for thrombotic disorders should be kept under careful observation. Subgroups of women who have underlying risk factors, or who are receiving relatively large doses of estrogens, may have increased risk. Therefore, estrogens should not be used in persons with active thrombophlebitis or thromboembolic disorders, and they should not be used (except in treatment of malignancy) in persons with a history of such disorders in association with estrogen use. They should be used with caution in patients with cerebral vascular or coronary artery disease and only for those in whom estrogens are clearly needed.

Large doses of estrogen (5 mg conjugated estrogens per day), comparable to those used to treat cancer of the prostate and breast, have been shown in a large prospective clinical trial in men[36] to increase the risk of nonfatal myocardial infarction, pulmonary embolism, and thrombophlebitis. When estrogen doses of this size are used, any of the thromboembolic and thrombotic adverse effects associated with oral contraceptives or estrogen replacement therapy should be considered a clear risk.

b. *Hepatic adenoma.* Benign hepatic adenomas appear to be associated with the use of oral contraceptives.[37–39] Although benign, and rare, these may rupture and may cause death through intra-abdominal hemorrhage. Such lesions have not yet been reported in association with other estrogen or progestogen preparations but should be considered in estrogen users having abdominal pain and tenderness, abdominal mass, or hypovolemic shock. Hepatocellular carcinoma has also been reported in women taking estrogen-containing oral contraceptives.[38] The relationship of this malignancy to these drugs is not known at this time.

c. *Elevated blood pressure.* Women using oral contraceptives sometimes experience increased blood pressure which, in most cases, returns to normal on discontinuing the drug. There is now a report that this may occur with use of estro-

gens in the menopause[40] and blood pressure should be monitored with estrogen use, especially if high doses are used.

d. *Glucose tolerance.* A worsening of glucose tolerance has been observed in a significant percentage of patients on estrogen-containing oral contraceptives. For this reason, diabetic patients should be carefully observed while receiving estrogen.

4. *Hypercalcemia.* Administration of estrogens may lead to severe hypercalcemia in patients with breast cancer and bone metastases. If this occurs, the drug should be stopped and appropriate measures taken to reduce the serum calcium level.

PRECAUTIONS

A. General Precautions.

1. A complete medical and family history should be taken prior to the initiation of any estrogen therapy. The pretreatment and periodic physical examinations should include special reference to blood pressure, breasts, abdomen, and pelvic organs, and should include a Papanicolaou smear. As a general rule, estrogens should not be prescribed for longer than one year without another physical examination being performed.

2. Fluid retention—Because estrogens may cause some degree of fluid retention, conditions which might be influenced by this factor, such as asthma, epilepsy, migraine, and cardiac or renal dysfunction, require careful observation.

3. Familial hyperlipoproteinemia—Estrogen therapy may be associated with massive elevations of plasma triglycerides leading to pancreatitis and other complications in patients with familial defects of lipoprotein metabolism.

4. Certain patients may develop undesirable manifestations of excessive estrogenic stimulation, such as abnormal or excessive uterine bleeding, mastodynia, etc.

5. Prolonged administration of unopposed estrogen therapy has been reported to increase the risk of endometrial hyperplasia in some patients.

6. Oral contraceptives appear to be associated with an increased incidence of mental depression.[24a] Although it is not clear whether this is due to the estrogenic or progestogenic component of the contraceptive, patients with a history of depression should be carefully observed.

7. Preexisting uterine leiomyomata may increase in size during estrogen use.

8. The pathologist should be advised of estrogen therapy when relevant specimens are submitted.

9. Patients with a past history of jaundice during pregnancy have an increased risk of recurrence of jaundice while receiving estrogen-containing oral-contraceptive therapy. If jaundice develops in any patient receiving estrogen, the medication should be discontinued while the cause is investigated.

10. Estrogens may be poorly metabolized in patients with impaired liver function and should be administered with caution in such patients.

11. Because estrogens influence the metabolism of calcium and phosphorus, they should be used with caution in patients with metabolic bone diseases that are associated with hypercalcemia or in patients with renal insufficiency.

12. Because of the effects of estrogens on epiphyseal closure, they should be used judiciously in young patients in whom bone growth is not yet complete.

13. Barrier contraceptives - Premarin Vaginal Cream exposure has been reported to weaken latex condoms. The potential for Premarin Vaginal Cream to weaken and contribute to the failure of condoms, diaphragms, or cervical caps made of latex or rubber should be considered.

Concomitant Progestin Use:

The lowest effective dose appropriate for the specific indication should be utilized. Studies of the addition of a progestin for 7 or more days of a cycle of estrogen administration have reported a lowered incidence of endometrial hyperplasia. Morphological and biochemical studies of the endometrium suggest that 10 to 13 days of progestin are needed to provide maximal maturation of the endometrium and to eliminate any hyperplastic changes. Whether this will provide protection from endometrial carcinoma has not been clearly established. There are possible additional risks which may be associated with the inclusion of progestin in estrogen replacement regimens. If concomitant progestin therapy is used, potential risks may include adverse effects on carbohydrate and lipid metabolism. The choice of progestin and dosage may be important in minimizing these adverse effects.

B. Information For Patients

(See text which appears after the **PHYSICIAN REFERENCES.**)

C. Drug/Laboratory Test Interactions

Certain endocrine and liver function tests may be affected by estrogen-containing oral contraceptives. The following similar changes may be expected with larger doses of estrogen:

a. Increased sulfobromophthalein retention.

b. Increased prothrombin and factors VII, VIII, IX, and X; decreased antithrombin 3; increased norepinephrine-induced platelet aggregability.

c. Increased thyroid binding globulin (TBG) leading to increased circulating total thyroid hormone, as measured by PBI, T_4 by column, or T_4 by radioimmunoassay. Free T_3 resin uptake is decreased, reflecting the elevated TBG; free T_4 concentration is unaltered.
d. Impaired glucose tolerance.
e. Decreased pregnanediol excretion.
f. Reduced response to metyrapone test.
g. Reduced serum folate concentration.
h. Increased serum triglyceride and phospholipid concentration.

D. **Carcinogenesis, Mutagenesis, Impairment Of Fertility**
(See **WARNINGS** section for information on carcinogenesis.)

E. **Pregnancy Category X**
(See **CONTRAINDICATIONS** and Boxed Warning.)

F. **Nursing Mothers**
It is not known whether this drug is excreted in human milk. Because many drugs are excreted in human milk and because of the potential for serious adverse reactions in nursing infants from estrogens, a decision should be made whether to discontinue nursing or to discontinue the drug, taking into account the importance of the drug to the mother.

G. **Pediatric Use**
Safety and effectiveness in pediatric patients have not been established.

ADVERSE REACTIONS

(See **WARNINGS** regarding induction of neoplasia, adverse effects on the fetus, increased incidence of gallbladder disease, and adverse effects similar to those of oral contraceptives, including thromboembolism.) The following additional adverse reactions have been reported with estrogenic therapy, including oral contraceptives:

1. *Genitourinary system:* Breakthrough bleeding, spotting, change in menstrual flow; dysmenorrhea; premenstrual-like syndrome; amenorrhea during and after treatment; increase in size of uterine fibromyomata; vaginal candidiasis; change in cervical erosion and in degree of cervical secretion; cystitis-like syndrome.
2. *Breasts:* Tenderness, enlargement, secretion.
3. *Gastrointestinal:* Nausea, vomiting; abdominal cramps, bloating; cholestatic jaundice, pancreatitis.
4. *Skin:* Chloasma or melasma which may persist when drug is discontinued; erythema multiforme; erythema nodosum; hemorrhagic eruption; loss of scalp hair; hirsutism.
5. *Cardiovascular:* Venous thromboembolism, pulmonary embolism.
6. *Eyes:* Steepening of corneal curvature; intolerance to contact lenses.
7. *CNS:* Headache, migraine, dizziness; mental depression; chorea.
8. *Miscellaneous:* Increase or decrease in weight; reduced carbohydrate tolerance; aggravation of porphyria; edema; changes in libido.

OVERDOSAGE

Numerous reports of ingestion of large doses of estrogen-containing oral contraceptives by young children indicate that acute serious ill effects do not occur. Overdosage of estrogens may cause nausea, and withdrawal bleeding may occur in females.

DOSAGE AND ADMINISTRATION

Given cyclically for short-term use only:
For treatment of atrophic vaginitis, or kraurosis vulvae.
The lowest dose that will control symptoms should be chosen and medication should be discontinued as promptly as possible.
Administration should be cyclic (e.g., three weeks on and one week off).
Attempts to discontinue or taper medication should be made at three- to six-month intervals.

Usual Dosage Range:
$^1/_2$ to 2 g daily, intravaginally, depending on the severity of the condition.
Treated patients with an intact uterus should be monitored closely for signs of endometrial cancer, and appropriate diagnostic measures should be taken to rule out malignancy in the event of persistent or recurring abnormal vaginal bleeding.

Instructions for Use of Gentle Measure™ Applicator:
1. Remove cap from tube.
2. Screw nozzle end of applicator onto tube.
3. *Gently* squeeze tube from the *bottom* to force sufficient cream into the barrel to provide the prescribed dose. Use the marked stopping points on the applicator as a guideline to measure the correct dose.
4. Unscrew applicator from tube.
5. Lie on back with knees drawn up. To deliver medication, gently insert applicator deeply into vagina and press plunger downward to its original position.

TO CLEANSE: Pull plunger to remove it from barrel. Wash with mild soap and warm water.
DO NOT BOIL OR USE HOT WATER.

HOW SUPPLIED

Premarin® (conjugated estrogens) Vaginal Cream—Each gram contains 0.625 mg conjugated estrogens, USP.
Combination package: Each contains Net Wt. $1^1/_2$ oz (42.5 g) tube with one plastic applicator calibrated in $^1/_2$ g increments to a maximum of 2 g (NDC 0046-0872-93).
Also Available—Refill package: Each contains Net Wt. $1^1/_2$ oz (42.5 g) tube (NDC 0046-0872-01).
Store at room temperature (approximately 25° C).

PHYSICIAN REFERENCES

1. Ziel, H. K. et al: N. Engl. J. Med. *293* :1167–1170, 1975.
2. Smith, D. C. et al: N. Engl. J. Med. *293* :1164–1167, 1975.
3. Mack, T. M. et al: N. Engl. J. Med *294* :1262–1267, 1976.
4. Weiss, N. S. et al: N. Engl. J. Med. *294* :1259–1262, 1976.
5. Herbst, A. L. et al: N. Engl. J. Med. *284* :878–881, 1971.
6. Greenwald, P. et al: N. Engl. J. Med. *285* :390–392, 1971.
7. Lanier, A. et al: Mayo Clin. Proc. *48* :793–799, 1973.
8. Herbst, A. et al: Obstet. Gynecol. *40* :287–298, 1972.
9. Herbst, A. et al: Am. J. Obstet. Gynecol. *118* :607–615, 1974.
10. Herbst, A. et al: N. Engl. J. Med. *292* :334–339, 1975.
11. Stafl, A. et al: Obstet. Gynecol. *43* :118–128, 1974.
12. Sherman, A. I. et al: Obstet. Gynecol. *44* :531–545, 1974.
13. Gal, I. et al: Nature *216* :83, 1967.
14. Levy, E. P. et al: Lancet *1* :611, 1973.
15. Nora, J. et al: Lancet *1* :941–942, 1973.
16. Janerich, D. T. et al: N. Engl. J. Med. *291* :697–700, 1974.
17. Boston Collaborative Drug Surveillance Program: N. Engl. J. Med. *290* :15–19, 1974.
18. Hoover, R. et al: N. Engl. J. Med. *295* :401–405, 1976.
19. Boston Collaborative Drug Surveillance Program: Lancet *1* :1399–1404, 1973.
20. Daniel, D. G. et al: Lancet *2* :287–289, 1967.
21. The Veterans Administration Cooperative Urological Research Group: J. Urol. *98* :516–522, 1967.
22. Bailar, J. C.: Lancet *2* :560, 1967.
23. Blackard, C. et al: Cancer *26* :249–256, 1970.
24. Royal College of General Practitioners: J. R. Coll. Gen. Pract. *13* :267–279, 1967.
24a. Royal College of General Practitioners: Oral Contraceptives and Health, New York, Pitman Corp., 1974.
25. Inman, W. H. W. et al: Br. Med. J. *2* :193–199, 1968.
26. Vessey, M. P. et al: Br. Med. J. *2* :651–657, 1969.
27. Sartwell, P. E. et al: Am. J. Epidemiol. *90* :365–380, 1969.
28. Collaborative Group for the Study of Stroke in Young Women: N. Engl. J. Med. *288* :871–878, 1973.
29. Collaborative Group for the Study of Stroke in Young Women: J.A.M.A. *231* :718–722, 1975.
30. Mann, J. I. et al: Br. Med. J. *2* :245–248, 1975.
31. Mann, J. I. et al: Br. Med. J. *2* :241–245, 1975.
32. Inman, W. H. W. et al: Br. Med. J. *2* :203–209, 1970.
33. Stolley, P. D. et al: Am. J. Epidemiol. *102* :197–208, 1975.
34. Vessey, M. P. et al: Br. Med. J. *3* :123–126, 1970.
35. Greene, G. R. et al: Am. J. Public Health *62* :680–685, 1972.
36. Coronary Drug Project Research Group: J.A.M.A. *214* : 1303–1313, 1970.
37. Baum, J. et al: Lancet *2* :926–928, 1973.
38. Mays, E. T. et al: J.A.M.A. *235* :730–732, 1976.
39. Edmondson, H. A. et al: N. Engl. J. Med. *294* :470–472, 1976.
40. Pfeffer, R. I. et al: Am. J. Epidemiol. *103* :445–456, 1976.

INFORMATION FOR THE PATIENT

WHAT YOU SHOULD KNOW ABOUT ESTROGENS

Estrogens are female hormones produced by the ovaries. The ovaries make several different kinds of estrogens. In addition, scientists have been able to make a variety of synthetic estrogens. As far as we know, all these estrogens have similar properties and, therefore, much the same usefulness, side effects, and risks. This leaflet is intended to help you understand what estrogens are used for, the risks involved in their use, and how to use them as safely as possible.
This leaflet includes the most important information about estrogens, but not all the information. If you want to know more, you should ask your doctor for more information or you can ask your doctor or pharmacist to let you read the package insert prepared for the doctor.

USES OF ESTROGEN

THERE IS NO PROPER USE OF ESTROGENS IN A PREGNANT WOMAN.
Estrogens are prescribed by doctors for a number of purposes, including:
1. To provide estrogen during a period of adjustment when a woman's ovaries stop producing a majority of her estrogens, in order to prevent certain uncomfortable symptoms of estrogen deficiency. (With the menopause, which generally occurs between the ages of 45 and 55, women produce a much smaller amount of estrogens.)
2. To prevent symptoms of estrogen deficiency when a woman's ovaries have been removed surgically before the natural menopause.
3. To prevent pregnancy. (Estrogens are given along with a progestogen, another female hormone; these combinations are called oral contraceptives, or birth-control pills. Patient labeling is available to women taking oral contraceptives and they will not be discussed in this leaflet.)
4. To treat certain cancers in women and men.

ESTROGENS IN THE MENOPAUSE

In the natural course of their lives, all women eventually experience a decrease in estrogen production. This usually occurs between ages 45 and 55, but may occur earlier or later. Sometimes the ovaries may need to be removed before natural menopause by an operation, producing a "surgical menopause."
When the amount of estrogen in the blood begins to decrease, many women may develop typical symptoms: feelings of warmth in the face, neck, and chest, or sudden intense episodes of heat and sweating throughout the body (called "hot flashes" or "hot flushes"). These symptoms are sometimes very uncomfortable. Some women may also develop changes in the vagina (called "atrophic vaginitis") that cause discomfort, especially during and after intercourse.
Estrogens can be prescribed to treat these symptoms of the menopause. It is estimated that considerably more than half of all women undergoing the menopause have only mild symptoms or no symptoms at all and, therefore, do not need estrogens. Other women may need estrogens for a few months, while their bodies adjust to lower estrogen levels. Sometimes the need will be for periods longer than six months. In an attempt to avoid overstimulation of the uterus (womb), estrogens are usually given cyclically during each month of use, such as three weeks of pills followed by one week without pills.
Sometimes women experience nervous symptoms or depression during menopause. There is no evidence that estrogens are effective for such symptoms without associated vasomotor symptoms. In the absence of vasomotor symptoms, estrogens should not be used to treat nervous symptoms, although other treatment may be needed.
You may have heard that taking estrogens for long periods (years) after the menopause will keep your skin soft and supple and keep you feeling young. There is no evidence that this is so, however, and such long-term treatment carries important risks.

THE DANGERS OF ESTROGENS

1. *Endometrial cancer.* There are reports that if estrogens are used in the postmenopausal period for more than a year, there is an increased risk of *endometrial cancer* (cancer of the lining of the uterus). Women taking estrogens have roughly 5- to 10-times as great a chance of getting this cancer as women who take no estrogens. To put this another way, while a postmenopausal woman not taking estrogens has 1 chance in 1,000 each year of getting endometrial cancer, a woman taking estrogens has 5 to 10 chances in 1,000 each year. For this reason *it is important to take estrogens only when they are really needed.*
The risk of this cancer is greater the longer estrogens are used and when larger doses are taken. Therefore, you should not take more estrogen than your doctor prescribes. *It is important to take the lowest dose of estrogen that will control symptoms and to take it only as long as it is needed.* If estrogens are needed for longer periods of time, your doctor will want to reevaluate your need for estrogens at least every six months.
Women using estrogens should report any vaginal bleeding to their doctors; such bleeding may be of no importance, but it can be an early warning of endometrial cancer. If you have undiagnosed vaginal bleeding, you should not use estrogens until a diagnosis is made and you are certain there is no endometrial cancer.
Note: If you have had your uterus removed (total hysterectomy), there is no danger of developing endometrial cancer.
2. *Other possible cancers.* Estrogens can cause development of other tumors in animals, such as tumors of the breast, cervix, vagina, or liver, when given for a long time. At present there is no good evidence that women using estrogens in the menopause have an increased risk of such tumors, but there is no way yet to be sure they do not; and one study raises the possibility that use of estrogens in the menopause may increase the risk of breast cancer many years later. This is a further reason to use estrogens only when clearly needed. While you are taking estrogens, it is important that you go to your doctor at least once a year for a physical examination. Also, if members of your family have had breast cancers or if you have breast nodules, or abnormal mammograms (breast X rays), your doctor may wish to carry out more frequent examinations of your breasts.
3. *Gallbladder disease.* Women who use estrogens after menopause are more likely to develop gallbladder disease needing surgery than women who do not use estrogens. Birth-control pills have a similar effect.

Continued on next page

Premarin Vaginal Cream—Cont.

4. *Abnormal blood clotting.* Taking estrogens may increase the risk of blood clotting in various parts of the body. This can result in a stroke (if the clot is in the brain), a heart attack (a clot in a blood vessel of the heart), or a pulmonary embolus (a clot which forms in the legs or pelvis, then breaks off and travels to the lungs). Any of these can be fatal.

It is recommended that if you have had clotting in the legs or lungs, or a heart attack or stroke while you were using estrogens or birth-control pills, you should not use estrogens (unless they are being used to treat cancer of the breast or prostate). If you have had a stroke or heart attack, or if you have angina pectoris, estrogens should be used with great caution and only if clearly needed (for example, if you have severe symptoms of the menopause).

5. *Inflammation of the pancreas (Pancreatitis).* Women with high triglyceride levels may have increased risk of developing inflammation of the pancreas.

SPECIAL WARNING ABOUT PREGNANCY

You should not receive estrogen if you are pregnant. If this should occur, there is a greater than usual chance that the developing child will be born with a birth defect, although the possibility remains fairly small. A female child may have an increased risk of developing cancer of the vagina or cervix later in life (in the teens or twenties). Every possible effort should be made to avoid exposure to estrogens during pregnancy. If exposure occurs, see your doctor.

OTHER EFFECTS OF ESTROGENS

In addition to the serious known risks of estrogens described above, estrogens have the following side effects and potential risks:

1. *Nausea and vomiting.* The most common side effect of estrogen therapy is nausea. Vomiting is less common.
2. *Effects on breasts.* Estrogens may cause breast tenderness or enlargement and may cause the breasts to secrete a liquid. These effects are not dangerous.
3. *Effects on the uterus.* Estrogens may cause benign fibroid tumors of the uterus to get larger.
4. *Effects on liver.* Women taking oral contraceptives develop, on rare occasions, a tumor of the liver which can rupture and bleed into the abdomen and may cause death. So far, these tumors have not been reported in women using estrogens in the menopause, but you should report any swelling or unusual pain or tenderness in the abdomen to your doctor immediately.

Women with a past history of jaundice (yellowing of the skin and white parts of the eyes) may get jaundice again during estrogen use. If this occurs, stop taking estrogens and see your doctor.

5. *Other effects.* Estrogens may cause excess fluid to be retained in the body. This may make some conditions worse, such as asthma, epilepsy, migraine, heart disease, or kidney disease.

SUMMARY

Estrogens have important uses, but they have serious risks as well. You must decide, with your doctor, whether the risks are acceptable to you in view of the benefits of treatment. Except where your doctor has prescribed estrogens for use in special cases of cancer of the breast or prostate, you should not use estrogens if you have cancer of the breast or uterus, are pregnant, have undiagnosed abnormal vaginal bleeding, clotting in the legs or lungs, or have had a stroke, heart attack or angina, or clotting in the legs or lungs in the past while you were taking estrogens.

You can use estrogens as safely as possible by understanding that your doctor will require regular physical examinations while you are taking them, will try to discontinue the drug as soon as possible, and will use the smallest dose possible. Be alert for signs of trouble including:

1. Abnormal bleeding from the vagina.
2. Pains in the calves or chest, sudden shortness of breath, or coughing blood.
3. Severe headache, dizziness, faintness, or changes in vision.
4. Breast lumps (you should ask your doctor how to examine your own breasts).
5. Jaundice (yellowing of the skin).
6. Mental depression.

Your doctor has prescribed this drug for you and you alone. Do not give the drug to anyone else.

Premarin Vaginal Cream exposure has been reported to weaken latex condoms. The potential for Premarin Vaginal Cream to weaken and contribute to the failure of condoms, diaphragms, or cervical caps made of latex or rubber should be considered.

HOW SUPPLIED

Premarin® (conjugated estrogens) Vaginal Cream—Each gram contains 0.625 mg conjugated estrogens, USP.

Combination package: Each contains Net Wt. 1$^1/_2$ oz (42.5 g) tube with one plastic applicator calibrated in $^1/_2$ g increments to a maximum of 2 g (NDC 0046-0872-93).

Also Available —Refill package: Each contains Net Wt. 1$^1/_2$ oz (42.5 g) tube (NDC 0046-0872-01).

Store at room temperature (approximately 25° C).

Instructions FOR Use of Premarin® (conjugated estrogens) VAGINAL CREAM Gentle Measure™ Applicator:

The Gentle Measure Applicator has been specifically designed for comfortable, easy use.

1. Remove cap from tube.
2. Screw nozzle end of applicator onto tube.
3. *Gently* squeeze tube from the *bottom* to force sufficient cream into the barrel to provide the prescribed dose. Use the marked stopping points on the applicator as a guideline to measure the correct dose.
4. Unscrew applicator from tube.
5. Lie on back with knees drawn up. To deliver medication, gently insert applicator deeply into vagina and press plunger downward to its original position.

TO CLEANSE: Pull plunger to remove it from barrel. Wash with mild soap and warm water.

DO NOT BOIL OR USE HOT WATER.

Manufactured by:
Ayerst Laboratories Inc.
A Wyeth-Ayerst Company
Philadelphia, PA 19101

Shown in Product Identification Guide, page 344

PREMPRO™ ℞

(conjugated estrogens/medroxyprogesterone acetate tablets)

PREMPHASE®

(conjugated estrogens/medroxyprogesterone acetate tablets)

Caution: Federal law prohibits dispensing without prescription.

DESCRIPTION

PREMPRO therapy consists of a single tablet containing 0.625 mg of the conjugated estrogens found in Premarin® tablets and 2.5 mg or 5 mg of medroxyprogesterone acetate (MPA) for oral administration.

PREMPHASE therapy consists of two separate tablets, a maroon Premarin tablet containing 0.625 mg of conjugated estrogens which is taken orally on days 1 through 14 and a light-blue tablet containing 0.625 mg of the conjugated estrogens found in Premarin tablets and 5 mg of medroxyprogesterone acetate (MPA) which is taken orally on days 15 through 28.

The conjugated estrogens found in Premarin tablets are a mixture of sodium estrone sulfate and sodium equilin sulfate. They contain as concomitant components sodium sulfate conjugates, 17α-dihydroequilin, 17α-estradiol and 17β-dihydroequilin.

Medroxyprogesterone acetate is a derivative of progesterone. It is a white to off-white, odorless, crystalline powder, stable in air, melting between 200° C and 210° C. It is freely soluble in chloroform, soluble in acetone and in dioxane, sparingly soluble in alcohol and in methanol, slightly soluble in ether, and insoluble in water. The chemical name for MPA is pregn-4-ene-3,20-dione, 17-(acetyloxy)-6-methyl-, (6α)-. Its molecular formula is $C_{24}H_{34}O_4$, with a molecular weight of 386.53. Its structural formula is:

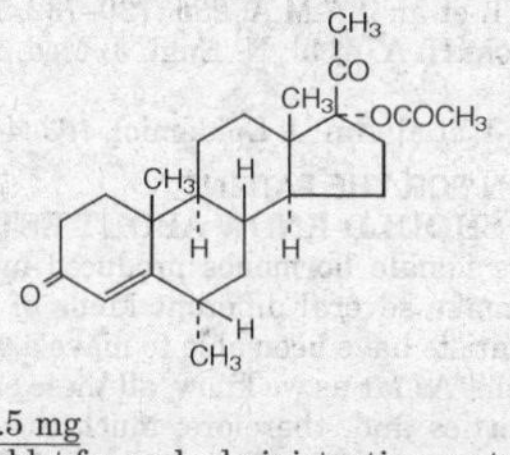

PREMPRO 2.5 mg

Each peach tablet for oral administration contains 0.625 mg conjugated estrogens, 2.5 mg of medroxyprogesterone acetate and the following inactive ingredients: calcium phosphate tribasic, calcium sulfate, carnauba wax, cellulose, glyceryl monooleate, lactose, magnesium stearate, methylcellulose, pharmaceutical glaze, polyethylene glycol, sucrose, povidone, titanium dioxide, and red ferric oxide.

PREMPRO 5.0 mg

Each light-blue tablet for oral administration contains 0.625 mg conjugated estrogens, 5 mg of medroxyprogesterone acetate and the following inactive ingredients: calcium phosphate tribasic, calcium sulfate, carnauba wax, cellulose, glyceryl monooleate, lactose, magnesium stearate, methylcellulose, pharmaceutical glaze, polyethylene glycol, sucrose, povidone, titanium dioxide, FD&C Blue No. 2.

PREMPHASE

Each maroon Premarin tablet for oral administration contains 0.625 mg of conjugated estrogens and the following inactive ingredients: calcium phosphate tribasic, calcium sulfate, carnauba wax, cellulose, glyceryl monooleate, lactose, magnesium stearate, methylcellulose, pharmaceutical glaze, polyethylene glycol, stearic acid, sucrose, titanium dioxide, FD&C Blue No.2, D&C Red No. 27, FD&C Red No. 40. These tablets comply with USP Drug Release Test 1.

Each light-blue tablet for oral administration contains 0.625 mg of conjugated estrogens and 5 mg of medroxyprogesterone acetate and the following inactive ingredients: calcium phosphate tribasic, calcium sulfate, carnauba wax, cellulose, glyceryl monooleate, lactose, magnesium stearate, methylcellulose, pharmaceutical glaze, polyethylene glycol, sucrose, povidone, titanium dioxide, FD&C Blue No.2.

CLINICAL PHARMACOLOGY

Estrogens are largely responsible for the development and maintenance of the female reproductive system and secondary sexual characteristics. By a direct action, they cause growth and development of the uterus, fallopian tubes, and vagina. With other hormones, such as pituitary hormones and progesterone, they cause enlargement of the breasts through promotion of ductal growth, stromal development, and the secretion of fat. Estrogens are intricately involved with other hormones, especially progesterone, in the processes of the ovulatory menstrual cycle and pregnancy and affect the release of pituitary gonadotropins. They also contribute to the shaping of the skeleton, maintenance of tone and elasticity of urogenital structures, changes in the epiphyses of the long bones that allow for the pubertal growth spurt and its termination, and pigmentation of the nipples and genitals.

Although circulating estrogens exist in a dynamic equilibrium of metabolic interconversions, estradiol is the principal intracellular human estrogen and is substantially more potent than its metabolites, estrone and estriol at the receptor level. The primary source of estrogen in normally cycling adult women is the ovarian follicle, which secretes 70 to 500 µg of estradiol daily, depending on the phase of the menstrual cycle. After menopause, most endogenous estrogen is produced by interconversion of androstenedione, secreted by the adrenal cortex, to estrone by peripheal tissues. Thus, estrone and the sulfate conjugated form, estrone sulfate, are the most abundant circulating estrogens in postmenopausal women.

Circulating estrogens modulate the pituitary secretion of gonadotropins, luteinizing hormone (LH) and follicle stimulating hormone (FSH) through a negative feedback mechanism. Estrogen replacement therapy acts to reduce the elevated levels of these hormones seen in postmenopausal women.

The pharmacologic effects of the administered conjugated estrogens are similar to those of endogenous estrogens. In responsive tissue (female genital organs, breasts, hypothalamus, pituitary) estrogens enter the cell and are transported into the nucleus. As a result of the estrogen action, specific RNA and protein synthesis occurs.

The use of unopposed estrogen therapy has been associated with an increased risk of endometrial hyperplasia, a possible precursor of endometrial adenocarcinoma. The results of clinical studies indicate that the addition of a progestin to an estrogen replacement regimen for more than 10 days per cycle reduces the incidence of endometrial hyperplasia and the attendant risk of adenocarcinoma in women with intact uteri. The addition of a progestin to an estrogen replacement regimen has not been shown to interfere with the efficacy of estrogen replacement therapy for its approved indications.

Androgenic and anabolic effects of medroxyprogesterone acetate (MPA) have been noted, but the drug is apparently devoid of significant estrogenic activity. Parenterally administered MPA inhibits gonadotropin production, which in turn prevents follicular maturation and ovulation, although available data indicate that this does not occur when the usually recommended oral dosage is given as single daily doses. MPA may achieve its beneficial effect on the endometrium in part by decreasing nuclear estradiol receptors and suppression of epithelial DNA synthesis in endometrial tissue.

PHARMACOKINETICS

Absorption

Conjugated estrogens are soluble in water and are well absorbed from the gastrointestinal tract after release from the drug formulation. However, PREMPRO and PREMPHASE contain a formulation of MPA that is immediately released and a modified-release formulation of conjugated estrogens that slowly releases estrogens over several hours. Maximum plasma concentrations of the various conjugated and unconjugated estrogens are attained within 4 to 10 hours after dose administration. MPA is well absorbed from the gastrointestinal tract, and maximum MPA plasma concentrations are attained within 2 to 4 hours after dose administration. Table 1 summarizes the mean pharmacokinetic parameters for unconjugated and conjugated estrogens, and medroxyprogesterone acetate following administration of 0.625 mg/2.5 mg and 0.625 mg/5mg tablets to healthy postmenopausal women.

Food-Effect: Single dose studies in healthy, postmenopausal women were conducted to investigate any potential

Table 1. PHARMACOKINETIC PARAMETERS FOR UNCONJUGATED AND CONJUGATED ESTROGENS (CE), AND MEDROXYPROGESTERONE ACETATE

DRUG	2 × 0.625 mg CE/2.5 mg MPA Combination Tablets (n=54)				2 × 0.625 mg CE/5 mg MPA Combination Tablets (n=51)			
PK Parameter Geometric Mean (SD)	C_{max} (pg/mL)	t_{max} (h)	$t_{1/2}$ (h)	AUC (pg•h/mL)	C_{max} (pg/mL)	t_{max} (h)	$t_{1/2}$ (h)	AUC (pg•h/mL)
Unconjugated Estrogens								
Estrone	175 (41)	7.6 (1.8)	31.6 (7.4)	5358 (1840)	124 (53)	10 (3.5)	62.2 (85.2)	6303 (2542)
BA*-Estrone	159 (41)	7.6 (1.8)	16.9 (5.8)	3313 (1310)	104 (51)	10 (3.5)	26.0 (25.9)	3136 (1598)
Equilin	71 (22)	5.8 (2.0)	9.9 (3.5)	951 (413)	52 (23)	8.9 (3.0)	15.5 (8.2)	1179 (540)
PK Parameter Geometric Mean (SD)	C_{max} (ng/mL)	t_{max} (h)	$t_{1/2}$ (h)	AUC (ng•h/mL)	C_{max} (ng/mL)	t_{max} (h)	$t_{1/2}$ (h)	AUC (ng•h/mL)
Conjugated Estrogens								
Total Estrone	6.6 (2.5)	6.1 (1.7)	20.7 (7.0)	116 (68)	6.3 (3.0)	9.1 (2.6)	23.6 (8.4)	151 (63)
BA*-Total Estrone	6.4 (2.5)	6.1 (1.7)	15.4 (5.2)	100 (57)	6.2 (3.0)	9.1 (2.6)	20.6 (7.3)	139 (56)
Total Equilin	5.1 (2.3)	4.6 (1.6)	11.4 (2.9)	50 (35)	4.2 (2.2)	7.0 (2.5)	17.2 (22.6)	72 (36)
Medroxyprogesterone Acetate	C_{max} (ng/mL)	t_{max} (h)	$t_{1/2}$ (h)	Cl/F (L/h/kg)	C_{max} (ng/mL)	t_{max} (h)	$t_{1/2}$ (h)	Cl/F (L/h/kg)
MPA	1.5 (0.6)	2.8 (1.5)	37.6 (11.2)	2.3 (0.7)	48 (1.5)	2.4 (1.2)	46.3 (18.0)	1.6 (0.5)

BA* = Baseline Adjusted
C_{max} = peak plasma concentration
t_{max} = time peak concentration occurs
$t_{1/2}$ = terminal-phase disposition half-life $(0.693/\lambda_z)$
AUC = total area under the curve
Cl/F = apparent oral clearance

drug interaction when PREMPRO or PREMPHASE is administered with a high fat breakfast. Administration with food decreased the C_{max} of total estrone by 18 to 34% and increased total equilin C_{max} by 38% compared to the fasting state, with no other effect on the rate or extent of absorption of other conjugated or unconjugated estrogens. Administration with food approximately doubles MPA C_{max} and increases MPA AUC by approximately 20 to 30%.

Dose Proportionality: The C_{max} and AUC values for MPA observed in two separate pharmacokinetic studies conducted with PREMPRO or PREMPHASE 2 × 0.625 mg/2.5 mg and 2 × 0.625 mg/5mg tablets exhibited nonlinear dose proportionality; doubling the MPA dose from 2 × 2.5 to 2 × 5.0 mg increased the mean C_{max} and AUC by 3.2 and 2.8 folds, respectively. The apparent clearance (Cl/F) of MPA obtained with 2 × 0.625 mg/5 mg tablets was lower than that observed with 2 × 0.625 mg/2.5 mg tablets.
[See table 1 above]

Distribution
The conjugated estrogens bind mainly to albumin, but the unconjugated estrogens bind to both albumin and sex-hormone-binding globulin (SHBG). MPA is approximately 90% bound to plasma proteins but does not bind to SHBG.

Metabolism
Metabolism and inactivation of estrogens occur primarily in the liver. Some estrogens are excreted into the bile; however, they are reabsorbed from the intestine and returned to the liver through the portal venous system. Metabolism and elimination of MPA occurs primarily in the liver via hydroxylation, with subsequent conjugation and elimination in the urine.

Excretion
Water-soluble estrogen conjugates are strongly acidic and are ionized in body fluids, which favor excretion through the kidneys since tubular reabsorption is minimal. The apparent terminal-phase disposition half-life ($t_{1/2}$) of the various estrogens is prolonged by the slow absorption from PREMPRO and PREMPHASE and ranges from 10 to 24 hours. Most metabolites of MPA are excreted as glucuronide conjugates with only minor amounts excreted as sulfates. MPA has a $t_{1/2}$ ranging from 38 to 46 hours.

Drug-Interactions
Coadministration of conjugated estrogens with MPA does not affect the pharmacokinetic profile of MPA. Similarly, MPA does not affect the pharmacokinetic profile of the conjugated or unconjugated estrogens.

CLINICAL STUDIES
In a 1-year clinical trial of 1376 women randomized to PREMPRO 0.625 mg/2.5 mg (Regimen A, n=340), PREMPRO 0.625 mg/5 mg (Regimen B, n=338), PREMPHASE 0.625 mg/5 mg (Regimen C, n=351), or Premarin 0.625 mg alone (n=347), results of evaluable biopsies at 12 months (n=279 for Regimen A, 274 for Regimen B, 277 for Regimen C, and 283 for Premarin alone) showed a reduced risk of endometrial hyperplasia in the two PREMPRO treatment groups (less than 1%) and in the PREMPHASE treatment group (less than 1%; 1% when focal hyperplasia was included) compared to the Premarin group (8%; 20% when focal hyperplasia was included). See Table 2.
[See table 2 at top of next page]
In this clinical trial the incidence of amenorrhea increased over time in both PREMPRO groups. Seventeen percent of

the patients randomized to Regimen A experienced amenorrhea during the entire 13 cycles of the study, and 15 percent of the patients on Regimen B experienced amenorrhea during the entire 13 cycles of the study. The following two figures describe cumulative amenorrhea which is defined as amenorrhea continuing from a given cycle to the end of the study.

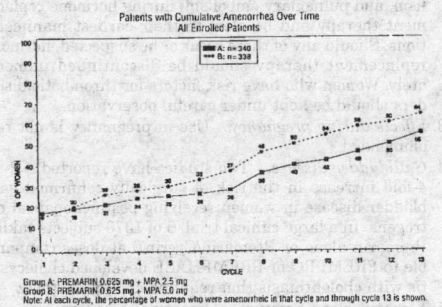

Group A: PREMARIN 0.625 mg + MPA 2.5 mg
Group B: PREMARIN 0.625 mg + MPA 5.0 mg
Note: At each cycle, the percentage of women who were amenorrheic in that cycle and through cycle 13 is shown.

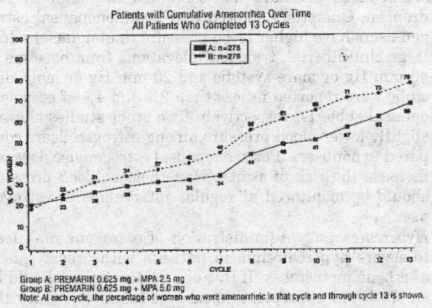

Group A: PREMARIN 0.625 mg + MPA 2.5 mg
Group B: PREMARIN 0.625 mg + MPA 5.0 mg
Note: At each cycle, the percentage of women who were amenorrheic in that cycle and through cycle 13 is shown.

Information Regarding Lipid Effects
The results of a clinical trial conducted in a 97% Caucasian population at low risk for cardiovascular disease, showed that the increases in HDL-C and HDL_2-C subfraction were significantly less for PREMPRO and PREMPHASE than Premarin alone, but decreases in LDL-C were comparable with Premarin alone. Compared with Premarin, total Cholesterol concentrations were significantly lower after 1 year of treatment than at baseline among patients receiving PREMPRO or PREMPHASE.
The following table summarizes mean percent changes from baseline lipid parameter values after 1 year of treatment with the combined regimens.
[See table 3 at top of next page]

INDICATIONS AND USAGE
PREMPRO or PREMPHASE therapy is indicated in women with an intact uterus for the:
1. Treatment of moderate to severe vasomotor symptoms associated with the menopause. There is no adequate evidence

that estrogens are effective for nervous symptoms or depression which might occur during menopause and they should not be used to treat these conditions.
2. Treatment of vulvar and vaginal atrophy.
3. Prevention of osteoporosis.
Since estrogen administration is associated with risks as well as benefits, selection of patients ideally should be based on prospective identification of risk factors for developing osteoporosis. Unfortunately, there is no certain way to identify those women who will develop osteoporotic fractures. Most prospective studies of efficacy for this indication have been carried out in white menopausal women, without stratification by other risk factors, and tend to show a universally salutary effect on bone. Thus, patient selection must be individualized based on the balance of risks and benefits.
Estrogen replacement therapy reduces bone resorption and retards or halts postmenopausal bone loss. Case-control studies have shown an approximately 60% reduction in hip and wrist fractures in women whose estrogen replacement was begun within a few years of menopause. Studies also suggest that estrogen reduces the rate of vertebral fractures. Even when started as late as 6 years after menopause, estrogen may prevent further loss of bone mass for as long as the treatment is continued. When estrogen therapy is discontinued, bone mass declines at a rate comparable to that in the immediate postmenopausal period. There is no evidence that estrogen replacement therapy restores bone mass to premenopausal levels.
At skeletal maturity there are sex and race differences in both the total amount of bone present and its density, in favor of men and blacks. Thus, women are at higher risk than men because they start with less bone mass and, for several years following natural or induced menopause, the rate of bone mass decline is accelerated. White and Asian women are at higher risk than black women.
Early menopause is one of the strongest predictors for the development of osteoporosis. In addition, other factors affecting the skeleton which are associated with osteoporosis include genetic factors (small build, family history), endocrine factors (nulliparity, thyrotoxicosis, hyperparathyroidism, Cushing's syndrome, hyperprolactinemia, type I diabetes), lifestyle (cigarette smoking, alcohol abuse, sedentary exercise habits) and nutrition (below average body weight, dietary calcium intake).
The mainstays of prevention and management of osteoporosis are estrogen, an adequate lifetime calcium intake, and exercise. Postmenopausal women absorb dietary calcium less efficiently than premenopausal women and require an average of 1500 mg/day of elemental calcium to remain in neutral calcium balance. By comparison, premenopausal women require about 1000 mg/day and the average calcium intake in the USA is 400–600 mg/day. Therefore, when not contraindicated, calcium supplementation may be helpful.
Weight-bearing exercise and nutrition may be important adjuncts to the prevention and management of osteoporosis. Immobilization and prolonged bed rest produce rapid bone loss, while weight-bearing exercise has been shown both to reduce bone loss and to increase bone mass. The optimal type and amount of physical activity that would prevent os-

Continued on next page

Prempro—Cont.

teoporosis have not been established; however, in two studies an hour of walking and running exercises twice or three times weekly significantly increased lumbar spine bone mass.

CONTRAINDICATIONS

Estrogens/progestins combined should not be used in women under any of the following conditions or circumstances:
1. Known or suspected pregnancy, including use for missed abortion or as a diagnostic test for pregnancy. Estrogen or progestin may cause fetal harm when administered to a pregnant woman.
2. Known or suspected cancer of the breast.
3. Known or suspected estrogen-dependent neoplasia.
4. Undiagnosed abnormal genital bleeding.
5. Active or past history of thrombophlebitis, thromboembolic disorders, or stroke.
6. Liver dysfunction or disease.
PREMPRO or PREMPHASE therapy should not be used in patients hypersensitive to the ingredients contained in the tablets.

WARNINGS

ALL WARNINGS BELOW PERTAIN TO THE USE OF THIS COMBINATION PRODUCT.

Based on experience with estrogens and/or progestins:
1. *Induction of malignant neoplasms*
Endometrial cancer. The reported endometrial cancer risk among users of unopposed estrogen was about 2- to 12-fold greater than in nonusers and appears dependent on duration of treatment and on estrogen dose. There is no significant increased risk associated with the use of estrogens for less than one year. The greatest risk appears associated with prolonged use, with increased risks of 15- to 24-fold for five years or more. In three studies, persistence of risk was demonstrated for 8 to over 15 years after cessation of estrogen treatment. In one study, a significant decrease in the incidence of endometrial cancer occurred six months after estrogen withdrawal.
A large clinical trial has demonstrated that when MPA is administered with Premarin, there is a markedly reduced incidence of endometrial hyperplasia, a possible precursor of endometrial cancer. Endometrial hyperplasia has been reported in a large clinical trial to occur at a rate of approximately 1% or less with PREMPRO and PREMPHASE. Studies have also demonstrated a reduced risk of endometrial cancer when a progestin is administered with estrogen replacement therapy. In the large clinical trial described above, only a single case of endometrial cancer was reported to occur among women taking combination Premarin/MPA therapy.
Clinical surveillance of all women taking estrogen/progestin combinations is important. Adequate diagnostic measures, including endometrial sampling when indicated, should be undertaken to rule out malignancy in all cases of undiagnosed persistent or recurring abnormal vaginal bleeding. There is no evidence that "natural" estrogens are more or less hazardous than "synthetic" estrogens at equivalent estrogen doses.
Breast cancer. Some studies have reported a moderately increased risk of breast cancer (relative risk of 1.3 to 2.0) in those women on estrogen replacement therapy taking higher doses, or in those taking lower doses for prolonged periods of time, especially in excess of 10 years. The majority of studies, however, have not shown an association in women who have ever used estrogen replacement therapy.
The effect of added progestins on the risk of breast cancer is unknown, although a moderately increased risk in those taking combination estrogen/progestin therapy has been reported. Other studies have not shown this relationship. In a one year clinical trial of PREMPRO, PREMPHASE and Premarin alone, 5 new cases of breast cancer were detected among 1377 women who received the combination treatments, while no new cases were detected among 347 women who received Premarin alone. The overall incidence of breast cancer in this clinical trial does not exceed that expected in the general population. In the three year clinical Postmenopausal Estrogen Progestin Intervention (PEPI) trial of 875 women to assess differences among placebo, unopposed Premarin, and three different combination hormone therapy regimens, one (1) new case of breast cancer was detected in the placebo group (n=174), one in the Premarin alone group (n=175), none in the continuous Premarin plus continuous medroxyprogesterone acetate group (n=174), and two (2) in the continuous Premarin plus cyclic medroxyprogesterone acetate group (n=174).
Women on hormone replacement therapy should have regular breast examinations and should be instructed in breast self-examination, and women over the age of 50 should have regular mammograms.

Table 2. INCIDENCE OF ENDOMETRIAL HYPERPLASIA AFTER ONE YEAR OF TREATMENT

	---- Groups ----			
Patient	PREMPRO 0.625 mg/2.5 mg	PREMPRO 0.625 mg/5 mg	PREMPHASE 0.625 mg/5 mg	Premarin 0.625 mg
Total number of patients	340	338	351	347
Number of patients with evaluable biopsies	279	274	277	283
No. (%) of patients with biopsies				
• all focal and non-focal hyperplasia	2 (<1)*	0 (0)*	3 (1)*	57 (20)
• excluding focal cystic hyperplasia	2 (<1)*	0 (0)*	1 (<1)*	25 (8)

*Significant ($p < 0.001$) in comparison with Premarin (0.625 mg) alone.

Table 3. MEAN PERCENT CHANGE FROM BASELINE LIPID PROFILE VALUES AFTER ONE YEAR OF TREATMENT

	------ Treatment Groups ------			
	PREMPRO 0.625 mg/2.5 mg n=90	PREMPRO 0.625 mg/5 mg n=84	PREMPHASE 0.625 mg/5 mg n=95	Premarin 0.625 mg n=86
Lipid Parameter				
Total Cholesterol	-4.7†	-4.2†	-3.5†	0.2
HDL-C	3.5†	3.7†	4.4†	14.1
HDL_2-C	34.7†	40.1†	30.3†	70.8
LDL-C	-10.3	-8.8	-8.7†	-7.7
Triglycerides	24.1†	19.1†	27.5†	39.4

†Significantly ($p \leq 0.05$) different from Premarin alone.

2. *Thromboembolic Disorders and Other Vascular Problems.* In some studies, women on estrogen replacement therapy, given alone or in combination with a progestin, have been reported to have an increased risk of thrombophlebitis, and/or thromboembolic disease. The physician should be aware of the possibility of thrombotic disorders (thrombophlebitis, retinal thrombosis, cerebral embolism, and pulmonary embolism) during hormone replacement therapy and be alert to their earliest manifestations. Should any of these occur or be suspected, hormone replacement therapy should be discontinued immediately. Women who have risk factors for thrombotic disorders should be kept under careful observation.
3. *Effects during pregnancy.* Use in pregnancy is not recommended.
4. *Gallbladder disease.* Two studies have reported a 2- to 4-fold increase in the risk of surgically confirmed gallbladder disease in women receiving postmenopausal estrogens. In a large clinical trial, 5 of 1376 subjects taking Premarin alone or Premarin/Cycrin® at doses comparable to PREMPRO or PREMPHASE developed cholecystitis with cholelithiasis that required cholecystectomy.
5. *Elevated blood pressure.* Occasional blood pressure increases during estrogen replacement therapy have been attributed to idiosyncratic reactions to estrogens. More often, blood pressure has remained the same or has dropped. One study showed that postmenopausal estrogen users have higher blood pressure than nonusers. In a large clinical trial, transient elevations from baseline of 40 mm Hg or more systolic and 20 mm Hg or more diastolic were reported in less than 2% and 4% of postmenopausal subjects, respectively. Two other studies showed slightly lower blood pressure among estrogen users compared to nonusers. Postmenopausal estrogen use does not increase the risk of stroke. Nonetheless, blood pressure should be monitored at regular intervals with estrogen use.
6. *Hypercalcemia.* Administration of estrogens may lead to severe hypercalcemia in patients with breast cancer and bone metastases. If this occurs, the drugs should be stopped and appropriate measures taken to reduce the serum calcium level.
7. *Visual abnormalities.* Discontinue medication pending examination if there is sudden partial or complete loss of vision, or a sudden onset of proptosis, diplopia, or migraine. If examination reveals papilledema or retinal vascular lesions, medication should be withdrawn.

PRECAUTIONS

GENERAL

Based on experience with estrogens and/or progestins:
1. *Cardiovascular risk.* A causal relationship between estrogen replacement therapy and reduction of cardiovascular disease in postmenopausal women has not been proven. Furthermore, the effect of added progestins on this putative benefit is not yet known.
In recent years many published studies have suggested that there may be a cause-effect relationship between postmenopausal oral estrogen replacement therapy *without added progestins* and a decrease in cardiovascular disease in women. Although most of the observational studies which assessed this statistical association have reported a 20% to 50% reduction in coronary heart disease risk and associated mortality in estrogen takers, the following should be considered when interpreting these reports.
Because only one of these studies was randomized and it was too small to yield statistically significant results, all relevant studies were subject to selection bias. Thus, the apparently reduced risk of coronary artery disease cannot be attributed with certainty to estrogen replacement therapy. It may instead have been caused by life-style and medical characteristics of the women studied with the result that healthier women were selected for estrogen therapy. In general, treated women were of higher socioeconomic and educational status, more slender, more physically active, more likely to have undergone surgical menopause, and less likely to have diabetes than the untreated women. Although some studies attempted to control for these selection factors, it is common for properly designed randomized trials to fail to confirm benefits suggested by less rigorous study designs. Thus, ongoing and future large-scale randomized trials may fail to confirm this apparent benefit.
Current medical practice often includes the use of concomitant progestin therapy in women with intact uteri. While the effects of added progestins on the risk of ischemic heart disease are not known, medroxyprogesterone acetate at the dose in PREMPRO or PREMPHASE attenuates much of the favorable effect of conjugated estrogens on HDL levels, although it maintains the favorable effect of conjugated estrogens on LDL levels (see **CLINICAL STUDIES**).
While the effects of added progestins on the risk of breast cancer are also unknown, available epidemiologic evidence suggests that progestins do not reduce, and may enhance, the moderately increased breast cancer risk that has been reported with prolonged estrogen replacement therapy (see **WARNINGS**).
The safety data regarding PREMPRO and PREMPHASE were obtained primarily from clinical trials and epidemiologic studies of postmenopausal Caucasian women, who were at generally low risk for cardiovascular disease and higher than average risk for osteoporosis. The safety profile of PREMPRO and PREMPHASE derived from these study populations cannot necessarily be extrapolated to other populations of diverse racial and/or demographic composition. When considering prescribing PREMPRO or PREMPHASE, physicians are advised to weigh the potential benefits and risks of therapy as applicable to each individual patient.
2. *Use in hysterectomized women.* Existing data do not support the use of the combination of estrogen and progestin in postmenopausal women without a uterus. There are possible risks which may be associated with the inclusion of progestin in estrogen replacement regimens. The potential risks include some deterioration in glucose tolerance, as reported in a large clinical trial of PREMPRO and PREMPHASE, and less favorable effects on lipid metabolism as compared to the lipid effects of Premarin alone (see **CLINICAL STUDIES**).
3. *Physical examination.* A complete medical and family history should be taken prior to the initiation of any estrogen/progestin therapy. The pretreatment and periodic physical examinations should include special reference to blood pressure, breasts, abdomen, and pelvic organs, and should include a Papanicolaou smear. As a general rule, estrogen should not be prescribed for longer than one year without another physical examination being performed.
4. *Fluid retention.* Because estrogens/progestins may cause some degree of fluid retention, conditions which

might be influenced by this factor, such as asthma, epilepsy, migraine, and cardiac or renal dysfunction, require careful observation.

5. *Uterine bleeding.* Certain patients may develop abnormal uterine bleeding. In cases of undiagnosed abnormal uterine bleeding, adequate diagnostic measures are indicated. (See **WARNINGS.**)

6. The pathologist should be advised of estrogen/progestin therapy when relevant specimens are submitted.

Based on experience with estrogens:

1. *Familial hyperlipoproteinemia.* Estrogen therapy may be associated with massive elevations of plasma triglycerides leading to pancreatitis and other complications in patients with familial defects of lipoprotein metabolism.

2. *Hypercoagulability.* Some epidemiological studies have shown that women taking estrogen replacement therapy have hypercoagulability primarily related to decreased antithrombin activity. This effect appears dose- and duration-dependent and is less pronounced than that associated with oral contraceptive use. Also, postmenopausal women tend to have changes in levels of coagulation parameters at baseline compared to premenopausal women. There is some suggestion that low-dose mestranol may increase the risk of thromboembolism in postmenopausal women. There is insufficient information on hypercoagulability in women who have had previous thromboembolic disease. In a clinical trial of 1724 patients, in which 204 PREMPRO™-treated patients and 107 PREMPHASE®-treated patients had metabolic studies performed, factors VII and X concentrations and plasminogen activity increased at the end of 1 year, and antithrombin III activity decreased in women receiving PREMPRO 0.625 mg/2.5 mg MPA or PREMPHASE 0.625 mg/5 mg MPA at the end of the year. At the end of the year, antithrombin III activity increased slightly in women receiving PREMPRO 0.625 mg/5.0 mg MPA.

3. *Mastodynia.* Certain patients may develop undesirable manifestations of estrogenic stimulation such as mastodynia. In a large clinical trial of PREMPRO, PREMPHASE, and Premarin®, approximately one third of the subjects receiving PREMPRO and approximately one third of the subjects receiving PREMPHASE reported breast pain during treatment versus 12% for Premarin alone.

Based on experience with progestins:

1. *Lipoprotein metabolism.* See **CLINICAL STUDIES.**

2. *Impaired glucose tolerance.* See *Use in hysterectomized women,* above.

3. *Depression.* Patients who have a history of depression should be observed and the drugs discontinued if the depression recurs to a serious degree.

Information for the Patient

See text of Patient Package Insert which appears after the **HOW SUPPLIED** section.

Drug/Laboratory Test Interactions

1. Accelerated prothrombin time, partial thromboplastin time, and platelet aggregation time; increased platelet count; increased factors II, VII antigen, VIII coagulant activity, IX, X, XII, VII-X complex, II-VII-X complex, and beta-thromboglobulin; decreased levels of anti-factor Xa and antithrombin III, decreased antithrombin III activity; increased levels of fibrinogen and fibrinogen activity; increased plasminogen antigen and activity.

2. Increased thyroid-binding globulin (TBG) leading to increased circulating total thyroid hormone, as measured by protein-bound iodine (PBI), T_4 levels (by column or by radioimmunoassay) or T_3 levels by radioimmunoassay, T_3 resin uptake is decreased, reflecting the elevated TBG. Free T_4 and free T_3 concentrations are unaltered.

3. Other binding proteins may be elevated in serum, i.e., corticosteroid binding globulin (CBG), sex hormone-binding globulin (SHBG), leading to increased circulating corticosteroids and sex steroids respectively. Free or biologically active hormone concentrations are unchanged. Other plasma proteins may be increased (angiotensinogen/renin substrate, alpha-1-antitrypsin, ceruloplasmin).

4. Increased plasma HDL and HDL-2 subfraction concentrations, reduced LDL cholesterol concentration, increased triglyceride levels.

5. Impaired glucose tolerance. For this reason, diabetic patients should be carefully observed while receiving estrogen/progestin therapy.

6. Reduced response to metyrapone test.

7. Reduced serum folate concentration.

8. Aminoglutethimide administered concomitantly with MPA may significantly depress the bioavailability of MPA.

Carcinogenesis, Mutagenesis, and Impairment of Fertility

Long term continuous administration of natural and synthetic estrogens in certain animal species increases the frequency of carcinomas of the breasts, uterus, cervix, vagina, testis, and liver. (See **CONTRAINDICATIONS** and **WARNINGS.**)

In a two-year oral study of MPA in which female rats were exposed to dosages of up to 5000 µg/kg/day in their diets (50 times higher—based on AUC—than the level observed experimentally in women taking 10 mg of MPA), a dose-related increase in pancreatic islet cell tumors (ad-

enomas and carcinomas) occurred. Pancreatic tumor incidence was increased at 1000 and 5000 µg/kg/day, but not at 200 µg/kg/day.

A decreased incidence of spontaneous mammary gland tumors was observed in all three MPA-treated groups, compared to controls, in the two-year rat study. The mechanism for the decreased incidence of mammary gland tumors observed in the MPA-treated rats may be linked to the significant decrease in serum prolactin concentration observed in rats.

Beagle dogs treated with MPA developed mammary nodules, some of which were malignant. Although nodules occasionally appeared in control animals, they were intermittent in nature, whereas the nodules in the drug-treated animals were larger, more numerous, persistent, and there were some breast malignancies with metastases. It is known that progestogens stimulate synthesis and release of growth hormone in dogs. The growth hormone, along with the progestogen, stimulates mammary growth and tumors. In contrast, growth hormone in humans is not increased, nor does growth hormone have any significant mammotrophic role. Therefore, the MPA-induced increase of mammary tumors in dogs probably has no significance to humans. No pancreatic tumors occurred in dogs.

Pregnancy Category X

Estrogens/progestins should not be used during pregnancy. See **CONTRAINDICATIONS.**

Nursing Mothers

As a general principle, the administration of any drug to nursing mothers should be done only when clearly necessary since many drugs are excreted in human milk. Estrogen administration to nursing mothers has been shown to decrease the quantity and quality of the milk. Detectable amounts of progestin have been identified in the milk of mothers receiving the drug. The effect of this on the nursing infant has not been determined.

ADVERSE REACTIONS

(See **WARNINGS** regarding induction of neoplasia, adverse effects on the fetus, increased incidence of gallbladder dis-

ease, elevated blood pressure, thromboembolic disorders, visual abnormalities, and hypercalcemia and **PRECAUTIONS** for cardiovascular disease.)

In a one year clinical trial that included 678 women treated with PREMPRO, 351 women treated with PREMPHASE, and 347 women treated with Premarin, the following adverse events occurred at a rate ≥ 5% (see Table 4):

[See table 4 above]

The following adverse reactions also have been reported with estrogen and/or progestin therapy:

Genitourinary system. Changes in vaginal bleeding pattern and abnormal withdrawal bleeding or flow, breakthrough bleeding, spotting, change in amount of cervical secretion, premenstrual-like syndrome, cystitis-like syndrome, increase in size of uterine leiomyomata, vaginal candidiasis, amenorrhea, changes in cervical erosion.

Breasts. Tenderness, enlargement, galactorrhea.

Gastrointestinal. Nausea, cholestatic jaundice, changes in appetite, vomiting, abdominal cramps, bloating, increased incidence of gallbladder disease, pancreatitis.

Skin. Chloasma or melasma that may persist when drug is discontinued, erythema multiforme, erythema nodosum, hemorrhagic eruption, loss of scalp hair, hirsutism, itching, urticaria, pruritus, generalized rash, rash (allergic) with and without pruritus, acne.

Cardiovascular. In susceptible individuals, change in blood pressure, thrombophlebitis, pulmonary embolism, cerebral thrombosis and embolism.

CNS. Headache, dizziness, mental depression, nervousness, migraine, chorea, insomnia, somnolence.

Eyes. Neuro-ocular lesions, e.g., retinal thrombosis and optic neuritis. Steepening of corneal curvature, intolerance of contact lenses.

Miscellaneous. Increase or decrease in weight, edema, changes in libido, fatigue, backache, reduced carbohydrate tolerance, aggravation of porphyria, pyrexia, anaphylactoid reactions, anaphylaxis.

Table 4. ALL TREATMENT EMERGENT STUDY EVENTS REGARDLESS OF DRUG RELATIONSHIP REPORTED AT A FREQUENCY ≥ 5%

	Regimen A PREMPRO 0.625 mg/2.5 mg continuous (n=340)	Regimen B PREMPRO 0.625 mg/5.0 mg continuous (n=338)	Regimen C PREMPHASE 0.625 mg/5.0 mg cyclic sequential (n=351)	Regimen E PREMARIN 0.625 mg (n=347)
Body as a whole				
abdominal pain	16%	21%	23%	17%
accidental injury	5%	4%	5%	5%
asthenia	6%	8%	10%	8%
back pain	14%	13%	16%	14%
flu syndrome	10%	13%	12%	14%
headache	36%	28%	37%	38%
infection	16%	16%	18%	14%
pain	11%	13%	12%	13%
pelvic pain	4%	5%	5%	5%
Digestive system				
diarrhea	6%	6%	5%	10%
dyspepsia	6%	6%	5%	5%
flatulence	8%	9%	8%	5%
nausea	11%	9%	11%	11%
Metabolic and Nutritional				
peripheral edema	4%	4%	3%	5%
Musculoskeletal system				
arthralgia	9%	7%	9%	7%
leg cramps	3%	4%	5%	4%
Nervous system				
depression	6%	11%	11%	10%
dizziness	5%	3%	4%	6%
hypertonia	4%	3%	3%	7%
Respiratory system				
pharyngitis	11%	11%	13%	12%
rhinitis	8%	6%	8%	7%
sinusitis	8%	7%	7%	5%
Skin and appendages				
pruritus	10%	8%	5%	4%
rash	4%	6%	4%	3%
Urogenital system				
breast pain	33%	38%	32%	12%
cervix disorder	4%	4%	5%	5%
dysmenorrhea	8%	5%	13%	5%
leukorrhea	6%	5%	9%	8%
vaginal hemorrhage	2%	1%	3%	6%
vaginitis	7%	7%	5%	3%

Continued on next page

Prempro—Cont.

ACUTE OVERDOSAGE

Serious ill effects have not been reported following acute ingestion of large doses of estrogen/progestin-containing oral contraceptives by young children. Overdosage may cause nausea and vomiting, and withdrawal bleeding may occur in females.

DOSAGE AND ADMINISTRATION

PREMPRO therapy consists of a single tablet to be taken once daily.

1. For treatment of moderate-to-severe vasomotor symptoms and vulval and vaginal atrophy associated with menopause, patients should be started at the lowest effective dose—PREMPRO 0.625 mg/2.5 mg daily. Patients should be reevaluated at 3-month to 6-month intervals to determine if treatment for symptoms is still necessary. Adequate diagnostic measures, including endometrial sampling when indicated, should be undertaken to rule out malignancy in cases of undiagnosed persistent or recurring abnormal vaginal bleeding. In patients where bleeding or spotting remains a problem, after appropriate evaluation, consideration should be given to increasing the MPA dose to PREMPRO 0.625 mg/5 mg daily. This dose can be periodically reassessed by the health care provider.
2. For prevention of osteoporosis—PREMPRO 0.625 mg/2.5 mg daily. Patients should be monitored closely for signs of endometrial cancer, and appropriate diagnostic measures should be taken to rule out malignancy in the event of persistent or recurring abnormal vaginal bleeding. In patients where bleeding or spotting remains a problem, after appropriate evaluation, consideration should be given to increasing the MPA dose to PREMPRO 0.625 mg/5 mg daily. This dose can be periodically reassessed by the health care provider.

PREMPHASE therapy consists of two separate tablets; one maroon 0.625 mg Premarin tablet taken daily on days 1 through 14 and one light-blue tablet, containing 0.625 mg conjugated estrogens and 5 mg of medroxyprogesterone acetate, taken on days 15 through 28.

1. For treatment of moderate to severe vasomotor symptoms and vulvar and vaginal atrophy associated with menopause. Patients should be reevaluated at 3-month to 6-month intervals to determine if treatment for symptoms is still necessary. Adequate diagnostic measures, including endometrial sampling when indicated, should be undertaken to rule out malignancy in cases of undiagnosed persistent or recurring abnormal vaginal bleeding.
2. For prevention of osteoporosis. Treated patients with an intact uterus should be monitored closely for signs of endometrial cancer, and appropriate diagnostic measures should be taken to rule out malignancy in the event of persistent or recurring abnormal vaginal bleeding.

HOW SUPPLIED

PREMPRO™ therapy consists of a single tablet to be taken once daily.

PREMPRO 0.625 mg/2.5 mg

Each carton includes 3 EZ DIAL™ dispensers containing 28 tablets. One EZ DIAL™ dispenser contains 28 oval, peach tablets containing 0.625 mg of the conjugated estrogens found in Premarin® tablets and 2.5 mg of medroxyprogesterone acetate for oral administration.

PREMPRO 0.625 mg/5 mg

Each carton includes 3 EZ DIAL™ dispensers containing 28 tablets. One EZ DIAL™ dispenser contains 28 oval, light-blue tablets containing 0.625 mg of the conjugated estrogens found in Premarin® tablets and 5 mg of medroxyprogesterone acetate for oral administration.

PREMPHASE® therapy consists of two separate tablets; one maroon Premarin® tablet taken daily on days 1 through 14 and one light-blue tablet taken on days 15 through 28.

Each carton includes 3 EZ DIAL™ dispensers containing 28 tablets. One EZ DIAL™ dispenser contains 14 oval, maroon Premarin tablets containing 0.625 mg of conjugated estrogens and 14 oval, light-blue tablets that contain 0.625 mg of the conjugated estrogens found in Premarin tablets and 5 mg of medroxyprogesterone acetate (MPA) for oral administration.

The appearance of PREMPRO™ tablets is a trademark of Wyeth-Ayerst Laboratories.

The appearance of Premarin® tablets is a trademark of Wyeth-Ayerst Laboratories. The appearance of the conjugated estrogens/medroxyprogesterone acetate combination tablets is a registered trademark.

Store at controlled room temperature, 20°C–25°C (68°F–77°F).

INFORMATION FOR THE PATIENT

Your physician has prescribed PREMPRO or PREMPHASE, a combination of two hormones, an estrogen and a progestin. This leaflet describes the major benefits and risks of your treatment, as well as how and when treatment should be taken.

PREMPRO and PREMPHASE replace the hormones in your body which naturally decrease at menopause. The hormone combination you will be taking has been shown to provide the benefits of estrogen replacement therapy while lowering the frequency of a possible precancerous condition of the uterine lining. This therapy is not intended for women who have had a hysterectomy (surgical removal of the uterus).

Estrogens have several important uses but also some risks. You must decide, with your doctor, whether the risks of estrogens are acceptable when weighed against their benefits. The length of treatment with estrogens can vary from woman to woman. Check with your doctor to make sure you are using the lowest possible effective dose.

With PREMPRO or PREMPHASE therapy several menstrual-like bleeding patterns may occur. These may range from absence of bleeding to irregular bleeding. If bleeding occurs, it is frequently light spotting or moderate menstrual-like bleeding, but it may be heavy. If you experience vaginal bleeding while taking PREMPRO or PREMPHASE, you should discuss your bleeding pattern with your doctor and set up an appropriate schedule for follow-up care.

USES OF ESTROGEN

To reduce moderate to severe menopausal symptoms. Estrogens are hormones produced by the ovaries of normal women. When a woman is between the ages of 45 and 55, the ovaries normally stop making estrogens. This leads to a drop in body estrogen levels that causes the "change of life" or menopause (the end of monthly menstrual periods). A sudden drop in estrogen levels also occurs if both ovaries are removed during an operation before natural menopause takes place. This is referred to as "surgical menopause."

When the estrogen levels begin dropping, some women develop very uncomfortable symptoms, such as feelings of warmth in the face, neck, and chest, or sudden intense episodes of heat and sweating ("hot flashes" or "hot flushes"). Using estrogen drugs can help the body adjust to lower estrogen levels and reduce these symptoms. In some women the symptoms are mild; in others they can be severe. These symptoms may last only a few months or longer. Taking PREMPRO or PREMPHASE can alleviate these symptoms. If you are not taking hormones for other reasons, such as the prevention of osteoporosis, you should take PREMPRO or PREMPHASE only as long as you need it for relief from your menopausal symptoms.

To prevent thinning of bones. Osteoporosis is a thinning of the bones that makes them weaker and allows them to break more easily. The bones of the spine, wrists, and hips break most often in osteoporosis. Both men and women start to lose bone mass after about age 40, but women lose bone mass faster after the menopause. Using estrogens after the menopause slows down bone thinning and may prevent bones from breaking. Lifelong adequate calcium intake, either from diet (such as dairy products) or from calcium supplements (to reach a total daily intake of 1000 milligrams per day before menopause or 1500 milligrams per day after menopause), may help to prevent osteoporosis. Regular weight-bearing exercise (like walking and running for an hour, two or three times a week) may also help to prevent osteoporosis. Before you change your calcium intake or exercise habits, it is important to discuss these lifestyle changes with your doctor to find out if they are safe for you.

Since estrogen use has some risks, only women who are likely to develop osteoporosis should use estrogens for prevention. Women who are likely to develop osteoporosis often have the following characteristics:

- White or Asian race
- Small, slim body frame
- Cigarette-smoking habit
- Family history of osteoporosis (in a mother, sister, or aunt)
- Early menopause either natural or because of surgical removal of ovaries ("surgical menopause")

To treat vulvar and vaginal atrophy (itching, burning, dryness in or around the vagina, difficulty or burning on urination) associated with menopause.

WHO SHOULD NOT USE ESTROGENS

During pregnancy. If you think you may be pregnant, do not use any form of estrogen-containing drug. Using estrogens while you are pregnant may cause your unborn child to have birth defects. Estrogens do not prevent miscarriage.

If you have unusual vaginal bleeding which has not been evaluated by your doctor. Unusual vaginal bleeding can be a warning sign of cancer of the uterus, especially if it happens after menopause. Your doctor must find out the cause of the bleeding so that he or she can recommend the proper treatment. Taking estrogens without visiting your doctor can cause you serious harm if your vaginal bleeding is caused by cancer of the uterus.

If you have had cancer. Since estrogens increase the risk of certain types of cancer, you should not use estrogens if you have ever had cancer of the breast or uterus.

If you have any circulation problems. Estrogen drugs should not be used except in unusually special situations in which your doctor decides that you need estrogen therapy so much that the risks are acceptable. Women with abnormal blood clotting conditions should avoid estrogen use (see **RISKS OF ESTROGENS AND/OR PROGESTINS**).

When they do not work. During menopause, some women develop nervous symptoms or depression. Estrogens do not relieve these symptoms. You may have heard that taking estrogens for years after menopause will keep your skin soft and supple and keep you feeling young. There is no evidence for these claims and such long-term estrogen use may have serious risks.

After childbirth or when breastfeeding a baby. Estrogen should not be used to try to stop the breast from filling with milk after a baby is born. Such treatment may increase the risk of developing blood clots (see **RISKS OF ESTROGENS AND/OR PROGESTINS**).

If you are breastfeeding, you should avoid using any drugs because many drugs pass through to the baby in the milk. While nursing a baby, you should take drugs only on the advice of your health-care provider.

RISKS OF ESTROGENS AND/OR PROGESTINS

Cancer of the uterus. If you use any drug which contains estrogen, it is important to visit your doctor regularly and report any unusual vaginal bleeding right away. Vaginal bleeding after menopause may be a warning sign of uterine cancer. Your doctor should evaluate any unusual vaginal bleeding to find out the cause.

The risk of cancer of the uterus increases when estrogens are used alone, the longer they are used, and when larger doses are taken. There is a higher risk of cancer of the uterus if you are overweight, diabetic, or have high blood pressure. The hormone combination you will be taking contains estrogen and progestin. This combination has been shown to provide the benefits of estrogen replacement therapy for the **USES OF ESTROGEN** listed above, while reducing the risk of a precancerous condition of the uterine lining (see **OTHER INFORMATION,** below).

However, additional risks may be associated with the inclusion of a progestin in estrogen treatment. The possible risks include less favorable effects on blood fats as compared to Premarin alone, unfavorable effects on blood sugars, and a possible increase in breast cancer risk (see *Cancer of the breast,* below). Usually, the smaller the dose and the shorter the duration of treatment, the more these effects are minimized. Check with your doctor to make sure you are using the lowest effective dose and only for as long as you need it. If you have had your uterus removed, there is no risk of developing cancer of the uterus and no benefit to be gained by using a combination estrogen/progestin product.

Cancer of the breast. Most studies have not shown a higher risk of breast cancer in women who have ever used estrogens. However, some studies have reported that breast cancer developed more often (up to twice the usual rate) in women who used estrogens for long periods of time (especially more than 10 years), or who used high doses for shorter time periods. The effects of added progestin on the risk of breast cancer are unknown. Some studies have reported a somewhat increased risk, even higher than the possible risk associated with estrogens alone. Others have not. Regular breast examinations by a health professional and monthly self-examination are recommended for all women. Regular mammograms are recommended for all women over 50 years of age.

Gallbladder disease. Women who use estrogens after menopause are more likely to develop gallbladder disease needing surgery than women who do not use estrogens.

Inflammation of the Pancreas. Women with high triglyceride levels may have an increased risk of developing inflammation of the pancreas.

Abnormal blood clotting. Taking estrogens may cause changes in your blood clotting system. These changes allow the blood to clot more easily, possibly allowing clots to form in your bloodstream. If blood clots do form in your bloodstream, they can cut off the blood supply to vital organs, causing serious problems. These problems may include a stroke (by cutting off blood to the brain), a heart attack (by cutting off blood to the heart), a pulmonary embolus (by cutting off blood to the lungs), or other problems. Any of these conditions may cause death or serious long-term disability.

Excess calcium in the blood. Taking estrogens may lead to severe hypercalcemia in women with breast and/or bone cancer.

During pregnancy. There is an increased risk of birth defects in children whose mothers take this drug during the first four months of pregnancy. Several reports suggest an association between mothers who take these drugs in the first trimester of pregnancy and genital abnormalities in male and female babies. The risk to the male baby is the possibility of being born with a condition in which the opening of the penis is on the underside rather than the tip of the penis (hypospadias). Hypospadias occurs in about 5 to 8 per 1,000 male births and is about doubled with exposure to these drugs. There is not enough information to quantify the risk to exposed female fetuses. However, enlargement of the clitoris and fusion of the labia may occur, although rarely.

Therefore, since drugs of this type may induce mild masculinization of the external genitalia of the female fetus, as well as hypospadias in the male fetus, it is wise to avoid using the drug during the first trimester of pregnancy. These drugs have been used as a test for pregnancy, but such use is no longer considered safe because of possible damage to a developing baby. Also, more rapid methods for testing for pregnancy are now available. If you take PREMPRO or PREMPHASE and later find you were pregnant when you took it, be sure to discuss this with your doctor as soon as possible.

SIDE EFFECTS WITH ESTROGENS AND/OR PROGESTINS

In addition to the risks listed above, the following side effects have been reported with estrogen and/or progestin use:

- Nausea, vomiting, pain, cramps, swelling, or tenderness in the abdomen.
- Yellowing of the skin and/or whites of the eyes.
- Breast tenderness or enlargement.
- Enlargement of benign tumors ("fibroids") of the uterus.
- Irregular bleeding or spotting.
- Change in amount of cervical secretion.
- Vaginal yeast infections.
- Retention of excess fluid. This may make some conditions worsen, such as asthma, epilepsy, migraine, heart disease, or kidney disease.
- A spotty darkening of the skin, particularly on the face; reddening of the skin; skin rashes.
- Worsening of porphyria.
- Headache, migraines, dizziness, faintness, or changes in vision (including intolerance to contact lenses).
- Mental depression.
- Involuntary muscle spasms.
- Hair loss or abnormal hairiness.
- Increase or decrease in weight.
- Changes in sex drive.
- Possible changes in blood sugar.

REDUCING THE RISKS OF ESTROGEN/PROGESTIN

If you decide to take an estrogen/progestin combination, you can reduce your risks by carefully monitoring your treatment.

See your doctor regularly. While you are taking PREMPRO or PREMPHASE, it is important to visit your doctor at least once a year for a checkup. If you develop vaginal bleeding while taking estrogens, you may need further evaluation. If members of your family have had breast cancer or if you have ever had breast lumps or an abnormal mammogram (breast X ray), you may need to have more frequent breast examinations.

Reassess your need for treatment. You and your doctor should reevaluate whether or not you still need estrogens at least every six months.

Be alert for signs of trouble. If any of these warning signals (or any other unusual symptoms) happen while you are using estrogen/progestin, call your doctor immediately:

- Abnormal bleeding from the vagina (possible uterine abnormality).
- Pains in the calves or chest, a sudden shortness of breath or coughing blood (indicating possible clots in the legs, heart, or lungs).
- Severe headache or vomiting, dizziness, faintness, or changes in vision or speech, weakness or numbness of an arm or leg (indicating possible clots in the brain or eye).
- Breast lumps (possible breast cancer; ask your doctor or health professional to show you how to examine your breasts monthly).
- Yellowing of the skin and/or whites of the eyes (possible liver problems).
- Pain, swelling, or tenderness in the abdomen (possible gallbladder problem).

OTHER INFORMATION

1. Estrogens increase the risk of developing a condition (endometrial hyperplasia) that may lead to cancer of the lining of the uterus. Taking progestins, another hormonal drug, with estrogens lowers the risk of developing this condition. Therefore, since your uterus has not been removed, your doctor has prescribed PREMPRO or PREMPHASE, which includes both a progestin and estrogens.

You should know, however, that taking estrogens *with* progestins may have unhealthy effects on blood sugar, which might make a diabetic condition worse. Additional risks include a possible further increase in breast cancer risk which may be associated with long-term estrogen use. Some research has shown that estrogens taken *without* progestins may protect women against developing heart disease. However, this is not certain. The protection shown may have been caused by the characteristics of the estrogen-treated women and not by the estrogen treatment itself. In general, treated women were slimmer, more physically active, and were less likely to have diabetes than the untreated women. These characteristics are known to protect against heart disease.

You are cautioned to discuss very carefully with your doctor or health-care provider all the possible risks and benefits of long-term estrogen and progestin treatment as they affect you personally.

2. Your doctor has prescribed this drug for you and you alone. Do not give the drug to anyone else.

3. If you will be taking calcium supplements as part of the treatment to help prevent osteoporosis, check with your doctor about the amounts recommended.

4. Keep this and all drugs out of the reach of children. In case of overdose, call your doctor, hospital, or poison control center immediately.

5. This leaflet provides the most important information about PREMPRO and PREMPHASE. If you want to read more, ask your doctor or pharmacist to let you read the professional labeling. The professional labeling is also published in a book called *The Physicians' Desk Reference*, which is available in bookstores and public libraries.

HOW SUPPLIED

PREMPRO™ is a combination of the conjugated estrogens found in Premarin® tablets and medroxyprogesterone acetate (MPA). Depending on the dosage strength, PREMPRO therapy consists of either a single peach tablet or a single light-blue tablet to be taken once daily.

PREMPRO 0.625 mg/2.5 mg

Each carton includes 3 EZ DIAL™ dispensers containing 28 tablets. One EZ DIAL™ dispenser contains 28 oval, peach tablets containing 0.625 mg of the conjugated estrogens found in Premarin® tablets and 2.5 mg of medroxyprogesterone acetate for oral administration.

PREMPRO 0.625 mg/5 mg

Each carton includes 3 EZ DIAL™ dispensers containing 28 tablets. One EZ DIAL™ dispenser contains 28 oval, light-blue tablets containing 0.625 mg of the conjugated estrogens found in Premarin® tablets and 5 mg of medroxyprogesterone acetate for oral administration.

The appearance of PREMPRO™ tablets is a trademark of Wyeth-Ayerst Laboratories.

PREMPHASE® is a combination of two separate tablets; one maroon Premarin® tablet taken daily on days 1 through 14 and one light-blue tablet taken on days 15 through 28. Each carton includes 3 EZ DIAL™ dispensers containing 28 tablets. One EZ DIAL™ dispenser contains 14 oval, maroon Premarin tablets containing 0.625 mg of conjugated estrogens and 14 oval, light-blue tablets that contain 0.625 mg of the conjugated estrogens found in Premarin tablets and 5 mg of medroxyprogesterone acetate (MPA) for oral administration.

The appearance of Premarin® tablets is a trademark of Wyeth-Ayerst Laboratories. The appearance of the conjugated estrogens/medroxyprogesterone acetate combination tablets is a registered trademark.

Keep out of reach of children.

Store at controlled room temperature, 20° C–25° C (68° F–77° F).

Manufactured by:
Ayerst Laboratories Inc.
A Wyeth-Ayerst Company
Philadelphia, PA 19101

Shown in Product Identification Guide, page 344

PROTOPAM® CHLORIDE ℞

(pralidoxime chloride)
Lyophilized Powder for Injection

Caution: Federal law prohibits dispensing without prescription.

DESCRIPTION

Chemical name: 2-formyl-1-methylpyridinium chloride oxime. Available in the United States as Protopam Chloride, pralidoxime chloride is frequently referred to as 2-PAM Chloride.

Structural formula:

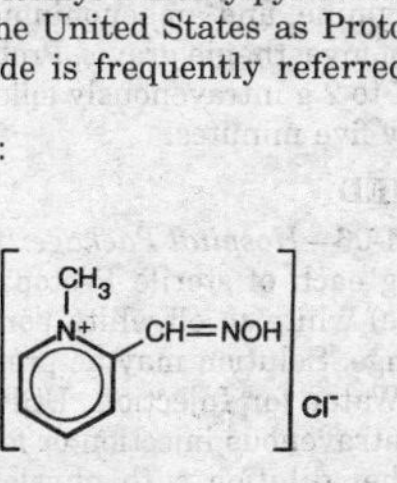

Pralidoxime chloride occurs as an odorless, white, nonhygroscopic, crystalline powder which is soluble in water to the extent of 1 g in less than 1 mL. Stable in air, it melts between 215° and 225°C, with decomposition.

The specific activity of the drug resides in the 2-formyl-1-methylpyridinium ion and is independent of the particular salt employed. The chloride is preferred because of physiologic compatibility, excellent water solubility at all temperatures, and high potency per gram, due to its low (173) molecular weight.

Pralidoxime chloride is a cholinesterase reactivator.

Protopam Chloride for intravenous injection or infusion is prepared by cryodesiccation. Each vial contains 1 g of sterile pralidoxime chloride, and NaOH to adjust pH, to be reconstituted with 20 mL of Sterile Water for Injection, USP. The pH of the reconstituted solution is 3.5 to 4.5. Intramuscular or subcutaneous injection may be used when intravenous injection is not feasible.

CLINICAL PHARMACOLOGY

The principal action of pralidoxime is to reactivate cholinesterase (mainly outside of the central nervous system) which has been inactivated by phosphorylation due to an organophosphate pesticide or related compound. The destruction of accumulated acetylcholine can then proceed, and neuromuscular junctions will again function normally. Pralidoxime also slows the process of "aging" of phosphorylated cholinesterase to a nonreactivatable form, and detoxifies certain organophosphates by direct chemical reaction. The drug has its most critical effect in relieving paralysis of the muscles of respiration. Because pralidoxime is less effective in relieving depression of the respiratory center, atropine is always required concomitantly to block the effect of accumulated acetylcholine at this site. Pralidoxime relieves muscarinic signs and symptoms, salivation, bronchospasm, etc., but this action is relatively unimportant since atropine is adequate for this purpose.

Pralidoxime is distributed throughout the extracellular water; it is not bound to plasma protein. The drug is rapidly excreted in the urine partly unchanged, and partly as a metabolite produced by the liver. Consequently, pralidoxime is relatively short acting, and repeated doses may be needed, especially where there is any evidence of continuing absorption of the poison.

The minimum therapeutic concentration of pralidoxime in plasma is 4 µg/mL; this level is reached in about 16 minutes after a single injection of 600 mg Protopam Chloride. The apparent half-life of Protopam Chloride is 74 to 77 minutes. It has been reported[1] that the supplemental use of oxime cholinesterase reactivators (such as pralidoxime) reduces the incidence and severity of developmental defects in chick embryos exposed to such known teratogens as parathion, bidrin, carbachol, and neostigmine. This protective effect of the oximes was shown to be dose related.

INDICATIONS AND USAGE

Protopam is indicated as an antidote: (1) in the treatment of poisoning due to those pesticides and chemicals of the organophosphate class which have anticholinesterase activity and (2) in the control of overdosage by anticholinesterase drugs used in the treatment of myasthenia gravis.

The principal indications for the use of pralidoxime are muscle weakness and respiratory depression. In severe poisoning, respiratory depression may be due to muscle weakness.

CONTRAINDICATIONS

There are no known absolute contraindications for the use of Protopam. Relative contraindications include known hypersensitivity to the drug and other situations in which the risk of its use clearly outweighs possible benefit (see "**Precautions**").

WARNINGS

Protopam is not effective in the treatment of poisoning due to phosphorus, inorganic phosphates, or organophosphates not having anticholinesterase activity

Protopam is **not** indicated as an antidote for intoxication by pesticides of the carbamate class since it may increase the toxicity of carbaryl.

PRECAUTIONS

GENERAL

Pralidoxime has been very well tolerated in most cases, but it must be remembered that the desperate condition of the organophosphate-poisoned patient will generally mask such minor signs and symptoms as have been noted in normal subjects.

Intravenous administration of Protopam should be carried out slowly and, preferably, by infusion, since certain side effects, such as tachycardia, laryngospasm, and muscle rigidity, have been attributed in a few cases to a too-rapid rate of injection. (See "**Dosage and Administration**".)

Protopam should be used with great caution in treating organophosphate overdosage in cases of myasthenia gravis since it may precipitate a myasthenic crisis.

Because pralidoxime is excreted in the urine, a decrease in renal function will result in increased blood levels of the drug. Thus, the dosage of pralidoxime should be reduced in the presence of renal insufficiency.

LABORATORY TESTS

Treatment of organophosphate poisoning should be instituted without waiting for the results of laboratory tests. Red blood cell, plasma cholinesterase, and urinary paranitrophenol measurements (in the case of parathion exposure) may be helpful in confirming the diagnosis and following

Continued on next page

Protopam—Cont.

the course of the illness. A reduction in red blood cell cholinesterase concentration to below 50% of normal has been seen only with organophosphate ester poisoning.

DRUG INTERACTIONS

When atropine and pralidoxime are used together, the signs of atropinization (flushing, mydriasis, tachycardia, dryness of the mouth and nose) may occur earlier than might be expected when atropine is used alone. This is especially true if the total dose of atropine has been large and the administration of pralidoxime has been delayed.[2-4]

The following precautions should be kept in mind in the treatment of anticholinesterase poisoning, although they do not bear directly on the use of pralidoxime: since barbiturates are potentiated by the anticholinesterases, they should be used cautiously in the treatment of convulsions; morphine, theophylline, aminophylline, succinylcholine, reserpine, and phenothiazine-type tranquilizers should be avoided in patients with organophosphate poisoning.

CARCINOGENESIS, MUTAGENESIS, IMPAIRMENT OF FERTILITY

Since pralidoxime chloride is indicated for short-term emergency use only, no investigations of its potential for carcinogenesis, mutagenesis, or impairment of fertility have been conducted by the manufacturer, or reported in the literature.

PREGNANCY

Teratogenic Effects —Pregnancy Category C:

Animal reproduction studies have not been conducted with pralidoxime. It is also not known whether pralidoxime can cause fetal harm when administered to a pregnant woman or can affect reproduction capacity. Pralidoxime should be given to a pregnant woman only if clearly needed.

NURSING MOTHERS

It is not known whether this drug is excreted in human milk. Because many drugs are excreted in human milk, caution should be exercised when pralidoxime is administered to a nursing woman.

PEDIATRIC USE

Safety and effectiveness in pediatric patients have not been established.

ADVERSE REACTIONS

Forty to 60 minutes after intramuscular injection, mild to moderate pain may be experienced at the site of injection. Pralidoxime may cause blurred vision, diplopia and impaired accommodation, dizziness, headache, drowsiness, nausea, tachycardia, increased systolic and diastolic blood pressure, hyperventilation, and muscular weakness when given parenterally to normal volunteers who have not been exposed to anticholinesterase poisoning. In patients, it is very difficult to differentiate the toxic effects produced by atropine or the organophosphate compounds from those of the drug.

Elevations in SGOT and/or SGPT enzyme levels were observed in 1 of 6 normal volunteers given 1200 mg of pralidoxime chloride intramuscularly, and in 4 of 6 volunteers given 1800 mg intramuscularly. Levels returned to normal in about 2 weeks. Transient elevations in creatine phosphokinase were observed in all normal volunteers given the drug. A single intramuscular injection of 330 mg in 1 mL in rabbits caused myonecrosis, inflammation, and hemorrhage.

When atropine and pralidoxime are used together, the signs of atropinization may occur earlier than might be expected when atropine is used alone. This is especially true if the total dose of atropine has been large and the administration of pralidoxime has been delayed.[2-4] Excitement and manic behavior immediately following recovery of consciousness have been reported in several cases. However, similar behavior has occurred in cases of organophosphate poisoning that were not treated with pralidoxime.[3,5,6]

DRUG ABUSE AND DEPENDENCE

Pralidoxime chloride is not subject to abuse and possesses no known potential for dependence.

OVERDOSAGE

MANIFESTATIONS OF OVERDOSAGE

Observed in normal subjects only: dizziness, blurred vision, diplopia, headache, impaired accommodation, nausea, slight tachycardia. In therapy it has been difficult to differentiate side effects due to the drug from those due to the effects of the poison.

TREATMENT OF OVERDOSAGE

Artificial respiration and other supportive therapy should be administered as needed.

ACUTE TOXICITY

IV—man TDLo: 14 mg/kg (toxic effects: CNS)
IV—rat LD50: 96 mg/kg
IM—rat LD50: 150 mg/kg
ORAL—mouse LD50: 4100 mg/kg
IP—mouse LD50: 155 mg/kg
IV—mouse LD50: 90 mg/kg
IM—mouse LD50: 180 mg/kg

IV—rabbit LD50: 95 mg/kg
IM—guinea pig LD50: 168 mg/kg

DOSAGE AND ADMINISTRATION

ORGANOPHOSPHATE POISONING

"Pralidoxime is most effective if administered immediately after poisoning. Generally, little is accomplished if the drug is given more than 36 hours after termination of exposure. When the poison has been ingested, however, exposure may continue for some time due to slow absorption from the lower bowel, and fatal relapses have been reported after initial improvement. Continued administration for several days may be useful in such patients. Close supervision of the patient is indicated for at least 48 to 72 hours. If dermal exposure has occurred, clothing should be removed and the hair and skin washed thoroughly with sodium bicarbonate or alcohol as soon as possible. Diazepam may be given cautiously if convulsions are not controlled by atropine."[7]

Severe poisoning (coma, cyanosis, respiratory depression) requires intensive management. This includes the removal of secretions, airway management, the correction of acidosis, and hypoxemia.

Atropine should be given as soon as possible after hypoxemia is improved. Atropine should not be given in the presence of significant hypoxia due to the risk of atropine-induced ventricular fibrillation. In adults, atropine may be given intravenously in doses of 2 to 4 mg. This should be repeated at 5- to 10-minute intervals until full atropinization (secretions are inhibited) or signs of atropine toxicity appear (delirium, hyperthermia, muscle twitching).

Some degree of atropinization should be maintained for at least 48 hours, and until any depressed blood cholinesterase activity is reversed.

Morphine, theophylline, aminophylline, and succinylcholine are contraindicated. Tranquilizers of the reserpine or phenothiazine type are to be avoided.

After the effects of atropine become apparent, Protopam may be administered.

PROTOPAM CHLORIDE INJECTION

Parenteral drug products should be inspected visually for particulate matter and discoloration prior to administration, whenever solution and container permit.

Discard unused solution after a dose has been withdrawn.

In adults, inject an initial dose of 1 to 2 g of Protopam, preferably as an infusion in 100 mL of saline, over a 15- to 30-minute period. If this is not practical or if pulmonary edema is present, the dose should be given slowly by intravenous injection as a 5 percent solution in water over not less than five minutes. After about an hour, a second dose of 1 to 2 g will be indicated if muscle weakness has not been relieved. Additional doses may be given cautiously if muscle weakness persists.

Too-rapid administration may result in temporary worsening of cholinergic manifestations. Injection rate should not exceed 200 mg/minute. If intravenous administration is not feasible, intramuscular or subcutaneous injection should be used.

In severe cases, especially after ingestion of the poison, it may be desirable to monitor the effect of therapy electrocardiographically because of the possibility of heart block due to the anticholinesterase. Where the poison has been ingested, it is particularly important to take into account the likelihood of continuing absorption from the lower bowel since this constitutes new exposure. In such cases, additional doses of Protopam (pralidoxime) may be needed every three to eight hours. In effect, the patient should be "titrated" with Protopam as long as signs of poisoning recur. As in all cases of organophosphate poisoning, care should be taken to keep the patient under observation for at least 24 hours.

If convulsions interfere with respiration, they may be controlled by the slow intravenous injection of diazepam, up to 20 mg in adults.

ANTICHOLINESTERASE OVERDOSAGE

As an antagonist to such anticholinesterases as neostigmine, pyridostigmine, and ambenonium, which are used in the treatment of myasthenia gravis, Protopam may be given in a dosage of 1 to 2 g intravenously followed by increments of 250 mg every five minutes.

HOW SUPPLIED

NDC 0046-0374-06—*Hospital Package:* This contains six 20 mL vials of 1 g each of sterile Protopam Chloride (pralidoxime chloride) white to off-white porous cake*, without diluent or syringe. Solution may be prepared by adding 20 mL of Sterile Water for Injection, USP. These are single-dose vials for intravenous injection or for intravenous infusion after further dilution with physiologic saline. Intramuscular or subcutaneous injection may be used when intravenous injection is not feasible.

*When necessary, sodium hydroxide is added during processing to adjust the pH.

Store at room temperature (approximately 25°C).

ANIMAL PHARMACOLOGY AND TOXICOLOGY

The following table lists chemical and trade or generic names of pesticides, chemicals, and drugs against which

Protopam (usually administered in conjunction with atropine) has been found to have antidotal activity on the basis of animal experiments. All compounds listed are organophosphates having anticholinesterase activity. A great many additional substances are in industrial use but have been omitted because of lack of special information.

AAT—see PARATHION

AFLIX®—see FORMOTHION

ALKRON®—See PARATHION

AMERICAN CYANAMID 3422—see PARATHION

AMITON—diethyl-S-(2-diethylaminoethyl)phosphorothiolate

ANTHIO®—see FORMOTHION

APHAMITE—see PARATHION

ARMIN—ethyl-4-nitrophenylethylphosphonate

AZINPHOS-METHYL—dimethyl-S-[(4-oxo-1,2,3,-benzotriazin-3 (4H)-yl)methyl] phosphorodithioate

MORPHOTHION—dimethyl-S-2-keto-2-(N-morpholyl)ethylphosphorodithioate

NEGUVON®—see TRICHLOROFON

NIRAN®—see PARATHION

NITROSTIGMINE—see PARATHION

O,O-DIETHYL-O-p-NITROPHENYL PHOSPHOROTHIOATE—see PARATHION

O,O-DIETHYL-O-p-NITROPHENYLTHIO PHOSPHATE—see PARATHION

OR 1191—see PHOSPHAMIDON

OS 1836—see VINYLPHOS

OXYDEMETONMETHYL—dimethyl-S-2-(ethylsulfinyl) ethyl phosphorothiolate

PARAOXON—diethyl (4-nitrophenyl) phosphate

PARATHION—diethyl (4-nitrophenyl) phosphorothionate

PENPHOS—see PARATHION

PHENCAPTON—diethyl-S-(2,5-dichlorophenylmercaptomethyl) phosphorodithioate

PHOSDRIN®—see MEVINPHOS

PHOS-KIL—see PARATHION

PHOSPHAMIDON—1-chloro-1-diethylcarbamoyl-1-propen-2-yl-dimethylphosphate

PHOSPHOLINE IODIDE®—see echothiophate iodide

PHOSPHOROTHIOIC ACID, O,O-DIETHYL-O-p-NITROPHENYL ESTER—see PARATHION

PLANTHION—see PARATHION

QUELETOX—see FENTHION

RHODIATOX®—see PARATHION

RUELENE®—4-tert-butyl-2-chlorophenylmethyl-N-methylphosphoroamidate

SARIN—isopropyl-methylphosphonofluoridate

SHELL OS 1836—see VINYLPHOS

SHELL 2046—see MEVINPHOS

SNP—see PARATHION

SOMAN—pinacolyl-methylphosphonofluoridate

SYSTOX®—diethyl-(2-ethylmercaptoethyl) phosphorothionate

TEP—see TEPP

TEPP—tetraethylpyro phosphate

THIOPHOS®—see PARATHION

TIGUVON—see FENTHION

TRICHLOROFON—dimethyl-1-hydroxy-2,2,2-trichloroethylphosphonate

VAPONA®—see DICHLORVOS

VAPOPHOS—see PARATHION

VINYLPHOS—diethyl-2-chloro-vinylphosphate

PROTOPAM appears to be ineffective, or marginally effective, against poisoning by:
CIODRIN® (alpha-methylbenzyl-3[dimethoxyphosphinyl-oxy]-ciscrotonate)
DIMEFOX (tetramethylphosphorodiamidic fluoride)
DIMETHOATE (dimethyl-S-[N-methylcarbamoylmethyl]phosphorodithioate)
METHYL DIAZINON (dimethyl-[2-isopropyl-4-methylpyrimidyl]-phosphorothionate)
METHYL PHENCAPTON (dimethyl-S-[2,5-dichlorophenylmercaptomethyl]phosphorodithioate)
PHORATE (diethyl-S-ethylmercaptomethylphosphorodithioate)
SCHRADAN (octamethylpyrophosphoramide)
WEPSYN® (5-amino-1-[bis-(dimethylamino) phosphinyl]-3-phenyl-1,2,4-triazole).
The use of Protopam should, nevertheless, be considered in any life-threatening situation resulting from poisoning by these compounds, since the limited and arbitrary conditions of pharmacologic screening do not always accurately reflect the usefulness of Protopam in the clinical situation.
CLINICAL STUDIES
The use of Protopam (pralidoxime) has been reported in the treatment of human cases of poisoning by the following substances:
Azodrin
Diazinon
Dichlorvos (DDVP) with chlordane
Disulfoton
EPN
Isoflurophate
Malathion
Metasystox I® and Fenthion
Methyldemeton
Methylparathion
Mevinphos
Parathion
Parathion and Mevinphos
Phosphamidon
Sarin
Systox®
TEPP
Of these cases, over 100 were due to parathion, about a dozen each to malathion, diazinon, and mevinphos, and a few to each of the other compounds.

REFERENCES

1. LANDAUER, W.: Cholinomimetic teratogens. V. The effect of oximes and related cholinesterase reactivators, *Teratology 15* :33 (Feb) 1977.
2. MOLLER, K.O., JENSEN-HOLM, J., and LAUSEN, H.H.: *Ugeskr. Laeg. 123* :501, 1961.
3. NAMBA, T., NOLTE, C.T., JACKREL, J. and GROB, D.: Poisoning due to organophosphate insecticides. Acute and chronic manifestations, *Amer. J. Med. 50* :475 (Apr), 1971.
4. ARENA, J.M.: Poisoning, Toxicology Symptoms, Treatments, ed. 4, Springfield, IL, Charles C. Thomas, 1979, p. 133.
5. BRACHFELD, J., and ZAVON, M.R.: Organic phosphate (Phosdrin®) intoxication. Report of a case and the results of treatment with 2-PAM, *Arch. Environ. Health 11* :859, 1965.
6. HAYES, W.J., Jr.: Toxicology of Pesticides, Baltimore, The Williams & Wilkins Company, 1975, p. 416.
7. AMA Department of Drugs: AMA Drug Evaluations, ed. 4, Chicago, American Medical Association, 1980, p. 1455.

Manufactured by:
Ayerst Laboratories Inc.
A Wyeth-Ayerst Company
Philadelphia, PA 19101

SECTRAL® ℞

[*sek 'tral*]
(acebutolol hydrochloride)
Capsules

DESCRIPTION

Sectral (acebutolol HCl) is a selective, hydrophilic beta-adrenoreceptor blocking agent with mild intrinsic sympathomimetic activity for use in treating patients with hypertension and ventricular arrhythmias. It is marketed in capsule form for oral administration. Sectral capsules are provided in two dosage strengths which contain 200 or 400 mg of acebutolol as the hydrochloride salt. The inactive ingredients present are D&C Red 22, FD&C Blue 1, FD&C Yellow 6, gelatin, povidone, starch, stearic acid, and titanium dioxide. The 200 mg dosage strength also contains D&C Red 28 and the 400 mg dosage strength also contains FD&C Red 40.
Acebutolol HCl has the following structural formula:

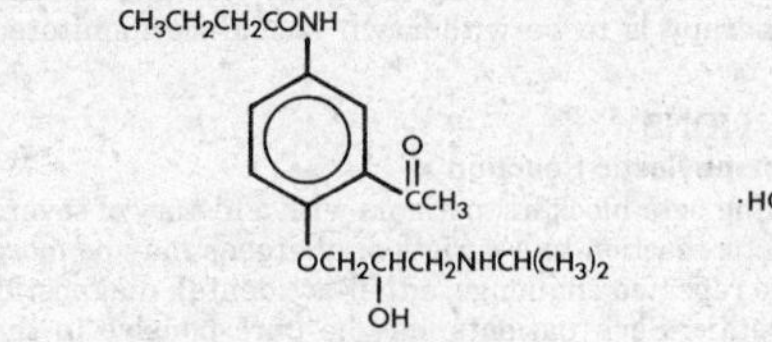

$C_{18}H_{28}N_2O_4 \cdot HCl$ M.W. 372.9

Acebutolol HCl is a white or slightly off-white powder freely soluble in water, and less soluble in alcohol. Chemically it is defined as the hydrochloride salt ±N-[3-Acetyl-4-[2-hydroxy-3-[(1-methylethyl)amino]propoxy]phenyl]butanamide, or (±)-3'-Acetyl-4'-[2-hydroxy -3- (isopropylamino) propoxy] butyranilide.

CLINICAL PHARMACOLOGY

Sectral is a cardioselective, β -adrenoreceptor blocking agent, which possesses mild intrinsic sympathomimetic activity (ISA) in its therapeutically effective dose range.

Pharmacodynamics

β_1-cardioselectivity has been demonstrated in experimental animal studies. In anesthetized dogs and cats, Sectral is more potent in antagonizing isoproterenol-induced tachycardia (β_1) than in antagonizing isoproterenol-induced vasodilatation (β_2). In guinea pigs and cats, it is more potent in antagonizing this tachycardia than in antagonizing isoproterenol-induced bronchodilatation (β_2). ISA of Sectral has been demonstrated in catecholamine-depleted rats by tachycardia induced by intravenous administration of this agent. A membrane-stabilizing effect has been detected in animals, but only with high concentrations of Sectral.
Clinical studies have demonstrated β_1-blocking activity at the recommended doses by: a) reduction in the resting heart rate and decrease in exercise-induced tachycardia; b) reduction in cardiac output at rest and after exercise; c) reduction of systolic and diastolic blood pressures at rest and postexercise; d) inhibition of isoproterenol-induced tachycardia.
The β_1-selectivity of Sectral has also been demonstrated on the basis of the following vascular and bronchial effects:
Vascular Effects: Sectral has less antagonistic effects on peripheral vascular β_2-receptors at rest and after epinephrine stimulation than nonselective β-antagonists.
Bronchial Effects: In single-dose studies in asthmatics examining effects of various beta-blockers on pulmonary function, low doses of acebutolol produce less evidence of bronchoconstriction and less reduction of beta$_2$ agonist, bronchodilating effects, than nonselective agents like propranolol but more than atenolol.
ISA has been observed with Sectral in man, as shown by a slightly smaller (about 3 beats per minute) decrease in resting heart rate when compared to equivalent β-blocking doses of propranolol, metoprolol or atenolol. Chronic therapy with Sectral induced no significant alteration in the blood lipid profile.
Sectral has been shown to delay AV conduction time and to increase the refractoriness of the AV node without significantly affecting sinus node recovery time, atrial refractory period, or the HV conduction time. The membrane-stabilizing effect of Sectral is not manifest at the doses used clinically.
Significant reductions in resting and exercise heart rates and systolic blood pressures have been observed 1.5 hours after Sectral administration with maximal effects occurring between 3 and 8 hours postdosing in normal volunteers. Sectral has demonstrated a significant effect on exercise-induced tachycardia 24 to 30 hours after drug administration.
There are significant correlations between plasma levels of acebutolol and both the reduction in resting heart rate and the percent of β-blockade of exercise-induced tachycardia.
The antihypertensive effect of Sectral has been shown in double-blind controlled studies to be superior to placebo and similar to propranolol and hydrochlorothiazide. In addition, patients responding to Sectral administered twice daily had a similar response whether the dosage regimen was changed to once daily administration or continued on a b.i.d. regimen. Most patients responded to 400 to 800 mg per day in divided doses.
The antiarrhythmic effect of Sectral was compared with placebo, propranolol, and quinidine. Compared with placebo, Sectral significantly reduced mean total ventricular ectopic beats (VEB), paired VEB, multiform VEB, R-on-T beats, and ventricular tachycardia (VT). Both Sectral and propranolol significantly reduced mean total and paired VEB and VT. Sectral and quinidine significantly reduced resting total and complex VEB; the antiarrhythmic efficacy of Sectral was also observed during exercise.

Pharmacokinetics and Metabolism

Sectral is well absorbed from the GI tract. It is subject to extensive first-pass hepatic biotransformation, with an absolute bioavailability of approximately 40% for the parent compound. The major metabolite, an N-acetyl derivative (diacetolol), is pharmacologically active. This metabolite is equipotent to Sectral and in cats is more cardioselective than Sectral; therefore, this first-pass phenomenon does not attenuate the therapeutic effect of Sectral. Food intake does not have a significant effect on the area under the plasma concentration-time curve (AUC) of Sectral although the rate of absorption and peak concentration decreased slightly.
The plasma elimination half-life of Sectral is approximately 3 to 4 hours, while that of its metabolite, diacetolol, is 8 to 13 hours. The time to reach peak concentration for Sectral is 2.5 hours and for diacetolol, after oral administration of Sectral, 3.5 hours.
Within the single oral dose range of 200 to 400 mg, the kinetics are dose proportional. However, this linearity is not seen at higher doses, probably due to saturation of hepatic biotransformation sites. In addition, after multiple dosing the lack of linearity is also seen by AUC increases of approximately 100% as compared to single oral dosing. Elimination via renal excretion is approximately 30% to 40% and by nonrenal mechanisms 50% to 60%, which includes excretion into the bile and direct passage through the intestinal wall.
Sectral has a low binding affinity for plasma proteins (about 26%). Sectral and its metabolite, diacetolol, are relatively hydrophilic and, therefore, only minimal quantities have been detected in the cerebrospinal fluid (CSF).
Drug interaction studies with tolbutamide and warfarin indicated no influence on the therapeutic effects of these compounds. Digoxin and hydrochlorothiazide plasma levels were not affected by concomitant Sectral administration. The kinetics of Sectral were not significantly altered by concomitant administration of hydrochlorothiazide, hydralazine, sulfinpyrazone, or oral contraceptives.
In patients with renal impairment, there is no effect on the elimination half-life of Sectral, but there is decreased elimination of the metabolite, diacetolol, resulting in a two- to three-fold increase in its half-life. For this reason, the drug should be administered with caution in patients with renal insufficiency (see **PRECAUTIONS**). Sectral and its major metabolite are dialyzable.
Sectral crosses the placental barrier and is secreted in breast milk.
In geriatric patients, the bioavailability of Sectral and its metabolite is increased, approximately two-fold, probably due to decreases in the first-pass metabolism and renal function in the elderly.

INDICATIONS AND USAGE

Hypertension

Sectral is indicated for the management of hypertension in adults. It may be used alone or in combination with other antihypertensive agents, especially thiazide-type diuretics.

Ventricular Arrhythmias

Sectral is indicated in the management of ventricular premature beats; it reduces the total number of premature beats, as well as the number of paired and multiform ventricular ectopic beats, and R-on-T beats.

CONTRAINDICATIONS

Sectral is contraindicated in: 1) persistently severe bradycardia; 2) second- and third-degree heart block; 3) overt cardiac failure; and 4) cardiogenic shock. (See **WARNINGS**.)

WARNINGS

Cardiac Failure

Sympathetic stimulation may be essential for support of the circulation in individuals with diminished myocardial contractility, and its inhibition by β-adrenergic receptor blockade may precipitate more severe failure. Although β-blockers should be avoided in overt cardiac failure, Sectral can be used with caution in patients with a history of heart failure who are controlled with digitalis and/or diuretics. Both digitalis and Sectral impair AV conduction. If cardiac failure persists, therapy with Sectral should be withdrawn.

In Patients Without A History of Cardiac Failure

In patients with aortic or mitral valve disease or compromised left ventricular function, continued depression of the myocardium with β-blocking agents over a period of time may lead to cardiac failure. At the first signs of failure, patients should be digitalized and/or be given a diuretic and the response observed closely. If cardiac failure continues despite adequate digitalization and/or diuretic, Sectral therapy should be withdrawn.

Exacerbation of Ischemic Heart Disease Following Abrupt Withdrawal

Following abrupt cessation of therapy with certain β-blocking agents in patients with coronary artery disease, exacer-

Continued on next page

Sectral—Cont.

bation of angina pectoris and, in some cases, myocardial infarction and death have been reported. Therefore, such patients should be cautioned against interruption of therapy without a physician's advice. Even in the absence of overt ischemic heart disease, when discontinuation of Sectral is planned, the patient should be carefully observed, and should be advised to limit physical activity to a minimum while Sectral is gradually withdrawn over a period of about two weeks. (If therapy with an alternative β-blocker is desired, the patient may be transferred directly to comparable doses of another agent without interruption of β-blocking therapy.) If an exacerbation of angina pectoris occurs, antianginal therapy should be restarted immediately in full doses and the patient hospitalized until his condition stabilizes.

Peripheral Vascular Disease
Treatment with β-antagonists reduces cardiac output and can precipitate or aggravate the symptoms of arterial insufficiency in patients with peripheral or mesenteric vascular disease. Caution should be exercised with such patients, and they should be observed closely for evidence of progression of arterial obstruction.

Bronchospastic Diseases
PATIENTS WITH BRONCHOSPASTIC DISEASE SHOULD, IN GENERAL, NOT RECEIVE A β-BLOCKER. Because of its relative β_1-selectivity, however, low doses of Sectral may be used with caution in patients with bronchospastic disease who do not respond to, or who cannot tolerate, alternative treatment. Since β_1-selectivity is not absolute and is dose-dependent, the lowest possible dose of Sectral should be used initially, preferably in divided doses to avoid the higher plasma levels associated with the longer dose-interval. A bronchodilator, such as a theophylline or a β_2-stimulant, should be made available in advance with instructions concerning its use.

Anesthesia and Major Surgery
The necessity, or desirability, of withdrawal of a β-blocking therapy prior to major surgery is controversial. β-adrenergic receptor blockade impairs the ability of the heart to respond to β-adrenergically mediated reflex stimuli. While this might be of benefit in preventing arrhythmic response, the risk of excessive myocardial depression during general anesthesia may be enhanced and difficulty in restarting and maintaining the heart beat has been reported with beta-blockers. If treatment is continued, particular care should be taken when using anesthetic agents which depress the myocardium, such as ether, cyclopropane and trichlorethylene, and it is prudent to use the lowest possible dose of Sectral. Sectral, like other β-blockers, is a competitive inhibitor of β-receptor agonists, and its effect on the heart can be reversed by cautious administration of such agents (e.g., dobutamine or isoproterenol—see **OVERDOSE**).

Manifestations of excessive vagal tone (e.g., profound bradycardia, hypotension) may be corrected with atropine 1 to 3 mg IV in divided doses.

Diabetes and Hypoglycemia
β-blockers may potentiate insulin-induced hypoglycemia and mask some of its manifestations such as tachycardia; however, dizziness and sweating are usually not significantly affected. Diabetic patients should be warned of the possibility of masked hypoglycemia.

Thyrotoxicosis
β-adrenergic blockade may mask certain clinical signs (tachycardia) of hyperthyroidism. Abrupt withdrawal of β-blockade may precipitate a thyroid storm; therefore, patients suspected of developing thyrotoxicosis from whom Sectral therapy is to be withdrawn should be monitored closely.

PRECAUTIONS

Risk of Anaphylactic Reaction
While taking beta-blockers, patients with a history of severe anaphylactic reaction to a variety of allergens may be more reactive to repeated challenge, either accidental, diagnostic, or therapeutic. Such patients may be unresponsive to the usual doses of epinephrine used to treat allergic reaction.

Impaired Renal or Hepatic Function
Studies on the effect of acebutolol in patients with renal insufficiency have not been performed in the U.S. Foreign published experience shows that acebutolol has been used successfully in chronic renal insufficiency. Acebutolol is excreted through the GI tract, but the active metabolite, diacetolol, is eliminated predominantly by the kidney. There is a linear relationship between renal clearance of diacetolol and creatinine clearance. Therefore, the daily dose of acebutolol should be reduced by 50% when the creatinine clearance is less than 50 mL/min and by 75% when it is less than 25 mL/min. Sectral should be used cautiously in patients with impaired hepatic function.

Sectral has been used successfully and without problems in elderly patients in the U.S. clinical trials without specific adjustment of dosage. However, elderly patients may require lower maintenance doses because the bioavailability of both Sectral and its metabolite are approximately doubled in this age group.

Information for Patients
Patients, especially those with evidence of coronary artery disease, should be warned against interruption or discontinuation of Sectral therapy without a physician's supervision. Although cardiac failure rarely occurs in properly selected patients, those being treated with β-adrenergic blocking agents should be advised to consult a physician if they develop signs or symptoms suggestive of impending CHF, or unexplained respiratory symptoms.

Patients should also be warned of possible severe hypertensive reactions from concomitant use of α-adrenergic stimulants, such as the nasal decongestants commonly used in OTC cold preparations and nasal drops.

Clinical Laboratory Findings
Sectral, like other β-blockers, has been associated with the development of antinuclear antibodies (ANA). In prospective clinical trials, patients receiving Sectral had a dose-dependent increase in the development of positive ANA ti-

ters, and the overall incidence was higher than that observed with propranolol. Symptoms (generally persistent arthralgias and myalgias) related to this laboratory abnormality were infrequent (less than 1% with both drugs). Symptoms and ANA titers were reversible upon discontinuation of treatment.

Drug Interactions
Catecholamine-depleting drugs, such as reserpine, may have an additive effect when given with β-blocking agents. Patients treated with Sectral plus catecholamine depletors should, therefore, be observed closely for evidence of marked bradycardia or hypotension which may present as vertigo, syncope/presyncope, or orthostatic changes in blood pressure without compensatory tachycardia. Exaggerated hypertensive responses have been reported from the combined use of β-adrenergic antagonists and α-adrenergic stimulants, including those contained in proprietary cold remedies and vasoconstrictive nasal drops. Patients receiving β-blockers should be warned of this potential hazard. Blunting of the antihypertensive effect of beta-adrenoceptor blocking agents by nonsteroidal anti-inflammatory drugs has been reported.

No significant interactions with digoxin, hydrochlorothiazide, hydralazine, sulfinpyrazone, oral contraceptives, tolbutamide, or warfarin have been observed.

Carcinogenesis, Mutagenesis, Impairment of Fertility
Chronic oral toxicity studies in rats and mice, employing dose levels as high as 300 mg/kg/day, which is equivalent to 15 times the maximum recommended (60 kg) human dose, did not indicate a carcinogenic potential for Sectral. Diacetolol, the major metabolite of Sectral in man, was without carcinogenic potential in rats when tested at doses as high as 1800 mg/kg/day. Sectral and diacetolol were also shown to be devoid of mutagenic potential in the Ames Test. Sectral, administered orally to two generations of male and female rats at doses of up to 240 mg/kg/day (equivalent to 12 times the maximum recommended therapeutic dose in a 60-kg human) and diacetolol, administered to two generations of male and female rats at doses of up to 1000 mg/kg/day, had no significant impact on reproductive performance or fertility.

Pregnancy
Teratogenic Effects
Pregnancy Category B: Reproduction studies have been performed with Sectral in rats (up to 630 mg/kg/day) and rabbits (up to 135 mg/kg/day). These doses are equivalent to approximately 31.5 and 6.8 times the maximum recommended therapeutic dose in a 60-kg human, respectively. The compound was not teratogenic in either species. In the rabbit, however, doses of 135 mg/kg/day caused slight fetal growth retardation; this effect was considered to be a result of maternal toxicity, as evidenced by reduced food intake, a lowered rate of body weight gain, and mortality. Studies have also been performed in these species with diacetolol (at doses of up to 450 mg/kg/day in rabbits and up to 1800 mg/kg/day in rats.) Other than a significant elevation in postimplantation loss with 450 mg/kg/day diacetolol, a level at which food consumption and body weight gain were reduced in rabbit dams and a nonstatistically significant increase in incidence of bilateral cataract in rat fetuses from dams treated with 1800 mg/kg/day diacetolol, there was no evidence of harm to the fetus. There are no adequate and well-controlled trials in pregnant women. Because animal teratology studies are not always predictive of the human response, Sectral should be used during pregnancy only if the potential benefit justifies the risk to the fetus.

Nonteratogenic Effects
Studies in humans have shown that both acebutolol and diacetolol cross the placenta. Neonates of mothers who have received acebutolol during pregnancy have reduced birth weight, decreased blood pressure, and decreased heart rate. In the newborn the elimination half-life of acebutolol was 6 to 14 hours, while the half-life of diacetolol was 24 to 30 hours for the first 24 hours after birth, followed by a half-life of 12 to 16 hours. Adequate facilities for monitoring these infants at birth should be available.

Labor and Delivery
The effect of Sectral on labor and delivery in pregnant women is unknown. Studies in animals have not shown any effect of Sectral on the usual course of labor and delivery.

Nursing Mothers
Acebutolol and diacetolol also appear in breast milk with a milk:plasma ratio of 7.1 and 12.2, respectively. Use in nursing mothers is not recommended.

Pediatric Use
Safety and effectiveness in pediatric patients have not been established.

ADVERSE REACTIONS
Sectral is well tolerated in properly selected patients. Most adverse reactions have been mild, not required discontinuation of therapy, and tended to decrease as duration of treatment increases.

The following table shows the frequency of treatment-related side effects derived from controlled clinical trials in

TOTAL VOLUNTEERED AND ELICITED (U.S. STUDIES)

Body System/ Adverse Reaction	SECTRAL (N=1002) %	Propranolol (N=424) %	Hydrochloro-thiazide (N=178) %	Placebo (N=314) %
Cardiovascular				
Chest Pain	2	4	4	1
Edema	2	2	4	1
Central Nervous System				
Depression	2	1	3	1
Dizziness	6	7	12	2
Fatigue	11	17	10	4
Headache	6	9	13	4
Insomnia	3	6	5	1
Abnormal dreams	2	3	0	1
Dermatologic				
Rash	2	2	4	1
Gastrointestinal				
Constipation	4	2	7	0
Diarrhea	4	5	5	1
Dyspepsia	4	6	3	1
Flatulence	3	4	7	1
Nausea	4	4	3	0
Genitourinary				
Micturition (frequency)	3	1	9	<1
Musculoskeletal				
Arthralgia	2	1	3	2
Myalgia	2	1	4	0
Respiratory				
Cough	1	1	2	0
Dyspnea	4	6	4	2
Rhinitis	2	1	4	<1
Special Senses				
Abnormal Vision	2	2	3	0

patients with hypertension, angina pectoris, and arrhythmia. These patients received Sectral, propranolol, or hydrochlorothiazide as monotherapy, or placebo.
[See table at bottom of previous page]

The following selected (potentially important) side effects were seen in up to 2% of Sectral patients:
Cardiovascular: hypotension, bradycardia, heart failure.
Central Nervous System: anxiety, hyper/hypoesthesia, impotence.
Dermatological: pruritus.
Gastrointestinal: vomiting, abdominal pain.
Genitourinary: dysuria, nocturia.
Liver and Biliary System: A small number of cases of liver abnormalities (increased SGOT, SGPT, LDH) have been reported in association with acebutolol therapy. In some cases increased bilirubin or alkaline phosphatase, fever, malaise, dark urine, anorexia, nausea, headache, and/or other symptoms have been reported. In some of the reported cases, the symptoms and signs were confirmed by rechallenge with acebutolol. The abnormalities were reversible upon cessation of acebutolol therapy.
Musculoskeletal: back pain, joint pain.
Respiratory: pharyngitis, wheezing.
Special Senses: conjunctivitis, dry eye, eye pain.
Autoimmune: In extremely rare instances, systemic lupus erythematosus has been reported.

The incidence of drug-related adverse effects (volunteered and solicited) according to Sectral dose is shown below. (Data from 266 hypertensive patients treated for 3 months on a constant dose.)

Body System	400 mg/day (N=132)	800 mg/day (N=63)	1200 mg/day (N=71)
Cardiovascular	5%	2%	1%
Gastrointstinal	3%	3%	7%
Musculoskeletal	2%	3%	4%
Central Nervous System	9%	13%	17%
Respiratory	1%	5%	6%
Skin	1%	2%	1%
Special Senses	2%	2%	6%
Genitourinary	2%	3%	1%

Potential Adverse Effects

In addition, certain adverse effects not listed above have been reported with other β-blocking agents and should also be considered as potential adverse effects of Sectral.
Central Nervous System: Reversible mental depression progressing to catatonia (an acute syndrome characterized by disorientation for time and place), short-term memory loss, emotional lability, slightly clouded sensorium, and decreased performance (neuropsychometrics).
Cardiovascular: Intensification of AV block (see **CONTRAINDICATIONS**).
Allergic: Erythematous rash, fever combined with aching and sore throat, laryngospasm, and respiratory distress.
Hematologic: Agranulocytosis, nonthrombocytopenic, and thrombocytopenic purpura.
Gastrointestinal: Mesenteric arterial thrombosis and ischemic colitis.
Miscellaneous: Reversible alopecia and Peyronie's disease.
The oculomucocutaneous syndrome associated with the β-blocker practolol has not been reported with Sectral during investigational use and extensive foreign clinical experience.

OVERDOSAGE

No specific information on emergency treatment of overdosage is available for Sectral. However, overdosage with other β-blocking agents has been accompanied by extreme bradycardia, advanced atrioventricular block, intraventricular conduction defects, hypotension, severe congestive heart failure, seizures, and in susceptible patients, bronchospasm and hypoglycemia. Although specific information on the emergency treatment of Sectral overdose is not available, on the basis of the pharmacological actions and the observations in treating overdoses with other β-blockers, the following general measures should be considered:

1. Empty stomach by emesis or lavage.
2. Bradycardia: IV atropine (1 to 3 mg in divided doses). If antivagal response is inadequate, administer isoproterenol cautiously since larger than usual doses of isoproterenol may be required.
3. Persistent hypotension in spite of correction of bradycardia: Administer vasopressor (e.g., epinephrine, levarterenol, dopamine, or dobutamine) with frequent monitoring of blood pressure and pulse rate.
4. Bronchospasm: A theophylline derivative, such as aminophylline and/or parenteral β_2-stimulant, such as terbutaline.
5. Cardiac failure: Digitalize the patient and/or administer a diuretic. It has been reported that glucagon is useful in this situation.

Sectral is dialyzable.

DOSAGE AND ADMINISTRATION

Hypertension

The initial dosage of Sectral in uncomplicated mild-to-moderate hypertension is 400 mg. This can be given as a single daily dose, but in occasional patients twice daily dosing may be required for adequate 24-hour blood-pressure control. An optimal response is usually achieved with dosages of 400 to 800 mg per day, although some patients have been maintained on as little as 200 mg per day. Patients with more severe hypertension or who have demonstrated inadequate control may respond to a total of 1200 mg daily (administered b.i.d.), or to the addition of a second antihypertensive agent. Beta-1 selectivity diminishes as dosage is increased.

Ventricular Arrhythmia

The usual initial dose of Sectral is 400 mg daily given as 200 mg b.i.d. Dosage should be increased gradually until an optimal clinical response is obtained, generally at 600 to 1200 mg per day. If treatment is to be discontinued, the dosage should be reduced gradually over a period of about two weeks.

Use in Older Patients

Older patients have an approximately 2-fold increase in bioavailability and may require lower maintenance doses. Doses above 800 mg/day should be avoided in the elderly.

HOW SUPPLIED

Sectral® (acebutolol HCl) is available in the following dosage strengths:
200 mg, opaque purple and orange capsule marked "WYETH 4177" and "Sectral 200"
NDC 0008-4177-01, in bottles of 100 capsules.
NDC 0008-4177-04, in Redipak® cartons of 100 capsules (10 blister strips of 10).
Keep tightly closed
Store at room temperature, approximately 25° C (77°F)
Protect from light
Dispense in a light-resistant, tight container
Use carton to protect contents from light
400 mg, opaque brown and orange capsule marked "WYETH 4179" and "Sectral 400"
NDC 0008-4179-01, in bottles of 100 capsules.
Keep tightly closed
Store at room temperature, approximately 25°C (77°F)
Dispense in a tight container
The appearance of these capsules is a trademark of Wyeth-Ayerst Laboratories.

by arrangement with Rhone-Poulenc Rorer France
Manufactured by:
Wyeth Laboratories Inc.
A Wyeth-Ayerst Company
Philadelphia, PA 19101

Shown in Product Identification Guide, page 345

SERAX® Ⓒ ℞

[ser 'aks]
(oxazepam)
CAPSULES • TABLETS

DESCRIPTION

Serax is the first of a chemical series of compounds known as the 3-hydroxybenzodiazepinones. A therapeutic agent providing versatility and flexibility in control of common emotional disturbances, this product exerts prompt action in a wide variety of disorders associated with anxiety, tension, agitation, and irritability, and anxiety associated with depression. In tolerance and toxicity studies on several animal species, this product reveals significantly greater safety factors than related compounds (chlordiazepoxide and diazepam) and manifests a wide separation of effective doses and doses inducing side effects.

Serax capsules contain 10 mg, 15 mg, or 30 mg oxazepam. The inactive ingredients present are gelatin, lactose, titanium dioxide, and other ingredients. Each dosage strength also contains the following:
10 mg—D&C Red 22, D&C Red 28, and FD&C Blue 1;
15 mg—FD&C Red 40 and FD&C Yellow 6;
30 mg—D&C Red 28, FD&C Red 40, and FD&C Blue 1.

Serax tablets contain 15 mg oxazepam. The inactive ingredients present are FD&C Yellow 5, lactose, magnesium stearate, methylcellulose, and polacrilin potassium.

Serax is 7-chloro-1,3,-dihydro-3-hydroxy-5-phenyl-2*H* -1,4-benzodiazepin-2-one, a white crystalline powder with a molecular weight of 286.7.

CLINICAL PHARMACOLOGY

Pharmacokinetic testing in twelve volunteers demonstrated that when given as a single 30 mg dose, the capsule, tablet, and suspension were equivalent in extent of absorption. For the capsule and tablet, peak plasma levels averaged 450 ng/mL and were observed to occur about 3 hours after dosing. The mean elimination half-life for oxazepam was approximately 8.2 hours (range 5.7 to 10.9 hours).

This product has a single, major inactive metabolite in man, a glucuronide excreted in the urine.

ANIMAL PHARMACOLOGY AND TOXICOLOGY

In mice, Serax exerts an anticonvulsant (anti-Metrazol®) activity at 50-percent-effective doses of about 0.6 mg/kg orally. (Such anticonvulsant activity of benzodiazepines correlates with their tranquilizing properties.) To produce ataxia (rotabar test) and sedation (abolition of spontaneous motor activity), the 50-percent-effective doses of this product are greater than 5 mg/kg orally. Thus, about ten times the therapeutic (anticonvulsant) dose must be given before ataxia ensues, indicating a wide separation of effective doses and doses inducing side effects.

In evaluation of antianxiety activity of compounds, conflict behavioral tests in rats differentiate continuous response for food in the presence of anxiety-provoking stress (shock) from drug-induced motor incoordination. This product shows significant separation of doses required to relieve anxiety and doses producing sedation or ataxia. Ataxia-producing doses exceed those of related CNS-acting drugs.

Acute oral LD_{50} in mice is greater than 5000 mg/kg, compared to 800 mg/kg for a related compound (chlordiazepoxide).

Subacute toxicity studies in dogs for four weeks at 480 mg/kg daily showed no specific changes; at 960 mg/kg two out of eight died with evidence of circulatory collapse. This wide margin of safety is significant compared to chlordiazepoxide HCl, which showed nonspecific changes in six dogs at 80 mg/ kg. On chlordiazepoxide, two out of six died with evidence of circulatory collapse at 127 mg/kg, and six out of six died at 200 mg/kg daily. Chronic toxicity studies of Serax in dogs at 120 mg/kg/day for 52 weeks produced no toxic manifestation.

Fatty metamorphosis of the liver has been noted in six-week toxicity studies in rats given this product at 0.5% of the diet. Such accumulations of fat are considered reversible, as there is no liver necrosis or fibrosis.

Breeding studies in rats through two successive litters did not produce fetal abnormality.

Oxazepam has not been adequately evaluated for mutagenic activity.

In a carcinogenicity study, oxazepam was administered with diet to rats for two years. Male rats receiving 30 times the maximum human dose showed a statistical increase, when compared to controls, in benign thyroid follicular cell tumors, testicular interstitial cell adenomas, and prostatic adenomas. An earlier published study reported that mice fed dietary dosages of 35 or 100 times the human daily dose of oxazepam for 9 months developed a dose-related increase in liver adenomas.[1] In an independent analysis of some of the microscopic slides from this mouse study, several of these tumors were classified as liver carcinomas. At this time, there is no evidence that clinical use of oxazepam is associated with tumors.

INDICATIONS

Serax (oxazepam) is indicated for the management of anxiety disorders or for the short-term relief of the symptoms of anxiety. Anxiety or tension associated with the stress of everyday life usually does not require treatment with an anxiolytic.

Anxiety associated with depression is also responsive to Serax therapy.

This product has been found particularly useful in the management of anxiety, tension, agitation, and irritability in older patients.

Alcoholics with acute tremulousness, inebriation, or with anxiety associated with alcohol withdrawal are responsive to therapy.

The effectiveness of Serax in long-term use, that is, more than 4 months, has not been assessed by systematic clinical studies. The physician should periodically reassess the usefulness of the drug for the individual patient.

CONTRAINDICATIONS

History of previous hypersensitivity reaction to oxazepam. Oxazepam is not indicated in psychoses.

WARNINGS

As with other CNS-acting drugs, patients should be cautioned against driving automobiles or operating dangerous machinery until it is known that they do not become drowsy or dizzy on oxazepam therapy.

Patients should be warned that the effects of alcohol or other CNS-depressant drugs may be additive to those of Serax, possibly requiring adjustment of dosage or elimination of such agents.

PHYSICAL AND PSYCHOLOGICAL DEPENDENCE

Withdrawal symptoms, similar in character to those noted with barbiturates and alcohol (convulsions, tremor, abdominal and muscle cramps, vomiting, and sweating), have occurred following abrupt discontinuance of oxazepam. The more severe withdrawal symptoms have usually been limited to those patients who received excessive doses over an extended period of time. Generally milder withdrawal symptoms (e.g., dysphoria and insomnia) have been reported following abrupt discontinuance of benzodiazepines

Continued on next page

Serax—Cont.

taken continuously at therapeutic levels for several months. Consequently, after extended therapy, abrupt discontinuation should generally be avoided and a gradual dosage-tapering schedule followed. Addiction-prone individuals (such as drug addicts or alcoholics) should be under careful surveillance when receiving oxazepam or other psychotropic agents because of the predisposition of such patients to habituation and dependence.

USE IN PREGNANCY

An increased risk of congenital malformations associated with the use of minor tranquilizers (chlordiazepoxide, diazepam, and meprobamate) during the first trimester of pregnancy has been suggested in several studies. Serax, a benzodiazepine derivative, has not been studied adequately to determine whether it, too, may be associated with an increased risk of fetal abnormality. Because use of these drugs is rarely a matter of urgency, their use during this period should almost always be avoided. The possibility that a woman of childbearing potential may be pregnant at the time of institution of therapy should be considered. Patients should be advised that if they become pregnant during therapy or intend to become pregnant they should communicate with their physician about the desirability of discontinuing the drug.

PRECAUTIONS

Although hypotension has occurred only rarely, oxazepam should be administered with caution to patients in whom a drop in blood pressure might lead to cardiac complications. This is particularly true in the elderly patient.

Serax 15 mg tablets, *but none of the other available dosage forms of this product,* contain FD&C Yellow 5 (tartrazine) which may cause allergic-type reactions (including bronchial asthma) in certain susceptible individuals. Although the overall incidence of FD&C Yellow 5 (tartrazine) sensitivity in the general population is low, it is frequently seen in patients who also have aspirin hypersensitivity.

INFORMATION FOR PATIENTS

To assure the safe and effective use of Serax (oxazepam), patients should be informed that, since benzodiazepines may produce psychological and physical dependence, it is advisable that they consult with their physician before either increasing the dose or abruptly discontinuing this drug.

PEDIATRIC USE

Safety and effectiveness in pediatric patients under 6 years of age have not been established. Absolute dosage for pediatric patients 6 to 12 years of age is not established.

ADVERSE REACTIONS

The necessity for discontinuation of therapy due to undesirable effects has been rare. Transient, mild drowsiness is commonly seen in the first few days of therapy. If it persists, the dosage should be reduced. In few instances, dizziness, vertigo, headache, and rarely syncope have occurred either alone or together with drowsiness. Mild paradoxical reactions, *i.e.,* excitement, stimulation of affect, have been reported in psychiatric patients; these reactions may be secondary to relief of anxiety and usually appear in the first two weeks of therapy.

Other side effects occurring during oxazepam therapy include rare instances of nausea, lethargy, edema, slurred speech, tremor, altered libido and minor diffuse skin rashes—morbilliform, urticarial, and maculopapular. Such side effects have been infrequent and are generally controlled with reduction of dosage. A case of an extensive fixed drug eruption also has been reported.

Although rare, leukopenia and hepatic dysfunction including jaundice have been reported during therapy. Periodic blood counts and liver-function tests are advisable.

Ataxia with oxazepam has been reported in rare instances and does not appear to be specifically related to dose or age. Although the following side reactions have not as yet been reported with oxazepam, they have occurred with related compounds (chlordiazepoxide and diazepam): paradoxical excitation with severe rage reactions, hallucinations, menstrual irregularities, change in EEG pattern, blood dyscrasias including agranulocytosis, blurred vision, diplopia, incontinence, stupor, disorientation, fever, and euphoria.

Transient amnesia or memory impairment has been reported in association with the use of benzodiazepines.

Overdosage

In the management of overdosage with any drug, it should be borne in mind that multiple agents may have been taken.

SYMPTOMS

Overdosage of benzodiazepines is usually manifested by varying degrees of central nervous system depression ranging from drowsiness to coma. In mild cases, symptoms include drowsiness, mental confusion and lethargy. In more serious cases, and especially when other drugs or alcohol were ingested, symptoms may include ataxia, hypotonia, hypotension, hypnotic state, stage one (1) to three (3) coma, and very rarely, death.

MANAGEMENT

Induced vomiting and/or gastric lavage should be undertaken, followed by general supportive care, monitoring of vital signs, and close observation of the patient. Hypotension, though unlikely, usually may be controlled with norepinephrine bitartrate injection. The value of dialysis has not been adequately determined for oxazepam.

The benzodiazepine antagonist flumazenil may be used in hospitalized patients as an adjunct to, not as a substitute for, proper management of benzodiazepine overdose. **The prescriber should be aware of a risk of seizure in association with flumazenil treatment, particularly in long-term benzodiazepine users and in cyclic antidepressant overdose.** The complete flumazenil package insert including **"Contraindications," "Warnings,"** and **"Precautions"** should be consulted prior to use.

DOSAGE AND ADMINISTRATION

Because of the flexibility of this product and the range of emotional disturbances responsive to it, dosage should be individualized for maximum beneficial effects.

[See table below]

This product is not indicated in pediatric patients under 6 years of age. Absolute dosage for pediatric patients 6 to 12 years of age is not established.

HOW SUPPLIED

Serax® (oxazepam) Capsules and Tablets are available in the following dosage strengths:

10 mg, NDC 0008-0051, white and pink capsule banded with Wyeth logo and marked "SERAX", "10", and "51", in bottles of 100 and 500 capsules.

15 mg, NDC 0008-0006, white and red capsule banded with Wyeth logo and marked "SERAX", "15", and "6", in bottles of 100 and 500 capsules.

30 mg, NDC 0008-0052, white and maroon capsule banded with Wyeth logo and marked "SERAX", "30", and "52", in bottles of 100 and 500 capsules.

15 mg, NDC 0008-0317, yellow, five-sided tablet with a raised "S" and a "15" on one side and "WYETH" and "317" on reverse side, in bottles of 100 tablets.

The appearance of SERAX capsules and tablets is a trademark of Wyeth-Ayerst Laboratories.

Store at room temperature, approximately 25°C (77°F).
Keep tightly closed.
Dispense in tight container.

REFERENCE

1. FOX, KA.; LAHCEN, R.B.: Liver-cell Adenomas and Peliosis Hepatis in Mice Associated with Oxazepam. Res. Commun. Chem. Pathol. Pharmacol. *8* :481–488, 1974.

Manufactured by:
Wyeth Laboratories Inc.
A Wyeth-Ayerst Company
Philadelphia, PA 19101

Shown in Product Identification Guide, page 345

SERAX (oxazepam)
USUAL DOSE

Mild-to-moderate anxiety, with associated tension, irritability, agitation, or related symptoms of functional origin or secondary to organic disease.	10 to 15 mg, 3 or 4 times daily
Severe anxiety syndromes, agitation, or anxiety associated with depression.	15 to 30 mg, 3 or 4 times daily
Older patients with anxiety, tension, irritability, and agitation.	Initial dosage: 10 mg, 3 times daily. If necessary, increase cautiously to 15 mg, 3 or 4 times daily
Alcoholics with acute inebriation, tremulousness, or anxiety on withdrawal.	15 to 30 mg, 3 or 4 times daily

SURMONTIL® ℞

[*sĭr 'mŏn "tĭll*]
(trimipramine maleate)

DESCRIPTION

Surmontil (trimipramine maleate) is 5-(3-dimethylamino-2-methylpropyl)-10,11-dihydro-5H-dibenz (b,f) azepine acid maleate (racemic form).

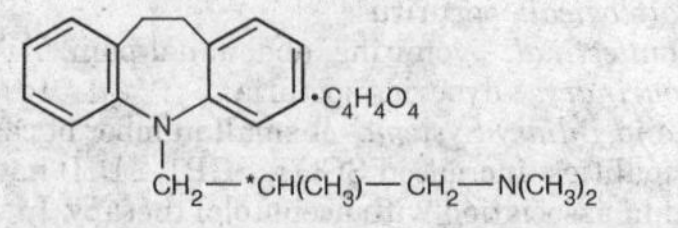

MOLECULAR FORMULA: $C_{20}H_{26}N_2 \cdot C_4H_4O_4$

MOLECULAR WEIGHT: 410.5

Surmontil capsules contain trimipramine maleate equivalent to 25 mg, 50 mg, or 100 mg of trimipramine as the base. The inactive ingredients present are FD&C Blue 1, gelatin, lactose, magnesium stearate, and titanium dioxide. The 25 mg dosage strength also contains D&C Yellow 10 and FD&C Yellow 6; the 50 mg dosage strength also contains D&C Red 28, FD&C Red 40, and FD&C Yellow 6.

Trimipramine maleate is prepared as a racemic mixture which can be resolved into levorotatory and dextrorotatory isomers. The asymmetric center responsible for optical isomerism is marked in the formula by an asterisk. Trimipramine maleate is an almost odorless, white or slightly cream-colored, crystalline substance, melting at 140–144°C. It is very slightly soluble in ether and water, is slightly soluble in ethyl alcohol and acetone, and freely soluble in chloroform and methanol at 20°C.

CLINICAL PHARMACOLOGY

Surmontil is an antidepressant with an anxiety-reducing sedative component to its action. The mode of action of Surmontil on the central nervous system is not known. However, unlike amphetamine-type compounds it does not act primarily by stimulation of the central nervous system. It does not act by inhibition of the monoamine oxidase system.

INDICATIONS AND USAGE

Surmontil is indicated for the relief of symptoms of depression. Endogenous depression is more likely to be alleviated than other depressive states. In studies with neurotic outpatients, the drug appeared to be equivalent to amitriptyline in the less-depressed patients but somewhat less effective than amitriptyline in the more severely depressed patients. In hospitalized depressed patients, trimipramine and imipramine were equally effective in relieving depression.

CONTRAINDICATIONS

Surmontil is contraindicated in cases of known hypersensitivity to the drug. The possibility of cross-sensitivity to other dibenzazepine compounds should be kept in mind. Surmontil should not be given in conjunction with drugs of the monoamine oxidase inhibitor class (e.g., tranylcypromine, isocarboxazid or phenelzine sulfate). The concomitant use of monoamine oxidase inhibitors (MAOI) and tricyclic compounds similar to Surmontil has caused severe hyperpyretic reactions, convulsive crises, and death in some patients. At least two weeks should elapse after cessation of therapy with MAOI before instituting therapy with Surmontil. Initial dosage should be low and increased gradually with caution and careful observation of the patient. The drug is contraindicated during the acute recovery period after a myocardial infarction.

WARNINGS

GENERAL CONSIDERATION FOR USE

Extreme caution should be used when this drug is given to patients with any evidence of cardiovascular disease because of the possibility of conduction defects, arrhythmias, myocardial infarction, strokes, and tachycardia.

Caution is advised in patients with increased intraocular pressure, history of urinary retention, or history of narrow-angle glaucoma because of the drug's anticholinergic properties; hyperthyroid patients or those on thyroid medication because of the possibility of cardiovascular toxicity; patients with a history of seizure disorder, because this drug has been shown to lower the seizure threshold; patients receiving guanethidine or similar agents, since Surmontil may block the pharmacologic effects of these drugs.

Since the drug may impair the mental and/or physical abilities required for the performance of potentially hazardous tasks, such as operating an automobile or machinery, the patient should be cautioned accordingly.

PRECAUTIONS

GENERAL

The possibility of suicide is inherent in any severely depressed patient and persists until a significant remission occurs. When a patient with a serious suicidal potential is not hospitalized, the prescription should be for the smallest amount feasible.

In schizophrenic patients activation of the psychosis may occur and require reduction of dosage or the addition of a major tranquilizer to the therapeutic regime.

Manic or hypomanic episodes may occur in some patients, in particular those with cyclic-type disorders. In some cases therapy with Surmontil must be discontinued until the episode is relieved, after which therapy may be reinstituted at lower dosages if still required.

Concurrent administration of Surmontil and electroshock therapy may increase the hazards of therapy. Such treatment should be limited to those patients for whom it is essential. When possible, discontinue the drug for several days prior to elective surgery.

Surmontil should be used with caution in patients with impaired liver function.

Chronic animal studies showed occasional occurrence of hepatic congestion, fatty infiltration, or increased serum liver enzymes at the highest dose of 60 mg/kg/day.

Both elevation and lowering of blood sugar have been reported with tricyclic antidepressants.

DRUG INTERACTIONS

Cimetidine

There is evidence that cimetidine inhibits the elimination of tricyclic antidepressants. Downward adjustment of Surmontil dosage may be required if cimetidine therapy is initiated; upward adjustment if cimetidine therapy is discontinued.

Alcohol

Patients should be warned that the concomitant use of alcoholic beverages may be associated with exaggerated effects.

Catecholamines/Anticholinergics

It has been reported that tricyclic antidepressants can potentiate the effects of catecholamines. Similarly, atropine-like effects may be more pronounced in patients receiving anticholinergic therapy. Therefore, particular care should be exercised when it is necessary to administer tricyclic antidepressants with sympathomimetic amines, local decongestants, local anesthetics containing epinephrine, atropine or drugs with an anticholinergic effect. In resistant cases of depression in adults, a dose of 2.5 mg/kg/day may have to be exceeded. If a higher dose is needed, ECG monitoring should be maintained during the initiation of therapy and at appropriate intervals during stabilization of dose.

Drugs Metabolized by P450 2D6

The biochemical activity of the drug metabolizing isozyme cytochrome P450 2D6 (debrisoquin hydroxylase) is reduced in a subset of the caucasian population (about 7–10% of caucasians are so called "poor metabolizers"); reliable estimates of the prevalence of reduced P450 2D6 isozyme activity among Asian, African, and other populations are not yet available. Poor metabolizers have higher than expected plasma concentrations of tricyclic antidepressants (TCAs) when given usual doses. Depending on the fraction of drug metabolized by P450 2D6, the increase in plasma concentration may be small, or quite large (8 fold increase in plasma AUC of the TCA).

In addition, certain drugs inhibit the activity of this isozyme and make normal metabolizers resemble poor metabolizers. An individual who is stable on a given dose of TCA may become abruptly toxic when given one of these inhibiting drugs as concomitant therapy. The drugs that inhibit cytochrome P450 2D6 include some that are not metabolized by the enzyme (quinidine; cimetidine) and many that are substrates for P450 2D6 (many other antidepressants, phenothiazines, and the Type 1C antiarrhythmics propafenone and flecainide). While all the selective serotonin reuptake inhibitors (SSRIs), e.g., fluoxetine, sertraline, and paroxetine, inhibit P450 2D6, they may vary in the extent of inhibition. The extent to which SSRI TCA interactions may pose clinical problems will depend on the degree of inhibition and the pharmacokinetics of the SSRI involved. Nevertheless, caution is indicated in the co-administration of TCAs with any of the SSRIs and also in switching from one class to the other. Of particular importance, sufficient time must elapse before initiating TCA treatment in a patient being withdrawn from fluoxetine, given the long half-life of the parent and active metabolite (at least 5 weeks may be necessary).

Concomitant use of tricyclic antidepressants with drugs that can inhibit cytochrome P450 2D6 may require lower doses than usually prescribed for either the tricyclic antidepressant or the other drug.

Furthermore, whenever one of these other drugs is withdrawn from co-therapy, an increased dose of tricyclic antidepressant may be required. It is desirable to monitor TCA plasma levels whenever a TCA is going to be co-administered with another drug known to be an inhibitor of P450 2D6.

CARCINOGENESIS, MUTAGENESIS, IMPAIRMENT OF FERTILITY

Semen studies in man (four schizophrenics and nine normal volunteers) revealed no significant changes in sperm morphology. It is recognized that drugs having a parasympathetic effect, including tricyclic antidepressants, may alter the ejaculatory response.

Chronic animal studies showed occasional evidence of degeneration of seminiferous tubules at the highest dose of 60 mg/kg/day.

PREGNANCY

Teratogenic Effects—Pregnancy Category C

Surmontil has shown evidence of embryo-toxicity and/or increased incidence of major anomalies in rats or rabbits at doses 20 times the human dose. There are no adequate and well-controlled studies in pregnant women. Surmontil® should be used during pregnancy only if the potential benefit justifies the potential risk to the fetus.

PEDIATRIC USE

This drug is not recommended for use in children, since safety and effectiveness in the pediatric age group have not been established.

ADVERSE REACTIONS

Note: The pharmacological similarities among the tricyclic antidepressants require that each of the reactions be considered when Surmontil is administered. Some of the adverse reactions included in this listing have not in fact been reported with Surmontil.

CARDIOVASCULAR

Hypotension, hypertension, tachycardia, palpitation, myocardial infarction, arrhythmias, heart block, stroke.

PSYCHIATRIC

Confusional states (especially the elderly) with hallucinations, disorientation, delusions; anxiety, restlessness, agitation; insomnia and nightmares; hypomania; exacerbation of psychosis.

NEUROLOGICAL

Numbness, tingling, paresthesias of extremities; incoordination, ataxia, tremors; peripheral neuropathy; extrapyramidal symptoms; seizures, alterations in EEG patterns; tinnitus; syndrome of inappropriate ADH (antidiuretic hormone) secretion.

ANTICHOLINERGIC

Dry mouth and, rarely, associated sublingual adenitis; blurred vision, disturbances of accommodation, mydriasis, constipation, paralytic ileus; urinary retention, delayed micturition, dilation of the urinary tract.

ALLERGIC

Skin rash, petechiae, urticaria, itching, photosensitization, edema of face and tongue.

HEMATOLOGIC

Bone-marrow depression including agranulocytosis, eosinophilia; purpura; thrombocytopenia. Leukocyte and differential counts should be performed in any patient who develops fever and sore throat during therapy; the drug should be discontinued if there is evidence of pathological neutrophil depression.

GASTROINTESTINAL

Nausea and vomiting, anorexia, epigastric distress, diarrhea, peculiar taste, stomatitis, abdominal cramps, black tongue.

ENDOCRINE

Gynecomastia in the male; breast enlargement and galactorrhea in the female; increased or decreased libido, impotence; testicular swelling; elevation or depression of blood-sugar levels.

OTHER

Jaundice (simulating obstructive); altered liver function; weight gain or loss; perspiration; flushing; urinary frequency; drowsiness, dizziness, weakness, and fatigue; headache; parotid swelling; alopecia.

WITHDRAWAL SYMPTOMS

Though not indicative of addiction, abrupt cessation of treatment after prolonged therapy may produce nausea, headache, and malaise.

DOSAGE AND ADMINISTRATION

Dosage should be initiated at a low level and increased gradually, noting carefully the clinical response and any evidence of intolerance.

Lower dosages are recommended for elderly patients and adolescents. Lower dosages are also recommended for outpatients as compared to hospitalized patients who will be under close supervision. It is not possible to prescribe a single dosage schedule of Surmontil that will be therapeutically effective in all patients. The physical psychodynamic factors contributing to depressive symptomatology are very complex; spontaneous remissions or exacerbations of depressive symptoms may occur with or without drug therapy. Consequently, the recommended dosage regimens are furnished as a guide which may be modified by factors such as the age of the patient, chronicity and severity of the disease, medical condition of the patient, and degree of psychotherapeutic support.

Most antidepressant drugs have a lag period of ten days to four weeks before a therapeutic response is noted. Increasing the dose will not shorten this period but rather increase the incidence of adverse reactions.

USUAL ADULT DOSE

Outpatients and Office Patients—Initially, 75 mg/day in divided doses, increased to 150 mg/day. Dosages over 200 mg/day are not recommended. Maintenance therapy is in the range of 50 to 150 mg/day. For convenient therapy and to facilitate patient compliance, the total dosage requirement may be given at bedtime.

Hospitalized Patients—Initially, 100 mg/day in divided doses. This may be increased gradually in a few days to 200 mg/day, depending upon individual response and tolerance. If improvement does not occur in 2 to 3 weeks, the dose may be increased to the maximum recommended dose of 250 to 300 mg/day.

Adolescent and Geriatric Patients—Initially, a dose of 50 mg/day is recommended, with gradual increments up to 100 mg/day, depending upon patient response and tolerance.

Maintenance—Following remission, maintenance medication may be required for a longer period of time, at the lowest dose that will maintain remission. Maintenance therapy is preferably administered as a single dose at bedtime. To minimize relapse, maintenance therapy should be continued for about three months.

OVERDOSAGE*

Deaths may occur from overdosage with this class of drugs. Multiple drug ingestion (including alcohol) is common in deliberate tricyclic antidepressant overdose. As the management is complex and changing, it is recommended that the physician contact a poison control center for current information on treatment. Signs and symptoms of toxicity develop rapidly after tricyclic antidepressant overdose, therefore, hospital monitoring is required as soon as possible.

MANIFESTATIONS

Critical manifestations of overdose include: cardiac dysrhythmias, severe hypotension, convulsions, and CNS depression, including coma. Changes in the electrocardiogram, particularly in QRS axis or width, are clinically significant indicators of tricyclic antidepressant toxicity.

Other signs of overdose may include: confusion, disturbed concentration, transient visual hallucinations, dilated pupils, agitation, hyperactive reflexes, stupor, drowsiness, muscle rigidity, vomiting, hypothermia, hyperpyrexia, or any of the symptoms listed under **Adverse Reactions**.

MANAGEMENT

General

Obtain an ECG and immediately initiate cardiac monitoring. Protect the patient's airway, establish an intravenous line and initiate gastric decontamination. A minimum of six hours of observation with cardiac monitoring and observation for signs of CNS or respiratory depression, hypotension, cardiac dysrhythmias and/or conduction blocks, and seizures is necessary. If signs of toxicity occur at any time during this period, extended monitoring is required. There are case reports of patients succumbing to fatal dysrhythmias late after overdose; these patients had clinical evidence of significant poisoning prior to death and most received inadequate gastrointestinal decontamination. Plasma drug levels may not reflect the severity of the poisoning. Therefore, monitoring of plasma drug levels alone should not guide management of the patient.

Gastrointestinal Decontamination

All patients suspected of tricyclic antidepressant overdose should receive gastrointestinal decontamination. This should include large volume gastric lavage followed by activated charcoal. If consciousness is impaired, the airway should be secured prior to lavage. Emesis is contraindicated.

Cardiovascular

A maximal limb-lead QRS duration of ≥0.10 seconds has been associated with an increased incidence of seizures. A QRS duration of ≥0.16 seconds has been associated with an increased incidence of ventricular dysrhythmias. Intravenous sodium bicarbonate should be used to maintain the serum pH in the range of 7.45 to 7.55. If the pH response is inadequate, hyperventilation may also be used. Concomitant use of hyperventilation and sodium bicarbonate should be done with extreme caution, with frequent pH monitoring. A pH >7.60 or a pCO₂ <20 mm Hg is undesirable. Dysrhythmias unresponsive to sodium bicarbonate therapy/hyperventilation may respond to lidocaine, bretylium or phenytoin. Type 1A and 1C antiarrhythmics are generally contraindicated (e.g., quinidine, disopyramide, and procainamide). In rare instances, hemoperfusion may be beneficial in acute refractory cardiovascular instability in patients with acute toxicity. However, hemodialysis, peritoneal dialysis, exchange transfusions, and forced diuresis generally have been reported as ineffective in tricyclic antidepressant poisoning.

CNS

In patients with CNS depression, early intubation is advised because of the potential for abrupt deterioration. Seizures should be controlled with benzodiazepines, or if these are ineffective, other anticonvulsants (e.g., phenobarbital, phenytoin). Physostigmine is not recommended except to treat life-threatening symptoms that have been unresponsive to other therapies, and then only in consultation with a poison control center.

Continued on next page

Surmontil—Cont.

Psychiatric Follow-up
Since overdosage is often deliberate, patients may attempt suicide by other means during the recovery phase. Psychiatric referral may be appropriate.

Pediatric Management
The principles of management of child and adult overdosages are similar. It is strongly recommended that the physician contact the local poison control center for specific pediatric treatment.

Poisindex® Toxicologic Management. Topic: Antidepressants, Tricyclic Micromedex Inc. Vol.85.

HOW SUPPLIED
Surmontil® (trimipramine maleate) Capsules are available in the following dosage strengths:
25 mg, NDC 0008-4132, opaque blue and yellow capsule marked "WYETH" and "4132", in bottles of 100 capsules.
50 mg, NDC 0008-4133, opaque blue and orange capsule marked "WYETH" and "4133", in bottles of 100 capsules.
100 mg, NDC 0008-4158, opaque blue and white capsule marked "WYETH" and "4158", in bottles of 100 capsules.
Store at room temperature, approximately 25°C (77°F).
Keep bottles tightly closed.
Dispense in tight container.
Protect capsules packaged in blister strips from moisture.
The appearance of these capsules is a trademark of Wyeth-Ayerst Laboratories.
by arrangement with Rhone-Poulenc Rorer France
Manufactured by:
Wyeth Laboratories Inc.
A Wyeth-Ayerst Company
Philadelphia, PA 19101
Shown in Product Identification Guide, page 345

SYNALGOS®-DC   ⓒ ℞
[sĭn 'al "gōs]
Capsules

DESCRIPTION
Each Synalgos-DC capsule contains 16 mg drocode (dihydrocodeine) bitartrate (Warning—may be habit-forming), 356.4 mg aspirin, and 30 mg caffeine.
The inactive ingredients present are alginic acid, cellulose, D&C Red 28, FD&C Blue 1, gelatin, iron oxides, stearic acid, and titanium dioxide.

HOW SUPPLIED
Synalgos®-DC Capsules are supplied in bottles of 100 and 500 capsules as follows:
NDC 0008-4191, blue and gray capsule marked "WYETH" and "4191".
Store at room temperature (approximately 25°C).
Keep tightly closed.
Dispense in tight container.
Manufactured by:
Wyeth Laboratories Inc.
A Wyeth-Ayerst Company
Philadelphia, PA 19101
For prescribing information write to Professional Service, Wyeth-Ayerst Laboratories, P.O. Box 8299, Philadelphia, PA 19101, or contact your local Wyeth-Ayerst representative.

SYNVISC®   ℞
[sĭn' vĭsk]
(Hylan G-F 20)

Caution: Federal law restricts this device to sale by or on the order of a physician (or properly licensed practitioner).

DESCRIPTION
Synvisc (hylan G-F 20) is an elastoviscous fluid containing hylan polymers produced from chicken combs. Hylans are derivatives of hyaluronan (sodium hyaluronate), a natural complex sugar of the glycosamino-glycan family. Hyaluronan is a long-chain polymer containing repeating disaccharide units of Na-glucuronate-N-acetylglucosamine.

INDICATIONS
Synvisc is indicated for the treatment of pain in osteoarthritis (OA) of the knee in patients who have failed to respond adequately to conservative nonpharmacologic therapy and simple analgesics, e.g., acetaminophen.

CONTRAINDICATIONS
- Do not administer to patients with known hypersensitivity (allergy) to hyaluronan (sodium hyaluronate) preparations.
- Do not inject Synvisc in the knees of patients having knee joint infections or skin diseases or infections in the area of the injection site.

WARNINGS
- Do not concomitantly use disinfectants containing quaternary ammonium salts for skin preparation because hyaluronan can precipitate in their presence.

TABLE 1
DEMOGRAPHIC DATA[1]

	DEMOGRAPHIC VARIABLE			
	Age	Gender [N[2] (%)]		Duration of Osteoarthritis (years)
		M	F	
German Multicenter[3]				
Synvisc®	62.3	21 (45%)	26 (55%)	5.4
Saline	64.7	13 (25%)	39 (75%)	5.6
P (Synvisc/Saline)	0.3	0.04		0.9
German Single Center				
Synvisc	59.8	10 (71%)	4 (29%)	2.4
Saline	59.5	8 (53%)	7 (47%)	2.5
P (Synvisc/Saline)	0.9	0.3		1.0
U.S. Multicenter[4]				
Synvisc	62.9	17 (39%)	27 (61%)	8.9
Arthrocentesis	67.1	12 (29%)	30 (71%)	7.9
P (Synvisc/Arthrocentesis)	0.06	0.3		0.5

Footnotes:
[1] Patients ≥40 years old and received the complete treatment course
[2] N = number of patients
[3] In addition, 1 male and 3 females were treated with Synvisc in one knee and saline in the other
[4] In addition, 4 females were treated with Synvisc in one knee and arthrocentesis in the other

TABLE 2
CONCURRENT OSTEOARTHRITIS THERAPIES[1]

CONCURRENT MEDICATIONS[2]	TREATED KNEES			p Synvisc/ Control
	TOTAL	Synvisc	Control	
German Multicenter	N[3]=109	N=52	N=57	
Medications [N (%)][4]	27 (25%)	5 (10%)	22 (39%)	0.001
NSAIDS	17 (16%)	4 (8%)	13 (23%)	0.03
Acetaminophen	7 (6%)	1 (2%)	6 (11%)	0.07
Other medications[5]	3 (3%)	3 (5%)	0 (0%)	0.09
German Single Center[6]	N=29	N=14	N=15	
Any concurrent medication [N (%)]	NA[7]	NA	NA	NA
U.S. Multicenter[8]	N=103	N=51	N=52	
Acetaminophen [N (%)]	100 (97%)	50 (98%)	50 (96%)	0.6

Footnotes:
[1] Patients ≥40 years old and received the complete treatment course
[2] Individual patients may be represented by more than one therapy
[3] N=number of knees
[4] Number and percentage of subjects
[5] Medications not approved in the U.S.
[6] No concurrent therapies were recorded
[7] Data not collected
[8] Only acetaminophen was allowed

- Do not inject Synvisc extra-articularly or into the synovial tissues and capsule. One such systemic adverse event occurred following extra-articular injections of Synvisc in clinical use outside the U.S.
- Intravascular injections of Synvisc may cause systemic adverse events.

PRECAUTIONS
General
- The effectiveness of a single treatment cycle of less than three injections of Synvisc has not been established.
- The safety and effectiveness of Synvisc in locations other than the knee and for conditions other than osteoarthritis have not been established.
- Do not inject anesthetics or other medications into the knee joint during Synvisc therapy. Such medications may dilute Synvisc and affect its safety and effectiveness.
- Use caution when injecting Synvisc into patients who are allergic to avian proteins, feathers, and egg products.
- The safety and effectiveness of Synvisc in severely inflamed knee joints have not been established.
- Strict aseptic administration technique must be followed.
- STERILE CONTENTS. The syringe is intended for single use. The contents of the syringe must be used immediately after its packaging is opened. Discard any unused Synvisc.

- Do not use Synvisc if package is opened or damaged. Store in original packaging (protected from light) at room temperature below 86°F (30°C). DO NOT FREEZE.
- Remove synovial fluid or effusion, if present, before injecting Synvisc.
- Synvisc should be used with caution when there is evidence of lymphatic or venous stasis in that leg.

Information for Patients
- Provide patients with a copy of the Patient Labeling prior to use.
- Transient pain and/or swelling of the injected joint may occur after intra-articular injection of Synvisc.
- As with any invasive joint procedure, it is recommended that the patient avoid any strenuous activities or prolonged weight-bearing activities such as jogging or tennis following the intra-articular injection.
- The safety and effectiveness of repeat treatment cycles of Synvisc have not been established.

Use in Specific Populations
- **Pregnancy:** The safety and effectiveness of Synvisc have not been established in pregnant women.
- **Nursing mothers:** It is not known if Synvisc is excreted in human milk. The safety and effectiveness of Synvisc have not been established in lactating women.
- The safety and effectiveness of Synvisc have not been established in children.

TABLE 3A
EFFECTIVENESS OF WEIGHT-BEARING PAIN[1]
EVALUATED BY PATIENTS

	Baseline	Improvement (Change from Baseline)					
Week	0	1	2	3	4	8	12
German Multicenter							
Synvisc-treated							
Mean[2]	69.7	12.0	26.5	37.9	NA[5]	45.9	46.5
p[3]		0.0001	0.0001	0.0001		0.0001	0.0001
Saline-treated							
Mean	75.1	9.0	17.0	23.0	NA	16.8	16.4
p[3]		0.0001	0.0001	0.0001		0.0001	0.0002
p[4]	0.1	0.3	0.01	0.0008	NA	<0.0001	<0.0001
German Single Center							
Synvisc-treated							
Mean	65.2	10.6	31.8	43.9	NA	51.7	53.5
p[3]		0.02	0.0001	0.0001		0.0001	0.0001
Saline-treated							
Mean	69.8	5.4	19.3	25.4	NA	24.4	26.8
p[3]		0.01	0.0001	0.0001		0.0001	0.0001
p[4]	0.4	0.2	0.03	0.01	NA	0.0001	0.0001
U.S. Multicenter							
Synvisc-treated							
Mean	67.3	12.9	18.9	NA	21.3	NA	NA
p[3]		0.0002	0.0001		0.0001		
Saline-treated							
Mean	69.4	9.4	21.2	NA	19.1	NA	NA
p[3]		0.01	0.0001		0.0002		
p[4]	0.6	0.5	0.7	NA	0.7	NA	NA

Footnotes:
1. Patients ≥40 years old and received the complete treatment course
2. Mean of assessments on VAS of 0 to 100 mm
3. Significance from baseline
4. Significance between Synvisc and control
5. NA =no measurement taken

TABLE 3B
EFFECTIVENESS OF NIGHT PAIN[1]
EVALUATED BY PATIENTS

	Baseline	Improvement (Change from Baseline)					
Week	0	1	2	3	4	8	12
German Multicenter							
Synvisc-treated							
Mean[2]	41.6	9.2	20.0	26.4	NA[5]	28.3	29.8
p[3]		0.0001	0.0001	0.0001		0.0001	0.0001
Saline-treated							
Mean	45.7	9.5	15.2	21.2	NA	18.4	17.3
p[3]		0.0001	0.0001	0.0001		0.0001	0.0001
p[4]	0.5	0.9	0.2	0.3	NA	0.05	0.02
German Single Center							
Synvisc-treated							
Mean	31.8	8.4	17.7	24.8	NA	28.9	29.5
p[3]		0.04	0.005	0.004		0.005	0.005
Saline-treated							
Mean	33.3	4.5	13.1	16.1	NA	16.1	17.9
p[3]		0.1	0.001	0.0007		0.0001	0.0001
p[4]	0.9	0.4	0.4	0.3	NA	0.1	0.2
U.S. Multicenter							
Synvisc-treated							
Mean	61.0	19.0	17.9	NA	22.8	NA	NA
p[3]		0.0001	0.0001		0.0001		
Saline-treated							
Mean	76.0	23.3	36.3	NA	29.8	NA	NA
p[3]		0.0001	0.0001		0.0001		
p[4]	0.002	0.5	0.004	NA	0.3	NA	NA

Footnotes:
1. Patients ≥40 years old and received the complete treatment course
2. Mean of assessments on VAS of 0 to 100 mm
3. Significance from baseline
4. Significance between Synvisc and control
5. NA =no measurement taken

ADVERSE EVENTS

A total of 511 patients (559 knees) received 1771 injections in seven clinical trials of Synvisc. There were 39 reports in 37 patients (2.2% of injections, 7.2% of patients) of knee pain and/or swelling after these injections.

Ten patients (10 knees) were treated with arthrocentesis and removal of joint effusion. Two additional patients (two knees) received treatment with intra-articular steroids. Two patients (two knees) received NSAIDs. One of these patients also received arthrocentesis. One patient was treated with arthroscopy. The remaining patients with adverse events localized to the knee received no treatment or only analgesics. Systemic adverse events each occurred in 10 (2.0%) of the Synvisc-treated patients. There was one case each of rash (thorax and back) and itching of the skin following Synvisc injections in these studies. These symptoms did not recur when these patients received additional Synvisc injections. The remaining generalized adverse events reported were calf cramps, hemorrhoid problems, ankle edema, muscle pain, tonsillitis with nausea, tachyarrhythmia, phlebitis with varicosities and low back sprain.

In three concurrently controlled clinical trials with a total of 112 patients who received Synvisc and 110 patients who received either saline or arthrocentesis, there were no statistically significant differences in the numbers or types of adverse events between the group of patients that received Synvisc and the group that received control treatments.

In clinical use in Canada (since 1992) and Sweden (since 1995), the most common adverse events reported have been pain, swelling, and/or effusion in the injected knees. Other adverse events reported were one case each of: generalized urticaria; recurring small hives; pain on one side of the body with nausea, anxiety and listlessness; facial flush with swelling of lips; nausea with dizziness; and shivering with headache, nausea, respiratory difficulties; and prickling in body which did not recur after subsequent Synvisc injections. No cases of anaphylaxis or anaphylactoid reactions have been reported. No deaths have been associated with the use of Synvisc. Intra-articular infections did not occur in any of the clinical trials, but have occurred in clinical use following Synvisc injections.

CLINICAL STUDIES

The safety and effectiveness of Synvisc was studied in patients ≥40 years old in the three concurrently controlled clinical trials referred to in the "Adverse Events" section. The three studies investigated a total of 136 women and 81 men. The demographics of trial participants were comparable across treatment groups with regard to age, gender, and duration of osteoarthritis, except that there were a significantly greater (p=0.04) number of men in the Synvisc group and women in the control group in one study (see Table 1). [See table 1 at top of previous page]

One study was a multicenter study, conducted at four sites, in Germany. It was a randomized, double-blind prospective clinical trial with two treatment groups. The study compared the safety and effectiveness of three weekly intra-articular injections of Synvisc and of physiological saline in 103 subjects (109 knees) with osteoarthritis of the knee.

A significantly greater number of saline-treated patients took concurrent osteoarthritis medications than did patients treated with Synvisc (See Table 2). While both the Synvisc and the saline-treated groups improved significantly as compared to baseline in all effectiveness measures, the Synvisc group showed a significantly greater improvement in all outcome measures than did the saline-treated patients over a twelve-week period (See Table 3). [See table 2 at top of previous page]

A second study conducted at a single-center in Germany was a concurrently controlled, randomized, double-blind prospective clinical trial with two treatment groups. This study compared the safety and effectiveness over a 12-week period of three weekly intra-articular injections of Synvisc and of physiological saline in 29 subjects (29 knees) with osteoarthritis of the knee. The results of the study were similar to those in the German multicenter study, except that the significance levels in most comparisons were smaller (See Tables 3A and 3B).

A third study was a prospective, concurrently controlled, randomized, double-blinded multicenter study conducted in 90 subjects (103 knees) at five U.S. sites. The study compared the safety and effectiveness of three weekly intra-articular injections of Synvisc and of three weekly arthrocenteses in subjects with osteoarthritis of the knee over a four-week period after the first injection or arthrocentesis. Both the Synvisc- and the saline-treated groups improved significantly as compared to baseline in all effectiveness measures. However, there were no significant differences between the Synvisc-treated and arthrocentesis-treated patients at any time during the four-week evaluation period (See Tables 3A and 3B above).

Covariate analyses with the covariates of center, presence or absence of previous treatments, baseline levels of outcome measures, age, gender, body mass, effusion, baseline X-ray score, duration of osteoarthritis, treatment of contralateral knee, and presence or absence of concurrent therapies, did not reveal any factors that significantly affected the results of any of the three studies.

The German studies and the U.S. study differed in several respects, including inclusion of patients with effusions, length of no treatment period prior to Synvisc injection, nature of control treatment, final evaluation time, mean dura-

Continued on next page

Synvisc—Cont.

tion of disease, mean weight, prior treatments for OA, and pain and X-ray inclusion criteria. Thus, German and the U.S. studies, which gave different results, investigated different patient populations and compared Synvisc with different control treatments.

Although success criteria for safety were not specified in any of the three studies, adverse events were enumerated in each study. These events are included in the "Adverse Events" section.

DETAILED DEVICE DESCRIPTION

Synvisc contains hylan A (average molecular weight 6,000,000) and hylan B hydrated gel in a buffered physiological sodium chloride solution, pH 7.2. Synvisc has an elasticity (storage modulus G') at 2.5 Hz of 111 ± 13 Pascals (Pa) and a viscosity (loss modulus G") of 25 ± 2 Pa (elasticity and viscosity of knee synovial fluid of 18–27 year old humans measured with a comparable method at 2.5 Hz: $G' = 117 \pm 13$ Pa; $G'' = 45 \pm 8$ Pa.)

Each syringe of Synvisc contains:

Hylan polymers (hylan A + hylan B)	16 mg
Sodium chloride	17 mg
Disodium hydrogen phosphate	0.32 mg
Sodium dihydrogen phosphate monohydrate	0.08 mg
Water for injection	q.s. to 2.0 mL

HOW SUPPLIED

Synvisc® is supplied in a 2.25 mL glass syringe containing 2 mL Synvisc.
Product Number: 0008-9149-02   3 disposable syringes
The contents of the syringe are sterile and nonpyrogenic.

DIRECTIONS FOR USE

Synvisc is administered by intra-articular injection once a week (one week apart) for a total of three injections.

Precaution: Do not use Synvisc if the package has been opened or damaged. Store in original packaging (protected from light) at room temperature below 86°F (30°C). DO NOT FREEZE.

Precaution: Strict aseptic administration technique must be followed.

Precaution: Do not concomitantly use disinfectants containing quaternary ammonium salts for skin preparation because hyaluronan can precipitate in their presence.

Precaution: Remove synovial fluid or effusion, if present, before injecting Synvisc.

Do not use the same syringe for removing synovial fluid and for injecting Synvisc, but the same needle should be used. Take particular care to remove the tip cap of the syringe and needle aseptically.

Inject Synvisc into the knee joint through an 18 to 22 gauge needle.

Do not inject anesthetics or any other medications intra-articularly into the knee while administering Synvisc therapy. This may dilute Synvisc and affect its safety and effectiveness.

Precaution: The syringe containing Synvisc is intended for single use. The contents of the syringe must be used immediately after the syringe has been removed from its packaging. Inject the full 2 mL in one knee only. If treatment is bilateral, a separate syringe must be used for each knee. Discard any unused Synvisc.

DISTRIBUTED BY:

Wyeth Laboratories Inc.
A Wyeth-Ayerst Company
Philadelphia, Pennsylvania 19101
Telephone: 1-800-99-WYETH
Fax: (610) 964-5999

DEVELOPED BY:

Biomatrix, Inc.
65 Railroad Avenue
Ridgefield, New Jersey 07657
Telephone: (201)945-9550
Fax: (201)945-0363

MANUFACTURED BY:

Biomatrix Medical Canada Inc.
275, avenue Labrosse
Pointe-Claire, Québec
Canada H9R 1A3

Covered by U.S. patents #4,636,524, #4,713,448, #5,099,013, #5,143,724.
Synvisc is a registered trademark of Biomatrix, Inc.

REFERENCE

Scale D, Wobig M, and Wolpert W: Viscosupplementation of osteoarthritic knees with hylan: a treatment schedule study. Curr Ther Res; 55:220-232, 1994.

TRECATOR®-SC   ℞

[trĕk " ă ' tōre]
(ethionamide tablets, USP)
Sugar-Coated Tablets

DESCRIPTION

Trecator-SC (ethionamide tablets, USP) is used in the treatment of tuberculosis. The chemical name for ethionamide is 2-ethylthioisonicotinamide with the following structural formula:

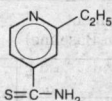

Ethionamide is a yellow crystalline, nonhygroscopic compound with a faint to moderate sulfide odor and a melting point of 162°C. It is practically insoluble in water and ether, but soluble in methanol and ethanol. It has a partition coefficient (octanol/water) Log P value of 0.3699.

Trecator-SC tablets contain 250 mg of ethionamide. The inactive ingredients present are lactose, methylcellulose, magnesium stearate, polacrilin potassium, pharmaceutical glaze, talc, gelatin, acacia, sucrose, calcium carbonate, confectioners sugar, FD&C Yellow #6, povidone, sodium benzoate, titanium dioxide, white wax, and carnauba wax.

CLINICAL PHARMACOLOGY

Ethionamide is essentially completely absorbed following oral administration and is not subjected to any appreciable first pass metabolism.[1] Following a single 250 mg oral dose of ethionamide in healthy volunteers, peak plasma concentrations of about 2 µg/mL were attained at 2 hours in most cases. Normal serum concentrations of 1 to 5 µg/mL are usually seen 2 hours following doses of 250 mg to 500 mg.[2] These concentrations approximate the therapeutic range for this drug when the therapeutic range is defined by those serum concentrations associated with a high probability of success and a low probability of dose-related toxicity. The drug is approximately 30 percent bound to plasma proteins. Trecator-SC is rapidly and widely distributed into body tissues and fluids, with concentrations in plasma and various organs being approximately equal. Significant concentrations also are present in cerebrospinal fluid.

Ethionamide is extensively metabolized to active and inactive metabolites with less than 1% excreted as the free form in urine. Metabolism is presumed to occur in the liver and thus far 6 metabolites have been isolated: 2-ethylisonicotinamide, carbamoyl-dihydropyridine, thiocarbamoyl-dihydropyridine, S-oxocarbamoyl dihydropyridine, 2-ethylthio-iso-nicotinamide, and ethionamide sulphoxide. The sulphoxide metabolite has been demonstrated to have antimicrobial activity against *Mycobacterium tuberculosis*. Trecator-SC has a plasma elimination half-life of approximately 2 hours after oral dosing.

Mechanism of Action

Ethionamide may be bacteriostatic or bactericidal in action, depending on the concentration of the drug attained at the site of infection and the susceptibility of the infecting organism. The exact mechanism of action of ethionamide has not been full elucidated, but the drug appears to inhibit peptide synthesis in susceptible organisms.

Microbiology

In Vitro Activity

Ethionamide exhibits bacteriostatic activity against extracellular and intracellular *Mycobacterium tuberculosis* organisms. The development of ethionamide resistant *M. tuberculosis* isolates can be obtained by repeated subculturing in liquid or on solid media containing increasing concentrations of ethionamide. Multi-drug resistant strains of *M. tuberculosis* may have acquired resistance to both isoniazid and ethionamide. However, the majority of *M. tuberculosis* isolates that are resistant to one are usually susceptible to the other. There is no evidence of cross-resistance between ethionamide and para-aminosalicylic acid (PAS), streptomycin, or cycloserine. However, limited data suggest that cross-resistance may exist between ethionamide and thiosemicarbazones (i.e., thiacetazone) as well as isoniazid.

In Vivo Activity

Ethionamide administered orally initially decreased the number of culturable *Mycobacterium tuberculosis* organisms from the lungs of H37Rv infected mice. Drug resistance developed with continued ethionamide monotherapy, but did not occur when mice received ethionamide in combination with streptomycin or isoniazid.

Susceptibility Testing

Ethionamide susceptibility testing should only be performed by qualified or reference laboratories.

Two standardized *in vitro* susceptibility methods are available for testing ethionamide against *M. tuberculosis* organisms. The modified proportion method (CDC or NCCLS M24-P) utilizes Middlebrook and Cohn 7H10 agar medium impregnated with ethionamide at a final concentration of 5.0 µg/mL. After 2 to 3 weeks of incubation, MIC_{99} values are calculated by comparing the quantity of organisms growing in the medium containing drug to the control cultures. Mycobacterial growth in the presence of drug, of at least 1% of the growth in the control culture, indicates resistance.

The radiometric broth method employs the BACTEC 460 machine to compare the growth index from untreated control cultures to cultures grown in the presence of 5.0 µg/mL of ethionamide. Strict adherence to the manufacturer's instructions for sample processing and data interpretation is required for this assay.

Susceptibility test results obtained by these two different methods cannot be compared unless equivalent drug concentrations are evaluated.

The clinical relevance of *in vitro* susceptibility test results for mycobacterial species other than *M. tuberculosis* using either the radiometric or the proportion method has not been determined.

INDICATIONS AND USAGE

Trecator-SC (ethionamide) is primarily indicated for the treatment of active tuberculosis in patients with *M. tuberculosis* resistant to isoniazid or rifampin, or when there is intolerance on the part of the patient to other drugs. Its use alone in the treatment of tuberculosis results in the rapid development of resistance. It is essential, therefore, to give a suitable companion drug or drugs, the choice being based on the results of susceptibility tests. If the susceptibility tests indicate that the patient's organism is resistant to one of the first-line antituberculosis drugs (i.e., isoniazid or rifampin) yet susceptible to ethionamide, ethionamide should be accompanied by at least one drug to which the *M. tuberculosis* is known to be susceptible.[6] If the tuberculosis is resistant to both isoniazid and rifampin, yet susceptible to ethionamide, ethionamide should be accompanied by at least two other drugs to which the *M. tuberculosis* isolate is known to be susceptible.[6]

Patient nonadherence to prescribed treatment can result in treatment failure and in the development of drug-resistant tuberculosis, which can be life-threatening and lead to other serious health risks. It is, therefore, essential that patients adhere to the drug regimen for the full duration of treatment. Directly observed therapy is recommended for all patients receiving treatment for tuberculosis. Patients in whom drug-resistant *M. tuberculosis* organisms are isolated should be managed in consultation with an expert in the treatment of drug-resistant tuberculosis.

CONTRAINDICATIONS

Ethionamide is contraindicated in patients with severe hepatic impairment and in patients who are hypersensitive to the drug.

WARNINGS

The use of Trecator-SC (ethionamide) alone in the treatment of tuberculosis results in rapid development of resistance. It is essential, therefore, to give a suitable companion drug or drugs, the choice being based on the results of susceptibility testing. However, therapy may be initiated prior to receiving the results of susceptibility tests as deemed appropriate by the physician. Ethionamide should be administered with at least one, sometimes two, other drugs to which the organism is known to be susceptible (see "**INDICATIONS AND USAGE**"). Drugs which have been used as companion agents are rifampin, ethambutol, pyrazinamide, cycloserine, kanamycin, streptomycin, and isoniazid. The usual warnings, precautions, and dosage regimens for these companion drugs should be observed.

Patient compliance is essential to the success of the antituberculosis therapy and to prevent the emergence of drug-resistant organisms. Therefore, patients should adhere to the drug regimen for the full duration of treatment. It is recommended that directly observed therapy be practiced when patients are receiving antituberculous medication. Additional consultation from experts in the treatment of drug-resistant tuberculosis is recommended when patients develop drug-resistant organisms.

PRECAUTIONS

General

Ethionamide may potentiate the adverse effects of the other anti-tuberculous drugs administered concomitantly (see "**Drug Interactions**"). Ophthalmologic examinations (including ophthalmoscopy) should be performed before and periodically during therapy with Trecator-SC.

Information For Patients

Patients should be advised to consult their physician should blurred vision or any loss of vision, with or without eye pain, occur during treatment.

Excessive ethanol ingestion should be avoided because a psychotic reaction has been reported.[3]

Laboratory Tests

Determination of serum transaminases (SGOT, SGPT) should be made prior to initiation of therapy and should be monitored monthly. If serum transaminases become elevated during therapy, ethionamide and the companion antituberculosis drug or drugs may be discontinued temporarily until the laboratory abnormalities have resolved. Ethionamide and the companion antituberculosis medication(s)

then should be reintroduced sequentially to determine which drug (or drugs) is (are) responsible for the hepatotoxicity.

Blood glucose determinations should be made prior to and periodically throughout therapy with Trecator®-SC. Diabetic patients should be particularly alert for episodes of hypoglycemia. Periodic monitoring of thyroid function tests is recommended as hypothyroidism, with or without goiter, has been reported with ethionamide therapy.

Drug Interactions

Trecator-SC has been found to temporarily raise serum concentrations of isoniazid. Trecator-SC may potentiate the adverse effects of other antituberculous drugs administered concomitantly. In particular, convulsions have been reported when ethionamide is administered with cycloserine and special care should be taken when the treatment regimen includes both of these drugs. Excessive ethanol ingestion should be avoided because a psychotic reaction has been reported.

Carcinogenesis, Mutagenesis, Impairment of Fertility
Teratogenic Effects: Pregnancy Category C

Animal studies conducted with Trecator (ethionamide) indicate that the drug has teratogenic potential in rabbits and rats. The doses used in these studies on a mg/kg basis were considerably in excess of those recommended in humans. There are no adequate and well-controlled studies in pregnant women. Because of these animal studies, however, it must be recommended that Trecator-SC (ethionamide) be withheld from women who are pregnant, or who are likely to become pregnant while under therapy, unless the prescribing physician considers it to be an essential part of the treatment.

Labor and Delivery

The effect of Trecator-SC on labor and delivery in pregnant women is unknown.

Nursing Mothers

Because no information is available on the excretion of ethionamide in human milk, Trecator-SC should be administered to nursing mothers only if the benefits outweigh the risks. Newborns who are breast-fed by mothers who are taking Trecator-SC should be monitored for adverse effects.

Pediatric Use

Due to the fact that pulmonary tuberculosis resistant to primary therapy is rarely found in neonates, infants, and children, investigations have been limited in these age groups. At present, the drug should not be used in pediatric patients under 12 years of age except when the organisms are definitely resistant to primary therapy and systemic dissemination of the disease, or other life-threatening complications of tuberculosis, is judged to be imminent.

ADVERSE REACTIONS

Gastrointestinal: The most common side effects of ethionamide are gastrointestinal disturbances including nausea, vomiting, diarrhea, abdominal pain, excessive salivation, metallic taste, stomatitis, anorexia and weight loss. Adverse gastrointestinal effects appear to be dose related, with approximately 50% of patients unable to tolerate 1 gm as a single dose. Gastrointestinal effects may be minimized by decreasing dosage, by changing the time of drug administration, or by the concurrent administration of an antiemetic agent.

Nervous System: Psychotic disturbances (including mental depression), drowsiness, dizziness, restlessness, headache, and postural hypotension have been reported with ethionamide. Rare reports of peripheral neuritis, optic neuritis, diplopia, blurred vision, and a pellagra-like syndrome also have been reported. Concurrent administration of pyridoxine has been recommended to prevent or relieve neurotoxic effects.

Hepatic: Transient increases in serum bilirubin, SGOT, SGPT; Hepatitis (with or without jaundice).

Other: Hypersensitivity reactions including rash, photosensitivity, thrombocytopenia and purpura have been reported rarely. Hypoglycemia, gynecomastia, impotence, and acne also have occurred. The management of patients with diabetes mellitus may become more difficult in those receiving ethionamide.

OVERDOSE

No specific information is available on the treatment of overdosage with Trecator-SC. If it should occur, standard procedures to evacuate gastric contents and to support vital functions should be employed.

DOSAGE AND ADMINISTRATION

In the treatment of tuberculosis, a major cause of the emergence of drug-resistant organisms, and thus treatment failure, is patient nonadherence to prescribed treatment. Treatment failure and drug-resistant organisms can be life-threatening and may result in other serious health risks. It is, therefore, important that patients adhere to the drug regimen for the full duration of treatment. Directly observed therapy is recommended when patients are receiving treatment for tuberculosis. Consultation with an expert in the treatment of drug-resistant tuberculosis is advised for patients in whom drug-resistant tuberculosis is suspected

or likely. Ethionamide should be administered with at least one, sometimes two, other drugs to which the organism is known to be susceptible (see **"INDICATIONS AND USAGE"**).

Trecator-SC (ethionamide) is administered orally. The usual adult dose is 15 to 20 mg/kg/day, administered once daily or, if patient exhibits poor gastrointestinal tolerance, in divided doses with a maximum daily dosage of 1 gram. Thus far, there is insufficient evidence to indicate the lowest effective dosage levels. Therefore, in order to minimize the risk of resistance developing to the drug or to the companion drug, the principle of giving the highest tolerated dose (based on gastrointestinal intolerance) has been followed. In the adult this would seem to be between 0.5 and 1.0 gm daily, with an average of 0.75 gm daily.

The optimum dosage for pediatric patients has not been established. However, pediatric dosages of 10 to 20 mg/kg p.o. daily in 2 or 3 divided doses given after meals or 15 mg/kg/24 hrs as a single daily dose have been recommended. [4,5] As with adults, ethionamide may be administered to pediatric patients once daily. It should be noted that in patients with concomitant tuberculosis and HIV infection, malabsorption syndrome may be present. Drug malabsorption should be suspected in patients who adhere to therapy, but who fail to respond appropriately. In such cases, consideration should be given to therapeutic drug monitoring (see **"CLINICAL PHARMACOLOGY"**).

The best times of administration are those which the individual patient finds most suitable in order to avoid or minimize gastrointestinal intolerance, which is usually at mealtimes. Every effort should be made to encourage patients to persevere with treatment when gastrointestinal side effects appear, since they may diminish in severity as treatment proceeds.

Initiation of therapy at a dose of 250 mg daily, with gradual titration to optimal doses as tolerated by the patient, also may be beneficial. A regimen of 250 mg daily for 1 or 2 days, followed by 250 mg twice daily for 1 or 2 days with a subsequent increase to 1 gm in 3 or 4 divided doses has been reported.[2]

Concomitant administration of pyridoxine is recommended. Duration of treatment should be based on individual clinical response. In general, continue therapy until bacteriological conversion has become permanent and maximal clinical improvement has occurred.

HOW SUPPLIED

Trecator®-SC (ethionamide tablets, USP) are supplied in bottles of 100 tablets as follows: 250 mg, NDC 0008-4130, reddish orange, sugar-coated tablet marked "WYETH" and "4130."

Store at room temperature, approximately 25°C (77°F). Dispense in a tight container.

REFERENCES

1) Jenner, P.J.: Plasma Levels of Ethionamide and Prothionamide in a Volunteer Following Intravenous and Oral Dosages, Lepr Rev 58:31–37, 1987.
2) Peloquin, C.A.: Pharmacology of the Antimycobacterial Drugs, Med Clin North Am 77(6):1253–1262, 1993.
3) Lansdown, F.S., Beran, M., Litwak, T.: Psychotoxic Reaction During Ethionamide Therapy, Am Rev Resp Dis 95(6):1053–1055, 1967.
4) Feigin, R.D., and Cherry, J.D.: Textbook of Pediatric Infectious Diseases, 2nd Edition. Philadelphia, W.B. Saunders Co., 1987, pp. 1371–1372.
5) Nelson, W.E., Behrman, R.E., Vaughan, V.C. (eds): Nelson Textbook of Pediatrics, 13th edition. Philadelphia, W.B. Saunders Co., 1987, p.636
6) Treatment of Tuberculosis and Tuberculosis Infection in Adults and Children, Am J Respiratory and Critical Care Medicine, 149:1359–1374. 1994.

Manufactured by:
Wyeth Laboratories Inc.
A Wyeth-Ayerst Company
Philadelphia, PA 19101

TRIPHASIL®–21   ℞
[tri-fa 'sil]
Tablets
(levonorgestrel and ethinyl estradiol tablets—triphasic regimen)

Patients should be counseled that this product does not protect against HIV infection (AIDS) and other sexually transmitted diseases.

DESCRIPTION

Each Triphasil cycle of 21 tablets consists of three different drug phases as follows: Phase 1 comprised of 6 brown tablets, each containing 0.050 mg of levonorgestrel (d(-)-13 beta-ethyl-17-alpha-ethinyl-17-beta-hydroxygon-4-en-3-one), a totally synthetic progestogen, and 0.030 mg of ethinyl estradiol (19-nor-17α-pregna-1,3,5(10)-trien -20- yne-3,17-diol); phase 2 comprised of 5 white tablets, each con-

taining 0.075 mg levonorgestrel and 0.040 mg ethinyl estradiol; and phase 3 comprised of 10 light-yellow tablets, each containing 0.125 mg levonorgestrel and 0.030 mg ethinyl estradiol. The inactive ingredients present are cellulose, iron oxides, lactose, magnesium stearate, polacrilin potassium, polyethylene glycol, titanium dioxide, and hydroxypropyl methylcellulose.

Levonorgestrel

Ethinyl Estradiol

CLINICAL PHARMACOLOGY

Combination oral contraceptives act by suppression of gonadotropins. Although the primary mechanism of this action is inhibition of ovulation, other alterations include changes in the cervical mucus (which increase the difficulty of sperm entry into the uterus) and the endometrium (which reduce the likelihood of implantation).

INDICATIONS AND USAGE

Oral contraceptives are indicated for the prevention of pregnancy in women who elect to use this product as a method of contraception.

Oral contraceptives are highly effective. Table I lists the typical accidental pregnancy rates for users of combination oral contraceptives and other methods of contraception. The efficacy of these contraceptive methods, except sterilization and the IUD, depends upon the reliability with which they are used. Correct and consistent use of methods can result in lower failure rates.

TABLE I
LOWEST EXPECTED AND TYPICAL FAILURE RATES
DURING THE FIRST YEAR OF CONTINUOUS USE OF
A METHOD

% of Women Experiencing an Accidental Pregnancy in the First Year of Continuous Use

Method	Lowest Expected*	Typical**
(No Contraception)	(85)	(85)
Oral contraceptives		3
combined	0.1	N/A***
progestin only	0.5	N/A***
Diaphragm with spermicidal cream or jelly	6	18
Spermicides alone (foams and vaginal suppositories)	3	21
Vaginal Sponge		
nulliparous	6	18
multiparous	9	28
DEPO-PROVERA® (injectable progestogen)	0.3	0.3
NORPLANT® SYSTEM (implants)	0.2#	0.2#
IUD		3
progesterone	2	N/A***
copper T 380A	0.8	N/A***
Condom without spermicides	2	12
Periodic abstinence (all methods)	1—9	20
Female sterilization	0.2	0.4
Male sterilization	0.1	0.15

Adapted from J. Trussell et al., Table 1, Studies in Family Planning, *21*(1): Jan.–Feb. 1990.

---

* The authors' best guess of the percentage of women expected to experience an accidental pregnancy among couples who initiate a method (not necessarily for the first time) and who use it consistently and correctly during the first year if they do not stop use for any other reason.

** This term represents "typical" couples who initiate use of a method (not necessarily for the first time), who experi-

Continued on next page

Triphasil-21—Cont.

ence an accidental pregnancy during the first year if they do not stop use for any other reason.
*** N/A—Data not available.
#This data is based on Norplant System clinical trials.

CONTRAINDICATIONS

Oral contraceptives should not be used in women with any of the following conditions:
Thrombophlebitis or thromboembolic disorders.
A past history of deep-vein thrombophlebitis or thromboembolic disorders.
Cerebral-vascular or coronary-artery disease.
Known or suspected carcinoma of the breast.
Carcinoma of the endometrium or other known or suspected estrogen-dependent neoplasia.
Undiagnosed abnormal genital bleeding.
Cholestatic jaundice of pregnancy or jaundice with prior pill use.
Hepatic adenomas or carcinomas.
Known or suspected pregnancy.

WARNINGS

Cigarette smoking increases the risk of serious cardiovascular side effects from oral-contraceptive use. This risk increases with age and with heavy smoking (15 or more cigarettes per day) and is quite marked in women over 35 years of age. Women who use oral contraceptives should be strongly advised not to smoke.

The use of oral contraceptives is associated with increased risks of several serious conditions including myocardial infarction, thromboembolism, stroke, hepatic neoplasia, gallbladder disease, and hypertension, although the risk of serious morbidity or mortality is very small in healthy women without underlying factors. The risk of morbidity and mortality increases significantly in the presence of other underlying risk factors such as hypertension, hyperlipidemias, obesity, and diabetes.
Practitioners prescribing oral contraceptives should be familiar with the following information relating to these risks.
The information contained in this package insert is based principally on studies carried out in patients who used oral contraceptives with higher formulations of estrogens and progestogens than those in common use today. The effect of long-term use of the oral contraceptives with lower formulations of both estrogens and progestogens remains to be determined.
Throughout this labeling, epidemiological studies reported are of two types: retrospective or case control studies and prospective or cohort studies. Case control studies provide a measure of the relative risk of disease, namely, a ratio of the incidence of a disease among oral-contraceptive users to that among nonusers. The relative risk does not provide information on the actual clinical occurrence of a disease. Cohort studies provide a measure of attributable risk, which is the difference in the incidence of disease between oral-contraceptive users and nonusers. The attributable risk does provide information about the actual occurrence of a disease in the population. For further information, the reader is referred to a text on epidemiological methods.

1. THROMBOEMBOLIC DISORDERS AND OTHER VASCULAR PROBLEMS

a. *Myocardial infarction*
An increased risk of myocardial infarction has been attributed to oral-contraceptive use. This risk is primarily in smokers or women with other underlying risk factors for coronary-artery disease such as hypertension, hypercholesterolemia, morbid obesity, and diabetes. The relative risk of heart attack for current oral-contraceptive users has been estimated to be two to six. The risk is very low under the age of 30.
Smoking in combination with oral-contraceptive use has been shown to contribute substantially to the incidence of myocardial infarctions in women in their mid-thirties or older with smoking accounting for the majority of excess cases. Mortality rates associated with circulatory disease have been shown to increase substantially in smokers over the age of 35 and nonsmokers over the age of 40 (Table II) among women who use oral contraceptives.
[See figure at top of next column]
Oral contraceptives may compound the effects of well-known risk factors, such as hypertension, diabetes, hyperlipidemias, age, and obesity. In particular, some progestogens are known to decrease HDL cholesterol and cause glucose intolerance, while estrogens may create a state of hyperinsulinism. Oral contraceptives have been shown to increase blood pressure among users (see section 9 in "Warnings"). Similar effects on risk factors have been associated with an increased risk of heart disease. Oral contraceptives must be used with caution in women with cardiovascular disease risk factors.

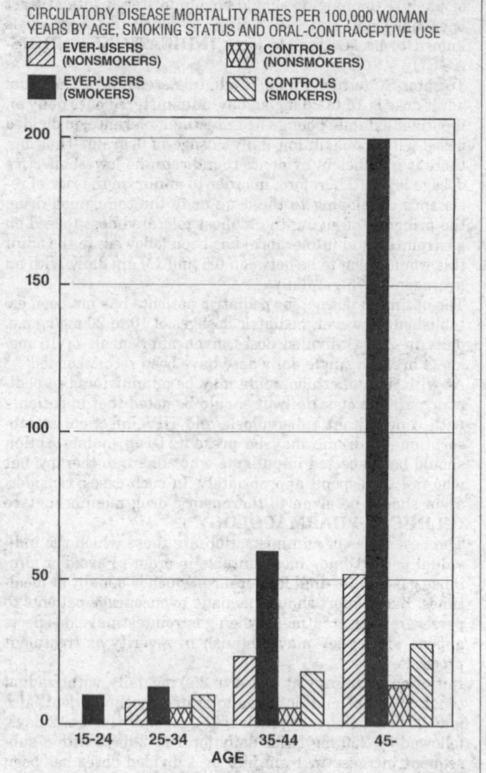
CIRCULATORY DISEASE MORTALITY RATES PER 100,000 WOMAN YEARS BY AGE, SMOKING STATUS AND ORAL-CONTRACEPTIVE USE
EVER-USERS (NONSMOKERS)
CONTROLS (NONSMOKERS)
EVER-USERS (SMOKERS)
CONTROLS (SMOKERS)
200
150
100
50
0
15-24
25-34
35-44
45-
AGE

TABLE II. (Adapted from P.M. Layde and V. Beral, Lancet, *1*:541–546, 1981.)

b. *Thromboembolism*
An increased risk of thromboembolic and thrombotic disease associated with the use of oral contraceptives is well established. Case control studies have found the relative risk of users compared to nonusers to be 3 for the first episode of superficial venous thrombosis, 4 to 11 for deep-vein thrombosis or pulmonary embolism, and 1.5 to 6 for women with predisposing conditions for venous thromboembolic disease. Cohort studies have shown the relative risk to be somewhat lower, about 3 for new cases and about 4.5 for new cases requiring hospitalization. The risk of thromboembolic disease due to oral contraceptives is not related to length of use and disappears after pill use is stopped.
A two- to four-fold increase in relative risk of postoperative thromboembolic complications has been reported with the use of oral contraceptives. The relative risk of venous thrombosis in women who have predisposing conditions is twice that of women without such medical conditions. If feasible, oral contraceptives should be discontinued at least four weeks prior to and for two weeks after elective surgery of a type associated with an increase in risk of thromboembolism and during and following prolonged immobilization. Since the immediate postpartum period is also associated with an increased risk of thromboembolism, oral contraceptives should be started no earlier than four to six weeks after delivery in women who elect not to breast-feed, or a midtrimester pregnancy termination.

c. *Cerebrovascular diseases*
Oral contraceptives have been shown to increase both the relative and attributable risks of cerebrovascular events (thrombotic and hemorrhagic strokes), although, in general, the risk is greatest among older (>35 years), hypertensive women who also smoke. Hypertension was found to be a risk factor for both users and nonusers, for both types of strokes, while smoking interacted to increase the risk for hemorrhagic strokes.
In a large study, the relative risk of thrombotic strokes has been shown to range from 3 for normotensive users to 14 for users with severe hypertension. The relative risk of hemorrhagic stroke is reported to be 1.2 for nonsmokers who used oral contraceptives, 2.6 for smokers who did not use oral contraceptives, 7.6 for smokers who used oral contraceptives, 1.8 for normotensive users, and 25.7 for users with severe hypertension. The attributable risk is also greater in older women.

d. *Dose-related risk of vascular disease from oral contraceptives*
A positive association has been observed between the amount of estrogen and progestogen in oral contraceptives and the risk of vascular disease. A decline in serum high-density lipoproteins (HDL) has been reported with many progestational agents. A decline in serum high-density lipoproteins has been associated with an increased incidence of ischemic heart disease. Because estrogens increase HDL cholesterol, the net effect of an oral contraceptive depends on a balance achieved between doses of estrogen and progestogen and the nature and absolute amount of progestogen used in the contraceptive. The amount of both hormones should be considered in the choice of an oral contraceptive.
Minimizing exposure to estrogen and progestogen is in keeping with good principles of therapeutics. For any particular estrogen/progestogen combination, the dosage regimen prescribed should be one which contains the least amount of estrogen and progestogen that is compatible with a low failure rate and the needs of the individual patient. New acceptors of oral-contraceptive agents should be started on preparations containing less than 50 mcg of estrogen.

e. *Persistence of risk of vascular disease*
There are two studies which have shown persistence of risk of vascular disease for ever-users of oral contraceptives. In a study in the United States, the risk of developing myocardial infarction after discontinuing oral contraceptives persists for at least 9 years for women 40 to 49 years who had used oral contraceptives for five or more years, but this increased risk was not demonstrated in other age groups. In another study in Great Britain, the risk of developing cerebrovascular disease persisted for at least 6 years after discontinuation of oral contraceptives, although excess risk was very small. However, both studies were performed with oral- contraceptive formulations containing 50 micrograms or higher of estrogens.

2. ESTIMATES OF MORTALITY FROM CONTRACEPTIVE USE

One study gathered data from a variety of sources which have estimated the mortality rate associated with different methods of contraception at different ages (Table III). These estimates include the combined risk of death associated with contraceptive methods plus the risk attributable to pregnancy in the event of method failure. Each method of contraception has its specific benefits and risks. The study concluded that with the exception of oral-contraceptive users 35 and older who smoke and 40 and older who do not smoke, mortality associated with all methods of birth control is less than that associated with childbirth. The observation of a possible increase in risk of mortality with age for oral-contraceptive users is based on data gathered in the 1970's—but not reported until 1983. However, current clinical practice involves the use of lower estrogen dose formulations combined with careful restriction of oral-contraceptive use to women who do not have the various risk factors listed in this labeling.
Because of these changes in practice and, also, because of some limited new data which suggest that the risk of cardiovascular disease with the use of oral contraceptives may now be less than previously observed, the Fertility and Maternal Health Drugs Advisory Committee was asked to review the topic in 1989. The Committee concluded that although cardiovascular-disease risks may be increased with oral-contraceptive use after age 40 in healthy nonsmoking women (even with the newer low-dose formulations), there are greater potential health risks associated with pregnancy in older women and with the alternative surgical and medical procedures which may be necessary if such women do not have access to effective and acceptable means of contraception.
Therefore, the Committee recommended that the benefits of oral-contraceptive use by healthy nonsmoking women over 40 may outweigh the possible risks. Of course, older women, as all women who take oral contraceptives, should take the lowest possible dose formulation that is effective.
[See table III at bottom of next page]

3. CARCINOMA OF THE REPRODUCTIVE ORGANS

Numerous epidemiological studies have been performed on the incidence of breast, endometrial, ovarian, and cervical cancer in women using oral contraceptives. The overwhelming evidence in the literature suggests that the use of oral contraceptives is not associated with an increase in the risk of developing breast cancer, regardless of the age and parity of first use or with most of the marketed brands and doses. The Cancer and Steroid Hormone (CASH) study also showed no latent effect on the risk of breast cancer for at least a decade following long-term use. A few studies have shown a slightly increased relative risk of developing breast cancer, although the methodology of these studies, which included differences in examination of users and nonusers and differences in age at start of use, has been questioned. Some studies suggest that oral-contraceptive use has been associated with an increase in the risk of cervical intraepithelial neoplasia in some populations of women. However, there continues to be controversy about the extent to which such findings may be due to differences in sexual behavior and other factors.
In spite of many studies of the relationship between oral-contraceptive use and breast and cervical cancers, a cause-and-effect relationship has not been established.

4. HEPATIC NEOPLASIA

Benign hepatic adenomas are associated with oral-contraceptive use, although the incidence of benign tumors is rare

in the United States. Indirect calculations have estimated the attributable risk to be in the range of 3.3 cases/100,000 for users, a risk that increases after four or more years of use. Rupture of rare, benign, hepatic adenomas may cause death through intra-abdominal hemorrhage.

Studies from Britain have shown an increased risk of developing hepatocellular carcinoma in long-term (>8 years) oral-contraceptive users. However, these cancers are extremely rare in the U.S., and the attributable risk (the excess incidence) of liver cancers in oral-contraceptive users approaches less than one per million users.

5. OCULAR LESIONS

There have been clinical case reports of retinal thrombosis associated with the use of oral contraceptives. Oral contraceptives should be discontinued if there is unexplained partial or complete loss of vision; onset of proptosis or diplopia; papilledema; or retinal vascular lesions. Appropriate diagnostic and therapeutic measures should be undertaken immediately.

6. ORAL-CONTRACEPTIVE USE BEFORE OR DURING EARLY PREGNANCY

Extensive epidemiological studies have revealed no increased risk of birth defects in women who have used oral contraceptives prior to pregnancy. Studies also do not suggest a teratogenic effect, particularly insofar as cardiac anomalies and limb-reduction defects are concerned, when taken inadvertently during early pregnancy.

The administration of oral contraceptives to induce withdrawal bleeding should not be used as a test for pregnancy. Oral contraceptives should not be used during pregnancy to treat threatened or habitual abortion.

It is recommended that for any patient who has missed two consecutive periods, pregnancy should be ruled out before continuing oral-contraceptive use. If the patient has not adhered to the prescribed schedule, the possibility of pregnancy should be considered at the time of the first missed period. Oral-contraceptive use should be discontinued if pregnancy is confirmed.

7. GALLBLADDER DISEASE

Earlier studies have reported an increased lifetime relative risk of gallbladder surgery in users of oral contraceptives and estrogens. More recent studies, however, have shown that the relative risk of developing gallbladder disease among oral-contraceptive users may be minimal. The recent findings of minimal risk may be related to the use of oral-contraceptive formulations containing lower hormonal doses of estrogens and progestogens.

8. CARBOHYDRATE AND LIPID METABOLIC EFFECTS

Oral contraceptives have been shown to cause glucose intolerance in a significant percentage of users. Oral contraceptives containing greater than 75 micrograms of estrogens cause hyperinsulinism, while lower doses of estrogen cause less glucose intolerance. Progestogens increase insulin secretion and create insulin resistance, this effect varying with different progestational agents. However, in the non-diabetic woman, oral contraceptives appear to have no effect on fasting blood glucose. Because of these demonstrated effects, prediabetic and diabetic women should be carefully observed while taking oral contraceptives.

A small proportion of women will have persistent hypertriglyceridemia while on the pill. As discussed earlier (see "WARNINGS" 1a. and 1d.), changes in serum triglycerides and lipoprotein levels have been reported in oral-contraceptive users.

9. ELEVATED BLOOD PRESSURE

An increase in blood pressure has been reported in women taking oral contraceptives, and this increase is more likely in older oral-contraceptive users and with continued use. Data from the Royal College of General Practitioners and subsequent randomized trials have shown that the incidence of hypertension increases with increasing quantities of progestations.

Women with a history of hypertension or hypertension-related diseases, or renal disease, should be encouraged to use another method of contraception. If women with hypertension elect to use oral contraceptives, they should be monitored closely, and if significant elevation of blood pressure occurs, oral contraceptives should be discontinued. For most women, elevated blood pressure will return to normal after stopping oral contraceptives, and there is no difference in the occurrence of hypertension between ever- and never- users.

10. HEADACHE

The onset or exacerbation of migraine or development of headache with a new pattern that is recurrent, persistent, or severe requires discontinuation of oral contraceptives and evaluation of the cause.

11. BLEEDING IRREGULARITIES

Breakthrough bleeding and spotting are sometimes encountered in patients on oral contraceptives, especially during the first three months of use. The type and dose of progestogen may be important. Nonhormonal causes should be considered and adequate diagnostic measures taken to rule out malignancy or pregnancy in the event of breakthrough bleeding, as in the case of any abnormal vaginal bleeding. If pathology has been excluded, time or a change to another formulation may solve the problem. In the event of amenorrhea, pregnancy should be ruled out.

Some women may encounter post-pill amenorrhea or oligomenorrhea, especially when such a condition was preexistent.

PRECAUTIONS

Patients should be counseled that this product does not protect against HIV infection (AIDS) and other sexually transmitted diseases.

1. PHYSICAL EXAMINATION AND FOLLOW-UP

A periodic history and physical examination is appropriate for all women, including women using oral contraceptives. The physical examination, however, may be deferred until after initiation of oral contraceptives if requested by the woman and judged appropriate by the clinician. The physical examination should include special reference to blood pressure, breasts, abdomen and pelvic organs, including cervical cytology, and relevant laboratory tests. In case of undiagnosed, persistent, or recurrent abnormal vaginal bleeding, appropriate measures should be conducted to rule out malignancy. Women with a strong family history of breast cancer or who have breast nodules should be monitored with particular care.

2. LIPID DISORDERS

Women who are being treated for hyperlipidemias should be followed closely if they elect to use oral contraceptives. Some progestogens may elevate LDL levels and may render the control of hyperlipidemias more difficult. (See "Warnings," 1d.)

3. LIVER FUNCTION

If jaundice develops in any woman receiving such drugs, the medication should be discontinued. Steroid hormones may be poorly metabolized in patients with impaired liver function.

4. FLUID RETENTION

Oral contraceptives may cause some degree of fluid retention. They should be prescribed with caution, and only with careful monitoring, in patients with conditions which might be aggravated by fluid retention.

5. EMOTIONAL DISORDERS

Patients becoming significantly depressed while taking oral contraceptives should stop the medication and use an alternate method of contraception in an attempt to determine whether the symptom is drug related.

Women with a history of depression should be carefully observed and the drug discontinued if depression recurs to a serious degree.

6. CONTACT LENSES

Contact-lens wearers who develop visual changes or changes in lens tolerance should be assessed by an ophthalmologist.

7. DRUG INTERACTIONS

Reduced efficacy and increased incidence of breakthrough bleeding and menstrual irregularities have been associated with concomitant use of rifampin. A similar association, though less marked, has been suggested with barbiturates, phenylbutazone, phenytoin sodium, and possibly with griseofulvin, ampicillin, and tetracyclines.

8. INTERACTIONS WITH LABORATORY TESTS

Certain endocrine- and liver-function tests and blood components may be affected by oral contraceptives:

a. Increased prothrombin and factors VII, VIII, IX, and X; decreased antithrombin 3; increased norepinephrine-induced platelet aggregability.

b. Increased thyroid-binding globulin (TBG) leading to increased circulating total thyroid hormone, as measured by protein-bound iodine (PBI), T4 by column or by radioimmunoassay. Free T3 resin uptake is decreased, reflecting the elevated TBG; free T4 concentration is unaltered.

c. Other binding proteins may be elevated in serum.

d. Sex-binding globulins are increased and result in elevated levels of total circulating sex steroids and corticoids; however, free or biologically active levels remain unchanged.

e. Triglycerides may be increased.

f. Glucose tolerance may be decreased.

g. Serum folate levels may be depressed by oral-contraceptive therapy. This may be of clinical significance if a woman becomes pregnant shortly after discontinuing oral contraceptives.

9. CARCINOGENESIS

See "Warnings" section.

10. PREGNANCY

Pregnancy Category X. See "Contraindications" and "Warnings" sections.

11. NURSING MOTHERS

Small amounts of oral-contraceptive steroids have been identified in the milk of nursing mothers, and a few adverse effects on the child have been reported, including jaundice and breast enlargement. In addition, oral contraceptives given in the postpartum period may interfere with lactation by decreasing the quantity and quality of breast milk. If possible, the nursing mother should be advised not to use oral contraceptives but to use other forms of contraception until she has completely weaned her child.

INFORMATION FOR THE PATIENT

See Patient Labeling Printed Below.

ADVERSE REACTIONS

An increased risk of the following serious adverse reactions has been associated with the use of oral contraceptives (see "Warnings" section):

Thrombophlebitis.
Arterial thromboembolism.
Pulmonary embolism.
Myocardial infarction.
Cerebral hemorrhage.
Cerebral thrombosis.
Hypertension.
Gallbladder disease.
Hepatic adenomas or benign liver tumors.

There is evidence of an association between the following conditions and the use of oral contraceptives, although additional confirmatory studies are needed:

Mesenteric thrombosis.
Retinal thrombosis.

The following adverse reactions have been reported in patients receiving oral contraceptives and are believed to be drug-related:

Nausea
Vomiting
Gastrointestinal symptoms (such as abdominal cramps and bloating).
Breakthrough bleeding.
Spotting.
Change in menstrual flow.
Amenorrhea.
Temporary infertility after discontinuation of treatment.
Edema.
Melasma which may persist.
Breast changes: tenderness, enlargement, secretion.
Change in weight (increase or decrease).
Change in cervical erosion and cervical secretion.
Diminution in lactation when given immediately postpartum.
Cholestatic jaundice.
Migraine.
Rash (allergic).
Mental depression.
Reduced tolerance to carbohydrates.

TABLE III
ANNUAL NUMBER OF BIRTH-RELATED OR METHOD-RELATED DEATHS ASSOCIATED WITH CONTROL OF FERTILITY PER 100,000 NONSTERILE WOMEN, BY FERTILITY-CONTROL METHOD ACCORDING TO AGE

Method of control and outcome	15–19	20–24	25–29	30–34	35–39	40–44
No fertility-control methods*	7.0	7.4	9.1	14.8	25.7	28.2
Oral contraceptives nonsmoker**	0.3	0.5	0.9	1.9	13.8	31.6
Oral contraceptives smoker**	2.2	3.4	6.6	13.5	51.1	117.2
IUD**	0.8	0.8	1.0	1.0	1.4	1.4
Condom*	1.1	1.6	0.7	0.2	0.3	0.4
Diaphragm/spermicide*	1.9	1.2	1.2	1.3	2.2	2.8
Periodic abstinence*	2.5	1.6	1.6	1.7	2.9	3.6

* Deaths are birth related
** Deaths are method related
Adapted from H.W. Ory, Family Planning Perspectives, 15:57–63, 1983.

Continued on next page

Triphasil-21—Cont.

Vaginal candidiasis.
Change in corneal curvature (steepening).
Intolerance to contact lenses.
The following adverse reactions have been reported in users of oral contraceptives, and the association has been neither confirmed nor refuted:

Congenital anomalies.
Premenstrual syndrome.
Cataracts.
Optic neuritis.
Changes in appetite.
Cystitis-like syndrome.
Headache.
Nervousness.
Dizziness.
Hirsutism.
Loss of scalp hair.
Erythema multiforme.
Erythema nodosum.
Hemorrhagic eruption.
Vaginitis.
Porphyria.
Impaired renal function.
Hemolytic uremic syndrome.
Budd-Chiari syndrome.
Acne.
Changes in libido.
Colitis.
Sickle-cell disease.
Cerebral-vascular disease with mitral valve prolapse.
Lupus-like syndromes.

OVERDOSAGE

Serious ill effects have not been reported following acute ingestion of large doses of oral contraceptives by young children. Overdosage may cause nausea, and withdrawal bleeding may occur in females.

NONCONTRACEPTIVE HEALTH BENEFITS

The following noncontraceptive health benefits related to the use of oral contraceptives are supported by epidemiological studies which largely utilized oral-contraceptive formulations containing doses exceeding 0.035 mg of ethinyl estradiol or 0.05 mg of mestranol.
Effects on menses:
Increased menstrual cycle regularity.
Decreased blood loss and decreased incidence of iron-deficiency anemia.
Decreased incidence of dysmenorrhea.
Effects related to inhibition of ovulation:
Decreased incidence of functional ovarian cysts.
Decreased incidence of ectopic pregnancies.
Effects from long-term use:
Decreased incidence of fibroadenomas and fibrocystic disease of the breast.
Decreased incidence of acute pelvic inflammatory disease.
Decreased incidence of endometrial cancer.
Decreased incidence of ovarian cancer.

DOSAGE AND ADMINISTRATION

To achieve maximum contraceptive effectiveness, Triphasil-21 Tablets (levonorgestrel and ethinyl estradiol tablets—triphasic regimen) must be taken exactly as directed and at intervals not exceeding 24 hours.
Triphasil-21 Tablets are a three-phase preparation. The dosage of Triphasil-21 Tablets is one tablet daily for 21 consecutive days per menstrual cycle in the following order: 6 brown tablets (phase 1), followed by 5 white tablets (phase 2), and then followed by the last 10 light-yellow tablets (phase 3), according to the prescribed schedule. Tablets are then discontinued for 7 days (three weeks on, one week off). It is recommended that Triphasil-21 Tablets be taken at the same time each day, preferably after the evening meal or at bedtime. During the first cycle of medication, the patient should be instructed to take one Triphasil-21 Tablet daily in the order of 6 brown, 5 white and, finally, 10 light-yellow tablets for twenty-one (21) consecutive days, beginning on day one (1) of her menstrual cycle. (The first day of menstruation is day one.) The tablets are then discontinued for one week (7 days). Withdrawal bleeding usually occurs within 3 days following discontinuation of Triphasil-21 Tablets. (If Triphasil-21 Tablets are first taken later than the first day of the first menstrual cycle of medication or postpartum, contraceptive reliance should not be placed on Triphasil-21 Tablets until after the first 7 consecutive days of administration. The possibility of ovulation and conception prior to initiation of medication should be considered.)
When switching from another oral contraceptive, Triphasil-21 Tablets should be started on the first day of bleeding following the last tablet taken of the previous oral contraceptive.
The patient begins her next and all subsequent 21-day courses of Triphasil-21 Tablets on the same day of the week that she began her first course, following the same schedule: 21 days on—7 days off. She begins taking her brown tablets

on the 8th day after discontinuance regardless of whether or not a menstrual period has occurred or is still in progress. Any time the next cycle of Triphasil-21 Tablets is started later than the 8th day, the patient should be protected by another means of contraception until she has taken a tablet daily for seven consecutive days.
If spotting or breakthrough bleeding occurs, the patient is instructed to continue on the same regimen. This type of bleeding is usually transient and without significance; however, if the bleeding is persistent or prolonged, the patient is advised to consult her physician. Although the occurrence of pregnancy is highly unlikely if Triphasil-21 Tablets are taken according to directions, if withdrawal bleeding does not occur, the possibility of pregnancy must be considered. If the patient has not adhered to the prescribed schedule (missed one or more tablets or started taking them on a day later than she should have), the probability of pregnancy should be considered at the time of the first missed period and appropriate diagnostic measures taken before the medication is resumed. If the patient has adhered to the prescribed regimen and misses two consecutive periods, pregnancy should be ruled out before continuing the contraceptive regimen.
The risk of pregnancy increases with each tablet missed. For additional patient instructions regarding missed pills, see the "WHAT TO DO IF YOU MISS PILLS" section in the DETAILED PATIENT LABELING below. If breakthrough bleeding occurs following missed tablets, it will usually be transient and of no consequence.
In the nonlactating mother, Triphasil-21 may be initiated postpartum, for contraception. When the tablets are administered in the postpartum period, the increased risk of thromboembolic disease associated with the postpartum period must be considered (See "Contraindications", "Warnings", and "Precautions" concerning thromboembolic disease). It is to be noted that early resumption of ovulation may occur if Parlodel® (bromocriptine mesylate) has been used for the prevention of lactation.

HOW SUPPLIED

Triphasil®-21 Tablets (levonorgestrel and ethinyl estradiol tablets—triphasic regimen) NDC 0008-2535, are available in packages of 3 dial dispensers. Each cycle contains 21 round, coated tablets as follows:
NDC 0008-0641, six brown tablets marked "W" and "641", each containing 0.050 mg levonorgestrel and 0.030 mg ethinyl estradiol;
NDC 0008-0642, five white to off-white tablets marked "W" and "642", each containing 0.075 mg levonorgestrel and 0.040 mg ethinyl estradiol; and
NDC 0008-0643, ten light-yellow tablets marked "W" and "643", each containing 0.125 mg levonorgestrel and 0.030 mg ethinyl estradiol.
References available upon request.

Brief Summary Patient Package Insert

This product (like all oral contraceptives) is intended to prevent pregnancy. It does not protect against HIV infection (AIDS) and other sexually transmitted diseases.
Oral contraceptives, also known as "birth-control pills" or "the pill," are taken to prevent pregnancy, and when taken correctly, have a failure rate of less than 1.0% per year when used without missing any pills. The typical failure rate of large numbers of pill users is less than 3.0% per year when women who miss pills are included. For most women oral contraceptives are also free of serious or unpleasant side effects. However, forgetting to take pills considerably increases the chances of pregnancy.
For the majority of women, oral contraceptives can be taken safely. But there are some women who are at high risk of developing certain serious diseases that can be life-threatening or may cause temporary or permanent disability or death. The risks associated with taking oral contraceptives increase significantly if you:
• smoke.
• have high blood pressure, diabetes, high cholesterol.
• have or have had clotting disorders, heart attack, stroke, angina pectoris, cancer of the breast or sex organs, jaundice or malignant or benign liver tumors.
You should not take the pill if you suspect you are pregnant or have unexplained vaginal bleeding.

Cigarette smoking increases the risk of serious adverse effects on the heart and blood vessels from oral-contraceptive use. This risk increases with age and with heavy smoking (15 or more cigarettes per day) and is quite marked in women over 35 years of age. Women who use oral contraceptives should not smoke.

Most side effects of the pill are not serious. The most common such effects are nausea, vomiting, bleeding between menstrual periods, weight gain, breast tenderness, and difficulty wearing contact lenses. These side effects, especially nausea and vomiting, may subside within the first three months of use.

The serious side effects of the pill occur very infrequently, especially if you are in good health and do not smoke. However, you should know that the following medical conditions have been associated with or made worse by the pill:
1. Blood clots in the legs (thrombophlebitis), lungs (pulmonary embolism), stoppage or rupture of a blood vessel in the brain (stroke), blockage of blood vessels in the heart (heart attack and angina pectoris) or other organs of the body. As mentioned above, smoking increases the risk of heart attacks and strokes and subsequent serious medical consequences.
2. Liver tumors, which may rupture and cause severe bleeding. A possible but not definite association has been found with the pill and liver cancer. However, liver cancers are extremely rare. The chance of developing liver cancer from using the pill is thus even rarer.
3. High blood pressure, although blood pressure usually returns to normal when the pill is stopped.
The symptoms associated with these serious side effects are discussed in the detailed leaflet given to you with your supply of pills. Notify your doctor or health-care provider if you notice any unusual physical disturbances while taking the pill. In addition, drugs such as rifampin, as well as some anti-convulsants and some antibiotics, may decrease oral-contraceptive effectiveness.
Studies to date of women taking the pill have not shown an increase in the incidence of cancer of the breast or cervix. There is, however, insufficient evidence to rule out the possibility that pills may cause such cancers.
Taking the pill provides some important noncontraceptive benefits. These include less painful menstruation, less menstrual blood loss and anemia, fewer pelvic infections, and fewer cancers of the ovary and the lining of the uterus.
Be sure to discuss any medical condition you may have with your health care provider. Your health-care provider will take a medical and family history before prescribing oral contraceptives and will examine you. The physical examination may be delayed to another time if you request it and the health-care provider believes that it is appropriate to postpone it. You should be reexamined at least once a year while taking oral contraceptives. The detailed patient information leaflet gives you further information which you should read and discuss with your health-care provider.

DETAILED PATIENT LABELING

This product (like all oral contraceptives) is intended to prevent pregnancy. It does not protect against HIV infection (AIDS) and other sexually transmitted diseases.
INTRODUCTION
Any woman who considers using oral contraceptives (the birth control pill or the pill) should understand the benefits and risks of using this form of birth control. This leaflet will give you much of the information you will need to make this decision and will also help you determine if you are at risk of developing any of the serious side effects of the pill. It will tell you how to use the pill properly so that it will be as effective as possible. However, this leaflet is not a replacement for a careful discussion between you and your health-care provider. You should discuss the information provided in this leaflet with him or her, both when you first start taking the pill and during your revisits. You should also follow your health-care provider's advice with regard to regular check-ups while you are on the pill.
EFFECTIVENESS OF ORAL CONTRACEPTIVES
Oral contraceptives or "birth-control pills" or "the pill" are used to prevent pregnancy and are more effective than other nonsurgical methods of birth control. When they are taken correctly, the chance of becoming pregnant is less than 1.0% when used perfectly, without missing any pills. Typical failure rates are actually 3.0% per year. The chance of becoming pregnant increases with each missed pill during the menstrual cycle.
In comparison, typical failure rates for other nonsurgical methods of birth control during the first year of use are as follows:
IUD: 3%.
DEPO-PROVERA® (injectable progestogen): 0.3%.
NORPLANT® SYSTEM (implants): 0.2%.
Diaphragm with spermicides: 18%.
Spermicides alone: 21%.
Vaginal sponge: 18 to 28%.
Condom alone: 12%.
Periodic abstinence: 20%.
No methods: 85%.
WHO SHOULD NOT TAKE ORAL CONTRACEPTIVES

Cigarette smoking increases the risk of serious adverse effects on the heart and blood vessels from oral-contraceptive use. This risk increases with age and with heavy smoking (15 or more cigarettes per day) and is quite marked in women over 35 years of age. Women who use oral contraceptives should not smoke.

Some women should not use the pill. For example, you should not take the pill if you are pregnant or think you may be pregnant. You should also not use the pill if you have any of the following conditions:

- Heart attack or stroke.
- Blood clots in the legs (thrombophlebitis), lungs (pulmonary embolism), or eyes.
- Blood clots in the deep veins of your legs.
- Known or suspected breast cancer or cancer of the lining of the uterus, cervix, or vagina.
- Liver tumor (benign or cancerous).

Or, if you have any of the following:

- Chest pain (angina pectoris).
- Unexplained vaginal bleeding (until a diagnosis is reached by your doctor).
- Yellowing of the whites of the eyes or of the skin (jaundice) during pregnancy or during previous use of the pill.
- Known or suspected pregnancy.

Tell your health-care provider if you have ever had any of these conditions. Your health-care provider can recommend another method of birth control.

OTHER CONSIDERATIONS BEFORE TAKING ORAL CONTRACEPTIVES

Tell your health-care provider if you or any family member has ever had:

- Breast nodules, fibrocystic disease of the breast, an abnormal breast X-ray or mammogram.
- Diabetes.
- Elevated cholesterol or triglycerides.
- High blood pressure.
- Migraine or other headaches or epilepsy.
- Mental depression.
- Gallbladder, heart or kidney disease.
- History of scanty or irregular menstrual periods.

Women with any of these conditions should be checked often by their health-care provider if they choose to use oral contraceptives. Also, be sure to inform your doctor or health-care provider if you smoke or are on any medications.

RISKS OF TAKING ORAL CONTRACEPTIVES

1. *Risk of developing blood clots*

Blood clots and blockage of blood vessels are the most serious side effects of taking oral contraceptives and can be fatal. In particular, a clot in the legs can cause thrombophlebitis and a clot that travels to the lungs can cause a sudden blocking of the vessel carrying blood to the lungs. Rarely, clots occur in the blood vessels of the eye and may cause blindness, double vision, or impaired vision.

If you take oral contraceptives and need elective surgery, need to stay in bed for a prolonged illness, or have recently delivered a baby, you may be at risk of developing blood clots. You should consult your doctor about stopping oral contraceptives three to four weeks before surgery and not taking oral contraceptives for two weeks after surgery or during bed rest. You should also not take oral contraceptives soon after delivery of a baby or a midtrimester pregnancy termination. It is advisable to wait for at least four weeks after delivery if you are not breast-feeding. If you are breast-feeding, you should wait until you have weaned your child before using the pill. (See also the section on breast-feeding in "General Precautions".)

2. *Heart attacks and strokes*

Oral contraceptives may increase the tendency to develop strokes (stoppage or rupture of blood vessels in the brain) and angina pectoris and heart attacks (blockage of blood vessels in the heart). Any of these conditions can cause death or serious disability.

Smoking greatly increases the possibility of suffering heart attacks and strokes. Furthermore, smoking and the use of oral contraceptives greatly increase the chances of developing and dying of heart disease.

3. *Gallbladder disease*

Oral-contraceptive users probably have a greater risk than nonusers of having gallbladder disease, although this risk may be related to pills containing high doses of estrogens.

4. *Liver tumors*

In rare cases, oral contraceptives can cause benign but dangerous liver tumors. These benign liver tumors can rupture and cause fatal internal bleeding. In addition, a possible but not definite association has been found with the pill and liver cancers in two studies in which a few women who developed these very rare cancers were found to have used oral contraceptives for long periods. However, liver cancers are extremely rare. The chance of developing liver cancer from using the pill is thus even rarer.

5. *Cancer of the reproductive organs*

There is, at present, no confirmed evidence that oral contraceptives increase in the risk of cancer of the reproductive organs in human studies. Several studies have found no overall increase in the risk of developing breast cancer. However, women who use oral contraceptives and have a strong family history of breast cancer or who have breast nodules or abnormal mammograms should be closely followed by their doctors.

ANNUAL NUMBER OF BIRTH-RELATED OR METHOD-RELATED DEATHS ASSOCIATED WITH CONTROL OF FERTILITY PER 100,000 NONSTERILE WOMEN, BY FERTILITY-CONTROL METHOD ACCORDING TO AGE

Method of control and outcome	15–19	20–24	25–29	30–34	35–39	40–44
No fertility-control methods*	7.0	7.4	9.1	14.8	25.7	28.2
Oral contraceptives nonsmoker**	0.3	0.5	0.9	1.9	13.8	31.6
Oral contraceptives smoker**	2.2	3.4	6.6	13.5	51.1	117.2
IUD**	0.8	0.8	1.0	1.0	1.4	1.4
Condom*	1.1	1.6	0.7	0.2	0.3	0.4
Diaphragm/spermicide*	1.9	1.2	1.2	1.3	2.2	2.8
Periodic abstinence*	2.5	1.6	1.6	1.7	2.9	3.6

* Deaths are birth related
** Deaths are method related

Some studies have found an increase in the incidence of cancer of the cervix in women who use oral contraceptives. However, this finding may be related to factors other than the use of oral contraceptives.

ESTIMATED RISK OF DEATH FROM A BIRTH-CONTROL METHOD OR PREGNANCY

All methods of birth control and pregnancy are associated with a risk of developing certain diseases which may lead to disability or death. An estimate of the number of deaths associated with different methods of birth control and pregnancy has been calculated and is shown in the following table.

[See table above]

In the above table, the risk of death from any birth-control method is less than the risk of childbirth, except for oral-contraceptive users over the age of 35 who smoke and pill users over the age of 40 even if they do not smoke. It can be seen in the table that for women aged 15 to 39, the risk of death was highest with pregnancy (7 to 26 deaths per 100,000 women, depending on age). Among pill users who do not smoke, the risk of death was always lower than that associated with pregnancy for any age group, except for those women over the age of 40, when the risk increases to 32 deaths per 100,000 women, compared to 28 associated with pregnancy at that age. However, for pill users who smoke and are over the age of 35, the estimated number of deaths exceeds those for other methods of birth control. If a woman is over the age of 40 and smokes, her estimated risk of death is four times higher (117/100,000 women) than the estimated risk associated with pregnancy (28/100,000 women) in that age group.

The suggestion that women over 40 who don't smoke should not take oral contraceptives is based on information from older high-dose pills and on less-selective use of pills than is practiced today. An Advisory Committee of the FDA discussed this issue in 1989 and recommended that the benefits of oral-contraceptive use by healthy, nonsmoking women over 40 years of age may outweigh the possible risks. However, all women, especially older women, are cautioned to use the lowest-dose pill that is effective.

WARNING SIGNALS

If any of these adverse effects occur while you are taking oral contraceptives, call your doctor immediately:

- Sharp chest pain, coughing of blood, or sudden shortness of breath (indicating a possible clot in the lung).
- Pain in the calf (indicating a possible clot in the leg).
- Crushing chest pain or heaviness in the chest (indicating a possible heart attack).
- Sudden severe headache or vomiting, dizziness or fainting, disturbances of vision or speech, weakness, or numbness in an arm or leg (indicating a possible stroke).
- Sudden partial or complete loss of vision (indicating a possible clot in the eye).
- Breast lumps (indicating possible breast cancer or fibrocystic disease of the breast; ask your doctor or health care provider to show you how to examine your breasts).
- Severe pain or tenderness in the stomach area (indicating a possibly ruptured liver tumor).
- Difficulty in sleeping, weakness, lack of energy, fatigue, or change in mood (possibly indicating severe depression).
- Jaundice or a yellowing of the skin or eyeballs, accompanied frequently by fever, fatigue, loss of appetite, dark colored urine, or light-colored bowel movements (indicating possible liver problems).

SIDE EFFECTS OF ORAL CONTRACEPTIVES

1. *Vaginal bleeding*

Irregular vaginal bleeding or spotting may occur while you are taking the pills. Irregular bleeding may vary from slight staining between menstrual periods to breakthrough bleeding which is a flow much like a regular period. Irregular bleeding occurs most often during the first few months of oral-contraceptive use, but may also occur after you have been taking the pill for some time. Such bleeding may be temporary and usually does not indicate any serious problems. It is important to continue taking your pills on schedule. If the bleeding occurs in more than one cycle or lasts for more than a few days, talk to your doctor or health-care provider.

2. *Contact lenses*

If you wear contact lenses and notice a change in vision or an inability to wear your lenses, contact your doctor or health-care provider.

3. *Fluid retention*

Oral contraceptives may cause edema (fluid retention) with swelling of the fingers or ankles and may raise your blood pressure. If you experience fluid retention, contact your doctor or health-care provider.

4. *Melasma*

A spotty darkening of the skin is possible, particularly of the face.

5. *Other side effects*

Other side effects may include change in appetite, headache, nervousness, depression, dizziness, loss of scalp hair, rash, and vaginal infections.

If any of these side effects bother you, call your doctor or health-care provider.

GENERAL PRECAUTIONS

1. *Missed periods and use of oral contraceptives before or during early pregnancy*

There may be times when you may not menstruate regularly after you have completed taking a cycle of pills. If you have taken your pills regularly and miss one menstrual period, continue taking your pills for the next cycle but be sure to inform your health-care provider before doing so. If you have not taken the pills daily as instructed and missed a menstrual period, or if you missed two consecutive menstrual periods, you may be pregnant. Check with your health-care provider immediately to determine whether you are pregnant. Do not continue to take oral contraceptives until you are sure you are not pregnant, but continue to use another method of contraception.

There is no conclusive evidence that oral-contraceptive use is associated with an increase in birth defects when taken inadvertently during early pregnancy. Previously, a few studies had reported that oral contraceptives might be associated with birth defects, but these studies have not been confirmed. Nevertheless, oral contraceptives or any other drugs should not be used during pregnancy unless clearly necessary and prescribed by your doctor. You should check with your doctor about risks to your unborn child of any medication taken during pregnancy.

2. *While breast-feeding*

If you are breast-feeding, consult your doctor before starting oral contraceptives. Some of the drug will be passed on to the child in the milk. A few adverse effects on the child have been reported, including yellowing of the skin (jaundice) and breast enlargement. In addition, oral contraceptives may decrease the amount and quality of your milk. If possible, do not use oral contraceptives while breast-feeding. You should use another method of contraception since breast-feeding provides only partial protection from becoming pregnant, and this partial protection decreases significantly as you breast-feed for longer periods of time. You should consider starting oral contraceptives only after you have weaned your child completely.

3. *Laboratory tests*

If you are scheduled for any laboratory tests, tell your doctor you are taking birth-control pills. Certain blood tests may be affected by birth-control pills.

4. *Drug interactions*

Certain drugs may interact with birth-control pills to make them less effective in preventing pregnancy or cause an increase in breakthrough bleeding. Such drugs include

Continued on next page

Triphasil-21—Cont.

rifampin, drugs used for epilepsy such as barbiturates (for example, phenobarbital) and phenytoin (Dilantin is one brand of this drug), phenylbutazolidin (Butazolidin is one brand), and possibly certain antibiotics. You may need to use an additional method of contraception during any cycle in which you take drugs that can make oral contraceptives less effective.

HOW TO TAKE THE PILL

This product (like all oral contraceptives) is intended to prevent pregnancy. It does not protect against transmission of HIV (AIDS) and other sexually transmitted diseases such as chlamydia, genital herpes, genital warts, gonorrhea, hepatitis B, and syphilis.

IMPORTANT POINTS TO REMEMBER

BEFORE YOU START TAKING YOUR PILLS:

1. BE SURE TO READ THESE DIRECTIONS:

Before you start taking your pills.

Anytime you are not sure what to do.

2. THE RIGHT WAY TO TAKE THE PILL IS TO TAKE ONE PILL EVERY DAY AT THE SAME TIME.

If you miss pills you could get pregnant. This includes starting the pack late. The more pills you miss, the more likely you are to get pregnant.

3. MANY WOMEN HAVE SPOTTING OR LIGHT BLEEDING, OR MAY FEEL SICK TO THEIR STOMACH DURING THE FIRST 1–3 PACKS OF PILLS.

If you feel sick to your stomach, do not stop taking the pill. The problem will usually go away. If it doesn't go away, check with your doctor or clinic.

4. MISSING PILLS CAN ALSO CAUSE SPOTTING OR LIGHT BLEEDING, even when you make up these missed pills.

On the days you take 2 pills to make up for missed pills, you could also feel a little sick to your stomach.

5. IF YOU HAVE VOMITING OR DIARRHEA, for any reason, or IF YOU TAKE SOME MEDICINES, including some antibiotics, your pills may not work as well.

Use a back-up method (such as condoms, foam, or sponge) until you check with your doctor or clinic.

6. IF YOU HAVE TROUBLE REMEMBERING TO TAKE THE PILL, talk to your doctor or clinic about how to make pill-taking easier or about using another method of birth control.

7. IF YOU HAVE ANY QUESTIONS OR ARE UNSURE ABOUT THE INFORMATION IN THIS LEAFLET, call your doctor or clinic.

BEFORE YOU START TAKING YOUR PILLS

1. DECIDE WHAT TIME OF DAY YOU WANT TO TAKE YOUR PILL. It is important to take it at about the same time every day.

2. LOOK AT YOUR PILL PACK TO SEE IF IT HAS 21 OR 28 PILLS:

The *21-pill pack* has 21 "active" brown, white or light-yellow pills (with hormones) to take for 3 weeks, followed by 1 week without pills.

The *28-pill pack* has 21 "active" brown, white or light-yellow pills (with hormones) to take for 3 weeks, followed by 1 week of reminder light-green pills (without hormones).

3. ALSO FIND:

1) where on the pack to start taking pills, and

2) in what order to take the pills (follow the arrows).

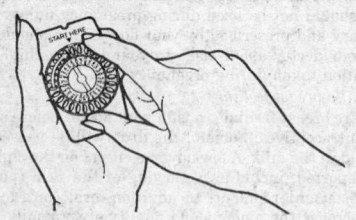

4. BE SURE YOU HAVE READY AT ALL TIMES:

ANOTHER KIND OF BIRTH CONTROL (such as condoms, foam or sponge) to use as a back-up in case you miss pills.

AN EXTRA, FULL PILL PACK.

WHEN TO START THE *FIRST* PACK OF PILLS

You have a choice of which day to start taking your first pack of pills. Decide with your doctor or clinic which is the best day for you. Pick a time of day which will be easy to remember.

DAY 1 START:

1. Take the first "active" brown pill of the first pack during the *first 24 hours of your period.*

2. You will not need to use a back-up method of birth control, since you are starting the pill at the beginning of your period.

SUNDAY START:

1. Take the first "active" brown pill of the first pack on the *Sunday after your period starts,* even if you are still bleeding. If your period begins on Sunday, start the pack that same day.

2. *Use another method of birth control* as a back-up method if you have sex anytime from the Sunday you start your first pack until the next Sunday (7 days). Condoms, foam, or the sponge are good back-up methods of birth control.

WHAT TO DO DURING THE MONTH:

1. **TAKE ONE PILL AT THE SAME TIME EVERY DAY UNTIL THE PACK IS EMPTY.**

Do not skip pills even if you are spotting or bleeding between monthly periods or feel sick to your stomach (nausea).

Do not skip pills even if you do not have sex very often.

2. **WHEN YOU FINISH A PACK OR SWITCH YOUR BRAND OF PILLS:**

21 pills: Wait 7 days to start the next pack. You will probably have your period during that week. Be sure that no more than 7 days pass between 21-day packs.

28 pills: Start the next pack on the day after your last "reminder" pill. Do not wait any days between packs.

WHAT TO DO IF YOU MISS PILLS

If you **MISS 1** brown, white or light-yellow "active" pill:

1. Take it as soon as you remember. Take the next pill at your regular time. This means you take 2 pills in 1 day.

2. You do not need to use a back-up birth-control method if you have sex.

If you **MISS 2** brown, white or light-yellow "active" pills in a row in **WEEK 1 OR WEEK 2** of your pack:

1. Take 2 pills on the day you remember and 2 pills the next day.

2. Then take 1 pill a day until you finish the pack.

3. You MAY BECOME PREGNANT if you have sex in the 7 *days* after you miss pills. You MUST use another birth-control method (such as condoms, foam, or sponge) as a back-up for those 7 days.

If you **MISS 2** brown, white or light-yellow "active" pills in a row in **THE 3rd WEEK:**

1. *If you are a Day 1 Starter:*

THROW OUT the rest of the pill pack and start a new pack that same day.

If you are a Sunday Starter:

Keep taking 1 pill every day until Sunday.

On Sunday, THROW OUT the rest of the pack and start a new pack of pills that same day.

2. You may not have your period this month but this is expected. However, if you miss your period 2 months in a row, call your doctor or clinic because you might be pregnant.

3. You MAY BECOME PREGNANT if you have sex in the 7 *days* after you miss pills. You MUST use another birth-control method (such as condoms, foam, or sponge) as a back-up for those 7 days.

If you **MISS 3 OR MORE** brown, white or light-yellow "active" pills in a row (during the first 3 weeks):

1. *If you are a Day 1 Starter:*

THROW OUT the rest of the pill pack and start a new pack that same day.

If you are a Sunday Starter:

Keep taking 1 pill every day until Sunday.

On Sunday, THROW OUT the rest of the pack and start a new pack of pills that same day.

2. You may not have your period this month but this is expected. However, if you miss your period 2 months in a row, call your doctor or clinic because you might be pregnant.

3. You MAY BECOME PREGNANT if you have sex in the 7 *days* after you miss pills. You MUST use another birth control method (such as condoms, foam, or sponge) as a back-up for those 7 days.

A REMINDER FOR THOSE ON 28-DAY PACKS:

If you forget any of the 7 light-green "reminder" pills in Week 4:

THROW AWAY the pills you missed.

Keep taking 1 pill each day until the pack is empty.

You do not need a back-up method if you start your next pack on time.

FINALLY, IF YOU ARE STILL NOT SURE WHAT TO DO ABOUT THE PILLS YOU HAVE MISSED:

Use a BACK-UP METHOD anytime you have sex.

KEEP TAKING ONE PILL EACH DAY until you can reach your doctor or clinic.

Pregnancy due to pill failure

The incidence of pill failure resulting in pregnancy is approximately less than 1.0% if taken every day as directed, but more typical failure rates are less than 3.0%. If failure does occur, the risk to the fetus is minimal.

RISKS TO THE FETUS

If you do become pregnant while using oral contraceptives, the risk to the fetus is small, on the order of no more than one per thousand. You should, however, discuss the risks to the developing child with your doctor.

Pregnancy after stopping the pill

There may be some delay in becoming pregnant after you stop using oral contraceptives, especially if you had irregular menstrual cycles before you used oral contraceptives. It may be advisable to postpone conception until you begin menstruating regularly once you have stopped taking the pill and desire pregnancy.

There does not appear to be any increase in birth defects in newborn babies when pregnancy occurs soon after stopping the pill.

Overdosage

Serious ill effects have not been reported following ingestion of large doses of oral contraceptives by young children. Overdosage may cause nausea and withdrawal bleeding in females. In case of overdosage, contact your health-care provider or pharmacist.

Other information

Your health-care provider will take a medical and family history before prescribing oral contraceptives and will examine you. The physical examination may be delayed to another time if you request it and the health-care provider believes that it is appropriate to postpone it. You should be reexamined at least once a year. Be sure to inform your health-care provider if there is a family history of any of the conditions listed previously in this leaflet. Be sure to keep all appointments with your health-care provider, because this is a time to determine if there are early signs of side effects of oral-contraceptive use.

Do not use the drug for any condition other than the one for which it was prescribed. This drug has been prescribed specifically for you; do not give it to others who may want birth-control pills.

HEALTH BENEFITS FROM ORAL CONTRACEPTIVES

In addition to preventing pregnancy, use of oral contraceptives may provide certain benefits. They are:

• Menstrual cycles may become more regular.

• Blood flow during menstruation may be lighter and less iron may be lost. Therefore, anemia due to iron deficiency is less likely to occur.

• Pain or other symptoms during menstruation may be encountered less frequently.

• Ovarian cysts may occur less frequently.

• Ectopic (tubal) pregnancy may occur less frequently.

• Noncancerous cysts or lumps in the breast may occur less frequently.

• Acute pelvic inflammatory disease may occur less frequently.

• Oral-contraceptive use may provide some protection against developing two forms of cancer: cancer of the ovaries and cancer of the lining of the uterus.

If you want more information about birth-control pills, ask your doctor or pharmacist. They have a more technical leaflet called the Professional Labeling which you may wish to read.

Manufactured by:

Wyeth Laboratories Inc.

A Wyeth-Ayerst Company

Philadelphia, PA 19101

Shown in Product Identification Guide, page 345

TRIPHASIL®—28

[*tri-fa 'sil*]

Tablets

(levonorgestrel and ethinyl estradiol tablets—triphasic regimen)

Patients should be counseled that this product does not protect against HIV infection (AIDS) and other sexually transmitted diseases.

DESCRIPTION

Each Triphasil cycle of 28 tablets consists of three different drug phases as follows: Phase 1 comprised of 6 brown tablets, each containing 0.050 mg of levonorgestrel (d(-)-13beta-ethy l -17- alpha-ethinyl- 17 -beta-hydroxygon-4-en-3-one), a totally synthetic progestogen, and 0.030 mg of ethinyl estradiol (19- nor- 17α-pregna -1,3,5(10)- trien -20- yne-3,17 -diol); phase 2 comprised of 5 white tablets, each containing 0.075 mg levonorgestrel and 0.040 mg ethinyl estradiol; and phase 3 comprised of 10 light-yellow tablets, each containing 0.125 mg levonorgestrel and 0.030 mg ethinyl estradiol; then followed by 7 light-green inert tablets. The inactive ingredients present are cellulose, FD&C Blue 1, iron oxides, lactose, magnesium stearate, polacrilin potassium, polyethylene glycol, titanium dioxide, and hydroxypropyl methylcellulose.

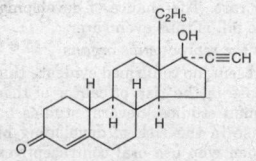

Levonorgestrel

[See chemical structure at top of next column]

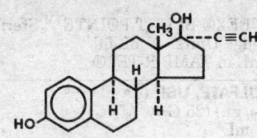

Ethinyl Estradiol

CLINICAL PHARMACOLOGY
See Triphasil®-21.

INDICATIONS AND USAGE
See Triphasil-21.

CONTRAINDICATIONS
See Triphasil-21.

WARNINGS
See Triphasil-21.

PRECAUTIONS
See Triphasil-21.

DRUG INTERACTIONS
See Triphasil-21.

CARCINOGENESIS
See Triphasil-21.

PREGNANCY
See Triphasil-21.

NURSING MOTHERS
See Triphasil-21.

INFORMATION FOR THE PATIENT
See Triphasil-21.

ADVERSE REACTIONS
See Triphasil-21.

OVERDOSAGE
See Triphasil-21.

NONCONTRACEPTIVE HEALTH BENEFITS
See Triphasil-21.

DOSAGE AND ADMINISTRATION
To achieve maximum contraceptive effectiveness, Triphasil-28 Tablets (levonorgestrel and ethinyl estradiol tablets—triphasic regimen) must be taken exactly as directed and at intervals not exceeding 24 hours.

Triphasil-28 Tablets are a three-phase preparation plus 7 inert tablets. The dosage of Triphasil-28 Tablets is **one tablet daily** for 28 consecutive days per menstrual cycle in the following order: 6 brown tablets (phase 1), followed by 5 white tablets (phase 2), followed by 10 light-yellow tablets (phase 3), plus 7 light-green inert tablets, according to the prescribed schedule.

It is recommended that Triphasil-28 Tablets be taken at the same time each day, preferably after the evening meal or at bedtime. During the first cycle of medication, the patient should be instructed to take one Triphasil-28 Tablet daily in the order of 6 brown, 5 white, 10 light-yellow, and then 7 light-green inert tablets for twenty-eight (28) consecutive days, beginning on day one (1) of her menstrual cycle. (The first day of menstruation is day one.) Withdrawal bleeding usually occurs within 3 days following the last light-yellow tablet. (If Triphasil-28 Tablets are first taken later than the first day of the first menstrual cycle of medication or postpartum, contraceptive reliance should not be placed on Triphasil-28 Tablets until after the first 7 consecutive days of administration. The possibility of ovulation and conception prior to initiation of medication should be considered.)

When switching from another oral contraceptive, Triphasil-28 Tablets should be started on the first day of bleeding following the last active tablet taken of the previous oral contraceptive.

The patient begins her next and all subsequent 28-day courses of Triphasil-28 Tablets on the same day of the week that she began her first course, following the same schedule. She begins taking her brown tablets on the next day after ingestion of the last light-green tablet, regardless of whether or not a menstrual period has occurred or is still in progress. Any time a subsequent cycle of Triphasil-28 Tablets is started later than the next day, the patient should be protected by another means of contraception until she has taken a tablet daily for seven consecutive days.

If spotting or breakthrough bleeding occurs, the patient is instructed to continue on the same regimen. This type of bleeding is usually transient and without significance; however, if the bleeding is persistent or prolonged, the patient is advised to consult her physician. Although the occurrence of pregnancy is highly unlikely if Triphasil-28 Tablets are taken according to directions, if withdrawal bleeding does not occur, the possibility of pregnancy must be considered. If the patient has not adhered to the prescribed schedule

(missed one or more tablets or started taking them on a day later than she should have), the probability of pregnancy should be considered at the time of the first missed period and appropriate diagnostic measures taken before the medication is resumed. If the patient has adhered to the prescribed regimen and misses two consecutive periods, pregnancy should be ruled out before continuing the contraceptive regimen.

The risk of pregnancy increases with each active (brown, white, or light-yellow) tablet missed. For additional patient instructions regarding missed pills, see the "WHAT TO DO IF YOU MISS PILLS" section in the DETAILED PATIENT LABELING below. If breakthrough bleeding occurs following missed active tablets, it will usually be transient and of no consequence. If the patient misses one or more light-green tablets, she is still protected against pregnancy **provided** she begins taking brown tablets again on the proper day.

In the nonlactating mother, Triphasil-28 may be initiated postpartum, for contraception. When the tablets are administered in the postpartum period, the increased risk of thromboembolic disease associated with the postpartum period must be considered (See "Contraindications", "Warnings", and "Precautions" concerning thromboembolic disease). It is to be noted that early resumption of ovulation may occur if Parlodel® (bromocriptine mesylate) has been used for the prevention of lactation.

HOW SUPPLIED
Triphasil®-28 Tablets (levonorgestrel and ethinyl estradiol tablets—triphasic regimen), NDC 0008-2536, are available in packages of 3 dial dispensers. Each cycle contains 28 round, coated tablets as follows:
NDC 0008-0641, six brown tablets marked "ᴡ" and "641", each containing 0.050 mg levonorgestrel and 0.030 mg ethinyl estradiol;
NDC 0008-0642, five white to off-white tablets marked "ᴡ" and "642", each containing 0.075 mg levonorgestrel and 0.040 mg ethinyl estradiol;
NDC 0008-0643, ten light-yellow tablets marked "ᴡ" and "643", each containing 0.125 mg levonorgestrel and 0.030 mg ethinyl estradiol; and
NDC 0008-0650, seven light-green inert tablets marked "ᴡ" and "650".
ALSO AVAILABLE:
Triphasil®-28 Tablets (levonorgestrel and ethinyl estradiol tablets—triphasic regimen), NDC 0008-2536, are available in packages of 12 Pilpak® dispensers for clinic use only. Each cycle contains 28 round, coated tablets as follows:
NDC 0008-0641, six brown tablets marked "ᴡ" and "641", each containing 0.050 mg levonorgestrel and 0.030 mg ethinyl estradiol;
NDC 0008-0642, five white to off-white tablets marked "ᴡ" and "642", each containing 0.075 mg levonorgestrel and 0.040 mg ethinyl estradiol;
NDC 0008-0643, ten light-yellow tablets marked "ᴡ" and "643", each containing 0.125 mg levonorgestrel and 0.030 mg ethinyl estradiol; and
NDC 0008-0650, seven light-green inert tablets marked " ᴡ" and "650".

REFERENCES
Available upon request.

Brief Summary Patient Package Insert: See Triphasil-21.
DETAILED PATIENT LABELING: See Triphasil-21.

HOW TO TAKE THE PILL

For Triphasil-28 Dial Dispenser: See Triphasil-21.
For Triphasil-28 Clinic Pilpak®, See below.
HOW TO TAKE THE PILL
This product (like all oral contraceptives) is intended to prevent pregnancy. It does not protect against transmission of HIV (AIDS) and other sexually transmitted diseases such as chlamydia, genital herpes, genital warts, gonorrhea, hepatitis B, and syphilis.
IMPORTANT POINTS TO REMEMBER
BEFORE YOU START TAKING YOUR PILLS:
1. BE SURE TO READ THESE DIRECTIONS:
Before you start taking your pills.
Anytime you are not sure what to do.
2. THE RIGHT WAY TO TAKE THE PILL IS TO TAKE ONE PILL EVERY DAY AT THE SAME TIME.
If you miss pills you could get pregnant. This includes starting the pack late. The more pills you miss, the more likely you are to get pregnant.
3. MANY WOMEN HAVE SPOTTING OR LIGHT BLEEDING, OR MAY FEEL SICK TO THEIR STOMACH DURING THE FIRST 1–3 PACKS OF PILLS.
If you feel sick to your stomach, do not stop taking the pill. The problem will usually go away. If it doesn't go away, check with your doctor or clinic.
4. MISSING PILLS CAN ALSO CAUSE SPOTTING OR LIGHT BLEEDING, even when you make up these missed pills.
On the days you take 2 pills to make up for missed pills, you could also feel a little sick to your stomach.

5. IF YOU HAVE VOMITING OR DIARRHEA, for any reason, or IF YOU TAKE SOME MEDICINES, including some antibiotics, your pills may not work as well.
Use a back-up method (such as condoms, foam, or sponge) until you check with your doctor or clinic.
6. IF YOU HAVE TROUBLE REMEMBERING TO TAKE THE PILL, talk to your doctor or clinic about how to make pill-taking easier or about using another method of birth control.
7. IF YOU HAVE ANY QUESTIONS OR ARE UNSURE ABOUT THE INFORMATION IN THIS LEAFLET, call your doctor or clinic.
BEFORE YOU START TAKING YOUR PILLS
1. DECIDE WHAT TIME OF DAY YOU WANT TO TAKE YOUR PILL.
It is important to take it about the same time every day.
2. LOOK AT YOUR PILL PACK TO SEE IF IT HAS 21 OR 28 PILLS:
The *21-pill pack* has 21 "active" brown, white or light-yellow pills (with hormones) to take for 3 weeks, followed by 1 week without pills.
The *28-pill pack* has 21 "active" brown, white or light-yellow pills (with hormones) to take for 3 weeks, followed by 1 week of reminder light-green pills (without hormones).
3. ALSO FIND:
1) where on the pack to start taking pills.
2) in what order to take the pills (follow the arrows), and
3) the week numbers as shown in the picture below.

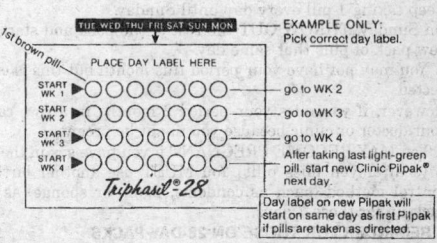

4. BE SURE YOU HAVE READY AT ALL TIMES:
ANOTHER KIND OF BIRTH CONTROL (such as condoms, foam or sponge) to use as a back-up in case you miss pills.
AN EXTRA, FULL PILL PACK.
WHEN TO START THE *FIRST* PACK OF PILLS
You have a choice of which day to start taking your first pack of pills. Decide with your doctor or clinic which is the best day for you. Pick a time of day which will be easy to remember.
DAY 1 START:
1. Take the first "active" brown pill of the first pack during the *first 24 hours of your period.*
2. You will not need to use a back-up method of birth control, since you are starting the pill at the beginning of your period.
SUNDAY START:
1. Take the first "active" brown pill of the first pack on the *Sunday after your period starts,* even if you are still bleeding. If your period begins on Sunday, start the pack that same day.
2. *Use another method of birth control* as a back-up method if you have sex anytime from the Sunday you start your first pack until the next Sunday (7 days). Condoms, foam or the sponge are good back-up methods of birth control.
WHAT TO DO DURING THE MONTH
1. TAKE ONE PILL AT THE SAME TIME EVERY DAY UNTIL THE PACK IS EMPTY.
Do not skip pills even if you are spotting or bleeding between monthly periods or feel sick to your stomach (nausea).
Do not skip pills even if you do not have sex very often.
2. WHEN YOU FINISH A PACK OR SWITCH YOUR BRAND OF PILLS:
21 pills: Wait 7 days to start the next pack. You will probably have your period during that week. Be sure that no more than 7 days pass between 21-day packs.
28 pills: Start the next pack on the day after your last "reminder" pill. Do not wait any days between packs.
WHAT TO DO IF YOU MISS PILLS
If you **MISS 1** brown, white or light-yellow "active" pill:
1. Take it as soon as you remember. Take the next pill at your regular time. This means you take 2 pills in 1 day.
2. You do not need to use a back-up birth-control method if you have sex.
If you **MISS 2** brown, white or light-yellow "active" pills in a row in **WEEK 1 OR WEEK 2** of your pack:
1. Take 2 pills on the day you remember and 2 pills the next day.
2. Then take 1 pill a day until you finish the pack.

Continued on next page

Triphasil-28—Cont.

3. You MAY BECOME PREGNANT if you have sex in the 7 *days* after you miss pills. You MUST use another birth-control method (such as condoms, foam, or sponge) as a back-up for those 7 days.

If you **MISS 2** brown, white or light-yellow "active" pills in a row in **THE 3rd WEEK**:

1. *If you are a Day 1 Starter.*
THROW OUT the rest of the pill pack and start a new pack that same day.

If you are a Sunday Starter:
Keep taking 1 pill every day until Sunday.
On Sunday, THROW OUT the rest of the pack and start a new pack of pills that same day.

2. You may not have your period this month but this is expected.
However, if you miss your period 2 months in a row, call your doctor or clinic because you might be pregnant.

3. You MAY BECOME PREGNANT if you have sex in the 7 *days* after you miss pills. You MUST use another birth-control method (such as condoms, foam, or sponge) as a back-up for those 7 days.

If you **MISS 3 OR MORE** brown, white or light-yellow "active" pills in a row (during the first 3 weeks):

1. *If you are a Day 1 Starter:*
THROW OUT the rest of the pill pack and start a new pack that same day.

If you are a Sunday Starter:
Keep taking 1 pill every day until Sunday.
On Sunday, THROW OUT the rest of the pack and start a new pack of pills that same day.

2. You may not have your period this month but this is expected.
However, if you miss your period 2 months in a row, call your doctor or clinic because you might be pregnant.

3. You MAY BECOME PREGNANT if you have sex in the 7 *days* after you miss pills. You MUST use another birth-control method (such as condoms, foam, or sponge) as a back-up for those 7 days.

A REMINDER FOR THOSE ON 28-DAY PACKS
If you forget any of the 7 light-green "reminder" pills in Week 4:
THROW AWAY the pills you missed.
Keep taking 1 pill each day until the pack is empty.
You do not need a back-up method if you start your next pack on time.

FINALLY, IF YOU ARE STILL NOT SURE WHAT TO DO ABOUT THE PILLS YOU HAVE MISSED
Use a BACK-UP METHOD anytime you have sex.
KEEP TAKING ONE PILL EACH DAY until you can reach your doctor or clinic.

Pregnancy due to pill failure
The incidence of pill failure resulting in pregnancy is approximately less than 1.0% if taken every day as directed, but more typical failure rates are less than 3.0%. If failure does occur, the risk to the fetus is minimal.

RISKS TO THE FETUS
If you do become pregnant while using oral contraceptives, the risk to the fetus is small, on the order of no more than one per thousand. You should, however, discuss the risks to the developing child with your doctor.

Pregnancy after stopping the pill
There may be some delay in becoming pregnant after you stop using oral contraceptives, especially if you had irregular menstrual cycles before you used oral contraceptives. It may be advisable to postpone conception until you begin menstruating regularly once you have stopped taking the pill and desire pregnancy.
There does not appear to be any increase in birth defects in newborn babies when pregnancy occurs soon after stopping the pill.

Overdosage
Serious ill effects have not been reported following ingestion of large doses of oral contraceptives by young children. Overdosage may cause nausea and withdrawal bleeding in females. In case of overdosage, contact your health-care provider or pharmacist.

Other information
Your health-care provider will take a medical and family history before prescribing oral contraceptives and will examine you. The physical examination may be delayed to another time if you request it and the health-care provider believes that it is appropriate to postpone it. You should be reexamined at least once a year. Be sure to inform your health-care provider if there is a family history of any of the conditions listed previously in this leaflet. Be sure to keep all appointments with your health-care provider, because this is a time to determine if there are early signs of side effects of oral-contraceptive use.

Do not use the drug for any condition other than the one for which it was prescribed. This drug has been prescribed specifically for you; do not give it to others who may want birth-control pills.

HEALTH BENEFITS FROM ORAL CONTRACEPTIVES: See Triphasil-21.
Manufactured by:
Wyeth Laboratories Inc.
A Wyeth-Ayerst Company
Philadelphia, PA 19101
Shown in Product Identification Guide, page 345

TUBEX® Closed Injection System
[tū 'beks]

The TUBEX® closed injection system delivers injectable medication in accurately machine-measured doses with each sterile, prefilled cartridge-needle unit permanently identified up to the moment of injection. Precisely calibrated single-use cartridge-needle units eliminate cross contamination and minimize dosage errors. Super-sharp, siliconized needles minimize penetration pressure. Medication is easily delivered via the TUBEX Injector.

TUBEX sterile cartridge-needle units are ready for instant use, fit easily into the physician's bag, and are readily stored and inventoried in the office.

TAMP-R-TEL® (tamper-resistant package) — a clear, sturdy plastic package for all TUBEX narcotics and barbiturates — adds a new dimension to the handling and record keeping of these controlled drugs. In TAMP-R-TEL, each TUBEX sterile cartridge-needle unit is locked into an individual slot within the package by its own end-lock tab, which is easily broken to release the unit for use. Once the end-lock tab is broken, it is almost impossible to replace it. TAMP-R-TEL thus enhances package integrity, discourages pilferage and facilitates "at a glance" drug count.

The following products are currently available in TUBEX closed injection system. *For prescribing information on products listed, write to Professional Service, Wyeth-Ayerst Laboratories, P.O. Box 8299, Philadelphia, PA 19101, or contact your local Wyeth-Ayerst representative.*

Product and Needle Size Units Per Pkg	NDC 0008-

NARCOTICS in TAMP-R-TEL®
(tamper-resistant package)

CODEINE PHOSPHATE, USP ⓒ•
| 30 mg ($^1/_2$ gr.) (25 G × $^5/_8$″) 10—1 mL | 0728-01 |

| 60 mg (1 gr.) (25 G × $^5/_8$″) 10—1 mL | 0729-01 |

HYDROMORPHONE HYDROCHLORIDE, USP ⓒ•
| 2 mg ($^1/_{30}$ gr.) (22 G × $1^1/_4$″) 10—1 mL fill in 2 mL | 0295-01 |

| 4 mg ($^1/_{15}$ gr.) (22 G × $1^1/_4$″) 10—1 mL fill in 2 mL | 0296-01 |

MEPERGAN® (Meperidine HCl and Promethazine HCl) 25 mg each/mL ⓒ•
| (22 G × $1^1/_4$″) 10—2 mL | 0235-01 |

| 10 TUBEX® BLUNT POINTE™ Sterile Cartridge Units in TAMP-R-TEL® | 0235-50 |

MEPERIDINE HYDROCHLORIDE, USP ⓒ•
| 25 mg (22 G × $1^1/_4$″) 10—1 mL fill in 2 mL | 0601-02 |

| 25 mg 10 TUBEX® BLUNT POINTE™ Sterile Cartridge Units—1 mL fill in 2 mL | 0601-50 |

| 50 mg (22 G × $1^1/_4$″) 10—1 mL fill in 2 mL | 0602-02 |

| 50 mg 10 TUBEX® BLUNT POINTE™ Sterile Cartridge Units—1 mL fill in 2 mL in TAMP-R-TEL® | 0602-50 |

| 75 mg (22 G × $1^1/_4$″) 10—1 mL fill in 2 mL | 0605-02 |

| 75 mg 10 TUBEX® BLUNT POINTE™ Sterile Cartridge Units—1 mL fill in 2 mL in TAMP-R-TEL® | 0605-50 |

| 100 mg (22 G × $1^1/_4$″) 10—1 mL fill in 2 mL | 0613-02 |

| 100 mg 10 TUBEX® BLUNT POINTE™ Sterile Cartridge Units—1 mL fill in 2 mL in TAMP-R-TEL® | 0613-50 |

MORPHINE SULFATE, USP ⓒ•
| 2 mg ($^1/_{30}$ gr.) (25 G × $^5/_8$″) 10—1 mL | 0649-01 |

| 2 mg ($^1/_{30}$ gr.) 10 TUBEX® BLUNT POINTE™ Sterile Cartridge Units—2 mL in TAMP-R-TEL® | 0649-50 |

| 4 mg ($^1/_{15}$ gr.) (25 G × $^5/_8$″) 10—1 mL | 0653-01 |

| 4 mg ($^1/_{15}$ gr.) 10 TUBEX® BLUNT POINTE™ Sterile Cartridge Units—1 mL in TAMP-R-TEL® | 0653-50 |

| 8 mg ($^1/_8$ gr.) (22 G × $1^1/_4$″) 10—1 mL fill in 2 mL | 0655-03 |

| 8 mg ($^1/_8$ gr.) 10 TUBEX® BLUNT POINTE™ Sterile Cartridge Units—1 mL fill in 2 mL in TAMP-R-TEL® | 0655-50 |

| 10 mg ($^1/_6$ gr.) (22 G × $1^1/_4$″) 10—1 mL fill in 1 mL | 0656-01 |

| 10 mg ($^1/_6$ gr.) 10 TUBEX® BLUNT POINTE™ Sterile Cartridge Units—1 mL fill in 2 mL in TAMP-R-TEL® | 0656-50 |

| 15 mg ($^1/_4$ gr.) (22 G × $1^1/_4$″) 10—1 mL fill in 2 mL | 0657-01 |

| 15 mg ($^1/_4$ gr.) 10 TUBEX® BLUNT POINTE™ Sterile Cartridge Units—1 mL fill in 2 mL in TAMP-R-TEL® | 0657-50 |

BARBITURATES in TAMP-R-TEL®
PENTOBARBITAL SODIUM, USP ⓒ•
| 100 mg ($1^1/_2$ gr.) (22 G × $1^1/_4$″) 10—2 mL | 0303-02 |

PHENOBARBITAL SODIUM, USP ⓥ•
| 30 mg ($^1/_2$ gr.) (22 G × $1^1/_4$″) 10—1 mL | 0499-01 |

| 60 mg (1 gr.) (22 G × $1^1/_4$″) 10—1 mL | 0747-01 |

| 130 mg (2 gr.) (22 G × $1^1/_4$″) 10—1 mL | 0304-01 |

SECOBARBITAL SODIUM, USP ⓒ•
| 100 mg ($1^1/_2$ gr.) (22 G × $1^1/_4$″) 10—2 mL | 0305-02 |

• Narcotic order blank required.

ANTIBIOTICS
BICILLIN® C-R (Penicillin G Benzathine and Penicillin G Procaine Suspension) 300,000 U each/mL
| 600,000 U (21 G x 1″) (Pediatric use) 10—1 mL | 0026-37 |

| 1,200,000 U (21 G x 1″) (Pediatric use) 10—2 mL | 0026-36 |

| 1,200,000 U (21 G x $1^1/_4$″) 10—2 mL | 0026-35 |

| 2,400,000 U (18 G × 2″) 10—4 mL (disposable syringe) | 0026-22 |

BICILLIN C-R 900/300
(900,000 units Penicillin G Benzathine and 300,000 units Penicillin G Procaine in suspension)
| 1,200,000 U (21 G x $1^1/_4$″) 10—2 mL | 0079-35 |

| 1,200,000 U (21 G x 1″) (Pediatric use) 10—2 mL | 0079-36 |

BICILLIN LONG-ACTING (Sterile Penicillin G Benzathine Suspension)
| 600,000 U (21 G × 1″) 10—1 mL | 0021-37 |

| 1,200,000 U (21 G × $1^1/_4$″) 10—2 mL | 0021-35 |

| 2,400,000 U (18 G × 2″) 10—4 mL (disposable syringe) | 0021-12 |

WYCILLIN® (Sterile Penicillin G Procaine Suspension)
600,000 U (20 G × 1¼″)
10—1 mL 0018-10

1,200,000 U (20 G × 1¼″)
10—2 mL 0018-08

2,400,000 U (18 G × 2″)
10—4 mL 0018-12
(disposable syringe)

BIOLOGICALS
FluShield®
INFLUENZA VIRUS VACCINE
Trivalent, Types A and B
(chromatograph- and filtered-purified subvirion antigen)
1998-1999 Formula
(25 G × ⁵⁄₈″)
10—0.5 mL 0981-02

CARDIOVASCULAR AGENTS
DIGOXIN, USP
0.25 mg (22 G × 1¼″)
10—1 mL 0480-02

0.5 mg (22 G × 1¼″)
10—2 mL 0480-01

EPINEPHRINE, USP (1:1000)
(25 G × ⁵⁄₈″)
10—1 mL 0263-01

HEPARIN SODIUM, USP
1,000 USP units (22 G × 1¼″)
10—1 mL 0275-01

1,000 USP units
10 TUBEX® BLUNT POINTE™ Sterile
Cartridge Units—1 mL
in TAMP-R-TEL® 0275-50

2,500 USP units (25 G × ⁵⁄₈″)
10—1 mL 0482-01

5,000 USP units (25 G × ⁵⁄₈″)
10—0.5 mL 0277-02

5,000 USP units (25 G × ⁵⁄₈″)
50—0.5 mL 0277-03

5,000 USP units (25 G × ⁵⁄₈″)
10—1.0 mL 0278-02

7,500 USP units (25 G × ⁵⁄₈″)
10—1 mL 0293-01

10,000 USP units (25 G × ⁵⁄₈″)
10—1 mL 0277-01

20,000 USP units (25 G × ⁵⁄₈″)
10—1 mL 0276-01

SPECIAL AGENTS
ATIVAN® (Lorazepam) Ⓒⓥ
2 mg/mL (22 G × 1¼″)
10—1 mL fill in 2 mL 0581-02

2 mg/mL (22 G × 1¼″)
10—1 mL fill in 2 mL
in TAMP-R-TEL® 0581-06

2 mg/mL
10 TUBEX® BLUNT POINTE™ Sterile
Cartridge Units—1 mL fill
in 2 mL 0581-52

2 mg/mL
10 TUBEX® BLUNT POINTE™ Sterile
Cartridge Units—1 mL fill
in 2 mL in TAMP-R-TEL® 0581-53

4 mg/mL (22 G × 1¼″)
10—1 mL fill in 2 mL 0570-02

4 mg/mL (22 G × 1¼″)
10—1 mL fill in 2 mL
in TAMP-R-TEL® 0570-05

4 mg/mL
10 TUBEX® BLUNT POINTE™ Sterile
Cartridge Units—1 mL fill
in 2 mL 0570-50

4 mg/mL
10 TUBEX® BLUNT POINTE™ Sterile
Cartridge Units—1 mL fill in 2 mL
in TAMP-R-TEL® 0570-51

DIMENHYDRINATE, USP
50 mg (22 G × 1¼″)
10—1 mL 0485-01

DIPHENHYDRAMINE HYDROCHLORIDE, USP
50 mg (22 G × 1¼″)
10—1 mL 0384-01

HEPARIN FLUSH 2.5 mL KITS
25 USP units
(25 G × ⁵⁄₈″)
30 Kits 2528-02
Each Unit of Use Kit contains:
One 2.5 mL size (25 G × ⁵⁄₈″) TUBEX Heparin Lock Flush Solution, USP, 10 USP units per mL and two 2.5 mL size (25 G × ⁵⁄₈″) TUBEX Bacteriostatic Sodium Chloride Injection, USP.

HEPARIN FLUSH 2.5 mL KITS
25 USP units per TUBEX® BLUNT POINTE™ Sterile Cartridge Unit
30 Kits 2528-51
Each Unit of Use Kit contains:
One TUBEX BLUNT POINTE (2.5 mL) Heparin Lock Flush Solution, USP, 25 USP units heparin sodium per TUBEX BLUNT POINTE or 10 USP units per mL. Two TUBEX BLUNT POINTE (2.5 mL) Bacteriostatic Sodium Chloride Injection, USP.

250 USP units
(25 G × ⁵⁄₈″)
30 Kits 2529-02
Each Unit of Use Kit contains:
One 2.5 mL size (25 G × ⁵⁄₈″) TUBEX Heparin Lock Flush Solution, USP, 100 USP units per mL and two 2.5 mL size (25 G × ⁵⁄₈″) TUBEX Bacteriostatic Sodium Chloride Injection, USP.

250 USP units per TUBEX® BLUNT POINTE™ Sterile Cartridge Unit
30 Kits 2529-51
Each Unit of Use Kit contains:
One TUBEX BLUNT POINTE (2.5 mL) Heparin Lock Flush Solution, USP, 250 USP units heparin sodium per TUBEX BLUNT POINTE or 100 USP units per mL. Two TUBEX BLUNT POINTE (2.5 mL) Bacteriostatic Sodium Chloride Injection, USP.

HEPARIN FLUSH KITS
10 USP units
(25 G × ⁵⁄₈″)
50 Kits 2528-01
Each Unit of Use Kit contains:
One 1 mL size (25 G × ⁵⁄₈″) TUBEX Heparin Lock Flush Solution, USP, 10 USP units per mL and two 2.5 mL size (25 G × ⁵⁄₈″) TUBEX Bacteriostatic Sodium Chloride Injection, USP.

10 USP units per TUBEX® BLUNT POINTE™ Sterile Cartridge Unit
50 Kits 2528-50
Each Unit of Use Kit contains:
One 1 mL size TUBEX BLUNT POINTE Heparin Lock Flush Solution, USP, 10 USP units per mL and two 2.5 mL size TUBEX BLUNT POINTE Bacteriostatic Sodium Chloride Injection, USP.

100 USP units
(25 G × ⁵⁄₈″)
50 Kits 2529-01
Each Unit of Use Kit contains:
One 1 mL size (25 G × ⁵⁄₈″) TUBEX Heparin Lock Flush Solution, USP, 100 USP units per mL and two 2.5 mL size (25 G × ⁵⁄₈″) TUBEX Bacteriostatic Sodium Chloride Injection, USP.

100 USP units per TUBEX® BLUNT POINTE™ Sterile Cartridge Unit
50 Kits 2529-50
Each Unit of Use Kit contains:
One 1 mL size TUBEX BLUNT POINTE Heparin Lock Flush Solution, USP, 100 USP units per mL and two 2.5 mL size TUBEX BLUNT POINTE Bacteriostatic Sodium Chloride Injection, USP.

HEPARIN FLUSH 1 mL KITS
10 USP units
(25 G × ⁵⁄₈″)
50 Kits 2528-03
Each Unit of Use Kit contains:
One 1 mL size (25 G × ⁵⁄₈″) TUBEX Heparin Lock Flush Solution, USP, 10 USP units per mL and two 1 mL size (25 G × ⁵⁄₈″) TUBEX Bacteriostatic Sodium Chloride Injection, USP.

10 USP units per TUBEX® BLUNT POINTE™ Sterile Cartridge Unit
50 Kits 2528-52
Each Unit of Use Kit contains:
One 1 mL size TUBEX BLUNT POINTE Heparin Lock Flush Solution, USP, 10 USP units per mL and two 1 mL size TUBEX BLUNT POINTE Bacteriostatic Sodium Chloride Injection, USP.

100 USP units
(25 G × ⁵⁄₈″)
50 Kits 2529-03
Each Unit of Use Kit contains:
One 1 mL size (25 G × ⁵⁄₈″) TUBEX Heparin Lock Flush Solution, USP, 100 USP units per mL and two 1 mL size (25 G × ⁵⁄₈″) TUBEX Bacteriostatic Sodium Chloride Injection, USP.

100 USP units per TUBEX® BLUNT POINTE™ Sterile Cartridge Unit
50 Kits 2529-52
Each Unit of Use Kit contains:
One 1 mL size TUBEX BLUNT POINTE Heparin Lock Flush Solution, USP, 100 USP units per mL and two 1 mL size TUBEX BLUNT POINTE Bacteriostatic Sodium Chloride Injection, USP.

HEPARIN LOCK FLUSH Solution, USP
10 USP units per mL (25 G × ⁵⁄₈″)
50—1 mL 0523-01

100 USP units per mL (25 G × ⁵⁄₈″)
50—1 mL 0487-01

10 USP units per mL—25 USP units per TUBEX
(25 G × ⁵⁄₈″)
50—2.5 mL 0523-02

100 USP units per mL—250 USP units per TUBEX
(25 G × ⁵⁄₈″)
50—2.5 mL 0487-03

10 USP units per mL
50 TUBEX® BLUNT POINTE™ Sterile
Cartridge Units—1 mL 0523-50

100 USP units per mL
50 TUBEX® BLUNT POINTE™ Sterile
Cartridge Units—1 mL 0487-50

10 USP units per mL—25 USP units per TUBEX
50 TUBEX® BLUNT POINTE™ Sterile
Cartridge Units—2.5 mL 0523-51

100 USP units per mL—250 USP units per TUBEX
50 TUBEX® BLUNT POINTE™ Sterile
Cartridge Units—2.5 mL 0487-51

NORMIFLO® (ardeparin sodium)
5,000 anti-Xa Units/0.5 mL
(25 G × ⁵⁄₈″)
10—0.5 mL fill in 1 mL TUBEX 0860-01

10,000 anti-Xa Units/0.5 mL
(25 G × ⁵⁄₈″)
10—0.5 mL fill in 1 mL TUBEX 0861-01

PHENERGAN® (Promethazine HCl)
25 mg (22 G × 1¼″)
10—1 mL 0416-01

50 mg (22 G × 1¼″)
10—1 mL 0417-01

SODIUM CHLORIDE, USP (Bacteriostatic)
(25 G × ⁵⁄₈″)
50—1 mL 0333-08

50 TUBEX® BLUNT POINTE™ Sterile
Cartridge Units—1 mL 0333-51

(22 G × 1¼″)
50—2.5 mL 0333-05

(25 G × ⁵⁄₈″)
50—2.5 mL 0333-02

50 TUBEX® BLUNT POINTE™ Sterile
Cartridge Units—2.5 mL 0333-50

Shown in Product Identification Guide, page 345
PLEASE NOTE: THE WYETH-AYERST METAL TUBEX HYPODERMIC SYRINGE AND TUBEX FAST-TRAK SYRINGE HAVE BEEN DISCONTINUED AND REPLACED BY THE TUBEX INJECTOR. EXCHANGE OF THESE DISCONTINUED SYRINGES IS AVAILABLE, FREE OF

Continued on next page

Tubex System—Cont.

CHARGE, FROM YOUR WYETH-AYERST AND/OR EL-KINS-SINN SALES REPRESENTATIVE, OR FROM WYETH-AYERST DIRECTLY. FOR LOADING AND UNLOADING INFORMATION OF THESE DISCONTINUED SYRINGES, CONTACT THE MEDICAL AFFAIRS DEPARTMENT, AT WYETH-AYERST LABORATORIES, P.O. BOX 8299, PHILADELPHIA, PA 19101.

TUBEX® Injector
NOTE: The TUBEX® Injector is reusable: do not discard.

DIRECTIONS FOR USE:

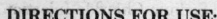
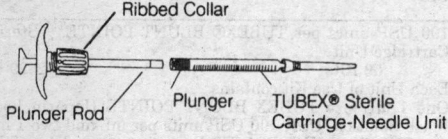

TUBEX® Sterile Cartridge-Needle Unit

TUBEX® BLUNT POINTE™ Sterile Cartridge Unit

DIRECTIONS FOR USE:

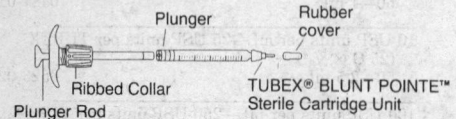

TUBEX® BLUNT POINTE™ Sterile Cartridge Unit is intended for use with injection sets specifically manufactured as "needle-less" injection systems. TUBEX® BLUNT POINTE™ Sterile Cartridge Unit is compatible with Abbott's LifeShield® prepierced reseal injection site, Baxter's Interlink® Injection Site and B. Braun Medical's SafSite® Reflux Valve. Consult manufacturer's recommendations regarding "Directions for Use" of the "needle-less" injection system.

To load a TUBEX® Sterile Cartridge-Needle Unit into the TUBEX® Injector
1. Turn the ribbed collar to the "OPEN" position until it stops.

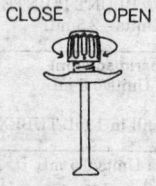

2. Hold the Injector with the open end up and fully insert the TUBEX® Sterile Cartridge Unit.
Firmly tighten the ribbed collar in the direction of the "CLOSE" arrow.

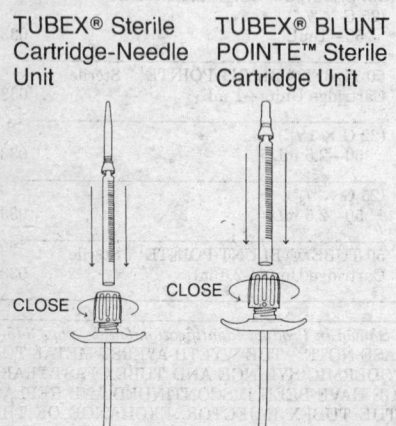

3. Thread the plunger rod into the plunger of the TUBEX® Sterile Cartridge Unit until slight resistance is felt.

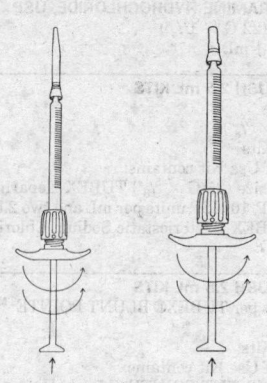

The Injector is now ready for use in the usual manner.

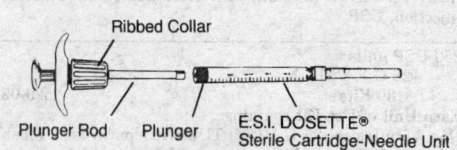

To load an E.S.I. DOSETTE® Sterile Cartridge-Needle Unit into the TUBEX® Injector
1. Turn the ribbed collar to the "OPEN" position until it stops.

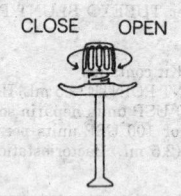

2. Hold the Injector with the open end up and fully insert the DOSETTE® Sterile Cartridge-Needle Unit.
Firmly tighten the ribbed collar in the direction of the "CLOSE" arrow.

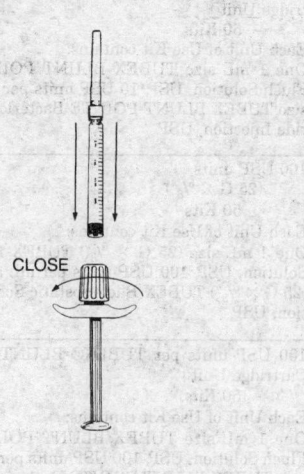

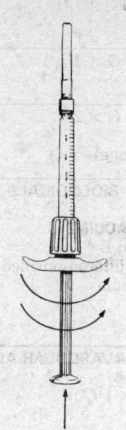

3. Thread the plunger rod into the plunger of the E.S.I. DOSETTE® Sterile Cartridge-Needle Unit until slight resistance is felt.

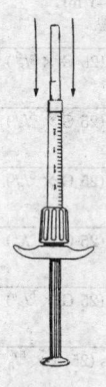

4. Engage the needle-cap assembly by pulling the cap down over the silver cartridge hub. The needle is fully engaged when the silver hub is completely covered.
The Injector is now ready for use in the usual manner.

To administer TUBEX®/DOSETTE® Sterile Cartridge-Needle Units
Method of administration is the same as with conventional syringe. Remove needle cover by grasping it securely; twist and pull. Introduce needle into patient, aspirate by pulling back slightly on the plunger, and inject.

To administer TUBEX® BLUNT POINTE™ Sterile Cartridge Units
"Needle-less" IV set administration is similar to administration with conventional syringes. Remove rubber cover by grasping it securely; twist and pull. For B. Braun Medical's SafSite® Reflux Valves, aseptically swab

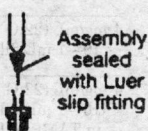

Assembly sealed with Luer slip fitting

the luer slip fitting of the BLUNT POINTE™ sterile cartridge tip assembly with a sterile, individually wrapped, saturated 70% Isopropyl Alcohol swab. This action will remove the lubricant coating from the tip to facilitate a tight seal. Introduce TUBEX® BLUNT POINTE™ Sterile Cartridge Unit into the "needle-less" IV set as per manufacturer's "Directions for Use."

To remove the empty TUBEX®/DOSETTE® Cartridge Unit and dispose into a vertical disposal container

1. Do not recap the needle/point. Disengage the plunger rod.

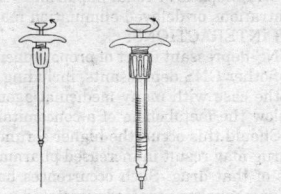

2. Hold the Injector, needle/point pointing down, over a verticle disposal container and loosen the ribbed collar. TUBEX®/DOSETTE® Cartridge Unit will drop into the container.

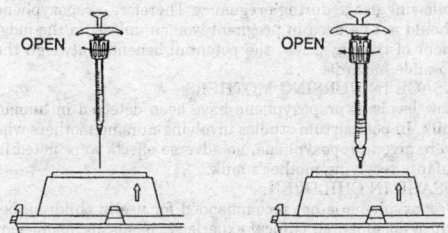

3. Discard the cover.

To remove the empty TUBEX®/DOSETTE® Cartridge Unit and dispose into a horizontal (mailbox) disposal container

1. Do not recap the needle/point. Disengage the plunger rod.
2. Open the horizontal (mailbox) disposal container. Insert TUBEX®/DOSETTE® Cartridge Unit, needle/point pointing down, halfway into container. Close the container lid on cartridge. Loosen ribbed collar; TUBEX®/DOSETTE® Cartridge Unit will drop into the container.

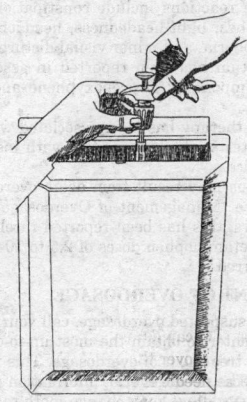

3. Discard the cover.

The TUBEX® Injector is reusable and should not be discarded.

Used TUBEX®/DOSETTE® Cartridge Units should not be employed for successive injections or as multiple-dose containers. They are intended to be used only once and discarded. **NOTE:** Any graduated markings on TUBEX®/DOSETTE® Sterile Cartridge Units are to be used only as a guide in mixing, withdrawing, or administering measured doses.

Wyeth-Ayerst does not recommend and will not accept responsibility for the use of any cartridge-needle units or needle-less system other than TUBEX® or E.S.I. DOSETTE® Cartridge Units in the TUBEX® Injector.

The ESI DOSETTE® cartridge holder has been discontinued. For instructions on its use, contact Medical Affairs, Wyeth-Ayerst Laboratories, P.O. Box 8299, Phila., PA 19101.
Manufactured by:
Wyeth Laboratories Inc.
A Wyeth-Ayerst Company
Philadelphia, Pa 19101
Shown in Product Identification Guide, page 345

TYPHOID VACCINE ℞
USP

DESCRIPTION

Typhoid Vaccine, USP is a saline suspension containing not more than 1000 million Salmonella typhosa (Ty-2 strain) organisms per mL. After growing on veal infusion agar (containing 0.5 percent sodium chloride, 2 percent peptone, and 5 percent agar), the bacteria are washed off the medium, suspended in buffered sodium chloride injection, and killed by a combination of phenol and heat. Phenol (0.5 percent) is added to the final vaccine as preservative. Typhoid Vaccine, USP is tested for safety, potency, and purity and standardized according to F.D.A. Additional Standards for Bacterial Vaccines, 21 C.F.R. 620.10-620.15.

INDICATIONS

Typhoid Vaccine, USP is indicated for active immunization against typhoid fever. Based on data obtained from field studies, it has been estimated that typhoid vaccine is 70% or more effective in preventing typhoid fever, depending in part on the degree of exposure.
Routine immunization against typhoid is no longer recommended for persons residing in the United States. Selective immunization is indicated in the following situations:
1. Intimate exposure to a known typhoid carrier, as would occur with continued household contact.
2. Foreign travel to areas where typhoid fever is endemic.
Although at one time typhoid immunization was suggested for persons attending summer camps or for residents of areas where flooding has occurred, there are no data to support continuation of such practices.[1,2]

CONTRAINDICATIONS

Administration should be postponed in the presence of acute respiratory or other active infection.
A severe systemic or allergic reaction following a prior dose is a contraindication to further use.[3]

PRECAUTIONS

A sterile syringe and needle should be used for each patient to prevent transmission of hepatitis B virus and other infectious agents from one person to another.
Specific information concerning use of typhoid vaccine during pregnancy is not available. However, as with other inactivated bacterial vaccines, its use is not contraindicated during pregnancy unless the intended recipient has manifested significant systemic or allergic reactions following administration of prior doses. Use of typhoid vaccine during pregnancy should be individualized to reflect actual need.
Before the injection of any biological, the physician should take all precautions known for prevention of allergic or any other side reactions. This should include: A review of the patient's history regarding possible sensitivity; the ready availability of epinephrine 1:1000 and other appropriate agents used for control of immediate allergic reactions; and a knowledge of the recent literature pertaining to use of the biological concerned.

REACTIONS

Most recipients of typhoid vaccine experience some degree of local and systemic response, usually beginning within 24 hours of administration and persisting for one or two days. Local reactions are usually manifested by erythema, induration, and tenderness and should be expected in all those injected intracutaneously.
Systemic manifestations may include malaise, headache, myalgia, and elevated temperature.

DOSAGE

PRIMARY IMMUNIZATION
1. Adults and children over 10 years of age:
Two doses of 0.5 mL each, administered subcutaneously, at an interval of four or more weeks.
2. Children less than 10 years of age:
Two doses of 0.25 mL, each administered subcutaneously, at an interval of four or more weeks.
In instances where there is insufficient time for two doses administered at the specified intervals, three doses of the appropriate volume may be given at weekly intervals.
BOOSTER DOSES
1. Adults and children over 10 years of age:
0.5 mL, administered subcutaneously, or 0.1 mL, injected intracutaneously (intradermally).
2. Children 6 months to 10 years of age:
0.25 mL, administered subcutaneously, or 0.1 mL, intracutaneously (intradermally)
Under conditions of continued or repeated exposure, a booster dose should be given at least every three years. In instances where an interval of more than three years has elapsed since primary immunization or the last booster dose, a single booster dose is considered sufficient; it is not necessary to repeat the primary immunizing series.

ADMINISTRATION

Shake vial vigorously before withdrawing each dose.
Before injection, the rubber diaphragm of the vial and the skin over the site to be injected should be cleansed and prepared with a suitable germicide.
After insertion of the needle, aspirate to help avoid inadvertent injection into a blood vessel.

HOW SUPPLIED

Typhoid Vaccine, USP is supplied in vials of 5 mL and 10 mL, each containing 8 units per mL.

REFERENCES

1. Recommendations of the Public Health Service Advisory Committee on Immunization Practices—Typhoid Vaccine. Morbidity and Mortality Weekly Report 27 (No. 27): 231, 1978.
2. Report of the Committee on Infectious Diseases, American Academy of Pediatrics, 1982 (Red Book).
3. Recommendations of the Public Health Service Advisory Committee on Immunization Practices—General Recommendations on Immunization. Morbidity and Mortality Weekly Report 29 (No.7): 76, 1980.
U.S. Gov't License No. 3
Manufactured by:
Wyeth Laboratories Inc.,
A Wyeth-Ayerst Company
Marietta, PA 17547.

WYCILLIN® ℞
[wi-sil´in]
(penicillin G procaine suspension)
INJECTION

FOR DEEP INTRAMUSCULAR INJECTION ONLY

DESCRIPTION

This product is designed to provide a stable aqueous suspension of penicillin G procaine, ready for immediate use. This eliminates the necessity for addition of any diluent, required for the usual dry formulation of injectable penicillin. Each TUBEX Sterile Cartridge-Needle Unit, 1,200,000 units (2 mL size) or 600,000 units (1 mL size), or disposable syringe, 2,400,000 units (4 mL size), contains penicillin G procaine in a stabilized aqueous suspension with sodium citrate buffer; and as w/v, approximately 0.5% lecithin, 0.5% carboxymethylcellulose, 0.5% povidone, 0.1% methylparaben, and 0.01% propylparaben.
Wycillin must be stored in a refrigerator. Keep from freezing. This will prevent deterioration and assure that no significant loss of potency occurs within the expiration date.
Wycillin suspension in the TUBEX and disposable syringe formulations is viscous and opaque. Read "**Contraindications**," "**Warnings**," "**Precautions**," and "**Dosage and Administration**" sections prior to use.

HOW SUPPLIED

Wycillin® (penicillin G procaine suspension) is supplied in packages of 10 TUBEX® Sterile Cartridge-Needle Units (21 gauge, thin wall, 1¼ inch needle), as follows:
1 mL size, containing 600,000 units per TUBEX, NDC 0008-0018-34.
2 mL size, containing 1,200,000 units per TUBEX, NDC 0008-0018-35.
Store in a refrigerator.
Keep from freezing.
ALSO AVAILABLE:
Wycillin (penicillin G procaine suspension) is also available in packages of 10 disposable syringes as follows:
4 mL size, containing 2,400,000 units per syringe (18 gauge × 2 inch needle), NDC 0008-0018-12.
Manufactured by:
Wyeth Laboratories Inc.
A Wyeth-Ayerst Company
Philadelphia, PA 19101
For prescribing information write to Professional Service, Wyeth-Ayerst Laboratories, P.O. Box 8299, Philadelphia, PA 19101, or contact your local Wyeth-Ayerst representative.

WYDASE® ℞
[wi-dās]
(hyaluronidase)

DESCRIPTION

Wydase, a protein enzyme, is a preparation of highly purified bovine testicular hyaluronidase. The exact chemical structure of this enzyme is unknown. Wydase is available in two dosage forms:
WYDASE LYOPHILIZED
Hyaluronidase, dehydrated in the frozen state under high vacuum, with lactose and thimerosal (mercury derivative), is supplied as a sterile, white, odorless, amorphous solid and is to be reconstituted with Sodium Chloride Injection, USP, before use, usually in the proportion of one mL per 150 USP units of hyaluronidase (Wydase Lyophilized).
Each vial of 1,500 USP units contains 1.0 mg thimerosal (mercury derivative), added as a preservative, and 13.3 mg

Continued on next page

Wydase—Cont.

lactose. Each vial of 150 USP units contains 0.075 mg thimerosal (mercury derivative), added as a preservative, and 2.66 mg lactose.

WYDASE STABILIZED SOLUTION

A hyaluronidase injection solution ready for use, colorless and odorless, containing 150 USP units of hyaluronidase per mL with 8.5 mg sodium chloride, 1 mg edetate disodium, 0.4 mg calcium chloride, monobasic sodium phosphate buffer, and not more than 0.1 mg thimerosal (mercury derivative).

The USP and the NF hyaluronidase units are the equivalent to the turbidity-reducing (TR) unit and to the International Unit.

HOW SUPPLIED

Wydase® Lyophilized is supplied as follows:
150 USP (TR) units of hyaluronidase
NDC 0008-0121-01, 1 mL vial, as single vials.
Not Recommended for IV Use.
Store at controlled room temperature in a dry place. Store sterile reconstituted solution below 30°C (86°F). Use within 24 hours.
Following reconstitution, store vial in upright position.
1,500 USP (TR) units of hyaluronidase
NDC 0008-0149-01, 10 mL vial, as single vials.
Not Recommended for IV Use.
Store at controlled room temperature in a dry place. Store sterile reconstituted solution below 30°C (86°F). Use within 14 days.
Following reconstitution, store vial in upright position.
Wydase® Stabilized Solution is supplied as follows:
150 USP (TR) units of hyaluronidase per mL
NDC 0008-0170-01, 1 mL vial, as single vials.
NDC 0008-0170-02, 10 mL vial, as single vials.
Not Recommended for IV Use.
Store in a refrigerator.
Do not use if solution is discolored or contains a precipitate.

Manufactured by:
Wyeth Laboratories Inc.
A Wyeth-Ayerst Company
Philadelphia, PA 19101

For prescribing information write to Professional Service, Wyeth-Ayerst Laboratories, P.O. Box 8299, Philadelphia, PA 19101, or contact your local Wyeth-Ayerst representative.

WYGESIC® Ⓒ ℞

[wi-je 'zik]
(propoxyphene HCl and acetaminophen)
Tablets

DESCRIPTION

Wygesic tablets contain 65 mg propoxyphene HCl and 650 mg acetaminophen. The inactive ingredients present are cellulose, D&C Yellow 10, FD&C Blue 1, FD&C Yellow 6, hydrogenated vegetable oil, hydroxypropyl methylcellulose, methylcellulose, polacrilin potassium, polyethylene glycol, and titanium dioxide.

Propoxyphene hydrochloride is an odorless white crystalline powder with a bitter taste. It is freely soluble in water. Chemically, it is [S-(R*,S*)]-α-[2-(dimethylamino)-1-methylethyl]-α-phenylbenzeneethanol, propanoate (ester), hydrochloride, which can be represented by the following structural formula:

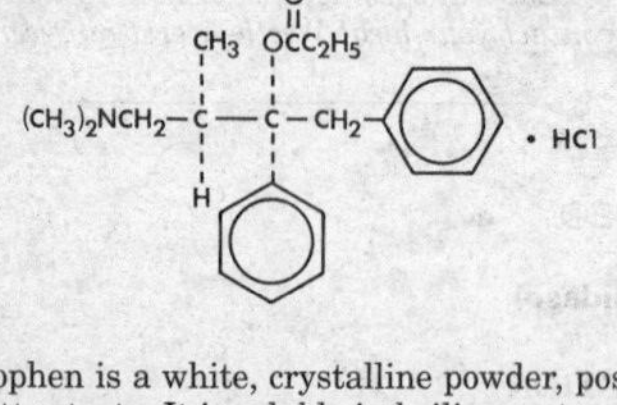

Acetaminophen is a white, crystalline powder, possessing a slightly bitter taste. It is soluble in boiling water and freely soluble in alcohol. Chemically, it is N-Acetyl-p-aminophenol, which can be presented by the following structural formula:

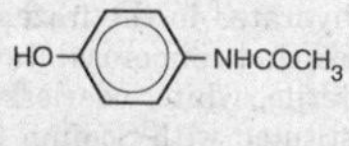

CLINICAL PHARMACOLOGY

Propoxyphene is a centrally acting narcotic analgesic agent. Equimolar doses of propoxyphene hydrochloride provide similar plasma concentrations. Following administration of 65, 130, or 195 mg of propoxyphene hydrochloride, the bioavailability of propoxyphene is equivalent to that of 100, 200, or 300 mg respectively of propoxyphene napsylate. Peak plasma concentrations of propoxyphene are reached in 2 to $2^1/_2$ hours. After a 65 mg oral dose of propoxyphene hydrochloride, peak plasma levels of 0.05 to 0.1 mcg/mL are achieved.

Repeated doses of propoxyphene at 6-hour intervals lead to increasing plasma concentrations, with a plateau after the ninth dose at 48 hours.

Propoxyphene is metabolized in the liver to yield norpropoxyphene. Propoxyphene has a half-life of 6 to 12 hours, whereas that of norpropoxyphene is 30 to 36 hours.

Norpropoxyphene has substantially less central nervous system depressant effect than propoxyphene, but a greater local anesthetic effect, which is similar to that of amitriptyline and antiarrhythmic agents, such as lidocaine and quinidine.

In animal studies in which propoxyphene and norpropoxyphene were continuously infused in large amounts, intracardiac conduction time (P-R and QRS intervals) was prolonged. Any intracardiac conduction delay attributable to high concentrations of norpropoxyphene may be of relatively long duration.

ACTIONS

Propoxyphene is a mild narcotic analgesic structurally related to methadone. The potency of propoxyphene hydrochloride is from two-thirds to equal that of codeine.

Propoxyphene hydrochloride and acetaminophen provide the analgesic activity of propoxyphene napsylate and the antipyretic-analgesic activity of acetaminophen.

The combination of propoxyphene and acetaminophen produces greater analgesia than that produced by either propoxyphene or acetaminophen alone.

INDICATIONS

Wygesic is indicated for the relief of mild-to-moderate pain, either when pain is present alone or when it is accompanied by fever.

CONTRAINDICATIONS

Hypersensitivity to propoxyphene or to acetaminophen.

WARNINGS

Do not prescribe propoxyphene for patients who are suicidal or addiction-prone.

Prescribe propoxyphene with caution for patients taking tranquilizers or antidepressant drugs and patients who use alcohol in excess.

Tell your patients not to exceed the recommended dose and to limit their intake of alcohol.

Propoxyphene products in excessive doses, either alone or in combination with other CNS depressants, including alcohol, are a major cause of drug-related deaths. Fatalities within the first hour of overdosage are not uncommon. In a survey of deaths due to overdosage conducted in 1975, in approximately 20% of the fatal cases, death occurred within the first hour (5% occurred within 15 minutes). Propoxyphene should not be taken in doses higher than those recommended by the physician. The judicious prescribing of propoxyphene is essential to the safe use of this drug. With patients who are depressed or suicidal, consideration should be given to the use of nonnarcotic analgesics. Patients should be cautioned about the concomitant use of propoxyphene products and alcohol because of potentially serious CNS-additive effects of these agents. Because of its added depressant effects, propoxyphene should be prescribed with caution for those patients whose medical condition requires the concomitant administration of sedatives, tranquilizers, muscle relaxants, antidepressants, or other CNS-depressant drugs. Patients should be advised of the additive depressant effects of these combinations.

Many of the propoxyphene-related deaths have occurred in patients with previous histories of emotional disturbances or suicidal ideation or attempts as well as histories of misuse of tranquilizers, alcohol, and other CNS-active drugs. Some deaths have occurred as a consequence of the accidental ingestion of excessive quantities of propoxyphene alone or in combination with other drugs. Patients taking propoxyphene should be warned not to exceed the dosage recommended by the physician.

DRUG DEPENDENCE:

Propoxyphene, when taken in higher-than-recommended doses over long periods of time, can produce drug dependence characterized by psychic dependence and, less frequently, physical dependence and tolerance. Propoxyphene will only partially suppress the withdrawal syndrome in individuals physically dependent on morphine or other narcotics. The abuse liability of propoxyphene is qualitatively similar to that of codeine although quantitatively less, and propoxyphene should be prescribed with the same degree of caution appropriate to the use of codeine.

USAGE IN AMBULATORY PATIENTS:

Propoxyphene may impair the mental and/or physical abilities required for the performance of potentially hazardous tasks, such as driving a car or operating machinery. The patient should be cautioned accordingly.

PRECAUTIONS

GENERAL:

Propoxyphene should be administered with caution to patients with hepatic or renal impairment since higher serum concentrations or delayed elimination may occur.

DRUG INTERACTIONS:

The CNS-depressant effect of propoxyphene is additive with that of other CNS depressants, including alcohol.

As is the case with many medicinal agents, propoxyphene may slow the metabolism of a concomitantly administered drug. Should this occur, the higher serum concentrations of that drug may result in increased pharmacologic or adverse effects of that drug. Such occurrences have been reported when propoxyphene was administered to patients on antidepressants, anticonvulsants, or warfarin-like drugs.

USAGE IN PREGNANCY:

Safe use in pregnancy has not been established relative to possible adverse effects on fetal development. Instances of withdrawal symptoms in the neonate have been reported following usage during pregnancy. Therefore, propoxyphene should not be used in pregnant women unless, in the judgment of the physician, the potential benefits outweigh the possible hazards.

USAGE IN NURSING MOTHERS:

Low levels of propoxyphene have been detected in human milk. In postpartum studies involving nursing mothers who were given propoxyphene, no adverse effects were noted in infants receiving mother's milk.

USAGE IN CHILDREN:

Propoxyphene is not recommended for use in children, because documented clinical experience has been insufficient to establish safety and a suitable dosage regimen in the pediatric age group.

A Patient Information Sheet is available for this product. See text following "How Supplied" section below.

ADVERSE REACTIONS

In a survey conducted in hospitalized patients, less than 1% of patients taking propoxyphene hydrochloride at recommended doses experienced side effects. The most frequently reported have been dizziness, sedation, nausea, and vomiting. Some of these adverse reactions may be alleviated if the patient lies down.

Other adverse reactions include constipation, abdominal pain, skin rashes, light-headedness, headache, weakness, euphoria, dysphoria, and minor visual disturbances.

Liver dysfunction has been reported in association with both active components of propoxyphene and acetaminophen tablets.

Propoxyphene therapy has been associated with abnormal liver-function tests and, more rarely, with instances of reversible jaundice.

Hepatic necrosis may result from acute overdoses of acetaminophen (see "Management of Overdosage"). In chronic ethanol abusers, this has been reported rarely with short-term use of acetaminophen doses of 2.5 to 10 g/day. Fatalities have occurred.

MANAGEMENT OF OVERDOSAGE

In all cases of suspected overdosage, call your regional Poison Control Center to obtain the most up-to-date information about the treatment of overdosage. This recommendation is made because, in general, information regarding the treatment of overdosage may change more rapidly than do package inserts.

Initial consideration should be given to the management of the CNS effects of propoxyphene overdosage. Resuscitative measures should be initiated promptly.

SYMPTOMS OF PROPOXYPHENE OVERDOSAGE:

The manifestations of acute overdosage with propoxyphene are those of narcotic overdosage. The patient is usually somnolent, but may be stuporous or comatose and convulsing. Respiratory depression is characteristic. The ventilatory rate and/or tidal volume is decreased, which results in cyanosis and hypoxia. Pupils, initially pinpoint, may become dilated as hypoxia increases. Cheyne-Stokes respiration and apnea may occur. Blood pressure and heart rate are usually normal initially, but blood pressure falls and cardiac performance deteriorates, which ultimately results in pulmonary edema and circulatory collapse unless the respiratory depression is corrected and adequate ventilation is restored promptly. Cardiac arrhythmias and conduction delay may be present. A combined respiratory-metabolic acidosis occurs, owing to retained CO_2 (hypercapnea) and to lactic acid formed during anaerobic glycolysis. Acidosis may be severe if large amounts of salicylates have also been ingested. Death may occur.

TREATMENT OF PROPOXYPHENE OVERDOSAGE:

Attention should be directed first to establishing a patent airway and to restoring ventilation. Mechanically assisted ventilation, with or without oxygen, may be required, and positive-pressure respiration may be desirable if pulmonary edema is present.

The narcotic antagonist naloxone hydrochloride will markedly reduce the degree of respiratory depression, and 0.4 to 2 mg should be administered promptly, preferably intrave-

nously. If the desired degree of counteraction with improvement in respiratory function is not obtained, naloxone should be repeated at 2- to 3-minute intervals. The duration of action of the antagonist may be brief. If no response is observed after 10 mg of naloxone have been administered, the diagnosis of propoxyphene toxicity should be questioned. Naloxone hydrochloride may also be administered by continuous intravenous infusion.

TREATMENT OF PROPOXYPHENE OVERDOSAGE IN CHILDREN:

The usual initial dose of naloxone in children is 0.01 mg/kg body weight given intravenously. If this dose does not result in the desired degree of clinical improvement, a subsequent increased dose of 0.1 mg/kg body weight may be administered. If an IV route of administration is not available, naloxone may be administered IM or subcutaneously in divided doses. If necessary, naloxone can be diluted with sterile water for injection.

Blood gases, pH, and electrolytes should be monitored in order that acidosis and any electrolyte disturbance present may be corrected promptly. Acidosis, hypoxia, and generalized CNS depression predispose to the development of cardiac arrhythmias. Ventricular fibrillation or cardiac arrest may occur and necessitate the full complement of cardiopulmonary resuscitation (CPR) measures. Respiratory acidosis rapidly subsides as ventilation is restored and hypercapnea eliminated, but lactic acidosis may require intravenous bicarbonate for prompt correction.

Electrocardiographic monitoring is essential. Prompt correction of hypoxia, acidosis, and electrolyte disturbance (when present) will help prevent these cardiac complications and will increase the effectiveness of agents administered to restore normal cardiac function.

In addition to the use of a narcotic antagonist, the patient may require careful titration with an anticonvulsant to control convulsions. Analeptic drugs (for example, caffeine or amphetamine) should not be used because of their tendency to precipitate convulsions.

General supportive measures, in addition to oxygen, include, when necessary, intravenous fluids, vasopressor-inotropic compounds, and, when infection is likely, anti-infective agents. Gastric lavage may be useful, and activated charcoal can adsorb a significant amount of ingested propoxyphene. Dialysis is of little value in poisoning due to propoxyphene. Efforts should be made to determine whether other agents, such as alcohol, barbiturates, tranquilizers, or other CNS depressants, were also ingested, since these increase CNS depression as well as cause specific toxic effects.

SYMPTOMS OF ACETAMINOPHEN OVERDOSAGE:

Shortly after oral ingestion of an overdosage of acetaminophen and for the next 24 hours, anorexia, nausea, vomiting, and abdominal pain have been noted. The patient may then present no symptoms, but evidence of liver dysfunction may be apparent during the next 24 to 48 hours, with elevated serum transaminase and lactic dehydrogenase levels, an increase in serum bilirubin concentrations, and a prolonged prothrombin time. Death from hepatic failure may result 3 to 7 days after overdosage.

Acute renal failure may accompany the hepatic dysfunction and has been noted in patients who do not exhibit signs of fulminant hepatic failure. Typically, renal impairment is more apparent 6 to 9 days after ingestion of the overdose.

TREATMENT OF ACETAMINOPHEN OVERDOSAGE: Acetaminophen in massive overdosage may cause hepatic toxicity in some patients. In all cases of suspected overdose, you may wish to call your regional poison center for assistance in diagnosis and for directions in the use of N-acetylcysteine as an antidote.

In adults, hepatic toxicity has rarely been reported with acute overdoses of less than 10 g and fatalities with less than 15 g. Importantly, young children seem to be more resistant than adults to the hepatotoxic effect of an acetaminophen overdose. Despite this, the measures outlined below should be initiated in any adult or child suspected of having ingested an acetaminophen overdose. Clinical and laboratory evidence of hepatic toxicity may not be apparent until 48 to 72 hours postingestion. Early symptoms following a potentially hepatotoxic overdose may include: nausea, vomiting, diaphoresis, and general malaise.

The stomach should be emptied promptly by lavage or by induction of emesis with syrup of ipecac. Patients' estimates of the quantity of a drug ingested are notoriously unreliable. Therefore, if an acetaminophen overdose is suspected, a serum acetaminophen assay should be obtained as early as possible, but no sooner than four hours following ingestion. Liver-function studies should be obtained initially and repeated at 24-hour intervals.

The antidote, N-acetylcysteine, should be administered as early as possible, preferably within 16 hours of the overdose ingestion for optimal results, but in any case, within 24 hours. Following recovery, there are no residual, structural or functional hepatic abnormalities.

ANIMAL TOXICOLOGY:

The acute lethal doses of the hydrochloride and napsylate salts of propoxyphene were determined in 4 species. The results shown in Figure 1 indicate that on a molar basis, the napsylate salt is less toxic than the hydrochloride. This may be due to the relative insolubility and retarded absorption of propoxyphene napsylate.

FIGURE 1
ACUTE ORAL TOXICITY OF PROPOXYPHENE
LD_{50} (mg/kg)±SE
LD_{50} (mMole/kg)

Species	Propoxyphene Hydrochloride	Propoxyphene Napsylate
Mouse	282 ± 39	915 ± 163
	0.75	1.62
Rat	230 ± 44	647 ± 95
	0.61	1.14
Rabbit	ca. 82	>183
	0.22	>0.32
Dog	ca. 100	>183
	0.27	>0.32

Some indication of the relative insolubility and retarded absorption of propoxyphene napsylate was obtained by measuring plasma propoxyphene levels in 2 groups of 4 dogs following oral administration of equimolar doses of the 2 salts. Although none of the animals in this experiment died, 3 of the 4 dogs given propoxyphene hydrochloride exhibited convulsive seizures during the time interval corresponding to the peak plasma levels. The 4 animals receiving the napsylate salt were ataxic but not acutely ill.

DOSAGE AND ADMINISTRATION

The product is given orally. The usual dose is 65 mg propoxyphene HCl and 650 mg acetaminophen every 4 hours as needed for pain. The maximum recommended dose of propoxyphene HCl is 390 mg per day.

Consideration should be given to a reduced total daily dosage in patients with hepatic or renal impairment.

HOW SUPPLIED

Wygesic® (propoxyphene HCl and acetaminophen) Tablets, 65 mg propoxyphene and 650 mg acetaminophen, are available as follows:

NDC 0008-0085, green, capsule-shaped, scored, film-coated tablet marked "WYETH" and "85", in bottles of 100 and 500 tablets, and in REDIPAK® cartons of 100 tablets (10 blister strips of 10).

Keep tightly closed.
Protect from light.
Store at controlled room temperature, 20°–25°C (68°–77°F).
Dispense in tight, light-resistant container as defined in the USP.

PATIENT INFORMATION

Summary

Products containing propoxyphene are used to relieve pain. LIMIT YOUR INTAKE OF ALCOHOL WHILE TAKING THIS DRUG. Make sure your doctor knows if you are taking tranquilizers, sleep aids, antidepressants, antihistamines, or any other drugs that make you sleepy. Combining propoxyphene with alcohol or these drugs in excessive doses is dangerous.

Use care while driving a car or using machines until you see how the drug affects you, because propoxyphene can make you sleepy. Do not take more of the drug than your doctor prescribed. Dependence has occurred when patients have taken propoxyphene for a long period of time at doses greater than recommended.

The rest of this leaflet gives you more information about propoxyphene. Please read it and keep it for further use.

Uses for Propoxyphene

Products containing propoxyphene are used for the relief of mild to moderate pain. Products which contain propoxyphene plus acetaminophen are prescribed for the relief of pain or pain associated with fever.

Before taking Propoxyphene

Make sure your doctor knows if you have ever had an allergic reaction to propoxyphene or acetaminophen.

The effect of propoxyphene in children under 12 has not been studied. Therefore, use of the drug in this age group is not recommended.

How to take Propoxyphene

Follow your doctor's directions exactly. Do not increase the amount you take without your doctor's approval. If you miss a dose of the drug, do not take twice as much the next time.

Pregnancy

Do not take propoxyphene during pregnancy unless your doctor knows you are pregnant and specifically recommends its use. Cases of temporary dependence in the newborn have occurred when the mother has taken propoxyphene consistently in the weeks before delivery. As a general principle, no drug should be taken during pregnancy unless it is clearly necessary.

General Caution

Heavy use of alcohol with propoxyphene is hazardous and may lead to overdosage symptoms (see "Overdosage" below); THEREFORE, LIMIT YOUR INTAKE OF ALCOHOL WHILE TAKING PROPOXYPHENE.

Combinations of excessive doses of propoxyphene, alcohol, and tranquilizers are dangerous. Make sure your doctor knows if you are taking tranquilizers, sleep aids, antidepressant drugs, antihistamines, or any other drugs that make you sleepy. The use of these drugs with propoxyphene increases their sedative effects and may lead to overdosage symptoms, including death (see "Overdosage" below).

Propoxyphene may cause drowsiness or impair your mental and/or physical abilities; therefore, use caution when driving a vehicle or operating dangerous machinery. DO NOT perform any hazardous task until you have seen your response to this drug.

Propoxyphene may increase the concentration in the body of medications such as anticoagulants ("blood thinners"), antidepressants, or drugs used for epilepsy. The result may be excessive or adverse effects of these medications. Make sure your doctor knows if you are taking any of these medications.

Dependence

You can become dependent on propoxyphene if you take it in higher than recommended doses over a long period of time. Dependence is a feeling of need for the drug and a feeling that you cannot perform normally without it.

Overdosage

An overdosage of propoxyphene, alone or in combination with other drugs, including alcohol, may cause weakness, difficulty in breathing, confusion, anxiety, and more severe drowsiness and dizziness. Extreme overdosage may lead to unconsciousness and death.

If the propoxyphene product contains acetaminophen, the overdosage symptoms include nausea, vomiting, lack of appetite, and abdominal pain. Liver damage may occur.

In any suspected overdosage situation, contact your doctor or nearest hospital emergency room. GET EMERGENCY HELP IMMEDIATELY. KEEP THIS AND ALL DRUGS OUT OF THE REACH OF CHILDREN.

Possible Side Effects

When propoxyphene is taken as directed, side effects are infrequent. Among those reported are drowsiness, dizziness, nausea, and vomiting. If these effects occur, it may help if you lie down and rest.

Less frequently reported side effects are constipation, abdominal pain, skin rashes, light-headedness, headache, weakness, minor visual disturbances, and feelings of elation or discomfort.

If side effects occur and concern you, contact your doctor.

Other Information

The safe and effective use of propoxyphene depends on your taking it exactly as directed. This drug has been prescribed specifically for you and your present condition. Do not give this drug to others who may have similar symptoms. Do not use it for any other reason.

If you would like more information about propoxyphene, ask your doctor or pharmacist. They have a more technical leaflet (professional labeling) you may read.

Manufactured by:
Wyeth Laboratories Inc.
A Wyeth-Ayerst Company
Philadelphia, PA 19101

Shown in Product Identification Guide, page 345

WYMOX® ℞

[wi 'moks]
(amoxicillin)
Capsules and Oral Suspension

DESCRIPTION

Wymox (amoxicillin) is a semisynthetic penicillin, an analog of ampicillin, with a broad spectrum of bactericidal activity against many gram-positive and gram-negative microorganisms. Chemically, it is D-(-)-a-amino-p-hydroxybenzyl penicillin trihydrate.

Wymox capsules contain amoxicillin as the trihydrate equivalent to 250 mg or 500 mg amoxicillin. The inactive ingredients present are colloidal silicon dioxide, D&C Yellow 10, FD&C Blue 1, gelatin, iron oxide, magnesium stearate, sodium lauryl sulfate, and titanium dioxide.

Wymox oral suspension is a powder which when reconstituted as directed yields a suspension of amoxicillin trihydrate equivalent to 125 mg or 250 mg amoxicillin per 5 mL.

Continued on next page

Wymox—Cont.

The inactive ingredients present are artificial flavors, carboxymethylcellulose sodium, cellulose, citric acid, D&C Red 28, FD&C Red 40, mannitol, sodium citrate, sucrose, and water.

HOW SUPPLIED

Wymox® (amoxicillin) Capsules contain amoxicillin as the trihydrate equivalent to 250 mg or 500 mg amoxicillin and are supplied as follows:

250 mg, NDC 0008-0559, grey and green capsule marked "WYETH" and "559", in bottles of 100 and 500 capsules.
500 mg, NDC 0008-0560, grey and green capsule marked "WYETH" and "560", in bottles of 50 and 500 capsules.

Store at room temperature, approximately 25°C (77°F).
Keep tightly closed.
Protect from light.
Dispense in light-resistant, tight container.

Wymox® (amoxicillin) Oral Suspension is available as a pink powder which when reconstituted as directed yields a palatable, pink suspension of amoxicillin trihydrate equivalent to 125 mg or 250 mg amoxicillin per 5 mL and is supplied as follows:

125 mg per 5 mL, NDC 0008-0557, in bottles to make 100 mL or 150 mL.
250 mg per 5 mL, NDC 0008-0558, in bottles to make 100 mL or 150 mL.

Store at room temperature, [approximately 25°C (77°F)] before reconstitution.
Keep tightly closed.
Shake well before using.
Store under refrigeration. Discard any unused portion after 14 days.

Manufactured by:
Wyeth Laboratories
A Wyeth-Ayerst Company
Philadelphia, PA 19101

For prescribing information write to Professional Service, Wyeth-Ayerst Laboratories, P.O. Box 8299, Philadelphia, PA 19101, or contact your local Wyeth-Ayerst representative.
Shown in Product Identification Guide, page 345

WYTENSIN®   ℞
[wi-ten 'sin]
(guanabenz acetate)

DESCRIPTION

Wytensin (guanabenz acetate), an antihypertensive agent for oral administration, is an aminoguanidine derivative, 2,6-dichlorobenzylideneaminoguanidine acetate, and its structural formula is:

It is an odorless, white to off-white, crystalline substance, sparingly soluble in water and soluble in alcohol, with a molecular weight of 291.14. Each tablet of Wytensin is equivalent to 4 mg or 8 mg of free guanabenz base. The inactive ingredients present are cellulose, iron oxide, lactose, and magnesium stearate. The 8 mg dosage strength also contains FD&C Blue 2.

Wytensin is available as 4 mg or 8 mg tablets for oral administration.

HOW SUPPLIED

Wytensin® (guanabenz acetate) Tablets are available in the following dosage strengths:

4 mg, orange, five-sided tablet with a raised "W"and a "4" under the "W" on one side and "WYETH 73" on reverse side, in bottles of 100 tablets (NDC 0008-0073-01) and 500 tablets (NDC 0008-0073-04) and in Redipak® cartons of 100 tablets (10 blister strips of 10–NDC 0008-0073-05).
8 mg, gray, five-sided tablet with a raised "W" and an "8" under the "W" on one side and "WYETH 74" on scored reverse side, in bottles of 100 tablets (NDC 0008-0074-01).
The appearance of these tablets is a trademark of Wyeth-Ayerst Laboratories.

Keep tightly closed.
Store at room temperature, approximately 25°C (77°F).
Protect from light.
Dispense in light-resistant, tight container.

Manufactured by:
Wyeth Laboratories Inc.
A Wyeth-Ayerst Company
Philadelphia, PA 19101

For prescribing information write to Professional Service, Wyeth-Ayerst Laboratories, P.O. Box 8299, Philadelphia, PA 19101, or contact your local Wyeth-Ayerst representative.

Zeneca Pharmaceuticals
A Business Unit of Zeneca Inc.
WILMINGTON, DE 19850-5437 USA

For Medical Information Contact:
Generally:
(302) 886-8000

After Hours and Weekend Emergencies:
(302) 886-3000

Adverse Drug Experiences:
(302) 886-8100

ACCOLATE®   ℞
[acc '-late]
(ZAFIRLUKAST)
TABLETS

DESCRIPTION

Zafirlukast is a synthetic, selective peptide leukotriene receptor antagonist (LTRA), with the chemical name 4-(5-cyclopentyloxy-carbonylamino -1-methyl-indol -3-ylmethyl)-3-methoxy-N-o-tolylsulfonylbenzamide. The molecular weight of zafirlukast is 575.7 and the structural formula is:

The empirical formula is: $C_{31}H_{33}N_3O_6S$

Zafirlukast, a fine white to pale yellow amorphous powder, is practically insoluble in water. It is slightly soluble in methanol and freely soluble in tetrahydrofuran, dimethylsulfoxide, and acetone.

ACCOLATE is supplied as a 20 mg tablet for oral administration.

Inactive Ingredients:
Film-coated tablets containing croscarmellose sodium, lactose, magnesium stearate, microcrystalline cellulose, povidone, hydroxypropylmethylcellulose and titanium dioxide.

CLINICAL PHARMACOLOGY

General: Zafirlukast is a selective and competitive receptor antagonist of leukotriene D_4 and E_4 (LTD_4 and LTE_4), components of slow-reacting substance of anaphylaxis (SRSA). Cysteinyl leukotriene production and receptor occupation have been correlated with the pathophysiology of asthma, including airway edema, smooth muscle constriction, and altered cellular activity associated with the inflammatory process, which contribute to the signs and symptoms of asthma. Patients with asthma were found in one study to be 25-100 times more sensitive to the bronchoconstricting activity of inhaled LTD_4 than nonasthmatic subjects.

In vitro studies demonstrated that zafirlukast antagonized the contractile activity of three leukotrienes (LTC_4, LTD_4 and LTE_4) in conducting airway smooth muscle from laboratory animals and humans. Zafirlukast prevented intradermal LTD_4-induced increases in cutaneous vascular permeability and inhibited inhaled LTD_4-induced influx of eosinophils into animal lungs. Inhalational challenge studies in sensitized sheep showed that zafirlukast suppressed the airway responses to antigen; this included both the early- and late-phase response and the nonspecific hyperresponsiveness.

In humans, zafirlukast inhibited bronchoconstriction caused by several kinds of inhalational challenges. Pretreatment with single oral doses of zafirlukast inhibited the bronchoconstriction caused by sulfur dioxide and cold air in patients with asthma. Pretreatment with single doses of zafirlukast attenuated the early- and late-phase reaction caused by inhalation of various antigens such as grass, cat dander, ragweed, and mixed antigens in patients with asthma. Zafirlukast also attenuated the increase in bronchial hyperresponsiveness to inhaled histamine that followed inhaled allergen challenge.

Clinical Pharmacokinetics and Bioavailability:
Zafirlukast is rapidly absorbed following oral administration. The absolute bioavailability of zafirlukast is unknown. Peak plasma concentrations are achieved 3 hours after dosing.
The mean terminal elimination half-life of zafirlukast is approximately 10 hours in both normal subjects and patients

with asthma. Steady-state plasma concentrations of zafirlukast are proportional to the dose and predictable from single-dose pharmacokinetic data.

Zafirlukast is extensively metabolized. Following oral administration of a radiolabeled dose, urinary excretion accounts for approximately 10% of the dose and the remainder is excreted in feces. Unmetabolized zafirlukast is not detected in urine. In vitro studies using human liver microsomes showed that the hydroxylated metabolites of zafirlukast are formed through the cytochrome P450 2C9 (CYP2C9) enzyme pathway. Additional in vitro studies utilizing human liver microsomes show that zafirlukast inhibits the cytochrome P450 CYP3A4 and CYP2C9 isoenzymes at concentrations close to the clinically achieved plasma concentrations. The metabolites of zafirlukast found in plasma are at least 90 times less potent as LTD_4 receptor antagonists than zafirlukast in a standard in vitro test of activity.

Cross-study comparisons in patients ranging from 7 years to greater than 65 years of age show that mean dose (mg/kg) normalized AUC and Cmax increase and plasma clearance (CL) decreases with increasing age. In patients above 65 years of age, there is an approximately 2-3 fold greater Cmax and AUC compared to young adult patients.

In a study of patients with hepatic impairment (biopsy-proven cirrhosis), there was a 50–60% greater C_{max} and AUC compared to normal subjects.

Based on a cross-study comparison, there are no apparent differences in the pharmacokinetics of zafirlukast between renally impaired patients and normal subjects.

In two separate studies, one using a high fat and the other a high protein meal, administration of ACCOLATE with food reduced the mean bioavailability by approximately 40%.

In the concentration range of 0.25–10 μg/mL, zafirlukast is >99% bound to plasma proteins, predominantly albumin.

Clinical Studies: Three U.S. double-blind, randomized, placebo-controlled, 13-week clinical trials in 1,380 patients with mild-to-moderate asthma demonstrated that ACCOLATE improved daytime asthma symptoms, nighttime awakenings, mornings with asthma symptoms, rescue beta₂-agonist use, FEV₁, and morning peak expiratory flow rate. In these studies, the patients had a mean baseline FEV₁ of approximately 75% of predicted normal and a mean baseline beta-agonist requirement of approximately 4-5 puffs of albuterol per day. The results of the largest of the trials are shown in the table below.

Table 1
Mean Change from Baseline at Study Endpoint

	ACCOLATE 20 mg twice daily N=514	Placebo N=248
Daytime Asthma symptom score (0–3 scale)	−0.44*	−0.25
Nighttime Awakenings (number per week)	−1.27*	−0.43
Mornings with Asthma Symptoms (days per week)	−1.32*	−0.75
Rescue β₂-agonist use (puffs per day)	−1.15*	−0.24
FEV₁ (L)	+0.15*	+0.05
Morning PEFR (L/min)	+22.06*	+7.63
Evening PEFR (L/min)	+13.12	+10.14

*p<0.05, compared to placebo

In a second and smaller study, the effect of ACCOLATE on most efficacy parameters was comparable to the active control (inhaled cromolyn sodium 1600 μg four times per day) and superior to placebo at endpoint for decreasing rescue beta-agonist use (figure below).

Mean β₂ - agonist use (puffs/day)

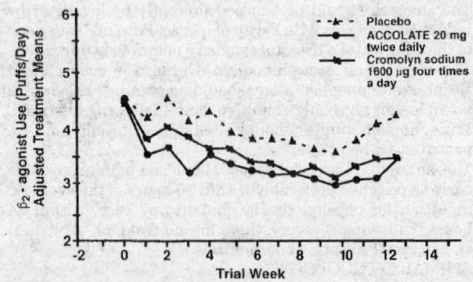

In these trials, improvement in asthma symptoms occurred within one week of initiating treatment with ACCOLATE.

The role of ACCOLATE in the management of patients with more severe asthma, patients receiving antiasthma therapy other than as-needed, inhaled beta$_2$-agonists, or as an oral or inhaled corticosteroid-sparing agent remains to be fully characterized.

INDICATIONS AND USAGE

ACCOLATE is indicated for the prophylaxis and chronic treatment of asthma in adults and children 12 years of age and older.

CONTRAINDICATIONS

ACCOLATE is contraindicated in patients who are hypersensitive to zafirlukast or any of its inactive ingredients.

WARNINGS

ACCOLATE is not indicated for use in the reversal of bronchospasm in acute asthma attacks, including status asthmaticus. Therapy with ACCOLATE can be continued during acute exacerbations of asthma.

Coadministration of zafirlukast with warfarin results in a clinically significant increase in prothrombin time (PT). Patients on oral warfarin anticoagulant therapy and ACCOLATE should have their prothrombin times monitored closely and anticoagulant dose adjusted accordingly. (See PRECAUTIONS, Drug Interactions.)

PRECAUTIONS

Information for Patients:

ACCOLATE is indicated for the chronic treatment of asthma and should be taken regularly as prescribed, even during symptom-free periods. ACCOLATE is not a bronchodilator and should not be used to treat acute episodes of asthma. Patients receiving ACCOLATE should be instructed not to decrease the dose or stop taking any other antiasthma medications unless instructed by a physician. Women who are breast-feeding should be instructed not to take ACCOLATE (see PRECAUTIONS, Nursing Mothers). Alternative antiasthma medication should be considered in such patients.

The bioavailability of ACCOLATE may be decreased when taken with food. Patients should be instructed to take ACCOLATE at least 1 hour before or 2 hours after meals.

Patients should be told that a rare side effect of ACCOLATE is elevation of liver enzymes and that if they experience signs and/or symptoms of liver dysfunction (e.g., right upper quadrant abdominal pain, nausea, fatigue, lethargy, pruritus, jaundice, and flu-like symptoms), they should contact their physician immediately.

Hepatic: Rarely, elevations of one or more liver enzymes may occur during ACCOLATE therapy. Most of these have been observed in clinical trials with ACCOLATE at doses four times higher than the recommended dose. The clinical signficance of these elevations are unknown. If clinical signs or symptoms of liver dysfunction (e.g., right upper quadrant abdominal pain, nausea, fatigue, lethargy, pruritus, jaundice, and flu-like symptoms) are noted, it is reasonable to recommend that standard liver tests be obtained and the patient managed accordingly. A decision to discontinue ACCOLATE should be individualized to the patient's condition weighing the risk of hepatic dysfunction against the clinical benefit of ACCOLATE to the patient. (See PRECAUTIONS-Information for Patients and ADVERSE REACTIONS sections.)

Eosinophilic Conditions: In rare cases, patients on ACCOLATE therapy may present with systemic eosinophilia, sometimes presenting with clinical features of vasculitis consistent with Churg-Strauss syndrome, a condition which is often treated with systemic steroid therapy. These events usually, but not always, have been associated with the reduction of oral steroid therapy. Physicians should be alert to eosinophilia, vasculitic rash, worsening pulmonary symptoms, cardiac complications, and/or neuropathy presenting in their patients. A casual association between ACCOLATE and these underlying conditions has not been established. (See ADVERSE REACTIONS).

Drug Interactions: In a drug interaction study in 16 healthy male volunteers, coadministration of multiple doses of zafirlukast (160 mg/day) to steady state with a single 25-mg dose of warfarin resulted in a significant increase in the mean AUC (+ 63%) and half-life (+36%) of S-warfarin. The mean prothrombin time (PT) increased by approximately 35%. This interaction is probably due to an inhibition by zafirlukast of the cytochrome P450 2C9 isoenzyme system. Patients on oral warfarin anticoagulant therapy and ACCOLATE should have their prothrombin times monitored closely and anticoagulant dose adjusted accordingly (see WARNINGS). No formal drug-drug interaction studies with ACCOLATE and other drugs known to be metabolized by the cytochrome P450 2C9 isoenzyme (e.g., tolbutamide, phenytoin, carbamazepine) have been conducted; however, care should be exercised when ACCOLATE is co-administered with these drugs.

In a drug interaction study in 16 healthy male volunteers, co-administration of zafirlukast (320 mg/day), with terfenadine (60 mg twice daily) to steady state resulted in a decrease in the mean C_{max} (−66%) and AUC (−54%) of ACCOLATE. No effect of zafirlukast on terfenadine plasma concentrations or ECG parameters (i.e., QTc interval) was seen. No formal drug-drug interaction studies between ACCOLATE and other drugs known to be metabolized by the P450 3A4 (CYP 3A4) isoenzyme (e.g., dihydropyridine calcium-channel blockers, cyclosporin, cisapride, astemizole) have been conducted. As ACCOLATE is known to be an inhibitor of CYP 3A4 in vitro, it is reasonable to employ appropriate clinical monitoring when these drugs are coadministered with ACCOLATE.

In a drug interaction study in 11 asthmatic patients, coadministration of a single dose of zafirlukast (40 mg) with erythromycin (500 mg three times daily for 5 days) to steady state resulted in decreased mean plasma levels of zafirlukast by approximately 40% due to a decrease in zafirlukast bioavailability.

Co-administration of zafirlukast (80 mg/day) at steady state with a single dose of a liquid theophylline preparation (6 mg/kg) in 13 asthmatic patients resulted in decreased mean plasma levels of zafirlukast by approximately 30%, but no effect on plasma theophylline levels was observed. Rare cases of patients experiencing increased theophylline levels with or without clinical signs or symptoms or theophylline toxicity after the addition of ACCOLATE to an existing theophylline regimen have been reported. The mechanism of the interaction between ACCOLATE and theophylline in these patients is unknown (see ADVERSE REACTIONS).

Co-administration of zafirlukast (40 mg/day) with aspirin (650 mg four times daily) resulted in mean increased plasma levels of zafirlukast by approximately 45%.

In a single-blind, parallel-group, 3-week study in 39 healthy female subjects taking oral contraceptives, 40 mg twice daily of zafirlukast had no significant effect on ethinyl estradiol plasma concentrations or contraceptive efficacy.

Carcinogenesis, Mutagenesis, Impairment of Fertility:

In two-year carcinogenicity studies, zafirlukast was administered at oral daily doses of 10, 100, and 300 mg/kg to mice and 40, 400, and 2000 mg/kg to rats. Male mice given 300 mg/kg/day of zafirlukast had a greater incidence of hepatocellular adenomas as compared to concurrent controls; female mice at this dose showed a greater incidence of whole body histocytic sarcomas. Male and female rats given 2000 mg/kg/day of zafirlukast had a greater incidence of urinary bladder transitional cell papillomas as compared to concurrent controls. Pharmacokinetic data show that the plasma concentrations in mice at non-tumorigenic (100 mg/kg) and tumorigenic (300 mg/kg) doses of zafirlukast were approximately 70 times and 220 times, respectively, the plasma concentrations at the maximum recommended human daily oral dose. For rats, plasma concentrations at the non-tumorigenic (400 mg/kg) and tumorigenic (2000 mg/kg) doses of zafirlukast were approximately 170 times and 200 times, respectively, the plasma concentrations in humans at the maximum recommended human daily oral dose. The clinical significance of these findings for the long-term use of ACCOLATE is unknown.

In mutagenicity studies, there was no evidence of mutagenic potential in reverse (*S. typhimurium* and *E. coli*) or forward point mutation (CHO-HGPRT and mouse lymphoma) assays or in two assays for chromosomal aberrations (human peripheral blood lymphocyte clastogenic assay and the rat bone marrow micronucleus assay).

Reproduction and fertility studies in rats showed no effect on fertility due to zafirlukast at doses up to 2000 mg/kg (approximately 400 times the maximum recommended human daily oral dose on mg/m^2 basis). In the one-year toxicity studies in dogs, zafirlukast produced an increase in absolute and relative uterine and ovarian weights at an oral dose of 150 mg/kg, resulting in approximately 85 times the systemic exposure (AUC_{0-12h}) in humans at the maximum recommended human oral daily dose.

Pregnancy Category B:

No teratogenicity was observed at oral doses up to 1600 mg/kg/day in mice (approximately 160 times the maximum recommended human daily oral dose on a mg/m^2 basis), 2000 mg/kg/day in rats (approximately 400 times the maximum recommended human daily oral dose on a mg/m^2 basis) and 2000 mg/kg/day in cynomolgus monkeys (approximately 800 times the maximum recommended human daily oral dose on a mg/m^2 basis). At 2000 mg/kg/day in rats, maternal toxicity and deaths were seen with increased incidence of early fetal resorption. Spontaneous abortions occurred in cynomolgus monkeys at a maternally toxic dose of 2000 mg/kg/day orally. There are no adequate and well-controlled trials in pregnant women. Because animal reproduction studies are not always predictive of human response, ACCOLATE should be used during pregnancy only if clearly needed.

Nursing Mothers:

Zafirlukast is excreted in breast milk. Following repeated 40-mg twice-a-day dosing in healthy women, average steady-state concentrations of zafirlukast in breast milk were 50 ng/mL compared to 255 ng/mL in plasma. Because of the potential for tumorigenicity shown for zafirlukast in mouse and rat studies and the enhanced sensitivity of neonatal rats and dogs to the adverse effects of zafirlukast, ACCOLATE should not be administered to mothers who are breast-feeding.

Pediatric Use:

The safety and effectiveness of ACCOLATE in pediatric patients below the age of 12 years have not been established.

ADVERSE REACTIONS

The safety database for ACCOLATE consists of more than 4,000 healthy volunteers and patients who received ACCOLATE, of which 1723 were asthmatics enrolled in trials of 13 weeks duration or longer. A total of 671 patients received ACCOLATE for 1 year or longer. The majority of the patients were 18 years of age or older; however 222 patients between the age of 12 and 18 years received ACCOLATE.

A comparison of adverse events reported by ≥ 1% of zafirlukast-treated patients, and at rates numerically greater than in placebo-treated patients, is shown for all trials in the table below.

Table 2

Adverse Event	ACCOLATE N=4058	PLACEBO N=2032
Headache	12.9%	11.7%
Infection	3.5%	3.4%
Nausea	3.1%	2.0%
Diarrhea	2.8%	2.1%
Pain (generalized)	1.9%	1.7%
Asthenia	1.8%	1.6%
Abdominal Pain	1.8%	1.1%
Accidental Injury	1.6%	1.5%
Dizziness	1.6%	1.5%
Myalgia	1.6%	1.5%
Fever	1.6%	1.1%
Back Pain	1.5%	1.2%
Vomiting	1.5%	1.1%
SGPT Elevation	1.5%	1.1%
Dyspepsia	1.3%	1.2%

The frequency of less common adverse events was comparable between ACCOLATE and placebo.

Rarely, elevations of one or more liver enzymes have occurred in patients receiving ACCOLATE in controlled clinical trials. Most of these have been observed in asymptomatic patients at doses four times higher than the recommended dose and returned to the normal range after a variable period of time upon discontinuation of ACCOLATE therapy. Rare cases of symptomatic hepatitis and hyperbilirubinemia, without other attributable cause, have occurred in patients who had received the recommended doses of ACCOLATE (40 mg/day). In these patients, the liver enzymes returned to normal or near-normal after stopping ACCOLATE.

In clinical trials, an increased proportion of zafirlukast patients over the age of 55 years reported infections as compared to placebo-treated patients. A similar finding was not observed in other age groups studied. These infections were mostly mild or moderate in intensity and predominantly affected the respiratory tract. Infections occurred equally in both sexes, were dose-proportional to total milligrams of zafirlukast exposure, and were associated with coadministration of inhaled corticosteroids. The clinical significance of this finding is unknown.

In rare cases, patients on ACCOLATE therapy may present with systemic eosinophilia, sometimes presenting with clinical features of vasculitis consistent with Churg-Strauss syndrome, a condition which is often treated with systemic steroid therapy. These events usually, but not always, have been associated with the reduction of oral steroid therapy. Physicians should be alert to eosinophilia, vasculitic rash, worsening pulmonary symptoms, cardiac complications, and/or neuropathy presenting in their patients. A causal association between ACCOLATE and these underlying conditions has not been established. (See PRECAUTIONS, Eosinophilic Conditions).

Hypersensitivity reactions, including urticaria angioedema and rashes, with or without blistering, have been reported in association with ACCOLATE therapy.

Rare cases of patients experiencing increased theophylline levels with or without clinical signs or symptoms of theophylline toxicity after the addition of ACCOLATE to an existing theophylline regimen have been reported. The mechanism of the interaction between ACCOLATE and theophylline in these patients is unknown and not predicted by available *in vitro* metabolism data and the results of a clinical drug interaction study (see CLINICAL PHARMACOLOGY and PRECAUTIONS - Drug Interactions sections).

OVERDOSAGE

No deaths occurred at oral zafirlukast doses of 2000 mg/kg in mice (approximately 200 times the maximum recommended human daily oral dose on a mg/m^2 basis), 2000 mg/kg in rats (approximately 400 times the maximum recommended human daily oral dose on a mg/m^2 basis), and 500 mg/kg in dogs (approximately 330 times the maximum recommended human daily oral dose on a mg/m^2 basis).

Continued on next page

Accolate—Cont.

There is no experience to date with zafirlukast overdose in humans. It is reasonable to employ the usual supportive measures in the event of an overdose; e.g., remove unabsorbed material from the gastrointestinal tract, employ clinical monitoring, and institute supportive therapy, if required.

DOSAGE AND ADMINISTRATION

The recommended dose of ACCOLATE is 20 mg twice daily in adults and children 12 years and older. Since food reduces the bioavailability of zafirlukast, ACCOLATE should be taken at least 1 hour before or 2 hours after meals.

Elderly Patients:

Based on cross-study comparisons, the clearance of zafirlukast is reduced in elderly patients (65 years of age and older), such that C_{max} and AUC are approximately twice those of younger adults. In clinical trials, a dose of 20 mg twice daily was not associated with an increase in the overall incidence of adverse events or withdrawals because of adverse events in elderly patients.

Patients with Hepatic Impairment:

The clearance of zafirlukast is reduced in patients with stable alcoholic cirrhosis such that the C_{max} and AUC are approximately 50–60% greater than those of normal adults. ACCOLATE has not been evaluated in patients with hepatitis or in long-term studies of patients with cirrhosis.

Patients with Renal Impairment:

Dosage adjustment is not required for patients with renal impairment.

Pediatric Patients:

The safety and effectiveness of ACCOLATE in pediatric patients below the age of 12 years have not been established.

HOW SUPPLIED

20 mg Tablets, (NDC 0310-0402) white, round, biconvex, coated tablets identified with "ZENECA" debossed on one side and "ACCOLATE 20" debossed on the other side are supplied in opaque HDPE bottles of 60 tablets and hospital Unit Dose blister packages of 100 tablets.

Store at controlled room temperature, (20°–25° C) (68°–77°F) [see USP]. Protect from light and moisture. Dispense in the original air-tight container.

Manufactured for:
Zeneca Pharmaceuticals
A Business Unit of Zeneca Inc.
Wilmington, Delaware 19850-5437
By: IPR Pharmaceuticals Inc.
Carolina, Puerto Rico
670005 G 06/98

Shown in Product Identification Guide, page 345

ARIMIDEX® ℞
anastrozole
TABLETS

DESCRIPTION

ARIMIDEX® (anastrozole) tablets for oral administration contain 1 mg of anastrozole, a non-steroidal aromatase inhibitor. It is chemically described as 1,3-Benzenediacetonitrile, α, α, α', α'-tetramethyl-5-(1H-1,2,4-triazol-1-ylmethyl). Its molecular formula is $C_{17}H_{19}N_5$ and its structural formula is:

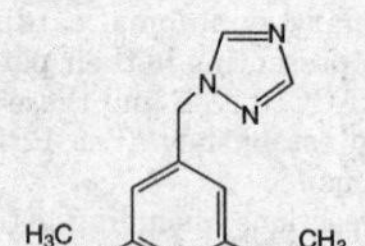

Anastrozole is an off-white powder with a molecular weight of 293.4. Anastrozole has moderate aqueous solubility (0.5 mg/mL at 25°C); solubility is independent of pH in the physiological range. Anastrozole is freely soluble in methanol, acetone, ethanol, and tetrahydrofuran, and very soluble in acetonitrile.

Each tablet contains as inactive ingredients: lactose, magnesium stearate, hydroxypropylmethylcellulose, polyethylene glycol, povidone, sodium starch glycolate, and titanium dioxide.

CLINICAL PHARMACOLOGY

Mechanism of Action

Many breast cancers have estrogen receptors and growth of these tumors can be stimulated by estrogens. In post-menopausal women, the principal source of circulating estrogen (primarily estradiol) is conversion of adrenally-generated androstenedione to estrone by aromatase in peripheral tissues, such as adipose tissue, with further conversion of estrone to estradiol. Many breast cancers also contain aromatase; the importance of tumor-generated estrogens is uncertain.

Treatment of breast cancer has included efforts to decrease estrogen levels by ovariectomy premenopausally and by use of antiestrogens and progestational agents both pre- and post-menopausally, and these interventions lead to decreased tumor mass or delayed progression of tumor growth in some women.

Anastrozole is a potent and selective non-steroidal aromatase inhibitor. It significantly lowers serum estradiol concentrations and has no detectable effect on formation of adrenal corticosteroids or aldosterone.

Pharmacokinetics

Inhibition of aromatase activity is primarily due to anastrozole, the parent drug. Studies with radiolabeled drug have demonstrated that orally administered anastrozole is well absorbed into the systemic circulation with 83 to 85% of the radiolabel recovered in urine and feces. Food does not affect the extent of absorption. Elimination of anastrozole is primarily via hepatic metabolism (approximately 85%) and to a lesser extent, renal excretion (approximately 11%), and anastrozole has a mean terminal elimination half-life of approximately 50 hours in postmenopausal women. The major circulating metabolite of anastrozole, triazole, lacks pharmacologic activity. The pharmacokinetic parameters are similar in patients and in healthy postmenopausal volunteers. The pharmacokinetics of anastrozole are linear over the dose range of 1 to 20 mg and do not change with repeated dosing. Consistent with the approximately 2-day terminal elimination half-life, plasma concentrations approach steady-state levels at about 7 days of once daily dosing and steady-state levels are approximately three- to four-fold higher than levels observed after a single dose of ARIMIDEX. Anastrozole is 40% bound to plasma proteins in the therapeutic range.

Metabolism and Excretion: Studies of postmenopausal women demonstrated that anastrozole is extensively metabolized with about 10% of the dose excreted in the urine as unchanged drug within 72 hours of dosing, and the remainder (about 60% of the dose) excreted in the urine as metabolites. Metabolism of anastrozole occurs by N-dealkylation, hydroxylation and glucoronidation. Three metabolites of anastrozole have been identified in human plasma and urine. The known metabolites are triazole, a glucuronide conjugate of hydroxy-anastrozole, and a glucuronide of anastrozole itself. Several minor (less than 5% of the radioactive dose) metabolites have not been identified.

Because renal elimination is not a significant pathway of elimination, total body clearance of anastrozole is unchanged even in severe (creatinine clearance less than 30 mL/min/1.73m^2) renal impairment; dosing adjustment in patients with renal dysfunction is not necessary (see Special Populations and DOSAGE AND ADMINISTRATION sections). Dosage adjustment is also unnecessary in patients with stable hepatic cirrhosis (see Special Populations and DOSAGE AND ADMINISTRATION sections).

Special Populations

Geriatric: Anastrozole pharmacokinetics have been investigated in postmenopausal female volunteers and patients with breast cancer. No age related effects were seen over the range <50 to >80 years.

Race: Anastrozole pharmacokinetic differences due to race have not been studied.

Renal Insufficiency: Anastrozole pharmacokinetics have been investigated in subjects with renal insufficiency. Anastrozole renal clearance decreased proportionally with creatinine clearance and was approximately 50% lower in volunteers with severe renal impairment (creatinine clearance less than 30 mL/min/1.73m^2) compared to controls. Since only about 10% of anastrozole is excreted unchanged in the urine, the reduction in renal clearance did not influence the total body clearance (see DOSAGE AND ADMINISTRATION).

Hepatic Insufficiency: Hepatic metabolism accounts for approximately 85% of anastrozole elimination. Anastrozole pharmacokinetics have been investigated in subjects with hepatic cirrhosis related to alcohol abuse. The apparent oral clearance (CL/F) of anastrozole was approximately 30% lower in subjects with stable hepatic cirrhosis than in control subjects with normal liver function. However, plasma anastrozole concentrations in the subjects with hepatic cirrhosis were within the range of concentrations seen in normal subjects across all clinical trials (see DOSAGE AND ADMINISTRATION), so that no dosage adjustment is needed.

Drug-Drug Interactions: Anastrozole inhibited reactions catalyzed by cytochrome P450 1A2, 2C8/9, and 3A4 *in vitro* with Ki values which were approximately 30 times higher than the mean steady-state C_{max} values observed following a 1-mg daily dose. Anastrozole had no inhibitory effect on reactions catalyzed by cytochrome P450 2A6 or 2D6 *in vitro*. Administration of a single 30 mg/kg or multiple 10 mg/kg doses of anastrozole to subjects had no effect on the clearance of antipyrine or urinary recovery of antipyrine metabolites. Based on these *in vitro* and *in vivo* results, it is unlikely that co-administration of ARIMIDEX 1 mg with other drugs will result in clinically significant inhibition of cytochrome P450 mediated metabolism.

Pharmacodynamics

Effect on Estradiol: Mean serum concentrations of estradiol were evaluated in multiple daily dosing trials with 0.5, 1, 3, 5, and 10 mg if ARIMIDEX in postmenopausal women with advanced breast cancer. Clinically significant suppression of serum estradiol was seen with all doses. Doses of 1 mg and higher resulted in suppression of mean serum concentrations of estradiol to the lower limit of detection (3.7 pmol/L). The recommended daily dose, ARIMIDEX 1 mg, reduced estradiol by approximately 70% within 24 hours and by approximately 80% after 14 days of daily dosing. Suppression of serum estradiol was maintained for up to 6 days after cessation of daily dosing with ARIMIDEX 1 mg.

Effect on Corticosteroids: In multiple daily dosing trials with 3, 5, and 10 mg, the selectivity of anastrozole was assessed by examining the effects on corticosteroid synthesis. For all doses, anastrozole did not effect cortisol or aldosterone secretion at baseline or in response to ACTH. No glucocorticoid or mineralocorticoid replacement therapy is necessary with anastrozole.

Other Endocrine Effects: In multiple daily dosing trials with 5 and 10 mg, thyroid stimulation hormone (TSH) was measured; there was no increase in TSH during the administration of ARIMIDEX. ARIMIDEX does not possess direct progestogenic, androgenic, or estrogenic activity in animals, but does perturb the circulating levels of progesterone, androgens, and estrogens.

Clinical Studies

Anastrozole was studied in two well-controlled clinical trials (0004, a North American study; 0005, a predominately European study) in postmenopausal women with advanced breast cancer who had disease progression following tamoxifen therapy for either advanced or early breast cancer. Some of the patients had also received previous cytotoxic treatment. Most patients were ER-positive; a smaller fraction were ER-unknown or ER-negative (the ER-negative patients were eligible only if they had had a positive response to tamoxifen). Eligible patients with measurable and non-measurable disease were randomized to receive either a single daily dose of 1 mg or 10 mg of ARIMIDEX or megestrol acetate 40 mg four times a day. The studies were double-blinded with respect to ARIMIDEX. Time to progression and objective response (only patients with measurable disease could be considered partial responders) rates were the primary efficacy variables. Objective response rates were calculated based on the Union Internationale Contre le Cancer (UICC) criteria. The rate of prolonged (more than 24 weeks) stable disease, the rate of progression, and survival were also calculated.

Both trials included over 375 patients; demographics and other baseline characteristics were similar for the three treatment groups in each trial. Patients in the 0005 trial had responded better to prior tamoxifen treatment. Of the patients entered who had prior tamoxifen therapy for advanced disease (58% in Trial 0004; 57% in Trial 0005), 18% of these patients in Trial 0004 and 42% in Trial 0005 were reported by the primary investigator to have responded. In Trial 0004, 81% of patients were ER-positive, 13% were ER-unknown, and 6% were ER-negative. In Trial 0005, 58% of patients were ER-positive, 37% were ER-unknown, and 5% were ER-negative. In Trial 0004, 62% of patients had measurable disease compared to 79% in Trial 0005. The sites of metastatic disease were similar among treatment groups for each trial. On average, 40% of the patients had soft tissue metastases, 60% had bone metastases, and 40% had visceral (15% liver) metastases.

As shown in the table below, similar results were observed among treatment groups and between the two trials. None of the within-trial differences were statistically significant.

	ARIMIDEX 1 mg	ARIMIDEX 10 mg	Megestrol Acetate 160 mg
Trial 0004 (N. America)	(n=128)	(n=130)	(n=128)
Median Follow-up (months)*	31.3	30.9	32.9
Median Time to Death (months)	29.6	25.7	26.7
2 Year Survival Probability (%)	62.0	58.0	53.1
Median Time to Progression (months)	5.7	5.3	5.1
Objective Response (all patients) (%)	12.5	10.0	10.2
Stable Disease for >24 weeks (%)	35.2	29.2	32.8
Progression (%)	86.7	85.4	90.6

Trial 0005 (Europe, Australia, S.Africa)	(n=135)	(n=118)	(n=125)
Median Follow-up (months)*	31.0	30.9	31.5
Median Time to Death (months)	24.3	24.8	19.8
2 Year Survival Probability (%)	50.5	50.9	39.1
Median Time to Progression (months)	4.4	5.3	3.9
Objective Response (all patients) (%)	12.6	15.3	14.4
Stable Disease for >24 weeks (%)	24.4	25.4	23.2
Progression (%)	91.9	89.8	92.0

* Surviving Patients

More than 1/3 of the patients in each treatment group in both studies had either an objective response or stabilization of their disease for greater than 24 weeks. Among the 263 patients who received ARIMIDEX 1 mg, there were 11 complete responders and 22 partial responders. In patients who had an objective response, more than 80% were still responding at 6 months from randomization and more than 45% were still responding at 12 months from randomization.

When data from the two controlled trials are pooled, the objective response rates and median times to progression and death were similar for patients randomized to ARIMIDEX 1 mg and megestrol acetate. There is, in this data, no indication that ARIMIDEX 10 mg is superior to ARIMIDEX 1 mg.

	ARIMIDEX 1 mg	ARIMIDEX 10 mg	Megestrol Acetate 160 mg
Trials 0004 & 0005 (Pooled Data)	(n=263)	(n=248)	(n=253)
Median Time to Death (months)	26.7	25.5	22.5
2 Year Survival Probability (%)	56.1	54.6	46.3
Median Time to Progression (months)	4.8	5.3	4.6
Objective Respose (all patients) (%)	12.5	12.5	12.3

Objective response rates and median times to progression and death for ARIMIDEX 1 mg were similar to megestrol acetate for women over or under 65. There were too few non-white patients studied to draw conclusions about racial differences in response.

INDICATIONS AND USAGE

ARIMIDEX is indicated for the treatment of advanced breast cancer in postmenopausal women with disease progression following tamoxifen therapy.

Patients with ER-negative disease and patients who did not respond to previous tamoxifen therapy rarely responded to ARIMIDEX.

CONTRAINDICATIONS

None known.

WARNINGS

ARIMIDEX can cause fetal harm when administered to a pregnant woman. Anastrozole has been found to cross the placenta following oral administration of 0.1 mg/kg in rats and rabbits (about 3/4 and 1.5 times the recommended human dose, respectively, on a mg/m^2 basis. Studies in both rats and rabbits at doses equal to or greater than 0.1 and 0.02 mg/kg/day, respectively (about 3/4 and 1/3, respectively, the recommended human dose on a mg/m^2 basis), administration during the period of organogenesis showed that anastrozole increased pregnancy loss (increased pre- and/or post-implantation loss, increased resorption, and decreased numbers of live fetuses); effects were dose-related in rats. Placental weights were significantly increased in rats at doses of 0.1 mg/kg/day or more.

Evidence of fetotoxicity, including delayed fetal development (i.e., incomplete ossification and depressed fetal body weights), was observed in rats administered doses of 1 mg/kg/day (which produced plasma anastrozole C_{ssmax} and $AUC_{0-24\ hr}$ that were 19 times and 9 times higher than the respective values found in healthy post-menopausal humans at the recommended dose). There was no evidence of teratogenicity in rats administered doses up to 1.0 mg/kg/day. In rabbits, anastrozole caused pregnancy failure at doses equal to or greater than 1.0 mg/kg/day (about 16 times the recommended human dose on a mg/m^2 basis); there was no evidence of teratogenicity in rabbits administered 0.2 mg/kg/day (about 3 times the recommended human dose on a mg/m^2 basis).

There are no adequate and well-controlled studies in pregnant women using ARIMIDEX. If ARIMIDEX is used during pregnancy or if the patient becomes pregnant while receiving this drug, the patient should be apprised of the potential hazard to the fetus or potential risk for loss of the pregnancy.

PRECAUTIONS

General: Before starting treatment with ARIMIDEX, pregnancy must be excluded (see WARNINGS).

ARIMIDEX should be administered under the supervision of a qualified physician experienced in the use of anticancer agents.

Laboratory Tests: Three-fold elevations of mean serum gamma glutamyl transferase (GT) levels have been observed among patients with liver metastases receiving ARIMIDEX or megestrol acetate. These changes were likely related to the progression of liver metastases in these patients, although other contributing factors could not be ruled out.

Drug Interactions: (See CLINICAL PHARMACOLOGY)

Anastrozole inhibited *in vitro* metabolic reactions catalyzed by cytochromes P450 1A2, 2C8/9, and 3A4 but only at relatively high concentrations. Anastrozole did not inhibit P450 2A6 or the polymorphic P450 2D6 in human liver microsomes. Anastrozole did not alter the pharmacokinetics of antipyrine. Although there have been no formal interaction studies other than with antipyrine, based on these *in vivo* and *in vitro* studies, it is unlikely that co-administration of a 1-mg dose of ARIMIDEX with other drugs will result in clinically significant drug inhibition of cytochrome P450-mediated metabolism of the other drugs.

Drug/Laboratory Test Interactions: No clinically significant changes in the results of clinical laboratory tests have been observed.

Carcinogenesis: No long-term animal studies have been conducted to assess the carcinogenic potential of ARIMIDEX.

Mutagenesis: ARIMIDEX has not been shown to be mutagenic in *in vitro* tests (Ames and E. coli bacterial tests, CHO-K1 gene mutation assay) or clastogenic either *in vitro* (chromosome aberrations in human lymphocytes) or *in vivo* (micronucleus test in rats).

Impairment of Fertility: Studies to investigate the effect of ARIMIDEX on fertility have not been conducted; however, chronic studies indicated hypertrophy of the ovaries and the presence of follicular cysts in rats administered doses equal to or greater than 1 mg/kg/day (which produced plasma anastrozole C_{ssmax} and $AUC_{0-24\ hr}$ that were 19 and 9 times higher than the respective values found in healthy post-menopausal humans at the recommended dose). In addition, hyperplastic uteri were observed in chronic studies of female dogs administered doses equal to or greater than 1 mg/kg/day (which produced plasma anastrozole C_{ssmax} and $AUC_{0-24\ hr}$ that were 22 times and 16 times higher than the respective values found in post-menopausal humans at the recommended dose). It is not known whether these effects on the reproductive organs of animals are associated with impaired fertility in humans.

Pregnancy: Pregnancy Category D: (See WARNINGS).

Nursing Mothers: It is not known if anastrozole is excreted in human milk. Because many drugs are excreted in human milk, caution should be exercised when ARIMIDEX is administered to a nursing woman (see WARNINGS and PRECAUTIONS).

Pediatric Use: The safety and efficacy of ARIMIDEX in pediatric patients have not been established.

Geriatric Use: Fifty percent of patients in studies 0004 and 0005 were 65 or older. Response rates and time to progression were similar for the over 65 and younger patients.

ADVERSE REACTIONS

ARIMIDEX was generally well tolerated in two well-controlled clinical trials (i.e., Trials 0004 and 0005), with less than 3.3% of the ARIMIDEX-treated patients and 4.0% of the megestrol acetate-treated patients withdrawing due to an adverse event.

The principal adverse event more common with ARIMIDEX than megestrol acetate was diarrhea. Adverse events reported in greater than 5% of the patients in any of the treatment groups in these two well-controlled clinical trials, regardless of causality, are presented below:

Number (n) and Percentage of Patients with Adverse Event †

	ARIMIDEX 1 mg (n=262)		ARIMIDEX 10 mg (n=246)		Megestrol Acetate 160 mg (n=253)	
Adverse Event	n	%	n	%	n	%
Asthenia	42	(16.0)	33	(13.4)	47	(18.6)
Nausea	41	(15.6)	48	(19.5)	28	(11.1)
Headache	34	(13.0)	44	(17.9)	24	(9.5)
Hot Flushes	32	(12.2)	29	(10.6)	21	(8.3)
Pain	28	(10.7)	38	(15.4)	29	(11.5)
Back Pain	28	(10.7)	26	(10.6)	19	(7.5)
Dyspnea	24	(9.2)	27	(11.0)	53	(20.9)
Vomiting	24	(9.2)	26	(10.6)	16	(6.3)
Cough Increased	22	(8.4)	18	(7.3)	19	(7.5)
Diarrhea	22	(8.4)	18	(7.3)	7	(2.8)
Constipation	18	(6.9)	18	(7.3)	21	(8.3)
Abdominal Pain	18	(6.9)	14	(5.7)	18	(7.1)
Anorexia	18	(6.9)	19	(7.7)	11	(4.3)
Bone Pain	17	(6.5)	26	(11.8)	19	(7.5)
Pharyngitis	16	(6.1)	23	(9.3)	15	(5.9)
Dizziness	16	(6.1)	12	(4.9)	15	(5.9)
Rash	15	(5.7)	15	(6.1)	19	(7.5)
Dry Mouth	15	(5.7)	11	(4.5)	13	(5.1)
Peripheral Edema	14	(5.3)	21	(8.5)	28	(11.1)
Pelvic Pain	14	(5.3)	17	(6.9)	13	(5.1)
Depression	14	(5.3)	6	(2.4)	5	(2.0)
Chest Pain	13	(5.0)	18	(7.3)	13	(5.1)
Paresthesia	12	(4.6)	15	(6.1)	9	(3.6)
Vaginal Hemorrhage	6	(2.3)	4	(1.6)	13	(5.1)
Weight Gain	4	(1.5)	9	(3.7)	30	(11.9)
Sweating	4	(1.5)	3	(1.2)	16	(6.3)
Increased Appetite	0	(0)	1	(0.4)	13	(5.1)

† A patient may have more than one adverse event.

Other less frequent (2% to 5%) adverse experiences reported in patients receiving ARIMIDEX 1 mg in either Trial 0004 or Trial 0005 are listed below. These adverse experiences are listed by body system and are in order of decreasing frequency within each body system regardless of assessed causality.

Body as a Whole: Flu syndrome; fever; neck pain; malaise; accidental injury; infection

Cardiovascular: Hypertension; thrombophlebitis

Hepatic: Gamma GT increased; SGOT increased; SGPT increased

Hematologic: Anemia; leukopenia

Metabolic and Nutritional: Alkaline phosphatase increased; weight loss

Mean serum total cholesterol levels increased by 0.5 mmol/L among patients receiving ARIMIDEX. Increases in LDL cholesterol have been shown to contribute to these changes.

Musculoskeletal: Myalgia; arthralgia; pathological fracture

Nervous: Somnolence; confusion; insomnia; anxiety; nervousness

Respiratory: Sinusitis; bronchitis; rhinitis

Skin and Appendages: Hair thinning; pruritus

Urogenital: Urinary tract infection; breast pain

Vaginal bleeding has been reported infrequently, mainly in patients during the first few weeks after changing from existing hormonal therapy to treatment with ARIMIDEX. If bleeding persists, further evaluation should be considered.

The incidences of the following adverse event groups, potentially causally related to one or both of the therapies because of their pharmacology, were statistically analyzed: weight gain, edema, thromboembolic disease, gastrointestinal disturbance, hot flushes, and vaginal dryness. These six groups, and the adverse events captured in the groups, were prospectively defined. The results are shown in the table below.

Number (n) and Percentage of Patients

	ARIMIDEX 1 mg (n=262)		ARIMIDEX 10 mg (n=246)		Megestrol Acetate 160 mg (n=253)	
Adverse Event Group	n	%	n	%	n	%
Gastrointestinal Disturbance	77	(29.4)	81	(32.9)	54	(21.3)
Hot Flushes	33	(12.6)	29	(11.8)	35	(13.8)
Edema	19	(7.3)	28	(11.4)	35	(13.8)
Thomboembolic Disease	9	(3.4)	4	(1.6)	12	(4.7)
Vaginal Dryness	5	(1.9)	3	(1.2)	2	(0.8)
Weight Gain	4	(1.5)	10	(4.1)	30	(11.9)

More patients treated with megestrol acetate reported weight gain as an adverse event compared to patients treated with ARIMIDEX 1 mg ($p<0.0001$). Other differences were not statistically significant.

An examination of the magnitude of change in weight in all patients was also conducted. Thirty-four percent (87/253) of the patients treated with megestrol acetate experienced weight gain of 5% or more and 11% (27/253) of the patients treated with megestrol acetate experienced weight gain of 10% or more. Among patients treated with ARIMIDEX 1

Continued on next page

Arimidex—Cont.

mg, 13 % (33/262) experienced weight gain of 5% or more and 3% (6/262) experienced weight gain of 10% or more. On average, this 5 to 10% weight gain represented between 6 and 12 pounds.

No patients receiving ARIMIDEX or megestrol acetate discontinued treatment due to drug-related weight gain.

OVERDOSAGE

Clinical trials have been conducted with ARIMIDEX, up to 60 mg in a single dose given to healthy male volunteers and up to 10 mg daily given to postmenopausal women with advanced breast cancer; these dosages were well tolerated. A single dose of ARIMIDEX that results in life-threatening symptoms has not been established. In rats, lethality was observed after single oral doses that were greater than 100 mg/kg (about 800 times the recommended human dose on a mg/m² basis) and was associated with severe irritation to the stomach (necrosis, gastritis, ulceration, and hemorrhage).

There is no specific antidote to overdosage and treatment must be symptomatic. In the management of an overdose, consider that multiple agents may have been taken. Vomiting may be induced if the patient is alert. Dialysis may be helpful because ARIMIDEX is not highly protein bound. General supportive care, including frequent monitoring of vital signs and close observation of the patient, is indicated.

DOSAGE AND ADMINISTRATION

The dose of ARIMIDEX is one 1-mg tablet taken once a day. Patients treated with ARIMIDEX do not require glucocorticoid or mineralocorticoid replacement therapy.

Patients with Hepatic Impairment: (See CLINICAL PHARMACOLOGY) Hepatic metabolism accounts for approximately 85% of anastrozole elimination. Although clearance of anastrozole was decreased in patients with cirrhosis due to alcohol abuse, plasma anastrozole concentrations stayed in the usual range seen in patients without liver disease. Therefore, no changes in dose are recommended for patients with mild-to-moderate hepatic impairment, although patients should be monitored for side effects. ARIMIDEX has not been studied in patients with severe hepatic impairment.

Patients with Renal Impairment: No changes in dose are necessary for patients with renal impairment.

HOW SUPPLIED

White, biconvex, film-coated tablets containing 1 mg of anastrozole. The tablets are impressed on one side with a logo consisting of a letter "A" (upper case) with an arrowhead attached to the foot of the extended right leg of the "A" and on the reverse with the tablet strength marking "Adx 1". These tablets are supplied in bottles of 30 tablets (NDC 0310-0201-30)

Store at controlled room temperature, 20°–25°C (68°–77°F) [see USP].

ZENECA Pharmaceuticals

A Business Unit of Zeneca Inc.
Wilmington, Delaware 19850-5437
64076-03   Rev E 02/98

Shown in Product Identification Guide, page 345

CASODEX®   ℞
bicalutamide tablets

DESCRIPTION

CASODEX® (bicalutamide) Tablets for oral administration contain 50 mg of bicalutamide, a non-steroidal antiandrogen with no other known endocrine activity. The chemical name is propanamide, N-[4-cyano-3-(trifluoromethyl)phenyl]-3-[(4-fluorophenyl)sulfonyl]-2-hydroxy-2-methyl-,(+ −). The structural and empirical formulas are:

$C_{18}H_{14}N_2O_4F_4S$

Bicalutamide has a molecular weight of 430.37. The pKa' is approximately 12. Bicalutamide is a fine white to off-white powder which is practically insoluble in water at 37°C (5 mg per 1000 mL), slightly soluble in chloroform and absolute ethanol, sparingly soluble in methanol, and soluble in acetone and tetrahydrofuran.

CASODEX is a racemate with its antiandrogenic activity being almost exclusively exhibited by the R-enantiomer of bicalutamide; the S-enantiomer is essentially inactive.

The inactive ingredients of CASODEX Tablets are lactose, magnesium stearate, methylhydroxypropylcellulose, polyethylene glycol, polyvidone, sodium starch glycollate, and titanium dioxide.

CLINICAL PHARMACOLOGY

Mechanism of Action: CASODEX is a non-steroidal antiandrogen. It competitively inhibits the action of androgens by binding to cytosol androgen receptors in the target tissue. Prostatic carcinoma is known to be androgen sensitive and responds to treatment that counteracts the effect of androgen and/or removes the source of androgen.

When CASODEX is combined with luteinizing hormone-releasing hormone (LHRH) analogue therapy, the suppression of serum testosterone induced by the LHRH analogue is not affected. However, in clinical trials with CASODEX as a single agent for prostate cancer, rises in serum testosterone and estradiol have been noted.

Pharmacokinetics

Absorption: Bicalutamide is well-absorbed following oral administration, although the absolute bioavailability is unknown. Co-administration of bicalutamide with food has no clinically significant effect on rate or extent of absorption.

Distribution: Bicalutamide is highly protein-bound (96%). See Drug-Drug Interactions below.

Metabolism/Elimination: Bicalutamide undergoes stereospecific metabolism. The S (inactive) isomer is metabolized primarily by glucuronidation. The R (active) isomer also undergoes glucuronidation but is predominantly oxidized to an inactive metabolite followed by glucuronidation. Both the parent and metabolite glucuronides are eliminated in the urine and feces. The S-enantiomer is rapidly cleared relative to the R-enantiomer, with the R-enantiomer accounting for about 99% of total steady-state plasma levels.

Special Populations

Geriatric: In two studies in patients given 50 or 150 mg daily, no significant relationship between age and steady-state levels of total bicalutamide or the active R-enantiomer has been shown.

Hepatic Insufficiency: No clinically significant difference in the pharmacokinetics of either enantiomer of bicalutamide was noted in patients with mild-to-moderate hepatic disease as compared to healthy controls. However, the half-life of the R-enantiomer was increased approximately 76% (5.9 and 10.4 days for normal and impaired patients, respectively) in patients with severe liver disease (n=4).

Renal Insufficiency: Renal impairment (as measured by creatinine clearance) had no significant effect on the elimination of total bicalutamide or the active R-enantiomer.

Women, Pediatrics: Bicalutamide has not been studied in women or pediatric subjects.

Drug-Drug Interactions: Clinical studies have not shown any drug interactions between bicalutamide and LHRH analogues (goserelin or leuprolide). There is no evidence that bicalutamide induces hepatic enzymes. *In vitro* protein-binding studies have shown that bicalutamide can displace coumarin anticoagulants from binding sites. Prothrombin times should be closely monitored in patients already receiving coumarin anticoagulants who are started on CASODEX.

Pharmacokinetics of the active enantiomer of CASODEX in normal males and patients with prostate cancer are presented in Table 1.

Table 1

Parameter	Mean	Standard Deviation
Normal Males (n=30)		
Apparent Oral Clearance (L/hr)	0.320	0.103
Single Dose Peak Concentration (µg/mL)	0.768	0.178
Single Dose Time to Peak Concentration (hours)	31.3	14.6
Half-Life (days)	5.8	2.29
Patients with Prostate Cancer (n=40)		
C_{SS} (µg/mL)	8.939	3.504

C_{SS} = Mean Steady-State Concentration

Clinical Studies

In a multicenter, double-blind, controlled clinical trial, 813 patients with previously untreated advanced prostate cancer were randomized to receive CASODEX 50 mg once daily (404 patients) or flutamide 250 mg (409 patients) three times a day, each in combination with LHRH analogues (either goserelin acetate implant or leuprolide acetate depot). In an analysis conducted after a median follow-up of 160 weeks was reached, 213 (52.7%) patients treated with

CASODEX-LHRH analogue therapy and 235 (57.5%) patients treated with flutamide-LHRH analogue therapy had died. There was no significant difference in survival between treatment groups (see Figure 1). The hazard ratio for time to death (survival) was 0.87 (95% confidence interval 0.72 to 1.05).

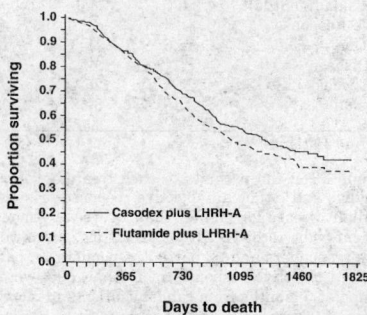

Figure 1
The Kaplan-Meier Probability of Death For Both Antiandrogen Treatment Groups

There was no significant difference in time to objective tumor progression between treatment groups (see Figure 2). Objective tumor progression was defined as the appearance of any bone metastases or the worsening of any existing bone metastases on bone scan attributable to metastatic disease, or an increase by 25% or more of any existing measurable extraskeletal metastases. The hazard ratio for time to progression of CASODEX plus LHRH analogue to that of flutamide plus LHRH analogue was 0.93 (95% confidence interval, 0.79 to 1.10).

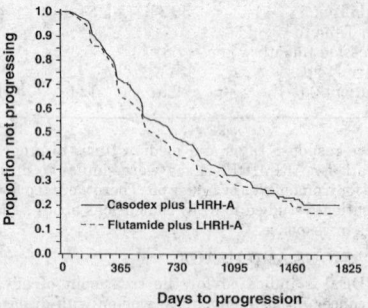

Figure 2
The Kaplan-Meier Curve For Time to Progression For Both Antiandrogen Treatment Groups

Quality of life was assessed with self-administered patient questionnaires on pain, social functioning, emotional well-being, vitality, activity limitation, bed disability, overall health, physical capacity, general symptoms, and treatment related symptoms. Assessment of the Quality of Life questionnaires did not indicate consistent significant differences between the two treatment groups.

INDICATIONS AND USAGE

CASODEX is indicated for use in combination therapy with a luteinizing hormone-releasing hormone (LHRH) analogue for the treatment of Stage D_2 metastatic carcinoma of the prostate.

CONTRAINDICATIONS

CASODEX is contraindicated in any patient who has shown a hypersensitivity reaction to the drug or any of the tablet's components.

CASODEX is not indicated in women. Further, CASODEX is contraindicated in women who are or may become pregnant. If this drug is used during pregnancy, or if the patient becomes pregnant while taking this drug, the patient should be apprised of the potential hazard to the fetus. CASODEX may cause fetal harm when administered to pregnant women. The male offspring of rats receiving doses of 10 mg/kg/day (plasma drug concentrations in rats equal to approximately 2/3 human therapeutic concentrations*) and above were observed to have reduced anogenital distance and hypospadias in reproductive toxicology studies. These pharmacological effects have been observed with other antiandrogens. No other teratogenic effects were observed in rabbits receiving doses up to 200 mg/kg/day (approximately 1/3 human therapeutic concentrations*) or rats receiving doses up to 250 mg/kg/day (approximately 2 times human therapeutic concentrations*).

*Based on a maximum dose of 50 mg/day of bicalutamide for an average 70 kg patient.

PRECAUTIONS

General

1. CASODEX should be used with caution in patients with moderate-to-severe hepatic impairment. CASODEX is extensively metabolized by the liver. Limited data in subjects with severe hepatic impairment suggest that excretion of CASODEX may be delayed and could lead to further accumulation. Periodic liver function tests should be considered for patients on long-term therapy.
2. In clinical trials with CASODEX as a single agent for prostate cancer, gynecomastia and breast pain have been reported in up to 38% and 39% of patients, respectively.
3. Regular assessments of serum Prostate Specific Antigen (PSA) may be helpful in monitoring the patient's response. If PSA levels rise during CASODEX therapy, the patient should be evaluated for clinical progression. For patients who have objective progression of disease together with an elevated PSA, a treatment-free period of antiandrogen, while continuing the LHRH analogue, may be considered.
4. Since transaminase abnormalities and, rarely, jaundice have been reported with the use of CASODEX, periodic liver function tests should be considered. If clinically indicated, eg, when the patient has jaundice or laboratory evidence of liver injury in the absence of liver metastases, CASODEX therapy should be discontinued. If transaminases increase over 2 times the upper limit of normal, treatment should be discontinued. Abnormalities are usually reversible upon discontinuation.

Information for Patients: Patients should be informed that therapy with CASODEX and the LHRH analogue should be initiated concomitantly, and that they should not interrupt or stop taking these medications without consulting their physician. Treatment with CASODEX should be started at the same time as treatment with an LHRH analogue.

Drug Interactions: *In vitro* studies have shown CASODEX can displace coumarin anticoagulants, such as warfarin, from their protein-binding sites. It is recommended that if CASODEX is started in patients already receiving coumarin anticoagulants, prothrombin times should be closely monitored and adjustment of the anticoagulant dose may be necessary (see CLINICAL PHARMACOLOGY, Drug-Drug Interactions).

Carcinogenesis, Mutagenesis, Impairment of Fertility: Two-year oral carcinogenicity studies were conducted in both male and female rats and mice at doses of 5, 15 or 75 mg/kg/day of bicalutamide. A variety of tumor target organ effects were identified and were attributed to the antiandrogenicity of bicalutamide, namely, testicular benign interstitial (Leydig) cell tumors in male rats at all dose levels (the steady-state plasma concentration with the 5 mg/kg/day dose is approximately 2/3 human therapeutic concentrations*) and uterine adenocarcinoma in female rats at 75 mg/kg/day (approximately 1 1/2 times the human therapeutic concentrations*). There is no evidence of Leydig cell hyperplasia in patients; uterine tumors are not relevant to the indicated patient population.

A small increase in the incidence of hepatocellular carcinoma in male mice given 75 mg/kg/day of bicalutamide (approximately 4 times human therapeutic concentrations*) and an increased incidence of benign thyroid follicular cell adenomas in rats given 5 mg/kg/day (approximately 2/3 human therapeutic concentrations*) and above were recorded. These neoplastic changes were progressions of non-neoplastic changes related to hepatic enzyme induction observed in animal toxicity studies. Enzyme induction has not been observed following bicalutamide administration in man. There were no tumorigenic effects suggestive of genotoxic carcinogenesis.

A comprehensive battery of both *in vitro* and *in vivo* genotoxicity tests (yeast gene conversion, Ames, *E. coli*, CHO/HGPRT, human lymphocyte cytogenetic, mouse micronucleus, and rat bone marrow cytogenetic tests) has demonstrated that CASODEX does not have genotoxic activity.

Administration of CASODEX may lead to inhibition of spermatogenesis. The long-term effects of CASODEX on male fertility have not been studied.

In male rats dosed at 250 mg/kg/day (approximately 2 times human therapeutic concentrations*), the precoital interval and time to successful mating were increased in the first pairing but no effects on fertility following successful mating were seen. These effects were reversed by 7 weeks after the end of an 11-week period of dosing.

No effects on female rats dosed at 10, 50 and 250 mg/kg/day (approximately 2/3, 1 and 2 times human therapeutic concentrations, respectively*) or their female offspring were observed. Administration of bicalutamide to pregnant females resulted in feminization of the male offspring leading to hypospadias at all dose levels. Affected male offspring were also impotent.

---

*Based on a maximum dose of 50 mg/day of bicalutamide for an average 70 kg patient.

Pregnancy: Pregnancy Category X (see CONTRAINDICATIONS).

Nursing Mothers: CASODEX is not indicated for use in women. It is not known whether this drug is excreted in human milk. Because many drugs are excreted in human milk, caution should be exercised when CASODEX is administered to a nursing woman.

Pediatric Use: Safety and effectiveness of CASODEX in pediatric patients have not been established.

ADVERSE REACTIONS

In patients with advanced prostate cancer treated with CASODEX in combination with an LHRH analogue, the most frequent adverse experience was hot flashes (53%).

In the multicenter, double-blind, controlled clinical trial comparing CASODEX 50 mg once daily with flutamide 250 mg three times a day, each in combination with an LHRH analogue, the following adverse experiences with an incidence of 5% or greater, regardless of causality, have been reported.

Table 2
Incidence of Adverse Events
(≥5% in Either Treatment Group)
Regardless of Causality

Body Systems Adverse Event	Treatment Group Number of Patients (%)			
	CASODEX Plus LHRH Analogue (n = 401)		Flutamide Plus LHRH Analogue (n = 407)	
Body as a Whole				
Pain (General)	142	(35)	127	(31)
Back Pain	102	(25)	105	(26)
Asthenia	89	(22)	87	(21)
Pelvic Pain	85	(21)	70	(17)
Infection	71	(18)	57	(14)
Abdominal Pain	46	(11)	46	(11)
Chest Pain	34	(8)	34	(8)
Headache	29	(7)	27	(7)
Flu Syndrome	28	(7)	30	(7)
Cardiovascular				
Hot Flashes	211	(53)	217	(53)
Hypertension	34	(8)	29	(7)
Digestive				
Constipation	87	(22)	69	(17)
Nausea	62	(15)	58	(14)
Diarrhea	49	(12)	107	(26)
Increased Liver Enzyme Test†	30	(7)	46	(11)
Dyspepsia	30	(7)	23	(6)
Flatulence	26	(6)	22	(5)
Anorexia	25	(6)	29	(7)
Vomiting	24	(6)	32	(8)
Hemic and Lymphatic				
Anemia††	45	(11)	53	(13)
Metabolic and Nutritional				
Peripheral Edema	53	(13)	42	(10)
Weight Loss	30	(7)	39	(10)
Hyperglycemia	26	(6)	27	(7)
Alkaline Phosphatase Increased	22	(5)	24	(6)
Weight gain	22	(5)	18	(4)
Musculoskeletal				
Bone Pain	37	(9)	43	(11)
Myastenia	27	(7)	19	(5)
Arthritis	21	(5)	29	(7)
Pathological Fracture	17	(4)	32	(8)
Nervous System				
Dizziness	41	(10)	35	(9)
Paresthesia	31	(8)	40	(10)
Insomnia	27	(7)	39	(10)
Anxiety	20	(5)	9	(2)
Depression	16	(4)	33	(8)
Respiratory System				
Dyspnea	51	(13)	32	(8)
Cough Increased	33	(8)	24	(6)
Pharyngitis	32	(8)	23	(6)
Bronchitis	24	(6)	22	(3)
Pneumonia	18	(4)	19	(5)
Rhinitis	15	(4)	22	(5)
Skin and Appendages				
Rash	35	(9)	30	(7)
Sweating	25	(6)	20	(5)
Urogenital				
Nocturia	49	(12)	55	(14)
Hematuria	48	(12)	26	(6)
Urinary Tract Infection	35	(9)	36	(9)
Gynecomastia	36	(9)	30	(7)
Impotence	27	(7)	35	(9)
Breast Pain	23	(6)	15	(4)
Urinary Frequency	23	(6)	29	(7)
Urinary Retention	20	(5)	14	(3)
Urination Impaired	19	(5)	15	(4)
Urinary Incontinence	15	(4)	32	(8)

† Increased liver enzyme test includes increases in AST, ALT or both.

†† Anemia includes anemia, hypochromic- and iron deficiency anemia.

Other adverse experiences (greater than or equal to 2%, but less than 5%) reported in the CASODEX-LHRH analogue treatment group are listed below by body system and are in order of decreasing frequency within each body system regardless of causality.

Body as a Whole: Neoplasm; Neck pain; Fever; Chills; Sepsis; Hernia; Cyst

Cardiovascular: Angina pectoris; Congestive heart failure; Myocardial infarct; Heart arrest; Coronary artery disorder; Syncope

Digestive: Melena; Rectal hemorrhage; Dry mouth; Dysphagia; Gastrointestinal disorder; Periodontal abscess; Gastrointestinal carcinoma

Metabolic and Nutritional: Edema; Bun increased; Creatinine increased; Dehydration; Gout; Hypercholesteremia

Musculoskeletal: Myalgia; Leg cramps

Nervous: Hypertonia; Confusion; Somnolence; Libido decreased; Neuropathy; Nervousness

Respiratory: Lung disorder; Asthma; Epistaxis; Sinusitis

Skin and Appendages: Dry skin; Alopecia; Pruritus; Herpes zoster; Skin carcinoma; Skin disorder

Special Senses: Cataract specified

Urogenital: Dysuria; Urinary urgency; Hydronephrosis; Urinary tract disorder

Abnormal Laboratory Test Values: Laboratory abnormalities including elevated AST, ALT, bilirubin, BUN, and creatinine and decreased hemoglobin and white cell count have been reported in both CASODEX-LHRH analogue treated and flutamide-LHRH analogue treated patients.

OVERDOSAGE

Long-term clinical trials have been conducted with dosages up to 200 mg of CASODEX daily and these dosages have been well tolerated. A single dose of CASODEX that results in symptoms of an overdose considered to be life-threatening has not been established.

There is no specific antidote; treatment of an overdose should be symptomatic.

In the management of an overdose with CASODEX, vomiting may be induced if the patient is alert. It should be remembered that, in this patient population, multiple drugs may have been taken. Dialysis is not likely to be helpful since CASODEX is highly protein bound and is extensively metabolized. General supportive care, including frequent monitoring of vital signs and close observation of the patient, is indicated.

DOSAGE AND ADMINISTRATION

The recommended dose for CASODEX therapy in combination with an LHRH analogue is one 50 mg tablet once daily (morning or evening), with or without food. It is recommended that CASODEX be taken at the same time each day. Treatment with CASODEX should be started at the same time as treatment with an LHRH analogue.

Dosage Adjustment in Renal Impairment: No dosage adjustment is necessary for patients with renal impairment (see CLINICAL PHARMACOLOGY, Special Populations, Renal Insufficiency).

Dosage Adjustment in Hepatic Impairment: No dosage adjustment is necessary for patients with mild to moderate hepatic impairment. Although there is a 76% (5.9 and 10.4 days for normal and impaired patients, respectively) increase in the half-life of the active enantiomer of bicalutamide in patients with severe liver impairment (n=4), no dosage adjustment is necessary (see CLINICAL PHARMACOLOGY, Special Populations, Hepatic Impairment and PRECAUTIONS sections).

HOW SUPPLIED

50 mg Tablets. (NDC 0310-0705) White, film-coated tablets (identified on one side with "CDX50" and on the reverse with the "CASODEX logo") are supplied in unit dose blisters of 30 tablets per carton (0310-0705-39), bottles of 30 tablets (0310-0705-30) and bottles of 100 tablets (0310-0705-10).

Store at controlled room temperature, 20°-25°C (68°-77°F).

Made in Germany

Manufactured for

Zeneca Pharmaceuticals
A Business Unit of Zeneca Inc.
Wilmington, Delaware 19850-5437 USA
by Zeneca GmbH, Plankstadt, Germany

64066-05 Rev J 03/98

Shown in Product Identification Guide, page 345

Continued on next page

CEFOTAN® ℞
[cef 'o-tan]
cefotetan disodium for injection
For Intravenous or Intramuscular Use

CEFOTAN® ℞
cefotetan injection
In GALAXY® Plastic Container (PL 2040)
For Intravenous Use Only

DESCRIPTION

CEFOTAN (cefotetan disodium for injection) and CEFOTAN (cefotetan injection) in Galaxy®* plastic container (PL 2040) as cefotetan disodium are sterile, semisynthetic, broad-spectrum, beta-lactamase resistant, cephalosporin (cephamycin) antibiotics for parenteral administration. It is the disodium salt of [6R-(6a,7a)]-7-[[[4-(2-amino-1-carboxy-2-oxoethylidene)-1,3-dithietan-2-yl]carbonyl]amino]-7-methoxy-3-[[(1-methyl-1*H*-tetrazol-5-yl)thio]methyl]-8-oxo-5-thia-1-azabicyclo[4.2.0]oct-2-ene-2-carboxylic acid. Its molecular formula is $C_{17}H_{15}N_7Na_2O_8S_4$ with a molecular weight of 619.57.

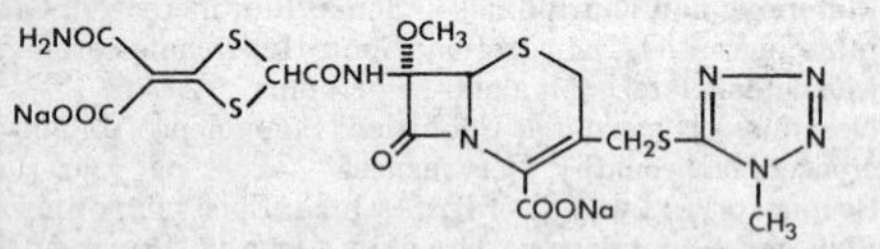

CEFOTAN (cefotetan disodium for injection) is supplied in vials containing 80 mg (3.5 mEq) of sodium per gram of cefotetan activity. It is a white to pale yellow powder which is very soluble in water. Reconstituted solutions of CEFOTAN (cefotetan disodium for injection) are intended for intravenous and intramuscular administration. The solution varies from colorless to yellow depending on the concentration. The pH of freshly reconstituted solutions is usually between 4.5 to 6.5.

CEFOTAN in the ADD-Vantage Vial† is intended for intravenous use only after dilution with the appropriate volume of ADD-Vantage diluent solution.

CEFOTAN is available in two vial strengths. Each CEFOTAN 1 g vial contains cefotetan disodium equivalent to 1 g cefotetan activity. Each CEFOTAN 2 g vial contains cefotetan disodium equivalent to 2 g cefotetan activity.

CEFOTAN (cefotetan injection) in the Galaxy® plastic container (PL 2040) is a frozen, iso-osmotic, sterile, nonpyrogenic premixed 50 mL solution containing 1 g or 2 g cefotetan as cefotetan disodium. Dextrose, USP has been added to adjust the osmolality to 300 mOsmol/kg (approximately 1.9 g and 1.1 g to the 1 g and 2 g dosages, respectively); sodium bicarbonate has been added to convert cefotetan free acid to the sodium salt. The pH has been adjusted between 4 and 6.5 with sodium bicarbonate and may have been adjusted with hydrochloric acid. CEFOTAN (cefotetan injection) in the Galaxy® plastic container (PL 2040) contains 80 mg (3.5 mEq) of sodium per gram of cefotetan activity. After thawing to room temperature, the solution is intended for intravenous use only.

This Galaxy® container is fabricated from a specially designed multilayer plastic (PL 2040). Solutions are in contact with the polyethylene layer of this container and can leach out certain chemical components of the plastic in very small amounts within the expiration dating period. The suitability of the plastic has been confirmed in tests in animals according to the USP biological tests for plastic containers as well as by tissue culture toxicity.

CLINICAL PHARMACOLOGY

High plasma levels of cefotetan are attained after intravenous and intramuscular administration of single doses to normal volunteers.

PLASMA CONCENTRATIONS AFTER 1 GRAM IV [a] OR IM DOSE
Mean Plasma Concentration (µg/mL)
Time After Injection

Route	15 min	30 min	1h	2h	4h	8h	12h
IV	92	158	103	72	42	18	9
IM	34	56	71	68	47	20	9

[a]30-minute infusion

PLASMA CONCENTRATIONS AFTER 2 GRAM IV [a] OR IM DOSE
Mean Plasma Concentration (µg/mL)
Time After Injection

Route	5 min	10 min	1h	3h	5h	9h	12h
IV	237	223	135	74	48	22	12[b]
IM	—	20	75	91	69	33	19

[a] Injected over 3 minutes
[b] Concentrations estimated from regression line

The plasma elimination half-life of cefotetan is 3 to 4.6 hours after either intravenous or intramuscular administration.

Repeated administration of CEFOTAN does not result in accumulation of the drug in normal subjects.

Cefotetan is 88% plasma protein bound.

No active metabolites of cefotetan have been detected; however, small amounts (less than 7%) of cefotetan in plasma and urine may be converted to its tautomer, which has antimicrobial activity similar to the parent drug.

In normal patients, from 51% to 81% of an administered dose of CEFOTAN is excreted unchanged by the kidneys over a 24 hour period, which results in high and prolonged urinary concentrations. Following intravenous doses of 1 gram and 2 grams, urinary concentrations are highest during the first hour and reach concentrations of approximately 1700 and 3500 µg/mL respectively.

In volunteers with reduced renal function, the plasma half-life of cefotetan is prolonged. The mean terminal half-life increases with declining renal function, from approximately 4 hours in volunteers with normal renal function to about 10 hours in those with moderate renal impairment. There is a linear correlation between the systemic clearance of cefotetan and creatinine clearance. When renal function is impaired, a reduced dosing schedule based on creatinine clearance must be used. (see DOSAGE AND ADMINISTRATION).

Therapeutic levels of cefotetan are achieved in many body tissues and fluids including:

skin	ureter
muscle	bladder
fat	maxillary sinus mucosa
myometrium	tonsil
endometrium	bile
cervix	peritoneal fluid
ovary	umbilical cord serum
kidney	amniotic fluid

Microbiology

The bactericidal action of cefotetan results from inhibition of cell wall synthesis. Cefotetan has *in vitro* activity against a wide range of aerobic and anaerobic gram-positive and gram-negative organisms. The methoxy group in the 7-alpha position provides cefotetan with a high degree of stability in the presence of beta-lactamases including both penicillinases and cephalosporinase of gram-negative bacteria. Cefotetan has been shown to be active against most strains of the following organisms **both *in vitro* and in clinical infections** (see **INDICATIONS AND USAGE**).

Gram-Negative Aerobes
Escherichia coli
Haemophilus influenzae (including ampicillin-resistant strains)
Klebsiella species (including *K. pneumoniae*)
Morganella morganii
Neisseria gonorrhoeae (nonpenicillinase-producing strains)
Proteus mirabilis
Proteus vulgaris
Providencia rettgeri
Serratia marcescens

NOTE: Approximately one-half of the usually clinically significant strains of *Enterobacter* species (e.g., *E. aerogenes* and *E. cloacae*) are resistant to cefotetan. Most strains of *Pseudomonas aeruginosa* and *Acinetobacter* species are resistant to cefotetan.

Gram-Positive Aerobes
Staphylococcus aureus (including penicillinase- and non-penicillinase-producing strains)
Staphylococcus epidermidis
Streptococcus agalactiae (group B beta-hemolytic streptococcus)
Streptococcus pneumoniae
Streptococcus pyogenes

NOTE: Methicillin-resistant staphylococci are resistant to cephalosporins. Some strains of *Staphylococcus epidermidis* and most strains of enterococci, e.g., *Enterococcus faecalis* (formerly *Streptococcus faecalis*) are resistant to cefotetan.

Anaerobes
Prevotella bivia (formerly *Bacteroides bivius*)
Prevotella disiens (formerly *Bacteroides disiens*)
Bacteroides fragilis
Prevotella melaninogenica (formerly Bacteroides melaninogenicus)
Bacteroides vulgatus
Fusobacterium species
Gram-positive bacilli (including *Clostridium* species; see WARNINGS)
NOTE: Most strains of *C. difficile* are resistant (see WARNINGS).
Peptococcus niger
Peptostreptococcus species

NOTE: Many strains of *B. distasonis*, *B. ovatus* and *B. thetaiotaomicron* are resistant to cefotetan *in vitro*. However, the therapeutic utility of cefotetan against these organisms cannot be accurately predicted on the basis of *in vitro* susceptibility tests alone.

The following *in vitro* data are available but their clinical significance is unknown. Cefotetan has been shown to be active *in vitro* against most strains of the following organisms:

Gram-Negative Aerobes
Citrobacter species (including *C. diversus* and *C. freundii*)
Klebsiella oxytoca
Moraxella (Branhamella) catarrhalis
Neisseria gonorrhoeae (penicillinase-producing strains)
Salmonella species
Serratia species
Shigella species
Yersinia enterocolitica

Anaerobes
Porphyromonas asaccharolytica (formerly *Bacteroides asaccharolyticus)*
Prevotella oralis (formerly *Bacteroides oralis)*
Bacteroides splanchnicus
Clostridium difficile (see WARNINGS)
Propionibacterium species
Veillonella species

Susceptibility Tests

Dilution Techniques: Quantitative methods are used to determine antimicrobial minimal inhibitory concentrations (MIC's). These MIC's provide estimates of the susceptibility of bacteria to antimicrobial compounds. The MICs should be determined using a standardized procedure. Standardized procedures are based on a dilution method[1] (broth or agar) or equivalent with standardized inoculum concentrations and standardized concentrations or cefotetan powder. The MIC values should be interpreted according to the following criteria:

MIC (µg/mL)	Interpretation
≤16	Susceptible (S)
32	Intermediate (I)
≥64	Resistant (R)

A report of 'Susceptible' indicates that the pathogen is likely to be inhibited if the antimicrobial compound in the blood reaches the concentrations usually achievable. A report of 'Intermediate' indicates that the result should be considered equivocal, and if the microorganism is not fully susceptible to alternative, clinically feasible drugs, the test should be repeated. This category implies possible clinical applicability in body sites where the drug is physiologically concentrated or in situations where high dosage of drug can be used. This category also provides a buffer zone which prevents small uncontrolled technical factors from causing major discrepancies in interpretation. A report of 'Resistant' indicates that the pathogen is not likely to be inhibited if the antimicrobial compound in the blood reaches the concentrations usually achievable; other therapy should be selected.

Standardized susceptibility test procedures require the use of laboratory control microorganisms to control the technical aspects of the laboratory procedures. Standard cefotetan powder should provide the following MIC values:

Microorganism	MIC (µg/mL)
E. coli ATCC 25922	0.06–0.25
S. aureus ATCC 29213	4–16

Diffusion Techniques: Quantitative methods that require measurement of zone diameters also provide reproducible estimates of the susceptibility of bacteria to antimicrobial compounds. One such standardized procedure[2] requires the use of the standardized inoculum concentrations. This procedure uses paper disks impregnated with 30 µg cefotetan to test the susceptibility of microorganisms to cefotetan.

Reports from the laboratory providing results of the standard single-disk susceptibility test with a 30 µg cefotetan disk should be interpreted according to the following criteria:

Zone Diameter (mm)	Interpretation
≥16	Susceptible (S)
13–15	Intermediate (I)
≤12	Resistant (R)

Interpretation should be as stated above for results using dilution techniques. Interpretation involves correlation of the diameter obtained in the disk test with the MIC for cefotetan.

As with standardized dilution techniques, diffusion methods require the use of laboratory control microorganisms that are used to control the technical aspects of the laboratory procedures. For the diffusion technique, the 30 µg cefotetan disk should provide the following zone diameters in these laboratory test quality control strains.

Microorganism	Zone Diameter (mm)
E. coli ATCC 25922	28–34
S. aureus ATCC 25923	17–23

Anaerobic Techniques: For anaerobic bacteria, the susceptibility to cefotetan as MIC's can be determined by standardized test methods[3]. The MIC values obtained should be interpreted according to the following criteria:

MIC (μg/mL)	Interpretation
≤16	Susceptible (S)
32	Intermediate (I)
≥64	Resistant (R)

Interpretation is identical to that stated above for results using dilution techniques.

As with other susceptibility techniques, the use of laboratory control microorganisms is required to control the technical aspects of the laboratory standardized procedures. Standardized cefotetan powder should provide the following MIC values:

Microorganism	MIC (μg/mL)
Bacteroides fragilis ATCC 25285	4–16
Bacteroides thetaiotaomicron ATCC 29741	32–128
Eubacterium lentum ATCC 43055	32–128

INDICATIONS AND USAGE

Treatment

CEFOTAN is indicated for the therapeutic treatment of the following infections when caused by susceptible strains of the designated organisms:

Urinary Tract Infections caused by *E. coli, Klebsiella* spp (including *K. pneumoniae*), *Proteus mirabilis* and *Proteus* spp (which may include the organisms now called *Proteus vulgaris, Providencia rettgeri*, and *Morganella morganii*).

Lower Respiratory Tract Infections caused by *Streptococcus pneumoniae, Staphylococcus aureus* (penicillinase- and non-penicillinase-producing strains), *Haemophilus influenzae* (including ampicillin- resistant strains), *Klebsiella* species (including *K. pneumoniae*), *E. coli, Proteus mirabilis*, and *Serratia marcescens**.

Skin and Skin Structure Infections due to *Staphylococcus aureus* (penicillinase- and nonpenicillinase-producing strains), *Staphylococcus epidermidis, Streptococcus pyogenes, Streptococcus* species (excluding enterococci), *Escherichia coli, Klebsiella pneumoniae, Peptococcus niger**, *Peptostreptococcus species*.

Gynecologic Infections caused by *Staphylococcus aureus*, (including penicillinase- and nonpenicillinase-producing strains), *Staphylococcus epidermidis, Streptococcus* species (excluding enterococci), *Streptococcus agalactiae, E. coli, Proteus mirabilis, Neisseria gonorrhoeae*, Bacteroides species (excluding *B. distasonis, B. ovatus, B. thetaiotaomicron*), *Fusobacterium* species*, and gram-positive anaerobic cocci (including *Peptococcus niger* and *Peptostreptococcus* species).

Cefotetan, like other cephalosporins, has no activity against *Chlamydia trachomatis*. Therefore, when cephalosporins are used in the treatment of pelvic inflammatory disease, and *C. trachomatis* is one of the suspected pathogens, appropriate antichlamydial coverage should be added.

Intra-abdominal Infections caused by *E. coli, Klebsiella* species (including *K. pneumoniae*), *Streptococcus* species (excluding enterococci), *Bacteroides* species (excluding *B. distasonis, B. ovatus, B. thetaiotaomicron*) and *Clostridium* species*.

Bone and Joint Infections caused by *Staphylococcus aureus*.*

*Efficacy for this organism in this organ system was studied in fewer than ten infections.

Specimens for bacteriological examination should be obtained in order to isolate and identify causative organisms and to determine their susceptibilities to cefotetan. Therapy may be instituted before results of susceptibility studies are known; however, once these results become available, the antibiotic treatment should be adjusted accordingly.

In cases of confirmed or suspected gram-positive or gram-negative sepsis or in patients with other serious infections in which the causative organism has not been identified, it is possible to use CEFOTAN concomitantly with an aminoglycoside. Cefotetan combinations with aminoglycosides have been shown to be synergistic *in vitro* against many Enterobacteriaceae and also some other gram-negative bacteria. The dosage recommended in the labeling of both antibiotics may be given and depends on the severity of the infection and the patient's condition.

NOTE: Increases in serum creatinine have occurred when CEFOTAN was given alone. If CEFOTAN and an aminoglycoside are used concomitantly, renal function should be carefully monitored, because nephrotoxicity may be potentiated.

Prophylaxis

The preoperative administration of CEFOTAN may reduce the incidence of certain postoperative infections in patients undergoing surgical procedures that are classified as clean contaminated or potentially contaminated (e.g., cesarean section, abdominal or vaginal hysterectomy, transurethral surgery, biliary tract surgery, and gastrointestinal surgery).

General Guidelines for Dosage of CEFOTAN

Type of Infection	Daily Dose	Frequency and Route
Urinary Tract	1–4 grams	500 mg every 12 hours IV or IM 1 or 2 g every 24 hours IV or IM 1 or 2 g every 12 hours IV or IM
Skin & Skin Structure		
Mild–Moderate[a]	2 grams	2 g every 24 hours IV 1 g every 12 hours IV or IM
Severe	4 grams	2 g every 12 hours IV
Other Sites	2–4 grams	1 or 2 g every 12 hours IV or IM
Severe	4 grams	2 g every 12 hours IV
Life-Threatening	6 grams[b]	3 g every 12 hours IV

[a] *Klebsiella pneumoniae* skin and skin structure infections should be treated with 1 or 2 grams every 12 hours IV or IM.
[b] Maximum daily dosage should not exceed 6 grams.

If there are signs and symptoms of infection, specimens for culture should be obtained for identification of the causative organism so that appropriate therapeutic measures may be initiated.

CONTRAINDICATIONS

CEFOTAN is contraindicated in patients with known allergy to the cephalosporin group of antibiotics and in those individuals who have experienced a cephalosporin associated hemolytic anemia.

WARNINGS

BEFORE THERAPY WITH CEFOTAN IS INSTITUTED, CAREFUL INQUIRY SHOULD BE MADE TO DETERMINE WHETHER THE PATIENT HAS HAD PREVIOUS HYPERSENSITIVITY REACTIONS TO CEFOTETAN, CEPHALOSPORINS, PENICILLINS, OR OTHER DRUGS. IF THIS PRODUCT IS TO BE GIVEN TO PENICILLIN-SENSITIVE PATIENTS, CAUTION SHOULD BE EXERCISED BECAUSE CROSS-HYPERSENSITIVITY AMONG BETA-LACTAM ANTIBIOTICS HAS BEEN CLEARLY DOCUMENTED AND MAY OCCUR IN UP TO 10% OF PATIENTS WITH A HISTORY OF PENICILLIN ALLERGY. IF AN ALLERGIC REACTION TO CEFOTAN OCCURS, DISCONTINUE THE DRUG. SERIOUS ACUTE HYPERSENSITIVITY REACTIONS MAY REQUIRE TREATMENT WITH EPINEPHRINE AND OTHER EMERGENCY MEASURES, INCLUDING OXYGEN, INTRAVENOUS FLUIDS, INTRAVENOUS ANTIHISTAMINES, CORTICOSTEROIDS, PRESSOR AMINES, AND AIRWAY MANAGEMENT, AS CLINICALLY INDICATED.

AN IMMUNE MEDIATED HEMOLYTIC ANEMIA HAS BEEN OBSERVED IN PATIENTS RECEIVING CEPHALOSPORIN CLASS ANTIBIOTICS. RARE CASES OF SEVERE HEMOLYTIC ANEMIA, INCLUDING FATALITIES, HAVE BEEN REPORTED IN ASSOCIATION WITH CEFOTETAN AND OTHER CEPHALOSPORINS. IF A PATIENT DEVELOPS ANEMIA ANYTIME WITHIN 2–3 WEEKS SUBSEQUENT TO THE ADMINISTRATION OF CEFOTETAN, THE DIAGNOSIS OF A CEPHALOSPORIN ASSOCIATED ANEMIA SHOULD BE CONSIDERED AND THE DRUG STOPPED UNTIL THE ETIOLOGY IS DETERMINED WITH CERTAINTY. BLOOD TRANSFUSIONS MAY BE CONSIDERED AS NEEDED (See CONTRAINDICATIONS).

PATIENTS WHO RECEIVE PROLONGED COURSES OF CEFOTETAN FOR TREATMENT OF INFECTIONS SHOULD HAVE PERIODIC MONITORING FOR SIGNS AND SYMPTOMS OF HEMOLYTIC ANEMIA INCLUDING A MEASUREMENT OF HEMATOLOGICAL PARAMETERS WHERE APPROPRIATE.

Pseudomembranous colitis has been reported with nearly all antibacterial agents, including cefotetan, and may range in severity from mild to life-threatening. Therefore, it is important to consider this diagnosis in patients who present with diarrhea subsequent to the administration of antibacterial agents.

Treatment with antibacterial agents alters the normal flora of the colon and may permit overgrowth of clostridia. Studies indicate that a toxin produced by *Clostridium difficile* is a primary cause of "antibiotic-associated colitis".

After the diagnosis of pseudomembranous colitis has been established, appropriate therapeutic measures should be initiated. Mild cases of pseudomembranous colitis usually respond to drug discontinuation alone. In moderate to severe cases, consideration should be given to management with fluids and electrolytes, protein supplementation, and treatment with an antibacterial drug clinically effective against *Clostridium difficile* colitis. (See ADVERSE REACTIONS.)

In common with many other broad-spectrum antibiotics, CEFOTAN may be associated with a fall in prothrombin activity and, possibly, subsequent bleeding. Those at increased risk include patients with renal or hepatobiliary impairment or poor nutritional state, the elderly, and patients with cancer. Prothrombin time should be monitored and exogenous vitamin K administered as indicated.

PRECAUTIONS

General: As with other broad-spectrum antibiotics, prolonged use of CEFOTAN may result in overgrowth of nonsusceptible organisms. Careful observation of the patient is essential. If superinfection does occur during therapy, appropriate measures should be taken.

CEFOTAN should be used with caution in individuals with a history of gastrointestinal disease, particularly colitis.

Information for Patients: As with some other cephalosporins, a disulfiram-like reaction characterized by flushing, sweating, headache, and tachycardia may occur when alcohol (beer, wine, etc.) is ingested within 72 hours after CEFOTAN administration. Patients should be cautioned about the ingestion of alcoholic beverages following the administration of CEFOTAN.

Drug Interactions: Increases in serum creatinine have occurred when CEFOTAN was given alone. If CEFOTAN and an aminoglycoside are used concomitantly, renal function should be carefully monitored, because nephrotoxicity may be potentiated.

Drug/Laboratory Test Interactions: The administration of CEFOTAN may result in a false positive reaction for glucose in the urine using Clinitest®‡, Benedict's solution, or Fehling's solution. It is recommended that glucose tests based on enzymatic glucose oxidase be used.

As with other cephalosporins, high concentrations of cefotetan may interfere with measurement of serum and urine creatinine levels by Jaffe' reaction and produce false increases in the levels of creatinine reported.

Carcinogenesis, Mutagenesis, Impairment of Fertility: Although long-term studies in animals have not been performed to evaluate carcinogenic potential, no mutagenic potential of cefotetan was found in standard laboratory tests. Cefotetan has adverse effects on the testes of prepubertal rats. Subcutaneous administration of 500 mg/kg/day (approximately 8-16 times the usual adult human dose) on days 6-35 of life (thought to be developmentally analogous to late childhood and prepuberty in humans) resulted in reduced testicular weight and seminiferous tubule degeneration in 10 of 10 animals. Affected cells included spermatogonia and spermatocytes; Sertoli and Leydig cells were unaffected. Incidence and severity of lesions were dose-dependent; at 120 mg/kg/day (approximately 2-4 times the usual human dose) only 1 of 10 treated animals was affected, and the degree of degeneration was mild.

Similar lesions have been observed in experiments of comparable design with other methylthiotetrazole-containing antibiotics and impaired fertility has been reported, particularly at high dose levels. No testicular effects were observed in 7-week-old rats treated with up to 1000 mg/kg/day SC for 5 weeks, or in infant dogs (3 weeks old) that received up to 300 mg/kg/day IV for 5 weeks. The relevance of these findings to humans is unknown.

Pregnancy: Teratogenic Effects. Pregnancy Category B: Reproduction studies have been performed in rats and monkeys at doses up to 20 times the human dose and have revealed no evidence of impaired fertility or harm to the fetus due to cefotetan. There are, however, no adequate and well-controlled studies in pregnant women. Because animal reproductive studies are not always predictive of human response, this drug should be used during pregnancy only if clearly needed.

Nursing Mothers: Cefotetan is excreted in human milk in very low concentrations. Caution should be exercised when cefotetan is administered to a nursing woman.

Pediatric Use: Safety and effectiveness in children have not been established.

ADVERSE REACTIONS

In clinical studies, the following adverse effects were considered related to CEFOTAN therapy. Those appearing in italics have been reported during postmarketing experience.

Gastrointestinal symptoms occurred in 1.5% of patients, the most frequent were diarrhea (1 in 80) and nausea (1 in 700);

Continued on next page

Cefotan—Cont.

pseudomembranous colitis. Onset of pseudomembranous colitis symptoms may occur during or after antibiotic treatment or surgical prophylaxis. (See **WARNINGS.**)

Hematologic laboratory abnormalities occurred in 1.4% of patients and included eosinophilia (1 in 200), positive direct Coombs' test (1 in 250), and thrombocytosis (1 in 300); *agranulocytosis, hemolytic anemia, leukopenia, thrombocytopenia,* and *prolonged prothrombin time with or without bleeding.*

Hepatic enzyme elevations occurred in 1.2% of patients and included a rise in ALT (SGPT) (1 in 150), AST (SGOT) (1 in 300), alkaline phosphatase (1 in 700), and LDH (1 in 700).

Hypersensitivity reactions were reported in 1.2% of patients and included rash (1 in 150) and itching (1 in 700); *anaphylactic reactions and urticaria.*

Local effects were reported in less than 1% of patients and included phlebitis at the site of injection (1 in 300), and discomfort (1 in 500).

Renal: *Elevations in BUN and serum creatinine have been reported.*

Urogenital: *Nephrotoxicity has rarely been reported.*

Miscellaneous: *Fever*

In addition to the adverse reactions listed above which have been observed in patients treated with cefotetan, the following adverse reactions and altered laboratory tests have been reported for cephalosporin-class antibiotics: pruritus, Stevens-Johnson syndrome, erythema multiforme, toxic epidermal necrolysis, vomiting, abdominal pain, colitis, superinfection, vaginitis including vaginal candidiasis, renal dysfunction, toxic nephropathy, hepatic dysfunction including cholestasis, aplastic anemia, hemorrhage, elevated bilirubin, pancytopenia, and neutropenia.

Several cephalosporins have been implicated in triggering seizures, particularly in patients with renal impairment, when the dosage was not reduced. (See DOSAGE AND ADMINISTRATION and OVERDOSAGE.) If seizures associated with drug therapy occur, the drug should be discontinued. Anticonvulsant therapy can be given if clinically indicated.

OVERDOSAGE

Information on overdosage with CEFOTAN in humans is not available. If overdosage should occur, it should be treated symptomatically and hemodialysis considered, particularly if renal function is compromised.

DOSAGE AND ADMINISTRATION

Treatment

Cefotetan injection in Galaxy® plastic container should not be used for intramuscular administration.

CEFOTAN in the ADD-Vantage Vial is intended for intravenous infusion only, after dilution with the appropriate volume of ADD-Vantage diluent solution.

The usual adult dosage is 1 or 2 grams of CEFOTAN (cefotetan disodium for injection) administered intravenously or intramuscularly or CEFOTAN (cefotetan injection) in the Galaxy® plastic container (PL 2040) administered intravenously every 12 hours for 5 to 10 days. Proper dosage and route of administration should be determined by the condition of the patient, severity of the infection, and susceptibility of the causative organism.

[See table at top of previous page]

If *Chlamydia trachomatis* is a suspected pathogen in gynecologic infections, appropriate antichlamydial coverage should be added, since cefotetan has no activity against this organism.

Prophylaxis:

To prevent postoperative infection in clean contaminated or potentially contaminated surgery in adults, the recommended dosage is 1 or 2 g of CEFOTAN administered once, intravenously, 30 to 60 minutes prior to surgery. In patients undergoing cesarean section, the dose should be administered as soon as the umbilical cord is clamped.

Impaired Renal Function:

When renal function is impaired, a reduced dosage schedule must be employed. The following dosage guidelines may be used.

[See table at bottom of next page]

Alternatively, the dosing interval may remain constant at 12 hour intervals, but the dose reduced to one-half the usual recommended dose for patients with a creatinine clearance of 10-30 mL/min, and one-quarter the usual recommended dose for patients with a creatinine clearance of less than 10 mL/min.

When only serum creatinine levels are available, creatinine clearance may be calculated from the following formula. The serum creatinine level should represent a steady state of renal function.

Males: $\dfrac{\text{Weight (kg)} \times (140 - \text{age})}{72 \times \text{serum creatinine (mg/100 mL)}}$

Females: $0.9 \times \text{value for males}$

Cefotetan is dialyzable and it is recommended that for patients undergoing intermittent hemodialysis, one-quarter

---

the usual recommended dose be given every 24 hours on days between dialysis and one-half the usual recommended dose on the day of dialysis.

CEFOTETAN DISODIUM FOR INJECTION

Preparation of Solution From Cefotetan Disodium For Injection

For Intravenous Use: Reconstitute with Sterile Water for Injection. Shake to dissolve and let stand until clear.

Vial Size	Amount of Diluent Added (mL)	Approximate Withdrawable Vol (mL)	Approximate Average Concentration (mg/mL)
1 gram	10	10.5	95
2 gram	10–20	11–21	182–95

Infusion bottles (100 mL) may be reconstituted with 50 to 100 mL of Dextrose Injection 5% or Sodium Chloride Injection 0.9%.

NOTE: ADD-VANTAGE VIALS ARE NOT TO BE USED IN THIS MANNER

For ADD-Vantage Vials: ADD-Vantage Vials of CEFOTAN are to be reconstituted only with Sodium Chloride Injection 0.9% or Dextrose Injection 5% in the 50 mL, 100 mL or 250 mL Flexible Diluent Containers. CEFOTAN supplied in single-use ADD-Vantage Vials should be prepared as directed.

Directions for Use of CEFOTAN (cefotetan disodium for injection) in ADD-Vantage Vials:

To Open Diluent Container: Peel overwrap from the corner and remove container. Some opacity of the plastic due to moisture absorption during the sterilization process may be observed. This is normal and does not affect the solution quality or safety. The opacity will diminish gradually.

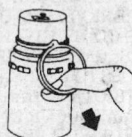

Figure 1

To Assemble ADD-Vantage Vial and Flexible Diluent Container: (Use Aseptic Technique)

1. Remove the protective covers from the top of the vial and the vial port on the diluent container as follows:

   a. To remove the breakaway vial cap, swing the pull ring over the top of the vial and pull down far enough to start the opening (See Figure 1), then pull straight up to remove the cap. (See Figure 2.) **NOTE:** Once the breakaway cap has been removed, do not access vial with syringe.

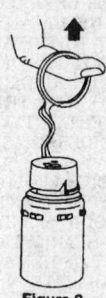

Figure 2

   b. To remove the vial port cover, grasp the tab on the pull ring, pull up to break the three tie strings, then pull back to remove the cover. (See Figure 3.)

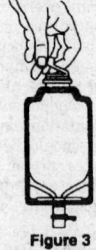

Figure 3

2. Screw the vial into the vial port until it will go no further. **THE VIAL MUST BE SCREWED IN TIGHTLY TO ASSURE A SEAL.** This occurs approximately 1/2 turn (180°) after the first audible click. (See Figure 4.) The clicking sound does not assure a seal; the vial must be turned as

---

far as it will go. **NOTE: ONCE VIAL IS SEATED, DO NOT ATTEMPT TO REMOVE. (See Figure 4.)**

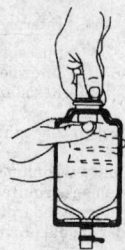

Figure 4

3. Recheck the vial to assure that it is tight by trying to turn it further in the direction of assembly.
4. Label appropriately.

To Prepare Admixture:

1. Squeeze the bottom of the diluent container gently to inflate the portion of the container surrounding the end of the drug vial.
2. With the other hand, push the drug vial down into the container telescoping the walls of the container. Grasp the inner cap of the vial through the walls of the container. (See Figure 5.)

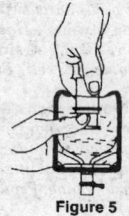

Figure 5

3. Pull the inner cap from the drug vial. (See Figure 6.) Verify that the rubber stopper has been pulled out and invert the system several times, allowing the drug and diluent to mix.

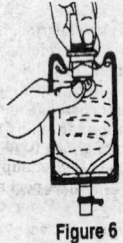

Figure 6

4. Mix contents thoroughly and use within the specified time.

Preparation For Administration: (Use Aseptic Technique)

1. Confirm the activation and admixture of vial contents.
2. Check for leaks by squeezing container firmly. If leaks are found, discard unit as sterility may be impaired.
3. Close flow control clamp of administration set.
4. Remove cover from outlet port at bottom of container.
5. Insert piercing pin of administration set into port with a twisting motion until the pin is firmly seated. **NOTE:** See full directions on administration set carton.
6. Lift the free end of the hanger loop on the bottom of the vial, breaking the two tie strings. Bend the loop outward to lock it in the upright position, then suspend container from hanger.
7. Squeeze and release drip chamber to establish proper fluid level in chamber.
8. Open flow control clamp and clear air from set. Close clamp.
9. Attach set to venipuncture device. If device is not indwelling, prime and make venipuncture.
10. Regulate rate of administration with flow control clamp.

WARNING: Do not use flexible container in series connections.

For Intramuscular Use: Reconstitute with Sterile Water for Injection; Bacteriostatic Water for Injection; Sodium Chloride Injection 0.9%, USP; 0.5% Lidocaine HCl; or 1% Lidocaine HCl. Shake to dissolve and let stand until clear.

Vial Size	Amount of Diluent Added (mL)	Approximate Withdrawable Vol (mL)	Average Concentration (mg/mL)
1 gram	2	2.5	400
2 gram	3	4	500

Intravenous Administration:
The intravenous route is preferable for patients with bacteremia, bacterial septicemia, or other severe or life-threatening infections, or for patients who may be poor risks because of lowered resistance resulting from such debilitating conditions as malnutrition, trauma, surgery, diabetes, heart failure, or malignancy, particularly if shock is present or impending.

For intermittent intravenous administration, a solution containing 1 gram or 2 grams of CEFOTAN (cefotetan disodium for injection) in Sterile Water for Injection can be injected over a period of three to five minutes. Using an infusion system, the solution may also be given over a longer period of time through the tubing system by which the patient may be receiving other intravenous solutions. Butterfly® or scalp vein- type needles are preferred for this type of infusion. However, during infusion of the solution containing CEFOTAN (cefotetan disodium for injection), it is advisable to discontinue temporarily the administration of other solutions at the same site.

NOTE: Solutions of CEFOTAN must not be admixed with solutions containing aminoglycosides. If CEFOTAN and aminoglycosides are to be administered to the same patient, they must be administered separately and not as a mixed injection.

Intramuscular Administration:
As with all intramuscular preparations, (cefotetan disodium for injection) should be injected well within the body of a relatively large muscle such as the upper outer quadrant of the buttock (i.e., gluteus maximus); aspiration is necessary to avoid inadvertent injection into a blood vessel.

CEFOTETAN INJECTION

Directions for Use of CEFOTAN (cefotetan injection) in Galaxy® Plastic Container (PL2040)
CEFOTAN (cefotetan injection) in Galaxy® plastic container (PL 2040) is for intravenous administration only.

Storage: Store in a freezer capable of maintaining a temperature of -20°C/-4°F.

Thawing of Plastic Container: Thaw frozen container at room temperature (25°C/77°F) or in a refrigerator (5°C/41°F). **[DO NOT FORCE THAW BY IMMERSION IN WATER BATHS OR BY MICROWAVE IRRADIATION.]**

Check for minute leaks by squeezing container firmly. If leaks are detected, discard solution as sterility may be impaired.

The container should be visually inspected. Components of the solution may precipitate in the frozen state and will dissolve upon reaching room temperature with little or no agitation. Potency is not affected. Agitate after solution has reached room temperature. If after visual inspection the solution remains cloudy or if an insoluble precipitate is noted or if any seals or outlet ports are not intact, the container should be discarded.

Preparation of Intravenous Use (Use aseptic technique):
1. Suspend container from eyelet support.
2. Remove protector from outlet port at bottom of container.
3. Attach administration set. Refer to complete directions accompanying set.

Caution: Do not use plastic containers in series connections. Such use could result in air embolism due to residual air being drawn from the primary container before administration of the fluid from the secondary container is complete.

Intravenous Administration:
The intravenous route is preferable for patients with bacteremia, bacterial septicemia, or other severe or life threatening infections, or for patients who may be poor risks because of lowered resistance resulting from such debilitating conditions as malnutrition, trauma, surgery, diabetes, heart failure, or malignancy, particularly if shock is present or impending.

Using an infusion system, CEFOTAN (cefotetan injection) in Galaxy® plastic container (PL 2040) should be given over 20 to 60 minutes through the tubing system by which the patient may be receiving other intravenous solutions. Butterfly® or scalp vein-type needles are preferred for this type of infusion. However, during infusion of the solution containing CEFOTAN (cefotetan injection) in Galaxy® plastic container (PL 2040), it is advisable to discontinue temporarily the administration of other solutions at the same site.

Compatibility and Stability of CEFOTAN Products:
Frozen samples should be thawed at room temperature before use. After the periods mentioned below, any unused solutions or frozen material should be discarded. **DO NOT REFREEZE.**

NOTE: Solutions of CEFOTAN must not be admixed-with solutions containing aminoglycosides. If CEFOTAN and aminoglycosides are to be administered to the same patient, they must be administered separately and not as a mixed injection. **DO NOT ADD SUPPLEMENTARY MEDICATION.**

CEFOTETAN DISODIUM FOR INJECTION
CEFOTAN (cefotetan disodium for injection) reconstituted as described above (PREPARATION OF SOLUTION) maintains satisfactory potency for 24 hours at room temperature (25°C/77°F), for 96 hours under refrigeration (5°C/41°F), and for at least 1 week in the frozen state (-20°C/-4°F). After reconstitution and subsequent storage in disposable glass or plastic syringes, CEFOTAN (cefotetan disodium for injection) is stable for 24 hours at room temperature and 96 hours under refrigeration.

ADD-Vantage Vials:
Ordinarily, ADD-Vantage Vials should be reconstituted only when it is certain that the patient is ready to receive the drug. However, ADD-Vantage Vials of CEFOTAN reconstituted as described in Preparation of Solution, for ADD-Vantage Vials, maintains satisfactory potency for 24 hours at room temperature (25°C/77°F).
(DO NOT REFRIGERATE OR FREEZE CEFOTAN IN ADD-VANTAGE VIALS.)

CEFOTETAN INJECTION
The thawed solution in Galaxy® plastic container (PL 2040) remains chemically stable for 48 hours at room temperature (25°C/77°F) or for 21 days under refrigeration (5°C/41°F).

NOTE: Parenteral drug products should be inspected visually for particulate matter and discoloration prior to administration whenever solution and container permit.

HOW SUPPLIED

CEFOTAN (cefotetan disodium for injection) is a dry, white to pale yellow powder supplied in vials containing cefotetan disodium equivalent to 1 g and 2 g cefotetan activity for intravenous and intramuscular administration. The vials should not be stored at temperatures above 22° C (72° F) and should be protected from light.
1 g ADD-Vantage Vial (NDC 0310-0376-31)
2 g ADD-Vantage Vial (NDC 0310-0377-32)
1 g Vial (NDC 0310-0376-10)
2 g Vial (NDC 0310-0377-20)
1 g Piggyback Vial (NDC 0310-0376-11)
2 g Piggyback Vial (NDC 0310-0377-21)
CEFOTAN is also available as a 10 g pharmacy bulk package.
10g in 100 mL Vial (NDC 0310-0375-10)
CEFOTAN (cefotetan injection) is supplied as a frozen, iso-osmotic, premixed solution in single dose Galaxy® plastic containers (PL 2040) as follows:
1 g in 50 mL plastic container (NDC 0310-0378-51)
2 g in 50 mL plastic container (NDC 0310-0379-51)
Store containers at or below -20°C/-4°F. **[See DIRECTIONS FOR USE OF CEFOTAN (cefotetan injection) IN GALAXY® PLASTIC CONTAINER (PL 2040)].**

REFERENCES

1. National Committee for Clinical Laboratory Standards. Methods for Dilution Antimicrobial Susceptibility Tests for Bacteria that Grow Aerobically—Third Edition. Approved Standard NCCLS Document M7-A3, Vol. 13, No. 25, NCCLS, Villanova, PA, December, 1993.
2. National Committee for Clinical Laboratory Standards. Performance Standards for antimicrobial Disk Susceptibility Tests—Fifth Edition. Approved Standard NCCLS Document M2-A5, Vol. 13, No. 24, NCCLS, Villanova, PA, December 1993.
3. National Committee for Clinical Laboratory Standards. Methods for Antimicrobial Susceptibility Testing of Anaerobic Bacteria—Third Edition. Approved Standard NCCLS Document M11-A3, Vol 13, No. 26, NCCLS, Villanova, PA, December 1993.

*Galaxy® is a registered trademark of Baxter Healthcare Corporation.
†ADD-Vantage is a registered trademark of Abbott Laboratories Inc.
‡ Clinitest® is a registered trademark of Ames Division, Miles Laboratories, Inc.

CEFOTAN® (cefotetan injection) in Galaxy® plastic container (PL 2040) is manufactured by Baxter Healthcare Corporation, Deerfield, Illinois 60015 USA for Zeneca Pharmaceuticals.
CEFOTAN® (cefotetan disodium for injection) is manufactured by SmithKline Beecham Corporation for:
Zeneca Pharmaceuticals
A Business Unit of Zeneca Inc.
Wilmington, Delaware 19850-5437
Rev G 2/97 SIC 64065-03
Shown in Product Identification Guide, page 345

DIPRIVAN® 1% ℞
INJECTABLE EMULSION
10 mg/mL propofol
FOR I.V. ADMINISTRATION

DESCRIPTION

DIPRIVAN® Injectable Emulsion is a sterile, nonpyrogenic emulsion containing 10mg/mL of propofol suitable for intravenous administration. Propofol is chemically described as 2,6-diisopropylphenol and has a molecular weight of 178.27. The structural and molecular formulas are:

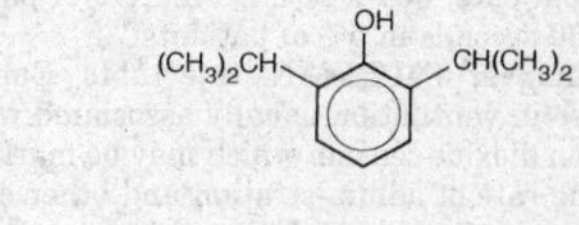
OH
(CH3)2CH
CH(CH3)2

$C_{12}H_{18}O$

Propofol is very slightly soluble in water and, thus, is formulated in a white, oil-in-water emulsion. The pKa is 11. The octanol/water partition coefficient for propofol 6761:1 at a pH of 6–8.5. In addition to the active component, propofol, the formulation also contains soybean oil (100 mg/mL), glycerol (22.5 mg/mL), egg lecithin (12 mg/mL), and disodium edetate (0.005%); with sodium hydroxide to adjust pH. The DIPRIVAN Injectable emulsion is isotonic and has a pH of 7–8.5.

STRICT ASEPTIC TECHNIQUE MUST ALWAYS BE MAINTAINED DURING HANDLING. DIPRIVAN INJECTABLE EMULSION IS A SINGLE-USE PARENTERAL PRODUCT WHICH CONTAINS 0.005% DISODIUM EDETATE TO RETARD THE RATE OF GROWTH OF MICROORGANISMS IN THE EVENT OF ACCIDENTAL EXTRINSIC CONTAMINATION. HOWEVER, DIPRIVAN INJECTABLE EMULSION CAN STILL SUPPORT THE GROWTH OF MICROORGANISMS AS IT IS NOT AN ANTIMICROBIALLY PRESERVED PRODUCT UNDER USP STANDARDS. ACCORDINGLY, STRICT ASEPTIC TECHNIQUE MUST STILL BE ADHERED TO. DO NOT USE IF CONTAMINATION IS SUSPECTED. DISCARD UNUSED PORTIONS AS DIRECTED WITHIN THE REQUIRED TIME LIMITS (SEE DOSAGE AND ADMINISTRATION, HANDLING PROCEDURES). THERE HAVE BEEN REPORTS IN WHICH FAILURE TO USE ASEPTIC TECHNIQUE WHEN HANDLING DIPRIVAN INJECTABLE EMULSION WAS ASSOCIATED WITH MICROBIAL CONTAMINATION OF THE PRODUCT AND WITH FEVER, INFECTION/SEPSIS, OTHER LIFE-THREATENING ILLNESS, AND/OR DEATH.

CLINICAL PHARMACOLOGY

General
DIPRIVAN Injectable Emulsion is an intravenous sedative-hypnotic agent for use in the induction and maintenance of anesthesia or sedation. Intravenous injection of a therapeutic dose of propofol produces hypnosis rapidly with minimal excitation, usually within 40 seconds from the start of an injection (the time for one arm-brain circulation). As with other rapidly acting intravenous anesthetic agents, the half-time of the blood-brain equilibration is approximately 1 to 3 minutes, and this accounts for the rapid induction of anesthesia.

Pharmacodynamics
Pharmacodynamic properties of propofol are dependent upon the therapeutic blood propofol concentrations. Steady state propofol blood concentrations are generally proportional to infusion rates, especially within an individual patient. Undesirable side effects such as cardiorespiratory depression are likely to occur at higher blood concentrations which result from bolus dosing or rapid increase in infusion rate. An adequate interval (3 to 5 minutes) must be allowed between clinical dosage adjustments in order to assess drug effects.

The hemodynamic effects of DIPRIVAN Injectable Emulsion during induction of anesthesia vary. If spontaneous ventilation is maintained, the major cardiovascular effects are arterial hypotension (sometimes greater than a 30% decrease) with little or no change in heart rate and no appreciable decrease in cardiac output. If ventilation is assisted or controlled (positive pressure ventilation), the degree and inci-

DOSAGE GUIDELINES FOR PATIENTS WITH IMPAIRED RENAL FUNCTION

Creatinine Clearance mL/min	Dose	Frequency
>30	Usual Recommended Dosage*	Every 12 hours
10–30	Usual Recommended Dosage*	Every 24 hours
<10	Usual Recommended Dosage*	Every 48 hours

* Dose determined by the type and severity of infection, and susceptibility of the causative organism.

Continued on next page

Diprivan—Cont.

dence of decrease in cardiac output are accentuated. Addition of a potent opioid (e.g., fentanyl) when used as a premedicant further decreases cardiac output and respiratory drive.

If anesthesia is continued by infusion of DIPRIVAN Injectable Emulsion, the stimulation of endotracheal intubation and surgery may return arterial pressure towards normal. However, cardiac output may remain depressed. Comparative clinical studies have shown that the hemodynamic effects of DIPRIVAN Injectable Emulsion during induction of anesthesia are generally more pronounced than with other IV induction agents traditionally used for this purpose.

Clinical and preclinical studies suggest that DIPRIVAN Injectable Emulsion is rarely associated with elevation of plasma histamine levels.

Induction of anesthesia with DIPRIVAN Injectable Emulsion is frequently associated with apnea in both adults and children. In 1573 adult patients who received DIPRIVAN Injectable Emulsion (2 to 2.5 mg/kg), apnea lasted less than 30 seconds in 7% of patients, 30-60 seconds in 24% of patients, and more than 60 seconds in 12% of patients. In the 213 pediatric patients between the ages of 3 and 12 years assessable for apnea who received DIPRIVAN Injectable Emulsion (1 to 3.6 mg/kg), apnea lasted less than 30 seconds in 12% of patients, 30-60 seconds in 10% of patients, and more than 60 seconds in 5% of patients.

During maintenance, DIPRIVAN Injectable Emulsion causes a decrease in ventilation usually associated with an increase in carbon dioxide tension which may be marked depending upon the rate of administration and other concurrent medications (e.g., opioids, sedatives, etc.).

During monitored anesthesia care (MAC) sedation, attention must be given to the cardiorespiratory effects of DIPRIVAN Injectable Emulsion. Hypotension, oxyhemoglobin desaturation, apnea, airway obstruction, and/or oxygen desaturation can occur, especially following a rapid bolus of DIPRIVAN Injectable Emulsion. During initiation of MAC sedation, slow infusion or slow injection techniques are preferable over rapid bolus administration, and during maintenance of MAC sedation, a variable rate infusion is preferable over intermittent bolus administration in order to minimize undesirable cardiorespiratory effects. In the elderly, debilitated, or ASA III/IV patients, rapid (single or repeated) bolus dose administration should not be used for MAC sedation. (See WARNINGS.) DIPRIVAN Injectable Emulsion is not recommended for MAC Sedation in children because safety and effectiveness have not been established. Clinical studies in humans and studies in animals show that DIPRIVAN Injectable Emulsion does not suppress the adrenal response to ACTH. Preliminary findings in patients with normal intraocular pressure indicate that DIPRIVAN Injectable Emulsion anesthesia produces a decrease in intraocular pressure which may be associated with a concomitant decrease in systemic vascular resistance.

Animal studies and limited experience in susceptible patients have not indicated any propensity of DIPRIVAN Injectable Emulsion to induce malignant hyperthermia.

Studies to date indicate that DIPRIVAN Injectable Emulsion when used in combination with hypocarbia increases cerebrovascular resistance and decreases cerebral blood flow, cerebral metabolic oxygen consumption, and intracranial pressure. DIPRIVAN Injectable Emulsion does not affect cerebrovascular reactivity to changes in arterial carbon dioxide tension. (see Clinical Trials-Neuroanesthesia).

Hemosiderin deposits have been observed in the liver of dogs receiving DIPRIVAN Injectable Emulsion containing 0.005% disodium edetate over a four week period; the clinical significance is unknown.

Pharmacokinetics

The proper use of DIPRIVAN Injectable Emulsion requires an understanding of the disposition and elimination characteristics of propofol.

The pharmacokinetics of propofol are well described by a three compartment linear model with compartments representing the plasma, rapidly equilibrating tissues, and slowly equilibrating tissues.

Following an IV bolus dose, there is rapid equilibration between the plasma and the highly perfused tissue of the brain, thus accounting for the rapid onset of anesthesia. Plasma levels initially decline rapidly as a result of both rapid distribution and high metabolic clearance. Distribution accounts for about half of this decline following a bolus of propofol.

However, distribution is not constant over time, but decreases as body tissues equilibrate with plasma and become

saturated. The rate at which equilibration occurs is a function of the rate and duration of the infusion. When equilibration occurs there is no longer a net transfer of propofol between tissues and plasma.

Discontinuation of the recommended doses of DIPRIVAN Injectable Emulsion after the maintenance of anesthesia for approximately one-hour, or for sedation in the ICU for one-day, results in a prompt decrease in blood propofol concentrations and rapid awakening. Longer infusions (10 days of ICU sedation) result in accumulation of significant tissue stores of propofol, such that the reduction in circulating propofol is slowed and the time to awakening is increased.

By daily titration of DIPRIVAN Injectable Emulsion dosage to achieve only the minimum effective therapeutic concentration, rapid awakening within 10 to 15 minutes will occur even after long term administration. If, however, higher than necessary infusion levels have been maintained for a long time, propofol will be redistributed from fat and muscle to the plasma, and this return of propofol from peripheral tissues will slow recovery.

The figure below illustrates the fall of plasma propofol levels following ICU sedation infusions of various durations.

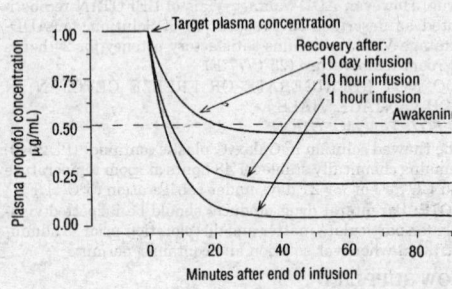

The large contribution of distribution (about 50%) to the fall of propofol plasma levels following brief infusions means that after very long infusions (at steady state), about half the initial rate will maintain the same plasma levels. Failure to reduce the infusion rate in patients receiving DIPRIVAN Injectable Emulsion for extended periods may result in excessively high blood concentrations of the drug. Thus, titration to clinical response and daily evaluation of sedation levels are important during use of DIPRIVAN Injectable Emulsion infusion for ICU sedation, especially of long duration.

Adults:

Propofol clearance ranges from 23–50mL/kg/min (1.6 to 3.4 L/min in 70 kg adults). It is chiefly eliminated by hepatic conjugation to inactive metabolites which are excreted by the kidney. A glucuronide conjugate accounts for about 50% of the administered dose. Propofol has a steady state volume of distribution (10-day infusion) approaching 60 L/kg in healthy adults. A difference in pharmacokinetics due to gender has not been observed. The terminal half-life of propofol after a 10-day infusion is 1 to 3 days.

Geriatrics:

With increasing patient age, the dose of propofol needed to achieve a defined anesthetic endpoint (dose-requirement) decreases. This does not appear to be an age-related change of pharmacodynamics or brain sensitivity, as measured by EEG burst suppression. With increasing patient age pharmacokinetic changes are such that for a given IV bolus dose, higher peak plasma concentrations occur, which can explain the decreased dose requirement. These higher peak plasma concentrations in the elderly can predispose patients to cardiorespiratory effects including hypotension, apnea, airway obstruction and/or oxygen desaturation. The higher plasma levels reflect an age-related decrease in volume of distribution and reduced intercompartmental clearance. Lower doses are thus recommended for initiation and maintenance of sedation/anesthesia in elderly patients. (See CLINICAL PHARMACOLOGY - Individualization of Dosage.)

Pediatrics:

The pharmacokinetics of propofol were studied in 53 children between the ages of 3 and 12 years who received DIPRIVAN Injectable Emulsion for periods of approximately 1-2 hours. The observed distribution and clearance of propofol in these children was similar to adults.

Organ Failure:

The pharmacokinetics of propofol do not appear to be different in people with chronic hepatic cirrhosis or chronic renal

impairment compared to adults with normal hepatic and renal function. The effects of acute hepatic or renal failure on the pharmacokinetics of propofol have not been studied.

Clinical Trials

Anesthesia and Monitored Anesthesia Care (MAC) Sedation

DIPRIVAN Injectable Emulsion was compared to intravenous and inhalational anesthetic or sedative agents in 91 trials involving a total of 5,135 patients. Of these 3,354 received DIPRIVAN Injectable Emulsion and comprised the overall safety database for anesthesia and MAC sedation. Fifty-five of these trials, 20 for anesthesia induction and 35 for induction and maintenance of anesthesia or MAC sedation, were carried out in the US or Canada and provided the basis for dosage recommendations and the adverse event profile during anesthesia or MAC sedation.

Pediatric Anesthesia

DIPRIVAN Injectable Emulsion was compared to standard anesthetic agents in 12 clinical trials involving 534 patients receiving DIPRIVAN Injectable Emulsion. Of these, 349 were from US/Canadian clinical trials and comprised the overall safety database for Pediatric Anesthesia.

TABLE 1. PEDIATRIC ANESTHESIA CLINICAL TRIALS
Patients Receiving DIPRIVAN Injectable Emulsion
Median and (Range)

	Induction Only	Induction and Maintenance
Number of Patients*	243	105
Induction Bolus Dosages	2.5 mg/kg (1–3.5)	3 mg/kg (2–3.6)
Injection Duration	20 sec (6–45)	
Maintenance Dosage	—	181 µg/kg/min (107–418)
Maintenance Duration	—	78 min (29–268)

*Body weight not recorded for one patient.

Neuroanesthesia

DIPRIVAN Injectable Emulsion was studied in 50 patients undergoing craniotomy for supratentorial tumors in two clinical trials. The mean lesion size (anterior/posterior and lateral) was 31 mm and 32 mm in one trial and 55 mm and 42 mm in the other trial respectively.

[See table 2 below]

In ten of these patients, DIPRIVAN Injectable Emulsion was administered by infusion in a controlled clinical trial to evaluate the effect of DIPRIVAN Injectable Emulsion on cerebrospinal fluid pressure (CSFP). The mean arterial pressure was maintained relatively constant over 25 minutes with a change from baseline of $-4\% \pm 17\%$ (mean $\pm$ SD), whereas the percent change in cerebrospinal fluid pressure (CSFP) was $-46\% \pm 14\%$. As CSFP is an indirect measure of intracranial pressure (ICP), when given by infusion or slow bolus, DIPRIVAN Injectable Emulsion, in combination with hypocarbia, is capable of decreasing ICP independent of changes in arterial pressure.

Intensive Care Unit (ICU) Sedation

DIPRIVAN Injectable Emulsion was compared to benzodiazepines and/or opioids in 14 clinical trials involving a total of 550 ICU patients. Of these, 302 received DIPRIVAN Injectable Emulsion and comprise the overall safety database for ICU sedation. Six of these studies were carried out in the US or Canada and provide the basis for dosage recommendations and the adverse event profile.

Information from 193 literature reports of DIPRIVAN Injectable Emulsion used for ICU sedation in over 950 patients and information from the clinical trials are summarized below:

[See table 3 at top of next page]

Cardiac Anesthesia

DIPRIVAN Injectable Emulsion was evaluated in 5 clinical trials conducted in the US and Canada, involving a total of 569 patients undergoing coronary artery bypass graft (CABG). Of these, 301 patients received DIPRIVAN Injectable Emulsion. They comprise the safety database for cardiac anesthesia and provide the basis for dosage recommendations in this patient population, in conjunction with reports in the published literature.

Individualization of Dosage

General:

STRICT ASEPTIC TECHNIQUE MUST ALWAYS BE MAINTAINED DURING HANDLING. DIPRIVAN INJECTABLE EMULSION IS A SINGLE-USE PARENTERAL PRODUCT WHICH CONTAINS 0.005% DISODIUM EDETATE TO RETARD THE RATE OF GROWTH OF MICROORGANISMS IN THE EVENT OF ACCIDENTAL EXTRINSIC CONTAMINATION. HOWEVER, DIPRIVAN INJECTABLE EMULSION CAN STILL SUPPORT THE GROWTH OF MICROORGANISMS AS IT IS NOT AN ANTIMICROBIALLY PRESERVED PRODUCT UNDER USP STANDARDS. ACCORDINGLY, STRICT ASEPTIC TECHNIQUE MUST STILL BE ADHERED TO. DO NOT USE IF CONTAMINATION IS SUSPECTED. DISCARD UN-

TABLE 2. NEUROANESTHESIA CLINICAL TRIALS
Patients Receiving DIPRIVAN Injectable Emulsion Median and (Range)

Patient Type	No. of Patients	Induction Bolus Dosages (mg/kg)	Maintenance Dosage (µg/kg/min)	Maintenance Duration (min)
Craniotomy patients	50	136 (0.9–6.9)	146 (68–425)	285 (48–622)

TABLE 3. ICU SEDATION CLINICAL TRIALS AND LITERATURE
Patients receiving DIPRIVAN Injectable Emulsion Median and (Range)

ICU Patient Type	Number of Patients Trials	Number of Patients Literature	Sedation Dose µg/kg/min	Sedation Dose mg/kg/h	Sedation Duration Hours
Post-CABG	41	—	11	.66	10
			(0.1–30)	(0.006–1.8)	(2–14)
	—	334	(5–100)	(0.3–6)	(4–24)
Post-Surgical	60	—	20	1.2	18
			(6–53)	(0.4–3.2)	(0.3–187)
	—	142	(23–82)	(1.4–4.9)	(6–96)
Neuro/Head Trauma	7	—	25	1.5	168
			(13–37)	(0.8–2.2)	(112–282)
	—	184	(8.3–87)	(0.5–5.2)	(8 hr–5 days)
Medical	49	—	41	2.5	72
			(9–131)	(0.5–7.9)	(0.4–337)
	—	76	(3.3–62)	(0.2–3.7)	(4–96)
Special Patients					
ARDS/Resp. Failure	—	56	(10–142)	(0.6–8.5)	(1 hr–8 days)
COPD/Asthma	—	49	(17–75)	(1.4–5)	(1–8 days)
Status Epilepticus	—	15	(25–167)	(1.5–10)	(1–21 days)
Tetanus	—	11	(5–100)	(0.3–6)	(1–25 days)

Trials (Individual patients from clinical studies)
Literature (Individual patients from published reports)
CABG (Coronary Artery Bypass Graft)
ARDS (Adult Respiratory Distress Syndrome)

Table 4. Cardiac Anesthesia Techniques

Primary Agent	Rate	Secondary Agent/Rate (Following Induction with Primary Agent)
DIPRIVAN Injectable Emulsion		OPIOID[a]/0.05–0.075 µg/kg/min (no bolus)
Preinduction anxiolysis	25 µg/kg/min	
Induction	0.5–1.5 mg/kg over 60 sec	
Maintenance (Titrated to Clinical Response)	100–150 µg/kg/min	
OPIOID[b]		DIPRIVAN Injectable Emulsion/50–100 µg/kg/min (no bolus)
Induction	25–50 µg/kg	
Maintenance	0.2–0.3 µg/kg/min	

[a] OPIOID is defined in terms of fentanyl equivalents, i.e.
1 µg of fentanyl =5 µg of alfentanil (for bolus)
             =10 µg of alfentanil (for maintenance)
             or
             =0.1 µg of sufentanil
[b] Care should be taken to ensure amnesia with concomitant benzodiazepine therapy

USED PORTIONS AS DIRECTED WITHIN THE REQUIRED TIME LIMITS (SEE DOSAGE AND ADMINISTRATION, HANDLING PROCEDURES). THERE HAVE BEEN REPORTS IN WHICH FAILURE TO USE ASEPTIC TECHNIQUE WHEN HANDLING DIPRIVAN INJECTABLE EMULSION WAS ASSOCIATED WITH MICROBIAL CONTAMINATION OF THE PRODUCT AND WITH FEVER, INFECTION/SEPSIS, OTHER LIFE-THREATENING ILLNESS, AND/OR DEATH.

Propofol blood concentrations at steady state are generally proportional to infusion rates, especially in individual patients. Undesirable effects such as cardiorespiratory depression are likely to occur at higher blood concentrations which result from bolus dosing or rapid increases in the infusion rate. An adequate interval (3 to 5 minutes) must be allowed between clinical dosage adjustments in order to assess drug effects.

When administering DIPRIVAN Injectable Emulsion by infusion, syringe pumps or volumetric pumps are recommended to provide controlled infusion rates. When infusing DIPRIVAN Injectable Emulsion to patients undergoing magnetic resonance imaging, metered control devices may be utilized if mechanical pumps are impractical.

Changes in vital signs (increases in pulse rate, blood pressure, sweating and/or tearing) that indicate a response to surgical stimulation or lightening of anesthesia may be controlled by the administration of DIPRIVAN Injectable Emulsion 25 mg (2.5 mL) to 50 mg (5 mL) incremental boluses and/or by increasing the infusion rate.

For minor surgical procedures (e.g. body surface) nitrous oxide (60%-70%) can be combined with a variable rate DIPRIVAN Injectable Emulsion infusion to provide satisfactory anesthesia. With more stimulating surgical procedures (e.g. intra-abdominal), or if supplementation with nitrous oxide is not provided, administration rate(s) of DIPRIVAN Injectable Emulsion and/or opioids should be increased in order to provide adequate anesthesia.

Infusion rates should always be titrated downward in the absence of clinical signs of light anesthesia until a mild response to surgical stimulation is obtained in order to avoid administration of DIPRIVAN Injectable Emulsion at rates higher than are clinically necessary. Generally, rates of 50 to 100 µg/kg/min in adults, should be achieved during maintenance in order to optimize recovery times.

Other drugs that cause CNS depression (hypnotics/sedatives, inhalational anesthetics and opioids) can increase CNS depression induced by propofol. Morphine premedication (0.15 mg/kg) with nitrous oxide 67% in oxygen has been shown to decrease the necessary propofol injection maintenance infusion rate and therapeutic blood concentrations when compared to non narcotic (lorazepam) premedication.

Induction of General Anesthesia
Adult Patients:
Most adult patients under 55 years of age and classified ASA I/II require 2 to 2.5 mg/kg of DIPRIVAN Injectable Emulsion for induction when unpremedicated or when premedicated with oral benzodiazepines or intramuscular opioids. For induction, DIPRIVAN Injectable Emulsion should be titrated (approximately 40 mg every 10 seconds) against the response of the patient until the clinical signs show the onset of anesthesia. As with other sedative-hypnotic agents, the amount of intravenous opioid and/or benzodiazepine premedication will influence the response of the patient to an induction dose of DIPRIVAN Injectable Emulsion.

Elderly, Debilitated, or ASA III/IV Patients:
It is important to be familiar and experienced with the intravenous use of DIPRIVAN Injectable Emulsion before treating elderly, debilitated or ASA III/IV patients. Due to the reduced clearance and higher blood concentrations, most of these patients require approximately 1 to 1.5 mg/kg (approximately 20 mg every 10 seconds) of DIPRIVAN Injectable Emulsion for induction of anesthesia according to their condition and responses. A rapid bolus should not be used as this will increase the likelihood of undesirable cardiorespiratory depression including hypotension, apnea, airway obstruction and/or oxygen desaturation. (See DOSAGE AND ADMINISTRATION.)

Neurosurgical Patients:
Slower induction is recommended using boluses of 20 mg every 10 seconds. Slower boluses or infusions of DIPRIVAN Injectable Emulsion for induction of anesthesia, titrated to clinical responses, will generally result in reduced induction dosage requirements (1 to 2 mg/kg). (See PRECAUTIONS and DOSAGE AND ADMINISTRATION.)

Cardiac Anesthesia:
DIPRIVAN Injectable Emulsion has been well studied in patients with coronary artery disease, but experience in patients with hemodynamically significant valvular or congenital heart disease is limited. As with other anesthetic and sedative-hypnotic agents, DIPRIVAN Injectable Emulsion in healthy patients causes a decrease in blood pressure that is secondary to decreases in preload (ventricular filling volume at the end of the diastole) and afterload (arterial resistance at the beginning of the systole). The magnitude of these changes is proportional to the blood and effect site concentrations achieved. These concentrations depend upon the dose and speed of the induction and maintenance infusion rates.

In addition, lower heart rates are observed during maintenance with DIPRIVAN Injectable Emulsion, possibly due to reduction of the sympathetic activity and/or resetting of the baroreceptor reflexes. Therefore, anticholinergic agents should be administered when increases in vagal tone are anticipated.

As with other anesthetic agents, DIPRIVAN Injectable Emulsion reduces myocardial oxygen consumption. Further studies are needed to confirm and delineate the extent of these effects on the myocardium and the coronary vascular system.

Morphine premedication (0.15 mg/kg) with nitrous oxide 67% in oxygen has been shown to decrease the necessary DIPRIVAN Injectable Emulsion maintenance infusion rates and therapeutic blood concentrations when compared to non narcotic (lorazepam) premedication. The rate of DIPRIVAN Injectable Emulsion administration should be determined based on the patient's premedication and adjusted according to clinical responses.

A rapid bolus induction should be avoided. A slow rate of approximately 20 mg every 10 seconds until induction onset (0.5 to 1.5 mg/kg) should be used. In order to assure adequate anesthesia, when DIPRIVAN Injectable Emulsion is used as the primary agent, maintenance infusion rates should not be less than 100 µg/kg/min and should be supplemented with analgesic levels of continuous opioid administration. When an opioid is used as the primary agent, DIPRIVAN Injectable Emulsion maintenance rates should not be less than 50 µg/kg/min and care should be taken to insure amnesia with concomitant benzodiazepines. Higher doses of DIPRIVAN Injectable Emulsion will reduce the opioid requirements (see Table 4). When DIPRIVAN Injectable Emulsion is used as the primary anesthetic, it should not be administered with the high-dose opioid technique as this may increase the likelihood of hypotension (see PRECAUTIONS - Cardiac Anesthesia).

[See table 4 at left]

Maintenance of General Anesthesia
In adults, anesthesia can be maintained by administering DIPRIVAN Injectable Emulsion by infusion or intermittent IV bolus injection. The patient's clinical response will determine the infusion rate or the amount and frequency of incremental injections.

Continuous Infusion:
DIPRIVAN Injectable Emulsion 100 to 200 µg/kg/min administered in a variable rate infusion with 60%–70% nitrous oxide and oxygen provides anesthesia for patients undergoing general surgery. Maintenance by infusion of DIPRIVAN Injectable Emulsion should immediately follow the induction dose in order to provide satisfactory or continuous anesthesia during the induction phase. During this initial period following the induction dose higher rates of infusion are generally required (150 to 200 µg/kg/min) for the first 10 to 15 minutes. Infusion rates should subsequently be decreased 30%–50% during the first half-hour of maintenance.

Other drugs that cause CNS depression (hypnotics/sedatives, inhalational anesthetics and opioids) can increase the CNS depression induced by propofol.

Intermittent Bolus:
Increments of DIPRIVAN Injectable Emulsion 25 mg (2.5 mL) to 50mg (5mL) may be administered with nitrous oxide in adult patients undergoing general surgery. The incremental boluses should be administered when changes in vital signs indicate a response to surgical stimulation or light anesthesia.

DIPRIVAN Injectable Emulsion has been used with a variety of agents commonly used in anesthesia such as atropine, scopolamine, glycopyrrolate, diazepam, depolarizing and nondepolarizing muscle relaxants, and opioid analgesics, as well as with inhalational and regional anesthetic agents.

In the elderly, debilitated or ASA III/IV patients, rapid bolus doses should not be used as this will increase cardiorespiratory effects including hypotension, apnea, airway obstruction and/or oxygen desaturation.

Pediatric Anesthesia
Induction of General Anesthesia:
Most pediatric patients 3 years of age or older and classified ASA I or II require 2.5 to 3.5 mg/kg of DIPRIVAN Injectable Emulsion for induction when unpremedicated or when lightly premedicated with oral benzodiazepines or intramuscular opioids. Within this dosage range, younger children may require larger induction doses than older children. As with other sedative hypnotic agents, the amount of intravenous opioid and/or benzodiazepine premedication will influence the response of the patient to an induction dose of DIPRIVAN Injectable Emulsion. In addition, a lower

Continued on next page

Diprivan—Cont.

dosage is recommended for children classified ASA III or IV. Attention should be paid to minimize pain on injection when administering DIPRIVAN Injectable Emulsion to pediatric patients. Rapid boluses of DIPRIVAN Injectable Emulsion may be administered if small veins are pretreated with lidocaine or when antecubital or larger veins are utilized (See PRECAUTIONS - General).

DIPRIVAN Injectable Emulsion administered in a variable rate infusion with nitrous oxide 60-70% provides satisfactory anesthesia for most pediatric patients 3 years of age or older, ASA I or II, undergoing general anesthesia.

Maintenance of General Anesthesia:

Maintenance by infusion of DIPRIVAN Injectable Emulsion at a rate of 200–300 µg/kg/min should immediately follow the induction dose. Following the first half hour of maintenance, if clinical signs of light anesthesia are not present, the infusion rate should be decreased; during this period, infusion rates of 125–150 µg/kg/min are typically needed. However, younger children (5 years of age or less) may require larger maintenance infusion rates than older children.

Monitored Anesthesia Care (MAC) Sedation in Adults

When DIPRIVAN Injectable Emulsion is administered for MAC sedation, rates of administration should be individualized and titrated to clinical response. In most patients the rates of DIPRIVAN Injectable Emulsion administration will be in the range of 25–75 µg/kg/min.

During initiation of MAC sedation, slow infusion or slow injection techniques are preferable over rapid bolus administration. During maintenance of MAC sedation, a variable rate infusion is preferable over intermittent bolus dose administration. In the elderly, debilitated, or ASA III/IV patients, rapid (single or repeated) bolus dose administration should not be used for MAC sedation. (See WARNINGS.) **A rapid bolus injection can result in undesirable cardiorespiratory depression including hypotension, apnea, airway obstruction, and/or oxygen desaturation.**

Initiation of MAC Sedation:

For initiation of MAC sedation, either an infusion or a slow injection method may be utilized while closely monitoring cardiorespiratory function. With the infusion method, sedation may be initiated by infusing DIPRIVAN Injectable Emulsion at 100 to 150 µg/kg/min (6 to 9 mg/kg/h) for a period of 3 to 5 minutes and titrating to the desired level of sedation while closely monitoring respiratory function. With the slow injection method for initiation, patients will require approximately 0.5 mg/kg administered over 3 to 5 minutes and titrated to clinical responses. When DIPRIVAN Injectable Emulsion is administered slowly over 3 to 5 minutes, most patients will be adequately sedated and the peak drug effect can be achieved while minimizing undesirable cardiorespiratory effects occurring at high plasma levels.

In the elderly, debilitated, or ASA III/IV patients, rapid (single or repeated) bolus dose administration should not be used for MAC sedation. (See WARNINGS.) The rate of administration should be over 3-5 minutes and the dosage of DIPRIVAN Injectable Emulsion should be reduced to approximately 80% of the usual adult dosage in these patients according to their condition, responses, and changes in vital signs. (See DOSAGE AND ADMINISTRATION.)

Maintenance of MAC Sedation:

For maintenance of sedation, a variable rate infusion method is preferable over an intermittent bolus dose method. With the variable rate infusion method, patients will generally require maintenance rates of 25 to 75 µg/kg/min (1.5 to 4.5 mg/kg/h) during the first 10 to 15 minutes of sedation maintenance. Infusion rates should subsequently be decreased over time to 25 to 50 µg/kg/min and adjusted to clinical responses. In titrating to clinical effect, allow approximately 2 minutes for onset of peak drug effect.

Infusion rates should always be titrated downward in the absence of clinical signs of light sedation until mild responses to stimulation are obtained in order to avoid sedative administration of DIPRIVAN Injectable Emulsion at rates higher than are clinically necessary.

If the intermittent bolus dose method is used, increments of DIPRIVAN Injectable Emulsion 10 mg (1 mL) or 20 mg (2 mL) can be administered and titrated to desired level of sedation. With the intermittent bolus method of sedation maintenance there is the potential for respiratory depression, transient increases in sedation depth, and/or prolongation of recovery.

In the elderly, debilitated, or ASA III/IV patients, rapid (single or repeated) bolus dose administration should not be used for MAC sedation. (See WARNINGS.) The rate of administration and the dosage of DIPRIVAN Injectable Emulsion should be reduced to approximately 80% of the usual adult dosage in these patients according to their condition, responses, and changes in vital signs. (See DOSAGE AND ADMINISTRATION.)

DIPRIVAN Injectable Emulsion can be administered as the sole agent for maintenance of MAC sedation during surgical/diagnostic procedures. When DIPRIVAN Injectable Emulsion sedation is supplemented with opioid and/or ben-

zodiazepine medications, these agents increase the sedative and respiratory effects of DIPRIVAN Injectable Emulsion and may also result in a slower recovery profile. (See PRECAUTIONS, Drug Interactions.)

ICU Sedation:

(See WARNINGS and DOSAGE AND ADMINISTRATION, Handling Procedures.) For intubated, mechanically ventilated adult patients, Intensive Care Unit (ICU) sedation should be initiated slowly with a continuous infusion in order to titrate to desired clinical effect and minimize hypotension. (See DOSAGE AND ADMINISTRATION.)

Across all 6 US/Canadian clinical studies, the mean infusion maintenance rate for all DIPRIVAN Injectable Emulsion patients was 27± 21 µg/kg/min. The maintenance infusion rates required to maintain adequate sedation ranged from 2.8 µg/kg/min to 130 µg/kg/min. The infusion rate was lower in patients over 55 years of age (approximately 20 µg/kg/min) compared to patients under 55 years of age (approximately 38 µg/kg/min). In these studies, morphine or fentanyl was used as needed for analgesia.

Most adult ICU patients recovering from the effects of general anesthesia or deep sedation will require maintenance rates of 5 to 50 µg/kg/min (0.3 to 3 mg/kg/h) individualized and titrated to clinical response. (See DOSAGE AND ADMINISTRATION.) With medical ICU patients or patients who have recovered from the effects of general anesthesia or deep sedation, the rate of administration of 50 µg/kg/min or higher may be required to achieve adequate sedation. These higher rates of administration may increase the likelihood of patients developing hypotension.

Although there are reports of reduced analgesic requirements, most patients received opioids for analgesia during maintenance of ICU sedation. Some patients also received benzodiazepines and/or neuromuscular blocking agents. During long term maintenance of sedation, some ICU patients were awakened once or twice every 24 hours for assessment of neurologic or respiratory function. (See Clinical Trials, Table 3.)

In post-CABG (coronary artery bypass graft) patients, the maintenance rate of propofol administration was usually low (median 11 µg/kg/min) due to the intraoperative administration of high opioid doses. Patients receiving DIPRIVAN Injectable Emulsion required 35% less nitroprusside than midazolam patients; this difference was statistically significant (P<0.05). During initiation of sedation in Post-CABG patients, a 15% to 20% decrease in blood pressure was seen in the first 60 minutes. It was not possible to determine cardiovascular effects in patients with severely compromised ventricular function (See Clinical Trials, Table 3).

In Medical or Postsurgical ICU studies comparing DIPRIVAN Injectable Emulsion to benzodiazepine infusion or bolus, there were no apparent differences in maintenance of adequate sedation, mean arterial pressure, or laboratory findings. Like the comparators, DIPRIVAN Injectable Emulsion reduced blood cortisol during sedation while maintaining responsivity to challenges with adrenocorticotropic hormone (ACTH). Case reports from the published literature generally reflect that DIPRIVAN Injectable Emulsion has been used safely in patients with a history of porphyria or malignant hyperthermia.

In hemodynamically stable head trauma patients ranging in age from 19–43 years, adequate sedation was maintained with DIPRIVAN Injectable Emulsion or morphine (N=7 in each group). There were no apparent differences in adequacy of sedation, intracranial pressure, cerebral perfusion pressure, or neurologic recovery between the treatment groups. In literature reports from Neurosurgical ICU and severely head-injured patients DIPRIVAN Injectable Emulsion infusion with or without diuretics and hyperventilation controlled intracranial pressure while maintaining cerebral perfusion pressure. In some patients bolus doses resulted in decreased blood pressure and compromised cerebral perfusion pressure. (See Clinical Trials, Table 3.)

DIPRIVAN Injectable Emulsion was found to be effective in status epilepticus which was refractory to the standard anticonvulsant therapies. For these patients as well as for ARDS/respiratory failure and tetanus patients sedation maintenance dosages were generally higher than those for other critically ill patient populations. (See Clinical Trials, Table 3.)

Abrupt discontinuation of DIPRIVAN Injectable Emulsion prior to weaning or for daily evaluation of sedation levels should be avoided. This may result in rapid awakening with associated anxiety, agitation and resistance to mechanical ventilation. Infusions of DIPRIVAN Injectable Emulsion should be adjusted to maintain a light level of sedation through the weaning process or evaluation of sedation level. (See PRECAUTIONS.)

INDICATIONS AND USAGE

DIPRIVAN Injectable Emulsion is an IV sedative-hypnotic agent that can be used for both induction and/or maintenance of anesthesia as part of a balanced anesthetic technique for inpatient and outpatient surgery in adults and in children 3 years of age or older.

DIPRIVAN Injectable Emulsion, when administered intravenously as directed, can be used to initiate and maintain monitored anesthesia care (MAC) sedation during diagnostic procedures in adults. DIPRIVAN Injectable Emulsion may also be used for MAC sedation in conjunction with local/regional anesthesia in patients undergoing surgical procedures. (See PRECAUTIONS.)

DIPRIVAN Injectable Emulsion should only be administered to intubated, mechanically ventilated adult patients in the Intensive Care Unit (ICU) to provide continuous sedation and control of stress responses. In this setting, DIPRIVAN Injectable Emulsion should be administered only by persons skilled in the medical management of critically ill patients and trained in cardiovascular resuscitation and airway management.

DIPRIVAN Injectable Emulsion is not recommended for obstetrics, including cesarean section deliveries. DIPRIVAN Injectable Emulsion crosses the placenta, and as with other general anesthetic agents, the administration of DIPRIVAN Injectable Emulsion may be associated with neonatal depression. (See PRECAUTIONS.)

DIPRIVAN Injectable Emulsion is not recommended for use in nursing mothers because DIPRIVAN Injectable Emulsion has been reported to be excreted in human milk and the effects of oral absorption of small amounts of propofol are not known. (See PRECAUTIONS.)

DIPRIVAN Injectable Emulsion is not recommended for anesthesia in children below the age of 3 years because safety and effectiveness have not been established. DIPRIVAN Injectable Emulsion is not recommended for MAC sedation in children because safety and effectiveness have not been established. DIPRIVAN Injectable Emulsion is not recommended for pediatric ICU sedation because safety and effectiveness have not been established.

CONTRAINDICATIONS

DIPRIVAN Injectable Emulsion is contraindicated in patients with a known hypersensitivity to DIPRIVAN Injectable Emulsion or its components, or when general anesthesia or sedation are contraindicated.

WARNINGS

For general anesthesia or monitored anesthesia care (MAC) sedation, DIPRIVAN Injectable Emulsion should be administered only by persons trained in the administration of general anesthesia and not involved in the conduct of the surgical/diagnostic procedure. Patients should be continuously monitored, and facilities for maintenance of a patent airway, artificial ventilation, and oxygen enrichment and circulatory resuscitation must be immediately available.

For sedation of intubated, mechanically ventilated adult patients in the Intensive Care Unit (ICU), DIPRIVAN Injectable Emulsion should be administered only by persons skilled in the management of critically ill patients and trained in cardiovascular resuscitation and airway management.

In the elderly, debilitated or ASA III/IV patients, rapid (single or repeated) bolus administration should not be used during general anesthesia or MAC sedation in order to minimize undesirable cardiorespiratory depression including hypotension, apnea, airway obstruction and/or oxygen desaturation.

MAC sedation patients should be continuously monitored by persons not involved in the conduct of the surgical or diagnostic procedure; oxygen supplementation should be immediately available and provided where clinically indicated; and oxygen saturation should be monitored in all patients. Patients should be continuously monitored for early signs of hypotension, apnea, airway obstruction and/or oxygen desaturation. These cardiorespiratory effects are more likely to occur following rapid initiation (loading) boluses or during supplemental maintenance boluses, especially in the elderly, debilitated, or ASA III/IV patients.

DIPRIVAN Injectable Emulsion should not be coadministered through the same IV catheter with blood or plasma because compatibility has not been established. *In vitro* tests have shown that aggregates of the globular component of the emulsion vehicle have occurred with blood/plasma/serum from humans and animals. The clinical significance is not known.

STRICT ASEPTIC TECHNIQUE MUST ALWAYS BE MAINTAINED DURING HANDLING. DIPRIVAN INJECTABLE EMULSION IS A SINGLE-USE PARENTERAL PRODUCT WHICH CONTAINS 0.005% DISODIUM EDETATE TO RETARD THE RATE OF GROWTH OF MICROORGANISMS IN THE EVENT OF ACCIDENTAL EXTRINSIC CONTAMINATION. HOWEVER, DIPRIVAN INJECTABLE EMULSION CAN STILL SUPPORT THE GROWTH OF MICROORGANISMS AS IT IS NOT AN ANTIMICROBIALLY PRESERVED PRODUCT UNDER USP STANDARDS. ACCORDINGLY, STRICT ASEPTIC TECHNIQUE MUST STILL BE ADHERED TO. DO NOT USE IF CONTAMINATION IS SUSPECTED. DISCARD UNUSED PORTIONS AS DIRECTED WITHIN THE REQUIRED TIME LIMITS (SEE DOSAGE AND ADMINISTRATION, HANDLING PROCEDURES). THERE HAVE BEEN REPORTS IN WHICH FAILURE TO USE ASEPTIC TECHNIQUE WHEN HANDLING DIPRIVAN INJECTABLE EMULSION WAS AS-

SOCIATED WITH MICROBIAL CONTAMINATION OF THE PRODUCT AND WITH FEVER, INFECTION/SEPSIS, OTHER LIFE-THREATENING ILLNESS, AND/OR DEATH.

PRECAUTIONS

General:

A lower induction dose and a slower maintenance rate of administration should be used in elderly, debilitated, or ASA III/IV patients. (See CLINICAL PHARMACOLOGY - Individualization of Dosage.) Patients should be continuously monitored for early signs of significant hypotension and/or bradycardia. Treatment may include increasing the rate of intravenous fluid, elevation of lower extremities, use of pressor agents, or administration of atropine. Apnea often occurs during induction and may persist for more than 60 seconds. Ventilatory support may be required. Because DIPRIVAN Injectable Emulsion is an emulsion, caution should be exercised in patients with disorders of lipid metabolism such as primary hyperlipoproteinemia, diabetic hyperlipemia, and pancreatitis.

The clinical criteria for discharge from the recovery/day surgery area established for each institution should be satisfied before discharge of the patient from the care of the anesthesiologist.

When DIPRIVAN Injectable Emulsion is administered to an epileptic patient, there may be a risk of seizure during the recovery phase.

In adults and children, attention should be paid to minimize pain on administration of DIPRIVAN Injectable Emulsion. Transient local pain can be minimized if the larger veins of the forearm or antecubital fossa are used. Pain during intravenous injection may also be reduced by prior injection of IV lidocaine (1 mL of a 1% solution). Pain on injection occurred frequently in pediatric patients (45%) when a small vein of the hand was utilized without lidocaine pretreatment. With lidocaine pretreatment or when antecubital veins were utilized, pain was minimal (incidence less than 10%) and well tolerated.

Venous sequelae (phlebitis or thrombosis) have been reported rarely (<1%). In two well-controlled clinical studies using dedicated intravenous catheters, no instances of venous sequelae were observed up to 14 days following induction.

Intra-arterial injection in animals did not induce local tissue effects. Accidental intra-arterial injection has been reported in patients, and, other than pain, there were no major sequelae.

Intentional injection into subcutaneous or perivascular tissues of animals caused minimal tissue reaction. During the post-marketing period there have been rare reports of local pain, swelling, blisters, and/or tissue necrosis following accidental extravasation of DIPRIVAN Injectable Emulsion.

Perioperative myoclonia, rarely including convulsions and opisthotonos, has occurred in temporal relationship in cases in which DIPRIVAN Injectable Emulsion has been administered.

Clinical features of anaphylaxis, which may include angioedema, bronchospasm, erythema and hypotension, occur rarely following DIPRIVAN Injectable Emulsion administration, although use of other drugs in most instances makes the relationship to DIPRIVAN Injectable Emulsion unclear.

There have been rare reports of pulmonary edema in temporal relationship to the administration of DIPRIVAN Injectable Emulsion, although a causal relationship is unknown.

Very rarely, cases of unexplained postoperative pancreatitis (requiring hospital admission) have been reported after anesthesia in which DIPRIVAN Injectable Emulsion was one of the induction agents used. Due to a variety of confounding factors in these cases, including concomitant medications, a causal relationship to DIPRIVAN Injectable Emulsion is unclear.

DIPRIVAN Injectable Emulsion has no vagolytic activity. Reports of bradycardia, asystole, and rarely, cardiac arrest have been associated with DIPRIVAN Injectable Emulsion. The intravenous administration of anticholinergic agents (e.g., atropine or glycopyrrolate) should be considered to modify potential increases in vagal tone due to concomitant agents (e.g., succinylcholine) or surgical stimuli.

Intensive Care Unit Sedation:

(See WARNINGS and DOSAGE AND ADMINISTRATION, Handling Procedures.) The administration of DIPRIVAN Injectable Emulsion should be initiated as a continuous infusion and changes in the rate of administration made slowly (>5 min) in order to minimize hypotension and avoid acute overdosage. (See CLINICAL PHARMACOLOGY- Individualization of Dosage.)

Patients should be monitored for early signs of significant hypotension and/or cardiovascular depression, which may be profound. These effects are responsive to discontinuation of DIPRIVAN Injectable Emulsion, IV fluid administration, and/or vasopressor therapy.

As with other sedative medications, there is wide interpatient variability in DIPRIVAN Injectable Emulsion dosage requirements, and these requirements may change with time.

Failure to reduce the infusion rate in patients receiving DIPRIVAN Injectable Emulsion for extended periods may result in excessively high blood concentrations of the drug. Thus, titration to clinical response and daily evaluation of sedation levels are important during use of DIPRIVAN Injectable Emulsion infusion for ICU sedation, especially of long duration.

Opioids and paralytic agents should be discontinued and respiratory function optimized prior to weaning patients from mechanical ventilation. Infusions of DIPRIVAN Injectable Emulsion should be adjusted to maintain a light level of sedation prior to weaning patients from mechanical ventilatory support. Throughout the weaning process this level of sedation may be maintained in the absence of respiratory depression. Because of the rapid clearance of DIPRIVAN Injectable Emulsion, abrupt discontinuation of a patient's infusion may result in rapid awakening of the patient with associated anxiety, agitation, and resistance to mechanical ventilation, making weaning from mechanical ventilation difficult. It is therefore recommended that administration of DIPRIVAN Injectable Emulsion be continued in order to maintain a light level of sedation throughout the weaning process until 10-15 minutes prior to extubation at which time the infusion can be discontinued.

Since DIPRIVAN Injectable Emulsion is formulated in an oil-in-water emulsion, elevations in serum triglycerides may occur when DIPRIVAN Injectable Emulsion is administered for extended periods of time. Patients at risk of hyperlipidemia should be monitored for increases in serum triglycerides or serum turbidity. Administration of DIPRIVAN Injectable Emulsion should be adjusted if fat is being inadequately cleared from the body. A reduction in the quantity of concurrently administered lipids is indicated to compensate for the amount of lipid infused as part of the DIPRIVAN Injectable Emulsion formulation; 1 mL of DIPRIVAN Injectable Emulsion contains approximately 0.1 g of fat (1.1 kcal).

In patients who are predisposed to zinc deficiency, such as those with burns, diarrhea, and/or major sepsis, the need for supplemental zinc should be considered during prolonged therapy with DIPRIVAN Injectable Emulsion.

EDTA is a strong chelator of trace metals—including zinc. Calcium disodium edetate has been used in gram quantities to treat heavy metal toxicity. When used in this manner it is possible that as much as 10 mg of elemental zinc can be lost per day via this mechanism. Although with DIPRIVAN Injectable Emulsion there are no reports of decreased zinc levels or zinc deficiency-related adverse events, DIPRIVAN Injectable Emulsion should not be infused for longer than 5 days without providing a drug holiday to safely replace estimated or measured urine zinc losses.

At high doses (2–3 grams per day), EDTA has been reported, on rare occasions, to be toxic to the renal tubules. Studies to-date, in patients with normal or impaired renal function have not shown any alteration in renal function with DIPRIVAN Injectable Emulsion containing 0.005% disodium edetate. In patients at risk for renal impairment, urinalysis and urine sediment should be checked before initiation of sedation and then be monitored on alternate days during sedation.

The long-term administration of DIPRIVAN Injectable Emulsion to patients with renal failure and/or hepatic insufficiency has not been evaluated.

Neurosurgical Anesthesia:

When DIPRIVAN Injectable Emulsion is used in patients with increased intracranial pressure or impaired cerebral circulation, significant decreases in mean arterial pressure should be avoided because of the resultant decreases in cerebral perfusion pressure. To avoid significant hypotension and decreases in cerebral perfusion pressure, an infusion or slow bolus of approximately 20 mg every 10 seconds should be utilized instead of rapid, more frequent, and/or larger boluses of DIPRIVAN Injectable Emulsion. Slower induction titrated to clinical responses, will generally result in reduced induction dosage requirements (1 to 2 mg/kg). When increased ICP is suspected, hyperventilation and hypocarbia should accompany the administration of DIPRIVAN Injectable Emulsion. (See DOSAGE AND ADMINISTRATION.)

Cardiac Anesthesia:

Slower rates of administration should be utilized in premedicated patients, geriatric patients, patients with recent fluid shifts, or patients who are hemodynamically unstable. Any fluid deficits should be corrected prior to administration of DIPRIVAN Injectable Emulsion. In those patients where additional fluid therapy may be contraindicated, other measures, e.g., elevation of lower extremities, or use of pressor agents, may be useful to offset the hypotension which is associated with the induction of anesthesia with DIPRIVAN Injectable Emulsion.

Information for Patients:

Patients should be advised that performance of activities requiring mental alertness, such as operating a motor vehicle, or hazardous machinery or signing legal documents may be impaired for some time after general anesthesia or sedation.

Drug Interactions:

The induction dose requirements of DIPRIVAN Injectable Emulsion may be reduced in patients with intramuscular or intravenous premedication, particularly with narcotics (e.g., morphine, meperidine, and fentanyl, etc.) and combinations of opioids and sedatives (e.g., benzodiazepines, barbiturates, chloral hydrate, droperidol, etc.). These agents may increase the anesthetic or sedative effects of DIPRIVAN Injectable Emulsion and may also result in more pronounced decreases in systolic, diastolic, and mean arterial pressures and cardiac output.

During maintenance of anesthesia or sedation, the rate of DIPRIVAN Injectable Emulsion administration should be adjusted according to the desired level of anesthesia or sedation and may be reduced in the presence of supplemental analgesic agents (e.g., nitrous oxide or opioids). The concurrent administration of potent inhalational agents (e.g., isoflurane, enflurane, and halothane) during maintenance with DIPRIVAN Injectable Emulsion has not been extensively evaluated. These inhalational agents can also be expected to increase the anesthetic or sedative and cardiorespiratory effects of DIPRIVAN Injectable Emulsion.

DIPRIVAN Injectable Emulsion does not cause a clinically significant change in onset, intensity or duration of action of the commonly used neuromuscular blocking agents (e.g., succinylcholine and nondepolarizing muscle relaxants).

No significant adverse interactions with commonly used premedications or drugs used during anesthesia or sedation (including a range of muscle relaxants, inhalational agents, analgesic agents, and local anesthetic agents) have been observed.

Carcinogenesis, Mutagenesis, Impairment of Fertility:

Animal carcinogenicity studies have not been performed with propofol.

In vitro and *in vivo* animal tests failed to show any potential for mutagenicity by propofol. Tests for mutagenicity included the Ames (using *Salmonella* sp) mutation test, gene mutation/gene conversion using Saccharomyces cerevisiae, invitro cytogenetic studies in Chinese hamsters and a mouse micronucleus test.

Studies in female rats at intravenous doses up to 15 mg/kg/day (6 times the maximum recommended human induction dose) for 2 weeks before pregnancy to day 7 of gestation did not show impaired fertility. Male fertility in rats was not affected in a dominant lethal study at intravenous doses up to 15 mg/kg/day for 5 days.

Pregnancy Category B:

Reproduction studies have been performed in rats and rabbits at intravenous doses of 15 mg/kg/day (6 times the recommended human induction dose) and have revealed no evidence of impaired fertility or harm to the fetus due to propofol. Propofol, however, has been shown to cause maternal deaths in rats and rabbits and decreased pup survival during the lactating period in dams treated with 15 mg/kg/day (or 6 times the recommended human induction dose). The pharmacological activity (anesthesia) of the drug on the mother is probably responsible for the adverse effects seen in the offspring. There are, however, no adequate and well-controlled studies in pregnant women. Because animal reproduction studies are not always predictive of human responses, this drug should be used during pregnancy only if clearly needed.

Labor and Delivery:

DIPRIVAN Injectable Emulsion is not recommended for obstetrics, including cesarean section deliveries. DIPRIVAN Injectable Emulsion crosses the placenta, and as with other general anesthetic agents, the administration of DIPRIVAN Injectable Emulsion may be associated with neonatal depression.

Nursing Mothers:

DIPRIVAN Injectable Emulsion is not recommended for use in nursing mothers because DIPRIVAN Injectable Emulsion has been reported to be excreted in human milk and the effects of oral absorption of small amounts of propofol are not known.

Pediatrics:

DIPRIVAN Injectable Emulsion is not recommended for use in pediatric patients for ICU or MAC sedation. In addition, DIPRIVAN Injectable Emulsion is not recommended for general anesthesia for children below the age of 3 years because safety and effectiveness have not been established.

Although no causal relationship has been established, serious adverse events (including fatalities) have been reported in children given DIPRIVAN Injectable Emulsion for ICU sedation. These events were seen most often in children with respiratory tract infections given doses in excess of those recommended for adults.

Geriatric use: A lower induction dose and a slower maintenance rate of administration of DIPRIVAN Injectable Emulsion should be used in elderly patients. In this group of patients, rapid (single or repeated) bolus administration should not be used in order to minimize undesirable cardiorespiratory depression including hypotension, apnea, airway obstruction and/or oxygen desaturation. All dosing should be titrated according to patient condition and response. (See DOSAGE AND ADMINISTRATION—Elderly,

Continued on next page

Diprivan—Cont.

debilitated or ASA III/IV patients and CLINICAL PHARMACOLOGY—Geriatrics.)

ADVERSE REACTIONS

General

Adverse event information is derived from controlled clinical trials and worldwide marketing experience. In the description below, rates of the more common events represent US/Canadian clinical study results. Less frequent events are also derived from publications and marketing experience in over 8 million patients; there are insufficient data to support an accurate estimate of their incidence rates. These studies were conducted using a variety of premedicants, varying lengths of surgical/diagnostic procedures and various other anesthetic/sedative agents. Most adverse events were mild and transient.

Anesthesia and MAC Sedation in Adults

The following estimates of adverse events for DIPRIVAN Injectable Emulsion include data from clinical trials in general anesthesia/MAC sedation (N=2889 adult patients). The adverse events listed below as probably causally related are those events in which the actual incidence rate in patients treated with DIPRIVAN Injectable Emulsion was greater than the comparator incidence rate in these trials. Therefore, incidence rates for anesthesia and MAC sedation in adults generally represent estimates of the percentage of clinical trial patients which appeared to have probable causal relationship.

The adverse experience profile from reports of 150 patients in the MAC sedation clinical trials is similar to the profile established with DIPRIVAN Injectable Emulsion during anesthesia (see below). During MAC sedation clinical trials, significant respiratory events included cough, upper airway obstruction, apnea, hypoventilation, and dyspnea.

Anesthesia in Children

Generally the adverse experience profile from reports of 349 DIPRIVAN Injectable Emulsion pediatric patients between the ages of 3 and 12 years in the US/Canadian anesthesia clinical trials is similar to the profile established with DIPRIVAN Injectable Emulsion during anesthesia in adults (see Pediatric percentages [Peds %] below). Although not reported as an adverse event in clinical trials, apnea is frequently observed in pediatric patients.

ICU Sedation in Adults

The following estimates of adverse events include data from clinical trials in ICU sedation (N=159) patients. Probably related incidence rates for ICU sedation were determined by individual case report form review. Probable causality was based upon an apparent dose response relationship and/or positive responses to rechallenge. In many instances the presence of concomitant disease and concomitant therapy made the causal relationship unknown. Therefore, incidence rates for ICU sedation generally represent estimates of the percentage of clinical trial patients which appeared to have a probable causal relationship.

[See table at left]

DRUG ABUSE AND DEPENDENCE

Rare cases of self administration of DIPRIVAN Injectable Emulsion by health care professionals have been reported, including some fatalities. DIPRIVAN Injectable Emulsion should be managed to prevent the risk of diversion, including restriction of access and accounting procedures as appropriate to the clinical setting.

OVERDOSAGE

If overdosage occurs, DIPRIVAN Injectable Emulsion administration should be discontinued immediately. Overdosage is likely to cause cardiorespiratory depression. Respiratory depression should be treated by artificial ventilation with oxygen. Cardiovascular depression may require repositioning of the patient by raising the patient's legs, increasing the flow rate of intravenous fluids and administering pressor agents and/or anticholinergic agents.

DOSAGE AND ADMINISTRATION

Dosage and rate of administration should be individualized and titrated to the desired effect, according to clinically relevant factors including preinduction and concomitant medications, age, ASA physical classification and level of debilitation of the patient.

The following is abbreviated dosage and administration information which is only intended as a general guide in the use of DIPRIVAN Injectable Emulsion. Prior to administering DIPRIVAN Injectable Emulsion, it is imperative that the physician review and be completely familiar with the specific dosage and administration information detailed in the CLINICAL PHARMACOLOGY - Individualization of Dosage section. In the elderly, debilitated , or ASA III/IV patients, rapid bolus doses should not be the method of administration. (See WARNINGS.)

Intensive Care Unit Sedation:

STRICT ASEPTIC TECHNIQUE MUST ALWAYS BE MAINTAINED DURING HANDLING. DIPRIVAN INJECTABLE EMULSION IS A SINGLE-USE PARENTERAL PRODUCT WHICH CONTAINS 0.005% DISODIUM EDETATE TO RETARD THE RATE OF GROWTH OF MICROORGANISMS IN THE EVENT OF ACCIDENTAL EXTRINSIC CONTAMINATION. HOWEVER, DIPRIVAN INJECTABLE EMULSION CAN STILL SUPPORT THE GROWTH OF MICROORGANISMS AS IT IS NOT AN ANTIMICROBIALLY PRESERVED PRODUCT UNDER USP STANDARDS. ACCORDINGLY, STRICT ASEPTIC TECHNIQUE MUST STILL BE ADHERED TO. DO NOT USE IF CONTAMINATION IS SUSPECTED. (See DOSAGE AND ADMINISTRATION, Handling Procedures.) DIPRIVAN Injectable Emulsion should be individualized according to the patient's condition and response, blood lipid profile, and vital signs. (See PRECAUTIONS- ICU sedation.) For intubated, mechanically ventilated adult patients, Intensive Care Unit (ICU) sedation should be initiated slowly with a continuous infusion in order to titrate to desired clinical effect and minimize hypotension. When indicated, initiation of sedation should begin at 5 μg/kg/min (0.3 mg/kg/h). The infusion rate should be increased by increments of 5 to 10 μg/kg/min (0.3 to 0.6 mg/kg/h) until the desired level of sedation is achieved. A minimum period of 5 minutes between adjustments should be allowed for onset of peak drug effect. Most adult patients require maintenance rates of 5 to 50 μg/kg/min (0.3 to 3 mg/kg/h) or higher. Dosages of DIPRIVAN Injectable Emulsion should be reduced in patients who have received large dosages of narcotics. Conversely, the DIPRIVAN Injectable Emulsion dosage requirement may be reduced by adequate management of pain with analgesic agents. As with other sedative medications, there is interpatient variability in dosage require-

Incidence greater than 1%—Probably Causally Related

	Anesthesia/MAC Sedation	ICU Sedation
Cardiovascular:	Bradycardia Hypotension* [Peds: 17%] [Hypertension Peds: 8%] (see also CLINICAL PHARMACOLOGY)	Bradycardia, Decreased Cardiac Output, Hypotension 26%
Central Nervous System:	Movement* [Peds: 17%]	
Injection Site:	Burning/Stinging or Pain, 17.6% [Peds: 10%]	
Metabolic/Nutritional:		Hyperlipemia*
Respiratory:	Apnea (see also CLINICAL PHARMACOLOGY)	Respiratory Acidosis During Weaning*
Skin and Appendages:	Rash [Peds: 5%]	

Events without an * or % had an incidence of 1%–3%
* Incidence of events 3% to 10%

Incidence less than 1%—Probably Causally Related

	Anesthesia/MAC Sedation	ICU Sedation
Body as a Whole:	Anaphylaxis/Anaphylactoid Reaction, Perinatal Disorder	
Cardiovascular:	Premature Atrial Contractions, Syncope	
Central Nervous System:	Hypertonia/Dystonia, Paresthesia	Agitation
Digestive:	Hypersalivation	
Musculoskeletal:	Myalgia	
Respiratory:	Wheezing	Decreased Lung Function
Skin and Appendages:	Flushing, Pruritus	
Special Senses:	Amblyopia	
Urogenital:	Cloudy Urine	Green Urine

Incidence less than 1%—Causal Relationship Unknown

	Anesthesia/MAC Sedation	ICU Sedation
Body as a Whole:	Asthenia, Awareness, Chest Pain Extremities Pain, Fever, Increased Drug Effect, Neck Rigidity/Stiffness, Trunk Pain	Fever, Sepsis, Trunk Pain, Whole Body Weakness
Cardiovascular:	Arrhythmia, Atrial Fibrillation, Atrioventricular Heart Block, Bigeminy, Bleeding, Bundle Branch Block, Cardiac Arrest, ECG Abnormal, Edema, Extrasystole, Heart Block, Hypertension, Myocardial Infarction, Myocardial Ischemia, Premature Ventricular Contractions, ST Segment Depression, Supraventricular Tachycardia, Tachycardia, Ventricular Fibrillation	Arrhythmia, Atrial Fibrillation, Bigeminy, Cardiac Arrest Extrasystole, Right Heart Failure, Ventricular Tachycardia
Central Nervous System:	Abnormal Dreams, Agitation, Amorous Behavior, Anxiety, Bucking/Jerking/Thrashing, Chills/Shivering, Clonic Myoclonic Movement, Combativeness, Confusion, Delirium, Depression, Dizziness, Emotional Lability, Euphoria, Fatigue, Hallucinations, Headache, Hypotonia, Hysteria, Insomnia, Moaning, Neuropathy, Opisthotonos, Rigidity, Seizures, Somnolence, Tremor, Twitching	Chills/Shivering, Intracranial Hypertension, Seizures, Somnolence, Thinking Abnormal
Digestive:	Cramping, Diarrhea, Dry Mouth, Enlarged Parotid, Nausea, Swallowing, Vomiting	Ileus, Liver Function Abnormal
Hematologic/Lymphatic:	Coagulation Disorder, Leukocytosis	
Injection Site:	Hives/Itching, Phlebitis, Redness/Discoloration	
Metabolic/Nutritional:	Hyperkalemia, Hyperlipemia	BUN Increased, Creatinine Increased, Dehydration, Hyperglycemia, Metabolic Acidosis, Osmolality Increased
Respiratory:	Bronchospasm, Burning in Throat, Cough, Dyspnea, Hiccough, Hyperventilation, Hypoventilation, Hypoxia, Laryngospasm, Pharyngitis, Sneezing, Tachypnea, Upper Airway Obstruction	Hypoxia
Skin and Appendages:	Conjunctival Hyperemia, Diaphoresis, Urticaria	Rash
Special Senses:	Diplopia, Ear Pain, Eye Pain, Nystagmus, Taste Perversion, Tinnitus	
Urogenital:	Oliguria, Urine Retention	Kidney Failure

INDICATION	DOSAGE AND ADMINISTRATION
Induction of General Anesthesia	**Healthy Adults Less Than 55 Years of Age:** 40 mg every 10 seconds until induction onset (2 to 2.5 mg/kg). **Elderly, Debilitated, or ASA III/IV Patients:** 20 mg every 10 seconds until induction onset (1 to 1.5 mg/kg). **Cardiac Anesthesia:** 20 mg every 10 seconds until induction onset (0.5 to 1.5 mg/kg). **Neurosurgical Patients:** 20 mg every 10 seconds until induction onset (1 to 2 mg/kg). **Pediatric —healthy, 3 years of age or older:** 2.5 to 3.5 mg/kg administered over 20–30 seconds.
Maintenance of General Anesthesia:	**Infusion** **Healthy Adults Less Than 55 Years of Age:** 100 to 200 µg/kg/min (6 to 12 mg/kg/h). **Elderly, Debilitated, ASA III/IV Patients:** 50 to 100 µg/kg/min (3 to 6 mg/kg/h). **Cardiac Anesthesia:** Most patients require: Primary DIPRIVAN Injectable Emulsion with Secondary Opioid—100–105 µg/kg/min Low Dose DIPRIVAN Injectable Emulsion with Primary Opioid—50–100 µg/kg/min (See CLINICAL PHARMACOLOGY—Table 4) **Neurosurgical Patients:** 100 to 200 µg/kg/min (6 to 12 mg/kg/h). **Pediatric—healthy, 3 years of age or older:** 125 to 300 µg/kg/min (7.5 to 18 mg/kg/h)
Maintenance of General Anesthesia:	**Intermittent Bolus** **Healthy Adults Less Than 55 Years of Age:** Increments of 20 to 50 mg as needed.
Initiation of MAC Sedation	**Healthy Adults Less Than 55 Years of Age:** Slow infusion or slow injection techniques are recommended to avoid apnea or hypotension. Most patients require an infusion of 100 to 150 µg/kg/min (6 to 9 mg/kg/h) for 3 to 5 minutes or a slow injection of 0.5 mg/kg over 3 to 5 minutes followed immediately by a maintenance infusion. **Elderly, Debilitated, Neurological, or ASA III/IV Patients:** Most patients require dosages similar to healthy adults. Rapic boluses are to be avoided. (See WARNINGS.)
Maintenance of MAC Sedation	**Healthy Adults Less Than 55 Years of Age:** A variable rate infusion technique is preferable over an intermittent bolus technique. Most patients require an infusion of 25 to 75 µg/kg/min (1.5 to 4.5 mg/kg/h) or incremental bolus doses of 10 mg or 20 mg. **In Elderly, Debilitated, Neurological, or ASA III/IV Patients:** Most patients require 80% of the usual adult dose. A rapid (single or repeated) bolus dose should not be used. (See WARNINGS.)
Initiation and Maintenance of ICU Sedation in Intubated, Mechanically Ventilated	**Adult Patients**—Because of the lingering effects of previous anesthetic or sedative agents, in most patients the initial infusion should be 5 µg/kg/min (0.3 mg/kg/h) for at least 5 minutes. Subsequent increments of 5 to 10 µg/kg/min (0.3 to 0.6 mg/kg/h) over 5 to 10 minutes may be used until desired level of sedation is achieved. Maintenance rates of 5 to 50 µg/kg/min (0.3 to 3 mg/kg/h) or higher may be required. **Evaluation of level of sedation and assessment of CNS function should be carried out daily throughout maintenance to determine the minimum dose of DIPRIVAN Injectable Emulsion required for sedation.** **The tubing and any unused portions of DIPRIVAN Injectable Emulsion should be discarded after 12 hours because DIPRIVAN Injectable Emulsion contains no preservatives and is capable of supporting growth of microorganisms. (See WARNINGS, and DOSAGE AND ADMINISTRATION.)**

— 5% Dextrose Injection, USP
— Lactated Ringers Injection, USP
— Lactated Ringers and 5% Dextrose Injection
— 5% Dextrose and 0.45% Sodium Chloride Injection, USP
— 5% Dextrose and 0.2% Sodium Chloride Injection, USP

Assembly Instructions for Pre-Filled Syringe

1. Remove the Luer connector from packaging.
2. Remove glass syringe barrel from tray and check for cracks or leaks. Shake. Remove the blue plastic cover. Disinfect the rubber stopper using alcohol swab provided in package. Allow to dry.
3. Pull off needle cover from Luer connector. The bevel of the needle spike is slightly bent (c-tip) to prevent potential coring.
4. Stand the syringe barrel vertically on a hard surface and push Luer connector on to syringe barrel so needle penetrates rubber seal and connector slides over the blue seal until firmly seated. (Fig. 1)

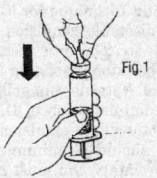
Fig.1

5. Add plunger rod by screwing clockwise. CAUTION: the rod must be fully screwed on, otherwise it may detach which could result in siphoning of the syringe contents. (Fig. 2)

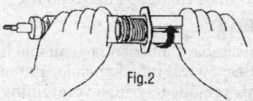
Fig.2

6. Unscrew Luer cover remove excess nitrogen gas from the syringe (a small nitrogen gas bubble may remain). Assemble administration line and connect syringe.

Handling Procedures

General

Parenteral drug products should be inspected visually for particulate matter and discoloration prior to administration whenever solution and container permit.

Clinical experience with the use of in-line filters and DIPRIVAN Injectable Emulsion during anesthesia or ICU/MAC sedation is limited. DIPRIVAN Injectable Emulsion should only be administered through a filter with a pore size of 5 microns or greater unless it has been demonstrated that the filter does not restrict the flow of DIPRIVAN Injectable Emulsion and/or cause the breakdown of the emulsion. Filters should be used with caution and where clinically appropriate. Continuous monitoring is necessary due to the potential for restricted flow and/or breakdown of the emulsion. Do not use if there is evidence of separation of the phases of the emulsion.

Rare cases of self administration of DIPRIVAN Injectable Emulsion, by health care professionals have been reported, including some fatalities (See DRUG ABUSE AND DEPENDENCE).

STRICT ASEPTIC TECHNIQUE MUST ALWAYS BE MAINTAINED DURING HANDLING. DIPRIVAN INJECTABLE EMULSION IS A SINGLE-USE PARENTERAL PRODUCT; WHICH CONTAINS 0.005% DISODIUM EDETATE TO RETARD THE RATE OF GROWTH OF MICROORGANISMS IN THE EVENT OF ACCIDENTAL EXTRINSIC CONTAMINATION. HOWEVER, DIPRIVAN INJECTABLE EMULSION CAN STILL SUPPORT THE GROWTH OF MICROORGANISMS AS IT IS NOT AN ANTIMICROBIALLY PRESERVED PRODUCT UNDER USP STANDARDS. ACCORDINGLY, STRICT ASEPTIC TECHNIQUE MUST STILL BE ADHERED TO. DO NOT USE IF CONTAMINATION IS SUSPECTED. DISCARD UNUSED PORTIONS AS DIRECTED WITHIN THE REQUIRED TIME LIMITS (SEE DOSAGE AND ADMINISTRATION, HANDLING PROCEDURES). THERE HAVE BEEN REPORTS IN WHICH FAILURE TO USE ASEPTIC TECHNIQUE WHEN HANDLING DIPRIVAN INJECTABLE EMULSION WAS ASSOCIATED WITH MICROBIAL CONTAMINATION OF THE PRODUCT AND WITH FEVER, INFECTION/SEPSIS, OTHER LIFE-THREATENING ILLNESS, AND/OR DEATH.

Guideline for Aseptic Technique for General Anesthesia/MAC Sedation

DIPRIVAN Injectable Emulsion should be prepared for use just prior to initiation of each individual anesthetic/sedative procedure. The ampoule neck surface, or vial/pre-filled syringe rubber stopper should be disinfected using 70% isopropyl alcohol. DIPRIVAN Injectable Emulsion should be

ments, and these requirements may change with time. (See DOSAGE GUIDE.) EVALUATION OF LEVEL OF SEDATION AND ASSESSMENT OF CNS FUNCTION SHOULD BE CARRIED OUT DAILY THROUGHOUT MAINTENANCE TO DETERMINE THE MINIMUM DOSE OF DIPRIVAN INJECTABLE EMULSION REQUIRED FOR SEDATION (See CLINICAL TRIALS, ICU Sedation). Bolus administration of 10 or 20 mg should only be used to rapidly increase depth of sedation in patients where hypotension is not likely to occur. Patients with compromised myocardial function, intravascular volume depletion, or abnormally low vascular tone (e.g., sepsis) may be more susceptible to hypotension. (See PRECAUTIONS.)

EDTA is a strong chelator of trace metals — including zinc. Calcium disodium edetate has been used in gram quantities to treat heavy metal toxicity. When used in this manner it is possible that as much as 10 mg of elemental zinc can be lost per day via this mechanism. Although with DIPRIVAN Injectable Emulsion there are no reports of decreased zinc levels or zinc deficiency-related adverse events, DIPRIVAN Injectable Emulsion should not be infused for longer than 5 days without providing a drug holiday to safely replace estimated or measured urine zinc losses.

At high doses (2–3 grams per day), EDTA has been reported, on rare occasions, to be toxic to the renal tubules. Studies to-date, in patients with normal or impaired renal function have not shown any alteration in renal function with DIPRIVAN Injectable Emulsion containing 0.005% disodium edetate. In patients at risk for renal impairment, urinalysis and urine sediment should be checked before initiation of sedation and then be monitored on alternate days during sedation.

SUMMARY OF DOSAGE GUIDELINES - Dosages and rates of administration in the following table should be individualized and titrated to clinical response. Safety and dosage requirements in pediatric patients have only been established for induction and maintenance of anesthesia. For complete dosage information, see CLINICAL PHARMACOLOGY - Individualization of Dosage.

[See table above]

Compatibility and Stability: DIPRIVAN Injectable Emulsion should not be mixed with other therapeutic agents prior to administration.

Dilution Prior to Administration: When DIPRIVAN Injectable Emulsion is diluted prior to administration, it should only be diluted with 5% Dextrose Injection, USP, and it should not be diluted to a concentration less than 2 mg/mL because it is an emulsion. In diluted form it has been shown to be more stable when in contact with glass than with plastic (95% potency after 2 hours of running infusion in plastic).

Administration with Other Fluids: Compatibility of DIPRIVAN Injectable Emulsion with the coadministration of blood/serum/plasma has not been established. (See WARNINGS.) DIPRIVAN Injectable Emulsion has been shown to be compatible when administered with the following intravenous fluids.

Continued on next page

Diprivan—Cont.

drawn into sterile syringes immediately after ampoules or vials are opened. When withdrawing DIPRIVAN Injectable Emulsion from vials, a sterile vent spike should be used. The syringe(s) should be labeled with appropriate information including the date and time the ampoule or vial was opened. Administration should commence promptly and be completed within 6 hours after the ampoules, vials, prefilled syringes have been opened.

DIPRIVAN Injectable Emulsion should be prepared for single patient use only. Any unused portions of DIPRIVAN Injectable Emulsion, reservoirs, dedicated administration tubing and/or solutions containing DIPRIVAN Injectable Emulsion must be discarded at the end of the anesthetic procedure or at 6 hours, whichever occurs sooner. The IV line should be flushed every 6 hours and at the end of the anesthetic procedure to remove residual DIPRIVAN Injectable Emulsion.

Guidelines for Aseptic Technique for ICU Sedation

When DIPRIVAN Injectable Emulsion is administered directly from the vial, strict aseptic techniques must be followed. The vial rubber stopper should be disinfected using 70% isopropyl alcohol. A sterile vent spike and sterile tubing must be used for administration of DIPRIVAN Injectable Emulsion. As with other lipid emulsions the number of IV line manipulations should be minimized. Administration should commence promptly and must be completed within 12 hours after the vial has been spiked. The tubing and any unused portions of DIPRIVAN Injectable Emulsion must be discarded after 12 hours.

If DIPRIVAN Injectable Emulsion is transferred to a syringe or other container prior to administration, the handling procedures for General anesthesia/MAC sedation should be followed, and the product should be discarded and administration lines changed after 6 hours.

HOW SUPPLIED

DIPRIVAN Injectable Emulsion is available in ready to use 20 mL ampoules, 50 mL infusion vials, 100 mL infusion vials, and 50 mL pre-filled syringes containing 10 mg/mL of propofol.

20 mL ampoules (NDC 0310-0300-20)
50 mL infusion vials (NDC 0310-0300-50)
100 mL infusion vials (NDC 0310-0300-11)
50 mL pre-filled syringes (NDC 0310-300-54)

Propofol undergoes oxidative degradation, in the presence of oxygen, and is therefore packaged under nitrogen to eliminate this degradation path.

Store between 4–22°C (40–72°F). Do not freeze. Shake well before use.

Manufactured by Zeneca S.p.A. for:
ZENECA
Pharmaceuticals
A Business Unit of Zeneca Inc.
Wilmington, Delaware 19850-5437
64104-02 Rev A 1/98

Shown in Product Identification Guide, page 345

ELAVIL® ℞
(AMITRIPTYLINE HCl)
Tablets and Injection

DESCRIPTION

Amitriptyline HCl is 3-(10,11-dihydro-5*H*-dibenzo [a,*d*] cycloheptene-5-ylidene)-*N*,*N*-dimethyl-1-propanamine hydrochloride. Its empirical formula is $C_{20}H_{23}N{\cdot}HCl$ and its structural formula is:

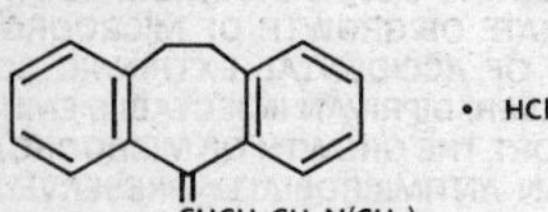

Amitriptyline HCl, a dibenzocycloheptadiene derivative, has a molecular weight of 313.87. It is a white, odorless, crystalline compound which is freely soluble in water.

ELAVIL* (Amitriptyline HCl) is supplied as 10 mg, 25 mg, 50 mg, 75 mg, 100 mg, and 150mg tablets and as a sterile solution for intramuscular use. Inactive ingredients of the tablets are calcium phosphate, cellulose, colloidal silicon dioxide, hydroxypropyl cellulose, hydroxypropyl methylcellulose, lactose, magnesium stearate, starch, stearic acid, talc, and titanium dioxide. Tablets ELAVIL 10 mg also contain FD&C Blue 1. Tablets ELAVIL 25 mg also contain D&C Yellow 10, FD&C Blue 1, and FD&C Yellow 6. Tablets ELAVIL 50 mg also contain D&C Yellow 10, FD&C Yellow 6 and iron oxide. Tablets ELAVIL 75 mg also contain FD&C Yellow 6. Tablets ELAVIL 100 mg also contain FD&C Blue 2 and FD&C Red 40. Tablets ELAVIL 150 mg also contain FD&C Blue 2 and FD&C Yellow 6. Each milliliter of the sterile solution contains:

Amitriptyline hydrochloride	10 mg
Dextrose	44 mg
Water for Injection, q.s	1 mL
Added as preservatives:	
Methylparaben	1.5 mg
Propylparaben	0.2 mg

ACTIONS

ELAVIL is an antidepressant with sedative effects. Its mechanism of action in man is not known. It is not a monoamine oxidase inhibitor and it does not act primarily by stimulation of the central nervous system.

Amitriptyline inhibits the membrane pump mechanism responsible for uptake of norepinephrine and serotonin in adrenergic and serotonergic neurons. Pharmacologically this action may potentiate or prolong neuronal activity since reuptake of these biogenic amines is important physiologically in terminating transmitting activity. This interference with the reuptake of norepinephrine and/or serotonin is believed by some to underlie the antidepressant activity of amitriptyline.

INDICATIONS

For the relief of symptoms of depression. Endogenous depression is more likely to be alleviated than are other depressive states.

CONTRAINDICATIONS

ELAVIL is contraindicated in patients who have shown prior hypersensitivity to it.

It should not be given concomitantly with monoamine oxidase inhibitors. Hyperpyretic crises, severe convulsions, and deaths have occurred in patients receiving tricyclic antidepressant and monoamine oxidase inhibiting drugs simultaneously. When it is desired to replace a monoamine oxidase inhibitor with ELAVIL, a minimum of 14 days should be allowed to elapse after the former is discontinued. ELAVIL should then be initiated cautiously with gradual increase in dosage until optimum response is achieved.

This drug is not recommended for use during the acute recovery phase following myocardial infarction.

WARNINGS

ELAVIL may block the antihypertensive action of guanethidine or similarly acting compounds.

It should be used with caution in patients with a history of seizures and, because of its atropine-like action, in patients with a history of urinary retention, angle-closure glaucoma or increased intraocular pressure. In patients with angle-closure glaucoma, even average doses may precipitate an attack.

Patients with cardiovascular disorders should be watched closely. Tricyclic antidepressant drugs, including ELAVIL, particularly when given in high doses, have been reported to produce arrhythmias, sinus tachycardia, and prolongation of the conduction time. Myocardial infarction and stroke have been reported with drugs of this class.

Close supervision is required when ELAVIL is given to hyperthyroid patients or those receiving thyroid medication.

ELAVIL may enhance the response to alcohol and the effects of barbiturates and other CNS depressants. In patients who may use alcohol excessively, it should be borne in mind that the potentiation may increase the danger inherent in any suicide attempt or overdosage. Delirium has been reported with concurrent administration of amitriptyline and disulfiram.

Usage in Pregnancy: Teratogenic effects were not observed in mice, rats, or rabbits when amitriptyline was given orally at doses of 2 to 40 mg/kg/day (up to 13 times the maximum recommended human dose**). Studies in literature have shown amitriptyline to be teratogenic in mice and hamsters when given by various routes of administration at doses of 28 to 100 mg/kg/day (9 to 33 times the maximum recommended human dose), producing multiple malformations. Another study in the rat reported that an oral dose of 25 mg/kg/day (8 times the maximum recommended human dose) produced delays in ossification of fetal vertebral bodies without other signs of embryotoxicity. In rabbits, an oral dose of 60 mg/kg/day (20 times the maximum recommended human dose) was reported to cause incomplete ossification of the cranial bones.

Amitriptyline has been shown to cross the placenta. Although a causal relationship has not been established, there have been a few reports of adverse events, including CNS effects, limb deformities, or developmental delay, in infants whose mothers had taken amitriptyline during pregnancy.

There are no adequate and well-controlled studies in pregnant women. ELAVIL should be used during pregnancy only if the potential benefit to the mother justifies the potential risk to the fetus.

Nursing Mothers: Amitriptyline is excreted into breast milk. In one report in which a patient received amitriptyline 100 mg/day while nursing her infant, levels of 83–141 ng/mL were detected in the mother's serum. Levels of 135–151 ng/mL were found in the breast milk, but no trace of the drug could be detected in the infant's serum.

Because of the potential for serious adverse reactions in nursing infants from amitriptyline, a decision should be made whether to discontinue nursing or to discontinue the drug, taking into account the importance of the drug to the mother.

Usage in Pediatric Patients: In view of the lack of experience with the use of this drug in pediatric patients, it is not recommended at the present time for patients under 12 years of age.

PRECAUTIONS

Schizophrenic patients may develop increased symptoms of psychosis; patients with paranoid symptomatology may have an exaggeration of such symptoms. Depressed patients, particularly those with known manic-depressive illness, may experience a shift to mania or hypomania. In these circumstances the dose of amitriptyline may be reduced or a major tranquilizer such as perphenazine may be administered concurrently.

The possibility of suicide in depressed patients remains until significant remission occurs. Potentially suicidal patients should not have access to large quantities of this drug. Prescriptions should be written for the smallest amount feasible.

Concurrent administration of ELAVIL and electroshock therapy may increase the hazards associated with such therapy. Such treatment should be limited to patients for whom it is essential.

When possible, the drug should be discontinued several days before elective surgery.

Both elevation and lowering of blood sugar levels have been reported.

ELAVIL should be used with caution in patients with impaired liver function.

Drug Interactions: Drugs Metabolized by P450 2D6—The biochemical activity of the drug metabolizing isozyme cytochrome P450 2D6 (debrisoquin hydroxylase) is reduced in a subset of the caucasian population (about 7–10% of Caucasians are so called "poor metabolizers"); reliable estimates of the prevalence of reduced P450 2D6 isozyme activity among Asian, African and other populations are not yet available. Poor metabolizers have higher than expected plasma concentrations of tricyclic antidepressants (TCAs) when given usual doses. Depending on the fraction of drug metabolized by P450 2D6, the increase in plasma concentration may be small, or quite large (8-fold increase in plasma AUC of the TCA).

In addition, certain drugs inhibit the activity of this isozyme and make normal metabolizers resemble poor metabolizers. An individual who is stable on a given dose of TCA may become abruptly toxic when given one of these inhibiting drugs as concomitant therapy. The drugs that inhibit cytochrome P450 2D6 include some that are not metabolized by the enzyme (quinidine; cimetidine) and many that are substrates for P450 2D6 (many other antidepressants, phenothiazines, and the Type 1C antiarrhythmics propafenone and flecainide). While all the selective serotonin reuptake inhibitors (SSRIs), e.g., fluoxetine, sertraline, and paroxetine, inhibit P450 2D6, they may vary in the extent of inhibition. The extent to which SSRI-TCA interactions may pose clinical problems will depend on the degree of inhibition and the pharmacokinetics of the SSRI involved. Nevertheless, caution is indicated in the coadministration of TCAs with any of the SSRIs and also in switching from one class to the other. Of particular importance, sufficient time must elapse before initiating TCA treatment in a patient being withdrawn from fluoxetine, given the long half-life of the parent and active metabolite (at least 5 weeks may be necessary).

Concomitant use of tricyclic antidepressants with drugs that can inhibit cytochrome P450 2D6 may require lower doses than usually prescribed for either the tricyclic antidepressant or the other drug. Furthermore, whenever one of these other drugs is withdrawn from co-therapy, an increased dose of tricyclic antidepressant may be required. It is desirable to monitor TCA plasma levels whenever a TCA is going to be coadministered with another drug known to be an inhibitor of P450 2D6.

Monoamine oxidase inhibitors—see CONTRAINDICATIONS section. Guanethidine or similarly acting compounds; thyroid medication; alcohol, barbiturates and other CNS depressants; and disulfiram— see WARNINGS section.

When ELAVIL is given with anticholinergic agents or sympathomimetic drugs, including epinephrine combined with local anesthetics, close supervision and careful adjustment of dosages are required.

Hyperpyrexia has been reported when ELAVIL is administered with anticholinergic agents or with neuroleptic drugs, particularly during hot weather.

Paralytic ileus may occur in patients taking tricyclic antidepressants in combination with anticholinergic-type drugs.

Cimetidine is reported to reduce hepatic metabolism of certain tricyclic antidepressants, thereby delaying elimination and increasing steady-state concentrations of these drugs. Clinically significant effects have been reported with the tricyclic antidepressants when used concomitantly with cime-

tidine. Increases in plasma levels of tricyclic antidepressants, and in the frequency and severity of side effects, particularly anticholinergic, have been reported when cimetidine was added to the drug regimen. Discontinuation of cimetidine in well-controlled patients receiving tricyclic antidepressants and cimetidine may decrease the plasma levels and efficacy of the antidepressants.

Caution is advised if patients receive large doses of ethchlorvynol concurrently. Transient delirium has been reported in patients who were treated with one gram of ethchlorvynol and 75–150mg of ELAVIL.

Information for Patients: While on therapy with ELAVIL, patients should be advised as to the possible impairment of mental and/or physical abilities required for performance of hazardous tasks, such as operating machinery or driving a motor vehicle.

ADVERSE REACTIONS

Within each category the following adverse reactions are listed in order of decreasing severity. Included in the listing are a few adverse reactions which have not been reported with this specific drug. However, pharmacological similarities among the tricyclic antidepressant drugs require that each of the reactions be considered when amitriptyline is administered.

Cardiovascular: Myocardial infarction; stroke; nonspecific ECG changes and changes in AV conduction; heart block; arrhythmias; hypotension, particularly orthostatic hypotension; syncope; hypertension; tachycardia; palpitation.

CNS and Neuromuscular: Coma; seizures; hallucinations; delusions; confusional states; disorientation; incoordination; ataxia; tremors; peripheral neuropathy; numbness, tingling, and paresthesias of the extremities; extrapyramidal symptoms including abnormal involuntary movements and tardive dyskinesia; dysarthria; disturbed concentration; excitement; anxiety; insomnia; restlessness; nightmares; drowsiness; dizziness; weakness; fatigue; headache; syndrome of inappropriate ADH (antidiuretic hormone) secretion; tinnitus; alteration in EEG patterns.

Anticholinergic: Paralytic ileus; hyperpyrexia; urinary retention; dilatation of the urinary tract; constipation; blurred vision, disturbance of accommodation, increased ocular pressure, mydriasis; dry mouth.

Allergic: Skin rash; urticaria; photosensitization; edema of face and tongue.

Hematologic: Bone marrow depression including agranulocytosis, leukopenia, thrombocytopenia; purpura; eosinophilia.

Gastrointestinal: Rarely hepatitis (including altered liver function and jaundice); nausea; epigastric distress; vomiting; anorexia; stomatitis; peculiar taste; diarrhea; parotid swelling; black tongue.

Endocrine: Testicular swelling and gynecomastia in the male; breast enlargement and galactorrhea in the female; increased or decreased libido; impotence; elevation and lowering of blood sugar levels.

Other: Alopecia; edema; weight gain or loss; urinary frequency; increased perspiration.

Withdrawal Symptoms: After prolonged administration, abrupt cessation of treatment may produce nausea, headache, and malaise. Gradual dosage reduction has been reported to produce, within two weeks, transient symptoms including irritability, restlessness, and dream and sleep disturbance.

These symptoms are not indicative of addiction. Rare instances have been reported of mania or hypomania occurring within 2–7 days following cessation of chronic therapy with tricyclic antidepressants.

Causal Relationship Unknown: Other reactions, reported under circumstances where a causal relationship could not be established, are listed to serve as alerting information to physicians:

Body as a Whole: Lupus-like syndrome (migratory arthritis, positive ANA and rheumatoid factor).

Digestive: Hepatic failure, ageusia.

DOSAGE AND ADMINISTRATION
Oral Dosage

Dosage should be initiated at a low level and increased gradually, noting carefully the clinical response and any evidence of intolerance.

Initial Dosage for Adults: For outpatients 75 mg of amitriptyline HCl a day in divided doses is usually satisfactory. If necessary, this may be increased to a total of 150 mg per day. Increases are made preferably in the late afternoon and/or bedtime doses. A sedative effect may be apparent before the antidepressant effect is noted, but an adequate therapeutic effect may take as long as 30 days to develop.

An alternate method of initiating therapy in outpatients is to begin with 50 to 100mg amitriptyline HCl at bedtime. This may be increased by 25 or 50 mg as necessary in the bedtime dose to a total of 150 mg per day.

Hospitalized patients may require 100 mg a day initially. This can be increased gradually to 200 mg a day if necessary. A small number of hospitalized patients may need as much as 300 mg a day.

Adolescent and Elderly Patients: In general, lower dosages are recommended for these patients. Ten mg 3 times a day with 20 mg at bedtime may be satisfactory in adolescent and elderly patients who do not tolerate higher dosages.

Maintenance: The usual maintenance dosage of amitriptyline HCl is 50 to 100 mg per day. In some patients 40 mg per day is sufficient. For maintenance therapy the total daily dosage may be given in a single dose preferably at bedtime. When satisfactory improvement has been reached, dosage should be reduced to the lowest amount that will maintain relief of symptoms. It is appropriate to continue maintenance therapy 3 months or longer to lessen the possibility of relapse.

Intramuscular Dosage

Initially, 20 to 30 mg (2 to 3 mL) four times a day.

When ELAVIL Injection is administered intramuscularly, the effects may appear more rapidly than with oral administration.

When ELAVIL Injection is used for initial therapy in patients unable or unwilling to take ELAVIL Tablets, the tablets should replace the injection as soon as possible.

Usage in Pediatric Patients

In view of the lack of experience with the use of this drug in pediatric patients, it is not recommended at the present time for patients under 12 years of age.

Plasma Levels

Because of the wide variation in the absorption and distribution of tricyclic antidepressants in body fluids, it is difficult to directly correlate plasma levels and therapeutic effect. However, determination of plasma levels may be useful in identifying patients who appear to have toxic effects and may have excessively high levels, or those in whom lack of absorption or noncompliance is suspected. Adjustments in dosage should be made according to the patient's clinical response and not on the basis of plasma levels.***

OVERDOSAGE

Deaths may occur from overdosage with this class of drugs. Multiple drug ingestion (including alcohol) is common in deliberate tricyclic antidepressant overdose. As the management is complex and changing, it is recommended that the physician contact a poison control center for current information on treatment. Signs and symptoms of toxicity develop rapidly after tricyclic antidepressant overdose, therefore, hospital monitoring is required as soon as possible.

Manifestations: Critical manifestations of overdose include: cardiac dysrhythmias, severe hypotension, convulsions, and CNS depression, including coma. Changes in the electrocardiogram, particularly in QRS axis or width, are clinically significant indicators of tricyclic antidepressant toxicity.

Other signs of overdose may include: impaired myocardial contractility, confusion, disturbed concentration, transient visual hallucinations, dilated pupils, disorders of ocular motility, agitation, hyperactive reflexes, polyradiculoneuropathy, stupor, drowsiness, muscle rigidity, vomiting, hypothermia, hyperpyrexia, or any of the symptoms listed under ADVERSE REACTIONS.

Management:

General: Obtain an ECG and immediately initiate cardiac monitoring. Protect the patient's airway, establish an intravenous line and initiate gastric decontamination. A minimum of six hours of observation with cardiac monitoring and observation for signs of CNS or respiratory depression, hypotension, cardiac dysrhythmias and/or conduction blocks, and seizures is necessary. If signs of toxicity occur at any time during the period, extended monitoring is required. There are case reports of patients succumbing to fatal dysrhythmias late after overdose; these patients had clinical evidence of significant poisoning prior to death and most received inadequate gastrointestinal decontamination. Monitoring of plasma drug levels should not guide management of the patient.

Gastrointestinal Decontamination: All patients suspected of tricyclic antidepressant overdose should receive gastrointestinal decontamination. This should include large volume gastric lavage followed by activated charcoal. If consciousness is impaired, the airway should be secured prior to lavage. EMESIS IS CONTRAINDICATED.

Cardiovascular: A maximal limb-lead QRS duration of ≥ 0.10 seconds may be the best indication of the severity of the overdose. Intravenous sodium bicarbonate should be used to maintain the serum pH in the range of 7.45 to 7.55. If the pH response is inadequate, hyperventilation may also be used. Concomitant use of hyperventilation and sodium bicarbonate should be done with extreme caution, with frequent pH monitoring. A pH > 7.60 or a pCO_2 < 20mm Hg is undesirable. Dysrhythmias unresponsive to sodium bicarbonate therapy/hyperventilation may respond to lidocaine, bretylium or phenytoin. Type 1A and 1C antiarrhythmics are generally contraindicated (e.g., quinidine, disopyramide, and procainamide).

In rare instances, hemoperfusion may be beneficial in acute refractory cardiovascular instability in patients with acute toxicity. However, hemodialysis, peritoneal dialysis, exchange transfusions, and forced diuresis generally have been reported as ineffective in tricyclic antidepressant poisoning.

CNS: In patients with CNS depression, early intubation is advised because of the potential for abrupt deterioration. Seizures should be controlled with benzodiazepines, or if these are ineffective, other anticonvulsants (e.g., phenobarbital, phenytoin). Physostigmine is not recommended except to treat life-threatening symptoms that have been unresponsive to other therapies, and then only in consultation with a poison control center.

Psychiatric Follow-up: Since overdosage is often deliberate, patients may attempt suicide by other means during the recovery phase. Psychiatric referral may be appropriate.

Pediatric Management: The principles of management of pediatric and adult overdosages are similar. It is strongly recommended that the physician contact the local poison control center for specific pediatric treatment.

HOW SUPPLIED

Tablets ELAVIL, 10 mg, are blue, round, film coated tablets, identified with "40" debossed on one side and "ELAVIL" on the other side. They are supplied as follows:
NDC 0310-0040-10 bottles of 100
NDC 0310-0040-34 bottles of 1000

Tablets ELAVIL, 25 mg, are yellow, round, film coated tablets, identified with "45" debossed on one side and "ELAVIL" on the other side. They are supplied as follows:
NDC 0310-0045-10 bottles of 100
NDC 0310-0045-39 unit dose packages of 100
NDC 0310-0045-34 bottles of 1000
NDC 0310-0045-50 bottles of 5000

Tablets ELAVIL, 50 mg, are beige, round, film coated tablets, identified with "41" debossed on one side and "ELAVIL" on the other side. They are supplied as follows:
NDC 0310-0041-10 bottles of 100
NDC 0310-0041-39 unit dose packages of 100
NDC 0310-0041-34 bottles of 1000

Tablets ELAVIL, 75 mg, are orange, round, film coated tablets, identified with "42" debossed on one side and "ELAVIL" on the other side. They are supplied as follows:
NDC 0310-0042-10 bottles of 100

Tablets ELAVIL, 100 mg, are mauve, round, film coated tablets, identified with "43" debossed on one side and "ELAVIL" on the other side. They are supplied as follows:
NDC 0310-0043-10 bottles of 100

Tablets ELAVIL, 150 mg, are blue, capsule shaped, film coated tablets, identified with "47" debossed on one side and "ELAVIL" on the other side. They are supplied as follows:
NDC 0310-0047-30 bottles of 30
NDC 0310-0047-10 bottles of 100

Injection ELAVIL, 10 mg/mL, is a clear, colorless solution, and is supplied as follows:
NDC 0310-0049-10 in 10 mL vials

Storage: Store Tablets ELAVIL in a well-closed container. Avoid storage at temperatures above 30°C (86°F). In addition, Tablets ELAVIL 10 mg must be protected from light and stored in a well-closed, light-resistant container.

Protect ELAVIL Injection from freezing and avoid storage above 30°C (86°F).

METABOLISM

Studies in man following oral administration of ^{14}C-labeled drug indicated that amitriptyline is rapidly absorbed and metabolized. Radioactivity of the plasma was practically negligible, although significant amounts of radioactivity appeared in the urine by 4 to 6 hours and one-half to one-third of the drug was excreted within 24 hours.

Amitriptyline is metabolized by N-demethylation and bridge hydroxylation in man, rabbit, and rat. Virtually the entire dose is excreted as glucuronide or sulfate conjugate of metabolites, with little unchanged drug appearing in the urine. Other metabolic pathways may be involved.

REFERENCES

Ayd FJ Jr: Amitriptyline (ELAVIL) therapy for depressive reactions. Psychosomatics 1960;1:320-325.
Diamond S: Human metabolizer of amitriptyline tagged with carbon 14. Curr Ther Res, Mar 1965, pp 170-175.
Dorfman W: Clinical experiences with amitriptyline (ELAVIL): A preliminary report. Psychosomatics 1960;1:153-155.
Fallette JM, Stasney CR, Mintz AA: Amitriptyline poisoning treated with physostigmine. South Med J 1970;63:1492-1493.
Hollister LE, Overall JE, Johnson M, et al: Controlled comparison of amitriptyline, imipramine and placebo in hospitalized depressed patients. J Nerv Ment Dis 1964;139:370-375.
Hordern A, Burt CG, Holt NF: Depressive states: A pharmacotherapeutic study, Springfield study. Springfield, Ill, Charles C. Thomas, 1965.
Klerman GL, Cole JO: Clinical pharmacology of imipramine and related antidepressant compounds. Int J Psychiatry 1976;3:267-304.

Continued on next page

Elavil—Cont.

McConaghy N, Joffe AD, Kingston WR, et al: Correlation of clinical features of depressed out-patients with response to amitriptyline and protriptyline. Br J Psychiatry 1968;114: 103-106.
McDonald IM, Perkins M, Marjerrison G, et al: A controlled comparison of amitriptyline and electroconvulsive therapy in the treatment of depression. Am J Psychiatry 1966;122: 1427-1431.
Slovis T, Ott J, Teitelbaum, et al: Physostigmine therapy in acute tricyclic antidepressant poisoning. Clin Toxicol 1971;4:451-459.
Symposium on depression with special studies of a new antidepressant, amitriptyline. Dis Nerv Syst, (Sect 2) May 1961, pp 5-56.

* Registered trademark of ZENECA Inc.
** Based on a maximum recommended amitriptyline dose of 150 mg/day or 3mg/kg/day for a 50 kg patient.
*** Hollister LE: JAMA 1979;241:2350-2533.

Manufactured for
Zeneca Pharmaceuticals
A Business Unit of Zeneca Inc
Wilmington, DE 19850-5437
by MERCK & CO., INC. West Point, PA 19846 USA
64059-03 Rev G 12/96

Shown in Product Identification Guide, page 346

HIBICLENS® Antiseptic/Antimicrobial **OTC**
[*hi 'bi-klenz*]
Skin Cleanser
(chlorhexidine gluconate)

DESCRIPTION

HIBICLENS is an antiseptic antimicrobial skin cleanser possessing bactericidal activities. HIBICLENS contains 4% w/v HIBITANE® (chlorhexidine gluconate), a chemically unique hexamethylenebis biguanide with inactive ingredients: Fragrance, isopropyl alcohol 4%, purified water, Red 40, and other ingredients, in a mild, sudsing base adjusted to pH 5.0–6.5 for optimal activity and stability as well as compatibility with the normal pH of the skin.

ACTION

HIBICLENS is bactericidal on contact. It has antiseptic activity and a persistent antimicrobial effect with rapid bactericidal activity against a wide range of microorganisms, including gram-positive bacteria, and gram-negative bacteria such as *Pseudomonas aeruginosa*. The effectiveness of HIBICLENS is not signficantly reduced by the presence of organic matter, such as blood.[1]

In a study[2] simulating surgical use, the immediate bactericidal effect of HIBICLENS after a single six-minute scrub resulted in a 99.9% reduction in resident bacterial flora, with a reduction of 99.98% after the eleventh scrub. Reductions on surgically gloved hands were maintained over the six-hour test period.

HIBICLENS displays persistent antimicrobial action. In one study[2], 93% of a radiolabeled formulation of HIBICLENS remained present on uncovered skin after five hours.

HIBICLENS prevents skin infection thereby reducing the risk of cross-infection.

INDICATIONS

HIBICLENS is indicated for use as a surgical scrub, as a health-care personnel handwash, for patient preoperative showering and bathing, as a patient preoperative skin preparation, and as a skin wound cleanser and general skin cleanser.

SAFETY

The extensive use of chlorhexidine gluconate for over 20 years outside the United States has produced no evidence of absorption of the compound through intact skin. The potential for producing skin reactions is extremely low. HIBICLENS can be used many times a day without causing irritation, dryness, or discomfort. Experimental studies indicate that when used for cleaning superficial wounds, HIBICLENS will neither cause additional tissue injury nor delay healing.

WARNINGS

FOR EXTERNAL USE ONLY. KEEP OUT OF EYES, EARS AND MOUTH. HIBICLENS SHOULD NOT BE USED AS A PREOPERATIVE SKIN PREPARATION OF THE FACE OR HEAD. MISUSE OF HIBICLENS HAS BEEN REPORTED TO CAUSE SERIOUS AND PERMANENT EYE INJURY WHEN IT HAS BEEN PERMITTED TO ENTER AND REMAIN IN THE EYE DURING SURGICAL PROCEDURES. IF HIBICLENS SHOULD CONTACT THESE AREAS, RINSE OUT PROMPTLY AND THOROUGHLY WITH WATER. Avoid contact with meninges. HIBICLENS should not be used by persons who have a sensitivity to it or its components. Chlorhexidine gluconate has been reported to cause deafness when instilled in the middle ear through perforated ear drums. Irritation, sensitization and generalized allergic reactions have been reported with chlorhexidine-containing products, especially in the genital areas. If adverse reactions occur, discontinue use immediately and if severe, contact a physician. Keep this and all drugs out of the reach of children. In case of accidental ingestion, seek professional assistance or contact a Poison Control Center immediately.

Accidental ingestion: Chlorhexidine gluconate taken orally is poorly absorbed. Treat with gastric lavage using milk, egg white, gelatin or mild soap. Employ supportive measures as appropriate.

Avoid excessive heat (above 104°F).

DIRECTIONS FOR USE

Skin Wound and General skin Cleansing

Wounds which involve more than the superficial layers of the skin should not be routinely treated with HIBICLENS. HIBICLENS should not be used for repeated general skin cleansing of large body areas except in those patients whose underlying condition makes it necessary to reduce the bacterial population of the skin. To use, thoroughly rinse the area to be cleansed with water. Apply the minimum amount of HIBICLENS necessary to cover the skin or wound area and wash gently. Rinse again thoroughly.

Preoperative Skin Preparation

Apply HIBICLENS liberally to surgical site and swab for at least two minutes. Dry with a sterile towel. Repeat procedure for an additional two minutes and dry with a sterile towel.

Preoperative Showering and Whole-Body bathing

The patient should be instructed to wash the entire body, including the scalp, on two consecutive occasions immediately prior to surgery. Each procedure should consist of two consecutive thorough applications of HIBICLENS followed by thorough rinsing. If the patient's condition allows, showering is recommended for whole-body bathing. The recommended procedure is: Wet the body, including hair. Wash the hair using 25 mL of HIBICLENS and the body with another 25 mL of HIBICLENS. Rinse. Repeat. Rinse thoroughly after second application.

HEALTH-CARE PERSONNEL USE

Surgical Hand Scrub

Directions for use of HIBICLENS Liquid: Wet hands and forearms with water. Scrub for 3 minutes with about 5 mL of HIBICLENS and a wet brush, paying particular attention to the nails, cuticles, and interdigital spaces. A separate nail cleaner may be used. Rinse thoroughly. Wash for an additional 3 minutes with 5 mL of HIBICLENS and rinse under running water. Dry thoroughly.

Personnel Hand Wash

Wet hands with warm water. (Avoid using very cold or very hot water.) Dispense about 5 mL of HIBICLENS into cupped hands. Wash for 15 seconds. (Do not use excessive pressure to produce additional lather.) Rinse thoroughly with warm water. Dry thoroughly.

Directions for use of HIBICLENS® Sponge/Brush: Open package and remove nail cleaner. Wet hands. Use nail cleaner under fingernails and to clean cuticles. Wet hands and forearms to the elbow with warm water. (Avoid using very cold or very hot water.) Wet sponge side of sponge/brush. Squeeze and pump immediately to work up adequate lather. Apply lather to hands and forearms using *sponge* side of the product. *Start 3 minute scrub* by using the brush side of the product to scrub *only* nails, cuticles, and interdigital areas. Use sponge side for scrubbing hands and forearms. (Avoid using brush on these more sensitive areas.) Rinse thoroughly with warm water. Scrub for an additional 3 minutes *using sponge side* only. To produce additional lather, add a small amount of water and pump the sponge. (While scrubbing, do not use excessive pressure to produce lather—a small amount of lather is all that is required to adequately cleanse skin with HIBICLENS.) Rinse and dry thoroughly, blotting hands and forearms with a soft sterile towel.

IMPORTANT LAUNDERING ADVICE FOR HOSPITAL STAFF AND OTHER USERS OF ANTISEPTIC PATIENT SKIN PREPARATIONS CONTAINING CHLORHEXIDINE GLUCONATE

Chlorhexidine gluconate is a unique agent that most closely fits the definition of an ideal antimicrobial agent, having (among others) one of the most important characteristics of persistent activity. This persistence is due to chlorhexidine gluconate binding to the protein of the skin and, thus, being available for residual activity over a relatively long period of time.

Chlorhexidine gluconate, however, binds not only to protein of the skin, but also to many fabrics, particularly cotton. Thus, special laundering procedures should be considered when such products contact these fabrics. As a result of such contact, chlorhexidine gluconate may become adsorbed onto the fabric and not be removed by washing. If sufficient available chlorine is present during the washing procedure, a fast brown stain may develop due to a chemical reaction between chlorhexidine gluconate and chlorine.

SUGGESTED LAUNDERING PROCEDURES TO LIMIT STAINING

1. **Not Aging.** Avoid allowing the product to age (set) on unwashed linens.
2. **Flushing and Washing.** A flush operation as the initial step in the wash process is helpful in the laundering of linen exposed to chlorhexidine gluconate. Such flushing is also important in the laundering of linen which contains organic materials such as blood or pus. For best results, warm water flushes (90°–100°F) are recommended. After a number of initial flushings followed by a washing with a low alkaline/nonchlorine detergent, most articles which come in contact with chlorhexidine gluconate should have an acceptable level of whiteness. If a rewash process using bleach is necessary to achieve a greater degree of whiteness, the bleach used should be a nonchlorine bleach.
3. **Not Using Chlorine Bleach.** Modern laundering methods often make the use of chlorine bleach unnecessary. It is worthwhile trying to wash without chlorine to ascertain if the resulting degree of whiteness is acceptable. Omission of chlorine from the laundering process can extend the useful life of cotton articles since oxidizing bleaches such as chlorine may cause some damage to cellulose even when used in low concentration.
4. **Changing to a Peroxide-Type Bleach, Such as Sodium Perborate, Sodium Percarbonate or Hydrogen Peroxide.** This should eliminate the reaction which could occur with the use of chlorine bleaches. If a chlorine bleach must be used, a concentration of less than 7 ppm available chlorine ($^{1}/_{10}$ the normal bleach level) is suggested to minimize possible staining.

A NOTE ON LAUNDERING OF PERSONAL CLOTHING

The laundering procedures set forth above using low alkaline, nonchlorinated laundry detergents are also applicable to laundering of uniforms and lab coats. Commercially available laundry detergents which do not contain chlorine include Borax, Borateem, Dreft, Oxydol, and Ivory Snow. These products, however, will not remove stains previously set into the fabric.

RECLAMATION OF STAINED LINENS

For those linens which previously have been stained due to the chemical reaction between chlorhexidine gluconate and chlorine, the following laundering procedure may be helpful in reducing the visible stain:
[See table at left]

Operation	Water Level	Temperature	Time (Min)	Supplies/ 100 lb
Break	Low	180°F	20	1.5 lb oxalic acid
Flush	High	Cold	1	—
Emulsify	Low	160°F	5	18 oz emulsifier
Flush	High	Cold	1	—
Bleach	Low	180°F	20	2 lb alkali builder and 1 lb organic bleach
Rinse	High	Cold	1	—
Antichlor	High	Cold	2	4 oz antichlor
Rinse	High	Cold	1	—
Rinse	High	Cold	1	—
Sour	Low	Cold	4	2 oz rust removing sour

HOW SUPPLIED

For general handwashing locations: pocket-size, 15 mL foil Packettes; plastic disposable bottles of 4 oz and 8 oz with dispenser caps; and 16 oz filled globes. *For surgical scrub areas:* disposable, unit-of-use 22 mL impregnated Sponge/Brushes with nail cleaner; plastic disposable bottles of 32 oz and 1 gal. The 32-oz bottle is designed for a special foot-operated wall dispenser. A hand-operated wall dispenser is available for the 16-oz globe. Hand pumps are available for 16 oz, 32 oz, and 1 gal sizes. Liquid: NDC 0310-0575. Sponge/Brush: NDC 0310-0577.

Store at controlled room temperature, 20–25°C (68–77°F) [see USP].

REFERENCES

1. Lowbury, EJL and Lilly, HA: The effect of blood on disinfection of surgeons' hands, Brit. J. Surg. 61:19–21 (Jan.) 1974.
2. Peterson AF, Rosenberg A, Alatary SD: Comparative evaluation of surgical scrub preparations, Surg. Gynecol. Obstet. 146:63–65 (Jan.) 1978.
Zeneca Pharmaceuticals
A Business Unit of Zeneca Inc.
Wilmington, DE 19850-5437 USA
  Shown in Product Identification Guide, page 346

HIBISTAT® Germicidal Hand Rinse   OTC
HIBISTAT® TOWELETTE
Germicidal Handwipe
[hi 'bi-stat]
(chlorhexidine gluconate)

DESCRIPTION

HIBISTAT is a germicidal hand rinse which provides rapid bactericidal action and has a persistent antimicrobial effect against a wide range of microorganisms. HIBISTAT is a clear, colorless liquid containing 0.5% w/w HIBITANE® (chlorhexidine gluconate) with inactive ingredients: emollients, isopropyl alcohol 70%, purified water.

INDICATIONS

HIBISTAT is indicated for health-care personnel use as a germicidal hand rinse. HIBISTAT is for hand hygiene on physically clean hands. It is used in those situations where hands are physically clean, but in need of degerming, when routine handwashing is not convenient or desirable. HIBISTAT provides rapid germicidal action and has a persistent effect.
HIBISTAT should be used in-between patients and procedures where there are no sinks available or continued return to the sink area is inconvenient. HIBISTAT can be used as an alternative to detergent-based products when hands are physically clean. Also, HIBISTAT is an effective germicidal hand rinse following a soap and water handwash.

WARNINGS

Flammable. This product is alcohol based. Alcohol is extremely flammable. It should be kept away from flame or devices which may generate an electrical spark.
FOR EXTERNAL USE ONLY. KEEP OUT OF EYES, EARS AND MOUTH. HIBISTAT SHOULD NOT BE USED AS A PRE-OPERATIVE SKIN PREPARATION OF THE FACE OR HEAD. MISUSE OF CHLORHEXIDINE-CONTAINING PRODUCTS HAS BEEN REPORTED TO CAUSE SERIOUS AND PERMANENT EYE INJURY WHEN IT HAS BEEN PERMITTED TO ENTER AND REMAIN IN THE EYE DURING SURGICAL PROCEDURES. IF HIBISTAT SHOULD CONTACT THESE AREAS, RINSE OUT PROMPTLY AND THOROUGHLY WITH WATER.
Avoid contact with meninges. HIBISTAT should not be used by persons who have a sensitivity to it or its components. Chlorhexidine gluconate has been reported to cause deafness when instilled in the middle ear through perforated ear drums. Irritation, sensitization, and generalized allergic reactions have been reported with chlorhexidine-containing products, especially in the genital areas. If adverse reactions occur, discontinue use immediately and if severe, contact a physician. Keep this and all drugs out of the reach of children. In case of accidental ingestion, seek professional assistance or contact a Poison Control Center immediately. Avoid excessive heat (above 104°F).
Accidental ingestion: Chlorhexidine gluconate taken orally is poorly absorbed. Treat with gastric lavage using milk, egg white, gelatin or mild soap avoiding pulmonary aspiration. Do not use apomorphine. Assist respiration if necessary and keep patient warm. Intravenous levulose can accelerate alcohol metabolism. In severe cases, hemodialysis or peritoneal dialysis may be appropriate.

DIRECTIONS FOR USE

HIBISTAT Towelette: Rub hands vigorously with HIBISTAT Towelette for approximately 15 seconds, paying particular attention to nails and interdigital spaces. HIBISTAT dries rapidly in use. No water or towel drying are necessary. The emollients contained in the HIBISTAT Towelette protect the hands from the potential drying effect of alcohol.
HIBISTAT Liquid: Dispense about 5 mL of HIBISTAT into cupped hands and rub vigorously until dry (about 15 seconds), paying particular attention to nails and interdigital spaces. HIBISTAT dries rapidly in use. No water or toweling are necessary. The emollients contained in HIBISTAT protect the hands from the potential drying effect of alcohol.

LAUNDERING

Chlorhexidine gluconate chemically reacts with chlorine to form a brown stain on fabric. Fabric which has come in contact with chlorhexidine gluconate should be rinsed well and washed without the addition of chlorine products. If bleach is desired, only nonchlorine bleach should be used. Full laundering instructions are packed with each case of HIBISTAT. (Please see HIBICLENS® for full laundering instructions.)

HOW SUPPLIED

In plastic disposable bottles of 4 oz and 8 oz with flip-top cap, and in disposable towelettes containing 5 mL, packaged 50 towelettes to a carton.
NDC 0310-0585 (bottles)
NDC 0310-0587 (towelettes)
Manufactured For:
Zeneca Pharmaceuticals
A Business Unit of Zeneca Inc.
Wilmington, DE 19850-5437 USA
by ACCUPAC, Inc
  Shown in Product Identification Guide, page 346

MERREM® I.V.   ℞
(meropenem for injection)
For Intravenous Use Only

DESCRIPTION

MERREM® I.V. (meropenem for injection) is a sterile, pyrogen-free, synthetic, broad-spectrum, carbapenem antibiotic for intravenous administration. It is (4R,5S,6S)-3-[[(3S,5S)-5-(Dimethylcarbamoyl)- 3-pyrrolidinyl]thio]-6-[(1R)-1-hydroxyethyl]-4-methyl-7-oxo-1-azabicyclo[3.2.0]hept-2-ene-2-carboxylic acid trihydrate. Its empirical formula is $C_{17}H_{25}N_3O_5S \cdot 3H_2O$ with a molecular weight of 437.52. Its structural formula is:

MERREM I.V. is a white to pale yellow crystalline powder. The solution varies from colorless to yellow depending on the concentration. The pH of freshly constituted solutions is between 7.3 and 8.3. Meropenem is soluble in 5% monobasic potassium phosphate solution, sparingly soluble in water, very slightly soluble in hydrated ethanol, and practically insoluble in acetone or ether.
When constituted as instructed (See **DOSAGE AND ADMINISTRATION; PREPARATION OF SOLUTION**), each 1 g MERREM I.V. vial will deliver 1 g of meropenem and 90.2 mg of sodium as sodium carbonate (3.92 mEq). Each 500 mg MERREM I.V. vial will deliver 500 mg meropenem and 45.1 mg of sodium as sodium carbonate (1.96 mEq).
MERREM I.V. in the ADD-Vantage† vial is intended for intravenous use only after dilution with the appropriate volume of diluent solution in the Abbott ADD-Vantage® diluent container (See **DOSAGE AND ADMINISTRATION-PREPARATION OF SOLUTION**). MERREM I.V. in the ADD-Vantage vial is available in two strengths. Each 1 g ADD-Vantage vial of MERREM I.V. will deliver 90.2 mg of sodium as sodium carbonate (3.92 mEq), and each 500 mg ADD-Vantage vial will deliver 45.1 mg of sodium as sodium carbonate (1.96 mEq).

CLINICAL PHARMACOLOGY

At the end of a 30-minute intravenous infusion of a single dose of MERREM I.V. in normal volunteers, mean peak plasma concentrations are approximately 23 µg/mL (range 14–26) for the 500 mg dose and 49 µg/mL (range 39–58) for the 1 g dose. A 5-minute intravenous bolus injection of MERREM I.V. in normal volunteers results in mean peak plasma concentrations of approximately 45 µg/mL (range 18–65) for the 500 mg dose and 112 µg/mL (range 83–140) for the 1 g dose.
Following intravenous doses of 500 mg, mean plasma concentrations of meropenem usually decline to approximately 1 µg/mL at 6 hours after administration.
In subjects with normal renal function, the elimination half-life of MERREM I.V. is approximately 1 hour. Approximately 70% of the intravenously administered dose is recovered as unchanged meropenem in the urine over 12 hours, after which little further urinary excretion is detectable. Urinary concentrations of meropenem in excess of 10 µg/mL are maintained for up to 5 hours after a 500 mg dose. No accumulation of meropenem in plasma or urine was observed with regimens using 500 mg administered every 8 hours or 1 g administered every 6 hours in volunteers with normal renal function.
Plasma protein binding of meropenem is approximately 2%. There is one metabolite which is microbiologically inactive. Meropenem penetrates well into most body fluids and tissues including cerebrospinal fluid, achieving concentrations matching or exceeding those required to inhibit most susceptible bacteria. After a single intravenous dose of MERREM I.V., the highest mean concentrations of meropenem were found in tissues and fluids at 1 hour (0.5 to 1.5 hours) after the start of infusion, except where indicated in the tissues and fluids listed in the table below.
[See table below]

The pharmacokinetics of MERREM I.V. in pediatric patients 2 years of age or older are essentially similar to those in adults. The elimination half-life for meropenem was approximately 1.5 hours in pediatric patients of age 3 months to 2 years. The pharmacokinetics are linear over the dose range from 10 to 40 mg/kg.
Pharmacokinetic studies with MERREM I.V. in patients with renal insufficiency have shown that the plasma clearance of meropenem correlates with creatinine clearance. Dosage adjustments are necessary in subjects with renal impairment. (See **DOSAGE AND ADMINISTRATION-Use in Adults with Renal Impairment.**) A pharmacokinetic study with MERREM I.V. in elderly patients with renal insufficiency has shown a reduction in plasma clearance of meropenem that correlates with age-associated reduction in creatinine clearance.
Meropenem I.V. is hemodialyzable. However, there is no information on the usefulness of hemodialysis to treat overdosage. (See **OVERDOSAGE**.)
A pharmacokinetic study with MERREM I.V. in patients with hepatic impairment has shown no effects of liver disease on the pharmacokinetics of meropenem.

MICROBIOLOGY

The bactericidal activity of meropenem results from the inhibition of cell wall synthesis. Meropenem readily pen-

Continued on next page

Meropenem Concentrations in Selected Tissues (Highest Concentrations Reported)

Tissue	I.V. Dose (g)	Number of Samples	Mean [µg/mL or µg/(g)]***	Range [µg/mL or µg/(g)]
Endometrium	0.5	7	4.2	1.7–10.2
Myometrium	0.5	15	3.8	0.4–8.1
Ovary	0.5	8	2.8	0.8–4.8
Cervix	0.5	2	7.0	5.4–8.5
Fallopian tube	0.5	9	1.7	0.3–3.4
Skin	0.5	22	5.3	0.5–12.6
Skin	1.0	10	5.3	1.3–16.7
Colon	1.0	2	2.6	2.5–2.7
Bile	1.0	7	14.6 (3 h)	4.0–25.7
Gallbladder	1.0	1	—	3.9
Interstitial fluid	1.0	5	26.3	20.9–37.4
Peritoneal fluid	1.0	9	30.2	7.4–54.6
Lung	1.0	2	4.8 (2 h)	1.4–8.2
Bronchial mucosa	1.0	7	4.5	1.3–11.1
Muscle	1.0	2	6.1 (2 h)	5.3–6.9
Fascia	1.0	9	8.8	1.5–20
Heart valves	1.0	7	9.7	6.4–12.1
Myocardium	1.0	10	15.5	5.2–25.5
CSF (inflamed)	20 mg/kg*	8	1.1 (2 h)	0.2–2.8
	40 mg/kg**	5	3.3 (3 h)	0.9–6.5
CSF (uninflamed)	1.0	4	0.2 (1 h)	0.1–0.3

* in pediatric patients of age 5 months to 8 years
** in pediatric patients of age 1 month to 15 years
*** at 1 hour unless otherwise noted

Merrem—Cont.

etrates the cell wall of most gram-positive and gram-negative bacteria to reach penicillin-binding-protein (PBP) targets. Its strongest affinities are toward PBPs 2, 3 and 4 of *Escherichia coli* and *Pseudomonas aeruginosa*; and PBPs 1, 2 and 4 of *Staphylococcus aureus*. Bactericidal concentrations (defined as a 3 $\log_{10}$ reduction in cell counts within 12 to 24 hours) are typically 1–2 times the bacteriostatic concentrations of meropenem, with the exception of *Listeria monocytogenes*, against which lethal activity is not observed.

Meropenem has significant stability to hydrolysis by β-lactamases of most categories, both penicillinases and cephalosporinases produced by gram-positive and gram-negative bacteria, with the exception of metallo-β-lactamases. Meropenem should not be used to treat methicillin-resistant staphylococci. Cross-resistance is sometimes observed with strains resistant to other carbapenems.

In vitro tests show meropenem to act synergistically with aminoglycoside antibiotics against some isolates of *Pseudomonas aeruginosa*.

Meropenem has been shown to be active against most strains of the following microorganisms, both *in vitro* and in clinical infections as described in the **INDICATIONS AND USAGE** section.

Gram-Positive Aerobes
Streptococcus pneumoniae (excluding penicillin-resistant strains)
Viridans group streptococci
NOTE: Penicillin-resistant strains had meropenem MIC90 values of 1 or 2 μg/mL, which is above the 0.12 μg/mL susceptible breakpoint for this species.

Gram-Negative Aerobes
Escherichia coli
Haemophilus influenzae (β-lactamase and non-β-lactamase-producing)
Klebsiella pneumoniae
Neisseria meningitidis
Pseudomonas aeruginosa

Anaerobes
Bacteroides fragilis
Bacteroides thetaiotaomicron
Peptostreptococcus species

The following *in vitro* data are available, **but their clinical significance is unknown.**

Meropenem exhibits *in vitro* minimum inhibitory concentrations (MICs) of 0.12 μg/mL against most (≥ 90%) strains of *Streptococcus pneumoniae*, 0.5 μg/mL or less against most (≥ 90%) strains of *Haemophilus influenzae*, and 4 μg/mL or less against most (≥ 90%) strains of the other microorganisms in the following list; however, the safety and effectiveness of meropenem in treating clinical infections due to these microorganisms have not been established in adequate and well-controlled clinical trials.

Gram-Positive Aerobes
Staphylococcus aureus (β-lactamase and non β-lactamase producing)
Staphylococcus epidermidis (β-lactamase and non β-lactamase-producing)
NOTE: Staphylococci which are resistant to methicillin/oxacillin must be considered resistant to meropenem.

Gram-Negative Aerobes
Acinetobacter species
Aeromonas hydrophila
Campylobacter jejuni
Citrobacter diversus
Citrobacter freundii
Enterobacter cloacae
Haemophilus influenzae (ampicillin-resistant, non-β-lactamase producing strains [BLNAR strains])
Hafnia alvei
Klebsiella oxytoca
Moraxella catarrhalis (β-lactamase and non-β-lactamase-producing strains)
Morganella morganii
Pasteurella multocida
Proteus mirabilis
Proteus vulgaris
Salmonella species
Serratia marcescens
Shigella species
Yersinia enterocolitica

Anaerobes
Bacteroides distasonis
Bacteroides ovatus
Bacteroides uniformis
Bacteroides ureolyticus
Bacteroides vulgatus
Clostridium difficile
Clostridium perfringens
Eubacterium lentum
Fusobacterium species
Prevotella bivia
Prevotella intermedia
Prevotella melaninogenica
Porphyromonas asaccharolytica
Propionibacterium acnes

SUSCEPTIBILITY TESTS

Dilution Techniques:
Quantitative methods are used to determine antimicrobial minimal inhibitory concentrations (MICs). These MICs provide estimates of the susceptibility of bacteria to antimicrobial compounds. The MIC's should be determined using a standardized procedure. Standardized procedures are based on a dilution method[1] (broth or agar) or equivalent with standardized inoculum concentrations and standardized concentrations of meropenem powder. The MIC values should be interpreted according to the following criteria for indicated aerobic organisms other than *Haemophilus* species and streptococci:

MIC (μg/mL)	Interpretation
≤ 4	(S) Susceptible
8	(I) Intermediate
≥ 16	(R) Resistant

Haemophilus Test Media (HTM) and the following interpretive criteria should be used when testing *Haemophilus* species:

MIC (μg/mL)	Interpretation
≤ 0.5	(S) Susceptible

The current absence of resistant strains precludes defining any categories other than "Susceptible". Strains yielding results suggestive of a "Nonsusceptible" category should be submitted to a reference laboratory for further testing.
The following criteria should be used when testing streptococci and *Streptococcus pneumoniae*.
When testing *S. pneumoniae*:

MIC (μg/mL)	Interpretation
≤ 0.12	(S) Susceptible

When testing viridans group streptococci:

MIC (μg/mL)	Interpretation
≤ 0.5	(S) Susceptible

The current absence of resistant strains precludes defining any categories other than "Susceptible". Strains yielding results suggestive of a "Nonsusceptible" category should be submitted to a reference laboratory for further testing.
A report of 'Susceptible' indicates that the pathogen is likely to be inhibited if the antimicrobial compound in the blood reaches the concentrations usually achievable. A report of 'Intermediate' indicates that the result should be considered equivocal, and, if the microorganism is not fully susceptible to alternative, clinically feasible drugs, the test should be repeated. This category implies possible clinical applicability in body sites where the drug is physiologically concentrated or in situations where high dosage of drug can be used. This category also provides a buffer zone which prevents small uncontrolled technical factors from causing major discrepancies in interpretation. A report of 'Resistant' indicates that the pathogen is not likely to be inhibited if the antimicrobial compound in the blood reaches the concentrations usually achievable; other therapy should be selected. Standardized susceptibility test procedures require the use of laboratory control microorganisms to control the technical aspects of the laboratory procedures. Standard meropenem powder should provide the following MIC values:

Microorganism	ATCC	MIC (μg/mL)
Enterococcus faecalis	29212	2.0–8.0
Escherichia coli	25922	0.008–0.06
Haemophilus influenzae	49247	0.06–0.25
Pseudomonas aeruginosa	27853	0.25–1.0
Streptococcus pneumoniae	49619	0.06–0.25

Diffusion Techniques:
Quantitative methods that require measurement of zone diameters also provide reproducible estimates of the susceptibility of bacteria to antimicrobial compounds. One such standardized procedure[2] requires the use of standardized inoculum concentrations. This procedure uses paper disks impregnated with 10-μg of meropenem to test the susceptibility of microorganisms to meropenem.
Reports from the laboratory providing results of the standard single-disk susceptibility test with a 10-μg disk should be interpreted according to the following criteria for indicated aerobic organisms other than *Haemophilus* species and streptococci:

Zone Diameter (mm)	Interpretation
≥ 16	(S) Susceptible
14–15	(I) Intermediate
≤ 13	(R) Resistant

Haemophilus Test Media and the following criteria should be used when testing *Haemophilus* species:

Zone Diameter (mm)	Interpretation
≥ 20	(S) Susceptible

The current absence of resistant strains precludes defining any categories other than "Susceptible". Strains yielding results suggestive of a "Nonsusceptible" category should be submitted to a reference laboratory for further testing.

Streptococcus pneumoniae isolates should be tested using 1 μg/mL oxacillin disk. Isolates with oxacillin zone sizes of ≥ 20 mm are susceptible (MIC ≤ 0.06 μg/mL) to penicillin and can be considered susceptible to meropenem for approved indications, and meropenem need not be tested. A meropenem MIC should be determined on isolates of *S. pneumoniae* with oxacillin zone sizes of ≤ 19 mm. The disk test does not distinguish penicillin intermediate strains (i.e., MICs = 0.12–1.0 μg/mL) from strains that are penicillin resistant (i.e., MICs ≥ 2 μg/mL). Viridans group streptococci should be tested for meropenem susceptibility using an MIC method. Reliable disk diffusion tests for meropenem do not yet exist for testing streptococci.
Interpretation should be as stated above for results using dilution techniques. Interpretation involves correlation of the diameter obtained in the disk test with the MIC for meropenem.
As with standardized dilution techniques, diffusion methods require the use of laboratory control microorganisms that are used to control the technical aspects of the laboratory procedures. For the diffusion technique, the 10-μg meropenem disk should provide the following zone diameters in these laboratory test quality control strains:

Microorganism	ATCC	Zone Diameter (mm)
Escherichia coli	25922	28–34
Haemophilus influenzae	49247	20–28
Pseudomonas aeruginosa	27853	27–33

Anaerobic Techniques:
for anaerobic bacteria, susceptibility to meropenem as MICs can be determined by standardized test methods.[3] The MIC values obtained should be interpreted according to the following criteria:

MIC (μg/mL)	Interpretation
≤ 4	(S) Susceptible
8	(I) Intermediate
≥ 16	(R) Resistant

Interpretation is identical to that stated above for results using dilution techniques.
As with other susceptibility techniques, the use of laboratory control microorganisms is required to control the technical aspects of the laboratory standardized procedures. Standardized meropenem powder should provide the following MIC values:

Microorganism	ATCC	MIC (μg/mL)
Bacteroides fragilis	25285	0.06–0.25
Bacteroides thetaiotaomicron	29741	0.125–0.5

INDICATIONS AND USAGE

MERREM I.V. is indicated as single agent therapy for the treatment of the following infections when caused by susceptible strains of the designated microorganisms:

Intra-abdominal Infections
Complicated appendicitis and peritonitis caused by viridans group streptococci, *Escherichia coli*, *Klebsiella pneumoniae*, *Pseudomonas aeruginosa*, *Bacteroides fragilis*, *B. thetaiotaomicron*, and *Peptostreptococcus* species.

Bacterial Meningitis (pediatric patients ≥ 3 months only)
Bacterial meningitis caused by *Streptococcus pneumoniae*‡, *Haemophilus influenzae* (β-lactamase and non-β-lactamase-producing strains), and *Neisseria meningitidis*.
‡Penicillin-resistant strains have not been studied in clinical trials.

MERREM I.V. has been found to be effective in eliminating concurrent bacteremia in association with bacteria meningitis.
For information regarding use in pediatric patients (3 months of age and older) See **PRECAUTIONS - Pediatrics**, **ADVERSE REACTIONS**, and **DOSAGE AND ADMINISTRATION** sections.
Appropriate cultures should usually be performed before initiating antimicrobial treatment in order to isolate and identify the organisms causing infection and determine their susceptibility to MERREM I.V.
MERREM I.V. is useful as presumptive therapy in the indicated condition (i.e., intra-abdominal infections) prior to the identification of the causative organisms because of its broad spectrum of bactericidal activity.
Antimicrobial therapy should be adjusted, if appropriate, once the results of culture(s) and antimicrobial susceptibility testing are known.

CONTRAINDICATIONS

MERREM I.V. is contraindicated in patients with known hypersensitivity to any component of this product or to other drugs in the same class or in patients who have demonstrated anaphylactic reactions to β-lactams.

WARNINGS

SERIOUS AND OCCASIONALLY FATAL HYPERSENSITIVITY (ANAPHYLACTIC) REACTIONS HAVE BEEN REPORTED IN PATIENTS RECEIVING THERAPY WITH

β-LACTAMS. THESE REACTIONS ARE MORE LIKELY TO OCCUR IN INDIVIDUALS WITH A HISTORY OF SENSITIVITY TO MULTIPLE ALLERGENS.

THERE HAVE BEEN REPORTS OF INDIVIDUALS WITH A HISTORY OF PENICILLIN HYPERSENSITIVITY WHO HAVE EXPERIENCED SEVERE HYPERSENSITIVITY REACTIONS WHEN TREATED WITH ANOTHER β-LACTAM. BEFORE INITIATING THERAPY WITH MERREM I.V., CAREFUL INQUIRY SHOULD BE MADE CONCERNING PREVIOUS HYPERSENSITIVITY REACTIONS TO PENICILLINS, CEPHALOSPORINS, OTHER β-LACTAMS, AND OTHER ALLERGENS. IF AN ALLERGIC REACTION TO MERREM I.V. OCCURS, DISCONTINUE THE DRUG IMMEDIATELY. **SERIOUS ANAPHYLACTIC REACTIONS REQUIRE IMMEDIATE EMERGENCY TREATMENT WITH EPINEPHRINE, OXYGEN, INTRAVENOUS STEROIDS, AND AIRWAY MANAGEMENT, INCLUDING INTUBATION. OTHER THERAPY MAY ALSO BE ADMINISTERED AS INDICATED.**

Seizures and other CNS adverse experiences have been reported during treatment with MERREM I.V. (See **PRECAUTIONS** and **ADVERSE REACTIONS**.)

Pseudomembranous colitis has been reported with nearly all antibacterial agents, including meropenem, and may range in severity from mild to life-threatening. Therefore, it is important to consider this diagnosis in patients who present with diarrhea subsequent to the administration of antibacterial agents.

Treatment with antibacterial agents alters the normal flora of the colon and may permit overgrowth of clostridia. Studies indicate that a toxin produced by *Clostridium difficile* is a primary cause of "antibiotic-associated colitis".

After the diagnosis of pseudomembranous colitis has been established, appropriate therapeutic measures should be initiated. Mild cases of pseudomembranous colitis usually respond to drug discontinuation alone. In moderate-to-severe cases, consideration should be given to management with fluids and electrolytes, protein supplementation, and treatment with an antibacterial drug clinically effective against *Clostridium difficile* colitis.

PRECAUTIONS

General: Seizures and other CNS adverse experiences have been reported during treatment with MERREM I.V. These adverse experiences have occurred most commonly in patients with CNS disorders (e.g., brain lesions or history of seizures) or with bacterial meningitis and/or compromised renal function.

During the initial clinical investigations, 2038 immunocompetent adult patients were treated for infections outside the CNS with MERREM I.V. (500 mg or 1000 mg q 8 hours). Overall seizures, whether drug related or not, occurred in 0.5% of the meropenem-treated patients. All meropenem-treated patients with seizures had pre-existing contributing factors. Among these are included prior history of seizures or CNS abnormality and concomitant medications with seizure potential. Dosage adjustment is recommended in patients with advanced age and/or reduced renal function. (See **DOSAGE AND ADMINISTRATION - Use in Adults with Renal Impairment.**)

Close adherence to the recommended dosage regimens is urged, especially in patients with known factors that predispose to convulsive activity. Anticonvulsant therapy should be continued in patients with known seizure disorders. If focal tremors, myoclonus, or seizures occur, patients should be evaluated neurologically, placed on anticonvulsant therapy if not already instituted, and the dosage of MERREM I.V. re-examined to determine whether it should be decreased or the antibiotic discontinued.

In patients with renal dysfunction, thrombocytopenia has been observed but no clinical bleeding reported. (See **DOSAGE AND ADMINISTRATION - Use in Adults with Renal Impairment.**)

There is inadequate information regarding the use of MERREM I.V. in patients on hemodialysis.

As with other broad-spectrum antibiotics, prolonged use of meropenem may result in overgrowth of nonsusceptible organisms. Repeated evaluation of the patient is essential. If superinfection does occur during therapy, appropriate measures should be taken.

Laboratory Tests: While MERREM I.V. possesses the characteristic low toxicity of the beta-lactam group of antibiotics, periodic assessment of organ system functions, including renal, hepatic, and hematopoietic, is advisable during prolonged therapy.

Drug Interactions: Probenecid competes with meropenem for active tubular secretion and thus inhibits the renal excretion of meropenem. This led to statistically significant increases in the elimination half-life (38%) and in the extent of systemic exposure (56%). Therefore, the coadministration of probenecid with meropenem is not recommended.

Other than probenecid, no specific drug interaction studies were conducted.

Carcinogenesis, Mutagenesis, Impairment of Fertility:

Carcinogenesis: Carcinogenesis studies have not been performed.

Mutagenesis: Genetic toxicity studies were performed with meropenem using the bacterial reverse mutation test, the Chinese hamster ovary HGPRT assay, cultured human lymphocytes cytogenic assay, and the mouse micronucleus test. There was no evidence of mutagenic potential found in any of these tests.

Impairment of fertility: Reproductive studies were performed with meropenem in rats at doses up to 1000 mg/kg/day, and cynomolgus monkeys at doses up to 360 mg/kg/day (on the basis of AUC comparisons, approximately 1.8 times and 3.7 times, respectively, to the human exposure at the usual dose of 1 g every 8 hours). There was no reproductive toxicity seen.

Pregnancy Category B: Reproductive studies have been performed with meropenem in rats at doses of up to 1000 mg/kg/day, and cynomolgus monkeys at doses of up to 360 mg/kg/day (on the basis of AUC comparisons, approximately 1.8 times and 3.7 times respectively, to the human exposure at the usual dose of 1 g every 8 hours). These studies revealed no evidence of impaired fertility or harm to the fetus due to meropenem, although there were slight changes in fetal body weight at doses of 250 mg/kg/day (on the basis of AUC comparisons, 0.4 times the human exposure at a dose of 1 g every 8 hours) and above in rats. There are, however, no adequate and well-controlled studies in pregnant women. Because animal reproduction studies are not always predictive of human response, this drug should be used during pregnancy only if clearly needed.

Pediatrics: The safety and effectiveness of MERREM I.V. have been established for pediatric patients ≥ 3 months of age. Use of MERREM I.V. in pediatric patients with bacterial meningitis is supported by evidence from adequate and well-controlled studies in the pediatric population. Use of MERREM I.V. in pediatric patients with intra-abdominal infections is supported by evidence from adequate and well-controlled studies with adults with additional data from pediatric pharmacokinetics studies and controlled clinical trials in pediatric patients. (See **CLINICAL PHARMACOLOGY, INDICATIONS AND USAGE, ADVERSE REACTIONS, DOSAGE AND ADMINISTRATION,** and **CLINICAL STUDIES** sections.)

Nursing Mothers: It is not known whether this drug is excreted in human milk. Because many drugs are excreted in human milk, caution should be exercised when MERREM I.V. is administered to a nursing woman.

ADVERSE REACTIONS

Adult Patients:

During the initial clinical investigations, 2038 immunocompetent adult patients were treated for infections outside the CNS with MERREM I.V. (500 mg or 1000 mg q 8 hours). Deaths in 3 patients were assessed as possibly related to meropenem; 28 (1.4%) patients had meropenem discontinued because of adverse events. Many patients in these trials were severely ill and had multiple background diseases, physiological impairments and were receiving multiple other drug therapies. In the seriously ill population, it was not possible to determine the relationship between observed adverse events and therapy with MERREM I.V.

The following adverse reaction frequencies were derived from the clinical trials in the 2038 patients treated with MERREM I.V.

Local Adverse Reactions

Local adverse reactions that were reported irrespective of the relationship to therapy with MERREM I.V. were as follows:

Inflammation at the injection site	3.0%
Phlebitis/thrombophlebitis	1.2%
Injection site reaction	1.1%
Pain at the injection site	0.4%
Edema at the injection site	0.2%

Systemic Adverse Reactions

Systemic adverse clinical reactions that were reported irrespective of the relationship to MERREM I.V. occurring in greater than 1.0% of the patients with diarrhea (5.0%), nausea/vomiting (3.9%), headache (2.8%), rash (1.7%), pruritus (1.6%), apnea (1.2%), and constipation (1.2%).

Additional adverse systemic clinical reactions that were reported irrespective of relationship to therapy with MERREM I.V. and occurring in less than 1.0% but greater than 0.1% of the patients are listed below within each body system in order of decreasing frequency:

Bleeding events [gastrointestinal hemorrhage, melena, epistaxis, and hemoperitoneum] occurred in 0.7% of meropenem patients.

Body as a Whole: pain, abdominal pain, chest pain, sepsis, shock, fever, abdominal enlargement, back pain, hepatic failure

Cardiovascular: heart failure, heart arrest, tachycardia, hypertension, myocardial infarction, pulmonary embolus, bradycardia, hypotension, syncope

Digestive: oral moniliasis, anorexia, cholestatic jaundice/jaundice, flatulence, ileus

Hemic/lymphatic: anemia

Metabolic/nutritional: peripheral edema, hypoxia

Nervous system: insomnia, agitation/delirium, confusion, dizziness, seizure (See **PRECAUTIONS**), nervousness, paresthesia, hallucinations, somnolence, anxiety, depression

Respiratory: respiratory disorder, dyspnea

Skin and Appendages: urticaria, sweating

Urogenital system: dysuria, kidney failure

Adverse Laboratory Changes

Adverse laboratory changes that were reported irrespective of relationship to MERREM I.V. occurring in greater than 0.2% of the patients were as follows:

Hepatic: increased SGPT (ALT), SGOT (AST), alkaline phosphatase, LDH, and bilirubin

Hematologic: increased platelets, increased eosinophils, prolonged prothrombin time, prolonged partial thromboplastin time, decreased platelets, positive direct or indirect Coombs test, decreased hemoglobin, decreased hematocrit, decreased WBC, shortened prothrombin time and shortened partial thromboplastin time.

Renal: increased creatinine and increased BUN

NOTE: It is not known if the safety profile of MERREM I.V. is changed in patients with varying degrees of renal impairment.

Urinalysis: presence of urine red blood cells

Pediatric Patients:

Clinical Adverse Reactions

MERREM I.V. was studied in 417 pediatric patients (≥ 3 months to <13 years of age) with serious bacterial infections at dosages of 10 to 20 mg/kg every 8 hours. The types of clinical adverse events seen in these patients are similar to the adults, with the most common adverse events reported as possibly, probably or definitely related to MERREM I.V. and their rates of occurrence as follows:

Diarrhea	4.3%
Rash	1.4%
Vomiting	1.0%

MERREM I.V. was studied in 198 pediatric patients (≥ 3 months to <17 years of age) with meningitis at a dosage of 40 mg/kg every 8 hours. The types of clinical adverse events seen in these patients are similar to the adults, with the most common adverse events reported as possibly, probably, or definitely related to MERREM I.V. and their rates of occurrence as follows:

Rash (mostly diaper area moniliasis)	3.5%
Diarrhea	3.5%
Oral Moniliasis	2.0%
Glossitis	1.0%

In the meningitis studies the rates of seizure activity during therapy were comparable between patients with no CNS abnormalities who received meropenem and those who received comparator agents (either cefotaxime or ceftriaxone). In the MERREM I.V. treated group, 12/15 patients with seizures had late onset seizures (defined as occurring on day 3 or later) versus 7/20 in the comparator arm.

Adverse Laboratory Changes:

Laboratory abnormalities seen in the pediatric-aged patients in both the pediatric and the meningitis studies are similar to those reported in adult patients.

There is no experience in pediatric patients with renal impairment.

Post-marketing Experience:

No post-marketing experience is available.

OVERDOSAGE

In mice and rats, large intravenous doses of meropenem (2200-4000 mg/kg) have been associated with ataxia, dyspnea, convulsions, and mortalities.

Intentional overdosing of MERREM I.V. is unlikely, although accidental overdosing might occur if large doses are given to patients with reduced renal function. The largest dose of meropenem administered in clinical trials has been 2 g given intravenously every 8 hours. At this dosage, no adverse pharmacological effects or increased safety risks have been observed.

No specific information is available for the treatment of MERREM I.V. overdosage. In the event of an overdose, MERREM I.V. should be discontinued and general supportive treatment given until renal elimination takes place. Meropenem and its metabolite are readily dialyzable and effectively removed by hemodialysis; however, no information is available on the use of hemodialysis to treat overdosage.

CLINICAL STUDIES

Intra-abdominal:

One controlled clinical study of complicated intra-abdominal infection was performed in the United States where meropenem was compared to clindamycin/tobramycin. Three controlled clinical studies of complicated intra-abdominal infections were performed in Europe; meropenem was compared to imipenem (two trials) and cefotaxime/metronidazole (one trial).

Using strict evaluability criteria and microbiologic eradication and clinical cures at follow-up which occurred 7 or more

Continued on next page

Merrem—Cont.

days after completion of therapy, the following presumptive microbiologic eradication/clinical cure rates and statistical findings were obtained:
[See table at bottom of page]

The finding that meropenem was not statistically equivalent of cefotaxim/metronidazole may have been due to uneven assignment of more seriously ill patients to the meropenem arm. Currently there is no additional information available to further interpret this observation.

Bacterial Meningitis:

Four hundred forty-six patients (397 pediatric patients ≥ 3 months to < 17 years of age) were enrolled in 4 separate clinical trials and randomized to treatment with meropenem (n=225) at a dose of 40 mg/kg q 8 hours or a comparator drug, i.e., cefotaxime (n=187) or ceftriaxone (n=34) at the approved dosing regimens. A comparable number of patients were found to be clinically evaluable (ranging from 61–68%) and with a similar distribution of pathogens isolated on initial CSF culture.

Patients were defined as clinically not cured if any one of the following three criteria were met:

1. At the 5–7 week post-completion of therapy visit, the patient had any one of the following: moderate to severe motor, behavior or development deficits, hearing loss of >60 decibels in one or both ears, or blindness.
2. During therapy the patient's clinical status necessitated the addition of other antibiotics.
3. Either during or post-therapy, the patient developed a large subdural effusion needing surgical drainage, or a cerebral abscess, or a bacteriologic relapse.

Using the definition, the following efficacy rates were obtained, per organism. The values represent the number of patients clinically cured/number of clinically evaluable patients, with the percent cure in parentheses.

MICROORGANISM	MERREM I.V.	COMPARATOR
S. pneumoniae	17/24 (71)	19/30 (63)
H. influenzae (+)	8/10 (80)	6/6 (100)
H. influenzae (-/NT)	44/59 (75)	44/60 (73)
N. meningitidis	30/35 (86)	35/39 (90)
TOTAL (including others)	102/131 (78)	108/140 (77)

(+) β-lactamase-producing; (-/NT) non-β-lactamase-producing or not tested

Sequelae were the most common reason patients were assessed as clinically not cured.

Five patients were found to be bacteriologically not cured, 3 in the comparator group (1 relapse and 2 patients with cerebral abscesses) and 2 in the meropenem group (1 relapse and 1 with continued growth of Pseudomonas aeruginosa). The adverse events seen were comparable between the two treatment groups both in type and frequency. The meropenem group did have a statistically higher number of patients with transient elevation of liver enzymes. (See **ADVERSE REACTIONS**.) Rates of seizure activity during therapy were comparable between patients with no CNS abnormalities who received meropenem and those who received comparator agents. In the MERREM I.V. treated group, 12/15 patients with seizures had late onset seizures (defined as occurring on day 3 or later) versus 7/20 in the comparator arm.

With respect to hearing loss, 263 of the 271 evaluable patients had at least one hearing test performed post-therapy. The following table shows the degree of hearing loss between the meropenem-treated patients and the comparator-treated patients.

Degree of Hearing Loss (in one or both ears)	Meropenem n=128	Comparator n=135
No loss	61%	56%
20–40 decibels	20%	24%
>40–60 decibels	8%	7%
>60 decibels	9%	10%

DOSAGE AND ADMINISTRATION

Adults: One gram (1 g) by intravenous administration every 8 hours. MERREM I.V. should be given by intravenous infusion, over approximately 15 to 30 minutes or as an intravenous bolus injection (5 to 20 mL) over approximately 3–5 minutes.

Use in Adults with Renal Impairment: Dosage should be reduced in patients with creatinine clearance less than 51 mL/min. (See dosing table below).

Recommended MERREM I.V. Dosage Schedule for Adults With Impaired Renal Function

Creatinine Clearance (mL/min)	Dose (dependent on type of infection)	Dosing Interval
26–50	recommended dose (1000 mg)	every 12 hours
10–25	one-half recommended dose	every 12 hours
<10	one-half recommended dose	every 24 hours

When only serum creatinine is available, the following formula (Cockcroft and Gault equation)[4] may be used to estimate creatinine clearance.

Males: Creatinine Clearance (mL/min) =

$$\frac{Weight\ (kg) \times (140 - age)}{72 \times serum\ creatinine\ (mg/dL)}$$

Females: 0.85 × above value

There is inadequate information regarding the use of MERREM I.V. in patients on hemodialysis.

There is no experience with peritoneal dialysis.

Use in Adults With Hepatic Insufficiency: No dosage adjustment is necessary in patients with impaired hepatic function.

Use in Elderly Patients: No dosage adjustment is required for elderly patients with creatinine clearance values above 50 mL/min.

Use in Pediatric Patients: For pediatric patients from 3 months of age and older, the MERREM I.V. dose is 20 or 40 mg/kg every 8 hours (maximum dose is 2 g every 8 hours), depending on the type of infection (intra-abdominal or meningitis). (See Dosing Table Below). Pediatric patients weighing over 50 kg should be administered MERREM I.V. at a dose of 1 g every 8 hours for intra-abdominal infections and 2 g every 8 hours for meningitis. MERREM I.V. should be given as intravenous infusion over approximately 15 to 30 minutes or as an intravenous bolus injection (5 to 20 mL) over approximately 3–5 minutes.

Recommended MERREM I.V. Dosage Schedule for Pediatrics With Normal Renal Function

Type of Infection	Dose (mg/kg)	Dosing Interval
Intra-abdominal	20	every 8 hours
Meningitis	40	every 8 hours

There is no experience in pediatric patients with renal impairment.

PREPARATION OF SOLUTION

For Intravenous Bolus Administration

Constitute injection vials (500 mg/20 mL and 1 g/30 mL) with sterile Water for Injection (See table below.) Shake to dissolve and let stand until clear.

Vial Size	Amount of Diluent Added (mL)	Approximate Withdrawable Volume (mL)	Approximate Average Concentration (mg/mL)
500 mg/20 mL	10	10	50
1 g/30 mL	20	20	50

For Infusion

Infusion vials (500 mg/100 mL and 1 g/100 mL) may be directly constituted with a compatible infusion fluid. (See **COMPATIBILITY AND STABILITY**). Alternatively, an injection vial may be constituted, then the resulting solution added to an I.V. container and further diluted with an appropriate infusion fluid. (See **COMPATIBILITY AND STABILITY**).

NOTE: ADD-VANTAGE VIALS ARE NOT TO BE USED IN THIS MANNER.

For ADD-Vantage Vials

ADD-Vantage vials of MERREM I.V. are to be constituted only with Sodium Chloride Injection 0.45%, Sodium Chloride Injection 0.9% or Dextrose Injection 5% in the 50, 100, and 250 mL Abbott ADD-Vantage® flexible diluent containers. MERREM I.V. supplied in single-use ADD-Vantage vials should be prepared as directed.

DIRECTIONS FOR USE OF MERREM I.V. (meropenem for injection) IN ADD-VANTAGE VIALS:

To Open Diluent Container: Peel overwrap from the corner and remove from container. Some opacity of the plastic due to moisture absorption during the sterilization process may be observed. This is normal and does not affect the solution quality or safety. The opacity will diminish gradually.

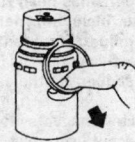

Figure 1

To Assemble ADD-Vantage Vial and Flexible Diluent Container: (Use Aseptic Technique)

1. Remove the protective covers from the top of the vial and the vial port on the diluent container as follows:
   a. To remove the breakaway vial cap, swing the pull ring over the top of the vial and pull down far enough to start the opening (See Figure 1), then pull straight up to remove the cap. (See Figure 2.)
   NOTE: Once the breakaway cap has been removed, do not access vial with syringe.

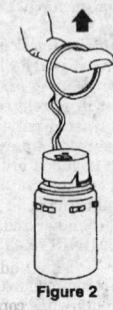

Figure 2

   b. To remove the vial port cover, grasp the tab on the pull ring, pull up to break the three tie strings, then pull back to remove the cover. (See Figure 3.)

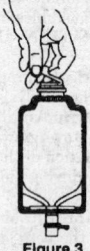

Figure 3

2. Screw the vial into the vial port until it will go no further. THE VIAL MUST BE SCREWED IN TIGHTLY TO ASSURE A SEAL. This occurs approximately $^1/_2$ turn (180°) after the first audible click. (See Figure 4.) The clicking sound does not assure a seal; the vial must be turned as far as it will go.
   NOTE: ONCE VIAL IS SEATED, DO NOT ATTEMPT TO REMOVE.
3. Recheck the vial to assure that it is tight by trying to turn it further in the direction of assembly.
4. Label appropriately.

Treatment Arm	No. evaluable/ No. enrolled (%)	Microbiologic Eradication Rate	Clinical Cure Rate	Outcome
meropenem	146/516 (28%)	98/146 (67%)	101/146 (69%)	
imipenem	65/220 (30%)	40/65 (62%)	42/65 (65%)	Meropenem equivalent to control
cefotaxime/ metronidazole	26/85 (30%)	22/26 (85%)	22/26 (85%)	Meropenem not equivalent to control
clindamycin/ tobramycin	50/212 (24%)	38/50 (76%)	38/50 (76%)	Meropenem equivalent to control

To Prepare Admixture:

1. Squeeze the bottom of the diluent container gently to inflate the portion of the container surrounding the end of the drug vial.

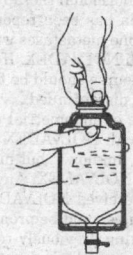

Figure 4

2. With the other hand, push the drug vial down into the container telescoping the walls of the container. Grasp the inner cap of the vial through the walls of the container. (See Figure 5.)

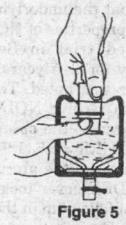

Figure 5

3. Pull the inner cap from the drug vial. (See Figure 6.) Verify that the rubber stopper has been pulled out and invert the system several times, allowing the drug and diluent to mix.

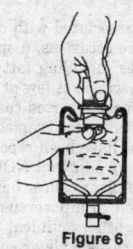

Figure 6

4. Mix contents thoroughly and use within the specified time.

Preparation For Administration: (Use Aseptic Technique)

1. Confirm the activation and admixture of vial contents.
2. Check for leaks by squeezing container firmly. If leaks are found, discard unit as sterility may be impaired.
3. Close flow control clamp of administration set.
4. Remove cover from outlet port at bottom of container.
5. Insert piercing pin of administration set into port with a twisting motion until the pin is firmly seated. **NOTE:** See full directions on administration set carton.
6. Lift the free end of the hanger loop on the bottom of the vial, breaking the two tie strings. Bend the loop outward to lock it in the upright position, then suspend container from hanger.
7. Squeeze and release drip chamber to establish proper fluid level in chamber.
8. Open flow control clamp and clear air from set. Close clamp.
9. Attach set to venipuncture device. If device is not indwelling, prime and make venipuncture.
10. Regulate rate of administration with flow control clamp.

WARNING: Do not use flexible container in series connections.

COMPATIBILITY AND STABILITY

Compatibility of MERREM I.V. with other drugs has not been established. MERREM I.V. should not be mixed with or physically added to solutions containing other drugs. Freshly prepared solutions of MERREM I.V. should be used whenever possible. However, constituted solutions of MERREM I.V. maintain satisfactory potency at controlled room temperature 15–25°C (59–77°F) or under refrigeration at 4°C (39°F) as described below. Solutions of intravenous MERREM I.V. should not be frozen.

Intravenous Bolus Administration

MERREM I.V. injection vials constituted with sterile Water for Injection for bolus administration (up to 50 mg/mL of MERREM I.V.) may be stored for up to 2 hours at controlled room temperature 15–25°C (59–77°F) or for up to 12 hours at 4°C (39°F).

Intravenous Infusion Administration

Stability in Infusion Vials: MERREM I.V. infusion vials constituted with Sodium Chloride Injection 0.9% (MERREM I.V. concentrations ranging from 2.5 to 50 mg/mL) are stable for up to 2 hours at controlled room temperature 15–25°C (55–77°F) or for up to 18 hours at 4°C (39°F). Infusion vials of MERREM I.V. constituted with Dextrose Injection 5% (MERREM I.V. concentrations ranging from 2.5 to 50 mg/mL) are stable for up to 1 hour at controlled room temperature 15–25°C (59–77°F) or for up to 8 hours at 4°C (39°F).

Stability in Plastic I.V. Bags: Solutions prepared for infusion (MERREM I.V. concentrations ranging from 1 to 20 mg/mL) may be stored in plastic intravenous bags with diluents as shown below:

	Number of Hours Stable at Controlled Room Temperature 15–25°C (59–77°F)	Number of Hours Stable at 4°C (39°F)
Sodium Chloride Injection 0.9%	4	24
Dextrose Injection 5.0%	1	4
Dextrose Injection 10.0%	1	2
Dextrose and Sodium Chloride Injection 5.0%/0.9%	1	2
Dextrose and Sodium Chloride Injection 5.0%/0.2%	1	4
Potassium Chloride in Dextrose Injection 0.15%/5.0%	1	6
Sodium Bicarbonate in Dextrose Injection 0.02%/5.0%	1	6
Dextrose Injection 5.0% in Normosol®-M	1	8
Dextrose Injection 5.0% in Ringers Lactate Injection	1	4
Dextrose and Sodium Chloride Injection 2.5%/0.45%	3	12
Mannitol Injection 2.5%	2	16
Ringers Injection	4	24
Ringers Lactate Injection	4	12
Sodium Lactate Injection 1/6 N	2	24
Sodium Bicarbonate Injection 5.0%	1	4

Stability in Baxter Minibag Plus: Solutions of MERREM I.V. (MERREM I.V. concentrations ranging from 2.5 to 20 mg/mL) in Baxter Minibag Plus bags with Sodium Chloride Injection 0.9% may be stored for up to 4 hours at controlled room temperatures 15–25°C (59–77°F) or for up to 24 hours at 4°C (39°F). Solutions of MERREM I.V. (MERREM I.V. concentrations ranging from 2.5 to 20 mg/mL) in Baxter Minibag Plus bags with Dextrose Injection 5.0% may be stored up to 1 hour at controlled room temperatures 15–25°C (59–77°F) or for up to 6 hours at 4°C (39°F).

Stability in Plastic Syringes, Tubing and Intravenous Infusion Sets: Solutions of MERREM I.V. (MERREM I.V. concentrations ranging from 1 to 20 mg/mL) in Water for Injection or Sodium Chloride Injection 0.9% (for up to 4 hours) or in Dextrose Injection 5.0% (for up to 2 hours) at controlled room temperatures 15–25°C (59–77°F) are stable in plastic syringes, plastic tubing, drip chambers, and volume control devices of common intravenous infusion sets.

ADD-Vantage Vials: ADD-Vantage vials diluted in Sodium Chloride Injection 0.45% (MERREM I.V. concentrations ranging from 5 to 20 mg/mL) may be stored for up to 6 hours at controlled room temperature 15–25°C (59–77°F) or for 24 hours at 4°C (39°F). ADD-Vantage vials diluted in Sodium Chloride Injection 0.9% (MERREM I.V. concentrations ranging from 1–20 mg/mL) may be stored for up to 4 hours at controlled room temperature 15–25°C (59–77°F) or for 24 hours at 4°C (39°F). ADD-Vantage vials diluted with Dextrose Injection 5.0% (MERREM I.V. concentrations ranging from 1–20 mg/mL) may be stored for up to 1 hour at controlled room temperature 15–25°C (59–77°F) or for 8 hours at 4°C (39°F).

NOTE: Parenteral drug products should be inspected visually for particulate matter and discoloration prior to administration, whenever solution and container permit.

HOW SUPPLIED

MERREM I.V. is supplied in 20 mL and 30 mL injection vials containing sufficient meropenem to deliver 500 mg or 1 g for intravenous administration, respectively. MERREM I.V. is supplied in 100 mL infusion vials containing sufficient meropenem to deliver 500 mg or 1 g for intravenous administration. The dry powder should be stored at controlled room temperature 20–25°C (68–77°F) [see USP].

MERREM I.V. is also supplied as ADD-Vantage Vials containing sufficient meropenem to deliver 500 mg or 1 g for intravenous administration.

500 mg/20 mL Injection Vial (NDC 0310-0325-20)
500 mg/100 mL Infusion Vial (NDC 0310-0325-11)
1 g/30 mL Injection Vial (NDC 0310-0321-30)
1 g/100 mL Infusion Vial (NDC 0310-0321-11)
500 mg/15 mL ADD-Vantage (NDC 0310-0325-15)
1 g/15 mL ADD-Vantage (NDC 0310-0321-15)

REFERENCES

1. National Committee for Clinical Laboratory Standards. Methods for Dilution Antimicrobial Susceptibility Tests for Bacteria that Grow Aerobically — Third Edition. Approved Standard NCCLS Document M7-A3, Vol. 13, No. 25, NCCLS, Villanova, PA, December, 1993.
2. National Committee for Clinical Laboratory Standards. Performance Standards for Antimicrobial Disk Susceptibility Tests — Fifth Edition. Approved Standard NCCLS Document M2-A5, Vol. 13, No. 24, NCCLS, Villanova, PA. December 1993.
3. National Committee for Clinical Laboratory Standards. Methods for Antimicrobial Susceptibility Testing of Anaerobic Bacteria – Third Edition. Approved Standard NCCLS Document M11-A3, Vol. 13, No. 26, NCCLS, Villanova, PA. December 1993.
4. Cockcroft DW, Gault MH. Prediction of creatinine clearance from serum creatinine. Nephron. 1976; 16.31-41.

†ADD-Vantage is a registered trademark of Abbott Laboratories Inc.

MERREM® (meropenem for injection) is manufactured by:
Sumitomo Pharmaceuticals Co. Ltd
Oita Works
Tsurusaki 2200
Oita-shi
Oita
Japan

Manufactured for:
Zeneca Pharmaceuticals
A business unit of Zeneca Inc.
Wilmington, DE 19850-5437
Rev F 07/96   SIC 64041-00

Shown in Product Identification Guide, page 346

NOLVADEX®   ℞
[nol 'va-dex]
tamoxifen citrate

DESCRIPTION

NOLVADEX® (tamoxifen citrate) Tablets, a nonsteroidal antiestrogen, are for oral administration. NOLVADEX Tablets are available as:

10 mg Tablets. Each tablet contains 15.2 mg of tamoxifen citrate which is equivalent to 10 mg of tamoxifen.

20 mg Tablets. Each tablet contains 30.4 mg of tamoxifen citrate which is equivalent to 20 mg of tamoxifen.

Inactive Ingredients: carboxymethylcellulose calcium, magnesium stearate, mannitol and starch.

Chemically, NOLVADEX is the trans-isomer of a triphenylethylene derivative. The chemical name is (Z)2-[4-(1,2-diphenyl-1-butenyl) phenoxy]-N, N-dimethylethanamine 2-hydroxy-1,2,3-propanetricarboxylate (1:1). The structural and empirical formulas are:

$$(CH_3)_2N(CH_2)_2O\text{—} \cdots C{=}C \cdots C_2H_5 \cdot C_6H_8O_7$$

$$(C_{32}H_{37}NO_8)$$

Tamoxifen citrate has a molecular weight of 563.62, the pKa' is 8.85, the equilibrium solubility in water at 37°C is 0.5 mg/mL and in 0.02 N HCl at 37°C, it is 0.2 mg/mL.

CLINICAL PHARMACOLOGY

NOLVADEX is a nonsteroidal agent which has demonstrated potent antiestrogenic properties in animal test systems. The antiestrogenic effects may be related to its ability to compete with estrogen for binding sites in target tissues such as breast. Tamoxifen inhibits the induction of rat mammary carcinoma induced by dimethylbenzanthracene (DMBA) and causes the regression of already established DMBA-induced tumors. In this rat model, tamoxifen appears to exert its antitumor effects by binding the estrogen receptors.

In cytosols derived from human breast adenocarcinomas, tamoxifen competes with estradiol for estrogen receptor protein.

Continued on next page

Nolvadex—Cont.

Tamoxifen is extensively metabolized after oral administration. Studies in women receiving 20 mg of ^{14}C tamoxifen have shown that approximately 65% of the administered dose was excreted from the body over a period of 2 weeks with fecal excretion as the primary route of elimination. The drug was excreted mainly as polar conjugates, with unchanged drug and unconjugated metabolites accounting for less than 30% of the total fecal radioactivity.
N-desmethyl tamoxifen was the major metabolite found in patients' plasma. The biological activity of N-desmethyl tamoxifen appears to be similar to tamoxifen. 4-Hydroxytamoxifen and a side chain primary alcohol derivative of tamoxifen have been identified as minor metabolities in plasma.
Following a single oral dose of 20 mg tamoxifen, an average peak plasma concentration of 40 ng/mL (range 35 to 45 ng/mL) occurred approximately 5 hours after dosing. The decline in plasma concentrations of tamoxifen is biphasic with a terminal elimination half-life of about 5 to 7 days. The average peak plasma concentration for N-desmethyl tamoxifen is 15 ng/mL (range 10 to 20 ng/mL). Chronic administration of 10 mg tamoxifen given twice daily for three months to patients results in average steady-state plasma concentrations of 120 ng/mL (range 67–183 ng/mL) for tamoxifen and 336 ng/mL (range 148–654 ng/mL) for N-desmethyl tamoxifen. The average steady-state plasma concentrations of tamoxifen and N-desmethyl tamoxifen after administration of 20 mg tamoxifen once daily for three months are 122 ng/mL (range 71–183 ng/mL) and 353 ng/mL (range 152–706 ng/mL), respectively. After initiation of therapy, steady state concentrations for tamoxifen are achieved in about 4 weeks and steady state concentrations for N-desmethyl tamoxifen are achieved in about 8 weeks, suggesting a half-life of approximately 14 days for this metabolite.
In a 3-month crossover steady-state bioavailability study with NOLVADEX 10 mg twice a day versus NOLVADEX 20 mg given once daily, the results deomonstrated that NOLVADEX 20 mg taken once daily has comparable bioavailability to NOLVADEX 10 mg taken twice a day.
Clinical Studies: The Early Breast Cancer Trialists' Collaborative Group (EBCTCG) conducted worldwide overviews of systemic adjuvant therapy for early breast cancer in 1985 and again in 1990. In 1992, 10-year outcome data were reported for 29,892 women in 40 randomized trials of adjuvant tamoxifen using doses of 20–40 mg/day for 1–5+ years (median 2 years). Fifty-one percent were entered into trials comparing tamoxifen to no adjuvant therapy and 49% were entered into trials of tamoxifen in combination with chemotherapy vs. the same chemotherapy alone. Twenty-nine percent were <50 years of age and 71% were ≥50 years. Fifty-seven percent were node-positive and 43% were node-negative. Fifty percent of the tumors were estrogen receptor (ER) positive (≥10 fmol/mg), 18% were ER poor (<10 fmol/mg), and 32% were ER unknown.
The overall recurrence-free survival at 10 years of follow-up was 51.2% for tamoxifen versus 44.7% for control (logrank 2p <0.00001). Overall survival at 10 years was 58.8% for tamoxifen versus 52.6% for control (logrank 2p <0.00001). Both the absolute risk of relapse and the absolute benefit of treatment with tamoxifen were greater in women with positive nodes than in women with negative nodes. In women with positive nodes, 10-year recurrence-free survival was 41.9% for tamoxifen versus 33.1% for control (logrank 1p <0.00001). Ten-year survival was 50.4% for tamoxifen versus 42.2% for control (logrank 1p <0.00001). In women with negative nodes, recurrence-free survival was 68.1% for tamoxifen versus 63.1% for control (logrank 1p <0.00001). Survival at 10 years was 74.5% for tamoxifen versus 71.0% for control (logrank 1p = 0.0002).
The reduction in the annual odds of recurrence with tamoxifen was 12% in women <50 years of age versus 29% in women ≥50 years. Similarly, the reduction in the annual odds of death was 6% versus 20%. The reduction in the annual odds of recurrence with tamoxifen was significantly greater in ER positive (32%) than in ER poor (13%) tumors (1p <0.00001). The reduction in recurrence and mortality was greater in those studies that used tamoxifen for longer (≥2 years) rather than shorter (<2 years) periods. There was no indication that doses greater than 20 mg per day were more effective.
Two studies (Hubay and NSABP B-09) demonstrated an improved disease-free survival following radical or modified radical mastectomy in postmenopausal women or women 50 years of age or older with surgically curable breast cancer with positive axillary nodes when NOLVADEX was added to adjuvant cytotoxic chemotherapy. In the Hubay study, NOLVADEX was added to "low-dose" CMF (cyclophosphamide, methotrexate and fluorouracil). In the NSABP B-09 study, NOLVADEX was added to melphalan [L-phenylalanine mustard (P)] and fluorouracil (F).
In the Hubay study, patients with a positive (more than 3 fmol) estrogen receptor were more likely to benefit. In the NSABP B-09 study in women age 50–59 years, only women with both estrogen and progesterone receptor levels 10 fmol or greater clearly benefited, while there was a nonstatistically significant trend toward adverse effect in women with both estrogen and progesterone receptor levels less than 10 fmol. In women age 60–70 years, there was a trend toward a beneficial effect of NOLVADEX without any clear relationship to estrogen or progesterone receptor status.
Three prospective studies (ECOG-1178, Toronto, NATO) using NOLVADEX adjuvantly as a single agent demonstrated an improved disease-free survival following total mastectomy and axillary dissection for postmenopausal women with positive axillary nodes compared to placebo/no treatment controls. The NATO study also demonstrated an overall survival benefit.
NSABP B-14, a prospective, double-blind, randomized study, evaluated NOLVADEX versus placebo in the treatment of women with axillary node-negative, estrogen-receptor positive (≥ 10 fmol/mg cytosol protein) breast cancer (as adjuvant therapy, following total mastectomy and axillary dissection, or segmental resection, axillary dissection, and breast radiation). After five years of treatment, a significant improvement in disease-free survival was demonstrated in women receiving NOLVADEX. This benefit was apparent both in women under age 50 and in women at or beyond age 50. In this trial women who received tamoxifen for five years and were disease-free at the end of this 5-year period were offered an additional five years of NOLVADEX, or placebo in a double-blind randomized scheme. With four years of follow-up after this rerandomization, 92% of the women that received five years of NOLVADEX followed by placebo are alive and disease-free, compared to 86% of the women scheduled to receive 10 years of NOLVADEX. This difference was not statistically significant. One additional randomized study (NATO) demonstrated improved disease-free survival for NOLVADEX compared to no adjuvant therapy following total mastectomy and axillary dissection in postmenopausal women with axillary node-negative breast cancer. In this study, the benefits of NOLVADEX appeared to be independent of estrogen receptor status.
Three prospective, randomized studies (Ingle, Pritchard, Buchanan) compared NOLVADEX to ovarian ablation (oophorectomy or ovarian irradiation) in premenopausal women with advanced breast cancer. Although the objective response rate, time to treatment failure, and survival were similar with both treatments, the limited patient accrual prevented a demonstration of equivalence. In an overview analysis of survival data from the three studies, the hazard ratio for death (NOLVADEX/ovarian ablation) was 1.00 with two-sided 95% confidence intervals of 0.73 to 1.37. Elevated serum and plasma estrogens have been observed in premenopausal women receiving NOLVADEX. However, the data from the randomized studies do not suggest an adverse effect. A limited number of premenopausal patients with disease progression during NOLVADEX therapy responded to subsequent ovarian ablation.
In a large randomized trial in Sweden of adjuvant NOLVADEX 40 mg/day for 2–5 years, the incidence of second primary breast tumors was reduced in the tamoxifen arm (p<0.05). In the NSABP B-14 trial in which patients were randomized to NOLVADEX 20 mg/day for 5 years versus placebo, the incidence of second primary breast cancers is also reduced.
Published results from 122 patients (119 evaluable) and case reports in 16 patients (13 evaluable) treated with NOLVADEX have shown that NOLVADEX is effective for the palliative treatment of male breast cancer. Sixty-six of these 132 evaluable patients responded to NOLVADEX which constitutes a 50% objective response rate.

INDICATIONS AND USAGE

Adjuvant Therapy: NOLVADEX is indicated for the treatment of axillary node-negative breast cancer in women following total mastectomy or segmental mastectomy, axillary dissection, and breast irradiation. Data are insufficient to predict which women are most likely to benefit and to determine if NOLVADEX provides any benefit in women with tumors less than 1 cm.
NOLVADEX is indicated for the treatment of node-positive breast cancer in postmenopausal women following total mastectomy, or segmental mastectomy, axillary dissection, and breast irradiation. In some NOLVADEX adjuvant studies, most of the benefit to date has been in the subgroup with 4 or more positive axillary nodes.
The estrogen and progesterone receptor values may help to predict whether adjuvant NOLVADEX therapy is likely to be beneficial.
Therapy for Advanced Disease: NOLVADEX is effective in the treatment of metastatic breast cancer in women and men. In premenopausal women with metastatic breast cancer, NOLVADEX is an alternative to oophorectomy or ovarian irradiation. Available evidence indicates that patients whose tumors are estrogen receptor positive are more likely to benefit from NOLVADEX therapy.

CONTRAINDICATIONS

NOLVADEX is contraindicated in patients with known hypersensitivity to the drug.

WARNINGS

Visual disturbance including corneal changes, cataracts and retinopathy have been reported in patients receiving NOLVADEX.
As with other additive hormonal therapy (estrogens and androgens), hypercalcemia has been reported in some breast cancer patients with bone metastases within a few weeks of starting treatment with NOLVADEX. If hypercalcemia does occur, appropriate measures should be taken and, if severe, NOLVADEX should be discontinued.
An increased incidence of endometrial cancer has been reported in association with NOLVADEX treatment. The underlying mechanism is unknown, but may be related to the estrogen-like effect of NOLVADEX. Any patients receiving or having previously received NOLVADEX, who report abnormal vaginal bleeding should be promptly evaluated. Patients receiving or having previously received NOLVADEX should have routine gynecological care and they should promptly inform their physician if they experience any abnormal gynecological symptoms, eg, menstrual irregularities, abnormal vaginal bleeding, changes in vaginal discharge, or pelvic pain or pressure.
An increased incidence of endometrial changes including hyperplasia and polyps have been reported in association with NOLVADEX treatment. The incidence and pattern of this increase suggest that the underlying mechanism is related to the estrogenic properties of NOLVADEX.
In a large randomized trial in Sweden of adjuvant NOLVADEX 40 mg/day for 2–5 years, an increased incidence of uterine cancer was noted. Twenty-three of 1,372 patients randomized to receive NOLVADEX versus 4 of 1,357 patients randomized to the observation group developed cancer of the uterus [RR = 5.6 (1.9–16.2), p<.001]. One of the patients with cancer of the uterus who was randomized to receive NOLVADEX never took the drug. After approximately 6.8 years of follow-up in the NSABP B-14 trial, 15 of 1,419 women randomized to receive NOLVADEX 20 mg/day for 5 years developed uterine cancer and 2 of the 1,424 women randomized to receive placebo, who subsequently were treated with NOLVADEX, also developed uterine cancer. Most of the uterine cancers were diagnosed at an early stage, but deaths from uterine cancer have been reported.
NOLVADEX has been associated with changes in liver enzyme levels, and on rare occasions, a spectrum of more severe liver abnormalities including fatty liver, cholestasis, hepatitis and hepatic necrosis. A few of these serious cases included fatalities. In most reported cases the relationship to NOLVADEX is uncertain. However, some positive rechallenges and dechallenges have been reported.
In the Swedish trial using adjuvant NOLVADEX 40 mg/day for 2–5 years, 3 cases of liver cancer have been reported in the NOLVADEX-treated group versus 1 case in the observation group. In other clinical trials evaluating NOLVADEX, no other cases of liver cancer have been reported to date.
Data from the NSABP B-14 study show no increase in other (non-uterine) cancers among patients receiving NOLVADEX. However, a number of second primary tumors, occurring at sites other than the endometrium, have been reported following the treatment of breast cancer with NOLVADEX in clinical trials. Whether an increased risk for other (non-uterine) cancers is associated with NOLVADEX is still uncertain and continues to be evaluated.
Pregnancy Category D: NOLVADEX may cause fetal harm when administered to a pregnant woman. Women should be advised not to become pregnant while taking NOLVADEX and should use barrier or nonhormonal contraceptive measures if sexually active. Effects on reproductive functions are expected from the antiestrogenic properties of the drug. In reproductive studies in rats at dose levels equal to or below the human dose, nonteratogenic developmental skeletal changes were seen and were found reversible. In addition, in fertility studies in rats and in teratology studies in rabbits using doses at or below those used in humans, a lower incidence of embryo implantation and a higher incidence of fetal death or retarded in utero growth were observed, with slower learning behavior in some rat pups when compared to historical controls. Several pregnant marmosets were dosed during organogenesis or in the last half of pregnancy. No deformations were seen and, although the dose was high enough to terminate pregnancy in some animals, those that did maintain pregnancy showed no evidence of teratogenic malformations.
In rodent models of fetal reproductive tract development, tamoxifen (at doses 0.3 to 2.4-fold the human maximum recommended dose on a mg/m^2 basis) caused changes in both sexes that are similar to those caused by estradiol, ethynylestradiol and diethylstilbestrol. Although the clinical relevance of these changes is unknown, some of these changes, especially vaginal adenosis, are similar to those seen in young women who were exposed to diethylstilbestrol *in utero* and who have a 1 in 1000 risk of developing clear-cell adenocarcinoma of the vagina or cervix. To date, *in utero* exposure to tamoxifen has not been shown to cause vaginal adenosis, or clear-cell adenocarcinoma of the vagina or cer-

vix, in young women. However, only a small number of young women have been exposed to tamoxifen *in utero*, and a smaller number have been followed long enough (to age 15–20) to determine whether vaginal or cervical neoplasia could occur as a result of this exposure.

There are no adequate and well controlled trials of tamoxifen in pregnant women. There have been a small number of reports of vaginal bleeding, spontaneous abortions, birth defects, and fetal deaths in pregnant women. If this drug is used during pregnancy, or the patient becomes pregnant while taking this drug, or within approximately two months after discontinuing therapy, the patient should be apprised of the potential risks to the fetus including the potential long term risk of a DES-like syndrome.

PRECAUTIONS

General: Decreases in platelet counts, usually to 50,000–100,000/mm^3, infrequently lower, have been occasionally reported in patients taking NOLVADEX for breast cancer. In patients with significant thrombocytopenia, rare hemorrhagic episodes have occurred, but it is uncertain if these episodes are due to NOLVADEX therapy. Leukopenia has been observed, sometimes in association with anemia and/or thrombocytopenia. There have been rare reports of neutropenia and pancytopenia in patients receiving NOLVADEX; this can sometimes be severe.

Information for Patients: Women taking or having previously taken NOLVADEX should be instructed to report abnormal vaginal bleeding which should be promptly investigated.

Laboratory Tests: Periodic complete blood counts, including platelet counts, and periodic liver function tests should be obtained.

Drug Interactions: When NOLVADEX is used in combination with coumarin-type anticoagulants, a significant increase in anticoagulant effect may occur. Where such coadministration exists, careful monitoring of the patient's prothrombin time is recommended.

There is an increased risk of thromboembolic events occurring when cytotoxic agents are used in combination with NOLVADEX.

Tamoxifen, N-desmethyl tamoxifen and 4-Hydroxytamoxifen have been found to be potent inhibitors of hepatic cytochrome p-450 mixed function oxidases. The effect of tamoxifen on metabolism and excretion of other antineoplastic drugs, such as cyclophosphamide and other drugs that require mixed function oxidases for activation, is not known.

One patient receiving NOLVADEX with concomitant phenobarbital exhibited a steady state serum level of tamoxifen lower than that observed for other patients (ie, 26 ng/mL vs. mean value of 122 ng/mL). However, the clinical significance of this finding is not known.

Concomitant bromocriptine therapy has been shown to elevate serum tamoxifen and N-desmethyltamoxifen.

Drug/Laboratory Testing Interactions: During postmarketing surveillance, T_4 elevations were reported for a few postmenopausal patients which may be explained by increases in thyroid-binding globulin. These elevations were not accompanied by clinical hyperthyroidism.

Variations in the karyopyknotic index on vaginal smears and various degrees of estrogen effect on Pap smears have been infrequently seen in postmenopausal patients given NOLVADEX.

In the postmarketing experience with NOLVADEX, infrequent cases of hyperlipidemias have been reported. Periodic monitoring of plasma triglycerides and cholesterol may be indicated in patients with pre-existing hyperlipidemias.

Carcinogenesis: A conventional carcinogenesis study in rats, (doses of 5, 20, and 35 mg/kg/day for up to 2 years) revealed hepatocellular carcinoma at all doses, and the incidence of these tumors was significantly greater among rats given 20 or 35 mg/kg/day (69%) than those given 5 mg/kg/day (14%). The incidence of these tumors in rats given 5 mg/kg/day (29.5 mg/m^2) was significantly greater than in controls.

In addition, preliminary data from 2 independent reports of 6-month studies in rats reveal liver tumors which in one study are classified as malignant. (See WARNINGS.)

Endocrine changes in immature and mature mice were investigated in a 13-month study. Granulosa cell ovarian tumors and interstitial cell testicular tumors were found in mice receiving NOLVADEX, but not in the controls.

Mutagenesis: Although no genotoxic potential was found in a conventional battery of *in vivo* and *in vitro* tests with pro- and eukaryotic test systems with drug metabolizing systems present, increased levels of DNA adducts have been found in the livers of rats exposed to tamoxifen. Tamoxifen also has been found to increase levels of micronucleus formation *in vitro* in human lymphoblastoid cell line (MCL-5). Based on these findings, tamoxifen is genotoxic in rodent and human MCL-5 cells.

Impairment of Fertility: Fertility in female rats was decreased following administration of 0.04 mg/kg for two weeks prior to mating through day 7 of pregnancy. There was a decreased number of implantations, and all fetuses were found dead.

Following administration to rats of 0.16 mg/kg from days 7–17 of pregnancy, there were increased numbers of fetal deaths. Administration of 0.125 mg/kg to rabbits during days 6–18 of pregnancy resulted in abortion or premature delivery. Fetal deaths occurred at higher doses. There were no teratogenic changes in either rat or rabbit segment II studies. Several pregnant marmosets were dosed with 10 mg/kg/day either during organogenesis or in the last half of pregnancy. No deformations were seen, and although the dose was high enough to terminate pregnancy in some animals, those that did maintain pregnancy showed no evidence of teratogenic malformations. Rats given 0.16 mg/kg from day 17 of pregnancy to 1 day before weaning demonstrated increased numbers of dead pups at parturition. It was reported that some rat pups showed slower learning behavior, but this did not achieve statistical significance in one study, and in another study where significance was reported, this was obtained by comparing dosed animals with controls of another study.

The recommended daily human dose of 20–40 mg corresponds to 0.4–0.8 mg/kg for an average 50 kg woman.

Pregnancy Category D: See WARNINGS.

Nursing Mothers: It is not known whether this drug is excreted in human milk. Because many drugs are excreted in human milk and because of the potential for serious adverse reactions in nursing infants from NOLVADEX, a decision should be made whether to discontinue nursing or to discontinue the drug, taking into account the importance of the drug to the mother.

Pediatric Use: The safety and efficacy of NOLVADEX in pediatric patients have not been established.

ADVERSE REACTIONS

Adverse reactions to NOLVADEX are relatively mild and rarely severe enough to require discontinuation of treatment.

In patients treated with NOLVADEX for metastatic breast cancer, the most frequent adverse reactions to NOLVADEX are hot flashes and nausea and/or vomiting. These may occur in up to one-fourth of patients.

Less frequently reported adverse reactions are vaginal bleeding, vaginal discharge, menstrual irregularities and skin rash. Usually these have not been of sufficient severity to require dosage reduction or discontinuation of treatment.

Very rare reports of erythema multiforme, Stevens-Johnson Syndrome and bullous pemphigoid have been reported with NOLVADEX therapy.

Increased bone and tumor pain and, also, local disease flare have occurred, which are sometimes associated with a good tumor response. Patients with increased bone pain may require additional analgesics. Patients with soft tissue disease may have sudden increases in the size of preexisting lesions, sometimes associated with marked erythema within and surrounding the lesions and/or the development of new lesions. When they occur, the bone pain or disease flare are seen shortly after starting NOLVADEX and generally subside rapidly.

Other adverse reactions which are seen infrequently are hypercalcemia, peripheral edema, distaste for food, pruritus vulvae, depression, dizziness, light-headedness, headache, hair thinning and/or partial hair loss, and vaginal dryness.

NOLVADEX has been associated with changes in liver enzyme levels, and on rare occasions, a spectrum of more severe liver abnormalities including fatty liver, cholestasis, hepatitis and hepatic necrosis. A few of these serious cases included fatalities. In most reported cases the relationship to NOLVADEX is uncertain. However, some positive rechallenges and dechallenges have been reported.

There have been a few reports of endometriosis and uterine fibroids in women receiving NOLVADEX. The underlying mechanism may be due to the partial estrogenic effect of NOLVADEX. Ovarian cysts have been observed in a small number of premenopausal patients with advanced breast cancer who have been treated with NOLVADEX.

Continued clinical studies have resulted in further information which better indicates the incidence of adverse reactions with NOLVADEX as compared to placebo.

In the NSABP study B-14, women with axillary node-negative breast cancer were randomized to 5 years of NOLVADEX 20 mg/day or placebo following primary surgery. The reported adverse effects are tabulated below (mean follow-up of approximately 6.8 years). The incidence of hot flashes (64% v 48%), vaginal discharge (30% v 15%), and irregular menses (25% v 19%) were higher with NOLVADEX compared with placebo. All other adverse effects occurred with similar frequency in the two treatment groups, with the exception of thrombotic events which although rare, were more common with NOLVADEX than with placebo. Two of the patients treated with NOLVADEX who had thrombotic events died.

NSABP B-14 STUDY

Adverse Effect	% of Women NOLVADEX (n=1424)	Placebo (n=1440)
Hot Flashes	63.9	47.6
Weight Gain (>5%)	38.1	40.1
Fluid Retention	32.4	29.7
Vaginal Discharge	29.6	15.2
Nausea	25.7	23.9
Irregular Menses	24.6	18.8
Weight Loss (>5%)	22.6	18.0
Skin Changes	18.7	15.3
Increased BUN	18.1	20.2
Diarrhea	11.2	14.0
Increased SGOT	4.8	2.8
Increased Alkaline Phosphatase	3.0	4.6
Vomiting	2.1	1.7
Increased Bilirubin	1.8	1.2
Increased Creatinine	1.7	1.0
Thrombocytopenia*	1.5	1.2
Leukopenia**	0.4	1.1
Thrombotic Events		
Deep Vein Thrombosis	0.8	0.3
Pulmonary Embolism	0.4	0.1
Superficial Phlebitis	0.3	0.0

* Defined as a platelet count of <100,000/mm^3
** Defined as a white blood cell count of <3000/mm^3

In the Eastern Cooperative Oncology Group (ECOG) adjuvant breast cancer trial, NOLVADEX or placebo was administered for 2 years to women following mastectomy. When compared to placebo, NOLVADEX showed a significantly higher incidence of hot flashes (19% versus 8% for placebo). The incidence of all other adverse reactions was similar in the 2 treatment groups with the exception of thrombocytopenia where the incidence for NOLVADEX was 10% versus 3% for placebo, an observation of borderline statistical significance.

The other adverse reactions reported equally in the ECOG study for NOLVADEX and placebo include abnormal renal function tests, fatigue, dyspnea, anorexia, cough, and abdominal cramps. A relationship of these reactions to the administration of NOLVADEX has not been demonstrated since the frequency was not significantly different from that reported in placebo treated women.

In other adjuvant studies, Toronto and NOLVADEX Adjuvant Trial Organization (NATO), women received either NOLVADEX or no therapy. In the Toronto study, hot flashes and nausea and/or vomiting were observed in 29% and 19% of patients, respectively, for NOLVADEX versus 1% and 0% in the untreated group. In the NATO trial, hot flashes, nausea and/or vomiting and vaginal bleeding were reported in 2.8%, 2.1%, and 2.0% of women, respectively, for NOLVADEX versus 0.2% for each in the untreated group.

The following table summarizes the incidence of adverse reactions reported at a frequency of 2% or greater from clinical trials (Ingle, Pritchard, Buchanan) which compared NOLVADEX therapy to ovarian ablation in premenopausal patients with metastatic breast cancer.

	NOLVADEX All Effects Number of Women (%)		OVARIAN ABLATION All Effects Number of Women (%)	
Adverse Reactions*	n=104		n=100	
Flush	34	(32.7)	46	(46)
Amenorrhea	17	(16.3)	69	(69)
Altered Menses	13	(12.5)	5	(5)
Oligomenorrhea	9	(8.7)	1	(1)
Bone Pain	6	(5.7)	6	(6)
Menstrual Disorder	6	(5.7)	4	(4)
Nausea	5	(4.8)	4	(4)
Cough/Coughing	4	(3.8)	1	(1)
Edema	4	(3.8)	1	(1)
Fatigue	4	(3.8)	1	(1)
Musculoskeletal Pain	3	(2.8)	0	(0)
Pain	3	(2.8)	4	(4)
Ovarian Cyst(s)	3	(2.8)	2	(2)
Depression	2	(1.9)	2	(2)
Abdominal Cramps	1	(1)	2	(2)
Anorexia	1	(1)	2	(2)

* Some women had more than one adverse reaction.

Continued on next page

Nolvadex—Cont.

NOLVADEX is well tolerated in males with breast cancer. Reports from the literature and case reports suggest that the safety profile of NOLVADEX in males is similar to that seen in women. Loss of libido and impotence have resulted in discontinuation of tamoxifen therapy in male patients. Also, in oligospermic males treated with tamoxifen, LH, FSH, testosterone and estrogen levels were elevated. No significant clinical changes were reported.

OVERDOSAGE

Signs observed at the highest doses following studies to determine LD_{50} in animals were respiratory difficulties and convulsions.

Acute overdosage in humans has not been reported. In a study of advanced metastatic cancer patients which specifically determined the maximum tolerated dose of NOLVADEX in evaluating the use of very high doses to reverse multidrug resistance, acute neurotoxicity manifested by tremor, hyperreflexia, unsteady gait and dizziness were noted. These symptoms occurred within 3–5 days of beginning NOLVADEX and cleared within 2–5 days after stopping therapy. No permanent neurologic toxicity was noted. One patient experienced a seizure several days after NOLVADEX was discontinued and neurotoxic symptoms had resolved. The causal relationship of the seizure to NOLVADEX therapy is unknown. Doses given in these patients were all greater than 400 mg/m^2 loading dose, followed by maintenance doses of 150 mg/m^2 of NOLVADEX given twice a day.

In the same study, prolongation of the QT interval on the electrocardiogram was noted when patients were given doses higher than 250 mg/m^2 loading dose, followed by maintenance doses of 80 mg/m^2 of NOLVADEX given twice a day. For a woman with a body surface area of 1.5 m^2 the minimal loading dose and maintenance doses given at which neurological symptoms and QT changes occurred were at least 6 fold higher in respect to the maximum recommended dose.

No specific treatment for overdosage is known; treatment must be symptomatic.

DOSAGE AND ADMINISTRATION

For patients with breast cancer, the recommended daily dose is 20–40 mg. Dosages greater than 20 mg per day should be given in divided doses (morning and evening).

In three single agent adjuvant studies in women, one 10 mg NOLVADEX tablet was administered two (ECOG and NATO) or three (Toronto) times a day for two years. In the EBCTCG 1990 overview, the reduction in recurrence and mortality was greater in those studies that used tamoxifen for two years or longer than in those that used tamoxifen for less than two years. There was no indication that doses greater than 20 mg per day were more effective. In B-14, the NSABP adjuvant study in women with node-negative breast cancer, one 10 mg NOLVADEX tablet was given twice a day for at least five years. Results of the B-14 study suggest that continuation of therapy beyond five years does not provide additional benefit (see CLINICAL PHARMACOLOGY). The optimal duration of adjuvant NOLVADEX therapy remains to be determined.

HOW SUPPLIED

10 mg Tablets containing tamoxifen as the citrate in an amount equivalent to 10 mg of tamoxifen (round, biconvex, uncoated, white tablet identified with NOLVADEX 600 debossed on one side and a cameo debossed on the other side) are supplied in bottles of 60 tablets and 250 tablets. NDC 0310-0600.

20 mg Tablets containing tamoxifen as the citrate in an amount equivalent to 20 mg of tamoxifen (round, biconvex, uncoated, white tablet identified with NOLVADEX 604 debossed on one side and a cameo debossed on the other side) are supplied in bottles of 30 tablets. NDC 0310-0604.

Store at controlled room temperature, 20–25° C (68–77° F) [see USP]. Dispense in a well-closed, light-resistant container.

ZENECA Pharmaceuticals
A Business Unit of ZENECA Inc.
Wilmington, DE 19850-5437 USA
SIC 64130-00 Rev S 02/98

Shown in Product Identification Guide, page 346

SEROQUEL® ℞

[serō-quĕl]
(quetiapine fumarate)
tablets

DESCRIPTION

SEROQUEL (quetiapine fumarate) is an antipsychotic drug belonging to a new chemical class, the dibenzothiazepine derivatives. The chemical designation is 2-[2-(4-dibenzo *[b,f]* [1,4]thiazepin-11-yl-1-piperazinyl)ethoxy]-ethanol fumarate (2:1) (salt). It is present in tablets as the fumarate salt. All doses and tablet strengths are expressed as milligrams of base, not as fumarate salt. Its molecular formula is $C_{42}H_{50}N_6O_4S_2{\cdot}C_4H_4O_4$ and it has a molecular weight of 883.11 (fumarate salt). The structural formula is:

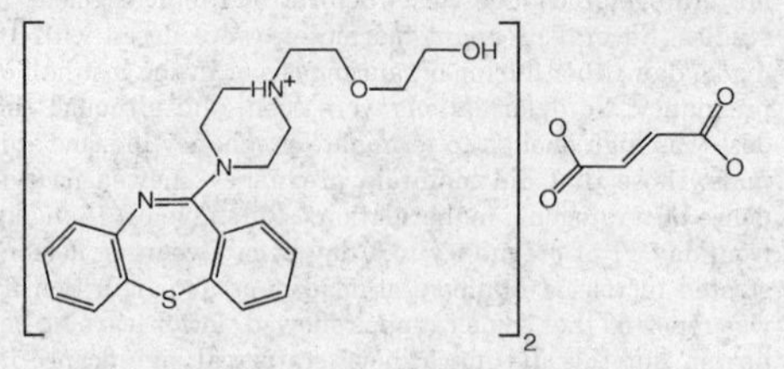

Quetiapine fumarate is a white to off-white crystalline powder which is moderately soluble in water.

SEROQUEL is supplied for oral administration as 25 mg (peach), 100 mg (yellow) and 200 mg (white) tablets.

Inactive ingredients are povidone, dibasic dicalcium phosphate dihydrate, microcrystalline cellulose, sodium starch glycolate, lactose monohydrate, magnesium stearate, hydroxypropyl methylcellulose, polyethylene glycol, and titanium dioxide.

The 25 mg tablets contain red ferric oxide and yellow ferric oxide and the 100 mg tablets contain only yellow ferric oxide.

CLINICAL PHARMACOLOGY

Pharmacodynamics

SEROQUEL is an antagonist at multiple neurotransmitter receptors in the brain; serotonin $5HT_{1A}$ and $5HT_2$ (IC_{50s}=717 & 148nM respectively), dopamine D_1 and D_2 (IC_{50s}= 1268 & 329nM respectively), histamine H_1 (IC_{50}=30nM), and adrenergic α_1 and α_2 receptors (IC_{50s}=94 & 271nM, respectively). SEROQUEL has no appreciable affinity at cholinergic muscarinic and benzodiazepine receptors (IC_{50s}>5000 nM).

The mechanism of action of SEROQUEL, as with other antipsychotic drugs, is unknown. However, it has been proposed that this drug's antipsychotic activity is mediated through a combination of dopamine type 2 (D_2) and serotonin type 2 ($5\text{-}HT_2$) antagonism. Antagonism at receptors other than dopamine and $5HT_2$ with similar receptor affinities may explain some of the other effects of SEROQUEL.

SEROQUEL'S antagonism of histamine H_1 receptors may explain the somnolence observed with this drug.

SEROQUEL'S antagonism of adrenergic α_1 receptors may explain the orthostatic hypotension observed with this drug.

Pharmacokinetics

Quetiapine fumarate activity is primarily due to the parent drug. The multiple-dose pharmacokinetics of quetiapine are dose-proportional within the proposed clinical dose range, and quetiapine accumulation is predictable upon multiple dosing. Elimination of quetiapine is mainly via hepatic metabolism with a mean terminal half-life of about 6 hours within the proposed clinical dose range. Steady state concentrations are expected to be achieved within two days of dosing. Quetiapine is unlikely to interfere with the metabolism of drugs metabolized by cytochrome P450 enzymes.

Absorption: Quetiapine fumarate is rapidly absorbed after oral administration, reaching peak plasma concentrations in 1.5 hours. The tablet formulation is 100% bioavailable relative to solution. The bioavailability of quetiapine is marginally affected by administration with food, with C_{max} and AUC values increased by 25% and 15%, respectively.

Distribution: Quetiapine is widely distributed throughout the body with an apparent volume of distribution of 10 ± 4 L/kg. It is 83% bound to plasma proteins at therapeutic concentrations. *In vitro,* quetiapine did not affect the binding of warfarin or diazepam to human serum albumin. In turn, neither warfarin nor diazepam altered the binding of quetiapine.

Metabolism and Elimination: Following a single oral dose of ^{14}C-quetiapine, less than 1% of the administered dose was excreted as unchanged drug, indicating that quetiapine is highly metabolized. Approximately 73% and 20% of the dose and was recovered in the urine and feces, respectively. Quetiapine is extensively metabolized by the liver. The major metabolic pathways are sulfoxidation to the sulfoxide metabolite and oxidation to the parent acid metabolite; both metabolites are pharmacologically inactive. *In vitro* studies using human liver microsomes revealed that the cytochrome P450 3A4 isoenzyme is involved in the metabolism of quetiapine to its major, but inactive, sulfoxide metabolite.

Population Subgroups

Age: Oral clearance of quetiapine was reduced by 40% in elderly patients (≥ 65 years, n=9) compared to young patients (n=12), and dosing adjustment may be necessary (See **DOSAGE AND ADMINISTRATION**).

Gender: There is no gender effect on the pharmacokinetics of quetiapine.

Race: There is no race effect on the pharmacokinetics of quetiapine.

Smoking: Smoking has no effect on the oral clearance of quetiapine.

Renal Insufficiency: Patients with severe renal impairment (Clcr=10–30 mL/min/1.73 m^2, n=8) had a 25% lower mean oral clearance than normal subjects (Clcr > 80 mL/min/1.73 m^2, n=8), but plasma quetiapine concentrations in the subjects with renal insufficiency were within the range of concentrations seen in normal subjects receiving the same dose. Dosage adjustment is therefore not needed in these patients.

Hepatic Insufficiency: Hepatically impaired patients (n=8) had a 30% lower mean oral clearance of quetiapine than normal subjects. In two of the 8 hepatically impaired patients, AUC and C_{max} were 3-times higher than those observed typically in healthy subjects. Since quetiapine is extensively metabolized by the liver, higher plasma levels are expected in the hepatically impaired population, and dosage adjustment may be needed. (See **DOSAGE AND ADMINISTRATION**).

Drug-Drug Interactions: *In vitro* enzyme inhibition data suggest that quetiapine and 9 of its metabolites would have little inhibitory effect on *in vivo* metabolism mediated by cytochromes P450 1A2, 2C9, 2C19, 2D6, and 3A4.

Quetiapine oral clearance is induced by the prototype cytochrome P450 3A4 inducer, phenytoin. Dose adjustment of quetiapine will be necessary if it is coadministered with phenytoin (See **DRUG INTERACTIONS** under **PRECAUTIONS** and **DOSAGE AND ADMINISTRATION**).

Quetiapine oral clearance is not inhibited by the non-specific enzyme inhibitor, cimetidine.

Quetiapine at doses of 750 mg/day did not affect the single dose pharmacokinetics of antipyrine, lithium, or lorazepam. (See **DRUG INTERACTIONS** under **PRECAUTIONS**).

Clinical Efficacy Data

The efficacy of SEROQUEL in the management of the manifestations of psychotic disorders was established in 3 short-term (6-week) controlled trials of psychotic inpatients who met DSM III-R criteria for schizophrenia. Although a single fixed dose haloperidol arm was included as a comparative treatment in one of the three trials, this single haloperidol dose group was inadequate to provide a reliable and valid comparison of SEROQUEL and haloperidol.

Several instruments were used for assessing psychiatric signs and symptoms in these studies, among them the Brief Psychiatric Rating Scale (BPRS), a multi-item inventory of general psychopathology traditionally used to evaluate the effects of drug treatment in psychosis. The BPRS psychosis cluster (conceptual disorganization, hallucinatory behavior, suspiciousness, and unusual thought content) is considered a particularly useful subset for assessing actively psychotic schizophrenic patients. A second traditional assessment, the Clinical Global Impression (CGI), reflects the impression of a skilled observer, fully familiar with the manifestations of schizophrenia, about the overall clinical state of the patient. In addition, the Scale for Assessing Negative Symptoms (SANS), a more recently developed but less well evaluated scale, was employed for assessing negative symptoms.

The results of the trials follow:

(1) In a 6-week, placebo-controlled trial (n=361) involving 5 fixed doses of SEROQUEL (75, 150, 300, 600, and 750 mg/day on a tid schedule), the 4 highest doses of SEROQUEL were generally superior to placebo on the BPRS total score, the BPRS psychosis cluster, and the CGI severity score, with the maximum effect seen at 300 mg/day, and the effects of doses of 150 to 750 were generally indistinguishable. SEROQUEL, at a dose of 300 mg/day, was superior to placebo on the SANS.

(2) In a 6-week, placebo-controlled trial (n=286) involving titration of SEROQUEL in high (up to 750 mg/day on a tid schedule) and low (up to 250 mg/day on a tid schedule) doses, only the high dose of SEROQUEL group (mean dose, 500 mg/day) was generally superior to placebo on the BPRS total score, the BPRS psychosis cluster, the CGI severity score, and the SANS.

(3) In a 6-week dose and dose regimen comparison trial (n=618) involving two fixed doses of SEROQUEL (450 mg/day on both bid and tid schedules and 50 mg/day on a bid schedule), only the 450 mg/day (225 mg bid schedule) dose group was generally superior to the 50 mg/day (25 mg bid) SEROQUEL dose group on the BPRS total score, the BPRS psychosis cluster, the CGI severity score, and on the SANS.

Examination of population subsets (race, gender, and age) did not reveal any differential responsiveness on the basis of race or gender, with an apparently greater effect in patients under the age of 40 compared to those older than 40. The clinical significance of this finding is unknown.

INDICATIONS AND USAGE

SEROQUEL is indicated for the management of the manifestations of psychotic disorders.

The antipsychotic efficacy of SEROQUEL was established in short-term (6-week) controlled trials of schizophrenic inpatients (See **CLINICAL PHARMACOLOGY**).

The effectiveness of SEROQUEL in long-term use, that is, for more than 6 weeks, has not been systematically evaluated in controlled trials. Therefore, the physician who elects

to use SEROQUEL for extended periods should periodically reevaluate the long-term usefulness of the drug for the individual patient (See **DOSAGE AND ADMINISTRATION**).

CONTRAINDICATIONS

SEROQUEL is contraindicated in individuals with a known hypersensitivity to this medication or any of its ingredients.

WARNINGS

Neuroleptic Malignant Syndrome (NMS)

A potentially fatal symptom complex sometimes referred to as Neuroleptic Malignant Syndrome (NMS) has been reported in association with administration of antipsychotic drugs. Two possible cases of NMS [2/2387 (0.1%)] have been reported in clinical trials with SEROQUEL. Clinical manifestations of NMS are hyperpyrexia, muscle rigidity, altered mental status, and evidence of autonomic instability (irregular pulse or blood pressure, tachycardia, diaphoresis, and cardiac dysrhythmia). Additional signs may include elevated creatinine phosphokinase, myoglobinuria (rhabdomyolysis), and acute renal failure.

The diagnostic evaluation of patients with this syndrome is complicated. In arriving at a diagnosis, it is important to exclude cases where the clinical presentation includes both serious medical illness (e.g., pneumonia, systemic infection, etc.) and untreated or inadequately treated extrapyramidal signs and symptoms (EPS). Other important considerations in the differential diagnosis include central anticholinergic toxicity, heat stroke, drug fever, and primary central nervous system (CNS) pathology.

The management of NMS should include: 1) immediate discontinuation of antipsychotic drugs and other drugs not essential to concurrent therapy; 2) intensive symptomatic treatment and medical monitoring; and 3) treatment of any concomitant serious medical problems for which specific treatments are available. There is no general agreement about specific pharmacological treatment regimens for NMS.

If a patient requires antipsychotic drug treatment after recovery from NMS, the potential reintroduction of drug therapy should be carefully considered. The patient should be carefully monitored since recurrences of NMS have been reported.

Tardive Dyskinesia

A syndrome of potentially irreversible, involuntary, dyskinetic movements may develop in patients treated with antipsychotic drugs. Although the prevalence of the syndrome appears to be highest among the elderly, especially elderly women, it is impossible to rely upon prevalence estimates to predict, at the inception of antipsychotic treatment, which patients are likely to develop the syndrome. Whether antipsychotic drug products differ in their potential to cause tardive dyskinesia is unknown.

The risk of developing tradive dyskinesia and the likelihood that it will become irreversible are believed to increase as the duration of treatment and the total cumulative dose of antipsychotic drugs administered to the patient increase. However, the syndrome can develop, although much less commonly, after relatively brief treatment periods at low doses.

There is no known treatment for established cases of tardive dyskinesia, although the syndrome may remit, partially or completely, if antipsychotic treatment is withdrawn. Antipsychotic treatment, itself, however, may suppress (or partially suppress) the signs and symptoms of the syndrome and thereby may possibly mask the underlying process. The effect that symptomatic suppression has upon the long-term course of the syndrome is unknown.

Given these considerations, SEROQUEL should be prescribed in a manner that is most likely to minimize the occurrence of tardive dyskinesia. Chronic antipsychotic treatment should generally be reserved for patients who appear to suffer from a chronic illness that (1) is known to respond to antipsychotic drugs, and (2) for whom alternative, equally effective, but potentially less harmful treatments are not available or appropriate. In patients who do require chronic treatment, the smallest dose and the shortest duration of treatment producing a satisfactory clinical response should be sought. The need for continued treatment should be reassessed periodically.

If signs and symptoms of tardive dyskinesia appear in a patient on SEROQUEL, drug discontinuation should be considered. However, some patients may require treatment with SEROQUEL despite the presence of the syndrome.

PRECAUTIONS

General

Orthostatic Hypotension: SEROQUEL may induce orthostatic hypotension associated with dizziness, tachycardia and, in some patients, syncope, especially during the initial dose-titration period, probably reflecting its α1-adrenergic antagonist properties. Syncope was reported in 1% (22/2162) of the patients treated with SEROQUEL, compared with 0% (0/206) on placebo and about 0.5% (2/420) on active control drugs. The risk of orthostatic hypotension and syncope may be minimized by limiting the initial dose to 25 mg bid (See **DOSAGE AND ADMINISTRATION**). If hypotension occurs during titration to the target dose, a return to the previous dose in the titration schedule is appropriate.

SEROQUEL should be used with particular caution in patients with known cardiovascular disease (history of myocardial infarction or ischemic heart disease, heart failure or conduction abnormalities), cerebrovascular disease or conditions which would predispose patients to hypotension (dehydration, hypovolemia, and treatment with antihypertensive medications).

Cataracts: The development of cataracts was observed in association with quetiapine treatment in chronic dog studies (see Animal Toxicology). Lens changes have also been observed in patients during long-term SEROQUEL treatment, but a causal relationship to SEROQUEL use has not been established. Nevertheless, the possibility of lenticular changes cannot be excluded at this time. Therefore, examination of the lens by methods adequate to defect cataract formation, such as slit lamp exam or other appropriately sensitive methods, is recommended at initiation of treatment or shortly thereafter, and at 6 month intervals during chronic treatment.

Seizures: During clinical trials, seizures occurred in 0.8% (18/2387) of patients treated with SEROQUEL compared 0.5% (1/206) on placebo and 1% (4/420) on active control drugs. As with other antipsychotics, SEROQUEL should be used cautiously in patients with a history of seizures or with conditions that potentially lower the seizure threshold, e.g., Alzheimer's dementia. Conditions that lower the seizure threshold may be more prevalent in a population of 65 years or older.

Hypothyroidism: Clinical trials with SEROQUEL demonstrated a dose-related decrease in total and free thyroxine (T4) of approximately 20% at the higher end of the therapeutic dose range that was apparent early on during treatment and maintained without adaptation or progression during more chronic therapy. Generally, these changes were of no clinical significance and TSH was unchanged in most patients, but about 0.4% (10/2386) of SEROQUEL patients did experience TSH increases. Six of the patients with TSH increases needed replacement thyroid treatment.

Cholesterol and Triglyceride Elevations: In a pool of 3- to 6-week placebo-controlled trials, SEROQUEL-treated patients had increases from baseline in cholesterol and triglyceride of 11% and 17%, respectively, compared to slight decreases for placebo patients. These changes were only weakly related to the increases in weight observed in SEROQUEL-treated patients.

Hyperprolactinemia: Although an elevation of prolactin levels was not demonstrated in clinical trials with SEROQUEL, increased prolactin levels were observed in rat studies with this compound and were associated with an increase in mammary gland neoplasia in rats (see Carcinogenesis). Tissue culture experiments indicate that approximately one-third of human breast cancers are prolactin dependent *in vitro*, a factor of potential importance if the prescription of these drugs is contemplated in a patient with previously detected breast cancer. Although disturbances such as galactorrhea, amenorrhea, gynecomastia, and impotence have been reported with prolactin-elevating compounds, the clinical significance of elevated serum prolactin levels is unknown for most patients. Neither clinical studies nor epidemiologic studies conducted to date have shown as association between chronic administration of this class of drugs and tumorigenesis in humans; the available evidence is considered too limited to be conclusive at this time.

Transaminase Elevations: Asymptomatic, transient, and reversible elevations in serum transaminases (primarily ALT) have been reported. The proportions of patients with transaminase elevations of > 3 times the upper limits of the normal reference range in a pool of 3- to 6-week placebo-controlled trials were approximately 6% for SEROQUEL compared to 1% for placebo. These hepatic enzyme elevations usually occurred within the first 3 weeks of drug treatment and promptly returned to prestudy levels with ongoing treatment with SEROQUEL.

Potential for Cognitive and Motor Impairment: Somnolence was a commonly reported adverse event reported in patients treated with SEROQUEL especially during the 3-5 day period of initial dose-titration. In the 3- to 6-week placebo-controlled trials, somnolence was reported in 18% of patients on SEROQUEL compared to 11% of placebo patients. Since SEROQUEL has the potential to impair judgment, thinking, or motor skills, patients should be cautioned about performing activities requiring mental alertness, such as operating a motor vehicle (including automobiles) or operating hazardous machinery until they are reasonably certain that SEROQUEL therapy does not affect them adversely.

Priapism: One case of priapism in a patient receiving SEROQUEL has been reported prior to market introduction. While a causal relationship to use of SEROQUEL has not been established, other drugs with alpha-adrenergic blocking effects have been reported to induce priapism, and it is possible that SEROQUEL may share this capacity. Severe priapism may require surgical intervention.

Body Temperature Regulation: Although not reported with SEROQUEL, disruption of the body's ability to reduce core body temperature has been attributed to antipsychotic agents. Appropriate care is advised when prescribing SEROQUEL for patients who will be experiencing conditions which may contribute to an elevation in core body temperature, e.g., exercising strenuously, exposure to extreme heat, receiving concomitant medication with anticholinergic activity, or being subject to dehydration.

Dysphagia: Esophageal dysmotility and aspiration have been associated with antipsychotic drug use. Aspiration pneumonia is a common cause of morbidity and mortality in elderly patients, in particular those with advanced Alzheimer's dementia. SEROQUEL and other antipsychotic drugs should be used cautiously in patients at risk for aspiration pneumonia.

Suicide: The possibility of a suicide attempt is inherent in schizophrenia, and close supervision of high-risk patients should accompany drug therapy. Prescriptions for SEROQUEL should be written for the smallest quantity of tablets consistent with good patient management in order to reduce the risk of overdose.

Use in Patients with Concomitant Illness: Clinical experience with SEROQUEL in patients with certain concomitant systemic illnesses (see Renal and Impairment and Hepatic Impairment under **CLINICAL PHARMACOLOGY**, Special Populations) is limited.

SEROQUEL has not been evaluated or used to any appreciable extent in patients with a recent history of myocardial infarction or unstable heart disease. Patients with these diagnoses were excluded from premarketing clinical studies. Because of the risk of orthostatic hypotension with SEROQUEL, caution should be observed in cardiac patients (see Orthostatic Hypotension).

Information for Patients

Physicians are advised to discuss the following issues with patients for whom they prescribe SEROQUEL.

Orthostatic Hypotension: Patients should be advised of the risk of orthostatic hypotension, especially during the 3–5 day period of initial dose titration, and also at times of reinitiating treatment or increases in dose.

Interference with Cognitive and Motor Performance: Since somnolence was a commonly reported adverse event associated with SEROQUEL treatment, patients should be advised of the risk of somnolence, especially during the 3–5 day period of initial dose titration. Patients should be cautioned about performing any activity requiring mental altertness, such as operating a motor vehicle (including automobiles) or operating hazardous machinery, until they are reasonably certain that SEROQUEL therapy does not affect them adversely.

Pregnancy: Patients should be advised to notify their physician if they become pregnant or intend to become pregnant during therapy.

Nursing: Patients should be advised not to breast feed if they are taking SEROQUEL.

Concomitant Medication: As with other medications, patients should be advised to notify their physicians if they are taking, or plan to take, any prescription or over-the-counter drugs.

Alcohol: Patients should be advised to avoid consuming alcoholic beverages while taking SEROQUEL.

Heat Exposure and Dehydration: Patients should be advised regarding appropriate care in avoiding overheating and dehydration.

Laboratory Tests

No specific laboratory tests are recommended.

Drug Interactions

The risks of using SEROQUEL in combination with other drugs have not been extensively evaluated in systematic studies. Given the primary CNS effects of SEROQUEL, caution should be used when it is taken in combination with other centrally acting drugs. SEROQUEL potentiated the cognitive and motor effects of alcohol in a clinical trial in subjects with selected psychotic disorders, and alcoholic beverages should be avoided while taking SEROQUEL.

Because of its potential for inducing hypotension, SEROQUEL may enhance the effects of certain antihypertensive agents.

SEROQUEL may antagonize the effects of levodopa and dopamine agonists.

The Effect of Other Drugs on SEROQUEL

Phenytoin: Coadministration of quetiapine (250 mg tid) and phenytoin (100 mg tid) increased the mean oral clearance of quetiapine by 5-fold. Increased doses of SEROQUEL may be required to maintain control of psychotic symptoms in patients receiving quetiapine and phenytoin, or other hepatic enzyme inducers (e.g., carbamazepine, barbiturates, rifampin, glucocorticoids). Caution should be taken if phenytoin is withdrawn and replaced with a noninducer (e.g., valproate) (see **DOSAGE AND ADMINISTRATION**).

Thioridazine: Thioridazine (200 mg bid) increased the oral clearance of quetiapine (300 mg bid) by 65%.

Continued on next page

Seroquel—Cont.

Cimetidine: Administration of multiple daily doses of cimetidine (400 mg tid for 4 days) resulted in a 20% decrease in the mean oral clearance of quetiapine (150 mg tid). Dosage adjustment for quetiapine is not required when it is given with cimetidine.

P450 3A Inhibitors: Although data are not available from clinical studies, caution is indicated when SEROQUEL is administered with a potent enzyme inhibitor of cytochrome P450 3A (e.g., ketoconazole, itraconzaole, fluconazole, and erythromycin).

Fluoxetine, Imipramine, Haloperidol, and Risperidone: Coadministration of fluoxetine (60 mg once daily); imipramine (75 mg bid), haloperidol (7.5 mg bid), or risperidone (3 mg bid) with quetiapine (300 mg bid) did not alter the steady state pharmacokinetics of quetiapine.

Effect of Quetiapine on Other Drugs:

Lorazepam: The mean oral clearance of lorazepam (2 mg, single dose) was reduced by 20% in the presence of quetiapine administered as 250 mg tid dosing.

Lithium: Concomitant administration of quetiapine (250 mg tid) with lithium had no effect on any of the steady state pharmacokinetic parameters of lithium.

Antipyrine: Administration of multiple daily doses up to 750 mg/day (one a tid schedule) of quetiapine to subjects with selected psychotic disorders had no clinically relevant effect on the clearance of antipyrine or urinary recovery of antipyrine metabolites. These results indicate that quetiapine does not significantly induce hepatic enzymes responsible for cytochrome P450 mediated metabolism of antipyrine.

Carcinogenesis, Mutagenesis, Impairment of Fertility

Carcinogenesis: Carcinogenicity studies were conducted in C57BL mice and Wistar rats. Quetiapine was administered in the diet to mice at doses of 20, 75, 250, and 750 mg/kg and to rats by gavage at doses of 25, 75, and 250 mg/kg for two years. These doses are equivalent to 0.1, 0.5, 1.5, and 4.5 times the maximum human dose (800 mg/kg) on a mg/m^2 basis (mice) or 0.3, 0.9, and 3.0 times the maximum human dose on a mg/m^2 basis (rats). There were statistically significant increases in thyroid gland follicular adenomas in male mice at doses of 250 and 750 mg/kg or 1.5 and 4.5 times the maximum human dose on a mg/m^2 basis and in male rats at a dose of 250 mg/kg or 3.0 times the maximum human dose on a mg/m^2 basis. Mammary gland adenocarcinomas were statistically significantly increased in female rats at all doses tested (25, 75, and 250 mg/kg or 0.3, 0.9, and 3.0 times the maximum recommended human dose on a mg/m^2 basis).

Thyroid follicular cell adenomas may have resulted from chronic stimulation of the thyroid gland by thyroid stimulating hormone (TSH) resulting from enhanced metabolism and clearance of thyroxine by rodent liver. Changes in TSH, thyroxine, and thyroxine clearance consistent with this mechanism were observed in subchronic toxicity studies in rat and mouse and in a 1-year toxicity study in rat; however, the result of these studies were not definitive. The relevance of the increases in thyroid follicular cell adenomas to human risk, through whatever mechanism, is unknown.

Antipsychotic drugs have been shown to chronically elevate prolactin levels in rodents. Serum measurements in a 1-yr toxicity study showed that quetiapine increased median serum prolactin levels a maximum of 32- and 13-fold in male and female rats, respectively. Increases in mammary neoplasms have been found in rodents after chronic administration of other antipsychotic drugs and are considered to be prolactin-mediated. The relevance of this increased incidence of prolactin-mediated mammary gland tumors in rats to human risk is unknown (see Hyperprolactinemia in **PRECAUTIONS, General**).

Mutagenesis: The mutagenic potential of quetiapine was tested in six *in vitro* bacterial gene mutation assays and in an *in vitro* mammalian gene mutation assay in Chinese Hamster Ovary cells. However, sufficiently high concentrations of quetiapine may not have been used for all tester strains. Quetiapine did produce a reproducible increase in mutations in one *Salmonella typhimurium* tester strain in the presence of metabolic activation. No evidence of clastogenic potential was obtained in an *in vitro* chromosomal aberration assay in cultured human lymphocytes or in the *in vivo* micronucleus assay in rats.

Impairment of Fertility: Quetiapine decreased mating and fertility in male Sprague-Dawley rats at oral doses of 50 and 150 mg/kg or 0.6 and 1.8 times the maximum human dose on a mg/m^2 basis. Drug-related effects included increases in interval to mate and in the number of matings required for successful impregnation. These effects continued to be observed at 150 mg/kg even after a two-week period without treatment. The no-effect dose for impaired mating and fertility in male rats was 25 mg/kg, or 0.3 times the maximum human dose on a mg/m^2 basis. Quetiapine adversely affected mating and fertility in female Sprague-Dawley rats at an oral dose of 50 mg/kg, or 0.6 times the maximum human dose on a mg/m^2 basis. Drug-related effects included decreases in matings and in matings resulting in pregnancy, and an increase in the interval to mate. An increase in irregular estrus cycles was observed at doses of 10 and 50 mg/kg, or 0.1 and 0.6 times the maximum human dose on a mg/m^2 basis. The no-effect dose in female rats was 1 mg/kg, or 0.01 times the maximum human dose on a mg/m^2 basis.

Pregnancy

Pregnancy Category C

The teratogenic potential of quetiapine was studied in Wistar rats and Dutch Belted rabbits dosed during the period of organogenesis. No evidence of a teratogenic effect was detected in rats at doses of 25 to 200 mg/kg or 0.3 to 2.4 times the maximum human dose on a mg/m^2 basis or in rabbits at 25 to 100 mg/kg or 0.6 to 2.4 times the maximum human dose on a mg/m^2 basis. There was, however, evidence of embryo/fetal toxicity. Delays in skeletal ossification were detected in rat fetuses at doses of 50 and 200 mg/kg (0.6 and 2.4 times the maximum human dose on a mg/m^2 basis) and in rabbits at 50 and 100 mg/kg (1.2 and 2.4 times the maximum human dose on a mg/m^2 basis). Fetal body weight was reduced in rat fetuses at 200 mg/kg and rabbit fetuses at 100 mg/kg (2.4 times the maximum human dose on a mg/m^2 basis for both species). There was an increased incidence of a minor soft tissue anomaly (carpal/tarsal flexure) in rabbit fetuses at a dose of 100 mg/kg (2.4 times the maximum human dose on a mg/m^2 basis). Evidence of maternal toxicity (i.e., decreases in body weight gain and/or death) was observed at the high dose in the rat study and at all doses in the rabbit study. In a peri/postnatal reproductive study in rats, no drug-related effects were observed at doses of 1, 10, and 20 mg/kg or 0.01, 0.12, and 0.24 times the maximum human dose on a mg/m^2 basis. However, in a preliminary peri/postnatal study, there were increases in fetal and pup death, and decreases in mean litter weight at 150 mg/kg, or 3.0 times the maximum human dose on a mg/m^2 basis.

There are no adequate and well-controlled studies in pregnant women, and quetiapine should be used during pregnancy only if the potential benefit justifies the potential risk to the fetus.

Labor and Delivery: The effect of SEROQUEL on labor and delivery in humans is unknown.

Nursing Mothers: SEROQUEL was excreted in milk of treated animals during lactation. It is not known if SEROQUEL is excreted in human milk. It is recommended that women receiving SEROQUEL should not breast feed.

Pediatric Use: The safety and effectiveness of SEROQUEL in pediatric patients have not been established.

Geriatric Use: Of the approximately 2400 patients in clinical studies with SEROQUEL, 8% (190) were 65 years of age or over. In general, there was no indication of any different tolerability of SEROQUEL in the elderly compared to younger adults. Nevertheless, the presence of factors that might decrease pharmacokinetic clearance, increase the pharmacodynamic response to SEROQUEL, or cause poorer tolerance or orthostasis, should lead to consideration of a lower starting dose, slower titration, and careful monitoring during the initial dosing period in the elderly. The mean plasma clearance of SEROQUEL was reduced by 30% to 50% in elderly patients when compared to younger patients. (see Pharmacokinetics under **CLINICAL PHARMACOLOGY** and **DOSAGE AND ADMINISTRATION**).

ADVERSE REACTIONS

The premarketing development program for SEROQUEL included over 2600 patients and/or normal subjects exposed to 1 or more doses of SEROQUEL. Of these 2600 subjects, approximately 2300 were patients who participated in multiple-dose effectiveness trials, and their experience corresponded to approximately 865 patient-years. The conditions and duration of treatment with SEROQUEL varied greatly and included (in overlapping categories) open-label and double-blind phases of studies, inpatients and outpatients, fixed-dose and dose-titration studies, and short-term or longer-term exposure. Adverse reactions were assessed by collecting adverse events, results of physical examinations, vital signs, weights, laboratory analyses, ECGs, and results of ophthalmologic examinations.

Adverse events during exposure were obtained by general inquiry and recorded by clinical investigators using terminology of their own choosing. Consequently, it is not possible to provide a meaningful estimate of the proportion of individuals experiencing adverse events without first grouping similar types of events into a smaller number of standardized event categories. In the tables and tabulations that follow, standard COSTART terminology has been used to classify reported adverse events.

The stated frequencies of adverse events represent the proportion of individuals who experienced, at least once, a treatment-emergent adverse event of the type listed. An event was considered treatment emergent if it occurred for the first time of worsened while receiving therapy following baseline evaluation.

Adverse Findings Observed in Short-Term, Controlled Trials

Adverse Events Associated with Discontinuation of Treatment in Short-Term, Placebo-Controlled Trials

Overall, there was little difference in the incidence of discontinuation due to adverse events (4% of SEROQUEL vs. 3% for placebo) in a pool of controlled trials. However, discontinuations due to somnolence and hypotension were considered to be drug related (see **PRECAUTIONS**):

Adverse Event	SEROQUEL	Placebo
Somnolence	0.8%	0%
Hypotension	0.4%	0%

Adverse Events Occurring at an Incidence of 1% or More Among SEROQUEL Treated Patients in Short-Term, Placebo-Controlled Trials: Table 1 enumerates the incidence, rounded in the nearest percent, of treatment-emergent adverse events that occurred during acute therapy (up to 6 weeks) of schizophrenia in 1% or more of patients treated with SEROQUEL (doses ranging from 75 to 750 mg/day) where the incidence in patients treated with SEROQUEL was greater than the incidence in placebo-treated patients. The prescriber should be aware that the figures in the tables and tabulations cannot be used to predict the incidence of side effects in the course of usual medical practice where patient characteristics and other factors differ from those that prevailed in the clinical trials. Similarly, the cited frequencies cannot be compared with figures obtained from other clinical investigations involving different treatments, uses, and investigators. The cited figures, however, do provide the prescribing physician with some basis for estimating the relative contribution of drug and nondrug factors to the side effect incidence in the population studied.

In these studies, the most commonly observed adverse events associated with the use of SEROQUEL (incidence of 5% or greater) and observed at a rate on SEROQUEL at least twice that of placebo were dizziness (10%), postural hypotension (7%), dry mouth (7%), and dyspepsia (6%).

[See table 1 at bottom of next page]

Explorations for interactions on the basis of gender, age, and race did not reveal any clinically meaningful differences in the adverse event occurrence on the basis of these demographic factors.

Dose Dependency of Adverse Events in Short-Term, Placebo-Controlled Trials

Dose-related Adverse Events: Spontaneously elicited adverse event data from a study comparing five fixed doses of SEROQUEL (75 mg, 150 mg, 300 mg, 600 mg, and 750 mg/day) to placebo were explored for dose-relatedness of adverse events. Logistic regression analyses revealed a positive dose response ($p<0.05$) for the following adverse events: dyspepsia, abdominal pain, and weight gain.

Extrapyramidal Symptoms: Data from one 6-week clinical trial comparing five fixed doses of SEROQUEL (75, 150, 300, 600, 750 mg/day) provided evidence for the lack of treatment-emergent extrapyramidal symptoms (EPS) and dose-relatedness of EPS associated with SEROQUEL treatment. Three methods were used to measure EPS (1) Simpson-Angus total score (mean change from baseline) which evaluates parkinsonism and akathisia, (2) incidence of spontaneous complaints of EPS (akathisia, akinesia, cogwheel rigidity, extrapydramidal syndrome, hypertonia, hypokinesia, neck rigidity, and tremor), and (3) use of anticholinergic medications to treat emergent EPS.

[See table at bottom of next page]

In three additional placebo-controlled clinical trials using variable doses of SEROQUEL, there were no differences between the SEROQUEL and placebo treatment groups in the incidence of EPS, as assessed by Simpson-Angus total scores, spontaneous complaints of EPS, and the use of concomitant anticholinergic medications to treat EPS.

Vital Sign Changes: SEROQUEL is associated with orthostatic hypotension (see **PRECAUTIONS**).

Weight Gain: The proportions of patients meeting a weight gain criterion of ≥7% of body weight were compared in a pool of four 3- to 6-week placebo-controlled clinical trials, revealing a statistically significantly greater incidence of weight gain for SEROQUEL (23%) compared to placebo (6%).

Laboratory Changes: An assessment of the premarketing experience for SEROQUEL suggested that it is associated with asymptomatic increases in SGPT and increases in both total cholesterol and triglycerides (see **PRECAUTIONS**).

An assessment of hematological parameters in short-term, placebo-controlled trials revealed no clinical important differences between SEROQUEL and placebo.

ECG Changes: Between group comparisons for pooled placebo-controlled trials revealed no statistically significant SEROQUEL/placebo differences in the proportions of patients experiencing potentially important changes in ECG parameters, including QT, QTc, and PR intervals. However, the proportions of patients meeting the criteria for tachycardia were compared in four 3- 6-week-placebo-controlled clinical trials revealing a 1% (4/399) incidence for SEROQUEL compared to 0.6% (1/156) incidence for placebo. SEROQUEL use was associated with a mean increase in heart rate, assessed by ECG, of 7 beats per minute compared to a mean increase of 1 beat per minute among placebo patients. This slight tendency to tachycardia may be related to SEROQUEL's potential for inducing orthostatic changes (see **PRECAUTIONS**).

Other Adverse Events Observed During the Premarketing Evaluation of SEROQUEL

Following is a list of COSTART terms that reflect treatment-emergent adverse events as defined in the introduction to the ADVERSE REACTIONS section reported by patients treated with SEROQUEL at multiple doses ≥ 75 mg/day during any phase of a trial within the premarketing database of approximately 2200 patients. All reported events are included except those already listed in Table 1 or elsewhere in labeling, those events for which a drug cause was remote, and those event terms which were so general as to be uninformative. It is important to emphasize that, although the events reported occurred during treatment with SEROQUEL, they were not necessarily caused by it.

Events are further categorized by body system and listed in order of decreasing frequency according to the following definitions: frequent adverse events are those occurring in at least 1/100 patients (only those not already listed in the tabulated results from placebo-controlled trials appear in this listing); infrequent adverse events are those occurring in 1/100 to 1/1000 patients; rare events are those occurring in fewer than 1/1000 patients.

Nervous System: ***Frequent:*** hypertonia, dysarthria; ***Infrequent:*** abnormal dreams, dyskinesia, thinking abnormal, tardive dyskinesia, vertigo, involuntary movements, confusion, amnesia, psychosis, hallucinations, hyperkinesia, libido increased* urinary retention, incoordination, paranoid reaction, abnormal gait, myoclonus, delusions, manic reaction, apathy, ataxia, depersonalization, stupor, bruxism, catatonic reaction, hemiplegia; ***Rare:*** aphasia, buccoglossal syndrome, choreoathetosis, delirium, emotional lability, euphoria, libido decreased*, neuralgia, stuttering, subdural hematoma.

Body as a Whole: ***Frequent:*** flu syndrome; ***Infrequent:*** neck pain, pelvic pain*, suicide attempt, malaise, photosensitivity reaction, chills face edema, moniliasis; ***Rare:*** abdomen enlarged.

Digestive System: ***Frequent:*** anorexia; ***Infrequent:*** increased salivation, increased appetite, gamma glutamyl transpeptidase increased, gingivitis, dysphagia, flatulence, gastroenteritis, gastritis, hemorrhoids, stomatitis, thirst, tooth caries, fecal incontinence, gastroesophageal reflux, gum hemorrhage, mouth ulceration, rectal hemorrhage, tongue edema; ***Rare:*** glossitis, hematemesis, intestinal obstruction, melena, pancreatitis.

Cardiovascular System: ***Frequent:*** palitation; ***Infrequent:*** vasodilatation, QT interval prolonged, migraine, bradycardia, cerebral ischemia, irregular pulse, T wave abnormality, bundle branch block, cerebrovascular accident, deep thrombophlebitis, T wave inversion; ***Rare:*** angina pectoris, atrial fibrillation, AV block first degree, congestive heart failure, ST elevated, thrombophlebitis, T wave flattening, ST abnormality, increased QRS duration.

Respiratory System: ***Frequent:*** pharyngitis, rhinitis, cough increased, dyspnea; ***Infrequent:*** pneumonia, epistaxis, asthma; ***Rare:*** hiccup, hyperventilation.

Metabolic and Nutritional System: ***Frequent:*** peripheral edema; ***Infrequent:*** weight loss, alkaline phosphatase increased, hyperlipemia, alcohol intolerance, dehydration, hyperglycemia, creatinine increased, hypoglycemia; ***Rare:*** glycosuria, gout, hand edema, hypokalemia, water intoxication.

Skin and Appendages System: ***Frequent:*** sweating; ***Infrequent:*** pruritis, acne, eczema, contact dermatitis, maculopapular rash, seborrhea, skin ulcer; ***Rare:*** exfoliative dermatitis, psoriasis, skin discoloration.

Urogenital System: ***Infrequent:*** dysmenorrhea*, vaginitis*, urinary incontinence, metorrhagia*, impotence*, dysuria, vaginal moniliasis*, abnormal ejaculation*, cystitis, urinary frequency, amenorrhea*, female lactation*, leukorrhea*, vaginal hemorrhage*, vulvovaginitis* orchitis*; ***Rare:*** gynecomastia*, nocturia, polyuria, acute kidney failure.

Special Senses: ***Infrequent:*** conjunctivitis, abnormal vision, dry eyes, tinnitus, taste perversion, blepharitis, eye pain; ***Rare:*** abnormality of accommodation, deafness, glaucoma.

Musculoskeletal System: ***Infrequent:*** pathological fracture, myasthenia, twitching, arthralgia, arthritis, leg cramps, bone pain.

Hemic and Lymphatic System: ***Frequent:*** leukopenia; ***Infrequent:*** leukocytosis, anemia, ecchymosis, eosinophilia, hypochromic anemia; lymphadenopathy, cyanosis; ***Rare:*** hemolysis, thrombocytopenia.

Endorcine System: ***Infrequent:*** hypothyroidism, diabetes mellitus; ***Rare:*** hyperthyroidism.

*adjusted for gender

DRUG ABUSE AND DEPENDENCE

Controlled Substance Class: SEROQUEL is not a controlled substance.

Physical and Psychologic dependence: SEROQUEL has not been systematically studied, in animals or humans, for its potential for abuse, tolerance, or physical dependence. While the clinical trials did not reveal any tendency for any drug-seeking behavior, these observations were not systematic, and it is not possible to predict on the basis of this limited experience the extent to which a CNS-active drug will be misused, diverted, and/or abused once marketed. Consequently, patients should be evaluated carefully for a history of drug abuse, and such patients should be observed closely for signs of misuse or abuse of SEROQUEL, e.g., development of tolerance, increases in dose, drug-seeking behavior.

Table 1. Treatment-Emergent Adverse Experience Incidence in 3- to 6-Week Placebo-Controlled Clinical Trials[1]

Body System/ Preferred Term	SEROQUEL (n=510)	Placebo (n=206)
Body as a Whole		
Headache	19%	18%
Asthenia	4%	3%
Abdominal pain	3%	1%
Back pain	2%	1%
Fever	2%	1%
Nervous System		
Somnolence	18%	11%
Dizziness	10%	4%
Digestive System		
Constipation	9%	5%
Dry Mouth	7%	3%
Dyspepsia	6%	2%
Cardiovascular System		
Postural hypotension	7%	2%
Tachycardia	7%	5%
Metabolic and Nutritional Disorders		
Weight gain	2%	0%
Skin and Appendages		
Rash	4%	3%
Respiratory System		
Rhinitis	3%	1%
Special Senses		
Ear pain	1%	0%

[1] Events for which the SEROQUEL incidence was equal to or less than placebo are not listed in the table, but included the following: pain, infection, chest pain, hostility, accidental injury, hypertension, hypotension, nausea, vomiting, diarrhea, myalgia, agitation, insomnia, anxiety, nervousness, akathisia, hypertonia, tremor, depression, paresthesia, pharyngitis, dry skin, amblyopia, and urinary tract infection.

Dose Groups	Placebo	SEROQUEL 75 mg	150 mg	300 mg	600 mg	750 mg
Parkinsonism	-0.6	-1.0	-1.2	-1.6	-1.8	-1.8
EPS incidence	16%	6%	6%	4%	8%	6%
Anticholinergic Medications	14%	11%	10%	8%	12%	11%

OVERDOSAGE

Human experience: Experience with SEROQUEL® (quetiapine fumarate) in acute overdosage was limited in the clinical trial database (6 reports) with estimated doses ranging from 1200 mg to 9600 mg and no fatalities. In general, reported signs and symptoms were those resulting from an exaggeration of the drug's known pharmacological effects, i.e., drowsiness and sedation, tachycardia and hypotension. One case, involving an estimated overdose of 9600 mg, was associated with hypokalemia and first degree heart block.

Management of Overdosage: In case of acute overdosage, establish and maintain an airway and ensure adequate oxygenation and ventilation. Gastric lavage (after intubation, if patient is unconscious) and administration of activated charcoal together with a laxative should be considered. The possibility of obtundation, seizure or dystonic reaction of the head and neck following overdose may create a risk of aspiration with induced emesis. Cardiovascular monitoring should commence immediately and should include continuous electrocardiographic monitoring to detect possible arrhythmias. If antiarrhythmic therapy is administered, disopyramide, procainamide and quinidine carry a theoretical hazard of additive QT-prolonging effects when administered in patients with acute overdosage of SEROQUEL. Similarly it is reasonable to expect that the alpha-adrenergic-blocking properties of bretylium might be additive to those of quetiapine, resulting in problematic hypotension.

There is no specific antidote to SEROQUEL. Therefore appropriate supportive measures should be instituted. The possibility of multiple drug involvement should be considered. Hypotension and circulatory collapse should be treated with appropriate measures such as intravenous fluids and/or sympathomimetic agents (epinephrine and dopamine should not be used, since beta stimulation may worsen hypotension in the setting of quetiapine-induced alpha blockade). In case of severe extrapyramidal symptoms, anticholinergic medication should be administered. Close medical supervision and monitoring should continue until the patient recovers.

DOSAGE AND ADMINISTRATION

Usual Dose: SEROQUEL should generally be administered with an initial dose of 25 mg bid, with increases in increments of 25–50 mg bid or tid on the second and third day, as tolerated, to a target dose range of 300 to 400 mg daily by the fourth day, given bid or tid. Further dosage adjustments, if indicated, should generally occur at intervals of not less than 2 days, as steady state for SEROQUEL would not be achieved for approximately 1–2 days in the typical patient. When dosage adjustments are necessary, dose increments/decrements of 25–50 mg bid are recommended. Most efficacy data with SEROQUEL were obtained using tid regimens, but in one controlled trial 225 mg bid was also effective.

Antipsychotic efficacy was demonstrated in a dose range of 150 to 750 mg/day in the clinical trials supporting the effectiveness of SEROQUEL. In a dose response study, doses above 300 mg/day were not demonstrated to be more efficacious than the 300 mg/day dose. In other studies, however, doses in the range of 400–500 mg/day appeared to be needed. The safety of doses above 800 mg/day has not been evaluated in clinical trials.

Dosing in Special Populations

Consideration should be given to a slower rate of dose titration and a lower target dose in the elderly, in patients with hepatic impairment, and in patients who are debilitated or who had a predisposition to hypotensive reactions (see **CLINICAL PHARMACOLOGY**). When indicated, dose escalation should be performed with caution in these patients. The elimination of quetiapine was enhanced in the presence of phenytoin. Higher maintenance doses of quetiapine may be required when it is coadministered with phenytoin and other enzyme inducers such as carbamazepine and phenobarbital. (See Drug Interactions under **PRECAUTIONS**)

Maintenance Treatment: While there is no body of evidence available to answer the question of how long the patient treated with SEROQUEL should remain on it, the effectiveness of maintenance treatment is well established for many other antipsychotic drugs. It is recommended that responding patients be continued on SEROQUEL, but at the lowest dose needed to maintain remission. Patients should be periodically reassessed to determine the need for maintenance treatment.

Reinitiation of Treatment in Patients Previously Discontinued: Although there are no data to specifically address reinitiation of treatment, it is recommended that when restarting patients who have had an interval of less than one week off SEROQUEL, titration of SEROQUEL is not required, and the maintenance dose may be reinitiated. When restarting therapy of patients who have been off SEROQUEL for more than one week, the initial titration schedule should be followed.

Switching from Other Antipsychotics: There are no systematically collected data to specifically address switching from other antipsychotics to SEROQUEL.

Continued on next page

Seroquel—Cont.

HOW SUPPLIED

25 mg Tablets (NDC 0310-0275) peach, round, biconvex, film coated tablets, identified with 'SEROQUEL' and '25' on one side and plain on the other side, are supplied in bottles of 100 tablets and hospital unit dose packages of 100 tablets.

100 mg Tablets (NDC 0310-0271) yellow, round, biconvex film coated tablets, identified with 'SEROQUEL' and '100' on one side and plain on the other side, are supplied in bottles of 100 tablets and hospital unit dose packages of 100 tablets.

200 mg Tablets (NDC 0310-0272) white, round, biconvex, film coated tablets, identified with 'SEROQUEL' and '200' on one side and plain on the other side, are supplied in bottles of 100 tablets and hospital unit dose packages of 100 tablets.

Store at 25°C (77°F) excursions permitted to 15–30°C (59–86°F). [See USP]

ANIMAL TOXICOLOGY

Quetiapine caused a dose-related increase in pigment deposition in thyroid gland in rat toxicity studies which were 4 weeks in duration or longer and in a mouse 2-year carcinogenicity study. Doses were 10–250 mg/kg in rats, 75–750 mg/kg in mice; these doses are 0.1–3.0, and 0.1–4.5 times the maximum recommended human dose (on a mg/m^2 basis), respectively. Pigment deposition was shown to be irreversible in rats. The identity of the pigment could not be determined, but was found to be co-localized with quetiapine in thyroid gland follicular epithelial cells. The functional effects and the relevance of this finding to human risk are unknown.

In dogs receiving quetiapine for 6 or 12 months, but not for 1 month, focal triangular cataracts occurred at the junction of posterior sutures in the outer cortex of the lens at a dose of 100 mg/kg, or 4 times the maximum recommended human dose on a mg/m^2 basis. This finding may be due to inhibition of cholesterol biosynthesis by quetiapine. Quetiapine caused a dose related reduction in plasma cholesterol levels in repeat-dose dog and monkey studies; however, there was no correlation between plasma cholesterol and the presence of cataracts in individual dogs. The appearance of delta-8-cholestanol in plasma is consistent with inhibition of a late stage in cholesterol biosynthesis in these species. There also was a 25% reduction in cholesterol content of the outer cortex of the lens observed in a special study in quetiapine treated female dogs. Drug-related cataracts have not been seen in any other species; however, in a 1-year study in monkeys, a striated appearance of the anterior lens surface was detected in 2/7 females at a dose of 225 mg/kg or 5.5 times the maximum recommended human dose on a mg/m^2 basis.

Manufactured by:
ZENECA
Pharmaceuticals
A Business Unit of Zeneca Inc.
Wilmington, Delaware 19850-5347
64122-00 Rev C 11/97

Shown in Product Identification Guide, page 346

SORBITRATE® ℞

[*sorb 'i-trate*]
(Isosorbide Dinitrate)

DESCRIPTION

Isosorbide dinitrate (ISDN) is 1,4:3,6-dianhydro-D-glucitol 2,5-dinitrate, an organic nitrate whose structural formula is:

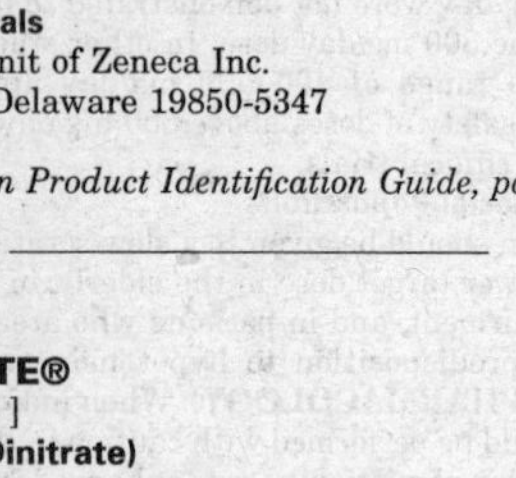

and whose molecular weight is 236.14. The organic nitrates are vasodilators, active on both arteries and veins.

Isosorbide dinitrate is a white, crystalline, odorless compound which is stable in air and in solution, has a melting point of 70°C and has an optical rotation of +134° (c = 1.0, alcohol, 20°C). Isosorbide dinitrate is freely soluble in organic solvents such as acetone, alcohol, and ether; but is only sparingly soluble in water.

SORBITRATE is available as:

SORBITRATE® CHEWABLE TABLETS USP

5 mg Chewable Tablet. Each tablet contains 5 mg of isosorbide dinitrate. Inactive Ingredients: Blue 1, confectioner's sugar, corn starch, flavor, hydrogenated vegetable oil, magnesium stearate, mannitol, povidone, Yellow 10.

SORBITRATE® ORAL TABLETS USP

5 mg Oral Tablet. Each tablet contains 5 mg of isosorbide dinitrate. Inactive Ingredients: Blue 1, corn starch, lactose (hydrous), magnesium stearate, pregelatinized starch, Yellow 10.

10 mg Oral Tablet. Each tablet contains 10 mg of isosorbide dinitrate. Inactive Ingredients: corn starch, lactose (hydrous), magnesium stearate, pregelatinized starch, Yellow 10.

20 mg Oral Tablet. Each tablet contains 20 mg of isosorbide dinitrate. Inactive Ingredients: Blue 1, corn starch, lactose (hydrous), magnesium stearate, pregelatinized starch.

30 mg Oral Tablet. Each tablet contains 30 mg of isosorbide dinitrate. Inactive Ingredients: corn starch, lactose (hydrous), magnesium stearate, pregelatinized starch.

40 mg Oral Tablet. Each tablet contains 40 mg of isosorbide dinitrate. Inactive Ingredients: Blue 1, corn starch, lactose (hydrous), magnesium stearate, pregelatinized starch.

CLINICAL PHARMACOLOGY

The principal pharmacological action of isosorbide dinitrate is relaxation of vascular smooth muscle and consequent dilatation of peripheral arteries and veins, especially the latter. Dilatation of the veins promotes peripheral pooling of blood and decreases venous return to the heart, thereby reducing left ventricular end-diastolic pressure and pulmonary capillary wedge pressure (preload). Arteriolar relaxation reduces systemic vascular resistance, systolic arterial pressure, and mean arterial pressure (afterload). Dilatation of the coronary arteries also occurs. The relative importance of preload reduction, afterload reduction, and coronary dilatation remains undefined.

Dosing regimens for most chronically used drugs are designed to provide plasma concentrations that are continuously greater than a minimally effective concentration. This strategy is inappropriate for for organic nitrates. Several well-controlled clinical trials have used exercise testing to assess the anti-anginal efficacy of continuously-delivered nitrates. In the large majority of these trials, active agents were no more effective than placebo after 24 hours (or less) of continuous therapy. Attempts to overcome nitrate tolerance by dose escalation, even to doses far in excess of those used acutely, have consistently failed. Only after nitrates have been absent from the body for several hours has their anti-anginal efficacy been restored.

Pharmacokinetics: Once absorbed, the distribution volume of isosorbide dinitrate is 2–4 L/kg, and this volume is cleared at the rate of 2–4 L/min, so ISDN's half-life in serum is about an hour. Since the clearance exceeds hepatic blood flow, considerable extrahepatic metabolism must also occur. Clearance is effected primarily by denitration to the 2-mononitrate (15%–25%) and the 5-mononitrate (75%–85%).

Both metabolites have biological activity, especially the 5-mononitrate. With an overall half-life of about 5 hours, the 5-mononitrate is cleared from the serum by denitration to isosorbide; glucuronidation to the 5-mononitrate glucuronide; and denitration/hydration to sorbitol. The 2-mononitrate has been less well studied, but it appears to participate in the same metabolic pathways, with a half-life of about 2 hours.

The daily dose-free interval sufficient to avoid tolerance to organic nitrates has not been well defined. Studies of nitroglycerin (an organic nitrate with a very short half-life) have shown that daily dose-free intervals of 10–12 hours are usually sufficient to minimize tolerance. Daily dose-free intervals that have succeeded in avoiding tolerance during trials of moderate doses (eg, 30 mg) of immediate-release ISDN have generally been somewhat longer (at least 14 hours), but this is consistent with the longer half-lives of ISDN and its active metabolites.

Few well-controlled clinical trials of organic nitrates have been designed to detect rebound or withdrawal effects. In one such trial, however, subjects receiving nitrogylcerin had *less* exercise tolerance at the end of the daily dose-free interval than the parallel group receiving placebo. The incidence, magnitude, and clinical significance of similar phenomena in patients receiving ISDN have not been studied.

Bioavailability of ISDN after single sublingual doses is 40%–50%. Multiple-dose studies of sublingual ISDN pharmacokinetics have not been reported; multiple-dose studies of ingested ISDN have observed progressive increases in bioavailability during chronic therapy. Serum levels of ISDN reach their maxima 10–15 minutes after sublingual dosing.

Absorption of isosorbide dinitrate after oral dosing is nearly complete, but bioavailability is highly varible (10%–90%), with extensive first-pass metabolism in the liver. Serum levels reach their maxima about an hour after ingestion. The average bioavailability of ISDN is about 25%; most studies have observed progressive increases in bioavailability during chronic therapy.

The absorption kinetics of chewable isosorbide dinitrate tablets have not been studied. Absorption of ingested ISDN is known to be nearly complete, although bioavailability is highly variable. Ingested ISDN undergoes extensive first-pass metabolism in the liver; it is not known what portion of this first-pass effect is avoided by buccal absorption of the chewable formulation.

Kinetic studies of absorption of immediate-release formulations of ISDN have found highly variable bioavailability with extensive first-pass metabolism in the liver. Most such studies have observed progressive increases in bioavailability during chronic therapy.

Clinical Trials: In a controlled trial in which 0.4 mg of sublingual nitroglycerin took 1.9 minutes to begin to produce an anti-anginal effect, 5 mg of sublingual ISDN took 3.4 minutes to begin to produce a similar effect. In the same trial, the anti-anginal effect of the sublingual nitrogylcerin was evident for about an hour, while that of the sublingual ISDN lasted about 2 hours.

In other controlled trials, the anti-anginal efficacy of sublingual ISDN has persisted for periods ranging from 30 minutes up to 4 hours.

Multiple-dose trials of sublingual ISDN have not been reported. Multiple-dose trials of ingested formulations of ISDN have shown that ISDN's anti-anginal efficacy is substantially attenuated by tolerance unless the daily regimen does not include at least one interdosing interval of at least 14 hours. The daily interdosing interval necessary in any chronic regimen using sublingual ISDN is not known.

In clinical trials, immediate-release oral isosorbide dinitrate has been administered in a variety of regimens, with total daily doses ranging from 30 mg to 480 mg.

Controlled trials of single oral doses of isosorbide dinitrate have demonstrated effective reductions in exercise-related angina for up to 8 hours. Anti-anginal activity is present about 1 hour after dosing.

Most controlled trials of multiple-dose oral ISDN taken every 12 hours (or more frequently) for several weeks have shown statistically significant anti-anginal efficacy for only 2 hours after dosing. Once-daily regimens, and regimens with at least one daily interval of at least 14 hours (eg, a regimen providing doses at 0800, 1400 and 1800) have shown efficacy after the first dose of each day that was similar to that shown in the single-dose studies cited above.

In controlled trials in which sublingual nitroglycerin took $1\frac{1}{2}$–2 minutes to begin to produce an anti-anginal effect, chewable ISDN tablets took $2\frac{1}{2}$–3 minutes to begin to produce a similar effect. In these same trials, the anti-anginal effect of sublingual nitroglycerin was evident for about 1–$1\frac{1}{2}$ hours, while that of chewable ISDN lasted about an hour longer.

Clinical trials of chewable ISDN have used doses of 5 and 10 mg. It is not known whether lower doses would be equally effective.

Multiple-dose trials of chewable ISDN have not been reported. Multiple-dose trials of ingested formulations of ISDN have shown that ISDN's anti-anginal efficacy is substantially attenuated by tolerance unless the daily regimen does not include at least one interdosing interval of at least 14 hours. The daily interdosing interval necessary in any chronic regimen using chewable ISDN is, because of the rapid onset of action of this formulation, probably somewhat longer.

From large, well-controlled studies of other nitrates, it is reasonable to believe that the maximal achievable daily duration of anti-anginal effect from isosorbide dinitrate is about 12 hours. No dosing regimen for isosorbide dinitrate has, however, ever actually been shown to achieve this duration of effect. In the absence of data from multiple-dose trials, and considering the capacity of organic nitrates to induce tolerance, it is not reasonable to assume that multiple sublingual ISDN tablets taken during the course of a day will all have similar effects.

INDICATIONS AND USAGE

SORBITRATE sublingual tablets and chewable tablets are indicated for the prevention and treatment of angina pectoris due to coronary artery disease. However, because the onset of action of these tablets is significantly slower than that of sublingual nitroglycerin, they are not the drug of first choice for abortion of an acute anginal episode.

SORBITRATE oral tablets are indicated for the prevention of angina pectoris due to coronary artery disease. The onset of action of immediate release oral isosorbide dinitrate is not sufficiently rapid for this product to be useful in aborting an acute anginal episode.

CONTRAINDICATIONS

Allergic reactions to organic nitrates are extremely rare, but they do occur. Isosorbide dinitrate is contraindicated in patients who are allergic to it or other nitrates.

WARNINGS

The benefits of isosorbide dinitrate in patients with acute myocardial infarction or congestive heart failure have not been established. If one elects to use isosorbide dinitrate in these conditions, careful clinical or hemodynamic monitor-

ing must be used to avoid the hazards of hypotension and tachycardia. Because the effects of oral and chewable ISDN tablets are so difficult to terminate rapidly, this formulation is not recommended in these settings.

PRECAUTIONS

General: Severe hypotension, particularly with upright posture, may occur with even small doses of isosorbide dinitrate. This drug should therefore be used with caution in patients who may be volume depleted or who, for whatever reason (eg, diuretics), are already hypotensive. Hypotension induced by isosorbide dinitrate may be accompanied by paradoxical bradycardia and increased angina pectoris.

Nitrate therapy may aggravate the angina caused by hypertrophic cardiomyopathy.

As tolerance to isosorbide dinitrate develops, the effect of sublingual nitroglycerin on exercise tolerance, allthough still observable, is somewhat blunted.

In industrial workers who have had long-term exposure to unknown (presumably high) doses of organic nitrates, tolerance clearly occurs. Chest pain, acute myocardial infarction, and even sudden death have occurred during temporary withdrawal of nitrates from these workers, demonstrating the existence of true physical dependence.

Some clinical trials in angina patients have provided nitroglycerin for about 12 continuous hours of every 24-hour day. During the daily dose-free intervals in some of these trials, anginal attacks have been more easily provoked than before treatment, and patients have demonstrated hemodynamic rebound and decreased exercise tolerance. The importance of these observations to the routine, clinical use of isosorbide dinitrate is not known. It may be prudent to gradually withdraw patients from ISDN when the therapy is being terminated, rather than stopping the drug abruptly.

Information for Patients: Patients should be told that the anti-anginal efficacy of isosorbide dinitrate is strongly related to its dosing regimen, so the prescribed schedule of dosing should be followed carefully. In particular, daily headaches sometimes accompany treatment with isosorbide dinitrate. In patients who get these headaches, the headaches are a marker of the activity of the drug. Patients should resist the temptation to avoid headaches by altering the schedule of their treatment with isosorbide dinitrate, since loss of headache may be associated with simultaneous loss of anti-anginal efficacy. Aspirin and/or acetaminophen, on the other hand, often successfully relieve isosorbide dinitrate-induced headaches with no deleterious effect on isosorbide dinitrate's anti-anginal efficacy.

Treatment with isosorbide dinitrate may be associated with lightheadedness on standing, especially just after rising from a recumbent or seated position. This effect may be more frequent in patients who have also consumed alcohol.

DRUG INTERACTIONS

The vasodilating effects of isosorbide dinitrate may be additive with those of other vasodilators. Alcohol, in particular, has been found to exhibit additive effects of this variety.

ISDN acts directly on vascular smooth muscle; therefore, any other agent that acts on vascular smooth muscle can be expected to have decreased or increased effect depending on the agents.

Marked symptomatic, orthostatic hypotension has been reported when calcium channel blockers and organic nitrates were used in combination. Dose adjustment of either class of agents may be necessary.

Carcinogenesis, Mutagenesis, and Impairment of Fertility: No long-term studies in animals have been performed to evaluate the carcinogenic potential of isosorbide dinitrate. In a modified two-litter reproduction study, there was no remarkable gross pathology and no altered fertility or gestation among rats fed isosorbide dinitrate at 25 or 100 mg/kg/day.

Pregnancy: Pregnancy Category C: At oral doses 35 and 150 times the maximum recommended human daily dose, isosorbide dinitrate has been shown to cause a dose-related increase in embryotoxicity (increase in mummified pups) in rabbits. There are no adequate, well-controlled studies in pregnant women. Isosorbide dinitrate should be used during pregnancy only if the potential benefit justifies the potential risk to the fetus.

Nursing Mothers: It is not known whether isosorbide dinitrate is excreted is human milk. Because many drugs are excreted in human milk, caution should be exercised when isosorbide dinitrate is administered to a nursing woman.

Pediatric Use: Safety and effectiveness in pediatric patients have not been established.

ADVERSE REACTIONS

Adverse reactions to isosorbide dinitrate are generally dose-related, and almost all of these reactions are the result of isosorbide dinitrate's activity as a vasodilator. Headache, which may be severe and persistent, is the most commonly reported side effect. Headache may be recurrent with each daily dose, especially at higher doses. Cutaneous vasodilation with flushing may occur. Transient episodes of lightheadedness, dizziness, and weakness, as well as other signs of cerebral ischemia associated with postural hypotension, may also occur. Hypotension occurs infrequently, but in some patients it may be severe enough to warrant discontinuation of therapy. (See OVERDOSAGE.)

Syncope, crescendo angina, and rebound hypertension have been reported but are uncommon.

Extremely rarely, ordinary doses of organic nitrates have caused methemoglobinemia in normal seeming patients. Methemoglobinemia is so infrequent at these doses that further discussion of its diagnosis and treatment is deferred. (See OVERDOSAGE.)

Data are not available to allow estimation of the frequency of adverse reactions during treatment with SORBITRATE tablets.

OVERDOSAGE

Hemodynamic Effects: The ill effects of isosorbide dinitrate overdose are generally the results of isosorbide dinitrate's capacity to induce vasodilatation, venous pooling, reduced cardiac output, and hypotension. These hemodynamic changes may have protean manifestations, including increased intracranial pressure, with any or all of the following: persistent throbbing headache, confusion, and moderate fever; vertigo; palpitations; visual disturbances; nausea and vomiting (possibly with colic and even bloody diarrhea); syncope (especially in the upright posture); initial hyperpnea; air hunger; and dyspnea, later followed by slow breathing and/or reduced ventilatory effort; diaphoresis, with the skin either flushed or cold and clammy; heart block and bradycardia; paralysis; coma; seizures; and death.

Laboratory determinations of serum levels of isosorbide dinitrate and its metabolites are not widely available, and such determinations have, in any event, no established role in the management of isosorbide dinitrate overdose.

There are no data suggesting what dose of isosorbide dinitrate is likely to be life-threatening in humans. In rats, the median acute lethal dose (LD_{50}) was found to be 1100 mg/kg (approximately 500 times the recommended therapeutic dose in humans).

No data are available to suggest physiological maneuvers (eg, maneuvers to change the pH of the urine) that might accelerate elimination of isosorbide dinitrate and its active metabolites. Similarly, it is not known which—if any—of these substances can usefully be removed from the body by hemodialysis.

No specific antagonist to the vasodilator effects of isosorbide dinitrate is known, and no intervention has been subject to controlled study as a therapy of isosorbide dinitrate overdose. Because the hypotension associated with isosorbide dinitrate overdose is the result of venodilatation and arterial hypovolemia, prudent therapy in this situation should be directed toward increase in central fluid volume. Passive elevation of the patient's legs and passive movement of extremities may be sufficient, but intravenous infusion of normal saline or similar fluid may also be necessary.

The use epinephrine or other arterial vasoconstrictors in this setting is likely to do more harm than good.

In patients with renal disease or congestive heart failure, therapy resulting in central volume expansion is not without hazard. Treatment of isosorbide dinitrate overdose in these patients may be subtle and difficult, and invasive monitoring may be required.

Methemoglobinemia: Nitrate ions liberated during metabolism of isosorbide dinitrate can oxidize hemoglobin into methemoglobin. Even in patients totally without cytochrome b_5 reductase activity, however, and even assuming that the nitrate moieties of isosorbide dinitrate are quantitatively applied to oxidation of hemoglobin, about 1 mg/kg of isosorbide dinitrate should be required before any of these patients manifests clinically significant ($\geq$10%) methemoglobinemia. In patients with normal reductase function, significant production of methemoglobin should require even larger doses of isosorbide dinitrate. In one study in which 36 patients received 2–4 weeks of continuous nitroglycerin therapy at 3.1 to 4.4 mg/hr (equivalent, in total administered dose of nitrate ions, to 4.8–6.9 mg of bioavailable isosorbide dinitrate per hour), the average methemoglobin level measured was 0.2%; this was comparable to that observed in parallel patients who received placebo.

Notwithstanding these observations, there are case reports of significant methemoglobinemia in association with moderate overdoses of organic nitrates. None of the affected patients had been thought to be unusually susceptible.

Methemoglobin levels are available from most clinical laboratories. The diagnosis should be suspected in patients who exhibit signs of impaired oxygen delivery despite adequate cardiac output and adequate arterial pO_2. Classically, methemoglobinemic blood is described as chocolate brown, without color change on exposure to air.

When methemoglobinemia is diagnosed, the treatment of choice is methylene blue, 1–2 mg/kg intravenously.

DOSAGE AND ADMINISTRATION

As noted above (**CLINICAL PHARMACOLOGY**), multiple studies with ISDN and other nitrates have shown that maintenance of continuous 24-hour plasma levels results in refractory tolerance. Every dosing regimen for ISDN must provide a daily dose-free interval to minimize the development of this tolerance. To achieve the necessary nitrate-free interval with immediate-release oral ISDN, it appears that at least one of the daily dose-free intervals must be at least 14 hours long. In the case of sublingual and chewable tablets, it is probably true that one of the daily dose-free intervals must be somewhat longer than 14 hours.

As also noted above (**CLINICAL PHARMACOLOGY**), the effects of the second and later doses have been smaller and shorter-lasting than the effects of the first.

Large controlled studies with other nitrates suggest that no dosing regimen with SORBITRATE Tablets should be expected to provide more than about 12 hours of continuous anti-anginal efficacy per day.

A patient anticipating activity likely to cause angina should take one SORBITRATE Chewable Tablet, 5 mg, about 15 minutes before the activity is expected to begin. SORBITRATE Sublingual Tablet, 2.5 mg to 5 mg, may be used to abort an acute anginal episode, but this use is recommended only in patients who fail to respond to sublingual nitroglycerin.

In clinical trials, immediate-release oral isosorbide dinitrate has been administered in a variety of regimens, with total daily doses ranging from 30 mg to 480 mg.

As with all titratable drugs, it is important to administer the minimum dose that produces the desired effect. The usual starting dose of SORBITRATE Oral Tablets is 5 mg to 20 mg, two or three times daily. For maintenance therapy, 10 mg to 40 mg, two to three times daily is recommended. Some patients may require higher doses. A daily dose-free interval of at least 14 hours is advisable to minimize tolerance. The optimal interval will vary with the individual patient, dose and regimen.

HOW SUPPLIED

SORBITRATE®Chewable Tablets USP

5 mg Chewable Tablets. (NDC-0310-0810) Green, round, scored tablets (identified front "S", reverse "810") are supplied in bottles of 100 and 500.

SORBITRATE Oral Tablets USP

5 mg Oral Tablets. (NDC-0310-0770) Green, oval-shaped, scored tablets (identified front "S", reverse "770") are supplied in bottles of 100 and 500 and Unit Dose 100.

10 mg Oral Tablets. (NDC-0310-0780) Yellow, oval-shaped, scored tablets (identified front "S", reverse "780") are supplied in bottles of 100, 500 and Unit Dose 100.

20 mg Oral Tablets. (NDC-0310-0820) Blue, oval-shaped, scored tablets (identified front "S", reverse "820") are supplied in bottles of 100 and Unit Dose 100.

30 mg Oral Tablets. (NDC-0310-0773) White, oval-shaped, scored tablets (identified front "S", reverse "773") are supplied in bottles of 100 and Unit Dose 100.

40 mg Oral Tablets. (NDC-0310-0774) Light Blue, oval-shaped, scored tablets (identified front "S", reverse "774") are supplied in bottles of 100 and Unit Dose 100.

Avoid storage at temperatures above 25°C (77°F).

Zeneca Pharmaceuticals
A Business Unit of Zeneca Inc.
Wilmington, DE 19850-5437

Rev P 02/98 SIC No. 64119-00

Shown in Product Identification Guide, page 346

SULAR® ℞

(Nisoldipine)
Extended Release Tablets
For Oral Use

DESCRIPTION

SULAR® (nisoldipine) is an extended release tablet dosage form of the dihydropyridine calcium channel blocker nisoldipine. Nisoldipine is 3,5-pyridinedicarboxylic acid, 1,4-dihydro-2,6-dimethyl-4-(2-nitrophenyl)-, methyl 2-methylpropyl ester, $C_{20}H_{24}N_2O_6$, and has the structural formula:

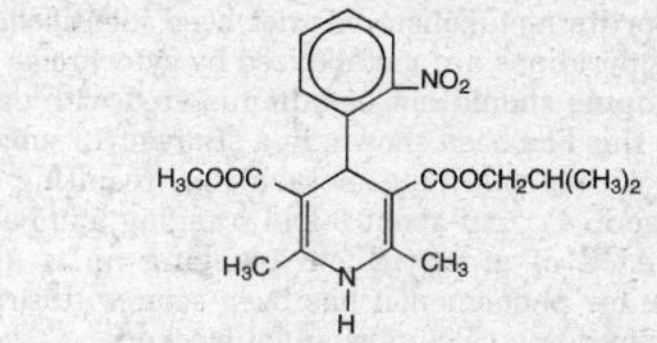

Nisoldipine is a yellow crystalline substance, practically insoluble in water but soluble in ethanol. It has a molecular weight of 388.4. SULAR tablets consist of an external coat and an internal core. Both coat and core contain nisoldipine, the coat as a slow release formulation and the core as a fast release formulation. SULAR tablets contain either 10, 20, 30 or 40 mg of nisoldipine for once-a-day oral administration.

Continued on next page

Sular—Cont.

Inert ingredients in the formulation are: hydroxypropylcellulose, lactose, corn starch, crospovidone, microcrystalline cellulose, sodium lauryl sulfate, povidone and magnesium stearate. The inert ingredients in the film coating are: hydroxypropylmethylcellulose, polyethylene glycol, ferric oxide, and titanium dioxide.

CLINICAL PHARMACOLOGY

Mechanism of Action

Nisoldipine is a member of the dihydropyridine class of calcium channel antagonists (calcium ion antagonists or slow channel blockers) that inhibit the transmembrane influx of calcium into vascular smooth muscle and cardiac muscle. It reversibly competes with other dihydropyridines for binding to the calcium channel. Because the contractile process of vascular smooth muscle is dependent upon the movement of extracellular calcium into the muscle through specific ion channels, inhibition of the calcium channel results in dilation of the arterioles. *In vitro* studies show that the effects of nisoldipine on contractile processes are selective, with greater potency on vascular smooth muscle than on cardiac muscle. Although, like other dihydropyridine calcium channel blockers, nisoldipine has negative inotropic effects *in vitro*, studies conducted in intact anesthetized animals have shown that the vasodilating effect occurs at doses lower than those that affect cardiac contractility.

The effect of nisoldipine on blood pressure is principally a consequence of a dose-related decrease of peripheral vascular resistance. While nisoldipine, like other dihydropyridines, exhibits a mild diuretic effect, most of the antihypertensive activity is attributed to its effect on peripheral vascular resistance.

Pharmacokinetics and Metabolism

Nisoldipine pharmacokinetics are independent of the dose in the range of 20 to 60 mg, with plasma concentrations proportional to dose. Nisoldipine accumulation, during multiple dosing, is predictable from a single dose.

Nisoldipine is relatively well absorbed into the systemic circulation with 87% of the radiolabeled drug recovered in urine and feces. The absolute bioavailability of nisoldipine is about 5%. Nisoldipine's low bioavailability is due, in part, to pre-systemic metabolism in the gut wall, and this metabolism decreases from the proximal to the distal parts of the intestine. Food with a high fat content has a pronounced effect on the release of of nisoldipine from the coat-core formulation and results in a significant increase in peak concentration (C_{max}) by up to 300%. Total exposure, however, is decreased about 25%, presumably because more of the drug is released proximally. This effect appears to be specific for nisoldipine in the controlled release formulation, as a less pronounced food effect was seen with the immediate release tablet. Concomitant intake of a high fat meal with SULAR should be avoided.

Maximal plasma concentrations of nisoldipine are reached 6 to 12 hours after dosing. The terminal elimination half-life (reflecting post absorption clearance of nisoldipine) ranges from 7 to 12 hours. C_{max} and AUC increase by factors of approximately 1.3 and 1.5, respectively, from first dose to steady state. After oral administration, the concentration of (+) nisoldipine, the active enantiomer, is about 6 times higher than the (−) inactive enantiomer. The plasma protein binding of nisoldipine is very high, with less than 1% unbound over the plasma concentration range of 100 ng/mL to 10 mcg/mL.

Nisoldipine is highly metabolized; 5 major urinary metabolites have been identified. Although 60–80% of an oral dose undergoes urinary excretion, only traces of unchanged nisoldipine are found in urine. The major biotransformation pathway appears to be the hydroxylation of the isobutyl ester. A hydroxylated derivative of the side chain, present in plasma at concentrations approximately equal to the parent compound, appears to be the only active metabolite, and has about 10% of the activity of the parent compound. Cytochrome P_{450} enzymes are believed to play a major role in the metabolism of nisoldipine. The particular isoenzyme system responsible for its metabolism has not been identified, but other dihydropyridines are metabolized by cytochrome P_{450} IIIA4. Nisoldipine should not be administered with grapefruit juice as this has been shown, in a study of 12 subjects, to interfere with nisoldipine metabolism, resulting in a mean increase in C_{max} of about 3-fold (ranging up to about 7-fold) and AUC of almost 2-fold (ranging up to about 5-fold). A similar phenomenon has been seen with several other dihydropyridine calcium channel blockers.

Special Populations

Renal dysfunction: Because renal elimination is not an important pathway, bioavailability and pharmacokinetics of SULAR were not significantly different in patients with various degrees of renal impairment. Dosing adjustments in patients with mild to moderate renal impairment are not necessary.

Geriatric: Elderly patients have been found to have 2 to 3 fold higher plasma concentrations (C_{max} and AUC) than young subjects. This should be reflected in more cautious dosing (See DOSAGE AND ADMINISTRATION).

Hepatic Insufficiency: In patients with liver cirrhosis given 10 mg SULAR, plasma concentrations of the parent compound were 4 to 5 times higher than those in healthy young subjects. Lower starting and maintenance doses should be used in cirrhotic patients (See DOSAGE AND ADMINISTRATION).

Gender and Race: The effect of gender or race on the pharmacokinetics of nisoldipine has not been investigated.

Disease States: Hypertension does not significantly alter the pharmacokinetics of nisoldipine.

Pharmacodynamics

Hemodynamic Effects

Administration of a single dose of nisoldipine leads to decreased systemic vascular resistance and blood pressure with a transient increase in heart rate. The change in heart rate is greater with immediate release nisoldipine preparations. The effect on blood pressure is directly related to the initial degree of elevation above normal. Chronic administration of nisoldipine results in a sustained decrease in vascular resistance and small increases in stroke index and left ventricular ejection fraction. A study of the immediate release formulation showed no effect of nisoldipine on the renin-angiotensin-aldosterone system or on plasma norepinephrine concentration in normals. Changes in blood pressure in hypertensive patients given SULAR were dose related over the range of 10–60 mg/day.

Nisoldipine does not appear to have significant negative inotropic activity in intact animals or humans, and did not lead to worsening of clinical heart failure in three small studies of patients with asymptomatic and symptomatic left ventricular dysfunction. There is little information, however, in patients with severe congestive heart failure, and all calcium channel blockers should be used with caution in any patient with heart failure.

Electropyhysiologic Effects

Nisoldipine has no clinically important chronotropic effects. Except for mild shortening of sinus cycle, SA conduction time and AH intervals, single oral doses up to 20 mg of immediate release nisoldipine did not significantly change other conduction parameters. Similar electrophysiologic effects were seen with single iv doses, which could be blunted in patients pre-treated with beta-blockers. Dose and plasma level related flattening or inversion of T-waves have been observed in a few small studies. Such reports were concentrated in patients receiving rapidly increased high doses in one study; the phenomenon has not been a cause of safety concern in large clinical trials.

Clinical Studies In Hypertension

The antihypertensive efficacy of SULAR was studied in 5 double-blind, placebo-controlled, randomized studies, in which over 600 patients were treated with SULAR as monotherapy and about 300 with placebo; 4 of the five studies compared 2 or 3 fixed doses while the fifth allowed titration from 10–40 mg. Once daily administration of SULAR produced sustained reductions in systolic and diastolic blood pressures over the 24 hour dosing interval in both supine and standing positions. The mean placebo-subtracted reductions in supine systolic and diastolic blood pressure at trough, 24 hours post-dose, in these studies, are shown below. Changes in standing blood pressure were similar:

MEAN SUPINE TROUGH SYSTOLIC AND DIASTOLIC BLOOD PRESSURE CHANGES (mm Hg)

SULAR Dose (mg/day)	10 mg	20 mg	30 mg	40 mg	60 mg	10–40 mg titrated
Systolic	8	11	11	14	15	15
Diastolic	3	5	7	7	10	8

In patients receiving atenolol, supine blood pressure reductions with SULAR at 20, 40 and 60 mg once daily were $^{12}/_{6}$, $^{19}/_{8}$ and $^{22}/_{10}$ mm Hg, respectively. The sustained antihypertensive effect of SULAR was demonstrated by 24 hour blood pressure monitoring and examination of peak and trough effects. The trough/peak ratios ranged from 70 to 100% for diastolic and systolic blood pressure. The mean change in heart rate in these studies was less than one beat per minute. In 4 of the 5 studies, patients received initial doses of 20–30 mg SULAR without incident (excessive effects on blood pressure or heart rate). The fifth study started patients on lower doses of SULAR.

Patient race and gender did not influence the blood pressure lowering effect of SULAR. Despite the higher plasma concentration of nisoldipine in the elderly, there was no consistent difference in their blood pressure response except that the 10 mg dose was somewhat more effective than in nonelderly patients. No postural effect on blood pressure was apparent and there was no evidence of tolerance to the antihypertensive effect of SULAR in patients treated for up to one year.

INDICATIONS AND USAGE

SULAR is indicated for the treatment of hypertension. It may be used alone or in combination with other antihypertensive agents.

CONTRAINDICATIONS

SULAR is contraindicated in patients with known hypersensitivity to dihydropyridine calcium channel blockers.

WARNINGS

Increased angina and/or myocardial infarction in patients with coronary artery disease: Rarely, patients, particularly those with severe obstructive coronary artery disease, have developed increased frequency, duration and/or severity of angina, or acute myocardial infarction on starting calcium channel blocker therapy or at the time of dosage increase. The mechanism of this effect has not been established. In controlled studies of SULAR in patients with angina this was seen about 1.5% of the time in patients given nisoldipine, compared with 0.9% in patients given placebo.

PRECAUTIONS

General

Hypotension: Because nisoldipine, like other vasodilators, decreases peripheral vascular resistance, careful monitoring of blood pressure during the initial administration and titration of SULAR is recommended. Close observation is especially important for patients already taking medications that are known to lower blood pressure. Although in most patients the hypotensive effect of SULAR is modest and well tolerated, occasional patients have had excessive and poorly tolerated hypotension. These responses have usually occurred during initial titration or at the time of subsequent upward dosage adjustment.

Congestive Heart Failure: Although acute hemodynamic studies of nisoldipine in patients with NYHA Class II–IV heart failure have not demonstrated negative inotropic effects, safety of SULAR in patients with heart failure has not been established. Caution therefore should be exercised when using SULAR in patients with heart failure or compromised ventricular function, particularly in combination with a beta-blocker.

Patients with Hepatic Impairment: Because nisoldipine is extensively metabolized by the liver and, in patients with cirrhosis, it reaches blood concentrations about 5 times those in normals, SULAR should be administered cautiously in patients with severe hepatic dysfunction (See DOSAGE AND ADMINISTRATION).

Information for Patients: SULAR is an extended release tablet and should be swallowed whole. Tablets should not be chewed, divided or crushed. SULAR should not be administered with a high fat meal. Grapefruit juice, which has been shown to increase significantly the bioavailability of nisoldipine and other dihydropyridine type calcium channel blockers, should not be taken with SULAR.

Laboratory Tests: SULAR is not known to interfere with the interpretation of laboratory tests.

Drug Interactions: A 30 to 45% increase in AUC and C_{max} of nisoldipine was observed with concomitant administration of cimetidine 400 mg twice daily. Ranitidine 150 mg twice daily did not interact significantly with nisoldipine (AUC was decreased by 15–20%). No pharmacodynamic effects of either histamine H_2 receptor antagonist were observed.

Pharmacokinetic interactions between nisoldipine and beta-blockers (atenolol, propranolol) were variable and not significant. Propranolol attenuated the heart rate increase following administration of immediate release nisoldipine. The blood pressure effect of SULAR tended to be greater in patients on atenolol than in patients on no other anithypertensive therapy.

Quinidine at 648 mg bid decreased the bioavailability (AUC) of nisoldipine by 26%, but not the peak concentration. The immediate release, but not the coat-core formulation of nisoldipine increased plasma quinidine concentrations by about 20%. This interaction was not accompanied by ECG changes and its clinical significance is not known. No significant interactions were found between nisoldipine and warfarin or digoxin.

Carcinogenesis, Mutagenesis, Impairment of Fertility: Dietary administration of nisoldipine to male and female rats for up to 24 months (mean doses up to 82 and 111 mg/kg/day, 16 and 19 times the maximum recommended human dose on a mg/m^2 basis, respectively) and female mice for up to 21 months (mean doses of up to 217 mg/kg/day, 20 times the MRHD on a mg/m^2 basis) revealed no evidence of tumorigenic effect of nisoldipine. In male mice receiving a mean dose of 163 mg nisolipine/kg/day (16 times the MRHD of 60 mg/day on a mg/m^2 basis), an increased frequency of stomach papilloma, but still within the historical range, was observed. No evidence of stomach neoplasia was observed at lower doses (up to 58 mg/kg/day). Nisoldipine was negative when tested in a battery of genotoxicity assays including the Ames test and the CHO/HGRPT assay for mutagenicity and the *in vivo* mouse micronucleus test and *in vitro* CHO cell test for clastogenicity.

When administered to male and female rats at doses of up to 30 mg/kg/day (about 5 times the MRHD on a mg/m^2 basis) nisoldipine had no effect on fertility.

Pregnancy Category C: Nisoldipine was neither teratogenic nor fetotoxic at doses that were not maternally toxic.

Nisoldipine was fetotoxic but not teratogenic in rats and rabbits at doses resulting in maternal toxicity (reduced maternal body weight gain). In pregnant rats, increased fetal resorption (post-implantation loss) was observed at 100 mg/kg/day and decreased fetal weight was observed at both 30 and 100 mg/kg/day. These doses are, respectively, about 5 and 16 times the MRHD when compared on a mg/m^2 basis. In pregnant rabbits, decreased fetal and placental weights were observed at a dose of 30 mg/kg/day, about 10 times the MRHD when compared on a mg/m^2 basis. In a study in which pregnant monkeys (both treated and control) had high rates of abortion and mortality, the only surviving fetus from a group exposed to a maternal dose of 100 mg nisoldipine/kg/day (about 30 times the MRHD when compared on a mg/m^2 basis) presented with forelimb and vertebral abnormalities not previously seen in control monkeys of the same strain. There are no adequate and well controlled studies in pregnant women. SULAR should be used in pregnancy only if the potential benefit justifies the potential risk to the fetus.

Nursing Mothers: It is not known whether nisoldipine is excreted in human milk. Because many drugs are excreted in human milk, a decision should be made to discontinue nursing, or to discontinue SULAR, taking into account the importance of the drug to the mother.

Pediatric Use: Safety and effectiveness in pediatric patients have not been established.

ADVERSE EXPERIENCES

More than 6000 patients world-wide have received nisoldipine in clinical trials for the treatment of hypertension, either as the immediate release or the SULAR extended release formulation. Of about 1,500 patients who received SULAR in hypertension studies, about 55% were exposed for at least 2 months and about one third were exposed for over 6 months, the great majority at doses of 20 to 60 mg daily.

SULAR is generally well-tolerated. In the U.S. clinical trials of SULAR in hypertension, 10.9% of the 921 SULAR patients discontinued treatment due to adverse events compared with 2.9% of 280 placebo patients. The frequency of discontinuations due to adverse experiences was related to dose, with a 5.4% discontinuation rate at 10 mg daily and a 10.9% discontinuation rate at 60 mg daily.

The most frequently occurring adverse experiences with SULAR are those related to its vasodilator properties; these are generally mild and only occasionally lead to patient withdrawal from treatment. The table below, from U.S. placebo-controlled parallel dose response trials of SULAR using doses from 10–60 mg once daily in patients with hypertension, lists all of the adverse events, regardless of the causal relationship to SULAR, for which the overall incidence on SULAR was both >1% and greater with SULAR than with placebo.

Adverse Event	Nisoldipine (%) (n=663)	Placebo (%) (n=280)
Peripheral Edema	22	10
Headache	22	15
Dizziness	5	4
Pharyngitis	5	4
Vasodilation	4	2
Sinusitis	3	2
Palpitation	3	1
Chest Pain	2	1
Nausea	2	1
Rash	2	1

Only peripheral edema and possibly dizziness appear to be dose related.

Adverse Event		SULAR				
(Rates in %)	Placebo	10 mg	20 mg	30 mg	40 mg	60 mg
	N=280	N=30	N=170	N=105	N=139	N=137
Peripheral Edema	10	7	15	20	27	29
Dizziness	4	4	3	3	4	10

The common adverse events occurred at about the same rate in men as in women, and at a similar rate in patients over age 65 as in those under that age, except that headache was much less common in older patients. Except for peripheral edema and vasodilation, which were more common in whites, adverse event rates were similar in blacks and whites.

The following adverse events occurred in ≤1% of all patients treated for hypertension in U.S. and foreign clinical trials, or with unspecified incidence in other studies. Although a causal relationship of SULAR to these events cannot be established, they are listed to alert the physician to a possible relationship with SULAR treatment.

Body As A Whole: cellulitis, chills, facial edema, fever, flu syndrome, malaise

Cardiovascular: atrial fibrillation, cerebrovascular accident, congestive heart failure, first degree AV block, hypertension, hypotension, jugular venous distension, migraine, myocardial infarction, postural hypotension, ventricular extrasystoles, supraventricular tachycardia, syncope, systolic ejection murmur, T wave abnormalities on ECG (flattening, inversion, nonspecific changes), venous insufficiency

Digestive: abnormal liver function tests, anorexia, colitis, diarrhea, dry mouth, dyspepsia, dysphagia, flatulence, gastritis, gastrointestinal hemorrhage, gingival hyperplasia, glossitis, hepatomegaly, increased appetite, melena, mouth ulceration

Endocrine: diabetes mellitus, thyroiditis

Hemic and Lymphatic: anemia, ecchymoses, leukopenia, petechiae

Metabolic and Nutritional: gout, hypokalemia, increased serum creatine kinase, increased nonprotein nitrogen, weight gain, weight loss

Musculoskeletal: arthralgia, arthritis, leg cramps, myalgia, myasthenia, myositis, tenosynovitis

Nervous: abnormal dreams, abnormal thinking and confusion, amnesia, anxiety, ataxia, cerebral ischemia, decreased libido, depression, hypesthesia, hypertonia, insomnia, nervousness, paresthesia, somnolence, tremor, vertigo

Respiratory: asthma, dyspnea, end inspiratory wheeze and fine rales, epistaxis, increased cough, laryngitis, pharyngitis, pleural effusion, rhinitis, sinusitis

Skin and Appendages: acne, alopecia, dry skin, exfoliative dermatitis, fungal dermatitis, herpes simplex, herpes zoster, maculopapular rash, pruritus, pustular rash, skin discoloration, skin ulcer, sweating, urticaria

Special senses: abnormal vision, amblyopia, blepharitis, conjunctivitis, ear pain, glaucoma, itchy eyes, keratoconjunctivitis, otitis media, retinal detachment, tinnitus, watery eyes, taste disturbance, temporary unilateral loss of vision, vitreous floater, watery eyes

Urogenital: dysuria, hematuria, impotence, nocturia, urinary frequency, increased BUN and serum creatinine, vaginal hemorrhage, vaginitis.

The following postmarketing event has been reported very rarely in patients receiving SULAR: systemic hypersensitivity reaction which may include one or more of the following: angioedema, shortness of breath, tachycardia, chest tightness, hypotension, and rash. A definite causal relationship with SULAR has not been established. An unusual event observed with immediate release nisoldipine but not observed with SULAR was one case of photosensitivity.

OVERDOSAGE

There is no experience with nisoldipine overdosage. Generally, overdosage with other dihydropyridines leading to pronounced hypotension calls for active cardiovascular support including monitoring of cardiovascular and respiratory function, elevation of extremities, judicious use of calcium infusion, pressor agents and fluids. Clearance of nisoldipine would be expected to be slowed in patients with impaired liver function. Since nisoldipine is highly protein bound, dialysis is not likely to be of any benefit; however, plasmapheresis may be beneficial.

DOSAGE AND ADMINISTRATION

The dosage of SULAR must be adjusted to each patient's needs. Therapy usually should be initiated with 20 mg orally once daily, then increased by 10 mg per week or longer intervals, to attain adequate control of blood pressure. Usual maintenance dosage is 20 to 40 mg once daily. Blood pressure response increases over the 10–60 mg daily dose range but adverse event rates also increase. Doses beyond 60 mg once daily are not recommended. SULAR has been used safely with diuretics, ACE inhibitors, and beta-blocking agents.

Patients over age 65, or patients with impaired liver function are expected to develop higher plasma concentrations of nisoldipine. Their blood pressure should be monitored closely during any dosage adjustment. A starting dose not exceeding 10 mg daily is recommended in these patient groups.

SULAR tablets should be administered orally once daily. Administration with a high fat meal can lead to excessive peak drug concentration and should be avoided. Grapefruit products should be avoided before and after dosing. SULAR is an extended release dosage form and tablets should be swallowed whole, not bitten, divided or crushed.

HOW SUPPLIED

SULAR extended release tablets are supplied at 10 mg, 20 mg, 30 mg, and 40 mg round film coated tablets. The different strengths can be identified as follows:

Strength	Color	Markings
10 mg	Oyster	891 on one side and ZENECA 10 on the other side.
20 mg	Yellow Cream	892 on one side and ZENECA 20 on the other side.
30 mg	Mustard	893 on one side and ZENECA 30 on the other side.
40 mg	Burnt Orange	894 on one side and ZENECA 40 on the other side.

SULAR Tablets are supplied in:

	Strength	NDC Code
Bottles of 100	10 mg	0310-0891-10
	20 mg	0310-0892-10
	30 mg	0310-0893-10
	40 mg	0310-0894-10
Unit Dose Packages of 100	10 mg	0310-0891-39
	20 mg	0310-0892-39
	30 mg	0310-0893-39

The tablets should be protected from light and moisture and stored below 86°F (30°C). Dispense in tight, light-resistant containers.

SULAR® is a trademark of Bayer AG, used under license by Zeneca Inc.

Manufactured AG for
ZENECA Pharmaceuticals
A Business Unit of Zeneca Inc.
Wilmington, Delaware 19850-5437
By Bayer AG
Made in Germany
64088-02   Rev H 12/96
Shown in Product Identification Guide, page 346

TENORETIC®   R
(atenolol and chlorthalidone) R
[ten "o-ret 'ic]

DESCRIPTION

TENORETIC® (atenolol and chlorthalidone) is for the treatment of hypertension. It combines the antihypertensive activity of two agents: a beta$_1$-selective (cardioselective) hydrophilic blocking agent (atenolol, TENORMIN®) and a monosulfonamyl diuretic (chlorthalidone). Atenolol is Benzeneacetamide, 4-[2′-hydroxy-3′-[(1-methylethyl) amino] propoxy].-.

$C_{14}H_{22}N_2O_3$

Atenolol (free base) is a relatively polar hydrophilic compound with a water solubility of 26.5 mg/mL at 37°C. It is freely soluble in 1N HCl (300 mg/mL at 25°C) and less soluble in chloroform (3 mg/mL at 25°C).

Chlorthalidone is 2-Chloro-5-(1-hydroxy-3-oxo-1-isoindolinyl) benzene sulfonamide:

$C_{14}H_{11}ClN_2O_4S$

Chlorthalidone has a water solubility of 12 mg/100 mL at 20°C.

Each TENORETIC 100 Tablet contains:
Atenolol (TENORMIN®) .... 100 mg
Chlorthalidone .... 25 mg
Each TENORETIC 50 Tablet contains:
Atenolol (TENORMIN®) .... 50 mg
Chlorthalidone .... 25 mg

Inactive ingredients: magnesium stearate, microcrystalline cellulose, povidone, sodium starch glycolate.

CLINICAL PHARMACOLOGY
TENORETIC

Atenolol and chlorthalidone have been used singly and concomitantly for the treatment of hypertension. The antihypertensive effects of these agents are additive, and studies have shown that there is no interference with bioavailabil-

Continued on next page

Tenoretic—Cont.

ity when these agents are given together in the single combination tablet. Therefore, this combination provides a convenient formulation for the concomitant administration of these two entities. In patients with more severe hypertension, TENORETIC may be administered with other antihypertensives such as vasodilators.

Atenolol

Atenolol is a $beta_1$-selective (cardioselective) beta-adrenergic receptor blocking agent without membrane stabilizing or intrinsic sympathomimetic (partial agonist) activities. This preferential effect is not absolute, however, and at higher doses, atenolol inhibits $beta_2$-adrenoreceptors, chiefly located in the bronchial and vascular musculature.

Pharmacodynamics: In standard animal or human pharmacological tests, beta-adrenoreceptor blocking activity of atenolol has been demonstrated by: (1) reduction in resting and exercise heart rates and cardiac output, (2) reduction of systolic and diastolic blood pressure at rest and on exercise, (3) inhibition of isoproterenol induced tachycardia and (4) reduction in reflex orthostatic tachycardia.

A significant beta-blocking effect of atenolol, as measured by reduction of exercise tachycardia, is apparent within one hour following oral administration of a single dose. This effect is maximal at about 2 to 4 hours and persists for at least 24 hours. The effect at 24 hours is dose related and also bears a linear relationship to the logarithm of plasma atenolol concentration. However, as has been shown for all beta-blocking agents, the antihypertensive effect does not appear to be related to plasma level.

In normal subjects, the $beta_1$-selectivity of atenolol has been shown by its reduced ability to reverse the $beta_2$-mediated vasodilating effect of isoproterenol as compared to equivalent beta-blocking doses of propranolol. In asthmatic patients, a dose of atenolol producing a greater effect on resting heart rate than propranolol resulted in much less increase in airway resistance. In a placebo controlled comparison of approximately equipotent oral doses of several beta blockers, atenolol produced a significantly smaller decrease of FEV_1 than nonselective beta blockers, such as propranolol and unlike those agents did not inhibit bronchodilation in response to isoproterenol.

Consistent with its negative chronotropic effect due to beta blockade of the SA node, atenolol increases sinus cycle length and sinus node recovery time. Conduction in the AV node is also prolonged. Atenolol is devoid of membrane stabilizing activity, and increasing the dose well beyond that producing beta blockade does not further depress myocardial contractility. Several studies have demonstrated a moderate (approximately 10%) increase in stroke volume at rest and exercise.

In controlled clinical trials, atenolol given as a single daily dose, was an effective antihypertensive agent providing 24-hour reduction of blood pressure. Atenolol has been studied in combination with thiazide-type diuretics and the blood pressure effects of the combination are approximately additive. Atenolol is also compatible with methyldopa, hydralazine and prazosin, the combination resulting in a larger fall in blood pressure than with the single agents. The dose range of atenolol is narrow, and increasing the dose beyond 100 mg once daily is not associated with increased antihypertensive effect. The mechanisms of the antihypertensive effects of beta-blocking agents have not been established. Several mechanisms have been proposed and include: (1) competitive antagonism of catecholamines at peripheral (especially cardiac) adrenergic neuron sites, leading to decreased cardiac output, (2) a central effect leading to reduced sympathetic outflow to the periphery and (3) suppression of renin activity. The results from long-term studies have not shown any diminution of the antihypertensive efficacy of atenolol with prolonged use.

Pharmacokinetics and Metabolism: In man, absorption of an oral dose is rapid and consistent but incomplete. Approximately 50% of an oral dose is absorbed from the gastrointestinal tract, the remainder being excreted unchanged in the feces. Peak blood levels are reached between 2 and 4 hours after ingestion. Unlike propranolol or metoprolol, but like nadolol, hydrophilic atenolol undergoes little or no metabolism by the liver, and the absorbed portion is eliminated primarily by renal excretion. Atenolol also differs from propranolol in that only a small amount (6–16%) is bound to proteins in the plasma. This kinetic profile results in relatively consistent plasma drug levels with about a fourfold interpatient variation. There is no information as to the pharmacokinetic effect of atenolol on chlorthalidone.

The elimination half-life of atenolol is approximately 6 to 7 hours and there is no alteration of the kinetic profile of the drug by chronic administration. Following doses of 50 mg or 100 mg, both beta-blocking and antihypertensive effects persist for at least 24 hours. When renal function is impaired, elimination of atenolol is closely related to the glomerular filtration rate; but significant accumulation does not occur until the creatinine clearance falls below 35 mL/min/1.73m^2 (see circular for atenolol [TENORMIN®]).

Chlorthalidone

Chlorthalidone is a monosulfonamyl diuretic which differs chemically from thiazide diuretics in that a double ring system is incorporated in its structure. It is an oral diuretic with prolonged action and low toxicity. The diuretic effect of the drug occurs within 2 hours of an oral dose. It produces diuresis with greatly increased excretion of sodium and chloride. At maximal therapeutic dosage, chlorthalidone is approximately equal in its diuretic effect to comparable maximal therapeutic doses of benzothiadiazine diuretics. The site of action appears to be the cortical diluting segment of the ascending limb of Henle's loop of the nephron.

INDICATIONS AND USAGE

TENORETIC is indicated in the treatment of hypertension. This fixed dose combination drug is not indicated for initial therapy of hypertension. If the fixed dose combination represents the dose appropriate to the individual patient's needs, it may be more convenient than the separate components.

CONTRAINDICATIONS

TENORETIC is contraindicated in patients with: sinus bradycardia; heart block greater than first degree; cardiogenic shock; overt cardiac failure (see WARNINGS); anuria; hypersensitivity to this product or to sulfonamide-derived drugs.

WARNINGS

Cardiac Failure: Sympathetic stimulation is necessary in supporting circulatory function in congestive heart failure, and beta blockade carries the potential hazard of further depressing myocardial contractility and precipitating more severe failure. In patients who have congestive heart failure controlled by digitalis and/or diuretics, TENORETIC should be administered cautiously. Both digitalis and atenolol slow AV conduction.

IN PATIENTS WITHOUT A HISTORY OF CARDIAC FAILURE, continued depression of the myocardium with beta-blocking agents over a period of time can, in some cases, lead to cardiac failure. At the first sign or symptom of impending cardiac failure, patients receiving TENORETIC should be digitalized and/or be given additional diuretic therapy. Observe the patient closely. If cardiac failure continues despite adequate digitalization and diuretic therapy, TENORETIC therapy should be withdrawn.

Renal and Hepatic Disease and Electrolyte Disturbances: Since atenolol is excreted via the kidneys, TENORETIC should be used with caution in patients with impaired renal function.

In patients with renal disease, thiazides may precipitate azotemia. Since cumultive effects may develop in the presence of impaired renal function, if progressive renal impairment becomes evident, TENORETIC should be discontinued.

In patients with impaired hepatic function or progressive liver disease, minor alterations in fluid and electrolyte balance may precipitate hepatic coma. TENORETIC should be used with caution in these patients.

Ischemic Heart Disease: Following abrupt cessation of therapy with certain beta-blocking agents in patients with coronary artery disease, exacerbations of angina pectoris and, in some cases, myocardial infarction have been reported. Therefore, such patients should be cautioned against interruption of therapy without the physician's advice. Even in the absence of overt angina pectoris, when discontinuation of TENORETIC is planned, the patient should be carefully observed and should be advised to limit physical activity to a minimum. TENORETIC should be reinstated if withdrawal symptoms occur. Because coronary artery disease is common and may be unrecognized, it may be prudent not to discontinue TENORETIC therapy abruptly even in patients treated only for hypertension.

Concomitant Use of Calcium Channel Blockers: Bradycardia and heart block can occur and the left ventricular end diastolic pressure can rise when beta blockers are administered with verapamil or diltiazem. Patients with pre-existing conduction abnormalities or left ventricular dysfunction are particularly susceptible (see PRECAUTIONS).

Bronchospastic Diseases: PATIENTS WITH BRONCHOSPASTIC DISEASE SHOULD, IN GENERAL, NOT RECEIVE BETA BLOCKERS. Because of its relative $beta_1$-selectivity, however, TENORETIC may be used with caution in patients with bronchospastic disease who do not respond to or cannot tolerate, other antihypertensive treatment. Since $beta_1$-selectivity is not absolute, the lowest possible dose of TENORETIC should be used and a $beta_2$-stimulating agent (bronchodilator) should be made available. If dosage must be increased, dividing the dose should be considered in order to achieve lower peak blood levels.

Anesthesia and Major Surgery: It is not advisable to withdraw beta-adrenoreceptor blocking drugs prior to surgery in the majority of patients. However, care should be taken when using anesthetic agents such as those which may depress the myocardium. Vagal dominance, if it occurs, may be corrected with atropine (1–2 mg IV).

Beta blockers are competitive inhibitors of beta-receptor agonists and their effects on the heart can be reversed by administration of such agents; eg, dobutamine or isoproterenol with caution (see section on Overdosage).

Metabolic and Endocrine Effects: TENORETIC may be used with caution in diabetic patients. Beta blockers may mask tachycardia occurring with hypoglycemia, but other manifestations such as dizziness and sweating may not be significantly affected. At recommended doses atenolol does not potentiate insulin-induced hypoglycemia and, unlike nonselective beta blockers, does not delay recovery of blood glucose to normal levels.

Insulin requirements in diabetic patients may be increased, decreased or unchanged; latent diabetes mellitus may become manifest during chlorthalidone administration.

Beta-adrenergic blockade may mask certain clinical signs (eg, tachycardia) of hyperthyroidism. Abrupt withdrawal of beta blockade might precipitate a thyroid storm; therefore, patients suspected of developing thyrotoxicosis from whom TENORETIC therapy is to be withdrawn should be monitored closely.

Because calcium excretion is decreased by thiazides, TENORETIC should be discontinued before carrying out tests for parathyroid function. Pathologic changes in the parathyroid glands, with hypercalcemia and hypophosphatemia, have been observed in a few patients on prolonged thiazide therapy; however, the common complications of hyperparathyroidism such as renal lithiasis, bone resorption, and peptic ulceration have not been seen.

Hyperuricemia may occur, or acute gout may be precipitated in certain patients receiving thiazide therapy.

Pregnancy and Fetal Injury: Atenolol can cause fetal harm when administered to a pregnant woman. Atenolol crosses the placental barrier and appears in cord blood. Administration of atenolol, starting in the second trimester of pregnancy, has been associated with the birth of infants that are small for gestational age. No studies have been performed on the use of atenolol in the first trimester and the possibility of fetal injury cannot be excluded. If this drug is used during pregnancy, or if the patient becomes pregnant while taking this drug, the patient should be apprised of the potential hazard to the fetus.

TENORETIC was studied for teratogenic potential in the rat and rabbit. Doses of atenolol/chlorthalidone of 8/2, 80/20, and 240/60 mg/kg/day were administered orally to pregnant rats with no evidence of embryofetotoxicity observed. Two studies were conducted in rabbits. In the first study, pregnant rabbits were dosed with 8/2, 80/20, and 160/40 mg/kg/day of atenolol/chlorthalidone. No teratogenic effects were noted, but embryonic resorptions were observed at all dose levels (ranging from approximately 5 times to 100 times the maximum recommended human dose*). In the second rabbit study, doses of atenolol/chlorthalidone were 4/1, 8/2, and 20/5 mg/kg/day. No teratogenic or embryotoxic effects were demonstrated.

Atenolol—Atenolol has been shown to produce a dose-related increase in embryo/fetal resorptions in rats at doses equal to or greater than 50 mg/kg/day or 25 or more times the maximum recommended human antihypertensive dose.* Although similar effects were not seen in rabbits, the compound was not evaluated in rabbits at doses above 25 mg/kg/day or 12.5 times the maximum recommended human antihypertensive dose.*

*Based on the maximum dose of 100 mg/day in a 50 kg patient.

Chlorthalidone—Thiazides cross the placental barrier and appear in cord blood. The use of chlorthalidone and related drugs in pregnant women requires that the anticipated benefits of the drug be weighed against possible hazards to the fetus. These hazards include fetal or neonatal jaundice, thrombocytopenia and possibly other adverse reactions which have occurred in the adult.

PRECAUTIONS

General: TENORETIC may aggravate peripheral arterial circulatory disorders.

Electrolyte and Fluid Balance Status: Periodic determination of serum electrolytes to detect possible electrolyte imbalance should be performed at appropriate intervals.

Patients should be observed for clinical signs of fluid or electrolyte imbalance; ie, hyponatremia, hypochloremic alkalosis, and hypokalemia. Serum and urine electrolyte determinations are particularly important when the patient is vomiting excessively or receiving parenteral fluids. Warning signs or symptoms of fluid and electrolyte imbalance include dryness of the mouth, thirst, weakness, lethargy, drowsiness, restlessness, muscle pains or cramps, muscular fatigue, hypotension, oliguria, tachycardia, and gastrointestinal disturbances such as nausea and vomiting.

Measurement of potassium levels is appropriate especially in elderly patients, those receiving digitalis preparations for cardiac failure, patients whose dietary intake of potassium is abnormally low, or those suffering from gastrointestinal complaints.

Hypokalemia may develop especially with brisk diuresis, when severe cirrhosis is present, or during concomitant use of corticosteroids or ACTH.

Interference with adequate oral electrolyte intake will also contribute to hypokalemia. Hypokalemia can sensitize or exaggerate the response of the heart to the toxic effects of digitalis (eg, increased ventricular irritability). Hypokalemia may be avoided or treated by use of potassium supplements or foods with a high potassium content.

Any chloride deficit during thiazide therapy is generally mild and usually does not require specific treatment except under extraordinary circumstances (as in liver disease or renal disease). Dilutional hyponatremia may occur in edematous patients in hot weather; appropriate therapy is water restriction rather than administration of salt except in rare instances when the hyponatremia is life-threatening. In actual salt depletion, appropriate replacement is the therapy of choice.

Drug Interactions: TENORETIC may potentiate the action of other antihypertensive agents used concomitantly. Patients treated with TENORETIC plus a catecholamine depletor (eg, reserpine) should be closely observed for evidence of hypotension and/or marked bradycardia which may produce vertigo, syncope or postural hypotension.

Calcium channel blockers may also have an additive effect when given with TENORETIC. (See WARNINGS.)

Thiazides may decrease arterial responsiveness to norepinephrine. This diminution is not sufficient to preclude the therapeutic effectiveness of norepinephrine. Thiazides may increase the responsiveness to tubocurarine.

Lithium generally should not be given with diuretics because they reduce its renal clearance and add a high risk of lithium toxicity. Read circulars for lithium preparations before use of such preparations with TENORETIC.

Beta blockers may exacerbate the rebound hypertension which can follow the withdrawal of cloridine. If the two drugs are coadministered, the beta blocker should be withdrawn several days before the gradual withdrawal of clonidine. If replacing clonidine by beta-blocker therapy, the introduction of beta blockers should be delayed for several days after clonidine administration has stopped.

While taking beta blockers, patients with a history of anaphylactic reaction to a variety of allergens may have a more severe reaction on repeated challenge, either accidental, diagnostic or therapeutic. Such patients may be unresponsive to the usual doses of epinephrine used to treat the allergic reaction.

Other Precautions: In patients receiving thiazides, sensitivity reactions may occur with or without a history of allergy or bronchial asthma. The possible exacerbation or activation of systemic lupus erythematosus has been reported. The antihypertensive effects of thiazides may be enhanced in the postsympathectomy patient.

Carcinogenesis, Mutagenesis, Impairment of Fertility: Two long-term (maximum dosing duration of 18 or 24 months) rat studies and one long-term (maximum dosing duration of 18 months) mouse study, each employing dose levels as high as 300 mg/kg/day or 150 times the maximum recommended human antihypertensive dose,* did not indicate a carcinogenic potential of atenolol. A third (24 month) rat study, employing doses of 500 and 1,500 mg/kg/day (250 and 750 times the maximum recommended human antihypertensive dose*) resulted in increased incidences of benign adrenal medullary tumors in males and females, mammary fibroadenomas in females, and anterior pituitary adenomas and thyroid parafollicular cell carcinomas in males. No evidence of a mutagenic potential of atenolol was uncovered in the dominant lethal test (mouse), in vivo cytogenetics test (Chinese hamster) or Ames test (*S typhimurium*).

Fertility of male or female rats (evaluated at dose levels as high as 200 mg/kg/day or 100 times the maximum recommended human dose*) was unaffected by atenolol administration.

Animal Toxicology: Six month oral administration studies were conducted in rats and dogs using TENORETIC doses up to 12.5 mg/kg/day (atenolol/chlorthalidone 10/2.5 mg/kg/day—approximately five times the maximum recommended human antihypertensive dose*). There were no functional or morphological abnormalities resulting from dosing either compound alone or together other than minor changes in heart rate, blood pressure and urine chemistry which were attributed to the known pharmacologic properties of atenolol and/or chlorthalidone.

Chronic studies of atenolol performed in animals have revealed the occurrence of vacuolation of epithelial cells of Brunner's glands in the duodenum of both male and female dogs at all tested dose levels (starting at 15 mg/kg/day or 7.5 times the maximum recommended human antihypertensive dose*) and increased incidence of atrial degeneration of hearts of male rats at 300 but not 150 mg atenolol/kg/day (150 and 75 times the maximum recommended human antihypertensive dose*, respectively).

*Based on the maximum dose of 100 mg/day in a 50 kg patient.

Use in Pregnancy: Pregnancy Category D. See WARNINGS—Pregnancy and Fetal Injury.

Nursing Mothers: Atenolol is excreted in human breast milk at a ratio of 1.5 to 6.8 when compared to the concentration in plasma. Caution should be exercised when atenolol is administered to a nursing woman. Clinically significant bradycardia has been reported in breast fed infants. Premature infants, or infants with impaired renal function, may be more likely to develop adverse effects.

	Volunteered (US Studies)		Total—Volunteered and Elicited (Foreign + US Studies)	
	Atenolol n=164 %	Placebo n=206 %	Atenolol n=399 %	Placebo n=407 %
CARDIOVASCULAR				
Bradycardia	3	0	3	0
Cold Extremities	0	0.5	12	5
Postural Hypotension	2	1	4	5
Leg Pain	0	0.5	3	1
CENTRAL NERVOUS SYSTEM/ NEUROMUSCULAR				
Dizziness	4	1	13	6
Vertigo	2	0.5	2	0.2
Light-Headedness	1	0	3	0.7
Tiredness	0.6	0.5	26	13
Fatigue	3	1	6	5
Lethargy	1	0	3	0.7
Drowsiness	0.6	0	2	0.5
Depression	0.6	0.5	12	9
Dreaming	0	0	3	1
GASTROINTESTINAL				
Diarrhea	2	0	3	2
Nausea	4	1	3	1
RESPIRATORY (see Warnings)				
Wheeziness	0	0	3	3
Dyspnea	0.6	1	6	4

Pediatric Use: Safety and effectiveness in pediatric patients have not been established.

ADVERSE REACTIONS

TENORETIC is usually well tolerated in properly selected patients. Most adverse effects have been mild and transient. The adverse effects observed for TENORETIC are essentially the same as those seen with the individual components.

Atenolol: The frequency estimates in the following table were derived from controlled studies in which adverse reactions were either volunteered by the patient (US studies) or elicited, eg, by checklist (foreign studies). The reported frequency of elicited adverse effects was higher for both atenolol and placebo-treated patients than when these reactions were volunteered. Where frequency of adverse effects for atenolol and placebo is similar, causal relationship to atenolol is uncertain.

[See table above]

During postmarketing experience, the following have been reported in temporal relationship to the use of the drug: elevated liver enzymes and/or billirubin, hallucinations, headache, impotence, Peyronie's disease, postural hypotension which may be associated with syncope, psoriasiform rash or exacerbation of psoriasis, psychoses, purpura, reversible alopecia, thrombocytopenia and visual disturbances. TENORETIC, like other beta blockers, has been associated with the development of antinuclear antibodies (ANA) and lupus syndrome.

Chlorthalidone: Cardiovascular: orthostatic hypotension; Gastrointestinal: anorexia, gastric irritation, vomiting, cramping, constipation, jaundice (intrahepatic cholestatic jaundice), pancreatitis; CNS: vertigo, paresthesias, xanthopsia; Hematologic: leukopenia, agranulocytosis, thrombocytopenia, aplastic anemia; Hypersensitivity: purpura, photosensitivity, rash, urticaria, necrotizing angiitis (vasculitis) (cutaneous vasculitis), Lyell's syndrome (toxic epidermal necrolysis); Miscellaneous: hyperglycemia, glycosuria, hyperuricemia, muscle spasm, weakness, restlessness. Clinical trials of TENORETIC conducted in the United States (89 patients treated with TENORETIC) revealed no new or unexpected adverse effects.

POTENTIAL ADVERSE EFFECTS: In addition, a variety of adverse effects not observed in clinical trials with atenolol but reported with other beta-adrenergic blocking agents should be considered potential adverse effects of atenolol. Nervous System: Reversible mental depression progressing to catatonia; an acute reversible syndrome characterized by disorientation for time and place, short-term memory loss, emotional lability, slightly clouded sensorium, decreased performance on neuropsychometrics; Cardiovascular: Intensification of AV block (see CONTRAINDICATIONS); Gastrointestinal: Mesenteric arterial thrombosis, ischemic colitis; Hematologic: Agranulocytosis; Allergic: Erythematous rash, fever combined with aching and sore throat, laryngospasm and respiratory distress; Other: Raynaud's phenomenon.

MISCELLANEOUS: There have been reports of skin rashes and/or dry eyes associated with the use of beta-adrenergic blocking drugs. The reported incidence is small, and, in most cases, the symptoms have cleared when treatment was withdrawn. Discontinuance of the drug should be considered if any such reaction is not otherwise explicable. Patients should be closely monitored following cessation of therapy. (See DOSAGE AND ADMINISTRATION.)

The oculomucocutaneous syndrome associated with the beta blocker practolol has not been reported with atenolol (TENORMIN). Furthermore, a number of patients who had previously demonstrated established practolol reactions were transferred to atenolol (TENORMIN) therapy with subsequent resolution or quiescence of the reaction.

Clinical Laboratory Test Findings: Clinically important changes in standard laboratory parameters were rarely associated with the administration of TENORETIC. The changes in laboratory parameters were not progressive and usually were not associated with clinical manifestations. The most common changes were increases in uric acid and decreases in serum potassium.

OVERDOSAGE

No specific information is available with regard to overdosage and TENORETIC in humans. Treatment should be symptomatic and supportive and directed to the removal of any unabsorbed drug by induced emesis, or administration or activated charcoal. Atenolol can be removed from the general circulation by hemodialysis. Further consideration should be given to dehydration, electrolyte imbalance and hypotension by established procedures.

Atenolol: Overdosage with atenolol has been reported with patients surviving acute doses as high as 5 g. One death was reported in a man who may have taken as much as 10 g acutely.

The predominant symptoms reported following atenolol overdose are lethargy, disorder of respiratory drive, wheezing, sinus pause, and bradycardia. Additionally, common effects associated with overdosage of any beta-adrenergic blocking agent are congestive heart failure, hypotension, bronchospasm, and/or hypoglycemia. Other treatment modalities should be employed at the physician's discretion and may include:

BRADYCARDIA: Atropine 1–2 mg intravenously. If there is no response to vagal blockade, give isoproterenol cautiously. In refractory cases, a transvenous cardiac pacemaker may be indicated. Glucagon in a 10 mg intravenous bolus has been reported to be useful. If required, this may be repeated or followed by an intravenous infusion of glucagon 1–10 mg/h depending on response.

HEART BLOCK (SECOND OR THIRD DEGREE): Isoproterenol or transvenous pacemaker.

CONGESTIVE HEART FAILURE: Digitalize the patient and administer a diuretic. Glucagon has been reported to be useful.

HYPOTENSION: Vasopressors such as dopamine or norepinephrine (levarterenol). Monitor blood pressure continuously.

BRONCHOSPASM: A $beta_2$-stimulant such as isoproterenol or terbutaline and/or aminophylline.

HYPOGLYCEMIA: Intravenous glucose.

ELECTROLYTE DISTURBANCE: Monitor electrolyte levels and renal function. Institute measures to maintain hydration and electrolytes.

Based on the severity of symptoms, management may require intensive support care and facilities for applying cardiac and respiratory support.

Continued on next page

Tenoretic—Cont.

Chlorthalidone: Symptoms of chlorthalidone overdose include nausea, weakness, dizziness and disturbances of electrolyte balance.

DOSAGE AND ADMINISTRATION

DOSAGE MUST BE INDIVIDUALIZED (See INDICATIONS AND USAGE)

Chlorthalidone is usually given at a dose of 25 mg daily; the usual initial dose of atenolol is 50 mg daily. Therefore, the initial dose should be one TENORETIC 50 tablet given once a day. If an optimal response is not achieved, the dosage should be increased to one TENORETIC 100 tablet given once a day.

When necessary, another antihypertensive agent may be added gradually beginning with 50 percent of the usual recommended starting dose to avoid an excessive fall in blood pressure.

Since atenolol is excreted via the kidneys, dosage should be adjusted in cases of severe impairment of renal function. No significant accumulation of atenolol occurs until creatinine clearance falls below 35 mL/min/1.73m^2 (normal range is 100–150 mL/min/1.73m^2); therefore, the following maximum dosages are recommended for patients with renal impairment.

Creatinine Clearance (mL/min/1.73m^2)	Atenolol Elimination Half-life (hrs)	Maximum Dosage
15–35	16–27	50 mg daily
<15	>27	50 mg every other day

HOW SUPPLIED

TENORETIC 50 Tablets (atenolol 50 mg and chlorthalidone 25 mg), NDC 0310-0115, (white, round, biconvex, uncoated tablets with TENORETIC on one side and 115 on the other side, bisected) are supplied in bottles of 100 tablets.

TENORETIC 100 Tablets (atenolol 100 mg and chlorthalidone 25 mg), NDC 0310-0117, (white, round, biconvex, uncoated tablets with TENORETIC on one side and 117 on the other side) are supplied in bottles of 100 tablets.

Store at controlled room temperature, 20–25°C (68–77°F) [see USP]. Dispense in well-closed, light-resistant containers.

Manufactured by IPR Pharmaceuticals Inc.

Distributed by:
ZENECA Pharmaceuticals
A Business Unit of Zeneca Inc.
Wilmington, Delaware 19850-5437 USA
64112-00 Rev B 08/96

Shown in Product Identification Guide, page 346

TENORMIN® Tablets ℞
TENORMIN® I.V. Injection

[ten-or 'min]
(atenolol)

DESCRIPTION

TENORMIN (atenolol), a synthetic, beta$_1$-selective (cardioselective) adrenoreceptor blocking agent, may be chemically described as benzeneacetamide, 4-[2'-hydroxy-3'-[(1-methylethyl)amino]propoxy]-. The molecular and structural formulas are:

$C_{14}H_{22}N_2O_3$

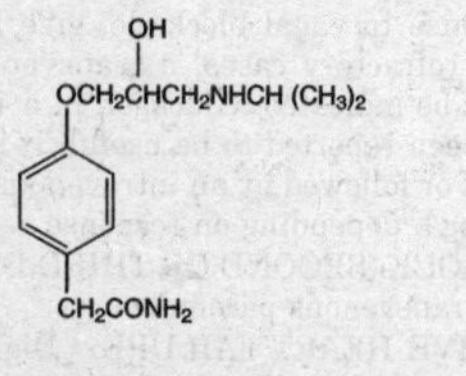
OH
OCH2CHCH2NHCH (CH3)2
CH2CONH2

Atenolol (free base) has a molecular weight of 266. It is a relatively polar hydrophilic compound with a water solubility of 26.5 mg/mL at 37°C and a log partition coefficient (octanol/ water) of 0.23. It is freely soluble in 1N HCl (300 mg/mL at 25°C) and less soluble in chloroform (3 mg/mL at 25°C).

TENORMIN is available as 25, 50 and 100 mg tablets for oral administration. TENORMIN for parenteral administration is available as TENORMIN I.V. Injection containing 5 mg atenolol in 10 mL sterile, isotonic, citrate-buffered, aqueous solution. The pH of the solution is 5.5–6.5.

Inactive Ingredients: TENORMIN Tablets: Magnesium stearate, microcrystalline cellulose, povidone, sodium starch glycolate. TENORMIN I.V. Injection: Sodium chloride for isotonicity and citric acid and sodium hydroxide to adjust pH.

CLINICAL PHARMACOLOGY

TENORMIN is a beta$_1$-selective (cardioselective) beta-adrenergic receptor blocking agent without membrane stabilizing or intrinsic sympathomimetic (partial agonist) activities. This preferential effect is not absolute, however, and at higher doses, TENORMIN inhibits beta$_2$-adrenoreceptors, chiefly located in the bronchial and vascular musculature.

Pharmacokinetics and Metabolism: In man, absorption of an oral dose is rapid and consistent but incomplete. Approximately 50% of an oral dose is absorbed from the gastrointestinal tract, the remainder being excreted unchanged in the feces. Peak blood levels are reached between two (2) and four (4) hours after ingestion. Unlike propranolol or metoprolol, but like nadolol, TENORMIN undergoes little or no metabolism by the liver, and the absorbed portion is eliminated primarily by renal excretion. Over 85% of an intravenous dose is excreted in urine within 24 hours compared with approximately 50% for an oral dose. TENORMIN also differs from propranolol in that only a small amount (6%–16%) is bound to proteins in the plasma. This kinetic profile results in relatively consistent plasma drug levels with about a fourfold interpatient variation.

The elimination half-life of oral TENORMIN is approximately 6 to 7 hours, and there is no alteration of the kinetic profile of the drug by chronic administration. Following intravenous administration, peak plasma levels are reached within 5 minutes. Declines from peak levels are rapid (5- to 10-fold) during the first 7 hours; thereafter, plasma levels decay with a half-life similar to that of orally administered drug. Following oral doses of 50 mg or 100 mg, both beta-blocking and antihypertensive effects persist for at least 24 hours. When renal function is impaired, elimination of TENORMIN is closely related to the glomerular filtration rate; significant accumulation occurs when the creatinine clearance falls below 35 mL/min/1.73m^2. (See DOSAGE AND ADMINISTRATION).

Pharmacodynamics: In standard animal or human pharmacological tests, beta-adrenoreceptor blocking activity of TENORMIN has been demonstrated by: (1) reduction in resting and exercise heart rate and cardiac output, (2) reduction of systolic and diastolic blood pressure at rest and on exercise, (3) inhibition of isoproterenol induced tachycardia, and (4) reduction in reflex orthostatic tachycardia.

A significant beta-blocking effect of TENORMIN, as measured by reduction of exercise tachycardia, is apparent within one hour following oral administration of a single dose. This effect is maximal at about 2 to 4 hours, and persists for at least 24 hours. Maximum reduction in exercise tachycardia occurs within 5 minutes of an intravenous dose. For both orally and intravenously administered drug, the duration of action is dose related and also bears a linear relationship to the logarithm of plasma TENORMIN concentration. The effect on exercise tachycardia of a single 10 mg intravenous dose is largely dissipated by 12 hours, whereas beta-blocking activity of single oral doses of 50 mg and 100 mg is still evident beyond 24 hours following administration. However, as has been shown for all beta-blocking agents, the antihypertensive effect does not appear to be related to plasma level.

In normal subjects, the beta$_1$-selectivity of TENORMIN has been shown by its reduced ability to reverse the beta$_2$-mediated vasodilating effect of isoproterenol as compared to equivalent beta-blocking doses of propranolol. In asthmatic patients, a dose of TENORMIN producing a greater effect on resting heart rate than propranolol resulted in much less increase in airway resistance. In a placebo controlled comparison of approximately equipotent oral doses of several beta blockers, TENORMIN produced a significantly smaller decrease of FEV$_1$ than nonselective beta blockers such as propranolol and, unlike those agents, did not inhibit bronchodilation in response to isoproterenol.

Consistent with its negative chronotropic effect due to beta blockade of the SA node, TENORMIN increases sinus cycle length and sinus node recovery time. Conduction in the AV node is also prolonged. TENORMIN is devoid of membrane stabilizing activity, and increasing the dose well beyond that producing beta blockade does not further depress myocardial contractility. Several studies have demonstrated a moderate (approximately 10%) increase in stroke volume at rest and during exercise.

In controlled clinical trials, TENORMIN, given as a single daily oral dose, was an effective antihypertensive agent providing 24-hour reduction of blood pressure. TENORMIN has been studied in combination with thiazide-type diuretics, and the blood pressure effects of the combination are approximately additive. TENORMIN is also compatible with methyldopa, hydralazine, and prazosin, each combination resulting in a larger fall in blood pressure than with the single agents. The dose range of TENORMIN is narrow and increasing the dose beyond 100 mg once daily is not associated with increased antihypertensive effect. The mechanisms of the antihypertensive effects of beta-blocking agents have not been established. Several possible mechanisms have been proposed and include: (1) competitive antagonism of catecholamines at peripheral (especially cardiac) adrenergic neuron sites, leading to decreased cardiac output, (2) a central effect leading to reduced sympathetic outflow to the periphery, and (3) suppression of renin activity. The results from long-term studies have not shown any diminution of the antihypertensive efficacy of TENORMIN with prolonged use.

By blocking the positive chronotropic and inotropic effects of catecholamines and by decreasing blood pressure, atenolol generally reduces the oxygen requirements of the heart at any given level of effort, making it useful for many patients in the long-term management of angina pectoris. On the other hand, atenolol can increase oxygen requirements by increasing left ventricular fiber length and end diastolic pressure, particularly in patients with heart failure.

In a multicenter clinical trial (ISIS-1) conducted in 16,027 patients with suspected myocardial infarction, patients presenting within 12 hours (mean = 5 hours) after the onset of pain were randomized to either conventional therapy plus TENORMIN (n = 8,037), or conventional therapy alone (n = 7,990). Patients with a heart rate of <50 bpm or systolic blood pressure <100 mm Hg, or with other contraindications to beta blockade, were excluded. Thirty-eight percent of each group were treated within 4 hours of onset of pain. The mean time from onset of pain to entry was 5.0 ± 2.7 hours in both groups. Patients in the TENORMIN group were to receive TENORMIN I.V. Injection 5–10 mg given over 5 minutes plus TENORMIN Tablets 50 mg every 12 hours orally on the first study day (the first oral dose administered about 15 minutes after the IV dose) followed by either TENORMIN Tablets 100 mg once daily or TENORMIN Tablets 50 mg twice daily on days 2–7. The groups were similar in demographic and medical history characteristics and in electrocardiographic evidence of myocardial infarction, bundle branch block, and first degree atrioventricular block at entry.

During the treatment period (days 0–7), the vascular mortality rates were 3.89% in the TENORMIN group (313 deaths) and 4.57% in the control group (365 deaths). This absolute difference in rates, 0.68%, is statistically significant at the P <0.05 level. The absolute difference translates into a proportional reduction of 15% (3.89-4.57/4.57 = −0.15). The 95% confidence limits are 1%–27%. Most of the difference was attributed to mortality in days 0-1 (TENORMIN—121 deaths; control—171 deaths).

Despite the large size of the ISIS-1 trial, it is not possible to identify clearly subgroups of patients most likely or least likely to benefit from early treatment with atenolol. Good clinical judgment suggests, however, that patients who are dependent on sympathetic stimulation for maintenance of adequate cardiac output and blood pressure are not good candidates for beta blockade. Indeed, the trial protocol reflected that judgment by excluding patients with blood pressure consistently below 100 mm Hg systolic. The overall results of the study are compatible with the possibility that patients with borderline blood pressure (less than 120 mm Hg systolic), especially if over 60 years of age, are less likely to benefit.

The mechanism through which atenolol improves survival in patients with definite or suspected acute myocardial infarction is unknown, as is the case for other beta blockers in the postinfarction setting. Atenolol, in addition to its effects on survival, has shown other clinical benefits including reduced frequency of ventricular premature beats, reduced chest pain, and reduced enzyme elevation.

INDICATIONS AND USAGE

Hypertension: TENORMIN is indicated in the management of hypertension. It may be used alone or concomitantly with other antihypertensive agents, particularly with a thiazide-type diuretic.

Angina Pectoris Due to Coronary Atherosclerosis: TENORMIN is indicated for the long-term management of patients with angina pectoris.

Acute Myocardial Infarction: TENORMIN is indicated in the management of hemodynamically stable patients with definite or suspected acute myocardial infarction to reduce cardiovascular mortality. Treatment can be initiated as soon as the patient's clinical condition allows. (See DOSAGE AND ADMINISTRATION, CONTRAINDICATIONS, AND WARNINGS.) In general, there is no basis for treating patients like those who were excluded from the ISIS-1 trial (blood pressure less than 100 mm Hg systolic, heart rate less than 50 bpm) or have other reasons to avoid beta blockade. As noted above, some subgroups (eg, elderly patients with systolic blood pressure below 120 mm Hg) seemed less likely to benefit.

CONTRAINDICATIONS

TENORMIN is contraindicated in sinus bradycardia, heart block greater than first degree, cardiogenic shock, and overt cardiac failure. (See WARNINGS.)

WARNINGS

Cardiac Failure: Sympathetic stimulation is necessary in supporting circulatory function in congestive heart failure, and beta blockade carries the potential hazard of further depressing myocardial contractility and precipitating more se-

vere failure. In patients who have congestive heart failure controlled by digitalis and/or diuretics, TENORMIN should be administered cautiously. Both digitalis and atenolol slow AV conduction.

In patients with acute myocardial infarction, cardiac failure which is not promptly and effectively controlled by 80 mg of intravenous furosemide or equivalent therapy is a contraindication to beta-blocker treatment.

In Patients Without a History of Cardiac Failure: Continued depression of the myocardium with beta-blocking agents over a period of time can, in some cases, lead to cardiac failure. At the first sign or symptom of impending cardiac failure, patients should be fully digitalized and/or be given a diuretic and the response observed closely. If cardiac failure continues despite adequate digitalization and diuresis, TENORMIN should be withdrawn. (SEE DOSAGE AND ADMINISTRATION.)

Cessation of Therapy with TENORMIN: Patients with coronary artery disease, who are being treated with TENORMIN, should be advised against abrupt discontinuation of therapy. Severe exacerbation of angina and the occurrence of myocardial infarction and ventricular arrhythmias have been reported in angina patients following the abrupt discontinuation of therapy with beta blockers. The last two complications may occur with or without preceding exacerbation of the angina pectoris. As with other beta blockers, when discontinuation of TENORMIN is planned, the patients should be carefully observed and advised to limit physical activity to a minimum. If the angina worsens or acute coronary insufficiency develops, it is recommended that TENORMIN be promptly reinstituted, at least temporarily. Because coronary artery disease is common and may be unrecognized, it may be prudent not to discontinue TENORMIN therapy abruptly even in patients treated only for hypertension. (See DOSAGE and ADMINISTRATION.)

Concomitant Use of Calcium Channel Blockers: Bradycardia and heart block can occur and the left ventricular end diastolic pressure can rise when beta blockers are administered with verapamil or diltiazem. Patients with pre-existing conduction abnormalities or left ventricular dysfunction are particularly susceptible. (See PRECAUTIONS.)

Bronchospastic Diseases: PATIENTS WITH BRONCHOSPASTIC DISEASE SHOULD, IN GENERAL, NOT RECEIVE BETA BLOCKERS. Because of its relative beta$_1$ selectivity, however, TENORMIN may be used with caution in patients with bronchospastic disease who do not respond to, or cannot tolerate, other antihypertensive treatment. Since beta$_1$ selectivity is not absolute, the lowest possible dose of TENORMIN should be used with therapy initiated at 50 mg and a beta$_2$-stimulating agent (bronchodilator) should be made available. If dosage must be increased, dividing the dose should be considered in order to achieve lower peak blood levels.

Anesthesia and Major Surgery: It is not advisable to withdraw beta-adrenoreceptor blocking drugs prior to surgery in the majority of patients. However, care should be taken when using anesthetic agents such as those which may depress the myocardium. Vagal dominance, if it occurs, may be corrected with atropine (1-2 mg IV).

Additionally, caution should be used when TENORMIN I.V. Injection is administered concomitantly with such agents. TENORMIN, like other beta blockers, is a competitive inhibitor of beta-receptor agonists and its effects on the heart can be reversed by administration of such agents: eg, dobutamine or isoproterenol with caution (see section on OVERDOSAGE).

Diabetes and Hypoglycemia: TENORMIN should be used with caution in diabetic patients if a beta-blocking agent is required. Beta blockers may mask tachycardia occurring with hypoglycemia, but other manifestations such as dizziness and sweating may not be significantly affected. At recommended doses TENORMIN does not potentiate insulin-induced hypoglycemia and, unlike nonselective beta blockers, does not delay recovery of blood glucose to normal levels.

Thyrotoxicosis: Beta-adrenergic blockade may mask certain clinical signs (eg, tachycardia) of hyperthyroidism. Patients suspected of having thyroid disease should be monitored closely when adminstering TENORMIN I.V. Injection. Abrupt withdrawal of beta blockade might precipitate a thyroid storm; therefore, patients suspected of developing thyrotoxicosis from whom TENORMIN therapy is to be withdrawn should be monitored closely. (See DOSAGE AND ADMINISTRATION.)

Pregnancy and Fetal Injury: Atenolol can cause fetal harm when administered to a pregnant woman. Atenolol crosses the placental barrier and appears in cord blood. Administration of atenolol, starting in the second trimester of pregnancy, has been associated with the birth of infants that are small for gestational age. No studies have been performed on the use of atenolol in the first trimester and the possibility of fetal injury cannot be excluded. If this drug is used during pregnancy, or if the patient becomes pregnant while taking this drug, the patient should be apprised of the potential hazard to the fetus.

Atenolol has been shown to produce a dose-related increase in embryo/fetal resorptions in rats at doses equal to or greater than 50 mg/kg/day or 25 or more times the maximum recommended human antihypertensive dose*. Although similar effects were not seen in rabbits, the compound was not evaluated in rabbits at doses above 25 mg/kg/day or 12.5 times the maximum recommended human antihypertensive dose*.

*Based on the maximum dose of 100 mg/day in a 50 kg patient.

PRECAUTIONS

General: Patients already on a beta blocker must be evaluated carefully before TENORMIN is administered. Initial and subsequent TENORMIN dosages can be adjusted downward depending on clinical observations including pulse and blood pressure. TENORMIN may aggravate peripheral arterial circulatory disorders.

Impaired Renal Function: The drug should be used with caution in patients with impaired renal function. (See DOSAGE AND ADMINISTRATION.)

Drug Interactions: Catecholamine-depleting drugs (eg, reserpine) may have an additive effect when given with beta-blocking agents. Patients treated with TENORMIN plus a catecholamine depletor should therefore be closely observed for evidence of hypotension and/or marked bradycardia which may produce vertigo, syncope or postural hypotension.

Calcium channel blockers may also have an additive effect when given with TENORMIN (See WARNINGS.).

Beta blockers may exacerbate the rebound hypertension which can follow the withdrawal of clonidine. If the two

	Volunteered (US Studies)		Total—Volunteered and Elicited (Foreign + US Studies)	
	Atenolol (n = 164) %	Placebo (n = 206) %	Atenolol (n = 399) %	Placebo (n = 407) %
CARDIOVASCULAR				
Bradycardia	3	0	3	0
Cold Extremities	0	0.5	12	5
Postural Hypotension	2	1	4	5
Leg Pain	0	0.5	3	1
CENTRAL NERVOUS SYSTEM/NEUROMUSCULAR				
Dizziness	4	1	13	6
Vertigo	2	0.5	2	0.2
Light-headedness	1	0	3	0.7
Tiredness	0.6	0.5	26	13
Fatigue	3	1	6	5
Lethargy	1	0	3	0.7
Drowsiness	0.6	0	2	0.5
Depression	0.6	0.5	12	9
Dreaming	0	0	3	1
GASTROINTESTINAL				
Diarrhea	2	0	3	2
Nausea	4	1	3	1
RESPIRATORY (see WARNINGS)				
Wheeziness	0	0	3	3
Dyspnea	0.6	1	6	4

	Conventional Therapy Plus Atenolol (n=244)		Conventional Therapy Alone (n=233)	
Bradycardia	43	(18%)	24	(10%)
Hypotension	60	(25%)	34	(15%)
Bronchospasm	3	(1.2%)	2	(0.9%)
Heart Failure	46	(19%)	56	(24%)
Heart Block	11	(4.5%)	10	(4.3%)
BBB + Major Axis Deviation	16	(6.6%)	28	(12%)
Supraventricular Tachycardia	28	(11.5%)	45	(19%)
Atrial Fibrillation	12	(5%)	29	(11%)
Atrial Flutter	4	(1.6%)	7	(3%)
Ventricular Tachycardia	39	(16%)	52	(22%)
Cardiac Reinfarction	0	(0%)	6	(2.6%)
Total Cardiac Arrests	4	(1.6%)	16	(6.9%)
Nonfatal Cardiac Arrests	4	(1.6%)	12	(5.1%)
Deaths	7	(2.9%)	16	(6.9%)
Cardiogenic Shock	1	(0.4%)	4	(1.7%)
Development of Ventricular Septal Defect	0	(0%)	2	(0.9%)
Development of Mitral Regurgitation	0	(0%)	2	(0.9%)
Renal Failure	1	(0.4%)	0	(0%)
Pulmonary Emboli	3	(1.2%)	0	(0%)

Reasons for Reduced Dosage	IV Atenolol Reduced Dose (<5 mg)*		Oral Partial Dose	
Hypotension/Bradycardia	105	(1.3%)	1168	(14.5%)
Cardiogenic Shock	4	(.04%)	35	(.44%)
Reinfarction	0	(0%)	5	(.06%)
Cardiac Arrest	5	(.06%)	28	(.34%)
Heart Block (> first degree)	5	(.06%)	143	(1.7%)
Cardiac Failure	1	(.01%)	233	(2.9%)
Arrhythmias	3	(.04%)	22	(.27%)
Bronchospasm	1	(.01%)	50	(.62%)

* Full dosage was 10 mg and some patients received less than 10 mg but more than 5 mg.

Continued on next page

Tenormin—Cont.

drugs are coadministered, the beta blocker should be withdrawn several days before the gradual withdrawal of clonidine. If replacing clonidine by beta-blocker therapy, the introduction of beta blockers should be delayed for several days after clonidine administration has stopped.

Caution should be exercised with TENORMIN I.V. Injection when given in close proximity with drugs that may also have a depressant effect on myocardial contractility. On rare occasions, concomitant use of intravenous beta blockers and intravenous verapamil has resulted in serious adverse reactions, especially in patients with severe cardiomyopathy, congestive heart failure, or recent myocardial infarction.

Information on concurrent usage of atenolol and aspirin is limited. Data from several studies, ie, TIMI-II, ISIS-2, currently do not suggest any clinical interaction between aspirin and beta blockers in the acute myocardial infarction setting.

While taking beta blockers, patients with a history of anaphylactic reaction to a variety of allergens may have a more severe reaction on repeated challenge, either accidental, diagnostic or therapeutic. Such patients may be unresponsive to the usual doses of epinephrine used to treat the allergic reaction.

Carcinogenesis, Mutagenesis, Impairment of Fertility: Two long-term (maximum dosing duration of 18 or 24 months) rat studies and one long-term (maximum dosing duration of 18 months) mouse study, each employing dose levels as high as 300 mg/kg/day or 150 times the maximum recommended human antihypertensive dose,* did not indicate a carcinogenic potential of atenolol. A third (24 month) rat study, employing doses of 500 and 1,500 mg/kg/day (250 and 750 times the maximum recommended human antihypertensive dose*) resulted in increased incidences of benign adrenal medullary tumors in males and females, mammary fibroadenomas in females, and anterior pituitary adenomas and thyroid parafollicular cell carcinomas in males. No evidence of a mutagenic potential of atenolol was uncovered in the dominant lethal test (mouse), in vivo cytogenetics test (Chinese hamster) or Ames test (*S typhimurium*).

Fertility of male or female rats (evaluated at dose levels as high as 200 mg/kg/day or 100 times the maximum recommended human dose*) was unaffected by atenolol administration.

Animal Toxicology: Chronic studies employing oral atenolol performed in animals have revealed the occurrence of vacuolation of epithelial cells of Brunner's glands in the duodenum of both male and female dogs at all tested dose levels of atenolol (starting at 15 mg/kg/day or 7.5 times the maximum recommended human antihypertensive dose*) and increased incidence of atrial degeneration of hearts of male rats at 300 but not 150 mg atenolol/kg/day (150 and 75 times the maximum recommended human antihypertensive dose,* respectively).

*Based on the maximum dose of 100 mg/day in a 50 kg patient.

Usage in Pregnancy: Pregnancy Category D: See WARNINGS—Pregnancy and Fetal Injury.

Nursing Mothers: Atenolol is excreted in human breast milk at a ratio of 1.5 to 6.8 when compared to the concentration in plasma. Caution should be exercised when TENORMIN is administered to a nursing woman. Clinically significant bradycardia has been reported in breast fed infants. Premature infants, or infants with impaired renal function, may be more likely to develop adverse effects.

Pediatric Use: Safety and effectiveness in pediatric patients have not been established.

ADVERSE REACTIONS

Most adverse effects have been mild and transient.

The frequency estimates in the following table were derived from controlled studies in hypertensive patients in which adverse reactions were either volunteered by the patient (US studies) or elicited, eg, by checklist (foreign studies). The reported frequency of elicited adverse effects was higher for both TENORMIN and placebo-treated patients than when these reactions were volunteered. Where frequency of adverse effects of TENORMIN and placebo is similar, causal relationship to TENORMIN is uncertain.

[See first table at top of previous page]

Acute Myocardial Infarction: In a series of investigations in the treatment of acute myocardial infarction, bradycardia and hypotension occurred more commonly, as expected for any beta blocker, in atenolol-treated patients than in control patients. However, these usually responded to atropine and/or to withholding further dosage of atenolol. The incidence of heart failure was not increased by atenolol. Inotropic agents were infrequently used. The reported frequency of these and other events occurring during these investigations is given in the following table.

In a study of 477 patients, the following adverse events were reported during either intravenous and/or oral atenolol administration:

[See second table on previous page]

In the subsequent International Study of Infarct Survival (ISIS-1) including over 16,000 patients of whom 8,037 were randomized to receive TENORMIN treatment, the dosage of intravenous and subsequent oral TENORMIN was either discontinued or reduced for the following reasons:

[See third table on previous page]

During postmarketing experience with TENORMIN, the following have been reported in temporal relationship to the use of the drug: elevated liver enzymes and/or bilirubin, hallucinations, headache, impotence, Peyronie's disease, postural hypotension which may be associated with syncope, psoriasiform rash or exacerbation of psoriasis, psychoses, purpura, reversible alopecia, thrombocytopenia and visual disturbances. TENORMIN, like other beta blockers, has been associated with the development of antinuclear antibodies (ANA) and lupus syndrome.

POTENTIAL ADVERSE EFFECTS

In addition, a variety of adverse effects have been reported with other beta-adrenergic blocking agents, and may be considered potential adverse effects of TENORMIN.

Hematologic: Agranulocytosis.

Allergic: Fever, combined with aching and sore throat, laryngospasm, and respiratory distress.

Central Nervous System: Reversible mental depression progressing to catatonia; an acute reversible syndrome characterized by disorientation of time and place; short-term memory loss; emotional lability with slightly clouded sensorium; and decreased performance on neuropsychometrics.

Gastrointestinal: Mesenteric arterial thrombosis, ischemic colitis.

Other: Erythematous rash, Raynaud's phenomenon.

Miscellaneous: There have been reports of skin rashes and/ or dry eyes associated with the use of beta-adrenergic blocking drugs. The reported incidence is small, and in most cases, the symptoms have cleared when treatment was withdrawn. Discontinuance of the drug should be considered if any such reaction is not otherwise explicable. Patients should be closely monitored following cessation of therapy. (See DOSAGE AND ADMINISTRATION.)

The oculomucocutaneous syndrome associated with the beta blocker practolol has not been reported with TENORMIN. Furthermore, a number of patients who had previously demonstrated established practolol reactions were transferred to TENORMIN therapy with subsequent resolution or quiescence of the reaction.

OVERDOSAGE

Overdosage with TENORMIN has been reported with patients surviving acute doses as high as 5 g. One death was reported in a man who may have taken as much as 10 g acutely.

The predominant symptoms reported following TENORMIN overdose are lethargy, disorder of respiratory drive, wheezing, sinus pause and bradycardia. Additionally, common effects associated with overdosage of any beta-adrenergic blocking agent and which might also be expected in TENORMIN overdose are congestive heart failure, hypotension, bronchospasm and/or hypoglycemia.

Treatment of overdose should be directed to the removal of any unabsorbed drug by induced emesis, gastric lavage, or administration of activated charcoal. TENORMIN can be removed from the general circulation by hemodialysis. Other treatment modalities should be employed at the physician's discretion and may include:

BRADYCARDIA: Atropine intravenously. If there is no response to vagal blockade, give isoproterenol cautiously. In refractory cases, a transvenous cardiac pacemaker may be indicated.

HEART BLOCK (SECOND OR THIRD DEGREE): Isoproterenol or transvenous cardiac pacemaker.

CARDIAC FAILURE: Digitalize the patient and administer a diuretic. Glucagon has been reported to be useful.

HYPOTENSION: Vasopressors such as dopamine or norepinephrine (levarterenol). Monitor blood pressure continuously.

BRONCHOSPASM: A beta$_2$ stimulant such as isoproterenol or terbutaline and/or aminophylline.

HYPOGLYCEMIA: Intravenous glucose.

Based on the severity of symptoms, management may require intensive support care and facilities for applying cardiac and respiratory support.

DOSAGE AND ADMINISTRATION

Hypertension: The initial dose of TENORMIN is 50 mg given as one tablet a day either alone or added to diuretic therapy. The full effect of this dose will usually be seen within one to two weeks. If an optimal response is not achieved, the dosage should be increased to TENORMIN 100 mg given as one tablet a day. Increasing the dosage beyond 100 mg a day is unlikely to produce any further benefit.

TENORMIN may be used alone or concomitantly with other antihypertensive agents including thiazide-type diuretics, hydralazine, prazosin, and alpha-methyldopa.

Angina Pectoris: The initial dose of TENORMIN is 50 mg given as one tablet a day. If an optimal response is not achieved within one week, the dosage should be increased to TENORMIN 100 mg given as one tablet a day. Some patients may require a dosage of 200 mg once a day for optimal effect.

Twenty-four hour control with once daily dosing is achieved by giving doses larger than necessary to achieve an imme-

diate maximum effect. The maximum early effect on exercise tolerance occurs with doses of 50 to 100 mg, but at these doses the effect at 24 hours is attenuated, averaging about 50% to 75% of that observed with once a day oral doses of 200 mg.

Acute Myocardial Infarction: In patients with definite or suspected acute myocardial infarction, treatment with TENORMIN I.V. Injection should be initiated as soon as possible after the patient's arrival in the hospital and after eligibility is established. Such treatment should be initiated in a coronary care or similar unit immediately after the patient's hemodynamic condition has stabilized. Treatment should begin with the intravenous administration of 5 mg TENORMIN over 5 minutes followed by another 5 mg intravenous injection 10 minutes later. TENORMIN I.V. Injection should be administered under carefully controlled conditions including monitoring of blood pressure, heart rate, and electrocardiogram. Dilutions of TENORMIN I.V. Injection in Dextrose Injection USP, Sodium Chloride Injection USP, or Sodium Chloride and Dextrose Injection may be used. These admixtures are stable for 48 hours if they are not used immediately.

In patients who tolerate the full intravenous dose (10 mg), TENORMIN Tablets 50 mg should be initiated 10 minutes after the last intravenous dose followed by another 50 mg oral dose 12 hours later. Thereafter, TENORMIN can be given orally either 100 mg once daily or 50 mg twice a day for a further 6–9 days or until discharge from the hospital. If bradycardia or hypotension requiring treatment or any other untoward effects occur, TENORMIN should be discontinued. (See full prescribing information prior to initiating therapy with TENORMIN tablets.)

Data from other beta blocker trials suggest that if there is any question concerning the use of IV beta blocker or clinical estimate that there is a contraindication, the IV beta blocker may be eliminated and patients fulfilling the safety criteria may be given TENORMIN Tablets 50 mg twice daily or 100 mg once a day for at least seven days (if the IV dosing is excluded).

Although the demonstration of efficacy of TENORMIN is based entirely on data from the first seven postinfarction days, data from other beta blocker trials suggest that treatment with beta blockers that are effective in the postinfarction setting may be continued for one to three years if there are no contraindications.

TENORMIN is an additional treatment to standard coronary care unit therapy.

Elderly Patients or Patients with Renal Impairment: TENORMIN is excreted by the kidneys; consequently dosage should be adjusted in cases of severe impairment of renal function. Some reduction in dosage may also be appropriate for the elderly, since decreased kidney function is a physiologic consequence of aging. Atenolol excretion would be expected to decrease with advancing age.

No significant accumulation of TENORMIN occurs until creatinine clearance falls below 35 mL/min/1.73 m^2. Accumulation of atenolol and prolongation of its half-life were studied in subjects with creatinine clearance between 5 and 105 mL/min. Peak plasma levels were significantly increased in subjects with creatinine clearances below 30 mL/min.

The following maximum oral dosages are recommended for elderly, renally-impaired patients and for patients with renal impairment due to other causes:

Creatinine Clearance (mL/min/1.73m^2)	Atenolol Elimination Half-Life (h)	Maximum Dosage
15–35	16–27	50 mg daily
<15	>27	25 mg daily

Some renally-impaired or elderly patients being treated for hypertension may require a lower starting dose of TENORMIN: 25 mg given as one tablet a day. If this 25 mg dose is used, assessment of efficacy must be made carefully. This should include measurement of blood pressure just prior to the next dose ("trough" blood pressure) to ensure that the treatment effect is present for a full 24 hours.

Although a similar dosage reduction may be considered for elderly and/or renally-impaired patients being treated for indications other than hypertension, data are not available for these patient populations.

Patients on hemodialysis should be given 25 mg or 50 mg after each dialysis; this should be done under hospital supervision as marked falls in blood pressure can occur.

Cessation of Therapy in Patients with Angina Pectoris: If withdrawal of TENORMIN therapy is planned, it should be achieved gradually and patients should be carefully observed and advised to limit physical activity to a minimum. Parenteral drug products should be inspected visually for particulate matter and discoloration prior to administration, whenever solution and container permit.

HOW SUPPLIED

TENORMIN Tablets: Tablets of 25 mg atenolol, NDC 0310-0107 (round, flat, uncoated white tablets identified with "T" debossed on one side and 107 debossed on the other side) are supplied in bottles of 100 tablets.

Tablets of 50 mg atenolol, NDC 0310-0105 (round, flat, uncoated white tablets identified with "TENORMIN" debossed on one side and 105 debossed on the other side, bisected) are supplied in bottles of 100 tablets and 1000 tablets, and unit dose packages of 100 tablets.
Tablets of 100 mg atenolol, NDC 0310-0101 (round, flat, uncoated white tablets identified with "TENORMIN" debossed on one side and 101 debossed on the other side) are supplied in bottles of 100 tablets and unit dose packages of 100 tablets.
Store at controlled room temperature, 20–25°C (68–77°F) [see USP]. Dispense in well-closed, light resistant containers.

TENORMIN I.V. Injection:*
TENORMIN I.V. Injection, NDC 0310-0108, is supplied as 5 mg atenolol in 10 mL ampules of isotonic citrate-buffered aqueous solution.
Protect from light. Keep ampules in outer packaging until time of use. Store at room temperature 20–25°C (68–77°F) [see USP].
*Manufactured By:
Marsam Pharmaceuticals Inc.
Cherry Hill, NJ 08034
For: Zeneca Pharmaceuticals
A Business Unit of Zeneca Inc.
Wilmington, Delaware 19850-5437
64108-00 Rev I 08/96
*64124-00 *Rev J 02/97

Shown in Product Identification Guide, page 346

ZESTORETIC® ℞
[*zes 'tor-etic*]
LISINOPRIL/HYDROCHLOROTHIAZIDE

USE IN PREGNANCY
When used in pregnancy during the second and third trimesters, ACE inhibitors can cause injury and even death to the developing fetus. When pregnancy is detected, ZESTORETIC should be discontinued as soon as possible. See WARNINGS, Pregnancy, Lisinopril, Fetal/Neonatal Morbidity and Mortality.

DESCRIPTION
ZESTORETIC® (Lisinopril and Hydrochlorothiazide) combines an angiotensin converting enzyme inhibitor, lisinopril, and a diuretic, hydrochlorothiazide.
Lisinopril, a synthetic peptide derivative, is an oral long-acting angiotensin converting enzyme inhibitor. It is chemically described as (S)-1-[N^2-(1-carboxy-3-phenylpropyl)-L-lysyl]-L-proline dihydrate. Its empirical formula is $C_{21}H_{31}N_3O_5 \cdot 2H_2O$ and its structural formula is:

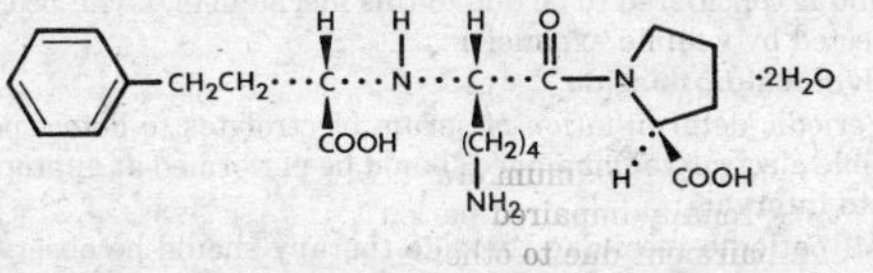

Lisinopril is a white to off-white, crystalline powder, with a molecular weight of 441.53. It is soluble in water, sparingly soluble in methanol, and practically insoluble in ethanol.
Hydrochlorothiazide is 6-chloro-3,4-dihydro-2H-1,2,4-benzothiadiazine-7-sulfonamide 1,1-dioxide. Its empirical formula is $C_7H_8ClN_3O_4S_2$ and its structural formula is:

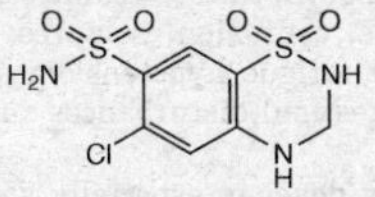

Hydrochlorothiazide is a white, or practically white, crystalline powder with a molecular weight of 297.72, which is slightly soluble in water, but freely soluble in sodium hydroxide solution.
ZESTORETIC is available for oral use in three tablet combinations of lisinopril with hydrochlorothiazide: ZESTORETIC 10-12.5 containing 10 mg lisinopril and 12.5 mg hydrochlorothiazide; ZESTORETIC 20-12.5 containing 20 mg lisinopril and 12.5 mg hydrochlorothiazide; and, ZESTORETIC 20–25 containing 20 mg lisinopril and 25 mg hydrochlorothiazide.
Inactive Ingredients:
10–12.5 Tablets—calcium phosphate, magnesium stearate, mannitol, red ferric oxide, starch, yellow ferric oxide.
20-12.5 Tablets—calcium phosphate, magnesium stearate, mannitol, starch.
20-25 Tablets—calcium phosphate, magnesium stearate, mannitol, red ferric oxide, starch, yellow ferric oxide.

CLINICAL PHARMACOLOGY
Lisinopril and Hydrochlorothiazide
As a result of its diuretic effects, hydrochlorothiazide increases plasma renin activity, increases aldosterone secretion, and decreases serum potassium. Administration of lisinopril blocks the renin-angiotensin aldosterone axis and tends to reverse the potassium loss associated with the diuretic.
In clinical studies, the extent of blood pressure reduction seen with the combination of lisinopril and hydrochlorothiazide was approximately additive. The ZESTORETIC 10–12.5 combination worked equally well in black and white patients. The ZESTORETIC 20–12.5 and ZESTORETIC 20–25 combinations appeared somewhat less effective in black patients, but relatively few black patients were studied. In most patients, the antihypertensive effect of ZESTORETIC was sustained for at least 24 hours.
In a randomized, controlled comparison, the mean antihypertensive effects of ZESTORETIC 20-12.5 and ZESTORETIC 20-25 were similar, suggesting that many patients who respond adequately to the latter combination may be controlled with ZESTORETIC 20-12.5. (See DOSAGE AND ADMINISTRATION.)
Concomitant administration of lisinopril and hydrochlorothiazide has little or no effect on the bioavailability of either drug. The combination tablet is bioequivalent to concomitant administration of the separate entities.
Lisinopril
Mechanism of Action: Lisinopril inhibits angiotensin-converting enzyme (ACE) in human subjects and animals. ACE is a peptidyl dipeptidase that catalyzes the conversion of angiotensin I to the vasoconstrictor substance, angiotensin II. Angiotensin II also stimulates aldosterone secretion by the adrenal cortex. Inhibition of ACE results in decreased plasma angiotensin II which leads to decreased vasopressor activity and to decreased aldosterone secretion. The latter decrease may result in a small increase of serum potassium. Removal of angiotensin II negative feedback on renin secretion leads to increased plasma renin activity. In hypertensive patients with normal renal function treated with lisinopril alone for up to 24 weeks, the mean increase in serum potassium was less than 0.1 mEq/L; however, approximately 15 percent of patients had increases greater than 0.5 mEq/L and approximately six percent had a decrease greater than 0.5 mEq/L. In the same study, patients treated with lisinopril plus a thiazide diuretic showed essentially no change in serum potassium. (See PRECAUTIONS.)
ACE is identical to kininase, an enzyme that degrades bradykinin. Whether increased levels of bradykinin, a potent vasodepressor peptide, play a role in the therapeutic effects of lisinopril remains to be elucidated.
While the mechanism through which lisinopril lowers blood pressure is believed to be primarily suppression of the renin-angiotensin-aldosterone system, lisinopril is antihypertensive even in patients with low-renin hypertension. Although lisinopril was antihypertensive in all races studied, black hypertensive patients (usually a low-renin hypertensive population) had a smaller average response to lisinopril monotherapy than non-black patients.
Pharmacokinetics and Metabolism: Following oral administration of lisinopril, peak serum concentrations occur within about 7 hours. Declining serum concentrations exhibit a prolonged terminal phase which does not contribute to drug accumulation. This terminal phase probably represents saturable binding to ACE and is not proportional to dose. Lisinopril does not appear to be bound to other serum proteins.
Lisinopril does not undergo metabolism and is excreted unchanged entirely in the urine. Based on urinary recovery, the mean extent of absorption of lisinopril is approximately 25 percent, with large intersubject variability (6%–60%) at all doses tested (5–80 mg). Lisinopril absorption is not influenced by the presence of food in the gastrointestinal tract.
Upon multiple dosing, lisinopril exhibits an effective half-life of accumulation of 12 hours.
Impaired renal function decreases elimination of lisinopril, which is excreted principally through the kidneys, but this decrease becomes clinically important only when the glomerular filtration rate is below 30 mL/min. Above this glomerular filtration rate, the elimination half-life is little changed. With greater impairment, however, peak and trough lisinopril levels increase, time to peak concentration increases and time to attain steady state is prolonged. Older patients, on average, have (approximately doubled) higher blood levels and area under the plasma concentration time curve (AUC) than younger patients. (See DOSAGE AND ADMINISTRATION.) Lisinopril can be removed by hemodialysis.
Studies in rats indicate that lisinopril crosses the blood-brain barrier poorly. Multiple doses of lisinopril in rats do not result in accumulation in any tissues. However, milk of lactating rats contains radioactivity following administration of ^{14}C lisinopril. By whole body autoradiography, radioactivity was found in the placenta following administration of labeled drug to pregnant rats, but none was found in the fetuses.
Pharmacodynamics: Administration of lisinopril to patients with hypertension results in a reduction of supine and standing blood pressure to about the same extent with no compensatory tachycardia. Symptomatic postural hypotension is usually not observed although it can occur and should be anticipated in volume and/or salt-depleted patients. (See WARNINGS.)
In most patients studied, onset of antihypertensive activity was seen at one hour after oral administration of an individual dose of lisinopril, with peak reduction of blood pressure achieved by six hours.
In some patients achievement of optimal blood pressure reduction may require two to four weeks of therapy.
At recommended single daily doses, antihypertensive effects have been maintained for at least 24 hours, after dosing, although the effect at 24 hours was substantially smaller than the effect six hours after dosing.
The antihypertensive effects of lisinopril have continued during long term therapy. Abrupt withdrawal of lisinopril has not been associated with a rapid increase in blood pressure; nor with a significant overshoot of pretreatment blood pressure.
In hemodynamic studies in patients with essential hypertension, blood pressure reduction was accompanied by a reduction in peripheral arterial resistance with little or no change in cardiac output and in heart rate. In a study in nine hypertensive patients, following administration of lisinopril, there was an increase in mean renal blood flow that was not significant. Data from several small studies are inconsistent with respect to the effect of lisinopril on glomerular filtration rate in hypertensive patients with normal renal function, but suggest that changes, if any, are not large.
In patients with renovascular hypertension lisinopril has been shown to be well tolerated and effective in controlling blood pressure. (See PRECAUTIONS.)
Hydrochlorothiazide
The mechanism of the antihypertensive effect of thiazides is unknown. Thiazides do not usually affect normal blood pressure.
Hydrochlorothiazide is a diuretic and antihypertensive. It affects the distal renal tubular mechanism of electrolyte reabsorption. Hydrochlorothiazide increases excretion of sodium and chloride in approximately equivalent amounts. Natriuresis may be accompanied by some loss of potassium and bicarbonate.
After oral use diuresis begins within two hours, peaks in about four hours and lasts about 6 to 12 hours.
Hydrochlorothiazide is not metabolized but is eliminated rapidly by the kidney. When plasma levels have been followed for at least 24 hours, the plasma half-life has been observed to vary between 5.6 and 14.8 hours. At least 61 percent of the oral dose is eliminated unchanged within 24 hours. Hydrochlorothiazide crosses the placental but not the blood-brain barrier.

INDICATIONS AND USAGE
ZESTORETIC is indicated for the treatment of hypertension. These fixed-dose combinations are not indicated for initial therapy (see DOSAGE AND ADMINISTRATION).
In using ZESTORETIC, consideration should be given to the fact that an angiotensin converting enzyme inhibitor, captopril, has caused agranulocytosis, particularly in patients with renal impairment or collagen vascular disease, and that available data are insufficient to show that lisinopril does not have a similar risk. (See WARNINGS.)
In considering the use of ZESTORETIC, it should be noted that ACE inhibitors have been associated with a higher rate of angioedema in black than in nonblack patients (see WARNINGS, Lisinopril, Angioedema).

CONTRAINDICATIONS
ZESTORETIC is contraindicated in patients who are hypersensitive to any component of this product and in patients with a history of angioedema related to previous treatment with an angiotensin converting enzyme inhibitor. Because of the hydrochlorothiazide component, this product is contraindicated in patients with anuria or hypersensitivity to other sulfonamide-derived drugs.

WARNINGS
Lisinopril
Anaphylactoid and Possibly Related Reactions: Presumably because angiotensin-converting enzyme inhibitors affect the metabolism of eicosanoids and polypeptides, including endogenous bradykinin, patients receiving ACE inhibitors (including ZESTORETIC) may be subject to a variety of adverse reactions, some of them serious.
Angioedema: Angioedema of the face, extremities, lips, tongue, glottis and/or larynx has been reported rarely in patients treated with angiotensin converting enzyme inhibitors, including lisinopril. This may occur at any time during treatment. ACE inhibitors have been associated with a higher rate of angioedema in black than in nonblack patients. ZESTORETIC should be promptly discontinued and the appropriate therapy and monitoring should be provided until complete and sustained resolution of signs and symptoms has occurred. In instances where swelling has been confined to the face and lips the condition has generally re-

Continued on next page

Zestoretic—Cont.

solved without treatment, although antihistamines have been useful in relieving symptoms. Angioedema associated with laryngeal edema may be fatal. **Where there is involvement of the tongue, glottis or larynx, likely to cause airway obstruction, subcutaneous epinephrine solution 1:1000 (0.3 mL to 0.5 mL) and/or measures necessary to ensure a patent airway should be promptly provided. (See ADVERSE REACTIONS.)**

Patients with a history or angioedema unrelated to ACE inhibitor therapy may be at increased risk of angioedema while receiving an ACE inhibitor (see also INDICATIONS AND USAGE and CONTRAINDICATIONS).

Anaphylactoid Reactions During Desensitization: Two patients undergoing desensitizing treatment with hymenoptra venom while receiving ACE inhibitors sustained life-threatening anaphylactoid reactions. In the same patients, these reactions were avoided when ACE inhibitors were temporarily withheld, but they reappeared upon inadvertent rechallenge.

Anaphylactoid Reactions During Membrane Exposure: Thiazide-containing combination products are not recommended in patients with severe renal dysfunction. Sudden and potentially life-threatening anaphylactoid reactions have been reported in some patients dialyzed with high-flux membranes (eg, AN69¶) and treated concomitantly with an ACE inhibitor. In such patients, dialysis must be stopped immediately, and aggressive therapy for anaphylactoid reactions be initiated. Symptoms have not been relieved by antihistamines in these situations. In these patients, consideration should be given to using a different type of dialysis membrane or a different class of antihypertensive agent. Anaphylactoid reactions have also been reported in patients undergoing low-density lipoprotein apheresis with dextran sulfate absorption.

Hypotension and Related Effects: Excessive hypotension was rarely seen in uncomplicated hypertensive patients but is a possible consequence of lisinopril use in salt/volume-depleted persons such as those treated vigorously with diuretics or patients on dialysis. (See PRECAUTIONS, Drug Interactions and ADVERSE REACTIONS.)

Syncope has been reported in 0.8 percent of patients receiving ZESTORETIC. In patients with hypertension receiving lisinopril alone, the incidence of syncope was 0.1 percent. The overall incidence of syncope may be reduced by proper titration of the individual components. (See PRECAUTIONS, Drug Interactions, ADVERSE REACTIONS and DOSAGE AND ADMINISTRATION.)

In patients with severe congestive heart failure, with or without associated renal insufficiency, excessive hypotension has been observed and may be associated with oliguria and/or progressive azotemia, and rarely with acute renal failure and/or death. Because of the potential fall in blood pressure in these patients, therapy should be started under very close medical supervision. Such patients should be followed closely for the first two weeks of treatment and whenever the dose of lisinopril and/or diuretic is increased. Similar considerations apply to patients with ischemic heart or cerebrovascular disease in whom an excessive fall in blood pressure could result in a myocardial infarction or cerebrovascular accident.

If hypotension occurs, the patient should be placed in supine position and, if necessary, receive an intravenous infusion of normal saline. A transient hypotensive response is not a contraindication to further doses which usually can be given without difficulty once the blood pressure has increased after volume expansion.

Leukopenia/Neutropenia/Agranulocytosis: Another angiotensin converting enzyme inhibitor, captopril, has been shown to cause agranulocytosis and bone marrow depression, rarely in uncomplicated patients but more frequently in patients with renal impairment, especially if they also have a collagen vascular disease. Available data from clinical trials of lisinopril are insufficient to show that lisinopril does not cause agranulocytosis at similar rates. Marketing experience has revealed rare cases of leukopenia/neutropenia and bone marrow depression in which a causal relationship to lisinopril cannot be excluded. Periodic monitoring of white blood cell counts in patients with collagen vascular disease and renal disease should be considered.

Hepatic Failure: Rarely, ACE inhibitors have been associated with a syndrome that starts with cholestatic jaundice and progresses to fulminant hepatic necrosis and (sometimes) death. The mechanism of this syndrome is not understood. Patients receiving ACE inhibitors who develop jaundice or marked elevations of hepatic enzymes should discontinue the ACE inhibitor and receive appropriate medical follow-up.

Pregnancy

Lisinopril and Hydrochlorothiazide: Teratogenicity studies were conducted in mice and rats with up to 90 mg/ kg/day of lisinopril (56 times the maximum recommended human dose) in combination with 10 mg/kg/day of hydrochlorothiazide (2.5 times the maximum recommended human dose). Maternal or fetotoxic effects were not seen in mice with the combination. In rats decreased maternal weight gain and decreased fetal weight occurred down to $^{3}/_{10}$ mg/kg/day (the lowest dose tested). Associated with the decreased fetal weight was a delay in fetal ossification. The decreased fetal weight and delay in fetal ossification were not seen in saline-supplemented animals given 90/10 mg/kg/day.

When used in pregnancy during the second and third trimesters, ACE inhibitors can cause injury and even death to the developing fetus. When pregnancy is detected ZESTORETIC should be discontinued as soon as possible. (See Lisinopril, Fetal/Neonatal Morbidity and Mortality below.)

Lisinopril

Fetal/Neonatal Morbidity and Mortality: ACE inhibitors can cause fetal and neonatal morbidity and death when administered to pregnant women. Several dozen cases have been reported in the world literature. When pregnancy is detected, ACE inhibitor therapy should be discontinued as soon as possible.

The use of ACE inhibitors during the second and third trimesters of pregnancy has been associated with fetal and neonatal injury, including hypotension, neonatal skull hypoplasia, anuria, reversible or irreversible renal failure, and death. Oligohydramnios has also been reported, presumably resulting from decreased fetal renal function; oligohydramnios in this setting has been associated with fetal limb contractures, craniofacial deformation, and hypoplastic lung development. Prematurity, intrauterine growth retardation, and patent ductus arteriosus have also been reported, although it is not clear whether these occurrences were due to the ACE-inhibitor exposure.

These adverse effects do not appear to have resulted from intrauterine ACE-inhibitor exposure that has been limited to the first trimester. Mothers whose embryos and fetuses are exposed to ACE inhibitors only during the first trimester should be so informed. Nonetheless, when patients become pregnant, physicians should make every effort to discontinue the use of ZESTORETIC as soon as possible.

Rarely (probably less often than once in every thousand pregnancies), no alternative to ACE inhibitors will be found. In these rare cases, the mothers should be apprised of the potential hazards to their fetuses, and serial ultrasound examinations should be performed to assess the intraamniotic environment.

If oligohydramnios is observed, ZESTORETIC should be discontinued unless it is considered lifesaving for the mother. Contraction stress testing (CST), a nonstress test (NST), or biophysical profiling (BPP) may be appropriate, depending upon the week of pregnancy. Patients and physicians should be aware, however, that oligohydramnios may not appear until after the fetus has sustained irreversible injury.

Infants with histories of in utero exposure to ACE inhibitors should be closely observed for hypotension, oliguria, and hyperkalemia. If oliguria occurs, attention should be directed toward support of blood pressure and renal perfusion. Exchange transfusion or dialysis may be required as means of reversing hypotension and/or substituting for disordered renal function. Lisinopril, which crosses the placenta, has been removed from neonatal circulation by peritoneal dialysis with some clinical benefit, and theoretically may be removed by exchange transfusion, although there is no experience with the latter procedure.

No teratogenic effects of lisinopril were seen in studies of pregnant rats, mice, and rabbits. On a mg/kg basis, the doses used were up to 625 times (in mice), 188 times (in rats), 0.6 times (in rabbits) the maximum recommended human dose.

Hydrochlorothiazide

Teratogenic Effects: Reproduction studies in the rabbit, the mouse and the rat at doses up to 100 mg/kg/day (50 times the human dose) showed no evidence of external abnormalities of the fetus due to hydrochlorothiazide. Hydrochlorothiazide given in a two-litter study in rats at doses of 4–5.6 mg/kg/day (approximately 1–2 times the usual daily human dose) did not impair fertility or produce birth abnormalities in the offspring. Thiazides cross the placental barrier and appear in cord blood.

Nonteratogenic Effects: These may include fetal or neonatal jaundice, thrombocytopenia, and possibly other adverse reactions have occurred in the adult.

Hydrochlorothiazide

Thiazides should be used with caution in severe renal disease. In patients with renal disease, thiazides may precipitate azotemia. Cumulative effects of the drug may develop in patients with impaired renal function.

Thiazides should be used with caution in patients with impaired hepatic function or progressive liver disease, since minor alterations of fluid and electrolyte balance may precipitate hepatic coma.

Sensitivity reactions may occur in patients with or without a history of allergy or bronchial asthma.

The possibility of exacerbation or activation of systemic lupus erythematosus has been reported.

Lithium generally should not be given with thiazides. (See PRECAUTIONS, Drug Interactions, Lisinopril and Hydrochlorothiazide.)

PRECAUTIONS

General

Lisinopril

Impaired Renal Function: As a consequence of inhibiting the renin-angiotensin-aldosterone system, changes in renal function may be anticipated in susceptible individuals. In patients with severe congestive heart failure whose renal function may depend on the activity of the renin-angiotensin-aldosterone system, treatment with angiotensin converting enzyme inhibitors, including lisinopril, may be associated with oliguria and/or progressive azotemia and rarely with acute renal failure and/or death.

In hypertensive patients with unilateral or bilateral renal artery stenosis, increases in blood urea nitrogen and serum creatinine may occur. Experience with another angiotensin converting enzyme inhibitor suggests that these increases are usually reversible upon discontinuation of lisinopril and/or diuretic therapy. In such patients renal function should be monitored during the first few weeks of therapy.

Some hypertensive patients with no apparent pre-existing renal vascular disease have developed increases in blood urea and serum creatinine, usually minor and transient, especially when lisinopril has been given concomitantly with a diuretic. This is more likely to occur in patients with pre-existing renal impairment. Dosage reduction of lisinopril and/or discontinuation of the diuretic may be required.

Evaluation of the hypertensive patient should always include assessment of renal function. (See DOSAGE and ADMINISTRATION.)

Hyperkalemia: In clinical trials hyperkalemia (serum potassium greater than 5.7 mEq/L) occurred in approximately 1.4 percent of hypertensive patients treated with lisinopril plus hydrochlorothiazide. In most cases these were isolated values which resolved despite continued therapy. Hyperkalemia was not a cause of discontinuation of therapy. Risk factors for the development of hyperkalemia include renal insufficiency, diabetes mellitus, and the concomitant use of potassium-sparing diuretics, potassium supplements and/or potassium-containing salt substitutes, which should be used cautiously if at all with ZESTORETIC. (See Drug Interactions.)

Cough: Presumably due to the inhibition of the degradation of endogenous bradykinin, persistent nonproductive cough has been reported with all ACE inhibitors, almost always resolving after discontinuation of therapy. ACE inhibitor-induced cough should be considered in the differential diagnosis of cough.

Surgery/Anesthesia: In patients undergoing major surgery or during anesthesia with agents that produce hypotension, lisinopril may block angiotensin II formation secondary to compensatory renin release. If hypotension occurs and is considered to be due to this mechanism, it can be corrected by volume expansion.

Hydrochlorothiazide

Periodic determination of serum electrolytes to detect possible electrolyte imbalance should be performed at appropriate intervals.

All patients receiving thiazide therapy should be observed for clinical signs of fluid or electrolyte imbalance: namely, hyponatremia, hypochloremic alkalosis, and hypokalemia. Serum and urine electrolyte determinations are particularly important when the patient is vomiting excessively or receiving parenteral fluids. Warning signs or symptoms of fluid and electrolyte imbalance, irrespective of cause, include dryness of mouth, thirst, weakness, lethargy, drowsiness, restlessness, confusion, seizures, muscle pains or cramps, muscular fatigue hypotension, oliguria, tachycardia, and gastrointestinal disturbances such as nausea and vomiting.

Hypokalemia may develop, especially with brisk diuresis, when severe cirrhosis is present, or after prolonged therapy. Interference with adequate oral electrolyte intake will also contribute to hypokalemia. Hypokalemia may cause cardiac arrhythmia and may also sensitize or exaggerate the response of the heart to the toxic effects of digitalis (eg, increased ventricular irritability). Because lisinopril reduces the production of aldosterone, concomitant therapy with lisinopril attenuates the diuretic-induced potassium loss. (See Drug Interactions, Agents Increasing Serum Potassium.)

Although any chloride deficit is generally mild and usually does not require specific treatment, except under extraordinary circumstances (as in liver disease or renal disease), chloride replacement may be required in the treatment of metabolic alkalosis.

Dilutional hyponatremia may occur in edematous patients in hot weather; appropriate therapy is water restriction, rather than administration of salt except in rare instances when the hyponatremia is life-threatening. In actual salt depletion, appropriate replacement is the therapy of choice.

Hyperuricemia may occur or frank gout may be precipitated in certain patients receiving thiazide therapy.

In diabetic patients dosage adjustments of insulin or oral hypoglycemic agents may be required. Hyperglycemia may occur with thiazide diuretics. Thus latent diabetes mellitus may become manifest during thiazide therapy.

The antihypertensive effects of the drug may be enhanced in the postsympathectomy patient.

If progressive renal impairment becomes evident consider withholding or discontinuing diuretic therapy.

Thiazides have been shown to increase the urinary excretion of magnesium; this may result in hypomagnesemia. Thiazides may decrease urinary calcium excretion. Thiazides may cause intermittent and slight elevation of serum calcium in the absence of known disorders of calcium metabolism. Marked hypercalcemia may be evidence of hidden hyperparathyroidism. Thiazides should be discontinued before carrying out tests for parathyroid function.

Increases in cholesterol and triglyceride levels may be associated with thiazide diuretic therapy.

Information for Patients

Angioedema: Angioedema, including laryngeal edema, may occur at any time during treatment with angiotensin converting enzyme inhibitors, including ZESTORETIC. Patients should be so advised and told to report immediately any signs or symptoms suggesting angioedema (swelling of face, extremities, eyes, lips, tongue, difficulty in swallowing or breathing) and to take no more drug until they have consulted with the prescribing physician.

Symptomatic Hypotension: Patients should be cautioned to report lightheadedness especially during the first few days of therapy. If actual syncope occurs, the patients should be told to discontinue the drug until they have consulted with the prescribing physician.

All patients should be cautioned that excessive perspiration and dehydration may lead to an excessive fall in blood pressure because of reduction in fluid volume. Other causes of volume depletion such as vomiting or diarrhea may also lead to a fall in blood pressure; patients should be advised to consult with their physician.

Hyperkalemia: Patients should be told not to use salt substitutes containing potassium without consulting their physician.

Leukopenia/Neutropenia: Patients should be told to report promptly any indication of infection (eg, sore throat, fever) which may be a sign of leukopenia/neutropenia.

Pregnancy: Female patients of childbearing age should be told about the consequences of second- and third-trimester exposure to ACE inhibitors, and they should also be told that these consequences do not appear to have resulted from intrauterine ACE-inhibitor exposure that has been limited to the first trimester. These patients should be asked to report pregnancies to their physicians as soon as possible.

NOTE: As with many other drugs, certain advice to patients being treated with ZESTORETIC is warranted. This information is intended to aid in the safe and effective use of this medication. It is not a disclosure of all possible adverse or intended effects.

Drug Interactions

Lisinopril

Hypotension—Patients on Diuretic Therapy: Patients on diuretics and especially those in whom diuretic therapy was recently instituted, may occasionally experience an excessive reduction of blood pressure after initiation of therapy with lisinopril. The possibility of hypotensive effects with lisinopril can be minimized by either discontinuing the diuretic or increasing the salt intake prior to initiation of treatment with lisinopril. If it is necessary to continue the diuretic, initiate therapy with lisinopril at a dose of 5 mg daily, and provide close medical supervision after the initial dose for at least two hours and until blood pressure has stabilized for at least an additional hour. (See WARNINGS, and DOSAGE AND ADMINISTRATION.) When a diuretic is added to the therapy of a patient receiving lisinopril, an additional antihypertensive effect is usually observed. (See DOSAGE AND ADMINISTRATION.)

Indomethacin: In a study in 36 patients with mild to moderate hypertension where the antihypertensive effects of lisinopril alone were compared to lisinopril given concomitantly with indomethacin, the use of indomethacin was associated with a reduced effect, although the difference between the two regimens was not significant.

Other Agents: Lisinopril has been used concomitantly with nitrates and/or digoxin without evidence of clinically significant adverse interactions. No meaningful clinically important pharmacokinetic interactions occurred when lisinopril was used concomitantly with propranolol, digoxin, or hydrochlorothiazide. The presence of food in the stomach does not alter the bioavailability of lisinopril.

Agents Increasing Serum Potassium: Lisinopril attenuates potassium loss caused by thiazide-type diuretics. Use of lisinopril with potassium-sparing diuretics (eg, spironolactone, triamterene, or amiloride), potassium supplements, or potassium-containing salt substitutes may lead to significant increases in serum potassium. Therefore, if concomitant use of these agents is indicated, because of demonstrated hypokalemia, they should be used with caution and with frequent monitoring of serum potassium.

Lithium: Lithium toxicity has been reported in patients receiving lithium concomitantly with drugs which cause elimination of sodium, including ACE inhibitors. Lithium toxicity was usually reversible upon discontinuation of lithium and the ACE inhibitor. It is recommended that serum lithium levels be monitored frequently if lisinopril is administered concomitantly with lithium.

Hydrochlorothiazide

When administered concurrently the following drugs may interact with thiazide diuretics.

Alcohol, barbiturates, or narcotics—potentiation of orthostatic hypotension may occur.

Antidiabetic drugs (oral agents and insulin)—dosage adjustment of the antidiabetic drug may be required.

Other antihypertensive drugs—additive effect or potentiation.

Cholestyramine and colestipol resins- Absorbtion of hydrochlorothiazide is impaired in the presence of anionic exchange resins. Single doses of either cholestyramine or colestipol resins bind the hydrochlorothiazide and reduce its absorption from the gastrointestinal tract by up to 85 and 43 percent, respectively.

Corticosteroids, ACTH—intensified electrolyte depletion, particularly hypokalemia.

Pressor amines (eg, norepinephrine)—possible decreased response to pressor amines but not sufficient to preclude their use.

Skeletal muscle relaxants, nondepolarizing (eg, tubocurarine)—possible increased responsiveness to the muscle relaxant.

Lithium—should not generally be given with diuretics. Diuretic agents reduce the renal clearance of lithium and add a high risk of lithium toxicity. Refer to the package insert for lithium preparations before use of such preparations with ZESTORETIC.

Non-Steroidal Anti-inflammatory Drugs—In some patients, the administration of a non-steroidal anti-inflammatory agent can reduce the diuretic, natriuretic, and antihypertensive effects of loop, potassium-sparing and thiazide diuretics. Therefore, when ZESTORETIC and non-steroidal anti-inflammatory agents are used concomitantly, the patient should be observed closely to determine if the desired effect of ZESTORETIC is obtained.

Carcinogenesis, Mutagenesis, Impairment of Fertility

Lisinopril and Hydrochlorothiazide: Lisinopril in combination with hydrochlorothiazide was not mutagenic in a microbial mutagen test using *Salmonella typhimurium* (Ames test) or *Escherichia coli* with or without metabolic activation or in a forward mutation assay using Chinese hamster lung cells. Lisinopril and hydrochlorothiazide did not produce DNA single strand breaks in an *in vitro* alkaline elution rat hepatocyte assay. In addition, it did not produce increases in chromosomal aberrations in an *in vitro* test in Chinese hamster ovary cells or in an *in vivo* study in mouse bone marrow.

Lisinopril: There was no evidence of a tumorigenic effect when lisinopril was administered for 105 weeks to male and female rats at doses up to 90 mg/kg/day (about 56 or 9 times* the maximum daily human dose, based on body weight and body surface area, respectively). There was no evidence of carcinogenicity when lisinopril was administered for 92 weeks to (male and female) mice at doses up to 135 mg/kg/day (about 84 times* the maximum recommended daily human dose). This dose was 6.8 times the maximum human dose based on body surface area in mice.

* Calculations assume a human weight of 50 kg and human body surface area of 1.62 m^2.

Lisinopril was not mutagenic in the Ames microbial mutagen test with or without metabolic activation. It was also negative in a forward mutation assay using Chinese hamster lung cells. Lisinopril did not produce single strand DNA breaks in an *in vitro* alkaline elution rat hepatocyte assay. In addition, lisinopril did not produce increases in chromosomal aberrations in an *in vitro* test in Chinese hamster ovary cells or in an *in vivo* study in mouse bone marrow.

There were no adverse effects on reproductive performance in male and female rats treated with up to 300 mg/kg/day of lisinopril. This dose is 188 times and 30 times the maximum daily human dose based on mg/kg and mg/m^2, respectively.

Hydrochlorothiazide: Two-year feeding studies in mice and rats conducted under the auspices of the National Toxicology Program (NTP) uncovered no evidence of a carcinogenic potential of hydrochlorothiazide in female mice (at doses of up to approximately 600 mg/kg/day) or in male and female rats (at doses of up to approximately 100 mg/kg/day). These doses are 150 times and 12 times for mice and 25 times and 4 times for rats the maximum human daily dose based on mg/kg and mg/m^2, respectively. The NTP, however, found equivocal evidence for hepatocarcinogenicity in male mice.

Hydrochlorothiazide was not genotoxic *in vitro* in the Ames mutagenicity assay of *Salmonella typhimurium* strains TA 98, TA 100, TA 1535, TA 1537, and TA 1538 and in the Chinese Hamster Ovary (CHO) test for chromosomal aberrations, or *in vivo* in assays using mouse germinal cell chromosomes. Chinese hamster bone marrow chromosomes, and the *Drosophila* sex-linked recessive lethal trait gene. Positive test results were obtained only in the *in vitro* CHO Sister Chromatid Exchange (clastogenicity) and in the Mouse Lymphoma Cell (mutagenicity) assays, using concentrations of hydrochlorothiazide from 43 to 1300 μg/mL, and in the *Aspergillus nidulans* nondisjunction assay at an unspecified concentration.

Hydrochlorothiazide had no adverse effects on the fertility of mice and rats of either sex in studies wherein these species were exposed, via their diet, to doses of up to 100 and 4 mg/kg, respectively, prior to conception and throughout gestation. In mice this dose is 25 times and 2 times the maximum daily human dose based on mg/kg and mg/m^2, respectively. In rats this dose is 1 times and 0.2 times the maximum daily human dose based on mg/kg and mg/m^2, respectively.

Pregnancy

Pregnancy Categories C (first trimester) and D (second and third trimesters). See WARNINGS, Pregnancy, Lisinopril, Fetal/Neonatal Morbidity and Mortality.

Nursing Mothers

It is not known whether lisinopril is excreted in human milk. However, milk of lactating rats contains radioactivity following administration of ^{14}C lisinopril. In another study, lisinopril was present in rat milk at levels similar to plasma levels in the dams. Thiazides do appear in human milk. Because of the potential for serious adverse reactions in nursing infants from ACE inhibitors and hydrochlorothiazide, a decision should be made whether to discontinue nursing and/or discontinue ZESTORETIC, taking into account the importance of the drug to the mother.

Pediatric Use

Safety and effectiveness in pediatric patients have not been established.

ADVERSE REACTIONS

ZESTORETIC has been evaluated for safety in 930 patients including 100 patients treated for 50 weeks or more.

In clinical trials with ZESTORETIC no adverse experiences peculiar to this combination drug have been observed. Adverse experiences that have occurred have been limited to those that have been previously reported with lisinopril or hydrochlorothiazide.

The most frequent clinical adverse experiences in controlled trials (including open label extensions) with any combination of lisinopril and hydrochlorothiazide were: dizziness (7.5%), headache (5.2%), cough (3.9%), fatigue (3.7%) and orthostatic effects (3.2%) all of which were more common than in placebo-treated patients. Generally, adverse experiences were mild and transient in nature, but see WARNINGS regarding angioedema and excessive hypotension or syncope. Discontinuation of therapy due to adverse effects was required in 4.4% of patients principally because of dizziness, cough, fatigue and muscle cramps.

Adverse experiences occurring in greater than one percent of patients treated with lisinopril plus hydrochlorothiazide in controlled clinical trials are shown below.

Percent of Patients in Controlled Studies

	Lisinopril and Hydrochlorothiazide (n=930) Incidence (discontinuation)		Placebo (n=207) Incidence
Dizziness	7.5	(0.8)	1.9
Headache	5.2	(0.3)	1.9
Cough	3.9	(0.6)	1.0
Fatigue	3.7	(0.4)	1.0
Orthostatic Effects	3.2	(0.1)	1.0
Diarrhea	2.5	(0.2)	2.4
Nausea	2.2	(0.1)	2.4
Upper Respiratory Infection	2.2	(0.0)	0.0
Muscle Cramps	2.0	(0.4)	0.5
Asthenia	1.8	(0.2)	1.0
Paresthesia	1.5	(0.1)	0.0
Hypotension	1.4	(0.3)	0.5
Vomiting	1.4	(0.1)	0.5
Dyspepsia	1.3	(0.0)	0.0
Rash	1.2	(0.1)	0.5
Impotence	1.2	(0.3)	0.0

Clinical adverse experiences occurring in 0.3% to 1.0% of patients in controlled trials included:

Body as a Whole: Chest pain, abdominal pain, syncope, chest discomfort, fever, trauma, virus infection. **Cardiovascular:** Palpitation, orthostatic hypotension. **Digestive:** Gastrointestinal cramps, dry mouth, constipation, heartburn. **Musculoskeletal:** Back pain, shoulder pain, knee pain, back strain, myalgia, foot pain. **Nervous/Psychiatric:** Decreased libido, vertigo, depression, somnolence. **Respiratory:** Common cold, nasal congestion, influenza, bronchitis, pharyngeal pain, dyspnea, pulmonary congestion, chronic sinusitis,

Continued on next page

Zestoretic—Cont.

allergic rhinitis, pharyngeal discomfort. **Skin:** Flushing, pruritus, skin inflammation, diaphoresis. **Special Senses:** Blurred vision, tinnitus, otalgia. **Urogenital:** Urinary tract infection.

Angioedema: Angioedema of the face, extremities, lips, tongue, glottis and/or larynx has been reported rarely. (See WARNINGS.)

Hypotension: In clinical trials, adverse effects relating to hypotension occurred as follows: hypotension (1.4%), orthostatic hypotension (0.5%), other orthostatic effects (3.2%). In addition syncope occurred in 0.8% of patients. (See WARNINGS.)

Cough: See PRECAUTIONS-Cough.

Clinical Laboratory Test Findings

Serum Electrolytes: (See PRECAUTIONS.)

Creatinine, Blood Urea Nitrogen: Minor reversible increases in blood urea nitrogen and serum creatinine were observed in patients with essential hypertension treated with ZESTORETIC. More marked increases have also been reported and were more likely to occur in patients with renal artery stenosis. (See PRECAUTIONS.)

Serum Uric Acid, Glucose, Magnesium, Cholesterol, Triglycerides and Calcium: (See PRECAUTIONS).

Hemoglobin and Hematocrit: Small decreases in hemoglobin and hematocrit (mean decreases of approximately 0.5 g% and 1.5 vol%, respectively) occurred frequently in hypertensive patients treated with ZESTORETIC but were rarely of clinical importance unless another cause of anemia coexisted. In clinical trials, 0.4% of patients discontinued therapy due to anemia.

Liver Function Tests: Rarely, elevations of liver enzymes and/or serum bilirubin have occurred. (See WARNINGS, Hepatic Failure.)

Other adverse reactions that have been reported with the individual components are listed below:

Lisinopril—In clinical trials adverse reactions which occurred with lisinopril were also seen with ZESTORETIC. In addition, and since lisinopril has been marketed, the following adverse reactions have been reported with lisinopril and should be considered potential adverse reactions for ZESTORETIC: **Body as a Whole:** Anaphylactoid reactions (see WARNINGS, Anaphylactoid Reactions During Membrane Exposure), malaise, edema, facial edema, pain, pelvic pain, flank pain, chills; **Cardiovascular:** Cardiac arrest, myocardial infarction or cerebrovascular accident, possibly secondary to excessive hypotension in high risk patients (see WARNINGS, Hypotension), pulmonary embolism and infarction, worsening of heart failure, arrhythmias (including tachycardia, ventricular tachycardia, atrial tachycardia, atrial fibrillation, bradycardia, and premature ventricular contractions), angina pectoris, transient ischemic attacks, paroxysmal nocturnal dyspnea, decreased blood pressure, peripheral edema, vasculitis; **Digestive:** Pancreatitis, hepatitis (hepatocellular or cholestatic jaundice) (see WARNINGS, Hepatic Failure), gastritis, anorexia, flatulence, increased salivation; **Endocrine:** Diabetes mellitus; **Hematologic:** Rare cases of bone marrow depression, hemolytic anemia, leukopenia/Neutropenia, and thrombocytopenia, have been reported in which a casual relationship to lisinopril can not be excluded; **Metabolic:** Gout, weight loss, dehydration, fluid overload, weight gain; **Musculoskeletal:** Arthritis, arthralgia, neck pain, hip pain, joint pain, leg pain, arm pain, lumbago; **Nervous System/Psychiatric:** Ataxia, memory impairment, tremor, insomnia, stroke, nervousness, confusion, peripheral neuropathy (eg, paresthesia, dysesthesia), spasm, hypersomnia, irritability; **Respiratory:** Malignant lung neoplasms, hemoptysis, pulmonary edema, pulmonary infiltrates, bronchospasm, asthma, pleural effusion, pneumonia, eosinophilic pneumonitis, wheezing, orthopnea, painful respiration, epistaxis, laryngitis, sinusitis, pharyngitis, rhinitis, rhinorrhea, chest sound abnormalities; **Skin:** Urticaria, alopecia, herpes zoster, photosensitivity, skin lesions, skin infections, pemphiqus, erythema, rare cases of other severe skin reactions including toxic epidermal necrolysis and Stevens-Johnson syndrome, (causal relationship has not been established); **Special Senses:** Visual loss, diplopia, photophobia, taste alteration; **Urogenital:** Acute renal failure, oliguria, anuria, uremia, progressive azotemia, renal dysfunction (see PRECAUTIONS and DOSAGE AND ADMINISTRATION), pyelonephritis, dysuria, breast pain.

Miscellaneous: A symptom complex has been reported which may include a positive ANA, an elevated erythrocyte sedimentation rate, arthralgia/arthritis, myalgia, fever, vasculitis, eosinophilia and leukocytosis. Rash, photosensitivity or other dermatological manifestations may occur alone or in combination with these symptoms.

Fetal/Neonatal Morbidity and Mortality

See WARNINGS—Pregnancy, Lisinopril, Fetal/Neonatal Morbidity and Mortality.

Hydrochlorothiazide—Body as a Whole: Weakness **Digestive:** Anorexia, gastric irritation, cramping, jaundice (intrahepatic cholestatic jaundice) (see WARNINGS, Hepatic Failure), pancreatitis, sialoadenitis, constipation; **Hematologic:** Leukopenia, agranulocytosis, thrombocytopenia, aplastic anemia, hemolytic anemia; **Musculoskeletal:** Muscle spasm; **Nervous System/Psychiatric:** Restlessness; **Renal:** Renal failure, renal dysfunction, interstitial nephritis (see WARNINGS): **Skin:** Erythema multiforme including Stevens-Johnson syndrome, exfoliative dermatitis including toxic epidermal necrolysis, alopecia; **Special Senses:** Xanthopsia; **Hypersensitivity:** Purpura, photosensitivity, urticaria, necrotizing angitis (vasculitis and cutaneous vasculitis), respiratory distress including pneumonitis and pulmonary edema, anaphylactic reactions.

OVERDOSAGE

No specific information is available on the treatment of overdosage with ZESTORETIC. Treatment is symptomatic and supportive. Therapy with ZESTORETIC should be discontinued and the patient observed closely. Suggested measures include induction of emesis and/or gastric lavage, and correction of dehydration, electrolyte imbalance and hypotension by established procedures.

Lisinopril: Following a single oral dose of 20 g/kg no lethality occurred in rats and death occurred in one of 20 mice receiving the same dose. The most likely manifestation of overdosage would be hypotension, for which the usual treatment would be intravenous infusion of normal saline solution.

Lisinopril can be removed by hemodialysis.

Hydrochlorothiazide: Oral administration of a single oral dose of 10 g/kg to mice and rats was not lethal. The most common signs and symptoms observed are those caused by electrolyte depletion (hypokalemia, hypochloremia, hyponatremia) and dehydration resulting from excessive diuresis. If digitalis has also been administered, hypokalemia may accentuate cardiac arrhythmias.

DOSAGE AND ADMINISTRATION

Lisinopril monotherapy is an effective treatment of hypertension in once-daily doses of 10-80 mg, while hydrochlorothiazide monotherapy is effective in doses of: 12.5–50 mg per day. In clinical trials of lisinopril/hydrochlorothiazide combination therapy using lisinopril doses of 10-80 mg and hydrochlorothiazide doses of 6.25-50 mg, the antihypertensive response rates generally increased with increasing dose of either component.

The side effects (see WARNINGS) of lisinopril are generally rare and apparently independent of dose; those of hydrochlorothiazide are a mixture of dose-dependent phenomena (primarily hypokalemia) and dose-independent phenomena (eg., pancreatitis), the former much more common than the latter. Therapy with any combination of lisinopril and hydrochlorothiazide may be associated with either or both dose-independent or dose-dependent side effects, but addition of lisinopril in clinical trials blunted the hypokalemia normally seen with diuretics.

To minimize dose-dependent side effects, it is usually appropriate to begin combination therapy only after a patient has failed to achieve the desired effect with monotherapy.

Dose Titration Guided by Clinical Effect: A patient whose blood pressure is not adequately controlled with either lisinopril or hydrochlorothiazide monotherapy may be switched to lisinopril/HCTZ 10/12.5 or lisinopril/HCTZ 20/12.5, depending on current monotherapy dose. Further increases of either or both components should depend on clinical response with blood pressure measured at the interdosing interval to ensure that there is an adequate antihypertensive effect at that time. The hydrochlorothiazide dose should generally not be increased until 2-3 weeks have elapsed. After addition of the diuretic it may be possible to reduce the dose of lisinopril. Patients whose blood pressures are adequately controlled with 25 mg of daily hydrochlorothiazide, but who experience significant potassium loss with this regimen may achieve similar or greater blood-pressure control without electrolyte disturbance if they are switched to lisinopril/HCTZ 10/12.5.

In patients who are currrently being treated with a diuretic, symptomatic hypotension occasionally may occur following the initial dose of lisinopril. The diuretic should, if possible, be discontinued for two to three days before beginning therapy with lisinopril to reduce the likelihood of hypotension. (See WARNINGS.) If the patient's blood pressure is not controlled with lisinopril alone, diuretic therapy may be resumed.

If the diuretic cannot be discontinued, an initial dose of 5 mg of lisinopril should be used under medical supervision for at least two hours and until blood pressure has stabilized for at least an additional hour. (See WARNINGS AND PRECAUTIONS, Drug Interactions.)

Concomitant administration of ZESTORETIC with potassium supplements, potassium salt substitutes or potassium-sparing diuretics may lead to increases of serum potassium. (See PRECAUTIONS.)

Replacement Therapy: The combination may be substituted for the titrated individual components.

Use in Elderly: In general, blood pressure response and adverse experiences were similar in younger and older patients given ZESTORETIC. However, in a multiple dose pharmacokinetic study in elderly versus young patients using the lisinopril/hydrochlorothiazide combination, area under the plasma concentration time curve (AUC) increased approximately 120% for lisinopril and approximately 80% for hydrochlorothiazide in older patients. Therefore, dosage adjustments in elderly patients should be made with particular caution.

Use in Renal Impairment: Regimens of therapy with lisinopril/HCTZ need not take account of renal function as long as the patient's creatinine clearance is >30 mL/min/1.7m² (serum creatinine roughly ≤3 mg/dL or 265 μmol/L). In patients with more severe renal impairment, loop diuretics are preferred to thiazides, so lisinopril/HCTZ is not recommended (see WARNINGS, Anaphylactoid Reactions During Membrane Exposure).

HOW SUPPLIED

ZESTORETIC 10–12.5 Tablets (NDC 0310–0141) Peach, round, biconvex, uncoated tablets identified with "141" debossed on one side and "ZESTORETIC" on the other side are supplied in bottles of 100 tablets.

ZESTORETIC 20-12.5 Tablets (NDC 0310-0142) White, round, biconvex, uncoated tablets identified with "142" debossed on one side and "ZESTORETIC" on the other side are supplied in bottles of 100 tablets.

ZESTORETIC 20-25 Tablets (NDC 0310-0145) Peach, round, biconvex, uncoated tablets identified with "145" debossed on one side and "ZESTORETIC" on the other side are supplied in bottles of 100 tablets.

Store at controlled room temperature, 20°–25° C (68°–77° F). [see USP]

Protect from excessive light and humidity.

¶Registered trademark of Hospal Ltd.

Manufactured by: IPR Pharmaceuticals Inc.

Distributed by:

ZENECA PHARMACEUTICALS

A Business Unit of Zeneca Inc.

Wilmington, DE 19850-5437

SIC 64110-01 Rev P 01/98

Shown in Product Identification Guide, page 346

ONCE-DAILY
ZESTRIL® (LISINOPRIL) ℞

USE IN PREGNANCY

When used in pregnancy during the second and third trimesters, ACE inhibitors can cause injury and even death to the developing fetus. When pregnancy is detected, ZESTRIL should be discontinued as soon as possible. See WARNINGS, Fetal/Neonatal Morbidity and Mortality.

DESCRIPTION

Lisinopril is an oral long-acting angiotensin converting enzyme inhibitor. Lisinopril, a synthetic peptide derivative, is chemically described as (S)-1-[N^2-(1-Carboxy-3-phenylpropyl)-L-lysyl]-L-proline dihydrate. Its empirical formula is $C_{21}H_{31}N_3O_5 \cdot 2H_2O$ and its structural formula is:

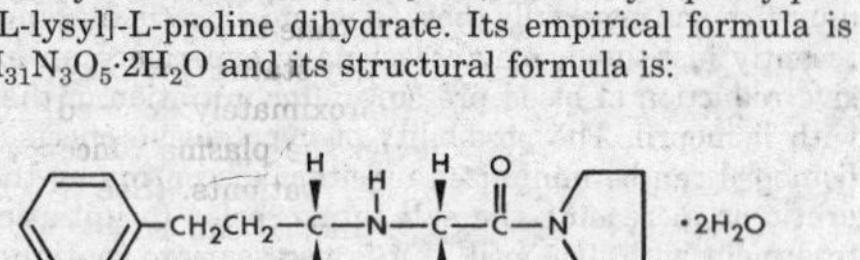

Lisinopril is a white to off-white, crystalline powder, with a molecular weight of 441.53. It is soluble in water and sparingly soluble in methanol and practically insoluble in ethanol.

ZESTRIL is supplied as 2.5 mg, 5 mg, 10 mg, 20 mg and 40 mg tablets for oral administration.

Inactive Ingredients:

2.5 mg tablets—calcium phosphate, magnesium stearate, mannitol, starch.

5, 10 and 20 mg tablets—calcium phosphate, magnesium stearate, mannitol, red ferric oxide, starch.

40 mg tablets—calcium phosphate, magnesium stearate, mannitol, starch, yellow ferric oxide.

CLINICAL PHARMACOLOGY

Mechanism of Action: Lisinopril inhibits angiotensin converting enzyme (ACE) in human subjects and animals. ACE is a peptidyl dipeptidase that catalyzes the conversion of angiotensin I to the vasoconstrictor substance, angiotensin II. Angiotensin II also stimulates aldosterone secretion by the adrenal cortex. The beneficial effects of lisinopril in hypertension and heart failure appear to result primarily from suppression of the renin-angiotensin-aldosterone system. Inhibition of ACE results in decreased plasma angiotensin II which leads to decreased vasopressor activity and to decreased aldosterone secretion. The latter decrease may result in a small increase of serum potassium. In hypertensive

patients with normal renal function treated with ZESTRIL alone for up to 24 weeks, the mean increase in serum potassium was approximately 0.1 mEq/L; however, approximately 15% of patients had increases greater than 0.5 mEq/L and approximately 6% had a decrease greater than 0.5 mEq/L. In the same study, patients treated with ZESTRIL and hydrochlorothiazide for up to 24 weeks had a mean decrease in serum potassium of 0.1 mEq/L; approximately 4% of patients had increases greater than 0.5 mEq/L and approximately 12% had a decrease greater than 0.5 mEq/L. (See PRECAUTIONS.) Removal of angiotensin II negative feedback on renin secretion leads to increased plasma renin activity.

ACE is identical to kininase, an enzyme that degrades bradykinin. Whether increased levels of bradykinin, a potent vasodepressor peptide, play a role in the therapeutic effects of ZESTRIL remains to be elucidated.

While the mechanism through which ZESTRIL lowers blood pressure is believed to be primarily suppression of the renin-angiotensin-aldosterone system, ZESTRIL is antihypertensive even in patients with low-renin hypertension. Although ZESTRIL was antihypertensive in all races studied, black hypertensive patients (usually a low-renin hypertensive population) had a smaller average response to monotherapy than nonblack patients.

Concomitant administration of ZESTRIL and hydrochlorothiazide further reduced blood pressure in black and nonblack patients and any racial differences in blood pressure response were no longer evident.

Pharmacokinetics and Metabolism: Following oral administration of ZESTRIL, peak serum concentrations of lisinopril occur within about 7 hours, although there was a trend to a small delay in time taken to reach peak serum concentrations in acute myocardial infarction patients. Declining serum concentrations exhibit a prolonged terminal phase which does not contribute to drug accumulation. This terminal phase probably represents saturable binding to ACE and is not proportional to dose.

Lisinopril does not appear to be bound to other serum proteins. Lisinopril does not undergo metabolism and is excreted unchanged entirely in the urine. Based on urinary recovery, the mean extent of absorption of lisinopril is approximately 25%, with large intersubject variability (6%–60%) at all doses tested (5–80 mg). Lisinopril absorption is not influenced by the presence of food in the gastrointestinal tract. The absolute bioavailability of lisinopril is reduced to 16% in patients with stable NYHA Class II-IV congestive heart failure, and the volume of distribution appears to be slightly smaller than that in normal subjects. The oral bioavailability of lisinopril in patients with acute myocardial infarction is similar to that in healthy volunteers.

Upon multiple dosing, lisinopril exhibits an effective half-life of accumulation of 12 hours.

Impaired renal function decreases elimination of lisinopril, which is excreted principally through the kidneys, but this decrease becomes clinically important only when the glomerular filtration rate is below 30 mL/min. Above this glomerular filtration rate, the elimination half-life is little changed. With greater impairment, however, peak and trough lisinopril levels increase, time to peak concentration increases and time to attain steady state is prolonged. Older patients, on average, have (approximately doubled) higher blood levels and the area under the plasma concentration time curve (AUC) than younger patients. (See DOSAGE AND ADMINISTRATION.) Lisinopril can be removed by hemodialysis.

Studies in rats indicate that lisinopril crosses the blood-brain barrier poorly. Multiple doses of lisinopril in rats do not result in accumulation in any tissues. Milk of lactating rats contains radioactivity following administration of ^{14}C lisinopril. By whole body autoradiography, radioactivity was found in the placenta following administration of labeled drug to pregnant rats, but none was found in the fetuses.

Pharmacodynamics and Clinical Effects

Hypertension: Administration of ZESTRIL to patients with hypertension results in a reduction of both supine and standing blood pressure to about the same extent with no compensatory tachycardia. Symptomatic postural hypotension is usually not observed although it can occur and should be anticipated in volume and/or salt-depleted patients. (See WARNINGS.) When given together with thiazide-type diuretics, the blood pressure lowering effects of the two drugs are approximately additive.

In most patients studied, onset of antihypertensive activity was seen at one hour after oral administration of an individual dose of ZESTRIL, with peak reduction of blood pressure achieved by 6 hours. Although an antihypertensive effect was observed 24 hours after dosing with recommended single daily doses, the effect was more consistent and the mean effect was considerably larger in some studies with doses of 20 mg or more than with lower doses. However, at all doses studied, the mean antihypertensive effect was substantially smaller 24 hours after dosing than it was 6 hours after dosing.

In some patients achievement of optimal blood pressure reduction may require two to four weeks of therapy.

The antihypertensive effects of ZESTRIL are maintained during long-term therapy. Abrupt withdrawal of ZESTRIL has not been associated with a rapid increase in blood pressure, or a significant increase in blood pressure compared to pretreatment levels.

Two dose-response studies utilizing a once daily regimen were conducted in 438 mild to moderate hypertensive patients not on a diuretic. Blood pressure was measured 24 hours after dosing. An antihypertensive effect of ZESTRIL was seen with 5 mg in some patients. However, in both studies blood pressure reduction occurred sooner and was greater in patients treated with 10, 20 or 80 mg of ZESTRIL. In controlled clinical studies, ZESTRIL 20–80 mg has been compared in patients with mild to moderate hypertension to hydrochlorothiazide 12.5–50 mg and with atenolol 50–200 mg; and in patients with moderate to severe hypertension to metoprolol 100–200 mg. It was superior to hydrochlorothiazide in effects on systolic and diastolic pressure in a population that was $^3/_4$ caucasian. ZESTRIL was approximately equivalent to atenolol and metoprolol in effects on diastolic blood pressure, and had somewhat greater effects on systolic blood pressure.

ZESTRIL had similar effectiveness and adverse effects in younger and older (>65 years) patients. It was less effective in blacks than in caucasians.

In hemodynamic studies in patients with essential hypertension, blood pressure reduction was accompanied by a reduction in peripheral arterial resistance with little or no change in cardiac output and in heart rate. In a study in nine hypertensive patients, following administration of ZESTRIL, there was an increase in mean renal blood flow that was not significant. Data from several small studies are inconsistent with respect to the effect of lisinopril on glomerular filtration rate in hypertensive patients with normal renal function, but suggest that changes, if any, are not large.

In patients with renovascular hypertension ZESTRIL has been shown to be well tolerated and effective in controlling blood pressure. (See PRECAUTIONS.)

Heart Failure: During baseline-controlled clinical trials, in patients receiving digitalis and diuretics, single doses of ZESTRIL resulted in decreases in pulmonary capillary wedge pressure, systemic vascular resistance and blood pressure accompanied by an increase in cardiac output and no change in heart rate.

In two placebo controlled, 12-week clinical studies, ZESTRIL as adjunctive therapy to digitalis and diuretics improved the following signs and symptoms due to congestive heart failure: edema, rales, paroxysmal nocturnal dyspnea and jugular venous distention. In one of the studies, beneficial response was also noted for: orthopnea, presence of third heart sound and the number of patients classified as NYHA Class III and IV. Exercise tolerance was also improved in this study. The effect of lisinopril on mortality in patients with heart failure has not been evaluated. The once daily dosing for the treatment of congestive heart failure was the only dosage regimen used during clinical trial development and was determined by the measurement of hemodynamic response.

Acute Myocardial Infarction: The Gruppo Italiano per lo Studio della Sopravvienza nell'Infarto Miocardico (GISSI-3) study was a multicenter, controlled, randomized, unblinded clinical trial conducted in 19,394 patients with acute myocardial infarction admitted to a coronary care unit. It was designed to examine the effects of short-term (6 week) treatment with lisinopril, nitrates, their combination, or no therapy on short-term (6 week) mortality and on longer-term death and markedly impaired cardiac function. Patients presenting within 24 hours of the onset of symptoms who were hemodynamically stable were randomized, in a 2 × 2 factorial design, to six weeks of either 1) ZESTRIL alone (n=4841), 2) nitrates alone (n=4869), 3) ZESTRIL plus nitrates (n=4841), or 4) open control (n=4843). All patients received routine therapies, including thrombolytics (72%), aspirin (84%), and a beta-blocker (31%), as appropriate, normally utilized in acute myocardial infarction (MI) patients.

The protocol excluded patients with hypotension (systolic blood pressure ≤100 mmHg), severe heart failure, cardiogenic shock, and renal dysfunction (serum creatinine >2 mg/dL and/or proteinuria >500 mg/24h). Doses of ZESTRIL were adjusted as necessary according to protocol (see DOSAGE AND ADMINISTRATION).

Study treatment was withdrawn at six weeks except where clinical conditions indicated continuation of treatment.

The primary outcomes of the trial were the overall mortality at 6 weeks and a combined endpoint at 6 months after the myocardial infarction, consisting of a number of patients who died, had late (day 4) clinical congestive heart failure, or had extensive left ventricular damage defined as ejection fraction ≤35% or an akinetic-dyskinetic [A–D] score ≥45%. Patients receiving ZESTRIL (n=9646), alone or with nitrates, had an 11% lower risk of death (2p [two-tailed] =0.04) compared to patients receiving no ZESTRIL (n=9672) (6.4% vs. 7.2%, respectively) at six weeks. Although patients randomized to receive ZESTRIL for up to six weeks also fared numerically better on the combined end-point at 6 months, the open nature of the assessment of heart failure, substantial loss to follow-up echocardiography, and substantial excess use of lisinopril between 6 weeks and 6 months in the group randomized to 6 weeks of lisinopril, preclude any conclusion about this endpoint.

Patients with acute myocardial infarction, treated with ZESTRIL, had a higher (9.0% versus 3.7%) incidence of persistent hypotension (systolic blood pressure <90 mmHg for more than 1 hour) and renal dysfunction (2.4% versus 1.1%) in-hospital and at six weeks (increasing creatinine concentration to over 3 mg/dL or a doubling or more of the baseline serum creatinine concentration). See ADVERSE REACTIONS—Acute Myocardial infarction.

INDICATIONS AND USAGE

Hypertension: ZESTRIL is indicated for the treatment of hypertension. It may be used alone as initial therapy or concomitantly with other classes of antihypertensive agents.

Heart Failure: ZESTRIL is indicated as adjunctive therapy in the management of heart failure in patients who are not responding adequately to diuretics and digitalis.

Acute Myocardial Infarction: ZESTRIL is indicated for the treatment of hemodynamically stable patients within 24 hours of acute myocardial infarction, to improve survival. Patients should receive, as appropriate, the standard recommended treatments such as thrombolytics, aspirin and beta-blockers.

In using ZESTRIL, consideration should be given to the fact that another angiotensin converting enzyme inhibitor, captopril, has caused agranulocytosis, particularly in patients with renal impairment or collagen vascular disease, and that available data are insufficient to show that ZESTRIL does not have a similar risk. (See WARNINGS.)

In considering the use of ZESTRIL, it should be noted that in controlled trials ACE inhibitors have an effect on blood pressure that is less in black patients than in nonblacks. In addition, ACE inhibitors have been associated with a higher rate of angioedema in black than in nonblack patients (see WARNINGS, Angioedema).

CONTRAINDICATIONS

ZESTRIL is contraindicated in patients who are hypersensitive to this product and in patients with a history of angioedema related to previous treatment with an angiotensin converting enzyme inhibitor.

WARNINGS

Anaphylactoid and Possibly Related Reactions: Presumably because angiotensin-converting enzyme inhibitors affect the metabolism of eicosanoids and polypeptides, including endogenous bradykinin, patients receiving ACE inhibitors (including ZESTRIL) may be subject to a variety of adverse reactions, some of them serious.

Angioedema: Angioedema of the face, extremities, lips, tongue, glottis and/or larynx has been reported in patients treated with angiotensin converting enzyme inhibitors, including ZESTRIL. This may occur at any time during treatment. ACE inhibitors have been associated with a higher rate of angioedema in black than in nonblack patients. ZESTRIL should be promptly discontinued and appropriate therapy and monitoring should be provided until complete and sustained resolution of signs and symptoms has occurred. In instances where swelling has been confined to the face and lips the condition has generally resolved without treatment, although antihistamines have been useful in relieving symptoms. Angioedema associated with laryngeal edema may be fatal. **Where there is involvement of the tongue, glottis or larynx, likely to cause airway obstruction, appropriate therapy, e.g., subcutaneous epinephrine solution 1:1000 (0.3 mL to 0.5 mL) and/or measures necessary to ensure a patent airway should be promptly provided. (See ADVERSE REACTIONS.)**

Patients with a history of angioedema unrelated to ACE inhibitor therapy may be at increased risk of angioedema while receiving an ACE inhibitor. (See also INDICATIONS AND USAGE and CONTRAINDICATIONS.)

Anaphylactoid Reactions During Desensitization: Two patients undergoing desensitizing treatment with hymenoptera venom while receiving ACE inhibitors sustained life-threatening anaphylactoid reactions. In the same patients, these reactions were avoided when ACE inhibitors were temporarily withheld, but they reappeared upon inadvertent rechallenge.

Anaphylactoid Reactions During Membrane Exposure: Sudden and potentially life-threatening anaphylactoid reactions have been reported in some patients dialyzed with high-flux membranes (e.g., AN69¶) and treated concomitantly with an ACE inhibitor. In such patients, dialysis must be stopped immediately, and aggressive therapy for anaphylactoid reactions be initiated. Symptoms have not been relieved by antihistamines in these situations. In these patients, consideration should be given to using a different type of dialysis membrane or a different class of antihyper-

Continued on next page

Zestril—Cont.

tensive agent. Anaphylactoid reactions have also been reported in patients undergoing low-density lipoprotein apheresis with dextran sulfate absorption.

Hypotension: Excessive hypotension is rare in patients with uncomplicated hypertension treated with ZESTRIL alone.

Patients with heart failure given ZESTRIL commonly have some reduction in blood pressure, with peak blood pressure reduction occurring 6 to 8 hours post dose, but discontinuation of therapy because of continuing symptomatic hypotension usually is not necessary when dosing instructions are followed; caution should be observed when initiating therapy. (See DOSAGE AND ADMINISTRATION.)

Patients at risk of excessive hypotension, sometimes associated with oliguria and/or progressive azotemia, and rarely with acute renal failure and/or death, include those with the following conditions or characteristics: heart failure with systolic blood pressure below 100 mmHg, hyponatremia, high dose diuretic therapy, recent intensive diuresis or increase in diuretic dose, renal dialysis, or severe volume and/or salt depletion of any etiology. It may be advisable to eliminate the diuretic (except in patients with heart failure), reduce the diuretic dose or increase salt intake cautiously before initiating therapy with ZESTRIL in patients at risk for excessive hypotension who are able to tolerate such adjustments. (See PRECAUTIONS, Drug Interactions and ADVERSE REACTIONS.)

Patients with acute myocardial infarction in the GISSI-3 trial had a higher (9.0% versus 3.7%) incidence of persistent hypotension (systolic blood pressure <90 mmHg for more than 1 hour) when treated with ZESTRIL. Treatment with ZESTRIL must not be initiated in acute myocardial infarction patients at risk of further serious hemodynamic deterioration after treatment with a vasodilator (systolic blood pressure of 100 mmHg or lower) or cardiogenic shock.

In patients at risk of excessive hypotension, therapy should be started under very close medical supervision and such patients should be followed closely for the first two weeks of treatment and whenever the dose of ZESTRIL and/or diuretic is increased. Similar considerations may apply to patients with ischemic heart or cerebrovascular disease, or in patients with acute myocardial infarction, in whom an excessive fall in blood pressure could result in a myocardial infarction or cerebrovascular accident.

If excessive hypotension occurs, the patient should be placed in the supine position and, if necessary, receive an intravenous infusion of normal saline. A transient hypotensive response is not a contraindication to further doses of ZESTRIL which usually can be given without difficulty once the blood pressure has stabilized. If symptomatic hypotension develops, a dose reduction or discontinuation of ZESTRIL or concomitant diuretic may be necessary.

Leukopenia/Neutropenia/Agranulocytosis: Another angiotensin converting enzyme inhibitor, captopril, has been shown to cause agranulocytosis and bone marrow depression, rarely in uncomplicated patients but more frequently in patients with renal impairment especially if they also have a collagen vascular disease. Available data from clinical trials of ZESTRIL are insufficient to show that ZESTRIL does not cause agranulocytosis at similar rates. Marketing experience has revealed rare cases of leukopenia/neutropenia and bone marrow depression in which a causal relationship to lisinopril cannot be excluded. Periodic monitoring of white blood cell counts in patients with collagen vascular disease and renal disease should be considered.

Hepatic Failure: Rarely, ACE inhibitors have been associated with a syndrome that starts with cholestatic jaundice and progresses to fulminant hepatic necrosis and (sometimes) death. The machanism of this syndrome is not understood. Patients receiving ACE inhibitors who develop jaundice or marked elevations of hepatic enzymes should discontinue the ACE inhibitor and receive appropriate medical follow-up.

Fetal/Neonatal Morbidity and Mortality: ACE inhibitors can cause fetal and neonatal morbidity and death when administered to pregnant women. Several dozen cases have been reported in the world literature. When pregnancy is detected, ACE inhibitors should be discontinued as soon as possible.

The use of ACE inhibitors during the second and third trimesters of pregnancy has been associated with fetal and neonatal injury, including hypotension, neonatal skull hypoplasia, anuria, reversible or irreversible renal failure, and death. Oligohydramnios has also been reported, presumably resulting from decreased fetal renal function; oligohydramnios in this setting has been associated with fetal limb contractures, craniofacial deformation, and hypoplastic lung development. Prematurity, intrauterine growth retardation, and patent ductus arteriosus have also been reported, although it is not clear whether these occurrences were due to the ACE-inhibitor exposure.

These adverse effects do not appear to have resulted from intrauterine ACE-inhibitor exposure that has been limited to the first trimester. Mothers whose embryos and fetuses are exposed to ACE inhibitors only during the first trimester should be so informed. Nonetheless, when patients become pregnant, physicians should make every effort to discontinue the use of ZESTRIL as soon as possible.

Rarely (probably less often than once in every thousand pregnancies), no alternative to ACE inhibitors will be found. In these rare cases, the mothers should be apprised of the potential hazards to their fetuses, and serial ultrasound examinations should be performed to assess the intraamniotic environment.

If oligohydramnios is observed, ZESTRIL should be discontinued unless it is considered lifesaving for the mother. Contraction stress testing (CST), a nonstress test (NST), or biophysical profiling (BPP) may be appropriate, depending upon the week of pregnancy. Patients and physicians should be aware, however, that oligohydramnios may not appear until after the fetus has sustained irreversible injury.

Infants with histories of *in utero* exposure to ACE inhibitors should be closely observed for hypotension, oliguria, and hyperkaliemia. If oliguria occurs, attention should be directed toward support of blood pressure and renal perfusion. Exchange transfusion or dialysis may be required as means of reversing hypotension and/or substituting for disordered renal function. Lisinopril, which crosses the placenta, has been removed from neonatal circulation by peritoneal dialysis with some clinical benefit, and theoretically may be removed by exchange transfusion, although there is no experience with the latter procedure.

No teratogenic effects of lisinopril were seen in studies of pregnant rats, mice, and rabbits. On a mg/kg basis, the doses used were up to 625 times (in mice), 188 times (in rats), and 0.6 times (in rabbits) the maximum recommended human dose.

PRECAUTIONS

General

Impaired Renal Function: As a consequence of inhibiting the renin-angiotensin-aldosterone system, changes in renal function may be anticipated in susceptible individuals. In patients with severe congestive heart failure whose renal function may depend on the activity of the renin-angiotensin-aldosterone system, treatment with angiotensin converting enzyme inhibitors, including ZESTRIL, may be associated with oliguria and/or progressive azotemia and rarely with acute renal failure and/or death.

In hypertensive patients with unilateral or bilateral renal artery stenosis, increases in blood urea nitrogen and serum creatinine may occur. Experience with another angiotensin converting enzyme inhibitor suggests that these increases are usually reversible upon discontinuation of ZESTRIL and/or diuretic therapy. In such patients, renal function should be monitored during the first few weeks of therapy.

Some patients with hypertension or heart failure with no apparent preexisting renal vascular disease have developed increases in blood urea nitrogen and serum creatinine, usually minor and transient, especially when ZESTRIL has been given concomitantly with a diuretic. This is more likely to occur in patients with pre-existing renal impairment. Dosage reduction and/or discontinuation of the diuretic and/or ZESTRIL may be required.

Patients with acute myocardial infarction in the GISSI-3 trial, treated with ZESTRIL had a higher (2.4% versus 1.1%) incidence of renal dysfunction in-hospital and at six weeks (increasing creatinine concentration to over 3 mg/dL or a doubling or more of the baseline serum creatinine concentration). In acute myocardial infarction, treatment with ZESTRIL should be initiated with caution in patients with evidence of renal dysfunction, defined as serum creatinine concentration exceeding 2 mg/dL. If renal dysfunction develops during treatment with ZESTRIL (serum creatinine concentration exceeding 3 mg/dL or a doubling from the pretreatment value) then the physician should consider withdrawal of ZESTRIL.

Evaluation of patients with hypertension, heart failure, or myocardial infarction should always include assessment of renal function. (See DOSAGE AND ADMINISTRATION.)

Hyperkalemia: In clinical trials hyperkalemia (serum potassium greater than 5.7 mEq/L) occurred in approximately 2.2% of hypertensive patients and 4.8% of patients with heart failure. In most cases these were isolated values which resolved despite continued therapy. Hyperkalemia was a cause of discontinuation of therapy in approximately 0.1% of hypertensive patients; 0.6% of patients with heart failure and 0.1% of patients with myocardial infarction. Risk factors for the development of hyperkalemia include renal insufficiency, diabetes mellitus, and the concomitant use of potassium-sparing diuretics, potassium supplements and/or potassium-containing salt substitutes, which should be used cautiously, if at all, with ZESTRIL. (See Drug Interactions.)

Cough: Presumably due to the inhibition of the degradation of endogenous bradykinin, persistent nonproductive cough has been reported with all ACE inhibitors, almost always resolving after discontinuation of therapy. ACE inhibitor-induced cough should be considered in the differential diagnosis of cough.

Surgery/Anesthesia: In patients undergoing major surgery or during anesthesia with agents that produce hypotension, ZESTRIL may block angiotensin II formation secondary to compensatory renin release. If hypotension occurs and is considered to be due to this mechanism, it can be corrected by volume expansion.

Information for Patients

Angioedema: Angioedema, including laryngeal edema, may occur at any time during treatment with angiotensin converting enzyme inhibitors, including ZESTRIL. Patients should be so advised and told to report immediately any signs or symptoms suggesting angioedema (swelling of face, extremities, eyes, lips, tongue, difficulty in swallowing or breathing) and to take no more drug until they have consulted with the prescribing physician.

Symptomatic Hypotension: Patients should be cautioned to report lightheadedness especially during the first few days of therapy. If actual syncope occurs, the patient should be told to discontinue the drug until they have consulted with the prescribing physician.

All patients should be cautioned that excessive perspiration and dehydration may lead to an excessive fall in blood pressure because of reduction in fluid volume. Other causes of volume depletion such as vomiting or diarrhea may also lead to a fall in blood pressure; patients should be advised to consult with their physician.

Hyperkalemia: Patients should be told not to use salt substitutes containing potassium without consulting their physician.

Leukopenia/Neutropenia: Patients should be told to report promptly any indication of infection (e.g., sore throat, fever) which may be a sign of leukopenia/neutropenia.

Pregnancy: Female patients of childbearing age should be told about the consequences of second- and third-trimester exposure to ACE inhibitors, and they should also be told that these consequences do not appear to have resulted from intrauterine ACE-inhibitor exposure that has been limited to the first trimester. These patients should be asked to report pregnancies to their physicians as soon as possible.

NOTE: As with many other drugs, certain advice to patients being treated with ZESTRIL is warranted. This information is intended to aid in the safe and effective use of this medication. It is not a disclosure of all possible adverse or intended effects.

Drug Interactions

Hypotension—Patients on Diuretic Therapy: Patients on diuretics and especially those in whom diuretic therapy was recently instituted, may occasionally experience an excessive reduction of blood pressure after initiation of therapy with ZESTRIL. The possibility of hypotensive effects with ZESTRIL can be minimized by either discontinuing the diuretic or increasing the salt intake prior to initiation of treatment with ZESTRIL. If it is necessary to continue the diuretic, initiate therapy with ZESTRIL at a dose of 5 mg daily, and provide close medical supervision after the initial dose until blood pressure has stabilized. (See WARNINGS, and DOSAGE AND ADMINISTRATION.) When a diuretic is added to the therapy of a patient receiving ZESTRIL, an additional antihypertensive effect is usually observed. Studies with ACE inhibitors in combination with diuretics indicate that the dose of the ACE inhibitor can be reduced when it is given with a diuretic. (See DOSAGE AND ADMINISTRATION.)

Indomethacin: In a study in 36 patients with mild to moderate hypertension where the antihypertensive effects of ZESTRIL alone were compared to ZESTRIL given concomitantly with indomethacin, the use of indomethacin was associated with a reduced effect, although the difference between the two regimens was not significant.

Other Agents: ZESTRIL has been used concomitantly with nitrates and/or digoxin without evidence of clinically significant adverse interactions. This included post myocardial infarction patients who were receiving intravenous or transdermal nitroglycerin. No clinically important pharmacokinetic interactions occurred when ZESTRIL was used concomitantly with propranolol or hydrochlorothiazide. The presence of food in the stomach does not alter the bioavailability of ZESTRIL.

Agents Increasing Serum Potassium: ZESTRIL attenuates potassium loss caused by thiazide-type diuretics. Use of ZESTRIL with potassium-sparing diuretics (e.g., spironolactone, triamterene or amiloride), potassium supplements, or potassium-containing salt substitutes may lead to significant increases in serum potassium. Therefore, if concomitant use of these agents is indicated because of demonstrated hypokalemia, they should be used with caution and with frequent monitoring of serum potassium. Potassium sparing agents should generally not be used in patients with heart failure who are receiving ZESTRIL.

Lithium: Lithium toxicity has been reported in patients receiving lithium concomitantly with drugs which cause elimination of sodium, including ACE inhibitors. Lithium toxicity was usually reversible upon discontinuation of lithium and the ACE inhibitor. It is recommended that serum lithium levels be monitored frequently if ZESTRIL is administered concomitantly with lithium.

PERCENT OF PATIENTS IN CONTROLLED STUDIES

	ZESTRIL (n=1349) Incidence (discontinuation)		ZESTRIL/ Hydrochlorothiazide (n=629) Incidence (discontinuation)		PLACEBO (n=207) Incidence (discontinuation)	
Body as a Whole						
Fatigue	2.5	(0.3)	4.0	(0.5)	1.0	(0.0)
Asthenia	1.3	(0.5)	2.1	(0.2)	1.0	(0.0)
Orthostatic Effects	1.2	(0.0)	3.5	(0.2)	1.0	(0.0)
Cardiovascular						
Hypotension	1.2	(0.5)	1.6	(0.5)	0.5	(0.5)
Digestive						
Diarrhea	2.7	(0.2)	2.7	(0.3)	2.4	(0.0)
Nausea	2.0	(0.4)	2.5	(0.2)	2.4	(0.0)
Vomiting	1.1	(0.2)	1.4	(0.1)	0.5	(0.0)
Dyspepsia	0.9	(0.0)	1.9	(0.0)	0.0	(0.0)
Musculoskeletal						
Muscle Cramps	0.5	(0.0)	2.9	(0.8)	0.5	(0.0)
Nervous/Psychiatric						
Headache	5.7	(0.2)	4.5	(0.5)	1.9	(0.0)
Dizziness	5.4	(0.4)	9.2	(1.0)	1.9	(0.0)
Paresthesia	0.8	(0.1)	2.1	(0.2)	0.0	(0.0)
Decreased Libido	0.4	(0.1)	1.3	(0.1)	0.0	(0.0)
Vertigo	0.2	(0.1)	1.1	(0.2)	0.0	(0.0)
Respiratory						
Cough	3.5	(0.7)	4.6	(0.8)	1.0	(0.0)
Upper Respiratory Infection	2.1	(0.1)	2.7	(0.1)	0.0	(0.0)
Common Cold	1.1	(0.1)	1.3	(0.1)	0.0	(0.0)
Nasal Congestion	0.4	(0.1)	1.3	(0.1)	0.0	(0.0)
Influenza	0.3	(0.1)	1.1	(0.1)	0.0	(0.0)
Skin						
Rash	1.3	(0.4)	1.6	(0.2)	0.5	(0.5)
Urogenital						
Impotence	1.0	(0.4)	1.6	(0.5)	0.0	(0.0)

Carcinogenesis, Mutagenesis, Impairment of Fertility: There was no evidence of a tumorigenic effect when lisinopril was administered for 105 weeks to male and female rats at doses up to 90 mg/kg/day (about 56 or 9 times* the maximum recommended daily human dose, based on body weight and body surface area, respectively). There was no evidence of carcinogenicity when lisinopril was administered for 92 weeks to (male and female) mice at doses up to 135 mg/kg/day (about 84 times* the maximum recommended daily human dose). This dose was 6.8 times the maximum human dose based on body surface area in mice. *Calculations assume a human weight of 50 kg and human body surface area of 1.62 m².

Lisinopril was not mutagenic in the Ames microbial mutagen test with or without metabolic activation. It was also negative in a forward mutation assay using Chinese hamster lung cells. Lisinopril did not produce single strand DNA breaks in an *in vitro* alkaline elution rat hepatocyte assay. In addition, lisinopril did not produce increases in chromosomal aberrations in an *in vitro* test in Chinese hamster ovary cells or in an *in vivo* study in mouse bone marrow.

There were no adverse effects on reproductive performance in male and female rats treated with up to 300 mg/kg/day of lisinopril. This dose is 188 times and 30 times the maximum human dose when based on mg/kg and mg/m², respectively.

Pregnancy

Pregnancy Categories C (first trimester) and D (second and third trimesters). See WARNINGS, Fetal/Neonatal Morbidity and Mortality.

Nursing Mothers: Milk of lactating rats contains radioactivity following administration of ¹⁴C lisinopril. It is not known whether this drug is excreted in human milk. Because many drugs are excreted in human milk and because of the potential for serious adverse reactions in nursing infants from ACE inhibitors, a decision should be made whether to discontinue nursing and/or discontinue ZESTRIL, taking into account the importance of the drug to the mother.

Pediatric Use: Safety and effectiveness in pediatric patients have not been established.

ADVERSE REACTIONS

ZESTRIL has been found to be generally well tolerated in controlled clinical trials involving 1969 patients with hypertension or heart failure. For the most part, adverse experiences were mild and transient.

Hypertension:

In clinical trials in patients with hypertension treated with ZESTRIL, discontinuation of therapy due to clinical adverse experiences occurred in 5.7% of patients. The overall frequency of adverse experiences could not be related to total daily dosage within the recommended therapeutic dosage range.

For adverse experiences occurring in greater than 1% of patients with hypertension treated with ZESTRIL or ZESTRIL plus hydrochlothiazide in controlled clinical trials, and more frequently with ZESTRIL and/or ZESTRIL plus hydrochlorothiazide than placebo, comparative incidence data are listed in the table below:

[See table above]

Chest pain and back pain were also seen, but were more common on placebo than ZESTRIL.

Heart Failure:

In patients with heart failure treated with ZESTRIL for up to four years, discontinuation of therapy due to clinical adverse experiences occurred in 11.0% of patients. In controlled studies in patients with heart failure, therapy was discontinued in 8.1% of patients treated with ZESTRIL for 12 weeks, compared to 7.7% of patients treated with placebo for 12 weeks.

The following table lists those adverse experiences which occurred in greater than 1% of patients with heart failure treated with ZESTRIL or placebo for up to 12 weeks in controlled clinical trials, and more frequently on ZESTRIL than placebo.

	Controlled Trials			
	ZESTRIL (n=407) Incidence (discontinuation) 12 weeks		Placebo (n=155) Incidence (discontinuation) 12 weeks	
Body as a Whole				
Chest Pain	3.4	(0.2)	1.3	(0.0)
Abdominal Pain	2.2	(0.7)	1.9	(0.0)
Cardiovascular				
Hypotension	4.4	(1.7)	0.6	(0.6)
Digestive				
Diarrhea	3.7	(0.5)	1.9	(0.0)
Nervous/Psychiatric				
Dizziness	11.8	(1.2)	4.5	(1.3)
Headache	4.4	(0.2)	3.9	(0.0)
Respiratory				
Upper Respiratory Infection	1.5	(0.0)	1.3	(0.0)
Skin				
Rash	1.7	(0.5)	0.6	(0.6)

Also observed at >1% with ZESTRIL but more frequent or as frequent on placebo than ZESTRIL in controlled trials were asthenia, angina pectoris, nausea, dyspnea, cough, and pruritus.

Worsening of heart failure, anorexia, increased salivation, muscle cramps, back pain, myalgia, depression, chest sound abnormalities, and pulmonary edema were also seen in controlled clinical trials, but were more common on placebo than ZESTRIL.

Acute Myocardial Infarction: In the GISSI-3 trial, in patients treated with ZESTRIL for six weeks following acute myocardial infarction, discontinuation of therapy occurred in 17.6% of patients.

Patients treated with ZESTRIL had a significantly higher incidence of hypotension and renal dysfunction compared with patients not taking ZESTRIL.

In the GISSI-3 trial, hypotension (9.7%), renal dysfunction (2.0%), cough (0.5%), post infarction angina (0.3%), skin rash and generalized edema (0.01%), and angioedema (0.01%) resulted in withdrawal of treatment. In elderly patients treated with ZESTRIL, discontinuation due to renal dysfunction was 4.2%.

Other clinical adverse experiences occurring in 0.3% to 1.0% of patients with hypertension or heart failure treated with ZESTRIL in controlled clinical trials and rarer, serious, possibly drug-related events reported in uncontrolled studies or marketing experience are listed below, and within each category are in order of decreasing severity:

Body as a Whole: Anaphylactoid reactions (see WARNINGS, Anaphylactoid Reactions During Membrane Exposure), syncope, orthostatic effects, chest discomfort, pain, pelvic pain, flank pain, edema, facial edema, virus infection, fever, chills, malaise.

Cardiovascular: Cardiac arrest; myocardial infarction or cerebrovascular accident possibly secondary to excessive hypotension in high risk patients (see WARNINGS, Hypotension); pulmonary embolism and infarction, arrhythmias (including ventricular tachycardia, atrial tachycardia, atrial fibrillation, bradycardia and premature ventricular contractions), palpitations, transient ischemic attacks, paroxysmal nocturnal dyspnea, orthostatic hypotension, decreased blood pressure, peripheral edema, vasculitis.

Digestive: Pancreatitis, hepatitis (hepatocellular or cholestatic jaundice) (see WARNINGS, Hepatic Failure), vomiting, gastritis, dyspepsia, heartburn, gastrointestinal cramps, constipation, flatulence, dry mouth.

Hematologic: Rare cases of bone marrow depression, hemolytic anemia, leukopenia/neutropenia and thrombocytopenia.

Endocrine: Diabetes mellitus.

Metabolic: Weight loss, dehydration, fluid overload, gout, weight gain.

Musculoskeletal: Arthritis, arthralgia, neck pain, hip pain, low back pain, joint pain, leg pain, knee pain, shoulder pain, arm pain, lumbago.

Nervous System/Psychiatric: Stroke, ataxia, memory impairment, tremor, peripheral neuropathy (e.g., dysesthesia), spasm, paresthesia, confusion, insomnia, somnolence, hypersomnia, irritability and nervousness.

Respiratory System: Malignant lung neoplasms, hemoptysis, pulmonary infiltrates, bronchospasm, asthma, pleural effusion, pneumonia, eosinophilic pneumonitis, bronchitis, wheezing, orthopnea, painful respiration, epistaxis, laryngitis, sinusitis, pharyngeal pain, pharyngitis, rhinitis, rhinorrhea.

Skin: Urticaria, alopecia, herpes zoster, photosensitivity, skin lesions, skin infections, pemphigus, erythema, flushing, diaphoresis. Other severe skin reactions have been reported rarely, including toxic epidermal necrolysis and Stevens-Johnson syndrome; causal relationship has not been established.

Special Senses: Visual loss, diplopia, blurred vision, tinnitus, photophobia, taste alteration.

Urogenital System: Acute renal failure, oliguria, anuria, uremia, progressive azotemia, renal dysfunction. (see PRECAUTIONS and DOSAGE AND ADMINISTRATION), pyelonephritis, dysuria, urinary tract infection, breast pain.

Miscellaneous: A symptom complex has been reported which may include a positive ANA, an elevated erythrocyte sedimentation rate, arthralgia/arthritis, myalgia, fever, vasculitis, eosinophilia and leukocytosis. Rash, photosensitivity or other dermatological manifestations may occur alone or in combination with these symptoms.

ANGIOEDEMA: Angioedema has been reported in patients receiving ZESTRIL (0.1%). Angioedema associated with laryngeal edema may be fatal. If angioedema of the face, extremities, lips, tongue, glottis and/or larynx occurs, treatment with ZESTRIL should be discontinued and appropriate therapy instituted immediately. (See WARNINGS.)

HYPOTENSION: In hypertensive patients, hypotension occurred in 1.2% and syncope occurred in 0.1% of patients. Hypotension or syncope was a cause of discontinuation of therapy in 0.5% of hypertensive patients. In patients with heart failure, hypotension occurred in 5.3% and syncope occurred in 1.8% of patients. These adverse experiences were causes for discontinuation of therapy in 1.8% of these patients. In patients treated with ZESTRIL for six weeks after acute myocardial infarction, hypotension (systolic blood pressure ≤100 mmHg) resulted in discontinuation of therapy in 9.7% of the patients. (See WARNINGS.)

Fetal/Neonatal Morbidity and Mortality: See WARNINGS, Fetal/Neonatal Morbidity and Mortality.

Cough: See PRECAUTIONS—Cough

Clinical Laboratory Test Findings

Serum Electrolytes: Hyperkalemia (See PRECAUTIONS), hyponatremia.

Creatinine, Blood Urea Nitrogen: Minor increases in blood urea nitrogen and serum creatinine, reversible upon discontinuation of therapy, were observed in about 2.0% of patients with essential hypertension treated with ZESTRIL

Continued on next page

Zestril—Cont.

alone. Increases were more common in patients receiving concomitant diuretics and in patients with renal artery stenosis. (See PRECAUTIONS.) Reversible minor increases in blood urea nitrogen and serum creatinine were observed in approximately 11.6% of patients with heart failure on concomitant diuretic therapy. Frequently, these abnormalities resolved when the dosage of the diuretic was decreased.

Hemoglobin and Hematocrit: Small decreases in hemoglobin and hematocrit (mean decreases of approximately 0.4 g% and 1.3 vol%, respectively) occurred frequently in patients treated with ZESTRIL but were rarely of clinical importance in patients without some other cause of anemia. In clinical trials, less than 0.1% of patients discontinued therapy due to anemia.

Liver Function Tests: Rarely, elevations of liver enzymes and/or serum bilirubin have occurred. (See WARNINGS, Hepatic Failure.)

In hypertensive patients, 2.0% discontinued therapy due to laboratory adverse experiences, principally elevations in blood urea nitrogen (0.6%), serum creatinine (0.5%) and serum potassium (0.4%).

In the heart failure trials, 3.4% of patients discontinued therapy due to laboratory adverse experiences; 1.8% due to elevations in blood urea nitrogen and/or creatinine and 0.6% due to elevations in serum potassium.

In the myocardial infarction trial, 2.0% of patients receiving ZESTRIL discontinued therapy due to renal dysfunction (increasing creatinine concentration to over 3 mg/dL or a doubling or more of the baseline serum creatinine concentration); less than 1.0% of patients discontinued therapy due to other laboratory adverse experiences: 0.1% with hyperkalemia and less than 0.1% with hepatic enzyme alterations.

OVERDOSAGE

Following a single oral dose of 20 g/kg no lethality occurred in rats, and death occurred in one of 20 mice receiving the same dose. The most likely manifestation of overdosage would be hypotension, for which the usual treatment would be intravenous infusion of normal saline solution.

Lisinopril can be removed by hemodialysis.

DOSAGE AND ADMINISTRATION

Hypertension

Initial Therapy: In patients with uncomplicated essential hypertension not on diuretic therapy, the recommended initial dose is 10 mg once a day. Dosage should be adjusted according to blood pressure response. The usual dosage range is 20 to 40 mg per day administered in a single daily dose. The antihypertensive effect may diminish toward the end of the dosing interval regardless of the administered dose, but most commonly with a dose of 10 mg daily. This can be evaluated by measuring blood pressure just prior to dosing to determine whether satisfactory control is being maintained for 24 hours. If it is not, an increase in dose should be considered. Doses up to 80 mg have been used but do not appear to give greater effect. If blood pressure is not controlled with ZESTRIL alone, a low dose of a diuretic may be added. Hydrochlorothiazide, 12.5 mg has been shown to provide an additive effect. After the addition of a diuretic, it may be possible to reduce the dose of ZESTRIL.

Diuretic Treated Patients: In hypertensive patients who are currently being treated with a diuretic, symptomatic hypotension may occur occasionally following the initial dose of ZESTRIL. The diuretic should be discontinued, if possible, for two to three days before beginning therapy with ZESTRIL to reduce the likelihood of hypotension. (See WARNINGS.) The dosage of ZESTRIL should be adjusted according to blood pressure response. If the patient's blood pressure is not controlled with ZESTRIL alone, diuretic therapy may be resumed as described above.

If the diuretic cannot be discontinued, an initial dose of 5 mg should be used under medical supervision for at least two hours and until blood pressure has stabilized for at least an additional hour. (See WARNINGS and PRECAUTIONS, Drug Interactions.)

Concomitant administration of ZESTRIL with potassium supplements, potassium salt substitutes, or potassium-sparing diuretics may lead to increases of serum potassium. (See PRECAUTIONS.)

Dosage Adjustment in Renal Impairment: The usual dose of ZESTRIL (10 mg) is recommended for patients with creatinine clearance >30 mL/min (serum creatinine of up to approximately 3 mg/dL). For patients with creatinine clearance ≥10 mL/min ≤30 mL/min (serum creatinine ≥3 mg/dL), the first dose is 5 mg once daily. For patients with creatinine clearance <10 mL/min (usually on hemodialysis) the recommended initial dose is 2.5 mg. The dosage may be titrated upward until blood pressure is controlled or to a maximum of 40 mg daily.

Renal Status	Creatinine Clearance mL/min	Initial Dose mg/day
Normal Renal Function to Mild Impairment	>30	10
Moderate to Severe Impairment	≥10 ≤30	5
Dialysis Patients*	<10	2.5**

* See WARNINGS, Anaphylactoid Reactions During Membrane Exposure.

** Dosage interval should be adjusted depending on the blood pressure response.

Heart Failure

ZESTRIL is indicated as adjunctive therapy with diuretics and digitalis. The recommended starting dose is 5 mg once a day. When initiating treatment with lisinopril in patients with heart failure, the initial dose should be administered under medical observation, especially in those patients with low blood pressure (systolic blood pressure below 100 mmHg). The mean peak blood pressure lowering occurs six to eight hours after dosing. Observation should continue until blood pressure is stable. The concomitant diuretic dose should be reduced, if possible, to help minimize hypovolemia which may contribute to hypotension. (See WARNINGS and PRECAUTIONS, Drug Interactions.) The appearance of hypotension after the initial dose of ZESTRIL does not preclude subsequent careful dose titration with the drug, following effective management of the hypotension.

The usual effective dosage range is 5 to 20 mg per day administered as a single daily dose.

Dosage Adjustment in Patients with Heart Failure and Renal Impairment or Hyponatremia: In patients with heart failure who have hyponatremia (serum sodium <130 mEq/L) or moderate to severe renal impairment (creatinine clearance ≤30 mL/min or serum creatinine >3 mg/dL), therapy with ZESTRIL should be initiated at a dose of 2.5 mg once a day under close medical supervision. (See WARNINGS and PRECAUTIONS, Drug Interactions.).

Acute Myocardial Infarction: In hemodynamically stable patients within 24 hours of the onset of symptoms of acute myocardial infarction, the first dose of ZESTRIL is 5 mg given orally, followed by 5 mg after 24 hours, 10 mg after 48 hours and then 10 mg of ZESTRIL once daily. Dosing should continue for six weeks. Patients should receive, as appropriate, the standard recommended treatments such as thrombolytics, aspirin, and beta-blockers.

Patients with a low systolic blood pressure (≤120 mmHg) when treatment is started or during the first 3 days after the infarct should be given a lower 2.5 mg oral dose of ZESTRIL (see WARNINGS). If hypotension occurs (systolic blood pressure ≤100 mmHg) a daily maintenance dose of 5 mg may be given with temporary reductions to 2.5 mg if needed. If prolonged hypotension occurs (systolic blood pressure <90 mmHg for more than 1 hour) ZESTRIL should be withdrawn. For patients who develop symptoms of heart failure, see DOSAGE AND ADMINISTRATION, Heart Failure.

Dosgae Adjustment in Patients With Myocardial Infarction with Renal Impairment: In acute myocardial infarction, treatment with ZESTRIL should be initiated with caution in patients with evidence of renal dysfunction, defined as serum creatinine concentration exceeding 2 mg/dL. No evaluation of dosing adjustments in myocardial infarction patients with severe renal impairment has been performed.

Use in Elderly: In general, blood pressure response and adverse experiences were similar in younger and older patients given similar doses of ZESTRIL. Pharmacokinetic studies, however, indicate that maximum blood levels and area under the plasma concentration time curve (AUC) are doubled in older patients, so that dosage adjustments should be made with particular caution.

HOW SUPPLIED

2.5 mg Tablets (NDC 0310-0135) white, oval, biconvex, uncoated tablets identifed as "ZESTRIL 2 1/2" on one side and "135" on the other side are supplied in bottles of 100 tablets. ZESTRIL 2.5 mg tablets are manufactured by Zeneca Pharmaceuticals.

5 mg Tablets (NDC 0310-0130) pink, capsule-shaped, biconvex, bisected, uncoated tablets, identified "ZESTRIL" on one side and "130" on the other side are supplied in bottles of 100 tablets and 1000 tablets, and unit dose packages of 100 tablets.

10 mg Tablets (NDC 0310-0131) pink, round, biconvex, uncoated tablets identified "ZESTRIL 10" debossed on one side, and "131" debossed on the other side are supplied in bottles of 100 tablets, 1000 tablets, 3000 tablets, and unit dose packages of 100 tablets.

20 mg Tablets (NDC 0310-0132) red, round, biconvex, uncoated tablets identified "ZESTRIL 20" debossed on one side and "132" debossed on the other side are supplied in bottles of 100 tablets, 1000 tablets, 3000 tablets, and unit dose packages of 100 tablets.

40 mg Tablets (NDC 0310-0134) yellow, round, biconvex, uncoated tablets identified "ZESTRIL 40" debossed on one side, and "134" debossed on the other side are supplied in bottles of 100 tablets.

Store at controlled room temperature, 20–25°C (68–77°F) [see USP]. Protect from moisture, freezing and excessive heat. Dispense in a tight container.

¶Registered trademark of Hospal Ltd.

Manufactured by: IPR Pharmaceuticals Inc.
Distributed by:
ZENECA Pharmaceuticals
A Business Unit of Zeneca Inc.
Wilmington, Delaware 19850-5437
64113-01 Rev O 12/97

Shown in Product Identification Guide, page 346

ZOLADEX® 3.6 mg ℞
GOSERELIN ACETATE IMPLANT
Equivalent to 3.6 mg goserelin

DESCRIPTION

ZOLADEX® (goserelin acetate implant), contains a potent synthetic decapeptide analogue of luteinizing hormone-releasing hormone (LHRH), also known as a gonadotropin releasing hormone (GnRH) agonist analogue. Goserelin acetate is chemically described as an acetate salt of [D-Ser(Bu^t)^6,Azgly^{10}]LHRH. Its chemical structure is pyro-Glu-His-Trp-Ser-Tyr-D-Ser(Bu^t)-Leu-Arg-Pro-Azgly-NH_2 acetate [$C_{59}H_{84}N_{18}O_{14} \cdot (C_2H_4O_2)_x$ where x = 1 to 2.4].

Goserelin acetate is an off-white powder with a molecular weight of 1269 Daltons (free base). It is freely soluble in glacial acetic acid. It is soluble in water, 0.1M hydrochloric acid, 0.1M sodium hydroxide, dimethylformamide and dimethyl sulfoxide. Goserelin acetate is practically insoluble in acetone, chloroform and ether.

ZOLADEX is supplied as a sterile, biodegradable product containing goserelin acetate equivalent to 3.6 mg of goserelin. ZOLADEX is designed for subcutaneous injection with continuous release over a 28-day period. Goserelin acetate is dispersed in a matrix of D,L-lactic and glycolic acids copolymer (13.3-14.3 mg/dose) containing less than 2.5% acetic acid and up to 12% goserelin-related substances and presented as a sterile, white to cream colored 1-mm diameter cylinder, preloaded in a special single use syringe with a 16-gauge needle and overwrapped in a sealed, light and moisture proof, aluminum foil laminate pouch containing a desiccant capsule. Studies of the D,L-lactic and glycolic acids copolymer have indicated that it is completely biodegradable and has no demonstrable antigenic potential.

CLINICAL PHARMACOLOGY

Mechanism of Action: ZOLADEX is a synthetic decapeptide analogue of LHRH. ZOLADEX acts as a potent inhibitor of pituitary gonadotropin secretion when administered in the biodegradable formulation.

Following initial administration in males, ZOLADEX causes an initial increase in serum luteinizing hormone (LH) and follicle stimulating hormone (FSH) levels with subsequent increases in serum levels of testosterone. Chronic administration of ZOLADEX leads to sustained suppression of pituitary gonadotropins, and serum levels of testosterone consequently fall into the range normally seen in surgically castrated men approximately 2–4 weeks after initiation of therapy. This leads to accessory sex organ regression. In animal and in vitro studies, administration of goserelin resulted in the regression or inhibition of growth of the hormonally sensitive dimethylbenzanthracene (DMBA)-induced rat mammary tumor and Dunning R3327 prostate tumor. In clinical trials with follow-up of more than 2 years, suppression of serum testosterone to castrate levels has been maintained for the duration of therapy.

In females, a similar down-regulation of the pituitary gland by chronic exposure to ZOLADEX leads to suppression of gonadotropin secretion, a decrease in serum estradiol to levels consistent with the postmenopausal state, and would be expected to lead to a reduction of ovarian size and function, reduction in the size of the uterus and mammary gland, as well as a regression of sex hormone-responsive tumors, if present. Serum estradiol is suppressed to levels similar to those observed in postmenopausal women within 3 weeks following initial administration; however, after suppression was attained, isolated elevations of estradiol were seen in 10% of the patients enrolled in clinical trials. Serum LH and FSH are suppressed to follicular phase levels within four weeks after initial administration of drug and are usually maintained at that range with continued use of ZOLADEX. In 5% or less of women treated with ZOLADEX, FSH and LH levels may not be suppressed to follicular phase levels on day 28 post treatment with use of a single 3.6 mg depot injection. In certain individuals, suppression of any of these hormones to such levels may not be achieved with ZOLADEX. Estradiol, LH and FSH levels return to pretreatment values within 12 weeks following the last implant administration in all but rare cases.

Pharmacokinetics:

Absorption: The pharmacokinetics of ZOLADEX have been determined in both male and female healthy volunteers and patients. In these studies, ZOLADEX was administered as a single 250 µg (aqueous solution) dose and as a single or multiple 3.6 mg depot dose by subcutaneous route. The absorption of radiolabeled drug was rapid, and the peak blood radioactivity levels occurred between 0.5 and 1.0 hour after dosing. The mean (± standard deviation) pharmacokinetic parameter estimates of ZOLADEX after administration of 3.6 mg depot for 2 months in males and females are presented in the following table.

[See table at right]

Parameters (Units)	Males n=7	Females n=9
Peak Plasma Concentration (ng/mL)	2.84 ± 1.81	1.46 ± 0.82
Time to Peak Concentration (days)	12–15	8–22
Area Under the Curve (0–28 days) (ng.h/mL)	27.8 ± 15.3	18.5 ± 10.3
Systemic Clearance (mL/min)	110.5 ± 47.5	163.9 ± 71.0
*Apparent Volume of Distribution (L)	44.1 ± 13.6	20.3 ± 4.1
*Elimination Half-life (h)	4.2 ± 1.1	2.3 ± 0.6

* The apparent volume of distribution and the elimination half-life were determined after subcutaneous administration of 250 µg aqueous solution of goserelin.

Pharmacokinetic data were obtained using a nonspecific RIA method.

Goserelin is released from the depot at a much slower rate initially for the first 8 days, and then there is more rapid and continuous release for the remainder of the 28-day dosing period. Despite the change in the releasing rate of goserelin, administration of ZOLADEX every 28 days resulted in testosterone levels that were suppressed to and maintained in the range normally seen in surgically castrated men.

When ZOLADEX 3.6 mg depot was used for treating male and female patients with normal renal and hepatic function, there was no significant evidence of drug accumulation. However, in clinical trials the minimum serum levels of a few patients were increased. These levels can be attributed to interpatient variation.

Distribution: The apparent volumes of distribution determined after subcutaneous administration of 250 µg aqueous solution of goserelin were 44.1 and 20.3 liters for males and females, respectively. The plasma protein binding of goserelin obtained from one sample was found to be 27.3%.

Metabolism: Metabolism of goserelin, by hydrolysis of the C-terminal amino acids, is the major clearance mechanism. The major circulating component in serum appeared to be 1–7 fragment, and the major component presented in urine of one healthy male volunteer was 5–10 fragment. The metabolism of goserelin in humans yields a similar but narrow profile of metabolites to that found in other species. All metabolites found in humans have also been found in toxicology species.

Excretion: Clearance of goserelin following subcutaneous administration of the solution formulation of goserelin is very rapid and occurs via a combination of hepatic metabolism and urinary excretion. More than 90% of a subcutaneous radiolabeled solution formulation dose of goserelin is excreted in urine. Approximately 20% of the dose in urine is accounted for by unchanged goserelin. The total body clearance of goserelin (administered subcutaneously as a 3.6 mg depot) was significantly ($p<0.05$) greater (163.9 versus 110.5 L/min) in females compared to males.

Special Populations: In clinical trials with the solution formulation of goserelin, male patients with impaired renal function (creatinine clearance < 20 mL/min) had a total body clearance and serum elimination half-life of 31.5 mL/min and 12.1 hours, respectively, compared to 133 mL/min and 4.2 hours for subjects with normal renal function (creatinine clearance > 70 mL/min). In females, the effects of reduced goserelin clearance due to impaired renal function on drug efficacy and toxicity are unknown. The total body clearances and serum elimination half-lives were similar between normal and hepatic impaired patients receiving 250 µg solution formulation of goserelin. Pharmacokinetic studies using the aqueous formulation of goserelin in patients with renal and hepatic impairment do not indicate a need for dose adjustment with the use of the depot formulation.

Drug-Drug Interactions: No formal drug-drug interaction studies have been performed.

Clinical Studies - Prostatic Carcinoma: In controlled studies of patients with advanced prostatic cancer comparing ZOLADEX to orchiectomy, the long-term endocrine responses and objective responses were similar between the two treatment arms. Additionally, duration of survival was similar between the two treatment arms in a comparative trial.

Clinical Studies - Endometriosis: In controlled clinical studies using the 3.6 mg formulation every 28 days for 6 months, ZOLADEX was shown to be as effective as danazol therapy in relieving clinical symptoms (dysmenorrhea, dyspareunia and pelvic pain) and signs (pelvic tenderness, pelvic induration) of endometriosis and decreasing the size of endometrial lesions as determined by laparoscopy. In one study comparing ZOLADEX with danazol (800 mg/day), 63% of ZOLADEX-treated patients and 42% of danazol-treated patients had a greater than or equal to 50% reduction in the extent of endometrial lesions. In the second study comparing ZOLADEX with danazol (600 mg/day), 62% of ZOLADEX-treated and 51% of danazol-treated patients had a greater than or equal to 50% reduction in the extent of endometrial lesions. The clinical significance of a decrease in endometriotic lesions is not known at this time; and in addition, laparoscopic staging of endometriosis does not necessarily correlate with severity of symptoms.

In these two studies, ZOLADEX led to amenorrhea in 92% and 80%, respectively, of all treated women within 8 weeks after initial administration. Menses usually resumed within 8 weeks following completion of therapy.

Within 4 weeks following initial administration, clinical symptoms were significantly reduced, and at the end of treatment were, on average, reduced by approximately 84%.

During the first two months of ZOLADEX use, some women experience vaginal bleeding of variable duration and intensity. In all likelihood, this bleeding represents estrogen withdrawal bleeding, and is expected to stop spontaneously.

There is insufficient evidence to determine whether pregnancy rates are enhanced or adversely affected by the use of ZOLADEX.

Clinical Studies - Breast Cancer: The Southwest Oncology Group conducted a prospective, randomized clinical trial (SWOG-8692 [INT-0075]) in premenopausal women with advanced estrogen receptor positive or progesterone receptor positive breast cancer which compared ZOLADEX with oophorectomy. On the basis of interim data from 124 women, the best objective response (CR+PR) for the ZOLADEX group is 22% versus 12% for the oophorectomy group. The median time to treatment failure is 6.7 months for patients treated with ZOLADEX and 5.5 months for patients treated with oophorectomy. The median survival time for the ZOLADEX arm is 33.2 months and for the oophorectomy arm is 33.6 months.

Subjective responses based on measures of pain control and performance status were observed with both treatments; 48% of the women in the ZOLADEX treatment group and 50% in the oophorectomy group had subjective responses. In the clinical trial (SWOG-8692 [INT 0075]), the mean post treatment estradiol level was reported as 17.8 pg/mL. (The mean estradiol level in post-menopausal women as reported in the literature is 13 pg/mL). During the conduct of the clinical trial, women whose estradiol levels were not reduced to the postmenopausal range, received two ZOLADEX depots, thus, increasing the dose of ZOLADEX from 3.6 mg to 7.2 mg.

Findings were similar in uncontrolled clinical trials involving patients with hormone receptor positive and negative breast cancer. Premenopausal women with estrogen receptor (ER) status of positive, negative, or unknown participated in the uncontrolled (Phase II and Trial 2302) clinical trials. Objective tumor responses were seen regardless of ER status, as shown in the following table.

OBJECTIVE RESPONSE BY ER STATUS

	CR + PR/Total No. (%)			
ER status	Phase II (N = 228)		Trial 2302 (N = 159)	
Positive	43/119	(36)	31/86	(36)
Negative	6/33	(18)	3/26	(10)
Unknown	20/76	(26)	18/44	(41)

Clinical Studies-Endometrial Thinning: Two trials were conducted with ZOLADEX prior to endometrial ablation for dysfunctional uterine bleeding.

Trial 0022, was a double-blind, prospective, randomized, parallel-group multicenter trial conducted in 358 premenopausal women with dysfunctional uterine bleeding. Eligible patients were randomized to receive either two depots of ZOLADEX 3.6 mg (n=180) or two placebo injections (n=178) administered four weeks apart. 175 patients in each group underwent endometrial ablation using either diathermy loop alone or in combination with rollerball approximately 2 weeks after the second injection. Endometrial thickness was assessed immediately before surgery using a transvaginal ultrasonic probe. The incidence of amenorrhea was compared between the ZOLADEX and placebo groups at 24 weeks after endometrial ablation.

The median endometrial thickness before surgery was significantly less in the ZOLADEX treatment group (1.50 mm) compared to the placebo group (3.55 mm). Six months after surgery, 40% of patients (70/175) treated with ZOLADEX in Trial 0022 reported amenorrhea as compared with 26% who had received placebo injections (44/171), a difference that was statistically significant.

Trial 0003, was a single center, open-label, randomized trial in premenopausal women with dysfunctional uterine bleeding. The trial allowed for a comparison of 1 depot of ZOLADEX and 2 depots of ZOLADEX administered 4 weeks apart with ablation using Nd: YAG laser occurring 4 weeks after ZOLADEX administration. Forty patients were randomized into each of the ZOLADEX treatment groups.

The median endometrial thickness before surgery was significantly less in the group treated with two depots (0.5 mm) compared to the group treated with one depot (1 mm). No difference in the incidence of amenorrhea was found at 24 weeks (24% in both groups). Of the 74 patients that completed the trial, 53 % reported hypomenorrhea and 20% reported normal menses six months after surgery.

INDICATIONS AND USAGE

Prostatic Carcinoma: ZOLADEX is indicated in the palliative treatment of advanced carcinoma of the prostate.

Endometriosis: ZOLADEX is indicated for the management of endometriosis, including pain relief and reduction of endometriotic lesions for the duration of therapy. Experience with ZOLADEX for the management of endometriosis has been limited to women 18 years of age and older treated for 6 months.

Advanced Breast Cancer: ZOLADEX is indicated for use in the palliative treatment of advanced breast cancer in pre- and perimenopausal women.

The estrogen and progesterone receptor values may help to predict whether ZOLADEX therapy is likely to be beneficial. (See CLINICAL PHARMACOLOGY.)

Endometrial Thinning: ZOLADEX is indicated for use as an endometrial-thinning agent prior to endometrial ablation for dysfunctional uterine bleeding.

CONTRAINDICATIONS

ZOLADEX is contraindicated in those patients who have a known hypersensitivity to LHRH, LHRH agonist analogues or any of the components in ZOLADEX.

ZOLADEX is contraindicated in women being treated for endometriosis or endometrial thinning who are or may become pregnant while receiving the drug. ZOLADEX can cause fetal harm when administered to a pregnant woman. Effects on reproductive function, as a result of antigonadotrophic properties of the drug, are expected to occur on chronic administration.

Effective nonhormonal contraception must be used by all premenopausal women during ZOLADEX therapy and for 12 weeks following discontinuation of therapy. There are no adequate and well-controlled studies in pregnant women using ZOLADEX. If this drug is used during pregnancy, or the patient being treated for endometriosis or endometrial thinning becomes pregnant while taking this drug, the patient should be apprised of the potential hazard to the fetus or potential risk for loss of the pregnancy. Women of childbearing potential should be advised to avoid becoming pregnant.

For a description of findings in animal reproductive toxicity studies, see **WARNINGS**.

ZOLADEX is contraindicated in women who are breast feeding (see Nursing Mothers Section).

WARNINGS

Before starting treatment with ZOLADEX, pregnancy must be excluded. Safe use of ZOLADEX in pregnancy has not been established. ZOLADEX can cause fetal harm when administered to a pregnant woman. ZOLADEX has been found to cross the placenta following subcutaneous administration of 50 and 1000 µg/kg in rats and rabbits, respectively. Studies in both rats and rabbits at doses equal to or greater than 2 and 20 µg/kg/day, respectively (about 1/10 and 2 times the daily maximum recommended human dose, respectively, on a mg/m^2 basis), administered during the period of organogenesis, have confirmed that ZOLADEX will increase pregnancy loss, and is embryotoxic/fetotoxic (characterized by increased preimplantation loss, increased resorption and an increase in umbilical hernia in rats at a dose of ≥ 10 µg/kg/day [about 1/2 the recommended human dose on a mg/m^2 basis]); effects were dose-related. In additional reproduction studies in rats, ZOLADEX was found to decrease fetus and pup survival.

There are no adequate and well-controlled studies in pregnant women using ZOLADEX. Women of childbearing potential should be advised to avoid becoming pregnant.

Continued on next page

Zoladex 3.6 mg—Cont.

When used every 28 days, ZOLADEX usually inhibits ovulation and stops menstruation. Contraception is not ensured, however, by taking ZOLADEX. During treatment, pregnancy must be avoided by the use of nonhormonal methods of contraception. If ZOLADEX is used during pregnancy (in a patient with advanced breast cancer) or the patient becomes pregnant while receiving this drug, the patient must be apprised of the potential risk for loss of the pregnancy due to possible hormonal imbalance as a result of the expected pharmacologic action of ZOLADEX treatment. Following the last ZOLADEX injection, nonhormonal methods of contraception must be continued until the return of menses or for at least 12 weeks. (See **CONTRAINDICATIONS**.)

Prostate and Breast Cancer: Initially, ZOLADEX, like other LHRH agonists, causes transient increases in serum levels of testosterone in men with prostate cancer, and estrogen in women with breast cancer. Transient worsening of symptoms, or the occurrence of additional signs and symptoms of prostate or breast cancer, may occasionally develop during the first few weeks of ZOLADEX treatment. A small number of patients may experience a temporary increase in bone pain, which can be managed symptomatically. As with other LHRH agonists, isolated cases of ureteral obstruction and spinal cord compression have been observed in patients with prostate cancer. If spinal cord compression or renal impairment develops, standard treatment of these complications should be instituted. For extreme cases in prostate cancer patients, an immediate orchiectomy should be considered.

As with other LHRH agonists or hormonal therapies (antiestrogens, estrogens, etc.), hypercalcemia has been reported in some prostate and breast cancer patients with bone metastases after starting treatment with ZOLADEX. If hypercalcemia does occur, appropriate treatment measures should be initiated.

PRECAUTIONS

General: Hypersensitivity, antibody formation and acute anaphylactic reactions have been reported with LHRH agonist analogues.

Of 115 women worldwide treated with ZOLADEX and tested for development of binding to goserelin following treatment with ZOLADEX, one patient showed low-titer binding to goserelin. On further testing of this patient's plasma obtained following treatment, her goserelin binding component was found not to be precipitated with rabbit antihuman immunoglobulin polyvalent sera. These findings suggest the possibility of antibody formation.

The pharmacologic action of ZOLADEX on the uterus and cervix may cause an increase in cervical resistance. Therefore, care should be taken when dilating the cervix for endometrial ablation.

Information for Patients

Males: The use of ZOLADEX in patients at particular risk of developing ureteral obstruction or spinal cord compression should be considered carefully and the patients monitored closely during the first month of therapy. Patients with ureteral obstruction or spinal cord compression should have appropriate treatment prior to initiation of ZOLADEX therapy.

Females: Patients must be made aware of the following information:

1. Since menstruation should stop with effective doses of ZOLADEX the patient should notify her physician if regular menstruation persists. Patients missing one or more successive doses of ZOLADEX may experience breakthrough menstrual bleeding.
2. ZOLADEX should not be prescribed if the patient is pregnant, breast feeding, lactating, has nondiagnosed abnormal vaginal bleeding, or is allergic to any of the components of ZOLADEX.
3. Use of ZOLADEX in pregnancy is contraindicated in women being treated for endometriosis or endometrial thinning. Therefore, a nonhormonal method of contraception should be used during treatment. Patients should be advised that if they miss one or more successive doses of ZOLADEX, breakthrough menstrual bleeding or ovulation may occur with the potential for conception. If a patient becomes pregnant during treatment for endometriosis or endometrial thinning, ZOLADEX treatment should be discontinued and the patient should be advised of the possible risks to the pregnancy and fetus. (see **CONTRAINDICATIONS**.)
   For patients being treated for advanced breast cancer, see **WARNINGS**.
4. Those adverse events occurring most frequently in clinical studies with ZOLADEX are associated with hypoestrogenism; of these, the most frequently reported are hot flashes (flushes), headaches, vaginal dryness, emotional lability, change in libido, depression, sweating and change in breast size. Clinical studies in endometriosis suggest the addition of Hormone Replacement Therapy (estrogens and/or progestins) to ZOLADEX may decrease the occurrence of vasomotor symptoms and vaginal dryness associated with hypoestrogenism without compromising the efficacy of ZOLADEX in relieving pelvic symptoms. The optimal drugs, dose and duration of treatment has not been established.
5. As with other LHRH agonist analogues, treatment with ZOLADEX induces a hypoestrogenic state which results in a loss of bone mineral density (BMD) over the course of treatment, some of which may not be reversible. In patients with a history of prior treatment that may have resulted in bone mineral density loss and/or in patients with major risk factors for decreased bone mineral density such as chronic alcohol abuse and/or tobacco abuse, significant family history of osteoporosis, or chronic use of drugs that can reduce bone density such as anticonvulsants or corticosteroids, ZOLADEX therapy may pose an additional risk. In these patients the risks and benefits must be weighed carefully before therapy with ZOLADEX is instituted. Clinical studies suggest the addition of Hormone Replacement Therapy (estrogens and/or progestins) to ZOLADEX is effective in reducing the bone mineral loss which occurs with ZOLADEX alone. The optimal drugs, dose and duration of treatment has not been established.
6. Currently, there are no clinical data on the effects of retreatment or treatment of benign gynecological conditions with ZOLADEX for periods in excess of 6 months.
7. As with other hormonal interventions that disrupt the pituitary-gonadal axis, some patients may have delayed return to menses. The rare patient, however, may experience persistent amenorrhea.

Drug Interactions: No formal drug-drug interaction studies have been performed. No confirmed interactions have been reported between ZOLADEX and other drugs.

Drug/Laboratory Test Interactions: Administration of ZOLADEX in therapeutic doses results in suppression of the pituitary-gonadal system. Because of this suppression, diagnostic tests of pituitary-gonadotropic and gonadal functions conducted during treatment and until the resumption of menses may show results which are misleading. Normal function is usually restored within 12 weeks after treatment is discontinued.

Carcinogenesis, Mutagenesis, Impairment of Fertility: Subcutaneous implant of ZOLADEX in male and female rats once every 4 weeks for 1 year and recovery for 23 weeks at doses of about 80 and 150 µg/kg (males) and 50 and 100 µg/kg (females) daily (about 3 to 9 times the recommended human dose on a mg/m^2 basis) resulted in an increased incidence of pituitary adenomas. An increased incidence of pituitary adenomas was also observed following subcutaneous implant of ZOLADEX in rats at similar dose levels for a period of 72 weeks in males and 101 weeks in females. The relevance of the rat pituitary adenomas to humans has not been established. Subcutaneous implants of ZOLADEX every 3 weeks for 2 years delivered to mice at doses of up 2400 µg/kg/day (about 70 times the recommended human dose on a mg/m^2 basis) resulted in an increased incidence of histiocytic sarcoma of the vertebral column and femur.

Mutagenicity tests using bacterial and mammalian systems for point mutations and cytogenetic effects have provided no evidence for mutagenic potential.

Administration of goserelin led to changes that were consistent with gonadal suppression in both male and female rats as a result of its endocrine action. In male rats administered 500–1000 µg/kg/day (about 30–60 times the recommended human dose on a mg/m^2 basis), a decrease in weight and atrophic histological changes were observed in the testes, epididymis, seminal vesicle and prostate gland with complete suppression of spermatogenesis. In female rats administered 50–1000 µg/kg/day (about 3–60 times the recommended daily human dose on a mg/m^2 basis), suppression of ovarian function led to decreased size and weight of ovaries and secondary sex organs; follicular development was arrested at the antral stage and the corpora lutea were reduced in size and number. Except for the testes, almost complete histologic reversal of these effects in males and females was observed several weeks after dosing was stopped; however, fertility and general reproductive performance were reduced in those that became pregnant after goserelin was discontinued. Fertile matings occurred within 2 weeks after cessation of dosing, even though total recovery of reproductive function may not have occurred before mating took place; and, the ovulation rate, the corresponding implantation rate, and number of live fetuses were reduced.

Based on histological examination, drug effects on reproductive organs were reversible in male and female dogs administered 107–214 µg/kg/day ZOLADEX (about 20–40 times the recommended daily human dose on a mg/m^2 basis) when drug treatment was stopped after continuous administration for 1 year.

Pregnancy: Pregnancy Category X for treatment of endometriosis and endometrial thinning. See **CONTRAINDICATIONS** and **WARNINGS** sections. **Pregnancy Category D** for treatment of advanced breast cancer in pre- and perimenopausal women. See WARNINGS section.

Nursing Mothers: ZOLADEX has been shown to be excreted in the milk of lactating rats. It is not known if this drug is excreted in human milk. Because many drugs are excreted in human milk, and because of the potential for serious adverse reactions from ZOLADEX in nursing infants, mothers should discontinue nursing prior to taking the drug.

Pediatric Use: The safety and efficacy of ZOLADEX in pediatric patients have not been established.

ADVERSE REACTIONS

General: Rarely, hypersensitivity reactions (including urticaria and anaphylaxis) have been reported in patients receiving ZOLADEX.

Males: ZOLADEX has been found to be generally well tolerated in clinical trials. Adverse reactions reported in these trials were rarely severe enough to result in the patients' withdrawal from ZOLADEX treatment. As seen with other hormonal therapies, the most commonly observed adverse events during ZOLADEX therapy were due to the expected physiological effects from decreased testosterone levels. These included hot flashes, sexual dysfunction and decreased erections.

Initially, ZOLADEX, like other LHRH agonists, causes transient increases in serum levels of testosterone. A small percentage of patients experienced a temporary worsening of signs and symptoms (see WARNINGS section), usually manifested by an increase in cancer-related pain which was managed symptomatically. Isolated cases of exacerbation of disease symptoms, either ureteral obstruction or spinal cord compression, occurred at similar rates in controlled clinical trials with both ZOLADEX and orchiectomy. The relationship of these events to therapy is uncertain.

In the controlled clinical trials of ZOLADEX versus orchiectomy, the following events were reported as adverse reactions in greater than 5% of the patients.

[See table at left]

	TREATMENT RECEIVED				
ADVERSE EVENT	ZOLADEX (n=242) %	ORCHIECTOMY (n=254) %	ADVERSE EVENT	ZOLADEX (n=242) %	ORCHIECTOMY (n=254) %
Hot Flashes	62	53	Rash	6	1
Sexual Dysfunction	21	15	Sweating	6	4
Decreased Erections	18	16	Anorexia	5	2
Lower Urinary Tract Symptoms	13	8	Chronic Obstructive Pulmonary Disease	5	3
Lethargy	8	4	Congestive Heart Failure	5	1
Pain (worsened in the first 30 days)	8	3	Dizziness	5	4
Edema	7	8	Insomnia	5	1
Upper Respiratory Infection	7	2	Nausea	5	2
			Complications of Surgery	0	18†

† Complications related to surgery were reported in 18% of the orchiectomy patients, while only 3% of ZOLADEX patients reported adverse reactions at the injection site. The surgical complications included scrotal infection (5.9%), groin pain (4.7%), wound seepage (3.1%) scrotal hematoma (2.8%), incisional discomfort (1.6%) and skin necrosis (1.2%).

The following additional adverse reactions were reported in greater than 1% but less than 5% of the patients treated with ZOLADEX: CARDIOVASCULAR - arrhythmia, cerebrovascular accident, hypertension, myocardial infarction, peripheral vascular disorder, chest pain; CENTRAL NERVOUS SYSTEM - anxiety, depression, headache; GASTROINTESTINAL - constipation, diarrhea, ulcer, vomiting; HEMATOLOGIC - anemia; METABOLIC/NUTRITIONAL - gout, hyperglycemia, weight increase; MISCELLANEOUS - chills, fever; UROGENITAL - renal insufficiency, urinary obstruction, urinary tract infection, breast swelling and tenderness.

Females: As would be expected with a drug that results in hypoestrogenism, the most frequently reported adverse reactions were those related to this effect.

Endometriosis: In controlled clinical trials comparing ZOLADEX every 28 days and danazol daily for the treat-

	TREATMENT RECEIVED					
ADVERSE EVENT	ZOLADEX (n=411) %	DANAZOL (n=207) %	ADVERSE EVENT	ZOLADEX (n=411) %	DANAZOL (n=207) %	
Hot Flushes	96	67	Hirsutism	7	15	
Vaginitis	75	43	Insomnia	11	4	
Headache	75	63	Breast Pain	7	4	
Emotional Lability	60	56	Abdominal Pain	7	7	
Libido Decreased	61	44	Back Pain	7	13	
Sweating	45	30	Flu Syndrome	5	5	
Depression	54	48	Dizziness	6	4	
Acne	42	55	Application Site Reaction	6	-	
Breast Atrophy	33	42	Voice Alterations	3	8	
Seborrhea	26	52	Pharyngitis	5	2	
Peripheral Edema	21	34	Hair Disorders	4	11	
Breast Enlargement	18	15	Myalgia	3	11	
Pelvic Symptoms	18	23	Nervousness	3	5	
Pain	17	16	Weight Gain	3	23	
Dyspareunia	14	5	Leg Cramps	2	6	
Libido Increased	12	19	Increased Appetite	2	5	
Infection	13	11	Pruritus	2	6	
Asthenia	11	13	Hypertonia	1	10	
Nausea	8	14				

ment of endometriosis, the following events were reported at a frequency of 5% or greater:
[See table above]
The following adverse events not already listed above were reported at a frequency of 1% or greater, regardless of causality, in ZOLADEX-treated women from all clinical trials: WHOLE BODY - allergic reaction, chest pain, fever, malaise; CARDIOVASCULAR - hemorrhage, hypertension, migraine, palpitations, tachycardia; DIGESTIVE - anorexia, constipation, diarrhea, dry mouth, dyspepsia, flatulence; HEMATOLOGIC - ecchymosis; METABOLIC AND NUTRITIONAL - edema; MUSCULOSKELETAL - arthralgia, joint disorder; CNS - anxiety, paresthesia, somnolence, thinking abnormal; RESPIRATORY - bronchitis, cough increased, epistaxis, rhinitis, sinusitis; SKIN - alopecia, dry skin, rash, skin discoloration; SPECIAL SENSES - amblyopia, dry eyes; UROGENITAL - dysmenorrhea, urinary frequency, urinary tract infection, vaginal hemorrhage.

Hormone Replacement Therapy: Clinical studies suggest the addition of Hormone Replacement Therapy (estrogens and/or progestins) to ZOLADEX may decrease the occurrence of vasomotor symptoms and vaginal dryness associated with hypoestrogenism without compromising the efficacy of ZOLADEX in relieving pelvic symptoms. The optimal drugs, dose and duration of treatment has not been established.

Changes in Bone Mineral Density: After 6 months of ZOLADEX treatment, 109 female patients treated with ZOLADEX showed an average 4.3% decrease of vertebral trabecular bone mineral density (BMD) as compared to pretreatment values. BMD was measured by dual-photon absorptiometry or dual energy x-ray absorptiometry. Sixty-six of these patients were assessed for BMD loss 6 months after the completion (posttherapy) of the 6-month therapy period. Data from these patients showed an average 2.4% BMD loss compared to pretreatment values. Twenty-eight of the 109 patients were assessed for BMD at 12 months posttherapy. Data from these patients showed an average decrease of 2.5% in BMD compared to pretreatment values. These data suggest a possibility of partial reversibility. Clinical studies suggest the addition of Hormone Replacement Therapy (estrogens and/or progestins) to ZOLADEX is effective in reducing the bone mineral loss which occurs with ZOLADEX alone without compromising the efficacy of ZOLADEX in relieving the symptoms of endometriosis. The optimal drugs, dose and duration of treatment has not been established.

Changes in Laboratory Values During Treatment
Plasma Enzymes. Elevation of liver enzymes (AST, ALT) have been reported in female patients exposed to ZOLADEX (representing less than 1% of all patients).

Lipids. In a controlled trial, ZOLADEX therapy resulted in a minor, but statistically significant effect on serum lipids. In patients treated for endometriosis at 6 months following initiation of therapy, danazol treatment resulted in a mean increase in LDL cholesterol of 33.3 mg/dL and a decrease in HDL cholesterol of 21.3 mg/dL compared to increases of 21.3 and 2.7 mg/dL in LDL cholesterol and HDL cholesterol, respectively, for ZOLADEX-treated patients. Triglycerides increased by 8.0 mg/dL in ZOLADEX-treated patients compared to a decrease of 8.9 mg/dL in danazol-treated patients.
In patients treated for endometriosis, ZOLADEX increased total cholesterol and LDL cholesterol during 6 months of treatment. However, ZOLADEX therapy resulted in HDL cholesterol levels which were significantly higher relative to danazol therapy. At the end of 6 months of treatment, HDL cholesterol fractions (HDL_2 and HDL_3) were decreased by 13.5 and 7.7 mg/dL, respectively, for danazol-treated patients compared to treatment increases of 1.9 and 0.8 mg/dL, respectively, for ZOLADEX treated patients.

Breast Cancer: The adverse event profile for women with advanced breast cancer treated with ZOLADEX is consistent with the profile described above for women treated with ZOLADEX for endometriosis. In a controlled clinical trial (SWOG-8692) comparing ZOLADEX with oophorectomy in premenopausal and perimenopausal women with advanced breast cancer, the following events were reported at a frequency of 5% or greater in either treatment group regardless of causality.

	TREATMENT RECEIVED	
ADVERSE EVENT	ZOLADEX (n=57) % of Pts.	OOPHORECTOMY (n=55) % of Pts.
Hot Flashes	70	47
Tumor Flare	23	4
Nausea	11	7
Edema	5	0
Malaise/Fatigue/Lethargy	5	2
Vomiting	4	7

In the Phase II clinical trial program in 333 pre- and perimenopausal women with advanced breast cancer, hot flashes were reported in 75.9% of patients and decreased libido was noted in 47.7% of patients. These two adverse events reflect the pharmacological actions of ZOLADEX. Injection site reactions were reported in less than 1% of patients.

ADVERSE EVENTS REPORTED AT A FREQUENCY OF 5% OR GREATER IN ZOLADEX AND PLACEBO TREATMENT GROUPS OF TRIAL 0022					
ADVERSE EVENT	ZOLADEX 3.6 mg (n=180) %	placebo (n=177) %	ADVERSE EVENT	ZOLADEX 3.6 mg (n=180) %	placebo (n=177) %
Whole body			**Respiratory**		
Headache	32	22	Pharyngitis	6	9
Abdominal Pain	11	10	Sinusitis	3	6
Pelvic Pain	9	6	**Skin and appendages**		
Back Pain	4	7	Sweating	16	5
Cardiovascular			**Urogenital**		
Vasodilatation	57	18	Dysmenorrhea	7	9
Migraine	7	4	Uterine Hemorrhage	6	4
Hypertension	6	2	Vulvovaginitis	5	1
Digestive			Menorrhagia	4	5
Nausea	5	6	Vaginitis	1	6
Nervous					
Nervousness	5	3			
Depression	3	7			

Endometrial Thinning: The following adverse events were reported at a frequency of 5% or greater in premenopausal women presenting with dysfunctional uterine bleeding in Trial 0022 for endometrial thinning. These results indicate that headache, hot flushes and sweating, were more common in the ZOLADEX group than in the placebo group.
[See table at bottom of page]

OVERDOSAGE
The pharmacologic properties of ZOLADEX and its mode of administration make accidental or intentional overdosage unlikely. There is no experience of overdosage from clinical trials. Animal studies indicate that no increased pharmacologic effect occurred at higher doses or more frequent administration. Subcutaneous doses of the drug as high as 1 mg/kg/day in rats and dogs did not produce any nonendocrine related sequelae; this dose is greater than 400 times that proposed for human use. If overdosage occurs, it should be managed symptomatically.

DOSAGE AND ADMINISTRATION
ZOLADEX, at a dose of 3.6 mg, should be administered subcutaneously every 28 days into the upper abdominal wall using an aseptic technique under the supervision of a physician.
While a delay of a few days is permissible, every effort should be made to adhere to the 28-day schedule.
Prostate Cancer and Breast Cancer: For the management of advanced prostate cancer and breast cancer, ZOLADEX is intended for long-term administration unless clinically inappropriate.
Endometriosis: For the management of endometriosis, the recommended duration of administration is 6 months. Currently, there are no clinical data on the effect of treatment of benign gynecological conditions with ZOLADEX for periods in excess of 6 months.
Retreatment cannot be recommended for the management of endometriosis since safety data for retreatment are not available. If the symptoms of endometriosis recur after a course of therapy, and further treatment with ZOLADEX is contemplated, consideration should be given to monitoring bone mineral density. Clinical studies suggest the addition of Hormone Replacement Therapy (estrogens and/or progestins) to ZOLADEX is effective in reducing the bone mineral loss which occurs with ZOLADEX alone without compromising the efficacy of ZOLADEX in relieving the symptoms of endometriosis. The addition of Hormone Replacement Therapy may also reduce the occurrence of vasomotor symptoms and vaginal dryness associated with hypoestrogenism. The optimal drugs, dose and duration of treatment has not been established.
Endometrial Thinning: For use as an endometrial-thinning agent prior to endometrial ablation, the dosing recommendation is one or two depots (with each depot given four weeks apart). When one depot is administered, surgery should be performed at four weeks. When two depots are administered, surgery should be performed within two to four weeks following administration of the second depot.
Renal or Hepatic Impairment: No dosage adjustment is necessary for patients with renal or hepatic impairment.
Administration Technique: The proper method of administration of ZOLADEX is described in the instructions that follow.
1. The package should be inspected for damage prior to opening. If the package is damaged, the syringe should not be used. Do not remove the sterile syringe from the package until immediately before use. Examine the syringe for damage, and check that ZOLADEX is visible in the translucent chamber.
2. Clean an area of the upper abdominal wall with an alcohol swab. (A local anesthetic may be used in the normal fashion at the option of the administrator or patient.)
3. Grasp red plastic safety clip tab, pull out and away from needle, and discard immediately. Then remove needle cover.
4. Using an aseptic technique, stretch or pinch the patient's skin with one hand, and grip syringe barrel. Insert the hypodermic needle into the subcutaneous tissue.
NOTE: The ZOLADEX syringe cannot be used for aspiration. If the hypodermic needle penetrates a large vessel, blood will be seen instantly in the syringe chamber. If a vessel is penetrated, withdraw the needle and inject with a new syringe elsewhere.
5. Change the direction of the needle so it parallels the abdominal wall. Push the needle in until the barrel hub touches the patient's skin. Withdraw the needle one centimeter to create a space to discharge ZOLADEX. Fully depress the plunger to discharge ZOLADEX.
6. Withdraw the needle. Then bandage the site. Confirm discharge of ZOLADEX by ensuring tip of the plunger is visible within the tip of the needle. Dispose of the used needle and syringe in a safe manner.
NOTE: In the unlikely event of the need to surgically remove ZOLADEX, it may be localized by ultrasound.

Continued on next page

Zoladex 3.6 mg—Cont.

HOW SUPPLIED

ZOLADEX is supplied as a sterile and totally biodegradable D,L-lactic and glycolic acids copolymer (13.3–14.3 mg/dose) impregnated with goserelin acetate equivalent to 3.6 mg of goserelin in a disposable syringe device fitted with a 16 gauge hypodermic needle (NDC 0310-0960). The unit is sterile and comes in a sealed, light and moisture proof, aluminum foil laminate pouch containing a desiccant capsule. Store at room temperature (do not exceed 25°C).

Manufactured for:
Zeneca Pharmaceuticals
A business unit of ZENECA Inc.
Wilmington, DE 19850-5437
By: Zeneca Limited, Macclesfield, England
Made in the United Kingdom

64132-00 Rev Z 04/98

Shown in Product Identification Guide, page 346

ZOLADEX® 3-MONTH ℞

GOSERELIN ACETATE IMPLANT 10.8 mg
Equivalent to 10.8 mg goserelin

FOR USE IN MEN WITH PROSTATE CANCER

DESCRIPTION

ZOLADEX® (goserelin acetate implant), contains a potent synthetic decapeptide analogue of luteinizing hormone-releasing hormone (LHRH), also known as a gonadotropin releasing hormone (GnRH) agonist analogue. Goserelin acetate is chemically described as an acetate salt of [D-Ser(Bu^t)^6,Azgly^{10}]LHRH. Its chemical structure is pyro-Glu-His-Trp-Ser-Tyr-D-Ser(Bu^t)-Leu-Arg-Pro-Azgly-NH_2 acetate [$C_{59}H_{84}N_{18}O_{14} \cdot (C_2H_4O_2)_x$ where x = 1 to 2.4].

Goserelin acetate is an off-white powder with a molecular weight of 1269 Daltons (free base). It is freely soluble in glacial acetic acid. It is soluble in water, 0.1M hydrochloric acid, 0.1M sodium hydroxide, dimethylformamide and dimethyl sulfoxide. Goserelin acetate is practically insoluble in acetone, chloroform and ether.

ZOLADEX 10.8 mg implant is supplied as a sterile, biodegradable product containing goserelin acetate equivalent to 10.8 mg of goserelin. ZOLADEX is designed for subcutaneous implantation with continuous release over a 12-week period. Goserelin acetate is dispersed in a matrix of D,L-lactic and glycolic acids copolymer (12.82–14.76 mg/dose) containing less than 2% acetic acid and up to 10% goserelin-related substances and presented as a sterile, white to cream colored 1.5 mm diameter cylinder, preloaded in a special single–use syringe with a 14–gauge needle and overwrapped in a sealed, light–and moisture proof, aluminum foil laminate pouch containing a desiccant capsule.

Studies of the D,L-lactic and glycolic acids copolymer have indicated that it is completely biodegradable and has no demonstrable antigenic potential.

ZOLADEX is also supplied as a sterile, biodegradable product containing goserelin acetate equivalent to 3.6 mg of goserelin designed for administration every 28 days.

CLINICAL PHARMACOLOGY

Mechanism of Action: ZOLADEX is a synthetic decapeptide analogue of LHRH. ZOLADEX acts as a potent inhibitor of pituitary gonadotropin secretion when administered in the biodegradable formulation.

Following initial administration, ZOLADEX causes an initial increase in serum–luteinizing hormone (LH) and follicle–stimulating hormone (FSH) levels with subsequent increases in serum levels of testosterone. Chronic administration of ZOLADEX leads to sustained suppression of pituitary gonadotropins, and serum levels of testosterone consequently fall into the range normally seen in surgically castrated men approximately 21 days after initiation of therapy. This leads to accessory sex organ regression.

In animal and in *in vitro* studies, administration of goserelin resulted in the regression or inhibition of growth of the hormonally sensitive dimethylbenzanthracene (DMBA)-induced rat mammary tumor and Dunning R3327 prostate tumor.

In clinical trials using ZOLADEX 3.6 mg with follow-up of more than 2 years, suppression of serum testosterone to castrate levels has been maintained for the duration of therapy.

Pharmacokinetics: The pharmacokinetics of goserelin have been determined in healthy male volunteers and prostate cancer patients using an RIA method, which has been shown to be specific for goserelin in the presence of its metabolites.

Serum goserelin concentrations in prostate cancer patients administered three 3.6 mg depots followed by one 10.8 mg depot are displayed in Figure 1. The profiles for both formulations are primarily dependent upon the rate of drug release from the depots. For the 3.6 mg depot, mean concentrations gradually rise to reach a peak of about 3 ng/mL at around 15 days after administration and then decline to approximately 0.5 ng/mL by the end of the treatment period. For the 10.8 mg depot, mean concentrations increase to reach a peak of about 8 ng/mL within the first 24 hours and then decline rapidly up to Day 4. Thereafter, mean concentrations remain relatively stable in the range of about 0.3 to 1 ng/mL up to the end of the treatment period.

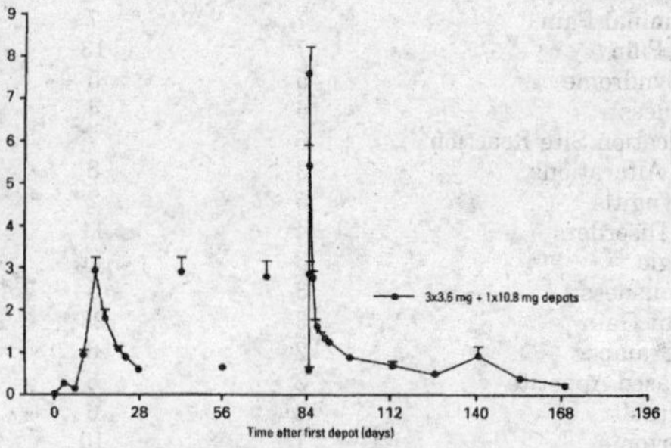

Figure 1: Goserelin serum concentrations during dosing three ZOLADEX 3.6 mg depots (0, 28, 56 days) then one ZOLADEX 10.8 mg depot (84 days) to prostate cancer patients.

Absorption: The absorption of radiolabelled drug was rapid following administration as a single 250 µg (aqueous solution) dose to volunteers by the subcutaneous route. The pharmacokinetics of goserelin following administration of a ZOLADEX 10.8 mg depot to patients with prostate cancer are determined by the release of drug from the depot; representative data are summarized in Table 1.

Release of goserelin from the depot was relatively rapid shortly after administration resulting in a peak concentration being observed 2 hours after dosing. Sustained release of goserelin produced a reasonably stable systemic exposure from Day 4 until the end of the 12-week dosing interval. This overall profile resulted in testosterone levels that were suppressed to and maintained within the range normally observed in surgically castrated men (0–1.73 nmol/L or 0–50 ng/dL), over the dosing interval in approximately 91% (145/160) of patients studied. In 6 of 15 patients that escaped from castrate range, serum testosterone levels were maintained below 2.0 nmol/L (58 ng/dL) and in only one of the 15 patients did the depot completely fail to maintain serum testosterone levels to within the recognized castrate range over a 336-day period (4 depot injections). In the 8 additional patients, a transient escape was followed 14 days later by a level within the castrate range. There is no clinically significant accumulation of goserelin following administration of four depots administered at 12-week intervals.

Distribution: The plasma protein-binding of goserelin is low (<30%).

Metabolism/Elimination: Clearance of goserelin following subcutaneous administration of the solution formulation of goserelin is very rapid and occurs via a combination of hepatic metabolism and urinary excretion. The metabolism of goserelin in humans yields a similar but narrow profile of metabolites to that found in other species. All the human metabolites have also been found in the toxicology species. The major component in serum was the 1–7 fragment formed by hydrolysis of the C-terminal amino acids.

Excretion: More than 90% of a subcutaneous radiolabelled solution formulation dose of goserelin is excreted in urine. Approximately 20% of the dose recovered in urine is accounted for by unchanged goserelin.

Special Populations

Renal Insufficiency: In clinical trials with the solution formulation of goserelin, subjects with impaired renal function (creatinine clearance less than 20 mL/min) had a serum elimination half-life of 12.1 hours compared to 4.2 hours for subjects with normal renal function (creatinine clearance greater than 70 mL/min). However, there was no evidence for any accumulation of goserelin on multiple dosing of the ZOLADEX 10.8 mg depot to subjects with impaired renal function. There was no evidence for any increase in incidence of adverse events in renally impaired patients administered the 10.8 mg depot. These data indicate that there is no need for any dosage adjustment when administering ZOLADEX 10.8 mg to subjects with impaired renal function.

Hepatic Insufficiency: The clearance and half-life of goserelin administered as an aqueous solution are not affected by hepatic impairment. These data indicate that there is no need for any dosage adjustment when administering ZOLADEX 10.8 mg to subjects with impaired hepatic function.

Geriatric: There is no need for any dosage adjustment when administering ZOLADEX 10.8 mg to geriatric patients.

Body Weight: A decline of approximately 1 to 2.5% in the AUC after administration of a 10.8 mg depot was observed with a kilogram increase in body weight. In obese patients who have not responded clinically, testosterone levels should be monitored closely.

Drug-Drug Interactions: No formal drug-drug interaction studies have been performed.

Table 1
Goserelin pharmacokinetic parameters
for the 10.8 mg depot

Parameter	n	Mean	SE	95% Cl Lower	95% Cl Upper
Systemic clearance (mL/min)	41	121	6.6	108	134
C_{max} (ng/mL)	41	8.85	0.44	7.96	9.74
T_{max}(h)	41	1.80	0.05	1.70	1.92
C_{min} (ng/mL)	44	0.37	0.03	0.30	0.43
Elimination Half-life (h) ¶	7	4.16	0.40	3.12	5.20

¶ = determined after subcutaneous administration of 250 µg aqueous solution of goserelin.
SE = standard error of the mean
95% Cl = 95% confidence interval

Clinical Studies: In two controlled clinical trials, 160 patients with advanced prostate cancer were randomized to receive either one 3.6 mg ZOLADEX implant every four weeks or a single 10.8 mg ZOLADEX implant every 12 weeks. Mean serum testosterone suppression was similar between the two arms. PSA falls at three months were 94% in patients who received the 10.8 mg implant and 92.5% in patients that received three 3.6 mg implants.

Periodic monitoring of serum testosterone levels should be considered if the anticipated clinical or biochemical response to treatment has not been achieved. A clinical outcome similar to that produced with the use of the 3.6 mg implant administered every 28 days is predicted with ZOLADEX 10.8 mg implant administered every 12 weeks (84 days). Total testosterone was measured by the DPC Coat-A-Count radioimmunoassay method which, as defined by the manufacturers, is highly specific and accurate. Acceptable variability of approximately 20% at low testosterone levels has been demonstrated in the clinical studies performed with the ZOLADEX 10.8 mg depot.

INDICATIONS AND USAGE

Prostatic Carcinoma: ZOLADEX is indicated in the palliative treatment of advanced carcinoma of the prostate. ZOLADEX offers an alternative treatment of prostatic cancer when orchiectomy or estrogen administration are either not indicated or unacceptable to the patient.

In controlled studies of patients with advanced prostatic cancer comparing ZOLADEX 3.6 mg to orchiectomy, the long-term endocrine responses and objective responses were similar between the two treatment arms. Additionally, duration of survival was similar between the two treatment arms in a major comparative trial.

In controlled studies of patients with advanced prostatic cancer, ZOLADEX 10.8 mg implant produced pharmacodynamically similar effect in terms of suppression of serum testosterone to that achieved with ZOLADEX 3.6 mg implant. Clinical outcome similar to that produced with the use of the ZOLADEX 3.6 mg implant administered every 28 days is predicted with the ZOLADEX 10.8 mg implant administered every 12 weeks.

CONTRAINDICATIONS

A report of an anaphylactic reaction to synthetic GnRH (Factrel) has been reported in the medical literature. ZOLADEX is contraindicated in those patients who have a known hypersensitivity to LHRH, LHRH agonist analogues or any of the components in ZOLADEX.

ZOLADEX 10.8 mg implant is not indicated in women as the data are insufficient to support reliable suppression of serum estradiol. For female patients requiring treatment with goserelin, refer to the prescribing information for ZOLADEX 3.6 mg implant.

ZOLADEX is contraindicated in women who are or may become pregnant while receiving the drug. In studies in rats and rabbits, ZOLADEX increased preimplantation loss, resorptions, and abortions (see Pregnancy section). In rats and dogs, ZOLADEX suppressed ovarian function, decreased ovarian weight and size, and led to atrophic changes in secondary sex organs. Further evidence suggests that fertility was reduced in female rats that became pregnant after ZOLADEX was stopped. These effects are an expected consequence of the hormonal alterations produced by ZOLADEX in humans. If a patient becomes pregnant during treatment, the drug must be discontinued and the patient must be apprised of the potential risk for loss of the pregnancy due to possible hormonal imbalance as a result of the expected pharmacologic action of ZOLADEX treatment. In animal studies, there was no evidence that ZOLADEX possessed the potential to cause teratogenicity in rabbits;

however, in rats the incidence of umbilical hernia was significantly increased with treatment. (See Pregnancy, Teratogenic Effects.)

WARNINGS

Initially, ZOLADEX, like other LHRH agonists, causes transient increases in serum levels of testosterone. Transient worsening of symptoms, or the occurrence of additional signs and symptoms of prostatic cancer, may occasionally develop during the first few weeks of ZOLADEX treatment. A small number of patients may experience a temporary increase in bone pain, which can be managed symptomatically. As with other LHRH agonists, isolated cases of ureteral obstruction and spinal cord compression have been observed. If spinal cord compression or renal impairment develops, standard treatment of these complications should be instituted, and in extreme cases an immediate orchiectomy considered.

PRECAUTIONS

General: Hypersensitivity, antibody formation and acute anaphylactic reactions have been reported with LHRH agonist analogues.

Of 115 women worldwide treated with ZOLADEX 3.6 mg and tested for development of binding to goserelin following treatment with ZOLADEX, one patient showed low-titer binding to goserelin. On further testing of this patient's plasma obtained following treatment, her goserelin binding component was found not to be precipitated with rabbit antihuman immunoglobulin polyvalent sera. These findings suggest the possibility of anitbody formation.

Information for Patients: The use of ZOLADEX in patients at particular risk of developing ureteral obstruction or spinal cord compression should be considered carefully and the patients monitored closely during the first month of therapy. Patients with ureteral obstruction or spinal cord compression should have appropriate treatment prior to initiation of ZOLADEX therapy.

Drug Interactions: No drug interaction studies with other drugs have been conducted with ZOLADEX. No confirmed interactions have been reported between ZOLADEX and other drugs.

Drug/Laboratory Test Interactions: Administration of ZOLADEX in therapeutic doses results in suppression of the pituitary-gonadal system. Because of this suppression, diagnostic tests of pituitary-gonadotropic and gonadal functions conducted during treatment may show results which are misleading.

Carcinogenesis, Mutagenesis, Impairment of Fertility: Subcutaneous implant of ZOLADEX in male and female rats once every 4 weeks for 1 year and recovery for 23 weeks at doses of about 80 and 150 µg/kg (males) and 50 and 100 µg/kg (females) daily (about 3 to 9 times the recommended human dose on a mg/m^2 basis) resulted in an increased incidence of pituitary adenomas. An increased incidence of pituitary adenomas was also observed following subcutaneous implant of ZOLADEX in rats at similar dose levels for a period of 72 weeks in males and 101 weeks in females. The relevance of the rat pituitary adenomas to humans has not been established. Subcutaneous implants of ZOLADEX every 3 weeks for 2 years delivered to mice at doses of up 2400 µg/kg/day (about 70 times the recommended human dose on a mg/m^2 basis) resulted in an increased incidence of histiocytic sarcoma of the vertebral column and femur.

Mutagenicity tests using bacterial and mammalian systems for point mutations and cytogenetic effects have provided no evidence for mutagenic potential.

Administration of goserelin led to changes that were consistent with gonadal suppression in both male and female rats as a result of its endocrine action. In male rats administered 500–1000 µg/kg/day (about 30–60 times the recommended human dose on a mg/m^2 basis), a decrease in weight and atrophic histological changes were observed in the testes, epididymis, seminal vesicle and prostate gland with complete suppression of spermatogenesis. In female rats administered 50–1000 µg/ky/day (about 3–60 times the recommended daily human dose on a mg/m^2 basis), suppression of ovarian function led to decreased size and weight of ovaries and secondary sex organs; follicular development was arrested at the antral stage and the corpora lutea were reduced in size and number. Except for the testes, almost complete histologic reversal of these effects in males and females was observed several weeks after dosing was stopped; however, fertility and general reproductive performance were reduced in those that became pregnant after goserelin was discontinued. Fertile matings occurred within 2 weeks after cessation of dosing, even though total recovery of reproductive function may not have occurred before mating took place; and, the ovulation rate, the corresponding implantation rate, and number of live fetuses were reduced.

Based on histological examination, drug effects on reproductive organs seem to be completely reversible in male and female dogs when drug treatment was stopped after continuous administration for 1 year at 100 times the recommended monthly dose.

Pregnancy, Teratogenic Effects: Pregnancy Category X. See CONTRAINDICATIONS section. ZOLADEX 10.8 mg is not indicated in women as the data are insufficient to support reliable suppression of serum estradiol. Studies in both rats and rabbits at doses of 2, 10, 20, and 50 µg/kg/day and 20, 250, and 1,000 µg/kg/day, respectively (about $^1/_{10}$ to 3 times and 2 to 100 times the daily maximum recommended human dose, respectively, on a mg/m^2 basis), administered during the period of organogenesis, have confirmed that ZOLADEX will increase pregnancy loss in a dose-related manner. While there was no evidence that ZOLADEX possessed the potential to cause teratogenicity in rabbits, in rats the incidence of umbilical hernia was significantly increased at doses greater than 10 mg/kg/day (about $^1/_2$ the recommended dose on a mg/m^2 basis).

Nursing Mothers: It is not known if this drug is excreted in human milk. Many drugs are excreted in human milk and there is a potential for serious adverse reactions in nursing infants of mothers receiving ZOLADEX (See CONTRAINDICATIONS).

Pediatric Use: Safety and efficacy of ZOLADEX in pediatric patients have not been established.

ADVERSE REACTIONS

General: Rarely, hypersensitivity reactions (including urticaria and anaphylaxis) have been reported in patients receiving ZOLADEX.

As with other endocrine therapies, hypercalcemia (increased calcium) has rarely been reported in cancer patients with bone metastases following initiation of treatment with ZOLADEX or other LHRH agonists.

ZOLADEX has been found to be generally well tolerated in clinical trials. Adverse reactions reported in these trials were rarely severe enough to result in the patients' withdrawal from ZOLADEX treatment. As seen with other hormonal therapies, the most commonly observed adverse events during ZOLADEX therapy were due to the expected physiological effects from decreased testosterone levels. These included hot flashes, sexual dysfunction and decreased erections.

Initially, ZOLADEX, like other LHRH agonists, causes transient increases in serum levels of testosterone. A small percentage of patients experienced a temporary worsening of signs and symptoms (see WARNINGS section), usually manifested by an increase in cancer-related pain which was managed symptomatically. Isolated cases of exacerbation of disease symptoms, either ureteral obstruction or spinal cord compression, occurred at similar rates in controlled clinical trials with both ZOLADEX and orchiectomy. The relationship of these events to therapy is uncertain.

Two controlled clinical trials using ZOLADEX 10.8 mg versus ZOLADEX 3.6 mg were conducted. During a comparative phase, patients were randomized to receive either a single 10.8 mg implant or three consecutive 3.6 mg implants every 4 weeks over weeks 0–12. During this phase, the only adverse event reported in greater than 5% of patients was hot flashes, with an incidence of 47% in the ZOLADEX 10.8 mg group and 48% in the ZOLADEX 3.6 mg group.

From weeks 12–48 all patients were treated with a 10.8 mg implant every 12 weeks. During this noncomparative phase, the following adverse events were reported in greater than 5% of patients:

Adverse Event	ZOLADEX 10.8 mg (n=157) %
Hot Flashes	64
Pain (General)	14
Gynecomastia	8
Pelvic Pain	6
Bone Pain	6
Asthenia	5

The following adverse events were reported in greater than 1%, but less than 5% of patients treated with ZOLADEX 10.8 mg implant every 12 weeks. Some of these are commonly reported in elderly patients.

WHOLE BODY—Abdominal pain, Back pain, Flu syndrome, Headache, Sepsis, Aggravation reaction
CARDIOVASCULAR—Angina pectoris, Cerebral ischemia, Cerebrovascular accident, Heart failure, Pulmonary embolus, Varicose veins
DIGESTIVE—Diarrhea, Hematemesis
ENDOCRINE—Diabetes mellitus
HEMATOLOGIC—Anemia
METABOLIC—Peripheral edema
NERVOUS SYSTEM—Dizziness, Paresthesis, Urinary retention
RESPIRATORY—Cough increased, Dyspnea, Pneumonia
SKIN—Herpes simplex, Pruritus
UROGENITAL—Bladder neoplasm, Breast pain, Hematuria, Impotence, Urinary frequency, Urinary incontinence, Urinary tract disorder, Urinary tract infection, Urination impaired.

The following adverse events not already listed above were reported in patients receiving ZOLADEX 3.6 mg in other clinical trials. Inclusion does not necessarily represent a causal relationship to ZOLADEX 10.8 mg.

WHOLE BODY—Allergic reaction, Chills, Fever, Infection, Injection site reaction, Lethargy, Malaise
CARDIOVASCULAR—Arrhythmia, Chest pain, Hemorrhage, Hypertension, Migraine, Myocardial infarction, Palpitations, Peripheral vascular disorder, Tachycardia
DIGESTIVE—Anorexia, Constipation, Dry mouth, Dyspepsia, Flatulence, Increased appetite, Nausea, Ulcer, Vomiting
HEMATOLOGIC—Ecchymosis
METABOLIC—Edema, Gout, Hyperglycemia, Weight increase
MUSCULOSKELETAL—Arthraliga, Hypertonia, Joint disorder, Leg cramps, Myalgia, Osteoporosis
NERVOUS SYSTEM—Anxiety, Depression, Emotional lability, Headache, Insomnia, Nervousness, Somnolence, Thinking abnormal
RESPIRATORY—Bronchitis, Chronic obstructive pulmonary disease, Epistaxis, Rhinitis, Sinusitis, Upper respiratory infection, Voice alterations
SKIN—Acne, Alopecia, Dry skin, Hair disorders, Rash, Seborrhea, Skin discoloration, Sweating
SPECIAL SENSES—Amblyopia, Dry eyes
UROGENITAL—Breast tenderness, Decreased erections, Renal insufficiency, Sexual dysfunction, Urinary obstruction

Changes in Laboratory Values During Treatment

Plasma Enzymes: Elevation of liver enzymes (AST, ALT) have been reported in female patients exposed to ZOLADEX 3.6 mg (representing less than 1% of all patients). There was no other evidence of abnormal liver function. Causality between these changes and ZOLADEX have not been established.

Lipids: In a controlled trial in females, ZOLADEX 3.6 mg implant therapy resulted in a minor, but statistically significant effect on serum lipids (ie, increases in I.DL cholesterol of 21.3 mg/dL, increases in HDL cholesterol of 2.7 mg/dL; and triglycerides increased by 8.0 mg/dL).

OVERDOSAGE

The pharmacologic properties of ZOLADEX and its mode of administration make accidental or intentional overdosage unlikely. There is no experience of overdosage from clinical trials. Animal studies indicate that no increased pharmacologic effect occurred at higher doses or more frequent administration. Subcutaneous doses of the drug as high as 1 mg/kg/day in rats and dogs did not produce any nonendocrine related sequelae; this dose is greater than 400 times that proposed for human use. If overdosage occurs, it should be managed symptomatically.

DOSAGE AND ADMINISTRATION

ZOLADEX, at a dose of 10.8 mg, should be administered subcutaneously every 12 weeks into the upper abdominal wall using an aseptic technique under the supervision of a physician.

While a delay of a few days is permissible, every effort should be made to adhere to the 12-week schedule.

For the management of advanced prostate cancer, ZOLADEX is intended for long-term administration unless clinically inappropriate.

No dosage adjustment is necessary for patients with renal or hepatic impairment.

ZOLADEX 10.8 mg implant is not indicated in women as the data are insufficient to support reliable suppression of serum estradiol. For female patients requiring treatment with goserelin, refer to the prescribing information for ZOLADEX 3.6 mg implant.

Administration Technique: The proper method of administration of ZOLADEX is described in the instructions that follow.

1. The package should be inspected for damage prior to opening. If the package is damaged, the syringe should not be used. Do not remove the sterile syringe from the package until immediately before use. Examine the syringe for damage, and check that ZOLADEX is visible in the translucent chamber.
2. Clean an area of the upper abdominal wall with an alcohol swab. (A local anesthetic may be used in the normal fashion at the option of the administrator or patient.)
3. Grasp blue plastic safety clip tab, pull out and away from needle, and discard immediately. Then remove needle cover.
4. Using an aseptic technique, stretch or pinch the patient's skin with one hand, and grip the syringe barrel. Insert the hypodermic needle into the subcutaneous tissue.
   NOTE: The ZOLADEX syringe cannot be used for aspiration. If the hypodermic needle penetrates a large vessel, blood will seen be instantly in the syringe chamber. If a vessel is penetrated, withdraw the needle and inject with a new syringe elsewhere.
5. Change the direction of the needle so it parallels the abdominal wall. Push the needle in until the barrel hub touches the patient's skin. Withdraw the needle one centimeter to create a space to discharge ZOLADEX. Fully depress the plunger to discharge ZOLADEX.

Continued on next page

Zoladex 3-month—Cont.

6. Withdraw the needle. Then bandage the site. Confirm discharge of ZOLADEX by ensuring tip of the plunger is visible within the tip of the needle. Dispose of the used needle and syringe in a safe manner.

NOTE: In the unlikely event of the need to surgically remove ZOLADEX, it may be localized by ultrasound.

HOW SUPPLIED

ZOLADEX 10.8 mg implant is supplied as a sterile and totally biodegradable D,L-lactic and glycolic acids copolymer (12.82–14.76 mg/dose) impregnated with goserelin acetate equivalent to 10.8 mg of goserelin in a disposable syringe device fitted with a 14-gauge hypodermic needle (NDC 0310-0961). The unit is sterile and comes in a sealed, light– and moisture–proof, aluminum foil laminate pouch containing a desiccant capsule. Store at room temperature (do not exceed 25°C).

Made in the United Kingdom
Manufactured for
ZENECA Pharmaceuticals
A Business Unit of Zeneca Inc.
Wilmington, Delaware 19850-5437 USA
by Zeneca Limited, Macclesfield, England
64114-00 Rev C 04/96

Shown in Product Identification Guide, page 346

ZOMIG
[zō-mĭg]
(ZOLMITRIPTAN)
TABLETS

DESCRIPTION

ZOMIG™ (zolmitriptan) Tablets contain zolmitriptan, which is a selective 5-hydroxytryptamine $_{1B/1D}$ (5-HT$_{1B/1D}$) receptor agonist. Zolmitriptan is chemically designated as (S)-4-[[3-[2-(Dimethylamino)ethyl]-1H-indol-5-yl]-methyl]-2-oxazolidinone and has the following chemical structure:

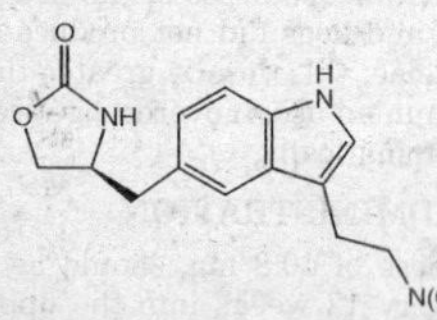

The empirical formula is $C_{16}H_{21}N_3O_2$, representing a molecular weight of 287.36. Zolmitriptan is a white to almost white powder that is readily soluble in water. ZOMIG is supplied as 2.5 mg (yellow) and 5 mg (pink) tablets for oral administration. The film-coated tablets contain anhydrous lactose NF, microcrystalline cellulose NF, sodium starch glycolate NF, magnesium stearate NF, hydroxypropyl methylcellulose USP, titanium dioxide USP, polyethylene glycol 400 NF, yellow iron oxide NF (2.5 mg tablet), red iron oxide NF (5 mg tablet), and polyethylene glycol 8000 NF.

CLINICAL PHARMACOLOGY

Mechanism of Action: Zolmitriptan binds with high affinity to human recombinant 5-HT$_{1D}$ and 5-HT$_{1B}$ receptors. Zolmitriptan exhibits modest affinity for 5-HT$_{1A}$ receptors, but has no significant affinity (as measured by radioligand binding assays) or pharmacological activity at 5-HT$_2$, 5-HT$_3$, 5-HT$_4$, alpha$_1$, alpha$_2$, or beta$_1$, -adrenergic; H$_1$, H$_2$, histaminic; muscarinic; dopamine$_1$, or dopamine$_2$ receptors. The N-desmethyl metabolite also has high affinity for 5-HT$_{1B/1D}$ and modest affinity for 5-HT$_{1A}$ receptors.

Current theories proposed to explain the etiology of migraine headache suggest that symptoms are due to local cranial vasodilatation and/or to the release of sensory neuropeptides (vasoactive intestinal peptide, substance P and calcitonin gene-related peptide) through nerve endings in the trigeminal system. The therapeutic activity of zolmitriptan for the treatment of migraine headache can most likely be attributed to the agonist effects at the 5-HT$_{1B/1D}$ receptors on intracranial blood vessels (including the arterio-venous anastomoses) and sensory nerves of the trigeminal system which result in cranial vessel constriction and inhibition of pro-inflammatory neuropeptide release.

Pharmacokinetics: Zolmitriptan is well absorbed after oral administration with peak plasma concentrations occurring in 2 hours. Mean absolute bioavailability is approximately 40%. Zolmitriptan displays linear kinetics over the dose range of 2.5 to 50 mg. The mean elimination half-life of zolmitriptan and of the active N-desmethyl metabolite is 3 hours. Zolmitriptan is converted to an active N-desmethyl metabolite such that the metabolite concentrations are about two thirds that of zolmitriptan. Because the 5HT$_{1B/1D}$ potency of the metabolite is 2 to 6 times that of the parent, the metabolite may contribute a substantial portion of the overall effect after zolmitriptan administration. The T_{max} for this metabolite is approximately 2 to 3 hours. No accumulation occurred on multiple dosing. Food has no significant effect on the bioavailability of zolmitriptan.

The mean apparent volume of distribution is 7.0 L/kg. Plasma protein binding of zolmitriptan is 25% over the concentration range of 10 – 1000 ng/mL.

Total radioactivity recovered in urine and feces was 65% and 30% of the administered dose, respectively. About 8% of the dose was recovered in the urine as unchanged zolmitriptan. Indole acetic acid metabolite accounted for 31% of the dose, followed by N-oxide (7%) and N-desmethyl (4%) metabolites. The indole acetic acid and N-oxide metabolites are inactive.

Mean total plasma clearance is 31.5 mL/min/kg, of which one-sixth is renal clearance. The renal clearance is greater than the glomerular filtration rate suggesting renal tubular secretion.

During a moderate to severe migraine attack, mean AUC_{0-4} and C_{max} for zolmitriptan were decreased by 40% and 25%, respectively, and mean T_{max} was delayed by one-half hour compared to the same patients during a migraine free period.

Special Populations

Age: Zolmitriptan pharmacokinetics in healthy elderly non-migraineur volunteers (age 65 – 76 yrs) were similar to those in younger non-migraineur volunteers (age 18 – 39 yrs).

Gender: Mean plasma concentrations of zolmitriptan were up to 1.5-fold higher in females than males.

Renal Impairment: Clearance of zolmitriptan was reduced by 25% in patients with severe renal impairment (Clcr ≥ 5 ≤ 25 mL/min) compared to the normal group (Clcr > = 70 mL/min); no significant change in clearance was observed in the moderately renally impaired group (Clcr ≥ 26 ≤ 50 mL/min).

Hepatic Impairment: In severely hepatically impaired patients, the mean C_{max}, T_{max}, and $AUC_{0-\infty}$ of zolmitriptan were increased 1.5, 2 (2 vs 4 hrs), and 3 fold, respectively, compared to normals. Seven out of 27 patients experienced 20 to 80 mm Hg elevations in systolic and/or diastolic blood pressure after a 10 mg dose. Zolmitriptan should be administered with caution in subjects with liver disease, generally using doses less than 2.5 mg (See WARNINGS and PRECAUTIONS).

Hypertensive Patients: No differences in the pharmacokinetics of zolmitriptan or its effects on blood pressure were seen in mild to moderate hypertensive volunteers compared to normotensive controls.

Race: Retrospective analysis of pharmacokinetic data between Japanese and Caucasians revealed no significant differences.

Drug Interactions: All drug interaction studies were performed in healthy volunteers using a single 10 mg dose of zolmitriptan and a single dose of the other drug except where otherwise noted.

Fluoxetine: The pharmacokinetics of zolmitriptan as well as its effect on blood pressure were unaffected by 4-weeks of pretreatment with oral fluoxetine (20 mg/day).

MAO Inhibitors: Following one week of administration of 150 mg bid moclobemide, a specific MAO-A inhibitor, there was an increase of about 25% in both C_{max} and AUC for zolmitriptan and a 3-fold increase in the C_{max} and AUC of the active N-desmethyl metabolite of zolmitriptan (see CONTRAINDICATIONS and PRECAUTIONS).

Selegiline, a selective MAO-B inhibitor, at a dose of 10 mg/day for 1 week, had no effect on the pharmacokinetics of Zolmitriptan and its metabolite.

Propranolol: C_{max} and AUC of Zolmitriptan increased 1.5-fold after one week of dosing with propranolol (160 mg/day). C_{max} and AUC of the N-desmethyl metabolite were reduced by 30% and 15%, respectively. There were no interactive effects on blood pressure or pulse rate following administration of propranolol with zolmitriptan.

Acetaminophen: A single 1 g dose of acetaminophen does not alter the pharmacokinetics of zolmitriptan and its N-desmethyl metabolite. However, zolmitriptan delayed the T_{max} of acetaminophen by one hour.

Metoclopramide: A single 10 mg dose of metoclopramide had no effect on the pharmacokinetics of zolmitriptan or its metabolites.

Oral Contraceptives: Retrospective analysis of pharmacokinetic data across studies indicated that mean plasma concentrations of zolmitriptan were generally higher in females taking oral contraceptives compared to those not taking oral contraceptives. Mean C_{max} and AUC of zolmitriptan were found to be higher by 30% and 50%, respectively, and T_{max} was delayed by one-half hour in females taking oral contraceptives. The effect of zolmitriptan on the pharmacokinetics of oral contraceptives has not been studied.

Cimetidine: Following the administration of cimetidine, the half life and AUC of a 5 mg dose of zolmitriptan and its active metabolite were approximately doubled (see PRECAUTIONS).

Clinical Studies: The efficacy of ZOMIG Tablets in the acute treatment of migraine headaches was demonstrated in five randomized, double blind, placebo controlled studies, of which 2 utilized the 1 mg dose, 2 utilized the 2.5 mg dose and 4 utilized the 5 mg dose; all studies used the marketed formulation. In study 1, patients treated their headaches in a clinic setting. In the other studies, patients treated their headaches as outpatients. In study 4, patients who had previously used sumatriptan were excluded, whereas in the other studies no such exclusion was applied. Patients enrolled in these 5 studies were predominantly female (82%) and Caucasian (97%) with a mean age of 40 years (range 12–65). Patients were instructed to treat a moderate to severe headache. Headache response, defined as a reduction in headache severity from moderate or severe pain to mild or no pain, was assessed at 1, 2, and, in most studies, 4 hours after dosing. Associated symptoms such as nausea, photophobia and phonophobia were also assessed. Maintenance of response was assessed for up to 24 hours post dose. A second dose of ZOMIG Tablets or other medication was allowed 2 to 24 hours after the initial treatment for persistent and recurrent headaches. The frequency and time to use of these additional treatments were also recorded. In all studies, the effect of zolmitriptan was compared to placebo in the treatment of a single migraine attack.

In all five studies, the percentage of patients achieving headache response 2 hours after treatment was significantly greater among patients receiving ZOMIG Tablets at all doses (except for the 1 mg dose in the smallest study) compared to those who received placebo. In the two studies that evaluated the 1 mg dose, there was a statistically significant greater percentage of patients with headache response at 2 hours in the higher dose groups (2.5 and/or 5 mg) compared to the 1 mg dose group. There were no statistically significant differences between the 2.5 and 5 mg dose groups (or of doses up to 20 mg) for the primary endpoint of headache response at 2 hours in any study. The results of these controlled clinical studies are summarized in Table 1.

Comparisons of drug performance based upon results obtained in different clinical trials are never reliable. Because studies are conducted at different times, with different samples of patients, by different investigators, employing different criteria and/or different interpretations of the same criteria, under different conditions (dose, dosing regimen, etc.), quantitative estimates of treatment response and the timing of response may be expected to vary considerably from study to study.

Table 1: Percentage of Patients with Headache Response (Mild or no Headache) 2 Hours Following Treatment (n=number of patients randomized).

	Placebo	ZOMIG 1.0 mg	ZOMIG 2.5 mg	ZOMIG 5 mg
Study 1[a]	16% (n=19)	27% (n=22)	NA	60%*# (n=20)
Study 2	19% (n=88)	NA	NA	66%* (n=179)
Study 3	34% (n=121)	50%* (n=140)	65%*# (n=260)	67%*# (n=245)
Study 4[b]	44% (n=55)	NA	NA	59%* (n=491)
Study 5	36% (n=92)	NA	62%* (n=178)	NA

* $p<0.05$ in comparison with placebo.
\# $p<0.05$ in comparison with 1 mg
a This was the only study in which patients treated the headache in a clinic setting.
b This was the only study where patients were excluded who had previously used sumatriptan
NA - not applicable

The estimated probability of achieving an initial headache response by 4 hours following treatment is depicted in Figure 1.

[See table 1 at top of next column]

For patients with migraine associated photophobia, phonophobia, and nausea at baseline, there was a decreased incidence of these symptoms following administration of ZOMIG as compared to placebo.

Two to 24 hours following the initial dose of study treatment, patients were allowed to use additional treatment for pain relief in the form of a second dose of study treatment or other medication. The estimated probability of patients taking a second dose or other medication for migraine over the 24 hours following the initial dose of study treatment is summarized in Figure 2.

[See figure 2 in next column]

The efficacy of ZOMIG was unaffected by presence of aura; duration of headache prior to treatment; relationship to menses; gender, age or weight of the patient, pretreatment nausea or concomitant use of common migraine prophylactic drugs.

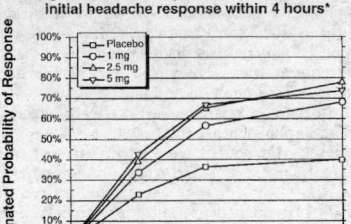

Figure 1: Estimated probability of Achieving Initial headache response within 4 hours*

*Figure 1 shows the Kaplan Meier plot of the probability over time of obtaining headache response (no or mild pain) following treatment with zolmitriptan. The averages displayed are based on pooled data from 3 placebo controlled, outpatient, trials providing evidence of efficacy (Trials 2, 3 and 5). Patients not achieving headache response or taking additional treatment prior to 4 hours were censored at 4 hours.

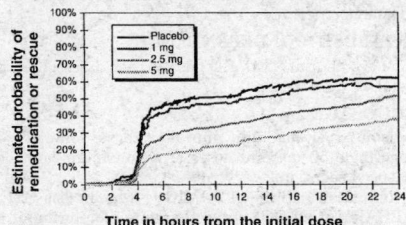

Figure 2: The Estimated Probability Of Patients Taking A Second Dose Or Other Medication For Migraines Over The 24 Hours Following The Initial Dose Of Study Treatment*

*This Kaplan-Meier plot is based on data obtained in 3 placebo controlled clinical trials (Study 2, 3 and 5). Patients not using additional treatments were censored at 24 hours. The plot includes both patients who had headache response at 2 hours and those who had no response to the initial dose. It should be noted that the protocols did not allow remedication within 2 hours post dose.

INDICATIONS AND USAGE

ZOMIG is indicated for the acute treatment of migraine with or without aura in adults.

ZOMIG is not intended for the prophylactic therapy of migraine or for use in the management of hemiplegic or basilar migraine (see CONTRAINDICATIONS). Safety and effectiveness of ZOMIG have not been established for cluster headache, which is present in an older, predominantly male population.

CONTRAINDICATIONS

ZOMIG should not be given to patients with ischemic heart disease (angina pectoris, history of myocardial infarction, or documented silent ischemia) or to patients who have symptoms or findings consistent with ischemic heart disease, coronary artery vasospasm, including Prinzmetal's variant angina, or other significant underlying cardiovascular disease (see WARNINGS).

Because ZOMIG may increase blood pressure, it should not be given to patients with uncontrolled hypertension (see WARNINGS).

ZOMIG should not be used within 24 hours of treatment with another 5HT$_1$ agonist, or an ergotamine-containing or ergot-type medication like dihydroergotamine or methysergide.

ZOMIG should not be administered to patients with hemiplegic or basilar migraine.

Concurrent administration of MAO A inhibitors or use of zolmitriptan within 2 weeks of discontinuation of MAO A inhibitor therapy is contraindicated (see CLINICAL PHARMACOLOGY: Drug Interactions and PRECAUTIONS: Drug Interactions).

ZOMIG is contraindicated in patients who are hypersensitive to zolmitriptan or any of its inactive ingredients.

WARNINGS

ZOMIG should only be used where a clear diagnosis of migraine has been established.

Risk of Myocardial Ischemia and/or Infarction and Other Adverse Cardiac Events: Because of the potential of this class of compounds (5-HT$_{1B/1D}$ agonists) to cause coronary vasospasm, ZOMIG should not be given to patients with documented ischemic or vasospastic coronary artery disease (see CONTRAINDICATIONS). It is strongly recommended that zolmitriptan not be given to patients in whom unrecognized coronary artery disease (CAD) is predicted by the presence of risk factors (e.g., hypertension, hypercholesterolemia, smoker, obesity, diabetes, strong family history of CAD, female with surgical or physiological menopause, or male over 40 years of age) unless a cardiovascular evaluation provides satisfactory clinical evidence that the patient is reasonably free of coronary artery and ischemic myocardial disease or other significant underlying cardiovascular disease. **The sensitivity of cardiac diagnostic procedures to detect cardiovascular disease or predisposition to coronary artery vasospasm is modest, at best.** If, during the cardiovascular evaluation, the patient's medical history, electrocardiographic or other investigations reveal findings indicative of, or consistent with, coronary artery vasospasm or myocardial ischemia, zolmitriptan should not be administered (see CONTRAINDICATIONS). Among the more than 2,500 patients with migraine who participated in premarketing controlled clinical trials of ZOMIG Tablets, no documented episodes of myocardial ischemia or infarction were reported. For patients with risk factors predictive of CAD, who are determined to have a satisfactory cardiovascular evaluation, it is strongly recommended that administration of the first dose of zolmitriptan take place in the setting of a physician's office or similar medically staffed and equipped facility unless the patient has previously received zolmitriptan. Because cardiac ischemia can occur in the absence of clinical symptoms, consideration should be given to obtaining on the first occasion of use an electrocardiogram (ECG) during the interval immediately following ZOMIG, in these patients with risk factors.

It is recommended that patients who are intermittent long-term users of ZOMIG and who have or acquire risk factors predictive of CAD, as described above, undergo periodic interval cardiovascular evaluation as they continue to use ZOMIG.

The systematic approach described above is intended to reduce the likelihood that patients with unrecognized cardiovascular disease will be inadvertently exposed to zolmitriptan.

Cardiac Events and Fatalities associated with 5HT$_1$ agonists: Among the more than 2,500 patients with migraine who participated in premarketing controlled clinical trials of ZOMIG Tablets, no deaths or serious cardiac events were reported. However, the potential for adverse cardiac events exists. Serious adverse cardiac events, including acute myocardial infarction, life-threatening disturbances of cardiac rhythm, and death have been reported within a few hours following the administration of 5HT$_1$ agonists. Considering the extent of use of 5HT$_1$ agonists in patients with migraine, the incidence of these events is extremely low.

Patients with symptomatic Wolff-Parkinson-White syndrome or arrhythmias associated with other cardiac accessory conduction pathway disorders should not receive ZOMIG.

Cerebrovascular Events and Fatalities with 5HT$_1$ agonists: Cerebral hemorrhage, subarachnoid hemorrhage, stroke, and other cerebrovascular events have been reported in patients treated with 5-HT$_1$ agonists; and some have resulted in fatalities. In a number of cases, it appears possible that the cerebrovascular events were primary, the agonist having been administered in the incorrect belief that the symptoms experienced were a consequence of migraine, when they were not. It should be noted that patients with migraine may be at increased risk of certain cerebrovascular events (e.g. Stroke, hemorrhage, transient ischemic attack).

Other Vasospasm-Related Events: 5HT$_1$ agonists may cause vasospastic reactions other than coronary artery vasospasm. Both peripheral vascular ischemia and colonic ischemia with abdominal pain and bloody diarrhea have been reported with 5HT$_1$ agonists.

Increase in Blood Pressure: Significant elevations in systemic blood pressure have been reported on rare occasions in patients with and without a history of hypertension treated with 5-HT$_1$ agonists. Zolmitriptan is contraindicated in patients with uncontrolled hypertension. In volunteers, an increase of 1 and 5 mmHg in the systolic and diastolic blood pressure, respectively, was seen at 5 mg. In the headache trials, vital signs were measured only in the small inpatient study and no effect on blood pressure was seen. In a study of patients with moderate to severe liver disease, 7 of 27 experienced 20 to 80 mm Hg elevations in systolic and/or diastolic blood pressure after a dose of 10 mg of zolmitriptan. (see CONTRAINDICATIONS).

An 18% increase in mean pulmonary artery pressure was seen following dosing with another 5 HT$_1$ agonist in a study evaluating subjects undergoing cardiac catheterization.

PRECAUTIONS

General: As with other 5-HT$_{1B/1D}$ agonists, sensations of tightness, pain, pressure, and heaviness have been reported after treatment with ZOMIG tablets in the precordium, throat, neck and jaw. These events have not been associated with arrhythmias or ischemic ECG changes in clinical trials. Because drugs in this class may cause coronary artery vasospasm, patients who experience signs or symptoms suggestive of angina following dosing should be evaluated for the presence of CAD or a predisposition to Prinzmetal's variant angina before receiving additional doses of medication, and should be monitored electrocardiographically if dosing is resumed and similar symptoms recur. Similarly, patients who experience other symptoms or signs suggestive of decreased arterial flow, such as ischemic bowel syndrome or Raynaud's syndrome following the use of any 5-HT agonist are candidates for further evaluation. (see WARNINGS).

Zolmitriptan should also be administered with caution to patients with diseases that may alter the absorption, metabolism, or excretion of drugs, such as impaired hepatic function (see CLINICAL PHARMACOLOGY).

For a given attack, if a patient does not respond to the first dose of zolmitriptan, the diagnosis of migraine headache should be reconsidered before administration of a second dose.

Binding to Melanin-Containing Tissues: When pigmented rats were given a single oral dose of 10 mg/kg of radiolabeled zolmitriptan the radioactivity in the eye after 7 days, the latest time point examined, was still 75% of the value measured after 4 hours. This suggests that zolmitriptan and/or its metabolites may bind to the melanin of the eye. Because there could be accumulation in melanin rich tissues over time, this raises the possibility that zolmitriptan could cause toxicity in these tissues after extended use. However, no effects on the retina related to treatment with zolmitriptan were noted in any of the toxicity studies. Although no systematic monitoring of ophthalmologic function was undertaken in clinical trials, and no specific recommendations for ophthalmologic monitoring are offered, prescribers should be aware of the possibility of long-term ophthalmologic effects.

Information for Patients: See PATIENT INFORMATION at the end of this labeling for the text of the separate leaflet provided for patients.

Laboratory Tests: No monitoring of specific laboratory tests is recommended.

Drug Interactions: Ergot-containing drugs have been reported to cause prolonged vasospastic reactions. Because there is a theoretical basis that these effects may be additive, use of ergotamine-containing or ergot-type medications (like dihydroergotamine or methysergide) and zolmitriptan within 24 hours of each other should be avoided (see CONTRAINDICATIONS).

MAO-A inhibitors increase the systemic exposure of zolmitriptan. Therefore, the use of zolmitriptan in patients receiving MAO-A inhibitors is contraindicated (see CLINICAL PHARMACOLOGY and CONTRAINDICATIONS).

Concomitant use of other 5-HT$_{1B/1D}$ agonists within 24 hours of ZOMIG treatment is not recommended. (see CONTRAINDICATIONS).

Following administration of cimetidine, the half life and AUC of zolmitriptan and its active metabolites were approximately doubled (see CLINICAL PHARMACOLOGY).

Selective serotonin reuptake inhibitors (SSRIs) (e.g., fluoxetine, fluvoxamine, paroxetine, sertraline) have been reported, rarely, to cause weakness, hyperreflexia, and incoordination when coadministered with 5HT$_1$ agonists. If concomitant treatment with zolmitriptan and an SSRI is clinically warranted, appropriate observation of the patient is advised.

Drug/Laboratory Test Interactions: Zolmitriptan is not known to interfere with commonly employed clinical laboratory tests.

Carcinogenesis, Mutagenesis, Impairment of Fertility:

Carcinogenesis: Carcinogenicity studies by oral gavage were carried out in mice and rats at doses up to 400 mg/kg/day. Mice were dosed for 85 weeks (males) and 92 weeks (females). The exposure (plasma AUC of parent drug) at the highest dose level was approximately 800 times that seen in humans after a single 10 mg dose (the maximum recommended total daily dose). There was no effect of zolmitriptan on tumor incidence. Control, low dose and middle dose rats were dosed for 104–105 weeks; the high dose group was sacrificed after 101 weeks (males) and 86 weeks (females) due to excess mortality. Aside from an increase in the incidence of thyroid follicular cell hyperplasia and thyroid follicular cell adenomas seen in male rats receiving 400 mg/kg/day, an exposure approximately 3000 times that seen in humans after dosing with 10 mg, no tumors were noted.

Mutagenesis: Zolmitriptan was mutagenic in an Ames test, in 2 of 5 strains of S. typhimurium tested, in the presence of, but not in the absence of, metabolic activation. It was not mutagenic in an *in vitro* mammalian gene cell mutation (CHO/HGPRT) assay. Zolmitriptan was clastogenic in an *in vitro* human lymphocyte assay both in the absence of and the presence of metabolic activation; it was not clastogenic in an *in vivo* mouse micronucleus assay. It was also not genotoxic in an unscheduled DNA synthesis study.

Impairment of Fertility: Studies of male and female rats administered zolmitriptan prior to and during mating and up to implantation have shown no impairment of fertility at doses up to 400 mg/kg/day. Exposure at this dose was approximately 3000 times exposure at the maximum recommended human dose of 10 mg/day.

Pregnancy: Pregnancy Category C: There are no adequate and well controlled studies in pregnant women; therefore, zolmitriptan should be used during pregnancy only if the potential benefit justifies the potential risk to the fetus.

Continued on next page

Zomig—Cont.

In reproductive toxicity studies in rats and rabbits, oral administration of zolmitriptan to pregnant animals was associated with embryolethality and fetal abnormalities. When pregnant rats were administered oral zolmitriptan during the period of organogenesis at doses of 100, 400 and 1200 mg/kg/day, there was a dose related increase in embryolethality which became statistically significant at the high dose. The maternal plasma exposures at these doses were approximately 280, 1100 and 5000 times the exposure in humans receiving the maximum recommended total daily dose of 10 mg. The high dose was maternally toxic, as evidenced by a decreased maternal body weight gain during gestation. In a similar study in rabbits, embryolethality was increased at the maternally toxic doses of 10 and 30 mg/kg/day (maternal plasma exposures equivalent to 11 and 42 times exposure in humans receiving the maximum recommended total daily dose of 10 mg), and increased incidences of fetal malformations (fused sternebrae, rib anomalies) and variations (major blood vessel variations, irregular ossification pattern of ribs) were observed at 30 mg/kg/day. Three mg/kg/day was a no effect dose (equivalent to human exposure at a dose of 10 mg). When female rats were given zolmitriptan during gestation, parturition, and lactation, an increased incidence of hydronephrosis was found in the offspring at the maternally toxic dose of 400 mg/kg/day (1100 times human exposure)

Nursing Mothers: It is not known whether zolmitriptan is excreted in human milk. Because many drugs are excreted in human milk, caution should be exercised when zolmitriptan is administered to a nursing woman. Lactating rats dosed with zolmitriptan had milk levels equivalent to maternal plasma levels at 1 hour and 4 times higher than plasma levels at 4 hours.

Pediatric Use: Safety and effectiveness of ZOMIG in pediatric patients have not been established.

Use in the Elderly: Although the pharmacokinetic disposition of the drug in the elderly is similar to that seen in younger adults, there is no information about the safety and effectiveness of zolmitriptan in this population because patients over age 65 were excluded from the controlled clinical trials. (see CLINICAL PHARMACOLOGY: Special Populations)

ADVERSE REACTIONS

Although not reported with zolmitriptan in clinical trials, serious cardiac events, including some that have been fatal, have rarely occurred following use of 5-HT$_1$ agonists. Events reported have included coronary artery vasospasm, transient myocardial ischemia, myocardial infarction, ventricular tachycardia, and ventricular fibrillation (see CONTRAINDICATIONS, WARNINGS, and PRECAUTIONS).

Incidence in Controlled Clinical Trials: Among 2,633 patients treated with ZOMIG in the active and placebo controlled trials, no patients withdrew for reasons related to adverse events, but as patients treated a single headache in these trials, the opportunity for discontinuation was limited. In a long-term, open label study where patients were allowed to treat multiple migraine attacks for up to 1 year, 8% (167 out of 2,058) withdrew from the trial because of adverse experience. The most common events were paresthesia, asthenia, nausea, dizziness, pain, chest or neck tightness or heaviness, somnolence and warm sensation.

Table 2 lists the adverse events that occurred in ≥ 2% of the 2,074 patients in any one of the ZOMIG 1 mg, ZOMIG 2.5 mg or ZOMIG 5 mg dose groups of the controlled clinical trials. Only events that were more frequent in a ZOMIG group compared to the placebo groups are included. The events cited reflect experience gained under closely monitored conditions of clinical trials in a highly selected patient population. In actual clinical practice or in other clinical trials, these frequency estimates may not apply, as the conditions of use, reporting behavior, and the kinds of patients treated may differ.

Several of the adverse events appear dose related, notably paresthesia, sensation of heaviness or tightness in chest, neck, jaw, and throat, dizziness, somnolence, and possibly asthenia and nausea.

[See table 2 below]

ZOMIG is generally well tolerated. Across all doses, most adverse reactions were mild and transient and did not lead to long-lasting effects. The incidence of adverse events in controlled clinical trials was not affected by gender, weight, or age of the patients; use of prophylactic medications; or presence of aura. There were insufficient data to assess the impact of race on the incidence of adverse events.

Other Events: In the paragraphs that follow, the frequencies of less commonly reported adverse clinical events are presented. Because the reports include events observed in the open and uncontrolled studies, the role of ZOMIG in their causation cannot be reliably determined. Furthermore, variability associated with adverse event reporting, the terminology used to describe adverse events, etc., limit the value of the quantitative frequency estimates provided. Event frequencies are calculated as the number of patients who used ZOMIG (n=4,027) and reported an event divided by the total number of patients exposed to ZOMIG. All reported events are included except those already listed in the previous table, those too general to be informative, and those not reasonably associated with the use of the drug. Events are further classified within body system categories and enumerated in order of decreasing frequency using the following definitions: infrequent adverse events are those occurring in 1/100 to 1/1,000 patients and rare adverse events are those occurring in fewer than 1/1,000 patients.

Atypical sensation: Infrequent was hyperesthesia

General: Infrequent were allergy reaction, chills, facial edema, fever, malaise and photosensitivity.

Cardiovascular: Infrequent were arrhythmias, hypertension and syncope. Rare were bradycardia, extrasystoles, postural hypotension, QT prolongation, tachycardia and thrombophlebitis.

Digestive: Infrequent were increased appetite, tongue edema, esophagitis, gastroenteritis, liver function abnormality and thirst. Rare were anorexia, constipation, gastritis, hematemesis, pancreatitis, melena and ulcer.

Hemic: Infrequent was ecchymosis. Rare was cyanosis, thrombocytopenia, eosinophilia and leukopenia.

Metabolic: Infrequent was edema. Rare were hyperglycemia and alkaline phosphatase increased.

Musculoskeletal: Infrequent were back pain, leg cramps and tenosynovitis. Rare were arthritis, tetany and twitching.

Neurological: Infrequent were agitation, anxiety, depression, emotional lability and insomnia; Rare were akathesia, amnesia, apathy, ataxia, dystonia, euphoria, hallucinations, cerebral ischemia, hyperkinesia, hypotonia, hypertonia and irritability.

Respiratory: Infrequent were bronchitis, bronchospasm, epistaxis, hiccup, laryngitis and yawn. Rare were apnea and voice alteration.

Skin: Infrequent were pruritus, rash and urticaria.

Special Senses: Infrequent were dry eye, eye pain, hyperacusis, ear pain, parosmia, and tinnitus. Rare were diplopia and lacrimation.

Urogenital: Infrequent were hematuria, cystitis, polyuria, urinary frequency, urinary urgency. Rare were miscarriage and dysmenorrhea.

DRUG ABUSE AND DEPENDENCE

The abuse potential of ZOMIG has not been assessed in clinical trials.

OVERDOSAGE

There is no experience with clinical overdose. Volunteers receiving single 50 mg oral doses of zolmitriptan commonly experienced sedation.

The elimination half-life of ZOMIG is 3 hours (see CLINICAL PHARMACOLOGY), and therefore monitoring of patients after overdose with ZOMIG should continue for at least 15 hours or while symptoms or signs persist.

There is no specific antidote to zolmitriptan. In cases of severe intoxication, intensive care procedures are recommended, including establishing and maintaining a patent airway, ensuring adequate oxygenation and ventilation, and monitoring and support of the cardiovascular system.

It is unknown what effect hemodialysis or peritoneal dialysis has on the plasma concentrations of zolmitriptan.

DOSAGE AND ADMINISTRATION

In controlled clinical trials, single doses of 1, 2.5 and 5 mg of zolmitriptan were effective for the acute treatment of migraines in adults. A greater proportion of patients had headache response following a 2.5 or 5 mg dose than following a 1 mg dose (see Table 1). In the only direct comparison of 2.5 and 5 mg, there was little added benefit from the larger dose but side effects are generally increased at 5 mg (see Table 2). Patients should, therefore, be started on 2.5 mg or lower. A dose lower than 2.5 mg can be achieved by manually breaking a 2.5 mg tablet in half.

If the headache returns, the dose may be repeated after 2 hours, not to exceed 10 mg within a 24 hour period. Controlled trials have not adequately established the effectiveness of a second dose if the initial dose is ineffective.

The safety of treating an average of more than three headaches in a 30 day period has not been established.

Hepatic Impairment: Patients with moderate to severe hepatic impairment have decreased clearance of zolmitriptan and significant elevation of blood pressure was observed in some patients. Use of a low dose with blood pressure monitoring is recommended (see CLINICAL PHARMACOLOGY AND WARNINGS).

HOW SUPPLIED

2.5 mg Tablets — Yellow, biconvex, film-coated scored tablets containing 2.5 mg of zolmitriptan identified with "ZOMIG" and "2.5" debossed on one side are supplied in cartons containing a blister pack of 6 tablets. (NDC 0310-0210-20).

5 mg Tablets — Pink, biconvex, film-coated tablets containing 5 mg of zolmitriptan identified with "ZOMIG" and "5" debossed on one side are supplied in cartons containing a blister pack of 3 tablets. (NDC 0310-0211-25).

Store at controlled room temperature, 20–25°C (68–77°F) [see USP]. Protect from light and moisture.

PATIENT INFORMATION

The following wording is contained in a separate leaflet provided for patients.

ZOMIG™ (zolmitriptan) Tablets

Patient Information about ZOMIG (Zo-mig) for Migraines

Generic Name: zolmitriptan (zol-mi-trip-tan)

Information for the Consumer on ZOMIG (zolmitriptan) Tablets: Please read this leaflet carefully before you administer ZOMIG Tablets. This provides a summary of the information available on your medicine. Please do not throw away this leaflet until you have finished your medicine. You may need to read this leaflet again. This leaflet does not contain all the information on ZOMIG Tablets. For further information or advice, ask your doctor or pharmacist.

Table 2: Adverse Experience Incidence in Five Placebo-Controlled Migraine Clinical Trials: Events Reported By ≥2% Patients Treated With ZOMIG

Adverse Event Type	Placebo (n=401)	ZOMIG 1 mg (n=163)	ZOMIG 2.5 mg (n=498)	ZOMIG 5 mg (n=1012)
ATYPICAL SENSATIONS	**6%**	**12%**	**12%**	**18%**
Hypesthesia	1%	1%	1%	2%
Paresthesia (all types)	2%	5%	7%	9%
Sensation warm/cold	4%	6%	5%	7%
PAIN AND PRESSURE SENSATIONS	**7%**	**13%**	**14%**	**22%**
Chest-pain/tightness/pressure and/or heaviness	1%	2%	3%	4%
Neck/throat/jaw-pain/tightness/ pressure	3%	4%	7%	10%
Heaviness other than chest or neck	1%	1%	2%	5%
Pain-location specified	1%	2%	2%	3%
Other-Pressure/tightness/ heaviness	0%	2%	2%	2%
DIGESTIVE	**8%**	**11%**	**16%**	**14%**
Dry Mouth	2%	5%	3%	3%
Dyspepsia	1%	3%	2%	1%
Dysphagia	0%	0%	0%	2%
Nausea	4%	4%	9%	6%
NEUROLOGICAL	**10%**	**11%**	**17%**	**21%**
Dizziness	4%	6%	8%	10%
Somnolence	3%	5%	6%	8%
Vertigo	0%	0%	0%	2%
OTHER				
Asthenia	3%	5%	3%	9%
Palpitations	1%	0%	<1%	2%
Myalgia	<1%	1%	1%	2%
Myasthenia	<1%	0%	1%	2%
Sweating	1%	0%	2%	3%

Information About Your Medicine: The name of your medicine is ZOMIG Tablets. It can be obtained only by prescription from your doctor. The decision to use ZOMIG Tablets is one that you and your doctor should make jointly, taking into account your individual preferences and medical circumstances. If you have risk factors for heart disease (such as high blood pressure, high cholesterol, obesity, diabetes, smoking, strong family history of heart disease, or you are postmenopausal or a male over the age of 40), you should tell your doctor, who should evaluate you for heart disease in order to determine if ZOMIG Tablets are appropriate for you.

1. **The Purpose of Your Medicine**: ZOMIG Tablets are intended to relieve your migraine, but not to prevent or reduce the number of attacks you experience. Use ZOMIG Tablets only to treat an actual migraine attack.
2. **Important Questions to Consider Before Using ZOMIG Tablets**: If the answer to any of the following questions is **YES** or if you do not know the answer, then you must discuss it with your doctor before you use ZOMIG Tablets.
   - Do you have any chest pain, heart disease, shortness of breath, or irregular heartbeats? Have you had a heart attack?
   - Do you have risk factors for heart disease (such as high blood pressure, high cholesterol, obesity, diabetes, smoking, strong family history of heart disease, or you are postmenopausal or a male over the age of 40)?
   - Do you have high blood pressure?
   - Are you pregnant? Do you think you might be pregnant? Are you trying to become pregnant? Are you not using adequate contraception? Are you breast feeding an infant?
   - Have you ever had to stop taking this or any other medication because of an allergy or other problems?
   - Are you taking any other migraine medications, including $5HT_1$ agonist or migraine medications containing ergotamine, dihydroergotamine, or methysergide?
   - Are you taking any medication for depression (monoamine oxidase inhibitors or selective serotonin reuptake inhibitors [SSRIs])?
   - Have you had, or do you have, any disease of the liver or kidney?
   - Have you had, or do you have, epilepsy or seizures?
   - Is this headache different from your usual migraine attacks?

   Remember, if you answered **YES** to any of the above questions, then you must discuss it with your doctor.
3. **The Use of ZOMIG Tablets During Pregnancy**: Do not use ZOMIG Tablets if you are pregnant, think you might be pregnant, are trying to become pregnant, or are not using adequate contraception, unless you have discussed this with your doctor.
4. **How to Use ZOMIG Tablets**: Adults should be started on a 2.5 mg dose or lower administered by mouth. A dose lower than 2.5 mg can be achieved by manually breaking a 2.5 mg tablet in half. If your headache comes back after your initial dose, a second dose may be administered anytime after 2 hours of administering the dose. For any attack where you have no response to the first dose, do not take a second dose without first consulting with your doctor. Do not administer more than a total of 10 mg of ZOMIG Tablets in any 24-hour period. Discard any unused tablets or its portion that have been removed from the blister packaging.
5. **Side Effects to Watch For**:
   - Some patients experience pain or tightness in the chest or throat when using ZOMIG Tablets. If this happens to you, then discuss it with your doctor before using any more ZOMIG Tablets. If the chest pain is severe or does not go away, call your doctor immediately.
   - Shortness of breath; wheeziness; heart throbbing; swelling of eyelids, face, or lips; or a skin rash, skin lumps, or hives happens rarely. If it happens to you, then tell your doctor immediately. Do not take any more ZOMIG Tablets unless your doctor tells you to do so.
   - Some people may have feelings of tingling, heat, heaviness or pressure after treatment with ZOMIG Tablets. A few people may feel drowsy, dizzy, tired, or sick. Tell your doctor immediately if you have symptoms that you do not understand.
6. **What To Do If An Overdose is Taken**: If you have taken more medication than you have been told, contact either your doctor, hospital emergency department, or nearest poison control center immediately. This medicine was prescribed for your particular condition and should not be used by others or for any other condition.
7. **Storing Your Medicine**: Keep your medicine in a safe place where children cannot reach it. It may be harmful to children. Store your medication away from heat, light, moisture and at a controlled room temperature. If your medication has expired (the expiration date is printed on the treatment pack), throw it away as instructed. If your doctor decides to stop your treatment, do not keep any leftover medicine unless your doctor tells you to. Throw away your medicine as instructed. Be sure that discarded tablets are out of the reach of children.

Manufactured For:
ZENECA Pharmaceuticals
A Business Unit of ZENECA Inc.
Wilmington, Delaware 19850-5437
By: IPR Pharmaceuticals Inc.
Rev F 03/98 SIC 680001

Shown in Product Identification Guide, page 346

Celgene Corporation

7 POWDER HORN DRIVE
WARREN, NJ 07059

Direct Inquiries to:
Ph: 1-888-423-5436

THALOMID™ ℞

[*thălō-mĭd*]
(thalidomide)
Capsules

WARNING: SEVERE, LIFE-THREATENING HUMAN BIRTH DEFECTS
IF THALIDOMIDE IS TAKEN DURING PREGNANCY, IT CAN CAUSE SEVERE BIRTH DEFECTS OR DEATH TO AN UNBORN BABY. THALIDOMIDE SHOULD NEVER BE USED BY WOMEN WHO ARE PREGNANT OR WHO COULD BECOME PREGNANT WHILE TAKING THE DRUG. EVEN A SINGLE DOSE [1 CAPSULE (50 mg)] TAKEN BY A PREGNANT WOMEN DURING HER PREGNANCY CAN CAUSE SEVERE BIRTH DEFECTS.
BECAUSE OF THIS TOXICITY AND IN AN EFFORT TO MAKE THE CHANCE OF FETAL EXPOSURE TO THALOMID™ (thalidomide) AS NEGLIGIBLE AS POSSIBLE, THALOMID™ (thalidomide) IS APPROVED FOR MARKETING ONLY UNDER A SPECIAL RESTRICTED DISTRIBUTION PROGRAM APPROVED BY THE FOOD AND DRUG ADMINISTRATION. THIS PROGRAM IS CALLED THE "SYSTEM FOR THALIDOMIDE EDUCATION AND PRESCRIBING SAFETY (*S.T.E.P.S.*)".
UNDER THIS RESTRICTED DISTRIBUTION PROGRAM, ONLY PRESCRIBERS AND PHARMACISTS REGISTERED WITH THE PROGRAM ARE ALLOWED TO PRESCRIBE AND DISPENSE THE PRODUCT. IN ADDITION, PATIENTS MUST BE ADVISED OF, AGREE TO, AND COMPLY WITH THE REQUIREMENTS OF THE (*S.T.E.P.S.*) PROGRAM IN ORDER TO RECEIVE PRODUCT.
PLEASE SEE THE FOLLOWING BOXED WARNINGS CONTAINING SPECIAL INFORMATION FOR PRESCRIBERS, FEMALE PATIENTS, AND MALE PATIENTS ABOUT THIS RESTRICTED DISTRIBUTION PROGRAM.

PRESCRIBERS

THALOMID™ (thalidomide) may be prescribed only by licensed prescribers who are registered in the *S.T.E.P.S.* program and understand the risk of teratogenicity if thalidomide is used during pregnancy.
Major human fetal abnormalities related to thalidomide administration during pregnancy have been documented: amelia (absence of limbs), phocomelia (short limbs), hypoplasticity of the bones, absence of bones, external ear abnormalities (including anotia, micro pinna, small or absent external auditory canals), facial palsy, eye abnormalities (anophthalmos, microphthalmos), and congenital heart defects. Alimentary tract, urinary tract, and genital malformations have also been documented.[1] Mortality at or shortly after birth has been reported at about 40%.[2]
Effective contraception (see **CONTRAINDICATIONS**) must be used for at least 1 month before beginning thalidomide therapy, during thalidomide therapy, and for 1 month following discontinuation of thalidomide therapy. Reliable contraception is indicated even where there has been a history of infertility, unless due to hysterectomy or because the patient has been post-menopausal for at least 24 months. Two reliable forms of contraception must be used simultaneously unless continuous abstinence from reproductive heterosexual sexual intercourse is the chosen method. Women of childbearing potential should be referred to a qualified provider of contraceptive methods, if needed. Sexually mature women who have not undergone a hysterectomy or who have not been post-menopausal for at least 24 consecutive months (i.e., who have had menses at some time in the preceding 24 consecutive months) are considered to be women of child-bearing potential.
Before starting treatment, women of childbearing potential should have a pregnancy test (sensitivity of at least 50 mIU/mL). The test should be performed within the 24 hours prior to beginning therapy. A prescription for thalidomide for a woman of childbearing potential must not be issued by the prescriber until a written report of a negative pregnancy test has been obtained by the prescriber.
Once treatment has started, pregnancy testing should occur weekly during the first month of use, then monthly thereafter in women with regular menstrual cycles. If menstrual cycles are irregular, the pregnancy testing should occur every 2 weeks. Pregnancy testing and counseling should be performed if a patient misses her period or if there is any abnormality in menstrual bleeding.
If pregnancy does occur during thalidomide treatment, thalidomide must be discontinued immediately.
Any suspected fetal exposure to THALOMID™ (thalidomide) must be reported immediately to the FDA *via* the MedWATCH number at 1-800-FDA-1088 and also to Celgene Corporation. The patient should be referred to an obstetrician/gynecologist experienced in reproductive toxicity for further evaluation and counseling.

FEMALE PATIENTS

Thalidomide is contraindicated in WOMEN of childbearing potential unless alternative therapies are considered inappropriate AND the patient MEETS ALL OF THE FOLLOWING CONDITIONS (i.e., she is essentially unable to become pregnant while on thalidomide therapy):
- she understands and can reliably carry out instructions.
- she is capable of complying with the mandatory contraceptive measures, pregnancy testing, patient registration, and patient survey as described in the System for Thalidomide Education and Prescribing Safety (*S.T.E.P.S.*) program.
- she has received both oral and written warnings of the hazards of taking thalidomide during pregnancy and of exposing a fetus to the drug.
- she has received both oral and written warnings of the risk of possible contraception failure and of the need to use two reliable forms of contraception simultaneously (see **CONTRAINDICATIONS**), unless continuous abstinence from reproductive heterosexual intercourse is the chosen method. (Sexually mature women who have not undergone a hysterectomy or who have not been post-menopausal for at least 24 consecutive months (i.e., who have had menses at some time in the preceding 24 consecutive months) are considered to be women of childbearing potential.).
- she acknowledges, in writing, her understanding of these warnings and of the need for using two reliable methods of contraception for one month prior to starting thalidomide therapy, during thalidomide therapy, and for one month after stopping thalidomide therapy.
- she has had a negative pregnancy test with a sensitivity of at least 50 mIU/mL, within the 24 hours prior to beginning therapy. (See **PRECAUTIONS, CONTRAINDICATIONS**.)
- if the patient is between 12 and 18 years of age, her parent or legal guardian must have read this material and agreed to ensure compliance with the above.

MALE PATIENTS

Thalidomide is contraindicated in sexually mature MALES unless the PATIENT MEETS ALL OF THE FOLLOWING CONDITIONS:
- he understands and can reliably carry out instructions.
- he is capable of complying with the mandatory contraceptive measures that are appropriate for men, patient registration, and patient survey as described in the *S.T.E.P.S.* program.
- he has received both oral and written warnings of the hazards of taking thalidomide and exposing a fetus to the drug.
- he has received both oral and written warnings of the risk of possible contraception failure and of the need to use barrier contraception when having sexual intercourse with women of childbearing potential, even if he has undergone successful vasectomy.
- he acknowledges, in writing, his understanding of these warnings and of the need for using barrier contraception (latex condom), even if he has undergone successful vasectomy, when having sexual intercourse

Continued on next page

Thalomid—Cont.

with women of childbearing potential. Sexually mature women who have not undergone a hysterectomy or who have not been post-menopausal for at least 24 consecutive months (i.e., who have had menses at some time in the preceding 24 consecutive months) are considered to be women of childbearing potential.

• if the patient is between 12 and 18 years of age, his parent or legal guardian must have read this material and agreed to ensure compliance with the above.

DESCRIPTION

THALOMID™ (thalidomide), α-(N-phthalimido)glutarimide, is an immunomodulatory agent. The empirical formula for thalidomide is $C_{13}H_{10}N_2O_4$ and the gram molecular weight is 258.2. The CAS number of thalidomide is 50-35-1.

Note: • = asymmetric carbon

Thalidomide is an off-white to white, nearly odorless, crystalline powder that is soluble at 25°C in dimethyl sulfoxide and sparingly soluble in water and ethanol. The glutarimide moiety contains a single asymmetric center and, therefore, may exist in either of two optically active forms designated S-(-) or R-(+). THALOMID™ (thalidomide) is an equal mixture of the S-(-) and R-(+) forms, therefore, and has a net optical rotation of zero.

THALOMID™ (thalidomide) is available in 50 mg capsules for oral administration. Active ingredient: thalidomide. Inactive ingredients: anhydrous lactose, microcrystalline cellulose, polyvinylpyrrolidone, stearic acid, colloidal anhydrous silica, and gelatin.

CLINICAL PHARMACOLOGY

Mechanism of Action

Thalidomide is an immunomodulatory agent with a spectrum of activity that is not fully characterized. In patients with erythema nodosum leprosum (ENL) the mechanism of action is not fully understood.

Available data from in vitro studies and preliminary clinical trials suggest that the immunologic effects of this compound can vary substantially under different conditions, but, may be related to suppression of excessive tumor necrosis factor-alpha (TNF-α) production and down-modulation of selected cell surface adhesion molecules involved in leukocyte migration[3,4,5,6]. For example, administration of thalidomide has been reported to decrease circulating levels of TNF-α in patients with ENL[3], however, it has also been shown to increase plasma TNF-α levels in HIV-seropositive patients[7].

Pharmacokinetics and Drug Metabolism

Absorption

The absolute bioavailability of thalidomide from THALOMID™ (thalidomide) capsules has not yet been characterized in human subjects due to its poor aqueous solubility. In studies of both healthy volunteers and subjects with Hansen's disease, the mean time to peak plasma concentrations (T_{max}) of THALOMID™ (thalidomide) ranged from 2.9 to 5.7 hours indicating that THALOMID™ (thalidomide) is slowly absorbed from the gastrointestinal tract. While the extent of absorption (as measured by area under the curve [AUC]) is proportional to dose in healthy subjects, the observed peak concentration (C_{max}) increased in a less than proportional manner (see Table 1 below). This lack of C_{max} dose proportionality, coupled with the observed increase in T_{max} values, suggests that the poor solubility of thalidomide in aqueous media may be hindering the rate of absorption.

Co-administration of THALOMID™ (thalidomide) with a high fat meal causes minor (<10%) changes in the observed AUC and C_{max} values: however, it causes an increase in T_{max} to approximately 6 hours.

[See table 1 above]

Distribution

It is not known whether thalidomide is present in the ejaculate of males. The extent of plasma protein binding of thalidomide is unknown.

Metabolism

At the present time, the exact metabolic route and fate of thalidomide is not known in humans. Thalidomide itself does not appears to be hepatically metabolized to any large extent, but appears to undergo non-enzymatic hydrolysis in plasma to multiple metabolites. In a repeat dose study in which THALOMID™ (thalidomide) 200 mg was administered to 10 healthy females for 18 days, thalidomide displayed similar pharmacokinetic profiles on the first and last day of dosing. This suggests that thalidomide does not induce or inhibit its own metabolism.

Elimination

As indicated in Table 1 (above) the mean half-life of elimination ranges from approximately 5 to 7 hours following a

Table 1
Pharmacokinetic Parameter Values for THALOMID™ (thalidomide) Mean (%CV)

Population/ Single Dose	AUC_{0-4} (μg-hr/mL)	C_{max} (μg/mL)	T_{max} (hrs)	Half-life (hrs)
Healthy Subjects (n=14)				
50 mg	4.9 (16%)	0.62 (52%)	2.9 (66%)	5.52 (37%)
200 mg	18.9 (17%)	1.76 (30%)	3.5 (57%)	5.53 (25%)
400 mg	36.4 (26%)	2.82 (28%)	4.3 (37%)	7.29 (36%)
Patients with Hansen's Disease (n=6)				
400 mg	46.4 (44.1%)	3.44 (52.6%)	5.7 (27%)	6.86 (17%)

Table 2
Double Blind, Controlled Clinical Trials of Thalidomide in Patients with ENL: Cutaneous Response

Reference	No. of Patients	No. Treatment Courses*	Percent Responding**	
Iyer et al.[9] Bull World Health Organization 1971; 45:719	92	204	Thalidomide 75%	Aspirin 25%
Sheskin et al.[10] Int J Lep 1969; 37:135	52	173	Thalidomide 66%	Placebo 10%

*In patients with cutaneous lesions
**Iyer: Complete response or lesions absent
**Sheskin: Complete Improvement + "striking" improvement (i.e., >50% improvement)

Table 3
Double Blind, Controlled Trial of Thalidomide in Patients with ENL: Reduction in Steroid Dosage

Reference	Duration of Treatment	No. of Patients	Number Responding	
			Thalidomide	Placebo
Waters[11] Lep Rev 1971; 42:26	4 weeks	9	4/5	0/4
	6 weeks (crossover)	8	8/8	1/8

single dose and is not altered upon multiple dosing. As noted in the metabolism subsection, the precise metabolic fate and route of elimination of thalidomide in humans is not known at this time. Thalidomide itself has a renal clearance of 1.15 mL/minute with less than 0.7% of the dose excreted in the urine as unchanged drug. Following a single dose, urinary levels of thalidomide were undetectable 48 hrs after dosing. Although thalidomide is thought to be hydrolyzed to a number of metabolites[8], only a very small amount (0.02% of the administered dose) of 4-OH-thalidomide was identified in the urine of subjects 12 to 24 hours after dosing.

Pharmacokinetic Data in Special Populations

HIV-seropositive Subjects: There is no apparent significant difference in measured pharmacokinetic parameter values between healthy human subjects and HIV-seropositive subjects following single dose administration of THALOMID™ (thalidomide) capsules.

Patients with Hansen's Disease: Analysis of data from a small study in Hansen's patients suggests that these patients, relative to healthy subjects, may have an increased bioavailability of THALOMID™ (thalidomide). The increase is reflected both in an increased area under the curve and in increased peak plasma levels. The clinical significance of this increase is unknown.

Patients with Renal Insufficiency: The pharmacokinetics of thalidomide in patients with renal dysfunction have not been determined.

Patients with Hepatic Disease: The pharmacokinetics of thalidomide in patients with hepatic impairment have not been determined.

Age: Analysis of the data from pharmacokinetic studies in healthy volunteers and patients with Hansen's disease ranging in age from 20 to 69 years does not reveal any age-related changes.

Pediatric: No pharmacokinetic data are available in subjects below the age of 18 years.

Gender: While a comparative trial of the effects of gender on thalidomide pharmacokinetics has not been conducted, examination of the data for thalidomide does not reveal any significant gender differences in pharmacokinetic parameter values.

Race: Pharmacokinetic differences due to race have not been studied.

Clinical Studies

The primary data demonstrating the efficacy of thalidomide in the treatment of the cutaneous manifestations of moderate to severe ENL are derived from the published medical literature and from a retrospective study of 102 patients treated by the U.S. Public Health Service.

Two double blind, randomized, controlled trials reported the dermatologic response to a 7 day course of 100 mg thalidomide (four times daily) or control. Dosage was lower for patients under 50 kg in weight.

[See table 2 above]

Waters[11] reported the results of two studies, both double blind, randomized, placebo controlled, crossover trials in a total of 10 hospitalized, steroid-dependent patients with chronic ENL treated with 100 mg thalidomide or placebo (three times daily). All patients also received dapsone. The primary endpoint was reduction in weekly steroid dosage.

[See table 3 above]

Data on the efficacy of thalidomide in prevention of ENL relapse were derived from a retrospective evaluation of 102 patients treated under the auspices of the U.S. Public Health Service. A subset of patients with ENL controlled on thalidomide demonstrated repeated relapse upon drug withdrawal and remission with reinstitution of therapy.

Twenty U.S. patients between the ages of 11 and 17 years were treated with thalidomide, generally at 100 mg daily. Response rates and safety profiles were similar to that observed in the adult population.

Thirty-two other published studies containing over 1600 patients consistently report generally successful treatment of the cutaneous manifestations of moderate to severe ENL with thalidomide.

INDICATIONS AND USAGE

THALOMID™ (thalidomide) is indicated for the acute treatment of the cutaneous manifestations of moderate to severe erythema nodosum leprosum (ENL).

THALOMID™ (thalidomide) is not indicated as monotherapy for such ENL treatment in the presence of moderate to severe neuritis.

THALOMID™ (thalidomide) is also indicated as maintenance therapy for prevention and suppression of the cutaneous manifestations of ENL recurrence.

CONTRAINDICATIONS (See BOXED WARNINGS.)
Pregnancy: Category X

Due to its known human teratogenicity, even following a single dose, thalidomide is contraindicated in pregnant women and women capable of becoming pregnant. (See **BOXED WARNINGS**.) When there is no alternative treatment, women of childbearing potential may be treated with thalidomide provided adequate precautions are taken to avoid pregnancy. Women must commit either to abstain con-

tinuously from heterosexual sexual intercourse or to use two methods of reliable birth control, including at least one highly effective method (*e.g.*, IUD, hormonal contraception, tubal ligation, or partner's vasectomy) and one additional effective method (*e.g.*, latex condom, diaphragm, or cervical cap), beginning 4 weeks prior to initiating treatment with thalidomide, during therapy with thalidomide, and continuing for 4 weeks following discontinuation of thalidomide therapy. If hormonal IUD contraception is medically contraindicated (see also **PRECAUTIONS: DRUG INTERACTIONS**), two other effective or highly effective methods may be used.

Women of childbearing potential being treated with thalidomide should have pregnancy testing (sensitivity of at least 50 mIU/mL). The test should be performed within the 24 hours before beginning thalidomide therapy and then weekly during the first month of thalidomide therapy, then monthly thereafter in women with regular menstrual cycles or every 2 weeks in women with irregular menstrual cycles. Pregnancy testing and counseling should be performed if a patient misses her period or if there is any abnormality in menstrual bleeding. If pregnancy occurs during thalidomide treatment, thalidomide must be immediately discontinued. Under these conditions, the patient should be referred to an obstetrician/gynecologist experienced in reproductive toxicity for further evaluation and counseling.

THALOMID™ (thalidomide) is contraindicated in patients who have demonstrated hypersensitivity to the drug and its components.

WARNINGS (See BOXED WARNINGS.)
Birth defects:
Thalidomide can cause severe birth defects in humans. (See **BOXED WARNINGS** and **CONTRAINDICATIONS**.) Patients should be instructed to take thalidomide only as prescribed and not to share their thalidomide with anyone else. Because it is not known whether or not thalidomide is present in the ejaculate of males receiving the drug, males receiving thalidomide must always use a latex condom when engaging in sexual activity with women of childbearing potential.

Drowsiness and somnolence:
Thalidomide frequently causes drowsiness and somnolence. Patients should be instructed to avoid situations where drowsiness may be a problem and not to take other medications that may cause drowsiness without adequate medical advice. Patients should be advised as to the possible impairment of mental and/or physical abilities required for the performance of hazardous tasks, such as driving a car or operating other complex or dangerous machinery.

Peripheral neuropathy:
Thalidomide is known to cause nerve damage that may be permanent. Peripheral neuropathy is a common, potentially severe, side effect of treatment with thalidomide that may be irreversible. Peripheral neuropathy generally occurs following chronic use over a period of months, however, reports following relatively short term use also exist. The correlation with cumulative dose is unclear. Symptoms may occur some time after thalidomide treatment has been stopped and may resolve slowly or not at all. Few reports of neuropathy have arisen in the treatment of ENL despite long-term thalidomide treatment. However, the inability clinically to differentiate thalidomide neuropathy from the neuropathy often seen in Hansen's disease makes it difficult to determine accurately the incidence of thalidomide-related neuropathy in ENL patients treated with thalidomide.

Patients should be examined at monthly intervals for the first 3 months of thalidomide therapy to enable the clinician to detect early signs of neuropathy, which include numbness, tingling or pain in the hands and feet. Patients should be evaluated periodically thereafter during treatment. Patients should be regularly counseled, questioned, and evaluated for signs or symptoms of peripheral neuropathy. Consideration should be given to electrophysiological testing, consisting of measurement of sensory nerve action potential (SNAP) amplitudes at baseline and thereafter every 6 months in an effort to detect asymptomatic neuropathy. If symptoms of drug-induced neuropathy develop, thalidomide should be discontinued immediately to limit further damage, if clinically appropriate. Usually, treatment with thalidomide should only be reinitiated if the neuropathy returns to baseline status. Medications known to be associated with neuropathy should be used with caution in patients receiving thalidomide.

Dizziness and orthostatic hypotension:
Patients should also be advised that thalidomide may cause dizziness and orthostatic hypotension and that, therefore, they should sit upright for a few minutes prior to standing up from a recumbent position.

Neutropenia:
Decreased white blood cell counts, including neutropenia, have been reported in association with the clinical use of thalidomide. Treatment should not be initiated with an absolute neutrophil count (ANC) of <750/mm³. White blood cell count and differential should be monitored on an ongoing basis, especially in patients who may be more prone to

neutropenia, such as patients who are HIV-seropositive. If ANC decreases to below 750/mm³ while on treatment, the patient's medication regimen should be re-evaluated and, if the neutropenia persists, consideration should be given to withholding thalidomide if clinically appropriate.

Increased HIV-Viral Load:
In a randomized, placebo controlled trial of thalidomide in an HIV-seropositive patient population, plasma HIV RNA levels were found to increase (median change=0.42 $\log_{10}$ copies HIV RNA/mL, p = 0.04 compared to placebo).[7] A similar trend was observed in a second, unpublished study conducted in patients who were HIV-seropositive[12]. The clinical significance of this increase is unknown. Both studies were conducted prior to availability of highly active antiretroviral therapy. Until the clinical significance of this finding is further understood, in HIV-seropositive patients, viral load should be measured after the first and third months of treatment and every 3 months thereafter.

PRECAUTIONS
Hypersensitivity:
Hypersensitivity to THALOMID™ (thalidomide) has been reported. Signs and symptoms have included the occurrence of erythematous macular rash, possibly associated with fever, tachycardia, and hypotension, and if severe, may necessitate interruption of therapy. If the reaction recurs when dosing is resumed, THALOMID™ (thalidomide) should be discontinued.

Bradycardia:
Bradycardia in association with thalidomide use has been reported. At present there have been no reports of bradycardia requiring medical or other intervention. The clinical significance and underlying etiology of the bradycardia noted in some thalidomide-treated patients are presently unknown.

Information for Patients (See BOXED WARNINGS.)
Patients should be instructed about the potential teratogenicity of thalidomide and the precautions that must be taken to preclude fetal exposure as per the *S.T.E.P.S.* program and boxed warnings in this package insert. Patients should be instructed to take thalidomide only as prescribed in compliance with all of the provisions of the *S.T.E.P.S.* Restricted Distribution Program.

Patients should be instructed not to share medication with anyone else.

Patients should be instructed that thalidomide frequently causes drowsiness and somnolence. Patients should be instructed to avoid situations where drowsiness may be a problem and not to take other medications that may cause drowsiness without adequate medical advice. Patients should be advised as to the possible impairment of mental and/or physical abilities required for the performance of hazardous tasks, such as driving a car or operating other complex machinery. Patients should be instructed that thalidomide may potentiate the somnolence caused by alcohol. Patients should be instructed that thalidomide can cause peripheral neuropathies that may be initially signaled by numbness, tingling, or pain or a burning sensation in the feet or hands. Patients should be instructed to report such occurrences to their prescriber immediately.

Patients should also be instructed that thalidomide may cause dizziness and orthostatic hypotension and that, therefore, they should sit upright for a few minutes prior to standing up from a recumbent position.

Patients should be instructed that they are not permitted to donate blood while taking thalidomide. In addition, male patients should be instructed that they are not permitted to donate sperm while taking thalidomide.

Laboratory Tests
Pregnancy Testing: **(See BOXED WARNINGS.)** Women of childbearing potential should have pregnancy testing performed (sensitivity of at least 50 mIU/mL). The test should be performed within the 24 hours prior to beginning thalidomide therapy and then weekly during the first month of use, then monthly thereafter in women with regular menstrual cycles or every 2 weeks in women with irregular menstrual cycles. Pregnancy testing should also be performed if a patient misses her period or if there is any abnormality in menstrual bleeding.

Neutropenia: **(See WARNINGS.)**

HIV Viral Load: **(See WARNINGS.)**

Drug Interactions
Thalidomide has been reported to enhance the sedative activity of barbiturates, alcohol, chlorpromazine, and reserpine.

Peripheral Neuropathy: Medications known to be associated with peripheral neuropathy should be used with caution in patients receiving thalidomide.

Oral Contraceptives: In 10 healthy women, the pharmacokinetic profiles of norethindrone and ethinyl estradiol following administration of a single dose containing 1.0 mg of norethindrone acetate and 75 μg of ethinyl estradiol were studied. The results were similar with and without coadministration of thalidomide 200 mg/day to steady-state levels.

Important Non-Thalidomide Drug Interactions
Drugs That Interfere with Hormonal Contraceptives: Concomitant use of HIV-protease inhibitors, griseofulvin, rifampin, rifabutin, phenytoin, or carbamazepine with hormonal contraceptive agents, may reduce the effectiveness of the contraception. Therefore, women requiring treatment with one or more of these drugs must use two OTHER effective or highly effective methods of contraception or abstain from reproductive heterosexual sexual intercourse.

Carcinogenesis, Mutagenesis, Impairment of Fertility
Long-term carcinogenicity tests have not been conducted using thalidomide. Thalidomide gave no evidence of mutagenic effects when assayed in *in vitro* bacterial (*Salmonella typhimurium* and *Escherichia coli*; Ames mutagenicity test), *in vitro* mammalian (AS52 Chinese hamster ovary cells; AS52/XPRT mammalian cell forward gene mutation assay) and *in vivo* mammalian (CD-1 mice; *in vivo* micronucleus test) test systems.

Animal studies to characterize the effects of thalidomide on fertility have not been conducted.

Pregnancy
Pregnancy Category X: See **BOXED WARNINGS** and **CONTRAINDICATIONS**.

Because of the known human teratogenicity of thalidomide, thalidomide is contraindicated in women who are or may become pregnant and who are not using the two required types of birth control or who are not continually abstaining from reproductive heterosexual sexual intercourse. If thalidomide is taken during pregnancy, it can cause severe birth defects or death to an unborn baby. Thalidomide should never be used by women who are pregnant or who could become pregnant while taking the drug. Even a single dose [1 capsule (50 mg)] taken by a pregnant woman can cause birth defects. If pregnancy does occur during treatment, the drug should be immediately discontinued. Under these conditions, the patient should be referred to an obstetrician/gynecologist experienced in reproductive toxicity for further evaluation and counseling. Any suspected fetal exposure to THALOMID™ (thalidomide) must be reported to the FDA *via* the MedWatch program at 1-800-FDA-1088 and also to Celgene Corporation.

Animal studies to characterize the effects of thalidomide on late stage pregnancy have not been conducted.

Use in Nursing Mothers
It is not known whether thalidomide is excreted in human milk. Because many drugs are excreted in human milk and because of the potential for serious adverse reactions in nursing infants from thalidomide, a decision should be made whether to discontinue nursing or to discontinue the drug, taking into account the importance of the drug to the mother.

Pediatric Use
Safety and effectiveness in pediatric patients below the age of 12 years have not been established.

Geriatric Use
No systematic studies in geriatric patients have been conducted. Thalidomide has been used in clinical trials in patients up to 90 years of age. Adverse events in patients over the age of 65 years did not appear to differ in kind from those reported for younger individuals.

ADVERSE REACTIONS

The most serious toxicity associated with thalidomide is its documented human teratogenicity. (See **BOXED WARNINGS** and **CONTRAINDICATIONS**.) The risk of severe birth defects, primarily phocomelia or death to the fetus, is extremely high during the critical period of pregnancy. The critical period is estimated, depending on the source of information, to range from 35 to 50 days after the last menstrual period. The risk of other potentially severe birth defects outside this critical period is unknown, but may be significant. Based on present knowledge, thalidomide must not be used at any time during pregnancy.

Thalidomide is associated with drowsiness / somnolence, peripheral neuropathy, dizziness / orthostatic hypotension, neutropenia, and HIV viral load increase. **(See WARNINGS.)**

Hypersensitivity to THALOMID™ (thalidomide) and bradycardia in patients treated with thalidomide have been reported. **(See PRECAUTIONS.)**

Somnolence, dizziness, and rash are the most commonly observed adverse events associated with the use of thalidomide. Thalidomide has been studied in controlled and uncontrolled clinical trials in patients with ENL and in people who are HIV-seropositive. In addition, thalidomide has been administered investigationally for more than 20 years in numerous indications. Adverse event profiles from these uses are summarized in the sections that follow.

Other Adverse Events:
Due to the nature of the longitudinal data that form the basis of this product's safety evaluation, no determination has been made of the causal relationship between the reported

Continued on next page

Thalomid—Cont.

adverse events listed below and thalidomide. These lists are of various adverse events noted by investigators in patients to whom they had administered thalidomide under various conditions.

Incidence in Controlled Clinical Trials

Table 4 lists treatment-emergent signs and symptoms that occurred in THALOMID™ (thalidomide)-treated patients in controlled clinical trials in ENL. Doses ranged from 50 to 300 mg/day. All adverse events were mild to moderate in severity, and none resulted in discontinuation. Table 4 also lists treatment-emergent adverse events that occurred in at least 3 of the THALOMID™ (thalidomide)-treated HIV-seropositive patients who participated in an 8-week, placebo controlled clinical trial. Events that were more frequent in the placebo-treated group are not included. (See **WARNINGS**, **PRECAUTIONS**, and **DRUG INTERACTIONS**.)

[See table 4 at right and on next page]

Other Adverse Events Observed in ENL Patients

Thalidomide in doses up to 400 mg/day has been administered investigationally in the United States over a 19-year period in 1465 patients with ENL. The published literature describes the treatment of an additional 1678 patients. To provide a meaningful estimate of the proportion of the individuals having adverse events, similar types of events were grouped into a smaller number of standardized categories using a modified COSTART dictionary / terminology. These categories are used in the listing below. All reported events are included except those already listed in the previous table. Due to the fact that these data were collected from uncontrolled studies, the incidence rate cannot be determined. As mentioned previously, **no causal relationship between thalidomide and these events can be conclusively determined at this time.** These are reports of all adverse events noted by investigators in patients to whom they had administered thalidomide.

Body as a Whole: Abdomen enlarged, fever, photosensitivity, upper extremity pain.

Cardiovascular System: Bradycardia, hypertension, hypotension, peripheral vascular disorder, tachycardia.

Digestive System: Anorexia, appetite increase/weight gain, dry mouth, dyspepsia, enlarged liver, eructation, flatulence, increased liver function tests, intestinal obstruction, vomiting.

Hemic and Lymphatic: ESR decrease, eosinophilia, granulocytopenia, hypochromic anemia, leukemia, leukocytosis, leukopenia, MCV elevated, RBC abnormal, spleen palpable thrombocytopenia.

Metabolic and Endocrine: ADH inappropriate, alkaline phosphatase, amyloidosis, bilirubinemia, BUN increased, creatinine increased, cyanosis, diabetes, edema, electrolyte abnormalities, hyperglycemia, hyperkalemia, hyperuricemia, hypocalcemia, hypoproteinemia, LDH increased, phosphorus decreased, SGPT increased.

Muscular Skeletal: Arthritis, bone tenderness, hypertonia, joint disorder, leg cramps, myalgia, myasthenia, periosteal disorder.

Nervous System: Abnormal thinking, agitation, amnesia, anxiety, causalgia, circumoral paresthesia, confusion, depression, euphoria, hyperesthesia, insomnia, nervousness, neuralgia, neuritis, neuropathy, paresthesia, peripheral neuritis, psychosis, vasodilation.

Respiratory System: Cough, emphysema, epistaxis, pulmonary embolus, rales, upper respiratory infection, voice alteration.

Skin and Appendages: Acne, alopecia, dry skin, eczematous rash, exfoliative dermatitis, ichthyosis, perifollicular thickening, skin necrosis, seborrhea, sweating, urticaria, vesiculobullous rash.

Special Senses: Amblyopia, deafness, dry eye, eye pain, tinnitus.

Urogenital: Decreased creatinine clearance, hematuria, orchitis, proteinuria, pyuria, urinary frequency.

Other Adverse Events Observed in HIV-seropositive Patients

In addition to controlled clinical trials, THALOMID™ (thalidomide) has been used in uncontrolled studies in 145 patients. Less frequent adverse events that have been reported in these HIV-seropositive patients treated with THALOMID™ (thalidomide) were grouped into a smaller number of standardized categories using modified COSTART dictionary / terminology and these categories are used in the listing below. Adverse events that have already been included in the tables and narrative above, or that are too general to be informative are not listed.

Body as a Whole: Ascites, AIDS, allergic reaction, cellulitis, chest pain, chills and fever, cyst, decreased CD4 count, facial edema, flu syndrome, hernia, hormone level altered, moniliasis, photosensitivity reaction, sarcoma, sepsis, viral infection.

Cardiovascular System: Angina pectoris, arrhythmia, atrial fibrillation, bradycardia, cerebral ischemia, cerebrovascular accident, congestive heart failure, deep thrombophlebitis, heart arrest, heart failure, hypertension, hypoten-

Table 4
Summary of Adverse Events (AEs)
Reported in Celgene-sponsored Controlled Clinical Trials

Body System/Adverse Event	All AEs Reported in ENL Patients	AEs Reported in 3 HIV-seropositive Patients		Placebo
		Thalidomide		
	50 to 300 mg/day (N=24)	100 mg/day (N=36)	200 mg/day (N=32)	(N=35)
Body as a Whole	16 (66.7%)	18 (50.0%)	19 (59.4%)	13 (37.1%)
Abdominal pain	1 (4.2%)	1 (2.8%)	1 (3.1%)	4 (11.4%)
Accidental injury	1 (4.2%)	2 (5.6%)	0	1 (2.9%)
Asthenia	2 (8.3%)	2 (5.6%)	7 (21.9%)	1 (2.9%)
Back pain	1 (4.2%)	2 (5.6%)	0	0
Chills	1 (4.2%)	0	3 (9.4%)	4 (11.4%)
Facial edema	1 (4.2%)	0	0	0
Fever	0	7 (19.4%)	7 (21.9%)	6 (17.1%)
Headache	3 (12.5%)	6 (16.7%)	6 (18.7%)	4 (11.4%)
Infection	0	3 (8.3%)	2 (6.3%)	1 (2.9%)
Malaise	2 (8.3%)	0	0	0
Neck pain	1 (4.2%)	0	0	0
Neck rigidity	1 (4.2%)	0	0	0
Pain	2 (8.3%)	0	1 (3.1%)	2 (5.7%)
Digestive System	5 (20.8%)	16 (44.4%)	16 (50.0%)	15 (42.9%)
Anorexia	0	1 (2.8%)	3 (9.4%)	2 (5.7%)
Constipation	1 (4.2%)	1 (2.8%)	3 (9.4%)	0
Diarrhea	1 (4.2%)	4 (11.1%)	6 (18.7%)	6 (17.1%)
Dry mouth	0	3 (8.3%)	3 (9.4%)	2 (5.7%)
Flatulence	0	3 (8.3%)	0	2 (5.7%)
Liver function tests multiple abnormalities	0	0	3 (9.4%)	0
Nausea	1 (4.2%)	0	4 (12.5%)	1 (2.9%)
Oral moniliasis	1 (4.2%)	4 (11.1%)	2 (6.3%)	0
Tooth pain	1 (4.2%)	0	0	0
Hemic and Lymphatic	0	8 (22.2%)	13 (40.6%)	10 (28.6%)
Anemia	0	2 (5.6%)	4 (12.5%)	3 (8.6%)
Leukopenia	0	6 (16.7%)	8 (25.0%)	3 (8.6%)
Lymphadenopathy	0	2 (5.6%)	4 (12.5%)	3 (8.6%)
Metabolic and Endocrine Disorders	1 (4.2%)	8 (22.2%)	12 (37.5%)	8 (22.9%)
Edema peripheral	1 (4.2%)	3 (8.3%)	1 (3.1%)	0
Hyperlipemia	0	2 (5.6%)	3 (9.4%)	1 (2.9%)
SGOT increased	0	1 (2.8%)	4 (12.5%)	2 (5.7%)
Nervous System	13 (54.2%)	19 (52.8%)	18 (56.3%)	12 (34.3%)
Agitation	0	0	3 (9.4%)	0
Dizziness	1 (4.2%)	7 (19.4%)	6 (18.7%)	0
Insomnia	0	0	3 (9.4%)	2 (5.7%)
Nervousness	0	1 (2.8%)	3 (9.4%)	0
Neuropathy	0	3 (8.3%)	0	0
Paresthesia	0	2 (5.6%)	5 (15.6%)	4 (11.4%)
Somnolence	9 (37.5%)	13 (36.1%)	12 (37.5%)	4 (11.4%)
Tremor	1 (4.2%)	0	0	0
Vertigo	2 (8.3%)	0	0	0

Continued on next page

Table 4 (Continued)
Summary of Adverse Events (AEs)
Reported in Celgene-sponsored Controlled Clinical Trials

Body System/Adverse Event	All AEs Reported in ENL Patients	AEs Reported in 3 HIV-seropositive Patients		Placebo
		Thalidomide		
	50 to 300 mg/day (N=24)	100 mg/day (N=36)	200 mg/day (N=32)	(N=35)
Respiratory System	3 (12.5%)	9 (25.0%)	6 (18.7%)	9 (25.7%)
Pharyngitis	1 (4.2%)	3 (8.3%)	2 (6.3%)	2 (5.7%)
Rhinitis	1 (4.2%)	0	0	4 (11.4%)
Sinusitis	1 (4.2%)	3 (8.3%)	1 (3.1%)	2 (5.7%)
Skin and Appendages	10 (41.7%)	17 (47.2%)	18 (56.3%)	19 (54.3%)
Acne	0	4 (11.1%)	1 (3.1%)	0
Dermatitis fungal	1 (4.2%)	2 (5.6%)	3 (9.4%)	0
Nail disorder	1 (4.2%)	0	1 (3.1%)	0
Pruritus	2 (8.3%)	1 (2.8%)	2 (6.3%)	2 (5.7%)
Rash	5 (20.8%)	9 (25.0%)	8 (25.0%)	11 (31.4%)
Rash maculo-papular	1 (4.2%)	6 (16.7%)	6 (18.7%)	2 (5.7%)
Sweating	0	0	4 (12.5%)	4 (11.4%)
Urogenital System	2 (8.3%)	6 (16.7%)	2 (6.3%)	4 (11.4%)
Albuminuria	0	3 (8.3%)	1 (3.1%)	2 (5.7%)
Hematuria	0	4 (11.1%)	0	1 (2.9%)
Impotence	2 (8.3%)	1 (2.8%)	0	0

sion, murmur, myocardial infarct, palpitation, pericarditis, peripheral vascular disorder, postural hypotension, syncope, tachycardia, thrombophlebitis, thrombosis.

Digestive System: Cholangitis, cholestatic jaundice, colitis, dyspepsia, dysphagia, esophagitis, gastroenteritis, gastrointestinal disorder, gastrointestinal hemorrhage, gum disorder, hepatitis, pancreatitis, parotid gland enlargement, periodontitis, stomatitis, tongue discoloration, tooth disorder.

Hemic and Lymphatic: Aplastic anemia, macrocytic anemia, megaloblastic anemia, microcytic anemia.

Metabolic and Endocrine: Avitaminosis, bilirubinemia, dehydration, hypercholesteremia, hypoglycemia, increased alkaline phosphatase, increased lipase, increased serum creatinine, peripheral edema.

Muscular Skeletal: Myalgia, myasthenia.

Nervous System: Abnormal gait, ataxia, decreased libido, decreased reflexes, dementia, dysesthesia, dyskinesia, emotional lability, hostility, hypalgesia, hyperkinesia, incoordination, meningitis, neurologic disorder, tremor, vertigo.

Respiratory System: Apnea, bronchitis, lung disorder, lung edema, pneumonia (including *Pneumocystis carinii* pneumonia), rhinitis.

Skin and Appendages: Angioedema, benign skin neoplasm, eczema, herpes simplex, incomplete Stevens-Johnson syndrome, nail disorder, pruritus, psoriasis, skin discoloration, skin disorder.

Special Senses: Conjunctivitis, eye disorder, lacrimation disorder, retinitis, taste perversion.

Other Adverse Events in the Published Literature or Reported from Other Sources

The following additional events have been identified either in the published literature or from spontaneous reports from other sources: acute renal failure, amenorrhea, aphthous stomatitis, bile duct obstruction, carpal tunnel, chronic myelogenous leukemia, diplopia, dysesthesia, dyspnea, enuresis, erythema nodosum, erythroleukemia, foot drop, galactorrhea, gynecomastia, hangover effect, hypomagnesemia, hypothyroidism, lymphedema, lymphopenia, metrorrhagia, migraine, myxedema, nodular sclerosing Hodgkin's disease, nystagmus, oliguria, pancytopenia, petechiae, purpura, Raynaud's syndrome, stomach ulcer, and suicide attempt.

DRUG ABUSE AND DEPENDENCE

Physical and psychological dependence has not been reported in patients taking thalidomide. However, as with other tranquilizers / hypnotics, thalidomide too has been reported to create in patients habituation to its soporific effects.

OVERDOSAGE

There have been three cases of overdose reported, all attempted suicides. There have been no reported fatalities in doses of up to 14.4 grams, and all patients recovered without reported sequelae.

DOSAGE AND ADMINISTRATION

THALOMID™ (thalidomide) MUST ONLY BE ADMINISTERED IN COMPLIANCE WITH ALL OF THE TERMS OUTLINED IN THE *S.T.E.P.S.* PROGRAM. THALOMID™ (thalidomide) MAY ONLY BE PRESCRIBED BY PRESCRIBERS REGISTERED WITH THE *S.T.E.P.S.* PROGRAM AND MAY ONLY BE DISPENSED BY PHARMACISTS REGISTERED WITH THE *S.T.E.P.S.* PROGRAM.

Drug prescribing to women of childbearing potential should be contingent upon initial and continued confirmed negative results of pregnancy testing.

For an episode of cutaneous ENL, THALOMID™ (thalidomide) dosing should be initiated at 100 to 300 mg/day, administered once daily with water, preferably at bedtime and at least 1 hour after the evening meal. Patients weighing less than 50 kilograms should be started at the low end of the dose range.

In patients with a severe cutaneous ENL reaction, or in those who have previously required higher doses to control the reaction, THALOMID™ (thalidomide) dosing may be initiated at higher doses up to 400 mg/day once daily at bedtime or in divided doses with water, at least 1 hour after meals.

In patients with moderate to severe neuritis associated with a severe ENL reaction, corticosteroids may be started concomitantly with THALOMID™ (thalidomide). Steroid usage can be tapered and discontinued when the neuritis has ameliorated.

Dosing with THALOMID™ (thalidomide) should usually continue until signs and symptoms of active reaction have subsided, usually a period of at least 2 weeks. Patients may then be tapered off medication in 50 mg decrements every 2 to 4 weeks.

Patients who have a documented history of requiring prolonged maintenance treatment to prevent the recurrence of cutaneous ENL or who flare during tapering, should be maintained on the minimum dose necessary to control the reaction. Tapering off medication should be attempted every 3 to 6 months, in decrements of 50 mg every 2 to 4 weeks.

HOW SUPPLIED

(THIS PRODUCT IS ONLY SUPPLIED TO PHARMACISTS REGISTERED WITH THE *S.T.E.P.S.* PROGRAM - See BOXED WARNINGS.)

THALOMID™ (thalidomide) is supplied in hard gelatin, 50 mg capsules [white opaque], imprinted "Celgene" with a "do not get pregnant" logo. Boxes containing six prescription packs of 14 capsules each (84 capsules total).
NDC Number(s)
59572-105-11

STORAGE AND DISPENSING

PHARMACISTS NOTE:

DRUG MUST ONLY BE DISPENSED IN NO MORE THAN A 1-MONTH SUPPLY AND ONLY ON PRESENTATION OF A NEW PRESCRIPTION WRITTEN WITHIN THE PREVIOUS 7 DAYS. SPECIFIC INFORMED CONSENT (copy attached as part of this package insert) AND COMPLIANCE WITH THE MANDATORY PATIENT REGISTRY AND SURVEY ARE REQUIRED FOR ALL PATIENTS (MALE AND FEMALE) PRIOR TO DISPENSING BY THE PHARMACIST.

This drug must not be repackaged.
Store at 59 to 86°F; 15 to 30°C. Protect from light.
Rx only and only able to be prescribed and dispensed under the terms of the *S.T.E.P.S.* Restricted Distribution Program
Manufactured for Celgene Corporation
7 Powder Horn Drive
Warren, New Jersey 07059

Important Information and Warnings For All Patients Taking THALOMID™ (thalidomide)

> **WARNING: SERIOUS HUMAN BIRTH DEFECTS**
> IF THALIDOMIDE IS TAKEN DURING PREGNANCY, IT CAN CAUSE SEVERE BIRTH DEFECTS OR DEATH TO AN UNBORN BABY. THALIDOMIDE SHOULD NEVER BE USED BY WOMEN WHO ARE PREGNANT OR WHO COULD BECOME PREGNANT WHILE TAKING THE DRUG. EVEN A SINGLE DOSE [1 CAPSULE (50 mg)] TAKEN BY A PREGNANT WOMAN CAN CAUSE SEVERE BIRTH DEFECTS.

CONSENT FOR WOMEN:

INIT:_____ 1. I understand that I must not take THALOMID™ (thalidomide) if I am pregnant, breast-feeding a baby, or able to get pregnant and not using the required two methods of birth control.

INIT:_____ 2. I understand that severe birth defects can occur with the use of THALOMID™ (thalidomide). I have been warned by my doctor that my unborn baby will almost certainly have serious birth defects or may even die if I am pregnant or become pregnant while taking THALOMID™ (thalidomide).

INIT:_____ 3. I understand that if I am able to become pregnant, I must use at least one highly effective method and one additional effective method of birth control (contraception) AT THE SAME TIME:

At least one highly effective method		One additional effective method
IUD	**AND**	Latex condom
Hormonal (Birth control pills, injections, or implants)		Diaphragm
		Cervical cap
Tubal ligation		
Partner's vasectomy		

These birth control methods must be used for at least 4 weeks before starting THALOMID™ (thalidomide) therapy, all during THALOMID™ (thalidomide) therapy, and for at least 4 weeks after THALOMID™ (thalidomide) therapy has stopped. I must use these methods even if I am infertile, unless I have had a hysterectomy or because I have been post-menopausal for at least 24 months (been through the changes of life). The only exception is if I completely avoid heterosexual sexual intercourse. If a hormonal (birth control pills, injections, or implants) or IUD method is not medically possible for me, I may use another highly effective method or two barrier methods AT THE SAME TIME.

INIT:_____ 4. I know that I must have a pregnancy test done by my doctor within the 24 hours prior to starting THALOMID™ (thalidomide) therapy, then every week during the first 4 weeks of THALOMID™ (thalidomide) therapy. I will then have a pregnancy test every 4 weeks if I have regular menstrual cycles, or every 2 weeks if my cycles are irregular while I am taking THALOMID™ (thalidomide).

Continued on next page

Thalomid—Cont.

INIT:____ 5. I know that I must immediately stop taking THALOMID™ (thalidomide) and inform my doctor if I become pregnant while taking the drug; if I miss my menstrual period, or experience unusual menstrual bleeding; stop using birth control; or think, FOR ANY REASON, that I may be pregnant. If my doctor is not available, I can call 1-888-668-2528 for information on emergency contraception.

INIT:____ 6. I am not now pregnant, nor will I try to become pregnant for at least 4 weeks after I have completely finished taking THALOMID™ (thalidomide).

INIT:____ 7. I understand that THALOMID™ (thalidomide) will be prescribed ONLY for me. I must NOT share it with ANYONE, even someone who has symptoms similar to mine. It must be kept out of the reach of children and should never be given to women who are able to have children.

INIT:____ 8. I have read the THALOMID™ (thalidomide) patient brochure and/or viewed the videotape, "Important Information for Men and Women Taking THALOMID™ (thalidomide)". I understand the contents, including other possible health problems from THALOMID™ (thalidomide), so-called "side effects". I know that I cannot donate blood while taking THALOMID™ (thalidomide).

INIT:____ 9. My doctor has answered any questions I have asked.

INIT:____ 10. I understand that I must participate in a survey and patient registry while I am on THALOMID™ (thalidomide), which will require completing additional forms.

CONSENT FOR MEN:

INIT:____ 1. I understand that I must not take THALOMID™ (thalidomide) if I cannot avoid unprotected sex with a woman, even if I have had a successful vasectomy.

INIT:____ 2. I understand that severe birth defects or death to an unborn baby have occurred when women took thalidomide during pregnancy.

INIT:____ 3. I have been told by my doctor that I must NEVER have unprotected sex with a woman because it is not known if the drug is present in semen or sperm. My doctor has explained that I must either completely avoid heterosexual sexual intercourse or I must use a latex condom EVERY TIME I have sexual intercourse with a female partner while I am taking THALOMID™ (thalidomide) - and for 4 weeks after I stop taking the drug, even if I have had a successful vasectomy.

INIT:____ 4. I also know that I must inform my doctor if I have had unprotected sex with a woman; or if I think, FOR ANY REASON, that my sexual partner may be pregnant. If my doctor is not available, I can call 1-888-668-2528 for information on emergency contraception.

INIT:____ 5. I understand that THALOMID™ (thalidomide) will be prescribed ONLY for me. I must NOT share it with ANYONE, even someone who has symptoms similar to mine. It must be kept out of the reach of children and should never be given to women who are able to have children.

INIT:____ 6. I have read the THALOMID™ (thalidomide) patient brochure and/or viewed the videotape, "Important Information for Men and Women Taking THALOMID™ (thalidomide)". I understand the contents, including other possible health problems from THALOMID™ (thalidomide), so-called "side effects". I know that I cannot donate blood or semen while taking THALOMID™ (thalidomide).

INIT:____ 7. My doctor has answered any questions I have asked.

INIT:____ 8. I understand that I must participate in a survey and patient registry while I am on THALOMID™ (thalidomide), which will require completing additional forms.

Authorization:

This information has been read aloud to me in the language of my choice. I understand that if I do not follow all of my doctor's instructions, I will not be able to receive THALOMID™ (thalidomide). I now authorize my doctor to begin my treatment with THALOMID™ (thalidomide).

Patient Name (please print)	Social Security No. (Only last six digits required)	Date of Birth (mo./day/yr.)

Patient, Parent/ Guardian Signature	Date (mo./day/yr.)

I have fully explained to the patient the nature, purpose, and risks of the treatment described above, especially the risks to women of childbearing potential. I have asked the patient if she/he has any questions regarding her/his treatment with THALOMID™ (thalidomide) and have answered those questions to the best of my ability. I will ensure that the appropriate components of the patient consent form are completed. In addition, I will comply with all of my obligations and responsibilities as a prescriber registered under the *S.T.E.P.S.* restricted distribution program.

Physician Name (please print)	DEA No.

Physician Signature	Date (mo./day/yr.)

REFERENCES

1. Manson JM. 1986. Teratogenicity. Cassarett and Doull's Toxicology: The Basic Science of Poisons. Third Edition. Pages 195–220. New York: MacMillan Publishing Co.
2. Smithels RW and Newman CG. 1992. J. Med. Genet. 29(10):716–723.
3. Sampaio EP, Kaplan G, Miranda A, *et al.* 1993. J. Infect. Dis. 168(2):408–414.
4. Sarno EN, Grau GE, Vieira LM, *et al.* 1991. Clin. Exp. Immunol. 84:103–108.
5. Sampaio EP, Moreira AL, Sarno EN, *et al.* 1992. J. Exp. Med. 175:1729–1737.
6. Nogueira AC, Neubert R, Helge H, *et al.* 1994. Life Sciences. 55(2):77–92.
7. Jacobson JM, Greenspan JS, Spritzler J, *et al.* 1997. New Eng. J. Med. 336(21):1487–1493.
8. Schumaker H, Smith RL, and Williams RT. 1965. Br. J. Pharmacol. 25:324–337.
9. Iyer CGS, Languillon J, Ramanujam K, *et al.* 1971. Bull. WHO. 45:719–732.
10. Sheskin J and Convit J. 1969. Intl. J. Leprosy. 37:135–146.
11. Waters MFR. 1971. Lepr. Rev. 42:26–42.
12. Unpublished data, on file at Celgene.

Shown in Product Identification Guide, page 309

Medeva Pharmaceuticals, Inc.
P.O. Box 1710
ROCHESTER, NY 14603

Direct Inquiries to:
Customer Service Department
P.O. Box 1766
Rochester, NY 14603
(716) 274-5300
(888) 9-MEDEVA
In Emergencies:
(800) 932-1950 (24 hours)

INFLUENZA VIRUS VACCINE
(FLUVIRIN™)   ℞
Purified Surface Antigen Vaccine, Trivalent, Types A and B
1998–1999 FORMULA

DESCRIPTION

Influenza Virus Vaccine, **FLUVIRIN™**, Types A and B (Surface Antigen) is a sterile parenteral for intramuscular use only. It is a purified split-virus preparation. The vaccine is a slightly opalescent liquid.

FLUVIRIN™ is prepared from the extraembryonic fluid of embryonated chicken eggs inoculated with a specific type of influenza virus suspension containing neomycin and polymyxin. The fluid containing the virus is harvested and clarified by centrifugation and filtration prior to inactivation with betapropiolactone. The inactivated virus is concentrated and purified by zonal centrifugation. The surface antigens, hemagglutinin and neuraminidase, are obtained from the influenza virus particle by further centrifugation in the presence of Triton® N101, a process which removes most of the internal proteins. The Triton® N101 is removed from the surface antigen preparation and the antigens are suspended in 0.01M phosphate buffered saline. The hemagglutinin content is standardized according to current US Public Health Service requirements. Each 0.5 mL contains the recommended ratio of 15µg each of A/Beijing/262/95-like (H1N1), A/Sydney/5/97-like (H3N2), B/Harbin/07/94 (B/Beijing/184/93-like) hemagglutinin antigens.

Thimerosal (mercury derivative) 0.01% is added as a preservative. Polymyxin, neomycin, and betapropiolactone cannot be detected in the final product by current assay procedures. This vaccine is manufactured and released by Evans Medical Limited.

CLINICAL PHARMACOLOGY

Influenza A viruses are classified into subtypes on the basis of two surface antigens: hemagglutinin (H) and neuraminidase (N). Three subtypes of hemagglutinin (H1, H2 and H3) and two subtypes of neuraminidase (N1 and N2) are recognized among influenza A viruses that have caused widespread human disease. Immunity to these antigens—especially the hemagglutinin—reduces the likelihood of infection and lessens the severity of the disease if infection occurs. Infection with a virus of one subtype confers little or no protection against viruses of other subtypes. Furthermore, over time, antigenic variation (antigenic drift) within a subtype may be so marked that infection or vaccination with one strain may not induce immunity to distantly related strains of the same subtype. Although influenza B viruses have shown more antigenic stability than influenza A viruses, antigenic variation does occur. For these reasons, major epidemics of respiratory disease caused by new variants of influenza continue to occur. The antigenic characteristics of circulating strains provide the basis for selecting the virus strains included in each year's vaccine.[1]

Typical influenza illness is characterized by abrupt onset of fever, myalgia, sore throat, and nonproductive cough. Unlike other common respiratory illnesses, influenza can cause severe malaise lasting several days. More severe illness can result if either primary influenza pneumonia or secondary bacterial pneumonia occurs. During influenza epidemics, high attack rates of acute illness result in both increased numbers of visits to physicians' offices, walk-in clinics, and emergency rooms and increased hospitalizations for management of lower respiratory tract complications.[1]

Elderly persons and persons with underlying health problems are at increased risk of complications from influenza infection. If they become ill with influenza, such members of high risk goups are more likely than the general population to require hospitalization.

During major epidemics, hospitalization rates for persons at high risk may increase substantially, depending on the age group. Previously healthy children and younger adults also may require hospitalization for influenza-related complications, but the relative increase in their hospitalization rates during epidemics is less than for persons who belong to high risk groups.[1]

Estimates of hospitalization rates for persons age 65 or older have ranged from approximately 200 to greater than 1000 per 100,000 population during different epidemics.[1] Even for persons 45–64 years of age, estimates of hospitalization rates due to influenza range from approximately 80 to 400 per 100,000 population for persons with high-risk medical conditions, and from approximately 20 to 40 per 100,000 for those without high-risk conditions.[1] Hospitalization rates for persons aged 15 to 44 years have ranged from approximately 40 to greater than 60 per 100,000 population for those with high risk-conditions and from approximately 20 to 30 per 100,000 population for those without high-risk conditions.[1]

For children aged 5 to 14 years hospitalization rates have ranged from approximately 200 per 100,000 population for those with high-risk conditions to 20 per 100,000 population for those without high-risk conditions.[1] For children aged from 0 to 4 years, hospitalization rates have ranged from approximately 500 per 100,000 population for those with high-risk conditions to 100 per 100,000 population for those without high-risk conditions.[1]

It has been estimated that during influenza epidemic in recent decades the number of excess hospitalizations has ranged from approximately 20,000 to greater than 300,000 per epidemic, with an average of approximately 130,000–170,000 per epidemic. The greatest numbers of influenza-associated hospitalizations have occurred during epidemics

cause by type A (H3N2) viruses, with an estimated average of 160,000–200,000 excess hospitalizations per epidemic.[1]
An increase in mortality further indicates the impact of influenza epidemics. Increased mortality results from not only influenza and pneumonia, but also cardiopulmonary or other chronic diseases that can be exacerbated by influenza infection. It is estimated that greater than 20,000 influenza related deaths occurred during each of eleven different US epidemics from 1972–73 to 1994–95, and greater than 40,000 influenza related deaths occurred during each of six of these eleven epidemics. More than 90% of the deaths attributed to pneumonia and influenza occurred among persons greater than or equal to 65 years of age. Increased pneumonia and influenza mortality may be related to the fact that the number of elderly persons in the U.S. population is increasing, as well as the number of persons aged less than 65 years at increased risk for influenza-related complications. Longer life expectancy for a) organ-transplant recipients, b) neonates in intensive-care units, and c) persons who have cystic fibrosis and acquired immunodeficiency syndrome (AIDS) results in a higher survival rate for younger persons at high risk for influenza.[1]
The effectiveness of influenza vaccine in preventing or attenuating illness varies, depending primarily on the age and immunocompetence of the vaccine recipient and the degree of similarity between the virus strains included in the vaccine and those that circulate during the influenza season. When there is a good match between vaccine and circulating viruses, influenza vaccine has been shown to prevent illness in approximately 70%–90% of healthy persons less than 65 years of age. In these circumstances, studies have also indicated that the effectiveness of influenza vaccine in preventing hospitalization for pneumonia and influenza among elderly persons living in settings other than nursing homes or similar chronic-care facilities ranges from 30%–70%.[1]
Among elderly persons residing in nursing homes, influenza vaccine is most effective in preventing severe illness, secondary complications, and death. Studies of this population have indicated that the vaccine can be 50%–60% effective in preventing hospitalization and pneumonia and 80% effective in preventing death, even though efficacy in preventing influenza illness may often be in the range of 30%–40% among the frail elderly. Achieving a high rate of vaccination among nursing home residents may reduce the spread of infection in a facility, thus preventing disease through herd immunity. Vaccination of health care workers in nursing homes has also been effective in reducing the impact of influenza among residents.[1]
Based upon epidemiological studies of circulating influenza virus strains, the Public Health Service has recommended that the 1998–1999 vaccine will be trivalent and contain 15μg of hemagglutinin of each strain:
A/Beijing/262/95-like (H1N1), A/Sydney/5/97-like (H3N2), B/Harbin/7/94 (B/Beijing/184/93-like) per each 0.5 mL.[1]

INDICATIONS AND USAGE

FLUVIRIN™ is indicated for immunization of persons 4 years of age and older against influenza viruses containing antigens related to those in the vaccine. The safety and efficacy in children between the ages 6 months through to 4 years has not been established for this product. However, the Advisory Committee on Immunization Practices (ACIP) of the US Public Health Service strongly recommends vaccination for any person greater than or equal to 6 months of age, who because of age or underlying medical condition, is at increased risk of complications from influenza.[1]
Health care workers and others (including household members) in close contact with persons in high-risk groups should be vaccinated.[1] Guidelines for the use of vaccine among different segments of the population are given below.[1]
Although the current influenza Virus Vaccine can contain one or more of the antigens administered in previous years, annual vaccination with the current vaccine is necessary because immunity declines in the year following vaccination.[1]
Therefore, a history of immunization in any previous year with a vaccine containing one or more antigens included in the current vaccine does not preclude the need to be reimmunized for the 1998–1999 influenza season.
Remaining 1997–1998 vaccine should not be used to provide protection for the 1998–1999 influenza season.[1]

TARGET GROUPS FOR SPECIAL IMMUNIZATION PROGRAMS

To maximize protection of high-risk persons, both they and their close contacts should be targeted for organized immunization programs.

Groups at increased risk for influenza-related complications

1. Persons 65 years of age or older.[1]
2. Residents of nursing homes and other chronic-care facilities housing patients of any age with chronic medical conditions.[1]
3. Adults and children with chronic disorders of the pulmonary or cardiovascular systems, including children with asthma.[1]
4. Adults and children who have required regular medical follow-up or hospitalization during the preceding year because of chronic metabolic diseases (including diabetes mellitus), renal dysfunction, hemoglobinopathies, or immunosuppression (including immunosuppression caused by medications).[1]
5. Children and teenagers (6 months through 18 years of age) who are receiving long-term aspirin therapy and, therefore, may be at risk of developing Reye syndrome after influenza.[1] Refer to (**Indications and Usage**) and (**Warnings**) sections for use of this product in children under the age of 4 years.
6. Women who will be in the second or third trimester of pregnancy during the influenza season.[1] Refer to **Immunization of Other Groups for use of this product in pregnant women.**

Groups that can transmit influenza to persons at high risk

Persons who are clinically or subclinically infected and who care for or live with members of high risk groups and can transmit influenza virus to them. Some persons at high risk (e.g., the elderly, transplant recipients, and persons with acquired immunodeficiency syndrome [AIDS]) can have low antibody responses to influenza vaccine. Efforts to protect these members of high risk groups against influenza may be improved by reducing the likelihood of influenza exposure from their caregivers. Therefore, the following groups should be immunized: [1]

1. Physicians, nurses, and other personnel in both hospital and outpatient care settings.[1]
2. Employees of nursing homes and chronic-care facilities who have contact with patients or residents.[1]
3. Providers of home care to persons at high risk (e.g., visiting nurses, volunteer workers).[1]
4. Household members (including children) of persons in high risk groups.[1]

IMMUNIZATION OF OTHER GROUPS

General Population

Physicians should administer influenza vaccine to any person greater than or equal to age 6 months who wishes to reduce the likelihood of becoming ill with influenza. Persons who provide essential community services may be considered for vaccination to minimize disruption of essential activities during influenza outbreaks. Students or other persons in institutional settings (e.g., those who reside in dormitories) should be encouraged to receive vaccine to minimize the disruption of routine activities during epidemics.[1]

Pregnant Women

Influenza-associated excess mortality among pregnant women has not been documented except during the pandemics of 1918–19 and 1957–58. However, because death-certificate data often do not indicate whether a woman was pregnant at the time of death, studies conducted during interpandemic periods may underestimate the impact of influenza in this population. Case reports and limited studies suggest that pregnancy may increase the risk for serious medical complications of influenza as a result of increases in heart rate, stroke volume and oxygen consumption, decreases in lung capacity and changes in immunologic function. A recent study of the impact of influenza during 17 interpandemic influenza seasons documented that the relative risk of hospitalization for selected cardiorespiratory conditions among pregnant women increased from 1.4 during weeks 14–20 of gestation to 4.7 during weeks 37–42 compared with rates among women who were 1–6 months postpartum. Women in their third trimester of pregnancy were hospitalized at a rate comparable to that of nonpregnant women who have high-risk medical conditions for whom influenza vaccine has traditionally been recommended. Using data from this study, it was estimated that an average of 1 to 2 hospitalizations among pregnant women could be prevented for every 1,000 pregnant women immunized.[1]
On the basis of these and other data that suggest that influenza infection may cause increased morbidity in women during the second and third trimesters of pregnancy, the ACIP recommends that women who will be beyond the first trimester of pregnancy (greater than, or equal to 14 weeks' gestation) during the influenza season be vaccinated. Pregnant women who have medical conditions that increase their risk for complications from influenza should be vaccinated before the influenza season—regardless of the stage of pregnancy. Studies of influenza immunization of more than 2,000 pregnant women have demonstrated no adverse fetal effects associated with influenza vaccine; however, more data are needed.[1] Because influenza vaccine is not a live virus vaccine and major systemic reactions to it are rare, many experts consider influenza vaccination safe during any stage of pregnancy.[1] However, because spontaneous abortion is common in the first trimester and unnecessary exposures have traditionally been avoided during this time, some experts prefer influenza vaccination during the second trimester to avoid coincidental association of the vaccine with early pregnancy loss.[1]
Controlled studies on Fluvirin™ have not been conducted to demonstrate safety in pregnant women.
The clinical judgment of the attending physician should prevail at all times in determining whether to administer the vaccine to a pregnant woman (see PRECAUTIONS, Use in Pregnancy).

Breast feeding mothers

ACIP states that influenza vaccine does not affect the safety of breast feeding for mothers or infants. Breast feeding does not adversely affect immunization and is not a contraindication for vaccination.[1]

Persons infected with Human Immunodeficiency Virus (HIV)

Limited information exists regarding the frequency and severity for influenza illness among HIV-infected persons, but reports suggest that symptoms may be prolonged and the risk of complications increased for some HIV-infected persons. Influenza vaccine has produced protective antibody titres against influenza in vaccinated HIV infected persons who have minimal AIDS-related symptoms and high CD4+ T-lymphocyte cell counts.[1] In patients who have advanced HIV disease and low CD4+ T-lymphocyte cell counts, however influenza vaccine may induce protective antibody titers; a second dose of vaccine does not improve the immune response for these persons.[1] Recent studies have examined the effect of influenza vaccination on replication of HIV type 1 (HIV-1). Although some studies have demonstrated a transient (i.e., 2- to 4-week) increase in replication of HIV-1 in the plasma or peripheral blood mononuclear cells of HIV-infected persons after vaccine administration, other studies using similar laboratory techniques have not indicated any substantial increase in replication. Deterioration of CD4+ T-lymphocyte cell counts and progression of clinical HIV disease have not been demonstrated among HIV-infected persons who receive vaccine. Because influenza can result in serious illness and complications and because influenza vaccination may result in protective antibody titers, vaccination will benefit many HIV-infected patients.[1]

Persons Traveling to Foreign Countries

The risk of exposure to influenza during foreign travel varies, depending on season and destination. In the tropics, influenza can occur throughout the year; in the Southern Hemisphere, the most activity occurs from April through September. Because of the short incubation period for influenza, exposure to the virus during travel can result in clinical illness that begins while traveling, which is an inconvenience or potential danger, especially for those at increased risk for complications. Persons preparing to travel to the tropics at any time of year or to the Southern Hemisphere from April through September should review their influenza immunization histories. If not immunized the previous fall/winter, they should consider influenza immunization prior to travel.[1] Persons in the high risk category should be especially encouraged to receive the most current vaccine. Persons at high risk who received the previous season's vaccine before travel should be revaccinated in the fall or winter with the current vaccine.[1]

TIMING OF IMMUNISATION

Beginning each September, when vaccine for the upcoming influenza season becomes available, persons at high risk who are seen by health-care providers for routine care or as a result of hospitalization should be offered influenza vaccine.
Opportunities to vaccinate persons at high risk for complications of influenza should not be missed.
The optimal time for organized vaccination compaigns for persons in high-risk groups is usually the period from October through mid-November. In the United States, influenza activity generally peaks between late December and early March. High levels of influenza activity infrequently occur in the contiguous 48 states before December. Administering vaccine too far in advance of the influenza season should be avoided in facilities such as nursing homes because antibody levels may begin to decline within a few months of vaccination. Vaccination programs can be undertaken as soon as current vaccine is available if regional influenza activity is expected to begin earlier than December.[1]
Children under 9 years of age who have not been immunized previously should receive two doses of vaccine at least 1 month apart to maximise the likelihood of a satisfactory antibody response to all three vaccine antigens. The second dose should be given before December, if possible. Vaccine should be offered to both children and adults up to and even after influenza virus activity is documented in a community.[1]

CONTRAINDICATIONS

INFLUENZA VIRUS IS PROPAGATED IN EGGS FOR THE PREPARATION OF INFLUENZA VIRUS VACCINE.

Continued on next page

Information on the Medeva Pharmaceuticals, Inc. products listed on these pages contains the full prescribing information from product circulars in use as of July 1998. For further information, please consult the package insert currently accompanying the product.

Fluvirin—Cont.

THUS, THIS VACCINE SHOULD NOT BE ADMINISTERED TO ANYONE WITH A HISTORY OF HYPERSITIVITY (ALLERGY) TO CHICKEN EGGS, CHICKEN, CHICKEN FEATHERS OR CHICKEN DANDER.

THE VACCINE IS ALSO CONTRAINDICATED IN INDIVIDUALS HYPERSENSITIVE TO ANY COMPONENT OF THE VACCINE INCLUDING THIMEROSAL (A MERCURY DERIVATIVE) (SEE ADVERSE REACTIONS). EPINEPHRINE INJECTION (1:1000) MUST BE IMMEDIATELY AVAILABLE SHOULD AN ACUTE ANAPHYLACTIC REACTION OCCUR DUE TO ANY COMPONENT OF THE VACCINE.

IMMUNIZATION SHOULD BE DELAYED IN PERSONS WITH AN ACTIVE NEUROLOGICAL DISORDER CHARACTERIZED BY CHANGING NEUROLOGICAL FINDINGS, BUT SHOULD BE CONSIDERED WITH THE DISEASE PROCESS HAS BEEN STABILIZED.

THE OCCURRENCE OF ANY NEUROLOGICAL SYMPTOMS OR SIGNS FOLLOWING ADMINISTRATION OF ANY VACCINE IS A CONTRAINDICATION TO FURTHER USE.

THE VACCINE SHOULD NOT BE ADMINISTERED TO PERSONS WITH ACUTE FEBRILE ILLNESSES UNTIL THEIR TEMPORARY SYMPTOMS AND/OR SIGNS HAVE ABATED.

The clinical judgment of the attending physician should prevail at all times.

WARNINGS

The safety and efficacy in children between the ages 6 months through to 4 years has not been established for this product. Influenza Virus Vaccine (Fluvirin™) should not be given to these children unless, in the judgement of the physician, the potential benefits clearly outweigh the risk of administration. In any case THIS PRODUCT SHOULD NOT BE ADMINISTERED TO CHILDREN YOUNGER THAN 6 MONTHS OF AGE.

THE OCCURRENCE OF A NEUROLOGICAL OR SEVERE HYPERSENSITIVITY REACTION FOLLOWING PREVIOUS IMMUNIZATION WITH INFLUENZA VIRUS VACCINE IS A CONTRAINDICATION TO FURTHER USE OF THIS PRODUCT.

Influenza Virus Vaccine should not be given to individuals with thrombocytopenia or any coagulation disorder that would contraindicate intramuscular injection unless, in the judgment of the physician, the potential benefits clearly outweigh the risk of administration.

Patients with impaired immune responsiveness, whether due to the use of immunosuppressive therapy (including irradiation, corticosteroids, antimetabolites, alkylating agents, and cytotoxic agents), a genetic defect, human immunodeficiency virus (HIV) infection, or other causes, may have a reduced antibody response in active immunization procedures.

Since the likelihood of febrile convulsions from any cause is greater in children between 6 and 35 months, special care should be taken in weighing the relative risks and benefits of immunization in this age group.

This product contains dry natural rubber or latex (see **Precautions** section) in the syringe stopper but not in the multi dose vial stopper.

As with any vaccine, immunization with influenza Virus Vaccine may not result in seroconversion of all individuals given the vaccine.

Special care should be taken to prevent injection into a blood vessel.

PRECAUTIONS

General

1. PRIOR TO ADMINISTRATION OF ANY DOSE OF INFLUENZA VIRUS VACCINE, THE PARENT, GUARDIAN, OR ADULT PATIENT SHOULD BE ASKED ABOUT THE RECENT HEALTH STATUS, MEDICAL AND IMMUNIZATION HISTORY OF THE PATIENT TO BE IMMUNIZED IN ORDER TO DETERMINE THE EXISTENCE OF ANY CONTRAINDICATION TO IMMUNIZATION WITH INFLUENZA VIRUS VACCINE (see **CONTRAINDICATIONS**, **WARNINGS**).
2. BEFORE ADMINISTRATION OF ANY BIOLOGICAL, THE PHYSICIAN SHOULD TAKE ALL PRECAUTIONS KNOWN FOR PREVENTION OF ALLERGIC OR ANY OTHER SIDE REACTIONS. This should include: a review of the patient's history regarding possible sensitivity (including to dry natural rubber or latex), the ready availability of epinephrine 1:1,000 and other appropriate agents used for control of immediate allergic reactions, and a knowledge of the recent literature pertaining to use of the biological concerned, including the nature of side effects and adverse reactions that may follow its use.
3. A separate sterile syringe and needle or a sterile disposable unit must be used for each individual patient to prevent transmission of infectious agents from one person to another.

Information for the Patient

PRIOR TO ADMINISTRATION OF THIS VACCINE, HEALTH CARE PERSONNEL SHOULD INFORM THE PARENT, GUARDIAN, OR ADULT PATIENT OF THE BENEFITS AND RISKS OF IMMUNIZATION AGAINST INFLUENZA.

Drug Interactions

Although influenza immunization can inhibit the clearance of warfarin and theophylline, studies have not established any adverse clinical effects attributable to these drugs in patients receiving influenza vaccine.

Use in Pregnancy

Pregnancy Category C

Animal reproduction studies have not been conducted with Influenza Virus Vaccine (Fluvirin™). It is also not known whether Influenza Virus Vaccine (Fluvirin™) can cause fetal harm when administered to a pregnant woman or can affect reproduction capacity. Influenza Virus Vaccine (Fluvirin™) should be given to a pregnant woman only if clearly needed.

See **INDICATIONS AND USAGE, Pregnant Women.**

The clinical judgment of the attending physician should prevail at all times in determining whether to administer Influenza Virus Vaccine to a pregnant woman.

ADVERSE REACTIONS

Because purified surface antigen influenza vaccine contains only noninfectious purified viral proteins, it cannot cause influenza. Respiratory disease after vaccination represents coincidental illness unrelated to influenza vaccination.[1]

Local Symptoms

The most frequent side effects of vaccination are slight tenderness, redness or induration at the site of injection lasting for up to 2 days.[1] These local reactions are generally mild and rarely interfere with the ability to carry out usual daily activities.[1]

Systemic Symptoms

Fever, malaise, myalgia, and other systemic symptoms can occur following vaccination, but most often affect persons who have had no exposure to the influenza virus antigens in the vaccine (e.g., young children). These reactions begin 6–12 hours after vaccination and can persist for 1 or 2 days. Recent placebo-controlled trials suggest that in elderly persons and healthy younger adults, split-virus influenza vaccine is not associated with higher rates of systemic symptoms such as fever, malaise, myalgia and headache when compared to placebo injections.[1]

Immediate—presumably allergic—reactions (such as hives, angioedema, allergic asthma, or systemic anaphylaxis) occur rarely after influenza vaccination. These reactions probably result from hypersensitivity to some vaccine component—the majority of reactions are most likely related to residual egg protein. Although current influenza vaccines contain only a small quantity of egg protein, this protein may induce immediate hypersensitivity reactions among persons with severe egg allergy. Persons who have developed hives, had swelling of the lips or tongue, or experienced acute respiratory distress or collapse after eating eggs should consult a physician for appropriate evaluation to help determine if vaccine should be administered. Persons with documented immunoglobulin E (IgE)-mediated hypersensitivity to eggs—including those who have had occupational asthma or other allergic responses from expsure to egg protein—may also be at increased risk for reactions from influenza vaccine, and similar consultation should be considered. The ACIP suggest that the protocol for influenza vaccination developed by Murphy and Strunk[2] may be considered for patients who have egg allergies and medical conditions that place them at increased risk for influenza-associated complications.[1] Hypersensitivity reactions to any vaccine component can occur. Although exposure to vaccines containing thimerosal can lead to induction of hypersensitivity, most patients do not develop reactions to thimerosal when administered as a component of vaccines—even when patch or intradermal tests for thimerosal indicate hypersensitivity. When resported, hypersensitivity to thimerosal usually has consisted of local, delayed-type hypersensitivity reactions.[1]

Unlike the 1976 swine influenza vaccine, evidence for a causal relationship of Gulliain-Barre syndrome (GBS) with subsequent vaccines prepared from other virus strains is less clear. However, it is difficult to obtain strong evidence for a possible small increase in risk for a rare condition such as GBS, which has an annual background incidence of only 10 to 20 cases per million adult population. During three of four seasons studied between 1977 and 1991, the point estimates of the overall relative risks of GBS after influenza vaccination were slightly elevated but were not statistically significant in any of these studies. However, a recent study of the 1992–3 and 1993–4 seasons found and elevation in the overall relative risk for GBS of 1.83 (95% Confidence interval 1.12–3.00) during the 6 weeks following vaccination, representing an excess of an estimated 1–2 cases of GBS per million persons vaccinated; the combined number of GBS cases peaked 2 weeks after vaccination. The increase in the relative risks and the increased number of cases in the second week after vaccination may be the result of vaccination but also could be due to other factors (e.g., confounding or diagnostic bias) rather than a true vaccine related risk.[1]

Among persons who received the swine influenza vaccine in 1976, the rate of GBS that exceeded the background rate was slightly less than 10 cases per million vaccinations. Even if GBS were a true side effect in subsequent years, the estimated risk for GBS of 1–2 cases per million vaccinations is substantially less than that for severe influenza, which could be prevented by vaccination among all age groups, especially among persons aged greater than or equal to 65 years and those who have medical indications for influenza vaccination.[1]

Estimates of excess hospitalization rates during different influenza epidemics have ranged from approximately 200 to 300 hospitalizations per million population for previously healthy persons aged 5–44 years to 2000 to greater than 10,000 hospitalizations per million for persons aged 65 years and older. Estimates of influenza-associated death rates during epidemics have ranged from approximately 300 to greater than 1500 per million persons aged 65 and older, which accound for more than 90% of all influenza-associated deaths. The average case-fatality ratio for GBS is approximately 6% and increases with age. There is no indication that the case-fatality ratio for GBS differs by influenza vaccination status. More detailed information about influenza-associated morbidity and mortality can be found in the section **Clinical Pharmacology**. The potential benefits of influenza vaccination clearly outweigh the possible risks for vaccine-associated GBS.[1]

Whereas the incidence of GBS in the general population is very low, persons with a history of GBS have a substantially greater likelihood of subsequently developing GBS than persons without such a history. Thus, the likelihood of coincidentally developing GBS after influenza vaccination is expected to be greater among persons with a history of GBS than among persons with no history of this syndrome. Whether influenza vaccination might be causally associated with this risk for recurrence is not known. Although avoiding a subsequent influenza vaccination in persons known to have developed GBS within 6 weeks of a previous influenza vaccination seems prudent, for most persons with a history of GBS who are at high risk for severe complications from influenza, many experts believe the established benefits of influenza vaccination justify yearly vaccination.[1]

Other neurological disorders, including encephalopathies not defined as GBS, have been temporally associated with influenza immunization, but no causal link has been established.[3,4]

DOSAGE AND ADMINISTRATION

For Intramuscular Use Only. Shake well before withdrawing each dose. DO NOT INJECT INTRAVENOUSLY.

Parenteral drug products should be inspected visually for particulate matter and discoloration prior to administration (see **DESCRIPTION**).

Remaining 1997–1998 influenza vaccine should not be used.

Although Influenza Virus Vaccine often contains one or more antigens used in previous years, immunity declines during the year following immunization. Therefore, a history of immunization in any previous year with a vaccine containing one or more antigens included in the current vaccine does NOT preclude the need for reimmunization for the 1998–1999 influenza season in order to provide optimal protection.

See **INDICATIONS AND USAGE** section for information regarding the optimal time of administration of this vaccine.

During recent decades, data on influenza vaccine immunogenicity and side effects have generally been obtained when vaccine has been administered intramuscularly. Because recent influenza vaccines have not been adequately evaluated when administered by other routes, the intramuscular route is recommended. Adults and older children should be immunized in the deltoid muscle; infants and young children in the anterolateral aspect of the thigh.

Before immunization, the skin over the site to be injected should be cleansed with a suitable germicide. After insertion of the needle, aspirate to help avoid inadvertent injection into a blood vessel.

Age Group	Dose	No. of Doses (See below for details)
6 to 35 months*	0.25 mL	1 or 2 Doses
3 years*	0.5 mL	1 or 2 Doses
4 to 8 years	0.5 mL	1 or 2 Doses
9 years and older	0.5 mL	1 Dose

*Refer to **Warnings** section for use of this product in these age ranges of children.

Two doses administered at least 1 month apart may be required for a satisfactory antibody response among previously unvaccinated children aged less than 9 months of age; however, studies of vaccines similar to those being used currently have indicated little or no improvement in antibody responses when a second dose is administered to adults during the same season.[1]

It is recommended that only a purified surface antigen or subvirion vaccine be administered to children under 12 years of age because of lower potential for causing febrile reactions.[1]

The 0.5 mL pre-filled syringe presentation is intended for single use only and must not be used in more than one individual. Do not reuse empty syringe.

Evans Medical Limited does not recommend the use of needleless injections for administration of Fluvirin™.

Simultaneous Administration with Other Vaccines

The target groups for influenza and pneumococcal immunization overlap considerably. Both vaccines may be given at the same time at different sites without increasing side effects. However, influenza vaccine must be administered each year, whereas pneumococcal vaccine is not.[1]

Physicians may prefer not to administer influenza vaccine within 3 days of administration of pertussis containing vaccines. However, the American Academy of Pediatrics now recommends that influenza vaccine may be administered simultaneously (but at a different site and with a different syringe) with other routine vaccinations in children, including pertussis vaccine.

(DTP or DTaP). Since influenza vaccine in young children can cause fever, DTaP may be preferable in those children 15 months and older who are receiving the fourth (or fifth) dose of pertussis vaccine.[5]

HOW SUPPLIED

NDC 19650-101-10 5 mL multi dose vial

NDC 19650-101-01 0.5 mL pre filled syringe

STORAGE

DO NOT FREEZE. STORE REFRIGERATED, AWAY FROM FREEZER COMPARTMENT, AT 2°C to 8°C (36°F to 46°F).

Vaccine must be transported under refrigeration temperatures.

REFERENCES

1. Prevention and control of influenza. Recommendations of the immunization Practices Advisory Committee (ACIP). MMWR 1998; 47(RR-6) 1–26.
2. Murphy KR, et al.: Safe administration of influenza vaccine in asthmatic children hypersensitive to egg proteins. J. Pediatr 1985; 105:931–3.
3. Center for Disease Control: December 1986; Adverse events following immunization: Report No. 2, 1982–1984.
4. Retalliou H, et al.: Illness after influenza vaccination reported through a nation-wide surveillance system, 1976–1977. Am J Epidemiol 1980; 111:270–278.
5. American Academy of Pediatrics: Report of the Committee on Infectious Diseases, ed. 23, 1994, Page 281.

IMPORTANT INFORMATION for Group Immunization Programs: If this vaccine is to be used in an immunization program sponsored by any organization WHERE A TRADITIONAL PHYSICIAN/PATIENT RELATIONSHIP DOES NOT EXIST, each recipient (or legal guardian) must be made aware of the benefits and risks of immunization, and informed consent should be obtained from the recipient (or legal guardian) before immunization. Risks of immunization are summarized in the current labeling. PLEASE CONTACT CDC, or your local State Department of Health to obtain important information about influenza and a sample Influenza Consent Form.

Triton® is a registered Trademark of Rohm & Haas Corp.

Manufactured by:

EVANS MEDICAL LIMITED

Leatherhead, England

An affiliate of:

Medeva Pharmaceuticals, Inc.,

755 Jefferson Road,

Rochester, NY 14623 USA

1-800-234-5535

REV: 5-98

SECTION 6

DIAGNOSTIC PRODUCT INFORMATION

This section is made possible through the courtesy of the manufacturers whose products appear on the following pages. The information concerning each product has been prepared, edited, and approved by the medical department, medical director, and/or medical counsel of its manufacturer.

When a product appearing in PHYSICIANS' DESK REFERENCE has an official package circular, its description must be in full compliance with Food and Drug Administration (FDA) regulations pertaining to labeling for prescription drugs. These regulations require that in PDR "indications, effects, dosages, routes, methods, and frequency and duration of administration, and any relevant warnings, hazards, contraindications, side effects, and precautions" must be *"same in language and emphasis"* as the approved labeling for the product. The FDA regards the words *"same in language and emphasis"* as requiring VERBATIM use of the approved labeling providing such information. Furthermore, information that is emphasized in the approved labeling by the use of type set in a box, or in capitals, boldface, or italics, must be given the same emphasis in PDR.

For products that do not have official package circulars, the publisher has emphasized the necessity of describing such products comprehensively, so that physicians can have access to all information essential for intelligent and informed decision-making.

The product descriptions in PHYSICIANS' DESK REFERENCE include all information made available to PDR by the manufacturer. The publisher does not warrant or guarantee any product, and does not perform any independent analysis of the information provided. Inclusion of a product in PDR does not represent an endorsement, and the publisher does not necessarily advocate the use of any product listed.

This edition of PHYSICIANS' DESK REFERENCE contains the latest information available when the book went to press. As new drugs are released and new research data and clinical findings become available throughout the year, the information in the PDR database is revised accordingly. These revisions are published twice annually in the PDR Supplements and are then incorporated in the following edition of the book. To be certain that you have the most current data, always consult the supplements or the latest edition before administering any product described in the following pages.

Ferring Pharmaceuticals Inc.
**120 WHITE PLAINS ROAD, SUITE # 400
TARRYTOWN, NY 10591**

Direct Inquiries to:
Ferring Pharmaceuticals Inc.
Customer Service Department
120 White Plains Road, Suite #400
Tarrytown, NY 10591
1-(888)-FERRING (337-7464)

**For Medical Information Contact:
In Emergencies:**
Ferring Pharmaceuticals Inc.
Professional Services Department
120 White Plains Road, Suite #400
Tarrytown, NY 10591
(800) 822-8214

ACTHREL®   Rx
(corticorelin ovine triflutate for injection)
For intravenous injection only
DIAGNOSTIC USE ONLY

DESCRIPTION
ACTHREL® (corticorelin ovine triflutate for injection) is a sterile, nonpyrogenic, lyophilized white cake powder, containing corticorelin ovine triflutate, a trifluoroacetate salt of a synthetic peptide that is used for the determination of pituitary corticotroph responsiveness. Corticorelin ovine has an amino acid sequence identical to ovine corticotropin-releasing hormone (oCRH). Corticorelin ovine is an analogue of the naturally occurring human CRH (hCRH) peptide. Both peptides are potent stimulators of adrenocorticotropic hormone (ACTH) release from the anterior pituitary. ACTH stimulates cortisol production from the adrenal cortex. The structural formula for corticorelin ovine triflutate is described below:

Ser-Gln-Glu-Pro-Pro-Ile-Ser-Leu-Asp-Leu-Thr-Phe-His-Leu-Leu-Arg-Glu-Val-Leu-Glu-Met-Thr-Lys-
Ala-Asp-Gln-Leu-Ala-Gln-Gln-Ala-His-Ser-Asn-Arg-Lys-Leu-Leu-Asp-Ile-Ala-NH$_2$·$_x$COOH

whereas $x = 4-8$.

The empirical formula of corticorelin ovine is $C_{205}H_{339}N_{59}O_{63}S$ with a molecular weight of 4670.35 Daltons.
ACTHREL® for Injection is available in vials containing 100 mcg corticorelin ovine (as the trifluoroacetate), 0.88 mg ascorbic acid, 10 mg lactose, and 26 mg cysteine hydrochloride monohydrate. Trace amounts of chloride ion may be present from the manufacturing process. The preparation is intended for intravenous administration.

CLINICAL PHARMACOLOGY
Pharmacodynamics: In normal subjects, intravenous administration of corticorelin results in a rapid and sustained increase of plasma ACTH levels and a near parallel increase of plasma cortisol. In addition, intravenous administration of corticorelin to normal subjects causes a concomitant and prolonged release of the related proopiomelanocortin peptides β- and γ-lipotropins (β- and γ-LPH) and β-endorphin (β-END). A number of dose-response studies have been performed on normal subjects using a range of corticorelin doses. In one study, doses of corticorelin ranging from 0.001 to 30 mcg/kg body weight were administered to 29 healthy volunteers. Blood samples were taken over a 2-hour period for determination of plasma ACTH and cortisol concentrations. There was a direct dose-dependent relationship that was more pronounced for ACTH than for cortisol. The threshold dose was 0.03 mcg/kg, the half-maximal dose was 0.3–1.0 mcg/kg and the maximally effective dose was 3–10 mcg/kg.
Plasma ACTH levels in normal subjects increased 2 minutes after injection of corticorelin doses of ≥0.3 mcg/kg and reached peak levels after 10–15 minutes. Plasma cortisol levels increased within 10 minutes and reached peak levels at 30 to 60 minutes. As the dose of corticorelin was increased, the rises in plasma ACTH and cortisol were more sustained, showing a biphasic response with a second lower

peak at 2–3 hours after injection. Similar results were found in another study using 0.3, 3.0, and 30 mcg/kg doses. The duration of mean plasma ACTH increase after injection of 0.3, 3.0, and 30 mcg/kg was 4, 7, and 8 hours, respectively. The effect on plasma cortisol was similar, but more prolonged. Because there are differences in basal levels and peak response levels following a.m. or p.m. administration, it is recommended that subsequent evaluations in the same patient using the corticorelin stimulation test be carried out at the same time of day as the original evaluation.
Baseline ACTH and cortisol levels are usually higher in the morning. Pooled ACTH values from normal unstressed subjects (n=119) were 25 ± 7 pg/mL in the a.m. and 10 ± 3 in the p.m.; similar pooled cortisol values (n=170) were 11 ± 3 mcg/dL in the a.m. and 4 ± 2 mcg/dL in the p.m. The normal unstressed person has about seven to ten secretory episodes of ACTH each day. Most of them occur in the early morning hours and are responsible for the morning plasma cortisol surge. The following figure shows the daily circadian rhythm of ACTH and cortisol secretions in a normal unstressed person. Insulin, plasma renin activity, prolactin, and growth hormone release are not affected by corticorelin administration in humans.

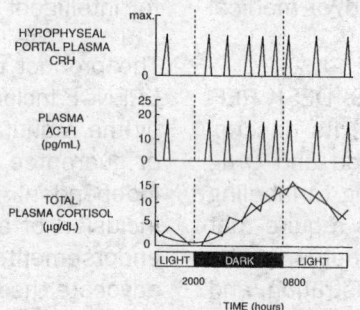

Continuous 24-hour infusion of corticorelin (0.5, 1.0, and 3.0 mcg/kg/hr) increased plasma ACTH concentrations to a plateau of 15–20 pg/mL by the third hour and urinary-free cortisol reaches 173 ± 43 mcg/dL by 24 hours, comparable to those levels observed in patients with major depression, but less than levels noted in Cushing's disease. Continuous infusion did not abolish the circadian rhythm of plasma ACTH and cortisol, but did appear to desensitize the corticotroph. Intermittent doses of corticorelin (25 mcg every 4 hours for 72 hours), however, continued to elicit the expected ACTH and cortisol responses. Intravenous administration of 1 mcg/kg corticorelin in combination with 10 pressor units intramuscular vasopressin had a synergistic effect on ACTH and a less marked synergistic effect on cortisol secretion.
The basal and peak response levels of ACTH and cortisol to a 1 mcg/kg or 100 mcg dose of corticorelin administered to normal volunteers in the morning and the evening are given below. These values were obtained by combining the results from 9 clinical trials conducted in the a.m. and 4 clinical trials conducted in the p.m.
The following table is to be used only as a general guide.
[See table below]
Pharmacokinetics: Following a single intravenous injection of 1 mcg/kg of corticorelin to normal men, the disappearance of immunoreactive corticorelin (IR-corticorelin from plasma follows a biexponential decay curve. Plasma half-lives for IR corticorelin are 11.6 ± 1.5 minutes (mean ± SE) for the fast component and 73 ± 8 minutes for the slow component. The mean volume of distribution for IR-corticorelin is 6.2 ± 0.5 L with an approximate metabolic clearance rate of 95 ± 11 L/m^2/day. Graded intravenous doses of corticorelin (0.01, 0.03, 0.1, 0.3, 1, 3, 10, 30 mcg/kg) produced a linear increase in plasma IR-corticorelin. Corticorelin does not appear to be bound specifically by a circulating plasma protein.

INDICATIONS AND USAGE
ACTHREL® is indicated for use in differentiating pituitary and ectopic production of ACTH in patients with ACTH-dependent Cushing's syndrome.
Differential Diagnosis: There are two forms of Cushing's syndrome:
(a) ACTH-dependent (83%), in which hypercortisolism is due either to pituitary hypersecretion of ACTH (Cushing's disease) resulting from an adenoma (40%, usually microadenomas) or nonadenomatous hyperplasia, possibly of hypothalamic origin (28%), or to hypercortisolism that is secondary to ectopic secretion of ACTH (15%) and,
(b) ACTH-independent (17%), in which hypercortisolism is due to autonomous cortisol secretion by an adrenal tumor (9% adenomas, 8% carcinomas).
After the establishment of hypercortisolism consistent with the presence of Cushing's syndrome, and following the elimination of autonomous adrenal hyperfunction as its cause, the corticorelin test is used to aid in establishing the source of excessive ACTH secretion.
The corticorelin stimulation test helps to differentiate between the etiologies of ACTH-dependent hypercortisolism as follows:
1. High basal plasma ACTH plus high basal plasma cortisol (20–40 mcg/dL). ACTHREL® injection (1 mcg/kg) results in:
   a. Increased plasma ACTH levels
   b. Increased plasma cortisol levels
      Diagnosis: Cushing's disease (ACTH of pituitary origin)
2. High basal plasma ACTH (may be very high) plus high basal plasma cortisol (20–40 mcg/dL).
   ACTHREL® injection (1 mcg/kg) results in:
   a. Little or no response of plasma ACTH levels
   b. Little or no response of plasma cortisol levels
      Diagnosis: Ectopic ACTH syndrome
Test Methodology: To evaluate the status of the pituitary-adrenal axis in the differentiation of a pituitary source from an ectopic source of excessive ACTH secretion, a corticorelin test procedure requires a minimum of five blood samples.
Procedure
1. Venous blood samples should be drawn 15 minutes before and immediately prior to ACTHREL® administration. The ACTH baseline is obtained by averaging the values of the two samples.
2. Administer ACTHREL® as an intravenous infusion over a 30- to 60- second interval at a dose of 1 mcg/kg body weight. Higher dosages are not recommended (see **PRECAUTIONS** and **ADVERSE REACTIONS**).
3. Draw venous blood samples at 15, 30, and 60 minutes after administration.
4. Blood samples should be handled as recommended by the laboratory that will determine their ACTH content. It is extremely important to recognize that the reliability of the ACTHREL® test is directly related to the inter-assay and intra-assay variability of the laboratory performing the assay.
Cortisol determinations may be performed on the same blood samples for the same time points as outlined above. The blood sample handling precautions noted for ACTH should be followed for cortisol.
Interpretation of Test Results: The interpretation of the ACTH and cortisol responses following ACTHREL® administration requires a knowledge of the clinical status of the individual patient, understanding of hypothalamic-pituitary-adrenal physiology, and familiarity with the normal hormonal ranges and the standards used by the laboratory that performs the ACTH and cortisol assays.
Cushing's Disease
The results of challenge with corticorelin injection have been reported in approximately 300 patients with Cushing's disease. Although the ACTH and cortisol responses were variable, a hyper-response to corticorelin was seen in a majority of patients, despite high basal cortisol levels. This response pattern indicates an impairment of the negative feedback of cortisol on the pituitary. Patients with pituitary-dependent Cushing's disease tested with corticorelin do not show the negative correlation between basal and stimulated levels of ACTH and cortisol that is found in normal subjects. A positive correlation between basal ACTH levels and maximum ACTH increments after corticorelin administration has been found in Cushing's disease patients.
Ectopic ACTH Secretion
Patients with Cushing's syndrome due to ectopic ACTH secretion (N=32) were found to have very high basal levels of ACTH and cortisol, which were not further stimulated by corticorelin. However, there have been rare instances of patients with ectopic sources of ACTH that have responded to the corticorelin test.

Time of Day	No. of Subjects	ACTH Concentration mean (range) pg/mL		Cortisol Concentration mean (range) mcg/dL	
		Basal	Peak	Basal	Peak
a.m.	143	28 (16-65)	68 (39-114)	11 (8-13)	21 (17-25)
p.m.	70	9 (8-13)	30 (25-42)	4 (2-6)	16 (15-18)

Basal Concentrations and Peak Responses of ACTH and Cortisol in Normal Subjects after 1 mcg/kg or 100 mcg of ACTHREL®

SUMMARY OF ACTH RESPONSES IN PATIENTS WITH HIGH BASAL CORTISOL

	High ACTH Response	Low ACTH Response
High Basal ACTH	Cushing's Disease	Ectopic ACTH Secretion

CUSHING'S DISEASE ACTH RESPONSES
(mean of 181 patients)
Basal ACTH 63 ± 72 pg/mL (mean ± SD)
Peak ACTH 189 ± 262 pg/mL (mean ± SD)
Mean of individual change from baseline +227%

ECTOPIC ACTH SECRETION RESPONSES
(mean for 31 patients)
Basal ACTH 266 ± 464 pg/mL (mean ± SD)
Peak ACTH 276 ±466 pg/mL (mean ± SD)
Mean of individual change from baseline +15%

False negative responses to the corticorelin test in Cushing's disease patients occur approximately 5 to 10% of the time, which may lead the clinician to an incorrect diagnosis of ectopic production of ACTH at that frequency. (See INDICATIONS AND USAGE, Differential Diagnosis)

PRECAUTIONS
General: The severity of adverse effects to a corticorelin injection appear to be dose-dependent. Dosages above 1 mcg/kg are not recommended. While few adverse effects have been observed at the 1 mcg/kg or 100 mcg dose, higher doses have been associated with transient tachycardia, decreased blood pressure, loss of consciousness, and asystole (see ADVERSE REACTIONS). These symptoms can be substantially reduced by administering the drug as a 30-second intravenous infusion instead of a bolus injection. At a dose of 200 mcg corticorelin, 4 of 60 volunteers and patients with disturbances of the hypothalamic-pituitary-adrenal (HPA) axis were reported to have had decreased blood pressures. One patient had a severe hypotensive reaction with asystole. Three other patients had an "absence-like" loss of consciousness lasting approximately 5 minutes. In subsequent investigations by the same researchers over a 3-year period using 100 mcg of corticorelin, one patient in approximately 150 to 200 experienced a severe drop in blood pressure and loss of sinus rhythm after receiving 55 mcg of corticorelin, which may have been due to interaction with heparin. (See Drug Interactions)
Drug Interactions: The plasma ACTH response to corticorelin injection is inhibited or blunted in normal subjects pretreated with dexamethasone. The use of a heparin solution to maintain i.v. cannula patency during the corticorelin test is not recommended. A possible interaction between corticorelin and heparin may have been responsible for a major hypotensive reaction that occurred after corticorelin administration. (See ADVERSE REACTIONS)
Carcinogenesis, Mutagenesis, Impairment of Fertility: Animal studies have not been conducted with corticorelin to evaluate carcinogenic potential, mutagenicity, or effect on fertility.
Pregnancy (Pregnancy Category C): Animal reproduction studies have not been conducted with corticorelin. It is also not known whether corticorelin can cause fetal harm when administered to a pregnant woman or can affect reproductive capacity. ACTHREL® should be given to a pregnant woman only if clearly needed.
Nursing Mothers: It is not known whether corticorelin is secreted in human milk. Because many drugs are excreted in human milk, caution should be exercised when ACTHREL® is administered to a nursing woman.

PEDIATRIC USE
Only a few tests have been performed on children. Dosages were 1 mcg/kg body weight. Patient studies have involved only children with multiple hypothalamic and/or pituitary hormone deficiencies, or tumors. Only two studies with normal pediatric subjects have been conducted. No differences in response to the corticorelin test have been reported in the children studied.

ADVERSE REACTIONS
Adverse effects reported with 1 mcg/kg or 100 mcg/patient include flushing of the face, neck, and upper chest (16%; 45/276), beginning almost immediately and lasting 3 to 5 minutes. Recipients have also reported an urge to take a deep breath (6%; 3/49), which occurs with a timing similar to, but less frequently than, that of flushing. Higher doses (≥3 mcg/kg) are associated with more prolonged flushing, tachycardia, hypotension, dyspnea, and "chest compression" or tightness. In addition, at doses of ≥5 mcg/kg, significant increases in heart rate and decreases in blood pressure were observed. The cardiovascular effects occurred 2–3 minutes after injection and lasted for 30–60 minutes. The facial flushing was more prolonged, lasting up to 4 hours in some subjects. All signs and symptoms could be reduced by administering the drug as a 30-second infusion instead of by bolus injection.

Total doses of up to 200 mcg of corticorelin were administered as a bolus injection to 60 men and women, including both healthy normal subjects and patients with endocrine disorders. In most cases, only minor adverse effects, such as transient flushing and feelings of dyspnea, were noted. However, a few patients with disorders of the pituitary-adrenal axis had major symptoms. One patient had a precipitous fall in blood pressure and pulse rate and developed asystole, which required resuscitation. In two patients with Cushing's disease and in one with secondary adrenal insufficiency, an "absence-like" loss of consciousness occurred, which started within a few seconds after injection of corticorelin and lasted from 10 seconds to 5 minutes. This was accompanied by a slight fall in blood pressure. One patient with a well documented seizure diathesis experienced a grand mal epileptic seizure following ACTHREL® administration. The patient had discontinued anti-convulsant therapy the day of the procedure. (See PRECAUTIONS and Drug Interactions)

OVERDOSAGE
Symptoms of overdose include severe facial flushing, cardiovascular changes and dyspnea. In the event of toxic overdose (see ADVERSE REACTIONS), adverse effects should be treated symptomatically.

DOSAGE AND ADMINISTRATION
Dosage: A single intravenous dose of ACTHREL® at 1 mcg/kg is recommended for the testing of pituitary corticotrophin function. A dose of 1 mcg/kg is the lowest dose that produces maximal cortisol responses and significant (though apparently sub-maximal) ACTH responses. Doses above 1 mcg/kg are not recommended. (See PRECAUTIONS and ADVERSE REACTIONS)
At a dose of 1 mcg/kg, the ACTH and cortisol responses to ACTHREL® are prolonged and remain elevated for up to 2 hours. The maximum increment in plasma ACTH occurs between 15 and 60 minutes after ACTHREL® administration, whereas the maximum increment in plasma cortisol occurs between 30 and 120 minutes. In a clinical study of 30 normal healthy men, the peak plasma ACTH and cortisol responses to ACTHREL® administration in the early afternoon occurred at 42 ± 29 minutes and 65 ± 26 minutes (average ± SD), respectively. **If a repeat evaluation using the corticorelin stimulation test with ACTHREL® is needed, it is recommended that the repeat test be carried out at the same time of day as the original test because there are differences in basal levels and peak response levels following a.m. or p.m. administration to normal humans.**
Administration: ACTHREL® is to be reconstituted aseptically with 2 mL of Sodium Chloride Injection, USP (0.9% sodium chloride), at the time of use by injecting 2 mL of the saline diluent into the lyophilized drug product cake. To avoid bubble formation, DO NOT SHAKE the vial; instead, roll the vial to dissolve the drug product. The sterile solution containing 50 mcg corticorelin/mL is then ready for injection by the intravenous route. The dosage to be administered is determined by the patient's weight (1 mcg corticorelin/kg). Some of the adverse effects can be reduced by administering the drug as an infusion over 30 seconds instead of as a bolus injection.
Parenteral drug products should be inspected visually for particulate matter and discoloration prior to administration, whenever solution and container permit.

HOW SUPPLIED
ACTHREL® is supplied as a sterile, nonpyrogenic, lyophilized, white cake containing 100 mcg corticorelin ovine (as the trifluoroacetate), 0.88 mg ascorbic acid, 10 mg lactose, and 26 mg cysteine hydrochloride monohydrate. Trace amounts of chloride ion may be present from the manufacturing process. The package provides a single-dose, rubber-capped, 5-mL, brown-glass vial (NDC 55566-0302-1) containing 100 mcg corticorelin ovine (as the trifluoroacetate). ACTHREL® is stable in the lyophilized form when stored refrigerated at 2°C to 8°C (36°F to 45°F) and protected from light. The reconstituted solution is stable up to 8 hours under refrigerated conditions. Discard unused reconstituted solution.
Manufactured for:
Ferring Pharmaceuticals Inc.
Tarrytown, New York 10591
By:
Ben Venue Laboratories, Inc.
Bedford, OH 44146
Caution: Federal law prohibits dispensing without a prescription
©1997 FERRING PHARMACEUTICALS INC.
01/97   OIDC171

SECRETIN–FERRING   Rx
secretin
For diagnostic use in pancreatic dysfunction

DESCRIPTION
Secretin is a gastrointestinal peptide hormone that was first extracted from porcine duodenum by Jorpes & Mutt (1961).

The heptacosa - peptide was subsequently sequenced and synthesized by Mutt, Bodansky and their co-workers at the Karolinska Institute. Secretin-Ferring is a highly purified naturally occurring porcine hormone with a potency of not less than 3000 clinical units (CU) per mg peptide. Secretin is chemically defined as follows:
Mol.Wt. 3055.5
Empirical Formula: $C_{130}H_{220}N_{44}O_{41}$
Structural Formula: H-His-Ser-Asp-Gly-Thr-Phe-Thr-Ser-Glu-Leu-Ser-Arg-Leu-Arg-Asp-Ser-Ala-Arg-Leu-Gln-Arg-Leu-Leu-Gln-Gly-Leu-Val-NH_2
Secretin-Ferring contains 75 CU of lyophilized, sterile purified secretin, 1 mg of L-cysteine hydrochloride, and 20 mg of mannitol per vial. When reconstituted with 7.5 ml of Sodium Chloride Injection USP, each ml of solution contains 10 CU secretion for intravenous use. The pH of the reconstituted solution has a range of 2.5–5.0.

CLINICAL PHARMACOLOGY
The primary action of secretin is to increase the volume and bicarbonate content of secreted pancreatic juices. The standard unit of activity used for Secretin-Ferring is the clinical unit defined by Jorpes & Mutt in 1966. In a study of 6 healthy subjects the $t(^1/_2)$ for secretin approximated 4 minutes with a clearance rate of 540 ml/min (Kolts and McGuigan, 1977). Normal ranges for pancreatic secretory response to intravenous secretin in patients with defined pancreatic diseases have been shown to vary. The variation is related to the secretin product used as well as inter-investigator differences in operative technique. However, it has been demonstrated that properly performed tests with secretin will identify pancreatic disease (Gutierrez and Baron, 1972, Lagerlöf et al., 1967).
The pancreatic secretory responses to secretin in normal subjects and patients with well-documented pancreatitis are shown in Table 1 (Gutierrez and Baron, 1972).

Table 1

	Normal male subjects (10)a	Chronic Pancreatitis (5)
Volume secreted (ml/kg/hr)	3.6 ± 0.8 b	1.1 ± 0.6
HCO₃ content (mEq/l)	114 ± 20	71 ± 33
HCO₃ output (mEq/kg/hr)	0.436 ± 0.141	0.105 ± 0.093

a number of subjects.
b x̄ ± S.D.

The values obtained for Table 1 are derived from a single study by investigators skilled in performing the secretin test and are to be taken only as guidelines. These results should not be generalized to results of secretin testing conducted in other laboratories. However, a volume response of less than 2.0 ml/kg/hr, bicarbonate concentration of less than 90 mEq/liter and bicarbonate output of less than 0.2 mEq/kg/hr are consistent with impaired pancreatic function. A physician or institution planning to perform secretin testing for diagnosis of pancreatic disease should begin by assessing enough normal subjects (≥ 5) to develop proficiency in proper technique and to generate normal response ranges for the three commonly assessed parameters of pancreatic exocrine response to Secretin-Ferring.
Proper technique for carrying out the secretin test of pancreatic function is described in DOSAGE AND ADMINISTRATION.
Secretin-Ferring administered intravenously stimulates gastrin release in patients with gastrinoma (Zollinger-Ellison syndrome), whereas no or only small changes in serum gastrin concentrations occur in normal subjects. Secretin-Ferring may produce a small decrease in serum gastrin levels in patients with duodenal ulcer disease. This gastrin response is the basis for the use of Secretin-Ferring as a provocative test in the evaluation of patients in whom gastrinoma is a diagnostic consideration. Accepted technique for carrying out the secretin provocation test is detailed in DOSAGE AND ADMINISTRATION.

INDICATIONS AND USAGE
Secretin-Ferring (secretin) is indicated for:
(1) Diagnosis of pancreatic exocrine disease.
(2) As an adjunct in obtaining desquamated pancreatic cells for cytopathologic examination.
(3) Diagnosis of gastrinoma (Zollinger-Ellison syndrome).

CONTRAINDICATIONS
Patients suffering from acute pancreatitis should not receive Secretin-Ferring until the attack has subsided.

WARNING
Because of a potential allergic reaction to secretin, patients should receive an initial intravenous test dose of 0.1–1.0

Continued on next page

Secretin-Ferring—Cont.

CU. If no allergic reaction is noted after one minute the recommended dose may be injected slowly over 1 minute. A test dose is especially important in patients with a history of atopic allergy and/or asthma. Appropriate measures for the treatment of acute hypersensitivity reactions should be immediately available.

PRECAUTIONS

GENERAL: Patients who have undergone vagotomy, or are receiving anticholinergics at the time of secretin testing, or who have inflammatory bowel disease may be hyporesponsive to secretin stimulation. This response does not indicate pancreatic disease. A greater than normal volume response to secretin stimulation, which can mask coexisting pancreatic disease, is occasionally encountered in patients with alcoholic or other liver disease.

DRUG/LABORATORY TEST INTERACTION: The concomitant use of anticholinergic agents may make patients hyporesponsive (false positive)

CARCINOGENESIS, MUTAGENESIS, IMPAIRMENT OF FERTILITY: Long-term studies in animals have not been performed to evaluate the carcinogenic, mutagenic potential or possible impairment of fertility effects of secretin.

PREGNANCY CATEGORY C: Animal reproduction studies have not been conducted with Secretin-Ferring. It is also not known whether Secretin-Ferring can cause fetal harm when administered to a pregnant woman or can affect reproductive capacity. Secretin-Ferring should be given to a pregnant woman for diagnosis of gastrinoma (Zollinger-Ellison syndrome) only if clearly needed. Insofar as fluoroscopic guidance is usually necessary to position the double-lumen tube used in the pancreatic function test, this test should be postponed until after delivery.

NURSING MOTHERS: It is not known whether secretin is excreted in human milk. Because many drugs are excreted in human milk, caution is advised when Secretin-Ferring is administered to a nursing woman. Further, normal values for pancreatic secretory response to Secretin-Ferring and for serum gastrin response have not been established for nursing women.

PEDIATRIC USE: Safety and effectiveness in children have not been established.

ADVERSE REACTIONS

No adverse reactions to Secretin-Ferring have been reported.

DOSAGE AND ADMINISTRATION

Secretin-Ferring should be prepared immediately prior to use. The contents of a vial are dissolved in 7.5 ml of Sodium Chloride Injection USP, to yield a concentration of 10 CU per ml. Avoid vigorous shaking. Discard any unused portion after reconstitution.

The reconstituted drug product should be inspected visually prior to administration. If particulate matter or discoloration are seen, the product should be discarded.

Dosage

PANCREATIC FUNCTION TESTING AND PROCEDURE FOR OBTAINING DESQUAMATED PANCREATIC CELLS FOR CYTOPATHOLOGY: 1 CU per kg body weight by slow intravenous injection over 1 minute.

DIAGNOSIS OF GASTRINOMA (Zollinger-Ellison syndrome): 2 CU per kg body weight by slow intravenous injection over 1 minute.

Administration

1. PANCREATIC FUNCTION TESTING: A Dreiling type, radioopaque, double-lumen tube is passed through the mouth following a 12–15 hour fast. The proximal lumen of the tube is placed in the gastric antrum and the distal lumen just beyond the papilla of Vater with the aid of fluoroscopic guidance. The positioning of the tube must be confirmed and the tube secured prior to secretin testing. A negative pressure of 25–40 mm Hg is applied to both lumens and maintained throughout the test. Interruption of suction at 1 minute intervals improves the reliability of fluid collections. When uncontaminated duodenal contents are obtained–i.e., when these secretions are clear, although possibly bile stained, and have a pH of ≥6.0–a baseline sample of duodenal fluids is collected for 2 consecutive 10 minute periods. Subsequent to the baseline collections, Secretin-Ferring at a dose of 1 CU/kg of body weight is injected intravenously in approximately 1 minute. Duodenal fluid is then collected for 60 minutes after secretin administration. The aspirate is fractioned into four collection periods, the first two at 10 minute intervals, and the last two at 20 minute intervals. The duodenal lumen of the tube is cleared with an injection of air after collection of each fraction. Wide variations in volume of the aspirate will be indicative of incomplete aspiration or contamination. Each fraction of duodenal fluid is to be chilled and subsequently analyzed for volume and bicarbonate concentration.

2. PROCEDURE FOR OBTAINING DESQUAMATED PANCREATIC CELLS FOR CYTOPATHOLOGY: A duodenal aspirate obtained as under Pancreatic Function Testing is submitted for cytopathological examination.

3. SECRETIN TESTING FOR GASTRINOMA (Zollinger-Ellison syndrome). The patient should have fasted for at least 12 hours prior to beginning the test. Prior to injection of Secretin-Ferring, two blood samples are drawn for determination of fasting serum gastrin levels (baseline values). Subsequently, 2 CU of Secretin-Ferring per kg of body weight are administered intravenously over 1 minute; post-injection blood samples are collected after 1,2,5,10 and 30 minutes for determination of serum gastrin concentrations. Gastrinoma is strongly indicated in patients with elevated fasting serum gastrin concentrations in the 120–500 pg/ml range (determined by RIA using an antibody to gastrin similar to that prepared by Rehfeld) and in patients who show an increase in serum gastrin concentration of more than 110 pg per ml over basal level.

HOW SUPPLIED

Secretin-Ferring is supplied as a lyophilized sterile powder in 10 mL vials (NDC 55566-1075-01) containing 75 CU. The unreconstituted product should be stored at −20°C (freezer). However, the biological activity of Secretin-Ferring will not be significantly decreased by storage at temperatures up to 25°C for up to 3 weeks. Expiration date is marked on the label.

Caution: Federal (USA) law prohibits dispensing without prescription.

REFERENCES

Jorpes, E., and Mutt, V.
On the biological activity and amino acid composition of secretin.
Acta Chem Scand 15 (1961) 1790–1791.

Jorpes, E., and Mutt V.
On the biological assay of secretin. The reference standard.
Acta Physiol Scand 66 (1966) 316–325.

Kolts, B.E. and Mc Guigan, J.E.
Radioimmunoassay Measurement of Secretin Half-Life in Man.
Gastroenterol. 72 (1977) 55–60.

Lagerlöf, H.O., et al.
A secretin test with high doses of secretin and correction for incomplete recovery of duodenal juice.
Gastroenterol 52 (1967) 67–77.

Gutierrez, L.V., and Baron, J.H.
A comparison of Boots and GIH secretin as stimuli of pancreatic secretion in human subjects with or without chronic pancreatitis.
Gut 13 (1972) 721–725.

41 42 83

Manufactured by Ferring AB, Malmö, Sweden, for
Ferring Pharmaceuticals, Inc.
120 White Plains Rd., Suite 400
Tarrytown, NY 10591
Revision dat June '88

THYREL® TRH ℞

(protirelin)
Injection
FOR INTRAVENOUS ADMINISTRATION

DESCRIPTION

Chemically, Thyrel® TRH (protirelin) is identified as 5-oxo-L-prolyl-L-histidyl-L-proline amide. It is a synthetic tripeptide that is believed to be structurally identical to the naturally-occurring thyrotropin-releasing hormone produced by the hypothalamus. The CAS Registry Number is 24305-27-9. The structural formula is:

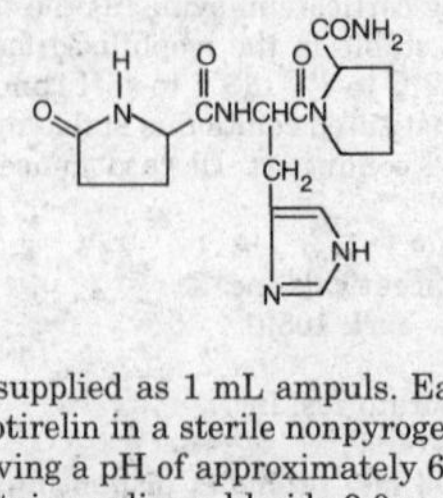

Thyrel TRH is supplied as 1 mL ampuls. Each ampul contains 500 µg protirelin in a sterile nonpyrogenic isotonic saline solution having a pH of approximately 6.5. In addition, each ampul contains sodium chloride 9.0 mg, Water for Injection, hydrochloric acid and sodium hydroxide as needed to adjust pH. Thyrel TRH is intended for intravenous administration.

CLINICAL PHARMACOLOGY

Pharmacologically, Thyrel TRH increases the release of the thyroid stimulating hormone (TSH) from the anterior pituitary. Prolactin release is also increased. It has recently been observed that approximately 65% of acromegalic patients tested respond with a rise in circulating growth hormone levels; the clinical significance is as yet not clear. Following intravenous administration, the mean plasma half-life of protirelin in normal subjects is approximately five minutes. TSH levels rise rapidly and reach a peak at 20 to 30 minutes. The decline in TSH levels takes place more slowly, approaching baseline levels after approximately three hours.

INDICATIONS AND USAGE

Thyrel TRH is indicated as an adjunctive agent in the diagnostic assessment of thyroid function. As an adjunct to other diagnostic procedures, testing with Thyrel® TRH (protirelin) may yield useful information in patients with pituitary and hypothalamic dysfunction.

Thyrel TRH is indicated as an adjunct to evaluate the effectiveness of thyrotropin suppression with a particular dose of T4 in patients with nodular or diffuse goiter. A normal TSH baseline value and a minimal difference between the 30 minute and baseline response to Thyrel TRH injection would indicated adequate suppression of the pituitary secretion of TSH.

Thyrel TRH may be used, adjunctively, for adjustment of thyroid hormone dosage given to patients with primary hypothyroidism. A normal or slightly blunted TSH response, thirty minutes following Thyrel TRH injection, would indicate adequate replacement therapy.

CONTRAINDICATIONS

Thyrel TRH is contraindicated in patients with a known hypersensitivity to the drug.

WARNINGS

Transient changes in blood pressure, either increases or decreases, frequently occur immediately following administration of Thyrel TRH. Blood pressure should therefore be measured before Thyrel TRH is administered and at frequent intervals during the first 15 minutes after its administration.

Increases in systolic pressure (usually less than 30 mm Hg) and/or increases in diastolic pressure (usually less than 20 mm Hg) have been observed more frequently than decreases in pressure. These changes have not ordinarily persisted for more than 15 minutes nor have they required therapy. More severe degrees of hypertension or hypotension with or without syncope have been reported in a few patients. To minimize the incidence and/or severity of hypotension, the patient should be supine before, during, and after Thyrel TRH administration. If a clinically important change in blood pressure occurs, monitoring of blood pressure should be continued until it returns to baseline levels. Thyrel TRH should not be administered to patients in whom marked, rapid changes in blood pressure would be dangerous unless the potential benefit clearly outweighs the potential risk.

PRECAUTIONS

Thyroid hormones reduce the TSH response to Thyrel® TRH. Accordingly, patients in whom Thyrel TRH is to be used diagnostically should be taken off liothyronine (T3) approximately seven days prior to testing and should be taken off thyroid medications containing levothyroxine (T4), e.g., desiccated thyroid, thyroglobulin, or liotrix, at least 14 days before testing. Hormone therapy is NOT to be discontinued when the test is used to evaluate the effectiveness of thyroid suppression with a particular dose of T4 in patients with nodular or diffuse goiter, or for adjustment of thyroid hormone dosage given to patients with primary hypothyroidism.

Chronic administration of levodopa has been reported to inhibit the TSH response to Thyrel TRH.

It is not advisable to withdraw maintenance doses of adrenocortical drugs used in the therapy of known hypopituitarism. Several published reported have shown that prolonged treatment with glucocorticosteroids at physiologic doses has no significant effect on the TSH response to thyrotropin releasing hormone, but that the administration of pharmacologic doses of steroids reduces the TSH response.

Therapeutic doses of acetylsalicylic acid (2 to 3.6 g/day) have been reported to inhibit the TSH response to protirelin. The ingestion of acetylsalicylic acid caused the peak level of TSH to decrease approximately 30% as compared to values obtained without acetylsalicylic acid administration. In both cases, the TSH peak occurred 30 minutes post-administration of protirelin.

Carcinogenesis, Mutagenesis, Impairment of Fertility

Long-term animal studies have not been performed to evaluate the carcinogenic potential of protirelin. Studies to determine potential effects concerning mutagenesis or impairment of fertility have also not been performed.

Pregnancy (Category C)

Protirelin has been shown to increase the number of resorptions in rabbits, but not in rats, when given in doses 1 $^{1}/_{2}$ and 6 times the human dose. There are no adequate and well-controlled studies in pregnant women. Thyrel TRH should be used during pregnancy only if the potential benefit justifies the potential risk to the fetus.

Nursing Mothers

It is not known whether this drug is excreted in human milk. Because many drugs are excreted in human milk, caution should be exercised when Thyrel® TRH is administered to a nursing woman.

ADVERSE REACTIONS

Side effects have been reported in about 50% of the patients tested with Thyrel TRH. Generally, the side effects are minor, have occurred promptly, and have persisted for only a few minutes following injection.

Cardiovascular reactions:

Marked changes in blood pressure, including both hypertension and hypotension with or without syncope, have been reported in a small number of patients.

Endocrine reaction:

Breast enlargement and leakage in lactating women for up to two or three days.

Other reactions:

Headaches, sometimes severe, and transient amaurosis in patients with pituitary tumors. Rarely, convulsions may occur in patients with predisposing conditions, e.g., epilepsy, brain damage.

Nausea; urge to urinate; flushed sensation; light-headedness; bad taste in mouth; abdominal discomfort; and dry mouth. Less frequently reported were: Anxiety; sweating; tightness in throat; pressure in chest; tingling sensation; drowsiness; and allergic reactions.

Pituitary apoplexy requiring acute neurosurgical intervention has been reported infrequently for patients with pituitary macroadenomas following the acute administration of protirelin injection in the setting of combined anterior pituitary function testing in conjunction with LHRH and insulin.

DOSAGE AND ADMINISTRATION

Thyrel TRH is intended for intravenous administration with the patient in the supine position. The drug is administered as a bolus over a period of 15 to 30 seconds, with the patient remaining supine until all scheduled postinjection blood samples have been taken. Blood pressure should be measured before Thyrel TRH is administered and at frequent intervals during the first 15 minutes thereafter (see **WARNINGS**). Have the patient urinate before injecting Thyrel TRH.

Dosage:

Adults: 500 µg. Doses between 200 and 500 µg have been used. 500 µg is considered the optimum dose to give the maximum response in the greatest number of patients. Doses greater than 500 µg are unlikely to elicit a greater TSH response.

Children age 6 to 16 years: 7 µg/kg body weight up to a dose of 500 µg.

Infants and children up to 6 years: Experience is limited in this age group; doses of 7 µg/kg have been administered.

One blood sample for TSH assay should be drawn immediately prior to the injection of Thyrel® TRH, and a second sample should be obtained 30 minutes after injection.

The TSH response to Thyrel TRH is reduced by repetitive administration of the drug. Accordingly, if the Thyrel TRH test is repeated, an interval of seven days before testing is recommended.

Elevated serum lipids may interfere with the TSH assay. Thus, fasting (except in patients with hypopituitarism) or a low-fat meal is recommended prior to the test.

INTERPRETATION OF TEST RESULTS

Interpretation of the TSH response to Thyrel TRH requires an understanding of thyroid-pituitary-hypothalamic physiology and knowledge of the clinical status of the individual patient.

Because the TSH test results may vary with the laboratory, the physician should be familiar with the TSH assay method used and the normal range for the laboratory performing the assay. TSH response 30 minutes after Thyrel TRH adminstration in normal subjects and in patients with hyperthyroidism and hypothyroidism are presented in Figure 1. The diagnoses were established prior to the administration of Thyrel TRH on the basis of the clinical history, physical examination, and the results of other thyroid and/or pituitary function tests.

Among the normal euthyroid subjects, women and children were found to have higher levels of TSH at 30 minutes than men.

[See figure 1 at top of next column]

Among the patients with hyperthyroidism or primary (thyroidal), secondary (pituitary), or tertiary (hypothalamic) hypothyroidism, no significant differences in TSH levels by age or sex were found.

Normal: Baseline TSH levels of less than 10 microunits/mL (µU/mL) were observed in 97% of euthyroid normal subjects tested. Thirty minutes after Thyrel TRH, the serum TSH increased by 2.0 µU/mL in 95% of euthyroid subjects.

Hyperthyroidism: All hyperthyroid patients tested had baseline TSH levels of less than 10 µU/mL and a rise of less than 2 µU/mL 30 minutes after Thyrel TRH.

Primary (thyroidal) hypothyroidism: The diagnosis of primary hypothyroidism is frequently supported by finding clearly elevated baseline TSH levels; 93% of patients tested had levels above 10 µU/mL. Thyrel TRH administration to these patients generally would not be expected to yield additional useful information. Ninety-four percent of patients with primary hypothyroidism given Thyrel® TRH in clinical

Figure 1

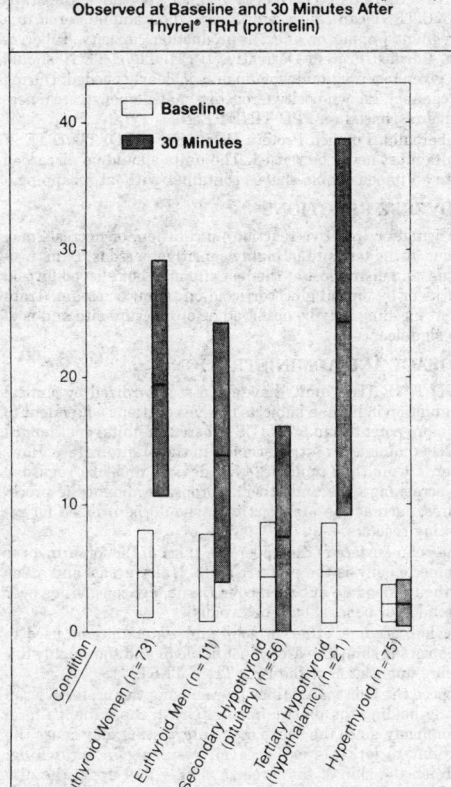

Mean ± One Standard Deviation of TSH Levels (µU/mL) Observed at Baseline and 30 Minutes After Thyrel® TRH (protirelin)

□ Baseline
■ 30 Minutes

(n = number of patients)

trials responded with a rise of TSH of 2.0 µU/mL or rise greater, since this response is also found in normal subjects. Thyrel TRH testing does not differentiate primary hypothyroidism from normal.

Table 1

Characterization Based on Serum TSH Levels at Baseline and 30 Minutes After Thyrel® TRH (protirelin)

	Baseline Serum TSH (µU/mL)	Change of Serum TSH (µU/mL) at 30 minutes
Euthyroidism (normal thryoid function)	10 or less (usually 6 or less; 20% have <1.5µU/mL)	2 or more (usually 6 to 30)
Hyperthyroidism	10 or less (usually 4 or less)	less than 2
Primary Hypothyroidism (thyroidal)	more than 10 (usually 15 to 100)	2 or more (usually 20 or more)
Secondary Hypothyroidism (pituitary)	10 or less (usually 6 or less)	less than 2 (59%) 2 to 50 (41%)
Tertiary Hypothyroidism (hypothalamic)	10 or less (often less than 2)	2 or more

Secondary (pituitary) and tertiary (hypothalamic) hypothyroidism: In the presence of clinical and other laboratory evidence of hypothyroidism, the finding of a baseline TSH levels less than 10 µU/mL should suggest secondary or tertiary hypothyroidism. In this situation, a response to Thyrel TRh of less than 2 µU/mL suggests secondary hypothyroidism since this response was observed in about 60% of patients with secondary hypothyroidism and only approximately 5% of patients with tertiary hypothyroidism. A TSH response to Thyrel TRH greater than 2 µU/mL is not helpful in differentiating between secondary and tertiary hypothyroidism since this response was noted in about 40% of the former and about 95% of the latter.

Establishing the diagnosis of secondary or tertiary hypothyroidism requires a careful history and physical examination along with appropriate tests of anterior pituitary and/or target gland function. The Thyrel® TRH test should not be used as the only laboratory determinant for establishing these diagnoses.

HOW SUPPLIED

As 1 mL ampuls—boxes of 5 (NDC 55566-081-5). Each mL contains Thyrel TRH 0.50 mg (500 µg), sodium chloride 9.0 mg for isotonicity, hydrochloric acid and sodium hydroxide as needed to adjust pH.

Store at controlled room temperature (59° to 86°F).

Caution: Federal law prohibits dispensing without a prescription.

Manufactured for:

FERRING PHARMACEUTICALS Inc.

120 White Plains Rd., Suite 400

Tarrytown, NY 10591

By: Taylor Pharmaceuticals

Decatur, IL 62525

0081-5-DC-115B   (3/94)

LEDERLE LABORATORIES

Division American Cyanamid Company

PEARL RIVER, NY 10965

US Gov't. License No. 17

For Medical Information Contact:

MARKETED ONCOLOGY PRODUCTS:

Immunex Corporation

Professional Services Department

51 University Street

Seattle, WA 98101

(800) IMMUNEX

OTHER MARKETED DRUG PRODUCTS:

Lederle Laboratories/Wyeth-Ayerst Laboratories

Medical Affairs Department

P.O. Box 8299

Philadelphia, PA 19101

Day: (800) 934-5556

8:30 AM to 4:30 PM

(Eastern Standard Time),

Weekdays only

Night: (610) 688-4400 (Emergencies only; non-emergencies should wait until the next day)

MARKETED VACCINES AND TINE TESTS:

Lederle Laboratories/Wyeth-Ayerst Laboratories

Medical Affairs Department

P.O. Box 8299

Philadelphia, PA 19101

Day: (800) 934-5556

8:30 AM to 4:30 PM

(Eastern Standard Time),

Weekdays only

Night: (610) 688-4400 (Emergencies only; non-emergencies should wait until the next day)

PPD TINE TEST®   ℞

[tīne tĕst]

Tuberculin, Purified Protein Derivative

DESCRIPTION

The Tuberculin, Purified Protein Derivative (PPD) TINE TEST is a simple, multiple-puncture, disposable intradermal test device for the detection of tuberculin reactivity. These convenient devices are especially useful in mass tuberculosis screening programs.

Each test unit consists of a stainless steel disc attached to a light blue plastic handle. Projecting from the disc are four triangular-shaped prongs (tines) which are 2 mm long and approximately 4 mm apart. The tines have been mechanically dipped into a concentrated solution of PPD. The PPD concentrate is prepared by the Seibert Process[1,2] and is stabilized with 7% acacia (gum arabic), 30% dextrose, and 5% glycerol. The glycerol also acts as a humectant preventing the film on the tines from becoming brittle-dry. The final PPD concentrate is standardized against U.S. Standard PPD. Following dipping, the tines are capped and sterilized with ethylene oxide. No preservative has been added. The unit is disposable and there is no need for syringes, needles, and other equipment necessary for the standard intradermal tests.

PPD TINE TEST units have been standardized by clinical evaluation in human subjects to give reactions equivalent to or more potent than 5 TU (US tuberculin units) of standard PPD administered intradermally in the Mantoux test. However, all multiple-puncture-type devices must be regarded as screening tools, and other appropriate diagnostic procedures such as the Mantoux test should be utilized for retesting individuals with positive reactions.

CLINICAL PHARMACOLOGY

Tuberculin deposited in the skin of tuberculin reactive individuals reacts with sensitized lymphocytes to effect the re-

Continued on next page

PPD Tine Test—Cont.

lease of mediators of cellular hypersensitivity. Some of these mediators (eg, skin reactive factor) induce an inflammatory response in the skin causing the induration and erythema characteristic of a "positive" reaction.[3,4]

INDICATIONS AND USAGE

Tuberculin, Purified Protein Derivative (PPD) TINE TEST is indicated to detect tuberculin-sensitive individuals. PPD TINE TEST units are also useful in programs to determine priorities for additional testing (eg, chest X-rays) and in epidemiological surveys to identify those areas having high levels of infection.

Data obtained from clinical studies with a total of 3,062 volunteer subjects (males and females), ranging in age from 4 to 96 years, of which 47.5% (1,443) were Mantoux positive, clearly demonstrates that PPD TINE TEST, when used as a screening test to determine tuberculin reactivity, is associated with very little, if any, adverse reactivity. Other than the skin test reaction itself, slight vesiculation and slight ulceration were the only adverse experiences reported. The slight to mild vesiculation was equally divided between the two tests (TINE TEST, 54/3,062, 1.78%; and PPD-T Mantoux, 55/3,062, 1.81%). The slight ulceration observed with one subject at 72 hours was associated with the TINE TEST site. Of the subjects classified as positive or intermediate by PPD-T Mantoux, 93.8% were classified similarly with the TINE TEST. The results of the clinical trials revealed a 72-hour false positive rate of 10.9% and a false negative rate of 6.2%.

In clinical studies of more than 1,800 PPD-S Mantoux positive subjects, only 6.3% gave negative PPD TINE TEST reactions at 72 hours; of more than 1,900 PPD TINE TEST positive tests, less than 11% gave negative Mantoux results. The frequency of repeated tuberculin tests depends on risk of exposure of the individual and on the prevalence of tuberculosis in the population group. The repeated testing of uninfected individuals does not sensitize to tuberculin. Among individuals with waning sensitivity to homologous or heterologous mycobacterial antigens, however, the stimulus of a tuberculin test may "boost" or increase the size of the reaction to a second test, even causing an apparent development of sensitivity in some cases.[3]

Tuberculin testing should be done with caution in individuals with active tuberculosis. (See PRECAUTIONS.)

CONTRAINDICATIONS

There are no known contraindications for use of Tuberculin, Purified Protein Derivative (PPD) TINE TEST. See PRECAUTIONS for information regarding special care to be exercised for safe and effective use.

WARNINGS

There are no known serious adverse reactions or potential safety hazards associated with the use of Tuberculin, Purified Protein Derivative (PPD) TINE TEST. However, as with the use of any biological product, the possibility of anaphylactic reaction should be considered. See PRECAUTIONS for information regarding special care to be exercised for safe and effective use.

PRECAUTIONS

Tuberculin testing should be done with caution in individuals with active tuberculosis. Although activation of quiescent lesions is rare, if a patient has a history of occurrence of vesiculation and necrosis with a previous tuberculin test by any method, tuberculin testing should be avoided.

Although clinical allergy to acacia is very rare, this product contains some acacia as stabilizer and should be used with caution in patients with known allergy to this component. In these instances remedial measures for anaphylactoid reactions, including epinephrine injection (1:1,000), must be available for immediate use.

Reactivity to the test may be suppressed in patients who are receiving corticosteroids or immunosuppressive agents, or those who have recently been immunized with live virus vaccines such as measles, mumps, rubella, polio. If tuberculin skin testing is indicated it should be done preceding, or at the time of such immunization, and read 48 to 72 hours later. If the test is not administered in the time suggested, an interval of 4 to 6 weeks should be allowed between tuberculin skin testing and immunization with live virus vaccines to prevent suppression of tuberculin reactivity.[5]

With a positive reaction further diagnostic procedures must be considered. These may include X-ray of the chest, microbiological examinations of sputa and other specimens, and confirmation of the positive TINE TEST reaction (except vesiculation reactions) using the Mantoux method. In general, the TINE TEST does not need to be repeated.

Antituberculous chemotherapy should not be instituted solely on the basis of a single positive TINE TEST.

When vesiculation occurs, the reaction is to be interpreted as strongly positive and a repeat test by the Mantoux method must not be attempted. Similar or more severe vesiculation with or without necrosis is likely to occur.

Pregnancy Category C. Animal reproduction studies have not been conducted with Tuberculin, Purified Protein Derivative (PPD) TINE TEST. It is also not known whether PPD TINE TEST can cause fetal harm when administered to a pregnant woman or affect reproduction capacity. Tuberculin, Purified Protein Derivative (PPD) TINE TEST should be given to a pregnant woman only if clearly needed. During pregnancy, known positive reactors may demonstrate a negative response to a PPD TINE TEST.

Tuberculin, Purified Protein Derivative (PPD) TINE TEST units must never be reused. The units should be discarded into an impenetrable sharps container without recapping.

ADVERSE REACTIONS

Vesiculation (positive reaction), ulceration, or necrosis may occur at the test site in highly sensitive persons. Pain, pruritus, and discomfort at the test site may be relieved by cold packs or by topical glucocorticoid ointment or cream. Transient bleeding may be observed at a puncture site and is of no significance.

DOSAGE AND ADMINISTRATION

PPD TINE TEST units have been standardized by clinical evaluation in human subjects to give reactions equivalent to or more potent than 5 TU (US tuberculin units) of standard PPD administered intradermally in the Mantoux test. However, all multiple puncture-type devices must be regarded as screening tools and other appropriate diagnostic procedures, such as the Mantoux test, should be utilized for retesting reactors.

The volar surface of the upper one-third of the forearm, over a muscle belly, is the preferred site. Hairy areas, and areas without adequate subcutaneous tissue, eg, concavities over a tendon or bone, should be avoided.

Alcohol, acetone, ether, or soap and water may be used to cleanse the skin. The area must be clean and thoroughly dry before application of the PPD TINE TEST.

Expose the four coated tines by removing the protective cap while holding the plastic handle. Grasp the patient's forearm firmly, since the sharp momentary sting may cause the patient to jerk his or her arm, resulting in scratching. Stretch the skin of the forearm tightly and apply the disc with the other hand. **Hold at least one second.** Release tension grip on forearm. Withdraw tine unit.

Sufficient pressure should be exerted so that the four puncture sites, and circular depression of the skin from the plastic base are visible.

After administration of the test, local care of the skin is not necessary.

Tuberculin, Purified Protein Derivative (PPD) TINE TEST units *must never be reused.* The units should be discarded into an impenetrable sharps container without recapping.

Reading Reactions: Tests should be read at 48 to 72 hours. Vesiculation or the extent of induration are the determining factors; erythema without induration is of no significance. Readings should be made in good light with the forearm slightly flexed. The size of the induration in millimeters should be determined by inspection, measuring, and palpation with gentle finger stroking. Identification of the application site is usually easy because of the distinct four-point pattern. The diameter of the largest single reaction around one of the puncture sites should be measured. With pronounced reactions, the areas of induration around the puncture sites may coalesce.

Interpretation:
Positive Reactions

A. Vesiculation. If vesiculation is present the test may be interpreted as positive, in which case the management of the patient is the same as that for one classified as positive to the Mantoux test.[3]

B. Induration, 2 mm or greater. The test may be interpreted as positive but further diagnostic procedures must be considered. These may include X-ray of the chest, microbiological examination of sputa and other specimens, and confirmation of the positive TINE TEST reaction using the Mantoux method.

Negative Reaction

Induration less than 2 mm. With a negative reaction there is no need for retesting unless the person is a contact of a patient with tuberculosis or there is clinical evidence suggestive of the disease.[3]

Induration indicator cards illustrating typical reactions are enclosed.

HOW SUPPLIED

Tuberculin, Purified Protein Derivative (PPD) TINE TEST is supplied as follows:

NDC 0005-2720-25   25 individual tests
NDC 0005-2720-28   100 individual tests

STORAGE

STORE AT CONTROLLED ROOM TEMPERATURE 15°C TO 30°C (59°F TO 86°F).
DO NOT REFRIGERATE.

REFERENCES

1. Seibert FB. Isolation and properties of purified protein derivative of tuberculin. *Am Rev Tuberc.* 1934;30:713–720.
2. Seibert FB, Glenn JF. Tuberculin purified protein derivative—preparation and analysis of a large quantity for standard. *Amer Rev Tuberc.* 1941;44:9–25.
3. Comstock CW, Daniel TM, Snider DE Jr, et al. The tuberculin skin test. *Amer Rev Resp Dis.* 1981;124:356–363.
4. Freeman BA. *Burrows Textbook of Microbiology.* 22nd ed. Philadelphia, Pa: W. B. Saunders Company; 1985: 295–299.
5. American Academy of Pediatrics. *Report of the Committee on Infectious Diseases.* 21st ed. Elk Grove Village, Ill: American Academy of Pediatrics. 1988:429–447.

Manufactured by:
LEDERLE LABORATORIES
Division American Cyanamid Company
Pearl River, NY 10965
US Gov't. License No. 17
Marketed by:
WYETH-LEDERLE VACCINES
Wyeth-Ayerst Laboratories
Philadelphia, PA 19101
Shown in Product Identification Guide, page 320

TUBERCULIN, OLD, TINE TEST®   ℞
[too-ber-cu-lĭn]

DESCRIPTION

The Tuberculin, Old, TINE TEST is a sterile, simple, multiple-puncture, disposable intradermal test device for the detection of tuberculin reactivity. These convenient devices are especially useful in mass tuberculosis screening programs.

Each test unit consists of a stainless steel disc attached to a white plastic handle. Projecting from the disc are four triangular-shaped prongs (tines) which are 2 mm long and approximately 4 mm apart. The tines have been mechanically dipped into a solution of Old Tuberculin, containing 7% acacia (gum arabic) and 8.5% lactose as stabilizers, and then dried. The entire unit has been sterilized by Cobalt 60 irradiation. No preservative has been added. The unit is disposable and there is no need for syringes, needles, and other equipment necessary for the standard intradermal tests.

Tuberculin, Old, TINE TEST units have been standardized by clinical evaluation in human subjects to give reactions equivalent to or more potent than 5 TU (US tuberculin units) of standard Old Tuberculin administered intradermally in the Mantoux test. However, all multiple-puncture-type devices must be regarded as screening tools, and other appropriate diagnostic procedures, such as the Mantoux test, should be utilized for retesting individuals with positive reactions.

CLINICAL PHARMACOLOGY

Tuberculin deposited in the skin of tuberculin reactive individuals reacts with sensitized lymphocytes to effect the release of mediators of cellular hypersensitivity. Some of these mediators (eg, skin reactive factor) induce an inflammatory response in the skin causing the induration and erythema characteristic of a "positive" reaction.[1,2]

INDICATIONS AND USAGE

Tuberculin, Old, TINE TEST is indicated to detect tuberculin-sensitive individuals. Tuberculin, Old, TINE TEST units are also useful in programs to determine priorities for additional testing (eg, chest X-rays) and in epidemiological surveys to identify those areas having high levels of infection.

In clinical studies covering various geographical areas of the US and all age groups, with a total of 30,588 test subjects, there were 911 (4%) false positive reactors among 26,236 subjects who were Mantoux negative, and 342 (8%) false negative reactors among 4,352 subjects who were Mantoux positive.

The frequency of repeated tuberculin tests depends on risk of exposure of the individual and on the prevalence of tuberculosis in the population group. The repeated testing of uninfected individuals does not sensitize to tuberculin. Among individuals with waning sensitivity to homologous or heterologous mycobacterial antigens, however, the stimulus of a tuberculin test may "boost" or increase the size of the reaction to a second test, even causing an apparent development of sensitivity in some cases.[1]

Tuberculin testing should be done with caution in individuals with active tuberculosis (see PRECAUTIONS).

CONTRAINDICATIONS

There are no known contraindications for use of Tuberculin, Old, TINE TEST. See PRECAUTIONS for information regarding special care to be exercised for safe and effective use.

WARNINGS

There are no known serious adverse reactions or potential safety hazards associated with the use of Tuberculin, Old, TINE TEST. However, as with the use of any biological product, the possibility of anaphylactic reaction should be considered. See **PRECAUTIONS** for information regarding special care to be exercised for safe and effective use.

PRECAUTIONS

Tuberculin testing should be done with caution in individuals with active tuberculosis. Although activation of quiescent lesions is rare, if a patient has a history of occurrence of vesiculation and necrosis with a previous tuberculin test by any method, tuberculin testing should be avoided.

Although clinical allergy to acacia is very rare, this product contains some acacia as stabilizer and should be used with caution in patients with known allergy to this component. In these instances, remedial measures for anaphylactoid reactions, including epinephrine injection (1:1000), must be available for immediate use.

Reactivity to the test may be suppressed in patients who are receiving corticosteroids or immunosuppressive agents, or those who have recently been immunized with live virus vaccines such as measles, mumps, rubella, polio. If tuberculin skin testing is indicated it should be done preceding, or at the time of such immunization, and read 48 to 72 hours later. If the test is not administered in the time suggested, an interval of 4 to 6 weeks should be allowed between tuberculin skin testing and immunization with live virus vaccines to prevent suppression of tuberculin reactivity.[3]

With a positive reaction further diagnostic procedures must be considered. These may include X-ray of the chest, microbiological examinations of sputa and other specimens, and confirmation of the positive TINE TEST reaction (except vesiculation reactions) using the Mantoux method. In general, the TINE TEST does not need to be repeated.

Antituberculous chemotherapy should not be instituted solely on the basis of a single positive TINE TEST.

When vesiculation occurs, the reaction is to be interpreted as strongly positive and a repeat test by the Mantoux method must not be attempted. Similar or more severe vesiculation with or without necrosis is likely to occur.

Pregnancy Category C: Animal reproduction studies have not been conducted with Tuberculin, Old, TINE TEST. It is also not known whether Tuberculin, Old, TINE TEST can cause fetal harm when administered to a pregnant woman or affect reproduction capacity. Tuberculin, Old, TINE TEST should be given to a pregnant woman only if clearly needed. During pregnancy, known positive reactors may demonstrate a negative response to a Tuberculin, Old, TINE TEST.

Tuberculin, Old, TINE TEST units must never be reused. The units should be discarded into an impenetrable sharps container without recapping.

ADVERSE REACTIONS

Vesiculation (positive reaction), ulceration, or necrosis may occur at the test site in highly sensitive persons. Pain, pruritus, and discomfort at the test site may be relieved by cold packs or by topical glucocorticoid ointment or cream. Transient bleeding may be observed at a puncture site and is of no significance.

DOSAGE AND ADMINISTRATION

Tuberculin, Old, TINE TEST units have been standardized by clinical evaluation in human subjects to give reactions equivalent to or more potent than 5 TU (US tuberculin units) of standard Old Tuberculin administered intradermally in the Mantoux test. However, all multiple-puncture-type devices must be regarded as screening tools, and other appropriate diagnostic procedures, such as the Mantoux test, should be utilized for retesting reactors.

The volar surface of the upper one-third of the forearm, over a muscle belly, is the preferred site. Hairy areas, and areas without adequate subcutaneous tissue, eg, concavities over a tendon or bone, should be avoided.

Alcohol, acetone, ether, or soap and water may be used to cleanse the skin. The area must be clean and thoroughly dry before application of the Tuberculin, Old, TINE TEST.

Expose the four coated tines by removing the protective cap while holding the plastic handle. Grasp the patient's forearm firmly, since the sharp momentary sting may cause the patient to jerk his or her arm, resulting in scratching. Stretch the skin of the forearm tightly and apply the disc with the other hand. **Hold at least one second.** Release tension grip on forearm. Withdraw tine unit.

Sufficient pressure should be exerted so that the four puncture sites, and circular depression of the skin from the plastic base are visible.

After administration of the test, local care of the skin is not necessary.

Tuberculin, Old, TINE TEST units *must never be reused.* The units should be discarded into an impenetrable sharps container without recapping.

Reading Reactions: Tests should be read at 48 to 72 hours. Vesiculation or the extent of induration are the determining factors; erythema without induration is of no significance. Readings should be made in good light with the forearm slightly flexed. The size of the induration in millimeters should be determined by inspection, measuring, and palpation with gentle finger stroking. Identification of the application site is usually easy because of the distinct four-point pattern. The diameter of the largest single reaction around one of the puncture sites should be measured. With pronounced reactions, the areas of induration around the puncture sites may coalesce.

INTERPRETATION

Positive Reactions:

A. Vesiculation. If vesiculation is present, the test may be interpreted as positive, in which case the management of the patient is the same as that for one classified as positive to the Mantoux test.[1]

B. Induration, 2 mm or greater. The test may be interpreted as positive but further diagnostic procedures must be considered. These may include X-ray of the chest, microbiological examination of sputa and other specimens, and confirmation of the positive TINE TEST reaction using the Mantoux method.

Negative Reaction:

Induration less than 2 mm. With a negative reaction there is no need for retesting unless the person is a contact of a patient with tuberculosis or there is clinical evidence suggestive of the disease.[1]

Induration indicator cards illustrating typical reactions are enclosed.

HOW SUPPLIED

Tuberculin, Old, TINE TEST is supplied as follows:
NDC 0005-2722-25 25 individual tests
NDC 0005-2722-28 100 individual tests
NDC 0005-2722-34 250 individual tests

STORAGE

STORE AT CONTROLLED ROOM TEMPERATURE 15°C to 30°C (59°F to 86°F). DO NOT REFRIGERATE.

REFERENCES

1. Comstock GW, Daniel TM, Snider DE Jr, et al. The tuberculin skin test. *Am Rev Respir Dis.* 1981;124:356–363.
2. Freeman BA. *Burrows Textbook of Microbiology,* 22nd ed. Philadelphia, Pa: W. B. Saunders Company; 1985:295–299.
3. *American Academy of Pediatrics. Report of the Committee on Infectious Diseases.* 21st ed. Elk Grove Village, Ill: American Academy of Pediatrics; 1988:429–447.

Manufactured by:
LEDERLE LABORATORIES
Division American Cyanamid Company
Pearl River, NY 10965
US Gov't. License No. 17
Marketed by:
WYETH-LEDERLE VACCINES
Wyeth-Ayerst Laboratories
Philadelphia, PA 19101

Shown in Product Identification Guide, page 320

Pasteur Mérieux Connaught
SWIFTWATER, PA 18370

For Medical Information Contact:
Generally:
Medical Affairs
(800) VACCINE
(800) 822-2463
Adverse Drug Experiences:
Medical Director
(717) 839-7187
(800) 835-3592

Sales and Ordering:
Pasteur Mérieux Connaught
Customer Service
(800) VACCINE
(800) 822-2463
(717) 839-7187

MONO-VACC® TEST (O.T.) ℞
[mon 'ō-vak]
TUBERCULIN, OLD,
Multiple Puncture Device

DESCRIPTION

The Tuberculin, Old, Mono-Vacc® Test (O.T.) is a sterile, multiple puncture intradermal test for the detection of tuberculin sensitivity. It provides a convenient and reliable method for determining tuberculin sensitivity of individuals in tuberculosis screening programs or for office or clinical use.

The Mono-Vacc® Test (O.T.) unit consists of a sterile, disposable, multi-puncture plastic scarifier with liquid old tuberculin on the points. No preservative has been added. A plastic cap provides an airtight seal over the points assuring sterility of the points and tuberculin until the unit is used. Tuberculin color variation may occur between different lots without alteration of potency or stability.

The preloaded test unit is disposable.

HOW SUPPLIED

Tamperproof.
Box of 25 tests.

Shown in Product Identification Guide, page 330

MUMPS SKIN TEST ANTIGEN USP ℞
MSTA®
NOT FOR IMMUNIZATION, DIAGNOSIS, OR TREATMENT
NOT FOR DIAGNOSIS OF IMMUNITY TO MUMPS

Caution: Federal (USA) law prohibits dispensing without prescription.

DESCRIPTION

MSTA®, Mumps Skin Test Antigen, is a sterile suspension of killed mumps virus for intradermal use. It is prepared from the extraembryonic fluid of the virus-infected chicken embryo and is concentrated and purified by differential centrifugation. The virus is killed with formaldehyde solution, 1:1000, and is then diluted with isotonic sodium chloride solution. The resultant product contains approximately 0.012 molar glycine and less than 1:8,000 formaldehyde solution. Thimerosal (mercury derivative) 1:10,000 is added as a preservative. The skin test antigen is formulated to contain at least 40 complement fixing units (CFU) per mL, at the time of release, as determined by the Complement-Fixation Test. This product, after shaking, is slightly opalescent in color.

CLINICAL PHARMACOLOGY

Information is available concerning the pharmacologic mode of action of skin test antigens.[1] Skin testing is a widely employed and readily available method of clinically assessing the cellular immune response. A positive skin-test reaction indicates previous antigenic exposure, T-cell competence, an intact inflammatory response, and is an assessment of the cellular integrity of the immune response.

Skin testing with MSTA detects delayed-hypersensitivity.[2] Since most of the population (except for the very young) have had contact or infection with mumps virus,[3] they usually demonstrate a delayed-hypersensitivity reaction to MSTA if an adequate cellular immune system exists.[4]

A single masked placebo-controlled study involving 90 cancer subjects was performed using MSTA, Tetanus Toxoid Fluid, Mixed Respiratory Vaccine, Dermatophyton O. staphage lysate and PPD (Tubersol®). The injection sites were read at 48 and 72 hours. The number of positive reactors to MSTA was greater than the number of positive subjects receiving the other antigens. None of the patients experienced any sloughing, necrosis, abscess formation, or painful lymphadenopathy as a result of the MSTA skin test. This study demonstrated that MSTA evoked a positive delayed-hypersensitivity (DH) reaction in immunocompetent individuals. The frequency of reactions in subjects with an impaired immune system was reduced. The sensitivity of MSTA has been demonstrated by the fact that: 1) in all instances when any of the other test antigens were positive, MSTA was also positive; and 2) several subjects showed a DH reaction to MSTA but did not show a DH reaction to the other antigens.[2]

INDICATIONS AND USAGE

MSTA, Mumps Skin Test Antigen, is indicated when detection of a delayed-hypersensitivity (DH) reaction is desired. MSTA has not been tested in persons immunized with live mumps vaccine; therefore, its safety and efficacy in this population group has not been established.

MSTA is not indicated for the immunization, diagnosis, or treatment of mumps virus infection, or determination of immune status to mumps virus.

CONTRAINDICATIONS

MUMPS VIRUS FOR THE PREPARATION OF MUMPS SKIN TEST ANTIGEN IS PROPAGATED IN EGGS. THEREFORE, THIS PRODUCT SHOULD NOT BE ADMINISTERED TO ANYONE WITH A HISTORY OF HYPERSENSITIVITY (ALLERGY), ESPECIALLY ANAPHYLACTIC REACTIONS TO EGGS OR EGG PRODUCTS. IT IS ALSO A CONTRAINDICATION TO ADMINISTER MSTA TO INDIVIDUALS KNOWN TO BE SENSITIVE TO THIMEROSAL. IN ANY CASE, EPINEPHRINE INJECTION (1:1000) MUST BE IMMEDIATELY AVAILABLE TO COMBAT UNEXPECTED ANAPHYLACTIC OR OTHER ALLERGIC REACTIONS.

WARNINGS

Neurologic complications, such as encephalopathies or peripheral-nervous systems disorders, or anaphylactic reac-

Continued on next page

MSTA—Cont.

tions have followed the administration of almost all biologics, although these have not been reported after the injection of MSTA.

PRECAUTIONS

GENERAL

Care is to be taken by the health-care provider for the safe and effective use of this product.

EPINEPHRINE INJECTION (1:1000) MUST BE IMMEDIATELY AVAILABLE TO COMBAT UNEXPECTED ANAPHYLACTIC OR OTHER ALLERGIC REACTIONS.

A separate, sterile syringe and needle or a sterile disposable unit should be used for each patient to prevent transmission of hepatitis or other infectious agents from person to person. Needles should not be recapped and should be disposed of according to biohazard waste guidelines.

Special care should be taken to ensure the product is not injected into a blood vessel.

The antigen must be given intradermally. If it is injected subcutaneously, no reaction or an unreliable reaction may occur.

DRUG INTERACTIONS

MSTA has not been tested in persons immunized with live mumps vaccine; therefore, its safety and efficacy in this population has not been established.

CARCINOGENESIS, MUTAGENESIS, IMPAIRMENT OF FERTILITY

MSTA has not been evaluated for its carcinogenic, mutagenic potentials or impairment of fertility.

PREGNANCY

REPRODUCTIVE STUDIES – PREGNANCY CATEGORY C

Animal reproduction studies have not been conducted with Mumps Skin Test Antigen. It is not known whether Mumps Skin Test Antigen can cause fetal harm when administered to a pregnant woman or can affect reproduction capacity. Mumps Skin Test Antigen should be given to a pregnant woman only if clearly needed. There are no carefully done studies available on the effect of the drug on later growth, development and functional maturation of the child.

USAGE IN NURSING MOTHERS

It is not known whether this drug is excreted in human milk. Because many drugs are excreted in human milk, caution should be exercised when Mumps Skin Test Antigen is administered to a nursing woman.

PEDIATRIC USE

SAFETY AND EFFECTIVENESS OF MSTA IN CHILDREN HAVE NOT BEEN ESTABLISHED.

USAGE IN YOUNG ADULTS

SAFETY AND EFFECTIVENESS HAVE NOT BEEN ESTABLISHED IN YOUNG ADULTS WHO HAVE BEEN IMMUNIZED WITH MUMPS VACCINE.

ADVERSE REACTIONS

Local reactions may include tenderness, pruritus, vesiculation and rash. Sloughing, necrosis, abscess formation, and/or regional lymphadenopathy may be associated with unusually large DH reactions. Adverse reactions may include nausea, anorexia, headache, unsteadiness, drowsiness, sweating, sensation of warmth and lymphadenopathy. None of these reactions were noted in this clinical study.[2] Epinephrine Injection (1:1000) must be immediately available to combat unexpected anaphylactic and other allergic reactions.

DOSAGE AND ADMINISTRATION

Parenteral drug products should be inspected visually for extraneous particulate matter and/or discoloration prior to administration. If these conditions exist, Mumps Skin Test Antigen should not be administered.

SHAKE VIAL WELL before withdrawing each dose.

A separate, sterile syringe and needle or a sterile disposable unit should be used for each patient to prevent transmission of hepatitis or other infectious agents from person to person. Needles should not be recapped and should be disposed of according to biohazard waste guidelines.

An injection of 0.1 mL of the antigen is made on the inner surface of the forearm. Before injection, the skin over the site to be injected should be cleansed with a suitable germicide. Care should be taken to inject the test antigen intradermally.

Interpretation of Reactions — The reaction should be examined in 48 to 72 hours. A mean diameter (i.e., the longest width plus the longest length, divided by 2) of induration of 5 mm or more indicates a positive DH reaction to the antigen. A negative reaction, if the test dose has been given correctly, usually indicates either anergy or nonsensitivity. Pseudopositive reactions may develop in persons highly sensitive to egg protein.

HOW SUPPLIED

Vial, 1 mL (10 tests) – Product No. 49281-240-10

STORAGE

Store between 2° – 8°C (35° – 46°F). DO NOT FREEZE.

REFERENCES

1. Holborow EJ, et al. Immunology in Medicine. Second Edition, pp 19 and 121. Grune & Stratton, 1983
2. Unpublished data available from Connaught Laboratories, Inc.
3. Petersdorf RG. Mumps. in Harrison's Principles of Internal Medicine, Ed. 7 (edited by M.M. Wintrobe, G.W. Thorn, R.D. Adams, E. Braunwald, K.J. Isselbacher, and R.G. Petersdorf) p 985. New York: McGraw-Hill Book Company, 1974
4. Dempster G. Mumps in Textbook of Virology, Ed. 5 (edited by A.J. Rhodes and C.E. Van Rooyen) p 461 Baltimore: The Williams & Wilkins Co., 1968

Product information
as of February 1997

Manufactured by:
CONNAUGHT LABORATORIES, INC.
Swiftwater, Pennsylvania 18370, USA   3343
Shown in Product Identification Guide, page 330

TUBERSOL®   ℞
[tū '-bur-sŏl]
TUBERCULIN PURIFIED PROTEIN DERIVATIVE (MANTOUX)
Diagnostic Antigen

DESCRIPTION

Tuberculin PPD (Mantoux)—Tubersol® for intracutaneous (Mantoux) tuberculin testing is available in stabilized solutions bio-equivalent to 5 U.S. units (TU) PPD-S per test dose (0.1 ml) and stabilized solutions diluted to a calculated bio-equivalence of 1 TU and 250 TU strengths per test dose (0.1 ml).

Tubersol® is prepared by the Connaught Laboratories Limited from a large Master Batch, Connaught Tuberculin (CT68), which has been obtained from a human strain of *Mycobacterium tuberculosis* grown on a protein-free synthetic medium. The use of a standard preparation derived from a single batch (CT68) has been recommended[2] in order to eliminate batch to batch variation by the same manufacturer.

Tubersol is a sterile isotonic solution of Tuberculin in phosphate buffered saline containing Tween 80 (0.0005%) as a stabilizer. Phenol 0.28% is added as a preservative.[3,4,5]

Independent studies conducted by the U.S. Public Health Service in humans have determined the amount of CT68 in stabilized solution necessary to produce bio-equivalency with Tuberculin PPD-S (in phosphate buffer without Tween 80) using 5 U.S. units (TU) Tuberculin PPD-S as the standard.

Prior to release, each successive lot is tested for potency in sensitized guinea pigs in comparison with the House Standard prepared from Batch CT68 and with the U.S. Standard Tuberculin PPD-S distributed by the Office of Biologics, Food and Drug Administration, Bethesda, Maryland, U.S.A.[6]

CLINICAL PHARMACOLOGY

Intracutaneous tuberculin testing is an accepted aid in the diagnosis of tuberculosis infection.

The reaction to intracutaneously injected tuberculin is a delayed (cellular) hypersensitivity reaction. The reaction which characteristically shows a delayed course, reaching its peak more than 24 hours after administration, consists of induration due to cell infiltration and occasionally vesiculation and necrosis. Clinically, a delayed hypersensitivity reaction to tuberculin is a manifestation of previous infection with *M. tuberculosis* or a variety of non-tuberculosis bacteria. In most cases sensitization is induced by natural mycobacterial infection or by vaccination with BCG Vaccine. The sensitization following infection with mycobacteria occurs primarily in the regional lymph nodes. Small lymphocytes (T lymphocytes) proliferate in response to the antigenic stimulus to give rise to specifically sensitized lymphocytes. After several weeks, these lymphocytes enter the blood stream and circulate for long periods of time. Subsequent restimulation of these sensitized lymphocytes with the same or a similar antigen, such as the intradermal injection of tuberculin, evokes a local reaction mediated by these cells. The tuberculin reaction is characterized by the early predominance of mononuclear cells (small and medium sized lymphocytes and monocytes). Only a small proportion of these cells appear to be lymphocytes sensitized to tuberculin. Most cells are brought into the reaction through the release of biologically active substances by sensitized lymphocytes. An increase in vascular permeability leading to erythema and edema also occurs in tuberculin reactions. Characteristically, delayed hypersensitivity reactions to tuberculin begin at 5 to 6 hours, are maximal at 48 to 72 hours and subside over a period of days. In those who are elderly or those who are being tested for the first time reactions may develop slowly and may not peak until after 72 hours. Immediate hypersensitivity reactions to tuberculin or to constituents of the diluent can also occur.

Not all infected persons will have a delayed hypersensitivity reaction to a tuberculin test. A large number of factors has been reported to cause a decreased ability to respond to the tuberculin test in the presence of tuberculous infection including viral infections (measles, mumps, chickenpox), live virus vaccinations (measles, mumps, polio), overwhelming tuberculosis, other bacterial infections, drugs (corticosteroids and many other immunosuppressive agents), and malignancy.[7]

INDICATIONS AND USAGE

Tubersol is indicated as an aid in the detection of infection with *Mycobacterium tuberculosis*.

For the initial intracutaneous (Mantoux) tuberculin test it is customary to use 5 U.S. units (TU) per test dose of 0.1 ml. The 1 TU per test dose (0.1 ml) preparation is used for individuals suspected of being highly sensitized since larger initial doses may result in severe skin reactions. The preparation containing **250 TU per test dose (0.1 ml), should be used exclusively for the testing of individuals who fail to react to a previous injection of 5 TU and under no circumstance is it to be used for the initial injection.**

CONTRAINDICATIONS

Tubersol should not be administered to known tuberculin positive reactors because of the severity of reactions (eg. vesiculation, ulceration or necrosis) that may occur at the test site in highly sensitive persons.

WARNINGS

Tuberson 250 TU per test dose (0.1 ml) is not, under any circumstances, to be used for the initial injection.

Avoid injecting Tubersol subcutaneously. Of this occurs, no local reaction will develop, but a general febrile reaction and/or acute inflammation around old tuberculosis lesions may occur in highly sensitive individuals.

PRECAUTIONS

a) General

A separate **sterile** syringe and needle must be used for each individual injection to prevent possibility of transmission of viral hepatitis or other infectious agents from one person to another.

The possibility of allergic reactions in individuals sensitive to the components of the product should be borne in mind. Epinephrine Hydrochloride Solution (1:1000) should be readily available for use in case an anaphylactic or acute hypersensitivity reaction occurs.

Failure to store and handle Tubersol as recommended will result in a loss of potency and inaccurate test results.

b) Information For Patients

Reactivity to the test may be depressed or suppressed for as long as 5 to 6 weeks in individuals who have received concurrent or recent immunization with certain virus vaccines (measles, influenza), who have had viral infections (rubeola, influenza, mumps and probably others) or who are receiving corticosteroids or immunosuppressive agents.

In those who are elderly or being tested for the first time reactions may develop slowly and may not peak until after 72 hours.

Vesiculation, ulceration or necrosis may appear at the test site in highly sensitive persons. Pain, pruritus and discomfort at the test site may also occur.

c) Laboratory Tests

Since a positive tuberculin reaction (10 mm or more) does not necessarily indicate the presence of active tuberculous disease, individuals showing such positive tuberculin reactions should be subjected to other diagnostic procedures, such as X-ray examination of the chest and microbiological examination of the sputum.

In the case of doubtful tuberculin reactions (5 to 9 mm) to 5 TU, the possibility should not be excluded that the skin sensitivity is due to previous contact with atypical mycobacteria or previous BCG vaccination. In the absence of signs of tuberculous disease, differential diagnosis by means of intracutaneous skin tests with PPD's derived from atypical mycobacteria may be indicated.

d) Drug Interactions

Reactivity to the test may be depressed or suppressed in individuals who are receiving corticosteroids or immunosuppressive agents.

Reactivity to PPD may be temporarily depressed by certain live virus vaccines (measles, mumps, rubella). Therefore, if a tuberculin test is to be performed, it should be administered either before or simultaneously with the injection of measles, mumps and rubella vaccines in combined form or as separate antigens.

e) Carcinogenesis, Mutagenesis, Impairment of Fertility

The product is not used for extended treatment over a long period of time.

f) Pregnancy Category C (Tuberculin)

Animal reproduction studies have not been conducted with Tubersol. It is also not known whether Tubersol can cause fetal harm when administered to a pregnant woman or can affect reproduction capacity. Tubersol should be given to a pregnant woman only if clearly needed.

However, the risk of unrecognized tuberculosis and the close post partum contact between a mother with active disease

and an infant leaves the infant in grave danger of tuberculosis and complications such as tuberculous meningitis. Therefore, the prescribing physician will want to consider if the potential benefits outweigh the possible risks for performing the tuberculin test on a pregnant woman or a woman of childbearing age, particularly in certain high risk populations.

ADVERSE REACTIONS

In highly sensitized individuals, strongly positive reactions including vesiculation, ulceration or necrosis may occur at the test site. Cold packs or topical steroid preparations may be employed for symptomatic relief of the associated pain, pruritus and discomfort.

Strongly positive reactions may result in scarring at the test site.

Immediate erythematous or other reactions may occur at the injection site. The reason(s) for these infrequent occurrences are presently unknown.

DOSAGE AND ADMINISTRATION

The Test: The Mantoux test is performed by intracutaneously injecting, with a syringe and needle, 0.1 ml of Tubersol. It is customary to use 5 TU per test dose. The 1 TU per test dose preparation is used for individuals suspected of being highly sensitized since larger initial doses may result in severe skin reactions. **The preparation containing 250 TU per test dose should be used exclusively for the testing of individuals who fail to react to a previous injection of 5 TU and under no circumstances is it to be used for the initial injection.**

The result is read 48 to 72 hours after administration and induration only is considered in interpreting the test.

Method of Administration: The following procedure is recommended for performing the Mantoux test:

1. The site of the test is the flexor surface of the forearm about 4 inches below the bend of the elbow.
2. The skin of the forearm is first cleansed with alcohol and allowed to dry.
3. The test dose (0.1 ml) of Tuberculin PPD is administered with a 1 ml syringe calibrated in tenths and fitted with a short, one-half inch, 26 or 27 gauge needle.
4. Disposable sterile syringes and needles may be used. Glass syringes and needles should be sterilized by autoclaving (121°C for 30 minutes), by boiling or by the use of dry heat. Do not sterilize by means of alcohol.
5. The rubber cap of the vial should be wiped with a sterile piece of cotton moistened with alcohol and allowed to dry. The needle is then inserted gently through the cap and the required amount of the Tuberculin PPD is drawn into the syringe.
6. The point of the needle is inserted into the most superficial layers of the skin with the needle bevel pointing upward. If the intracutaneous injection is performed properly, a definite white bleb will rise at the needle point, about 10 mm ($^3/_8$") in diameter. This will disappear within minutes. No dressing is required.

In the event of a subcutaneous injection (i.e. no bleb formed), the test should be repeated immediately at another site.

Tubersol is a stabilized solution of Tuberculin PPD. Data indicate that Tubersol will remain stable for at least four weeks when prefilled into syringes and stored between 2° and 8°C.[4] However, in order to avoid possible contamination of the product this practice is not recommended.

Parenteral drug products should be inspected visually for particulate matter and discoloration prior to administration, whenever solutions and container permit.

Interpretation of the Test: The test should be read 48 to 72 hours after administration of Tubersol. Sensitivity is indicated by induration, usually accompanied by erythema. The widest diameter of distinctly palpable induration should be recorded in millimeters (mm). Presence of edema and necrosis should also be recorded.

A positive reaction indicates a sensitivity to tuberculin, which may be the result of a previous infection with mycobacteria. This infection, likely due to *Mycobacterium tuberculosis,* may have occurred years ago or may be of recent origin.

Reactions should be interpreted as follows:

Positive Reaction—Any palpable induration measuring 10 mm or more is considered a positive reaction. In the case of tuberculosis suspects or close contacts of individuals with tuberculosis an induration of 5 mm or even smaller should be interpreted as a positive reaction and appropriate additional follow-up measures initiated.

Doubtful Reaction—Induration measuring 5 to 9 mm indicates a doubtful reaction. Retesting is indicated using a different site and 5 TU per test dose.

The possibility should not be excluded that the skin sensitivity is due to previous contact with atypical mycobacteria or previous BCG vaccination.

Negative Reaction—Induration of less than 5 mm is considered negative. An individual who does not show a positive reaction to either 1 TU or 5 TU on the first test may be retested with 5 TU and if still found negative further testing

with 0.1 ml containing 250 TU of Tuberculin PPD (Mantoux) is suggested. If the latter test is employed, it may be given in the other forearm.

An individual who does not show a positive reaction to an initial injection of either 1 TU and 5 TU or 5 TU alone, and to a subsequent injection of 250 TU of Tuberculin PPD may be considered as tuberculin negative.

Booster Effect—Infection of an individual with tubercle bacilli or other mycobacteria results in a delayed hypersensitivity response to tuberculin which is demonstrated by the skin test. The delayed hypersensitivity response may gradually wane over a period of years. If a person receives a tuberculin test at this time (after several years) the response may be a reaction that is not significant. The stimulus of the test may boost or increase the size of the reaction to a second test, sometimes causing an apparent conversion or development of sensitivity. The booster effect can be seen on a second test done as soon as a week after the initial stimulating test and can persist for a year, and perhaps longer. When routine periodic tuberculin testing of adults is done, two stage testing should be used to minimize the likelihood of interpreting a boosted reaction as a conversion.[7,8]

Since a positive tuberculin reaction does not necessarily indicate the presence of active tuberculosis disease, individuals showing a positive tuberculin reaction should be subjected to other diagnostic procedures.

Those individuals giving a positive tuberculin reaction may or may not show evidence of tuberculosis disease. Chest X-ray examination and microbiological examination of the sputum in these cases are recommended as a means of determining the presence or absence of pulmonary tuberculosis.

HOW SUPPLIED

Tubersol bioequivalent to 5 U.S. units (TU) PPD-S per test dose (0.1 ml) is available in 1 ml and 5 ml vials.

Tubersol 1 TU and 250 TU per test dose (0.1 ml) are available in 1 ml vials. Tubersol solutions are ready for immediate use without any further dilution.

Storage

Tubersol should be stored between 2° and 8°C (35° and 46°F).[5,9] Tuberculin solutions can be adversely affected by exposure to light. The product should be stored in the dark except when doses are actually being withdrawn from vial.[10]

A vial of Tuberculin PPD which has been opened and in use for one month should be discarded because oxidation and degradation may have reduced the potency.[11]

REFERENCES

1. Landi, S.: Preparation, purification, and stability of tuberculin. Appl. Microbiol. **11**: 408–412, 1963.
2. Canadian Tuberculosis and Respiratory Disease Association: Classification and reporting of tuberculosis in Canada, Ottawa, the Association, 1972 p. 42.
3. Landi, S., Held H. R., Hauschild, A. H. W., Hilsheimer, R.: Adsorption of tuberculin PPD to glass and plastic surfaces. Bull. W.H.O. **35**: 593–602, 1966.
4. Landi, S., Held, H. R., Tseng, M. D.: Disparity of potency between stabilized and nonstabilized dilute tuberculin solutions. Am. Rev. Respir. Dis. **104**: 385–393, 1971.
5. Landi, S., Held, H. R.: Stability of dilute solutions of tuberculin purified protein derivative. Tubercle **59**: 121–133, 1978.
6. U.S. Code of Federal Regulations, Title 21, Part 650, Subpart B—tuberculin, 144–146, April 1, 1981.
7. The Tuberculin Skin Test. Am. Rev. Respir. Dis. **124**: 356–363, 1981.
8. American Thoracic Society: Diagnostic Standards and Classification of Tuberculosis and Other Mycobacterial Diseases (14th ed.), 1980. Am. Rev. Respir. Dis. **123**: 343–358, 1981.
9. Landi, S., Held, H. R.: Stability of dilute solution of tuberculin purified protein derivative at extreme temperatures. J. Biol. Stand. **9**: 195–199, 1981.
10. Landi, S., Held, H. R.: Effect of light on tuberculin purified protein derivative solutions. Am. Rev. Respir. Dis. **111**: 52–61, 1975.

11. Landi, S., Held, H. R.: Effect of oxidation on the stability of tuberculin purified protein derivative (PPD) In: International Symposium on Tuberculins and BCG Vaccine. Basel: International Association of Biological Standardization, 1983. (Developments in Biological Standardization) In press.

Manufactured by:
**CONNAUGHT
LABORATORIES LIMITED
A POSTEUR MÉRIEUX COMPANY
WILLOWDALE, ONTARIO, CANADA**
Distributed by:
CONNAUGHT LABORATORIES INC.
Swiftwater, Pennsylvania 18370,
U.S.A.
01-686 CLI
Shown in Product Identification Guide, page 330

Wyeth-Ayerst Laboratories
**Division of American Home
Products Corporation
P.O. BOX 8299
PHILADELPHIA, PA 19101**

Direct General Inquiries to:
(610) 688-4400

For Medical Information Contact:
Medical Affairs
Day: (800) 934-5556
8:30 AM to 4:30 PM (Eastern Standard Time),
Weekdays only
In Emergencies:
Day: (800) 934-5556
Night: (610) 688-4400
(Emergencies only; non-emergencies should wait until the next day)

FACTREL® ℞
[*făc 'trel*]
**(gonadorelin hydrochloride)
Synthetic Luteinizing Hormone Releasing
Hormone (LH-RH)
DIAGNOSTIC USE ONLY**

Caution: Federal law prohibits dispensing without prescription.

DESCRIPTION

An agent for use in evaluating hypothalamic-pituitary gonadotropic function. Factrel (gonadorelin hydrochloride) injectable is available as a sterile lyophilized powder for reconstitution and administration by subcutaneous or intravenous routes.

Chemical Name: 5-oxo-L-prolyl-L-histidyl-L-tryptophyl-L-seryl -L- tyrosyl-glycyl -L- leucyl-L-arginyl-L-prolyl glycinamide hydrochloride
[See chemical structure below]

Factrel is $C_{55}H_{75}N_{17}O_{13}HCl$, as the mono- or dihydrochloride, or their mixture. The gonadorelin base has a molecular weight of 1182.33. It is a white powder, soluble in alcohol and water, hygroscopic and moisture-sensitive, and stable at room temperature. The synthetic decapeptide, Factrel, has a chemical composition and structure identical to the natural hormone, identified from porcine or ovine hypothalami.

Each Secule® vial of Factrel contains 100 or 500 mcg gonadorelin as the hydrochloride, with 100 mg lactose, USP. Each ampul of sterile diluent contains 2% benzyl alcohol in sterile water.

Continued on next page

Structural Formula:

Factrel—Cont.

CLINICAL PHARMACOLOGY

Factrel has been shown to have gonadotropin-releasing effects upon the anterior pituitary. The range for normal baseline LH levels, as determined from the literature, is 5–25 mIU/mL in postpubertal males, and postpubertal and premenopausal females. The standard used is the Second International Reference Preparation—HMC. This range may not correspond in each laboratory performing the assay since the concentration of LH in normal individuals varies with different assay methods. The normal responses to Factrel analyzed from the results of clinical studies included:
(1) LH peak (mIU/mL)
(highest LH value post-Factrel administration)
(2) Maximum LH increase (mIU/mL)
(peak LH value—LH baseline value)
(3) LH percent response
$$\frac{\text{peak LH—baseline LH}}{\text{baseline LH}} \times 100\%$$
(4) Time to peak (minutes)
(time required to reach LH peak value)
Normal adult subjects were shown to have these LH responses following Factrel administration by subcutaneous or intravenous routes.
I. MALE ADULTS:
A) Subcutaneous Administration
The results are based on 18 tests in males between the ages of 18–42 years, inclusive:
(1) LH peak: mean 60.3 ± 26.2 mIU/mL
100% ≥ 24.0 mIU/mL
90% ≥ 32.8 mIU/mL
(2) Maximum LH increase: mean 46.7 ± 20.8 mIU/mL
100% ≥ 12.3 mIU/mL
90% ≥ 20.9 mIU/mL
(3) LH percent response: mean 437 ± 245% range: 66–1853%
90% ≥ 188%
(4) Time to peak: mean 34 ± 13 min
B) Intravenous Administration
The results are based on 26 tests in males between the ages of 19–58 years, inclusive:
(1) LH peak: mean 63.8 ± 40.3 mIU/mL
100% ≥ 12.6 mIU/mL
90% ≥ 26.0 mIU/mL
(2) Maximum LH increase: mean 51.3 ± 35.2 mIU/mL
100% ≥ 7.4 mIU/mL
90% ≥ 14.8 mIU/mL
(3) LH percent response: mean 481 ± 184% range: 67–2139%
90% ≥ 142%
(4) Time to peak: mean 27 ± 14 min
In males older than 50 years, the LH baseline and peak levels tend to be higher; however, the maximum LH increases do not differ in regard to age.
II. FEMALE ADULTS:
A) Subcutaneous Administration
The results are based on 38 tests in females between the ages of 19–36 years, inclusive:
(1) LH peak: mean 67.9 ± 27.5 mIU/mL
100% ≥ 12.5 mIU/mL
90% ≥ 39.0 mIU/mL
(2) Maximum LH increase: mean 52.8 ± 26.4 mIU/mL
100% ≥ 7.5 mIU/mL
90% ≥ 23.8 mIU/mL
(3) LH percent response: mean 374 ± 221% range: 108–981%
90% ≥ 185%
(4) Time to peak: mean 71.5 ± 49.6 min
B) Intravenous Administration
The results are based on 31 tests in females between the ages of 20–35 years, inclusive:
(1) LH peak: mean 57.6 ± 36.7 mIU/mL
100% ≥ 20.0 mIU/mL
90% ≥ 24.6 mIU/mL
(2) Maximum LH increase: mean 44.5 ± 31.8 mIU/mL
100% ≥ 7.5 mIU/mL
90% ≥ 16.2 mIU/mL
(3) LH percent response: mean 356 ± 282% range: 60–1300%
90% ≥ 142%
(4) Time to peak: mean 36 ± 24 min
The Factrel tests on which the normal female responses are based were performed in the early follicular phase of the menstrual cycle (Days 1–7).

In menopausal and postmenopausal females, the baseline LH levels are elevated and the maximum LH increases are exaggerated when compared with the premenopausal levels.

Patients with clinically diagnosed or suspected pituitary and/or hypothalamic dysfunction were often shown to have subnormal or no LH responses following Factrel administration. For example, in clinical tests of 6 patients with known postpubertal panhypopituitarism, and 11 patients with Prader-Willi syndrome, 100% showed subnormal responses or no rise in LH. Subnormal responses to the Factrel test also were observed in 21 (95%) of 22 patients with prepubertal panhypopituitarism. In 19 patients with Sheehan's syndrome, 16 (84%) had a subnormal response. In the Factrel test in 44 patients with Kallmann's syndrome, 33 (77%) had subnormal LH responses.

INDICATIONS AND USAGE

Factrel as a single injection is indicated for evaluating the functional capacity and response of the gonadotropes of the anterior pituitary. This single-injection test does not measure pituitary gonadotropic reserve, for which more prolonged or repeated administration may be required. The LH response is useful in testing patients with suspected gonadotropin deficiency, whether due to the hypothalamus alone or in combination with anterior pituitary failure. Factrel is also indicated for evaluating residual gonadotropic function of the pituitary following removal of a pituitary tumor by surgery and/or irradiation. In clinical studies to date, however, the single-injection test has not been useful in differentiating pituitary disorders from hypothalamic disorders. The Factrel test can be performed concomitantly with other post-treatment evaluations. The results of the Factrel test complement the clinical examination and other laboratory tests used to confirm or substantiate hypogonadotropic hypogonadism.
In cases where there is a normal response, it indicates the presence of functional pituitary gonadotropes. The single-injection test does not measure pituitary gonadotropic reserve.

CONTRAINDICATIONS

Hypersensitivity to gonadorelin hydrochloride or any of the components.

PRECAUTIONS

A. General

Although allergic and hypersensitivity reactions have been observed with other polypeptide hormones, and rarely with multiple doses of Factrel, to date no such reactions have been reported following the administration of a single 100 mcg dose of Factrel.
Antibody formation has been reported rarely after chronic administration of large doses of Factrel.

B. Drug Interactions

The Factrel test should be conducted in the absence of other drugs which directly affect the pituitary secretion of the gonadotropins. These would include a variety of preparations which contain androgens, estrogens, progestins, or glucocorticoids. The gonadotropin levels may be transiently elevated by spironolactone, minimally elevated by levodopa, and suppressed by oral contraceptives and digoxin. The response to Factrel may be blunted by phenothiazine and dopamine antagonists which cause a rise in prolactin.

C. Carcinogenesis, Mutagenesis, Impairment of Fertility

Repetitive, high doses of Factrel may cause luteolysis and inhibition of spermatogenesis. No long-term animal studies have been done to evaluate carcinogenic potential.

D. Pregnancy Category B

Reproduction studies have been performed in mice, rats, and rabbits at doses up to 50 times the human dose, and have revealed no evidence of harm to the fetus due to Factrel. There are, however, no adequate and well-controlled studies in pregnant women. Because animal reproduction studies are not always predictive of human response, this drug should be used during pregnancy only if clearly needed.
Appropriate precautions should be taken because the effects of LH-RH on the fetus and developing offspring have not been adequately evaluated.
Nursing Mothers: It is not known whether this drug is excreted in human milk. Because many drugs are excreted in human milk, caution should be exercised when Factrel is administered to a nursing woman.
Pediatric Use: Safety and effectiveness in pediatric patients have not been established.

ADVERSE REACTIONS

Systemic effects have been reported rarely following administration of 100 mcg of Factrel.
CNS: headache, light-headedness.
GI: nausea, abdominal discomfort.
Dermatologic: local swelling, occasionally with pain and pruritis, at the injection site may occur following subcutaneous administration; local and generalized skin rash have been noted after chronic subcutaneous administration.
Cardiovascular: flushing.
Rare instances of hypersensitivity reaction (bronchospasm, tachycardia, flushing, urticaria, induration at injection site) and anaphylactic reactions have been reported following multiple-dose administration.

There has been a report of pituitary apoplexy and sudden blindness following gonadotropin-releasing hormone administration to a patient with a gonadotropin-secreting adenoma.

OVERDOSAGE

Factrel has been administered parenterally in doses up to 3 mg b.i.d. for 28 days without any signs or symptoms of overdosage. In case of overdosage or idiosyncrasy, symptomatic treatment should be administered as required.

DOSAGE AND ADMINISTRATION

Parenteral drug products should be inspected visually for particulate matter and discoloration prior to administration, whenever solution and container permit.
Adults: 100 mcg dose, subcutaneously or intravenously. In females for whom the phase of the menstrual cycle can be established, the test should be performed in the early follicular phase (Days 1–7).

TEST METHODOLOGY

To determine the status of the gonadotropin secretory capacity of the anterior pituitary, a test procedure requiring seven venous blood samples for LH is recommended.
Procedure:
1. Venous blood samples should be drawn at -15 minutes and immediately prior to Factrel administration. The LH baseline is obtained by averaging the LH values of the two samples.
2. Administer a bolus of 100 mcg of Factrel subcutaneously or intravenously.
3. Draw venous blood samples at 15, 30, 45, 60, and 120 minutes after administration.
4. Blood samples should be handled as recommended by the laboratory that will determine the LH content. It must be emphasized that the reliability of the test is directly related to the inter-assay and intra-assay reliability of the laboratory performing the assay.

INTERPRETATION OF TEST RESULTS

Interpretation of the LH response to Factrel requires an understanding of the hypothalamic-pituitary physiology,

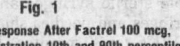

Fig. 1
Normal Male LH Response After Factrel 100 mcg, Subcutaneous Administration 10th and 90th percentiles.

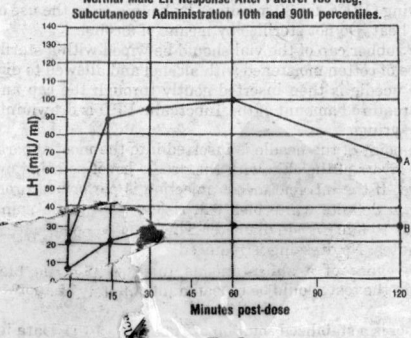

Fig. 2
Normal Male LH Response After Factrel 100 mcg, Intravenous Administration 10th and 90th percentiles.

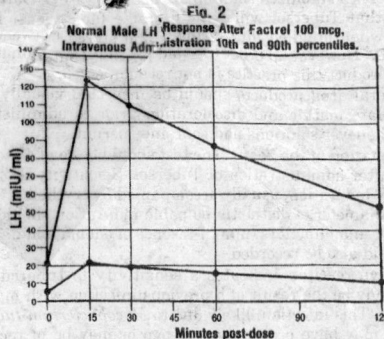

Fig. 3
Normal Female LH Response After Factrel 100 mcg, Subcutaneous Administration 10th and 90th percentiles.

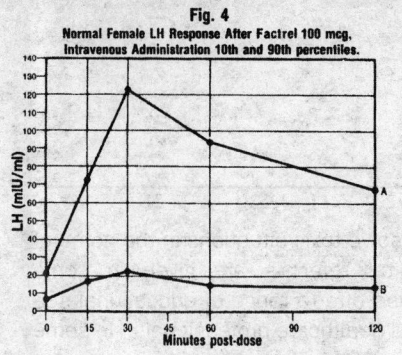

Fig. 4
Normal Female LH Response After Factrel 100 mcg,
Intravenous Administration 10th and 90th percentiles.

knowledge of the clinical status of the individual patient, and familiarity with the normal ranges and the standards used in the laboratory performing the LH assays.

Figures 1 through 4 represent the LH response curves after Factrel administration in normal subjects. The normal LH response curves were established between the 10th percentile (B line) and 90th percentile (A line) of all LH responses in normal subjects analyzed from the results of clinical studies. LH values are reported in units of mIU/mL and time is displayed in minutes. Individual patient responses should be plotted on the appropriate curve. A subnormal response in patients is defined as three or more LH values which fall below the B line of the normal LH response curve. In cases where there is a blunted or borderline response, the Factrel test should be repeated.

The Factrel test complements the clinical assessment of patients with a variety of endocrine disorders involving the hypothalamic-pituitary axis. In cases where there is a normal response, it indicates the presence of functional pituitary gonadotropes. The single-injection test does not determine the pathophysiological cause for the subnormal response and does not measure pituitary gonadotropic reserve.

HOW SUPPLIED

Lyophilized Powder—in single-dose Secule® vials containing 100 mcg (NDC 0046-0507-05) and 500 mcg (NDC 0046-0509-05) gonadorelin as the hydrochloride with 100 mg lactose, USP. Each Secule vial is accompanied by one ampul containing 2 mL sterile diluent of 2% benzyl alcohol in sterile water.

DIRECTIONS

Store at room temperature (approximately 25°C).

Reconstitute 100 mcg Secule® vial with 1.0 mL of the accompanying sterile diluent.

Reconstitute 500 mcg Secule® vial with 2.0 mL of the accompanying sterile diluent.

Prepare solution immediately before use. After reconstitution, store at room temperature and use within 1 day.

Discard unused reconstituted solution and diluent.

Secule®—Registered trademark to designate a vial containing an injectable preparation in dry form.

Manufactured by:
Ayerst Laboratories Inc.
A Wyeth-Ayerst Company
Philadelphia, PA 19101

POISON CONTROL CENTERS

Many of the centers listed below are certified by the American Association of Poison Control Centers. Certified centers are marked by an asterisk after the name. Each has to meet certain criteria. It must, for example, serve a large geographic area; it must be open 24 hours a day and provide direct-dial or toll-free access; it must be supervised by a medical director; and it must have registered pharmacists or nurses available to answer questions from the public.

The centers have a wide variety of toxicology resources, including a computerized database of some 750,000 substances maintained by MICROMEDEX, INC., an affiliate of PDR. Staff members are trained to resolve toxic situations in the home of the caller, though hospital referrals are given in some instances. The centers also offer a range of educational services to both the public and healthcare professionals. In some states, these larger centers exist side by side with smaller centers offering a more limited range of services.

Within each state, centers are listed alphabetically by city. Telephone numbers designated "TTY" are teletype lines for the hearing-impaired. "TDD" numbers reach a telecommunication device for the deaf.

ALABAMA

BIRMINGHAM

Regional Poison Control Center, The Children's Hospital of Alabama (*)
1600 7th Ave. South
Birmingham, AL 35233-1711
Business: 205-939-9720
Emergency: 205-933-4050
    205-939-9201
    800-292-6678 (AL)
Fax: 205-939-9245

TUSCALOOSA

Alabama Poison Center, Tuscaloosa (*)a
2503 Phoenix Dr.
Tuscaloosa, AL 35405
Business: 205-345-0600
Emergency: 205-345-0600a
    800-462-0800 (AL)
Fax: 205-759-7994

ALASKA

ANCHORAGE

Anchorage Poison Center, Providence Hospital
P.O. Box 196604
3200 Providence Dr.
Anchorage, AK 99519-6604
Business: 907-562-2211
    ext. 3633
Emergency: 907-261-3193
    800-478-3193 (AK)
Fax: 907-261-3645

FAIRBANKS

Fairbanks Poison Control Center
1650 Cowles St.
Fairbanks, AK 99701
Business: 907-456-7182
Emergency: 907-456-7182
Fax: 907-458-5553

ARIZONA

PHOENIX

Samaritan Regional Poison Center (*)
Good Samaritan Regional Medical Center
Ancillary-1
1111 East McDowell Rd.
Phoenix, AZ 85006
Business: 602-495-4884
Emergency: 602-253-3334
    800-362-0101 (AZ)
Fax: 602-256-7579

TUCSON

Arizona Poison and Drug Information Center (*)
Arizona Health Sciences Center
1501 North Campbell Ave.
Rm. #1156
Tucson, AZ 85724
Emergency: 520-626-6016
    800-322-0101 (AZ)
Fax: 520-626-2720

ARKANSAS

LITTLE ROCK

Arkansas Poison and Drug Information Center, College of Pharmacy - UAMS
4301 West Markham St.
Slot 522-2
Little Rock, AR 72205
Business: 501-661-6161
Emergency: 800-376-4766 (AR)

CALIFORNIA

FRESNO

California Poison Control System-Fresno (*)
Valley Children's Hospital
3151 North Millbrook, IN31
Fresno, CA 93703
Business: 209-241-6040
Emergency: 800-876-4766 (CA)
Fax: 209-241-6050

SACRAMENTO

California Poison Control System-Sacramento (*)
UCDMC-HSF Room 1024
2315 Stockton Blvd.
Sacramento, CA 95817
Business: 916-734-3415
Emergency: 800-876-4766 (CA)
Fax: 916-734-7796

SAN DIEGO

California Poison Control System-San Diego (*)
UCSD Medical Center
200 West Arbor Dr.
San Diego, CA 92103-8925
Business: 619-543-3666
Emergency: 800-876-4766 (CA)
Fax: 619-692-1867

SAN FRANCISCO

San Francisco Bay Area Regional Poison Control Center, SF General Hospital
1001 Potrero Ave.
Bldg. 80, Rm. 230
San Francisco, CA 94110
Business:
Emergency:
Fax: 415-821-8513

COLORADO

DENVER

Rocky Mountain Poison and Drug Center (*)
8802 East 9th Ave.
Denver, CO 80220-6800
Business: 303-739-1100
Emergency: 303-739-1123
    800-332-3073 (CO)
Fax: 303-739-1119

CONNECTICUT

FARMINGTON

Connecticut Regional Poison Center (*)
University of Connecticut Health Center
263 Farmington Ave.
Farmington, CT 06030
Emergency: 800-343-2722 (CT)
Fax: 203-679-1623

DELAWARE

PHILADELPHIA, PA

The Poison Control Center
3600 Market St.
Suite 220
Philadelphia, PA 19104
Emergency: 800-722-7112 (PA)
    215-386-2100

DISTRICT OF COLUMBIA

WASHINGTON, DC

National Capital Poison Center (*)
3201 New Mexico Ave., NW
Suite 310
Washington, DC 20016
Business: 202-362-3867
Emergency: 202-625-3333
TTY: 202-362-8563
Fax: 202-362-8377

FLORIDA

JACKSONVILLE

Florida Poison Information Center-Jacksonville (*)
University Medical Center
University of Florida Health Science Center-Jacksonville
655 W. 8th St.
Jacksonville, FL 32209
Emergency: 904-549-4480
    800-282-3171 (FL)
Fax: 904-549-4063

MIAMI

Florida Poison Information Center-Miami (*)
University of Miami, School of Medicine
Department of Pediatrics
P.O. Box 016960 (R-131)
Miami, FL 33101
Emergency: 305-585-5253
    800-282-3171 (FL)
Fax: 305-242-9762

TAMPA

The Florida Poison Information Center
Tampa General Hospital
P.O. Box 1289
Tampa, FL 33601
Emergency: 813-253-4444
    (Tampa)
    800-282-3171 (FL)
Fax: 813-253-4443

GEORGIA

ATLANTA

Georgia Poison Center (*)
Hughes Spalding Children's Hospital, Grady Health System
80 Butler St. SE
P.O. Box 26066
Atlanta, GA 30335-3801
Emergency: 404-616-9000
    800-282-5846 (GA)
Fax: 404-616-6657

MACON

Regional Poison Control Center, Medical Center of Central Georgia
777 Hemlock St.
Macon, GA 31201
Poison Ctr: 912-633-1427
Fax: 912-633-5082

IDAHO

DENVER, CO

Rocky Mountain Poison & Drug Center
8802 E. 9th Ave.
Denver, CO 80220-6800
Emergency: 800-860-0620 (ID)
    303-739-1123

ILLINOIS

CHICAGO

Illinois Poison Control Center
222 South Riverside Plaza
Suite 1900
Chicago, IL 60606
Business: 312-942-7064
Emergency: 800-942-5969 (IL)
Fax: 312-803-5400

URBANA

ASPCA/National Animal Poison Control Center
1717 Philo Rd., Suite 36
Urbana, IL 61802
Business: 800-548-2423
(24-hour subscribers)
Fax: 217-337-0599

INDIANA

INDIANAPOLIS

Indiana Poison Center (*) Methodist Hospital of Indiana
I-65 at 21st St.
Indianapolis, IN 46206-1367
Emergency: 317-929-2323
800-382-9097 (IN)
Fax: 317-929-2337

IOWA

SIOUX CITY

Iowa Poison Center
2720 Stone Park Blvd.
Sioux City, IA 51104
Business: 712-277-2222
Emergency: 800-352-2222 (IA)
Fax: 712-279-7852

KANSAS

KANSAS CITY

Mid-America Poison Control Center, University of Kansas Medical Center
3901 Rainbow Blvd.
Room B-400
Kansas City, KS 66160-7231
Business & 913-588-6633
Emergency: 800-332-6633 (KS)
Fax: 913-588-2350

TOPEKA

Stormont-Vail Regional Medical Center Emergency Department
1500 S.W. 10th
Topeka, KS 66604-1353
Business: 913-354-6000
Emergency: 913-354-6100
Fax: 913-354-5004

KENTUCKY

LOUISVILLE

Kentucky Regional Poison Center
Medical Towers S.
Suite 572
234 E. Gray St.
Louisville, KY 40202
Business: 502-629-7264
Emergency: 502-589-8222
Fax: 502-629-7277

LOUISIANA

MONROE

Louisiana Drug and Poison Information Center (*)
Northeast Louisiana University Sugar Hall
Monroe, LA 71209-6430
Business: 318-342-1710
Emergency: 800-256-9822 (LA)
Fax: 318-342-1744

MAINE

PORTLAND

Maine Poison Center
Maine Medical Center
22 Bramhall St.
Portland, ME 04102
Business: 207-871-2950
Emergency: 800-442-6305 (ME)
Fax: 207-871-6226

MARYLAND

BALTIMORE

Maryland Poison Center (*)
20 North Pine St.
Baltimore, MD 21201
Business: 410-706-7604
Emergency: 410-706-7701
800-492-2414 (MD)
Fax: 410-706-7184

MASSACHUSETTS

BOSTON

Massachusetts Poison Control System (*)
300 Longwood Ave.
Boston, MA 02115
Emergency: 617-232-2120
800-682-9211 (MA)
Fax: 617-738-0032

MICHIGAN

DETROIT

Poison Control Center (*) Children's Hospital of Michigan
4160 John R.,
Harper Office Bldg.
Suite 616
Detroit, MI 48201
Business: 313-745-5335
Emergency: 313-745-5711
800-764-7661 (MI)
Fax: 313-745-5493

GRAND RAPIDS

Spectrum Health Regional Poison Center (*)
1840 Wealthy SE
Grand Rapids, MI 49506-2968
Business: 616-774-5329
Emergency: 800-764-7661 (MI)
Fax: 616-774-7204

MINNESOTA

MINNEAPOLIS

Hennepin Regional Poison Center (*) Hennepin County Medical Center
701 Park Ave.
Minneapolis, MN 55415
Business: 612-347-3144
Emergency: 800-764-7661 (MN)
612-347-3141
Fax: 612-904-4289

Minnesota Regional Poison Center (*)
8100 34th Ave. South
P.O. Box 1309
Minneapolis, MN 55440-1309
Business: 612-851-8100
Emergency: 612-221-2113
800-222-1222 (MN)
Fax: 612-851-8166

MISSISSIPPI

HATTIESBURG

Poison Center, Forrest General Hospital
400 South 28th Ave.
Hattiesburg, MS 39401
Business: 601-288-4221
Emergency: 601-288-2100

JACKSON

Mississippi Regional Poison Control, University of Mississippi Medical Center
2500 North State St.
Jackson, MS 39216
Business: 601-984-1675
Emergency: 601-354-7660
Fax: 601-984-1676

MISSOURI

KANSAS CITY

Poison Control Center, Children's Mercy Hospital
2401 Gillham Rd.
Kansas City, MO 64108
Business: 816-234-3053
Emergency: 816-234-3430
Fax: 816-234-3421

ST. LOUIS

Cardinal Glennon Children's Hospital Regional Poison Center (*)
1465 South Grand Blvd.
St. Louis, MO 63104
Emergency: 800-366-8888 (MO)
314-772-5200
Fax: 314-577-5355

MONTANA

DENVER, CO

Rocky Mountain Poison and Drug Center (*)
8802 East 9th Ave.
Denver, CO 80220-6800
Emergency: 800-525-5042 (MT)
Fax: 303-739-1119

NEBRASKA

OMAHA

The Poison Center (*)
8301 Dodge St.
Omaha, NE 68114
Emergency: 402-354-5555
(Omaha)
800-955-9119
(NE & WY)

NEVADA

DENVER, CO

Rocky Mountain Poison and Drug Center (*)
8802 East 9th Ave.
Denver, CO 80220-6800
Emergency: 800-446-6179 (NV)
303-739-1123
Fax: 303-739-1119

RENO

Poison Center, Washoe Medical Center
77 Pringle Way
Reno, NV 89520
Business: 702-328-4129
Emergency: 702-328-4129
Fax: 702-328-5555

NEW HAMPSHIRE

LEBANON

New Hampshire Poison Information Center, Dartmouth-Hitchcock Medical Center
1 Medical Center Dr.
Lebanon, NH 03756
Emergency: 603-650-5000
(ask for Poison Center)
800-562-8236 (NH)
Fax: 603-650-8986

NEW JERSEY

NEWARK

New Jersey Poison Information and Education System (*)
201 Lyons Ave.
Newark, NJ 07112
Emergency: 800-764-7661 (NJ)
Fax: 201-705-8098

PHILLIPSBURG

Warren Hospital Poison Control Center
185 Roseberry St.
Phillipsburg, NJ 08865
Business: 908-859-6768
Emergency: 908-859-6767
800-962-1253 (NJ)
Fax: 908-859-6812

NEW MEXICO

ALBUQUERQUE

New Mexico Poison and Drug Information Center (*)
University of New Mexico
Health Sciences Library, Rm. 125
Albuquerque, NM 87131-1076
Emergency: 505-272-2222
800-432-6866 (NM)
Fax: 505-277-5892

NEW YORK

BUFFALO

Western New York Regional Poison Control Center Children's Hospital of Buffalo
219 Bryant St.
Buffalo, NY 14222
Business: 716-878-7657
Emergency: 716-878-7654
800-888-7655
(NY Western Regions Only)

MINEOLA

Long Island Regional Poison Control Center (*)
Winthrop University Hospital
259 First St.
Mineola, NY 11501
Emergency: 516-542-2323
Fax: 516-739-2070

NEW YORK

New York City Poison Control Center (*)
NYC Dept. of Health
455 First Ave., Room 123
New York, NY 10016
Business: 212-447-8154
Emergency: 212-340-4494
212-POISONS
212-447-2205
Fax: 212-447-8223

ROCHESTER

Finger Lakes Regional Poison Center (*)
University of Rochester Medical Center
601 Elmwood Ave.
Box 321
Rochester, NY 14642
Business: 716-273-4155
Emergency: 716-275-3232
800-333-0542 (NY)
Fax: 716-244-1677

SLEEPY HOLLOW

Hudson Valley Regional Poison Center (*) Phelps Memorial Hospital Center
701 N. Broadway
Sleepy Hollow, NY 10590
Emergency: 914-366-3030
800-336-6997 (NY)
Fax: 914-353-1050

SYRACUSE

Central New York Poison Control Center (*)
SUNY Health Science Center
750 East Adams St.
Syracuse, NY 13210
Business: 315-464-7073
Emergency: 315-476-4766
800-252-5655 (NY)
Fax: 315-464-7077

NORTH CAROLINA

ASHEVILLE
**Western North Carolina
Poison Control Center,
Memorial Mission Hospital**
509 Biltmore Ave.
Asheville, NC 28801
Emergency: 704-255-4490
                800-542-4225 (NC)
Fax: 704-255-4467

CHARLOTTE
**Carolinas Poison Center
Carolinas Medical Center**
5000 Airport Center Pkwy.
Suite B
P.O. Box 32861
Charlotte, NC 28232
Business: 704-355-3054
Emergency: 704-355-4000
              800-848-6946 (NC)

NORTH DAKOTA

FARGO
**North Dakota Poison Information Center,
Meritcare Medical Center**
720 North 4th St.
Fargo, ND 58122
Business: 701-234-6062
Emergency: 701-234-5575
            800-732-2200 (ND)
Fax: 701-234-5090

OHIO

CINCINNATI
**Cincinnati Drug & Poison Information
Center and Regional Poison Control
System (*)**
2368 Victory Pkwy.
Suite 300
Cincinnati, OH 45206
Emergency: 513-558-5111
           800-872-5111 (OH)
Fax: 513-558-5301

CLEVELAND
Greater Cleveland Poison Control Center
11100 Euclid Ave.
Cleveland, OH 44106
Emergency: 216-231-4455
          888-231-4455
Fax: 216-844-3242

COLUMBUS
Central Ohio Poison Center (*)
700 Children's Dr.
Columbus, OH 43205-2696
Business: 614-722-2635
Emergency: 614-228-1323
          800-682-7625 (OH)
Fax: 614-221-2672
**Greater Dayton Area Hospital
Association at Central Ohio Poison
Center**
700 Children's Dr.
Columbus, OH 43205
Business: 614-722-2635
Emergency: 937-222-2227
          800-762-0727 (OH)

TOLEDO
**Poison Information Center of NW Ohio,
Medical College of Ohio Hospital**
3000 Arlington Ave.
Toledo, OH 43614
Business: 419-383-3897
Emergency: 419-381-3897
          800-589-3897 (OH)
Fax: 419-381-6066

OKLAHOMA

OKLAHOMA CITY
**Oklahoma Poison Control Center,
University of Oklahoma and Children's
Hospital of Oklahoma**
940 Northeast 13th St.
Oklahoma City, OK 73104
Emergency: 405-271-5454 (Bus.)
          800-764-7661
          (Bus.) (OK)
TDD: 405-271-1122
Fax: 405-271-1816

OREGON

PORTLAND
**Oregon Poison Center (*)
Oregon Health Sciences University**
3181 S.W. Sam Jackson Park Rd.
Portland, OR 97201
Emergency: 503-494-8968
          800-452-7165 (OR)
Fax: 503-494-4980

PENNSYLVANIA

HERSHEY
**Central Pennsylvania
Poison Center (*)
University Hospital
Milton S. Hershey Medical Center**
Hershey, PA 17033
Emergency: 800-521-6110 (PA)
          717-531-6111
Fax: 717-531-6932

PHILADELPHIA
The Poison Control Center (*)
3600 Market St., Suite 220
Philadelphia, PA 19104-2641
Business: 215-590-2003
Emergency: 215-386-2100
          800-722-7112 (PA)
Fax: 215-590-4419

PITTSBURGH
Pittsburgh Poison Center (*)
3705 Fifth Ave.
Pittsburgh, PA 15213
Business: 412-692-5600
Emergency: 412-681-6669
Fax: 412-692-7497

RHODE ISLAND

PROVIDENCE
**Lifespan Poison Center
Rhode Island Hospital**
593 Eddy St.
Providence, RI 02903
Emergency: 401-444-5727
Fax: 401-444-8062

SOUTH CAROLINA

COLUMBIA
**Palmetto Poison Center,
College of Pharmacy,
University of South Carolina**
Columbia, SC 29208
Business: 803-777-7909
Emergency: 803-777-1117
          800-922-1117 (SC)
Fax: 803-777-6127

SOUTH DAKOTA

ABERDEEN
**Poison Control Center,
St. Luke's Midland Regional Medical
Center**
305 South State St.
Aberdeen, SD 57401
Business: 605-622-5000
Emergency: 605-622-5100
          800-592-1889
           (SD, MN, ND, WY)

TENNESSEE

MEMPHIS
Southern Poison Center
875 Monroe Ave.
Suite 104
Memphis, TN 38163
Business: 901-448-6800
Emergency: 901-528-6048
          800-288-9999 (TN)
Fax: 901-448-5419

NASHVILLE
**Middle Tennessee Poison Center (*)
The Center for Clinical Toxicology,
Vanderbilt University
Medical Center**
1161 21st Ave. South
501 Oxford House
Nashville, TN 37232-4632
Business: 615-936-0760
Emergency: 615-936-2034
          800-288-9999 (TN)
Fax: 615-936-2046

TEXAS

DALLAS
North Texas Poison Center (*)
5201 Harry Hines Blvd.
P.O. Box 35926
Dallas, TX 75235
Business: 214-590-6625
Emergency: 800-764-7661 (TX)
Fax: 214-590-5008

GALVESTON
**Southeast Texas Poison Center (*)
The University of Texas
Medical Branch**
301 University Ave.
Galveston, TX 77555-1175
Emergency: 409-765-1420
          800-764-7661 (TX)
Fax: 409-772-3917

TEMPLE
**Central Texas Poison Center (*) Scott &
White Memorial Hospital**
2401 South 31st St.
Temple, TX 76508
Business: 254-724-4636
Emergency: 800-764-7661 (TX)
          254-724-7401
Fax: 254-724-1731

UTAH

SALT LAKE CITY
Utah Poison Control Center (*)
410 Chipeta Way
Suite 230
Salt Lake City, UT 84108
Emergency: 801-581-2151
          800-456-7707 (UT)
Fax: 801-581-4199

VERMONT

BURLINGTON
**Vermont Poison Center,
Fletcher Allen Health Care**
111 Colchester Ave.
Burlington, VT 05401
Business: 802-656-2721
Emergency: 802-658-3456
Fax: 802-656-4802

VIRGINIA

CHARLOTTESVILLE
**Blue Ridge Poison Center (*)
Blue Ridge University of
Virginia Medical Center**
Box 437
Charlottesville, VA 22908
Emergency: 804-924-5543
          800-451-1428 (VA)
Fax: 804-971-8657

RICHMOND
**Virginia Poison Center,
Virginia Commonwealth University**
P.O. Box 980522
Richmond, VA 23298-0522
Emergency: 800-552-6337 (VA)
          804-828-9123
Fax: 804-828-5291

WASHINGTON

SEATTLE
Washington Poison Center (*)
155 N.E. 100th St.
Suite 400
Seattle, WA 98125-8012
Business: 206-517-2351
Emergency: 206-526-2121
          800-732-6985 (WA)
Fax: 206-526-8490

WEST VIRGINIA

CHARLESTON
West Virginia Poison Center (*)
3110 MacCorkle Ave. S.E.
Charleston, WV 25304
Business: 304-347-1212
Emergency: 304-348-4211
          800-642-3625 (WV)
Fax: 304-348-9560

WISCONSIN

MADISON
**Poison Control Center, University of
Wisconsin Hospital and Clinics**
600 Highland Ave.
F6-133
Madison, WI 53792
Business: 608-262-7537
Emergency: 608-262-3702
          800-815-8855 (WI)

MILWAUKEE
**Children's Hospital
Poison Center,
Children's Hospital of Wisconsin**
9000 W. Wisconsin Ave.
P.O. Box 1997
Milwaukee, WI 53201
Business: 414-266-2000
Emergency: 414-266-2222
          800-815-8855 (WI)
Fax: 414-266-2820

WYOMING

OMAHA, NE
The Poison Center (*)
8301 Dodge St.
Omaha, NE 68114
Emergency: 402-354-5555
          (Omaha)
          800-955-9119
          (WY & NE)

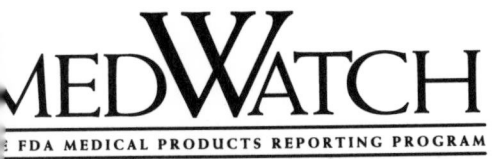

FDA MEDICAL PRODUCTS REPORTING PROGRAM

For **VOLUNTARY** reporting
by health professionals of adverse
events and product problems

Page ____ of ____

Form Approved: OMB No. 0910-0291 Expires: 4/30/96
See OMB statement on reverse

FDA Use Only

Triage unit
sequence #

Patient information

Patient identifier	2. **Age at time of event:** or ———————— **Date of birth:**	3. **Sex** ☐ female ☐ male	4. **Weight** ——— lbs or ——— kgs

In confidence

Adverse event or product problem

☐ **Adverse event** and/or   ☐ **Product problem** (e.g., defects/malfunctions)

Outcomes attributed to adverse event (check all that apply)

☐ death ————————— (mo/day/yr)
☐ life-threatening
☐ hospitalization – initial or prolonged

☐ disability
☐ congenital anomaly
☐ required intervention to prevent permanent impairment/damage
☐ other: ————————

Date of event (mo/day/yr)	4. **Date of this report** (mo/day/yr)

Describe event or problem

Relevant tests/laboratory data, including dates

Other relevant history, including preexisting medical conditions (e.g., allergies, race, pregnancy, smoking and alcohol use, hepatic/renal dysfunction, etc.)

C. Suspect medication(s)

1. **Name** (give labeled strength & mfr/labeler, if known)

#1 _____

#2 _____

2. **Dose, frequency & route used** #1 #2	3. **Therapy dates** (if unknown, give duration) from/to (or best estimate) #1 #2

4. **Diagnosis for use** (indication) #1 #2	5. **Event abated after use stopped or dose reduced** #1 ☐yes ☐no ☐doesn't apply #2 ☐yes ☐no ☐doesn't apply

6. **Lot #** (if known) #1 #2	7. **Exp. date** (if known) #1 #2	8. **Event reappeared after reintroduction** #1 ☐yes ☐no ☐doesn't apply #2 ☐yes ☐no ☐doesn't apply

9. **NDC #** (for product problems only)
___ — ___ — ___

10. **Concomitant medical products** and therapy dates (exclude treatment of event)

D. Suspect medical device

1. **Brand name**

2. **Type of device**

3. **Manufacturer name & address**	4. **Operator of device** ☐ health professional ☐ lay user/patient ☐ other: ————————
6. model # ————————— catalog # ————————— serial # ————————— lot # ————————— other #	5. **Expiration date** (mo/day/yr) 7. **If implanted, give date** (mo/day/yr) 8. **If explanted, give date** (mo/day/yr)

9. **Device available for evaluation?** (Do not send to FDA)
☐ yes   ☐ no   ☐ returned to manufacturer on ——————— (mo/day/yr)

10. **Concomitant medical products** and therapy dates (exclude treatment of event)

E. Reporter (see confidentiality section on back)

1. **Name & address**	phone #

2. **Health professional?** ☐ yes ☐ no	3. **Occupation**	4. **Also reported to** ☐ manufacturer ☐ user facility ☐ distributor

5. **If you do NOT want your identity disclosed to the manufacturer, place an " X " in this box.** ☐

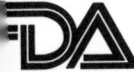

Mail to: MEDWATCH
5600 Fishers Lane
Rockville, MD 20852-9787

or **FAX to:**
1-800-FDA-0178

Submission of a report does not constitute an admission that medical personnel or the product caused or contributed to the event.

ADVICE ABOUT VOLUNTARY REPORTING

Report experiences with:
- medications (drugs or biologics)
- medical devices (including in-vitro diagnostics)
- special nutritional products (dietary supplements, medical foods, infant formulas)
- other products regulated by FDA

Report SERIOUS adverse events. An event is serious when the patient outcome is:
- death
- life-threatening (real risk of dying)
- hospitalization (initial or prolonged)
- disability (significant, persistent or permanent)
- congenital anomaly
- required intervention to prevent permanent impairment or damage

Report even if:
- you're not certain the product caused the event
- you don't have all the details

Report product problems – quality, performance or safety concerns such as:
- suspected contamination
- questionable stability
- defective components
- poor packaging or labeling
- therapeutic failures

How to report:
- just fill in the sections that apply to your report
- use section C for all products except medical devices
- attach additional blank pages if needed
- use a separate form for each patient
- report either to FDA or the manufacturer (or both)

Important numbers:
- 1-800-FDA-0178 to FAX report
- 1-800-FDA-7737 to report by modem
- 1-800-FDA-1088 to report by phone or for more information
- 1-800-822-7967 for a VAERS form for vaccines

If your report involves a serious adverse event with a device and it occurred in a facility outside a doctor's office, that facility may be legally required to report to FDA and/or the manufacturer. Please notify the person in that facility who would handle such reporting.

Confidentiality: The patient's identity is held in strict confidence by FDA and protected to the fullest extent of the law. The reporter's identity, including the identity of a self-reporter, may be shared with the manufacturer unless requested otherwise. However, FDA will not disclose the reporter's identity in response to a request from the public, pursuant to the Freedom of Information Act.

FDA Form 3500-back **Please Use Address Provided Below – Just Fold In Thirds, Tape and Mail**

**Department of
Health and Human Services**

Public Health Service
Food and Drug Administration
Rockville, MD 20857

Official Business
Penalty for Private Use $300

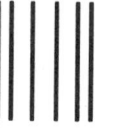

NO POSTAGE
NECESSARY
IF MAILED
IN THE
UNITED STATES
OR APO/FPO

BUSINESS REPLY MAIL
FIRST CLASS MAIL   PERMIT NO. 946   ROCKVILLE, MD

POSTAGE WILL BE PAID BY FOOD AND DRUG ADMINISTRATION

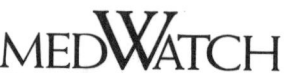
MedWatch

**The FDA Medical Products Reporting Program
Food and Drug Administration
5600 Fishers Lane
Rockville, MD 20852-9787**